BNF

90

September 2025 – March 2026

BMJ Group

PHARMACEUTICAL PRESS
Essential Knowledge

Published jointly by
BMJ
Tavistock Square
London
WC1H 9JP
UK

and

Pharmaceutical Press
66-68 East Smithfield
London
E1W 1AW
UK

Pharmaceutical Press is the publishing division of the Royal Pharmaceutical Society.

BNF 90 ISBN: 978 0 85711 490 7

Printed by GGP Media GmbH, Pößneck, Germany

Typeset by Data Standards Ltd, UK

Text design by Peter Burgess

A catalogue record for this book is available from the British Library.

Requesting copies of BNF Publications
Paper copies may be obtained through any bookseller or direct from:
Pharmaceutical Press
c/o Macmillan Distribution (MDL)
Hampshire International Business Park
Lime Tree Way
Basingstoke
Hampshire
RG24 8YJ
Tel: +44 (0) 1256 302 699
Fax: +44 (0) 1256 812 521
direct@macmillan.co.uk

or via our website www.PharmaceuticalPress.com/shop/

For all bulk orders of more than 20 copies:
Tel: +44 (0) 207 572 2266
pharmpress-support@rpharms.com

The BNF is available as a mobile app, online (bnf.nice.org.uk/) and also through MedicinesComplete. In addition, BNF content can be integrated into a local formulary by using BNF on FormularyComplete; see www.bnf.org for details.

About BNF content
The BNF is designed as a digest for rapid reference and it may not always include all the information necessary for prescribing and dispensing. Also, less detail is given on areas such as obstetrics, malignant disease, and anaesthesia since it is expected that those undertaking treatment will have specialist knowledge and access to specialist literature. BNF for Children should be consulted for detailed information on the use of medicines in children. The BNF should be interpreted in the light of professional knowledge and supplemented as necessary by specialised publications and by reference to the product literature. Information is also available from Medicines Information Services.

Please refer to digital versions of BNF for the most up-to-date content. BNF is published in print but interim updates are issued and published in the digital versions of BNF. The publishers work to ensure that the information is as accurate and up-to-date as possible at the date of publication, but knowledge and best practice in this field change regularly. BNF's accuracy and currency cannot be guaranteed and neither the publishers nor the authors accept any responsibility for errors or omissions. While considerable efforts have been made to check the material in this publication, it should be treated as a guide only. Prescribers, pharmacists and other healthcare professionals are advised to check www.bnf.org/ for information about key updates and corrections.

Pharmaid
Numerous requests have been received from developing countries for BNFs. The Pharmaid scheme of the Commonwealth Pharmacists Association will dispatch old BNFs to certain Commonwealth countries. For more information on this scheme see commonwealthpharmacy.org/what-we-do/pharmaid/.
If you would like to donate your copy email: admin@commonwealthpharmacy.org

Preface

The BNF is a joint publication of BMJ and the Royal Pharmaceutical Society. It is published under the authority of a Joint Formulary Committee which comprises representatives of the two professional bodies, the UK Health Departments, the Medicines and Healthcare products Regulatory Agency, and a national guideline producer. The Dental Advisory Group oversees the preparation of advice on the drug management of dental and oral conditions; the Group includes representatives of the British Dental Association and a representative from the UK Health Departments. The Nurse Prescribers' Advisory Group advises on the content relevant to nurses and includes representatives from different parts of the nursing community and from the UK Health Departments.

The BNF aims to provide prescribers, pharmacists, and other healthcare professionals with sound up-to-date information about the use of medicines.

The BNF includes key information on the selection, prescribing, dispensing and administration of medicines. Medicines generally prescribed in the UK are covered and those considered less suitable for prescribing are clearly identified. Little or no information is included on medicines promoted for purchase by the public.

Information on drugs is drawn from the manufacturers' product literature, medical and pharmaceutical literature, UK health departments, regulatory authorities, and professional bodies. Advice is constructed from clinical literature and reflects, as far as possible, an evaluation of the evidence from diverse sources. The BNF also takes account of authoritative national guidelines and emerging safety concerns. In addition, the editorial team receives advice on all therapeutic areas from expert clinicians; this ensures that the BNF's recommendations are relevant to practice.

The BNF is designed as a digest for rapid reference and it may not always include all the information necessary for prescribing and dispensing. Also, less detail is given on areas such as obstetrics, malignant disease, and anaesthesia since it is expected that those undertaking treatment will have specialist knowledge and access to specialist literature. Similarly, little or no information is included on medicines for very rare conditions. BNF for Children should be consulted for detailed information on the use of medicines in children. The BNF should be interpreted in the light of professional knowledge and supplemented as necessary by specialised publications and by reference to the product literature. Information is also available from medicines information services, see Medicines Information Services (see inside front cover).

It is **important** to use the most recent BNF information for making clinical decisions. The print edition of the BNF is updated in March and September each year. Monthly updates are provided online via MedicinesComplete and NICE (www.nice.org.uk). The more important changes listed under Changes p. xvi are cumulative (from one print edition to the next), and can be printed off each month to show the main changes since the last print edition as an aide memoire for those using print copies.

The BNF Publications website (www.bnf.org) includes additional information of relevance to healthcare professionals. Other digital formats of the BNF—including versions for mobile devices and integration into local formularies—are also available.

BNF Publications welcomes comments from healthcare professionals. Comments and constructive criticism should be sent to:

British National Formulary
Royal Pharmaceutical Society
66–68 East Smithfield
London
E1W 1AW
editor@bnf.org

The contact email for manufacturers or pharmaceutical companies wishing to contact BNF Publications is manufacturerinfo@bnf.org

Contents

NOTES ON DRUGS AND PREPARATIONS

APPENDICES AND INDICES

Acknowledgements

The Joint Formulary Committee is grateful to individuals and organisations that have provided advice and information to British National Formulary (BNF).

Contributors for this update were:

K.W. Ah-See, A.K. Bahl, D. Bilton, M.F. Bultitude, I.F. Burgess, C.E. Dearden, D.W. Denning, D.A.C. Elliman, P. Emery, A. Freyer, N.J.L. Gittoes, M. Gupta, T.L. Hawkins, S.P. Higgins, T.H. Lee, A. Lekkas, D.N.J. Lockwood, A.M. Lovering, M.G. Lucas, P.D. Mason, D.A. McArthur, L.M. Melvin, R.M. Mirakian, P. Morrison, S.M.S. Nasser, C. Nelson-Piercy, D.J. Nutt, R. Patel, A.B. Provan, A.S.C. Rice, D.J. Rowbotham, S.E. Slater, J. Soar, M.D. Stewart, S. Thomas, A.D. Weeks, A. Wilcock.

Expert advice on the management of oral and dental conditions was kindly provided by A. Crighton, C. Scully, R.A. Seymour, and R. Welbury. S. Kaur provided valuable advice on dental prescribing policy.

Valuable advice has been provided by the following expert groups: Advisory Committee on Malaria Prevention, Association of British Neurologists, British Association of Dermatologists' Therapy & Guidelines Sub-committee, British Association for Sexual Health and HIV, British Association of Urological Surgeons, British Geriatrics Society, British Inherited Metabolic Disease Group, British Menopause Society, British Oncology Pharmacy Association, British Pain Society, British Society for Allergy & Clinical Immunology, British Society for Antimicrobial Chemotherapy, British Society of Gastroenterology, British Society for Haematology, British Society of Rheumatology, British Thoracic Society, College of Mental Health Pharmacy, ENT UK, Faculty of Sexual and Reproductive Healthcare, National Poisons Information Service & TOXBASE, Public Health England, Renal Association, Royal College of Anaesthetists, Royal College of Obstetricians and Gynaecologists, Royal College of Ophthalmologists, Royal College of Pathologists, Royal College of Physicians, Royal College of Psychiatrists, Society for Endocrinology, UK Clinical Pharmacy Association, UK Drugs in Lactation Advisory Service, UK Teratology Information Service, Vascular Society.

We also value the contribution made by clinical pharmacology trainees A. Daneshmend from Imperial College Healthcare NHS Trust and M. Amran from University College London Hospitals NHS Foundation Trust.

The MHRA have provided valuable assistance.

Correspondents in the pharmaceutical industry have provided information on new products and commented on products in BNF.

Numerous doctors, pharmacists, nurses, and others have sent comments and suggestions.

The BNF team are grateful for the support and access to in-house expertise at Pharmaceutical Press and acknowledge the assistance of K. Baxter, A. Chester, D. Gordon, N. Potter, D. Wright and their teams.

F. Aimufua, R. Akinnawonu, S. Aldwinckle, S. Amin, M. Bradbury, A. Chiu, F. Colclough, S. Janarthan, S. Khan, M. Kolapo, C. Kwofie, C. Lam, M. Quansah, A. Sekiwano, and O. Seymour provided considerable assistance during the production of this update of BNF.

BNF Staff

CONTENT DIRECTOR (BNF PUBLICATIONS)
Kate Towers *BPharm (AU), GCClinPharm (AU)*

SENIOR EDITORIAL STAFF

Kiri Aikman *BPharm (NZ), PGDipClinPharm (NZ), ARPharmS*

Hannah Arnold *BPharm (NZ)*

Rosalind Barker *BMus, MA*

Alison Brayfield *BPharm, MRPharmS*

Catherine Cadart *BPharm (AU), BA(Hons), GradDipHospPharm (AU), MRPharmS*

Darren Chan *BSc, MSc*

Mahinaz Harrison *BPharm, DipPharmPract, IP, MRPharmS*

Emily Henderson *BPharm (NZ), PGCertClinPharm (NZ)*

Jean MacKershan *BSc, PgDip*

Angela McFarlane *BSc, DipClinPharm*

Anna McLachlan *BPharm (NZ), PGCertClinPharm (NZ)*

Laura Pham *BPharm(Hons) (AU)*

Claire Preston *BPharm, PGDipMedMan, MRPharmS*

India Smith *MPharm, PGCert*

EDITORIAL STAFF

Natasha Bell-Asher *BPharm (NZ), PGDipClinPharm (NZ)*

Adam Brelsford *MPharm, PhD*

Charlotte Clark *MPharm*

Molly Dennis *MPharm, PGDipClinPharm, IP*

Naira Ghanem *MPharm, PGCertClinPharm*

Sue Wend Ho *BPharm (AU), MRPharmS*

Emma Jones *MPharm*

Elizabeth King *MAPharmT*

Julia Lacey *BPharm, PGDipClinPharm, PharmD*

Anne Lee *MPhil, FRPharmS*

David Lipanovic *BPharm (NZ), PGCertClinPharm (NZ)*

Sorcha McCann *MPharm, PGDipClinPharm, IPresc, MRPharmS*

Marie McIlwain *MPharm, PGDipPharmPrac, MRPharmS*

Lona Mehta *MPharm, MRPharmS*

Navpreet Mittal *MPharm, PGCert*

Faye Morley *MPharm, PGCertClinPharm*

Nalwenga Mutambo *MPharm*

Barbara Okpala *MPharm, PGDipGPP*

Heenaben Patel *MPharm, PGDipClinPharm, MRPharmS*

Leah Richardson *BPharm (NZ)*

Punam Solanki *MPharm, PGCertClinPharm*

Renee Spriggs *BPharm (NZ), PGCertClinPharm (NZ)*

Miranda Stuart *BPharm(Hons) (NZ), PGCertClinPharm (NZ)*

Paula Sutton *BPharm (NZ), PGCertPharm (NZ)*

Shaunagh Swain *BPharm(Hons) (AU)*

Jodie-Anne Swatton *BSc(Hons)*

Harpreet Takhar *MPharm, MRPharmS*

Iris Yapp *MPharm, PGClinDip, GDL, MRPharmS*

Jennifer Yick *MPharm*

SUPPORT STAFF

Libby Achilles *BSc(Hons)*

Sophia Aldwinckle *BSc(Hons)*

Lauren Cheetham *BA(Hons)*

Clare Dunne *BSc(Hons), PhD, DIC, ARCS, MRSC*

Melanie Eustace

Ella Farrelly *BSc(Hons), MSc*

Rebecca Harwood *BSc(Hons), MRSB*

Rhiann Jhaj *MPharm*

Jonathan Law *BSc(Hons), MSc*

Philip Lee *BSc(Hons), PhD*

Rebecca Luckhurst *BSc(Hons), MSc*

Hang Nguyen *BSc(Hons)*

Jessica Nguyen *BPharm(Hons) (AU), GradCertPharmPrac (AU)*

Yvette Palmer *BSc(Hons)*

Bhavini Patel *MPharm(Hons), PGDipClinPharm, IP*

Philip Shaw *BSc(Hons), MPhil*

Enikő Steiner *BSc (HU)*

Najwa Zaman *BSc(Hons), MSc*

Joint Formulary Committee

CHAIR
Fraz A. Mir
BSc, MA, MBBS, FRCP

COMMITTEE MEMBERS
Andy Burman (lay member)
CMgr, FCMI, FRSA, FIAM

Daniel Burrage
MRCP, MSc, PhD, FHEA

Rima Chauhan
MPharm (Hons), MSc, IP, MRPharmS

Carmel M. Darcy
BSc, MSc, IP, MPSNI, MRPharmS

Sue Faulding
BPharm, MSc, FRPharmS

Daniel Greenwood
MPharm(Hons), PgCertMedEd, PgDip(ClinPharm), PhD

Tracy Hall
BSc, MSc, RN, DN, NIP, Dip N, Cert N, QN

Simon Hurding
MB, ChB, MRCGP

Valerie Joynson
BSc, PGCE, PGCert

Sandeep Kapur
BSc(Hons), MB BS, MRCGP(Dist)

Mark P. Lythgoe
MB BS, MRPharmS

Louise Picton
BSc, DipCommPharm, MSc, MRPharmS

Bernadette Rae
Pg Cert Ed, Fellow HEA, MSc Nursing, Pg CertANP, BSc(Hons), Grad Cert NMP, RGN

Fiona Raje (lay member)
DPhil, MSc, BA, FRGS

Muhammad Magdi Yaqoob
MD, FRCP

Dental Advisory Group

CHAIR
Sarah Manton
BDS, FDSRCS Ed, FHEA, PhD, FDFTEd

COMMITTEE MEMBERS
Natasha Bell-Asher
BPharm (NZ), PGDipClinPharm (NZ)

Elaine Boylan (observer)
PhD

Andrew K. Brewer
BSc, BchD, MFDS (Glas)

Alexander Crighton
BDS, MB, ChB, FDS, OM

Angela McFarlane
BSc, DipClinPharm

Faye Morley
MPharm, PGCertClinPharm

Monica Neil
BDS, MFDS RCS, MSc, MPaed Dent RCS, FDS RCS, MBA

Suzanne Sykes
BDS (Hons), MSc Adv HCP (Open), MFGDP (UK) MJDF, PG Cert Dental Sedation and Pain Management (UCL), Dip FMS (FMS), Dip Spec Care Dent RCSEd

Adrian Thorp
BDS, LLB (Hons), MFDS RCS (Eng), M Surg Dent RCS (Eng), MAcadMEd, FDS RCSEd, FDTFEd, FFGDP (UK), FCGDent, PG Cert

ADVICE ON DENTAL PRACTICE
The **British Dental Association** has contributed to the advice on medicines for dental practice through its representatives on the Dental Advisory Group.

Nurse Prescribers' Advisory Group

COMMITTEE MEMBERS
Penny M. Franklin
RN, RCN, RSCPHN(HV), MA, PGCE

Matt Griffiths
BA(Hons), FAETC, RGN, Cert A&E, NISP, PHECC

Tracy Hall
BSc, MSc, RN, DN, NIP, Dip N, Cert N, QN

Angela McFarlane
BSc, DipClinPharm

Stacey Moss
BSc, RGN

Fiona Peniston-Bird
BSc(Hons), NIP, RHV, RGN

Kathy Radley
BSc, RGN

Neil Thomas (representative of Chief Nursing Officer for Wales)

How BNF Publications are constructed

Overview

The BNF is an independent professional publication that addresses the day-to-day prescribing information needs of healthcare professionals. Use of this resource throughout the health service helps to ensure that medicines are used safely, effectively, and appropriately.

Hundreds of changes are made between print editions, and are published monthly in a number of digital formats. The most clinically significant updates are listed under Changes p. xvi.

The BNF is unique in bringing together authoritative, independent guidance on best practice with clinically validated drug information. Validation of information follows a standardised process, reviewing emerging evidence, best-practice guidelines, and advice from a network of clinical experts. Where the evidence base is weak, further validation may be undertaken through a process of peer review. The process and its governance are outlined in greater detail in the sections that follow.

Joint Formulary Committee

The Joint Formulary Committee (JFC) is responsible for the content of the BNF. The JFC includes pharmacy, medical, nursing, and lay representatives; there are also representatives from the Medicines and Healthcare products Regulatory Agency (MHRA), the UK Health Departments, and a national guideline producer. The JFC decides on matters of policy and reviews amendments to the BNF in the light of new complex or contentious evidence and expert advice.

Dental Advisory Group

The Dental Advisory Group oversees the preparation of advice on the drug management of dental and oral conditions; the group includes representatives from the British Dental Association and a representative from the UK Health Departments.

Nurse Prescribers' Advisory Group

The Nurse Prescribers' Advisory Group oversees the list of drugs approved for inclusion in the Nurse Prescribers' Formulary; the group includes representatives from a range of nursing disciplines and stakeholder organisations.

Expert advisers

The BNF uses representatives from expert groups (professional societies and advisory bodies) to provide expert advice on clinical content. These expert advisers are practice-based healthcare professionals (including doctors, pharmacists, nurses, and dentists), and are regarded as specialists in their field. The role of these expert advisers is to provide independent advice on their area of expertise by reviewing existing text and commenting on amendments drafted by the clinical writers. These clinical experts help to ensure that the BNF remains reliable by:

- commenting on the relevance of the text in the context of best clinical practice in the UK;
- checking draft amendments for appropriate interpretation of any new evidence;
- providing expert opinion in areas of controversy or when reliable evidence is lacking.

The BNF may also call on other clinical specialists for specific developments when particular expertise is required.

The BNF works closely with a number of expert bodies that produce clinical guidelines. Drafts or pre-publication copies of guidelines are often received for comment and assimilation into the BNF.

Editorial team

BNF clinical writers have worked as pharmacists or possess a pharmacy degree and many have a further, relevant post-graduate qualification; they therefore have a sound understanding of how drugs are used in clinical practice. As a team, the clinical writers are responsible for editing, maintaining, and updating BNF content. They follow a systematic prioritisation process in response to updates to the evidence base in order to ensure the most clinically important topics are reviewed as quickly as possible. In addition, review of content is carried out proactively, with the aim of considering all recommendations for review every 3 to 4 years.

Amendments to the text are drafted when the clinical writers are satisfied that any new information is reliable and relevant. A set of standard criteria defines when content is referred to expert advisers, the Joint Formulary Committee or other advisory groups, or submitted for peer review.

Clinical writers prepare the text for publication and undertake a number of validation checks at various stages of the content creation process.

Sources of BNF information

The BNF uses a variety of sources for its information; the main ones are shown below.

Summaries of product characteristics

The BNF reviews summaries of product characteristics (SPCs) of all new products as well as revised SPCs for existing products. The SPCs are the principal source of product information and are carefully processed. Such processing involves:

- verifying the approved names of all relevant ingredients including 'non-active' ingredients (the BNF is committed to using approved names and descriptions as laid down by the Human Medicine Regulations 2012);
- comparing the indications, cautions, contra-indications, and side-effects with similar existing drugs. Where these are different from the expected pattern, justification is sought for their inclusion or exclusion;
- seeking independent data on the use of drugs in pregnancy and breast-feeding;
- incorporating the information into the BNF using established criteria for the presentation and inclusion of the data;
- checking interpretation of the information by a second clinical writer before submitting to a content approver; changes relating to doses receive a further check;
- identifying potential clinical problems or omissions and seeking further information from manufacturers or from expert advisers;
- constructing, with the help of expert advisers, a comment on the role of the drug in the context of similar drugs.

Much of this processing is applicable to the following sources as well.

Literature

Clinical writers monitor and process various sources of information on a regular basis. When a difference between the advice in the BNF and the source is noted, the new information is assessed for reliability (using tools based on SIGN methodology if appropriate) and relevance to UK clinical practice. If necessary, new text is drafted and discussed with expert advisers and the Joint Formulary Committee. The BNF enjoys a close working relationship with a number of national information providers.

In addition to the routine process, which is used to identify 'triggers' for changing the content, systematic literature searches are used to identify the best quality evidence available to inform an update. Clinical writers receive training in critical appraisal, literature evaluation, and search strategies.

Consensus guidelines

The advice in the BNF is checked against consensus guidelines produced by expert bodies. The quality of the guidelines is assessed using adapted versions of the AGREE II tool. A number of bodies make drafts or pre-publication copies of the guidelines available to the BNF; it is therefore possible to ensure that a consistent message is disseminated. The BNF routinely processes guidelines from the National Institute for Health and Care Excellence (NICE), the All Wales Medicines Strategy Group (AWMSG), the Scottish Medicines Consortium (SMC), and the Scottish Intercollegiate Guidelines Network (SIGN).

Reference sources

Textbooks and reference sources are used to provide background information for the review of existing text or for the construction of new text. The BNF team works closely with the editorial team that produces *Martindale: The Complete Drug Reference*. The BNF has access to *Martindale* information resources and each team keeps the other informed of significant developments and shifts in the trends of drug usage.

Peer review
Although every effort is made to identify the most robust data available, inevitably there are areas where the evidence base is weak or contradictory. While the BNF has the valuable support of expert advisers and the Joint Formulary Committee, the recommendations made may be subject to a further level of scrutiny through peer review to ensure they reflect best practice.

Content for open peer review is posted on bnf.org and interested parties are notified via a number of channels, including the BNF e-newsletter.

Statutory information
The BNF routinely processes relevant information from various Government bodies including Statutory Instruments and regulations affecting the Prescription Only Medicines Order. Official compendia such as the British Pharmacopoeia and its addenda are processed routinely to ensure that the BNF complies with the relevant sections of the Human Medicines Regulations 2012.

The BNF maintains close links with the Home Office (in relation to controlled drug regulations) and the Medicines and Healthcare products Regulatory Agency (including the British Pharmacopoeia Commission). Safety warnings issued by the Commission on Human Medicines (CHM) and guidelines on drug use issued by the UK health departments are processed as a matter of routine.

Relevant professional statements issued by the Royal Pharmaceutical Society are included in the BNF as are guidelines from bodies such as the Royal College of General Practitioners.

Medicines and devices
NHS Prescription Services (from the NHS Business Services Authority) provides non-clinical, categorical information (including prices) on the medicines and devices included in the BNF.

Comments from readers
Readers of the BNF are invited to send in comments. Numerous letters and emails are received by the BNF team. Such feedback helps to ensure that the BNF provides practical and clinically relevant information. Many changes in the presentation and scope of the BNF have resulted from comments sent in by users.

Comments from industry
Close scrutiny of BNF by the manufacturers provides an additional check and allows them an opportunity to raise issues about BNF's presentation of the role of various drugs; this is yet another check on the balance of BNF's advice. All comments are looked at with care and, where necessary, additional information and expert advice are sought.

Market research
Market research is conducted at regular intervals to gather feedback on specific areas of development.

Assessing the evidence
From January 2016, recommendations made in the BNF have been evidence graded to reflect the strength of the recommendation. The addition of evidence grading is to support clinical decision-making based on the best available evidence.

Recommendations from summaries of product characteristics
Recommendations from summaries of product characteristics (SPCs) and other product literature are either preceded by "manufacturer advises" or have the symbol M (manufacturer information) displayed next to the recommendation within the text.

Grading system
The BNF has adopted a five-level grading system from A to E, based on the former SIGN grading system. This grade is displayed next to the recommendation within the text.

Evidence used to make a recommendation is assessed for validity using standardised methodology tools based on AGREE II or SIGN and then assigned a level of evidence. The recommendation is given a grade that is extrapolated from the level of evidence, and an assessment of the body of evidence and its applicability.

Evidence assigned a level 1- or 2- score has an unacceptable level of bias or confounding and is not used to form recommendations.

Levels of evidence
- **Level 1++**
  High quality meta-analyses, systematic reviews of randomised controlled trials (RCTs), or RCTs with a very low risk of bias.

- **Level 1+**
  Well-conducted meta-analyses, systematic reviews, or RCTs with a low risk of bias.

- **Level 1-**
  Meta-analyses, systematic reviews, or RCTs with a high risk of bias.

- **Level 2++**
  High quality systematic reviews of case control or cohort studies; or high quality case control or cohort studies with a very low risk of confounding or bias and a high probability that the relationship is causal.

- **Level 2+**
  Well-conducted case control or cohort studies with a low risk of confounding or bias and a moderate probability that the relationship is causal.

- **Level 2-**
  Case control or cohort studies with a high risk of confounding or bias and a significant risk that the relationship is not causal.

- **Level 3**
  Non-analytic studies, e.g. case reports, case series.

- **Level 4**
  Expert advice or clinical experience from respected authorities.

Grades of recommendation
- **Grade A: High strength**
  NICE-accredited guidelines; or other guidelines, assessed using AGREE II, that meet the grade A threshold; or at least one meta-analysis, systematic review, or RCT rated as 1++, and directly applicable to the target population; or a body of evidence consisting principally of studies rated as 1+, directly applicable to the target population, and demonstrating overall consistency of results.

- **Grade B: Moderate strength**
  Guidelines, assessed using AGREE II, that meet the grade B threshold; or a body of evidence including studies rated as 2++, directly applicable to the target population, and demonstrating overall consistency of results; or extrapolated evidence from studies rated as 1++ or 1+.

- **Grade C: Low strength**
  Guidelines, assessed using AGREE II, that meet the grade C threshold; or a body of evidence including studies rated as 2+, directly applicable to the target population and demonstrating overall consistency of results; or extrapolated evidence from studies rated as 2++.

- **Grade D: Very low strength**
  Guidelines, assessed using AGREE II, that meet the grade D threshold; or evidence level 3; or extrapolated evidence from studies rated as 2+; or tertiary reference source created by a transparent, defined methodology, where the basis for recommendation is clear.

- **Grade E: Practice point**
  Evidence level 4.

How to use BNF Publications in print

Introduction

In order to achieve the safe, effective, and appropriate use of medicines, healthcare professionals must be able to use the BNF effectively, and keep up to date with significant changes in the BNF that are relevant to their clinical practice. This *How to Use the BNF* is key to understanding the structure of the BNF for all healthcare professionals involved with prescribing, monitoring, supplying, and administering medicines, as well as supporting the learning of students training to join these professions.

Structure of the BNF

The BNF print edition is structured as follows:

Front matter, comprising information on how to use the BNF, the significant content changes in each edition, and guidance on various prescribing matters (e.g. prescription writing, the use of intravenous drugs, particular considerations for special patient populations).

Chapters, containing drug monographs describing the uses, safety issues and other considerations involved in the use of drugs; drug class monographs; and treatment summaries, covering guidance on the selection of drugs. Monographs and treatment summaries are divided into chapters based on specific aspects of medical care, such as Chapter 5, Infections, or Chapter 16, Emergency treatment of poisoning; or drug use related to a particular system of the body, such as Chapter 2, Cardiovascular.

Within each chapter, content is organised alphabetically by therapeutic use (e.g. Airways disease, obstructive), with the treatment summaries first, (e.g. asthma), followed by the monographs of the drugs used to manage the conditions discussed in the treatment summary. Within each therapeutic use, the drugs are organised alphabetically by classification (e.g. Antimuscarinics, Beta$_2$-agonist bronchodilators) and then alphabetically within each classification (e.g. Aclidinium bromide, Glycopyrronium bromide, Ipratropium bromide).

Appendices, covering interactions, borderline substances, cautionary and advisory labels, and wound care.

Back matter, covering the lists of medicines approved by the NHS for Dental and Nurse Practitioner prescribing, proprietary and specials manufacturers' contact details, and the index. Quick reference guides for life support and key drug doses in medical emergencies are also included, for ease of access.

Navigating the BNF

The contents page provides the high-level layout of information within the BNF; and in addition, each chapter begins with a small contents section, describing the therapeutic uses covered within that chapter. Once in a chapter, location is guided by the side of the page showing the chapter number (the *thumbnail*), alongside the chapter title. The top of the page includes the therapeutic use (the *running head*) alongside the page number.

Once on a page, visual cues aid navigation: treatment summary information is in black type, with therapeutic use titles similarly styled in black, whereas the use of colour indicates drug-related information, including drug classification titles, drug class monographs, and drug monographs.

Although navigation is possible by browsing, primarily access to the information is via the index, which covers the titles of drug class monographs, drug monographs, and treatment summaries. The index also includes the names of branded medicines and other topics of relevance, such as abbreviations, guidance sections, tables, and images.

Content types

Treatment summaries

Treatment summaries are of three main types;

- an overview of delivering a drug to a particular body system (e.g. Skin conditions, management p. 1386)
- a comparison between a group or groups of drugs (e.g. Beta-adrenoceptor blocking drugs p. 173)
- an overview of the drug management or prophylaxis of common conditions intended to facilitate rapid appraisal of options (e.g. Hypertension p. 166, or Malaria, prophylaxis p. 702).

In order to select safe and effective medicines for individual patients, information in the treatment summaries must be used in conjunction with other prescribing details about the drugs and knowledge of the patient's medical and drug history.

Monographs

Overview

All of the information for the systemic use of a drug is contained within one monograph. Where a drug has systemic and local uses, for example, chloramphenicol, and the considerations around drug use are markedly different according to the route of administration, the monograph is split into the relevant chapters.

Monographs used within specialist settings (such as drugs used for malignancy and drugs given via intravitreal injection) contain less detail than regular monographs within the BNF since it is expected that those undertaking treatment will have specialist knowledge and access to specialist literature. These monographs include the words [Specialist drug] alongside the monograph title, and so are easily identifiable in content. Specialist monographs will continue to include information to support patient safety and non-specialist patient care (allergy and cross-sensitivity, conception and contraception, contra-indications, important safety information, indications (high-level), interactions, medicinal forms, patient and carer advice, side-effects, synonyms, and unlicensed use), but will not contain information which is within the remit of specialist care (breast feeding, cautions, directions for administration, doses, drug action, effects on laboratory tests, exception to legal category, handling and storage, hepatic impairment, less suitable for prescribing, monitoring requirements, palliative care, pregnancy, prescribing and dispensing information, pre-treatment screening, profession-specific information, renal impairment, and treatment cessation). The current level of additional prescribing information has been retained for drug monographs that have a mix of specialist and non-specialist uses (such as methotrexate that is used for both malignancy and rheumatological conditions), although specialist indications within these monographs will no longer include doses.

Monographs may include over 20 sections; the number of sections included within an individual monograph is dependent on whether relevant information has been identified and whether it is used within specialist settings. The following information describes these sections and their uses in more detail.

Nomenclature

Monograph titles follow the convention of recommended international non-proprietary names (rINNs), or, in the absence of a rINN, British Approved Names. Relevant synonyms are included below the title and, in some instances a brief description of the drug action is included.

In some monographs, immediately below the nomenclature or drug action, there are cross references or flags used to signpost the user to any additional information they need to consider about a drug. This is most common for drugs formulated in combinations, where users will be signposted to the monographs for the individual ingredients to access full prescribing information for the combination drug (e.g. senna with ispaghula husk p. 69) or for drugs that are related to a drug class monograph (see Drug class monographs, below).

Indication and dose
User feedback has highlighted that one of the main uses of the BNF is identifying indications and doses of drugs. Therefore, indication and dose information appears towards the top of the monograph and is highlighted by a coloured panel to aid quick reference.

The indication and dose section is highly structured, giving clarity around which doses should be used for which indications and by which route. Where a dose varies with a specific preparation or formulation, dosing information appears under a heading of the preparation name.

Doses are either expressed in terms of a definite frequency (e.g. 1 g 4 times daily) or in the total daily dose format (e.g. 6 g daily in 3 divided doses); the total daily dose should be divided into individual doses (in the second example, the patient should receive 2 g 3 times daily).

Doses for specific patient groups (e.g. the elderly) may be included if they are different to the standard dose. Doses for children can be identified by the relevant age range and may vary according to their age or body-weight.

Wherever possible age and weight ranges do not overlap. When interpreting age ranges it is important to understand that a patient is considered to be 64 up until the point of their 65th birthday, meaning that an age range of adult 18 to 64 is applicable to a patient from the day of their 18th birthday until the day before their 65th birthday. All age ranges should be interpreted in this way. Similarly, when interpreting weight ranges, it should be understood that a weight of up to 30 kg is applicable to a patient up to, but not including, the point that they tip the scales at 30 kg and a weight range of 35 to 59 kg is applicable to a patient as soon as they tip the scales at 35 kg right up until, but not including, the point that they tip the scales at 60 kg. All weight ranges should be interpreted in this way.

In all circumstances, it is important to consider the patient in question and their physical condition, and select the dose most appropriate for the individual.

Other information relevant to Indication and dose
The dose panel also contains, where known, an indication of **pharmacokinetic considerations** that may affect the choice of dose, and **dose equivalence** information, which may aid the selection of dose when switching between drugs or preparations.

The BNF includes **unlicensed use** of medicines when the clinical need cannot be met by licensed medicines; such use should be supported by appropriate evidence and experience. When the BNF recommends an unlicensed medicine or the 'off-label' use of a licensed medicine, this is shown below the indication and dose panel in the unlicensed use section.

Minimising harm and drug safety
The drug chosen to treat a particular condition should minimise the patient's susceptibility to adverse effects and, where co-morbidities exist, have minimal detrimental effects on the patient's other diseases. To achieve this, the *Contra-indications, Cautions* and *Side-effects* of the relevant drug should be reviewed.

The information under Cautions can be used to assess the risks of using a drug in a patient who has co-morbidities that are also included in the Cautions for that drug—if a safer alternative cannot be found, the drug may be prescribed while monitoring the patient for adverse effects or deterioration in the co-morbidity. Contra-indications are far more restrictive than Cautions and mean that the drug

should be avoided in a patient with a condition that is contra-indicated.

The impact that potential side-effects may have on a patient's quality of life should also be assessed. For instance, in a patient who has difficulty sleeping, it may be preferable to avoid a drug that frequently causes insomnia.

The *Important safety information* section in the BNF, delineated by a coloured outline box, highlights important safety concerns, often those raised by regulatory authorities or guideline producers. Safety warnings issued by the Commission on Human Medicines (CHM) or Medicines and Healthcare products Regulatory Agency (MHRA) are found here.

Drug selection should aim to minimise drug interactions. If it is necessary to prescribe a potentially serious combination of drugs, patients should be monitored appropriately. The mechanisms underlying drug interactions are explained in Appendix 1, followed by details of drug interactions.

Use of drugs in specific patient populations
Drug selection should aim to minimise the potential for drug accumulation, adverse drug reactions, and exacerbation of pre-existing hepatic or renal disease. If it is necessary to prescribe drugs whose effect is altered by hepatic or renal disease, appropriate drug dose adjustments should be made, and patients should be monitored adequately. The general principles for prescribing are outlined under Prescribing in hepatic impairment p. 20, and Prescribing in renal impairment p. 21. Information about drugs that should be avoided or used with caution in hepatic disease or renal impairment can be found in drug monographs under *Hepatic impairment* and *Renal impairment* (e.g. fluconazole p. 690).

Similarly, drug selection should aim to minimise harm to the fetus, nursing infant, and mother. The infant should be monitored for potential side-effects of drugs used by the mother during pregnancy or breast-feeding. The general principles for prescribing are outlined under Prescribing in pregnancy p. 24 and Prescribing in breast-feeding p. 25. The Treatment summaries provide guidance on the drug treatment of common conditions that can occur during pregnancy or breast feeding (e.g. Venous thromboembolism p. 134). Information about the use of specific drugs during pregnancy and breast feeding can be found in their drug monographs under *Pregnancy*, and *Breast feeding* (e.g. fluconazole p. 690).

The section *Conception and contraception* contains information around considerations for females of childbearing potential or men who might father a child (e.g. isotretinoin p. 1443).

Administration and monitoring
When selecting the most appropriate drug, it may be necessary to screen the patient for certain genetic markers or metabolic states. This information is included within a section called *Pre-treatment screening* (e.g. abacavir p. 744). This section covers one-off tests required to assess the suitability of a patient for a particular drug.

Once the drug has been selected, it needs to be given in the most appropriate manner. The *Directions for administration* section provides practical information on the preparation of intravenous drug infusions, including compatibility of drugs with standard intravenous infusion fluids, method of dilution or reconstitution, and administration rates. In addition, general advice relevant to other routes of administration is provided within this section (e.g. fentanyl p. 520).

Typical layout of a monograph and associated medicinal forms

❶ Class monographs and Drug monographs

In most cases, all information that relates to an individual drug is contained within its drug monograph

Some drugs formulated in combinations include cross reference links that signpost to component drug monographs. Cross reference links are preceded by the following statement, which appears below the title of relevant monographs: The properties listed below are those particular to the combination only. For the properties of the components please consider, ...

Class monographs have been created where substantial amounts of information are common to all drugs in a drug class; these are indicated by a flag symbol in a circle: ⊖

Drug monographs with a corresponding class monograph are indicated by a tab with a flag symbol; the tab includes the page number of the corresponding class monograph: ⚑ 1234

Drug monographs that are used within specialist settings include [Specialist drug] alongside the monograph title. These monographs contain less detail, however, information to support patient safety and non-specialist patient care is included where relevant information has been identified

For further information, see How to use BNF Publications

❷ Drug classifications

Used to inform users of the class of a drug and to assist in finding other drugs of the same class. May be based on pharmacological class (e.g. opioids) but can also be associated with the use of the drug (e.g. cough suppressants)

❸ Review date

The date of last review of the content

❹ Specific preparation name

If the dose varies with a specific preparation or formulation it appears under a heading of the preparation name

---

Class monograph ❶ 

CLASSIFICATION ❷

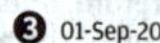

Drug monograph ❶   ❸ 01-Sep-2023

(Synonym) another name by which a drug may be known

- **DRUG ACTION** how a drug exerts its effect in the body

- **INDICATIONS AND DOSE**

Indications are the clinical reasons a drug is used. The dose of a drug will often depend on the indications

Indication

▸ ROUTE

▸ Age groups: [Child/Adult/Elderly]
  Dose and frequency of administration (max. dose)

SPECIFIC PREPARATION NAME ❹

Indication

▸ ROUTE

▸ Age groups: [Child/Adult/Elderly]
  Dose and frequency of administration (max. dose)

DOSE ADJUSTMENTS DUE TO INTERACTIONS dosing information when used concurrently with other drugs

DOSES AT EXTREMES OF BODY-WEIGHT dosing information for patients who are overweight or underweight

DOSE EQUIVALENCE AND CONVERSION information around the bioequivalence between formulations of the same drug, or equivalent doses of drugs that are members of the same class

PHARMACOKINETICS how the body affects a drug (absorption, distribution, metabolism, and excretion)

POTENCY a measure of drug activity expressed in terms of the concentration required to produce an effect of given intensity

- **UNLICENSED USE** describes the use of medicines outside the terms of their UK licence (off-label use), or use of medicines that have no licence for use in the UK

> **IMPORTANT SAFETY INFORMATION**
> Information produced and disseminated by drug regulators often highlights serious risks associated with the use of a drug, and may include advice that is mandatory

- **CONTRA-INDICATIONS** circumstances when a drug should be avoided

- **CAUTIONS** details of precautions required

- **INTERACTIONS** when one drug changes the effects of another drug; the mechanisms underlying drug interactions are explained in Appendix 1

- **SIDE-EFFECTS** listed in order of frequency, where known, and arranged alphabetically

- **ALLERGY AND CROSS-SENSITIVITY** for drugs that carry an increased risk of hypersensitivity reactions

- **CONCEPTION AND CONTRACEPTION** potential for a drug to have harmful effects on an unborn child when prescribing for a woman of childbearing age or for a man trying to father a child; information on the effect of drugs on the efficacy of latex condoms or diaphragms

- PREGNANCY advice on the use of a drug during pregnancy
- BREAST FEEDING EvGr advice on the use of a drug during breast feeding Ⓐ ❺
- HEPATIC IMPAIRMENT advice on the use of a drug in hepatic impairment
- RENAL IMPAIRMENT advice on the use of a drug in renal impairment
- PRE-TREATMENT SCREENING covers one off tests required to assess the suitability of a patient for a particular drug
- MONITORING REQUIREMENTS specifies any special monitoring requirements, including information on monitoring the plasma concentration of drugs with a narrow therapeutic index
- EFFECTS ON LABORATORY TESTS for drugs that can interfere with the accuracy of seemingly unrelated laboratory tests
- TREATMENT CESSATION specifies whether further monitoring or precautions are advised when the drug is withdrawn
- DIRECTIONS FOR ADMINISTRATION practical information on the preparation of intravenous drug infusions; general advice relevant to other routes of administration
- PRESCRIBING AND DISPENSING INFORMATION practical information around how a drug can be prescribed and dispensed including details of when brand prescribing is necessary
- HANDLING AND STORAGE includes information on drugs that can cause adverse effects to those who handle them before they are taken by, or administered to, a patient; advice on storage conditions
- PATIENT AND CARER ADVICE for drugs with a special need for counselling
- PROFESSION SPECIFIC INFORMATION provides details of the restrictions certain professions such as dental practitioners or nurse prescribers need to be aware of when prescribing on the NHS
- NATIONAL FUNDING/ACCESS DECISIONS references to NICE Technology Appraisals, SMC advice and AWMSG advice
- LESS SUITABLE FOR PRESCRIBING preparations that are considered by the Joint Formulary Committee to be less suitable for prescribing
- EXCEPTION TO LEGAL CATEGORY advice and information on drugs which may be sold without a prescription under specific conditions

---

- MEDICINAL FORMS

Form

CAUTIONARY AND ADVISORY LABELS if applicable
EXCIPIENTS clinically important but not comprehensive [consult manufacturer information for full details]
ELECTROLYTES if clinically significant quantities occur

▸ Preparation name (Manufacturer/Non-proprietary)
  Drug name and strength pack sizes PoM ❻ Prices

Combinations available this indicates a combination preparation is available and a cross reference page number is provided to locate this preparation

❺ **Evidence grading**

Evidence grading to reflect the strengths of recommendations will be applied as content goes through the revalidation process. A five level evidence grading system based on the former SIGN grading system has been adopted. The grades Ⓐ Ⓑ Ⓒ Ⓓ Ⓔ are displayed next to the recommendations within the text, and are preceded by the symbol: EvGr

The symbol ⟨M⟩ indicates manufacturer information

For further information, see How BNF Publications are constructed

❻ **Legal categories**

PoM This symbol has been placed against those preparations that are available only on a prescription issued by an appropriate practitioner. For more detailed information see *Medicines, Ethics and Practice*, London, Pharmaceutical Press (always consult latest edition)

CD1 CD2 CD3 CD4-1 CD4-2 CD5 These symbols indicate that the preparations are subject to the prescription requirements of the Misuse of Drugs Act

For regulations governing prescriptions for such preparations, see Controlled Drugs and Drug Dependence

Not all monographs include all possible sections; sections are only included when relevant information has been identified

After selecting and administering the most appropriate drug by the most appropriate route, patients should be monitored to ensure they are achieving the expected benefits from drug treatment without any unwanted side-effects. The *Monitoring* section specifies any special monitoring requirements, including information on monitoring the plasma concentration of drugs with a narrow therapeutic index (e.g. theophylline p. 313). Monitoring may, in certain cases, be affected by the impact of a drug on laboratory tests (e.g. hydroxocobalamin p. 1162), and this information is included in *Effects on laboratory tests*.

In some cases, when a drug is withdrawn, further monitoring or precautions may be advised (e.g. clonidine hydrochloride p. 172): these are covered under *Treatment cessation*.

Choice and supply

The prescriber and the patient should agree on the health outcomes that the patient desires and on the strategy for achieving them. Taking the time to explain to the patient (and carers) the rationale and the potential adverse effects of treatment may improve adherence. For some medicines there is a special need for counselling (e.g. appropriate posture during administration of doxycycline p. 655); this is shown in *Patient and carer advice*.

Other information contained in the latter half of the monograph also helps prescribers and those dispensing medicines choose medicinal forms (by indicating information such as flavour or when branded products may not be interchangeable (e.g. diltiazem hydrochloride p. 185), assess the suitability of a drug for prescribing, understand the NHS funding status for a drug (e.g. sildenafil p. 940), or assess when a patient may be able to purchase a drug without prescription (e.g. loperamide hydrochloride p. 74).

Medicinal forms

In the BNF, preparations follow immediately after the monograph for the drug that is their main ingredient.

The medicinal forms section provides information on the type of formulation (e.g. tablet), the amount of active drug in a solid dosage form, and the concentration of active drug in a liquid dosage form. The legal status is shown for prescription-only medicines and controlled drugs, as well as pharmacy medicines and medicines on the general sales list. Practitioners are reminded, by a statement under the heading of "Medicinal Forms" that not all products containing a specific drug ingredient may be similarly licensed. To be clear on the precise licensing status of specific medicinal forms, practitioners should check the product literature for the particular product being prescribed or dispensed.

Details of all medicinal forms available on the dm+d for each drug in BNF Publications appears in this section. In print editions, due to space constraints, only certain branded products are included in detail. Where medicinal forms are listed they should not be inferred as equivalent to the other brands listed under the same form heading. For example, all the products listed under a heading of "Modified release capsule" will be available as modified release capsules, however, the brands listed under that form heading may have different release profiles, the available strengths may vary and/or the products may have different licensing information. Practitioners must ensure that the particular product being prescribed or dispensed is appropriate.

Patients should be prescribed a preparation that complements their daily routine, and that provides the right dose of drug for the right indication and route of administration. When dispensing liquid preparations, a sugar-free preparation should always be used in preference to one containing sugar. Patients receiving medicines containing cariogenic sugars should be advised of appropriate dental hygiene measures to prevent caries.

Information on possible inclusion of excipients and electrolytes is covered at the level of the dose form (e.g.

tablet). It is not possible to keep abreast of all of the generic products available on the UK market, and so this information serves as a reminder to the healthcare professional that, if the presence of a particular excipient is of concern, they should check the product literature for the particular product being prescribed or dispensed.

Cautionary and advisory labels that pharmacists are recommended to add when dispensing are included in the medicinal forms section. Details of these labels can be found in Appendix 3, Guidance for cautionary and advisory labels p. 1925.

In the case of compound preparations, the prescribing information for all constituents should be taken into account.

Prices in the BNF

Basic NHS **net prices** are given in the BNF to provide an indication of relative cost. Where there is a choice of suitable preparations for a particular disease or condition the relative cost may be used in making a selection. Cost-effective prescribing must, however, take into account other factors (such as dose frequency and duration of treatment) that affect the total cost. The use of more expensive drugs is justified if it will result in better treatment of the patient, or a reduction of the length of an illness, or the time spent in hospital.

Prices are regularly updated using the Drug Tariff and proprietary price information published by the NHS dictionary of medicines and devices (dm+d, www.nhsbsa.nhs. uk/pharmacies-gp-practices-and-appliance-contractors/ dictionary-medicines-and-devices-dmd). The weekly updated dm+d data (including prices) can be accessed using the dm+d browser of the NHS Business Services Authority (services. nhsbsa.nhs.uk/dmd-browser/). Prices have been calculated from the net cost used in pricing NHS prescriptions and generally reflect whole dispensing packs. Prices for extemporaneously prepared preparations are not provided in the BNF as prices vary between different manufacturers. In Appendix 4, prices stated are per dressing or bandage.

BNF prices are not suitable for quoting to patients seeking private prescriptions or contemplating over-the-counter purchases because they do not take into account VAT, professional fees, and other overheads.

A fuller explanation of costs to the NHS may be obtained from the Drug Tariff. Separate drug tariffs are applicable to England and Wales (www.nhsbsa.nhs.uk/pharmacies-gp-practices-and-appliance-contractors/drug-tariff), Scotland (publichealthscotland.scot/resources-and-tools/medical-practice-and-pharmaceuticals/scottish-drug-tariff/), and Northern Ireland (www.hscbusiness.hscni.net/services/2034.htm); prices in the different tariffs may vary.

Drug class monographs

Drug class monographs contain information relating to a class of drugs sharing the same properties (e.g. tetracyclines p. 655); this ensures information is easier to find, and has a regularised structure.

For consistency and ease of use, the class monograph follows the same structure as a drug monograph. Class monographs are indicated by the presence of a flag ⊖ (e.g. beta-adrenoceptor blockers (systemic) p. 175). If a drug monograph has a corresponding class monograph, that needs to be considered in tandem, in order to understand the full information about a drug, the monograph is also indicated by a flag ⊩ 1234 (e.g. metoprolol tartrate p. 182). Within this flag, the page number of the drug class monograph is provided (e.g. 1234), to help navigate the user to this information. This is particularly useful where occasionally, due to differences in therapeutic use, the drug monograph may not directly follow the drug class monograph (e.g. sotalol hydrochloride p. 124).

Other content

Nutrition

Appendix 2, Borderline substances p. 1878, includes tables of ACBS-approved enteral feeds and nutritional supplements based on their energy and protein content. Sections on foods for special diets, specialised formulae for specific clinical conditions, and nutritional supplements for metabolic diseases are also included.

Wound dressings

A table on wound dressings in Appendix 4, Wound management products and elasticated garments p. 1928, allows an appropriate dressing to be selected based on the appearance and condition of the wound. Further information about the dressing can be found by following the cross-reference to the relevant classified section in the Appendix.

Advanced wound contact dressings have been classified in order of increasing absorbency.

Other useful information

Finding significant changes in the BNF

- *Changes*, provides a list of significant changes, dose changes, classification changes, new names, and new preparations that have been incorporated into the BNF, as well as a list of preparations that have been discontinued and removed from the BNF. Changes listed online are cumulative (from one print edition to the next), and can be printed off each month to show the main changes since the last print edition as an aide memoire for those using print copies. So many changes are made for each update of the BNF, that not all of them can be accommodated in the *Changes* section. We encourage healthcare professionals to regularly review the prescribing information on drugs that they encounter frequently;
- *Changes to the Dental Practioners' Formulary*, are located at the end of the Dental List;
- *E-newsletter*, the BNF & BNF for Children e-newsletter service is available free of charge. It alerts healthcare professionals to details of significant changes in the clinical content of these publications and to the way that this information is delivered. Newsletters also provide tips on using these publications effectively, and highlight forthcoming changes to the publications. To sign up for e-newsletters go to www.bnf.org.

Using other sources for medicines information

The BNF is designed as a digest for rapid reference. Less detail is given on areas such as obstetrics, malignant disease, and anaesthesia. The BNF should be interpreted in the light of professional knowledge and supplemented as necessary by specialised publications and by reference to the product literature. Information is also available from medicines information services. BNF for Children should be consulted for detailed information on the use of medicines in children.

Changes

Monthly updates are provided online via Medicines Complete and the NICE BNF website. The changes listed below are cumulative (from one print edition to the next).

Significant changes

Significant changes that appear in the print edition of BNF 90 (September 2025 — March 2026):

- Amphotericin B p. 689: review of indications and dose for liposomal preparations, as well as updates to directions for administration, breast-feeding, pregnancy, cautions, and monitoring advice.
- Andexanet alfa p. 165 [therapeutic use changed to reversal of anticoagulation].
- Apixaban p. 145: update to structure of dosing for prophylaxis of stroke and systemic embolism in non-valvular atrial fibrillation and at least one risk factor.
- Asthma, chronic p. 271: updated guidance on management.
- Bempedoic acid p. 238: new indication and dose for established or at high-risk of atherosclerotic cardiovascular disease.
- Bimekizumab p. 1422: new indication and dose for hidradenitis suppurativa.
- Budesonide with formoterol p. 298 (*DuoResp Spiromax*®160 micrograms/4.5 micrograms): new indication and dose for mild asthma, reliever therapy.
- Budesonide with formoterol p. 298 (*Fobumix*®160/4.5 Easyhaler): new indication and dose for mild asthma, reliever therapy.
- Cardiovascular disease risk assessment and prevention p. 219: updated guidance.
- Chloroquine p. 710: updated pregnancy and breast-feeding advice when used for rheumatic disease.
- Contraceptives, hormonal p. 912: inclusion of guidance for use of combined oral contraceptives for preventive treatment of ovarian cancer in at-risk females.
- Dupilumab p. 1423: new indication and dose for chronic obstructive pulmonary disease.
- Emtricitabine with tenofovir alafenamide p. 749: new indication and dose for pre-exposure prophylaxis of HIV-1.
- Fezolinetant p. 869: risk of drug-induced liver injury and new recommendations on monitoring of liver function before and during treatment [MHRA/CHM advice].
- GLP-1 and dual GIP/GLP-1 receptor agonists: potential risk of pulmonary aspiration during general anaesthesia or deep sedation [MHRA/CHM advice] (advice in dulaglutide, exenatide, liraglutide, lixisenatide, semaglutide, tirzepatide; see example in liraglutide p. 816).
- Hydroxychloroquine sulfate p. 1253: updated pregnancy and breast-feeding advice.
- Idarucizumab p. 166 [therapeutic use changed to reversal of anticoagulation].
- Immunisation schedule p. 1472: updated guidance for immunisation against diphtheria, tetanus, pertussis and poliomyelitis in children aged 3 years and 4 months.
- Malaria, prophylaxis p. 702: updated guidance.
- Naltrexone hydrochloride p. 564: new indication and dose for gambling-related harm.
- Pneumococcal polysaccharide conjugate vaccine (adsorbed) p. 1510: name change of *Apexxnar*® to *Prevenar 20*®.
- Prolonged-release opioids: removal of indication for relief of post-operative pain [MHRA/CHM advice] (advice in all opioids; see Opioids p. 510).
- Sepsis p. 579: updated guidance on management.
- Smoking cessation p. 565: updated drug treatment guidance.
- Sodium valproate p. 378: new advice for male patients already taking sodium valproate [MHRA/CHM advice].
- Sympathomimetics p. 214: updated guidance for septic shock.
- Tuberculosis p. 670: updated guidance for multi-drug resistant tuberculosis.
- Valproic acid p. 409: new advice for male patients already taking valproic acid [MHRA/CHM advice].
- *Wegovy*® (semaglutide p. 819): new indication and dose for cardiovascular risk reduction.

Dose changes

Changes in dose statements that appear in the print edition of BNF 90 (September 2025 — March 2026):

- Colchicine p. 1279 [update to dosing for prophylaxis of familial Mediterranean fever].
- Ferrous fumarate p. 1158 [update to dosing for iron-deficiency anaemia using oral solution].
- *Fobumix*®80/4.5 Easyhaler (budesonide with formoterol p. 298) [update to dosing for asthma, maintenance therapy].
- *Fobumix*®160/4.5 Easyhaler (budesonide with formoterol p. 298) [update to dosing for asthma, maintenance therapy].
- *Fobumix*®320/9 Easyhaler (budesonide with formoterol p. 298) [update to dosing for asthma, maintenance therapy].
- Glyceryl trinitrate p. 252 [update to dosing for treatment of angina using sublingual tablets or spray].
- Medical emergencies in the community p. 2028 [update to dosing of glyceryl trinitrate for acute coronary syndromes].
- *Ozempic*® (semaglutide p. 819) [update to indications and dosing].
- Rilpivirine p. 743 [update to dosing for HIV-1 infection].
- Rosuvastatin p. 235 [update to dose adjustments due to interactions].
- Sodium feredetate p. 1160 [update to dosing for iron-deficiency anaemia using oral solution].
- Sodium hyaluronate with trehalose p. 1331 [update to dosing for dry eye conditions].
- *Vocabria*® (cabotegravir p. 737) [update to dosing for HIV-1 infection].

Classification changes

Classification changes that appear in the print edition of BNF 90 (September 2025 — March 2026):

New monographs

New monographs that appear in the print edition of BNF 90 (September 2025 — March 2026):

- *Agamree*® [vamorolone p. 1283].
- *Anzupgo*® [delgocitinib p. 1431].
- *Balversa*® [erdafitinib p. 1108].
- *Briumvi*® [ublituximab p. 995].
- *Duvyzat*® [givinostat p. 1284].
- *Fruzaqla*® [fruquintinib p. 1111].
- *Imdylltra*® [tarlatamab p. 1023].
- *Joenja*® [leniolisib p. 964].
- *Kisunla*® [donanemab p. 344].
- *Loargys*® [pegzilarginase p. 1224].
- *Lunivia*® [eszopiclone p. 554].
- *Vafseo*® [vadadustat p. 1149].
- *Wainzua*® [eplontersen p. 1205].
- *Winlevi*® [clascoterone p. 1440].
- *Yorvipath*® [palopegteriparatide p. 1186].

New preparations

New preparations that appear in the print edition of BNF 90 (September 2025 — March 2026):

- *Abilify Maintena*®720 mg or 960 mg prolonged-release suspension for injection [aripiprazole p. 454].
- *Apretude*®30 mg film-coated tablets [cabotegravir p. 737].
- *Apretude*®600 mg prolonged-release suspension for injection [cabotegravir p. 737].

- *Bibecfo*®100/6 [beclometasone with formoterol p. 294].
- *Bibecfo*®200/6 [beclometasone with formoterol p. 294].
- *Budenofalk*®suppositories [budesonide p. 47].
- *Cequa*® [ciclosporin p. 1326].
- *Hyftor*® [sirolimus p. 1387].
- *Luforbec*®200/6 [beclometasone with formoterol p. 294].
- *Netildex*®eye gel [dexamethasone with netilmicin p. 1326].
- *Proxor*®100/6 [beclometasone with formoterol p. 294].
- *Proxor*®200/6 [beclometasone with formoterol p. 294].
- *Verorab*® [rabies vaccine p. 1511].
- *Vivaire*®100/6 [beclometasone with formoterol p. 294].
- *Vivaire*®200/6 [beclometasone with formoterol p. 294].

Deleted monographs
Deleted monographs since the print edition of BNF 89
(March — September 2025):
- Co-flumactone.
- Co-simalcite.

Deleted preparations
Deleted preparations since the print edition of BNF 89
(March — September 2025):
- *Ambisome*® [amphotericin B p. 689].

Guidance on prescribing

General guidance

Medicines should be prescribed only when they are necessary, and in all cases the benefit of administering the medicine should be considered in relation to the risk involved. This is particularly important during pregnancy, when the risk to both mother and fetus must be considered.

It is important to discuss treatment options carefully with the patient to ensure that the patient is content to take the medicine as prescribed. In particular, the patient should be helped to distinguish the adverse effects of prescribed drugs from the effects of the medical disorder. When the beneficial effects of the medicine are likely to be delayed, the patient should be advised of this.

For guidance on medicines optimisation, see Medicines optimisation p. 16.

Never Events Never events are serious and avoidable medical errors for which there should be preventative measures in place to stop their occurrence.

The NHS Never Events policy and framework can be viewed at: www.england.nhs.uk/publication/never-events/.

For never events related to single drugs or drug classes, BNF Publications contain information within the monographs, in the important safety information section.

Prescribing competency framework The Royal Pharmaceutical Society has published a Prescribing Competency Framework that includes a common set of competencies that form the basis for prescribing, regardless of professional background. The competencies have been developed to help healthcare professionals to be safe and effective prescribers, with the aim of supporting patients to get the best outcomes from their medicines. It is available at www.rpharms.com/resources/frameworks/prescribers-competency-framework.

Biological medicines

Biological medicines are medicines that are made by or derived from a biological source using biotechnology processes, such as recombinant DNA technology. The size and complexity of biological medicines, as well as the way they are produced, may result in a degree of natural variability in molecules of the same active substance, particularly in different batches of the medicine. This variation is maintained within strict acceptable limits. Examples of biological medicines include insulins and monoclonal antibodies. [EvGr] Biological medicines must be prescribed by brand name and the brand name specified on the prescription should be dispensed in order to avoid inadvertent switching. Automatic substitution of brands at the point of dispensing is not appropriate for biological medicines. ⟨A⟩

Biosimilar medicines

A **biosimilar medicine** is a biological medicine that is highly similar and clinically equivalent (in terms of quality, safety, and efficacy) to an existing biological medicine that has already been authorised in the European Union (known as the reference biological medicine or originator medicine). The active substance of a biosimilar medicine is similar, but not identical, to the originator biological medicine. Once the patent for a biological medicine has expired, a biosimilar medicine may be authorised by the European Medicines Agency (EMA). A biosimilar medicine is not the same as a generic medicine, which contains a simpler chemical structure and a molecular structure that is identical to the originator medicine.

Therapeutic equivalence [EvGr] Biosimilar medicines should be considered to be therapeutically equivalent to the originator biological medicine within their authorised indications. ⟨A⟩ Biosimilar medicines are usually licensed for all the indications of the originator biological medicine, but this depends on the evidence submitted to the EMA for authorisation and must be scientifically justified on the basis of demonstrated or extrapolated equivalence.

Prescribing and dispensing The choice of whether to prescribe a biosimilar medicine or the originator biological medicine rests with the clinician in consultation with the patient. [EvGr] Biological medicines (including biosimilar medicines) must be prescribed by brand name and the brand name specified on the prescription should be dispensed in order to avoid inadvertent switching. Automatic substitution of brands at the point of dispensing is not appropriate for biological medicines. ⟨A⟩

Safety monitoring Biosimilar medicines are subject to a black triangle status (▼) at the time of initial authorisation. [EvGr] It is important to report suspected adverse reactions using the Yellow Card scheme (see Adverse reactions to drugs p. 11). For all biological medicines, adverse reaction reports should clearly state the brand name and the batch number of the suspected medicine. ⟨A⟩

National funding/access decisions The Department of Health and Social Care has confirmed that, in England, NICE can decide to apply the same remit, and the resulting technology appraisal guidance, to relevant biosimilar medicines which appear on the market subsequent to their originator biological medicine.

National information In England, see www.nice.org.uk/About/What-we-do/Our-Programmes/NICE-guidance/NICE-technology-appraisal-guidance.

In Northern Ireland, see niformulary.hscni.net/managed-entry/biosimilars/.

In Scotland, see www.scottishmedicines.org.uk/about-us/policies-publications/.

In Wales, see awttc.nhs.wales/accessing-medicines/make-a-submission/pharmaceutical-industry-submissions/submit-for-awmsg-appraisal/invisible/appraisal-of-biosimilar-medicines-cell-therapies-and-gene-therapies/.

Availability The following are examples of drugs available as a biosimilar medicine (this list is not exhaustive):

- Adalimumab p. 1269
- Bevacizumab p. 999
- Enoxaparin sodium p. 155
- Epoetin alfa p. 1144
- Epoetin zeta p. 1146
- Etanercept p. 1273
- Filgrastim p. 1166
- Follitropin alfa p. 857
- Infliximab p. 1275
- Insulin glargine p. 839
- Insulin lispro p. 836
- Rituximab p. 1019
- Somatropin p. 861
- Teriparatide p. 776
- Trastuzumab p. 1023

Complementary and alternative medicine

An increasing amount of information on complementary and alternative medicine is becoming available. The scope of the BNF is restricted to the discussion of conventional medicines but reference is made to complementary treatments if they affect conventional therapy (e.g. interactions with St John's wort). Further information on herbal medicines is available at www.gov.uk/government/organisations/medicines-and-healthcare-products-regulatory-agency.

Abbreviation of titles

In general, titles of drugs and preparations should be written in full. Unofficial abbreviations should not be used as they may be misinterpreted.

Non-proprietary titles

Where non-proprietary ('generic') titles are given, they should be used in prescribing. This will enable any suitable product to be dispensed, thereby saving delay to the patient and sometimes expense to the health service. The only exception is where there is a demonstrable difference in clinical effect between each manufacturer's version of the formulation, making it important that the patient should always receive the same brand; in such cases, the brand name or the manufacturer should be stated. Non-proprietary titles should not be invented for the purposes of prescribing generically since this can lead to confusion, particularly in the case of compound and modified-release preparations.

Titles used as headings for monographs may be used freely in the United Kingdom but in other countries may be subject to restriction.

Many of the non-proprietary titles used in this book are titles of monographs in the European Pharmacopoeia, British Pharmacopoeia, or British Pharmaceutical Codex 1973. In such cases the preparations must comply with the standard (if any) in the appropriate publication, as required by the Human Medicines Regulations 2012.

Proprietary titles

Names followed by the symbol ® are or have been used as proprietary names in the United Kingdom. These names may in general be applied only to products supplied by the owners of the trade marks.

Marketing authorisation and BNF advice

In general the *doses, indications, cautions, contra-indications,* and *side-effects* in the BNF reflect those in the manufacturers' data sheets or Summaries of Product Characteristics (SPCs) which, in turn, reflect those in the corresponding marketing authorisations (formerly known as Product Licences). The BNF does not generally include proprietary medicines that are not supported by a valid Summary of Product Characteristics or when the marketing authorisation holder has not been able to supply essential information. When a preparation is available from more than one manufacturer, the BNF reflects advice that is the most clinically relevant regardless of any variation in the marketing authorisations. Unlicensed products can be obtained from 'special-order' manufacturers or specialist importing companies.

Where an unlicensed drug is included in the BNF, this is indicated in the unlicensed use section of the drug monograph. When the BNF suggests a use that is outside the terms defined by the licence ('off-label' use), this too is indicated. Unlicensed or off-label use may be necessary if the clinical need cannot be met by licensed medicines; such use should be supported by appropriate evidence and experience.

The doses stated in the BNF are intended for general guidance and represent, unless otherwise stated, the usual range of doses that are generally regarded as being suitable for adults.

Prescribing unlicensed medicines

Prescribing medicines outside the recommendations of their marketing authorisation alters (and probably increases) the prescriber's professional responsibility and potential liability. The prescriber should be able to justify and feel competent in using such medicines, and also inform the patient or the patient's carer that the prescribed medicine is unlicensed.

Oral syringes

An **oral syringe** is supplied when oral liquid medicines are prescribed in doses other than multiples of 5 mL. The oral syringe is marked in 0.5 mL divisions from 1 to 5 mL to measure doses of less than 5 mL (other sizes of oral syringe may also be available). It is provided with an adaptor and an instruction leaflet. The 5–*mL spoon* is used for doses of 5 mL (or multiples thereof).

Important To avoid inadvertent intravenous administration of oral liquid medicines, only an appropriate oral or enteral syringe should be used to measure an oral liquid medicine (if a medicine spoon or graduated measure cannot be used); these syringes should not be compatible with intravenous or other parenteral devices. Oral or enteral syringes should be clearly labelled 'Oral' or 'Enteral' in a large font size; it is the healthcare practitioner's responsibility to label the syringe with this information if the manufacturer has not done so.

Excipients

Branded oral liquid preparations that do not contain *fructose, glucose,* or *sucrose* are described as 'sugar-free' in the BNF. Preparations containing hydrogenated glucose syrup, mannitol, maltitol, sorbitol, or xylitol are also marked 'sugar-free' since there is evidence that they do not cause dental caries. Patients receiving medicines containing cariogenic sugars should be advised of appropriate dental hygiene measures to prevent caries. Sugar-free preparations should be used whenever possible.

Where information on the presence of *aspartame, gluten, sulfites, tartrazine, arachis (peanut) oil* or *sesame oil* is available, this is indicated in the BNF against the relevant preparation.

Information is provided on selected excipients in skin preparations, in vaccines, and on *selected preservatives* and *excipients* in eye drops and injections.

The presence of *benzyl alcohol* and *polyoxyl castor oil* (polyethoxylated castor oil) in injections is indicated in the BNF. Benzyl alcohol has been associated with a fatal toxic syndrome in preterm neonates, and therefore, parenteral preparations containing the preservative should not be used in neonates. Polyoxyl castor oils, used as vehicles in intravenous injections, have been associated with severe anaphylactoid reactions.

The presence of *propylene glycol* in oral or parenteral medicines is indicated in the BNF; it can cause adverse effects if its elimination is impaired, e.g. in renal failure, in neonates and young children, and in slow metabolisers of the substance. It may interact with disulfiram p. 563 and metronidazole p. 628.

The *lactose* content in most medicines is too small to cause problems in most lactose-intolerant patients. However in severe lactose intolerance, the lactose content should be determined before prescribing. The amount of lactose varies according to manufacturer, product, formulation, and strength.

Electrolytes

The *sodium* content of medicines should be considered for all patients, especially those with cardiovascular disease or on a reduced sodium diet, or those requiring long-term or regular medication.

Some formulations of medicines, especially those that are effervescent, dispersible or soluble, can contain high levels of sodium as an excipient and this may be associated with an increased risk of cardiovascular events, including hypertension.

The sodium content of a medicine is provided in the product literature for all medicines containing ≥ 1 mmol sodium per dose; below this level is considered essentially sodium-free. Medicines containing ≥ 17 mmol sodium in the total daily dose are considered to have a high sodium content and this is highlighted for medicines intended to be taken regularly (repeated use for more than 2 days every week) or long-term (continuous daily use for more than 1 month). 17 mmol sodium is approximately 20% of the WHO recommended maximum daily dietary intake of sodium for an adult.

Important In the absence of information on excipients or electrolytes in the BNF and in the product literature (available at www.medicines.org.uk/emc), contact the manufacturer (see Index of Manufacturers) if it is essential to check details.

Extemporaneous preparation

A product should be dispensed extemporaneously only when no product with a marketing authorisation is available.

The BP direction that a preparation must be *freshly prepared* indicates that it must be made not more than 24 hours before it is issued for use. The direction that a preparation should be *recently prepared* indicates that deterioration is likely if the preparation is stored for longer than about 4 weeks at 15–25° C.

The term **water** used without qualification means either potable water freshly drawn direct from the public supply and suitable for drinking or freshly boiled and cooled purified water. The latter should be used if the public supply is from a local storage tank or if the potable water is unsuitable for a particular preparation (Water for injections).

Drugs and driving

Prescribers and other healthcare professionals should advise patients if treatment is likely to affect their ability to perform skilled tasks (e.g. driving). This applies especially to drugs with sedative effects; patients should be warned that these effects are increased by alcohol. General information about a patient's fitness to drive is available from the Driver and Vehicle Licensing Agency at www.gov.uk/government/ organisations/driver-and-vehicle-licensing-agency.

A new offence of driving, attempting to drive, or being in charge of a vehicle, with certain specified controlled drugs in excess of specified limits, came into force on 2nd March 2015. This offence is an addition to the existing rules on drug impaired driving and fitness to drive, and applies to two groups of drugs—commonly abused drugs, including amfetamines, cannabis, cocaine, and ketamine p. 1539, and drugs used mainly for medical reasons, such as opioids and benzodiazepines. Anyone found to have any of the drugs (including related drugs, for example, apomorphine hydrochloride p. 481) above specified limits in their blood will be guilty of an offence, whether their driving was impaired or not. This also includes prescribed drugs which metabolise to those included in the offence, for example, selegiline hydrochloride p. 490. However, the legislation provides a statutory "medical defence" for patients taking drugs for medical reasons in accordance with instructions, *if their driving was not impaired*—it continues to be an offence to drive if actually impaired. Patients should therefore be advised to continue taking their medicines as prescribed, and when driving, to carry suitable evidence that the drug was prescribed, or sold, to treat a medical or dental problem, and that it was taken according to the instructions given by the prescriber, or information provided with the medicine (e.g. a repeat prescription form or the medicine's patient information leaflet). Further information is available from the Department for Transport at www.gov.uk/government/ collections/drug-driving.

Patents

In the BNF, certain drugs have been included notwithstanding the existence of actual or potential patent rights. In so far as such substances are protected by Letters Patent, their inclusion in this Formulary neither conveys, nor implies, licence to manufacture.

Health and safety

When handling chemical or biological materials particular attention should be given to the possibility of allergy, fire, explosion, radiation, or poisoning. Substances such as corticosteroids, some antimicrobials, phenothiazines, and many cytotoxics, are irritant or very potent and should be handled with caution. Contact with the skin and inhalation of dust should be avoided.

Safety in the home

Patients must be warned to keep all medicines out of the reach of children. All solid dose and all oral and external liquid preparations must be dispensed in a reclosable *child-resistant container* unless:

- the medicine is in an original pack or patient pack such as to make this inadvisable;
- the patient will have difficulty in opening a child-resistant container;
- a specific request is made that the product shall not be dispensed in a child-resistant container;
- no suitable child-resistant container exists for a particular liquid preparation.

All patients should be advised to dispose of *unwanted medicines* by returning them to a supplier for destruction.

Labelling of prescribed medicines

There is a legal requirement for the following to appear on the label of any prescribed medicine:

- name of the patient;
- name and address of the supplying pharmacy;
- date of dispensing;
- name of the medicine;
- directions for use of the medicine;
- precautions relating to the use of the medicine.

The Royal Pharmaceutical Society recommends that the following also appears on the label:

- the words 'Keep out of the sight and reach of children';
- where applicable, the words 'Use this medicine only on your skin'.

A pharmacist can exercise professional skill and judgement to amend or include more appropriate wording for the name of the medicine, the directions for use, or the precautions relating to the use of the medicine.

Non-proprietary names of compound preparations

Non-proprietary names of **compound preparations** which appear in the BNF are those that have been compiled by the British Pharmacopoeia Commission or another recognised body; whenever possible they reflect the names of the active ingredients.

Prescribers should avoid creating their own compound names for the purposes of generic prescribing; such names do not have an approved definition and can be misinterpreted.

Special care should be taken to avoid errors when prescribing compound preparations; in particular the hyphen in the prefix 'co-' should be retained.

Special care should also be taken to avoid creating generic names for **modified-release** preparations where the use of these names could lead to confusion between formulations with different lengths of action.

EEA and Swiss prescriptions

Pharmacists can dispense prescriptions issued by doctors, dentists, and nurse prescribers from the European Economic Area (EEA) or Switzerland (except prescriptions for

Prescription writing

controlled drugs in Schedules 1, 2, or 3, or for drugs without a UK marketing authorisation). Prescriptions should be written in ink or otherwise so as to be indelible, should be dated, should state the name of the patient, should state the address of the prescriber, should contain particulars indicating whether the prescriber is a doctor, dentist, or nurse, and should be signed by the prescriber.

Security and validity of prescriptions

The Councils of the British Medical Association and the Royal Pharmaceutical Society have issued a joint statement on the security and validity of prescriptions.

In particular, prescription forms should:

- not be left unattended at reception desks;
- not be left in a car where they may be visible; and
- when not in use, be kept in a locked drawer within the surgery and at home.

Where there is any doubt about the authenticity of a prescription, the pharmacist should contact the prescriber. If this is done by telephone, the number should be obtained from the directory rather than relying on the information on the prescription form, which may be false.

Patient group direction (PGD)

In most cases, the most appropriate clinical care will be provided on an individual basis by a prescriber to a specific individual patient. However, a Patient Group Direction for supply and administration of medicines by other healthcare professionals can be used where it would benefit patient care without compromising safety.

A Patient Group Direction is a written direction relating to the supply and administration (or administration only) of a licensed prescription-only medicine (including some

Controlled Drugs in specific circumstances) by certain classes of healthcare professionals; the Direction is signed by a doctor (or dentist) and by a pharmacist. Further information on Patient Group Directions is available in Health Service Circular HSC 2000/026 (England), HDL (2001) 7 (Scotland), and WHC (2000) 116 (Wales); see also the Human Medicines Regulations 2012.

NICE, Scottish Medicines Consortium and All Wales Medicines Strategy Group

Advice issued by the National Institute for Health and Care Excellence (NICE), the Scottish Medicines Consortium (SMC) and the All Wales Medicines Strategy Group (AWMSG) is referenced in the BNF when relevant. Full details of this advice together with updates can be obtained from the funding body websites: www.nice.org.uk, www.scottishmedicines.org.uk and awttc.nhs.wales/.

Specialised commissioning decisions

NHS England develops specialised commissioning policies that define access to specialised services for particular groups of patients to ensure consistency in access to treatments nationwide. For further information, see www.england.nhs.uk/specialised-commissioning-document-library/routinely-commissioned-policies/.

National genomic test directory

The *National genomic test directory* specifies which genomic tests are commissioned by the NHS in England, the technology by which they are available, and the patients who will be eligible to access a test. For further information, see www.england.nhs.uk/publication/national-genomic-test-directories/.

Prescription writing

Shared care

In its guidelines on responsibility for prescribing (circular EL (91) 127) between hospitals and general practitioners, the Department of Health has advised that legal responsibility for prescribing lies with the doctor who signs the prescription.

Requirements

Prescriptions should be written legibly in ink or otherwise so as to be indelible (it is permissible to issue carbon copies of NHS prescriptions as long as they are signed in ink), should be dated, should state the name and address of the patient, the address of the prescriber, an indication of the type of prescriber, and should be signed in ink by the prescriber (computer-generated facsimile signatures do not meet the legal requirement). The age and the date of birth of the patient should preferably be stated, and it is a legal requirement in the case of prescription-only medicines to state the age for children under 12 years. These recommendations are acceptable for **prescription-only medicines**. Prescriptions for controlled drugs have additional legal requirements.

Wherever appropriate the prescriber should state the current weight of the child to enable the dose prescribed to be checked. Consideration should also be given to including the dose per unit mass e.g. mg/kg or the dose per m^2 body-surface area e.g. mg/m^2 where this would reduce error.

The following should be noted:

- The strength or quantity to be contained in capsules, lozenges, tablets etc. should be stated by the prescriber. In particular, strength of liquid preparations should be clearly stated (e.g. 125 mg/5 mL).

- Quantities of 1 gram or more should be written as 1 g, 1.5 g etc. Quantities less than 1 gram should be written in milligrams, e.g. 500 mg, not 0.5 g. Quantities less than 1 mg should be written in micrograms, e.g. 100 micrograms, not 0.1 mg. The unnecessary use of decimal points should be avoided, e.g. 3 mg, not 3.0 mg. When decimals are unavoidable a zero should be written in front of the decimal point where there is no other figure, e.g. 0.5 mL, not .5 mL. Use of the decimal point is acceptable to express a range, e.g. 0.5 to 1 g.
- 'Micrograms' and 'nanograms' should **not** be abbreviated. Similarly 'units' should **not** be abbreviated.
- The term 'millilitre' (ml or mL) is used in medicine and pharmacy, and cubic centimetre, c.c., or cm^3 should not be used. (The use of capital 'L' in mL is a printing convention throughout the BNF; both 'mL' and 'ml' are recognised SI abbreviations).
- Dose and dose frequency should be stated; in the case of preparations to be taken 'as required' a **minimum dose interval** should be specified. Care should be taken to ensure children receive the correct dose of the active drug. Therefore, the dose should normally be stated in terms of the mass of the active drug (e.g. '125 mg 3 times daily'); terms such as '5 mL' or '1 tablet' should be avoided except for compound preparations. When doses other than multiples of 5 mL are prescribed for *oral liquid preparations* the dose-volume will be provided by means of an **oral syringe**, (except for preparations intended to be measured with a pipette). Suitable quantities:
- Elixirs, Linctuses, and Paediatric Mixtures (5-mL dose), 50, 100, or 150 mL
- Adult Mixtures (10 mL dose), 200 or 300 mL

- Ear Drops, Eye drops, and Nasal Drops, 10 mL (or the manufacturer's pack)
- Eye Lotions, Gargles, and Mouthwashes, 200 mL

- The names of drugs and preparations should be written clearly and **not** abbreviated, using approved titles **only**; **avoid** creating generic titles for modified-release preparations.
- The quantity to be supplied may be stated by indicating the number of days of treatment required in the box provided on NHS forms. In most cases the exact amount will be supplied. This does not apply to items directed to be used as required—if the dose and frequency are not given then the quantity to be supplied needs to be stated. When several items are ordered on one form the box can be marked with the number of days of treatment provided the quantity is added for any item for which the amount cannot be calculated.
- Although directions should preferably be in **English without abbreviation**, it is recognised that some Latin abbreviations are used.

Sample prescription

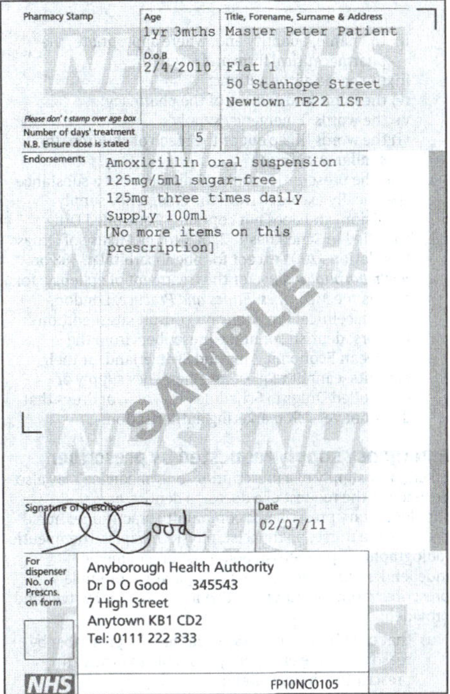

Prescribing by dentists

Until new prescribing arrangements are in place for NHS prescriptions, dentists should use form FP10D (GP14 in Scotland, WP10D in Wales) to prescribe only those items listed in the Dental Practitioners' Formulary. The Human Medicines Regulations 2012 does not set any limitations upon the number and variety of substances which the dentist may administer to patients in the surgery or may order by private prescription—provided the relevant legal requirements are observed the dentist may use or order whatever is required for the clinical situation. There is no statutory requirement for the dentist to communicate with a patient's medical practitioner when prescribing for dental use. There are, however, occasions when this would be in the patient's interest and such communication is to be encouraged. For legal requirements relating to prescriptions of Controlled Drugs, see Controlled drugs and drug dependence p. 7.

Computer-issued prescriptions

For computer-issued prescriptions the following advice, based on the recommendations of the Joint GP Information Technology Committee, should also be noted:

1. The computer must print out the date, the patient's surname, one forename, other initials, and address, and may also print out the patient's title and date of birth. The age of children under 12 years and of adults over 60 years must be printed in the box available; the age of children under 5 years should be printed in years and months. A facility may also exist to print out the age of patients between 12 and 60 years.
2. The doctor's name must be printed at the bottom of the prescription form; this will be the name of the doctor responsible for the prescription (who will normally sign it). The doctor's surgery address, reference number, and Primary Care Trust (PCT, Health Board in Scotland, Local Health Board in Wales) are also necessary. In addition, the surgery telephone number should be printed.
3. When prescriptions are to be signed by general practitioner registrars, assistants, locums, or deputising doctors, the name of the doctor printed at the bottom of the form must still be that of the responsible principal.
4. Names of medicines must come from a dictionary held in the computer memory, to provide a check on the spelling and to ensure that the name is written in full. The computer can be programmed to recognise both the non-proprietary and the proprietary name of a particular drug and to print out the preferred choice, but must not print out both names. For medicines not in the dictionary, separate checks are required—the user must be warned that no check was possible and the entire prescription must be entered in the lexicon.
5. The dictionary may contain information on the usual doses, formulations, and pack sizes to produce standard predetermined prescriptions for common preparations, and to provide a check on the validity of an individual prescription on entry.
6. The prescription must be printed in English without abbreviation; information may be entered or stored in abbreviated form. The dose must be in numbers, the frequency in words, and the quantity in numbers in brackets, thus: 40 mg four times daily (112). It must also be possible to prescribe by indicating the length of treatment required.
7. The BNF recommendations should be followed as listed above.
8. Checks may be incorporated to ensure that all the information required for dispensing a particular drug has been filled in. For instructions such as 'as directed' and 'when required', the maximum daily dose should normally be specified.
9. Numbers and codes used in the system for organising and retrieving data must never appear on the form.
10. Supplementary warnings or advice should be written in full, should not interfere with the clarity of the prescription itself, and should be in line with any warnings or advice in the BNF; numerical codes should not be used.
11. A mechanism (such as printing a series of nonspecific characters) should be incorporated to cancel out unused space, or wording such as 'no more items on this prescription' may be added after the last item. Otherwise the doctor should delete the space manually.

12 To avoid forgery the computer may print on the form the number of items to be dispensed (somewhere separate from the box for the pharmacist). The number of items per form need be limited only by the ability of the printer to produce clear and well-demarcated instructions with sufficient space for each item and a spacer line before each fresh item.

13 Handwritten alterations should only be made in exceptional circumstances—it is preferable to print out a new prescription. Any alterations must be made in the doctor's own handwriting and countersigned; computer records should be updated to fully reflect any alteration. Prescriptions for drugs used for contraceptive purposes (but which are not promoted as contraceptives) may need to be marked in handwriting with the symbol ♀, (or endorsed in another way to indicate that the item is prescribed for contraceptive purposes).

14 Prescriptions for controlled drugs can be printed from the computer, but the prescriber's signature must be handwritten (See Controlled Drugs and Drug Dependence; the prescriber may use a date stamp).

15 The strip of paper on the side of the FP10SS (GP10SS in Scotland, WP10SS in Wales) may be used for various purposes but care should be taken to avoid including confidential information. It may be advisable for the patient's name to appear at the top, but this should be preceded by 'confidential'.

16 In rural dispensing practices prescription requests (or details of medicines dispensed) will normally be entered in one surgery. The prescriptions (or dispensed medicines) may then need to be delivered to another surgery or location; if possible the computer should hold up to 10 alternatives.

17 Prescription forms that are reprinted or issued as a duplicate should be labelled clearly as such.

Emergency supply of medicines

Emergency supply requested by member of the public

Pharmacists are sometimes called upon by members of the public to make an emergency supply of medicines. The Human Medicines Regulations 2012 allows exemptions from the Prescription Only requirements for emergency supply to be made by a person lawfully conducting a retail pharmacy business provided:

a) that the pharmacist has interviewed the person requesting the prescription-only medicine and is satisfied:

  i) that there is immediate need for the prescription-only medicine and that it is impracticable in the circumstances to obtain a prescription without undue delay;

  ii) that treatment with the prescription-only medicine has on a previous occasion been prescribed for the person requesting it;

  iii) as to the dose that it would be appropriate for the person to take;

b) that no greater quantity shall be supplied than will provide 5 days' treatment of phenobarbital p. 388, *phenobarbital sodium*, or Controlled Drugs in Schedules 4 or 5 (doctors, dentists, or nurse prescribers from the European Economic Area and Switzerland, or their patients, cannot request an emergency supply of Controlled Drugs in Schedules 1, 2, or 3, or drugs that do not have a UK marketing authorisation) or 30 days' treatment for other prescription-only medicines, except when the prescription-only medicine is:

  i) insulin, an ointment or cream, or a preparation for the relief of asthma in an aerosol dispenser when the smallest pack can be supplied;

  ii) an oral contraceptive when a full cycle may be supplied;

  iii) an antibiotic in liquid form for oral administration when the smallest quantity that will provide a full course of treatment can be supplied;

c) that an entry shall be made by the pharmacist in the prescription book stating:

  i) the date of supply;

  ii) the name, quantity and, where appropriate, the pharmaceutical form and strength;

  iii) the name and address of the patient;

  iv) the nature of the emergency;

d) that the container or package must be labelled to show:

  i) the date of supply;

  ii) the name, quantity and, where appropriate, the pharmaceutical form and strength;

  iii) the name of the patient;

  iv) the name and address of the pharmacy;

  v) the words 'Emergency supply';

  vi) the words 'Keep out of the reach of children' (or similar warning);

e) that the prescription-only medicine is not a substance specifically excluded from the emergency supply provision, and does not contain a Controlled Drug specified in Schedules 1, 2, or 3 to the Misuse of Drugs Regulations 2001 except for phenobarbital p. 388 or *phenobarbital sodium* for the treatment of epilepsy: for details see *Medicines, Ethics and Practice*, London, Pharmaceutical Press (always consult latest edition). Doctors, dentists, or nurse prescribers from the European Economic Area and Switzerland, or their patients, cannot request an emergency supply of Controlled Drugs in Schedules 1, 2, or 3, or drugs that do not have a UK marketing authorisation.

Emergency supply requested by prescriber

Emergency supply of a prescription-only medicine may also be made at the request of a doctor, a dentist, a supplementary prescriber, a community practitioner nurse prescriber, a nurse, pharmacist, physiotherapist, therapeutic radiographer, optometrist, podiatrist or paramedic independent prescriber; or a doctor, dentist, or nurse prescriber from the European Economic Area or Switzerland, provided:

a) that the pharmacist is satisfied that the prescriber by reason of some emergency is unable to furnish a prescription immediately;

b) that the prescriber has undertaken to furnish a prescription within 72 hours;

c) that the medicine is supplied in accordance with the directions of the prescriber requesting it;

d) that the medicine is not a Controlled Drug specified in Schedules 1, 2, or 3 to the Misuse of Drugs Regulations 2001 except for phenobarbital p. 388 or *phenobarbital sodium* for the treatment of epilepsy: for details see *Medicines, Ethics and Practice*, London, Pharmaceutical Press (always consult latest edition); (Doctors, dentists, or nurse prescribers from the European Economic Area and Switzerland, or their patients, cannot request an emergency supply of Controlled Drugs in Schedules 1, 2, or 3, or drugs that do not have a UK marketing authorisation).

e) that an entry shall be made in the prescription book stating:
- i) the date of supply;
- ii) the name, quantity and, where appropriate, the pharmaceutical form and strength;
- iii) the name and address of the practitioner requesting the emergency supply;
- iv) the name and address of the patient;
- v) the date on the prescription;
- vi) when the prescription is received the entry should be amended to include the date on which it is received.

Royal Pharmaceutical Society's guidelines

1. The pharmacist should consider the medical consequences of not supplying a medicine in an emergency.
2. If the pharmacist is unable to make an emergency supply of a medicine the pharmacist should advise the patient how to obtain essential medical care.

For conditions that apply to supplies made at the request of a patient see Medicines, Ethics and Practice, London Pharmaceutical Press, (always consult latest edition).

Controlled drugs and drug dependence

Regulations and classification

The Misuse of Drugs Act, 1971 as amended prohibits certain activities in relation to 'Controlled Drugs', in particular their manufacture, supply, and possession (except where permitted by the 2001 Regulations or under licence from the Secretary of State). The penalties applicable to offences involving the different drugs are graded broadly according to the *harmfulness attributable to a drug when it is misused* and for this purpose the drugs are defined in the following three classes:

- **Class A** includes: alfentanil p. 1537, cocaine, diamorphine hydrochloride p. 518 (heroin), dipipanone hydrochloride, fentanyl p. 520, lysergide (LSD), methadone hydrochloride p. 570, 3,4-methylenedioxymethamfetamine (MDMA, 'ecstasy'), morphine p. 525, opium, oxycodone hydrochloride p. 528, pethidine hydrochloride p. 531, phencyclidine, remifentanil p. 1538, and class B substances when prepared for injection.
- **Class B** includes: oral amfetamines, barbiturates, cannabis, *Sativex®*, codeine phosphate p. 517, dihydrocodeine tartrate p. 518, ethylmorphine, glutethimide, ketamine p. 1539, nabilone p. 493, pentazocine, phenmetrazine, and pholcodine.
- **Class C** includes: certain drugs related to the amfetamines such as benzfetamine and chlorphentermine, buprenorphine p. 511, mazindol, meprobamate, pemoline, pipradrol, most benzodiazepines, tramadol hydrochloride p. 534, zaleplon, zolpidem tartrate, zopiclone, androgenic and anabolic steroids, clenbuterol, chorionic gonadotrophin (HCG), non-human chorionic gonadotrophin, somatotropin, somatrem, somatropin p. 861, gabapentin p. 362, pregabalin and nitrous oxide.

The Misuse of Drugs (Safe Custody) Regulations 1973 as amended details the storage and safe custody requirements for Controlled Drugs.

The Misuse of Drugs Regulations 2001 (and subsequent amendments) defines the classes of person who are authorised to supply and possess Controlled Drugs while acting in their professional capacities and lays down the conditions under which these activities may be carried out. In the 2001 regulations, drugs are divided into five Schedules, each specifying the requirements governing such activities as import, export, production, supply, possession, prescribing, and record keeping which apply to them.

- **Schedule 1** includes drugs not used medicinally such as hallucinogenic drugs (e.g. LSD), ecstasy-type substances, raw opium, and cannabis. A Home Office licence is generally required for their production, possession, or supply. A Controlled Drug register must be used to record details of any Schedule 1 Controlled Drugs received or supplied by a pharmacy.
- **Schedule 2** includes opiates (e.g. diamorphine hydrochloride p. 518 (heroin), morphine p. 525, methadone hydrochloride p. 570, oxycodone hydrochloride p. 528, pethidine hydrochloride p. 531), major stimulants (e.g. amfetamines), quinalbarbitone (secobarbital), cocaine, ketamine p. 1539, and cannabis-based products for medicinal use in humans. Schedule 2 Controlled Drugs are subject to the full Controlled Drug requirements relating to prescriptions, safe custody (except for quinalbarbitone (secobarbital) and some liquid preparations), and the need to keep a Controlled Drug register, (unless exempted in Schedule 5). Possession, supply and procurement is authorised for pharmacists and other classes of persons named in the 2001 Regulations.
- **Schedule 3** includes the barbiturates (except secobarbital, now Schedule 2), buprenorphine p. 511, gabapentin p. 362, mazindol, meprobamate, midazolam p. 394, pentazocine, phentermine, pregabalin, temazepam p. 552, and tramadol hydrochloride p. 534. They are subject to the special prescription requirements. Safe custody requirements do apply, except for any 5,5 disubstituted barbituric acid (e.g. phenobarbital), gabapentin p. 362, mazindol, meprobamate, midazolam p. 394, pentazocine, phentermine, pregabalin, tramadol hydrochloride p. 534, or any stereoisomeric form or salts of the above. Records in registers do not need to be kept (although there are requirements for the retention of invoices for 2 years).
- **Schedule 4** includes in Part I drugs that are subject to minimal control, such as benzodiazepines (except temazepam p. 552 and midazolam p. 394, which are in Schedule 3), non-benzodiazepine hypnotics (zaleplon, zolpidem tartrate, and zopiclone) and *Sativex®*. Part II includes androgenic and anabolic steroids, clenbuterol, chorionic gonadotrophin (HCG), non-human chorionic gonadotrophin, somatotropin, somatrem, and somatropin p. 861. Controlled drug prescription requirements do not apply and Schedule 4 Controlled Drugs are not subject to safe custody requirements. Records in registers do not need to be kept (except in the case of *Sativex®*).
- **Schedule 5** includes preparations of certain Controlled Drugs (such as codeine, pholcodine, or morphine p. 525) which due to their low strength, are exempt from virtually all Controlled Drug requirements other than retention of invoices for two years, and nitrous oxide.

Since the Responsible Pharmacist Regulations were published in 2008, standing operation procedures for the management of Controlled Drugs, are required in registered pharmacies.

The Health Act 2006 introduced the concept of the 'accountable officer' with responsibility for the management

Controlled drugs and drug dependence

of Controlled Drugs and related governance issues in their organisation. Most recently, in 2013 The Controlled Drugs (Supervision of Management and Use) Regulations were published to ensure good governance concerning the safe management and use of Controlled Drugs in England and Scotland.

Prescriptions

Preparations in Schedules 1, 2, 3, 4 and 5 of the Misuse of Drugs Regulations 2001 (and subsequent amendments) are identified throughout the BNF and BNF for Children using the following symbols:

CD1	for preparations in Schedule 1
CD2	for preparations in Schedule 2
CD3	for preparations in Schedule 3
CD4–1	for preparations in Schedule 4 (Part I)
CD4–2	for preparations in Schedule 4 (Part II)
CD5	for preparations in Schedule 5

The principal legal requirements relating to medical prescriptions are listed below (see also Department of Health Guidance at www.gov.uk/dh).

Prescription requirements Prescriptions for Controlled Drugs that are subject to prescription requirements (all preparations in Schedules 2 and 3) must be indelible, must be *signed* by the prescriber, include the *date* on which they were signed, and specify the prescriber's *address* (must be within the UK). A computer-generated prescription is acceptable, but the prescriber's signature must be handwritten. Advanced electronic signatures can be accepted for Schedule 2 and 3 Controlled Drugs where the Electronic Prescribing Service (EPS) is used. All prescriptions for Controlled Drugs that are subject to the prescription requirements must always state:

- the name and address of the patient (use of a PO Box is acceptable);
- in the case of a preparation, the form (the dosage form e.g. tablets must be included on a Controlled Drugs prescription irrespective of whether it is implicit in the proprietary name e.g. *MST Continus*, or whether only one form is available), and, where appropriate, the strength of the preparation (when more than one strength of a preparation exists the strength required must be specified); to avoid ambiguity, where a prescription requests multiple strengths of a medicine, each strength should be prescribed separately (i.e. separate dose, total quantity, etc);
- for liquids, the total volume in millilitres (in both words and figures) of the preparation to be supplied; for dosage units (tablets, capsules, ampoules), state the total number (in both words and figures) of dosage units to be supplied (e.g. 10 tablets [of 10 mg] rather than 100 mg total quantity);
- the dose, which must be clearly defined (i.e. the instruction 'one as directed' constitutes a dose but 'as directed' does not); it is not necessary that the dose is stated in both words and figures;
- the words 'for dental treatment only' if issued by a dentist.

A pharmacist is **not** allowed to dispense a Controlled Drug unless all the information required by law is given on the prescription. In the case of a prescription for a Controlled Drug in Schedule 2 or 3, a pharmacist can amend the prescription *if* it specifies the total quantity only in words or in figures or if it contains minor typographical errors, provided that such amendments are indelible and clearly attributable to the pharmacist (e.g. name, date, signature and GPhC registration number). The prescription should be

marked with the date of supply at the time the Controlled Drug supply is made.

The Department of Health and the Scottish Government have issued a strong recommendation that the maximum quantity of Schedule 2, 3 or 4 Controlled Drugs prescribed should not exceed 30 days; exceptionally, to cover a justifiable clinical need and after consideration of any risk, a prescription can be issued for a longer period, but the reasons for the decision should be recorded on the patient's notes.

A prescription for a Controlled Drug in Schedules 2, 3, or 4 is valid for 28 days after the date stated thereon (the prescriber may forward-date the prescription; the start date may also be specified in the body of the prescription). Schedule 5 prescriptions are valid for 6 months from the appropriate date.

See sample prescription:

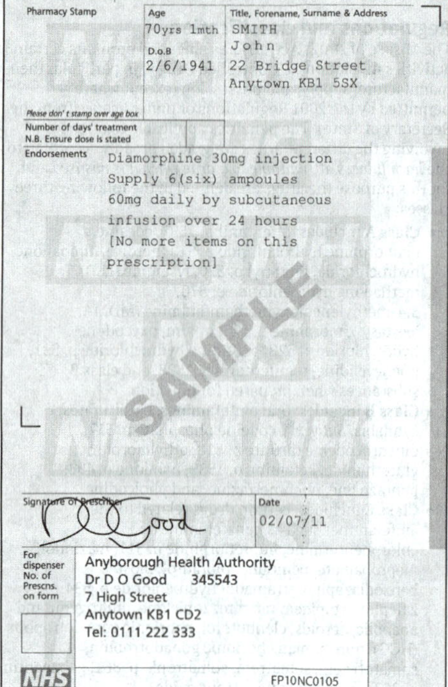

Instalments and repeatable prescriptions Prescriptions for Schedule 2 or 3 Controlled Drugs can be dispensed by instalments. An instalment prescription must have an instalment direction including both the dose and the instalment amount specified separately on the prescription, and it must also state the interval between each time the medicine can be supplied.

The first instalment must be dispensed no later than 28 days after the appropriate day (i.e. date of signing unless the prescriber indicates a date before which the Controlled Drug should not be dispensed) and the remainder should be dispensed in accordance with the instructions on the prescription. The prescription must be marked with the date of each supply.

The instalment direction is a legal requirement and needs to be complied with, however, for certain situations (e.g. if a pharmacy is closed on the day an instalment is due) the Home Office has approved specific wording which provides pharmacists some flexibility for supply. For details, see

Medicines, Ethics and Practice, London, Pharmaceutical Press (always consult latest edition) or see Home Office approved wording for instalment prescribing (Circular 027/2015), available at www.gov.uk/.

Repeatable prescriptions are prescriptions which contain a direction that they can be dispensed more than once (e.g. repeat × 3). Only Schedule 4 and 5 Controlled Drugs are permitted on repeatable prescriptions.

Private prescriptions Private prescriptions for Controlled Drugs in Schedules 2 and 3 must be written on specially designated forms which are provided by local NHS England area teams in England (form FP10PCD), local NHS Health Boards in Scotland (form PPCD) and Wales (form W10PCD); in addition, prescriptions must specify the *prescriber's identification number* (or a NHS prescriber code in Scotland). Prescriptions to be supplied by a pharmacist in hospital are exempt from the requirements for private prescriptions.

Medicines that are not Controlled Drugs should not be prescribed on the same form as a Schedule 2 or 3 Controlled Drug. This is because the form needs to be sent to the relevant NHS agency so the pharmacist would be unable to comply with the requirement to keep private prescriptions for a POM for two years.

Prescription security Prescribers are responsible for the security of prescription forms once issued to them. The stealing and misuse of prescription forms could be minimised by the following precautions:

- records of serial numbers received and issued should be retained for at least three years;
- blank prescriptions should never be pre-signed;
- prescription forms should not be left unattended and should be locked in a secure drawer, cupboard, or carrying case when not in use;
- doctors', dentists' and surgery stamps should be kept in a secure location separate from the prescription forms;
- alterations are best avoided but if any are made and the prescription is to be used, best practice is for the prescriber to cross out the error, initial and date the error, then write the correct information;
- if an error made in a prescription cannot be corrected, best practice for the prescriber is to put a line through the script and write 'spoiled' on the form, or destroy the form and start writing a new prescription;
- prescribers and pharmacists dispensing drugs prone to abuse should ensure compliance with all relevant legal requirements specially when dealing with prescriptions for Controlled Drugs (see *Prescription requirements* and *Instalments* above);
- at the time of dispensing, prescriptions should be stamped with the pharmacy stamp and endorsed by the pharmacist or pharmacy technician with what has been supplied; where loss or theft is suspected, the police should be informed immediately.

Prescribing of drugs associated with dependence and withdrawal symptoms

Drugs such as benzodiazepines, Z-drugs (e.g. zopiclone, zolpidem), opioids, gabapentin, and pregabalin are associated with dependence, however this is not a reason in itself to avoid their use. When prescribing or continuing these drugs, ensure that all suitable management options, including non-pharmacological approaches, have been discussed with and offered to patients. The risk of developing problems associated with dependence and potential difficulty with stopping treatment should also be discussed, where appropriate. A written management plan should be agreed with the patient and include information such as the intended outcomes of treatment, the dose and how it will be titrated, the risks of taking more than the prescribed dose, how long they might be taking the medicine for, and the duration of each prescription that will be issued.

A minimal amount should be prescribed in the first instance, or when seeing a patient for the first time.

Regular treatment reviews should be offered, and at each review the benefits and risks of continuing, adjusting or stopping treatment should be discussed, and the patient's management plan updated as agreed and the date of the next review documented. Recognition of dependence is not easy and it may be difficult to distinguish between the re-emergence of underlying conditions and the emergence of withdrawal symptoms. Signs that may indicate that a patient is developing problems associated with dependence include running out of a medicine early, making frequent requests for dose increases or reporting loss of efficacy of a medicine that was previously working well. Prescribers should avoid being used as an unwitting source of supply for patients with problems associated with dependence and be vigilant to methods for obtaining medicines. Methods include visiting more than one doctor, fabricating stories, and forging prescriptions. Patients under temporary care should be given only small supplies of drugs unless they present an unequivocal letter from their own doctor. Prescribers should also remember that their own patients may be attempting to collect prescriptions from other prescribers, especially in hospitals.

Abrupt discontinuation of these drugs should be avoided in most cases, and a withdrawal or dose reduction schedule should be agreed with the patient, and modified according to the individual's need.

For further guidance on the prescribing of drugs associated with dependence, and management of withdrawal, see NICE guideline: **Medicines associated with dependence or withdrawal symptoms: safe prescribing and withdrawal management for adults** (available at: www.nice.org.uk/ guidance/ng215).

Dependence and misuse

The most common drugs of addiction are **crack cocaine** and **opioids**, particularly **diamorphine hydrochloride p. 518 (heroin)**. For arrangements for prescribing of diamorphine hydrochloride, dipipanone, or cocaine for addicts, see *Prescribing of diamorphine (heroin), dipipanone, and cocaine for addicts* below.

Along with traditional stimulants, such as amfetamine and cocaine, there has been an emerging use of methamphetamine and a range of psychoactive substances with stimulant, depressant or hallucinogenic properties such as lysergide (lysergic acid diethylamide, LSD), ketamine or gamma-hydroxybutyrate (sodium oxybate, GHB).

Benzodiazepines and Z-drugs (i.e. zopiclone p. 557, zolpidem tartrate p. 556) have their own potential for misuse and dependence and are often taken in combination with opiates or stimulants.

Cannabis-based products for medicinal use are Schedule 2 Controlled Drugs and can be prescribed only by clinicians listed on the Specialist Register of the General Medical Council. Cannabis with no approved medicinal use is a Schedule 1 Controlled Drug and cannot be prescribed. It remains the most frequently used illicit drug by young people and dependence can develop in around 10% of users. Cannabis use can exacerbate depression and it may cause an acute short-lived toxic psychosis which resolves with cessation, however paranoid symptoms may persist in chronic users; withdrawal symptoms can occur in some users and these can contribute to sleep problems, agitation and risk of self-harm.

Prescribing of diamorphine (heroin), dipipanone, and cocaine for addicts

The Misuse of Drugs (Supply to Addicts) Regulations 1997 require that **only** medical practitioners who hold a special licence issued by the Home Secretary (or Scottish Government's Chief Medical Officer) may prescribe, administer, or supply diamorphine hydrochloride p. 518, dipipanone, or cocaine for *the treatment of drug addiction*. Medical prescribers, pharmacists independent prescribers, nurses independent prescribers and supplementary prescribers do not require a special licence for prescribing diamorphine hydrochloride p. 518, dipipanone, or cocaine for patients (including addicts) for relieving pain from organic disease or injury.

Supervised consumption

Supervised consumption is not a legal requirement under the 2001 Regulations. Nevertheless, when supervised consumption is directed on the prescription, the Department of Health recommends that any deviation from the prescriber's intended method of supply should be documented and the justification for this recorded.

Individuals prescribed opioid substitution therapy can take their daily dose under the supervision of a doctor, nurse, or pharmacist during the dose stabilisation phase (usually the first 3 months of treatment), after a relapse or period of instability, or if there is a significant increase in the dose of methadone. Supervised consumption should continue (in accordance with local protocols) until the prescriber is confident that the patient is compliant with their treatment. It is good practice for pharmacists to alert the prescriber when a patient has missed consecutive daily doses.

Notification of patients receiving structured drug treatment for substance dependence

In **England**, doctors should report cases where they are providing structured drug treatment for substance dependence to their local National Drug Treatment Monitoring System (NDTMS) Team. General information about NDTMS can be found at www.gov.uk/government/collections/alcohol-and-drug-misuse-prevention-and-treatment-guidance.

Enquiries about NDTMS, and how to submit data, should initially be directed to:

- EvidenceApplicationteam@phe.gov.uk

In **Scotland**, doctors should report cases to the Substance Drug Misuse Database. General information about the Scottish Drug Misuse Database can be found in www.isdscotland.org/Health-Topics/Drugs-and-Alcohol-Misuse/Drugs-Misuse/Scottish-Drug-Misuse-Database/. Enquiries about reporting can be directed to:

- nss.isdsubstancemisuse@nhs.net

In **Northern Ireland**, the Misuse of Drugs (Notification of and Supply to Addicts) (Northern Ireland) Regulations 1973 require doctors to send particulars of persons whom they consider to be addicted to certain Controlled Drugs to the Chief Medical Officer of the Ministry of Health and Social Services. The Northern Ireland contact is:

Public Health Information & Research Branch
Department of Health
Annexe 2
Castle Buildings
Stormont
Belfast
BT4 3SQ
028 9052 2340
phirb@health-ni.gov.uk

Public Health Information & Research Branch also maintains the Northern Ireland Drug Misuse Database (NIDMD) which collects detailed information on those presenting for treatment, on drugs misused and injecting behaviour; participation is not a statutory requirement.

In **Wales**, doctors should report cases where they are providing structured drug treatment for substance dependence on the Welsh National Database for Substance Misuse; enquiries should be directed to:
substancemisuse-queries@wales.nhs.uk.

Travelling abroad

Prescribed drugs listed in Schedule 4 Part II (CD Anab) for self-administration and Schedule 5 of the Misuse of Drugs Regulations 2001 (and subsequent amendments) are not subject to export or import licensing. A personal import/export licence is required for patients travelling abroad with Schedules 2, 3, or 4 Part I (CD Benz) and Part II (CD Anab) Controlled Drugs if, they are carrying more than 3 months' supply or are travelling for 3 calendar months or more. A Home Office licence is required for any amount of a Schedule 1 Controlled Drug imported into the UK for personal use regardless of the duration of travel. Further details can be obtained at www.gov.uk/guidance/controlled-drugs-licences-fees-and-returns or from the Home Office by contacting DFLU.ie@homeoffice.gsi.gov.uk. In cases of emergency, telephone (020) 7035 6330.

Applications for obtaining a licence must be supported by a cover letter signed by the prescribing doctor or drug worker, which must confirm:

- the patient's name and address;
- the travel itinerary;
- the names of the prescribed Controlled Drug(s), doses and total amounts to be carried.

Applications for licences should be sent to the Home Office, Drugs & Firearms Licensing Unit, Fry Building, 2 Marsham Street, London, SW1P 4DF.

Alternatively, completed application forms can be emailed to DFLU.ie@homeoffice.gsi.gov.uk. A minimum of 10 days should be allowed for processing the application.

Patients travelling for less than 3 months or carrying less than 3 months supply of Controlled Drugs do not require a personal export/import licence, but are advised to carry a cover letter signed by the prescribing doctor or drug worker. Those travelling for more than 3 months are advised to make arrangements to have their medication prescribed by a practitioner in the country they are visiting.

Doctors who want to take Controlled Drugs abroad while accompanying patients may similarly be issued with licences. Licences are not normally issued to doctors who want to take Controlled Drugs abroad solely in case a family emergency should arise.

Personal export/import licences do not have any legal status outside the UK and are issued only to comply with the Misuse of Drugs Act 2001 and to facilitate passage through UK Customs and Excise control. For clearance in the country to be visited it is necessary to approach that country's consulate in the UK.

Adverse reactions to drugs

Yellow Card scheme

Any drug may produce unwanted or unexpected adverse reactions. Rapid detection and recording of adverse drug reactions is of vital importance so that unrecognised hazards are identified promptly and appropriate regulatory action is taken to ensure that medicines are used safely.

Healthcare professionals and coroners are urged to report suspected adverse drug reactions directly to the Medicines and Healthcare products Regulatory Agency (MHRA) through the Yellow Card scheme using the online form on the Yellow Card website (yellowcard.mhra.gov.uk), or by downloading and using the Yellow Card app. Reporting is also integrated into some clinical systems such as EMIS, SystmOne, Vision, MiDatabank, and Ulysses.

Suspected adverse drug reactions to any therapeutic agent should be reported, including drugs (*self-medication* as well as those *prescribed*), blood products, vaccines, radiographic contrast media, complementary, homeopathic and herbal products. This includes suspected adverse drug reactions associated with misuse, overdose, medication errors or from use of unlicensed and off-label medicines. For biological or biosimilar medicines and vaccines, adverse reaction reports should clearly state the brand name and the batch number of the suspected medicine or vaccine.

The Yellow Card scheme can also be used to report medical device adverse incidents, defective medicines, suspected falsified (fake) medicines, as well as safety concerns associated with e-cigarettes and their refill containers (e-liquids).

Spontaneous reporting is particularly valuable for recognising possible new hazards rapidly. An adverse reaction should be reported even if it is not certain that the drug has caused it, or if the reaction is well recognised, or if other drugs have been given at the same time. Reports of overdoses (deliberate or accidental) can complicate the assessment of adverse drug reactions, but provide important information on the potential toxicity of drugs.

A freephone service is available to all parts of the UK for advice and information on suspected adverse drug reactions; contact the National Yellow Card Information Service at the MHRA on 0800 731 6789 (9am to 5pm Monday to Friday only). Outside office hours a telephone-answering machine will take messages.

The MHRA commissions six regional Yellow Card Centres to increase awareness as well as to educate and promote the reporting of suspected side-effects to the Yellow Card scheme from healthcare professionals, patients, and their representative organisations. The following Yellow Card Centres can be contacted for further information:

Yellow Card Centre North West
2nd Floor
70 Pembroke Place
Liverpool
L69 3GF
0151 794 8117
yccnorthwest@rlbuht.nhs.net

Yellow Card Centre Northern & Yorkshire
Regional Drug and Therapeutics Centre
16/17 Framlington Place
Newcastle upon Tyne
NE2 4AB
0191 213 7855
yccnorthernandyorkshire@nuth.nhs.uk

Yellow Card Centre West Midlands
City Hospital
Dudley Road
Birmingham
B18 7QH
0121 507 5672
swb-tr.swbh-team-yccwestmidlands@nhs.net

Yellow Card Centre Northern Ireland
Northern Ireland Medicines and Poisons Advice Service
Belfast Health and Social Care Trust
Pharmacy Department
Building 36
Knockbracken Clinic
Knockbracken Healthcare Park
Saintfield Road
Belfast
BT8 8BH
028 9504 0558
medicineinfo@belfasttrust.hscni.net

Yellow Card Centre Scotland
51 Little France Crescent
Old Dalkeith Road
Edinburgh
EH16 4SA
0131 242 2919
yccscotland@nhslothian.scot.nhs.uk

Yellow Card Centre Wales
All Wales Therapeutics and Toxicology Centre
Academic Building
University Hospital Llandough
Penlan Road
Penarth
Vale of Glamorgan
CF64 2XX
029 2074 5831
yccwales@wales.nhs.uk

The MHRA's database facilitates the monitoring of adverse drug reactions. More detailed information on reporting and a list of products currently under additional monitoring can be found on the MHRA website: www.gov.uk/government/organisations/medicines-and-healthcare-products-regulatory-agency.

MHRA Drug Safety Update *Drug Safety Update* is a monthly newsletter from the MHRA and the Commission on Human Medicines (CHM); it is available at www.gov.uk/drug-safety-update. Drug Safety Update is also available to access from the Yellow Card app, which allows users to create a watchlist of medicines.

Interactive Drug Analysis Profiles *interactive Drug Analysis Profiles* (iDAPs) are available on the Yellow Card website (yellowcard.mhra.gov.uk) under *What is being reported*. Each iDAP contains complete data for all spontaneous suspected adverse drug reactions, or side-effects, which have been reported on that drug substance to the MHRA via the Yellow Card scheme, from healthcare professionals and members of the public. iDAPs are also available to access from the Yellow Card app.

Yellow Card biobank Yellow Card biobank is a collaboration between the MHRA and Genomics England that aims to improve understanding of how a patient's genetic makeup may increase their risk of harm from side-effects. Through the collection of genetic samples from patients who have experienced suspected side-effects, the Yellow Card biobank will create a repository of genetic information that can be used to help determine whether a suspected side-effect was caused by a specific genetic trait. Further information (including current topics) can be found on the Yellow Card website (yellowcard.mhra.gov.uk).

Self-reporting

Patients and their carers can also report suspected adverse drug reactions to the MHRA. Healthcare professionals are encouraged to discuss side-effects with patients and carers and encourage them to self-report if side-effects occur.

Reports can be submitted directly to the MHRA through the Yellow Card scheme using the online form, by downloading a copy of the form from the Yellow Card website, using the Yellow Card app, or by freephone on 0800 731 6789. Alternatively, patient Yellow Cards may be available from pharmacies and GP surgeries. Information for patients about the Yellow Card scheme is available in other languages from the Yellow Card website (yellowcard.mhra.gov. uk).

Prescription-event monitoring

In addition to the MHRA's Yellow Card scheme, an independent scheme monitors the safety of new medicines using a different approach. The Drug Safety Research Unit identifies patients who have been prescribed selected new medicines and collects data on clinical events in these patients. The data are submitted on a voluntary basis by general practitioners on green forms. More information about the scheme and the Unit's educational material is available from www.dsru.org.

Newer drugs and vaccines

Only limited information is available from clinical trials on the safety of new medicines. Further understanding about the safety of medicines depends on the availability of information from routine clinical practice.

The black triangle symbol (▼) identifies newly licensed medicines that require additional monitoring, such as new active substances and biosimilar medicines. The black triangle symbol also appears in the Patient Information Leaflets for relevant medicines, with a brief explanation of what it means. Products usually retain a black triangle for 5 years, but this can be extended if required.

Spontaneous reporting is particularly valuable for recognising possible new hazards rapidly. For medicines showing the black triangle symbol, the MHRA asks that **all** suspected reactions (including those considered not to be serious) are reported through the Yellow Card scheme. An adverse reaction should be reported even if it is not certain that the drug has caused it, or if the reaction is well recognised, or if other drugs have been given at the same time.

A list of products under additional monitoring can be found on the MHRA's website (www.gov.uk/guidance/the-yellow-card-scheme-guidance-for-healthcare-professionals#black-triangle-scheme).

Established drugs and vaccines

Healthcare professionals and coroners are asked to report all suspected reactions to established drugs (including over-the-counter, herbal, homeopathic, and unlicensed medicines and medicines used off-label) and vaccines that are **serious, medically significant, or result in harm**. Serious reactions include those that are fatal, life-threatening, disabling, incapacitating, or which result in or prolong hospitalisation, or a congenital abnormality; they should be reported even if the effect is well recognised. Examples include anaphylaxis, blood disorders, endocrine disturbances, effects on fertility, haemorrhage from any site, renal impairment, jaundice, ophthalmic disorders, severe CNS effects, severe skin reactions, reactions in pregnant women, and any drug interactions. Reports of serious adverse reactions are required to enable comparison with other drugs of a similar class. Reports of overdoses (deliberate or accidental) can

complicate the assessment of adverse drug reactions, but provide important information on the potential toxicity of drugs.

For established drugs there is no need to report well-known, relatively minor side-effects, such as dry mouth with tricyclic antidepressants or constipation with opioids.

Medication errors

Adverse drug reactions where harm occurs as a result of a medication error are reportable through the Yellow Card scheme or through a local risk management system (LRMS).

In England, medication errors reported via a LRMS are uploaded to the national Learn From Patient Safety Events service (LFPSE); if a LRMS is not available, medication errors can also be reported directly via the LFPSE online service (record.learn-from-patient-safety-events.nhs.uk). If incidents are uploaded into the LFPSE, these will be shared with the MHRA. (This service is being rolled out across England, Wales, and Northern Ireland—speak to your local safety team about which system you should currently be using.) If the LFPSE is not available and harm occurs, report through the Yellow Card scheme.

In Scotland, local incident/event management systems with a focus on quality improvement and learning are promoted. The Healthcare Improvement Scotland *Adverse Events National Framework: Learning from adverse events through reporting and review - A national framework for Scotland: December* 2019 (www.healthcareimprovementscotland.org/our_work/governance_and_assurance/learning_from_adverse_events/national_framework.aspx) provides useful context to the management of adverse events.

Adverse reactions to medical devices

Suspected adverse reactions to medical devices including dental or surgical materials, intra-uterine devices, and contact lens fluids should be reported. Information about reporting medical device adverse incidents can be found at: yellowcard.mhra.gov.uk/medicaldevices.

Side-effects in the BNF

The BNF includes clinically relevant side-effects for most drugs; an exhaustive list is not included for drugs that are used by specialists (e.g. cytotoxic drugs and drugs used in anaesthesia). Where causality has not been established, side-effects in the manufacturers' literature may be omitted from the BNF.

Recognising that hypersensitivity reactions (including anaphylactic and anaphylactoid reactions) can occur with virtually all drugs, this effect is not generally listed, unless the drug carries an increased risk of such reactions or specific management advice is provided by the manufacturer. Administration site reactions have been omitted from the BNF (e.g. pain at injection site). The BNF also omits effects that are likely to have little clinical consequence (e.g. transient increase in liver enzymes). Drugs that are applied locally or topically carry a theoretical or low risk of systemic absorption and therefore systemic side-effects for these drugs are not listed in the BNF unless they are associated with a high risk to patient safety. Infections are a known complication of treatment with drugs that affect the immune system (e.g. corticosteroids or immunosuppressants); this side-effect is listed in the BNF as 'increased risk of infection'. Symptoms of drug withdrawal reactions are not individually listed, but are collectively termed 'withdrawal syndrome'.

Side-effects are generally listed alphabetically in order of frequency. In the product literature the frequency of side-effects is generally described as follows:

Description of the frequency of side-effects

Very common	greater than 1 in 10
Common	1 in 100 to 1 in 10
Uncommon [formerly 'less commonly' in BNF publications]	1 in 1000 to 1 in 100
Rare	1 in 10 000 to 1 in 1000
Very rare	less than 1 in 10 000
Frequency not known	frequency is not defined by product literature or the side-effect has been reported from post-marketing surveillance data

The BNF might not use the same wording as manufacturers' literature because, for consistency, the terms used to describe side-effects are standardised using a defined vocabulary across all of the drug monographs in the BNF (e.g. postural hypotension is used for the term orthostatic hypotension). In addition, individual side-effects are often grouped together in the BNF where there are two or more similar side-effects (e.g. hepatitis, hepatic failure, and jaundice are grouped together as 'hepatic disorders').

Some drug monographs in the BNF include information that is common across the drug class. If a side-effect is associated with at least 60% of the drugs in a class then it will appear as a class side-effect for all drugs in the class, and the frequency of the side-effect will be the highest of all the drugs in that class.

Special problems

Delayed drug effects Some reactions (e.g. cancers, chloroquine retinopathy, and retroperitoneal fibrosis) may become manifest months or years after exposure. Any suspicion of such an association should be reported through the Yellow Card scheme.

The elderly Particular vigilance is required to identify adverse reactions in the elderly, especially if taking multiple medicines.

Congenital abnormalities When an infant is born with a congenital abnormality or there is a malformed aborted fetus doctors are asked to consider whether this might be an adverse reaction to a drug and to report all drugs (including self-medication) taken during pregnancy.

Children Particular vigilance is required to identify and report adverse reactions in children, including those resulting from the unlicensed or off-label use of medicines; suspected reactions should be reported through the Yellow Card scheme (see also *Adverse drug reactions in children* under Prescribing in children p. 19).

Prevention of adverse reactions

Adverse reactions may be prevented as follows:

- never use any drug unless there is a good indication. If the patient is pregnant do not use a drug unless the need for it is imperative;
- allergy and idiosyncrasy are important causes of adverse drug reactions. Ask if the patient had previous reactions to the drug or formulation;
- ask if the patient is already taking other drugs including self-medication drugs, health supplements, complementary and alternative therapies; interactions may occur;
- age and hepatic or renal disease may alter the metabolism or excretion of drugs, so that much smaller doses may be needed. Genetic factors may also be responsible for variations in metabolism, and therefore for the adverse effect of the drug; notably of isoniazid p. 679 and the tricyclic antidepressants;
- prescribe as few drugs as possible and give very clear instructions to the elderly or any patient likely to misunderstand complicated instructions;
- whenever possible use a familiar drug; with a new drug, be particularly alert for adverse reactions or unexpected events;
- consider if excipients (e.g. colouring agents) may be contributing to the adverse reaction. If the reaction is minor, a trial of an alternative formulation of the same drug may be considered before abandoning the drug;
- warn the patient if serious adverse reactions are liable to occur.

Drug allergy (suspected or confirmed)

Suspected drug allergy is any reaction caused by a drug with clinical features compatible with an immunological mechanism. All drugs have the potential to cause adverse drug reactions, but not all of these are allergic in nature. A reaction is more likely to be caused by drug allergy if:

- The reaction occurred while the patient was being treated with the drug, or
- The drug is known to cause this pattern of reaction, or
- The patient has had a similar reaction to the same drug or drug-class previously.

A suspected reaction is less likely to be caused by a drug allergy if there is a possible non-drug cause or if there are only gastro-intestinal symptoms present.

The following signs, allergic patterns and timing of onset can be used to help decide whether to suspect drug allergy:
Immediate, rapidly-evolving reactions (onset usually less than 1 hour after drug exposure)

- Anaphylaxis, with erythema, urticaria or angioedema, and hypotension and/or bronchospasm. See also Antihistamines, allergen immunotherapy and allergic emergencies p. 316
- Urticaria or angioedema without systemic features
- Exacerbation of asthma e.g. with non-steroidal anti-inflammatory drugs (NSAIDs)

*Non-immediate reactions, **without** systemic involvement* (onset usually 6–10 days after first drug exposure or 3 days after second exposure)

- Cutaneous reactions, e.g. widespread red macules and/or papules, or, fixed drug eruption (localised inflamed skin)

*Non-immediate reactions, **with** systemic involvement* (onset may be variable, usually 3 days to 6 weeks after first drug exposure, depending on features, or 3 days after second exposure)

- Cutaneous reactions with systemic features, e.g. drug reaction with eosinophilia and systemic signs (DRESS) or drug hypersensitivity syndrome (DHS), characterised by widespread red macules, papules or erythroderma, fever, lymphadenopathy, liver dysfunction or eosinophilia
- Toxic epidermal necrolysis or Stevens–Johnson syndrome
- Acute generalised exanthematous pustulosis (AGEP)

EvGr Suspected drug allergy information should be clearly and accurately documented in clinical notes and prescriptions, and shared among all healthcare professionals. Patients should be given information about which drugs and drug-classes to avoid and encouraged to share their drug allergy status.

If a drug allergy is suspected, consider stopping the suspected drug and advising the patient or carer to avoid this drug in future. Symptoms of the acute reaction should be treated, in hospital if severe. Patients presenting with a suspected anaphylactic reaction, or a severe or non-immediate cutaneous reaction, should be referred to a specialist drug allergy service. Patients presenting with a suspected drug allergic reaction or anaphylaxis to NSAIDs, and local and general anaesthetics may also need to be referred to a specialist drug allergy service, e.g. in cases of anaphylactoid reactions or to determine future treatment options. Patients presenting with a suspected drug allergic reaction or anaphylaxis associated with beta-lactam antibiotics should be referred to a specialist drug allergy service if their disease or condition can only be treated by a beta-lactam antibiotic or they are likely to need beta-lactam antibiotics frequently in the future (e.g. immunodeficient patients). Ⓐ For further information see Drug allergy: diagnosis and management. NICE Clinical Guideline 183 (September 2014) www.nice.org.uk/guidance/cg183.

Oral side-effects of drugs

Drug-induced disorders of the mouth may be due to a local action on the mouth or to a systemic effect manifested by oral changes. In the latter case urgent referral to the patient's medical practitioner may be necessary.

Oral mucosa Medicaments left in contact with or applied directly to the oral mucosa can lead to inflammation or ulceration; the possibility of allergy should also be borne in mind.

Aspirin tablets p. 142 allowed to dissolve in the sulcus for the treatment of toothache can lead to a white patch followed by ulceration.

Flavouring agents, particularly **essential oils**, may sensitise the skin, but mucosal swelling is not usually prominent.

The oral mucosa is particularly vulnerable to ulceration in patients treated with cytotoxic drugs, e.g. methotrexate p. 1048. Other drugs capable of causing oral ulceration include **ACE inhibitors**, **gold**, nicorandil p. 246, **NSAIDs**, pancreatin p. 76, penicillamine p. 1255, **proguanil hydrochloride**, and **protease inhibitors**.

Erythema multiforme or Stevens-Johnson syndrome may follow the use of a wide range of drugs including **antibacterials, antiretrovirals, sulfonamide derivatives,** and **anticonvulsants**; the oral mucosa may be extensively ulcerated, with characteristic target lesions on the skin. Oral lesions of toxic epidermal necrolysis have been reported with a similar range of drugs.

Lichenoid eruptions are associated with **ACE inhibitors, NSAIDs**, methyldopa p. 172, chloroquine p. 710, **oral antidiabetics, thiazide diuretics**, and **gold**.

Candidiasis can complicate treatment with **antibacterials** and **immunosuppressants** and is an occasional side-effect of **corticosteroid inhalers**.

Teeth and jaw *Brown staining* of the teeth frequently follows the use of chlorhexidine mouthwash, spray or gel p. 1377, but can readily be removed by polishing. **Iron** salts in liquid form can stain the enamel black. Superficial staining has been reported rarely with co-amoxiclav suspension p. 638.

Intrinsic staining of the teeth is most commonly caused by **tetracyclines**. They will affect the teeth if given at any time from about the fourth month *in utero* until the age of twelve years; they are contra-indicated during pregnancy, in breast-feeding women, and in children under 12 years. All tetracyclines can cause permanent, unsightly staining in children, the colour varying from yellow to grey.

Excessive ingestion of **fluoride** leads to *dental fluorosis* with mottling of the enamel and areas of hypoplasia or pitting; fluoride supplements occasionally cause mild mottling (white patches) if the dose is too large for the child's age (taking into account the fluoride content of the local drinking water and of toothpaste).

The risk of *osteonecrosis of the jaw* is substantially greater for patients receiving intravenous bisphosphonates in the treatment of cancer than for patients receiving oral bisphosphonates for osteoporosis or Paget's disease. All patients receiving bisphosphonates should have a dental check-up (and any necessary remedial work should be performed) before bisphosphonate treatment, or as soon as possible after starting treatment. Patients with cancer receiving bevacizumab p. 999 or sunitinib p. 1128 may also be at risk of osteonecrosis of the jaw.

Periodontium *Gingival overgrowth* (gingival hyperplasia) is a side-effect of phenytoin p. 372 and sometimes of ciclosporin p. 966 or of nifedipine p. 189 (and some other calcium-channel blockers).

Thrombocytopenia may be drug related and may cause bleeding at the gingival margins, which may be spontaneous or may follow mild trauma (such as toothbrushing).

Salivary glands The most common effect that drugs have on the salivary glands is to *reduce flow* (xerostomia). Patients with a persistently dry mouth may have poor oral hygiene; they are at an increased risk of dental caries and oral infections (particularly candidiasis). Many drugs have been implicated in xerostomia, particularly **antimuscarinics** (anticholinergics), **antidepressants** (including tricyclic antidepressants, and selective serotonin re-uptake inhibitors), **alpha-blockers, antihistamines, antipsychotics, baclofen p. 1289, bupropion hydrochloride p. 566, clonidine hydrochloride p. 172, 5HT$_1$ agonists, opioids**, and tizanidine p. 1291. Excessive use of **diuretics** can also result in xerostomia.

Some drugs (e.g. clozapine p. 457, neostigmine p. 1286) can *increase saliva production* but this is rarely a problem unless the patient has associated difficulty in swallowing.

Pain in the salivary glands has been reported with some **antihypertensives** (e.g. clonidine hydrochloride p. 172, methyldopa p. 172) and with **vinca alkaloids**.

Swelling of the salivary glands can occur with **iodides, antithyroid drugs, phenothiazines**, and **sulfonamides**.

Taste There can be *decreased* taste acuity or *alteration* in taste sensation. Many drugs are implicated, including amiodarone hydrochloride p. 120, **calcitonin, ACE inhibitors**, carbimazole p. 887, clarithromycin p. 621, **gold**, griseofulvin p. 697, **lithium salts**, metformin hydrochloride p. 807, metronidazole p. 628, penicillamine p. 1255, phenindione p. 164, propafenone hydrochloride p. 119, **protease inhibitors**, terbinafine p. 1401, and zopiclone p. 557.

Defective medicines

During the manufacture or distribution of a medicine an error or accident may occur whereby the finished product does not conform to its specification. While such a defect may impair the therapeutic effect of the product and could adversely affect the health of a patient, it should **not** be confused with an adverse drug reaction where the product conforms to its specification. Reports of a defective medicine can be made online through the Yellow Card scheme.

The Defective Medicines Report Centre (DMRC) assists with the investigation of problems arising from licensed medicinal products thought to be defective and co-ordinates any necessary protective action. Reports on suspect defective medicinal products should include the brand or the non-proprietary name, the name of the manufacturer or supplier, the strength and dosage form of the product, the product licence number, the batch number or numbers of the product, the nature of the defect, and an account of any action already taken in consequence. The Centre can be contacted at:

The Defective Medicines Report Centre
Medicines and Healthcare products Regulatory Agency
10 South Colonnade
Canary Wharf
London
E14 4PU
dmrc@mhra.gov.uk

During office hours (8:45am to 4:45pm Monday to Friday), contact DMRC on 020 3080 6574.

Out of hours (urgent reports outside of normal working hours, at weekends or on public holidays), contact DMRC on 07795 641 532.

Guidance on intravenous infusions

Intravenous additives policies

A local policy on the addition of drugs to intravenous fluids should be drawn up by a multi-disciplinary team and issued as a document to the members of staff concerned.

Centralised additive services are provided in a number of hospital pharmacy departments and should be used in preference to making additions on wards.

The information that follows should be read in conjunction with local policy documents.

Guidelines

- Drugs should only be added to infusion containers when constant plasma concentrations are needed or when the administration of a more concentrated solution would be harmful.
- In general, only one drug should be added to any infusion container and the components should be compatible. Ready-prepared solutions should be used whenever possible. Drugs should not normally be added to blood products, mannitol, or sodium bicarbonate. Only specially formulated additives should be used with fat emulsions or amino-acid solutions.
- Solutions should be thoroughly mixed by shaking and checked for absence of particulate matter before use.
- Strict asepsis should be maintained throughout and in general the giving set should not be used for more than 24 hours (for drug admixtures).
- The infusion container should be labelled with the patient's name, the name and quantity of additives, and the date and time of addition (and the new expiry date or time). Such additional labelling should not interfere with information on the manufacturer's label that is still valid. When possible, containers should be retained for a period after use in case they are needed for investigation.
- It is good practice to examine intravenous infusions from time to time while they are running. If cloudiness, crystallisation, change of colour, or any other sign of interaction or contamination is observed the infusion should be discontinued.

Problems

Microbial contamination The accidental entry and subsequent growth of micro-organisms converts the infusion fluid pathway into a potential vehicle for infection with micro-organisms, particularly species of *Candida*, *Enterobacter*, and *Klebsiella*. Ready-prepared infusions containing the additional drugs, or infusions prepared by an additive service (when available) should therefore be used in preference to making extemporaneous additions to infusion containers on wards etc. However, when this is necessary strict aseptic procedure should be followed.

Incompatibility Physical and chemical incompatibilities may occur with loss of potency, increase in toxicity, or other adverse effect. The solutions may become opalescent or precipitation may occur, but in many instances there is no visual indication of incompatibility. Interaction may take place at any point in the infusion fluid pathway, and the potential for incompatibility is increased when more than one substance is added to the infusion fluid.

Common incompatibilities Precipitation reactions are numerous and varied and may occur as a result of pH, concentration changes, 'salting-out' effects, complexation or other chemical changes. Precipitation or other particle formation must be avoided since, apart from lack of control of dosage on administration, it may initiate or exacerbate adverse effects. This is particularly important in the case of drugs which have been implicated in either thrombophlebitis (e.g. diazepam) or in skin sloughing or necrosis caused by extravasation (e.g. sodium bicarbonate and certain cytotoxic drugs). It is also especially important to effect solution of colloidal drugs and to prevent their subsequent precipitation in order to avoid a pyrogenic reaction (e.g. amphotericin B).

It is considered undesirable to mix beta-lactam antibiotics, such as semi-synthetic penicillins and cephalosporins, with proteinaceous materials on the grounds that immunogenic and allergenic conjugates could be formed.

A number of preparations undergo significant loss of potency when added singly or in combination to large volume infusions. Examples include ampicillin in infusions that contain glucose or lactates. The breakdown products of dacarbazine have been implicated in adverse effects.

Blood Because of the large number of incompatibilities, drugs should not normally be added to blood and blood products for infusion purposes. Examples of incompatibility with blood include hypertonic mannitol solutions (irreversible crenation of red cells), dextrans (rouleaux formation and interference with cross-matching), glucose (clumping of red cells), and oxytocin (inactivated).

If the giving set is not changed after the administration of blood, but used for other infusion fluids, a fibrin clot may form which, apart from blocking the set, increases the likelihood of microbial growth.

Intravenous fat emulsions These may break down with coalescence of fat globules and separation of phases when additions such as antibacterials or electrolytes are made, thus increasing the possibility of embolism. Only specially formulated products such as *Vitlipid N*® may be added to appropriate intravenous fat emulsions.

Other infusions Infusions that frequently give rise to incompatibility include amino acids, mannitol, and sodium bicarbonate.

Bactericides Bactericides such as chlorocresol 0.1% or phenylmercuric nitrate 0.001% are present in some injection solutions. The total volume of such solutions added to a container for infusion on one occasion should not exceed 15 mL.

Method

Ready-prepared infusions should be used whenever available. **Potassium chloride** is usually available in concentrations of 20, 27, and 40 mmol/litre in sodium chloride intravenous infusion (0.9%), glucose intravenous infusion (5%) or sodium chloride and glucose intravenous infusion. **Lidocaine hydrochloride** is usually available in concentrations of 0.1 or 0.2% in glucose intravenous infusion (5%).

When addition is required to be made extemporaneously, any product reconstitution instructions such as those relating to concentration, vehicle, mixing, and handling precautions should be strictly followed using an aseptic technique throughout. Once the product has been reconstituted, addition to the infusion fluid should be made immediately in order to minimise microbial contamination and, with certain products, to prevent degradation or other formulation change which may occur; e.g. reconstituted ampicillin injection degrades rapidly on standing, and also may form polymers which could cause sensitivity reactions.

It is also important in certain instances that an infusion fluid of specific pH be used (e.g. **furosemide** injection requires dilution in infusions of pH greater than 5.5).

When drug additions are made it is important to mix thoroughly; additions should not be made to an infusion container that has been connected to a giving set, as mixing is hampered. If the solutions are not thoroughly mixed a concentrated layer of the additive may form owing to differences in density. **Potassium chloride** is particularly prone to this 'layering' effect when added without adequate mixing to infusions packed in non-rigid infusion containers; if such a mixture is administered it may have a serious effect on the heart.

A time limit between addition and completion of administration must be imposed for certain admixtures to guarantee satisfactory drug potency and compatibility. For admixtures in which degradation occurs without the formation of toxic substances, an acceptable limit is the time taken for 10% decomposition of the drug. When toxic substances are produced stricter limits may be imposed. Because of the risk of microbial contamination a maximum time limit of 24 hours may be appropriate for additions made elsewhere than in hospital pharmacies offering central additive service.

Certain injections must be protected from light during continuous infusion to minimise oxidation, e.g. dacarbazine and sodium nitroprusside.

Dilution with a small volume of an appropriate vehicle and administration using a motorised infusion pump is advocated for preparations such as unfractionated heparin where strict control over administration is required. In this case the appropriate dose may be dissolved in a convenient volume (e.g. 24–48 mL) of sodium chloride intravenous infusion (0.9%).

Information provided in the BNF

The BNF gives information about preparations given by three methods:

- continuous infusion;
- intermittent infusion;
- addition via the drip tubing.

Drugs for **continuous infusion** must be diluted in a large volume infusion. Penicillins and cephalosporins are not usually given by continuous infusion because of stability problems and because adequate plasma and tissue concentrations are best obtained by intermittent infusion. Where it is necessary to administer them by continuous infusion, detailed literature should be consulted.

Drugs that are both compatible and clinically suitable may be given by **intermittent infusion** in a relatively small volume of infusion over a short period of time, e.g. 100 mL in 30 minutes. The method is used if the product is incompatible or unstable over the period necessary for continuous infusion; the limited stability of ampicillin or amoxicillin in large volume glucose or lactate infusions may be overcome in this way.

Intermittent infusion is also used if adequate plasma and tissue concentrations are not produced by continuous infusion as in the case of drugs such as dacarbazine, gentamicin, and ticarcillin.

An in-line burette may be used for intermittent infusion techniques in order to achieve strict control over the time and rate of administration, especially for infants and children and in intensive care units. Intermittent infusion may also make use of the 'piggy-back' technique provided that no additions are made to the primary infusion. In this method the drug is added to a small secondary container connected to a Y-type injection site on the primary infusion giving set; the secondary solution is usually infused within 30 minutes.

Addition *via* the drip tubing is indicated for a number of cytotoxic drugs in order to minimise extravasation. The preparation is added aseptically via the rubber septum of the injection site of a fast-running infusion. In general, drug preparations intended for a bolus effect should be given directly into a separate vein where possible. Failing this, administration may be made via the drip tubing provided that the preparation is compatible with the infusion fluid when given in this manner.

Drugs given by intravenous infusion The BNF includes information on addition to *Glucose intravenous infusion* 5 and 10%, and *Sodium chloride intravenous infusion* 0.9%. Compatibility with glucose 5% and with sodium chloride 0.9% indicates compatibility with *Sodium chloride and glucose intravenous infusion*. Infusion of a large volume of hypotonic solution should be avoided therefore care should be taken if water for injections is used. The information relates to the proprietary preparations indicated; for other preparations suitability should be checked with the manufacturer.

Medicines optimisation

Overview

Medicines are the most common intervention in healthcare for the prevention, treatment and/or management of many illnesses. As life expectancy increases and as the population ages, more people are living with several long-term conditions that are being managed with an increasing number of medicines. Medicines use can be complex and how patients can take their medicines safely and effectively is a challenge for the health service.

Multimorbidity (the presence of 2 or more long-term conditions) is associated with a greater use of health services, higher mortality, higher treatment burden (due to polypharmacy or multiple appointments), and reduced quality of life. The risk of patients suffering harm from their medicines increases with polypharmacy, and treatment regimens (including non-pharmacological treatments) can very easily become burdensome for patients with multimorbidity and can lead to care becoming fragmented and uncoordinated. Prescribers should consider the risks and benefits of treatments recommended from guidance for single health conditions, as the evidence for these recommendations is regularly drawn from patients without multimorbidity and who are taking fewer prescribed regular medicines. The management of risk factors for future disease can also be a major treatment burden for patients with multimorbidity and should be taken into consideration.

Medicines optimisation encompasses many aspects of medicines use and helps to ensure that they are taken as intended, thus supporting the management of long-term conditions, multimorbidities, and appropriate polypharmacy. It focuses on actions taken by all health and social care practitioners, and requires greater patient engagement and professional collaboration across health and social care settings. Through the adoption of a patient-focused approach to safe and effective medicines use, medicines optimisation changes the way patients are supported to get the best possible outcomes from their medicines. The use of shared decision-making informed by the best available evidence to guide decisions, ensures all patients have the opportunity to be involved in decisions about their medicines, taking into account their needs, preferences and values.

Overprescribing in the NHS has been reviewed by the Department of Health and Social Care in order to reduce the risk of harm, manage the spend on medicines, and ensure patients taking multiple medicines are receiving the most appropriate treatments for their needs. The national overprescribing review report is available at: www.gov.uk/government/publications/national-overprescribing-review-report.

Medicines optimisation

Optimisation tools

Medicines optimisation includes aspects of care such as clinical assessment, clinical audits, disease prevention, health education, individual reviews and monitoring, and risk management. Having effective processes and systems in place can minimise the risk of preventable medicines-related problems (such as interactions with other medicines or comorbidities, and side-effects). Health and social care organisations should consider the use of multiple methods for identifying medicines-related patient safety incidents; learning from these incidents is important for guiding practice and minimising patient harm.

When optimising patient care, areas of intervention to consider include: deprescribing; medicines reconciliation, reviews and repeat prescribing; problematic polypharmacy; reducing medication waste and errors; and self-management plans. Self-management plans can be patient or health professional led and vary in their content depending on the individual needs of the patient, with the aim of supporting both their involvement and empowerment in managing their condition.

Medicines optimisation services such as Structured Medication Reviews (SMRs), the Discharge Medicines Service (DMS), and New Medicines Service (NMS) are available to support individuals with their medicines. These can be undertaken in different care settings, such as community pharmacies or Primary Care Networks, and should be led by an appropriate health professional with effective communication skills, technical knowledge in the processes for managing medicines, and therapeutic knowledge on medicines use. Further information about these services is available from the Pharmaceutical Services Negotiating Committee, available at: psnc.org.uk/services-commissioning/; NHS England, available at: www.england.nhs.uk/primary-care/ pharmacy/community-pharmacy-contractual-framework/; Community Pharmacy Wales, available at: cpwales.org.uk/ Services-and-commissioning-d54; Community Pharmacy Northern Ireland, available at: www.communitypharmacyni.co. uk/services/; and Community Pharmacy Scotland, available at: www.cps.scot/core.

To support the medicines optimisation agenda, The Royal Pharmaceutical Society have produced good practice guidance for health professionals, which details four guiding principles for medicines optimisation. These are:

- Aim to understand the patient's experience;
- Evidence-based choice of medicines;
- Ensure medicines use is as safe as possible;
- Make medicines optimisation part of routine practice.

For further guidance around medicines optimisation and tools to use, NHS England have compiled useful links; NICE have produced guidelines on **Medicines optimisation**, **Medicines adherence**, and **Multimorbidity**; and the Scottish Government have produced a guideline on **Polypharmacy**, see *Useful resources*.

Communication

As health professionals from various disciplines and specialties may be caring for the same patient at the same time, good communication is required between health professionals in order to avoid fragmentation of care. Medication reviews may be carried out by health professionals other than the prescriber, therefore the prescriber should be informed of the review and its outcome—particularly if difficulties with adherence were discussed and further review is required.

There is a greater risk of poor communication and unintended medication changes when patients transfer between different care providers (such as when a person is admitted to or discharged from hospital). To support high-quality care when moving from one care setting to another, relevant information about medicines should be shared with patients, their family members/carers (if appropriate), and between health and social care practitioners using robust and transparent processes. Information should be securely shared between health and social care practitioners ideally within 24 hours of patient transfer.

Good communication between health professionals and patients, and their family members/carers (if appropriate) is needed for shared decision-making and supporting adherence. Information about their condition and possible treatments should be provided in a format that meets a patient's (and carer's) individual needs and preferences. The use of patient decision aids during consultations can help support a shared decision-making approach, and ensure patients and their family members/carers (where appropriate) are able to make well-informed choices that are consistent with their values and preferences.

For further guidance around communication between health professionals and patients (and carers), NICE have produced guidelines on **Medicines optimisation**, **Medicines adherence**, **Shared decision making**, and **Supporting adult carers** (see *Useful resources*).

Organisations such as the 'NHS Specialist Pharmacy Service' help support medicines optimisation across the NHS by joining health professionals together through online networks (e.g. Regional Medicines Optimisation Committees and the English Deprescribing Network). This is available at: www.sps.nhs.uk/.

Useful resources

Medicines optimisation: the safe and effective use of medicines to enable the best possible outcomes. National Institute for Health and Care Excellence. NICE guideline 5. March 2015.

www.nice.org.uk/guidance/ng5

Multimorbidity: clinical assessment and management. National Institute for Health and Care Excellence. NICE guideline 56. September 2016.

www.nice.org.uk/guidance/ng56

Medicines adherence: involving patients in decisions about prescribed medicines and supporting adherence. National Institute for Health and Care Excellence. Clinical guideline 76. January 2009.

www.nice.org.uk/guidance/cg76

Medicines Optimisation. NHS England.

www.england.nhs.uk/medicines-2/medicines-optimisation/

Polypharmacy Guidance, Realistic Prescribing. Scottish Government Polypharmacy Model of Care Group. 3rd Edition. 2018.

www.therapeutics.scot.nhs.uk/polypharmacy/

Shared decision making. National Institute for Health and Care Excellence. NICE Guideline 197. June 2021.

www.nice.org.uk/guidance/ng197

Supporting adult carers. National Institute for Health and Care Excellence. NICE Guideline 150. January 2020.

www.nice.org.uk/guidance/ng150

Medicines Optimisation: Helping patients to make the most of medicines. Royal Pharmaceutical Society. May 2013.

www.rpharms.com/resources/pharmacy-guides/medicines-optimisation-hub

Antimicrobial stewardship

Overview

Effective antimicrobials are required for preventive and curative measures, protecting patients from potentially fatal diseases, and ensuring that complex procedures can be provided at low risk of infection. Antimicrobial resistance (AMR) is the loss of antimicrobial effectiveness, and although it evolves naturally, this process is accelerated by the inappropriate or incorrect use of antimicrobials. Direct consequences of infection with resistant microorganisms can be severe and affect all areas of health, such as prolonged illnesses and hospital stays, increased costs and mortality, and reduced protection for patients undergoing operations or procedures. AMR is an international problem with an increasing prevalence that has consequences for the whole of society. The UK Government has recognised AMR as a significant area of concern and have committed global action to address this as a priority. For information and resources on the UK's plans for AMR, see the Public Health England (PHE) collection: **Antimicrobial resistance** (www.gov.uk/ government/collections/antimicrobial-resistance-amr- information-and-resources).

Antimicrobial stewardship (AMS) refers to an organisational or healthcare system-wide approach to promoting and monitoring judicious use of antimicrobials to preserve their future effectiveness. Addressing AMR through improving stewardship is a national medicines optimisation priority, led by NHS England and supported by PHE.

AMR can be managed by a combination of interventions that address:

- A political commitment to prioritise AMR;
- Monitoring antimicrobial use and resistance in microbes;
- Development of new drugs, treatments, and diagnostics;
- Individuals' behaviour relating to infection prevention and control, antimicrobial use, and AMR;
- Healthcare professionals' prescribing decisions.

Guidance for organisations (commissioners and providers)

Commissioners (clinical commissioning groups and local authorities) and providers (e.g. hospitals, GPs, out-of-hours services, dentists, and social enterprises) of health or social care services should establish an AMS programme, taking into account the resources needed to support AMS across all care settings. An AMS programme should take into consideration monitoring and evaluating antimicrobial prescribing, regular feedback to individual prescribers, education and training for health and social care staff, and integrating audits into existing quality improvement programmes.

Commissioners should work collaboratively to provide consistent information and advice to the public and health professionals that reduces inappropriate antimicrobial demand and use, and limits the spread of infection. Local authority public health teams should ensure that information and resources (such as posters, leaflets and digital resources) are made available through multiple routes to provide a coordinated system of information. Information should include simple and practical steps such as scrupulous personal and safe food hygiene practices.

Organisations should involve lead health and social care staff in establishing processes for developing, reviewing, updating, and implementing local antimicrobial guidelines in line with national guidance and informed by local prescribing data and resistance patterns.

Organisations should also consider establishing processes for reviewing national horizon scanning to plan for the availability of new antimicrobials and to use an existing local decision-making group to consider the introduction of new antimicrobials locally.

Guidance for health and social care staff

Health and social care staff should assist with the implementation of local or national guidelines and recognise the significance of them for AMS.

Health professionals should be familiar with current AMS campaigns and programmes. For further information, see PHE and Health Education England's e-learning session **All Our Health: Antimicrobial Resistance** (portal.e-lfh.org.uk/ Component/Details/571263), PHE guidance **Health matters: antimicrobial resistance** (www.gov.uk/government/ publications/health-matters-antimicrobial-resistance), and the PHE campaigns **Antibiotic Guardian** (antibioticguardian.com/) and **Keep Antibiotics Working** (campaignresources.phe.gov. uk/resources/campaigns/58-keep-antibiotics-working).

Health professionals should be aware of resources and services that can help individuals minimise infections such as travel vaccination clinics, screening programmes, sexual health services, immunisation programmes, and other local referral pathways or schemes. The benefits of good hygiene, vaccination, and other preventative measures to reduce the risk of acquiring infections should be discussed with individuals, and individuals referred to further information or services if necessary.

Those involved in providing care should be educated about the standard principles of infection prevention and control. They should be trained in hand decontamination, the use of personal protective equipment, and the safe use and disposal of sharps. For further information, see NICE guideline: **Healthcare-associated infections** (see *Useful resources*).

Guidance on antimicrobial prescribing

National antimicrobial prescribing and stewardship competencies have been developed to improve the quality of antimicrobial treatment and stewardship. For further information, see Antimicrobial Resistance and Healthcare Associated Infections and PHE guidance: **Antimicrobial prescribing and stewardship competencies** (see *Useful resources*).

National toolkits to support the implementation of AMS best practice include the Royal College of General Practitioners' **TARGET antibiotics toolkit** (www.rcgp.org.uk/ TARGETantibiotics) for primary care, and PHE's **Start smart – then focus** (www.gov.uk/government/publications/ antimicrobial-stewardship-start-smart-then-focus) for secondary care, and **Dental antimicrobial stewardship: toolkit** (www.gov.uk/guidance/dental-antimicrobial-stewardship-toolkit) for dentists.

Clinical syndrome-specific guidance and advice to help slow the development of AMR have been developed by NICE, in collaboration with PHE, and are available at www.nice.org. uk/.

Considerations for antimicrobial prescribing When deciding whether or not to prescribe an antimicrobial, undertake a clinical assessment and consider the risk of AMR for individual patients and the population as a whole. An immediate antimicrobial prescription for a patient who is likely to have a self-limiting condition is not recommended.

Document in the patient's records (electronically wherever possible) the decisions related to antimicrobial use, including the plan as discussed with the patient, and their family and/or carers (if appropriate), and reason for prescribing/not prescribing an antimicrobial.

In hospital, microbiological samples should be taken before initiating an antimicrobial for patients with suspected infection. In primary care, consider taking microbiological samples when prescribing an antimicrobial for patients with recurrent or persistent infections. The choice of antimicrobial should be reviewed when microbiological results are available. For non-severe infections, consider taking microbiological samples before making a decision about prescribing an antimicrobial, providing it is safe to withhold treatment until the results are available.

Follow local or national guidelines on prescribing the shortest effective course and most appropriate dose and route of administration. Review intravenous antimicrobials within 48 hours (taking into account response to treatment and microbiological results) and consider stepping down to oral antimicrobials where possible. If prescribing outside of local or national guidelines, document in the patient's records the reasons for the decision.

Patients on antimicrobial treatment should be appropriately monitored to reduce side-effects and be assessed on the continued need for treatment. Repeat antimicrobial prescriptions are not recommended, unless needed for a particular clinical condition or indication. Avoid issuing a repeat prescription for longer than 6 months without review.

Advice for patients and their family and/or carers

Prescribers, primary care and community pharmacy teams should provide patients with resources educating them about not asking for antimicrobials as a preventive measure against becoming ill or as a stand-by measure, unless the patient has a specific condition or a specific risk that requires antimicrobial prophylaxis.

Prescribers should discuss with patients, and their family and/or carers (if appropriate) the likely nature of the condition, their views on antimicrobials, benefits and harms of antimicrobial prescribing, and why prescribing an antimicrobial may not always be the best option. Information should be provided about what to do if their symptoms worsen or if problems arise as a result of treatment. Written information should be provided if needed.

If antimicrobial treatment is not the most appropriate option, prescribers should advise patients, and their family and/or carers (if appropriate) about other options (as appropriate), such as self-care with over-the-counter preparations, back-up (delayed) prescribing, or other non-pharmacological interventions. Prescribers, primary care and community pharmacy teams should verbally emphasise and provide written advice about managing self-limiting infections.

If antimicrobials are prescribed or supplied, prescribers, primary care and community pharmacy teams should provide patients with verbal and written information on the correct use of antimicrobials. Advice should encourage people to:

- Take, or use antimicrobials only when recommended by a suitably qualified health professional;
- Obtain antimicrobials only from a health professional;
- Take, or use antimicrobials as instructed (right dose for the duration specified and via the right route);
- Return any unused antimicrobials to a pharmacy for safe disposal.

Useful resources

Antimicrobial prescribing and stewardship competencies. Antimicrobial Resistance and Healthcare Associated Infections (ARHAI) and Public Health England guideline. October 2013.

www.gov.uk/government/publications/antimicrobial-prescribing-and-stewardship-competencies

Antimicrobial resistance (AMR): applying All Our Health. Public Health England guideline. April 2015 (updated June 2019).

www.gov.uk/government/publications/antimicrobial-resistance-amr-applying-all-our-health

Antimicrobial stewardship: systems and processes for effective antimicrobial medicine use. National Institute for Health and Care Excellence. NICE guideline 15. August 2015.

www.nice.org.uk/guidance/NG15

Antimicrobial stewardship: changing risk-related behaviours in the general population. National Institute for Health and Care Excellence. NICE guideline 63. January 2017.

www.nice.org.uk/guidance/NG63

Healthcare-associated infections: prevention and control in primary and community care. National Institute for Health and Care Excellence. Clinical guideline 139. March 2012 (updated February 2017).

www.nice.org.uk/guidance/cg139

Prescribing in children

Overview

For detailed advice on medicines used for children, consult BNF for Children.

Children, and particularly neonates, differ from adults in their response to drugs. Special care is needed in the neonatal period (first 28 days of life) and doses should always be calculated with care. At this age, the risk of toxicity is increased by reduced drug clearance and differing target organ sensitivity.

Whenever possible, intramuscular injections should be **avoided** in children because they are painful.

Where possible, medicines for children should be prescribed within the terms of the marketing authorisation (product licence). However, many children may require medicines not specifically licensed for paediatric use.

Although medicines cannot be promoted outside the limits of the licence, the Human Medicines Regulations 2012 does not prohibit the use of unlicensed medicines. It is recognised that the informed use of unlicensed medicines or of licensed medicines for unlicensed applications ('off-label' use) is often necessary in paediatric practice.

Adverse drug reactions in children

Suspected adverse drug reactions in children and young adults under 18 years should be reported through the Yellow Card scheme at: yellowcard.mhra.gov.uk/. For detailed advice on adverse drug reactions in children, consult BNF for Children.

Prescription writing

Prescriptions should be written according to the guidelines in Prescription Writing. Inclusion of age is a legal requirement in the case of prescription-only medicines for children under 12 years of age, but it is preferable to state the age for **all** prescriptions for children.

It is particularly important to state the strengths of capsules or tablets. Although liquid preparations are particularly suitable for children, they may contain sugar which encourages dental decay. Sugar-free medicines are preferred for long-term treatment.

Many children are able to swallow tablets or capsules and may prefer a solid dose form; involving the child and parents in choosing the formulation is helpful.

When a prescription for a liquid oral preparation is written and the dose ordered is smaller than 5 mL an **oral syringe** will be supplied. Parents should be advised not to add any medicines to the infant's feed, since the drug may interact with the milk or other liquid in it; moreover the ingested dosage may be reduced if the child does not drink all the contents.

Parents must be warned to keep **all** medicines out of reach of children.

Rare paediatric conditions

Information on substances such as *biotin* and *sodium benzoate* used in rare metabolic conditions is included in BNF for Children; further information can be obtained from:

Alder Hey Children's Hospital
Drug Information Centre
Liverpool
L12 2AP
(0151) 252 5837

Great Ormond Street Hospital for Children
Pharmacy
Great Ormond St
London
WC1N 3JH
(020) 7405 9200

Dosage in children

Children's doses in the BNF are stated in the individual drug entries.

Doses are generally based on body-weight (in kilograms) or specific age ranges. In the BNF and BNF for Children, the term neonate is used to describe a newborn infant aged 0–28 days. The terms child or children are used generically to describe the entire range from infant to adolescent (1 month–17 years). An age range is specified when the dose information applies to a narrower age range than a child from 1 month–17 years.

Dose calculation

Many children's doses are standardised by **weight** (and therefore require multiplying by the body-weight in kilograms to determine the child's dose); occasionally, the doses have been standardised by **body surface area** (in m^2). These methods should be used rather than attempting to calculate a child's dose on the basis of doses used in adults.

For most drugs the adult maximum dose should not be exceeded. For example if the dose is stated as 8 mg/kg (max. 300 mg), a child weighing 10 kg should receive 80 mg but a child weighing 40 kg should receive 300 mg (rather than 320 mg).

Young children may require a higher dose per kilogram than adults because of their higher metabolic rates. Other problems need to be considered. For example, calculation by body-weight in the overweight child may result in much higher doses being administered than necessary; in such cases, dose should be calculated from an ideal weight, related to height and age.

Body surface area (BSA) estimates are sometimes preferable to body-weight for calculation of paediatric doses since many physiological phenomena correlate better with body surface area. Body surface area can be estimated from weight. For more information, refer to BNF for Children.

Where the dose for children is not stated, prescribers should consult BNF for Children or seek advice from a medicines information centre.

Dose frequency

Antibacterials are generally given at regular intervals throughout the day. Some flexibility should be allowed in children to avoid waking them during the night. For example, the night-time dose may be given at the child's bedtime.

Where new or potentially toxic drugs are used, the manufacturers' recommended doses should be carefully followed.

Prescribing in hepatic impairment

Overview

Liver disease may alter the response to drugs in several ways as indicated below, and drug prescribing should be kept to a minimum in all patients with severe liver disease. The main problems occur in patients with jaundice, ascites, or evidence of encephalopathy.

Impaired drug metabolism

Metabolism by the liver is the main route of elimination for many drugs, but hepatic reserve is large and liver disease has to be severe before important changes in drug metabolism occur. Routine liver-function tests are a poor guide to the capacity of the liver to metabolise drugs, and in the individual patient it is not possible to predict the extent to which the metabolism of a particular drug may be impaired.

A few drugs, e.g. rifampicin p. 674 and fusidic acid p. 663, are excreted in the bile unchanged and can accumulate in patients with intrahepatic or extrahepatic obstructive jaundice.

Hypoproteinaemia

The hypoalbuminaemia in severe liver disease is associated with reduced protein binding and increased toxicity of some highly protein-bound drugs such as phenytoin p. 372 and prednisolone p. 791.

Reduced clotting

Reduced hepatic synthesis of blood-clotting factors, indicated by a prolonged prothrombin time, increases the sensitivity to oral anticoagulants such as warfarin sodium p. 165 and phenindione p. 164.

Hepatic encephalopathy

In severe liver disease many drugs can further impair cerebral function and may precipitate hepatic encephalopathy. These include all sedative drugs, opioid analgesics, those diuretics that produce hypokalaemia, and drugs that cause constipation.

Fluid overload

Oedema and ascites in chronic liver disease can be exacerbated by drugs that give rise to fluid retention e.g. NSAIDs and corticosteroids.

Hepatotoxic drugs

Hepatotoxicity is either dose-related or unpredictable (idiosyncratic). Drugs that cause dose-related toxicity may do so at lower doses in the presence of hepatic impairment than in individuals with normal liver function, and some drugs that produce reactions of the idiosyncratic kind do so more frequently in patients with liver disease. These drugs should be avoided or used very carefully in patients with liver disease.

Where care is needed when prescribing in hepatic impairment, this is indicated under the relevant drug in the BNF.

Prescribing in renal impairment

Issues encountered in renal impairment

The use of drugs in patients with reduced renal function can give rise to problems for several reasons:

- reduced renal excretion of a drug or its metabolites may cause toxicity;
- sensitivity to some drugs is increased even if elimination is unimpaired;
- many side-effects are tolerated poorly by patients with renal impairment;
- some drugs are not effective when renal function is reduced.

Many of these problems can be avoided by reducing the dose or by using alternative drugs.

If even mild renal impairment is considered likely on clinical grounds, renal function should be checked before prescribing any drug which requires dose modification.

General guidance

Drugs eliminated via the kidneys can accumulate during acute kidney injury (AKI) or chronic kidney disease (CKD) and this can lead to further renal impairment or adverse effects. EvGr A review of these drugs is therefore required; any drug which can cause or exacerbate renal impairment should be avoided in AKI, and the appropriateness reviewed in CKD. E

Where care is needed when prescribing in renal impairment, this is indicated under the relevant drug monograph in the BNF. Dose recommendations are based on the severity of renal impairment.

When both efficacy and toxicity are closely related to plasma-drug concentration, recommended regimens should be regarded only as a guide to initial treatment; subsequent doses must be adjusted according to clinical response and plasma-drug concentration.

The total daily maintenance dose of a drug can be reduced either by reducing the size of the individual doses or by increasing the interval between doses.

For some drugs, although the size of the maintenance dose is reduced it is important to give a loading dose if an immediate effect is required. This is because it takes about five times the half-life of the drug to achieve steady-state plasma concentration. Because the plasma half-life of drugs excreted by the kidney is prolonged in renal impairment, it can take many doses at the reduced dosage to achieve a therapeutic plasma concentration.

For information on prescribing in renal impairment in children, see BNF for Children.

Important: dosage adjustment advice in the BNF Clinical laboratories routinely report renal function in adults based on *estimated glomerular filtration rate* (eGFR) normalised to a body surface area of 1.73 m^2—this is derived from either the Chronic Kidney Disease Epidemiology Collaboration (CKD-EPI) formula or the Modification of Diet in Renal disease (MDRD) formula.

However, in product literature, the effects of renal impairment on drug elimination is usually stated in terms of *creatinine clearance* (CrCl) as a surrogate for GFR.

EvGr Although eGFR and CrCl are not interchangeable, for most drugs and for most adult patients of average build and height, eGFR (rather than CrCl) can be used to determine dosage adjustments. Exceptions to the use of eGFR include toxic drugs, in elderly patients and in patients at extremes of muscle mass (see *Estimating renal function in patients at extremes of muscle mass* and *Estimating renal function in elderly patients*, below) where calculation of CrCl is recommended. E

MHRA/CHM advice: Prescribing medicines in renal impairment: using the appropriate estimate of renal function to avoid the risk of adverse drug reactions (October 2019) For cases where CrCl, calculated using the Cockcroft and Gault formula, should be used to determine renal dose adjustments, see *Important: dosage adjustment advice in the BNF*, above. In addition, the MHRA advises that CrCl should be used as an estimate of renal function for direct-acting oral anticoagulants (DOACs), and drugs with a narrow therapeutic index that are mainly renally excreted.

If dose adjustment based on CrCl is important and no advice is provided in the relevant BNF drug monograph, prescribers should consult product literature.

Renal function and drug dosing should be reassessed in situations where eGFR and/or CrCl change rapidly, such as in patients with AKI.

Acute kidney injury EvGr Caution is advised when using eGFR or CrCl to estimate renal function during AKI, as serum creatinine levels lag behind the development of the injury and progress of recovery. As creatinine rises, estimates of GFR will overestimate renal function and as creatinine falls and kidney function improves, estimates of GFR will underestimate renal function. This should be considered when using estimates of renal function to inform dose adjustments. E

During intercurrent illness the risk of AKI is increased in patients with an eGFR of less than 60 mL/min/1.73 m^2. EvGr Renally excreted drugs or those that can cause renal impairment may require dose reduction or temporary discontinuation. E

For information and advice on the prevention, detection, and management of acute kidney injury, see NICE clinical guideline: **Acute Kidney Injury** (www.nice.org.uk/guidance/ng148).

Renal replacement therapy and transplantation For prescribing in patients who have received a renal transplant or who are on renal replacement therapy (peritoneal dialysis or haemodialysis), consult specialist literature.

Estimating renal function

Direct measure of Glomerular filtration rate (GFR) using plasma or urinary clearance is considered the best overall index of renal function. However, this is difficult to do in practice.

As an alternative, the *estimated* Glomerular filtration rate (eGFR) based on serum creatinine is used to assess renal function. Creatinine clearance (CrCl) is also used as an estimate of GFR.

Various equations for estimating glomerular filtration rate exist, however there is no compelling evidence to support the superiority of any given method for drug dosing in *all* patient populations or clinical situations. There is also insufficient evidence to provide *definitive* guidance about dosage adjustment of all drugs in patients with reduced renal function. Therefore, an understanding of drug pharmacokinetics is necessary in order to make appropriate dosing decisions.

Using serum creatinine to derive eGFR has a number of limitations; serum creatinine levels are dependent on muscle mass and diet, therefore estimates should be interpreted with caution in certain individuals (such as the elderly, body builders, amputees, in muscle-wasting disorders and vegans)—estimates will be higher or lower than the true value. Creatinine-derived measurements are also **not** accurate in periods of rapidly changing renal function or in patients with AKI.

Estimated glomerular filtration rate Chronic Kidney Disease Epidemiology Collaboration (CKD-EPI) formula The CKD-EPI formula is the recommended method for estimating GFR and calculating drug doses in **most** patients with renal impairment.

CKD-EPI is adjusted for body surface area (BSA) and utilises serum creatinine, age, and sex as variables. Clinical laboratories should use the CKD-EPI formula to routinely report eGFR.

CKD-EPI equation

$$\text{eGFR (ml/min/1.73 m}^2) = 141 \times \min(S_{Cr}/K, 1)^{\alpha} \times \max(S_{Cr}/K, 1)^{-1.209} \times 0.993^{Age}[\times 1.018 \text{ if female}]$$

Where:

- S_{Cr} = serum creatinine in mg/dL;
- K = 0.7 for females and 0.9 for males;
- α = -0.329 for females and -0.411 for males;
- $\min(S_{Cr}/K, 1)$ indicates the minimum of S_{Cr}/K or 1;
- $\max(S_{Cr}/K, 1)$ indicates the maximum of S_{Cr}/K or 1.

Modification of Diet in Renal Disease (MDRD) The MDRD formula, like CKD-EPI, is expressed in terms of body surface area. It is less accurate than the CKD-EPI formula when eGFR is greater than 60 mL/min/1.73 m². It also overestimates GFR in elderly patients.

Estimated creatinine clearance Cockcroft and Gault The Cockcroft and Gault formula is the preferred method for estimating renal function or calculating drug doses in patients with renal impairment who are elderly or at extremes of muscle mass (see below); it provides an estimate of CrCl (which is not equivalent to eGFR, see *Important: dosage adjustment advice in the BNF above*).

$$\text{Estimated Creatinine Clearance in mL/minute} = \frac{(140 - \text{Age}) \times \text{Weight} \times \text{Constant}}{\text{Serum creatinine}}$$

- Age in years
- Weight in kilograms (use ideal body weight where fat is likely to be the major contributor to body mass)
- Serum creatinine in micromol/litre
- Constant = 1.23 for men; 1.04 for women

Estimating renal function in patients at extremes of muscle mass In patients at both extremes of muscle mass, eGFR should be interpreted with caution. Reduced muscle mass will lead to overestimation of GFR and increased muscle mass will lead to underestimation of the GFR.

Creatinine clearance or *absolute glomerular filtration rate* should be used to adjust drug doses in patients with a BMI less than 18 kg/m² or greater than 40 kg/m².

Ideal body weight should be used to calculate the CrCl. Where the patient's actual body weight is less than their ideal body weight, actual body weight should be used instead.

The absolute glomerular filtration rate is determined by removing the normalisation for BSA from the eGFR using the following formula:

GFR (Absolute) = eGFR × (individual's body surface area / 1.73)

The ideal body weight is calculated as follows:

Ideal body weight (kilograms) = Constant + 0.91 (Height - 152.4)

Where:

- Constant = 50 for men; 45.5 for women
- Height in centimetres

Estimating renal function in elderly patients EvGr The Cockcroft and Gault formula is the preferred method for estimating renal function in elderly patients aged 75 years and over.

The use of CKD-EPI may be appropriate in patients over 75 years, however muscle mass should be taken into consideration (see *Estimating renal function in patients at extremes of muscle mass*, above). E Using CKD-EPI to calculate eGFR has the potential to overestimate renal function progressively as age increases, which can increase the risk of adverse effects due to higher than recommended doses being prescribed.

Chronic kidney disease

For guidance on the management of patients with, or who are at risk of, chronic kidney disease, see NICE guideline: **Chronic kidney disease: assessment and management** (available at: www.nice.org.uk/guidance/ng203).

Classification of chronic kidney disease using GFR and ACR categories Chronic kidney disease is classified using a combination of GFR and albumin:creatinine ratio (ACR). A decreased GFR and an increased ACR is associated with an increased risk of adverse outcomes.

For example, a person with an eGFR of 25 ml/min/1.73 m² and an ACR of 15 mg/mmol has a CKD classification of G4A2.

Classification of chronic kidney disease using GFR and ACR categories

<table>
<tr><td rowspan="2" colspan="2">GFR and ACR categories and risk of adverse outcomes</td><td colspan="3">ACR categories (mg/mmol), description and range</td></tr>
<tr><td><3 Normal to mild increase</td><td>3–30 Moderate increase</td><td>>30 Severe increase</td></tr>
<tr><td></td><td></td><td>A1</td><td>A2</td><td>A3</td></tr>
<tr><td>≥90 Normal or high</td><td>G1</td><td rowspan="2">No CKD in the absence of markers of kidney damage</td><td></td><td></td></tr>
<tr><td>60–89 Mild reduction relative to normal range for a young adult</td><td>G2</td><td></td><td></td></tr>
<tr><td>45–59 Mild-moderate reduction</td><td>G3a</td><td></td><td></td><td></td></tr>
<tr><td>30–44 Moderate-severe reduction</td><td>G3b</td><td></td><td></td><td></td></tr>
<tr><td>15–29 Severe reduction</td><td>G4</td><td></td><td></td><td></td></tr>
<tr><td><15 Kidney failure</td><td>G5</td><td></td><td></td><td></td></tr>
</table>

GFR categories (ml/min/1.73m²), description and range

Increasing risk

Increasing risk

Abbreviations: ACR, albumin:creatinine ratio; CKD, chronic kidney disease; GFR, glomerular filtration rate

Adapted with the kind permission of the Kidney Disease: Improving Global Outcomes (KDIGO) CKD Work Group, 2013.

Prescribing in pregnancy

Overview

Drugs can have harmful effects on the embryo or fetus at any time during pregnancy. It is important to bear this in mind when prescribing for a woman of *childbearing age* or for men *trying* to *father* a child.

During the *first trimester* drugs can produce congenital malformations (teratogenesis), and the period of greatest risk is from the third to the eleventh week of pregnancy.

During the *second* and *third trimesters* drugs can affect the growth or functional development of the fetus, or they can have toxic effects on fetal tissues.

Drugs given shortly before term or during labour can have adverse effects on labour or on the neonate after delivery.

Not all the damaging effects of intra-uterine exposure to drugs are obvious at birth, some may only manifest later in life. Such late-onset effects include malignancy, e.g. adenocarcinoma of the vagina after puberty in females exposed to diethylstilbestrol in the womb, and adverse effects on intellectual, social, and functional development.

The BNF and BNF for Children identify drugs which:

- may have harmful effects in pregnancy and indicate the trimester of risk
- are not known to be harmful in pregnancy

The information is based on human data, but information from *animal* studies has been included for some drugs when its omission might be misleading. Maternal drug doses may require adjustment during pregnancy due to changes in maternal physiology but this is beyond the scope of the BNF and BNF for Children.

Where care is needed when prescribing in pregnancy, this is indicated under the relevant drug in the BNF and BNF for Children.

Important

Drugs should be prescribed in pregnancy only if the expected benefit to the mother is thought to be greater than the risk to the fetus, and all drugs should be avoided if possible during the first trimester. Drugs which have been extensively used in pregnancy and appear to be usually safe should be prescribed in preference to new or untried drugs; and the smallest effective dose should be used. Few drugs have been shown conclusively to be teratogenic in humans, but no drug is safe beyond all doubt in early pregnancy. Screening procedures are available when there is a known risk of certain defects.

Absence of information does not imply safety. It should be noted that the BNF and BNF for Children provide independent advice and may not always agree with the product literature.

Information on drugs and pregnancy is also available from the UK Teratology Information Service at: www.uktis.org.

MHRA/CHM advice: Medicines in pregnancy and breastfeeding: new initiative for consistent guidance; report on optimising data for medicines used during pregnancy (February 2021)

The Safer Medicines in Pregnancy and Breastfeeding Consortium, formed of the MHRA and partner organisations, aims to improve the health information available to women who are thinking about becoming pregnant, are pregnant, or are breast-feeding, and ensure that they can make informed decisions about their healthcare, particularly about medicines. To support this, healthcare professionals are requested to report inconsistencies in UK advice on the use of individual or classes of medicines during pregnancy or breast-feeding via the consortium at: www.gov.uk/government/publications/safer-medicines-in-pregnancy-and-breastfeeding-consortium.

The Report of the CHM Expert Working Group on Optimising Data on Medicines used During Pregnancy provides recommendations on ways in which data on medicines used during pregnancy and breast-feeding can be better collected and made available for analysis. This will enable more robust evidence to be generated through research and will help to develop clear and consistent advice about medicines used during pregnancy and breast-feeding. The report is available at: www.gov.uk/government/publications/report-of-the-commission-on-human-medicines-expert-working-group-on-optimising-data-on-medicines-used-during-pregnancy.

Prescribing in breast-feeding

Overview

Breast-feeding is beneficial; the immunological and nutritional value of breast milk to the infant is greater than that of formula feeds.

Although there is concern that drugs taken by the mother might affect the infant, there is very little information on this. In the absence of evidence of an effect, the potential for harm to the infant can be inferred from:

- the amount of drug or active metabolite of the drug delivered to the infant (dependent on the pharmacokinetic characteristics of the drug in the mother);
- the efficiency of absorption, distribution, and elimination of the drug by the infant (infant pharmacokinetics);
- the nature of the effect of the drug on the infant (pharmacodynamic properties of the drug in the infant).

The amount of drug transferred in breast milk is rarely sufficient to produce a discernible effect on the infant. This applies particularly to drugs that are poorly absorbed and need to be given parenterally. However, there is a theoretical possibility that a small amount of drug present in breast milk can induce a hypersensitivity reaction.

A clinical effect can occur in the infant if a pharmacologically significant quantity of the drug is present in milk. For some drugs (e.g. fluvastatin p. 234), the ratio between the concentration in milk and that in maternal plasma may be high enough to expose the infant to adverse effects. Some infants, such as those born prematurely or who have jaundice, are at a slightly higher risk of toxicity.

Some drugs inhibit the infant's sucking reflex (e.g. phenobarbital p. 388) while others can affect lactation (e.g. bromocriptine p. 482).

The BNF identifies drugs:

- that should be used with caution or are contra-indicated in breast-feeding;
- that can be given to the mother during breast-feeding because they are present in milk in amounts which are too small to be harmful to the infant;
- that might be present in milk in significant amount but are not known to be harmful.

Where care is needed when prescribing in breast-feeding, this is indicated under the relevant drug in the BNF.

Important

For many drugs insufficient evidence is available to provide guidance and it is advisable to administer only essential drugs to a mother during breast-feeding. Because of the inadequacy of information on drugs in breast-feeding, absence of information does not imply safety.

MHRA/CHM advice: Medicines in pregnancy and breastfeeding: new initiative for consistent guidance; report on optimising data for medicines used during pregnancy (February 2021)

The Safer Medicines in Pregnancy and Breastfeeding Consortium, formed of the MHRA and partner organisations, aims to improve the health information available to women who are thinking about becoming pregnant, are pregnant, or are breast-feeding, and ensure that they can make informed decisions about their healthcare, particularly about medicines. To support this, healthcare professionals are requested to report inconsistencies in UK advice on the use of individual or classes of medicines during pregnancy or breast-feeding via the consortium at: www.gov.uk/government/publications/safer-medicines-in-pregnancy-and-breastfeeding-consortium.

The Report of the CHM Expert Working Group on Optimising Data on Medicines used During Pregnancy provides recommendations on ways in which data on medicines used during pregnancy and breast-feeding can be better collected and made available for analysis. This will enable more robust evidence to be generated through research and will help to develop clear and consistent advice about medicines used during pregnancy and breast-feeding. The report is available at: www.gov.uk/government/publications/report-of-the-commission-on-human-medicines-expert-working-group-on-optimising-data-on-medicines-used-during-pregnancy.

Prescribing in palliative care

Overview

Palliative care is the active holistic care of an individual with a life-limiting or life-threatening condition provided by a multidisciplinary team. Palliative care aims to prevent and relieve suffering by managing pain and other distressing symptoms, in addition to identifying and addressing other physical, psychological, social, and spiritual needs. It focuses on enhancing quality of life, supporting individuals to live as actively as possible, and addressing both their needs and those of their families.

Palliative care may be provided for months or years. The terms 'end-of-life-care' usually refers to the care of individuals in their last 12 months of life, and 'terminal care' to the care of those in their last few weeks or days of life.

The place of care can vary based on the patient's needs and preference, and may be the patient's home, nursing or care home, hospice, or hospital. For patients who wish to remain at home with their families, support can be provided by community nurses, social care staff, volunteers and hospices, together with the patient's general practitioner and palliative care team.

Bereavement care is a core element of palliative care. It encompasses both care and support of the patient and their families throughout their illness, and after the patient's death. Bereavement care is facilitated by good communication and the rapport built up with the family—various bereavement organisations and health professionals can offer support to individuals following the loss of a loved one.

For information on end-of-life care and support for carers, see NICE guidelines: **Care of dying adults in the last days of life; End of life care for adults;** and **Supporting adult carers** (see *Useful resources*).

Non-drug treatment

The use of non-drug treatment options for symptom management are an important part of palliative care. For example, pain or breathlessness can be managed by using positioning, relaxation, controlled breathing, and anxiety management techniques. Guidance on non-drug treatments for specific symptoms can be found in the Palliative Care Formulary, and the Scottish Palliative Care Guidelines (see *Useful resources*).

Drug treatment

Medicines used in the palliative care setting are often unlicensed or used off-label (outside of the recommendations of their marketing authorisation, such as an unapproved route, indication, or dose).

Close collaboration between health professionals in different care settings is essential, especially for controlled drugs and special-order preparations, to ensure continuity of supply when transferring between care locations. For information on obtaining special-order preparations, see Special-order manufacturers p. 1967.

For prescription requirements for controlled drugs, see Controlled drugs and drug dependence p. 7. Information on available strengths, formulations, and pack sizes can be found under medicinal forms in drug monographs. Systems should be in place to ensure the safe use and management of controlled drugs in an individual's home.

For parenteral drug administration, appropriate diluents and flushes may also need to be prescribed.

Particular care should be taken when prescribing for elderly or frail patients, and for patients who are malnourished, cachectic and/or oedematous, as for these patients, renal function tests may underestimate the actual degree of renal impairment. For further information on prescribing considerations in renal and/or hepatic impairment, or in the elderly, see Prescribing in renal impairment p. 21, Prescribing in hepatic impairment p. 20, and Prescribing in the elderly p. 31.

Deprescribing in palliative care The use of multiple medicines concurrently is common in palliative care, as patients may already be taking medicines for chronic conditions in addition to an increasing number of treatments for symptom management, therefore deprescribing of medicines should be considered where appropriate. Deprescribing is a collaborative process of the safe withdrawal of medicines that are no longer appropriate, beneficial or wanted (patient preference), to improve quality of life and reduce the burden of unnecessary treatments, particularly in the final months of life. Medication reviews within all specialties should be undertaken regularly to meet the changing needs of the patient, and to reduce potential harm from previously well tolerated medicines due to factors such as the patient's age, comorbidities, and the number of and types of medication they are taking. After discussion and in agreement with the patient and those important to the patient, any prescribed medicines that are not providing symptomatic benefit, are causing harm, or are deemed no longer necessary should be stopped. This may include long-term prophylaxis medication such as statins and antihypertensives.

Anticipatory prescribing and last days of life EvGr Using an individualised approach, assess which medicines may be needed to manage symptoms likely to occur in the patient's last days of life (such as morphine for pain and breathlessness; midazolam for agitation; levomepromazine or haloperidol for nausea and vomiting and delirium; or hyoscine butylbromide for respiratory secretions). D Ensure that the prescribing of anticipatory drugs (with specification of indication, route, dose, frequency, and maximum dosage) is done as early as possible and reviewed as the patient's needs change. Individuals may also benefit from a dose range to allow flexibility for administration by community teams, especially out of hours.

The hydration status of the patient should also be assessed in their last days of life, and the need for clinically-assisted hydration reviewed, taking into consideration the patient's preference and wishes.

Routes of administration

Where possible, the oral route is the preferred method of drug administration. For patients with swallowing difficulties, reducing the number of drugs and frequency of administration should be considered where possible. A speech and language therapist (SALT) assessment can help to determine the feasibility of using alternative oral formulations, e.g. dispersible or soluble tablets, or oral liquids, and a pharmacist can advise on the advantages and disadvantages of the potential options. However, the oral administration of drugs may not always be possible, such as when there is persistent nausea and vomiting, dysphagia, bowel obstruction, poor absorption of oral drugs, or patient preference, therefore alternative routes of administration (such as buccal or sublingual, intranasal, rectal, transdermal, subcutaneous, and enteral feeding tube) may be necessary. If drugs are required to be given via an enteral feeding tube, advice should be obtained from a pharmacist to ensure suitable formulations are chosen to minimise the risks associated with administration.

Parenteral administration For patients who are unable to take or tolerate oral medicines, subcutaneous or intravenous administration should be considered, although the subcutaneous route is the preferred choice. The use of continuous subcutaneous infusions (CSCIs) is common within palliative care in the UK, particularly for patients where swallowing medication has become increasingly difficult or impossible. CSCIs reduce the need for bolus injections, provide comfort from stable drug plasma concentrations, and allow control of multiple symptoms with a combination of drugs. CSCIs are usually administered via a portable continuous infusion device (such as a syringe driver or pump), thus supporting patient independence and mobility. The use of intramuscular injections is not recommended.

Continuous subcutaneous infusions CSCIs over 24 hours are generally considered satisfactory in terms of sterility, practicality, and stability (if there is adequate stability data for 24 hours). The dilution of CSCIs minimises the risk of injection-site reactions and drug incompatibility, and reduces the impact of priming the infusion line. 20 mL syringes are generally recommended as the minimum size for use with a syringe driver or pump.

Water for injection is usually the standard diluent used for CSCIs as there is more compatibility data available. Large volumes of water for injection are hypotonic, which can cause infusion site pain or skin reactions, although this is not usually a problem with slow infusion rates. Sodium chloride 0.9% is isotonic and is preferred for diluting irritant drugs or if inflammatory skin reactions occur at the injection site, but incompatibility can be a problem with some drugs. Some parenteral drug formulations (e.g. chlorpromazine, diazepam) are too irritant to be given by CSCI and alternatives should be used (for further guidance, see the Palliative Care Formulary, or seek specialist advice if unsure).

It is common practice for two or three different drugs to be mixed in a CSCI (unlicensed product), although the greater the number of drugs mixed, the greater the potential for compatibility issues. Physical and/or chemical changes can occur when mixing drugs that may lead to reduced efficacy. It is therefore essential to consider drug compatibility when mixing drugs in a CSCI.

For specialist resources with information on drug compatibility, see *Appendix 3: Compatibility charts* in the Palliative Care Formulary (see *Useful resources*), the Palliative Care Formulary Syringe Driver Database on Drug Compatibility Checker, available at: www.medicinescomplete. com/#/compatibility, and the Scottish Palliative Care Guidelines (see *Useful resources*).

Management of pain

Non-opioid analgesics (such as paracetamol and NSAIDs), opioids (such as codeine or morphine), and adjuvant analgesics (such as antidepressants and antiepileptics) are used in conjunction with non-drug measures for pain relief in palliative care. Depending on the type of pain and response to treatment, drugs from the different classes may be used alone or in combination.

EvGr For cancer pain, consider a stepwise approach using the World Health Organization analgesic ladder. Paracetamol p. 507 or a NSAID can be given to manage mild pain. If non-opioid analgesics alone are not sufficient, then an opioid analgesic, alone or in combination with a non-opioid analgesic, can be given to control the pain. A EvGr For cancer pain however, there is no pharmacological rationale for using a weak opioid as the benefits from a low dose of a strong opioid are greater and more rapidly achieved. D

EvGr Adjuvant analgesics should be considered at any stage for individuals with specific pain types, such as muscle spasm or neuropathic pain. For further guidance on the use of adjuvant analgesics, see the relevant sections below. A

EvGr For chronic non-cancer pain, alternatives to opioids are often more appropriate. Consider seeking specialist advice before using opioids for chronic non-cancer pain, even if the therapeutic aim is palliation. E

Opioid analgesics EvGr For most patients, morphine p. 525 is the strong opioid of choice. A EvGr Patients should be commenced on a regular oral modified-release morphine preparation, with rescue doses of 'as required' oral immediate-release morphine for breakthrough pain. E EvGr The initial oral dose is based on previous medication use, pain severity, and other factors (such as the presence of renal or hepatic impairment, increasing age, or frailty). D EvGr The standard 'rescue dose' of morphine for breakthrough pain is usually one-tenth to one-sixth of the regular 24-hour dose, repeated every 2–4 hours as required (up to hourly may be needed). A EvGr If in doubt, seek specialist advice before prescribing strong opioids for patients with moderate-to-severe renal or hepatic impairment. E

EvGr Regular pain management reviews should be undertaken, particularly in the titration phase, and the patient's dose adjusted until a good balance exists between acceptable pain control and side-effects. Specialist advice should be sought if pain control is proving difficult to achieve. A EvGr The use of rescue doses twice daily or more should prompt a pain management review. When adjusting the regular dose of morphine take into account the number of rescue doses required and the patient's response (with careful assessment of the pain). Dose increments of morphine should not exceed one-third to one-half of the total daily dose every 24 hours. D

Patients receiving opioids should be monitored closely for efficacy and side-effects, particularly constipation, nausea and vomiting, and respiratory depression (rare). EvGr A regular laxative should be prescribed and, where appropriate, anti-emetics prescribed regularly or 'as required' (see *Constipation* and *Nausea and vomiting*). A

Alternatives to morphine The pharmacokinetics of the various opioids differ, with marked differences in bioavailability, metabolism, and response among patients. A suitable opioid should be selected for each patient and the dose individually titrated as effective and safe titration has a major impact on patient comfort.

EvGr In patients in whom morphine is not tolerated or is ineffective despite dose titration and appropriate use of adjuvant analgesics, seek specialist advice on the use of oxycodone, buprenorphine, fentanyl, or hydromorphone. A

If the oral route is unsuitable, alternatives include subcutaneous or transdermal opioids; prescribers should be sufficiently experienced *and* able to closely monitor the patient, otherwise specialist advice should be sought.

Transdermal fentanyl p. 520 and buprenorphine p. 511 are not suitable for the management of acute pain, or for use in patients whose pain requirements are changing rapidly— these take a long time for plasma concentrations to reach steady state, which prevents rapid titration of the dose. Transdermal fentanyl is also not generally recommended for use in opioid-naïve patients or as a first-line strong opioid; use in opioid-naive patients with non-cancer pain is contra-indicated. For information on the approximate dose equivalence of oral morphine to fentanyl and buprenorphine patches, see the dose equivalence tables below.

EvGr Transmucosal formulations of fentanyl p. 520 administered by the nasal, buccal, or sublingual route are only used for breakthrough pain in patients with chronic cancer pain who are on regular strong opioids. They should only be initiated by palliative care specialists. These products are not interchangeable on a microgram per microgram basis; dose titration when switching to a new formulation is necessary. ⓓ

Opioid dose conversion Prior to switching treatment, consider whether other options may be more appropriate (such as the use of adjuvant analgesics or modifying the management of undesirable effects). Conversion ratios between opioids vary in the literature and product information, and are only ever an approximate guide; careful monitoring when switching from one opioid to another is therefore necessary to avoid under or over-dosing. Explicit guidance on switching between opioids is difficult as each patient's reasons for switching and their circumstances differ. When reviewing or changing opioid prescriptions ensure that the total dose of opioid taken in a 24-hour period has been considered. When switching between different opioids, the calculated equivalent dose should be reduced in most cases to prevent patients from receiving too much opioid during this period. Guidance from the Royal College of Anaesthetists (UK) suggests that the starting point for dose reduction from the calculated equivalent dose is around 25–50%. Patient factors such as pain severity, age, frailty, tolerability, and current opioid dose are then taken into account to modify the reduction as appropriate. EvGr Specialist advice should be sought before switching opioids in patients receiving high doses of oral morphine ($\geq$ 120 mg/24 hours) or equivalent doses of other opioids; significantly lower-than-predicted doses and close monitoring will be required. Rescue doses can make up for any deficit while re-titrating to a suitable dose of the new opioid. Ⓔ The half-life and time to onset of action of each drug should also be considered when stopping one opioid and starting a new one so that the patient does not experience breakthrough pain or receive too much opioid during the conversion period.

Equivalent doses of opioid analgesics to oral morphine

Equivalent doses of opioid analgesics to 10 mg of oral morphine sulfate. The equivalent doses in the table are an *approximate* guide and should be adjusted according to individual patient factors (see *Opioid dose conversion* guidance above) and response. These figures are based on the Palliative Care Formulary 8th edition.

Analgesic/Route	Equivalent dose to 10 mg of oral morphine sulfate
This table is intended to be used as an approximate guide for equivalence to PO morphine only. It is *not* meant to be used to derive conversion ratios between other drugs (or their routes) within the table.	
Codeine: PO	100 mg
Diamorphine: IV, SC	3.3 mg
Dihydrocodeine: PO	100 mg
Hydromorphone: PO	2 mg
Morphine: IV, SC	5 mg
Oxycodone: PO	6.6 mg
Oxycodone: IV, SC	5 mg
Tramadol: PO	100 mg
PO = by mouth; IV = intravenous; SC = subcutaneous.	

Note: 10 mg **PO** oxycodone is approximately equivalent to 6.6 mg **IV/SC oxycodone**. This is based on the Palliative Care Formulary 8th edition ratio of 1.5:1 for PO oxycodone: IV/SC oxycodone.

Conversion from oral administration to continuous subcutaneous infusion EvGr Many palliative care units use morphine p. 525 as the parenteral opioid of choice unless there is a more appropriate option. Diamorphine hydrochloride p. 518 is recommended as an alternative if high opioid doses are being given, as it has a higher solubility and larger doses can be diluted in a smaller volume; but also see the cautions above regarding converting higher-doses of opioids.

Rescue doses given as a subcutaneous bolus equivalent to one-tenth to one-sixth of the total 24-hour subcutaneous infusion dose should be prescribed for breakthrough pain. ⓓ

Equivalent doses of morphine sulfate, diamorphine hydrochloride, and oxycodone hydrochloride given over 24 hours. These equivalences are an *approximate* guide and should be adjusted according to individual patient factors (see *Opioid dose conversion* guidance above) and response. These figures are based on the Palliative Care Formulary 8th edition.

Oral morphine sulfate over 24 hours	Subcutaneous infusion of morphine sulfate over 24 hours	Subcutaneous infusion of diamorphine hydrochloride over 24 hours	Subcutaneous infusion of oxycodone hydrochloride over 24 hours
30 mg	15 mg	10 mg	15 mg
60 mg	30 mg	20 mg	30 mg
90 mg	45 mg	30 mg	45 mg
120 mg	60 mg	40 mg	60 mg
Always seek specialist advice before titrating opioids above this level; pain is often opioid-poorly responsive and adjuvant analgesics may be required.			
180 mg	90 mg	60 mg	90 mg
240 mg	120 mg	80 mg	120 mg
360 mg	180 mg	120 mg	180 mg

Note: A 1:1 dose equivalence ratio between parenteral morphine and parenteral oxycodone is also recommended by the manufacturers of oxycodone.

Conversion from oral to transdermal administration For guidance on the use of transdermal buprenorphine and fentanyl, see *Alternatives to morphine* above.

EvGr Immediate-release morphine can be given for breakthrough pain at one-tenth to one-sixth of the regular 24-hour equivalent morphine dose, repeated every 2–4 hours as required (up to hourly may be needed). ⓓ

The following 24-hour oral doses of morphine are considered to be approximately equivalent to the buprenorphine and fentanyl transdermal patches shown.

Prescribing in palliative care

Buprenorphine transdermal patches are *approximately* equivalent to the following 24-hour doses of oral morphine; patient factors (see *Opioid dose conversion* guidance above) and response should be taken into account and doses adjusted accordingly. These figures are based on the Palliative Care Formulary 8th edition.

morphine salt 12 mg daily	≡ buprenorphine 5 micrograms/hour transdermal patch
morphine salt 24 mg daily	≡ buprenorphine 10 micrograms/hour transdermal patch
morphine salt 36 mg daily	≡ buprenorphine 15 micrograms/hour transdermal patch
morphine salt 48 mg daily	≡ buprenorphine 20 micrograms/hour transdermal patch
morphine salt 84 mg daily	≡ buprenorphine 35 micrograms/hour transdermal patch
morphine salt 126 mg daily	≡ buprenorphine 52.5 micrograms/hour transdermal patch

Always seek specialist advice before titrating opioids above this level; pain is often opioid-poorly responsive and adjuvant analgesics may be required.

morphine salt 168 mg daily	≡ buprenorphine 70 micrograms/hour transdermal patch

Formulations of transdermal patches are available as 7-day, 72-hourly, and 96-hourly patches; strengths are written as micrograms/hour; for further information see buprenorphine p. 511. To avoid confusion, patches should be prescribed by brand, dose, and duration. Morphine equivalences have been approximated to allow comparison with available preparations of buprenorphine patches.

Fentanyl transdermal patches are *approximately* equivalent to the following 24-hour doses of oral morphine; patient factors (see *Opioid dose conversion* guidance above) and response should be taken into account and doses adjusted accordingly. These figures are based on the *Palliative Care Formulary* 8th edition.

morphine salt 30 mg daily	≡ fentanyl 12 micrograms/hour transdermal patch
morphine salt 60 mg daily	≡ fentanyl 25 micrograms/hour transdermal patch
morphine salt 90 mg daily	≡ fentanyl 37.5 micrograms/hour transdermal patch
morphine salt 120 mg daily	≡ fentanyl 50 micrograms/hour transdermal patch

Always seek specialist advice before titrating opioids above this level; pain is often opioid-poorly responsive and adjuvant analgesics may be required.

morphine salt 180 mg daily	≡ fentanyl 75 micrograms/hour transdermal patch
morphine salt 240 mg daily	≡ fentanyl 100 micrograms/hour transdermal patch

Formulations of transdermal patches are available as 72-hourly patches; strengths are written as micrograms/hour. To avoid confusion, patches should be prescribed by brand, dose, and duration. Morphine equivalences have been approximated to allow comparison with available preparations of fentanyl patches.

Cancer-related bone pain [EvGr] When opioids, NSAIDs, radiotherapy, and/or orthopaedic interventions have been unsuccessful at managing bone pain or are unsuitable, advice should be sought from a palliative care specialist for other treatment options. ⟨D⟩

Neuropathic pain [EvGr] Antidepressants (such as amitriptyline hydrochloride p. 431, nortriptyline p. 437 and duloxetine), and gabapentinoids (such as gabapentin p. 362 and pregabalin p. 374) are used as first-line adjuvant analgesics for both cancer-related and non-cancer neuropathic pain. Due to a similar mechanism of action, only switch between antidepressants if the first choice was poorly tolerated (but not if it was ineffective). Combination therapy, using drugs which act via different mechanisms (e.g. an antidepressant and a gabapentinoid), can be considered if pain remains uncontrolled with a single drug. Systemic corticosteroids can be used as an alternative for cancer-related neuropathic pain, particularly for pain associated with spinal cord or nerve compression. ⟨D⟩ If pain persists, seek specialist advice; specialist options include non-gabapentinoid antiepileptics, ketamine, and methadone.

Muscle spasm, spasticity, and cramp Painful chronic muscle spasm and spasticity (associated with neural injury), and troublesome cramp can be treated with skeletal muscle relaxants. [EvGr] Baclofen p. 1289 is generally considered to be the first-line option. Benzodiazepines, such as diazepam p. 398 or midazolam p. 394 can be used as alternatives, particularly if the anticipated duration of use is less than 4 weeks. ⟨D⟩

Gastro-intestinal disorders and symptoms

Anorexia Anorexia is common in patients with advanced disease. [EvGr] For patients with early satiety due to delayed gastric emptying, a trial of a prokinetic drug such as metoclopramide hydrochloride or domperidone (if benefits outweigh risks) can be considered. Dexamethasone p. 786, prednisolone p. 791, or a progestogen (such as megestrol acetate) may also be considered as treatment options to stimulate appetite, although there is no evidence that they improve muscle mass/strength, and corticosteroids themselves can cause myopathy. Thus, treatment should be closely monitored and stopped if no benefit is achieved after 1–2 weeks. If longer term treatment (beyond 2-3 weeks) is being contemplated, a progestogen may be more appropriate than a corticosteroid. ⟨D⟩

Bowel colic Bowel colic can occur with conditions such as bowel obstruction, or as a side-effect of some drugs. [EvGr] Bowel colic may be reduced by hyoscine butylbromide p. 96. If bowel colic is related to constipation, it is also important to ensure stool is adequately softened. ⟨D⟩

Constipation Constipation can cause psychological distress and agitation in patients, and is common with the use of opioid analgesics. [EvGr] All patients prescribed a strong opioid should be given a regular laxative. ⟨A⟩

[EvGr] A stimulant laxative (such as bisacodyl p. 67 or senna p. 69) is recommended, with the dose adjusted according to response. If there is a lack of response at the highest dose of a stimulant laxative and/or there has been no bowel movement within 3–4 days, an osmotic laxative (such as macrogol 3350 p. 62 or lactulose p. 61) should be added to the regimen with further titration as needed. For patients with a history of colic with stimulant laxatives, initial treatment with an osmotic laxative is preferable. Docusate sodium p. 66 may also be considered as an option in some patients who have failed to respond or have bowel colic. If oral laxatives are ineffective or unsuitable, suppositories of bisacodyl p. 67 or glycerol p. 68, or a micro-enema of sodium citrate p. 909 should be offered. If these options are also ineffective, an enema of sodium acid phosphate with sodium phosphate p. 64 should be offered. The use of methylnaltrexone bromide p. 71 is reserved for opioid-induced constipation when optimal use of other laxatives is ineffective. ⟨D⟩

Prescribing in palliative care

Dry mouth [EvGr] Certain drugs can cause dry mouth, including opioids, antimuscarinics, some antidepressants, and some antiemetics; if possible, alternative options should be considered. Dry mouth may be relieved by good mouth care, and measures such as sucking crushed ice and taking frequent sips of water. Chewing sugar-free gum acts as a saliva stimulant and is as effective as, and for some patients is preferred to, the use of artificial saliva. Artificial saliva may be considered for those who do not respond to non-drug measures; specialist options include systemic salivary stimulants.

Dry mouth associated with candidiasis can be treated with oral preparations of miconazole p. 1384 or nystatin p. 1385. Fluconazole p. 690 is preferred for moderate-to-severe infections, or with concurrent odynophagia (suggesting oesophageal candidiasis), or if nystatin or miconazole are unsuitable or ineffective. ⓓ

Dysphagia [EvGr] A corticosteroid such as dexamethasone p. 786 may be used if there is an obstruction due to a tumour. Dysphagia caused by oesophagitis and oesophageal spasm may be treated with sublingual glyceryl trinitrate used before meals. ⓓ

Nausea and vomiting Causes of nausea and vomiting include gastric stasis, bowel obstruction, bio-chemical abnormalities, and drug treatment. [EvGr] The most appropriate cause-specific antiemetic should be prescribed regularly and 'as required'. ⓓ[EvGr] Patients should be advised that nausea may occur when starting (and titrating) strong opioids, but it is likely to be transient and improve after 5-7 days. Ⓐ

[EvGr] Metoclopramide hydrochloride p. 494 or alternatively domperidone p. 494 is commonly used for nausea and vomiting associated with gastritis, gastric stasis, and functional bowel obstruction, because of their prokinetic action. Drugs with antimuscarinic effects antagonise prokinetic drugs and, if possible, should not be used concurrently.

Haloperidol p. 445 is commonly used for most chemical causes of vomiting (such as hypercalcaemia, morphine use, and renal failure).

Cyclizine p. 492 is commonly used for nausea and vomiting due to raised intracranial pressure (in conjunction with dexamethasone p. 786), and/or vestibular dysfunction. ⓓ

The patient's regular antiemetic dose and 'as required' use should initially be reviewed daily and adjusted accordingly. For patients who have little benefit from antiemetic therapy despite upward titration of the dose, review the likely cause(s), antiemetic choice and route of administration. [EvGr] Changing to a broad-spectrum antiemetic (such as levomepromazine p. 502) may sometimes be necessary, and dual therapy with antiemetics with different mechanisms (e.g. levomepromazine and ondansetron) may occasionally be required. ⓓ

For the treatment of nausea and vomiting associated with cancer chemotherapy, see Cytotoxic drugs p. 1027.

Mental health conditions

Agitation The non-pharmacological management of agitation should be considered, and any reversible causes treated. [EvGr] A benzodiazepine should be considered for managing agitation where anxiety is prominent, or an antipsychotic (such as haloperidol) for managing agitation where delirium is prominent. Ⓐ Specialist advice should be sought if the agitation or delirium diagnosis is uncertain, is not responding to treatment, or if treatment causes unwanted sedation.

Anxiety In the management of anxiety (and panic disorder), there is comparable efficacy between drug treatment and cognitive behavioural therapy. For drug treatment, the choice of drug is largely influenced by the likely duration of use. [EvGr] For patients with a prognosis of days to weeks, a benzodiazepine (such as diazepam p. 398, lorazepam p. 393 or midazolam p. 394) can be used; and for patients with a prognosis of months, a selective serotonin reuptake inhibitor (SSRI) with or without a benzodiazepine initially, can be used. ⓓ

Depression There is comparable efficacy between drug treatment and cognitive behavioural therapy, with treatment choice based on the severity of symptoms, their functional impact, and patient preference, with frequent reviews of the patient's response, concordance, and other sources of distress. [EvGr] When antidepressant treatment is considered, SSRIs are usually considered as first-line drug treatment for most patients, with citalopram p. 422 or sertraline p. 425 being the first-line drugs of choice, due to their lower risk in overdose and being better tolerated. Mirtazapine p. 431 may be preferred for patients who also suffer from nausea, insomnia, or a reduced appetite. A serotonin-norepinephrine reuptake inhibitor (SNRI) (such as duloxetine p. 426) may be considered if depression and neuropathic pain co-exist. ⓓ

Insomnia Some patients may have difficulty falling or staying asleep, which can impair daytime functioning. Contributing factors may include pain, certain drugs (such as corticosteroids or diuretics), or conditions such as delirium, depression, anxiety, or obstructive sleep apnoea. [EvGr] Initial treatment involves correction of any contributing factors (where possible) and non-drug measures (such as sleep hygiene techniques) before drug treatments are considered. When drug treatment is required, consider the use of a drug to help the underlying cause, which may include the use of a benzodiazepine, Z-drug, melatonin, antidepressant, or antipsychotic. ⓓ

Neurological disorders

Raised intracranial pressure [EvGr] A corticosteroid (such as dexamethasone p. 786) can provide temporary symptomatic relief from pain (or headaches) due to raised intracranial pressure from cerebral oedema. ⓓ

Seizures There are many potential causes of seizures in advanced disease (such as brain tumours or biochemical abnormalities) and specialist advice should be sought where the diagnosis of seizures, or choice or dose of antiepileptic drug is in doubt. [EvGr] Antiepileptic drugs should not be used prophylactically in the absence of a history of seizures. In palliative care, levetiracetam p. 368 is generally preferred as a first-line option as the dose can be titrated rapidly and there are fewer drug interactions. In the last days of life, midazolam p. 394 may be preferred due to benefit in concurrent symptoms and compatibility with other drugs in a CSCI. ⓓ For guidance on the initial management and doses of benzodiazepines for the management of status epilepticus, see Medical emergencies in the community p. 2028.

Respiratory symptoms

Breathlessness In advanced disease, breathlessness is often multifactorial, and management involves correcting causes where possible (such as anxiety or heart failure), the use of non-drug treatments (such as breathing control, positioning, relaxation techniques, and the use of a hand-held or electric fan), and/or symptomatic drug treatment.

[EvGr] When airflow obstruction (expiratory wheeze) is suspected, a one-to-two-week trial of a bronchodilator, with evaluation of the impact on symptoms may be a more pragmatic approach than undertaking objective tests of ventilatory function. Standard inhaled or nebulised beta$_2$ agonists alone or in combination with an antimuscarinic such as ipratropium bromide p. 281 improves breathlessness in most lung cancer patients with chronic obstructive pulmonary disease. An 'as required' dose of a short-acting beta₂ agonist should be encouraged prior to exertion.

In symptom-focused care, where underlying causes cannot be corrected, moderate to severe breathlessness at rest may be relieved by an opioid, namely morphine p. 525, in carefully titrated doses (note that breathlessness often responds to lower doses than those used for pain relief). A benzodiazepine or an SSRI may be helpful for managing breathlessness associated with (or exacerbated by) anxiety that has not responded to non-drug measures or an opioid. A corticosteroid can be tried if breathlessness is caused by airway obstruction, pneumonitis (after radiation therapy), tracheal compression/stridor, or lymphangitic carcinomatosis.

In the last days of life, for patients with distressing breathlessness at rest, the combination of an opioid with a benzodiazepine is more effective than monotherapy. ◇D

Hiccups EvGr In patients with hiccup due to gastric distension with or without gastro-oesophageal reflux, a prokinetic (such as metoclopramide), an antiflatulent (such as peppermint oil or simeticone), or a proton pump inhibitor (such as lansoprazole or omeprazole) can be given. ◇D

Intractable cough Where possible, the underlying cause of the cough should be treated. A wet cough is generally encouraged as it helps to clear the central airways of foreign matter, secretions, or pus. EvGr If sputum is sticky, expectorants (such as nebulised sodium chloride 0.9%) and/or mucolytics (such as acetylcysteine p. 333) help loosen secretions. Non-drug treatment, provided by physiotherapists and speech and language therapists, should also be considered. However, a dry cough adversely affects sleep, rest, eating, or social activities, and causes complications (such as muscular strain, rib fractures, and vomiting), thus, symptomatic relief is appropriate. In patients with a dry cough, a demulcent (such as simple linctus, citric acid p. 340) can be tried. If a demulcent is not effective, addition of an opioid (such as morphine p. 525 can be considered, particularly if needed for concurrent symptoms. ◇D If cough persists, seek advice; specialist options include gabapentinoids.

Noisy respiratory secretions Fluid collection in the upper airway (most commonly from saliva) can cause a rattling noise (also known as 'death rattle'). EvGr If this causes distress in the patient's last days of life, consider non-drug measures (such as positioning) or a trial of drug treatment (medicines may take up to 12 hours to become effective). An antimuscarinic (such as hyoscine butylbromide p. 96 or glycopyrronium bromide p. 1527) given subcutaneously as soon as the rattle begins may be of benefit. ◇A

Other disorders

Capillary bleeding EvGr Capillary bleeding can be treated with oral tranexamic acid p. 127; treatment is usually

discontinued one week after the bleeding has stopped, or if necessary, it can be continued at a reduced dose. Consider specialist referral to address the underlying cause and/or for advice on specialist measures, e.g. topical preparations. ◇D

Malodourous fungating tumours EvGr Malodourous (or infected) fungating tumours can be treated with topical or systemic metronidazole. Systemic treatment is often required to reduce malodour, but topical metronidazole p. 1398 can be considered when systemic treatment is impractical or causes unacceptable side-effects, the cancer is relatively small and easily accessible for topical application, and/or the cancer is poorly vascularised and very sloughy. ◇D

Pruritus Pruritus occurs commonly, and for some patients it can be very severe and distressing. Causes may include dry skin (very common in advanced cancer), other conditions such as renal or hepatic failure, or be drug-induced (e.g. opioid-induced). Whenever possible, the treatment of pruritus should be cause-specific; where a drug is the likely cause this should be reviewed, and where possible stopped and an alternative prescribed. EvGr Even when there is a probable endogenous cause, pruritus often responds to the application of an emollient. A topical antipruritic cream (such as levomenthol p. 1438) can be used to relieve pruritus unresponsive to an emollient and/or cause-specific treatment. A trial of an antihistamine can also be considered. ◇D If pruritus persists, seek advice; specialist options include SSRIs (cholestatic pruritus) and gabapentinoids (uraemic pruritus).

Useful resources

Care of dying adults in the last days of life. National Institute for Health and Care Excellence. NICE guideline 31. December 2015.
www.nice.org.uk/guidance/ng31
End of life care for adults: service delivery. National Institute for Health and Care Excellence. NICE guideline 142. October 2019.
www.nice.org.uk/guidance/ng142
Palliative care for adults: strong opioids for pain relief. National Institute for Health and Care Excellence. Clinical guideline 140. May 2012 (updated August 2016).
www.nice.org.uk/guidance/cg140
Supporting adults carers. National Institute for Health and Care Excellence. NICE guideline 150. January 2020.
www.nice.org.uk/guidance/ng150
Wilcock A, Howard P (Eds.). Palliative Care Formulary (8th ed). Pharmaceutical Press.
www.medicinescomplete.com
NHS Scotland. Scottish Palliative Care Guidelines.
www.palliativecareguidelines.scot.nhs.uk/

Prescribing in the elderly

Overview

Old people, especially the very old, require special care and consideration from prescribers. *Medicines for Older People*, a component document of the National Service Framework for Older People (Department of Health. National Service Framework for Older People. London: Department of Health, March 2001), describes how to maximise the benefits of medicines and how to avoid excessive, inappropriate, or inadequate consumption of medicines by older people.

Appropriate prescribing

Elderly patients often receive multiple drugs for their multiple diseases. This greatly increases the risk of drug interactions as well as adverse reactions, and may affect compliance. The balance of benefit and harm of some medicines may be altered in the elderly. Therefore, elderly patients' medicines should be reviewed regularly and medicines which are not of benefit should be stopped.

Non-pharmacological measures may be more appropriate for symptoms such as headache, sleeplessness, and light-headedness when associated with social stress as in widowhood, loneliness, and family dispersal.

In some cases prophylactic drugs are inappropriate if they are likely to complicate existing treatment or introduce unnecessary side-effects, especially in elderly patients with poor prognosis or with poor overall health. However, elderly patients should not be denied medicines which may help them, such as anticoagulants or antiplatelet drugs for atrial fibrillation, antihypertensives, statins, and drugs for osteoporosis.

STOPP/START criteria STOPP/START criteria are evidence-based criteria used to review medication regimens in elderly people. STOPP (Screening Tool of Older Persons' potentially inappropriate Prescriptions) aims to reduce the incidence of medicines-related adverse events from potentially inappropriate prescribing and polypharmacy. START (Screening Tool to Alert to Right Treatment) can be used to prevent omissions of indicated, appropriate medicines in older patients with specific conditions.

For STOPP criteria related to single drugs or drug classes, BNF Publications contain information within the monographs, in the cautions section. Where criteria relate to a drug class without a class monograph, information is outlined in the relevant treatment summaries. START criteria are not included within the monographs, however further information can be found in:

- Gallagher, P. et al. (2008). STOPP (Screening Tool of Older Persons' Prescriptions) and START (Screening Tool to Alert Doctors to Right Treatment): Consensus Validation. Int J Clin Pharmacol Ther 46(2):72–83.
- O'Mahony, D. et al. (2015). STOPP/START criteria for potentially inappropriate prescribing in older people: version 2. Age Ageing 44(2):213–8.

Form of medicine

Frail elderly patients may have difficulty swallowing tablets; if left in the mouth, ulceration may develop. They should always be encouraged to take their tablets or capsules with enough fluid, and whilst in an upright position to avoid the possibility of oesophageal ulceration. It can be helpful to discuss with the patient the possibility of taking the drug as a liquid if available.

Manifestations of ageing

In the very old, manifestations of normal ageing may be mistaken for disease and lead to inappropriate prescribing. In addition, age-related muscle weakness and difficulty in maintaining balance should not be confused with neurological disease. Disorders such as light-headedness not associated with postural or postprandial hypotension are unlikely to be helped by drugs.

Sensitivity

The nervous system of elderly patients is more sensitive to many commonly used drugs, such as opioid analgesics, benzodiazepines, antipsychotics, and antiparkinsonian drugs, all of which must be used with caution. Similarly, other organs may also be more susceptible to the effects of drugs such as anti-hypertensives and NSAIDs.

Pharmacokinetics

Pharmacokinetic changes can markedly increase the tissue concentration of a drug in the elderly, especially in debilitated patients.

The most important effect of age is reduced renal clearance. Many aged patients thus *excrete drugs slowly*, and are *highly susceptible to nephrotoxic drugs*. Acute illness can lead to rapid reduction in renal clearance, especially if accompanied by dehydration. Hence, a patient stabilised on a drug with a narrow margin between the therapeutic and the toxic dose (e.g. digoxin p. 125) can rapidly develop adverse effects in the aftermath of a myocardial infarction or a respiratory-tract infection. The hepatic metabolism of lipid soluble drugs is reduced in elderly patients because there is a reduction in liver volume. This is important for drugs with a narrow therapeutic window.

Adverse reactions

Adverse reactions often present in the elderly in a vague and non-specific fashion. *Confusion* is often the presenting symptom (caused by almost any of the commonly used drugs). Other common manifestations are *constipation* (with antimuscarinics and many tranquillisers) and postural *hypotension* and *falls* (with diuretics and many psychotropics).

Hypnotics

Many hypnotics with long half-lives have serious hangover effects, including drowsiness, unsteady gait, slurred speech, and confusion. Hypnotics with short half-lives should be used but they too can present problems. Short courses of hypnotics are occasionally useful for helping a patient through an acute illness or some other crisis but every effort must be made to avoid dependence. Benzodiazepines impair balance, which can result in falls.

Diuretics

Diuretics are overprescribed in old age and should **not** be used on a long-term basis to treat simple gravitational oedema which will usually respond to increased movement, raising the legs, and support stockings. A few days of diuretic treatment may speed the clearing of the oedema but it should rarely need continued drug therapy.

NSAIDs

Bleeding associated with aspirin and other NSAIDs is more common in the elderly who are more likely to have a fatal or serious outcome. NSAIDs are also a special hazard in patients with cardiac disease or renal impairment which may again place older patients at particular risk.

Owing to the *increased susceptibility of the elderly* to the *side-effects of NSAIDs* the following recommendations are made:

- for *soft-tissue lesions,* and *back pain,* first try measures such as weight reduction (if obese), warmth, exercise, and use of a walking stick;
- for *soft-tissue lesions, back pain*, and *pain in rheumatoid arthritis*, paracetamol p. 507 should be used first and can often provide adequate pain relief;
- alternatively, a low-dose NSAID (e.g. ibuprofen p. 1302 up to 1.2 g daily) may be given;
- for pain relief when either drug is inadequate, paracetamol in a full dose plus a low-dose NSAID may be given;
- if necessary, the NSAID dose can be increased or an opioid analgesic given with paracetamol p. 507;
- do not give two NSAIDs at the same time.

Prophylaxis of NSAID-induced peptic ulcers may be required if continued NSAID treatment is necessary. For further information, see Peptic ulcer disease p. 81.

Other drugs

Other drugs which commonly cause adverse reactions are *antiparkinsonian drugs, antihypertensives, psychotropics*, and digoxin p. 125. The usual maintenance dose of digoxin in very old patients is 125 micrograms daily (62.5 micrograms in those with renal disease); lower doses are often inadequate but toxicity is common in those given 250 micrograms daily.

Drug-induced blood disorders are much more common in the elderly. Therefore drugs with a tendency to cause bone marrow depression (e.g. co-trimoxazole p. 652, mianserin hydrochloride p. 430) should be avoided unless there is no acceptable alternative.

The elderly generally require a lower maintenance dose of warfarin sodium p. 165 than younger adults; once again, the outcome of bleeding tends to be more serious.

Guidelines

Always consider whether a drug is indicated at all.

Limit range It is a sensible policy to prescribe from a limited range of drugs and to be thoroughly familiar with their effects in the elderly.

Reduce dose Dosage should generally be substantially lower than for younger patients and it is common to start with about 50% of the adult dose. Some drugs (e.g. long-acting antidiabetic drugs such as glibenclamide) should be avoided altogether.

Review regularly Review repeat prescriptions regularly. In many patients it may be possible to stop some drugs, provided that clinical progress is monitored. It may be

necessary to reduce the dose of some drugs as renal function declines.

Simplify regimens Elderly patients benefit from simple treatment regimens. Only drugs with a clear indication should be prescribed and whenever possible given once or twice daily. In particular, regimens which call for a confusing array of dosage intervals should be avoided.

Explain clearly Write full instructions on every prescription (*including* repeat prescriptions) so that containers can be properly labelled with full directions. Avoid imprecisions like 'as directed'. Child-resistant containers may be unsuitable.

Repeats and disposal Instruct patients what to do when drugs run out, and also how to dispose of any that are no longer necessary. Try to prescribe matching quantities.

If these guidelines are followed most elderly people will cope adequately with their own medicines. If not then it is essential to enrol the help of a third party, usually a relative or a friend.

Drugs and sport

Anti-doping

UK Anti-Doping, the national body responsible for the UK's anti-doping policy, advises that athletes are personally responsible should a prohibited substance be detected in their body. Information regarding the use of medicines in sport is available from:

UK Anti-doping
Fleetbank House
2-6 Salisbury Square
London
EC4Y 8AE
(020) 7842 3450
ukad@ukad.org.uk
www.ukad.org.uk

Information about the prohibited status of specific medications based on the current World Anti-Doping Agency Prohibited List is available from Global Drug Reference Online: www.globaldro.com/UK/search

General Medical Council's advice

Doctors who prescribe or collude in the provision of drugs or treatment with the intention of improperly enhancing an individual's performance in sport contravene the GMC's guidance, and such actions would usually raise a question of a doctor's continued registration. This does not preclude the provision of any care or treatment where the doctor's intention is to protect or improve the patient's health.

Prescribing in dental practice

General guidance

Advice on the drug management of dental and oral conditions has been integrated into the main text. For ease of access, guidance on such conditions is usually identified by means of a relevant heading (e.g. Dental and Orofacial Pain) in the appropriate sections of the BNF.

The following is a list of topics of particular relevance to dentists.

- Prescribing by dentists, see Prescription writing p. 4
- Oral side-effects of drugs, see Adverse reactions to drugs p. 11
- Medical emergencies in dental practice, see below
- Medical problems in dental practice, see below

Drug management of dental and oral conditions

Dental and orofacial pain

- Neuropathic pain p. 547
- Non-opioid analgesics and compound analgesic preparations, see Analgesics p. 505
- Opioid analgesics, see Analgesics p. 505
- Non-steroidal anti-inflammatory drugs p. 1292

Oral infections

Bacterial infections, see Antibacterials, principles of therapy p. 573

- Phenoxymethylpenicillin p. 634

- Broad-spectrum penicillins (amoxicillin p. 635 and ampicillin p. 637)
- Cephalosporins (cefalexin p. 603 and cefradine p. 605)
- Tetracyclines p. 655
- Macrolides (clarithromycin p. 621, erythromycin p. 624 and azithromycin p. 620)
- Clindamycin p. 618
- Metronidazole p. 628
- Fusidic acid p. 663

Fungal infections, see Antifungals, systemic use p. 685

- Local treatment, see Oropharyngeal fungal infections p. 1384
- Systemic treatment, see Antifungals, systemic use p. 685

Viral infections

- Herpetic gingivostomatitis, local treatment, see Oropharyngeal viral infections p. 1385
- Herpetic gingivostomatitis, systemic treatment, see Oropharyngeal viral infections p. 1385 and Herpesvirus infections p. 727
- Herpes labialis, see Skin infections p. 1395

Anaesthetics, anxiolytics and hypnotics

- Sedation, anaesthesia, and resuscitation in dental practice p. 1521
- Hypnotics, see Hypnotics and anxiolytics p. 549

- Sedation for dental procedures, see Hypnotics and anxiolytics p. 549
- Anaesthesia (local) p. 1542

Minerals
- Fluoride p. 1378

Oral ulceration and inflammation
- See Oral ulceration and inflammation p. 1379

Mouthwashes, gargles and dentifrices
- See Mouthwashes and other preparations for oropharyngeal use p. 1376

Dry mouth
- See Dry mouth p. 1374

Aromatic inhalations
- See Aromatic inhalations, cough preparations and systemic nasal decongestants p. 339

Nasal decongestants
- See Aromatic inhalations, cough preparations and systemic nasal decongestants p. 339

Dental Practitioners' Formulary
- See Dental Practitioners' Formulary p. 1951

Medical emergencies in dental practice

This section provides guidelines on the management of the more common medical emergencies which may arise in dental practice. Dentists and their staff should be familiar with standard resuscitation procedures, but in all circumstances it is advisable to summon medical assistance as soon as possible. See also **algorithm** of the procedure for Cardiopulmonary resuscitation p. 256.

The drugs referred to in this section include:
- Adrenaline/epinephrine Injection, adrenaline 1 in 1000, (adrenaline 1 mg/mL as acid tartrate), 1 mL amps p. 256
- Aspirin Dispersible Tablets 300 mg p. 142
- Glucagon Injection, glucagon (as hydrochloride), 1-unit vial (with solvent) p. 845
- Glucose p. 1182 (for administration by mouth)
- Glyceryl trinitrate Spray p. 252
- Midazolam Oromucosal Solution p. 394
- Oxygen
- Salbutamol Aerosol Inhalation, salbutamol 100 micrograms/metered inhalation p. 287

Adrenal insufficiency

Adrenal insufficiency may follow prolonged therapy with corticosteroids and can persist for years after stopping. A patient with adrenal insufficiency may become hypotensive under the stress of a dental visit (important: see individual monographs for details of corticosteroid cover before dental surgical procedures under general anaesthesia).

Management
- Lay the patient flat
- Give **oxygen**
- Transfer patient urgently to hospital

Anaphylaxis

A severe allergic reaction may follow oral or parenteral administration of a drug. Anaphylactic reactions in dentistry may follow the administration of a drug or contact with substances such as latex in surgical gloves. In general, the more rapid the onset of the reaction the more profound it tends to be. Symptoms may develop within minutes and rapid treatment is essential.

Anaphylactic reactions may also be associated with *additives* and *excipients* in foods and medicines. Refined arachis (peanut) oil, which may be present in some medicinal products, is unlikely to cause an allergic reaction—nevertheless it is wise to check the full formula of preparations which may contain allergens (including those for topical application, particularly if they are intended for use in the mouth or for application to the nasal mucosa).

Symptoms and signs
- Paraesthesia, flushing, and swelling of face
- Generalised itching, especially of hands and feet
- Bronchospasm and laryngospasm (with wheezing and difficulty in breathing)
- Rapid weak pulse together with fall in blood pressure and pallor; finally cardiac arrest

Management
For a quick reference resource with doses for intramuscular adrenaline/epinephrine p. 256, see *Anaphylaxis* in Medical emergencies in the community p. 2028.

EvGr Immediately call for an ambulance and begin initial anaphylaxis treatment.

Remove the trigger causing the anaphylactic reaction if possible. Place the patient in a comfortable position based on their signs and symptoms—lay the patient flat (with or without legs raised) to aid in the restoration of blood pressure, or in a semi-recumbent position for patients with airway and breathing problems (and no evidence of cardiovascular instability) to make breathing easier, or in the recovery position for patients who are unconscious and breathing normally; pregnant females should lie on their left side to prevent aortocaval compression.

Give intramuscular adrenaline/epinephrine as first line treatment for anaphylaxis, and assess response to treatment by monitoring vital signs (such as blood pressure, pulse, respiratory function, and level of consciousness) and auscultate for wheeze. A repeat dose of intramuscular adrenaline/epinephrine should be given after a 5-minute interval if there is no improvement in the patient's condition. Patients who have no improvement in respiratory and/or cardiovascular problems despite 2 appropriate doses of intramuscular adrenaline/epinephrine should have their care escalated quickly. Continue to give intramuscular adrenaline/epinephrine at 5-minute intervals while life-threatening cardiovascular and/or respiratory features persist. Ⓐ

High-flow oxygen and intravenous fluids are also used for initial treatment of anaphylaxis. For further information on the management of anaphylaxis, see Antihistamines, allergen immunotherapy and allergic emergencies p. 316.

Asthma

Patients with asthma may have an attack while at the dental surgery. Most attacks will respond to 2 puffs of the patient's short-acting beta$_2$ agonist inhaler such as salbutamol 100 micrograms/puff p. 287; further puffs are required if the patient does not respond rapidly. If the patient is unable to use the inhaler effectively, further puffs should be given through a large-volume spacer device (or, if not available, through a plastic or paper cup with a hole in the bottom for the inhaler mouthpiece). If the patient has features of severe or life-threatening acute asthma, or the response remains unsatisfactory, or if further deterioration occurs, then the patient should be transferred urgently to hospital. Whilst awaiting transfer, **oxygen** should be given with salbutamol 5 mg p. 287 or terbutaline sulfate 10 mg p. 290 by nebuliser; if a nebuliser is unavailable, then 2−10 puffs of salbutamol 100 micrograms/metered inhalation should be given (preferably by a large-volume spacer), and repeated every 10−20 minutes if necessary. If asthma is part of a more generalised anaphylactic reaction, an intramuscular injection of adrenaline/epinephrine p. 256 (as detailed under Anaphylaxis) should be given.

Patients with severe chronic asthma or whose asthma has deteriorated previously during a dental procedure may require an increase in their prophylactic medication before a dental procedure. This should be discussed with the patient's medical practitioner and may include increasing the dose of inhaled or oral corticosteroid.

Cardiac emergencies

If there is a history of *angina* the patient will probably carry glyceryl trinitrate spray or tablets p. 252 (or isosorbide dinitrate tablets p. 254) and should be allowed to use them. Hospital admission is not necessary if symptoms are mild and resolve rapidly with the patient's own medication. See also Coronary Artery Disease below.

Arrhythmias may lead to a sudden reduction in cardiac output with loss of consciousness. Medical assistance should be summoned. For advice on pacemaker interference, see also Pacemakers below.

The pain of *myocardial infarction* is similar to that of angina but generally more severe and more prolonged. For general advice see also Coronary Artery Disease below.

Symptoms and signs of myocardial infarction:

- Progressive onset of severe, crushing pain across front of chest; pain may radiate towards the shoulder and down arm, or into neck and jaw
- Skin becomes pale and clammy
- Nausea and vomiting are common
- Pulse may be weak and blood pressure may fall
- Breathlessness

Initial management of myocardial infarction: Call immediately for medical assistance and an ambulance, as appropriate.

Allow the patient to rest in the position that feels most comfortable; in the presence of breathlessness this is likely to be sitting position, whereas the syncopal patient should be laid flat; often an intermediate position (dictated by the patient) will be most appropriate.

Sublingual glyceryl trinitrate p. 252 may relieve pain. Intramuscular injection of drugs should be avoided because absorption may be too slow (particularly when cardiac output is reduced) and pain relief is inadequate. Intramuscular injection also increases the risk of local bleeding into the muscle if the patient is given a thrombolytic drug.

Reassure the patient as much as possible to relieve further anxiety. If available, aspirin p. 142 in a single dose of 300 mg should be given. A note (to say that aspirin has been given) should be sent with the patient to the hospital.

High flow **oxygen** (15 L/min) may be administered if the patient is cyanosed (blue lips) or conscious level deteriorates.

If the patient collapses and loses consciousness attempt standard resuscitation measures. See also **algorithm** of the procedure for Cardiopulmonary resuscitation p. 256.

Epileptic seizures

Patients with epilepsy must continue with their normal dosage of anticonvulsant drugs when attending for dental treatment. It is not uncommon for epileptic patients not to volunteer the information that they are epileptic but there should be little difficulty in recognising a tonic-clonic (grand mal) seizure.

Symptoms and signs

- There may be a brief warning (but variable)
- Sudden loss of consciousness, the patient becomes rigid, falls, may give a cry, and becomes cyanotic (tonic phase)
- After 30 seconds, there are jerking movements of the limbs; the tongue may be bitten (clonic phase)
- There may be frothing from mouth and urinary incontinence
- The seizure typically lasts a few minutes; the patient may then become flaccid but remain unconscious. After a variable time the patient regains consciousness but may remain confused for a while

Management

During a convulsion try to ensure that the patient is not at risk from injury but make no attempt to put anything in the mouth or between the teeth (in mistaken belief that this will protect the tongue). Give **oxygen** to support respiration if necessary.

Do not attempt to restrain convulsive movements.

After convulsive movements have subsided place the patient in the coma (recovery) position and check the airway.

After the convulsion the patient may be confused ('post-ictal confusion') and may need reassurance and sympathy. The patient should not be sent home until fully recovered. Seek medical attention or transfer the patient to hospital if it was the first episode of epilepsy, or if the convulsion was atypical, prolonged (or repeated), or if injury occurred.

Medication should only be given if convulsive seizures are prolonged (convulsive movements lasting 5 minutes or longer) or repeated rapidly. Midazolam oromucosal solution p. 394 can be given by the buccal route. For a quick reference resource with doses of benzodiazepines for the management of convulsive status epilepticus, see *Seizures* in Medical emergencies in the community p. 2028. For further information on the management of convulsive status epilepticus, see Status epilepticus p. 392.

Focal seizures similarly need very little active management (in an automatism only a minimum amount of restraint should be applied to prevent injury). Again, the patient should be observed until post-ictal confusion has completely resolved.

Hypoglycaemia

Insulin-treated diabetic patients attending for dental treatment under local anaesthesia should inject insulin and eat meals as normal. If food is omitted the blood glucose will fall to an abnormally low level (hypoglycaemia). Patients can often recognise the symptoms themselves and this state responds to fast-acting carbohydrates. Children may not have such prominent changes but may appear unduly lethargic.

Symptoms and signs Hypoglycaemia should be excluded in any person with diabetes who is acutely unwell, drowsy, unconscious, unable to co-operate, or presenting with aggressive behaviour or seizures. Symptoms of hypoglycaemia in children include shakiness, pounding heart, sweatiness, headache, drowsiness, and difficulty concentrating. In young children, behavioural changes such as irritability, agitation, quietness, and tantrums, may be prominent.

Management of adults

For a quick reference resource with doses for the treatment of hypoglycaemia, see *Hypoglycaemia* in Medical emergencies in the community p. 2028.

EvGr Any patient with a blood-glucose concentration less than 4 mmol/litre, with or without symptoms, and who is **conscious and able to swallow**, should be treated with a fast-acting carbohydrate by mouth. Fast-acting carbohydrates include *Lift*® glucose liquid (previously *Glucojuice*®), glucose tablets, glucose 40% gels (e.g. *Glucogel*®, *Dextrogel*®, or *Rapilose*®), pure fruit juice, and sugar (sucrose) dissolved in an appropriate volume of water. Oral glucose formulations p. 1182 are preferred as absorption occurs more quickly. Orange juice should not be given to patients following a low-potassium diet due to chronic kidney disease, and sugar dissolved in water will not be effective in patients taking acarbose.

If necessary, repeat treatment after 15 minutes, up to a maximum of 3 treatments in total. Once blood-glucose concentration is above 4 mmol/litre and the patient has recovered, a snack providing a long-acting carbohydrate should be given to prevent blood-glucose concentration from falling again (e.g. two biscuits, one slice of bread, 200–300 mL milk (not soya or other forms of 'alternative' milk, e.g. almond or coconut), or a normal carbohydrate-containing meal if due).

If hypoglycaemia is unresponsive, or the oral route cannot be used, intramuscular glucagon p. 845 should be given. Once blood-glucose concentration is above 4 mmol/litre and the patient has recovered, a snack providing a long-acting carbohydrate should be given. Patients who have received glucagon require a larger portion of long-acting carbohydrate to replenish glycogen stores (e.g. four biscuits, two slices of bread, 400–600 mL of milk (not soya or other forms of 'alternative' milk, e.g. almond or coconut) or a normal carbohydrate containing meal if due).

Glucagon may be less effective in patients taking a sulfonylurea or under the influence of alcohol; in these cases, intravenous glucose 10% will be required. If glucagon is unsuitable or ineffective after 10 minutes, the patient should be transferred urgently to hospital. Ⓔ The patient must also be admitted to hospital if hypoglycaemia is caused by an oral antidiabetic drug.

Management of children
For a quick reference resource with doses for the treatment of hypoglycaemia, see *Hypoglycaemia* in Medical emergencies in the community p. 2028.

ⒺⒼ In children who are **conscious and able to swallow**, non-severe hypoglycaemia is treated with a fast-acting carbohydrate by mouth, preferably in liquid form. Ⓐ ⒺⒼ Fast-acting carbohydrates include *Lift*® glucose liquid (previously *Glucojuice*®), glucose tablets, glucose 40% gels (e.g. *Glucogel*®, *Dextrogel*®, or *Rapilose*®), and sugar (sucrose) dissolved in an appropriate volume of water. Oral glucose formulations p. 1182 are preferred as absorption occurs more quickly. Glucose 40% gel may be given buccally in children who are uncooperative, but are conscious and able to swallow. Ⓔ

Blood-glucose concentrations should rise within 5–15 minutes; ⒺⒼ if hypoglycaemia persists after 15 minutes, repeat the fast-acting glucose. As symptoms improve or normoglycaemia is restored, a long-acting carbohydrate snack (e.g. two biscuits, one banana) or a meal, can be given to prevent blood-glucose concentration from falling again. Ⓐ

ⒺⒼ Severe hypoglycaemia may be treated with concentrated oral glucose solution, as long as the child is **conscious and able to swallow**. Ⓔ Proprietary products of fast-acting carbohydrate, as glucose 40% gel (e.g. *Glucogel*®, *Dextrogel*®, or *Rapilose*®) are available for use in severe hypoglycaemia.

ⒺⒼ If hypoglycaemia is unresponsive, or the oral route cannot be used, intramuscular glucagon p. 845 should be given. As symptoms improve or normoglycaemia is restored, and the child is sufficiently awake, a long-acting carbohydrate snack (e.g. two biscuits, one banana) or a meal should be given. Ⓐ

ⒺⒼ Glucagon may be less effective in patients taking a sulfonylurea or under the influence of alcohol; in these cases, intravenous glucose 10% will be required. ⒺⒺⒼ If glucagon is unsuitable or ineffective after 10 minutes, the child should be transferred urgently to hospital. Ⓐ The child must also be admitted to hospital if hypoglycaemia is caused by an oral antidiabetic drug.

Syncope
Insufficient blood supply to the brain results in loss of consciousness. The commonest cause is a vasovagal attack or simple faint (syncope) due to emotional stress.

Symptoms and signs
- Patient feels faint
- Low blood pressure
- Pallor and sweating
- Yawning and slow pulse
- Nausea and vomiting

- Dilated pupils
- Muscular twitching

Management
- Lay the patient as flat as is reasonably comfortable and, in the absence of associated breathlessness, raise the legs to improve cerebral circulation
- Loosen any tight clothing around the neck
- Once consciousness is regained, give sugar in water or a cup of sweet tea

Other possible causes
Postural hypotension can be a consequence of rising abruptly or of standing upright for too long; antihypertensive drugs predispose to this. When rising, susceptible patients should take their time. Management is as for a vasovagal attack.

Under stressful circumstances, some patients hyperventilate. This gives rise to feelings of faintness but does not usually result in syncope. In most cases reassurance is all that is necessary; rebreathing from cupped hands or a bag may be helpful but calls for careful supervision.

Adrenal insufficiency or arrhythmias are other possible causes of syncope.

Medical problems in dental practice
Individuals presenting at the dental surgery may also suffer from an unrelated medical condition; this may require modification to the management of their dental condition. If the patient has systemic disease or is taking other medication, the matter may need to be discussed with the patient's general practitioner or hospital consultant.

Allergy
Patients should be asked about any history of allergy; those with a history of atopic allergy (asthma, eczema, hay fever, etc.) are at special risk. Those with a history of a severe allergy or of anaphylactic reactions are at high risk—it is essential to confirm that they are not allergic to any medication, or to any dental materials or equipment (including latex gloves). See also Anaphylaxis above.

Arrhythmias
Patients, especially those who suffer from heart failure or who have sustained a myocardial infarction, may have irregular cardiac rhythm. Atrial fibrillation is a common arrhythmia even in patients with normal hearts and is of little concern except that dentists should be aware that such patients may be receiving anticoagulant therapy. The patient's medical practitioner should be asked whether any special precautions are necessary. Premedication (e.g. with temazepam p. 552) may be useful in some instances for very anxious patients.

See also Cardiac emergencies above, and Dental Anaesthesia (Anaesthesia (local) p. 1542).

Cardiac prostheses
For an account of the risk of infective endocarditis in patients with prosthetic heart valves, see Infective Endocarditis below. For advice on patients receiving anticoagulants, see Thromboembolic disease below.

Coronary artery disease
Patients are vulnerable for at least 4 weeks following a myocardial infarction or following any sudden increase in the symptoms of angina. It would be advisable to check with the patient's medical practitioner before commencing treatment. See also Cardiac Emergencies above.

Treatment with low-dose aspirin (75 mg daily), clopidogrel p. 143, or dipyridamole p. 144 should not be stopped routinely nor should the dose be altered before dental procedures.

A Working Party of the British Society for Antimicrobial Chemotherapy has not recommended antibiotic prophylaxis for patients following coronary artery bypass surgery.

Cyanotic heart disease

Patients with cyanotic heart disease are at risk in the dental chair, particularly if they have pulmonary hypertension. In such patients a syncopal reaction increases the shunt away from the lungs, causing more hypoxia which worsens the syncopal reaction—a vicious circle that may prove fatal. The advice of the cardiologist should be sought on any patient with congenital cyanotic heart disease. Treatment in hospital is more appropriate for some patients with this condition.

Hypertension

Patients with hypertension are likely to be receiving antihypertensive drugs. Their blood pressure may fall dangerously low under general anaesthesia, see also under Dental Anaesthesia (Anaesthesia (local) p. 1542).

Immunosuppression and indwelling intraperitoneal catheters

Advice of a Working Party of the British Society for Antimicrobial Chemotherapy is that patients who are immunosuppressed (including transplant patients) and patients with indwelling intraperitoneal catheters do not require antibiotic prophylaxis for dental treatment provided there is no other indication for prophylaxis.

The Working Party has commented that there is little evidence that dental treatment is followed by infection in immunosuppressed and immunodeficient patients nor is there evidence that dental treatment is followed by infection in patients with indwelling intraperitoneal catheters.

Infective endocarditis

While almost any dental procedure can cause bacteraemia, there is no clear association with the development of infective endocarditis. Routine daily activities such as tooth brushing also produce a bacteraemia and may present a greater risk of infective endocarditis than a single dental procedure.

Antibacterial prophylaxis and chlorhexidine mouthwash p. 1377 are **not** recommended for the prevention of endocarditis in patients undergoing dental procedures. Such prophylaxis may expose patients to the adverse effects of antimicrobials when the evidence of benefit has not been proven.

Reduction of oral bacteraemia Patients at risk of endocarditis including those with valve replacement, acquired valvular heart disease with stenosis or regurgitation, structural congenital heart disease (including surgically corrected or palliated structural conditions, but excluding isolated atrial septal defect, fully repaired ventricular septal defect, fully repaired patent ductus arteriosus, and closure devices considered to be endothelialised), hypertrophic cardiomyopathy, or a previous episode of infective endocarditis, should be advised to maintain the highest possible standards of oral hygiene in order to reduce the:

- need for dental extractions or other surgery;
- chances of severe bacteraemia if dental surgery is needed;
- possibility of 'spontaneous' bacteraemia.

Postoperative care Patients at risk of endocarditis including those with valve replacement, acquired valvular heart disease with stenosis or regurgitation, structural congenital heart disease (including surgically corrected or palliated structural conditions, but excluding isolated atrial septal defect, fully repaired ventricular septal defect, fully repaired patent ductus arteriosus, and closure devices considered to

be endothelialised), hypertrophic cardiomyopathy, or a previous episode of infective endocarditis, should be warned to report to the doctor or dentist any unexplained illness that develops after dental treatment.

Any infection in patients at risk of endocarditis should be investigated promptly and treated appropriately to reduce the risk of endocarditis.

Patients on anticoagulant therapy

For general advice on dental surgery in patients receiving oral anticoagulant therapy see Thromboembolic Disease below.

Joint prostheses

Advice of a Working Party of the British Society for Antimicrobial Chemotherapy is that patients with prosthetic joint implants (including total hip replacements) do not require antibiotic prophylaxis for dental treatment. The Working Party considers that it is unacceptable to expose patients to the adverse effects of antibiotics when there is no evidence that such prophylaxis is of any benefit, but that those who develop any intercurrent infection require prompt treatment with antibiotics to which the infecting organisms are sensitive.

The Working Party has commented that joint infections have rarely been shown to follow dental procedures and are even more rarely caused by oral streptococci.

Pacemakers

Pacemakers prevent asystole or severe bradycardia. Some ultrasonic scalers, electronic apex locators, electro-analgesic devices, and electrocautery devices interfere with the normal function of pacemakers (including shielded pacemakers) and should not be used. The manufacturer's literature should be consulted whenever possible. If severe bradycardia occurs in a patient fitted with a pacemaker, electrical equipment should be switched off and the patient placed supine with the legs elevated. If the patient loses consciousness and the pulse remains slow or is absent, cardiopulmonary resuscitation may be needed. Call immediately for medical assistance and an ambulance, as appropriate.

A Working Party of the British Society for Antimicrobial Chemotherapy does not recommend antibacterial prophylaxis for patients with pacemakers.

Thromboembolic disease

Patients receiving a **heparin** or an oral anticoagulant such as warfarin sodium p. 165, acenocoumarol p. 164 (nicoumalone), phenindione p. 164, apixaban p. 145, dabigatran etexilate p. 159 or rivaroxaban p. 149 may be liable to excessive bleeding after extraction of teeth or other dental surgery. Often dental surgery can be delayed until the anticoagulant therapy has been completed.

For a patient requiring long-term therapy with warfarin sodium, the patient's medical practitioner should be consulted and the International Normalised Ratio (INR) should be assessed 72 hours before the dental procedure. This allows sufficient time for dose modification if necessary. In those with an unstable INR (including those who require weekly monitoring of their INR, or those who have had some INR measurements greater than 4.0 in the last 2 months), the INR should be assessed within 24 hours of the dental procedure. Patients requiring minor dental procedures (including extractions) who have an INR below 4.0 may continue warfarin sodium without dose adjustment. There is no need to check the INR for a patient requiring a non-invasive dental procedure.

If it is necessary to remove several teeth, a single extraction should be done first; if this goes well further teeth may be extracted at subsequent visits (two or three at a time). Measures should be taken to minimise bleeding during and after the procedure. This includes the use of sutures and a haemostatic such as oxidised cellulose, collagen sponge or resorbable gelatin sponge. Scaling and root planing should initially be restricted to a limited area to assess the potential for bleeding.

For a patient on long-term warfarin sodium, the advice of the clinician responsible for the patient's anticoagulation should be sought if:

- the INR is unstable, or if the INR is greater than 4.0;
- the patient has thrombocytopenia, haemophilia, or other disorders of haemostasis, or suffers from liver impairment, alcoholism, or renal failure;
- the patient is receiving antiplatelet drugs, cytotoxic drugs or radiotherapy.

Intramuscular injections are *contra-indicated* in patients taking anticoagulants with an INR above the therapeutic range, and in those with any disorder of haemostasis. In patients taking anticoagulants who have a stable INR within the therapeutic range, intramuscular injections should be avoided if possible; if an intramuscular injection is necessary, the patient should be informed of the increased risk of localised bleeding and monitored carefully.

A local anaesthetic containing a vasoconstrictor should be given by infiltration, or by intraligamentary or mental nerve injection if possible. If regional nerve blocks cannot be avoided the local anaesthetic should be given cautiously using an aspirating syringe.

Drugs which have potentially serious interactions with anticoagulants include aspirin and other NSAIDs, carbamazepine p. 355, imidazole and triazole antifungals (including miconazole p. 1384), erythromycin p. 624, clarithromycin p. 621, and metronidazole p. 628; for details of these and other interactions with anticoagulants, see Appendix 1 (dabigatran etexilate, heparins, phenindione, rivaroxaban, and coumarins).

Although studies have failed to demonstrate an interaction, common experience in anticoagulant clinics is that the INR can be altered following a course of an oral broad-spectrum antibiotic, such as ampicillin p. 637 or amoxicillin p. 635.

Information on the treatment of patients who take anticoagulants is available at www.sdcep.org.uk/published-guidance/anticoagulants-and-antiplatelets/.

Liver disease

Liver disease may alter the response to drugs and drug prescribing should be kept to a minimum in patients with severe liver disease. Problems are likely mainly in patients with *jaundice, ascites,* or evidence of *encephalopathy.*

For guidance on prescribing for patients with hepatic impairment, see Prescribing in hepatic impairment p. 20. Where care is needed when prescribing in hepatic impairment, this is indicated under the relevant drug in the BNF.

Renal impairment

The use of drugs in patients with reduced renal function can give rise to many problems. Many of these problems can be avoided by reducing the dose or by using alternative drugs.

Special care is required in renal transplantation and immunosuppressed patients; if necessary such patients should be referred to specialists.

For guidance on prescribing in patients with renal impairment, see Prescribing in renal impairment p. 21. Where care is needed when prescribing in renal impairment, this is indicated under the relevant drug in the BNF.

Pregnancy

Drugs taken during pregnancy can be harmful to the fetus and should be prescribed only if the expected benefit to the mother is thought to be greater than the risk to the fetus; all drugs should be avoided if possible during the first trimester.

For guidance on prescribing in pregnancy, see Prescribing in pregnancy p. 24. Where care is needed when prescribing in pregnancy, this is indicated under the relevant drug in the BNF.

Breast-feeding

Some drugs taken by the mother whilst breast-feeding can be transferred to the breast milk, and may affect the infant.

For guidance on prescribing in breast-feeding, see Prescribing in breast-feeding p. 25. Where care is needed when prescribing in breast-feeding, this is indicated under the relevant drug in the BNF.

Chapter 1
Gastro-intestinal system

CONTENTS

1   Chronic bowel disorders
1.1   Coeliac disease

Coeliac disease
25-Jul-2016

Description of condition

Coeliac disease is an autoimmune condition which is associated with chronic inflammation of the small intestine. Dietary proteins known as gluten, which are present in wheat, barley and rye, activate an abnormal immune response in the intestinal mucosa, which can lead to malabsorption of nutrients.

Aims of treatment

The management of coeliac disease is aimed at eliminating symptoms (such as diarrhoea, bloating and abdominal pain) and reducing the risk of complications, including those resulting from malabsorption.

Non-drug treatment

EvGr The only effective treatment for coeliac disease is a strict, life-long, gluten-free diet. A range of gluten-free products is available for prescription (see *Borderline substances*). ⓐ

Drug treatment

EvGr Patients who have coeliac disease are at an increased risk of malabsorption of key nutrients (such as calcium and vitamin D). Their risk of osteoporosis and the need for active treatment of bone disease should form part of the ongoing management of coeliac disease. Supplementation of key nutrients may be required if dietary intake is insufficient.

Patients who have coeliac disease should be advised **not** to self-medicate with over-the-counter vitamins or mineral supplements. Initiation of supplementation should involve a discussion with a member of the patient's healthcare team in order to identify the individual needs of the patient and to allow for appropriate ongoing monitoring.

Confirmed cases of refractory coeliac disease should be referred to a specialist centre. Treatment with prednisolone p. 791 can be considered for initial management while awaiting specialist advice. ⓐ

Useful Resources

Coeliac disease: recognition, assessment and management. National Institute for Health and Care Excellence. Clinical guideline 20. September 2015.
www.nice.org.uk/guidance/ng20

1.2   Diverticular disease and diverticulitis

Diverticular disease and diverticulitis
20-Feb-2020

Description of condition

Diverticulosis is an asymptomatic condition characterised by the presence of diverticula (small pouches protruding from the walls of the large intestine). Its prevalence is difficult to determine but it is age dependent, with the majority of patients aged 40 years and over.

Diverticular disease is a condition where diverticula are present with symptoms such as abdominal tenderness and/or mild, intermittent lower abdominal pain with constipation, diarrhoea, or occasional large rectal bleeds. Symptoms of diverticular disease may overlap with other conditions such as Irritable bowel syndrome p. 52, colitis (bowel inflammation related to Crohn's disease p. 40, Ulcerative colitis p. 41, ischaemia or microscopic colitis), and malignancy.

Acute diverticulitis occurs when diverticula suddenly become inflamed or infected. Signs and symptoms include constant lower abdominal pain (usually severe) together with features such as fever, a sudden change in bowel habits and significant rectal bleeding, lower abdominal tenderness, or a palpable abdominal mass. **Complicated acute diverticulitis** refers to diverticulitis associated with complications such as abscess, bowel perforation and peritonitis, fistula, intestinal obstruction, haemorrhage, or sepsis. For further information on signs and symptoms of acute diverticulitis or complicated acute diverticulitis, see NICE clinical guideline: **Diverticular disease** (see *Useful resources*).

Aims of treatment

Treatment aims to relieve symptoms of diverticular disease, improve quality of life, manage episodes of acute diverticulitis, and reduce the risk of recurrence and complications.

Non drug management

[EvGr] Patients and their family and/or carers, where appropriate, should be provided with information about diet and lifestyle changes, the course of the disease and likelihood of progression, symptoms and symptom management, investigations and treatment options, and when and how to seek further medical advice.

Patients with diverticulosis or diverticular disease should be advised to eat a healthy, balanced diet including whole grains, fruit and vegetables. In patients with constipation and on a low fibre diet, a gradual increase of dietary fibre may minimise flatulence and bloating. Patients increasing dietary fibre should be advised to drink an adequate amount of fluid, especially if dehydration is a risk. Advice should also be given about the benefits of exercise, weight loss (if overweight or obese), and Smoking cessation p. 565, in reducing the risk of symptomatic disease and acute diverticulitis.

Patients with diverticular disease should also be informed that it may take several weeks for the benefits of increasing fibre in their diet to be achieved and that if a high-fibre diet is tolerated, it should be continued for life.

In patients with complicated acute diverticulitis, emergency or elective surgical management may be required. (A) For information on surgical management, see NICE clinical guideline: **Diverticular disease** (see *Useful resources*).

Drug treatment

Diverticulosis

[EvGr] As diverticulosis is an asymptomatic condition, specific treatments are not recommended. Bulk-forming laxatives can be considered for patients with constipation. (A)

Diverticular disease

[EvGr] Antibacterials are not recommended for patients with diverticular disease.

Bulk-forming laxatives should be considered when a high-fibre diet is unsuitable, or for patients with persistent constipation or diarrhoea.

Consider the use of simple analgesia such as paracetamol p. 507 in patients with ongoing abdominal pain, and antispasmodics in those with abdominal cramps. Non-steroidal anti-inflammatory drugs and opioid analgesics are not recommended as their use may increase the risk of diverticular perforation.

For patients with persistent symptoms or symptoms that do not respond to treatment, consider an alternative diagnosis. (A)

Acute diverticulitis

[EvGr] Offer simple analgesia such as paracetamol to patients with acute diverticulitis who are systemically well. Consider a watchful waiting and a no antibacterial prescribing strategy, and advise patients to re-present if symptoms persist or worsen. (A)

For guidance on antibacterial management, see *Diverticulitis, acute* in Gastro-intestinal system infections, antibacterial therapy p. 582.

[EvGr] Patients with persistent or worsening symptoms should be reassessed in primary care and considered for referral to hospital for further assessment.

Refer patients with suspected complicated acute diverticulitis and uncontrolled abdominal pain for same-day hospital assessment. Those presenting with significant rectal bleeding should be referred to hospital urgently.

Treatment with aminosalicylates or prophylactic antibacterials are not recommended to prevent recurrent acute diverticulitis. (A)

Useful Resources

Diverticular disease: diagnosis and management. National Institute for Health and Care Excellence. NICE guideline 147. November 2019.
www.nice.org.uk/guidance/ng147

1.3   Inflammatory bowel disease

Crohn's disease
25-Sep-2023

Description of condition

Crohn's disease is a chronic, inflammatory bowel disease that mainly affects the gastro-intestinal tract. It is characterised by thickened areas of the gastro-intestinal wall with inflammation extending through all layers, deep ulceration and fissuring of the mucosa, and the presence of granulomas; affected areas may occur in any part of the gastro-intestinal tract, interspersed with areas of relatively normal tissue. Crohn's disease may present as recurrent attacks, with acute exacerbations combined with periods of remission or less active disease. Symptoms depend on the site of disease but may include abdominal pain, diarrhoea, fever, weight loss and rectal bleeding.

Complications of Crohn's disease include intestinal strictures, abscesses in the wall of the intestine or adjacent structures, fistulae, anaemia, malnutrition, colorectal and small bowel cancers, and growth failure and delayed puberty in children. Crohn's disease may also be associated with extra-intestinal manifestation: the most common are arthritis and abnormalities of the joints, eyes, liver and skin. Crohn's disease is also a cause of secondary osteoporosis and those at greatest risk should be monitored for osteopenia and assessed for the risk of fractures.

Fistulating Crohn's disease

Fistulating Crohn's disease is a complication that involves the formation of a fistula between the intestine and adjacent structures, such as perianal skin, bladder, and vagina. It occurs in about one quarter of patients, mostly when the disease involves the ileocolonic area.

Aims of treatment

Treatment is largely directed at the induction and maintenance of remission and the relief of symptoms. Active treatment of acute Crohn's disease should be distinguished from preventing relapse. The aims of drug treatment are to reduce symptoms and maintain or improve quality of life, while minimising toxicity related to drugs over both the short and long term.

In fistulating Crohn's disease, surgery and medical treatment aim to close and maintain closure of the fistula.

Non-drug treatment

[EvGr] In addition to drug treatment, management options for Crohn's disease include Smoking cessation p. 565 and attention to nutrition, which plays an important role in supportive care. Surgery may be considered in certain patients with early disease limited to the distal ileum and in severe or chronic active disease. (A)

Drug treatment

Treatment of acute disease

Monotherapy

EvGr A corticosteroid (either prednisolone p. 791 or methylprednisolone p. 790 or intravenous hydrocortisone p. 787), is used to induce remission in patients with a first presentation or a single inflammatory exacerbation of Crohn's disease in a 12-month period.

In patients with distal ileal, ileocaecal or right-sided colonic disease, in whom a conventional corticosteroid is unsuitable or contra-indicated, budesonide p. 47 may be considered. Budesonide is less effective but may cause fewer side-effects than other corticosteroids, as systemic exposure is limited. Aminosalicylates (such as sulfasalazine p. 46 and mesalazine p. 43) are an alternative option in these patients. They are less effective than a corticosteroid or budesonide, but may be preferred because they have fewer side-effects. Aminosalicylates and budesonide are not appropriate for severe presentations or exacerbations. Ⓐ

Add-on treatment

EvGr Add on treatment is prescribed if there are two or more inflammatory exacerbations in a 12-month period, or the corticosteroid dose cannot be reduced.

Azathioprine p. 965 or mercaptopurine p. 1047 [unlicensed indications] can be added to a corticosteroid or budesonide to induce remission. In patients who cannot tolerate azathioprine or mercaptopurine or in whom thiopurine methyltransferase (TPMT) activity is deficient, methotrexate p. 1048 can be added to a corticosteroid.

Under specialist care, certain tumour necrosis factor alpha inhibitors may be used for the treatment of severe, active Crohn's disease, and for moderate to severely active disease, other biologics (such as certain anti-lymphocyte monoclonal antibodies or interleukin inhibitors), or certain Janus kinase inhibitors may be used. Ⓐ

Maintenance of remission

EvGr Patients who choose not to receive maintenance treatment during remission should be made aware of the symptoms that may suggest a relapse (most frequently unintended weight loss, abdominal pain, diarrhoea and general ill-health). For those who choose not to receive maintenance treatment during remission, a suitable follow up plan should be agreed upon and information provided on how to access healthcare if a relapse should occur.

Azathioprine or mercaptopurine [unlicensed indications] as monotherapy can be used to maintain remission when previously used with a corticosteroid to induce remission. They may also be used in patients who have not previously received these drugs (particularly those with adverse prognostic factors such as early age of onset, perianal disease, corticosteroid use at presentation, and severe presentations). Methotrexate can be used to maintain remission only in patients who required methotrexate to induce remission, or who are intolerant of or are not suitable for azathioprine or mercaptopurine for maintenance. Corticosteroids or budesonide should not be used. Ⓐ

Maintaining remission following surgery

EvGr Azathioprine in combination with up to 3 months' postoperative metronidazole p. 628 [unlicensed indication] should be considered to maintain remission in patients with ileocolonic Crohn's disease who have had complete macroscopic resection within the previous 3 months. Azathioprine alone should be considered for patients who cannot tolerate metronidazole p. 628. Ⓐ Aminosalicylates are no longer recommended due to the lack of clinical efficacy. NICE do not consider mercaptopurine to be a cost-effective treatment and do not recommend its use.

EvGr Biologic therapies should no longer be used to maintain remission after complete macroscopic resection of ileocolonic Crohn's disease because of limited evidence. Budesonide should also not be used in these patients. Ⓐ

Other treatments

EvGr Loperamide hydrochloride p. 74 or codeine phosphate p. 517 can be used to manage diarrhoea associated with Crohn's disease in those who do not have colitis. Ⓐ Colestyramine p. 229 is licensed for the relief of diarrhoea associated with Crohn's disease. See also Diarrhoea (acute) p. 72.

Fistulating Crohn's disease

Perianal fistulae are the most common occurrence in patients with fistulating Crohn's disease. EvGr Treatment may not be necessary for simple, asymptomatic perianal fistulae. When fistulae are symptomatic, local drainage and surgery may be required in conjunction with the medical therapy.

Metronidazole p. 628 or ciprofloxacin p. 648 [unlicensed indications], alone or in combination, can improve symptoms of fistulating Crohn's disease but complete healing occurs rarely. Metronidazole is usually given for 1 month, but no longer than 3 months because of concerns about peripheral neuropathy. Other antibacterials should be given if specifically indicated (e.g. in sepsis associated with fistulae and perianal disease) and for managing bacterial overgrowth in the small bowel.

Either azathioprine or mercaptopurine [unlicensed indications] is used to control the inflammation in fistulating Crohn's disease and they are continued for maintenance.

Infliximab p. 1275 is recommended for patients with active fistulating Crohn's disease who have not responded to conventional therapy (including antibacterials, drainage and immunosuppressive treatments), or who are intolerant of or have contra-indications to conventional therapy. Infliximab p. 1275 should be used after ensuring that all sepsis is actively draining.

Abscess drainage, fistulotomy, and seton insertion may be appropriate, particularly before infliximab treatment.

Azathioprine p. 965, mercaptopurine p. 1047, or infliximab should be continued as maintenance treatment for at least one year.

For the management of non-perianal fistulating Crohn's disease (including entero-gynaecological and enterovesical fistulae) surgery is the only recommended approach. Ⓐ

Useful Resources

Crohn's disease: management. National Institute for Health and Care Excellence. Clinical guideline 129. May 2019. www.nice.org.uk/guidance/ng129

Ulcerative colitis

03-May-2024

Description of condition

Ulcerative colitis is a chronic inflammatory condition, characterised by diffuse mucosal inflammation—it has a relapsing-remitting pattern. It is a life-long disease that is associated with significant morbidity. It most commonly presents between the ages of 15 and 25 years, although diagnosis can be made at any age.

The pattern of inflammation is continuous, extending from the rectum upwards to a varying degree. Inflammation of the rectum is referred to as **proctitis**, and inflammation of the rectum and sigmoid colon as **proctosigmoiditis**. **Left-sided colitis** refers to disease involving the colon distal to the splenic flexure. **Extensive colitis** affects the colon proximal to the splenic flexure, and includes pan-colitis, where the whole colon is involved. Common symptoms of active disease or relapse include bloody diarrhoea, an urgent need to defaecate, and abdominal pain.

Complications associated with ulcerative colitis include an increased risk of colorectal cancer, secondary osteoporosis, venous thromboembolism, and toxic megacolon.

Aims of treatment

Treatment is focused on treating active disease to manage symptoms and to induce and maintain remission.

Drug treatment

Overview

Management of ulcerative colitis is dependent on factors such as clinical severity, extent of disease, and patient preference. Clinical and laboratory investigations are used to determine the extent and severity of disease and to guide treatment. Severity is classified as mild, moderate or severe by using the Truelove and Witts' Severity Index to assess bowel movements, heart rate, erythrocyte sedimentation rate and the presence of pyrexia, melaena or anaemia—see the NICE guideline for Ulcerative Colitis for further information (see *Useful resources*).

[EvGr] The extent of disease should be considered when choosing the route of administration for aminosalicylates and corticosteroids; whether oral treatment, topical treatment or both are to be used. If the inflammation is distal, a rectal preparation is adequate but if the inflammation is extended, systemic medication is required. Either suppositories or enemas can be offered, taking into account the patient's preferences. (A)

[EvGr] Rectal foam preparations and suppositories can be used when patients have difficulty retaining liquid enemas.

Diarrhoea associated with ulcerative colitis is sometimes treated with anti-diarrhoeal drugs (such as loperamide hydrochloride p. 74 or codeine phosphate p. 517) on the advice of a specialist; however their use is contra-indicated in acute ulcerative colitis as they can increase the risk of toxic megacolon.

A macrogol-containing osmotic laxative (such as macrogol 3350 with potassium chloride, sodium bicarbonate and sodium chloride p. 62) may be useful for proximal faecal loading in proctitis. (E)

Oral aminosalicylates for the treatment of ulcerative colitis are available in different preparations and release forms. [EvGr] The preparation and dosing schedule should be chosen taking into account the delivery characteristics and suitability for the patient. When used to maintain remission, single daily doses of oral aminosalicylates can be more effective than multiple daily dosing, but may result in more side-effects.

The duration of corticosteroid course (usually 4 to 8 weeks) depends on the corticosteroid chosen. (A)

Treatment of acute mild-to-moderate ulcerative colitis

Proctitis

[EvGr] A topical aminosalicylate is recommended as first-line treatment for patients with a mild-to-moderate initial presentation or inflammatory exacerbation of proctitis. If remission is not achieved within 4 weeks, adding an oral aminosalicylate should be considered. If response remains inadequate, consider addition of a topical or an oral corticosteroid for 4 to 8 weeks.

Monotherapy with an oral aminosalicylate can be considered for patients who prefer not to use enemas or suppositories, although this may not be as effective. If remission is not achieved within 4 weeks, adding a topical or an oral corticosteroid for 4 to 8 weeks should be considered.

A topical or an oral corticosteroid for 4 to 8 weeks should be considered for patients in whom aminosalicylates are unsuitable. (A)

Proctosigmoiditis and left-sided ulcerative colitis

[EvGr] A topical aminosalicylate is recommended as first-line treatment for patients with a mild-to-moderate initial presentation or inflammatory exacerbation of proctosigmoiditis or left-sided ulcerative colitis. If remission is not achieved within 4 weeks, consider adding a high-dose oral aminosalicylate, or switching to a high-dose oral aminosalicylate and 4 to 8 weeks of a topical corticosteroid.

If response remains inadequate, stop topical treatment and offer an oral aminosalicylate and 4 to 8 weeks of an oral corticosteroid.

Monotherapy with a high-dose oral aminosalicylate can be considered for patients who prefer not to use enemas or suppositories, although this may not be as effective. If remission is not achieved within 4 weeks, an oral corticosteroid for 4 to 8 weeks in addition to the high-dose aminosalicylate should be offered.

A topical or an oral corticosteroid for 4 to 8 weeks should be considered for patients in whom aminosalicylates are unsuitable. (A)

Extensive ulcerative colitis

[EvGr] A topical aminosalicylate and a high-dose oral aminosalicylate are recommended as first-line treatment for patients with a mild-to-moderate initial presentation or inflammatory exacerbation of extensive ulcerative colitis. If remission is not achieved within 4 weeks, stop topical aminosalicylate treatment and offer a high-dose oral aminosalicylate and 4 to 8 weeks of an oral corticosteroid. An oral corticosteroid for 4 to 8 weeks should be considered for patients in whom aminosalicylates are unsuitable. (A)

Treatment of acute moderate-to-severe ulcerative colitis

[EvGr] Under specialist care, certain Janus kinase inhibitors, sphingosine-1-phosphate receptor modulators, and biological drugs (such as anti-lymphocyte monoclonal antibodies, interleukin inhibitors, and tumor necrosis factor alpha (TNF-a) inhibitors) may be used for the treatment of moderate-to-severe active ulcerative colitis. (A)

Treatment of acute severe ulcerative colitis

Acute severe ulcerative colitis of any extent can be life-threatening and is regarded as a medical emergency. [EvGr] Immediate hospital admission is required for treatment.

Intravenous corticosteroids (such as hydrocortisone p. 787 or methylprednisolone p. 790) should be given to induce remission in patients with acute severe ulcerative colitis (at first presentation or an exacerbation) while assessing the need for surgery. If intravenous corticosteroids are contra-indicated, declined or cannot be tolerated, then intravenous ciclosporin p. 966 [unlicensed indication] or surgery should be considered. A combination of intravenous ciclosporin with intravenous corticosteroids, or surgery is second line therapy for patients who have little or no improvement within 72 hours of starting intravenous corticosteroids or whose symptoms worsen despite treatment.

Infliximab p. 1275 can be used to treat acute exacerbations of severely active ulcerative colitis if ciclosporin is contra-indicated or clinically inappropriate. (A)

[EvGr] In patients who experience an initial response to steroids followed by deterioration, stool cultures should be taken to exclude the presence of pathogens; cytomegalovirus activation should be considered. (E)

Maintaining remission in mild, moderate or severe ulcerative colitis

[EvGr] To reduce the chances of relapse occurring, maintenance therapy with an aminosalicylate is recommended in most patients. Corticosteroids are **not** suitable for maintenance treatment because of their side-effects.

After a mild-to-moderate inflammatory exacerbation of *proctitis* or *proctosigmoiditis*, a rectal aminosalicylate can be started alone or in combination with an oral aminosalicylate, administered daily or as part of an intermittent regimen (such as twice to three times weekly or the first seven days of each month). An oral aminosalicylate can be used alone in patients who prefer not to use enemas or suppositories, although this may not be as effective.

A low-dose of oral aminosalicylate is given to maintain remission in patients after a mild-to-moderate inflammatory exacerbation of left-sided or extensive ulcerative colitis.

1

Gastro-intestinal system

When used to maintain remission, single daily doses of oral aminosalicylates can be more effective than multiple daily dosing, but may result in more side-effects.

Oral azathioprine p. 965 or mercaptopurine p. 1047 [unlicensed indications] can be considered to maintain remission, if there has been two or more inflammatory exacerbations in a 12-month period that required treatment with systemic corticosteroids, or if remission is not maintained by aminosalicylates, or following a single acute severe episode. Ⓐ

There is no evidence to support the use of methotrexate p. 1048 to induce or maintain remission in ulcerative colitis, though its use is common in clinical practice.

Treatment with certain Janus kinase inhibitors, sphingosine-1-phosphate receptor modulators, anti-lymphocyte monoclonal antibodies, interleukin inhibitors, and tumor necrosis factor alpha (TNF-a) inhibitors may be continued into the maintenance phase.

Non-drug treatment

EvGr Surgery may be necessary as emergency treatment for severe ulcerative colitis that does not respond to drug treatment. Patients can also choose to have elective surgery for unresponsive or frequently relapsing disease that is affecting their quality of life. Ⓐ

Useful Resources

Ulcerative colitis: management. National Institute for Health and Care Excellence. Clinical guideline 130. May 2019.
www.nice.org.uk/guidance/NG130

> **Other drugs used for Inflammatory bowel disease**
> Adalimumab, p. 1269 · Filgotinib, p. 1263 · Golimumab, p. 1274 · Ozanimod, p. 988 · Risankizumab, p. 1427 · Tofacitinib, p. 1265 · Upadacitinib, p. 1267 · Ustekinumab, p. 1260

AMINOSALICYLATES

Aminosalicylates 🏴

- **SIDE-EFFECTS**
- ▸ **Common or very common** Arthralgia · cough · diarrhoea · dizziness · fever · gastrointestinal discomfort · headache · leucopenia · nausea · proteinuria · skin reactions · vomiting
- ▸ **Uncommon** Alopecia · depression · dyspnoea · myalgia · pancreatitis · paraesthesia · photosensitivity reaction · thrombocytopenia
- ▸ **Rare or very rare** Agranulocytosis · blood disorder · bone marrow disorders · cardiac inflammation · hepatitis · nephrotic syndrome · neutropenia · peripheral neuropathy · renal impairment · respiratory disorders
- ▸ **Frequency not known** Angioedema · eosinophilia · haematuria · haemolytic anaemia · interstitial lung disease · lupus-like syndrome · nephritis tubulointerstitial · oligozoospermia (reversible) · severe cutaneous adverse reactions (SCARs) · ulcerative colitis aggravated

  SIDE-EFFECTS, FURTHER INFORMATION A blood count should be performed and the drug stopped immediately if there is suspicion of a blood dyscrasia.

- **ALLERGY AND CROSS-SENSITIVITY** EvGr Contra-indicated in salicylate hypersensitivity Ⓜ.
- **MONITORING REQUIREMENTS** Renal function should be monitored before starting an oral aminosalicylate, at 3 months of treatment, and then annually during treatment.
- **PATIENT AND CARER ADVICE**
  Blood disorders Patients receiving aminosalicylates, and their carers, should be advised to report any unexplained bleeding, bruising, purpura, sore throat, fever or malaise that occurs during treatment.

◄ above

Balsalazide sodium
24-Jun-2021

- **INDICATIONS AND DOSE**

Treatment of mild to moderate ulcerative colitis, acute attack
- ▸ BY MOUTH
- ▸ Adult: 2.25 g 3 times a day until remission occurs or for up to maximum of 12 weeks

Maintenance of remission of ulcerative colitis
- ▸ BY MOUTH
- ▸ Adult: 1.5 g twice daily (max. per dose 3 g), adjusted according to response; maximum 6 g per day

- **CAUTIONS** History of asthma
- **INTERACTIONS** → Appendix 1: balsalazide
- **SIDE-EFFECTS** Cholelithiasis
- **PREGNANCY** Manufacturer advises avoid.
- **BREAST FEEDING** Diarrhoea may develop in the infant. **Monitoring** Monitor breast-fed infants for diarrhoea.
- **HEPATIC IMPAIRMENT** Manufacturer advises caution; avoid in severe impairment (no information available).
- **RENAL IMPAIRMENT** EvGr Use with caution in mild impairment; avoid in moderate to severe impairment. Ⓜ

- **MEDICINAL FORMS** There can be variation in the licensing of different medicines containing the same drug.
  Oral capsule
  CAUTIONARY AND ADVISORY LABELS 21, 25
  - ▸ **Colazide** (Almirall Ltd)
    Balsalazide disodium 750 mg Colazide 750mg capsules | 130 capsule PoM £30.42 DT = £30.42

◄ above

Mesalazine
22-Nov-2023

- **INDICATIONS AND DOSE**
  DOSE EQUIVALENCE AND CONVERSION
  There is no evidence to show that any one oral preparation of mesalazine is more effective than another; however, the delivery characteristics of oral mesalazine preparations may vary.

  ASACOL® MR 400MG TABLETS

Treatment of mild to moderate ulcerative colitis, acute attack
- ▸ BY MOUTH
- ▸ Child 12-17 years: 800 mg 3 times a day
- ▸ Adult: 2.4 g daily in divided doses

Maintenance of remission of ulcerative colitis and Crohn's ileo-colitis
- ▸ BY MOUTH
- ▸ Child 12-17 years: 400–800 mg 2–3 times a day
- ▸ Adult: 1.2–2.4 g daily in divided doses

  ASACOL® MR 800MG TABLETS

Treatment of mild to moderate ulcerative colitis, acute attack
- ▸ BY MOUTH
- ▸ Adult: 2.4–4.8 g daily in divided doses

Maintenance of remission of ulcerative colitis
- ▸ BY MOUTH
- ▸ Adult: Up to 2.4 g once daily, alternatively up to 2.4 g daily in divided doses

Maintenance of remission of Crohn's ileo-colitis
- ▸ BY MOUTH
- ▸ Adult: Up to 2.4 g daily in divided doses   continued →

ASACOL® FOAM ENEMA

Treatment of acute attack of mild to moderate ulcerative colitis affecting the rectosigmoid region
- BY RECTUM
- Adult: 1 g daily for 4–6 weeks, to be administered into the rectum

Treatment of acute attack of mild to moderate ulcerative colitis, affecting the descending colon
- BY RECTUM
- Adult: 2 g once daily for 4–6 weeks, to be administered into the rectum

ASACOL® SUPPOSITORIES

Treatment of acute attack of mild to moderate ulcerative colitis and maintenance of remission
- BY RECTUM
- Adult: 0.75–1.5 g daily in divided doses, last dose to be administered at bedtime

MEZAVANT® XL

Treatment of mild to moderate ulcerative colitis, acute attack
- BY MOUTH
- Adult: 2.4 g once daily, increased if necessary to 4.8 g once daily, review treatment at 8 weeks

Maintenance of remission of ulcerative colitis
- BY MOUTH
- Adult: 2.4 g once daily

OCTASA® MR 1600MG TABLETS

Treatment of mild to moderate ulcerative colitis, acute attack
- BY MOUTH
- Adult: Up to 4.8 g once daily, dose to be adjusted according to response, alternatively up to 4.8 g daily in 2–3 divided doses, dose to be adjusted according to response

Maintenance of remission of ulcerative colitis
- BY MOUTH
- Adult: 1.6 g once daily

OCTASA® MR 400MG AND 800MG TABLETS

Treatment of mild to moderate ulcerative colitis, acute attack
- BY MOUTH
- Adult: 2.4–4.8 g daily in divided doses, alternatively dose of 2.4 g daily may be given as a single dose

Maintenance of remission of ulcerative colitis and Crohn's ileo-colitis
- BY MOUTH
- Adult: 1.2–2.4 g once daily, alternatively 1.2–2.4 g daily in divided doses

OCTASA® SUPPOSITORIES

Treatment of mild to moderate ulcerative proctitis, acute attack | Maintenance of remission of ulcerative proctitis
- BY RECTUM
- Adult: 1 g once daily, to be administered preferably at bedtime

PENTASA® GRANULES

Treatment of mild to moderate ulcerative colitis, acute attack
- BY MOUTH
- Child 5-17 years (body-weight up to 40 kg): 10–20 mg/kg 3 times a day
- Child 5-17 years (body-weight 40 kg and above): 1–2 g twice daily, total daily dose may alternatively be given in 3–4 divided doses
- Adult: Up to 4 g once daily, alternatively up to 4 g daily in 2–4 divided doses

Maintenance of remission of ulcerative colitis
- BY MOUTH
- Child 5-17 years (body-weight up to 40 kg): 7.5–15 mg/kg twice daily, total daily dose may alternatively be given in 3 divided doses
- Child 5-17 years (body-weight 40 kg and above): 2 g once daily
- Adult: 2 g once daily

PENTASA® RETENTION ENEMA

Treatment of acute attack of mild to moderate ulcerative colitis or maintenance of remission
- BY RECTUM
- Adult: 1 g once daily, dose to be administered at bedtime

Treatment of acute attack of mild to moderate ulcerative colitis affecting the rectosigmoid region
- BY RECTUM
- Child 12-17 years: 1 g once daily, dose to be administered at bedtime

PENTASA® SUPPOSITORIES

Treatment of acute attack, ulcerative proctitis
- BY RECTUM
- Adult: 1 g daily for 2–4 weeks

Maintenance, ulcerative proctitis
- BY RECTUM
- Adult: 1 g daily

PENTASA® TABLETS

Treatment of mild to moderate ulcerative colitis, acute attack
- BY MOUTH
- Adult: Up to 4 g once daily, alternatively up to 4 g daily in 2–3 divided doses

Maintenance of remission of ulcerative colitis
- BY MOUTH
- Adult: 2 g once daily

SALOFALK® ENEMA

Treatment of acute attack of mild to moderate ulcerative colitis or maintenance of remission
- BY RECTUM
- Adult: 2 g once daily, dose to be administered at bedtime

SALOFALK® GRANULES

Treatment of mild to moderate ulcerative colitis, acute attack
- BY MOUTH
- Child 5-17 years (body-weight up to 40 kg): 30–50 mg/kg once daily, dose preferably given in the morning, alternatively 10–20 mg/kg 3 times a day
- Child 5-17 years (body-weight 40 kg and above): 1.5–3 g once daily, dose preferably given in the morning, alternatively 0.5–1 g 3 times a day
- Adult: 1.5–3 g once daily, dose preferably taken in the morning, alternatively 0.5–1 g 3 times a day

Maintenance of remission of ulcerative colitis
- BY MOUTH
- Child 5-17 years (body-weight up to 40 kg): 7.5–15 mg/kg twice daily, total daily dose may alternatively be given in 3 divided doses
- Child 5-17 years (body-weight 40 kg and above): 500 mg 3 times a day
- Adult: 500 mg 3 times a day

SALOFALK ® RECTAL FOAM

Treatment of mild ulcerative colitis affecting sigmoid colon and rectum

▸ BY RECTUM

▸ Child 12-17 years: 2 g once daily, dose to be administered into the rectum at bedtime, alternatively 2 g daily in 2 divided doses

▸ Adult: 2 g once daily, dose to be administered into the rectum at bedtime, alternatively 2 g daily in 2 divided doses

SALOFALK ® SUPPOSITORIES

Treatment of acute attack of mild to moderate ulcerative colitis affecting the rectum

▸ BY RECTUM

▸ Adult: 0.5–1 g 2–3 times a day, adjusted according to response, dose to be given using 500 mg suppositories, alternatively 1 g once daily, preferably at bedtime, dose to be given using 1 g suppositories

SALOFALK ® TABLETS

Treatment of mild to moderate ulcerative colitis, acute attack

▸ BY MOUTH

▸ Child 5-17 years (body-weight up to 40 kg): 10–20 mg/kg 3 times a day

▸ Child 5-17 years (body-weight 40 kg and above): 0.5–1 g 3 times a day

▸ Adult: 0.5–1 g 3 times a day

Maintenance of remission of ulcerative colitis

▸ BY MOUTH

▸ Child 5-17 years (body-weight up to 40 kg): 7.5–15 mg/kg twice daily, total daily dose may alternatively be given in 3 divided doses

▸ Child 5-17 years (body-weight 40 kg and above): 500 mg 3 times a day

▸ Adult: 500 mg 3 times a day

● **UNLICENSED USE**

▸ With oral use in children *Asacol* ® (all preparations) not licensed for use in children under 18 years. *Pentasa* ® granules and *Salofalk* ® tablets and granules not licensed for use in children under 6 years.

▸ With rectal use in children *Salofalk* ® rectal foam no dose recommendations for children (age range not specified by manufacturer).

● **CONTRA-INDICATIONS**

▸ With oral use Blood clotting abnormalities

● **CAUTIONS** Elderly · maintain adequate fluid intake · pulmonary disease

● **INTERACTIONS** → Appendix 1: mesalazine

● **SIDE-EFFECTS**

GENERAL SIDE-EFFECTS

▸ **Uncommon** Flatulence

▸ **Rare or very rare** Nephritis · pulmonary fibrosis

▸ **Frequency not known** Nephrolithiasis

SPECIFIC SIDE-EFFECTS

▸ **Uncommon**

▸ With oral use Chest pain · hepatic disorders

▸ **Rare or very rare**

▸ With oral use Asthenia

▸ With rectal use Cholestasis exacerbated · constipation

▸ **Frequency not known**

▸ With oral use Condition aggravated · ketonuria · weight decreased

SIDE-EFFECTS, FURTHER INFORMATION Discontinue immediately if symptoms of acute intolerance syndrome occur such as abdominal pain, fever, severe headache and rash. Worsening abdominal pain and diarrhoea may be difficult to distinguish from an exacerbation of ulcerative colitis.

● **PREGNANCY** Negligible quantities cross placenta.

● **BREAST FEEDING** Diarrhoea reported in breast-fed infants, but negligible amounts of mesalazine detected in breast milk.

Monitoring Monitor breast-fed infant for diarrhoea.

● **HEPATIC IMPAIRMENT** Manufacturer advises caution in mild to moderate impairment; avoid in severe impairment.

● **RENAL IMPAIRMENT** EvGr Use with caution in mild to moderate impairment (risk of toxicity including crystalluria); avoid in severe impairment. ⬧

● **DIRECTIONS FOR ADMINISTRATION**

PENTASA ® **GRANULES** Manufacturer advises granules should be placed on tongue and washed down with water or orange juice without chewing.

▸ In children Expert sources advise contents of one sachet should be weighed and divided immediately before use; discard any remaining granules.

PENTASA ® **TABLETS** Manufacturer advises tablets may be halved, quartered, or dispersed in water, but should not be chewed.

SALOFALK ® **GRANULES** Manufacturer advises granules should be placed on tongue and washed down with water without chewing.

● **PRESCRIBING AND DISPENSING INFORMATION** There is no evidence to show that any one oral preparation of mesalazine is more effective than another; however, the delivery characteristics of oral mesalazine preparations may vary.

Flavours of granule formulations of *Salofalk* ® may include vanilla.

● **PATIENT AND CARER ADVICE** If it is necessary to switch a patient to a different brand of mesalazine, the patient should be advised to report any changes in symptoms. Some products may require special administration advice; patients and carers should be informed.

Medicines for Children leaflet: Mesalazine (oral) for inflammatory bowel disease www.medicinesforchildren.org.uk/medicines/mesalazine-oral-for-inflammatory-bowel-disease/

Medicines for Children leaflet: Mesalazine foam enema for inflammatory bowel disease www.medicinesforchildren.org.uk/medicines/mesalazine-foam-enema-for-inflammatory-bowel-disease/

Medicines for Children leaflet: Mesalazine liquid enema for inflammatory bowel disease www.medicinesforchildren.org.uk/medicines/mesalazine-liquid-enema-for-inflammatory-bowel-disease/

● **MEDICINAL FORMS** There can be variation in the licensing of different medicines containing the same drug.

Modified-release tablet

CAUTIONARY AND ADVISORY LABELS 21(does not apply to Pentasa ® tablets), 25 (does not apply to Pentasa ® tablets)

▸ **Mezavant XL** (Takeda UK Ltd)

Mesalazine 1.2 gram Mezavant XL 1200mg tablets | 60 tablet PoM £42.95 DT = £42.95

▸ **Pentasa** (Ferring Pharmaceuticals Ltd)

Mesalazine 500 mg Pentasa 500mg modified-release tablets | 100 tablet PoM £30.74 DT = £30.74

Mesalazine 1 gram Pentasa 1g modified-release tablets | 60 tablet PoM £36.89 DT = £36.89

Gastro-resistant tablet

CAUTIONARY AND ADVISORY LABELS 5, 25

▸ **Asacol** (AbbVie Ltd)

Mesalazine 800 mg Asacol 800mg MR gastro-resistant tablets | 84 tablet PoM £54.90 DT = £54.90

▸ **Octasa MR** (Tillotts Pharma UK Ltd)

Mesalazine 400 mg Octasa 400mg MR gastro-resistant tablets | 90 tablet PoM £19.50 DT = £19.50 | 120 tablet PoM £26.00

Mesalazine 800 mg Octasa 800mg MR gastro-resistant tablets | 90 tablet PoM £40.38 | 180 tablet PoM £80.75 DT = £80.75

Mesalazine 1.6 gram Octasa 1600mg MR gastro-resistant tablets | 30 tablet PoM £30.08 DT = £30.08

1 Gastro-intestinal system

▶ **Salofalk** (Dr. Falk Pharma UK Ltd)
Mesalazine 500 mg Salofalk 500mg gastro-resistant tablets |
100 tablet PoM £32.38 DT = £32.38

Suppository
▶ **Octasa** (Tillotts Pharma UK Ltd)
Mesalazine 1 gram Octasa 1g suppositories | 30 suppository PoM
£29.62
▶ **Pentasa** (Ferring Pharmaceuticals Ltd)
Mesalazine 1 gram Pentasa 1g suppositories | 28 suppository PoM
£40.01 DT = £40.01
▶ **Salofalk** (Dr. Falk Pharma UK Ltd)
Mesalazine 500 mg Salofalk 500mg suppositories |
30 suppository PoM £14.81 DT = £14.81
Mesalazine 1 gram Salofalk 1g suppositories | 30 suppository PoM
£29.62

Rectal foam
EXCIPIENTS: May contain Cetostearyl alcohol (including cetyl and
stearyl alcohol), disodium edetate, hydroxybenzoates (parabens),
polysorbates, propylene glycol, sodium metabisulfite
▶ **Salofalk** (Dr. Falk Pharma UK Ltd)
Mesalazine 1 gram per 1 application Salofalk 1g/application foam
enema | 14 actuation PoM £30.17 DT = £30.17

Modified-release granules
CAUTIONARY AND ADVISORY LABELS 25 (does not apply to Pentasa ®
granules)
EXCIPIENTS: May contain Aspartame
▶ **Pentasa** (Ferring Pharmaceuticals Ltd)
Mesalazine 1 gram Pentasa 1g modified-release granules sachets |
50 sachet PoM £30.74 DT = £30.74 SF
Mesalazine 2 gram Pentasa 2g modified-release granules sachets |
60 sachet PoM £73.78 DT = £73.78 SF
▶ **Salofalk** (Dr. Falk Pharma UK Ltd)
Mesalazine 1 gram Salofalk 1g gastro-resistant modified-release
granules sachets | 50 sachet PoM £28.74 DT = £28.74 SF
Mesalazine 1.5 gram Salofalk 1.5g gastro-resistant modified-release
granules sachets | 60 sachet PoM £48.85 DT = £48.85 SF
Mesalazine 3 gram Salofalk 3g gastro-resistant modified-release
granules sachets | 60 sachet PoM £97.70 DT = £97.70 SF

Enema
▶ **Pentasa** (Ferring Pharmaceuticals Ltd)
Mesalazine 10 mg per 1 ml Pentasa Mesalazine 1g/100ml enema |
7 enema PoM £17.73 DT = £17.73
▶ **Salofalk** (Dr. Falk Pharma UK Ltd)
Mesalazine 33.9 mg per 1 ml Salofalk 2g/59ml enema |
7 enema PoM £29.92 DT = £29.92

⊩ 43

Olsalazine sodium
24-Jun-2021

● INDICATIONS AND DOSE
Treatment of acute attack of mild ulcerative colitis
▶ BY MOUTH
▶ Adult: 1 g daily in divided doses, doses to be taken after
meals, then increased if necessary up to 3 g daily in
divided doses (max. per dose 1 g), dose to be increased
over 1 week

Maintenance of remission of mild ulcerative colitis
▶ BY MOUTH
▶ Adult: Maintenance 500 mg twice daily, dose to be
taken after food

● **SIDE-EFFECTS**
▶ **Uncommon** Tachycardia
▶ **Frequency not known** Palpitations · vision blurred

● **PREGNANCY** Manufacturer advises avoid unless potential
benefit outweighs risk.

● **BREAST FEEDING**
Monitoring Monitor breast-fed infants for diarrhoea.

● **RENAL IMPAIRMENT** EvGr Use with caution in mild to
moderate impairment; avoid in significant impairment.
Ⓜ

● **DIRECTIONS FOR ADMINISTRATION** Expert sources advise
capsules can be opened and contents sprinkled on food.

● **MEDICINAL FORMS** There can be variation in the licensing of
different medicines containing the same drug. Forms available
from special-order manufacturers include: oral suspension, oral
solution

Oral tablet
CAUTIONARY AND ADVISORY LABELS 21
▶ **Olsalazine sodium (Non-proprietary)**
Olsalazine sodium 500 mg Olsalazine 500mg tablets |
60 tablet PoM £161.00 DT = £161.00

Oral capsule
CAUTIONARY AND ADVISORY LABELS 21
▶ **Olsalazine sodium (Non-proprietary)**
Olsalazine sodium 250 mg Olsalazine 250mg capsules |
112 capsule PoM £144.00 DT = £144.00

⊩ 43

Sulfasalazine
24-Jun-2021
(Sulphasalazine)

● INDICATIONS AND DOSE
**Treatment of acute attack of mild to moderate and severe
ulcerative colitis | Active Crohn's disease**
▶ BY MOUTH
▶ Adult: 1–2 g 4 times a day until remission occurs,
corticosteroids may also be given, if necessary
▶ BY RECTUM
▶ Adult: 0.5–1 g twice daily, administered alone or in
conjunction with oral therapy, morning and night after
a bowel movement

**Maintenance of remission of mild to moderate and severe
ulcerative colitis**
▶ BY MOUTH
▶ Adult: 500 mg 4 times a day
▶ BY RECTUM
▶ Adult: 0.5–1 g twice daily, administered alone or in
conjunction with oral therapy, morning and night after
a bowel movement

**Active rheumatoid arthritis (administered on expert
advice)**
▶ BY MOUTH
▶ Adult: Initially 500 mg daily, increased in steps of
500 mg every week, increased to 2–3 g daily in divided
doses, enteric coated tablets to be administered

> **IMPORTANT SAFETY INFORMATION**
> **SAFE PRACTICE**
> Sulfasalazine has been confused with sulfadiazine; care
> must be taken to ensure the correct drug is prescribed
> and dispensed.

● **CAUTIONS** Acute porphyrias p. 1202 · G6PD deficiency ·
history of allergy · history of asthma · maintain adequate
fluid intake · risk of haematological toxicity · risk of hepatic
toxicity · slow acetylator status

● **INTERACTIONS** → Appendix 1: sulfasalazine

● **SIDE-EFFECTS**

GENERAL SIDE-EFFECTS
▶ **Common or very common** Insomnia · stomatitis · taste
altered · tinnitus
▶ **Uncommon** Face oedema · seizure · vasculitis · vertigo
▶ **Frequency not known** Anaemia · appetite decreased · ataxia
· crystalluria · cyanosis · encephalopathy · hallucination ·
hepatic failure · hypoprothrombinaemia ·
lymphadenopathy · macrocytosis · meningitis aseptic ·
methaemoglobinaemia · parotitis · periorbital oedema ·
pseudomembranous enterocolitis · serum sickness · smell
disorders · systemic lupus erythematosus (SLE) · yellow
discolouration of body fluids

SPECIFIC SIDE-EFFECTS
▶ With oral use Urine discolouration

1

Gastro-intestinal system

SIDE-EFFECTS, FURTHER INFORMATION Incidence of side-effects increases with higher doses.

Blood disorders Haematological abnormalities occur usually in the first 3 to 6 months of treatment—discontinue if these occur.

- **PREGNANCY** Theoretical risk of neonatal haemolysis in third trimester; adequate folate supplements should be given to mother.

- **BREAST FEEDING** Small amounts in milk (1 report of bloody diarrhoea); theoretical risk of neonatal haemolysis especially in G6PD-deficient infants.

- **HEPATIC IMPAIRMENT** Manufacturer advises caution.

- **RENAL IMPAIRMENT** [EvGr] Use with caution in mild to moderate impairment (risk of toxicity including crystalluria); avoid in severe impairment. Ⓜ

- **MONITORING REQUIREMENTS**
- Blood disorders Close monitoring of full blood counts (including differential white cell count and platelet count) is necessary initially, and at monthly intervals during the first 3 months.
- Renal function Although the manufacturer recommends renal function tests in rheumatic diseases, evidence of practical value is unsatisfactory.
- Liver function Liver function tests should be performed at monthly intervals for first 3 months.

- **PATIENT AND CARER ADVICE**
Contact lenses Some soft contact lenses may be stained.

- **MEDICINAL FORMS** There can be variation in the licensing of different medicines containing the same drug. Forms available from special-order manufacturers include: oral suspension

Oral tablet
CAUTIONARY AND ADVISORY LABELS 14
- **Sulfasalazine (Non-proprietary)**
  Sulfasalazine 500 mg Sulfasalazine 500mg tablets | 112 tablet [PoM] £14.42 DT = £5.13
- **Salazopyrin** (Pfizer Ltd)
  Sulfasalazine 500 mg Salazopyrin 500mg tablets | 112 tablet [PoM] £6.97 DT = £5.13

Oral suspension
CAUTIONARY AND ADVISORY LABELS 14
EXCIPIENTS: May contain Alcohol
- **Sulfasalazine (Non-proprietary)**
  Sulfasalazine 50 mg per 1 ml Sulfasalazine 250mg/5ml oral suspension sugar free | 500 ml [PoM] £63.56–£147.00 DT = £147.00 [SF]

Gastro-resistant tablet
CAUTIONARY AND ADVISORY LABELS 5, 14, 25
- **Sulfasalazine (Non-proprietary)**
  Sulfasalazine 500 mg Sulfasalazine 500mg gastro-resistant tablets | 112 tablet [PoM] £70.17 DT = £21.76
- **Salazopyrin EN** (Pfizer Ltd)
  Sulfasalazine 500 mg Salazopyrin EN-Tabs 500mg | 112 tablet [PoM] £8.43 DT = £21.76

Suppository
CAUTIONARY AND ADVISORY LABELS 14
- **Sulfasalazine (Non-proprietary)**
  Sulfasalazine 500 mg Sulfasalazine 500mg suppositories | 10 suppository [PoM] £3.30 DT = £3.30
- **Salazopyrin** (Pfizer Ltd)
  Sulfasalazine 500 mg Salazopyrin 500mg suppositories | 10 suppository [PoM] £3.30 DT = £3.30

CORTICOSTEROIDS

▼ 783

Beclometasone dipropionate
08-Oct-2024
(Beclomethasone dipropionate)

- **INDICATIONS AND DOSE**
Adjunct to aminosalicylates in acute mild to moderate ulcerative colitis
- BY MOUTH
- Adult: 5 mg once daily maximum duration of treatment of 4 weeks, dose to be taken in the morning

- **INTERACTIONS** → Appendix 1: corticosteroids
- **SIDE-EFFECTS**
- **Uncommon** Constipation · idiopathic intracranial hypertension · muscle cramps
- **HEPATIC IMPAIRMENT** Manufacturer advises avoid in severe impairment (no information available).

- **MEDICINAL FORMS** There can be variation in the licensing of different medicines containing the same drug.
Modified-release tablet
CAUTIONARY AND ADVISORY LABELS 25
- **Clipper** (Chiesi Ltd)
  Beclometasone dipropionate 5 mg Clipper 5mg gastro-resistant modified-release tablets | 30 tablet [PoM] £56.56 DT = £56.56

▼ 783

Budesonide
10-Feb-2025

- **DRUG ACTION** Budesonide is a glucocorticoid, which exerts significant local anti-inflammatory effects.

- **INDICATIONS AND DOSE**
Microscopic colitis, induction of remission
- BY MOUTH USING MODIFIED-RELEASE CAPSULES
- Adult: 9 mg once daily, to be taken in the morning, when stopping treatment, consider reducing dose for the last 2–4 weeks of therapy

Microscopic colitis, maintenance
- BY MOUTH USING MODIFIED-RELEASE CAPSULES
- Adult: 6 mg once daily, to be taken in the morning, alternatively, the lowest effective dose should be given, when stopping treatment, consider reducing dose for the last 2–4 weeks of therapy

Mild to moderate Crohn's disease affecting the ileum and/or ascending colon
- BY MOUTH USING MODIFIED-RELEASE CAPSULES
- Adult: 9 mg once daily for up to 8 weeks, to be taken in the morning, when stopping treatment, reduce dose for the last 2–4 weeks of therapy

BUDENOFALK SUPPOSITORIES ®

Treatment of mild-to-moderate acute ulcerative proctitis
- BY RECTUM
- Adult: 4 mg once daily for up to 8 weeks, to be administered at bedtime

BUDENOFALK ® **CAPSULES**

Mild to moderate Crohn's disease affecting the ileum and/or ascending colon
- BY MOUTH
- Adult: 9 mg once daily for up to 8 weeks, to be taken in the morning, alternatively 3 mg 3 times a day for up to 8 weeks, reduce dose gradually over 2 weeks following treatment course before stopping

Microscopic colitis, induction of remission
- BY MOUTH
- Adult: 9 mg once daily for up to 8 weeks, to be taken in the morning, reduce dose gradually over 2 weeks following treatment course before stopping continued →

Microscopic colitis, maintenance
▶ BY MOUTH
▶ Adult: 6 mg once daily, to be taken in the morning, alternatively 6 mg once daily and 3 mg once daily, to be taken on alternate mornings, review treatment regularly and no later than 12 months after initiation of maintenance treatment, treatment may be extended to beyond 12 months if required, when stopping treatment, reduce dose gradually over 2 weeks

Autoimmune hepatitis, induction of remission
▶ BY MOUTH
▶ Adult: 3 mg 3 times a day until remission is achieved, reduce dose gradually over 2 weeks following treatment course before stopping

Autoimmune hepatitis, maintenance
▶ BY MOUTH
▶ Adult: 3 mg twice daily for at least 24 months, when stopping treatment, reduce dose gradually over 2 weeks

BUDENOFALK ® GRANULES

Mild to moderate Crohn's disease affecting the ileum and/or ascending colon | Microscopic colitis, induction of remission
▶ BY MOUTH
▶ Adult: 9 mg once daily for up to 8 weeks, to be taken in the morning, reduce dose over 2 weeks by giving doses on alternate days following treatment course before stopping

BUDENOFALK ® RECTAL FOAM

Ulcerative colitis affecting sigmoid colon and rectum
▶ BY RECTUM
▶ Adult: 1 metered application once daily for up to 8 weeks

DOSE EQUIVALENCE AND CONVERSION
▶ For *Budenofalk* ® rectal foam: 1 metered application is equivalent to budesonide 2 mg.

CORTIMENT ®

Induction of remission of mild to moderate active ulcerative colitis | Induction of remission of active microscopic colitis
▶ BY MOUTH
▶ Adult: 9 mg once daily for up to 8 weeks, dose to be taken in the morning

ENTOCORT ® ENEMA

Ulcerative colitis involving rectal and recto-sigmoid disease
▶ BY RECTUM
▶ Adult: 1 enema daily for 4 weeks, to be administered at bedtime

JORVEZA ®

Eosinophilic oesophagitis, induction of remission (initiated by a specialist)
▶ BY MOUTH USING ORODISPERSIBLE TABLET
▶ Adult: 1 mg twice daily for 6 weeks; treatment may be extended to up to 12 weeks if required, to be taken after food

Eosinophilic oesophagitis, maintenance (initiated by a specialist)
▶ INITIALLY BY MOUTH USING ORODISPERSIBLE TABLET
▶ Adult: 0.5 mg twice daily, to be taken after food, alternatively (by mouth) 1 mg twice daily, to be taken after food, use higher dose option for patients with long-term disease and/or with extensive oesophageal inflammation in the acute phase

KINPEYGO ®

Primary immunoglobulin A (IgA) nephropathy
▶ BY MOUTH
▶ Adult: 16 mg once daily for 9 months, to be taken in the morning; reduced to 8 mg once daily for 2 weeks, to be taken in the morning, dose to be reduced when stopping treatment, dose may be further reduced to 4 mg once daily for another 2 weeks if required

● INTERACTIONS → Appendix 1: corticosteroids

● SIDE-EFFECTS
▶ **Common or very common**
▶ With oral use Dry mouth · fatigue · insomnia · muscle complaints · oedema · oral disorders
▶ With rectal use Arthralgia · depression · gastrointestinal disorders · muscle complaints · muscle weakness
▶ **Uncommon**
▶ With oral use Back pain · dizziness · flatulence
▶ With rectal use Adrenal hypofunction · akathisia · altered smell sensation · asthenia · dizziness · flushing · insomnia · oral ulceration · paraesthesia
▶ **Rare or very rare**
▶ With oral use Malaise
▶ With rectal use Constipation · increased risk of thrombosis · malaise

SIDE-EFFECTS, FURTHER INFORMATION Systemic absorption can follow rectal administration, therefore also consider the side-effects of systemic corticosteroids.

● ALLERGY AND CROSS-SENSITIVITY

CORTIMENT ® EvGr Avoid in patients with hypersensitivity to peanuts or soya (contains soya lecithin). Ⓜ

● HEPATIC IMPAIRMENT For *Budenofalk* ® manufacturer advises avoid in cirrhosis (risk of increased exposure, limited information available).

JORVEZA ® Manufacturer advises avoid (no information available).

● RENAL IMPAIRMENT

JORVEZA ® Manufacturer advises caution in mild to moderate impairment; avoid in severe impairment (no information available).

● MONITORING REQUIREMENTS EvGr When used in autoimmune hepatitis, liver-function tests should be monitored every 2 weeks for first month, then at least every 3 months. Ⓜ

● DIRECTIONS FOR ADMINISTRATION
▶ With oral use Manufacturer advises granules should be placed on tongue and washed down with water without chewing.

JORVEZA ® Manufacturer advises the tablet should be placed on the tip of the tongue, gently pressed against the roof of the mouth to dissolve, and the dissolved material swallowed with saliva as the tablet disintegrates. Patients should avoid eating, drinking or performing oral hygiene for at least 30 minutes after taking the tablet. Oral solutions, sprays or chewable tablets should be avoided for at least 30 minutes before and after taking the tablet.

KINPEYGO ® Capsules should be taken at least 1 hour before food.

● PRESCRIBING AND DISPENSING INFORMATION
▶ With oral use Dispense modified-release capsules in original container (contains desiccant).

BUDENOFALK ® GRANULES Flavours of granule formulations may include lemon.

● PATIENT AND CARER ADVICE Patients or carers should be given advice on how to administer budesonide granules.

JORVEZA ® Manufacturer advises patients or carers should be given advice on how to administer orodispersible tablets.

- **NATIONAL FUNDING/ACCESS DECISIONS**
  For full details see funding body website
  NICE decisions
- ▶ Budesonide orodispersible tablet for inducing remission of eosinophilic oesophagitis (June 2021) NICE TA708 Recommended
- ▶ Targeted-release budesonide for treating primary IgA nephropathy (December 2023) NICE TA937 Recommended with restrictions

  Scottish Medicines Consortium (SMC) decisions
- ▶ Budesonide 3 mg gastro-resistant capsules (*Budenofalk*®) for autoimmune hepatitis (May 2015) SMC No. 1043/15 Recommended with restrictions
- ▶ Budesonide (*Cortiment*®) in adults for induction of remission in patients with mild to moderate active ulcerative colitis (UC) where aminosalicylate (5-ASA) treatment is not sufficient (October 2016) SMC No. 1093/15 Recommended with restrictions
- ▶ Budesonide (*Jorveza*®) for the treatment of eosinophilic oesophagitis in adults (October 2020) SMC No. SMC2158 Recommended with restrictions
- ▶ Budesonide (*Cortiment*®) for induction of remission in patients with active microscopic colitis (January 2022) SMC No. SMC2448 Recommended

- **MEDICINAL FORMS** There can be variation in the licensing of different medicines containing the same drug.
  Modified-release tablet
  CAUTIONARY AND ADVISORY LABELS 10, 25
  EXCIPIENTS: May contain Lecithin
  - ▶ Cortiment (Ferring Pharmaceuticals Ltd)
    Budesonide 9 mg Cortiment 9mg modified-release tablets | 30 tablet [PoM] £75.00 DT = £75.00

  Gastro-resistant capsule
  CAUTIONARY AND ADVISORY LABELS 5, 10, 22, 25
  - ▶ Budenofalk (Dr. Falk Pharma UK Ltd)
    Budesonide 3 mg Budenofalk 3mg gastro-resistant capsules | 100 capsule [PoM] £75.05 DT = £75.05

  Suppository
  - ▶ Budenofalk (Dr. Falk Pharma UK Ltd)
    Budesonide 4 mg Budenofalk 4mg suppositories | 30 suppository [PoM] £198.00 DT = £198.00

  Modified-release capsule
  CAUTIONARY AND ADVISORY LABELS 10, 25
  - ▶ Budesonide (Non-proprietary)
    Budesonide 3 mg Budesonide 3mg gastro-resistant modified-release capsules | 100 capsule [PoM] £75.05 DT = £75.05
  - ▶ Kinpeygo (Genus Pharmaceuticals Holdings Ltd) ▼
    Budesonide 4 mg Kinpeygo 4mg modified-release capsules | 120 capsule [PoM] £4,681.24 (Hospital only)

  Rectal foam
  EXCIPIENTS: May contain Cetostearyl alcohol (including cetyl and stearyl alcohol), disodium edetate, propylene glycol, sorbic acid
  - ▶ Budenofalk (Dr. Falk Pharma UK Ltd)
    Budesonide 2 mg per 1 actuation Budenofalk 2mg/application foam enema | 14 dose [PoM] £57.11 DT = £57.11

  Gastro-resistant granules
  CAUTIONARY AND ADVISORY LABELS 5, 10, 22, 25
  - ▶ Budenofalk (Dr. Falk Pharma UK Ltd)
    Budesonide 9 mg Budenofalk 9mg gastro-resistant granules sachets | 60 sachet [PoM] £135.00 DT = £135.00

  Orodispersible tablet
  CAUTIONARY AND ADVISORY LABELS 10
  ELECTROLYTES: May contain Sodium
  - ▶ Jorveza (Dr. Falk Pharma UK Ltd)
    Budesonide 500 microgram Jorveza 0.5mg orodispersible tablets | 60 tablet [PoM] £214.80 DT = £214.80 [SF]
    Budesonide 1 mg Jorveza 1mg orodispersible tablets | 90 tablet [PoM] £323.00 DT = £323.00 [SF]

  Enema
  - ▶ Entocort (Tillotts Pharma UK Ltd)
    Budesonide 20 microgram per 1 ml Entocort 2mg/100ml enema | 7 enema [PoM] £33.66 DT = £33.66

IMMUNOSUPPRESSANTS ›
IMMUNOMODULATING DRUGS

| Etrasimod   25-Jun-2024

- **DRUG ACTION** Etrasimod is a sphingosine-1-phosphate receptor modulator, which prevents movement of lymphocytes out of lymph nodes, thereby limiting inflammation in the intestine.

- **INDICATIONS AND DOSE**
  Ulcerative colitis (initiated under specialist supervision)
  - ▶ BY MOUTH
  - ▶ Adult: 2 mg once daily

- **CONTRA-INDICATIONS** Active malignancy · decompensated heart failure (requiring inpatient treatment) in the previous 6 months · heart failure (New York Heart Association class III or IV) in the previous 6 months · immunodeficiency · myocardial infarction in the previous 6 months · phototherapy with UV-B radiation or PUVA-photochemotherapy (increased risk of cutaneous neoplasm) · posterior reversible encephalopathy syndrome (suspected or confirmed) · progressive multifocal leukoencephalopathy · second-degree Mobitz type II AV block, third-degree AV block, sick sinus syndrome or sino-atrial block, if the patient does not have a pacemaker · severe active infection · stroke (including transient ischaemic attack) in the previous 6 months · unstable angina in the previous 6 months

- **CAUTIONS** Administration of vaccinations · arrhythmias requiring treatment with Class Ia or Class III anti-arrhythmic drugs · asthma · body-weight less than 40 kg (increased risk of exposure) · cerebrovascular disease · chronic obstructive pulmonary disease · diabetes mellitus (increased risk of macular oedema) · elderly (limited information available) · heart failure · immunosuppression or other risk factors for infection · myocardial infarction · patients receiving QT-prolonging or heart rate-lowering drugs, including beta-blockers and heart rate-lowering calcium-channel blockers · pulmonary fibrosis · recurrent syncope · retinal disease (increased risk of macular oedema) · second-degree Mobitz type I AV block · severe respiratory disease · severe untreated sleep apnoea · significant QT prolongation (QTc equal to or greater than 470 milliseconds in females, or QTc equal to or greater than 450 milliseconds in males) · sinus bradycardia (heart rate below 50 beats per minute) · uncontrolled hypertension · uveitis (increased risk of macular oedema)

  CAUTIONS, FURTHER INFORMATION
- ▶ Bradycardia and cardiac rhythm disturbance [EvGr] Etrasimod may cause transient bradycardia, AV conduction delays and heart block after the first dose. It is not recommended in patients with a history of cardiac arrest, cerebrovascular disease, symptomatic bradycardia or recurrent syncope, unstable ischaemic heart disease, uncontrolled hypertension, severe untreated sleep apnoea, or significant QT prolongation or other risk factors for QT prolongation unless the anticipated benefits outweigh the potential risks, and advice from a cardiologist (including monitoring advice) is sought before initiation. ⟨M⟩
- ▶ Vaccinations [EvGr] Vaccination may be less effective during and for up to 2 weeks after stopping treatment. Live attenuated vaccines should be avoided during and for 2 weeks after stopping treatment; if they are required they should be given at least 1 month prior to initiation. ⟨M⟩

- **INTERACTIONS** → Appendix 1: etrasimod

- **SIDE-EFFECTS**
- ▶ **Common or very common** Arrhythmias · cystitis · dizziness · headache · hypercholesterolaemia · hypertension · increased risk of infection · lymphopenia · neutropenia · visual impairment

▸ **Uncommon** Atrioventricular block · macular oedema
▸ **Frequency not known** Hepatic disorders

● **CONCEPTION AND CONTRACEPTION** [EvGr] Exclude pregnancy before treatment; females of childbearing potential should use effective contraception during treatment and for at least 14 days after last dose. ⟨M⟩

● **PREGNANCY** [EvGr] Avoid (toxicity in *animal* studies and limited human data suggests increased risk of abnormal pregnancy outcomes). ⟨M⟩

● **BREAST FEEDING** Specialist sources indicate use with caution, especially if breast-feeding a newborn or preterm infant (no information available). High plasma-protein binding suggests limited excretion into milk.

● **HEPATIC IMPAIRMENT** [EvGr] Caution when history of significant liver disease (no information available); avoid in severe impairment. ⟨M⟩

● **MONITORING REQUIREMENTS**
▸ [EvGr] ECG should be obtained for all patients prior to treatment initiation. Patients with certain pre-existing cardiac conditions should be monitored for bradycardia for 4 hours after the first dose, and another ECG obtained after this 4-hour period ⟨M⟩—consult product literature for further information.
▸ [EvGr] Monitor blood pressure regularly during treatment.
▸ Monitor hepatic transaminases and bilirubin before initiation of treatment and then at months 1, 3, 6, 9, 12, and periodically thereafter (interrupt treatment if significant liver injury occurs: liver transaminases above 3 times the upper limit of normal and total bilirubin above 2 times the upper limit of normal).
▸ Monitor full blood count before initiation and periodically during treatment (interrupt treatment if lymphocyte count reduced) ⟨M⟩—consult product literature.
▸ [EvGr] Eye examination recommended in all patients at initiation of treatment and then as clinically indicated (interrupt treatment if macular oedema occurs); patients with history of diabetes or uveitis or retinal disease to have eye examination periodically during treatment. ⟨M⟩

● **DIRECTIONS FOR ADMINISTRATION** [EvGr] Tablet should be taken with food for the first 3 days of treatment to reduce potential transient heart rate lowering effects, after which it can be taken with or without food. ⟨M⟩

● **PRESCRIBING AND DISPENSING INFORMATION** The manufacturer of *Velsipity* ® has provided a *Checklist for Prescribers*.

● **PATIENT AND CARER ADVICE** Patients and carers should be given advice on how to administer etrasimod tablets. Patients and carers should be advised to avoid exposure to sunlight without protection. Patients and carers should be advised to promptly report symptoms of infection during and for up to 2 weeks after stopping treatment.
Patient card and guide Patients and carers should be given a *Patient/Caregiver Guide*.
Female patients of childbearing potential should be given a *Patient card*.
Missed doses If treatment is interrupted for 7 or more consecutive days, resume treatment with food for the first 3 doses.
Driving and skilled tasks Patients and carers should be counselled on the effects on driving and performance of skilled tasks—increased risk of dizziness.

● **NATIONAL FUNDING/ACCESS DECISIONS**
For full details see funding body website

NICE decisions
▸ Etrasimod for treating moderately to severely active ulcerative colitis in people aged 16 and over **(March 2024)** NICE TA956 Recommended

Scottish Medicines Consortium (SMC) decisions
▸ Etrasimod (*Velsipity* ®) for the treatment of patients 16 years of age and older with moderately to severely active ulcerative

colitis who have had an inadequate response, lost response, or were intolerant to either conventional therapy, or a biological agent **(June 2024)** SMC No. SMC2655 Recommended

● **MEDICINAL FORMS** There can be variation in the licensing of different medicines containing the same drug.
Oral tablet
EXCIPIENTS: May contain Tartrazine
▸ **Velsipity** (Pfizer Ltd) ▼
  Etrasimod (as Etrasimod arginine) 2 mg Velsipity 2mg tablets | 28 tablet [PoM] £843.84 (Hospital only)

IMMUNOSUPPRESSANTS ⟩ INTERLEUKIN INHIBITORS

Mirikizumab
03-May-2024

● **DRUG ACTION** Mirikizumab is a humanised monoclonal antibody that selectively binds to cytokine interleukin-23 (IL-23) and inhibits the release of pro-inflammatory cytokines.

● **INDICATIONS AND DOSE**
Ulcerative colitis (under expert supervision)
▸ INITIALLY BY INTRAVENOUS INFUSION
▸ Adult: Initially 300 mg every 4 weeks for 3 doses, if an adequate therapeutic response is not achieved after 12 weeks, the induction regimen can be extended for an additional 12 weeks, discontinue treatment if no response after 24 weeks, then (by subcutaneous injection) maintenance 200 mg every 4 weeks, if response is lost, consider re-induction—consult product literature

● **CONTRA-INDICATIONS** Active infection

● **CAUTIONS** Chronic infection · history of recurrent infection
CAUTIONS, FURTHER INFORMATION
▸ Risk of infection [EvGr] Patients must be screened for tuberculosis before starting treatment. Consider anti-tuberculosis therapy before initiation of mirikizumab in patients with a history of latent or active tuberculosis in whom an adequate course of treatment cannot be confirmed.
  Patients should be brought up to date with current immunisation schedule before initiating treatment. ⟨M⟩

● **INTERACTIONS** → Appendix 1: monoclonal antibodies

● **SIDE-EFFECTS**
▸ **Common or very common** Arthralgia · headache · increased risk of infection · oropharyngeal complaints · skin reactions
▸ **Uncommon** Infusion related hypersensitivity reaction
▸ **Frequency not known** Drug-induced liver injury · hypersensitivity

● **CONCEPTION AND CONTRACEPTION** [EvGr] Females of childbearing potential should use effective contraception during treatment and for at least 10 weeks after last treatment. ⟨M⟩

● **PREGNANCY** [EvGr] Avoid (limited information available). ⟨M⟩

● **BREAST FEEDING** [EvGr] Avoid (no information available). ⟨M⟩

● **MONITORING REQUIREMENTS**
▸ [EvGr] Monitor for signs and symptoms of active tuberculosis during and after treatment.
▸ Monitor liver enzymes and bilirubin before starting treatment, then every month during induction phase, and every 1–4 months during maintenance phase or as clinically indicated—interrupt treatment if transaminases are elevated and drug-induced liver injury suspected. ⟨M⟩

● **DIRECTIONS FOR ADMINISTRATION** For *intermittent intravenous infusion* (*Omvoh* ®), dilute in 50–250 mL of

Glucose 5% or Sodium Chloride 0.9%; give over 30 minutes.

For *subcutaneous injection* (*Omvoh*®), remove pre-filled pen from the refrigerator 30 minutes before administration. Inject into the thigh or abdomen (except for the 5 cm around the navel), or back of upper arm (if not self-administered); rotate injection site and avoid skin that is tender, bruised, red, or hardened. Patients may self-administer pre-filled pens after appropriate training in subcutaneous injection technique.

- **PRESCRIBING AND DISPENSING INFORMATION** Mirikizumab is a biological medicine. Biological medicines must be prescribed and dispensed by brand name, see *Biological medicines* and *Biosimilar medicines*, under Guidance on prescribing p. 1; record the brand name and batch number after each administration.

- **HANDLING AND STORAGE** Store in a refrigerator (2–8°C) and protect from light—consult product literature for further information regarding storage outside refrigerator.

- **PATIENT AND CARER ADVICE** Patients or their carers should be advised to seek medical attention if signs or symptoms of infection occur.
  Self administration Patients or their carers should be given training in subcutaneous injection technique.
  A patient leaflet and user manual should be provided.

- **NATIONAL FUNDING/ACCESS DECISIONS**
  For full details see funding body website
  NICE decisions
  ▸ Mirikizumab for treating moderately to severely active ulcerative colitis (October 2023) NICE TA925 Recommended with restrictions
  Scottish Medicines Consortium (SMC) decisions
  ▸ Mirikizumab (*Omvoh*®) for the treatment of adults with moderately to severely active ulcerative colitis who are intolerant of, or whose disease has had an inadequate response or loss of response to, either conventional therapy or a biologic or have medical contra-indications to such therapies (April 2024) SMC No. SMC2650 Recommended

- **MEDICINAL FORMS** There can be variation in the licensing of different medicines containing the same drug.
  Solution for injection
  EXCIPIENTS: May contain Polysorbates
  ▸ Omvoh (Eli Lilly and Company Ltd) ▼
    Mirikizumab 100 mg per 1 ml Omvoh 100mg/1ml solution for injection pre-filled pens | 2 pre-filled disposable injection [PoM] £2,056.56 (Hospital only)
  Solution for infusion
  EXCIPIENTS: May contain Polysorbates
  ELECTROLYTES: May contain Sodium
  ▸ Omvoh (Eli Lilly and Company Ltd) ▼
    Mirikizumab 20 mg per 1 ml Omvoh 300mg/15ml concentrate for solution for infusion vials | 1 vial [PoM] £2,056.56 (Hospital only)

IMMUNOSUPPRESSANTS › MONOCLONAL ANTIBODIES, ANTI-LYMPHOCYTE

Vedolizumab

24-Mar-2021

- **DRUG ACTION** Vedolizumab is a monoclonal antibody that binds specifically to the $\alpha_4\beta_7$ integrin, which is expressed on gut homing T helper lymphocytes and causes a reduction in gastrointestinal inflammation.

- **INDICATIONS AND DOSE**
  Ulcerative colitis (under expert supervision)
  ▸ BY INTRAVENOUS INFUSION
  ▸ Adult: Initially 300 mg, then 300 mg after 2 weeks, followed by 300 mg after 4 weeks, followed by 300 mg every 8 weeks, dose to be given over 30 minutes, if treatment is interrupted or response decreases, dosing frequency may be increased—consult product

literature; review treatment if no response within 10 weeks of initial dose
▸ BY SUBCUTANEOUS INJECTION
▸ Adult: Maintenance 108 mg every 2 weeks, following at least 2 intravenous infusions; the first subcutaneous dose should be administered in place of the next scheduled intravenous dose

Crohn's disease (under expert supervision)
▸ BY INTRAVENOUS INFUSION
▸ Adult: Initially 300 mg, then 300 mg after 2 weeks, followed by 300 mg after 4 weeks, followed by 300 mg every 8 weeks, dose to be given over 30 minutes, if no response is observed, an additional dose of 300 mg may be given 10 weeks after initial dose; if treatment is interrupted or response decreases, dosing frequency may be increased—consult product literature; review treatment if no response within 14 weeks of initial dose
▸ BY SUBCUTANEOUS INJECTION
▸ Adult: Maintenance 108 mg every 2 weeks, following at least 2 intravenous infusions; the first subcutaneous dose should be administered in place of the next scheduled intravenous dose

- **CONTRA-INDICATIONS** Severe active infection

- **CAUTIONS** Controlled chronic severe infection · history of recurring severe infection · previous treatment with natalizumab (wait at least 12 weeks between natalizumab use and initiation of vedolizumab unless potential benefit outweighs risk) · previous treatment with rituximab
  CAUTIONS, FURTHER INFORMATION
  ▸ Risk of infection [EvGr] Patients must be screened for tuberculosis before starting treatment; if latent tuberculosis is diagnosed, appropriate treatment must be initiated prior to vedolizumab treatment; if tuberculosis is diagnosed during treatment, discontinue vedolizumab until infection is resolved.
    Patients should be brought up to date with current immunisation schedule before initiating treatment. ◈M◈

- **INTERACTIONS** → Appendix 1: monoclonal antibodies

- **SIDE-EFFECTS**
  ▸ **Common or very common** Arthralgia · constipation · cough · fatigue · fever · gastrointestinal discomfort · gastrointestinal disorders · headache · hypertension · increased risk of infection · muscle spasms · muscle weakness · nasal congestion · nausea · night sweats · oropharyngeal pain · pain · paraesthesia · skin reactions
  ▸ **Uncommon** Chills · feeling cold · infusion related reaction
  ▸ **Rare or very rare** Hypersensitivity · vision blurred
  ▸ **Frequency not known** Meningitis listeria · sepsis
  SIDE-EFFECTS, FURTHER INFORMATION Infusion-related and hypersensitivity reactions have been reported. Patients should be observed continuously during each infusion for signs and symptoms of acute hypersensitivity reactions; they should also be observed for 2 hours after the initial two infusions, and for 1 hour after subsequent infusions. Discontinue treatment if a severe infusion-related or other severe reaction occurs and initiate appropriate treatment (e.g. adrenaline and antihistamines); if a mild to moderate infusion-related reaction occurs, interrupt infusion or reduce infusion rate and initiate appropriate treatment (if reaction subsides the infusion may be continued)—consider pretreatment with an antihistamine, hydrocortisone, and/or paracetamol prior to subsequent infusions in patients who experience mild to moderate infusion-related reactions.

- **CONCEPTION AND CONTRACEPTION** Manufacturer advises effective contraception required during and for at least 18 weeks after treatment.

- **PREGNANCY** Manufacturer advises use only if potential benefit outweighs risk.

1 Gastro-intestinal system

- **BREAST FEEDING** [EvGr] Specialist sources indicate use with caution—present in milk. ⓓ

- **MONITORING REQUIREMENTS**
- ▸ Manufacturer advises monitor closely for infection before, during and after treatment—potential increased risk of opportunistic infection.
- ▸ Manufacturer advises monitor for new onset or worsening neurological signs and symptoms (withhold treatment if progressive multifocal leukoencephalopathy (PML) is suspected).

- **DIRECTIONS FOR ADMINISTRATION** For *intravenous infusion* (*Entyvio* ®), manufacturer advises give intermittently *in* Sodium Chloride 0.9%; allow vial to reach room temperature then reconstitute with 4.8 mL of Water for Injections (using a syringe with a 21–25 gauge needle); gently swirl vial for at least 15 seconds, do not shake vigorously or invert; allow to stand for up to 20 minutes (gently swirl vial if needed), leave for an additional 10 minutes if not dissolved; gently invert vial three times, withdraw 5 mL of reconstituted solution (using a syringe with a 21–25 gauge needle), and add to 250 mL of infusion fluid; gently mix and give over 30 minutes.

- **PRESCRIBING AND DISPENSING INFORMATION** Vedolizumab is a biological medicine. Biological medicines must be prescribed and dispensed by brand name, see *Biological medicines* and *Biosimilar medicines*, under Guidance on prescribing p. 1; manufacturer advises to record the brand name and batch number after each administration.

- **PATIENT AND CARER ADVICE**
Self-administration Manufacturer advises patients and their carers should be given training in subcutaneous injection technique if appropriate.
Alert card Patients should be provided with a patient alert card.

- **NATIONAL FUNDING/ACCESS DECISIONS**
For full details see funding body website
  NICE decisions
- ▸ **Vedolizumab for treating moderately to severely active Crohn's disease after prior therapy (August 2015)** NICE TA352 Recommended with restrictions
- ▸ **Vedolizumab for treating moderately to severely active ulcerative colitis (June 2015)** NICE TA342 Recommended
  Scottish Medicines Consortium (SMC) decisions
- ▸ **Vedolizumab powder for concentrate for solution for infusion (*Entyvio* ®) for the treatment of adult patients with moderately to severely active Crohn's disease who have had an inadequate response with, lost response to, or were intolerant to either conventional therapy or a tumour necrosis factor-alpha antagonist (July 2015)** SMC No. 1064/15 Recommended with restrictions
- ▸ **Vedolizumab solution for injection (*Entyvio* ®) for the treatment of adult patients with moderately to severely active Crohn's disease who have had an inadequate response with, lost response to, or were intolerant to either conventional therapy or a tumour necrosis factor-alpha antagonist (August 2020)** SMC No. SMC2277 Recommended with restrictions
- ▸ **Vedolizumab powder for concentrate for solution for infusion (*Entyvio* ®) for the treatment of adult patients with moderately to severely active ulcerative colitis who have had an inadequate response with, lost response to, or were intolerant to either conventional therapy or a tumour necrosis factor-alpha antagonist (May 2015)** SMC No. 1045/15 Recommended
- ▸ **Vedolizumab solution for injection (*Entyvio* ®) for the treatment of adult patients with moderately to severely active ulcerative colitis who have had an inadequate response with, lost response to, or were intolerant to either conventional therapy or a tumour necrosis factor-alpha antagonist (August 2020)** SMC No. SMC2276 Recommended

- **MEDICINAL FORMS** There can be variation in the licensing of different medicines containing the same drug.
  Solution for injection
  CAUTIONARY AND ADVISORY LABELS 10
  EXCIPIENTS: May contain Polysorbates
- ▸ **Entyvio** (Takeda UK Ltd)
  Vedolizumab 158.82 mg per 1 ml Entyvio 108mg/0.68ml solution for injection pre-filled pens | 1 pre-filled disposable injection [PoM] £512.50 (Hospital only) | 2 pre-filled disposable injection [PoM] £1,025.00 (Hospital only)
  Entyvio 108mg/0.68ml solution for injection pre-filled syringes | 2 pre-filled disposable injection [PoM] £1,025.00 (Hospital only)
  Powder for solution for infusion
  CAUTIONARY AND ADVISORY LABELS 10
  EXCIPIENTS: May contain Polysorbates
- ▸ **Entyvio** (Takeda UK Ltd)
  Vedolizumab 300 mg Entyvio 300mg powder for concentrate for solution for infusion vials | 1 vial [PoM] £2,050.00 (Hospital only)

1.4 Irritable bowel syndrome

Irritable bowel syndrome
02-May-2020

Description of condition

Irritable bowel syndrome (IBS) is a common, chronic, relapsing, and often life-long condition, mainly affecting people aged between 20 and 30 years. It is more common in women. Symptoms include abdominal pain or discomfort, disordered defaecation (either diarrhoea, or constipation with straining, urgency, and incomplete evacuation), passage of mucus, and bloating. Symptoms are usually relieved by defaecation. Obtaining an accurate clinical diagnosis of IBS prior to treatment is crucial.

Aims of treatment

The treatment of IBS is focused on symptom control, in order to improve quality of life.

Non-drug treatment

[EvGr] Diet and lifestyle changes are important for effective self-management of IBS. Patients should be encouraged to increase physical activity, and advised to eat regularly, without missing meals or leaving long gaps between meals. Dietary advice should also include, limiting fresh fruit consumption to no more than 3 portions per day. The fibre intake of patients with IBS should be reviewed. If an increase in dietary fibre is required, soluble fibre such as ispaghula husk p. 60, or foods high in soluble fibre such as oats, are recommended. Intake of insoluble fibre (e.g. bran) and 'resistant starch' should be reduced or discouraged as they may exacerbate symptoms. Fluid intake (mostly water) should be increased to at least 8 cups each day and the intake of caffeine, alcohol and fizzy drinks reduced. The artificial sweetener sorbitol should be avoided in patients with diarrhoea. Where probiotics are being used, continue for at least 4 weeks while monitoring the effect.

If a patient's symptoms persist following lifestyle and dietary advice, single food avoidance and exclusion diets may be an option under the supervision of a dietitian or medical specialist. Ⓐ

Drug treatment

[EvGr] The choice of drug treatment depends on the nature and severity of the symptoms. Many drug treatment options for IBS are available over-the-counter.

Antispasmodic drugs (such as alverine citrate p. 97, mebeverine hydrochloride p. 98 and peppermint oil p. 53) can be taken in addition to dietary and lifestyle changes. A laxative (excluding lactulose p. 61 as it may cause bloating) can be used to treat constipation. Patients who have not responded to laxatives from the different classes and who have had constipation for at least 12 months, can be treated with linaclotide p. 54. Loperamide hydrochloride p. 74 is the first-line choice of anti-motility drug for relief of diarrhoea. Patients with IBS should be advised how on to adjust their dose of laxative or anti-motility drug according to stool consistency, with the aim of achieving a soft, well-formed stool. ⟨A⟩ See Constipation p. 58, for information on other drugs used for chronic constipation.

⟨EvGr⟩ A low-dose tricyclic antidepressant, such as amitriptyline hydrochloride p. 431 [unlicensed indication], can be used for abdominal pain or discomfort as a second-line option in patients who have not responded to antispasmodics, anti-motility drugs, or laxatives. A selective serotonin reuptake inhibitor may be considered in those who do not respond to a tricyclic antidepressant [unlicensed indication].

Psychological intervention can be offered to patients who have no relief of IBS symptoms after 12 months of drug treatment. ⟨A⟩

Useful Resources

Irritable bowel syndrome in adults: diagnosis and management. National Institute for Health and Care Excellence. Clinical guideline 61. February 2008 (updated April 2017).

www.nice.org.uk/guidance/cg61

ANTISPASMODICS

Alverine with simeticone
27-Mar-2024

The properties listed below are those particular to the combination only. For the properties of the components please consider, alverine citrate p. 97.

- **INDICATIONS AND DOSE**

Abdominal pain in irritable bowel syndrome
- ▶ BY MOUTH
- ▸ Adult: 60/300 mg 2–3 times a day, to be taken at the beginning of meals

DOSE EQUIVALENCE AND CONVERSION
- ▸ Dose expressed as x/y mg alverine citrate/simeticone.

- **ALLERGY AND CROSS-SENSITIVITY** ⟨EvGr⟩ Contra-indicated in patients with hypersensitivity to peanuts or soya (external lubricant contains soya lecithin). ⟨M⟩

- **MEDICINAL FORMS** There can be variation in the licensing of different medicines containing the same drug.
Oral capsule
- ▸ SimAlvia (Mayoly UK Ltd)
Alverine citrate 60 mg, Simeticone 300 mg SimAlvia 60mg/300mg capsules | 90 capsule [PoM] £11.00 DT = £11.00

Mebeverine with ispaghula husk

09-Nov-2020

The properties listed below are those particular to the combination only. For the properties of the components please consider, mebeverine hydrochloride p. 98, ispaghula husk p. 60.

- **INDICATIONS AND DOSE**

Irritable bowel syndrome
- ▶ BY MOUTH
- ▸ Child 12–17 years: 1 sachet twice daily, in water, morning and evening, 30 minutes before food and 1 sachet daily if required, taken 30 minutes before midday meal
- ▸ Adult: 1 sachet twice daily, in water, morning and evening, 30 minutes before food and 1 sachet daily if required, taken 30 minutes before midday meal

- **DIRECTIONS FOR ADMINISTRATION** Manufacturer advises contents of one sachet should be stirred into a glass (approx. 150 mL) of cold water and drunk immediately.

- **PATIENT AND CARER ADVICE** Patients or carers should be given advice on how to administer ispaghula husk with mebeverine granules.

- **MEDICINAL FORMS** There can be variation in the licensing of different medicines containing the same drug.
Effervescent granules
CAUTIONARY AND ADVISORY LABELS 13, 22
EXCIPIENTS: May contain Aspartame
ELECTROLYTES: May contain Potassium
- ▸ Fybogel Mebeverine (Reckitt Benckiser Healthcare (UK) Ltd)
Mebeverine hydrochloride 135 mg, Ispaghula husk 3.5 gram Fybogel Mebeverine effervescent granules sachets orange | 10 sachet [P] £9.16 DT = £9.16 [SF]

Peppermint oil
19-Nov-2020

- **INDICATIONS AND DOSE**
COLPERMIN ®

Relief of abdominal colic and distension, particularly in irritable bowel syndrome
- ▶ BY MOUTH
- ▸ Child 15-17 years: 1–2 capsules 3 times a day for up to 3 months if necessary, capsule to be swallowed whole with water
- ▸ Adult: 1–2 capsules 3 times a day for up to 3 months if necessary, capsule to be swallowed whole with water

MINTEC ®

Relief of abdominal colic and distension, particularly in irritable bowel syndrome
- ▶ BY MOUTH
- ▸ Adult: 1–2 capsules 3 times a day for up to 2–3 months if necessary, dose to be taken before meals, swallowed whole with water

- **CAUTIONS** Sensitivity to menthol

- **INTERACTIONS** → Appendix 1: peppermint

- **SIDE-EFFECTS** Ataxia · bradycardia · gastrointestinal discomfort · gastrooesophageal reflux disease · headache · nausea · paraesthesia · rash erythematous · tremor · vomiting

- **PREGNANCY** Not known to be harmful.

- **BREAST FEEDING** Significant levels of menthol in breast milk unlikely.

- **DIRECTIONS FOR ADMINISTRATION** Manufacturer advises capsules should not be broken or chewed because peppermint oil may irritate mouth or oesophagus.

- **MEDICINAL FORMS** There can be variation in the licensing of different medicines containing the same drug.
Gastro-resistant capsule
CAUTIONARY AND ADVISORY LABELS 5, 22, 25
- ▸ Mintec (Teofarma S.r.l.)
Peppermint oil 200 microlitre Mintec 0.2ml gastro-resistant capsules | 84 capsule [GSL] £7.04 DT = £7.04
Modified-release capsule
CAUTIONARY AND ADVISORY LABELS 5, 22, 25
EXCIPIENTS: May contain Arachis (peanut) oil
- ▸ Colpermin (Johnson & Johnson Ltd)
Peppermint oil 200 microlitre Colpermin IBS Relief gastro-resistant modified-release capsules | 20 capsule [GSL] £4.90 | 100 capsule [GSL] £18.46 DT = £18.46

1

Gastro-intestinal system

LAXATIVES > GUANYLATE CYCLASE-C RECEPTOR AGONISTS

Linaclotide

10-Nov-2020

● INDICATIONS AND DOSE

Moderate to severe irritable bowel syndrome with constipation
▸ BY MOUTH
▸ **Adult:** 290 micrograms once daily, dose to be taken at least 30 minutes before meals, review treatment if no response after 4 weeks

● **CONTRA-INDICATIONS** Gastro-intestinal obstruction · inflammatory bowel disease

● **CAUTIONS** Predisposition to fluid and electrolyte disturbances

● **SIDE-EFFECTS**
▸ **Common or very common** Diarrhoea · dizziness · gastrointestinal discomfort · gastrointestinal disorders
▸ **Uncommon** Appetite decreased · dehydration · haemorrhage · hypokalaemia · nausea · postural hypotension · vomiting
▸ **Frequency not known** Rash

SIDE-EFFECTS, FURTHER INFORMATION Manufacturer advises if diarrhoea severe or prolonged, consider suspending treatment.

● **PREGNANCY** Manufacturer advises avoid.

● **BREAST FEEDING** Unlikely to be present in milk in significant amounts, but manufacturer advises avoid.

● **PRESCRIBING AND DISPENSING INFORMATION** Dispense capsules in original container (contains desiccant); discard any capsules remaining 18 weeks after opening.

● **NATIONAL FUNDING/ACCESS DECISIONS**
For full details see funding body website
Scottish Medicines Consortium (SMC) decisions
▸ Linaclotide (*Constella*®) for the symptomatic treatment of moderate to severe irritable bowel syndrome with constipation (IBS-C) in adults (June 2013) SMC No. 869/13 Recommended with restrictions

● **MEDICINAL FORMS** There can be variation in the licensing of different medicines containing the same drug.
Oral capsule
CAUTIONARY AND ADVISORY LABELS 22
▸ **Constella** (AbbVie Ltd)
  Linaclotide 290 microgram Constella 290microgram capsules | 28 capsule [PoM] £37.56 DT = £37.56

1.5 Short bowel syndrome

Short bowel syndrome

31-Aug-2016

Description of condition

Patients with a shortened bowel due to large surgical resection (with or without stoma formation) may require medical management to ensure adequate absorption of nutrients and fluid. Absorption of oral medication is also often impaired.

Aims of treatment

The management of short bowel syndrome focuses on ensuring adequate nutrition and drug absorption, thereby reducing the risk of complications resulting from these effects.

Drug treatment

Nutritional deficiencies

[EvGr] Patients with a short bowel may require replacement of vitamins and minerals depending on the extent and position of the bowel resection. Deficiencies in vitamins A, B_{12}, D, E, and K, essential fatty acids, zinc, and selenium can occur.

Hypomagnesaemia is common and is treated with oral or intravenous magnesium supplementation (see Magnesium imbalance p. 1191), though administration of oral magnesium may cause diarrhoea. Occasionally the use of oral alfacalcidol p. 1240 and correction of sodium depletion may be useful. Nutritional support can range from oral supplements to parenteral nutrition, depending on the severity of intestinal failure. (A)

Diarrhoea and high output stomas

Diarrhoea is common in short bowel syndrome and can be due to multiple factors. [EvGr] The use of oral rehydration salts can be considered in order to promote adequate hydration. Oral intake influences the volume of stool passed, so reducing food intake will lessen diarrhoea, but will also exacerbate the problems of undernutrition. A patient may require parenteral nutrition to allow them to eat less, if the extent of diarrhoea is unacceptable.

Pharmacological treatment may be necessary, with the choice of drug depending on the potential for side-effects and the degree of resection. (A)

Antimotility drugs

[EvGr] Loperamide hydrochloride p. 74 and codeine phosphate p. 517 reduce intestinal motility and thus exert antidiarrhoeal actions. Loperamide hydrochloride is preferred as it is not sedative and does not cause dependence or fat malabsorption. High doses of loperamide hydrochloride [unlicensed] may be required in patients with a short bowel due to disrupted enterohepatic circulation and rapid gastrointestinal transit time. If the desired response is not obtained with loperamide hydrochloride, codeine phosphate may be added to therapy.

Co-phenotrope p. 73 has traditionally been used alone or in combination with other medications to help decrease faecal output. Co-phenotrope crosses the blood–brain barrier and can produce central nervous system side-effects, which may limit its use; the potential for dependence and anticholinergic effects may also restrict its use. (A)

Colestyramine

[EvGr] In patients with an intact colon and less than 100 cm of ileum resected, colestyramine p. 229 can be used to bind the unabsorbed bile salts and reduce diarrhoea. When colestyramine is given to these patients, it is important to monitor for evidence of fat malabsorption (steatorrhoea) or fat-soluble vitamin deficiencies. (A)

Antisecretory drugs

[EvGr] Drugs that reduce gastric acid secretion reduce jejunostomy output. Omeprazole p. 89 is readily absorbed in the duodenum and upper small bowel, but if less than 50 cm of jejunum remains, it may need to be given intravenously. Use of a proton pump inhibitor alone does not eliminate the need for further intervention for fluid control (such as antimotility agents, intravenous fluids, or oral rehydration salts).

Octreotide [unlicensed indication] reduces ileostomy diarrhoea and large volume jejunostomy output by inhibiting multiple pro-secretory substances. There is insufficient evidence to establish its role in the management of short bowel syndrome. (A)

Growth factors

Growth factors can be used to facilitate intestinal adaptation after surgery in patients with short bowel syndrome, thus enhancing fluid, electrolyte, and micronutrient absorption.

Teduglutide p. 55 is an analogue of endogenous human glucagon-like peptide 2 (GLP-2) which is licensed for use in the management of short bowel syndrome. It may be considered after a period of stabilisation following surgery, during which intravenous fluids and nutritional support should have been optimised.

Drug absorption

For *Prescribing in patients with stoma*, see Stoma care p. 112. [EvGr] Many drugs are incompletely absorbed by patients with a short bowel and may need to be prescribed in much higher doses than usual (such as levothyroxine, warfarin, oral contraceptives, and digoxin) or may need to be given intravenously. Ⓐ

Several factors can alter the absorption of drugs taken by mouth in patients with a compromised gastrointestinal system. The most important factors are the length of intestine available for drug absorption, and which section has been removed. The small intestine, with its large surface area and high blood flow, is the most important site of drug absorption. The larger the amount of the small intestine that has been removed, the higher the possibility that drug absorption will be affected. Other factors, such as gastric emptying and gastric transit time, also affect drug handling. [EvGr] Enteric-coated and modified-release preparations are unsuitable for use in patients with short bowel syndrome, particularly in patients with an ileostomy, as there may not be sufficient release of the active ingredient.

Dosage forms with quick dissolution (soluble tablets) should be used. Uncoated tablets and liquid formulations may also be suitable. Ⓐ[EvGr] Before prescribing liquid formulations, prescribers should consider the osmolarity, excipient content and volume required. Hyperosmolar liquids and some excipients (such as sorbitol) can result in fluid loss. The calorie density of oral supplements should also be considered, as it will influence the volume to be taken. Ⓔ

> **Other drugs used for Short bowel syndrome** Cimetidine, p. 83

AMINO ACIDS AND DERIVATIVES

Teduglutide

07-Jul-2022

- **DRUG ACTION** Teduglutide is an analogue of human glucagon-like peptide-2 (GLP-2), which preserves mucosal integrity by promoting growth and repair of the intestine.

- **INDICATIONS AND DOSE**

  Short bowel syndrome (initiated under specialist supervision)
  - ▸ BY SUBCUTANEOUS INJECTION
  - ▸ Adult: 0.05 mg/kg once daily, dose to be administered to alternating quadrants of the abdomen; alternatively the thigh can be used, for optimal injection volume per body weight, consult product literature. Review treatment after 6 months

- **CONTRA-INDICATIONS** Active or suspected malignancy · history of gastro-intestinal malignancy (in previous 5 years)

- **CAUTIONS** Abrupt withdrawal of parenteral support (reduce gradually with concomitant monitoring of fluid status) · cardiac insufficiency · cardiovascular disease · colo-rectal polyps · hypertension

- **SIDE-EFFECTS**
  - ▸ **Common or very common** Anxiety · appetite decreased · congestive heart failure · cough · dyspnoea · fluid imbalance · gallbladder disorders · gastrointestinal discomfort · gastrointestinal disorders · gastrointestinal stoma complication · headache · influenza like illness · insomnia · nausea · pancreatitis · peripheral oedema · respiratory tract infection · vomiting
  - ▸ **Uncommon** Syncope

- **ALLERGY AND CROSS-SENSITIVITY** Manufacturer advises caution in patients with tetracycline hypersensitivity.

- **PREGNANCY** [EvGr] Specialist sources indicate use if necessary—no human data available. Ⓓ

- **BREAST FEEDING** Manufacturer advises avoid—toxicity in *animal* studies.

- **RENAL IMPAIRMENT**
  Dose adjustments [EvGr] Use half the daily dose if creatinine clearance is less than 50 mL/minute, Ⓜ see p. 21.

- **MONITORING REQUIREMENTS** Manufacturer advises monitoring of small bowel function, gall bladder, bile ducts and pancreas during treatment.

- **TREATMENT CESSATION** Caution when discontinuing treatment—risk of dehydration.

- **PATIENT AND CARER ADVICE** Patients with cardiovascular disease should seek medical attention if they notice sudden weight gain, swollen ankles or dyspnoea—may indicate increased fluid absorption.

- **NATIONAL FUNDING/ACCESS DECISIONS** For full details see funding body website
  NICE decisions
  - ▸ Teduglutide for treating short bowel syndrome (June 2022) NICE TA804 Recommended

  Scottish Medicines Consortium (SMC) decisions
  - ▸ Teduglutide (*Revestive*®) for the treatment of adults with short bowel syndrome (SBS). Patients should be stable following a period of intestinal adaptation after surgery (February 2020) SMC No. SMC2225 Recommended

- **MEDICINAL FORMS** There can be variation in the licensing of different medicines containing the same drug.
  Powder and solvent for solution for injection
  - ▸ Revestive (Takeda UK Ltd) ▼
    Teduglutide 1.25 mg Revestive 1.25mg powder and solvent for solution for injection vials | 28 vial [PoM] £7,307.70 (Hospital only)
    Teduglutide 5 mg Revestive 5mg powder and solvent for solution for injection vials | 28 vial [PoM] £14,615.39 (Hospital only)

2   Constipation and bowel cleansing

2.1   Bowel cleansing

> **Other drugs used for Bowel cleansing** Bisacodyl, p. 67 · Docusate sodium, p. 66 · Magnesium sulfate, p. 1193

LAXATIVES ⟩ OSMOTIC LAXATIVES

Citric acid with magnesium carbonate

09-May-2024

- **DRUG ACTION** Formulated as a bowel cleansing preparation

- **INDICATIONS AND DOSE**

  Bowel evacuation for surgery, colonoscopy or radiological examination
  - ▸ BY MOUTH
  - ▸ Child 5-9 years: One-third of a sachet to be given at 8 a.m. the day before the procedure and, one-third of a sachet to be given between 2 and 4 p.m. the day before the procedure
  - ▸ Child 10-17 years: 0.5–1 sachet, given at 8 a.m. the day before the procedure and 0.5–1 sachet, given between 2 and 4 p.m. the day before the procedure
  - ▸ Adult: 1 sachet, given 8 a.m. the day before the procedure and 1 sachet, given between continued →

2 and 4 p.m. the day before the procedure, use half the dose in frail elderly patients

● **CONTRA-INDICATIONS** Acute intestinal or gastric ulceration · acute severe colitis · gastric retention · gastro-intestinal obstruction · gastro-intestinal perforation · toxic megacolon

● **CAUTIONS** Debilitated · elderly · hypovolaemia (should be corrected before administration of bowel cleansing preparations) · patients with fluid and electrolyte disturbances

CAUTIONS, FURTHER INFORMATION Adequate hydration should be maintained during treatment.

● **INTERACTIONS** → Appendix 1: bowel cleansing preparations

● **SIDE-EFFECTS**

▶ **Common or very common** Gastrointestinal discomfort · nausea · vomiting

▶ **Uncommon** Dehydration · dizziness · electrolyte imbalance · headache

SIDE-EFFECTS, FURTHER INFORMATION Abdominal pain is usually transient and can be reduced by taking preparation more slowly.

● **PREGNANCY** Use with caution.

● **BREAST FEEDING** Use with caution.

● **RENAL IMPAIRMENT** EvGr Caution in mild to moderate impairment; avoid in severe impairment (risk of hypermagnesaemia). ⓜ

● **MONITORING REQUIREMENTS** Renal function should be measured before starting treatment in patients at risk of fluid and electrolyte disturbances.

● **DIRECTIONS FOR ADMINISTRATION** Manufacturer advises one sachet should be reconstituted with 200 mL of hot water; the solution should be allowed to cool for approx. 30 minutes before drinking.

● **PRESCRIBING AND DISPENSING INFORMATION** Reconstitution of one sachet containing 11.57 g magnesium carbonate and 17.79 g anhydrous citric acid produces a solution containing magnesium citrate with 118 mmol Mg^{2+}.
   Flavours of oral powders may include lemon and lime.

● **PATIENT AND CARER ADVICE** Low residue or fluid only diet (e.g. water, fruit squash, clear soup, black tea or coffee) recommended before procedure (according to prescriber's advice) and copious intake of clear fluids recommended until procedure. Patient or carers should be given advice on how to administer oral powder.

● **MEDICINAL FORMS** There can be variation in the licensing of different medicines containing the same drug.

Effervescent powder
CAUTIONARY AND ADVISORY LABELS 13, 10
ELECTROLYTES: May contain Magnesium
▶ Citramag (Cambridge Healthcare Supplies Ltd)
   Magnesium carbonate heavy 11.57 gram, Citric acid anhydrous 17.79 gram Citramag effervescent powder sachets | 10 sachet P
   £20.50 DT = £20.50 SF

Macrogol 3350 with anhydrous sodium sulfate, ascorbic acid, potassium chloride, sodium ascorbate and sodium chloride

17-Aug-2021

(Polyethylene glycols)

● **INDICATIONS AND DOSE**

MOVIPREP ®

Bowel cleansing [before any procedure requiring a clean bowel]
▶ BY MOUTH
▶ Adult: 1 litre daily for 2 doses; first dose of reconstituted solution taken on the evening before procedure and the second dose on the morning of procedure, alternatively 2 litres daily for 1 dose; reconstituted solution to be taken on the evening before the procedure, or on the morning of the procedure, treatment should be completed at least 1 hour before clinical procedures conducted without general anaesthesia, and at least 2 hours before clinical procedures conducted under general anaesthesia

PLENVU ®

Bowel cleansing [before any procedure requiring a clean bowel]
▶ BY MOUTH
▶ Adult: 500 mL daily for 2 doses; first dose of reconstituted solution taken on the evening before procedure and the second dose on the morning of procedure, alternatively 1 litre daily in 2 divided doses, reconstituted solution to be taken either on the evening before the procedure, or in the morning of the procedure—separate doses by at least 1 hour, treatment should be completed at least 1 hour before clinical procedures conducted without general anaesthesia, and at least 2 hours before clinical procedures conducted under general anaesthesia

---

IMPORTANT SAFETY INFORMATION

MHRA/CHM ADVICE: POLYETHYLENE GLYCOL (PEG) LAXATIVES AND STARCH-BASED THICKENERS: POTENTIAL INTERACTIVE EFFECT WHEN MIXED, LEADING TO AN INCREASED RISK OF ASPIRATION (APRIL 2021)
Addition of a macrogol (PEG)-based laxative to a liquid that has been thickened with a starch-based thickener may counteract the thickening action, resulting in a thin watery liquid that, when swallowed, increases the risk of potentially fatal aspiration in patients with dysphagia. Healthcare professionals are advised to avoid directly mixing macrogol-based laxatives with starch-based thickeners, especially for patients with dysphagia who are considered at risk of aspiration.

● **CONTRA-INDICATIONS** Disorders of gastric emptying · G6PD deficiency · gastro-intestinal obstruction · gastro-intestinal perforation · ileus · toxic megacolon

● **CAUTIONS** Debilitated patients · dehydration (correct before administration) · impaired consciousness · impaired gag reflex or possibility of regurgitation or aspiration · moderate-to-severe cardiac impairment · patients at risk of arrhythmia (including those with thyroid disease or electrolyte imbalance) · severe acute inflammatory bowel disease

● **INTERACTIONS** → Appendix 1: bowel cleansing preparations

● **SIDE-EFFECTS**

▶ **Common or very common** Chills · dehydration · dizziness · fever · gastrointestinal discomfort · headaches · hunger · malaise · nausea · sleep disorder · thirst · vomiting

▶ **Uncommon** Arrhythmias · asthenia · drowsiness · dry mouth · dry throat · dysphagia · electrolyte imbalance · hot flush · pain · palpitations · temperature sensation altered

▶ **Frequency not known** Flatulence · hyponatraemic seizure

SIDE-EFFECTS, FURTHER INFORMATION Abdominal pain is usually transient and can be reduced by taking preparation more slowly.

- **PREGNANCY** Manufacturer advises use only if essential—no or limited information available.
- **BREAST FEEDING** Manufacturer advises use only if essential—no information available.
- **RENAL IMPAIRMENT** Manufacturer advises caution if creatinine clearance less than 30 mL/minute. See p. 21.
- **MONITORING REQUIREMENTS** Manufacturer advises consider monitoring baseline and post-treatment electrolytes, renal function and ECG as appropriate, in debilitated patients, those with significant renal impairment, arrhythmia, or at risk of electrolyte imbalance.
- **DIRECTIONS FOR ADMINISTRATION**

  MOVIPREP® Manufacturer advises one pair of sachets (A and B) should be made up to 1 litre with water and taken over 1–2 hours; 1 litre of other clear fluid should also be taken during treatment.

  PLENVU® Manufacturer advises the contents of the single sachet for Dose 1 should be made up to 500 mL with water and taken over 30 minutes; the contents of the 2 sachets (A and B) for Dose 2 should be made up to 500 mL with water and taken over 30 minutes. Each dose should be followed by 500 mL of clear fluid taken over 30 minutes.
- **PRESCRIBING AND DISPENSING INFORMATION**

  MOVIPREP® 1 pair of sachets (A+B) when reconstituted up to 1 litre with water provides Na^+ 181.6 mmol (Na^+ 56.2 mmol absorbable), K^+ 14.2 mmol, Cl^- 59.8 mmol.

  PLENVU® Dose 1 (single sachet) when reconstituted up to 500 mL with water provides Na^+ 160.9 mmol, K^+ 13.3 mmol, Cl^- 47.6 mmol; Dose 2 (sachets A and B) when reconstituted up to 500 mL with water provides Na^+ 297.6 mmol, K^+ 16.1 mmol, Cl^- 70.9 mmol.
- **PATIENT AND CARER ADVICE** Manufacturer advises solid food should not be taken during treatment until procedure completed.

- **MEDICINAL FORMS** There can be variation in the licensing of different medicines containing the same drug.

  Form unstated

  CAUTIONARY AND ADVISORY LABELS 10, 13
  EXCIPIENTS: May contain Aspartame
  ELECTROLYTES: May contain Chloride, potassium, sodium
  ▸ Moviprep (Forum Health Products Ltd)
    Moviprep oral powder sachets | 4 sachet [P] £14.92 [SF]
  ▸ Plenvu (Forum Health Products Ltd)
    Plenvu oral powder sachets | 3 sachet [P] £12.43 [SF]

Macrogol 3350 with anhydrous sodium sulfate, potassium chloride, sodium bicarbonate and sodium chloride

09-May-2024

- **DRUG ACTION** Formulated as a bowel cleansing preparation

- **INDICATIONS AND DOSE**

  Bowel cleansing before radiological examination, colonoscopy, or surgery
  ▸ INITIALLY BY MOUTH
  ▸ Adult: Initially 2 litres daily for 2 doses: first dose of reconstituted solution taken on the evening before procedure and the second dose on the morning of procedure, alternatively (by mouth) initially 250 mL every 10–15 minutes, reconstituted solution to be administered, alternatively (by nasogastric tube)

initially 20–30 mL/minute, starting on the day before procedure until 4 litres have been consumed

> **IMPORTANT SAFETY INFORMATION**
>
> MHRA/CHM ADVICE: POLYETHYLENE GLYCOL (PEG) LAXATIVES AND STARCH-BASED THICKENERS: POTENTIAL INTERACTIVE EFFECT WHEN MIXED, LEADING TO AN INCREASED RISK OF ASPIRATION (APRIL 2021)
>
> Addition of a macrogol (PEG)-based laxative to a liquid that has been thickened with a starch-based thickener may counteract the thickening action, resulting in a thin watery liquid that, when swallowed, increases the risk of potentially fatal aspiration in patients with dysphagia. Healthcare professionals are advised to avoid directly mixing macrogol-based laxatives with starch-based thickeners, especially for patients with dysphagia who are considered at risk of aspiration.

- **CONTRA-INDICATIONS** Acute severe colitis · gastric retention · gastro-intestinal obstruction · gastro-intestinal perforation · toxic megacolon
- **CAUTIONS** Colitis · debilitated patients · fluid and electrolyte disturbances · heart failure (avoid if moderate to severe) · hypovolaemia (should be corrected before administration of bowel cleansing preparations) · impaired gag reflex or possibility of regurgitation or aspiration
- **INTERACTIONS** → Appendix 1: bowel cleansing preparations
- **SIDE-EFFECTS** Angioedema · arrhythmia · chills · confusion · dehydration · dizziness · dyspnoea · electrolyte imbalance · fever · flatulence · gastrointestinal discomfort · headache · malaise · nausea · palpitations · seizure · skin reactions · thirst · vomiting

  SIDE-EFFECTS, FURTHER INFORMATION Abdominal pain is usually transient and can be reduced by taking preparation more slowly.
- **PREGNANCY** Manufacturers advise use only if essential—no information available.
- **BREAST FEEDING** Manufacturers advise use only if essential—no information available.
- **MONITORING REQUIREMENTS** Renal function should be measured before starting treatment in patients at risk of fluid and electrolyte disturbances.
- **DIRECTIONS FOR ADMINISTRATION** [EvGr] 1 sachet should be reconstituted with 1 litre of water. After reconstitution the solution should be kept in a refrigerator and discarded if unused after 24 hours. Ⓜ
- **PRESCRIBING AND DISPENSING INFORMATION** Each *Klean-Prep*® sachet provides Na^+ 125 mmol, K^+ 10 mmol, Cl^- 35 mmol and HCO_3^- 20 mmol when reconstituted with 1 litre of water.
- **PATIENT AND CARER ADVICE** Solid food should not be taken for 2 hours before starting treatment. Adequate hydration should be maintained during treatment. Treatment can be stopped if bowel motions become watery and clear.

- **MEDICINAL FORMS** No licensed medicines listed.

LAXATIVES > STIMULANT LAXATIVES

Magnesium citrate with sodium picosulfate

09-May-2024

- **DRUG ACTION** Formulated as a bowel cleansing preparation

- **INDICATIONS AND DOSE**

CITRAFLEET ® SACHETS

Bowel evacuation on day before radiological examination, endoscopy, or surgery
▶ BY MOUTH
- Adult: 1 sachet taken before 8 a.m, then 1 sachet after 6–8 hours

PHARMACOKINETICS
▶ For *CitraFleet®*: Acts within 3 hours of first dose.

PICOLAX ® SACHETS

Bowel evacuation on day before radiological procedure, endoscopy, or surgery
▶ BY MOUTH
- Child 1 year: 0.25 sachet taken before 8 a.m, then 0.25 sachet after 6–8 hours
- Child 2-3 years: 0.5 sachet taken before 8 a.m, then 0.5 sachet after 6–8 hours
- Child 4-8 years: 1 sachet taken before 8 a.m, then 0.5 sachet after 6–8 hours
- Child 9-17 years: 1 sachet taken before 8 a.m, then 1 sachet after 6–8 hours
- Adult: 1 sachet taken before 8 a.m, then 1 sachet after 6–8 hours

PHARMACOKINETICS
▶ For *Picolax®*: Acts within 3 hours of first dose.

- **CONTRA-INDICATIONS** Acute severe colitis · ascites · congestive cardiac failure · gastric retention · gastro-intestinal obstruction · gastro-intestinal perforation · gastro-intestinal ulceration · toxic megacolon

- **CAUTIONS** Cardiac disease · children · colitis · debilitated patients · elderly · fluid and electrolyte disturbances (avoid in severe dehydration or hypermagnesaemia) · hypovolaemia (should be corrected before administration) · recent gastro-intestinal surgery

- **INTERACTIONS** → Appendix 1: bowel cleansing preparations

- **SIDE-EFFECTS**
▶ **Common or very common** Gastrointestinal discomfort · headache · nausea
▶ **Uncommon** Confusion · electrolyte imbalance · gastrointestinal disorders · seizures · skin reactions · vomiting

- **PREGNANCY** Caution.

- **BREAST FEEDING** Caution.

- **HEPATIC IMPAIRMENT** Avoid in hepatic coma if risk of renal failure.

- **RENAL IMPAIRMENT** EvGr Caution in mild to moderate impairment; avoid in severe impairment (risk of hypermagnesaemia). M

- **DIRECTIONS FOR ADMINISTRATION** Manufacturer advises one sachet of sodium picosulfate with magnesium citrate powder should be reconstituted with 150 mL (approx. half a glass) of cold water; patients should be wearned that heat is generated during reconstitution and that the solution should be allowed to cool before drinking.

- **PRESCRIBING AND DISPENSING INFORMATION** Flavours of oral powder formulations may include lemon.

CITRAFLEET ® SACHETS One reconstituted sachet contains K⁺ 5 mmol and Mg²⁺ 86 mmol.

PICOLAX ® SACHETS One reconstituted sachet contains K⁺ 5 mmol and Mg²⁺ 87 mmol.

- **PATIENT AND CARER ADVICE** Low residue diet recommended on the day before procedure and copious intake of water or other clear fluids recommended during treatment. Patients and carers should be given advice on how to administer oral powder; they should be warned that heat is generated during reconstitution and that the solution should be allowed to cool before drinking.

- **MEDICINAL FORMS** There can be variation in the licensing of different medicines containing the same drug.
Powder for oral solution
CAUTIONARY AND ADVISORY LABELS 10, 13
ELECTROLYTES: May contain Magnesium, potassium
▶ **CitraFleet** (Recordati Pharmaceuticals Ltd)
Sodium picosulfate 10 mg, Magnesium oxide light 3.5 gram, Citric acid anhydrous 10.97 gram CitraFleet oral powder 15.08g sachets | 2 sachet PoM £3.25 SF
▶ **Picolax** (Ferring Pharmaceuticals Ltd)
Sodium picosulfate 10 mg, Magnesium oxide 3.5 gram, Citric acid anhydrous 12 gram Picolax oral powder 16.1g sachets | 20 sachet PoM £33.90 SF

2.2 Constipation

Constipation

10-May-2023

Description of condition

Constipation is defaecation that is unsatisfactory because of infrequent stools, difficult stool passage, or seemingly incomplete defaecation. It can occur at any age and is commonly seen in women, the elderly, and during pregnancy.

It is important for those who complain of constipation to understand that bowel habit can vary considerably in frequency without doing harm. Some people erroneously consider themselves constipated if they do not have a bowel movement each day.

New onset constipation, especially in patients over 50 years of age, or accompanying symptoms such as anaemia, abdominal pain, weight loss, or overt or occult blood in the stool should provoke urgent investigation because of the risk of malignancy or other serious bowel disorder. In those patients with secondary constipation caused by a drug, the drug should be reviewed.

Overview

EvGr In all patients with constipation, an increase in dietary fibre, adequate fluid intake and exercise is advised. Diet should be balanced and contain whole grains, fruits and vegetables. Fibre intake should be increased gradually (to minimise flatulence and bloating). The effects of a high-fibre diet may be seen in a few days although it can take as long as 4 weeks. Adequate fluid intake is important (particularly with a high-fibre diet or fibre supplements), but can be difficult for some people (for example, the frail or elderly). Fruits high in fibre and sorbitol, and fruit juices high in sorbitol, can help prevent and treat constipation. A

Misconceptions about bowel habits have led to excessive laxative use. Laxative abuse may lead to hypokalaemia. Before prescribing laxatives it is important to be sure that the patient is constipated and that the constipation is not secondary to an underlying undiagnosed complaint.

Laxatives
Bulk-forming laxatives
Bulk-forming laxatives include bran, ispaghula husk p. 60, methylcellulose and sterculia p. 61. They are of particular value in adults with small hard stools if fibre cannot be increased in the diet. Onset of action is up to 72 hours. Symptoms of flatulence, bloating, and cramping may be

exacerbated. Adequate fluid intake must be maintained to avoid intestinal obstruction.

Methylcellulose, ispaghula husk and sterculia may be used in patients who cannot tolerate bran. Methylcellulose also acts as a faecal softener.

Stimulant laxatives

Stimulant laxatives include bisacodyl p. 67, sodium picosulfate p. 70, and members of the anthraquinone group (senna p. 69, co-danthramer p. 67 and co-danthrusate p. 68). Stimulant laxatives increase intestinal motility and often cause abdominal cramp; manufacturer advises they should be avoided in intestinal obstruction.

The use of co-danthramer and co-danthrusate is limited to constipation in terminally ill patients because of potential carcinogenicity (based on animal studies) and evidence of genotoxicity.

Docusate sodium p. 66 is believed to act as both a stimulant laxative and as a faecal softener (below). Glycerol suppositories act as a lubricant and as a rectal stimulant by virtue of the mildly irritant action of glycerol.

Faecal softeners

Faecal softeners are claimed to act by decreasing surface tension and increasing penetration of intestinal fluid into the faecal mass. Docusate sodium and glycerol suppositories p. 68 have softening properties. Enemas containing arachis oil p. 66 (ground-nut oil, peanut oil) lubricate and soften impacted faeces and promote a bowel movement. Liquid paraffin p. 66 has also been used as a lubricant for the passage of stools but manufacturer advises that it should be used with caution because of its adverse effects, which include anal seepage and the risks of granulomatous disease of the gastro-intestinal tract or of lipoid pneumonia on aspiration.

Osmotic laxatives

Osmotic laxatives increase the amount of water in the large bowel, either by drawing fluid from the body into the bowel or by retaining the fluid they were administered with. Lactulose p. 61 is a semi-synthetic disaccharide which is not absorbed from the gastro-intestinal tract. It produces an osmotic diarrhoea of low faecal pH, and discourages the proliferation of ammonia-producing organisms. It is therefore useful in the treatment of hepatic encephalopathy. Macrogols (such as macrogol 3350 with potassium chloride, sodium bicarbonate and sodium chloride p. 62) are inert polymers of ethylene glycol which sequester fluid in the bowel; giving fluid with macrogols may reduce the dehydrating effect sometimes seen with osmotic laxatives.

Other drugs used in constipation

Linaclotide p. 54 is a guanylate cyclase-C receptor agonist that is licensed for the treatment of moderate to severe irritable bowel syndrome associated with constipation. It increases intestinal fluid secretion and transit, and decreases visceral pain.

Prucalopride p. 65 is a selective serotonin $5HT_4$-receptor agonist with prokinetic properties. It is licensed for the treatment of chronic constipation in adults, when other laxatives have failed to provide an adequate response.

Bowel cleansing preparations

Bowel cleansing preparations are used before colonic surgery, colonoscopy or radiological examination to ensure the bowel is free of solid contents; examples include macrogol 3350 with anhydrous sodium sulfate, potassium chloride, sodium bicarbonate and sodium chloride p. 57, citric acid with magnesium carbonate p. 55, magnesium citrate with sodium picosulfate p. 58 and sodium acid phosphate with sodium phosphate p. 64. Bowel cleansing treatments are not treatments for constipation.

Management

Short-duration constipation

[EvGr] In the management of short-duration constipation (where dietary measures are ineffective) treatment should be started with a bulk-forming laxative, ensuring adequate fluid intake. If stools remain hard, add or switch to an osmotic laxative. If stools are soft but difficult to pass or the person complains of inadequate emptying, a stimulant laxative should be added. (A)

Opioid-induced constipation

For guidance on the management of constipation in palliative care, see Prescribing in palliative care p. 26.

[EvGr] In patients with opioid-induced constipation, an osmotic laxative (or docusate sodium to soften the stools) and a stimulant laxative is recommended. Bulk-forming laxatives should be avoided.

Naloxegol p. 72 is recommended for the treatment of opioid-induced constipation when response to other laxatives is inadequate. (A)

Methylnaltrexone bromide p. 71 is licensed for the treatment of opioid-induced constipation when response to other laxatives is inadequate.

Faecal impaction

The treatment of faecal impaction depends on the stool consistency. [EvGr] In patients with hard stools, a high dose of an oral macrogol (such as macrogol 3350 with potassium chloride, sodium bicarbonate and sodium chloride) may be considered. In those with soft stools, or with hard stools after a few days treatment with a macrogol, an oral stimulant laxative should be started or added to the previous treatment. If the response to oral laxatives is inadequate, for soft stools consider rectal administration of bisacodyl, and for hard stools rectal administration of glycerol alone, or glycerol plus bisacodyl. Alternatively, an enema of docusate sodium or sodium citrate p. 909 may be tried.

If the response is still insufficient, a sodium acid phosphate with sodium phosphate or arachis oil retention enema may be necessary. For hard faeces it can be helpful to give the enema of arachis oil overnight before giving an enema of sodium acid phosphate with sodium phosphate p. 64 or sodium citrate p. 909 the following day. Enemas may need to be repeated several times to clear hard impacted faeces. (A)

Chronic constipation

[EvGr] In the management of chronic constipation, treatment should be started with a bulk-forming laxative, whilst ensuring good hydration. If stools remain hard, add or change to an osmotic laxative such as a macrogol. Lactulose p. 61 is an alternative if macrogols are not effective, or not tolerated. If the response is inadequate, a stimulant laxative can be added. The dose of laxative should be adjusted gradually to produce one or two soft, formed stools per day.

If at least two laxatives (from different classes) have been tried at the highest tolerated recommended doses for at least 6 months, the use of prucalopride p. 65 (in women only) should be considered. If treatment with prucalopride is not effective after 4 weeks, the patient should be re-examined and the benefit of continuing treatment reconsidered.

Laxatives can be slowly withdrawn when regular bowel movements occur without difficulty, according to the frequency and consistency of the stools. If a combination of laxatives has been used, reduce and stop one laxative at a time; if possible, the stimulant laxative should be reduced first. However, it may be necessary to also adjust the dose of the osmotic laxative to compensate. (A)

Constipation in pregnancy and breast-feeding

[EvGr] If dietary and lifestyle changes fail to control constipation in pregnancy, fibre supplements in the form of bran or wheat are likely to help women experiencing constipation in pregnancy, and raise no serious concerns about side-effects to the mother or fetus.

A bulk-forming laxative is the first choice during pregnancy if fibre supplements fail. An osmotic laxative, such as lactulose, can also be used. Bisacodyl p. 67 or senna

1

p. 69 may be suitable if a stimulant effect is necessary but use of senna should be avoided near term or if there is a history of unstable pregnancy. Stimulant laxatives are more effective than bulk-forming laxatives but are more likely to cause side-effects (diarrhoea and abdominal discomfort), reducing their acceptability to patients. Docusate sodium p. 66 and glycerol suppositories p. 68 can also be used.

A bulk-forming laxative is the first choice during breast-feeding, if dietary measures fail. Lactulose or a macrogol may be used if stools remain hard. As an alternative, a short course of a stimulant laxative such as bisacodyl or senna can be considered. Ⓐ

Constipation in children

Early identification of constipation and effective treatment can improve outcomes for children. Without early diagnosis and treatment, an acute episode of constipation can lead to anal fissure and become chronic.

EvGr The first-line treatment for children with constipation requires the use of a laxative in combination with dietary modification and behavioural interventions. Diet modification alone is not recommended as first-line treatment.

In children, an increase in dietary fibre, adequate fluid intake, and exercise is advised. Diet should be balanced and contain fruits, vegetables, high-fibre bread, baked beans, and wholegrain breakfast cereals. Unprocessed bran (which may cause bloating and flatulence and reduces the absorption of micronutrients) is **not** recommended.

If faecal impaction is not present (or has been treated), the child should be treated promptly with a laxative. A macrogol (such as macrogol 3350 with potassium chloride, sodium bicarbonate and sodium chloride p. 62) is preferred as first-line management, with the dose adjusted according to symptoms and response. If the response is inadequate add a stimulant laxative, or change to a stimulant laxative if the first-line therapy is not tolerated. If stools remain hard, lactulose or another laxative with softening effects, such as docusate sodium should be added.

In children with chronic constipation, laxatives should be continued for several weeks after a regular pattern of bowel movements or toilet training is established. The dose of laxatives should then be tapered gradually, over a period of months, according to response. Some children may require laxative therapy for several years.

A shorter duration of laxative treatment may be possible in some children with a very short history of constipation, but they should be carefully monitored for a relapse of constipation.

Laxatives should be administered at a time that produces an effect that is likely to fit in with the child's toilet routine. Ⓐ

Faecal impaction in children

EvGr Treatment of faecal impaction may initially increase symptoms of soiling and abdominal pain. An oral preparation containing a macrogol (such as macrogol 3350 with potassium chloride, sodium bicarbonate and sodium chloride) is used first-line for all children to clear faecal mass and to establish and maintain soft well-formed stools. In children over 1 year of age with faecal impaction, an escalating dose regimen should be used. If disimpaction does not occur after 2 weeks of macrogol treatment, a stimulant laxative should be added. If macrogol therapy is not tolerated, change to a stimulant laxative alone or, if stools are hard, use in combination with an osmotic laxative such as lactulose. Long-term regular use of laxatives is essential to maintain well-formed stools and prevent recurrence of faecal impaction; intermittent use may provoke relapses. Ⓐ

LAXATIVES > BULK-FORMING LAXATIVES

Ispaghula husk
27-Jul-2020

- **DRUG ACTION** Bulk-forming laxatives relieve constipation by increasing faecal mass which stimulates peristalsis.

- **INDICATIONS AND DOSE**

Constipation
▸ BY MOUTH
- Child 1 month-5 years: 2.5–5 mL twice daily, dose to be taken only when prescribed by a doctor, as half or whole level spoonful in water, preferably after meals, morning and evening
- Child 6-11 years: 2.5–5 mL twice daily, dose to be given as a half or whole level spoonful in water, preferably after meals, morning and evening
- Child 12-17 years: 1 sachet twice daily, dose to be given in water preferably after meals, morning and evening
- Adult: 1 sachet twice daily, dose to be given in water preferably taken after food, morning and evening

Constipation (dose approved for use by community practitioner nurse prescribers)
▸ BY MOUTH
- Child 6-11 years: 2.5–5 mL twice daily, dose to be given as a half or whole level spoonful in water, preferably after meals, morning and evening
- Child 12-17 years: 1 sachet twice daily, dose to be given in water preferably after meals, morning and evening
- Adult: 1 sachet twice daily, dose to be given in water preferably taken after food, morning and evening

DOSE EQUIVALENCE AND CONVERSION
▸ 1 sachet equivalent to 2 level 5 ml spoonsful.

- **CONTRA-INDICATIONS** Colonic atony · faecal impaction · intestinal obstruction · reduced gut motility · sudden change in bowel habit that has persisted more than two weeks · undiagnosed rectal bleeding

- **CAUTIONS** Adequate fluid intake should be maintained to avoid oesophageal or intestinal obstruction

- **SIDE-EFFECTS** Abdominal distension · bronchospasm · conjunctivitis · gastrointestinal disorders · hypersensitivity · rhinitis · skin reactions

- **DIRECTIONS FOR ADMINISTRATION** Manufacturer advises dose to be taken with at least 150 mL liquid.

- **PRESCRIBING AND DISPENSING INFORMATION** Flavours of soluble granules formulations may include plain, lemon, or orange.

- **HANDLING AND STORAGE** Ispaghula husk contains potent allergens. Individuals exposed to the product (including those handling the product) can develop hypersensitivity reactions such as rhinitis, conjunctivitis, bronchospasm and in some cases, anaphylaxis.

- **PATIENT AND CARER ADVICE** Manufacturer advises that preparations that swell in contact with liquid should always be carefully swallowed with water and should not be taken immediately before going to bed. Patients and their carers should be advised that the full effect may take some days to develop and should be given advice on how to administer ispaghula husk.

- **MEDICINAL FORMS** There can be variation in the licensing of different medicines containing the same drug.

Effervescent granules
CAUTIONARY AND ADVISORY LABELS 13
EXCIPIENTS: May contain Aspartame
▸ Fybogel (Reckitt Benckiser Healthcare (UK) Ltd)
  Ispaghula husk 3.5 gram Fybogel 3.5g effervescent granules sachets plain SF | 30 sachet GSL £5.49 DT = £5.49 SF
  Fybogel Orange 3.5g effervescent granules sachets SF | 30 sachet GSL £5.49 DT = £5.49 SF

Fybogel Lemon 3.5g effervescent granules sachets SF |
30 sachet [GSL] £5.49 DT = £5.49 [SF]
- ▶ **Fybogel Hi-Fibre** (Reckitt Benckiser Healthcare (UK) Ltd)
  Ispaghula husk 3.5 gram Fybogel Hi-Fibre Orange 3.5g effervescent granules sachets | 10 sachet [GSL] £3.55 [SF] | 30 sachet [GSL] £9.70 DT = £5.49 [SF]
  Fybogel Hi-Fibre Lemon 3.5g effervescent granules sachets | 10 sachet [GSL] £3.55 [SF]
- ▶ **Ispagel** (Bristol Laboratories Ltd)
  Ispaghula husk 3.5 gram Ispagel Orange 3.5g effervescent granules sachets | 10 sachet [GSL] £4.50 [SF] | 30 sachet [GSL] £6.50 DT = £5.49 [SF]

Granules for oral suspension
CAUTIONARY AND ADVISORY LABELS 13
EXCIPIENTS: May contain Aspartame
- ▶ **Ispaghula husk (Non-proprietary)**
  Ispaghula husk 3.5 gram Ispaghula husk 3.5g granules for oral suspension sachets gluten free | 30 sachet [GSL] £5.49
  Ispaghula husk 3.5g granules for oral suspension sachets gluten free sugar free | 30 sachet [GSL] [▣] [SF]

Combinations available: *Senna with ispaghula husk,* p. 69

Sterculia

12-Aug-2020

- ● DRUG ACTION Sterculia is a bulk-forming laxative. It relieves constipation by increasing faecal mass which stimulates peristalsis.

- ● **INDICATIONS AND DOSE**

Constipation
- ▶ BY MOUTH
  - ▶ Child 6–11 years: 0.5–1 sachet 1–2 times a day, alternatively, half to one heaped 5-mL spoonful once or twice a day; washed down without chewing with plenty of liquid after meals
  - ▶ Child 12–17 years: 1–2 sachets 1–2 times a day, alternatively, one to two heaped 5-mL spoonfuls once or twice a day; washed down without chewing with plenty of liquid after meals
  - ▶ Adult: 1–2 sachets 1–2 times a day, alternatively, one to two heaped 5-mL spoonfuls once or twice a day; washed down without chewing with plenty of liquid after meals

- ● CONTRA-INDICATIONS Colonic atony · difficulty swallowing · faecal impaction · intestinal obstruction
- ● CAUTIONS Adequate fluid intake should be maintained to avoid oesophageal or intestinal obstruction

  CAUTIONS, FURTHER INFORMATION It may be necessary to supervise elderly or debilitated patients or those with intestinal narrowing or decreased motility to ensure adequate fluid intake.

- ● SIDE-EFFECTS Diarrhoea · gastrointestinal discomfort · gastrointestinal disorders · nausea
- ● DIRECTIONS FOR ADMINISTRATION Manufacturer advises may be mixed with soft food (e.g. yoghurt) before swallowing, followed by plenty of liquid.
- ● PATIENT AND CARER ADVICE Patients and their carers should be advised that the full effect may take some days to develop. Preparations that swell in contact with liquid should always be carefully swallowed with water and should not be taken immediately before going to bed.

- ● MEDICINAL FORMS No licensed medicines listed.

Sterculia with frangula

The properties listed below are those particular to the combination only. For the properties of the components please consider, sterculia above.

- ● **INDICATIONS AND DOSE**

After haemorrhoidectomy
- ▶ BY MOUTH
  - ▶ Adult: 1–2 sachets 1–2 times a day, alternatively, 1–2 heaped 5 mL spoonfuls once or twice a day; washed down without chewing with plenty of liquid after meals

Constipation
- ▶ BY MOUTH
  - ▶ Adult: 1–2 sachets 1–2 times a day, alternatively, 1–2 heaped 5 mL spoonfuls once or twice a day; washed down without chewing with plenty of liquid after meals

- ● PREGNANCY Manufacturer advises avoid.
- ● BREAST FEEDING Manufacturer advises avoid.
- ● PATIENT AND CARER ADVICE Patients and their carers should be advised that the full effect may take some days to develop. Preparations that swell in contact with liquid should always be carefully swallowed with water and should not be taken immediately before going to bed.

- ● MEDICINAL FORMS No licensed medicines listed.

LAXATIVES › OSMOTIC LAXATIVES

Lactulose

10-Nov-2021

- ● **INDICATIONS AND DOSE**

Constipation
- ▶ BY MOUTH
  - ▶ Child 1–11 months: 2.5 mL twice daily, to be adjusted according to response
  - ▶ Child 1–4 years: 2.5–10 mL twice daily, to be adjusted according to response
  - ▶ Child 5–17 years: 5–20 mL twice daily, to be adjusted according to response
  - ▶ Adult: Initially 15 mL twice daily, to be adjusted according to response

Hepatic encephalopathy (portal systemic encephalopathy)
- ▶ BY MOUTH
  - ▶ Adult: 30–50 mL 3 times a day, dose subsequently adjusted to produce 2–3 soft stools per day

Constipation (dose approved for use by community practitioner nurse prescribers)
- ▶ BY MOUTH
  - ▶ Child 1–11 months: 2.5 mL twice daily, to be adjusted according to response
  - ▶ Child 1–4 years: 5 mL twice daily, to be adjusted according to response
  - ▶ Child 5–10 years: 10 mL twice daily, to be adjusted according to response
  - ▶ Child 11–17 years: Initially 15 mL twice daily, to be adjusted according to response
  - ▶ Adult: Initially 15 mL twice daily, to be adjusted according to response

PHARMACOKINETICS
- ▶ Lactulose may take up to 48 hours to act.

- ● UNLICENSED USE
- ▶ In adults Lactulose doses in the BNF may differ from those in product literature.

- ● CONTRA-INDICATIONS Galactosaemia · gastro-intestinal obstruction · gastro-intestinal perforation · risk of gastro-intestinal perforation

- **CAUTIONS** Lactose intolerance
- **SIDE-EFFECTS**
- ▶ **Common or very common** Abdominal pain · diarrhoea · flatulence · nausea · vomiting
- ▶ **Uncommon** Electrolyte imbalance
- **PREGNANCY** Not known to be harmful.
- **PATIENT AND CARER ADVICE**
  Medicines for Children leaflet: Lactulose for constipation
  www.medicinesforchildren.org.uk/medicines/lactulose-for-constipation/
- **MEDICINAL FORMS** There can be variation in the licensing of different medicines containing the same drug.
  Oral solution
  - ▶ Lactulose (Non-proprietary)
    Lactulose 666.667 mg per 1 ml Lactulose 10g/15ml oral solution 15ml sachets sugar free | 10 sachet P £3.65 DT = £3.65 SF
    Lactulose 10g/15ml oral solution 15ml sachets sugar free unflavoured | 10 sachet P £2.50 DT = £3.65 SF
    Lactulose 10g/15ml oral solution 15ml sachets sugar free plum | 10 sachet P £2.60 DT = £3.65 SF
    Lactulose 680 mg per 1 ml Lactulose 3.1-3.7g/5ml oral solution | 300 ml P £2.44–£7.72 | 500 ml P £12.72 DT = £4.92

Macrogol 3350

05-May-2021

- **INDICATIONS AND DOSE**

Chronic constipation
- ▶ BY MOUTH
- ▶ Adult: 2 sachets once daily usually for up to 2 weeks, dose to be taken preferably in the morning

PHARMACOKINETICS
- ▶ Onset of action 24–48 hours.

IMPORTANT SAFETY INFORMATION

MHRA/CHM ADVICE: POLYETHYLENE GLYCOL (PEG) LAXATIVES AND STARCH-BASED THICKENERS: POTENTIAL INTERACTIVE EFFECT WHEN MIXED, LEADING TO AN INCREASED RISK OF ASPIRATION (APRIL 2021)

Addition of a macrogol (PEG)-based laxative to a liquid that has been thickened with a starch-based thickener may counteract the thickening action, resulting in a thin watery liquid that, when swallowed, increases the risk of potentially fatal aspiration in patients with dysphagia. Healthcare professionals are advised to avoid directly mixing macrogol-based laxatives with starch-based thickeners, especially for patients with dysphagia who are considered at risk of aspiration.

- **CONTRA-INDICATIONS** Ileus · intestinal obstruction · intestinal perforation · risk of intestinal perforation · severe inflammatory bowel disease · toxic megacolon
- **INTERACTIONS** → Appendix 1: macrogol 3350
- **SIDE-EFFECTS**
- ▶ **Common or very common** Flatulence · gastrointestinal discomfort · nausea · vomiting
- ▶ **Uncommon** Anaemia · angioedema · appetite disorder · dehydration · dizziness · fatigue · hiccups · hypertension · hypoglycaemia · hypothyroidism · increased risk of infection · local swelling · migraine · muscle twitching · neuritis · oedema · pain · pelvic pain · sinus congestion · skin reactions · tachycardia · taste altered
- **PREGNANCY** Limited data, but manufacturer advises no effects anticipated as systemic exposure is negligible.
- **DIRECTIONS FOR ADMINISTRATION** Manufacturer advises contents of each sachet to be dissolved in half a glass (approx. 100 mL) of water just before administration.

- **MEDICINAL FORMS** There can be variation in the licensing of different medicines containing the same drug.
  Powder for oral solution
  CAUTIONARY AND ADVISORY LABELS 13
  - ▶ TransiSoft (Mayoly UK Ltd)
    Macrogol '3350' 85 gram per 1 litre TransiSoft oral powder 8.5g sachets | 28 sachet P £217.17 DT = £188.84 SF

Macrogol 3350 with potassium chloride, sodium bicarbonate and sodium chloride

27-Jan-2025

- **INDICATIONS AND DOSE**

Chronic constipation (dose for 'paediatric' sachets) | Prevention of faecal impaction (dose for 'paediatric' sachets)
- ▶ BY MOUTH
- ▶ Child 2–5 years: 1 sachet daily in 1–2 divided doses, adjust dose to produce regular soft stools; maximum 4 sachets per day
- ▶ Child 6–11 years: 2 sachets daily in 1–2 divided doses, adjust dose to produce regular soft stools; maximum 4 sachets per day

Faecal impaction (dose for 'paediatric' sachets)
- ▶ BY MOUTH
- ▶ Child 5–11 years: 4 sachets on first day, dose then increased in steps of 2 sachets per day up to maximum 12 sachets per day, total daily dose to be taken within a 12-hour period, after disimpaction, switch to maintenance laxative therapy

Chronic constipation (dose for 'half-strength' sachets)
- ▶ BY MOUTH
- ▶ Child 12–17 years: 2 sachets 1–3 times a day usually for up to 2 weeks; maintenance 2 sachets 1–2 times a day
- ▶ Adult: 2 sachets 1–3 times a day usually for up to 2 weeks; maintenance 2 sachets 1–2 times a day

Faecal impaction (dose for 'half-strength' sachets)
- ▶ BY MOUTH
- ▶ Child 12–17 years: 8 sachets on first day, dose then increased in steps of 4 sachets per day up to maximum 16 sachets per day, total daily dose to be taken within a 6-hour period, after disimpaction, switch to maintenance laxative therapy if required
- ▶ Adult: 8 sachets on first day, dose then increased in steps of 4 sachets per day up to maximum 16 sachets per day, total daily dose to be taken within a 6-hour period, after disimpaction, switch to maintenance laxative therapy if required

Chronic constipation (dose for 'full-strength' sachets)
- ▶ BY MOUTH
- ▶ Child 12–17 years: 1 sachet 1–3 times a day usually for up to 2 weeks; maintenance 1 sachet 1–2 times a day
- ▶ Adult: 1 sachet 1–3 times a day usually for up to 2 weeks; maintenance 1 sachet 1–2 times a day

Faecal impaction (dose for 'full-strength' sachets)
- ▶ BY MOUTH
- ▶ Child 12–17 years: 4 sachets on first day, dose then increased in steps of 2 sachets per day up to maximum 8 sachets per day, total daily dose to be taken within a 6-hour period, after disimpaction, switch to maintenance laxative therapy if required
- ▶ Adult: 4 sachets on first day, dose then increased in steps of 2 sachets per day up to maximum 8 sachets per day, total daily dose to be taken within a 6-hour period, after disimpaction, switch to maintenance laxative therapy if required

DOSE EQUIVALENCE AND CONVERSION
- ▶ Each 'paediatric' sachet contains 6.563 g of macrogol 3350; each 'half-strength' sachet contains 6.563 g of

macrogol 3350; each 'full-strength' sachet contains 13.125 g of macrogol 3350.

MOVICOL® READY TO TAKE SACHETS

Chronic constipation

▶ BY MOUTH

▶ Child 12–17 years: 1 sachet 1–3 times a day usually for up to 2 weeks; maintenance 1 sachet 1–2 times a day

▶ Adult: 1 sachet 1–3 times a day usually for up to 2 weeks; maintenance 1 sachet 1–2 times a day

Faecal impaction

▶ BY MOUTH

▶ Child 12–17 years: 4 sachets on first day, dose then increased in steps of 2 sachets per day up to maximum 8 sachets per day, total daily dose to be taken within a 6-hour period; patients should also take an additional 1 litre of fluid daily, after disimpaction, switch to maintenance laxative therapy if required

▶ Adult: 4 sachets on first day, dose then increased in steps of 2 sachets per day up to maximum 8 sachets per day, total daily dose to be taken within a 6-hour period; patients should also take an additional 1 litre of fluid daily, after disimpaction, switch to maintenance laxative therapy if required

MOVICOL® LIQUID

Chronic constipation

▶ BY MOUTH

▶ Child 12–17 years: 25 mL 1–3 times a day usually for up to 2 weeks; maintenance 25 mL 1–2 times a day

▶ Adult: 25 mL 1–3 times a day usually for up to 2 weeks; maintenance 25 mL 1–2 times a day

VISTAPREP® ORAL POWDER

Bowel cleansing before colonoscopy

▶ BY MOUTH

▶ Adult: 3–4 litres, reconstituted solution taken over 4 hours, generally on the day of procedure; alternatively, it can be taken on the evening before procedure *or* started on the evening before procedure and completed on the morning of procedure

● **UNLICENSED USE**

▶ In children Macrogol 3350 with potassium chloride, sodium bicarbonate and sodium chloride may be used as detailed below, although these situations are considered outside the scope of its licence:
  ● EvGr dose for chronic constipation/prevention of faecal impaction in children aged 6 years;
  ● dose titration schedule for faecal impaction in children aged 12–17 years Ⓐ.
▶ In adults Macrogol 3350 with potassium chloride, sodium bicarbonate and sodium chloride may be used as detailed below, although this is considered outside the scope of its licence: EvGr dose titration schedule for faecal impaction Ⓔ

> **IMPORTANT SAFETY INFORMATION**
>
> **MHRA/CHM ADVICE: POLYETHYLENE GLYCOL (PEG) LAXATIVES AND STARCH-BASED THICKENERS: POTENTIAL INTERACTIVE EFFECT WHEN MIXED, LEADING TO AN INCREASED RISK OF ASPIRATION (APRIL 2021)**
>
> Addition of a macrogol (PEG)-based laxative to a liquid that has been thickened with a starch-based thickener may counteract the thickening action, resulting in a thin watery liquid that, when swallowed, increases the risk of potentially fatal aspiration in patients with dysphagia. Healthcare professionals are advised to avoid directly mixing macrogol-based laxatives with starch-based thickeners, especially for patients with dysphagia who are considered at risk of aspiration.

● **CONTRA-INDICATIONS** Intestinal obstruction · intestinal perforation · paralytic ileus · severe inflammatory conditions of the intestinal tract (including Crohn's disease, ulcerative colitis and toxic megacolon) · use of 'paediatric' sachets for faecal impaction in impaired cardiovascular function (no information available)

VISTAPREP® ORAL POWDER Impaired consciousness · impaired swallowing reflex · moderate-to-severe heart failure—limited safety information available · risk of regurgitation or aspiration · severe dehydration—limited safety information available

● **CAUTIONS** Cardiovascular impairment (should not take more than 2 'full-strength' sachets or 4 'half-strength' sachets in any one hour) · impaired consciousness (with high doses) · impaired gag reflex (with high doses) · reflux oesophagitis (with high doses)

VISTAPREP® ORAL POWDER Chronic inflammatory bowel disease · elderly · heart rhythm abnormalities · reflux oesophagitis

● **INTERACTIONS** → Appendix 1: macrogol 3350

● **SIDE-EFFECTS** Electrolyte imbalance (discontinue if symptoms occur) · flatulence · gastrointestinal discomfort · nausea · vomiting

● **PREGNANCY** Manufacturers advise may be used—limited data available.

● **HEPATIC IMPAIRMENT**

VISTAPREP® ORAL POWDER Manufacturer advises avoid (limited information available).

● **RENAL IMPAIRMENT**

▶ In children Manufacturers advise avoid use of 'paediatric' sachets for faecal impaction—no information available.

VISTAPREP® ORAL POWDER Manufacturer advises avoid—limited safety information available.

● **DIRECTIONS FOR ADMINISTRATION** Manufacturers advise dissolve contents of each 'half-strength' sachet of oral powder in 62.5 mL of water, and each 'full-strength' sachet of oral powder in 125 mL of water; after reconstitution the solution should be kept in a refrigerator—for further information consult product literature.

▶ In children Manufacturers advise dissolve contents of each 'paediatric' sachet of oral powder in 62.5 mL of water; after reconstitution the solution should be kept in a refrigerator—for further information consult product literature.

MOVICOL® LIQUID Manufacturer advises dilute 25 mL of oral concentrate with 100 mL of water; after dilution the solution should be discarded if unused after 24 hours.

VISTAPREP® ORAL POWDER Manufacturer advises dissolve the contents of each sachet in 1 L water; if not consumed immediately, the reconstituted solution should be kept in a refrigerator and discarded if unused after 48 hours.

● **PATIENT AND CARER ADVICE** Patients or carers should be counselled on how to take the oral powder and oral solution.

Medicines for Children leaflet: Movicol for constipation www.medicinesforchildren.org.uk/medicines/movicol-for-constipation/

VISTAPREP® ORAL POWDER Manufacturer advises treatment can be stopped if bowel motions become watery and clear.

● **MEDICINAL FORMS** There can be variation in the licensing of different medicines containing the same drug.

Oral solution

CAUTIONARY AND ADVISORY LABELS 13

ELECTROLYTES: May contain Bicarbonate, chloride, potassium, sodium

▶ Movicol (Forum Health Products Ltd)
  Macrogol '3350' 13.125 gram, Potassium 27 mmol per 1 litre, Bicarbonate 85 mmol per 1 litre, Chloride 267 mmol per 1 litre, Sodium 325 mmol per 1 litre Movicol Ready to Take oral solution 25ml sachets | 30 sachet Ⓟ £9.89 DT = £8.59 SF

Powder for oral solution
CAUTIONARY AND ADVISORY LABELS 10, 13
ELECTROLYTES: May contain Bicarbonate, chloride, potassium, sodium

▸ **Macrogol 3350 with potassium chloride, sodium bicarbonate and sodium chloride (Non-proprietary)**
Macrogol '3350' 105 gram per 1 litre, Potassium 5.4 mmol per 1 litre, Bicarbonate 17 mmol per 1 litre, Chloride 53 mmol per 1 litre, Sodium 65 mmol per 1 litre Macrogol compound oral powder sachets sugar free | 20 sachet P £4.45 SF | 30 sachet P £6.68 DT = £5.97 SF

▸ **CosmoCol** (Stirling Anglian Pharmaceuticals Ltd)
Macrogol '3350' 105 gram per 1 litre, Potassium 5.4 mmol per 1 litre, Bicarbonate 17 mmol per 1 litre, Chloride 53 mmol per 1 litre, Sodium 65 mmol per 1 litre CosmoCol Paediatric oral powder 6.9g sachets | 30 sachet PoM £3.76 DT = £4.38 SF CosmoCol Orange Flavour oral powder sachets | 20 sachet P £4.18 SF | 30 sachet P £5.97 DT = £5.97 SF CosmoCol Lemon and Lime Flavour oral powder sachets | 20 sachet P £4.18 SF | 30 sachet P £5.97 DT = £5.97 SF CosmoCol Orange Lemon and Lime oral powder sachets | 30 sachet P £5.97 DT = £5.97 SF CosmoCol Plain oral powder sachets | 30 sachet P £5.97 DT = £5.97 SF

▸ **Laxido** (Galen Ltd)
Macrogol '3350' 105 gram per 1 litre, Potassium 5.4 mmol per 1 litre, Bicarbonate 17 mmol per 1 litre, Chloride 53 mmol per 1 litre, Sodium 65 mmol per 1 litre Laxido Orange oral powder sachets sugar free | 20 sachet P £4.18 SF | 30 sachet P £5.97 DT = £5.97 SF Laxido Paediatric Plain oral powder 6.9g sachets | 30 sachet PoM £4.38 DT = £4.38 SF

▸ **Molaxole** (Viatris UK Healthcare Ltd)
Macrogol '3350' 105 gram per 1 litre, Potassium 5.4 mmol per 1 litre, Bicarbonate 17 mmol per 1 litre, Chloride 53 mmol per 1 litre, Sodium 65 mmol per 1 litre Molaxole oral powder sachets | 20 sachet P £3.78 SF | 30 sachet P £5.68 DT = £5.97 SF

▸ **Movicol** (Forum Health Products Ltd, Norgine Pharmaceuticals Ltd)
Macrogol '3350' 105 gram per 1 litre, Potassium 5.4 mmol per 1 litre, Bicarbonate 17 mmol per 1 litre, Chloride 53 mmol per 1 litre, Sodium 65 mmol per 1 litre Movicol Chocolate oral powder 13.9g sachets | 30 sachet P £9.45 DT = £5.97 SF Movicol Paediatric Plain oral powder 6.9g sachets | 30 sachet PoM £4.38 DT = £4.38 SF Movicol oral powder 13.8g sachets lemon & lime | 20 sachet P £6.61 SF | 30 sachet P £9.45 DT = £5.97 SF | 50 sachet P £14.29 SF Movicol Paediatric Chocolate oral powder 6.9g sachets | 30 sachet PoM £4.38 DT = £4.38 SF Movicol Plain oral powder 13.7g sachets | 30 sachet P £9.45 DT = £5.97 SF | 50 sachet P £14.29 SF

▸ **Strigol** (Strides Pharma UK Ltd)
Macrogol '3350' 105 gram per 1 litre, Potassium 5.4 mmol per 1 litre, Bicarbonate 17 mmol per 1 litre, Chloride 53 mmol per 1 litre, Sodium 65 mmol per 1 litre Strigol oral powder 13.72g sachets plain | 20 sachet P £3.50 SF | 30 sachet P £4.99 DT = £5.97 SF Strigol Paediatric oral powder 6.86g sachets | 30 sachet PoM £3.15 DT = £4.38 SF Strigol oral powder 13.72g sachets orange | 30 sachet P £4.99 DT = £5.97 SF

Magnesium hydroxide
01-Dec-2021

● **INDICATIONS AND DOSE**
Constipation
▸ BY MOUTH
▸ Child 3-11 years: 5–10 mL as required, dose to be given mixed with water at bedtime
▸ Child 12-17 years: 30–45 mL as required, dose to be given mixed with water at bedtime
▸ Adult: 30–45 mL as required, dose to be given mixed with water at bedtime

● **CONTRA-INDICATIONS** Acute gastro-intestinal conditions
● **CAUTIONS** Debilitated patients · elderly
● **INTERACTIONS** → Appendix 1: magnesium

● **HEPATIC IMPAIRMENT** Avoid in hepatic coma if risk of renal failure.
● **RENAL IMPAIRMENT** EvGr Caution (risk of hypermagnesaemia); avoid in severe renal failure. ◈ M
● **PRESCRIBING AND DISPENSING INFORMATION** When prepared extemporaneously, the BP states Magnesium Hydroxide Mixture, BP consists of an aqueous suspension containing about 8% hydrated magnesium oxide.

● **MEDICINAL FORMS** There can be variation in the licensing of different medicines containing the same drug.
Oral suspension
▸ **Magnesium hydroxide (Non-proprietary)**
Magnesium hydroxide 79 mg per 1 ml Magnesium hydroxide 7.45-8.35% oral suspension BP | 500 ml GSL £5.31
▸ Brands may include Phillips' Milk of Magnesia

Sodium acid phosphate with sodium phosphate
18-Oct-2021

● **INDICATIONS AND DOSE**

Constipation (using Phosphates Enema BP Formula B) | Bowel evacuation before abdominal radiological procedures, endoscopy, and surgery (using Phosphates Enema BP Formula B)
▸ BY RECTUM
▸ Child 3-6 years: 45–65 mL once daily
▸ Child 7-11 years: 65–100 mL once daily
▸ Child 12-17 years: 100–128 mL once daily
▸ Adult: 128 mL daily

Constipation, using Phosphates Enema BP Formula B (dose approved for use by community practitioner nurse prescribers)
▸ BY RECTUM
▸ Child 3-17 years: Reduced according to body-weight
▸ Adult: 128 mL daily

Constipation, using Phosphates Enema (Cleen Ready-to-Use) (dose approved for use by community practitioner nurse prescribers)
▸ BY RECTUM
▸ Child 3-11 years: On doctor's advice only
▸ Child 12-17 years: 118 mL
▸ Adult: 118 mL

FLEET ® READY-TO-USE ENEMA

Constipation | Bowel evacuation before abdominal radiological procedures | Bowel evacuation before endoscopy | Bowel evacuation before surgery
▸ BY RECTUM
▸ Adult: 118 mL

FLEET ® PHOSPHO-SODA

Bowel evacuation before colonic surgery | Bowel evacuation before colonoscopy | Bowel evacuation before radiological examination
▸ BY MOUTH
▸ Adult: 45 mL twice daily, each dose must be diluted with half a glass (120 mL) of cold water, followed by one full glass (240 mL) of cold water, timing of doses is dependent on the time of the procedure, for morning procedure, the first dose should be taken at 7 a.m. and second at 7 p.m. on day before the procedure; for afternoon procedure, first dose should be taken at 7 p.m. on day before and second dose at 7 a.m. on day of the procedure

PHARMACOKINETICS
▸ For *Fleet ® Phospho-soda*: onset of action is within half to 6 hours of first dose.

● **CONTRA-INDICATIONS**
▸ With oral use Acute severe colitis · ascites · congestive cardiac failure · gastric retention · gastro-intestinal

obstruction · gastro-intestinal perforation · toxic megacolon
▸ **With rectal use** Conditions associated with increased colonic absorption · gastro-intestinal obstruction · inflammatory bowel disease

● **CAUTIONS**
▸ **With oral use** Cardiac disease · colitis · debilitated patients · elderly · fluid and electrolyte disturbances · hypovolaemia (should be corrected before administration)
▸ **With rectal use** Ascites · congestive heart failure · debilitated patients · elderly · fluid and electrolyte disturbances · uncontrolled hypertension

● **INTERACTIONS** → Appendix 1: bowel cleansing preparations

● **SIDE-EFFECTS**

GENERAL SIDE-EFFECTS
▸ **Common or very common** Chills · gastrointestinal discomfort · nausea · vomiting
▸ **Uncommon** Dehydration
▸ **Rare or very rare** Electrolyte imbalance · metabolic acidosis

SPECIFIC SIDE-EFFECTS
▸ **Common or very common**
▸ With oral use Asthenia · chest pain · dizziness · headache
▸ **Rare or very rare**
▸ With oral use Allergic dermatitis · arrhythmia · hypotension · loss of consciousness · muscle cramps · myocardial infarction · nephrocalcinosis · paraesthesia · renal impairment · tetany
▸ With rectal use Pain

● **PREGNANCY**
▸ With oral use Caution.

● **BREAST FEEDING**
▸ With oral use Caution.

● **RENAL IMPAIRMENT**
▸ With oral use [EvGr] Avoid. ⟨M⟩
▸ With rectal use [EvGr] Caution; avoid in significant impairment. ⟨M⟩

● **MONITORING REQUIREMENTS**
▸ With oral use Renal function should be measured before starting treatment in patients at risk of fluid and electrolyte disturbances.

● **DIRECTIONS FOR ADMINISTRATION**
FLEET ® PHOSPHO-SODA Manufacturer advises copious intake of water or other clear fluids (e.g. clear soup, strained fruit juice without pulp, black tea or coffee) recommended until midnight before morning procedure and until 8 a.m. before afternoon procedure. At least one glass (approx 240 mL) of water or other clear fluid should also be taken immediately before each dose.

● **PRESCRIBING AND DISPENSING INFORMATION** When prepared extemporaneously, the BP states Phosphates Enema BP Formula B consists of sodium dihydrogen phosphate dihydrate 12.8 g, disodium phosphate dodecahydrate 10.24 g, purified water, freshly boiled and cooled, to 128 mL.

● **PATIENT AND CARER ADVICE**
FLEET ® PHOSPHO-SODA Intake of solid food should be stopped for at least 6 hours before starting treatment and until procedure completed. Patients or carers should be advised that adequate hydration should be maintained during treatment. Patients or carers should be given advice on administration of *Fleet* ® *Phospho-soda* oral solution.

● **MEDICINAL FORMS** There can be variation in the licensing of different medicines containing the same drug.
Oral solution
CAUTIONARY AND ADVISORY LABELS 10
ELECTROLYTES: May contain Phosphate, sodium
▸ Fleet Phospho-soda (Recordati Pharmaceuticals Ltd)
Disodium hydrogen phosphate dodecahydrate 240 mg per 1 ml, Sodium dihydrogen phosphate dihydrate 542 mg per 1 ml Phospho-soda 24.4g/10.8g oral solution | 90 ml [P] £4.79 DT = £4.79 [SF]
Enema
▸ Sodium acid phosphate with sodium phosphate (Non-proprietary)
Disodium hydrogen phosphate dodecahydrate 80 mg per 1 ml, Sodium dihydrogen phosphate dihydrate 100 mg per 1 ml Phosphates enema (Formula B) 128ml long tube | 1 enema [P] £41.29-£75.40 DT = £75.40
Phosphates enema (Formula B) 128ml standard tube | 1 enema [P] £55.46 DT = £55.46
▸ Fleet Ready-to-use (Recordati Pharmaceuticals Ltd)
Disodium hydrogen phosphate dodecahydrate 80 mg per 1 ml, Sodium dihydrogen phosphate dihydrate 181 mg per 1 ml Cleen Ready-to-use 133ml enema | 1 enema [P] £3.51 DT = £3.51

LAXATIVES ⟩ SELECTIVE 5-HT₄ RECEPTOR AGONISTS

Prucalopride   09-Aug-2021

● **DRUG ACTION** A selective serotonin 5HT₄-receptor agonist with prokinetic properties.

● **INDICATIONS AND DOSE**
Chronic constipation when other laxatives fail to provide an adequate response
▸ BY MOUTH
▸ Adult: 2 mg once daily, review treatment if no response after 4 weeks
▸ Elderly: Initially 1 mg once daily, increased if necessary to 2 mg once daily, review treatment if no response after 4 weeks

● **CONTRA-INDICATIONS** Crohn's disease · intestinal obstruction · intestinal perforation · toxic megacolon · ulcerative colitis

● **CAUTIONS** History of arrhythmias · history of ischaemic heart disease

● **SIDE-EFFECTS**
▸ **Common or very common** Appetite decreased · diarrhoea · dizziness · fatigue · gastrointestinal discomfort · gastrointestinal disorders · headache · nausea · vomiting
▸ **Uncommon** Anorectal haemorrhage · fever · malaise · palpitations · tremor · urinary frequency increased
SIDE-EFFECTS, FURTHER INFORMATION Side-effects generally occur at the start of treatment and are usually transient.

● **CONCEPTION AND CONTRACEPTION** Manufacturer recommends effective contraception during treatment.

● **PREGNANCY** Manufacturer advises avoid—limited data available.

● **BREAST FEEDING** Manufacturer advises avoid—present in milk.

● **HEPATIC IMPAIRMENT** Manufacturer advises caution in severe impairment (risk of increased exposure, limited information available).
Dose adjustments Manufacturer advises initial dose of 1 mg once daily in severe impairment; if tolerated this may be increased to 2 mg once daily.

● **RENAL IMPAIRMENT**
Dose adjustments [EvGr] Reduce dose to 1 mg daily if eGFR less than 30 mL/minute/1.73 m². ⟨M⟩ See p. 21.

- **PATIENT AND CARER ADVICE**
Driving and skilled tasks Manufacturer advises that dizziness and fatigue may initially affect ability to drive or operate machinery.
- **NATIONAL FUNDING/ACCESS DECISIONS**
For full details see funding body website
NICE decisions
▶ Prucalopride for the treatment of chronic constipation in women (December 2010) NICE TA211 Recommended with restrictions

Scottish Medicines Consortium (SMC) decisions
▶ Prucalopride (*Resolor*®) for chronic constipation (July 2011) SMC No. 653/10 Not recommended

- **MEDICINAL FORMS** There can be variation in the licensing of different medicines containing the same drug.
Oral tablet
▶ Prucalopride (Non-proprietary)
Prucalopride (as Prucalopride succinate) 1 mg Prucalopride 1mg tablets | 28 tablet PoM £38.69 DT = £15.44
Prucalopride (as Prucalopride succinate) 2 mg Prucalopride 2mg tablets | 28 tablet PoM £59.52 DT = £7.86
▶ Resolor (Takeda UK Ltd)
Prucalopride (as Prucalopride succinate) 1 mg Resolor 1mg tablets | 28 tablet PoM £38.69 DT = £15.44
Prucalopride (as Prucalopride succinate) 2 mg Resolor 2mg tablets | 28 tablet PoM £59.52 DT = £7.86

LAXATIVES > SOFTENING LAXATIVES

Arachis oil

18-Nov-2020

- **INDICATIONS AND DOSE**
To soften impacted faeces
▶ BY RECTUM
▶ Adult: 130 mL as required

- **CONTRA-INDICATIONS** Inflammatory bowel disease (except under medical supervision)
- **CAUTIONS** Hypersensitivity to soya · intestinal obstruction
- **ALLERGY AND CROSS-SENSITIVITY** EvGr Contra-indicated if history of hypersensitivity to arachis oil or peanuts. ⟨M⟩
- **DIRECTIONS FOR ADMINISTRATION** Manufacturer advises warm enema in warm water before use.

- **MEDICINAL FORMS** There can be variation in the licensing of different medicines containing the same drug.
Enema
▶ Arachis oil (Non-proprietary)
Arachis oil 1 ml per 1 ml Arachis oil 130ml enema | 1 enema P £54.66 DT = £54.66

Docusate sodium

12-Apr-2023

(Dioctyl sodium sulphosuccinate)

- **INDICATIONS AND DOSE**
Chronic constipation
▶ BY MOUTH
▶ Child 6-23 months: 12.5 mg 3 times a day, use paediatric oral solution, dose to be adjusted according to response
▶ Child 2-11 years: 12.5–25 mg 3 times a day, use paediatric oral solution, dose to be adjusted according to response
▶ Child 12-17 years: 100 mg 3 times a day, dose can be increased if necessary up to maximum 500 mg daily in divided doses
▶ Adult: 100 mg 3 times a day, dose can be increased if necessary up to maximum 500 mg daily in divided doses

▶ BY RECTUM
▶ Child 12-17 years: 120 mg for 1 dose
▶ Adult: 120 mg for 1 dose
Adjunct in abdominal radiological procedures
▶ BY MOUTH
▶ Adult: 400 mg for 1 dose, to be administered with barium meal
▶ BY RECTUM
▶ Adult: 120 mg for 1 dose

PHARMACOKINETICS
▶ Oral preparations act within 1–2 days; response to rectal administration usually occurs within 20 minutes.

- **UNLICENSED USE** *Adult oral solution and capsules* not licensed for use in children under 12 years.
- **CONTRA-INDICATIONS** Avoid in intestinal obstruction
- **CAUTIONS** Do not give with liquid paraffin · excessive use of stimulant laxatives can cause diarrhoea and related effects such as hypokalaemia
▶ With rectal use Rectal preparations not indicated if haemorrhoids or anal fissure
- **INTERACTIONS** → Appendix 1: docusates
- **SIDE-EFFECTS**
▶ **Rare or very rare**
▶ With oral use Abdominal cramps · nausea · rash
- **PREGNANCY** Not known to be harmful—manufacturer advises caution.
- **BREAST FEEDING**
▶ With oral use Manufacturer advises caution—present in milk following oral administration.
▶ With rectal use Rectal administration not known to be harmful.
- **DIRECTIONS FOR ADMINISTRATION**
▶ With oral use in children For administration *by mouth*, manufacturer advises solution may be mixed with milk or squash.

- **MEDICINAL FORMS** There can be variation in the licensing of different medicines containing the same drug.
Oral solution
▶ Docusate sodium (Non-proprietary)
Docusate sodium 2.5 mg per 1 ml Docusate 12.5mg/5ml oral solution sugar free | 300 ml P £21.20–£32.43 DT = £32.43 SF
Docusate sodium 10 mg per 1 ml Docusate 50mg/5ml oral solution sugar free | 300 ml P £29.00 DT = £18.67 SF
Docusate sodium 20 mg per 1 ml Docusate 100mg/5ml oral solution sugar free | 150 ml P £28.00 SF | 300 ml P £33.34 DT = £33.34 SF
▶ Docusol (Typharm Ltd)
Docusate sodium 2.5 mg per 1 ml Docusol Paediatric 12.5mg/5ml oral solution | 125 ml P £4.46 SF
Oral capsule
▶ Dioctyl (Teofarma S.r.l.)
Docusate sodium 100 mg Dioctyl 100mg capsules | 30 capsule P £2.50 DT = £2.50 | 100 capsule P £8.76 DT = £8.76
Enema
▶ Norgalax (Essential Pharma Ltd)
Docusate sodium 12 mg per 1 gram Norgalax 120mg/10g enema | 6 enema P £28.00 DT = £28.00

Combinations available: *Co-danthrusate*, p. 68

Liquid paraffin

01-May-2020

- **INDICATIONS AND DOSE**
Constipation
▶ BY MOUTH
▶ Adult: 10–30 mL daily if required, to be administered at night

- **CONTRA-INDICATIONS** Children under 3 years
- **CAUTIONS** Avoid prolonged use

- **SIDE-EFFECTS** Anal irritation · contact dermatitis · granuloma · pneumonia lipoid · rectal discharge of drug
- **PATIENT AND CARER ADVICE** Oral emulsion should not be taken immediately before going to bed.

- **MEDICINAL FORMS** There can be variation in the licensing of different medicines containing the same drug.

  Oral liquid
  - ▸ Liquid paraffin (Non-proprietary)
    Liquid paraffin 1 ml per 1 ml Liquid paraffin liquid | 150 ml ⓟ £2.77 DT = £2.77

LAXATIVES › STIMULANT LAXATIVES

| Bisacodyl
10-Sep-2020

- **INDICATIONS AND DOSE**

Constipation
- ▸ BY MOUTH
- ▸ Child 4-17 years: 5–20 mg once daily, dose to be taken at night, dose to be adjusted according to response
- ▸ Adult: 5–10 mg once daily, dose to be taken at night; increased if necessary up to 20 mg once daily, dose to be taken at night
- ▸ BY RECTUM
- ▸ Child 2-17 years: 5–10 mg once daily, dose to be adjusted according to response
- ▸ Adult: 10 mg once daily, dose to be taken in the morning

Bowel clearance before radiological procedures and surgery
- ▸ INITIALLY BY MOUTH
- ▸ Adult: 10 mg for 1 dose, dose to be taken in the morning on the day before procedure, then (by mouth) 10 mg for 1 dose, dose to be taken in the evening on the day before procedure, then (by rectum) 10 mg for 1 dose, dose to be administered 1–2 hours before procedure

Constipation (dose approved for use by community practitioner nurse prescribers)
- ▸ BY MOUTH
- ▸ Child 4-17 years: 5–20 mg once daily, dose to be taken at night, dose to be adjusted according to response (on doctor's advice only)
- ▸ Adult: 5–10 mg once daily, dose to be taken at night; increased if necessary up to 20 mg once daily, dose to be taken at night
- ▸ BY RECTUM
- ▸ Child 4-9 years: 5 mg once daily, dose to be adjusted according to response
- ▸ Child 10-17 years: 10 mg once daily, dose to be taken in the morning
- ▸ Adult: 10 mg once daily, dose to be taken in the morning

PHARMACOKINETICS
- ▸ Tablets act in 10–12 hours; suppositories act in 20–60 minutes.

- **UNLICENSED USE**
- ▸ With rectal use in children [EvGr] Bisacodyl may be used in children aged under 10 years for the management of constipation, ⓐ but the higher dose option is not licensed in this age group.

- ▸ With oral use in children [EvGr] Bisacodyl may be used in children for the management of constipation, ⓐ but the higher dose option is not licensed.

> **IMPORTANT SAFETY INFORMATION**
>
> MHRA/CHM ADVICE: STIMULANT LAXATIVES (BISACODYL, SENNA AND SENNOSIDES, SODIUM PICOSULFATE) AVAILABLE OVER-THE-COUNTER: NEW MEASURES TO SUPPORT SAFE USE (AUGUST 2020)
>
> Following a national safety review and concerns over misuse and abuse, the MHRA has introduced new pack size restrictions, revised recommended ages for use, and new safety warnings for over-the-counter stimulant laxatives (administered orally and rectally). Patients should be advised that dietary and lifestyle measures should be used first-line for relieving short-term occasional constipation, and that stimulant laxatives should only be used if these measures and other laxatives (bulk-forming and osmotic) are ineffective.
>
> Smaller packs will remain available for general sale for the treatment of short-term, occasional constipation in adults only, and will be limited to a pack size of two short treatment courses. Stimulant laxatives should not be used in children under 12 years of age without advice from a prescriber; in children aged 12 to 17 years, products can be supplied under the supervision of a pharmacist.

- **CONTRA-INDICATIONS** Acute abdominal conditions · acute inflammatory bowel disease · intestinal obstruction · severe dehydration
- **CAUTIONS** Excessive use of stimulant laxatives can cause diarrhoea and related effects such as hypokalaemia · prolonged use may harm intestinal function · risk of electrolyte imbalance with prolonged use
- **SIDE-EFFECTS**
- ▸ **Common or very common** Gastrointestinal discomfort · nausea
- ▸ **Uncommon** Haematochezia · vomiting
- ▸ **Rare or very rare** Angioedema · colitis · dehydration
- **PREGNANCY** May be suitable for constipation in pregnancy, if a stimulant effect is necessary.

- **MEDICINAL FORMS** There can be variation in the licensing of different medicines containing the same drug. Forms available from special-order manufacturers include: oral suspension, suppository

  Gastro-resistant tablet
  CAUTIONARY AND ADVISORY LABELS 5, 25
  - ▸ Bisacodyl (Non-proprietary)
    Bisacodyl 5 mg Bisacodyl 5mg gastro-resistant tablets | 60 tablet ⓟ £6.50 DT = £3.24 | 100 tablet ⓟ £5.40-£10.83 | 500 tablet ⓟ £25.73 | 1000 tablet ⓟ £51.45
  - ▸ Dulco-Lax (bisacodyl) (Opella Healthcare UK Ltd)
    Bisacodyl 5 mg Dulcolax Twelve Plus 5mg gastro-resistant tablets | 40 tablet ⓟ £3.39 | 100 tablet ⓟ £8.14

  Suppository
  - ▸ Dulco-Lax (bisacodyl) (Opella Healthcare UK Ltd)
    Bisacodyl 5 mg Dulcolax 5mg suppositories | 5 suppository [PoM] £1.11 DT = £1.11
    Bisacodyl 10 mg Dulcolax Twelve Plus 10mg suppositories | 12 suppository ⓟ £3.32 DT = £3.32

| Co-danthramer
16-Mar-2020

- **INDICATIONS AND DOSE**

Constipation in palliative care (standard strength capsules)
- ▸ BY MOUTH USING CAPSULES
- ▸ Child 6-11 years: 1 capsule once daily, dose should be taken at night
- ▸ Child 12-17 years: 1–2 capsules once daily, dose should be taken at night

continued →

1

Gastro-intestinal system

▸ Adult: 1–2 capsules once daily, dose should be taken at night

Constipation in palliative care (strong capsules)
▸ BY MOUTH USING CAPSULES
▸ Child 12-17 years: 1–2 capsules once daily, dose should be given at night
▸ Adult: 1–2 capsules once daily, dose should be given at night

Constipation in palliative care (standard strength suspension)
▸ BY MOUTH USING ORAL SUSPENSION
▸ Child 2-11 years: 2.5–5 mL once daily, dose should be taken at night
▸ Child 12-17 years: 5–10 mL once daily, dose should be taken at night
▸ Adult: 5–10 mL once daily, dose should be taken at night

Constipation in palliative care (strong suspension)
▸ BY MOUTH USING ORAL SUSPENSION
▸ Child 12-17 years: 5 mL once daily, dose should be taken at night
▸ Adult: 5 mL once daily, dose should be taken at night

DOSE EQUIVALENCE AND CONVERSION
▸ Co-danthramer (standard strength) capsules contain dantron 25 mg with poloxamer '188' 200 mg per capsule.
▸ Co-danthramer (standard strength) oral suspension contains dantron 25 mg with poloxamer '188' 200 mg per 5 mL.
▸ Co-danthramer **strong** capsules contain dantron 37.5 mg with poloxamer '188' 500 mg.
▸ Co-danthramer **strong** oral suspension contains dantron 75 mg with poloxamer '188' 1 g per 5 mL.
▸ Co-danthramer suspension 5 mL = one co-danthramer capsule, **but** strong co-danthramer suspension 5 mL = two strong co-danthramer capsules.

● **CONTRA-INDICATIONS** Acute abdominal conditions · acute inflammatory bowel disease · intestinal obstruction · severe dehydration

● **CAUTIONS** Excessive use of stimulant laxatives can cause diarrhoea and related effects such as hypokalaemia · may cause local irritation · *rodent* studies indicate potential carcinogenic risk

CAUTIONS, FURTHER INFORMATION
▸ Local irritation Avoid prolonged contact with skin (incontinent patients or infants wearing nappies—risk of irritation and excoriation).

● **SIDE-EFFECTS** Abdominal cramps · asthenia · gastrointestinal disorders · hypermagnesaemia · skin reactions · urine discolouration

● **PREGNANCY** Manufacturers advise avoid—limited information available.

● **BREAST FEEDING** Manufacturers advise avoid—no information available.

● **PRESCRIBING AND DISPENSING INFORMATION**
Palliative care For further information on the use of co-danthramer in palliative care, see www.medicinescomplete. com/#/content/palliative/stimulant-laxatives.

● **MEDICINAL FORMS** There can be variation in the licensing of different medicines containing the same drug.
Oral suspension
CAUTIONARY AND ADVISORY LABELS 14 (urine red)
▸ Co-danthramer (Non-proprietary)
Dantron 5 mg per 1 ml, Poloxamer 188 40 mg per 1 ml Co-danthramer 25mg/200mg/5ml oral suspension sugar free | 300 ml [PoM] [⚠] [SF]
Dantron 15 mg per 1 ml, Poloxamer 188 200 mg per 1 ml Co-danthramer 75mg/1000mg/5ml oral suspension sugar free | 300 ml [PoM] £503.98 [SF]

Co-danthrusate

16-Mar-2020

● **INDICATIONS AND DOSE**
Constipation in palliative care
▸ BY MOUTH USING ORAL SUSPENSION
▸ Child 6-11 years: 5 mL once daily, to be taken at night
▸ Child 12-17 years: 5–15 mL once daily, to be taken at night
▸ Adult: 5–15 mL once daily, to be taken at night

DOSE EQUIVALENCE AND CONVERSION
▸ Co-danthrusate suspension contains dantron 50 mg and docusate sodium 60 mg per 5 mL.

● **CONTRA-INDICATIONS** Acute abdominal conditions · acute inflammatory bowel disease · intestinal obstruction · severe dehydration

● **CAUTIONS** Excessive use of stimulant laxatives can cause diarrhoea and related effects such as hypokalaemia · may cause local irritation · *rodent* studies indicate potential carcinogenic risk

CAUTIONS, FURTHER INFORMATION
▸ Local irritation Avoid prolonged contact with skin (incontinent patients—risk of irritation and excoriation).

● **INTERACTIONS** → Appendix 1: docusates

● **SIDE-EFFECTS** Gastrointestinal disorders · skin reactions · urine discolouration

● **PREGNANCY** Manufacturers advise avoid—limited information available.

● **BREAST FEEDING** Manufacturers advise avoid—no information available.

● **MEDICINAL FORMS** There can be variation in the licensing of different medicines containing the same drug.
Oral suspension
CAUTIONARY AND ADVISORY LABELS 14 (urine orange)
▸ Co-danthrusate (Non-proprietary)
Dantron 10 mg per 1 ml, Docusate sodium 12 mg per 1 ml Co-danthrusate 50mg/60mg/5ml oral suspension sugar free | 200 ml [PoM] [⚠] [SF]

Glycerol

10-Nov-2021

(Glycerin)

● **INDICATIONS AND DOSE**
Constipation
▸ BY RECTUM
▸ Child 1-11 months: 1 g as required
▸ Child 1-11 years: 2 g as required
▸ Child 12-17 years: 4 g as required
▸ Adult: 4 g as required

● **DIRECTIONS FOR ADMINISTRATION** Manufacturer advises moisten suppositories with water before insertion.

● **PRESCRIBING AND DISPENSING INFORMATION** When prepared extemporaneously, the BP states Glycerol Suppositories, BP consists of gelatin 140 mg, glycerol 700 mg, purified water to 1 g.

● **PATIENT AND CARER ADVICE**
Medicines for Children leaflet: Glycerin (glycerol) suppositories for constipation www.medicinesforchildren.org.uk/medicines/glycerin-glycerol-suppositories-for-constipation/

● **MEDICINAL FORMS** There can be variation in the licensing of different medicines containing the same drug. Forms available from special-order manufacturers include: suppository
Suppository
▸ Glycerol (Non-proprietary)
Glycerol 700 mg Glycerol 1g suppositories | 12 suppository [GSL]
£4.32 DT = £3.64

Glycerol **1400 mg** Glycerol 2g suppositories | 12 suppository [GSL]
£3.35 DT = £3.25
Glycerol **2800 mg** Glycerol 4g suppositories | 12 suppository [GSL]
£3.31 DT = £2.12

Senna
03-May-2023

- **DRUG ACTION** Senna is a stimulant laxative. After metabolism of sennosides in the gut the anthrone component stimulates peristalsis thereby increasing the motility of the large intestine.

- **INDICATIONS AND DOSE**

Constipation
- ▶ BY MOUTH USING TABLETS
- ▸ **Child 6-17 years:** 7.5–30 mg once daily, to be adjusted according to response
- ▸ **Adult:** 7.5–15 mg once daily, dose usually taken at bedtime, initial dose should be low then gradually increased, higher doses up to 30 mg once daily may be prescribed under medical supervision
- ▶ BY MOUTH USING SYRUP
- ▸ **Child 1 month-3 years:** 3.75–15 mg once daily, to be adjusted according to response
- ▸ **Child 4-17 years:** 3.75–30 mg once daily, to be adjusted according to response
- ▸ **Adult:** 7.5–15 mg once daily, dose usually taken at bedtime, higher doses up to 30 mg once daily may be prescribed under medical supervision

Constipation (dose approved for use by community practitioner nurse prescribers)
- ▶ BY MOUTH USING TABLETS
- ▸ **Child 6-17 years:** 7.5–30 mg once daily, to be adjusted according to response
- ▸ **Adult:** 15–30 mg once daily, dose usually taken at night, initial dose should be low then gradually increased
- ▶ BY MOUTH USING SYRUP
- ▸ **Child 2-3 years:** 3.75–15 mg once daily, to be adjusted according to response
- ▸ **Child 4-17 years:** 3.75–30 mg once daily, to be adjusted according to response
- ▸ **Adult:** 15–30 mg once daily, dose usually taken at bedtime

PHARMACOKINETICS
- ▸ Onset of action 8–12 hours.

- **UNLICENSED USE** *Tablets* and *syrup* not licensed for use in children under 12 years.
  Doses in BNF Publications adhere to national guidelines and may differ from those in product literature.

> **IMPORTANT SAFETY INFORMATION**
>
> **MHRA/CHM ADVICE: STIMULANT LAXATIVES (BISACODYL, SENNA AND SENNOSIDES, SODIUM PICOSULFATE) AVAILABLE OVER-THE-COUNTER: NEW MEASURES TO SUPPORT SAFE USE (AUGUST 2020)**
> Following a national safety review and concerns over misuse and abuse, the MHRA has introduced new pack size restrictions, revised recommended ages for use, and new safety warnings for over-the-counter stimulant laxatives (administered orally and rectally). Patients should be advised that dietary and lifestyle measures should be used first-line for relieving short-term occasional constipation, and that stimulant laxatives should only be used if these measures and other laxatives (bulk-forming and osmotic) are ineffective.
> Smaller packs will remain available for general sale for the treatment of short-term, occasional constipation in adults only, and will be limited to a pack size of two short treatment courses. Stimulant laxatives should not be used in children under 12 years of age without advice from a prescriber; in children aged 12 to 17 years, products can be supplied under the supervision of a pharmacist.

- **CONTRA-INDICATIONS** Atony · intestinal obstruction · undiagnosed abdominal pain
- **SIDE-EFFECTS** Albuminuria · diarrhoea · electrolyte imbalance · fluid imbalance · gastrointestinal discomfort · haematuria · pseudomelanosis coli · skin reactions · urine discolouration

  SIDE-EFFECTS, FURTHER INFORMATION Prolonged or excessive use can cause hypokalaemia.
- **PREGNANCY** [EvGr] Specialist sources indicate suitable for use in pregnancy. ⟨D⟩
- **BREAST FEEDING** [EvGr] Specialist sources indicate suitable for use in breast-feeding in infants over 1 month. ⟨D⟩
- **PATIENT AND CARER ADVICE**
  Medicines for Children leaflet: Senna for constipation
  www.medicinesforchildren.org.uk/medicines/senna-for-constipation/
- **NATIONAL FUNDING/ACCESS DECISIONS**
  NHS restrictions *Senokot* ® tablets are not prescribable in NHS primary care.
- **EXCEPTIONS TO LEGAL CATEGORY** Senna is on sale to the public for use in children over 12 years; doses on packs may vary from those in BNF Publications.

- **MEDICINAL FORMS** There can be variation in the licensing of different medicines containing the same drug.

Oral tablet
- ▸ **Senna (Non-proprietary)**
  Sennoside B (as Sennosides) 7.5 mg Sennosides 7.5mg tablets 12 Years Plus | 20 tablet [P] [⊠]
- ▸ **Cenlax** (Manx Healthcare Ltd)
  Sennoside B (as Sennosides) 7.5 mg Cenlax 7.5mg tablets 12 Years Plus | 20 tablet [P] £0.80 | 60 tablet [P] £1.70
- ▸ **Senease Twelve Years Plus** (RX Farma)
  Sennoside B (as Sennosides) 7.5 mg Senease Twelve Years Plus 7.5mg tablets | 60 tablet [P] £2.99 | 100 tablet [P] £4.98
- ▸ **Senokot** (Reckitt Benckiser Healthcare (UK) Ltd)
  Sennoside B (as Senna fruit) 7.5 mg Senokot 7.5mg tablets 12 Years Plus | 500 tablet [PoM] £12.50
  Sennoside B (as Senna fruit) 15 mg Senokot Max Strength tablets 12 Years Plus | 24 tablet [P] £4.17 | 48 tablet [P] £6.63 DT = £6.63

Oral solution
- ▸ **Senokot** (Reckitt Benckiser Healthcare (UK) Ltd)
  Sennoside B (as Sennosides) 1.5 mg per 1 ml Senokot 7.5mg/5ml Syrup 12 Years Plus | 150 ml [P] £4.89 [SF] | 500 ml [P] £10.09 DT = £10.09 [SF]

Senna with ispaghula husk
11-Nov-2020

The properties listed below are those particular to the combination only. For the properties of the components please consider, senna above, ispaghula husk p. 60.

- **INDICATIONS AND DOSE**

Constipation
- ▶ BY MOUTH
- ▸ **Child 12-17 years:** 5–10 g once daily, to be taken at night, up to 2–3 times a week
- ▸ **Adult:** 5–10 g once daily, to be taken at night, up to 2–3 times a week

DOSE EQUIVALENCE AND CONVERSION
- ▸ 5 g equivalent to one level spoonful of granules.

- **PREGNANCY** Manufacturer advises avoid during first trimester. To be used only intermittently and only if dietary and lifestyle changes fail.
- **DIRECTIONS FOR ADMINISTRATION** [EvGr] Take at night with at least 150 mL liquid. ⟨M⟩

- **MEDICINAL FORMS** There can be variation in the licensing of different medicines containing the same drug.

Oral granules

CAUTIONARY AND ADVISORY LABELS 25
EXCIPIENTS: May contain Sucrose

▸ **Manevac** (Ceuta Healthcare Ltd)
  Senna fruit 124 mg per 1 gram, Ispaghula 542 mg per 1 gram Manevac granules | 400 gram PoM £9.50

Sodium acid phosphate with sodium bicarbonate

03-Dec-2020

The properties listed below are those particular to the combination only. For the properties of the components please consider, sodium bicarbonate p. 1178.

- **INDICATIONS AND DOSE**

LECICARBON A ®

Constipation | Bowel evacuation [before diagnostic or therapeutic procedures in the rectum]
▸ BY RECTUM
▸ Child 12-17 years: 1 suppository as required, dose may be repeated after 30–60 minutes
▸ Adult: 1 suppository as required, dose may be repeated after 30–60 minutes

PHARMACOKINETICS
▸ Onset of action 15–30 minutes.

LECICARBON C ®

Constipation | Bowel evacuation [before diagnostic or therapeutic procedures in the rectum]
▸ BY RECTUM
▸ Child 1-11 years: 1 suppository as required, dose may be repeated after 30–60 minutes

PHARMACOKINETICS
▸ Onset of action 15–30 minutes.

- **CONTRA-INDICATIONS** Anal and rectal region diseases (risk of excessive absorption of carbon dioxide, particularly in infants and children) · ileus · toxic megacolon (except with explicit permission of the physician)

- **INTERACTIONS** → Appendix 1: bowel cleansing preparations · sodium bicarbonate

- **ALLERGY AND CROSS-SENSITIVITY** EvGr Contra-indicated in patients with peanut or soya hypersensitivity. ⟨M⟩

- **PREGNANCY** EvGr Use only if potential benefit outweighs risk—effect of the expanding volume of carbon dioxide may be negligible. ⟨M⟩

- **BREAST FEEDING** EvGr Suitable for use in breast-feeding—the developed carbon dioxide will not be excreted in milk. ⟨M⟩

- **DIRECTIONS FOR ADMINISTRATION** EvGr Moisten suppositories with water before insertion if needed. ⟨M⟩

- **MEDICINAL FORMS** There can be variation in the licensing of different medicines containing the same drug.

Suppository
▸ **Lecicarbon A** (Aspire Pharma Ltd)
  Sodium bicarbonate 500 mg, Sodium dihydrogen phosphate anhydrous 680 mg Lecicarbon A suppositories | 10 suppository P £8.20 DT = £8.20
▸ **Lecicarbon C** (Aspire Pharma Ltd)
  Sodium bicarbonate 250 mg, Sodium dihydrogen phosphate anhydrous 340 mg Lecicarbon C suppositories | 10 suppository P £8.20 DT = £8.20

Sodium picosulfate

11-Nov-2021

(Sodium picosulphate)

- **DRUG ACTION** Sodium picosulfate is a stimulant laxative. After metabolism in the colon it stimulates the mucosa thereby increasing the motility of the large intestine.

- **INDICATIONS AND DOSE**

Constipation
▸ BY MOUTH
▸ Child 1 month-3 years: 2.5–10 mg once daily, dose to be adjusted according to response
▸ Child 4-17 years: 2.5–20 mg once daily, dose to be adjusted according to response
▸ Adult: 5–10 mg once daily, dose to be taken at bedtime

Constipation (dose approved for use by community practitioner nurse prescribers)
▸ BY MOUTH
▸ Child 1 month-3 years: 250 micrograms/kg once daily (max. per dose 5 mg), dose to be taken at night, dose to be adjusted according to response (on doctor's advice only)
▸ Child 4-10 years: 2.5–5 mg once daily, dose to be taken at night, dose to be adjusted according to response (on doctor's advice only)
▸ Child 11-17 years: 5–10 mg once daily, dose to be taken at night, dose to be adjusted according to response
▸ Adult: 5–10 mg once daily, dose to be taken at night

PHARMACOKINETICS
▸ Onset of action 6–12 hours.

- **UNLICENSED USE** Sodium picosulfate doses in BNF Publications adhere to national guidelines and may differ from those in product literature.

> **IMPORTANT SAFETY INFORMATION**
>
> MHRA/CHM ADVICE: STIMULANT LAXATIVES (BISACODYL, SENNA AND SENNOSIDES, SODIUM PICOSULFATE) AVAILABLE OVER-THE-COUNTER: NEW MEASURES TO SUPPORT SAFE USE (AUGUST 2020)
> Following a national safety review and concerns over misuse and abuse, the MHRA has introduced new pack size restrictions, revised recommended ages for use, and new safety warnings for over-the-counter stimulant laxatives (administered orally and rectally). Patients should be advised that dietary and lifestyle measures should be used first-line for relieving short-term occasional constipation, and that stimulant laxatives should only be used if these measures and other laxatives (bulk-forming and osmotic) are ineffective.
>
> Smaller packs will remain available for general sale for the treatment of short-term, occasional constipation in adults only, and will be limited to a pack size of two short treatment courses. Stimulant laxatives should not be used in children under 12 years of age without advice from a prescriber; in children aged 12 to 17 years, products can be supplied under the supervision of a pharmacist.

- **CONTRA-INDICATIONS** Intestinal obstruction · undiagnosed abdominal pain

- **INTERACTIONS** → Appendix 1: sodium picosulfate

- **SIDE-EFFECTS**
▸ **Common or very common** Diarrhoea · gastrointestinal discomfort
▸ **Uncommon** Dizziness · nausea · vomiting
▸ **Frequency not known** Angioedema · skin reactions · syncope

SIDE-EFFECTS, FURTHER INFORMATION Prolonged or excessive use can cause diarrhoea and related effects such as hypokalaemia.

Gastro-intestinal system

- **PREGNANCY** Manufacturer states evidence limited but not known to be harmful.
- **BREAST FEEDING** [EvGr] Specialist sources indicate suitable for use in breast-feeding in infants over 1 month—not known to be present in milk. ◇D◇
- **PATIENT AND CARER ADVICE**
  Medicines for Children leaflet: Sodium picosulfate for constipation
  www.medicinesforchildren.org.uk/medicines/sodium-picosulfate-for-constipation/

- **MEDICINAL FORMS** There can be variation in the licensing of different medicines containing the same drug.
  Oral solution
  EXCIPIENTS: May contain Alcohol
  ▸ **Sodium picosulfate (Non-proprietary)**
    Sodium picosulfate 1 mg per 1 ml Sodium picosulfate 5mg/5ml oral solution sugar free | 100 ml [P] £1.56-£17.32 [SF] | 300 ml [P] £50.00 DT = £39.33 [SF]
  ▸ **Dulco-Lax (sodium picosulfate)** (Opella Healthcare UK Ltd)
    Sodium picosulfate 1 mg per 1 ml Dulcolax Pico Twelve Plus 5mg/5ml liquid | 300 ml [P] £7.23 DT = £39.33 [SF]

OPIOID RECEPTOR ANTAGONISTS

Methylnaltrexone bromide
29-Jul-2021

- **DRUG ACTION** Methylnaltrexone bromide is a peripherally acting opioid-receptor antagonist. It therefore blocks the gastro-intestinal (constipating) effects of opioids without altering their central analgesic effects.

- **INDICATIONS AND DOSE**

Opioid-induced constipation in patients with chronic pain (except palliative care patients with advanced illness)
▸ BY SUBCUTANEOUS INJECTION
▸ Adult: 12 mg once daily if required, to be given as 4–7 doses weekly

Adjunct to other laxatives in opioid-induced constipation in palliative care
▸ BY SUBCUTANEOUS INJECTION
▸ Adult (body-weight up to 38 kg): 150 micrograms/kg once daily on alternate days for maximum duration of treatment 4 months, two consecutive doses may be given 24 hours apart if no response to treatment on the preceding day
▸ Adult (body-weight 38-61 kg): 8 mg once daily on alternate days for maximum duration of treatment 4 months, two consecutive doses may be given 24 hours apart if no response to treatment on the preceding day
▸ Adult (body-weight 62-114 kg): 12 mg once daily on alternate days for maximum duration of treatment 4 months, two consecutive doses may be given 24 hours apart if no response to treatment on the preceding day
▸ Adult (body-weight 115 kg and above): 150 micrograms/kg once daily on alternate days for maximum duration of treatment 4 months, two consecutive doses may be given 24 hours apart if no response to treatment on the preceding day

PHARMACOKINETICS
▸ May act within 30–60 minutes.

- **CONTRA-INDICATIONS** Acute surgical abdominal conditions · gastro-intestinal obstruction
- **CAUTIONS** Diverticular disease (when active) · faecal impaction · gastro-intestinal tract lesions (known or suspected) · patients with colostomy · patients with peritoneal catheter
- **SIDE-EFFECTS**
▸ **Common or very common** Abdominal pain · diarrhoea · dizziness · gastrointestinal disorders · nausea · opioid withdrawal-like syndrome · vomiting

Overdose Symptoms of overdosage include orthostatic hypotension.
- **PREGNANCY** Manufacturer advises avoid unless essential—toxicity at high doses in *animal* studies.
- **BREAST FEEDING** Manufacturer advises use only if potential benefit outweighs risk—present in milk in *animal* studies.
- **HEPATIC IMPAIRMENT** Manufacturer advises avoid in severe impairment (no information available).
- **RENAL IMPAIRMENT**
  Dose adjustments [EvGr] If creatinine clearance less than 30 mL/minute, reduce dose as follows: body-weight up to 62 kg, 75 micrograms/kg; body-weight 62–114 kg, 8 mg; body-weight 115 kg and above, 75 micrograms/kg. ⓜ See p. 21.
- **DIRECTIONS FOR ADMINISTRATION** Rotate injection site.
- **PRESCRIBING AND DISPENSING INFORMATION**
  Palliative care For further information on the use of methylnaltrexone in palliative care, see
  www.medicinescomplete.com/#/content/palliative/opioid-antagonists-therapeutic-target-outside-the-cns.
- **HANDLING AND STORAGE** Protect from light.

- **MEDICINAL FORMS** There can be variation in the licensing of different medicines containing the same drug.
  Solution for injection
  ▸ **Relistor** (Alliance Pharmaceuticals Ltd)
    Methylnaltrexone bromide 20 mg per 1 ml Relistor 12mg/0.6ml solution for injection vials | 1 vial [PoM] £21.05 | 7 vial [PoM] £147.35 DT = £147.35

Naldemedine
10-Dec-2020

- **DRUG ACTION** Naldemedine is a peripherally acting opioid receptor antagonist. It therefore decreases the constipating effects of opioids without altering their central analgesic effects.

- **INDICATIONS AND DOSE**

Opioid-induced constipation [previous treatment with a laxative]
▸ BY MOUTH
▸ Adult: 200 micrograms once daily

- **CONTRA-INDICATIONS** Increased risk of recurrent obstruction (risk of gastro-intestinal perforation) · known or suspected gastro-intestinal obstruction (risk of gastro-intestinal perforation)
- **CAUTIONS** Conditions with impaired integrity of the gastro-intestinal wall (risk of gastro-intestinal perforation) · treatment initiation in patients aged 75 years and over (limited information available)
  CAUTIONS, FURTHER INFORMATION
▸ Disruptions to blood-brain barrier Manufacturer advises caution in patients with clinically important disruptions to the blood-brain barrier (e.g. advanced Alzheimer's disease, active multiple sclerosis, primary brain malignancies)—risk of opioid withdrawal or reduced analgesia.
▸ Cardiovascular disorders Safety and efficacy has not been established in patients with these conditions.
- **INTERACTIONS** → Appendix 1: naldemedine
- **SIDE-EFFECTS**
▸ **Common or very common** Diarrhoea · gastrointestinal discomfort · nausea · vomiting
- **PREGNANCY** Manufacturer advises avoid unless potential benefit outweighs risk— *animal* studies do not indicate toxicity; risk of opioid withdrawal in fetus.
- **BREAST FEEDING** Manufacturer advises avoid—present in milk in *animal* studies; theoretical risk of opioid withdrawal in breast-fed neonate.

- **HEPATIC IMPAIRMENT** Manufacturer advises avoid in severe impairment (no information available).
- **PATIENT AND CARER ADVICE** Manufacturer advises patients and carers to report severe, persistent or worsening gastro-intestinal effects (such as abdominal pain) to their prescriber. Manufacturer advises patients and carers should be counselled on the risk of opioid withdrawal syndrome and to seek medical advice if this occurs.
- **NATIONAL FUNDING/ACCESS DECISIONS** For full details see funding body website

  NICE decisions
  - ▸ Naldemedine for treating opioid-induced constipation (September 2020) NICE TA651 Recommended

  Scottish Medicines Consortium (SMC) decisions
  - ▸ Naldemedine (*Rizmoic*®) for the treatment of opioid-induced constipation (OIC) in adult patients who have previously been treated with a laxative (April 2020) SMC No. SMC2242 Recommended

- **MEDICINAL FORMS** There can be variation in the licensing of different medicines containing the same drug.
  Oral tablet
  - ▸ Rizmoic (Viatris UK Healthcare Ltd)
    Naldemedine (as Naldemedine tosylate) 200 microgram Rizmoic 200microgram tablets | 30 tablet PoM £44.70

Naloxegol

26-Apr-2021

- **DRUG ACTION** Naloxegol is a peripherally acting opioid receptor antagonist. It therefore decreases the constipating effects of opioids without altering their central analgesic effects.

- **INDICATIONS AND DOSE**

  Opioid-induced constipation when response to laxatives inadequate
  - ▸ BY MOUTH
  - ▸ Adult: 25 mg once daily, to be taken in the morning

  DOSE ADJUSTMENTS DUE TO INTERACTIONS
  - ▸ Manufacturer advises reduce initial dose to 12.5 mg daily with concurrent use of moderate inhibitors of CYP3A4, increasing to 25 mg daily if well tolerated.

- **CONTRA-INDICATIONS** Gastro-intestinal or peritoneum malignancy (risk of gastro-intestinal perforation) · known or suspected gastro-intestinal obstruction · patients at risk of recurrent gastro-intestinal obstruction · recurrent or advanced ovarian cancer (risk of gastro-intestinal perforation) · vascular endothelial growth factor (VEGF) inhibitor treatment (risk of gastro-intestinal perforation)

- **CAUTIONS** Alzheimer's disease (advanced) · cardiovascular disease · CNS metastases · congestive heart failure (symptomatic) · Crohn's disease · diverticulitis (active or recurrent) · multiple sclerosis (active) · peptic ulcer disease (severe) · primary brain malignancies · QT interval over 500 milliseconds · recent history of myocardial infarction (within 6 months)

  CAUTIONS, FURTHER INFORMATION
  - ▸ Disruptions to blood-brain barrier Manufacturer advises caution in patients with clinically important disruptions to the blood-brain barrier (e.g. advanced Alzheimer's disease, active multiple sclerosis, primary brain malignancies)— risk of uptake into the CNS.
  - ▸ Cardiovascular disorders Safety and efficacy has not been established in patients with these conditions.

- **INTERACTIONS** → Appendix 1: naloxegol
- **SIDE-EFFECTS**
  - ▸ **Common or very common** Abdominal pain · diarrhoea · flatulence · headache · hyperhidrosis · nasopharyngitis · nausea · vomiting

- ▸ **Uncommon** Withdrawal syndrome

  SIDE-EFFECTS, FURTHER INFORMATION Manufacturer advises that gastrointestinal side-effects typically occur shortly after initiation of treatment — consider reducing the dose.

- **PREGNANCY** Manufacturer advises avoid—limited data available but toxicity at high doses in *animal* studies; theoretical risk of opioid withdrawal in fetus.

- **BREAST FEEDING** Manufacturer advises avoid—present in milk in *animal* studies and theoretical risk of opioid withdrawal in breast-fed infants.

- **HEPATIC IMPAIRMENT** Manufacturer advises avoid in severe impairment (no information available).

- **RENAL IMPAIRMENT**
  Dose adjustments Manufacturer advises lower initial dose in moderate to severe impairment—initially 12.5 mg daily, increase to 25 mg if well tolerated.

- **DIRECTIONS FOR ADMINISTRATION** Manufacturer advises tablets can be crushed, mixed with 120 mL of water and taken immediately if patients are unable to swallow tablets whole. The mixture may be administered via a nasogastric tube, if required.

- **PATIENT AND CARER ADVICE** Manufacturer advises patients report severe, persistent or worsening gastro-intestinal effects (such as abdominal pain) to their prescriber.

- **NATIONAL FUNDING/ACCESS DECISIONS** For full details see funding body website

  NICE decisions
  - ▸ Naloxegol for treating opioid-induced constipation (July 2015) NICE TA345 Recommended

- **MEDICINAL FORMS** There can be variation in the licensing of different medicines containing the same drug.
  Oral tablet
  CAUTIONARY AND ADVISORY LABELS 23
  - ▸ Moventig (Kyowa Kirin International UK NewCo Ltd)
    Naloxegol (as Naloxegol oxalate) 12.5 mg Moventig 12.5mg tablets | 30 tablet PoM £55.20 DT = £55.20
    Naloxegol (as Naloxegol oxalate) 25 mg Moventig 25mg tablets | 30 tablet PoM £55.20 DT = £55.20

3 Diarrhoea

Diarrhoea (acute)

08-Mar-2022

Description of condition

Diarrhoea is the abnormal passing of loose or liquid stools, with increased frequency, increased volume, or both. Acute diarrhoea is that which lasts less than 14 days, but symptoms usually improve within 2–4 days. It can result from infection, as a side-effect of a drug, or as an acute symptom of a chronic gastro-intestinal disorder (such as Crohn's disease p. 40, Irritable bowel syndrome p. 52, or Ulcerative colitis p. 41). It may also result from the accumulation of non-absorbed osmotically active solutes in the gastro-intestinal lumen (e.g. in lactase deficiency) or from the gastro-intestinal effects of secretory stimuli (other than the enterotoxins from an infection). It may also occur when intestinal motility or morphology is altered.

Prompt investigation is required to identify or exclude any serious underlying cause if the patient has any red flag symptoms such as unexplained weight loss, rectal bleeding, persistent diarrhoea, a systemic illness, has received recent hospital treatment or antibiotic treatment, or following foreign travel (other than to Western Europe, North America, Australia or New Zealand).

Aims of treatment

The priority of acute diarrhoea treatment, as in gastro-enteritis, is the prevention or reversal of fluid and electrolyte depletion and the management of dehydration when it is present. This is particularly important in infants, frail and elderly patients, when excessive water and electrolyte loss and dehydration can be life-threatening.

Treatment

Most episodes of acute diarrhoea will settle spontaneously without the need for any medical treatment. EvGr Oral rehydration therapy (ORT, such as disodium hydrogen citrate with glucose, potassium chloride and sodium chloride p. 1183; potassium chloride with sodium chloride p. 1180; potassium chloride with rice powder, sodium chloride and sodium citrate p. 1183) is the mainstay of treatment for acute diarrhoea to prevent or correct diarrhoea dehydration and to maintain the appropriate fluid intake once rehydration is achieved—see Fluids and electrolytes p. 1175.

However, in patients with severe dehydration and in those unable to drink, immediate admission to hospital and urgent replacement treatment with an intravenous rehydration fluid is recommended—see Fluids and electrolytes p. 1175.

The antimotility drug loperamide hydrochloride p. 74 is usually considered to be the standard treatment when rapid control of symptoms is required. It can also be used for mild-to-moderate travellers' diarrhoea (e.g. where toilet amenities are limited or unavailable) but should be avoided in bloody or suspected inflammatory diarrhoea (febrile patients) and in cases of significant abdominal pain (which also suggests inflammatory diarrhoea).

Loperamide hydrochloride is also the first-line treatment for patients with faecal incontinence [unlicensed indication] after the underlying cause of incontinence has been addressed. Ⓐ

Racecadotril is licensed as an adjunct to rehydration for the symptomatic treatment of uncomplicated acute diarrhoea in adults and children over 3 months.

There is insufficient evidence to recommend adsorbent preparations (such as kaolin) in acute diarrhoea.

Antibacterial drugs for acute diarrhoea

EvGr Ciprofloxacin p. 648 is occasionally used for prophylaxis against travellers' diarrhoea, but routine use is **not** recommended. Ⓐ For guidance on antibacterial treatment for infections that cause acute diarrhoea, see Gastro-intestinal system infections, antibacterial therapy p. 582.

Related drugs

Other drugs used for diarrhoea: codeine phosphate p. 517, co-phenotrope below, methylcellulose, rifaximin p. 667.

> **Other drugs used for Diarrhoea** Colesevelam hydrochloride, p. 228 · Colestyramine, p. 229

ANTIDIARRHOEALS > ANTIPROPULSIVES

ꜰ 510

Co-phenotrope

25-Nov-2020

● INDICATIONS AND DOSE

Adjunct to rehydration in acute diarrhoea
▸ BY MOUTH
▸ Child 4-8 years: 1 tablet 3 times a day
▸ Child 9-11 years: 1 tablet 4 times a day
▸ Child 12-15 years: 2 tablets 3 times a day
▸ Child 16-17 years: Initially 4 tablets, followed by 2 tablets every 6 hours until diarrhoea controlled
▸ Adult: Initially 4 tablets, followed by 2 tablets every 6 hours until diarrhoea controlled

Control of faecal consistency after colostomy or ileostomy
▸ BY MOUTH
▸ Child 4-8 years: 1 tablet 3 times a day
▸ Child 9-11 years: 1 tablet 4 times a day
▸ Child 12-15 years: 2 tablets 3 times a day
▸ Child 16-17 years: Initially 4 tablets, then 2 tablets 4 times a day
▸ Adult: Initially 4 tablets, then 2 tablets 4 times a day

● CONTRA-INDICATIONS Antibiotic-associated colitis · gastro-intestinal obstruction · intestinal atony · myasthenia gravis (but some antimuscarinics may be used to decrease muscarinic side-effects of anticholinesterases) · paralytic ileus · prostatic enlargement (in adults) · pyloric stenosis · severe ulcerative colitis · significant bladder outflow obstruction · toxic megacolon · urinary retention

● CAUTIONS Presence of subclinical doses of atropine may give rise to atropine side-effects in susceptible individuals or in overdosage · young children are particularly susceptible to **overdosage**—symptoms may be delayed and observation is needed for at least 48 hours after ingestion

● INTERACTIONS → Appendix 1: atropine · opioids

● SIDE-EFFECTS Abdominal discomfort · angioedema · angle closure glaucoma · appetite decreased · cardiac disorder · depression · dysuria · fever · gastrointestinal disorders · malaise · mucosal dryness · mydriasis · restlessness · vision disorders

● PREGNANCY Manufacturer advises caution.

● BREAST FEEDING May be present in milk.

● HEPATIC IMPAIRMENT Manufacturer advises caution; avoid in jaundice.

● DIRECTIONS FOR ADMINISTRATION Expert sources advise for administration *by mouth* tablets may be crushed.

● PRESCRIBING AND DISPENSING INFORMATION A mixture of diphenoxylate hydrochloride and atropine sulfate in the mass proportions 100 parts to 1 part respectively.

● EXCEPTIONS TO LEGAL CATEGORY Co-phenotrope 2.5/0.025 can be sold to the public for adults and children over 16 years (provided packs do not contain more than 20 tablets) as an adjunct to rehydration in acute diarrhoea (max. daily dose 10 tablets).

● MEDICINAL FORMS There can be variation in the licensing of different medicines containing the same drug. Forms available from special-order manufacturers include: oral tablet

Oral tablet
▸ Co-phenotrope (Non-proprietary)
Atropine sulfate 25 microgram, Diphenoxylate hydrochloride 2.5 mg Lomotil 2.5mg/25microgram tablets | 100 tablet PoM Ⓢ CD5
Lofenoxal 2.5mg/25microgram tablets | 20 tablet PoM Ⓢ DT = £38.50 CD5

ꜰ 510

Kaolin with morphine

31-Aug-2023

● INDICATIONS AND DOSE

Acute diarrhoea
▸ BY MOUTH
▸ Adult: 10 mL every 6 hours, dose to be given in water

● CONTRA-INDICATIONS Acute abdomen · delayed gastric emptying · heart failure secondary to chronic lung disease · phaeochromocytoma

● CAUTIONS Cardiac arrhythmias · pancreatitis · severe cor pulmonale

● INTERACTIONS → Appendix 1: kaolin · opioids

● BREAST FEEDING Therapeutic doses unlikely to affect infant.

● HEPATIC IMPAIRMENT EvGr Avoid in acute impairment. 

- **RENAL IMPAIRMENT** Avoid use or reduce dose; opioid effects increased and prolonged, and increased cerebral sensitivity occurs.
- **PRESCRIBING AND DISPENSING INFORMATION** When prepared extemporaneously, the BP states Kaolin and Morphine Mixture, BP consists of light kaolin or light kaolin (natural) 20%, sodium bicarbonate 5%, and chloroform and morphine tincture 4% in a suitable vehicle. Contains anhydrous morphine 550–800 micrograms/10 mL.
- **LESS SUITABLE FOR PRESCRIBING** Kaolin and Morphine Mixture, BP (Kaolin and Morphine Oral Suspension) is less suitable for prescribing.
- **MEDICINAL FORMS** No licensed medicines listed.

Loperamide hydrochloride
10-Nov-2021

- **INDICATIONS AND DOSE**

Symptomatic treatment of acute diarrhoea

▶ BY MOUTH

- Child 4-7 years: 1 mg 3–4 times a day for up to 3 days only
- Child 8-11 years: 2 mg 4 times a day for up to 5 days
- Child 12-17 years: Initially 4 mg, followed by 2 mg for up to 5 days, dose to be taken after each loose stool; usual dose 6–8 mg daily; maximum 16 mg per day
- Adult: Initially 4 mg, followed by 2 mg for up to 5 days, dose to be taken after each loose stool; usual dose 6–8 mg daily; maximum 16 mg per day

Chronic diarrhoea

▶ BY MOUTH

- Adult: Initially 4–8 mg daily in divided doses, adjusted according to response; maintenance up to 16 mg daily in 2 divided doses

Faecal incontinence

▶ BY MOUTH

- Adult: Initially 500 micrograms daily, adjusted according to response, maximum daily dose to be given in divided doses; maximum 16 mg per day

Pain of bowel colic in palliative care

▶ BY MOUTH

- Adult: 2–4 mg 4 times a day

- **UNLICENSED USE**
▶ In children *Capsules* not licensed for use in children under 8 years.
▶ In adults Use for faecal incontinence is an unlicensed indication.

> **IMPORTANT SAFETY INFORMATION**
>
> **MHRA/CHM ADVICE: REPORTS OF SERIOUS CARDIAC ADVERSE REACTIONS WITH HIGH DOSES OF LOPERAMIDE ASSOCIATED WITH ABUSE OR MISUSE (SEPTEMBER 2017)**
>
> Serious cardiovascular events (such as QT prolongation, torsades de pointes, and cardiac arrest), including fatalities, have been reported in association with large overdoses of loperamide.
>
> Healthcare professionals are reminded that if symptoms of overdose occur, naloxone can be given as an antidote. The duration of action of loperamide is longer than that of naloxone (1–3 hours), so repeated treatment with naloxone might be indicated; patients should be monitored closely for at least 48 hours to detect possible CNS depression.
>
> Pharmacists should remind patients not to take more than the recommended dose on the label.

- **CONTRA-INDICATIONS** Active ulcerative colitis · antibiotic-associated colitis · bacterial enterocolitis · conditions where abdominal distension develops · conditions where inhibition of peristalsis should be avoided
- **CAUTIONS** Not recommended for children under 12 years
- **INTERACTIONS** → Appendix 1: loperamide
- **SIDE-EFFECTS**
▶ **Common or very common** Gastrointestinal disorders · headache · nausea
▶ **Uncommon** Dizziness · drowsiness · dry mouth · gastrointestinal discomfort · skin reactions · vomiting
▶ **Rare or very rare** Angioedema · consciousness impaired · coordination abnormal · fatigue · miosis · muscle tone increased · severe cutaneous adverse reactions (SCARs) · urinary retention
- **PREGNANCY** Manufacturers advise avoid—no information available.
- **BREAST FEEDING** Amount probably too small to be harmful.
- **HEPATIC IMPAIRMENT** Manufacturer advises caution—risk of reduced first pass metabolism leading to central nervous system toxicity.
- **PRESCRIBING AND DISPENSING INFORMATION**

Palliative care For further information on the use of loperamide in palliative care, see www.medicinescomplete. com/#/content/palliative/loperamide.

- **PATIENT AND CARER ADVICE**
Medicines for Children leaflet: Loperamide for diarrhoea www.medicinesforchildren.org.uk/medicines/loperamide-for-diarrhoea/

- **EXCEPTIONS TO LEGAL CATEGORY** Loperamide can be sold to the public, for use in adults and children over 12 years, provided it is licensed and labelled for the treatment of acute diarrhoea.
▶ In adults Loperamide can be sold to the public, provided it is licensed and labelled for the treatment of acute diarrhoea associated with irritable bowel syndrome (after initial diagnosis by a doctor) in adults over 18 years of age.

- **MEDICINAL FORMS** There can be variation in the licensing of different medicines containing the same drug. Forms available from special-order manufacturers include: oral suspension, oral solution

Oral tablet

▶ Loperamide hydrochloride (Non-proprietary)
Loperamide hydrochloride 2 mg Loperamide 2mg tablets | 30 tablet PoM £2.34 DT = £2.21
▶ Norimode (Tillomed Laboratories Ltd)
Loperamide hydrochloride 2 mg Norimode 2mg tablets | 30 tablet PoM £2.15 DT = £2.21

Oral capsule

▶ Loperamide hydrochloride (Non-proprietary)
Loperamide hydrochloride 2 mg Loperamide 2mg capsules | 30 capsule PoM £1.44 DT = £0.75

Oral lyophilisate

▶ Loperamide hydrochloride (Non-proprietary)
Loperamide hydrochloride 2 mg Loperamide 2mg oral lyophilisates sugar free | 12 tablet P £4.14-£6.62 DT = £4.14 SF

Orodispersible tablet

▶ Imodium (McNeil Products Ltd)
Loperamide hydrochloride 2 mg Imodium Instant Melts 2mg orodispersible tablets | 12 tablet P £4.89 SF | 18 tablet P £6.76 DT = £6.76 SF

Loperamide with simeticone

24-Apr-2020

The properties listed below are those particular to the combination only. For the properties of the components please consider, loperamide hydrochloride p. 74, simeticone p. 80.

● **INDICATIONS AND DOSE**

Acute diarrhoea with abdominal colic

▶ BY MOUTH

▶ Child 12-17 years: Initially 1 tablet, then 1 tablet, after each loose stool, for up to 2 days; maximum 4 tablets per day

▶ Adult: Initially 2 tablets, then 1 tablet, after each loose stool, for up to 2 days; maximum 4 tablets per day

● **INTERACTIONS** → Appendix 1: loperamide

● **MEDICINAL FORMS** There can be variation in the licensing of different medicines containing the same drug.

Oral tablet

▶ **Imodium Plus** (McNeil Products Ltd)
Loperamide hydrochloride 2 mg, Dimeticone (as Simeticone) **125 mg** Imodium Dual Action Relief tablets | 12 tablet P £4.40 DT = £4.40

⊏ 510

Opium

10-Aug-2021

● **DRUG ACTION** Opium is obtained from *Papaver somniferum* and contains various active alkaloids, mainly morphine.

● **INDICATIONS AND DOSE**

Severe acute diarrhoea [when other treatments ineffective] (specialist use only)

▶ BY MOUTH USING ORAL DROPS

▶ Adult: Initially 5–10 drops 2–3 times a day (max. per dose 20 drops), adjust dose according to response; use the lowest effective dose for the shortest possible duration, a lower initial dose should be used for elderly patients; maximum 120 drops per day

DOSE EQUIVALENCE AND CONVERSION

▶ 1 drop contains 50 mg opium tincture corresponding to 0.5 mg morphine; 20 drops equals 1 mL.

● **CONTRA-INDICATIONS** Glaucoma · heart failure secondary to chronic lung disease (cor pulmonale)

● **CAUTIONS** Gastrointestinal haemorrhage · pancreatitis

● **INTERACTIONS** → Appendix 1: opioids

● **SIDE-EFFECTS**

▶ **Common or very common** Appetite decreased · asthenia · bronchospasm · cough decreased · gastrointestinal discomfort · taste altered

▶ **Uncommon** Urethral spasm

▶ **Rare or very rare** Allodynia · amenorrhoea · biliary colic · chills · dyspnoea · hyperalgesia · ileus · malaise · muscle cramps · nystagmus · pancreatitis · peripheral oedema · renal colic · SIADH · vision disorders

▶ **Frequency not known** Addiction · adrenal insufficiency · hyperthermia · libido decreased · muscle contractions involuntary · restlessness

● **PREGNANCY** EvGr Avoid unless potential benefit outweighs risk—toxicity in *animal* studies; limited information available in pregnant women. Ⓜ

● **BREAST FEEDING** EvGr Avoid—present in milk in higher concentrations than maternal plasma. If use cannot be avoided, closely monitor infant for respiratory depression and sedation. Ⓜ

● **HEPATIC IMPAIRMENT** EvGr Caution in mild or moderate impairment (may precipitate coma); avoid in severe impairment Ⓜ
Dose adjustments EvGr Consider dose reduction in mild or moderate impairment. Ⓜ

● **RENAL IMPAIRMENT** EvGr Caution in mild or moderate impairment; avoid in severe impairment. Ⓜ
Dose adjustments EvGr Consider dose reduction in mild or moderate impairment. Ⓜ

● **DIRECTIONS FOR ADMINISTRATION** *Dropizol* ® oral drops may be taken undiluted or mixed in a glass of water immediately before taking.

● **MEDICINAL FORMS** There can be variation in the licensing of different medicines containing the same drug.

Oral drops

CAUTIONARY AND ADVISORY LABELS 2
EXCIPIENTS: May contain Ethanol

▶ **Dropizol** (Atnahs Pharma UK Ltd)
Morphine anhydrous 10 mg per 1 ml Dropizol 10mg/ml oral drops | 10 ml PoM £41.00 CD2 SF

4   Exocrine pancreatic insufficiency

Exocrine pancreatic insufficiency

20-Aug-2024

Description of condition

Exocrine pancreatic insufficiency is characterised by reduced secretion of pancreatic enzymes into the duodenum.

The main clinical manifestations are maldigestion and malnutrition, associated with low circulating levels of micronutrients, fat-soluble vitamins and lipoproteins. Patients also present with gastro-intestinal symptoms such as diarrhoea, abdominal cramps and steatorrhoea.

Exocrine pancreatic insufficiency can result from chronic pancreatitis, cystic fibrosis, obstructive pancreatic tumours, coeliac disease, Zollinger-Ellison syndrome, and gastro-intestinal or pancreatic surgical resection.

Aims of treatment

The aim of treatment is to relieve gastro-intestinal symptoms and to achieve a normal nutritional status.

Drug treatment

Pancreatic enzyme replacement therapy with pancreatin p. 76 is the mainstay of treatment for exocrine pancreatic insufficiency.

Pancreatin contains the three main groups of digestive enzymes: lipase, amylase and protease. These enzymes respectively digest fats, carbohydrates and proteins into their basic components so that they can be absorbed and utilised by the body. EvGr Pancreatin should be administered with meals and snacks. The dose should be adjusted, as necessary, to the lowest effective dose according to the symptoms of maldigestion and malabsorption. Ⓐ

Fibrosing colonopathy has been reported in patients with cystic fibrosis taking high dose pancreatic enzyme replacement therapy (in excess of 10 000 units/kg/day of lipase). Possible risk factors are sex (in children, boys are at greater risk than girls), more severe cystic fibrosis, and concomitant use of laxatives. The peak age for developing fibrosing colonopathy is between 2 and 8 years. The manufacturer of *Nutrizym 22* ® recommend that the total dose of pancreatin used in patients with cystic fibrosis should not usually exceed 10 000 units/kg/day of lipase. Manufacturers of pancreatin recommend that if a patient taking pancreatin develops new abdominal symptoms (or any change in existing abdominal symptoms) the patient should be reviewed to exclude the possibility of colonic damage.

There is limited evidence that acid suppression may improve the effectiveness of pancreatin. EvGr Acid-suppressing drugs (proton pump inhibitors or H$_2$-receptor antagonists) may be trialled in patients who continue to experience symptoms despite high doses of pancreatin.

Levels of fat-soluble vitamins and micronutrients (such as zinc and selenium) should be routinely assessed and supplementation advised whenever necessary. Ⓐ

Pancreatin preparations			
Preparation	Protease units	Amylase units	Lipase units
Creon® 10 000 capsule, e/c granules	600	8000	10 000
Creon® Micro e/c granules (per 100 mg)	200	3600	5000
Pancrex V® capsule, powder	430	9000	8000
Pancrex V '125'® capsule, powder	160	3300	2950
Pancrex V® powder (per gram)	1400	30 000	25 000

Higher-strength pancreatin preparations			
Preparation	Protease units	Amylase units	Lipase units
Creon® 25 000 capsule, e/c pellets	1000	18 000	25 000
Nutrizym 22® capsule, e/c minitablets	1100	19 800	22 000

Non-drug treatment

EvGr Dietary advice should be provided. Food intake should be distributed between three main meals per day, and two or three snacks. Food that is difficult to digest should be avoided, such as legumes (peas, beans, lentils) and high-fibre foods. Alcohol should be avoided completely. Reduced fat diets are not recommended. Ⓐ

Medium-chain triglycerides (see MCT oil, in *Borderline substances*), which are directly absorbed by the intestinal mucosa, were thought to be useful in some patients. However evidence has shown that MCT-enriched preparations offer no advantage over a normal balanced diet.

PANCREATIC ENZYMES

Pancreatin

15-Aug-2024

● **DRUG ACTION** Supplements of pancreatin are given to compensate for reduced or absent exocrine secretion. They assist the digestion of starch, fat, and protein.

● **INDICATIONS AND DOSE**

CREON® 10000

Pancreatic insufficiency
▸ BY MOUTH
▸ Child: Initially 1–2 capsules, dose to be taken with each meal either taken whole or contents mixed with acidic fluid or soft food (then swallowed immediately without chewing)
▸ Adult: Initially 1–2 capsules, dose to be taken with each meal either taken whole or contents mixed with acidic fluid or soft food (then swallowed immediately without chewing)

CREON® 25000

Pancreatic insufficiency
▸ BY MOUTH
▸ Child 2-17 years: Initially 1–2 capsules, dose to be taken with each meal either taken whole or contents mixed with acidic fluid or soft food (then swallowed immediately without chewing)
▸ Adult: Initially 1–2 capsules, dose to be taken with each meal either taken whole or contents mixed with

acidic fluid or soft food (then swallowed immediately without chewing)

CREON® MICRO

Pancreatic insufficiency
▸ BY MOUTH
▸ Child: Initially 100 mg, for administration advice, see *Directions for administration*
▸ Adult: Initially 100 mg, for administration advice, see *Directions for administration*

DOSE EQUIVALENCE AND CONVERSION
▸ For *Creon® Micro* : 100 mg granules = one measured scoopful (scoop supplied with product).

NUTRIZYM 22® GASTRO-RESISTANT CAPSULES

Pancreatic insufficiency
▸ BY MOUTH
▸ Adult: Initially 1–2 capsules, dose to be taken with meals and 1 capsule as required, dose to be taken with snacks, doses should be swallowed whole or contents taken with water, or mixed with acidic fluid or soft food (then swallowed immediately without chewing)

PANCREX® V

Pancreatic insufficiency
▸ BY MOUTH
▸ Child 1-11 months: 1–2 capsules, contents of capsule to be mixed with feeds
▸ Child 1-17 years: 2–6 capsules, dose to be taken with each meal either swallowed whole or sprinkled on food
▸ Adult: 2–6 capsules, dose to be taken with each meal either swallowed whole or sprinkled on food

PANCREX® V POWDER

Pancreatic insufficiency
▸ BY MOUTH
▸ Child: 0.5–2 g, to be taken before or with meals, washed down or mixed with milk or water
▸ Adult: 0.5–2 g, to be taken before or with meals, washed down or mixed with milk or water

● CAUTIONS Can irritate the perioral skin and buccal mucosa if retained in the mouth · excessive doses can cause perianal irritation

● INTERACTIONS → Appendix 1: pancreatin

● SIDE-EFFECTS
▸ **Common or very common** Abdominal distension · constipation · nausea · vomiting
▸ **Uncommon** Skin reactions
▸ **Frequency not known** Fibrosing colonopathy

● PREGNANCY Not known to be harmful.

● DIRECTIONS FOR ADMINISTRATION Pancreatin is inactivated by gastric acid therefore manufacturer advises pancreatin preparations are best taken with food (or immediately before or after food). Since pancreatin is inactivated by heat, excessive heat should be avoided if preparations are mixed with liquids or food; manufacturer advises the resulting mixtures should not be kept for more than one hour and any left-over food or liquid containing pancreatin should be discarded. Enteric-coated preparations deliver a higher enzyme concentration in the duodenum (provided the capsule contents are swallowed whole without chewing). Manufacturer advises gastro-resistant granules should be mixed with slightly acidic soft food or liquid such as apple juice, and then swallowed immediately without chewing. Capsules containing enteric-coated granules can be opened and the granules administered in the same way. For infants, *Creon® Micro* granules can be mixed with a small amount of milk on a spoon and administered immediately—granules should not be added to the baby's bottle. Manufacturer advises *Pancrex® V* powder may be administered via nasogastric tube or gastrostomy tube—consult local and national official guidelines.

- **PRESCRIBING AND DISPENSING INFORMATION** Preparations may contain pork pancreatin—consult product literature.
- **HANDLING AND STORAGE** Hypersensitivity reactions have occasionally occurred in those handling the powder.
- **PATIENT AND CARER ADVICE** Patients or carers should be given advice on administration. It is important to ensure adequate hydration at all times in patients receiving higher-strength pancreatin preparations.
  Medicines for Children leaflet: Pancreatin for pancreatic insufficiency www.medicinesforchildren.org.uk/medicines/pancreatin-for-pancreatic-insufficiency/

- **MEDICINAL FORMS** There can be variation in the licensing of different medicines containing the same drug.
  Gastro-resistant capsule
  - ► Creon (Viatris UK Healthcare Ltd)
    Protease 600 unit, Amylase 8000 unit, Lipase 10000 unit Creon 10000 gastro-resistant capsules | 100 capsule [P] £12.93
    Protease 1000 unit, Amylase 18000 unit, Lipase 25000 unit Creon 25000 gastro-resistant capsules | 100 capsule [PoM] £28.25
  - ► Nutrizym (Zentiva Pharma UK Ltd)
    Protease 1100 unit, Amylase 19800 unit, Lipase 22000 unit Nutrizym 22 gastro-resistant capsules | 100 capsule [PoM] £36.20
  Gastro-resistant granules
  CAUTIONARY AND ADVISORY LABELS 25
  - ► Creon (Viatris UK Healthcare Ltd)
    Protease 200 unit, Amylase 3600 unit, Lipase 5000 unit Creon Micro Pancreatin 60.12mg gastro-resistant granules | 20 gram [P] £31.50
  Oral capsule
  - ► Pancrex (Essential Pharmaceuticals Ltd)
    Protease 430 unit, Lipase 8000 unit, Amylase 9000 unit Pancrex V capsules | 300 capsule [P] £55.86
  Powder for gastroenteral or oral liquid
  - ► Pancrex (Essential Pharmaceuticals Ltd)
    Protease 1400 unit, Lipase 25000 unit, Amylase 30000 unit Pancrex V oral powder | 300 gram [P] £246.40 [SF]

5   Food allergy

Food allergy

02-Aug-2022

Description of condition

Food allergy is an adverse immune response to a food, commonly associated with cutaneous and gastro-intestinal reactions, and less frequently associated with respiratory reactions and anaphylaxis. It is distinct from food intolerance which is non-immunological. Cow's milk, hen's eggs, soy, wheat, peanuts, tree nuts, fish, and shellfish are the most common allergens. Cross-reactivity between similar foods can occur (e.g. allergy to other mammalian milk in patients with cow's milk allergy).

Management of food allergy

[EvGr] Allergy caused by specific foods should be managed by strict avoidance of the causal food. Educating patients about appropriate nutrition, food preparation, and the risks of accidental exposure is recommended, such as food and drinks to avoid, ensuring adequate nutritional intake, and interpreting food labels. ⟨A⟩

Sodium cromoglicate below is licensed as an adjunct to dietary avoidance in patients with food allergy.

[EvGr] Peanut protein p. 328 may be offered as an adjunct to dietary avoidance to patients with peanut allergy in childhood, and treatment can be continued into adulthood. ⟨A⟩

Drug treatment

[EvGr] There is low quality evidence to support the use of antihistamines to treat acute, **non-life-threatening** symptoms (such as flushing and urticaria) if accidental ingestion of allergenic food has occurred. Chlorphenamine maleate p. 323 is licensed for the symptomatic control of food allergy. In case of food-induced anaphylaxis, intramuscular adrenaline/epinephrine p. 256 is the first-line immediate treatment. Patients who are at risk of anaphylaxis should be trained to use self-injectable adrenaline/epinephrine. ⟨A⟩ For further guidance, see Antihistamines, allergen immunotherapy and allergic emergencies p. 316.

MAST-CELL STABILISERS

Sodium cromoglicate

03-Aug-2023

(Sodium cromoglycate)

- **INDICATIONS AND DOSE**
  Food allergy (in conjunction with dietary restriction)
  - ► BY MOUTH
  - ► Child 2–13 years: Initially 100 mg 4 times a day for 2–3 weeks, to be taken before meals, dose then increased if necessary up to 40 mg/kg per day, then reduced according to response
  - ► Child 14–17 years: Initially 200 mg 4 times a day for 2–3 weeks, to be taken before meals, dose then increased if necessary up to 40 mg/kg per day, then reduced according to response
  - ► Adult: Initially 200 mg 4 times a day for 2–3 weeks, to be taken before meals, dose then increased if necessary up to 40 mg/kg per day, then reduced according to response

- **SIDE-EFFECTS** Arthralgia · nausea · rash
- **PREGNANCY** Not known to be harmful.
- **BREAST FEEDING** Unlikely to be present in milk.
- **DIRECTIONS FOR ADMINISTRATION** Expert sources advise capsules may be swallowed whole or the contents dissolved in hot water and diluted with cold water before taking.
- **PATIENT AND CARER ADVICE** Patient counselling is advised for sodium cromoglicate capsules (administration).

- **MEDICINAL FORMS** There can be variation in the licensing of different medicines containing the same drug. Forms available from special-order manufacturers include: oral solution
  Oral solution
  - ► Sodium cromoglicate (Non-proprietary)
    Sodium cromoglicate 20 mg per 1 ml Sodium cromoglicate 100mg/5ml oral solution 5ml unit dose ampoules sugar free | 96 unit dose [PoM] £121.86 DT = £121.86 [SF]
  Oral capsule
  CAUTIONARY AND ADVISORY LABELS 22
  - ► Sodium cromoglicate (Non-proprietary)
    Sodium cromoglicate 100 mg Sodium cromoglicate 100mg capsules | 100 capsule [PoM] £110.00-£262.00 DT = £218.56

6 Gastric acid disorders and ulceration

6.1 Dyspepsia

Dyspepsia

31-Oct-2019

Description of condition

Dyspepsia describes a range of upper gastro-intestinal symptoms, which are typically present for 4 or more weeks. Symptoms include but are not limited to upper abdominal pain or discomfort, heartburn, gastric reflux, bloating, nausea and/or vomiting. Symptoms can be attributed to an underlying cause (e.g. Gastro-oesophageal reflux disease p. 92, Peptic ulcer disease p. 81, gastro-oesophageal malignancy, or side effects from drugs), but the majority of patients are likely to have functional dyspepsia, where an underlying cause cannot be identified and endoscopy findings are normal. Uninvestigated dyspepsia describes symptoms in patients who have not had an endoscopy.

Dyspepsia symptoms in pregnancy are commonly due to gastro-oesophageal reflux disease (GORD), for management see *GORD in pregnancy* in Gastro-oesophageal reflux disease p. 92.

Aims of treatment

The aim of treatment is to manage symptoms, and where possible, to treat the underlying cause of dyspepsia.

Non-drug treatment

[EvGr] Lifestyle measures, such as healthy eating, weight loss (if obese), avoiding any trigger foods, eating smaller meals, eating the evening meal 3–4 hours before going to bed, raising the head of the bed, Smoking cessation p. 565, and reducing alcohol consumption may improve symptoms. Assess the patient for stress, anxiety, or depression, as these conditions may exacerbate symptoms.

Urgent endoscopic investigation is required for patients with dysphagia, significant acute gastrointestinal bleeding, or in those aged 55 years and over with unexplained weight loss and symptoms of upper abdominal pain, reflux or dyspepsia. (A)

Drug treatment

[EvGr] Drugs that may cause dyspepsia, such as alpha-blockers, antimuscarinics, aspirin, benzodiazepines, beta-blockers, bisphosphonates, calcium-channel blockers, corticosteroids, nitrates, non-steroidal anti-inflammatory drugs (NSAIDs), theophyllines, and tricyclic antidepressants, should be reviewed. The lowest effective dose should be used and if possible, stopped.

Antacids and/or alginates may be used for short-term symptom control, but long-term, continuous use is not recommended. (A)

Initial management

Uninvestigated dyspepsia

[EvGr] A proton pump inhibitor should be taken for 4 weeks. Patients with dyspepsia should be tested for *Helicobacter pylori* (*H. pylori*) infection, and treated if positive. (A) Public Health England recommends that patients who are at high risk for *H. pylori* infection should be tested for *H. pylori* first, or in parallel with a course of proton pump inhibitor. For treatment regimens, see Helicobacter pylori infection p. 93.

Functional dyspepsia

[EvGr] Patients should be tested for *H. pylori* infection and treated if positive. (A) See Helicobacter pylori infection p. 93 for testing and management of *H. pylori* infection. [EvGr] In patients not infected with *H. pylori*, a proton pump inhibitor or a histamine₂-receptor antagonist (H₂-receptor antagonist) should be taken for 4 weeks. (A)

Follow up management

Uninvestigated and functional dyspepsia

[EvGr] For patients with refractory dyspepsia symptoms, new alarm symptoms should be assessed and alternative diagnoses should be considered. The patient's adherence to initial management should be checked and lifestyle advice reinforced.

If symptoms persist or recur following initial management, a proton pump inhibitor or H₂-receptor antagonist therapy should be used at the lowest dose needed to control symptoms. The patient may use the treatment on an 'as-needed' basis.

In patients with uninvestigated dyspepsia taking an NSAID and unable to stop the drug, consider reducing the NSAID dose and using long-term gastro-protection with acid suppression therapy, or switching to an alternative to the NSAID, such as paracetamol p. 507 or a selective cyclo-oxygenase (COX)-2 inhibitor (but see *Cardiovascular Events* under Non-steroidal anti-inflammatory drugs p. 1292).

In patients with uninvestigated dyspepsia taking aspirin and unable to stop the drug, consider switching from aspirin to an alternative antiplatelet drug.

Patients treated with *H. pylori* eradication therapy do not require routine retesting. (A) There are specific situations where retesting may be appropriate, see *Retesting for Helicobacter pylori*, under Helicobacter pylori infection p. 93. [EvGr] If retesting is positive, second-line eradication therapy should be prescribed.

An annual review should be performed for patients with dyspepsia to assess their symptoms and treatment. A 'step down' approach, or stopping treatment, should be encouraged if possible and clinically appropriate. A return to self-treatment with antacid and/or alginate therapy may be appropriate.

Referral to a specialist for further investigations should occur in patients of any age with gastro-oesophageal symptoms that are unexplained or non-responsive to treatment, or in patients with *H. pylori* infection that has not responded to second-line eradication therapy—see Helicobacter pylori infection p. 93. (A)

Useful Resources

Gastro-oesophageal reflux disease and dyspepsia in adults: investigation and management. National Institute for Health and Care Excellence. NICE guideline 184. September 2014, reviewed October 2019.
www.nice.org.uk/guidance/cg184

ANTACIDS › ALGINATE

Alginic acid

09-Nov-2021

● **INDICATIONS AND DOSE**

GAVISCON INFANT ® POWDER SACHETS

Management of gastro-oesophageal reflux disease

▶ BY MOUTH

▶ Child 1-23 months (body-weight up to 4.5 kg): 1 sachet as required, to be mixed with feeds (or water, for breast-fed infants); maximum 6 sachets per day

▶ Child 1-23 months (body-weight 4.5 kg and above): 2 sachets as required, to be mixed with feeds (or water, for breast-fed infants); maximum 12 sachets per day

● **CONTRA-INDICATIONS** Intestinal obstruction · preterm neonates · where excessive water loss likely (e.g. fever, diarrhoea, vomiting, high room temperature)

GAVISCON INFANT ® POWDER SACHETS Concurrent use of preparations containing thickening agents

● RENAL IMPAIRMENT ⟨EvGr⟩ Avoid (risk of hypernatraemia).
Ⓜ

● MEDICINAL FORMS There can be variation in the licensing of
different medicines containing the same drug.

Oral powder
ELECTROLYTES: May contain Sodium
▸ Gaviscon Infant (Reckitt Benckiser Healthcare (UK) Ltd)
   Magnesium alginate 87.5 mg, Sodium alginate 225 mg Gaviscon
   Infant oral powder sachets | 30 sachet Ⓟ £7.64 DT = £7.64 ⓈⒻ

Sodium alginate with potassium bicarbonate

The properties listed below are those particular to the
combination only. For the properties of the components
please consider, alginic acid p. 78.

● **INDICATIONS AND DOSE**

**Management of mild symptoms of dyspepsia and gastro-
oesophageal reflux disease**
▸ BY MOUTH USING CHEWABLE TABLETS
▸ Child 6-11 years (under medical advice only): 1 tablet, to
  be chewed after meals and at bedtime
▸ Child 12-17 years: 1–2 tablets, to be chewed after meals
  and at bedtime
▸ Adult: 1–2 tablets, to be chewed after meals and at
  bedtime
▸ BY MOUTH USING ORAL SUSPENSION
▸ Child 2-11 years (under medical advice only): 2.5–5 mL, to
  be taken after meals and at bedtime
▸ Child 12-17 years: 5–10 mL, to be taken after meals and
  at bedtime
▸ Adult: 5–10 mL, to be taken after meals and at bedtime

● PRESCRIBING AND DISPENSING INFORMATION Flavours of
oral liquid formulations may include aniseed or
peppermint.

● MEDICINAL FORMS There can be variation in the licensing of
different medicines containing the same drug.

Oral suspension
ELECTROLYTES: May contain Potassium, sodium
▸ Acidex Advance (Wockhardt UK Ltd)
   **Potassium bicarbonate 20 mg per 1 ml, Sodium alginate 100 mg
   per 1 ml** Acidex Advance oral suspension peppermint | 250 ml Ⓟ
   £1.92 ⓈⒻ | 500 ml Ⓟ £3.84 DT = £7.59 ⓈⒻ
   Acidex Advance oral suspension aniseed | 250 ml Ⓟ £1.92 ⓈⒻ |
   500 ml Ⓟ £3.84 DT = £7.59 ⓈⒻ
▸ Gaviscon Advance (Reckitt Benckiser Healthcare (UK) Ltd)
   **Potassium bicarbonate 20 mg per 1 ml, Sodium alginate 100 mg
   per 1 ml** Gaviscon Advance oral suspension aniseed | 250 ml Ⓟ
   £3.79 ⓈⒻ | 500 ml Ⓟ £7.59 DT = £7.59 ⓈⒻ | 600 ml Ⓟ
   £12.75 ⓈⒻ
   Gaviscon Advance oral suspension peppermint | 250 ml Ⓟ
   £3.79 ⓈⒻ | 500 ml Ⓟ £7.59 DT = £7.59 ⓈⒻ

Chewable tablet
EXCIPIENTS: May contain Aspartame
ELECTROLYTES: May contain Potassium, sodium
▸ Gaviscon Advance (Reckitt Benckiser Healthcare (UK) Ltd)
   **Potassium bicarbonate 100 mg, Sodium alginate
   500 mg** Gaviscon Advance Mint chewable tablets | 24 tablet ⒼⓈⓁ
   £4.85 ⓈⒻ | 60 tablet ⒼⓈⓁ £6.32 DT = £6.32 ⓈⒻ

Co-magaldrox
15-Dec-2020

The properties listed below are those particular to the
combination only. For the properties of the components
please consider, magnesium hydroxide p. 64.

● **INDICATIONS AND DOSE**
MAALOX ®
Dyspepsia
▸ BY MOUTH
▸ Child 14-17 years: 10–20 mL, to be taken 20–60 minutes
  after meals, and at bedtime or when required
▸ Adult: 10–20 mL, to be taken 20–60 minutes after
  meals, and at bedtime or when required
MUCOGEL ®
Dyspepsia
▸ BY MOUTH
▸ Child 12-17 years: 10–20 mL 3 times a day, to be taken
  20–60 minutes after meals, and at bedtime, or when
  required
▸ Adult: 10–20 mL 3 times a day, to be taken
  20–60 minutes after meals, and at bedtime, or when
  required

● INTERACTIONS → Appendix 1: aluminium hydroxide ·
magnesium

● SIDE-EFFECTS
▸ **Uncommon** Constipation · diarrhoea
▸ **Rare or very rare** Electrolyte imbalance
▸ **Frequency not known** Abdominal pain · hyperaluminaemia

● RENAL IMPAIRMENT There is a risk of accumulation and
aluminium toxicity with antacids containing aluminium
salts. Absorption of aluminium from aluminium salts is
increased by citrates, which are contained in many
effervescent preparations (such as effervescent
analgesics).

● PRESCRIBING AND DISPENSING INFORMATION Co-
magaldrox is a mixture of aluminium hydroxide and
magnesium hydroxide; the proportions are expressed in
the form x/y where x and y are the strengths in milligrams
per unit dose of magnesium hydroxide and aluminium
hydroxide respectively.

MAALOX ® *Maalox*® suspension is low in sodium.
MUCOGEL ® *Mucogel*® suspension is low in sodium.

● MEDICINAL FORMS There can be variation in the licensing of
different medicines containing the same drug.

Oral suspension
▸ Mucogel (Rosemont Pharmaceuticals Ltd)
   **Magnesium hydroxide 39 mg per 1 ml, Aluminium hydroxide gel
   dried 44 mg per 1 ml** Mucogel oral suspension | 500 ml ⒼⓈⓁ £2.99
   DT = £2.99 ⓈⒻ

Simeticone with aluminium hydroxide and magnesium hydroxide
04-May-2020

The properties listed below are those particular to the
combination only. For the properties of the components
please consider, simeticone p. 80.

● **INDICATIONS AND DOSE**

Dyspepsia
▸ BY MOUTH
▸ Child 12-17 years: 5–10 mL 4 times a day, to be taken
  after meals and at bedtime, or when required
▸ Adult: 5–10 mL 4 times a day, to be taken after meals
  and at bedtime, or when required

- INTERACTIONS → Appendix 1: aluminium hydroxide · antacids · magnesium
- SIDE-EFFECTS
- ▶ **Uncommon** Constipation · diarrhoea
- ▶ **Rare or very rare** Electrolyte imbalance
- ▶ **Frequency not known** Abdominal pain · hyperaluminaemia
- RENAL IMPAIRMENT There is a risk of accumulation and aluminium toxicity with antacids containing aluminium salts. Absorption of aluminium from aluminium salts is increased by citrates, which are contained in many effervescent preparations (such as effervescent analgesics).

- MEDICINAL FORMS There can be variation in the licensing of different medicines containing the same drug.

Oral suspension
- ▶ Maalox Plus (Opella Healthcare UK Ltd)
  Simeticone 5 mg per 1 ml, Aluminium hydroxide gel dried 35 mg per 1 ml, Magnesium hydroxide 40 mg per 1 ml Maalox Plus oral suspension | 250 ml [GSL] £3.84 [SF]

ANTACIDS > MAGNESIUM

Magnesium carbonate

- INDICATIONS AND DOSE

Dyspepsia
- ▶ BY MOUTH USING ORAL SUSPENSION
- ▶ Adult: 10 mL 3 times a day, dose to be taken in water

- CONTRA-INDICATIONS Hypophosphataemia
- INTERACTIONS → Appendix 1: magnesium
- SIDE-EFFECTS Diarrhoea
- HEPATIC IMPAIRMENT In patients with fluid retention, avoid antacids containing large amounts of sodium. Avoid antacids containing magnesium salts in hepatic coma if there is a risk of renal failure.
- RENAL IMPAIRMENT Magnesium carbonate mixture has a high sodium content; avoid in patients with fluid retention.
  Dose adjustments Avoid or use at a reduced dose; increased risk of toxicity.
- PRESCRIBING AND DISPENSING INFORMATION When prepared extemporaneously, the BP states Aromatic Magnesium Carbonate Mixture, BP consists of light magnesium carbonate 3%, sodium bicarbonate 5%, in a suitable vehicle containing aromatic cardamom tincture.

- MEDICINAL FORMS No licensed medicines listed.

Magnesium trisilicate

- INDICATIONS AND DOSE

Dyspepsia
- ▶ BY MOUTH USING CHEWABLE TABLETS
- ▶ Adult: 1–2 tablets as required

- CONTRA-INDICATIONS Hypophosphataemia
- INTERACTIONS → Appendix 1: magnesium
- SIDE-EFFECTS Diarrhoea · nephrolithiasis (long term use)
- HEPATIC IMPAIRMENT Avoid in hepatic coma; risk of renal failure.
- RENAL IMPAIRMENT
  Dose adjustments Avoid or used at a reduced dose (increased risk of toxicity).

- MEDICINAL FORMS No licensed medicines listed.

Magnesium trisilicate with magnesium carbonate and sodium bicarbonate

30-Nov-2021

The properties listed below are those particular to the combination only. For the properties of the components please consider, magnesium trisilicate above, magnesium carbonate above, sodium bicarbonate p. 1178.

- INDICATIONS AND DOSE

Dyspepsia
- ▶ BY MOUTH
- ▶ Child 5–11 years: 5–10 mL 3 times a day, alternatively as required, dose to be made up with water
- ▶ Child 12–17 years: 10–20 mL 3 times a day, alternatively as required, dose to be made up with water
- ▶ Adult: 10–20 mL 3 times a day, alternatively as required, dose to be made up with water

- CONTRA-INDICATIONS Hypophosphataemia · severe renal failure
- CAUTIONS Heart failure · hypermagnesaemia · hypertension · metabolic alkalosis · respiratory alkalosis
- INTERACTIONS → Appendix 1: magnesium · sodium bicarbonate
- HEPATIC IMPAIRMENT In patients with fluid retention avoid antacids containing large amounts of sodium. Avoid antacids containing magnesium salts in hepatic coma if there is a risk of renal failure.
- RENAL IMPAIRMENT [EvGr] Extreme caution (high sodium content); avoid in severe renal failure. ⓜ
- PRESCRIBING AND DISPENSING INFORMATION When prepared extemporaneously, the BP states Magnesium Trisilicate Mixture, BP consists of 5% each of magnesium trisilicate, light magnesium carbonate, and sodium bicarbonate in a suitable vehicle with a peppermint flavour.

- MEDICINAL FORMS No licensed medicines listed.

ANTIFOAMING DRUGS

Simeticone

05-Jun-2020

(Activated dimeticone)

- DRUG ACTION Simeticone (activated dimeticone) is an antifoaming agent.

- INDICATIONS AND DOSE

DENTINOX ®

Colic | Wind pains
- ▶ BY MOUTH
- ▶ Child 1 month–1 year: 2.5 mL, to be taken with or after each feed; may be added to bottle feed; maximum 6 doses per day

INFACOL ®

Colic | Wind pains
- ▶ BY MOUTH
- ▶ Child 1 month–1 year: 0.5–1 mL, to be taken before feeds

- PRESCRIBING AND DISPENSING INFORMATION

  DENTINOX ® The brand name *Dentinox* ® is also used for other preparations including teething gel.
- PATIENT AND CARER ADVICE

  INFACOL ® Patients or carers should be given advice on use of the *Infacol* ® dropper.

• LESS SUITABLE FOR PRESCRIBING

DENTINOX ® *Dentinox*® colic drops are less suitable for prescribing (evidence of benefit in infantile colic uncertain).

INFACOL ® *Infacol*® is less suitable for prescribing (evidence of benefit in infantile colic uncertain).

• MEDICINAL FORMS There can be variation in the licensing of different medicines containing the same drug.

Oral suspension

▸ Infacol (Dendron Brands Ltd)
Simeticone 40 mg per 1 ml Infacol 40mg/ml oral suspension | 55 ml GSL £3.48 DT = £3.48 SF | 85 ml GSL £5.12 DT = £5.12 SF

Oral drops

▸ Dentinox Infant (Dendron Brands Ltd)
Simeticone 8.4 mg per 1 ml Dentinox Infant colic drops | 100 ml GSL £2.13 DT = £2.13

Combinations available: *Simeticone with aluminium hydroxide and magnesium hydroxide,* p. 79

6.2 Gastric and duodenal ulceration

Peptic ulcer disease
01-May-2025

Description of condition

Peptic ulcer disease includes gastric or duodenal ulceration, which is a breach in the epithelium of the gastric or duodenal mucosa. The main symptom of peptic ulcer disease is upper abdominal pain but other less common symptoms include nausea, indigestion, heartburn, loss of appetite, weight loss and a bloated feeling. The use of non-steroidal anti-inflammatory drugs (NSAIDs), and *Helicobacter pylori* (*H. pylori*) infection are the most common causes of peptic ulcer disease. Smoking, alcohol consumption, and stress may also contribute to the development of peptic ulcer disease.

NSAIDs may have an additive effect if there is co-existent *H. pylori* infection, further increasing the risk of peptic ulceration. The risk of upper gastro-intestinal side-effects varies between individual NSAIDs and is influenced by the dose and duration of use. For recommendations on individual NSAID choice, see under *NSAIDs and gastro-intestinal events* in Non-steroidal anti-inflammatory drugs p. 1292.

Complications of peptic ulcer disease include gastric outlet obstruction and potentially life-threatening gastro-intestinal perforation and haemorrhage. Patients at high risk of developing gastro-intestinal complications with an NSAID include those with a history of complicated peptic ulcer, or those with more than 2 of the following risk factors:

- age over 65 years;
- high dose NSAIDs;
- other drugs that increase the risk of gastro-intestinal adverse-effects (e.g. anticoagulants, corticosteroids, selective serotonin reuptake inhibitors);
- serious co-morbidity (e.g. cardiovascular disease, hypertension, diabetes, renal or hepatic impairment);
- heavy smoker;
- excessive alcohol consumption;
- previous adverse reaction to NSAIDs;
- prolonged requirement for NSAIDs.

Aims of treatment

The aims of treatment are to promote ulcer healing, manage symptoms, treat *H. pylori* infection if detected and reduce the risk of ulcer complications and recurrence.

Non-drug treatment

EvGr Lifestyle measures, such as healthy eating, weight loss (if obese), avoiding trigger foods, eating smaller meals, eating the evening meal 3–4 hours before going to bed, raising the head of the bed, Smoking cessation p. 565, and reducing alcohol consumption may improve symptoms. Assess the patient for stress, anxiety, or depression, as these conditions may exacerbate symptoms.

Urgent endoscopic investigation is required for patients with dysphagia, significant acute gastrointestinal bleeding, or in those aged 55 years and over with unexplained weight loss and symptoms of upper abdominal pain, reflux or dyspepsia. Ⓐ

Initial management

EvGr Drugs that induce peptic ulcers, such as NSAIDs, aspirin, bisphosphonates, immunosuppressive agents (e.g. corticosteroids), potassium chloride, selective serotonin reuptake inhibitors (SSRIs) and recreational drugs such as crack cocaine should be reviewed and stopped, if clinically appropriate. Antacids and/or alginates may be used for short-term symptom control, but long-term, continuous use is not recommended. Ⓐ

The treatment strategy in peptic ulcer disease can vary depending on whether a patient has *H. pylori* infection, or has recently taken NSAIDs.

EvGr The patient should be tested for *H. pylori* infection. In patients who have tested positive and have no history of NSAID use, *H. pylori* infection should be eradicated. Ⓐ For guidance on *H. pylori* testing and eradication treatment, see Helicobacter pylori infection p. 93.

EvGr If the ulcer is associated with NSAID use, a proton pump inhibitor or histamine$_2$-receptor antagonist (H$_2$-receptor antagonist) should be used for 8 weeks, followed by *H. pylori* infection eradication treatment if the patient has tested positive for *H. pylori*.

In patients who have tested negative for *H. pylori* and have no history of NSAID use, a proton pump inhibitor or H$_2$-receptor antagonist should be used for 4–8 weeks. Ⓐ

Follow-up management

EvGr Patients with peptic ulcers (gastric or duodenal) who tested positive for *H. pylori* should be reviewed 6–8 weeks after starting eradication treatment and re-tested, depending on the size of the lesion. Patients with a gastric ulcer who tested positive for *H. pylori* should also have a repeat endoscopy 6–8 weeks after treatment to confirm ulcer healing, depending on the size of the lesion.

If the ulcer is healed and the patient is to continue taking NSAIDs, the potential harm from NSAID treatment should be discussed. The need for NSAIDs should be reviewed at least every 6 months, and use on a limited, 'as-needed' basis trialled. Consider reducing the dose, substituting the NSAID with paracetamol p. 507, or use of an alternative analgesic or low dose ibuprofen.

In patients with previous ulceration, for whom NSAID continuation is necessary, or those at high risk of gastro-intestinal side effects, consider a cyclo-oxygenase (COX)-2 inhibitor instead of a standard NSAID (but see *Cardiovascular Events* under Non-steroidal anti-inflammatory drugs p. 1292). Gastro-protection with acid suppression therapy should always be co-prescribed. A proton pump inhibitor is the preferred choice for gastro-protection; other options include a H$_2$-receptor antagonist or misoprostol, but the side effects of misoprostol limit its use.

If symptoms recur after initial treatment, a proton pump inhibitor may be taken at the lowest dose possible to control symptoms. Treatment should be used on an 'as-needed' basis with patients managing their own symptoms.

In cases where there are persistent symptoms or an unhealed ulcer, the patient's adherence to initial management should be checked and lifestyle advice reinforced. Other causes, such as malignancy, failure to detect *H. pylori*, inadvertent NSAID use, other ulcer-inducing medication, and rare causes such as Zollinger-Ellison syndrome or Crohn's disease should be considered.

Switching to an alternative acid suppression therapy, e.g. a H_2-receptor antagonist, may be beneficial if the response to proton pump inhibitor therapy is inadequate.

Referral to a specialist for investigations and management should occur in refractory or recurrent peptic ulcer cases with gastro-oesophageal symptoms that are unexplained, or non-responsive to treatment.

Patients with peptic ulcer disease who are on long-term treatment should receive an annual review of their symptoms and treatment. A step down approach, or stopping treatment, should be encouraged if possible and clinically appropriate. Ⓐ

Useful Resources

Gastro-oesophageal reflux disease and dyspepsia in adults: investigation and management. National Institute for Health and Care Excellence. NICE guideline 184. September 2014, reviewed October 2019.
www.nice.org.uk/guidance/cg184

> **Other drugs used for Gastric and duodenal ulceration**
> Misoprostol, p. 85

GASTROPROTECTIVE COMPLEXES AND CHELATORS

Sucralfate

19-Nov-2021

● **DRUG ACTION** Sucralfate is a complex of aluminium hydroxide and sulfated sucrose which forms a barrier to protect the mucosa from acid, pepsin and bile attack in gastric and duodenal ulcers.

● **INDICATIONS AND DOSE**

Benign gastric ulceration | Benign duodenal ulceration
▸ BY MOUTH
▸ Child 15-17 years: 2 g twice daily, dose to be taken on rising and at bedtime, alternatively 1 g 4 times a day for 4–6 weeks, or in resistant cases up to 12 weeks, dose to be taken 1 hour before meals and at bedtime; maximum 8 g per day
▸ Adult: 2 g twice daily, dose to be taken on rising and at bedtime, alternatively 1 g 4 times a day for 4–6 weeks, or in resistant cases up to 12 weeks, dose to be taken 1 hour before meals and at bedtime; maximum 8 g per day

Chronic gastritis
▸ BY MOUTH
▸ Adult: 2 g twice daily, dose to be taken on rising and at bedtime, alternatively 1 g 4 times a day for 4–6 weeks or in resistant cases up to 12 weeks, dose to be taken 1 hour before meals and at bedtime; maximum 8 g per day

Prophylaxis of stress ulceration in child under intensive care
▸ BY MOUTH
▸ Child 15-17 years: 1 g 6 times a day; maximum 8 g per day

Prophylaxis of stress ulceration
▸ BY MOUTH
▸ Adult: 1 g 6 times a day; maximum 8 g per day

● **UNLICENSED USE**
▸ In children Tablets not licensed for prophylaxis of stress ulceration.

● **CAUTIONS** Patients under intensive care (**Important: reports of bezoar formation**)

CAUTIONS, FURTHER INFORMATION
▸ Bezoar formation Following reports of bezoar formation associated with sucralfate, caution is advised in seriously ill patients, especially those receiving concomitant enteral feeds or those with predisposing conditions such as delayed gastric emptying.

● **INTERACTIONS** → Appendix 1: sucralfate

● **SIDE-EFFECTS**
▸ **Common or very common** Constipation
▸ **Uncommon** Dry mouth · nausea
▸ **Rare or very rare** Bezoar · rash
▸ **Frequency not known** Back pain · bone disorders · diarrhoea · dizziness · drowsiness · encephalopathy · flatulence · headache · vertigo

● **PREGNANCY** No evidence of harm; absorption from gastro-intestinal tract negligible.

● **BREAST FEEDING** Amount probably too small to be harmful.

● **RENAL IMPAIRMENT** EvGr Caution (aluminium is absorbed and may accumulate). Ⓜ

● **DIRECTIONS FOR ADMINISTRATION** Expert sources advise administration of sucralfate and enteral feeds should be separated by 1 hour. EvGr For administration by *mouth*, sucralfate should be given 1 hour before meals. Ⓜ *Oral suspension* blocks fine-bore feeding tubes. Expert sources advise crushed *tablets* may be dispersed in water.

● **PRESCRIBING AND DISPENSING INFORMATION** Flavours of oral liquid formulations may include aniseed and caramel.

● **MEDICINAL FORMS** There can be variation in the licensing of different medicines containing the same drug. Forms available from special-order manufacturers include: oral tablet, oral suspension

Oral tablet
CAUTIONARY AND ADVISORY LABELS 5
▸ Sucralfate (Non-proprietary)
  Sucralfate 1 gram Sulcrate 1g tablets | 100 tablet 🅧
  Carafate 1g tablets | 100 tablet 🅧

Oral suspension
CAUTIONARY AND ADVISORY LABELS 5
▸ Sucralfate (Non-proprietary)
  Sucralfate 100 mg per 1 ml Carafate 1g/10ml oral suspension | 420 ml PoM 🅧 (Hospital only) SF
  Sucralfate 200 mg per 1 ml Sucralfate 1g/5ml oral suspension sugar free | 200 ml PoM £288.48-£426.26 DT = £288.48 SF

H_2-RECEPTOR ANTAGONISTS

H_2-receptor antagonists

● **CAUTIONS** Signs and symptoms of gastric cancer (in adults)

CAUTIONS, FURTHER INFORMATION
▸ Gastric cancer
▸ In adults H_2-receptor antagonists might mask symptoms of gastric cancer; particular care is required in patients presenting with 'alarm features' in such cases gastric malignancy should be ruled out before treatment.

● **SIDE-EFFECTS**
▸ **Common or very common** Constipation · diarrhoea · dizziness · fatigue · headache · myalgia · skin reactions
▸ **Uncommon** Confusion · depression · erectile dysfunction · gynaecomastia · hallucination · hepatic disorders · leucopenia · nausea · tachycardia
▸ **Rare or very rare** Agranulocytosis · alopecia · arthralgia · atrioventricular block · fever · galactorrhoea · pancytopenia · thrombocytopenia · vasculitis

📙 82

Cimetidine

23-Jul-2021

● **INDICATIONS AND DOSE**

Benign duodenal ulceration

▸ BY MOUTH

▸ Adult: 400 mg twice daily for at least 4 weeks, to be taken with breakfast and at night, alternatively 800 mg once daily for at least 4 weeks, to be taken at night; increased if necessary up to 400 mg 4 times a day; maintenance 400 mg once daily, to be taken at night, alternatively maintenance 400 mg twice daily, to be taken in the morning and at night

Benign gastric ulceration

▸ BY MOUTH

▸ Adult: 400 mg twice daily for 6 weeks, to be taken with breakfast and at night, alternatively 800 mg daily for 6 weeks, to be taken at night; increased if necessary up to 400 mg 4 times a day; maintenance 400 mg once daily, to be taken at night, alternatively maintenance 400 mg twice daily, to be taken in the morning and at night

NSAID-associated ulceration

▸ BY MOUTH

▸ Adult: 400 mg twice daily for 8 weeks, to be taken with breakfast and at night, alternatively 800 mg daily for 8 weeks, to be taken at night; increased if necessary up to 400 mg 4 times a day; maintenance 400 mg daily, to be taken at night, alternatively maintenance 400 mg twice daily, to be taken in the morning and at night

Reflux oesophagitis

▸ BY MOUTH

▸ Adult: 400 mg 4 times a day for 4–8 weeks

Prophylaxis of stress ulceration

▸ BY MOUTH

▸ Adult: 200–400 mg every 4–6 hours

Gastric acid reduction in obstetrics

▸ BY MOUTH

▸ Adult: Initially 400 mg, to be administered at start of labour, then increased if necessary up to 400 mg every 4 hours, do not use syrup in prophylaxis of acid aspiration; maximum 2.4 g per day

Gastric acid reduction during surgical procedures

▸ BY MOUTH

▸ Adult: 400 mg, to be given 90–120 minutes before induction of general anaesthesia

Short-bowel syndrome

▸ BY MOUTH

▸ Adult: 400 mg twice daily, adjusted according to response, to be taken with breakfast and at bedtime

To reduce degradation of pancreatic enzyme supplements

▸ BY MOUTH

▸ Adult: 0.8–1.6 g daily in 4 divided doses, dose to be taken 1–1½ hours before meals

● **INTERACTIONS** → Appendix 1: H_2 receptor antagonists

● **SIDE-EFFECTS**

▸ **Rare or very rare** Anaphylactic reaction · aplastic anaemia · nephritis tubulointerstitial · pancreatitis · sinus bradycardia

● **PREGNANCY** Manufacturer advises avoid unless essential.

● **BREAST FEEDING** Significant amount present in milk—not known to be harmful but manufacturer advises avoid.

● **HEPATIC IMPAIRMENT** Increased risk of confusion.
Dose adjustments Reduce dose.

● **RENAL IMPAIRMENT**
Dose adjustments [EvGr] Reduce dose to 200 mg 4 times a day if creatinine clearance 30–50 mL/minute.
    Reduce dose to 200 mg 3 times a day if creatinine clearance 15–30 mL/minute.

Reduce dose to 200 mg twice daily if creatinine clearance less than 15 mL/minute. ⟨M⟩
    See p. 21.

● **EXCEPTIONS TO LEGAL CATEGORY** Cimetidine can be sold to the public for adults and children over 16 years (provided packs do not contain more than 2 weeks' supply) for the short-term symptomatic relief of heartburn, dyspepsia, and hyperacidity (max. single dose 200 mg, max. daily dose 800 mg), and for the prophylactic management of nocturnal heartburn (single night-time dose 100 mg).

● **MEDICINAL FORMS** There can be variation in the licensing of different medicines containing the same drug. Forms available from special-order manufacturers include: oral suspension

Oral tablet

▸ Cimetidine (Non-proprietary)
    Cimetidine 200 mg Cimetidine 200mg tablets | 60 tablet [PoM] £19.00 DT = £10.04
    Cimetidine 400 mg Cimetidine 400mg tablets | 60 tablet [PoM] £16.60 DT = £5.55
    Cimetidine 800 mg Cimetidine 800mg tablets | 30 tablet [PoM] £25.90 DT = £21.25

Oral solution
EXCIPIENTS: May contain Propylene glycol

▸ Cimetidine (Non-proprietary)
    Cimetidine 40 mg per 1 ml Cimetidine 200mg/5ml oral solution sugar free | 300 ml [PoM] £48.75-£48.80 DT = £48.75 [SF]

▸ Tagamet (Rosemont Pharmaceuticals Ltd)
    Cimetidine 40 mg per 1 ml Tagamet 200mg/5ml syrup | 600 ml [PoM] £28.49 DT = £28.49

📙 82

Famotidine

07-Jul-2023

● **INDICATIONS AND DOSE**

Treatment of benign gastric and duodenal ulceration

▸ BY MOUTH

▸ Adult: 40 mg once daily for 4–8 weeks, dose to be taken at night

Maintenance treatment of duodenal ulceration

▸ BY MOUTH

▸ Adult: 20 mg once daily, dose to be taken at night

Reflux oesophagitis

▸ BY MOUTH

▸ Adult: 20–40 mg twice daily for 6–12 weeks; maintenance 20 mg twice daily

● **INTERACTIONS** → Appendix 1: H_2 receptor antagonists

● **SIDE-EFFECTS**

▸ **Uncommon** Appetite decreased · dry mouth · taste altered · vomiting

▸ **Rare or very rare** Anxiety · chest tightness · drowsiness · insomnia · interstitial pneumonia · libido decreased · muscle cramps · neutropenia · paraesthesia · psychiatric disorder · seizures · severe cutaneous adverse reactions (SCARs)

● **PREGNANCY** Manufacturer advises avoid unless potential benefit outweighs risk.

● **BREAST FEEDING** Present in milk—not known to be harmful but manufacturer advises avoid.

● **RENAL IMPAIRMENT** [EvGr] Use with caution. ⟨M⟩
Dose adjustments [EvGr] Use half of normal dose if creatinine clearance less than 30 mL/minute. Consider reducing dose to 20 mg once daily at night if creatinine clearance less than 10 mL/minute. ⟨M⟩ See p. 21.

● **EXCEPTIONS TO LEGAL CATEGORY** Famotidine can be sold to the public for adults and children over 16 years (provided packs do not contain more than 2 weeks' supply) for the short-term symptomatic relief of heartburn, dyspepsia, and hyperacidity, and for the prevention of these symptoms when associated with consumption of

Gastro-intestinal system

food or drink including when they cause sleep disturbance (max. single dose 10 mg, max. daily dose 20 mg).

- **MEDICINAL FORMS** There can be variation in the licensing of different medicines containing the same drug.
  Oral tablet
  - Famotidine (Non-proprietary)
    Famotidine 20 mg Famotidine 20mg tablets | 28 tablet PoM
    £28.59 DT = £14.32 | 56 tablet PoM £25.00–£57.18
    Famotidine 40 mg Famotidine 40mg tablets | 28 tablet PoM
    £50.69 DT = £24.85 | 56 tablet PoM £74.56–£101.38

⮕ 82

Nizatidine

09-Jul-2021

- **INDICATIONS AND DOSE**

Benign gastric, duodenal or NSAID-associated ulceration
- BY MOUTH
  - Adult: 300 mg once daily for 4–8 weeks, dose to be taken in the evening, alternatively 150 mg twice daily for 4–8 weeks; maintenance 150 mg once daily, dose to be taken at night

Gastro-oesophageal reflux disease
- BY MOUTH
  - Adult: 150–300 mg twice daily for up to 12 weeks

- **INTERACTIONS** → Appendix 1: H₂ receptor antagonists
- **SIDE-EFFECTS**
- **Rare or very rare** Anaemia · hyperuricaemia · serum sickness
- **Frequency not known** Hyperhidrosis
- **PREGNANCY** Manufacturer advises avoid unless essential.
- **BREAST FEEDING** Amount too small to be harmful.
- **HEPATIC IMPAIRMENT** Manufacturer advises caution.
- **RENAL IMPAIRMENT** EvGr Use with caution. Ⓜ
  Dose adjustments EvGr Use half normal dose if creatinine clearance 20–50 mL/minute.
    Use one-quarter normal dose if creatinine clearance less than 20 mL/minute. Ⓜ
    See p. 21.
- **EXCEPTIONS TO LEGAL CATEGORY** Nizatidine can be sold to the public for the prevention and treatment of symptoms of food-related heartburn and meal-induced indigestion in adults and children over 16 years; max. single dose 75 mg, max. daily dose 150 mg for max. 14 days.

- **MEDICINAL FORMS** There can be variation in the licensing of different medicines containing the same drug. Forms available from special-order manufacturers include: oral suspension, oral solution
  Oral capsule
  - Nizatidine (Non-proprietary)
    Nizatidine 150 mg Nizatidine 150mg capsules | 30 capsule PoM
    £36.00 DT = £17.96
    Nizatidine 300 mg Nizatidine 300mg capsules | 30 capsule PoM
    £72.00 DT = £63.77

⮕ 82

Ranitidine

09-Aug-2023

- **INDICATIONS AND DOSE**

Benign gastric ulceration | Duodenal ulceration
- BY MOUTH
  - Child 1-5 months: 1 mg/kg 3 times a day (max. per dose 3 mg/kg 3 times a day)
  - Child 6 months-2 years: 2–4 mg/kg twice daily
  - Child 3-11 years: 2–4 mg/kg twice daily (max. per dose 150 mg)
  - Child 12-17 years: 150 mg twice daily, alternatively 300 mg once daily, dose to be taken at night

- Adult: 150 mg twice daily for 4–8 weeks, alternatively 300 mg once daily for 4–8 weeks, dose to be taken at night

Chronic episodic dyspepsia
- BY MOUTH
  - Adult: 150 mg twice daily for 6 weeks, alternatively 300 mg once daily for 6 weeks, dose to be taken at night

NSAID-associated gastric ulceration
- BY MOUTH
  - Adult: 150 mg twice daily for up to 8 weeks, alternatively 300 mg once daily for up to 8 weeks, dose to be taken at night

NSAID-associated duodenal ulcer
- BY MOUTH
  - Adult: 300 mg twice daily for 4 weeks, to achieve a higher healing rate

Prophylaxis of NSAID-associated gastric ulcer |
Prophylaxis of NSAID-associated duodenal ulcer
- BY MOUTH
  - Adult: 300 mg twice daily

Gastro-oesophageal reflux disease
- BY MOUTH
  - Adult: 150 mg twice daily for up to 8 weeks or if necessary 12 weeks, alternatively 300 mg once daily for up to 8 weeks or if necessary 12 weeks, dose to be taken at night

Moderate to severe gastro-oesophageal reflux disease
- BY MOUTH
  - Adult: 600 mg daily in 2–4 divided doses for up to 12 weeks

Long-term treatment of healed gastro-oesophageal reflux disease
- BY MOUTH
  - Adult: 150 mg twice daily

Gastric acid reduction (prophylaxis of acid aspiration) in obstetrics
- BY MOUTH
  - Adult: 150 mg, dose to be given at onset of labour, then 150 mg every 6 hours

Gastric acid reduction (prophylaxis of acid aspiration) in surgical procedures
- INITIALLY BY INTRAMUSCULAR INJECTION, OR BY SLOW INTRAVENOUS INJECTION
  - Adult: 50 mg, to be given 45–60 minutes before induction of anaesthesia, intravenous injection diluted to 20 mL and given over at least 2 minutes, alternatively (by mouth) 150 mg, to be given 2 hours before induction of anaesthesia and also when possible on the preceding evening

Prophylaxis of stress ulceration
- INITIALLY BY SLOW INTRAVENOUS INJECTION
  - Adult: 50 mg every 8 hours, dose to be diluted to 20 mL and given over at least 2 minutes, then (by mouth) 150 mg twice daily, may be given when oral feeding commences

Reflux oesophagitis and other conditions where gastric acid reduction is beneficial
- BY MOUTH
  - Child 1-5 months: 1 mg/kg 3 times a day (max. per dose 3 mg/kg 3 times a day)
  - Child 6 months-2 years: 2–4 mg/kg twice daily
  - Child 3-11 years: 2–4 mg/kg twice daily (max. per dose 150 mg); increased to up to 5 mg/kg twice daily (max. per dose 300 mg), dose increase for severe gastro-oesophageal disease
  - Child 12-17 years: 150 mg twice daily, alternatively 300 mg once daily, dose to be taken at night, then increased if necessary to 300 mg twice daily for up to 12 weeks in moderate to severe gastro-oesophageal

reflux disease, alternatively increased if necessary to 150 mg 4 times a day for up to 12 weeks in moderate to severe gastro-oesophageal reflux disease

Conditions where reduction of gastric acidity is beneficial and oral route not available
▶ BY INTRAMUSCULAR INJECTION
▶ Adult: 50 mg every 6–8 hours
▶ BY SLOW INTRAVENOUS INJECTION
▶ Adult: 50 mg, dose to be diluted to 20 mL and given over at least 2 minutes; may be repeated every 6–8 hours

● UNLICENSED USE
▶ In children *Oral* preparations not licensed for use in children under 3 years.
▶ In adults Doses given for prophylaxis of NSAID-associated gastric or duodenal ulcer, and prophylaxis of stress ulceration, are not licensed.

> **IMPORTANT SAFETY INFORMATION**
> MHRA: RANITIDINE: ALL FORMULATIONS—SUPPLY DISRUPTION (NOVEMBER 2019)
> Due to ongoing safety concerns about a contaminant, all formulations of ranitidine are currently unavailable in the UK; it is not known when they will become available.
> No new patients should be initiated on treatment with ranitidine. All patients should be reviewed as repeat prescriptions are requested and, if ongoing treatment is required, switched to a suitable alternative. Local specialists should be consulted for advice on alternative treatment in specialist or unlicensed indications and high-risk cohorts of patients, including children.
> For further information, see: www.cas.mhra.gov.uk/ ViewandAcknowledgment/ViewAlert.aspx?AlertID=102934.

● INTERACTIONS → Appendix 1: H_2 receptor antagonists
● SIDE-EFFECTS
GENERAL SIDE-EFFECTS
▶ **Rare or very rare** Bone marrow depression · bradycardia · breast conditions · dyskinesia · nephritis acute interstitial · pancreatitis acute · vision blurred
▶ **Frequency not known** Dyspnoea
SPECIFIC SIDE-EFFECTS
▶ **Rare or very rare**
▶ With parenteral use Anaphylactic shock · cardiac arrest
● PREGNANCY Manufacturer advises avoid unless essential, but not known to be harmful.
● BREAST FEEDING Significant amount present in milk, but not known to be harmful.
● RENAL IMPAIRMENT
Dose adjustments
▶ In adults Use half normal dose if eGFR less than 50 mL/minute/1.73 m^2.
▶ In children Use half normal dose if estimated glomerular filtration rate less than 50 mL/minute/1.73 m^2.
● DIRECTIONS FOR ADMINISTRATION For *intravenous infusion* (*Zantac*®), manufacturer advises give intermittently in Glucose 5% or Sodium Chloride 0.9%.
● PATIENT AND CARER ADVICE In fat malabsorption syndrome, give oral doses 1–2 hours before food to enhance effects of pancreatic enzyme replacement.
Medicines for Children leaflet: Ranitidine for acid reflux www.medicinesforchildren.org.uk/medicines/ranitidine-for-acid-reflux/
● EXCEPTIONS TO LEGAL CATEGORY Ranitidine can be sold to the public for adults and children over 16 years (provided packs do not contain more than 2 weeks' supply) for the short-term symptomatic relief of heartburn, dyspepsia, and hyperacidity, and for the prevention of these symptoms when associated with consumption of food or drink (max. single dose 75 mg, max. daily dose 300 mg).

● MEDICINAL FORMS There can be variation in the licensing of different medicines containing the same drug. Forms available from special-order manufacturers include: oral suspension, oral solution, infusion
Oral solution
EXCIPIENTS: May contain Alcohol

PROSTAGLANDINS AND ANALOGUES

Misoprostol
10-Jan-2025

● DRUG ACTION Misoprostol is a synthetic prostaglandin analogue that has antisecretory and protective properties, promoting healing of gastric and duodenal ulcers.

● INDICATIONS AND DOSE
CYTOTEC®
Benign gastric ulcer | Benign duodenal ulcer | NSAID-induced peptic ulcer
▶ BY MOUTH
▶ Adult: 400 micrograms twice daily, alternatively 200 micrograms 4 times a day continued for at least 4 weeks or may be continued for up to 8 weeks if required, dose to be taken with breakfast (or main meals) and at bedtime
Prophylaxis of NSAID-induced peptic ulcer
▶ BY MOUTH
▶ Adult: 200 micrograms 2–4 times a day

● CAUTIONS
CYTOTEC® Conditions where hypotension might precipitate severe complications (e.g. cerebrovascular disease, cardiovascular disease) · conditions which predispose to diarrhoea (e.g. inflammatory bowel disease)
● INTERACTIONS → Appendix 1: misoprostol
● SIDE-EFFECTS
▶ **Common or very common** Chills · constipation · diarrhoea · dizziness · fever · flatulence · gastrointestinal discomfort · haemorrhage · headache · muscle cramps · nausea · post abortion infection · skin reactions · uterine cramps · vomiting
▶ **Uncommon** Menstrual cycle irregularities · postmenopausal haemorrhage
▶ **Rare or very rare** Angioedema · erythema nodosum · malaise · toxic epidermal necrolysis · uterine rupture
▶ **Frequency not known** Back pain · cardiac arrest · cardiovascular event · coronary vasospasm · hypotension · myocardial infarction

SIDE-EFFECTS, FURTHER INFORMATION Diarrhoea may occasionally be severe and require withdrawal, reduced by giving single doses not exceeding 200 micrograms and by avoiding magnesium-containing antacids.
● CONCEPTION AND CONTRACEPTION
CYTOTEC® Manufacturer advises do not use in women of childbearing potential unless pregnancy has been excluded; patients must use effective contraception during treatment, and be informed of the risks of taking misoprostol if pregnant.
● PREGNANCY
CYTOTEC® Manufacturer advises avoid—induces uterine contractions, and associated with abortion and birth defects; teratogenic in first trimester.
● BREAST FEEDING Manufacturer advises avoid—present in milk, and may cause diarrhoea in nursing infants. EvGr Tertiary sources state present in milk but amount probably too small to be harmful.
● PATIENT AND CARER ADVICE
Driving and skilled tasks Patients should be cautioned on the effects on driving and performance of skilled tasks—increased risk of dizziness.

1

Gastro-intestinal system

- **MEDICINAL FORMS** There can be variation in the licensing of different medicines containing the same drug.

Oral tablet

CAUTIONARY AND ADVISORY LABELS 21 (applies to Cytotec ® only)

▶ Cytotec (Pfizer Ltd)
Misoprostol 200 microgram Cytotec 200microgram tablets |
60 tablet [PoM] £10.03 DT = £10.03

PROTON PUMP INHIBITORS

Proton pump inhibitors

Overview

Proton pump inhibitors are effective short-term treatments for *gastric* and *duodenal ulcers*; they are also used in combination with antibacterials for the eradication of *Helicobacter pylori* (see specific regimens). Following endoscopic treatment of severe peptic ulcer bleeding, an intravenous, high-dose proton pump inhibitor reduces the risk of rebleeding and the need for surgery. Proton pump inhibitors can be used for the treatment of *dyspepsia* and *gastro-oesophageal reflux disease*.

Proton pump inhibitors are also used for the prevention and treatment of NSAID-associated ulcers. In patients who need to continue NSAID treatment after an ulcer has healed, the dose of proton pump inhibitor should normally not be reduced because asymptomatic ulcer deterioration may occur.

A proton pump inhibitor can be used to reduce the degradation of pancreatic enzyme supplements in patients with cystic fibrosis. They can also be used to control excessive secretion of gastric acid in *Zollinger–Ellison syndrome*; high doses are often required.

Proton pump inhibitors 

- **DRUG ACTION** Proton pump inhibitors inhibit gastric acid secretion by blocking the hydrogen-potassium adenosine triphosphatase enzyme system (the 'proton pump') of the gastric parietal cell.

> **IMPORTANT SAFETY INFORMATION**
>
> MHRA ADVICE: PROTON PUMP INHIBITORS (PPIS): VERY LOW RISK OF SUBACUTE CUTANEOUS LUPUS ERYTHEMATOSUS (SEPTEMBER 2015)
>
> Very infrequent cases of subacute cutaneous lupus erythematosus (SCLE) have been reported in patients taking PPIs. Drug-induced SCLE can occur weeks, months or even years after exposure to the drug.
>
> If a patient treated with a PPI develops lesions—especially in sun-exposed areas of the skin—and it is accompanied by arthralgia:
> - advise them to avoid exposing the skin to sunlight;
> - consider SCLE as a possible diagnosis;
> - consider discontinuing PPI treatment unless it is imperative for a serious acid-related condition; a patient who develops SCLE with a particular PPI may be at risk of the same reaction with another;
> - in most cases, symptoms resolve on PPI withdrawal; topical or systemic steroids might be necessary for treatment of SCLE only if there are no signs of remission after a few weeks or months.

- **CAUTIONS** Can increase the risk of fractures (particularly when used at high doses for over a year in the elderly) · may increase the risk of gastro-intestinal infections (including *Clostridioides difficile* infection) · may mask the symptoms of gastric cancer (in adults) · may reduce absorption of vitamin B_{12} with long-term treatment · patients at risk of osteoporosis

▶ Risk of osteoporosis Patients at risk of osteoporosis should maintain an adequate intake of calcium and vitamin D, and if necessary, receive other preventative therapy.
▶ Gastric cancer
▶ In adults Particular care is required in those presenting with 'alarm features', in such cases gastric malignancy should be ruled out before treatment.
▶ Elderly Screening Tool of Older Persons' potentially inappropriate Prescriptions (STOPP) criteria to aid medication reviews (see Prescribing in the elderly p. 31 for information): potentially inappropriate for uncomplicated peptic ulcer disease or erosive peptic oesophagitis at full therapeutic dosage for longer than 8 weeks (dose reduction or earlier discontinuation indicated).

- **SIDE-EFFECTS**
▶ **Common or very common** Abdominal pain · constipation · diarrhoea · dizziness · dry mouth · gastrointestinal disorders · headache · insomnia · nausea · skin reactions · vomiting
▶ **Uncommon** Arthralgia · bone fractures · confusion · depression · drowsiness · leucopenia · malaise · myalgia · paraesthesia · peripheral oedema · thrombocytopenia · vertigo · vision disorders
▶ **Rare or very rare** Agranulocytosis · alopecia · gynaecomastia · hallucination · hepatic disorders · hyperhidrosis · hyponatraemia · nephritis tubulointerstitial · pancytopenia · photosensitivity reaction · severe cutaneous adverse reactions (SCARs) · stomatitis · taste altered
▶ **Frequency not known** Gastrointestinal infection · hypomagnesaemia (more common after 1 year of treatment, but sometimes after 3 months of treatment) · subacute cutaneous lupus erythematosus

- **MONITORING REQUIREMENTS** Measurement of serum-magnesium concentrations should be considered before and during prolonged treatment with a proton pump inhibitor, especially when used with other drugs that cause hypomagnesaemia or with digoxin.

- **PRESCRIBING AND DISPENSING INFORMATION** A proton pump inhibitor should be prescribed for appropriate indications at the lowest effective dose for the shortest period; the need for long-term treatment should be reviewed periodically.

⚑ above

Esomeprazole

10-Apr-2024

- **INDICATIONS AND DOSE**

Peptic ulcer disease
▶ BY MOUTH
▶ Adult: 20 mg once daily for 4–8 weeks

NSAID-associated gastric ulcer
▶ BY MOUTH
▶ Adult: 20 mg once daily for 4–8 weeks
▶ BY INTRAVENOUS INJECTION, OR BY INTRAVENOUS INFUSION
▶ Adult: 20 mg once daily until oral administration possible

Prophylaxis of NSAID-associated gastric ulcer in patients with an increased risk of gastroduodenal complications who require continued NSAID treatment
▶ BY MOUTH
▶ Adult: 20 mg once daily

Prophylaxis of NSAID-associated gastric or duodenal ulcer
▶ BY INTRAVENOUS INJECTION, OR BY INTRAVENOUS INFUSION
▶ Adult: 20 mg once daily until oral administration possible

Gastro-oesophageal reflux disease (in the presence of erosive reflux oesophagitis)
▶ BY MOUTH
▶ Child 1–11 years (body-weight 10–19 kg): 10 mg once daily for 8 weeks
▶ Child 1–11 years (body-weight 20 kg and above): 10–20 mg once daily for 8 weeks
▶ Child 12–17 years: 40 mg once daily for 4 weeks, continued for further 4 weeks if not fully healed or symptoms persist; maintenance 20 mg once daily
▶ BY INTRAVENOUS INJECTION, OR BY INTRAVENOUS INFUSION
▶ Adult: 40 mg once daily until oral administration possible

Severe oesophagitis
▶ BY MOUTH
▶ Adult: 40 mg once daily for 8 weeks, continue as maintenance treatment if appropriate

Severe oesophagitis, refractory to initial treatment
▶ BY MOUTH
▶ Adult: 40 mg twice daily

Gastro-oesophageal reflux disease (in the absence of oesophagitis)
▶ BY MOUTH
▶ Child 1–11 years (body-weight 10 kg and above): 10 mg once daily for up to 8 weeks
▶ Child 12–17 years: 20 mg once daily for up to 4 weeks
▶ Adult: 20 mg once daily for 4 or 8 weeks, then 20 mg once daily as required
▶ BY INTRAVENOUS INJECTION, OR BY INTRAVENOUS INFUSION
▶ Adult: 20 mg once daily until oral administration possible

Uninvestigated dyspepsia
▶ BY MOUTH
▶ Adult: 20 mg once daily for 4 weeks

Zollinger–Ellison syndrome
▶ BY MOUTH
▶ Adult: Initially 40 mg twice daily, to be adjusted according to response; usual dose 80–160 mg per day, doses above 80 mg per day should be given in 2 divided doses

Severe peptic ulcer bleeding (following endoscopic treatment)
▶ INITIALLY BY INTRAVENOUS INFUSION
▶ Adult: Initially 80 mg for 1 dose, to be given over 30 minutes, then (by continuous intravenous infusion) 8 mg/hour for 72 hours, then (by mouth) 40 mg once daily for 4 weeks

***Helicobacter pylori* eradication [in combination with other drugs]**
▶ BY MOUTH
▶ Adult: 20 mg twice daily for 7 days for first- and second-line eradication therapy; 10 days for third-line eradication therapy

● UNLICENSED USE
▶ In adults [EvGr] Combination regimens and durations for *Helicobacter pylori* eradication may differ from product literature but adhere to national guidelines. (A) See Helicobacter pylori infection p. 93 for further information. Esomeprazole may be used as detailed below, although these situations are considered outside the scope of its licence:
  ● [EvGr] treatment of peptic ulcer disease, (A) see Peptic ulcer disease p. 81 for further information;
  ● [EvGr] treatment of severe oesophagitis, refractory to initial treatment, (A) see Gastro-oesophageal reflux disease p. 92 for further information;
  ● [EvGr] treatment of uninvestigated dyspepsia, (A) see Dyspepsia p. 78 for further information.
▶ With oral use in adults [EvGr] Duration of treatment of gastro-oesophageal reflux disease (in the absence of oesophagitis)

differs from product literature but adheres to national guidelines. (A) See Gastro-oesophageal reflux disease p. 92 for further information.

● INTERACTIONS → Appendix 1: proton pump inhibitors
● SIDE-EFFECTS
  GENERAL SIDE-EFFECTS
▶ Rare or very rare Aggression · agitation · bronchospasm · gastrointestinal candidiasis · muscle weakness · renal failure

  SPECIFIC SIDE-EFFECTS
▶ Rare or very rare
▶ With parenteral use Encephalopathy

● PREGNANCY Manufacturer advises caution—no information available.

● BREAST FEEDING Specialist sources indicate use with caution—limited human data available. Likely to be present in milk, but amount probably too small to be harmful.

● HEPATIC IMPAIRMENT Manufacturer advises caution in severe impairment.
  Dose adjustments
▶ With oral use in adults Manufacturer advises max. 20 mg daily in severe impairment.
▶ With intravenous use in adults Manufacturer advises for gastro-oesophageal reflux disease, max. 20 mg daily in severe impairment. Manufacturer advises for bleeding ulcers, by intravenous infusion, initially 80 mg, then 4 mg/hour for 72 hours in severe impairment.
▶ In children Manufacturer advises in children 1–11 years, max. 10 mg daily in severe impairment. Manufacturer advises in children 12–17 years, max. 20 mg daily in severe impairment.

● RENAL IMPAIRMENT Manufacturer advises caution in severe renal insufficiency.

● DIRECTIONS FOR ADMINISTRATION
▶ With intravenous use For *intravenous injection*, give over at least 3 minutes. For *intravenous infusion* (*Nexium* ®), give continuously *or* intermittently in Sodium Chloride 0.9%; reconstitute 40–80 mg with up to 100 ml infusion fluid; for intermittent infusion, give requisite dose over 10–30 minutes; stable for 12 hours in Sodium Chloride 0.9%.
▶ With oral use [EvGr] Do not chew or crush capsules; swallow whole *or* mix capsule contents in water and drink within 30 minutes. Do not crush or chew tablets; swallow whole *or* disperse in water and drink within 30 minutes. Disperse the contents of each sachet of gastro-resistant granules in approx. 15 mL water. Stir and leave to thicken for a few minutes; stir again before administration and use within 30 minutes; rinse container with 15 mL water to obtain full dose. (M) For administration through a gastric tube, consult product literature.

● PATIENT AND CARER ADVICE Counselling on administration of gastro-resistant capsules, tablets, and granules advised.

● MEDICINAL FORMS There can be variation in the licensing of different medicines containing the same drug. Forms available from special-order manufacturers include: oral suspension

Gastro-resistant capsule
▶ **Esomeprazole (Non-proprietary)**
  Esomeprazole 20 mg Esomeprazole 20mg gastro-resistant capsules | 28 capsule [PoM] £12.95 DT = £1.36
  Esomeprazole 40 mg Esomeprazole 40mg gastro-resistant capsules | 28 capsule [PoM] £17.63 DT = £1.89
▶ **Emozul** (Krka UK Ltd)
  Esomeprazole 20 mg Emozul 20mg gastro-resistant capsules | 28 capsule [PoM] £5.30 DT = £1.36
  Esomeprazole 40 mg Emozul 40mg gastro-resistant capsules | 28 capsule [PoM] £6.37 DT = £1.89

1

Gastro-intestinal system

Gastro-resistant tablet

▶ **Esomeprazole** (Non-proprietary)
Esomeprazole 20 mg Esomeprazole 20mg gastro-resistant tablets | 28 tablet `PoM` £4.40 DT = £3.28
Esomeprazole 40 mg Esomeprazole 40mg gastro-resistant tablets | 28 tablet `PoM` £4.40 DT = £3.29
▶ **Nexium** (Grunenthal Ltd)
Esomeprazole 20 mg Nexium 20mg gastro-resistant tablets | 28 tablet `PoM` £18.50 DT = £3.28
Esomeprazole 40 mg Nexium 40mg gastro-resistant tablets | 28 tablet `PoM` £25.19 DT = £3.29

Powder for solution for injection

▶ **Esomeprazole** (Non-proprietary)
Esomeprazole (as Esomeprazole sodium) 40 mg Esomeprazole 40mg powder for solution for injection vials | 1 vial `PoM` £2.53–£4.25 (Hospital only)
▶ **Nexium** (Grunenthal Ltd)
Esomeprazole (as Esomeprazole sodium) 40 mg Nexium I.V 40mg powder for solution for injection vials | 10 vial `PoM` £42.50 (Hospital only)

Gastro-resistant granules

CAUTIONARY AND ADVISORY LABELS 25

▶ **Esomeprazole** (Non-proprietary)
Esomeprazole (as Esomeprazole magnesium trihydrate) 10 mg Esomeprazole 10mg gastro-resistant granules sachets | 28 sachet `PoM` £25.19 DT = £25.19
▶ **Nexium** (Grunenthal Ltd)
Esomeprazole (as Esomeprazole magnesium trihydrate) 10 mg Nexium 10mg gastro-resistant granules sachets | 28 sachet `PoM` £25.19 DT = £25.19

🖙 86

Lansoprazole

17-Apr-2024

● INDICATIONS AND DOSE

Helicobacter pylori eradication [in combination with other drugs]
▶ BY MOUTH
▶ Adult: 30 mg twice daily for 7 days for first- and second-line eradication therapy; 10 days for third-line eradication therapy

Benign gastric ulcer
▶ BY MOUTH
▶ Adult: 30 mg once daily for 8 weeks, dose to be taken in the morning

Duodenal ulcer
▶ BY MOUTH
▶ Adult: 30 mg once daily for 4 weeks, dose to be taken in the morning; maintenance 15 mg once daily, dose to be taken in the morning

NSAID-associated duodenal ulcer | NSAID-associated gastric ulcer
▶ BY MOUTH
▶ Adult: 30 mg once daily for 4 weeks, continued for further 4 weeks if not fully healed

Prophylaxis of NSAID-associated duodenal ulcer | Prophylaxis of NSAID-associated gastric ulcer
▶ BY MOUTH
▶ Adult: 15–30 mg once daily

Zollinger–Ellison syndrome
▶ BY MOUTH
▶ Adult: Initially 60 mg once daily, to be adjusted according to response, dose can be increased if necessary up to 180 mg per day, doses above 120 mg per day should be given in 2 divided doses

Gastro-oesophageal reflux disease
▶ BY MOUTH
▶ Adult: 30 mg once daily for 4 weeks, continued for further 4 weeks if not fully healed, dose to be taken in the morning; maintenance 15–30 mg once daily, dose to be taken in the morning

Severe oesophagitis
▶ BY MOUTH
▶ Adult: 30 mg once daily for 8 weeks, continue as maintenance treatment if appropriate

Severe oesophagitis, refractory to initial treatment
▶ BY MOUTH
▶ Adult: 30 mg twice daily

Functional dyspepsia
▶ BY MOUTH
▶ Adult: 15 mg once daily for 4 weeks

Uninvestigated dyspepsia
▶ BY MOUTH
▶ Adult: 30 mg once daily for 4 weeks

● **UNLICENSED USE** Lansoprazole doses in BNF may differ from those in product literature. `EvGr` Combination regimens and durations for _Helicobacter pylori_ eradication may differ from product literature but adhere to national guidelines. Ⓐ See Helicobacter pylori infection p. 93 for further information. Lansoprazole may be used as detailed below, although these situations are considered outside the scope of its licence:
  ● `EvGr` treatment of severe oesophagitis, refractory to initial treatment, Ⓐ see Gastro-oesophageal reflux disease p. 92 for further information;
  ● `EvGr` treatment of functional and uninvestigated dyspepsia, Ⓐ see Dyspepsia p. 78 for further information.

● **INTERACTIONS** → Appendix 1: proton pump inhibitors

● **SIDE-EFFECTS**
▶ **Common or very common** Dry throat · fatigue
▶ **Uncommon** Eosinophilia · oedema
▶ **Rare or very rare** Anaemia · angioedema · appetite decreased · erectile dysfunction · fever · glossitis · oesophageal candidiasis · pancreatitis · restlessness · tremor

● **PREGNANCY** Manufacturer advises avoid.

● **BREAST FEEDING** Specialist sources indicate use with caution—no human data available. Likely to be present in milk, but amount probably too small to be harmful.

● **HEPATIC IMPAIRMENT** Manufacturer advises caution in moderate to severe impairment (risk of increased exposure).
Dose adjustments Manufacturer advises dose reduction of 50% in moderate to severe impairment.

● **DIRECTIONS FOR ADMINISTRATION** Manufacturer advises orodispersible tablets should be placed on the tongue, allowed to disperse and swallowed, or may be swallowed whole with a glass of water. Alternatively, tablets can be dispersed in a small amount of water and administered by an oral syringe or nasogastric tube.

● **PATIENT AND CARER ADVICE** Counselling on administration of orodispersible tablet advised.

● **PROFESSION SPECIFIC INFORMATION**
Dental practitioners' formulary Lansoprazole capsules may be prescribed.

● **MEDICINAL FORMS** There can be variation in the licensing of different medicines containing the same drug. Forms available from special-order manufacturers include: oral suspension, oral solution, oral powder

Gastro-resistant capsule

CAUTIONARY AND ADVISORY LABELS 5, 22, 25

▶ **Lansoprazole** (Non-proprietary)
Lansoprazole 15 mg Lansoprazole 15mg gastro-resistant capsules | 28 capsule `PoM` £15.79 DT = £0.84
Lansoprazole 30 mg Lansoprazole 30mg gastro-resistant capsules | 28 capsule `PoM` £28.36 DT = £1.13

Orodispersible tablet

CAUTIONARY AND ADVISORY LABELS 5, 22

EXCIPIENTS: May contain Aspartame

▸ Lansoprazole (Non-proprietary)
  Lansoprazole 15 mg Lansoprazole 15mg orodispersible tablets |
  28 tablet [PoM] £3.00 DT = £2.28
  Lansoprazole 30 mg Lansoprazole 30mg orodispersible tablets |
  28 tablet [PoM] £5.80 DT = £4.15
▸ Zoton FasTab (Pfizer Ltd)
  Lansoprazole 15 mg Zoton FasTab 15mg | 28 tablet [PoM] £2.99 DT
  = £2.28
  Lansoprazole 30 mg Zoton FasTab 30mg | 28 tablet [PoM] £5.50 DT
  = £4.15

F 86

Omeprazole

09-Apr-2024

● **INDICATIONS AND DOSE**

Helicobacter pylori eradication [in combination with other drugs]
▸ BY MOUTH
▸ Adult: 20–40 mg twice daily for 7 days for first- and
  second-line eradication therapy; 10 days for third-line
  eradication therapy

Benign gastric ulceration
▸ BY MOUTH
▸ Adult: 20 mg once daily for 8 weeks, dose can be
  increased if necessary to 40 mg once daily in severe or
  recurrent cases

Duodenal ulceration
▸ BY MOUTH
▸ Adult: 20 mg once daily for 4 weeks, dose can be
  increased if necessary to 40 mg once daily in severe or
  recurrent cases

Prevention of relapse in gastric ulcer
▸ BY MOUTH
▸ Adult: 20 mg once daily, increased if necessary to
  40 mg once daily

Prevention of relapse in duodenal ulcer
▸ BY MOUTH
▸ Adult: 20 mg once daily, adjusted according to
  response to 10–40 mg once daily

**NSAID-associated duodenal ulcer | NSAID-associated
gastric ulcer | NSAID-associated gastroduodenal erosions**
▸ BY MOUTH
▸ Adult: 20 mg once daily for 4 weeks, continued for a
  further 4 weeks if not fully healed

**Prophylaxis in patients with a history of NSAID-associated
duodenal ulcer who require continued NSAID treatment |
Prophylaxis in patients with a history of NSAID-
associated gastric ulcer who require continued NSAID
treatment | Prophylaxis in patients with a history of
NSAID-associated gastroduodenal lesions who require
continued NSAID treatment | Prophylaxis in patients with
a history of NSAID-associated dyspeptic symptoms who
require continued NSAID treatment**
▸ BY MOUTH
▸ Adult: 20 mg once daily

Zollinger–Ellison syndrome
▸ BY MOUTH
▸ Adult: Initially 60 mg once daily, usual dose 20–120 mg
  per day, doses above 80 mg per day should be given in
  2 divided doses
▸ BY INTRAVENOUS INFUSION
▸ Adult: Initially 60 mg once daily, infusion to be given
  over 20–30 minutes, dose to be adjusted according to
  response, doses above 60 mg per day should be given in
  2 divided doses

Gastro-oesophageal reflux disease
▸ BY MOUTH
▸ Adult: 20 mg once daily for 4 or 8 weeks

Severe oesophagitis
▸ BY MOUTH
▸ Adult: 40 mg once daily for 8 weeks, continue as
  maintenance treatment if appropriate

Severe oesophagitis, refractory to initial treatment
▸ BY MOUTH
▸ Adult: 40 mg twice daily

Acid reflux disease (long-term management)
▸ BY MOUTH
▸ Adult: 10 mg once daily, increased if necessary up to
  40 mg once daily, dose only increased if symptoms
  return

Functional dyspepsia
▸ BY MOUTH
▸ Adult: 10 mg once daily for 4 weeks

Uninvestigated dyspepsia
▸ BY MOUTH
▸ Adult: 20 mg once daily for 4 weeks

**Treatment and prevention of benign gastric ulcers |
Treatment and prevention of duodenal ulcers |
Treatment and prevention of NSAID-associated ulcers |
Treatment and prevention of gastro-oesophageal reflux
disease**
▸ BY INTRAVENOUS INFUSION
▸ Adult: 40 mg once daily until oral administration
  possible

**Major peptic ulcer bleeding (following endoscopic
treatment)**
▸ INITIALLY BY INTRAVENOUS INFUSION
▸ Adult: Initially 80 mg for 1 dose, to be given over
  40–60 minutes, then (by continuous intravenous
  infusion) 8 mg/hour for 72 hours, subsequent dose
  then changed to oral therapy

● **UNLICENSED USE** [EvGr] Combination regimens and
durations for _Helicobacter pylori_ eradication may differ
from product literature but adhere to national guidelines.
Ⓐ See Helicobacter pylori infection p. 93 for further
information. Omeprazole may be used as detailed below,
although these situations are considered outside the scope
of its licence:
  ● [EvGr] treatment of severe oesophagitis, refractory to
    initial treatment, Ⓐ see Gastro-oesophageal reflux
    disease p. 92 for further information;
  ● [EvGr] treatment of functional and uninvestigated
    dyspepsia, Ⓐ see Dyspepsia p. 78 for further
    information;
  ● treatment of major peptic ulcer bleeding (following
    endoscopic treatment).
Oral suspension not licensed for use in Zollinger-Ellison
syndrome.
▸ With oral use [EvGr] Duration of treatment for gastro-
oesophageal reflux disease differs from product literature
and adheres to national guidelines. Ⓐ See Gastro-
oesophageal reflux disease p. 92 for further information.

● **INTERACTIONS** → Appendix 1: proton pump inhibitors

● **SIDE-EFFECTS**
▸ **Rare or very rare** Aggression · agitation · bronchospasm ·
gastrointestinal candidiasis · muscle weakness

● **PREGNANCY** Not known to be harmful.

● **BREAST FEEDING** Specialist sources indicate amount in
milk is small and not known to be harmful; [EvGr]
therapeutic doses unlikely to affect infant. Ⓜ

● **HEPATIC IMPAIRMENT**
Dose adjustments Not more than 20 mg daily should be
needed.

● **DIRECTIONS FOR ADMINISTRATION** For administration by
mouth using tablets or capsules:
  ● Tablets (_Losec MUPS®_, _Mezzopram®_) or capsules (_Losec®_)
    containing enteric-coated pellets can be dispersed in

non-carbonated water or a slightly acidic liquid e.g. fruit juice or apple sauce; do **not** use milk or carbonated water. The dispersion should be stirred just before drinking and taken immediately, rinsed down with half a glass of water. The enteric-coated pellets must not be chewed.

- Enteric-coated tablets (*Dexcel*®) must be swallowed whole and not chewed or crushed.

For instructions on reconstitution of oral suspension, consult product literature.

[EvGr] For *continuous or intermittent intravenous infusion*, reconstitute each 40 mg vial with infusion fluid and dilute to 100 mL with Glucose 5% or Sodium Chloride 0.9%; for *intermittent infusion* give 40 mg over 20–30 minutes; stable for 6 hours in Glucose 5% or 12 hours in Sodium Chloride 0.9%. ⟨M⟩

- **PATIENT AND CARER ADVICE**
▸ With oral use Counselling on administration advised.

- **PROFESSION SPECIFIC INFORMATION**

Dental practitioners' formulary Gastro-resistant omeprazole capsules may be prescribed.

- **EXCEPTIONS TO LEGAL CATEGORY** Omeprazole 20 mg tablets can be sold to the public for the short-term relief of reflux-like symptoms (e.g. heartburn, acid regurgitation) in adults over 18 years, max. daily dose 20 mg for max. 14 days, and a pack size of 14 tablets.

- **MEDICINAL FORMS** There can be variation in the licensing of different medicines containing the same drug. Forms available from special-order manufacturers include: oral suspension, oral solution

Gastro-resistant capsule
CAUTIONARY AND ADVISORY LABELS 25
▸ Omeprazole (Non-proprietary)
Omeprazole 10 mg Omeprazole 10mg gastro-resistant capsules | 28 capsule [PoM] £9.30 DT = £1.01
Omeprazole 20 mg Omeprazole 20mg gastro-resistant capsules | 28 capsule [PoM] £11.14 DT = £0.85 | 100 capsule [PoM] £3.07 | 250 capsule [PoM] £7.59–£11.00
Omeprazole 40 mg Omeprazole 40mg gastro-resistant capsules | 7 capsule [PoM] £4.93 DT = £0.68 | 28 capsule [PoM] £1.88–£19.72
▸ Losec (Neon Healthcare Ltd)
Omeprazole 10 mg Losec 10mg gastro-resistant capsules | 28 capsule [PoM] £11.16 DT = £1.01
Omeprazole 20 mg Losec 20mg gastro-resistant capsules | 28 capsule [PoM] £16.70 DT = £0.85
Omeprazole 40 mg Losec 40mg gastro-resistant capsules | 7 capsule [PoM] £8.35 DT = £0.68

Gastro-resistant tablet
CAUTIONARY AND ADVISORY LABELS 25
▸ Omeprazole (Non-proprietary)
Omeprazole 10 mg Omeprazole 10mg gastro-resistant tablets | 28 tablet [PoM] £18.91 DT = £10.73
Omeprazole 20 mg Omeprazole 20mg gastro-resistant tablets | 28 tablet [PoM] £28.56 DT = £6.46
Omeprazole 40 mg Omeprazole 40mg gastro-resistant tablets | 7 tablet [PoM] £14.28 DT = £10.36
▸ Losec MUPS (Neon Healthcare Ltd)
Omeprazole (as Omeprazole magnesium) 10 mg Losec MUPS 10mg gastro-resistant tablets | 28 tablet [PoM] £9.30 DT = £9.30
Omeprazole (as Omeprazole magnesium) 20 mg Losec MUPS 20mg gastro-resistant tablets | 28 tablet [PoM] £13.92 DT = £13.92
Omeprazole (as Omeprazole magnesium) 40 mg Losec MUPS 40mg gastro-resistant tablets | 7 tablet [PoM] £6.96 DT = £6.96
▸ Mezzopram (Sandoz Ltd)
Omeprazole (as Omeprazole magnesium) 10 mg Mezzopram 10mg dispersible gastro-resistant tablets | 28 tablet [PoM] £6.58 DT = £9.30
Omeprazole (as Omeprazole magnesium) 20 mg Mezzopram 20mg dispersible gastro-resistant tablets | 28 tablet [PoM] £9.86 DT = £13.92
Omeprazole (as Omeprazole magnesium) 40 mg Mezzopram 40mg dispersible gastro-resistant tablets | 7 tablet [PoM] £4.93 DT = £6.96

Oral suspension
▸ Omeprazole (Non-proprietary)
Omeprazole 1 mg per 1 ml Omeprazole 1mg/ml oral suspension sugar free | 75 ml [PoM] £111.00 DT = £111.00 [SF]
Omeprazole 2 mg per 1 ml Omeprazole 10mg/5ml oral suspension sugar free | 75 ml [PoM] £124.00 DT = £124.00 [SF]
Omeprazole 4 mg per 1 ml Omeprazole 20mg/5ml oral suspension sugar free | 75 ml [PoM] £234.00 DT = £234.00 [SF]

Oral solution
▸ Omeprazole (Non-proprietary)
Omeprazole 670 microgram per 1 ml Omeprazole 10mg/15ml oral solution unit dose sugar free | 14 unit dose [PoM] £115.73–£183.18 DT = £115.73 [SF]
Omeprazole 1.33 mg per 1 ml Omeprazole 20mg/15ml oral solution unit dose sugar free | 14 unit dose [PoM] £218.40–£349.44 DT = £218.40 [SF]

Powder for solution for infusion
▸ Omeprazole (Non-proprietary)
Omeprazole (as Omeprazole sodium) 40 mg Omeprazole 40mg powder for solution for infusion vials | 5 vial [PoM] £27.50 DT = £26.00 | 5 vial [PoM] £26.00–£29.23 DT = £26.00 (Hospital only) | 10 vial [PoM] £55.08 (Hospital only)

⟨⟩ 86

Pantoprazole

10-Apr-2024

- **INDICATIONS AND DOSE**

Helicobacter pylori **eradication [in combination with other drugs]**
▸ BY MOUTH
▸ Adult: 40 mg twice daily for 7 days for first- and second-line eradication therapy; 10 days for third-line eradication therapy

Benign gastric ulcer
▸ BY MOUTH
▸ Adult: 40 mg once daily for 8 weeks, dose can be increased if necessary up to 80 mg per day in severe cases

Gastric ulcer
▸ BY INTRAVENOUS INJECTION, OR BY INTRAVENOUS INFUSION
▸ Adult: 40 mg once daily until oral administration can be resumed

Duodenal ulcer
▸ BY MOUTH
▸ Adult: 40 mg once daily for 4 weeks, dose can be increased if necessary up to 80 mg per day in severe cases
▸ BY INTRAVENOUS INJECTION, OR BY INTRAVENOUS INFUSION
▸ Adult: 40 mg once daily until oral administration can be resumed

NSAID-associated peptic ulcer disease
▸ BY MOUTH
▸ Adult: 40 mg once daily for 8 weeks

Prophylaxis of NSAID-associated gastric ulcer in patients with an increased risk of gastroduodenal complications who require continued NSAID treatment | Prophylaxis of NSAID-associated duodenal ulcer in patients with an increased risk of gastroduodenal complications who require continued NSAID treatment
▸ BY MOUTH
▸ Adult: 20 mg once daily

Gastro-oesophageal reflux disease
▸ BY MOUTH
▸ Adult: 40 mg once daily for 4 or 8 weeks
▸ BY INTRAVENOUS INJECTION, OR BY INTRAVENOUS INFUSION
▸ Adult: 40 mg once daily until oral administration can be resumed

Severe oesophagitis
▸ BY MOUTH
▸ Adult: 40 mg once daily for 8 weeks, continue as maintenance treatment if appropriate

Severe oesophagitis, refractory to initial treatment
▶ BY MOUTH
▸ Adult: 40 mg twice daily

Functional dyspepsia
▶ BY MOUTH
▸ Adult: 20 mg once daily for 4 weeks

Uninvestigated dyspepsia
▶ BY MOUTH
▸ Adult: 40 mg once daily for 4 weeks

Zollinger–Ellison syndrome (and other hypersecretory conditions)
▶ BY MOUTH
▸ Adult: Initially 80 mg once daily, dose to be adjusted according to response, doses above 80 mg per day should be given in 2 divided doses
▶ BY INTRAVENOUS INJECTION, OR BY INTRAVENOUS INFUSION
▸ Adult: Initially 80 mg for 1 dose, alternatively initially 160 mg for 1 dose, to be used if rapid acid control required, then 80 mg once daily, dose to be adjusted according to response, doses above 80 mg per day should be given in 2 divided doses

● **UNLICENSED USE** EvGr Combination regimens and durations for *Helicobacter pylori* eradication may differ from product literature but adhere to national guidelines. (A) See Helicobacter pylori infection p. 93 for further information.

Pantoprazole may be used as detailed below, although these situations are considered outside the scope of its licence:
- EvGr treatment of severe oesophagitis, refractory to initial treatment, (A) see Gastro-oesophageal reflux disease p. 92 for further information;
- EvGr treatment of NSAID-associated peptic ulcer disease, (A) see Peptic ulcer disease p. 81 for further information;
- EvGr treatment of functional and uninvestigated dyspepsia, (A) see Dyspepsia p. 78 for further information.

▸ With oral use EvGr Dose for the treatment of gastro-oesophageal reflux disease differs from product literature and adheres to national guidelines. (A)

● **INTERACTIONS** → Appendix 1: proton pump inhibitors

● **SIDE-EFFECTS**

GENERAL SIDE-EFFECTS
▶ **Uncommon** Asthenia · gastrointestinal discomfort · sleep disorder
▶ **Rare or very rare** Angioedema · hyperlipidaemia · weight change

SPECIFIC SIDE-EFFECTS
▸ With intravenous use Electrolyte imbalance · muscle spasms

● **PREGNANCY** Manufacturer advises avoid unless potential benefit outweighs risk—fetotoxic in *animals*.

● **BREAST FEEDING** Specialist sources indicate amount in milk is small and not known to be harmful.

● **HEPATIC IMPAIRMENT** Manufacturer advises caution in severe impairment (increased half-life)—monitor liver function and discontinue if deterioration.
Dose adjustments Manufacturer advises maximum dose of 20 mg daily in severe impairment.

● **RENAL IMPAIRMENT** EvGr Avoid in combination therapy for *Helicobacter pylori* eradication (no information available). (M)

● **DIRECTIONS FOR ADMINISTRATION** For *intravenous infusion* (*Protium*®), manufacturer advises give intermittently in Glucose 5% or Sodium Chloride 0.9%; reconstitute 40 mg with 10 mL Sodium Chloride 0.9% and dilute with 100 mL of infusion fluid; give 40 mg over 15 minutes.

For *intravenous injection*, give over at least 2 minutes.

● **EXCEPTIONS TO LEGAL CATEGORY** Pantoprazole 20 mg tablets can be sold to the public for the short-term treatment of reflux symptoms (e.g. heartburn) in adults over 18 years, max. daily dose 20 mg for max. 4 weeks.

● **MEDICINAL FORMS** There can be variation in the licensing of different medicines containing the same drug. Forms available from special-order manufacturers include: oral suspension

Gastro-resistant tablet
CAUTIONARY AND ADVISORY LABELS 25
▸ Pantoprazole (Non-proprietary)
Pantoprazole (as Pantoprazole sodium sesquihydrate)
20 mg Pantoprazole 20mg gastro-resistant tablets | 28 tablet PoM £5.40 DT = £0.99
Pantoprazole (as Pantoprazole sodium sesquihydrate)
40 mg Pantoprazole 40mg gastro-resistant tablets | 28 tablet PoM £11.10 DT = £1.04

Powder for solution for injection
▸ Pantoprazole (Non-proprietary)
Pantoprazole (as Pantoprazole sodium sesquihydrate)
40 mg Pantoprazole 40mg powder for solution for injection vials | 1 vial PoM £5.00 DT = £5.00 (Hospital only) | 1 vial PoM £5.00 DT = £5.00 | 5 vial PoM £22.50 DT = £22.50 (Hospital only)
▸ Protium (Takeda UK Ltd)
Pantoprazole (as Pantoprazole sodium sesquihydrate)
40 mg Protium I.V. 40mg powder for solution for injection vials | 1 vial PoM £5.10 DT = £5.00 (Hospital only)

F 86

Rabeprazole sodium

20-May-2021

● **INDICATIONS AND DOSE**

Benign gastric ulcer
▶ BY MOUTH
▸ Adult: 20 mg daily for 8 weeks, dose to be taken in the morning

Duodenal ulcer
▶ BY MOUTH
▸ Adult: 20 mg daily for 4 weeks, dose to be taken in the morning

NSAID-associated peptic ulcer disease
▶ BY MOUTH
▸ Adult: 20 mg once daily for 8 weeks

Gastro-oesophageal reflux disease
▶ BY MOUTH
▸ Adult: 20 mg once daily for 4–8 weeks; maintenance 10–20 mg daily

Gastro-oesophageal reflux disease (symptomatic treatment in the absence of oesophagitis)
▶ BY MOUTH
▸ Adult: 10 mg daily for up to 4 weeks, then 10 mg daily if required

Severe oesophagitis
▶ BY MOUTH
▸ Adult: 20 mg once daily for 8 weeks, continue as maintenance treatment if appropriate

Severe oesophagitis, refractory to initial treatment
▶ BY MOUTH
▸ Adult: 20 mg twice daily

Functional dyspepsia
▶ BY MOUTH
▸ Adult: 10 mg once daily for 4 weeks

Uninvestigated dyspepsia
▶ BY MOUTH
▸ Adult: 20 mg once daily for 4 weeks

Zollinger–Ellison syndrome
▶ BY MOUTH
▸ Adult: Initially 60 mg once daily, adjusted according to response, doses above 100 mg daily given in 2 divided doses; maximum 120 mg per day

continued →

Gastro-intestinal system

1

***Helicobacter pylori* eradication [in combination with other drugs (see Helicobacter pylori infection p. 93)]**
▶ BY MOUTH
▶ Adult: 20 mg twice daily for 7 days for first- and second-line eradication therapy; 10 days for third-line eradication therapy

● UNLICENSED USE Rabeprazole may be used as detailed below, although these situations are considered outside the scope of its licence:
  ● [EvGr] treatment of NSAID-associated peptic ulcer disease, ⒶA see Peptic ulcer disease p. 81 for further information;
  ● [EvGr] treatment of severe oesophagitis and severe oesophagitis, refractory to initial treatment, ⒶA see Gastro-oesophageal reflux disease below for further information;
  ● [EvGr] treatment of functional and uninvestigated dyspepsia, ⒶA see Dyspepsia p. 78 for further information.
  [EvGr] Combination regimens and durations for *Helicobacter pylori* eradication may differ from product literature but adhere to national guidelines. ⒶA See Helicobacter pylori infection p. 93 for further information.

● INTERACTIONS → Appendix 1: proton pump inhibitors

● SIDE-EFFECTS
▶ **Common or very common** Asthenia · cough · increased risk of infection · influenza like illness · pain
▶ **Uncommon** Burping · dyspepsia · leg cramps · nervousness
▶ **Rare or very rare** Appetite decreased · hepatic encephalopathy · leucocytosis · neutropenia · weight increased
▶ **Frequency not known** Chest pain · chills · fever

● PREGNANCY Manufacturer advises avoid—no information available.

● BREAST FEEDING Specialist sources indicate use with caution—no human data available. Likely to be present in milk, but amount probably too small to be harmful.

● HEPATIC IMPAIRMENT Manufacturer advises caution in severe impairment (no information available).

● MEDICINAL FORMS There can be variation in the licensing of different medicines containing the same drug.
Gastro-resistant tablet
CAUTIONARY AND ADVISORY LABELS 25
▶ **Rabeprazole sodium (Non-proprietary)**
  Rabeprazole sodium 10 mg Rabeprazole 10mg gastro-resistant tablets | 28 tablet [PoM] £13.87 DT = £1.30
  Rabeprazole sodium 20 mg Rabeprazole 20mg gastro-resistant tablets | 28 tablet [PoM] £23.46 DT = £2.09
▶ **Pariet** (Eisai Ltd)
  Rabeprazole sodium 10 mg Pariet 10mg gastro-resistant tablets | 28 tablet [PoM] £5.78 DT = £1.30
  Rabeprazole sodium 20 mg Pariet 20mg gastro-resistant tablets | 28 tablet [PoM] £11.34 DT = £2.09

6.3 Gastro-oesophageal reflux disease

Gastro-oesophageal reflux disease

01-Oct-2021

Description of condition

Gastro-oesophageal reflux disease (GORD) is usually a chronic condition where there is reflux of gastric contents (particularly acid, bile, and pepsin) back into the oesophagus, causing symptoms of heartburn and acid regurgitation. Less common symptoms such as chest pain, hoarseness, cough, wheezing, asthma and dental erosions can also occur if acid reflux reaches the oropharynx and/or respiratory tract.

GORD can be classified as non-erosive when a person has symptoms of GORD but the endoscopy is normal or erosive oesophagitis when oesophageal inflammation and mucosal erosions are seen at endoscopy.

Certain factors may contribute to the risk of developing GORD. These include consumption of trigger and fatty foods, pregnancy, hiatus hernia, family history of GORD, increased intra-gastric pressure from straining and coughing, stress, anxiety, obesity, drug side-effects, smoking and alcohol consumption.

Complications of GORD include oesophageal inflammation (oesophagitis), ulceration, haemorrhage and stricture formation, anaemia due to chronic blood loss, aspiration pneumonia, and Barrett's oesophagus.

Aims of treatment

The aim of treatment is to manage the symptoms of GORD and reduce the risk of recurrence and complications associated with the disease.

Non-drug treatment

[EvGr] Lifestyle measures, such as healthy eating, weight loss (if obese), avoiding trigger foods, eating smaller meals, eating the evening meal 3–4 hours before going to bed, raising the head of the bed, Smoking cessation p. 565, and reducing alcohol consumption may improve symptoms. Assess the patient for stress and anxiety as these conditions may exacerbate symptoms.

Urgent endoscopic investigation is required for patients with dysphagia, significant acute gastrointestinal bleeding, or in those aged 55 years and over with unexplained weight loss and symptoms of upper abdominal pain, reflux or dyspepsia. Endoscopy can be considered to diagnose Barrett's oesophagus if the patient has GORD. Patient preference and individual risk factors should be taken into account. ⒶA

Drug treatment

Initial management

[EvGr] Drugs that may cause or exacerbate the symptoms of GORD, such as alpha-blockers, anticholinergics, benzodiazepines, beta-blockers, bisphosphonates, calcium-channel blockers, corticosteroids, non-steroidal anti-inflammatory drugs (NSAIDs), nitrates, theophyllines, and tricyclic antidepressants should be reviewed. The lowest effective dose should be used and if appropriate, stopped.

Long term continuous use of antacids is not recommended for the treatment of GORD.

Patients with uninvestigated symptoms which suggest GORD should be managed as uninvestigated Dyspepsia p. 78.

In patients with an endoscopy confirmed diagnosis of GORD, a proton pump inhibitor (PPI), should be offered for 4 or 8 weeks. ⒶA If there is no response to a PPI, then offer a histamine$_2$-receptor antagonist (H$_2$-receptor antagonist).

[EvGr] Severe oesophagitis should be treated with a PPI for 8 weeks, taking into consideration patient preference and factors such as underlying health conditions and possible interactions with other drugs. ⒶA

Follow up management

[EvGr] For patients with refractory GORD, new alarm symptoms should be assessed and alternate diagnoses considered. Other options include prescribing a further course of the initial PPI dose for 1 month, double the initial PPI dose for 1 month or the addition of a H$_2$-receptor antagonist at bedtime for nocturnal symptoms or for short term use. The patient's adherence to initial management should also be checked and lifestyle advice reinforced.

For patients diagnosed with GORD in whom symptoms recur after initial treatment, a PPI should be given at the lowest dose that can achieve symptom control and self management on an "as-needed" basis should be discussed.

If treatment for severe oesophagitis fails, a higher dose of the same PPI should be used or switching to another PPI should be considered taking into account patient preference, tolerability, underlying health conditions and possible interactions with other drugs.

For patients with severe oesophagitis that fail to respond to long term maintenance PPI therapy a clinical review and switching to another PPI can be considered and/or specialist advice can be sought.

Patients with severe oesophagitis or who have had dilatation of an oesophageal stricture should remain on long-term PPI therapy taking into consideration the factors mentioned above. Ⓐ

GORD in pregnancy

[EvGr] Heartburn and acid reflux are symptoms of Dyspepsia p. 78 in pregnancy commonly caused by GORD. Dietary and lifestyle advice should be given as first-line management. If this approach fails to control symptoms, an antacid or an alginate can be used. If this is ineffective or symptoms are severe omeprazole p. 89 or ranitidine p. 84 (unlicensed) may help to control symptoms. Ⓐ

Useful Resources

Gastro-oesophageal reflux disease and dyspepsia in adults: investigation and management. National Institute for Health and Care Excellence. NICE clinical guideline 184. September 2014, updated October 2019.
www.nice.org.uk/guidance/cg184

NICE Patient Decision Aid: Option grid to help people make decisions about long term heartburn treatment
www.nice.org.uk/about/what-we-do/our-programmes/nice-guidance/nice-guidelines/shared-decision-making

> **Other drugs used for Gastro-oesophageal reflux disease**
> Cimetidine, p. 83 · Esomeprazole, p. 86 · Famotidine, p. 83 · Lansoprazole, p. 88 · Nizatidine, p. 84 · Pantoprazole, p. 90 · Rabeprazole sodium, p. 91

ANTACIDS ⟩ ALGINATE

Sodium alginate with calcium carbonate and sodium bicarbonate

11-Nov-2021

The properties listed below are those particular to the combination only. For the properties of the components please consider, alginic acid p. 78, sodium bicarbonate p. 1178, calcium carbonate p. 1188.

- ● **INDICATIONS AND DOSE**
  Gastro-oesophageal reflux disease
  ▸ BY MOUTH
  ▸ Child 6-11 years: 5–10 mL, to be taken after meals and at bedtime
  ▸ Child 12-17 years: 10–20 mL, to be taken after meals and at bedtime
  ▸ Adult: 10–20 mL, to be taken after meals and at bedtime

- ● INTERACTIONS → Appendix 1: calcium salts · sodium bicarbonate

- ● PRESCRIBING AND DISPENSING INFORMATION Flavours of oral liquid formulations may include aniseed or peppermint.

- ● PATIENT AND CARER ADVICE
  Medicines for Children leaflet: Gaviscon for gastro-oesophageal reflux disease www.medicinesforchildren.org.uk/medicines/gaviscon-for-gastro-oesophageal-reflux-disease/

- ● MEDICINAL FORMS There can be variation in the licensing of different medicines containing the same drug.
  Oral suspension
  ELECTROLYTES: May contain Sodium
  ▸ Sodium alginate with calcium carbonate and sodium bicarbonate (Non-proprietary)
  Calcium carbonate 16 mg per 1 ml, Sodium bicarbonate 26.7 mg per 1 ml, Sodium alginate 50 mg per 1 ml Care Heartburn Relief oral suspension | 500 ml [GSL] £4.69 DT = £4.69 [SF]
  ▸ Brands may include Peptac, Rennie

6.4 Helicobacter pylori infection

Helicobacter pylori infection   14-Jun-2022

Description of condition

Helicobacter pylori (*H. pylori*) infection is one of the most common causes of peptic ulcer disease, with 95% of duodenal and 70–80% of gastric ulcers associated with it. The use of NSAIDs may have an additive effect if there is co-existent *H. pylori* infection, further increasing the risk of peptic ulceration and bleeding. *H. pylori* is also associated with acute and chronic gastritis, gastric cancer, and gastric mucosa associated lymphoid tissue (MALT) lymphoma.

Aims of treatment

Treatment aims to eradicate *H. pylori*, reduce the risk of peptic ulcer disease, ulcer bleeding and gastric malignancy, and the recurrence of gastritis and peptic ulcers.

Testing for *Helicobacter pylori*

[EvGr] The presence of *H. pylori* should be confirmed before starting eradication treatment ('test and treat' strategy). Ⓐ

Testing for *H. pylori* is recommended in the following patients in line with PHE guidance:

- Patients with uncomplicated dyspepsia and no alarm symptoms who are unresponsive to lifestyle changes and antacids, following a single one month treatment course with a proton pump inhibitor;
- Patients considered to be at high risk of *H. pylori* infection (such as older people, individuals of North African ethnicity, and those living in a known high risk area) should be tested for *H. pylori* infection first, or in parallel with a course of a proton pump inhibitor;
- Previously untested patients with a history of peptic ulcers or bleeds;
- Prior to initiating NSAIDs in patients with a prior history of peptic ulcers or bleeds;
- Patients with unexplained iron-deficiency anaemia after endoscopic investigation has excluded malignancy, and other causes have been investigated.

[EvGr] The urea (13C) breath test p. 95, Stool Helicobacter Antigen Test (SAT), or laboratory-based serology where its performance has been locally validated, are recommended for the diagnosis of gastro-duodenal infection with *H. pylori*. Ⓐ PHE advises that the urea (13C) breath test and SAT should not be performed within 2 weeks of treatment with a proton pump inhibitor or within 4 weeks of antibacterial treatment, as this can lead to false negatives.
[EvGr] Office based serological tests for *H. pylori* are not recommended due to their inadequate performance. Ⓐ

Retesting for *Helicobacter pylori*

[EvGr] In patients with functional dyspepsia, routine retesting after *H. pylori* eradication is not recommended. Retesting may be considered in patients who would value the information. Ⓐ

PHE recommends retesting in the following circumstances:

- If compliance is poor, or there are high local resistance rates;
- The patient has persistent symptoms and the initial test was performed within 2 weeks of treatment with a proton pump inhibitor, or within 4 weeks of antibacterial treatment;
- In patients with an associated peptic ulcer, MALT lymphoma, or after resection of an early gastric carcinoma;
- Patients taking aspirin without concomitant treatment with a proton pump inhibitor;
- Patients with severe persistent or recurrent symptoms, particularly if not typical of gastro-oesophageal reflux disease.

Retesting should be performed at least 4 weeks (ideally 8 weeks) after treatment. In patients requiring gastric acid suppression, histamine$_2$-receptor antagonists should be used.

EvGr The urea (13C) breath test should be used for retesting. A

Drug treatment

Treatment of *H. pylori* usually involves a triple-therapy regimen that comprises a proton pump inhibitor (such as esomeprazole p. 86, lansoprazole p. 88, omeprazole p. 89, pantoprazole p. 90, or rabeprazole sodium p. 91) **and** two antibacterials. PHE advises that the choice of antibacterials should take into consideration the patient's antibacterial treatment history, as each additional course of clarithromycin, metronidazole, or quinolone increases the risk of resistance.

EvGr Consider referral to a specialist in patients who remain *H. pylori* positive after second-line eradication therapy. A PHE also advises that patients should be referred for an endoscopy, culture and susceptibility testing if the choice of antibacterial treatment is reduced due to hypersensitivity, there are known high local resistance rates, or patients have previously received treatment with clarithromycin, metronidazole, and a quinolone.

PHE advises that if diarrhoea develops, *Clostridioides difficile* infection should be considered and the need for treatment reviewed. For guidance on *Clostridioides difficile* infection, see Gastro-intestinal system infections, antibacterial therapy p. 582.

EvGr The importance of adherence to treatment should be discussed and emphasised to the patient. A

Choice of treatment regimen
No penicillin allergy

- **Oral** first line for 7 days:
  - EvGr A proton pump inhibitor, plus amoxicillin p. 635, and *either* clarithromycin p. 621 or metronidazole p. 628 (treatment choice should take into account previous treatment with clarithromycin or metronidazole). A
- **Oral** second line for 7 days (if ongoing symptoms after first line treatment):
  - EvGr A proton pump inhibitor, plus amoxicillin, and *either* clarithromycin or metronidazole (whichever was not used first line). A
- **Oral** alternative second line for 7 days (for patients who have received previous treatment with clarithromycin and metronidazole):
  - EvGr A proton pump inhibitor, plus amoxicillin, and tetracycline p. 659 [unlicensed] (or, if a tetracycline cannot be used, levofloxacin p. 650 [unlicensed]). A
- **Oral** third line for 10 days **on specialist advice only** in line with PHE guidance:
  - A proton pump inhibitor, plus bismuth subsalicylate p. 95 [unlicensed], and *either* two antibacterials from those mentioned above not previously used, or rifabutin p. 673 [unlicensed], or furazolidone [unlicensed].

Penicillin allergy

- **Oral** first line for 7 days:
  - EvGr A proton pump inhibitor, plus clarithromycin, and metronidazole. A
- **Oral** alternative first line for 7 days (for patients previously treated with clarithromycin):
  - EvGr A proton pump inhibitor, plus bismuth subsalicylate [unlicensed], plus metronidazole, and tetracycline [unlicensed]. A
- **Oral** second line for 7 days (if ongoing symptoms after first line treatment in patients who have **not** received previous treatment with a fluoroquinolone):
  - EvGr A proton pump inhibitor, plus metronidazole, and levofloxacin [unlicensed]. A
- **Oral** alternative second line for 7 days (in patients who have received previous treatment with a fluoroquinolone):
  - EvGr A proton pump inhibitor, plus bismuth subsalicylate [unlicensed], plus metronidazole, and tetracycline [unlicensed]. A
- **Oral** third line for 10 days **on specialist advice only** in line with PHE guidance:
  - A proton pump inhibitor, plus bismuth subsalicylate [unlicensed], and *either* rifabutin [unlicensed] or furazolidone [unlicensed].

For any advice, consult a local microbiologist or the Helicobacter Reference Laboratory at: www.gov.uk/guidance/gbru-reference-and-diagnostic-services.

For additional information on the management of patients with *H. pylori* infection and peptic ulcer disease or dyspepsia, see Peptic ulcer disease p. 81 and Dyspepsia p. 78.

Useful Resources

Gastro-oesophgeal reflux disease and dyspepsia in adults: investigation and management. National Institute for Health and Care Excellence. NICE guideline 184. September 2014, updated October 2019.
www.nice.org.uk/guidance/cg184

Test and treat for *Helicobacter pylori* (HP) in dyspepsia; Quick reference guide for primary care: For consultation and local adaptation. Public Health England. July 2017, updated August 2019.
www.gov.uk/government/publications/helicobacter-pylori-diagnosis-and-treatment

ANTIBACTERIALS

Bismuth potassium with metronidazole and tetracycline hydrochloride

26-Nov-2024

The properties listed below are those particular to the combination only. For the properties of the components please consider, metronidazole p. 628, tetracycline p. 659.

● INDICATIONS AND DOSE

Helicobacter pylori eradication [doses for 140/125/125 mg capsules in combination with omeprazole] | Prevention of relapse of *Helicobacter pylori*-associated peptic ulcers [doses for 140/125/125 mg capsules in combination with omeprazole]

- BY MOUTH
- Adult: 3 capsules 4 times a day for 10 days

DOSE EQUIVALENCE AND CONVERSION

- Capsule strength expressed as *x/y/z* mg representing bismuth subcitrate potassium/metronidazole/tetracycline hydrochloride, respectively.
- Bismuth subcitrate potassium 140 mg is equivalent to bismuth oxide 40 mg.

- **CAUTIONS** Gastro-intestinal tract x-ray (bismuth absorbs x-rays and may interfere with such diagnostic procedures) · low-potassium diet (*Pylera*® is high in potassium)
- **INTERACTIONS** → Appendix 1: bismuth · metronidazole · tetracyclines
- **SIDE-EFFECTS**
- ▸ **Common or very common** Appetite decreased · asthenic conditions · constipation · diarrhoea · dizziness · drowsiness · dry mouth · gastrointestinal discomfort · gastrointestinal disorders · headache · increased risk of infection · nausea · skin reactions · taste altered · urine discolouration · vomiting
- ▸ **Uncommon** Anxiety · burping · chest discomfort · depression · insomnia · memory loss · oral disorders · sensation abnormal · tongue discolouration · tremor · vertigo · vision blurred
- ▸ **Frequency not known** Encephalopathy · meningitis aseptic · peripheral neuropathy · pseudomembranous enterocolitis · severe cutaneous adverse reactions (SCARs)
- **PREGNANCY** [EvGr] Avoid (no information available). ⟨M⟩
- **BREAST FEEDING** [EvGr] Avoid (presence of bismuth potassium in milk unknown). ⟨M⟩
- **HEPATIC IMPAIRMENT** [EvGr] Avoid (no information available). ⟨M⟩
- **RENAL IMPAIRMENT** [EvGr] Avoid (no information available). ⟨M⟩
- **DIRECTIONS FOR ADMINISTRATION** Capsules should be swallowed whole with plenty of fluid, after a meal, while sitting; patients should be advised not to lie down immediately afterwards.
- **PRESCRIBING AND DISPENSING INFORMATION** For choice of antibacterial therapy, see Helicobacter pylori infection p. 93.
- **PATIENT AND CARER ADVICE** Patients or carers should be given advice on how to administer *Pylera*® capsules.
- **NATIONAL FUNDING/ACCESS DECISIONS** For full details see funding body website

    Scottish Medicines Consortium (SMC) decisions
- ▸ **Bismuth subcitrate potassium with metronidazole and tetracycline hydrochloride (*Pylera*®) in combination with omeprazole for the eradication of *Helicobacter pylori* and prevention of relapse of peptic ulcers in patients with active or a history of *H. pylori* associated ulcers (November 2024) SMC No. SMC2701 Recommended with restrictions**

- **MEDICINAL FORMS** There can be variation in the licensing of different medicines containing the same drug.

    Oral capsule
    CAUTIONARY AND ADVISORY LABELS 4, 7, 9, 27
    ELECTROLYTES: May contain Potassium
- ▸ Pylera (Flynn Pharma Ltd)
    Metronidazole 125 mg, Tetracycline hydrochloride 125 mg, Bismuth subcitrate potassium 140 mg Pylera 140mg/125mg/125mg capsules | 120 capsule [PoM] £40.14

Bismuth subsalicylate
27-Aug-2024

- **INDICATIONS AND DOSE**

Helicobacter pylori eradication [in combination with other drugs (see Helicobacter pylori infection p. 93)]
- ▸ BY MOUTH
- ▸ Adult: 525 mg 4 times a day for 7 days for first- and second-line eradication therapy; 10 days for third-line eradication therapy

- **UNLICENSED USE** [EvGr] Bismuth subsalicylate is used for the eradication of *Helicobacter pylori*, ⟨A⟩ but is not licensed for this indication.
- **CONTRA-INDICATIONS** Children under 16 years (risk of Reye's syndrome)

- **CAUTIONS** Blood clotting disorders · gout
- **INTERACTIONS** → Appendix 1: bismuth
- **SIDE-EFFECTS**
- ▸ **Common or very common** Black tongue · faeces black

    Overdose The main features of salicylate poisoning are hyperventilation, tinnitus, deafness, vasodilatation, and sweating. Bismuth overdose may present as acute encephalopathy with confusion, myoclonus, tremor, dysarthria and gait disturbances. Gastrointestinal disturbances, skin reactions, discolouration of mucous membranes and renal impairment may also be present.
- **ALLERGY AND CROSS-SENSITIVITY** Contra-indicated in patients with a history of hypersensitivity to aspirin or other salicylates.
- **PREGNANCY** Manufacturer advises avoid unless essential—no information available.
- **BREAST FEEDING** Manufacturer advises avoid unless essential—no information available.

- **MEDICINAL FORMS** There can be variation in the licensing of different medicines containing the same drug.
    Oral suspension
    CAUTIONARY AND ADVISORY LABELS 12
- ▸ Pepto-Bismol (Procter & Gamble (Health & Beauty Care) Ltd)
    Bismuth subsalicylate 17.5 mg per 1 ml Pepto-Bismol 17.5mg/1ml oral suspension | 120 ml [P] [℞] [SF]
    Chewable tablet
    CAUTIONARY AND ADVISORY LABELS 12, 24
- ▸ Pepto-Bismol (Procter & Gamble (Health & Beauty Care) Ltd)
    Bismuth subsalicylate 262.5 mg Pepto-Bismol 262.5mg chewable tablets | 12 tablet [P] [℞] [SF]

DIAGNOSTIC AGENTS

Urea (13C)

- **INDICATIONS AND DOSE**

Diagnosis of gastro-duodenal *Helicobacter pylori* infection
- ▸ BY MOUTH
- ▸ Adult: (consult product literature)

- **MEDICINAL FORMS** There can be variation in the licensing of different medicines containing the same drug.
    Oral tablet
- ▸ Diabact UBT (Mayoly UK Ltd)
    Urea [13-C] 50 mg diabact UBT 50mg tablets | 1 tablet [PoM] £21.25 DT = £21.25 | 10 tablet [PoM] £78.75 (Hospital only)
    Powder for oral solution
- ▸ Helicobacter Test INFAI (INFAI UK Ltd)
    Urea [13-C] 45 mg Helicobacter Test INFAI for children breath test kit | 1 kit [PoM] £19.20 DT = £19.20 [SF]
    Urea [13-C] 75 mg Helicobacter Test INFAI breath test kit | 1 kit [PoM] £21.70 DT = £21.70 [SF] | 50 kit [PoM] £950.00 [SF]

7   Gastro-intestinal smooth muscle spasm

Antispasmodics
02-May-2020

Overview

Antispasmodics can be divided into two main classifications: antimuscarinics and smooth muscle relaxants.

Antimuscarinics (formerly termed 'anticholinergics') reduce intestinal motility and are used for gastro-intestinal smooth muscle spasm. They include the tertiary amines atropine sulfate p. 1526 and dicycloverine hydrochloride p. 96, and the quaternary ammonium compounds propantheline bromide p. 97 and hyoscine butylbromide p. 96. The quaternary ammonium compounds are less lipid soluble than tertiary amines and are less likely to cross the blood–brain barrier; therefore have a lower risk for central nervous system side-effects. They are also less well absorbed from the gastro-intestinal tract.

Dicycloverine hydrochloride has a much less marked antimuscarinic action than atropine sulfate and may also have some direct action on smooth muscle. Hyoscine butylbromide is advocated as a gastro-intestinal antispasmodic, but is poorly absorbed.

Alverine citrate p. 97, mebeverine hydrochloride p. 98, and peppermint oil p. 53 are direct-acting intestinal smooth muscle relaxants and may relieve abdominal pain or spasm in Irritable bowel syndrome p. 52.

ANTIMUSCARINICS

Dicycloverine hydrochloride
23-Apr-2020

(Dicyclomine hydrochloride)

● INDICATIONS AND DOSE

Symptomatic relief of gastro-intestinal disorders characterised by smooth muscle spasm
▶ BY MOUTH
▶ Child 6-23 months: 5–10 mg 3–4 times a day, dose to be taken 15 minutes before feeds
▶ Child 2-11 years: 10 mg 3 times a day
▶ Child 12-17 years: 10–20 mg 3 times a day
▶ Adult: 10–20 mg 3 times a day

● INTERACTIONS → Appendix 1: dicycloverine

● SIDE-EFFECTS Appetite decreased · fatigue · thirst

● PREGNANCY Not known to be harmful; manufacturer advises use only if essential.

● BREAST FEEDING Avoid—present in milk; apnoea reported in infant.

● EXCEPTIONS TO LEGAL CATEGORY Dicycloverine hydrochloride can be sold to the public provided that max. single dose is 10 mg and max. daily dose is 60 mg.

● MEDICINAL FORMS There can be variation in the licensing of different medicines containing the same drug.
Oral tablet
▶ Dicycloverine hydrochloride (Non-proprietary)
Dicycloverine hydrochloride 10 mg Dicycloverine 10mg tablets | 100 tablet [PoM] £212.24 DT = £28.67
Dicycloverine hydrochloride 20 mg Dicycloverine 20mg tablets | 84 tablet [PoM] £226.57 DT = £30.04
Oral solution
▶ Dicycloverine hydrochloride (Non-proprietary)
Dicycloverine hydrochloride 2 mg per 1 ml Dicycloverine 10mg/5ml oral solution sugar free | 120 ml [PoM] [E] [SF] Dicycloverine 10mg/5ml oral solution | 120 ml [PoM] £174.11 DT = £174.11

Dicycloverine hydrochloride with aluminium hydroxide, magnesium oxide and simeticone
28-Apr-2020

The properties listed below are those particular to the combination only. For the properties of the components please consider, dicycloverine hydrochloride above, simeticone p. 80.

● INDICATIONS AND DOSE

Symptomatic relief of gastro-intestinal disorders characterised by smooth muscle spasm
▶ BY MOUTH
▶ Child 12-17 years: 10–20 mL every 4 hours as required
▶ Adult: 10–20 mL every 4 hours as required

● INTERACTIONS → Appendix 1: aluminium hydroxide · antacids · dicycloverine · magnesium

● SIDE-EFFECTS Anticholinergic syndrome

● RENAL IMPAIRMENT There is a risk of accumulation and aluminium toxicity with antacids containing aluminium salts. Absorption of aluminium from aluminium salts is increased by citrates, which are contained in many effervescent preparations (such as effervescent analgesics).

● MEDICINAL FORMS No licensed medicines listed.

Hyoscine butylbromide
03-Apr-2024

● INDICATIONS AND DOSE

Symptomatic relief of gastro-intestinal or genito-urinary disorders characterised by smooth muscle spasm
▶ BY MOUTH
▶ Child 6-11 years: 10 mg 3 times a day
▶ Child 12-17 years: 20 mg 4 times a day
▶ Adult: 20 mg 4 times a day

Irritable bowel syndrome
▶ BY MOUTH
▶ Adult: 10 mg 3 times a day; increased if necessary up to 20 mg 4 times a day

Acute spasm | Spasm in diagnostic procedures
▶ BY INTRAMUSCULAR INJECTION, OR BY SLOW INTRAVENOUS INJECTION
▶ Adult: 20 mg for 1 dose, dose can be repeated after 30 minutes if required (may be repeated more frequently in endoscopy); maximum 100 mg per day

Excessive respiratory secretions in palliative care
▶ BY MOUTH
▶ Child 1 month-1 year: 300–500 micrograms/kg 3–4 times a day (max. per dose 5 mg)
▶ Child 2-4 years: 5 mg 3–4 times a day
▶ Child 5-11 years: 10 mg 3–4 times a day
▶ Child 12-17 years: 10–20 mg 3–4 times a day
▶ BY INTRAMUSCULAR INJECTION, OR BY SLOW INTRAVENOUS INJECTION
▶ Child 1 month-4 years: 300–500 micrograms/kg 3–4 times a day (max. per dose 5 mg)
▶ Child 5-11 years: 5–10 mg 3–4 times a day
▶ Child 12-17 years: 10–20 mg 3–4 times a day
▶ BY SUBCUTANEOUS INJECTION
▶ Adult: 20 mg every 4 hours as required, dose to be adjusted according to response up to 20 mg every 1 hour
▶ BY CONTINUOUS SUBCUTANEOUS INFUSION
▶ Adult: 20–120 mg/24 hours

Bowel colic in palliative care
▶ BY MOUTH
▶ Child 1 month-1 year: 300–500 micrograms/kg 3–4 times a day (max. per dose 5 mg)
▶ Child 2-4 years: 5 mg 3–4 times a day
▶ Child 5-11 years: 10 mg 3–4 times a day
▶ Child 12-17 years: 10–20 mg 3–4 times a day
▶ BY INTRAMUSCULAR INJECTION, OR BY SLOW INTRAVENOUS INJECTION
▶ Child 1 month-4 years: 300–500 micrograms/kg 3–4 times a day (max. per dose 5 mg)
▶ Child 5-11 years: 5–10 mg 3–4 times a day
▶ Child 12-17 years: 10–20 mg 3–4 times a day
▶ BY SUBCUTANEOUS INJECTION
▶ Adult: 20 mg every 4 hours as required, dose to be adjusted according to response up to 20 mg every 1 hour
▶ BY CONTINUOUS SUBCUTANEOUS INFUSION
▶ Adult: 60–300 mg/24 hours

PHARMACOKINETICS
▶ Administration by mouth is associated with poor absorption.

● UNLICENSED USE *Tablets* not licensed for use in children under 6 years. *Injection* not licensed for use in children (age range not specified by manufacturer).

IMPORTANT SAFETY INFORMATION

MHRA/CHM ADVICE: HYOSCINE BUTYLBROMIDE (*BUSCOPAN*®) INJECTION: RISK OF SERIOUS ADVERSE EFFECTS IN PATIENTS WITH UNDERLYING CARDIAC DISEASE (FEBRUARY 2017)

The MHRA advises that hyoscine butylbromide injection can cause serious adverse effects including tachycardia, hypotension, and anaphylaxis; several reports have noted that anaphylaxis is more likely to be fatal in patients with underlying coronary heart disease. Hyoscine butylbromide injection is contra-indicated in patients with tachycardia and should be used with caution in patients with cardiac disease; the MHRA recommends that these patients are monitored and that resuscitation equipment and trained personnel are readily available.

INTRAVENOUS ADMINISTRATION

Healthcare professionals are reminded that intravenous hyoscine butylbromide must be given slowly to reduce the risk of marked hypotension and anaphylactic shock.

● CONTRA-INDICATIONS
▶ With parenteral use Tachycardia

● INTERACTIONS → Appendix 1: hyoscine

● SIDE-EFFECTS

GENERAL SIDE-EFFECTS Dyspnoea

SPECIFIC SIDE-EFFECTS
▶ With parenteral use Anaphylactic reaction · feeling hot · hypotension · mydriasis · sweat changes

● PREGNANCY Manufacturer advises avoid.

● BREAST FEEDING Amount too small to be harmful.

● DIRECTIONS FOR ADMINISTRATION
▶ With intravenous use in adults EvGr For *slow intravenous injection*, dilute with Glucose 5% or Sodium Chloride 0.9%. Ⓜ
▶ With intravenous use in children For *slow intravenous injection*, expert sources advise may be diluted with Glucose 5% or Sodium Chloride 0.9%.
▶ With oral use in children For administration by *mouth*, expert sources advise injection solution may be used; content of ampoule may be stored in a refrigerator for up to 24 hours after opening.

● PRESCRIBING AND DISPENSING INFORMATION

Palliative care, For further information on the use of hyoscine butylbromide in palliative care, see www.medicinescomplete.com/#/content/palliative/hyoscine-butylbromide.

● EXCEPTIONS TO LEGAL CATEGORY Hyoscine butylbromide tablets can be sold to the public for medically confirmed irritable bowel syndrome, provided single dose does not exceed 20 mg, daily dose does not exceed 80 mg, and pack does not contain a total of more than 240 mg.

● MEDICINAL FORMS There can be variation in the licensing of different medicines containing the same drug. Forms available from special-order manufacturers include: oral suspension, oral solution

Solution for injection

▶ Hyoscine butylbromide (Non-proprietary)
  Hyoscine butylbromide 20 mg per 1 ml Hyoscine butylbromide 20mg/1ml solution for injection ampoules | 10 ampoule PoM £2.92 DT = £4.08 (Hospital only)
▶ Buscopan (Opella Healthcare UK Ltd)
  Hyoscine butylbromide 20 mg per 1 ml Buscopan 20mg/1ml solution for injection ampoules | 10 ampoule PoM £4.08 DT = £4.08

Oral tablet

▶ Hyoscine butylbromide (Non-proprietary)
  Hyoscine butylbromide 10 mg Hyoscine butylbromide 10mg tablets | 56 tablet PoM £4.02–£6.70 DT = £4.02 | 100 tablet PoM £7.06–£11.62
  Hyoscine butylbromide 20 mg Hyoscine butylbromide 20mg tablets | 56 tablet PoM £6.43–£11.84 | 100 tablet PoM £20.76 DT = £15.95
▶ Buscopan (Opella Healthcare UK Ltd)
  Hyoscine butylbromide 10 mg Buscopan 10mg tablets | 56 tablet PoM £4.02 DT = £4.02

F 896

Propantheline bromide
27-Apr-2021

● **INDICATIONS AND DOSE**

Adult enuresis | Hyperhidrosis | Symptomatic relief of gastro-intestinal disorders characterised by smooth muscle spasm
▶ BY MOUTH
▶ Adult: 15 mg 3 times a day, dose to be taken at least one hour before food and 30 mg, dose to be taken at bedtime; maximum 120 mg per day

● INTERACTIONS → Appendix 1: propantheline

● SIDE-EFFECTS Arrhythmias · bronchial secretion decreased · mydriasis

● PREGNANCY Manufacturer advises avoid unless essential—no information available.

● BREAST FEEDING May suppress lactation.

● HEPATIC IMPAIRMENT Manufacturer advises caution.

● RENAL IMPAIRMENT Manufacturer advises caution.

● MEDICINAL FORMS There can be variation in the licensing of different medicines containing the same drug. Forms available from special-order manufacturers include: oral suspension, oral solution

Oral tablet
CAUTIONARY AND ADVISORY LABELS 23
▶ Propantheline bromide (Non-proprietary)
  Propantheline bromide 15 mg Propantheline bromide 15mg tablets | 112 tablet PoM £103.33–£195.14 DT = £20.74
▶ Pro-Banthine (Kyowa Kirin International UK NewCo Ltd)
  Propantheline bromide 15 mg Pro-Banthine 15mg tablets | 112 tablet PoM £20.74 DT = £20.74

ANTISPASMODICS

Alverine citrate
28-Aug-2020

● **INDICATIONS AND DOSE**

Symptomatic relief of gastro-intestinal disorders characterised by smooth muscle spasm | Dysmenorrhoea
▶ BY MOUTH
▶ Child 12-17 years: 60–120 mg 1–3 times a day
▶ Adult: 60–120 mg 1–3 times a day

● CONTRA-INDICATIONS Intestinal obstruction · paralytic ileus

● SIDE-EFFECTS Dizziness · dyspnoea · headache · jaundice (reversible on discontinuation) · nausea · skin reactions · wheezing

● PREGNANCY Manufacturer advises avoid—limited information available

● BREAST FEEDING Manufacturer advises avoid—limited information available.

● PATIENT AND CARER ADVICE

Driving and skilled tasks Dizziness may affect performance of skilled tasks (e.g. driving).

- **MEDICINAL FORMS** There can be variation in the licensing of different medicines containing the same drug.

Oral capsule

► **Alverine citrate (Non-proprietary)**
Alverine citrate 60 mg Alverine 60mg capsules | 100 capsule P £16.45 DT = £5.79
Alverine citrate 120 mg Alverine 120mg capsules | 60 capsule P £19.42 DT = £6.57

► **Audmonal** (Teva UK Ltd)
Alverine citrate 120 mg Audmonal Forte 120mg capsules | 60 capsule P £17.75 DT = £6.57

► **Spasmonal** (Ceuta Healthcare Ltd)
Alverine citrate 60 mg Spasmonal 60mg capsules | 20 capsule P £3.29 | 100 capsule P £16.45 DT = £5.79
Alverine citrate 120 mg Spasmonal Forte 120mg capsules | 60 capsule P £19.42 DT = £6.57

Mebeverine hydrochloride
10-Nov-2021

● **INDICATIONS AND DOSE**

Adjunct in gastro-intestinal disorders characterised by smooth muscle spasm

► BY MOUTH USING IMMEDIATE-RELEASE MEDICINES
► Child 10-17 years: 135–150 mg 3 times a day, dose preferably taken 20 minutes before meals
► Adult: 135–150 mg 3 times a day, dose preferably taken 20 minutes before meals

Irritable bowel syndrome

► BY MOUTH USING MODIFIED-RELEASE MEDICINES
► Child 12-17 years: 200 mg twice daily
► Adult: 200 mg twice daily

● **UNLICENSED USE** *Tablets* and *modified-release capsules* not licensed for use in children.

● **CONTRA-INDICATIONS** Paralytic ileus

● **SIDE-EFFECTS** Angioedema · face oedema · skin reactions

● **PREGNANCY** Not known to be harmful—manufacturers advise avoid.

● **BREAST FEEDING** Manufacturers advise avoid—no information available.

● **PATIENT AND CARER ADVICE** Patients or carers should be given advice on the timing of administration of mebeverine hydrochloride tablets and oral suspension. Medicines for Children leaflet: Mebeverine hydrochloride for intestinal spasm www.medicinesforchildren.org.uk/medicines/mebeverine-hydrochloride-for-intestinal-spasm/

● **EXCEPTIONS TO LEGAL CATEGORY**
► In adults Mebeverine hydrochloride can be sold to the public for symptomatic relief of irritable bowel syndrome provided that max. single dose is 135 mg and max. daily dose is 405 mg; for uses other than symptomatic relief of irritable bowel syndrome provided that max. single dose is 100 mg and max. daily dose is 300 mg.

● **MEDICINAL FORMS** There can be variation in the licensing of different medicines containing the same drug. Forms available from special-order manufacturers include: oral suspension

Oral tablet

► **Mebeverine hydrochloride (Non-proprietary)**
Mebeverine hydrochloride 135 mg Mebeverine 135mg tablets | 100 tablet PoM £9.02 DT = £2.79

► **Colofac** (Ceuta Healthcare Ltd)
Mebeverine hydrochloride 135 mg Colofac 135mg tablets | 100 tablet PoM £9.02 DT = £2.79

Oral suspension

► **Mebeverine hydrochloride (Non-proprietary)**
Mebeverine hydrochloride (as Mebeverine pamoate) 10 mg per 1 ml Mebeverine 50mg/5ml oral suspension sugar free | 300 ml PoM £260.00 DT = £205.70 SF

Modified-release capsule

CAUTIONARY AND ADVISORY LABELS 25

► **Mebeverine hydrochloride (Non-proprietary)**
Mebeverine hydrochloride 200 mg Mebeverine 200mg modified-release capsules | 60 capsule PoM £18.44 DT = £13.76

► **Aurobeverine MR** (Milpharm Ltd)
Mebeverine hydrochloride 200 mg Aurobeverine MR 200mg capsules | 60 capsule PoM £6.92 DT = £13.76

► **Colofac MR** (Ceuta Healthcare Ltd)
Mebeverine hydrochloride 200 mg Colofac MR 200mg capsules | 60 capsule PoM £6.92 DT = £13.76

8 Liver disorders and related conditions

8.1 Biliary disorders

Cholestasis
01-May-2017

Description of condition

Cholestasis is an impairment of bile formation and/or bile flow, which may clinically present with fatigue, pruritus, dark urine, pale stools and, in its most overt form, jaundice and signs of fat soluble vitamin deficiencies.

Treatment of cholestatic pruritus

Several drugs are used to relieve cholestatic pruritus, even if evidence to support their use is limited.

EvGr Colestyramine p. 229 is the drug of choice for treating cholestatic pruritus. It is an anion-exchange resin that is not absorbed from the gastro-intestinal tract. It relieves pruritus by forming an insoluble complex in the intestine with bile acids and other compounds—the reduction of serum bile acid levels reduces excess deposition in the dermal tissue with a resultant decrease in pruritus. A

EvGr Ursodeoxycholic acid p. 100 has a small and variable impact on cholestatic pruritus. E

EvGr Rifampicin p. 674 [unlicensed indication] can be used as an alternative treatment for pruritus, but should be used with caution in patients with pre-existing liver disease because of possible hepatotoxicity. A

EvGr Where previous therapy has proved ineffective or was not tolerated, other drugs including sertraline p. 425 [unlicensed indication] and naltrexone hydrochloride p. 564 [unlicensed indication], may be used to treat cholestatic pruritus. However, their use is limited due to significant side-effects. E

Intrahepatic cholestasis in pregnancy

EvGr Ursodeoxycholic acid is effective for the treatment of pruritus associated with intrahepatic cholestasis in pregnancy. E

Intrahepatic cholestasis usually occurs in late pregnancy and is associated with adverse fetal outcomes. EvGr There is no evidence that ursodeoxycholic acid used in late pregnancy affects birth weight in the infant or the risk of preterm delivery. There is limited data about the effect of fetal exposure during the first trimester. D

Gallstones
01-May-2017

Description of condition

Gallstones (cholelithiases) occur when hard mineral or fatty deposits form in the gallbladder. Gallstone disease is a general term that describes the presence of one or more stones in the gallbladder or in the bile duct, and the symptoms and complications that they may cause.

The majority of patients with gallstones remain asymptomatic. When the stones irritate the gallbladder or block part of the biliary system, the patient can experience symptoms such as pain, or infection and inflammation that if left untreated, can lead to severe complications such as biliary colic, acute cholecystitis, cholangitis, pancreatitis, and obstructive jaundice.

Non-drug treatment

EvGr Asymptomatic gallbladder stones do not need to be treated unless symptoms develop.

The definitive treatment of symptomatic gallstones (and all bile duct stones) is surgical removal by laparoscopic cholecystectomy. Ⓐ

Drug treatment

EvGr Analgesia should be offered to control pain symptoms. Paracetamol p. 507 or a nonsteroidal anti-inflammatory drug (see Non-steroidal anti-inflammatory drugs p. 1292) is recommended for intermittent mild-to-moderate pain. Intramuscular diclofenac sodium p. 1297 can be given for severe pain or, if not suitable, an intramuscular opioid (such as morphine p. 525 or pethidine hydrochloride p. 531). Ⓐ

Although ursodeoxycholic acid p. 100 has been used for the management of gallstone disease, there is no evidence to support its use.

Useful Resources

Gallstone disease: diagnosis and management. National Institute for Health and Care Excellence. Clinical guideline 188. October 2014.
www.nice.org.uk/guidance/cg188

Inborn errors of primary bile acid synthesis
27-Apr-2018

Description of condition

Inborn errors of primary bile acid synthesis are a group of diseases in which the liver does not produce enough primary bile acids due to enzyme deficiencies. These acids are the main components of the bile, and include cholic acid and chenodeoxycholic acid.

Treatment

Cholic acid below is licensed for the treatment of inborn errors in primary bile acid synthesis due to an inborn deficiency of two specific liver enzymes. It acts by replacing some of the missing bile acids, therefore relieving the symptoms of the disease.

Chenodeoxycholic acid below is licensed for the treatment of inborn errors of primary bile acid synthesis due to a deficiency of one specific enzyme in the bile acid synthesis pathway when presenting as cerebrotendinous xanthomatosis.

Ursodeoxycholic acid p. 100 [unlicensed indication] has been used to treat inborn errors of primary bile acid synthesis, but there is an absence of evidence to recommend its use.

Primary biliary cholangitis
28-Nov-2024

Description of condition

Primary biliary cholangitis (or primary biliary cirrhosis) is a chronic cholestatic disease which develops due to progressive destruction of small and intermediate bile ducts within the liver, subsequently evolving to fibrosis and cirrhosis.

Treatment

EvGr Ursodeoxycholic acid p. 100 is recommended for the management of primary biliary cholangitis, including those with asymptomatic disease. It slows disease progression, but the effect on overall survival is uncertain. Elafibranor p. 102 or obeticholic acid p. 100 may be used as monotherapy for the treatment of primary biliary cholangitis in patients who are unable to tolerate ursodeoxycholic acid, or as an adjunct to ursodeoxycholic acid in patients who have had an inadequate response to ursodeoxycholic acid monotherapy. Liver transplantation can be considered in patients with advanced primary biliary cholangitis. Ⓐ

BILE ACIDS

Chenodeoxycholic acid
05-Apr-2018

- **INDICATIONS AND DOSE**

Cerebrotendinous xanthomatosis (specialist use only)
▸ BY MOUTH
▸ Adult: Initially 750 mg daily in 3 divided doses, increased if necessary up to 1000 mg daily in divided doses

- **CONTRA-INDICATIONS** Non-functioning gall bladder · radio-opaque stones
- **INTERACTIONS** → Appendix 1: chenodeoxycholic acid
- **SIDE-EFFECTS** Constipation
- **PREGNANCY** Manufacturer advises avoid—fetotoxicity reported in *animal* studies.
- **HEPATIC IMPAIRMENT** Manufacturer advises monitor—no information available.
- **RENAL IMPAIRMENT** Manufacturer advises monitor—no information available.
- **MONITORING REQUIREMENTS** Manufacturer advises to monitor serum cholestanol levels and/or urine bile alcohols every 3 months during the initiation of therapy and dose adjustment, and then at least annually; liver function should also be monitored during initiation of therapy and then at least annually; additional or more frequent investigations may need to be undertaken to monitor therapy during periods of fast growth or concomitant disease.
- **DIRECTIONS FOR ADMINISTRATION** For administration *by mouth* in patients who are unable to swallow capsules and/or need to take a dose below 250 mg, manufacturer advises to add capsule contents to sodium bicarbonate solution 8.4%—for further information, consult product literature.
- **MEDICINAL FORMS** There can be variation in the licensing of different medicines containing the same drug.

Oral capsule
▸ Chenodeoxycholic acid (non-proprietary) ▼
Chenodeoxycholic acid 250 mg Chenodeoxycholic acid 250mg capsules | 100 capsule PoM £14,000.00 DT = £14,000.00

Cholic acid
04-Sep-2020

- **DRUG ACTION** Cholic acid is the predominant primary bile acid in humans, which can be used to provide a source of bile acid in patients with inborn deficiencies in bile acid synthesis.

- **INDICATIONS AND DOSE**

Inborn errors of primary bile acid synthesis (initiated by a specialist)
▸ BY MOUTH
▸ Adult: Usual dose 5–15 mg/kg daily; increased in steps of 50 mg daily in divided doses if required, continued →

dose to be given with food at the same time each day; Usual maximum 500 mg/24 hours

- **INTERACTIONS** → Appendix 1: cholic acid
- **SIDE-EFFECTS** Cholelithiasis (long term use) · diarrhoea · pruritus
  SIDE-EFFECTS, FURTHER INFORMATION Patients presenting with pruritus and/or persistent diarrhoea should be investigated for potential overdose by a serum and/or urine bile acid assay.
- **PREGNANCY** Limited data available—not known to be harmful, manufacturer advises continue treatment. **Monitoring** Manufacturer advises monitor patient parameters more frequently in pregnancy.
- **BREAST FEEDING** Present in milk but not known to be harmful.
- **HEPATIC IMPAIRMENT** Manufacturer advises caution and stop treatment if there are signs of severe hepatic failure—limited information available (no experience with impairment from causes not related to inborn errors of primary bile acid synthesis).
  Dose adjustments Manufacturer advises adjust dose as the degree of impairment improves during treatment.
- **MONITORING REQUIREMENTS** Manufacturer advises monitor serum and/or urine bile-acid concentrations every 3 months for the first year, then every 6 months for three years, then annually; monitor liver function tests at the same or greater frequency.
- **DIRECTIONS FOR ADMINISTRATION** Manufacturer advises capsules may be opened and the content added to infant formula, juice, fruit compote, or yoghurt for administration.
- **PATIENT AND CARER ADVICE** Counselling advised on administration.

- **MEDICINAL FORMS** There can be variation in the licensing of different medicines containing the same drug.
  Oral capsule
  CAUTIONARY AND ADVISORY LABELS 25
  - Orphacol (Abacus Medicine Pharma Services Ltd) ▼
    Cholic acid 50 mg Orphacol 50mg capsules | 30 capsule PoM £1,860.00
    Cholic acid 250 mg Orphacol 250mg capsules | 30 capsule PoM £6,630.00

Obeticholic acid

26-Aug-2020

- **DRUG ACTION** Obeticholic acid is a selective farnesoid X receptor agonist, which decreases circulating bile acid.

- **INDICATIONS AND DOSE**
  Primary biliary cholangitis in combination with ursodeoxycholic acid when response to ursodeoxycholic acid has been inadequate, or as monotherapy in patients intolerant of ursodeoxycholic acid
  - BY MOUTH
    - Adult: Initially 5 mg once daily for 6 months, then increased to 10 mg once daily if necessary and if tolerated, for dose adjustments due to severe pruritus, consult product literature

IMPORTANT SAFETY INFORMATION
MHRA/CHM ADVICE: OBETICHOLIC ACID (*OCALIVA*®): RISK OF SERIOUS LIVER INJURY IN PATIENTS WITH PRE-EXISTING MODERATE OR SEVERE HEPATIC IMPAIRMENT; REMINDER TO ADJUST DOSING ACCORDING TO LIVER FUNCTION MONITORING (APRIL 2018)
The MHRA is aware of reports of serious liver injuries and deaths in patients with primary biliary cholangitis with pre-existing moderate or severe liver impairment who were not adequately dose-adjusted. Follow dose

reduction and monitoring advice in these patients to reduce the risk of serious liver injury; for further information, see *Hepatic impairment* and *Monitoring*.

- **CONTRA-INDICATIONS** Complete biliary obstruction
- **INTERACTIONS** → Appendix 1: obeticholic acid
- **SIDE-EFFECTS**
  - **Common or very common** Arthralgia · constipation · dizziness · fatigue · fever · gastrointestinal discomfort · oropharyngeal pain · palpitations · peripheral oedema · skin reactions
  - **Frequency not known** Hepatic failure
- **PREGNANCY** No evidence of harm but manufacturer advises avoid.
- **BREAST FEEDING** Not known to be harmful but manufacturer advises avoid.
- **HEPATIC IMPAIRMENT** Manufacturer advises caution in moderate to severe impairment or decompensated cirrhosis (risk of increased exposure).
  Dose adjustments Manufacturer advises initial dose reduction to 5 mg once weekly in moderate to severe impairment or decompensated cirrhosis; titrate dose according to alkaline phosphatase and/or total bilirubin level—consult product literature.
- **MONITORING REQUIREMENTS** Manufacturer advises assess hepatic status before treatment initiation and then monitor for progression of primary biliary cholangitis with laboratory and clinical assessment to evaluate the need for dose reduction; patients at an increased risk of hepatic decompensation, including those with laboratory evidence of worsening liver function and/or progression to cirrhosis, should be monitored more closely.
- **NATIONAL FUNDING/ACCESS DECISIONS**
  For full details see funding body website
  NICE decisions
  - **Obeticholic acid for treating primary biliary cholangitis (April 2017) NICE TA443 Recommended with restrictions**
  Scottish Medicines Consortium (SMC) decisions
  - **Obeticholic acid (*Ocaliva*®) for the treatment of primary biliary cholangitis in combination with ursodeoxycholic acid in adults with an inadequate response to ursodeoxycholic acid or as monotherapy in adults unable to tolerate ursodeoxycholic acid (June 2017) SMC No. 1232/17 Recommended**

- **MEDICINAL FORMS** There can be variation in the licensing of different medicines containing the same drug.
  Oral tablet
  - Ocaliva (Advanz Pharma) ▼
    Obeticholic acid 5 mg Ocaliva 5mg tablets | 30 tablet PoM £2,384.04
    Obeticholic acid 10 mg Ocaliva 10mg tablets | 30 tablet PoM £2,384.04

Ursodeoxycholic acid

02-Sep-2020

- **INDICATIONS AND DOSE**
  Dissolution of gallstones
  - BY MOUTH
    - Adult: 8–12 mg/kg once daily for up to 2 years, dose to be taken at bedtime, treatment is continued for 3–4 months after stones dissolve, alternatively 8–12 mg/kg daily in 2 divided doses for up to 2 years, treatment is continued for 3–4 months after stones dissolve

  Primary biliary cirrhosis
  - BY MOUTH
    - Adult: 12–16 mg/kg daily in 3 divided doses for 3 months, then 12–16 mg/kg once daily, dose to be taken at bedtime

Gall reflux gastritis
▶ BY MOUTH
▶ Adult (body-weight 47 kg and above): 250 mg once daily for 10–14 days, dose to be taken at bedtime

● **CONTRA-INDICATIONS** Acute inflammation of the gall bladder · frequent episodes of biliary colic · inflammatory diseases and other conditions of the colon, liver or small intestine which interfere with enterohepatic circulation of bile salts · non-functioning gall bladder · radio-opaque stones

● **INTERACTIONS** → Appendix 1: ursodeoxycholic acid

● **SIDE-EFFECTS**
▶ **Common or very common** Diarrhoea · pale faeces
▶ **Rare or very rare** Abdominal pain upper · cholelithiasis calcification · hepatic cirrhosis exacerbated · skin reactions
▶ **Frequency not known** Nausea · vomiting

● **PREGNANCY** No evidence of harm but manufacturer advises avoid.

● **BREAST FEEDING** Not known to be harmful but manufacturer advises avoid.

● **HEPATIC IMPAIRMENT** Avoid in chronic liver disease (but used in primary biliary cirrhosis).

● **MONITORING REQUIREMENTS** In primary biliary cirrhosis, monitor liver function every 4 weeks for 3 months, then every 3 months.

● **PATIENT AND CARER ADVICE** Patients should be given dietary advice (including avoidance of excessive cholesterol and calories).

● **MEDICINAL FORMS** There can be variation in the licensing of different medicines containing the same drug. Forms available from special-order manufacturers include: oral suspension, oral solution

Oral tablet
CAUTIONARY AND ADVISORY LABELS 21
▶ Ursodeoxycholic acid (Non-proprietary)
  Ursodeoxycholic acid 150 mg Ursodeoxycholic acid 150mg tablets | 60 tablet [PoM] £78.00 DT = £52.81
  Ursodeoxycholic acid 300 mg Ursodeoxycholic acid 300mg tablets | 60 tablet [PoM] £90.00 DT = £79.92
▶ Cholurso (Mayoly UK Ltd)
  Ursodeoxycholic acid 250 mg Cholurso 250mg tablets | 60 tablet [PoM] £18.00 DT = £18.00
  Ursodeoxycholic acid 500 mg Cholurso 500mg tablets | 60 tablet [PoM] £45.00
▶ Ursofalk (Dr. Falk Pharma UK Ltd)
  Ursodeoxycholic acid 500 mg Ursofalk 500mg tablets | 100 tablet [PoM] £80.00 DT = £80.00
▶ Ursonorm (PRO.MED.CS Praha a.s.)
  Ursodeoxycholic acid 500 mg Ursonorm 500mg tablets | 60 tablet [PoM] £45.00 | 100 tablet [PoM] £79.00 DT = £80.00

Oral suspension
CAUTIONARY AND ADVISORY LABELS 21
▶ Ursofalk (Dr. Falk Pharma UK Ltd)
  Ursodeoxycholic acid 50 mg per 1 ml Ursofalk 250mg/5ml oral suspension | 250 ml [PoM] £26.98 DT = £26.98 [SF]

Oral capsule
CAUTIONARY AND ADVISORY LABELS 21
▶ Ursodeoxycholic acid (Non-proprietary)
  Ursodeoxycholic acid 250 mg Ursodeoxycholic acid 250mg capsules | 60 capsule [PoM] £29.00 DT = £8.37 | 100 capsule [PoM] £45.00
▶ Ursofalk (Dr. Falk Pharma UK Ltd)
  Ursodeoxycholic acid 250 mg Ursofalk 250mg capsules | 60 capsule [PoM] £30.17 DT = £8.37 | 100 capsule [PoM] £31.88
▶ Ursonorm (PRO.MED.CS Praha a.s.)
  Ursodeoxycholic acid 250 mg Ursonorm 250mg capsules | 60 capsule [PoM] £29.00 DT = £8.37

ILEAL BILE ACID TRANSPORTER INHIBITORS

Maralixibat
02-Feb-2024

● **DRUG ACTION** Maralixibat is an inhibitor of the ileal bile acid transporter that acts locally in the ileum to reduce re-uptake of bile acids from the intestines into the liver, thereby preventing their accumulation.

● **INDICATIONS AND DOSE**
Cholestatic pruritus [associated with Alagille syndrome] (under expert supervision)
▶ BY MOUTH
▶ Adult: Initially 190 micrograms/kg once daily (max. per dose 14.25 mg) for 7 days, dose to be taken up to 30 minutes before or with a meal in the morning, then increased to 380 micrograms/kg once daily (max. per dose 28.5 mg), dose to be taken up to 30 minutes before or with a meal in the morning, reduce dose to 190 micrograms/kg once daily or interrupt treatment if poor tolerability; consider alternative treatment if no benefit after 3 months

● **SIDE-EFFECTS**
▶ **Common or very common** Abdominal pain · diarrhoea
● **PREGNANCY** [EvGr] Avoid (no information available). [M]
● **BREAST FEEDING** [EvGr] Present in milk but amount probably too small to be harmful [M] (recommendation also supported by tertiary sources).
● **MONITORING REQUIREMENTS**
▶ [EvGr] Monitor liver function tests before starting and during treatment.
▶ Monitor INR and fat-soluble vitamin levels before starting treatment. [M]
● **HANDLING AND STORAGE** Protect from light and discard within 130 days after first opening.
● **PATIENT AND CARER ADVICE**
Missed doses If a dose is more than 12 hours late, the missed dose should not be taken and the next dose should be taken at the normal time.

● **MEDICINAL FORMS** There can be variation in the licensing of different medicines containing the same drug.
Oral solution
EXCIPIENTS: May contain Disodium edetate, propylene glycol
▶ Livmarli (Mirum Pharmaceuticals International BV) ▼
  Maralixibat (as Maralixibat chloride) 9.5 mg per 1 ml Livmarli 9.5mg/ml oral solution | 30 ml [PoM] £43,970.00 (Hospital only) [SF]

Odevixibat
22-Jul-2022

● **DRUG ACTION** Odevixibat is an inhibitor of the ileal bile acid transporter that acts locally in the ileum to reduce re-uptake of bile acids from the intestines into the liver, thereby preventing their accumulation and resultant damage to liver tissue.

● **INDICATIONS AND DOSE**
Progressive familial intrahepatic cholestasis (under expert supervision)
▶ BY MOUTH
▶ Adult: 40 micrograms/kg once daily (max. per dose 2.4 mg), to be taken in the morning, increased if necessary up to 120 micrograms/kg once daily (max. per dose 7.2 mg), to be taken in the morning, dose to be increased if adequate clinical response not achieved after 3 months at initial dose. Consider alternative treatment if no benefit after 6 months

● **CAUTIONS** Impaired gastrointestinal motility or enterohepatic circulation (potential for reduced efficacy)

- **SIDE-EFFECTS**
▶ **Common or very common** Diarrhoea · diarrhoea haemorrhagic · faeces soft · gastrointestinal discomfort · hepatomegaly
- **CONCEPTION AND CONTRACEPTION** EvGr Effective contraception required during treatment in females of childbearing potential (important: effectiveness of some oral contraceptives may be reduced; barrier contraception should be used). M
- **PREGNANCY** EvGr Avoid—reproductive toxicity in *animal* studies. M
- **BREAST FEEDING** EvGr Avoid—no information available. M
- **MONITORING REQUIREMENTS** EvGr Monitor liver function tests, INR and fat-soluble vitamins before starting treatment, and then as clinically indicated. M
- **DIRECTIONS FOR ADMINISTRATION** EvGr Capsules may be swallowed whole with water. Alternatively, capsules may be opened and the contents mixed into approximately 2 tablespoons of soft food (e.g. yoghurt, apple sauce) at or below room temperature, and administered immediately. M
- **PATIENT AND CARER ADVICE** Patients or carers should be given advice on how to administer *Bylvay*® capsules.
- **NATIONAL FUNDING/ACCESS DECISIONS** For full details see funding body website
NICE decisions
▶ Odevixibat for treating progressive familial intrahepatic cholestasis (February 2022) NICE HST17 Recommended

- **MEDICINAL FORMS** There can be variation in the licensing of different medicines containing the same drug.
Oral capsule
▶ Bylvay (Ipsen Ltd) ▼
Odevixibat (as Odevixibat sesquihydrate) 200 microgram Bylvay 200microgram capsules | 30 capsule PoM £3,085.00 (Hospital only)
Odevixibat (as Odevixibat sesquihydrate) 400 microgram Bylvay 400microgram capsules | 30 capsule PoM £6,170.00 (Hospital only)
Odevixibat (as Odevixibat sesquihydrate) 600 microgram Bylvay 600microgram capsules | 30 capsule PoM £9,255.00 (Hospital only)
Odevixibat (as Odevixibat sesquihydrate) 1.2 mg Bylvay 1200microgram capsules | 30 capsule PoM £18,510.00 (Hospital only)

PEROXISOME PROLIFERATOR-ACTIVATED RECEPTOR AGONISTS

Elafibranor

25-Apr-2025

- **DRUG ACTION** Elafibranor is a peroxisome proliferator-activated receptor (PPAR) alpha and delta agonist that decreases synthesis, increases detoxification, and modulates output of bile acid, and also reduces hepatic inflammation.

- **INDICATIONS AND DOSE**
Primary biliary cholangitis [in combination with ursodeoxycholic acid when response to ursodeoxycholic acid has been inadequate, or as monotherapy in patients intolerant of ursodeoxycholic acid]
▶ BY MOUTH
▶ Adult: 80 mg once daily

- **CAUTIONS** Risk factors for elevated creatine kinase concentration
- **INTERACTIONS** → Appendix 1: elafibranor
- **SIDE-EFFECTS**
▶ **Common or very common** Cholelithiasis · constipation · diarrhoea · gastrointestinal discomfort · headache · myalgia · nausea · vomiting
▶ **Uncommon** Pruritic rash
▶ **Frequency not known** Bone fracture

- **CONCEPTION AND CONTRACEPTION** EvGr Females of childbearing potential should use effective contraception during treatment and for at least 3 weeks after last treatment. M
- **PREGNANCY** EvGr Avoid (toxicity in *animal* studies). M
- **BREAST FEEDING** EvGr Avoid during treatment and for at least 3 weeks after last treatment (toxicity in *animal* studies). M
- **HEPATIC IMPAIRMENT** EvGr Avoid in severe impairment (risk of increased exposure). M
- **MONITORING REQUIREMENTS**
▶ EvGr Assess hepatic status before treatment initiation and thereafter as clinically indicated.
▶ Assess creatine kinase concentration before treatment initiation and periodically thereafter or as clinically indicated. M
- **PATIENT AND CARER ADVICE** Patients and their carers should be advised to promptly report any unexplained muscle pain, soreness, or weakness, especially if accompanied by malaise or fever.
- **NATIONAL FUNDING/ACCESS DECISIONS** For full details see funding body website
NICE decisions
▶ Elafibranor for previously treated primary biliary cholangitis (November 2024) NICE TA1016 Recommended
Scottish Medicines Consortium (SMC) decisions
▶ Elafibranor (*Iqirvo*®) for the treatment of primary biliary cholangitis in combination with ursodeoxycholic acid (UDCA) in adults with an inadequate response to UDCA, or as monotherapy in adults unable to tolerate UDCA (April 2025) SMC No. SMC2714 Recommended

- **MEDICINAL FORMS** There can be variation in the licensing of different medicines containing the same drug.
Oral tablet
▶ Iqirvo (Ipsen Ltd) ▼
Elafibranor 80 mg Iqirvo 80mg tablets | 30 tablet PoM £2,867.00

TERPENES

Borneol with camphene, cineole, menthol, menthone and pinene

- **INDICATIONS AND DOSE**
Biliary disorders
▶ BY MOUTH
▶ Adult: 1–2 capsules 3 times a day, to be taken before food

- **LESS SUITABLE FOR PRESCRIBING** *Rowachol*® is less suitable for prescribing.

- **MEDICINAL FORMS** No licensed medicines listed.

8.2 Oesophageal varices

Other drugs used for Oesophageal varices Carvedilol, p. 175 · Propranolol hydrochloride, p. 178 · Vasopressin, p. 766

PITUITARY AND HYPOTHALAMIC HORMONES AND ANALOGUES > VASOPRESSIN AND ANALOGUES

Terlipressin acetate

14-Apr-2023

● INDICATIONS AND DOSE

GLYPRESSIN ® INJECTION

Bleeding from oesophageal varices
▶ BY INTRAVENOUS INJECTION
▶ Adult (body-weight up to 50 kg): Initially 2 mg every 4 hours until bleeding controlled, then reduced to 1 mg every 4 hours if required, maximum duration 48 hours
▶ Adult (body-weight 50 kg and above): Initially 2 mg every 4 hours until bleeding controlled, reduced if not tolerated to 1 mg every 4 hours, maximum duration 48 hours

VARIQUEL ® INJECTION

Bleeding from oesophageal varices
▶ BY INTRAVENOUS INJECTION
▶ Adult (body-weight up to 50 kg): Initially 1 mg, then 1 mg every 4–6 hours for up to 72 hours
▶ Adult (body-weight 50-69 kg): Initially 1.5 mg, then 1 mg every 4–6 hours for up to 72 hours
▶ Adult (body-weight 70 kg and above): Initially 2 mg, then 1 mg every 4–6 hours for up to 72 hours

Type 1 hepatorenal syndrome
▶ BY INTRAVENOUS INJECTION
▶ Adult: 1 mg every 4–6 hours, increased if necessary up to 2 mg every 4 hours for a usual total duration of 7 days (up to a max. of 14 days), dose to be increased if serum-creatinine does not decrease by at least 25% after 3 days, discontinue treatment when serum-creatinine falls below 133 micromol/litre (1.5 mg/dL)

IMPORTANT SAFETY INFORMATION

MHRA/CHM ADVICE: TERLIPRESSIN: NEW RECOMMENDATIONS TO REDUCE RISKS OF RESPIRATORY FAILURE AND SEPTIC SHOCK IN PATIENTS WITH TYPE 1 HEPATORENAL SYNDROME (MARCH 2023)
The CONFIRM trial has shown that terlipressin was associated with increased mortality from respiratory disorders and an increased risk of sepsis and septic shock in type 1 hepatorenal syndrome patients. A subsequent EU-wide review has concluded that further measures are required to reduce such risks in this patient group.
  Healthcare professionals are advised to:
● avoid use in patients with severe liver disease (Acute-on-Chronic Liver Failure [ACLF] grade 3, a Model for End-stage Liver Disease [MELD] score $\geq$ 39, or both) unless benefit outweighs potential risk;
● avoid use in patients with advanced renal dysfunction (baseline serum-creatinine $\geq$ 442 micromol/litre [5 mg/dL]) unless benefit outweighs potential risk;
● stabilise patients with new-onset breathing difficulties or worsening of existing respiratory disease before administration and monitor closely during treatment;
● consider a reduction in albumin dose in patients with signs or symptoms of respiratory failure or fluid overload—discontinue terlipressin if symptoms are severe or do not resolve;
● monitor patients daily for signs and symptoms of infection;
● monitor blood pressure, heart rate, oxygen saturation, serum-sodium and -potassium levels, and fluid balance—terlipressin may induce myocardial ischaemia and pulmonary vascular congestion, especially in those with pre-existing cardiopulmonary disease;

● consider administration by continuous intravenous infusion as this may be associated with lower rates of severe adverse events than bolus injection;
● counsel patients and carers on the benefits and risks, even if that counselling occurs after administration.
This advice is not relevant to the use of terlipressin for bleeding from oesophageal varices.

● **CAUTIONS** Arrhythmia · elderly · electrolyte and fluid disturbances · heart disease · history of QT-interval prolongation · respiratory disease · septic shock · uncontrolled hypertension · vascular disease

● **SIDE-EFFECTS**
▶ **Common or very common** Abdominal cramps · arrhythmias · diarrhoea · headache · hypertension · hypotension · nausea · pallor · peripheral ischaemia · vasoconstriction
▶ **Uncommon** Chest pain · cyanosis · fluid overload · heart failure · hot flush · hyponatraemia · injection site necrosis · intestinal ischaemia · ischaemic heart disease · lymphangitis · myocardial infarction · pulmonary oedema · respiratory disorders · seizure · skin reactions · uterine ischaemia · vomiting
▶ **Rare or very rare** Dyspnoea · stroke
▶ **Frequency not known** QT interval prolongation · sepsis

SIDE-EFFECTS, FURTHER INFORMATION In those with type 1 hepatorenal syndrome, terlipressin acetate can cause serious or fatal respiratory failure, and can increase the risk of sepsis and septic shock.

● **PREGNANCY** Avoid unless benefits outweigh risk—uterine contractions and increased intra-uterine pressure in early pregnancy, and decreased uterine blood flow reported.

● **BREAST FEEDING** Avoid unless benefits outweigh risk—no information available.

● **HEPATIC IMPAIRMENT**
VARIQUEL ® INJECTION
▶ When used for Type 1 hepatorenal syndrome MHRA advises avoid in severe impairment—see *Important safety information*.

● **RENAL IMPAIRMENT** [EvGr] Use with caution in chronic renal failure. Ⓜ
VARIQUEL ® INJECTION
▶ When used for Type 1 hepatorenal syndrome MHRA advises avoid in severe impairment—see *Important safety information*.

● **DIRECTIONS FOR ADMINISTRATION**
VARIQUEL ® INJECTION For *intravenous injection*, give undiluted over at least 1 minute.

● **HANDLING AND STORAGE** Store solutions for injection in a refrigerator (2–8°C) and protect from light.

● **MEDICINAL FORMS** There can be variation in the licensing of different medicines containing the same drug.

Solution for injection

▶ Terlipressin acetate (Non-proprietary)
 Terlipressin acetate 120 microgram per 1 ml Terlipressin 1mg/8.5ml solution for injection ampoules | 5 ampoule [PoM] £96.95 (Hospital only)
 Terlipressin acetate 200 microgram per 1 ml Terlipressin 1mg/5ml solution for injection vials | 5 vial [PoM] £96.95 (Hospital only)

Powder and solvent for solution for injection

▶ Terlipressin acetate (Non-proprietary)
 Terlipressin acetate 1 mg Terlipressin 1mg powder and solvent for solution for injection vials | 5 vial [PoM] £92.33 (Hospital only)
▶ Glypressin (Ferring Pharmaceuticals Ltd)
 Terlipressin acetate 1 mg Glypressin 1mg powder and solvent for solution for injection vials | 5 vial [PoM] £92.33

9 Obesity

Obesity

29-Nov-2023

Description of condition

Overweight, obesity, or increased central adiposity are associated with an increased risk of developing a number of health conditions, including type 2 diabetes, hypertension, cardiovascular disease, dyslipidaemia, fatty liver disease, gallstones, some types of cancers, reproductive problems, respiratory and musculoskeletal conditions, and gastro-oesophageal reflux disease. They are also associated with psychological and psychiatric morbidities.

BMI and waist-to-height ratio are measures of obesity and central adiposity, respectively. Both these measures aid the evaluation of health risks in overweight and obese individuals, although BMI alone should be interpreted with caution as it is not a direct measure of central adiposity, particularly in individuals who are very muscular or have muscle weakness or atrophy, and in those aged 65 years and over. When assessing health risks, measurement of BMI is advised; in addition, in individuals with a BMI below $35\,kg/m^2$, waist-to-height ratio should also be measured, including in those whose BMI is in the healthy weight category.

In individuals from a white family background, overweight or obesity is defined as follows:

- healthy weight: BMI $18.5\,kg/m^2$ to $24.9\,kg/m^2$
- overweight: BMI $25\,kg/m^2$ to $29.9\,kg/m^2$
- obesity class 1: BMI $30\,kg/m^2$ to $34.9\,kg/m^2$
- obesity class 2: BMI $35\,kg/m^2$ to $39.9\,kg/m^2$
- obesity class 3: BMI $40\,kg/m^2$ or more

Individuals with a Black African, African-Caribbean, South Asian, Chinese, other Asian, or Middle Eastern family background are at increased risk of chronic health conditions at lower BMI thresholds. Overweight or obesity in these individuals is defined as:

- overweight: BMI $23\,kg/m^2$ to $27.4\,kg/m^2$
- obesity: BMI $27.5\,kg/m^2$ or above—classes 2 and 3 are usually identified by reducing the thresholds above by $2.5\,kg/m^2$

In all individuals with a BMI below $35\,kg/m^2$, central adiposity based on waist-to-height ratio is defined as:

- increased central adiposity: waist-to-height ratio 0.5 to 0.59
- high central adiposity: waist-to-height ratio 0.6 or more

Individuals with a BMI of $35\,kg/m^2$ or more are at very high risk of obesity related-health problems, regardless of waist-to-height ratio.

Aims of treatment

Management should be aimed at modest, sustainable weight loss and maintenance of a healthy weight, to reduce the risk factors associated with obesity.

Overview

EvGr Weight management interventions should be delivered by staff experienced in the management of overweight and obesity. Realistic weight loss goals should be discussed and agreed with the individual.

An initial assessment should consider potential underlying causes (e.g. hypothyroidism) and a review of the appropriateness of current medications which are known to cause weight gain, e.g. atypical antipsychotics, beta-adrenoceptor blocking drugs, insulin (when used in the treatment of type 2 diabetes), lithium carbonate, lithium citrate, sodium valproate, sulphonylureas, thiazolidinediones, and tricyclic antidepressants. Individuals should be assessed for comorbidities such as type 2 diabetes, hypertension, cardiovascular disease, dyslipidaemia, osteoarthritis, and sleep apnoea. A

Lifestyle changes

EvGr Individuals who are overweight or obese should be encouraged to engage in a sustainable weight management programme which includes behavioural change strategies to increase physical activity and improve diet and eating behaviour. A

Drug treatment

EvGr Drug treatment should **never** be used as the sole element of treatment and should be used as part of an overall weight management plan. Orlistat p. 105 may be considered for individuals with a BMI of $\geq 30\,kg/m^2$ in whom diet, exercise and behavioural changes fail to achieve an adequate reduction in weight, or for individuals with a BMI $\geq 28\,kg/m^2$ in the presence of associated risk factors. Under specialist care, liraglutide p. 816 or semaglutide p. 819 may be considered for certain patients. Drug treatment may also be used to maintain weight loss rather than to continue to lose weight.

The effect of drug treatment should be monitored on a regular basis with reinforcement of supporting lifestyle advice. Rates of weight loss may be slower in patients with type 2 diabetes, so less strict goals than in those without diabetes may be appropriate.

Setmelanotide p. 106 may be considered under expert supervision in individuals with specific genetic conditions. A

Drugs which produce a feeling of satiety (such as methylcellulose and sterculia p. 61 [unlicensed indications]) have been used in an attempt to control appetite, but there is little evidence for their efficacy. Various other centrally acting appetite suppressants, including stimulants and serotonergic drugs (such as dexfenfluramine, fenfluramine, sibutramine, and rimonabant), have been used in the management of obesity but have been withdrawn or are no longer recommended due to serious safety concerns or their addictive potential.

Surgery

EvGr Bariatric surgery may be considered for patients who have a BMI of $\geq 40\,kg/m^2$, or between $35–39.9\,kg/m^2$ and a significant disease (such as cardiovascular disease, non-alcoholic fatty liver disease, obstructive sleep apnoea, type 2 diabetes or hypertension) which could be improved with weight loss. Bariatric surgery may also be considered for patients with a BMI of $30–34.9\,kg/m^2$ who have recent-onset type 2 diabetes. A

Useful Resources

Obesity: identification, assessment and management. National Institute for Health and Care Excellence. Clinical guideline 189. November 2014 (updated July 2023). www.nice.org.uk/guidance/cg189

> **Other drugs used for Obesity** Tirzepatide, p. 822

ANTIDEPRESSANTS › SEROTONIN AND NORADRENALINE RE-UPTAKE INHIBITORS

Naltrexone with bupropion
21-Apr-2021

The properties listed below are those particular to the combination only. For the properties of the components please consider, bupropion hydrochloride p. 566, naltrexone hydrochloride p. 564.

● INDICATIONS AND DOSE

Adjunct in obesity (in conjunction with dietary measures and increased physical activity in individuals with a body mass index (BMI) of 30 kg/m^2 or more or in individuals with a BMI of 27 kg/m^2 or more in the presence of one or more weight related co-morbidity)
▸ BY MOUTH
▸ Adult 18-75 years: Initially 1 tablet daily for 7 days, then increased to 1 tablet twice daily for 7 days, then increased to 3 tablets daily in divided doses for 7 days, two tablets to be taken in the morning, and one tablet to be taken in the evening, then maintenance 2 tablets twice daily, review treatment after 16 weeks and then annually

DOSE EQUIVALENCE AND CONVERSION
▸ Each tablet contains 8 mg naltrexone with 90 mg bupropion.

IMPORTANT SAFETY INFORMATION

MHRA/CHM ADVICE: NALTREXONE/BUPROPION (*MYSIMBA*®): RISK OF ADVERSE REACTIONS THAT COULD AFFECT ABILITY TO DRIVE (AUGUST 2019)
An EU cumulative review of worldwide data has found naltrexone with bupropion to be commonly associated with dizziness or somnolence, and rarely with loss of consciousness or seizure. These can affect the ability of patients to drive, operate machinery, or perform dangerous tasks, particularly at the start of treatment or during the dose titration phase. Healthcare professionals are advised to inform patients of these adverse effects and to avoid such tasks until they are resolved.

● **CONTRA-INDICATIONS** Uncontrolled hypertension

● **CAUTIONS** History of mania · hypertension

● **INTERACTIONS** → Appendix 1: bupropion · naltrexone

● **HEPATIC IMPAIRMENT** Manufacturer advises avoid (no information available).

● **RENAL IMPAIRMENT** EvGr Avoid in end-stage renal disease. Ⓜ
Dose adjustments EvGr Max. 1 tablet twice daily in moderate to severe impairment. Ⓜ

● **PRESCRIBING AND DISPENSING INFORMATION** Prescribers should consult the *Mysimba*® *Physician Prescribing Checklist* provided by the manufacturer, before initiation of treatment.

● **NATIONAL FUNDING/ACCESS DECISIONS**
For full details see funding body website
NICE decisions
▸ Naltrexone–bupropion for managing overweight and obesity (December 2017) NICE TA494 Not recommended

---

● **MEDICINAL FORMS** There can be variation in the licensing of different medicines containing the same drug.
Modified-release tablet
CAUTIONARY AND ADVISORY LABELS 21, 25
▸ Mysimba (Orexigen Therapeutics Ireland Ltd) ▼
Naltrexone hydrochloride 8 mg, Bupropion hydrochloride 90 mg Mysimba 8mg/90mg prolonged-release tablets | 112 tablet PoM £73.00 DT = £73.00

ANTIOBESITY DRUGS

Orlistat
11-Nov-2022

● **DRUG ACTION** Orlistat, a lipase inhibitor, reduces the absorption of dietary fat.

● INDICATIONS AND DOSE

Adjunct in obesity (in conjunction with a mildly hypocaloric diet in individuals with a body mass index (BMI) of 30 kg/m^2 or more or in individuals with a BMI of 28 kg/m^2 or more in the presence of other risk factors such as type 2 diabetes, hypertension, or hypercholesterolaemia)
▸ BY MOUTH
▸ Adult: 120 mg up to 3 times a day, dose to be taken immediately before, during, or up to 1 hour after each main meal, continue treatment beyond 12 weeks only if weight loss since start of treatment exceeds 5% (target for initial weight loss may be lower in patients with type 2 diabetes), if a meal is missed or contains no fat, the dose of orlistat should be omitted

● **CONTRA-INDICATIONS** Cholestasis · chronic malabsorption syndrome

● **CAUTIONS** Chronic kidney disease · may impair absorption of fat-soluble vitamins · volume depletion

CAUTIONS, FURTHER INFORMATION Vitamin supplementation (especially of vitamin D) may be considered if there is concern about deficiency of fat-soluble vitamins.

● **INTERACTIONS** → Appendix 1: orlistat

● **SIDE-EFFECTS**
▸ **Common or very common** Abdominal pain (may be minimised by reduced fat intake) · anxiety · diarrhoea · gastrointestinal disorders
▸ **Frequency not known** Anorectal haemorrhage · bullous dermatitis · cholelithiasis · diverticulitis · hepatitis · oxalate nephropathy · pancreatitis · renal failure

● **PREGNANCY** Use with caution.

● **BREAST FEEDING** Avoid—no information available.

● **MEDICINAL FORMS** There can be variation in the licensing of different medicines containing the same drug.
Oral capsule
▸ Orlistat (Non-proprietary)
Orlistat 120 mg Orlistat 120mg capsules | 84 capsule PoM £38.66 DT = £22.13
▸ Alli (Haleon UK Trading Ltd)
Orlistat 60 mg Alli 60mg capsules | 84 capsule P £33.77 DT = £33.77
▸ Orlos (Crescent Pharma Ltd)
Orlistat 60 mg Orlos 60mg capsules | 84 capsule P £24.56 DT = £33.77
▸ Xenical (Neon Healthcare Ltd)
Orlistat 120 mg Xenical 120mg capsules | 84 capsule PoM £31.63 DT = £22.13

Setmelanotide

05-Aug-2024

- **DRUG ACTION** Setmelanotide is a centrally-acting selective melanocortin-4 receptor agonist that regulates hunger, satiety, and energy expenditure, thereby promoting weight loss.

- **INDICATIONS AND DOSE**

Obesity with underlying genetic aetiology [pro-opiomelanocortin (POMC), proprotein convertase subtilisin/kexin type 1 (PCSK1), or leptin receptor (LEPR) deficiency] (under expert supervision)
- ▶ BY SUBCUTANEOUS INJECTION
- ▶ Adult: 1 mg once daily for 2 weeks, to be administered in the morning, then increased if tolerated to 2 mg once daily, to be administered in the morning; increased if necessary to 2.5 mg once daily, to be administered in the morning, then increased if necessary up to 3 mg once daily, to be administered in the morning

Obesity with underlying genetic aetiology [Bardet-Biedl syndrome (BBS)] (under expert supervision)
- ▶ BY SUBCUTANEOUS INJECTION
- ▶ Adult: 2 mg once daily for 2 weeks, to be administered in the morning, if not tolerated, reduce dose to 1 mg once daily; then if tolerated, increase dose to 2 mg once daily, then increased if tolerated to 3 mg once daily, to be administered in the morning

- **CAUTIONS** Contains benzyl alcohol as an excipient (risk of allergic reactions, and of metabolic acidosis due to accumulation over time)

- **SIDE-EFFECTS**
- ▶ **Common or very common** Alopecia · asthenia · constipation · depression · diarrhoea · dizziness · dry mouth · gastrointestinal discomfort · headaches · hot flush · hyperhidrosis · muscle complaints · nausea · neoplasms · pain · sexual dysfunction · skin reactions · sleep disorders · vertigo · vomiting
- ▶ **Uncommon** Altered smell sensation · anxiety · arthralgia · chest pain · chills · cough · drowsiness · eye naevus · gastrointestinal disorders · genital abnormalities · genital disorder female · hair colour changes · hyperaesthesia · jaundice ocular · mood altered · nail discolouration · nail disorder · oral disorders · rhinorrhoea · scleral discolouration · taste altered · temperature sensation altered · yawning
- ▶ **Frequency not known** Hyperpigmentation disorders · tongue discolouration

- **PREGNANCY** EvGr No evidence of teratogenicity in *animal* studies, but lack of information in pregnant women. Avoid initiation during pregnancy—weight loss during pregnancy may cause fetal harm. If pregnancy occurs during treatment in a patient who is still losing weight, consider reducing dose or discontinuing treatment. If pregnancy occurs during treatment in a patient who has reached a stable weight, consider continuing treatment. Ⓜ
Monitoring EvGr Monitor weight against recommended weight gain if treatment is continued during pregnancy. Ⓜ

- **BREAST FEEDING** EvGr Avoid—present in milk in *animal* studies. Ⓜ

- **HEPATIC IMPAIRMENT** EvGr Avoid (no information available). Ⓜ

- **RENAL IMPAIRMENT** EvGr Avoid in end-stage renal disease (no information available). Ⓜ
Dose adjustments EvGr Start with reduced dose in severe impairment (risk of increased exposure—consult product literature). Ⓜ

- **MONITORING REQUIREMENTS**
- ▶ EvGr Full body examination of pre-existing and new skin pigmentary lesions is advised at baseline and annually during treatment.
- ▶ Monitor heart rate and blood pressure at least every 6 months during treatment.
- ▶ Monitor patients with depression during treatment for signs of suicidal thoughts or behaviours. Ⓜ

- **DIRECTIONS FOR ADMINISTRATION** EvGr Allow the vial to reach room temperature prior to administration. Inject into the abdomen (except for the 5 cm around the navel); rotate injection site and avoid skin that is red, swollen, or irritated. Ⓜ Patients may self-administer *Imcivree*® after appropriate training in preparation and administration.

- **HANDLING AND STORAGE** Store unopened vials in a refrigerator (2–8°C) and protect from light; may be stored at room temperature (below 30°C) for up to 30 days. Once opened, vials may be stored for a maximum of 28 days at 2–30°C.

- **PATIENT AND CARER ADVICE** Patients who have a penile erection lasting longer than 4 hours should be advised to seek emergency medical attention for potential priapism.
Self-administration Patients and their carers should be given training in subcutaneous injection technique.
Missed doses If a dose is missed, the missed dose should be omitted and the next dose administered at the normal time.

- **NATIONAL FUNDING/ACCESS DECISIONS**
For full details see funding body website
NICE decisions
- ▶ **Setmelanotide for treating obesity caused by LEPR or POMC deficiency (July 2022)** NICE HST21 Recommended
- ▶ **Setmelanotide for treating obesity and hyperphagia in Bardet-Biedl syndrome (May 2024)** NICE HST31 Recommended with restrictions

- **MEDICINAL FORMS** There can be variation in the licensing of different medicines containing the same drug.
Solution for injection
EXCIPIENTS: May contain Benzyl alcohol, disodium edetate
- ▶ **Imcivree** (Rhythm Pharmaceuticals UK Ltd) ▼
Setmelanotide 10 mg per 1 ml Imcivree 10mg/1ml solution for injection vials | 1 vial PoM £2,376.00 (Hospital only)

10 Rectal and anal disorders

10.1 Anal fissures

Anal fissure

31-Aug-2016

Description of condition

An anal fissure is a tear or ulcer in the lining of the anal canal, immediately within the anal margin. Clinical features of anal fissure include bleeding and persistent pain on defecation, and a linear split in the anal mucosa.

Aims of treatment

The aim of treatment is to relieve pain and promote healing of the fissure.

Drug treatment

Acute anal fissure

EvGr Initial management of acute anal fissures (present for less than 6 weeks) should focus on ensuring that stools are soft and easily passed. Bulk-forming laxatives (such as ispaghula husk p. 60) are recommended and an osmotic laxative (such as lactulose p. 61) can be considered as an alternative—see also Constipation p. 58, for further information about these laxatives. Short-term use of a

topical preparation containing a local anaesthetic (such as lidocaine hydrochloride p. 1547) or a simple analgesic (such as paracetamol p. 507 or ibuprofen p. 1302) may be offered for prolonged burning pain following defecation. If these measures are inadequate, the patient should be referred for specialist treatment in hospital. Ⓐ

Chronic anal fissure

EvGr Chronic anal fissures (present for 6 weeks or longer), and associated pain, may be treated with glyceryl trinitrate rectal ointment 0.4% or 0.2% p. 252 [unlicensed] (available from Special-order manufacturers p. 1967 or specialist importing companies). Limited evidence suggests that the strength used does not influence the effectiveness, but that the higher strength potentially increases the incidence of side-effects. Healing rates with topical glyceryl trinitrate are marginally superior to placebo, but the incidence of headache as an adverse effect is quite high (about 20-30% of patients). Recurrence of the fissure after treatment is common.

As an alternative to glyceryl trinitrate rectal ointment, chronic anal fissure may also be treated with topical diltiazem hydrochloride 2% p. 185 [unlicensed] or nifedipine 0.2-0.5% p. 189 [unlicensed] (available from Special-order manufacturers p. 1967 or specialist importing companies), which have a lower incidence of adverse effects than topical glyceryl trinitrate. Oral nifedipine [unlicensed indication] and oral diltiazem hydrochloride [unlicensed indication] may be as effective as topical treatment, but the incidence of adverse effects are likely to be higher and topical preparations are preferred.

Patients who do not respond to first-line treatment may be referred to a specialist for local injection of botulinum toxin type A [unlicensed indication]. Ⓐ

Non-drug treatment

EvGr Surgery is an effective option for the management of chronic anal fissure in adults but is generally reserved for those who do not respond to drug treatment. Ⓐ

10.2 Haemorrhoids

Haemorrhoids

05-Feb-2024

Description of condition

Haemorrhoids, or piles, are abnormal swellings of the vascular mucosal anal cushions around the anus. Internal haemorrhoids arise above the dentate line and are usually painless unless they become strangulated. External haemorrhoids originate below the dentate line and can be itchy or painful. Women are predisposed to developing haemorrhoids during pregnancy.

Aims of treatment

The aims of treatment are to reduce the symptoms (pain, bleeding and swelling), promote healing, and prevent recurrence.

Non-drug treatment

EvGr Stools should be kept soft and easy to pass (to minimise straining) by increasing dietary fibre and fluid intake. Advice about perianal hygiene is helpful to aid healing and reduce irritation and itching. Ⓐ

Drug treatment

EvGr If constipation is reported, it should be treated. A bulk-forming laxative can be prescribed (see Constipation p. 58)

A simple analgesic such as paracetamol p. 507 can be used for pain relief. Opioid analgesics should be avoided as they can cause constipation, and NSAIDs should be avoided if rectal bleeding is present. Ⓐ

Topical preparations that contain a combination of local anaesthetics, corticosteroids, astringents, lubricants, and antiseptics are available—see *Related drugs* below. EvGr They can offer symptomatic relief of local pain and itching but evidence does not suggest that any preparation is more effective than any other.

Topical preparations containing local anaesthetics (lidocaine, benzocaine, cinchocaine and pramocaine) should only be used for a few days as they may cause sensitisation of the anal skin. Local anaesthetics can be absorbed through the rectal mucosa (with a theoretical risk of systemic side effects) and very rarely may cause increased irritation; therefore excessive application should be **avoided**. Ⓐ

Topical preparations combining corticosteroids with local anaesthetics and soothing agents are available for the management of haemorrhoids. They may ameliorate local perianal inflammation, but no data suggest that they actually reduce haemorrhoidal swelling, bleeding, or protrusion.

EvGr Topical corticosteroids are suitable for occasional short-term use (no more than 7 days) after exclusion of infections (such as perianal streptococcal infection, *herpes simplex* or perianal thrush). Long-term use of corticosteroid creams can cause ulceration or permanent damage due to thinning of the perianal skin and should be avoided. Ⓐ Continuous or excessive use carries a risk of adrenal suppression and systemic corticosteroid effects.

EvGr Recurrent symptoms, should be referred to secondary care for further investigation and management.

Treatments available from *specialists* include rubber band ligation, injection sclerotherapy (using phenol p. 111 in oil), infrared coagulation/photocoagulation, bipolar diathermy and direct-current electrotherapy, haemorrhoidectomy, stapled haemorrhoidectomy, and haemorrhoidal artery ligation. Ⓐ

Pregnancy

EvGr Bulk forming laxatives are not absorbed, and are therefore safe for use in pregnant women (see Pregnancy, under Constipation p. 58). Ⓐ No topical haemorrhoidal preparations are licensed for use during pregnancy.

EvGr If treatment with a topical haemorrhoidal preparation is required, a soothing preparation containing simple, soothing products (**not** local anaesthetics or corticosteroids) can be considered. Ⓐ

Related drugs

Topical preparations used for haemorrhoids: lidocaine hydrochloride p. 1547, benzyl benzoate with bismuth oxide, bismuth subgallate, hydrocortisone acetate, peru balsam and zinc oxide below, cinchocaine with hydrocortisone p. 108, cinchocaine with prednisolone p. 110.

CORTICOSTEROIDS

Benzyl benzoate with bismuth oxide, bismuth subgallate, hydrocortisone acetate, peru balsam and zinc oxide

05-Jun-2024

● INDICATIONS AND DOSE

Haemorrhoids | Pruritus ani

▸ BY RECTUM USING OINTMENT

▸ Adult: Apply twice daily for no longer than 7 days, to be applied morning and night, an additional dose should be applied after a bowel movement

continued →

1

Gastro-intestinal system

▸ BY RECTUM USING SUPPOSITORIES
▸ Adult: 1 suppository twice daily for no longer than 7 days, to be inserted night and morning, additional dose after a bowel movement

IMPORTANT SAFETY INFORMATION

MHRA/CHM ADVICE: CORTICOSTEROIDS: RARE RISK OF CENTRAL SEROUS CHORIORETINOPATHY WITH LOCAL AS WELL AS SYSTEMIC ADMINISTRATION (AUGUST 2017)
See Corticosteroids, general use p. 780.

NHS IMPROVEMENT PATIENT SAFETY ALERT: STEROID EMERGENCY CARD TO SUPPORT EARLY RECOGNITION AND TREATMENT OF ADRENAL CRISIS IN ADULTS (AUGUST 2020)
See Adrenal insufficiency p. 781.

MHRA/CHM ADVICE: TOPICAL CORTICOSTEROIDS: INFORMATION ON THE RISK OF TOPICAL STEROID WITHDRAWAL REACTIONS (SEPTEMBER 2021)
Rarely, long-term continuous or inappropriate use of topical corticosteroids, particularly those of moderate to high potency, can result in the development of rebound flares, reported as dermatitis with intense redness, stinging, and burning that can spread beyond the initial treatment area.

The MHRA advises that the lowest potency topical corticosteroid needed should be used. For patients who are currently on long-term topical corticosteroid treatment, consider reducing potency or frequency of application (or both). Healthcare professionals should also be vigilant for the signs and symptoms of topical corticosteroid withdrawal reactions and review the position statement from the National Eczema Society and British Association of Dermatologists eczema.org/wp-content/uploads/Topical-Steroid-Withdrawal-position-statement.pdf.

Healthcare professionals should inform patients:
- how much should be applied, as under-use can prolong treatment duration;
- how long they should use a topical corticosteroid for, especially on sensitive areas such as the face and genitals;
- to always apply topical corticosteroids as instructed and consult the patient information leaflet provided;
- to seek medical advice before using a topical corticosteroid on a new body area, as some areas of the body are more prone to side-effects;
- to return for medical advice if their skin condition worsens while using topical corticosteroid, and advise them when it would be appropriate to re-treat without a consultation and;
- if their skin worsens within 2 weeks of stopping a topical corticosteroid, treatment should not be started again without consulting their doctor unless they have previously been advised to do so

The MHRA advises healthcare professionals to report any suspected adverse effects, via the Yellow Card Scheme, even when the adverse affects occur after stopping corticosteroid treatment.

MHRA/CHM ADVICE: TOPICAL STEROIDS: INTRODUCTION OF NEW LABELLING AND A REMINDER OF THE POSSIBILITY OF SEVERE SIDE EFFECTS, INCLUDING TOPICAL STEROID WITHDRAWAL REACTIONS (MAY 2024)
The risk of serious side-effects, such as Topical Steroid Withdrawal Reactions (TSW), thinning of the skin, and systemic effects, increases with prolonged use of higher potency topical corticosteroids. Regulatory action has resulted in new labelling for topical corticosteroids with information on their potency to assist with patient counselling and correct selection. The MHRA continue to receive reports regarding TSW, particularly associated with eczema treatment; healthcare professionals are reminded to continue to follow the advice issued in 2021 (see above). In addition, healthcare professionals are advised that alternative treatments should be considered if previous discontinuation of a topical corticosteroid was associated with a reaction suspicious of TSW, and that they should support patients living with symptoms of TSW and review treatment plans alongside them.

Healthcare professionals should review the position statement from the National Eczema Society, the British Dermatological Nursing Group, and the British Association of Dermatologists: www.bad.org.uk/topical-steroid-withdrawal-joint-statement/.

The MHRA Patient Safety Leaflet on topical corticosteroids and withdrawal reactions can be used to aid patient counselling: www.gov.uk/guidance/topical-corticosteroids-and-withdrawal-reactions.

- **CONTRA-INDICATIONS** Infection—consult product literature
- **SIDE-EFFECTS** Skin reactions · vision disorders
- **PREGNANCY** Manufacturer advises avoid—toxicity in animal studies.
- **BREAST FEEDING** Manufacturer advises avoid.
- **PRESCRIBING AND DISPENSING INFORMATION** A proprietary brand *Anusol Plus HC*® (ointment and suppositories) is on sale to the public.
- **PATIENT AND CARER ADVICE** If systemic absorption occurs following topical or local use, side-effects applicable to systemic corticosteroids may apply; a patient information leaflet should be supplied and the need for a Steroid Treatment Card and a Steroid Emergency Card considered, see Corticosteroids, general use p. 780.

- **MEDICINAL FORMS** There can be variation in the licensing of different medicines containing the same drug.
Rectal ointment
▸ Anusol-Hc (Church & Dwight UK Ltd)
Hydrocortisone acetate 2.5 mg per 1 gram, Bismuth oxide 8.75 mg per 1 gram, Benzyl benzoate 12.5 mg per 1 gram, Peru Balsam 18.75 mg per 1 gram, Bismuth subgallate 22.5 mg per 1 gram, Zinc oxide 107.5 mg per 1 gram Anusol HC ointment | 30 gram [PoM] £6.00
Suppository
▸ Anusol-Hc (Church & Dwight UK Ltd)
Hydrocortisone acetate 10 mg, Bismuth oxide 24 mg, Benzyl benzoate 33 mg, Peru Balsam 49 mg, Bismuth subgallate 59 mg, Zinc oxide 296 mg Anusol HC suppositories | 12 suppository [PoM] £4.24

Cinchocaine with hydrocortisone

05-Jun-2024

- **INDICATIONS AND DOSE**

PROCTOSEDYL ® **OINTMENT**

Haemorrhoids | Pruritus ani
▸ TO THE SKIN, OR BY RECTUM
▸ Child: Apply twice daily, to be administered morning and night and after a bowel movement. Apply externally or by rectum. Do not use for longer than 7 days
▸ Adult: Apply twice daily, to be administered morning and night and after a bowel movement. Apply externally or by rectum. Do not use for longer than 7 days

PROCTOSEDYL ® **SUPPOSITORIES**

Haemorrhoids | Pruritus ani
▸ BY RECTUM
▸ Child 12-17 years: 1 suppository, insert suppository night and morning and after a bowel movement. Do not use for longer than 7 days

▸ Adult: 1 suppository, insert suppository night and morning and after a bowel movement. Do not use for longer than 7 days

UNIROID-HC® OINTMENT

Haemorrhoids | Pruritus ani

▸ TO THE SKIN, OR BY RECTUM

▸ Child 12–17 years: Apply twice daily, and apply after a bowel movement, apply externally or by rectum, do not use for longer than 7 days

▸ Adult: Apply twice daily, and apply after a bowel movement, apply externally or by rectum, do not use for longer than 7 days

UNIROID-HC® SUPPOSITORIES

Haemorrhoids | Pruritus ani

▸ BY RECTUM

▸ Child 12–17 years: 1 suppository, insert twice daily and after a bowel movement. Do not use for longer than 7 days

▸ Adult: 1 suppository, insert twice daily and after a bowel movement. Do not use for longer than 7 days

---

IMPORTANT SAFETY INFORMATION

MHRA/CHM ADVICE: CORTICOSTEROIDS: RARE RISK OF CENTRAL SEROUS CHORIORETINOPATHY WITH LOCAL AS WELL AS SYSTEMIC ADMINISTRATION (AUGUST 2017)

See Corticosteroids, general use p. 780.

NHS IMPROVEMENT PATIENT SAFETY ALERT: STEROID EMERGENCY CARD TO SUPPORT EARLY RECOGNITION AND TREATMENT OF ADRENAL CRISIS IN ADULTS (AUGUST 2020)

▸ In adults

See Adrenal insufficiency p. 781.

MHRA/CHM ADVICE: TOPICAL CORTICOSTEROIDS: INFORMATION ON THE RISK OF TOPICAL STEROID WITHDRAWAL REACTIONS (SEPTEMBER 2021)

Rarely, long-term continuous or inappropriate use of topical corticosteroids, particularly those of moderate to high potency, can result in the development of rebound flares, reported as dermatitis with intense redness, stinging, and burning that can spread beyond the initial treatment area.

The MHRA advises that the lowest potency topical corticosteroid needed should be used. For patients who are currently on long-term topical corticosteroid treatment, consider reducing potency or frequency of application (or both). Healthcare professionals should also be vigilant for the signs and symptoms of topical corticosteroid withdrawal reactions and review the position statement from the National Eczema Society and British Association of Dermatologists eczema.org/wp-content/uploads/Topical-Steroid-Withdrawal-position-statement.pdf.

Healthcare professionals should inform patients:

● how much should be applied, as under-use can prolong treatment duration;

● how long they should use a topical corticosteroid for, especially on sensitive areas such as the face and genitals;

● to always apply topical corticosteroids as instructed and consult the patient information leaflet provided;

● to seek medical advice before using a topical corticosteroid on a new body area, as some areas of the body are more prone to side-effects;

● to return for medical advice if their skin condition worsens while using topical corticosteroid, and advise them when it would be appropriate to re-treat without a consultation and;

● if their skin worsens within 2 weeks of stopping a topical corticosteroid, treatment should not be started again without consulting their doctor unless they have previously been advised to do so

---

The MHRA advises healthcare professionals to report any suspected adverse effects, via the Yellow Card Scheme, even when the adverse affects occur after stopping corticosteroid treatment.

ADRENAL INSUFFICIENCY CARD (APRIL 2023)

The British Society for Paediatric Endocrinology and Diabetes (BSPED) has developed an Adrenal Insufficiency Card which should be issued to children with adrenal insufficiency and steroid dependence. The card includes a management summary for the emergency treatment of adrenal crisis and sick day dosing, and can be issued by any healthcare professional managing such patients. The BSPED Adrenal Insufficiency Card is available at: www.bsped.org.uk/adrenal-insufficiency.

MHRA/CHM ADVICE: TOPICAL STEROIDS: INTRODUCTION OF NEW LABELLING AND A REMINDER OF THE POSSIBILITY OF SEVERE SIDE EFFECTS, INCLUDING TOPICAL STEROID WITHDRAWAL REACTIONS (MAY 2024)

The risk of serious side-effects, such as Topical Steroid Withdrawal Reactions (TSW), thinning of the skin, and systemic effects, increases with prolonged use of higher potency topical corticosteroids. Regulatory action has resulted in new labelling for topical corticosteroids with information on their potency to assist with patient counselling and correct selection. The MHRA continue to receive reports regarding TSW, particularly associated with eczema treatment; healthcare professionals are reminded to continue to follow the advice issued in 2021 (see above). In addition, healthcare professionals are advised that alternative treatments should be considered if previous discontinuation of a topical corticosteroid was associated with a reaction suspicious of TSW, and that they should support patients living with symptoms of TSW and review treatment plans alongside them.

Healthcare professionals should review the position statement from the National Eczema Society, the British Dermatological Nursing Group, and the British Association of Dermatologists: www.bad.org.uk/topical-steroid-withdrawal-joint-statement/.

The MHRA Patient Safety Leaflet on topical corticosteroids and withdrawal reactions can be used to aid patient counselling: www.gov.uk/guidance/topical-corticosteroids-and-withdrawal-reactions.

● **CONTRA-INDICATIONS** Infection—consult product literature

● **CAUTIONS** Local anaesthetic component can be absorbed through the rectal mucosa (avoid excessive application, particularly in children and infants) · local anaesthetic component may cause sensitisation (use for short periods only—no longer than a few days)

● **SIDE-EFFECTS** Adrenal suppression · skin reactions · vision disorders

● **PATIENT AND CARER ADVICE** If systemic absorption occurs following topical and local use, side-effects applicable to systemic corticosteroids may apply; a patient information leaflet should be supplied and the need for a Steroid Treatment Card and a Steroid Emergency Card considered, see Corticosteroids, general use p. 780.

● **MEDICINAL FORMS** There can be variation in the licensing of different medicines containing the same drug.

Rectal ointment

▸ **Proctosedyl** (Phoenix Labs Ltd)
Cinchocaine hydrochloride 5 mg per 1 gram, Hydrocortisone 5 mg per 1 gram Proctosedyl ointment | 30 gram [PoM] £10.34 DT = £10.34

▸ **Uniroid HC** (Essential Generics Ltd)
Cinchocaine hydrochloride 5 mg per 1 gram, Hydrocortisone 5 mg per 1 gram Uniroid HC ointment | 30 gram [PoM] £5.91 DT = £10.34

1 Gastro-intestinal system

Suppository

▸ **Proctosedyl** (Phoenix Labs Ltd)
**Cinchocaine hydrochloride 5 mg, Hydrocortisone
5 mg** Proctosedyl suppositories | 12 suppository PoM £5.08 DT =
£5.08

▸ **Uniroid HC** (Essential Generics Ltd)
Cinchocaine hydrochloride 5 mg, Hydrocortisone 5 mg Uniroid HC
suppositories | 12 suppository PoM £2.67 DT = £5.08

Cinchocaine with prednisolone
05-Jun-2024

● **INDICATIONS AND DOSE**

Haemorrhoids | Pruritus ani

▸ BY RECTUM USING OINTMENT

▸ Adult: Apply twice daily for 5–7 days, apply 3–4 times a
day on the first day if necessary, then apply once daily
for a few days after symptoms have cleared

▸ BY RECTUM USING SUPPOSITORIES

▸ Adult: 1 suppository daily for 5–7 days, to be inserted
after a bowel movement

Haemorrhoids (severe cases) | Pruritus ani (severe cases)

▸ BY RECTUM USING SUPPOSITORIES

▸ Adult: Initially 1 suppository 2–3 times a day, then
1 suppository daily for a total of 5–7 days, to be
inserted after a bowel movement

IMPORTANT SAFETY INFORMATION

MHRA/CHM ADVICE: CORTICOSTEROIDS: RARE RISK OF CENTRAL
SEROUS CHORIORETINOPATHY WITH LOCAL AS WELL AS SYSTEMIC
ADMINISTRATION (AUGUST 2017)
See Corticosteroids, general use p. 780.

NHS IMPROVEMENT PATIENT SAFETY ALERT: STEROID
EMERGENCY CARD TO SUPPORT EARLY RECOGNITION AND
TREATMENT OF ADRENAL CRISIS IN ADULTS (AUGUST 2020)
See Adrenal insufficiency p. 781.

MHRA/CHM ADVICE: TOPICAL CORTICOSTEROIDS: INFORMATION
ON THE RISK OF TOPICAL STEROID WITHDRAWAL REACTIONS
(SEPTEMBER 2021)
Rarely, long-term continuous or inappropriate use of
topical corticosteroids, particularly those of moderate to
high potency, can result in the development of rebound
flares, reported as dermatitis with intense redness,
stinging, and burning that can spread beyond the initial
treatment area.

The MHRA advises that the lowest potency topical
corticosteroid needed should be used. For patients who
are currently on long-term topical corticosteroid
treatment, consider reducing potency or frequency of
application (or both). Healthcare professionals should
also be vigilant for the signs and symptoms of topical
corticosteroid withdrawal reactions and review the
position statement from the National Eczema Society
and British Association of Dermatologists eczema.org/wp-
content/uploads/Topical-Steroid-Withdrawal-position-
statement.pdf.

Healthcare professionals should inform patients:

● how much should be applied, as under-use can
prolong treatment duration;

● how long they should use a topical corticosteroid for,
especially on sensitive areas such as the face and
genitals;

● to always apply topical corticosteroids as instructed
and consult the patient information leaflet provided;

● to seek medical advice before using a topical
corticosteroid on a new body area, as some areas of the
body are more prone to side-effects;

● to return for medical advice if their skin condition
worsens while using topical corticosteroid, and advise
them when it would be appropriate to re-treat without
a consultation and;

● if their skin worsens within 2 weeks of stopping a
topical corticosteroid, treatment should not be started
again without consulting their doctor unless they have
previously been advised to do so

The MHRA advises healthcare professionals to report
any suspected adverse effects, via the Yellow Card
Scheme, even when the adverse affects occur after
stopping corticosteroid treatment.

MHRA/CHM ADVICE: TOPICAL STEROIDS: INTRODUCTION OF NEW
LABELLING AND A REMINDER OF THE POSSIBILITY OF SEVERE
SIDE EFFECTS, INCLUDING TOPICAL STEROID WITHDRAWAL
REACTIONS (MAY 2024)
The risk of serious side-effects, such as Topical Steroid
Withdrawal Reactions (TSW), thinning of the skin, and
systemic effects, increases with prolonged use of higher
potency topical corticosteroids. Regulatory action has
resulted in new labelling for topical corticosteroids with
information on their potency to assist with patient
counselling and correct selection. The MHRA continue
to receive reports regarding TSW, particularly associated
with eczema treatment; healthcare professionals are
reminded to continue to follow the advice issued in 2021
(see above). In addition, healthcare professionals are
advised that alternative treatments should be considered
if previous discontinuation of a topical corticosteroid
was associated with a reaction suspicious of TSW, and
that they should support patients living with symptoms
of TSW and review treatment plans alongside them.

Healthcare professionals should review the position
statement from the National Eczema Society, the British
Dermatological Nursing Group, and the British
Association of Dermatologists: www.bad.org.uk/topical-
steroid-withdrawal-joint-statement/.

The MHRA Patient Safety Leaflet on topical
corticosteroids and withdrawal reactions can be used to
aid patient counselling: www.gov.uk/guidance/topical-
corticosteroids-and-withdrawal-reactions.

● **CONTRA-INDICATIONS** Infection—consult product
literature

● **CAUTIONS** Local anaesthetic component can be absorbed
through the rectal mucosa (avoid excessive application) ·
local anaesthetic component may cause sensitisation (use
for short periods only—no longer than a few days)

● **PATIENT AND CARER ADVICE** If systemic absorption occurs
following topical and local use, side-effects applicable to
systemic corticosteroids may apply; a patient information
leaflet should be supplied and the need for a Steroid
Treatment Card and a Steroid Emergency Card considered,
see Corticosteroids, general use p. 780.

● **MEDICINAL FORMS** There can be variation in the licensing of
different medicines containing the same drug.

Rectal ointment

▸ **Scheriproct** (Karo Healthcare UK Ltd)
**Prednisolone hexanoate 1.9 mg per 1 gram, Cinchocaine
hydrochloride 5 mg per 1 gram** Scheriproct ointment |
30 gram PoM £3.23 DT = £3.23

Suppository

▸ **Scheriproct** (Karo Healthcare UK Ltd)
**Cinchocaine hydrochloride 1 mg, Prednisolone hexanoate
1.3 mg** Scheriproct suppositories | 12 suppository PoM £1.52 DT =
£1.52

Hydrocortisone with lidocaine
05-Jun-2024

● **INDICATIONS AND DOSE**

Haemorrhoids | Pruritus ani

▶ BY RECTUM USING AEROSOL SPRAY
▸ Adult: 1 spray up to 3 times a day for no longer than 7 days without medical advice, spray once over the affected area
▶ BY RECTUM USING OINTMENT
▸ Adult: Apply several times daily, for short term use only

IMPORTANT SAFETY INFORMATION

MHRA/CHM ADVICE: CORTICOSTEROIDS: RARE RISK OF CENTRAL SEROUS CHORIORETINOPATHY WITH LOCAL AS WELL AS SYSTEMIC ADMINISTRATION (AUGUST 2017)
See Corticosteroids, general use p. 780.

NHS IMPROVEMENT PATIENT SAFETY ALERT: STEROID EMERGENCY CARD TO SUPPORT EARLY RECOGNITION AND TREATMENT OF ADRENAL CRISIS IN ADULTS (AUGUST 2020)
See Adrenal insufficiency p. 781.

MHRA/CHM ADVICE: TOPICAL CORTICOSTEROIDS: INFORMATION ON THE RISK OF TOPICAL STEROID WITHDRAWAL REACTIONS (SEPTEMBER 2021)
Rarely, long-term continuous or inappropriate use of topical corticosteroids, particularly those of moderate to high potency, can result in the development of rebound flares, reported as dermatitis with intense redness, stinging, and burning that can spread beyond the initial treatment area.

The MHRA advises that the lowest potency topical corticosteroid needed should be used. For patients who are currently on long-term topical corticosteroid treatment, consider reducing potency or frequency of application (or both). Healthcare professionals should also be vigilant for the signs and symptoms of topical corticosteroid withdrawal reactions and review the position statement from the National Eczema Society and British Association of Dermatologists eczema.org/wp-content/uploads/Topical-Steroid-Withdrawal-position-statement.pdf.

Healthcare professionals should inform patients:
● how much should be applied, as under-use can prolong treatment duration;
● how long they should use a topical corticosteroid for, especially on sensitive areas such as the face and genitals;
● to always apply topical corticosteroids as instructed and consult the patient information leaflet provided;
● to seek medical advice before using a topical corticosteroid on a new body area, as some areas of the body are more prone to side-effects;
● to return for medical advice if their skin condition worsens while using topical corticosteroid, and advise them when it would be appropriate to re-treat without a consultation and;
● if their skin worsens within 2 weeks of stopping a topical corticosteroid, treatment should not be started again without consulting their doctor unless they have previously been advised to do so

The MHRA advises healthcare professionals to report any suspected adverse effects, via the Yellow Card Scheme, even when the adverse affects occur after stopping corticosteroid treatment.

MHRA/CHM ADVICE: TOPICAL STEROIDS: INTRODUCTION OF NEW LABELLING AND A REMINDER OF THE POSSIBILITY OF SEVERE SIDE EFFECTS, INCLUDING TOPICAL STEROID WITHDRAWAL REACTIONS (MAY 2024)
The risk of serious side-effects, such as Topical Steroid Withdrawal Reactions (TSW), thinning of the skin, and systemic effects, increases with prolonged use of higher potency topical corticosteroids. Regulatory action has resulted in new labelling for topical corticosteroids with information on their potency to assist with patient counselling and correct selection. The MHRA continue to receive reports regarding TSW, particularly associated with eczema treatment; healthcare professionals are reminded to continue to follow the advice issued in 2021 (see above). In addition, healthcare professionals are advised that alternative treatments should be considered if previous discontinuation of a topical corticosteroid was associated with a reaction suspicious of TSW, and that they should support patients living with symptoms of TSW and review treatment plans alongside them.

Healthcare professionals should review the position statement from the National Eczema Society, the British Dermatological Nursing Group, and the British Association of Dermatologists: www.bad.org.uk/topical-steroid-withdrawal-joint-statement/.

The MHRA Patient Safety Leaflet on topical corticosteroids and withdrawal reactions can be used to aid patient counselling: www.gov.uk/guidance/topical-corticosteroids-and-withdrawal-reactions.

● **CONTRA-INDICATIONS** Infection—consult product literature

● **CAUTIONS** Local anaesthetic component can be absorbed through the rectal mucosa (avoid excessive application) · local anaesthetic component may cause sensitisation (use for short periods only—no longer than a few days)

● **SIDE-EFFECTS** Adrenal suppression · paraesthesia · skin reactions · vision disorders

● **PATIENT AND CARER ADVICE** If systemic absorption occurs following topical and local use, side-effects applicable to systemic corticosteroids may apply; a patient information leaflet should be supplied and the need for a Steroid Treatment Card and a Steroid Emergency Card considered, see Corticosteroids, general use p. 780.

● **MEDICINAL FORMS** There can be variation in the licensing of different medicines containing the same drug.

Cutaneous ointment
▸ Xyloproct (Aspen Pharma Trading Ltd)
  Hydrocortisone acetate 2.75 mg per 1 gram, Lidocaine 50 mg per 1 gram Xyloproct 5%/0.275% ointment | 20 gram PoM £4.19 DT = £4.19

SCLEROSANTS

Phenol

● **INDICATIONS AND DOSE**

Haemorrhoids (particularly when unprolapsed)
▶ BY SUBMUCOSAL INJECTION
▸ Adult: 2–3 mL, dose (using phenol 5%) to be injected into the submucosal layer at the base of the pile; several injections may be given at different sites, max. total injected 10 mL at any one time

● **SIDE-EFFECTS** Abdominal sepsis · abscess · dizziness · erectile dysfunction · fever · hepatitis · increased risk of infection · injection site necrosis · ulcer · urinary disorders

● **PRESCRIBING AND DISPENSING INFORMATION** When prepared extemporaneously, the BP states Oily Phenol Injection, BP consists of phenol 5% in a suitable fixed oil.

● **MEDICINAL FORMS** There can be variation in the licensing of different medicines containing the same drug. Forms available from special-order manufacturers include: solution for injection

Solution for injection
▸ Phenol (Non-proprietary)
  Phenol 50 mg per 1 ml Oily phenol 5% solution for injection 5ml ampoules | 10 ampoule PoM £93.80-£140.60 DT = £113.50

Gastro-intestinal system · 1

11   Stoma care

Stoma care

17-Mar-2021

Description of condition

A stoma is an artificial opening on the abdomen to divert flow of faeces or urine into an external pouch located outside of the body. This procedure may be temporary or permanent. Colostomy and ileostomy are the most common forms of stoma but a gastrostomy, jejunostomy, duodenostomy, or caecostomy may also be performed. Understanding the type and extent of surgical intervention in each patient is crucial in managing the patient's pharmaceutical needs correctly.

Prescribing in patients with stoma

Prescribing for patients with a stoma calls for special care due to modifications in drug delivery, resulting in a higher risk of sub-optimal absorption. The following is a brief account of some of the main points to be borne in mind.

Enteric-coated and modified-release medicines are **unsuitable**, particularly in patients with an ileostomy, as there may be insufficient release of the active ingredient. Preparation forms with quick dissolution and absorption should be used. Liquids, capsules, and uncoated or soluble tablets are usually well absorbed. When a solid-dose form such as a capsule or a tablet is given, the contents of the stoma bag should be checked for any remnants.

Preparations containing sorbitol as an excipient may have a laxative effect.

Opioid **analgesics** may cause constipation in colostomy patients. Aspirin and NSAIDs may cause gastric irritation and bleeding; faecal output should be monitored for traces of blood.

The effect of **antacids** in patients with a stoma is dependent on the class of antacids and the type of stoma. Calcium-containing antacids can cause constipation and magnesium-containing antacids can cause diarrhoea, especially in patients with an ileostomy as they can cause osmotic diarrhoea. The aluminium hydroxide antacids can cause constipation and may be of concern in colostomy patients.

The **antidiarrhoeal** drugs, loperamide hydrochloride p. 74 and codeine phosphate p. 517, reduce intestinal motility and decrease water and sodium output from an ileostomy. Loperamide hydrochloride circulates through the enterohepatic circulation, which is disrupted in patients with a short bowel.

Patients with a stoma are particularly susceptible to fluid and sodium depletion which can often lead to hypokalaemia; potassium supplements are not usually required. Hypokalaemia may cause an increased sensitivity to digoxin p. 125.

Diuretics may cause excessive dehydration in patients with an ileostomy or with urostomy and potassium depletion may easily occur; potassium-sparing diuretics are available.

Iron preparations may cause diarrhoea in ileostomy patients, constipation in colostomy patients, and sore skin if output leaks; stools may also appear black. Parenteral iron is licensed for use in patients who are unable to tolerate gastro-intestinal adverse effects of oral iron.

Laxatives may cause rapid and severe loss of water and electrolytes in ileostomy patients and are, therefore, used with caution. In colostomy patients, bulk-forming laxatives may provide more benefit than a stimulant laxative; they aid in the formation of solid stools and promote regularity. Stool softeners can also help with constipation.

Liquid formulations of potassium supplements are preferred to modified-release formulations; to avoid osmotic diarrhoea, the daily dose is split into divided doses.

Care of stoma

Patients and their carers are usually given advice about the use of cleansing agents, protective creams, lotions, deodorants, or sealants whilst in hospital, either by the surgeon or by stoma care nurses. Voluntary organisations offer help and support to patients with stoma.

Chapter 2
Cardiovascular system

CONTENTS

1   Arrhythmias

Arrhythmias
06-Jun-2023

Overview

Management of an arrhythmia requires precise diagnosis of the type of arrhythmia, and electrocardiography is essential; underlying causes such as heart failure require appropriate treatment.

Ectopic beats

If ectopic beats are spontaneous and the patient has a normal heart, treatment is rarely required and reassurance to the patient will often suffice. If they are particularly troublesome, beta-blockers are sometimes effective and may be safer than other suppressant drugs.

Atrial fibrillation

Treatment of patients with atrial fibrillation aims to reduce symptoms and prevent complications, especially stroke. All patients with atrial fibrillation should be assessed for their risk of stroke and thromboembolism. Atrial fibrillation can be managed by either controlling the ventricular rate ('rate control') or by attempting to restore and maintain sinus rhythm ('rhythm control'). If treatment fails to control symptoms or if symptoms reoccur after cardioversion and specialised management is required, referral should be made within 4 weeks. Where drug treatment has failed to control the symptoms of atrial fibrillation or is unsuitable, ablation strategies can be considered.

Acute presentation

[EvGr] All patients with life-threatening haemodynamic instability caused by new-onset atrial fibrillation should undergo emergency electrical cardioversion, without delaying to achieve anticoagulation.

In patients presenting acutely but without life-threatening haemodynamic instability, rate or rhythm control can be offered if the onset of arrhythmia is less than 48 hours; rate control is preferred if onset is more than 48 hours or is uncertain. ⒶIf urgent rate control is required, a beta-blocker can be given intravenously; a rate-limiting calcium channel blocker such as verapamil hydrochloride p. 191 (if left ventricular ejection fraction (LVEF) is $\geq$40%) may also be given. [EvGr] In patients with suspected concomitant acute decompensated heart failure, calcium-channel blockers should be avoided and senior specialist advice sought on the use of beta-blockers.

Consideration of pharmacological or electrical cardioversion should be based on clinical circumstances in patients with new-onset atrial fibrillation who are to be treated with a rhythm-control strategy. If pharmacological cardioversion has been agreed, flecainide acetate p. 119 (if no structural or ischaemic heart disease present) or amiodarone hydrochloride p. 120 can be used. Ⓐ

Cardioversion

Sinus rhythm can be restored by electrical cardioversion or by pharmacological cardioversion with an anti-arrhythmic drug such as flecainide acetate or amiodarone hydrochloride. [EvGr] If atrial fibrillation has been present for more than 48 hours, electrical cardioversion is preferred to pharmacological cardioversion, but should be delayed until the patient has been fully anticoagulated for at least 3 weeks. If this is not possible, a left atrial thrombus should be ruled out and parenteral anticoagulation (heparin) commenced immediately before cardioversion; oral anticoagulation should be given after cardioversion and continued for at least 4 weeks. During the period prior to cardioversion, offer rate control as appropriate. Amiodarone hydrochloride started 4 weeks before and continued for up to 12 months after electrical cardioversion to maintain sinus rhythm, may also be considered. Ⓐ

Drug treatment

[EvGr] *Rate control* is the preferred first-line treatment strategy for atrial fibrillation except in patients with new-onset atrial fibrillation, with atrial flutter suitable for an ablation strategy, with atrial fibrillation with a reversible cause, or with heart failure primarily caused by atrial fibrillation, or if rhythm control is more suitable based on clinical judgement. Ventricular rate can be controlled with a standard beta-blocker (not sotalol hydrochloride), or with a rate-limiting calcium channel blocker such as diltiazem hydrochloride p. 185 [unlicensed indication] or verapamil hydrochloride as monotherapy. Choice of drug should be based on individual symptoms, heart rate, comorbidities, and patient preference; Ⓐ for guidance on the use of rate-control drugs in patients with concomitant heart failure, see Chronic heart failure p. 222.

[EvGr] Digoxin p. 125 monotherapy should only be considered for initial rate control in patients with non-paroxysmal atrial fibrillation who are predominantly sedentary, or in those where other rate-limiting drugs are unsuitable.

When monotherapy fails to adequately control the ventricular rate, consider combination therapy with any 2 of the following drugs: a beta-blocker, digoxin, diltiazem hydrochloride. If symptoms are not controlled with a combination of 2 drugs, a rhythm-control strategy should be considered. Ⓐ If ventricular function is diminished (LVEF <40%), the combination of a beta-blocker (that is licensed for use in heart failure) and digoxin is preferred. Digoxin is also used when atrial fibrillation is accompanied by congestive heart failure.

[EvGr] If drug treatment is required to maintain sinus rhythm ('rhythm control') post-cardioversion, consider a standard beta-blocker (not sotalol hydrochloride) as first-line treatment. If a standard beta-blocker is not appropriate or is ineffective, consider an alternative anti-arrhythmic drug (such as amiodarone hydrochloride, flecainide acetate, propafenone hydrochloride p. 119, or sotalol hydrochloride p. 124) taking into consideration patient comorbidities: flecainide acetate and propafenone hydrochloride should be avoided in patients with known ischaemic or structural heart disease and, for patients with left ventricular impairment or heart failure, consider amiodarone hydrochloride. Dronedarone p. 122 may be considered as a second-line treatment option in patients with persistent or paroxysmal atrial fibrillation. In selected patients with infrequent episodes of symptomatic paroxysmal atrial fibrillation, sinus rhythm can be restored using the 'pill-in-the-pocket' approach; this involves the patient taking an oral anti-arrhythmic drug to self-treat an episode of atrial fibrillation when it occurs. Ⓐ

Anticoagulation and stroke prevention

For guidance on the management of patients with stroke and atrial fibrillation, see Stroke p. 137.

Anticoagulants are indicated during cardioversion procedures, for further information, see *Cardioversion*

[EvGr] All patients with atrial fibrillation (including those with continuing risk of arrhythmia recurrence after cardioversion back to sinus rhythm or catheter ablation) should be assessed for their risk of stroke and the need for thromboprophylaxis; this needs to be balanced with the patient's risk of bleeding. Anticoagulation treatment should not be withheld solely because of the patient's age or risk of falls. The decision to stop anticoagulation should be based on patient preference and a reassessment of the patient's stroke and bleeding risk, and not solely due to the arrhythmia no longer being detectable. Prior to and during anticoagulation treatment, assess stroke risk using the CHA_2DS_2-VASc risk tool and bleeding risk using the ORBIT bleeding risk tool (the ORBIT risk tool has a higher accuracy in predicting absolute bleeding risk than other risk tools, however, these may be used if the ORBIT tool is inaccessible). Risk factors for stroke taken into account by CHA_2DS_2-VASc include age, sex, and prior history of congestive heart failure, hypertension, stroke, transient ischaemic attacks (TIA), thromboembolic events, vascular disease, or diabetes mellitus. Anticoagulation should be offered for stroke prevention to all patients with a CHA_2DS_2-VASc score of 2 or above, and be considered in men with a CHA_2DS_2-VASc score of 1; these scores should be reviewed at least annually. Patients with a very low risk of stroke (CHA_2DS_2-VASc score of 0 for men or 1 for women) do not require anticoagulation for stroke prevention, but should have their stroke risk reviewed when they reach 65 years of age, or, at any age, if they develop diabetes, heart failure, peripheral arterial disease, coronary heart disease, stroke, TIA, or systemic thromboembolism. For those not taking an anticoagulant because of bleeding risk or other factors, review risks annually.

Parenteral anticoagulation (heparin) should be offered to patients with new-onset atrial fibrillation who are receiving subtherapeutic or no anticoagulation therapy, until assessment is made and appropriate anticoagulation is started. Oral anticoagulation should be offered to patients with a confirmed diagnosis of atrial fibrillation in whom a stable sinus rhythm has not been successfully restored within 48 hours of onset; or where their risk of stroke outweighs their risk of bleeding; or who have had, or are at high risk of, recurrence of atrial fibrillation such as those with structural heart disease, a prolonged history of atrial fibrillation (more than 12 months), or a history of failed attempts at cardioversion.

Oral anticoagulation with a direct-acting oral anticoagulant such as apixaban p. 145, dabigatran etexilate p. 159, edoxaban p. 147, or rivaroxaban p. 149, is recommended in non-valvular atrial fibrillation. If direct-acting oral anticoagulants are contra-indicated or unsuitable, offer a vitamin K antagonist such as warfarin sodium p. 165. For patients already taking a vitamin K antagonist and who are stable, continue current treatment and discuss the option of switching treatment at their next clinic review (taking into account the patients' time in therapeutic range). The use of aspirin p. 142 monotherapy solely for stroke prevention in patients with atrial fibrillation is not recommended. Ⓐ For further information on the use of anticoagulants for stroke prevention, see NICE guideline: **Atrial fibrillation: diagnosis and management** (see *Useful resources*).

[EvGr] If anticoagulant treatment is contra-indicated or not tolerated, left atrial appendage occlusion can be considered. Ⓐ

Atrial flutter

Like atrial fibrillation, treatment options for atrial flutter involve either controlling the ventricular rate or attempting to restore and maintain sinus rhythm. However, atrial flutter generally responds less well to drug treatment than atrial fibrillation.

Control of the ventricular rate is usually an interim measure pending restoration of sinus rhythm. Ventricular rate can be controlled by administration of a beta-blocker, diltiazem hydrochloride p. 185 [unlicensed indication], or verapamil hydrochloride p. 191; an intravenous beta-blocker or verapamil hydrochloride is preferred for rapid control. Digoxin p. 125 can be added if rate control remains inadequate, and may be particularly useful in those with heart failure.

Conversion to sinus rhythm can be achieved by electrical cardioversion (by cardiac pacing or direct current), pharmacological cardioversion, or catheter ablation. If the duration of atrial flutter is unknown, or it has lasted for over 48 hours, cardioversion should not be attempted until the patient has been fully anticoagulated for at least 3 weeks; if this is not possible, parenteral anticoagulation should be commenced and a left atrial thrombus ruled out immediately before cardioversion; oral anticoagulation should be given after cardioversion and continued for at least 4 weeks.

Direct current cardioversion is usually the treatment of choice when rapid conversion to sinus rhythm is necessary (e.g. when atrial flutter is associated with haemodynamic compromise); catheter ablation is preferred for the treatment of recurrent atrial flutter. There is a limited role for anti-arrhythmic drugs as their use is not always successful. Flecainide acetate p. 119 or propafenone hydrochloride p. 119 can slow atrial flutter, resulting in 1:1 conduction to the ventricles, and should therefore be prescribed in conjunction with a ventricular rate controlling drug such as a beta-blocker, diltiazem hydrochloride [unlicensed indication], or verapamil hydrochloride. Amiodarone hydrochloride p. 120 can be used when other drug treatments are contra-indicated or ineffective.

All patients should be assessed for their risk of stroke and the need for thromboprophylaxis; the choice of anticoagulant is based on the same criteria as for atrial fibrillation.

Paroxysmal supraventricular tachycardia

This will often terminate spontaneously or with reflex vagal stimulation such as a Valsalva manoeuvre, immersing the face in ice-cold water, or carotid sinus massage; such manoeuvres should be performed with ECG monitoring.

If the effects of reflex vagal stimulation are transient or ineffective, or if the arrhythmia is causing severe symptoms, intravenous adenosine p. 122 should be given. If adenosine is ineffective or contra-indicated, intravenous verapamil hydrochloride is an alternative, but it should be avoided in patients recently treated with beta-blockers.

Failure to terminate paroxysmal supraventricular tachycardia with reflex vagal stimulation or drug treatment may suggest an arrhythmia of atrial origin, such as focal atrial tachycardia or atrial flutter.

Treatment with direct current cardioversion is needed in haemodynamically unstable patients or when the above measures have failed to restore sinus rhythm (and an alternative diagnosis has not been found).

Recurrent episodes of paroxysmal supraventricular tachycardia can be treated by catheter ablation, or prevented with drugs such as diltiazem hydrochloride, verapamil hydrochloride, beta-blockers including sotalol hydrochloride p. 124, flecainide acetate or propafenone hydrochloride.

Arrhythmias after myocardial infarction

In patients with a paroxysmal tachycardia or rapid irregularity of the pulse it is best not to administer an anti-arrhythmic until an ECG record has been obtained. Bradycardia, particularly if complicated by hypotension, should be treated with an intravenous dose of atropine sulfate p. 1526 the dose may be repeated if necessary. If there is a risk of asystole, or if the patient is unstable and has failed to respond to atropine sulfate, adrenaline/epinephrine p. 256 should be given by intravenous infusion, and the dose adjusted according to response.

For further advice, refer to the most recent recommendations of the Resuscitation Council (UK) available at www.resus.org.uk.

Ventricular tachycardia

Pulseless ventricular tachycardia or ventricular fibrillation require resuscitation (see Life support algorithm (image) Inside back cover).

Patients with unstable sustained ventricular tachycardia, who continue to deteriorate with signs of hypotension or reduced cardiac output, should receive direct current cardioversion to restore sinus rhythm. If this fails, intravenous amiodarone hydrochloride should be administered and direct current cardioversion repeated.

Patients with sustained ventricular tachycardia who are haemodynamically stable can be treated with intravenous anti-arrhythmic drugs. Amiodarone hydrochloride is the preferred drug. Flecainide acetate, propafenone hydrochloride, and, although less effective, lidocaine hydrochloride p. 117 have all been used. If sinus rhythm is not restored, direct current cardioversion or pacing should be considered. Catheter ablation is an alternative if cessation of the arrhythmia is not urgent. Non-sustained ventricular tachycardia can be treated with a beta-blocker.

All patients presenting with ventricular tachycardia should be referred to a specialist. Following restoration of sinus rhythm, patients who remain at high risk of cardiac arrest will require maintenance therapy. Most patients will be treated with an implantable cardioverter defibrillator. Beta-blockers or sotalol hydrochloride p. 124 (in place of a standard beta-blocker), or amiodarone hydrochloride p. 120 (in combination with a standard beta-blocker), can be used in addition to the device in some patients; alternatively, they can be used alone when use of an implantable cardioverter defibrillator is not appropriate.

Torsade de pointes

Torsade de pointes is a form of ventricular tachycardia associated with a long QT syndrome (usually drug-induced, but other factors including hypokalaemia, severe bradycardia, and genetic predisposition are also implicated). Episodes are usually self-limiting, but are frequently recurrent and can cause impairment or loss of consciousness. If not controlled, the arrhythmia can progress to ventricular fibrillation and sometimes death. Intravenous infusion of magnesium sulfate p. 1193 is usually effective. A beta-blocker (but not sotalol hydrochloride) and atrial (or ventricular) pacing can be considered. Anti-arrhythmics can further prolong the QT interval, thus worsening the condition.

Anti-arrhythmic drugs

Anti-arrhythmic drugs can be classified clinically into those that act on supraventricular arrhythmias (e.g. verapamil hydrochloride p. 191), those that act on both supraventricular and ventricular arrhythmias (e.g. amiodarone hydrochloride), and those that act on ventricular arrhythmias (e.g. lidocaine hydrochloride p. 117).

Anti-arrhythmic drugs can also be classified according to their effects on the electrical behaviour of myocardial cells during activity (the Vaughan Williams classification) although this classification is of less clinical significance:

- Class I: membrane stabilising drugs (e.g. lidocaine, flecainide)
- Class II: beta-blockers
- Class III: amiodarone; sotalol (also Class II)
- Class IV: calcium-channel blockers (includes verapamil but not dihydropyridines)

The negative inotropic effects of anti-arrhythmic drugs tend to be additive. Therefore special care should be taken if two or more are used, especially if myocardial function is impaired. Most drugs that are effective in countering arrhythmias can also provoke them in some circumstances; moreover, hypokalaemia enhances the arrhythmogenic (pro-arrhythmic) effect of many drugs.

Supraventricular arrhythmias

Adenosine p. 122 is usually the treatment of choice for terminating paroxysmal supraventricular tachycardia. As it has a very short duration of action (half-life only about 8 to 10 seconds, but prolonged in those taking dipyridamole p. 144), most side-effects are short lived. Unlike verapamil hydrochloride, adenosine can be used after a beta-blocker. Verapamil hydrochloride may be preferable to adenosine in asthma.

Oral administration of a **cardiac glycoside** (such as digoxin p. 125) slows the ventricular response in cases of atrial fibrillation and atrial flutter. However, intravenous infusion of digoxin is rarely effective for rapid control of ventricular rate. Cardiac glycosides are contra-indicated in supraventricular arrhythmias associated with accessory conducting pathways (e.g. Wolff- Parkinson-White syndrome).

Verapamil hydrochloride is usually effective for supraventricular tachycardias. An initial intravenous dose (**important:** serious beta-blocker interaction hazard) may be followed by oral treatment; hypotension may occur with large doses. It should not be used for tachyarrhythmias where the QRS complex is wide (i.e. broad complex) unless a supraventricular origin has been established beyond reasonable doubt. It is also contra-indicated in atrial fibrillation or atrial flutter associated with accessory conducting pathways (e.g. Wolff-Parkinson-White syndrome). It should not be used in children with arrhythmias without specialist advice; some supraventricular arrhythmias in childhood can be accelerated by verapamil hydrochloride with dangerous consequences.

Intravenous administration of a **beta-blocker** such as esmolol hydrochloride p. 182 or propranolol hydrochloride p. 178, can achieve rapid control of the ventricular rate.

Drugs for both supraventricular and ventricular arrhythmias include amiodarone hydrochloride, **beta-blockers**, disopyramide below, flecainide acetate p. 119, **procainamide** (available from 'special-order' manufacturers or specialist importing companies), and propafenone hydrochloride p. 119.

Supraventricular and ventricular arrhythmias

Amiodarone hydrochloride is used in the treatment of arrhythmias, particularly when other drugs are ineffective or contra-indicated. It can be used for paroxysmal supraventricular, nodal and ventricular tachycardias, atrial fibrillation and flutter, and ventricular fibrillation. It can also be used for tachyarrhythmias associated with Wolff-Parkinson-White syndrome. It should be initiated only under hospital or specialist supervision. Amiodarone hydrochloride may be given by intravenous infusion as well as by mouth, and has the advantage of causing little or no myocardial depression. Unlike oral amiodarone hydrochloride, intravenous amiodarone hydrochloride acts relatively rapidly.

Intravenous injection of amiodarone hydrochloride is given in cardiopulmonary resuscitation for ventricular fibrillation or pulseless tachycardia refractory to defibrillation.

Amiodarone hydrochloride has a very long half-life (extending to several weeks) and only needs to be given once daily (but high doses can cause nausea unless divided). Many weeks or months may be required to achieve steady-state plasma-amiodarone concentration; this is particularly important when drug interactions are likely.

Beta-blockers act as anti-arrhythmic drugs principally by attenuating the effects of the sympathetic system on automaticity and conductivity within the heart. Sotalol hydrochloride has a role in the management of ventricular arrhythmias.

Disopyramide can be given by intravenous injection to control arrhythmias after myocardial infarction (including those not responding to lidocaine hydrochloride), but it impairs cardiac contractility. Oral administration of disopyramide is useful, but it has an antimuscarinic effect which limits its use in patients susceptible to angle-closure glaucoma or with prostatic hyperplasia.

Flecainide acetate belongs to the same general class as lidocaine hydrochloride and may be of value for serious symptomatic ventricular arrhythmias. It may also be indicated for junctional re-entry tachycardias and for paroxysmal atrial fibrillation. However, it can precipitate serious arrhythmias in a small minority of patients (including those with otherwise normal hearts).

Propafenone hydrochloride is used for the prophylaxis and treatment of ventricular arrhythmias and also for some supraventricular arrhythmias. It has complex mechanisms of action, including weak beta-blocking activity (therefore caution is needed in obstructive airways disease—contra-indicated if severe).

Drugs for supraventricular arrhythmias include adenosine, **cardiac glycosides**, and verapamil hydrochloride. Drugs for ventricular arrhythmias include lidocaine hydrochloride.

Procainamide is available from 'special-order' manufacturers or specialist importing companies. Mexiletine p. 118 can be used for life-threatening ventricular

arrhythmias; procainamide is given by intravenous injection to control ventricular arrhythmias.

Ventricular arrhythmias

Intravenous lidocaine hydrochloride can be used for the treatment of ventricular tachycardia in haemodynamically stable patients, and ventricular fibrillation and pulseless ventricular tachycardia in cardiac arrest refractory to defibrillation, however it is no longer the anti-arrhythmic drug of first choice.

Drugs for both supraventricular and ventricular arrhythmias include amiodarone hydrochloride, **beta-blockers**, disopyramide, flecainide acetate, **procainamide** (available from 'special- order' manufacturers or specialist importing companies), and propafenone hydrochloride.

Mexiletine can be used for the treatment of life-threatening ventricular arrhythmias.

Useful resources

Atrial fibrillation: diagnosis and management. National Institute for Health and Care Excellence. NICE guideline NG196. June 2021.
www.nice.org.uk/guidance/ng196

> **Other drugs used for Arrhythmias** Acebutolol, p. 179 · Metoprolol tartrate, p. 182 · Nadolol, p. 177

ANTIARRHYTHMICS 〉 CLASS IA

Disopyramide

29-Jun-2021

● **INDICATIONS AND DOSE**

Prevention and treatment of ventricular and supraventricular arrhythmias, including after myocardial infarction | Maintenance of sinus rhythm after cardioversion

▸ BY MOUTH USING IMMEDIATE-RELEASE MEDICINES
▸ Adult: 300–800 mg daily in divided doses
▸ BY MOUTH USING MODIFIED-RELEASE MEDICINES
▸ Adult: 250–375 mg every 12 hours

● **CONTRA-INDICATIONS** Bundle-branch block associated with first-degree AV block · pre-existing long QT syndrome · second- and third-degree AV block or bifascicular block (unless pacemaker fitted) · severe heart failure (unless secondary to arrhythmia) · severe sinus node dysfunction

● **CAUTIONS** Atrial flutter or atrial tachycardia with partial block · avoid in Acute porphyrias p. 1202 · elderly · heart failure (avoid if severe) · myasthenia gravis · prostatic enlargement · structural heart disease · susceptibility to angle-closure glaucoma

● **INTERACTIONS** → Appendix 1: antiarrhythmics

● **SIDE-EFFECTS** Abdominal pain · appetite decreased · arrhythmias · cardiac conduction disorders · cardiogenic shock · cognitive disorder · constipation · diarrhoea · dizziness · dry mouth · erectile dysfunction · headache · heart failure · hyperhidrosis · hypoglycaemia · hypotension · jaundice cholestatic · nausea · neutropenia · psychotic disorder · QT interval prolongation · rash · urinary disorders · vision disorders · vomiting

● **PREGNANCY** Manufacturer advises use only if potential benefit outweighs risk; may induce labour if used in third trimester.

● **BREAST FEEDING** Present in milk—use only if essential. **Monitoring** Monitor infant for antimuscarinic effects.

● **HEPATIC IMPAIRMENT** For *immediate-release capsules*, manufacturer advises caution (risk of increased half-life). For *modified-release tablets*, manufacturer advises avoid. **Dose adjustments** For *immediate-release capsules*, manufacturer advises consider dose reduction.

2

Cardiovascular system

- **RENAL IMPAIRMENT** [EvGr] Avoid *modified-release tablets.* ⟨M⟩

  Dose adjustments [EvGr] For *immediate-release capsules,* reduce dose by increasing dose interval; adjust according to response. ⟨M⟩

- **MONITORING REQUIREMENTS**
  ‣ Monitor for hypotension, hypoglycaemia, ventricular tachycardia, ventricular fibrillation or torsade de pointes (discontinue if occur).
  ‣ Monitor serum potassium.

- **MEDICINAL FORMS** There can be variation in the licensing of different medicines containing the same drug. Forms available from special-order manufacturers include: oral capsule, oral suspension, oral solution

  Modified-release tablet
  CAUTIONARY AND ADVISORY LABELS 25
  ‣ Rythmodan Retard (Neon Healthcare Ltd)
  Disopyramide (as Disopyramide phosphate) 250 mg Rythmodan Retard 250mg tablets | 60 tablet [PoM] £32.08 DT = £32.08

  Oral capsule
  ‣ Rythmodan (Neon Healthcare Ltd)
  Disopyramide 100 mg Rythmodan 100mg capsules | 84 capsule [PoM] £14.14 DT = £14.14

ANTIARRHYTHMICS ⟩ CLASS IB

Lidocaine hydrochloride
10-Nov-2020

(Lignocaine hydrochloride)

- **INDICATIONS AND DOSE**

Cardiopulmonary resuscitation (as an alternative if amiodarone is not available)
‣ BY INTRAVENOUS INJECTION
‣ Adult: 1 mg/kg, do not exceed 3 mg/kg over the first hour

Ventricular arrhythmias, especially after myocardial infarction in patients without gross circulatory impairment
‣ INITIALLY BY INTRAVENOUS INJECTION
‣ Adult: 100 mg, to be given as a bolus dose over a few minutes, followed immediately by (by intravenous infusion) 4 mg/minute for 30 minutes, then (by intravenous infusion) 2 mg/minute for 2 hours, then (by intravenous infusion) 1 mg/minute, reduce concentration further if infusion continued beyond 24 hours (ECG monitoring and specialist advice for infusion), following intravenous injection lidocaine has a short duration of action (lasting for 15–20 minutes). If an intravenous infusion is not immediately available the initial intravenous injection of 100 mg can be repeated if necessary once or twice at intervals of not less than 10 minutes

Ventricular arrhythmias, especially after myocardial infarction in lighter patients or those whose circulation is severely impaired
‣ INITIALLY BY INTRAVENOUS INJECTION
‣ Adult: Initially 50 mg, to be given as a bolus dose over a few minutes, followed immediately by (by intravenous infusion) 4 mg/minute for 30 minutes, then (by intravenous infusion) 2 mg/minute for 2 hours, then (by intravenous infusion) 1 mg/minute, reduce concentration further if infusion continued beyond 24 hours (ECG monitoring and specialist advice for infusion), following intravenous injection lidocaine has a short duration of action (lasting for 15–20 minutes). If an intravenous infusion is not immediately available the initial intravenous injection of 50 mg can be repeated if necessary once or twice at intervals of not less than 10 minutes

- **CONTRA-INDICATIONS** All grades of atrioventricular block · severe myocardial depression · sino-atrial disorders

- **CAUTIONS** Acute porphyrias p. 1202 (consider infusion with glucose for its anti-porphyrinogenic effects) · congestive cardiac failure (consider lower dose) · post cardiac surgery (consider lower dose)

- **INTERACTIONS** → Appendix 1: antiarrhythmics

- **SIDE-EFFECTS** Anxiety · arrhythmias · atrioventricular block · cardiac arrest · circulatory collapse · confusion · dizziness · drowsiness · euphoric mood · headache · hypotension (may lead to cardiac arrest) · loss of consciousness · methaemoglobinaemia · muscle twitching · myocardial contractility decreased · nausea · neurological effects · nystagmus · pain · psychosis · respiratory disorders · seizure · sensation abnormal · temperature sensation altered · tinnitus · tremor · vision blurred · vomiting

SIDE-EFFECTS, FURTHER INFORMATION
Methaemoglobinaemia Methylthioninium chloride is licensed for the acute symptomatic treatment of drug-induced methaemoglobinaemia.

- **PREGNANCY** Crosses the placenta but not known to be harmful in *animal* studies—use if benefit outweighs risk.

- **BREAST FEEDING** Present in milk but amount too small to be harmful.

- **HEPATIC IMPAIRMENT** Manufacturer advises caution (risk of increased exposure).
  Dose adjustments Manufacturer advises slower infusion rate.

- **RENAL IMPAIRMENT** Possible accumulation of lidocaine and active metabolite; caution in severe impairment.

- **MONITORING REQUIREMENTS** Monitor ECG and have resuscitation facilities available.

- **MEDICINAL FORMS** There can be variation in the licensing of different medicines containing the same drug. Forms available from special-order manufacturers include: solution for injection

  Solution for injection
  ‣ Lidocaine hydrochloride (Non-proprietary)
  Lidocaine hydrochloride 5 mg per 1 ml Lidocaine 50mg/10ml (0.5%) solution for injection ampoules | 10 ampoule [PoM] £10.00 DT = £10.00
  Lidocaine hydrochloride 10 mg per 1 ml Lidocaine 100mg/10ml (1%) solution for injection Mini-Plasco ampoules | 20 ampoule [PoM] £13.80
  Lidocaine 100mg/10ml (1%) solution for injection ampoules | 10 ampoule [PoM] £5.00-£7.00 DT = £7.00 | 20 ampoule [PoM] £14.00-£234.00 (Hospital only)
  Lidocaine 200mg/20ml (1%) solution for injection vials | 10 vial [PoM] £26.40 DT = £26.40
  Lidocaine 200mg/20ml (1%) solution for injection ampoules | 1 ampoule [PoM] £25.07 (Hospital only) | 10 ampoule [PoM] £10.00-£14.00 DT = £14.00 | 20 ampoule [PoM] £19.00-£501.40 (Hospital only)
  Lidocaine 50mg/5ml (1%) solution for injection ampoules | 1 ampoule [PoM] £8.28 (Hospital only) | 10 ampoule [PoM] £3.10-£6.23 DT = £6.23 | 20 ampoule [PoM] £12.40-£165.60 (Hospital only)
  Lidocaine 20mg/2ml (1%) solution for injection ampoules | 10 ampoule [PoM] £5.03 DT = £5.03
  Lidocaine 50mg/5ml (1%) solution for injection Mini-Plasco ampoules | 20 ampoule [PoM] £8.05
  Lidocaine hydrochloride 20 mg per 1 ml Lidocaine 100mg/5ml (2%) solution for injection ampoules | 10 ampoule [PoM] £3.80-£6.00 DT = £6.00 | 20 ampoule [PoM] £15.60-£165.00 (Hospital only)
  Lidocaine 400mg/20ml (2%) solution for injection vials | 10 vial [PoM] £27.50 DT = £27.50
  Lidocaine 40mg/2ml (2%) solution for injection ampoules | 10 ampoule [PoM] £5.20 DT = £5.20
  Lidocaine 100mg/5ml (2%) solution for injection Mini-Plasco ampoules | 20 ampoule [PoM] £12.00
  Lidocaine 200mg/10ml (2%) solution for injection ampoules | 20 ampoule [PoM] £14.95-£382.80 (Hospital only)
  Lidocaine 400mg/20ml (2%) solution for injection ampoules | 10 ampoule [PoM] £11.00-£15.00 DT = £15.00 | 20 ampoule [PoM] £31.00-£521.80 (Hospital only)

Mexiletine

04-Jan-2022

- **DRUG ACTION** Mexiletine is a sodium channel blocker with anti-arrhythmic and muscle relaxant properties.

- **INDICATIONS AND DOSE**

Life-threatening ventricular arrhythmias (specialist use only)

▶ BY MOUTH
▶ Adult: Loading dose 400 mg, followed by maintenance 150–300 mg 2–3 times a day, dose may be adjusted if necessary in steps of 50 or 100 mg at intervals of at least 2 to 3 days, according to response and tolerance, at least 1 week is recommended between dose adjustments in patients who are poor CYP2D6 metabolisers; maximum 1200 mg per day

DOSE EQUIVALENCE AND CONVERSION
▶ Dose expressed as mexiletine hydrochloride.
▶ Mexiletine hydrochloride 100 mg is approximately equivalent to mexiletine 83.1 mg.

NAMUSCLA ®

Myotonia in non-dystrophic myotonic disorders

▶ BY MOUTH
▶ Adult: 167 mg once daily for at least 1 week, then increased if necessary to 333 mg daily in divided doses for at least another week, then increased if necessary to 500 mg daily in divided doses; maintenance 167–500 mg daily; maximum 500 mg per day

DOSE EQUIVALENCE AND CONVERSION
▶ *Namuscla* ® contains mexiletine hydrochloride; doses are expressed as mexiletine base.

- **CONTRA-INDICATIONS**
▶ When used for Myotonia Abnormal Q-waves · atrial tachyarrhythmia, fibrillation, or flutter · complete heart block or any heart block susceptible to evolve to complete heart block · heart failure (with ejection fraction less than 50%) · history of myocardial infarction · sinus node dysfunction · symptomatic coronary artery disease · ventricular tachyarrhythmia
▶ When used for Ventricular arrhythmias Cardiogenic shock · inherited long QT syndrome (other than LQTS3) · reduced left ventricular ejection fraction · severe AV conduction disturbances (unless pacemaker fitted) · severe heart failure · sinus node dysfunction (unless pacemaker fitted)

- **CAUTIONS**

GENERAL CAUTIONS Epilepsy or history of seizures (increased risk of seizures) · poor CYP2D6 metabolisers (increased plasma levels)

SPECIFIC CAUTIONS
▶ When used for Myotonia Cardiac disorders other than those contra-indicated
▶ When used for Ventricular arrhythmias Congestive heart failure · first-degree AV block or intraventricular conduction abnormalities · hypotension

- **INTERACTIONS** → Appendix 1: mexiletine

- **SIDE-EFFECTS**
▶ **Common or very common** Angina pectoris · arrhythmias · asthenia · ataxia · chest discomfort · constipation · dizziness · drowsiness · dry mouth · gastrointestinal discomfort · headache · hypotension · insomnia · malaise · nausea · pain in extremity · palpitations · paraesthesia · skin reactions · tinnitus · tremor · vasodilation · vertigo · vision disorders
▶ **Uncommon** Alopecia · arthralgia · erectile dysfunction · hiccups · loss of consciousness · memory loss · seizure · speech disorder
▶ **Rare or very rare** Agranulocytosis · heart failure · hepatic disorders · neutropenia · severe cutaneous adverse reactions (SCARs)

▶ **Frequency not known** Atrioventricular block · circulatory collapse · confusion · diarrhoea · gastrointestinal disorders · hallucination · leucopenia · lupus-like syndrome · pulmonary fibrosis · taste altered · thrombocytopenia · vomiting

- **ALLERGY AND CROSS-SENSITIVITY** [EvGr] Avoid if hypersensitivity to any local anaesthetic. ⓜ

- **PREGNANCY** Specialist sources indicate use with caution—limited human and animal data available.

- **BREAST FEEDING** Specialist sources indicate use with caution—limited data show present in breast milk; monitor breast-fed infants for adverse reactions.

- **HEPATIC IMPAIRMENT** [EvGr] Caution in mild or moderate impairment; avoid in severe impairment (limited information available). ⓜ
Dose adjustments [EvGr] Any dose increase should only be made after at least 2 weeks of treatment in mild or moderate impairment. ⓜ

- **RENAL IMPAIRMENT** [EvGr] Avoid in severe impairment (limited information available). ⓜ

- **MONITORING REQUIREMENTS**
▶ [EvGr] Monitor electrolytes before starting treatment and during treatment—imbalances should be corrected. ⓜ
▶ When used for Ventricular arrhythmias [EvGr] Monitor platelets and white blood cell count before starting treatment and during treatment—consult product literature. ⓜ
▶ When used for Myotonia [EvGr] Perform cardiac evaluation before starting treatment, within 48 hours of starting treatment, and during treatment—consult product literature. ⓜ

- **DIRECTIONS FOR ADMINISTRATION** [EvGr] Capsules should be swallowed whole with water, while in an upright position. If digestive intolerance occurs, capsules should be taken with food. ⓜ

- **PRESCRIBING AND DISPENSING INFORMATION**
NAMUSCLA ® The manufacturer has provided a *Guide for Healthcare Professionals*.

- **PATIENT AND CARER ADVICE** Patient and carers should be given advice on how to administer mexiletine capsules.
Driving and skilled tasks Patients and carers should be counselled on the effects on driving and performance of skilled tasks—increased risk of fatigue, confusion, and blurred vision.

NAMUSCLA ® Patients and carers should be informed about the presenting symptoms of arrhythmias (e.g. fainting, palpitation, chest pain, shortness of breath, light-headedness, lipothymia, and syncope) and advised to seek immediate medical attention if symptoms develop.
Alert card An alert card should be provided.

- **NATIONAL FUNDING/ACCESS DECISIONS**
For full details see funding body website

NICE decisions
▶ **Mexiletine for treating the symptoms of myotonia in non-dystrophic myotonic disorders (December 2021)** NICE TA748 Recommended

Scottish Medicines Consortium (SMC) decisions
▶ **Mexiletine (*Namuscla* ®) for the symptomatic treatment of myotonia in adult patients with non-dystrophic myotonic disorders (December 2020)** SMC No. SMC2307 Recommended

- **MEDICINAL FORMS** There can be variation in the licensing of different medicines containing the same drug. Forms available from special-order manufacturers include: oral capsule

Oral capsule
EXCIPIENTS: May contain Gelatin
▶ **Mexiletine (Non-proprietary)**
Mexiletine hydrochloride 50 mg Mexiletine 50mg capsules | 84 capsule [PoM] £185.00
Mexiletine hydrochloride 100 mg Mexiletine 100mg capsules | 84 capsule [PoM] £375.00

2

Cardiovascular system

Mexiletine (as Mexiletine hydrochloride) 167 mg Ritalmex 200mg
capsules | 100 capsule [PoM] [Ⅹ] DT = £5,000.00
Mexiletine hydrochloride 200mg (Mexiletine 167mg) capsules |
100 capsule [PoM] £875.00 DT = £5,000.00
► Namuscla (Lupin Healthcare (UK) Ltd)
Mexiletine (as Mexiletine hydrochloride) 167 mg Namuscla 167mg
capsules | 100 capsule [PoM] £5,000.00 DT = £5,000.00

ANTIARRHYTHMICS 〉 CLASS IC

Flecainide acetate
03-Apr-2025

● **INDICATIONS AND DOSE**

**Supraventricular arrhythmias (initiated under direction
of hospital consultant)**
► BY MOUTH
► Adult: Initially 50 mg twice daily, dose can be increased
  if necessary up to 300 mg per day

**Ventricular arrhythmias (initiated under direction of
hospital consultant)**
► BY MOUTH
► Adult: Initially 100 mg twice daily for 3–5 days,
  maximum dose of 400 mg per day can be used for rapid
  control or in heavily built patients; for maintenance,
  reduce to the lowest dose that controls the arrhythmia

DOSE ADJUSTMENTS DUE TO INTERACTIONS
► Manufacturer advises reduce dose by half with
  concurrent use of amiodarone.

● **CONTRA-INDICATIONS** Abnormal left ventricular function ·
atrial conduction defects (unless pacing rescue available) ·
bundle branch block (unless pacing rescue available) ·
distal block (unless pacing rescue available) ·
haemodynamically significant valvular heart disease ·
heart failure · history of myocardial infarction and either
asymptomatic ventricular ectopics or asymptomatic non-
sustained ventricular tachycardia · long-standing atrial
fibrillation where conversion to sinus rhythm not
attempted · second-degree or greater AV block (unless
pacing rescue available) · sinus node dysfunction (unless
pacing rescue available)

● **CAUTIONS** Atrial fibrillation following heart surgery ·
elderly (accumulation may occur) · patients with
pacemakers (especially those who may be pacemaker
dependent because stimulation threshold may rise
appreciably)

● **INTERACTIONS** → Appendix 1: antiarrhythmics

● **SIDE-EFFECTS**
► **Common or very common** Arrhythmias · asthenia · dizziness
  · dyspnoea · fever · oedema · vision disorders
► **Uncommon** Alopecia · appetite decreased · constipation ·
  diarrhoea · flatulence · gastrointestinal discomfort · nausea
  · skin reactions · vomiting
► **Rare or very rare** Anxiety · confusion · corneal deposits ·
  depression · drowsiness · flushing · hallucination ·
  headache · hepatic disorders · hyperhidrosis · inflammation
  · insomnia · interstitial lung disease · memory loss ·
  movement disorders · peripheral neuropathy ·
  photosensitivity reaction · seizure · sensation abnormal ·
  syncope · tinnitus · tremor · vertigo
► **Frequency not known** Altered pacing threshold ·
  atrioventricular block · cardiac arrest · chest pain · heart
  failure · hypotension · palpitations · pulmonary fibrosis ·
  QT interval prolongation

● **PREGNANCY** Used in pregnancy to treat maternal and fetal
arrhythmias in specialist centres; toxicity reported in
animal studies; infant hyperbilirubinaemia also reported.

● **BREAST FEEDING** Significant amount present in milk but
not known to be harmful.

● **HEPATIC IMPAIRMENT**
Dose adjustments Avoid or reduce dose in severe
impairment.

● **RENAL IMPAIRMENT**
Dose adjustments Reduce initial oral dose to max. 100 mg
daily if eGFR less than 35 mL/minute/1.73 m^2.

● **MEDICINAL FORMS** There can be variation in the licensing of
different medicines containing the same drug. Forms available
from special-order manufacturers include: oral suspension, oral
solution
Oral tablet
► Flecainide acetate (Non-proprietary)
Flecainide acetate 50 mg Flecainide 50mg tablets | 60 tablet [PoM]
£7.68 DT = £2.24
Flecainide acetate 100 mg Flecainide 100mg tablets |
60 tablet [PoM] £8.06 DT = £3.29
Oral solution
► Flecainide acetate (Non-proprietary)
Flecainide acetate 5 mg per 1 ml Flecainide 25mg/5ml oral solution
sugar free | 300 ml [PoM] £375.00 [SF]

Propafenone hydrochloride
03-Feb-2020

● **INDICATIONS AND DOSE**

**Ventricular arrhythmias (specialist supervision in
hospital) | Paroxysmal supraventricular
tachyarrhythmias which include paroxysmal atrial
flutter or fibrillation and paroxysmal re-entrant
tachycardias involving the AV node or accessory
pathway, where standard therapy ineffective or contra-
indicated (specialist supervision in hospital)**
► BY MOUTH
► Adult: Initially 150 mg 3 times a day, dose to be taken
  after food, monitor ECG and blood pressure, if QRS
  interval prolonged by more than 20%, reduce dose or
  discontinue until ECG returns to normal limits;
  increased if necessary to 300 mg twice daily (max. per
  dose 300 mg 3 times a day), dose to be increased at
  intervals of at least 3 days, reduce total daily dose for
  patients under 70 kg
► Elderly: Initially 150 mg 3 times a day, dose to be taken
  after food, monitor ECG and blood pressure, if QRS
  interval prolonged by more than 20%, reduce dose or
  discontinue until ECG returns to normal limits;
  increased if necessary to 300 mg twice daily (max. per
  dose 300 mg 3 times a day), dose to be increased at
  intervals of at least 5 days, reduce total daily dose for
  patients under 70 kg

● **CONTRA-INDICATIONS** Atrial conduction defects (unless
adequately paced) · Brugada syndrome · bundle branch
block (unless adequately paced) · cardiogenic shock
(except arrhythmia induced) · distal block (unless
adequately paced) · electrolyte disturbances · marked
hypotension · myasthenia gravis · myocardial infarction
within last 3 months · second degree or greater AV block
(unless adequately paced) · severe bradycardia · severe
obstructive pulmonary disease (due to weak beta-blocking
activity) · sinus node dysfunction (unless adequately
paced) · uncontrolled congestive heart failure with left
ventricular ejection fraction less than 35%

● **CAUTIONS** Elderly · heart failure · mild to moderate
obstructive airways disease owing to beta-blocking activity
· pacemaker patients · potential for conversion of
paroxysmal atrial fibrillation to atrial flutter with 2:1
conduction block or 1:1 conduction

● **INTERACTIONS** → Appendix 1: antiarrhythmics

● **SIDE-EFFECTS**
► **Common or very common** Anxiety · arrhythmias · asthenia ·
  cardiac conduction disorder · chest pain · constipation ·
  diarrhoea · dizziness · dry mouth · dyspnoea · fever ·

gastrointestinal discomfort · headache · hepatic disorders · nausea · palpitations · sleep disorders · taste altered · vision blurred · vomiting

▸ **Uncommon** Appetite decreased · erectile dysfunction · gastrointestinal disorders · hypotension · movement disorders · paraesthesia · skin reactions · syncope · thrombocytopenia · vertigo

▸ **Frequency not known** Agranulocytosis · confusion · granulocytopenia · heart failure · leucopenia · lupus-like syndrome · seizure

● PREGNANCY Use only if potential benefit outweighs risk.

● BREAST FEEDING Use with caution—present in milk.

● PATIENT AND CARER ADVICE
Driving and skilled tasks May affect performance of skilled tasks e.g. driving.

● MEDICINAL FORMS There can be variation in the licensing of different medicines containing the same drug. Forms available from special-order manufacturers include: oral suspension, oral solution

Oral tablet
CAUTIONARY AND ADVISORY LABELS 21, 25

▸ **Propafenone hydrochloride (Non-proprietary)**
Propafenone hydrochloride 150 mg Propafenone 150mg tablets | 90 tablet PoM £10.73-£12.46 DT = £12.46
Propafenone hydrochloride 300 mg Propafenone 300mg tablets | 60 tablet PoM £9.34 DT = £9.34

▸ **Arythmol** (Viatris UK Healthcare Ltd)
Propafenone hydrochloride 150 mg Arythmol 150mg tablets | 90 tablet PoM £7.37 DT = £12.46
Propafenone hydrochloride 300 mg Arythmol 300mg tablets | 60 tablet PoM £9.34 DT = £9.34

ANTIARRHYTHMICS > CLASS III

Amiodarone hydrochloride

15-Apr-2024

● INDICATIONS AND DOSE

Treatment of arrhythmias, particularly when other drugs are ineffective or contra-indicated (including paroxysmal supraventricular, nodal and ventricular tachycardias, atrial fibrillation and flutter, ventricular fibrillation, and tachyarrhythmias associated with Wolff-Parkinson-White syndrome) (initiated in hospital or under specialist supervision)

▸ BY MOUTH
▸ Adult: 200 mg 3 times a day for 1 week, then reduced to 200 mg twice daily for a further week, followed by maintenance dose, usually 200 mg daily or the minimum dose required to control arrhythmia

▸ BY INTRAVENOUS INFUSION
▸ Adult: Initially 5 mg/kg, to be given over 20–120 minutes with ECG monitoring, subsequent infusions given if necessary according to response; maximum 1.2 g per day

Ventricular fibrillation or pulseless ventricular tachycardia refractory to defibrillation (for cardiopulmonary resuscitation)

▸ BY INTRAVENOUS INJECTION
▸ Adult: Initially 300 mg, dose should be given from a pre-filled syringe or diluted in 20 mL Glucose 5%, then 150 mg if required, consult Resuscitation Council (UK) guidelines for further details

IMPORTANT SAFETY INFORMATION

MHRA/CHM ADVICE: SOFOSBUVIR WITH DACLATASVIR; SOFOSBUVIR AND LEDIPASVIR (MAY 2015); SIMEPREVIR WITH SOFOSBUVIR (AUGUST 2015): RISK OF SEVERE BRADYCARDIA AND HEART BLOCK WHEN TAKEN WITH AMIODARONE
Avoid concomitant use unless other antiarrhythmics cannot be given.

MHRA/CHM ADVICE: AMIODARONE (*CORDARONE X* ®): REMINDER OF RISKS OF TREATMENT AND NEED FOR PATIENT MONITORING AND SUPERVISION (MARCH 2022)
Healthcare professionals are reminded that amiodarone can cause serious adverse reactions affecting the eyes, heart, lung, liver, thyroid gland, skin, and peripheral nervous system that may persist for a month or longer after treatment discontinuation. Some of these reactions may be life-threatening but onset can be delayed; patients should be supervised and reviewed regularly, especially those on long-term treatment. Liver and thyroid function tests should be performed—see *Monitoring requirements*.

Patients and carers should be counselled to seek medical advice if new or worsening respiratory symptoms develop; healthcare professionals should consider using computerised tomography (CT) scans if pulmonary toxicity is suspected. Patients and carers should also be advised to seek immediate medical attention if other symptoms of serious adverse reactions develop during or after stopping treatment.

● CONTRA-INDICATIONS

GENERAL CONTRA-INDICATIONS Avoid in severe conduction disturbances (unless pacemaker fitted) · avoid in sinus node disease (unless pacemaker fitted) · iodine sensitivity · sino-atrial heart block (except in cardiac arrest) · sinus bradycardia (except in cardiac arrest) · thyroid dysfunction
SPECIFIC CONTRA-INDICATIONS
▸ With intravenous use Avoid bolus injection in cardiomyopathy · avoid bolus injection in congestive heart failure · avoid in circulatory collapse · avoid in severe arterial hypotension · avoid in severe respiratory failure

● CAUTIONS

GENERAL CAUTIONS Acute porphyrias p. 1202 · conduction disturbances (in excessive dosage) · elderly · heart failure · hypokalaemia · severe bradycardia (in excessive dosage)
SPECIFIC CAUTIONS
▸ With intravenous use Moderate and transient fall in blood pressure (circulatory collapse precipitated by rapid administration or overdosage) · severe hepatocellular toxicity

CAUTIONS, FURTHER INFORMATION
▸ Elderly Screening Tool of Older Persons' potentially inappropriate Prescriptions (STOPP) criteria to aid medication reviews (see Prescribing in the elderly p. 31 for information): potentially inappropriate as first-line antiarrhythmic therapy in supraventricular tachyarrhythmias (higher risk of side-effects than beta-blockers, digoxin, verapamil, or diltiazem).

● INTERACTIONS → Appendix 1: antiarrhythmics

● SIDE-EFFECTS

GENERAL SIDE-EFFECTS
▸ **Common or very common** Arrhythmias · hepatic disorders · hyperthyroidism · nausea · pulmonary fibrosis · skin reactions
▸ **Rare or very rare** Bronchospasm (in patients with severe respiratory failure) · headache · idiopathic intracranial hypertension · nerve disorders · SIADH
▸ **Frequency not known** Angioedema · confusion · delirium · pancreatitis · severe cutaneous adverse reactions (SCARs)

SPECIFIC SIDE-EFFECTS
▸ **Common or very common**
▸ With oral use Constipation · corneal deposits · hypothyroidism · interstitial lung disease · movement disorders · photosensitivity reaction · respiratory disorders · sleep disorders · taste altered · vomiting
▸ With parenteral use Hypotension (following rapid injection)

▶ **Uncommon**
▶ With oral use Cardiac conduction disorders · dry mouth · myopathy (usually reversible on discontinuation) · peripheral neuropathy (usually reversible on discontinuation)
▶ **Rare or very rare**
▶ With oral use Alopecia · aplastic anaemia · epididymo-orchitis · erectile dysfunction · haemolytic anaemia · pulmonary haemorrhage · thrombocytopenia · vertigo
▶ With parenteral use Hot flush · hyperhidrosis · interstitial pneumonitis · pulmonary toxicity
▶ **Frequency not known**
▶ With oral use Altered smell sensation · appetite decreased · parkinsonism · vasculitis
▶ With parenteral use Agranulocytosis · libido decreased · neutropenia

SIDE-EFFECTS, FURTHER INFORMATION Side-effects can occur at any time during treatment with, or in the months after stopping amiodarone.

Corneal microdeposits Patients taking amiodarone may develop corneal microdeposits (reversible on withdrawal of treatment). However, if vision is impaired or if optic neuritis or optic neuropathy occur, amiodarone must be stopped to prevent blindness and expert advice sought.

Thyroid function Amiodarone contains iodine and can cause disorders of thyroid function; both hypothyroidism and hyperthyroidism can occur. Hypothyroidism can be treated with replacement therapy without withdrawing amiodarone if it is essential; careful supervision is required.

Hepatotoxicity Amiodarone is also associated with hepatotoxicity and treatment should be discontinued if severe liver function abnormalities or clinical signs of liver disease develop.

Pulmonary toxicity If new or progressive shortness of breath or cough develops in patients taking amiodarone (or recently stopped), pulmonary toxicity should always be suspected. Pulmonary toxicity is usually reversible following early withdrawal of amiodarone.

● **PREGNANCY** Possible risk of neonatal goitre; use only if no alternative.

● **BREAST FEEDING** Avoid; present in milk in significant amounts; theoretical risk of neonatal hypothyroidism from release of iodine.

● **MONITORING REQUIREMENTS**
▶ EvGr Liver function tests required before treatment and then every 6 months.
▶ Serum potassium concentration should be measured before treatment.
▶ Chest x-ray required before treatment.
▶ Thyroid function tests should be performed before treatment, then at 6-monthly intervals, and for several months after stopping treatment (particularly in the elderly). Thyroid stimulating hormone levels should be measured if thyroid dysfunction is suspected. ◈M̂◈ Consult specialist if thyroid function is abnormal.
▶ EvGr If concomitant use of amiodarone with sofosbuvir and daclatasvir, simeprevir and sofosbuvir, or sofosbuvir and ledipasvir cannot be avoided because other anti-arrhythmics are not tolerated or contra-indicated, patients should be closely monitored, particularly during the first weeks of treatment. Patients at high risk of bradycardia should be monitored continuously for 48 hours in an appropriate clinical setting after starting concomitant treatment. Patients who have stopped amiodarone within the last few months and need to start sofosbuvir and daclatasvir, simeprevir and sofosbuvir, or sofosbuvir and ledipasvir should be monitored. ◈M̂◈
▶ With intravenous use EvGr ECG monitoring and resuscitation facilities must be available. Monitor liver transaminases closely. ◈M̂◈

● **DIRECTIONS FOR ADMINISTRATION**
▶ With intravenous use EvGr Intravenous infusion via central venous catheter recommended if repeated or continuous infusion required, as infusion via peripheral veins may cause pain and inflammation. In emergency use for cardiopulmonary resuscitation, a peripheral venous route can be used if central venous access is not available; the peripheral line should be flushed liberally. ◈M̂◈

For *intravenous infusion* (*Cordarone X*®), manufacturer advises give continuously or intermittently in Glucose 5%. Suggested initial infusion volume 250 mL given over 20–120 minutes; for repeat infusions up to 1.2 g in max. 500 mL; should not be diluted to less than 600 micrograms/mL. See cardiopulmonary resuscitation for details of administration in extreme emergency. Incompatible with Sodium Chloride infusion fluids; avoid equipment containing the plasticizer di-2-ethylhexphthalate (DEHP).
▶ With oral use For administration *by mouth*, expert sources advise tablets may be crushed and dispersed in water; injection solution should **not** be given orally (irritant).

● **PATIENT AND CARER ADVICE**
Phototoxicity Because of the possibility of phototoxic reactions, patients should be advised to shield the skin from light during treatment and for several months after discontinuing amiodarone; a wide-spectrum sunscreen to protect against both long-wave ultraviolet and visible light should be used.
Concurrent sofosbuvir-containing regimens If taking amiodarone with concurrent sofosbuvir-containing regimens, patients and their carers should be told how to recognise signs and symptoms of bradycardia and heart block and advised to seek immediate medical attention if symptoms such as shortness of breath, light-headedness, palpitations, fainting, unusual tiredness or chest pain develop.
Alert card A patient alert card should be provided.
Driving and skilled tasks Patients and carers should be cautioned on the effects on driving and performance of skilled tasks—corneal microdeposits may be associated with blurred vision (see *Side-effects, further information*).

● **MEDICINAL FORMS** There can be variation in the licensing of different medicines containing the same drug. Forms available from special-order manufacturers include: oral suspension, oral solution

Oral tablet
CAUTIONARY AND ADVISORY LABELS 11
▶ **Amiodarone hydrochloride (Non-proprietary)**
  Amiodarone hydrochloride 100 mg Amiodarone 100mg tablets | 28 tablet PoM £3.42 DT = £1.92
  Amiodarone hydrochloride 200 mg Amiodarone 200mg tablets | 28 tablet PoM £5.59 DT = £1.84
Solution for injection
EXCIPIENTS: May contain Benzyl alcohol
▶ **Amiodarone hydrochloride (Non-proprietary)**
  Amiodarone hydrochloride 30 mg per 1 ml Amiodarone 300mg/10ml solution for injection pre-filled syringes | 1 pre-filled disposable injection PoM £30.39-£60.30
  Amiodarone hydrochloride 50 mg per 1 ml Amiodarone 150mg/3ml concentrate for solution for injection ampoules | 5 ampoule PoM £7.75 (Hospital only) | 10 ampoule PoM £25.00

2 Cardiovascular system

Dronedarone
04-Aug-2021

- **DRUG ACTION** Dronedarone is a multi-channel blocking anti-arrhythmic drug.

- **INDICATIONS AND DOSE**

Maintenance of sinus rhythm after cardioversion in clinically stable patients with paroxysmal or persistent atrial fibrillation, when alternative treatments are unsuitable (initiated under specialist supervision)
▸ BY MOUTH
▸ Adult: 400 mg twice daily

- **CONTRA-INDICATIONS** Atrial conduction defects · bradycardia · complete bundle branch block · distal block · existing or previous heart failure or left ventricular systolic dysfunction · haemodynamically unstable patients · liver toxicity associated with previous amiodarone use · lung toxicity associated with previous amiodarone use · permanent atrial fibrillation · prolonged QT interval · second- or third- degree AV block · sick sinus syndrome (unless pacemaker fitted) · sinus node dysfunction

- **CAUTIONS** Coronary artery disease · correct hypokalaemia and hypomagnesaemia before starting and during treatment

- **INTERACTIONS** → Appendix 1: antiarrhythmics

- **SIDE-EFFECTS**
▸ **Common or very common** Asthenia · bradycardia · congestive heart failure · diarrhoea · gastrointestinal discomfort · nausea · QT interval prolongation · skin reactions · vomiting
▸ **Uncommon** Interstitial lung disease · photosensitivity reaction · pulmonary fibrosis · taste altered
▸ **Rare or very rare** Hepatic disorders · vasculitis

  SIDE-EFFECTS, FURTHER INFORMATION **Liver injury** Liver injury including life-threatening acute liver failure reported rarely; discontinue treatment if 2 consecutive alanine aminotransferase concentrations exceed 3 times upper limit of normal.
  Heart failure New onset or worsening heart failure reported. If heart failure or left ventricular systolic dysfunction develops, discontinue treatment.
  Pulmonary toxicity Interstitial lung disease, pneumonitis and pulmonary fibrosis reported. Investigate if symptoms such as dyspnoea or dry cough develop and discontinue if confirmed.

- **PREGNANCY** Manufacturer advises avoid—toxicity in *animal* studies.

- **BREAST FEEDING** Manufacturer advises avoid—present in milk in *animal* studies.

- **HEPATIC IMPAIRMENT** Manufacturer advises avoid in severe impairment.

- **RENAL IMPAIRMENT** EvGr Avoid if creatinine clearance less than 30 mL/minute. Ⓜ See p. 21.

- **MONITORING REQUIREMENTS**
▸ Ongoing monitoring should occur under specialist supervision.
▸ Monitor for heart failure.
▸ Perform ECG at least every 6 months—consider discontinuation if atrial fibrillation reoccurs.
▸ Measure serum creatinine before treatment and 7 days after initiation—if raised, measure again after a further 7 days and consider discontinuation if creatinine continues to rise.
▸ Monitor liver function before treatment, 1 week and 1 month after initiation of treatment, then monthly for 6 months, then every 3 months for 6 months and periodically thereafter.

- **PATIENT AND CARER ADVICE**
Heart failure Patients or their carers should be told how to recognise signs of heart failure and advised to seek prompt medical attention if symptoms such as weight gain, dependent oedema, or dyspnoea develop or worsen.
Hepatic disorders Patients or their carers should be told how to recognise signs of liver disorder and advised to seek prompt medical attention if symptoms such as abdominal pain, anorexia, nausea, vomiting, fever, malaise, itching, dark urine, or jaundice develop.

- **NATIONAL FUNDING/ACCESS DECISIONS**
For full details see funding body website
NICE decisions
▸ **Dronedarone for the treatment of non-permanent atrial fibrillation (updated December 2012)** NICE TA197 Recommended

- **MEDICINAL FORMS** There can be variation in the licensing of different medicines containing the same drug.
Oral tablet
CAUTIONARY AND ADVISORY LABELS 21
▸ **Dronedarone (Non-proprietary)**
  Dronedarone (as Dronedarone hydrochloride)
  400 mg Dronedarone 400mg tablets | 20 tablet PoM £22.49 DT = £19.53 | 60 tablet PoM £58.59–£67.49
▸ **Multaq** (Sanofi)
  Dronedarone (as Dronedarone hydrochloride) 400 mg Multaq 400mg tablets | 60 tablet PoM £67.50

ANTIARRHYTHMICS › OTHER

Adenosine
28-Jul-2020

- **INDICATIONS AND DOSE**

Rapid reversion to sinus rhythm of paroxysmal supraventricular tachycardias, including those associated with accessory conducting pathways (e.g. Wolff-Parkinson-White syndrome) | Used to aid to diagnosis of broad or narrow complex supraventricular tachycardias
▸ BY RAPID INTRAVENOUS INJECTION
▸ Adult: Initially 6 mg, administer into central or large peripheral vein and give over 2 seconds, cardiac monitoring required, followed by 12 mg after 1–2 minutes if required, then 12 mg after 1–2 minutes if required, increments should not be given if high level AV block develops at any particular dose

Rapid reversion to sinus rhythm of paroxysmal supraventricular tachycardias, including those associated with accessory conducting pathways (e.g. Wolff-Parkinson-White syndrome) in patients with a heart transplant | Aid to diagnosis of broad or narrow complex supraventricular tachycardias in patients with a heart transplant
▸ BY RAPID INTRAVENOUS INJECTION
▸ Adult: Initially 3 mg, administer into a central or large peripheral vein and give over 2 seconds, followed by 6 mg after 1–2 minutes if required, then 12 mg after 1–2 minutes if required, patients with a heart transplant are very sensitive to the effects of adenosine

Used in conjunction with radionuclide myocardial perfusion imaging in patients who cannot exercise adequately or for whom exercise is inappropriate
▸ BY INTRAVENOUS INFUSION
▸ Adult: (consult product literature)

- **UNLICENSED USE** Adenosine doses in the BNF may differ from those in the product literature.

- **CONTRA-INDICATIONS** Asthma · chronic obstructive lung disease · decompensated heart failure · long QT syndrome · second- or third-degree AV block and sick sinus syndrome (unless pacemaker fitted) · severe hypotension

- **CAUTIONS** Atrial fibrillation · atrial fibrillation with accessory pathway (conduction down anomalous pathway may increase) · atrial flutter · atrial flutter with accessory pathway (conduction down anomalous pathway may increase) · autonomic dysfunction · bundle branch block · first-degree AV block · heart transplant · left main coronary artery stenosis · left to right shunt · pericardial effusion · pericarditis · QT-interval prolongation · recent myocardial infarction · severe heart failure · stenotic carotid artery disease with cerebrovascular insufficiency · stenotic valvular heart disease · uncorrected hypovolaemia

- **INTERACTIONS** → Appendix 1: antiarrhythmics
- **SIDE-EFFECTS**
  ▸ **Common or very common** Abdominal discomfort · arrhythmias · atrioventricular block · chest discomfort · chest pain (discontinue) · dizziness · dry mouth · dyspnoea · flushing · headache · hypotension (discontinue if severe) · pain · paraesthesia · throat discomfort
  ▸ **Uncommon** Asthenia · back discomfort · bradycardia (discontinue if asystole or severe bradycardia occur) · hyperhidrosis · limb discomfort · nervousness · taste metallic
  ▸ **Rare or very rare** Drowsiness · nasal congestion · nipple tenderness · respiratory disorders · respiratory failure (discontinue) · tinnitus · tremor · urinary urgency · vision blurred
  ▸ **Frequency not known** Apnoea · cardiac arrest · loss of consciousness · nausea · seizure · syncope · vomiting

- **PREGNANCY** Large doses may produce fetal toxicity; manufacturer advises use only if potential benefit outweighs risk.

- **BREAST FEEDING** No information available—unlikely to be present in milk owing to short half-life.

- **MONITORING REQUIREMENTS** Monitor ECG and have resuscitation facilities available.

- **DIRECTIONS FOR ADMINISTRATION** For *rapid intravenous injection*, expert sources advise give over 2 seconds into central or large peripheral vein followed by rapid Sodium Chloride 0.9% flush; injection solution may be diluted with Sodium Chloride 0.9% if required.

- **MEDICINAL FORMS** There can be variation in the licensing of different medicines containing the same drug. Forms available from special-order manufacturers include: solution for injection, infusion, solution for infusion

Solution for injection
ELECTROLYTES: May contain Sodium
  ▸ **Adenosine (Non-proprietary)**
    Adenosine 3 mg per 1 ml Adenosine 6mg/2ml solution for injection vials | 5 vial [PoM] £33.00 (Hospital only) | 6 vial [PoM] £26.70–£29.24 (Hospital only)
    Adenosine 6mg/2ml solution for injection ampoules | 10 ampoule [PoM] £44.50 (Hospital only)
  ▸ **Adenocor (Sanofi)**
    Adenosine 3 mg per 1 ml Adenocor 6mg/2ml solution for injection vials | 6 vial [PoM] £6.45 (Hospital only)

Solution for infusion
ELECTROLYTES: May contain Sodium
  ▸ **Adenosine (Non-proprietary)**
    Adenosine 3 mg per 1 ml Adenosine 30mg/10ml solution for infusion vials | 5 vial [PoM] £93.50 (Hospital only) | 6 vial [PoM] £70.00–£85.57 (Hospital only)
  ▸ **Adenoscan (Sanofi)**
    Adenosine 3 mg per 1 ml Adenoscan 30mg/10ml solution for infusion vials | 6 vial [PoM] £16.05 (Hospital only)

Vernakalant

15-Jul-2019

- **DRUG ACTION** Vernakalant is an anti-arrhythmic drug that blocks potassium and sodium channels in the atria, thereby restoring normal heart rhythm.

- **INDICATIONS AND DOSE**

Rapid conversion of recent onset atrial fibrillation to sinus rhythm (specialist supervision in hospital)
  ▸ BY INTRAVENOUS INFUSION
  ▸ **Adult:** Initially 3 mg/kg (max. per dose 339 mg), followed by 2 mg/kg (max. per dose 226 mg), if conversion to sinus rhythm does not occur within 15 minutes after the end of initial infusion, maximum 5 mg/kg per 24 hours; maximum 565 mg per day

DOSE EQUIVALENCE AND CONVERSION
  ▸ Doses expressed as vernakalant hydrochloride.

- **CONTRA-INDICATIONS** Acute coronary syndrome within the last 30 days · baseline QT interval 440 milliseconds or greater · congestive heart failure with left ventricular ejection fraction $\leq 35\%$ · heart failure (New York Heart Association class III/IV) · second- or third-degree heart block (unless pacemaker fitted) · severe aortic stenosis · severe bradycardia · sinus node dysfunction · systolic blood pressure less than 100 mmHg

- **CAUTIONS** Haemodynamically stable patients with congestive heart failure (increased risk of hypotension and ventricular arrhythmia) · patients receiving oral anti-arrhythmics (class I or III) (risk of atrial flutter) · valvular heart disease (increased incidence of ventricular arrhythmia)

- **INTERACTIONS** → Appendix 1: antiarrhythmics

- **SIDE-EFFECTS**
  ▸ **Common or very common** Arrhythmias · cough · dizziness · feeling hot · headache · hypotension · nasal complaints · nausea · oral disorders · sensation abnormal · skin reactions · sweat changes · taste altered · vomiting
  ▸ **Uncommon** Altered smell sensation · cardiac conduction disorders · cardiogenic shock · chest discomfort · choking sensation · defaecation urgency · diarrhoea · drowsiness · dry mouth · dyspnoea · excessive tearing · eye irritation · fatigue · malaise · pain in extremity · pallor · palpitations · QT interval prolongation · suffocation feeling · syncope · throat irritation · vasodilation · visual impairment

SIDE-EFFECTS, FURTHER INFORMATION Discontinue and initiate appropriate treatment if hypotension, bradycardia, ECG changes, or a sudden drop in blood pressure or heart rate occur.

- **PREGNANCY** Manufacturer advises avoid—no information available.

- **BREAST FEEDING** Manufacturer advises caution—no information available.

- **MONITORING REQUIREMENTS** Manufacturer advises monitor blood pressure and ECG during and for at least 15 minutes after completion of the infusion.

- **DIRECTIONS FOR ADMINISTRATION** Manufacturer advises for *intermittent intravenous infusion* in patients with body-weight up to and including 100 kg, dilute to a concentration of 4 mg/mL with 100 mL of Glucose 5% *or* Sodium Chloride 0.9% *or* Lactated Ringer's Solution; give over 10 minutes. Manufacturer advises for *intermittent intravenous infusion* in patients with body-weight more than 100 kg, dilute to a concentration of 4 mg/mL with 120 mL of Glucose 5% *or* Sodium Chloride 0.9% *or* Lactated Ringer's Solution; give over 10 minutes.

- **PRESCRIBING AND DISPENSING INFORMATION** The manufacturer of *Brinavess*® has provided a *Pre-infusion Checklist* and a *Healthcare Professional Card*.

- **PATIENT AND CARER ADVICE**
Driving and skilled tasks Manufacturer advises patients and carers should be counselled on the effects on driving and performance of skilled tasks—increased risk of dizziness.

- **MEDICINAL FORMS** There can be variation in the licensing of different medicines containing the same drug.
Solution for infusion
ELECTROLYTES: May contain Sodium
  ‣ Brinavess (Advanz Pharma)
  Vernakalant hydrochloride 20 mg per 1 ml Brinavess 500mg/25ml concentrate for solution for infusion vials | 1 vial [PoM] £290.00 (Hospital only)

BETA-ADRENOCEPTOR BLOCKERS > NON-SELECTIVE

F 175

Sotalol hydrochloride
26-Jul-2021

- **INDICATIONS AND DOSE**
Symptomatic non-sustained ventricular tachyarrhythmias | Prophylaxis of paroxysmal atrial tachycardia or fibrillation, paroxysmal AV re-entrant tachycardias (both nodal and involving accessory pathways), and paroxysmal supraventricular tachycardia after cardiac surgery | Maintenance of sinus rhythm following cardioversion of atrial fibrillation or flutter
  ‣ BY MOUTH
  ‣ Adult: Initially 80 mg daily in 1–2 divided doses, then increased to 160–320 mg daily in 2 divided doses, dose to be increased gradually at intervals of 2–3 days
Life-threatening arrhythmias including ventricular tachyarrhythmias
  ‣ BY MOUTH
  ‣ Adult: Initially 80 mg daily in 1–2 divided doses, then increased to 160–320 mg daily in 2 divided doses, dose to be increased gradually at intervals of 2–3 days, higher doses of 480–640 mg daily may be required for life-threatening ventricular arrhythmias (under specialist supervision)

IMPORTANT SAFETY INFORMATION
Sotalol may prolong the QT interval, and it occasionally causes life threatening ventricular arrhythmias (**important**: manufacturer advises particular care is required to avoid hypokalaemia in patients taking sotalol—electrolyte disturbances, particularly hypokalaemia and hypomagnesaemia should be corrected before sotalol started and during use).
  Manufacturer advises reduce dose or discontinue if corrected QT interval exceeds 550 msec.

- **CONTRA-INDICATIONS** Long QT syndrome (congenital or acquired) · torsade de pointes
- **CAUTIONS** Diarrhoea (severe or prolonged)
- **INTERACTIONS** → Appendix 1: beta blockers, non-selective
- **SIDE-EFFECTS**
  ‣ **Common or very common** Anxiety · arrhythmia · chest pain · dyspepsia · fever · flatulence · hearing impairment · mood altered · muscle spasms · oedema · palpitations · sexual dysfunction · taste altered · torsade de pointes (increased risk in females)
- **BREAST FEEDING** Water soluble beta-blockers such as sotalol are present in breast milk in greater amounts than other beta blockers.
- **RENAL IMPAIRMENT** Manufacturer advises avoid if creatinine clearance less than 10 mL/minute.
Dose adjustments See p. 21.
  Manufacturer advises use half normal dose if creatinine clearance 30–60 mL/minute; use one-quarter normal dose if creatinine clearance 10–30 mL/minute.

- **MONITORING REQUIREMENTS** Measurement of corrected QT interval, and monitoring of ECG and electrolytes required; correct hypokalaemia, hypomagnesaemia, or other electrolyte disturbances.

- **MEDICINAL FORMS** There can be variation in the licensing of different medicines containing the same drug. Forms available from special-order manufacturers include: oral suspension, oral solution
Oral tablet
CAUTIONARY AND ADVISORY LABELS 8
  ‣ Sotalol hydrochloride (Non-proprietary)
  Sotalol hydrochloride 40 mg Sotalol 40mg tablets | 28 tablet [PoM] £6.74 DT = £0.94
  Sotalol hydrochloride 80 mg Sotalol 80mg tablets | 28 tablet [PoM] £7.24 DT = £1.16
  Sotalol hydrochloride 160 mg Sotalol 160mg tablets | 28 tablet [PoM] £7.55 DT = £7.55

BETA-ADRENOCEPTOR BLOCKERS > SELECTIVE

F 175

Landiolol hydrochloride
07-Jun-2023

- **INDICATIONS AND DOSE**
Supraventricular arrhythmias [for short-term use in atrial fibrillation or atrial flutter] (under expert supervision) | Sinus tachycardia [for short-term use] (under expert supervision)
  ‣ BY CONTINUOUS INTRAVENOUS INFUSION
  ‣ Adult: 10–40 micrograms/kg/minute, heart rate-lowering effect usually occurs within 10–20 minutes, for rapid onset (within 2–4 minutes), dose titration, or reduced-dose regimen for use in patients with impaired left ventricular function—consult product literature

DOSE EQUIVALENCE AND CONVERSION
  ‣ Doses are expressed as landiolol hydrochloride; landiolol hydrochloride 300 mg ≡ landiolol base 280 mg.

- **CONTRA-INDICATIONS** Pre-excitation syndrome in combination with atrial fibrillation
- **INTERACTIONS** → Appendix 1: beta blockers, selective
- **SIDE-EFFECTS**
  ‣ **Common or very common** Hypotension
  ‣ **Uncommon** Arrhythmias · cardiac arrest · cerebrovascular insufficiency · hypertension · hyponatraemia · liver disorder · pneumonia · pulmonary oedema
  ‣ **Rare or very rare** Asthma · bundle branch block · chest discomfort · chills · cold sweat · erythema · fever · hot flush · hyperbilirubinaemia · hyperglycaemia · hypoxia · low cardiac output syndrome · muscle spasms · myocardial infarction · oral disorders · platelet disorder · renal impairment · respiratory disorders · seizure · shock · thrombocytopenia
  ‣ **Frequency not known** Sensation of pressure
- **PREGNANCY** [EvGr] Avoid unless potential benefit outweighs risk—limited information available. ⓜ
- **BREAST FEEDING** [EvGr] Avoid—present in milk in *animal* studies. ⓜ
- **HEPATIC IMPAIRMENT** [EvGr] Caution (limited information available). ⓜ
Dose adjustments [EvGr] Use lowest starting dose. ⓜ For patients with impaired left ventricular function—consult product literature.
- **RENAL IMPAIRMENT** [EvGr] Use with caution. ⓜ
- **DIRECTIONS FOR ADMINISTRATION** [EvGr] For *continuous intravenous infusion*, reconstitute with Glucose 5% *or* Sodium Chloride 0.9%. ⓜ

● **MEDICINAL FORMS** There can be variation in the licensing of different medicines containing the same drug.

Powder for solution for infusion
▸ **Rapibloc** (AOP Orphan Ltd)
  Landiolol hydrochloride 300 mg Rapibloc 300mg powder for solution for infusion vials | 1 vial PoM £248.54 (Hospital only)

CARDIAC GLYCOSIDES

Cardiac glycosides

Digoxin-specific antibody

Serious cases of digoxin toxicity should be discussed with the National Poisons Information Service (see further information, under Poisoning, emergency treatment p. 1554). Digoxin-specific antibody fragments p. 1564 are indicated for the treatment of known or strongly suspected life-threatening digoxin toxicity associated with ventricular arrhythmias or bradyarrhythmias unresponsive to atropine sulfate p. 1526 and when measures beyond the withdrawal of digoxin below and correction of any electrolyte abnormalities are considered necessary.

Digoxin

Digoxin is most useful for controlling ventricular response in persistent and permanent atrial fibrillation and atrial flutter. Digoxin also has a role in heart failure.

For management of atrial fibrillation the maintenance dose of digoxin can usually be determined by the ventricular rate at rest, which should not usually be allowed to fall persistently below 60 beats per minute.

Digoxin is now rarely used for rapid control of heart rate (see management of supraventricular arrhythmias). Even with intravenous administration, response may take many hours; persistence of tachycardia is therefore not an indication for exceeding the recommended dose. The intramuscular route is **not** recommended.

In patients with heart failure who are in sinus rhythm a loading dose is not required, and a satisfactory plasma-digoxin concentration can be achieved over a period of about a week.

Digoxin has a long half-life and maintenance doses need to be given only once daily (although higher doses may be divided to avoid nausea); renal function is the most important determinant of digoxin dosage.

Unwanted effects depend both on the concentration of digoxin in the plasma and on the sensitivity of the conducting system or of the myocardium, which is often increased in heart disease. It can sometimes be difficult to distinguish between toxic effects and clinical deterioration because symptoms of both are similar. The plasma concentration alone cannot indicate toxicity reliably, but the likelihood of toxicity increases progressively through the range 1.5 to 3 micrograms/litre for digoxin. Digoxin should be used with special care in the elderly, who may be particularly susceptible to digitalis toxicity.

Regular monitoring of plasma-digoxin concentration during maintenance treatment is not necessary unless problems are suspected. Hypokalaemia predisposes the patient to digitalis toxicity; it is managed by giving a potassium-sparing diuretic or, if necessary, potassium supplementation.

If toxicity occurs, digoxin should be withdrawn; serious manifestations require urgent specialist management. Digoxin-specific antibody fragments are available for reversal of life-threatening overdosage.

Digoxin   15-Apr-2024

● **DRUG ACTION** Digoxin is a cardiac glycoside that increases the force of myocardial contraction and reduces conductivity within the atrioventricular (AV) node.

● **INDICATIONS AND DOSE**

Rapid digitalisation, for atrial fibrillation or flutter
▸ BY MOUTH
▸ Adult: 0.75–1.5 mg in divided doses, dose to be given over 24 hours, reduce dose in the elderly

Maintenance, for atrial fibrillation or flutter
▸ BY MOUTH
▸ Adult: Maintenance 125–250 micrograms daily, dose according to renal function and initial loading dose, reduce dose in the elderly

Heart failure (for patients in sinus rhythm)
▸ BY MOUTH
▸ Adult: 62.5–125 micrograms once daily, reduce dose in the elderly

Emergency loading dose, for atrial fibrillation or flutter
▸ INITIALLY BY INTRAVENOUS INFUSION
▸ Adult: Loading dose 0.75–1 mg, to be given over at least 2 hours, then (by mouth) maintenance, loading dose is rarely necessary, maintenance dose to be started on the day following the loading dose, reduce dose in the elderly

DOSE ADJUSTMENTS DUE TO INTERACTIONS
▸ Manufacturer advises reduce dose by half with concurrent use of amiodarone, dronedarone and quinine.

DOSE EQUIVALENCE AND CONVERSION
▸ Dose may need to be reduced if digoxin (or another cardiac glycoside) has been given in the preceding 2 weeks.
▸ When switching from intravenous to oral route may need to increase dose by 20–33% to maintain the same plasma-digoxin concentration.

● **UNLICENSED USE** Digoxin doses in the BNF may differ from those in product literature.

● **CONTRA-INDICATIONS** Constrictive pericarditis (unless to control atrial fibrillation or improve systolic dysfunction—but use with caution) · hypertrophic cardiomyopathy (unless concomitant atrial fibrillation and heart failure—but use with caution) · intermittent complete heart block · myocarditis · second degree AV block · supraventricular arrhythmias associated with accessory conducting pathways e.g. Wolff-Parkinson-White syndrome (although can be used in infancy) · ventricular tachycardia or fibrillation

● **CAUTIONS** Hypercalcaemia (risk of digitalis toxicity) · hypokalaemia (risk of digitalis toxicity) · hypomagnesaemia (risk of digitalis toxicity) · hypoxia (risk of digitalis toxicity) · recent myocardial infarction · severe respiratory disease · sick sinus syndrome · thyroid disease

CAUTIONS, FURTHER INFORMATION
▸ Elderly Screening Tool of Older Persons' potentially inappropriate Prescriptions (STOPP) criteria to aid medication reviews (see Prescribing in the elderly p. 31 for information). Potentially inappropriate:
  ● in heart failure with normal systolic ventricular function (no clear evidence of benefit)
  ● at a long-term dose greater than 125 micrograms daily if eGFR less than 30 mL/minute/1.73 m^2 (risk of digoxin toxicity if plasma levels not measured)

● **INTERACTIONS** → Appendix 1: digoxin

● **SIDE-EFFECTS**
▸ **Common or very common** Arrhythmias · cardiac conduction disorder · cerebral impairment · diarrhoea · dizziness ·

eosinophilia · nausea · skin reactions · vision disorders · vomiting
▶ **Uncommon** Depression
▶ **Rare or very rare** Appetite decreased · asthenia · confusion · gastrointestinal disorders · gynaecomastia · headache · malaise · psychosis · thrombocytopenia

Overdose If toxicity occurs, digoxin should be withdrawn; serious manifestations require urgent specialist management.

● PREGNANCY
Dose adjustments May need dosage adjustment.
● BREAST FEEDING Amount too small to be harmful.
● RENAL IMPAIRMENT
Dose adjustments EvGr Consider reducing initial and maintenance doses. Ⓜ
● MONITORING REQUIREMENTS
▶ For plasma-digoxin concentration assay, blood should be taken at least 6 hours after a dose.
▶ Monitor serum electrolytes and renal function. Toxicity increased by electrolyte disturbances.
● DIRECTIONS FOR ADMINISTRATION
▶ With intravenous use Avoid rapid intravenous administration (risk of hypertension and reduced coronary flow). For *intravenous infusion* (*Lanoxin*®), give intermittently in Glucose 5% or Sodium chloride 0.9%; dilute to a concentration of not more than 62.5 micrograms/mL. To be given over at least 2 hours.
▶ With oral use For *oral* administration, oral solution must **not** be diluted.
● PATIENT AND CARER ADVICE Patient counselling is advised for digoxin elixir (use pipette).

● MEDICINAL FORMS There can be variation in the licensing of different medicines containing the same drug. Forms available from special-order manufacturers include: oral suspension, oral solution, solution for injection

Oral tablet
▶ Digoxin (Non-proprietary)
Digoxin 62.5 microgram Digoxin 62.5microgram tablets | 28 tablet PoM £2.65 DT = £1.78 | 30 tablet PoM £1.91-£2.45
Digoxin 125 microgram Digoxin 125microgram tablets | 28 tablet PoM £2.53 DT = £1.70 | 30 tablet PoM £2.37-£2.45
Digoxin 250 microgram Digoxin 250microgram tablets | 28 tablet PoM £2.37 DT = £1.73 | 30 tablet PoM £1.85-£2.45

Solution for injection
EXCIPIENTS: May contain Alcohol, propylene glycol
▶ Digoxin (Non-proprietary)
Digoxin 100 microgram per 1 ml Lanoxin Injection Pediatric 100micrograms/1ml solution for injection ampoules | 10 ampoule PoM Ⓢ

Solution for infusion
▶ Digoxin (Non-proprietary)
Digoxin 250 microgram per 1 ml Digoxin 500micrograms/2ml solution for infusion ampoules | 5 ampoule PoM £4.95 (Hospital only)

Oral solution
▶ Digoxin (Non-proprietary)
Digoxin 50 microgram per 1 ml Digoxin 50micrograms/ml oral solution | 60 ml PoM £6.95 DT = £6.95

SYMPATHOMIMETICS > INOTROPIC

Isoprenaline hydrochloride

28-Aug-2024

● **INDICATIONS AND DOSE**

Emergency treatment of life-threatening bradycardia [when treatment with atropine is ineffective] (under expert supervision)
▶ BY INTRAVENOUS INFUSION
▶ Adult: Initially 5 micrograms/minute, adjust dose according to response. Consult Resuscitation Council (UK) guidance for further information

Severe or permanent bradycardia (under expert supervision) | Stokes-Adams syndrome (under expert supervision)
▶ BY INTRAVENOUS INFUSION
▶ Adult: Carefully titrate dose according to heart rate and response—consult local protocols or product literature

● CONTRA-INDICATIONS Acute coronary insufficiency, especially acute myocardial infarction (except in complete atrioventricular block with extreme bradycardia) · angina pectoris · digitalis intoxication · pre-existing ventricular arrhythmias · tachycardia (heart rate >130 beats per minute) · uncontrolled hyperthyroidism
● CAUTIONS Cardiovascular disorders e.g. chronic coronary insufficiency, arrhythmias and hypertension · controlled hyperthyroidism · convulsive disorders · diabetes mellitus · hypovolaemia
● INTERACTIONS → Appendix 1: isoprenaline
● SIDE-EFFECTS Angina pectoris · arrhythmias · headache · hot flush · hypotension · nausea · tremor
● PREGNANCY EvGr Avoid unless potential benefit outweighs risk. Ⓜ
● BREAST FEEDING Specialist sources indicate probably compatible—careful monitoring of infant recommended. Risk is low if infant is breastfed at least half an hour after administration of isoprenaline.
● MONITORING REQUIREMENTS EvGr Continuous monitoring of ECG and other cardiovascular parameters required—reduce dose in cases of ventricular myocardial hyperexcitability (polymorphic extrasystoles, repetitive burst pacing or ventricular tachycardia); discontinue if heart rate ≥130 beats per minute. Ⓜ
● DIRECTIONS FOR ADMINISTRATION EvGr For *intravenous infusion*, give in Glucose 5% *or* Sodium Chloride 0.9% into a central line or large peripheral vein (to avoid venous irritation from low pH). For *Midomil*®, reconstitute each vial with the requisite volume of infusion fluid to a final concentration of 2-20 micrograms/mL—consult product literature. For *Isoprenaline Macure*®, reconstitute 10 mL in 500 mL of infusion fluid to a final concentration of 4 micrograms/mL. Ⓜ
● HANDLING AND STORAGE Protect from light. Reconstituted solution may be stored at room temperature for up to 25°C for 24 hours. For *Isoprenaline Macure*®: Store and transport in a refrigerator (2-8°C).

● MEDICINAL FORMS There can be variation in the licensing of different medicines containing the same drug. Forms available from special-order manufacturers include: solution for injection

Solution for injection
EXCIPIENTS: May contain Edetic acid (edta)
▶ Isoprenaline hydrochloride (Non-proprietary)
Isoprenaline hydrochloride 200 microgram per 1 ml Isuprel 200micrograms/1ml solution for injection ampoules | 25 ampoule PoM Ⓢ (Hospital only)
Isuprel 1mg/5ml solution for injection ampoules | 10 ampoule PoM Ⓢ (Hospital only)
Isoprenaline hydrochloride 1mg/5ml concentrate for solution for infusion ampoules | 5 ampoule PoM £275.00 (Hospital only)

Solution for infusion
EXCIPIENTS: May contain Edetic acid (edta)
▶ Midomil (Macure Pharma UK Ltd)
Isoprenaline hydrochloride 200 microgram per 1 ml Midomil 1mg/5ml solution for infusion vials | 5 vial PoM £275.00 (Hospital only)

2   Bleeding disorders

ANTIHAEMORRHAGICS > ANTIFIBRINOLYTICS

| Tranexamic acid
05-Jan-2024

- **DRUG ACTION** Tranexamic acid is an antifibrinolytic that prevents or reduces bleeding by impairing fibrin dissolution.

● INDICATIONS AND DOSE
Local fibrinolysis
- ▸ BY MOUTH
- ▸ Adult: 1–1.5 g 2–3 times a day, alternatively 15–25 mg/kg 2–3 times a day
- ▸ INITIALLY BY SLOW INTRAVENOUS INJECTION
- ▸ Adult: 0.5–1 g 2–3 times a day, followed by (by continuous intravenous infusion) 25–50 mg/kg/24 hours, infusion to be given if required

Menorrhagia
- ▸ BY MOUTH
- ▸ Adult: 1 g 3 times a day for up to 4 days, to be initiated when menstruation has started, dose can be increased if necessary up to maximum 4 g per day

Hereditary angioedema
- ▸ BY MOUTH
- ▸ Adult: 1–1.5 g 2–3 times a day, for short-term prophylaxis of hereditary angioedema, tranexamic acid is started several days before planned procedures which may trigger an acute attack of hereditary angioedema (e.g. dental work) and continued for 2–5 days afterwards

Epistaxis
- ▸ BY MOUTH
- ▸ Adult: 1 g 3 times a day for 7 days

General fibrinolysis
- ▸ BY SLOW INTRAVENOUS INJECTION
- ▸ Adult: 1 g every 6–8 hours, alternatively 15 mg/kg every 6–8 hours

Prevention and treatment of significant haemorrhage following major trauma
- ▸ INITIALLY BY SLOW INTRAVENOUS INJECTION
- ▸ Adult: Loading dose 1 g for 1 dose, given as soon as possible within 3 hours of injury (unless there is evidence of hyperfibrinolysis), followed by (by intravenous infusion) 1 g for 1 dose, dose to be infused over 8 hours

Prevention and treatment of haemorrhage following head injury [Glasgow Coma Scale score of 12 or less, and without active extracranial bleeding]
- ▸ BY SLOW INTRAVENOUS INJECTION
- ▸ Adult: 2 g for 1 dose, given as soon as possible within 2 hours of the injury

Treatment of postpartum haemorrhage
- ▸ BY SLOW INTRAVENOUS INJECTION
- ▸ Adult: 1 g for 1 dose, to be repeated if necessary after at least 30 minutes

- **UNLICENSED USE** [EvGr] Tranexamic acid is used in the doses provided in the BNF for the treatment of postpartum haemorrhage, ⟨A⟩ but these may differ from those licensed.

  Tranexamic acid may be used as detailed below, although these situations are considered unlicensed:
  - treatment of local fibrinolysis by continuous intravenous infusion
  - [EvGr] prevention and treatment of significant haemorrhage following major trauma
  - prevention and treatment of haemorrhage following head injury ⟨A⟩

- **CONTRA-INDICATIONS** Fibrinolytic conditions following disseminated intravascular coagulation (unless predominant activation of fibrinolytic system with severe bleeding) · history of convulsions · thromboembolic disease

- **CAUTIONS** Irregular menstrual bleeding (establish cause before initiating therapy) · massive haematuria (avoid if risk of ureteric obstruction) · patients receiving oral contraceptives (increased risk of thrombosis)

  ### CAUTIONS, FURTHER INFORMATION
  - ▸ Menorrhagia Before initiating treatment for menorrhagia, exclude structural or histological causes or fibroids causing distortion of uterine cavity.

- **SIDE-EFFECTS**

  ### GENERAL SIDE-EFFECTS
  - ▸ **Common or very common** Diarrhoea (reduce dose) · nausea · vomiting
  - ▸ **Uncommon** Allergic dermatitis
  - ▸ **Rare or very rare** Colour vision change (discontinue) · embolism and thrombosis
  - ▸ **Frequency not known** Seizure (more common at high doses) · visual impairment (discontinue)

  ### SPECIFIC SIDE-EFFECTS
  - ▸ With intravenous use Hypotension · malaise (on rapid intravenous injection)

- **PREGNANCY** No evidence of teratogenicity in *animal* studies; manufacturer advises use only if potential benefit outweighs risk—crosses the placenta.

- **BREAST FEEDING** Small amount present in milk— antifibrinolytic effect in infant unlikely.

- **RENAL IMPAIRMENT**
  Dose adjustments Reduce dose—consult product literature for details.

- **MONITORING REQUIREMENTS** Regular liver function tests in long-term treatment of hereditary angioedema.

- **DIRECTIONS FOR ADMINISTRATION** [EvGr] Give by slow intravenous injection or infusion at a maximum rate of 100 mg/minute; can be diluted in Glucose 5% *or* Sodium Chloride 0.9%. ⟨M⟩

- **MEDICINAL FORMS** There can be variation in the licensing of different medicines containing the same drug. Forms available from special-order manufacturers include: oral suspension, oral solution

Oral tablet
- ▸ **Tranexamic acid (Non-proprietary)**
  Tranexamic acid 500 mg Tranexamic acid 500mg tablets | 60 tablet [PoM] £35.43 DT = £4.71
- ▸ **Cyklokapron** (Viatris UK Healthcare Ltd)
  Tranexamic acid 500 mg Cyklokapron 500mg tablets | 60 tablet [PoM] £14.30 DT = £4.71

Solution for injection
- ▸ **Tranexamic acid (Non-proprietary)**
  Tranexamic acid 100 mg per 1 ml Tranexamic acid 500mg/5ml solution for injection ampoules | 5 ampoule [PoM] £7.50 DT = £7.50 (Hospital only) | 10 ampoule [PoM] £15.47 DT = £15.47 (Hospital only) Tranexamic acid 1g/10ml solution for injection ampoules | 5 ampoule [PoM] £15.00 (Hospital only)
- ▸ **Cyklokapron** (Pfizer Ltd)
  Tranexamic acid 100 mg per 1 ml Cyklokapron 500mg/5ml solution for injection ampoules | 10 ampoule [PoM] £15.47 DT = £15.47 (Hospital only)

2 Cardiovascular system

ANTIHAEMORRHAGICS > HAEMOSTATICS

Emicizumab

09-May-2018

- **DRUG ACTION** Emicizumab is a monoclonal antibody that bridges activated factor IX and factor X to restore function of missing activated factor VIII, which is needed for haemostasis.

- **INDICATIONS AND DOSE**

Prophylaxis of haemorrhage in haemophilia A (initiated by a specialist)
- ▸ BY SUBCUTANEOUS INJECTION
- ▸ Adult: Initially 3 mg/kg once weekly for 4 weeks, then maintenance 1.5 mg/kg once weekly, alternatively maintenance 3 mg/kg every 2 weeks, alternatively maintenance 6 mg/kg every 4 weeks

- **CAUTIONS** Concomitant bypassing agent · risk factors for thrombotic microangiopathy
  CAUTIONS, FURTHER INFORMATION
- ▸ Concomitant bypassing agent Manufacturer advises discontinue bypassing agents the day before starting emicizumab; if a bypassing agent is required—consult product literature.
- **SIDE-EFFECTS**
- ▸ **Common or very common** Arthralgia · diarrhoea · fever · headache · myalgia
- ▸ **Uncommon** Cavernous sinus thrombosis · embolism and thrombosis · skin necrosis · thrombotic microangiopathy
- **CONCEPTION AND CONTRACEPTION** Manufacturer advises effective contraception during and for 6 months after treatment in women of childbearing potential.
- **PREGNANCY** Manufacturer advises use only if potential benefit outweighs risk—no information available.
- **BREAST FEEDING** Manufacturer advises avoid—no information available.
- **EFFECT ON LABORATORY TESTS** Manufacturer advises to avoid intrinsic pathway clotting-based laboratory tests or use with caution as results may be misinterpreted—consult product literature.
- **DIRECTIONS FOR ADMINISTRATION** Manufacturer advises max. 2 mL per injection site; rotate injection site and avoid skin that is tender, damaged or scarred. Patients or their caregivers may self-administer *Hemlibra*® after appropriate training.
- **PRESCRIBING AND DISPENSING INFORMATION** Emicizumab is a biological medicine. Biological medicines must be prescribed and dispensed by brand name, see *Biological medicines* and *Biosimilar medicines*, under Guidance on prescribing p. 1; manufacturer advises to record the brand name and batch number after each administration.
- **PATIENT AND CARER ADVICE**
  Missed doses Manufacturer advises if a dose is missed, the missed dose may be taken up to a day before the next scheduled dose. The next dose should then be taken on the usual scheduled dosing day.

- **MEDICINAL FORMS** There can be variation in the licensing of different medicines containing the same drug.
  Solution for injection
  - ▸ Hemlibra (Roche Products Ltd)
    Emicizumab 30 mg per 1 ml Hemlibra 12mg/0.4ml solution for injection vials | 1 vial PoM £966.12 (Hospital only)
    Hemlibra 30mg/1ml solution for injection vials | 1 vial PoM £2,415.30 (Hospital only)
    Emicizumab 150 mg per 1 ml Hemlibra 150mg/1ml solution for injection vials | 1 vial PoM £12,076.50 (Hospital only)
    Hemlibra 105mg/0.7ml solution for injection vials | 1 vial PoM £8,453.55 (Hospital only)
    Hemlibra 60mg/0.4ml solution for injection vials | 1 vial PoM £4,830.60 (Hospital only)

2.1 Coagulation factor deficiencies

BLOOD AND RELATED PRODUCTS > COAGULATION PROTEINS

Dried prothrombin complex

20-Nov-2020

(Human prothrombin complex)

- **INDICATIONS AND DOSE**

Congenital deficiency of factors II, VII, IX, or X if purified specific coagulation factors not available (specialist use only) | Acquired deficiency of factors II, VII, IX, or X (e.g. during warfarin treatment) (specialist use only)
- ▸ BY INTRAVENOUS INFUSION
- ▸ Adult: Specialist indication – access specialist resources for dosing information

Major bleeding in patients on warfarin [following phytomenadione] (initiated under specialist supervision)
- ▸ BY INTRAVENOUS INFUSION
- ▸ Adult: 25–50 units/kg

- **CONTRA-INDICATIONS** History of heparin induced thrombocytopenia · myocardial infarction within the last 3 months (no information available) · unstable angina within the last 3 months (no information available)
- **CAUTIONS** Disseminated intravascular coagulation · history of myocardial infarction or coronary heart disease · postoperative use · risk of thrombosis · vaccination against hepatitis A and hepatitis B may be required
- **SIDE-EFFECTS**
- ▸ **Common or very common** Embolism and thrombosis
- ▸ **Uncommon** Anxiety · device thrombosis · haemorrhage · hepatic function abnormal · hypertension · respiratory disorders
- ▸ **Frequency not known** Cardiac arrest · chills · circulatory collapse · disseminated intravascular coagulation · dyspnoea · heparin-induced thrombocytopenia · hypotension · nausea · skin reactions · tachycardia · tremor
- **HEPATIC IMPAIRMENT** Manufacturer advises caution (risk of thromboembolic complications).
  Monitoring Monitor closely in hepatic impairment (risk of thromboembolic complications).
- **PRESCRIBING AND DISPENSING INFORMATION** Dried prothrombin complex is prepared from human plasma by a suitable fractionation technique, and contains factor IX, together with variable amounts of factors II, VII, and X.

- **MEDICINAL FORMS** There can be variation in the licensing of different medicines containing the same drug.
  Powder and solvent for solution for injection
  - ▸ Beriplex P/N (CSL Behring UK Ltd)
    Factor VII 175 unit, Protein S 195 unit, Factor IX 255 unit, Protein C 300 unit, Factor II 340 unit, Factor X 410 unit Beriplex P/N 250 powder and solvent for solution for injection vials | 1 vial PoM £150.00 (Hospital only)
    Factor VII 350 unit, Protein S 390 unit, Factor IX 510 unit, Protein C 600 unit, Factor II 680 unit, Factor X 820 unit Beriplex P/N 500 powder and solvent for solution for injection vials | 1 vial PoM £300.00 (Hospital only)
    Factor VII 700 unit, Protein S 1000 unit, Factor IX 1020 unit, Protein C 1200 unit, Factor II 1360 unit, Factor X 1640 unit Beriplex P/N 1,000 powder and solvent for solution for injection vials | 1 vial PoM £600.00 (Hospital only)
  Powder and solvent for solution for infusion
  - ▸ Octaplex (Octapharma Ltd)
    Factor VII 330 unit, Protein C 380 unit, Protein S 390 unit, Factor X 480 unit, Factor II 490 unit, Factor IX 500 unit Octaplex 500unit

powder and solvent for solution for infusion vials | 1 vial [PoM]
£245.00 (Hospital only)
Octaplex 1,000unit powder and solvent for solution for infusion vials |
1 vial [PoM] £490.00 (Hospital only)

Factor VIIa (recombinant)   26-Mar-2024

● INDICATIONS AND DOSE

**Congenital haemophilia [with inhibitors to, or high
anamnestic response to, factors VIII or IX] (specialist use
only) | Acquired haemophilia (specialist use only) |
Congenital factor VII deficiency (specialist use only) |
Glanzmann's thrombasthenia (specialist use only)**
▶ BY INTRAVENOUS INJECTION
▶ Adult: Specialist indication – access specialist
resources for dosing information

NOVOSEVEN ®

Postpartum haemorrhage (under expert supervision)
▶ BY INTRAVENOUS INJECTION
▶ Adult: 60–90 micrograms/kg for 1 dose, peak
coagulation activity can be expected at 10 minutes,
dose can be repeated after 30 minutes if insufficient
haemostatic response

● **CAUTIONS** Disseminated intravascular coagulation · risk of
thrombosis

● **SIDE-EFFECTS**
▶ **Common or very common** Dizziness · headache · injection
related reaction
▶ **Uncommon** Embolism and thrombosis · fever · hepatic
disorders · intestinal ischaemia · skin reactions
▶ **Rare or very rare** Angina pectoris · cerebrovascular
insufficiency · coagulation disorders · myocardial
infarction · nausea · peripheral ischaemia
▶ **Frequency not known** Angioedema · flushing

● **ALLERGY AND CROSS-SENSITIVITY** For *Cevenfacta* ®,
contra-indicated if hypersensitivity to rabbits or rabbit
protein. For *NovoSeven* ®, contra-indicated if
hypersensitivity to mouse, hamster or bovine protein.

● **PREGNANCY**

NOVOSEVEN ® [EvGr] Avoid (limited information available).
Ⓜ

● **BREAST FEEDING**

NOVOSEVEN ® Specialist source suggest probably safe in
breast-feeding; unlikely to enter milk or be absorbed from
infants gastro-intestinal tract.

● **PRESCRIBING AND DISPENSING INFORMATION** The
available preparations may not be licensed for all
indications or all age-groups—further information can be
found in the product literature.
    NovoSeven ® contains eptacog alfa.
    Cevenfacta ® contains eptacog beta.
    Factor VIIa (recombinant) is a biological medicine.
Biological medicines must be prescribed and dispensed by
brand name, see Biological medicines and Biosimilar
medicines, under Guidance on prescribing p. 1; record the
brand name and batch number after each administration.

● **MEDICINAL FORMS** There can be variation in the licensing of
different medicines containing the same drug.
Powder and solvent for solution for injection
EXCIPIENTS: May contain Polysorbates
▶ Cevenfacta (LFB Biopharmaceuticals Ltd) ▼
Eptacog beta activated 1 mg Cevenfacta 1mg (45,000units) powder
and solvent for solution for injection vials | 1 vial [PoM] £525.20
Eptacog beta activated 2 mg Cevenfacta 2mg (90,000units) powder
and solvent for solution for injection vials | 1 vial [PoM] £1,050.40
Eptacog beta activated 5 mg Cevenfacta 5mg (225,000units)
powder and solvent for solution for injection vials | 1 vial [PoM]
£2,626.00

▶ NovoSeven (Novo Nordisk Ltd)
Eptacog alfa activated 1 mg NovoSeven 1mg (50,000units) powder
and solvent for solution for injection pre-filled syringes | 1 pre-filled
disposable injection [PoM] £525.20 (Hospital only)
Eptacog alfa activated 2 mg NovoSeven 2mg (100,000units) powder
and solvent for solution for injection pre-filled syringes | 1 pre-filled
disposable injection [PoM] £1,050.40 (Hospital only)
Eptacog alfa activated 5 mg NovoSeven 5mg (250,000units) powder
and solvent for solution for injection pre-filled syringes | 1 pre-filled
disposable injection [PoM] £2,626.00 (Hospital only)
Eptacog alfa activated 8 mg NovoSeven 8mg (400,000units) powder
and solvent for solution for injection pre-filled syringes | 1 pre-filled
disposable injection [PoM] £4,201.60 (Hospital only)

Factor VIII fraction, dried [Specialist drug]

25-Apr-2025

(Human coagulation factor VIII, dried)

● INDICATIONS AND DOSE

**Congenital factor VIII deficiency (haemophilia A),
acquired factor VIII deficiency | Von Willebrand's disease**
▶ BY INTRAVENOUS INJECTION, OR BY INTRAVENOUS INFUSION,
OR BY CONTINUOUS INTRAVENOUS INFUSION
▶ Adult: Specialist drug – access specialist resources for
dosing information

● **SIDE-EFFECTS**
▶ **Common or very common** Anamnestic reaction · cough ·
device thrombosis · diarrhoea · factor VIII inhibition · fever
· flushing · haemorrhage · headaches · infusion related
reaction · joint disorders · nausea · pain · skin reactions ·
thrombophlebitis · vomiting
▶ **Uncommon** Dizziness · fatigue · feeling hot · hyperaemia ·
hypersensitivity · hypertension · insomnia · lymphoedema ·
musculoskeletal stiffness · myocardial infarction ·
peripheral oedema · sinus tachycardia

● **NATIONAL FUNDING/ACCESS DECISIONS**
For full details see funding body website
NICE decisions
▶ **Efanesoctocog alfa for treating and preventing bleeding
episodes in haemophilia A in people 2 years and over (April
2025)** NICE TA1051 Recommended with restrictions

● **MEDICINAL FORMS** There can be variation in the licensing of
different medicines containing the same drug.
Powder and solvent for solution for injection
EXCIPIENTS: May contain Polysorbates, sucrose
▶ Factor viii fraction, dried (Non-proprietary)
Dried Factor VIII Fraction type 8Y 250unit powder and solvent for
solution for injection vials | 1 vial [PoM] £137.00
Factor VIII 500 unit, von Willebrand factor 1000 unit Dried Factor
VIII Fraction type 8Y 500unit powder and solvent for solution for
injection vials | 1 vial [PoM] £274.00
▶ Advate (Takeda UK Ltd)
Octocog alfa 250 unit Advate 250unit powder and 2ml solvent for
solution for injection vials | 1 vial [PoM] £177.50
Advate 250unit powder and 5ml solvent for solution for injection vials
| 1 vial [PoM] £177.50
Octocog alfa 500 unit Advate 500unit powder and 5ml solvent for
solution for injection vials | 1 vial [PoM] £355.00
Advate 500unit powder and 2ml solvent for solution for injection vials
| 1 vial [PoM] £355.00
Octocog alfa 1000 unit Advate 1,000unit powder and solvent for
solution for injection vials | 1 vial [PoM] £710.00
Octocog alfa 2000 unit Advate 2,000unit powder and solvent for
solution for injection vials | 1 vial [PoM] £1,420.00
▶ Adynovi (Takeda UK Ltd) ▼
Rurioctocog alfa pegol 250 unit Adynovi 250unit powder and
solvent for solution for injection vials | 1 vial [PoM] £212.50 (Hospital
only)
Rurioctocog alfa pegol 1000 unit Adynovi 1,000unit powder and
solvent for solution for injection vials | 1 vial [PoM] £850.00 (Hospital
only)

Rurioctocog alfa pegol 2000 unit Adynovi 2,000unit powder and solvent for solution for injection vials | 1 vial [PoM] £1,700.00 (Hospital only)

▸ **Altuvoct** (Swedish Orphan Biovitrum Ltd) ▼
Efanesoctocog alfa 250 unit Altuvoct 250unit powder and solvent for solution for injection vials | 1 vial [PoM] £600.00 (Hospital only)
Efanesoctocog alfa 500 unit Altuvoct 500unit powder and solvent for solution for injection vials | 1 vial [PoM] £1,200.00 (Hospital only)
Efanesoctocog alfa 1000 unit Altuvoct 1,000unit powder and solvent for solution for injection vials | 1 vial [PoM] £2,400.00 (Hospital only)
Efanesoctocog alfa 2000 unit Altuvoct 2,000unit powder and solvent for solution for injection vials | 1 vial [PoM] £4,800.00 (Hospital only)
Efanesoctocog alfa 3000 unit Altuvoct 3,000unit powder and solvent for solution for injection vials | 1 vial [PoM] £7,200.00 (Hospital only)
Efanesoctocog alfa 4000 unit Altuvoct 4,000unit powder and solvent for solution for injection vials | 1 vial [PoM] £9,600.00 (Hospital only)

▸ **Elocta** (Swedish Orphan Biovitrum Ltd)
Efmoroctocog alfa 250 unit Elocta 250unit powder and solvent for solution for injection vials | 1 vial [PoM] £212.50 (Hospital only)
Efmoroctocog alfa 500 unit Elocta 500unit powder and solvent for solution for injection vials | 1 vial [PoM] £425.00 (Hospital only)
Efmoroctocog alfa 750 unit Elocta 750unit powder and solvent for solution for injection vials | 1 vial [PoM] £637.50 (Hospital only)
Efmoroctocog alfa 1000 unit Elocta 1,000unit powder and solvent for solution for injection vials | 1 vial [PoM] £850.00 (Hospital only)
Efmoroctocog alfa 1500 unit Elocta 1,500unit powder and solvent for solution for injection vials | 1 vial [PoM] £1,275.00 (Hospital only)
Efmoroctocog alfa 2000 unit Elocta 2,000unit powder and solvent for solution for injection vials | 1 vial [PoM] £1,700.00 (Hospital only)
Efmoroctocog alfa 3000 unit Elocta 3,000unit powder and solvent for solution for injection vials | 1 vial [PoM] £2,550.00 (Hospital only)
Efmoroctocog alfa 4000 unit Elocta 4,000unit powder and solvent for solution for injection vials | 1 vial [PoM] [S] (Hospital only)

▸ **Esperoct** (Novo Nordisk Ltd) ▼
Turoctocog alfa pegol 500 unit Esperoct 500unit powder and solvent for solution for injection vials | 1 vial [PoM] £425.00 (Hospital only)
Turoctocog alfa pegol 1000 unit Esperoct 1,000unit powder and solvent for solution for injection vials | 1 vial [PoM] £850.00 (Hospital only)
Turoctocog alfa pegol 1500 unit Esperoct 1,500unit powder and solvent for solution for injection vials | 1 vial [PoM] £1,275.00 (Hospital only)
Turoctocog alfa pegol 2000 unit Esperoct 2,000unit powder and solvent for solution for injection vials | 1 vial [PoM] £1,700.00 (Hospital only)
Turoctocog alfa pegol 3000 unit Esperoct 3,000unit powder and solvent for solution for injection vials | 1 vial [PoM] £2,550.00 (Hospital only)

▸ **Haemoctin** (Grifols UK Ltd)
Factor VIII high purity 1000 unit Haemoctin 1,000unit powder and solvent for solution for injection vials | 1 vial [PoM] £600.00 (Hospital only)

▸ **NovoEight** (Novo Nordisk Ltd)
Turoctocog alfa 250 unit NovoEight 250unit powder and solvent for solution for injection vials | 1 vial [PoM] £138.59 (Hospital only)
Turoctocog alfa 500 unit NovoEight 500unit powder and solvent for solution for injection vials | 1 vial [PoM] £277.18 (Hospital only)
Turoctocog alfa 1000 unit NovoEight 1,000unit powder and solvent for solution for injection vials | 1 vial [PoM] £554.37 (Hospital only)
Turoctocog alfa 1500 unit NovoEight 1,500unit powder and solvent for solution for injection vials | 1 vial [PoM] £831.55 (Hospital only)
Turoctocog alfa 2000 unit NovoEight 2,000unit powder and solvent for solution for injection vials | 1 vial [PoM] £1,108.74 (Hospital only)
Turoctocog alfa 3000 unit NovoEight 3,000unit powder and solvent for solution for injection vials | 1 vial [PoM] £1,663.11 (Hospital only)

▸ **Nuwiq** (Octapharma Ltd)
Simoctocog alfa 250 unit Nuwiq 250unit powder and solvent for solution for injection vials | 1 vial [PoM] £190.00 (Hospital only)
Simoctocog alfa 500 unit Nuwiq 500unit powder and solvent for solution for injection vials | 1 vial [PoM] £380.00 (Hospital only)
Simoctocog alfa 1000 unit Nuwiq 1,000unit powder and solvent for solution for injection vials | 1 vial [PoM] £760.00 (Hospital only)
Simoctocog alfa 1500 unit Nuwiq 1,500unit powder and solvent for solution for injection vials | 1 vial [PoM] £1,140.00 (Hospital only)
Simoctocog alfa 2000 unit Nuwiq 2,000unit powder and solvent for solution for injection vials | 1 vial [PoM] £1,520.00 (Hospital only)

▸ **Obizur** (Takeda UK Ltd) ▼
Susoctocog alfa 500 unit Obizur 500unit powder and solvent for solution for injection vials | 1 vial [PoM] £1,145.00 (Hospital only)

▸ **Octanate LV** (Octapharma Ltd)
von Willebrand factor 600 unit, Factor VIII 1000 unit Octanate LV 1,000unit powder and solvent for solution for injection vials | 1 vial [PoM] £600.00 (Hospital only)

▸ **ReFacto** (Pfizer Ltd)
Moroctocog alfa 250 unit ReFacto AF 250unit powder and solvent for solution for injection vials | 1 vial [PoM] £125.55 (Hospital only)
ReFacto AF 250unit powder and solvent for solution for injection pre-filled syringes | 1 pre-filled disposable injection [PoM] £125.55 (Hospital only)
Moroctocog alfa 500 unit ReFacto AF 500unit powder and solvent for solution for injection vials | 1 vial [PoM] £251.10 (Hospital only)
ReFacto AF 500unit powder and solvent for solution for injection pre-filled syringes | 1 pre-filled disposable injection [PoM] £251.10 (Hospital only)
Moroctocog alfa 1000 unit ReFacto AF 1,000unit powder and solvent for solution for injection vials | 1 vial [PoM] £502.20 (Hospital only)
ReFacto AF 1,000unit powder and solvent for solution for injection pre-filled syringes | 1 pre-filled disposable injection [PoM] £502.20 (Hospital only)
Moroctocog alfa 2000 unit ReFacto AF 2,000unit powder and solvent for solution for injection pre-filled syringes | 1 pre-filled disposable injection [PoM] £1,004.40 (Hospital only)
ReFacto AF 2,000unit powder and solvent for solution for injection vials | 1 vial [PoM] £1,004.40 (Hospital only)
Moroctocog alfa 3000 unit ReFacto AF 3,000unit powder and solvent for solution for injection pre-filled syringes | 1 pre-filled disposable injection [PoM] £1,506.60 (Hospital only)

▸ **Voncento** (CSL Behring UK Ltd)
Factor VIII 500 unit, von Willebrand factor 1200 unit Voncento 500unit/1,200unit powder and solvent for solution for injection vials | 1 vial [PoM] £385.00
Factor VIII 1000 unit, von Willebrand factor 2400 unit Voncento 1,000unit/2,400unit powder and solvent for solution for injection vials | 1 vial [PoM] £770.00

Powder and solvent for solution for infusion

▸ **Advate** (Takeda UK Ltd)
Octocog alfa 1500 unit Advate 1,500unit powder and solvent for solution for infusion vials | 1 vial [PoM] £1,065.00
Octocog alfa 3000 unit Advate 3,000unit powder and solvent for solution for infusion vials | 1 vial [PoM] £2,130.00

▸ **Wilate 1000** (Octapharma Ltd)
Factor VIII 1000 unit, von Willebrand factor 1000 unit Wilate 1000 powder and solvent for solution for infusion vials | 1 vial [PoM] £500.00 (Hospital only)

▸ **Wilate 500** (Octapharma Ltd)
Factor VIII 500 unit, von Willebrand factor 500 unit Wilate 500 powder and solvent for solution for infusion vials | 1 vial [PoM] £250.00 (Hospital only)

Factor IX [Specialist drug]

22-Nov-2023

● **INDICATIONS AND DOSE**

Congenital factor IX deficiency (haemophilia B)

▸ BY INTRAVENOUS INJECTION, OR BY INTRAVENOUS INFUSION
▸ Adult: Specialist drug – access specialist resources for dosing information

● **CONTRA-INDICATIONS** Disseminated intravascular coagulation

● **SIDE-EFFECTS**

▸ **Common or very common** Anxiety · dizziness · dyspnoea · ear pruritus · factor IX inhibition · fatigue · feeling cold · headache · hot flush · hyperaesthesia · hypersensitivity · nausea · oral disorders · pain · skin reactions · taste altered · urinary tract obstruction

▸ **Uncommon** Appetite decreased · haematuria · hypotension · palpitations · renal colic

▸ **Frequency not known** Disseminated intravascular coagulation · embolism and thrombosis · myocardial infarction · nephrotic syndrome

● **ALLERGY AND CROSS-SENSITIVITY** EvGr For *BeneFIX*®, *Idelvion*®, *Refixia*®, and *Rixubis*®, contra-indicated if hypersensitivity to hamster protein. Ⓜ

● **MEDICINAL FORMS** There can be variation in the licensing of different medicines containing the same drug.

Powder and solvent for solution for injection
EXCIPIENTS: May contain Polysorbates

▸ **Alprolix** (Swedish Orphan Biovitrum Ltd)

Eftrenonacog alfa 250 unit Alprolix 250unit powder and solvent for solution for injection vials | 1 vial PoM £300.00 (Hospital only)

Eftrenonacog alfa 500 unit Alprolix 500unit powder and solvent for solution for injection vials | 1 vial PoM £600.00 (Hospital only)

Eftrenonacog alfa 1000 unit Alprolix 1,000unit powder and solvent for solution for injection vials | 1 vial PoM £1,200.00 (Hospital only)

Eftrenonacog alfa 2000 unit Alprolix 2,000unit powder and solvent for solution for injection vials | 1 vial PoM £2,400.00 (Hospital only)

Eftrenonacog alfa 3000 unit Alprolix 3,000unit powder and solvent for solution for injection vials | 1 vial PoM £3,600.00 (Hospital only)

▸ **Haemonine** (Grifols UK Ltd)

Factor IX high purity 1000 unit Haemonine 1,000unit powder and solvent for solution for injection vials | 1 vial PoM £600.00 (Hospital only)

▸ **Idelvion** (CSL Behring UK Ltd)

Albutrepenonacog alfa 250 unit Idelvion 250unit powder and solvent for solution for injection vials | 1 vial PoM £522.50 (Hospital only)

Albutrepenonacog alfa 500 unit Idelvion 500unit powder and solvent for solution for injection vials | 1 vial PoM £1,045.00 (Hospital only)

Albutrepenonacog alfa 1000 unit Idelvion 1,000unit powder and solvent for solution for injection vials | 1 vial PoM £2,090.00 (Hospital only)

Albutrepenonacog alfa 2000 unit Idelvion 2,000unit powder and solvent for solution for injection vials | 1 vial PoM £4,180.00 (Hospital only)

▸ **Refixia** (Novo Nordisk Ltd) ▼

Nonacog beta pegol 500 unit Refixia 500unit powder and solvent for solution for injection vials | 1 vial PoM £1,221.50 (Hospital only)

Nonacog beta pegol 1000 unit Refixia 1,000unit powder and solvent for solution for injection vials | 1 vial PoM £2,443.00 (Hospital only)

Nonacog beta pegol 2000 unit Refixia 2,000unit powder and solvent for solution for injection vials | 1 vial PoM £4,886.00 (Hospital only)

Nonacog beta pegol 3000 unit Refixia 3,000unit powder and solvent for solution for injection vials | 1 vial PoM £7,329.00 (Hospital only)

▸ **Replenine-VF** (Bio Products Laboratory Ltd)

Factor IX high purity 500 unit Replenine-VF 500unit powder and solvent for solution for injection vials | 1 vial PoM £265.00 (Hospital only)

Factor IX high purity 1000 unit Replenine-VF 1,000unit powder and solvent for solution for injection vials | 1 vial PoM £530.00 (Hospital only)

▸ **Rixubis** (Takeda UK Ltd)

Nonacog gamma 1000 unit Rixubis 1,000unit powder and solvent for solution for injection vials | 1 vial PoM £607.20 (Hospital only)

Nonacog gamma 2000 unit Rixubis 2,000unit powder and solvent for solution for injection vials | 1 vial PoM £1,214.40 (Hospital only)

Powder and solvent for solution for infusion
EXCIPIENTS: May contain Polysorbates

▸ **BeneFIX** (Pfizer Ltd)

Nonacog alfa 250 unit BeneFIX 250unit powder and solvent for solution for infusion vials | 1 vial PoM £151.80 (Hospital only)

Nonacog alfa 500 unit BeneFIX 500unit powder and solvent for solution for infusion vials | 1 vial PoM £303.60 (Hospital only)

Nonacog alfa 1000 unit BeneFIX 1,000unit powder and solvent for solution for infusion vials | 1 vial PoM £607.20 (Hospital only)

Nonacog alfa 2000 unit BeneFIX 2,000unit powder and solvent for solution for infusion vials | 1 vial PoM £1,214.40 (Hospital only)

Nonacog alfa 3000 unit BeneFIX 3,000unit powder and solvent for solution for infusion vials | 1 vial PoM £1,821.60 (Hospital only)

Factor XIII A-subunit (recombinant)
[Specialist drug]   27-Jul-2022

(Catridecacog)

● **INDICATIONS AND DOSE**

Congenital factor XIII A-subunit deficiency

▸ BY INTRAVENOUS INJECTION

▸ Adult: Specialist drug – access specialist resources for dosing information

● **SIDE-EFFECTS**

▸ **Common or very common** Headache · leucopenia · neutropenia · pain in extremity

● **MEDICINAL FORMS** There can be variation in the licensing of different medicines containing the same drug.

Powder and solvent for solution for injection
EXCIPIENTS: May contain Polysorbates

▸ **NovoThirteen** (Novo Nordisk Ltd)

Catridecacog 2500 unit NovoThirteen 2,500unit powder and solvent for solution for injection vials | 1 vial PoM £15,918.13

Factor XIII fraction, dried [Specialist drug]
30-Jan-2020

(Human fibrin-stabilising factor, dried)

● **INDICATIONS AND DOSE**

Congenital factor XIII deficiency

▸ BY INTRAVENOUS INJECTION, OR BY INTRAVENOUS INFUSION

▸ Adult: Specialist drug – access specialist resources for dosing information

● **SIDE-EFFECTS**

▸ **Rare or very rare** Anaphylactoid reaction · dyspnoea · skin reactions

● **MEDICINAL FORMS** There can be variation in the licensing of different medicines containing the same drug.

Powder and solvent for solution for injection

▸ **Fibrogammin P** (CSL Behring UK Ltd)

Factor XIII 250 unit Fibrogammin 250unit powder and solvent for solution for injection vials | 1 vial PoM £152.50

Factor XIII 1250 unit Fibrogammin 1,250unit powder and solvent for solution for injection vials | 1 vial PoM £762.50

Fibrinogen, dried [Specialist drug]
13-Mar-2024

(Human fibrinogen)

● **INDICATIONS AND DOSE**

Hypofibrinogenaemia or afibrinogenaemia

▸ BY INTRAVENOUS INJECTION, OR BY INTRAVENOUS INFUSION

▸ Adult: Specialist drug – access specialist resources for dosing information

● **SIDE-EFFECTS**

▸ **Common or very common** Headache

▸ **Uncommon** Asthma · dizziness · embolism and thrombosis · feeling hot · night sweats · skin reactions · tinnitus · vomiting

● **MEDICINAL FORMS** There can be variation in the licensing of different medicines containing the same drug.

Powder for solution for infusion

▸ **Riastap** (CSL Behring UK Ltd)

Human fibrinogen 1 gram Riastap 1g powder for solution for infusion vials | 1 vial PoM £400.00 (Hospital only)

Powder and solvent for solution for infusion
ELECTROLYTES: May contain Sodium
▸ **FibCLOT** (LFB Biopharmaceuticals Ltd)
   Human fibrinogen 1.5 gram FibCLOT 1.5g powder and solvent for
   solution for infusion vials | 1 vial [PoM] £600.00 (Hospital only)
▸ **Fibryga** (Octapharma Ltd)
   Human fibrinogen 1 gram Fibryga 1g powder and solvent for
   solution for infusion bottles | 1 bottle [PoM] £400.00 (Hospital only)

Protein C concentrate [Specialist drug]

30-Jan-2020

● **INDICATIONS AND DOSE**
Congenital protein C deficiency
▸ BY INTRAVENOUS INJECTION
▸ Adult: Specialist drug – access specialist resources for
   dosing information

● **SIDE-EFFECTS**
▸ **Rare or very rare** Dizziness · fever · skin reactions
▸ **Frequency not known** Haemothorax · hyperhidrosis ·
   restlessness

● **MEDICINAL FORMS** There can be variation in the licensing of
   different medicines containing the same drug.
   Powder and solvent for solution for injection
   ▸ **Ceprotin** (Takeda UK Ltd)
   Protein C human 500 unit Ceprotin 500unit powder and solvent for
   solution for injection vials | 1 vial [PoM] £1,000.00
   Protein C human 1000 unit Ceprotin 1000unit powder and solvent
   for solution for injection vials | 1 vial [PoM] £2,000.00

Von Willebrand factor [Specialist drug]

03-Mar-2021

● **INDICATIONS AND DOSE**
von Willebrand disease
▸ BY SLOW INTRAVENOUS INJECTION
▸ Adult: Specialist drug – access specialist resources for
   dosing information

● **SIDE-EFFECTS**
▸ **Common or very common** Chest discomfort · dizziness ·
   embolism and thrombosis · hypertension · nausea · skin
   reactions · tachycardia · taste altered · tremor · vasodilation
   · vertigo · vomiting
▸ **Uncommon** Angioedema · chills · headache · hypotension ·
   lethargy · paraesthesia · restlessness · wheezing
▸ **Rare or very rare** Fever
▸ **Frequency not known** Dyspnoea · infusion related reaction ·
   vision blurred

● **MEDICINAL FORMS** There can be variation in the licensing of
   different medicines containing the same drug.
   Powder and solvent for solution for injection
   EXCIPIENTS: May contain Polysorbates
   ELECTROLYTES: May contain Sodium
   ▸ **Veyvondi** (Takeda UK Ltd)
   Vonicog alfa 650 unit Veyvondi 650unit powder and solvent for
   solution for injection vials | 1 vial [PoM] £598.00 (Hospital only)
   Vonicog alfa 1300 unit Veyvondi 1,300unit powder and solvent for
   solution for injection vials | 1 vial [PoM] £1,196.00 (Hospital only)
   ▸ **Willfact** (LFB Biopharmaceuticals Ltd)
   von Willebrand factor 1000 unit Willfact 1,000unit powder and
   solvent for solution for injection vials | 1 vial [PoM] £922.00 (Hospital
   only)

BLOOD AND RELATED PRODUCTS ＞
HAEMOSTATIC PRODUCTS

Factor VIII inhibitor bypassing fraction [Specialist drug]

30-Jan-2020

● **INDICATIONS AND DOSE**
**Congenital factor VIII deficiency (haemophilia A) and
factor VIII inhibitors | Non-haemophiliac patients with
acquired factor VIII inhibitors**
▸ BY INTRAVENOUS INFUSION, OR BY INTRAVENOUS INJECTION
▸ Adult: Specialist drug – access specialist resources for
   dosing information

● **CONTRA-INDICATIONS** Disseminated intravascular
   coagulation

● **SIDE-EFFECTS**
▸ **Common or very common** Dizziness · headache ·
   hypersensitivity · hypotension · skin reactions
▸ **Frequency not known** Abdominal discomfort · anamnestic
   reaction · angioedema · chest discomfort · chills · cough ·
   diarrhoea · disseminated intravascular coagulation ·
   drowsiness · dyspnoea · embolism and thrombosis · fever ·
   flushing · hypertension · ischaemic stroke · malaise ·
   myocardial infarction · nausea · paraesthesia · respiratory
   disorders · restlessness · tachycardia · taste altered ·
   vomiting

● **MEDICINAL FORMS** There can be variation in the licensing of
   different medicines containing the same drug.
   Powder and solvent for solution for infusion
   ▸ **FEIBA Imuno** (Takeda UK Ltd)
   Factor VIII inhibitor bypassing fraction 500 unit FEIBA 50units/ml
   (500unit) powder and 10ml solvent for solution for infusion vials |
   1 vial [PoM] £390.00 (Hospital only)
   FEIBA 25units/ml (500unit) powder and 20ml solvent for solution for
   infusion vials | 1 vial [PoM] £390.00 (Hospital only)
   Factor VIII inhibitor bypassing fraction 1000 unit FEIBA
   50units/ml (1,000unit) powder and 20ml solvent for solution for
   infusion vials | 1 vial [PoM] £780.00 (Hospital only)

BLOOD AND RELATED PRODUCTS ＞ PLASMA PRODUCTS

Fresh frozen plasma

13-Jan-2021

● **INDICATIONS AND DOSE**
**Replacement of coagulation factors or other plasma
proteins (specialist use only)**
▸ BY INTRAVENOUS INFUSION
▸ Adult: Specialist indication – access specialist
   resources for dosing information

**Major bleeding in patients on warfarin [following
phytomenadione if dried prothrombin complex is
unavailable]**
▸ BY INTRAVENOUS INFUSION
▸ Adult: 15 mL/kilogram

● **CONTRA-INDICATIONS** Avoid use as a volume expander ·
   IgA deficiency with confirmed antibodies to IgA

● **CAUTIONS** Cardiac decompensation · pulmonary oedema ·
   risk of thrombosis · severe protein S deficiency (avoid
   products with low protein S activity e.g. *OctaplasLG*®) ·
   vaccination against hepatitis A and hepatitis B may be
   required

● **SIDE-EFFECTS**
▸ **Common or very common** Skin reactions
▸ **Uncommon** Fever · hypersensitivity · hypoxia · nausea ·
   sensation abnormal · vomiting
▸ **Rare or very rare** Abdominal pain · anxiety · arrhythmias ·
   back pain · cardiac arrest · chest discomfort · chills ·

circulatory collapse · citrate toxicity · dizziness · dyspnoea · flushing · haemolytic anaemia · haemorrhage · hyperhidrosis · hypertension · hypotension · localised oedema · malaise · procedural complications · pulmonary oedema · respiratory disorders · thromboembolism

- **PRESCRIBING AND DISPENSING INFORMATION** Fresh frozen plasma is prepared from the supernatant liquid obtained by centrifugation of one donation of whole blood.
  A preparation of solvent/detergent treated human plasma (frozen) from pooled donors is available from Octapharma (*OctaplasLG*®).

- **MEDICINAL FORMS** There can be variation in the licensing of different medicines containing the same drug.
  Infusion
  ▸ **OctaplasLG** (Octapharma Ltd)
  Human plasma proteins 57.5 mg per 1 ml OctaplasLG Blood Group A infusion 200ml bags | 1 bag [PoM] £75.00 (Hospital only)
  OctaplasLG Blood Group B infusion 200ml bags | 1 bag [PoM] £75.00 (Hospital only)
  OctaplasLG Blood Group AB infusion 200ml bags | 1 bag [PoM] £75.00 (Hospital only)
  OctaplasLG Blood Group O infusion 200ml bags | 1 bag [PoM] £75.00 (Hospital only)

2.2 Subarachnoid haemorrhage

CALCIUM-CHANNEL BLOCKERS

[F 183]

Nimodipine

01-Dec-2021

- **DRUG ACTION** Nimodipine is a dihydropyridine calcium-channel blocker.

● INDICATIONS AND DOSE

Prevention of ischaemic neurological defects following aneurysmal subarachnoid haemorrhage
▸ BY MOUTH
▸ Adult: 60 mg every 4 hours, to be started within 4 days of aneurysmal subarachnoid haemorrhage and continued for 21 days

Treatment of ischaemic neurological defects following aneurysmal subarachnoid haemorrhage
▸ BY INTRAVENOUS INFUSION
▸ Adult (body-weight up to 70 kg): Initially up to 0.5 mg/hour, increased after 2 hours if no severe fall in blood pressure; increased to 2 mg/hour and continue for at least 5 days (max. 14 days); if surgical intervention during treatment, continue for at least 5 days after surgery; max. total duration of nimodipine use 21 days, to be given via central catheter
▸ Adult (body-weight 70 kg and above): Initially 1 mg/hour, increased after 2 hours if no severe fall in blood pressure; increased to 2 mg/hour and continue for at least 5 days (max. 14 days); if surgical intervention during treatment, continue for at least 5 days after surgery; max. total duration of nimodipine use 21 days, to be given via central catheter

Treatment of ischaemic neurological defects following aneurysmal subarachnoid haemorrhage in patients with unstable blood pressure
▸ BY INTRAVENOUS INFUSION
▸ Adult: Initially up to 0.5 mg/hour, increased after 2 hours if no severe fall in blood pressure; increased to 2 mg/hour and continue for at least 5 days (max. 14 days); if surgical intervention during treatment, continue for at least 5 days after surgery; max. total

duration of nimodipine use 21 days, to be given via central catheter

> **IMPORTANT SAFETY INFORMATION**
> **SAFE PRACTICE**
> Nimodipine has been confused with amlodipine; care must be taken to ensure the correct drug is prescribed and dispensed.

- **CONTRA-INDICATIONS** Unstable angina · within 1 month of myocardial infarction
- **CAUTIONS** Cerebral oedema · hypotension · severely raised intracranial pressure
- **INTERACTIONS** → Appendix 1: calcium channel blockers
- **SIDE-EFFECTS**
  ▸ **Uncommon** Thrombocytopenia · vasodilation
  ▸ **Rare or very rare** Bradycardia · ileus
- **PREGNANCY** Manufacturer advises use only if potential benefit outweighs risk.
- **BREAST FEEDING** Manufacturer advises avoid—present in milk.
- **HEPATIC IMPAIRMENT**
  ▸ With oral use Manufacturer advises consider avoiding in severe impairment.
  Dose adjustments
  ▸ With oral use Manufacturer advises dose reduction, if used in severe impairment.
- **DIRECTIONS FOR ADMINISTRATION** [EvGr] Avoid concomitant administration of nimodipine infusion and tablets. Ⓜ
  ▸ With oral use For administration *by mouth*, expert sources advise tablets may be crushed but are light sensitive.
  ▸ With intravenous use [EvGr] For *continuous intravenous infusion*, administer undiluted via an infusion pump and three-way stopcock on a central venous catheter connected to a running infusion of Glucose 5%, or Sodium Chloride 0.9% (consult product literature); not to be added to an infusion container; incompatible with polyvinyl chloride giving sets or containers; protect infusion from light. Ⓜ Polyethylene, polypropylene, or glass apparatus should be used.

- **MEDICINAL FORMS** There can be variation in the licensing of different medicines containing the same drug. Forms available from special-order manufacturers include: oral suspension
  Solution for infusion
  ▸ **Nimotop** (Bayer Plc)
  Nimodipine 200 microgram per 1 ml Nimotop 0.02% solution for infusion 50ml vials | 1 vial [PoM] £13.60 (Hospital only)
  Oral tablet
  ▸ **Nimotop** (Bayer Plc)
  Nimodipine 30 mg Nimotop 30mg tablets | 100 tablet [PoM] £40.00 DT = £40.00

3   Blood clots

3.1 Blocked catheters and lines

> **Other drugs used for Blocked catheters and lines** Heparin (unfractionated), p. 156 · Urokinase, p. 162

Cardiovascular system

2

PROSTAGLANDINS AND ANALOGUES

Epoprostenol

25-Jan-2021

(Prostacyclin)

- **DRUG ACTION** Epoprostenol is a prostaglandin and a potent vasodilator. It is also a powerful inhibitor of platelet aggregation.

- **INDICATIONS AND DOSE**

Inhibition of platelet aggregation during renal dialysis when heparins are unsuitable or contra-indicated | Treatment of primary pulmonary hypertension resistant to other treatments, usually with oral anti-coagulation (initiated by a specialist)

▸ BY CONTINUOUS INTRAVENOUS INFUSION
▸ Adult: (consult product literature)

PHARMACOKINETICS
▸ Short half-life of approximately 3 minutes, therefore it must be administered by continuous intravenous infusion.

- **CONTRA-INDICATIONS** Severe left ventricular dysfunction

- **CAUTIONS** Avoid abrupt withdrawal when used for primary pulmonary hypertension (risk of rebound pulmonary hypertension) · extreme caution in coronary artery disease · haemorrhagic diathesis · pulmonary veno-occlusive disease · reconstituted solution highly alkaline—avoid extravasation (irritant to tissues) · risk of pulmonary oedema (dose titration for pulmonary hypertension should be in hospital)

- **INTERACTIONS** → Appendix 1: epoprostenol

- **SIDE-EFFECTS**
▸ **Common or very common** Abdominal pain · anxiety · arrhythmias · arthralgia · chest discomfort · diarrhoea · flushing · haemorrhage · headache · intracranial haemorrhage · nausea · pain · rash · sepsis · vomiting
▸ **Uncommon** Dry mouth · hyperhidrosis
▸ **Rare or very rare** Fatigue · hyperthyroidism · intravenous catheter occlusion · local infection · pallor
▸ **Frequency not known** Ascites · pulmonary oedema (avoid chronic use if occurs during dose titration) · spleen abnormalities

- **PREGNANCY** Use if potential benefit outweighs risk.

- **BREAST FEEDING** Manufacturer advises avoid—no information available.

- **MONITORING REQUIREMENTS** Anticoagulant monitoring required when given with anticoagulants.

- **TREATMENT CESSATION** Avoid abrupt withdrawal when used for primary pulmonary hypertension (risk of rebound pulmonary hypertension).

- **DIRECTIONS FOR ADMINISTRATION** Directions for administration vary depending on the preparation used—consult product literature.

- **MEDICINAL FORMS** There can be variation in the licensing of different medicines containing the same drug.

Powder for solution for infusion
▸ Epoprostenol (Non-proprietary)
Epoprostenol (as Epoprostenol sodium) 1.5 mg Epoprostenol 1.5mg powder (pH12) for solution for infusion vials | 1 vial [PoM] Ⓢ (Hospital only)
▸ Veletri (Janssen-Cilag Ltd)
Epoprostenol (as Epoprostenol sodium) 500 microgram Veletri 500microgram powder for solution for infusion vials | 1 vial [PoM] £24.44 (Hospital only)
Epoprostenol (as Epoprostenol sodium) 1.5 mg Veletri 1.5mg powder for solution for infusion vials | 1 vial [PoM] £49.24

Powder and solvent for solution for infusion
ELECTROLYTES: May contain Sodium
▸ Flolan (GlaxoSmithKline UK Ltd)
Epoprostenol (as Epoprostenol sodium) 500 microgram Flolan 500microgram powder and solvent for solution for infusion vials | 1 vial [PoM] £22.22
Epoprostenol (as Epoprostenol sodium) 1.5 mg Flolan 1.5mg powder and solvent for solution for infusion vials | 1 vial [PoM] £44.76 (Hospital only)

3.2 Thromboembolism

Venous thromboembolism

10-Aug-2022

Description of condition

Venous thromboembolism (VTE) includes both deep-vein thrombosis (DVT) and pulmonary embolism (PE), and refers to a blood clot that forms in a vein which partially or completely obstructs blood flow. Hospital-acquired venous thromboembolism refers to a VTE that occurs within 90 days of hospital admission. It is a common and potentially preventable problem.

Risk factors for VTE include surgery, trauma, significant immobility, malignancy, obesity, acquired or inherited hypercoagulable states, pregnancy and the postpartum period, and hormonal therapy (combined hormonal contraception or hormone replacement therapy).

A DVT, the most common form of VTE, usually occurs in the deep veins of the legs or pelvis but may affect other sites such as the upper limbs, and the intracranial and splanchnic veins. Symptoms of a DVT include unilateral localised pain, swelling, tenderness, skin changes, and/or vein distension.

A PE most commonly occurs when a thrombus, usually from a DVT, travels in the blood (embolus) and obstructs blood flow to the lungs causing respiratory dysfunction. Symptoms of a PE include chest pain, shortness of breath, and/or haemoptysis.

Venous thromboembolism prophylaxis

For guidance on reducing the risk of venous thromboembolism in individuals with COVID-19, see NICE rapid guideline: **Managing COVID-19** (available at: www.nice.org.uk/guidance/ng191), and SIGN rapid guideline: **Prevention and management of venous thromboembolism in patients with COVID-19** (available at: www.sign.ac.uk/our-guidelines/prevention-and-management-of-venous-thromboembolism-in-covid-19/). For further information on COVID-19, see COVID-19 p. 714.

[EvGr] All patients should undergo a risk assessment to identify their risk of venous thromboembolism (VTE) and bleeding on admission to hospital. Ⓐ Commonly used risk assessment tools can be found at: www.nice.org.uk/guidance/ng89/resources.

There are two methods of thromboprophylaxis: mechanical and pharmacological. Options for mechanical prophylaxis are anti-embolism stockings that provide graduated compression and produce a calf pressure of 14–15 mmHg, and intermittent pneumatic compression. [EvGr] Anti-embolism stockings should be worn day and night until the patient is sufficiently mobile; they should not be offered to patients admitted with acute stroke or those with conditions such as peripheral arterial disease, peripheral neuropathy, severe leg oedema, or local conditions (e.g. gangrene, dermatitis).

When using pharmacological prophylaxis, in most cases, it should start as soon as possible or within 14 hours of admission. Patients with risk factors for bleeding (e.g. acute stroke, thrombocytopenia, acquired or untreated inherited bleeding disorders) should *only* receive pharmacological prophylaxis when their risk of VTE outweighs their risk of bleeding. Patients receiving anticoagulant treatment who are at high risk of VTE should be considered for prophylaxis if their anticoagulant treatment is interrupted, for example during the peri-operative period. ⓐ

For full guidance on the prophylaxis of VTE, see NICE guideline: **Venous thromboembolism in over 16s** (see *Useful resources*).

Surgical patients

EvGr To reduce the risk of VTE in surgical patients, regional anaesthesia over general anaesthesia should be used if possible.

Mechanical prophylaxis (e.g. anti-embolism stockings or intermittent pneumatic compression) should be offered to patients with major trauma, or undergoing cranial, abdominal, bariatric, thoracic, maxillofacial, ear, nose, and throat, cardiac or elective spinal surgery. Prophylaxis should continue until the patient is sufficiently mobile or discharged from hospital (or for 30 days in spinal injury, elective spinal surgery or cranial surgery). ⓐ Choice of mechanical prophylaxis depends on factors such as the type of surgery, suitability for the patient, and their condition.

EvGr Pharmacological prophylaxis should be considered in patients undergoing general or orthopaedic surgery when the risk of VTE outweighs the risk of bleeding. ⓐ The choice of prophylaxis will depend on the type of surgery, suitability for the patient, and local policy. EvGr A low molecular weight heparin is suitable in all types of general and orthopaedic surgery; heparin (unfractionated) p. 156 is preferred in patients with renal impairment. Fondaparinux sodium p. 148 is an option for patients undergoing abdominal, bariatric, thoracic or cardiac surgery, or for patients with lower limb immobilisation or fragility fractures of the pelvis, hip or proximal femur.

Pharmacological prophylaxis in general surgery should usually continue for at least 7 days post-surgery, or until sufficient mobility has been re-established. Pharmacological prophylaxis should be extended to 28 days after major cancer surgery in the abdomen, and to 30 days in spinal surgery.

Mechanical prophylaxis with intermittent pneumatic compression should be considered when pharmacological prophylaxis is contra-indicated in patients undergoing lower limb amputation, or those with major trauma or fragility fractures of the pelvis, hip or proximal femur.

Patients undergoing an *elective hip replacement* should be given thromboprophylaxis with either a low molecular weight heparin administered for 10 days followed by low-dose aspirin p. 142 for a further 28 days, or a low molecular weight heparin administered for 28 days in combination with anti-embolism stockings until discharge, or rivaroxaban p. 149. If these options are unsuitable, apixaban p. 145 or dabigatran etexilate p. 159 can be considered as alternatives. If pharmacological prophylaxis is contra-indicated, anti-embolism stockings can be used until discharge.

Patients undergoing an *elective knee replacement* should be given thromboprophylaxis with either low-dose aspirin p. 142 for 14 days, or a low molecular weight heparin administered for 14 days in combination with anti-embolism stockings until discharge, or rivaroxaban. If these options are unsuitable, apixaban or dabigatran etexilate can be considered as alternatives. If pharmacological prophylaxis is contra-indicated, intermittent pneumatic compression can be used until the patient is mobile. ⓐ

Medical patients

The choice of prophylaxis will depend on the medical condition, suitability for the patient, and local policy. EvGr Acutely ill medical patients who are at high risk of VTE should be offered pharmacological prophylaxis. Patients should be given either a low molecular weight heparin as a first-line option, or fondaparinux sodium as an alternative, for a minimum of 7 days. Patients with renal impairment should be given either a low molecular weight heparin or heparin (unfractionated) and the dose should be adjusted as necessary.

Mechanical prophylaxis can be considered when pharmacological prophylaxis is contra-indicated; their use should be continued until the patient is sufficiently mobile. In patients admitted with acute stroke, mechanical prophylaxis with intermittent pneumatic compression should be considered, as anti-embolism stockings are unsuitable in these patients; their use should be started within 3 days of the acute stroke and continued for 30 days, or until the patient is sufficiently mobile or discharged from hospital. ⓐ

Thromboprophylaxis in pregnancy

EvGr All pregnant women (who are not in active labour), or women who have given birth, had a miscarriage or termination of pregnancy during the past 6 weeks, with a risk of VTE that outweighs the risk of bleeding should be considered for pharmacological prophylaxis with a low molecular weight heparin during hospital admission. In pregnant women, prophylaxis should be continued until there is no longer a risk of VTE, or until discharge from hospital. Women who have given birth, had a miscarriage or termination of pregnancy during the past 6 weeks, should start thromboprophylaxis with a low molecular weight heparin 4–8 hours after the event, unless contra-indicated, and continue for a minimum of 7 days.

Additional mechanical prophylaxis should be considered for women who are likely to be immobilised or have significantly reduced mobility and continued until the woman is sufficiently mobile or discharged from hospital. Intermittent pneumatic compression should be used as the first-line option and anti-embolism stockings as an alternative. ⓐ

Venous thromboembolism treatment

For guidance on the management of venous thromboembolism (VTE) in individuals with COVID-19, see SIGN rapid guideline: **Prevention and management of venous thromboembolism in patients with COVID-19** (available at: www.sign.ac.uk/our-guidelines/prevention-and-management-of-venous-thromboembolism-in-covid-19/). For further information on COVID-19, see COVID-19 p. 714.

For full guidance on assessment and diagnostic investigations for a deep-vein thrombosis (DVT) or a pulmonary embolism (PE), see NICE guideline: **Venous thromboembolic diseases** (see *Useful resources*).

EvGr Immediately refer patients for hospital admission if they have a suspected PE and signs of haemodynamic instability (including pallor, tachycardia, hypotension, shock, and collapse). ⓐ

Non-drug treatment

EvGr Elastic graduated compression stockings may be used to manage leg symptoms after a DVT. Patients should be given information about their correct use, duration of application, and replacement. Elastic graduated compression stockings are not recommended to prevent post-thrombotic syndrome or venous thromboembolism (VTE) recurrence after a DVT.

Mechanical interventions (such as inferior vena caval filters or percutaneous mechanical thrombectomy) can be considered in certain patients. ⓐ For further information, see NICE guideline: **Venous thromboembolic diseases** (see *Useful resources*).

Drug treatment

EvGr Thrombolytic treatment may be appropriate for selected patients with a symptomatic iliofemoral DVT or a PE with haemodynamic instability. ⓐ For full guidance, see NICE guideline: **Venous thromboembolic diseases** (see *Useful resources*).

EvGr Offer interim therapeutic anticoagulation [unlicensed use for some options] to patients in whom diagnostic investigations cannot be completed or results obtained within the required time frame. If possible, the choice of interim therapeutic anticoagulant should be one that can be continued if a proximal DVT and/or PE is confirmed.

When offering anticoagulation treatment, take into account comorbidities, contra-indications, and the patient's preferences. When starting treatment, carry out baseline blood tests (including full blood count, renal and hepatic function, prothrombin time and activated partial thromboplastin time).

Offer either apixaban p. 145 or rivaroxaban p. 149 for patients with a confirmed proximal DVT or PE (see below for guidance on specific population groups). If apixaban or rivaroxaban are unsuitable, offer either a:

- low molecular weight heparin (LMWH) for at least 5 days followed by dabigatran etexilate p. 159 or edoxaban p. 147; **or**
- LMWH given concurrently with a vitamin K antagonist for at least 5 days or until the INR is at least 2.0 for 2 consecutive readings, followed by a vitamin K antagonist on its own.

The use of heparin (unfractionated) p. 156 with a vitamin K antagonist to treat a confirmed proximal DVT or PE is not routinely recommended, unless the patient has renal impairment, established renal failure, or an increased risk of bleeding.

For renally impaired patients (estimated creatinine clearance between 15–50 mL/min) with a confirmed proximal DVT or PE, follow locally agreed protocols, or advice from a specialist or multidisciplinary team, and offer one of the following options:

- Apixaban;
- Rivaroxaban;
- LMWH for at least 5 days followed by either dabigatran etexilate (if estimated creatinine clearance is 30 mL/min or above) or edoxaban;
- LMWH or heparin (unfractionated), given concurrently with a vitamin K antagonist for at least 5 days or until the INR is at least 2.0 for 2 consecutive readings, followed by a vitamin K antagonist on its own. Ⓐ

For guidance on anticoagulation treatment for patients with established renal failure (estimated creatinine clearance less than 15 mL/min), see NICE guideline: **Venous thromboembolic diseases** (see *Useful resources*).

For further information on anticoagulation treatment for patients at extremes of body weight (less than 50 kg or more than 120 kg), and for guidance on anticoagulation treatment in those with active cancer, triple positive antiphospholipid syndrome, or confirmed PE with haemodynamic instability, see NICE guideline: **Venous thromboembolic diseases** (see *Useful resources*).

EvGr Provide patients initiated on anticoagulation treatment with verbal and written information. This should include how to take anticoagulants and for how long, possible side-effects, interactions, monitoring requirements, affect on activities (such as sports or travel) and on dental treatments, and when and how to seek medical help. In addition, women should be provided with advice on the use of anticoagulants if planning a pregnancy or they become pregnant. An 'anticoagulant alert card' that is specific to the patient's treatment should also be provided—advise patients to carry this at all times.

If anticoagulation treatment fails, assess adherence and other potential sources of hypercoagulability; increase the dose of the anticoagulant or change to an anticoagulant with a different mode of action as appropriate. Ⓐ

Duration of anticoagulation treatment and long-term anticoagulation for secondary prevention

EvGr Patients with a confirmed proximal DVT or PE should be offered anticoagulation treatment for at least 3 months (3 to 6 months for those with active cancer). The benefits and risks of continuing, stopping, or changing anticoagulation treatment should be assessed and discussed with the patient after this duration.

Consider stopping anticoagulation treatment 3 months (3 to 6 months for those with active cancer) after a provoked DVT or PE if the provoking factor is no longer present and the clinical course has been uncomplicated. Patients should be given advice about the risk of recurrence; written information on symptoms or signs to look out for; and who to contact to discuss any new signs, symptoms or other concerns.

For patients with an unprovoked DVT or PE, consider continuing anticoagulation beyond 3 months (beyond 6 months for those with active cancer). Discuss with the patient their preferences, and risk of VTE recurrence and bleeding—explain to patients with low bleeding risk that the benefits of continuing anticoagulation treatment are likely to outweigh the risks. If there is a plan to stop anticoagulation treatment, consider testing for hereditary thrombophilia in patients with a first-degree relative who has had a DVT or PE, and testing for antiphospholipid antibodies—these tests can be affected by anticoagulants and specialist advice may be needed.

Consider the patient's preferences and their clinical situation when selecting an anticoagulant for long-term treatment. Predictive risk tools (such as HAS-BLED score) can be considered to assess whether long-term anticoagulation is appropriate, but relying on them solely is not recommended.

Offer continued treatment with the anticoagulant used for initial treatment if it is well tolerated for patients who do not have renal impairment, active cancer, established triple positive antiphospholipid syndrome, or are not at extremes of body weight. If the current treatment is not well tolerated, or the clinical situation or patient's preferences has changed, consider switching to apixaban p. 145 if the current treatment is a direct-acting anticoagulant other than apixaban.

For patients with renal impairment, active cancer, established triple positive antiphospholipid syndrome, or are at extremes of body weight, consider continuing current anticoagulation treatment if it is well tolerated.

Consider aspirin p. 142 [unlicensed] for patients who decline continued anticoagulation treatment.

Patients on long-term anticoagulation or aspirin treatment should be reviewed at least once a year for general health, risk of VTE recurrence, bleeding risk, and treatment preferences. Ⓐ

Venous thromboembolism treatment in pregnancy

EvGr Women with a suspected deep-vein thrombosis (DVT) and/or pulmonary embolism (PE) who are pregnant or who have given birth during the past 6 weeks, should be referred immediately to hospital for assessment and management.

Before initiating pharmacological anticoagulation treatment for venous thromboembolism (VTE), carry out baseline blood tests (including full blood count, coagulation screen, urea and electrolytes, and liver function tests).

A low molecular weight heparin (LMWH) should be started immediately for suspected VTE (until VTE has been excluded) and be continued as maintenance treatment in patients with confirmed DVT or PE. Routine measurements of peak anti-Xa activity is recommended for women on LMWH who are at extremes of body weight (less than 50 kg or 90 kg or more) or those with complicating factors (such as renal impairment or recurrent VTE).

In the initial management of a DVT, an elastic graduated compression stocking should be applied on the affected leg as an additional treatment to manage symptoms such as pain and swelling.

Women considered to be at high risk of haemorrhage and in whom continued heparin treatment is essential, should be treated with intravenous heparin (unfractionated) p. 156

until the risk factors for haemorrhage have resolved. If VTE occurs at term, consider using intravenous heparin (unfractionated).

Pregnant women who develop heparin-induced thrombocytopenia or are heparin allergic should be managed with an alternative anticoagulant under specialist advice. Ⓐ

For further guidance on anticoagulation treatment during pregnancy and labour or prior to planned delivery; and for full guidance on anticoagulation treatment postnatally, and duration of treatment, see Royal College of Obstetricians and Gynaecologists guideline: **Thromboembolic Disease in Pregnancy and the Puerperium** (see *Useful resources*).

Extracorporeal circuits

Heparin (unfractionated) is also used in the maintenance of extracorporeal circuits in cardiopulmonary bypass and haemodialysis.

Haemorrhage

If haemorrhage occurs, it is usually sufficient to withdraw unfractionated or low molecular weight heparin, but if rapid reversal of the effects of the heparin is required, protamine sulfate p. 1564 is a specific antidote (but only partially reverses the effects of low molecular weight heparins).

For information on the management of haemorrhage in patients on oral anticoagulants, see Oral anticoagulants p. 138.

Useful Resources

Thromboembolic Disease in Pregnancy and the Puerperium: Acute Management. Royal College of Obstetricians and Gynaecologists guidelines. Green-top Guideline 37b. April 2015.
www.rcog.org.uk/en/guidelines-research-services/guidelines/gtg37b/

Venous thromboembolic diseases: diagnosis, management and thrombophilia testing. National Institute for Health and Care Excellence. NICE guideline 158. March 2020.
www.nice.org.uk/guidance/ng158

Venous thromboembolism in over 16s: reducing the risk of hospital-acquired deep vein thrombosis or pulmonary embolism. National Institute for Health and Care Excellence. NICE guideline 89. March 2018 (updated August 2019).
www.nice.org.uk/guidance/ng89

Stroke

01-Oct-2024

Overview

Stroke is associated with a significant risk of morbidity and mortality. Patients presenting with acute symptoms should be immediately transferred to hospital for accurate diagnosis of stroke type, and urgent initiation of appropriate treatment; patients should be managed by a specialist multidisciplinary stroke team.

The following section gives an overview of the initial and long-term management of transient ischaemic attack, ischaemic stroke, and intracerebral haemorrhage. For information on the management of other conditions (such as cerebral amyloid angiopathy, cerebral venous thrombosis, cervical artery dissection, intracranial artery stenosis, and subarachnoid haemorrhage) see **National Clinical Guideline for Stroke for the UK and Ireland** (see *Useful resources*).

Transient ischaemic attack and minor ischaemic stroke

EvGr Patients suspected of having a transient ischaemic attack should immediately receive aspirin p. 142, unless contra-indicated. Patients with aspirin hypersensitivity, or those intolerant of aspirin despite the addition of a proton

pump inhibitor, should receive a suitable alternative antiplatelet.

Patients presenting within 24 hours of transient ischaemic attack or minor stroke who have a low risk of bleeding, should be considered for dual antiplatelet therapy with clopidogrel p. 143 plus aspirin followed by clopidogrel monotherapy. Ticagrelor p. 249 [unlicensed use] plus aspirin dual antiplatelet therapy followed by either ticagrelor [unlicensed use] or clopidogrel [unlicensed use] monotherapy is also an option. For patients who are not appropriate for dual antiplatelet therapy, clopidogrel monotherapy [unlicensed use] should be given.

A proton pump inhibitor should be considered for patients with a history of dyspepsia associated with aspirin, or for concurrent use with dual antiplatelet therapy to reduce the risk of gastrointestinal haemorrhage.

Following a confirmed diagnosis, patients should receive treatment for secondary prevention (see *Long-term Management*, under *Ischaemic Stroke*). Ⓐ

Ischaemic stroke

Initial management

EvGr Alteplase p. 250 or tenecteplase p. 251 are recommended in the treatment of acute ischaemic stroke if it can be administered within 4.5 hours of symptom onset and if intracranial haemorrhage has been excluded by appropriate imaging techniques. It should be given by medical staff experienced in the administration of thrombolytics and the treatment of acute stroke, within a specialist stroke centre. Some patients may also be eligible for surgical management. Provided that intracranial haemorrhage has been excluded, patients who received thrombolysis should be started on an antiplatelet after 24 hours, unless contra-indicated.

Patients with disabling acute ischaemic stroke should be started on aspirin (unless contra-indicated) as soon as possible within 24 hours and continued for 2 weeks after stroke onset, when long-term antithrombotic treatment should be started. Patients being transferred to care at home before 2 weeks should be started on long-term antithrombotic treatment earlier.

A proton pump inhibitor should be considered for patients with a history of dyspepsia associated with aspirin, or for concurrent use with dual antiplatelet therapy to reduce the risk of gastrointestinal haemorrhage. Patients with aspirin hypersensitivity, or those intolerant of aspirin despite the addition of a proton pump inhibitor, should receive an alternative antiplatelet (such as clopidogrel p. 143).

Anticoagulants are not recommended as an alternative to antiplatelet drugs in acute ischaemic stroke in patients who are in sinus rhythm. However, anticoagulants may be indicated in patients with ischaemic stroke and symptomatic deep vein thrombosis or pulmonary embolism. Patients with immobility after acute stroke should not be routinely given low molecular weight heparin or graduated compression stockings for the prevention of deep vein thrombosis. Ⓐ Warfarin sodium p. 165 should not be given in the acute phase of an ischaemic stroke.

EvGr Patients already receiving anticoagulation for a prosthetic heart valve who experience a disabling ischaemic stroke and are at significant risk of haemorrhagic transformation, should have their anticoagulant treatment stopped for 7 days and substituted with aspirin.

Treatment of hypertension in the acute phase of ischaemic stroke can result in reduced cerebral perfusion, and should therefore only be instituted in the event of a hypertensive emergency, or in those patients considered for thrombolysis. Ⓐ

For further information on initial management (such as thrombolysis beyond 4.5 hours of symptom onset, surgical management, and management when anticoagulants are considered inappropriate), see **National Clinical Guideline for Stroke for the UK and Ireland** (see *Useful resources*).

Long-term management

EvGr Patients should receive long-term treatment following a transient ischaemic attack or an ischaemic stroke to reduce the risk of further cardiovascular events.

Long-term treatment with clopidogrel [unlicensed in transient ischaemic attack] monotherapy is recommended in patients who presented with transient ischaemic attack or ischaemic stroke (not associated with atrial fibrillation). If clopidogrel is contra-indicated or not tolerated, aspirin should be used.

A proton pump inhibitor should be considered for patients with a history of dyspepsia associated with aspirin, or for concurrent use with dual antiplatelet therapy to reduce the risk of gastrointestinal haemorrhage.

Anticoagulants are not routinely recommended in the long-term prevention of recurrent stroke, except when atrial fibrillation or other indications (such as a cardiac source of embolism, cerebral venous thrombosis or arterial dissection) are present. Patients with ischaemic stroke or transient ischaemic attack associated with atrial fibrillation or atrial flutter should be reviewed for long-term anticoagulant treatment, the timing of anticoagulant treatment depends on stroke severity and individual patient factors. (A) For guidance on long-term anticoagulation in patients with atrial fibrillation, see *Atrial fibrillation* in Arrhythmias p. 113.

EvGr A high-intensity statin (such as atorvastatin p. 234) should be initiated in patients not already taking a statin as soon as they can swallow medication safely, irrespective of the patient's serum-cholesterol concentration. Patients with ischaemic stroke who are already taking a statin can continue statin treatment. If investigation confirms no evidence of atherosclerosis, patients should be assessed for lipid-lowering therapy on the basis of their overall cardiovascular risk. (A) For further information, see Cardiovascular disease risk assessment and prevention p. 219.

EvGr Beta-blockers should not be used in the management of hypertension following a stroke, unless they are indicated for a co-existing condition. (A) For guidance on blood pressure lowering therapy and treatment targets, see Hypertension p. 166.

EvGr All patients should be advised to make lifestyle modifications that include beneficial changes to diet, physical activity, weight, alcohol intake, and Smoking cessation p. 565. (A)

For further information on long-term management (such as anticoagulation and management when anticoagulants are considered inappropriate, and management of post-stroke complications) see **National Clinical Guideline for Stroke for the UK and Ireland** (see *Useful resources*).

Intracerebral haemorrhage

Initial Management

EvGr Surgical intervention may be required following intracerebral haemorrhage to remove the haematoma and relieve intracranial pressure.

Rapid blood pressure lowering treatment should not be given to patients who have an underlying structural cause, have a score on the Glasgow Coma Scale of below 6, are going to have early neurosurgery to evacuate the haematoma, or who have a very large haematoma with a poor expected prognosis.

Consider rapid blood pressure lowering for patients who present within 6 hours of symptom onset with a systolic blood pressure between 150 and 220 mmHg and who do not fit any exclusion criteria. Aim for a systolic blood pressure target of 130 to 139 mmHg within 1 hour and sustained for at least 7 days, ensuring that the magnitude drop does not exceed 60 mmHg within 1 hour of starting treatment. Rapid blood pressure lowering should also be considered on a case-by-case basis for patients who present beyond 6 hours of symptom onset or who have a systolic blood pressure greater than 220 mmHg and who do not fit any exclusion criteria. Seek specialist paediatric advice if considering blood pressure lowering in patients aged 16 or 17 years who do not fit any exclusion criteria.

Patients taking anticoagulants should have this treatment stopped and reversed. Anticoagulant therapy has, however, been used in patients with intracerebral haemorrhage who are symptomatic of deep vein thrombosis or pulmonary embolism; placement of a caval filter is an alternative in this situation.

Patients with immobility after acute stroke should not be routinely given low molecular weight heparin or graduated compression stockings for the prevention of deep vein thrombosis. (A)

Long-term management

EvGr Specialist advice should be sought for patients with atrial fibrillation and those at a high risk of ischaemic stroke or cardiac ischaemic events, as aspirin p. 142 and anticoagulant therapy are not normally recommended following an intracerebral haemorrhage.

Blood pressure should be measured and treatment initiated where appropriate, taking care to avoid hypoperfusion. (A) For guidance on blood pressure lowering therapy and treatment targets, see Hypertension p. 166.

EvGr Statins should be avoided following intracerebral haemorrhage, however they can be used with caution when the risk of a vascular event outweighs the risk of further haemorrhage. (M)(EvGr) Patients should be assessed for lipid-lowering therapy on the basis of their overall cardiovascular risk and the underlying cause of the haemorrhage. (A) For further information, see Cardiovascular disease risk assessment and prevention p. 219.

For further information on long-term management (such as post-stroke complications), see **National Clinical Guideline for Stroke for the UK and Ireland** (see *Useful resources*).

Useful resources

National Clinical Guideline for Stroke for the United Kingdom and Ireland. Scottish Intercollegiate Guidelines Network and Royal College of Physicians. April 2023.
www.strokeguideline.org/

Oral anticoagulants

10-Aug-2022

Overview

The main use of anticoagulants is to prevent thrombus formation or extension of an existing thrombus in the slower-moving venous side of the circulation, where the thrombus consists of a fibrin web enmeshed with platelets and red cells. For further information on prevention and treatment of venous thromboembolism, see Venous thromboembolism p. 134.

Anticoagulants are of less use in preventing thrombus formation in arteries, for in faster-flowing vessels thrombi are composed mainly of platelets with little fibrin.

Patients prescribed an anticoagulant should be provided with verbal and written information about their treatment, including how and when to seek medical attention. Immediate medical attention is required in certain patients, such as in those with bleeding that is severe, does not stop or recurs, or who have other signs or symptoms of concern (e.g. sudden severe back pain or breathlessness); in particular, patients who have sustained a head injury should be referred to a hospital emergency department.

Vitamin K antagonists

The oral anticoagulants warfarin sodium p. 165, acenocoumarol p. 164 and phenindione p. 164, antagonise the effects of vitamin K, and take at least 48 to 72 hours for the anticoagulant effect to develop fully; warfarin sodium is the drug of choice. If an immediate effect is required, unfractionated or low molecular weight heparin must be given concomitantly.

These oral anticoagulants should not be used in cerebral artery thrombosis or peripheral artery occlusion as first-line therapy; aspirin p. 142 is more appropriate for reduction of risk in transient ischaemic attacks. Unfractionated or a low molecular weight heparin (see under Parenteral anticoagulants p. 140) is usually preferred for the prophylaxis of venous thromboembolism in patients undergoing surgery; alternatively, warfarin sodium can be continued in selected patients currently taking long-term warfarin sodium and who are at high risk of thromboembolism (seek expert advice).

Dose
The base-line prothrombin time should be determined but the initial dose should not be delayed whilst awaiting the result.

Target INR
The following indications and target INRs for adults for warfarin take into account recommendations of the British Society for Haematology guidelines on oral anticoagulation with warfarin—fourth edition. *Br J Haematol* 2011; **154**: 311–324:

An INR which is within 0.5 units of the target value is generally satisfactory; larger deviations require dosage adjustment. Target values (rather than ranges) are now recommended.

INR 2.5 for:

- treatment of deep-vein thrombosis or pulmonary embolism (including those associated with antiphospholipid syndrome or for recurrence in patients no longer receiving warfarin sodium)
- atrial fibrillation
- cardioversion—target INR should be achieved at least 3 weeks before cardioversion and anticoagulation should continue for at least 4 weeks after the procedure (higher target values, such as an INR of 3, can be used for up to 4 weeks before the procedure to avoid cancellations due to low INR)
- dilated cardiomyopathy
- mitral stenosis or regurgitation in patients with either atrial fibrillation, a history of systemic embolism, a left atrial thrombus, or an enlarged left atrium
- bioprosthetic heart valves in the mitral position (treat for 3 months), or in patients with a history of systemic embolism (treat for at least 3 months), or with a left atrial thrombus at surgery (treat until clot resolves), or with other risk factors (e.g. atrial fibrillation or a low ventricular ejection fraction) *[note: NICE guideline NG208 (Heart valve disease presenting in adults: investigation and management, November 2021) does not recommend anticoagulation after surgical biological heart valve replacement unless there is another indication for anticoagulation.]*
- acute arterial embolism requiring embolectomy (consider long-term treatment)
- myocardial infarction

INR 3.5 for:

- recurrent deep-vein thrombosis or pulmonary embolism in patients currently receiving anticoagulation and with an INR above 2;

Mechanical prosthetic heart valves:

- the recommended target INR depends on the type and location of the valve, and patient-related risk factors

- consider increasing the INR target or adding an antiplatelet drug, if an embolic event occurs whilst anticoagulated at the target INR.

Duration
The risks of thromboembolism recurrence and anticoagulant-related bleeding should be considered when deciding the duration of anticoagulation.

The British Society for Haematology (Guidelines on Oral Anticoagulation with Warfarin—fourth edition. *Br J Haematol* 2011; **154**: 311–324) recommend 6 weeks of warfarin sodium for isolated calf-vein deep-vein thrombosis.

For information on duration of anticoagulant treatment following a confirmed proximal deep-vein thrombosis or pulmonary embolism, see Venous thromboembolism p. 134.

Haemorrhage
The main adverse effect of all oral anticoagulants is haemorrhage. Checking the INR and omitting doses when appropriate is essential; if the anticoagulant is stopped but not reversed, the INR should be measured 2–3 days later to ensure that it is falling. The cause of an elevated INR should be investigated. The following recommendations (which take into account the recommendations of the British Society for Haematology Guidelines on Oral Anticoagulation with Warfarin—fourth edition. *Br J Haematol* 2011; **154**: 311–324) are based on the result of the INR and whether there is major or minor bleeding; the recommendations apply to adults taking warfarin:

- Major bleeding—stop warfarin sodium; give phytomenadione p. 1248 (vitamin K₁) by slow intravenous injection; give dried prothrombin complex p. 128 (factors II, VII, IX, and X); if dried prothrombin complex unavailable, fresh frozen plasma can be given but is less effective; recombinant factor VIIa is not recommended for emergency anticoagulation reversal
- INR >8.0, minor bleeding—stop warfarin sodium; give phytomenadione (vitamin K₁) by slow intravenous injection; repeat dose of phytomenadione if INR still too high after 24 hours; restart warfarin sodium when INR <5.0
- INR >8.0, no bleeding—stop warfarin sodium; give phytomenadione (vitamin K₁) by mouth using the intravenous preparation orally [unlicensed use]; repeat dose of phytomenadione if INR still too high after 24 hours; restart warfarin when INR <5.0
- INR 5.0–8.0, minor bleeding—stop warfarin sodium; give phytomenadione (vitamin K₁) by slow intravenous injection; restart warfarin sodium when INR <5.0
- INR 5.0–8.0, no bleeding—withhold 1 or 2 doses of warfarin sodium and reduce subsequent maintenance dose
- Unexpected bleeding at therapeutic levels—always investigate possibility of underlying cause e.g. unsuspected renal or gastro-intestinal tract pathology

Peri-operative anticoagulation
Warfarin sodium should usually be stopped 5 days before elective surgery; phytomenadione (vitamin K₁) by mouth (using the intravenous preparation orally [unlicensed use]) should be given the day before surgery if the INR is ≥1.5. If haemostasis is adequate, warfarin sodium can be resumed at the normal maintenance dose on the evening of surgery or the next day.

Patients stopping warfarin sodium p. 165 prior to surgery who are considered to be at high risk of thromboembolism (e.g. those with a venous thromboembolic event within the last 3 months, atrial fibrillation with previous stroke or transient ischaemic attack, or mitral mechanical heart valve) may require interim therapy ('bridging') with a low molecular weight heparin (using treatment dose). The low molecular weight heparin should be stopped at least 24 hours before surgery; if the surgery carries a high risk of bleeding, the low molecular weight heparin should not be restarted until at least 48 hours after surgery.

Patients on warfarin sodium who require emergency surgery that can be delayed for 6–12 hours can be given intravenous phytomenadione p. 1248 (vitamin K_1) to reverse the anticoagulant effect. If surgery cannot be delayed, dried prothrombin complex p. 128 can be given in addition to intravenous phytomenadione (vitamin K_1) and the INR checked before surgery.

Combined anticoagulant and antiplatelet therapy

Existing antiplatelet therapy following an acute coronary syndrome or percutaneous coronary intervention should be continued for the necessary duration according to the indication being treated. The addition of warfarin sodium, when indicated (e.g. for venous thromboembolism or atrial fibrillation) should be considered following an assessment of the patient's risk of bleeding and discussion with a cardiologist. The duration of treatment with dual therapy (e.g. aspirin p. 142 and warfarin sodium) or triple therapy (e.g. aspirin with clopidogrel p. 143 and warfarin sodium) should be kept to a minimum where possible. The risk of bleeding with aspirin and warfarin sodium dual therapy is lower than with clopidogrel and warfarin sodium. Depending on the indications being treated and the patient's risk of thromboembolism, it may be possible to withhold antiplatelet therapy until warfarin sodium therapy is complete, or *vice versa* (on specialist advice) in order to reduce the length of time on dual or triple therapy.

Direct-acting oral anticoagulants

Direct-acting oral anticoagulants (DOACs) include apixaban p. 145, dabigatran etexilate p. 159, edoxaban p. 147, and rivaroxaban p. 149. Dabigatran etexilate is a reversible inhibitor of free thrombin, fibrin-bound thrombin, and thrombin-induced platelet aggregation. Apixaban, edoxaban, and rivaroxaban are reversible inhibitors of activated factor X (factor Xa) which prevents thrombin generation and thrombus development.

Indications

Apixaban, dabigatran etexilate, edoxaban, and rivaroxaban are used for the prevention of stroke and systemic embolism in patients with non-valvular atrial fibrillation in specific circumstances, and for the treatment and secondary prevention of deep-vein thrombosis and/or pulmonary embolism. For guidance on the management of these conditions, see *Stroke prevention* in Arrhythmias p. 113, and Venous thromboembolism p. 134.

Apixaban, dabigatran etexilate, and rivaroxaban are also used for the prevention of venous thromboembolism after elective hip or knee replacement surgery. For guidance on venous thromboembolism prevention, see Venous thromboembolism p. 134.

Rivaroxaban is also used for the prevention of atherothrombotic events in patients with coronary or peripheral artery disease, and following an acute coronary syndrome with raised biomarkers in specific circumstances— for guidance, see *Secondary prevention of cardiovascular events* in Acute coronary syndromes p. 247.

Monitoring

Routine anticoagulant monitoring is not required with direct-acting oral anticoagulant (DOAC) treatment. For further information on other monitoring parameters, see *Monitoring requirements* in individual drug monographs. The anticoagulant effects of DOACs diminish 12 to 24 hours after the last dose is taken, therefore omitted or delayed doses could lead to a reduction in anticoagulant effect.

Haemorrhage

Reversal agents are available for dabigatran etexilate, apixaban, and rivaroxaban.

Idarucizumab p. 166 is licensed for the rapid reversal of dabigatran etexilate in life-threatening or uncontrolled bleeding, or for emergency surgery or urgent procedures.

Andexanet alfa p. 165 is licensed for the reversal of apixaban or rivaroxaban in life-threatening or uncontrolled bleeding.

Parenteral anticoagulants

12-Feb-2021

Overview

The main use of anticoagulants is to prevent thrombus formation or extension of an existing thrombus in the slower-moving venous side of the circulation, where the thrombus consists of a fibrin web enmeshed with platelets and red cells. For information on the prevention and treatment of venous thromboembolism, see Venous thromboembolism p. 134.

Anticoagulants are of less use in preventing thrombus formation in arteries, for in faster-flowing vessels thrombi are composed mainly of platelets with little fibrin.

Patients prescribed an anticoagulant should be provided with verbal and written information about their treatment, including how and when to seek medical attention. Immediate medical attention is required in certain patients, such as in those with bleeding that is severe, does not stop or recurs, or who have other signs or symptoms of concern; in particular, patients who have sustained a head injury should be referred to a hospital emergency department.

Heparin

Heparin initiates anticoagulation rapidly but has a short duration of action. It is often referred to as **'standard'** or heparin (unfractionated) p. 156 to distinguish it from the **low molecular weight heparins**, which have a longer duration of action. Although a low molecular weight heparin is generally preferred for routine use, heparin (unfractionated) can be used in those at high risk of bleeding because its effect can be terminated rapidly by stopping the infusion.

Low molecular weight heparins

Low molecular weight heparins (dalteparin sodium p. 153, enoxaparin sodium p. 155, and tinzaparin sodium p. 157) are usually preferred over heparin (unfractionated) in the *prevention* of venous thromboembolism because they are as effective and they have a lower risk of heparin-induced thrombocytopenia. The standard prophylactic regimen does not require anticoagulant monitoring. The duration of action of low molecular weight heparins is longer than that of heparin (unfractionated) and *once-daily subcutaneous* administration is possible for some indications, making them convenient to use.

Low molecular weight heparins are generally preferred over heparin (unfractionated) in the *treatment* of deep vein thrombosis and pulmonary embolism, and are also used for the prevention of clotting in extracorporeal circuits.

Low molecular weight heparins may be used in the treatment of acute coronary syndromes, however other agents are preferred. For further information, see Acute coronary syndromes p. 247.

Heparinoids

Danaparoid sodium p. 152 is a heparinoid used for prophylaxis of deep-vein thrombosis in patients undergoing general or orthopaedic surgery. Providing there is no evidence of cross-reactivity, it also has a role in patients who develop heparin-induced thrombocytopenia.

Argatroban

An oral anticoagulant can be given with argatroban monohydrate p. 158, but it should only be started once thrombocytopenia has substantially resolved.

Hirudins

Bivalirudin, a hirudin analogue, is a thrombin inhibitor which is licensed for unstable angina or non-ST-segment elevation myocardial infarction in patients planned for urgent or early intervention, and as an anticoagulant for patients undergoing percutaneous coronary intervention (including patients with ST-segment elevation myocardial infarction undergoing primary percutaneous coronary intervention—see also *ST-segment elevation myocardial infarction (STEMI)* in Acute coronary syndromes p. 247).

Heparin flushes

The use of heparin flushes should be kept to a minimum. For maintaining patency of peripheral venous catheters, sodium chloride injection 0.9% is as effective as heparin flushes. The role of heparin flushes in maintaining patency of arterial and central venous catheters is unclear.

Epoprostenol

Epoprostenol (prostacyclin) can be given to inhibit platelet aggregation during renal dialysis when heparins are unsuitable or contra-indicated. It is also licensed for the treatment of primary pulmonary hypertension resistant to other treatment, usually with oral anticoagulation; it should be initiated by specialists in pulmonary hypertension. Epoprostenol is a potent vasodilator. It has a short half-life of approximately 3 minutes and therefore it must be administered by continuous intravenous infusion.

Fondaparinux

Fondaparinux sodium is a synthetic pentasaccharide that inhibits activated factor X.

> **Other drugs used for Thromboembolism** Streptokinase, p. 251

ANTITHROMBOTIC DRUGS > ANTIPLATELET DRUGS

Antiplatelet drugs
06-Jun-2023

Overview

Antiplatelet drugs decrease platelet aggregation and inhibit thrombus formation in the arterial circulation, because in faster-flowing vessels, thrombi are composed mainly of platelets with little fibrin.

[EvGr] Use of aspirin p. 142 in primary prevention of cardiovascular disease, in patients with or without diabetes, or hypertension, is not recommended. Long-term use of low-dose aspirin is recommended in patients with established cardiovascular disease (secondary prevention); (A) unduly high blood pressure must be controlled before aspirin is given. If the patient is at a high risk of gastro-intestinal bleeding, a proton pump inhibitor can be added. For full guidance on the assessment and prevention of cardiovascular disease risk, see Cardiovascular disease risk assessment and prevention p. 219.

Aspirin is given following coronary bypass surgery. It is also used for intermittent claudication, for stable angina and acute coronary syndromes, for use following placement of coronary stents and for use in stroke.

[EvGr] Following transcatheter aortic valve implantation (TAVI), consider aspirin monotherapy [unlicensed] rather than dual antiplatelet therapy. If aspirin is not tolerated, clopidogrel [unlicensed] should be considered as an alternative. (A)

Clopidogrel p. 143 is used for the prevention of atherothrombotic events in patients with a history of symptomatic ischaemic disease (e.g. ischaemic stroke).

Clopidogrel is also used, in combination with low-dose aspirin, for the prevention of atherothrombotic and thromboembolic events in patients with atrial fibrillation (and at least one risk factor for a vascular event), and for whom warfarin sodium p. 165 is unsuitable.

Use of clopidogrel with aspirin increases the risk of bleeding. Clopidogrel monotherapy may be an alternative when aspirin is contra-indicated, for example in patients with aspirin hypersensitivity, or when aspirin is not tolerated despite the addition of a proton pump inhibitor.

Dipyridamole p. 144 is licensed for secondary prevention of ischaemic stroke and transient ischaemic attacks.

Prasugrel p. 248, in combination with aspirin, is licensed for the prevention of atherothrombotic events in patients with acute coronary syndrome undergoing percutaneous coronary intervention; the combination is usually given for up to 12 months.

Ticagrelor p. 249, in combination with aspirin, is licensed for the prevention of atherothrombotic events in patients with acute coronary syndrome; the combination is usually given for up to 12 months.

Cangrelor p. 243, in combination with aspirin, is licensed for the reduction of thrombotic cardiovascular events in patients with coronary artery disease undergoing percutaneous coronary intervention (PCI) who have not received treatment with oral clopidogrel, prasugrel or ticagrelor prior to the procedure and in whom oral therapy with these drugs is not suitable. Cangrelor is to be used under expert supervision only.

For recommendations on the use of antiplatelet drugs following an acute coronary syndrome, see Acute coronary syndromes p. 247, and for further information on the use of antiplatelet drugs in stroke and transient ischaemic attack, see Stroke p. 137.

Antiplatelet drugs and coronary stents

Patients selected for percutaneous coronary intervention (PCI), with the placement of a coronary stent, will require dual antiplatelet therapy with aspirin and either cangrelor, clopidogrel, prasugrel, or ticagrelor. Aspirin therapy should continue indefinitely. [EvGr] Following PCI in patients with stable angina, clopidogrel is recommended in addition to aspirin for at least 1 month after placement of a bare-metal stent, and for at least 6 months if a drug-eluting stent is used. (A) Clopidogrel should not be discontinued prematurely in patients with a drug-eluting stent—there is an increased risk of stent thrombosis as a result of the eluted drug slowing the re-endothelialisation process. Patients considered to be at high-risk of developing late stent thrombosis with a drug-eluting stent may require a longer duration of treatment with clopidogrel combined with aspirin. Prasugrel or ticagrelor are alternatives to clopidogrel in certain patients undergoing PCI. For information on the use of antiplatelet drugs in patients with an acute coronary syndrome who are undergoing PCI with placement of a coronary stent, see Acute coronary syndromes p. 247.

Glycoprotein IIb/IIIa inhibitors

Glycoprotein IIb/IIIa inhibitors prevent platelet aggregation by blocking the binding of fibrinogen to receptors on platelets. Abciximab is a monoclonal antibody which binds to glycoprotein IIb/IIIa receptors and to other related sites; it is licensed as an adjunct to heparin (unfractionated) p. 156 and aspirin for the prevention of ischaemic complications in high-risk patients undergoing percutaneous transluminal coronary intervention. Abciximab should be used once only (to avoid additional risk of thrombocytopenia). Eptifibatide p. 244 (in combination with heparin (unfractionated) and aspirin) and tirofiban p. 244 (in combination with heparin (unfractionated), aspirin, and clopidogrel) also inhibit glycoprotein IIb/IIIa receptors; they are licensed for use to prevent early myocardial infarction in patients with unstable angina or non-ST-segment-elevation myocardial infarction. Tirofiban is also licensed for use in combination with heparin (unfractionated), aspirin, and clopidogrel, for the reduction of major cardiovascular events in patients with ST-segment elevation myocardial infarction intended for primary percutaneous coronary intervention. Abciximab, eptifibatide and tirofiban should be used by specialists only.

Aspirin

15-Apr-2024

(Acetylsalicylic Acid)

● INDICATIONS AND DOSE

Cardiovascular disease (secondary prevention)
▶ BY MOUTH
▹ Adult: 75 mg once daily

Secondary prevention of deep-vein thrombosis (in patients who decline continued anticoagulation treatment) | Secondary prevention of pulmonary embolism (in patients who decline continued anticoagulation treatment)
▶ BY MOUTH
▹ Adult: 75 mg once daily, alternatively 150 mg once daily

Management of unstable angina and non-ST-segment elevation myocardial infarction (NSTEMI) | Management of ST-segment elevation myocardial infarction (STEMI)
▶ BY MOUTH
▹ Adult: 300 mg for 1 dose, dose to be chewed or dispersed in water

Suspected transient ischaemic attack
▶ BY MOUTH
▹ Adult: 300 mg once daily until diagnosis established

Disabling acute ischaemic stroke
▶ BY MOUTH, OR BY RECTUM
▹ Adult: 300 mg once daily for 14 days, to be started 24 hours after thrombolysis or as soon as possible within 24 hours of symptom onset in patients not receiving thrombolysis

Transient ischaemic attack [in combination with clopidogrel in patients with a low risk of bleeding] | Minor ischaemic stroke [in combination with clopidogrel in patients with a low risk of bleeding]
▶ BY MOUTH
▹ Adult: Initially 300 mg for 1 dose, to be started within 24 hours of onset of symptoms, then 75 mg once daily for 21 days

Transient ischaemic attack [in combination with ticagrelor in patients with a low risk of bleeding] | Minor ischaemic stroke [in combination with ticagrelor in patients with a low risk of bleeding]
▶ BY MOUTH
▹ Adult: Initially 300 mg for 1 dose, to be started within 24 hours of onset of symptoms, then 75 mg once daily for 30 days

Ischaemic stroke [in patients with atrial fibrillation or flutter]
▶ BY MOUTH
▹ Adult: 300 mg once daily until anticoagulant treatment is started

Following disabling ischaemic stroke in patients receiving anticoagulation for a prosthetic heart valve and who are at significant risk of haemorrhagic transformation
▶ BY MOUTH
▹ Adult: 300 mg once daily, anticoagulant treatment stopped for 7 days and to be substituted with aspirin

Secondary prevention of transient ischaemic attack [in patients without atrial fibrillation and when clopidogrel contra-indicated or not tolerated] | Secondary prevention of ischaemic stroke [in patients without atrial fibrillation and when clopidogrel contra-indicated or not tolerated]
▶ BY MOUTH
▹ Adult: 75 mg once daily

Following coronary by-pass surgery
▶ BY MOUTH
▹ Adult: 75–300 mg once daily

Mild to moderate pain | Pyrexia
▶ BY MOUTH
▹ Adult: 300–900 mg every 4–6 hours as required; maximum 4 g per day
▶ BY RECTUM
▹ Adult: 450–900 mg every 4 hours; maximum 3.6 g per day

Acute migraine
▶ BY MOUTH
▹ Adult: 900 mg for 1 dose, to be taken as soon as migraine symptoms develop

Prevention of pre-eclampsia in women at moderate or high risk
▶ BY MOUTH
▹ Adult: 75–150 mg once daily from 12 weeks gestation until the birth of the baby

Mild to moderate pain (dose approved for use by community practitioner nurse prescribers) | Pyrexia (dose approved for use by community practitioner nurse prescribers)
▶ BY MOUTH
▹ Child 16-17 years: 300–600 mg every 4–6 hours as required, maximum 2.4 g per day without doctor's advice
▹ Adult: 300–600 mg every 4–6 hours as required, maximum 2.4 g per day without doctor's advice

● UNLICENSED USE Aspirin may be used as detailed below, although these situations are considered unlicensed:
  ● EvGr secondary prevention of deep-vein thrombosis in patients who decline continued anticoagulation treatment
  ● secondary prevention of pulmonary embolism in patients who decline continued anticoagulation treatment
  ● prevention of pre-eclampsia in women at moderate or high risk Ⓐ

● CONTRA-INDICATIONS Active peptic ulceration · bleeding disorders · children under 16 years (risk of Reye's syndrome) · haemophilia · previous peptic ulceration (analgesic dose) · severe cardiac failure (analgesic dose)
CONTRA-INDICATIONS, FURTHER INFORMATION
▶ Reye's syndrome Owing to an association with Reye's syndrome, manufacturer advises aspirin-containing preparations should not be given to children under 16 years, unless specifically indicated, e.g. for Kawasaki disease.

● CAUTIONS Allergic disease · anaemia · asthma · dehydration · elderly · G6PD deficiency · history of gout · hypertension · may mask symptoms of infection · preferably avoid during fever or viral infection in children (risk of Reye's syndrome) · previous peptic ulceration (but manufacturers may advise avoidance of aspirin in history of peptic ulceration) · thyrotoxicosis
CAUTIONS, FURTHER INFORMATION
▶ Elderly Screening Tool of Older Persons' potentially inappropriate Prescriptions (STOPP) criteria to aid medication reviews (see Prescribing in the elderly p. 31 for information). Potentially inappropriate:

- at long-term doses greater than 160 mg daily (increased risk of bleeding, no evidence for increased efficacy)
- with a past history of peptic ulcer disease without concomitant proton pump inhibitor use (risk of recurrent peptic ulcer)
- with concurrent significant bleeding risk, such as uncontrolled severe hypertension, bleeding diathesis, or recent non-trivial spontaneous bleeding (high risk of bleeding)
- when used with clopidogrel as secondary stroke prevention unless the patient has a coronary stent(s) inserted in the previous 12 months, or concurrent acute coronary syndrome, or has a high grade symptomatic carotid arterial stenosis (no evidence of added benefit over clopidogrel monotherapy)
- when used with vitamin K antagonists, direct thrombin inhibitors, or factor Xa inhibitors in patients with chronic atrial fibrillation (no added benefit from aspirin)

- **INTERACTIONS** → Appendix 1: aspirin

- **SIDE-EFFECTS**
  GENERAL SIDE-EFFECTS
  ▸ **Rare or very rare** Asthmatic attack · bronchospasm
  SPECIFIC SIDE-EFFECTS
  ▸ **Common or very common**
  ▸ With oral use Dyspepsia · haemorrhage
  ▸ **Uncommon**
  ▸ With oral use Dyspnoea · rhinitis · severe cutaneous adverse reactions (SCARs) · skin reactions
  ▸ **Rare or very rare**
  ▸ With oral use Aplastic anaemia · erythema nodosum · gastrointestinal haemorrhage (severe) · granulocytosis · haemorrhagic vasculitis · intracranial haemorrhage · menorrhagia · nausea · thrombocytopenia · vomiting
  ▸ **Frequency not known**
  ▸ With oral use Fluid retention · gastrointestinal disorders · headache · hearing loss · hepatic failure · hyperuricaemia · iron deficiency anaemia · renal impairment · sodium retention · tinnitus · vertigo

  Overdose The main features of salicylate poisoning are hyperventilation, tinnitus, deafness, vasodilatation, and sweating. Coma is uncommon but indicates very severe poisoning.
  For specific details on the management of poisoning, see Aspirin, under Emergency treatment of poisoning p. 1554.

- **ALLERGY AND CROSS-SENSITIVITY** EvGr Aspirin is **contra-indicated** in history of hypersensitivity to aspirin or any other NSAID—which includes those in whom attacks of asthma, angioedema, urticaria, or rhinitis have been precipitated by aspirin or any other NSAID. Ⓜ

- **PREGNANCY** Use antiplatelet doses with caution during third trimester; impaired platelet function and risk of haemorrhage; delayed onset and increased duration of labour with increased blood loss; avoid analgesic doses if possible in last few weeks (low doses probably not harmful); high doses may be related to intra-uterine growth restriction, teratogenic effects, closure of fetal ductus arteriosus in utero and possibly persistent pulmonary hypertension of newborn; kernicterus may occur in jaundiced neonates.

- **BREAST FEEDING** Avoid—possible risk of Reye's syndrome; regular use of high doses could impair platelet function and produce hypoprothrombinaemia in infant if neonatal vitamin K stores low.

- **HEPATIC IMPAIRMENT** Manufacturer advises use with caution in mild-to-moderate impairment; avoid in severe impairment.

- **RENAL IMPAIRMENT** EvGr Caution in mild to moderate impairment (risk of fluid retention, further renal impairment, and gastro-intestinal bleeding); avoid in severe impairment. Ⓜ

- **PRESCRIBING AND DISPENSING INFORMATION** BP directs that when no strength is stated the 300 mg strength should be dispensed, and that when soluble aspirin tablets are prescribed, dispersible aspirin tablets shall be dispensed.

- **PROFESSION SPECIFIC INFORMATION**
  Dental practitioners' formulary Aspirin Dispersible Tablets 300 mg may be prescribed.

- **EXCEPTIONS TO LEGAL CATEGORY** Can be sold to the public provided packs contain no more than 32 capsules or tablets; pharmacists can sell multiple packs up to a total quantity of 100 capsules or tablets in justifiable circumstances.

- **MEDICINAL FORMS** There can be variation in the licensing of different medicines containing the same drug. Forms available from special-order manufacturers include: oral capsule, oral suspension, oral solution

  Oral tablet
  CAUTIONARY AND ADVISORY LABELS 21, 32
  ▸ Aspirin (Non-proprietary)
    Aspirin 75 mg Aspirin 75mg tablets | 28 tablet PoM £1.12 DT = £0.73
    Aspirin 300 mg Aspirin 300mg tablets | 100 tablet PoM £7.08 DT = £6.09

  Gastro-resistant tablet
  CAUTIONARY AND ADVISORY LABELS 5, 25, 32
  ▸ Aspirin (Non-proprietary)
    Aspirin 75 mg Aspirin 75mg gastro-resistant tablets | 28 tablet P £0.76 DT = £0.76 | 56 tablet P £1.52–£2.40
    Aspirin 300 mg Aspirin 300mg gastro-resistant tablets | 100 tablet PoM £87.00 DT = £63.85
  ▸ Nu-Seals (Alliance Pharmaceuticals Ltd)
    Aspirin 75 mg Nu-Seals 75 gastro-resistant tablets | 56 tablet P £3.12

  Suppository
  CAUTIONARY AND ADVISORY LABELS 32
  ▸ Aspirin (Non-proprietary)
    Aspirin 150 mg Aspirin 150mg suppositories | 10 suppository P £28.97 DT = £28.97
    Aspirin 300 mg Aspirin 300mg suppositories | 10 suppository P £55.68 DT = £55.68

  Dispersible tablet
  CAUTIONARY AND ADVISORY LABELS 13, 21, 32
  ▸ Aspirin (Non-proprietary)
    Aspirin 75 mg Aspirin 75mg dispersible tablets | 1000 tablet PoM ⓧ
    Aspirin 300 mg Aspirin 300mg dispersible tablets | 32 tablet P £1.01 DT = £0.94
  ▸ Disprin (Reckitt Benckiser Healthcare (UK) Ltd)
    Aspirin 300 mg Disprin 300mg dispersible tablets | 32 tablet P £2.65 DT = £0.94

Clopidogrel

16-Oct-2024

- **INDICATIONS AND DOSE**

Prevention of atherothrombotic events in percutaneous coronary intervention (adjunct with aspirin) in patients not already on clopidogrel
▸ BY MOUTH
▸ Adult: Loading dose 300 mg for 1 dose, to be taken prior to the procedure, alternatively loading dose 600 mg for 1 dose, to be taken prior to the procedure, higher dose may produce a greater and more rapid inhibition of platelet aggregation

Transient ischaemic attack [in combination with aspirin in patients with a low risk of bleeding or as monotherapy when dual antiplatelet therapy inappropriate] | Minor ischaemic stroke [in combination with aspirin in patients with a low risk of bleeding or as monotherapy when dual antiplatelet therapy inappropriate]
▸ BY MOUTH
▸ Adult: Initially 300 mg for 1 dose, to be started within 24 hours of onset of symptoms, then 75 mg once daily

continued →

2

Cardiovascular system

Secondary prevention of transient ischaemic attack [in patients without atrial fibrillation] | Secondary prevention of ischaemic stroke [in patients without atrial fibrillation]
▶ BY MOUTH
▶ Adult: 75 mg once daily

Prevention of atherothrombotic events in peripheral arterial disease or within 35 days of myocardial infarction
▶ BY MOUTH
▶ Adult: 75 mg once daily

Prevention of atherothrombotic events in acute coronary syndrome without ST-segment elevation (given with aspirin)
▶ BY MOUTH
▶ Adult: Initially 300 mg for 1 dose, then 75 mg once daily for up to 12 months

Prevention of atherothrombotic events in acute myocardial infarction with ST-segment elevation (given with aspirin)
▶ BY MOUTH
▶ Adult 18-75 years: Initially 300 mg for 1 dose, then 75 mg once daily for at least 4 weeks
▶ Adult 76 years and over: 75 mg once daily for at least 4 weeks

Prevention of atherothrombotic and thromboembolic events in patients with atrial fibrillation and at least one risk factor for a vascular event (with aspirin) and for whom warfarin is unsuitable
▶ BY MOUTH
▶ Adult: 75 mg once daily

● UNLICENSED USE 600 mg loading dose prior to percutaneous coronary intervention is an unlicensed dose.

● CONTRA-INDICATIONS Active bleeding

● CAUTIONS Discontinue 7 days before elective surgery if antiplatelet effect not desirable · patients at risk of increased bleeding from trauma, surgery, or other pathological conditions

CAUTIONS, FURTHER INFORMATION
▶ Elderly Screening Tool of Older Persons' potentially inappropriate Prescriptions (STOPP) criteria to aid medication reviews (see Prescribing in the elderly p. 31 for information): potentially inappropriate with concurrent significant bleeding risk, such as uncontrolled severe hypertension, bleeding diathesis, or recent non-trivial spontaneous bleeding (high risk of bleeding).

● INTERACTIONS → Appendix 1: clopidogrel

● SIDE-EFFECTS
▶ Common or very common Diarrhoea · gastrointestinal discomfort · haemorrhage · skin reactions
▶ Uncommon Constipation · dizziness · eosinophilia · gastrointestinal disorders · headache · intracranial haemorrhage · leucopenia · nausea · paraesthesia · thrombocytopenia · vomiting
▶ Rare or very rare Acquired haemophilia · agranulocytosis · anaemia · angioedema · arthralgia · arthritis · bone marrow disorders · confusion · fever · glomerulonephritis · gynaecomastia · hallucination · hepatic disorders · hypersensitivity · hypotension · interstitial pneumonitis · myalgia · neutropenia · pancreatitis · respiratory disorders · severe cutaneous adverse reactions (SCARs) · stomatitis · taste altered · ulcerative colitis · vasculitis · vertigo · wound haemorrhage
▶ Frequency not known Kounis syndrome

● ALLERGY AND CROSS-SENSITIVITY EvGr Caution with history of hypersensitivity reactions to thienopyridines (e.g. prasugrel). Ⓜ

● PREGNANCY Manufacturer advises avoid—no information available.

● BREAST FEEDING Manufacturer advises avoid.

● HEPATIC IMPAIRMENT Manufacturer advises caution in moderate impairment in patients with an increased risk of bleeding—limited information available; avoid in severe impairment.

● RENAL IMPAIRMENT Manufacturer advises caution.

● PRE-TREATMENT SCREENING NICE is working with NHS England to deliver a national pilot to produce an implementation guide and information to support future commissioning decisions on CYP2C19 genotype testing to guide clopidogrel use after ischaemic stroke or transient ischaemic attack. Testing is only available as part of the pilot, which is running from October 2024 to April 2025. For more information, see www.nice.org.uk/guidance/dg59.

● NATIONAL FUNDING/ACCESS DECISIONS
For full details see funding body website
NICE decisions
▶ Clopidogrel and modified-release dipyridamole for the prevention of occlusive vascular events (December 2010) NICE TA210 Recommended

Scottish Medicines Consortium (SMC) decisions
▶ Clopidogrel (*Plavix*®) for the prevention of atherothrombotic events in acute coronary syndrome (without ST-segment elevation) in combination with aspirin (March 2004) SMC No. 88/04 Recommended with restrictions
▶ Clopidogrel (*Plavix*®) for ST-segment elevation myocardial infarction (STEMI), in combination with aspirin (August 2007) SMC No. 390/07 Recommended with restrictions

● MEDICINAL FORMS There can be variation in the licensing of different medicines containing the same drug. Forms available from special-order manufacturers include: oral suspension, oral solution
Oral tablet
▶ Clopidogrel (Non-proprietary)
  Clopidogrel 75 mg Clopidogrel 75mg tablets | 28 tablet PoM £40.73 DT = £1.10 | 30 tablet PoM £1.18-£44.34
▶ Plavix (Sanofi)
  Clopidogrel 75 mg Plavix 75mg tablets | 30 tablet PoM £35.64
  Clopidogrel (as Clopidogrel hydrogen sulfate) 300 mg Plavix 300mg tablets | 30 tablet PoM £142.54 DT = £142.54

Dipyridamole
15-Apr-2024

● INDICATIONS AND DOSE
Secondary prevention of ischaemic stroke (not associated with atrial fibrillation) and transient ischaemic attacks (used alone or with aspirin) | Adjunct to oral anticoagulation for prophylaxis of thromboembolism associated with prosthetic heart valves
▶ BY MOUTH USING MODIFIED-RELEASE MEDICINES
▶ Adult: 200 mg twice daily, to be taken preferably with food

Adjunct to oral anticoagulation for prophylaxis of thromboembolism associated with prosthetic heart valves
▶ BY MOUTH USING IMMEDIATE-RELEASE MEDICINES
▶ Adult: 300–600 mg daily in 3–4 divided doses

● CAUTIONS Coagulation disorders · heart failure · hypotension · left ventricular outflow obstruction · myasthenia gravis (risk of exacerbation) · rapidly worsening angina · recent myocardial infarction · severe coronary artery disease

CAUTIONS, FURTHER INFORMATION
▶ Elderly Screening Tool of Older Persons' potentially inappropriate Prescriptions (STOPP) criteria to aid medication reviews (see Prescribing in the elderly p. 31 for information): potentially inappropriate with concurrent significant bleeding risk, such as uncontrolled severe

hypertension, bleeding diathesis, or recent non-trivial spontaneous bleeding (high risk of bleeding).

- INTERACTIONS → Appendix 1: dipyridamole
- SIDE-EFFECTS
- ▶ **Common or very common** Angina pectoris · diarrhoea · dizziness · headache · myalgia · nausea · skin reactions · vomiting
- ▶ **Frequency not known** Angioedema · bronchospasm · haemorrhage · hot flush · hypotension · tachycardia · thrombocytopenia
- PREGNANCY Not known to be harmful.
- BREAST FEEDING Manufacturers advise use only if essential—small amount present in milk.
- PRESCRIBING AND DISPENSING INFORMATION Modified-release capsules should be dispensed in original container (pack contains a desiccant) and any capsules remaining should be discarded 6 weeks after opening.
- NATIONAL FUNDING/ACCESS DECISIONS For full details see funding body website

  NICE decisions
- ▶ **Clopidogrel and modified-release dipyridamole for the prevention of occlusive vascular events (December 2010)** NICE TA210 Recommended with restrictions

- MEDICINAL FORMS There can be variation in the licensing of different medicines containing the same drug. Forms available from special-order manufacturers include: oral suspension, oral solution

  Oral tablet
  CAUTIONARY AND ADVISORY LABELS 22
  - ▶ Dipyridamole (Non-proprietary)
    Dipyridamole 25 mg Dipyridamole 25mg tablets | 84 tablet [PoM] £12.28 DT = £8.67
    Dipyridamole 100 mg Dipyridamole 100mg tablets | 84 tablet [PoM] £49.08 DT = £47.27

  Oral suspension
  - ▶ Dipyridamole (Non-proprietary)
    Dipyridamole 10 mg per 1 ml Dipyridamole 50mg/5ml oral suspension sugar free | 150 ml [PoM] £369.72 DT = £211.27 [SF]

  Modified-release capsule
  CAUTIONARY AND ADVISORY LABELS 21, 25
  - ▶ Dipyridamole (Non-proprietary)
    Dipyridamole 200 mg Dipyridamole 200mg modified-release capsules | 60 capsule [PoM] £22.00 DT = £13.15
  - ▶ Attia (Dr Reddy's Laboratories (UK) Ltd)
    Dipyridamole 200 mg Attia 200mg modified-release capsules | 60 capsule [PoM] £13.15 DT = £13.15

ANTITHROMBOTIC DRUGS › FACTOR XA INHIBITORS

Apixaban
21-Feb-2025

- DRUG ACTION Apixaban is a direct inhibitor of activated factor X (factor Xa).

- **INDICATIONS AND DOSE**

  Prophylaxis of venous thromboembolism following knee replacement surgery
  - ▶ BY MOUTH
  - ▶ Adult: 2.5 mg twice daily for 10–14 days, to be started 12–24 hours after surgery

  Prophylaxis of venous thromboembolism following hip replacement surgery
  - ▶ BY MOUTH
  - ▶ Adult: 2.5 mg twice daily for 32–38 days, to be started 12–24 hours after surgery

  Treatment of deep-vein thrombosis | Treatment of pulmonary embolism
  - ▶ BY MOUTH
  - ▶ Adult: Initially 10 mg twice daily for 7 days, then maintenance 5 mg twice daily

  Prophylaxis of recurrent deep-vein thrombosis | Prophylaxis of recurrent pulmonary embolism
  - ▶ BY MOUTH
  - ▶ Adult: 2.5 mg twice daily, following completion of 6 months anticoagulant treatment

  Prophylaxis of stroke and systemic embolism in non-valvular atrial fibrillation and at least one risk factor [such as previous stroke or transient ischaemic attack, symptomatic heart failure, diabetes mellitus, hypertension, or age 75 years and over]
  - ▶ BY MOUTH
  - ▶ Adult: 5 mg twice daily, reduce dose to 2.5 mg twice daily in patients with at least two of the following characteristics: age 80 years and over, weight 60 kg or less, or serum-creatinine 133 micromol/litre and over

  DOSE EQUIVALENCE AND CONVERSION
  - ▶ For information on changing from, or to, other anticoagulants, consult product literature.

IMPORTANT SAFETY INFORMATION

MHRA/CHM ADVICE: NEW ORAL ANTICOAGULANTS APIXABAN (*ELIQUIS*®), DABIGATRAN (*PRADAXA*®) AND RIVAROXABAN (*XARELTO*®) (OCTOBER 2013)
The following contra-indications now apply to all new oral anticoagulants, for all indications and doses:
- a lesion or condition, if considered a significant risk factor for major bleeding—see *Contra-indications* for further information;
- concomitant treatment with any other anticoagulant agent—see *Contra-indications* for further information.

Healthcare professionals are advised to take caution when deciding to prescribe these anticoagulants to patients with other conditions, undergoing other procedures, and on other treatments, which may increase the risk of major bleeding. The renal function of patients should also be considered.

MHRA/CHM ADVICE: DIRECT-ACTING ORAL ANTICOAGULANTS (DOACS): INCREASED RISK OF RECURRENT THROMBOTIC EVENTS IN PATIENTS WITH ANTIPHOSPHOLIPID SYNDROME (JUNE 2019)
A clinical trial has shown an increased risk of recurrent thrombotic events associated with rivaroxaban compared with warfarin, in patients with antiphospholipid syndrome and a history of thrombosis. There may be a similar risk associated with other DOACs. Healthcare professionals are advised that DOACs are not recommended in patients with antiphospholipid syndrome, particularly high-risk patients who test positive for all three antiphospholipid tests—lupus anticoagulant, anticardiolipin antibodies, and anti-beta$_2$ glycoprotein I antibodies. Continued treatment should be reviewed in these patients to determine if appropriate, and switching to a vitamin K antagonist such as warfarin should be considered.

MHRA/CHM ADVICE: DIRECT-ACTING ORAL ANTICOAGULANTS (DOACS): REMINDER OF BLEEDING RISK, INCLUDING AVAILABILITY OF REVERSAL AGENTS (JUNE 2020)
The MHRA reminds healthcare professionals to remain vigilant for signs and symptoms of bleeding complications during treatment with apixaban after ongoing reports of serious, potentially fatal bleeds associated with the use of DOACs. Healthcare professionals are also advised to use apixaban with caution in patients with increased bleeding risk, and to ensure that those with renal impairment are dosed appropriately and their renal function monitored during treatment. Patients should be counselled on the signs and symptoms of bleeding, and encouraged to read the patient information leaflet. The apixaban reversal agent andexanet alfa (*Ondexxya*®) is available if required; its reversal effects should be monitored using clinical

parameters, as anti-FXa assay results may not be reliable.

MHRA/CHM ADVICE: WARFARIN AND OTHER ANTICOAGULANTS: MONITORING OF PATIENTS DURING THE COVID-19 PANDEMIC (OCTOBER 2020)

Healthcare professionals are reminded that:
- direct-acting oral anticoagulants (DOACs), such as apixaban, may interact with other medicines (including antibacterials and antivirals)—advice in product literature should be followed to minimise the risk of potential interactions;
- if patients are switched from warfarin to apixaban, warfarin treatment should be stopped before apixaban treatment is started to reduce the risk of over-anticoagulation and bleeding.

MHRA/CHM ADVICE: DIRECT-ACTING ORAL ANTICOAGULANTS (DOACS): REMINDER OF DOSE ADJUSTMENTS IN PATIENTS WITH RENAL IMPAIRMENT (MAY 2023)

Healthcare professionals are reminded that:
- exposure to DOACs, such as apixaban, is increased in patients with renal impairment, and these patients should receive an appropriately adjusted dose—see *Renal impairment* for further information;
- such patients should be reviewed regularly during treatment to ensure the dose remains appropriate;
- renal function should be assessed by calculating creatinine clearance using the Cockcroft and Gault formula.

- **CONTRA-INDICATIONS** Active, clinically significant bleeding · antiphospholipid syndrome (increased risk of recurrent thrombotic events) · prosthetic heart valve (efficacy not established) · significant risk of major bleeding · use with any other anticoagulant

CONTRA-INDICATIONS, FURTHER INFORMATION
- Significant risk of major bleeding [EvGr] Avoid in conditions with significant risk factors for major bleeding, including current or recent gastrointestinal ulceration, malignant neoplasms at high risk of bleeding, recent brain or spinal injury, recent brain, spinal or ophthalmic surgery, recent intracranial haemorrhage, known or suspected oesophageal varices, arteriovenous malformations, vascular aneurysms or major intraspinal or intracerebral vascular abnormalities. Ⓜ
- Use with any other anticoagulant [EvGr] Concomitant use with any other anticoagulant is contra-indicated, except when switching therapy, or when unfractionated heparin is given at doses necessary to maintain an open central venous or arterial catheter or for catheter ablation—use with caution. Ⓜ

- **CAUTIONS** Anaesthesia with postoperative indwelling epidural catheter (risk of paralysis—monitor neurological signs and wait 20–30 hours after apixaban dose before removing catheter and do not give next dose until at least 5 hours after catheter removal) · elderly · low body-weight · risk of bleeding

CAUTIONS, FURTHER INFORMATION
- Elderly For factor Xa inhibitors, Screening Tool of Older Persons' potentially inappropriate Prescriptions (STOPP) criteria to aid medication reviews (see Prescribing in the elderly p. 31 for information). Potentially inappropriate:
  - with concurrent significant bleeding risk, such as uncontrolled severe hypertension, bleeding diathesis or recent non-trivial spontaneous bleeding (high risk of bleeding)
  - for first deep venous thrombosis without continuing provoking risk factors (e.g. thrombophilia) for greater than 6 months (no proven added benefit)
  - for first pulmonary embolus without continuing provoking risk factors for greater than 12 months (no proven added benefit)

- as part of dual therapy with an antiplatelet agent in patients with stable coronary, cerebrovascular or peripheral arterial disease, without a clear indication for anticoagulant therapy (no added benefit)
- if eGFR less than 15 mL/min/1.73 m² (contra-indicated in kidney failure; risk of bleeding)

- **INTERACTIONS** → Appendix 1: factor XA inhibitors

- **SIDE-EFFECTS**
- **Common or very common** Anaemia · haemorrhage · nausea · skin reactions
- **Uncommon** CNS haemorrhage · hypotension · post procedural haematoma · thrombocytopenia · wound complications

- **PREGNANCY** Manufacturer advises avoid—no information available.

- **BREAST FEEDING** Manufacturer advises avoid—present in milk in *animal* studies.

- **HEPATIC IMPAIRMENT** Manufacturer advises caution in mild to moderate impairment (or if hepatic transaminases greater than 2 times the upper limit of normal, or if bilirubin is equal or greater than 1.5 times the upper limit of normal); avoid in severe impairment or impairment associated with coagulopathy and clinically relevant bleeding risk.

- **RENAL IMPAIRMENT** See p. 21. [EvGr] Avoid if creatinine clearance less than 15 mL/minute (no information available). Ⓜ
- When used for Prophylaxis of venous thromboembolism following knee or hip replacement surgery or Prophylaxis of recurrent deep-vein thrombosis or pulmonary embolism or Treatment of deep-vein thrombosis or pulmonary embolism [EvGr] Use with caution if creatinine clearance 15–29 mL/minute. Ⓜ
  Dose adjustments
  - When used for Prophylaxis of stroke and systemic embolism in non-valvular atrial fibrillation and at least one risk factor [EvGr] Reduce dose to 2.5 mg twice daily if creatinine clearance 15–29 mL/minute (regardless of age or body-weight). Ⓜ For other patient groups that require a reduced dose, see *Indications and dose*.

- **MONITORING REQUIREMENTS**
- Patients should be monitored for signs of bleeding or anaemia; treatment should be stopped if severe bleeding occurs.
- No routine anticoagulant monitoring required (INR tests are unreliable).

- **PRESCRIBING AND DISPENSING INFORMATION** Duration of treatment should be determined by balancing the benefit of treatment with the bleeding risk; shorter duration of treatment (at least 3 months) should be based on transient risk factors i.e recent surgery, trauma, immobilisation.

  Apixaban should not be used as an alternative to unfractionated heparin in pulmonary embolism in patients with haemodynamic instability, or who may receive thrombolysis or pulmonary embolectomy.

- **PATIENT AND CARER ADVICE** Patients should be provided with an alert card and advised to keep it with them at all times.

- **NATIONAL FUNDING/ACCESS DECISIONS**
  For full details see funding body website
  NICE decisions
- **Apixaban for the prevention of venous thromboembolism after total hip or knee replacement in adults (January 2012)** NICE TA245 Recommended
- **Apixaban for preventing stroke and systemic embolism in people with non-valvular atrial fibrillation (updated July 2021)** NICE TA275 Recommended
- **Apixaban for the treatment and secondary prevention of deep vein thrombosis and/or pulmonary embolism (June 2015)** NICE TA341 Recommended

● **MEDICINAL FORMS** There can be variation in the licensing of different medicines containing the same drug.

Oral tablet

CAUTIONARY AND ADVISORY LABELS 10

▸ **Apixaban (Non-proprietary)**
Apixaban 2.5 mg Apixaban 2.5mg tablets | 10 tablet [PoM] £0.50–£9.50 | 20 tablet [PoM] £0.99–£19.00 | 60 tablet [PoM] £57.00 DT = £2.97
Apixaban 5 mg Apixaban 5mg tablets | 28 tablet [PoM] £1.42–£26.60 | 56 tablet [PoM] £53.20 DT = £2.84

▸ **Eliquis** (Bristol-Myers Squibb Pharmaceuticals Ltd)
Apixaban 2.5 mg Eliquis 2.5mg tablets | 10 tablet [PoM] £9.50 | 20 tablet [PoM] £19.00 | 60 tablet [PoM] £57.00 DT = £2.97
Apixaban 5 mg Eliquis 5mg tablets | 28 tablet [PoM] £26.60 | 56 tablet [PoM] £53.20 DT = £2.84

Edoxaban

15-Apr-2024

● **DRUG ACTION** Edoxaban is a direct and reversible inhibitor of activated factor X (factor Xa), which prevents conversion of prothrombin to thrombin and prolongs clotting time, thereby reducing the risk of thrombus formation.

● **INDICATIONS AND DOSE**

Prophylaxis of stroke and systemic embolism in non-valvular atrial fibrillation, in patients with at least one risk factor (such as congestive heart failure, hypertension, aged 75 years and over, diabetes mellitus, previous stroke or transient ischaemic attack)

▸ BY MOUTH
▸ Adult (body-weight up to 61 kg): 30 mg once daily
▸ Adult (body-weight 61 kg and above): 60 mg once daily

Treatment of deep-vein thrombosis | Prophylaxis of recurrent deep-vein thrombosis | Treatment of pulmonary embolism | Prophylaxis of recurrent pulmonary embolism

▸ BY MOUTH
▸ Adult (body-weight up to 61 kg): 30 mg once daily, duration of treatment adjusted according to risk factors—consult product literature, treatment should follow initial use of parenteral anticoagulant for at least 5 days
▸ Adult (body-weight 61 kg and above): 60 mg once daily, duration of treatment adjusted according to risk factors—consult product literature, treatment should follow initial use of parenteral anticoagulant for at least 5 days

DOSE ADJUSTMENTS DUE TO INTERACTIONS

▸ Manufacturer advises max. dose of 30 mg once daily with concurrent ciclosporin, dronedarone, erythromycin, or ketoconazole.

DOSE EQUIVALENCE AND CONVERSION

▸ For information on changing from, or to, other anticoagulants, consult product literature.

IMPORTANT SAFETY INFORMATION

MHRA/CHM ADVICE: NEW ORAL ANTICOAGULANTS APIXABAN (*ELIQUIS*®), DABIGATRAN (*PRADAXA*®) AND RIVAROXABAN (*XARELTO*®) (OCTOBER 2013)

The following contra-indications now apply to all new oral anticoagulants (including edoxaban (*Lixiana*®) which was not launched at the release of this advice), for all indications and doses:
● a lesion or condition, if considered a significant risk factor for major bleeding—see *Contra-indications* for further information;
● concomitant treatment with any other anticoagulant agent—see *Contra-indications* for further information.
Healthcare professionals are advised to take caution when deciding to prescribe these anticoagulants to patients with other conditions, undergoing other procedures, and on other treatments, which may increase the risk of major bleeding. The renal function of patients should also be considered.

MHRA/CHM ADVICE: DIRECT-ACTING ORAL ANTICOAGULANTS (DOACS): INCREASED RISK OF RECURRENT THROMBOTIC EVENTS IN PATIENTS WITH ANTIPHOSPHOLIPID SYNDROME (JUNE 2019)

A clinical trial has shown an increased risk of recurrent thrombotic events associated with rivaroxaban compared with warfarin, in patients with antiphospholipid syndrome and a history of thrombosis. There may be a similar risk associated with other DOACs. Healthcare professionals are advised that DOACs are not recommended in patients with antiphospholipid syndrome, particularly high-risk patients who test positive for all three antiphospholipid tests—lupus anticoagulant, anticardiolipin antibodies, and anti-beta$_2$ glycoprotein I antibodies. Continued treatment should be reviewed in these patients to determine if appropriate, and switching to a vitamin K antagonist such as warfarin should be considered.

MHRA/CHM ADVICE: DIRECT-ACTING ORAL ANTICOAGULANTS (DOACS): REMINDER OF BLEEDING RISK, INCLUDING AVAILABILITY OF REVERSAL AGENTS (JUNE 2020)

The MHRA reminds healthcare professionals to remain vigilant for signs and symptoms of bleeding complications during treatment with edoxaban after ongoing reports of serious, potentially fatal bleeds associated with the use of DOACs. Healthcare professionals are also advised to use edoxaban with caution in patients with increased bleeding risk, and to ensure that those with renal impairment are dosed appropriately and their renal function monitored during treatment. Patients should be counselled on the signs and symptoms of bleeding, and encouraged to read the patient information leaflet. There is currently no specific authorised reversal agent available for edoxaban.

MHRA/CHM ADVICE: WARFARIN AND OTHER ANTICOAGULANTS: MONITORING OF PATIENTS DURING THE COVID-19 PANDEMIC (OCTOBER 2020)

Healthcare professionals are reminded that:
● direct-acting oral anticoagulants (DOACs), such as edoxaban, may interact with other medicines (including antibacterials and antivirals)—advice in product literature should be followed to minimise the risk of potential interactions;
● if patients are switched from warfarin to edoxaban, warfarin treatment should be stopped before edoxaban treatment is started to reduce the risk of over-anticoagulation and bleeding.

MHRA/CHM ADVICE: DIRECT-ACTING ORAL ANTICOAGULANTS (DOACS): REMINDER OF DOSE ADJUSTMENTS IN PATIENTS WITH RENAL IMPAIRMENT (MAY 2023)

Healthcare professionals are reminded that:
● exposure to DOACs, such as edoxaban, is increased in patients with renal impairment, and these patients should receive an appropriately adjusted dose—see *Renal impairment* for further information;
● such patients should be reviewed regularly during treatment to ensure the dose remains appropriate;
● renal function should be assessed by calculating creatinine clearance using the Cockcroft and Gault formula.

● **CONTRA-INDICATIONS** Active bleeding · antiphospholipid syndrome (increased risk of recurrent thrombotic events) · arteriovenous malformations · current or recent gastro-intestinal ulceration · hepatic disease (associated with coagulopathy and clinically relevant bleeding risk) · known or suspected oesophageal varices · major intraspinal or intracerebral vascular abnormalities · presence of malignant neoplasms at high risk of bleeding · prosthetic heart valve (safety and efficacy not established) · recent brain or spinal injury · recent brain, spinal or ophthalmic surgery · recent intracranial haemorrhage · significant risk of major bleeding · uncontrolled severe hypertension · use with any other anticoagulant · vascular aneurysms

CONTRA-INDICATIONS, FURTHER INFORMATION

▸ Use with any other anticoagulant [EvGr] Concomitant use with any other anticoagulant is contra-indicated, except when switching therapy, or when unfractionated heparin is given at doses necessary to maintain an open central venous or arterial catheter or for catheter ablation—use with caution. (M)

● **CAUTIONS**

GENERAL CAUTIONS Edoxaban should not be used as an alternative to unfractionated heparin in pulmonary embolism in patients with haemodynamic instability, or who may receive thrombolysis or pulmonary embolectomy · moderate to severe mitral stenosis (safety and efficacy not established) · risk of bleeding · surgery

SPECIFIC CAUTIONS

▸ When used for Prophylaxis of stroke and systemic embolism in non-valvular atrial fibrillation Creatinine clearance more than 100 mL/minute (potential for reduced efficacy—evaluate thromboembolic and bleeding risk)

CAUTIONS, FURTHER INFORMATION

▸ Surgery [EvGr] Discontinue treatment at least 24 hours before a surgical procedure; the risk of bleeding should be weighed against the urgency of the intervention (M)— consult product literature.

▸ Elderly For factor Xa inhibitors, Screening Tool of Older Persons' potentially inappropriate Prescriptions (STOPP) criteria to aid medication reviews (see Prescribing in the elderly p. 31 for information). Potentially inappropriate:
  ● with concurrent significant bleeding risk, such as uncontrolled severe hypertension, bleeding diathesis or recent non-trivial spontaneous bleeding (high risk of bleeding)
  ● for first deep venous thrombosis without continuing provoking risk factors (e.g. thrombophilia) for greater than 6 months (no proven added benefit)
  ● for first pulmonary embolus without continuing provoking risk factors for greater than 12 months (no proven added benefit)
  ● as part of dual therapy with an antiplatelet agent in patients with stable coronary, cerebrovascular or peripheral arterial disease, without a clear indication for anticoagulant therapy (no added benefit)
  ● if eGFR less than 15 mL/min/1.73 m^2 (contra-indicated in kidney failure; risk of bleeding)

● **INTERACTIONS** → Appendix 1: factor XA inhibitors

● **SIDE-EFFECTS**

▸ **Common or very common** Abdominal pain · anaemia · dizziness · haemorrhage · headache · nausea · skin reactions

▸ **Uncommon** CNS haemorrhage · thrombocytopenia

SIDE-EFFECTS, FURTHER INFORMATION Should a bleeding complication arise in a patient receiving edoxaban, the manufacturer recommends to delay the next dose or treatment should be discontinued as appropriate.

● **PREGNANCY** Manufacturer advises avoid—toxicity in *animal* studies.

● **BREAST FEEDING** Manufacturer advises avoid—present in milk in *animal* studies.

● **HEPATIC IMPAIRMENT** Manufacturer advises caution in mild to moderate impairment, or if liver transaminases greater than 2 times the upper limit of normal, or total bilirubin 1.5 times the upper limit of normal or greater; avoid in severe impairment or hepatic disease associated with coagulopathy and clinically relevant bleeding risk.

● **RENAL IMPAIRMENT** [EvGr] Avoid if creatinine clearance less than 15 mL/minute. (M)
Dose adjustments [EvGr] Use a dose of 30 mg once daily if creatinine clearance 15–50 mL/minute. (M) See p. 21.

● **MONITORING REQUIREMENTS**

▸ Manufacturer advises monitor renal function before treatment and when clinically indicated during treatment; monitor hepatic function before treatment and repeat periodically if treatment duration longer than 1 year.

▸ Manufacturer advises monitor for signs of mucosal bleeding and anaemia in patients at increased risk; treatment should be stopped if severe bleeding occurs.

▸ No routine anticoagulant monitoring required (INR tests are unreliable).

● **PATIENT AND CARER ADVICE** Patients should be provided with an alert card and advised to keep it with them at all times.

● **NATIONAL FUNDING/ACCESS DECISIONS** For full details see funding body website

NICE decisions

▸ **Edoxaban for treating and preventing deep vein thrombosis and pulmonary embolism (August 2015)** NICE TA354 Recommended

▸ **Edoxaban for preventing stroke and systemic embolism in people with non-valvular atrial fibrillation (updated July 2021)** NICE TA355 Recommended

● **MEDICINAL FORMS** There can be variation in the licensing of different medicines containing the same drug.
Oral tablet
CAUTIONARY AND ADVISORY LABELS 10
▸ Lixiana (Daiichi Sankyo UK Ltd)
  Edoxaban (as Edoxaban tosilate) 15 mg Lixiana 15mg tablets | 10 tablet [PoM] £17.50 DT = £17.50
  Edoxaban (as Edoxaban tosilate) 30 mg Lixiana 30mg tablets | 28 tablet [PoM] £49.00 DT = £49.00
  Edoxaban (as Edoxaban tosilate) 60 mg Lixiana 60mg tablets | 28 tablet [PoM] £49.00 DT = £49.00

Fondaparinux sodium

30-Aug-2023

● **DRUG ACTION** Fondaparinux sodium is a synthetic pentasaccharide that inhibits activated factor X.

● **INDICATIONS AND DOSE**

Prophylaxis of venous thromboembolism in patients after undergoing major orthopaedic surgery of the hip or leg, or abdominal surgery

▸ BY SUBCUTANEOUS INJECTION

▸ Adult: Initially 2.5 mg for 1 dose, dose to be given 6 hours after surgery, then 2.5 mg once daily

Prophylaxis of venous thromboembolism in medical patients immobilised because of acute illness

▸ BY SUBCUTANEOUS INJECTION

▸ Adult: 2.5 mg once daily

Treatment of superficial-vein thrombosis

▸ BY SUBCUTANEOUS INJECTION

▸ Adult (body-weight 50 kg and above): 2.5 mg once daily for at least 30 days (max. 45 days if high risk of thromboembolic complications), treatment should be stopped 24 hours before surgery and restarted at least 6 hours post operatively

Treatment of unstable angina and non-ST-segment elevation myocardial infarction

▸ BY SUBCUTANEOUS INJECTION

▸ Adult: 2.5 mg once daily for up to 8 days (or until hospital discharge if sooner), treatment should be stopped 24 hours before coronary artery bypass graft surgery (where possible) and restarted 48 hours post operatively

Treatment of ST-segment elevation myocardial infarction

► INITIALLY BY INTRAVENOUS INJECTION, OR BY INTRAVENOUS INFUSION

► Adult: Initially 2.5 mg for 1 dose on the first day, then (by subcutaneous injection) 2.5 mg once daily, total treatment for up to 8 days (or until hospital discharge if sooner), treatment should be stopped 24 hours before coronary artery bypass graft surgery (where possible) and restarted 48 hours post operatively

Treatment of deep-vein thrombosis and pulmonary embolism

► BY SUBCUTANEOUS INJECTION

► Adult (body-weight up to 50 kg): 5 mg once daily for at least 5 days and until adequate oral anticoagulation established

► Adult (body-weight 50-100 kg): 7.5 mg once daily for at least 5 days and until adequate oral anticoagulation established

► Adult (body-weight 101 kg and above): 10 mg once daily for at least 5 days and until adequate oral anticoagulation established

● CONTRA-INDICATIONS Active bleeding · bacterial endocarditis

● CAUTIONS Active gastro-intestinal ulcer disease · bleeding disorders · brain surgery · elderly patients · low body-weight · ophthalmic surgery · recent intracranial haemorrhage · risk of catheter thrombus during percutaneous coronary intervention · spinal or epidural anaesthesia (risk of spinal haematoma—avoid if using treatment doses for venous thromboembolism) · spinal surgery

● INTERACTIONS → Appendix 1: factor XA inhibitors

● SIDE-EFFECTS

► **Common or very common** Anaemia · haemorrhage

► **Uncommon** Chest pain · coagulation disorder · dyspnoea · fever · hepatic function abnormal · nausea · oedema · platelet abnormalities · skin reactions · thrombocytopenia · vomiting · wound secretion

► **Rare or very rare** Anxiety · confusion · constipation · cough · diarrhoea · dizziness · drowsiness · fatigue · gastritis · gastrointestinal discomfort · genital oedema · headache · hyperbilirubinaemia · hypersensitivity · hypokalaemia · hypotension · leg pain · post procedural infection · syncope · vasodilation · vertigo

● PREGNANCY Manufacturer advises avoid unless potential benefit outweighs possible risk—no information available.

● BREAST FEEDING Present in milk in *animal* studies—manufacturer advises avoid.

● HEPATIC IMPAIRMENT

► When used for Prophylaxis of venous thromboembolism or Treatment of unstable angina and non-ST-segment elevation myocardial infarction or Treatment of ST-segment elevation myocardial infarction or Treatment of deep-vein thrombosis and pulmonary embolism ⬦EvGr⬦ Caution in severe impairment (increased risk of bleeding). ⬦M⬦

► When used for Treatment of superficial-vein thrombosis ⬦EvGr⬦ Avoid in severe impairment (no information available). ⬦M⬦

● RENAL IMPAIRMENT Increased risk of bleeding in renal impairment.

► When used for Prophylaxis of venous thromboembolism or Treatment of superficial-vein thrombosis or Treatment of unstable angina and non-ST-segment elevation myocardial infarction or Treatment of ST-segment elevation myocardial infarction ⬦EvGr⬦ Avoid if creatinine clearance less than 20 mL/minute. ⬦M⬦

► When used for Treatment of deep-vein thrombosis and pulmonary embolism ⬦EvGr⬦ Use with caution if creatinine clearance 30–50 mL/minute; avoid if creatinine clearance less than 30 mL/minute. ⬦M⬦

Dose adjustments See p. 21.

► When used for Prophylaxis of venous thromboembolism or Treatment of superficial-vein thrombosis ⬦EvGr⬦ Reduce dose to 1.5 mg once daily if creatinine clearance 20–50 mL/minute. ⬦M⬦

● DIRECTIONS FOR ADMINISTRATION For *intravenous infusion* (*Arixtra* ®), give intermittently in Sodium Chloride 0.9%. For ST-segment elevation myocardial infarction, add requisite dose to 25-50 mL infusion fluid and give over 1-2 minutes.

● MEDICINAL FORMS There can be variation in the licensing of different medicines containing the same drug.

Solution for injection

► **Fondaparinux sodium** (Non-proprietary)

Fondaparinux sodium 5 mg per 1 ml Fondaparinux sodium 2.5mg/0.5ml solution for injection pre-filled syringes | 10 pre-filled disposable injection ⟨PoM⟩ £62.79 DT = £62.79

Fondaparinux sodium 12.5 mg per 1 ml Fondaparinux sodium 5mg/0.4ml solution for injection pre-filled syringes | 10 pre-filled disposable injection ⟨PoM⟩ £110.70 DT = £116.53
Fondaparinux sodium 10mg/0.8ml solution for injection pre-filled syringes | 10 pre-filled disposable injection ⟨PoM⟩ £110.70 DT = £116.53
Fondaparinux sodium 7.5mg/0.6ml solution for injection pre-filled syringes | 10 pre-filled disposable injection ⟨PoM⟩ £110.70 DT = £116.53 (Hospital only)

► **Arixtra** (Viatris UK Healthcare Ltd)

Fondaparinux sodium 5 mg per 1 ml Arixtra 2.5mg/0.5ml solution for injection pre-filled syringes | 10 pre-filled disposable injection ⟨PoM⟩ £62.79 DT = £62.79 (Hospital only)
Arixtra 1.5mg/0.3ml solution for injection pre-filled syringes | 10 pre-filled disposable injection ⟨PoM⟩ £62.79 (Hospital only)

Fondaparinux sodium 12.5 mg per 1 ml Arixtra 7.5mg/0.6ml solution for injection pre-filled syringes | 10 pre-filled disposable injection ⟨PoM⟩ £116.53 DT = £116.53 (Hospital only)
Arixtra 5mg/0.4ml solution for injection pre-filled syringes | 10 pre-filled disposable injection ⟨PoM⟩ £116.53 DT = £116.53 (Hospital only)
Arixtra 10mg/0.8ml solution for injection pre-filled syringes | 10 pre-filled disposable injection ⟨PoM⟩ £116.53 DT = £116.53 (Hospital only)

Rivaroxaban
15-Apr-2024

● DRUG ACTION Rivaroxaban is a direct inhibitor of activated factor X (factor Xa).

● INDICATIONS AND DOSE

Prophylaxis of venous thromboembolism following knee replacement surgery

► BY MOUTH

► Adult: 10 mg once daily for 2 weeks, to be started 6–10 hours after surgery

Prophylaxis of venous thromboembolism following hip replacement surgery

► BY MOUTH

► Adult: 10 mg once daily for 5 weeks, to be started 6–10 hours after surgery

Treatment of deep-vein thrombosis | Treatment of pulmonary embolism

► BY MOUTH

► Adult: Initially 15 mg twice daily for 21 days, to be taken with food, then maintenance 20 mg once daily, to be taken with food, for duration of treatment—consult product literature

Prophylaxis of recurrent deep-vein thrombosis | Prophylaxis of recurrent pulmonary embolism

► BY MOUTH

► Adult: 10 mg once daily, to be given following completion of at least 6 months of anticoagulant treatment, consider 20 mg once daily, to be taken with food, in those at high risk of recurrence (such as complicated comorbidities, or previous recurrence with rivaroxaban 10 mg once daily)

continued →

Prophylaxis of stroke and systemic embolism in patients with non-valvular atrial fibrillation and with at least one of the following risk factors: congestive heart failure, hypertension, previous stroke or transient ischaemic attack, age ≥ 75 years, or diabetes mellitus
▸ BY MOUTH
▸ Adult: 20 mg once daily, to be taken with food

Prophylaxis of atherothrombotic events following an acute coronary syndrome with elevated cardiac biomarkers (in combination with aspirin alone or aspirin and clopidogrel)
▸ BY MOUTH
▸ Adult: 2.5 mg twice daily usual duration 12 months

Prophylaxis of atherothrombotic events in patients with coronary artery disease or symptomatic peripheral artery disease at high risk of ischaemic events (in combination with aspirin)
▸ BY MOUTH
▸ Adult: 2.5 mg twice daily

DOSE EQUIVALENCE AND CONVERSION
▸ For information on changing from, or to, other anticoagulants—consult product literature.

IMPORTANT SAFETY INFORMATION

MHRA/CHM ADVICE: NEW ORAL ANTICOAGULANTS APIXABAN (*ELIQUIS* ®), DABIGATRAN (*PRADAXA* ®) AND RIVAROXABAN (*XARELTO* ®) (OCTOBER 2013)
The following contra-indications now apply to all new oral anticoagulants, for all indications and doses:
● a lesion or condition, if considered a significant risk factor for major bleeding—see *Contra-indications* for further information;
● concomitant treatment with any other anticoagulant agent—see *Contra-indications* for further information.
Healthcare professionals are advised to take caution when deciding to prescribe these anticoagulants to patients with other conditions, undergoing other procedures, and on other treatments, which may increase the risk of major bleeding. The renal function of patients should also be considered.

MHRA/CHM ADVICE: RIVAROXABAN (*XARELTO* ®) AFTER TRANSCATHETER AORTIC VALVE REPLACEMENT: INCREASE IN ALL-CAUSE MORTALITY, THROMBOEMBOLIC AND BLEEDING EVENTS IN A CLINICAL TRIAL (OCTOBER 2018)
A phase 3 clinical trial showed that the risk of all-cause death and bleeding after transcatheter aortic valve replacement (TAVR) approximately doubled in patients assigned to a rivaroxaban-based anticoagulation strategy compared with those receiving an antiplatelet-based strategy (clopidogrel and aspirin). The MHRA reminds healthcare professionals that rivaroxaban should not be used for thromboprophylaxis in patients with prosthetic heart valves, including patients who have undergone TAVR. Rivaroxaban treatment in patients who undergo TAVR should be stopped and switched to standard care.

MHRA/CHM ADVICE: DIRECT-ACTING ORAL ANTICOAGULANTS (DOACS): INCREASED RISK OF RECURRENT THROMBOTIC EVENTS IN PATIENTS WITH ANTIPHOSPHOLIPID SYNDROME (JUNE 2019)
A clinical trial has shown an increased risk of recurrent thrombotic events associated with rivaroxaban compared with warfarin, in patients with antiphospholipid syndrome and a history of thrombosis. There may be a similar risk associated with other DOACs. Healthcare professionals are advised that DOACs are not recommended in patients with antiphospholipid syndrome, particularly high-risk patients who test positive for all three antiphospholipid tests—lupus anticoagulant, anticardiolipin antibodies, and anti-beta$_2$ glycoprotein I antibodies. Continued treatment should be reviewed in these patients to determine if

appropriate, and switching to a vitamin K antagonist such as warfarin should be considered.

MHRA/CHM ADVICE: RIVAROXABAN (*XARELTO* ®): REMINDER THAT 15 MG AND 20 MG TABLETS SHOULD BE TAKEN WITH FOOD (JULY 2019)
The MHRA has received a small number of reports suggesting a lack of efficacy (thromboembolic events) in patients taking 15 mg or 20 mg rivaroxaban tablets on an empty stomach. Healthcare professionals are advised to remind patients to take rivaroxaban 15 mg or 20 mg tablets with food. In those who have difficulty swallowing, these tablets can be crushed and mixed with water or apple puree immediately before, and followed by food immediately after, ingestion.

MHRA/CHM ADVICE: DIRECT-ACTING ORAL ANTICOAGULANTS (DOACS): REMINDER OF BLEEDING RISK, INCLUDING AVAILABILITY OF REVERSAL AGENTS (JUNE 2020)
The MHRA reminds healthcare professionals to remain vigilant for signs and symptoms of bleeding complications during treatment with rivaroxaban after ongoing reports of serious, potentially fatal bleeds associated with the use of DOACs. Healthcare professionals are also advised to use rivaroxaban with caution in patients with increased bleeding risk, and to ensure that those with renal impairment are dosed appropriately and their renal function monitored during treatment. Patients should be counselled on the signs and symptoms of bleeding, and encouraged to read the patient information leaflet. The rivaroxaban reversal agent andexanet alfa (*Ondexxya* ®) is available if required; its reversal effects should be monitored using clinical parameters, as anti-FXa assay results may not be reliable.

MHRA/CHM ADVICE: WARFARIN AND OTHER ANTICOAGULANTS: MONITORING OF PATIENTS DURING THE COVID-19 PANDEMIC (OCTOBER 2020)
Healthcare professionals are reminded that:
● direct-acting oral anticoagulants (DOACs), such as rivaroxaban, may interact with other medicines (including antibacterials and antivirals)—advice in product literature should be followed to minimise the risk of potential interactions;
● if patients are switched from warfarin to rivaroxaban, warfarin treatment should be stopped before rivaroxaban treatment is started to reduce the risk of over-anticoagulation and bleeding.

MHRA/CHM ADVICE: DIRECT-ACTING ORAL ANTICOAGULANTS (DOACS): REMINDER OF DOSE ADJUSTMENTS IN PATIENTS WITH RENAL IMPAIRMENT (MAY 2023)
Healthcare professionals are reminded that:
● exposure to DOACs, such as rivaroxaban, is increased in patients with renal impairment, and these patients should receive an appropriately adjusted dose—see *Renal impairment* for further information;
● such patients should be reviewed regularly during treatment to ensure the dose remains appropriate;
● renal function should be assessed by calculating creatinine clearance using the Cockcroft and Gault formula.

● **CONTRA-INDICATIONS**

GENERAL CONTRA-INDICATIONS Active bleeding · antiphospholipid syndrome (increased risk of recurrent thrombotic events) · arteriovenous malformation · major intraspinal or intracerebral vascular abnormalities · malignant neoplasms at high risk of bleeding · oesophageal varices · prosthetic heart valve (efficacy not established) · recent brain or spinal injury · recent brain surgery · recent gastro-intestinal ulcer · recent intracranial haemorrhage · recent ophthalmic surgery · recent spine surgery · significant risk of major bleeding · use with any other anticoagulant · vascular aneurysm

SPECIFIC CONTRA-INDICATIONS
▸ When used for Prophylaxis of atherothrombotic events following an acute coronary syndrome Previous stroke · transient ischaemic attack
▸ When used for Prophylaxis of atherothrombotic events in patients with coronary artery disease or symptomatic peripheral artery disease Previous stroke (no information available—consult product literature)

CONTRA-INDICATIONS, FURTHER INFORMATION
▸ Use with any other anticoagulant [EvGr] Concomitant use with any other anticoagulant is contra-indicated, except when switching therapy, or when unfractionated heparin is given at doses necessary to maintain an open central venous or arterial catheter or for catheter ablation—use with caution. ⟨M⟩

● **CAUTIONS**
GENERAL CAUTIONS Anaesthesia with postoperative indwelling epidural catheter (risk of paralysis—monitor neurological signs and wait at least 18 hours after rivaroxaban dose before removing catheter and do not give next dose until at least 6 hours after catheter removal) · bronchiectasis · elderly · risk of bleeding · rivaroxaban should not be used as an alternative to unfractionated heparin in pulmonary embolism in patients with haemodynamic instability, or who may receive thrombolysis or pulmonary embolectomy · severe hypertension · vascular retinopathy

SPECIFIC CAUTIONS
▸ When used for Prophylaxis of atherothrombotic events following an acute coronary syndrome or Prophylaxis of atherothrombotic events in patients with coronary artery disease or symptomatic peripheral artery disease Body-weight less than 60 kg

CAUTIONS, FURTHER INFORMATION
▸ Elderly For factor Xa inhibitors, Screening Tool of Older Persons' potentially inappropriate Prescriptions (STOPP) criteria to aid medication reviews (see Prescribing in the elderly p. 31 for information). Potentially inappropriate:
 ● with concurrent significant bleeding risk, such as uncontrolled severe hypertension, bleeding diathesis or recent non-trivial spontaneous bleeding (high risk of bleeding)
 ● for first deep venous thrombosis without continuing provoking risk factors (e.g. thrombophilia) for greater than 6 months (no proven added benefit)
 ● for first pulmonary embolus without continuing provoking risk factors for greater than 12 months (no proven added benefit)
 ● as part of dual therapy with an antiplatelet agent in patients with stable coronary, cerebrovascular or peripheral arterial disease, without a clear indication for anticoagulant therapy (no added benefit)
 ● if eGFR less than 15 mL/min/1.73 m^2 (contra-indicated in kidney failure; risk of bleeding)

● **INTERACTIONS** → Appendix 1: factor XA inhibitors

● **SIDE-EFFECTS**
▸ **Common or very common** Anaemia · asthenia · constipation · diarrhoea · dizziness · fever · gastrointestinal discomfort · haemorrhage · headache · hypotension · menorrhagia · nausea · oedema · pain in extremity · post procedural anaemia · renal impairment · skin reactions · vomiting · wound complications
▸ **Uncommon** Angioedema · dry mouth · hepatic disorders · hypersensitivity · intracranial haemorrhage · malaise · syncope · tachycardia · thrombocytopenia · thrombocytosis
▸ **Rare or very rare** Severe cutaneous adverse reactions (SCARs) · vascular pseudoaneurysm

● **PREGNANCY** Manufacturer advises avoid—toxicity in *animal* studies.

● **BREAST FEEDING** Manufacturer advises avoid—present in milk in *animal* studies.

● **HEPATIC IMPAIRMENT** Manufacturer advises avoid in hepatic disease with coagulopathy and clinically-relevant bleeding risk including patients with moderate to severe cirrhosis.

● **RENAL IMPAIRMENT** See p. 21. [EvGr] Use with caution if concomitant use of drugs that increase plasma-rivaroxaban concentration (consult product literature). Caution if creatinine clearance 15–29 mL/minute; avoid if creatinine clearance less than 15 mL/minute. ⟨M⟩
Dose adjustments
▸ When used for Treatment of deep-vein thrombosis or pulmonary embolism [EvGr] Following the first 21 days of treatment for deep-vein thrombosis or pulmonary embolism, the usual dose of 20 mg once daily can be given, but consider reducing to 15 mg once daily if creatinine clearance 15–49 mL/minute and the risk of bleeding outweighs the risk of recurrent deep-vein thrombosis or pulmonary embolism. ⟨M⟩
▸ When used for Prophylaxis of recurrent deep-vein thrombosis or pulmonary embolism [EvGr] When the recommended dose is 20 mg once daily, consider reducing to 15 mg once daily if creatinine clearance 15–49 mL/minute and the risk of bleeding outweighs the risk of recurrent deep-vein thrombosis or pulmonary embolism. ⟨M⟩
▸ When used for Prophylaxis of stroke and systemic embolism in patients with non-valvular atrial fibrillation [EvGr] Reduce dose to 15 mg once daily if creatinine clearance 15–49 mL/minute. ⟨M⟩

● **MONITORING REQUIREMENTS**
▸ Patients should be monitored for signs of bleeding or anaemia; treatment should be stopped if severe bleeding occurs.
▸ No routine anticoagulant monitoring required (INR tests are unreliable).

● **DIRECTIONS FOR ADMINISTRATION** Manufacturer advises tablets may be crushed and mixed with water or apple puree just before administration.

● **PRESCRIBING AND DISPENSING INFORMATION** The manufacturer of *Xarelto*® has provided a *Prescriber Guide*.
 Low-dose rivaroxaban, in combination with aspirin alone *or* aspirin and clopidogrel, is licensed for the prevention of atherothrombotic events following an acute coronary syndrome with elevated cardiac biomarkers. Treatment should be started as soon as possible after the patient has been stabilised following the acute coronary event, at the earliest 24 hours after admission to hospital, and at the time when parenteral anticoagulation therapy would normally be discontinued; the usual duration of treatment is 12 months.

● **PATIENT AND CARER ADVICE** Patients and their carers should be provided with an alert card and advised to keep it with them at all times.

● **NATIONAL FUNDING/ACCESS DECISIONS**
For full details see funding body website
NICE decisions
▸ **Rivaroxaban for the prevention of venous thromboembolism after total hip or total knee replacement in adults (April 2009)** NICE TA170 Recommended
▸ **Rivaroxaban for the prevention of stroke and systemic embolism in people with atrial fibrillation (updated July 2021)** NICE TA256 Recommended
▸ **Rivaroxaban for the treatment of deep-vein thrombosis and prevention of recurrent deep-vein thrombosis and pulmonary embolism (July 2012)** NICE TA261 Recommended
▸ **Rivaroxaban for treating pulmonary embolism and preventing recurrent venous thromboembolism (June 2013)** NICE TA287 Recommended
▸ **Rivaroxaban for preventing adverse outcomes after acute management of acute coronary syndrome (March 2015)** NICE TA335 Recommended

▸ Rivaroxaban for preventing atherothrombotic events in people with coronary or peripheral artery disease (October 2019) NICE TA607 Recommended

Scottish Medicines Consortium (SMC) decisions

▸ Rivaroxaban (*Xarelto*®) for the prevention of venous thromboembolism in elective hip or knee replacement surgery (December 2008) SMC No. 519/08 Recommended

▸ Rivaroxaban (*Xarelto*®) for the prevention of stroke and systemic embolism in patients with atrial fibrillation (February 2012) SMC No. 756/12 Recommended with restrictions

▸ Rivaroxaban (*Xarelto*®) for the treatment of deep-vein thrombosis (DVT) and prevention of recurrent DVT and pulmonary embolism following acute DVT in adults (February 2012) SMC No. 755/12 Recommended

▸ Rivaroxaban (*Xarelto*®) for the treatment of pulmonary embolism (PE), and prevention of recurrent deep-vein thrombosis (DVT) and PE in adults (March 2013) SMC No. 852/13 Recommended

▸ Rivaroxaban (*Xarelto*®) co-administered with acetylsalicylic acid [aspirin] for the prevention of atherothrombotic events in adult patients with coronary artery disease or symptomatic peripheral artery disease at high risk of ischaemic events (February 2019) SMC No. SMC2128 Recommended with restrictions

● **MEDICINAL FORMS** There can be variation in the licensing of different medicines containing the same drug.

Oral tablet

CAUTIONARY AND ADVISORY LABELS 10, 21 (15 and 20 mg tablets)

▸ **Rivaroxaban (non-proprietary)** ▼
Rivaroxaban 2.5 mg Rivaroxaban 2.5mg tablets | 56 tablet PoM £3.18 DT = £3.28 (Hospital only) | 56 tablet PoM £60.48 DT = £3.28
Rivaroxaban 10 mg Rivaroxaban 10mg tablets | 10 tablet PoM £1.03–£18.00 | 30 tablet PoM £54.00 DT = £3.10 | 100 tablet PoM £18.00–£180.00
Rivaroxaban 15 mg Rivaroxaban 15mg tablets | 14 tablet PoM £1.28–£25.20 | 28 tablet PoM £50.40 DT = £2.55 | 42 tablet PoM £3.83–£75.60 | 100 tablet PoM £10.14–£180.00
Rivaroxaban 20 mg Rivaroxaban 20mg tablets | 28 tablet PoM £50.40 DT = £2.34 | 100 tablet PoM £8.36–£180.00

▸ **Xarelto** (Bayer Plc)
Rivaroxaban 2.5 mg Xarelto 2.5mg tablets | 56 tablet PoM £50.40 DT = £3.28
Rivaroxaban 10 mg Xarelto 10mg tablets | 10 tablet PoM £18.00 | 30 tablet PoM £54.00 DT = £3.10 | 100 tablet PoM £180.00
Rivaroxaban 15 mg Xarelto 15mg tablets | 14 tablet PoM £25.20 | 28 tablet PoM £50.40 DT = £2.55 | 42 tablet PoM £75.60 | 100 tablet PoM £180.00
Rivaroxaban 20 mg Xarelto 20mg tablets | 28 tablet PoM £50.40 DT = £2.34 | 100 tablet PoM £180.00

ANTITHROMBOTIC DRUGS ⟩ HEPARINOIDS

Danaparoid sodium
13-Jan-2021

● **INDICATIONS AND DOSE**

Prevention of deep-vein thrombosis in general or orthopaedic surgery

▸ BY SUBCUTANEOUS INJECTION
▸ Adult: 750 units twice daily for 7–10 days, initiate treatment before operation, with last pre-operative dose 1–4 hours before surgery

Thromboembolic disease in patients with history of heparin-induced thrombocytopenia

▸ INITIALLY BY INTRAVENOUS INJECTION
▸ Adult (body-weight up to 55 kg): Initially 1250 units, then (by continuous intravenous infusion) 400 units/hour for 2 hours, then (by continuous intravenous infusion) 300 units/hour for 2 hours, then (by continuous intravenous infusion) 200 units/hour for 5 days
▸ Adult (body-weight 55–89 kg): Initially 2500 units, then

(by continuous intravenous infusion) 400 units/hour for 2 hours, then (by continuous intravenous infusion) 300 units/hour for 2 hours, then (by continuous intravenous infusion) 200 units/hour for 5 days

▸ Adult (body-weight 90 kg and above): Initially 3750 units, then (by continuous intravenous infusion) 400 units/hour for 2 hours, then (by continuous intravenous infusion) 300 units/hour for 2 hours, then (by continuous intravenous infusion) 200 units/hour for 5 days

● **CONTRA-INDICATIONS** Active peptic ulcer (unless this is the reason for operation) · acute bacterial endocarditis · diabetic retinopathy · epidural anaesthesia (with treatment doses) · haemophilia and other haemorrhagic disorders · recent cerebral haemorrhage · severe uncontrolled hypertension · spinal anaesthesia (with treatment doses) · thrombocytopenia (unless patient has heparin-induced thrombocytopenia)

● **CAUTIONS** Antibodies to heparins (risk of antibody-induced thrombocytopenia) · body-weight over 90 kg · recent bleeding · risk of bleeding

● **INTERACTIONS** → Appendix 1: danaparoid

● **SIDE-EFFECTS**
▸ **Common or very common** Haemorrhage · heparin-induced thrombocytopenia · skin reactions · thrombocytopenia
▸ **Uncommon** Post procedural haematoma
▸ **Rare or very rare** Anastomotic haemorrhage

● **PREGNANCY** Manufacturer advises avoid—limited information available but not known to be harmful.

● **BREAST FEEDING** Amount probably too small to be harmful but manufacturer advises avoid.

● **HEPATIC IMPAIRMENT** Manufacturer advises caution in moderate impairment with impaired haemostasis—increased risk of bleeding; avoid in severe hepatic failure unless patient has heparin-induced thrombocytopenia and no alternative available.

● **RENAL IMPAIRMENT** Use with caution in moderate impairment. Avoid in severe impairment unless patient has heparin-induced thrombocytopenia and no alternative available.
Monitoring Increased risk of bleeding in renal impairment, monitor anti-Factor Xa activity.

● **MONITORING REQUIREMENTS** Monitor anti factor Xa activity in patients with body-weight over 90 kg.

● **DIRECTIONS FOR ADMINISTRATION** Manufacturer advises for *intravenous infusion*, give continuously in Glucose 5% or Sodium Chloride 0.9%.

● **MEDICINAL FORMS** There can be variation in the licensing of different medicines containing the same drug.

Solution for injection

▸ **Danaparoid sodium (Non-proprietary)**
Danaparoid sodium 1250 unit per 1 ml Danaparoid sodium 750units/0.6ml solution for injection ampoules | 10 ampoule PoM £599.99 (Hospital only)

ANTITHROMBOTIC DRUGS ⟩ HEPARINS

Heparins

● **CONTRA-INDICATIONS** Acute bacterial endocarditis · after major trauma · avoid injections containing benzyl alcohol in neonates · epidural anaesthesia with treatment doses · haemophilia or other haemorrhagic disorders · peptic ulcer · recent cerebral haemorrhage · recent surgery to eye · recent surgery to nervous system · spinal anaesthesia with treatment doses · thrombocytopenia (including history of heparin-induced thrombocytopenia)

● **CAUTIONS** Elderly · risk of bleeding · severe hypertension

- **SIDE-EFFECTS**
- **Common or very common** Haemorrhage · heparin-induced thrombocytopenia · skin reactions
- **Rare or very rare** Alopecia · hyperkalaemia · osteoporosis (following long term use) · spinal haematoma

  SIDE-EFFECTS, FURTHER INFORMATION **Haemorrhage** If haemorrhage occurs it is usually sufficient to withdraw unfractionated or low molecular weight heparin, but if rapid reversal of the effects of the heparin is required, protamine sulfate is a specific antidote (but only partially reverses the effects of low molecular weight heparins).

  Heparin-induced thrombocytopenia Clinically important heparin-induced thrombocytopenia is immune-mediated and can be complicated by thrombosis. Signs of heparin-induced thrombocytopenia include a 30% reduction of platelet count, thrombosis, or skin allergy. If heparin-induced thrombocytopenia is strongly suspected or confirmed, the heparin should be stopped and an alternative anticoagulant, such as danaparoid, should be given. Ensure platelet counts return to normal range in those who require warfarin.

  Hyperkalaemia Inhibition of aldosterone secretion by unfractionated or low molecular weight heparin can result in hyperkalaemia; patients with diabetes mellitus, chronic renal failure, acidosis, raised plasma potassium or those taking potassium-sparing drugs seem to be more susceptible. The risk appears to increase with duration of therapy.

- **MONITORING REQUIREMENTS**
- Heparin-induced thrombocytopenia Platelet counts should be measured just before treatment with unfractionated or low molecular weight heparin, and regular monitoring of platelet counts may be required if given for longer than 4 days. See the British Society for Haematology's Guidelines on the diagnosis and management of heparin-induced thrombocytopenia: second edition. *Br J Haematol* 2012; **159**: 528–540.
- Hyperkalaemia Plasma-potassium concentration should be measured in patients at risk of hyperkalaemia before starting the heparin and monitored regularly thereafter, particularly if treatment is to be continued for longer than 7 days.

Bemiparin sodium

06-Jul-2021

- **INDICATIONS AND DOSE**

Prophylaxis of deep-vein thrombosis [general surgery]
- BY SUBCUTANEOUS INJECTION
- Adult: 2500 units for 1 dose, dose to be given 2 hours before or 6 hours after surgery, then 2500 units every 24 hours

Prophylaxis of deep-vein thrombosis [orthopaedic surgery]
- BY SUBCUTANEOUS INJECTION
- Adult: 3500 units for 1 dose, dose to be given 2 hours before or 6 hours after surgery, then 3500 units every 24 hours

Prevention of clotting in extracorporeal circuits
- TO THE DEVICE AS A FLUSH
- Adult: (consult product literature)

- **CONTRA-INDICATIONS** Recent surgery to ear · severe impairment of pancreatic function

- **INTERACTIONS** → Appendix 1: low molecular-weight heparins

- **SIDE-EFFECTS** Epidural haematoma

- **ALLERGY AND CROSS-SENSITIVITY** EvGr Contra-indicated in hypersensitivity to unfractionated or low molecular weight heparin. M

- **PREGNANCY** EvGr Caution—limited information available (no toxicity in *animal* studies and not known if bemiparin sodium crosses the placenta). M

- **BREAST FEEDING** EvGr Avoid—no information available. M

- **HEPATIC IMPAIRMENT** EvGr Avoid in severe impairment. M

- **RENAL IMPAIRMENT**
- When used for Prophylaxis of deep-vein thrombosis [general and orthopaedic surgery] EvGr Caution if creatinine clearance less than 80 mL/minute (limited information available). Consider measuring anti-Factor Xa levels at about 4 hours after dosing if creatinine clearance less than 30 mL/minute. M

  Dose adjustments See p. 21.
- When used for Prophylaxis of deep-vein thrombosis [orthopaedic surgery] EvGr A dose of 2500 units once daily could be considered if creatinine clearance less than 30 mL/minute (limited information available). M

- **MEDICINAL FORMS** No licensed medicines listed.

Dalteparin sodium

01-Feb-2024

- **INDICATIONS AND DOSE**

FRAGMIN ®

Treatment of deep-vein thrombosis | Treatment of pulmonary embolism
- BY SUBCUTANEOUS INJECTION
- Adult: 200 units/kg daily (max. per dose 18 000 units) until adequate oral anticoagulation with vitamin K antagonist established (at least 5 days of combined treatment is usually required)

Treatment of deep-vein thrombosis (in patients at increased risk of haemorrhage) | Treatment of pulmonary embolism (in patients at increased risk of haemorrhage)
- BY SUBCUTANEOUS INJECTION
- Adult: 100 units/kg twice daily until adequate oral anticoagulation with vitamin K antagonist established (at least 5 days of combined treatment is usually required)

Unstable coronary artery disease
- BY SUBCUTANEOUS INJECTION
- Adult: 120 units/kg every 12 hours (max. per dose 10 000 units twice daily) for 5–8 days

Prevention of clotting in extracorporeal circuits
- TO THE DEVICE AS A FLUSH
- Adult: (consult product literature)

FRAGMIN ® **GRADUATED SYRINGES**

Unstable coronary artery disease (including non-ST-segment-elevation myocardial infarction)
- BY SUBCUTANEOUS INJECTION
- Adult: 120 units/kg every 12 hours (max. per dose 10 000 units twice daily) for up to 8 days

Patients with unstable coronary artery disease (including non-ST-segment-elevation thyocardial infarction) awaiting angiography or revascularisation and having already had 8 days treatment with dalteparin
- BY SUBCUTANEOUS INJECTION
- Adult (body-weight up to 70 kg and male): 5000 units every 12 hours until the day of the procedure (max. 45 days).
- Adult (body-weight up to 80 kg and female): 5000 units every 12 hours until the day of the procedure (max. 45 days).
- Adult (body-weight 70 kg and above and male): 7500 units every 12 hours until the day of the procedure (max. 45 days).

continued →

▸ Adult (body-weight 80 kg and above and female): 7500 units every 12 hours until the day of the procedure (max. 45 days).

FRAGMIN® SINGLE-DOSE SYRINGES

Prophylaxis of deep-vein thrombosis in surgical patients—moderate risk

▸ BY SUBCUTANEOUS INJECTION

▸ Adult: Initially 2500 units for 1 dose, dose to be given 1–2 hours before surgery, then 2500 units every 24 hours

Prophylaxis of deep-vein thrombosis in surgical patients—high risk

▸ BY SUBCUTANEOUS INJECTION

▸ Adult: Initially 2500 units for 1 dose, dose to be administered 1–2 hours before surgery, followed by 2500 units after 8–12 hours, then 5000 units every 24 hours, alternatively initially 5000 units for 1 dose, dose to be given on the evening before surgery, followed by 5000 units after 24 hours, then 5000 units every 24 hours

Prophylaxis of deep-vein thrombosis in medical patients

▸ BY SUBCUTANEOUS INJECTION

▸ Adult: 5000 units every 24 hours

Treatment of deep-vein thrombosis | Treatment of pulmonary embolism

▸ BY SUBCUTANEOUS INJECTION

▸ Adult (body-weight up to 46 kg): 7500 units once daily until adequate oral anticoagulation with vitamin K antagonist established (at least 5 days of combined treatment is usually required)

▸ Adult (body-weight 46-56 kg): 10 000 units once daily until adequate oral anticoagulation with vitamin K antagonist established (at least 5 days of combined treatment is usually required)

▸ Adult (body-weight 57-68 kg): 12 500 units once daily until adequate oral anticoagulation with vitamin K antagonist established (at least 5 days of combined treatment is usually required)

▸ Adult (body-weight 69-82 kg): 15 000 units once daily until adequate oral anticoagulation with vitamin K antagonist established (at least 5 days of combined treatment is usually required)

▸ Adult (body-weight 83 kg and above): 18 000 units once daily until adequate oral anticoagulation with vitamin K antagonist established (at least 5 days of combined treatment is usually required)

Extended treatment of venous thromboembolism and prevention of recurrence in patients with solid tumours

▸ BY SUBCUTANEOUS INJECTION

▸ Adult (body-weight 40-45 kg): 7500 units once daily for 30 days, then 7500 units once daily for a further 5 months, interrupt treatment or reduce dose in chemotherapy-induced thrombocytopenia—consult product literature

▸ Adult (body-weight 46-56 kg): 10 000 units once daily for 30 days, then 7500 units once daily for a further 5 months, interrupt treatment or reduce dose in chemotherapy-induced thrombocytopenia—consult product literature

▸ Adult (body-weight 57-68 kg): 12 500 units once daily for 30 days, then 10 000 units once daily for a further 5 months, interrupt treatment or reduce dose in chemotherapy-induced thrombocytopenia—consult product literature

▸ Adult (body-weight 69-82 kg): 15 000 units once daily for 30 days, then 12 500 units once daily for a further 5 months, interrupt treatment or reduce dose in chemotherapy-induced thrombocytopenia—consult product literature

▸ Adult (body-weight 83-98 kg): 18 000 units once daily for 30 days, then 15 000 units once daily for a further 5 months, interrupt treatment or reduce dose in chemotherapy-induced thrombocytopenia—consult product literature

▸ Adult (body-weight 99 kg and above): 18 000 units once daily for 30 days, then 18 000 units once daily for a further 5 months, interrupt treatment or reduce dose in chemotherapy-induced thrombocytopenia—consult product literature

Treatment of venous thromboembolism in pregnancy

▸ BY SUBCUTANEOUS INJECTION

▸ Adult (body-weight up to 50 kg): 5000 units twice daily, use body-weight in early pregnancy to calculate the dose

▸ Adult (body-weight 50-69 kg): 6000 units twice daily, use body-weight in early pregnancy to calculate the dose

▸ Adult (body-weight 70-89 kg): 8000 units twice daily, use body-weight in early pregnancy to calculate the dose

▸ Adult (body-weight 90 kg and above): 10 000 units twice daily, use body-weight in early pregnancy to calculate the dose

● UNLICENSED USE Dalteparin sodium is used for the treatment of venous thromboembolism in pregnancy, but is not licensed for this indication.

● CONTRA-INDICATIONS Mechanical prosthetic heart valve

● INTERACTIONS → Appendix 1: low molecular-weight heparins

● SIDE-EFFECTS Epidural haematoma · hypoaldosteronism · intracranial haemorrhage · prosthetic cardiac valve thrombosis

● ALLERGY AND CROSS-SENSITIVITY EvGr Contra-indicated in hypersensitivity to unfractionated or low molecular weight heparin. Ⓜ

● PREGNANCY Not known to be harmful, low molecular weight heparins do not cross the placenta. Multidose vial contains benzyl alcohol—manufacturer advises avoid.

● BREAST FEEDING Due to the relatively high molecular weight and inactivation in the gastro-intestinal tract, passage into breast-milk and absorption by the nursing infant are likely to be negligible, however manufacturers advise avoid.

● HEPATIC IMPAIRMENT Manufacturer advises caution in severe impairment (increased risk of bleeding complications).
Dose adjustments Manufacturer advises consider dose reduction in severe impairment.

● RENAL IMPAIRMENT Use of unfractionated heparin may be preferable.
Dose adjustments Risk of bleeding may be increased—dose reduction may be required.

● MONITORING REQUIREMENTS

▸ For monitoring during treatment of deep-vein thrombosis and of pulmonary embolism, blood should be taken 3–4 hours after a dose (recommended plasma concentration of anti-Factor Xa 0.5–1 unit/mL); monitoring not required for once-daily treatment regimen and not generally necessary for twice-daily regimen.

▸ Routine monitoring of anti-Factor Xa activity during treatment with dalteparin may be necessary in patients at increased risk of bleeding (e.g. in renal impairment and those who are underweight or overweight).

● DIRECTIONS FOR ADMINISTRATION For *subcutaneous injection*, administration into the anterolateral or posterolateral aspect of the abdomen, or the lateral part of the thigh is preferred.

- **NATIONAL FUNDING/ACCESS DECISIONS**
  For full details see funding body website
  Scottish Medicines Consortium (SMC) decisions
  - Dalteparin (*Fragmin*®) for use in patients with solid tumours: extended treatment of symptomatic VTE and prevention of recurrence (March 2011) SMC No. 683/11 Recommended with restrictions

- **MEDICINAL FORMS**　There can be variation in the licensing of different medicines containing the same drug.
  Solution for injection
  EXCIPIENTS:　May contain Benzyl alcohol
  - Fragmin (Pfizer Ltd)
    Dalteparin sodium 2500 unit per 1 ml　Fragmin 10,000units/4ml solution for injection ampoules | 10 ampoule [PoM] £51.22 DT = £51.22
    Dalteparin sodium 10000 unit per 1 ml　Fragmin Graduated Syringe 10,000units/1ml solution for injection pre-filled syringes | 5 pre-filled disposable injection [PoM] £29.06 DT = £28.23
    Fragmin 10,000units/1ml solution for injection ampoules | 10 ampoule [PoM] £51.22 DT = £51.22
    Dalteparin sodium 12500 unit per 1 ml　Fragmin 2,500units/0.2ml solution for injection pre-filled syringes | 10 pre-filled disposable injection [PoM] £19.59 DT = £18.58
    Dalteparin sodium 25000 unit per 1 ml　Fragmin 18,000units/0.72ml solution for injection pre-filled syringes | 5 pre-filled disposable injection [PoM] £50.82 DT = £50.82
    Fragmin 15,000units/0.6ml solution for injection pre-filled syringes | 5 pre-filled disposable injection [PoM] £42.42 DT = £42.34
    Fragmin 5,000units/0.2ml solution for injection pre-filled syringes | 10 pre-filled disposable injection [PoM] £29.82 DT = £28.23
    Fragmin 12,500units/0.5ml solution for injection pre-filled syringes | 5 pre-filled disposable injection [PoM] £35.44 DT = £35.29
    Fragmin 7,500units/0.3ml solution for injection pre-filled syringes | 10 pre-filled disposable injection [PoM] £42.77 DT = £42.34
    Fragmin 100,000units/4ml solution for injection vials | 1 vial [PoM] £48.66 DT = £48.66
    Fragmin 10,000units/0.4ml solution for injection pre-filled syringes | 5 pre-filled disposable injection [PoM] £34.11 DT = £28.23

⯈ 152

Enoxaparin sodium

10-Mar-2024

- **INDICATIONS AND DOSE**

Treatment of venous thromboembolism in pregnancy
- BY SUBCUTANEOUS INJECTION
- Adult (body-weight up to 50 kg):　40 mg twice daily, dose based on early pregnancy body-weight
- Adult (body-weight 50–69 kg):　60 mg twice daily, dose based on early pregnancy body-weight
- Adult (body-weight 70–89 kg):　80 mg twice daily, dose based on early pregnancy body-weight
- Adult (body-weight 90 kg and above):　100 mg twice daily, dose based on early pregnancy body-weight

Prophylaxis of deep-vein thrombosis, especially in surgical patients—moderate risk
- BY SUBCUTANEOUS INJECTION
- Adult:　20 mg for 1 dose, dose to be given approximately 2 hours before surgery, then 20 mg every 24 hours

Prophylaxis of deep-vein thrombosis, especially surgical patients—high risk (e.g. orthopaedic surgery)
- BY SUBCUTANEOUS INJECTION
- Adult:　40 mg for 1 dose, dose to be given 12 hours before surgery, then 40 mg every 24 hours

Prophylaxis of deep-vein thrombosis in medical patients
- BY SUBCUTANEOUS INJECTION
- Adult:　40 mg every 24 hours

Treatment of deep-vein thrombosis in uncomplicated patients with low risk of recurrence | Treatment of pulmonary embolism in uncomplicated patients with low risk of recurrence
- BY SUBCUTANEOUS INJECTION
- Adult:　1.5 mg/kg every 24 hours until adequate oral anticoagulation established

Treatment of deep-vein thrombosis in patients with risk factors such as obesity, cancer, recurrent VTE, or proximal thrombosis | Treatment of pulmonary embolism in patients with risk factors such as obesity, symptomatic pulmonary embolism, cancer, or recurrent VTE
- BY SUBCUTANEOUS INJECTION
- Adult:　1 mg/kg every 12 hours until adequate oral anticoagulation established

Treatment of acute ST-segment elevation myocardial infarction (patients not undergoing percutaneous coronary intervention)
- INITIALLY BY INTRAVENOUS INJECTION
- Adult 18–74 years:　Initially 30 mg for 1 dose, followed immediately by (by subcutaneous injection) 1 mg/kg for 1 dose (max. per dose 100 mg), then (by subcutaneous injection) 1 mg/kg for 1 dose (max. per dose 100 mg), to be administered 12 hours after initial subcutaneous dose, then (by subcutaneous injection) 1 mg/kg every 12 hours, total treatment for up to 8 days or until hospital discharge, whichever is sooner
- BY SUBCUTANEOUS INJECTION
- Adult 75 years and over:　750 micrograms/kg every 12 hours (max. per dose 75 mg) for 2 doses, then 750 micrograms/kg every 12 hours, total treatment for up to 8 days or until hospital discharge, whichever is sooner

Treatment of acute ST-segment elevation myocardial infarction (patients undergoing percutaneous coronary intervention)
- INITIALLY BY INTRAVENOUS INJECTION
- Adult 18–74 years:　Initially 30 mg for 1 dose, followed immediately by (by subcutaneous injection) 1 mg/kg for 1 dose (max. per dose 100 mg), then (by subcutaneous injection) 1 mg/kg for 1 dose (max. per dose 100 mg), to be administered 12 hours after initial subcutaneous dose, then (by subcutaneous injection) 1 mg/kg every 12 hours, total treatment for up to 8 days or until hospital discharge, whichever is sooner, then (by intravenous injection) 300 micrograms/kg for 1 dose, dose only to be given at the time of procedure if the last subcutaneous dose was given more than 8 hours previously
- INITIALLY BY SUBCUTANEOUS INJECTION
- Adult 75 years and over:　750 micrograms/kg every 12 hours (max. per dose 75 mg) for 2 doses, then (by subcutaneous injection) 750 micrograms/kg every 12 hours, total treatment for up to 8 days or until hospital discharge, whichever is sooner, then (by intravenous injection) 300 micrograms/kg for 1 dose, dose only to be given at the time of procedure if the last subcutaneous dose was given more than 8 hours previously

Unstable angina | Non-ST-segment-elevation myocardial infarction
- BY SUBCUTANEOUS INJECTION
- Adult:　1 mg/kg every 12 hours usually for 2–8 days (minimum 2 days)

Prevention of clotting in extracorporeal circuits
- TO THE DEVICE AS A FLUSH
- Adult:　(consult product literature)
- DOSE EQUIVALENCE AND CONVERSION
- 1 mg equivalent to 100 units.

- **UNLICENSED USE**　Not licensed for treatment of venous thromboembolism in pregnancy.
- **CONTRA-INDICATIONS**　Mechanical prosthetic heart valve
- **CAUTIONS**　Low body-weight (increased risk of bleeding) · Obesity (increased risk of thromboembolism)
- **INTERACTIONS**　→ Appendix 1: low molecular-weight heparins

- **SIDE-EFFECTS**
  - ▶ **Common or very common** Haemorrhagic anaemia · headache · hypersensitivity · thrombocytopenia · thrombocytosis
  - ▶ **Uncommon** Hepatic disorders · injection site necrosis · intracranial haemorrhage
  - ▶ **Rare or very rare** Cutaneous vasculitis · eosinophilia
  - ▶ **Frequency not known** Acute generalised exanthematous pustulosis (AGEP)

- **ALLERGY AND CROSS-SENSITIVITY** [EvGr] Contra-indicated in hypersensitivity to unfractionated or low molecular weight heparin. ⟨M⟩

- **PREGNANCY** Not known to be harmful, low molecular weight heparins do not cross the placenta. Multidose vial contains benzyl alcohol—avoid.

- **BREAST FEEDING** Manufacturer advises suitable for use during breast feeding—passage into breast milk and absorption by the nursing infant considered to be negligible due to the relatively high molecular weight of enoxaparin and inactivation in the gastro-intestinal tract.

- **HEPATIC IMPAIRMENT** Manufacturer advises caution—no information available.

- **RENAL IMPAIRMENT** Risk of bleeding increased; use of unfractionated heparin may be preferable. Manufacturer advises avoid if creatinine clearance less than 15 mL/minute.
  Dose adjustments Manufacturer advises reduce dose if creatinine clearance 15–30 mL/minute—consult product literature for details.

- **MONITORING REQUIREMENTS** Routine monitoring of anti-Factor Xa activity is not usually required during treatment with enoxaparin, but may be necessary in patients at increased risk of bleeding (e.g. in renal impairment and those who are underweight or overweight).

- **DIRECTIONS FOR ADMINISTRATION** When administered in conjunction with a thrombolytic, manufacturer advises enoxaparin should be given between 15 minutes before and 30 minutes after the start of thrombolytic therapy.

- **PRESCRIBING AND DISPENSING INFORMATION** Enoxaparin sodium is a biological medicine. Biological medicines must be prescribed and dispensed by brand name, see *Biological medicines* and *Biosimilar medicines*, under Guidance on prescribing p. 1.

- **MEDICINAL FORMS** There can be variation in the licensing of different medicines containing the same drug.

  Solution for injection
  EXCIPIENTS: May contain Benzyl alcohol

  - ▶ **Arovi** (ROVI Biotech Ltd) ▼
    Enoxaparin sodium 100 mg per 1 ml Arovi 20mg/0.2ml solution for injection pre-filled syringes | 10 pre-filled disposable injection [PoM] £15.65 DT = £20.86
    Arovi 60mg/0.6ml solution for injection pre-filled syringes | 10 pre-filled disposable injection [PoM] £29.45 DT = £39.26
    Arovi 40mg/0.4ml solution for injection pre-filled syringes | 10 pre-filled disposable injection [PoM] £22.70 DT = £30.27
    Arovi 80mg/0.8ml solution for injection pre-filled syringes | 10 pre-filled disposable injection [PoM] £41.35 DT = £55.13
    Arovi 100mg/1ml solution for injection pre-filled syringes | 10 pre-filled disposable injection [PoM] £54.23 DT = £72.30
    Enoxaparin sodium 150 mg per 1 ml Arovi 150mg/1ml solution for injection pre-filled syringes | 10 pre-filled disposable injection [PoM] £74.93 DT = £99.91
    Arovi 120mg/0.8ml solution for injection pre-filled syringes | 10 pre-filled disposable injection [PoM] £65.95 DT = £87.93

  - ▶ **Clexane** (Sanofi)
    Enoxaparin sodium 100 mg per 1 ml Clexane 60mg/0.6ml solution for injection pre-filled syringes | 10 pre-filled disposable injection [PoM] £39.26 DT = £39.26
    Clexane 300mg/3ml solution for injection multidose vials | 1 vial [PoM] £21.33 DT = £21.33
    Clexane 80mg/0.8ml solution for injection pre-filled syringes | 10 pre-filled disposable injection [PoM] £55.13 DT = £55.13

Clexane 40mg/0.4ml solution for injection pre-filled syringes | 10 pre-filled disposable injection [PoM] £30.27 DT = £30.27
Clexane 100mg/1ml solution for injection pre-filled syringes | 10 pre-filled disposable injection [PoM] £72.30 DT = £72.30
Clexane 20mg/0.2ml solution for injection pre-filled syringes | 10 pre-filled disposable injection [PoM] £20.86 DT = £20.86
Enoxaparin sodium 150 mg per 1 ml Clexane Forte 120mg/0.8ml solution for injection pre-filled syringes | 10 pre-filled disposable injection [PoM] £87.93 DT = £87.93
Clexane Forte 150mg/1ml solution for injection pre-filled syringes | 10 pre-filled disposable injection [PoM] £99.91 DT = £99.91

- ▶ **Inhixa** (Techdow Pharma England Ltd)
  Enoxaparin sodium 100 mg per 1 ml Inhixa 40mg/0.4ml solution for injection pre-filled syringes | 10 pre-filled disposable injection [PoM] £22.70 DT = £30.27
  Inhixa 80mg/0.8ml solution for injection pre-filled syringes | 10 pre-filled disposable injection [PoM] £41.35 DT = £55.13
  Inhixa 60mg/0.6ml solution for injection pre-filled syringes | 10 pre-filled disposable injection [PoM] £29.45 DT = £39.26
  Inhixa 100mg/1ml solution for injection pre-filled syringes | 10 pre-filled disposable injection [PoM] £54.23 DT = £72.30
  Inhixa 20mg/0.2ml solution for injection pre-filled syringes | 10 pre-filled disposable injection [PoM] £15.65 DT = £20.86
  Enoxaparin sodium 150 mg per 1 ml Inhixa 120mg/0.8ml solution for injection pre-filled syringes | 10 pre-filled disposable injection [PoM] £65.95 DT = £87.93
  Inhixa 150mg/1ml solution for injection pre-filled syringes | 10 pre-filled disposable injection [PoM] £74.93 DT = £99.91

- ▶ **Ledraxen** (Venipharm Ltd) ▼
  Enoxaparin sodium 100 mg per 1 ml Ledraxen 20mg/0.2ml solution for injection pre-filled syringes | 10 pre-filled disposable injection [PoM] £20.86 DT = £20.86
  Ledraxen 40mg/0.4ml solution for injection pre-filled syringes | 10 pre-filled disposable injection [PoM] £30.27 DT = £30.27
  Ledraxen 100mg/1ml solution for injection pre-filled syringes | 10 pre-filled disposable injection [PoM] £72.30 DT = £72.30
  Ledraxen 60mg/0.6ml solution for injection pre-filled syringes | 10 pre-filled disposable injection [PoM] £39.26 DT = £39.26
  Ledraxen 80mg/0.8ml solution for injection pre-filled syringes | 10 pre-filled disposable injection [PoM] £55.13 DT = £55.13

◀ 152

Heparin (unfractionated)

18-Feb-2022

- **INDICATIONS AND DOSE**

Treatment of mild to moderate pulmonary embolism | Treatment of unstable angina | Treatment of acute peripheral arterial occlusion
  - ▶ INITIALLY BY INTRAVENOUS INJECTION
  - ▶ Adult: Loading dose 5000 units, alternatively (by intravenous injection) loading dose 75 units/kg, followed by (by continuous intravenous infusion) 18 units/kg/hour, laboratory monitoring essential—preferably on a daily basis, and dose adjusted accordingly

Treatment of severe pulmonary embolism
  - ▶ INITIALLY BY INTRAVENOUS INJECTION
  - ▶ Adult: Loading dose 10 000 units, followed by (by continuous intravenous infusion) 18 units/kg/hour, laboratory monitoring essential—preferably on a daily basis, and dose adjusted accordingly

Treatment of deep-vein thrombosis
  - ▶ INITIALLY BY INTRAVENOUS INJECTION
  - ▶ Adult: Loading dose 5000 units, alternatively (by intravenous injection) loading dose 75 units/kg, followed by (by continuous intravenous infusion) 18 units/kg/hour, alternatively (by subcutaneous injection) 15 000 units every 12 hours, laboratory monitoring essential—preferably on a daily basis, and dose adjusted accordingly

Thromboprophylaxis in medical patients
  - ▶ BY SUBCUTANEOUS INJECTION
  - ▶ Adult: 5000 units every 8–12 hours

2

Cardiovascular system

Thrombophylaxis in surgical patients
▶ BY SUBCUTANEOUS INJECTION
▸ Adult: 5000 units for 1 dose, to be taken 2 hours before surgery, then 5000 units every 8–12 hours

Thromboprophylaxis during pregnancy
▶ BY SUBCUTANEOUS INJECTION
▸ Adult: 5000–10 000 units every 12 hours, to be administered with monitoring, **Important**: prevention of prosthetic heart-valve thrombosis in pregnancy calls for **specialist management**

Haemodialysis
▶ INITIALLY BY INTRAVENOUS INJECTION
▸ Adult: Initially 1000–5000 units, followed by (by continuous intravenous infusion) 250–1000 units/hour

Prevention of clotting in extracorporeal circuits
▶ TO THE DEVICE AS A FLUSH
▸ Adult: (consult product literature)

To maintain patency of catheters, cannulas, other indwelling intravenous infusion devices
▶ TO THE DEVICE AS A FLUSH
▸ Adult: 10–200 units, to be flushed through every 4–8 hours, not for therapeutic use

● **INTERACTIONS** → Appendix 1: heparin

● **SIDE-EFFECTS** Adrenal hypofunction · hypokalaemia · priapism · rebound hyperlipidaemia · thrombocytopenia

● **ALLERGY AND CROSS-SENSITIVITY** [EvGr] Caution in hypersensitivity to low molecular weight heparin. ⟨M⟩

● **PREGNANCY** Does not cross the placenta; maternal osteoporosis reported after prolonged use; multidose vials may contain benzyl alcohol—some manufacturers advise avoid.

● **BREAST FEEDING** Not excreted into milk due to high molecular weight.

● **HEPATIC IMPAIRMENT** Manufacturer advises caution; consider avoiding in severe impairment (increased risk of bleeding complications).
Dose adjustments Manufacturer advises consider dose reduction if used in severe impairment.

● **RENAL IMPAIRMENT** [EvGr] Use with caution. ⟨M⟩
Dose adjustments [EvGr] Consider dose reduction in severe impairment (increased risk of bleeding). ⟨M⟩

● **DIRECTIONS FOR ADMINISTRATION** For *intravenous infusion*, give continuously in Glucose 5% or Sodium Chloride 0.9%; administration with a motorised pump is advisable.

● **PRESCRIBING AND DISPENSING INFORMATION** Doses listed take into account the guidelines of the British Society for Haematology.

● **MEDICINAL FORMS** There can be variation in the licensing of different medicines containing the same drug. Forms available from special-order manufacturers include: solution for injection, solution for infusion

Solution for injection
EXCIPIENTS: May contain Benzyl alcohol

▶ Heparin (unfractionated) (Non-proprietary)
Heparin sodium 1000 unit per 1 ml Heparin sodium 1,000units/1ml solution for injection ampoules | 10 ampoule [PoM] £20.05 DT = £20.05
Heparin sodium 5,000units/5ml solution for injection vials | 10 vial [PoM] £16.50-£49.76 DT = £16.50
Heparin sodium 20,000units/20ml solution for injection ampoules | 10 ampoule [PoM] £99.94 DT = £99.94
Heparin sodium 5,000units/5ml solution for injection ampoules | 10 ampoule [PoM] £49.76-£52.46 DT = £52.46
Heparin sodium 10,000units/10ml solution for injection ampoules | 10 ampoule [PoM] £93.66 DT = £93.66
Heparin sodium 5000 unit per 1 ml Heparin sodium 25,000units/5ml solution for injection ampoules | 10 ampoule [PoM] £98.51 DT = £98.51 (Hospital only) | 10 ampoule [PoM] £98.51 DT = £98.51

Heparin sodium 5,000units/1ml solution for injection ampoules | 10 ampoule [PoM] £28.90-£39.20 DT = £39.20 | 10 ampoule [PoM] £39.20 DT = £39.20 (Hospital only)
Heparin sodium 25,000units/5ml solution for injection vials | 10 vial [PoM] £45.00-£114.21 DT = £45.00
Heparin calcium 25000 unit per 1 ml Heparin calcium 5,000units/0.2ml solution for injection ampoules | 10 ampoule [PoM] £64.82 DT = £64.82
Heparin sodium 25000 unit per 1 ml Heparin sodium 25,000units/1ml solution for injection ampoules | 10 ampoule [PoM] £111.58 DT = £111.58
Heparin sodium 5,000units/0.2ml solution for injection ampoules | 10 ampoule [PoM] £54.16 DT = £54.16

Form unstated
EXCIPIENTS: May contain Benzyl alcohol

▶ Heparin (unfractionated) (Non-proprietary)
Heparin sodium 10 unit per 1 ml Heparin sodium 50units/5ml patency solution ampoules | 10 ampoule [PoM] £20.20 DT = £20.20
Heparin sodium 50units/5ml I.V. flush solution ampoules | 10 ampoule [PoM] £20.20 DT = £20.20 | 10 ampoule [PoM] £20.20 DT = £20.20 (Hospital only)
Heparin sodium 100 unit per 1 ml Heparin sodium 200units/2ml I.V. flush solution ampoules | 10 ampoule [PoM] £21.17 DT = £21.17 (Hospital only) | 10 ampoule [PoM] £21.17 DT = £21.17
Heparin sodium 200units/2ml patency solution ampoules | 10 ampoule [PoM] £21.17 DT = £21.17

Infusion

▶ Heparin (unfractionated) (Non-proprietary)
Heparin sodium 1 unit per 1 ml Heparin sodium 500units/500ml infusion Viaflex bags | 1 bag [PoM] £13.44 (Hospital only) | 20 bag [PoM] £268.80 (Hospital only)
Heparin sodium 2 unit per 1 ml Heparin sodium 1,000units/500ml infusion Viaflex bags | 1 bag [PoM] £13.44 (Hospital only) | 20 bag [PoM] £268.80 (Hospital only)
Heparin sodium 2,000units/1litre infusion Viaflex bags | 1 bag [PoM] £13.44 (Hospital only) | 10 bag [PoM] £134.40 (Hospital only)
Heparin sodium 5 unit per 1 ml Heparin sodium 5,000units/1litre infusion Viaflex bags | 1 bag [PoM] £12.79 (Hospital only) | 10 bag [PoM] £127.90 (Hospital only)

⯅ 152

Tinzaparin sodium
27-Aug-2021

● **INDICATIONS AND DOSE**

INNOHEP ® 10,000 UNITS/ML

Prophylaxis of deep-vein thrombosis (general surgery)
▶ BY SUBCUTANEOUS INJECTION
▸ Adult: 3500 units for 1 dose, dose to be given 2 hours before surgery, then 3500 units every 24 hours

Prophylaxis of deep-vein thrombosis (orthopaedic surgery)
▶ BY SUBCUTANEOUS INJECTION
▸ Adult: Initially 50 units/kg for 1 dose, dose to be given 2 hours before surgery, then 50 units/kg every 24 hours, alternatively initially 4500 units for 1 dose, dose to be given 12 hours before surgery, then 4500 units every 24 hours

Prevention of clotting in extracorporeal circuits
▶ TO THE DEVICE AS A FLUSH
▸ Adult: (consult product literature)

INNOHEP ® 20,000 UNITS/ML

Extended treatment of venous thromboembolism and prevention of recurrence in patients with active cancer
▶ BY SUBCUTANEOUS INJECTION
▸ Adult: 175 units/kg once daily for 6 months; the benefit of continued treatment beyond 6 months should be evaluated

Treatment of deep-vein thrombosis | Treatment of pulmonary embolism
▶ BY SUBCUTANEOUS INJECTION
▸ Adult: 175 units/kg once daily until adequate oral anticoagulation established, treatment regimens do not require anticoagulation monitoring   continued →

Treatment of venous thromboembolism in pregnancy
▸ BY SUBCUTANEOUS INJECTION
▸ Adult: 175 units/kg once daily, dose based on early pregnancy body-weight, treatment regimens do not require anticoagulation monitoring

● UNLICENSED USE Not licensed for the treatment of venous thromboembolism in pregnancy.

● CONTRA-INDICATIONS Mechanical prosthetic heart valve

● INTERACTIONS → Appendix 1: low molecular-weight heparins

● SIDE-EFFECTS
▸ **Common or very common** Anaemia
▸ **Rare or very rare** Angioedema · priapism · Stevens-Johnson syndrome · thrombocytosis

● ALLERGY AND CROSS-SENSITIVITY [EvGr] Contra-indicated in hypersensitivity to unfractionated or low molecular weight heparin. ⓜ

● PREGNANCY Not known to be harmful, low molecular weight heparins do not cross the placenta. Vials contain benzyl alcohol—manufacturer advises avoid.

● BREAST FEEDING Due to the relatively high molecular weight of tinzaparin and inactivation in the gastro-intestinal tract, passage into breast-milk and absorption by the nursing infant are likely to be negligible; however manufacturer advise avoid.

● RENAL IMPAIRMENT Risk of bleeding may be increased. Unfractionated heparin may be preferable. Manufacturer advises caution if eGFR less than 30 mL/minute/1.73 m^2.
Monitoring In renal impairment monitoring of anti-Factor Xa may be required if eGFR less than 30 mL/minute/1.73 m^2.

● MONITORING REQUIREMENTS Routine monitoring of anti-Factor Xa activity is not usually required during treatment with tinzaparin, but may be necessary in patients at increased risk of bleeding (e.g. in renal impairment and those who are underweight or overweight).

● MEDICINAL FORMS There can be variation in the licensing of different medicines containing the same drug.
Solution for injection
EXCIPIENTS: May contain Benzyl alcohol, sulfites
▸ Tinzaparin sodium (Non-proprietary)
Tinzaparin sodium 10000 unit per 1 ml Tinzaparin sodium 3,500units/0.35ml solution for injection pre-filled syringes | 10 pre-filled disposable injection [PoM] £29.79 DT = £29.79
Tinzaparin sodium 4,500units/0.45ml solution for injection pre-filled syringes | 10 pre-filled disposable injection [PoM] £38.30 DT = £38.30
Tinzaparin sodium 2,500units/0.25ml solution for injection pre-filled syringes | 10 pre-filled disposable injection [PoM] £21.29 DT = £21.29
Tinzaparin sodium 20,000units/2ml solution for injection vials | 10 vial [PoM] £110.94 DT = £110.94
Tinzaparin sodium 20000 unit per 1 ml Tinzaparin sodium 8,000units/0.4ml solution for injection pre-filled syringes | 10 pre-filled disposable injection [PoM] £49.98 DT = £49.98
Tinzaparin sodium 14,000units/0.7ml solution for injection pre-filled syringes | 10 pre-filled disposable injection [PoM] £87.36 DT = £87.36
Tinzaparin sodium 16,000units/0.8ml solution for injection pre-filled syringes | 10 pre-filled disposable injection [PoM] £99.96 DT = £99.96
Tinzaparin sodium 40,000units/2ml solution for injection vials | 10 vial [PoM] £359.10 DT = £359.10
Tinzaparin sodium 12,000units/0.6ml solution for injection pre-filled syringes | 10 pre-filled disposable injection [PoM] £74.97 DT = £74.97
Tinzaparin sodium 10,000units/0.5ml solution for injection pre-filled syringes | 10 pre-filled disposable injection [PoM] £62.48 DT = £62.48
Tinzaparin sodium 18,000units/0.9ml solution for injection pre-filled syringes | 10 pre-filled disposable injection [PoM] £112.46 DT = £112.46

ANTITHROMBOTIC DRUGS > THROMBIN INHIBITORS, DIRECT

Argatroban monohydrate
12-Jan-2021

● INDICATIONS AND DOSE
Anticoagulation in patients with heparin-induced thrombocytopenia type II who require parenteral antithrombotic treatment
▸ INITIALLY BY CONTINUOUS INTRAVENOUS INFUSION
▸ Adult: Initially 2 micrograms/kg/minute, dose to be adjusted according to activated partial thromboplastin time, (by intravenous infusion) increased to up to 10 micrograms/kg/minute maximum duration of treatment 14 days

Anticoagulation in patients with heparin-induced thrombocytopenia type II who require parenteral antithrombotic treatment (for dose in cardiac surgery, percutaneous coronary intervention, or critically ill patients)
▸ BY CONTINUOUS INTRAVENOUS INFUSION
▸ Adult: (consult product literature)

Anticoagulation in patients with heparin-induced thrombocytopenia type II who require parenteral antithrombotic treatment (when initiating concomitant warfarin treatment)
▸ BY CONTINUOUS INTRAVENOUS INFUSION
▸ Adult: Reduced to 2 micrograms/kg/minute, dose should be temporarily reduced and INR measured after 4–6 hours; warfarin should be initiated at intended maintenance dose (do not give loading dose of warfarin); consult product literature for further details

● CAUTIONS Bleeding disorders · diabetic retinopathy · gastro-intestinal ulceration · immediately after lumbar puncture · major surgery (especially of brain, spinal cord, or eye) · risk of bleeding · severe hypertension · spinal anaesthesia

● INTERACTIONS → Appendix 1: thrombin inhibitors

● SIDE-EFFECTS
▸ **Common or very common** Anaemia · haemorrhage · nausea · skin reactions
▸ **Uncommon** Alopecia · appetite decreased · arrhythmias · cardiac arrest · confusion · constipation · deafness · diarrhoea · dizziness · dysphagia · dyspnoea · fatigue · fever · gastritis · headache · hepatic disorders · hiccups · hyperbilirubinaemia · hyperhidrosis · hypertension · hypoglycaemia · hyponatraemia · hypotension · hypoxia · increased risk of infection · leucopenia · muscle tone decreased · muscle weakness · myalgia · myocardial infarction · pain · pericardial effusion · peripheral ischaemia · peripheral oedema · pleural effusion · renal failure · shock · speech disorder · stroke · syncope · thrombocytopenia · tongue disorder · visual impairment · vomiting · wound secretion

● PREGNANCY Manufacturer advises avoid unless essential—limited information available.

● BREAST FEEDING Avoid—no information available.

● HEPATIC IMPAIRMENT Manufacturer advises caution in mild to moderate impairment—monitor aPTT; avoid in severe impairment or in patients with impairment undergoing percutaneous coronary intervention.
Dose adjustments Manufacturer advises reduce initial dose to 0.5 micrograms/kg/minute in moderate impairment; adjust dose according to aPTT and as clinically indicated—consult product literature.

● MONITORING REQUIREMENTS Determine activated partial thromboplastin time 2 hours after start of treatment, then 2 or 4 hours after infusion rate altered (consult product literature), and at least once daily thereafter.

- **DIRECTIONS FOR ADMINISTRATION** For *intravenous infusion* (*Exembol - Ready to use®*), manufacturer advises administer 1 mg/mL solution via a syringe driver. For *intravenous infusion* (*Exembol - Multidose®*), manufacturer advises give continuously in Glucose 5%, Sodium Chloride 0.9% *or* Sodium Lactate Intravenous Infusion Compound; dilute to a concentration of 1 mg/mL prior to use.

- **MEDICINAL FORMS** There can be variation in the licensing of different medicines containing the same drug.
  Solution for infusion
  EXCIPIENTS: May contain Ethanol
  ▸ Exembol (Ethypharm UK Ltd)
  Argatroban monohydrate 1 mg per 1 ml Exembol 50mg/50ml solution for infusion vials | 4 vial [PoM] £198.80 (Hospital only)
  Argatroban monohydrate 100 mg per 1 ml Exembol Multidose 250mg/2.5ml concentrate for solution for infusion vials | 1 vial [PoM] £248.50 (Hospital only)

Bivalirudin
16-Sep-2021

- **DRUG ACTION** Bivalirudin, a hirudin analogue, is a thrombin inhibitor.

- **INDICATIONS AND DOSE**

Unstable angina or non-ST-segment elevation myocardial infarction in patients planned for urgent or early intervention (in addition to aspirin and clopidogrel)
▸ INITIALLY BY INTRAVENOUS INJECTION
▸ Adult: Initially 100 micrograms/kg, then (by intravenous infusion) 250 micrograms/kg/hour (for up to 72 hours in medically managed patients)

Unstable angina or non-ST-segment elevation myocardial infarction (in addition to aspirin and clopidogrel) in patients proceeding to percutaneous coronary intervention or coronary artery bypass surgery without cardiopulmonary bypass
▸ INITIALLY BY INTRAVENOUS INJECTION
▸ Adult: Initially 100 micrograms/kg for 1 dose, then (by intravenous injection) 500 micrograms/kg for 1 dose, then (by intravenous infusion) 1.75 mg/kg/hour for duration of procedure; (by intravenous infusion) reduced to 250 micrograms/kg/hour for 4–12 hours as necessary following percutaneous coronary intervention, for patients proceeding to coronary artery bypass surgery with cardiopulmonary bypass, discontinue intravenous infusion 1 hour before procedure and treat with unfractionated heparin

Anticoagulation in patients undergoing percutaneous coronary intervention including patients with ST-segment elevation myocardial infarction undergoing primary percutaneous coronary intervention (in addition to aspirin and clopidogrel)
▸ INITIALLY BY INTRAVENOUS INJECTION
▸ Adult: Initially 750 micrograms/kg, followed immediately by (by intravenous infusion) 1.75 mg/kg/hour during procedure and for up to 4 hours after procedure, then (by intravenous infusion) reduced to 250 micrograms/kg/hour for a further 4–12 hours if necessary

- **CONTRA-INDICATIONS** Bleeding (active) · bleeding disorders · hypertension (severe) · subacute bacterial endocarditis

- **CAUTIONS** Brachytherapy procedures · previous exposure to lepirudin (theoretical risk from lepirudin antibodies)

- **INTERACTIONS** → Appendix 1: thrombin inhibitors

- **SIDE-EFFECTS**
▸ **Common or very common** Procedural complications · skin reactions
▸ **Uncommon** Anaemia · headache · hypersensitivity · hypotension · nausea · shock · thrombocytopenia

▸ **Rare or very rare** Arrhythmias · cardiac tamponade · chest pain · compartment syndrome · dyspnoea · embolism and thrombosis · intracranial haemorrhage · pain · vascular disorders · vomiting

- **PREGNANCY** Manufacturer advises avoid unless potential benefit outweighs risk—no information available.

- **BREAST FEEDING** Manufacturer advises caution—no information available.

- **RENAL IMPAIRMENT** [EvGr] Avoid if eGFR less than 30 mL/minute/1.73 m^2. ⟨M⟩
  Dose adjustments
  ▸ When used for Percutaneous coronary intervention [EvGr] Use initial dose then reduce rate of infusion to 1.4 mg/kg/hour if eGFR 30–60 mL/minute/1.73 m^2—monitor blood clotting parameters. ⟨M⟩ See p. 21.

- **DIRECTIONS FOR ADMINISTRATION** For *intravenous infusion*, manufacturer advises give continuously in Glucose 5% *or* Sodium Chloride 0.9%. Reconstitute each 250-mg vial with 5 mL Water for Injections then withdraw 5 mL and dilute to 50 mL with infusion fluid.

- **NATIONAL FUNDING/ACCESS DECISIONS**
  For full details see funding body website
  Scottish Medicines Consortium (SMC) decisions
  ▸ Bivalirudin (*Angiox®*) for acute coronary syndromes (December 2008) SMC No. 516/08 Recommended with restrictions
  ▸ Bivalirudin (*Angiox®*) as an anticoagulant in adult patients undergoing PCI, including patients with ST-segment elevation myocardial infarction (STEMI) undergoing primary PCI (September 2010) SMC No. 638/10 Recommended with restrictions

- **MEDICINAL FORMS** There can be variation in the licensing of different medicines containing the same drug.
  Powder for solution for infusion
  ▸ Bivalirudin (Non-proprietary)
  Bivalirudin 250 mg Bivalirudin 250mg powder for concentrate for solution for infusion vials | 1 vial [PoM] £180.00 (Hospital only) | 5 vial [PoM] £875.00 (Hospital only) | 10 vial [PoM] £1,250.00 (Hospital only)

Dabigatran etexilate
10-May-2024

- **DRUG ACTION** Dabigatran etexilate is a direct thrombin inhibitor with a rapid onset of action.

- **INDICATIONS AND DOSE**

Prophylaxis of venous thromboembolism following total knee replacement surgery
▸ BY MOUTH
▸ Adult 18-74 years: 110 mg for 1 dose, to be taken 1–4 hours after surgery, followed by 220 mg once daily for 10 days, to be taken on the first day after surgery
▸ Adult 75 years and over: 75 mg for 1 dose, to be taken 1–4 hours after surgery, followed by 150 mg once daily for 10 days, to be taken on the first day after surgery

Prophylaxis of venous thromboembolism following total knee replacement surgery in patients receiving concomitant treatment with amiodarone or verapamil
▸ BY MOUTH
▸ Adult 18-74 years: 75 mg for 1 dose, to be taken 1–4 hours after surgery, followed by 150 mg once daily for 10 days, to be taken on the first day after surgery
▸ Adult 75 years and over: 75 mg for 1 dose, to be taken 1–4 hours after surgery, followed by 150 mg once daily for 10 days, to be taken on the first day after surgery

continued →

Prophylaxis of venous thromboembolism following total hip replacement surgery
▸ BY MOUTH
▸ Adult 18-74 years: 110 mg for 1 dose, to be taken 1–4 hours after surgery, followed by 220 mg once daily for 28–35 days, to be taken on the first day after surgery
▸ Adult 75 years and over: 75 mg for 1 dose, to be taken 1–4 hours after surgery, followed by 150 mg once daily for 28–35 days, to be taken on the first day after surgery

Prophylaxis of venous thromboembolism following total hip replacement surgery in patients receiving concomitant treatment with amiodarone or verapamil
▸ BY MOUTH
▸ Adult 18-74 years: 75 mg for 1 dose, to be taken 1–4 hours after surgery, followed by 150 mg once daily for 28–35 days, to be taken on the first day after surgery
▸ Adult 75 years and over: 75 mg for 1 dose, to be taken 1–4 hours after surgery, followed by 150 mg once daily for 28–35 days, to be taken on the first day after surgery

Treatment of deep-vein thrombosis | Treatment of pulmonary embolism | Prophylaxis of recurrent deep-vein thrombosis | Prophylaxis of recurrent pulmonary embolism
▸ BY MOUTH
▸ Adult 18-74 years: 150 mg twice daily, to be given following at least 5 days treatment with a parenteral anticoagulant
▸ Adult 75-79 years: 110–150 mg twice daily, to be given following at least 5 days treatment with a parenteral anticoagulant
▸ Adult 80 years and over: 110 mg twice daily, to be given following at least 5 days treatment with a parenteral anticoagulant

Treatment of deep-vein thrombosis in patients with moderate renal impairment | Treatment of deep-vein thrombosis in patients at increased risk of bleeding | Treatment of pulmonary embolism in patients with moderate renal impairment | Treatment of pulmonary embolism in patients at increased risk of bleeding | Prophylaxis of recurrent deep-vein thrombosis in patients with moderate renal impairment | Prophylaxis of recurrent deep-vein thrombosis in patients at increased risk of bleeding | Prophylaxis of recurrent pulmonary embolism in patients with moderate renal impairment | Prophylaxis of recurrent pulmonary embolism in patients at increased risk of bleeding
▸ BY MOUTH
▸ Adult: 110–150 mg twice daily, to be given following at least 5 days treatment with a parenteral anticoagulant

Treatment of deep-vein thrombosis in patients receiving concomitant treatment with verapamil | Treatment of pulmonary embolism in patients receiving concomitant treatment with verapamil | Prophylaxis of recurrent deep-vein thrombosis in patients receiving concomitant treatment with verapamil | Prophylaxis of recurrent pulmonary embolism in patients receiving concomitant treatment with verapamil
▸ BY MOUTH
▸ Adult: 110 mg twice daily, to be given following at least 5 days treatment with a parenteral anticoagulant

Prophylaxis of stroke and systemic embolism in non-valvular atrial fibrillation and with one or more risk factors such as previous stroke or transient ischaemic attack, symptomatic heart failure, age $\geq$ 75 years, diabetes mellitus, or hypertension
▸ BY MOUTH
▸ Adult 18-74 years: 150 mg twice daily
▸ Adult 75-79 years: 110–150 mg twice daily
▸ Adult 80 years and over: 110 mg twice daily

Prophylaxis of stroke and systemic embolism in non-valvular atrial fibrillation and with one or more risk factors such as previous stroke or transient ischaemic attack, symptomatic heart failure, age $\geq$ 75 years, diabetes mellitus, or hypertension in patients receiving concomitant treatment with verapamil
▸ BY MOUTH
▸ Adult: 110 mg twice daily

Prophylaxis of stroke and systemic embolism in non-valvular atrial fibrillation and with one or more risk factors such as previous stroke or transient ischaemic attack, symptomatic heart failure, age $\geq$ 75 years, diabetes mellitus, or hypertension, in patients at increased risk of bleeding | Prophylaxis of stroke and systemic embolism in non-valvular atrial fibrillation and with one or more risk factors such as previous stroke or transient ischaemic attack, symptomatic heart failure, age $\geq$ 75 years, diabetes mellitus, or hypertension, in patients with moderate renal impairment
▸ BY MOUTH
▸ Adult: 110–150 mg twice daily

DOSE EQUIVALENCE AND CONVERSION
▸ For information on changing between formulations, or changing from, or to, other anticoagulants—consult product literature.

IMPORTANT SAFETY INFORMATION

MHRA/CHM ADVICE: NEW ORAL ANTICOAGULANTS APIXABAN (*ELIQUIS*®), DABIGATRAN (*PRADAXA*®) AND RIVAROXABAN (*XARELTO*®) (OCTOBER 2013)

The following contra-indications now apply to all new oral anticoagulants, for all indications and doses:
● a lesion or condition, if considered a significant risk factor for major bleeding—see *Contra-indications* for further information;
● concomitant treatment with any other anticoagulant agent—see *Contra-indications* for further information.
Healthcare professionals are advised to take caution when deciding to prescribe these anticoagulants to patients with other conditions, undergoing other procedures, and on other treatments, which may increase the risk of major bleeding. The renal function of patients should also be considered.

MHRA/CHM ADVICE: DIRECT-ACTING ORAL ANTICOAGULANTS (DOACS): INCREASED RISK OF RECURRENT THROMBOTIC EVENTS IN PATIENTS WITH ANTIPHOSPHOLIPID SYNDROME (JUNE 2019)

A clinical trial has shown an increased risk of recurrent thrombotic events associated with rivaroxaban compared with warfarin, in patients with antiphospholipid syndrome and a history of thrombosis. There may be a similar risk associated with other DOACs. Healthcare professionals are advised that DOACs are not recommended in patients with antiphospholipid syndrome, particularly high-risk patients who test positive for all three antiphospholipid tests—lupus anticoagulant, anticardiolipin antibodies, and anti-beta$_2$ glycoprotein I antibodies. Continued treatment should be reviewed in these patients to determine if appropriate, and switching to a vitamin K antagonist such as warfarin should be considered.

MHRA/CHM ADVICE: DIRECT-ACTING ORAL ANTICOAGULANTS (DOACS): REMINDER OF BLEEDING RISK, INCLUDING AVAILABILITY OF REVERSAL AGENTS (JUNE 2020)

The MHRA reminds healthcare professionals to remain vigilant for signs and symptoms of bleeding complications during treatment with dabigatran after ongoing reports of serious, potentially fatal bleeds associated with the use of DOACs. Healthcare professionals are also advised to use dabigatran with caution in patients with increased bleeding risk, and to ensure that those with renal impairment are dosed appropriately and their renal function monitored during treatment. Patients should be counselled on the signs and symptoms of bleeding, and encouraged to read the patient information leaflet. The dabigatran reversal agent idarucizumab (*Praxbind*®) is available if required.

MHRA/CHM ADVICE: WARFARIN AND OTHER ANTICOAGULANTS: MONITORING OF PATIENTS DURING THE COVID-19 PANDEMIC (OCTOBER 2020)

Healthcare professionals are reminded that:
- direct-acting oral anticoagulants (DOACs), such as dabigatran, may interact with other medicines (including antibacterials and antivirals)—advice in product literature should be followed to minimise the risk of potential interactions;
- if patients are switched from warfarin to dabigatran, warfarin treatment should be stopped before dabigatran treatment is started to reduce the risk of over-anticoagulation and bleeding.

MHRA/CHM ADVICE: DIRECT-ACTING ORAL ANTICOAGULANTS (DOACS): REMINDER OF DOSE ADJUSTMENTS IN PATIENTS WITH RENAL IMPAIRMENT (MAY 2023)

Healthcare professionals are reminded that:
- exposure to DOACs, such as dabigatran, is increased in patients with renal impairment, and these patients should receive an appropriately adjusted dose—see *Renal impairment* for further information;
- such patients should be reviewed regularly during treatment to ensure the dose remains appropriate;
- renal function should be assessed by calculating creatinine clearance using the Cockcroft and Gault formula.

- **CONTRA-INDICATIONS** Active bleeding · antiphospholipid syndrome (increased risk of recurrent thrombotic events) · arteriovenous malformation · do not use as anticoagulant for prosthetic heart valve · major intraspinal or intracerebral vascular abnormalities · malignant neoplasms at high risk of bleeding · oesophageal varices · recent brain or spinal injury · recent brain surgery · recent gastro-intestinal ulcer · recent intracranial haemorrhage · recent ophthalmic surgery · recent spine surgery · significant risk of major bleeding · use with any other anticoagulant · vascular aneurysm

CONTRA-INDICATIONS, FURTHER INFORMATION
- Use with any other anticoagulant [EvGr] Concomitant use with any other anticoagulant is contra-indicated, except when switching therapy, or when unfractionated heparin is given at doses necessary to maintain an open central venous or arterial catheter or for catheter ablation—use with caution. ⟨M⟩

- **CAUTIONS** Anaesthesia with postoperative indwelling epidural catheter (risk of paralysis—give initial dose at least 2 hours after catheter removal and monitor neurological signs) · bacterial endocarditis · bleeding disorders · body-weight less than 50 kg · elderly · gastritis · gastro-oesophageal reflux · oesophagitis · recent biopsy · recent major trauma · risk of bleeding · thrombocytopenia

CAUTIONS, FURTHER INFORMATION
- Elderly For direct thrombin inhibitors, Screening Tool of Older Persons' potentially inappropriate Prescriptions (STOPP) criteria to aid medication reviews (see Prescribing

in the elderly p. 31 for information). Potentially inappropriate:
- with concurrent significant bleeding risk, such as uncontrolled severe hypertension, bleeding diathesis or recent non-trivial spontaneous bleeding (high risk of bleeding)
- for first deep venous thrombosis without continuing provoking risk factors (e.g. thrombophilia) for greater than 6 months (no proven added benefit)
- for first pulmonary embolus without continuing provoking risk factors for greater than 12 months (no proven added benefit)
- as part of dual therapy with an antiplatelet agent in patients with stable coronary, cerebrovascular or peripheral arterial disease, without a clear indication for anticoagulant therapy (no added benefit)
- if eGFR less than 30 mL/min/1.73 m^2 (contra-indicated in severe renal impairment; risk of bleeding)

- **INTERACTIONS** → Appendix 1: thrombin inhibitors

- **SIDE-EFFECTS**
- **Common or very common** Anaemia · diarrhoea · gastrointestinal discomfort · haemorrhage · hepatic function abnormal · nausea
- **Uncommon** Dysphagia · gastrointestinal disorders · hyperbilirubinaemia · intracranial haemorrhage · post procedural complications · skin reactions · thrombocytopenia · vomiting · wound complications
- **Rare or very rare** Angioedema · post procedural drainage · wound drainage
- **Frequency not known** Agranulocytosis · alopecia · bronchospasm · neutropenia

- **PREGNANCY** Manufacturer advises avoid unless essential—toxicity in *animal* studies.

- **BREAST FEEDING** Manufacturer advises avoid—no information available.

- **HEPATIC IMPAIRMENT** Manufacturer advises avoid in severe impairment; consider avoiding in those with liver enzymes greater than 2 times the upper limit of normal (no information available).

- **RENAL IMPAIRMENT** See p. 21. [EvGr] Avoid if creatinine clearance less than 30 mL/minute. ⟨M⟩
Dose adjustments [EvGr] When used for *prophylaxis of venous thromboembolism following knee or hip replacement surgery*, reduce initial dose to 75 mg and subsequent doses to 150 mg once daily if creatinine clearance 30–50 mL/minute; consider reducing dose to 75 mg once daily if creatinine clearance 30–50 mL/minute and patient receiving concomitant treatment with verapamil.

When used for *treatment of deep-vein thrombosis and pulmonary embolism, prophylaxis of recurrent deep-vein thrombosis and pulmonary embolism, prophylaxis of stroke and systemic embolism in non-valvular atrial fibrillation,* consider reduced dose of 110–150 mg twice daily if creatinine clearance 30–50 mL/minute, based on individual assessment of thromboembolic risk and risk of bleeding. ⟨M⟩

- **MONITORING REQUIREMENTS**
- Patients should be monitored for signs of bleeding or anaemia; treatment should be stopped if severe bleeding occurs.
- No routine anticoagulant monitoring required (INR tests are unreliable).
- Assess renal function (manufacturer recommends Cockroft and Gault formula to calculate creatinine clearance) before treatment in all patients and at least annually thereafter.

- **DIRECTIONS FOR ADMINISTRATION** [EvGr] When dose reduction recommended due to concurrent amiodarone or verapamil, doses should be taken at the same time ⟨M⟩(see *Indications and dose*).

Cardiovascular system

2

● **PRESCRIBING AND DISPENSING INFORMATION**

▶ When used for Treatment of deep-vein thrombosis and pulmonary embolism or Prophylaxis of recurrent deep-vein thrombosis and pulmonary embolism Duration of treatment should be determined by balancing the benefit of treatment with the bleeding risk. Shorter duration of treatment (at least 3 months) should be based on transient risk factors i.e. recent surgery, trauma, or immobilisation, and longer duration of treatment should be based on permanent risk factors, or idiopathic deep-vein thrombosis or pulmonary embolism.

The manufacturer of *Pradaxa*® has provided *Prescriber Guides*.

● **PATIENT AND CARER ADVICE** Patients and their carers should be advised to contact their doctor if gastro-intestinal symptoms such as dyspepsia develop during treatment.

Alert card Patients and their carers should be provided with a patient alert card and advised to keep it with them at all times.

Missed doses If a dose is more than 6 hours late, the missed dose should not be taken and the next dose should be taken at the normal time.

● **NATIONAL FUNDING/ACCESS DECISIONS**
For full details see funding body website

NICE decisions

▶ Dabigatran etexilate for the prevention of venous thromboembolism after hip or knee replacement surgery in adults (September 2008) NICE TA157 Recommended

▶ Dabigatran etexilate for the prevention of stroke and systemic embolism in atrial fibrillation (updated July 2021) NICE TA249 Recommended

▶ Dabigatran etexilate for the treatment and secondary prevention of deep vein thrombosis and/or pulmonary embolism (December 2014) NICE TA327 Recommended

● **MEDICINAL FORMS** There can be variation in the licensing of different medicines containing the same drug.

Oral capsule
CAUTIONARY AND ADVISORY LABELS 10, 25

▶ Dabigatran etexilate (Non-proprietary)
Dabigatran etexilate (as Dabigatran etexilate mesilate)
75 mg Dabigatran etexilate 75mg capsules | 10 capsule PoM £8.49 DT = £8.50 | 60 capsule PoM £51.00–£81.60 DT = £51.00
Dabigatran etexilate (as Dabigatran etexilate mesilate)
110 mg Dabigatran etexilate 110mg capsules | 10 capsule PoM £8.08–£18.97 DT = £5.05 | 60 capsule PoM £30.28–£51.00 DT = £30.28
Dabigatran etexilate 110mg capsule | 10 capsule PoM £7.65 DT = £5.05 | 60 capsule PoM £45.90 DT = £30.28
Dabigatran etexilate (as Dabigatran etexilate mesilate)
150 mg Dabigatran etexilate 150mg capsule | 60 capsule PoM £45.90 DT = £30.15
Dabigatran etexilate 150mg capsules | 60 capsule PoM £30.15–£51.00 DT = £30.15

▶ Pradaxa (Boehringer Ingelheim Ltd)
Dabigatran etexilate (as Dabigatran etexilate mesilate)
75 mg Pradaxa 75mg capsules | 10 capsule PoM £8.50 DT = £8.50 | 60 capsule PoM £51.00 DT = £51.00
Dabigatran etexilate (as Dabigatran etexilate mesilate)
110 mg Pradaxa 110mg capsules | 10 capsule PoM £8.50 DT = £5.05 | 60 capsule PoM £51.00 DT = £30.28
Dabigatran etexilate (as Dabigatran etexilate mesilate)
150 mg Pradaxa 150mg capsules | 60 capsule PoM £51.00 DT = £30.15

ANTITHROMBOTIC DRUGS ＞TISSUE PLASMINOGEN ACTIVATORS

☞ 249

Urokinase

04-Jan-2022

● **INDICATIONS AND DOSE**

Deep-vein thrombosis (thromboembolic occlusive vascular disease)
▶ INITIALLY BY INTRAVENOUS INFUSION
▶ Adult: Initially 4400 units/kg for 1 dose, to be given over 10–20 minutes, then (by continuous intravenous infusion) 100 000 units/hour for 2–3 days

Pulmonary embolism (thromboembolic occlusive vascular disease)
▶ INITIALLY BY INTRAVENOUS INFUSION
▶ Adult: Initially 4400 units/kg for 1 dose, to be given over 10–20 minutes, then (by continuous intravenous infusion) 4400 units/kg/hour for 12 hours

Occlusive peripheral arterial disease (thromboembolic occlusive vascular disease)
▶ BY INTRA-ARTERIAL INFUSION
▶ Adult: (consult product literature)

Occluded central venous catheters (blocked by fibrin clots)
▶ TO THE DEVICE AS A FLUSH
▶ Adult: Instil directly into occluded catheter **only**, to be dissolved in Sodium Chloride 0.9% to a concentration of 5000 units/mL; use a volume sufficient to fill the catheter lumen; leave for 20–60 minutes then aspirate the lysate; repeat if necessary

Occluded arteriovenous haemodialysis shunts (blocked by fibrin clots)
▶ TO THE DEVICE AS A FLUSH
▶ Adult: (consult product literature)

SYNER-KINASE ®

Deep-vein thrombosis (thromboembolic occlusive vascular disease)
▶ INITIALLY BY INTRAVENOUS INFUSION
▶ Adult: Initially 4400 units/kg for 1 dose, to be given over 10 minutes, dose to be made up in 15 mL Sodium Chloride 0.9%, then (by continuous intravenous infusion) 4400 units/kg/hour for 12–24 hours

Pulmonary embolism (thromboembolic occlusive vascular disease)
▶ INITIALLY BY INTRAVENOUS INFUSION
▶ Adult: Initially 4400 units/kg for 1 dose, to be given over 10 minutes, dose to be made up in 15 mL Sodium Chloride 0.9%, then (by continuous intravenous infusion) 4400 units/kg/hour for 12 hours, alternatively (by intra-arterial injection) initially 15 000 units/kg, to be injected into pulmonary artery, subsequent doses adjusted according to response; maximum 3 doses per day

Occlusive peripheral arterial disease
▶ BY INTRA-ARTERIAL INFUSION
▶ Adult: (consult product literature)

Occluded intravascular catheters and cannulas (blocked by fibrin clots)
▶ TO THE DEVICE AS A FLUSH
▶ Adult: 5000–25 000 units, instil directly into catheter or cannula lumen **only**, dose dissolved in suitable volume of Sodium Chloride 0.9% to fill the catheter or cannula lumen; leave for 20–60 minutes then aspirate the lysate; repeat if necessary, alternatively up to 250 000 units, instil directly into the catheter or cannula lumen **only**, dose dissolved in Sodium Chloride 0.9% to a concentration of 1000–2500 units/mL and infused over 90–180 minutes into the catheter or cannula

- **CAUTIONS** Cavernous pulmonary disease
- **INTERACTIONS** → Appendix 1: urokinase
- **SIDE-EFFECTS**
- ▸ **Common or very common** Artery dissection · embolism and thrombosis · stroke
- ▸ **Uncommon** Renal failure
- ▸ **Rare or very rare** Vascular pseudoaneurysm
- **BREAST FEEDING** Manufacturer advises avoid—no information available.
- **HEPATIC IMPAIRMENT** Manufacturer advises caution in mild to moderate impairment.
  Dose adjustments Manufacturer advises consider dose reduction in mild to moderate impairment.
- **RENAL IMPAIRMENT** [EvGr] Caution in mild to moderate impairment (fibrinogen level should not fall below 100 mg/dL); avoid in severe impairment. ⓜ
  Dose adjustments [EvGr] Consider dose reduction in mild to moderate impairment. ⓜ
- **DIRECTIONS FOR ADMINISTRATION** For *intravenous infusion* (*Syner-KINASE®*), give continuously or intermittently in Sodium Chloride 0.9%.

- **MEDICINAL FORMS** There can be variation in the licensing of different medicines containing the same drug.
  Powder for solution for injection
  - ▸ Syner-KINASE (Syner-Med (Pharmaceutical Products) Ltd)
    Urokinase 100000 unit Syner-KINASE 100,000unit powder for solution for injection vials | 1 vial [PoM] £112.95 (Hospital only)
    Urokinase 250000 unit Syner-KINASE 250,000unit powder for solution for injection vials | 1 vial [PoM] £140.00 (Hospital only)
    Urokinase 500000 unit Syner-KINASE 500,000unit powder for solution for injection vials | 1 vial [PoM] £270.00 (Hospital only)

ANTITHROMBOTIC DRUGS > VITAMIN K ANTAGONISTS

Vitamin K antagonists

IMPORTANT SAFETY INFORMATION

MHRA/CHM ADVICE: DIRECT-ACTING ANTIVIRALS TO TREAT CHRONIC HEPATITIS C: RISK OF INTERACTION WITH VITAMIN K ANTAGONISTS AND CHANGES IN INR (JANUARY 2017)

A EU-wide review has identified that changes in liver function, secondary to hepatitis C treatment with direct-acting antivirals, may affect the efficacy of vitamin K antagonists; the MHRA has advised that INR should be monitored closely in patients receiving concomitant treatment.

MHRA/CHM ADVICE: WARFARIN AND OTHER ANTICOAGULANTS: MONITORING OF PATIENTS DURING THE COVID-19 PANDEMIC (OCTOBER 2020)

Healthcare professionals are reminded that:
- acute illness (including COVID-19 infection) may exaggerate the effect of warfarin and necessitate a dose reduction;
- continued INR monitoring is important in patients taking warfarin or other vitamin K antagonists if they have suspected or confirmed COVID-19 infection, so they can be clinically managed at an early stage to reduce the risk of bleeding;
- vitamin K antagonists may interact with other medicines (including antibacterials and antivirals)—advice in product literature, such as INR monitoring in patients taking vitamin K antagonists who have recently started new medicines, should be followed to minimise the risk of potential interactions;
- if patients are switched from warfarin to a direct-acting oral anticoagulant (DOAC), warfarin treatment should be stopped before DOAC treatment is started to reduce the risk of over-anticoagulation and bleeding.

Patients on vitamin K antagonists should be reminded to carefully follow instructions for use (including the patient information leaflet) and advised to notify their GP or healthcare team if they:
- have symptoms of, or confirmed, COVID-19 infection;
- are otherwise unwell with sickness or diarrhoea, or have lost their appetite;
- have changed their diet, smoking habits, or alcohol consumption;
- are taking any new medicines or supplements;
- are unable to attend their next scheduled blood test for any reason.

- **CONTRA-INDICATIONS** Avoid use within 48 hours postpartum · haemorrhagic stroke · significant bleeding
- **CAUTIONS** Bacterial endocarditis (use only if warfarin otherwise indicated) · conditions in which risk of bleeding is increased · history of gastro-intestinal bleeding · hyperthyroidism · hypothyroidism · peptic ulcer · recent ischaemic stroke · recent surgery · uncontrolled hypertension

CAUTIONS, FURTHER INFORMATION
- ▸ Elderly Screening Tool of Older Persons' potentially inappropriate Prescriptions (STOPP) criteria to aid medication reviews (see Prescribing in the elderly p. 31 for information). Potentially inappropriate:
  - with concurrent significant bleeding risk, such as uncontrolled severe hypertension, bleeding diathesis, or recent non-trivial spontaneous bleeding (high risk of bleeding)
  - as part of dual therapy with an antiplatelet agent in patients with stable coronary, cerebrovascular, or peripheral arterial disease, without a clear indication for anticoagulant therapy (no added benefit)
  - for first deep venous thrombosis without continuing provoking risk factors (e.g. thrombophilia) for longer than 6 months (no proven added benefit)
  - for first pulmonary embolus without continuing provoking risk factors for longer than 12 months (no proven added benefit)

- **SIDE-EFFECTS**
- ▸ **Common or very common** Haemorrhage
- ▸ **Rare or very rare** Alopecia · nausea · vomiting
- ▸ **Frequency not known** Blue toe syndrome · CNS haemorrhage · diarrhoea · fever · haemothorax · jaundice · pancreatitis · skin necrosis (increased risk in patients with protein C or protein S deficiency) · skin reactions

- **CONCEPTION AND CONTRACEPTION** Women of child-bearing age should be warned of the danger of teratogenicity.
- **PREGNANCY** Should not be given in the first trimester of pregnancy. Warfarin, acenocoumarol, and phenindione cross the placenta with risk of congenital malformations, and placental, fetal, or neonatal haemorrhage, especially during the last few weeks of pregnancy and at delivery. Therefore, if at all possible, they should be avoided in pregnancy, especially in the first and third trimesters (difficult decisions may have to be made, particularly in women with prosthetic heart valves, atrial fibrillation, or with a history of recurrent venous thrombosis or pulmonary embolism). Stopping these drugs before the sixth week of gestation may largely avoid the risk of fetal abnormality.
- **HEPATIC IMPAIRMENT** In general, manufacturers advise caution in mild to moderate impairment; avoid in severe impairment.
- **MONITORING REQUIREMENTS**
- ▸ The base-line prothrombin time should be determined but the initial dose should not be delayed whilst awaiting the result.

- It is essential that the INR be determined daily or on alternate days in early days of treatment, *then* at longer intervals (depending on response), *then* up to every 12 weeks.
- Change in patient's clinical condition, particularly associated with liver disease, intercurrent illness, or drug administration, necessitates more frequent testing.
- **PATIENT AND CARER ADVICE** Anticoagulant treatment booklets should be issued to all patients or their carers; these booklets include advice for patients on anticoagulant treatment, an alert card to be carried by the patient at all times, and a section for recording of INR results and dosage information. In **England**, **Wales**, and **Northern Ireland**, they are available for purchase from:

3M Security Print and Systems Limited
Gorse Street, Chadderton
Oldham
OL9 9QH
Tel: 0845 610 1112

GP practices can obtain supplies through their Local Area Team stores. NHS Trusts can order supplies from cmswebshop.corp.xerox.com/NHS/Login.aspx.

In **Scotland**, treatment booklets and starter information packs can be obtained by emailing stockorders.DPPAS@apsgroup.co.uk or by fax on (0131) 6299 967

Electronic copies of the warfarin anticoagulant alert card and record booklet are also available as risk minimisation materials at www.medicines.org.uk/emc/rmm-directory/.

◄ 163

Acenocoumarol

07-Aug-2024

(Nicoumalone)

- **INDICATIONS AND DOSE**

Prophylaxis of embolisation in rheumatic heart disease and atrial fibrillation | Prophylaxis after insertion of prosthetic heart valve | Prophylaxis and treatment of venous thrombosis and pulmonary embolism | Transient ischaemic attacks
- BY MOUTH
- Adult: Initially 2–4 mg once daily for 2 days, alternatively initially 6 mg on day 1, then 4 mg on day 2; maintenance 1–8 mg daily, adjusted according to response, dose to be taken at the same time each day, lower doses may be required in patients over 65 years, severe heart failure with hepatic congestion, and malnutrition

IMPORTANT SAFETY INFORMATION

MHRA/CHM ADVICE: WARFARIN: BE ALERT TO THE RISK OF DRUG INTERACTIONS WITH TRAMADOL (JUNE 2024)

The MHRA has received a Coroner's report regarding the death of a patient from a bleed on the brain after taking warfarin with tramadol. Healthcare professionals are reminded that caution is advised when tramadol is prescribed alongside coumarin-derived anticoagulants, such as acenocoumarol. There is a risk of increased INR when these drugs are taken together which can lead to potentially life-threatening bruising and bleeding. Dose adjustments for acenocoumarol and/or additional INR monitoring should be considered when starting concomitant tramadol or other medicines.

Patients and carers should be advised of the increased risk of bleeding due to drug interactions with acenocoumarol, to inform their healthcare professional that they are on acenocoumarol treatment before taking any new medicines, and to discuss with their healthcare professional before stopping treatment. They should also be counselled to seek medical treatment and have

an urgent INR test if any signs or symptoms of a major bleeding event occur.

- **CAUTIONS** Patients over 65 years
- **INTERACTIONS** → Appendix 1: coumarins
- **SIDE-EFFECTS**
- **Rare or very rare** Appetite decreased · liver injury · skin necrosis haemorrhagic (increased risk in patients with protein C or protein S deficiency) · vasculitis
- **BREAST FEEDING** Risk of haemorrhage; increased by vitamin K deficiency—manufacturer recommends prophylactic vitamin K for the infant (consult product literature).
- **HEPATIC IMPAIRMENT**
Dose adjustments Manufacturer advises consider dose reduction in mild to moderate impairment.
- **RENAL IMPAIRMENT** [EvGr] Caution in mild to moderate impairment; avoid in severe impairment. [M]
- **PATIENT AND CARER ADVICE** Anticoagulant card to be provided.

- **MEDICINAL FORMS** There can be variation in the licensing of different medicines containing the same drug.
Oral tablet
CAUTIONARY AND ADVISORY LABELS 10
- Sinthrome (Norgine Pharmaceuticals Ltd)
Acenocoumarol 1 mg Sinthrome 1mg tablets | 100 tablet [PoM] £4.62 DT = £4.62

◄ 163

Phenindione

17-May-2021

- **INDICATIONS AND DOSE**

Prophylaxis of embolisation in rheumatic heart disease and atrial fibrillation | Prophylaxis after insertion of prosthetic heart valve | Prophylaxis and treatment of venous thrombosis and pulmonary embolism
- BY MOUTH
- Adult: Initially 200 mg on day 1, then 100 mg on day 2, then, adjusted according to response; maintenance 50–150 mg daily

- **INTERACTIONS** → Appendix 1: phenindione
- **SIDE-EFFECTS** Agranulocytosis · albuminuria · eosinophilia · hepatitis · increased leucocytes · kidney injury · leucopenia · lymphadenopathy · pancytopenia · renal tubular necrosis · taste altered · urine discolouration
- **BREAST FEEDING** Avoid. Risk of haemorrhage; increased by vitamin K deficiency.
- **RENAL IMPAIRMENT** [EvGr] Caution in mild to moderate impairment; avoid in severe impairment. [M]
Dose adjustments [EvGr] Dose reduction may be required in mild to moderate impairment. [M]
- **PATIENT AND CARER ADVICE** Patient counselling is advised for phenindione tablets (may turn urine pink or orange). Anticoagulant card to be provided.

- **MEDICINAL FORMS** There can be variation in the licensing of different medicines containing the same drug.
Oral tablet
CAUTIONARY AND ADVISORY LABELS 10, 14
- Phenindione (Non-proprietary)
Phenindione 10 mg Phenindione 10mg tablets | 28 tablet [PoM] £657.00 DT = £657.00
Phenindione 25 mg Phenindione 25mg tablets | 28 tablet [PoM] £657.00 DT = £657.00

Warfarin sodium
07-Aug-2024
F 163

- **INDICATIONS AND DOSE**

Prophylaxis of embolisation in rheumatic heart disease and atrial fibrillation | Prophylaxis after insertion of prosthetic heart valve | Prophylaxis and treatment of venous thrombosis and pulmonary embolism | Transient ischaemic attacks
▶ BY MOUTH
▶ Adult: Initially 5–10 mg, to be taken on day 1; subsequent doses dependent on the prothrombin time, reported as INR (international normalised ratio), a lower induction dose can be given over 3–4 weeks in patients who do not require rapid anticoagulation, elderly patients to be given a lower induction dose; maintenance 3–9 mg daily, to be taken at the same time each day

IMPORTANT SAFETY INFORMATION

MHRA/CHM ADVICE: WARFARIN: REPORTS OF CALCIPHYLAXIS (JULY 2016)

An EU-wide review has concluded that on rare occasions, warfarin use may lead to calciphylaxis—patients should be advised to consult their doctor if they develop a painful skin rash; if calciphylaxis is diagnosed, appropriate treatment should be started and consideration should be given to stopping treatment with warfarin. The MHRA has advised that calciphylaxis is most commonly observed in patients with known risk factors such as end-stage renal disease, however cases have also been reported in patients with normal renal function.

MHRA/CHM ADVICE: WARFARIN: BE ALERT TO THE RISK OF DRUG INTERACTIONS WITH TRAMADOL (JUNE 2024)

The MHRA has received a Coroner's report regarding the death of a patient from a bleed on the brain after taking warfarin with tramadol. Healthcare professionals are reminded that:
- there is a risk of increased INR when warfarin and tramadol are taken together which can lead to potentially life-threatening bruising and bleeding;
- caution should be exercised when warfarin is prescribed alongside other drugs due to the risk of drug interactions;
- dose adjustments for warfarin and/or additional INR monitoring should be considered when starting concomitant tramadol or other medicines.

Patients and carers should be advised of the increased risk of bleeding due to drug interactions with warfarin, to inform their healthcare professional that they are on warfarin treatment before taking any new medicines, and to discuss with their healthcare professional before stopping treatment. They should also be counselled to seek medical treatment and have an urgent INR test if any signs or symptoms of a major bleeding event occur.

- **CAUTIONS** Postpartum (delay warfarin until risk of haemorrhage is low—usually 5–7 days after delivery)
- **INTERACTIONS** → Appendix 1: coumarins
- **SIDE-EFFECTS** Calciphylaxis · hepatic function abnormal
- **PREGNANCY** Babies of mothers taking warfarin at the time of delivery need to be offered immediate prophylaxis with intramuscular phytomenadione (vitamin K_1).
- **BREAST FEEDING** Not present in milk in significant amounts and appears safe. Risk of haemorrhage which is increased by vitamin K deficiency.
- **RENAL IMPAIRMENT** Use with caution in mild to moderate impairment.

Monitoring In severe renal impairment, monitor INR more frequently.

- **PATIENT AND CARER ADVICE** Anticoagulant card to be provided.

- **MEDICINAL FORMS** There can be variation in the licensing of different medicines containing the same drug. Forms available from special-order manufacturers include: oral suspension, oral solution

Oral tablet
CAUTIONARY AND ADVISORY LABELS 10
▶ Warfarin sodium (Non-proprietary)
    Warfarin sodium 500 microgram Warfarin 500microgram tablets | 28 tablet [PoM] £1.90 DT = £1.89
    Warfarin sodium 1 mg Warfarin 1mg tablets | 28 tablet [PoM] £1.48 DT = £0.92
    Warfarin sodium 3 mg Warfarin 3mg tablets | 28 tablet [PoM] £1.81 DT = £0.94
    Warfarin sodium 4 mg Coumadin 4mg tablets | 100 tablet [PoM] [X]
    Warfarin sodium 5 mg Warfarin 5mg tablets | 28 tablet [PoM] £3.39 DT = £1.29

Oral suspension
CAUTIONARY AND ADVISORY LABELS 10
▶ Warfarin sodium (Non-proprietary)
    Warfarin sodium 1 mg per 1 ml Warfarin 1mg/ml oral suspension sugar free | 150 ml [PoM] £196.35 DT = £196.35 [SF]

3.2a Reversal of anticoagulation

ANTIDOTES AND CHELATORS

Andexanet alfa
14-Feb-2025

- **DRUG ACTION** Andexanet alfa is a recombinant form of human factor X_a protein which binds specifically to apixaban or rivaroxaban, thereby reversing their anticoagulant effects.

- **INDICATIONS AND DOSE**

Reversal of apixaban or rivaroxaban in life-threatening or uncontrolled bleeding (specialist supervision in hospital)
▶ BY INTRAVENOUS INFUSION
▶ Adult: (consult product literature)

IMPORTANT SAFETY INFORMATION

MRHA/CHM ADVICE: *ONDEXXYA*® (ANDEXANET ALFA): COMMERCIAL ANTI-FXA ACTIVITY ASSAYS ARE UNSUITABLE FOR MEASURING ANTI-FXA ACTIVITY FOLLOWING ADMINISTRATION OF ANDEXANET ALFA (JULY 2020)

Treatment monitoring after administration of andexanet alfa should not be based on anti-FXa activity assays. In these assays, the FXa inhibitor dissociates from andexanet alfa, resulting in the detection of falsely elevated anti-FXa activity levels, and consequently a substantial underestimation of the reversal activity of andexanet alfa. Healthcare professionals are advised to monitor treatment using clinical parameters indicative of appropriate response (i.e. achievement of haemostasis), lack of efficacy (i.e. re-bleeding), and adverse events (i.e. thromboembolic events).

MHRA/CHM ADVICE: *ONDEXXYA*® (ANDEXANET ALFA): AVOID USE OF ANDEXANET PRIOR TO HEPARINISATION (NOVEMBER 2020)

Off-label use of andexanet alfa to reverse FXa anticoagulation prior to surgery with intended heparin anticoagulation has been reported to cause unresponsiveness to heparin and healthcare professionals are advised to avoid such use. In-vitro data suggest binding of andexanet alfa to the heparin-antithrombin III (ATIII) complex and neutralisation of the anticoagulant effect of heparin. Results of coagulation tests might be misleading when andexanet alfa and heparin are given within a short time of one another. The effect of andexanet alfa has not been validated while heparin is active, and its use for anti-FXa reversal before urgent surgery has not been evaluated.

- **CAUTIONS** Risk of thrombosis

  CAUTIONS, FURTHER INFORMATION Manufacturer advises to consider re-starting anticoagulant therapy as soon as medically appropriate to reduce the risk of thrombosis.
- **INTERACTIONS** → Appendix 1: andexanet alfa
- **SIDE-EFFECTS**
► **Common or very common** Back pain · cerebrovascular insufficiency · chest discomfort · cough · dizziness postural · dry mouth · dyspnoea · feeling hot · fever · flushing · gastrointestinal discomfort · headache · hyperhidrosis · muscle spasms · nausea · palpitations · peripheral coldness · skin reactions · taste altered
► **Uncommon** Cardiac arrest · embolism and thrombosis · iliac artery occlusion · myocardial infarction

- **PREGNANCY** Manufacturer advises avoid—no information available.
- **BREAST FEEDING** Manufacturer advises discontinue breast-feeding—no information available.
- **HANDLING AND STORAGE** Manufacturer advises store in a refrigerator (2–8°C)—consult product literature about storage after reconstitution.
- **NATIONAL FUNDING/ACCESS DECISIONS**
  For full details see funding body website
  NICE decisions
► Andexanet alfa for reversing anticoagulation from apixaban or rivaroxaban (updated January 2025) NICE TA697 Recommended with restrictions
  Scottish Medicines Consortium (SMC) decisions
► Andexanet alfa (*Ondexxya*®) for adult patients treated with a direct factor Xa (FXa) inhibitor (apixaban or rivaroxaban) when reversal of anticoagulation is needed due to life-threatening or uncontrolled bleeding (September 2020) SMC No. SMC2273 Recommended

- **MEDICINAL FORMS** There can be variation in the licensing of different medicines containing the same drug.
  Powder for solution for infusion
  EXCIPIENTS: May contain Polysorbates, sucrose
► Ondexxya (AstraZeneca UK Ltd) ▼
  Andexanet alfa 200 mg Ondexxya 200mg powder for solution for infusion vials | 4 vial [PoM] £11,100.00 (Hospital only) | 5 vial [PoM] £13,875.00 (Hospital only)

Idarucizumab

14-Feb-2025

- **DRUG ACTION** Idarucizumab is a humanised monoclonal antibody fragment that binds specifically to dabigatran and its metabolites, thereby reversing the anticoagulant effect.

- **INDICATIONS AND DOSE**

Rapid reversal of dabigatran for emergency procedures, or in life-threatening or uncontrolled bleeding (specialist supervision in hospital)
► BY INTRAVENOUS INJECTION, OR BY INTRAVENOUS INFUSION
► Adult: 5 g, followed by 5 g if required

- **CAUTIONS** Risk of thrombosis

  CAUTIONS, FURTHER INFORMATION Manufacturer advises to consider re-starting anticoagulant therapy as soon as medically appropriate to reduce the risk of thrombosis. Dabigatran can be re-started 24 hours after administration of idarucizumab; other anticoagulant therapy can be started at any time.
- **PREGNANCY** Manufacturer advises use only if potential benefit outweighs risk—no information available.

- **DIRECTIONS FOR ADMINISTRATION** Manufacturer advises that one dose of *Praxbind*® is administered as either two consecutive intravenous infusions, each given over 5–10 minutes, *or* as a bolus injection.
- **HANDLING AND STORAGE** Manufacturer advises store in a refrigerator at 2–8°C.
- **NATIONAL FUNDING/ACCESS DECISIONS**
  For full details see funding body website
  Scottish Medicines Consortium (SMC) decisions
► Idarucizumab (*Praxbind*®) is a specific reversal agent for dabigatran and is indicated in adult patients treated with dabigatran etexilate when rapid reversal of its anticoagulant effects is required for emergency surgery/urgent procedures or in life-threatening or uncontrolled bleeding (September 2016) SMC No. 1178/16 Recommended

- **MEDICINAL FORMS** There can be variation in the licensing of different medicines containing the same drug.
  Solution for infusion
  EXCIPIENTS: May contain Polysorbates, sorbitol
  ELECTROLYTES: May contain Sodium
► **Praxbind** (Boehringer Ingelheim Ltd)
  Idarucizumab 50 mg per 1 ml Praxbind 2.5g/50ml solution for infusion vials | 2 vial [PoM] £2,400.00 (Hospital only)

4 Blood pressure conditions

4.1 Hypertension

Hypertension

18-Jun-2024

Description of condition

Hypertension is defined as persistently raised arterial blood pressure and is one of the most important treatable causes of premature morbidity and mortality. It is a major risk factor for stroke, myocardial infarction, heart failure, chronic kidney disease, cognitive decline, and premature death. Hypertension is more common in advancing age, in women aged between 65–74 years, and in people of black African or African-Caribbean origin. Other risk factors include social deprivation, lifestyle factors, anxiety, and emotional stress.

Aims of treatment

Treatment aims to reduce the risk of cardiovascular morbidity and mortality, including myocardial infarction and stroke, by lowering blood pressure.

Assessment of cardiovascular risk and target organ damage

[EvGr] In patients with suspected or diagnosed hypertension, carry out investigations for target organ damage, and assess cardiovascular disease risk using a cardiovascular risk assessment tool and clinic blood pressure measurements. △

For full guidance on the risk assessment and prevention of cardiovascular disease, see Cardiovascular disease risk assessment and prevention p. 219.

Non-drug treatment

[EvGr] In patients with suspected or diagnosed hypertension, offer lifestyle advice and support to enable patients to make healthy lifestyle changes.

Give advice about the benefits of regular exercise, a healthy diet, low dietary sodium intake, and reduced alcohol intake (if excessive) as these changes can reduce blood pressure.

Discourage excessive consumption of coffee and other caffeine-rich products, and offer advice to help smokers to stop smoking (see Smoking cessation p. 565). △

Hypertension thresholds for treatment

Recommendations on the management of hypertension and blood pressure thresholds are from *NICE—Hypertension in adults: diagnosis and management (NG136, November 2023)*, and *SIGN—A national clinical guideline: Risk estimation and the prevention of cardiovascular disease (SIGN 149, June 2017)*. These recommendations differ slightly. Recommendations are based on NICE guidelines, and differences with SIGN (2017) have been highlighted.

For blood pressure thresholds, targets, and the management of hypertension in patients with renal disease or diabetes, or during pregnancy, see *Hypertension in renal disease*, *Hypertension in diabetes*, and *Hypertension in pregnancy*.

[EvGr] Patients presenting with a blood pressure of 140/90 mmHg or higher when measured in a clinic setting, should be offered ambulatory blood pressure monitoring (ABPM), or home blood pressure monitoring if ABPM is unsuitable, to confirm the diagnosis and stage of hypertension. ◇A

Stage 1 hypertension is a clinic blood pressure ranging from 140/90 mmHg to 159/99 mmHg, and an ambulatory daytime average or home blood pressure average ranging from 135/85 mmHg to 149/94 mmHg.

[EvGr] Discuss starting antihypertensive drug treatment with patients aged under 80 years who have stage 1 hypertension if they have one or more of the following: target-organ damage (for example left ventricular hypertrophy, chronic kidney disease or hypertensive retinopathy), established cardiovascular disease, renal disease, diabetes, or a 10 year cardiovascular risk ≥10%.

Consider antihypertensive drug treatment for adults aged under 60 years with stage 1 hypertension and an estimated 10 year cardiovascular risk below 10%.

Antihypertensive drug treatment should also be considered for patients aged over 80 years with a clinic blood pressure of over 150/90 mmHg.

For patients aged under 40 years with stage 1 hypertension, consider seeking specialist advice for evaluation of secondary causes of hypertension.

SIGN (2017) recommends antihypertensive drug treatment be offered to patients at high cardiovascular risk or with evidence of cardiovascular disease, and a sustained clinic systolic blood pressure over 140 mmHg and/or diastolic blood pressure over 90 mmHg regardless of age. SIGN (2017) also recommends that antihypertensive drug treatment should be offered to patients who have had a haemorrhagic or ischaemic stroke, or transient ischaemic attack even when their baseline blood pressure is at a level that would be considered conventionally normotensive. ◇A

Stage 2 hypertension is a clinic blood pressure of 160/100 mmHg or higher but less than 180/120 mmHg, and an ambulatory daytime average or home blood pressure average of 150/95 mmHg or higher.

[EvGr] Treat all patients who have stage 2 hypertension, regardless of age. ◇A

Severe hypertension is a clinic systolic blood pressure of 180 mmHg or higher, or a clinic diastolic blood pressure of 120 mmHg or higher.

[EvGr] Treat severe hypertension promptly (see *Same-day specialist referral*). ◇A

Same-day specialist referral

[EvGr] Refer patients for specialist assessment, carried out on the same day, if they have suspected phaeochromocytoma (for example labile or postural hypotension, headache, palpitations, pallor, abdominal pain, or diaphoresis).

Patients should also be referred for specialist assessment, carried out on the same day, if they have a clinic blood pressure of 180/120 mmHg or higher with signs of retinal haemorrhage or papilloedema (accelerated hypertension), or life-threatening symptoms for example new onset confusion, chest pain, signs of heart failure, or acute kidney injury.

For patients with severe hypertension, but no symptoms or signs indicating the need for same-day referral, carry out investigations for target organ damage as soon as possible. If target organ damage is identified, consider starting antihypertensive drug treatment immediately, without waiting for the results of ambulatory or home blood pressure monitoring. If no target organ damage is identified, repeat clinic blood pressure measurement within 7 days. ◇A

Hypertension treatment targets

For blood pressure thresholds, targets and the management of hypertension in patients with renal disease or diabetes, or during pregnancy, see *Hypertension in renal disease*, *Hypertension in diabetes*, and *Hypertension in pregnancy*.

[EvGr] Clinic blood pressure should be reduced and maintained to below 140/90 mmHg for patients aged under 80 years, and to below 150/90 mmHg for patients aged over 80 years. For ambulatory or home blood pressure monitoring (during the patient's waking hours), the average blood pressure should be maintained at below 135/85 mmHg for patients aged under 80 years, and below 145/85 mmHg for patients aged over 80 years. SIGN (2017) instead recommends a target clinic blood pressure below 140/90 mmHg regardless of age, whilst patients with established cardiovascular disease and target organ damage should aim for a clinic blood pressure below 135/85 mmHg. These figures are a general guide and may be adapted depending on tolerability, especially in the frail or elderly.

Patients with symptoms of postural hypotension, or those aged over 80 years with a significant postural drop, should be treated to a blood pressure target based on standing blood pressure.

SIGN and the Royal College of Physicians—National Clinical Guideline for Stroke for the UK and Ireland (2023) recommends that for patients with stroke or transient ischaemic attack, clinic systolic blood pressure should be reduced and maintained to below 130 mmHg, equivalent to an average home systolic blood pressure below 125 mmHg. The exception is for patients with severe bilateral carotid artery stenosis, for whom a systolic blood pressure target of 140–150 mmHg is appropriate. ◇A

Drugs for hypertension

For patients with cardiovascular disease, condition-specific drug treatments may overlap with treatments for hypertension. Condition-specific recommendations should be initiated first. If blood pressure remains uncontrolled, offer further antihypertensive drug treatment in line with the recommendations below.

A single antihypertensive drug is often inadequate in the management of hypertension and additional antihypertensive drugs are usually added in a step-wise manner until control is achieved. Clinicians should ensure antihypertensive drugs are titrated to the optimum or maximum tolerated dose at each step of treatment along with support and discussions around adherence throughout treatment. Response to drug treatment may be affected by age and ethnicity.

Discuss treatment options, preferences for treatment and individual cardiovascular disease risk with the patient. Continue to offer lifestyle advice and support (see *Non-drug treatment*), whether or not they choose to start antihypertensive drug treatment.

Clinical judgement should be used for all patients with frailty or multimorbidity when starting antihypertensive drug treatment.

For females with diagnosed hypertension who are considering pregnancy or who are pregnant or breastfeeding, manage hypertension in line with the recommendations in *Hypertension in pregnancy*.

[EvGr] If an angiotensin-converting enzyme (ACE) inhibitor is not tolerated, for example because of cough, offer an angiotensin II receptor blocker (ARB) to treat hypertension.

The use of an ACE inhibitor with an ARB is not recommended in the treatment of hypertension.

When choosing antihypertensive drug treatment for adults of black African or African–Caribbean family origin, consider an ARB, in preference to an ACE inhibitor.

If a calcium channel blocker is not tolerated, for example because of oedema, offer a thiazide-like diuretic to treat hypertension.

If starting or changing diuretic treatment for hypertension, offer a thiazide-like diuretic such as indapamide p. 194 in preference to conventional thiazide diuretics, for example bendroflumethiazide p. 193 or hydrochlorothiazide p. 193. Continue current treatment in patients with hypertension who already have stable, well-controlled blood pressure whilst on bendroflumethiazide or hydrochlorothiazide. (A)

For blood pressure thresholds, targets, and the management of hypertension in patients with renal disease or diabetes, see *Hypertension in renal disease* and *Hypertension in diabetes*.

Isolated systolic hypertension
[EvGr] Offer patients with isolated systolic hypertension (systolic blood pressure of 160 mmHg or more) the same treatment as patients with both raised systolic and diastolic blood pressure. (A)

Hypertension with type 2 diabetes in all patients (any age or origin), or hypertension without type 2 diabetes in those aged 55 years or below and not of black African or African-Caribbean origin
[EvGr] **Step 1:** Offer an ACE inhibitor or ARB.

Step 2: In addition to an ACE inhibitor or ARB, add in a calcium channel blocker or thiazide-like diuretic. Offer a thiazide-like diuretic if there is evidence of heart failure. (A) For full guidance on the management of chronic heart failure, see Chronic heart failure p. 222.

[EvGr] **Step 3:** Offer an ACE inhibitor or ARB, a calcium channel blocker and a thiazide-like diuretic.

Step 4: Before considering further treatment for a person with resistant hypertension, confirm elevated clinic blood pressure measurements using ambulatory or home blood pressure recordings, assess for postural hypotension and discuss adherence. If further treatment is required, consider seeking specialist advice, or the addition of low-dose spironolactone [unlicensed indication] if potassium is 4.5 mmol/litre or less; or an alpha blocker or a beta blocker if potassium is greater than 4.5 mmol/litre.

When using further diuretic therapy for step 4 treatment of resistant hypertension, monitor blood sodium, potassium and renal function within 1 month of starting treatment and repeat as needed thereafter.

Seek specialist advice if blood pressure remains uncontrolled despite taking optimal tolerated doses of 4 drugs. (A)

Hypertension without type 2 diabetes in patients aged 55 and over, or all ages of black African or African-Caribbean origin patients without type 2 diabetes
[EvGr] **Step 1:** Offer a calcium channel blocker.

Step 2: In addition to a calcium channel blocker offer an ACE inhibitor, ARB or a thiazide-like diuretic.

Step 3: Offer an ACE inhibitor or ARB, a calcium channel blocker and a thiazide-like diuretic.

Step 4: Before considering further treatment for a person with resistant hypertension, confirm elevated clinic blood pressure measurements using ambulatory or home blood pressure recordings, assess for postural hypotension and discuss adherence. If further treatment is required, consider seeking specialist advice, or consider low-dose spironolactone [unlicensed indication] if potassium is

4.5 mmol/litre or less; or an alpha blocker or a beta blocker if potassium is greater than 4.5 mmol/litre.

When using further diuretic therapy for step 4 treatment of resistant hypertension, monitor blood sodium, potassium, and renal function within 1 month of starting treatment and repeat as needed thereafter.

Seek specialist advice if blood pressure remains uncontrolled despite taking optimal tolerated doses of 4 drugs. (A)

Hypertension in diabetes
[EvGr] Hypertension in patients with diabetes should be treated aggressively with lifestyle modification and drug treatment. Lowering blood pressure in patients with diabetes reduces the risk of macrovascular and microvascular complications. (A)

Hypertension in type 1 diabetes
Recommendations on the management of hypertension are from *NICE—Type 1 diabetes in adults: diagnosis and management (NG17, August 2022)*, *NICE—Hypertension in adults: diagnosis and management (NG136, November 2023)*, *SIGN—A national clinical guideline: Risk estimation and the prevention of cardiovascular disease (SIGN 149, June 2017)*, and *SIGN—A national clinical guideline: the management of diabetes (SIGN 116, updated November 2017)*. These recommendations differ slightly. Recommendations are based on NICE guidelines, and differences with SIGN (2017) have been highlighted.

[EvGr] In adults aged under 80 years with **type 1 diabetes**, aim for clinic blood pressure targets as follows: (A)
- If the urine albumin:creatinine ratio (ACR) is less than 70 mg/mmol: below 140/90 mmHg;
- If the ACR is 70 mg/mmol or more: below 130/80 mmHg.

[EvGr] In adults aged 80 years or over, aim for a clinic blood pressure below 150/90 mmHg, regardless of the patient's ACR.

SIGN (June 2017) recommends that adults with type 1 diabetes should be offered antihypertensive drug treatment if clinic systolic blood pressure is above 140 mmHg. Antihypertensive drug treatment should also be considered even if clinic systolic blood pressure is below 140 mmHg, with treatment targeted at individuals thought to be at greatest risk of complications such as stroke, progression of retinopathy and albuminuria. SIGN (November 2017) recommends a clinic target blood pressure of below 130/80 mmHg for patients with type 1 diabetes.

If drug treatment is required, start a trial of a renin–angiotensin system blocking drug as first-line treatment for hypertension in patients with type 1 diabetes. Potential side-effects should not prevent the use of a particular class of drug in order to control blood pressure, unless the side-effects become symptomatic or otherwise clinically significant. In particular:
- selective beta-blockers should not be avoided where indicated for adults on insulin;
- low-dose thiazides may be used in combination with beta-blockers;
- only long-acting preparations of calcium channel blockers should be used. (A)

Hypertension in type 2 diabetes
Recommendations on the management of hypertension and blood pressure thresholds are from *NICE—Hypertension in adults: diagnosis and management (NG136, November 2023)*, *SIGN—A national clinical guideline: Risk estimation and the prevention of cardiovascular disease (SIGN 149, June 2017)*, and *SIGN—A national clinical guideline: the management of diabetes (SIGN 116, updated November 2017)*. These recommendations differ slightly. Recommendations are based on NICE guidelines, and differences with SIGN (2017) have been highlighted.

EvGr NICE (November 2023) recommends that the same blood pressure thresholds and treatment targets are used for patients with or without type 2 diabetes, see *Hypertension thresholds for treatment* and *Hypertension treatment targets*.

SIGN (June 2017) instead recommends that regardless of age, adults with type 2 diabetes should be offered antihypertensive drug treatment if clinic systolic blood pressure is above 140 mmHg. Antihypertensive drug treatment should also be considered even if clinic systolic blood pressure is below 140 mmHg, with treatment targeted at individuals thought to be at greatest risk of complications such as stroke, progression of retinopathy and albuminuria. SIGN (November 2017) recommends a clinic target blood pressure of 130/80 mmHg.

Patients with type 2 diabetes who have symptoms of postural hypotension or who have a significant postural drop, should be treated to a blood pressure target based on standing blood pressure. Ⓐ

For the management of hypertension in patients with type 2 diabetes, see **Hypertension with type 2 diabetes in all patients (any age or origin), or hypertension without type 2 diabetes in those aged 55 years or below and not of black African or African-Caribbean origin** in *Drugs for hypertension*.

Hypertension in renal disease

Recommendations on the management of hypertension and blood pressure thresholds are from the *NICE—Hypertension in adults: diagnosis and management guideline (NG136, November 2023), NICE—Chronic kidney disease: assessment and management guideline (NG203, November 2021), and SIGN—A national clinical guideline: Risk estimation and the prevention of cardiovascular disease (SIGN 149, June 2017).* These recommendations differ slightly. Recommendations are based on NICE guidelines, and differences with SIGN (2017) have been highlighted.

EvGr SIGN (2017) recommends that all people with stage 3 or higher chronic kidney disease, or micro- or macroalbuminuria, or who are on dialysis should be offered blood pressure-lowering treatment.

A target clinic blood pressure below 140/90 mmHg is recommended in patients with renal disease (chronic kidney disease) and an albumin:creatinine ratio (ACR) less than 70 mg/mmol. A blood pressure below 130/80 mmHg is advised in patients with chronic kidney disease and an ACR of 70 mg/mmol or more. SIGN (2017) recommends a blood pressure below 135/85 mmHg should be considered in patients with established cardiovascular disease and chronic kidney disease.

If possible, offer treatment with drugs taken only once a day. Ⓐ For guidance on the choice of antihypertensive agent in patients with chronic kidney disease, see NICE guideline: **Chronic kidney disease** (see *Useful resources*).

Hypertension in pregnancy

Hypertensive disorders during pregnancy affect approximately 8% to 10% of all pregnant females and the complications can be associated with significant morbidity and mortality to the mother and baby. Hypertension can exist before pregnancy or it can be diagnosed in the first 20 weeks of gestation (known as chronic hypertension), it can occur as new-onset of hypertension after 20 weeks gestation (gestational hypertension) or it can occur after 20 weeks gestation with features of multi-organ involvement (pre-eclampsia). Symptoms of pre-eclampsia include severe headache, problems with vision, severe pain below ribs, vomiting and sudden swelling of hands, feet or face accompanied with significant proteinuria and blood pressure greater than 140/90 mmHg. EvGr Referral to a specialist is required in all pregnant females with hypertension. Pregnant females with a first episode of hypertension (blood pressure of 140/90 mmHg or higher) after 20 weeks gestation should be referred to secondary care to be seen within 24 hours. Urgent referral to secondary care for a same-day assessment is required for pregnant women with severe hypertension (blood pressure of 160/110 mmHg or higher); referral urgency should be determined by an overall clinical assessment.

Pregnant females are at high risk of developing pre-eclampsia if they have chronic kidney disease, diabetes mellitus, autoimmune disease, chronic hypertension, or if they have had hypertension during a previous pregnancy; these females are advised to take aspirin p. 142 [unlicensed indication] from week 12 of pregnancy until the baby is born. Females with more than one moderate risk factor for developing pre-eclampsia (first pregnancy, greater than 40 years of age, pregnancy interval of greater than 10 years, BMI above 35 kg/m² at first visit, multiple pregnancy, or family history of pre-eclampsia) are also advised to take aspirin [unlicensed indication] from week 12 of pregnancy until the baby is born.

Pregnant females with chronic hypertension who are already receiving antihypertensive treatment should be referred to a specialist and have their drug therapy reviewed. Stop ACE inhibitors, ARBs, thiazide or thiazide-like diuretics due to an increased risk of congenital abnormalities.

Females with pre-eclampsia, gestational or chronic hypertension who present with a sustained blood pressure of 140/90 mmHg or higher should be offered antihypertensive treatment. First-line treatment is with oral labetalol hydrochloride p. 176 to achieve a target blood pressure of less than 135/85 mmHg. If labetalol is unsuitable, consider nifedipine modified-release p. 189 [unlicensed] and if nifedipine and labetalol are both unsuitable consider methyldopa p. 172 [unlicensed].

Females with a blood pressure of greater than 160/110 mmHg who require critical care during pregnancy or after birth should receive immediate treatment with either oral or intravenous labetalol hydrochloride, intravenous hydralazine hydrochloride p. 207, or oral nifedipine modified-release to achieve a target blood pressure of 135/85 mmHg or less.

Give intravenous magnesium sulfate p. 1193 to females in a critical care setting with severe hypertension or severe pre-eclampsia or if they have or have previously had an eclamptic fit. Consider intravenous magnesium sulfate p. 1193 in severe pre-eclampsia if birth is planned within 24 hours.

In females with pre-eclampsia where early birth is considered likely within 7 days, consider a course of antenatal corticosteroids for fetal lung maturation.

Appropriate antihypertensive treatment should be continued if required after birth (with dose adjustment according to blood pressure).

Females who have been managed with methyldopa p. 172 during pregnancy should discontinue treatment within 2 days of the birth and switch to an alternative antihypertensive.

Post-birth, advise females with hypertension that the need to take antihypertensives does not prevent them from breastfeeding should they wish to do so, although very low levels of antihypertensive medicines can pass into breast milk and most medicines are not tested in pregnant or breastfeeding women. For females who decide to breastfeed, offer enalapril maleate p. 196 first-line to treat hypertension during the post-natal period, and monitor maternal renal function and serum potassium. In females of black African or African-Caribbean family origin consider nifedipine p. 189 or amlodipine p. 184 first line. If blood pressure is not controlled with a single drug consider a combination of nifedipine (or amlodipine) and enalapril. If this combination is not tolerated or ineffective consider either adding labetalol hydrochloride p. 176 or atenolol p. 180 to the combination treatment or swapping one of the medicines being used for atenolol or labetalol. Blood pressure monitoring should be considered in babies born to mothers taking antihypertensives who are breastfeeding, and females should be advised to monitor their babies for any adverse reactions (for example: drowsiness, lethargy, pallor, cold peripheries or poor feeding).

Females with hypertension in the postnatal period who are not and do not plan to breastfeed should be treated the same way as patients in the section *Drugs for hypertension*.

Following birth, females remaining on antihypertensives should have their treatment reviewed 2 weeks after the birth. Females treated for hypertension during pregnancy should have a medical review 6–8 weeks after birth with their GP or specialist. Ⓐ

Useful Resources

Hypertension in pregnancy: diagnosis and management. National Institute for Health and Care Excellence guideline NG133. June 2019 (updated April 2023). www.nice.org.uk/guidance/ng133

Hypertension in adults: diagnosis and management. National Institute for Health and Care Excellence guideline NG136. August 2019 (updated November 2023). www.nice.org.uk/guidance/ng136

Type 1 diabetes in adults: diagnosis and management. National Institute for Health and Care Excellence guideline NG17. August 2015 (updated August 2022). www.nice.org.uk/guidance/ng17

Chronic kidney disease: assessment and management. National Institute for Health and Care Excellence guideline NG203. November 2021. www.nice.org.uk/guidance/ng203

Risk estimation and the prevention of cardiovascular disease. Scottish Intercollegiate Guidelines Network. Clinical guideline 149. June 2017. www.sign.ac.uk/sign-149-risk-estimation-and-the-prevention-of-cardiovascular-disease

Management of diabetes. Scottish Intercollegiate Guidelines Network. Clinical guideline 116. March 2010 (updated November 2017). www.sign.ac.uk/our-guidelines/management-of-diabetes/

Antihypertensive drugs

Vasodilator antihypertensive drugs

Vasodilators have a potent hypotensive effect, especially when used in combination with a beta-blocker and a thiazide. **Important:** see Hypertension (hypertensive crises) for a warning on the hazards of a very rapid fall in blood pressure.

Hydralazine hydrochloride p. 207 is given by mouth as an adjunct to other antihypertensives for the treatment of resistant hypertension but is rarely used; when used alone it causes tachycardia and fluid retention.

Sodium nitroprusside p. 209 [unlicensed] is given by intravenous infusion to control severe hypertensive emergencies when parenteral treatment is necessary.

Minoxidil p. 207 should be reserved for the treatment of severe hypertension resistant to other drugs. Vasodilatation is accompanied by increased cardiac output and tachycardia and the patients develop fluid retention. For this reason the addition of a beta-blocker and a diuretic (usually furosemide p. 261, in high dosage) are mandatory. Hypertrichosis is troublesome and renders this drug unsuitable for females.

Prazosin p. 904, doxazosin p. 903, and terazosin p. 906 have alpha-blocking and vasodilator properties.

Ambrisentan p. 210, bosentan p. 211, iloprost p. 212, macitentan p. 211, sildenafil p. 940, and tadalafil p. 941 are licensed for the treatment of pulmonary arterial hypertension and should be used under specialist supervision. Epoprostenol p. 134 can be used in patients with primary pulmonary hypertension resistant to other treatments. Bosentan is also licensed to reduce the number of new digital ulcers in patients with systemic sclerosis and ongoing digital ulcer disease. Riociguat p. 212 is licensed for the treatment of pulmonary arterial hypertension and chronic thromboembolic pulmonary hypertension; it should be used under specialist supervision.

Sitaxentan has been withdrawn from the market because the benefit of treatment does not outweigh the risk of severe hepatotoxicity.

Centrally acting antihypertensive drugs

Methyldopa p. 172 is a centrally acting antihypertensive; it may be used for the management of hypertension in pregnancy.

Clonidine hydrochloride p. 172 has the disadvantage that sudden withdrawal of treatment may cause severe rebound hypertension.

Moxonidine p. 173, a centrally acting drug, is licensed for mild to moderate essential hypertension. It may have a role when thiazides, calcium-channel blockers, ACE inhibitors, and beta-blockers are not appropriate or have failed to control blood pressure.

Adrenergic neurone blocking drugs

Adrenergic neurone blocking drugs prevent the release of noradrenaline from postganglionic adrenergic neurones. These drugs do not control supine blood pressure and may cause postural hypotension. For this reason they have largely fallen from use, but may be necessary with other therapy in resistant hypertension.

Guanethidine monosulfate, which also depletes the nerve endings of noradrenaline, is licensed for rapid control of blood pressure, however alternative treatments are preferred.

Alpha-adrenoceptor blocking drugs

Prazosin has post-synaptic alpha-blocking and vasodilator properties and rarely causes tachycardia. It may, however, reduce blood pressure rapidly after the first dose and should be introduced with caution. Doxazosin, indoramin p. 903, and terazosin have properties similar to those of prazosin.

Alpha-blockers can be used with other antihypertensive drugs in the treatment of resistant hypertension.

Prostatic hyperplasia

Alfuzosin hydrochloride p. 902, doxazosin, indoramin, prazosin, tamsulosin hydrochloride p. 905, and terazosin are indicated for benign prostatic hyperplasia.

Drugs affecting the renin-angiotensin system

01-Mar-2022

Angiotensin-converting enzyme inhibitors

Angiotensin-converting enzyme inhibitors (ACE inhibitors) inhibit the conversion of angiotensin I to angiotensin II. They have many uses and are generally well tolerated. The main indications of ACE inhibitors are shown below.

Heart failure

ACE inhibitors are used in all grades of heart failure, usually combined with a beta-blocker. Potassium supplements and potassium-sparing diuretics should be discontinued before introducing an ACE inhibitor because of the risk of hyperkalaemia. However, a low dose of spironolactone p. 224 may be beneficial in severe heart failure and can be used with an ACE inhibitor provided serum potassium is monitored carefully. Profound first-dose hypotension may occur when ACE inhibitors are introduced to patients with heart failure who are already taking a high dose of a loop diuretic (e.g. furosemide 80 mg daily or more). Temporary withdrawal of the loop diuretic reduces the risk, but may cause severe rebound pulmonary oedema. Therefore, for patients on high doses of loop diuretics, the ACE inhibitor may need to be initiated under specialist supervision. An ACE inhibitor can be initiated in the community in patients who are receiving a low dose of a diuretic or who are not otherwise at risk of serious hypotension; nevertheless, care is required and a very low dose of the ACE inhibitor is given initially. For further guidance on the use of ACE inhibitors in heart failure, see Chronic heart failure p. 222.

Hypertension
An ACE inhibitor may be the most appropriate initial drug for hypertension in younger Caucasian patients; patients of black African or African-Caribbean origin, those aged over 55 years, and those with primary aldosteronism respond less well. ACE inhibitors are particularly indicated for hypertension in patients with type 1 diabetes with nephropathy. They may reduce blood pressure very rapidly in some patients particularly in those receiving diuretic therapy.

Diabetic nephropathy
ACE inhibitors have a role in the management of diabetic nephropathy.

Prophylaxis of cardiovascular events
ACE inhibitors are used in the early and long-term management of patients who have had a myocardial infarction. ACE inhibitors may also have a role in preventing cardiovascular events.

Initiation under specialist supervision
ACE inhibitors should be initiated under specialist supervision and with careful clinical monitoring in those with severe heart failure or in those:
- receiving multiple or high-dose diuretic therapy (e.g. more than 80 mg of furosemide daily or its equivalent);
- receiving concomitant angiotensin-II receptor antagonist or aliskiren;
- with hypovolaemia;
- with hyponatraemia (plasma-sodium concentration below 130 mmol/litre);
- with hypotension (systolic blood pressure below 90 mmHg);
- with unstable heart failure;
- with haemodynamically significant left ventricular inflow or outflow impediment (e.g. stenosis of the aortic or mitral valve);
- receiving high-dose vasodilator therapy;
- known renovascular disease.

Renal effects
Renal function and electrolytes should be checked before starting ACE inhibitors (or increasing the dose) and monitored during treatment (more frequently if features mentioned below present); hyperkalaemia and other side-effects of ACE inhibitors are more common in those with impaired renal function and the dose may need to be reduced. Although ACE inhibitors now have a specialised role in some forms of renal disease, including chronic kidney disease, they also occasionally cause impairment of renal function which may progress and become severe in other circumstances (at particular risk are the elderly). A specialist should be involved if renal function is significantly reduced as a result of treatment with an ACE inhibitor.

Concomitant treatment with NSAIDs increases the risk of renal damage, and potassium-sparing diuretics (or potassium-containing salt substitutes) increase the risk of hyperkalaemia.

In patients with severe bilateral renal artery stenosis (or severe stenosis of the artery supplying a single functioning kidney), ACE inhibitors reduce or abolish glomerular filtration and are likely to cause severe and progressive renal failure. They are therefore not recommended in patients known to have these forms of critical renovascular disease.

ACE inhibitor treatment is unlikely to have an adverse effect on overall renal function in patients with severe unilateral renal artery stenosis and a normal contralateral kidney, but glomerular filtration is likely to be reduced (or even abolished) in the affected kidney and the long-term consequences are unknown.

ACE inhibitors are therefore best avoided in patients with known or suspected renovascular disease, unless the blood pressure cannot be controlled by other drugs. If ACE inhibitors are used, they should be initiated only under specialist supervision and renal function should be monitored regularly.

ACE inhibitors should also be used with particular caution in patients who may have undiagnosed and clinically silent renovascular disease. This includes patients with peripheral vascular disease or those with severe generalised atherosclerosis.

ACE inhibitors in combination with other drugs
See also, *Concomitant use of drugs affecting the renin-angiotensin system*, p. 172.

Concomitant diuretics
ACE inhibitors can cause a very rapid fall in blood pressure in volume-depleted patients; treatment should therefore be initiated with very low doses. If the dose of diuretic is greater than 80 mg furosemide p. 261 or equivalent, the ACE inhibitor should be initiated under close supervision and in some patients the diuretic dose may need to be reduced or the diuretic discontinued at least 24 hours beforehand (may not be possible in heart failure—risk of pulmonary oedema). If high-dose diuretic therapy cannot be stopped, close observation is recommended after administration of the first dose of ACE inhibitor, for at least 2 hours or until the blood pressure has stabilised.

Combination products
Products incorporating an ACE inhibitor with a thiazide diuretic or a calcium-channel blocker are available for the management of hypertension. Use of these combination products should be reserved for patients whose blood pressure has not responded adequately to a single antihypertensive drug and who have been stabilised on the individual components of the combination in the same proportions.

Angiotensin-II receptor antagonists
Azilsartan medoxomil p. 202, candesartan cilexetil p. 202, eprosartan p. 202, irbesartan p. 203, losartan potassium p. 203, olmesartan medoxomil p. 204, telmisartan p. 205, and valsartan p. 206 are angiotensin-II receptor antagonists with many properties similar to those of the ACE inhibitors. However, unlike ACE inhibitors, they do not inhibit the breakdown of bradykinin and other kinins, and thus are less likely to cause the persistent dry cough which can complicate ACE inhibitor therapy. They are therefore a useful alternative for patients who have to discontinue an ACE inhibitor because of persistent cough.

An angiotensin-II receptor antagonist may be used as an alternative to an ACE inhibitor in the management of heart failure, acute coronary syndromes, or diabetic nephropathy. Candesartan cilexetil p. 202 and valsartan p. 206 are also licensed as adjuncts to ACE inhibitors under specialist supervision, in the management of heart failure when other treatments are unsuitable.

Renal effects
Angiotensin-II receptor antagonists should be used with caution in renal artery stenosis (see also Renal effects under Angiotensin-converting enzyme inhibitors, p. 170).

Renin inhibitor

Aliskiren is a renin inhibitor that is licensed for the treatment of hypertension.

Concomitant use of drugs affecting the renin-angiotensin system

Combination therapy with two drugs affecting the renin-angiotensin system (ACE inhibitors, angiotensin-II receptor antagonists, and aliskiren p. 207) is not recommended due to an increased risk of hyperkalaemia, hypotension, and renal impairment, compared to use of a single drug. Patients with diabetic nephropathy are particularly susceptible to developing hyperkalaemia and should not be given an ACE inhibitor with an angiotensin-II receptor antagonist. There is some evidence that the benefits of combination use of an ACE inhibitor with candesartan or valsartan may outweigh the risks in selected patients with heart failure for whom other treatments are unsuitable, however, the concomitant use of this combination, together with a mineralocorticoid receptor antagonist or a potassium-sparing diuretic is not recommended.

For patients currently taking combination therapy, the need for continued combined therapy should be reviewed. If combination therapy is considered essential, it should be carried out under specialist supervision, with close monitoring of blood pressure, renal function, and electrolytes (particularly potassium); monitoring should be considered at the start of treatment, then monthly, and also after any change in dose or during intercurrent illness.

> **Other drugs used for Hypertension** Amiloride hydrochloride, p. 263 · Chlortalidone, p. 264 · Metolazone, p. 264 · Torasemide, p. 262 · Triamterene with chlortalidone, p. 264 · Xipamide, p. 265

ANTIHYPERTENSIVES, CENTRALLY ACTING

Clonidine hydrochloride

15-Apr-2024

● **INDICATIONS AND DOSE**

Hypertension

▶ BY MOUTH
▶ Adult: Initially 50–100 micrograms 3 times a day, increase dose every second or third day, usual maximum dose 1.2 mg per day

Prevention of recurrent migraine | Prevention of vascular headache | Menopausal symptoms, particularly flushing and vasomotor conditions

▶ BY MOUTH
▶ Adult: Initially 50 micrograms twice daily for 2 weeks, then increased if necessary to 75 micrograms twice daily

● **CONTRA-INDICATIONS** Severe bradyarrhythmia secondary to second- or third-degree AV block or sick sinus syndrome

● **CAUTIONS** Cerebrovascular disease · constipation · heart failure · history of depression · mild to moderate bradyarrhythmia · polyneuropathy · Raynaud's syndrome or other occlusive peripheral vascular disease

CAUTIONS, FURTHER INFORMATION

▶ Elderly For centrally-acting antihypertensives, Screening Tool of Older Persons' potentially inappropriate Prescriptions (STOPP) criteria to aid medication reviews (see Prescribing in the elderly p. 31 for information): potentially inappropriate unless clear intolerance of, or lack of efficacy with, other classes of antihypertensives (generally less well tolerated by older people).

● **INTERACTIONS** → Appendix 1: clonidine

● **SIDE-EFFECTS**

▶ **Common or very common** Constipation · depression · dizziness · dry mouth · fatigue · headache · nausea · postural hypotension · salivary gland pain · sedation · sexual dysfunction · sleep disorders · vomiting
▶ **Uncommon** Delusions · hallucination · malaise · paraesthesia · Raynaud's phenomenon · skin reactions
▶ **Rare or very rare** Alopecia · atrioventricular block · dry eye · gynaecomastia · intestinal pseudo-obstruction · nasal dryness
▶ **Frequency not known** Accommodation disorder · arrhythmias · confusion

● **PREGNANCY** May lower fetal heart rate. Avoid oral use unless potential benefit outweighs risk. Avoid using injection.

● **BREAST FEEDING** Avoid—present in milk.

● **RENAL IMPAIRMENT** Manufacturer advises caution. **Dose adjustments** Manufacturer advises adjust dose according to response.

● **TREATMENT CESSATION** In hypertension, must be withdrawn gradually to avoid severe rebound hypertension.

● **PATIENT AND CARER ADVICE**
Driving and skilled tasks Drowsiness may affect performance of skilled tasks (e.g. driving); effects of alcohol may be enhanced.

● **LESS SUITABLE FOR PRESCRIBING** Clonidine is less suitable for prescribing.

● **MEDICINAL FORMS** There can be variation in the licensing of different medicines containing the same drug. Forms available from special-order manufacturers include: oral suspension, oral solution

Oral tablet
CAUTIONARY AND ADVISORY LABELS 3, 8
▶ **Clonidine hydrochloride (Non-proprietary)**
Clonidine hydrochloride 25 microgram Clonidine 25microgram tablets | 112 tablet [PoM] £20.40 DT = £11.62
▶ **Catapres** (Glenwood GmbH)
Clonidine hydrochloride 100 microgram Catapres 100microgram tablets | 100 tablet [PoM] £8.04 DT = £8.04

Oral solution
▶ **Clonidine hydrochloride (Non-proprietary)**
Clonidine hydrochloride 10 microgram per 1 ml Clonidine 50micrograms/5ml oral solution sugar free | 100 ml [PoM] £216.10 DT = £207.94 [SF]

Methyldopa

15-Apr-2024

● **INDICATIONS AND DOSE**

Hypertension

▶ BY MOUTH
▶ Adult: Initially 250 mg 2–3 times a day, dose should be increased gradually at intervals of at least 2 days; maximum 3 g per day
▶ Elderly: Initially 125 mg twice daily, dose should be increased gradually; maximum 2 g per day

● **CONTRA-INDICATIONS** Acute porphyrias p. 1202 · depression · paraganglioma · phaeochromocytoma

● **CAUTIONS** History of hepatic impairment

CAUTIONS, FURTHER INFORMATION

▶ Elderly For centrally-acting antihypertensives, Screening Tool of Older Persons' potentially inappropriate Prescriptions (STOPP) criteria to aid medication reviews (see Prescribing in the elderly p. 31 for information): potentially inappropriate unless clear intolerance of, or lack of efficacy with, other classes of antihypertensives (generally less well tolerated by older people).

● **INTERACTIONS** → Appendix 1: methyldopa

- **SIDE-EFFECTS** Abdominal distension · amenorrhoea · angina pectoris · angioedema · arthralgia · asthenia · atrioventricular block · bone marrow failure · bradycardia · breast enlargement · cardiac inflammation · carotid sinus syndrome · cerebrovascular insufficiency · choreoathetosis · cognitive impairment · constipation · depression · diarrhoea · dizziness · dry mouth · eosinophilia · facial paralysis · fever · gastrointestinal disorders · granulocytopenia · gynaecomastia · haemolytic anaemia · headache · hepatic disorders · hyperprolactinaemia · lactation disorder · leucopenia · lupus-like syndrome · myalgia · nasal congestion · nausea · nightmare · oedema · pancreatitis · paraesthesia · parkinsonism · postural hypotension · psychiatric disorder · psychosis · sedation · sexual dysfunction · sialadenitis · skin reactions · thrombocytopenia · tongue burning · tongue discolouration · toxic epidermal necrolysis · vomiting

  SIDE-EFFECTS, FURTHER INFORMATION Side-effects are minimised if the daily dose is kept below 1g; discontinue permanently if fever or hepatic disorders occur.

- **PREGNANCY** Not known to be harmful.

- **BREAST FEEDING** Amount too small to be harmful.

- **HEPATIC IMPAIRMENT** Manufacturer advises avoid in active disease.

- **RENAL IMPAIRMENT**
  Dose adjustments [EvGr] May respond to lower doses (increased sensitivity to hypotensive and sedative effect).
  Ⓜ

- **MONITORING REQUIREMENTS** Monitor blood counts and liver-function before treatment and at intervals during first 6–12 weeks or if unexplained fever occurs.

- **EFFECT ON LABORATORY TESTS** Interference with laboratory tests. Positive direct Coombs' test in up to 20% of patients (may affect blood cross-matching).

- **PATIENT AND CARER ADVICE**
  Driving and skilled tasks Drowsiness may affect performance of skilled tasks (e.g. driving); effects of alcohol may be enhanced.

- **MEDICINAL FORMS** There can be variation in the licensing of different medicines containing the same drug. Forms available from special-order manufacturers include: oral suspension, oral solution
  Oral tablet
  CAUTIONARY AND ADVISORY LABELS 3, 8
  ‣ Methyldopa (Non-proprietary)
    Methyldopa (anhydrous) 125 mg Methyldopa 125mg tablets | 56 tablet [PoM] £100.01 DT = £45.81
    Methyldopa (anhydrous) 250 mg Methyldopa 250mg tablets | 56 tablet [PoM] £21.96 DT = £10.41 | 60 tablet [PoM] £6.15
    Methyldopa (anhydrous) 500 mg Methyldopa 500mg tablets | 30 tablet [PoM] £4.55 | 56 tablet [PoM] £17.58 DT = £16.34

Moxonidine

15-Apr-2024

- **INDICATIONS AND DOSE**
  Mild to moderate essential hypertension
  ‣ BY MOUTH
  ‣ Adult: 200 micrograms once daily for 3 weeks, dose to be taken in the morning, then increased if necessary to 400 micrograms daily in 1–2 divided doses (max. per dose 400 micrograms), maximum daily dose to be given in 2 divided doses; maximum 600 micrograms per day

- **CONTRA-INDICATIONS** Bradycardia · second- or third-degree AV block · severe heart failure · sick sinus syndrome · sino-atrial block

- **CAUTIONS** First-degree AV block · moderate heart failure · severe coronary artery disease · unstable angina

CAUTIONS, FURTHER INFORMATION
‣ Elderly For centrally-acting antihypertensives, Screening Tool of Older Persons' potentially inappropriate Prescriptions (STOPP) criteria to aid medication reviews (see Prescribing in the elderly p. 31 for information): potentially inappropriate unless clear intolerance of, or lack of efficacy with, other classes of antihypertensives (generally less well tolerated by older people).

- **INTERACTIONS** → Appendix 1: moxonidine

- **SIDE-EFFECTS**
  ‣ **Common or very common** Asthenia · diarrhoea · dizziness · drowsiness · dry mouth · dyspepsia · headache · insomnia · nausea · pain · skin reactions · vertigo · vomiting
  ‣ **Uncommon** Angioedema · bradycardia · nervousness · oedema · syncope · tinnitus

- **PREGNANCY** Manufacturer advises avoid—no information available.

- **BREAST FEEDING** Present in milk—manufacturer advises avoid.

- **RENAL IMPAIRMENT** Avoid if eGFR less than 30 mL/minute/1.73 m^2.
  Dose adjustments Max. single dose 200 micrograms and max. daily dose 400 micrograms if eGFR 30–60 mL/minute/1.73 m^2.

- **TREATMENT CESSATION** Avoid abrupt withdrawal (if concomitant treatment with beta-blocker has to be stopped, discontinue beta-blocker first, then moxonidine after a few days).

- **MEDICINAL FORMS** There can be variation in the licensing of different medicines containing the same drug.
  Oral tablet
  CAUTIONARY AND ADVISORY LABELS 3
  ‣ Moxonidine (Non-proprietary)
    Moxonidine 200 microgram Moxonidine 200microgram tablets | 28 tablet [PoM] £8.40 DT = £5.37
    Moxonidine 300 microgram Moxonidine 300microgram tablets | 28 tablet [PoM] £6.79 DT = £3.96
    Moxonidine 400 microgram Moxonidine 400microgram tablets | 28 tablet [PoM] £6.64 DT = £3.93
  ‣ Physiotens (Viatris UK Healthcare Ltd)
    Moxonidine 200 microgram Physiotens 200microgram tablets | 28 tablet [PoM] £9.72 DT = £5.37
    Moxonidine 300 microgram Physiotens 300microgram tablets | 28 tablet [PoM] £11.49 DT = £3.96
    Moxonidine 400 microgram Physiotens 400microgram tablets | 28 tablet [PoM] £13.26 DT = £3.93

BETA-ADRENOCEPTOR BLOCKERS

Beta-adrenoceptor blocking drugs

11-Oct-2023

Overview

Beta-adrenoceptor blocking drugs (beta-blockers) block the beta-adrenoceptors in the heart, peripheral vasculature, bronchi, pancreas, and liver.

Many beta-blockers are now available and in general they are all equally effective. There are, however, differences between them, which may affect choice in treating particular diseases or individual patients.

Intrinsic sympathomimetic activity (ISA, partial agonist activity) represents the capacity of beta-blockers to stimulate as well as to block adrenergic receptors. Celiprolol hydrochloride p. 181, pindolol p. 177, acebutolol p. 179, and oxprenolol hydrochloride have intrinsic sympathomimetic activity; they tend to cause less bradycardia than the other beta-blockers and may also cause less coldness of the extremities.

Some beta-blockers are lipid soluble and some are water soluble. Water-soluble beta-blockers (such as atenolol p. 180, celiprolol hydrochloride, nadolol p. 177, and sotalol hydrochloride p. 124) are less likely to enter the brain, and may therefore cause less sleep disturbance and nightmares. Water-soluble beta-blockers are excreted by the kidneys and dosage reduction is often necessary in renal impairment.

Beta-blockers with a relatively short duration of action have to be given two or three times daily. Many of these are, however, available in modified-release formulations so that administration once daily is adequate for hypertension. For angina twice-daily treatment may sometimes be needed even with a modified-release formulation. Some beta-blockers, such as atenolol, bisoprolol fumarate p. 180, celiprolol hydrochloride, and nadolol, have an intrinsically longer duration of action and need to be given only once daily.

Beta-blockers slow the heart and can depress the myocardium; they are contra-indicated in patients with second- or third-degree heart block. Beta-blockers should also be avoided in patients with worsening unstable heart failure; care is required when initiating a beta-blocker in those with stable heart failure.

Labetalol hydrochloride p. 176, celiprolol hydrochloride, carvedilol p. 175, and nebivolol p. 183 are beta-blockers that have, in addition, an arteriolar vasodilating action, by diverse mechanisms, and thus lower peripheral resistance. There is no evidence that these drugs have important advantages over other beta-blockers in the treatment of hypertension.

Beta-blockers can precipitate bronchospasm and should therefore usually be avoided in patients with a history of asthma. When there is no suitable alternative, it may be necessary for a patient with well-controlled asthma, or chronic obstructive pulmonary disease (without significant reversible airways obstruction), to receive treatment with a beta-blocker for a co-existing condition (e.g. heart failure or following myocardial infarction). In this situation, a cardioselective beta-blocker should be selected and initiated at a low dose by a specialist; the patient should be closely monitored for adverse effects. Atenolol, bisoprolol fumarate, metoprolol tartrate p. 182, nebivolol, and (to a lesser extent) acebutolol, have less effect on the beta$_2$ (bronchial) receptors and are, therefore, relatively *cardioselective*, but they are not *cardiospecific*. They have a lesser effect on airways resistance but are not free of this side-effect.

Beta-blockers are also associated with fatigue, coldness of the extremities (may be less common with those with ISA), and sleep disturbances with nightmares (may be less common with the water-soluble beta-blockers).

Beta-blockers can affect carbohydrate metabolism, causing hypoglycaemia or hyperglycaemia in patients with or without diabetes; they can also interfere with metabolic and autonomic responses to hypoglycaemia, thereby masking symptoms such as tachycardia. However, beta-blockers are not contra-indicated in diabetes, although the cardioselective beta-blockers may be preferred. Beta-blockers should be avoided altogether in those with frequent episodes of hypoglycaemia. Beta-blockers, especially when combined with a thiazide diuretic, should be avoided for the routine treatment of uncomplicated hypertension in patients with diabetes or in those at high risk of developing diabetes.

Hypertension

The mode of action of beta-blockers in hypertension is not understood, but they reduce cardiac output, alter baroceptor reflex sensitivity, and block peripheral adrenoceptors. Some beta-blockers depress plasma renin secretion. It is possible that a central effect may also partly explain their mode of action.

Beta-blockers are effective for reducing blood pressure but other antihypertensives are usually more effective for reducing the incidence of stroke, myocardial infarction, and cardiovascular mortality, especially in the elderly. Other antihypertensives are therefore preferred for routine initial treatment of uncomplicated hypertension.

In general, the dose of a beta-blocker does not have to be high.

Beta-blockers can be used to control the pulse rate in patients with *phaeochromocytoma*. However, they should never be used alone as beta-blockade without concurrent alpha-blockade may lead to a hypertensive crisis. For this reason phenoxybenzamine hydrochloride p. 208 should always be used together with the beta-blocker.

Angina

By reducing cardiac work beta-blockers improve exercise tolerance and relieve symptoms in patients with *angina*. As with hypertension there is no good evidence of the superiority of any one drug, although occasionally a patient will respond better to one beta-blocker than to another. There is some evidence that sudden withdrawal may cause an exacerbation of angina and therefore gradual reduction of dose is preferable when beta-blockers are to be stopped. There is a risk of precipitating heart failure when beta-blockers and verapamil are used together in established ischaemic heart disease.

Myocardial infarction

For recommendations on the use of beta-blockers following a myocardial infarction, see *Secondary prevention of cardiovascular events* in Acute coronary syndromes p. 247.

Several studies have shown that some beta-blockers can reduce the recurrence rate of *myocardial infarction*. However, uncontrolled heart failure, hypotension, bradyarrhythmias, and obstructive airways disease render beta-blockers unsuitable in some patients following a myocardial infarction. Atenolol and metoprolol tartrate may reduce early mortality after intravenous and subsequent oral administration in the acute phase, while acebutolol, metoprolol tartrate, propranolol hydrochloride p. 178, and timolol maleate p. 179 have protective value when started in the early convalescent phase. The evidence relating to other beta-blockers is less convincing; some have not been tested in trials of secondary prevention.

Arrhythmias

Beta-blockers act as *anti-arrhythmic drugs* principally by attenuating the effects of the sympathetic system on automaticity and conductivity within the heart. They can be used in conjunction with digoxin to control the ventricular response in atrial fibrillation, especially in patients with thyrotoxicosis. Beta-blockers are also useful in the management of supraventricular tachycardias, and are used to control those following myocardial infarction.

Esmolol hydrochloride p. 182 is a relatively cardioselective beta-blocker with a very short duration of action, used intravenously for the short-term treatment of supraventricular arrhythmias, sinus tachycardia, or hypertension, particularly in the peri-operative period. It may also be used in other situations, such as acute myocardial infarction, when sustained beta-blockade might be hazardous.

Sotalol hydrochloride p. 124, a non-cardioselective beta-blocker with additional class III anti-arrhythmic activity, is used for prophylaxis in paroxysmal supraventricular arrhythmias. It also suppresses ventricular ectopic beats and non-sustained ventricular tachycardia. It has been shown to be more effective than lidocaine in the termination of spontaneous sustained ventricular tachycardia due to coronary disease or cardiomyopathy. However, it may induce torsade de pointes in susceptible patients.

Heart failure

Beta-blockers may produce benefit in heart failure by blocking sympathetic activity. Bisoprolol fumarate p. 180

and carvedilol below reduce mortality in any grade of stable heart failure; nebivolol p. 183 is licensed for stable mild to moderate heart failure in patients over 70 years. Ideally, treatment should be initiated by those experienced in the management of heart failure.

Thyrotoxicosis

Beta-blockers are used in pre-operative preparation for thyroidectomy. Administration of propranolol hydrochloride p. 178 can reverse clinical symptoms of *thyrotoxicosis* within 4 days. Routine tests of increased thyroid function remain unaltered. The thyroid gland is rendered less vascular thus making surgery easier.

Other uses

Beta-blockers have been used to alleviate some symptoms of *anxiety*; probably patients with palpitation, tremor, and tachycardia respond best. Beta-blockers are also used in the *prophylaxis of migraine*. Betaxolol p. 1342, levobunolol hydrochloride p. 1342, and timolol maleate p. 1342 are used topically in *glaucoma*.

[EvGr] Carvedilol [unlicensed use] and propranolol hydrochloride [unlicensed use] may be used for primary prevention of decompensated cirrhosis; carvedilol is considered first-choice as it has fewer side-effects and a greater effect on portal vein pressure. Carvedilol [unlicensed use] and propranolol hydrochloride are also used to prevent bleeding from oesophageal varices. ⒶFor further guidance see NICE guideline **Cirrhosis in over 16s: assessment and management** (available at: www.nice.org.uk/guidance/ng50).

Beta-adrenoceptor blockers (systemic)

- **CONTRA-INDICATIONS** Asthma · cardiogenic shock · hypotension · marked bradycardia · metabolic acidosis · phaeochromocytoma (apart from specific use with alpha-blockers) · Prinzmetal's angina · second-degree AV block · severe peripheral arterial disease · sick sinus syndrome · third-degree AV block · uncontrolled heart failure

  CONTRA-INDICATIONS, FURTHER INFORMATION
  ▸ Bronchospasm Beta-blockers, including those considered to be cardioselective, should usually be avoided in patients with a history of asthma, bronchospasm or a history of obstructive airways disease. However, when there is no alternative, a cardioselective beta-blocker can be given to these patients with caution and under specialist supervision. In such cases the risk of inducing bronchospasm should be appreciated and appropriate precautions taken.

- **CAUTIONS** Diabetes · first-degree AV block · history of obstructive airways disease (introduce cautiously) · myasthenia gravis · portal hypertension (risk of deterioration in liver function) · psoriasis · symptoms of hypoglycaemia may be masked · symptoms of thyrotoxicosis may be masked

  CAUTIONS, FURTHER INFORMATION
  ▸ Elderly Screening Tool of Older Persons' potentially inappropriate Prescriptions (STOPP) criteria to aid medication reviews (see Prescribing in the elderly p. 31 for information). Potentially inappropriate:
  - in combination with verapamil or diltiazem (risk of heart block)
  - with bradycardia (heart rate less than 50 beats per minute), or second- or third-degree AV block (contra-indicated; risk of complete heart block, asystole)
  - in diabetes mellitus patients with frequent hypoglycaemic episodes (risk of suppressing hypoglycaemic symptoms)

- if prescribed a **non-selective** beta-blocker (including topical beta-blockers) in a history of asthma requiring treatment (contra-indicated in asthma; risk of increased bronchospasm)

- **SIDE-EFFECTS**
▸ **Common or very common** Abdominal discomfort · bradycardia · confusion · depression · diarrhoea · dizziness · dry eye (reversible on discontinuation) · dyspnoea · erectile dysfunction · fatigue · headache · heart failure · nausea · paraesthesia · peripheral coldness · rash (reversible on discontinuation) · Raynaud's phenomenon · sleep disorders · syncope · visual impairment · vomiting
▸ **Uncommon** Alopecia · atrioventricular block · bronchospasm
▸ **Rare or very rare** Hallucination · psoriasis exacerbated

  SIDE-EFFECTS, FURTHER INFORMATION With administration by intravenous injection, excessive bradycardia can occur and may be countered with **intravenous injection** of atropine sulfate.

  Overdose Therapeutic overdosages with beta-blockers may cause lightheadedness, dizziness, and possibly syncope as a result of bradycardia and hypotension; heart failure may be precipitated or exacerbated. With administration by intravenous injection, excessive bradycardia can occur and may be countered with intravenous injection of atropine sulfate.

  For details on the management of poisoning, see Beta-blockers, under Emergency treatment of poisoning p. 1554.

- **ALLERGY AND CROSS-SENSITIVITY** [EvGr] Caution is advised in patients with a history of hypersensitivity—may increase sensitivity to allergens and result in more serious hypersensitivity response. ⓂFurthermore beta-adrenoceptor blockers may reduce response to adrenaline (epinephrine).

- **PREGNANCY** Beta-blockers may cause intra-uterine growth restriction, neonatal hypoglycaemia, and bradycardia; the risk is greater in severe hypertension.

- **BREAST FEEDING** With systemic use in the mother, infants should be monitored as there is a risk of possible toxicity due to beta-blockade. However, the amount of most beta-blockers present in milk is too small to affect infants.

- **MONITORING REQUIREMENTS** Monitor lung function (in patients with a history of obstructive airway disease).

- **TREATMENT CESSATION** Avoid abrupt withdrawal especially in ischaemic heart disease. Sudden cessation of a beta-blocker can cause a rebound worsening of myocardial ischaemia and therefore gradual reduction of dose is preferable when beta-blockers are to be stopped.

BETA-ADRENOCEPTOR BLOCKERS ❭ ALPHA- AND BETA-ADRENOCEPTOR BLOCKERS

⚑ above

Carvedilol

29-Sep-2023

- **INDICATIONS AND DOSE**
Hypertension
▸ BY MOUTH
▸ Adult: Initially 12.5 mg once daily for 2 days, then increased to 25 mg once daily; increased if necessary up to 50 mg daily, dose to be increased at intervals of at least 2 weeks and can be given as a single dose or in divided doses
▸ Elderly: Initially 12.5 mg daily, initial dose may provide satisfactory control

Angina
▸ BY MOUTH
▸ Adult: Initially 12.5 mg twice daily for 2 days, then increased to 25 mg twice daily   continued →

Adjunct to diuretics, digoxin, or ACE inhibitors in symptomatic chronic heart failure
▶ BY MOUTH
▶ Adult: Initially 3.125 mg twice daily, dose to be taken with food, then increased to 6.25 mg twice daily, then increased to 12.5 mg twice daily, then increased to 25 mg twice daily, dose should be increased at intervals of at least 2 weeks up to the highest tolerated dose, max. 25 mg twice daily in patients with severe heart failure or body-weight less than 85 kg; max. 50 mg twice daily in patients over 85 kg

Prevention of bleeding from medium or large oesophageal varices [in patients with cirrhosis]
▶ BY MOUTH
▶ Adult: 6.25 mg once daily, increased if necessary up to 12.5 mg once daily, dose to be adjusted gradually according to heart rate and blood pressure

Primary prevention of decompensated cirrhosis [in patients with clinically significant portal hypertension]
▶ BY MOUTH
▶ Adult: 6.25 mg once daily, dose to be adjusted gradually according to heart rate and blood pressure

● UNLICENSED USE Carvedilol may be used as detailed below, although these situations are considered unlicensed:
● EvGr prevention of bleeding from medium or large oesophageal varices;
● primary prevention of decompensated cirrhosis. Ⓐ

● CONTRA-INDICATIONS Acute or decompensated heart failure requiring intravenous inotropes

● INTERACTIONS → Appendix 1: beta blockers, non-selective

● SIDE-EFFECTS
▶ **Common or very common** Anaemia · asthma · dyspepsia · eye irritation · fluid imbalance · genital oedema · hypercholesterolaemia · hyperglycaemia · hypoglycaemia · increased risk of infection · oedema · peripheral vascular disease · postural hypotension · pulmonary oedema · renal impairment · urinary disorders · weight increased
▶ **Uncommon** Angina pectoris · constipation · hyperhidrosis · skin reactions
▶ **Rare or very rare** Dry mouth · hypersensitivity · leucopenia · nasal congestion · severe cutaneous adverse reactions (SCARs) · thrombocytopenia

● PREGNANCY Information on the safety of carvedilol during pregnancy is lacking. If carvedilol is used close to delivery, infants should be monitored for signs of alpha-blockade (as well as beta-blockade).

● BREAST FEEDING Infants should be monitored as there is a risk of possible toxicity due to alpha-blockade (in addition to beta-blockade).

● HEPATIC IMPAIRMENT EvGr Avoid in severe impairment. Ⓜ
▶ When used for Prevention of bleeding from medium or large oesophageal varices or Primary prevention of decompensated cirrhosis EvGr Caution in mild to moderate impairment (may have greater effect on heart rate and blood pressure). Ⓐ
Dose adjustments EvGr Dose adjustment may be required in moderate impairment. Ⓜ

● MONITORING REQUIREMENTS Monitor renal function during dose titration in patients with heart failure who also have renal impairment, low blood pressure, ischaemic heart disease, or diffuse vascular disease.

● MEDICINAL FORMS There can be variation in the licensing of different medicines containing the same drug. Forms available from special-order manufacturers include: oral suspension
Oral tablet
CAUTIONARY AND ADVISORY LABELS 8
▶ Carvedilol (Non-proprietary)
Carvedilol 3.125 mg Carvedilol 3.125mg tablets | 28 tablet PoM £1.20 DT = £0.78
Carvedilol 6.25 mg Carvedilol 6.25mg tablets | 28 tablet PoM £1.66 DT = £1.22
Carvedilol 12.5 mg Carvedilol 12.5mg tablets | 28 tablet PoM £1.93 DT = £1.20
Carvedilol 25 mg Carvedilol 25mg tablets | 28 tablet PoM £2.41 DT = £1.15

◀ 175

Labetalol hydrochloride

13-May-2021

● INDICATIONS AND DOSE
Controlled hypotension in anaesthesia
▶ BY INTRAVENOUS INFUSION, OR BY INTRAVENOUS INJECTION
▶ Adult: (consult product literature or local protocols)

Hypertension of pregnancy
▶ BY INTRAVENOUS INFUSION
▶ Adult: Initially 20 mg/hour, then increased if necessary to 40 mg/hour after 30 minutes, then increased if necessary to 80 mg/hour after 30 minutes, then increased if necessary to 160 mg/hour after 30 minutes, adjusted according to response; Usual maximum 160 mg/hour
▶ BY MOUTH
▶ Adult: Use dose for hypertension

Hypertension following myocardial infarction
▶ BY INTRAVENOUS INFUSION
▶ Adult: 15 mg/hour, then increased to up to 120 mg/hour, dose to be increased gradually

Hypertensive emergencies
▶ BY INTRAVENOUS INJECTION
▶ Adult: 50 mg, to be given over at least 1 minute, then 50 mg every 5 minutes if required until a satisfactory response occurs; maximum 200 mg per course
▶ BY INTRAVENOUS INFUSION
▶ Adult: Initially 2 mg/minute until a satisfactory response is achieved, then discontinue; usual dose 50–200 mg

Hypertension
▶ BY MOUTH
▶ Adult: Initially 100 mg twice daily, dose to be increased at intervals of 14 days; usual dose 200 mg twice daily, increased if necessary up to 800 mg daily in 2 divided doses, to be taken with food, higher doses to be given in 3–4 divided doses; maximum 2.4 g per day
▶ Elderly: Initially 50 mg twice daily, dose to be increased at intervals of 14 days; usual dose 200 mg twice daily, increased if necessary up to 800 mg daily in 2 divided doses, to be taken with food, higher doses to be given in 3–4 divided doses; maximum 2.4 g per day
▶ BY INTRAVENOUS INJECTION
▶ Adult: 50 mg, dose to be given over at least 1 minute, then 50 mg after 5 minutes if required; maximum 200 mg per course
▶ BY INTRAVENOUS INFUSION
▶ Adult: Initially 2 mg/minute until a satisfactory response is achieved, then discontinue; usual dose 50–200 mg

● CAUTIONS Liver damage

● INTERACTIONS → Appendix 1: beta blockers, non-selective

● SIDE-EFFECTS
GENERAL SIDE-EFFECTS
▶ **Common or very common** Drug fever · ejaculation failure · hypersensitivity · urinary disorders

2

Cardiovascular system

- ► **Rare or very rare** Hepatic disorders · systemic lupus erythematosus (SLE) · toxic myopathy · tremor
- ► **Frequency not known** Cyanosis · hyperhidrosis · hyperkalaemia · interstitial lung disease · lethargy · lichenoid keratosis · muscle cramps · nasal congestion · peripheral oedema · postural hypotension · psychosis · thrombocytopenia

  SPECIFIC SIDE-EFFECTS

- ► **Rare or very rare**
- ► With oral use Peripheral vascular disease
- ► **Frequency not known**
- ► With intravenous use Fever · hypoglycaemia masked · intermittent claudication exacerbated · thyrotoxicosis masked
- ► With oral use Photosensitivity reaction
- ● **PREGNANCY** The use of labetalol in maternal hypertension is not known to be harmful, except possibly in the first trimester. If labetalol is used close to delivery, infants should be monitored for signs of alpha-blockade (as well as beta blockade).
- ● **BREAST FEEDING** Infants should be monitored as there is a risk of possible toxicity due to alpha-blockade (in addition to beta-blockade).
- ● **HEPATIC IMPAIRMENT** Manufacturer advises caution (risk of slow metabolism).
  Dose adjustments Manufacturer advises consider dose reduction.
- ● **RENAL IMPAIRMENT**
  Dose adjustments Manufacturer advises consider dose reduction.
- ● **MONITORING REQUIREMENTS**
- ► Liver damage Severe hepatocellular damage reported after both short-term and long-term treatment. Appropriate laboratory testing needed at first symptom of liver dysfunction and if laboratory evidence of damage (or if jaundice) labetalol should be stopped and not restarted.
- ● **EFFECT ON LABORATORY TESTS** Interferes with laboratory tests for catecholamines.
- ● **DIRECTIONS FOR ADMINISTRATION** [EvGr] For *intravenous infusion*, give intermittently *in* Glucose 5% *or* Sodium Chloride and Glucose. Dilute to a concentration of 1 mg/mL; suggested volume 200 mL; adjust rate with in-line burette. Avoid upright position during and for 3 hours after intravenous administration. Ⓜ

- ● **MEDICINAL FORMS** There can be variation in the licensing of different medicines containing the same drug. Forms available from special-order manufacturers include: oral suspension, oral solution

  Solution for injection
  - ► Labetalol hydrochloride (Non-proprietary)
    Labetalol hydrochloride 5 mg per 1 ml Labetalol 50mg/10ml solution for injection ampoules | 5 ampoule [PoM] £60.00 (Hospital only) | 10 ampoule [PoM] £125.00 (Hospital only)
    Labetalol 100mg/20ml solution for injection ampoules | 5 ampoule [PoM] £69.00-£148.82 (Hospital only) | 5 ampoule [PoM] £168.60

  Oral tablet
  CAUTIONARY AND ADVISORY LABELS 8, 21
  - ► Labetalol hydrochloride (Non-proprietary)
    Labetalol hydrochloride 100 mg Labetalol 100mg tablets | 56 tablet [PoM] £19.64 DT = £4.98
    Labetalol hydrochloride 200 mg Labetalol 200mg tablets | 56 tablet [PoM] £25.34 DT = £15.63
    Labetalol hydrochloride 400 mg Labetalol 400mg tablets | 56 tablet [PoM] £35.90 DT = £21.12
  - ► Trandate (RPH Pharmaceuticals AB)
    Labetalol hydrochloride 50 mg Trandate 50mg tablets | 56 tablet [PoM] £3.79 DT = £3.79
    Labetalol hydrochloride 100 mg Trandate 100mg tablets | 56 tablet [PoM] £4.87 DT = £4.98
    Labetalol hydrochloride 200 mg Trandate 200mg tablets | 56 tablet [PoM] £8.72 DT = £15.63

BETA-ADRENOCEPTOR BLOCKERS ›
NON-SELECTIVE

[F 175]

Nadolol

26-Jun-2019

- ● **INDICATIONS AND DOSE**

  Hypertension
  - ► BY MOUTH
  - ► Adult: Initially 80 mg once daily, then increased in steps of up to 80 mg every week if required, doses higher than the maximum are rarely necessary; maximum 240 mg per day

  Angina
  - ► BY MOUTH
  - ► Adult: Initially 40 mg once daily, then increased if necessary up to 160 mg daily, doses should be increased at weekly intervals, maximum dose rarely is used; maximum 240 mg per day

  Arrhythmias
  - ► BY MOUTH
  - ► Adult: Initially 40 mg once daily, then increased if necessary up to 160 mg once daily, doses should be increased at weekly intervals; reduced to 40 mg daily if bradycardia occurs

  Migraine prophylaxis
  - ► BY MOUTH
  - ► Adult: Initially 40 mg once daily, then increased in steps of 40 mg every week, adjusted according to response; maintenance 80–160 mg once daily

  Thyrotoxicosis (adjunct)
  - ► BY MOUTH
  - ► Adult: 80–160 mg once daily

- ● **INTERACTIONS** → Appendix 1: beta blockers, non-selective
- ● **SIDE-EFFECTS**
- ► **Common or very common** Peripheral vascular disease
- ► **Uncommon** Appetite decreased · behaviour abnormal · constipation · cough · dry mouth · dyspepsia · facial swelling · flatulence · hyperhidrosis · nasal congestion · sedation · sexual dysfunction · skin reactions · speech slurred · tinnitus · vision blurred · weight increased
- ► **Frequency not known** Hypoglycaemia
- ● **BREAST FEEDING** Water soluble beta-blockers such as nadolol are present in breast milk in greater amounts than other beta blockers.
- ● **HEPATIC IMPAIRMENT** Manufacturer advises caution.
- ● **RENAL IMPAIRMENT**
  Dose adjustments Increase dosage interval if eGFR less than 50 mL/minute/1.73 m^2.

- ● **MEDICINAL FORMS** There can be variation in the licensing of different medicines containing the same drug. Forms available from special-order manufacturers include: oral tablet, oral suspension, oral solution

  Oral tablet
  CAUTIONARY AND ADVISORY LABELS 8
  - ► Nadolol (Non-proprietary)
    Nadolol 80 mg Nadolol 80mg tablets | 28 tablet [PoM] £19.45 DT = £19.45

[F 175]

Pindolol

05-May-2021

- ● **INDICATIONS AND DOSE**

  Hypertension
  - ► BY MOUTH
  - ► Adult: Initially 5 mg 2–3 times a day, alternatively 15 mg once daily, doses to be increased as required at weekly intervals; maintenance 15–30 mg daily; maximum 45 mg per day

continued →

2

Cardiovascular system

Angina
▶ BY MOUTH
▶ Adult: 2.5–5 mg up to 3 times a day

● INTERACTIONS → Appendix 1: beta blockers, non-selective
● SIDE-EFFECTS Agranulocytosis · arrhythmia · arthralgia · constipation · cutaneous lupus erythematosus · diabetes mellitus · dry mouth · dyspepsia · gastrointestinal disorders · glycosuria · hyperglycaemia · hyperhidrosis · hyperpyrexia · hypoglycaemia · hypoglycaemia masked · intermittent claudication · keratoconjunctivitis · muscle complaints · myasthenia gravis · psychosis · sexual dysfunction · skin reactions · thrombocytopenia · thyrotoxicosis masked · toxic epidermal necrolysis · tremor · vasculitis necrotising · vision blurred
● RENAL IMPAIRMENT [EvGr] Avoid (may adversely affect renal function in severe impairment). Ⓜ

● MEDICINAL FORMS No licensed medicines listed.

⚑ 175

Propranolol hydrochloride
03-Apr-2024

● INDICATIONS AND DOSE

Thyrotoxicosis (adjunct)
▶ BY MOUTH
▶ Adult: 10–40 mg 3–4 times a day

Thyrotoxic crisis
▶ BY INTRAVENOUS INJECTION
▶ Adult: 1 mg, to be given over 1 minute, dose may be repeated if necessary at intervals of 2 minutes, maximum total dose is 5 mg in anaesthesia; maximum 10 mg per course

Hypertension
▶ BY MOUTH
▶ Adult: Initially 80 mg twice daily, dose should be increased at weekly intervals as required; maintenance 160–320 mg daily

Prevention of bleeding from medium or large oesophageal varices [in patients with cirrhosis]
▶ BY MOUTH
▶ Adult: 40 mg twice daily, increased if necessary up to 160 mg twice daily, dose to be adjusted gradually according to heart rate and blood pressure

Primary prevention of decompensated cirrhosis [in patients with clinically significant portal hypertension]
▶ BY MOUTH
▶ Adult: 40 mg twice daily, dose to be adjusted gradually according to heart rate and blood pressure

Phaeochromocytoma (only with an alpha-blocker) in preparation for surgery
▶ BY MOUTH
▶ Adult: 60 mg daily for 3 days before surgery

Phaeochromocytoma (only with an alpha-blocker) in patients unsuitable for surgery
▶ BY MOUTH
▶ Adult: 30 mg daily

Angina
▶ BY MOUTH
▶ Adult: Initially 40 mg 2–3 times a day; maintenance 120–240 mg daily

Hypertrophic cardiomyopathy | Anxiety tachycardia
▶ BY MOUTH
▶ Adult: 10–40 mg 3–4 times a day

Anxiety with symptoms such as palpitation, sweating and tremor
▶ BY MOUTH
▶ Adult: 40 mg once daily, then increased if necessary to 40 mg 3 times a day

Prophylaxis after myocardial infarction
▶ BY MOUTH
▶ Adult: Initially 40 mg 4 times a day for 2–3 days, then 80 mg twice daily, start treatment 5 to 21 days after infarction

Essential tremor
▶ BY MOUTH
▶ Adult: Initially 40 mg 2–3 times a day; maintenance 80–160 mg daily

Migraine prophylaxis
▶ BY MOUTH
▶ Adult: 80–240 mg daily in divided doses

Arrhythmias
▶ BY MOUTH
▶ Adult: 10–40 mg 3–4 times a day
▶ BY INTRAVENOUS INJECTION
▶ Adult: 1 mg, to be given over 1 minute, dose may be repeated if necessary at intervals of 2 minutes, maximum 10 mg per course (5 mg in anaesthesia)

● UNLICENSED USE [EvGr] Propranolol hydrochloride may be used for primary prevention of decompensated cirrhosis Ⓐ, but is not licensed for this indication.

> **IMPORTANT SAFETY INFORMATION**
> SAFE PRACTICE
> Propranolol has been confused with prednisolone; care must be taken to ensure the correct drug is prescribed and dispensed.
>
> HEALTH SERVICES SAFETY INVESTIGATIONS BODY (HSSIB) PATIENT SAFETY INVESTIGATIONS: POTENTIAL UNDER-RECOGNISED RISK OF HARM FROM THE USE OF PROPRANOLOL (FEBRUARY 2020)
> A review of reported incidents identified an increase in deaths due to propranolol overdose between 2012 and 2017. To minimise the risk of harm from toxicity and rapid deterioration due to propranolol overdose, the HSSIB has issued advice: www.hssib.org.uk/patient-safety-investigations/potential-under-recognised-risk-of-harm-from-the-use-of-propranolol/.

● INTERACTIONS → Appendix 1: beta blockers, non-selective
● SIDE-EFFECTS
▶ **Rare or very rare** Intermittent claudication · memory loss · mood altered · neuromuscular dysfunction · postural hypotension · psychosis · skin reactions · thrombocytopenia
▶ **Frequency not known** Hypoglycaemia

Overdose Severe overdosages with propranolol may cause cardiovascular collapse, CNS depression, and convulsions.

● HEPATIC IMPAIRMENT [EvGr] Caution (increased risk of hepatic encephalopathy; risk of increased half-life). Ⓜ
▶ When used for Prevention of bleeding from medium or large oesophageal varices or Primary prevention of decompensated cirrhosis [EvGr] Caution (may have greater effect on heart rate and blood pressure). Ⓐ
Dose adjustments
▶ With oral use [EvGr] Consider dose reduction. Ⓜ

● RENAL IMPAIRMENT [EvGr] Use with caution (risk of increased half-life). Ⓜ
Dose adjustments [EvGr] Consider dose reduction. Ⓜ

● PRESCRIBING AND DISPENSING INFORMATION Modified-release preparations can be used for once daily administration.

- **MEDICINAL FORMS** There can be variation in the licensing of different medicines containing the same drug. Forms available from special-order manufacturers include: oral suspension, oral solution

Oral tablet

CAUTIONARY AND ADVISORY LABELS 8

▸ Propranolol hydrochloride (Non-proprietary)

Propranolol hydrochloride 10 mg Propranolol 10mg tablets | 28 tablet [PoM] £1.54 DT = £0.73 | 1000 tablet [PoM] £25.00–£30.71

Propranolol hydrochloride 40 mg Propranolol 40mg tablets | 28 tablet [PoM] £1.53 DT = £0.73 | 1000 tablet [PoM] £25.36–£30.00

Propranolol hydrochloride 80 mg Propranolol 80mg tablets | 56 tablet [PoM] £3.19 DT = £1.29

Propranolol hydrochloride 160 mg Propranolol 160mg tablets | 56 tablet [PoM] £5.88 DT = £5.87

Oral solution

CAUTIONARY AND ADVISORY LABELS 8

▸ Propranolol hydrochloride (Non-proprietary)

Propranolol hydrochloride 1 mg per 1 ml Propranolol 5mg/5ml oral solution sugar free | 150 ml [PoM] £23.50 DT = £18.77 [SF]

Propranolol hydrochloride 2 mg per 1 ml Propranolol 10mg/5ml oral solution sugar free | 150 ml [PoM] £29.54 DT = £28.30 [SF]

Propranolol hydrochloride 8 mg per 1 ml Propranolol 40mg/5ml oral solution sugar free | 150 ml [PoM] £36.50 DT = £27.53 [SF]

Propranolol hydrochloride 10 mg per 1 ml Propranolol 50mg/5ml oral solution sugar free | 150 ml [PoM] £38.50 DT = £38.50 [SF]

Modified-release capsule

CAUTIONARY AND ADVISORY LABELS 8, 25

▸ Propranolol hydrochloride (Non-proprietary)

Propranolol hydrochloride 80 mg Propranolol 80mg modified-release capsules | 28 capsule [PoM] £4.95 DT = £4.95

Propranolol hydrochloride 160 mg Propranolol 160mg modified-release capsules | 28 capsule [PoM] £4.88 DT = £4.88

▸ Bedranol SR (Sandoz Ltd, Almus Pharmaceuticals Ltd)

Propranolol hydrochloride 80 mg Bedranol SR 80mg capsules | 28 capsule [PoM] £4.16–£4.95 DT = £4.95

Propranolol hydrochloride 160 mg Bedranol SR 160mg capsules | 28 capsule [PoM] £4.59 DT = £4.88

▸ Beta-Prograne (Accord-UK Ltd)

Propranolol hydrochloride 160 mg Beta-Prograne 160mg modified-release capsules | 28 capsule [PoM] £6.11 DT = £4.88

▸ Half Beta-Prograne (Accord-UK Ltd)

Propranolol hydrochloride 80 mg Half Beta-Prograne 80mg modified-release capsules | 28 capsule [PoM] £4.95 DT = £4.95

⚑ 175

Timolol maleate

05-May-2021

● **INDICATIONS AND DOSE**

Hypertension

▸ BY MOUTH

▸ Adult: Initially 10 mg daily in 1–2 divided doses, then increased if necessary up to 60 mg daily, doses to be increased gradually. Doses above 30 mg daily given in divided doses, usual maintenance 10–30 mg daily; maximum 60 mg per day

Angina

▸ BY MOUTH

▸ Adult: Initially 5 mg twice daily, then increased in steps of 10 mg daily (max. per dose 30 mg twice daily), to be increased every 3–4 days

Prophylaxis after myocardial infarction

▸ BY MOUTH

▸ Adult: Initially 5 mg twice daily for 2 days, then increased if tolerated to 10 mg twice daily

Migraine prophylaxis

▸ BY MOUTH

▸ Adult: 10–20 mg daily in 1–2 divided doses

● **INTERACTIONS** → Appendix 1: beta blockers, non-selective

● **SIDE-EFFECTS**

▸ **Common or very common** Eye disorders · eye inflammation · vision disorders

▸ **Rare or very rare** Arthralgia · retroperitoneal fibrosis · skin reactions

▸ **Frequency not known** Angioedema · arrhythmia · asthenia · cardiac arrest · cerebrovascular insufficiency · chest pain · cough · cyanosis · drowsiness · dry mouth · eye irritation · gastrointestinal discomfort · hypoglycaemia · intermittent claudication exacerbated · memory loss · myalgia · myasthenia gravis · oedema · palpitations · psychotic disorder · sexual dysfunction · systemic lupus erythematosus (SLE) · taste altered · vertigo

● **BREAST FEEDING** Manufacturer advises avoidance.

● **HEPATIC IMPAIRMENT** Manufacturer advises caution. **Dose adjustments** Manufacturer advises consider dose reduction.

● **RENAL IMPAIRMENT** [EvGr] Use with caution. ⟨M⟩ **Dose adjustments** [EvGr] Consider dose reduction. ⟨M⟩

● **MEDICINAL FORMS** There can be variation in the licensing of different medicines containing the same drug.

Oral tablet

CAUTIONARY AND ADVISORY LABELS 8

▸ Timolol maleate (Non-proprietary)

Timolol maleate 10 mg Timolol 10mg tablets | 30 tablet [PoM] £69.53 DT = £69.53

Timolol with bendroflumethiazide

The properties listed below are those particular to the combination only. For the properties of the components please consider, timolol maleate above, bendroflumethiazide p. 193.

● **INDICATIONS AND DOSE**

Hypertension

▸ BY MOUTH

▸ Adult: 1–2 tablets daily; maximum 4 tablets per day

● **INTERACTIONS** → Appendix 1: beta blockers, non-selective · thiazide diuretics

● **MEDICINAL FORMS** There can be variation in the licensing of different medicines containing the same drug.

Oral tablet

CAUTIONARY AND ADVISORY LABELS 8

▸ Timolol with bendroflumethiazide (Non-proprietary)

Bendroflumethiazide 2.5 mg, Timolol maleate 10 mg Timolol 10mg / Bendroflumethiazide 2.5mg tablets | 30 tablet [PoM] £53.62–£63.08 DT = £63.08

BETA-ADRENOCEPTOR BLOCKERS ❯ SELECTIVE

⚑ 175

Acebutolol

19-Jul-2021

● **INDICATIONS AND DOSE**

Hypertension

▸ BY MOUTH

▸ Adult: Initially 400 mg daily for 2 weeks, alternatively initially 200 mg twice daily for 2 weeks, then increased if necessary to 400 mg twice daily; maximum 1.2 g per day

Angina

▸ BY MOUTH

▸ Adult: Initially 400 mg daily, alternatively initially 200 mg twice daily; maximum 1.2 g per day

Arrhythmias

▸ BY MOUTH

▸ Adult: 0.4–1.2 g daily in 2–3 divided doses

Severe angina

▸ BY MOUTH

▸ Adult: Initially 300 mg 3 times a day; maximum 1.2 g per day

● **INTERACTIONS** → Appendix 1: beta blockers, selective

Cardiovascular system

2

- SIDE-EFFECTS
  - ▶ **Common or very common** Gastrointestinal disorder
  - ▶ **Frequency not known** Cyanosis · hepatic disorders · intermittent claudication · lung infiltration · lupus-like syndrome · nervous system disorder · pneumonitis · psychosis · sexual dysfunction
- BREAST FEEDING Acebutolol and water soluble beta-blockers are present in breast milk in greater amounts than other beta-blockers.
- RENAL IMPAIRMENT [EvGr] Caution in severe impairment (risk of accumulation). ⟨M⟩
  Dose adjustments [EvGr] Halve dose if eGFR $25-50$ mL/minute/1.73 m^2; use quarter dose if eGFR less than 25 mL/minute/1.73 m^2; do not administer more than once daily. ⟨M⟩ See p. 21.

- MEDICINAL FORMS There can be variation in the licensing of different medicines containing the same drug.
  Oral tablet
  CAUTIONARY AND ADVISORY LABELS 8
  - ▶ **Acebutolol (Non-proprietary)**
    Acebutolol (as Acebutolol hydrochloride) 400 mg Acebutolol 400mg tablets | 28 tablet [PoM] £30.00 DT = £18.62

▶ 175

Atenolol

01-Dec-2023

- INDICATIONS AND DOSE
  Hypertension
  - ▶ BY MOUTH
  - ▶ Adult: 25–50 mg once daily, higher doses are rarely necessary

  Angina
  - ▶ BY MOUTH
  - ▶ Adult: 100 mg daily in 1–2 divided doses

  Arrhythmias
  - ▶ BY MOUTH
  - ▶ Adult: 50–100 mg once daily
  - ▶ BY INTRAVENOUS INJECTION
  - ▶ Adult: 2.5 mg every 5 minutes as required, to be given at a rate of 1 mg/minute, treatment course may be repeated every 12 hours if necessary; maximum 10 mg per course
  - ▶ BY INTRAVENOUS INFUSION
  - ▶ Adult: 150 micrograms/kg every 12 hours as required, to be given over 20 minutes

  Migraine prophylaxis
  - ▶ BY MOUTH
  - ▶ Adult: 50–200 mg daily in divided doses

  Early intervention within 12 hours of myocardial infarction
  - ▶ INITIALLY BY INTRAVENOUS INJECTION
  - ▶ Adult: 5–10 mg for 1 dose, to be given at a rate of 1 mg/minute, followed by (by mouth) 50 mg for 1 dose, to be given 15 minutes after intravenous dose, then (by mouth) 50 mg for 1 dose, to be given 12 hours after intravenous dose, then (by mouth) 100 mg for 1 dose, to be given 12 hours after previous oral dose, then (by mouth) 100 mg once daily

- UNLICENSED USE Use of atenolol for migraine prophylaxis is an unlicensed indication.

> **IMPORTANT SAFETY INFORMATION**
> **SAFE PRACTICE**
> Atenolol has been confused with amlodipine; care must be taken to ensure the correct drug is prescribed and dispensed.

- INTERACTIONS → Appendix 1: beta blockers, selective
- SIDE-EFFECTS
  - ▶ **Common or very common** Gastrointestinal disorder

- ▶ **Rare or very rare** Dry mouth · hepatic disorders · intermittent claudication · mood altered · postural hypotension · psychosis · skin reactions · thrombocytopenia
- ▶ **Frequency not known** Hypersensitivity · lupus-like syndrome
- BREAST FEEDING Water soluble beta-blockers such as atenolol are present in breast milk in greater amounts than other beta blockers.
- RENAL IMPAIRMENT
  Dose adjustments
  - ▶ With oral use Max. 50 mg daily if eGFR $15-35$ mL/minute/1.73 m^2; max. 25 mg daily or 50 mg on alternate days if eGFR less than 15 mL/minute/1.73 m^2.
  - ▶ With intravenous use Max. 10 mg on alternate days if eGFR $15-35$ mL/minute/1.73 m^2; max. 10 mg every 4 days if eGFR less than 15 mL/minute/1.73 m^2.
- DIRECTIONS FOR ADMINISTRATION For *intravenous infusion* (*Tenormin*®), manufacturer advises give intermittently in Glucose 5% or Sodium Chloride 0.9%. Suggested infusion time 20 minutes.

- MEDICINAL FORMS There can be variation in the licensing of different medicines containing the same drug. Forms available from special-order manufacturers include: oral suspension, oral solution
  Solution for injection
  - ▶ **Tenormin** (Atnahs Pharma UK Ltd)
    Atenolol 500 microgram per 1 ml Tenormin 5mg/10ml solution for injection ampoules | 10 ampoule [PoM] £34.45 (Hospital only)
  Oral tablet
  CAUTIONARY AND ADVISORY LABELS 8
  - ▶ **Atenolol (Non-proprietary)**
    Atenolol 25 mg Atenolol 25mg tablets | 28 tablet [PoM] £1.46 DT = £0.61
    Atenolol 50 mg Atenolol 50mg tablets | 28 tablet [PoM] £8.18 DT = £0.62
    Atenolol 100 mg Atenolol 100mg tablets | 28 tablet [PoM] £0.80 DT = £0.63
  - ▶ **Tenormin** (Atnahs Pharma UK Ltd)
    Atenolol 50 mg Tenormin LS 50mg tablets | 28 tablet [PoM] £10.22 DT = £0.62
  Oral solution
  CAUTIONARY AND ADVISORY LABELS 8
  - ▶ **Atenolol (Non-proprietary)**
    Atenolol 5 mg per 1 ml Atenolol 25mg/5ml oral solution sugar free | 300 ml [PoM] £10.48 DT = £7.44 [SF]
  Oral suspension
  CAUTIONARY AND ADVISORY LABELS 8

▶ 175

Bisoprolol fumarate

03-Mar-2022

- INDICATIONS AND DOSE
  Hypertension | Angina
  - ▶ BY MOUTH
  - ▶ Adult: Initially 5 mg once daily, usual maintenance 10 mg once daily; increased if necessary up to 20 mg once daily

  Adjunct in heart failure
  - ▶ BY MOUTH
  - ▶ Adult: Initially 1.25 mg once daily for 1 week, dose to be taken in the morning, then increased if tolerated to 2.5 mg once daily for 1 week, then increased if tolerated to 3.75 mg once daily for 1 week, then increased if tolerated to 5 mg once daily for 4 weeks, then increased if tolerated to 7.5 mg once daily for 4 weeks, then increased if tolerated to 10 mg once daily

- CONTRA-INDICATIONS Acute or decompensated heart failure requiring intravenous inotropes · sino–atrial block
- CAUTIONS Ensure heart failure not worsening before increasing dose

- **INTERACTIONS** → Appendix 1: beta blockers, selective
- **SIDE-EFFECTS**
  - **Common or very common** Constipation
  - **Uncommon** Muscle cramps · muscle weakness · postural hypotension
  - **Rare or very rare** Allergic rhinitis · auditory disorder · conjunctivitis · flushing · hepatitis · hypersensitivity · pruritus
- **HEPATIC IMPAIRMENT** Manufacturer advises caution.
  Dose adjustments
  - When used for Angina or Hypertension Manufacturer advises consider maximum dose of 10 mg once daily in severe impairment—consult product literature.
  - When used for Heart failure Manufacturer advises caution when titrating dose (no information available).
- **RENAL IMPAIRMENT**
  Dose adjustments
  - When used for Angina or Hypertension EvGr Max. 10 mg daily if creatinine clearance less than 20 mL/minute. (M) See p. 21.
  - When used for Heart failure EvGr Use with caution when titrating dose (no information available). (M)

- **MEDICINAL FORMS** There can be variation in the licensing of different medicines containing the same drug. Forms available from special-order manufacturers include: oral suspension, oral solution

Oral tablet

CAUTIONARY AND ADVISORY LABELS 8

- Bisoprolol fumarate (Non-proprietary)
  - **Bisoprolol fumarate 1.25 mg** Bisoprolol 1.25mg tablets | 28 tablet PoM £2.34 DT = £0.65 | 100 tablet PoM £3.60–£6.79
  - **Bisoprolol fumarate 2.5 mg** Bisoprolol 2.5mg tablets | 28 tablet PoM £2.34 DT = £0.68 | 100 tablet PoM £5.80–£6.39
  - **Bisoprolol fumarate 3.75 mg** Bisoprolol 3.75mg tablets | 28 tablet PoM £4.89 DT = £0.74
  - **Bisoprolol fumarate 5 mg** Bisoprolol 5mg tablets | 28 tablet PoM £6.00 DT = £0.66 | 100 tablet PoM £3.72–£4.25
  - **Bisoprolol fumarate 7.5 mg** Bisoprolol 7.5mg tablets | 28 tablet PoM £5.89 DT = £0.78
  - **Bisoprolol fumarate 10 mg** Bisoprolol 10mg tablets | 28 tablet PoM £2.89 DT = £0.68 | 100 tablet PoM £4.42–£4.50
- Cardicor (Merck Serono Ltd)
  - **Bisoprolol fumarate 1.25 mg** Cardicor 1.25mg tablets | 28 tablet PoM £2.35 DT = £0.65
  - **Bisoprolol fumarate 2.5 mg** Cardicor 2.5mg tablets | 28 tablet PoM £2.35 DT = £0.68
  - **Bisoprolol fumarate 3.75 mg** Cardicor 3.75mg tablets | 28 tablet PoM £4.90 DT = £0.74
  - **Bisoprolol fumarate 5 mg** Cardicor 5mg tablets | 28 tablet PoM £5.90 DT = £0.66
  - **Bisoprolol fumarate 7.5 mg** Cardicor 7.5mg tablets | 28 tablet PoM £5.90 DT = £0.78
  - **Bisoprolol fumarate 10 mg** Cardicor 10mg tablets | 28 tablet PoM £5.90 DT = £0.68

F 175

Celiprolol hydrochloride

27-Jul-2021

- **INDICATIONS AND DOSE**

Mild to moderate hypertension
- BY MOUTH
  - Adult: 200 mg once daily, dose to be taken in the morning, then increased if necessary to 400 mg once daily

- **INTERACTIONS** → Appendix 1: beta blockers, selective
- **SIDE-EFFECTS** Alveolitis allergic · dermatitis psoriasiform · drowsiness · hypoglycaemia masked · palpitations · thyrotoxicosis masked · tremor
- **BREAST FEEDING** Manufacturers advise avoidance.
- **HEPATIC IMPAIRMENT** Manufacturer advises caution.
  Dose adjustments Manufacturer advises consider dose reduction.
- **RENAL IMPAIRMENT** EvGr Avoid if creatinine clearance less than 15 mL/minute. (M)
  Dose adjustments EvGr Consider reducing dose by half if creatinine clearance 15–40 mL/minute. (M) See p. 21.

- **MEDICINAL FORMS** There can be variation in the licensing of different medicines containing the same drug. Forms available from special-order manufacturers include: oral suspension

Oral tablet

CAUTIONARY AND ADVISORY LABELS 8, 22

- Celiprolol hydrochloride (Non-proprietary)
  - **Celiprolol hydrochloride 200 mg** Celiprolol 200mg tablets | 28 tablet PoM £35.82 DT = £27.77
  - **Celiprolol hydrochloride 400 mg** Celiprolol 400mg tablets | 28 tablet PoM £62.78 DT = £49.45
- Celectol (Neon Healthcare Ltd)
  - **Celiprolol hydrochloride 200 mg** Celectol 200mg tablets | 28 tablet PoM £19.83 DT = £27.77

F 175 F 192

Co-tenidone

21-Jun-2021

- **INDICATIONS AND DOSE**

Hypertension
- BY MOUTH
  - Adult: 50/12.5 mg daily, alternatively increased if necessary to 100/25 mg daily, doses higher than 50 mg atenolol rarely necessary

DOSE EQUIVALENCE AND CONVERSION
- A mixture of atenolol and chlortalidone in mass proportions corresponding to 4 parts of atenolol and 1 part chlortalidone.

- **INTERACTIONS** → Appendix 1: beta blockers, selective · thiazide diuretics
- **SIDE-EFFECTS**
  - **Common or very common** Gastrointestinal disorder · glucose tolerance impaired
  - **Rare or very rare** Dry mouth · hepatic disorders · intermittent claudication · mood altered · neutropenia · psychosis
  - **Frequency not known** Lupus-like syndrome
- **PREGNANCY** Avoid. Diuretics not used to treat hypertension in pregnancy.
- **BREAST FEEDING** Atenolol present in milk in greater amounts than some other beta-blockers. Possible toxicity due to beta-blockade—monitor infant. Large doses of chlortalidone may suppress lactation.

- **MEDICINAL FORMS** There can be variation in the licensing of different medicines containing the same drug. Forms available from special-order manufacturers include: oral suspension, oral solution

Oral tablet

CAUTIONARY AND ADVISORY LABELS 8

- Co-tenidone (Non-proprietary)
  - **Chlortalidone 12.5 mg, Atenolol 50 mg** Co-tenidone 50mg/12.5mg tablets | 28 tablet PoM £9.64 DT = £9.64
  - **Chlortalidone 25 mg, Atenolol 100 mg** Co-tenidone 100mg/25mg tablets | 28 tablet PoM £1.83 DT = £1.55
- Tenoret (Atnahs Pharma UK Ltd)
  - **Chlortalidone 12.5 mg, Atenolol 50 mg** Tenoret 50mg/12.5mg tablets | 28 tablet PoM £10.36 DT = £9.64
- Tenoretic (Atnahs Pharma UK Ltd)
  - **Chlortalidone 25 mg, Atenolol 100 mg** Tenoretic 100mg/25mg tablets | 28 tablet PoM £10.36 DT = £1.55

Esmolol hydrochloride

05-May-2021

⚑ 175

● INDICATIONS AND DOSE

Short-term treatment of supraventricular arrhythmias (including atrial fibrillation, atrial flutter, sinus tachycardia) | Tachycardia and hypertension in peri-operative period

▸ BY INTRAVENOUS INFUSION
▸ Adult: 50–200 micrograms/kg/minute, consult product literature for details of dose titration and doses during peri-operative period

● INTERACTIONS → Appendix 1: beta blockers, selective

● SIDE-EFFECTS

▸ **Common or very common** Anxiety · appetite decreased · concentration impaired · drowsiness · hyperhidrosis
▸ **Uncommon** Arrhythmias · chills · constipation · costochondritis · dry mouth · dyspepsia · fever · flushing · nasal congestion · oedema · pain · pallor · peripheral vascular disease · pulmonary oedema · respiratory disorders · seizure · skin reactions · speech disorder · taste altered · thinking abnormal · urinary retention
▸ **Rare or very rare** Cardiac arrest · extravasation necrosis · thrombophlebitis
▸ **Frequency not known** Angioedema · coronary vasospasm · hyperkalaemia · metabolic acidosis

● BREAST FEEDING Manufacturer advises avoidance.

● RENAL IMPAIRMENT Manufacturer advises caution.

● MEDICINAL FORMS There can be variation in the licensing of different medicines containing the same drug.

Solution for injection

▸ **Esmolol hydrochloride (Non-proprietary)**
Esmolol hydrochloride 10 mg per 1 ml Esmolol hydrochloride 100mg/10ml solution for injection vials | 5 vial PoM £38.95 (Hospital only)
Esmolol 100mg/10ml solution for injection vials | 10 vial PoM £100.00 (Hospital only)
▸ **Brevibloc** (Baxter Healthcare Ltd)
Esmolol hydrochloride 10 mg per 1 ml Brevibloc Premixed 100mg/10ml solution for injection vials | 5 vial PoM £38.95 (Hospital only)

Solution for infusion

▸ **Esmolol hydrochloride (Non-proprietary)**
Esmolol hydrochloride 10 mg per 1 ml Esmolol 2.5g/250ml solution for infusion bottles | 1 bottle PoM £89.69 (Hospital only)

Infusion

▸ **Brevibloc** (Baxter Healthcare Ltd)
Esmolol hydrochloride 10 mg per 1 ml Brevibloc Premixed 2.5g/250ml infusion bags | 1 bag PoM £89.69 (Hospital only)

Metoprolol tartrate

02-Feb-2023

⚑ 175

● INDICATIONS AND DOSE

Hypertension

▸ BY MOUTH USING IMMEDIATE-RELEASE MEDICINES
▸ Adult: Initially 100 mg daily, increased if necessary to 200 mg daily in 1–2 divided doses, high doses are rarely required; maximum 400 mg per day
▸ BY MOUTH USING MODIFIED-RELEASE MEDICINES
▸ Adult: 200 mg once daily

Angina

▸ BY MOUTH USING IMMEDIATE-RELEASE MEDICINES
▸ Adult: 50–100 mg 2–3 times a day
▸ BY MOUTH USING MODIFIED-RELEASE MEDICINES
▸ Adult: 200–400 mg daily

Arrhythmias

▸ BY MOUTH USING IMMEDIATE-RELEASE MEDICINES
▸ Adult: Usual dose 50 mg 2–3 times a day, then increased if necessary up to 300 mg daily in divided doses
▸ BY INTRAVENOUS INJECTION
▸ Adult: Up to 5 mg, dose to be given at a rate of 1–2 mg/minute, then up to 5 mg after 5 minutes if required, total dose of 10–15 mg

Migraine prophylaxis

▸ BY MOUTH USING IMMEDIATE-RELEASE MEDICINES
▸ Adult: 100–200 mg daily in divided doses
▸ BY MOUTH USING MODIFIED-RELEASE MEDICINES
▸ Adult: 200 mg daily

Hyperthyroidism (adjunct)

▸ BY MOUTH USING IMMEDIATE-RELEASE MEDICINES
▸ Adult: 50 mg 4 times a day

In surgery

▸ BY SLOW INTRAVENOUS INJECTION
▸ Adult: Initially 2–4 mg, given at induction or to control arrhythmias developing during anaesthesia, then 2 mg, repeated if necessary; maximum 10 mg per course

Early intervention within 12 hours of infarction

▸ INITIALLY BY INTRAVENOUS INJECTION
▸ Adult: Initially 5 mg every 2 minutes, to a max. of 15 mg, followed by (by mouth) 50 mg every 6 hours for 48 hours, to be taken 15 minutes after intravenous injection; (by mouth) maintenance 200 mg daily in divided doses

● INTERACTIONS → Appendix 1: beta blockers, selective

● SIDE-EFFECTS

GENERAL SIDE-EFFECTS

▸ **Common or very common** Constipation · palpitations · postural disorders
▸ **Uncommon** Chest pain · drowsiness · dystrophic skin lesion · hyperhidrosis · muscle cramps · oedema · weight increased
▸ **Rare or very rare** Arrhythmia · conjunctivitis · dry mouth · eye irritation · gangrene · hepatitis · rhinitis · sexual dysfunction · thrombocytopenia

SPECIFIC SIDE-EFFECTS

▸ **Uncommon**
▸ With intravenous use Cardiogenic shock · concentration impaired · dermatitis psoriasiform
▸ **Rare or very rare**
▸ With intravenous use Anxiety · arthralgia · atrioventricular block exacerbated · intermittent claudication · memory loss · photosensitivity reaction · taste altered · tinnitus
▸ With oral use Alertness decreased · arthritis · auditory disorder · personality disorder · skin reactions
▸ **Frequency not known**
▸ With oral use Peyronie's disease · retroperitoneal fibrosis

● HEPATIC IMPAIRMENT Manufacturer advises caution in severe impairment (bioavailability may be increased in patients with liver cirrhosis).

Dose adjustments Manufacturer advises consider dose reduction in severe impairment.

● MEDICINAL FORMS There can be variation in the licensing of different medicines containing the same drug. Forms available from special-order manufacturers include: oral capsule, oral suspension, oral solution

Oral tablet

CAUTIONARY AND ADVISORY LABELS 8

▸ **Metoprolol tartrate (Non-proprietary)**
Metoprolol tartrate 25 mg Metoprolol 25mg tablets | 28 tablet PoM £18.75-£36.16 DT = £36.11
Metoprolol tartrate 50 mg Metoprolol 50mg tablets | 28 tablet PoM £3.76 DT = £2.37
Metoprolol tartrate 100 mg Metoprolol 100mg tablets | 28 tablet PoM £4.40 DT = £3.99

Solution for injection
▸ **Betaloc** (Recordati Pharmaceuticals Ltd)
Metoprolol tartrate 1 mg per 1 ml Betaloc I.V. 5mg/5ml solution for injection ampoules | 5 ampoule [PoM] £5.02 (Hospital only)

⟊ 175

Nebivolol
13-Dec-2021

● **INDICATIONS AND DOSE**
Essential hypertension
▸ BY MOUTH
▸ Adult: 5 mg daily
▸ Elderly: Initially 2.5 mg daily, then increased if necessary to 5 mg daily

Hypertension in patient with renal impairment
▸ BY MOUTH
▸ Adult: Initially 2.5 mg once daily, then increased if necessary to 5 mg once daily

Adjunct in stable mild to moderate heart failure
▸ BY MOUTH
▸ Adult 70 years and over: Initially 1.25 mg once daily for 1–2 weeks, then increased if tolerated to 2.5 mg once daily for 1–2 weeks, then increased if tolerated to 5 mg once daily for 1–2 weeks, then increased if tolerated to 10 mg once daily

● **CONTRA-INDICATIONS** Acute or decompensated heart failure requiring intravenous inotropes

● **INTERACTIONS** → Appendix 1: beta blockers, selective

● **SIDE-EFFECTS**
▸ **Common or very common** Constipation · oedema · postural hypertension
▸ **Uncommon** Dyspepsia · flatulence · intermittent claudication · skin reactions

● **BREAST FEEDING** Manufacturers advise avoidance.

● **HEPATIC IMPAIRMENT** Manufacturer advises avoid (limited information available).

● **RENAL IMPAIRMENT** [EvGr] Avoid in heart failure if severe renal insufficiency (serum creatinine greater than 250 micromol/litre; no information available). ⓜ

● **MEDICINAL FORMS** There can be variation in the licensing of different medicines containing the same drug.
Oral tablet
CAUTIONARY AND ADVISORY LABELS 8
▸ **Nebivolol (Non-proprietary)**
Nebivolol (as Nebivolol hydrochloride) 1.25 mg Nebivolol 1.25mg tablets | 28 tablet [PoM] £144.00 DT = £104.60
Nebivolol (as Nebivolol hydrochloride) 2.5 mg Nebivolol 2.5mg tablets | 28 tablet [PoM] £69.84 DT = £5.33
Nebivolol (as Nebivolol hydrochloride) 5 mg Nebivolol 5mg tablets | 28 tablet [PoM] £5.12 DT = £1.88
Nebivolol (as Nebivolol hydrochloride) 10 mg Nebivolol 10mg tablets | 28 tablet [PoM] £28.07 DT = £21.56
▸ **Nebilet** (A. Menarini Farmaceutica Internazionale SRL)
Nebivolol (as Nebivolol hydrochloride) 5 mg Nebilet 5mg tablets | 28 tablet [PoM] £9.23 DT = £1.88

CALCIUM-CHANNEL BLOCKERS

Calcium-channel blockers
24-Nov-2020

Overview

Calcium-channel blockers differ in their predilection for the various possible sites of action and, therefore, their therapeutic effects are disparate, with much greater variation than those of beta-blockers. There are important differences between verapamil hydrochloride p. 191, diltiazem hydrochloride p. 185, and the dihydropyridine calcium-channel blockers (amlodipine p. 184, felodipine p. 187, lacidipine p. 188, lercanidipine hydrochloride p. 188, nicardipine hydrochloride p. 188, nifedipine p. 189, and

nimodipine p. 133). [EvGr] Calcium channel blockers, with the exception of amlodipine, should be avoided in heart failure as they can further depress cardiac function and exacerbate symptoms. Ⓐ For further guidance on the management of heart failure, see Chronic heart failure p. 222. With the exception of amlodipine, they can also increase mortality after myocardial infarction in patients with left ventricular dysfunction and pulmonary congestion.

Verapamil hydrochloride is used for the treatment of angina, hypertension, and arrhythmias. It is a highly negatively inotropic calcium channel-blocker and it reduces cardiac output, slows the heart rate, and may impair atrioventricular conduction. It may precipitate heart failure, exacerbate conduction disorders, and cause hypotension at high doses and should **not** be used with beta-blockers. Constipation is the most common side-effect.

Nifedipine relaxes vascular smooth muscle and dilates coronary and peripheral arteries. It has more influence on vessels and less on the myocardium than does verapamil hydrochloride, and unlike verapamil hydrochloride has no anti-arrhythmic activity. It rarely precipitates heart failure because any negative inotropic effect is offset by a reduction in left ventricular work.

Nicardipine hydrochloride has similar effects to those of nifedipine and may produce less reduction of myocardial contractility. Amlodipine and felodipine also resemble nifedipine and nicardipine hydrochloride in their effects and do not reduce myocardial contractility and they do not produce clinical deterioration in heart failure. They have a longer duration of action and can be given once daily. Nifedipine, nicardipine hydrochloride, amlodipine, and felodipine are used for the treatment of angina or hypertension. All are valuable in forms of angina associated with coronary vasospasm. Side-effects associated with vasodilatation such as flushing and headache (which become less obtrusive after a few days), and ankle swelling (which may respond only partially to diuretics) are common.

Intravenous nicardipine hydrochloride is licensed for the treatment of acute life-threatening hypertension, for example in the event of malignant arterial hypertension or hypertensive encephalopathy; aortic dissection, when a short-acting beta-blocker is not suitable, or in combination with a beta-blocker when beta-blockade alone is not effective; severe pre-eclampsia, when other intravenous anti-hypertensives are not recommended or are contra-indicated; and for treatment of postoperative hypertension.

Lacidipine and lercanidipine hydrochloride have similar effects to those of nifedipine and nicardipine hydrochloride; they are indicated for hypertension only.

Nimodipine is related to nifedipine but the smooth muscle relaxant effect preferentially acts on cerebral arteries. Its use is confined to prevention and treatment of vascular spasm following aneurysmal subarachnoid haemorrhage.

Diltiazem hydrochloride is effective in most forms of angina; the longer-acting formulation is also used for hypertension. It may be used in patients for whom beta-blockers are contra-indicated or ineffective. It has a less negative inotropic effect than verapamil hydrochloride and significant myocardial depression occurs rarely. Nevertheless because of the risk of bradycardia it should be used with caution in association with beta-blockers.

Calcium-channel blockers 

● **DRUG ACTION** Calcium-channel blockers (less correctly called 'calcium-antagonists') interfere with the inward displacement of calcium ions through the slow channels of active cell membranes. They influence the myocardial cells, the cells within the specialised conducting system of the heart, and the cells of vascular smooth muscle. Thus, myocardial contractility may be reduced, the formation and propagation of electrical impulses within the heart

Cardiovascular system

Cardiovascular system

2

may be depressed, and coronary or systemic vascular tone may be diminished.

- CAUTIONS
- ► Elderly Screening Tool of Older Persons' potentially inappropriate Prescriptions (STOPP) criteria to aid medication reviews (see Prescribing in the elderly p. 31 for information): potentially inappropriate with persistent postural hypotension i.e. recurrent drop in systolic blood pressure ≥ 20 mmHg (risk of syncope and falls).

- SIDE-EFFECTS
- ► **Common or very common** Abdominal pain · dizziness · drowsiness · flushing · headache · nausea · palpitations · peripheral oedema · skin reactions · tachycardia · vomiting
- ► **Uncommon** Angioedema · depression · erectile dysfunction · gingival hyperplasia · myalgia · paraesthesia · syncope

Overdose Features of calcium-channel blocker poisoning include nausea, vomiting, dizziness, agitation, confusion, and coma in severe poisoning. Metabolic acidosis and hyperglycaemia may occur. In overdose, the dihydropyridine calcium-channel blockers cause severe hypotension secondary to profound peripheral vasodilatation. For details on the management of poisoning, see Calcium-channel blockers, under Emergency treatment of poisoning.

- HEPATIC IMPAIRMENT In general, manufacturers advise caution (risk of increased exposure).

- TREATMENT CESSATION There is some evidence that sudden withdrawal of calcium-channel blockers may be associated with an exacerbation of myocardial ischaemia.

◄ 183

Amlodipine

03-Mar-2022

- DRUG ACTION Amlodipine is a dihydropyridine calcium-channel blocker.

- **INDICATIONS AND DOSE**

Angina | Hypertension
- ► BY MOUTH
- ► Adult: Initially 5 mg once daily; increased if necessary up to 10 mg once daily

DOSE EQUIVALENCE AND CONVERSION
- ► Tablets from various suppliers may contain different salts (e.g. amlodipine besilate, amlodipine maleate, and amlodipine mesilate) but the strength is expressed in terms of amlodipine (base); tablets containing different salts are considered interchangeable.

IMPORTANT SAFETY INFORMATION

SAFE PRACTICE
Amlodipine has been confused with nimodipine and atenolol; care must be taken to ensure the correct drug is prescribed and dispensed.

- CONTRA-INDICATIONS Cardiogenic shock · significant aortic stenosis · unstable angina
- INTERACTIONS → Appendix 1: calcium channel blockers
- SIDE-EFFECTS
- ► **Common or very common** Asthenia · constipation · diarrhoea · dyspepsia · dyspnoea · gastrointestinal disorders · joint disorders · muscle cramps · oedema · vision disorders
- ► **Uncommon** Alopecia · anxiety · arrhythmias · chest pain · cough · dry mouth · gynaecomastia · hyperhidrosis · hypotension · insomnia · malaise · mood altered · numbness · pain · rhinitis · taste altered · tinnitus · tremor · urinary disorders · weight changes
- ► **Rare or very rare** Confusion · hepatic disorders · hyperglycaemia · leucopenia · muscle tone increased · myocardial infarction · pancreatitis · peripheral

neuropathy · photosensitivity reaction · severe cutaneous adverse reactions (SCARs) · thrombocytopenia · vasculitis
- ► **Frequency not known** Extrapyramidal symptoms · pulmonary oedema

- PREGNANCY No information available—manufacturer advises avoid, but risk to fetus should be balanced against risk of uncontrolled maternal hypertension.

- BREAST FEEDING Manufacturer advises avoid—no information available.

- HEPATIC IMPAIRMENT

Dose adjustments Manufacturer advises initiate at low dose and titrate slowly (limited information available).

- DIRECTIONS FOR ADMINISTRATION Expert sources advise tablets may be dispersed in water.

- MEDICINAL FORMS There can be variation in the licensing of different medicines containing the same drug. Forms available from special-order manufacturers include: oral suspension, oral solution

Oral tablet
- ► Amlodipine (Non-proprietary)
  Amlodipine 2.5 mg Amlodipine 2.5mg tablets | 28 tablet [PoM] £10.53 DT = £4.50
  Amlodipine 5 mg Amlodipine 5mg tablets | 28 tablet [PoM] £9.42 DT = £0.59 | 500 tablet [PoM] £9.87–£10.54
  Amlodipine 10 mg Amlodipine 10mg tablets | 28 tablet [PoM] £14.07 DT = £0.62 | 500 tablet [PoM] £10.17–£11.07
- ► Istin (Viatris UK Healthcare Ltd)
  Amlodipine 5 mg Istin 5mg tablets | 28 tablet [PoM] £11.08 DT = £0.59
  Amlodipine 10 mg Istin 10mg tablets | 28 tablet [PoM] £16.55 DT = £0.62

Oral solution
- ► Amlodipine (Non-proprietary)
  Amlodipine 1 mg per 1 ml Amlodipine 5mg/5ml oral solution sugar free | 150 ml [PoM] £72.00 DT = £70.96 [SF]
  Amlodipine 2 mg per 1 ml Amlodipine 10mg/5ml oral solution sugar free | 150 ml [PoM] £110.00 DT = £71.07 [SF]

Oral suspension
- ► Amlodipine (Non-proprietary)
  Amlodipine 1 mg per 1 ml Amlodipine 5mg/5ml oral suspension sugar free | 150 ml [PoM] £70.00 DT = £70.00 [SF]

Combinations available: *Olmesartan with amlodipine*, p. 204 · *Olmesartan with amlodipine and hydrochlorothiazide*, p. 205 · *Perindopril erbumine with amlodipine*, p. 199

Amlodipine with valsartan

22-Dec-2020

The properties listed below are those particular to the combination only. For the properties of the components please consider, amlodipine above, valsartan p. 206.

- **INDICATIONS AND DOSE**

Hypertension in patients stabilised on the individual components in the same proportions
- ► BY MOUTH
- ► Adult: (consult product literature)

- INTERACTIONS → Appendix 1: angiotensin-II receptor antagonists · calcium channel blockers

- MEDICINAL FORMS There can be variation in the licensing of different medicines containing the same drug.

Oral tablet
- ► Amlodipine with valsartan (Non-proprietary)
  Amlodipine (as Amlodipine besilate) 5 mg, Valsartan 80 mg Amlodipine 5mg / Valsartan 80mg tablets | 28 tablet [PoM] £19.10–£30.00 DT = £20.11
  Amlodipine (as Amlodipine besilate) 10 mg, Valsartan 160 mg Amlodipine 10mg / Valsartan 160mg tablets | 28 tablet [PoM] £21.58–£40.00 DT = £26.51
  Amlodipine (as Amlodipine besilate) 5 mg, Valsartan 160 mg Amlodipine 5mg / Valsartan 160mg tablets | 28 tablet [PoM] £25.18–£42.00 DT = £26.51

▸ Exforge (Novartis Pharmaceuticals UK Ltd)
**Amlodipine (as Amlodipine besilate) 5 mg, Valsartan
80 mg** Exforge 5mg/80mg tablets | 28 tablet [PoM] £20.11 DT =
£20.11
**Amlodipine (as Amlodipine besilate) 10 mg, Valsartan
160 mg** Exforge 10mg/160mg tablets | 28 tablet [PoM] £26.51 DT =
£26.51
**Amlodipine (as Amlodipine besilate) 5 mg, Valsartan
160 mg** Exforge 5mg/160mg tablets | 28 tablet [PoM] £26.51 DT =
£26.51

▶ 183

Diltiazem hydrochloride
15-Apr-2024

● **INDICATIONS AND DOSE**

Prophylaxis and treatment of angina
▸ BY MOUTH
▸ Adult: Initially 60 mg 3 times a day, adjusted according
to response; maximum 360 mg per day
▸ Elderly: Initially 60 mg twice daily, adjusted according
to response; maximum 360 mg per day

Chronic anal fissure
▸ BY RECTUM USING CREAM, OR BY RECTUM USING OINTMENT
▸ Adult: Apply twice daily until pain stops. Max. duration
of use 8 weeks, apply to the anal canal, using 2% topical
preparation
▸ BY MOUTH
▸ Adult: 60 mg twice daily until pain stops. Max. duration
of use 8 weeks

ADIZEM-SR ® CAPSULES

Mild to moderate hypertension
▸ BY MOUTH
▸ Adult: 120 mg twice daily, dose form not appropriate
for initial dose titration

Angina
▸ BY MOUTH
▸ Adult: Initially 90 mg twice daily; increased if necessary
to 180 mg twice daily, dose form not appropriate for
initial dose titration in the elderly

ADIZEM-XL ®

Angina | Mild to moderate hypertension
▸ BY MOUTH
▸ Adult: Initially 240 mg once daily, increased if
necessary to 300 mg once daily
▸ Elderly: Initially 120 mg once daily, increased if
necessary up to 300 mg once daily

ANGITIL ® SR

Angina | Mild to moderate hypertension
▸ BY MOUTH
▸ Adult: Initially 90 mg twice daily; increased if necessary
to 120–180 mg twice daily

ANGITIL ® XL

Angina | Mild to moderate hypertension
▸ BY MOUTH
▸ Adult: Initially 240 mg once daily; increased if
necessary to 300 mg once daily, dose form not
appropriate for initial dose titration in the elderly

DILCARDIA ® SR

Angina | Mild to moderate hypertension
▸ BY MOUTH
▸ Adult: Initially 90 mg twice daily; increased if necessary
to 180 mg twice daily
▸ Elderly: Initially 60 mg twice daily; increased if
necessary to 90 mg twice daily

DILZEM ® SR

Angina | Mild to moderate hypertension
▸ BY MOUTH
▸ Adult: Initially 90 mg twice daily; increased if necessary
up to 180 mg twice daily

▸ Elderly: Initially 60 mg twice daily; increased if
necessary up to 180 mg twice daily

DILZEM ® XL

Angina | Mild to moderate hypertension
▸ BY MOUTH
▸ Adult: Initially 180 mg once daily; increased if
necessary to 360 mg once daily
▸ Elderly: Initially 120 mg once daily; increased if
necessary to 360 mg once daily

SLOZEM ®

Angina | Mild to moderate hypertension
▸ BY MOUTH
▸ Adult: Initially 240 mg once daily; increased if
necessary to 360 mg once daily
▸ Elderly: Initially 120 mg once daily; increased if
necessary to 360 mg once daily

TILDIEM RETARD ®

Mild to moderate hypertension
▸ BY MOUTH
▸ Adult: Initially 90–120 mg twice daily; increased if
necessary to 360 mg daily in divided doses
▸ Elderly: Initially 120 mg once daily; increased if
necessary to 120 mg twice daily

Angina
▸ BY MOUTH
▸ Adult: Initially 90–120 mg twice daily; increased if
necessary to 480 mg daily in divided doses
▸ Elderly: Up to 120 mg twice daily, dose form not
appropriate for initial dose titration

TILDIEM ® LA

Angina | Mild to moderate hypertension
▸ BY MOUTH
▸ Adult: Initially 200 mg once daily, to be taken with or
before food, increased if necessary to 300–400 mg once
daily; maximum 500 mg per day
▸ Elderly: Initially 200 mg once daily, increased if
necessary to 300 mg once daily

VIAZEM ® XL

Angina | Mild to moderate hypertension
▸ BY MOUTH
▸ Adult: Initially 180 mg once daily, adjusted according
to response to 240 mg once daily; maximum 360 mg
per day
▸ Elderly: Initially 120 mg once daily, adjusted according
to response

ZEMTARD ®

Angina
▸ BY MOUTH
▸ Adult: 180–300 mg once daily, increased if necessary to
480 mg once daily
▸ Elderly: Initially 120 mg once daily, increased if
necessary to 480 mg once daily

Mild to moderate hypertension
▸ BY MOUTH
▸ Adult: 180–300 mg once daily, increased if necessary to
360 mg once daily
▸ Elderly: Initially 120 mg once daily, increased if
necessary to 360 mg once daily

● **UNLICENSED USE** [EvGr] Diltiazem is used for the treatment
of chronic anal fissures, ◇E◇ but it is not licensed for this
indication.

● **CONTRA-INDICATIONS**
▸ With systemic use Acute porphyrias p. 1202 · cardiogenic
shock · heart failure (with reduced ejection fraction) · left
ventricular failure with pulmonary congestion · second- or
third-degree AV block (unless pacemaker fitted) · severe
bradycardia · sick sinus syndrome · significant aortic
stenosis

Cardiovascular system

2

CONTRA-INDICATIONS, FURTHER INFORMATION Systemic absorption following rectal use is unknown, therefore consider the possibility of contra-indications listed for systemic use.

● CAUTIONS
▶ With systemic use Bradycardia (avoid if severe) · first degree AV block · prolonged PR interval · significantly impaired left ventricular function

CAUTIONS, FURTHER INFORMATION Systemic absorption following rectal use is unknown, therefore consider the possibility of cautions listed for systemic use.
▶ Elderly Screening Tool of Older Persons' potentially inappropriate Prescriptions (STOPP) criteria to aid medication reviews (see Prescribing in the elderly p. 31 for information): potentially inappropriate in patients with NYHA Class III or IV heart failure (contra-indicated in heart failure with reduced ejection fraction; may worsen heart failure).

● INTERACTIONS → Appendix 1: calcium channel blockers

● SIDE-EFFECTS
▶ **Common or very common** Cardiac conduction disorders · constipation · gastrointestinal discomfort · malaise
▶ **Uncommon** Arrhythmias · diarrhoea · insomnia · nervousness · postural hypotension
▶ **Rare or very rare** Dry mouth
▶ **Frequency not known** Cardiac arrest · congestive heart failure · extrapyramidal symptoms · fever · gynaecomastia · hepatitis · hyperglycaemia · hyperhidrosis · mood altered · photosensitivity reaction · severe cutaneous adverse reactions (SCARs) · thrombocytopenia · vasculitis

SIDE-EFFECTS, FURTHER INFORMATION Systemic absorption following rectal use is unknown, therefore consider the possibility of side-effects listed for oral use.

Overdose
▶ With oral use In overdose, diltiazem has a profound cardiac depressant effect causing hypotension and arrhythmias, including complete heart block and asystole.

● PREGNANCY
▶ With systemic use Avoid.

● BREAST FEEDING
▶ With systemic use Significant amount present in milk—no evidence of harm but avoid unless no safer alternative.

● HEPATIC IMPAIRMENT
Dose adjustments
▶ With systemic use In general, manufacturers advise initial dose reduction to 60 mg twice daily (or 120 mg daily if using a once daily formulation), increased gradually as required.

ADIZEM-SR ® CAPSULES Dose form not appropriate for initial dose titration.

ANGITIL ® SR Dose form not appropriate for initial dose titration.

ANGITIL ® XL Dose form not appropriate for initial dose titration.

DILCARDIA ® SR Dose form not appropriate for initial titration; manufacturer advises maximum 90 mg twice daily in hypertension.

TILDIEM RETARD ® For *treatment of angina*, dose form not appropriate for initial titration; manufacturer advises maximum 120 mg twice daily.

   For *mild to moderate hypertension*, manufacturer advises initial dose reduction to 120 mg once daily; maximum 120 mg twice daily.

TILDIEM ® LA Manufacturer advises initial dose 200 mg daily; maximum 300 mg daily.

● RENAL IMPAIRMENT
Dose adjustments
▶ With systemic use In general, manufacturers advise initial dose 60 mg twice daily (or 120 mg daily if using a once daily

formulation), increased gradually as required (risk of increased exposure).

ADIZEM-SR ® CAPSULES Dose form not appropriate for initial dose titration.

ANGITIL ® SR Dose form not appropriate for initial dose titration.

ANGITIL ® XL Dose form not appropriate for initial dose titration.

DILCARDIA ® SR Dose form not appropriate for initial titration; manufacturer advises max. dose 90 mg twice daily in hypertension.

TILDIEM RETARD ® For *mild to moderate hypertension*, manufacturer advises initial dose 120 mg once daily; max. dose 120 mg twice daily.

   For *treatment of angina*, dose form not appropriate for initial titration; manufacturer advises max. dose 120 mg twice daily.

TILDIEM ® LA Manufacturer advises initial dose 200 mg daily; max. dose 300 mg daily.

● PRESCRIBING AND DISPENSING INFORMATION
▶ With systemic use The standard formulations containing 60 mg diltiazem hydrochloride are licensed as generics and there is no requirement for brand name dispensing. Although their means of formulation has called for the strict designation 'modified-release', their duration of action corresponds to that of tablets requiring administration more frequently. Different versions of modified-release preparations containing more than 60 mg diltiazem hydrochloride may not have the same clinical effect. To avoid confusion between these different formulations of diltiazem, prescribers should specify the brand to be dispensed.

● PATIENT AND CARER ADVICE

TILDIEM RETARD ® Tablet membrane may pass through gastro-intestinal tract unchanged, but being porous has no effect on efficacy.

● MEDICINAL FORMS There can be variation in the licensing of different medicines containing the same drug. Forms available from special-order manufacturers include: oral suspension, oral solution

Modified-release tablet
CAUTIONARY AND ADVISORY LABELS 25
▶ Diltiazem hydrochloride (Non-proprietary)
   Diltiazem hydrochloride 60 mg Diltiazem 60mg modified-release tablets | 84 tablet [PoM] £12.59 DT = £6.28 | 90 tablet [PoM] £6.49 | 100 tablet [PoM] £29.01
▶ Retalzem (Kent Pharma (UK) Ltd)
   Diltiazem hydrochloride 60 mg Retalzem 60 modified-release tablets | 84 tablet [PoM] £7.43 DT = £6.28
▶ Tildiem (Sanofi)
   Diltiazem hydrochloride 60 mg Tildiem 60mg modified-release tablets | 90 tablet [PoM] £7.96
▶ Tildiem Retard (Sanofi)
   Diltiazem hydrochloride 90 mg Tildiem Retard 90mg tablets | 56 tablet [PoM] £7.27 DT = £7.27
   Diltiazem hydrochloride 120 mg Tildiem Retard 120mg tablets | 56 tablet [PoM] £7.15 DT = £7.15
▶ Zeyam (Ennogen Healthcare International Ltd)
   Diltiazem hydrochloride 60 mg Zeyam 60mg modified-release tablets | 84 tablet [PoM] £6.45 DT = £6.28

Modified-release capsule
CAUTIONARY AND ADVISORY LABELS 25
▶ Adizem-SR (Napp Pharmaceuticals Ltd)
   Diltiazem hydrochloride 90 mg Adizem-SR 90mg capsules | 56 capsule [PoM] £8.50 DT = £8.50
   Diltiazem hydrochloride 120 mg Adizem-SR 120mg capsules | 56 capsule [PoM] £9.45 DT = £9.45
   Diltiazem hydrochloride 180 mg Adizem-SR 180mg capsules | 56 capsule [PoM] £14.15 DT = £14.15
▶ Adizem-XL (Napp Pharmaceuticals Ltd)
   Diltiazem hydrochloride 120 mg Adizem-XL 120mg capsules | 28 capsule [PoM] £9.14 DT = £9.14

2

Cardiovascular system

Diltiazem hydrochloride 180 mg Adizem-XL 180mg capsules |
28 capsule [PoM] £10.37 DT = £10.37
Diltiazem hydrochloride 200 mg Adizem-XL 200mg capsules |
28 capsule [PoM] £6.30 DT = £6.29
Diltiazem hydrochloride 240 mg Adizem-XL 240mg capsules |
28 capsule [PoM] £11.52 DT = £11.52
Diltiazem hydrochloride 300 mg Adizem-XL 300mg capsules |
28 capsule [PoM] £9.14 DT = £9.01

► **Angitil SR** (Ethypharm UK Ltd)
Diltiazem hydrochloride 90 mg Angitil SR 90 capsules |
56 capsule [PoM] £7.03 DT = £8.50
Diltiazem hydrochloride 120 mg Angitil SR 120 capsules |
56 capsule [PoM] £6.91 DT = £9.45
Diltiazem hydrochloride 180 mg Angitil SR 180 capsules |
56 capsule [PoM] £13.27 DT = £14.15

► **Angitil XL** (Ethypharm UK Ltd)
Diltiazem hydrochloride 240 mg Angitil XL 240 capsules |
28 capsule [PoM] £7.94 DT = £11.52
Diltiazem hydrochloride 300 mg Angitil XL 300 capsules |
28 capsule [PoM] £6.98 DT = £9.01

► **Slozem** (Zentiva Pharma UK Ltd)
Diltiazem hydrochloride 120 mg Slozem 120mg capsules |
28 capsule [PoM] £5.49 DT = £9.14
Diltiazem hydrochloride 180 mg Slozem 180mg capsules |
28 capsule [PoM] £5.58 DT = £10.37
Diltiazem hydrochloride 240 mg Slozem 240mg capsules |
28 capsule [PoM] £5.67 DT = £11.52
Diltiazem hydrochloride 300 mg Slozem 300mg capsules |
28 capsule [PoM] £6.03 DT = £9.01

► **Tildiem LA** (Sanofi)
Diltiazem hydrochloride 200 mg Tildiem LA 200 capsules |
28 capsule [PoM] £6.29 DT = £6.29
Diltiazem hydrochloride 300 mg Tildiem LA 300 capsules |
28 capsule [PoM] £9.01 DT = £9.01

► **Viazem XL** (Thornton & Ross Ltd)
Diltiazem hydrochloride 120 mg Viazem XL 120mg capsules |
28 capsule [PoM] £6.60 DT = £9.14
Diltiazem hydrochloride 180 mg Viazem XL 180mg capsules |
28 capsule [PoM] £7.36 DT = £10.37
Diltiazem hydrochloride 240 mg Viazem XL 240mg capsules |
28 capsule [PoM] £7.74 DT = £11.52
Diltiazem hydrochloride 300 mg Viazem XL 300mg capsules |
28 capsule [PoM] £8.03 DT = £9.01
Diltiazem hydrochloride 360 mg Viazem XL 360mg capsules |
28 capsule [PoM] £13.85 DT = £13.85

► **Zemtard XL** (Galen Ltd)
Diltiazem hydrochloride 120 mg Zemtard 120 XL capsules |
28 capsule [PoM] £6.10 DT = £9.14
Diltiazem hydrochloride 180 mg Zemtard 180 XL capsules |
28 capsule [PoM] £6.20 DT = £10.37
Diltiazem hydrochloride 240 mg Zemtard 240 XL capsules |
28 capsule [PoM] £6.30 DT = £11.52
Diltiazem hydrochloride 300 mg Zemtard 300 XL capsules |
28 capsule [PoM] £6.70 DT = £9.01

⌐ 183

Felodipine

12-May-2023

● **DRUG ACTION** Felodipine is a dihydropyridine calcium-channel blocker.

● **INDICATIONS AND DOSE**

Prophylaxis of angina
► BY MOUTH
► Adult: Initially 5 mg once daily, to be taken in the morning; increased if necessary to 10 mg once daily
► Elderly: Initially 2.5 mg once daily, to be taken in the morning; increased if necessary up to 10 mg once daily

Hypertension
► BY MOUTH
► Adult: Initially 5 mg once daily, to be taken in the morning; usual maintenance 5–10 mg once daily, doses above 20 mg per day rarely needed
► Elderly: Initially 2.5 mg once daily, to be taken in the morning; usual maintenance 5–10 mg once daily, doses above 20 mg per day rarely needed

● **CONTRA-INDICATIONS** Cardiac outflow obstruction · significant cardiac valvular obstruction (e.g. aortic stenosis) · uncontrolled heart failure · unstable angina · within 1 month of myocardial infarction

● **CAUTIONS** Predisposition to tachycardia · severe left ventricular dysfunction

CAUTIONS, FURTHER INFORMATION Manufacturer advises discontinue if ischaemic pain occurs or existing pain worsens shortly after initiating treatment.

● **INTERACTIONS** → Appendix 1: calcium channel blockers

● **SIDE-EFFECTS**
► **Uncommon** Fatigue
► **Rare or very rare** Arthralgia · gingivitis · hypersensitivity vasculitis · photosensitivity reaction · sexual dysfunction · urinary frequency increased

● **PREGNANCY** Avoid; toxicity in *animal* studies; may inhibit labour.

● **BREAST FEEDING** Present in milk but amount probably too small to be harmful.

● **HEPATIC IMPAIRMENT**
Dose adjustments Manufacturer advises consider dose reduction.

● **MEDICINAL FORMS** There can be variation in the licensing of different medicines containing the same drug. Forms available from special-order manufacturers include: oral solution
Modified-release tablet
CAUTIONARY AND ADVISORY LABELS 25
► **Felodipine** (Non-proprietary)
Felodipine 2.5 mg Felodipine 2.5mg modified-release tablets |
28 tablet [PoM] £6.31 DT = £5.68
Felodipine 5 mg Felodipine 5mg modified-release tablets |
28 tablet [PoM] £1.99 DT = £3.87
Felodipine 10 mg Felodipine 10mg modified-release tablets |
28 tablet [PoM] £1.99 DT = £4.81
► **Cardioplen XL** (Chiesi Ltd)
Felodipine 2.5 mg Cardioplen XL 2.5mg tablets | 28 tablet [PoM]
£5.68 DT = £5.68
Felodipine 5 mg Cardioplen XL 5mg tablets | 28 tablet [PoM] £3.87
DT = £3.87
Felodipine 10 mg Cardioplen XL 10mg tablets | 28 tablet [PoM]
£4.81 DT = £4.81
► **Delofine XL** (Morningside Healthcare Ltd)
Felodipine 2.5 mg Delofine XL 2.5mg tablets | 28 tablet [PoM] £4.25
DT = £5.68
Felodipine 5 mg Delofine XL 5mg tablets | 28 tablet [PoM] £1.98 DT
= £3.87
Felodipine 10 mg Delofine XL 10mg tablets | 28 tablet [PoM] £1.98
DT = £4.81
► **Neofel XL** (Kent Pharma (UK) Ltd)
Felodipine 2.5 mg Neofel XL 2.5mg tablets | 28 tablet [PoM] £6.31
DT = £5.68
Felodipine 5 mg Neofel XL 5mg tablets | 28 tablet [PoM] £4.21 DT =
£3.87
Felodipine 10 mg Neofel XL 10mg tablets | 28 tablet [PoM] £5.66 DT
= £4.81
► **Parmid XL** (Sandoz Ltd)
Felodipine 2.5 mg Parmid XL 2.5mg tablets | 28 tablet [PoM] £5.36
DT = £5.68
► **Pinefeld XL** (Tillomed Laboratories Ltd)
Felodipine 10 mg Pinefeld XL 10mg tablets | 28 tablet [PoM] £11.98
DT = £4.81
► **Vascalpha** (Accord-UK Ltd)
Felodipine 5 mg Vascalpha 5mg modified-release tablets |
28 tablet [PoM] £1.99 DT = £3.87
Felodipine 10 mg Vascalpha 10mg modified-release tablets |
28 tablet [PoM] £1.99 DT = £4.81

Combinations available: *Ramipril with felodipine,* p. 200

Lacidipine

📖 183

22-Dec-2020

- **DRUG ACTION** Lacidipine is a dihydropyridine calcium-channel blocker.

● INDICATIONS AND DOSE

Hypertension
▶ BY MOUTH
▶ Adult: Initially 2 mg daily; increased if necessary to 4 mg daily, then increased if necessary to 6 mg daily, dose increases should occur at intervals of 3–4 weeks, to be taken preferably in the morning

- **CONTRA-INDICATIONS** Acute porphyrias p. 1202 · aortic stenosis · avoid within 1 month of myocardial infarction · cardiogenic shock · unstable angina

- **CAUTIONS** Cardiac conduction abnormalities · poor cardiac reserve

- **INTERACTIONS** → Appendix 1: calcium channel blockers

- **SIDE-EFFECTS**
▶ **Common or very common** Abdominal discomfort · asthenia · polyuria
▶ **Uncommon** Ischaemic heart disease
▶ **Rare or very rare** Muscle cramps · tremor

- **PREGNANCY** Manufacturer advises avoid; may inhibit labour.

- **BREAST FEEDING** Manufacturer advises avoid—no information available.

- **HEPATIC IMPAIRMENT**
Dose adjustments Manufacturer advises consider dose reduction if hypotension occurs.

- **MEDICINAL FORMS** There can be variation in the licensing of different medicines containing the same drug.
Oral tablet
▶ Lacidipine (Non-proprietary)
Lacidipine 2 mg Lacidipine 2mg tablets | 28 tablet [PoM] £3.00 DT = £2.37
Lacidipine 4 mg Lacidipine 4mg tablets | 28 tablet [PoM] £3.30 DT = £2.51
▶ Motens (GlaxoSmithKline UK Ltd)
Lacidipine 2 mg Motens 2mg tablets | 28 tablet [PoM] £2.95 DT = £2.37
Lacidipine 4 mg Motens 4mg tablets | 28 tablet [PoM] £3.10 DT = £2.51

Lercanidipine hydrochloride

📖 183

02-Aug-2021

- **DRUG ACTION** Lercanidipine is a dihydropyridine calcium-channel blocker.

● INDICATIONS AND DOSE

Mild to moderate hypertension
▶ BY MOUTH
▶ Adult: Initially 10 mg once daily; increased if necessary to 20 mg daily, dose can be adjusted after 2 weeks

- **CONTRA-INDICATIONS** Aortic stenosis · uncontrolled heart failure · unstable angina · within 1 month of myocardial infarction

- **CAUTIONS** Left ventricular dysfunction · sick sinus syndrome (if pacemaker not fitted)

- **INTERACTIONS** → Appendix 1: calcium channel blockers

- **SIDE-EFFECTS**
▶ **Rare or very rare** Angina pectoris · asthenia · chest pain · diarrhoea · dyspepsia · urinary disorders

- **PREGNANCY** Manufacturer advises avoid—no information available.

- **BREAST FEEDING** Manufacturer advises avoid.

- **HEPATIC IMPAIRMENT** Manufacturer advises avoid in severe impairment.

- **RENAL IMPAIRMENT** [EvGr] Caution in mild to moderate impairment; avoid if eGFR less than 30 mL/minute/1.73 m^2. Ⓜ See p. 21.

- **MEDICINAL FORMS** There can be variation in the licensing of different medicines containing the same drug.
Oral tablet
CAUTIONARY AND ADVISORY LABELS 22
▶ Lercanidipine hydrochloride (Non-proprietary)
Lercanidipine hydrochloride 10 mg Lercanidipine 10mg tablets | 28 tablet [PoM] £12.99 DT = £1.86
Lercanidipine hydrochloride 20 mg Lercanidipine 20mg tablets | 28 tablet [PoM] £15.99 DT = £2.98
▶ Zanidip (Recordati Pharmaceuticals Ltd)
Lercanidipine hydrochloride 10 mg Zanidip 10mg tablets | 28 tablet [PoM] £5.70 DT = £1.86
Lercanidipine hydrochloride 20 mg Zanidip 20mg tablets | 28 tablet [PoM] £10.82 DT = £2.98

Nicardipine hydrochloride

📖 183

04-Jan-2022

- **DRUG ACTION** Nicardipine is a dihydropyridine calcium-channel blocker.

● INDICATIONS AND DOSE

Prophylaxis of angina
▶ BY MOUTH USING IMMEDIATE-RELEASE MEDICINES
▶ Adult: Initially 20 mg 3 times a day, then increased to 30 mg 3 times a day, dose increased after at least 3 days; usual dose 60–120 mg daily

Mild to moderate hypertension
▶ BY MOUTH USING IMMEDIATE-RELEASE MEDICINES
▶ Adult: Initially 20 mg 3 times a day, then increased to 30 mg 3 times a day, dose increased after at least 3 days; usual dose 60–120 mg daily

Life-threatening hypertension (specialist use only) | Post-operative hypertension (specialist use only)
▶ BY CONTINUOUS INTRAVENOUS INFUSION
▶ Adult: Initially 3–5 mg/hour for 15 minutes, increased in steps of 0.5–1 mg every 15 minutes, adjusted according to response, maximum rate 15 mg/hour, reduce dose gradually when target blood pressure achieved; maintenance 2–4 mg/hour
▶ Elderly: Initially 1–5 mg/hour, then adjusted in steps of 500 micrograms/hour after 30 minutes, adjusted according to response, maximum rate 15 mg/hour

Life-threatening hypertension in patients with hepatic or renal impairment (specialist use only) | Postoperative hypertension in patients with hepatic or renal impairment (specialist use only)
▶ BY CONTINUOUS INTRAVENOUS INFUSION
▶ Adult: Initially 1–5 mg/hour, then adjusted in steps of 500 micrograms/hour after 30 minutes, adjusted according to response, maximum rate 15 mg/hour

Acute life-threatening hypertension in pregnancy (specialist use only)
▶ BY CONTINUOUS INTRAVENOUS INFUSION
▶ Adult: Initially 1–5 mg/hour, then adjusted in steps of 500 micrograms/hour after 30 minutes, adjusted according to response, usual maximum rate 4 mg/hour in treatment of pre-eclampsia (maximum rate 15 mg/hour)

- **CONTRA-INDICATIONS**
GENERAL CONTRA-INDICATIONS Acute porphyrias p. 1202 · cardiogenic shock · significant or advanced aortic stenosis · unstable or acute attacks of angina

SPECIFIC CONTRA-INDICATIONS
▶ With intravenous use Avoid within 8 days of myocardial infarction · compensatory hypertension

▶ **With oral use** Avoid within 1 month of myocardial infarction

● **CAUTIONS**

GENERAL CAUTIONS Congestive heart failure · elderly · increased risk of serious hypotension · ischaemic heart disease · pulmonary oedema · significantly impaired left ventricular function · stroke

SPECIFIC CAUTIONS

▶ **With intravenous use** Elevated intracranial pressure · portal hypertension

CAUTIONS, FURTHER INFORMATION Manufacturer advises discontinue if ischaemic pain occurs or existing pain worsens within 30 minutes of initiating treatment or increasing dose.

● **INTERACTIONS** → Appendix 1: calcium channel blockers

● **SIDE-EFFECTS**

GENERAL SIDE-EFFECTS

▶ **Common or very common** Hypotension

▶ **Frequency not known** Pulmonary oedema · thrombocytopenia

SPECIFIC SIDE-EFFECTS

▶ **With intravenous use** Atrioventricular block · hepatic disorders · ischaemic heart disease · paralytic ileus

▶ **With oral use** Abdominal distress · angina pectoris exacerbated · asthenia · dyspnoea · feeling hot · hepatic function abnormal · insomnia · nervous system disorder · renal impairment · tinnitus · urinary frequency increased

SIDE-EFFECTS, FURTHER INFORMATION Systemic hypotension and reflex tachycardia with rapid reduction of blood pressure may occur — during intravenous use consider stopping infusion or decreasing dose by half.

● **PREGNANCY** May inhibit labour. Not to be used in multiple pregnancy (twins or more) unless there is no other acceptable alternative. Toxicity in *animal* studies. Risk of severe maternal hypotension and fatal fetal hypoxia— avoid excessive decrease in blood pressure. For treatment of acute life-threatening hypertension only.

● **BREAST FEEDING** Manufacturer advises avoid—present in breast milk.

● **HEPATIC IMPAIRMENT**

Dose adjustments

▶ With oral use Manufacturer advises consider using lowest initial dose and extending dosing interval according to individual response.

▶ With intravenous use See *Indications and dose* section.

● **RENAL IMPAIRMENT** EvGr Caution (increased risk of serious hypotension). Ⓜ

Dose adjustments

▶ With oral use EvGr Consider using lowest initial dose and extending dosing interval according to individual response. Ⓜ

▶ With intravenous use See *Indications and dose* section.

● **MONITORING REQUIREMENTS** Monitor blood pressure and heart rate at least every 5 minutes during intravenous infusion, and then until stable, and continue monitoring for at least 12 hours after end of infusion.

● **DIRECTIONS FOR ADMINISTRATION** Intravenous nicardipine should only be administered under the supervision of a specialist and in a hospital or intensive care setting in which patients can be closely monitored. For *intravenous infusion*, manufacturer advises give continuously *in* Glucose 5%; dilute dose in infusion fluid to a final concentration of 100–200 micrograms/mL (undiluted solution *via* central venous line only) and give *via* volumetric infusion pump or syringe driver; protect from light; risk of adsorption on to plastic of infusion set in the presence of saline solutions; incompatible with bicarbonate or alkaline solutions—consult product

literature. To minimise peripheral venous irritation, expert sources advise change site of infusion every 12 hours.

● **MEDICINAL FORMS** There can be variation in the licensing of different medicines containing the same drug. Forms available from special-order manufacturers include: oral suspension, oral solution

Solution for infusion

▶ Nicardipine hydrochloride (Non-proprietary)

Nicardipine hydrochloride 1 mg per 1 ml Nicardipine 10mg/10ml solution for infusion ampoules | 5 ampoule [PoM] £85.00 (Hospital only)

Nicardipine hydrochloride 2.5 mg per 1 ml Cardene I.V. 25mg/10ml solution for infusion ampoules | 10 ampoule [PoM] Ⓢ (Hospital only)

Oral capsule

▶ Cardene (Laboratoire X.O)

Nicardipine hydrochloride 20 mg Cardene 20mg capsules | 56 capsule [PoM] £5.52 DT = £5.52

Nicardipine hydrochloride 30 mg Cardene 30mg capsules | 56 capsule [PoM] £6.40 DT = £6.40

▶ 183

Nifedipine
                                                                          24-Jul-2020

● **INDICATIONS AND DOSE**

Raynaud's syndrome

▶ BY MOUTH USING IMMEDIATE-RELEASE MEDICINES

▶ Adult: Initially 5 mg 3 times a day, then adjusted according to response to 20 mg 3 times a day

Angina prophylaxis (not recommended)

▶ BY MOUTH USING IMMEDIATE-RELEASE MEDICINES

▶ Adult: Initially 5 mg 3 times a day, then adjusted according to response to 20 mg 3 times a day

Postponement of premature labour

▶ BY MOUTH USING IMMEDIATE-RELEASE MEDICINES

▶ Adult: Initially 20 mg, followed by 10–20 mg 3–4 times a day, adjusted according to uterine activity

Hiccup in palliative care

▶ BY MOUTH USING IMMEDIATE-RELEASE MEDICINES

▶ Adult: 10 mg 3 times a day

Chronic anal fissure

▶ BY RECTUM USING OINTMENT

▶ Adult: Apply 2–3 times a day until pain stops. Max. duration of use 8 weeks, apply to anal canal, using 0.2%–0.5% topical preparation

▶ BY MOUTH USING MODIFIED-RELEASE MEDICINES

▶ Adult: 20 mg twice daily until pain stops. Max. duration of use 8 weeks

ADIPINE ® MR

Hypertension | Angina prophylaxis

▶ BY MOUTH

▶ Adult: 10 mg twice daily, adjusted according to response to 40 mg twice daily

ADIPINE ® XL

Hypertension | Angina prophylaxis

▶ BY MOUTH

▶ Adult: 30 mg daily, increased if necessary up to 90 mg daily

CORACTEN ® SR

Hypertension | Angina prophylaxis

▶ BY MOUTH

▶ Adult: Initially 10 mg twice daily, increased if necessary up to 40 mg twice daily

CORACTEN ® XL

Hypertension | Angina prophylaxis

▶ BY MOUTH

▶ Adult: Initially 30 mg daily, increased if necessary up to 90 mg daily
continued →

FORTIPINE® LA 40

Hypertension | Angina prophylaxis
▸ BY MOUTH
▸ Adult: Initially 40 mg once daily, increased if necessary to 80 mg daily in 1–2 divided doses

NIFEDIPRESS® MR

Hypertension | Angina prophylaxis
▸ BY MOUTH
▸ Adult: 10 mg twice daily, adjusted according to response to 40 mg twice daily

TENSIPINE® MR

Hypertension | Angina prophylaxis
▸ BY MOUTH
▸ Adult: Initially 10 mg twice daily, adjusted according to response to 40 mg twice daily

VALNI® XL

Severe hypertension | Prophylaxis of angina
▸ BY MOUTH
▸ Adult: 30 mg once daily, increased if necessary up to 90 mg once daily

● UNLICENSED USE Not licensed for use in postponing premature labour.
  EvGr Nifedipine is used for the treatment of chronic anal fissure, Ⓔ but is not licensed for this indication.

● CONTRA-INDICATIONS
▸ With systemic use Acute attacks of angina · cardiogenic shock · significant aortic stenosis · unstable angina · within 1 month of myocardial infarction

CONTRA-INDICATIONS, FURTHER INFORMATION Systemic absorption following rectal use is unknown, therefore consider the possibility of contra-indications listed for systemic use.

● CAUTIONS
▸ With systemic use Diabetes mellitus · elderly · heart failure · ischaemic pain · poor cardiac reserve · severe hypotension · short-acting formulations are not recommended for angina or long-term management of hypertension (their use may be associated with large variations in blood pressure and reflex tachycardia) · significantly impaired left ventricular function (heart failure deterioration observed)

CAUTIONS, FURTHER INFORMATION Systemic absorption following rectal use is unknown, therefore consider the possibility of cautions listed for systemic use.
▸ Ischaemic pain Manufacturer advises discontinue if ischaemic pain occurs or existing pain worsens shortly after initiating treatment.

VALNI® XL Dose form not appropriate for use where there is a history of oesophageal or gastro-intestinal obstruction, decreased lumen diameter of the gastro-intestinal tract, inflammatory bowel disease, or ileostomy after proctocolectomy.

● INTERACTIONS → Appendix 1: calcium channel blockers

● SIDE-EFFECTS
▸ **Common or very common** Constipation · malaise · oedema · vasodilation
▸ **Uncommon** Allergic oedema · anxiety · chills · diarrhoea · dry mouth · epistaxis · gastrointestinal discomfort · gastrointestinal disorders · hypotension · joint disorders · laryngeal oedema · migraine · muscle complaints · nasal congestion · pain · sleep disorders · tremor · urinary disorders · vertigo · vision disorders
▸ **Rare or very rare** Appetite decreased · burping · cardiovascular disorder · fever · hyperhidrosis · mood altered · sensation abnormal
▸ **Frequency not known** Agranulocytosis · bezoar · cerebral ischaemia · chest pain · dysphagia · dyspnoea · eye pain · gingival disorder · gynaecomastia (following long term

use) · hepatic disorders · hyperglycaemia · ischaemic heart disease · leucopenia · myasthenia gravis aggravated · photoallergic reaction · pulmonary oedema · telangiectasia · toxic epidermal necrolysis · weight decreased

SIDE-EFFECTS, FURTHER INFORMATION Systemic absorption following rectal use is unknown therefore consider the possibility of side-effects listed for oral use.

● PREGNANCY
▸ With systemic use May inhibit labour; manufacturer advises avoid before week 20, but risk to fetus should be balanced against risk of uncontrolled maternal hypertension. Use only if other treatment options are not indicated or have failed.

● BREAST FEEDING
▸ With systemic use Amount too small to be harmful but manufacturers advise avoid.

● HEPATIC IMPAIRMENT
▸ With oral use For once-daily preparations, manufacturers advise dose form not appropriate (owing to the duration of action of the formulation).
Dose adjustments
  ▸ With oral use Manufacturer advises consider dose reduction in severe impairment.

● DIRECTIONS FOR ADMINISTRATION

FORTIPINE® LA 40 Manufacturer advises take with or just after food, or a meal.

● PRESCRIBING AND DISPENSING INFORMATION Different versions of modified-release preparations may not have the same clinical effect. To avoid confusion between these different formulations of nifedipine, prescribers should specify the brand to be dispensed.

Palliative care For further information on the use of nifedipine in palliative care, see www.medicinescomplete.com/#/content/palliative/nifedipine.

● MEDICINAL FORMS There can be variation in the licensing of different medicines containing the same drug. Forms available from special-order manufacturers include: oral suspension, oral drops

Modified-release tablet
CAUTIONARY AND ADVISORY LABELS 25
▸ **Adalat LA** (Bayer Plc)
  Nifedipine 30 mg Adalat LA 30mg tablets | 28 tablet PoM £6.85 DT = £4.70
▸ **Adanif XL** (Advanz Pharma)
  Nifedipine 30 mg Adanif XL 30mg tablets | 28 tablet PoM £9.70 DT = £4.70
  Nifedipine 60 mg Adanif XL 60mg tablets | 28 tablet PoM £11.20 DT = £7.10
▸ **Adipine MR** (Chiesi Ltd)
  Nifedipine 10 mg Adipine MR 10 tablets | 56 tablet PoM £3.73 DT = £9.23
  Nifedipine 20 mg Adipine MR 20 tablets | 56 tablet PoM £5.21 DT = £10.06
▸ **Adipine XL** (Chiesi Ltd)
  Nifedipine 30 mg Adipine XL 30mg tablets | 28 tablet PoM £4.70 DT = £4.70
  Nifedipine 60 mg Adipine XL 60mg tablets | 28 tablet PoM £7.10 DT = £7.10
▸ **Dexipress MR** (Dexcel-Pharma Ltd)
  Nifedipine 20 mg Dexipress MR 20mg tablets | 56 tablet PoM £10.06 DT = £10.06
▸ **Fortipine LA** (Advanz Pharma)
  Nifedipine 40 mg Fortipine LA 40 tablets | 30 tablet PoM £14.40 DT = £14.40
▸ **Neozipine XL** (Kent Pharma (UK) Ltd)
  Nifedipine 30 mg Neozipine XL 30mg tablets | 28 tablet PoM £7.59 DT = £4.70
  Nifedipine 60 mg Neozipine XL 60mg tablets | 28 tablet PoM £9.03 DT = £7.10
▸ **Nifedipress MR** (Dexcel-Pharma Ltd)
  Nifedipine 10 mg Nifedipress MR 10 tablets | 56 tablet PoM £9.23 DT = £9.23

Nifedipine 20 mg Nifedipress MR 20 tablets | 56 tablet [PoM] £10.06 DT = £10.06
‣ Tensipine MR (Genus Pharmaceuticals Ltd)
  Nifedipine 10 mg Tensipine MR 10 tablets | 56 tablet [PoM] £4.30 DT = £9.23
  Nifedipine 20 mg Tensipine MR 20 tablets | 56 tablet [PoM] £5.49 DT = £10.06
‣ Valni Retard (Tillomed Laboratories Ltd)
  Nifedipine 20 mg Valni 20 Retard tablets | 56 tablet [PoM] £10.06 DT = £10.06

Modified-release capsule
CAUTIONARY AND ADVISORY LABELS 25
‣ Coracten SR (Teofarma S.r.l.)
  Nifedipine 10 mg Coracten SR 10mg capsules | 60 capsule [PoM] £3.90 DT = £3.90
  Nifedipine 20 mg Coracten SR 20mg capsules | 60 capsule [PoM] £5.41 DT = £5.41
‣ Coracten XL (Teofarma S.r.l.)
  Nifedipine 30 mg Coracten XL 30mg capsules | 28 capsule [PoM] £4.89 DT = £4.89
  Nifedipine 60 mg Coracten XL 60mg capsules | 28 capsule [PoM] £7.34 DT = £7.34

Oral capsule
‣ Nifedipine (Non-proprietary)
  Nifedipine 5 mg Nifedipine 5mg capsules | 90 capsule [PoM] £84.12 DT = £49.67
  Nifedipine 10 mg Nifedipine 10mg capsules | 90 capsule [PoM] £106.00 DT = £62.10

Oral drops
‣ Nifedipine (Non-proprietary)
  Nifedipine 20 mg per 1 ml Nifedipin-ratiopharm 20mg/ml oral drops | 30 ml [PoM] [⅀] DT = £26.34

[F 183]

Verapamil hydrochloride
15-Apr-2024

● **INDICATIONS AND DOSE**

Treatment of supraventricular arrhythmias
▶ BY MOUTH USING IMMEDIATE-RELEASE MEDICINES
‣ Adult: 40–120 mg 3 times a day
▶ BY SLOW INTRAVENOUS INJECTION
‣ Adult: 5–10 mg, to be given over 2 minutes, preferably with ECG monitoring
‣ Elderly: 5–10 mg, to be given over 3 minutes, preferably with ECG monitoring

Paroxysmal tachyarrhythmias
▶ BY SLOW INTRAVENOUS INJECTION
‣ Adult: Initially 5–10 mg, followed by 5 mg after 5–10 minutes if required, to be given over 2 minutes, preferably with ECG monitoring
‣ Elderly: Initially 5–10 mg, followed by 5 mg after 5–10 minutes if required, to be given over 3 minutes, preferably with ECG monitoring

Angina
▶ BY MOUTH USING IMMEDIATE-RELEASE MEDICINES
‣ Adult: 80–120 mg 3 times a day

Hypertension
▶ BY MOUTH USING IMMEDIATE-RELEASE MEDICINES
‣ Adult: 240–480 mg daily in 2–3 divided doses

Prophylaxis of cluster headache (initiated under specialist supervision)
▶ BY MOUTH USING IMMEDIATE-RELEASE MEDICINES
‣ Adult: 240–960 mg daily in 3–4 divided doses

HALF SECURON ® SR

Hypertension (in patients new to verapamil)
▶ BY MOUTH
‣ Adult: Initially 120 mg daily, increased if necessary up to 480 mg daily, doses above 240 mg daily as 2 divided doses

Hypertension
▶ BY MOUTH
‣ Adult: 240 mg daily, increased if necessary up to 480 mg daily, doses above 240 mg daily as 2 divided doses

Angina
▶ BY MOUTH
‣ Adult: 240 mg twice daily, may sometimes be reduced to once daily

Prophylaxis after myocardial infarction where beta-blockers not appropriate
▶ BY MOUTH
‣ Adult: 360 mg daily in divided doses, started at least 1 week after infarction, given as either 240 mg in the morning and 120 mg in the evening *or* 120 mg 3 times daily

SECURON ® SR

Hypertension (in patients new to verapamil)
▶ BY MOUTH
‣ Adult: Initially 120 mg daily, increased if necessary up to 480 mg daily, doses above 240 mg daily as 2 divided doses

Hypertension
▶ BY MOUTH
‣ Adult: 240 mg daily, increased if necessary up to 480 mg daily, doses above 240 mg daily as 2 divided doses

Angina
▶ BY MOUTH
‣ Adult: 240 mg twice daily, may sometimes be reduced to once daily

Prophylaxis after myocardial infarction where beta-blockers not appropriate
▶ BY MOUTH
‣ Adult: 360 mg daily in divided doses, started at least 1 week after infarction, given as either 240 mg in the morning and 120 mg in the evening *or* 120 mg 3 times daily

VERAPRESS ® MR

Hypertension
▶ BY MOUTH
‣ Adult: 240 mg daily, increased if necessary to 240 mg twice daily

Angina
▶ BY MOUTH
‣ Adult: 240 mg twice daily, may sometimes be reduced to once daily

VERTAB ® SR 240

Mild to moderate hypertension
▶ BY MOUTH
‣ Adult: 240 mg daily, increased if necessary to 240 mg twice daily

Angina
▶ BY MOUTH
‣ Adult: 240 mg twice daily, may sometimes be reduced to once daily

● **UNLICENSED USE** Prophylaxis of cluster headaches is an unlicensed indication.

● **CONTRA-INDICATIONS** Acute porphyrias p. 1202 · atrial flutter or fibrillation associated with accessory conducting pathways (e.g. Wolff-Parkinson-White-syndrome) · bradycardia · cardiogenic shock · heart failure (with reduced ejection fraction) · history of significantly impaired left ventricular function (even if controlled by therapy) · hypotension · second- and third-degree AV block · sick sinus syndrome · sino-atrial block

2

Cardiovascular system

- **CAUTIONS** Acute phase of myocardial infarction (avoid if bradycardia, hypotension, left ventricular failure) · first-degree AV block · neuromuscular disorders
  CAUTIONS, FURTHER INFORMATION
  ▸ Elderly Screening Tool of Older Persons' potentially inappropriate Prescriptions (STOPP) criteria to aid medication reviews (see Prescribing in the elderly p. 31 for information): potentially inappropriate in patients with NYHA Class III or IV heart failure (contra-indicated in heart failure with reduced ejection fraction; may worsen heart failure).
- **INTERACTIONS** → Appendix 1: calcium channel blockers
- **SIDE-EFFECTS**
  GENERAL SIDE-EFFECTS
  ▸ **Common or very common** Hypotension
  ▸ **Frequency not known** Atrioventricular block · extrapyramidal symptoms · gynaecomastia · Stevens-Johnson syndrome · vertigo
  SPECIFIC SIDE-EFFECTS
  ▸ **Common or very common**
  ▸ With intravenous use Bradycardia
  ▸ **Frequency not known**
  ▸ With intravenous use Cardiac arrest · hepatic impairment · hyperhidrosis · myocardial contractility decreased · nervousness · seizure
  ▸ With oral use Abdominal discomfort · alopecia · arrhythmias · arthralgia · constipation · erythromelalgia · fatigue · galactorrhoea · heart failure · ileus · muscle weakness · tinnitus · tremor

  Overdose In overdose, verapamil has a profound cardiac depressant effect causing hypotension and arrhythmias, including complete heart block and asystole.
- **PREGNANCY** May reduce uterine blood flow with fetal hypoxia. Manufacturer advises avoid in first trimester unless absolutely necessary. May inhibit labour.
- **BREAST FEEDING** Amount too small to be harmful.
- **HEPATIC IMPAIRMENT**
  Dose adjustments
  ▸ With oral use Manufacturer advises dose reduction.

- **MEDICINAL FORMS** There can be variation in the licensing of different medicines containing the same drug. Forms available from special-order manufacturers include: oral suspension, oral solution
  Oral tablet
  ▸ **Verapamil hydrochloride (Non-proprietary)**
  Verapamil hydrochloride 40 mg Verapamil 40mg tablets | 84 tablet PoM £1.90 DT = £1.43
  Verapamil hydrochloride 80 mg Verapamil 80mg tablets | 84 tablet PoM £3.70 DT = £2.17
  Verapamil hydrochloride 120 mg Verapamil 120mg tablets | 28 tablet PoM £3.31 DT = £3.31
  Verapamil hydrochloride 160 mg Verapamil 160mg tablets | 56 tablet PoM £44.20 DT = £31.53
  Modified-release tablet
  CAUTIONARY AND ADVISORY LABELS 25
  ▸ **Half Securon** (Viatris UK Healthcare Ltd)
  Verapamil hydrochloride 120 mg Half Securon SR 120mg tablets | 28 tablet PoM £7.71 DT = £7.71
  ▸ **Securon SR** (Viatris UK Healthcare Ltd)
  Verapamil hydrochloride 240 mg Securon SR 240mg tablets | 28 tablet PoM £5.55 DT = £5.55
  ▸ **Vera-Til SR** (Tillomed Laboratories Ltd, Accord-UK Ltd)
  Verapamil hydrochloride 120 mg Vera-Til SR 120mg tablets | 28 tablet PoM £6.98 DT = £7.71
  Verapamil hydrochloride 240 mg Vera-Til SR 240mg tablets | 28 tablet PoM £5.00–£10.00 DT = £5.55
  ▸ **Verapress MR** (Dexcel-Pharma Ltd)
  Verapamil hydrochloride 240 mg Verapress MR 240mg tablets | 28 tablet PoM £9.90 DT = £5.55

Solution for injection
▸ **Securon** (Viatris UK Healthcare Ltd)
Verapamil hydrochloride 2.5 mg per 1 ml Securon IV 5mg/2ml solution for injection ampoules | 5 ampoule PoM £5.41 DT = £5.41
Oral solution
▸ **Verapamil hydrochloride (Non-proprietary)**
Verapamil hydrochloride 8 mg per 1 ml Verapamil 40mg/5ml oral solution sugar free | 150 ml PoM £158.85 DT = £158.85 SF

DIURETICS > THIAZIDES AND RELATED DIURETICS

Thiazides and related diuretics 

- **CONTRA-INDICATIONS** Addison's disease · hypercalcaemia · hyponatraemia · refractory hypokalaemia · symptomatic hyperuricaemia
- **CAUTIONS** Diabetes · gout · risk of hypokalaemia · systemic lupus erythematosus
  CAUTIONS, FURTHER INFORMATION
  ▸ Existing conditions Thiazides and related diuretics can exacerbate diabetes, gout, and systemic lupus erythematosus.
  ▸ Potassium loss Hypokalaemia can occur with thiazides and related diuretics.
    Hypokalaemia is dangerous in severe cardiovascular disease and in patients also being treated with cardiac glycosides. Often the use of potassium-sparing diuretics avoids the need to take potassium supplements.
    In hepatic impairment, hypokalaemia caused by diuretics can precipitate encephalopathy.
  ▸ Elderly EvGr Lower initial doses of diuretics may be necessary in the elderly because they are particularly susceptible to the side-effects. The dose should then be adjusted according to renal function. M
    Screening Tool of Older Persons' potentially inappropriate Prescriptions (STOPP) criteria to aid medication reviews (see Prescribing in the elderly p. 31 for information). Potentially inappropriate:
    ● with current significant hypokalaemia (serum potassium less than 3 mmol/L), hyponatraemia (serum sodium less than 130 mmol/L), or hypercalcaemia (corrected serum calcium greater than 2.65 mmol/L)—contra-indicated; hypokalaemia, hyponatraemia, and hypercalcaemia can be precipitated by a thiazide diuretic
    ● with a history of gout (gout can be precipitated by a thiazide diuretic)
- **SIDE-EFFECTS**
  ▸ **Common or very common** Alkalosis hypochloraemic · constipation · diarrhoea · dizziness · electrolyte imbalance · erectile dysfunction · fatigue · headache · hyperglycaemia · hyperuricaemia · nausea · postural hypotension · skin reactions · vomiting
  ▸ **Uncommon** Agranulocytosis · aplastic anaemia · leucopenia · pancreatitis · photosensitivity reaction · thrombocytopenia
  ▸ **Rare or very rare** Paraesthesia
- **PREGNANCY** Thiazides and related diuretics should not be used to treat gestational hypertension. They may cause neonatal thrombocytopenia, bone marrow suppression, jaundice, electrolyte disturbances, and hypoglycaemia; placental perfusion may also be reduced. Stimulation of labour, uterine inertia, and meconium staining have also been reported.
- **HEPATIC IMPAIRMENT** In general, manufacturer advises caution in mild to moderate impairment; avoid in severe impairment.
- **RENAL IMPAIRMENT** In general, manufacturers advise caution in mild to moderate impairment (risk of electrolyte imbalance and reduced renal function); avoid in severe impairment (ineffective if creatinine clearance less than 30 mL/minute). See p. 21.

- **MONITORING REQUIREMENTS** Electrolytes should be monitored, particularly with high doses and long-term use.

Bendroflumethiazide

F 192

10-Jul-2023

(Bendrofluazide)

- **INDICATIONS AND DOSE**

Oedema
- ▸ BY MOUTH
- ▸ Adult: Initially 5–10 mg once daily or on alternate days, dose to be taken in the morning, then maintenance 5–10 mg 1–3 times a week

Hypertension
- ▸ BY MOUTH
- ▸ Adult: 2.5 mg once daily, dose to be taken in the morning, higher doses are rarely necessary

- **INTERACTIONS** → Appendix 1: thiazide diuretics

- **SIDE-EFFECTS** Blood disorder · cholestasis · gastrointestinal disorder · gout · neutropenia · pneumonitis · pulmonary oedema · severe cutaneous adverse reactions (SCARs)

- **BREAST FEEDING** The amount present in milk is too small to be harmful. Large doses may suppress lactation.

- **MEDICINAL FORMS** There can be variation in the licensing of different medicines containing the same drug. Forms available from special-order manufacturers include: oral suspension, oral solution

Oral tablet
- ▸ Bendroflumethiazide (Non-proprietary)
  Bendroflumethiazide 2.5 mg Bendroflumethiazide 2.5mg tablets | 28 tablet PoM £0.72 DT = £0.51
  Bendroflumethiazide 5 mg Bendroflumethiazide 5mg tablets | 28 tablet PoM £0.98 DT = £0.68

Combinations available: *Timolol with bendroflumethiazide*, p. 179

Co-amilozide

04-Oct-2021

The properties listed below are those particular to the combination only. For the properties of the components please consider, hydrochlorothiazide below.

- **INDICATIONS AND DOSE**

Hypertension
- ▸ BY MOUTH
- ▸ Adult: Initially 2.5/25 mg daily, increased if necessary up to 5/50 mg daily

Congestive heart failure
- ▸ BY MOUTH
- ▸ Adult: Initially 2.5/25 mg daily; increased if necessary up to 10/100 mg daily, reduce dose for maintenance if possible

Oedema and ascites in cirrhosis of the liver
- ▸ BY MOUTH
- ▸ Adult: Initially 5/50 mg daily; increased if necessary up to 10/100 mg daily, reduce dose for maintenance if possible

DOSE EQUIVALENCE AND CONVERSION
- ▸ A mixture of amiloride hydrochloride and hydrochlorothiazide in the mass proportions of 1 part amiloride hydrochloride to 10 parts hydrochlorothiazide.

- **CONTRA-INDICATIONS** Anuria · hyperkalaemia

- **CAUTIONS** Diabetes mellitus · elderly

- **INTERACTIONS** → Appendix 1: potassium-sparing diuretics · thiazide diuretics

- **SIDE-EFFECTS** Angina pectoris · appetite abnormal · arrhythmias · arthralgia · asthenia · chest pain · confusion · constipation · depression · diarrhoea · dizziness · drowsiness · dyspnoea · electrolyte imbalance · erectile dysfunction · flatulence · flushing · gastrointestinal discomfort · gastrointestinal haemorrhage · gout · headache · hiccups · hyperhidrosis · insomnia · malaise · muscle cramps · nasal congestion · nausea · nervousness · pain · paraesthesia · postural hypotension · renal impairment · skin reactions · stupor · syncope · taste unpleasant · urinary disorders · vertigo · visual impairment · vomiting

- **BREAST FEEDING** Avoid—no information regarding amiloride component available. Amount of hydrochlorothiazide in milk probably too small to be harmful. Large doses of hydrochlorothiazide may suppress lactation.

- **RENAL IMPAIRMENT** EvGr Caution in mild to moderate impairment—monitor plasma-potassium concentration (high risk of hyperkalaemia). Avoid in severe impairment. Ⓜ

- **MONITORING REQUIREMENTS** Monitor electrolytes.

- **MEDICINAL FORMS** There can be variation in the licensing of different medicines containing the same drug. Forms available from special-order manufacturers include: oral solution

Oral tablet
- ▸ Co-amilozide (Non-proprietary)
  Amiloride hydrochloride 2.5 mg, Hydrochlorothiazide 25 mg Co-amilozide 2.5mg/25mg tablets | 28 tablet PoM £28.00 DT = £12.90
  Amiloride hydrochloride 5 mg, Hydrochlorothiazide 50 mg Co-amilozide 5mg/50mg tablets | 28 tablet PoM £32.05 DT = £13.28

Hydrochlorothiazide

F 192

03-Dec-2018

- **INDICATIONS AND DOSE**

Indications listed in combination monographs (available in the UK only in combination with other drugs)
- ▸ BY MOUTH
- ▸ Adult: Doses listed in combination monographs

> **IMPORTANT SAFETY INFORMATION**
>
> MHRA/CHM ADVICE: HYDROCHLOROTHIAZIDE: RISK OF NON-MELANOMA SKIN CANCER, PARTICULARLY IN LONG-TERM USE (NOVEMBER 2018)
>
> The MHRA advises healthcare professionals to:
> - inform patients taking hydrochlorothiazide-containing products of the cumulative, dose-dependent increased risk of non-melanoma skin cancer, particularly in long-term use, and advise patients to regularly check for and report any new or changed skin lesions or moles;
> - advise patients to limit exposure to sunlight and UV rays and use adequate sun protection;
> - reconsider the use of hydrochlorothiazide in patients who have had previous skin cancer;
> - examine all suspicious moles or skin lesions (potentially including histological examination of biopsies).

- **INTERACTIONS** → Appendix 1: thiazide diuretics

- **SIDE-EFFECTS**
- ▸ **Uncommon** Appetite decreased · epigastric discomfort · fever · gastrointestinal spasm · glycosuria · haemolytic anaemia · insomnia · jaundice cholestatic · muscle cramps · nephritis tubulointerstitial · pneumonitis · pulmonary oedema · renal impairment · respiratory distress · sialadenitis · toxic epidermal necrolysis · vasculitis · vision disorders
- ▸ **Frequency not known** Basal cell carcinoma (particularly in long term use) · cutaneous lupus erythematosus ·

restlessness · squamous cell carcinoma (particularly in long term use)

- **MEDICINAL FORMS** No licensed medicines listed.

  Combinations available: *Enalapril with hydrochlorothiazide,* p. 196 · *Irbesartan with hydrochlorothiazide,* p. 203 · *Lisinopril with hydrochlorothiazide,* p. 198 · *Losartan with hydrochlorothiazide,* p. 204 · *Olmesartan with amlodipine and hydrochlorothiazide,* p. 205 · *Olmesartan with hydrochlorothiazide,* p. 205 · *Quinapril with hydrochlorothiazide,* p. 200 · *Telmisartan with hydrochlorothiazide,* p. 206 · *Valsartan with hydrochlorothiazide,* p. 206

◀ 192

Indapamide

24-Nov-2020

- **DRUG ACTION** Indapamide is a thiazide-like diuretic with antihypertensive effects. At lower doses, vasodilatation is more prominent than diuresis; the diuretic effect becomes more apparent with higher doses.

- **INDICATIONS AND DOSE**

  Essential hypertension
  - ▸ BY MOUTH USING IMMEDIATE-RELEASE MEDICINES
  - ▸ Adult: 2.5 mg daily, dose to be taken in the morning
  - ▸ BY MOUTH USING MODIFIED-RELEASE MEDICINES
  - ▸ Adult: 1.5 mg daily, dose to be taken preferably in the morning

- **CAUTIONS** Acute porphyrias p. 1202

- **INTERACTIONS** → Appendix 1: thiazide diuretics

- **SIDE-EFFECTS**
  - ▸ **Common or very common** Hypersensitivity
  - ▸ **Rare or very rare** Angioedema · arrhythmias · dry mouth · haemolytic anaemia · hepatic disorders · renal failure · severe cutaneous adverse reactions (SCARs) · vertigo
  - ▸ **Frequency not known** Hepatic encephalopathy · QT interval prolongation · rhabdomyolysis · syncope · systemic lupus erythematosus exacerbated · vision disorders

- **ALLERGY AND CROSS-SENSITIVITY** [EvGr] Contra-indicated if history of hypersensitivity to sulfonamides. [M]

- **BREAST FEEDING** Present in milk—manufacturer advises avoid.

- **MEDICINAL FORMS** There can be variation in the licensing of different medicines containing the same drug. Forms available from special-order manufacturers include: oral suspension

  Oral tablet
  - ▸ **Indapamide (Non-proprietary)**
    Indapamide hemihydrate 2.5 mg Indapamide 2.5mg tablets | 28 tablet [PoM] £6.34 DT = £0.73 | 56 tablet [PoM] £1.46–£12.68
  - ▸ **Natrilix** (Servier Laboratories Ltd)
    Indapamide hemihydrate 2.5 mg Natrilix 2.5mg tablets | 30 tablet [PoM] £3.40

  Modified-release tablet
  CAUTIONARY AND ADVISORY LABELS 25
  - ▸ **Indapamide (Non-proprietary)**
    Indapamide 1.5 mg Indapamide 1.5mg modified-release tablets | 30 tablet [PoM] £3.47 DT = £3.40
  - ▸ **Alkapamid XL** (HBS Healthcare Ltd)
    Indapamide 1.5 mg Alkapamid XL 1.5mg tablets | 30 tablet [PoM] £3.10 DT = £3.40
  - ▸ **Cardide SR** (Teva UK Ltd)
    Indapamide 1.5 mg Cardide SR 1.5mg tablets | 30 tablet [PoM] £1.99 DT = £3.40
  - ▸ **Lorvacs XL** (Torrent Pharma (UK) Ltd)
    Indapamide 1.5 mg Lorvacs XL 1.5mg tablets | 30 tablet [PoM] £3.40 DT = £3.40
  - ▸ **Natrilix SR** (Servier Laboratories Ltd)
    Indapamide 1.5 mg Natrilix SR 1.5mg tablets | 30 tablet [PoM] £3.40 DT = £3.40

  Combinations available: *Perindopril arginine with indapamide,* p. 198

DRUGS ACTING ON THE RENIN-ANGIOTENSIN SYSTEM > ACE INHIBITORS

Angiotensin-converting enzyme inhibitors

> **IMPORTANT SAFETY INFORMATION**
>
> MHRA/CHM ADVICE: ACE INHIBITORS AND ANGIOTENSIN II RECEPTOR ANTAGONISTS: NOT FOR USE IN PREGNANCY (DECEMBER 2014)
> See *Conception and contraception* and *Pregnancy*.
>
> MHRA/CHM ADVICE: ACE INHIBITORS AND ANGIOTENSIN II RECEPTOR ANTAGONISTS: RECOMMENDATIONS ON HOW TO USE FOR BREASTFEEDING (DECEMBER 2014)
> See *Breast feeding.*

- **CONTRA-INDICATIONS** Hereditary or idiopathic angioedema · history of angioedema associated with prior ACE inhibitor therapy · the combination of an ACE inhibitor with aliskiren is contra-indicated in patients with an eGFR less than 60 mL/minute/1.73 m^2 · the combination of an ACE inhibitor with aliskiren is contra-indicated in patients with diabetes mellitus

- **CAUTIONS** Concomitant diuretics · diabetes (may lower blood glucose; increased risk of hyperkalaemia) · first dose hypotension (especially in patients taking high doses of diuretics, on a low-sodium diet, on dialysis, dehydrated, or with cerebrovascular disease, ischaemic heart disease, or heart failure) · patients of black African or African-Caribbean origin (may respond less well to ACE inhibitors) · peripheral vascular disease or generalised atherosclerosis (risk of clinically silent renovascular disease) · primary aldosteronism (patients may respond less well to ACE inhibitors) · the risk of agranulocytosis is possibly increased in collagen vascular disease (blood counts recommended) · use with care in patients with aortic or mitral valve stenosis (risk of hypotension) · use with care in patients with hypertrophic cardiomyopathy

  CAUTIONS, FURTHER INFORMATION
  - ▸ Anaphylactoid reactions [EvGr] To prevent anaphylactoid reactions, ACE inhibitors should be avoided during dialysis with high-flux membranes (e.g. polyacrylonitrile) and during low-density lipoprotein apheresis with dextran sulfate; they should also be withheld before desensitisation with wasp or bee venom. [M]
  - ▸ Elderly Screening Tool of Older Persons' potentially inappropriate Prescriptions (STOPP) criteria to aid medication reviews (see Prescribing in the elderly p. 31 for information). Potentially inappropriate:
    - with hyperkalaemia
    - with persistent postural hypotension i.e. recurrent drop in systolic blood pressure ≥ 20 mmHg (risk of syncope and falls)

- **SIDE-EFFECTS**
  - ▸ **Common or very common** Alopecia · angina pectoris · angioedema (can be delayed; more common in black patients) · arrhythmias · asthenia · chest pain · constipation · cough · depression · diarrhoea · dizziness · drowsiness · dry mouth · dyspnoea · electrolyte imbalance · gastrointestinal discomfort · headache · hypotension · myalgia · nausea · palpitations · paraesthesia · renal impairment · rhinitis · skin reactions · sleep disorder · syncope · taste altered · tinnitus · vertigo · vomiting
  - ▸ **Uncommon** Arthralgia · confusion · eosinophilia · erectile dysfunction · fever · haemolytic anaemia · hyperhidrosis · myocardial infarction · pancreatitis · peripheral oedema · photosensitivity reaction · respiratory disorders · stroke
  - ▸ **Rare or very rare** Agranulocytosis · hepatitis · leucopenia · neutropenia · pancytopenia · Stevens-Johnson syndrome · thrombocytopenia

SIDE-EFFECTS, FURTHER INFORMATION In light of reports of cholestatic jaundice, hepatitis, fulminant hepatic necrosis, and hepatic failure, ACE inhibitors should be discontinued if marked elevation of hepatic enzymes or jaundice occur.

- ALLERGY AND CROSS-SENSITIVITY [EvGr] ACE inhibitors are contra-indicated in patients with hypersensitivity to ACE inhibitors (including angioedema). [M]
- CONCEPTION AND CONTRACEPTION [EvGr] Females planning pregnancy should be switched to alternative treatments that have an established safety profile for use in pregnancy, unless continued treatment with an angiotensin-converting enzyme inhibitor is considered essential [M](recommendation also supported by specialist sources).
- PREGNANCY [EvGr] Avoid (risk of teratogenicity in first trimester cannot be excluded; known risk of fetotoxicity (decreased renal function, oligohydramnios, skull ossification retardation) and neonatal toxicity (renal failure, hypotension, hyperkalaemia) in second and third trimesters); [M] recommendation also supported by specialist sources.
- BREAST FEEDING Information on the use of ACE inhibitors in breast-feeding is limited.
- RENAL IMPAIRMENT [EvGr] Caution (hyperkalaemia and other side-effects of ACE inhibitors are more common in those with impaired renal function). [M]
  Dose adjustments [EvGr] Start with low dose and adjust according to response. [M]
- MONITORING REQUIREMENTS Renal function and electrolytes should be checked before starting ACE inhibitors (or increasing the dose) and monitored during treatment (more frequently if side effects mentioned are present).
- DIRECTIONS FOR ADMINISTRATION For hypertension the first dose should preferably be given at bedtime.

◀ 194

Captopril

08-Jun-2021

- **INDICATIONS AND DOSE**

Hypertension
▶ BY MOUTH
▸ Adult: Initially 12.5–25 mg twice daily, then increased if necessary up to 150 mg daily in 2 divided doses, doses to be increased at intervals of at least 2 weeks, once-daily dosing may be appropriate if other concomitant antihypertensive drugs taken
▸ Elderly: Initially 6.25 mg twice daily, then increased if necessary up to 150 mg daily in 2 divided doses, doses to be increased at intervals of at least 2 weeks, once-daily dosing may be appropriate if other concomitant antihypertensive drugs taken

Essential hypertension if used in volume depletion, cardiac decompensation, or renovascular hypertension
▶ BY MOUTH
▸ Adult: Initially 6.25–12.5 mg for 1 dose (under close medical supervision), then 6.25–12.5 mg twice daily; increased if necessary up to 100 mg daily in 1–2 divided doses, doses to be increased at intervals of at least 2 weeks, once-daily dosing may be appropriate if other concomitant antihypertensive drugs taken

Heart failure
▶ BY MOUTH
▸ Adult (under close medical supervision): Initially 6.25–12.5 mg 2–3 times a day, then increased if tolerated to up to 150 mg daily in divided doses, dose to be increased gradually at intervals of at least 2 weeks

Short-term treatment within 24 hours of onset of myocardial infarction in clinically stable patients
▶ BY MOUTH
▸ Adult: Initially 6.25 mg, then increased to 12.5 mg after 2 hours, followed by 25 mg after 12 hours; increased if tolerated to 50 mg twice daily for 4 weeks

Prophylaxis of symptomatic heart failure after myocardial infarction in clinically stable patients with asymptomatic left ventricular dysfunction (starting 3–16 days after infarction) (under close medical supervision)
▶ BY MOUTH
▸ Adult: Initially 6.25 mg daily, then increased to 12.5 mg 3 times a day for 2 days, then increased if tolerated to 25 mg 3 times a day, then increased if tolerated to 75–150 mg daily in 2–3 divided doses, doses exceeding 75 mg per day to be increased gradually

Diabetic nephropathy in type 1 diabetes mellitus
▶ BY MOUTH
▸ Adult: 75–100 mg daily in divided doses

- INTERACTIONS → Appendix 1: ACE inhibitors
- SIDE-EFFECTS
▸ **Common or very common** Insomnia · peptic ulcer
▸ **Uncommon** Appetite decreased · flushing · malaise · pallor · Raynaud's phenomenon
▸ **Rare or very rare** Alveolitis allergic · anaemia · aplastic anaemia · autoimmune disorder · cardiac arrest · cardiogenic shock · cerebrovascular insufficiency · gynaecomastia · hepatic disorders · hypoglycaemia · lymphadenopathy · nephrotic syndrome · oral disorders · proteinuria · urinary disorders · vision blurred
- BREAST FEEDING Avoid in first few weeks after delivery, particularly in preterm infants—risk of profound neonatal hypotension; can be used in mothers breast-feeding older infants if essential but monitor infant's blood pressure.
- RENAL IMPAIRMENT
  Dose adjustments [EvGr] Max. initial dose 25 mg daily (do not exceed 100 mg daily) if creatinine clearance 20–40 mL/minute.
  Max. initial dose 12.5 mg daily (do not exceed 75 mg daily) if creatinine clearance 10–20 mL/minute.
  Max. initial dose 6.25 mg daily (do not exceed 37.5 mg daily) if creatinine clearance less than 10 mL/minute. [M] See p. 21.

- MEDICINAL FORMS There can be variation in the licensing of different medicines containing the same drug. Forms available from special-order manufacturers include: oral tablet, oral capsule, oral suspension, oral solution

Oral tablet
▸ Captopril (Non-proprietary)
  Captopril 12.5 mg Captopril 12.5mg tablets | 56 tablet [PoM] £39.76 DT = £39.76
  Captopril 25 mg Captopril 25mg tablets | 56 tablet [PoM] £38.94 DT = £38.94
  Captopril 50 mg Captopril 50mg tablets | 56 tablet [PoM] £57.30 DT = £22.39

Oral solution
ELECTROLYTES: May contain Sodium
▸ Captopril (Non-proprietary)
  Captopril 1 mg per 1 ml Captopril 5mg/5ml oral solution sugar free | 100 ml [PoM] £98.21 DT = £93.30 [SF]
  Captopril 5 mg per 1 ml Captopril 25mg/5ml oral solution sugar free | 100 ml [PoM] £108.94 DT = £101.00 [SF]

☞ 194

Enalapril maleate

30-May-2024

- **INDICATIONS AND DOSE**

Hypertension
▸ BY MOUTH
▸ Adult: Initially 5 mg once daily, lower initial doses may be required when used in addition to diuretic or in renal impairment; maintenance 20 mg once daily; maximum 40 mg per day

Heart failure
▸ BY MOUTH
▸ Adult (under close medical supervision): Initially 2.5 mg once daily, increased if tolerated to 10–20 mg twice daily, dose to be increased gradually over 2–4 weeks

Prevention of symptomatic heart failure in patients with asymptomatic left ventricular dysfunction
▸ BY MOUTH
▸ Adult (under close medical supervision): Initially 2.5 mg once daily, increased if tolerated to 10–20 mg twice daily, dose to be increased gradually over 2–4 weeks

- **INTERACTIONS** → Appendix 1: ACE inhibitors

- **SIDE-EFFECTS**
▸ **Common or very common** Hypersensitivity · vision blurred
▸ **Uncommon** Anaemia · appetite decreased · asthma · bone marrow disorders · flushing · gastrointestinal disorders · hoarseness · hypoglycaemia · malaise · muscle cramps · nervousness · proteinuria · rhinorrhoea · sleep disorders · throat pain
▸ **Rare or very rare** Alveolitis allergic · autoimmune disorder · gynaecomastia · hepatic disorders · lymphadenopathy · oral disorders · Raynaud's phenomenon · toxic epidermal necrolysis
▸ **Frequency not known** SIADH

- **BREAST FEEDING** Avoid in first few weeks after delivery, particularly in preterm infants—risk of profound neonatal hypotension; can be used in mothers breast-feeding older infants if essential but monitor infant's blood pressure.

- **HEPATIC IMPAIRMENT** Enalapril is a prodrug.

- **RENAL IMPAIRMENT**
Dose adjustments See p. 21.
EvGr Max. initial dose 2.5 mg daily if creatinine clearance less than 30 mL/minute. Ⓜ

- **DIRECTIONS FOR ADMINISTRATION** Expert sources advise oral tablets may be crushed and suspended in water immediately before use.

- **MEDICINAL FORMS** There can be variation in the licensing of different medicines containing the same drug. Forms available from special-order manufacturers include: oral suspension, oral solution
Oral tablet
▸ Enalapril maleate (Non-proprietary)
Enalapril maleate 2.5 mg Enalapril 2.5mg tablets | 28 tablet PoM £7.00 DT = £5.51
Enalapril maleate 5 mg Enalapril 5mg tablets | 28 tablet PoM £4.13 DT = £0.94
Enalapril maleate 10 mg Enalapril 10mg tablets | 28 tablet PoM £5.64 DT = £0.88
Enalapril maleate 20 mg Enalapril 20mg tablets | 28 tablet PoM £6.63 DT = £0.87
▸ Innovace (Organon Pharma (UK) Ltd)
Enalapril maleate 2.5 mg Innovace 2.5mg tablets | 28 tablet PoM £5.35 DT = £5.51
Enalapril maleate 5 mg Innovace 5mg tablets | 28 tablet PoM £7.51 DT = £0.94
Enalapril maleate 10 mg Innovace 10mg tablets | 28 tablet PoM £10.53 DT = £0.88
Enalapril maleate 20 mg Innovace 20mg tablets | 28 tablet PoM £12.51 DT = £0.87

Oral solution
▸ Enalapril maleate (Non-proprietary)
Enalapril maleate 1 mg per 1 ml Enalapril 5mg/5ml oral solution sugar free | 150 ml PoM £238.00 DT = £238.00 SF

Enalapril with hydrochlorothiazide

The properties listed below are those particular to the combination only. For the properties of the components please consider, enalapril maleate above, hydrochlorothiazide p. 193.

- **INDICATIONS AND DOSE**

Mild to moderate hypertension in patients stabilised on the individual components in the same proportions
▸ BY MOUTH
▸ Adult: (consult product literature)

- **INTERACTIONS** → Appendix 1: ACE inhibitors · thiazide diuretics

- **MEDICINAL FORMS** There can be variation in the licensing of different medicines containing the same drug.
Oral tablet
▸ Enalapril with hydrochlorothiazide (Non-proprietary)
Hydrochlorothiazide 12.5 mg, Enalapril maleate 20 mg Enalapril 20mg / Hydrochlorothiazide 12.5mg tablets | 28 tablet PoM £28.00 DT = £27.13
▸ Innozide (Organon Pharma (UK) Ltd)
Hydrochlorothiazide 12.5 mg, Enalapril maleate 20 mg Innozide 20mg/12.5mg tablets | 28 tablet PoM £13.90 DT = £27.13

☞ 194

Fosinopril sodium

10-Dec-2018

- **INDICATIONS AND DOSE**

Hypertension
▸ BY MOUTH
▸ Adult: Initially 10 mg daily for 4 weeks, then increased if necessary up to 40 mg daily, doses over 40 mg not shown to increase efficacy

Congestive heart failure (adjunct) (under close medical supervision)
▸ BY MOUTH
▸ Adult: Initially 10 mg once daily, then increased if tolerated to 40 mg once daily, doses to be increased gradually

- **INTERACTIONS** → Appendix 1: ACE inhibitors

- **SIDE-EFFECTS**
▸ **Common or very common** Eye disorder · increased risk of infection · mood altered · oedema · pain · sexual dysfunction · urinary disorder · visual impairment
▸ **Frequency not known** Appetite abnormal · arthritis · balance impaired · behaviour abnormal · cardiac arrest · cardiac conduction disorder · cerebrovascular insufficiency · dysphagia · dysphonia · ear pain · flatulence · flushing · gout · haemorrhage · hypertensive crisis · lymphadenopathy · memory loss · muscle weakness · oral disorders · prostatic disorder · tremor · weight changes

- **BREAST FEEDING** Not recommended; alternative treatment options, with better established safety information during breast-feeding, are available.

- **HEPATIC IMPAIRMENT** Fosinopril is a prodrug. Manufacturer advises caution (risk of increased exposure).

- **MEDICINAL FORMS** There can be variation in the licensing of different medicines containing the same drug. Forms available from special-order manufacturers include: oral suspension, oral solution
Oral tablet
▸ Fosinopril sodium (Non-proprietary)
Fosinopril sodium 10 mg Fosinopril 10mg tablets | 28 tablet PoM £5.11 DT = £5.11

Fosinopril sodium 20 mg Fosinopril 20mg tablets | 28 tablet PoM £5.27 DT = £2.93

⚑ 194

Imidapril hydrochloride

08-Jun-2021

- **INDICATIONS AND DOSE**

Essential hypertension
▸ BY MOUTH
▸ Adult: Initially 5 mg daily, increased if necessary to 10 mg daily, dose to be taken before food, doses to be increased at intervals of at least 3 weeks; maximum 20 mg per day
▸ Elderly: Initially 2.5 mg daily, increased if necessary to 10 mg daily, dose to be taken before food, doses to be increased at intervals of at least 3 weeks

Essential hypertension in patients with heart failure, angina or cerebrovascular disease
▸ BY MOUTH
▸ Adult: Initially 2.5 mg daily, increased if necessary to 10 mg daily, dose to be taken before food, dose to be increased at intervals of at least 3 weeks; maximum 20 mg per day

- **INTERACTIONS** → Appendix 1: ACE inhibitors

- **SIDE-EFFECTS**
▸ **Uncommon** Cerebrovascular disorder · increased risk of infection · joint swelling · limb pain · oedema
▸ **Rare or very rare** Anaemia

- **BREAST FEEDING** Not recommended; alternative treatment options, with better established safety information during breast-feeding, are available.

- **HEPATIC IMPAIRMENT** Imidapril is a prodrug. Manufacturer advises caution (risk of increased exposure). **Dose adjustments** Manufacturer advises initial dose of 2.5 mg daily.

- **RENAL IMPAIRMENT** EvGr Avoid if creatinine clearance less than 30 mL/minute. Ⓜ
Dose adjustments EvGr Initial dose 2.5 mg daily if creatinine clearance 30–80 mL/minute. Ⓜ See p. 21.

- **MEDICINAL FORMS** There can be variation in the licensing of different medicines containing the same drug.

Oral tablet
▸ Tanatril (Northumbria Pharma Ltd)
Imidapril hydrochloride 5 mg Tanatril 5mg tablets | 28 tablet PoM £10.88 DT = £10.88
Imidapril hydrochloride 10 mg Tanatril 10mg tablets | 28 tablet PoM £12.27 DT = £12.27
Imidapril hydrochloride 20 mg Tanatril 20mg tablets | 28 tablet PoM £14.74 DT = £14.74

⚑ 194

Lisinopril

08-Aug-2023

- **INDICATIONS AND DOSE**

Hypertension
▸ BY MOUTH
▸ Adult: Initially 10 mg once daily; usual maintenance 20 mg once daily; maximum 80 mg per day

Hypertension, when used in addition to diuretic, in cardiac decompensation or in volume depletion
▸ BY MOUTH
▸ Adult: Initially 2.5–5 mg once daily; usual maintenance 20 mg once daily; maximum 80 mg per day

Short-term treatment following myocardial infarction in haemodynamically stable patients—systolic blood pressure over 120 mmHg
▸ BY MOUTH
▸ Adult: Initially 5 mg, taken within 24 hours of myocardial infarction, followed by 5 mg, to be taken 24 hours after initial dose, then 10 mg, to be taken

24 hours after second dose, then 10 mg once daily for 6 weeks (or continued if heart failure), temporarily reduce maintenance dose to 5 mg and if necessary 2.5 mg daily if systolic blood pressure 100 mmHg or less during treatment; withdraw if prolonged hypotension occurs during treatment (systolic blood pressure less than 90 mmHg for more than 1 hour)

Short-term treatment following myocardial infarction in haemodynamically stable patients—systolic blood pressure 100–120 mmHg
▸ BY MOUTH
▸ Adult: Initially 2.5 mg once daily, maintenance 5 mg once daily, increase to maintenance dose only after at least 3 days of the initial dose, should not be started after myocardial infarction if systolic blood pressure less than 100 mmHg, temporarily reduce maintenance dose to 2.5 mg daily if systolic blood pressure 100 mmHg or less during treatment; withdraw if prolonged hypotension occurs (systolic blood pressure less than 90 mmHg for more than 1 hour)

Renal complications of diabetes mellitus
▸ BY MOUTH
▸ Adult: Initially 2.5–5 mg once daily, adjusted according to response; usual dose 10–20 mg once daily

Heart failure (adjunct) (under close medical supervision)
▸ BY MOUTH
▸ Adult: Initially 2.5 mg once daily; increased in steps of up to 10 mg at least every 2 weeks; maximum 35 mg per day

- **INTERACTIONS** → Appendix 1: ACE inhibitors

- **SIDE-EFFECTS**
▸ **Common or very common** Postural disorders
▸ **Uncommon** Hallucination · mood altered · Raynaud's phenomenon
▸ **Rare or very rare** Alveolitis allergic · anaemia · autoimmune disorder · azotaemia · bone marrow depression · gynaecomastia · hepatic disorders · hypersensitivity · hypoglycaemia · lymphadenopathy · olfactory nerve disorder · SIADH · sinusitis · toxic epidermal necrolysis
▸ **Frequency not known** Leucocytosis · vasculitis

- **BREAST FEEDING** Not recommended; alternative treatment options, with better established safety information during breast-feeding, are available.

- **RENAL IMPAIRMENT**
Dose adjustments See p. 21.
EvGr Max. initial doses 5–10 mg daily if creatinine clearance 30–80 mL/minute (max. 40 mg daily); 2.5–5 mg daily if creatinine clearance 10–30 mL/minute (max. 40 mg daily); 2.5 mg daily if creatinine clearance less than 10 mL/minute. Ⓜ

- **MEDICINAL FORMS** There can be variation in the licensing of different medicines containing the same drug. Forms available from special-order manufacturers include: oral suspension, oral solution

Oral tablet
▸ Lisinopril (Non-proprietary)
Lisinopril 2.5 mg Lisinopril 2.5mg tablets | 28 tablet PoM £8.02 DT = £0.60 | 500 tablet PoM £11.84-£12.80
Lisinopril 5 mg Lisinopril 5mg tablets | 28 tablet PoM £9.02 DT = £0.67 | 500 tablet PoM £10.93-£20.26
Lisinopril 10 mg Lisinopril 10mg tablets | 28 tablet PoM £11.81 DT = £0.72 | 500 tablet PoM £10.78-£22.96
Lisinopril 20 mg Lisinopril 20mg tablets | 28 tablet PoM £12.02 DT = £0.82 | 500 tablet PoM £12.75-£22.32
▸ Zestril (Atnahs Pharma UK Ltd)
Lisinopril 5 mg Zestril 5mg tablets | 28 tablet PoM £9.42 DT = £0.67
Lisinopril 10 mg Zestril 10mg tablets | 28 tablet PoM £14.76 DT = £0.72

Lisinopril 20 mg Zestril 20mg tablets | 28 tablet [PoM] £13.02 DT = £0.82

Oral solution

▸ Lisinopril (Non-proprietary)
Lisinopril 1 mg per 1 ml Lisinopril 5mg/5ml oral solution sugar free | 150 ml [PoM] £228.90 DT = £228.90 [SF]

Lisinopril with hydrochlorothiazide

The properties listed below are those particular to the combination only. For the properties of the components please consider, lisinopril p. 197, hydrochlorothiazide p. 193.

● **INDICATIONS AND DOSE**

Mild to moderate hypertension in patients stabilised on the individual components in the same proportions

▸ BY MOUTH
▸ Adult: (consult product literature)

● **INTERACTIONS** → Appendix 1: ACE inhibitors · thiazide diuretics

● **MEDICINAL FORMS** There can be variation in the licensing of different medicines containing the same drug.

Oral tablet

▸ Lisinopril with hydrochlorothiazide (Non-proprietary)
Lisinopril 10 mg, Hydrochlorothiazide 12.5 mg Lisinopril 10mg / Hydrochlorothiazide 12.5mg tablets | 28 tablet [PoM] £13.59 DT = £13.59
Hydrochlorothiazide 12.5 mg, Lisinopril 20 mg Lisinopril 20mg / Hydrochlorothiazide 12.5mg tablets | 28 tablet [PoM] £15.42 DT = £15.42

▸ Lisoretic (Bristol Laboratories Ltd)
Lisinopril 10 mg, Hydrochlorothiazide 12.5 mg Lisoretic 10mg/12.5mg tablets | 28 tablet [PoM] £2.36 DT = £13.59
Hydrochlorothiazide 12.5 mg, Lisinopril 20 mg Lisoretic 20mg/12.5mg tablets | 28 tablet [PoM] £2.33 DT = £15.42

▸ Zestoretic (Atnahs Pharma UK Ltd)
Lisinopril 10 mg, Hydrochlorothiazide 12.5 mg Zestoretic 10 tablets | 28 tablet [PoM] £13.62 DT = £13.59
Hydrochlorothiazide 12.5 mg, Lisinopril 20 mg Zestoretic 20 tablets | 28 tablet [PoM] £13.82 DT = £15.42

F 194

Perindopril arginine

28-Jan-2025

● **INDICATIONS AND DOSE**

Hypertension

▸ BY MOUTH
▸ Adult: Initially 5 mg once daily for 1 month, dose to be taken in the morning, then, adjusted according to response; maximum 10 mg per day
▸ Elderly: Initially 2.5 mg once daily for 1 month, dose to be taken in the morning, then, adjusted according to response; maximum 10 mg per day

Hypertension, if used in addition to diuretic, or in cardiac decompensation or volume depletion

▸ BY MOUTH
▸ Adult: Initially 2.5 mg once daily for 1 month, dose to be taken in the morning, then, adjusted according to response; maximum 10 mg per day

Symptomatic heart failure (adjunct) (under close medical supervision)

▸ BY MOUTH
▸ Adult: Initially 2.5 mg once daily for 2 weeks, then increased if tolerated to 5 mg once daily, dose to be taken in the morning

Prophylaxis of cardiac events following myocardial infarction or revascularisation in stable coronary artery disease

▸ BY MOUTH
▸ Adult: Initially 5 mg once daily for 2 weeks, then increased if tolerated to 10 mg once daily, dose to be taken in the morning
▸ Elderly: Initially 2.5 mg once daily for 1 week, then increased if tolerated to 5 mg once daily for 1 week, then increased if tolerated to 10 mg once daily, dose to be taken in the morning

● **INTERACTIONS** → Appendix 1: ACE inhibitors

● **SIDE-EFFECTS**

▸ **Common or very common** Muscle cramps · visual impairment
▸ **Uncommon** Fall · hypoglycaemia · malaise · mood altered · vasculitis
▸ **Rare or very rare** Cholestasis

● **BREAST FEEDING** [EvGr] Not recommended; alternative treatment options, with better established safety information during breast-feeding, are available. ⟨M⟩

● **HEPATIC IMPAIRMENT** Perindopril is a prodrug.

● **RENAL IMPAIRMENT**

Dose adjustments [EvGr] Max. initial dose 2.5 mg once daily if creatinine clearance 30–60 mL/minute; 2.5 mg once daily on alternate days if creatinine clearance 15–30 mL/minute. ⟨M⟩ See p. 21.

● **MEDICINAL FORMS** There can be variation in the licensing of different medicines containing the same drug.

Oral tablet

CAUTIONARY AND ADVISORY LABELS 22

▸ Coversyl Arginine (Servier Laboratories Ltd)
Perindopril arginine 2.5 mg Coversyl Arginine 2.5mg tablets | 30 tablet [PoM] £4.43 DT = £4.43
Perindopril arginine 5 mg Coversyl Arginine 5mg tablets | 30 tablet [PoM] £6.28 DT = £6.28
Perindopril arginine 10 mg Coversyl Arginine 10mg tablets | 30 tablet [PoM] £10.65 DT = £10.65

Perindopril arginine with indapamide

The properties listed below are those particular to the combination only. For the properties of the components please consider, perindopril arginine above, indapamide p. 194.

● **INDICATIONS AND DOSE**

Hypertension not adequately controlled by perindopril alone

▸ BY MOUTH
▸ Adult: (consult product literature)

● **INTERACTIONS** → Appendix 1: ACE inhibitors · thiazide diuretics

● **MEDICINAL FORMS** There can be variation in the licensing of different medicines containing the same drug.

Oral tablet

CAUTIONARY AND ADVISORY LABELS 22

▸ Coversyl Arginine Plus (Servier Laboratories Ltd)
Indapamide 1.25 mg, Perindopril arginine 5 mg Coversyl Arginine Plus 5mg/1.25mg tablets | 30 tablet [PoM] £9.51 DT = £9.51

Perindopril erbumine

▶ 194　　　28-Feb-2023

- **INDICATIONS AND DOSE**

Hypertension

▶ BY MOUTH

▸ **Adult:** Initially 4 mg once daily for 1 month, dose to be taken in the morning, then, adjusted according to response; maximum 8 mg per day

▸ **Elderly:** Initially 2 mg once daily for 1 month, dose to be taken in the morning, then, adjusted according to response; maximum 8 mg per day

Hypertension, if used in addition to diuretic, or in cardiac decompensation or volume depletion

▶ BY MOUTH

▸ **Adult:** Initially 2 mg once daily for 1 month, dose to be taken in the morning, then, adjusted according to response; maximum 8 mg per day

Heart failure (adjunct) (under close medical supervision)

▶ BY MOUTH

▸ **Adult:** Initially 2 mg once daily for at least 2 weeks, dose to be taken in the morning, then increased if tolerated to 4 mg once daily

Prophylaxis of cardiac events following myocardial infarction or revascularisation in stable coronary artery disease

▶ BY MOUTH

▸ **Adult:** Initially 4 mg once daily for 2 weeks, dose to be taken in the morning, then increased if tolerated to 8 mg once daily

▸ **Elderly:** Initially 2 mg once daily for 1 week, then increased if tolerated to 4 mg once daily for 1 week, then increased if tolerated to 8 mg once daily

- **INTERACTIONS** → Appendix 1: ACE inhibitors

- **SIDE-EFFECTS**
▶ **Common or very common** Muscle cramps · visual impairment
▶ **Uncommon** Anxiety · fall · hypoglycaemia · malaise · mood altered · vasculitis
▶ **Rare or very rare** Flushing · SIADH
▶ **Frequency not known** Cardiac arrest · Raynaud's phenomenon

- **BREAST FEEDING** Not recommended; alternative treatment options, with better established safety information during breast-feeding, are available.

- **HEPATIC IMPAIRMENT** Perindopril is a prodrug.

- **RENAL IMPAIRMENT**
Dose adjustments [EvGr] Max. initial dose 2 mg once daily if creatinine clearance 30–60 mL/minute; 2 mg once daily on alternate days if creatinine clearance 15–30 mL/minute. (M) See p. 21.

- **MEDICINAL FORMS** There can be variation in the licensing of different medicines containing the same drug. Forms available from special-order manufacturers include: oral suspension, oral solution
Oral tablet
CAUTIONARY AND ADVISORY LABELS 22
▸ Perindopril erbumine (Non-proprietary)
　Perindopril erbumine 2 mg Perindopril erbumine 2mg tablets |
　30 tablet [PoM] £13.14 DT = £1.25 | 56 tablet [PoM] £3.34 |
　60 tablet [PoM] £13.90
　Perindopril erbumine 4 mg Perindopril erbumine 4mg tablets |
　30 tablet [PoM] £13.14 DT = £1.56 | 56 tablet [PoM] £3.38 |
　60 tablet [PoM] £27.80
　Perindopril erbumine 8 mg Perindopril erbumine 8mg tablets |
　30 tablet [PoM] £13.14 DT = £2.43 | 56 tablet [PoM] £3.88 |
　60 tablet [PoM] £40.00

Perindopril erbumine with amlodipine

08-Mar-2023

The properties listed below are those particular to the combination only. For the properties of the components please consider, perindopril erbumine above, amlodipine p. 184.

- **INDICATIONS AND DOSE**

Hypertension [in patients stabilised on the individual components in the same proportions] | Coronary artery disease [in patients stabilised on the individual components in the same proportions]

▶ BY MOUTH

▸ **Adult:** Doses listed in individual monographs

- **INTERACTIONS** → Appendix 1: ACE inhibitors · calcium channel blockers

- **MEDICINAL FORMS** No licensed medicines listed.

Quinapril

▶ 194　　　28-Jan-2025

- **INDICATIONS AND DOSE**

Essential hypertension

▶ BY MOUTH

▸ **Adult:** Initially 10 mg once daily; maintenance 20–40 mg daily in up to 2 divided doses; maximum 80 mg per day

▸ **Elderly:** Initially 2.5 mg once daily; maintenance 20–40 mg daily in up to 2 divided doses; maximum 80 mg per day

Essential hypertension if used in addition to diuretic

▶ BY MOUTH

▸ **Adult:** Initially 2.5 mg once daily; maintenance 20–40 mg daily in up to 2 divided doses; maximum 80 mg per day

Heart failure (adjunct) (under close medical supervision)

▶ BY MOUTH

▸ **Adult:** Initially 2.5 mg daily, increased if tolerated to 10–20 mg daily in 1–2 divided doses, doses to be increased gradually; maximum 40 mg per day

- **INTERACTIONS** → Appendix 1: ACE inhibitors

- **SIDE-EFFECTS**
▶ **Common or very common** Back pain · increased risk of infection · insomnia
▶ **Uncommon** Dry throat · gastrointestinal disorders · generalised oedema · nervousness · proteinuria · transient ischaemic attack · vasodilation · vision disorders
▶ **Rare or very rare** Balance impaired · glossitis
▶ **Frequency not known** Arthritis · hypersensitivity · jaundice cholestatic · leucocytosis · pneumonitis · pulmonary oedema · serositis · toxic epidermal necrolysis · vasculitis necrotising

- **BREAST FEEDING** [EvGr] Avoid in the first few weeks after delivery, particularly in preterm infants—risk of profound neonatal hypotension; can be used in mothers breast-feeding older infants if essential but monitor infant's blood pressure. (M)

- **HEPATIC IMPAIRMENT** Quinapril is a prodrug. Manufacturer advises caution when used in combination with a diuretic.

- **RENAL IMPAIRMENT**
Dose adjustments [EvGr] Max. initial dose 2.5 mg once daily if creatinine clearance less than 40 mL/minute. (M) See p. 21.

- **MEDICINAL FORMS** No licensed medicines listed.

Quinapril with hydrochlorothiazide

The properties listed below are those particular to the combination only. For the properties of the components please consider, quinapril p. 199, hydrochlorothiazide p. 193.

● **INDICATIONS AND DOSE**

Hypertension in patients stabilised on the individual components in the same proportions
▶ BY MOUTH
▶ Adult: (consult product literature)

● INTERACTIONS → Appendix 1: ACE inhibitors · thiazide diuretics

● MEDICINAL FORMS No licensed medicines listed.

⚑ 194

Ramipril

19-Apr-2023

● **INDICATIONS AND DOSE**

Hypertension
▶ BY MOUTH
▶ Adult: Initially 1.25–2.5 mg once daily, increased if necessary up to 10 mg once daily, dose to be increased at intervals of 2–4 weeks

Symptomatic heart failure (adjunct) (under close medical supervision)
▶ BY MOUTH
▶ Adult: Initially 1.25 mg once daily, increased if tolerated to 10 mg daily in 1–2 divided doses, daily dose preferably taken in 2 divided doses, increase dose gradually at intervals of 1–2 weeks

Prophylaxis after myocardial infarction in patients with clinical evidence of heart failure (started at least 48 hours after infarction)
▶ BY MOUTH
▶ Adult: Initially 2.5 mg twice daily for 3 days, then increased to 5 mg twice daily

Prophylaxis after myocardial infarction in patients with clinical evidence of heart failure (started at least 48 hours after infarction) when initial dose of 2.5 mg not tolerated
▶ BY MOUTH
▶ Adult: 1.25 mg twice daily for 2 days, then increased to 2.5 mg twice daily, withdraw treatment if dose cannot be increased to 2.5 mg twice daily, then increased to 5 mg twice daily

Prevention of cardiovascular events in patients with atherosclerotic cardiovascular disease or with diabetes mellitus and at least one additional risk factor for cardiovascular disease
▶ BY MOUTH
▶ Adult: Initially 2.5 mg once daily for 1–2 weeks, then increased to 5 mg once daily for 2–3 weeks, then increased to 10 mg once daily

Nephropathy (consult product literature)
▶ BY MOUTH
▶ Adult: Initially 1.25 mg once daily for 2 weeks, then increased to 2.5 mg once daily for 2 weeks, then increased if tolerated to 5 mg once daily

● INTERACTIONS → Appendix 1: ACE inhibitors

● **SIDE-EFFECTS**
▶ **Common or very common** Gastrointestinal disorders · increased risk of infection · muscle spasms
▶ **Uncommon** Anxiety · appetite decreased · asthma exacerbated · flushing · libido decreased · myocardial ischaemia · nasal congestion · proteinuria aggravated · vision disorders
▶ **Rare or very rare** Conjunctivitis · hearing impairment · hepatic disorders · hypoperfusion · movement disorders · onycholysis · oral disorders · tremor · vascular stenosis · vasculitis
▶ **Frequency not known** Altered smell sensation · bone marrow failure · cerebrovascular insufficiency · concentration impaired · enanthema · gynaecomastia · hypersensitivity · Raynaud's phenomenon · SIADH · toxic epidermal necrolysis

● **BREAST FEEDING** Not recommended; alternative treatment options, with better established safety information during breast-feeding, are available.

● **HEPATIC IMPAIRMENT** Ramipril is a prodrug. Manufacturer advises caution.
Dose adjustments Manufacturer advises maximum 2.5 mg daily.

● **RENAL IMPAIRMENT**
Dose adjustments EvGr Max. daily dose 5 mg if creatinine clearance 30–60 mL/minute; max. initial dose 1.25 mg once daily (do not exceed 5 mg daily) if creatinine clearance less than 30 mL/minute. 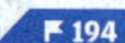 See p. 21.

● **MEDICINAL FORMS** There can be variation in the licensing of different medicines containing the same drug. Forms available from special-order manufacturers include: oral suspension, oral solution

Oral tablet
▶ Ramipril (Non-proprietary)
Ramipril 1.25 mg Ramipril 1.25mg tablets | 28 tablet PoM £4.74 DT = £1.47
Ramipril 2.5 mg Ramipril 2.5mg tablets | 28 tablet PoM £6.76 DT = £1.15
Ramipril 5 mg Ramipril 5mg tablets | 28 tablet PoM £9.42 DT = £0.94
Ramipril 10 mg Ramipril 10mg tablets | 28 tablet PoM £12.81 DT = £1.08
▶ Tritace (Sanofi)
Ramipril 2.5 mg Tritace 2.5mg tablets | 28 tablet PoM £7.22 DT = £1.15
Ramipril 5 mg Tritace 5mg tablets | 28 tablet PoM £10.05 DT = £0.94
Ramipril 10 mg Tritace 10mg tablets | 28 tablet PoM £13.68 DT = £1.08

Oral solution
▶ Ramipril (Non-proprietary)
Ramipril 500 microgram per 1 ml Ramipril 2.5mg/5ml oral solution sugar free | 150 ml PoM £205.80 DT = £205.80 SF
Ramipril 1 mg per 1 ml Ramipril 5mg/5ml oral solution sugar free | 150 ml PoM £411.60 SF
Ramipril 2 mg per 1 ml Ramipril 10mg/5ml oral solution sugar free | 150 ml PoM £823.20 SF

Oral capsule
▶ Ramipril (Non-proprietary)
Ramipril 1.25 mg Ramipril 1.25mg capsules | 28 capsule PoM £1.80 DT = £0.86
Ramipril 2.5 mg Ramipril 2.5mg capsules | 28 capsule PoM £1.90 DT = £0.78
Ramipril 5 mg Ramipril 5mg capsules | 28 capsule PoM £2.05 DT = £0.79
Ramipril 10 mg Ramipril 10mg capsules | 28 capsule PoM £2.20 DT = £0.86

Ramipril with felodipine

22-Dec-2020

The properties listed below are those particular to the combination only. For the properties of the components please consider, ramipril above, felodipine p. 187.

● **INDICATIONS AND DOSE**

Hypertension in patients stabilised on the individual components in the same proportions
▶ BY MOUTH
▶ Adult: (consult product literature)

● INTERACTIONS → Appendix 1: ACE inhibitors · calcium channel blockers

● MEDICINAL FORMS No licensed medicines listed.

Trandolapril

⬛ 194

11-Jun-2021

- **INDICATIONS AND DOSE**

Mild to moderate hypertension
▸ BY MOUTH
▸ Adult: Initially 500 micrograms once daily; increased to 1–2 mg once daily, dose to be increased at intervals of 2–4 weeks; maximum 4 mg per day

Prophylaxis after myocardial infarction in patients with left ventricular dysfunction (starting as early as 3 days after infarction)
▸ BY MOUTH
▸ Adult: Initially 500 micrograms once daily, then increased to up to 4 mg once daily, doses to be increased gradually

- **INTERACTIONS** → Appendix 1: ACE inhibitors

- **SIDE-EFFECTS**
▸ **Uncommon** Feeling abnormal · gastrointestinal disorders · hot flush · increased risk of infection · insomnia · libido decreased · malaise · muscle spasms · pain · rhinorrhoea
▸ **Rare or very rare** Anaemia · anxiety · appetite abnormal · azotaemia · cerebrovascular insufficiency · enzyme abnormality · eye disorder · eye inflammation · gout · haemorrhage · hallucination · hyperbilirubinaemia · hyperglycaemia · hypersensitivity · hyperuricaemia · migraine · movement disorders · myocardial ischaemia · oedema · osteoarthritis · platelet disorder · throat irritation · urinary disorders · vascular disorders · visual impairment · white blood cell disorder
▸ **Frequency not known** Atrioventricular block · cardiac arrest · jaundice · proteinuria · toxic epidermal necrolysis

  SIDE-EFFECTS, FURTHER INFORMATION If symptomatic hypotension develops during titration, do not increase dose further; if possible, reduce dose of any adjunctive treatment and if this is not effective or feasible, reduce dose of trandolapril.

- **BREAST FEEDING** Not recommended; alternative treatment options, with better established safety information during breast-feeding, are available.

- **HEPATIC IMPAIRMENT** Trandolapril is a prodrug. Manufacturer advises caution.
  Dose adjustments Manufacturer advises initiate under close supervision and adjust dose according to blood pressure response in severe impairment.

- **RENAL IMPAIRMENT**
  Dose adjustments [EvGr] Max. 1 mg once daily if creatinine clearance 10–30 mL/minute; max. 500 micrograms once daily if creatinine clearance less than 10 mL/minute. ⟨M⟩ See p. 21.

- **MEDICINAL FORMS** There can be variation in the licensing of different medicines containing the same drug. Forms available from special-order manufacturers include: oral suspension

  Oral capsule
  ▸ Trandolapril (Non-proprietary)
  Trandolapril 500 microgram Trandolapril 500microgram capsules | 14 capsule [PoM] £2.60 DT = £1.67
  Trandolapril 1 mg Trandolapril 1mg capsules | 28 capsule [PoM] £32.30 DT = £20.19
  Trandolapril 2 mg Trandolapril 2mg capsules | 28 capsule [PoM] £4.88 DT = £3.41
  Trandolapril 4 mg Trandolapril 4mg capsules | 28 capsule [PoM] £16.14 DT = £16.14

Angiotensin II receptor antagonists 

> **IMPORTANT SAFETY INFORMATION**
> MHRA/CHM ADVICE: ACE INHIBITORS AND ANGIOTENSIN II RECEPTOR ANTAGONISTS: NOT FOR USE IN PREGNANCY (DECEMBER 2014)
> See *Conception and contraception* and *Pregnancy*.
>
> MHRA/CHM ADVICE: ACE INHIBITORS AND ANGIOTENSIN II RECEPTOR ANTAGONISTS: RECOMMENDATIONS ON HOW TO USE FOR BREASTFEEDING (DECEMBER 2014)
> See *Breast feeding*.

- **CONTRA-INDICATIONS** The combination of an angiotensin-II receptor antagonist with aliskiren is contra-indicated in patients with an eGFR less than 60 mL/minute/1.73 m^2 · the combination of an angiotensin-II receptor antagonist with aliskiren is contra-indicated in patients with diabetes mellitus

- **CAUTIONS** Aortic or mitral valve stenosis · elderly (lower initial doses may be appropriate) · hypertrophic cardiomyopathy · patients of black African or African-Caribbean origin · patients with a history of angioedema · patients with primary aldosteronism (may not benefit from an angiotensin-II receptor antagonist) · renal artery stenosis

  CAUTIONS, FURTHER INFORMATION
  ▸ Elderly Screening Tool of Older Persons' potentially inappropriate Prescriptions (STOPP) criteria to aid medication reviews (see Prescribing in the elderly p. 31 for information). Potentially inappropriate:
    - with hyperkalaemia
    - with persistent postural hypotension i.e. recurrent drop in systolic blood pressure ≥ 20 mmHg (risk of syncope and falls)

- **SIDE-EFFECTS**
▸ **Common or very common** Abdominal pain · asthenia · back pain · cough · diarrhoea · dizziness · headache · hyperkalaemia · hypotension · nausea · postural hypotension (more common in patients with intravascular volume depletion, e.g. those taking high-dose diuretics) · renal impairment · vertigo · vomiting
▸ **Uncommon** Angioedema · myalgia · skin reactions · thrombocytopenia
▸ **Rare or very rare** Arthralgia · hepatic function abnormal

- **CONCEPTION AND CONTRACEPTION** [EvGr] Females planning pregnancy should be switched to alternative treatments that have an established safety profile for use in pregnancy, unless continued treatment with an angiotensin II receptor antagonist is considered essential ⟨M⟩ (recommendation also supported by specialist sources).

- **PREGNANCY** [EvGr] Avoid (risk of teratogenicity in first trimester cannot be excluded; known risk of fetotoxicity (decreased renal function, oligohydramnios, skull ossification retardation) and neonatal toxicity (renal failure, hypotension, hyperkalaemia) in second and third trimesters); ⟨M⟩ recommendation also supported by specialist sources.

- **BREAST FEEDING** [EvGr] Information on the use of angiotensin-II receptor antagonists in breast-feeding is limited. They are not recommended in breast-feeding. Alternative treatment options, with better established safety profile during breast-feeding, are preferable ⟨M⟩ (recommendation also supported by specialist sources).

- **HEPATIC IMPAIRMENT** In general, manufacturers advise caution in mild to moderate impairment (limited information available); avoid in severe impairment (no information available).
- **RENAL IMPAIRMENT**
Dose adjustments In general, manufacturers advise start with low dose and adjust according to response.
- **MONITORING REQUIREMENTS** Monitor plasma-potassium concentration, particularly in the elderly and in patients with renal impairment.

⚑ 201

Azilsartan medoxomil

09-Jun-2021

- **INDICATIONS AND DOSE**
Hypertension
▸ BY MOUTH
  ▸ Adult 18–74 years: Initially 40 mg once daily, increased if necessary to 80 mg once daily
  ▸ Adult 75 years and over: Initially 20–40 mg once daily, increased if necessary to 80 mg once daily

Hypertension with intravascular volume depletion
▸ BY MOUTH
  ▸ Adult: Initially 20–40 mg daily, increased if necessary to 80 mg daily

- **CAUTIONS** Heart failure
- **INTERACTIONS** → Appendix 1: angiotensin-II receptor antagonists
- **SIDE-EFFECTS**
▸ **Uncommon** Hyperuricaemia · muscle spasms · peripheral oedema
- **HEPATIC IMPAIRMENT**
Dose adjustments Manufacturer advises consider initial dose of 20 mg in mild to moderate impairment.
Monitoring Manufacturer advises monitor closely in mild to moderate hepatic impairment (limited information available).
- **RENAL IMPAIRMENT** Manufacturer advises caution in severe impairment—no information available.

- **MEDICINAL FORMS** There can be variation in the licensing of different medicines containing the same drug.
Oral tablet
▸ Edarbi (Takeda UK Ltd)
  Azilsartan medoxomil (as Azilsartan medoxomil potassium) 20 mg Edarbi 20mg tablets | 28 tablet PoM £16.80 DT = £16.80
  Azilsartan medoxomil (as Azilsartan medoxomil potassium) 40 mg Edarbi 40mg tablets | 28 tablet PoM £16.80 DT = £16.80
  Azilsartan medoxomil (as Azilsartan medoxomil potassium) 80 mg Edarbi 80mg tablets | 28 tablet PoM £19.95 DT = £19.95

⚑ 201

Candesartan cilexetil

28-Jan-2025

- **INDICATIONS AND DOSE**
Hypertension
▸ BY MOUTH
  ▸ Adult: Initially 8 mg once daily, increased if necessary up to 32 mg once daily, dose to be increased at intervals of 4 weeks; usual dose 8 mg once daily

Hypertension with intravascular volume depletion
▸ BY MOUTH
  ▸ Adult: Initially 4 mg once daily, increased if necessary up to 32 mg once daily, dose to be increased at intervals of 4 weeks; usual dose 8 mg once daily

Heart failure with impaired left ventricular systolic function when ACE inhibitors are not tolerated
▸ BY MOUTH
  ▸ Adult: Initially 4 mg once daily, increased to up to 32 mg once daily, dose to be increased at intervals of at least 2 weeks to 'target' dose of 32 mg once daily or to maximum tolerated dose

Heart failure with impaired left ventricular systolic function in conjunction with an ACE inhibitor (under expert supervision)
▸ BY MOUTH
  ▸ Adult: Initially 4 mg once daily, increased to up to 32 mg once daily, dose to be increased at intervals of at least 2 weeks to 'target' dose of 32 mg once daily or to maximum tolerated dose

Migraine prophylaxis
▸ BY MOUTH
  ▸ Adult: 16 mg once daily

- **UNLICENSED USE** EvGr Candesartan is used for migraine prophylaxis, Ⓐ but is not licensed for this indication.
- **CONTRA-INDICATIONS** Cholestasis
- **INTERACTIONS** → Appendix 1: angiotensin-II receptor antagonists
- **SIDE-EFFECTS**
▸ **Common or very common** Increased risk of infection
▸ **Rare or very rare** Agranulocytosis · hepatitis · hyponatraemia · leucopenia · neutropenia
- **CONCEPTION AND CONTRACEPTION**
▸ When used for Migraine prophylaxis EvGr Females of childbearing potential should be advised to seek advice about alternative treatments if they are planning a pregnancy. Ⓐ
- **HEPATIC IMPAIRMENT** Manufacturer advises avoid in severe impairment or cholestasis.
Dose adjustments Manufacturer advises initial dose reduction to 4 mg once daily in mild to moderate impairment; adjust according to response.
- **RENAL IMPAIRMENT** See p. 21. EvGr Caution if creatinine clearance less than 15 mL/minute (limited experience). Ⓜ
Dose adjustments EvGr Initially 4 mg daily. Ⓜ

- **MEDICINAL FORMS** There can be variation in the licensing of different medicines containing the same drug. Forms available from special-order manufacturers include: oral suspension, oral solution
Oral tablet
▸ Candesartan cilexetil (Non-proprietary)
  Candesartan cilexetil 2 mg Candesartan 2mg tablets | 7 tablet PoM £2.86 DT = £0.63 | 28 tablet PoM £2.52–£11.46
  Candesartan cilexetil 4 mg Candesartan 4mg tablets | 7 tablet PoM £3.10 DT = £0.53 | 28 tablet PoM £0.49–£11.74
  Candesartan cilexetil 8 mg Candesartan 8mg tablets | 28 tablet PoM £11.87 DT = £0.98
  Candesartan cilexetil 16 mg Candesartan 16mg tablets | 28 tablet PoM £15.26 DT = £1.02
  Candesartan cilexetil 32 mg Candesartan 32mg tablets | 28 tablet PoM £19.36 DT = £1.34
▸ Amias (Neon Healthcare Ltd)
  Candesartan cilexetil 2 mg Amias 2mg tablets | 7 tablet PoM £3.58 DT = £0.63
  Candesartan cilexetil 4 mg Amias 4mg tablets | 28 tablet PoM £9.78
  Candesartan cilexetil 8 mg Amias 8mg tablets | 28 tablet PoM £9.89 DT = £0.98
  Candesartan cilexetil 16 mg Amias 16mg tablets | 28 tablet PoM £12.72 DT = £1.02
  Candesartan cilexetil 32 mg Amias 32mg tablets | 28 tablet PoM £16.13 DT = £1.34

⚑ 201

Eprosartan

09-Jun-2021

- **INDICATIONS AND DOSE**
Hypertension
▸ BY MOUTH
  ▸ Adult: 600 mg once daily

- **INTERACTIONS** → Appendix 1: angiotensin-II receptor antagonists
- **SIDE-EFFECTS**
▶ **Common or very common** Gastrointestinal disorder · rhinitis
- **RENAL IMPAIRMENT** [EvGr] Caution if creatinine clearance less than 30 mL/minute. ⟨M⟩ See p. 21.

- **MEDICINAL FORMS** There can be variation in the licensing of different medicines containing the same drug. Forms available from special-order manufacturers include: oral suspension, oral solution
Oral tablet
CAUTIONARY AND ADVISORY LABELS 21
  ▶ Eprosartan (Non-proprietary)
   Eprosartan (as Eprosartan mesilate) 300 mg Eprosartan 300mg tablets | 28 tablet [PoM] £7.31
   Eprosartan (as Eprosartan mesilate) 400 mg Eprosartan 400mg tablets | 56 tablet [PoM] £26.57 DT = £26.57
   Eprosartan (as Eprosartan mesilate) 600 mg Eprosartan 600mg tablets | 28 tablet [PoM] £14.31 DT = £14.31
  ▶ Teveten (Viatris UK Healthcare Ltd)
   Eprosartan (as Eprosartan mesilate) 600 mg Teveten 600mg tablets | 28 tablet [PoM] £14.31 DT = £14.31

⊩ 201

Irbesartan
23-Nov-2022

- **INDICATIONS AND DOSE**
Hypertension
▶ BY MOUTH
▶ Adult 18–74 years: Initially 150 mg once daily, increased if necessary to 300 mg once daily
▶ Adult 75 years and over: Initially 75–150 mg once daily, increased if necessary to 300 mg once daily

Hypertension in patients receiving haemodialysis
▶ BY MOUTH
▶ Adult: Initially 75–150 mg once daily, increased if necessary to 300 mg once daily

Renal disease in hypertensive type 2 diabetes mellitus
▶ BY MOUTH
▶ Adult 18–74 years: Initially 150 mg once daily, increased if tolerated to 300 mg once daily
▶ Adult 75 years and over: Initially 75–150 mg once daily, increased if tolerated to 300 mg once daily

Renal disease in hypertensive type 2 diabetes mellitus in patients receiving haemodialysis
▶ BY MOUTH
▶ Adult: Initially 75–150 mg once daily, increased if tolerated to 300 mg once daily

- **INTERACTIONS** → Appendix 1: angiotensin-II receptor antagonists

- **SIDE-EFFECTS**
▶ **Common or very common** Musculoskeletal pain
▶ **Uncommon** Chest pain · dyspepsia · flushing · hepatic disorders · sexual dysfunction · tachycardia
▶ **Frequency not known** Hypersensitivity vasculitis · muscle cramps · taste altered · tinnitus

- **MEDICINAL FORMS** There can be variation in the licensing of different medicines containing the same drug. Forms available from special-order manufacturers include: oral suspension
Oral tablet
  ▶ Irbesartan (Non-proprietary)
   Irbesartan 75 mg Irbesartan 75mg tablets | 28 tablet [PoM] £9.88 DT = £1.03
   Irbesartan 150 mg Irbesartan 150mg tablets | 28 tablet [PoM] £12.07 DT = £1.20
   Irbesartan 300 mg Irbesartan 300mg tablets | 28 tablet [PoM] £16.25 DT = £2.07
  ▶ Aprovel (Sanofi)
   Irbesartan 150 mg Aprovel 150mg tablets | 28 tablet [PoM] £11.84 DT = £1.20

Irbesartan 300 mg Aprovel 300mg tablets | 28 tablet [PoM] £15.93 DT = £2.07

Irbesartan with hydrochlorothiazide

The properties listed below are those particular to the combination only. For the properties of the components please consider, irbesartan above, hydrochlorothiazide p. 193.

- **INDICATIONS AND DOSE**
Hypertension not adequately controlled with irbesartan alone
▶ BY MOUTH
▶ Adult: (consult product literature)

- **INTERACTIONS** → Appendix 1: angiotensin-II receptor antagonists · thiazide diuretics

- **MEDICINAL FORMS** There can be variation in the licensing of different medicines containing the same drug.
Oral tablet
  ▶ Irbesartan with hydrochlorothiazide (Non-proprietary)
   Hydrochlorothiazide 12.5 mg, Irbesartan 150 mg Irbesartan 150mg / Hydrochlorothiazide 12.5mg tablets | 28 tablet [PoM] £11.84 DT = £3.75
   Hydrochlorothiazide 25 mg, Irbesartan 300 mg Irbesartan 300mg / Hydrochlorothiazide 25mg tablets | 28 tablet [PoM] £16.93 DT = £3.66
   Hydrochlorothiazide 12.5 mg, Irbesartan 300 mg Irbesartan 300mg / Hydrochlorothiazide 12.5mg tablets | 28 tablet [PoM] £15.93 DT = £3.97
  ▶ CoAprovel (Sanofi)
   Hydrochlorothiazide 12.5 mg, Irbesartan 150 mg CoAprovel 150mg/12.5mg tablets | 28 tablet [PoM] £11.84 DT = £3.75
   Hydrochlorothiazide 12.5 mg, Irbesartan 300 mg CoAprovel 300mg/12.5mg tablets | 28 tablet [PoM] £15.93 DT = £3.97

⊩ 201

Losartan potassium
10-Jun-2021

- **INDICATIONS AND DOSE**
Diabetic nephropathy in type 2 diabetes mellitus
▶ BY MOUTH
▶ Adult 18-75 years: Initially 50 mg once daily for several weeks, then increased if necessary to 100 mg once daily
▶ Adult 76 years and over: Initially 25 mg once daily for several weeks, then increased if necessary up to 100 mg once daily

Chronic heart failure when ACE inhibitors are unsuitable or contra-indicated
▶ BY MOUTH
▶ Adult: Initially 12.5 mg once daily, increased if tolerated to up to 150 mg once daily, doses to be increased at weekly intervals

Hypertension (including reduction of stroke risk in hypertension with left ventricular hypertrophy)
▶ BY MOUTH
▶ Adult 18-75 years: Initially 50 mg once daily for several weeks, then increased if necessary to 100 mg once daily
▶ Adult 76 years and over: Initially 25 mg once daily for several weeks, then increased if necessary up to 100 mg once daily

Hypertension with intravascular volume depletion
▶ BY MOUTH
▶ Adult 18-75 years: Initially 25 mg once daily for several weeks, then increased if necessary up to 100 mg once daily

- **CAUTIONS** Severe heart failure
- **INTERACTIONS** → Appendix 1: angiotensin-II receptor antagonists

- **SIDE-EFFECTS**
▶ **Common or very common** Anaemia · hypoglycaemia · postural disorders
▶ **Uncommon** Angina pectoris · constipation · drowsiness · dyspnoea · oedema · palpitations · sleep disorder
▶ **Rare or very rare** Atrial fibrillation · hepatitis · hypersensitivity · paraesthesia · stroke · syncope · vasculitis
▶ **Frequency not known** Depression · erectile dysfunction · hyponatraemia · influenza like illness · malaise · migraine · pancreatitis · photosensitivity reaction · rhabdomyolysis · taste altered · tinnitus · urinary tract infection

- **HEPATIC IMPAIRMENT**
Dose adjustments Manufacturer advises consider dose reduction if history of impairment (risk of increased plasma concentrations).

- **PRESCRIBING AND DISPENSING INFORMATION** Flavours of oral liquid formulations may include berry-citrus.

- **MEDICINAL FORMS** There can be variation in the licensing of different medicines containing the same drug. Forms available from special-order manufacturers include: oral suspension, oral solution

Oral tablet
▶ Losartan potassium (Non-proprietary)
Losartan potassium 12.5 mg Losartan 12.5mg tablets | 28 tablet PoM £36.00 DT = £2.10
Losartan potassium 25 mg Losartan 25mg tablets | 28 tablet PoM £19.42 DT = £0.74
Losartan potassium 50 mg Losartan 50mg tablets | 28 tablet PoM £15.36 DT = £0.77 | 100 tablet PoM £3.19–£3.99 | 500 tablet PoM £13.74–£13.75
Losartan potassium 100 mg Losartan 100mg tablets | 28 tablet PoM £19.42 DT = £0.95 | 100 tablet PoM £3.68–£4.60 | 250 tablet PoM £8.38
▶ Cozaar (Organon Pharma (UK) Ltd)
Losartan potassium 12.5 mg Cozaar 12.5mg tablets | 28 tablet PoM £9.70 DT = £2.10
Losartan potassium 25 mg Cozaar 25mg tablets | 28 tablet PoM £16.18 DT = £0.74
Losartan potassium 50 mg Cozaar 50mg tablets | 28 tablet PoM £12.80 DT = £0.77
Losartan potassium 100 mg Cozaar 100mg tablets | 28 tablet PoM £16.18 DT = £0.95

Losartan with hydrochlorothiazide

The properties listed below are those particular to the combination only. For the properties of the components please consider, losartan potassium p. 203, hydrochlorothiazide p. 193.

- **INDICATIONS AND DOSE**
Hypertension not adequately controlled with losartan alone
▶ BY MOUTH
▶ Adult: (consult product literature)

- **INTERACTIONS** → Appendix 1: angiotensin-II receptor antagonists · thiazide diuretics

- **MEDICINAL FORMS** There can be variation in the licensing of different medicines containing the same drug.
Oral tablet
▶ Losartan with hydrochlorothiazide (Non-proprietary)
Hydrochlorothiazide 12.5 mg, Losartan potassium 50 mg Losartan 50mg / Hydrochlorothiazide 12.5mg tablets | 28 tablet PoM £15.36 DT = £3.26
Hydrochlorothiazide 25 mg, Losartan potassium 100 mg Losartan 100mg / Hydrochlorothiazide 25mg tablets | 28 tablet PoM £19.42 DT = £3.73
Hydrochlorothiazide 12.5 mg, Losartan potassium 100 mg Losartan 100mg / Hydrochlorothiazide 12.5mg tablets | 28 tablet PoM £19.42 DT = £4.50
▶ Cozaar-Comp (Organon Pharma (UK) Ltd)
Hydrochlorothiazide 12.5 mg, Losartan potassium 50 mg Cozaar-Comp 50mg/12.5mg tablets | 28 tablet PoM £12.80 DT = £3.26
Hydrochlorothiazide 25 mg, Losartan potassium 100 mg Cozaar-Comp 100mg/25mg tablets | 28 tablet PoM £16.18 DT = £3.73
Hydrochlorothiazide 12.5 mg, Losartan potassium 100 mg Cozaar-Comp 100mg/12.5mg tablets | 28 tablet PoM £16.18 DT = £4.50

◄ 201

Olmesartan medoxomil

17-Jun-2021

- **INDICATIONS AND DOSE**
Hypertension
▶ BY MOUTH
▶ Adult: Initially 10 mg daily, increased if necessary to 20 mg daily; maximum 40 mg per day

- **CONTRA-INDICATIONS** Biliary obstruction

- **INTERACTIONS** → Appendix 1: angiotensin-II receptor antagonists

- **SIDE-EFFECTS**
▶ **Common or very common** Arthritis · bone pain · chest pain · dyspepsia · haematuria · hypertriglyceridaemia · hyperuricaemia · increased risk of infection · influenza like illness · oedema
▶ **Uncommon** Angina pectoris · malaise
▶ **Rare or very rare** Lethargy · muscle spasms · sprue-like enteropathy

- **HEPATIC IMPAIRMENT** Manufacturer advises caution in moderate impairment; avoid in severe impairment (no information available).
Dose adjustments Manufacturer advises maximum 20 mg daily in moderate impairment.

- **RENAL IMPAIRMENT** EvGr Avoid if creatinine clearance less than 20 mL/minute. Ⓜ
Dose adjustments EvGr Max. 20 mg daily if creatinine clearance 20–60 mL/minute (limited experience). Ⓜ See p. 21.

- **MEDICINAL FORMS** There can be variation in the licensing of different medicines containing the same drug. Forms available from special-order manufacturers include: oral suspension, oral solution

Oral tablet
▶ Olmesartan medoxomil (Non-proprietary)
Olmesartan medoxomil 10 mg Olmesartan medoxomil 10mg tablets | 28 tablet PoM £10.95 DT = £1.07
Olmesartan medoxomil 20 mg Olmesartan medoxomil 20mg tablets | 28 tablet PoM £12.95 DT = £1.17
Olmesartan medoxomil 40 mg Olmesartan medoxomil 40mg tablets | 28 tablet PoM £17.50 DT = £1.82
▶ Olmetec (Daiichi Sankyo UK Ltd)
Olmesartan medoxomil 10 mg Olmetec 10mg tablets | 28 tablet PoM £10.95 DT = £1.07
Olmesartan medoxomil 20 mg Olmetec 20mg tablets | 28 tablet PoM £12.95 DT = £1.17
Olmesartan medoxomil 40 mg Olmetec 40mg tablets | 28 tablet PoM £17.50 DT = £1.82

Olmesartan with amlodipine

22-Dec-2020

The properties listed below are those particular to the combination only. For the properties of the components please consider, olmesartan medoxomil above, amlodipine p. 184.

- **INDICATIONS AND DOSE**
Hypertension in patients stabilised on the individual components in the same proportions
▶ BY MOUTH
▶ Adult: (consult product literature)

- **INTERACTIONS** → Appendix 1: angiotensin-II receptor antagonists · calcium channel blockers

● **MEDICINAL FORMS** There can be variation in the licensing of different medicines containing the same drug.
Oral tablet
▶ Sevikar (Daiichi Sankyo UK Ltd)
 Amlodipine (as Amlodipine besilate) 5 mg, Olmesartan medoxomil 20 mg Sevikar 20mg/5mg tablets | 28 tablet [PoM] £16.95 DT = £16.95
 Amlodipine (as Amlodipine besilate) 10 mg, Olmesartan medoxomil 40 mg Sevikar 40mg/10mg tablets | 28 tablet [PoM] £16.95 DT = £16.95
 Amlodipine (as Amlodipine besilate) 5 mg, Olmesartan medoxomil 40 mg Sevikar 40mg/5mg tablets | 28 tablet [PoM] £16.95 DT = £16.95

Olmesartan with amlodipine and hydrochlorothiazide
05-Oct-2021

The properties listed below are those particular to the combination only. For the properties of the components please consider, olmesartan medoxomil p. 204, amlodipine p. 184, hydrochlorothiazide p. 193.

● **INDICATIONS AND DOSE**

Hypertension in patients stabilised on the individual components in the same proportions, or for hypertension not adequately controlled with olmesartan and amlodipine
▶ BY MOUTH
▶ Adult: (consult product literature)

● INTERACTIONS → Appendix 1: angiotensin-II receptor antagonists · calcium channel blockers · thiazide diuretics

● **MEDICINAL FORMS** There can be variation in the licensing of different medicines containing the same drug.
Oral tablet
▶ Sevikar HCT (Daiichi Sankyo UK Ltd)
 Amlodipine besilate 5 mg, Hydrochlorothiazide 12.5 mg, Olmesartan medoxomil 20 mg Sevikar HCT 20mg/5mg/12.5mg tablets | 28 tablet [PoM] £16.95
 Amlodipine besilate 5 mg, Hydrochlorothiazide 25 mg, Olmesartan medoxomil 40 mg Sevikar HCT 40mg/5mg/25mg tablets | 28 tablet [PoM] £16.95
 Amlodipine besilate 10 mg, Hydrochlorothiazide 25 mg, Olmesartan medoxomil 40 mg Sevikar HCT 40mg/10mg/25mg tablets | 28 tablet [PoM] £16.95
 Amlodipine besilate 5 mg, Hydrochlorothiazide 12.5 mg, Olmesartan medoxomil 40 mg Sevikar HCT 40mg/5mg/12.5mg tablets | 28 tablet [PoM] £16.95
 Amlodipine besilate 10 mg, Hydrochlorothiazide 12.5 mg, Olmesartan medoxomil 40 mg Sevikar HCT 40mg/10mg/12.5mg tablets | 28 tablet [PoM] £16.95

Olmesartan with hydrochlorothiazide
05-Oct-2021

The properties listed below are those particular to the combination only. For the properties of the components please consider, olmesartan medoxomil p. 204, hydrochlorothiazide p. 193.

● **INDICATIONS AND DOSE**

Hypertension not adequately controlled with olmesartan alone
▶ BY MOUTH
▶ Adult: (consult product literature)

● INTERACTIONS → Appendix 1: angiotensin-II receptor antagonists · thiazide diuretics

● **MEDICINAL FORMS** There can be variation in the licensing of different medicines containing the same drug.
Oral tablet
▶ Olmesartan with hydrochlorothiazide (Non-proprietary)
 Hydrochlorothiazide 12.5 mg, Olmesartan medoxomil 20 mg Olmesartan medoxomil 20mg / Hydrochlorothiazide 12.5mg tablets | 28 tablet [PoM] £12.50-£12.95 DT = £12.95
 Olmesartan medoxomil 20 mg, Hydrochlorothiazide 25 mg Olmesartan medoxomil 20mg / Hydrochlorothiazide 25mg tablets | 28 tablet [PoM] £12.95 DT = £12.95
 Hydrochlorothiazide 12.5 mg, Olmesartan medoxomil 40 mg Olmesartan medoxomil 40mg / Hydrochlorothiazide 12.5mg tablets | 28 tablet [PoM] £17.50 DT = £17.50
▶ Olmetec Plus (Daiichi Sankyo UK Ltd)
 Hydrochlorothiazide 12.5 mg, Olmesartan medoxomil 20 mg Olmetec Plus 20mg/12.5mg tablets | 28 tablet [PoM] £12.95 DT = £12.95
 Olmesartan medoxomil 20 mg, Hydrochlorothiazide 25 mg Olmetec Plus 20mg/25mg tablets | 28 tablet [PoM] £12.95 DT = £12.95
 Hydrochlorothiazide 12.5 mg, Olmesartan medoxomil 40 mg Olmetec Plus 40mg/12.5mg tablets | 28 tablet [PoM] £17.50 DT = £17.50

F 201

Telmisartan
10-Jun-2021

● **INDICATIONS AND DOSE**

Hypertension
▶ BY MOUTH
▶ Adult: Initially 20–40 mg once daily for at least 4 weeks, increased if necessary up to 80 mg once daily

Prevention of cardiovascular events in patients with established atherosclerotic cardiovascular disease, or type 2 diabetes mellitus with target-organ damage
▶ BY MOUTH
▶ Adult: 80 mg once daily

● CONTRA-INDICATIONS Biliary obstructive disorders · cholestasis

● INTERACTIONS → Appendix 1: angiotensin-II receptor antagonists

● **SIDE-EFFECTS**
▶ **Uncommon** Anaemia · arrhythmias · chest pain · cystitis · depression · dyspnoea · flatulence · gastrointestinal discomfort · hyperhidrosis · increased risk of infection · insomnia · muscle spasms · sciatica · syncope
▶ **Rare or very rare** Anxiety · drowsiness · dry mouth · eosinophilia · hypoglycaemia · influenza like illness · interstitial lung disease · liver disorder · pain in extremity · sepsis · taste altered · tendon pain · visual impairment

● **HEPATIC IMPAIRMENT**
Dose adjustments Manufacturer advises maximum 40 mg daily in mild to moderate impairment.

● **RENAL IMPAIRMENT**
Dose adjustments Manufacturer advises initial dose of 20 mg once daily in severe impairment.

● **MEDICINAL FORMS** There can be variation in the licensing of different medicines containing the same drug.
Oral tablet
▶ Telmisartan (Non-proprietary)
 Telmisartan 20 mg Telmisartan 20mg tablets | 28 tablet [PoM] £9.99 DT = £2.36
 Telmisartan 40 mg Telmisartan 40mg tablets | 28 tablet [PoM] £17.36 DT = £1.55
 Telmisartan 80 mg Telmisartan 80mg tablets | 28 tablet [PoM] £21.43 DT = £7.91
▶ Micardis (Boehringer Ingelheim Ltd)
 Telmisartan 40 mg Micardis 40mg tablets | 28 tablet [PoM] £13.61 DT = £1.55
 Telmisartan 80 mg Micardis 80mg tablets | 28 tablet [PoM] £17.00 DT = £7.91

Telmisartan with hydrochlorothiazide

The properties listed below are those particular to the combination only. For the properties of the components please consider, telmisartan p. 205, hydrochlorothiazide p. 193.

- ● **INDICATIONS AND DOSE**

Hypertension not adequately controlled by telmisartan alone
▸ BY MOUTH
▸ Adult: (consult product literature)

- ● INTERACTIONS → Appendix 1: angiotensin-II receptor antagonists · thiazide diuretics

- ● MEDICINAL FORMS There can be variation in the licensing of different medicines containing the same drug.

Oral tablet
▸ **Telmisartan with hydrochlorothiazide (Non-proprietary)**
Hydrochlorothiazide 12.5 mg, Telmisartan 40 mg Telmisartan 40mg / Hydrochlorothiazide 12.5mg tablets | 28 tablet PoM £16.33 DT = £13.61
Hydrochlorothiazide 25 mg, Telmisartan 80 mg Telmisartan 80mg / Hydrochlorothiazide 25mg tablets | 28 tablet PoM £20.40 DT = £17.00
Hydrochlorothiazide 12.5 mg, Telmisartan 80 mg Telmisartan 80mg / Hydrochlorothiazide 12.5mg tablets | 28 tablet PoM £20.40 DT = £4.59
▸ **MicardisPlus** (Boehringer Ingelheim Ltd)
Hydrochlorothiazide 12.5 mg, Telmisartan 40 mg MicardisPlus 40mg/12.5mg tablets | 28 tablet PoM £13.61 DT = £13.61
Hydrochlorothiazide 12.5 mg, Telmisartan 80 mg MicardisPlus 80mg/12.5mg tablets | 28 tablet PoM £17.00 DT = £4.59
▸ **MicardisPlus 80/25** (Boehringer Ingelheim Ltd)
Hydrochlorothiazide 25 mg, Telmisartan 80 mg MicardisPlus 80mg/25mg tablets | 28 tablet PoM £17.00 DT = £17.00

▶ 201

Valsartan

10-Jun-2021

- ● **INDICATIONS AND DOSE**

Hypertension
▸ BY MOUTH
▸ Adult: Initially 80 mg once daily, increased if necessary up to 320 mg daily, doses to be increased at intervals of 4 weeks

Hypertension with intravascular volume depletion
▸ BY MOUTH
▸ Adult: Initially 40 mg once daily, increased if necessary up to 320 mg daily, doses to be increased at intervals of 4 weeks

Heart failure when ACE inhibitors cannot be used, or in conjunction with an ACE inhibitor when a beta-blocker cannot be used | Heart failure, in conjunction with an ACE inhibitor when a beta-blocker cannot be used (under expert supervision)
▸ BY MOUTH
▸ Adult: Initially 40 mg twice daily, increased to up to 160 mg twice daily, doses to be increased at intervals of at least 2 weeks

Myocardial infarction with left ventricular failure or left ventricular systolic dysfunction (adjunct)
▸ BY MOUTH
▸ Adult: Initially 20 mg twice daily, increased if necessary up to 160 mg twice daily, doses to be increased over several weeks if tolerated

- ● CONTRA-INDICATIONS Biliary cirrhosis · cholestasis
- ● INTERACTIONS → Appendix 1: angiotensin-II receptor antagonists
- ● **SIDE-EFFECTS**
▸ **Uncommon** Syncope

▸ **Frequency not known** Hyponatraemia · neutropenia · respiratory disorders · serum sickness · vasculitis
- ● **HEPATIC IMPAIRMENT**
Dose adjustments Manufacturer advises maximum 80 mg daily in mild to moderate impairment.
- ● **RENAL IMPAIRMENT** See p. 21. EvGr Caution if creatinine clearance less than 10 mL/minute (no information available). Ⓜ

- ● MEDICINAL FORMS There can be variation in the licensing of different medicines containing the same drug. Forms available from special-order manufacturers include: oral suspension, oral solution

Oral tablet
▸ **Valsartan (Non-proprietary)**
Valsartan 40 mg Valsartan 40mg tablets | 7 tablet PoM £7.55 DT = £6.95 | 28 tablet PoM £9.54-£27.80
Valsartan 80 mg Valsartan 80mg tablets | 28 tablet PoM £13.69 DT = £13.69
Valsartan 160 mg Valsartan 160mg tablets | 28 tablet PoM £14.69 DT = £13.25
Valsartan 320 mg Valsartan 320mg tablets | 28 tablet PoM £20.23 DT = £5.30

Oral solution
▸ **Diovan** (Novartis Pharmaceuticals UK Ltd)
Valsartan 3 mg per 1 ml Diovan 3mg/1ml oral solution | 160 ml PoM £7.20 DT = £7.20

Oral capsule
▸ **Valsartan (Non-proprietary)**
Valsartan 40 mg Valsartan 40mg capsules | 28 capsule PoM £13.97 DT = £3.30
Valsartan 80 mg Valsartan 80mg capsules | 28 capsule PoM £13.97 DT = £8.84
Valsartan 160 mg Valsartan 160mg capsules | 28 capsule PoM £18.41 DT = £9.39

Combinations available: *Amlodipine with valsartan,* p. 184

Valsartan with hydrochlorothiazide

The properties listed below are those particular to the combination only. For the properties of the components please consider, valsartan above, hydrochlorothiazide p. 193.

- ● **INDICATIONS AND DOSE**

Hypertension not adequately controlled by valsartan alone
▸ BY MOUTH
▸ Adult: (consult product literature)

- ● INTERACTIONS → Appendix 1: angiotensin-II receptor antagonists · thiazide diuretics

- ● MEDICINAL FORMS There can be variation in the licensing of different medicines containing the same drug.

Oral tablet
▸ **Valsartan with hydrochlorothiazide (Non-proprietary)**
Hydrochlorothiazide 12.5 mg, Valsartan 80 mg Valsartan 80mg / Hydrochlorothiazide 12.5mg tablets | 28 tablet PoM £24.34 DT = £23.35
Hydrochlorothiazide 25 mg, Valsartan 160 mg Valsartan 160mg / Hydrochlorothiazide 25mg tablets | 28 tablet PoM £34.31 DT = £31.07
Hydrochlorothiazide 12.5 mg, Valsartan 160 mg Valsartan 160mg / Hydrochlorothiazide 12.5mg tablets | 28 tablet PoM £18.77 DT = £13.35
▸ **Co-Diovan** (Novartis Pharmaceuticals UK Ltd)
Hydrochlorothiazide 12.5 mg, Valsartan 80 mg Co-Diovan 80mg/12.5mg tablets | 28 tablet PoM £16.76 DT = £23.35
Hydrochlorothiazide 25 mg, Valsartan 160 mg Co-Diovan 160mg/25mg tablets | 28 tablet PoM £22.09 DT = £31.07
Hydrochlorothiazide 12.5 mg, Valsartan 160 mg Co-Diovan 160mg/12.5mg tablets | 28 tablet PoM £22.09 DT = £13.35

DRUGS ACTING ON THE RENIN-ANGIOTENSIN SYSTEM > RENIN INHIBITORS

Aliskiren
24-Aug-2021

- **DRUG ACTION** Renin inhibitors inhibit renin directly; renin converts angiotensinogen to angiotensin I.

- **INDICATIONS AND DOSE**

Essential hypertension either alone or in combination with other antihypertensives
▸ BY MOUTH
▸ Adult: 150 mg once daily, increased if necessary to 300 mg once daily

- **CONTRA-INDICATIONS** Concomitant treatment with an ACE inhibitor or an angiotensin-II receptor antagonist in patients with an eGFR less than 60 mL/minute/1.73 m^2 · concomitant treatment with an ACE inhibitor or an angiotensin-II receptor antagonist in patients with diabetes mellitus · hereditary angioedema · idiopathic angioedema

- **CAUTIONS** Combination treatment with an ACE inhibitor · combination treatment with an angiotensin-II receptor antagonist · concomitant use of diuretics (first doses may cause hypotension—initiate with care) · history of angioedema · moderate to severe congestive heart failure · patients at risk of renal impairment · salt depletion (first doses may cause hypotension—initiate with care) · volume depletion (first doses may cause hypotension—initiate with care)

- **INTERACTIONS** → Appendix 1: aliskiren

- **SIDE-EFFECTS**
▸ **Common or very common** Arthralgia · diarrhoea · dizziness · electrolyte imbalance
▸ **Uncommon** Cough · oral disorder · palpitations · peripheral oedema · renal impairment · severe cutaneous adverse reactions (SCARs) · skin reactions
▸ **Rare or very rare** Angioedema · hypersensitivity
▸ **Frequency not known** Dyspnoea · hepatic disorders · nausea · vertigo · vomiting

SIDE-EFFECTS, FURTHER INFORMATION If diarrhoea is severe or persistent discontinue treatment.

- **PREGNANCY** Manufacturer advises avoid—no information available; other drugs acting on the renin-angiotensin system have been associated with fetal malformations and neonatal death.

- **BREAST FEEDING** Present in milk in *animal* studies—manufacturer advises avoid.

- **RENAL IMPAIRMENT** EvGr Avoid if eGFR is less than 30 mL/minute/1.73 m^2—no information available. ⟨M⟩ See p. 21. EvGr Use with caution in renal artery stenosis—no information available. ⟨M⟩

- **MONITORING REQUIREMENTS** Monitor patients with a history of angioedema closely during treatment.

- **NATIONAL FUNDING/ACCESS DECISIONS**
For full details see funding body website
Scottish Medicines Consortium (SMC) decisions
▸ Aliskiren (*Rasilez*®) for essential hypertension (February 2010) SMC No. 462/08 Not recommended

- **MEDICINAL FORMS** No licensed medicines listed.

VASODILATORS > POTASSIUM-CHANNEL OPENERS

Minoxidil
08-Nov-2021

- **INDICATIONS AND DOSE**

Severe hypertension, in addition to a diuretic and a beta-blocker
▸ BY MOUTH
▸ Adult: Initially 5 mg daily in 1–2 divided doses, then increased in steps of 5–10 mg, increased at intervals of at least 3 days; maximum 100 mg per day
▸ Elderly: Initially 2.5 mg daily in 1–2 divided doses, then increased in steps of 5–10 mg, increased at intervals of at least 3 days; maximum 100 mg per day

- **CONTRA-INDICATIONS** Phaeochromocytoma
- **CAUTIONS** Acute porphyrias p. 1202 · after myocardial infarction (until stabilised) · angina
- **INTERACTIONS** → Appendix 1: minoxidil
- **SIDE-EFFECTS**
▸ **Common or very common** Fluid retention · hair changes · oedema · pericardial disorders · pericarditis · tachycardia
▸ **Rare or very rare** Leucopenia · skin reactions · Stevens-Johnson syndrome · thrombocytopenia
▸ **Frequency not known** Angina pectoris · breast tenderness · gastrointestinal disorder · pleural effusion · sodium retention · weight increased
- **PREGNANCY** Avoid—possible toxicity including reduced placental perfusion. Neonatal hirsutism reported.
- **BREAST FEEDING** Present in milk but not known to be harmful.
- **RENAL IMPAIRMENT** EvGr Caution in significant impairment. ⟨M⟩
Dose adjustments EvGr Smaller doses may be required in renal failure. ⟨M⟩

- **MEDICINAL FORMS** There can be variation in the licensing of different medicines containing the same drug.
Oral tablet
▸ Minoxidil (Non-proprietary)
Minoxidil 2.5 mg Minoxidil 2.5mg tablets | 60 tablet [PoM] £8.88 DT = £8.88
Minoxidil 5 mg Minoxidil 5mg tablets | 60 tablet [PoM] £15.83 DT = £15.83
Minoxidil 10 mg Minoxidil 10mg tablets | 60 tablet [PoM] £30.68 DT = £30.68
▸ Loniten (Pfizer Ltd)
Minoxidil 2.5 mg Loniten 2.5mg tablets | 60 tablet [PoM] £8.88 DT = £8.88
Minoxidil 5 mg Loniten 5mg tablets | 60 tablet [PoM] £15.83 DT = £15.83
Minoxidil 10 mg Loniten 10mg tablets | 60 tablet [PoM] £30.68 DT = £30.68

VASODILATORS > VASODILATOR ANTIHYPERTENSIVES

Hydralazine hydrochloride
08-Dec-2021

- **INDICATIONS AND DOSE**

Moderate to severe hypertension (adjunct)
▸ BY MOUTH
▸ Adult: Initially 25 mg twice daily, increased if necessary up to 50 mg twice daily

Heart failure (with long acting nitrate) (initiated in hospital or under specialist supervision)
▸ BY MOUTH
▸ Adult: Initially 25 mg 3–4 times a day, subsequent doses to be increased every 2 days if necessary; usual maintenance 50–75 mg 4 times a day   continued →

Hypertensive emergencies (including during pregnancy) | Hypertension with renal complications
▶ BY INTRAVENOUS INFUSION
▶ Adult: Initially 200–300 micrograms/minute; usual maintenance 50–150 micrograms/minute
▶ BY SLOW INTRAVENOUS INJECTION
▶ Adult: 5–10 mg, to be diluted with 10 mL sodium chloride 0.9%; dose may be repeated after 20–30 minutes

● CONTRA-INDICATIONS Acute porphyrias p. 1202 · cor pulmonale · dissecting aortic aneurysm · high output heart failure · idiopathic systemic lupus erythematosus · myocardial insufficiency due to mechanical obstruction · severe tachycardia

● CAUTIONS Cerebrovascular disease · coronary artery disease (may provoke angina, avoid after myocardial infarction until stabilised) · occasionally blood pressure reduction too rapid even with low parenteral doses

● INTERACTIONS → Appendix 1: hydralazine

● SIDE-EFFECTS
▶ **Common or very common** Angina pectoris · diarrhoea · dizziness · flushing · gastrointestinal disorders · headache · hypotension · joint disorders · lupus-like syndrome (after long-term therapy with over 100 mg daily (or less in women and in slow acetylator individuals)) · myalgia · nasal congestion · nausea · palpitations · tachycardia · vomiting
▶ **Rare or very rare** Acute kidney injury · agranulocytosis · anaemia · anxiety · appetite decreased · conjunctivitis · depression · dyspnoea · eosinophilia · eye disorders · fever · glomerulonephritis · haematuria · haemolytic anaemia · hallucination · heart failure · hepatic disorders · leucocytosis · leucopenia · lymphadenopathy · malaise · nerve disorders · neutropenia · oedema · pancytopenia · paradoxical pressor response · paraesthesia · pleuritic pain · proteinuria · skin reactions · splenomegaly · thrombocytopenia · urinary retention · vasculitis · weight decreased

SIDE-EFFECTS, FURTHER INFORMATION The incidence of side-effects is lower if the dose is kept below 100mg daily, but systemic lupus erythematosus should be suspected if there is unexplained weight loss, arthritis, or any other unexplained ill health.

● PREGNANCY Neonatal thrombocytopenia reported, but risk should be balanced against risk of uncontrolled maternal hypertension. Manufacturer advises avoid before third trimester.

● BREAST FEEDING Present in milk but not known to be harmful.
Monitoring Monitor infant in breast-feeding.

● HEPATIC IMPAIRMENT Manufacturer advises caution (risk of accumulation).
Dose adjustments Manufacturer advises adjust dose or dosing interval according to clinical response.

● RENAL IMPAIRMENT
Dose adjustments See p. 21.
Manufacturer advises adjust dose or dosing interval according to clinical response if creatinine clearance less than 30 mL/minute (risk of accumulation).

● MONITORING REQUIREMENTS Manufacturer advises test for antinuclear factor and for proteinuria every 6 months and check acetylator status before increasing dose above 100 mg daily, but evidence of clinical value unsatisfactory.

● DIRECTIONS FOR ADMINISTRATION For *intravenous infusion* (*Apresoline*®) give continuously in Sodium Chloride 0.9%. Suggested infusion volume 500 mL.

● MEDICINAL FORMS There can be variation in the licensing of different medicines containing the same drug. Forms available from special-order manufacturers include: oral tablet, oral suspension, oral solution

Oral tablet
EXCIPIENTS: May contain Gluten, propylene glycol
▶ Hydralazine hydrochloride (Non-proprietary)
Hydralazine hydrochloride 10 mg Apo-Hydralazine 10mg tablets | 100 tablet [PoM] ⓧ
Hydralazine hydrochloride 25 mg Hydralazine 25mg tablets | 56 tablet [PoM] £16.00 DT = £3.48 | 84 tablet [PoM] £14.00
Hydralazine hydrochloride 50 mg Hydralazine 50mg tablets | 56 tablet [PoM] £15.46 DT = £3.89
▶ Apresoline (Advanz Pharma)
Hydralazine hydrochloride 25 mg Apresoline 25mg tablets | 84 tablet [PoM] £3.38

Powder for solution for injection
▶ Hydralazine hydrochloride (Non-proprietary)
Hydralazine hydrochloride 20 mg Hydralazine 20mg powder for concentrate for solution for injection ampoules | 5 ampoule [PoM] £74.17

4.1a Hypertension associated with phaeochromocytoma

Other drugs used for Hypertension associated with phaeochromocytoma Propranolol hydrochloride, p. 178

VASODILATORS ❯ PERIPHERAL VASODILATORS

Phenoxybenzamine hydrochloride
20-Sep-2021

● **INDICATIONS AND DOSE**
Hypertension in phaeochromocytoma
▶ BY MOUTH
▶ Adult: Initially 10 mg daily, increased in steps of 10 mg daily until hypertension controlled or treatment not tolerated; maintenance 1–2 mg/kg daily in 2 divided doses

● CONTRA-INDICATIONS During recovery period after myocardial infarction (usually 3–4 weeks) · history of cerebrovascular accident

● CAUTIONS Avoid in Acute porphyrias p. 1202 · carcinogenic in *animals* · cerebrovascular disease · congestive heart failure · elderly · severe ischaemic heart disease

● SIDE-EFFECTS Abdominal distress · dizziness · ejaculation failure · fatigue · miosis · nasal congestion · postural hypotension · reflex tachycardia

● PREGNANCY Hypotension may occur in newborn.

● BREAST FEEDING May be present in milk.

● RENAL IMPAIRMENT [EvGr] Use with caution. ⓜ

● HANDLING AND STORAGE Owing to risk of contact sensitisation healthcare professionals should avoid contamination of hands.

● MEDICINAL FORMS There can be variation in the licensing of different medicines containing the same drug. Forms available from special-order manufacturers include: oral suspension, oral solution

Oral capsule
▶ Phenoxybenzamine hydrochloride (Non-proprietary)
Phenoxybenzamine hydrochloride 10 mg Phenoxybenzamine 10mg capsules | 30 capsule [PoM] £129.21 DT = £129.21

4.1b Hypertensive crises

> **Other drugs used for Hypertensive crises** Hydralazine hydrochloride, p. 207 · Labetalol hydrochloride, p. 176

VASODILATORS > VASODILATOR ANTIHYPERTENSIVES

| Sodium nitroprusside

05-Oct-2021

● **INDICATIONS AND DOSE**

Hypertensive emergencies

▶ BY INTRAVENOUS INFUSION

▸ Adult: Initially 0.5–1.5 micrograms/kg/minute, adjusted in steps of 500 nanograms/kg/minute every 5 minutes, usual dose 0.5–8 micrograms/kg/minute, use lower doses if already receiving other antihypertensives, stop if response unsatisfactory with max. dose in 10 minutes, lower initial dose of 300 nanograms/kg/minute has been used

Maintenance of blood pressure at 30-40% lower than pretreatment diastolic blood pressure

▶ BY INTRAVENOUS INFUSION

▸ Adult: 20–400 micrograms/minute, use lower doses for patients being treated with other antihypertensives

Controlled hypotension in anaesthesia during surgery

▶ BY INTRAVENOUS INFUSION

▸ Adult: Up to 1.5 micrograms/kg/minute

Acute or chronic heart failure

▶ BY INTRAVENOUS INFUSION

▸ Adult: Initially 10–15 micrograms/minute, increased every 5–10 minutes as necessary; usual dose 10–200 micrograms/minute normally for max. 3 days

● UNLICENSED USE Not licensed for use in the UK.

● CONTRA-INDICATIONS Compensatory hypertension · impaired cerebral circulation · Leber's optic atrophy · severe vitamin B_{12} deficiency

● CAUTIONS Elderly · hyponatraemia · hypothermia · hypothyroidism · ischaemic heart disease

● INTERACTIONS → Appendix 1: nitroprusside

● SIDE-EFFECTS Abdominal pain · anaemia · arrhythmias · chest discomfort · cyanide toxicity · dizziness · flushing · headache · hyperhidrosis · hypothyroidism · hypovolaemia · ileus · intracranial pressure increased · methaemoglobinaemia · muscle twitching · nausea · palpitations · rash · thiocyanate toxicity

SIDE-EFFECTS, FURTHER INFORMATION Side-effects associated with over rapid reduction in blood pressure: Headache, dizziness, nausea, retching, abdominal pain, perspiration, palpitation, anxiety, retrosternal discomfort—reduce infusion rate if any of these side-effects occur.

Overdose Side-effects caused by excessive plasma concentration of the cyanide metabolite include tachycardia, sweating, hyperventilation, arrhythmias, marked metabolic acidosis (discontinue and give antidote, see cyanide in Emergency treatment of poisoning p. 1554).

● PREGNANCY Avoid prolonged use—potential for accumulation of cyanide in fetus.

● BREAST FEEDING No information available. Caution advised due to thiocyanate metabolite.

● HEPATIC IMPAIRMENT Use with caution. Avoid in hepatic failure—cyanide or thiocyanate metabolites may accumulate.

● RENAL IMPAIRMENT Avoid prolonged use—cyanide or thiocyanate metabolites may accumulate.

● MONITORING REQUIREMENTS Monitor blood pressure (including intra-arterial blood pressure) and blood-cyanide concentration, and if treatment exceeds 3 days, also blood thiocyanate concentration.

● TREATMENT CESSATION Avoid sudden withdrawal—terminate infusion over 15–30 minutes.

● DIRECTIONS FOR ADMINISTRATION For *continuous intravenous infusion* in Glucose 5%, manufacturer advises infuse *via* infusion device to allow precise control. For further details, consult product literature. Protect infusion from light.

● MEDICINAL FORMS There can be variation in the licensing of different medicines containing the same drug.

Powder and solvent for solution for infusion

▸ Sodium nitroprusside (Non-proprietary)
  Sodium nitroprusside dihydrate 50 mg Nitroprussiat Fides 50mg powder and solvent for solution for infusion vials | 1 vial [PoM] [Ⅹ] (Hospital only)
  Sodium nitroprusside 50mg powder and solvent for solution for infusion vials | 1 vial [PoM] [Ⅹ] (Hospital only)

4.1c Pulmonary hypertension

> **Other drugs used for Pulmonary hypertension** Epoprostenol, p. 134 · Sildenafil, p. 940 · Tadalafil, p. 941

ANTITHROMBOTIC DRUGS > ANTIPLATELET DRUGS

| Selexipag

19-Aug-2020

● DRUG ACTION Selexipag is a selective prostacyclin (IP) receptor agonist.

● **INDICATIONS AND DOSE**

Pulmonary arterial hypertension either as combination therapy (if insufficiently controlled with an endothelin receptor antagonist and/or a phosphodiesterase type-5 inhibitor), or as monotherapy (initiated under specialist supervision)

▶ BY MOUTH

▸ Adult: Initially 200 micrograms twice daily, increased in steps of 200 micrograms twice daily at weekly intervals up to the highest tolerated dose, usual maintenance 200–1600 micrograms twice daily, initial dose and first dose after each dose increase should be taken in the evening; maximum 3200 micrograms per day

DOSE ADJUSTMENTS DUE TO INTERACTIONS

▸ Manufacturer advises reduce dose frequency to once daily with concurrent use of clopidogrel or moderate CYP2C8 inhibitors.

● CONTRA-INDICATIONS Cerebrovascular event (within the last 3 months) · congenital or acquired valvular defects with myocardial function disorders (not related to pulmonary hypertension) · decompensated cardiac failure (unless under close medical supervision) · myocardial infarction (within last 6 months) · severe arrhythmias · severe coronary heart disease · unstable angina

● CAUTIONS Elderly (limited information available)

● INTERACTIONS → Appendix 1: selexipag

● SIDE-EFFECTS

▸ **Common or very common** Abdominal pain · anaemia · appetite decreased · arthralgia · diarrhoea · flushing · headache · hyperthyroidism · hypotension · myalgia · nasal congestion · nasopharyngitis · nausea · pain · skin reactions · vomiting · weight decreased

▸ **Uncommon** Sinus tachycardia

2
Cardiovascular system

- PREGNANCY Manufacturer advises avoid—no information available.
- BREAST FEEDING Manufacturer advises avoid—present in milk in *animal* studies.
- HEPATIC IMPAIRMENT Manufacturer advises caution in moderate impairment (risk of increased exposure); avoid in severe impairment (no information available). **Dose adjustments** Manufacturer advises initial dose reduction to 200 micrograms once daily in moderate impairment, increased in steps of 200 micrograms once daily at weekly intervals up to the highest tolerated dose.
- RENAL IMPAIRMENT Manufacturer advises caution with dose titration in severe impairment.
- PATIENT AND CARER ADVICE
  Missed doses Manufacturer advises if a dose is more than 6 hours late, the missed dose should not be taken and the next dose should be taken at the normal time; if a dose is missed for 3 days or more, treatment should be restarted at a lower dose and then increased—consult product literature.
- NATIONAL FUNDING/ACCESS DECISIONS
  For full details see funding body website
  Scottish Medicines Consortium (SMC) decisions
  ▸ Selexipag (*Uptravi®*) for the long-term treatment of pulmonary arterial hypertension (PAH) in adult patients with WHO functional class (FC) II-III, either as combination therapy in patients insufficiently controlled with an endothelin receptor antagonist (ERA) and/or a phosphodiesterase type-5 (PDE-5) inhibitor, or as monotherapy in patients who are not candidates for these therapies (May 2018) SMC No. 1235/17 Recommended with restrictions
  All Wales Medicines Strategy Group (AWMSG) decisions
  ▸ Selexipag (*Uptravi®*) for long-term treatment of pulmonary arterial hypertension (PAH) in adult patients with WHO functional class (FC) II-III, either as combination therapy in patients insufficiently controlled with an endothelin receptor antagonist (ERA) and/or a phosphodiesterase type-5 (PDE-5) inhibitor, or as monotherapy in patients who are not candidates for these therapies (June 2018) AWMSG No. 700 Recommended with restrictions

- MEDICINAL FORMS There can be variation in the licensing of different medicines containing the same drug.
  Oral tablet
  CAUTIONARY AND ADVISORY LABELS 21, 25
  ▸ Uptravi (Janssen-Cilag Ltd)
    Selexipag 200 microgram Uptravi 200microgram tablets | 60 tablet [PoM] £3,000.00 (Hospital only) | 140 tablet [PoM] £7,000.00 (Hospital only)
    Selexipag 400 microgram Uptravi 400microgram tablets | 60 tablet [PoM] £3,000.00 (Hospital only)
    Selexipag 600 microgram Uptravi 600microgram tablets | 60 tablet [PoM] £3,000.00 (Hospital only)
    Selexipag 800 microgram Uptravi 800microgram tablets | 60 tablet [PoM] £3,000.00 (Hospital only)
    Selexipag 1 mg Uptravi 1,000microgram tablets | 60 tablet [PoM] £3,000.00 (Hospital only)
    Selexipag 1.2 mg Uptravi 1,200microgram tablets | 60 tablet [PoM] £3,000.00 (Hospital only)
    Selexipag 1.4 mg Uptravi 1,400microgram tablets | 60 tablet [PoM] £3,000.00 (Hospital only)
    Selexipag 1.6 mg Uptravi 1,600microgram tablets | 60 tablet [PoM] £3,000.00 (Hospital only)

ENDOTHELIN RECEPTOR ANTAGONISTS

Ambrisentan
14-Apr-2023

- INDICATIONS AND DOSE
  Pulmonary arterial hypertension (initiated by a specialist)
  ▸ BY MOUTH
  ▸ Adult: 5 mg once daily, increased if necessary to 10 mg once daily
  DOSE ADJUSTMENTS DUE TO INTERACTIONS
  ▸ [EvGr] Max. dose 5 mg once daily with concurrent use of ciclosporin. Ⓜ

- CONTRA-INDICATIONS Idiopathic pulmonary fibrosis
- CAUTIONS Not to be initiated in significant anaemia · pulmonary veno-occlusive disease
- INTERACTIONS → Appendix 1: endothelin receptor antagonists
- SIDE-EFFECTS
  ▸ **Common or very common** Abdominal pain · anaemia · asthenia · chest discomfort · constipation · diarrhoea · dizziness · dyspnoea · epistaxis · fluid retention · flushing · headaches · heart failure · hypersensitivity · hypotension · increased risk of infection · nasal congestion · nausea · palpitations · peripheral oedema · skin reactions · syncope · tinnitus · upper respiratory tract congestion · vision disorders · vomiting
  ▸ **Uncommon** Hepatic disorders · sudden hearing loss
- ALLERGY AND CROSS-SENSITIVITY [EvGr] Contra-indicated in patients with soya or peanut hypersensitivity (film-coating contains soya lecithin). Ⓜ
- CONCEPTION AND CONTRACEPTION Exclude pregnancy before treatment and ensure effective contraception during treatment. Monthly pregnancy tests advised.
- PREGNANCY Avoid (teratogenic in *animal* studies).
- BREAST FEEDING Manufacturer advises avoid—no information available.
- HEPATIC IMPAIRMENT Manufacturer advises avoid in severe impairment or if baseline serum transaminases exceed 3 times the upper limit of normal.
- RENAL IMPAIRMENT [EvGr] Use with caution if creatinine clearance less than 30 mL/minute. Ⓜ See p. 21.
- MONITORING REQUIREMENTS
  ▸ Monitor haemoglobin concentration or haematocrit after 1 month and 3 months of starting treatment, and periodically thereafter (reduce dose or discontinue treatment if significant decrease in haemoglobin concentration or haematocrit observed).
  ▸ Monitor liver function before treatment, and monthly thereafter—discontinue if liver enzymes raised significantly or if symptoms of liver impairment develop.
- PATIENT AND CARER ADVICE
  Alert card A patient alert card should be provided.
  Driving and skilled tasks Patients and carers should be cautioned on the effects on driving and performance of skilled tasks—increased risk of dizziness, blurred vision, syncope, and fatigue.
- NATIONAL FUNDING/ACCESS DECISIONS
  For full details see funding body website
  Scottish Medicines Consortium (SMC) decisions
  ▸ Ambrisentan (*Volibris®*) for pulmonary arterial hypertension (November 2008) SMC No. 511/08 Recommended with restrictions
  All Wales Medicines Strategy Group (AWMSG) decisions
  ▸ Ambrisentan (*Volibris®*) for the treatment of pulmonary arterial hypertension in adults, adolescents and children (aged 8 to less than 18 years) of WHO Functional Class II to III including use in combination treatment (November 2022) AWMSG No. 4819 Recommended

● **MEDICINAL FORMS** There can be variation in the licensing of different medicines containing the same drug.

Oral tablet

EXCIPIENTS: May contain Lecithin

▸ **Ambrisentan (Non-proprietary)**

Ambrisentan 5 mg Ambrisentan 5mg tablets | 30 tablet PoM £1,375.37 DT = £1,618.08 | 30 tablet PoM £1,618.00-£1,618.08 DT = £1,618.08 (Hospital only)

Ambrisentan 10 mg Ambrisentan 10mg tablets | 30 tablet PoM £1,618.00-£1,618.08 DT = £1,618.08 (Hospital only) | 30 tablet PoM £1,375.37 DT = £1,618.08

▸ **Volibris** (GlaxoSmithKline UK Ltd)

Ambrisentan 2.5 mg Volibris 2.5mg tablets | 30 tablet PoM £1,618.08 (Hospital only)

Ambrisentan 5 mg Volibris 5mg tablets | 30 tablet PoM £1,618.08 DT = £1,618.08

Ambrisentan 10 mg Volibris 10mg tablets | 30 tablet PoM £1,618.08 DT = £1,618.08

Bosentan

05-Feb-2020

● **INDICATIONS AND DOSE**

Pulmonary arterial hypertension (initiated under specialist supervision)

▸ BY MOUTH

▸ Adult: Initially 62.5 mg twice daily for 4 weeks, then increased to 125 mg twice daily (max. per dose 250 mg); maximum 500 mg per day

Systemic sclerosis with ongoing digital ulcer disease (to reduce number of new digital ulcers)

▸ BY MOUTH

▸ Adult: Initially 62.5 mg twice daily for 4 weeks, then increased to 125 mg twice daily

● **CONTRA-INDICATIONS** Acute porphyrias p. 1202

● **CAUTIONS** Not to be initiated if systemic systolic blood pressure is below 85 mmHg · pulmonary veno-occlusive disease

● **INTERACTIONS** → Appendix 1: endothelin receptor antagonists

● **SIDE-EFFECTS**

▸ **Common or very common** Anaemia · diarrhoea · erythema · fluid retention · flushing · gastrooesophageal reflux disease · headache · hypotension · nasal congestion · oedema · palpitations · syncope

▸ **Uncommon** Hepatic disorders · leucopenia · neutropenia · thrombocytopenia

▸ **Rare or very rare** Angioedema

▸ **Frequency not known** Pulmonary oedema · vision blurred

● **CONCEPTION AND CONTRACEPTION** Effective contraception required during administration (hormonal contraception not considered effective). Monthly pregnancy tests advised.

● **PREGNANCY** Avoid (teratogenic in *animal* studies).

● **BREAST FEEDING** Manufacturer advises avoid—no information available.

● **HEPATIC IMPAIRMENT** Manufacturer advises avoid in moderate-to-severe impairment or if baseline serum transaminases exceed 3 times the upper limit of normal.

● **MONITORING REQUIREMENTS**

▸ Monitor haemoglobin before and during treatment (monthly for first 4 months, then 3-monthly).

▸ Monitor liver function before treatment, at monthly intervals during treatment, and 2 weeks after dose increase (reduce dose or suspend treatment if liver enzymes raised significantly)—discontinue if symptoms of liver impairment.

● **TREATMENT CESSATION** Avoid abrupt withdrawal—withdraw treatment gradually.

● **MEDICINAL FORMS** There can be variation in the licensing of different medicines containing the same drug.

Oral tablet

▸ **Bosentan (Non-proprietary)**

Bosentan (as Bosentan monohydrate) 62.5 mg Bosentan 62.5mg tablets | 56 tablet PoM £1,510.21 (Hospital only) | 56 tablet PoM £1,359.19

Bosentan (as Bosentan monohydrate) 125 mg Bosentan 125mg tablets | 56 tablet PoM £1,510.21 (Hospital only) | 56 tablet PoM £1,359.19-£1,510.21

Macitentan

16-Dec-2021

● **INDICATIONS AND DOSE**

Pulmonary arterial hypertension (initiated under specialist supervision)

▸ BY MOUTH

▸ Adult: 10 mg daily

● **CONTRA-INDICATIONS** Severe anaemia

● **CAUTIONS** Patients over 75 years · pulmonary veno-occlusive disease

● **INTERACTIONS** → Appendix 1: endothelin receptor antagonists

● **SIDE-EFFECTS**

▸ **Common or very common** Anaemia · fluid retention · flushing · headache · hypotension · increased risk of infection · leucopenia · nasal congestion · oedema · thrombocytopenia

● **CONCEPTION AND CONTRACEPTION** Manufacturer advises exclude pregnancy before treatment and ensure effective contraception during and for one month after stopping treatment. Monthly pregnancy tests advised.

● **PREGNANCY** Toxicity in *animal* studies.

● **BREAST FEEDING** Manufacturer advises avoid—present in milk in *animal* studies.

● **HEPATIC IMPAIRMENT** Manufacturer advises avoid in severe impairment or if hepatic transaminases are greater than 3 times the upper limit of normal.

● **RENAL IMPAIRMENT** EvGr Caution in severe impairment and avoid in patients undergoing dialysis (no information available). Consider monitoring blood pressure and haemoglobin (risk of hypotension and anaemia). ◈

● **MONITORING REQUIREMENTS**

▸ Monitor liver function before treatment, then monthly thereafter (discontinue if unexplained persistent raised serum transaminases or signs of hepatic injury—can restart on advice on hepatologist if liver function tests return to normal and no hepatic injury).

▸ Monitor haemoglobin concentration before treatment and then as indicated.

● **PATIENT AND CARER ADVICE** Patients should be told how to recognise signs of liver disorder and advised to seek immediate medical attention if symptoms such as dark urine, nausea, vomiting, fatigue, abdominal pain, or pruritus develop.

Patient card should be provided.

● **NATIONAL FUNDING/ACCESS DECISIONS**

For full details see funding body website

Scottish Medicines Consortium (SMC) decisions

▸ Macitentan (*Opsumit*®), as monotherapy or in combination, for the long-term treatment of pulmonary arterial hypertension in adult patients of World Health Organisation Functional Class II to III (April 2014) SMC No. 952/14 Recommended with restrictions

- **MEDICINAL FORMS** There can be variation in the licensing of different medicines containing the same drug.
Oral tablet
CAUTIONARY AND ADVISORY LABELS 25
  ▸ Opsumit (Janssen-Cilag Ltd)
    Macitentan 10 mg Opsumit 10mg tablets | 30 tablet [PoM]
    £2,306.00 (Hospital only)

GUANYLATE CYCLASE STIMULATORS

Riociguat

16-Aug-2021

- **INDICATIONS AND DOSE**

Chronic thromboembolic pulmonary hypertension that is recurrent or persistent following surgery, or is inoperable (initiated under specialist supervision) | Monotherapy or in combination with an endothelin receptor antagonist for idiopathic or hereditary pulmonary arterial hypertension, or pulmonary arterial hypertension associated with connective tissue disease (initiated under specialist supervision)

▸ BY MOUTH

▸ Adult: Initially 1 mg 3 times a day for 2 weeks, increased in steps of 0.5 mg 3 times a day, dose to be increased every 2 weeks, increased to up to 2.5 mg 3 times a day (max. per dose 2.5 mg 3 times a day), increase up to maximum dose only if systolic blood pressure $\geq$ 95 mmHg and no signs of hypotension, if treatment interrupted for 3 or more days, restart at 1 mg three times daily for 2 weeks and titrate as before, during titration, reduce dose by 0.5 mg three times daily if systolic blood pressure falls below 95 mmHg and patient shows signs of hypotension

DOSE ADJUSTMENTS DUE TO INTERACTIONS

▸ Manufacturer advises consider initial dose of 0.5 mg 3 times daily in those stable on a strong multi-pathway cytochrome P450 and P-glycoprotein (P-gp)/breast cancer resistance protein (BCRP) inhibitor.

IMPORTANT SAFETY INFORMATION

MHRA/CHM ADVICE: PULMONARY HYPERTENSION ASSOCIATED WITH IDIOPATHIC INTERSTITIAL PNEUMONIAS (PH-IIP) (AUGUST 2016)

Interim results from a terminated study to investigate the efficacy and safety of riociguat in patients with symptomatic PH-IIP, showed increased mortality and increased risk of serious adverse events in the riociguat group compared with the placebo group. The MHRA has advised that use of riociguat is contra-indicated in these patients and that existing treatment for this unauthorised indication should be discontinued.

- **CONTRA-INDICATIONS** History of serious haemoptysis · previous bronchial artery embolisation · pulmonary hypertension associated with idiopathic interstitial pneumonias · pulmonary veno-occlusive disease
- **CAUTIONS** Autonomic dysfunction · elderly (risk of hypotension) · hypotension (do not initiate if systolic blood pressure below 95 mmHg) · hypovolaemia · severe left ventricular outflow obstruction

CAUTIONS, FURTHER INFORMATION

▸ Smoking Smoking cessation advised (response possibly reduced); dose adjustment may be necessary if smoking started or stopped during treatment.

- **INTERACTIONS** → Appendix 1: riociguat
- **SIDE-EFFECTS**
▸ **Common or very common** Anaemia · constipation · diarrhoea · dizziness · dysphagia · gastroenteritis · gastrointestinal discomfort · gastrointestinal disorders · haemorrhage · headache · hypotension · nasal congestion · nausea · palpitations · peripheral oedema · vomiting

- **CONCEPTION AND CONTRACEPTION** Effective contraception required during treatment. Monthly pregnancy tests advised.
- **PREGNANCY** Avoid—toxicity in *animal* studies.
- **BREAST FEEDING** Manufacturer advises avoid—present in milk in *animal* studies.
- **HEPATIC IMPAIRMENT** Manufacturer advises caution in moderate impairment; avoid in severe impairment (no information available).
Dose adjustments Manufacturer advises cautious dose titration in moderate impairment.
- **RENAL IMPAIRMENT** [EvGr] Avoid if creatinine clearance less than 30 mL/minute (limited information available). Ⓜ
Dose adjustments [EvGr] Titrate dose cautiously if creatinine clearance 30–80 mL/minute (risk of hypotension), Ⓜ see p. 21.
- **DIRECTIONS FOR ADMINISTRATION** Manufacturer advises tablets may be crushed and mixed with water or soft foods and swallowed immediately.
- **PATIENT AND CARER ADVICE** Smoking cessation advised (response possibly reduced).
- **NATIONAL FUNDING/ACCESS DECISIONS**
For full details see funding body website
Scottish Medicines Consortium (SMC) decisions
▸ Riociguat (*Adempas*®) for chronic thromboembolic pulmonary hypertension (CTEPH) treatment in adult patients with World Health Organisation functional class II to III with inoperable CTEPH, persistent or recurrent CTEPH after surgical treatment, to improve exercise capacity (December 2014) SMC No. 1001/14 Recommended with restrictions
▸ Riociguat (*Adempas*®) for pulmonary arterial hypertension (PAH) as monotherapy or in combination with endothelin receptor antagonists, for the treatment of adult patients with PAH with World Health Organisation Functional Class II to III to improve exercise capacity (July 2015) SMC No. 1056/15 Recommended with restrictions

---

- **MEDICINAL FORMS** There can be variation in the licensing of different medicines containing the same drug.
Oral tablet
CAUTIONARY AND ADVISORY LABELS 5
  ▸ Adempas (Merck Sharp & Dohme (UK) Ltd)
    Riociguat 500 microgram Adempas 0.5mg tablets | 42 tablet [PoM] £997.36 DT = £997.36
    Riociguat 1 mg Adempas 1mg tablets | 42 tablet [PoM] £997.36 DT = £997.36
    Riociguat 1.5 mg Adempas 1.5mg tablets | 42 tablet [PoM] £997.36 DT = £997.36
    Riociguat 2 mg Adempas 2mg tablets | 42 tablet [PoM] £997.36 DT = £997.36 | 84 tablet [PoM] £1,994.72
    Riociguat 2.5 mg Adempas 2.5mg tablets | 42 tablet [PoM] £997.36 DT = £997.36 | 84 tablet [PoM] £1,994.72

PROSTAGLANDINS AND ANALOGUES

Iloprost

13-Jan-2021

- **INDICATIONS AND DOSE**

Idiopathic or familial pulmonary arterial hypertension (initiated under specialist supervision)

▸ BY INHALATION OF NEBULISED SOLUTION

▸ Adult: Initially 2.5 micrograms for 1 dose, increased to 5 micrograms for 1 dose, increased if tolerated to 5 micrograms 6–9 times a day, adjusted according to response; reduced if not tolerated to 2.5 micrograms 6–9 times a day, reduce to lower maintenance dose if high dose not tolerated

Severe Raynaud's phenomenon in patients with progressive trophic disorders
▸ BY INTRAVENOUS INFUSION
▸ Adult: Initially 0.5 nanogram/kg/minute for 30 minutes, then increased, if tolerated, in steps of 0.5 nanogram/kg/minute every 30 minutes (max. per dose 2 nanograms/kg/minute); usual dose 1.5–2 nanograms/kg/minute given over 6 hours daily for 5 days, repeat cycles should take place at intervals of at least 4 weeks (preferably 6–12 weeks)

Severe chronic lower limb ischaemia
▸ BY INTRAVENOUS INFUSION
▸ Adult: Initially 0.5 nanogram/kg/minute for 30 minutes, then increased, if tolerated, in steps of 0.5 nanogram/kg/minute every 30 minutes (max. per dose 2 nanograms/kg/minute); usual dose 0.5–2 nanograms/kg/minute given over 6 hours daily for up to 4 weeks

● CONTRA-INDICATIONS
GENERAL CONTRA-INDICATIONS Conditions which increase risk of haemorrhage · congenital or acquired valvular defects with myocardial function disorders (not related to pulmonary hypertension) · decompensated heart failure (unless under close medical supervision) · severe arrhythmias · severe coronary heart disease · unstable angina · within 3 months of cerebrovascular events · within 6 months of myocardial infarction

SPECIFIC CONTRA-INDICATIONS
▸ When used by inhalation Pulmonary veno-occlusive disease · systolic blood pressure below 85 mmHg · unstable pulmonary hypertension with advanced right heart failure
▸ With intravenous use Acute or chronic congestive heart failure (NYHA II-IV) · pulmonary oedema

● CAUTIONS
GENERAL CAUTIONS Hypotension
SPECIFIC CAUTIONS
▸ When used by inhalation Acute pulmonary infection · chronic obstructive pulmonary disease · severe asthma
▸ With intravenous use Significant heart disease

● INTERACTIONS → Appendix 1: iloprost

● SIDE-EFFECTS
GENERAL SIDE-EFFECTS
▸ **Common or very common** Cough · diarrhoea · dizziness · dyspnoea · haemorrhage · hypotension · nausea · pain · palpitations · syncope · vomiting
▸ **Uncommon** Taste altered · thrombocytopenia

SPECIFIC SIDE-EFFECTS
▸ **Common or very common**
▸ When used by inhalation Chest discomfort · headache · oral disorders · rash · tachycardia · throat complaints · vasodilation
▸ With intravenous use Angina pectoris · anxiety · appetite decreased · arrhythmias · arthralgia · asthenia · bradyphrenia · chills · confusion · drowsiness · feeling hot · fever · flushing · gastrointestinal discomfort · headaches · hyperhidrosis · muscle complaints · sensation abnormal · thirst · vertigo
▸ **Uncommon**
▸ With intravenous use Asthma · cerebrovascular insufficiency · constipation · depression · dry mouth · dysphagia · dysuria · embolism and thrombosis · eye discomfort · hallucination · heart failure · hepatic impairment · myocardial infarction · pruritus · pulmonary oedema · renal pain · seizure · tetany · tremor · vision blurred
▸ **Frequency not known**
▸ When used by inhalation Respiratory disorders

● PREGNANCY
▸ When used by inhalation Use if potential benefit outweighs risk.

▸ With intravenous use Manufacturer advises avoid—toxicity in *animal* studies.
● BREAST FEEDING Manufacturer advises avoid—no information available.
● HEPATIC IMPAIRMENT Manufacturer advises caution (risk of increased exposure).
Dose adjustments
▸ When used by inhalation Manufacturer advises initial dose reduction to 2.5 micrograms at intervals of 3–4 hours (max. 6 times daily), adjusted according to response—consult product literature.
▸ With intravenous use Manufacturer advises initial dose reduction in severe impairment, consider half the normal dose.

● MONITORING REQUIREMENTS
▸ With intravenous use Manufacturer advises monitor blood pressure and heart rate at the start of the infusion and at every dose increase.

● DIRECTIONS FOR ADMINISTRATION
▸ With intravenous use For *intravenous infusion* dilute to a concentration of 200 nanograms/mL with Glucose 5% or Sodium Chloride 0.9%; alternatively, may be diluted to a concentration of 2 micrograms/mL and given via syringe driver.
▸ When used by inhalation For *inhaled treatment*, to minimise accidental exposure use only with nebulisers listed in product literature in a well ventilated room.

● PRESCRIBING AND DISPENSING INFORMATION
▸ When used by inhalation Delivery characteristics of nebuliser devices may vary—only switch devices under medical supervision.
▸ With intravenous use Concentrate for infusion available on a named patient basis from Bayer Schering in 0.5 mL and 1 mL ampoules.

● HANDLING AND STORAGE Manufacturer advises avoid contact with skin and eyes.

● PATIENT AND CARER ADVICE
Driving and skilled tasks Manufacturer advises patients and carers should be counselled on the effects on driving and performance of skilled tasks—increased risk of dizziness.

● NATIONAL FUNDING/ACCESS DECISIONS
For full details see funding body website
Scottish Medicines Consortium (SMC) decisions
▸ **Iloprost trometamol (*Ventavis*®) for primary pulmonary hypertension (December 2005)** SMC No. 219/05 Recommended with restrictions

● MEDICINAL FORMS There can be variation in the licensing of different medicines containing the same drug.
Solution for infusion
EXCIPIENTS: May contain Ethanol
▸ Iloprost (Non-proprietary)
Iloprost (as Iloprost trometamol) 100 microgram per 1 ml Ilomedin 100micrograms/1ml solution for infusion ampoules | 1 ampoule [PoM] 💊
Iloprost 50micrograms/0.5ml concentrate for solution for infusion ampoules | 1 ampoule [PoM] £58.00-£75.00 (Hospital only) | 5 ampoule [PoM] £300.00 (Hospital only)

Nebuliser liquid
EXCIPIENTS: May contain Ethanol
▸ Iloprost (Non-proprietary)
Iloprost (as Iloprost trometamol) 10 microgram per 1 ml Iloprost 10micrograms/1ml nebuliser liquid ampoules | 30 ampoule [PoM] £300.00 | 160 ampoule [PoM] £1,700.00
Iloprost (as Iloprost trometamol) 20 microgram per 1 ml Iloprost 20micrograms/1ml nebuliser liquid ampoules | 30 ampoule [PoM] £375.00 (Hospital only) | 168 ampoule [PoM] £2,000.00 (Hospital only)
▸ Ventavis (Bayer Plc)
Iloprost (as Iloprost trometamol) 10 microgram per 1 ml Ventavis 10micrograms/ml nebuliser solution 1ml ampoules | 42 ampoule [PoM] £560.27 (Hospital only) | 168 ampoule [PoM] £2,241.08 (Hospital only)

Ventavis 10micrograms/ml nebuliser solution 1ml ampoules with
Breelib | 168 ampoule [PoM] £2,241.08
Iloprost (as Iloprost trometamol) 20 microgram per 1 ml Ventavis
20micrograms/ml nebuliser solution 1ml ampoules with Breelib |
168 ampoule [PoM] £2,241.08
Ventavis 20micrograms/ml nebuliser solution 1ml ampoules |
42 ampoule [PoM] £560.27

Treprostinil
19-Jan-2021

- **DRUG ACTION** Treprostinil is a prostacyclin analogue that
has a direct vasodilation effect on the pulmonary and
systemic arterial circulation and inhibits platelet
aggregation.

- **INDICATIONS AND DOSE**
**Idiopathic or hereditary pulmonary arterial hypertension
(specialist use only)**
  ▸ BY CONTINUOUS SUBCUTANEOUS INFUSION, OR BY
  CONTINUOUS INTRAVENOUS INFUSION
  ▸ Adult: (consult product literature)

- **CONTRA-INDICATIONS** Bleeding, such as active gastrointestinal ulcer, intracranial haemorrhage, or injury ·
cerebrovascular event (within the last 3 months) ·
congenital or acquired valvular defects with myocardial
function disorders (not related to pulmonary
hypertension) · congestive heart failure due to severe left
ventricular dysfunction · decompensated cardiac failure
(unless under close medical supervision) · myocardial
infarction (within the last 6 months) · pulmonary arterial
hypertension caused by veno-occlusive disease · severe
arrhythmias · severe coronary heart disease · unstable
angina

- **CAUTIONS** Avoid abrupt withdrawal or sudden marked
dose reductions (risk of rebound pulmonary hypertension)
· BMI greater than 30 kg/m^2 (slower clearance) · elderly
(limited information available) · systolic blood pressure
below 85 mmHg (increased risk of systemic hypotension)

- **INTERACTIONS** → Appendix 1: treprostinil

- **SIDE-EFFECTS**
  ▸ **Common or very common** Arthralgia · diarrhoea · dizziness ·
  haemorrhage · headache · hypotension · myalgia · nausea ·
  oedema · pain · skin reactions · vasodilation · vomiting
  ▸ **Frequency not known** Cardiac failure high output · catheter
  related infection · increased risk of infection · sepsis ·
  thrombocytopenia · thrombophlebitis

- **PREGNANCY** [EvGr] Use only if potential benefit outweighs
risk—limited information available. Ⓜ

- **BREAST FEEDING** [EvGr] Discontinue breast-feeding—no
information available. Ⓜ

- **HEPATIC IMPAIRMENT** [EvGr] Caution in mild to moderate
impairment; avoid in severe impairment (risk of increased
exposure). Ⓜ
  Dose adjustments [EvGr] Dose reduction (risk of increased
  exposure)—consult product literature. Ⓜ

- **RENAL IMPAIRMENT** [EvGr] Caution (risk of increased
exposure). Ⓜ

- **MONITORING REQUIREMENTS** [EvGr] Monitor blood pressure
and heart rate during any dose adjustment; stop infusion if
hypotension develops or systolic blood pressure is
85 mmHg or lower. Ⓜ

- **TREATMENT CESSATION** [EvGr] Avoid abrupt withdrawal
(risk of rebound pulmonary hypertension). Ⓜ

- **PATIENT AND CARER ADVICE**
  Driving and skilled tasks [EvGr] Patients and carers should be
  counselled on the effects on driving and performance of
  skilled tasks—increased risk of hypotension or dizziness at
  the start of treatment or dose adjustment. Ⓜ

- **MEDICINAL FORMS** There can be variation in the licensing of
different medicines containing the same drug.
Solution for infusion
ELECTROLYTES: May contain Sodium
  ▸ **Treprostinil (Non-proprietary)**
  Treprostinil (as Treprostinil sodium) 1 mg per 1 ml Treprostinil
  20mg/20ml solution for infusion vials | 1 vial [PoM] £1,338.00
  (Hospital only)
  Treprostinil (as Treprostinil sodium) 2.5 mg per 1 ml Treprostinil
  50mg/20ml solution for infusion vials | 1 vial [PoM] £2,998.75–
  £4,062.00 (Hospital only)
  Treprostinil (as Treprostinil sodium) 5 mg per 1 ml Treprostinil
  100mg/20ml solution for infusion vials | 1 vial [PoM] £6,222.50–
  £7,407.00 (Hospital only)
  Treprostinil (as Treprostinil sodium) 10 mg per 1 ml Treprostinil
  200mg/20ml solution for infusion vials | 1 vial [PoM] £11,417.50
  (Hospital only)
  ▸ **Treposuvi** (AOP Orphan Ltd)
  Treprostinil (as Treprostinil sodium) 1 mg per 1 ml Treposuvi
  10mg/10ml solution for infusion vials | 1 vial [PoM] £533.20 (Hospital
  only)
  Treprostinil (as Treprostinil sodium) 2.5 mg per 1 ml Treposuvi
  25mg/10ml solution for infusion vials | 1 vial [PoM] £1,333.00
  (Hospital only)
  Treprostinil (as Treprostinil sodium) 5 mg per 1 ml Treposuvi
  50mg/10ml solution for infusion vials | 1 vial [PoM] £2,666.00
  (Hospital only)
  Treprostinil (as Treprostinil sodium) 10 mg per 1 ml Treposuvi
  100mg/10ml solution for infusion vials | 1 vial [PoM] £5,332.00
  (Hospital only)
  ▸ **Trepulmix** (AOP Orphan Ltd)
  Treprostinil (as Treprostinil sodium) 1 mg per 1 ml Trepulmix
  10mg/10ml solution for infusion vials | 1 vial [PoM] £533.20 (Hospital
  only)
  Treprostinil (as Treprostinil sodium) 2.5 mg per 1 ml Trepulmix
  25mg/10ml solution for infusion vials | 1 vial [PoM] £1,333.00
  (Hospital only)
  Treprostinil (as Treprostinil sodium) 5 mg per 1 ml Trepulmix
  50mg/10ml solution for infusion vials | 1 vial [PoM] £2,666.00
  (Hospital only)
  Treprostinil (as Treprostinil sodium) 10 mg per 1 ml Trepulmix
  100mg/10ml solution for infusion vials | 1 vial [PoM] £5,332.00
  (Hospital only)

4.2 Hypotension and shock

Sympathomimetics
15-Jan-2025

Inotropic sympathomimetics

Shock

Shock is a medical emergency associated with a high
mortality. The underlying causes of shock such as
haemorrhage, sepsis, or myocardial insufficiency should be
corrected. The profound hypotension of shock must be
treated promptly to prevent tissue hypoxia and organ failure.
Volume replacement is essential to correct the hypovolaemia
associated with haemorrhage and sepsis but may be
detrimental in cardiogenic shock. Depending on
haemodynamic status, cardiac output may be improved by
the use of sympathomimetic inotropes such as
adrenaline/epinephrine p. 256, dobutamine p. 215 or
dopamine hydrochloride p. 216. In septic shock, when fluid
replacement fails to maintain blood pressure, the
vasoconstrictor noradrenaline/norepinephrine p. 217 may be
considered as the first-line agent. In cardiogenic shock
peripheral resistance is frequently high and to raise it further
may worsen myocardial performance and exacerbate tissue
ischaemia.

The use of sympathomimetic inotropes and
vasoconstrictors should preferably be confined to the
intensive care setting and undertaken with invasive
haemodynamic monitoring.

See also advice on the management of anaphylactic shock in Antihistamines, allergen immunotherapy and allergic emergencies p. 316.

Vasoconstrictor sympathomimetics

Vasoconstrictor sympathomimetics raise blood pressure transiently by acting on alpha-adrenergic receptors to constrict peripheral vessels. They are sometimes used as an emergency method of elevating blood pressure where other measures have failed.

The danger of vasoconstrictors is that although they raise blood pressure they also reduce perfusion of vital organs such as the kidney.

Spinal and epidural anaesthesia may result in sympathetic block with resultant hypotension. Management may include intravenous fluids (which are usually given prophylactically), oxygen, elevation of the legs, and injection of a pressor drug such as ephedrine hydrochloride p. 311. As well as constricting peripheral vessels ephedrine hydrochloride also accelerates the heart rate (by acting on beta receptors). Use is made of this dual action of ephedrine hydrochloride to manage associated bradycardia (although intravenous injection of atropine sulfate p. 1526 may also be required if bradycardia persists).

DRUGS ACTING ON THE RENIN-ANGIOTENSIN SYSTEM

Angiotensin II
30-Nov-2022

- **DRUG ACTION** Angiotensin II stimulates release of aldosterone. It also acts directly on vascular smooth muscle cells via angiotensin II receptor type 1 (AT1) to increase blood pressure by vasoconstriction.

- **INDICATIONS AND DOSE**
  Refractory hypotension in distributive shock (under expert supervision)
  ▸ BY CONTINUOUS INTRAVENOUS INFUSION
  ▸ Adult: 20 nanograms/kg/minute, dose to be adjusted according to response, titrated up to every 5 minutes in steps of up to 15 nanograms/kg/minute; maximum 80 nanograms/kg/minute in the first 3 hours of treatment. Maximum maintenance dose 40 nanograms/kg/minute

- **CAUTIONS** Peripheral ischaemia (use lowest effective dose) · thromboembolism

  CAUTIONS, FURTHER INFORMATION
  ▸ Venous thromboembolism (VTE) [EvGr] Pharmacological VTE prophylaxis is recommended during treatment; if contra-indicated, mechanical prophylaxis should be considered. Ⓜ

- **SIDE-EFFECTS**
  ▸ **Common or very common** Embolism and thrombosis · peripheral ischaemia · tachycardia

- **PREGNANCY** [EvGr] Avoid unless potential benefit outweighs risk—limited information available. Ⓜ

- **BREAST FEEDING** [EvGr] Avoid—no information available. Ⓜ

- **TREATMENT CESSATION** [EvGr] Avoid abrupt withdrawal—reduce dose gradually according to blood pressure to avoid rebound hypotension or worsening of underlying shock. Ⓜ

- **DIRECTIONS FOR ADMINISTRATION** [EvGr] For *intravenous infusion*, give continuously in Sodium Chloride 0.9% via central venous catheter; dilute to a concentration of 5000 nanograms/mL or 10 000 nanograms/mL. Ⓜ

- **HANDLING AND STORAGE** Store in a refrigerator (2–8°C)—consult product literature for storage conditions after dilution.

- **MEDICINAL FORMS** There can be variation in the licensing of different medicines containing the same drug.
  Solution for infusion
  ▸ **Giapreza** (PAION Deutschland GmbH) ▼
  Angiotensin II (as Angiotensin II acetate) 2.5 mg per 1 ml Giapreza 2.5mg/1ml concentrate for solution for infusion vials | 10 vial [PoM] £8,510.00 (Hospital only)

SYMPATHOMIMETICS › INOTROPIC

Dobutamine
30-May-2023

- **DRUG ACTION** Dobutamine is a cardiac stimulant which acts on beta$_1$ receptors in cardiac muscle, and increases contractility.

- **INDICATIONS AND DOSE**
  Inotropic support in infarction, cardiac surgery, cardiomyopathies, septic shock, cardiogenic shock, and during positive end expiratory pressure ventilation
  ▸ BY INTRAVENOUS INFUSION
  ▸ Adult: Usual dose 2.5–10 micrograms/kg/minute, adjusted according to response, alternatively 0.5–40 micrograms/kg/minute
  Cardiac stress testing
  ▸ BY INTRAVENOUS INFUSION
  ▸ Adult: (consult product literature)

- **CONTRA-INDICATIONS** Phaeochromocytoma
- **CAUTIONS** Acute heart failure · acute myocardial infarction · arrhythmias · correct hypercapnia before starting and during treatment · correct hypovolaemia before starting and during treatment · correct hypoxia before starting and during treatment · correct metabolic acidosis before starting and during treatment · diabetes mellitus · elderly · extravasation may cause tissue necrosis · extreme caution or avoid in marked obstruction of cardiac ejection (such as idiopathic hypertrophic subaortic stenosis) · hyperthyroidism · ischaemic heart disease · occlusive vascular disease · severe hypotension · susceptibility to angle-closure glaucoma · tachycardia · tolerance may develop with continuous infusions longer than 72 hours

- **INTERACTIONS** → Appendix 1: sympathomimetics, inotropic

- **SIDE-EFFECTS**
  ▸ **Common or very common** Arrhythmias · bronchospasm · chest pain · dyspnoea · eosinophilia · fever · headache · inflammation localised · ischaemic heart disease · nausea · palpitations · platelet aggregation inhibition (on prolonged administration) · skin reactions · urinary urgency · vasoconstriction
  ▸ **Uncommon** Myocardial infarction
  ▸ **Rare or very rare** Atrioventricular block · cardiac arrest · coronary vasospasm · hypertension exacerbated · hypokalaemia · hypotension exacerbated
  ▸ **Frequency not known** Anxiety · cardiomyopathy · feeling hot · myoclonus · paraesthesia · tremor

- **PREGNANCY** No evidence of harm in *animal* studies—manufacturers advise use only if potential benefit outweighs risk.

- **BREAST FEEDING** Manufacturers advise avoid—no information available.

- **MONITORING REQUIREMENTS** Monitor serum-potassium concentration.

- **DIRECTIONS FOR ADMINISTRATION** Manufacturer advises dobutamine *injection* should be diluted before use or given undiluted with syringe pump. Dobutamine *concentrate* for intravenous infusion should be diluted before use.

  For *intravenous infusion*, manufacturer advises give continuously in Glucose 5% or Sodium Chloride 0.9%. Dilute to a concentration of 0.5–1 mg/mL and give via an infusion pump; give higher concentration (max. 5 mg/mL) through central venous catheter; incompatible with bicarbonate and other strong alkaline solutions.

- **MEDICINAL FORMS** There can be variation in the licensing of different medicines containing the same drug. Forms available from special-order manufacturers include: solution for infusion

Solution for infusion
EXCIPIENTS: May contain Sulfites

▸ Dobutamine (Non-proprietary)
Dobutamine (as Dobutamine hydrochloride) 5 mg per 1 ml Dobutamine 250mg/50ml solution for infusion vials | 1 vial PoM £11.20
Dobutamine 250mg/50ml solution for infusion pre-filled syringes | 1 pre-filled disposable injection PoM £15.00 (Hospital only)
Dobutamine (as Dobutamine hydrochloride) 12.5 mg per 1 ml Dobutamine 250mg/20ml concentrate for solution for infusion ampoules | 10 ampoule PoM £63.50 | 10 ampoule PoM £52.50–£63.50 (Hospital only)

Dopamine hydrochloride

22-Feb-2021

- **DRUG ACTION** Dopamine is a cardiac stimulant which acts on beta$_1$ receptors in cardiac muscle, and increases contractility with little effect on rate.

- **INDICATIONS AND DOSE**

Cardiogenic shock in infarction or cardiac surgery
▸ BY CONTINUOUS INTRAVENOUS INFUSION
▸ Adult: Initially 2–5 micrograms/kg/minute

- **CONTRA-INDICATIONS** Phaeochromocytoma · tachyarrhythmia

- **CAUTIONS** Correct hypovolaemia · hypertension (may raise blood pressure) · hyperthyroidism · low dose in shock due to acute myocardial infarction

- **INTERACTIONS** → Appendix 1: sympathomimetics, inotropic

- **SIDE-EFFECTS** Angina pectoris · anxiety · arrhythmias · azotaemia · cardiac conduction disorder · dyspnoea · gangrene · headache · hypertension · mydriasis · nausea · palpitations · piloerection · polyuria · tremor · vasoconstriction · vomiting

- **PREGNANCY** No evidence of harm in *animal* studies—manufacturer advises use only if potential benefit outweighs risk.

- **BREAST FEEDING** May suppress lactation—not known to be harmful.

- **DIRECTIONS FOR ADMINISTRATION** EvGr Dopamine concentrate for intravenous infusion to be diluted before use; give via a large vein.
  For *intravenous infusion*, give continuously in Glucose 5% or Sodium Chloride 0.9%. Dilute to max. concentration of 3.2 mg/mL; incompatible with bicarbonate. Ⓜ

- **MEDICINAL FORMS** There can be variation in the licensing of different medicines containing the same drug. Forms available from special-order manufacturers include: solution for infusion

Solution for infusion

▸ Dopamine hydrochloride (Non-proprietary)
Dopamine hydrochloride 40 mg per 1 ml Dopamine 200mg/5ml solution for infusion ampoules | 10 ampoule PoM £14.78 | 10 ampoule PoM £14.78 (Hospital only)
Dopamine 200mg/5ml concentrate for solution for infusion ampoules | 10 ampoule PoM £20.00 (Hospital only)

Metaraminol

28-Apr-2020

- **INDICATIONS AND DOSE**

Emergency treatment of acute hypotension
▸ INITIALLY BY INTRAVENOUS INJECTION
▸ Adult: Initially 0.5–5 mg, then (by intravenous infusion) 15–100 mg, adjusted according to response

Acute hypotension
▸ BY INTRAVENOUS INFUSION
▸ Adult: 15–100 mg, adjusted according to response

- **CAUTIONS** Cirrhosis · coronary vascular thrombosis · diabetes mellitus · elderly · extravasation at injection site may cause necrosis · following myocardial infarction · hypercapnia · hypertension · hyperthyroidism · hypoxia · mesenteric vascular thrombosis · peripheral vascular thrombosis · Prinzmetal's variant angina · uncorrected hypovolaemia

CAUTIONS, FURTHER INFORMATION
▸ Hypertensive response Metaraminol has a longer duration of action than noradrenaline, and an excessive vasopressor response may cause a prolonged rise in blood pressure.

- **INTERACTIONS** → Appendix 1: sympathomimetics, vasoconstrictor

- **SIDE-EFFECTS**
▸ **Common or very common** Headache · hypertension
▸ **Rare or very rare** Skin exfoliation · soft tissue necrosis
▸ **Frequency not known** Abscess · arrhythmias · nausea · palpitations · peripheral ischaemia

- **PREGNANCY** May reduce placental perfusion—manufacturer advises use only if potential benefit outweighs risk.

- **BREAST FEEDING** Manufacturer advises caution—no information available.

- **MONITORING REQUIREMENTS** Monitor blood pressure and rate of flow frequently.

- **DIRECTIONS FOR ADMINISTRATION** For *intravenous infusion*, give continuously or via drip tubing in Glucose 5% or Sodium Chloride 0.9%. Suggested volume 500 mL.

- **MEDICINAL FORMS** There can be variation in the licensing of different medicines containing the same drug. Forms available from special-order manufacturers include: solution for injection

Solution for injection

▸ Metaraminol (Non-proprietary)
Metaraminol (as Metaraminol tartrate) 500 microgram per 1 ml Metaraminol 2.5mg/5ml solution for injection ampoules | 10 ampoule PoM £52.90 (Hospital only)
Metaraminol 5mg/10ml solution for injection ampoules | 10 ampoule PoM £107.40 (Hospital only)
Metaraminol 2.5mg/5ml solution for injection pre-filled syringes | 10 pre-filled disposable injection PoM £95.00 (Hospital only)
Metaraminol 5mg/10ml solution for injection vials | 10 vial PoM £55.00 (Hospital only)
Metaraminol (as Metaraminol tartrate) 10 mg per 1 ml Metaraminol 10mg/1ml solution for injection vials | 10 vial PoM £20.50 (Hospital only)
Metaraminol 10mg/1ml solution for injection ampoules | 5 ampoule PoM £25.00 | 10 ampoule PoM £70.60 | 10 ampoule PoM £21.50 (Hospital only)

Midodrine hydrochloride
11-May-2021

- **DRUG ACTION** Midodrine hydrochloride is a pro-drug of desglymidodrine. Desglymidodrine is a sympathomimetic agent, which acts on peripheral alpha-adrenergic receptors to increase arterial resistance, resulting in an increase in blood pressure.

● INDICATIONS AND DOSE

Severe orthostatic hypotension due to autonomic dysfunction when corrective factors have been ruled out and other forms of treatment are inadequate
- ▸ BY MOUTH
- ▸ Adult: Initially 2.5 mg 3 times a day, increased if necessary up to 10 mg 3 times a day, dose to be increased at weekly intervals, according to blood pressure measurements; usual maintenance 10 mg 3 times a day, avoid administration at night; the last daily dose should be taken at least 4 hours before bedtime

- **CONTRA-INDICATIONS** Aortic aneurysm · blood vessel spasm · bradycardia · cardiac conduction disturbances · cerebrovascular occlusion · congestive heart failure · hypertension · hyperthyroidism · myocardial infarction · narrow-angle glaucoma · phaeochromocytoma · proliferative diabetic retinopathy · serious obliterative blood vessel disease · serious prostate disorder · urinary retention

- **CAUTIONS** Atherosclerotic cardiovascular disease (especially with symptoms of intestinal angina or claudication of the legs) · autonomic dysfunction · elderly (manufacturer recommends cautious dose titration) · prostate disorders

- **INTERACTIONS** → Appendix 1: sympathomimetics, vasoconstrictor

- **SIDE-EFFECTS**
- ▸ **Common or very common** Chills · flushing · gastrointestinal discomfort · headache · nausea · paraesthesia · piloerection · scalp pruritus · skin reactions · stomatitis · supine hypertension (dose-dependent) · urinary disorders
- ▸ **Uncommon** Anxiety · arrhythmias · irritability · sleep disorders
- ▸ **Rare or very rare** Hepatic function abnormal · palpitations
- ▸ **Frequency not known** Confusion · diarrhoea · vomiting
- **SIDE-EFFECTS, FURTHER INFORMATION** Manufacturer advises that treatment must be stopped if supine hypertension is not controlled by reducing the dose.

- **CONCEPTION AND CONTRACEPTION** Manufacturer recommends effective contraception during treatment in women of childbearing potential.

- **PREGNANCY** Manufacturer advises avoid—toxicity in *animal* studies.

- **BREAST FEEDING** Manufacturer advises avoid—no information available.

- **RENAL IMPAIRMENT** Manufacturer advises avoid in severe or acute impairment.

- **MONITORING REQUIREMENTS**
- ▸ Manufacturer advises measure hepatic and renal function before treatment and at regular intervals during treatment.
- ▸ Manufacturer advises regular monitoring of supine and standing blood pressure due to the risk of hypertension in the supine position.

- **PATIENT AND CARER ADVICE** Manufacturer advises that patients report symptoms of supine hypertension (such as chest pain, palpitations, shortness of breath, headache and blurred vision) immediately. The risk of supine hypertension at night can be reduced by raising the head of the bed.

- **MEDICINAL FORMS** There can be variation in the licensing of different medicines containing the same drug.
Oral tablet
- ▸ **Midodrine hydrochloride (Non-proprietary)**
  Midodrine hydrochloride 2.5 mg Midodrine 2.5mg tablets | 100 tablet [PoM] £53.35 DT = £12.80
  Midodrine hydrochloride 5 mg Midodrine 5mg tablets | 100 tablet [PoM] £76.01 DT = £18.94
  Midodrine hydrochloride 10 mg Midodrine 10mg tablets | 100 tablet [PoM] £128.34 DT = £40.00
- ▸ **Bramox** (Brancaster Pharma Ltd)
  Midodrine hydrochloride 2.5 mg Bramox 2.5mg tablets | 100 tablet [PoM] £22.50 DT = £12.80
  Midodrine hydrochloride 5 mg Bramox 5mg tablets | 100 tablet [PoM] £30.00 DT = £18.94
  Midodrine hydrochloride 10 mg Bramox 10mg tablets | 100 tablet [PoM] £40.00 DT = £40.00

Noradrenaline/norepinephrine
13-May-2020

● INDICATIONS AND DOSE

Acute hypotension [initial and on-going treatment]
- ▸ BY INTRAVENOUS INFUSION
- ▸ Adult: Initially 0.16–0.33 mL/minute, adjusted according to response, dose applies to a solution containing noradrenaline 40 micrograms(base)/mL only; dilute the 1 mg/mL concentrate for infusion for this solution—consult product literature

On-going treatment of acute hypotension [with escalating dose requirements]
- ▸ BY INTRAVENOUS INFUSION
- ▸ Adult (body-weight 50 kg and above): Use the 0.08 mg/mL or 0.16 mg/mL solution for infusion (consult product literature)
- **DOSE EQUIVALENCE AND CONVERSION**
- ▸ 1 mg of noradrenaline base is equivalent to 2 mg of noradrenaline acid tartrate. **Doses expressed as the base.**

> **IMPORTANT SAFETY INFORMATION**
> ASSOCIATION OF NORADRENALINE/NOREPINEPHRINE 0.08 MG/ML (4 MG IN 50 ML) AND 0.16 MG/ML (8 MG IN 50 ML) SOLUTION FOR INFUSION WITH POTENTIAL RISK OF MEDICATION ERRORS
> Healthcare professionals should be aware of the differences in strength and presentation between noradrenaline/norepinephrine products—manufacturer advises noradrenaline 0.08 mg/mL solution for infusion and noradrenaline 0.16 mg/mL solution for infusion must **not** be diluted before use and should only be used for the on-going treatment of patients already established on noradrenaline therapy, whose dose requirements are clinically confirmed to be escalating.

- **CONTRA-INDICATIONS** Hypertension
- **CAUTIONS** Coronary vascular thrombosis · diabetes mellitus · elderly · extravasation at injection site may cause necrosis · following myocardial infarction · hypercapnia · hyperthyroidism · hypoxia · mesenteric vascular thrombosis · peripheral vascular thrombosis · Prinzmetal's variant angina · uncorrected hypovolaemia
- **INTERACTIONS** → Appendix 1: sympathomimetics, vasoconstrictor
- **SIDE-EFFECTS** Acute glaucoma · anxiety · arrhythmias · asthenia · cardiomyopathy · confusion · dyspnoea · extravasation necrosis · gangrene · headache · heart failure · hypovolaemia · hypoxia · injection site necrosis · insomnia · ischaemia · myocardial contractility increased · nausea · palpitations · peripheral ischaemia · psychotic

2
Cardiovascular system

disorder · respiratory failure · tremor · urinary retention · vomiting

- **PREGNANCY** Manufacturer advises use if potential benefit outweighs risk—may reduce placental perfusion and induce fetal bradycardia.

- **MONITORING REQUIREMENTS** Monitor blood pressure and rate of flow frequently.

- **DIRECTIONS FOR ADMINISTRATION** For *intravenous infusion* using a solution containing noradrenaline 40 micrograms (base)/mL, manufacturer advises give continuously in Glucose 5% or Sodium Chloride and Glucose via a controlled infusion device. For administration via syringe pump, dilute 2 mg (2 mL of 1 mg/mL concentrate for infusion) noradrenaline base with 48 mL infusion fluid. For administration via drip counter dilute 20 mg (20 mL of 1 mg/mL concentrate for infusion) noradrenaline base with 480 mL infusion fluid; give through a central venous catheter; incompatible with alkalis.

- **PRESCRIBING AND DISPENSING INFORMATION** For a period of time, preparations on the UK market may be described as either noradrenaline base or noradrenaline acid tartrate; doses in BNF Publications are expressed as the base.

- **MEDICINAL FORMS** There can be variation in the licensing of different medicines containing the same drug. Forms available from special-order manufacturers include: infusion, solution for infusion

Solution for infusion

▸ Noradrenaline/norepinephrine (Non-proprietary)
Noradrenaline (as Noradrenaline acid tartrate) 80 microgram per 1 ml Noradrenaline (base) 4mg/50ml solution for infusion vials | 10 vial PoM £111.00 (Hospital only)
Noradrenaline (as Noradrenaline acid tartrate) 1 mg per 1 ml Noradrenaline (base) 1mg/1ml concentrate for solution for infusion ampoules | 10 ampoule PoM ⚕ (Hospital only)
Noradrenaline (base) 8mg/8ml concentrate for solution for infusion ampoules | 10 ampoule PoM £116.00–£145.30 (Hospital only)
Noradrenaline (base) 2mg/2ml solution for infusion ampoules | 5 ampoule PoM £12.00 (Hospital only)
Noradrenaline (base) 2mg/2ml concentrate for solution for infusion ampoules | 10 ampoule PoM ⚕ (Hospital only)
Noradrenaline (base) 4mg/4ml concentrate for solution for infusion ampoules | 5 ampoule PoM £22.00 (Hospital only) | 10 ampoule PoM £22.00–£72.00 (Hospital only)
Noradrenaline (base) 10mg/10ml concentrate for solution for infusion ampoules | 10 ampoule PoM ⚕ (Hospital only)
▸ Sinora (Sandoz Ltd)
Noradrenaline (as Noradrenaline acid tartrate) 160 microgram per 1 ml Sinora 8mg/50ml solution for infusion vials | 1 vial PoM £14.22 (Hospital only)

Phenylephrine hydrochloride

- **INDICATIONS AND DOSE**

Acute hypotension
▸ BY SUBCUTANEOUS INJECTION, OR BY INTRAMUSCULAR INJECTION
▸ Adult: Initially 2–5 mg, followed by 1–10 mg, after at least 15 minutes if required
▸ BY SLOW INTRAVENOUS INJECTION
▸ Adult: 100–500 micrograms, repeated as necessary after at least 15 minutes
▸ BY INTRAVENOUS INFUSION
▸ Adult: Initially up to 180 micrograms/minute, reduced to 30–60 micrograms/minute, adjusted according to response

- **CONTRA-INDICATIONS** Hypertension · severe hyperthyroidism

- **CAUTIONS** Coronary disease · coronary vascular thrombosis · diabetes · elderly · extravasation at injection site may cause necrosis · following myocardial infarction ·

hypercapnia · hyperthyroidism · hypoxia · mesenteric vascular thrombosis · peripheral vascular thrombosis · Prinzmetal's variant angina · susceptibility to angle-closure glaucoma · uncorrected hypovolaemia

CAUTIONS, FURTHER INFORMATION

▸ Hypertensive response Phenylephrine has a longer duration of action than noradrenaline (norepinephrine), and an excessive vasopressor response may cause a prolonged rise in blood pressure.

- **INTERACTIONS** → Appendix 1: sympathomimetics, vasoconstrictor

- **SIDE-EFFECTS** Anxiety · arrhythmias · cardiac arrest · confusion · dizziness · dyspnoea · extravasation necrosis · flushing · glaucoma exacerbated · glucose tolerance impaired · headache · hyperhidrosis · hypersalivation · hypertensive crisis · hypotension · insomnia · intracranial haemorrhage · ischaemic heart disease · metabolic change · muscle weakness · mydriasis · nausea · pallor · palpitations · paraesthesia · peripheral coldness · piloerection · psychotic disorder · pulmonary oedema · soft tissue necrosis · syncope · tremor · urinary disorders · vomiting

- **PREGNANCY** Avoid if possible; malformations reported following use in first trimester; fetal hypoxia and bradycardia reported in late pregnancy and labour.

- **MONITORING REQUIREMENTS** Contra-indicated in hypertension—monitor blood pressure and rate of flow frequently.

- **DIRECTIONS FOR ADMINISTRATION** For *intravenous infusion* give intermittently in Glucose 5% or Sodium Chloride 0.9%. Dilute 10 mg in 500 mL infusion fluid.

- **MEDICINAL FORMS** There can be variation in the licensing of different medicines containing the same drug. Forms available from special-order manufacturers include: solution for injection

Solution for injection
▸ Phenylephrine hydrochloride (Non-proprietary)
Phenylephrine (as Phenylephrine hydrochloride) 50 microgram per 1 ml Phenylephrine 500micrograms/10ml solution for injection pre-filled syringes | 10 pre-filled disposable injection PoM £150.00 (Hospital only)
Phenylephrine hydrochloride 100 microgram per 1 ml Phenylephrine 1mg/10ml solution for injection ampoules | 10 ampoule PoM £47.59 (Hospital only)
Phenylephrine 2mg/20ml solution for injection vials | 10 vial PoM £110.00 (Hospital only)
Phenylephrine hydrochloride 10 mg per 1 ml Phenylephrine 10mg/1ml solution for injection ampoules | 10 ampoule PoM £99.00–£99.12 (Hospital only)
Phenylephrine 10mg/1ml concentrate for solution for injection ampoules | 10 ampoule PoM £102.09 (Hospital only)

5 Cardiomyopathy

CARDIAC MYOSIN INHIBITORS

Mavacamten

28-Nov-2024

- **DRUG ACTION** Mavacamten is a cardiac myosin inhibitor that acts to normalise cardiac contractility, reduce dynamic left ventricular outflow tract obstruction, and improve cardiac filling pressures.

- **INDICATIONS AND DOSE**

Symptomatic obstructive hypertrophic cardiomyopathy (initiated by a specialist)
▸ BY MOUTH
▸ Adult: (consult product literature)

DOSE EQUIVALENCE AND CONVERSION

▶ Bioequivalence between different capsule strengths has not been confirmed—consult product literature.

IMPORTANT SAFETY INFORMATION

Bioequivalence between different capsule strengths has not been confirmed, therefore only one capsule of the appropriate strength should be used to achieve the prescribed dose and not multiple capsules—consult product literature.

● **CONTRA-INDICATIONS** Left ventricular ejection fraction less than 55% (do not initiate)

● **CAUTIONS** Risk factors for systolic dysfunction

CAUTIONS, FURTHER INFORMATION

▶ Systolic dysfunction [EvGr] Patients with a serious intercurrent illness (e.g. infection or arrhythmia) or undergoing major cardiac surgery may be at greater risk of systolic dysfunction and progress to heart failure. ⟨M⟩ For treatment interruption due to systolic dysfunction— consult product literature.

● **INTERACTIONS** → Appendix 1: mavacamten

● **SIDE-EFFECTS**

▶ **Common or very common** Dizziness · dyspnoea · syncope · systolic dysfunction

● **CONCEPTION AND CONTRACEPTION** [EvGr] Females of childbearing potential should use effective contraception during treatment and for 6 months after last treatment. ⟨M⟩

● **PREGNANCY** [EvGr] Avoid (toxicity in *animal* studies). ⟨M⟩

● **BREAST FEEDING** [EvGr] Avoid (no information available). ⟨M⟩

● **HEPATIC IMPAIRMENT** [EvGr] Caution in severe impairment (no information available). ⟨M⟩
Dose adjustments For dose adjustments in mild to moderate impairment—consult product literature.

● **PRE-TREATMENT SCREENING** NHS England commissions genetic testing under the *National genomic test directory* indication: R454 - Mavacamten for treating symptomatic obstructive hypertrophic cardiomyopathy. The testing is available to individuals with symptomatic obstructive hypertrophic cardiomyopathy who have a New York Heart Association class of II to III and are eligible for treatment with mavacamten in line with NICE TA913. For further information, see www.england.nhs.uk/publication/national-genomic-test-directories/.

● **MONITORING REQUIREMENTS**

▶ [EvGr] Monitor left ventricular ejection fraction before starting and during treatment ⟨M⟩—consult product literature.

▶ [EvGr] Monitor left ventricular outflow tract gradient during treatment ⟨M⟩—consult product literature.

● **PRESCRIBING AND DISPENSING INFORMATION** The manufacturer of *Camzyos*® has provided a *Healthcare Professional Checklist.*

● **PATIENT AND CARER ADVICE** A patient card and patient guide should be provided.
Driving and skilled tasks Patients and carers should be counselled on the effects on driving and performance of skilled tasks—increased risk of dizziness.

● **NATIONAL FUNDING/ACCESS DECISIONS**
For full details see funding body website

NICE decisions

▶ Mavacamten for treating symptomatic obstructive hypertrophic cardiomyopathy (September 2023) NICE TA913 Recommended with restrictions

Scottish Medicines Consortium (SMC) decisions

▶ Mavacamten (*Camzyos*®) for the treatment of symptomatic (New York Heart Association class II to III) obstructive

hypertrophic cardiomyopathy in adult patients (April 2024) SMC No. SMC2618 Recommended

● **MEDICINAL FORMS** There can be variation in the licensing of different medicines containing the same drug.
Oral capsule

▶ Camzyos (Bristol-Myers Squibb Pharmaceuticals Ltd) ▼
Mavacamten 2.5 mg Camzyos 2.5mg capsules | 28 capsule [PoM] £1,073.20 (Hospital only)
Mavacamten 5 mg Camzyos 5mg capsules | 28 capsule [PoM] £1,073.20 (Hospital only)
Mavacamten 10 mg Camzyos 10mg capsules | 28 capsule [PoM] £1,073.20 (Hospital only)
Mavacamten 15 mg Camzyos 15mg capsules | 28 capsule [PoM] £1,073.20 (Hospital only)

---

6 Cardiovascular risk assessment and prevention

Cardiovascular disease risk assessment and prevention
12-Sep-2024

Description of condition

Cardiovascular disease (CVD) is a term that describes a group of disorders of the heart and blood vessels caused by atherosclerosis and thrombosis, which includes coronary heart disease, stroke, peripheral arterial disease, and aortic disease.

The risk of CVD is greater in males, individuals with a family history of CVD, and in certain ethnic backgrounds such as those from South Asian or sub-Saharan African origins. CVD risk is also greater in individuals aged over 50 years, and increases with age. CVD has several important and potentially modifiable risk factors such as hypertension, abnormal lipids, obesity, diabetes mellitus, and psychosocial factors such as depression, anxiety, and social isolation. Low physical activity, poor diet, smoking, and excessive alcohol intake are also modifiable risk factors.

Aims of treatment

The overall aim of treatment is to prevent the occurrence of a cardiovascular event by reducing modifiable risk factors through lifestyle changes and drug management.

Cardiovascular disease risk assessment

Recommendations on CVD risk assessment are from the *NICE—Cardiovascular disease: risk assessment and reduction, including lipid modification guideline (NG238, 2023)*, and *SIGN—Risk estimation and the prevention of cardiovascular disease guideline (SIGN 149, 2017)*. *SIGN* 149 uses risk assessment strategies outlined by the *Joint British Society (JBS)—Joint British Societies' consensus recommendations for the prevention of cardiovascular disease (2014)*. Recommendations where NICE and SIGN differ have been highlighted.

[EvGr] NICE (2023) recommends that for primary prevention of CVD in primary care, a systematic approach be used to identify those who are likely to be at high risk. Individuals should be prioritised based on an estimate of their CVD risk using risk factors already recorded in their medical records, before a full formal risk assessment. Priority for a full formal risk assessment should be given to those with an estimated 10-year risk of 10% or more. Individuals aged over 40 years should have their CVD risk estimated and reviewed on an ongoing basis. SIGN (2017) instead recommends that CVD risk assessments are offered at least every 5 years to all individuals aged 40 years and over with no history of CVD, familial hypercholesterolaemia, chronic kidney disease, or diabetes mellitus, and those not receiving treatment to reduce blood pressure or lipids. As well as to individuals with a first-degree relative who has premature atherosclerotic CVD or familial dyslipidaemia, regardless of their age.

Risk assessment with a calculator is not necessary in patients who are clearly at high risk of CVD. This includes individuals with an estimated glomerular filtration rate (eGFR) less than 60 mL/minute/1.73 m^2 or albuminuria, with type 1 diabetes mellitus, or those with familial hypercholesterolaemia or other inherited disorders of lipid metabolism. In addition to these patients, NICE (2023) states that individuals aged 85 years and over, particularly if they smoke or have hypertension, are considered to be at high risk of CVD because of age alone. SIGN (2017) states that use of a calculator to estimate CVD risk is not required for patients with diabetes mellitus aged 40 years and over, and in those aged under 40 years with diabetes mellitus who have either had it for more than 20 years, present with target organ damage (such as proteinuria, albuminuria, proliferative retinopathy, or autonomic neuropathy), or have other significantly elevated cardiovascular risk factors. Ⓐ

Risk calculators

Cardiovascular risk assessment calculators are used to predict the approximate likelihood of a cardiovascular event occurring over a given period of time. EvGr Standard risk scores may be underestimated in certain patient groups with additional risk due to existing conditions (e.g. patients being treated for HIV, or those with severe mental illness, autoimmune disorders, or other systemic inflammatory disorders), or those taking medications that can cause dyslipidaemia (e.g. immunosuppressants). CVD risk may also be underestimated in patients who are already taking antihypertensives or lipid-regulating drugs, or who have recently stopped smoking. Interpretation of risk scores as well as the need for further management of risk factors in those who fall below the CVD risk threshold, should always reflect informed clinical judgement. Ⓐ

QRISK® 3

The QRISK® 3 risk calculator (available at: www.qrisk.org/) is recommended by NICE (2023), and is used in England and Wales. It is used to estimate the risk of developing coronary heart disease (angina and myocardial infarction), stroke, and transient ischaemic attack (TIA) within the next 10 years in individuals aged 25–84 years without CVD (including those with type 2 diabetes mellitus). This is based on age, sex, ethnicity, social deprivation, lipid profile, systolic blood pressure (including variability), BMI, smoking status, diabetes mellitus, family history of premature CVD in a first-degree relative, chronic kidney disease (stage 3 or above), atrial fibrillation, treated hypertension, rheumatoid arthritis, systemic lupus erythematosus, severe mental illness, migraine, atypical antipsychotics use, corticosteroid use, and erectile dysfunction.

ASSIGN

The ASSIGN cardiovascular risk assessment calculator is tailored to the Scottish population and uses factors such as age, sex, smoking, systolic blood pressure, lipid profile, family history of premature CVD, diabetes mellitus, rheumatoid arthritis, and social deprivation to estimate cardiovascular risk. EvGr Other risk factors not included in this CVD risk assessment calculator (such as ethnicity, BMI, atrial fibrillation, psychological wellbeing, and physical inactivity) should also be taken into account when assessing and managing the individual's overall CVD risk.

SIGN (2017) recommends that asymptomatic individuals without established CVD (or other conditions that are automatically associated with a high CVD risk) should be considered at high risk if they are assessed as having a 20% or more risk of a first cardiovascular event within 10 years. Ⓐ

The online calculator tool can be found at: rightdecisions. scot.nhs.uk/assign-v20. Full details can be found in the *SIGN* 149 *clinical guideline* (see *Useful resources*).

Cardiovascular disease prevention

Recommendations on cardiovascular disease (CVD) prevention are from the *NICE—Cardiovascular disease: risk assessment and reduction, including lipid modification guideline (NG238, 2023)*, and *SIGN—Risk estimation and the prevention of cardiovascular disease guideline (SIGN 149, 2017)*. SIGN 149 uses strategies outlined by the *Joint British Society (JBS)— Joint British Societies' consensus recommendations for the prevention of cardiovascular disease (2014)*. Recommendations where NICE and SIGN differ have been highlighted.

EvGr All patients at any risk of CVD should be advised to make lifestyle modifications that may include beneficial changes to diet (such as increasing fruit and vegetable consumption, reducing saturated fat and dietary salt intake), increasing physical exercise, weight management, reducing alcohol consumption, and Smoking cessation p. 565.

Further preventative measures with drug treatment should be taken in individuals with a high risk of developing CVD (primary prevention), and to prevent recurrence of events in those with established CVD (secondary prevention). An annual review should be considered to discuss lifestyle modification, medication adherence and risk factors. The frequency of review may be tailored to the individual. Ⓐ

Primary prevention

Antiplatelet therapy

EvGr Aspirin p. 142 is not recommended for *primary prevention* of CVD due to the limited benefit gained versus risk of side-effects such as bleeding. Ⓐ

Antihypertensive therapy

EvGr Antihypertensive drug treatment should be offered to patients who are at high risk of CVD and have sustained elevated systolic blood pressure and/or diastolic blood pressure. For further guidance on prescribing antihypertensive drugs in patients without symptomatic CVD and for specific groups at high cardiovascular risk, see Hypertension p. 166. Ⓐ

Lipid-lowering therapy

EvGr A statin is recommended as the lipid-lowering drug of choice for primary prevention of CVD. All modifiable risk factors, comorbidities and secondary causes of dyslipidaemia (e.g. uncontrolled diabetes mellitus, hepatic disease, nephrotic syndrome, excessive alcohol consumption, or hypothyroidism) should be managed before starting treatment with a statin. Factors such as polypharmacy, frailty, and comorbidities should be taken into account before starting statin therapy.

NICE (2023) recommends low-dose atorvastatin p. 234 for all patients (including those with type 2 diabetes mellitus) who have a 10% or greater 10-year risk of developing CVD (using the QRISK3 calculator), and for patients with chronic kidney disease. Low-dose atorvastatin p. 234 can also be considered in individuals with a risk score less than 10% if there is a concern the risk has been underestimated. Low-dose atorvastatin p. 234 should be considered in all patients with type 1 diabetes mellitus aged 18–40 years, and should be offered to patients with type 1 diabetes mellitus who are aged over 40 years, or have had diabetes mellitus for more than 10 years, or have established nephropathy, or have other CVD risk factors. Patients aged 85 years and over may also benefit from low-dose atorvastatin p. 234 to reduce their risk of non-fatal myocardial infarction. SIGN (2017) recommends low-dose atorvastatin p. 234 for patients who are considered to be at high risk of CVD and not on dialysis.

Patients taking statins should have an annual medication review to discuss medication adherence, lifestyle modification, and CVD risk factors; a full lipid profile should be considered (total cholesterol, HDL-cholesterol, triglycerides, non-HDL-cholesterol and LDL-cholesterol). Liver transaminases and a full lipid profile should also be assessed 2–3 months after starting or changing lipid-lowering treatment; liver transaminases should be reassessed at 12 months, but not again unless clinically indicated.

For primary prevention of CVD, aim for a reduction in non-HDL-cholesterol concentration of greater than 40%. If this is not achieved, adherence to drug treatment should be checked, lifestyle modifications optimised, and increasing the statin intensity considered if the patient is not on a high-intensity statin at the maximum tolerated dose. The use of higher doses in those with chronic kidney disease with an eGFR less than 30mL/minute/1.73 m^2 should be discussed with a renal specialist. ⒶFor statin intensity categorisation, see Dyslipidaemias p. 227.

EvGr SIGN (2017) recommends that ezetimibe p. 229 and bile acid sequestrants, such as colestyramine p. 229 and colestipol hydrochloride p. 228, only be considered for primary prevention in patients with an elevated cardiovascular risk in whom statin therapy is contra-indicated, and in patients with familial hypercholesterolaemia.

NICE (TA385, 2016) recommends that ezetimibe p. 229 be considered for primary hypercholesterolaemia as monotherapy when statins are unsuitable or not tolerated, or in combination with a statin for patients in whom the maximum tolerated dose of initial statin therapy fails to adequately control lipid concentrations and an alternative statin is being considered. NICE (2023) does not recommend bile acid sequestrants for primary prevention of CVD.

Although fibrates are not routinely recommended for primary prevention of CVD, SIGN (2017) states that they should be considered in patients with a combination of high CVD risk, marked hypertriglyceridaemia and low HDL-cholesterol concentration. Ⓐ

For other lipid-lowering therapy options, see NICE guideline: **Cardiovascular disease: risk assessment and reduction, including lipid modification** and SIGN guideline: **Risk estimation and the prevention of cardiovascular disease** (see *Useful resources*).

Lipid-lowering therapy recommendations from NICE guideline 238 (2023), and SIGN Clinical guideline 149 (2017) differ in certain respects for prevention of CVD in patients with diabetes mellitus—see individual guidelines for further details.

For further information on lipid-lowering therapy and familial hypercholesterolaemia, see Dyslipidaemias p. 227.

Secondary prevention
Antiplatelet therapy
EvGr Antiplatelet therapy with low-dose daily aspirin p. 142 should be offered to patients with established atherosclerotic disease. Alternatively, clopidogrel p. 143 can be considered in patients who are intolerant to *aspirin* or in whom it is contra-indicated. Ⓐ

For guidance on the use of antiplatelet drugs in patients with a history of stroke or TIA, see Stroke p. 137. For guidance on the use of antiplatelet drugs in patients with acute coronary syndrome, see Acute coronary syndromes p. 247.

Antihypertensive therapy
EvGr Antihypertensive drug treatment is recommended in patients with established CVD and sustained elevated systolic blood pressure and/or diastolic blood pressure. For further guidance on prescribing antihypertensive drugs in patients with CVD, see Hypertension p. 166. Ⓐ

Lipid-lowering therapy
EvGr A statin is recommended as the lipid-lowering drug of choice for secondary prevention of CVD. Factors such as polypharmacy, frailty, and comorbidities should be taken into account when starting statin therapy.

Treatment with high-dose atorvastatin p. 234 should be offered to patients with CVD, regardless of their cholesterol concentration. However, a lower dose can be used if the patient is at an increased risk of side-effects or drug interactions. NICE (2023) recommends that low-dose

atorvastatin p. 234 should be offered to patients with CVD and chronic kidney disease.

High-dose simvastatin p. 237 is generally avoided due to the risk of myopathy, unless the patient has been stable on this regimen for at least one year. Ⓐ Furthermore, the MHRA advises that high-dose simvastatin p. 237 should only be considered for patients who have not achieved their treatment goals with lower doses and have severe hypercholesterolaemia and a high risk of cardiovascular complications; benefits should outweigh risks.

EvGr Patients taking statins should have an annual medication review to discuss medication adherence, lifestyle modification, and CVD risk factors; a full lipid profile should be considered (total cholesterol, HDL-cholesterol, triglycerides, non-HDL-cholesterol, and LDL-cholesterol). Liver transaminases and a full lipid profile should also be assessed 2–3 months after starting or changing lipid-lowering treatment; liver transaminases should be reassessed at 12 months, but not again unless clinically indicated. Patients who are stable on a low- or medium-intensity statin should discuss the benefits and risks of switching to a high-intensity statin at their next medication review. For statin intensity categorisation, see Dyslipidaemias p. 227.

NICE (2023) recommends a reduction of LDL-cholesterol concentration to 2.0 mmol/litre or less, or non-HDL-cholesterol concentration to 2.6 mmol/litre or less. SIGN (2017) instead recommends aiming for a reduction in non-HDL-cholesterol concentration of greater than 40%. Patients with ischaemic stroke or TIA and evidence of atherosclerosis should aim to reduce their fasting LDL-cholesterol to below 1.8 mmol/litre (equivalent to a non-HDL-cholesterol of below 2.5 mmol/litre in a non-fasting sample) as recommended in *SIGN and Royal College of Physicians' National Clinical Guideline for Stroke for the UK and Ireland (2023)*.

If these targets are not achieved, adherence to drug treatment should be checked, lifestyle modifications optimised, and increasing the statin intensity considered if the patient is not already taking a high-intensity statin at the maximum tolerated dose. NICE (2023) recommends that the use of higher doses in those with chronic kidney disease with an eGFR less than 30mL/minute/1.73 m^2 should be discussed with a renal specialist.

SIGN (2017) recommends that ezetimibe p. 229 and bile acid sequestrants such as colestyramine p. 229 and colestipol hydrochloride p. 228, can be considered for use in combination with a statin at the maximum tolerated dose if LDL-cholesterol remains inadequately controlled. NICE (2023) recommends that additional lipid-lowering treatments, such as alirocumab p. 238, bempedoic acid p. 238, evolocumab p. 239, ezetimibe p. 229, and inclisiran p. 240 can be considered for secondary prevention of CVD when the maximum tolerated dose of statin therapy fails to adequately control lipid concentrations. Ezetimibe in combination with the maximum tolerated dose of statin can also be considered to further reduce CVD risk, even if the lipid target is met. If statins are unsuitable or not tolerated, ezetimibe monotherapy can be considered for secondary prevention of CVD; alternative or additional lipid-lowering treatments such as alirocumab, bempedoic acid, evolocumab, and inclisiran can be considered if ezetimibe fails to adequately control lipid concentrations. NICE (2023) does not recommend bile acid sequestrants for the secondary prevention of CVD.

NICE (2023) does not routinely recommend omega-3 fatty acid compounds for the secondary prevention of CVD, however icosapent ethyl p. 240 is recommended in combination with a statin for patients with established CVD who have a raised fasting triglyceride concentration of 1.7 mmol/litre or above, and a LDL-cholesterol

2

Cardiovascular system

concentration above 1.04 mmol/litre and below or equal to 2.6 mmol/litre.

Although fibrates are not routinely recommended for secondary prevention of CVD, SIGN (2017) recommends that they be considered in patients with both marked hypertriglyceridaemia and low HDL-cholesterol concentration. Ⓐ

For other lipid-lowering therapy options, see NICE guideline: **Cardiovascular disease: risk assessment and reduction, including lipid modification** and SIGN guideline: **Risk estimation and the prevention of cardiovascular disease** (see *Useful resources*).

For further information on lipid-lowering therapy and familial hypercholesterolaemia, see Dyslipidaemias p. 227.

Psychological risk factors

[EvGr] Psychological treatment should be considered in patients with mood and anxiety disorders and comorbid CVD; complex patients may require referral to mental health services for assessment and delivery of high-intensity or specialist treatments. Selective serotonin re-uptake inhibitors (SSRIs) should be considered for treatment in patients with depression and coronary heart disease. Ⓐ For guidance on prescribing of antidepressant drugs, see Antidepressant drugs p. 417.

Useful Resources

Risk estimation and the prevention of cardiovascular disease. Scottish Intercollegiate Guidelines Network. Clinical guideline 149. June 2017.
www.sign.ac.uk/our-guidelines/risk-estimation-and-the-prevention-of-cardiovascular-disease/

Cardiovascular disease: risk assessment and reduction, including lipid modification. National Institute for Health and Care Excellence. Clinical guideline NG238. December 2023.
www.nice.org.uk/guidance/ng238

Lipid lowering to prevent cardiovascular disease. GP Evidence.
gpevidence.org/conditions/lipids/

7 Heart failure

Chronic heart failure

10-Aug-2022

Description of condition

Heart failure is a progressive clinical syndrome caused by structural or functional abnormalities of the heart, resulting in reduced cardiac output. It is characterised by symptoms such as shortness of breath, persistent coughing or wheezing, ankle swelling, reduced exercise tolerance, and fatigue. These symptoms may be accompanied by signs such as elevated jugular venous pressure, pulmonary crackles, and pulmonary oedema.

The risk of heart failure is greater in men, smokers and diabetic patients, and increases with age.

The most common cause of heart failure is coronary heart disease, however, patients of African or Afro-Caribbean origin are more likely to develop heart failure secondary to hypertension. In addition to coronary heart disease, heart failure often co-exists with other co-morbidities such as chronic kidney disease, atrial fibrillation, hypertension, dyslipidaemia, obesity, diabetes mellitus, and chronic obstructive pulmonary disease. Patients with co-morbidities have a worse prognosis, and the presence of atrial fibrillation or chronic kidney disease affects the management of heart failure in these patients. Complications of heart failure include chronic kidney disease, atrial fibrillation, depression, cachexia, sexual dysfunction, and sudden cardiac death.

Heart failure can be defined as either having a reduced or preserved ejection fraction. Both conditions present with signs and symptoms of heart failure. In heart failure with reduced ejection fraction, the left ventricle loses its ability to contract normally and therefore presents with an ejection fraction of less than 40%. In heart failure with preserved ejection fraction, the left ventricle loses its ability to relax normally therefore the ejection fraction is normal or only mildly reduced.

The New York Heart Association (NYHA) functional classification tool is used to define the progression of chronic heart failure according to severity of symptoms and limitation to physical activity. Heart failure is considered to be stable or chronic when symptoms remain unchanged for at least one month despite optimal management.

Aims of treatment

The aims of treatment are to reduce mortality, relieve symptoms, improve exercise tolerance, and reduce the incidence of acute exacerbations.

Non-drug treatment

[EvGr] Patients with heart failure should be advised to make lifestyle changes to reduce the risk of progression of their heart failure and associated co-morbidities. These include Smoking cessation p. 565, reducing alcohol consumption, increasing physical exercise if appropriate, weight control, and dietary changes such as increasing fruit and vegetable consumption and reducing saturated fat intake. Patients should be encouraged to weigh themselves daily at a set time of day and to report any weight gain of more than 1.5–2.0 kg in 2 days to their GP or heart failure specialist. Salt and fluid intake should only be restricted if these are high, and a salt intake of less than 6 g per day is advised. Patients with dilutional hyponatraemia should only restrict their fluid intake. Salt substitutes containing potassium should be avoided to reduce the risk of hyperkalaemia.

Contraception and pregnancy should be discussed with women of childbearing potential and heart failure. Advice from a heart failure specialist and an obstetrician should be sought if pregnancy occurs or is being considered.

Patients should be given the opportunity to join a personalised rehabilitation programme including education, psychological support, and exercise when appropriate.

Implantable cardioverter defibrillators and cardiac resynchronisation therapy are treatment options recommended in patients with heart failure and a reduced ejection fraction of less than 35%. If symptoms remain severe and unresponsive despite optimal drug treatment, specialist referral should be considered. Ⓐ

Drug treatment

[EvGr] The treatment of heart failure should include management of symptoms, risk factors and underlying causes and complications. Patients should have their medication reviewed, and any drugs that may cause or worsen their heart failure should be stopped if appropriate.

Vaccination against pneumococcal disease, and annual influenza vaccination is recommended. Ⓐ

Chronic heart failure with reduced ejection fraction

[EvGr] Rate-limiting calcium-channel blockers (verapamil hydrochloride p. 191, and diltiazem hydrochloride p. 185) and short-acting dihydropyridines (e.g. nifedipine p. 189, or nicardipine hydrochloride p. 188) should be avoided in patients who have heart failure with reduced ejection fraction as these drugs reduce cardiac contractility. Patients with heart failure and angina may safely be treated with amlodipine p. 184.

Diuretics are recommended for the relief of breathlessness and oedema in patients with fluid retention. Loop diuretics such as furosemide p. 261, bumetanide p. 260, or torasemide p. 262 are usually the diuretics of choice. Thiazide diuretics may only be of benefit in patients with mild fluid retention and an eGFR greater than 30 mL/minute/1.73 m^2. Diuretic doses should be titrated according to clinical response and adjusted if needed following the initiation of subsequent heart failure treatments, to minimise the risk of dehydration, renal impairment or hypotension. If symptoms persist despite optimal titration, advice from a heart failure specialist should be sought.

An angiotensin-converting enzyme (ACE) inhibitor (e.g. perindopril, ramipril p. 200, captopril p. 195, enalapril maleate p. 196, lisinopril p. 197, quinapril p. 199 or fosinopril sodium p. 196) and a beta-blocker licensed for heart failure (e.g. bisoprolol fumarate p. 180, carvedilol p. 175, or nebivolol p. 183) should be given as first-line treatment to reduce morbidity and mortality. Treatment with a beta-blocker should not be withheld because of age or the presence of diabetes, chronic obstructive pulmonary disease, peripheral vascular disease, erectile dysfunction, or interstitial pulmonary disease. Patients who are already taking a beta-blocker for co-morbidities (e.g. angina or hypertension) and whose condition is stable should be switched to a beta-blocker licensed for heart failure. Clinical judgement should be used when deciding whether to start an ACE inhibitor or beta blocker first. The additional drug should only be initiated when the patient is stable on their existing treatment. Treatment should be initiated at a low dose and slowly titrated up to the maximum tolerated dose. An angiotensin II receptor blocker (ARB) licensed for heart failure (e.g. candesartan cilexetil p. 202, losartan potassium p. 203, or valsartan p. 206) can be considered if ACE inhibitors are not tolerated.

If heart failure symptoms persist or worsen despite optimal first-line treatment, a mineralocorticoid receptor antagonist such as spironolactone p. 224 or eplerenone below should be offered as add-on therapy unless contra-indicated (e.g. due to hyperkalaemia or renal impairment). Hydralazine hydrochloride p. 207 combined with a nitrate can be considered under the advice of a heart failure specialist in patients who are intolerant of both ACE inhibitors and ARBs (in particular those of African or Caribbean origin with moderate to severe heart failure).

If symptoms persist despite optimal treatment, advice from a heart failure specialist should be sought on the use of amiodarone hydrochloride p. 120, digoxin p. 125, sacubitril with valsartan p. 225, ivabradine p. 245, empagliflozin p. 827, or dapagliflozin p. 826.

For patients in sinus rhythm, digoxin is recommended as add-on therapy in worsening or severe heart failure despite optimal treatment. Although digoxin does not reduce mortality, it may decrease symptoms and hospitalisation due to acute exacerbations. Routine monitoring of serum levels is not recommended in patients with heart failure. Anticoagulation should also be considered for patients in sinus rhythm with heart failure if they have a history of thromboembolism, left ventricular aneurysm or intracardiac thrombus. Ⓐ For guidance in patients with atrial fibrillation see Arrhythmias p. 113.

Monitoring drug treatment

EvGr When initiating ACE inhibitors, ARBs and mineralocorticoid receptor antagonists, serum potassium and sodium, renal function, and blood pressure should be checked prior to starting treatment, 1-2 weeks after starting treatment, and at each dose increment. Once the target, or maximum tolerated dose is achieved, treatment should be monitored monthly for 3 months and then at least every 6 months, and if the patient becomes acutely unwell.

When initiating beta blockers, heart rate, blood pressure and symptom control should be assessed at the start of treatment and after each dose change.

In patients with chronic kidney disease, lower doses and slower dose titrations of ACE inhibitors, ARBs, mineralocorticoid receptor antagonists and digoxin should

be considered. Advice from a renal specialist should be considered where appropriate. Ⓐ

Chronic heart failure with preserved ejection fraction

EvGr Patients with heart failure and preserved ejection fraction should be managed under the care of a heart failure specialist. For the relief of fluid retention symptoms, a low to medium dose loop diuretic should be prescribed. If the patient fails to respond to treatment, advice from a heart failure specialist should be sought. Ⓐ

Advanced heart failure

Breathlessness is a common symptom in advanced heart failure and may occur even with optimal management and in the absence of clinical pulmonary oedema. EvGr Long-term oxygen therapy is not recommended in advanced heart failure, although it may be considered in patients with heart failure and additional co-morbidities that would benefit from oxygen therapy such as chronic obstructive pulmonary disease. Ⓐ

Useful Resources

Chronic heart failure in adults: diagnosis and management. National Institute of Health and Care Excellence. Clinical guideline 106. September 2018.
www.nice.org.uk/guidance/ng106

Management of chronic heart failure. Scottish Intercollegiate Guidelines Network. Clinical guideline 147. March 2016.
www.sign.ac.uk/our-guidelines/management-of-chronic-heart-failure/

> **Other drugs used for Heart failure** Bendroflumethiazide, p. 193 · Chlortalidone, p. 264 · Co-amilozide, p. 193 · Glyceryl trinitrate, p. 252 · Isosorbide dinitrate, p. 254 · Isosorbide mononitrate, p. 254 · Perindopril arginine, p. 198 · Perindopril erbumine, p. 199 · Prazosin, p. 904 · Sodium nitroprusside, p. 209

DIURETICS > POTASSIUM-SPARING DIURETICS > MINERALOCORTICOID RECEPTOR ANTAGONISTS

Eplerenone　　　　　　　　　　　　　　15-Apr-2024

● **INDICATIONS AND DOSE**

Adjunct in stable patients with left ventricular ejection fraction ≤40% with evidence of heart failure, following myocardial infarction (start therapy within 3–14 days of event) | Adjunct in chronic mild heart failure with left ventricular ejection fraction ≤30%

▶ BY MOUTH

▶ Adult: Initially 25 mg daily, then increased to 50 mg daily, increased within 4 weeks of initial treatment

DOSE ADJUSTMENTS DUE TO INTERACTIONS

▶ Manufacturer advises max. dose 25 mg daily with concurrent use of amiodarone or moderate inhibitors of CYP3A4.

● **CONTRA-INDICATIONS** Hyperkalaemia

● **CAUTIONS**

▶ **Elderly** For mineralocorticoid receptor antagonists, Screening Tool of Older Persons' potentially inappropriate Prescriptions (STOPP) criteria to aid medication reviews (see Prescribing in the elderly p. 31 for information): potentially inappropriate with concurrent potassium-conserving drugs without monitoring of serum potassium (risk of dangerous hyperkalaemia).

● **INTERACTIONS** → Appendix 1: mineralocorticoid receptor antagonists

● **SIDE-EFFECTS**

▶ **Common or very common** Arrhythmias · asthenia · constipation · cough · diarrhoea · dizziness · dyslipidaemia ·

electrolyte imbalance · headache · insomnia · muscle spasms · nausea · pain · renal impairment · skin reactions · syncope · vomiting
▶ **Uncommon** Angioedema · arterial thrombosis · cholecystitis · eosinophilia · flatulence · gynaecomastia · hyperhidrosis · hypothyroidism · increased risk of infection · malaise · numbness · postural hypotension

● PREGNANCY Manufacturer advises caution—no information available.

● BREAST FEEDING Manufacturer advises use only if potential benefit outweighs risk.

● HEPATIC IMPAIRMENT Manufacturer advises avoid in severe impairment (no information available).

● RENAL IMPAIRMENT [EvGr] Avoid if creatinine clearance less than 30 mL/minute. ⓜ
Dose adjustments [EvGr] Initially 25 mg on alternate days if creatinine clearance 30–60 mL/minute, adjust dose according to serum-potassium concentration (consult product literature). ⓜ See p. 21.

● MONITORING REQUIREMENTS Monitor plasma-potassium concentration before treatment, during initiation, and when dose changed.

● MEDICINAL FORMS There can be variation in the licensing of different medicines containing the same drug.
Oral tablet
▶ Eplerenone (Non-proprietary)
Eplerenone 25 mg Eplerenone 25mg tablets | 28 tablet [PoM] £42.72 DT = £2.75 | 30 tablet [PoM] £32.33
Eplerenone 50 mg Eplerenone 50mg tablets | 28 tablet [PoM] £42.72 DT = £4.28 | 30 tablet [PoM] £25.32
▶ Inspra (Viatris UK Healthcare Ltd)
Eplerenone 25 mg Inspra 25mg tablets | 28 tablet [PoM] £42.72 DT = £2.75
Eplerenone 50 mg Inspra 50mg tablets | 28 tablet [PoM] £42.72 DT = £4.28

Spironolactone

14-May-2025

● INDICATIONS AND DOSE
Oedema in cirrhosis of the liver | Ascites in cirrhosis of the liver
▶ BY MOUTH
▶ Adult: 100–400 mg once daily, to be adjusted according to response

Malignant ascites
▶ BY MOUTH
▶ Adult: Initially 100–200 mg once daily, then increased if necessary up to 400 mg once daily, maintenance dose adjusted according to response

Nephrotic syndrome
▶ BY MOUTH
▶ Adult: 100–200 mg once daily

Oedema in congestive heart failure
▶ BY MOUTH
▶ Adult: Initially 100 mg once daily, dose may also be taken as divided doses, maintenance dose adjusted according to response, alternatively initially 25–200 mg once daily, dose may also be taken as divided doses, maintenance dose adjusted according to response

Moderate to severe heart failure (adjunct)
▶ BY MOUTH
▶ Adult: Initially 25 mg once daily, then adjusted according to response to 50 mg once daily

Resistant hypertension (adjunct)
▶ BY MOUTH
▶ Adult: 25 mg once daily

Primary hyperaldosteronism in patients awaiting surgery
▶ BY MOUTH
▶ Adult: 100–400 mg once daily, may be used for long-term maintenance if surgery inappropriate, use lowest effective dose

● UNLICENSED USE Resistant hypertension (adjunct) unlicensed indication.

● CONTRA-INDICATIONS Addison's disease · anuria · hyperkalaemia

● CAUTIONS Acute porphyrias p. 1202 · elderly · *rodent studies indicate potential carcinogenic risk*
CAUTIONS, FURTHER INFORMATION
▶ Elderly For mineralocorticoid receptor antagonists, Screening Tool of Older Persons' potentially inappropriate Prescriptions (STOPP) criteria to aid medication reviews (see Prescribing in the elderly p. 31 for information): potentially inappropriate with concurrent potassium-conserving drugs without monitoring of serum potassium (risk of dangerous hyperkalaemia).

● INTERACTIONS → Appendix 1: mineralocorticoid receptor antagonists

● SIDE-EFFECTS Acidosis hyperchloraemic · acute kidney injury · agranulocytosis · alopecia · breast neoplasm benign · breast pain · confusion · dizziness · electrolyte imbalance · gastrointestinal disorder · gynaecomastia · hepatic function abnormal · hyperkalaemia (discontinue) · hypertrichosis · leg cramps · leucopenia · libido disorder · malaise · menstrual disorder · nausea · severe cutaneous adverse reactions (SCARs) · skin reactions · thrombocytopenia

● PREGNANCY Use only if potential benefit outweighs risk—feminisation of male fetus in *animal* studies.

● BREAST FEEDING Metabolites present in milk, but amount probably too small to be harmful.

● RENAL IMPAIRMENT Avoid in acute renal insufficiency or severe impairment.
Monitoring Monitor plasma-potassium concentration (high risk of hyperkalaemia in renal impairment).

● MONITORING REQUIREMENTS Monitor electrolytes—discontinue if hyperkalaemia occurs (in *severe heart failure* monitor potassium and creatinine 1 week after initiation and after any dose increase, monthly for first 3 months, then every 3 months for 1 year, and then every 6 months).

● MEDICINAL FORMS There can be variation in the licensing of different medicines containing the same drug. Forms available from special-order manufacturers include: oral suspension, oral solution
Oral tablet
CAUTIONARY AND ADVISORY LABELS 21
▶ Spironolactone (Non-proprietary)
Spironolactone 12.5 mg Spironolactone 12.5mg tablets | 28 tablet [PoM] £25.23 DT = £25.23
Spironolactone 25 mg Spironolactone 25mg tablets | 28 tablet [PoM] £1.72 DT = £1.17
Spironolactone 50 mg Spironolactone 50mg tablets | 28 tablet [PoM] £4.26 DT = £2.91
Spironolactone 100 mg Spironolactone 100mg tablets | 28 tablet [PoM] £4.38 DT = £2.45
▶ Aldactone (Pfizer Ltd)
Spironolactone 25 mg Aldactone 25mg tablets | 100 tablet [PoM] £8.89
Spironolactone 50 mg Aldactone 50mg tablets | 100 tablet [PoM] £17.78
Spironolactone 100 mg Aldactone 100mg tablets | 28 tablet [PoM] £9.96 DT = £2.45
Oral solution
▶ Spironolactone (Non-proprietary)
Spironolactone 5 mg per 1 ml Spironolactone 25mg/5ml oral solution sugar free | 125 ml [PoM] £99.66 [SF]

▸ Urospir (Rosemont Pharmaceuticals Ltd)
Spironolactone 5 mg per 1 ml Urospir 25mg/5ml oral solution |
150 ml [PoM] £123.93 [SF]
Spironolactone 10 mg per 1 ml Urospir 50mg/5ml oral solution |
150 ml [PoM] £247.85 [SF]

Oral suspension
CAUTIONARY AND ADVISORY LABELS 21
▸ Qaialdo (Nova Laboratories Ltd)
Spironolactone 10 mg per 1 ml Qaialdo 10mg/ml oral suspension |
150 ml [PoM] £247.85

DRUGS ACTING ON THE RENIN-ANGIOTENSIN SYSTEM › ANGIOTENSIN II RECEPTOR ANTAGONISTS

Sacubitril with valsartan
03-Sep-2024

The properties listed below are those particular to the
combination only. For the properties of the components
please consider, valsartan p. 206.

● DRUG ACTION Sacubitril (a prodrug) inhibits the
breakdown of natriuretic peptides resulting in varied
effects including increased diuresis, natriuresis, and
vasodilation.

● **INDICATIONS AND DOSE**

**Symptomatic chronic heart failure with reduced ejection
fraction [in patients not currently taking an ACE
inhibitor or angiotensin II receptor antagonist, or
stabilised on low doses of either of these agents]**
▸ BY MOUTH
▸ Adult: Initially 50 mg twice daily for 3–4 weeks, dose to
be given using 24/26 mg strength tablet, increased if
tolerated to 100 mg twice daily for 3–4 weeks, dose to
be given using 49/51 mg strength tablet, then increased
if tolerated to 200 mg twice daily, dose to be given
using 97/103 mg strength tablet

**Symptomatic chronic heart failure with reduced ejection
fraction [in patients currently stabilised on an ACE
inhibitor or angiotensin II receptor antagonist]**
▸ BY MOUTH
▸ Adult: Initially 100 mg twice daily for 2–4 weeks, dose
to be given using 49/51 mg strength tablet, if systolic
blood pressure between 100–110 mmHg consider an
initial dose of 50 mg twice daily for 2–4 weeks (dose to
be given using 24/26 mg strength tablet), increased to
100 mg twice daily for 2–4 weeks (dose to be given
using 49/51 mg strength tablet), then increased if
tolerated to 200 mg twice daily, dose to be given using
97/103 mg strength tablet

DOSE EQUIVALENCE AND CONVERSION
▸ *Entresto* ® tablets and granules contain *x/y* mg of
sacubitril and valsartan, respectively.
▸ Doses in BNF Publications are expressed as the total of
both drug strengths.
▸ For *Entresto* ® tablets, used in patients weighing 40 kg
or more, the 24/26 mg strength equates to a dose of
50 mg, the 49/51 mg strength equates to a dose of
100 mg, and the 97/103 mg strength equates to a dose
of 200 mg.
▸ For *Entresto* ® granules in capsules for opening, used in
children weighing less than 40 kg, the 6/6 mg strength
equates to a dose of 12 mg and the 15/16 mg strength
equates to a dose of 31 mg.
▸ Valsartan in *Entresto* ® is more bioavailable than other
tablet formulations—26 mg, 51 mg, and 103 mg
valsartan in *Entresto* ® is equivalent to 40 mg, 80 mg,
and 160 mg, respectively, in other valsartan tablet
formulations.

● CONTRA-INDICATIONS Concomitant use with an ACE
inhibitor (risk of angioedema—do not initiate until at least
36 hours after the last dose when switching treatment) ·
concomitant use with an angiotensin II receptor
antagonist · hereditary or idiopathic angioedema · known
history of angioedema related to previous ACE inhibitor or
angiotensin II receptor antagonist

● CAUTIONS Serum-potassium concentration above
5.4 mmol/litre (do not initiate—may increase risk of
hyperkalaemia) · systolic BP less than 100 mmHg (do not
initiate—limited data available)

● INTERACTIONS → Appendix 1: angiotensin-II receptor
antagonists · sacubitril

● SIDE-EFFECTS
▸ **Common or very common** Anaemia · asthenia · cough ·
diarrhoea · dizziness · electrolyte imbalance · gastritis ·
headache · hypoglycaemia · hypotension · nausea · renal
impairment · syncope · vertigo
▸ **Uncommon** Angioedema · skin reactions
▸ **Rare or very rare** Hallucinations · paranoia · sleep disorder
▸ **Frequency not known** Psychiatric disorder

● PREGNANCY [EvGr] Avoid—toxicity with sacubitril in *animal*
studies. ⟨M⟩

● BREAST FEEDING [EvGr] Avoid—present in milk in *animal*
studies. ⟨M⟩

● HEPATIC IMPAIRMENT [EvGr] Caution in moderate
impairment or if hepatic transaminases exceed 2 times the
upper limit of normal (limited information available);
avoid in severe impairment, biliary cirrhosis, or cholestasis
(no information available). ⟨M⟩
Dose adjustments [EvGr] Start with 50 mg twice daily (dose
to be given using 24/26 mg strength tablet) in moderate
impairment or if hepatic transaminases exceed 2 times the
upper limit of normal. ⟨M⟩

● RENAL IMPAIRMENT [EvGr] Caution (increased risk of
hypotension; limited information available in severe
impairment); avoid in end-stage renal disease (no
information available). ⟨M⟩
Dose adjustments [EvGr] Start with 50 mg twice daily (dose
to be given using 24/26 mg strength tablet) if eGFR less
than 30 mL/minute/1.73m^2. Also consider this starting
dose if eGFR 30–60 mL/minute/1.73m^2. ⟨M⟩ See p. 21.

● NATIONAL FUNDING/ACCESS DECISIONS
For full details see funding body website
NICE decisions
▸ **Sacubitril valsartan for treating symptomatic chronic heart
failure with reduced ejection fraction (April 2016)** NICE TA388
Recommended with restrictions

● MEDICINAL FORMS There can be variation in the licensing of
different medicines containing the same drug.
Oral tablet
▸ Entresto (Novartis Pharmaceuticals UK Ltd)
Sacubitril 24 mg, Valsartan 26 mg Entresto 24mg/26mg tablets |
28 tablet [PoM] £45.78 DT = £45.78
Sacubitril 49 mg, Valsartan 51 mg Entresto 49mg/51mg tablets |
28 tablet [PoM] £45.78 | 56 tablet [PoM] £91.56 DT = £91.56
Sacubitril 97 mg, Valsartan 103 mg Entresto 97mg/103mg tablets
| 56 tablet [PoM] £91.56 DT = £91.56

2

Cardiovascular system

GUANYLATE CYCLASE STIMULATORS

Vericiguat

01-Sep-2021

- **DRUG ACTION** Vericiguat is a stimulator of soluble guanylate cyclase that augments levels of intracellular cyclic guanosine monophosphate, which may improve both myocardial and vascular function.

- **INDICATIONS AND DOSE**

Chronic heart failure with reduced ejection fraction [in patients stabilised after a recent decompensation event requiring intravenous therapy]
- ▸ BY MOUTH
- ▸ Adult: Initially 2.5 mg once daily, dose to be doubled approximately every 2 weeks if tolerated, to maintenance dose; maintenance 10 mg once daily

- **CONTRA-INDICATIONS** Hypotension (do not initiate if systolic blood pressure less than 100 mmHg)
- **CAUTIONS** Autonomic dysfunction · history of hypotension · hypovolaemia · resting hypotension · severe left ventricular outflow obstruction
  CAUTIONS, FURTHER INFORMATION
  - ▸ Hypotension EvGr If symptomatic hypotension or systolic blood pressure less than 90 mmHg is observed during treatment, temporary dose reduction or discontinuation of vericiguat is recommended. Ⓜ
- **INTERACTIONS** → Appendix 1: vericiguat
- **SIDE-EFFECTS**
  - ▸ **Common or very common** Anaemia · dizziness · dyspepsia · gastrooesophageal reflux disease · headache · hypotension · nausea · vomiting
- **PREGNANCY** EvGr Avoid—toxicity in *animal* studies. Ⓜ
- **BREAST FEEDING** EvGr Avoid—present in milk in *animal* studies. Ⓜ
- **HEPATIC IMPAIRMENT** EvGr Avoid in severe impairment (no information available). Ⓜ
- **RENAL IMPAIRMENT** EvGr Avoid if eGFR less than 15 mL/minute/1.73 m^2 at start of treatment, or in patients on dialysis (no information available). Ⓜ See p. 21.
- **DIRECTIONS FOR ADMINISTRATION** EvGr *Verquvo*® tablets may be crushed and mixed with water immediately before administration. Ⓜ
- **PATIENT AND CARER ADVICE**
  Driving and skilled tasks Patients and carers should be counselled on the effects on driving and performance of skilled tasks—increased risk of dizziness.

- **MEDICINAL FORMS** There can be variation in the licensing of different medicines containing the same drug.
  Oral tablet
  CAUTIONARY AND ADVISORY LABELS 21
  - ▸ **Verquvo** (Bayer Plc) ▼
    Vericiguat 2.5 mg Verquvo 2.5mg tablet | 14 tablet PoM £45.78 (Hospital only)
    Vericiguat 5 mg Verquvo 5mg tablets | 14 tablet PoM £45.78 (Hospital only)
    Vericiguat 10 mg Verquvo 10mg tablets | 28 tablet PoM £91.56 (Hospital only)

PHOSPHODIESTERASE TYPE-3 INHIBITORS

Enoximone

24-Jun-2021

- **DRUG ACTION** Enoximone is a phosphodiesterase type-3 inhibitor that exerts most effect on the myocardium; it has positive inotropic properties and vasodilator activity.

- **INDICATIONS AND DOSE**

Congestive heart failure where cardiac output reduced and filling pressures increased
- ▸ BY SLOW INTRAVENOUS INJECTION
- ▸ Adult: Initially 0.5–1 mg/kg, rate not exceeding 12.5 mg/minute, then 500 micrograms/kg every 30 minutes until satisfactory response or total of 3 mg/kg given; maintenance, initial dose of up to 3 mg/kg may be repeated every 3–6 hours as required
- ▸ BY INTRAVENOUS INFUSION
- ▸ Adult: Initially 90 micrograms/kg/minute, dose to be given over 10–30 minutes, followed by 5–20 micrograms/kg/minute, dose to be given as either a continuous or intermittent infusion; maximum 24 mg/kg per day

- **CAUTIONS** Heart failure associated with hypertrophic cardiomyopathy, stenotic or obstructive valvular disease or other outlet obstruction
- **SIDE-EFFECTS**
  - ▸ **Common or very common** Headache · hypotension · insomnia
  - ▸ **Uncommon** Arrhythmias · diarrhoea · dizziness · nausea · vomiting
  - ▸ **Rare or very rare** Chills · fever · fluid retention · myalgia · oliguria · urinary retention
- **PREGNANCY** Manufacturer advises use only if potential benefit outweighs risk.
- **BREAST FEEDING** Manufacturer advises caution—no information available.
- **RENAL IMPAIRMENT**
  Dose adjustments Manufacturer advises consider dose reduction.
- **MONITORING REQUIREMENTS** Monitor blood pressure, heart rate, ECG, central venous pressure, fluid and electrolyte status, renal function, platelet count and hepatic enzymes.
- **DIRECTIONS FOR ADMINISTRATION** Incompatible with glucose solutions. Use only plastic containers or syringes; crystal formation if glass used. Avoid extravasation.
  For *intravenous infusion* (*Perfan*®), give continuously or intermittently in Sodium Chloride 0.9% or Water for Injections; dilute to a concentration of 2.5 mg/mL.
- **PRESCRIBING AND DISPENSING INFORMATION** Sustained haemodynamic benefit has been observed after administration of phosphodiesterase type-3 inhibitors, but there is no evidence of any beneficial effect on survival.

- **MEDICINAL FORMS** There can be variation in the licensing of different medicines containing the same drug.
  Solution for injection
  EXCIPIENTS: May contain Alcohol, propylene glycol
  - ▸ **Perfan** (Macure Pharma UK Ltd)
    Enoximone 5 mg per 1 ml Perfan 100mg/20ml solution for injection ampoules | 10 ampoule PoM £150.15 (Hospital only)

Milrinone
27-Jan-2020

- **DRUG ACTION** Milrinone is a phosphodiesterase type-3 inhibitor that exerts most effect on the myocardium; it has positive inotropic properties and vasodilator activity.

- **INDICATIONS AND DOSE**

  Short-term treatment of severe congestive heart failure unresponsive to conventional maintenance therapy (not immediately after myocardial infarction) | Acute heart failure, including low output states following heart surgery
  - INITIALLY BY INTRAVENOUS INJECTION
  - Adult: Initially 50 micrograms/kg, given over 10 minutes, followed by (by intravenous infusion) 375–750 nanograms/kg/minute usually given following surgery for up to 12 hours or in congestive heart failure for 48-72 hours; maximum 1.13 mg/kg per day

- **CONTRA-INDICATIONS** Severe hypovolaemia

- **CAUTIONS** Correct hypokalaemia · heart failure associated with hypertrophic cardiomyopathy, stenotic or obstructive valvular disease or other outlet obstruction

- **SIDE-EFFECTS**
  - **Common or very common** Arrhythmia supraventricular (increased risk in patients with pre-existing arrhythmias) · arrhythmias · headache · hypotension
  - **Uncommon** Angina pectoris · chest pain · hypokalaemia · thrombocytopenia · tremor
  - **Rare or very rare** Anaphylactic shock · bronchospasm · skin eruption
  - **Frequency not known** Renal failure

- **PREGNANCY** Manufacturer advises use only if potential benefit outweighs risk.

- **BREAST FEEDING** Manufacturer advises avoid—no information available.

- **RENAL IMPAIRMENT**
  Dose adjustments Reduce dose and monitor response if eGFR less than 50 mL/minute/1.73 m^2—consult product literature for details.

- **MONITORING REQUIREMENTS** Monitor blood pressure, heart rate, ECG, central venous pressure, fluid and electrolyte status, renal function, platelet count and hepatic enzymes.

- **DIRECTIONS FOR ADMINISTRATION** Avoid extravasation.
  For *intravenous injection*, may be given either undiluted or diluted before use.
  For *intravenous infusion* (*Primacor*®) give continuously in Glucose 5% or Sodium chloride 0.9%; dilute to a suggested concentration of 200 micrograms/mL.

- **PRESCRIBING AND DISPENSING INFORMATION** Sustained haemodynamic benefit has been observed after administration of phosphodiesterase type-3 inhibitors, but there is no evidence of any beneficial effect on survival.

- **MEDICINAL FORMS** There can be variation in the licensing of different medicines containing the same drug. Forms available from special-order manufacturers include: solution for infusion

  Solution for injection
  - Milrinone (Non-proprietary)
    Milrinone (as Milrinone lactate) 1 mg per 1 ml Milrinone 10mg/10ml solution for injection vials | 10 vial [PoM] £179.06 (Hospital only)

  Solution for infusion
  - Milrinone (Non-proprietary)
    Milrinone 1 mg per 1 ml Milrinone 10mg/10ml solution for infusion ampoules | 10 ampoule [PoM] £149.50-£199.06 (Hospital only)
    Milrinone 10mg/10ml concentrate for solution for infusion ampoules | 10 ampoule [PoM] [S] (Hospital only)
  - Primacor (Sanofi)
    Milrinone 1 mg per 1 ml Primacor 10mg/10ml solution for injection ampoules | 10 ampoule [PoM] £199.06 (Hospital only)

8 Hyperlipidaemia

Dyslipidaemias
23-Mar-2018

Hypercholesterolaemia and hypertriglyceridaemia

Statins are the drugs of first choice for treating hypercholesterolaemia and moderate hypertriglyceridaemia. Severe hypercholesterolaemia or hypertriglyceridaemia not adequately controlled with a maximal dose of a statin may require the use of an additional lipid-regulating drug such as ezetimibe p. 229; such treatment should generally be supervised by a specialist.

A number of conditions, some familial, are characterised by very high LDL-cholesterol concentration, high triglyceride concentration, or both. Although statins are more effective than other lipid-regulating drugs at lowering LDL-cholesterol concentration, they are less effective than fibrates in reducing triglyceride concentration. Fenofibrate p. 231 may be added to statin therapy if triglycerides remain high even after the LDL-cholesterol concentration has been reduced adequately.

Familial hypercholesterolaemia

Patients with familial hypercholesterolaemia are at high risk of premature coronary heart disease. [EvGr] Lifelong lipid-modifying therapy and advice on lifestyle changes should be offered to all patients with familial hypercholesterolaemia.

A high-intensity statin, defined as the dose at which a reduction in LDL-cholesterol of greater than 40% is achieved, is recommended as first-line therapy in all patients with familial hypercholesterolaemia. The dose of the statin should be titrated to achieve a reduction in LDL-cholesterol concentration of greater than 50% from baseline.

Patients with primary *heterozygous familial hypercholesterolaemia* who have contra-indications to, or are intolerant of statins, can be considered for treatment with ezetimibe as monotherapy. A combination of a statin and ezetimibe is recommended if the maximum tolerated dose of a statin alone fails to provide adequate control of LDL-cholesterol, or a switch to an alternative statin is being considered. Treatment with a fibrate or a bile acid sequestrant (such as colestyramine p. 229 or colestipol hydrochloride p. 228) can be considered under specialist advice, in patients for whom statins or ezetimibe are inappropriate.

The combination of a statin with a fibrate carries an increased risk of muscle-related side-effects (including rhabdomyolysis) and should be used under specialist supervision. The concomitant administration of gemfibrozil with a statin increases the risk of rhabdomyolysis considerably—this combination should not be used.

Alirocumab p. 238 and evolocumab p. 239 can be considered for patients with primary heterozygous familial hypercholesterolaemia whose LDL-cholesterol has not been adequately controlled on maximum tolerated lipid-lowering therapy. Ⓐ See National funding/access decisions information for alirocumab p. 238 and evolocumab p. 239.

[EvGr] The prescribing of drug therapy in *homozygous familial hypercholesterolaemia* should be undertaken in a specialist centre. Ⓐ

Cardiovascular system

2

Reduction in low-density lipoprotein cholesterol

Therapy intensity	Drug	Daily dose (reduction in LDL cholesterol)
High-intensity	Atorvastatin	20 mg (43%)
		40 mg (49%)
		80 mg (55%)
	Rosuvastatin	10 mg (43%)
		20 mg (48%)
		40 mg (53%)
	Simvastatin	80 mg (42%)
Medium-intensity	Atorvastatin	10 mg (37%)
	Fluvastatin	80 mg (33%)
	Rosuvastatin	5 mg (38%)
	Simvastatin	20 mg (32%)
		40 mg (37%)
Low-intensity	Fluvastatin	20 mg (21%)
		40 mg (27%)
	Pravastatin	10 mg (20%)
		20 mg (24%)
		40 mg (29%)
	Simvastatin	10 mg (27%)

Advice from the MHRA: there is an increased risk of myopathy associated with high-dose (80 mg) simvastatin. The 80 mg dose should be considered only in patients with severe hypercholesterolaemia and high risk of cardiovascular complications who have not achieved their treatment goals on lower doses, when the benefits are expected to outweigh the potential risks.

LIPID MODIFYING DRUGS > BILE ACID SEQUESTRANTS

Bile acid sequestrants

- **DRUG ACTION** Bile acid sequestrants act by binding bile acids, preventing their reabsorption; this promotes hepatic conversion of cholesterol into bile acids; the resultant increased LDL-receptor activity of liver cells increases the clearance of LDL-cholesterol from the plasma.
- **CAUTIONS** Interference with the absorption of fat-soluble vitamins (supplements of vitamins A, D, K, and folic acid may be required when treatment is prolonged).
- **SIDE-EFFECTS**
- **Common or very common** Constipation · gastrointestinal discomfort · headache · nausea · vomiting
- **Uncommon** Appetite decreased · diarrhoea · gastrointestinal disorders
- **PREGNANCY** Bile acid sequestrants should be used with caution as although the drugs are not absorbed, they may cause fat-soluble vitamin deficiency on prolonged use.
- **BREAST FEEDING** Bile acid sequestrants should be used with caution as although the drugs are not absorbed, they may cause fat-soluble vitamin deficiency on prolonged use.

Colesevelam hydrochloride

04-Feb-2020

- **INDICATIONS AND DOSE**

Primary hypercholesterolaemia as an adjunct to dietary measures [monotherapy]
- ▶ BY MOUTH
- ▶ Adult: 3.75 g daily in 1–2 divided doses; maximum 4.375 g per day

Primary hypercholesterolaemia as an adjunct to dietary measures [in combination with a statin] | Primary and familial hypercholesterolaemia [in combination with ezetimibe, either with or without a statin]
- ▶ BY MOUTH
- ▶ Adult: 2.5–3.75 g daily in 1–2 divided doses, may be taken at the same time as the statin and ezetimibe

Bile acid malabsorption
- ▶ BY MOUTH
- ▶ Adult: 1.25–3.75 g daily in 2–3 divided doses

- **UNLICENSED USE** [EvGr] Colesevelam is used for the treatment of bile acid malabsorption,  but is not licensed for this indication.
- **CONTRA-INDICATIONS** Biliary obstruction · bowel obstruction
- **CAUTIONS** Gastro-intestinal motility disorders · inflammatory bowel disease · major gastro-intestinal surgery
- **INTERACTIONS** → Appendix 1: colesevelam
- **SIDE-EFFECTS**
- **Uncommon** Dysphagia · myalgia
- **Rare or very rare** Pancreatitis
- **HEPATIC IMPAIRMENT** Manufacturer advises caution in hepatic failure (no information available).
- **MONITORING REQUIREMENTS** Patients receiving ciclosporin should have their blood-ciclosporin concentration monitored before, during, and after treatment with colesevelam.
- **PATIENT AND CARER ADVICE** Patient counselling on administration is advised for colesevelam hydrochloride tablets (avoid other drugs at same time).
- **MEDICINAL FORMS** There can be variation in the licensing of different medicines containing the same drug.

Oral tablet
CAUTIONARY AND ADVISORY LABELS 21
- ▶ Colesevelam hydrochloride (Non-proprietary)
  Colesevelam hydrochloride 625 mg Colesevelam 625mg tablets | 90 tablet [PoM] £54.00–£57.66 | 120 tablet [PoM] £72.00–£76.88 | 180 tablet [PoM] £115.32 DT = £115.32
- ▶ Cholestagel (Neon Healthcare Ltd)
  Colesevelam hydrochloride 625 mg Cholestagel 625mg tablets | 180 tablet [PoM] £115.32 DT = £115.32

Colestipol hydrochloride

20-Jul-2020

- **INDICATIONS AND DOSE**

Hyperlipidaemias, particularly type IIa, in patients who have not responded adequately to diet and other appropriate measures
- ▶ BY MOUTH
- ▶ Adult: Initially 5 g 1–2 times a day, increased in steps of 5 g every month if required, total daily dose may be given in 1–2 divided doses; maximum 30 g per day

- **INTERACTIONS** → Appendix 1: colestipol
- **SIDE-EFFECTS** Angina pectoris · arthralgia · arthritis · asthenia · burping · chest pain · dizziness · dyspnoea · gallbladder disorders · headaches · inflammation · insomnia · pain · peptic ulcer haemorrhage · tachycardia

2 Cardiovascular system

- **DIRECTIONS FOR ADMINISTRATION** Manufacturer advises the contents of each sachet should be mixed with at least 100 mL of water or other suitable liquid such as fruit juice or skimmed milk; alternatively it can be mixed with thin soups, cereals, yoghurt, or pulpy fruits ensuring at least 100 mL of liquid is provided.

- **PATIENT AND CARER ADVICE** Patient counselling on administration is advised for colestipol hydrochloride granules (avoid other drugs at same time).

- **MEDICINAL FORMS** There can be variation in the licensing of different medicines containing the same drug. Forms available from special-order manufacturers include: oral tablet

Oral tablet
  ‣ Colestipol hydrochloride (Non-proprietary)
    Colestipol hydrochloride 1 gram Colestid 1g tablets | 120 tablet [PoM] Ⓢ

▸ 228

Colestyramine

(Cholestyramine)

20-Jul-2020

● INDICATIONS AND DOSE

Hyperlipidaemias, particularly type IIa, in patients who have not responded adequately to diet and other appropriate measures | Primary prevention of coronary heart disease in men aged 35–59 years with primary hypercholesterolaemia who have not responded to diet and other appropriate measures
  ▸ BY MOUTH
  ‣ Adult: Initially 4 g daily, increased in steps of 4 g every week; increased to 12–24 g daily in 1–4 divided doses, adjusted according to response; maximum 36 g per day

Pruritus associated with partial biliary obstruction and primary biliary cirrhosis
  ▸ BY MOUTH
  ‣ Adult: 4–8 g once daily

Diarrhoea associated with Crohn's disease, ileal resection, vagotomy, diabetic vagal neuropathy, and radiation
  ▸ BY MOUTH
  ‣ Adult: Initially 4 g daily, increased in steps of 4 g every week; increased to 12–24 g daily in 1–4 divided doses, adjusted according to response, if no response within 3 days an alternative therapy should be initiated; maximum 36 g per day

Accelerated elimination of teriflunomide
  ▸ BY MOUTH
  ‣ Adult: 8 g 3 times a day for 11 days; reduced to 4 g 3 times a day, dose should only be reduced if not tolerated

Accelerated elimination of leflunomide (washout procedure)
  ▸ BY MOUTH
  ‣ Adult: 8 g 3 times a day for 11 days

- **CONTRA-INDICATIONS** Complete biliary obstruction (not likely to be effective)

- **INTERACTIONS** → Appendix 1: colestyramine

- **SIDE-EFFECTS**
  ▸ **Uncommon** Bleeding tendency · hypoprothrombinaemia · night blindness · osteoporosis · skin reactions · tongue irritation · vitamin deficiencies

- **DIRECTIONS FOR ADMINISTRATION** Manufacturer advises the contents of each sachet should be mixed with at least 150 mL of water or other suitable liquid such as fruit juice, skimmed milk, thin soups, and pulpy fruits with a high moisture content.

- **PATIENT AND CARER ADVICE** Patient counselling on administration is advised for colestyramine powder (avoid other drugs at same time).

- **MEDICINAL FORMS** There can be variation in the licensing of different medicines containing the same drug. Forms available from special-order manufacturers include: oral suspension, oral solution

Powder for oral suspension
CAUTIONARY AND ADVISORY LABELS 13
EXCIPIENTS: May contain Aspartame, sucrose
  ‣ Colestyramine (Non-proprietary)
    Colestyramine anhydrous 4 gram Colestyramine 4g oral powder sachets sugar free | 50 sachet [PoM] £42.00 DT = £39.01 [SF]
  ‣ Questran (Neon Healthcare Ltd)
    Colestyramine anhydrous 4 gram Questran 4g oral powder sachets | 50 sachet [PoM] £10.76 DT = £10.76
  ‣ Questran Light (Neon Healthcare Ltd)
    Colestyramine anhydrous 4 gram Questran Light 4g oral powder sachets | 50 sachet [PoM] £16.15 DT = £39.01 [SF]

LIPID MODIFYING DRUGS > CHOLESTEROL ABSORPTION INHIBITORS

Ezetimibe

02-Jan-2024

- **DRUG ACTION** Ezetimibe inhibits the intestinal absorption of cholesterol. If used alone, it has a modest effect on lowering LDL-cholesterol, with little effect on other lipoproteins.

● INDICATIONS AND DOSE

Adjunct to dietary measures and statin treatment in primary hypercholesterolaemia | Adjunct to dietary measures and statin in homozygous familial hypercholesterolaemia | Primary hypercholesterolaemia (if statin inappropriate or not tolerated) | Adjunct to dietary measures in homozygous sitosterolaemia
  ▸ BY MOUTH
  ‣ Adult: 10 mg once daily

Prevention of cardiovascular events [in patients with coronary heart disease and a history of acute coronary syndrome, in combination with a statin]
  ▸ BY MOUTH
  ‣ Adult: 10 mg once daily

- **INTERACTIONS** → Appendix 1: ezetimibe

- **SIDE-EFFECTS**
  ▸ **Common or very common** Asthenia · diarrhoea · gastrointestinal discomfort · gastrointestinal disorders · headache · muscle complaints
  ▸ **Uncommon** Appetite decreased · arthralgia · chest pain · cough · dry mouth · hot flush · hypertension · muscle weakness · nausea · pain · paraesthesia · peripheral oedema · skin reactions
  ▸ **Frequency not known** Constipation · depression · dizziness · dyspnoea · hepatitis · myopathy · pancreatitis · thrombocytopenia

- **PREGNANCY** Manufacturer advises use only if potential benefit outweighs risk—no information available.

- **BREAST FEEDING** Manufacturer advises avoid—present in milk in *animal* studies.

- **HEPATIC IMPAIRMENT** Manufacturer advises avoid in moderate to severe impairment.

- **NATIONAL FUNDING/ACCESS DECISIONS** For full details see funding body website

NICE decisions
  ▸ **Ezetimibe for treating primary heterozygous-familial and non-familial hypercholesterolaemia (February 2016)** NICE TA385 Recommended with restrictions

- **MEDICINAL FORMS** There can be variation in the licensing of different medicines containing the same drug.
Oral tablet
  ‣ Ezetimibe (Non-proprietary)
    Ezetimibe 10 mg Ezetimibe 10mg tablets | 28 tablet [PoM] £26.31 DT = £2.53

▶ **Ezetrol** (Organon Pharma (UK) Ltd)
Ezetimibe 10 mg Ezetrol 10mg tablets | 28 tablet [PoM] £26.31 DT = £2.53

Combinations available: *Bempedoic acid with ezetimibe,* p. 239 · *Simvastatin with ezetimibe,* p. 237

LIPID MODIFYING DRUGS > FIBRATES

Bezafibrate

09-Aug-2021

● **DRUG ACTION** Fibrates act by decreasing serum triglycerides; they have variable effect on LDL-cholesterol.

● **INDICATIONS AND DOSE**

Adjunct to diet and other appropriate measures in mixed hyperlipidaemia if statin contra-indicated or not tolerated | Adjunct to diet and other appropriate measures in severe hypertriglyceridaemia

▶ BY MOUTH USING IMMEDIATE-RELEASE MEDICINES
▶ Adult: 200 mg 3 times a day
▶ BY MOUTH USING MODIFIED-RELEASE MEDICINES
▶ Adult: 400 mg once daily, modified-release dose form is not appropriate in patients with renal impairment

● **CONTRA-INDICATIONS** Gall bladder disease · hypoalbuminaemia · nephrotic syndrome · photosensitivity to fibrates

● **CAUTIONS** Correct hypothyroidism before initiating treatment · risk factors for myopathy

● **INTERACTIONS** → Appendix 1: fibrates

● **SIDE-EFFECTS**
▶ **Common or very common** Appetite decreased · gastrointestinal disorder
▶ **Uncommon** Acute kidney injury · alopecia · cholestasis · constipation · diarrhoea · dizziness · erectile dysfunction · gastrointestinal discomfort · headache · muscle complaints · muscle weakness · nausea · photosensitivity reaction · skin reactions
▶ **Rare or very rare** Cholelithiasis · depression · insomnia · interstitial lung disease · pancreatitis · pancytopenia · paraesthesia · peripheral neuropathy · rhabdomyolysis (increased risk in renal impairment) · severe cutaneous adverse reactions (SCARs) · thrombocytopenic purpura

● **PREGNANCY** Manufacturers advise avoid—no information available.

● **BREAST FEEDING** Manufacturer advises avoid—no information available.

● **HEPATIC IMPAIRMENT** Manufacturer advises avoid in significant impairment (except in fatty liver disease).

● **RENAL IMPAIRMENT** Manufacturer advises avoid *immediate-release* preparations if creatinine clearance less than 15 mL/minute. Manufacturer advises avoid *modified-release* preparations if creatinine clearance less than 60 mL/minute.
Myotoxicity Manufacturer advises special care needed in patients with renal disease, as progressive increases in serum creatinine concentration or failure to follow dosage guidelines may result in myotoxicity (rhabdomyolysis); discontinue if myotoxicity suspected or creatine kinase concentration increases significantly.
Dose adjustments See p. 21.
    Manufacturer advises reduce dose to 400 mg daily if creatinine clearance 40–60 mL/minute.
    Manufacturer advises reduce dose to 200 mg every 1–2 days if creatinine clearance 15–40 mL/minute.

● **MONITORING REQUIREMENTS** Consider monitoring of liver function and creatine kinase when fibrates used in combination with a statin.

● **PRESCRIBING AND DISPENSING INFORMATION** Fibrates are mainly used in those whose serum-triglyceride

concentration is greater than 10 mmol/litre or in those who cannot tolerate a statin (specialist use).

● **MEDICINAL FORMS** There can be variation in the licensing of different medicines containing the same drug. Forms available from special-order manufacturers include: oral suspension

Oral tablet
CAUTIONARY AND ADVISORY LABELS 21
▶ **Bezafibrate (Non-proprietary)**
Bezafibrate 200 mg Bezafibrate 200mg tablets | 100 tablet [PoM] £8.63 DT = £8.63
▶ **Bezalip** (Teva UK Ltd)
Bezafibrate 200 mg Bezalip 200mg tablets | 100 tablet [PoM] £8.63 DT = £8.63

Modified-release tablet
CAUTIONARY AND ADVISORY LABELS 21, 25
▶ **Bezalip Mono** (Teva UK Ltd)
Bezafibrate 400 mg Bezalip Mono 400mg modified-release tablets | 30 tablet [PoM] £7.63 DT = £7.63
▶ **Lipozate** (Noumed Life Sciences Ltd)
Bezafibrate 400 mg Lipozate 400mg modified-release tablets | 30 tablet [PoM] [£] DT = £7.63

Ciprofibrate

07-May-2021

● **DRUG ACTION** Fibrates act by decreasing serum triglycerides; they have variable effect on LDL-cholesterol.

● **INDICATIONS AND DOSE**

Adjunct to diet and other appropriate measures in mixed hyperlipidaemia if statin contra-indicated or not tolerated | Adjunct to diet and other appropriate measures in severe hypertriglyceridaemia

▶ BY MOUTH
▶ Adult: 100 mg daily

● **CONTRA-INDICATIONS** Gall bladder disease · hypoalbuminaemia · nephrotic syndrome · photosensitivity to fibrates

● **CAUTIONS** Correct hypothyroidism before initiating treatment · risk factors for myopathy

● **INTERACTIONS** → Appendix 1: fibrates

● **SIDE-EFFECTS**
▶ **Common or very common** Alopecia · diarrhoea · dizziness · drowsiness · fatigue · gastrointestinal discomfort · headache · myalgia · nausea · skin reactions · vertigo · vomiting
▶ **Frequency not known** Cholelithiasis · erectile dysfunction · hepatic disorders · leucopenia · myopathy · photosensitivity reaction · pneumonitis · pulmonary fibrosis · rhabdomyolysis (increased risk in renal impairment) · thrombocytopenia

● **PREGNANCY** Manufacturers advise avoid—toxicity in *animal* studies.

● **BREAST FEEDING** Manufacturer advises avoid—present in milk in *animal* studies.

● **HEPATIC IMPAIRMENT** Manufacturer advises use with caution in mild-to-moderate impairment; avoid in severe impairment

● **RENAL IMPAIRMENT** [EvGr] Avoid in severe impairment. ⓜ
Myotoxicity [EvGr] Special care needed in patients with renal disease, as progressive increases in serum creatinine concentration or failure to follow dosage guidelines may result in myotoxicity (rhabdomyolysis); discontinue if myotoxicity suspected or creatine kinase concentration increases significantly. ⓜ
Dose adjustments [EvGr] Reduce dose to 100 mg on alternate days in moderate impairment. ⓜ

● **MONITORING REQUIREMENTS**
▶ Liver function tests recommended every 3 months for first year (discontinue treatment if significantly raised).

▸ Consider monitoring liver function and creatine kinase when fibrates used in combination with a statin.

● **PRESCRIBING AND DISPENSING INFORMATION** Fibrates are mainly used in those whose serum-triglyceride concentration is greater than 10 mmol/litre or in those who cannot tolerate a statin (specialist use).

● **MEDICINAL FORMS** There can be variation in the licensing of different medicines containing the same drug.

Oral tablet

▸ Ciprofibrate (Non-proprietary)
Ciprofibrate 100 mg Ciprofibrate 100mg tablets | 28 tablet PoM £112.06 DT = £40.25

Fenofibrate
09-Aug-2021

● **DRUG ACTION** Fibrates act by decreasing serum triglycerides; they have variable effect on LDL-cholesterol.

● **INDICATIONS AND DOSE**

Adjunct to diet and other appropriate measures in mixed hyperlipidaemia if statin contra-indicated or not tolerated | Adjunct to diet and other appropriate measures in severe hypertriglyceridaemia | Adjunct to statin in mixed hyperlipidaemia if triglycerides and HDL-cholesterol inadequately controlled in patients at high cardiovascular risk

▸ BY MOUTH USING CAPSULES
▸ Adult: Initially 200 mg daily, then increased if necessary to 267 mg daily, maximum 200 mg daily with concomitant statin, 267 mg capsules not appropriate for initial dose titration
▸ BY MOUTH USING TABLETS
▸ Adult: 160 mg daily

DOSE ADJUSTMENTS DUE TO INTERACTIONS
▸ Manufacturer advises max. dose 200 mg daily with concurrent use of a statin.

● **CONTRA-INDICATIONS** Gall bladder disease · pancreatitis (unless due to severe hypertriglyceridaemia) · photosensitivity to fibrates · photosensitivity to ketoprofen

● **CAUTIONS** Correct hypothyroidism before initiating treatment · risk factors for myopathy

● **INTERACTIONS** → Appendix 1: fibrates

● **SIDE-EFFECTS**
▸ **Common or very common** Abdominal pain · diarrhoea · flatulence · nausea · vomiting
▸ **Uncommon** Cholelithiasis · embolism and thrombosis · headache · muscle complaints · muscle weakness · myopathy · pancreatitis · sexual dysfunction · skin reactions
▸ **Rare or very rare** Alopecia · hepatic disorders · photosensitivity reaction
▸ **Frequency not known** Fatigue · interstitial lung disease · rhabdomyolysis (increased risk in renal impairment) · severe cutaneous adverse reactions (SCARs)

● **PREGNANCY** Avoid—embryotoxicity in *animal* studies.

● **BREAST FEEDING** Manufacturers advise avoid—no information available.

● **HEPATIC IMPAIRMENT** Manufacturer advises avoid —no information available.

● **RENAL IMPAIRMENT** EvGr Use with caution in mild-to-moderate impairment; avoid if eGFR less than 30 mL/minute/1.73 m². Ⓜ
Myotoxicity EvGr Special care needed in patients with renal disease, as progressive increases in serum creatinine concentration or failure to follow dosage guidelines may result in myotoxicity (rhabdomyolysis); discontinue if myotoxicity suspected or creatine kinase concentration increases significantly. Ⓜ

Dose adjustments See p. 21.
EvGr Max. 67 mg daily if eGFR 30–59 mL/minute/1.73 m². Ⓜ

● **MONITORING REQUIREMENTS** Manufacturer advises monitor hepatic transaminases every 3 months during the first 12 months of treatment and periodically thereafter—discontinue treatment if levels increase to more than 3 times the upper limit of normal; monitor serum creatinine levels during the first 3 months of treatment and periodically thereafter—interrupt treatment if creatinine level is 50% above the upper limit of normal.

● **PRESCRIBING AND DISPENSING INFORMATION** Fibrates are mainly used in those whose serum-triglyceride concentration is greater than 10 mmol/litre or in those who cannot tolerate a statin (specialist use).

● **MEDICINAL FORMS** There can be variation in the licensing of different medicines containing the same drug.

Oral tablet
CAUTIONARY AND ADVISORY LABELS 21

▸ Fenofibrate (Non-proprietary)
Fenofibrate micronised 160 mg Fenofibrate micronised 160mg tablets | 28 tablet PoM £4.45 DT = £2.86 | 30 tablet PoM £2.87
▸ Supralip (Viatris UK Healthcare Ltd)
Fenofibrate micronised 160 mg Supralip 160mg tablets | 28 tablet PoM £6.69 DT = £2.86

Oral capsule
CAUTIONARY AND ADVISORY LABELS 21

▸ Fenofibrate (Non-proprietary)
Fenofibrate micronised 67 mg Fenofibrate micronised 67mg capsules | 90 capsule PoM £23.30 DT = £9.34
Fenofibrate micronised 200 mg Fenofibrate micronised 200mg capsules | 28 capsule PoM £5.04 DT = £3.95
Fenofibrate micronised 267 mg Fenofibrate micronised 267mg capsules | 28 capsule PoM £21.75 DT = £2.69
▸ Lipantil Micro (Viatris UK Healthcare Ltd)
Fenofibrate micronised 67 mg Lipantil Micro 67 capsules | 90 capsule PoM £23.30 DT = £9.34
Fenofibrate micronised 200 mg Lipantil Micro 200 capsules | 28 capsule PoM £14.23 DT = £3.95
Fenofibrate micronised 267 mg Lipantil Micro 267 capsules | 28 capsule PoM £21.75 DT = £2.69

Gemfibrozil
09-Aug-2021

● **DRUG ACTION** Fibrates act by decreasing serum triglycerides; they have variable effect on LDL-cholesterol.

● **INDICATIONS AND DOSE**

Adjunct to diet and other appropriate measures in mixed hyperlipidaemia if statin contra-indicated or not tolerated | Adjunct to diet and other appropriate measures in primary hypercholesterolaemia if statin contra-indicated or not tolerated | Adjunct to diet and other appropriate measures in severe hypertriglyceridaemia | Adjunct to diet and other appropriate measures in primary prevention of cardiovascular disease in men with hyperlipidaemias if statin contra-indicated or not tolerated

▸ BY MOUTH
▸ Adult: 1.2 g daily in 2 divided doses, maintenance 0.9–1.2 g daily

● **CONTRA-INDICATIONS** History of gall-bladder or biliary tract disease including gallstones · photosensitivity to fibrates

● **CAUTIONS** Correct hypothyroidism before initiating treatment · elderly · risk factors for myopathy

● **INTERACTIONS** → Appendix 1: fibrates

● **SIDE-EFFECTS**
▸ **Common or very common** Constipation · diarrhoea · fatigue · flatulence · gastrointestinal discomfort · headache · nausea · skin reactions · vertigo · vomiting

2 Cardiovascular system

▶ **Uncommon** Atrial fibrillation
▶ **Rare or very rare** Alopecia · anaemia · angioedema · appendicitis · bone marrow failure · depression · dizziness · drowsiness · eosinophilia · gallbladder disorders · hepatic disorders · joint disorders · laryngeal oedema · leucopenia · muscle weakness · myalgia · myopathy · pain in extremity · pancreatitis · paraesthesia · peripheral neuropathy · photosensitivity reaction · sexual dysfunction · thrombocytopenia · vision blurred

● **PREGNANCY** Manufacturers advise avoid unless essential— toxicity in *animal* studies.

● **BREAST FEEDING** Manufacturer advises avoid—no information available.

● **HEPATIC IMPAIRMENT** Manufacturer advises avoid.

● **RENAL IMPAIRMENT** [EvGr] Avoid if eGFR less than 30 mL/minute/1.73 m². Ⓜ
Myotoxicity [EvGr] Special care needed in patients with renal disease, as progressive increases in serum creatinine concentration or failure to follow dosage guidelines may result in myotoxicity (rhabdomyolysis); discontinue if myotoxicity suspected or creatine kinase concentration increases significantly. Ⓜ
Dose adjustments [EvGr] Initially 900 mg daily if eGFR 30–80 mL/minute/1.73 m². Ⓜ See p. 21.

● **MONITORING REQUIREMENTS**
▶ Monitor blood counts for first year.
▶ Monitor liver-function (discontinue treatment if abnormalities persist).
▶ Consider monitoring creatine kinase if used in combination with a statin.

● **PRESCRIBING AND DISPENSING INFORMATION** Fibrates are mainly used in those whose serum-triglyceride concentration is greater than 10 mmol/litre or in those who cannot tolerate a statin (specialist use).

● **MEDICINAL FORMS** There can be variation in the licensing of different medicines containing the same drug.
Oral tablet
CAUTIONARY AND ADVISORY LABELS 22
▶ **Gemfibrozil (Non-proprietary)**
Gemfibrozil 600 mg Gemfibrozil 600mg tablets | 56 tablet [PoM] £64.00 DT = £35.57
▶ **Lopid** (Pfizer Ltd)
Gemfibrozil 600 mg Lopid 600mg tablets | 56 tablet [PoM] £35.57 DT = £35.57
Oral capsule
CAUTIONARY AND ADVISORY LABELS 22
▶ **Lopid** (Pfizer Ltd)
Gemfibrozil 300 mg Lopid 300mg capsules | 100 capsule [PoM] £31.76 DT = £31.76

LIPID MODIFYING DRUGS › NICOTINIC ACID DERIVATIVES

│ Acipimox
19-Jul-2021

● **INDICATIONS AND DOSE**
Adjunct or alternative treatment in hyperlipidaemias of types IIb and IV in patients who have not responded adequately to other lipid-regulating drugs such as a statin or fibrate, and lifestyle changes (including diet, exercise, and weight reduction)
▶ BY MOUTH
▶ Adult: 250 mg 2–3 times a day

● **CONTRA-INDICATIONS** Peptic ulcer
● **INTERACTIONS** → Appendix 1: acipimox
● **SIDE-EFFECTS**
▶ **Common or very common** Asthenia · gastrointestinal discomfort · headache · skin reactions · vasodilation
▶ **Uncommon** Angioedema · arthralgia · feeling hot · malaise · myalgia · myositis · nausea

▶ **Frequency not known** Bronchospasm · diarrhoea · dry eye · eye disorder · eyes gritty

● **PREGNANCY** Manufacturer advises avoid—no information available.

● **BREAST FEEDING** Manufacturer advises avoid—no information available.

● **RENAL IMPAIRMENT** [EvGr] Avoid if creatinine clearance less than 30 mL/minute. Ⓜ
Dose adjustments [EvGr] Reduce dose to 250 mg 1–2 times daily if creatinine clearance 30–60 mL/minute, Ⓜ see p. 21.

● **MONITORING REQUIREMENTS** Monitor hepatic and renal function.

● **MEDICINAL FORMS** There can be variation in the licensing of different medicines containing the same drug.
Oral capsule
CAUTIONARY AND ADVISORY LABELS 21
▶ **Olbetam** (Pfizer Ltd)
Acipimox 250 mg Olbetam 250mg capsules | 90 capsule [PoM] £46.33 DT = £46.33

│ Nicotinic acid
07-Feb-2020

● **DRUG ACTION** In doses of 1.5 to 3 g daily, it lowers both cholesterol and triglyceride concentrations by inhibiting synthesis; it also increases HDL-cholesterol.

● **INDICATIONS AND DOSE**
Adjunct to statin in dyslipidaemia or used alone if statin not tolerated
▶ BY MOUTH
▶ Adult: (consult product literature)

● **CONTRA-INDICATIONS** Active peptic ulcer disease · arterial bleeding

● **CAUTIONS** Acute myocardial infarction · diabetes mellitus · gout · history of peptic ulceration · unstable angina

● **INTERACTIONS** → Appendix 1: nicotinic acid

● **SIDE-EFFECTS** Angioedema · arrhythmias · asthenia · burping · cough aggravated · diarrhoea · dizziness · dyspnoea · flushing · gastrointestinal disorders · gout · hepatic disorders · hyperhidrosis · hypotension · insomnia · macular oedema · migraine · myalgia · myopathy · nausea · nervousness · oedema · palpitations · paraesthesia · respiratory disorders · skin reactions · syncope · tongue oedema · vision blurred · vomiting

SIDE-EFFECTS, FURTHER INFORMATION Prostaglandin-mediated flushing is common, typically within an hour of dosing and lasting for 15–30 minutes (particularly with the initial doses). Taking after a meal or taking aspirin before dosing minimises flushing.

● **PREGNANCY** No information available—manufacturer advises avoid unless potential benefit outweighs risk.

● **BREAST FEEDING** Present in milk—avoid.

● **HEPATIC IMPAIRMENT** Avoid in severe impairment. Discontinue if severe abnormalities in liver function tests.
Monitoring Manufacturer advises monitor liver function in mild to moderate hepatic impairment.

● **RENAL IMPAIRMENT** Manufacturer advises use with caution—no information available.

● **MEDICINAL FORMS** There can be variation in the licensing of different medicines containing the same drug. Forms available from special-order manufacturers include: oral tablet, modified-release tablet, oral capsule
Oral capsule
▶ **Nicotinic acid (Non-proprietary)**
Nicotinic acid 500 mg Solgar Niacin 500mg capsules | 100 capsule 🅴

LIPID MODIFYING DRUGS › STATINS

Statins 

- **DRUG ACTION** Statins competitively inhibit 3-hydroxy-3-methylglutaryl coenzyme A (HMG CoA) reductase, an enzyme involved in cholesterol synthesis, especially in the liver.

> **IMPORTANT SAFETY INFORMATION**
>
> **MHRA/CHM ADVICE: STATINS: VERY INFREQUENT REPORTS OF MYASTHENIA GRAVIS (SEPTEMBER 2023)**
>
> There has been a very small number of reports of new-onset, or exacerbation of pre-existing, myasthenia gravis or ocular myasthenia associated with statin use, albeit very infrequent and no reported fatalities. In most cases, patients recovered after stopping statin treatment. However, a minority continued to experience symptoms, some of which recurred on rechallenge with the same, or an alternative, statin. Symptom onset ranged from a few days to 3 months after starting statin treatment.
>
> Healthcare professionals are advised to refer patients who present with suspected new-onset myasthenia gravis symptoms, after starting a statin, to a neurologist—the statin may need to be discontinued if its risks outweigh the benefits. Healthcare professionals are also advised to counsel patients and their carers to:
> - inform their doctor, before taking a statin, if they have a history of myasthenia gravis or ocular myasthenia as it may exacerbate their symptoms;
> - continue taking their statin unless they are advised to stop;
> - inform their doctor if they experience symptoms such as weakness in the arms or legs that worsens after activity, double vision, drooping of the eyelids, difficulty swallowing, or shortness of breath;
> - seek immediate medical attention if they develop severe breathing or swallowing problems.

- **CAUTIONS** Risk factors for muscle toxicity, including myopathy or rhabdomyolysis

  CAUTIONS, FURTHER INFORMATION
- ▸ Muscle effects `EvGr` Muscle toxicity can occur with all statins, however the likelihood increases with higher doses and in certain patients. Statins should be used with caution in patients at increased risk of muscle toxicity. This includes the elderly, those with a personal or family history of muscular disorders, history of muscular toxicity or unexplained persistent muscle pain, history of liver disease, a high alcohol intake, known genetic polymorphisms—consult product literature, renal impairment, hypothyroidism, or those who undertake strenuous exercise. Ⓜ See also *Monitoring requirements*.
- ▸ Hypothyroidism Hypothyroidism should be managed adequately before starting treatment with a statin.

- **SIDE-EFFECTS**
- ▸ **Common or very common** Arthralgia · asthenia · constipation · diarrhoea · dizziness · flatulence · gastrointestinal discomfort · headache · muscle complaints · nausea · sleep disorders · thrombocytopenia
- ▸ **Uncommon** Alopecia · hepatic disorders · memory loss · pancreatitis · paraesthesia · sexual dysfunction · skin reactions · vomiting
- ▸ **Rare or very rare** Lupus-like syndrome · myopathy · peripheral neuropathy · tendon disorders
- ▸ **Frequency not known** Depression · diabetes mellitus (in those at risk) · interstitial lung disease · neuromuscular dysfunction

  SIDE-EFFECTS, FURTHER INFORMATION **Muscle effects**
  Although myalgia has been reported commonly in patients receiving statins, muscle toxicity truly attributable to statin use is rare. The risk of myopathy, myositis, and rhabdomyolysis associated with statin use is also rare. If muscle pain, weakness, or cramps occur during treatment, creatine kinase concentrations should be measured; if the concentration is more than 5 times the ULN (in the absence of strenuous exercise), treatment should be discontinued. If muscular symptoms are severe and cause daily discomfort, treatment discontinuation should be considered, even if creatine kinase concentrations are less than 5 times the ULN. If symptoms resolve and creatine kinase concentrations return to normal, the statin can be reintroduced, or introduction of an alternative statin can be considered, at the lowest dose and the patient monitored closely.

  Diabetes Statins should not be discontinued if there is an increase in the blood-glucose concentration as the benefits continue to outweigh the risks.

  Interstitial lung disease If patients develop symptoms such as dyspnoea, cough, and weight loss, they should seek medical attention.

- **CONCEPTION AND CONTRACEPTION** Adequate contraception is required during treatment and for 1 month afterwards.

- **PREGNANCY** Statins should be avoided in pregnancy (discontinue 3 months before attempting to conceive) as congenital anomalies have been reported and the decreased synthesis of cholesterol possibly affects fetal development.

- **HEPATIC IMPAIRMENT** In general, manufacturers advise caution (risk of increased exposure); avoid in active disease or unexplained persistent elevations in serum transaminases.

- **MONITORING REQUIREMENTS**
- ▸ `EvGr` Before starting treatment with statins, at least one full lipid profile should be measured, including total cholesterol, triglycerides, HDL-cholesterol, non-HDL-cholesterol and LDL-cholesterol concentrations, and repeated 2–3 months after starting or changing treatment. Baseline thyroid-stimulating hormone (in patients with symptoms of underactive or overactive thyroid), and renal function should also be assessed. Ⓐ
- ▸ Liver function `EvGr` Liver transaminases should be measured before starting treatment with statins, repeated 2–3 months after starting or changing treatment, and then at 12 months, unless indicated at other times by signs or symptoms suggestive of hepatotoxicity. Patients with serum transaminases that are raised, but less than 3 times the upper limit of normal (ULN), should **not** be routinely excluded from statin therapy. Ⓐ`EvGr` Those with serum transaminases of more than 3 times the ULN should discontinue statin therapy. Ⓜ
- ▸ Muscle effects `EvGr` Before initiation of statin treatment, creatine kinase concentration should be measured in patients who have had persistent, generalised, unexplained muscle pain, tenderness or weakness (whether associated or not with previous lipid-regulating drugs); if the baseline concentration is more than 5 times the ULN, a repeat measurement should be taken after 7 days. If the repeat concentration remains above 5 times the ULN, statin treatment should not be started; if concentrations are still raised but less than 5 times the ULN, the statin should be started at a lower dose. During statin treatment, creatine kinase concentration should be measured in patients who develop unexplained muscle pain, tenderness or weakness. Ⓐ Some patients may present with an extremely elevated baseline creatine kinase concentration, for example because of a physical occupation or rigorous exercise—specialist advice should be sought regarding consideration of statin therapy in these patients.
- ▸ Diabetes Patients at high risk of diabetes mellitus should have fasting blood-glucose concentration or HbA$_{1C}$

checked before starting statin treatment, and then repeated after 3 months.

- **PRESCRIBING AND DISPENSING INFORMATION**
  Patient decision aid Taking a statin to reduce the risk of coronary heart disease and stroke. National Institute for Health and Care Excellence. November 2014.
  www.nice.org.uk/about/what-we-do/our-programmes/nice-guidance/nice-guidelines/shared-decision-making

- **PATIENT AND CARER ADVICE** Advise patients to report promptly unexplained muscle pain, tenderness, or weakness.

☞ 233

Atorvastatin

12-Sep-2024

- **INDICATIONS AND DOSE**

Primary hypercholesterolaemia in patients who have not responded adequately to diet and other appropriate measures | Combined (mixed) hyperlipidaemia in patients who have not responded adequately to diet and other appropriate measures
- ▸ BY MOUTH
- ▸ Adult: Usual dose 10 mg once daily; increased if necessary up to 80 mg once daily, dose to be increased at intervals of at least 4 weeks

Heterozygous familial hypercholesterolaemia in patients who have not responded adequately to diet and other appropriate measures | Homozygous familial hypercholesterolaemia in patients who have not responded adequately to diet and other appropriate measures
- ▸ BY MOUTH
- ▸ Adult: Initially 10 mg once daily, then increased to 40 mg once daily, dose to be increased at intervals of at least 4 weeks, then increased if necessary up to 80 mg once daily

Primary prevention of cardiovascular events in patients at high risk of a first cardiovascular event
- ▸ BY MOUTH
- ▸ Adult: 20 mg once daily; increased if necessary up to 80 mg once daily, dose to be increased at intervals of at least 4 weeks

Secondary prevention of cardiovascular events
- ▸ BY MOUTH
- ▸ Adult: 80 mg once daily

DOSE ADJUSTMENTS DUE TO INTERACTIONS
- ▸ Manufacturer advises if concurrent use of ciclosporin is unavoidable, max. dose cannot exceed 10 mg daily.
- ▸ Manufacturer advises max. dose 40 mg daily when combined with anion-exchange resin for heterozygous familial hypercholesterolaemia.
- ▸ Manufacturer advises max. dose 20 mg daily with concurrent use of elbasvir with grazoprevir.
- ▸ Manufacturer advises max. dose 20 mg daily with concurrent use of letermovir without ciclosporin.
- ▸ Manufacturer advises max. dose 20 mg daily with concurrent use of sofosbuvir with velpatasvir and voxilaprevir.

- **UNLICENSED USE** EvGr Atorvastatin is used in the doses provided in the BNF for primary prevention of cardiovascular events Ⓐ, but these may differ from those licensed. EvGr Atorvastatin is used for secondary prevention of cardiovascular events ⒶGr, but is not licensed for this indication.

- **CAUTIONS** Haemorrhagic stroke

- **INTERACTIONS** → Appendix 1: statins

- **SIDE-EFFECTS**
- ▸ **Common or very common** Epistaxis · hyperglycaemia · hypersensitivity · joint swelling · laryngeal pain · nasopharyngitis · pain

- ▸ **Uncommon** Appetite decreased · burping · chest pain · fever · hypoglycaemia · malaise · numbness · peripheral oedema · taste altered · tinnitus · vision disorders · weight increased
- ▸ **Rare or very rare** Angioedema · gynaecomastia · hearing loss · severe cutaneous adverse reactions (SCARs)

- **BREAST FEEDING** Manufacturer advises avoid—no information available.

- **RENAL IMPAIRMENT**
  Dose adjustments
- ▸ When used for Primary prevention of cardiovascular events or Secondary prevention of cardiovascular events EvGr In chronic kidney disease, initially 20 mg once daily, increased if necessary (on specialist advice if eGFR less than 30 mL/minute/1.73 m^2); max. 80 mg once daily. Ⓐ See p. 21.

- **PATIENT AND CARER ADVICE** Patient counselling is advised for atorvastatin tablets (muscle effects).

- **MEDICINAL FORMS** There can be variation in the licensing of different medicines containing the same drug. Forms available from special-order manufacturers include: oral suspension, oral solution

Oral tablet
- ▸ Atorvastatin (Non-proprietary)
  Atorvastatin (as Atorvastatin calcium trihydrate)
  10 mg Atorvastatin 10mg tablets | 28 tablet PoM £15.60 DT = £0.61 | 90 tablet PoM £35.52
  Atorvastatin (as Atorvastatin calcium trihydrate)
  20 mg Atorvastatin 20mg tablets | 28 tablet PoM £29.57 DT = £0.67 | 90 tablet PoM £3.85
  Atorvastatin (as Atorvastatin calcium trihydrate)
  30 mg Atorvastatin 30mg tablets | 28 tablet PoM £29.40 DT = £8.39
  Atorvastatin (as Atorvastatin calcium trihydrate)
  40 mg Atorvastatin 40mg tablets | 28 tablet PoM £29.57 DT = £0.77 | 90 tablet PoM £67.32
  Atorvastatin (as Atorvastatin calcium trihydrate)
  60 mg Atorvastatin 60mg tablets | 28 tablet PoM £33.60 DT = £8.24
  Atorvastatin (as Atorvastatin calcium trihydrate)
  80 mg Atorvastatin 80mg tablets | 28 tablet PoM £33.85 DT = £1.23
- ▸ Lipitor (Viatris UK Healthcare Ltd)
  Atorvastatin (as Atorvastatin calcium trihydrate) 10 mg Lipitor 10mg tablets | 28 tablet PoM £13.00 DT = £0.61
  Atorvastatin (as Atorvastatin calcium trihydrate) 20 mg Lipitor 20mg tablets | 28 tablet PoM £24.64 DT = £0.67
  Atorvastatin (as Atorvastatin calcium trihydrate) 40 mg Lipitor 40mg tablets | 28 tablet PoM £24.64 DT = £0.77
  Atorvastatin (as Atorvastatin calcium trihydrate) 80 mg Lipitor 80mg tablets | 28 tablet PoM £28.21 DT = £1.23

Oral suspension
- ▸ Atorvastatin (Non-proprietary)
  Atorvastatin (as Atorvastatin calcium trihydrate) 4 mg per 1 ml Atorvastatin 20mg/5ml oral suspension sugar free | 150 ml PoM £226.80 DT = £226.80 SF

Chewable tablet
CAUTIONARY AND ADVISORY LABELS 24
- ▸ Lipitor (Viatris UK Healthcare Ltd)
  Atorvastatin (as Atorvastatin calcium trihydrate) 10 mg Lipitor 10mg chewable tablets | 30 tablet PoM £13.80 DT = £13.80 SF
  Atorvastatin (as Atorvastatin calcium trihydrate) 20 mg Lipitor 20mg chewable tablets | 30 tablet PoM £26.40 DT = £26.40 SF

☞ 233

Fluvastatin

20-Jul-2021

- **INDICATIONS AND DOSE**

Adjunct to diet in primary hypercholesterolaemia or combined (mixed) hyperlipidaemia (types IIa and IIb)
- ▸ BY MOUTH USING IMMEDIATE-RELEASE MEDICINES
- ▸ Adult: Initially 20–40 mg daily, dose to be taken in the evening, increased if necessary up to 80 mg daily in 2 divided doses, dose to be adjusted at intervals of at least 4 weeks

▶ BY MOUTH USING MODIFIED-RELEASE MEDICINES
▶ Adult: 80 mg daily, dose form is not appropriate for initial dose titration

Prevention of coronary events after percutaneous coronary intervention
▶ BY MOUTH USING IMMEDIATE-RELEASE MEDICINES
▶ Adult: 80 mg daily
▶ BY MOUTH USING MODIFIED-RELEASE MEDICINES
▶ Adult: 80 mg daily, dose form is not appropriate for initial dose titration

DOSE ADJUSTMENTS DUE TO INTERACTIONS
▶ Max. dose 20 mg daily with concomitant elbasvir with grazoprevir.

● INTERACTIONS → Appendix 1: statins

● SIDE-EFFECTS
▶ **Rare or very rare** Angioedema · face oedema · muscle weakness · sensation abnormal · vasculitis

● **BREAST FEEDING** Manufacturer advises avoid—no information available.

● **RENAL IMPAIRMENT**
Dose adjustments EvGr Doses above 40 mg daily should be initiated with caution if creatinine clearance less than 30 mL/minute (limited information available), Ⓜ see p. 21.

● **PATIENT AND CARER ADVICE** Patient counselling is advised for fluvastatin tablets/capsules (muscle effects).

● **NATIONAL FUNDING/ACCESS DECISIONS**
For full details see funding body website
Scottish Medicines Consortium (SMC) decisions
▶ **Fluvastatin (*Lescol*®) for the secondary prevention of coronary events after percutaneous coronary intervention (February 2004)** SMC No. 76/04 Recommended with restrictions

● **MEDICINAL FORMS** There can be variation in the licensing of different medicines containing the same drug.
Modified-release tablet
CAUTIONARY AND ADVISORY LABELS 25
▶ Fluvastatin (Non-proprietary)
Fluvastatin (as Fluvastatin sodium) 80 mg Fluvastatin 80mg modified-release tablets | 28 tablet PoM £19.20–£37.00 DT = £19.20
Oral capsule
▶ Fluvastatin (Non-proprietary)
Fluvastatin (as Fluvastatin sodium) 20 mg Fluvastatin 20mg capsules | 28 capsule PoM £4.18 DT = £4.18
Fluvastatin (as Fluvastatin sodium) 40 mg Fluvastatin 40mg capsules | 28 capsule PoM £5.00 DT = £4.89

F 233

Pravastatin sodium
26-Apr-2021

● **INDICATIONS AND DOSE**
Adjunct to diet for primary hypercholesterolaemia or combined (mixed) hyperlipidaemias in patients who have not responded adequately to dietary control
▶ BY MOUTH
▶ Adult: 10–40 mg daily, dose to be taken at night, dose to be adjusted at intervals of at least 4 weeks

Prevention of cardiovascular events in patients with previous myocardial infarction or unstable angina | Adjunct to diet to prevent cardiovascular events in patients with hypercholesterolaemia
▶ BY MOUTH
▶ Adult: 40 mg daily, dose to be taken at night

Reduction of hyperlipidaemia in patients receiving immunosuppressive therapy following solid-organ transplantation
▶ BY MOUTH
▶ Adult: Initially 20 mg daily, then increased if necessary up to 40 mg daily, dose to be taken at night, close

medical supervision is required if dose is increased to maximum dose

DOSE ADJUSTMENTS DUE TO INTERACTIONS
▶ Manufacturer advises reduce dose by half with concurrent use of ombitasvir with paritaprevir and ritonavir.
▶ Manufacturer advises max. 20 mg daily with concurrent use of glecaprevir with pibrentasvir.
▶ Manufacturer advises max. 40 mg daily with concurrent use of sofosbuvir with velpatasvir and voxilaprevir.

● INTERACTIONS → Appendix 1: statins

● SIDE-EFFECTS
▶ **Uncommon** Hair abnormal · scalp abnormal · urinary disorders · vision disorders
▶ **Frequency not known** Muscle weakness · musculoskeletal pain

● **BREAST FEEDING** Manufacturer advises avoid—small amount of drug present in breast milk.

● **HEPATIC IMPAIRMENT**
Dose adjustments Manufacturer advises initial dose reduction to 10 mg daily; adjust according to response.

● **RENAL IMPAIRMENT**
Dose adjustments Manufacturer advises initial dose of 10 mg once daily in moderate to severe impairment.

● **PATIENT AND CARER ADVICE** Patient counselling is advised for pravastatin tablets (muscle effects).

● **MEDICINAL FORMS** There can be variation in the licensing of different medicines containing the same drug. Forms available from special-order manufacturers include: oral suspension, oral solution
Oral tablet
▶ Pravastatin sodium (Non-proprietary)
Pravastatin sodium 10 mg Pravastatin 10mg tablets | 28 tablet PoM £1.60 DT = £1.37
Pravastatin sodium 20 mg Pravastatin 20mg tablets | 28 tablet PoM £1.68 DT = £1.39
Pravastatin sodium 40 mg Pravastatin 40mg tablets | 28 tablet PoM £2.45 DT = £1.69

F 233

Rosuvastatin
24-Mar-2025

● **INDICATIONS AND DOSE**
Primary hypercholesterolaemia (type IIa including heterozygous familial hypercholesterolaemia), mixed dyslipidaemia (type IIb), or homozygous familial hypercholesterolaemia in patients who have not responded adequately to diet and other appropriate measures
▶ BY MOUTH
▶ Adult 18-69 years: Initially 5–10 mg once daily, then increased if necessary up to 20 mg once daily, dose to be increased gradually at intervals of at least 4 weeks
▶ Adult (patients of Asian origin): Initially 5 mg once daily, then increased if necessary up to 20 mg once daily, dose to be increased gradually at intervals of at least 4 weeks.
▶ Adult 70 years and over: Initially 5 mg once daily, then increased if necessary up to 20 mg once daily, dose to be increased gradually at intervals of at least 4 weeks

continued →

Primary hypercholesterolaemia (type IIa including heterozygous familial hypercholesterolaemia), mixed dyslipidaemia (type IIb), or homozygous familial hypercholesterolaemia in patients who have not responded adequately to diet and other appropriate measures and who have risk factors for myopathy or rhabdomyolysis
▶ BY MOUTH
▶ Adult: Initially 5 mg once daily, then increased if necessary up to 20 mg once daily, dose to be increased gradually at intervals of at least 4 weeks

Severe primary hypercholesterolaemia (type IIa including heterozygous familial hypercholesterolaemia), mixed dyslipidaemia (type IIb), or homozygous familial hypercholesterolaemia in patients with high cardiovascular risk who have not responded adequately to diet and other appropriate measures (specialist use only)
▶ BY MOUTH
▶ Adult 18-69 years: Initially 5–10 mg once daily, then increased if necessary up to 40 mg once daily, dose to be increased gradually at intervals of at least 4 weeks
▶ Adult (patients of Asian origin): Initially 5 mg once daily, then increased if necessary up to 20 mg once daily, dose to be increased gradually at intervals of at least 4 weeks.
▶ Adult 70 years and over: Initially 5 mg once daily, then increased if necessary up to 40 mg once daily, dose to be increased gradually at intervals of at least 4 weeks

Severe primary hypercholesterolaemia (type IIa including heterozygous familial hypercholesterolaemia), mixed dyslipidaemia (type IIb), or homozygous familial hypercholesterolaemia in patients with high cardiovascular risk who have not responded adequately to diet and other appropriate measures, and who have risk factors for myopathy or rhabdomyolysis (specialist use only)
▶ BY MOUTH
▶ Adult: Initially 5 mg once daily, then increased if necessary up to 20 mg once daily, dose to be increased gradually at intervals of at least 4 weeks

Prevention of cardiovascular events in patients at high risk of a first cardiovascular event
▶ BY MOUTH
▶ Adult 18-69 years: 20 mg once daily
▶ Adult (patients of Asian origin): Initially 5 mg once daily, then increased if tolerated to 20 mg once daily, dose to be increased gradually at intervals of at least 4 weeks.
▶ Adult 70 years and over: Initially 5 mg once daily, then increased if tolerated to 20 mg once daily, dose to be increased gradually at intervals of at least 4 weeks

Prevention of cardiovascular events in patients at high risk of a first cardiovascular event and with risk factors for myopathy or rhabdomyolysis
▶ BY MOUTH
▶ Adult: Initially 5 mg once daily, then increased if tolerated to 20 mg once daily, dose to be increased gradually at intervals of at least 4 weeks

DOSE ADJUSTMENTS DUE TO INTERACTIONS
▶ [EvGr] Initially 5 mg daily with concurrent use of bezafibrate, ciprofibrate, and fenofibrate—40 mg dose is contra-indicated.
▶ Initially 5 mg daily with concurrent use of gemfibrozil—max. dose 20 mg daily.
▶ Initially 5 mg daily with concurrent use of clopidogrel; for max. daily dose—consult product literature.
▶ Initially 5 mg daily with concurrent use of elbasvir with grazoprevir—max. dose 10 mg daily.
▶ Initially 5 mg daily with concurrent use of sofosbuvir with velpatasvir—max. dose 10 mg daily.

▶ Initially 5 mg daily, or reduce dose by half with concurrent use of teriflunomide.
▶ Max. dose 5 mg daily with concurrent use of glecaprevir with pibrentasvir.
▶ Initially 5 mg daily with concurrent use of regorafenib; for max. daily dose—consult product literature.
▶ Initially 5 mg daily with concurrent use of atazanavir boosted with ritonavir—max. dose 10 mg daily.
▶ Initially 5 mg daily with concurrent use of lopinavir boosted with ritonavir; for max. daily dose—consult product literature.
▶ Max. dose 10 mg daily with concurrent use of atazanavir boosted with cobicistat.
▶ Max. dose 10 mg daily with concurrent use of leflunomide.
▶ Initially 5 mg daily with concurrent use of darolutamide; for max. daily dose—consult product literature.
▶ Initially 5 mg daily with concurrent use of fostamatinib; for max. daily dose—consult product literature.
▶ Initially 5 mg daily with concurrent use of febuxostat; for max. daily dose—consult product literature. ⓜ

● INTERACTIONS → Appendix 1: statins
● SIDE-EFFECTS
▶ **Rare or very rare** Gynaecomastia · haematuria · polyneuropathy
▶ **Frequency not known** Cough · dyspnoea · oedema · proteinuria · severe cutaneous adverse reactions (SCARs)
● BREAST FEEDING Manufacturer advises avoid—no information available.
● RENAL IMPAIRMENT [EvGr] Avoid if creatinine clearance less than 30 mL/minute. ⓜ
  Dose adjustments See p. 21.
    [EvGr] Initially 5 mg once daily (avoid 40 mg daily) if creatinine clearance 30–60 mL/minute. ⓜ
● MONITORING REQUIREMENTS Manufacturer advises consider routine monitoring of renal function when using 40 mg daily dose.
● DIRECTIONS FOR ADMINISTRATION Capsules may be swallowed whole. Alternatively, capsules may be opened and the contents mixed into 1 teaspoonful of soft food (e.g. apple sauce) and swallowed within 1 hour without chewing, followed with a glass of water.
● PATIENT AND CARER ADVICE Patient counselling is advised for rosuvastatin tablets/capsules (muscle effects).

● MEDICINAL FORMS There can be variation in the licensing of different medicines containing the same drug. Forms available from special-order manufacturers include: oral suspension
Oral tablet
▶ Rosuvastatin (Non-proprietary)
  Rosuvastatin (as Rosuvastatin calcium) 5 mg Rosuvastatin 5mg tablets | 28 tablet [PoM] £21.64 DT = £0.76 | 250 tablet [PoM] £6.43
  Rosuvastatin (as Rosuvastatin calcium) 10 mg Rosuvastatin 10mg tablets | 28 tablet [PoM] £21.64 DT = £0.88 | 250 tablet [PoM] £8.04
  Rosuvastatin (as Rosuvastatin calcium) 15 mg Rosuvastatin 15mg tablets | 28 tablet [PoM] £3.47-£5.56 DT = £3.47
  Rosuvastatin (as Rosuvastatin calcium) 20 mg Rosuvastatin 20mg tablets | 28 tablet [PoM] £31.22 DT = £1.15 | 250 tablet [PoM] £6.99-£8.74
  Rosuvastatin (as Rosuvastatin calcium) 30 mg Rosuvastatin 30mg tablets | 28 tablet [PoM] £4.47-£7.16 DT = £4.47
  Rosuvastatin (as Rosuvastatin calcium) 40 mg Rosuvastatin 40mg tablets | 28 tablet [PoM] £35.63 DT = £1.55
▶ Crestor (AstraZeneca UK Ltd)
  Rosuvastatin (as Rosuvastatin calcium) 5 mg Crestor 5mg tablets | 28 tablet [PoM] £18.03 DT = £0.76
  Rosuvastatin (as Rosuvastatin calcium) 10 mg Crestor 10mg tablets | 28 tablet [PoM] £18.03 DT = £0.88
  Rosuvastatin (as Rosuvastatin calcium) 20 mg Crestor 20mg tablets | 28 tablet [PoM] £26.02 DT = £1.15

Rosuvastatin (as Rosuvastatin calcium) **40 mg** Crestor 40mg tablets | 28 tablet [PoM] £29.69 DT = £1.55

Oral capsule

▸ **Rosuvastatin (Non-proprietary)**
Rosuvastatin (as Rosuvastatin calcium) **5 mg** Rosuvastatin 5mg capsules | 28 capsule [PoM] £15.34 DT = £8.52
Rosuvastatin (as Rosuvastatin calcium) **10 mg** Rosuvastatin 10mg capsules | 28 capsule [PoM] £17.18 DT = £9.54
Rosuvastatin (as Rosuvastatin calcium) **20 mg** Rosuvastatin 20mg capsules | 28 capsule [PoM] £22.90 DT = £12.72
Rosuvastatin (as Rosuvastatin calcium) **40 mg** Rosuvastatin 40mg capsules | 28 capsule [PoM] £27.22 DT = £15.12

⚑ 233

Simvastatin
20-Jul-2021

● **INDICATIONS AND DOSE**

Primary hypercholesterolaemia, or combined (mixed) hyperlipidaemia in patients who have not responded adequately to diet and other appropriate measures
▸ BY MOUTH
▸ Adult: 10–20 mg once daily, dose to be taken at night, then increased if necessary up to 80 mg once daily, dose to be taken at night, adjusted at intervals of at least 4 weeks; 80 mg dose only for those with severe hypercholesterolaemia and at high risk of cardiovascular complications

Homozygous familial hypercholesterolaemia in patients who have not responded adequately to diet and other appropriate measures
▸ BY MOUTH
▸ Adult: Initially 40 mg once daily, dose to be taken at night, then increased if necessary up to 80 mg once daily, dose to be taken at night, adjusted at intervals of at least 4 weeks; 80 mg dose only for those with severe hypercholesterolaemia and at high risk of cardiovascular complications

Prevention of cardiovascular events in patients with atherosclerotic cardiovascular disease or diabetes mellitus
▸ BY MOUTH
▸ Adult: Initially 20–40 mg once daily, dose to be taken at night, then increased if necessary up to 80 mg once daily, dose to be taken at night, adjusted at intervals of at least 4 weeks; 80 mg dose only for those with severe hypercholesterolaemia and at high risk of cardiovascular complications

DOSE ADJUSTMENTS DUE TO INTERACTIONS
▸ Manufacturer advises max. 10 mg daily with concurrent use of bezafibrate or ciprofibrate.
▸ Manufacturer advises max. 20 mg daily with concurrent use of amiodarone, amlodipine, or ranolazine.
▸ Manufacturer advises reduce dose with concurrent use of some moderate inhibitors of CYP3A4 (max. 20 mg daily with verapamil and diltiazem).
▸ Manufacturer advises max. 40 mg daily with concurrent use of lomitapide or ticagrelor.
▸ Manufacturer advises max. 20 mg daily with concurrent use of elbasvir with grazoprevir.
▸ Manufacturer advises usual max. 20 mg daily with concurrent use of bempedoic acid or bempedoic acid with ezetimibe; max. dose 40 mg daily in patients with severe hypercholesterolaemia and at high risk of cardiovascular complications.

● **INTERACTIONS** → Appendix 1: statins

● **SIDE-EFFECTS**
▸ **Rare or very rare** Acute kidney injury · anaemia
▸ **Frequency not known** Cognitive impairment

● **BREAST FEEDING** Manufacturer advises avoid—no information available.

● **RENAL IMPAIRMENT**
Dose adjustments [EvGr] Doses above 10 mg daily should be used with caution if creatinine clearance less than 30 mL/minute, Ⓜ see p. 21.

● **PATIENT AND CARER ADVICE** Patient counselling is advised for simvastatin tablets/oral suspension (muscle effects).

● **EXCEPTIONS TO LEGAL CATEGORY** Simvastatin 10 mg tablets can be sold to the public to reduce risk of first coronary event in individuals at moderate risk of coronary heart disease (approx. 10–15 % risk of major event in 10 years), max. daily dose 10 mg and pack size of 28 tablets; treatment should form part of a programme to reduce risk of coronary heart disease.

● **MEDICINAL FORMS** There can be variation in the licensing of different medicines containing the same drug. Forms available from special-order manufacturers include: oral suspension, oral solution

Oral tablet
▸ **Simvastatin (Non-proprietary)**
Simvastatin **10 mg** Simvastatin 10mg tablets | 28 tablet [PoM] £14.42 DT = £0.62 | 500 tablet [PoM] £11.07-£13.04
Simvastatin **20 mg** Simvastatin 20mg tablets | 28 tablet [PoM] £23.75 DT = £0.84 | 500 tablet [PoM] £15.00-£16.07
Simvastatin **40 mg** Simvastatin 40mg tablets | 28 tablet [PoM] £23.75 DT = £0.84 | 500 tablet [PoM] £14.45-£15.00
Simvastatin **80 mg** Simvastatin 80mg tablets | 28 tablet [PoM] £6.00 DT = £1.76
▸ **Zocor** (Organon Pharma (UK) Ltd)
Simvastatin **10 mg** Zocor 10mg tablets | 28 tablet [PoM] £18.03 DT = £0.62
Simvastatin **20 mg** Zocor 20mg tablets | 28 tablet [PoM] £29.69 DT = £0.84
Simvastatin **40 mg** Zocor 40mg tablets | 28 tablet [PoM] £29.69 DT = £0.84

Oral suspension
EXCIPIENTS: May contain Propylene glycol
▸ **Simvastatin (Non-proprietary)**
Simvastatin **4 mg per 1 ml** Simvastatin 20mg/5ml oral suspension sugar free | 150 ml [PoM] £213.15 DT = £213.15 [SF]
Simvastatin **8 mg per 1 ml** Simvastatin 40mg/5ml oral suspension sugar free | 150 ml [PoM] £299.25 DT = £299.25 [SF]

Simvastatin with ezetimibe
10-Dec-2020

The properties listed below are those particular to the combination only. For the properties of the components please consider, simvastatin above, ezetimibe p. 229.

● **INDICATIONS AND DOSE**

Homozygous familial hypercholesterolaemia, primary hypercholesterolaemia, and mixed hyperlipidaemia in patients over 10 years stabilised on the individual components in the same proportions, or for patients not adequately controlled by statin alone
▸ BY MOUTH
▸ Adult: (consult product literature)

● **INTERACTIONS** → Appendix 1: ezetimibe · statins

● **MEDICINAL FORMS** There can be variation in the licensing of different medicines containing the same drug.
Oral tablet
▸ **Simvastatin with ezetimibe (Non-proprietary)**
Ezetimibe **10 mg**, Simvastatin **20 mg** Simvastatin 20mg / Ezetimibe 10mg tablets | 28 tablet [PoM] £33.42 DT = £33.42
Ezetimibe **10 mg**, Simvastatin **40 mg** Simvastatin 40mg / Ezetimibe 10mg tablets | 28 tablet [PoM] £38.98 DT = £38.98
Ezetimibe **10 mg**, Simvastatin **80 mg** Simvastatin 80mg / Ezetimibe 10mg tablets | 28 tablet [PoM] £41.21-£50.00 DT = £41.21
▸ **Inegy** (Organon Pharma (UK) Ltd)
Ezetimibe **10 mg**, Simvastatin **20 mg** Inegy 10mg/20mg tablets | 28 tablet [PoM] £33.42 DT = £33.42
Ezetimibe **10 mg**, Simvastatin **40 mg** Inegy 10mg/40mg tablets | 28 tablet [PoM] £38.98 DT = £38.98

Cardiovascular system

2

Ezetimibe 10 mg, Simvastatin 80 mg Inegy 10mg/80mg tablets | 28 tablet [PoM] £41.21 DT = £41.21

LIPID MODIFYING DRUGS > OTHER

Alirocumab

07-May-2021

- **DRUG ACTION** Alirocumab binds to a pro-protein involved in the regulation of LDL receptors on liver cells; receptor numbers are increased, which results in increased uptake of LDL-cholesterol from the blood.

- **INDICATIONS AND DOSE**

Primary hypercholesterolaemia or mixed dyslipidaemia in patients who have not responded adequately to other appropriate measures [in combination with a statin, or with a statin and other lipid-lowering therapies, or with other lipid-lowering therapies or alone if a statin contra-indicated or not tolerated] | Established atherosclerotic cardiovascular disease [in combination with the maximum tolerated dose of a statin with or without other lipid-lowering therapies, or with other lipid-lowering therapies or alone if a statin contra-indicated or not tolerated]

- BY SUBCUTANEOUS INJECTION
- Adult: Initially 75 mg every 2 weeks; increased if necessary to 150 mg every 2 weeks, alternatively 300 mg every 4 weeks, patients requiring an LDL-C reduction of greater than 60% may be initiated on 150 mg every 2 weeks or 300 mg every 4 weeks, dose adjustments should be made at 4 to 8 weekly intervals

- **SIDE-EFFECTS**
- **Common or very common** Nasal complaints · oropharyngeal pain · pulmonary reaction · skin reactions
- **Rare or very rare** Hypersensitivity · hypersensitivity vasculitis
- **Frequency not known** Angioedema · influenza like illness
- **PREGNANCY** Manufacturer advises avoid unless clinical condition requires treatment—maternal toxicity in *animal* studies.

- **BREAST FEEDING** Manufacturer advises avoid—no information available.

- **HEPATIC IMPAIRMENT** Manufacturer advises use with caution in severe impairment—no information available.

- **RENAL IMPAIRMENT** Manufacturer advises use with caution in severe impairment—limited information available.

- **HANDLING AND STORAGE** Manufacturer advises store in a refrigerator (2–8 °C)—consult product literature for further information regarding storage outside refrigerator.

- **NATIONAL FUNDING/ACCESS DECISIONS**
  For full details see funding body website
  NICE decisions
- Alirocumab for treating primary hypercholesterolaemia and mixed dyslipidaemia (June 2016) NICE TA393 Recommended with restrictions

  Scottish Medicines Consortium (SMC) decisions
- Alirocumab (*Praluent*®) for primary hypercholesterolaemia or mixed dyslipidaemia, as an adjunct to diet: in combination with a statin or statin with other lipid lowering therapies in patients unable to reach LDL-C goals with the maximum tolerated dose of a statin, or alone or in combination with other lipid-lowering therapies in patients who are statin-intolerant, or for whom a statin is contra-indicated (August 2016) SMC No. 1147/16 Recommended with restrictions

- **MEDICINAL FORMS** There can be variation in the licensing of different medicines containing the same drug.
  Solution for injection
  EXCIPIENTS: May contain Polysorbates
  - **Praluent** (Sanofi)
    Alirocumab 75 mg per 1 ml Praluent 75mg/1ml solution for injection pre-filled pens | 1 pre-filled disposable injection [PoM] £168.00 | 2 pre-filled disposable injection [PoM] £336.00 DT = £336.00
    Alirocumab 150 mg per 1 ml Praluent 150mg/1ml solution for injection pre-filled pens | 1 pre-filled disposable injection [PoM] £168.00 | 2 pre-filled disposable injection [PoM] £336.00 DT = £336.00 Praluent 300mg/2ml solution for injection pre-filled pens | 1 pre-filled disposable injection [PoM] £336.00 DT = £336.00

Bempedoic acid

03-Mar-2025

- **DRUG ACTION** Bempedoic acid is an adenosine triphosphate citrate lyase (ACL) inhibitor which inhibits cholesterol synthesis in the liver, thereby lowering LDL-cholesterol.

- **INDICATIONS AND DOSE**

Primary hypercholesterolaemia or mixed dyslipidaemia in patients who have not responded adequately to other appropriate measures [in combination with a statin, or with a statin and other lipid-lowering therapies, or with other lipid-lowering therapies or alone if a statin contra-indicated or not tolerated] | Established or at high-risk of atherosclerotic cardiovascular disease [in combination with the maximum tolerated dose of a statin with or without ezetimibe, or with ezetimibe or alone if a statin contra-indicated or not tolerated]

- BY MOUTH
- Adult: 180 mg once daily

- **INTERACTIONS** → Appendix 1: bempedoic acid
- **SIDE-EFFECTS**
- **Common or very common** Anaemia · gout · hyperuricaemia · pain in extremity
- **Frequency not known** Diarrhoea · muscle spasms · nausea

  SIDE-EFFECTS, FURTHER INFORMATION **Hepatic enzyme changes** Manufacturer advises discontinue treatment if transaminase levels at least 3 times the upper limit of normal, and persist.

  Hyperuricaemia Manufacturer advises discontinue treatment if hyperuricaemia accompanied with symptoms of gout occur.

- **PREGNANCY** Manufacturer advises avoid—toxicity in *animal* studies.

- **BREAST FEEDING** Manufacturer advises avoid—no information available.

- **NATIONAL FUNDING/ACCESS DECISIONS**
  For full details see funding body website
  NICE decisions
- Bempedoic acid with ezetimibe for treating primary hypercholesterolaemia or mixed dyslipidaemia (April 2021) NICE TA694 Recommended with restrictions

  Scottish Medicines Consortium (SMC) decisions
- Bempedoic acid (*Nilemdo*®) in adults with primary hypercholesterolaemia or mixed dyslipidaemia, as an adjunct to diet: in combination with a statin or statin with other lipid-lowering therapies; or alone or in combination with other lipid-lowering therapies in patients who are statin-intolerant, or for whom a statin is contra-indicated (July 2021) SMC No. SMC2363 Recommended with restrictions

- **MEDICINAL FORMS** There can be variation in the licensing of different medicines containing the same drug.
  Oral tablet
  - **Nilemdo** (Daiichi Sankyo UK Ltd)
    Bempedoic acid 180 mg Nilemdo 180mg tablets | 28 tablet [PoM] £55.44 DT = £55.44

Bempedoic acid with ezetimibe   07-Nov-2021

The properties listed below are those particular to the combination only. For the properties of the components please consider, bempedoic acid p. 238, ezetimibe p. 229.

- **INDICATIONS AND DOSE**
  Primary hypercholesterolaemia or mixed dyslipidaemia in patients who have not responded adequately to other appropriate measures [in combination with a statin, or alone if a statin is contra-indicated or not tolerated] | Primary hypercholesterolaemia or mixed dyslipidaemia in patients already taking bempedoic acid and ezetimibe as separate tablets with or without statin
  ▸ BY MOUTH
  ▸ Adult: 180/10 mg daily
  DOSE EQUIVALENCE AND CONVERSION
  ▸ Dose expressed as x/y mg bempedoic acid/ezetimibe.

- **INTERACTIONS** → Appendix 1: bempedoic acid · ezetimibe
- **NATIONAL FUNDING/ACCESS DECISIONS**
  For full details see funding body website
  NICE decisions
  ▸ Bempedoic acid with ezetimibe for treating primary hypercholesterolaemia or mixed dyslipidaemia (April 2021) NICE TA694 Recommended with restrictions
  Scottish Medicines Consortium (SMC) decisions
  ▸ Bempedoic acid with ezetimibe (*Nustendi*®) for use in adults with primary hypercholesterolaemia (heterozygous familial and non-familial) or mixed dyslipidaemia (October 2021) SMC No. SMC2406 Recommended with restrictions

- **MEDICINAL FORMS** There can be variation in the licensing of different medicines containing the same drug.
  Oral tablet
  ▸ Nustendi (Daiichi Sankyo UK Ltd)
    Ezetimibe 10 mg, Bempedoic acid 180 mg Nustendi 180mg/10mg tablets | 28 tablet PoM £55.44 DT = £55.44

Evinacumab   21-Feb-2025

- **DRUG ACTION** Evinacumab is a recombinant human monoclonal antibody that binds to and blocks the angiopoeitin-like 3 protein (ANGPTL3) to prevent its inhibition of lipoprotein and endothelial lipase, thereby lowering triglycerides and cholesterol.

- **INDICATIONS AND DOSE**
  Homozygous familial hypercholesterolaemia (under expert supervision)
  ▸ BY INTRAVENOUS INFUSION
  ▸ Adult: 15 mg/kg every 4 weeks

- **SIDE-EFFECTS**
- **Common or very common** Abdominal pain · asthenia · constipation · dizziness · increased risk of infection · influenza like illness · infusion related reaction · nausea · pain · rhinorrhoea
- **Uncommon** Hypersensitivity

- **CONCEPTION AND CONTRACEPTION** EvGr Females of childbearing potential should use effective contraception during treatment and for at least 5 months after last treatment. M

- **PREGNANCY** EvGr Avoid unless potential benefit outweighs risk (toxicity in *animal* studies). M

- **BREAST FEEDING** Specialist sources indicate use with caution, especially if breast-feeding a neonate or pre-term infant (no information available). Large molecular weight suggests limited excretion into milk and drug molecule likely to be partially destroyed in the infant's gastro-intestinal tract.

- **DIRECTIONS FOR ADMINISTRATION** For *intravenous infusion* (*Evkeeza*®), dilute requisite dose in Glucose 5% or Sodium Chloride 0.9% to a final concentration of 0.5–20 mg/mL (gently invert, do not shake); give over 60 minutes through an in-line or add-on filter (0.2–5 micron).

- **PRESCRIBING AND DISPENSING INFORMATION** Evinacumab is a biological medicine. Biological medicines must be prescribed and dispensed by brand name, see *Biological medicines* and *Biosimilar medicines*, under Guidance on prescribing p. 1; record the brand name and batch number after each administration.

- **HANDLING AND STORAGE** Store in a refrigerator (2–8°C) and protect from light—consult product literature about storage after dilution.

- **NATIONAL FUNDING/ACCESS DECISIONS**
  For full details see funding body website
  NICE decisions
  ▸ Evinacumab for treating homozygous familial hypercholesterolaemia in people 12 years and over (September 2024) NICE TA1002 Recommended

- **MEDICINAL FORMS** There can be variation in the licensing of different medicines containing the same drug.
  Solution for infusion
  EXCIPIENTS: May contain Polysorbates
  ▸ **Evkeeza** (Ultragenyx UK Ltd) ▼
    Evinacumab 150 mg per 1 ml Evkeeza 345mg/2.3ml concentrate for solution for infusion vials | 1 vial PoM £6,432.75 (Hospital only)

Evolocumab   14-Oct-2021

- **DRUG ACTION** Evolocumab binds to a pro-protein involved in the regulation of LDL receptors on liver cells; receptor numbers are increased, which results in increased uptake of LDL-cholesterol from the blood.

- **INDICATIONS AND DOSE**
  Primary hypercholesterolaemia or mixed dyslipidaemia in patients who have not responded adequately to other appropriate measures (in combination with a statin, or with a statin and other lipid-lowering therapies, or with other lipid-lowering therapies or alone if a statin contra-indicated or not tolerated) | Established atherosclerotic cardiovascular disease (in combination with the maximum tolerated dose of a statin with or without other lipid-lowering therapies, or with other lipid-lowering therapies or alone if a statin contra-indicated or not tolerated)
  ▸ BY SUBCUTANEOUS INJECTION
  ▸ Adult: 140 mg every 2 weeks, alternatively 420 mg every month, to be administered into the thigh, abdomen or upper arm
  Homozygous familial hypercholesterolaemia (in combination with other lipid-lowering therapies)
  ▸ BY SUBCUTANEOUS INJECTION
  ▸ Adult: Initially 420 mg every month; increased if necessary to 420 mg every 2 weeks, if inadequate response after 12 weeks of treatment, to be administered into the thigh, abdomen or upper arm
  Homozygous familial hypercholesterolaemia in patients on apheresis (in combination with other lipid-lowering therapies)
  ▸ BY SUBCUTANEOUS INJECTION
  ▸ Adult: 420 mg every 2 weeks, to correspond with apheresis schedule, to be administered into the thigh, abdomen or upper arm

- **SIDE-EFFECTS**
- **Common or very common** Arthralgia · back pain · hypersensitivity · increased risk of infection · nausea · skin reactions
- **Uncommon** Influenza like illness

▶ **Rare or very rare** Angioedema

● PREGNANCY Manufacturer advises avoid unless essential—limited information available.

● BREAST FEEDING Manufacturer advises avoid—no information available.

● HEPATIC IMPAIRMENT Manufacturer advises caution in moderate to severe impairment (risk of reduced efficacy; no information available in severe impairment).

● HANDLING AND STORAGE Manufacturer advises store in a refrigerator (2–8°C)—consult product literature for further information regarding storage outside refrigerator.

● PATIENT AND CARER ADVICE Patients and their carers should be given training in subcutaneous injection technique.

● NATIONAL FUNDING/ACCESS DECISIONS
For full details see funding body website
NICE decisions
▶ Evolocumab for treating primary hypercholesterolaemia and mixed dyslipidaemia (June 2016) NICE TA394 Recommended with restrictions

Scottish Medicines Consortium (SMC) decisions
▶ Evolocumab (*Repatha®*) for use in adults with primary hypercholesterolaemia (heterozygous familial hypercholesterolaemia and non-familial) or mixed dyslipidaemia (February 2017) SMC No. 1148/16 Recommended with restrictions

● MEDICINAL FORMS There can be variation in the licensing of different medicines containing the same drug.
Solution for injection
▶ Repatha SureClick (Amgen Ltd)
Evolocumab 140 mg per 1 ml Repatha SureClick 140mg/1ml solution for injection pre-filled pens | 2 pre-filled disposable injection PoM £340.20 DT = £340.20

Icosapent ethyl
21-Aug-2023

● **INDICATIONS AND DOSE**

Adjunct to statin in prevention of cardiovascular events in hyperlipidaemia [in patients with triglycerides ≥ 150 mg/dL (≥ 1.7 mmol/L) and either established cardiovascular disease, or diabetes with at least 1 other cardiovascular risk factor]
▶ BY MOUTH
▶ Adult: 1.996 g twice daily

● CAUTIONS Antithrombotic treatment (bleeding time increased) · history of atrial fibrillation or flutter

● INTERACTIONS → Appendix 1: eicosapentaenoic acid

● SIDE-EFFECTS
▶ **Common or very common** Arrhythmias · burping · constipation · gout · haemorrhage · pain · peripheral oedema · skin reactions
▶ **Uncommon** Taste altered
▶ **Frequency not known** Abdominal discomfort · arthralgia · diarrhoea · throat swelling

● ALLERGY AND CROSS-SENSITIVITY EvGr Caution in patients with known hypersensitivity to fish and/or shellfish (obtained from fish oil). Avoid in patients with hypersensitivity to soya or peanuts (contains soya lecithin). M

● PREGNANCY EvGr Avoid unless potential benefit outweighs risk—limited information available. M

● BREAST FEEDING EvGr Avoid—present in milk in *animal* studies. M

● PRESCRIBING AND DISPENSING INFORMATION Icosapent ethyl is an ethyl ester of the omega-3 fatty acid, eicosapentaenoic acid.

● NATIONAL FUNDING/ACCESS DECISIONS
For full details see funding body website
NICE decisions
▶ Icosapent ethyl with statin therapy for reducing the risk of cardiovascular events in people with raised triglycerides (July 2022) NICE TA805 Recommended with restrictions

Scottish Medicines Consortium (SMC) decisions
▶ Icosapent ethyl (*Vazkepa®*) to reduce the risk of cardiovascular events in adult statin-treated patients at high cardiovascular risk with elevated triglycerides (150 mg/dL or more [1.7 mmol/L or more]) and established cardiovascular disease, or diabetes, and at least one other cardiovascular risk factor (August 2023) SMC No. SMC2602 Recommended with restrictions

● MEDICINAL FORMS There can be variation in the licensing of different medicines containing the same drug.
Oral capsule
CAUTIONARY AND ADVISORY LABELS 21
EXCIPIENTS: May contain Gelatin, sorbitol
▶ Vazkepa (Amarin Pharmaceuticals Ireland Ltd) ▼
Icosapent ethyl 998 mg Vazkepa 998mg capsules | 120 capsule PoM £144.21 DT = £144.21

Inclisiran
12-Apr-2022

● DRUG ACTION Inclisiran is a small interfering RNA which limits production of PCSK9, increasing uptake of LDL-cholesterol and thereby lowering levels in blood.

● **INDICATIONS AND DOSE**

Primary hypercholesterolaemia or mixed dyslipidaemia [in combination with a statin, or with a statin and other lipid-lowering therapies, or with other lipid-lowering therapies or alone if a statin contra-indicated or not tolerated]
▶ BY SUBCUTANEOUS INJECTION
▶ Adult: Initially 284 mg for 1 dose, followed by 284 mg after 3 months for 1 dose, then 284 mg every 6 months

● PREGNANCY EvGr Avoid—no information available. M
● BREAST FEEDING EvGr Avoid—no information available. M
● HEPATIC IMPAIRMENT EvGr Caution in severe impairment—no information available. M
● RENAL IMPAIRMENT EvGr Caution in severe impairment—no information available. M
● DIRECTIONS FOR ADMINISTRATION EvGr Inject into the abdomen; alternatively inject into the thigh or upper arm. M

● PATIENT AND CARER ADVICE
Missed doses EvGr If a dose is more than 3 months late, treatment should be re-initiated. M

● NATIONAL FUNDING/ACCESS DECISIONS
For full details see funding body website
NICE decisions
▶ Inclisiran for treating primary hypercholesterolaemia or mixed dyslipidaemia (October 2021) NICE TA733 Recommended with restrictions

Scottish Medicines Consortium (SMC) decisions
▶ Inclisiran (*Leqvio®*) in adults with primary hypercholesterolaemia or mixed dyslipidaemia, as an adjunct to diet: in combination with a statin or statin with other lipid-lowering therapies; or alone or in combination with other lipid-lowering therapies in patients who are statin-intolerant, or for whom a statin is contra-indicated (August 2021) SMC No. SMC2358 Recommended with restrictions

All Wales Medicines Strategy Group (AWMSG) decisions
▶ Inclisiran (*Leqvio®*) in adults with primary hypercholesterolaemia or mixed dyslipidaemia, as an adjunct to diet: in combination with a statin or statin with other lipid-

lowering therapies; or alone or in combination with other lipid-lowering therapies in patients who are statin-intolerant, or for whom a statin is contra-indicated (February 2022) AWMSG No. 3746 Recommended with restrictions

● **MEDICINAL FORMS** There can be variation in the licensing of different medicines containing the same drug.
Solution for injection
▸ **Leqvio** (Novartis Pharmaceuticals UK Ltd) ▼
   Inclisiran (as Inclisiran sodium) 189 mg per 1 ml Leqvio 284mg/1.5ml solution for injection pre-filled syringes | 1 pre-filled disposable injection PoM £1,987.36 DT = £60.00

Lomitapide
07-May-2021

● **DRUG ACTION** Lomitapide, an inhibitor of microsomal triglyceride transfer protein (MTP), reduces lipoprotein secretion and circulating concentrations of lipoprotein-borne lipids such as cholesterol and triglycerides.

● **INDICATIONS AND DOSE**

Adjunct to dietary measures and other lipid-regulating drugs with or without low-density lipoprotein apheresis in homozygous familial hypercholesterolaemia (under expert supervision)
▸ BY MOUTH
▸ Adult: Initially 5 mg daily for 2 weeks, dose to be taken at least 2 hours after evening meal, then increased if necessary to 10 mg daily, for at least 4 weeks, then increased to 20 mg daily for at least 4 weeks, then increased in steps of 20 mg daily, adjusted at intervals of at least 4 weeks; maximum 60 mg per day

● **CONTRA-INDICATIONS** Significant or chronic bowel disease

● **CAUTIONS** Concomitant use of hepatotoxic drugs · lomitapide can interfere with the absorption of fat-soluble nutrients and supplementation of vitamin E and fatty acids is required · patients over 65 years

● **INTERACTIONS** → Appendix 1: lomitapide

● **SIDE-EFFECTS**
▸ **Common or very common** Aerophagia · appetite abnormal · asthenia · burping · constipation · diarrhoea · dizziness · gastrointestinal discomfort · gastrointestinal disorders · haemorrhage · headaches · hepatic disorders · increased risk of infection · muscle complaints · nausea · skin reactions · vomiting · weight decreased
▸ **Uncommon** Anaemia · chest pain · chills · dehydration · drowsiness · dry mouth · eye swelling · fever · gait abnormal · hyperhidrosis · joint disorders · malaise · pain in extremity · paraesthesia · throat lesion · upper-airway cough syndrome · vertigo
▸ **Frequency not known** Alopecia
   SIDE-EFFECTS, FURTHER INFORMATION Reduce dose if serum transaminases raised during treatment (consult product literature).

● **CONCEPTION AND CONTRACEPTION** Manufacturer advises exclude pregnancy before treatment and ensure effective contraception used.

● **PREGNANCY** Avoid—teratogenicity and embryotoxicity in *animal* studies.

● **BREAST FEEDING** Manufacturer advises avoid—no information available.

● **HEPATIC IMPAIRMENT** Manufacturer advises avoid in moderate to severe impairment, or if unexplained persistent abnormal liver function tests.
   Dose adjustments Manufacturer advises max. 40 mg daily in mild impairment.

● **RENAL IMPAIRMENT**
   Dose adjustments EvGr Max. 40 mg daily in end-stage renal disease. ⟨M⟩

● **MONITORING REQUIREMENTS**
▸ Monitor liver function tests before treatment, then at least monthly and before each dose increase for first year, then at least every 3 months and before each dose increase thereafter.
▸ Screen for hepatic steatosis and fibrosis before treatment, then annually thereafter.

● **MEDICINAL FORMS** There can be variation in the licensing of different medicines containing the same drug.
Oral capsule
▸ **Lojuxta** (Chiesi Ltd) ▼
   Lomitapide (as Lomitapide mesylate) 5 mg Lojuxta 5mg capsules | 28 capsule PoM £17,765.00 (Hospital only)
   Lomitapide (as Lomitapide mesylate) 10 mg Lojuxta 10mg capsules | 28 capsule PoM £17,765.00 (Hospital only)
   Lomitapide (as Lomitapide mesylate) 20 mg Lojuxta 20mg capsules | 28 capsule PoM £17,765.00 (Hospital only)

Omega-3-acid ethyl esters
26-Feb-2024

● **INDICATIONS AND DOSE**

Adjunct to diet and statin in type IIb or III hypertriglyceridaemia | Adjunct to diet in type IV hypertriglyceridaemia
▸ BY MOUTH
▸ Adult: Initially 2 capsules daily, dose to be taken with food, increased if necessary to 4 capsules daily

---

IMPORTANT SAFETY INFORMATION

MHRA/CHM ADVICE: OMEGA-3-ACID ETHYL ESTER MEDICINES (*OMACOR*®/ *TEROMEG*® 1000 MG CAPSULES): DOSE-DEPENDENT INCREASED RISK OF ATRIAL FIBRILLATION IN PATIENTS WITH ESTABLISHED CARDIOVASCULAR DISEASES OR CARDIOVASCULAR RISK FACTORS (JANUARY 2024)

Systematic reviews and meta-analyses of clinical trials have highlighted a dose-dependent increased risk of atrial fibrillation in patients with cardiovascular diseases or risk factors taking omega-3-acid ethyl ester medicines, compared with placebo; the observed risk was found to be highest at a dose of 4 g daily. Healthcare professionals are advised that atrial fibrillation is now listed as a common side-effect of oral medicines containing omega-3-acid ethyl esters licensed for the treatment of hypertriglyceridaemia. If a patient develops atrial fibrillation during treatment, it should be permanently discontinued.

Patients and their carers should be advised to inform their healthcare professional if they have any current or previous heart problems before taking these medicines for hypertriglyceridaemia. Patients should also be advised to seek medical attention if they develop symptoms of atrial fibrillation during treatment, and to continue treatment unless advised to stop.

● **CAUTIONS** Anticoagulant treatment (bleeding time increased) · haemorrhagic disorders

● **INTERACTIONS** → Appendix 1: omega-3-acid ethyl esters

● **SIDE-EFFECTS**
▸ **Common or very common** Atrial fibrillation · burping · constipation · diarrhoea · gastrointestinal discomfort · gastrointestinal disorders · nausea · vomiting
▸ **Uncommon** Dizziness · gout · haemorrhage · headache · hyperglycaemia · hypotension · skin reactions · taste altered
▸ **Rare or very rare** Liver disorder

● **ALLERGY AND CROSS-SENSITIVITY** EvGr Use with caution in patients with known hypersensitivity to fish. Avoid in patients with hypersensitivity to soya or peanuts (contains soya lecithin). ⟨M⟩

- **PREGNANCY** Manufacturers advise use only if potential benefit outweighs risk—no information available.
- **BREAST FEEDING** Manufacturers advise avoid—no information available.
- **NATIONAL FUNDING/ACCESS DECISIONS**
  For full details see funding body website
  Scottish Medicines Consortium (SMC) decisions
  ▸ Omega-3-acid ethyl esters (*Omacor*®) for hypertriglyceridaemia (November 2002) SMC No. 16/02 Not recommended

- **MEDICINAL FORMS** There can be variation in the licensing of different medicines containing the same drug.
  Oral capsule
  CAUTIONARY AND ADVISORY LABELS 21
  ▸ **Omega-3-acid ethyl esters (Non-proprietary)**
    Eicosapentaenoic acid 60 mg, Docosahexaenoic acid 300 mg Omega-3 600mg capsules | 28 capsule 🅔
    Docosahexaenoic acid 380 mg, Eicosapentaenoic acid 460 mg Omega 3-acid-ethyl esters 1000mg capsules | 28 capsule PoM £14.24 DT = £14.24
  ▸ **Teromeg** (Advanz Pharma)
    Docosahexaenoic acid 380 mg, Eicosapentaenoic acid 460 mg Teromeg 1000mg capsules | 28 capsule PoM £11.39 DT = £14.24

Volanesorsen

11-Nov-2020

- **DRUG ACTION** Volanesorsen is an antisense oligonucleotide which inhibits the formation of the apolipoprotein apoC−III, thereby lowering serum triglycerides.

- **INDICATIONS AND DOSE**
  Familial chylomicronaemia syndrome (specialist use only)
  ▸ BY SUBCUTANEOUS INJECTION
  ▸ Adult: Initially 285 mg once weekly for 3 months, then reduced to 285 mg every 2 weeks, review and adjust dosing based on serum triglycerides—consult product literature

- **CONTRA-INDICATIONS** Chronic or unexplained thrombocytopenia (platelet count less than 140 × 10^9/litre)
- **CAUTIONS** Body-weight less than 70 kg (increased risk of thrombocytopenia)
- **INTERACTIONS** → Appendix 1: volanesorsen
- **SIDE-EFFECTS**
  ▸ **Common or very common** Arthritis · asthenia · chills · cough · diabetes mellitus · diarrhoea · dizziness · dry mouth · dyspnoea · eosinophilia · facial swelling · feeling hot · fever · gastrointestinal discomfort · haemorrhage · headaches · hot flush · hypersensitivity · hypertension · immunisation reaction · influenza like illness · insomnia · joint disorders · leucopenia · malaise · muscle complaints · myositis · nasal congestion · nausea · numbness · oedema · oral disorders · pain · polymyalgia rheumatica · proteinuria · skin reactions · sweat changes · syncope · throat oedema · thrombocytopenia · tremor · vision blurred · vomiting · wheezing
  ▸ **Frequency not known** Nephrotoxicity
- **PREGNANCY** Manufacturer advises avoid—limited information; *animal* studies do not indicate toxicity.
- **BREAST FEEDING** Manufacturer advises avoid—present in very low levels in milk in *animal* studies.
- **MONITORING REQUIREMENTS**
  ▸ Manufacturer advises monitor platelet count before treatment and then at least every 2 weeks during treatment.

▸ Manufacturer advises monitor liver function, erythrocyte sedimentation rate, and urine dipstick every 3 months during treatment.
- **DIRECTIONS FOR ADMINISTRATION** Manufacturer advises administer injection into the upper thigh or abdomen, or upper arm (if not self-administered). Patients may self-administer *Waylivra*® after appropriate training in subcutaneous injection technique.
- **HANDLING AND STORAGE** Manufacturer advises store in a refrigerator (2°C–8°C) and protect from light—consult product literature about storage outside refrigerator.
- **PATIENT AND CARER ADVICE** Manufacturer advises patients should immediately report any signs of bleeding, neck stiffness, or atypical severe headache.
  Missed doses Manufacturer advises if a dose is more than 48 hours late, the missed dose should be omitted and the next dose given at the normal time.
- **NATIONAL FUNDING/ACCESS DECISIONS**
  For full details see funding body website
  NICE decisions
  ▸ Volanesorsen for treating familial chylomicronaemia syndrome (October 2020) NICE HST13 Recommended

- **MEDICINAL FORMS** There can be variation in the licensing of different medicines containing the same drug.
  Solution for injection
  ▸ **Waylivra** (Swedish Orphan Biovitrum Ltd) ▼
    Volanesorsen (as Volanesorsen sodium) 190 mg per 1 ml Waylivra 285mg/1.5ml solution for injection pre-filled syringes | 1 pre-filled disposable injection PoM £11,394.00 (Hospital only)

9 Myocardial ischaemia

Stable angina

10-Aug-2022

Description of condition

Stable angina is characterised by predictable chest pain or pressure, often precipitated by physical exertion or emotional stress causing an increase in myocardial oxygen demand. Although pain typically occurs in the front of the chest, it may also radiate to the neck, shoulders, jaw or arms; the pain is relieved with rest. Stable angina usually results from atherosclerotic plaques in the coronary arteries that restrict blood flow and oxygen supply to the heart; it can lead to cardiovascular complications such as stroke, unstable angina, myocardial infarction, and sudden cardiac death. For information about *unstable angina* and *myocardial infarction*, see Acute coronary syndromes p. 247.

Prinzmetal's or vasospastic angina is a rare form of angina caused by narrowing or occlusion of proximal coronary arteries due to spasm, in which pain is experienced at rest rather than during activity.

Aims of treatment

Antianginal drug therapy and revascularisation aims to prevent or minimise angina symptoms, in order to improve quality of life and long-term morbidity and mortality. The aim of drug therapy for secondary prevention is to minimise the risk of cardiovascular events such as myocardial infarction and stroke.

Drug treatment

Antianginal drug therapy

EvGr Acute attacks of stable angina should be managed with sublingual glyceryl trinitrate p. 252, which can also be used as a preventative measure immediately before performing activities that are known to bring on an attack.

For long-term prevention of chest pain in patients with stable angina, a beta-blocker (such as atenolol p. 180, bisoprolol fumarate p. 180, metoprolol tartrate p. 182 or propranolol hydrochloride p. 178) should be given as first-line therapy. A rate-limiting calcium-channel blocker (such as verapamil hydrochloride p. 191 or diltiazem hydrochloride p. 185) should be considered as an alternative if beta-blockers are contra-indicated, for example in patients with Prinzmetal's angina or decompensated heart failure. Dihydropyridine derivative calcium-channel blockers (such as amlodipine p. 184) may be effective in patients with Prinzmetal's angina.

If a beta-blocker alone fails to control symptoms adequately, a combination of a beta-blocker and a calcium-channel blocker should be considered. If this combination is not appropriate due to intolerance of, or contra-indication to, either beta-blockers or calcium-channel blockers, NICE CG126 recommends to consider addition of either a long-acting nitrate, ivabradine p. 245, nicorandil p. 246, or ranolazine p. 245.

A long-acting nitrate, ivabradine p. 245, nicorandil p. 246, or ranolazine p. 245, should also be considered as monotherapy in patients who cannot tolerate beta-blockers and calcium-channel blockers, if both are contra-indicated, or when they both fail to adequately control angina symptoms.

Response to treatment should be assessed every 2–4 weeks following initiation or change of drug therapy; drug doses should be titrated to the maximum tolerated effective dose.

If a combination of two drugs at a maximum therapeutic dose fails to control angina symptoms, patients should be considered for referral to a specialist. Ⓐ

Secondary prevention of cardiovascular events

All patients with angina are assumed to be at high-risk for cardiovascular events. The occurrence of cardiovascular events can be prevented by management of cardiovascular risk factors through lifestyle changes (such as smoking cessation, weight management, increased physical activity), psychological support, and drug treatment.

EvGr All patients with stable angina due to atherosclerotic disease should be given long-term treatment with low-dose aspirin p. 142 and a statin. Treatment with an ACE inhibitor should also be considered, particularly if the patient has diabetes. Ⓐ See also *Secondary prevention* in Cardiovascular disease risk assessment and prevention p. 219 for further information.

Non-drug treatment

EvGr Revascularisation by coronary artery bypass graft or percutaneous coronary intervention should be considered for patients with stable angina who remain symptomatic whilst on optimal drug therapy. Ⓐ See also *Antiplatelet drugs and coronary stents* in Antiplatelet drugs p. 141.

Useful Resources

Management of stable angina. Scottish Intercollegiate Guidelines Network. A national clinical guideline 151. April 2018.
www.sign.ac.uk/our-guidelines/management-of-stable-angina/

Stable angina: management. National Institute for Health and Care Excellence. Clinical guideline 126. July 2011 (updated August 2016).
www.nice.org.uk/guidance/cg126

Other drugs used for Myocardial ischaemia Acebutolol, p. 179 · Bivalirudin, p. 159 · Carvedilol, p. 175 · Felodipine, p. 187 · Fondaparinux sodium, p. 148 · Nadolol, p. 177 · Nicardipine hydrochloride, p. 188 · Nifedipine, p. 189 · Perindopril erbumine with amlodipine, p. 199 · Pindolol, p. 177 · Timolol maleate, p. 179

ANTITHROMBOTIC DRUGS › ANTIPLATELET DRUGS

Cangrelor
07-May-2021

- **DRUG ACTION** Cangrelor is a direct $P2Y_{12}$ platelet receptor antagonist that blocks adenosine diphosphate induced platelet activation and aggregation.

- **● INDICATIONS AND DOSE**

  In combination with aspirin for the reduction of thrombotic cardiovascular events in patients with coronary artery disease undergoing percutaneous coronary intervention (PCI) who have not received an oral $P2Y_{12}$ inhibitor (e.g. clopidogrel, prasugrel, ticagrelor) prior to the PCI procedure and in whom oral therapy with a $P2Y_{12}$ inhibitor is not suitable (under expert supervision)
  - ▸ INITIALLY BY INTRAVENOUS INJECTION
  - ▸ Adult: Initially 30 micrograms/kg, to be given as a bolus dose, followed immediately by (by intravenous infusion) 4 micrograms/kg/minute, start treatment before percutaneous coronary intervention and continue infusion for at least 2 hours or for the duration of intervention if longer; maximum duration of infusion 4 hours

- **CONTRA-INDICATIONS** Active bleeding · history of stroke · history of transient ischaemic attack · patients at increased risk of bleeding (e.g. impaired haemostasis, irreversible coagulation disorders, major surgery or trauma, uncontrolled severe hypertension)

- **CAUTIONS** Disease states associated with increased bleeding risk

- **INTERACTIONS** → Appendix 1: cangrelor

- **SIDE-EFFECTS**
  - ▸ **Common or very common** Dyspnoea · haemorrhage · skin reactions
  - ▸ **Uncommon** Cardiac tamponade · haemodynamic instability · renal impairment · retroperitoneal haemorrhage (including fatal cases)
  - ▸ **Rare or very rare** Anaemia · haematoma infection · intracranial haemorrhage · menorrhagia · skin neoplasm haemorrhage · stroke · thrombocytopenia · vascular pseudoaneurysm · wound haemorrhage

- **PREGNANCY** Manufacturer advises avoid—toxicity in *animal* studies.

- **BREAST FEEDING** Manufacturer advises potential risk to infant —no information available.

- **RENAL IMPAIRMENT** Manufacturer advises caution in severe renal impairment—increased risk of bleeding.

- **DIRECTIONS FOR ADMINISTRATION** For *intravenous bolus injection* and *intravenous infusion*, manufacturer advises reconstitute each 50 mg vial with 5 mL of water for injection and gently swirl, do not shake vigorously. Withdraw 5 mL of reconstituted solution, add to 250 mL of either Sodium Chloride 0.9% *or* Glucose 5% and mix thoroughly. The bolus injection and infusion should be administered from the infusion solution.

- **MEDICINAL FORMS** There can be variation in the licensing of different medicines containing the same drug.
  Powder for solution for injection
  - ▸ **Kengrexal** (Chiesi Ltd)
    Cangrelor (as Cangrelor tetrasodium) 50 mg Kengrexal 50mg powder for concentrate for solution for injection / infusion vials | 10 vial PoM £2,500.00 (Hospital only)

Cardiovascular system

2

Cardiovascular system

ANTITHROMBOTIC DRUGS > GLYCOPROTEIN IIB/IIIA INHIBITORS

Eptifibatide

16-Sep-2021

● **INDICATIONS AND DOSE**

In combination with aspirin and unfractionated heparin for the prevention of early myocardial infarction in patients with unstable angina or non-ST-segment-elevation myocardial infarction and with last episode of chest pain within 24 hours (specialist use only)
▸ INITIALLY BY INTRAVENOUS INJECTION
▸ Adult: Initially 180 micrograms/kg, then (by intravenous infusion) 2 micrograms/kg/minute for up to 72 hours (up to 96 hours if percutaneous coronary intervention during treatment)

● **CONTRA-INDICATIONS** Abnormal bleeding within 30 days · haemorrhagic diathesis · history of haemorrhagic stroke · increased INR · increased prothrombin time · intracranial disease · major surgery or severe trauma within 6 weeks · severe hypertension · stroke within last 30 days · thrombocytopenia

● **CAUTIONS** Discontinue if emergency cardiac surgery necessary · discontinue if intra-aortic balloon pump necessary · discontinue if thrombolytic therapy necessary · risk of bleeding—discontinue immediately if uncontrolled serious bleeding

● **INTERACTIONS** → Appendix 1: eptifibatide

● **SIDE-EFFECTS**
▸ **Common or very common** Arrhythmias · atrioventricular block · cardiac arrest · congestive heart failure · haemorrhage · hypotension · intracranial haemorrhage · procedural complications · shock
▸ **Uncommon** Cerebral ischaemia · thrombocytopenia
▸ **Rare or very rare** Rash

● **PREGNANCY** Manufacturer advises use only if potential benefit outweighs risk—no information available.

● **BREAST FEEDING** Manufacturer advises avoid—no information available.

● **HEPATIC IMPAIRMENT** Manufacturer advises caution; avoid in significant impairment (increased risk of bleeding complications, limited information available).

● **RENAL IMPAIRMENT** EvGr Avoid if creatinine clearance less than 30 mL/minute. Ⓜ
Dose adjustments EvGr Initially 180 micrograms/kg, then reduce infusion to 1 microgram/kg/minute if creatinine clearance 30–50 mL/minute (increased risk of bleeding; limited information available). Ⓜ See p. 21.

● **MONITORING REQUIREMENTS**
▸ Measure baseline prothrombin time, activated partial thromboplastin time, platelet count, haemoglobin, haematocrit and serum creatinine.
▸ Monitor haemoglobin, haematocrit and platelets within 6 hours after start of treatment, then at least once daily.

● **MEDICINAL FORMS** There can be variation in the licensing of different medicines containing the same drug.
Solution for injection
▸ Eptifibatide (Non-proprietary)
Eptifibatide 2 mg per 1 ml Eptifibatide 20mg/10ml solution for injection vials | 1 vial PoM £78.95 (Hospital only)
Solution for infusion
▸ Eptifibatide (Non-proprietary)
Eptifibatide 750 microgram per 1 ml Eptifibatide 75mg/100ml solution for infusion vials | 1 vial PoM £155.95 (Hospital only)

Tirofiban

16-Sep-2021

● **INDICATIONS AND DOSE**

In combination with unfractionated heparin, aspirin, and clopidogrel for prevention of early myocardial infarction in patients with unstable angina or non-ST-segment-elevation myocardial infarction (NSTEMI) and with last episode of chest pain within 12 hours (with angiography planned for 4–48 hours after diagnosis) (initiated under specialist supervision)
▸ BY INTRAVENOUS INFUSION
▸ Adult: Initially 400 nanograms/kg/minute for 30 minutes, then 100 nanograms/kg/minute for at least 48 hours (continue during and for 12–24 hours after percutaneous coronary intervention), maximum duration of treatment 108 hours

In combination with unfractionated heparin, aspirin, and clopidogrel for prevention of early myocardial infarction in patients with unstable angina or non-ST-segment-elevation myocardial infarction (NSTEMI) and with last episode of chest pain within 12 hours (with angiography within 4 hours of diagnosis) (initiated under specialist supervision)
▸ INITIALLY BY INTRAVENOUS INJECTION
▸ Adult: 25 micrograms/kg, to be given over 3 minutes at start of percutaneous coronary intervention, then (by intravenous infusion) 150 nanograms/kg/minute for 12–24 hours, maximum duration of treatment 48 hours

In combination with unfractionated heparin, aspirin, and clopidogrel for reduction of major cardiovascular events in patients with ST-segment elevation myocardial infarction (STEMI) intended for primary percutaneous coronary intervention (PCI) (initiated under specialist supervision)
▸ INITIALLY BY INTRAVENOUS INJECTION
▸ Adult: 25 micrograms/kg, to be given over 3 minutes at start of percutaneous coronary intervention, then (by intravenous infusion) 150 nanograms/kg/minute for 12–24 hours, maximum duration of treatment 48 hours

● **CONTRA-INDICATIONS** Abnormal bleeding within 30 days · history of haemorrhagic stroke · history of intracranial disease · increased INR · increased prothrombin time · severe hypertension · stroke within 30 days · thrombocytopenia

● **CAUTIONS** Active peptic ulcer (within 3 months) · acute pericarditis · anaemia · aortic dissection · cardiogenic shock · discontinue if intra-aortic balloon pump necessary · discontinue if thrombolytic therapy necessary · discontinue immediately if serious or uncontrollable bleeding occurs · discontiue if emergency cardiac surgery necessary · elderly · faecal occult blood · haematuria · haemorrhagic retinopathy · low body-weight · major surgery within 3 months (avoid if within 6 weeks) · organ biopsy or lithotripsy within last 2 weeks · puncture of non-compressible vessel within 24 hours · risk of bleeding · severe heart failure · severe trauma within 3 months (avoid if within 6 weeks) · traumatic or protracted cardiopulmonary resuscitation within last 2 weeks · uncontrolled severe hypertension · vasculitis

● **INTERACTIONS** → Appendix 1: tirofiban

● **SIDE-EFFECTS**
▸ **Common or very common** Ecchymosis · fever · haemorrhage · headache · nausea · thrombocytopenia
▸ **Frequency not known** Intracranial haemorrhage

● **PREGNANCY** Manufacturer advises use only if potential benefit outweighs risk—no information available.

● **BREAST FEEDING** Manufacturer advises avoid—no information available.

- **HEPATIC IMPAIRMENT** Manufacturer advises caution in mild to moderate hepatic failure; avoid in severe hepatic failure (no information available).
- **RENAL IMPAIRMENT** [EvGr] Monitor carefully if creatinine clearance less than 60 mL/minute (increased risk of bleeding). ⓜ
  Dose adjustments [EvGr] Use half normal dose if creatinine clearance less than 30 mL/minute (consult product literature). ⓜ See p. 21.
- **MONITORING REQUIREMENTS** Monitor platelet count, haemoglobin and haematocrit before treatment, 2–6 hours after start of treatment and then at least once daily.
- **DIRECTIONS FOR ADMINISTRATION** For *intravenous infusion* (*Aggrastat*®), manufacturer advises give continuously in Glucose 5% or Sodium Chloride 0.9%. Withdraw 50 mL infusion fluid from 250 mL bag and replace with 50 mL tirofiban concentrate (250 micrograms/mL) to give a final concentration of 50 micrograms/mL.

- **MEDICINAL FORMS** There can be variation in the licensing of different medicines containing the same drug.
  Solution for infusion
  ELECTROLYTES: May contain Sodium
  - ▸ Aggrastat (Advanz Pharma)
    Tirofiban 250 microgram per 1 ml Aggrastat 12.5mg/50ml concentrate for solution for infusion vials | 1 vial [PoM] £146.11 (Hospital only)
  Infusion
  ELECTROLYTES: May contain Sodium
  - ▸ Tirofiban (Non-proprietary)
    Tirofiban 50 microgram per 1 ml Tirofiban 12.5mg/250ml infusion bags | 1 bag [PoM] £159.00–£160.72 (Hospital only)
  - ▸ Aggrastat (Advanz Pharma)
    Tirofiban 50 microgram per 1 ml Aggrastat 12.5mg/250ml infusion bags | 1 bag [PoM] £160.72 (Hospital only)

PIPERAZINE DERIVATIVES

Ranolazine
06-Aug-2021

- **● INDICATIONS AND DOSE**
  As adjunctive therapy in the treatment of stable angina in patients inadequately controlled or intolerant of first-line antianginal therapies
  - ▸ BY MOUTH
  - ▸ Adult: Initially 375 mg twice daily for 2–4 weeks, then increased to 500 mg twice daily, then adjusted according to response to 750 mg twice daily; reduced if not tolerated to 375–500 mg twice daily

- **CAUTIONS** Body-weight less than 60 kg · elderly · moderate to severe congestive heart failure · QT interval prolongation
- **INTERACTIONS** → Appendix 1: ranolazine
- **SIDE-EFFECTS**
  - ▸ **Common or very common** Asthenia · constipation · headache · vomiting
  - ▸ **Uncommon** Anxiety · appetite decreased · confusion · cough · dehydration · dizziness postural · drowsiness · dry mouth · gastrointestinal discomfort · gastrointestinal disorders · haemorrhage · hallucination · hot flush · hypotension · insomnia · joint swelling · muscle cramps · muscle weakness · pain in extremity · peripheral oedema · QT interval prolongation · sensation abnormal · skin reactions · syncope · tinnitus · tremor · urinary disorders · urine discolouration · vertigo · vision disorders · weight decreased
  - ▸ **Rare or very rare** Acute kidney injury · altered smell sensation · angioedema · consciousness impaired · coordination abnormal · erectile dysfunction · gait abnormal · hearing impairment · hyponatraemia · memory loss · oral hypoaesthesia · pancreatitis · peripheral coldness

- **PREGNANCY** Manufacturer advises avoid unless essential—no information available.
- **BREAST FEEDING** Manufacturer advises avoid—no information available.
- **HEPATIC IMPAIRMENT** Manufacturer advises caution in mild impairment; avoid in moderate to severe impairment (risk of increased exposure).
  Dose adjustments Manufacturer advises careful dose titration in mild impairment.
- **RENAL IMPAIRMENT** [EvGr] Use with caution if creatinine clearance 30–80 mL/minute (risk of increased exposure); avoid if creatinine clearance less than 30 mL/minute. ⓜ See p. 21.
- **NATIONAL FUNDING/ACCESS DECISIONS**
  For full details see funding body website
  Scottish Medicines Consortium (SMC) decisions
  - ▸ Ranolazine (*Ranexa*®) as add-on therapy for the symptomatic treatment of patients with stable angina pectoris who are inadequately controlled or intolerant to first-line antianginal therapies (such as beta-blockers and/or calcium antagonists) (November 2012) SMC No. 565/09 Not recommended

- **MEDICINAL FORMS** There can be variation in the licensing of different medicines containing the same drug.
  Modified-release tablet
  CAUTIONARY AND ADVISORY LABELS 25
  - ▸ Ranolazine (Non-proprietary)
    Ranolazine 375 mg Ranolazine 375mg modified-release tablets | 60 tablet [PoM] £10.49–£48.98 DT = £10.49
    Ranolazine 500 mg Ranolazine 500mg modified-release tablets | 60 tablet [PoM] £10.54–£48.98 DT = £10.54
    Ranolazine 750 mg Ranolazine 750mg modified-release tablets | 60 tablet [PoM] £10.24–£48.98 DT = £10.24
  - ▸ Ranexa (A. Menarini Farmaceutica Internazionale SRL)
    Ranolazine 375 mg Ranexa 375mg modified-release tablets | 60 tablet [PoM] £48.98 DT = £10.49
    Ranolazine 500 mg Ranexa 500mg modified-release tablets | 60 tablet [PoM] £48.98 DT = £10.54
    Ranolazine 750 mg Ranexa 750mg modified-release tablets | 60 tablet [PoM] £48.98 DT = £10.24
  - ▸ Ranogelan (G.L. Pharma UK Ltd)
    Ranolazine 375 mg Ranogelan 375mg prolonged-release tablets | 60 tablet [PoM] £44.08 DT = £10.49
    Ranolazine 500 mg Ranogelan 500mg prolonged-release tablets | 60 tablet [PoM] £44.08 DT = £10.54
    Ranolazine 750 mg Ranogelan 750mg prolonged-release tablets | 60 tablet [PoM] £44.08 DT = £10.24

SELECTIVE SINUS NODE I$_F$ INHIBITORS

Ivabradine
02-Aug-2021

- **● INDICATIONS AND DOSE**
  Treatment of angina in patients in normal sinus rhythm
  - ▸ BY MOUTH
  - ▸ Adult 18-74 years: Initially 2.5–5 mg twice daily for 3–4 weeks, then increased if necessary up to 7.5 mg twice daily, dose to be increased gradually; reduced if not tolerated to 2.5–5 mg twice daily, heart rate at rest should not be allowed to fall below 50 beats per minute, discontinue treatment if no improvement in symptoms within 3 months
  - ▸ Adult 75 years and over: Initially 2.5 mg twice daily for 3–4 weeks, then increased if necessary up to 7.5 mg twice daily, dose to be increased gradually; reduced if not tolerated to 2.5–5 mg twice daily, heart rate at rest should not be allowed to fall below 50 beats per minute, discontinue treatment if no improvement in symptoms within 3 months
  Mild to severe chronic heart failure
  - ▸ BY MOUTH
  - ▸ Adult 18-74 years: Initially 5 mg twice daily for 2 weeks, then increased if necessary to 7.5 mg twice continued →

2
Cardiovascular system

daily; reduced if not tolerated to 2.5–5 mg twice daily, heart rate at rest should not be allowed to fall below 50 beats per minute
▸ Adult 75 years and over: Initially 2.5 mg twice daily for 2 weeks, then increased if necessary up to 7.5 mg twice daily, dose to be increased gradually; reduced if not tolerated to 2.5–5 mg twice daily, heart rate at rest should not be allowed to fall below 50 beats per minute

DOSE ADJUSTMENTS DUE TO INTERACTIONS
▸ Manufacturer advises reduce initial dose to 2.5 mg twice daily with concurrent use of moderate CYP3A4 inhibitors (except diltiazem, erythromycin and verapamil where concurrent use is contra-indicated).

● **CONTRA-INDICATIONS** Acute myocardial infarction · cardiogenic shock · congenital QT syndrome · do not initiate for angina if heart rate below 70 beats per minute · do not initiate for chronic heart failure if heart rate below 75 beats per minute · immediately after cerebrovascular accident · patients dependent on pacemaker · second- and third-degree heart block · severe hypotension · sick-sinus syndrome · sino-atrial block · unstable angina · unstable or acute heart failure

● **CAUTIONS** Atrial fibrillation or other arrhythmias (treatment ineffective) · elderly · in angina, consider stopping if there is no or limited symptom improvement after 3 months · intraventricular conduction defects · mild to moderate hypotension (avoid if severe) · retinitis pigmentosa

● **INTERACTIONS** → Appendix 1: ivabradine

● **SIDE-EFFECTS**
▸ **Common or very common** Arrhythmias · atrioventricular block · dizziness · headache · hypertension · vision disorders
▸ **Uncommon** Abdominal pain · angioedema · constipation · diarrhoea · eosinophilia · hyperuricaemia · hypotension · muscle cramps · nausea · QT interval prolongation · skin reactions · syncope · vertigo

● **PREGNANCY** Manufacturer advises avoid— *toxicity* in animal studies.

● **BREAST FEEDING** Present in milk in *animal* studies— manufacturer advises avoid.

● **HEPATIC IMPAIRMENT** Manufacturer advises caution in moderate impairment; avoid in severe impairment—no information available.

● **RENAL IMPAIRMENT** EvGr Caution if creatinine clearance less than 15 mL/minute (no information available). ⓜ See p. 21.

● **MONITORING REQUIREMENTS**
▸ Monitor regularly for atrial fibrillation (consider benefits and risks of continued treatment if atrial fibrillation occurs).
▸ Monitor for bradycardia, especially after any dose increase, and discontinue if resting heart rate persistently below 50 beats per minute or continued symptoms of bradycardia despite dose reduction.

● **NATIONAL FUNDING/ACCESS DECISIONS**
For full details see funding body website

NICE decisions
▸ Ivabradine for the treatment of chronic heart failure (November 2012) NICE TA267 Recommended with restrictions

Scottish Medicines Consortium (SMC) decisions
▸ Ivabradine (*Procoralan*®) for chronic heart failure New York Heart Association (NYHA) II to IV class with systolic dysfunction, in patients in sinus rhythm and whose heart rate is ≥75 beats per minute (bpm), in combination with standard therapy including beta-blocker therapy or when beta-blocker therapy is contra-indicated or not tolerated (October 2012) SMC No. 805/12 Recommended with restrictions

● **MEDICINAL FORMS** There can be variation in the licensing of different medicines containing the same drug.

Oral tablet
▸ Ivabradine (Non-proprietary)
Ivabradine (as Ivabradine hydrochloride) **2.5 mg** Ivabradine 2.5mg tablets | 56 tablet PoM £80.34 DT = £21.42
Ivabradine **5 mg** Ivabradine 5mg tablets | 56 tablet PoM £40.17 DT = £4.23
Ivabradine (as Ivabradine hydrochloride) **7.5 mg** Ivabradine 7.5mg tablets | 56 tablet PoM £40.17 DT = £3.29
▸ Procoralan (Servier Laboratories Ltd)
Ivabradine **5 mg** Procoralan 5mg tablets | 56 tablet PoM £40.17 DT = £4.23
Ivabradine (as Ivabradine hydrochloride) **7.5 mg** Procoralan 7.5mg tablets | 56 tablet PoM £40.17 DT = £3.29

VASODILATORS › POTASSIUM-CHANNEL OPENERS

Nicorandil

06-Feb-2020

● **INDICATIONS AND DOSE**

Prophylaxis and treatment of stable angina (second-line)
▸ BY MOUTH
▸ Adult: Initially 5–10 mg twice daily, then increased if tolerated to 40 mg twice daily; usual dose 10–20 mg twice daily, use lower initial dose regimen if patient susceptible to headache

● **CONTRA-INDICATIONS** Acute pulmonary oedema · hypovolaemia · left ventricular dysfunction with low filling pressure or cardiac decompensation · severe hypotension · shock (including cardiogenic shock)

● **CAUTIONS** Diverticular disease (risk of fistula formation or bowel perforation) · G6PD deficiency · heart failure (class III–IV) · hyperkalaemia

● **INTERACTIONS** → Appendix 1: nicorandil

● **SIDE-EFFECTS**
▸ **Common or very common** Asthenia · dizziness · haemorrhage · headache (more common on initiation, usually transitory) · nausea · vasodilation · vomiting
▸ **Rare or very rare** Abdominal pain · angioedema · conjunctivitis · eye disorders · gastrointestinal disorders · genital ulceration · hepatic disorders · hyperkalaemia · mucosal ulceration · myalgia · oral disorders · skin reactions · skin ulcer
▸ **Frequency not known** Diplopia

SIDE-EFFECTS, FURTHER INFORMATION Nicorandil can cause serious skin, mucosal, and eye ulceration; including gastrointestinal ulcers, which may progress to perforation, haemorrhage, fistula or abscess. Stop treatment if ulceration occurs and consider an alternative.

● **PREGNANCY** Manufacturer advises use only if potential benefit outweighs risk—no information available.

● **BREAST FEEDING** No information available—manufacturer advises avoid.

● **PATIENT AND CARER ADVICE**
Driving and skilled tasks Patients should be warned not to drive or operate machinery until it is established that their performance is unimpaired.

● **MEDICINAL FORMS** There can be variation in the licensing of different medicines containing the same drug.

Oral tablet
▸ Nicorandil (Non-proprietary)
Nicorandil **10 mg** Nicorandil 10mg tablets | 60 tablet PoM £8.00 DT = £6.92
Nicorandil **20 mg** Nicorandil 20mg tablets | 60 tablet PoM £16.00 DT = £12.62

9.1 Acute coronary syndromes

Acute coronary syndromes
10-Aug-2022

Description of condition

Acute coronary syndrome (ACS) encompasses a spectrum of conditions which include myocardial infarction with or without ST-segment-elevation (STEMI or NSTEMI respectively), and unstable angina. These result from the formation of a thrombus on an atheromatous plaque in a coronary artery, and while the presentation and management of these conditions is similar, there are important distinctions between them. A definitive diagnosis of ACS is based on clinical presentation, ECG changes, and measurement of biochemical cardiac markers.

A **STEMI** is generally caused by a *complete* and *persistent* blockage of the artery resulting in myocardial necrosis with ST-segment elevation seen on the ECG. In **NSTEMI** and **unstable angina** a *partial* or *intermittent* blockage of the artery occurs, which usually results in myocardial necrosis in NSTEMI but not in unstable angina. The ECG may show ST-segment depression, T-wave inversion, or may be normal. High-sensitivity blood tests for serum troponin are used to differentiate between NSTEMI and unstable angina.

For recommendations on the management of suspected or confirmed acute myocardial injury in patients with COVID-19, see NICE rapid guideline: **Managing COVID-19** (available at: www.nice.org.uk/guidance/ng191). For further information on COVID-19, see COVID-19 p. 714.

Non-drug treatment

Revascularisation procedures such as percutaneous coronary intervention (PCI) or coronary artery bypass graft (CABG) are often appropriate, alongside drug treatment, for patients with an ACS. The decision regarding choice of these management options depends on multiple factors such as the type of ACS, time since symptom onset, the patient's clinical condition, comorbidities, and their formally-assessed risk of future cardiovascular events. For further information, see NICE guideline: **Acute coronary syndrome** (see *Useful resources*).

Initial management

EvGr The management of ACS aims to provide supportive care and pain relief, and to prevent progression of cardiac injury. Treatment should be started as soon as an ACS is suspected but should not delay transfer to hospital.

Pain relief should be offered as soon as possible with glyceryl trinitrate p. 252 (sublingual or buccal). Intravenous opioids such as morphine p. 525 may also be administered, particularly if acute myocardial infarction (MI) is suspected.

A loading dose of aspirin p. 142 should be given as soon as possible. If aspirin is given before arrival at hospital, a note saying that it has been given should be sent with the patient. Other antiplatelet agents should only be offered once the patient is in hospital according to their diagnosis and risk factors (see *ST-segment elevation myocardial infarction (STEMI)* and *Unstable angina and non-ST-segment elevation myocardial infarction (NSTEMI)* for specific recommendations).

Oxygen should not be routinely administered, however the patient's oxygen saturation should be monitored (ideally before hospital admission) and supplemental oxygen offered if indicated. A For further information, see NICE clinical guideline: **Recent-onset chest pain of suspected cardiac origin** (see *Useful resources*).

EvGr All patients admitted to hospital should be closely monitored for hyperglycaemia. Those with a blood-glucose concentration greater than 11.0 mmol/litre should receive insulin p. 835—consider administration via a dose-adjusted infusion. A

ST-segment elevation myocardial infarction (STEMI)

The management of a STEMI aims to restore adequate coronary blood flow as quickly as possible and to reduce mortality.

EvGr Coronary reperfusion therapy (either primary PCI or fibrinolysis) should be delivered as soon as possible in eligible patients with a STEMI. Primary PCI (if within 12 hours of symptom onset and within 120 minutes of the time when fibrinolysis could have been given) is the preferred strategy for most patients.

In addition to aspirin, most patients with a STEMI should be offered a second antiplatelet agent (prasugrel p. 248, ticagrelor p. 249, or clopidogrel p. 143). The choice of second antiplatelet depends on the planned intervention (primary PCI, fibrinolysis or conservative management) and the patient's bleeding risk. Prasugrel is the preferred agent for most patients undergoing a primary PCI, unless the risk of bleeding outweighs its effectiveness. Aspirin alone may be appropriate for some patients with a high bleeding risk not undergoing a PCI.

For patients undergoing primary PCI with radial access, heparin (unfractionated) p. 156 should also be given. If femoral access is needed, bivalirudin p. 159 should be considered instead [unlicensed]. A bailout glycoprotein IIb/IIIa inhibitor may be given if indicated during the PCI.

For patients undergoing fibrinolysis, an antithrombin agent should be given at the same time. A

For further information on STEMI management, including use of drug-eluting stents, see NICE guideline: **Acute coronary syndrome** (see *Useful resources*).

Unstable angina and non-ST-segment elevation myocardial infarction (NSTEMI)

Unstable angina and NSTEMI are managed similarly and treatment aims to prevent further cardiac events and mortality.

EvGr Reperfusion therapy or medical management may be appropriate; the type of treatment is determined by the patient's risk of future adverse cardiovascular events.

In addition to aspirin, most patients with unstable angina or NSTEMI should be offered a second antiplatelet agent (prasugrel, ticagrelor, or clopidogrel). The choice of second antiplatelet depends on the planned intervention (angiography with follow-on PCI if indicated, or conservative management), and the patient's bleeding risk. Aspirin alone may be appropriate for some patients with a high bleeding risk.

Antithrombin therapy with fondaparinux sodium p. 148 should also be offered, unless the patient is undergoing immediate coronary angiography, or has a high bleeding risk. Heparin (unfractionated) may be used as an alternative in patients with significant renal impairment. For patients with a high bleeding risk associated with advancing age, known bleeding complications, renal impairment, and/or low body-weight, care should be taken when selecting the antithrombin agent and dose. Patients undergoing PCI should be offered heparin (unfractionated) in the cardiac catheter laboratory [unlicensed], regardless of whether or not they have already received fondaparinux. A

For further information on the management of unstable angina and NSTEMI, including use of drug-eluting stents, see NICE guideline: **Acute coronary syndrome** (see *Useful resources*).

Secondary prevention of cardiovascular events

EvGr Following an ACS, all patients should be offered a cardiac rehabilitation programme including advice for lifestyle changes, stress management and health education. Lifestyle-specific interventions to reduce their cardiovascular risk should include healthy eating, reducing alcohol consumption, regular physical exercise, smoking cessation and weight management. (A) For further information, see *Cardiovascular disease prevention* in Cardiovascular disease risk assessment and prevention p. 219.

Treatment for secondary prevention should be initiated in all patients following a STEMI and NSTEMI. Clinical judgement should be used in patients with unstable angina; the following treatment options may be appropriate for these patients, depending on their clinical history, other potential diagnoses, comorbidities, and discussion with the patient.

[EvGr] For secondary prevention, patients should be offered treatment with an **angiotensin-converting enzyme (ACE) inhibitor**, a **beta-blocker**, **dual antiplatelet therapy** (unless they have a separate indication for anticoagulation—see below), and a **statin**.

An ACE inhibitor should be started once the patient is haemodynamically stable and continued indefinitely. If intolerant to an ACE inhibitor, an angiotensin II receptor blocker (ARB) should be offered instead.

A beta-blocker should be started as soon as the patient is haemodynamically stable and continued indefinitely for patients *with* a reduced left ventricular ejection fraction (LVEF). In those *without* reduced LVEF, it may be appropriate to discontinue beta-blocker therapy after 12 months; this should be discussed with the patient and the potential benefits and risks of continuation taken into account. Diltiazem hydrochloride p. 185 or verapamil hydrochloride p. 191 may be considered as an alternative to beta-blocker therapy in patients who do *not* have pulmonary congestion or a reduced LVEF.

Treatment with aspirin p. 142 should continue indefinitely. Dual antiplatelet therapy (aspirin with a second antiplatelet) should be continued for up to 12 months unless contra-indicated. Clopidogrel p. 143 monotherapy should be considered as an alternative to aspirin in patients who have aspirin hypersensitivity. Rivaroxaban p. 149, in combination with either aspirin alone *or* aspirin and clopidogrel is also recommended as an option for preventing atherothrombotic events following an ACS with elevated cardiac biomarkers.

For patients with an ongoing separate indication for anticoagulation, the duration and type (dual or monotherapy) of antiplatelet therapy in the 12 months following an ACS should be considered, taking into account their bleeding, thromboembolic, and cardiovascular risks. (A) For specific recommendations on antiplatelet agents in people with an ongoing or new indication for anticoagulation, see NICE guideline: **Acute coronary syndrome** (see *Useful resources*).

[EvGr] A statin is recommended for patients with clinical evidence of cardiovascular disease. (A) For specific recommendations on statin choice, see *Cardiovascular disease prevention* in Cardiovascular disease risk assessment and prevention p. 219.

Useful Resources

Acute coronary syndromes. National Institute of Health and Care Excellence. NICE guideline 185. November 2020.
www.nice.org.uk/guidance/ng185

Recent-onset chest pain of suspected cardiac origin: assessment and diagnosis. National Institute of Health and Care Excellence. Clinical guideline 95. March 2010 (updated November 2016).
www.nice.org.uk/guidance/cg95

Other drugs used for Acute coronary syndromes
Captopril, p. 195 · Dalteparin sodium, p. 153 · Enoxaparin sodium, p. 155 · Lisinopril, p. 197 · Perindopril arginine, p. 198 · Perindopril erbumine, p. 199 · Ramipril, p. 200 · Trandolapril, p. 201 · Valsartan, p. 206

ANTITHROMBOTIC DRUGS ⟩ ANTIPLATELET DRUGS

Prasugrel
07-May-2021

● INDICATIONS AND DOSE

In combination with aspirin for the prevention of atherothrombotic events in patients with acute coronary syndrome undergoing percutaneous coronary intervention

▶ BY MOUTH
- Adult 18–74 years (body-weight up to 60 kg): Initially 60 mg for 1 dose, then 5 mg once daily usually for up to 12 months
- Adult 18–74 years (body-weight 60 kg and above): Initially 60 mg for 1 dose, then 10 mg once daily usually for up to 12 months
- Adult 75 years and over: Initially 60 mg for 1 dose, then 5 mg once daily usually for up to 12 months

Patients undergoing coronary angiography within 48 hours of admission for unstable angina or NSTEMI

▶ BY MOUTH
- Adult: Loading dose 60 mg, not to be administered until the time of percutaneous coronary intervention in order to minimise the risk of bleeding, maintenance dose of 10 mg or 5 mg daily should then be selected as appropriate based on age and weight

● **CONTRA-INDICATIONS** Active bleeding · history of stroke or transient ischaemic attack

● **CAUTIONS** Body-weight less than 60 kg · discontinue at least 7 days before elective surgery if antiplatelet effect not desirable · elderly · patients at increased risk of bleeding (e.g. from recent trauma, surgery, gastro-intestinal bleeding, or active peptic ulcer disease)

● **INTERACTIONS** → Appendix 1: prasugrel

● **SIDE-EFFECTS**
▶ **Common or very common** Anaemia · haemorrhage · skin reactions
▶ **Uncommon** Angioedema · hypersensitivity
▶ **Rare or very rare** Thrombocytopenia

● **ALLERGY AND CROSS-SENSITIVITY** [EvGr] Caution in patients with history of hypersensitivity reactions to thienopyridines (e.g. clopidogrel). (M)

● **PREGNANCY** Manufacturer advises use only if potential benefit outweighs risk.

● **BREAST FEEDING** Manufacturer advises avoid—no information available.

● **HEPATIC IMPAIRMENT** Manufacturer advises caution in moderate impairment (increased risk of bleeding, limited information available); avoid in severe impairment (no information available).

● **RENAL IMPAIRMENT** [EvGr] Use with caution (increased risk of bleeding, limited information available). (M)

● **NATIONAL FUNDING/ACCESS DECISIONS**
For full details see funding body website
NICE decisions
▶ Prasugrel with percutaneous coronary intervention for treating acute coronary syndromes (July 2014) NICE TA317 Recommended

● **MEDICINAL FORMS** There can be variation in the licensing of different medicines containing the same drug.
Oral tablet
▶ Prasugrel (Non-proprietary)
Prasugrel 5 mg Prasugrel 5mg tablets | 28 tablet [PoM] £57.07 DT = £28.09
Prasugrel 10 mg Prasugrel 10mg tablets | 28 tablet [PoM] £57.07 DT = £3.76

► **Efient** (Vygoris Ltd)
Prasugrel 5 mg Efient 5mg tablets | 28 tablet [PoM] £47.56 DT = £28.09
Prasugrel 10 mg Efient 10mg tablets | 28 tablet [PoM] £47.56 DT = £3.76

Ticagrelor
27-Jul-2023

- **DRUG ACTION** Ticagrelor is a $P2Y_{12}$ receptor antagonist that prevents ADP-mediated $P2Y_{12}$ dependent platelet activation and aggregation.

- **INDICATIONS AND DOSE**

Prevention of atherothrombotic events in patients with acute coronary syndrome [in combination with aspirin]
► BY MOUTH
► Adult: Initially 180 mg for 1 dose, then 90 mg twice daily usually for up to 12 months

Prevention of atherothrombotic events in patients with a history of myocardial infarction and a high risk of an atherothrombotic event [in combination with aspirin]
► BY MOUTH
► Adult: 60 mg twice daily, extended treatment may be started without interruption after the initial 12-month therapy for acute coronary syndrome. Treatment may also be initiated up to 2 years from the myocardial infarction, or within 1 year after stopping previous ADP receptor inhibitor treatment. There are limited data on the efficacy and safety of extended treatment beyond 3 years

Transient ischaemic attack [in patients with a low risk of bleeding] | Minor ischaemic stroke [in patients with a low risk of bleeding]
► BY MOUTH
► Adult: Initially 180 mg for 1 dose, to be started within 24 hours of onset of symptoms, then 90 mg twice daily, to be combined with aspirin for the first 30 days

- **UNLICENSED USE** [EvGr] Ticagrelor is used for transient ischaemic attack and minor ischaemic stroke, (A) but is not licensed for these indications.

- **CONTRA-INDICATIONS** Active bleeding · history of intracranial haemorrhage

- **CAUTIONS** Asthma · bradycardia (unless pacemaker fitted) · chronic obstructive pulmonary disease · discontinue 5 days before elective surgery if antiplatelet effect not desirable · history of hyperuricaemia · patients at increased risk of bleeding (e.g. from recent trauma, surgery, gastro-intestinal bleeding, or coagulation disorders) · second- or third-degree AV block (unless pacemaker fitted) · sick sinus syndrome (unless pacemaker fitted)

- **INTERACTIONS** → Appendix 1: ticagrelor

- **SIDE-EFFECTS**
► **Common or very common** Constipation · diarrhoea · dizziness · dyspepsia · dyspnoea · gout · gouty arthritis · haemorrhage · headache · hyperuricaemia · hypotension · nausea · skin reactions · syncope · vertigo
► **Uncommon** Angioedema · confusion · intracranial haemorrhage · tumour haemorrhage
► **Frequency not known** Thrombotic thrombocytopenic purpura

- **PREGNANCY** Manufacturer advises avoid—toxicity in *animal* studies.

- **BREAST FEEDING** Manufacturer advises avoid—present in milk in *animal* studies.

- **HEPATIC IMPAIRMENT** Manufacturer advises caution in moderate impairment (limited information available); avoid in severe impairment (no information available).

- **MONITORING REQUIREMENTS** Manufacturer advises monitor renal function 1 month after initiation in patients with acute coronary syndrome.

- **NATIONAL FUNDING/ACCESS DECISIONS**
For full details see funding body website
NICE decisions
► Ticagrelor for the treatment of acute coronary syndromes (October 2011) NICE TA236 Recommended
► Ticagrelor for preventing atherothrombotic events after myocardial infarction (December 2016) NICE TA420 Recommended

- **MEDICINAL FORMS** There can be variation in the licensing of different medicines containing the same drug.
Oral tablet
► **Brilique** (AstraZeneca UK Ltd)
Ticagrelor 60 mg Brilique 60mg tablets | 56 tablet [PoM] £54.60 DT = £54.60
Ticagrelor 90 mg Brilique 90mg tablets | 56 tablet [PoM] £54.60 DT = £54.60
Orodispersible tablet
► **Brilique** (AstraZeneca UK Ltd)
Ticagrelor 90 mg Brilique 90mg orodispersible tablets | 56 tablet [PoM] £54.60 DT = £54.60 [SF]

ANTITHROMBOTIC DRUGS > TISSUE PLASMINOGEN ACTIVATORS

Fibrinolytic drugs
01-Oct-2024

Overview

The value of thrombolytic drugs for the treatment of *myocardial infarction* has been established. Streptokinase p. 251 and alteplase p. 250 have been shown to reduce mortality. Reteplase and tenecteplase p. 251 are also licensed for acute myocardial infarction. Thrombolytic drugs are indicated for any patient with acute myocardial infarction for whom the benefit is likely to outweigh the risk of treatment. Trials have shown that the benefit is greatest in those with ECG changes that include ST segment elevation (especially in those with anterior infarction) and in patients with bundle branch block. Patients should not be denied thrombolytic treatment on account of age alone because mortality in the elderly is high and the reduction in mortality is the same as in younger patients. Alteplase should be given within 6–12 hours of symptom onset, reteplase and streptokinase within 12 hours of symptom onset, but ideally all should be given within 1 hour; use after 12 hours requires specialist advice. Tenecteplase should be given as early as possible and usually within 6 hours of symptom onset.

Alteplase, streptokinase and urokinase p. 162 can be used for other thromboembolic disorders such as deep-vein thrombosis and pulmonary embolism. Alteplase or tenecteplase are also used for acute ischaemic stroke.

Urokinase is also licensed to restore the patency of occluded intravenous catheters and cannulas blocked with fibrin clots.

Fibrinolytics

- **DRUG ACTION** Fibrinolytic drugs act as thrombolytics by activating plasminogen to form plasmin, which degrades fibrin and so breaks up thrombi.

- **CONTRA-INDICATIONS** Acute pancreatitis · aneurysm · aortic dissection · arteriovenous malformation · bacterial endocarditis · bleeding diatheses · coagulation defects · coma · heavy vaginal bleeding · history of cerebrovascular disease (especially recent events or with any residual disability) · neoplasm with risk of haemorrhage · oesophageal varices · pericarditis · recent gastro-intestinal ulceration · recent haemorrhage · recent surgery (including dental extraction) · recent trauma · severe hypertension

- **CAUTIONS** Conditions in which thrombolysis might give rise to embolic complications such as enlarged left atrium with atrial fibrillation (risk of dissolution of clot and subsequent embolisation) · elderly · external chest compression · hypertension · risk of bleeding (including that from venepuncture or invasive procedures)
- **SIDE-EFFECTS**
  ▶ **Common or very common** Anaphylactic reaction · angina pectoris · cardiac arrest · cardiogenic shock · chills · CNS haemorrhage · ecchymosis · fever · haemorrhage · heart failure · ischaemia recurrent (when used in myocardial infarction) · nausea · pulmonary oedema · vomiting
  ▶ **Uncommon** Mitral valve incompetence · reperfusion arrhythmia (when used in myocardial infarction)
  ▶ **Rare or very rare** Seizure

  SIDE-EFFECTS, FURTHER INFORMATION Serious bleeding calls for discontinuation of the thrombolytic and may require administration of coagulation factors and antifibrinolytic drugs.

- **PREGNANCY** Thrombolytic drugs can possibly lead to premature separation of the placenta in the first 18 weeks of pregnancy. There is also a risk of maternal haemorrhage throughout pregnancy and post-partum, and also a theoretical risk of fetal haemorrhage throughout pregnancy.
- **HEPATIC IMPAIRMENT** Manufacturers advise avoid in severe impairment.

F 249

Alteplase

27-Jul-2023

(rt-PA; Tissue-type plasminogen activator)

- **INDICATIONS AND DOSE**

Acute myocardial infarction, accelerated regimen
  ▶ INITIALLY BY INTRAVENOUS INJECTION
  ▶ Adult (body-weight up to 65 kg): Initially 15 mg, to be initiated within 6 hours of symptom onset, followed by (by intravenous infusion) 0.75 mg/kg, to be given over 30 minutes, then (by intravenous infusion) 0.5 mg/kg, to be given over 60 minutes, maximum total dose of 100 mg administered over 90 minutes
  ▶ Adult (body-weight 65 kg and above): Initially 15 mg, to be initiated within 6 hours of symptom onset, followed by (by intravenous infusion) 50 mg, to be given over 30 minutes, then (by intravenous infusion) 35 mg, to be given over 60 minutes, maximum total dose of 100 mg administered over 90 minutes

Acute myocardial infarction
  ▶ INITIALLY BY INTRAVENOUS INJECTION
  ▶ Adult: Initially 10 mg, to be initiated within 6–12 hours of symptom onset, followed by (by intravenous infusion) 50 mg, to be given over 60 minutes, then (by intravenous infusion) 10 mg for 4 infusions, each 10 mg infusion dose to be given over 30 minutes, total dose of 100 mg over 3 hours; maximum 1.5 mg/kg in patients less than 65 kg

Pulmonary embolism
  ▶ INITIALLY BY INTRAVENOUS INJECTION
  ▶ Adult: Initially 10 mg, to be given over 1–2 minutes, followed by (by intravenous infusion) 90 mg, to be given over 2 hours, maximum 1.5 mg/kg in patients less than 65 kg

Acute ischaemic stroke (under specialist neurology physician only)
  ▶ BY INTRAVENOUS INFUSION
  ▶ Adult: 900 micrograms/kg (max. per dose 90 mg), the initial 10% of dose is to be administered by intravenous

injection and the remainder by intravenous infusion over 60 minutes, treatment should begin as soon as possible within 4.5 hours of symptom onset and when intracranial haemorrhage excluded by imaging. For further information on thrombolysis beyond 4.5 hours of symptom onset, see *National Clinical Guideline for Stroke for the UK and Ireland*

ACTILYSE CATHFLO ®

Thrombolytic treatment of occluded central venous access devices (including those used for haemodialysis)
  ▶ BY INTRAVENOUS INJECTION
  ▶ Adult: (consult product literature)

- **CONTRA-INDICATIONS**
  GENERAL CONTRA-INDICATIONS Recent delivery
  SPECIFIC CONTRA-INDICATIONS
  ▶ When used for Acute ischaemic stroke Convulsion accompanying stroke · history of stroke in patients with diabetes · hyperglycaemia · hypoglycaemia · stroke in last 3 months
- **INTERACTIONS** → Appendix 1: alteplase
- **SIDE-EFFECTS**
  ▶ **Common or very common** Haemorrhagic stroke · hypotension
  ▶ **Uncommon** Haemothorax
  ▶ **Rare or very rare** Agitation · confusion · delirium · depression · epilepsy · psychosis · speech impairment
  ▶ **Frequency not known** Brain oedema (caused by reperfusion)
- **ALLERGY AND CROSS-SENSITIVITY** [EvGr] Contra-indicated if history of hypersensitivity to gentamicin (residue from manufacturing process). ⟨M⟩
- **MONITORING REQUIREMENTS**
  ▶ When used for Acute ischaemic stroke [EvGr] Monitor for intracranial haemorrhage. ⟨M⟩ [EvGr] Monitor blood pressure; ensure blood pressure reduced to below 185/110 mmHg before treatment. ⟨A⟩
- **DIRECTIONS FOR ADMINISTRATION** For *intravenous infusion* (*Actilyse ®*), manufacturer advises give intermittently in Sodium Chloride 0.9%; dissolve in Water for Injections to a concentration of 1 mg/mL or 2 mg/mL and infuse intravenously; alternatively dilute the solution further in the infusion fluid to a concentration of not less than 200 micrograms/mL; not to be infused in Glucose solution.
- **NATIONAL FUNDING/ACCESS DECISIONS**
  For full details see funding body website
  NICE decisions
  ▶ Alteplase for treating acute ischaemic stroke (September 2012) NICE TA264 Recommended

- **MEDICINAL FORMS** There can be variation in the licensing of different medicines containing the same drug. Forms available from special-order manufacturers include: solution for injection

Powder and solvent for solution for injection
  ▶ Actilyse (Boehringer Ingelheim Ltd)
    Alteplase 10 mg Actilyse 10mg powder and solvent for solution for injection vials | 1 vial [PoM] £172.80
    Alteplase 20 mg Actilyse 20mg powder and solvent for solution for injection vials | 1 vial [PoM] £259.20

Powder and solvent for solution for infusion
  ▶ Actilyse (Boehringer Ingelheim Ltd)
    Alteplase 50 mg Actilyse 50mg powder and solvent for solution for infusion vials | 1 vial [PoM] £432.00

Streptokinase
F 249   13-Apr-2021

- **INDICATIONS AND DOSE**

Acute myocardial infarction
- ▶ BY INTRAVENOUS INFUSION
- ▶ Adult: 1 500 000 units, to be initiated within 12 hours of symptom onset, dose to be given over 60 minutes

Deep-vein thrombosis | Central retinal venous or arterial thrombosis
- ▶ BY INTRAVENOUS INFUSION
- ▶ Adult: 250 000 units, dose to be given over 30 minutes, then 100 000 units every 1 hour for 12 hours for central retinal venous or arterial thrombosis, or for 72 hours for deep-vein thrombosis

Pulmonary embolism
- ▶ BY INTRAVENOUS INFUSION
- ▶ Adult: 250 000 units, dose to be given over 30 minutes, then 100 000 units every 1 hour for 24 hours, alternatively 1 500 000 units, dose to be given over 1–2 hours

Occlusive peripheral arterial disease
- ▶ BY INTRAVENOUS INFUSION
- ▶ Adult: 250 000 units, dose to be given over 30 minutes, then 100 000 units every 1 hour for up to 5 days
- ▶ BY INTRA-ARTERIAL INFUSION
- ▶ Adult: (consult product literature)

- **CAUTIONS** Cavernous pulmonary disease · recent streptococcal infections

- **INTERACTIONS** → Appendix 1: streptokinase

- **SIDE-EFFECTS**
- ▶ **Common or very common** Arrhythmias · asthenia · diarrhoea · epigastric pain · headache · malaise · pain · pericarditis
- ▶ **Uncommon** Myocardial rupture · pericardial disorders · respiratory arrest · splenic rupture
- ▶ **Rare or very rare** Arthritis · eye inflammation · hypersensitivity · nephritis · nerve disorders · neurological effects · pulmonary oedema non-cardiogenic (caused by reperfusion) · shock · vasculitis

- **ALLERGY AND CROSS-SENSITIVITY** Contra-indicated if previous allergic reaction to either streptokinase or anistreplase (no longer available). Prolonged persistence of antibodies to streptokinase and anistreplase (no longer available) can reduce the effectiveness of subsequent treatment; therefore, streptokinase should not be used again beyond 4 days of first administration of either streptokinase or anistreplase.

- **DIRECTIONS FOR ADMINISTRATION** Manufacturer advises for *intravenous infusion*, give continuously or intermittently; reconstitute with Sodium Chloride 0.9%, then dilute further with Glucose 5% or Sodium Chloride 0.9% or Compound Sodium Lactate after reconstitution.

- **MEDICINAL FORMS** There can be variation in the licensing of different medicines containing the same drug.
  ### Powder for solution for infusion
  - ▶ Streptokinase (Non-proprietary)
    Streptokinase 1.5 mega unit Streptokinase 1.5million unit powder for solution for infusion vials | 1 vial [PoM] £195.00 (Hospital only)
    Streptokinase 250000 unit Streptokinase 250,000unit powder for solution for infusion vials | 1 vial [PoM] £97.50 (Hospital only)

Tenecteplase
F 249   27-Nov-2024

- **INDICATIONS AND DOSE**

Acute myocardial infarction [using 50 mg (10 000 unit) vial] (under expert supervision)
- ▶ BY INTRAVENOUS INJECTION
- ▶ Adult (body-weight up to 60 kg): 30 mg for 1 dose, to be given over 10 seconds, treatment should begin as soon as possible within 6 hours of symptom onset
- ▶ Adult (body-weight 60-69 kg): 35 mg for 1 dose, to be given over 10 seconds, treatment should begin as soon as possible within 6 hours of symptom onset
- ▶ Adult (body-weight 70-79 kg): 40 mg for 1 dose, to be given over 10 seconds, treatment should begin as soon as possible within 6 hours of symptom onset
- ▶ Adult (body-weight 80-89 kg): 45 mg for 1 dose, to be given over 10 seconds, treatment should begin as soon as possible within 6 hours of symptom onset
- ▶ Adult (body-weight 90 kg and above): 50 mg for 1 dose, to be given over 10 seconds, treatment should begin as soon as possible within 6 hours of symptom onset

Acute ischaemic stroke [using 25 mg (5000 unit) vial] (under expert supervision)
- ▶ BY INTRAVENOUS INJECTION
- ▶ Adult (body-weight up to 60 kg): 15 mg for 1 dose, to be given over 5–10 seconds, treatment should begin as soon as possible within 4.5 hours of symptom onset and when intracranial haemorrhage excluded by imaging
- ▶ Adult (body-weight 60-69 kg): 17.5 mg for 1 dose, to be given over 5–10 seconds, treatment should begin as soon as possible within 4.5 hours of symptom onset and when intracranial haemorrhage excluded by imaging
- ▶ Adult (body-weight 70-79 kg): 20 mg for 1 dose, to be given over 5–10 seconds, treatment should begin as soon as possible within 4.5 hours of symptom onset and when intracranial haemorrhage excluded by imaging
- ▶ Adult (body-weight 80-89 kg): 22.5 mg for 1 dose, to be given over 5–10 seconds, treatment should begin as soon as possible within 4.5 hours of symptom onset and when intracranial haemorrhage excluded by imaging
- ▶ Adult (body-weight 90 kg and above): 25 mg for 1 dose, to be given over 5–10 seconds, treatment should begin as soon as possible within 4.5 hours of symptom onset and when intracranial haemorrhage excluded by imaging

- **DOSE EQUIVALENCE AND CONVERSION**
- ▶ Tenecteplase 25 mg is equivalent to 5000 units.

- **CONTRA-INDICATIONS**
- ▶ When used for Acute ischaemic stroke Acute ischaemic stroke without disabling neurological deficit or symptoms rapidly improving before start of injection · history of stroke and concomitant diabetes · hyperglycaemia · hypoglycaemia · platelet count less than 100,000 mm^3 · seizure accompanying stroke · stroke in last 3 months · symptoms suggestive of subarachnoid haemorrhage
- ▶ When used for Acute myocardial infarction Dementia

- **CAUTIONS**
- ▶ When used for Acute ischaemic stroke Severe stroke (National Institutes of Health Stroke Scale (NIHSS) > 25 and/or as assessed by imaging)

- **INTERACTIONS** → Appendix 1: tenecteplase

- **SIDE-EFFECTS** Fat embolism

- **ALLERGY AND CROSS-SENSITIVITY** [EvGr] Contra-indicated if history of hypersensitivity to gentamicin (residue from manufacturing process). ◈M◈

- **BREAST FEEDING** Manufacturer advises avoid breast-feeding for 24 hours after dose (express and discard milk during this time).

- **PRESCRIBING AND DISPENSING INFORMATION** Tenecteplase is a biological medicine. Biological medicines must be prescribed and dispensed by brand name, see *Biological medicines* and *Biosimilar medicines*, under Guidance on prescribing p. 1; record the brand name and batch number after each administration.

- **NATIONAL FUNDING/ACCESS DECISIONS** For full details see funding body website
  NICE decisions
  ▶ **Tenecteplase for treating acute ischaemic stroke (July 2024)** NICE TA990 Recommended
  Scottish Medicines Consortium (SMC) decisions
  ▶ Tenecteplase (*Metalyse*®) in adults for the thrombolytic treatment of acute ischaemic stroke within 4.5 hours from last known well and after exclusion of intracranial haemorrhage (November 2024) SMC No. SMC2697 Recommended

- **MEDICINAL FORMS** There can be variation in the licensing of different medicines containing the same drug.
  Powder and solvent for solution for injection
  EXCIPIENTS: May contain Gentamicin, polysorbates
  ▶ Metalyse (Boehringer Ingelheim Ltd)
  Tenecteplase 10000 unit Metalyse 10,000unit powder and solvent for solution for injection vials | 1 vial [PoM] £602.70
  Powder for solution for injection
  EXCIPIENTS: May contain Gentamicin, polysorbates
  ▶ Metalyse (Boehringer Ingelheim Ltd)
  Tenecteplase 5000 unit Metalyse 5,000unit powder for solution for injection vials | 1 vial [PoM] £602.70 (Hospital only)

NITRATES

Nitrates

16-Sep-2021

Overview

Nitrates have a useful role in *angina*, see Stable angina p. 242 and Acute coronary syndromes p. 247. Although they are potent coronary vasodilators, their principal benefit follows from a reduction in venous return which reduces left ventricular work. Unwanted effects (such as flushing, headache, and postural hypotension) may limit therapy, especially when angina is severe or when patients are unusually sensitive to the effects of nitrates.

Sublingual glyceryl trinitrate below provides rapid symptomatic relief of angina, but its effect lasts only for 20 to 30 minutes. The *aerosol* spray provides an alternative method of rapid relief of symptoms for those who find difficulty in dissolving sublingual preparations. *Transdermal* preparations are used for the prophylaxis of angina; duration of action may be prolonged (but tolerance may develop).

Isosorbide dinitrate p. 254 is effective by mouth for the prophylaxis and treatment of angina; although the effect is slower in onset, it may persist for several hours. *Modified-release* preparations can have a duration of action up to 12 hours. The activity of isosorbide dinitrate may depend on the production of active metabolites, the most important of which is isosorbide mononitrate p. 254. Isosorbide mononitrate itself is licensed for the prophylaxis of angina; *modified-release* preparations (for once daily administration) are available.

Glyceryl trinitrate *intravenous injection* is licensed for the treatment of unstable angina and coronary insufficiency when the sublingual form is ineffective. Glyceryl trinitrate and isosorbide dinitrate intravenous injections are licensed for the treatment of heart failure.

Nitrates 

- **CONTRA-INDICATIONS** Aortic stenosis · cardiac tamponade · constrictive pericarditis · hypertrophic cardiomyopathy · hypotensive conditions · hypovolaemia · marked anaemia · mitral stenosis · raised intracranial pressure due to cerebral haemorrhage · raised intracranial pressure due to head trauma · toxic pulmonary oedema

- **CAUTIONS** Heart failure due to obstruction · hypothermia · hypothyroidism · hypoxaemia · malnutrition · metal-containing transdermal systems should be removed before magnetic resonance imaging procedures, cardioversion, or diathermy · recent history of myocardial infarction · susceptibility to angle-closure glaucoma · tolerance · ventilation and perfusion abnormalities

  CAUTIONS, FURTHER INFORMATION
  ▶ Tolerance Many patients on long-acting or transdermal nitrates rapidly develop tolerance (with reduced therapeutic effects). Reduction of blood-nitrate concentrations to low levels for 4 to 12 hours each day usually maintains effectiveness in such patients. If tolerance is suspected during the use of transdermal patches they should be left off for 8–12 hours (usually overnight) in each 24 hours; in the case of modified-release tablets of isosorbide dinitrate (and conventional formulations of isosorbide mononitrate), the second of the two daily doses should be given after about 8 hours rather than after 12 hours. Conventional formulations of isosorbide mononitrate should not usually be given more than twice daily unless small doses are used; modified-release formulations of isosorbide mononitrate should only be given once daily, and used in this way do not produce tolerance.
  ▶ Elderly Screening Tool of Older Persons' potentially inappropriate Prescriptions (STOPP) criteria to aid medication reviews (see Prescribing in the elderly p. 31 for information): potentially inappropriate if prescribed a **long-acting** nitrate with persistent postural hypotension i.e. recurrent drop in systolic blood pressure ≥ 20 mmHg (risk of syncope and falls).

- **SIDE-EFFECTS**
  ▶ **Common or very common** Arrhythmias · asthenia · cerebral ischaemia · dizziness · drowsiness · flushing · headache · hypotension · nausea · vomiting
  ▶ **Uncommon** Circulatory collapse · diarrhoea · skin reactions · syncope

- **ALLERGY AND CROSS-SENSITIVITY** [EvGr] Contra-indicated in nitrate hypersensitivity. Ⓜ

- **BREAST FEEDING** No information available—manufacturers advise use only if potential benefit outweighs risk.

- **HEPATIC IMPAIRMENT** In general, manufacturers advise caution in severe impairment.

- **RENAL IMPAIRMENT** In general, manufacturers advise caution in severe impairment.

- **MONITORING REQUIREMENTS** Monitor blood pressure and heart rate during intravenous infusion.

- **TREATMENT CESSATION** Avoid abrupt withdrawal.

⚑ above

Glyceryl trinitrate

07-Jan-2025

- **INDICATIONS AND DOSE**
  Prophylaxis of angina
  ▶ BY SUBLINGUAL ADMINISTRATION USING SUBLINGUAL TABLETS
  ▶ Adult: 1 tablet, to be administered prior to activity likely to cause angina

Treatment of angina
▸ BY SUBLINGUAL ADMINISTRATION USING SUBLINGUAL TABLETS
▸ Adult: 1 tablet, dose may be repeated at 5 minute intervals if symptoms have not resolved, up to a maximum of 3 tablets in total; seek urgent medical attention if symptoms have not resolved 5 minutes after the second dose, or earlier if the pain is intensifying or the person is unwell

Prophylaxis of angina
▸ BY SUBLINGUAL ADMINISTRATION USING AEROSOL SPRAY
▸ Adult: 1–2 sprays, to be administered under the tongue and then close mouth prior to activity likely to cause angina

Treatment of angina
▸ BY SUBLINGUAL ADMINISTRATION USING AEROSOL SPRAY
▸ Adult: 1–2 sprays, to be administered under the tongue and then close mouth, dose may be repeated at 5 minute intervals if symptoms have not resolved, up to a maximum of 3 sprays in total; seek urgent medical attention if symptoms have not resolved 5 minutes after the second dose, or earlier if the pain is intensifying or the person is unwell

Control of hypertension and myocardial ischaemia during and after cardiac surgery | Induction of controlled hypotension during surgery | Congestive heart failure | Unstable angina
▸ BY INTRAVENOUS INFUSION
▸ Adult: 10–200 micrograms/minute (max. per dose 400 micrograms/minute), adjusted according to response, consult product literature for recommended starting doses specific to indication

Anal fissure
▸ BY RECTUM USING OINTMENT
▸ Adult: Apply 2.5 centimetres every 12 hours until pain stops. Max. duration of use 8 weeks, apply to anal canal, 2.5 cm of ointment contains 1.5 mg of glyceryl trinitrate

DOSE EQUIVALENCE AND CONVERSION
▸ With sublingual use
▸ 1 spray contains 400 micrograms glyceryl trinitrate. 1 tablet contains either 500 micrograms or 600 micrograms glyceryl trinitrate.

DEPONIT ®

Prophylaxis of angina
▸ BY TRANSDERMAL APPLICATION
▸ Adult: One '5' or one '10' patch to be applied to lateral chest wall, upper arm, thigh, abdomen, or shoulder; increase to two '10' patches every 24 hours if necessary, to be replaced every 24 hours, siting replacement patch on different area

MINITRAN ®

Prophylaxis of angina
▸ BY TRANSDERMAL APPLICATION
▸ Adult: One '5' patch to be applied to chest or upper arm; replace every 24 hours, siting replacement patch on different area, dose to be adjusted according to response

Maintenance of venous patency ('5' patch only)
▸ BY TRANSDERMAL APPLICATION
▸ Adult: (consult product literature)

NITRO-DUR ®

Prophylaxis of angina
▸ BY TRANSDERMAL APPLICATION
▸ Adult: One '0.2mg/h' patch to be applied to chest or outer upper arm and replaced every 24 hours, siting replacement patch on different area, dose adjusted according to response; maximum 15 mg per day

TRANSIDERM-NITRO ®

Prophylaxis of angina
▸ BY TRANSDERMAL APPLICATION
▸ Adult: One '5' or one '10' patch to be applied to lateral chest wall and replaced every 24 hours, siting replacement patch on different area, max. two '10' patches daily

Prophylaxis of phlebitis and extravasation ('5' patch only)
▸ BY TRANSDERMAL APPLICATION
▸ Adult: (consult product literature)

● INTERACTIONS → Appendix 1: nitrates

● SIDE-EFFECTS
▸ **Uncommon**
▸ With parenteral use Cardiac disorder · cyanosis
▸ With rectal use Anorectal disorder · anorectal haemorrhage · gastrointestinal discomfort
▸ With sublingual use Cyanosis
▸ **Rare or very rare**
▸ With parenteral or sublingual use Methaemoglobinaemia · respiratory disorder · restlessness
▸ With topical use Dyspepsia
▸ **Frequency not known**
▸ With parenteral use Hyperhidrosis
▸ With rectal use Vertigo
▸ With sublingual use Tongue blistering
▸ With transdermal use Palpitations

● PREGNANCY Not known to be harmful.

● DIRECTIONS FOR ADMINISTRATION For *intravenous infusion*, give continuously in Glucose 5% or Sodium Chloride 0.9%, suggested infusion concentration 100 micrograms/mL; incompatible with polyvinyl chloride infusion containers such as *Viaflex* ® or *Steriflex* ®; use glass or polyethylene containers or give via a syringe pump.
   Glass or polyethylene apparatus is preferable; loss of potency will occur if PVC is used. Glyceryl trinitrate 1 mg/mL to be diluted before use or given undiluted with syringe pump. Glyceryl trinitrate 5 mg/mL to be diluted before use.

● PRESCRIBING AND DISPENSING INFORMATION Glyceryl trinitrate tablets are available in strengths of 500- and 600-micrograms—tablets should be supplied in glass containers of not more than 100 tablets, closed with a foil-lined cap, and containing no cotton wool wadding; they should be discarded after 8 weeks in use.

● PATIENT AND CARER ADVICE Rectal ointment should be discarded 8 weeks after first opening.

● NATIONAL FUNDING/ACCESS DECISIONS
For full details see funding body website
Scottish Medicines Consortium (SMC) decisions
▸ Glyceryl trinitrate 0.4% ointment (*Rectogesic* ®) for relief of pain associated with chronic anal fissure (February 2008) SMC No. 200/05 Not recommended

● MEDICINAL FORMS There can be variation in the licensing of different medicines containing the same drug. Forms available from special-order manufacturers include: solution for infusion
Solution for infusion
EXCIPIENTS: May contain Ethanol, propylene glycol
▸ Glyceryl trinitrate (Non-proprietary)
   Glyceryl trinitrate 1 mg per 1 ml Glyceryl trinitrate 10mg/10ml solution for infusion ampoules | 10 ampoule PoM £34.80
   Glyceryl trinitrate 50mg/50ml solution for infusion vials | 1 vial PoM £21.00 (Hospital only) | 10 vial PoM £250.00
   Glyceryl trinitrate 5 mg per 1 ml Glyceryl trinitrate 50mg/10ml solution for infusion ampoules | 5 ampoule PoM £64.90 (Hospital only)
   Glyceryl trinitrate 25mg/5ml solution for infusion ampoules | 5 ampoule PoM £32.45 (Hospital only)
▸ Nitronal (Beaumont Pharma Ltd)
   Glyceryl trinitrate 1 mg per 1 ml Nitronal 50mg/50ml solution for infusion vials | 1 vial PoM £17.40

2

Cardiovascular system

Sublingual tablet
CAUTIONARY AND ADVISORY LABELS 16
- Glyceryl trinitrate (Non-proprietary)
  Glyceryl trinitrate 500 microgram Glyceryl trinitrate 500microgram sublingual tablets | 100 tablet P £10.51 DT = £10.51
  Glyceryl trinitrate 600 microgram Glyceryl trinitrate 600microgram sublingual tablets | 100 tablet P ⊠

Transdermal patch
- Deponit (Forum Health Products Ltd)
  Glyceryl trinitrate 5 mg per 24 hour Deponit 5 transdermal patches | 28 patch P £12.77 DT = £12.77
  Glyceryl trinitrate 10 mg per 24 hour Deponit 10 transdermal patches | 28 patch P £14.06 DT = £14.06
- Minitran (Viatris UK Healthcare Ltd)
  Glyceryl trinitrate 5 mg per 24 hour Minitran 5 transdermal patches | 30 patch P £11.62
  Glyceryl trinitrate 10 mg per 24 hour Minitran 10 transdermal patches | 30 patch P £12.87

Rectal ointment
EXCIPIENTS: May contain Propylene glycol, woolfat and related substances (including lanolin)
- Rectogesic (Kyowa Kirin International UK NewCo Ltd)
  Glyceryl trinitrate 4 mg per 1 gram Rectogesic 0.4% rectal ointment | 30 gram PoM £39.30 DT = £39.30

Sublingual spray
- Glyceryl trinitrate (Non-proprietary)
  Glyceryl trinitrate 400 microgram per 1 dose Glyceryl trinitrate 400micrograms/dose pump sublingual spray | 180 dose P £3.60 DT = £3.41 | 200 dose P £3.44–£3.90 DT = £3.78
- Nitrolingual (Beaumont Pharma Ltd)
  Glyceryl trinitrate 400 microgram per 1 dose Nitrolingual 400micrograms/dose pump sublingual spray | 75 dose P £2.75 DT = £2.75 (Hospital only) | 180 dose P £3.41 DT = £3.41 | 200 dose P £3.78 DT = £3.78

☞ 252

Isosorbide dinitrate

21-Jul-2020

● INDICATIONS AND DOSE
Prophylaxis and treatment of angina
- BY MOUTH USING IMMEDIATE-RELEASE MEDICINES
- Adult: 30–120 mg daily in divided doses
- BY INTRAVENOUS INFUSION
- Adult: 2–10 mg/hour, increased if necessary up to 20 mg/hour
- BY SUBLINGUAL ADMINISTRATION USING AEROSOL SPRAY
- Adult: 1–3 sprays, to be administered under tongue whilst holding breath, allow a 30 second interval between each dose

Left ventricular failure
- BY MOUTH USING IMMEDIATE-RELEASE MEDICINES
- Adult: 40–160 mg daily in divided doses, increased if necessary up to 240 mg daily in divided doses
- BY INTRAVENOUS INFUSION
- Adult: Initially 2–10 mg/hour, increased if necessary up to 20 mg/hour

Prophylaxis of angina
- BY MOUTH USING MODIFIED-RELEASE MEDICINES
- Adult: 40 mg daily in 1–2 divided doses, increased if necessary to 60–80 mg daily in 2–3 divided doses

- ● INTERACTIONS → Appendix 1: nitrates
- ● SIDE-EFFECTS
- **Common or very common**
- With oral use Peripheral oedema
- **Rare or very rare**
- With oral use Angioedema · angle closure glaucoma · hypoventilation · hypoxia · pituitary haemorrhage · Stevens-Johnson syndrome

- ● PREGNANCY May cross placenta—manufacturers advise avoid unless potential benefit outweighs risk.
- ● DIRECTIONS FOR ADMINISTRATION For *intravenous infusion*, manufacturer advises give continuously in Glucose 5% or Sodium Chloride 0.9%. Adsorbed to some

extent by polyvinyl chloride infusion containers; preferably use glass or polyethylene containers or give via a syringe pump; 0.05% strength can alternatively be administered undiluted using a syringe pump with a glass or rigid plastic syringe. Glass or polyethylene infusion apparatus is preferable; loss of potency if PVC used.

- ● MEDICINAL FORMS There can be variation in the licensing of different medicines containing the same drug. Forms available from special-order manufacturers include: oral suspension, oral solution

Oral tablet
- Isosorbide dinitrate (Non-proprietary)
  Isosorbide dinitrate 10 mg Isosorbide dinitrate 10mg tablets | 56 tablet P £34.00 DT = £17.56
  Isosorbide dinitrate 20 mg Isosorbide dinitrate 20mg tablets | 56 tablet P £70.00 DT = £17.74

Modified-release tablet
CAUTIONARY AND ADVISORY LABELS 25
- Isoket Retard (Forum Health Products Ltd)
  Isosorbide dinitrate 20 mg Isoket Retard 20 tablets | 60 tablet P £3.04 DT = £3.04

Solution for injection
- Isosorbide dinitrate (Non-proprietary)
  Isosorbide dinitrate 1 mg per 1 ml Isosorbide dinitrate 10mg/10ml concentrate for solution for injection ampoules | 10 ampoule £64.30 (Hospital only)
- Isoket (Forum Health Products Ltd)
  Isosorbide dinitrate 1 mg per 1 ml Isoket 0.1% solution for injection 10ml ampoules | 10 ampoule PoM £26.93 (Hospital only)

Solution for infusion
- Isosorbide dinitrate (Non-proprietary)
  Isosorbide dinitrate 500 microgram per 1 ml Isosorbide dinitrate 25mg/50ml solution for infusion vials | 10 vial PoM £109.30
  Isosorbide dinitrate 1 mg per 1 ml Isosorbide dinitrate 50mg/50ml concentrate for solution for infusion vials | 10 vial PoM £141.40

☞ 252

Isosorbide mononitrate

20-Feb-2021

● INDICATIONS AND DOSE
Prophylaxis of angina | Adjunct in congestive heart failure
- BY MOUTH USING IMMEDIATE-RELEASE MEDICINES
- Adult: Initially 20 mg 2–3 times a day, alternatively initially 40 mg twice daily, increased if necessary up to 120 mg daily in divided doses

Prophylaxis of angina (for patients who have not previously had a nitrate) | Adjunct in congestive heart failure (for patients who have not previously had a nitrate)
- BY MOUTH USING IMMEDIATE-RELEASE MEDICINES
- Adult: Initially 10 mg twice daily, increased if necessary up to 120 mg daily in divided doses

CHEMYDUR ® 60XL

Prophylaxis of angina
- BY MOUTH
- Adult: Initially 0.5 tablet daily for 2–4 days, to minimise possibility of headache, then 1 tablet daily, increased if necessary to 2 tablets daily, dose to be taken in the morning

ELANTAN ® LA

Prophylaxis of angina
- BY MOUTH
- Adult: 25–50 mg once daily, then increased if necessary to 50–100 mg once daily, dose to be taken in the morning, the lowest effective dose should be used

IMDUR ®

Prophylaxis of angina
- BY MOUTH
- Adult: Initially 0.5 tablet once daily, to minimise the occurrence of headache, then 1 tablet once daily, then

2

Cardiovascular system

increased if necessary to 2 tablets once daily, dose to be taken in the morning

ISIB ® 60XL

Prophylaxis of angina

▸ BY MOUTH

▸ Adult: Initially 0.5 tablet once daily for 2–4 days, to minimise the occurrence of headache, then 1 tablet once daily, increased if necessary to 2 tablets once daily, dose to be taken in the morning

ISMO RETARD ®

Prophylaxis of angina

▸ BY MOUTH

▸ Adult: 1 tablet once daily, dose to be taken in the morning

ISODUR ®

Prophylaxis of angina

▸ BY MOUTH

▸ Adult: 25–50 mg once daily, then increased if necessary to 50–100 mg once daily, dose to be taken in the morning

ISOTARD ®

Prophylaxis of angina

▸ BY MOUTH

▸ Adult: 25–60 mg once daily, if headaches occur with 60 mg tablet, half a 60 mg tablet may be given for 2–4 days, then increased if necessary to 50–120 mg once daily, dose to be taken in the morning

MODISAL ® XL

Prophylaxis of angina

▸ BY MOUTH

▸ Adult: Initially 0.5 tablet once daily for 2–4 days, to minimise the occurrence of headache, then 1 tablet once daily, increased if necessary to 2 tablets once daily, dose to be taken in the morning

MONOMAX ® XL

Prophylaxis of angina

▸ BY MOUTH

▸ Adult: Initially 0.5 tablet once daily for 2–4 days, to minimise occurrence of headache, then 1 tablet once daily, increased if necessary to 2 tablets once daily, dose to be taken in the morning

MONOMIL ® XL

Prophylaxis of angina

▸ BY MOUTH

▸ Adult: Initially 0.5 tablet daily for 2–4 days, to minimise possibility of headache, then 1 tablet daily, increased if necessary to 2 tablets once daily, to be taken in the morning

MONOSORB ® XL60

Prophylaxis of angina

▸ BY MOUTH

▸ Adult: Initially 0.5 tablet once daily for the first 2–4 days, to minimise the occurrence of headache, then 1 tablet once daily, increased if necessary to 2 tablets once daily, dose to be taken in the morning

ZEMON ®

Prophylaxis of angina

▸ BY MOUTH

▸ Adult: Initially 30 mg once daily for 2–4 days, to minimise the occurrence of headache, then 40–60 mg once daily, increased if necessary to 80–120 mg once daily, dose to be taken in the morning

● INTERACTIONS → Appendix 1: nitrates

● SIDE-EFFECTS

▸ **Rare or very rare** Myalgia

● PREGNANCY Manufacturers advise avoid unless potential benefit outweighs risk.

● MEDICINAL FORMS There can be variation in the licensing of different medicines containing the same drug. Forms available from special-order manufacturers include: oral suspension, oral solution

Oral tablet

CAUTIONARY AND ADVISORY LABELS 25

▸ **Isosorbide mononitrate (Non-proprietary)**
Isosorbide mononitrate 10 mg Isosorbide mononitrate 10mg tablets | 56 tablet [PoM] £13.10 DT = £1.19
Isosorbide mononitrate 20 mg Isosorbide mononitrate 20mg tablets | 56 tablet [PoM] £13.88 DT = £1.23
Isosorbide mononitrate 30 mg Isosorbide mononitrate 30mg tablets | 56 tablet [P] £6.00-£8.00 DT = £6.00
Isosorbide mononitrate 40 mg Isosorbide mononitrate 40mg tablets | 56 tablet [PoM] £2.55-£20.55 DT = £1.62

Modified-release tablet

CAUTIONARY AND ADVISORY LABELS 25

▸ **Chemydur 60XL** (Advanz Pharma)
Isosorbide mononitrate 60 mg Chemydur 60XL tablets | 28 tablet [P] £3.49 DT = £10.50

▸ **Imdur** (TopRidge Pharma (Ireland) Ltd)
Isosorbide mononitrate 60 mg Imdur 60mg modified-release tablets | 28 tablet [P] £10.50 DT = £10.50

▸ **Ismo Retard** (Esteve Pharmaceuticals Ltd)
Isosorbide mononitrate 40 mg Ismo Retard 40mg tablets | 30 tablet [P] £10.71

▸ **Isotard XL** (Evolan Pharma AB)
Isosorbide mononitrate 25 mg Isotard 25XL tablets | 28 tablet [P] £6.75 DT = £6.75
Isosorbide mononitrate 40 mg Isotard 40XL tablets | 28 tablet [P] £6.75 DT = £6.75
Isosorbide mononitrate 50 mg Isotard 50XL tablets | 28 tablet [P] £6.75 DT = £6.75
Isosorbide mononitrate 60 mg Isotard 60XL tablets | 28 tablet [P] £5.75 DT = £10.50

▸ **Modisal XL** (Ennogen Healthcare International Ltd)
Isosorbide mononitrate 40 mg Modisal XL 40mg tablets | 28 tablet [PoM] £5.40 DT = £6.75

▸ **Monomax XL** (Chiesi Ltd)
Isosorbide mononitrate 60 mg Monomax XL 60mg tablets | 28 tablet [P] £5.25 DT = £10.50

▸ **Monomil XL** (Teva UK Ltd)
Isosorbide mononitrate 60 mg Monomil XL 60mg tablets | 28 tablet [P] £3.49 DT = £10.50

▸ **Monosorb XL** (Dexcel-Pharma Ltd)
Isosorbide mononitrate 60 mg Monosorb XL 60 tablets | 28 tablet [P] £15.53 DT = £10.50

▸ **Relosorb XL** (Relonchem Ltd)
Isosorbide mononitrate 60 mg Relosorb XL 60mg tablets | 28 tablet [PoM] £22.45 DT = £10.50

▸ **Xismox XL** (Genus Pharmaceuticals Ltd)
Isosorbide mononitrate 60 mg Xismox XL 60 tablets | 28 tablet [PoM] £5.51 DT = £10.50

Modified-release capsule

CAUTIONARY AND ADVISORY LABELS 25

▸ **Elantan LA** (Forum Health Products Ltd)
Isosorbide mononitrate 25 mg Elantan LA25 capsules | 28 capsule [P] £4.22 DT = £4.22
Isosorbide mononitrate 50 mg Elantan LA50 capsules | 28 capsule [P] £5.53 DT = £5.53

▸ **Isodur XL** (Galen Ltd)
Isosorbide mononitrate 25 mg Isodur 25XL capsules | 28 capsule [P] £4.63 DT = £4.22
Isosorbide mononitrate 50 mg Isodur 50XL capsules | 28 capsule [P] £6.45 DT = £5.53

▸ **Monomax SR** (Martindale Pharmaceuticals Ltd)
Isosorbide mononitrate 40 mg Nyzamac SR 40mg capsules | 28 capsule [P] £6.52 DT = £6.52
Isosorbide mononitrate 60 mg Nyzamac SR 60mg capsules | 28 capsule [P] £8.86 DT = £8.86

9.1a Cardiac arrest

Cardiopulmonary resuscitation

05-May-2021

Overview

The algorithm for cardiopulmonary resuscitation (Life support algorithm (image) Inside back cover) reflects the most recent recommendations of the Resuscitation Council (UK); this has been reproduced with the kind permission of the Resuscitation Council (UK). The guidelines are available at www.resus.org.uk.

Cardiac arrest can be associated with ventricular fibrillation, pulseless ventricular tachycardia, asystole, and pulseless electrical activity. Adrenaline/epinephrine 1 in 10000 (100 micrograms/mL) below is recommended by intravenous injection repeated every 3–5 minutes if necessary. Intravenous injection of amiodarone hydrochloride p. 120 should also be given to treat ventricular fibrillation or pulseless ventricular tachycardia in cardiac arrest refractory to defibrillation. An additional dose of amiodarone hydrochloride can be given if necessary. Lidocaine hydrochloride p. 117, is an alternative if amiodarone is not available or a local decision has been made to use lidocaine instead.

During cardiopulmonary arrest if intravenous access cannot be obtained, the intraosseous route can be used instead.

For the management of acute anaphylaxis, see allergic emergencies under Antihistamines, allergen immunotherapy and allergic emergencies p. 316.

SYMPATHOMIMETICS › VASOCONSTRICTOR

Adrenaline/epinephrine

10-Apr-2025

● DRUG ACTION Acts on both alpha and beta receptors and increases both heart rate and contractility (beta$_1$ effects); it can cause peripheral vasodilation (a beta$_2$ effect) or vasoconstriction (an alpha effect).

● INDICATIONS AND DOSE

Cardiopulmonary resuscitation (specialist use only)
▶ BY SLOW INTRAVENOUS INJECTION
▶ Child: 10 micrograms/kg every 3–5 minutes (max. per dose 1 mg) as required, a 1 in 10 000 (100 micrograms/mL) solution is recommended, suitable syringe to be used for measuring small volume
▶ Adult: 1 mg every 3–5 minutes as required, a 1 in 10 000 (100 micrograms/mL) solution is recommended

Acute hypotension
▶ BY CONTINUOUS INTRAVENOUS INFUSION
▶ Neonate: Initially 100 nanograms/kg/minute, to be adjusted according to response, higher doses up to 1.5 micrograms/kg/minute have been used in acute hypotension.

▶ Child: Initially 100 nanograms/kg/minute, to be adjusted according to response, higher doses up to 1.5 micrograms/kg/minute have been used in acute hypotension

Emergency treatment of acute anaphylaxis (under expert supervision)
▶ BY INTRAMUSCULAR INJECTION
▶ Child up to 6 months: 100–150 micrograms, using adrenaline 1 in 1000 (1 mg/mL) injection, repeat dose after 5 minutes if no response; if life-threatening features persist, further doses can be given every

5 minutes until specialist critical care available, suitable syringe to be used for measuring small volume; injected preferably into the anterolateral aspect of the middle third of the thigh
▶ Child 6 months-5 years: 150 micrograms, using adrenaline 1 in 1000 (1 mg/mL) injection, repeat dose after 5 minutes if no response; if life-threatening features persist, further doses can be given every 5 minutes until specialist critical care available, suitable syringe to be used for measuring small volume; injected preferably into the anterolateral aspect of the middle third of the thigh
▶ Child 6-11 years: 300 micrograms, using adrenaline 1 in 1000 (1 mg/mL) injection, repeat dose after 5 minutes if no response; if life-threatening features persist, further doses can be given every 5 minutes until specialist critical care available, to be injected preferably into the anterolateral aspect of the middle third of the thigh
▶ Child 12-17 years: 500 micrograms, using adrenaline 1 in 1000 (1 mg/mL) injection, repeat dose after 5 minutes if no response; if life-threatening features persist, further doses can be given every 5 minutes until specialist critical care available, to be injected preferably into the anterolateral aspect of the middle third of the thigh, 300 micrograms to be administered if child is small or prepubertal
▶ Adult: 500 micrograms, using adrenaline 1 in 1000 (1 mg/mL) injection, repeat dose after 5 minutes if no response; if life-threatening features persist, further doses can be given every 5 minutes until specialist critical care available, to be injected preferably into the anterolateral aspect of the middle third of the thigh

Refractory anaphylaxis [persistent symptoms despite at least 2 appropriate doses of intramuscular adrenaline/epinephrine] (specialist use only)
▶ BY INTRAVENOUS INFUSION
▶ Adult: Consult Resuscitation Council (UK) emergency treatment of anaphylaxis guideline or local protocols

Control of bradycardia in patients with arrhythmias after myocardial infarction, if there is a risk of asystole, or if the patient is unstable and has failed to respond to atropine
▶ BY CONTINUOUS INTRAVENOUS INFUSION
▶ Adult: 2–10 micrograms/minute, to be adjusted according to response

EPIPEN ® AUTO-INJECTOR 0.3MG

Acute anaphylaxis (for self-administration at the first signs of anaphylaxis)
▶ BY INTRAMUSCULAR INJECTION
▶ Child (body-weight 25 kg and above): 300 micrograms, then 300 micrograms after 5 minutes as required
▶ Adult: 300 micrograms, then 300 micrograms after 5 minutes as required

EPIPEN ® JR AUTO-INJECTOR 0.15MG

Acute anaphylaxis (for self-administration at the first signs of anaphylaxis)
▶ BY INTRAMUSCULAR INJECTION
▶ Child (body-weight up to 15 kg): 150 micrograms, then 150 micrograms after 5 minutes as required
▶ Child (body-weight 15-24 kg): 150 micrograms, then 150 micrograms after 5 minutes as required, on the basis of a dose of 10 micrograms/kg, 300 micrograms may be more appropriate for some children

JEXT ® 150 MICROGRAMS

Acute anaphylaxis (for self-administration at the first signs of anaphylaxis)
▶ BY INTRAMUSCULAR INJECTION
▶ Child (body-weight up to 15 kg): 150 micrograms, then 150 micrograms after 5 minutes as required

▶ Child (body-weight 15-24 kg): 150 micrograms, then 150 micrograms after 5 minutes as required, on the basis of a dose of 10 micrograms/kg, 300 micrograms may be more appropriate for some children

JEXT ® 300 MICROGRAMS

Acute anaphylaxis (for self-administration at the first signs of anaphylaxis)
▶ BY INTRAMUSCULAR INJECTION
▶ Child (body-weight 25 kg and above): 300 micrograms, then 300 micrograms after 5 minutes as required
▶ Adult: 300 micrograms, then 300 micrograms after 5 minutes as required

● UNLICENSED USE
▶ With intramuscular use for Acute anaphylaxis (for self-administration at the first signs of anaphylaxis) in children EvGr Adrenaline, given via an auto-injector, is used in the doses provided in BNF Publications, but these may differ from those licensed. E
▶ With intravenous use in children EvGr Adrenaline is used for cardiopulmonary resuscitation in neonates and infants with body-weight under 5 kg, A but it is not licensed for this age group.
▶ With intravenous use for Acute hypotension in children Adrenaline 1 in 1000 (1 mg/mL) solution is not licensed for intravenous administration.
▶ With intramuscular use in children EvGr Adrenaline is used in the doses provided in BNF Publications for the emergency treatment of acute anaphylaxis in children up to 6 months, A but these may differ from those licensed.

IMPORTANT SAFETY INFORMATION

SAFE PRACTICE
Intravenous route should be used with **extreme care** by specialists only.

MHRA/CHM ADVICE: ADRENALINE AUTO-INJECTORS: UPDATED ADVICE AFTER EUROPEAN REVIEW (AUGUST 2017)
Following a European review of all adrenaline auto-injectors approved in the EU, the MHRA recommend that 2 adrenaline auto-injectors are prescribed, which patients should carry at all times. This is particularly important for patients with allergic asthma, who are at increased risk of a severe anaphylactic reaction. Patients with allergies and their carers should be trained to use the particular auto-injector they have been prescribed and encouraged to practise using a trainer device. Patients are advised to check the expiry date of the adrenaline auto-injectors and obtain replacements before they expire.

NATIONAL PATIENT SAFETY ALERT: RECALL OF *EMERADE*® 500 MICROGRAMS AND *EMERADE*® 300 MICROGRAMS AUTO-INJECTORS DUE TO THE POTENTIAL FOR DEVICE FAILURE (MAY 2023)
All unexpired batches of *Emerade*® 500 micrograms and *Emerade*® 300 micrograms adrenaline auto-injectors (also referred to as pens) have been recalled as a precautionary measure due to an issue identified by the manufacturer where some auto-injectors failed to deliver adrenaline or activated prematurely after being dropped. Future production of these preparations is on hold and no further supplies will be available; patients should be switched to an equivalent strength adrenaline auto-injector in an alternative brand— *EpiPen*® **300 micrograms** or *Jext*® **300 micrograms** are appropriate alternatives to *Emerade*® **500 micrograms**. This recall also applies to schools, and to adrenaline auto-injectors held by healthcare professionals, such as in emergency anaphylaxis kits and dental kits; anaphylaxis kits in the healthcare setting should be restocked with adrenaline ampoules (together with dosing charts for use of intramuscular adrenaline to treat

2

Cardiovascular system

anaphylaxis, needles and syringes) and **not** auto-injectors. Patients and their carers should be advised:
● to carry 2 in-date adrenaline auto-injectors with them at all times in case a second dose needs to be administered before the arrival of emergency services;
● that they need to receive training so that they are confident in using any new devices—instructions for use can be found in patient information leaflets and training videos on respective manufacturers' websites;
● of the signs and symptoms of anaphylaxis and the actions they should take immediately;
● that the risk of mishandling or failure exists with all adrenaline auto-injectors, and that a second adrenaline auto-injector should be used immediately if the first fails to activate, despite pressing firmly against the thigh. If the patient is not improving, further attempts to activate a failed auto-injector should be made even if one auto-injector has worked, as this may suggest a need for further doses while waiting for emergency services.
Healthcare professionals and patients are strongly recommended to order a trainer device from the manufacturer to ensure they are familiar with use and prepared for an emergency.
    For further information, refer to the National Patient Safety Alert available at: www.gov.uk/drug-device-alerts/national-patient-safety-alert-class-1-medicines-recall-notification-recall-of-emerade-500-micrograms-and-emerade-300-micrograms-auto-injectors-due-to-the-potential-for-device-failure-natpsa-slash-2023-slash-004-slash-mhra.

● CAUTIONS Arteriosclerosis (in adults) · arrhythmias · cerebrovascular disease · cor pulmonale · diabetes mellitus · elderly · hypercalcaemia · hyperreflexia · hypertension · hyperthyroidism · hypokalaemia · ischaemic heart disease · obstructive cardiomyopathy · occlusive vascular disease · organic brain damage · phaeochromocytoma · prostate disorders · psychoneurosis · severe angina · susceptibility to angle-closure glaucoma
CAUTIONS, FURTHER INFORMATION Cautions listed are only for non-life-threatening situations.
● INTERACTIONS → Appendix 1: sympathomimetics, vasoconstrictor
● SIDE-EFFECTS
GENERAL SIDE-EFFECTS
▶ **Rare or very rare** Cardiomyopathy
▶ **Frequency not known** Angina pectoris · angle closure glaucoma · anxiety · appetite decreased · arrhythmias · asthenia · CNS haemorrhage · confusion · dizziness · dry mouth · dyspnoea · headache · hepatic necrosis · hyperglycaemia · hyperhidrosis · hypersalivation · hypertension (increased risk of cerebral haemorrhage) · hypokalaemia · injection site necrosis · insomnia · intestinal necrosis · metabolic acidosis · mydriasis · myocardial infarction · nausea · pallor · palpitations · peripheral coldness · psychosis · pulmonary oedema (on excessive dosage or extreme sensitivity) · renal necrosis · soft tissue necrosis · tremor · urinary disorders · vomiting
SPECIFIC SIDE-EFFECTS
▶ With intramuscular use Muscle necrosis · necrotising fasciitis · peripheral ischaemia
▶ With intravenous use Hemiplegia · muscle rigidity
● PREGNANCY May reduce placental perfusion and cause tachycardia, cardiac irregularities, and extrasystoles in fetus. Can delay second stage of labour. Manufacturers advise use only if benefit outweighs risk.
● BREAST FEEDING Present in milk but unlikely to be harmful as poor oral bioavailability.
● RENAL IMPAIRMENT Manufacturers advise use with caution in severe impairment.

2

Cardiovascular system

- **MONITORING REQUIREMENTS** Monitor blood pressure and ECG.
- **DIRECTIONS FOR ADMINISTRATION**
  ▸ With intravenous use for Acute hypotension in children For *continuous intravenous infusion*, expert sources advise dilute with Glucose 5% or Sodium Chloride 0.9% and give through a central venous catheter. Incompatible with bicarbonate and alkaline solutions. *Neonatal intensive care*, expert sources advise dilute 3 mg/kg body-weight to a final volume of 50 mL with infusion fluid; an intravenous infusion rate of 0.1 mL/hour provides a dose of 100 nanograms/kg/minute; infuse through a central venous catheter. Incompatible with bicarbonate and alkaline solutions. Expert sources advise these infusions are usually made up with adrenaline 1 in 1000 (1 mg/mL) solution.
- **PRESCRIBING AND DISPENSING INFORMATION**
  ▸ With intramuscular use It is important, in acute anaphylaxis where intramuscular injection might still succeed, time should not be wasted seeking intravenous access. Great vigilance is needed to ensure that the *correct strength* of adrenaline injection is used; anaphylactic shock kits need to make a *very clear distinction* between the 1 in 10 000 strength and the 1 in 1000 strength. Patients with severe allergy should be instructed in the self-administration of adrenaline by intramuscular injection. Packs for self-administration need to be **clearly labelled with instructions** on how to administer adrenaline (intramuscularly, preferably at the midpoint of the outer thigh, through light clothing if necessary) so that in the case of rapid collapse someone else is able to give it. Adrenaline for administration by intramuscular injection is available in 'auto-injectors' (e.g. *EpiPen®* or *Jext®*), pre-assembled syringes fitted with a needle suitable for very rapid administration (if necessary by a bystander or a healthcare provider if it is the only preparation available); injection technique is device specific. To ensure patients receive the auto-injector device that they have been trained to use, prescribers should specify the brand to be dispensed. If switching between brands, patients should receive full training in use of the new auto-injector device. Licensed doses differ between brands of adrenaline auto-injectors. Adrenaline bioavailability has the potential to be influenced by a number of factors including formulation, propulsive force of the device, needle length and patient specific factors—consult product literature for further information.
- **PATIENT AND CARER ADVICE**
  ▸ With intramuscular use Patients and carers should be advised on the safe and effective use of adrenaline auto-injector devices in advance and to sign up for expiry alert services—see also *Important safety information*. For further information, see MHRA guidance: Adrenaline Auto-Injectors (AAIs) Safety Campaign at: www.gov.uk/government/publications/adrenaline-auto-injectors-aais-safety-campaign.

  At the first signs of anaphylaxis Patients and carers should be advised the following:
  - Use your adrenaline auto-injector immediately if you have any signs of anaphylaxis. Use even if in doubt of severity, don't delay;
  - Call 999 and say anaphylaxis ("ana-fill-axis")—straight after using your adrenaline auto-injector;
  - Lie down and raise your legs;
  - Use a second adrenaline auto-injector if your symptoms haven't improved after 5 minutes;
  - Lying down is important to keep blood flowing to your organs; you can sit up if you are struggling to breathe, but keep your legs elevated as far as possible and lie back down again as soon as you can. Young children may need to lie down first to help assist injection administration by carer;

- An ambulance should be called even if symptoms appear to be improving after using an adrenaline auto-injector and the individual should not be left alone. The purpose of adrenaline auto-injectors is to start treatment for anaphylaxis that is continued by the emergency services. Medicines for Children leaflet: Adrenaline auto-injector for anaphylaxis www.medicinesforchildren.org.uk/medicines/adrenaline-auto-injector-for-anaphylaxis/

  EPIPEN® AUTO-INJECTOR 0.3MG 1.7 mL of the solution remains in the auto-injector device after use.

  EPIPEN® JR AUTO-INJECTOR 0.15MG 1.7 mL of the solution remains in the auto-injector device after use.

  JEXT® 150 MICROGRAMS 1.25 mL of the solution remains in the auto-injector device after use.

  JEXT® 300 MICROGRAMS 1.1 mL of the solution remains in the auto-injector device after use.

- **EXCEPTIONS TO LEGAL CATEGORY** POM restriction does not apply to the intramuscular administration of up to 1 mg of adrenaline injection 1 in 1000 (1 mg/mL) for the emergency treatment of anaphylaxis.

- **MEDICINAL FORMS** There can be variation in the licensing of different medicines containing the same drug. Forms available from special-order manufacturers include: solution for injection

Solution for injection
EXCIPIENTS: May contain Sulfites
  ▸ **Adrenaline/epinephrine (Non-proprietary)**
    Adrenaline 100 microgram per 1 ml Adrenaline (base) 100micrograms/1ml (1 in 10,000) dilute solution for injection ampoules | 10 ampoule PoM £157.10 DT = £135.55
    Adrenaline (base) 1mg/10ml (1 in 10,000) dilute solution for injection pre-filled syringes | 1 pre-filled disposable injection PoM £7.21-£18.00 (Hospital only) | 10 pre-filled disposable injection PoM £180.00 (Hospital only)
    Adrenaline (as Adrenaline acid tartrate) 100 microgram per 1 ml Adrenaline (base) 1mg/10ml (1 in 10,000) dilute solution for injection ampoules | 10 ampoule PoM £178.37 DT = £157.08
    Adrenaline (base) 500micrograms/5ml (1 in 10,000) dilute solution for injection ampoules | 10 ampoule PoM £148.73 DT = £144.40
    Adrenaline 1 mg per 1 ml Adrenaline (base) 10mg/10ml (1 in 1,000) solution for injection ampoules | 10 ampoule PoM £162.98-£281.10 DT = £162.98
    Adrenaline (base) for anaphylaxis 1mg/1ml (1 in 1,000) solution for injection pre-filled syringes | 1 pre-filled disposable injection PoM £15.77 DT = £15.77
    Adrenaline (base) 1mg/1ml (1 in 1,000) solution for injection pre-filled syringes | 1 pre-filled disposable injection PoM £12.98-£15.77 DT = £15.77
    Adrenaline (as Adrenaline acid tartrate) 1 mg per 1 ml Adrenaline (base) 5mg/5ml (1 in 1,000) solution for injection ampoules | 10 ampoule PoM £199.90 DT = £166.15
    Adrenaline (base) 500micrograms/0.5ml (1 in 1,000) solution for injection ampoules | 10 ampoule PoM £333.46-£533.52 DT = £333.46
    Adrenaline (base) 1mg/1ml (1 in 1,000) solution for injection ampoules | 10 ampoule PoM £11.81 DT = £11.81 (Hospital only) | 10 ampoule PoM £6.00-£11.81 DT = £11.81
  ▸ **EpiPen** (Viatris UK Healthcare Ltd)
    Adrenaline 500 microgram per 1 ml EpiPen Jr. 150micrograms/0.3ml (1 in 2,000) solution for injection auto-injectors | 1 pre-filled disposable injection PoM £60.69 DT = £60.69 | 2 pre-filled disposable injection PoM £121.38 DT = £121.38
    Adrenaline 1 mg per 1 ml EpiPen 300micrograms/0.3ml (1 in 1,000) solution for injection auto-injectors | 1 pre-filled disposable injection PoM £60.69 DT = £60.69 | 2 pre-filled disposable injection PoM £121.38
  ▸ **Jext** (ALK-Abello Ltd)
    Adrenaline 1 mg per 1 ml Jext 300micrograms/0.3ml (1 in 1,000) solution for injection auto-injectors | 1 pre-filled disposable injection PoM £60.69 DT = £60.69
    Adrenaline (as Adrenaline acid tartrate) 1 mg per 1 ml Jext 150micrograms/0.15ml (1 in 1,000) solution for injection auto-injectors | 1 pre-filled disposable injection PoM £60.69 DT = £60.69

10 Oedema

Diuretics

10-Aug-2022

Overview

Thiazides are used to relieve oedema due to chronic heart failure and, in lower doses, to reduce blood pressure.

Loop diuretics are used in pulmonary oedema due to left ventricular failure and in patients with chronic heart failure.

Combination diuretic therapy may be effective in patients with oedema resistant to treatment with one diuretic. Vigorous diuresis, particularly with loop diuretics, may induce acute hypotension; rapid reduction of plasma volume should be avoided.

Thiazides and related diuretics

Thiazides and related compounds are moderately potent diuretics; they inhibit sodium reabsorption at the beginning of the distal convoluted tubule. They act within 1 to 2 hours of oral administration and most have a duration of action of 12 to 24 hours; they are usually administered early in the day so that the diuresis does not interfere with sleep.

In the management of *hypertension* a low dose of a thiazide produces a maximal or near-maximal blood pressure lowering effect, with very little biochemical disturbance. Higher doses cause more marked changes in plasma potassium, sodium, uric acid, glucose, and lipids, with little advantage in blood pressure control. Chlortalidone p. 264 and indapamide p. 194 are the preferred diuretics in the management of hypertension. Thiazides also have a role in chronic heart failure.

Bendroflumethiazide p. 193 can be used for mild or moderate heart failure; it is licensed for the treatment of hypertension but is no longer considered the first-line diuretic for this indication, although patients with stable and controlled blood pressure currently taking bendroflumethiazide can continue treatment.

Chlortalidone, a thiazide-related compound, has a longer duration of action than the thiazides and may be given on alternate days to control oedema. It is also useful if acute retention is liable to be precipitated by a more rapid diuresis or if patients dislike the altered pattern of micturition caused by other diuretics. Chlortalidone can also be used under close supervision for the treatment of ascites due to cirrhosis in stable patients.

Xipamide p. 265 and indapamide are chemically related to chlortalidone. Indapamide is claimed to lower blood pressure with less metabolic disturbance, particularly less aggravation of diabetes mellitus.

Metolazone p. 264 is particularly effective when combined with a loop diuretic (even in renal failure); profound diuresis can occur and the patient should therefore be monitored carefully.

The thiazide diuretics benzthiazide, clopamide, hydrochlorothiazide, and hydroflumethiazide do not offer any significant advantage over other thiazides and related diuretics.

Loop diuretics

Loop diuretics are used in pulmonary oedema due to left ventricular failure; intravenous administration produces relief of breathlessness and reduces pre-load sooner than would be expected from the time of onset of diuresis. Loop diuretics are also used in patients with chronic heart failure. Diuretic-resistant oedema (except lymphoedema and oedema due to peripheral venous stasis or calcium-channel blockers) can be treated with a loop diuretic combined with a thiazide or related diuretic (e.g. bendroflumethiazide or metolazone).

If necessary, a loop diuretic can be added to antihypertensive treatment to achieve better control of blood pressure in those with resistant hypertension, or in patients with impaired renal function or heart failure.

Loop diuretics can exacerbate diabetes (but hyperglycaemia is less likely than with thiazides) and gout. If there is an enlarged prostate, urinary retention can occur, although this is less likely if small doses and less potent diuretics are used initially.

Furosemide p. 261 and bumetanide p. 260 are similar in activity; both act within 1 hour of oral administration and diuresis is complete within 6 hours so that, if necessary, they can be given twice in one day without interfering with sleep. Following intravenous administration furosemide has a peak effect within 30 minutes. The diuresis associated with these drugs is dose related.

Torasemide p. 262 has properties similar to those of furosemide and bumetanide, and is indicated for oedema and for hypertension.

Potassium-sparing diuretics and mineralocorticoid receptor antagonists

Amiloride hydrochloride p. 263 and triamterene p. 264 on their own are weak diuretics. They cause retention of potassium and are therefore given with thiazide or loop diuretics as a more effective alternative to potassium supplements. See compound preparations with thiazides or loop diuretics.

Potassium supplements must **not** be given with potassium- sparing diuretics. Administration of a potassium sparing diuretic to a patient receiving an ACE inhibitor or an angiotensin-II receptor antagonist can also cause severe hyperkalaemia.

Mineralocorticoid receptor antagonists

Spironolactone p. 224 potentiates thiazide or loop diuretics by antagonising aldosterone; it is a potassium-sparing diuretic. Spironolactone is of value in the treatment of oedema and ascites caused by cirrhosis of the liver; furosemide can be used as an adjunct. Low doses of spironolactone are beneficial in moderate to severe heart failure and when used in resistant hypertension [unlicensed indication].

Spironolactone is also used in primary hyperaldosteronism (Conn's syndrome). It is given before surgery or if surgery is not appropriate, in the lowest effective dose for maintenance.

Eplerenone p. 223 is licensed for use as an adjunct in left ventricular dysfunction with evidence of heart failure after a myocardial infarction; it is also licensed as an adjunct in chronic mild heart failure with left ventricular systolic dysfunction.

Potassium supplements must **not** be given with mineralocorticoid receptor antagonists.

Potassium-sparing diuretics with other diuretics

Although it is preferable to prescribe thiazides and potassium-sparing diuretics separately, the use of fixed combinations may be justified if compliance is a problem. Potassium-sparing diuretics are not usually necessary in the routine treatment of hypertension, unless hypokalaemia develops.

Other diuretics

Mannitol p. 262 is an osmotic diuretic that can be used to treat cerebral oedema and raised intra-ocular pressure.

Mercurial diuretics are effective but are now almost never used because of their nephrotoxicity.

The carbonic anhydrase inhibitor acetazolamide p. 1343 is a weak diuretic and is little used for its diuretic effect. It is used for prophylaxis against mountain sickness [unlicensed indication] but is not a substitute for acclimatisation.

Eye drops of dorzolamide p. 1345 and brinzolamide p. 1344 inhibit the formation of aqueous humour and are used in glaucoma.

Diuretics with potassium

Many patients on diuretics do not need potassium supplements. For many of those who do, the amount of potassium in combined preparations may not be enough, and for this reason their use is to be discouraged.

Diuretics with potassium and potassium-sparing diuretics should **not** usually be given together. Diuretics and potassium supplements should be prescribed separately for children.

> **Other drugs used for Oedema** Diamorphine hydrochloride, p. 518

DIURETICS > LOOP DIURETICS

Loop diuretics

- **DRUG ACTION** Loop diuretics inhibit reabsorption from the ascending limb of the loop of Henlé in the renal tubule and are powerful diuretics.
- **CONTRA-INDICATIONS** Anuria · comatose and precomatose states associated with liver cirrhosis · renal failure due to nephrotoxic or hepatotoxic drugs · severe hypokalaemia · severe hyponatraemia
- **CAUTIONS** Can exacerbate diabetes (but hyperglycaemia less likely than with thiazides) · can excacerbate gout · hypotension should be corrected before initiation of treatment · hypovolaemia should be corrected before initiation of treatment · urinary retention can occur in prostatic hyperplasia

  CAUTIONS, FURTHER INFORMATION
  - Elderly EvGr Lower initial doses of diuretics may be necessary in the elderly because they are particularly susceptible to the side-effects. The dose should then be adjusted according to renal function. M

    Screening Tool of Older Persons' potentially inappropriate Prescriptions (STOPP) criteria to aid medication reviews (see Prescribing in the elderly p. 31 for information). Potentially inappropriate:
    - as a first-line treatment for hypertension (safer, more effective alternatives available)
    - for treatment of hypertension with concurrent urinary incontinence (may exacerbate incontinence)
    - for dependent ankle oedema without evidence of heart failure, liver failure, nephrotic syndrome, or renal failure (leg elevation and/or compression hosiery usually more appropriate)
  - Potassium loss Hypokalaemia can occur with loop diuretics. Hypokalaemia is dangerous in severe cardiovascular disease and in patients also being treated with cardiac glycosides. Often the use of potassium-sparing diuretics avoids the need to take potassium supplements.

    In hepatic impairment, hypokalaemia caused by diuretics can precipitate encephalopathy.
  - Urinary retention If there is an enlarged prostate, urinary retention can occur, although this is less likely if small doses and less potent diuretics are used initially; manufacturer advises adequate urinary output should be established before initiating treatment.

- **SIDE-EFFECTS**
  - **Common or very common** Dizziness · electrolyte imbalance · fatigue · headache · metabolic alkalosis · muscle spasms · nausea
  - **Uncommon** Diarrhoea
  - **Rare or very rare** Bone marrow depression · photosensitivity reaction
  - **Frequency not known** Deafness (more common in renal impairment) · leucopenia · paraesthesia · rash · severe cutaneous adverse reactions (SCARs) · thrombocytopenia · tinnitus (more common with rapid intravenous administration, and in renal impairment) · vomiting
- **HEPATIC IMPAIRMENT** Hypokalaemia induced by loop diuretics may precipitate hepatic encephalopathy and coma—potassium-sparing diuretics can be used to prevent this. Diuretics can increase the risk of hypomagnesaemia in alcoholic cirrhosis, leading to arrhythmias.
- **RENAL IMPAIRMENT** High doses or rapid intravenous administration can cause tinnitus and deafness. **Dose adjustments** High doses of loop diuretics may occasionally be needed in renal impairment.
- **MONITORING REQUIREMENTS** Monitor electrolytes during treatment.

> ⌐ above

Bumetanide

- **INDICATIONS AND DOSE**

Oedema
- ▸ BY MOUTH
- ▸ Adult: 1 mg, dose to be taken in the morning, then 1 mg after 6–8 hours if required
- ▸ Elderly: 500 micrograms daily, this lower dose may be sufficient in elderly patients

Oedema, severe cases
- ▸ BY MOUTH
- ▸ Adult: Initially 5 mg daily, increased in steps of 5 mg every 12–24 hours, adjusted according to response

- **INTERACTIONS** → Appendix 1: loop diuretics
- **SIDE-EFFECTS**
  - **Common or very common** Dehydration · hypotension · skin reactions
  - **Uncommon** Breast pain · chest discomfort · ear pain · vertigo
  - **Rare or very rare** Hearing impairment
  - **Frequency not known** Arthralgia · encephalopathy · gastrointestinal discomfort · gynaecomastia · hyperglycaemia · hyperuricaemia · muscle cramps · musculoskeletal pain (with high doses in renal failure)
- **PREGNANCY** Bumetanide should not be used to treat gestational hypertension because of the maternal hypovolaemia associated with this condition.
- **BREAST FEEDING** No information available. May inhibit lactation.

- **MEDICINAL FORMS** There can be variation in the licensing of different medicines containing the same drug. Forms available from special-order manufacturers include: oral suspension

Oral tablet
- ▸ Bumetanide (Non-proprietary)
  Bumetanide 1 mg Bumetanide 1mg tablets | 28 tablet PoM £6.00 DT = £2.60
  Bumetanide 5 mg Bumetanide 5mg tablets | 28 tablet PoM £51.20 DT = £41.81

Oral solution
- ▸ Bumetanide (Non-proprietary)
  Bumetanide 200 microgram per 1 ml Bumetanide 1mg/5ml oral solution sugar free | 150 ml PoM £270.90 DT = £270.90 SF

Combinations available: *Amiloride with bumetanide,* p. 263

Co-amilofruse

24-Sep-2020

● **INDICATIONS AND DOSE**

Oedema
▶ BY MOUTH
▶ Adult: 2.5/20–10/80 mg daily, dose to be taken in the morning

DOSE EQUIVALENCE AND CONVERSION
▶ A mixture of amiloride hydrochloride and furosemide (frusemide) in the mass proportions of 1 part amiloride hydrochloride to 8 parts furosemide (frusemide).

● **CONTRA-INDICATIONS** Addison's disease · anuria · comatose or precomatose states associated with liver cirrhosis · dehydration · hyperkalaemia · hypovolaemia · renal failure · severe hypokalaemia · severe hyponatraemia

● **CAUTIONS** Correct hypovolaemia · diabetes mellitus · elderly · gout · hepatorenal syndrome · hypoproteinaemia · hypotension · impaired micturition · prostatic enlargement

● **INTERACTIONS** → Appendix 1: loop diuretics · potassium-sparing diuretics

● **SIDE-EFFECTS**
▶ **Uncommon** Hearing impairment
▶ **Frequency not known** Acute urinary retention · agranulocytosis · aplastic anaemia · cholestasis · constipation · diarrhoea · dizziness · electrolyte imbalance · eosinophilia · epigastric discomfort · gout · haemolytic anaemia · headache · leucopenia · loss of consciousness · lupus erythematosus · malaise · nausea · nephritis tubulointerstitial · pancreatitis acute · paraesthesia · psychiatric disorder · renal failure · severe cutaneous adverse reactions (SCARs) · skin eruption · syncope · tetany · thrombocytopenia · tinnitus · vasculitis · vomiting

● **PREGNANCY** Not used to treat hypertension in pregnancy.

● **BREAST FEEDING** Manufacturers advise avoid—no information regarding amiloride component available. Amount of furosemide in milk too small to be harmful. Furosemide may inhibit lactation.

● **HEPATIC IMPAIRMENT** Manufacturer advises caution in hepatic cirrhosis with renal impairment.

● **RENAL IMPAIRMENT** Risk of hyperkalaemia in renal impairment but may need higher doses. Avoid if eGFR less than 30 mL/minute/1.73 m^2.
Monitoring Monitor plasma-potassium concentration.

● **MONITORING REQUIREMENTS** Monitor electrolytes.

● **MEDICINAL FORMS** There can be variation in the licensing of different medicines containing the same drug. Forms available from special-order manufacturers include: oral suspension, oral solution

Oral tablet
▶ Co-amilofruse (Non-proprietary)
Amiloride hydrochloride 2.5 mg, Furosemide 20 mg Co-amilofruse 2.5mg/20mg tablets | 28 tablet PoM £12.86 DT = £4.64
Amiloride hydrochloride 5 mg, Furosemide 40 mg Co-amilofruse 5mg/40mg tablets | 28 tablet PoM £8.30 DT = £5.19
▶ Frumil (Sanofi)
Amiloride hydrochloride 5 mg, Furosemide 40 mg Frumil 40mg/5mg tablets | 28 tablet PoM £5.29 DT = £5.19

F 260

Furosemide

24-Sep-2020

(Frusemide)

● **INDICATIONS AND DOSE**

Oedema
▶ BY MOUTH
▶ Adult: Initially 40 mg daily, dose to be taken in the morning, then maintenance 20–40 mg daily

▶ INITIALLY BY INTRAMUSCULAR INJECTION, OR BY SLOW INTRAVENOUS INJECTION, OR BY INTRAVENOUS INFUSION
▶ Adult: Initially 20–50 mg, then (by intramuscular injection or by intravenous injection or by intravenous infusion) increased in steps of 20 mg every 2 hours if required, doses greater than 50 mg given by intravenous infusion only; maximum 1.5 g per day

Resistant oedema
▶ BY MOUTH
▶ Adult: 80–120 mg daily
▶ INITIALLY BY INTRAMUSCULAR INJECTION, OR BY SLOW INTRAVENOUS INJECTION, OR BY INTRAVENOUS INFUSION
▶ Adult: Initially 20–50 mg, then (by intramuscular injection or by intravenous injection or by intravenous infusion) increased in steps of 20 mg every 2 hours if required, doses greater than 50 mg given by intravenous infusion only; maximum 1.5 g per day

Resistant hypertension
▶ BY MOUTH
▶ Adult: 40–80 mg daily
▶ INITIALLY BY INTRAMUSCULAR INJECTION, OR BY SLOW INTRAVENOUS INJECTION, OR BY INTRAVENOUS INFUSION
▶ Adult: Initially 20–50 mg, then (by intramuscular injection or by intravenous injection or by intravenous infusion) increased in steps of 20 mg every 2 hours if required, doses greater than 50 mg given by intravenous infusion only; maximum 1.5 g per day

● **CAUTIONS** Hepatorenal syndrome · hypoproteinaemia may reduce diuretic effect and increase risk of side-effects

● **INTERACTIONS** → Appendix 1: loop diuretics

● **SIDE-EFFECTS**
GENERAL SIDE-EFFECTS Agranulocytosis · aplastic anaemia · auditory disorder (more common with rapid intravenous administration, and in renal impairment) · diabetes mellitus · eosinophilia · fever · gout · haemolytic anaemia · malaise · mucosal reaction · nephritis tubulointerstitial · pancreatitis acute · shock · skin eruption · tetany · vasculitis

SPECIFIC SIDE-EFFECTS
▶ With oral use Acute kidney injury · hepatic disorders · metabolic acidosis · psychiatric disorder · urinary disorders
▶ With parenteral use Acute urinary retention · cholestasis

● **PREGNANCY** Furosemide should not be used to treat gestational hypertension because of the maternal hypovolaemia associated with this condition.

● **BREAST FEEDING** Amount too small to be harmful. May inhibit lactation.

● **DIRECTIONS FOR ADMINISTRATION** Intravenous administration rate should not usually exceed 4 mg/minute however single doses of up to 80 mg may be administered more rapidly; a lower rate of infusion may be necessary in renal impairment. For *intravenous infusion* (*Lasix*®), give continuously in Sodium chloride 0.9%; infusion pH must be above 5.5; glucose solutions are unsuitable.

● **MEDICINAL FORMS** There can be variation in the licensing of different medicines containing the same drug. Forms available from special-order manufacturers include: oral suspension, oral solution

Oral tablet
▶ Furosemide (Non-proprietary)
Furosemide 20 mg Furosemide 20mg tablets | 28 tablet PoM £0.68 DT = £0.59
Furosemide 40 mg Furosemide 40mg tablets | 28 tablet PoM £0.70 DT = £0.60 | 250 tablet PoM £5.36
Furosemide 500 mg Furosemide 500mg tablets | 28 tablet PoM £39.50 DT = £27.01

Solution for injection

▸ **Furosemide (Non-proprietary)**
Furosemide 10 mg per 1 ml Furosemide 250mg/25ml solution for injection ampoules | 10 ampoule [PoM] £40.00 DT = £40.00
Furosemide 40mg/4ml solution for injection ampoules | 10 ampoule [PoM] £12.19 (Hospital only)
Furosemide 50mg/5ml solution for injection ampoules | 10 ampoule [PoM] £17.00 DT = £7.00 | 10 ampoule [PoM] £15.40-£18.70 DT = £7.00 (Hospital only)
Furosemide 20mg/2ml solution for injection ampoules | 10 ampoule [PoM] £4.91-£13.20 DT = £13.20 | 10 ampoule [PoM] £16.50 DT = £13.20 (Hospital only)

Oral solution

EXCIPIENTS: May contain Alcohol

▸ **Furosemide (Non-proprietary)**
Furosemide 4 mg per 1 ml Furosemide 20mg/5ml oral solution sugar free | 150 ml [PoM] £15.99 DT = £15.99 [SF]
Furosemide 8 mg per 1 ml Furosemide 40mg/5ml oral solution sugar free | 150 ml [PoM] £20.87 DT = £20.29 [SF]
Furosemide 10 mg per 1 ml Furosemide 50mg/5ml oral solution sugar free | 150 ml [PoM] £21.51 DT = £20.99 [SF]

▸ **Frusol** (Rosemont Pharmaceuticals Ltd)
Furosemide 4 mg per 1 ml Frusol 20mg/5ml oral solution | 150 ml [PoM] £12.07 DT = £15.99 [SF]
Furosemide 8 mg per 1 ml Frusol 40mg/5ml oral solution | 150 ml [PoM] £15.58 DT = £20.29 [SF]
Furosemide 10 mg per 1 ml Frusol 50mg/5ml oral solution | 150 ml [PoM] £16.84 DT = £20.99 [SF]

Combinations available: *Spironolactone with furosemide,* p. 263

Furosemide with triamterene
16-Dec-2021

The properties listed below are those particular to the combination only. For the properties of the components please consider, furosemide p. 261, triamterene p. 264.

● **INDICATIONS AND DOSE**

Oedema
▸ BY MOUTH
▸ Adult: 0.5–2 tablets daily, dose to be taken in the morning

● **CONTRA-INDICATIONS** Anuria · dehydration · hyperkalaemia · hypovolaemia · renal failure · severe hypokalaemia · severe hyponatraemia

● **CAUTIONS** Diabetes mellitus · elderly · gout · hepatorenal syndrome · hypotension · impaired micturition · may cause blue fluorescence of urine · prostatic enlargement

● **INTERACTIONS** → Appendix 1: loop diuretics · potassium-sparing diuretics

● **BREAST FEEDING** Triamterene present in milk—manufacturer advises avoid. Furosemide may inhibit lactation.

● **HEPATIC IMPAIRMENT** Manufacturer advises caution; avoid in severe hepatic failure or hepatic coma.
Dose adjustments Manufacturer advises initial dose reduction.

● **RENAL IMPAIRMENT** [EvGr] Avoid if creatinine clearance less than 25 mL/minute (risk of accumulation of triamterene and hyperkalaemia). ⓜ See p. 21.

● **MONITORING REQUIREMENTS** Monitor electrolytes.

● **PATIENT AND CARER ADVICE** Urine may look slightly blue in some lights.

● **MEDICINAL FORMS** No licensed medicines listed.

▶ 260

Torasemide
05-Jun-2020

● **INDICATIONS AND DOSE**

Oedema
▸ BY MOUTH
▸ Adult: 5 mg once daily, to be taken preferably in the morning, then increased if necessary to 20 mg once daily; maximum 40 mg per day

Hypertension
▸ BY MOUTH
▸ Adult: 2.5 mg daily, then increased if necessary to 5 mg once daily

● **INTERACTIONS** → Appendix 1: loop diuretics

● **SIDE-EFFECTS**
▸ **Common or very common** Asthenia · gastrointestinal disorder
▸ **Uncommon** Bladder dilation · urinary retention
▸ **Rare or very rare** Allergic dermatitis
▸ **Frequency not known** Anaemia · cerebral ischaemia · confusion · dry mouth · embolism · ischaemic heart disease · myocardial infarction · pancreatitis · syncope · visual impairment

● **PREGNANCY** Manufacturer advises avoid—toxicity in *animal* studies.

● **BREAST FEEDING** Manufacturer advises avoid—no information available.

● **MEDICINAL FORMS** There can be variation in the licensing of different medicines containing the same drug.

Oral tablet

▸ **Torasemide (Non-proprietary)**
Torasemide 5 mg Torasemide 5mg tablets | 28 tablet [PoM] £14.50 DT = £10.67
Torasemide 10 mg Torasemide 10mg tablets | 28 tablet [PoM] £18.50 DT = £15.21

▸ **Torem** (Viatris UK Healthcare Ltd)
Torasemide 10 mg Torem 10mg tablets | 28 tablet [PoM] £8.14 DT = £15.21

DIURETICS > OSMOTIC DIURETICS

Mannitol
15-Oct-2021

● **INDICATIONS AND DOSE**

Cerebral oedema
▸ BY INTRAVENOUS INFUSION
▸ Adult: 0.25–2 g/kg, repeated if necessary, to be administered over 30-60 minutes, dose may be repeated 1–2 times after 4–8 hours

Raised intra-ocular pressure
▸ BY INTRAVENOUS INFUSION
▸ Adult: 0.25–2 g/kg, repeated if necessary, to be administered over 30–60 minutes, dose may be repeated 1–2 times after 4–8 hours

● **CONTRA-INDICATIONS** Anuria · intracranial bleeding (except during craniotomy) · severe cardiac failure · severe dehydration · severe pulmonary oedema

● **CAUTIONS** Extravasation causes inflammation and thrombophlebitis

● **INTERACTIONS** → Appendix 1: mannitol

● **SIDE-EFFECTS**
▸ **Common or very common** Cough · headache · vomiting
▸ **Uncommon** Dizziness · fever · malaise · nausea · pain · skin reactions
▸ **Frequency not known** Arrhythmia · asthenia · azotaemia · chest pain · chills · coma · compartment syndrome · confusion · congestive heart failure · dry mouth · electrolyte imbalance · fluid imbalance · hyperhidrosis · hypersensitivity · hypertension · lethargy · metabolic

acidosis · muscle complaints · musculoskeletal stiffness · nephrotic syndrome · neurotoxicity · peripheral oedema · pulmonary oedema · rebound intracranial pressure increase · renal impairment · rhinitis · seizure · thirst · urinary disorders · vision blurred

● **PREGNANCY** Manufacturer advises avoid unless essential— no information available.

● **BREAST FEEDING** Manufacturer advises avoid unless essential—no information available.

● **RENAL IMPAIRMENT** EvGr Caution in severe impairment (consult product literature). M

● **PRE-TREATMENT SCREENING** Assess cardiac function before treatment.

● **MONITORING REQUIREMENTS** Monitor fluid and electrolyte balance, serum osmolality, and cardiac, pulmonary and renal function.

● **DIRECTIONS FOR ADMINISTRATION** An in-line filter is recommended.

● **NATIONAL FUNDING/ACCESS DECISIONS** For full details see funding body website

● **MEDICINAL FORMS** There can be variation in the licensing of different medicines containing the same drug. Forms available from special-order manufacturers include: infusion, solution for infusion

Infusion

▸ Mannitol (Non-proprietary)
Mannitol 100 mg per 1 ml Mannitol 50g/500ml (10%) infusion Viaflo bags | 1 bag PoM ⚠
Mannitol 150 mg per 1 ml Mannitol 75g/500ml (15%) infusion Viaflo bags | 20 bag PoM ⚠ (Hospital only)
Mannitol 200 mg per 1 ml Polyfusor mannitol 20% infusion 500ml bottles | 12 bottle PoM £203.88

DIURETICS ⟩ POTASSIUM-SPARING DIURETICS ⟩ MINERALOCORTICOID RECEPTOR ANTAGONISTS

Spironolactone with furosemide

The properties listed below are those particular to the combination only. For the properties of the components please consider, spironolactone p. 224, furosemide p. 261.

● **INDICATIONS AND DOSE**

Resistant oedema
▸ BY MOUTH
▸ Adult: 20/50–80/200 mg daily

● **INTERACTIONS** → Appendix 1: loop diuretics · mineralocorticoid receptor antagonists

● **MEDICINAL FORMS** No licensed medicines listed.

DIURETICS ⟩ POTASSIUM-SPARING DIURETICS ⟩ OTHER

Amiloride hydrochloride　　　　11-Dec-2020

● **INDICATIONS AND DOSE**

Oedema (monotherapy)
▸ BY MOUTH
▸ Adult: Initially 10 mg daily, alternatively initially 5 mg twice daily, adjusted according to response; maximum 20 mg per day

Potassium conservation when used as an adjunct to thiazide or loop diuretics for hypertension or congestive heart failure
▸ BY MOUTH
▸ Adult: Initially 5–10 mg daily

Potassium conservation when used as an adjunct to thiazide or loop diuretics for hepatic cirrhosis with ascites
▸ BY MOUTH
▸ Adult: Initially 5 mg daily

● **CONTRA-INDICATIONS** Addison's disease · anuria · hyperkalaemia

● **CAUTIONS** Diabetes mellitus · elderly

● **INTERACTIONS** → Appendix 1: potassium-sparing diuretics

● **SIDE-EFFECTS** Alopecia · angina pectoris · aplastic anaemia · appetite decreased · arrhythmia · arthralgia · asthenia · atrioventricular block exacerbated · bladder spasm · chest pain · confusion · constipation · cough · depression · diarrhoea · dizziness · drowsiness · dry mouth · dyspnoea · dysuria · electrolyte imbalance · encephalopathy · gastrointestinal discomfort · gastrointestinal disorders · gastrointestinal haemorrhage · gout · headache · insomnia · jaundice · muscle cramps · nasal congestion · nausea · nervousness · neutropenia · pain · palpitations · paraesthesia · postural hypotension · sexual dysfunction · skin reactions · tinnitus · tremor · vertigo · visual impairment · vomiting

● **PREGNANCY** Not to be used to treat gestational hypertension.

● **BREAST FEEDING** Manufacturer advises avoid—no information available.

● **RENAL IMPAIRMENT** Manufacturers advise avoid in severe impairment.
Monitoring Monitor plasma-potassium concentration (high risk of hyperkalaemia in renal impairment).

● **MONITORING REQUIREMENTS** Monitor electrolytes.

● **MEDICINAL FORMS** There can be variation in the licensing of different medicines containing the same drug. Forms available from special-order manufacturers include: oral suspension, oral solution

Oral tablet

▸ Amiloride hydrochloride (Non-proprietary)
Amiloride hydrochloride 5 mg Amiloride 5mg tablets | 28 tablet PoM £39.82 DT = £16.73

Oral solution
EXCIPIENTS: May contain Propylene glycol
▸ Amiloride hydrochloride (Non-proprietary)
Amiloride hydrochloride 1 mg per 1 ml Amiloride 5mg/5ml oral solution sugar free | 150 ml PoM £158.85 DT = £158.85 SF

Combinations available: *Co-amilofruse,* p. 261

Amiloride with bumetanide

The properties listed below are those particular to the combination only. For the properties of the components please consider, amiloride hydrochloride above, bumetanide p. 260.

● **INDICATIONS AND DOSE**

Oedema
▸ BY MOUTH
▸ Adult: 1–2 tablets daily

● **INTERACTIONS** → Appendix 1: loop diuretics · potassium-sparing diuretics

● **MEDICINAL FORMS** There can be variation in the licensing of different medicines containing the same drug.

Oral tablet

▸ Amiloride with bumetanide (Non-proprietary)
Bumetanide 1 mg, Amiloride hydrochloride 5 mg Amiloride 5mg / Bumetanide 1mg tablets | 28 tablet PoM £59.74 DT = £59.74

Triamterene

03-Sep-2020

● **INDICATIONS AND DOSE**

Oedema | Potassium conservation with thiazide and loop diuretics

▸ BY MOUTH

▸ Adult: Initially 150–250 mg daily for 1 week, lower initial dose when given with other diuretics, then reduced to 150–250 mg daily on alternate days, to be taken in divided doses after breakfast and lunch

● **CONTRA-INDICATIONS** Addison's disease · anuria · hyperkalaemia

● **CAUTIONS** Diabetes mellitus · elderly · gout · may cause blue fluorescence of urine

● **INTERACTIONS** → Appendix 1: potassium-sparing diuretics

● **SIDE-EFFECTS**

▸ **Common or very common** Diarrhoea · hyperkalaemia · nausea · vomiting

▸ **Uncommon** Dry mouth · headache · hyperuricaemia · renal failure (reversible on discontinuation) · skin reactions

▸ **Rare or very rare** Megaloblastic anaemia · nephritis tubulointerstitial · pancytopenia · photosensitivity reaction · serum sickness · urolithiasis

▸ **Frequency not known** Asthenia · jaundice · metabolic acidosis · urine discolouration

● **PREGNANCY** Not used to treat gestational hypertension. Avoid unless essential.

● **BREAST FEEDING** Present in milk—manufacturer advises avoid.

● **HEPATIC IMPAIRMENT** Manufacturer advises caution; avoid in progressive impairment.

● **RENAL IMPAIRMENT** Avoid in progressive impairment. **Monitoring** Monitor plasma-potassium concentration (high risk of hyperkalaemia in renal impairment).

● **MONITORING REQUIREMENTS** Monitor electrolytes.

● **PATIENT AND CARER ADVICE** Urine may look slightly blue in some lights.

● **MEDICINAL FORMS** No licensed medicines listed.

Combinations available: *Furosemide with triamterene*, p. 262

Triamterene with chlortalidone

The properties listed below are those particular to the combination only. For the properties of the components please consider, triamterene above, chlortalidone below.

● **INDICATIONS AND DOSE**

Hypertension | Oedema

▸ BY MOUTH

▸ Adult: 50/50–100/100 mg once daily, dose to be taken in the morning

DOSE EQUIVALENCE AND CONVERSION

▸ Dose expressed as *x/y* mg of triamterene/chlortalidone.

● **INTERACTIONS** → Appendix 1: potassium-sparing diuretics · thiazide diuretics

● **MEDICINAL FORMS** There can be variation in the licensing of different medicines containing the same drug.

Oral tablet

CAUTIONARY AND ADVISORY LABELS 14, 21

▸ **Triamterene with chlortalidone (Non-proprietary)**
Chlortalidone 50 mg, Triamterene 50 mg Triamterene 50mg / Chlortalidone 50mg tablets | 28 tablet PoM £185.00-£323.74 DT = £185.00

DIURETICS > THIAZIDES AND RELATED DIURETICS

⚑ 192

Chlortalidone

(Chlorthalidone)

● **INDICATIONS AND DOSE**

Ascites due to cirrhosis in stable patients (under close supervision) | Oedema due to nephrotic syndrome

▸ BY MOUTH

▸ Adult: Up to 50 mg daily

Hypertension

▸ BY MOUTH

▸ Adult: 25 mg daily, dose to be taken in the morning, then increased if necessary to 50 mg daily

Mild to moderate chronic heart failure

▸ BY MOUTH

▸ Adult: 25–50 mg daily, dose to be taken in the morning, then increased if necessary to 100–200 mg daily, reduce to lowest effective dose for maintenance

Nephrogenic diabetes insipidus | Partial pituitary diabetes insipidus

▸ BY MOUTH

▸ Adult: Initially 100 mg twice daily, then reduced to 50 mg daily

● **INTERACTIONS** → Appendix 1: thiazide diuretics

● **SIDE-EFFECTS**

▸ **Common or very common** Appetite decreased · gastrointestinal discomfort

▸ **Uncommon** Gout

▸ **Rare or very rare** Arrhythmia · diabetes mellitus exacerbated · eosinophilia · glycosuria · hepatic disorders · nephritis tubulointerstitial · pulmonary oedema · respiratory disorder

● **BREAST FEEDING** The amount present in milk is too small to be harmful. Large doses may suppress lactation.

● **MEDICINAL FORMS** There can be variation in the licensing of different medicines containing the same drug. Forms available from special-order manufacturers include: oral suspension

Oral tablet

▸ **Chlortalidone (Non-proprietary)**
Chlortalidone 25 mg Chlortalidone 25mg tablets | 100 tablet PoM ⅀ (Hospital only)
Chlortalidone 50 mg Chlortalidone 50mg tablets | 30 tablet PoM £88.04 DT = £34.03

▸ **Hylaton** (Morningside Healthcare Ltd)
Chlortalidone 12.5 mg Hylaton 12.5mg tablets | 30 tablet PoM £42.00 DT = £42.00
Chlortalidone 50 mg Hylaton 50mg tablets | 30 tablet PoM £59.00 DT = £34.03

Combinations available: *Triamterene with chlortalidone*, above

⚑ 192

Metolazone

27-Mar-2025

● **INDICATIONS AND DOSE**

Oedema in congestive heart failure [using Xaqua ® tablets] | Oedema in renal disease [using Xaqua ® tablets] | Hypertension [using Xaqua ® tablets]

▸ BY MOUTH

▸ Adult: Initially 2.5 mg once daily, increased if necessary to 5 mg once daily

Oedema [using metolazone preparations with different bioavailability to Xaqua ® tablets]

▸ BY MOUTH

▸ Adult: 5–10 mg daily, dose to be taken in the morning; increased if necessary to 20 mg daily, dose to be taken in the morning, dose increased in resistant oedema; maximum 80 mg per day

Hypertension [using metolazone preparations with different bioavailability to Xaqua ® tablets]
▶ BY MOUTH
▶ Adult: Initially 5 mg daily, dose to be taken in the morning; maintenance 5 mg once daily on alternate days, dose to be taken in the morning

DOSE EQUIVALENCE AND CONVERSION
▶ Metolazone preparations are not interchangeable due to differences in bioavailability.

IMPORTANT SAFETY INFORMATION

MHRA/CHM ADVICE: *XAQUA*® (METOLAZONE) 5 MG TABLETS: EXERCISE CAUTION WHEN SWITCHING PATIENTS BETWEEN METOLAZONE PREPARATIONS (JANUARY 2023)

The MHRA advises caution if switching patients between different metolazone preparations because of potential differences in bioavailability and dosing instructions. Healthcare professionals are advised to:

- consider prescribing the licensed formulation (*Xaqua*®) over unlicensed imported preparations for new patients;
- assess individual patient factors before switching from unlicensed preparations to *Xaqua*®;
- consider adjusting the dose and monitor patients when switching to *Xaqua*®;
- only split *Xaqua*® tablets into halves using the tablet score-line;
- prescribe and supply metolazone by brand name, or manufacturer name, and document this clearly.

Healthcare professionals are advised to counsel patients or their carers:

- not to use different metolazone preparations at the same time;
- to be aware of the brand name, or manufacturer of the preparation prescribed, and specific dosing instructions;
- on the signs and symptoms of electrolyte imbalance that may occur when switching preparations, and to contact a healthcare professional if they develop;
- on the signs and symptoms of an inadequate dose, and to contact a healthcare professional if they occur;
- not to stop taking metolazone without discussion with their doctor.

● **CAUTIONS** Acute porphyrias p. 1202

● **INTERACTIONS** → Appendix 1: thiazide diuretics

● **SIDE-EFFECTS**
▶ **Common or very common** Azotaemia · glycosuria · hypotension · muscle complaints
▶ **Uncommon** Arthralgia · gout · vasculitis
▶ **Rare or very rare** Apathy · appetite decreased · asthenia · chest pain · chills · confusion · dehydration · drowsiness · gastrointestinal discomfort · haemoconcentration · hepatic disorders · hepatic encephalopathy · hypoplastic anaemia · palpitations · peripheral neuropathy · psychotic depression · renal impairment · restlessness · seizure · severe cutaneous adverse reactions (SCARs) · syncope · tachycardia · venous thrombosis · vertigo · vision blurred

● **BREAST FEEDING** Specialist sources indicate that levels in milk have not been determined, but are likely to be too low to affect the infant. Large doses may suppress lactation.

● **HEPATIC IMPAIRMENT**

XAQUA ® EvGr Caution in severe impairment. ⟨M⟩

● **RENAL IMPAIRMENT** See p. 21. Manufacturer advises metolazone remains effective if eGFR is less than 30 mL/minute/1.73 m² but is associated with a risk of excessive diuresis.

● **PATIENT AND CARER ADVICE**

XAQUA ® **Driving and skilled tasks** Patients and carers should be counselled on the effects on driving and performance of skilled tasks—increased risk of dizziness and fatigue.

● **MEDICINAL FORMS** There can be variation in the licensing of different medicines containing the same drug. Forms available from special-order manufacturers include: oral tablet, oral suspension, oral solution

Oral tablet
▶ **Metolazone (Non-proprietary)**
 Metolazone 2.5 mg Zaroxolyn 2.5mg tablets | 100 tablet PoM ⓢ
 Metolazone 5 mg Zaroxolyn 5mg tablets | 50 tablet PoM ⓢ
▶ **Xaqua** (Renascience Pharma Ltd)
 Metolazone 5 mg Xaqua 5mg tablets | 20 tablet PoM £110.00 DT = £110.00

⊩ 192

Xipamide
23-Sep-2020

● **INDICATIONS AND DOSE**

Oedema
▶ BY MOUTH
▶ Adult: Initially 40 mg daily, dose to be taken in the morning, increased if necessary to 80 mg daily, higher dose to be used in resistant cases; maintenance 20 mg daily, dose to be taken in the morning

Hypertension
▶ BY MOUTH
▶ Adult: 20 mg daily, dose to be taken in the morning

● **CAUTIONS** Acute porphyrias p. 1202

● **INTERACTIONS** → Appendix 1: thiazide diuretics

● **SIDE-EFFECTS**
▶ **Common or very common** Anxiety · dry mouth · gastrointestinal discomfort · gouty arthritis · hyperhidrosis · lethargy · muscle complaints · palpitations
▶ **Rare or very rare** Cholecystitis acute · hyperlipidaemia · jaundice · nephritis acute interstitial · pancreatitis haemorrhagic · vision disorders

● **BREAST FEEDING** No information available.

● **MEDICINAL FORMS** There can be variation in the licensing of different medicines containing the same drug.

Oral tablet
▶ **Diurexan** (Viatris UK Healthcare Ltd)
 Xipamide 20 mg Diurexan 20mg tablets | 140 tablet PoM £19.46

11   Vascular disease

Peripheral vascular disease
08-Aug-2023

Classification and management

Peripheral vascular disease can be either occlusive (e.g. *intermittent claudication*) in which occlusion of the peripheral arteries is caused by atherosclerosis, or vasospastic (e.g. *Raynaud's phenomenon*). Peripheral arterial occlusive disease is associated with an increased risk of cardiovascular events. This risk is reduced by measures such as Smoking cessation p. 565, effective control of blood pressure, regulating blood lipids, optimising glycaemic control in diabetes, antiplatelet therapy, diet and weight management, and increasing exercise.

EvGr A supervised exercise programme should be offered to all patients with *intermittent claudication*. Revascularisation procedures may be appropriate if other measures fail. Naftidrofuryl oxalate p. 267 can be considered if supervised exercise has not led to satisfactory improvement, and the patient prefers not to be referred for consideration of angioplasty or bypass surgery. Review treatment with naftidrofuryl oxalate after 3–6 months; discontinue if there has been no symptomatic benefit. (A)

Cilostazol below and pentoxifylline p. 267 are licensed for the treatment of intermittent claudication. Naftidrofuryl oxalate has shown a greater increase in maximum walking distance and pain-free walking distance than cilostazol and pentoxifylline.

Intravenous iloprost p. 212 is licensed for the treatment of severe chronic lower limb ischaemia in patients at risk of amputation where surgery has failed or is unsuitable.

[EvGr] Management of *Raynaud's phenomenon* includes avoidance of exposure to cold and Smoking cessation p. 565. If lifestyle modifications fail and symptoms are having a significant negative impact, a trial of nifedipine p. 189 as prophylaxis can be considered. (A)

Naftidrofuryl oxalate and prazosin p. 904 are licensed for the treatment of Raynaud's phenomenon. There is a lack of evidence for the use of vasodilators other than calcium-channel blockers in primary Raynaud's phenomenon.

The evidence for drug treatment in *chilblains* is limited and does not support its routine use.

ANTITHROMBOTIC DRUGS > ANTIPLATELET DRUGS

Cilostazol

19-Jul-2021

● **INDICATIONS AND DOSE**

Intermittent claudication in patients without rest pain and no peripheral tissue necrosis
▶ BY MOUTH
▶ Adult: 100 mg twice daily, to be taken 30 minutes before food, cilostazol should be initiated by those experienced in the management of intermittent claudication, patients receiving cilostazol should be assessed for improvement after 3 months; consider discontinuation of treatment if there is no clinically relevant improvement in walking distance

DOSE ADJUSTMENTS DUE TO INTERACTIONS
▶ Manufacturer advises reduce dose to 50 mg twice daily with concurrent use of potent inhibitors of CYP3A4, potent inhibitors of CYP2C19, omeprazole and erythromycin.

● **CONTRA-INDICATIONS** Active peptic ulcer · congestive heart failure · coronary intervention in previous 6 months · haemorrhagic stroke in previous 6 months · history of severe tachyarrhythmia · myocardial infarction in previous 6 months · poorly controlled hypertension · predisposition to bleeding · proliferative diabetic retinopathy · prolongation of QT interval · unstable angina · ventricular arrhythmia

● **CAUTIONS** Atrial fibrillation · atrial flutter · atrial or ventricular ectopy · diabetes mellitus (higher risk of intraocular bleeding) · stable coronary disease · surgery

● **INTERACTIONS** → Appendix 1: cilostazol

● **SIDE-EFFECTS**
▶ **Common or very common** Appetite decreased · arrhythmias · diarrhoea · dizziness · gastrointestinal discomfort · gastrointestinal disorders · headache · increased risk of infection · nausea · oedema · palpitations · skin reactions · vomiting
▶ **Uncommon** Anaemia · anxiety · congestive heart failure · cough · dyspnoea · haemorrhage · hyperglycaemia · hypotension · sleep disorders · syncope
▶ **Rare or very rare** Renal impairment · thrombocytosis
▶ **Frequency not known** Agranulocytosis · bone marrow disorders · conjunctivitis · fever · granulocytopenia · hepatic disorders · hot flush · hypertension · intracranial haemorrhage · leucopenia · paresis · severe cutaneous

adverse reactions (SCARs) · thrombocytopenia · tinnitus · urinary frequency increased

● **PREGNANCY** Avoid—toxicity in *animal* studies.

● **BREAST FEEDING** Present in milk in *animal* studies—manufacturer advises avoid.

● **HEPATIC IMPAIRMENT** Manufacturer advises avoid in moderate-to-severe impairment—no information available.

● **RENAL IMPAIRMENT** [EvGr] Avoid if creatinine clearance less than 25 mL/minute. (M) See p. 21.

● **PATIENT AND CARER ADVICE**
Blood disorders Patients should be advised to report any unexplained bleeding, bruising, sore throat, or fever.

● **NATIONAL FUNDING/ACCESS DECISIONS**
For full details see funding body website

NICE decisions
▶ Cilostazol, naftidrofuryl oxalate, pentoxifylline and inositol nicotinate for the treatment of intermittent claudication in people with peripheral arterial disease (May 2011) NICE TA223 Not recommended

● **MEDICINAL FORMS** There can be variation in the licensing of different medicines containing the same drug.
Oral tablet
▶ Cilostazol (Non-proprietary)
Cilostazol 50 mg Cilostazol 50mg tablets | 56 tablet [PoM] £65.40 DT = £35.31
Cilostazol 100 mg Cilostazol 100mg tablets | 56 tablet [PoM] £44.40 DT = £44.40

LIPID MODIFYING DRUGS > NICOTINIC ACID DERIVATIVES

Inositol nicotinate

10-May-2022

● **INDICATIONS AND DOSE**

Peripheral vascular disease
▶ BY MOUTH
▶ Adult: 3 g daily in 2–3 divided doses; maximum 4 g per day

● **CONTRA-INDICATIONS** Acute phase of a cerebrovascular accident · recent myocardial infarction

● **CAUTIONS** Cerebrovascular insufficiency · unstable angina

● **SIDE-EFFECTS**
▶ **Uncommon** Dizziness · flushing · headache · nausea · oedema · paraesthesia · postural hypotension · rash · syncope · vomiting
▶ **Frequency not known** Myalgia

● **PREGNANCY** No information available—manufacturer advises avoid unless potential benefit outweighs risk.

● **NATIONAL FUNDING/ACCESS DECISIONS**
For full details see funding body website

NICE decisions
▶ Cilostazol, naftidrofuryl oxalate, pentoxifylline and inositol nicotinate for the treatment of intermittent claudication in people with peripheral arterial disease (May 2011) NICE TA223 Not recommended

● **LESS SUITABLE FOR PRESCRIBING** Less suitable for prescribing.

● **MEDICINAL FORMS** There can be variation in the licensing of different medicines containing the same drug. Forms available from special-order manufacturers include: oral suspension
Oral capsule
▶ Inositol nicotinate (Non-proprietary)
Inositol nicotinate 500 mg Solgar No-Flush Niacin 500mg capsules | 50 capsule [£]

VASODILATORS > FLAVONOIDS

Oxerutins

- **INDICATIONS AND DOSE**

Relief of symptoms of oedema associated with chronic venous insufficiency
  - ▶ BY MOUTH
  - ▶ Adult: 500 mg twice daily

- **SIDE-EFFECTS**
- ▶ **Rare or very rare** Alopecia · arthralgia · diarrhoea · dizziness · fatigue · flushing · gastrointestinal discomfort · gastrointestinal disorders · headache · photosensitivity reaction · skin reactions

- **LESS SUITABLE FOR PRESCRIBING** Oxerutins (rutosides) are not vasodilators and are not generally regarded as effective preparations as capillary sealants or for the treatment of cramps; they are less suitable for prescribing.

- **MEDICINAL FORMS** There can be variation in the licensing of different medicines containing the same drug.
  Oral capsule
  - ▶ Paroven (Thornton & Ross Ltd)
    Oxerutins 250 mg Paroven 250mg capsules | 120 capsule [PoM] £27.70 DT = £27.70

VASODILATORS > PERIPHERAL VASODILATORS

Naftidrofuryl oxalate

- **INDICATIONS AND DOSE**

Peripheral vascular disease
  - ▶ BY MOUTH
  - ▶ Adult: 100–200 mg 3 times a day, patients taking naftidrofuryl should be assessed for improvement after 3–6 months

Cerebral vascular disease
  - ▶ BY MOUTH
  - ▶ Adult: 100 mg 3 times a day, patients taking naftidrofuryl should be assessed for improvement after 3–6 months

- **SIDE-EFFECTS**
- ▶ **Uncommon** Diarrhoea · epigastric pain · nausea · rash · vomiting
- ▶ **Rare or very rare** Liver injury · oxalate nephrolithiasis
- ▶ **Frequency not known** Oesophagitis

- **NATIONAL FUNDING/ACCESS DECISIONS**
  For full details see funding body website
  NICE decisions
- ▶ Cilostazol, naftidrofuryl oxalate, pentoxifylline and inositol nicotinate for the treatment of intermittent claudication in people with peripheral arterial disease (May 2011) NICE TA223 Recommended

- **MEDICINAL FORMS** There can be variation in the licensing of different medicines containing the same drug. Forms available from special-order manufacturers include: oral solution
  Oral capsule
  CAUTIONARY AND ADVISORY LABELS 25, 27
  - ▶ Naftidrofuryl oxalate (Non-proprietary)
    Naftidrofuryl oxalate 100 mg Naftidrofuryl 100mg capsules | 84 capsule [PoM] £20.98 DT = £10.65

Pentoxifylline
(Oxpentifylline)   23-Jul-2021

- **INDICATIONS AND DOSE**

Peripheral vascular disease | Venous leg ulcer (adjunct)
  - ▶ BY MOUTH
  - ▶ Adult: 400 mg 2–3 times a day

- **UNLICENSED USE** Use of pentoxifylline as adjunct therapy for venous leg ulcers is an unlicensed indication.

- **CONTRA-INDICATIONS** Acute myocardial infarction · cerebral haemorrhage · extensive retinal haemorrhage · severe cardiac arrhythmias

- **CAUTIONS** Avoid in Acute porphyrias p. 1202 · coronary artery disease · hypotension

- **INTERACTIONS** → Appendix 1: pentoxifylline

- **SIDE-EFFECTS** Agitation · angina pectoris · angioedema · arrhythmias · bronchospasm · cholestasis · constipation · diarrhoea · dizziness · gastrointestinal discomfort · gastrointestinal disorder · haemorrhage · headache · hot flush · hypersalivation · hypotension · leucopenia · meningitis aseptic · nausea · neutropenia · skin reactions · sleep disorder · thrombocytopenia · vomiting

- **PREGNANCY** Manufacturer advises avoid—no information available.

- **BREAST FEEDING** Present in milk—manufacturer advises use only if potential benefit outweighs risk.

- **HEPATIC IMPAIRMENT** Manufacturer advises caution in severe impairment.
  Dose adjustments Manufacturer advises consider dose reduction in severe impairment.

- **RENAL IMPAIRMENT**
  Dose adjustments [EvGr] Reduce dose by 30–50% if creatinine clearance less than 30 mL/minute. ⟨M⟩ See p. 21.

- **NATIONAL FUNDING/ACCESS DECISIONS**
  For full details see funding body website
  NICE decisions
- ▶ Cilostazol, naftidrofuryl oxalate, pentoxifylline and inositol nicotinate for the treatment of intermittent claudication in people with peripheral arterial disease (May 2011) NICE TA223 Not recommended

- **LESS SUITABLE FOR PRESCRIBING** Less suitable for prescribing.

- **MEDICINAL FORMS** There can be variation in the licensing of different medicines containing the same drug. Forms available from special-order manufacturers include: oral solution
  Modified-release tablet
  CAUTIONARY AND ADVISORY LABELS 21, 25
  - ▶ Trental (Neuraxpharm UK Ltd)
    Pentoxifylline 400 mg Trental 400 modified-release tablets | 90 tablet [PoM] £19.39 DT = £19.39

11.1 Vein malformations

SCLEROSANTS

Lauromacrogol 400
(Polidocanol)   16-Jan-2023

- **INDICATIONS AND DOSE**

Sclerotherapy of varicose veins in legs
  - ▶ BY INTRAVENOUS INJECTION
  - ▶ Adult: (consult product literature)

- **CONTRA-INDICATIONS** Asthma · blood disorders · high risk of thrombosis · hyperthyroidism · inability to walk · neoplasm · respiratory disease · severe occlusive arterial disease · skin disease · symptomatic right-to-left shunt e.g. patent foramen ovale (if administered as foam) · systemic infection · thromboembolism · uncontrolled diabetes mellitus

- **CAUTIONS** Asymptomatic patent foramen ovale (use smaller volumes and avoid Valsalva manoeuvre immediately after administration) · extravasation may cause necrosis of tissues · leg oedema · microangiopathy or neuropathy · occlusive arterial disease (when treating telangiectasias) · previous visual or neurological symptoms, e.g. migraine, with foam sclerotherapy (use smaller volumes and avoid Valsalva manoeuvre immediately after administration) · reduced mobility · resuscitation facilities must be available

- **SIDE-EFFECTS**
- ▶ **Common or very common** Haematoma · neovascularisation · skin reactions
- ▶ **Uncommon** Embolism and thrombosis · induration · nerve injury · soft tissue necrosis · swelling
- ▶ **Rare or very rare** Angioedema · aphasia · arrhythmias · asthenia · asthma · ataxia · cardiac arrest · cerebrovascular insufficiency · chest discomfort · circulatory collapse · confusion · cough · dizziness · dyspnoea · fever · headaches · hemiparesis · hot flush · loss of consciousness · malaise · nausea · oral hypoaesthesia · pain in extremity · palpitations · paraesthesia · stress cardiomyopathy · syncope · taste altered · vasculitis · visual impairment · vomiting

- **PREGNANCY** [EvGr] Avoid unless potential benefit outweighs risk—toxicity in *animal* studies. Ⓜ

- **BREAST FEEDING** Specialist sources indicate probably suitable for use—unlikely to be excreted into milk.

- **MEDICINAL FORMS** There can be variation in the licensing of different medicines containing the same drug.
  Solution for injection
  EXCIPIENTS: May contain Ethanol
  - ▶ **Lauromacrogol 400 (Non-proprietary)**
    Lauromacrogol 400 2.5 mg per 1 ml Aethoxysklerol 5mg/2ml solution for injection ampoules | 5 ampoule [PoM] Ⓢ (Hospital only)
    Lauromacrogol 400 20 mg per 1 ml Aethoxysklerol 40mg/2ml solution for injection ampoules | 5 ampoule [PoM] Ⓢ (Hospital only)
  - ▶ **Aethoxysklerol** (Kora Healthcare)
    Lauromacrogol 400 5 mg per 1 ml Aethoxysklerol 10mg/2ml solution for injection ampoules | 5 ampoule [PoM] £18.74 (Hospital only)
    Lauromacrogol 400 10 mg per 1 ml Aethoxysklerol 20mg/2ml solution for injection ampoules | 5 ampoule [PoM] £22.38 (Hospital only)
    Lauromacrogol 400 30 mg per 1 ml Aethoxysklerol 60mg/2ml solution for injection ampoules | 5 ampoule [PoM] £33.31 (Hospital only)

Sodium tetradecyl sulfate

24-Aug-2020

- **INDICATIONS AND DOSE**

Sclerotherapy of reticular veins and spider veins in legs and varicose veins
- ▶ BY INTRAVENOUS INJECTION
- ▶ Adult: Test dose recommended before each treatment (consult product literature)

- **CONTRA-INDICATIONS** Acute infection · asthma · blood disorders · deep vein thrombosis · high risk of thromboembolism · hyperthyroidism · inability to walk · neoplasm · occlusive arterial disease · phlebitis · pulmonary embolism · recent acute superficial thrombophlebitis · recent surgery · respiratory disease · significant valvular incompetence in deep veins · skin disease · symptomatic patent foramen ovale (if administered as foam) · uncontrolled diabetes mellitus · varicose veins caused by tumours (unless tumour removed)

- **CAUTIONS** Arterial disease · asymptomatic patent foramen ovale (use smaller volumes and avoid Valsalva manoeuvre immediately after administration) · extravasation may cause necrosis of tissues · history of migraine (use smaller volumes) · resuscitation facilities must be available · venous insufficiency with lymphoedema (pain and inflammation may worsen)

- **SIDE-EFFECTS**
- ▶ **Common or very common** Embolism and thrombosis · haematoma · skin reactions
- ▶ **Uncommon** Headaches · telangiectasia matting · vision disorders
- ▶ **Rare or very rare** Arterial spasm · asthenia · cerebrovascular insufficiency · chest pressure · circulatory collapse · cough · diarrhoea · dry mouth · dyspnoea · fever · hemiparesis · hemiplegia · hot flush · hypersensitivity · local exfoliation · nausea · nerve damage · palpitations · paraesthesia · presyncope · soft tissue necrosis · tongue swelling · vasculitis · vomiting

- **PREGNANCY** Avoid unless benefits outweigh risks—no information available.

- **BREAST FEEDING** Use with caution—no information available.

- **MEDICINAL FORMS** There can be variation in the licensing of different medicines containing the same drug.
  Solution for injection
  EXCIPIENTS: May contain Benzyl alcohol
  - ▶ **Fibro-Vein** (STD Pharmaceutical Products Ltd)
    Sodium tetradecyl sulfate 2 mg per 1 ml Fibrovein 0.2% solution for injection 5ml vials | 10 vial [PoM] £88.33
    Sodium tetradecyl sulfate 5 mg per 1 ml Fibrovein 0.5% solution for injection 2ml ampoules | 5 ampoule [PoM] £22.72
    Sodium tetradecyl sulfate 10 mg per 1 ml Fibrovein 1% solution for injection 2ml ampoules | 5 ampoule [PoM] £27.13
    Sodium tetradecyl sulfate 30 mg per 1 ml Fibrovein 3% solution for injection 2ml ampoules | 5 ampoule [PoM] £40.38

Chapter 3
Respiratory system

CONTENTS

Respiratory system, inhaled drug delivery

13-Mar-2025

Overview

The inhaled route delivers the drug directly to the airways; the dose required is smaller than when given by mouth and side-effects are reduced.

Inhaler devices

Different types of inhaler devices are available, these include *pressurised metered-dose inhalers*, *breath-actuated metered-dose inhalers*, *dry powder inhalers*, and *soft mist inhalers*. Their administration techniques vary and good technique is essential in ensuring optimum use of inhaler devices. Pressurised metered-dose inhalers (pMDIs) require dexterity and the ability to coordinate actuation with inhalation; a spacer device should usually be used with a pMDI, particularly in children (see *Spacer devices* for further information). Dry powder inhalers or breath-actuated metered-dose inhalers require a minimum inspiratory effort to be able to generate enough inspiratory flow to allow effective drug delivery, which may not be achievable for some children (generally younger ones) and some elderly patients. The patient's ability to achieve an effective technique with the inhaler device will therefore influence choice, as will the suitability of the inhaler device for the patient's lifestyle, their preference, the environmental impact of the device, the presence of an integral dose counter, concomitant prescribed inhaler devices, and the range of available inhaler device types for a specific drug.

The number and different types of inhalers given to a patient should be minimised. To help reduce confusion and ensure patients receive the inhaler they have been given training for, the brand and inhaler device should be specified when prescribing. The strength of inhaler device should also be considered and the one that uses the least amount of puffs to deliver the required dose is favourable.

Patients should be instructed carefully on the use of the inhaler device and be able to demonstrate satisfactory technique. It is important to check that the inhaler continues to be used correctly because inadequate inhalation technique may be mistaken for a lack of response to the drug. For information on the correct use of inhaler devices, see Asthma and Lung UK: **How to use your inhaler** (see *Useful resources*).

On changing from a pMDI inhaler to a dry powder inhaler, patients may notice a lack of sensation in the mouth and throat previously associated with each actuation; coughing may also occur.

⟨EvGr⟩ In adults with mild or moderate acute asthma attacks, a pMDI with a spacer is at least as effective as nebulisation. ⟨A⟩

For additional information on the delivery of inhaled medicines in the management of patients with COPD, see Chronic obstructive pulmonary disease p. 276.

Advice to be given to patients

Patients should be advised on how to check the number of medication doses in their inhaler device. For metered-dose inhalers, they should be informed that these inhaler devices deliver a fixed number of medication doses per canister, and that after these doses have been used up, the inhaler will continue to actuate, expelling propellant gas but no active ingredient. This may lead to patients inadvertently using 'empty' inhalers and inhaling propellant only instead of medication, which could lead to exacerbation and destabilisation of their condition, as well as unnecessary expulsion of harmful propellant gas into the environment. An inhaler with an integral dose counter which alerts patients when all therapeutic doses have been delivered should be used where possible. For inhalers without a dose counter, there is no accurate way to gauge the remaining number of therapeutic doses other than by either recording every actuation used, or by calculating when the inhaler is likely to become 'empty' according to their standard usage. Shaking, weighing, or floating the inhaler device, or using it until it no longer actuates are inaccurate and not recommended.

Patients should also be advised to follow manufacturers' instructions on the care and cleaning of their inhaler device, and to return empty or expired inhalers to pharmacies for correct disposal (and recycling where available).

For information on inhalers and their environmental impact, see British Thoracic Society, NICE, and SIGN patient decision aid: **Asthma inhalers and climate change** (see *Useful resources*).

MHRA/CHM advice: Pressurised metered dose inhalers (pMDI): risk of airway obstruction from aspiration of loose objects (July 2018)

The MHRA have received reports of patients who have inhaled objects into the back of the throat—in some cases objects were aspirated, causing airway obstruction. Patients should be reminded to remove the mouthpiece cover fully, shake the inhaler device and check that both the outside and inside of the mouthpiece are clear and undamaged before inhaling a dose, and to store the inhaler with the mouthpiece cover on.

Spacer devices

Spacer devices remove the need for coordination between actuation of a pMDI and inhalation. They reduce the velocity of the aerosol and subsequent impaction on the oropharynx, and allow more time for evaporation of the propellant so that a larger proportion of the particles can be inhaled and deposited in the lungs. A spacer device should usually be prescribed for use with a pMDI, particularly in children (with or without a face mask), the elderly, in patients requiring high doses of inhaled corticosteroids, and for those prone to candidiasis with inhaled corticosteroids. The spacer device used should be compatible with the prescribed inhaler. Spacer devices should not be regarded as interchangeable; patients should be advised not to switch between spacer devices. For information on the different types of spacer devices available, see Spacers p. 315.

Use and care of spacer devices

Patients should inhale from the spacer device as soon as possible after actuation because the drug aerosol is very short-lived. Single puffs should be inhaled (i.e. one puff at a time) using either the tidal (or multiple) breathing method or the single breath and hold method, until the total dose (which may be more than a single puff) has been administered. Tidal breathing is as effective as single breaths. The choice of breathing method is dependent on factors such as the patient's ability, inspiratory flow, and age. Patients should be counselled appropriately on the chosen breathing method.

The spacer device should be cleaned once a month by washing in mild detergent and allowed to air-dry; the mouthpiece should be wiped clean of detergent before use. Some manufacturers recommend more frequent cleaning, but this should be avoided since any electrostatic charge may affect drug delivery. Spacer devices should be replaced every 6–12 months.

For more information on the use of spacer devices, see Asthma and Lung UK: **Spacers** (see *Useful resources*).

Nebulisers

A nebuliser converts a solution of a drug into an aerosol for inhalation via a face mask or a mouthpiece. It delivers higher doses of drug to the airways than is usual with standard inhalers. Nebuliser solutions may be used undiluted or may require dilution; the usual diluent is sterile sodium chloride 0.9% (physiological saline). Indications for use of a nebuliser include:

- to deliver a beta$_2$ agonist or ipratropium bromide p. 281 to a patient with an *acute exacerbation* of asthma or of chronic obstructive pulmonary disease;
- to deliver a beta$_2$ agonist, corticosteroid, or ipratropium bromide on a *regular basis* to a patient with severe asthma or reversible airways obstruction when the patient is unable to use other inhalational devices;
- to deliver an antibacterial (such as colistimethate sodium p. 645) or a mucolytic to a patient with cystic fibrosis;
- to deliver pentamidine isetionate p. 698 for the prophylaxis of pneumocystis pneumonia.

NHS England and NHS Improvement have issued a national patient safety alert (NPSA) regarding the inadvertent use of piped medical air via a flowmeter to drive the administration of nebulised medication. For further information, see NHS England and NHS Improvement NPSA: **Eliminating the risk of inadvertent connection to medical air via a flowmeter** (available at: www.england.nhs.uk/publication/national-patient-safety-alert-eliminating-the-risk-of-inadvertent-connection-to-medical-air-via-a-flowmeter/).

The proportion of nebuliser solution that reaches the lungs depends on the type of nebuliser. The extent to which the nebulised solution is deposited in the airways or alveoli depends on the particle size, pattern of breath inhalation, and lung disease severity. Particles with a mass median diameter of 1–5 microns are deposited in the airways, and a particle size of 1–2 microns is needed for alveolar deposition. The type of nebuliser is therefore chosen according to the deposition required and according to the viscosity of the solution.

When a nebuliser is prescribed, the patient must:
- have clear instructions on how to use the nebuliser, and maintain and clean it;
- be instructed not to treat acute attacks without also seeking medical help;
- have regular reviews as appropriate.

Jet nebulisers

Jet nebulisers are more widely used than ultrasonic nebulisers. Most jet nebulisers require an optimum gas flow rate of 6–8 litres/minute and can be driven by air or oxygen. Domiciliary oxygen cylinders do not provide an adequate flow rate therefore an electrical compressor is required for domiciliary use.

For patients at risk of hypercapnia, such as those with chronic obstructive pulmonary disease, oxygen can be dangerous and the nebuliser should be driven by air. If oxygen is required, it should be given simultaneously by nasal cannula.

Some jet nebulisers are able to increase drug output during inspiration and hence increase efficiency.

Tubing

The Department of Health and Social Care has reminded users of the need to use the correct grade of tubing when connecting a nebuliser to a medical gas supply or compressor.

Ultrasonic nebulisers

Ultrasonic nebulisers produce an aerosol by ultrasonic vibration of the drug solution and therefore do not require a gas flow; they are not suitable for the nebulisation of some drugs, such as dornase alfa p. 335 or nebulised suspensions.

Vibrating mesh nebulisers

Vibrating mesh nebulisers produce an aerosol of consistently small sized particles by using the vibration of the mesh to act as a pump to push the liquid drug through the holes of the mesh. They do not require a compressed air source, can be battery operated, and are silent, small, and portable.

Peak flow meters

When used in addition to symptom-based monitoring, peak flow monitoring has not been proven to improve asthma control, however measurement of peak flow may be of benefit in adult patients who are 'poor perceivers' and hence slow to detect deterioration in their asthma, and for those with more severe asthma.

When peak flow meters are used, patients must be given clear guidelines as to the action they should take if their peak flow falls below a certain level. Patients can be encouraged to adjust some of their own treatment (within specified limits) according to changes in peak flow rate. Peak flow diaries are available for patients to use to record their peak flow scores.

For information on the types of peak flow meters available, see Peak flow meters: standard range p. 315.

Useful Resources

Patient decision aid: Asthma inhalers and climate change. British Thoracic Society, National Institute for Health and Care Excellence, and Scottish Intercollegiate Guidelines Network. NICE guideline NG245. November 2024. www.nice.org.uk/guidance/ng245/resources

Spacers. Asthma and Lung UK. January 2024. www.asthmaandlung.org.uk/symptoms-tests-treatments/treatments/spacers

How to use your inhaler. Asthma and Lung UK. www.asthmaandlung.org.uk/living-with/inhaler-videos

Resources for families and children, young people with asthma, schools, primary healthcare professionals, secondary healthcare professionals. Beat asthma. www.beatasthma.co.uk/resources/

1 Airways disease, obstructive

Asthma, chronic

13-Mar-2025

Description of condition

Asthma is a common chronic inflammatory condition of the airways, associated with airway hyperresponsiveness and variable airflow obstruction. The most frequent symptoms of asthma are cough, wheeze, chest tightness, and breathlessness. Asthma symptoms vary over time and in intensity and can gradually or suddenly worsen, provoking an acute asthma attack that, if severe, may require hospitalisation.

Aims of treatment

The aim of treatment is to achieve control of asthma. Complete control of asthma is defined as no daytime symptoms, no night-time awakening due to asthma, no asthma attacks, no need for rescue medication, no limitations on activity including exercise, normal lung function (in practical terms forced expiratory volume in 1 second (FEV_1) and/or peak expiratory flow (PEF) > 80% predicted or best), and minimal side-effects from treatment. Uncontrolled asthma refers to asthma symptoms that impact a person's lifestyle or restrict their normal activities; it includes any asthma exacerbation needing treatment with oral corticosteroids and/or frequent regular symptoms such as needing a reliever inhaler 3 or more days per week, or night-time awakening due to asthma symptoms at least once a week. For effective asthma management, the patient's/carer's concerns and expectations should also be considered as these may differ from clinical goals.

Lifestyle changes

EvGr Weight loss in overweight or obese patients may lead to an improvement in asthma symptoms and control. Patients should be advised on approaches for minimising exposure to air pollution and any other personal triggers which cause asthma symptoms and exacerbations. Patients with asthma and parents of children with asthma should also be advised about the dangers of smoking, to themselves and to their children, and be offered appropriate support to stop smoking. A For further information, see Smoking cessation p. 565.

EvGr Breathing exercise programmes (including physiotherapist-taught methods and audiovisual programmes) can be offered to adults as an adjuvant to drug treatment to improve quality of life and reduce symptoms. A

Principles of pharmacological management

EvGr A stepwise approach aims to stop symptoms quickly and to improve peak flow. Treatment should be started at the level most appropriate to initial severity of asthma. The aim is to achieve early control and to maintain it by stepping up treatment as necessary and decreasing treatment when control is good. Possible reasons for uncontrolled asthma (such as alternative diagnoses or co-morbidities, suboptimal adherence or inhaler technique, active or passive smoking, and psychosocial, seasonal, or environmental factors) should be taken into account or addressed before starting or adjusting treatment. The response should be reviewed 8 to 12 weeks after starting or adjusting asthma treatment.

Short-acting beta$_2$ agonists (SABAs) such as salbutamol or terbutaline should not be prescribed to patients with asthma without a concomitant prescription of an inhaled corticosteroid (ICS) as clinical outcomes are poorer when a SABA is used alone.

A self-management programme comprising of a written personalised action plan and education should be offered to all patients with asthma (and/or their family or carers), and should be supported with regular review by a healthcare professional. A

The following terms are used in *Drug treatment for adults and children aged* 12 *years and over*, *Drug treatment for children aged* 5 *to* 11 *years*, and *Decreasing treatment*:

- **Anti-inflammatory reliever (AIR) therapy**
  - AIR therapy is treatment with a reliever inhaler that contains a combination of an ICS and the fast-onset long-acting beta$_2$ agonist (LABA) formoterol. When this is used in response to symptoms without regular maintenance therapy, it is called **as-needed AIR** therapy. Currently, only budesonide with formoterol p. 298 is licensed for as-needed AIR therapy in mild asthma.
- **Maintenance and reliever therapy (MART)**
  - MART refers to treatment with a combination inhaler containing an ICS and formoterol used for daily maintenance therapy *and* the relief of symptoms as needed. The terms low-dose MART and moderate-dose MART refer to the ICS dosage of the maintenance component of MART. Currently, only beclometasone with formoterol p. 294 and budesonide with formoterol are licensed for MART.

For information on devices used for the delivery of inhaled medicines, see Respiratory system, inhaled drug delivery p. 269.

Drug treatment for adults and children aged 12 years and over

For definitions of terms used in the treatment pathways, see *Principles of pharmacological management*, and for guidance on ICS doses, see *Inhaled corticosteroid (ICS) doses for adults and children aged* 12 *years and over* table.

Initial treatment

EvGr The recommended first-line treatment for newly-diagnosed asthma is as-needed AIR therapy with a low-dose ICS and formoterol combination inhaler such as budesonide with formoterol. If the patient presents as highly symptomatic or with a severe exacerbation, start treatment with low-dose MART (a course of oral corticosteroids may also be needed to treat acute symptoms); consider stepping down to as-needed AIR therapy at a later date if their asthma is controlled. A

Further treatment

EvGr Offer low-dose MART to patients with asthma not controlled on as-needed AIR therapy.

If asthma is not controlled on low-dose MART, offer patients moderate-dose MART. A

For patients not controlled on moderate-dose MART despite good adherence:

- EvGr check their fractional exhaled nitric oxide (FeNO) level if available, and blood eosinophil count. If either of these is raised, refer to a specialist in asthma care;
- if neither FeNO nor eosinophil count is raised, consider a trial of either a leukotriene receptor antagonist (LTRA) such as montelukast p. 310 or a long-acting muscarinic receptor antagonist (LAMA) such as tiotropium p. 283 in addition to moderate-dose MART. Review after 8–12 weeks and:
  - if asthma is controlled, continue treatment;
  - if asthma control is improved, but still inadequate, continue the treatment and start a trial of the other drug (LTRA or LAMA);
  - if control has not improved, stop the LTRA or LAMA and start a trial of the alternative drug (LAMA or LTRA).

If asthma is not controlled despite treatment with moderate-dose MART and trials of an LTRA and a LAMA, refer the patient to a specialist in asthma care. A

Specialist treatments for severe or difficult asthma may include theophylline, high-dose ICS, continuous oral corticosteroids, immunotherapy, or monoclonal antibodies. For further information, see British Thoracic Society (BTS)/NICE/SIGN guidance NG244: **Asthma pathway** (available at: www.nice.org.uk/guidance/ng244), and BTS/SIGN guideline 158: **British guideline on the management of asthma** (see *Useful resources*).

Treatment pathways for patients with existing asthma
Many patients with existing asthma will be on treatment pathways recommended in previous BTS/SIGN and NICE asthma guidelines.

EvGr For patients with confirmed asthma who are currently receiving treatment with a SABA only, change to as-needed AIR therapy with a low-dose ICS and formoterol combination inhaler such as budesonide with formoterol p. 298.

Patients with asthma that is well controlled on their current regimen which includes an ICS can remain on their current treatment pathway.

For patients with uncontrolled asthma, consider changing treatment as follows: A

Transferring adults and children aged 12 years and over with uncontrolled asthma from other treatment pathways

Current treatment	Consider changing to
Regular low-dose ICS plus as-needed SABA	Low-dose MART
Regular low-dose ICS/LABA combination inhaler plus as-needed SABA	Low-dose MART
Regular low-dose ICS and LTRA plus as-needed SABA	Low-dose MART, +/- LTRA
Regular low-dose ICS/LABA combination inhaler and LTRA plus as-needed SABA	Low-dose MART, +/- LTRA
Regular moderate-dose ICS plus as-needed SABA	Moderate-dose MART
Regular moderate-dose ICS/LABA combination inhaler plus as-needed SABA	Moderate-dose MART
Regular moderate-dose ICS and LTRA or LAMA, or both, plus as-needed SABA	Moderate-dose MART, +/- LTRA, +/- LAMA
Regular moderate-dose ICS/LABA combination inhaler and LTRA or LAMA, or both, plus as-needed SABA	Moderate-dose MART, +/- LTRA, +/- LAMA
Any regimen including high-dose ICS	Refer to asthma specialist

Note: When changing from a regimen containing an LTRA or a LAMA, or both, to MART, consider whether to stop or continue the LAMA and/or LTRA based on the degree of benefit achieved when first introduced.

EvGr If asthma is still not controlled despite treatment with moderate-dose MART and trials of an LTRA and a LAMA, refer the patient to a specialist in asthma care. A

Drug treatment for children aged 5 to 11 years
For definitions of terms used in the treatment pathways, see *Principles of pharmacological management*, and for guidance on ICS doses, see *Inhaled corticosteroid (ICS) doses for children aged 5 to 11 years* table.

Initial treatment
EvGr Offer a twice-daily paediatric low-dose ICS, plus a SABA as needed. A

Further treatment
MART pathway
EvGr Consider paediatric low-dose MART [unlicensed use] for children with asthma that is not controlled on twice-daily paediatric low-dose ICS plus SABA as needed, as long as they are assessed to have the ability to manage a MART regimen (otherwise, see *Conventional pathway (if MART regimen is unsuitable)*).

Consider increasing to paediatric moderate-dose MART [unlicensed use] if asthma is not controlled on paediatric low-dose MART.

Children on MART do not normally need a SABA separately, however, an additional metered-dose SABA inhaler plus a spacer may be provided for emergency use in children aged under 12 years who may be unable to activate a dry powder inhaler during an acute asthma attack.

Refer children to a specialist in asthma care if asthma is not controlled on paediatric moderate-dose MART. A

Conventional pathway (if MART regimen is unsuitable)
EvGr In children with uncontrolled asthma, consider adding a leukotriene receptor antagonist (LTRA) such as montelukast p. 310 to twice-daily paediatric low-dose ICS plus SABA as needed. Stop the LTRA if it is ineffective after 8–12 weeks.

If asthma is not controlled on twice-daily paediatric low-dose ICS, plus SABA as needed, offer a twice-daily paediatric low-dose ICS and LABA combination inhaler plus SABA as needed (with or without an LTRA depending on previous response).

If asthma is not controlled on twice-daily paediatric low-dose ICS and LABA combination inhaler, plus SABA as needed, offer a twice-daily paediatric moderate-dose ICS and LABA combination inhaler plus SABA as needed (with or without an LTRA depending on previous response).

Refer children to a specialist in asthma care if asthma is not controlled on twice-daily paediatric moderate-dose ICS and LABA combination inhaler (with or without an LTRA depending on previous response). A

Drug treatment for children aged under 5 years

Differentiating asthma symptoms from those caused by recurrent viral infections in children aged under 5 years is challenging; children with recurrent wheeze and features suggesting asthma should be treated empirically as outlined below. EvGr Any pre-school child with an admission to hospital, or 2 or more admissions to an emergency department, with wheeze in a 12-month period should be referred to a specialist respiratory paediatrician.

For children with suspected asthma and symptoms that indicate the need for maintenance therapy or who have severe acute episodes of difficulty breathing and wheeze, consider an 8 to 12 week trial of twice-daily paediatric low-dose ICS plus SABA as needed. A

If symptoms do not resolve during the trial period:
- EvGr check inhaler technique and adherence;
- check if there is an environmental source for their symptoms (e.g. mould in the home, cold housing, smokers, or indoor air pollution);
- review whether an alternative diagnosis is likely;
- refer the child to a specialist in asthma care if none of these explain the failure to respond to treatment.

If symptoms do resolve after 8 to 12 weeks, consider stopping the ICS and SABA treatment, and review the symptoms after a further 3 months. If symptoms recur by the 3-month review, or if the child has an acute episode requiring systemic corticosteroids or hospitalisation, restart twice-daily paediatric low-dose ICS with as-needed SABA. Titrate up to twice-daily paediatric moderate-dose ICS if needed. Consider a further trial without treatment after reviewing the child within 12 months.

If suspected asthma is uncontrolled on paediatric moderate-dose ICS plus SABA as needed, consider adding a leukotriene receptor antagonist (LTRA) such as montelukast. Review after 8–12 weeks and stop the LTRA if ineffective.

If suspected asthma is uncontrolled on paediatric moderate-dose ICS and a trial of an LTRA has been unsuccessful or not tolerated, stop the LTRA and refer the child to a specialist in asthma care for further investigation and management. ⟨A⟩

Decreasing treatment

For definitions of terms used, see *Principles of pharmacological management*.

EvGr When the patient's asthma has been well controlled and maintained, the potential risks and benefits of decreasing their current maintenance treatment should be discussed. When deciding which drug to decrease first and at what rate, the severity of asthma, the side-effects of treatment, duration on current dose, the beneficial effect achieved, and the patient's preference should be considered. Patients should be regularly reviewed when decreasing treatment. Allow at least 8 to 12 weeks before considering further treatment reduction.

If considering step-down treatment for patients aged 12 years and over who are using low-dose regular ICS plus a SABA as needed or low-dose MART, step down to as-needed AIR therapy. ⟨A⟩

Pregnancy

EvGr Patients with asthma should be closely monitored during pregnancy. It is important that asthma is well controlled during pregnancy to avoid maternal or fetal complications.

Patients should be counselled about the importance and safety of taking their asthma medication during pregnancy to maintain good control. Patients who smoke should be advised about the dangers to themselves and to their baby and be offered appropriate support to stop smoking. ⟨A⟩ For further information, see Smoking cessation p. 565.

EvGr Short- and long-acting beta$_2$ agonists, inhaled corticosteroids, and oral theophylline can be used as normal during pregnancy. Oral corticosteroids should be offered if necessary as the benefits outweigh the risks. If leukotriene receptor antagonists or long-acting muscarinic receptor antagonists are required to achieve adequate control, they should not be withheld. ⟨A⟩

Inhaled corticosteroid dose tables

Inhaled corticosteroid (ICS) doses for adults and children aged 12 years and over		
Dose type	Corticosteroid and form (MDI = metered dose inhaler; DPI = dry powder inhaler)	Dose
Low dose	Beclometasone dipropionate standard particle MDI and DPI	200–500 micrograms per day in 2 divided doses
	Beclometasone dipropionate extra-fine particle MDI	100–200 micrograms per day in 2 divided doses
	Budesonide DPI	200–400 micrograms per day as a single dose or in 2 divided doses
	Ciclesonide MDI	80–160 micrograms per day as a single dose
	Fluticasone propionate MDI and DPI	100–250 micrograms per day in 2 divided doses
	Mometasone furoate DPI	200 micrograms per day as a single dose
	Mometasone furoate inhalation powder capsules	80 micrograms per day as a single dose
Moderate dose	Beclometasone dipropionate standard particle MDI and DPI	600–800 micrograms per day in 2 divided doses
	Beclometasone dipropionate extra-fine particle MDI	300–400 micrograms per day in 2 divided doses
	Budesonide DPI	600–800 micrograms per day as a single dose or in 2 divided doses
	Ciclesonide MDI	240–320 micrograms per day as a single dose or in 2 divided doses
	Fluticasone propionate MDI and DPI	300–500 micrograms per day in 2 divided doses
	Fluticasone furoate DPI	100 micrograms per day as a single dose
	Mometasone furoate DPI	400 micrograms per day as a single dose or in 2 divided doses
	Mometasone furoate inhalation powder capsules	160 micrograms per day as a single dose

Dose type	Corticosteroid and form (MDI = metered dose inhaler; DPI = dry powder inhaler)	Dose
High dose	Beclometasone dipropionate standard particle MDI and DPI	1–2 mg per day in 2 divided doses
	Beclometasone dipropionate extra-fine particle MDI	500–800 micrograms per day in 2 divided doses
	Budesonide DPI	1–1.6 mg per day in 2 divided doses
	Ciclesonide MDI	400–640 micrograms per day in 2 divided doses
	Fluticasone propionate MDI and DPI	600–1000 micrograms per day in 2 divided doses
	Fluticasone furoate DPI	200 micrograms per day as a single dose
	Mometasone furoate DPI	600–800 micrograms per day in 2 divided doses
	Mometasone furoate inhalation powder capsules	320 micrograms per day as a single dose

Notes: The dose relates to the metered ICS dose, which may be different to the dose that leaves the mouthpiece (delivered dose) and the labelled strength. If an ICS/LABA inhaler is used in a MART regimen, the dose relates to the regular ICS maintenance dose. Dosages in the table are not strict dose equivalences but a guide to similar clinical effectiveness; the smallest dosage should be used to obtain optimal control. Not all inhalers are licensed for use at all dosages or for all ages (see the respective drug monographs for further information). The dosages in this table are based on BTS/NICE/SIGN guidance NG245: Asthma: diagnosis, monitoring and chronic asthma management.

Inhaled corticosteroid (ICS) doses for children aged 5 to 11 years

Dose type	Corticosteroid and form (MDI = metered dose inhaler; DPI = dry powder inhaler)	Dose
Paediatric low dose	Beclometasone dipropionate standard particle MDI	100–200 micrograms per day in 2 divided doses
	Beclometasone dipropionate extra-fine particle MDI	100 micrograms per day in 2 divided doses
	Budesonide DPI	100–200 micrograms per day as a single dose or in 2 divided doses
	Ciclesonide MDI	80 micrograms per day as a single dose
	Fluticasone propionate MDI and DPI	100 micrograms per day in 2 divided doses

Dose type	Corticosteroid and form (MDI = metered dose inhaler; DPI = dry powder inhaler)	Dose
Paediatric moderate dose	Beclometasone dipropionate standard particle MDI	300–400 micrograms per day in 2–4 divided doses
	Beclometasone dipropionate extra-fine particle MDI	150–200 micrograms per day in 2 divided doses
	Budesonide DPI	300–400 micrograms per day as a single dose or in 2 divided doses
	Ciclesonide MDI	160 micrograms per day as a single dose or in 2 divided doses
	Fluticasone propionate MDI and DPI	150–200 micrograms per day in 2 divided doses
Paediatric high dose	Beclometasone dipropionate standard particle MDI	500–800 micrograms per day in 2–4 divided doses
	Beclometasone dipropionate extra-fine particle MDI	300–400 micrograms per day in 2 divided doses
	Budesonide DPI	500–800 micrograms per day in 2 divided doses
	Ciclesonide MDI	240–320 micrograms per day in 2 divided doses
	Fluticasone propionate MDI and DPI	250–400 micrograms per day in 2 divided doses

Notes: The dose relates to the metered ICS dose, which may be different to the dose that leaves the mouthpiece (delivered dose) and the labelled strength. If an ICS/LABA inhaler is used in a MART regimen, the dose relates to the regular ICS maintenance dose. Dosages in the table are not strict dose equivalences but a guide to similar clinical effectiveness; the smallest dosage should be used to obtain optimal control. Not all inhalers are licensed for use at all dosages or for all ages (see the respective drug monographs for further information). The dosages in this table are based on BTS/NICE/SIGN guidance NG245: Asthma: diagnosis, monitoring and chronic asthma management.

Useful Resources

Asthma: diagnosis, monitoring and chronic asthma management. British Thoracic Society, National Institute for Health and Care Excellence, and Scottish Intercollegiate Guidelines Network. NICE guideline NG245. November 2024. www.nice.org.uk/guidance/ng245

British guideline on the management of asthma. British Thoracic Society and Scottish Intercollegiate Guidelines Network. A national clinical guideline SIGN158. November 2024.
www.sign.ac.uk/sign-158-british-guideline-on-the-management-of-asthma

Asthma, acute

17-Jan-2023

Description of condition

Acute asthma is the progressive worsening of asthma symptoms, including breathlessness, wheeze, cough, and chest tightness. An acute exacerbation is marked by a reduction in baseline objective measures of pulmonary function, such as peak expiratory flow rate and FEV_1.

Most asthma attacks severe enough to require hospitalisation develop relatively slowly over a period of six hours or more. In children, intermittent wheezing attacks are usually triggered by viral infections and response to asthma medication may be inconsistent. Low birth weight and/or prematurity may be risk factors for recurrent wheeze.

An asthma care bundle is available to inform the management of patients discharged from hospital following an acute asthma attack. It aims to reduce the number of hospital admissions and improve patient outcomes. For more information, see British Thoracic Society: **Asthma care bundles** (available at: www.brit-thoracic.org.uk/quality-improvement/clinical-resources/asthma/bts-asthma-care-bundles/).

Aims of treatment

The aim of treatment is to relieve airflow obstruction and prevent future relapses. Early treatment is most advantageous.

Levels of severity

Adults

EvGr An acute exacerbation of asthma should be correctly differentiated from poor asthma control and its severity categorised in order to be appropriately treated. The categories are described as follows: ⓐ

Moderate acute asthma

- Increasing symptoms;
- Peak flow > 50-75% best or predicted;
- No features of acute severe asthma.

Severe acute asthma

Any one of the following:

- Peak flow 33-50% best or predicted;
- Respiratory rate $\geq$ 25/min;
- Heart rate $\geq$ 110/min;
- Inability to complete sentences in one breath.

Life-threatening acute asthma

Any one of the following in a patient with severe asthma:

- Peak flow < 33% best or predicted;
- Arterial oxygen saturation (SpO_2) < 92%;
- Partial arterial pressure of oxygen (PaO_2) < 8 kPa;
- Normal partial arterial pressure of carbon dioxide ($PaCO_2$) (4.6–6.0 kPa);
- Silent chest;
- Cyanosis;
- Poor respiratory effort;
- Arrhythmia;
- Exhaustion;
- Altered conscious level;
- Hypotension.

Near-fatal acute asthma

- Raised $PaCO_2$ and/or the need for mechanical ventilation with raised inflation pressures.

Children

EvGr An acute exacerbation of asthma should be correctly differentiated from poor asthma control and its severity categorised in order to be appropriately treated. The categories are described as follows: ⓐ

Moderate acute asthma

- Able to talk in sentences;
- Arterial oxygen saturation (SpO_2) $\geq$ 92%;
- Peak flow $\geq$ 50% best or predicted;
- Heart rate $\leq$ 140/minute in children aged 1–5 years; heart rate $\leq$ 125/minute in children aged over 5 years;
- Respiratory rate $\leq$ 40/minute in children aged 1–5 years; respiratory rate $\leq$ 30/minute in children aged over 5 years.

Severe acute asthma

- Can't complete sentences in one breath or too breathless to talk or feed;
- SpO_2 < 92%;
- Peak flow 33–50% best or predicted;
- Heart rate > 140/minute in children aged 1–5 years; heart rate > 125/minute in children aged over 5 years;

- Respiratory rate > 40/minute in children aged 1–5 years; respiratory rate > 30/minute in children aged over 5 years.

Life-threatening acute asthma

Any one of the following in a child with severe asthma:

- SpO_2 < 92%;
- Peak flow < 33% best or predicted;
- Silent chest;
- Cyanosis;
- Poor respiratory effort;
- Hypotension;
- Exhaustion;
- Confusion.

Management in adults

EvGr Patients with features of **severe** or **life-threatening** acute asthma should start treatment as soon as possible and be referred to hospital immediately following initial assessment. Patients with **moderate** acute asthma should be treated at home or in primary care and response to treatment assessed. Hospital referral may also be warranted depending on the patient's response to treatment, social circumstances or concomitant disease.

Supplementary oxygen should be given to all hypoxaemic patients with severe acute asthma to maintain an SpO_2 level between 94–98%. Do not delay if pulse oximetry is unavailable.

First-line treatment for acute asthma is a high-dose inhaled short-acting beta$_2$ agonist (such as salbutamol p. 287) given as soon as possible. For patients with mild to moderate acute asthma, a pressurised metered-dose inhaler and spacer can be used. For patients with acute severe or life-threatening symptoms, administration via an oxygen-driven nebuliser is recommended, if available. If the response to an initial dose of nebulised short-acting beta$_2$ agonist is poor, consider continuous nebulisation with an appropriate nebuliser. Intravenous beta$_2$ agonists are reserved for those patients in whom inhaled therapy cannot be used reliably.

In all cases of acute asthma, patients should be prescribed an adequate dose of oral prednisolone p. 791. Continue usual inhaled corticosteroid use during oral corticosteroid treatment. Parenteral hydrocortisone p. 787 or intramuscular methylprednisolone p. 790 are alternatives in patients who are unable to take oral prednisolone. ⓐ

For information on the general use and side-effects of corticosteroids, see Corticosteroids, general use p. 780. For information on the cessation of oral corticosteroid treatment, see *Treatment cessation* for systemic corticosteroids (such as prednisolone).

EvGr Nebulised ipratropium bromide p. 281 may be combined with a nebulised beta$_2$ agonist in patients with severe or life-threatening acute asthma, or in those with a poor initial response to beta$_2$ agonist therapy to provide greater bronchodilation. ⓐ

There is some evidence that magnesium sulfate p. 1193 has bronchodilator effects. EvGr A single intravenous dose of magnesium sulfate may be considered in patients with severe acute asthma (peak flow < 50% best or predicted) who have not had a good initial response to inhaled bronchodilator therapy [unlicensed use]. ⓐ In an acute asthma attack, intravenous aminophylline p. 312 is not likely to produce any additional bronchodilation compared to standard therapy with inhaled bronchodilators and corticosteroids. However, in some patients with near-fatal or life-threatening acute asthma with a poor response to initial therapy, intravenous aminophylline may provide some benefit. EvGr Magnesium sulfate by intravenous infusion or aminophylline should only be used after consultation with senior medical staff. ⓐ

Management in children aged 2 years and over

EvGr Children with features of **severe** or **life-threatening** acute asthma should start treatment as soon as possible and be referred to hospital immediately following initial assessment.

Any child who fails to respond to treatment adequately at any time should also be referred to hospital immediately.

Supplementary high flow oxygen (via a tight-fitting face mask or nasal cannula) should be given to all children with life-threatening acute asthma or $SpO_2 < 94\%$ to achieve normal saturations of 94–98%.

First-line treatment for acute asthma is an inhaled short-acting $beta_2$ agonist (such as salbutamol) given as soon as possible. For children with mild to moderate acute asthma, a pressurised metered-dose inhaler and spacer device is the preferred option. The dose given should be individualised according to severity and adjusted based on response. Parents/carers of children with acute asthma at home, should seek urgent medical attention if initial symptoms are not controlled with up to 10 puffs of salbutamol p. 287 via a spacer; if symptoms are severe, additional bronchodilator doses should be given as needed whilst awaiting medical attention. Urgent medical attention should also be sought if a child's symptoms return within 3-4 hours; if symptoms return within this time, a further or larger dose (maximum of 10 puffs of salbutamol via a spacer) should be given whilst awaiting medical attention. For children with acute severe or life-threatening symptoms, administration via an oxygen-driven nebuliser is recommended, if available. A Home use of nebulisers for the treatment of acute asthma in children should be initiated and managed by an appropriate specialist.

EvGr In all cases of acute asthma, children should be prescribed an adequate dose of oral prednisolone p. 791. Treatment for up to 3 days is usually sufficient, but the length of the course should be tailored to the number of days necessary to bring about recovery. Repeat the dose in children who vomit and consider the intravenous route in those who are unable to retain oral medication. It is considered good practice that inhaled corticosteroids are continued at their usual maintenance dose whilst receiving additional treatment for the attack, but they should not be used as a replacement for the oral corticosteroid. A

For information on the general use and side-effects of corticosteroids, see Corticosteroids, general use p. 780. For information on the cessation of oral corticosteroid treatment, see *Treatment cessation* for systemic corticosteroids (such as prednisolone).

EvGr Nebulised ipratropium bromide p. 281 can be combined with a nebulised $beta_2$ agonist for children with a poor initial response to $beta_2$ agonist therapy to provide greater bronchodilation. Consider adding magnesium sulfate p. 1193 [unlicensed use] to each nebulised salbutamol and ipratropium bromide in the first hour in children with a short duration of severe acute asthma symptoms presenting with an oxygen saturation less than 92%.

Children with continuing severe acute asthma despite frequent nebulised $beta_2$ agonists and ipratropium bromide plus oral corticosteroids, and those with life-threatening features, need urgent review by a specialist with a view to transfer to a high dependency unit or paediatric intensive care unit (PICU) to receive second-line intravenous therapies.

In children who respond poorly to first-line treatments, intravenous magnesium sulfate [unlicensed use] may be considered as first-line intravenous treatment. In a severe asthma attack where the child has not responded to initial inhaled therapy, early addition of a single bolus dose of intravenous salbutamol may be an option. Continuous intravenous infusion of salbutamol, administered under specialist supervision with continuous ECG and electrolyte monitoring, should be considered in children with unreliable inhalation or severe refractory asthma. Intravenous aminophylline p. 312 may be considered in children with severe or life-threatening acute asthma unresponsive to maximal doses of bronchodilators and corticosteroids. A

Management in children aged under 2 years

EvGr Acute asthma treatment for all children aged under 2 years should be given in the hospital setting. Treatment of children aged under 1 year should be under the direct guidance of a respiratory paediatrician.

For moderate and severe acute asthma attacks, immediate treatment with oxygen via a tight-fitting face mask or nasal prongs should be given to achieve normal SpO_2 saturations of 94-98%. Trial an inhaled short-acting $beta_2$ agonist and if response is poor, combine nebulised ipratropium bromide to each nebulised $beta_2$ agonist dose. Consider oral prednisolone daily for up to 3 days, early in the management of severe asthma attacks.

In children not responsive to first-line treatments or have life-threatening features, discuss management with a senior paediatrician or the PICU team. A

Follow up in all cases

EvGr Episodes of acute asthma may be a failure of preventative therapy, review is required to prevent further episodes. A careful history should be taken to establish the reason for the asthma attack. Inhaler technique should be checked and regular treatment should be reviewed. Patients should be given a written asthma action plan aimed at preventing relapse, optimising treatment, and preventing delay in seeking assistance in future attacks. It is essential that the patient's GP practice is informed within 24 hours of discharge from the emergency department or hospital following an asthma attack, and the patient be reviewed by their GP within 2 working days. Patients who have had a near-fatal asthma attack should be kept under specialist supervision indefinitely. A respiratory specialist should follow up all patients admitted with a severe asthma attack for at least one year after the admission. A

Useful Resources

British guideline on the management of asthma. British Thoracic Society and Scottish Intercollegiate Guidelines Network. Full guidance - A national clinical guideline 158. July 2019.
www.sign.ac.uk/sign-158-british-guideline-on-the-management-of-asthma

Chronic obstructive pulmonary disease

20-Aug-2023

Description of condition

Chronic obstructive pulmonary disease (COPD) is a common, largely preventable and treatable disease, characterised by persistent respiratory symptoms and airflow limitation that is usually progressive and not fully reversible. Airflow limitation is due to a combination of small airways disease (obstructive bronchiolitis) and parenchymal destruction (emphysema). Symptoms of COPD include dyspnoea, wheeze, chronic cough, and regular sputum production.

The main risk factor for development and exacerbations of COPD is tobacco smoking. Other risk factors include environmental pollution and occupational exposures, genetic factors (such as hereditary alpha-1 antitrypsin deficiency), and poor lung growth during childhood. Complications of COPD include cor pulmonale, depression, anxiety, type 2 respiratory failure, and secondary polycythaemia.

Asthma-COPD overlap syndrome (ACOS) is characterised by persistent airflow limitation that displays features of both asthma and COPD.

Aims of treatment

The primary aim of treatment is to reduce symptoms and exacerbations and improve quality of life.

Management of stable COPD

Non-drug treatment

[EvGr] Patients who are smokers should be encouraged to stop smoking and be offered help to do so. For further information, see Smoking cessation p. 565.

All patients should receive care delivered by a multidisciplinary team. Pulmonary rehabilitation should be offered to appropriate patients, including those who view themselves as being functionally disabled by COPD. Pulmonary rehabilitation programmes should be tailored to the patient's individual needs, and include physical training, disease education, and nutritional, psychological and behavioural intervention.

Patients with excessive sputum production should be taught active cycle of breathing techniques, and how to use positive expiratory pressure devices by a physiotherapist.

Refer patients with a BMI that is abnormal or changing over time for dietetic input, and be attentive to changes in weight in the elderly.

Interventional procedures including surgery may be deemed appropriate following a respiratory review and input from the multidisciplinary team. [A]

Vaccinations

[EvGr] All patients should be offered the pneumococcal vaccine and annual influenza vaccine (inactivated) p. 1508. [A]

Inhaled treatment

[EvGr] The choice of inhaler device should be based on the patient's preference and ability to use the inhaler. When prescribing an inhaler, patients should be trained on how to use the device and be able to demonstrate satisfactory inhaler technique, and continue to have their inhaler technique regularly assessed. Where appropriate a spacer can be provided. Nebulised treatment should be considered for patients with distressing or disabling breathlessness despite maximal use of inhalers, and continued if an improvement is seen in symptoms, ability to undertake activities of daily living, exercise capacity, or lung function. [A] For further information on devices used for the delivery of inhaled medicines, see Respiratory system, inhaled drug delivery p. 269.

Initial management for all patients

[EvGr] For initial empirical treatment, offer a short-acting bronchodilator as required to relieve breathlessness and exercise limitation. This can either be a short-acting beta$_2$ agonist (SABA) or a short-acting muscarinic antagonist (SAMA).

Before considering step-up treatment options, ensure that COPD is confirmed spirometrically, relevant vaccinations are given, non-drug treatment options have been optimised including smoking cessation, and that a short-acting bronchodilator is being used. [A]

Step-up treatment for patients without asthmatic features or features suggesting steroid responsiveness

[EvGr] In patients who continue to be breathless or have exacerbations, offer a long-acting beta$_2$ agonist (LABA) and a long-acting muscarinic antagonist (LAMA). Discontinue SAMA treatment if a LAMA is given. Treatment with a SABA as required may be continued in all stages of COPD.

In patients on a LAMA and LABA who have a severe exacerbation (requiring hospitalisation) or at least two moderate exacerbations (requiring systemic corticosteroids and/or antibacterial treatment) within a year, consider the addition of an inhaled corticosteroid (ICS)—triple therapy. If an ICS is given, review at least annually and document the reason for continuation.

In patients on a LAMA and LABA whose day-to-day symptoms continue to adversely impact their quality of life, consider trialling the addition of an ICS for 3 months. If symptoms have improved, continue triple therapy and review at least annually. If there has been no improvement, step back down to a LAMA and LABA combination. [A]

Step-up treatment for patients with asthmatic features or features suggesting steroid responsiveness

[EvGr] In patients who continue to be breathless or have exacerbations, consider treatment with a long-acting beta$_2$ agonist (LABA) and an inhaled corticosteroid (ICS). If an ICS is given, review annually documenting the reason for continuation.

In patients on a LABA and ICS who have a severe exacerbation (requiring hospitalisation) or at least two moderate exacerbations (requiring systemic corticosteroids and/or antibacterial treatment) within a year, or who continue to have day-to-day symptoms adversely impacting their quality of life, add a long-acting muscarinic antagonist (LAMA)—triple therapy. Discontinue SAMA treatment if a LAMA is given. Treatment with a SABA as required may be continued in all stages of COPD. [A]

Prophylactic antibiotics

[EvGr] After considering if respiratory specialist input is required, consider azithromycin p. 620 [unlicensed] prophylaxis to reduce the risk of exacerbations in patients who are non-smokers, have had all other treatment options optimised, and who continue to either have prolonged or frequent (4 or more per year) exacerbations with sputum production, or exacerbations resulting in hospitalisation. Ensure sputum culture and sensitivity testing, a CT scan of the thorax (to rule out other lung pathologies), a baseline ECG (to rule out QT prolongation), and LFTs are performed before offering prophylaxis. Review treatment after the first 3 months, then at least 6 monthly thereafter; only continue if benefits outweigh risks. [A]

Other treatments

[EvGr] Roflumilast p. 311 is recommended as add-on treatment to bronchodilator therapy in patients with severe COPD with chronic bronchitis (respiratory specialist initiation only), see *National funding/access decisions* for roflumilast. For guidance and the national funding access decision for roflumilast in Scotland, refer to the *Scottish Medicines Consortium*.

Consider mucolytic treatment in patients with chronic cough productive of sputum; only continue if symptomatic improvement is seen. Antitussive treatment should not be used in the management of stable COPD.

Modified-release theophylline p. 313 should only be used after a trial of short-acting and long-acting bronchodilators, or if the patient is unable to use inhaled treatment.

Be alert to the presence of anxiety or depression in patients, and manage accordingly. [A]

For information on oxygen therapy in COPD patients, see Oxygen p. 278.

For guidance on the management of COPD patients with cor pulmonale and/or pulmonary hypertension, see NICE guideline: **Chronic obstructive pulmonary disease in over 16s** (see *Useful resources*).

Management of exacerbations of COPD

[EvGr] Together with the patient, action plans should be created for those at risk of exacerbations. In patients who have had an exacerbation within the last year, a short course of antibacterials (non-macrolide if on prophylactic azithromycin) and oral corticosteroids should be kept at home. Patients should understand and be confident with when and how to take these medicines, and to report having taken them to their healthcare professional. Patients may continue prophylactic azithromycin during an acute exacerbation.

Action plans may also include information on adjusting the short-acting bronchodilator dose, and a cognitive behavioural plan to manage symptoms of anxiety and associated breathlessness. Ⓐ

For guidance on assessing the need for hospital referral, see NICE guideline: **Chronic obstructive pulmonary disease in over 16s** (see *Useful resources*).

For guidance on antibacterial treatment in acute exacerbations of COPD, see *Chronic obstructive pulmonary disease, acute exacerbations* in Respiratory system infections, antibacterial therapy p. 586.

Non-drug treatment
EvGr Where appropriate consider physiotherapy using positive expiratory pressure devices to help with sputum clearance. Ⓐ

Drug treatment
EvGr Give short-acting inhaled bronchodilators, usually at higher doses than the patient's maintenance treatment through a nebuliser or hand-held device to manage breathlessness. The choice should be dependant on the dose required, the patient's ability to use the device, and resources available to supervise administration. Withhold LAMA treatment if a SAMA is given.

In the absence of significant contra-indications in patients that present to hospital with an exacerbation, use a short course of prednisolone p. 791 along with other therapies. Consider a short course for patients in the community experiencing an exacerbation with a significant increase in breathlessness that interferes with daily activities. Consider osteoporosis prophylaxis for patients who require frequent courses of oral corticosteroids.

Long-term oral corticosteroid treatment is not usually recommended, however in some patients this may need to be continued when withdrawal following an exacerbation is not possible; the lowest dose possible should be used. Monitor patients for osteoporosis and give them appropriate prophylaxis. Start prophylaxis without monitoring for osteoporosis in patients aged over 65 years; for guidance on choice of therapy, see Osteoporosis p. 768. Ⓐ

For information on the general use and side effects of corticosteroids, see Corticosteroids, general use p. 780. For information on the cessation of oral corticosteroid treatment, see *Treatment cessation* for systemic corticosteroids (such as prednisolone).

EvGr Aminophylline p. 312 should only be used as add-on treatment when there is an inadequate response to nebulised bronchodilators; ensure therapeutic drug monitoring is performed and that previous oral theophylline use is considered to avoid toxicity.

If necessary, oxygen should be given to ensure oxygen saturation of arterial blood levels are kept within the target range for the patient. For further information, see Oxygen below.

For patients with persistant hypercapnic ventilatory failure, use non-invasive ventilation (NIV) if patients experience exacerbations despite the optimisation of medical treatment. If deemed necessary, invasive ventilation for COPD exacerbations should be given in an intensive care unit. Doxapram should only be given when NIV is inappropriate or unavailable in the clinical setting. Ⓐ

Useful Resources

Chronic obstructive pulmonary disease in over 16s: diagnosis and management. National Institute for Health and Care Excellence. NICE guideline 115; December 2018, updated July 2019.
www.nice.org.uk/guidance/ng115

Chronic obstructive pulmonary disease (acute exacerbation): antimicrobial prescribing. National Institute

for Health and Care Excellence. NICE guideline 114; December 2018.
www.nice.org.uk/guidance/ng114

Oxygen

29-Sep-2019

Overview

Oxygen should be regarded as a drug. It is prescribed for hypoxaemic patients to increase alveolar oxygen tension and decrease the work of breathing. The concentration of oxygen required depends on the condition being treated; the administration of an inappropriate concentration of oxygen can have serious or even fatal consequences.

Oxygen is probably the most common drug used in medical emergencies. It should be prescribed initially to achieve a normal or near–normal oxygen saturation; in most acutely ill patients with a normal or low arterial carbon dioxide ($P_a CO_2$), oxygen saturation should be 94–98% oxygen saturation. However, in some clinical situations such as cardiac arrest and carbon monoxide poisoning it is more appropriate to aim for the highest possible oxygen saturation until the patient is stable. A lower target of 88–92% oxygen saturation is indicated for patients at risk of hypercapnic respiratory failure.

High concentration oxygen therapy is safe in uncomplicated cases of conditions such as pneumonia, pulmonary thromboembolism, pulmonary fibrosis, shock, severe trauma, sepsis, or anaphylaxis. In such conditions low arterial oxygen ($P_a O_2$) is usually associated with low or normal arterial carbon dioxide ($P_a CO_2$), and therefore there is little risk of hypoventilation and carbon dioxide retention.

In acute severe asthma, the arterial carbon dioxide ($P_a CO_2$) is usually subnormal but as asthma deteriorates it may rise steeply (particularly in children). These patients usually require high concentrations of oxygen and if the arterial carbon dioxide ($P_a CO_2$) remains high despite other treatment, intermittent positive-pressure ventilation needs to be considered urgently.

Low concentration oxygen therapy (controlled oxygen therapy) is reserved for patients at risk of hypercapnic respiratory failure, which is more likely in those with:

- chronic obstructive pulmonary disease (COPD);
- advanced cystic fibrosis;
- severe non-cystic fibrosis bronchiectasis;
- severe kyphoscoliosis or severe ankylosing spondylitis;
- severe lung scarring caused by tuberculosis;
- musculoskeletal disorders with respiratory weakness, especially if on home ventilation;
- an overdose of opioids, benzodiazepines, or other drugs causing respiratory depression.

EvGr Until blood gases can be measured, initial oxygen should be given using a controlled concentration of 24% or 28%, titrated towards a target oxygen saturation of 88–92% or the level specified on the patient's *oxygen alert card* if available. Ⓐ The aim is to provide the patient with enough oxygen to achieve an acceptable arterial oxygen tension without worsening carbon dioxide retention and respiratory acidosis.

EvGr Patients with COPD and other at-risk conditions who have had an episode of hypercapnic respiratory failure, should be given a 24% or 28% Venturi mask and an oxygen alert card endorsed with the oxygen saturations required during previous exacerbations. Patients and their carers should be instructed to show the card to emergency healthcare providers in the event of an exacerbation. Ⓐ

The oxygen alert card template is available at www.brit-thoracic.org.uk.

Domiciliary oxygen

Oxygen should only be prescribed for use in the home after careful evaluation in hospital by respiratory experts. Patients should be advised of the risks of continuing to smoke when receiving oxygen therapy, including the risk of fire. Smoking cessation p. 565 therapy should be recommended before home oxygen prescription. EvGr In patients with COPD, it should only be provided if the patient has stopped smoking. Ⓐ

Air travel

Some patients with arterial hypoxaemia require supplementary oxygen for air travel. The patient's requirement should be discussed with the airline before travel.

Long-term oxygen therapy

Long-term administration of oxygen (usually at least 15 hours daily) improves survival in COPD patients with more severe hypoxaemia. EvGr The need for oxygen should be assessed in COPD patients with an FEV_1 less than 30% predicted (consider assessment if FEV_1 is 30-49%), cyanosis, polycythaemia, peripheral oedema, raised JVP, and when oxygen saturation levels are 92% or less breathing air. Ⓐ

Assessment for long-term oxygen therapy requires measurement of arterial blood gas tensions. Measurements should be taken on 2 occasions at least 3 weeks apart to demonstrate clinical stability. Long-term oxygen therapy should be considered for patients with:

- EvGr COPD with $P_a O_2 < 7.3$ kPa when stable and who do not smoke (minimum of 15 hours per day);
- COPD with $P_a O_2$ 7.3–8 kPa when stable and do not smoke, and also have either secondary polycythaemia, peripheral oedema, or evidence of pulmonary hypertension (minimum of 15 hours per day); Ⓐ
- severe chronic asthma with $P_a O_2 < 7.3$ kPa or persistent disabling breathlessness;
- interstitial lung disease with $P_a O_2 < 8$ kPa and in patients with $P_a O_2 > 8$ kPa with disabling dyspnoea;
- cystic fibrosis when $P_a O_2 < 7.3$ kPa or if $P_a O_2$ 7.3–8 kPa in the presence of secondary polycythaemia, nocturnal hypoxaemia, pulmonary hypertension, or peripheral oedema;
- pulmonary hypertension, without parenchymal lung involvement when $P_a O_2 < 8$ kPa;
- neuromuscular or skeletal disorders, after specialist assessment;
- obstructive sleep apnoea despite continuous positive airways pressure therapy, after specialist assessment;
- pulmonary malignancy or other terminal disease with disabling dyspnoea;
- heart failure with daytime $P_a O_2 < 7.3$ kPa when breathing air or with nocturnal hypoxaemia;
- paediatric respiratory disease, after specialist assessment.

Increased respiratory depression is seldom a problem in patients with stable respiratory failure treated with low concentrations of oxygen although it may occur during exacerbations; patients and relatives should be warned to call for medical help if drowsiness or confusion occur.

EvGr A risk assessment should be carried out for all COPD patients being considered for long-term oxygen therapy and if treatment is given, should be reviewed at least annually. Offer smoking cessation advice, treatment and specialist referral for people who smoke or smokers living with the patient with COPD. Do not offer long-term oxygen therapy to patients who continue to smoke despite being offered smoking cessation interventions. Ⓐ

Short-burst oxygen therapy

Oxygen is occasionally prescribed for short-burst (intermittent) use for episodes of breathlessness not relieved by other treatment in patients with interstitial lung disease, heart failure, and in palliative care. It is important, however, that the patient does not rely on oxygen instead of obtaining medical help or taking more specific treatment. Short-burst oxygen therapy can be used to improve exercise capacity and

recovery; it should only be continued if there is proven improvement in breathlessness or exercise tolerance. EvGr It is not recommended for COPD patients who have mild or no hypoxaemia at rest. Ⓐ

Ambulatory oxygen therapy

Ambulatory oxygen is prescribed for patients on long-term oxygen therapy who need to be away from home on a regular basis. Patients who are not on long-term oxygen therapy can be considered for ambulatory oxygen therapy if there is evidence of exercise-induced oxygen desaturation and of improvement in blood oxygen saturation and exercise capacity with oxygen. Ambulatory oxygen therapy is not recommended for patients with heart failure, COPD with mild or no hypoxaemia at rest, or those who smoke.

Oxygen therapy equipment

Under the NHS oxygen may be supplied as **oxygen cylinders**. Oxygen flow can be adjusted as the cylinders are equipped with an oxygen flow meter with 'medium' (2 litres/minute) and 'high' (4 litres/minute) settings. Oxygen delivered from a cylinder should be passed through a humidifier if used for long periods.

Oxygen concentrators are more economical for patients who require oxygen for long periods, and in England and Wales can be ordered on the NHS on a regional tendering basis. A concentrator is recommended for a patient who requires oxygen for more than 8 hours a day (or 21 cylinders per month). Exceptionally, if a higher concentration of oxygen is required the output of 2 oxygen concentrators can be combined using a 'Y' connection.

A nasal cannula is usually preferred for long-term oxygen therapy from an oxygen concentrator. It can, however, produce dermatitis and mucosal drying in sensitive individuals.

Giving oxygen by nasal cannula allows the patient to talk, eat, and drink, but the concentration of oxygen is not controlled; this may not be appropriate for acute respiratory failure. When oxygen is given through a nasal cannula at a rate of 1–2 litres/minute the inspiratory oxygen concentration is usually low, but it varies with ventilation and can be high if the patient is underventilating.

Arrangements for supplying oxygen

The following oxygen services may be ordered in England and Wales:

- emergency oxygen;
- short-burst (intermittent) oxygen therapy;
- long-term oxygen therapy;
- ambulatory oxygen.

The type of oxygen service (or combination of services) should be ordered on a Home Oxygen Order Form (HOOF); the amount of oxygen required (hours per day) and flow rate should be specified. The clinician will determine the appropriate equipment to be provided. Special needs or preferences should be specified on the HOOF.

The clinician should obtain the patient or carers consent, to pass on the patient's details to the supplier, the fire brigade, and other relevant organisations. The supplier will contact the patient to make arrangements for delivery, installation, and maintenance of the equipment. The supplier will also train the patient or carer to use the equipment.

The clinician should send the HOOF to the supplier who will continue to provide the service until a revised HOOF is received, or until notified that the patient no longer requires the home oxygen service.

- East of England, North East: BOC Medical: Tel: 0800 136 603 Fax: 0800 169 9989
- South West: Air Liquide: Tel: 0808 202 2229 Fax: 0191 497 4340

- London, East Midlands, North West: Air Liquide: Tel: 0500 823 773 Fax: 0800 781 4610
- Yorkshire and Humberside, West Midlands, Wales: Air Products: Tel: 0800 373 580 Fax: 0800 214 709
- South East Coast, South Central: Dolby Vivisol: Tel: 08443 814 402 Fax: 0800 781 4610

In **Scotland** refer the patient for assessment by a respiratory consultant. If the need for a concentrator is confirmed the consultant will arrange for the provision of a concentrator through the Common Services Agency. Prescribers should complete a Scottish Home Oxygen Order Form (SHOOF) and email it to Health Facilities Scotland. Health Facilities Scotland will then liaise with their contractor to arrange the supply of oxygen. Further information can be obtained at: www.dolbyvivisol.com/services/healthcare-professionals/.

In **Northern Ireland** oxygen concentrators and cylinders should be prescribed on form HS21; oxygen concentrators are supplied by a local contractor. Prescriptions for oxygen cylinders and accessories can be dispensed by pharmacists contracted to provide domiciliary oxygen services.

Croup

21-Oct-2020

Management

EvGr Mild croup is largely self-limiting, but treatment with a single dose of a corticosteroid (e.g. dexamethasone p. 786) by mouth may be of benefit.

Moderate to severe croup (or mild croup that might cause complications such as in those with chronic lung disease, immunodeficiency, impending respiratory failure, or in children aged under 3 months) calls for hospital admission; a single dose of a corticosteroid (e.g. dexamethasone or prednisolone p. 791 by mouth) should be administered while awaiting hospital admission. If the child is too unwell to receive oral medication, dexamethasone (by intramuscular injection) or budesonide p. 297 (by nebulisation) are suitable alternatives while awaiting hospital admission.

For severe croup not effectively controlled with corticosteroid treatment, nebulised adrenaline/epinephrine solution 1 in 1000 (1 mg/mL) p. 256 should be given with close clinical monitoring; Ⓐ the clinical effects of nebulised adrenaline/epinephrine last at least 1 hour, but usually subside 2 hours after administration. EvGr The child needs to be monitored carefully for recurrence of severe respiratory distress. Ⓐ

> **Other drugs used for Airways disease, obstructive**
> Dupilumab, p. 1423

ANTIMUSCARINICS

Antimuscarinics (inhaled)

09-Feb-2016

- **CAUTIONS** Bladder outflow obstruction · paradoxical bronchospasm · prostatic hyperplasia · susceptibility to angle-closure glaucoma

  CAUTIONS, FURTHER INFORMATION
  > Elderly Screening Tool of Older Persons' potentially inappropriate Prescriptions (STOPP) criteria to aid medication reviews (see Prescribing in the elderly p. 31 for information): potentially inappropriate with a history of angle-closure glaucoma (may exacerbate glaucoma) or bladder outflow obstruction (may cause urinary retention).

- **SIDE-EFFECTS**
  > **Common or very common** Arrhythmias · constipation · cough · dizziness · dry mouth · headache · nausea
  > **Uncommon** Dysphonia · glaucoma · palpitations · skin reactions · stomatitis · urinary disorders · vision blurred

Aclidinium bromide

⌐ above

17-Mar-2020

- **INDICATIONS AND DOSE**

Maintenance treatment of chronic obstructive pulmonary disease
> BY INHALATION OF POWDER
> Adult: 375 micrograms twice daily

DOSE EQUIVALENCE AND CONVERSION
> Each 375 microgram inhalation of aclidinium bromide delivers 322 micrograms of aclidinium.

- **CAUTIONS** Arrhythmia (when newly diagnosed within last 3 months) · heart failure (hospitalisation with moderate or severe heart failure within last 12 months) · myocardial infarction within last 6 months · unstable angina

- **INTERACTIONS** → Appendix 1: aclidinium

- **SIDE-EFFECTS**
  > **Common or very common** Diarrhoea · nasopharyngitis
  > **Uncommon** Angioedema
  > **Rare or very rare** Hypersensitivity

- **PREGNANCY** Manufacturer advises use only if potential benefit outweighs risk.

- **BREAST FEEDING** Manufacturer advises only use if potential benefits outweigh risks.

- **PATIENT AND CARER ADVICE** Patients or carers should be given advice on appropriate inhaler technique.

- **MEDICINAL FORMS** There can be variation in the licensing of different medicines containing the same drug.
  Inhalation powder
  > **Eklira** (Covis Pharma GmbH) ▼
  Aclidinium bromide 375 microgram per 1 dose Eklira 322micrograms/dose Genuair | 60 dose PoM £32.50 DT = £32.50

Aclidinium bromide with formoterol

16-Mar-2020

The properties listed below are those particular to the combination only. For the properties of the components please consider, aclidinium bromide above, formoterol fumarate p. 285.

- **INDICATIONS AND DOSE**

Maintenance treatment of chronic obstructive pulmonary disease
> BY INHALATION OF POWDER
> Adult: 1 inhalation twice daily

- **CAUTIONS** Convulsive disorders · phaeochromocytoma
- **INTERACTIONS** → Appendix 1: aclidinium · beta$_2$ agonists
- **PATIENT AND CARER ADVICE** Patients or carers should be given advice on appropriate inhaler technique.

- **MEDICINAL FORMS** There can be variation in the licensing of different medicines containing the same drug.
  Inhalation powder
  > **Duaklir** (Covis Pharma GmbH) ▼
  Formoterol fumarate dihydrate 11.8 microgram per 1 dose, Aclidinium bromide 396 microgram per 1 dose Duaklir 340micrograms/dose / 12micrograms/dose Genuair | 60 dose PoM £32.50 DT = £32.50

Respiratory system

3

Glycopyrronium bromide

F 280

17-Jan-2024

(Glycopyrrolate)

- **INDICATIONS AND DOSE**

Maintenance treatment of chronic obstructive pulmonary disease

- ▶ BY INHALATION OF POWDER
- ▶ Adult: 1 capsule once daily, each capsule delivers 55 micrograms of glycopyrronium bromide (equivalent to 44 micrograms of glycopyrronium)

- **CAUTIONS** Arrhythmia (excluding chronic stable atrial fibrillation) · history of myocardial infarction · history of QT-interval prolongation · left ventricular failure · unstable ischaemic heart disease

- **INTERACTIONS** → Appendix 1: glycopyrronium

- **SIDE-EFFECTS**
- ▶ **Common or very common** Increased risk of infection · insomnia · pain
- ▶ **Uncommon** Asthenia · cystitis · dental caries · dyspepsia · epistaxis · hyperglycaemia · numbness · respiratory disorders · throat irritation

- **PREGNANCY** Manufacturer advises use only if potential benefit outweighs risk.

- **BREAST FEEDING** Manufacturer advises use only if potential benefit outweighs risk.

- **RENAL IMPAIRMENT** See p. 21. Manufacturer advises use only if potential benefit outweighs risk if eGFR less than 30 mL/minute/1.73 m^2.

- **PATIENT AND CARER ADVICE** Patients or carers should be given advice on appropriate inhaler technique.

- **MEDICINAL FORMS** There can be variation in the licensing of different medicines containing the same drug.

Inhalation powder

- ▶ Seebri Breezhaler (Novartis Pharmaceuticals UK Ltd)
  Glycopyrronium bromide 55 microgram Seebri Breezhaler 44microgram inhalation powder capsules with device | 10 capsule [PoM] £9.17 | 30 capsule [PoM] £27.50 DT = £27.50

Combinations available: *Beclometasone with formoterol and glycopyrronium,* p. 296 · *Formoterol fumarate with glycopyrronium and budesonide,* p. 305 · *Mometasone furoate with glycopyrronium bromide and indacaterol,* p. 306

Glycopyrronium with formoterol fumarate

03-May-2024

The properties listed below are those particular to the combination only. For the properties of the components please consider, glycopyrronium bromide above, formoterol fumarate p. 285.

- **INDICATIONS AND DOSE**

Maintenance treatment of chronic obstructive pulmonary disease

- ▶ BY INHALATION OF AEROSOL
- ▶ Adult: 2 inhalations twice daily

- **INTERACTIONS** → Appendix 1: beta$_2$ agonists · glycopyrronium

- **HEPATIC IMPAIRMENT** [EvGr] Caution in severe impairment (no information available). ⟨M⟩

- **NATIONAL FUNDING/ACCESS DECISIONS**
  For full details see funding body website

Scottish Medicines Consortium (SMC) decisions

- ▶ Glycopyrronium with formoterol fumarate (*Bevespi Aerosphere*®) as a maintenance bronchodilator treatment to relieve symptoms in adult patients with chronic obstructive

pulmonary disease (April 2024) SMC No. SMC2652
Recommended

- **MEDICINAL FORMS** There can be variation in the licensing of different medicines containing the same drug.

Pressurised inhalation

- ▶ Bevespi Aerosphere (AstraZeneca UK Ltd)
  Formoterol fumarate dihydrate 5 microgram per 1 dose, Glycopyrronium (as Glycopyrronium bromide) 7.2 microgram per 1 dose Bevespi Aerosphere 7.2micrograms/dose / 5micrograms/dose pressurised inhaler | 120 dose [PoM] £32.50 DT = £32.50

Glycopyrronium with indacaterol

16-Mar-2020

The properties listed below are those particular to the combination only. For the properties of the components please consider, glycopyrronium bromide above, indacaterol p. 286.

- **INDICATIONS AND DOSE**

Maintenance treatment of chronic obstructive pulmonary disease

- ▶ BY INHALATION OF POWDER
- ▶ Adult: 1 inhalation daily

- **CAUTIONS** Convulsive disorders

- **INTERACTIONS** → Appendix 1: beta$_2$ agonists · glycopyrronium

- **PATIENT AND CARER ADVICE** Patients or carers should be given advice on appropriate inhaler technique and reminded that the capsules are not for oral administration.

- **MEDICINAL FORMS** There can be variation in the licensing of different medicines containing the same drug.

Inhalation powder

- ▶ Ultibro Breezhaler (Novartis Pharmaceuticals UK Ltd)
  Glycopyrronium bromide 54 microgram per 1 dose, Indacaterol (as Indacaterol maleate) 85 microgram per 1 dose Ultibro Breezhaler 85microgram/43microgram inhalation powder capsules with device | 10 capsule [PoM] £10.83 | 30 capsule [PoM] £32.50 DT = £32.50

Ipratropium bromide

F 280

13-Mar-2025

- **INDICATIONS AND DOSE**

Reversible airways obstruction

- ▶ BY INHALATION OF AEROSOL
- ▶ Child 1 month–5 years: 20 micrograms 3 times a day
- ▶ Child 6–11 years: 20–40 micrograms 3 times a day
- ▶ Child 12–17 years: 20–40 micrograms 3–4 times a day

Reversible airways obstruction, particularly in chronic obstructive pulmonary disease

- ▶ BY INHALATION OF AEROSOL
- ▶ Adult: 20–40 micrograms 3–4 times a day
- ▶ BY INHALATION OF NEBULISED SOLUTION
- ▶ Adult: 250–500 micrograms 3–4 times a day

Acute bronchospasm

- ▶ BY INHALATION OF NEBULISED SOLUTION
- ▶ Child 1 month–5 years: 125–250 micrograms as required; maximum 1 mg per day
- ▶ Child 6–11 years: 250 micrograms as required; maximum 1 mg per day
- ▶ Child 12-17 years: 500 micrograms as required, doses higher than max. can be given under medical supervision; maximum 2 mg per day
- ▶ Adult: 500 micrograms as required, doses higher than max. can be given under medical supervision; maximum 2 mg per day

continued →

Severe or life-threatening acute asthma
- ▶ BY INHALATION OF NEBULISED SOLUTION
- ▶ Child 1 month-11 years: 250 micrograms every 20–30 minutes for the first 2 hours, then 250 micrograms every 4–6 hours as required
- ▶ Child 12-17 years: 500 micrograms every 4–6 hours as required
- ▶ Adult: 500 micrograms every 4–6 hours as required

PHARMACOKINETICS
- ▶ The maximal effect of inhaled ipratropium occurs 30–60 minutes after use; its duration of action is 3 to 6 hours and bronchodilation can usually be maintained with treatment 3 times a day.

- ● UNLICENSED USE [EvGr] The dose of ipratropium for severe or life-threatening acute asthma is unlicensed. ⒶInhalvent ® not licensed for use in children under 6 years.

IMPORTANT SAFETY INFORMATION

MHRA/CHM ADVICE: PRESSURISED METERED DOSE INHALERS (PMDI): RISK OF AIRWAY OBSTRUCTION FROM ASPIRATION OF LOOSE OBJECTS (JULY 2018)
See Respiratory system, inhaled drug delivery p. 269.

MHRA/CHM ADVICE: NEBULISED ASTHMA RESCUE THERAPY IN CHILDREN: HOME USE OF NEBULISERS IN PAEDIATRIC ASTHMA SHOULD BE INITIATED AND MANAGED ONLY BY SPECIALISTS (AUGUST 2022)

The MHRA has reviewed the evidence regarding a number of deaths in children with asthma, where the clinically unsupervised use of a nebuliser to deliver asthma rescue medication was a potential contributory factor. Healthcare professionals are advised that home use of nebulisers for the acute treatment of asthma in children and adolescents should only be initiated and managed by asthma specialists. Home use of nebulisers for this purpose, without adequate medical supervision, can mask a deterioration in the underlying disease, which could result in delays in seeking medical attention and be fatal or have serious consequences. The purchase of nebulisers for this purpose, outside of medical advice, is not recommended. Patients and their carers should be advised to seek urgent medical attention if worsening asthma symptoms are not relieved by prescribed rescue medication, even if there is short-term recovery following its use. They should receive training from a healthcare professional on the usage and maintenance of the nebuliser, and be given advice on when to seek medical attention, so that deterioration in asthma control can be treated without delay. Patients (or their carers) who have been using a nebuliser at home without specialist management should contact their GP about referral to a specialist. The MHRA has produced videos to support this advice—guidance for healthcare professionals is available at: www.youtube.com/watch?v=qfppzpdeYmk and guidance for patients, parents, and carers is available at: www.youtube.com/watch?v=NO0ir0i043Q.

- ● CAUTIONS Avoid spraying near eyes · cystic fibrosis
  CAUTIONS, FURTHER INFORMATION
- ▶ Glaucoma *Acute angle-closure glaucoma* has been reported with nebulised ipratropium, particularly when given with nebulised salbutamol (and possibly other beta₂ agonists); care needed to protect the patient's eyes from nebulised drug or from drug powder.
- ● INTERACTIONS → Appendix 1: ipratropium
- ● SIDE-EFFECTS
- ▶ **Common or very common** Gastrointestinal motility disorder · throat complaints
- ▶ **Uncommon** Corneal oedema · diarrhoea · eye disorders · eye pain · respiratory disorders · vision disorders · vomiting

- ● ALLERGY AND CROSS-SENSITIVITY Contra-indicated in patients with hypersensitivity to atropine or its derivatives.
- ● PREGNANCY
- ▶ When used for Asthma Inhaled drugs can be taken as normal during pregnancy.
- ▶ When used for Reversible airways obstruction or Rhinorrhoea [EvGr] Use only if potential benefit outweighs the risk. ⓜ
- ● BREAST FEEDING No information available—manufacturer advises only use if potential benefit outweighs risk.
- ● DIRECTIONS FOR ADMINISTRATION Manufacturer advises if dilution of ipratropium bromide nebuliser solution is necessary use only sterile sodium chloride 0.9%.
- ● PRESCRIBING AND DISPENSING INFORMATION
- ▶ When used for Asthma For choice of therapy, see Asthma, acute p. 274 and Asthma, chronic p. 271.
- ● PATIENT AND CARER ADVICE Patients or carers should be counselled on appropriate administration technique and warned against accidental contact with the eye (due to risk of ocular complications).
  Driving and skilled tasks Manufacturer advises patients and carers should be counselled on the effects on driving and performance of skilled tasks—increased risk of dizziness and vision disorders.

- ● MEDICINAL FORMS There can be variation in the licensing of different medicines containing the same drug.
  Nebuliser liquid
- ▶ Ipratropium bromide (Non-proprietary)
  Ipratropium bromide 250 microgram per 1 ml Ipratropium bromide 500micrograms/2ml nebuliser liquid unit dose vials | 20 unit dose [PoM] £6.94 DT = £6.94
  Ipratropium bromide 250micrograms/1ml nebuliser liquid unit dose vials | 20 unit dose [PoM] £8.72 DT = £8.72
  Ipratropium 250micrograms/1ml nebuliser liquid Steri-Neb unit dose vials | 20 unit dose [PoM] £8.99 DT = £8.72
  Ipratropium 500micrograms/2ml nebuliser liquid Steri-Neb unit dose vials | 20 unit dose [PoM] £4.56 DT = £6.94
- ▶ Atrovent UDV (Boehringer Ingelheim Ltd)
  Ipratropium bromide 250 microgram per 1 ml Atrovent 500micrograms/2ml nebuliser liquid UDVs | 20 unit dose [PoM] £4.87 DT = £6.94
  Atrovent 250micrograms/1ml nebuliser liquid UDVs | 20 unit dose [PoM] £4.14 DT = £8.72
  Pressurised inhalation
- ▶ Atrovent (Boehringer Ingelheim Ltd)
  Ipratropium bromide 20 microgram per 1 dose Atrovent 20micrograms/dose inhaler CFC free | 200 dose [PoM] £5.56 DT = £5.56
- ▶ Inhalvent (Alissa Healthcare Research Ltd)
  Ipratropium bromide 20 microgram per 1 dose Inhalvent 20micrograms/dose inhaler | 200 dose [PoM] £5.56 DT = £5.56

Ipratropium with salbutamol
16-Mar-2020

The properties listed below are those particular to the combination only. For the properties of the components please consider, ipratropium bromide p. 281, salbutamol p. 287.

- ● INDICATIONS AND DOSE

Bronchospasm in chronic obstructive pulmonary disease
- ▶ BY INHALATION OF NEBULISED SOLUTION
- ▶ Adult: 0.5/2.5 mg 3–4 times a day

- ● INTERACTIONS → Appendix 1: beta₂ agonists · ipratropium
- ● PRESCRIBING AND DISPENSING INFORMATION A mixture of ipratropium bromide and salbutamol (as sulfate); the proportions are expressed in the form x/y where x and y are the strengths in milligrams of ipratropium and salbutamol respectively.

3

Respiratory system

● **MEDICINAL FORMS** There can be variation in the licensing of different medicines containing the same drug.

Nebuliser liquid

▶ Combiprasal (TriOn Pharma Ltd)

Ipratropium bromide 200 microgram per 1 ml, Salbutamol (as Salbutamol sulfate) 1 mg per 1 ml Combiprasal 0.5mg/2.5mg nebuliser solution 2.5ml unit dose vials | 60 unit dose PoM £18.98 DT = £24.10

▶ Combivent (Boehringer Ingelheim Ltd)

Ipratropium bromide 200 microgram per 1 ml, Salbutamol (as Salbutamol sulfate) 1 mg per 1 ml Combivent nebuliser liquid 2.5ml UDVs | 60 unit dose PoM £24.10 DT = £24.10

▶ Ipramol (Teva UK Ltd)

Ipratropium bromide 200 microgram per 1 ml, Salbutamol (as Salbutamol sulfate) 1 mg per 1 ml Ipramol nebuliser solution 2.5ml Steri-Neb unit dose vials | 60 unit dose PoM £23.83 DT = £24.10

◤ 280

Tiotropium

13-Mar-2025

● **INDICATIONS AND DOSE**

Maintenance treatment of chronic obstructive pulmonary disease

▶ BY INHALATION OF POWDER

▶ Adult: 1 capsule once daily

DOSE EQUIVALENCE AND CONVERSION

▶ For *Spiriva*® inhalation powder, 1 capsule contains a metered dose of 18 micrograms tiotropium; for *Braltus*® inhalation powder, 1 capsule contains a metered dose of 13 micrograms tiotropium.

▶ The delivered dose of *Spiriva*® and *Braltus*® inhalation powder products are the same (10 micrograms); no dose adjustment is necessary when switching between brands.

SPIRIVA RESPIMAT®

Maintenance treatment of chronic obstructive pulmonary disease | Severe asthma [add-on to inhaled corticosteroid (at least 800 micrograms budesonide daily or equivalent) and at least 1 controller in patients who have suffered one or more severe exacerbations in the last year]

▶ BY INHALATION

▶ Adult: 5 micrograms once daily

Severe asthma [add-on to inhaled corticosteroid (over 400 micrograms budesonide daily or equivalent) and 1 controller, or inhaled corticosteroid (200–400 micrograms budesonide daily or equivalent) and 2 controllers, in patients who have suffered one or more severe exacerbations in the last year]

▶ BY INHALATION

▶ Child 6-11 years: 5 micrograms once daily

Severe asthma [add-on to inhaled corticosteroid (over 800 micrograms budesonide daily or equivalent) and 1 controller, or inhaled corticosteroid (400–800 micrograms budesonide daily or equivalent) and 2 controllers, in patients who have suffered one or more severe exacerbations in the last year]

▶ BY INHALATION

▶ Child 12-17 years: 5 micrograms once daily

DOSE EQUIVALENCE AND CONVERSION

▶ For *Spiriva Respimat*®: 2 puffs of inhalation solution is equivalent to 5 micrograms tiotropium.

IMPORTANT SAFETY INFORMATION

MHRA/CHM ADVICE: *BRALTUS*® (TIOTROPIUM): RISK OF INHALATION OF CAPSULE IF PLACED IN THE MOUTHPIECE OF THE INHALER (MAY 2018)

The MHRA have received reports of patients who have inhaled a *Braltus*® capsule from the mouthpiece into the back of the throat, resulting in coughing and risking aspiration or airway obstruction. Patients should be trained in the correct use of their inhaler and told to

store capsules in the screw-top bottle provided (never in the inhaler) and to always check the mouthpiece is clear before inhaling. Pharmacists dispensing *Braltus*® capsules should remind patients always to read the instructions for use in the package leaflet and that they must never place a capsule directly into the mouthpiece.

MHRA/CHM ADVICE: PRESSURISED METERED DOSE INHALERS (PMDI): RISK OF AIRWAY OBSTRUCTION FROM ASPIRATION OF LOOSE OBJECTS (JULY 2018)

See Respiratory system, inhaled drug delivery p. 269.

● **CAUTIONS** Arrhythmia (unstable, life-threatening or requiring intervention in the previous 12 months) · heart failure (hospitalisation for moderate to severe heart failure in the previous 12 months) · myocardial infarction in the previous 6 months

● **INTERACTIONS** → Appendix 1: tiotropium

● **SIDE-EFFECTS**

▶ **Uncommon** Gastrointestinal disorders · increased risk of infection · taste altered

▶ **Rare or very rare** Bronchospasm · dysphagia · epistaxis · insomnia · oral disorders

▶ **Frequency not known** Dehydration · joint swelling · skin ulcer

● **PREGNANCY**

▶ When used for Chronic obstructive pulmonary disease in adults EvGr Avoid (limited data available). Ⓜ

▶ When used for Asthma Inhaled drugs can be taken as normal during pregnancy.

● **BREAST FEEDING** Manufacturer advises avoid—no information available.

● **RENAL IMPAIRMENT** Manufacturer advises use only if potential benefit outweighs risk if creatinine clearance less than or equal to 50 mL/minute—plasma-tiotropium concentration raised. See p. 21.

● **PRESCRIBING AND DISPENSING INFORMATION**

▶ When used for Asthma For choice of therapy, see Asthma, acute p. 274 and Asthma, chronic p. 271.

● **PATIENT AND CARER ADVICE** Patients or carers should be advised that the *Respimat*® inhaler device is re-usable and can be used with a total of 6 cartridges before it needs to be replaced. Refer patients or carers to the Instructions for Use for information on how and when to replace the cartridge.

▶ In adults Patients or carers should be given advice on appropriate inhaler technique and reminded that the powder inhalation capsules are not for oral administration; for *Braltus*®, see also *Important safety Information*.

▶ In children Patients or carers should be given advice on appropriate inhaler technique.

● **NATIONAL FUNDING/ACCESS DECISIONS**

For full details see funding body website

Scottish Medicines Consortium (SMC) decisions

▶ **Tiotropium (*Spiriva Respimat*®) as add-on maintenance bronchodilator treatment in adults with asthma who are currently treated with the maintenance combination of inhaled corticosteroids (at least 800 micrograms budesonide/day or equivalent) and long-acting beta$_2$ agonists and who experienced one or more severe exacerbations in the previous year (August 2015)** SMC No. 1028/15 Recommended

▶ **Tiotropium (*Spiriva Respimat*®) as a maintenance bronchodilator treatment to relieve symptoms of patients with chronic obstructive pulmonary disease (COPD) (December 2017)** SMC No. 411/07 Recommended

▶ **Tiotropium (*Spiriva Respimat*®) as add-on maintenance bronchodilator treatment in patients aged 6 years and older with severe asthma who experienced one or more severe asthma exacerbations in the preceding year (January 2019)** SMC No. SMC2118 Recommended

All Wales Medicines Strategy Group (AWMSG) decisions
▶ Tiotropium (*Spiriva Respimat®*) as add-on maintenance bronchodilator treatment in patients aged 6 years and older with severe asthma who experienced one or more severe asthma exacerbations in the preceding year (December 2018) AWMSG No. 1882 Recommended

● **MEDICINAL FORMS** There can be variation in the licensing of different medicines containing the same drug.

Inhalation powder
▶ **Acopair** (Viatris UK Healthcare Ltd)
Tiotropium (as Tiotropium bromide) **18 microgram** Acopair 18microgram inhalation powder capsules with NeumoHaler | 30 capsule [PoM] £19.99 DT = £34.87 | 60 capsule [PoM] £39.98
▶ **Braltus** (Teva UK Ltd)
Tiotropium (as Tiotropium bromide) **10 microgram** Braltus 10microgram inhalation powder capsules with Zonda inhaler | 30 capsule [PoM] £25.80 DT = £25.80
▶ **Spiriva** (Boehringer Ingelheim Ltd)
Tiotropium (as Tiotropium bromide) **18 microgram** Spiriva 18microgram inhalation powder capsules with HandiHaler | 30 capsule [PoM] £34.87 DT = £34.87
Spiriva 18microgram inhalation powder capsules | 30 capsule [PoM] £33.50 DT = £33.50
▶ **Tiogiva** (Glenmark Pharmaceuticals Europe Ltd)
Tiotropium (as Tiotropium bromide) **18 microgram** Tiogiva 18microgram inhalation powder capsules | 30 capsule [PoM] £19.20 DT = £33.50 | 60 capsule [PoM] £38.40
Tiogiva 18microgram inhalation powder capsules with device | 30 capsule [PoM] £19.99 DT = £34.87
▶ **Trokide** (Genus Pharmaceuticals Ltd)
Tiotropium (as Tiotropium bromide) **18 microgram** Trokide 18microgram inhalation powder capsules | 30 capsule [PoM] £8.50 DT = £33.50
Trokide 18microgram inhalation powder capsules with Vertical-Haler | 30 capsule [PoM] £12.50 DT = £34.87

Inhalation solution
▶ **Spiriva Respimat** (Boehringer Ingelheim Ltd)
Tiotropium (as Tiotropium bromide) **2.5 microgram per 1 dose** Spiriva Respimat 2.5micrograms/dose inhalation solution refill cartridge | 60 dose [PoM] £23.00 DT = £23.00
Spiriva Respimat 2.5micrograms/dose inhalation solution cartridge with device | 60 dose [PoM] £23.00 DT = £23.00

Tiotropium with olodaterol

03-Sep-2020

The properties listed below are those particular to the combination only. For the properties of the components please consider, tiotropium p. 283, olodaterol p. 286.

● **INDICATIONS AND DOSE**

Maintenance treatment of chronic obstructive pulmonary disease
▶ BY INHALATION
▶ Adult: 2 puffs once daily

DOSE EQUIVALENCE AND CONVERSION
▶ 2 puffs of inhalation solution is equivalent to 5 micrograms tiotropium and 5 micrograms olodaterol.

● **INTERACTIONS** → Appendix 1: beta₂ agonists · tiotropium

● **PATIENT AND CARER ADVICE** Patient or carers should be given advice on appropriate inhaler technique. Patients or carers should be advised that the *Respimat®* inhaler device is re-usable and can be used with a total of 6 cartridges before it needs to be replaced. Refer patients or carers to the Instructions for Use for information on how and when to replace the cartridge.

● **MEDICINAL FORMS** There can be variation in the licensing of different medicines containing the same drug.

Inhalation solution
▶ **Spiolto Respimat** (Boehringer Ingelheim Ltd)
Olodaterol (as Olodaterol hydrochloride) **2.5 microgram per 1 dose,** Tiotropium (as Tiotropium bromide) **2.5 microgram per 1 dose** Spiolto Respimat 2.5micrograms/dose / 2.5micrograms/dose

inhalation solution cartridge with device | 60 dose [PoM] £32.50 DT = £32.50
Spiolto Respimat 2.5micrograms/dose / 2.5micrograms/dose inhalation solution refill cartridge | 60 dose [PoM] £32.50 DT = £32.50

F 280

Umeclidinium

02-Sep-2020

● **INDICATIONS AND DOSE**

Maintenance treatment of chronic obstructive pulmonary disease
▶ BY INHALATION OF POWDER
▶ Adult: 55 micrograms once daily

DOSE EQUIVALENCE AND CONVERSION
▶ Each 65 microgram inhalation of umeclidinium bromide delivers 55 micrograms of umeclidinium.

● **CAUTIONS** Cardiac disorders (particularly cardiac rhythm disorders)

● **INTERACTIONS** → Appendix 1: umeclidinium

● **SIDE-EFFECTS**
▶ **Uncommon** Taste altered
▶ **Rare or very rare** Eye pain

● **PREGNANCY** Manufacturer advises use only if potential benefit outweighs risk.

● **BREAST FEEDING** Manufacturer advises avoid—no information available.

● **HEPATIC IMPAIRMENT** Manufacturer advises caution in severe impairment (no information available).

● **PATIENT AND CARER ADVICE** Patient or carers should be given advice on appropriate inhaler technique.

● **MEDICINAL FORMS** There can be variation in the licensing of different medicines containing the same drug.

Inhalation powder
▶ **Incruse Ellipta** (GlaxoSmithKline UK Ltd)
Umeclidinium bromide **65 microgram per 1 dose** Incruse Ellipta 55micrograms/dose dry powder inhaler | 30 dose [PoM] £27.50 DT = £27.50

Combinations available: *Fluticasone with umeclidinium and vilanterol,* p. 304

F 285

Umeclidinium with vilanterol

01-Feb-2022

The properties listed below are those particular to the combination only. For the properties of the components please consider, umeclidinium above.

● **INDICATIONS AND DOSE**

Maintenance treatment of chronic obstructive pulmonary disease
▶ BY INHALATION OF POWDER
▶ Adult: 1 inhalation once daily

● **INTERACTIONS** → Appendix 1: beta₂ agonists · umeclidinium

● **SIDE-EFFECTS**
▶ **Common or very common** Constipation · dry mouth · oropharyngeal pain · sinusitis
▶ **Uncommon** Dysphonia · taste altered
▶ **Rare or very rare** Glaucoma · urinary disorders · vision blurred
▶ **Frequency not known** Dizziness

● **PATIENT AND CARER ADVICE** Patient or carers should be given advice on appropriate inhaler technique.

● **MEDICINAL FORMS** There can be variation in the licensing of different medicines containing the same drug.

Inhalation powder
▶ **Anoro Ellipta** (GlaxoSmithKline UK Ltd)
Vilanterol (as Vilanterol trifenatate) **22 microgram per 1 dose,** Umeclidinium bromide **65 microgram per 1 dose** Anoro Ellipta 55micrograms/dose / 22micrograms/dose dry powder inhaler | 30 dose [PoM] £32.50 DT = £32.50

BETA₂-ADRENOCEPTOR AGONISTS, SELECTIVE

Beta₂-adrenoceptor agonists, selective

12-Feb-2016

- **CAUTIONS** Arrhythmias · cardiovascular disease · diabetes (risk of hyperglycaemia and ketoacidosis, especially with intravenous use) · hypertension · hyperthyroidism · hypokalaemia · susceptibility to QT-interval prolongation

CAUTIONS, FURTHER INFORMATION
▸ Hypokalaemia Potentially serious hypokalaemia may result from beta₂ agonist therapy. EvGr Particular caution is required in severe asthma or COPD, because this effect may be potentiated by concomitant treatment with theophylline and its derivatives, corticosteroids, diuretics, and by hypoxia. ⓜ

- **SIDE-EFFECTS**
▸ **Common or very common** Arrhythmias · headache · palpitations · tremor
▸ **Uncommon** Hyperglycaemia
▸ **Rare or very rare** Bronchospasm paradoxical (sometimes severe)

- **PREGNANCY** Inhaled drugs for asthma can be taken as normal during pregnancy.

- **MONITORING REQUIREMENTS**
▸ In severe asthma, plasma-potassium concentration should be monitored (risk of hypokalaemia).
▸ In patients with diabetes, monitor blood glucose (risk of hyperglycaemia and ketoacidosis, especially when beta₂ agonist given intravenously).

- **PATIENT AND CARER ADVICE**
▸ When used by inhalation The **dose**, the frequency, and the maximum number of inhalations in 24 hours of the beta₂ agonist should be **stated explicitly** to the patient or their carer. The patient or their carer should be advised to seek medical advice when the prescribed dose of beta₂ agonist fails to provide the usual degree of symptomatic relief because this usually indicates a worsening of the asthma and the patient may require a prophylactic drug. Patients or their carers should be advised to follow manufacturers' instructions on the care and cleansing of inhaler devices.

BETA₂-ADRENOCEPTOR AGONISTS, SELECTIVE > LONG-ACTING

ℱ above

Formoterol fumarate
17-Jan-2023

(Eformoterol fumarate)

- **INDICATIONS AND DOSE**

Reversible airways obstruction in patients requiring long-term regular bronchodilator therapy | Nocturnal asthma in patients requiring long-term regular bronchodilator therapy | Prophylaxis of exercise-induced bronchospasm in patients requiring long-term regular bronchodilator therapy | Chronic asthma in patients who regularly use an inhaled corticosteroid
▸ BY INHALATION OF POWDER
▸ Child 6-11 years: 12 micrograms twice daily, a daily dose of 24 micrograms of formoterol should be sufficient for the majority of children, particularly for younger age-groups; higher doses should be used rarely, and only when control is not maintained on the lower dose
▸ Child 12-17 years: 12 micrograms twice daily, dose may be increased in more severe airway obstruction; increased to 24 micrograms twice daily, a daily dose of 24 micrograms of formoterol should be sufficient for

the majority of children, particularly for younger age-groups; higher doses should be used rarely, and only when control is not maintained on the lower dose
▸ Adult: 12 micrograms twice daily, dose may be increased in more severe airway obstruction; increased to 24 micrograms twice daily
▸ BY INHALATION OF AEROSOL
▸ Child 12-17 years: 12 micrograms twice daily, dose may be increased in more severe airway obstruction; increased to 24 micrograms twice daily, a daily dose of 24 micrograms of formoterol should be sufficient for the majority of children, particularly for younger age-groups; higher doses should be used rarely, and only when control is not maintained on the lower dose
▸ Adult: 12 micrograms twice daily, dose may be increased in more severe airway obstruction; increased to 24 micrograms twice daily

Chronic obstructive pulmonary disease
▸ BY INHALATION OF POWDER
▸ Adult: 12 micrograms twice daily
▸ BY INHALATION OF AEROSOL
▸ Adult: 12 micrograms twice daily (max. per dose 24 micrograms), for symptom relief additional doses may be taken to maximum daily dose; maximum 48 micrograms per day

PHARMACOKINETICS
▸ At recommended inhaled doses, the duration of action of formoterol is about 12 hours.

OXIS ®

Chronic asthma
▸ BY INHALATION OF POWDER
▸ Child 6-17 years: 6–12 micrograms 1–2 times a day (max. per dose 12 micrograms), occasionally doses up to the maximum daily may be needed, reassess treatment if additional doses required on more than 2 days a week; maximum 48 micrograms per day
▸ Adult: 6–12 micrograms 1–2 times a day, increased if necessary up to 24 micrograms twice daily (max. per dose 36 micrograms), occasionally doses up to the maximum daily may be needed, reassess treatment if additional doses required on more than 2 days a week; maximum 72 micrograms per day

Relief of bronchospasm
▸ BY INHALATION OF POWDER
▸ Child 6-17 years: 6–12 micrograms
▸ Adult: 6–12 micrograms

Prophylaxis of exercise-induced bronchospasm
▸ BY INHALATION OF POWDER
▸ Child 6-17 years: 6–12 micrograms, dose to be taken before exercise
▸ Adult: 12 micrograms, dose to be taken before exercise

Chronic obstructive pulmonary disease
▸ BY INHALATION OF POWDER
▸ Adult: 12 micrograms 1–2 times a day (max. per dose 24 micrograms), for symptom relief additional doses up to maximum daily dose can be taken; maximum 48 micrograms per day

---

IMPORTANT SAFETY INFORMATION

CHM ADVICE

To ensure safe use, the CHM has advised that for the management of chronic asthma, long-acting beta₂ agonist (formoterol) should:
- be added only if regular use of standard-dose inhaled corticosteroids has failed to control asthma adequately;
- not be initiated in patients with rapidly deteriorating asthma;
- be introduced at a low dose and the effect properly monitored before considering dose increase;

3

- be discontinued in the absence of benefit;
- not be used for the relief of exercise-induced asthma symptoms unless regular inhaled corticosteroids are also used;
- be reviewed as clinically appropriate: stepping down therapy should be considered when good long-term asthma control has been achieved.

MHRA/CHM ADVICE: PRESSURISED METERED DOSE INHALERS (PMDI): RISK OF AIRWAY OBSTRUCTION FROM ASPIRATION OF LOOSE OBJECTS (JULY 2018)
See Respiratory system, inhaled drug delivery p. 269.

- **INTERACTIONS** → Appendix 1: beta₂ agonists
- **SIDE-EFFECTS**
▸ **Common or very common** Dizziness · muscle cramps · nausea
▸ **Uncommon** Angina pectoris · hypokalaemia · sleep disorder · taste altered
▸ **Rare or very rare** Anxiety · QT interval prolongation
- **PREGNANCY** Inhaled drugs for asthma can be taken as normal during pregnancy.
- **BREAST FEEDING** Inhaled drugs for asthma can be taken as normal during breast-feeding.
- **PRESCRIBING AND DISPENSING INFORMATION**
▸ When used for Asthma For choice of therapy, see Asthma, acute p. 274 and Asthma, chronic p. 271.
- **PATIENT AND CARER ADVICE** Advise patients not to exceed prescribed dose, and to follow manufacturer's directions; if a previously effective dose of inhaled formoterol fails to provide adequate relief, a doctor's advice should be obtained as soon as possible. Patients should be advised to report any deterioration in symptoms following initiation of treatment with a long-acting beta₂ agonist. Patient or carer should be given advice on how to administer formoterol fumarate inhalers.

- **MEDICINAL FORMS** There can be variation in the licensing of different medicines containing the same drug.
Inhalation powder
▸ **Easyhaler (formoterol)** (Orion Pharma (UK) Ltd)
Formoterol fumarate dihydrate 12 microgram per 1 dose Formoterol Easyhaler 12micrograms/dose dry powder inhaler | 120 dose [PoM] £23.75 DT = £23.75
▸ **Oxis Turbohaler** (AstraZeneca UK Ltd)
Formoterol fumarate dihydrate 6 microgram per 1 dose Oxis 6 Turbohaler | 60 dose [PoM] £24.80 DT = £24.80
Formoterol fumarate dihydrate 12 microgram per 1 dose Oxis 12 Turbohaler | 60 dose [PoM] £24.80 DT = £24.80
Pressurised inhalation
EXCIPIENTS: May contain Alcohol
▸ **Atimos Modulite** (Chiesi Ltd)
Formoterol fumarate dihydrate 12 microgram per 1 dose Atimos Modulite 12micrograms/dose inhaler | 100 dose [PoM] £30.06 DT = £30.06

Combinations available: *Aclidinium bromide with formoterol,* p. 280 · *Beclometasone with formoterol,* p. 294 · *Beclometasone with formoterol and glycopyrronium,* p. 296 · *Budesonide with formoterol,* p. 298 · *Fluticasone with formoterol,* p. 301 · *Formoterol fumarate with glycopyrronium and budesonide,* p. 305 · *Glycopyrronium with formoterol fumarate,* p. 281

▶ 285

Indacaterol

16-Jan-2021

- **INDICATIONS AND DOSE**
Maintenance treatment of chronic obstructive pulmonary disease
▸ BY INHALATION OF POWDER
▸ Adult: 150 micrograms once daily, then increased to 300 micrograms once daily

- **CAUTIONS** Convulsive disorders

- **INTERACTIONS** → Appendix 1: beta₂ agonists
- **SIDE-EFFECTS**
▸ **Common or very common** Chest pain · cough · dizziness · increased risk of infection · muscle complaints · oropharyngeal pain · peripheral oedema · rhinorrhoea · throat irritation
▸ **Uncommon** Diabetes mellitus · hypersensitivity · musculoskeletal pain · myocardial ischaemia · paraesthesia · skin reactions
- **PREGNANCY** Manufacturer advises use only if potential benefit outweighs risk.
- **BREAST FEEDING** Manufacturer advises avoid—present in milk in *animal* studies.
- **HEPATIC IMPAIRMENT** Manufacturer advises caution in severe impairment (no information available).
- **PATIENT AND CARER ADVICE** Patients or carers should be given advice on how to administer indacaterol inhalation powder.

- **MEDICINAL FORMS** There can be variation in the licensing of different medicines containing the same drug.
Inhalation powder
▸ **Onbrez Breezhaler** (Novartis Pharmaceuticals UK Ltd)
Indacaterol (as Indacaterol maleate) 150 microgram Onbrez Breezhaler 150microgram inhalation powder capsules with device | 30 capsule [PoM] £32.19 DT = £32.19
Indacaterol (as Indacaterol maleate) 300 microgram Onbrez Breezhaler 300microgram inhalation powder capsules with device | 30 capsule [PoM] £32.19 DT = £32.19

Combinations available: *Glycopyrronium with indacaterol,* p. 281 · *Mometasone furoate with glycopyrronium bromide and indacaterol,* p. 306

▶ 285

Olodaterol

17-Jan-2023

- **INDICATIONS AND DOSE**
Maintenance treatment of chronic obstructive pulmonary disease
▸ BY INHALATION
▸ Adult: 5 micrograms once daily
DOSE EQUIVALENCE AND CONVERSION
▸ 2 puffs is equivalent to 5 micrograms.

IMPORTANT SAFETY INFORMATION

MHRA/CHM ADVICE: PRESSURISED METERED DOSE INHALERS (PMDI): RISK OF AIRWAY OBSTRUCTION FROM ASPIRATION OF LOOSE OBJECTS (JULY 2018)
See Respiratory system, inhaled drug delivery p. 269.

- **CAUTIONS** Aneurysm · convulsive disorders
- **INTERACTIONS** → Appendix 1: beta₂ agonists
- **SIDE-EFFECTS**
▸ **Uncommon** Dizziness · nasopharyngitis · rash
▸ **Rare or very rare** Arthralgia · hypertension
▸ **Frequency not known** Dry mouth · fatigue · hypokalaemia · hypotension · insomnia · ischaemic heart disease · malaise · metabolic acidosis · muscle spasms · nausea · nervousness
- **PREGNANCY** Manufacturer advises avoid—no information available.
- **BREAST FEEDING** Manufacturer advises avoid— present in milk in *animal* studies.
- **HEPATIC IMPAIRMENT** Manufacturer advises caution in severe hepatic impairment (no information available).
- **PATIENT AND CARER ADVICE** Patients or carers should be given advice on how to administer olodaterol solution for inhalation. Patients or carers should be advised that the *Respimat®* inhaler device is re-usable and can be used with a total of 6 cartridges before it needs to be replaced. Refer

patients or carers to the Instructions for Use for information on how and when to replace the cartridge.

- **MEDICINAL FORMS** There can be variation in the licensing of different medicines containing the same drug.

Inhalation solution

▸ Striverdi Respimat (Boehringer Ingelheim Ltd)
Olodaterol (as Olodaterol hydrochloride) 2.5 microgram per 1 dose Striverdi Respimat 2.5micrograms/dose inhalation solution cartridge with device | 60 dose [PoM] £26.35 DT = £26.35
Striverdi Respimat 2.5micrograms/dose inhalation solution refill cartridge | 60 dose [PoM] £26.35 DT = £26.35

Combinations available: *Tiotropium with olodaterol,* p. 284

▶ 285

Salmeterol

17-Jan-2023

- **INDICATIONS AND DOSE**

Reversible airways obstruction in patients requiring long-term regular bronchodilator therapy | Nocturnal asthma in patients requiring long-term regular bronchodilator therapy | Prevention of exercise-induced bronchospasm in patients requiring long-term regular bronchodilator therapy | Chronic asthma only in patients who regularly use an inhaled corticosteroid (not for immediate relief of acute asthma)

▸ BY INHALATION OF AEROSOL, OR BY INHALATION OF POWDER
▸ Child 5–11 years: 50 micrograms twice daily
▸ Child 12–17 years: 50 micrograms twice daily, dose may be increased in more severe airway obstruction; increased to 100 micrograms twice daily
▸ Adult: 50 micrograms twice daily, dose may be increased in more severe airway obstruction; increased to 100 micrograms twice daily

Chronic obstructive pulmonary disease

▸ BY INHALATION OF AEROSOL, OR BY INHALATION OF POWDER
▸ Adult: 50 micrograms twice daily

PHARMACOKINETICS

▸ At recommended inhaled doses, the duration of action of salmeterol is about 12 hours.

- **UNLICENSED USE** *Neovent*® not licensed for use in children under 12 years.

> **IMPORTANT SAFETY INFORMATION**
>
> CHM ADVICE
>
> To ensure safe use, the CHM has advised that for the management of chronic asthma, long-acting beta$_2$ agonist (salmeterol) should:
> - be added only if regular use of standard-dose inhaled corticosteroids has failed to control asthma adequately;
> - not be initiated in patients with rapidly deteriorating asthma;
> - be introduced at a low dose and the effect properly monitored before considering dose increase;
> - be discontinued in the absence of benefit;
> - not be used for the relief of exercise-induced asthma symptoms unless regular inhaled corticosteroids are also used;
> - be reviewed as clinically appropriate: stepping down therapy should be considered when good long-term asthma control has been achieved.
>
> MHRA/CHM ADVICE: PRESSURISED METERED DOSE INHALERS (PMDI): RISK OF AIRWAY OBSTRUCTION FROM ASPIRATION OF LOOSE OBJECTS (JULY 2018)
> See Respiratory system, inhaled drug delivery p. 269.

- **INTERACTIONS** → Appendix 1: beta$_2$ agonists
- **SIDE-EFFECTS**
▸ **Common or very common** Muscle cramps
▸ **Uncommon** Nervousness · skin reactions

▸ **Rare or very rare** Arthralgia · bronchospasm · chest pain · dizziness · hypokalaemia · insomnia · nausea · oedema · oropharyngeal irritation

- **PREGNANCY** Inhaled drugs for asthma can be taken as normal during pregnancy.
- **BREAST FEEDING** Inhaled drugs for asthma can be taken as normal during breast-feeding.
- **PRESCRIBING AND DISPENSING INFORMATION**
▸ When used for Asthma For choice of therapy, see Asthma, acute p. 274 and Asthma, chronic p. 271.
- **PATIENT AND CARER ADVICE** Advise patients that salmeterol should **not** be used for relief of acute attacks, not to exceed prescribed dose, and to follow manufacturer's directions; if a previously effective dose of inhaled salmeterol fails to provide adequate relief, a doctor's advice should be obtained as soon as possible. Patients should be advised to report any deterioration in symptoms following initiation of treatment with a long-acting beta$_2$ agonist.
Medicines for Children leaflet: Salmeterol inhaler for asthma www.medicinesforchildren.org.uk/medicines/salmeterol-inhaler-for-asthma/

- **MEDICINAL FORMS** There can be variation in the licensing of different medicines containing the same drug.

Inhalation powder

▸ Serevent Accuhaler (GlaxoSmithKline UK Ltd)
Salmeterol (as Salmeterol xinafoate) 50 microgram per 1 dose Serevent 50micrograms/dose Accuhaler | 60 dose [PoM] £35.11 DT = £35.11

Pressurised inhalation

▸ Serevent Evohaler (GlaxoSmithKline UK Ltd)
Salmeterol (as Salmeterol xinafoate) 25 microgram per 1 dose Serevent 25micrograms/dose Evohaler | 120 dose [PoM] £29.26 DT = £29.26
▸ Soltel (Cipla EU Ltd)
Salmeterol (as Salmeterol xinafoate) 25 microgram per 1 dose Soltel 25micrograms/dose inhaler CFC free | 120 dose [PoM] £19.95 DT = £29.26

Combinations available: *Fluticasone with salmeterol,* p. 302

BETA$_2$-ADRENOCEPTOR AGONISTS, SELECTIVE > SHORT-ACTING

▶ 285

Salbutamol

13-Mar-2025

(Albuterol)

- **INDICATIONS AND DOSE**

Chronic asthma [in line with management advice for chronic asthma]

▸ BY INHALATION OF AEROSOL
▸ Child 1–17 years: 100–200 micrograms, to be taken when required for symptomatic relief, review prevention medication if salbutamol usage is 3 or more days per week, or if nocturnal symptoms occur
▸ Adult: 100–200 micrograms, to be taken when required for symptomatic relief, review prevention medication if salbutamol usage is 3 or more days per week, or if nocturnal symptoms occur
▸ BY INHALATION OF POWDER
▸ Child 6–17 years: 100–200 micrograms, to be taken when required for symptomatic relief, review prevention medication if salbutamol usage is 3 or more days per week, or if nocturnal symptoms occur
▸ Adult: 100–200 micrograms, to be taken when required for symptomatic relief, review prevention medication if salbutamol usage is 3 or more days per week, or if nocturnal symptoms occur

continued →

▸ BY INHALATION OF NEBULISED SOLUTION
▹ Child 1–4 years (initiated by a specialist): 2.5 mg, to be taken when required for symptomatic relief, review prevention medication if salbutamol usage is 3 or more days per week, or if nocturnal symptoms occur
▹ Child 5–17 years (initiated by a specialist): 2.5–5 mg, to be taken when required for symptomatic relief, review prevention medication if salbutamol usage is 3 or more days per week, or if nocturnal symptoms occur
▹ Adult (initiated by a specialist): 2.5–5 mg, to be taken when required for symptomatic relief, review prevention medication if salbutamol usage is 3 or more days per week, or if nocturnal symptoms occur

Acute asthma [in line with management advice for acute asthma]
▸ BY INHALATION OF AEROSOL
▹ Child 1–2 years: 100 micrograms every 0.5–1 minute for up to 10 doses, each dose to be inhaled separately via a spacer and a close-fitting face mask; repeat every 10–20 minutes or when required
▹ Child 3–17 years: 100 micrograms every 0.5–1 minute for up to 10 doses, each dose to be inhaled separately via a spacer; repeat every 10–20 minutes or when required
▹ Adult: 100 micrograms every 0.5–1 minute for up to 10 doses, each dose to be inhaled separately via a spacer; repeat every 10–20 minutes or when required
▸ BY INHALATION OF POWDER
▹ Child 6–17 years: 100 micrograms every 0.5–1 minute for up to 10 doses, each dose to be inhaled separately; repeat every 10–20 minutes or when required, alternatively 200 micrograms every 0.5–1 minute for up to 5 doses, each dose to be inhaled separately; repeat every 10–20 minutes or when required
▹ Adult: 100 micrograms every 0.5–1 minute for up to 10 doses, each dose to be inhaled separately; repeat every 10–20 minutes or when required, alternatively 200 micrograms every 0.5–1 minute for up to 5 doses, each dose to be inhaled separately; repeat every 10–20 minutes or when required
▸ BY INHALATION OF NEBULISED SOLUTION
▹ Child 1–4 years: 2.5 mg, repeat every 20–30 minutes or when required, give via oxygen-driven nebuliser if available
▹ Child 5–17 years: 2.5–5 mg, repeat every 20–30 minutes or when required, give via oxygen-driven nebuliser if available
▹ Adult: 2.5–5 mg, repeat every 15–30 minutes or when required, give via oxygen-driven nebuliser if available
▸ BY SLOW INTRAVENOUS INJECTION
▹ Child 12–23 months: 5 micrograms/kg for 1 dose, to be administered over 5–10 minutes
▹ Child 2–17 years: 15 micrograms/kg for 1 dose (max. per dose 250 micrograms), to be administered over 5–10 minutes
▹ Adult: 250 micrograms, to be administered over 5–10 minutes, dose can be repeated if necessary
▸ BY CONTINUOUS INTRAVENOUS INFUSION
▹ Adult: Initially 5 micrograms/minute, to be adjusted according to response and tolerance, usual dose 3–20 micrograms/minute, higher doses may be required in respiratory failure

Prophylaxis of allergen- or exercise-induced bronchospasm
▸ BY INHALATION OF AEROSOL
▹ Child: 100–200 micrograms, to be taken 10–15 minutes before challenge
▹ Adult: 200 micrograms, to be taken 10–15 minutes before challenge

▸ BY INHALATION OF POWDER
▹ Child 6–11 years: 100–200 micrograms, to be taken 10–15 minutes before challenge
▹ Child 12–17 years: 200 micrograms, to be taken 10–15 minutes before challenge
▹ Adult: 200 micrograms, to be taken 10–15 minutes before challenge

Other conditions associated with reversible airways obstruction
▸ BY INHALATION OF AEROSOL
▹ Adult: 100–200 micrograms, to be taken when required for symptomatic relief, up to 4 times a day, review maintenance treatment if usage is frequent
▸ BY INHALATION OF POWDER
▹ Adult: 100–200 micrograms, to be taken when required for symptomatic relief, up to 4 times a day, review maintenance treatment if usage is frequent
▸ BY INHALATION OF NEBULISED SOLUTION
▹ Adult: 2.5–5 mg, to be taken when required for symptomatic relief, up to 4 times a day, review maintenance treatment if usage is frequent

Exacerbation of reversible airways obstruction
▸ BY INHALATION OF AEROSOL
▹ Child: 100–200 micrograms, to be taken up to 4 times a day for persistent symptoms

Moderate to severe hyperkalaemia [adjuvant treatment]
▸ BY INHALATION OF NEBULISED SOLUTION
▹ Adult: 10 mg for 1 dose, alternatively 20 mg for 1 dose, consider a dose of 10 mg in patients with cardiac disease

Uncomplicated premature labour (between 22 and 37 weeks of gestation) (specialist supervision in hospital)
▸ BY CONTINUOUS INTRAVENOUS INFUSION
▹ Adult: Initially 10 micrograms/minute, rate increased gradually according to response at 10-minute intervals until contractions diminish then increase rate slowly until contractions cease (maximum rate 45 micrograms/minute), maintain rate for 1 hour after contractions have stopped, then gradually reduce by 50% every 6 hours, maximum duration 48 hours

PHARMACOKINETICS
▸ At recommended inhaled doses, the duration of action of salbutamol is about 3 to 5 hours.

● UNLICENSED USE
▸ When used for Asthma or Prophylaxis of allergen- or exercise-induced bronchospasm or Other conditions associated with reversible airways obstruction in adults National guidelines and expert advice recommend that salbutamol is used as detailed within the indications and dose section, but this may differ from licensed product information.
▸ When used for Asthma or Prophylaxis of allergen- or exercise-induced bronchospasm or Exacerbation of reversible airways obstruction in children National guidelines and expert advice recommend that salbutamol is used as detailed within the indications and dose section, but this may differ from licensed product information.
▸ When used by inhalation in adults EvGr Salbutamol is used for the treatment of hyperkalaemia, ⒶA but is not licensed for this indication.
▸ With intravenous use in children Injection and solution for intravenous infusion not licensed for use in children under 12 years.

▸ **With intravenous use in children** Administration of undiluted salbutamol injection through a central venous catheter is not licensed.

> **IMPORTANT SAFETY INFORMATION**
>
> MHRA/CHM ADVICE: PRESSURISED METERED DOSE INHALERS (PMDI): RISK OF AIRWAY OBSTRUCTION FROM ASPIRATION OF LOOSE OBJECTS (JULY 2018)
>
> See Respiratory system, inhaled drug delivery p. 269.
>
> MHRA/CHM ADVICE: NEBULISED ASTHMA RESCUE THERAPY IN CHILDREN: HOME USE OF NEBULISERS IN PAEDIATRIC ASTHMA SHOULD BE INITIATED AND MANAGED ONLY BY SPECIALISTS (AUGUST 2022)
>
> The MHRA has reviewed the evidence regarding a number of deaths in children with asthma, where the clinically unsupervised use of a nebuliser to deliver asthma rescue medication was a potential contributory factor. Healthcare professionals are advised that home use of nebulisers for the acute treatment of asthma in children and adolescents should only be initiated and managed by asthma specialists. Home use of nebulisers for this purpose, without adequate medical supervision, can mask a deterioration in the underlying disease, which could result in delays in seeking medical attention and be fatal or have serious consequences. The purchase of nebulisers for this purpose, outside of medical advice, is not recommended. Patients and their carers should be advised to seek urgent medical attention if worsening asthma symptoms are not relieved by prescribed rescue medication, even if there is short-term recovery following its use. They should receive training from a healthcare professional on the usage and maintenance of the nebuliser, and be given advice on when to seek medical attention, so that deterioration in asthma control can be treated without delay. Patients (or their carers) who have been using a nebuliser at home without specialist management should contact their GP about referral to a specialist. The MHRA has produced videos to support this advice—guidance for healthcare professionals is available at: www.youtube.com/watch?v=qfppzpdeYmk and guidance for patients, parents, and carers is available at: www.youtube.com/watch?v=N00ir0i043Q.

● **CONTRA-INDICATIONS**
▸ **When used for Uncomplicated premature labour** Abruptio placenta · antepartum haemorrhage · cord compression · eclampsia · history of cardiac disease · intra-uterine fetal death · intra-uterine infection · placenta praevia · pulmonary hypertension · severe pre-eclampsia · significant risk factors for myocardial ischaemia · threatened miscarriage

● **CAUTIONS**
▸ **With intravenous use** Mild to moderate pre-eclampsia (when used for uncomplicated premature labour) · suspected cardiovascular disease (should be assessed by a cardiologist before initiating therapy for uncomplicated premature labour)

● **INTERACTIONS** → Appendix 1: beta$_2$ agonists

● **SIDE-EFFECTS**

GENERAL SIDE-EFFECTS
▸ **Common or very common** Muscle cramps
▸ **Rare or very rare** Akathisia · hypokalaemia (with high doses) · vasodilation
▸ **Frequency not known** Metabolic change · myocardial ischaemia

SPECIFIC SIDE-EFFECTS
▸ **Uncommon**
▸ **When used by inhalation** Oral irritation · throat irritation
▸ **With parenteral use** Pulmonary oedema
▸ **Frequency not known**
▸ **When used by inhalation** Lactic acidosis (with high doses)

▸ **With parenteral use** Lactic acidosis (with high doses) · nausea · vomiting

● **BREAST FEEDING** Inhaled drugs for asthma can be taken as normal during breast-feeding.

● **MONITORING REQUIREMENTS** In uncomplicated premature labour it is important to monitor blood pressure, pulse rate (should not exceed 120 beats per minute), ECG (discontinue treatment if signs of myocardial ischaemia develop), blood glucose and lactate concentrations, and the patient's fluid and electrolyte status (avoid over-hydration—discontinue drug immediately and initiate diuretic therapy if pulmonary oedema occurs).

● **DIRECTIONS FOR ADMINISTRATION**
▸ **With intravenous use in children** For *continuous intravenous infusion*, dilute to a concentration of 200 micrograms/mL with Glucose 5% *or* Sodium Chloride 0.9%. If fluid-restricted, can be given undiluted through central venous catheter [unlicensed]. For *intravenous injection*, dilute to a concentration of 50 micrograms/mL with Glucose 5%, Sodium Chloride 0.9%, *or* Water for injections.
▸ **When used by inhalation** For *nebulisation*, dilute nebuliser solution with a suitable volume of sterile Sodium Chloride 0.9% solution according to nebuliser type and duration of administration; salbutamol and ipratropium bromide solutions are compatible and can be mixed for nebulisation.
▸ **With intravenous use in adults** For *bronchodilation* by *continuous intravenous infusion*, dilute to a concentration of 200 micrograms/mL with glucose 5% or sodium chloride 0.9%. For *premature labour* by *continuous intravenous infusion*, dilute with glucose 5% to a concentration of 200 micrograms/mL for use in a syringe pump *or* for other infusion methods (preferably *via* controlled infusion device), dilute to a concentration of 20 micrograms/mL; close attention to patient's fluid and electrolyte status essential.

● **PRESCRIBING AND DISPENSING INFORMATION** For information on devices used for the delivery of inhaled medicines, see Respiratory system, inhaled drug delivery p. 269.
▸ **When used for Asthma** For choice of therapy, see Asthma, acute p. 274 and Asthma, chronic p. 271.

● **PATIENT AND CARER ADVICE** *For inhalation by aerosol or dry powder*, advise patients and carers not to exceed prescribed dose and to follow manufacturer's directions; if a previously effective dose of inhaled salbutamol fails to provide at least 3 hours relief, a doctor's advice should be obtained as soon as possible. *For inhalation by nebuliser*, the dose given by nebuliser is substantially higher than that given by inhaler. Patients should therefore be warned that it is dangerous to exceed the prescribed dose and they should seek medical advice if they fail to respond to the usual dose of the respirator solution.
Medicines for Children leaflet: Salbutamol inhaler for asthma and wheeze www.medicinesforchildren.org.uk/medicines/salbutamol-inhaler-for-asthma-and-wheeze/

● **MEDICINAL FORMS** There can be variation in the licensing of different medicines containing the same drug.

Inhalation powder
▸ **Easyhaler (salbutamol)** (Orion Pharma (UK) Ltd)
Salbutamol 100 microgram per 1 dose Easyhaler Salbutamol sulfate 100micrograms/dose dry powder inhaler | 200 dose [PoM] £3.31 DT = £3.31
Salbutamol 200 microgram per 1 dose Easyhaler Salbutamol sulfate 200micrograms/dose dry powder inhaler | 200 dose [PoM] £6.63 DT = £6.63
▸ **Salbulin Novolizer** (Viatris UK Healthcare Ltd)
Salbutamol (as Salbutamol sulfate) 100 microgram per 1 dose Salbulin Novolizer 100micrograms/dose inhalation powder | 200 dose [PoM] £4.95 DT = £4.95
Salbulin Novolizer 100micrograms/dose inhalation powder refill | 200 dose [PoM] £2.75 DT = £2.75

▸ **Ventolin Accuhaler** (GlaxoSmithKline UK Ltd)
Salbutamol 200 microgram per 1 dose Ventolin 200micrograms/dose Accuhaler | 60 dose [PoM] £3.60 DT = £3.60

Solution for injection
▸ **Ventolin** (GlaxoSmithKline UK Ltd)
Salbutamol (as Salbutamol sulfate) 500 microgram per 1 ml Ventolin 500micrograms/1ml solution for injection ampoules | 5 ampoule [PoM] £1.91 DT = £1.91

Solution for infusion
▸ **Ventolin** (GlaxoSmithKline UK Ltd)
Salbutamol (as Salbutamol sulfate) 1 mg per 1 ml Ventolin 5mg/5ml solution for infusion ampoules | 10 ampoule [PoM] £24.81 DT = £24.81

Pressurised inhalation
▸ **Airomir Autohaler** (Teva UK Ltd)
Salbutamol (as Salbutamol sulfate) 100 microgram per 1 dose Airomir 100micrograms/dose Autohaler | 200 dose [PoM] £6.02 DT = £6.30
▸ **Salamol** (Teva UK Ltd)
Salbutamol (as Salbutamol sulfate) 100 microgram per 1 dose Salamol 100micrograms/dose inhaler CFC free | 200 dose [PoM] £1.46 DT = £1.50
▸ **Salamol Easi-Breathe** (Teva UK Ltd)
Salbutamol (as Salbutamol sulfate) 100 microgram per 1 dose Salamol 100micrograms/dose Easi-Breathe inhaler | 200 dose [PoM] £6.30 DT = £6.30
▸ **Ventolin Evohaler** (GlaxoSmithKline UK Ltd)
Salbutamol (as Salbutamol sulfate) 100 microgram per 1 dose Ventolin 100micrograms/dose Evohaler | 200 dose [PoM] £1.50 DT = £1.50

Nebuliser liquid
▸ **Salbutamol** (Non-proprietary)
Salbutamol (as Salbutamol sulfate) 830 microgram per 1 ml Salbutamol 2.5mg/3ml nebuliser liquid unit dose vials | 25 unit dose [PoM] [Σ] (Hospital only)
Salbutamol (as Salbutamol sulfate) 1 mg per 1 ml Salbutamol 2.5mg/2.5ml nebuliser liquid unit dose ampoules | 20 unit dose [PoM] £13.09–£17.86 | 30 unit dose [PoM] £24.00–£25.50
Salbutamol 2.5mg/2.5ml nebuliser liquid unit dose vials | 20 unit dose [PoM] £22.86 DT = £9.31
Salbutamol (as Salbutamol sulfate) 2 mg per 1 ml Salbutamol 5mg/2.5ml nebuliser liquid unit dose vials | 20 unit dose [PoM] £24.81 DT = £21.54
Salbutamol 5mg/2.5ml nebuliser liquid unit dose ampoules | 20 unit dose [PoM] £15.00–£22.00 | 30 unit dose [PoM] £30.00–£34.20
▸ **Ventolin** (GlaxoSmithKline UK Ltd)
Salbutamol (as Salbutamol sulfate) 5 mg per 1 ml Ventolin 5mg/ml respirator solution | 20 ml [PoM] £2.18 DT = £2.18

Combinations available: *Ipratropium with salbutamol*, p. 282

⮞ 285

Terbutaline sulfate
22-Nov-2023

● INDICATIONS AND DOSE

Asthma | Other conditions associated with reversible airways obstruction
▸ BY MOUTH
▸ Adult: Initially 2.5 mg 3 times a day for 1–2 weeks, then increased to up to 5 mg 3 times a day, use by inhalation preferred over by mouth
▸ BY SUBCUTANEOUS INJECTION, OR BY SLOW INTRAVENOUS INJECTION
▸ Adult: 250–500 micrograms up to 4 times a day, reserve intravenous beta₂ agonists for those in whom inhaled therapy cannot be used reliably or there is no current effect
▸ BY CONTINUOUS INTRAVENOUS INFUSION
▸ Adult: 90–300 micrograms/hour for 8-10 hours, to be administered as a solution containing 3–5 micrograms/mL, high doses require close monitoring, reserve intravenous beta₂ agonists for those in whom inhaled therapy cannot be used reliably or there is no current effect

▸ BY INHALATION OF POWDER
▸ Adult: 500 micrograms up to 4 times a day, for persistent symptoms
▸ BY INHALATION OF NEBULISED SOLUTION
▸ Adult: 5–10 mg 2–4 times a day, additional doses may be necessary in severe acute asthma

Acute asthma
▸ BY SUBCUTANEOUS INJECTION, OR BY SLOW INTRAVENOUS INJECTION
▸ Child 2-14 years: 10 micrograms/kg up to 4 times a day (max. per dose 300 micrograms), reserve intravenous beta₂ agonists for those in whom inhaled therapy cannot be used reliably or there is no current effect
▸ Child 15-17 years: 250–500 micrograms up to 4 times a day, reserve intravenous beta₂ agonists for those in whom inhaled therapy cannot be used reliably or there is no current effect
▸ BY CONTINUOUS INTRAVENOUS INFUSION
▸ Child: Loading dose 2–4 micrograms/kg, then 1–10 micrograms/kg/hour, dose to be adjusted according to response and heart rate, close monitoring is required for doses above 10 micrograms/kg/hour, reserve intravenous beta₂ agonists for those in whom inhaled therapy cannot be used reliably or there is no current effect

Moderate, severe, or life-threatening acute asthma
▸ BY INHALATION OF NEBULISED SOLUTION
▸ Child 1 month-4 years: 5 mg, repeat every 20–30 minutes or when required, give via oxygen-driven nebuliser if available
▸ Child 5-11 years: 5–10 mg, repeat every 20–30 minutes or when required, give via oxygen-driven nebuliser if available
▸ Child 12-17 years: 10 mg, repeat every 20–30 minutes or when required, give via oxygen-driven nebuliser if available
▸ Adult: 10 mg, repeat every 20–30 minutes or when required, give via oxygen-driven nebuliser if available

Exacerbation of reversible airways obstruction (including nocturnal asthma) | Prevention of exercise-induced bronchospasm
▸ BY INHALATION OF POWDER
▸ Child 5-17 years: 500 micrograms up to 4 times a day, for occasional use only
▸ BY MOUTH
▸ Child 1 month-6 years: 75 micrograms/kg 3 times a day (max. per dose 2.5 mg), administration by mouth is not recommended
▸ Child 7-14 years: 2.5 mg 2–3 times a day, administration by mouth is not recommended
▸ Child 15-17 years: Initially 2.5 mg 3 times a day, then increased if necessary to 5 mg 3 times a day, administration by mouth is not recommended

Uncomplicated premature labour (between 22 and 37 weeks of gestation) (specialist supervision in hospital)
▸ BY INTRAVENOUS INFUSION
▸ Adult: Initially 5 micrograms/minute for 20 minutes, then increased in steps of 2.5 micrograms/minute every 20 minutes until contractions have ceased (more than 10 micrograms/minute should **seldom** be given—20 micrograms/minute should **not** be exceeded), continue for 1 hour, then reduced in steps of 2.5 micrograms/minute every 20 minutes to lowest dose that maintains suppression (maximum total duration 48 hours)

PHARMACOKINETICS
▸ At recommended inhaled doses, the duration of action of terbutaline is about 3 to 5 hours.

- **UNLICENSED USE** Tablets not licensed for use in children under 7 years. Injection not licensed for use in children under 2 years.

IMPORTANT SAFETY INFORMATION

MHRA/CHM ADVICE: NEBULISED ASTHMA RESCUE THERAPY IN CHILDREN: HOME USE OF NEBULISERS IN PAEDIATRIC ASTHMA SHOULD BE INITIATED AND MANAGED ONLY BY SPECIALISTS (AUGUST 2022)

The MHRA has reviewed the evidence regarding a number of deaths in children with asthma, where the clinically unsupervised use of a nebuliser to deliver asthma rescue medication was a potential contributory factor. Healthcare professionals are advised that home use of nebulisers for the acute treatment of asthma in children and adolescents should only be initiated and managed by asthma specialists. Home use of nebulisers for this purpose, without adequate medical supervision, can mask a deterioration in the underlying disease, which could result in delays in seeking medical attention and be fatal or have serious consequences. The purchase of nebulisers for this purpose, outside of medical advice, is not recommended. Patients and their carers should be advised to seek urgent medical attention if worsening asthma symptoms are not relieved by prescribed rescue medication, even if there is short-term recovery following its use. They should receive training from a healthcare professional on the usage and maintenance of the nebuliser, and be given advice on when to seek medical attention, so that deterioration in asthma control can be treated without delay. Patients (or their carers) who have been using a nebuliser at home without specialist management should contact their GP about referral to a specialist. The MHRA has produced videos to support this advice—guidance for healthcare professionals is available at: www.youtube.com/watch? v=qfppzpdeYmk and guidance for patients, parents, and carers is available at: www.youtube.com/watch? v=NO0ir0i043Q.

- **CONTRA-INDICATIONS**
- When used for Uncomplicated premature labour Abruptio placenta · antepartum haemorrhage · cord compression · eclampsia · history of cardiac disease · intra-uterine fetal death · intra-uterine infection · placenta praevia · pulmonary hypertension · severe pre-eclampsia · significant risk factors for myocardial ischaemia · threatened miscarriage

- **CAUTIONS** Mild to moderate pre-eclampsia (when used for uncomplicated premature labour) · suspected cardiovascular disease (should be assessed by a cardiologist before initiating therapy for uncomplicated premature labour)

- **INTERACTIONS** → Appendix 1: beta$_2$ agonists

- **SIDE-EFFECTS**

  GENERAL SIDE-EFFECTS
- **Common or very common** Hypokalaemia · hypotension · muscle spasms · nausea
- **Rare or very rare** Myocardial ischaemia · vasodilation
- **Frequency not known** Angioedema · anxiety · behaviour abnormal · bronchospasm · circulatory collapse · oral irritation · skin reactions · sleep disorder · throat irritation

  SPECIFIC SIDE-EFFECTS
- **Uncommon**
- With parenteral use Pulmonary oedema
- **Rare or very rare**
- With parenteral use Lactic acidosis
- **Frequency not known**
- When used by inhalation Lactic acidosis (with high doses)
- With parenteral use Akathisia · bleeding tendency

- **PREGNANCY** Inhaled drugs for asthma can be taken as normal during pregnancy.

- **BREAST FEEDING** Inhaled drugs for asthma can be taken as normal during breast-feeding.

- **MONITORING REQUIREMENTS** In uncomplicated premature labour it is important to monitor blood pressure, pulse rate (should not exceed 120 beats per minute), ECG (discontinue treatment if signs of myocardial ischaemia develop), blood glucose and lactate concentrations, and the patient's fluid and electrolyte status (avoid over-hydration—discontinue drug immediately and initiate diuretic therapy if pulmonary oedema occurs).

- **DIRECTIONS FOR ADMINISTRATION**
- With intravenous use in children [EvGr] For *continuous intravenous infusion*, dilute to a concentration of 3–5 micrograms/mL with Glucose 5% *or* Sodium Chloride 0.9%. (M) If fluid-restricted, expert sources advise dilute to a concentration of 100 micrograms/mL; give via a syringe pump.
- When used by inhalation [EvGr] For *nebulisation*, dilute nebuliser solution with sterile Sodium Chloride 0.9% solution, if required, according to nebuliser type and duration of administration; terbutaline and ipratropium bromide solutions are compatible and may be mixed for nebulisation. (M)
- With intravenous use in adults [EvGr] For *bronchodilation* by *continuous intravenous infusion*, dilute 1.5–2.5 mg with 500 mL glucose 5% or sodium chloride 0.9% and give over 8–10 hours. For *premature labour* by *continuous intravenous infusion*, dilute in glucose 5% and give *via* controlled infusion device preferably a syringe pump; if syringe pump available dilute to a concentration of 100 micrograms/mL; if syringe pump not available dilute to a concentration of 10 micrograms/mL; close attention to patient's fluid and electrolyte status essential. (M)

- **PRESCRIBING AND DISPENSING INFORMATION**
- When used for Asthma For choice of therapy, see Asthma, acute p. 274 and Asthma, chronic p. 271.

- **PATIENT AND CARER ADVICE** *For inhalation by dry powder*, advise patients and carers not to exceed prescribed dose and to follow manufacturer's directions; if a previously effective dose of inhaled terbutaline fails to provide at least 3 hours relief, a doctor's advice should be obtained as soon as possible. *For inhalation by nebuliser*, the dose given by nebuliser is substantially higher than that given by inhaler. Patients should therefore be warned that it is dangerous to exceed the prescribed dose and they should seek medical advice if they fail to respond to the usual dose of the respirator solution.

- **MEDICINAL FORMS** There can be variation in the licensing of different medicines containing the same drug.

  Solution for injection
- Bricanyl (AstraZeneca UK Ltd)
  Terbutaline sulfate 500 microgram per 1 ml Bricanyl 2.5mg/5ml solution for injection ampoules | 10 ampoule [PoM] £20.09 DT = £20.09
  Bricanyl 500micrograms/1ml solution for injection ampoules | 5 ampoule [PoM] £6.48 DT = £6.48

  Inhalation powder
- Bricanyl Turbohaler (AstraZeneca UK Ltd)
  Terbutaline sulfate 500 microgram per 1 dose Bricanyl 500micrograms/dose Turbohaler | 120 dose [PoM] £8.30 DT = £8.30

  Nebuliser liquid
- Terbutaline sulfate (Non-proprietary)
  Terbutaline sulfate 2.5 mg per 1 ml Terbutaline 5mg/2ml nebuliser liquid unit dose vials | 20 unit dose [PoM] £8.91–£12.50 DT = £11.64
- Bricanyl Respules (AstraZeneca UK Ltd)
  Terbutaline sulfate 2.5 mg per 1 ml Bricanyl 5mg/2ml Respules | 20 unit dose [PoM] £11.64 DT = £11.64

CORTICOSTEROIDS

Corticosteroids (inhaled) 

> **IMPORTANT SAFETY INFORMATION**
>
> **MHRA/CHM ADVICE: CORTICOSTEROIDS: RARE RISK OF CENTRAL SEROUS CHORIORETINOPATHY WITH LOCAL AS WELL AS SYSTEMIC ADMINISTRATION (AUGUST 2017)**
>
> Central serous chorioretinopathy is a retinal disorder that has been linked to the systemic use of corticosteroids. Recently, it has also been reported after local administration of corticosteroids via inhaled and intranasal, epidural, intra-articular, topical dermal, and periocular routes. The MHRA recommends that patients should be advised to report any blurred vision or other visual disturbances with corticosteroid treatment given by any route; consider referral to an ophthalmologist for evaluation of possible causes if a patient presents with vision problems.
>
> **NHS IMPROVEMENT PATIENT SAFETY ALERT: STEROID EMERGENCY CARD TO SUPPORT EARLY RECOGNITION AND TREATMENT OF ADRENAL CRISIS IN ADULTS (AUGUST 2020)**
>
> A patient-held **Steroid Emergency Card** has been developed for patients with adrenal insufficiency and steroid dependence who are at risk of adrenal crisis. It aims to support healthcare staff with the early recognition of patients at risk of adrenal crisis and the emergency treatment of adrenal crisis. All eligible patients should be issued a Steroid Emergency Card. Providers that treat patients with acute physical illness or trauma, or who may require emergency treatment, elective surgery, or other invasive procedures, should establish processes to check for risk of adrenal crisis and confirm if the patient has a Steroid Emergency Card.
>
> **ADRENAL INSUFFICIENCY CARD (APRIL 2023)**
>
> The British Society for Paediatric Endocrinology and Diabetes (BSPED) has developed an Adrenal Insufficiency Card which should be issued to children with adrenal insufficiency and steroid dependence. The card includes a management summary for the emergency treatment of adrenal crisis and sick day dosing, and can be issued by any healthcare professional managing such patients. The BSPED Adrenal Insufficiency Card is available at: www.bsped.org.uk/ adrenal-insufficiency.

● **SIDE-EFFECTS**
▸ **Common or very common** Headache · oral candidiasis · pneumonia (in patients with COPD) · taste altered · voice alteration
▸ **Uncommon** Bronchospasm paradoxical · cataract · vision blurred
▸ **Rare or very rare** Adrenal suppression · anxiety · behaviour abnormal · glaucoma · growth retardation (in children) · sleep disorder

SIDE-EFFECTS, FURTHER INFORMATION Systemic absorption may follow inhaled administration particularly if high doses are used or if treatment is prolonged. Therefore also consider the side-effects of systemic corticosteroids.

Candidiasis The risk of oral candidiasis can be reduced by using a spacer device with the corticosteroid inhaler; rinsing the mouth with water after inhalation of a dose may also be helpful. An anti-fungal oral suspension or oral gel can be used to treat oral candidiasis without discontinuing corticosteroid therapy.

Paradoxical bronchospasm The potential for paradoxical bronchospasm (calling for discontinuation and alternative therapy) should be borne in mind. Mild bronchospasm may be prevented by inhalation of a short-acting beta₂ agonist beforehand (or by transfer from an aerosol inhalation to a dry powder inhalation).

● **PREGNANCY** Inhaled drugs for asthma can be taken as normal during pregnancy.

● **BREAST FEEDING** Inhaled corticosteroids for asthma can be taken as normal during breast-feeding.

● **MONITORING REQUIREMENTS**
▸ In children The height and weight of children receiving prolonged treatment with inhaled corticosteroids should be monitored annually; if growth is slowed, referral to a paediatrician should be considered.

● **PATIENT AND CARER ADVICE** If systemic absorption occurs following inhaled use, side-effects applicable to systemic corticosteroids may apply.
Steroid Emergency Card
▸ In adults Steroid Emergency Cards should be issued to patients with adrenal insufficiency and steroid dependence for whom missed doses, illness, or surgery puts them at risk of adrenal crisis. The Royal College of Physicians and the Society for Endocrinology advise that patients taking inhaled corticosteroids at doses greater than beclometasone 1000 micrograms daily (using traditional beclometasone dipropionate inhalers such as *Clenil Modulite®* or *Soprobec®*) or fluticasone 500 micrograms daily are considered at risk of adrenal insufficiency and should be given a Steroid Emergency Card. The card includes a management summary for the emergency treatment of adrenal crisis and can be issued by any healthcare professional managing such patients. Steroid Emergency Cards are available for purchase from the NHS Print online ordering portal cmswebshop.corp. xerox.com/NHS/Login.aspx or Primary Care Support England (PCSE) online.

● **NATIONAL FUNDING/ACCESS DECISIONS**
For full details see funding body website
NICE decisions
▸ **Inhaled corticosteroids for the treatment of chronic asthma in children under 12 years (November 2007) NICE TA131** Recommended
▸ **Inhaled corticosteroids for the treatment of chronic asthma in adults and children over 12 years (March 2008) NICE TA138** Recommended

⚑ above

Beclometasone dipropionate

08-Oct-2024

(Beclomethasone dipropionate)

● **INDICATIONS AND DOSE**
Prophylaxis of asthma
▸ BY INHALATION OF POWDER
▸ Child 5-11 years: 100–200 micrograms twice daily, dose to be adjusted as necessary
▸ Child 12-17 years: 200–400 micrograms twice daily; increased if necessary up to 800 micrograms twice daily, dose to be adjusted as necessary
▸ Adult: 200–400 micrograms twice daily; increased if necessary up to 800 micrograms twice daily, dose to be adjusted as necessary

DOSE EQUIVALENCE AND CONVERSION
▸ Dose adjustments may be required for some inhaler devices, see under individual preparations.

CLENIL MODULITE®
Prophylaxis of asthma
▸ BY INHALATION OF AEROSOL
▸ Child 2-11 years: 100–200 micrograms twice daily
▸ Child 12-17 years: 200–400 micrograms twice daily; increased if necessary up to 1 mg twice daily
▸ Adult: 200–400 micrograms twice daily; increased if necessary up to 1 mg twice daily

KELHALE ®
Prophylaxis of asthma
▶ BY INHALATION OF AEROSOL
▶ Adult: 50–200 micrograms twice daily; increased if necessary up to 400 micrograms twice daily

POTENCY
▶ *Kelhale* ® has extra-fine particles and is more potent than traditional beclometasone dipropionate CFC-containing inhalers.

QVAR ® PREPARATIONS
Prophylaxis of asthma
▶ BY INHALATION OF AEROSOL
▶ Child 5-11 years: 50–100 micrograms twice daily, using Autohaler or MDI device
▶ Child 12-17 years: 50–200 micrograms twice daily, using Autohaler, MDI, or Easi-Breathe device; increased if necessary up to 400 micrograms twice daily
▶ Adult: 50–200 micrograms twice daily, using Autohaler, MDI, or Easi-Breathe device; increased if necessary up to 400 micrograms twice daily

POTENCY
▶ *Qvar* ® has extra-fine particles, is more potent than traditional beclometasone dipropionate CFC-containing inhalers and is approximately twice as potent as *Clenil Modulite* ®.

SOPROBEC ®
Prophylaxis of asthma
▶ BY INHALATION OF AEROSOL
▶ Child: 100 micrograms twice daily; increased if necessary up to 400 micrograms daily in 2–4 divided doses
▶ Adult: 200 micrograms twice daily; increased if necessary up to 2 mg daily in 2–4 divided doses

● **UNLICENSED USE** *Easyhaler* ® *Beclometasone Dipropionate* is not licensed for use in children. *Clenil Modulite* ® 200 and 250 are not licensed for use in children.

> **IMPORTANT SAFETY INFORMATION**
> **MHRA/CHM ADVICE (JULY 2008)**
> Beclometasone dipropionate CFC-free pressurised metered-dose inhalers (*Qvar* ® and *Clenil Modulite* ®) are **not** interchangeable and should be prescribed by brand name; *Qvar* ® has extra-fine particles, is more potent than traditional beclometasone dipropionate CFC-containing inhalers, and is approximately twice as potent as *Clenil Modulite* ®.
>
> **MHRA/CHM ADVICE: PRESSURISED METERED DOSE INHALERS (PMDI): RISK OF AIRWAY OBSTRUCTION FROM ASPIRATION OF LOOSE OBJECTS (JULY 2018)**
> See Respiratory system, inhaled drug delivery p. 269.

● **INTERACTIONS** → Appendix 1: corticosteroids

● **SIDE-EFFECTS**
▶ **Common or very common** Throat irritation
▶ **Rare or very rare** Wheezing

● **PRESCRIBING AND DISPENSING INFORMATION** For choice of therapy, see Asthma, acute p. 274 and Asthma, chronic p. 271. The MHRA has advised (July 2008) that beclometasone dipropionate CFC-free inhalers should be prescribed by brand name. Pressurised metered-doses inhalers with extra-fine particles (*Qvar* ® and *Kelhale* ®) are more potent than, and not interchangeable with, traditional CFC-containing and CFC-free inhalers (*Clenil Modulite* ® and *Soprobec* ®).

KELHALE ® Manufacturer advises when switching a patient with well-controlled asthma from another corticosteroid inhaler, initially a 100-microgram metered dose of *Kelhale* ® should be prescribed for 200–250 micrograms of budesonide and for 100 micrograms of fluticasone propionate; the dose of *Kelhale* ® should be adjusted according to response, up to a maximum of 800 micrograms daily. Manufacturer advises when switching a patient with poorly-controlled asthma from another corticosteroid inhaler, initially a 100-microgram metered dose of *Kelhale* ® should be prescribed for 100 micrograms of budesonide or fluticasone propionate; the dose of *Kelhale* ® should be adjusted according to response, up to a maximum of 800 micrograms daily.

QVAR ® PREPARATIONS When switching a patient with well-controlled asthma from another corticosteroid inhaler, initially a 100-microgram metered dose of *Qvar* ® should be prescribed for 200–250 micrograms of beclometasone dipropionate or budesonide and for 100 micrograms of fluticasone propionate. When switching a patient with poorly controlled asthma from another corticosteroid inhaler, initially a 100-microgram metered dose of *Qvar* ® should be prescribed for 100 micrograms of beclometasone dipropionate, budesonide, or fluticasone propionate; the dose of *Qvar* ® should be adjusted according to response.

● **PROFESSION SPECIFIC INFORMATION**

Dental practitioners' formulary *Clenil Modulite* ® 50 micrograms/metered inhalation may be prescribed.

● **MEDICINAL FORMS** There can be variation in the licensing of different medicines containing the same drug.

Inhalation powder
CAUTIONARY AND ADVISORY LABELS 8, 10
▶ **Easyhaler (beclometasone)** (Orion Pharma (UK) Ltd)
Beclometasone dipropionate 200 microgram per 1 dose Easyhaler Beclometasone 200micrograms/dose dry powder inhaler | 200 dose PoM £14.93 DT = £14.93

Pressurised inhalation
CAUTIONARY AND ADVISORY LABELS 8, 10
▶ **Beclu** (Lupin Healthcare (UK) Ltd)
Beclometasone dipropionate 200 microgram per 1 dose Beclu 200micrograms/dose inhaler | 200 dose PoM £11.31 DT = £16.17
▶ **Clenil Modulite** (Chiesi Ltd)
Beclometasone dipropionate 50 microgram per 1 dose Clenil Modulite 50micrograms/dose inhaler | 200 dose PoM £3.70 DT = £3.70
Beclometasone dipropionate 100 microgram per 1 dose Clenil Modulite 100micrograms/dose inhaler | 200 dose PoM £7.42 DT = £7.42
Beclometasone dipropionate 200 microgram per 1 dose Clenil Modulite 200micrograms/dose inhaler | 200 dose PoM £16.17 DT = £16.17
Beclometasone dipropionate 250 microgram per 1 dose Clenil Modulite 250micrograms/dose inhaler | 200 dose PoM £16.29 DT = £16.29
▶ **Kelhale** (Cipla EU Ltd)
Beclometasone dipropionate 50 microgram per 1 dose Kelhale 50micrograms/dose inhaler | 200 dose PoM £5.20 DT = £3.70
Beclometasone dipropionate 100 microgram per 1 dose Kelhale 100micrograms/dose inhaler | 200 dose PoM £5.20 DT = £7.42
▶ **Qvar** (Teva UK Ltd)
Beclometasone dipropionate 50 microgram per 1 dose Qvar 50 inhaler | 200 dose PoM £7.87 DT = £3.70
Beclometasone dipropionate 100 microgram per 1 dose Qvar 100 inhaler | 200 dose PoM £17.21 DT = £7.42
▶ **Qvar Autohaler** (Teva UK Ltd)
Beclometasone dipropionate 50 microgram per 1 dose Qvar 50 Autohaler | 200 dose PoM £7.87 DT = £7.87
Beclometasone dipropionate 100 microgram per 1 dose Qvar 100 Autohaler | 200 dose PoM £17.21 DT = £17.21
▶ **Qvar Easi-Breathe** (Teva UK Ltd)
Beclometasone dipropionate 50 microgram per 1 dose Qvar 50micrograms/dose Easi-Breathe inhaler | 200 dose PoM £7.74 DT = £7.87
Beclometasone dipropionate 100 microgram per 1 dose Qvar 100micrograms/dose Easi-Breathe inhaler | 200 dose PoM £16.95 DT = £17.21
▶ **Soprobec** (Glenmark Pharmaceuticals Europe Ltd)
Beclometasone dipropionate 50 microgram per 1 dose Soprobec 50micrograms/dose inhaler | 200 dose PoM £2.41 DT = £3.70

Beclometasone dipropionate 100 microgram per 1 dose Soprobec 100micrograms/dose inhaler | 200 dose PoM £4.82 DT = £7.42
Beclometasone dipropionate 200 microgram per 1 dose Soprobec 200micrograms/dose inhaler | 200 dose PoM £10.51 DT = £16.17
Beclometasone dipropionate 250 microgram per 1 dose Soprobec 250micrograms/dose inhaler | 200 dose PoM £10.59 DT = £16.29

Beclometasone with formoterol   13-Jan-2025

The properties listed below are those particular to the combination only. For the properties of the components please consider, beclometasone dipropionate p. 292, formoterol fumarate p. 285.

● **INDICATIONS AND DOSE**

BIBECFO ® 100/6

Asthma maintenance therapy
▶ BY INHALATION OF AEROSOL
▸ Adult: 1–2 inhalations twice daily; maximum 4 inhalations per day

Asthma, maintenance and reliever therapy
▶ BY INHALATION OF AEROSOL
▸ Adult: Maintenance 1 inhalation twice daily; 1 inhalation as required, for relief of symptoms; maximum 8 inhalations per day

Chronic obstructive pulmonary disease with forced expiratory volume in 1 second < 50% of predicted
▶ BY INHALATION OF AEROSOL
▸ Adult: 2 inhalations twice daily

DOSE EQUIVALENCE AND CONVERSION
▸ 1 inhalation contains 100 micrograms beclometasone dipropionate and 6 micrograms formoterol fumarate, in extrafine particles.
▸ 100 micrograms of beclometasone dipropionate extrafine is equivalent to 250 micrograms of beclometasone dipropionate in a non-extrafine formulation. When switching patients from non-extrafine formulations to *Bibecfo*®, the dose should be reduced and adjusted according to response.

BIBECFO ® 200/6

Asthma maintenance therapy
▶ BY INHALATION OF AEROSOL
▸ Adult: 2 inhalations twice daily; maximum 4 inhalations per day

DOSE EQUIVALENCE AND CONVERSION
▸ 1 inhalation contains 200 micrograms beclometasone dipropionate and 6 micrograms formoterol fumarate, in extrafine particles.
▸ 100 micrograms of beclometasone dipropionate extrafine is equivalent to 250 micrograms of beclometasone dipropionate in a non-extrafine formulation. When switching patients from non-extrafine formulations to *Bibecfo*®, the dose should be reduced and adjusted according to response.

FOSTAIR NEXTHALER ® 100/6

Asthma maintenance therapy
▶ BY INHALATION OF POWDER
▸ Adult: 1–2 inhalations twice daily; maximum 4 inhalations per day

Asthma, maintenance and reliever therapy
▶ BY INHALATION OF POWDER
▸ Adult: Maintenance 1 inhalation twice daily; 1 inhalation as required, for relief of symptoms; maximum 8 inhalations per day

Chronic obstructive pulmonary disease with forced expiratory volume in 1 second < 50% of predicted
▶ BY INHALATION OF POWDER
▸ Adult: 2 inhalations twice daily

DOSE EQUIVALENCE AND CONVERSION
▸ 1 inhalation contains 100 micrograms beclometasone dipropionate and 6 micrograms formoterol fumarate, in extrafine particles.
▸ 100 micrograms of beclometasone dipropionate extrafine is equivalent to 250 micrograms of beclometasone dipropionate in a non-extrafine formulation. When switching from non-extrafine formulations to *Fostair NEXThaler*®, the dose should be reduced and adjusted according to response.

FOSTAIR NEXTHALER ® 200/6

Asthma maintenance therapy
▶ BY INHALATION OF POWDER
▸ Adult: 2 inhalations twice daily; maximum 4 inhalations per day

DOSE EQUIVALENCE AND CONVERSION
▸ 1 inhalation contains 200 micrograms beclometasone dipropionate and 6 micrograms formoterol fumarate, in extrafine particles.
▸ 100 micrograms of beclometasone dipropionate extrafine is equivalent to 250 micrograms of beclometasone dipropionate in a non-extrafine formulation. When switching patients from non-extrafine formulations to *Fostair NEXThaler*®, the dose should be reduced and adjusted according to response.

FOSTAIR ® 100/6

Asthma maintenance therapy
▶ BY INHALATION OF AEROSOL
▸ Adult: 1–2 inhalations twice daily; maximum 4 inhalations per day

Asthma, maintenance and reliever therapy
▶ BY INHALATION OF AEROSOL
▸ Adult: Maintenance 1 inhalation twice daily; 1 inhalation as required, for relief of symptoms; maximum 8 inhalations per day

Chronic obstructive pulmonary disease with forced expiratory volume in 1 second < 50% of predicted
▶ BY INHALATION OF AEROSOL
▸ Adult: 2 inhalations twice daily

DOSE EQUIVALENCE AND CONVERSION
▸ 1 inhalation contains 100 micrograms beclometasone dipropionate and 6 micrograms formoterol fumarate, in extrafine particles.
▸ 100 micrograms of beclometasone dipropionate extrafine is equivalent to 250 micrograms of beclometasone dipropionate in a non-extrafine formulation. When switching patients from non-extrafine formulations to *Fostair*®, the dose should be reduced and adjusted according to response.

FOSTAIR ® 200/6

Asthma maintenance therapy
▶ BY INHALATION OF AEROSOL
▸ Adult: 2 inhalations twice daily; maximum 4 inhalations per day

DOSE EQUIVALENCE AND CONVERSION
▸ 1 inhalation contains 200 micrograms beclometasone dipropionate and 6 micrograms formoterol fumarate, in extrafine particles.
▸ 100 micrograms of beclometasone dipropionate extrafine is equivalent to 250 micrograms of beclometasone dipropionate in a non-extrafine formulation. When switching patients from non-extrafine formulations to *Fostair*®, the dose should be reduced and adjusted according to response.

Respiratory system

3

LUFORBEC ® 100/6

Asthma maintenance therapy

▸ BY INHALATION OF AEROSOL

▸ Adult: 1–2 inhalations twice daily; maximum 4 inhalations per day

Asthma, maintenance and reliever therapy

▸ BY INHALATION OF AEROSOL

▸ Adult: Maintenance 1 inhalation twice daily; 1 inhalation as required, for relief of symptoms; maximum 8 inhalations per day

Chronic obstructive pulmonary disease with forced expiratory volume in 1 second < 50% of predicted

▸ BY INHALATION OF AEROSOL

▸ Adult: 2 inhalations twice daily

DOSE EQUIVALENCE AND CONVERSION

▸ 1 inhalation contains 100 micrograms beclometasone dipropionate and 6 micrograms formoterol fumarate, in extrafine particles.

▸ 100 micrograms of beclometasone dipropionate extrafine is equivalent to 250 micrograms of beclometasone dipropionate in a non-extrafine formulation. When switching from non-extrafine formulations to *Luforbec*®, the dose should be reduced and adjusted according to response.

LUFORBEC ® 200/6

Asthma maintenance therapy

▸ BY INHALATION OF AEROSOL

▸ Adult: 2 inhalations twice daily; maximum 4 inhalations per day

DOSE EQUIVALENCE AND CONVERSION

▸ 1 inhalation contains 200 micrograms beclometasone dipropionate and 6 micrograms formoterol fumarate, in extrafine particles.

▸ 100 micrograms of beclometasone dipropionate extrafine is equivalent to 250 micrograms of beclometasone dipropionate in a non-extrafine formulation. When switching patients from non-extrafine formulations to *Luforbec*®, the dose should be reduced and adjusted according to response.

PROXOR ® 100/6

Asthma maintenance therapy

▸ BY INHALATION OF AEROSOL

▸ Adult: 1–2 inhalations twice daily; maximum 4 inhalations per day

Asthma, maintenance and reliever therapy

▸ BY INHALATION OF AEROSOL

▸ Adult: Maintenance 1 inhalation twice daily; 1 inhalation as required, for relief of symptoms; maximum 8 inhalations per day

Chronic obstructive pulmonary disease with forced expiratory volume in 1 second < 50% of predicted

▸ BY INHALATION OF AEROSOL

▸ Adult: 2 inhalations twice daily

DOSE EQUIVALENCE AND CONVERSION

▸ 1 inhalation contains 100 micrograms beclometasone dipropionate and 6 micrograms formoterol fumarate, in extrafine particles.

▸ 100 micrograms of beclometasone dipropionate extrafine is equivalent to 250 micrograms of beclometasone dipropionate in a non-extrafine formulation. When switching patients from non-extrafine formulations to *Proxor*®, the dose should be reduced and adjusted according to response.

PROXOR ® 200/6

Asthma maintenance therapy

▸ BY INHALATION OF AEROSOL

▸ Adult: 2 inhalations twice daily; maximum 4 inhalations per day

---

DOSE EQUIVALENCE AND CONVERSION

▸ 1 inhalation contains 200 micrograms beclometasone dipropionate and 6 micrograms formoterol fumarate, in extrafine particles.

▸ 100 micrograms of beclometasone dipropionate extrafine is equivalent to 250 micrograms of beclometasone dipropionate in a non-extrafine formulation. When switching patients from non-extrafine formulations to *Proxor*®, the dose should be reduced and adjusted according to response.

VIVAIRE ® 100/6

Asthma maintenance therapy

▸ BY INHALATION OF AEROSOL

▸ Adult: 1–2 inhalations twice daily; maximum 4 inhalations per day

Asthma, maintenance and reliever therapy

▸ BY INHALATION OF AEROSOL

▸ Adult: Maintenance 1 inhalation twice daily; 1 inhalation as required, for relief of symptoms; maximum 8 inhalations per day

Chronic obstructive pulmonary disease with forced expiratory volume in 1 second < 50% of predicted

▸ BY INHALATION OF AEROSOL

▸ Adult: 2 inhalations twice daily

DOSE EQUIVALENCE AND CONVERSION

▸ 1 inhalation contains 100 micrograms beclometasone dipropionate and 6 micrograms formoterol fumarate, in extrafine particles.

▸ 100 micrograms of beclometasone dipropionate extrafine is equivalent to 250 micrograms of beclometasone dipropionate in a non-extrafine formulation. When switching patients from non-extrafine formulations to *Vivaire*®, the dose should be reduced and adjusted according to response.

VIVAIRE ® 200/6

Asthma maintenance therapy

▸ BY INHALATION OF AEROSOL

▸ Adult: 2 inhalations twice daily; maximum 4 inhalations per day

DOSE EQUIVALENCE AND CONVERSION

▸ 1 inhalation contains 200 micrograms beclometasone dipropionate and 6 micrograms formoterol fumarate, in extrafine particles.

▸ 100 micrograms of beclometasone dipropionate extrafine is equivalent to 250 micrograms of beclometasone dipropionate in a non-extrafine formulation. When switching patients from non-extrafine formulations to *Vivaire*®, the dose should be reduced and adjusted according to response.

IMPORTANT SAFETY INFORMATION

MHRA/CHM ADVICE (JULY 2008)

Fostair® contains extra-fine particles of beclometasone dipropionate and is more potent than traditional beclometasone dipropionate CFC-free inhalers. The dose of beclometasone dipropionate in *Fostair*® should be lower than non-extra-fine formulations of beclometasone dipropionate and will need to be adjusted to the individual needs of the patient.

● INTERACTIONS → Appendix 1: beta$_2$ agonists · corticosteroids

● PATIENT AND CARER ADVICE Patients or carers should be given advice on appropriate inhaler technique.

3

- **MEDICINAL FORMS** There can be variation in the licensing of different medicines containing the same drug.

Inhalation powder

CAUTIONARY AND ADVISORY LABELS 8, 10

▶ Fostair NEXThaler (Chiesi Ltd)
Formoterol fumarate dihydrate 6 microgram per 1 dose, Beclometasone dipropionate 100 microgram per 1 dose Fostair NEXThaler 100micrograms/dose / 6micrograms/dose dry powder inhaler | 120 dose [PoM] £29.32 DT = £29.32
Formoterol fumarate dihydrate 6 microgram per 1 dose, Beclometasone dipropionate 200 microgram per 1 dose Fostair NEXThaler 200micrograms/dose / 6micrograms/dose dry powder inhaler | 120 dose [PoM] £29.32 DT = £29.32

Pressurised inhalation

CAUTIONARY AND ADVISORY LABELS 8, 10

▶ Bibecfo (Cipla EU Ltd)
Formoterol fumarate dihydrate 6 microgram, Beclometasone dipropionate 200 microgram Bibecfo 200micrograms/dose / 6micrograms/dose inhaler | 120 dose [PoM] £13.98 DT = £29.32
Formoterol fumarate dihydrate 6 microgram per 1 dose, Beclometasone dipropionate 100 microgram per 1 dose Bibecfo 100micrograms/dose / 6micrograms/dose inhaler | 120 dose [PoM] £13.98 DT = £29.32

▶ Fostair (Chiesi Ltd)
Formoterol fumarate dihydrate 6 microgram, Beclometasone dipropionate 200 microgram Fostair 200micrograms/dose / 6micrograms/dose inhaler | 120 dose [PoM] £29.32 DT = £29.32
Formoterol fumarate dihydrate 6 microgram per 1 dose, Beclometasone dipropionate 100 microgram per 1 dose Fostair 100micrograms/dose / 6micrograms/dose inhaler | 120 dose [PoM] £29.32 DT = £29.32

▶ Luforbec (Lupin Healthcare (UK) Ltd)
Formoterol fumarate dihydrate 6 microgram, Beclometasone dipropionate 200 microgram Luforbec 200micrograms/dose / 6micrograms/dose inhaler | 120 dose [PoM] £13.98 DT = £29.32
Formoterol fumarate dihydrate 6 microgram per 1 dose, Beclometasone dipropionate 100 microgram per 1 dose Luforbec 100micrograms/dose / 6micrograms/dose inhaler | 120 dose [PoM] £13.98 DT = £29.32

▶ Proxor (Genus Pharmaceuticals Ltd)
Formoterol fumarate dihydrate 6 microgram, Beclometasone dipropionate 200 microgram Proxor 200micrograms/dose / 6micrograms/dose inhaler | 120 dose [PoM] £9.90 DT = £29.32
Formoterol fumarate dihydrate 6 microgram per 1 dose, Beclometasone dipropionate 100 microgram per 1 dose Proxor 100micrograms/dose / 6micrograms/dose inhaler | 120 dose [PoM] £9.90 DT = £29.32

▶ Vivaire (Zentiva Pharma UK Ltd)
Formoterol fumarate dihydrate 6 microgram, Beclometasone dipropionate 200 microgram Vivaire 200micrograms/dose / 6micrograms/dose inhaler | 120 dose [PoM] £9.85 DT = £29.32
Formoterol fumarate dihydrate 6 microgram per 1 dose, Beclometasone dipropionate 100 microgram per 1 dose Vivaire 100micrograms/dose / 6micrograms/dose inhaler | 120 dose [PoM] £9.85 DT = £29.32

Beclometasone with formoterol and glycopyrronium

23-Sep-2022

The properties listed below are those particular to the combination only. For the properties of the components please consider, beclometasone dipropionate p. 292, formoterol fumarate p. 285, glycopyrronium bromide p. 281.

- **INDICATIONS AND DOSE**

TRIMBOW 172/5/9 ®

Asthma maintenance therapy
▶ BY INHALATION OF AEROSOL
▶ Adult: 2 inhalations twice daily

TRIMBOW 87/5/9 ®

Moderate-to-severe chronic obstructive pulmonary disease | Asthma maintenance therapy
▶ BY INHALATION OF AEROSOL
▶ Adult: 2 inhalations twice daily

TRIMBOW NEXTHALER 88/5/9 ®

Moderate-to-severe chronic obstructive pulmonary disease
▶ BY INHALATION OF POWDER
▶ Adult: 2 inhalations twice daily

- **INTERACTIONS** → Appendix 1: beta₂ agonists · corticosteroids · glycopyrronium

- **PREGNANCY** [EvGr] Use only if potential benefit outweighs risk. ⓜ

- **BREAST FEEDING** [EvGr] Avoid—no information available. ⓜ

- **HEPATIC IMPAIRMENT** [EvGr] Use in severe impairment only if potential benefit outweighs risk (no information available). ⓜ

- **RENAL IMPAIRMENT** [EvGr] Use in severe impairment or end-stage renal disease requiring dialysis, especially if associated with significant weight loss, only if potential benefit outweighs risk. ⓜ

- **HANDLING AND STORAGE**
TRIMBOW 172/5/9 ® For *pressurised metered-dose inhalers (pMDI)*, store in a refrigerator (2–8°C)—consult product literature for further information regarding storage conditions outside refrigerator after dispensing.

- **PATIENT AND CARER ADVICE** Patients or carers should be given advice on appropriate inhaler technique.

- **NATIONAL FUNDING/ACCESS DECISIONS**
For full details see funding body website

Scottish Medicines Consortium (SMC) decisions
▶ Beclometasone with formoterol and glycopyrronium (*Trimbow 87/5/9*®) for maintenance treatment in adult patients with moderate to severe chronic obstructive pulmonary disease (COPD) who are not adequately treated by a combination of an inhaled corticosteroid and a long-acting beta₂-agonist (October 2017) SMC No. 1274/17 Recommended with restrictions
▶ Beclometasone with formoterol and glycopyrronium (*Trimbow 87/5/9*®) for maintenance treatment of asthma, in adults not adequately controlled with a maintenance combination of a long-acting beta₂-agonist and medium dose of inhaled corticosteroid, and who experienced one or more asthma exacerbations in the previous year (March 2021) SMC No. SMC2335 Recommended
▶ Beclometasone with formoterol and glycopyrronium (*Trimbow 172/5/9*®) for maintenance treatment of asthma, in adults not adequately controlled with a maintenance combination of a long-acting beta₂-agonist and high dose of inhaled corticosteroid, and who experienced one or more asthma exacerbations in the previous year (August 2022) SMC No. SMC2334 Recommended

- **MEDICINAL FORMS** There can be variation in the licensing of different medicines containing the same drug.

Inhalation powder

CAUTIONARY AND ADVISORY LABELS 8, 10

▶ Trimbow NEXThaler (Chiesi Ltd)
Formoterol fumarate dihydrate 5 microgram per 1 dose, Glycopyrronium (as Glycopyrronium bromide) 9 microgram per 1 dose, Beclometasone dipropionate 88 microgram per 1 dose Trimbow NEXThaler 88micrograms/dose / 5micrograms/dose / 9micrograms/dose dry powder inhaler | 120 dose [PoM] £44.50

Pressurised inhalation

CAUTIONARY AND ADVISORY LABELS 8, 10

EXCIPIENTS: May contain Ethanol

▶ Trimbow (Chiesi Ltd)
Formoterol fumarate dihydrate 5 microgram per 1 dose, Glycopyrronium (as Glycopyrronium bromide) 9 microgram per 1 dose, Beclometasone dipropionate 87 microgram per 1 dose Trimbow 87micrograms/dose / 5micrograms/dose / 9micrograms/dose inhaler | 120 dose [PoM] £44.50
Formoterol fumarate dihydrate 5 microgram per 1 dose, Glycopyrronium (as Glycopyrronium bromide) 9 microgram per

1 dose, Beclometasone dipropionate 172 microgram per
1 dose Trimbow 172micrograms/dose / 5micrograms/dose /
9micrograms/dose inhaler | 120 dose [PoM] £44.50

▶ 292

Budesonide
03-Apr-2024

- **DRUG ACTION** Budesonide is a glucocorticoid, which exerts
significant local anti-inflammatory effects.

- **INDICATIONS AND DOSE**

**Prophylaxis of mild to moderate asthma (in patients
stabilised on twice daily dose)**

▶ BY INHALATION OF POWDER

▸ Child 6-11 years: 200–400 micrograms once daily, dose
to be given in the evening

▸ Child 12-17 years: 200–400 micrograms once daily (max.
per dose 800 micrograms), dose to be given in the
evening

▸ Adult: 200–400 micrograms once daily (max. per dose
800 micrograms), dose to be given in the evening

Prophylaxis of asthma

▶ BY INHALATION OF POWDER

▸ Child 6-11 years: 100–400 micrograms twice daily, dose
to be adjusted as necessary

▸ Child 12-17 years: 100–800 micrograms twice daily, dose
to be adjusted as necessary

▸ Adult: 100–800 micrograms twice daily, dose to be
adjusted as necessary

▶ BY INHALATION OF NEBULISED SUSPENSION

▸ Child 6 months-11 years: 125–500 micrograms twice
daily, adjusted according to response; maximum 2 mg
per day

▸ Child 12-17 years: Initially 0.25–1 mg twice daily,
adjusted according to response, doses higher than
recommended max. may be used in severe disease;
maximum 2 mg per day

▸ Adult: Initially 0.25–1 mg twice daily, adjusted
according to response, doses higher than
recommended max. may be used in severe disease;
maximum 2 mg per day

POTENCY

▸ Dose adjustments may be required for some inhaler
devices, see under individual preparations.

BUDELIN NOVOLIZER ®

Prophylaxis of asthma

▶ BY INHALATION OF POWDER

▸ Adult: 200–800 micrograms twice daily, dose is
adjusted as necessary

**Alternative in mild to moderate asthma, for patients
previously stabilised on a twice daily dose**

▶ BY INHALATION OF POWDER

▸ Adult: 200–400 micrograms once daily (max. per dose
800 micrograms), to be taken in the evening

PULMICORT ® RESPULES

Prophylaxis of asthma

▶ BY INHALATION OF NEBULISED SUSPENSION

▸ Child 3 months-11 years: Initially 0.5–1 mg twice daily,
reduced to 250–500 micrograms twice daily

▸ Child 12-17 years: Initially 1–2 mg twice daily, reduced
to 0.5–1 mg twice daily

▸ Adult: Initially 1–2 mg twice daily, reduced to 0.5–1 mg
twice daily

PULMICORT ® TURBOHALER

Prophylaxis of asthma

▶ BY INHALATION OF POWDER

▸ Adult: 100–800 micrograms twice daily, dose to be
adjusted as necessary

**Alternative in mild to moderate asthma, for patients
previously stabilised on a twice daily dose**

▶ BY INHALATION OF POWDER

▸ Adult: 200–400 micrograms once daily (max. per dose
800 micrograms), to be taken in the evening

- **INTERACTIONS** → Appendix 1: corticosteroids

- **SIDE-EFFECTS**

▶ **Common or very common** Cough · throat irritation

▶ **Uncommon** Muscle spasms · tremor

▶ **Rare or very rare** Akathisia

- **DIRECTIONS FOR ADMINISTRATION** Budesonide nebuliser
suspension is not suitable for use in ultrasonic nebulisers.

- **PRESCRIBING AND DISPENSING INFORMATION** For choice
of therapy, see Asthma, acute p. 274 and Asthma, chronic
p. 271.

- **PATIENT AND CARER ADVICE** Patients or carers should be
given advice on how to administer budesonide dry powder
inhaler and nebuliser suspension.
Medicines for Children leaflet: Budesonide inhaler for asthma
prevention www.medicinesforchildren.org.uk/medicines/
budesonide-inhaler-for-asthma-prevention/

BUDELIN NOVOLIZER ® Patients or carers should be given
advice on administration of *Budelin Novolizer* ®.

- **MEDICINAL FORMS** There can be variation in the licensing of
different medicines containing the same drug.

Inhalation powder

CAUTIONARY AND ADVISORY LABELS 8, 10

▸ Budelin Novolizer (Viatris UK Healthcare Ltd)
Budesonide 200 microgram per 1 dose Budelin Novolizer
200micrograms/dose inhalation powder | 100 dose [PoM] £14.86 DT =
£14.86
Budelin Novolizer 200micrograms/dose inhalation powder refill |
100 dose [PoM] £9.59 DT = £9.59

▸ Easyhaler (budesonide) (Orion Pharma (UK) Ltd)
Budesonide 100 microgram per 1 dose Easyhaler Budesonide
100micrograms/dose dry powder inhaler | 200 dose [PoM] £8.86 DT =
£14.25
Budesonide 200 microgram per 1 dose Easyhaler Budesonide
200micrograms/dose dry powder inhaler | 200 dose [PoM] £17.71
Budesonide 400 microgram per 1 dose Easyhaler Budesonide
400micrograms/dose dry powder inhaler | 100 dose [PoM] £17.71

▸ Pulmicort Turbohaler (AstraZeneca UK Ltd)
Budesonide 100 microgram per 1 dose Pulmicort 100 Turbohaler
| 200 dose [PoM] £14.25 DT = £14.25
Budesonide 200 microgram per 1 dose Pulmicort 200 Turbohaler
| 100 dose [PoM] £14.25 DT = £14.25
Budesonide 400 microgram per 1 dose Pulmicort 400 Turbohaler
| 50 dose [PoM] £14.25 DT = £14.25

Nebuliser liquid

CAUTIONARY AND ADVISORY LABELS 8, 10

▸ Budesonide (Non-proprietary)
Budesonide 250 microgram per 1 ml Budesonide
500micrograms/2ml nebuliser suspension unit dose ampoules |
20 unit dose [PoM] £30.12
Budesonide 500micrograms/2ml nebuliser liquid unit dose vials |
20 unit dose [PoM] £29.41 DT = £28.71
Budesonide 500 microgram per 1 ml Budesonide 1mg/2ml
nebuliser suspension unit dose ampoules | 20 unit dose [PoM] £45.60
Budesonide 1mg/2ml nebuliser liquid unit dose vials | 20 unit
dose [PoM] £40.13 DT = £36.60

▸ Pulmicort Respules (AstraZeneca UK Ltd)
Budesonide 250 microgram per 1 ml Pulmicort 0.5mg Respules |
20 unit dose [PoM] £31.70 DT = £28.71
Budesonide 500 microgram per 1 ml Pulmicort 1mg Respules |
20 unit dose [PoM] £48.00 DT = £36.60

Budesonide with formoterol

10-Apr-2025

The properties listed below are those particular to the combination only. For the properties of the components please consider, budesonide p. 297, formoterol fumarate p. 285.

● INDICATIONS AND DOSE

DUORESP SPIROMAX ® 160MICROGRAMS/4.5MICROGRAMS

Asthma, maintenance therapy
▶ BY INHALATION OF POWDER
▸ Child 12–17 years: Initially 1–2 inhalations twice daily; reduced to 1 inhalation daily, dose reduced only if control is maintained
▸ Adult: Initially 1–2 inhalations twice daily, increased if necessary up to 4 inhalations twice daily; reduced to 1 inhalation daily, dose reduced only if control is maintained

Asthma, maintenance and reliever therapy
▶ BY INHALATION OF POWDER
▸ Child 12–17 years: Maintenance 2 inhalations daily in 1–2 divided doses, increased if necessary to 2 inhalations twice daily; 1 inhalation as required, for relief of symptoms, increased if necessary up to 6 inhalations as required, max. 8 inhalations per day; up to 12 inhalations daily can be used for a limited time but medical assessment is recommended
▸ Adult: Maintenance 2 inhalations daily in 1–2 divided doses, increased if necessary to 2 inhalations twice daily; 1 inhalation as required, for relief of symptoms, increased if necessary up to 6 inhalations as required, max. 8 inhalations per day; up to 12 inhalations daily can be used for a limited time but medical assessment is recommended

Mild asthma, reliever therapy
▶ BY INHALATION OF POWDER
▸ Child 12–17 years: 1 inhalation as required, for relief of symptoms, increased if necessary up to 6 inhalations as required, max. 8 inhalations per day; up to 12 inhalations daily can be used for a limited time but medical assessment is recommended
▸ Adult: 1 inhalation as required, for relief of symptoms, increased if necessary up to 6 inhalations as required, max. 8 inhalations per day; up to 12 inhalations daily can be used for a limited time but medical assessment is recommended

Chronic obstructive pulmonary disease with forced expiratory volume in 1 second < 70% of predicted (post-bronchodilator)
▶ BY INHALATION OF POWDER
▸ Adult: 2 inhalations twice daily

DUORESP SPIROMAX ® 320MICROGRAMS/9MICROGRAMS

Asthma, maintenance therapy
▶ BY INHALATION OF POWDER
▸ Child 12–17 years: Initially 1 inhalation twice daily; reduced to 1 inhalation daily, dose reduced only if control is maintained
▸ Adult: Initially 1 inhalation twice daily, increased if necessary up to 2 inhalations twice daily; reduced to 1 inhalation daily, dose reduced only if control is maintained

Chronic obstructive pulmonary disease with forced expiratory volume in 1 second < 70% of predicted (post-bronchodilator)
▶ BY INHALATION OF POWDER
▸ Adult: 1 inhalation twice daily

FOBUMIX ® 160/4.5 EASYHALER

Asthma, maintenance therapy
▶ BY INHALATION OF POWDER
▸ Child 12–17 years: Initially 1–2 inhalations twice daily; reduced to 1 inhalation daily, dose reduced only if control is maintained
▸ Adult: Initially 1–2 inhalations twice daily, increased if necessary up to 4 inhalations twice daily; reduced to 1 inhalation daily, dose reduced only if control is maintained

Asthma, maintenance and reliever therapy
▶ BY INHALATION OF POWDER
▸ Child 12–17 years: Maintenance 2 inhalations daily in 1–2 divided doses, increased if necessary to 2 inhalations twice daily; 1 inhalation as required, for relief of symptoms, increased if necessary up to 6 inhalations as required, max. 8 inhalations per day; up to 12 inhalations daily can be used for a limited time but medical assessment is recommended
▸ Adult: Maintenance 2 inhalations daily in 1–2 divided doses, increased if necessary to 2 inhalations twice daily; 1 inhalation as required, for relief of symptoms, increased if necessary up to 6 inhalations as required, max. 8 inhalations per day; up to 12 inhalations daily can be used for a limited time but medical assessment is recommended

Mild asthma, reliever therapy
▶ BY INHALATION OF POWDER
▸ Child 12–17 years: 1 inhalation as required, for relief of symptoms, increased if necessary up to 6 inhalations as required, max. 8 inhalations per day; up to 12 inhalations daily can be used for a limited time but medical assessment is recommended
▸ Adult: 1 inhalation as required, for relief of symptoms, increased if necessary up to 6 inhalations as required, max. 8 inhalations per day; up to 12 inhalations daily can be used for a limited time but medical assessment is recommended

Chronic obstructive pulmonary disease with forced expiratory volume in 1 second < 70% of predicted (post-bronchodilator)
▶ BY INHALATION OF POWDER
▸ Adult: 2 inhalations twice daily

FOBUMIX ® 320/9 EASYHALER

Asthma, maintenance therapy
▶ BY INHALATION OF POWDER
▸ Child 12–17 years: Initially 1 inhalation twice daily; reduced to 1 inhalation daily, dose reduced only if control is maintained
▸ Adult: Initially 1 inhalation twice daily, increased if necessary up to 2 inhalations twice daily; reduced to 1 inhalation daily, dose reduced only if control is maintained

Chronic obstructive pulmonary disease with forced expiratory volume in 1 second < 70% of predicted (post-bronchodilator)
▶ BY INHALATION OF POWDER
▸ Adult: 1 inhalation twice daily

FOBUMIX ® 80/4.5 EASYHALER

Asthma, maintenance therapy
▶ BY INHALATION OF POWDER
▸ Child 6–17 years: Initially 1–2 inhalations twice daily; reduced to 1 inhalation daily, dose reduced only if control is maintained
▸ Adult: Initially 1–2 inhalations twice daily, increased if necessary up to 4 inhalations twice daily; reduced to 1 inhalation daily, dose reduced only if control is maintained

Asthma, maintenance and reliever therapy
▸ BY INHALATION OF POWDER
▸ Child 12–17 years: Maintenance 2 inhalations daily in 1–2 divided doses; 1 inhalation as required, for relief of symptoms, increased if necessary up to 6 inhalations as required, max. 8 inhalations per day; up to 12 inhalations daily can be used for a limited time but medical assessment is recommended
▸ Adult: Maintenance 2 inhalations daily in 1–2 divided doses; 1 inhalation as required, for relief of symptoms, increased if necessary up to 6 inhalations as required, max. 8 inhalations per day; up to 12 inhalations daily can be used for a limited time but medical assessment is recommended

SYMBICORT 100/6 TURBOHALER ®

Asthma, maintenance therapy
▸ BY INHALATION OF POWDER
▸ Child 6-17 years: Initially 1–2 inhalations twice daily; reduced to 1 inhalation daily, dose reduced only if control is maintained
▸ Adult: Initially 1–2 inhalations twice daily, increased if necessary up to 4 inhalations twice daily; reduced to 1 inhalation daily, dose reduced only if control is maintained

Asthma, maintenance and reliever therapy
▸ BY INHALATION OF POWDER
▸ Child 12–17 years: Maintenance 2 inhalations daily in 1–2 divided doses; 1 inhalation as required, for relief of symptoms, increased if necessary up to 6 inhalations as required, max. 8 inhalations per day; up to 12 inhalations daily can be used for a limited time but medical assessment is recommended
▸ Adult: Maintenance 2 inhalations daily in 1–2 divided doses; 1 inhalation as required, for relief of symptoms, increased if necessary up to 6 inhalations as required, max. 8 inhalations per day; up to 12 inhalations daily can be used for a limited time but medical assessment is recommended

SYMBICORT 200/6 TURBOHALER ®

Asthma, maintenance therapy
▸ BY INHALATION OF POWDER
▸ Child 12-17 years: Initially 1–2 inhalations twice daily; reduced to 1 inhalation daily, dose reduced only if control is maintained
▸ Adult: Initially 1–2 inhalations twice daily, increased if necessary up to 4 inhalations twice daily; reduced to 1 inhalation daily, dose reduced only if control is maintained

Asthma, maintenance and reliever therapy
▸ BY INHALATION OF POWDER
▸ Child 12-17 years: Maintenance 2 inhalations daily in 1–2 divided doses, increased if necessary to 2 inhalations twice daily; 1 inhalation as required, for relief of symptoms, increased if necessary up to 6 inhalations as required, max. 8 inhalations per day; up to 12 inhalations daily can be used for a limited time but medical assessment is recommended
▸ Adult: Maintenance 2 inhalations daily in 1–2 divided doses, increased if necessary to 2 inhalations twice daily; 1 inhalation as required, for relief of symptoms, increased if necessary up to 6 inhalations as required, max. 8 inhalations per day; up to 12 inhalations daily can be used for a limited time but medical assessment is recommended

Mild asthma, reliever therapy
▸ BY INHALATION OF POWDER
▸ Child 12-17 years: 1 inhalation as required, for relief of symptoms, increased if necessary up to 6 inhalations as required, max. 8 inhalations per day; up to 12 inhalations daily can be used for a limited time but medical assessment is recommended
▸ Adult: 1 inhalation as required, for relief of symptoms, increased if necessary up to 6 inhalations as required, max. 8 inhalations per day; up to 12 inhalations daily can be used for a limited time but medical assessment is recommended

Chronic obstructive pulmonary disease with forced expiratory volume in 1 second < 70% of predicted (post-bronchodilator)
▸ BY INHALATION OF POWDER
▸ Adult: 2 inhalations twice daily

SYMBICORT 400/12 TURBOHALER ®

Asthma, maintenance therapy
▸ BY INHALATION OF POWDER
▸ Child 12-17 years: Initially 1 inhalation twice daily; reduced to 1 inhalation daily, dose reduced only if control is maintained
▸ Adult: Initially 1 inhalation twice daily, increased if necessary up to 2 inhalations twice daily; reduced to 1 inhalation daily, dose reduced only if control is maintained

Chronic obstructive pulmonary disease with forced expiratory volume in 1 second < 70% of predicted (post-bronchodilator)
▸ BY INHALATION OF POWDER
▸ Adult: 1 inhalation twice daily

SYMBICORT ® 100/3 PRESSURISED INHALER

Asthma, maintenance therapy
▸ BY INHALATION OF AEROSOL
▸ Child 12-17 years: Initially 2–4 inhalations twice daily; reduced to 1 inhalation daily, dose reduced only if control is maintained
▸ Adult: Initially 2–4 inhalations twice daily, increased if necessary up to 8 inhalations twice daily; reduced to 1 inhalation daily, dose reduced only if control is maintained

Asthma, maintenance and reliever therapy
▸ BY INHALATION OF AEROSOL
▸ Child 12-17 years: Maintenance 4 inhalations daily in 1–2 divided doses, increased if necessary up to 4 inhalations twice daily; 2 inhalations as required for relief of symptoms, increased if necessary up to 12 inhalations as required, usual max. 16 inhalations per day; up to 24 inhalations daily can be used for a limited time but medical assessment is recommended
▸ Adult: Maintenance 4 inhalations daily in 1–2 divided doses, increased if necessary up to 4 inhalations twice daily; 2 inhalations as required for relief of symptoms, increased if necessary up to 12 inhalations as required, usual max. 16 inhalations per day; up to 24 inhalations daily can be used for a limited time but medical assessment is recommended

SYMBICORT ® 200/6 PRESSURISED INHALER

Chronic obstructive pulmonary disease with forced expiratory volume in 1 second < 70% of predicted (post bronchodilator)
▸ BY INHALATION OF AEROSOL
▸ Adult: 2 inhalations twice daily

WOCKAIR ® 160MICROGRAMS/4.5MICROGRAMS

Asthma, maintenance therapy
▸ BY INHALATION OF POWDER
▸ Child 12-17 years: Initially 1–2 inhalations twice daily; reduced to 1 inhalation daily, dose reduced only if control is maintained
▸ BY INHALATION OF POWDER
▸ Adult: Initially 1–2 inhalations twice daily, increased if necessary up to 4 inhalations twice daily; continued →

reduced to 1 inhalation daily, dose reduced only if control is maintained

Asthma, maintenance and reliever therapy
▸ BY INHALATION OF POWDER
▸ Child 12-17 years: Maintenance 2 inhalations daily in 1–2 divided doses, increased if necessary to 2 inhalations twice daily; 1 inhalation as required, for relief of symptoms, increased if necessary up to 6 inhalations as required, max. 8 inhalations per day; up to 12 inhalations daily can be used for a limited time but medical assessment is recommended
▸ BY INHALATION OF POWDER
▸ Adult: Maintenance 2 inhalations daily in 1–2 divided doses, increased if necessary to 2 inhalations twice daily; 1 inhalation as required, for relief of symptoms, increased if necessary up to 6 inhalations as required, max. 8 inhalations per day; up to 12 inhalations daily can be used for a limited time but medical assessment is recommended

Mild asthma, reliever therapy
▸ BY INHALATION OF POWDER
▸ Child 12-17 years: 1 inhalation as required, for relief of symptoms, increased if necessary up to 6 inhalations as required, max. 8 inhalations per day; up to 12 inhalations daily can be used for a limited time but medical assessment is recommended
▸ Adult: 1 inhalation as required, for relief of symptoms, increased if necessary up to 6 inhalations as required, max. 8 inhalations per day; up to 12 inhalations daily can be used for a limited time but medical assessment is recommended

Chronic obstructive pulmonary disease with forced expiratory volume in 1 second < 70% of predicted (post-bronchodilator)
▸ BY INHALATION OF POWDER
▸ Adult: 2 inhalations twice daily

WOCKAIR ® 320MICROGRAMS/9MICROGRAMS

Asthma, maintenance therapy
▸ BY INHALATION OF POWDER
▸ Child 12-17 years: Initially 1 inhalation twice daily; reduced to 1 inhalation daily, dose reduced only if control is maintained
▸ Adult: Initially 1 inhalation twice daily, increased if necessary up to 2 inhalations twice daily; reduced to 1 inhalation daily, dose reduced only if control is maintained

Chronic obstructive pulmonary disease with forced expiratory volume in 1 second < 70% of predicted (post-bronchodilator)
▸ BY INHALATION OF POWDER
▸ Adult: 1 inhalation twice daily

● INTERACTIONS → Appendix 1: beta₂ agonists · corticosteroids

● PATIENT AND CARER ADVICE Patient counselling is advised for budesonide with formoterol inhalation (administration).

● NATIONAL FUNDING/ACCESS DECISIONS
For full details see funding body website
Scottish Medicines Consortium (SMC) decisions
▸ Budesonide/formoterol 100/6, 200/6 inhalation powder turbohaler (*Symbicort* ® SMART ®) for asthma in adults (June 2007) SMC No. 362/07 Recommended
▸ Budesonide/formoterol 100/6, 200/6 inhalation powder turbohaler (*Symbicort* ® SMART ®) for asthma in adolescents aged 12 years and over (June 2017) SMC No. 1244/17 Recommended
▸ Budesonide/formoterol 200/6 inhalation powder (*Symbicort* ® Turbohaler ®) as reliever therapy for adults and adolescents 12 years and older with mild asthma (May 2024) SMC No. SMC2622 Recommended with restrictions

● MEDICINAL FORMS There can be variation in the licensing of different medicines containing the same drug.

Inhalation powder
CAUTIONARY AND ADVISORY LABELS 8, 10 (high doses)
▸ **DuoResp Spiromax** (Teva UK Ltd)
Formoterol fumarate dihydrate 6 microgram per 1 dose, Budesonide 200 microgram per 1 dose DuoResp Spiromax 160micrograms/dose / 4.5micrograms/dose dry powder inhaler | 120 dose PoM £27.97 DT = £28.00
Formoterol fumarate dihydrate 12 microgram per 1 dose, Budesonide 400 microgram per 1 dose DuoResp Spiromax 320micrograms/dose / 9micrograms/dose dry powder inhaler | 60 dose PoM £27.97 DT = £28.00
▸ **Fobumix Easyhaler** (Orion Pharma (UK) Ltd)
Formoterol fumarate dihydrate 6 microgram per 1 dose, Budesonide 100 microgram per 1 dose Fobumix Easyhaler 80micrograms/dose / 4.5micrograms/dose dry powder inhaler | 120 dose PoM £21.50 DT = £28.00
Formoterol fumarate dihydrate 6 microgram per 1 dose, Budesonide 200 microgram per 1 dose Fobumix Easyhaler 160micrograms/dose / 4.5micrograms/dose dry powder inhaler | 60 dose PoM £10.75 | 120 dose PoM £21.50 DT = £28.00
Formoterol fumarate dihydrate 12 microgram per 1 dose, Budesonide 400 microgram per 1 dose Fobumix Easyhaler 320micrograms/dose / 9micrograms/dose dry powder inhaler | 60 dose PoM £21.50 DT = £28.00
▸ **Symbicort Turbohaler** (AstraZeneca UK Ltd)
Formoterol fumarate dihydrate 6 microgram per 1 dose, Budesonide 100 microgram per 1 dose Symbicort 100/6 Turbohaler | 120 dose PoM £28.00 DT = £28.00
Formoterol fumarate dihydrate 6 microgram per 1 dose, Budesonide 200 microgram per 1 dose Symbicort 200/6 Turbohaler | 120 dose PoM £28.00 DT = £28.00
Formoterol fumarate dihydrate 12 microgram per 1 dose, Budesonide 400 microgram per 1 dose Symbicort 400/12 Turbohaler | 60 dose PoM £28.00 DT = £28.00
▸ **WockAIR** (Wockhardt UK Ltd)
Formoterol fumarate dihydrate 6 microgram per 1 dose, Budesonide 200 microgram per 1 dose WockAIR 160micrograms/dose / 4.5micrograms/dose dry powder inhaler | 120 dose PoM £19.00 DT = £28.00
Formoterol fumarate dihydrate 12 microgram per 1 dose, Budesonide 400 microgram per 1 dose WockAIR 320micrograms/dose / 9micrograms/dose dry powder inhaler | 60 dose PoM £19.00 DT = £28.00

Pressurised inhalation
CAUTIONARY AND ADVISORY LABELS 8, 10 (high doses)
▸ **Symbicort** (AstraZeneca UK Ltd)
Formoterol fumarate dihydrate 3 microgram per 1 dose, Budesonide 100 microgram per 1 dose Symbicort 100micrograms/dose / 3micrograms/dose pressurised inhaler | 120 dose PoM £14.00 DT = £14.00
Formoterol fumarate dihydrate 6 microgram per 1 dose, Budesonide 200 microgram per 1 dose Symbicort 200micrograms/dose / 6micrograms/dose pressurised inhaler | 120 dose PoM £28.00 DT = £28.00

F 292

Ciclesonide

20-Jul-2023

● INDICATIONS AND DOSE
Prophylaxis of asthma
▸ BY INHALATION OF AEROSOL
▸ Child 12-17 years: 160 micrograms once daily, increased if necessary up to 320 micrograms twice daily, dose increased in severe asthma; reduced to 80 micrograms once daily, dose reduced only if control is maintained
▸ Adult: 160 micrograms once daily, increased if necessary up to 320 micrograms twice daily, dose

increased in severe asthma; reduced to 80 micrograms once daily, dose reduced only if control is maintained

---

IMPORTANT SAFETY INFORMATION

MHRA/CHM ADVICE: PRESSURISED METERED DOSE INHALERS (PMDI): RISK OF AIRWAY OBSTRUCTION FROM ASPIRATION OF LOOSE OBJECTS (JULY 2018)

See Respiratory system, inhaled drug delivery p. 269.

- **INTERACTIONS** → Appendix 1: corticosteroids
- **SIDE-EFFECTS** Cushing's syndrome
- **HEPATIC IMPAIRMENT** Manufacturer advises caution in severe impairment (risk of increased exposure, no information available).
- **PRESCRIBING AND DISPENSING INFORMATION** For choice of therapy, see Asthma, acute p. 274 and Asthma, chronic p. 271.
- **PATIENT AND CARER ADVICE** Patients or carers should be given advice on how to administer ciclesonide aerosol inhaler.

- **MEDICINAL FORMS** There can be variation in the licensing of different medicines containing the same drug.

Pressurised inhalation

CAUTIONARY AND ADVISORY LABELS 8

- ▸ Ciclesonide (Non-proprietary)
  Ciclesonide 80 microgram per 1 dose Ciclesonide 80micrograms/dose inhaler CFC free | 120 dose PoM £29.55-£42.00 DT = £32.83
  Ciclesonide 160 microgram per 1 dose Ciclesonide 160micrograms/dose inhaler CFC free | 120 dose PoM £32.83-£55.60 DT = £38.62
- ▸ Alvesco (Covis Pharma GmbH)
  Ciclesonide 80 microgram per 1 dose Alvesco 80 inhaler | 120 dose PoM £32.83 DT = £32.83
  Ciclesonide 160 microgram per 1 dose Alvesco 160 inhaler | 60 dose PoM £19.31 DT = £19.31 | 120 dose PoM £38.62 DT = £38.62

▶ 292

Fluticasone

08-Oct-2024

- **INDICATIONS AND DOSE**

Prophylaxis of asthma

- ▸ BY INHALATION OF POWDER
- ▸ Child 5-15 years: Initially 50–100 micrograms twice daily, increased if necessary up to 200 micrograms twice daily, dose to be adjusted as necessary
- ▸ Child 16-17 years: Initially 100–500 micrograms twice daily, increased if necessary up to 1 mg twice daily, doses above 500 micrograms twice daily to be initiated by a specialist, dose to be adjusted as necessary
- ▸ Adult: Initially 100–500 micrograms twice daily, increased if necessary up to 1 mg twice daily, doses above 500 micrograms twice daily to be initiated by a specialist, dose to be adjusted as necessary
- ▸ BY INHALATION OF AEROSOL
- ▸ Child 4-15 years: Initially 50–100 micrograms twice daily, increased if necessary up to 200 micrograms twice daily, dose to be adjusted as necessary
- ▸ Child 16-17 years: Initially 100–500 micrograms twice daily, increased if necessary up to 1 mg twice daily, doses above 500 micrograms twice daily to be initiated by a specialist, dose to be adjusted as necessary
- ▸ Adult: Initially 100–500 micrograms twice daily, increased if necessary up to 1 mg twice daily, doses above 500 micrograms twice daily to be initiated by a specialist, dose to be adjusted as necessary
- ▸ BY INHALATION OF NEBULISED SUSPENSION
- ▸ Child 4-15 years: 1 mg twice daily
- ▸ Child 16-17 years: 0.5–2 mg twice daily

- ▸ Adult: 0.5–2 mg twice daily

IMPORTANT SAFETY INFORMATION

MHRA/CHM ADVICE: PRESSURISED METERED DOSE INHALERS (PMDI): RISK OF AIRWAY OBSTRUCTION FROM ASPIRATION OF LOOSE OBJECTS (JULY 2018)

See Respiratory system, inhaled drug delivery p. 269.

- **INTERACTIONS** → Appendix 1: corticosteroids
- **SIDE-EFFECTS**
- ▸ **Rare or very rare** Dyspepsia
- **DIRECTIONS FOR ADMINISTRATION** EvGr Fluticasone nebuliser liquid may be diluted with sterile sodium chloride 0.9%. It is not suitable for use in ultrasonic nebulisers. ◈M◈
- **PRESCRIBING AND DISPENSING INFORMATION** For choice of therapy, see Asthma, acute p. 274 and Asthma, chronic p. 271.
- **PATIENT AND CARER ADVICE** Patients or carers should be given advice on how to administer all fluticasone inhalation preparations.
  Medicines for Children leaflet: Fluticasone inhaler for asthma prevention (prophylaxis) www.medicinesforchildren.org.uk/medicines/fluticasone-inhaler-for-asthma-prevention-prophylaxis/

- **MEDICINAL FORMS** There can be variation in the licensing of different medicines containing the same drug.

Inhalation powder

CAUTIONARY AND ADVISORY LABELS 8, 10

- ▸ Flixotide Accuhaler (GlaxoSmithKline UK Ltd)
  Fluticasone propionate 50 microgram per 1 dose Flixotide 50micrograms/dose Accuhaler | 60 dose PoM £4.00 DT = £4.00
  Fluticasone propionate 100 microgram per 1 dose Flixotide 100micrograms/dose Accuhaler | 60 dose PoM £8.00 DT = £8.00
  Fluticasone propionate 250 microgram per 1 dose Flixotide 250micrograms/dose Accuhaler | 60 dose PoM £25.51 DT = £25.51
  Fluticasone propionate 500 microgram per 1 dose Flixotide 500micrograms/dose Accuhaler | 60 dose PoM £43.37 DT = £43.37

Pressurised inhalation

CAUTIONARY AND ADVISORY LABELS 8, 10

- ▸ Flixotide Evohaler (GlaxoSmithKline UK Ltd)
  Fluticasone propionate 50 microgram per 1 dose Flixotide 50micrograms/dose Evohaler | 120 dose PoM £6.53 DT = £6.53
  Fluticasone propionate 125 microgram per 1 dose Flixotide 125micrograms/dose Evohaler | 120 dose PoM £21.26 DT = £21.26
  Fluticasone propionate 250 microgram per 1 dose Flixotide 250micrograms/dose Evohaler | 120 dose PoM £36.14 DT = £36.14

Fluticasone with formoterol

20-Apr-2021

The properties listed below are those particular to the combination only. For the properties of the components please consider, fluticasone above, formoterol fumarate p. 285.

- **INDICATIONS AND DOSE**

FLUTIFORM ® 125

Prophylaxis of asthma

- ▸ BY INHALATION OF AEROSOL
- ▸ Child 12-17 years: 2 puffs twice daily
- ▸ Adult: 2 puffs twice daily

FLUTIFORM ® 250

Prophylaxis of asthma

- ▸ BY INHALATION OF AEROSOL
- ▸ Adult: 2 puffs twice daily

FLUTIFORM ® 50

Prophylaxis of asthma

- ▸ BY INHALATION OF AEROSOL
- ▸ Child 5-17 years: 2 puffs twice daily
- ▸ Adult: 2 puffs twice daily

continued →

FLUTIFORM ® K-HALER 125

Prophylaxis of asthma
▶ BY INHALATION OF AEROSOL
▶ Child 12-17 years: 2 puffs twice daily
▶ Adult: 2 puffs twice daily

FLUTIFORM ® K-HALER 50

Prophylaxis of asthma
▶ BY INHALATION OF AEROSOL
▶ Child 12-17 years: 2 puffs twice daily
▶ Adult: 2 puffs twice daily

● INTERACTIONS → Appendix 1: beta$_2$ agonists · corticosteroids

● SIDE-EFFECTS
▶ **Uncommon** Dry mouth · rash · sleep disorders
▶ **Rare or very rare** Asthenia · cough · diarrhoea · dyspepsia · hypertension · muscle spasms · oral fungal infection · peripheral oedema · vertigo

● PATIENT AND CARER ADVICE Patients or carers should be given advice on how to administer fluticasone with formoterol aerosol inhalation.

● NATIONAL FUNDING/ACCESS DECISIONS For full details see funding body website
Scottish Medicines Consortium (SMC) decisions
▶ Fluticasone propionate with formoterol fumarate (*Flutiform*®) for the regular treatment of asthma (October 2012) SMC No. 736/11 Recommended
▶ Fluticasone propionate with formoterol fumarate (*Flutiform*® 50/5 metered dose inhaler) for the regular treatment of asthma in children aged 5 to 12 years (June 2019) SMC No. SMC2178 Recommended

● MEDICINAL FORMS There can be variation in the licensing of different medicines containing the same drug.
Pressurised inhalation
CAUTIONARY AND ADVISORY LABELS 8, 10 (high doses)
▶ Flutiform (Napp Pharmaceuticals Ltd)
Formoterol fumarate dihydrate 5 microgram per 1 dose, Fluticasone propionate 50 microgram per 1 dose Flutiform 50micrograms/dose / 5micrograms/dose inhaler | 120 dose PoM £14.40 DT = £14.40
Formoterol fumarate dihydrate 5 microgram per 1 dose, Fluticasone propionate 125 microgram per 1 dose Flutiform 125micrograms/dose / 5micrograms/dose inhaler | 120 dose PoM £28.00 DT = £28.00
Formoterol fumarate dihydrate 10 microgram per 1 dose, Fluticasone propionate 250 microgram per 1 dose Flutiform 250micrograms/dose / 10micrograms/dose inhaler | 120 dose PoM £45.56 DT = £45.56

Fluticasone with salmeterol
13-Oct-2022

The properties listed below are those particular to the combination only. For the properties of the components please consider, fluticasone p. 301, salmeterol p. 287.

● INDICATIONS AND DOSE
AIRFLUSAL FORSPIRO ®

Chronic obstructive pulmonary disease with forced expiratory volume in 1 second <60% of predicted |
Prophylaxis of asthma
▶ BY INHALATION OF POWDER
▶ Adult: 1 inhalation twice daily

AIRFLUSAL ® 125

Prophylaxis of moderate-to-severe asthma
▶ BY INHALATION OF AEROSOL
▶ Adult: 2 inhalations twice daily

AIRFLUSAL ® 250

Prophylaxis of moderate-to-severe asthma
▶ BY INHALATION OF AEROSOL
▶ Adult: 2 inhalations twice daily

ALOFLUTE ® 25/125

Prophylaxis of moderate-to-severe asthma
▶ BY INHALATION OF AEROSOL
▶ Adult: 2 inhalations twice daily

ALOFLUTE ® 25/250

Prophylaxis of moderate-to-severe asthma
▶ BY INHALATION OF AEROSOL
▶ Adult: 2 inhalations twice daily

AVENOR ® 25/125

Prophylaxis of asthma
▶ BY INHALATION OF AEROSOL
▶ Child 12-17 years: 2 inhalations twice daily
▶ Adult: 2 inhalations twice daily

AVENOR ® 25/250

Prophylaxis of asthma
▶ BY INHALATION OF AEROSOL
▶ Child 12-17 years: 2 inhalations twice daily
▶ Adult: 2 inhalations twice daily

AVENOR ® 25/50

Prophylaxis of asthma
▶ BY INHALATION OF AEROSOL
▶ Child 4-17 years: 2 inhalations twice daily, reduced to 2 inhalations once daily, use reduced dose only if control maintained
▶ Adult: 2 inhalations twice daily, reduced to 2 inhalations once daily, use reduced dose only if control maintained

COMBISAL ® 25/125

Prophylaxis of asthma
▶ BY INHALATION OF AEROSOL
▶ Child 12-17 years: 2 inhalations twice daily
▶ Adult: 2 inhalations twice daily

COMBISAL ® 25/250

Prophylaxis of asthma
▶ BY INHALATION OF AEROSOL
▶ Child 12-17 years: 2 inhalations twice daily
▶ Adult: 2 inhalations twice daily

COMBISAL ® 25/50

Prophylaxis of asthma
▶ BY INHALATION OF AEROSOL
▶ Child 4-17 years: 2 inhalations twice daily, reduced to 2 inhalations once daily, use reduced dose only if control maintained
▶ Adult: 2 inhalations twice daily, reduced to 2 inhalations once daily, use reduced dose only if control maintained

FIXKOH AIRMASTER ® 50/100

Prophylaxis of asthma
▶ BY INHALATION OF POWDER
▶ Child 12-17 years: 1 inhalation twice daily, reduced to 1 inhalation once daily, use reduced dose only if control maintained
▶ Adult: 1 inhalation twice daily, reduced to 1 inhalation once daily, use reduced dose only if control maintained

FIXKOH AIRMASTER ® 50/250

Prophylaxis of asthma
▶ BY INHALATION OF POWDER
▶ Child 12-17 years: 1 inhalation twice daily
▶ Adult: 1 inhalation twice daily

FIXKOH AIRMASTER ® 50/500

Prophylaxis of asthma

▸ BY INHALATION OF POWDER
▸ Child 12-17 years: 1 inhalation twice daily
▸ Adult: 1 inhalation twice daily

Chronic obstructive pulmonary disease [with forced expiratory volume in 1 second <60% of predicted]

▸ BY INHALATION OF POWDER
▸ Adult: 1 inhalation twice daily

FUSACOMB 50/250 EASYHALER ®

Prophylaxis of asthma

▸ BY INHALATION OF POWDER
▸ Child 12-17 years: 1 inhalation twice daily, reduced to 1 inhalation once daily, use reduced dose only if control maintained
▸ Adult: 1 inhalation twice daily, reduced to 1 inhalation once daily, use reduced dose only if control maintained

FUSACOMB 50/500 EASYHALER ®

Prophylaxis of asthma

▸ BY INHALATION OF POWDER
▸ Child 12-17 years: 1 inhalation twice daily
▸ Adult: 1 inhalation twice daily

Chronic obstructive pulmonary disease [with forced expiratory volume in 1 second <60% of predicted]

▸ BY INHALATION OF POWDER
▸ Adult: 1 inhalation twice daily

SEFFALAIR SPIROMAX ® 12.75/100

Prophylaxis of asthma

▸ BY INHALATION OF POWDER
▸ Child 12-17 years: 1 inhalation twice daily
▸ Adult: 1 inhalation twice daily

SEFFALAIR SPIROMAX ® 12.75/202

Prophylaxis of asthma

▸ BY INHALATION OF POWDER
▸ Child 12-17 years: 1 inhalation twice daily
▸ Adult: 1 inhalation twice daily

SEREFLO CIPHALER ® 50/250

Prophylaxis of asthma

▸ BY INHALATION OF POWDER
▸ Child 12-17 years: 1 inhalation twice daily, reduced to 1 inhalation once daily, use reduced dose only if control maintained
▸ Adult: 1 inhalation twice daily, reduced to 1 inhalation once daily, use reduced dose only if control maintained

SEREFLO ® 125

Moderate-to-severe asthma

▸ BY INHALATION OF AEROSOL
▸ Adult: 2 inhalations twice daily

SEREFLO ® 250

Moderate-to-severe asthma

▸ BY INHALATION OF AEROSOL
▸ Adult: 2 inhalations twice daily

SERETIDE 100 ACCUHALER ®

Prophylaxis of asthma

▸ BY INHALATION OF POWDER
▸ Child 4-17 years: 1 inhalation twice daily, reduced to 1 inhalation once daily, use reduced dose only if control maintained
▸ Adult: 1 inhalation twice daily, reduced to 1 inhalation once daily, use reduced dose only if control maintained

SERETIDE 125 EVOHALER ®

Prophylaxis of asthma

▸ BY INHALATION OF AEROSOL
▸ Child 12-17 years: 2 puffs twice daily
▸ Adult: 2 puffs twice daily

SERETIDE 250 ACCUHALER ®

Prophylaxis of asthma

▸ BY INHALATION OF POWDER
▸ Child 12-17 years: 1 inhalation twice daily
▸ Adult: 1 inhalation twice daily

SERETIDE 250 EVOHALER ®

Prophylaxis of asthma

▸ BY INHALATION OF AEROSOL
▸ Child 12-17 years: 2 puffs twice daily
▸ Adult: 2 puffs twice daily

SERETIDE 50 EVOHALER ®

Prophylaxis of asthma

▸ BY INHALATION OF AEROSOL
▸ Child 4-17 years: 2 puffs twice daily, reduced to 2 puffs once daily, use reduced dose only if control maintained
▸ Adult: 2 puffs twice daily, reduced to 2 puffs once daily, use reduced dose only if control maintained

SERETIDE 500 ACCUHALER ®

Prophylaxis of asthma

▸ BY INHALATION OF POWDER
▸ Child 12-17 years: 1 inhalation twice daily
▸ Adult: 1 inhalation twice daily

Chronic obstructive pulmonary disease with forced expiratory volume in 1 second <60% of predicted

▸ BY INHALATION OF POWDER
▸ Adult: 1 inhalation twice daily

STALPEX ® 50/500

Prophylaxis of severe asthma

▸ BY INHALATION OF POWDER
▸ Child 12-17 years: 1 inhalation twice daily
▸ Adult: 1 inhalation twice daily

Chronic obstructive pulmonary disease with forced expiratory volume in 1 second <60% of predicted

▸ BY INHALATION OF POWDER
▸ Adult: 1 inhalation twice daily

IMPORTANT SAFETY INFORMATION

EvGr *Seffalair Spiromax* ® 12.75/100 and 12.75/202 *dry powder inhalers* are not interchangeable with other fluticasone with salmeterol preparations, as the delivered doses differ. ⓜ

● INTERACTIONS → Appendix 1: beta₂ agonists · corticosteroids

● PRESCRIBING AND DISPENSING INFORMATION
▸ In children EvGr *Volumatic* ® spacer devices are compatible with *Seretide Evohaler* ® pressurised metered-dose inhalers. Only the *AeroChamber Plus* ® spacer device is compatible with *Avenor* ® and *Combisal* ® pressurised metered-dose inhalers. ⓜ
▸ In adults EvGr *Volumatic* ® spacer devices are compatible with *Seretide Evohaler* ® pressurised metered-dose inhalers. *Volumatic* ® and *AeroChamber Plus* ® spacer devices are compatible with *Airflusal* ® pressurised metered-dose inhalers. Only the *AeroChamber Plus* ® spacer device is compatible with *Aloflute* ®, *Avenor* ® and *Combisal* ® pressurised metered-dose inhalers. Spacer devices are not compatible with *Sereflo* ® 125 pressurised metered-dose inhaler—if spacer device required, switch to alternative fixed-dose combination preparation. *Volumatic* ® and *AeroChamber Plus* ® spacer devices are compatible with *Sereflo* ® 250 pressurised metered-dose inhaler. ⓜ

● PATIENT AND CARER ADVICE Patients or carers should be given advice on how to administer fluticasone with salmeterol dry powder inhalation and aerosol inhalation.

● **NATIONAL FUNDING/ACCESS DECISIONS**
For full details see funding body website
Scottish Medicines Consortium (SMC) decisions
▸ Fluticasone with salmeterol combination inhaler (*Seretide 500 Accuhaler*®) for symptomatic treatment of patients with chronic obstructive pulmonary disease (January 2009) SMC No. 450/08 Not recommended

● **MEDICINAL FORMS** There can be variation in the licensing of different medicines containing the same drug.

Inhalation powder
CAUTIONARY AND ADVISORY LABELS 8, 10
▸ **AirFluSal Forspiro** (Sandoz Ltd)
Salmeterol (as Salmeterol xinafoate) 50 microgram per 1 dose, Fluticasone propionate 500 microgram per 1 dose AirFluSal Forspiro 50micrograms/dose / 500micrograms/dose dry powder inhaler | 60 dose PoM £29.97 DT = £32.74
▸ **Fixkoh Airmaster** (Genus Pharmaceuticals Holdings Ltd)
Salmeterol (as Salmeterol xinafoate) 50 microgram per 1 dose, Fluticasone propionate 100 microgram per 1 dose Fixkoh Airmaster 50micrograms/dose / 100micrograms/dose dry powder inhaler | 60 dose PoM £14.47 DT = £17.46
Salmeterol (as Salmeterol xinafoate) 50 microgram per 1 dose, Fluticasone propionate 250 microgram per 1 dose Fixkoh Airmaster 50micrograms/dose / 250micrograms/dose dry powder inhaler | 60 dose PoM £19.29 DT = £33.95
Salmeterol (as Salmeterol xinafoate) 50 microgram per 1 dose, Fluticasone propionate 500 microgram per 1 dose Fixkoh Airmaster 50micrograms/dose / 500micrograms/dose dry powder inhaler | 60 dose PoM £16.12 DT = £32.74
▸ **Fusacomb Easyhaler** (Orion Pharma (UK) Ltd)
Salmeterol (as Salmeterol xinafoate) 50 microgram per 1 dose, Fluticasone propionate 250 microgram per 1 dose Fusacomb Easyhaler 50micrograms/dose / 250micrograms/dose dry powder inhaler | 60 dose PoM £21.50 DT = £33.95
Salmeterol (as Salmeterol xinafoate) 50 microgram per 1 dose, Fluticasone propionate 500 microgram per 1 dose Fusacomb Easyhaler 50micrograms/dose / 500micrograms/dose dry powder inhaler | 60 dose PoM £26.99 DT = £32.74
▸ **Sereflo Ciphaler** (Cipla EU Ltd)
Salmeterol (as Salmeterol xinafoate) 50 microgram per 1 dose, Fluticasone propionate 250 microgram per 1 dose Sereflo Ciphaler 50micrograms/dose / 250micrograms/dose dry powder inhaler | 60 dose PoM £10.99 DT = £33.95
▸ **Seretide Accuhaler** (GlaxoSmithKline UK Ltd)
Salmeterol (as Salmeterol xinafoate) 50 microgram per 1 dose, Fluticasone propionate 100 microgram per 1 dose Seretide 100 Accuhaler | 60 dose PoM £17.46 DT = £17.46
Salmeterol (as Salmeterol xinafoate) 50 microgram per 1 dose, Fluticasone propionate 250 microgram per 1 dose Seretide 250 Accuhaler | 60 dose PoM £33.95 DT = £33.95
Salmeterol (as Salmeterol xinafoate) 50 microgram per 1 dose, Fluticasone propionate 500 microgram per 1 dose Seretide 500 Accuhaler | 60 dose PoM £32.74 DT = £32.74
▸ **Stalpex** (Glenmark Pharmaceuticals Europe Ltd)
Salmeterol (as Salmeterol xinafoate) 50 microgram per 1 dose, Fluticasone propionate 500 microgram per 1 dose Stalpex 50micrograms/dose / 500micrograms/dose dry powder inhaler | 60 dose PoM £16.12 DT = £32.74

Pressurised inhalation
CAUTIONARY AND ADVISORY LABELS 8, 10
▸ **AirFluSal** (Sandoz Ltd)
Salmeterol (as Salmeterol xinafoate) 25 microgram per 1 dose, Fluticasone propionate 125 microgram per 1 dose AirFluSal 25micrograms/dose / 125micrograms/dose inhaler | 120 dose PoM £16.42 DT = £23.45
Salmeterol (as Salmeterol xinafoate) 25 microgram per 1 dose, Fluticasone propionate 250 microgram per 1 dose AirFluSal 25micrograms/dose / 250micrograms/dose inhaler | 120 dose PoM £20.52 DT = £29.32
▸ **Aloflute** (Viatris UK Healthcare Ltd)
Salmeterol (as Salmeterol xinafoate) 25 microgram per 1 dose, Fluticasone propionate 125 microgram per 1 dose Aloflute 25micrograms/dose / 125micrograms/dose inhaler | 120 dose PoM £22.45 DT = £23.45
Salmeterol (as Salmeterol xinafoate) 25 microgram per 1 dose, Fluticasone propionate 250 microgram per 1 dose Aloflute 25micrograms/dose / 250micrograms/dose inhaler | 120 dose PoM £28.32 DT = £29.32

▸ **Avenor** (Zentiva Pharma UK Ltd)
Salmeterol (as Salmeterol xinafoate) 25 microgram per 1 dose, Fluticasone propionate 50 microgram per 1 dose Avenor 25micrograms/dose / 50micrograms/dose inhaler | 120 dose PoM £12.99 DT = £17.46
Salmeterol (as Salmeterol xinafoate) 25 microgram per 1 dose, Fluticasone propionate 125 microgram per 1 dose Avenor 25micrograms/dose / 125micrograms/dose inhaler | 120 dose PoM £10.33 DT = £23.45
Salmeterol (as Salmeterol xinafoate) 25 microgram per 1 dose, Fluticasone propionate 250 microgram per 1 dose Avenor 25micrograms/dose / 250micrograms/dose inhaler | 120 dose PoM £13.66 DT = £29.32
▸ **Combisal** (Aspire Pharma Ltd)
Salmeterol (as Salmeterol xinafoate) 25 microgram per 1 dose, Fluticasone propionate 50 microgram per 1 dose Combisal 25micrograms/dose / 50micrograms/dose inhaler | 120 dose PoM £13.50 DT = £17.46
Salmeterol (as Salmeterol xinafoate) 25 microgram per 1 dose, Fluticasone propionate 125 microgram per 1 dose Combisal 25micrograms/dose / 125micrograms/dose inhaler | 120 dose PoM £10.48 DT = £23.45
Salmeterol (as Salmeterol xinafoate) 25 microgram per 1 dose, Fluticasone propionate 250 microgram per 1 dose Combisal 25micrograms/dose / 250micrograms/dose inhaler | 120 dose PoM £13.99 DT = £29.32
▸ **Sereflo** (Cipla EU Ltd)
Salmeterol (as Salmeterol xinafoate) 25 microgram per 1 dose, Fluticasone propionate 125 microgram per 1 dose Sereflo 25micrograms/dose / 125micrograms/dose inhaler | 120 dose PoM £14.99 DT = £23.45
Salmeterol (as Salmeterol xinafoate) 25 microgram per 1 dose, Fluticasone propionate 250 microgram per 1 dose Sereflo 25micrograms/dose / 250micrograms/dose inhaler | 120 dose PoM £19.99 DT = £29.32
▸ **Seretide Evohaler** (GlaxoSmithKline UK Ltd)
Salmeterol (as Salmeterol xinafoate) 25 microgram per 1 dose, Fluticasone propionate 50 microgram per 1 dose Seretide 50 Evohaler | 120 dose PoM £17.46 DT = £17.46
Salmeterol (as Salmeterol xinafoate) 25 microgram per 1 dose, Fluticasone propionate 125 microgram per 1 dose Seretide 125 Evohaler | 120 dose PoM £23.45 DT = £23.45
Salmeterol (as Salmeterol xinafoate) 25 microgram per 1 dose, Fluticasone propionate 250 microgram per 1 dose Seretide 250 Evohaler | 120 dose PoM £29.32 DT = £29.32

⬈ 285

Fluticasone with umeclidinium and vilanterol

06-Nov-2020

The properties listed below are those particular to the combination only. For the properties of the components please consider, fluticasone p. 301, umeclidinium p. 284.

● **INDICATIONS AND DOSE**

Maintenance of moderate-to-severe chronic obstructive pulmonary disease
▸ BY INHALATION OF POWDER
▸ Adult: 1 inhalation once daily, dose should be taken at the same time each day

● **CAUTIONS** Convulsive disorders · pulmonary tuberculosis · thyrotoxicosis
● **INTERACTIONS** → Appendix 1: beta₂ agonists · corticosteroids · umeclidinium
● **SIDE-EFFECTS**
▸ **Common or very common** Arthralgia · back pain · constipation · cough · increased risk of infection · oropharyngeal pain
▸ **Uncommon** Bone fracture · dry mouth · dysphonia
▸ **Frequency not known** Vision disorders
● **HEPATIC IMPAIRMENT** Manufacturer advises caution in moderate to severe impairment.
● **PATIENT AND CARER ADVICE** Patients or carers should be given advice on appropriate inhaler technique.

- **NATIONAL FUNDING/ACCESS DECISIONS**
  For full details see funding body website
  Scottish Medicines Consortium (SMC) decisions
  ▶ Fluticasone furoate with umeclidinium and vilanterol
  (*Trelegy® Ellipta®*) for maintenance treatment in adult
  patients with moderate to severe chronic obstructive
  pulmonary disease who are not adequately treated by a
  combination of an inhaled corticosteroid and a long-acting
  beta$_2$-agonist (February 2018) SMC No. 1303/18 Recommended
  with restrictions

- **MEDICINAL FORMS** There can be variation in the licensing of
  different medicines containing the same drug.
  Inhalation powder
  CAUTIONARY AND ADVISORY LABELS 8, 10
  ▶ Trelegy Ellipta (GlaxoSmithKline UK Ltd)
    Vilanterol (as Vilanterol trifenatate) 22 microgram per 1 dose,
    Umeclidinium (as Umeclidinium bromide) 55 microgram per
    1 dose, Fluticasone furoate 92 microgram per 1 dose Trelegy
    Ellipta 92micrograms/dose / 55micrograms/dose /
    22micrograms/dose dry powder inhaler | 30 dose PoM £44.50

Fluticasone with vilanterol   ◤ 285

20-Apr-2021

The properties listed below are those particular to the
combination only. For the properties of the components
please consider, fluticasone p. 301.

- **INDICATIONS AND DOSE**
  RELVAR ELLIPTA® 184 MICROGRAMS/22 MICROGRAMS
  Prophylaxis of asthma
  ▶ BY INHALATION OF POWDER
  ▶ Child 12–17 years: 1 inhalation once daily
  ▶ Adult: 1 inhalation once daily

  RELVAR ELLIPTA® 92 MICROGRAMS/22 MICROGRAMS
  Prophylaxis of asthma
  ▶ BY INHALATION OF POWDER
  ▶ Child 12–17 years: 1 inhalation once daily
  ▶ Adult: 1 inhalation once daily

  **Chronic obstructive pulmonary disease with forced
  expiratory volume in 1 second < 70% of predicted**
  ▶ BY INHALATION OF POWDER
  ▶ Adult: 1 inhalation once daily

- **INTERACTIONS** → Appendix 1: beta$_2$ agonists ·
  corticosteroids

- **SIDE-EFFECTS**
  ▶ **Common or very common** Abdominal pain · arthralgia · back
  pain · bone fracture · cough · dysphonia · fever · increased
  risk of infection · muscle spasms · oropharyngeal pain
  ▶ **Uncommon** Vision blurred
  ▶ **Rare or very rare** Angioedema · anxiety

- **PREGNANCY** Manufacturer advises use only if potential
  benefit outweighs risk.

- **BREAST FEEDING** Manufacturer advises avoid—no
  information available.

- **HEPATIC IMPAIRMENT** Manufacturer advises caution.
  Dose adjustments Manufacturer advises maximum dose of
  92 microgram/22 microgram once daily in moderate to
  severe impairment.

- **PATIENT AND CARER ADVICE** Patients or carers should be
  given advice on how to administer fluticasone with
  vilanterol powder for inhalation.

- **NATIONAL FUNDING/ACCESS DECISIONS**
  For full details see funding body website
  Scottish Medicines Consortium (SMC) decisions
  ▶ Fluticasone furoate with vilanterol (*Relvar® Ellipta®*) for
  symptomatic treatment of adults with chronic obstructive
  pulmonary disease with a forced expiratory volume in
  1 second (FEV$_1$) less than 70% predicted normal (post-

bronchodilator) with an exacerbation history despite regular
bronchodilator therapy (April 2014) SMC No. 953/14
Recommended with restrictions

- **MEDICINAL FORMS** There can be variation in the licensing of
  different medicines containing the same drug.
  Inhalation powder
  CAUTIONARY AND ADVISORY LABELS 8, 10
  ▶ Relvar Ellipta (GlaxoSmithKline UK Ltd)
    Vilanterol 22 microgram per 1 dose, Fluticasone furoate
    92 microgram per 1 dose Relvar Ellipta 92micrograms/dose /
    22micrograms/dose dry powder inhaler | 30 dose PoM £22.00 DT =
    £22.00
    Vilanterol 22 microgram per 1 dose, Fluticasone furoate
    184 microgram per 1 dose Relvar Ellipta 184micrograms/dose /
    22micrograms/dose dry powder inhaler | 30 dose PoM £29.50 DT =
    £29.50

Formoterol fumarate with glycopyrronium and budesonide

26-Feb-2021

The properties listed below are those particular to the
combination only. For the properties of the components
please consider, formoterol fumarate p. 285, glycopyrronium
bromide p. 281, budesonide p. 297.

- **INDICATIONS AND DOSE**
  **Maintenance treatment of moderate-to-severe chronic
  obstructive pulmonary disease**
  ▶ BY INHALATION OF AEROSOL
  ▶ Adult: 2 inhalations twice daily

- **INTERACTIONS** → Appendix 1: beta$_2$ agonists ·
  corticosteroids · glycopyrronium

- **PREGNANCY** [EvGr] Use only if potential benefit outweighs
  risk—limited information available. ◈M◈

- **BREAST FEEDING** [EvGr] Use only if potential benefit
  outweighs risk—limited information available. ◈M◈

- **HEPATIC IMPAIRMENT** [EvGr] Use only if potential benefit
  outweighs risk in severe impairment. ◈M◈

- **NATIONAL FUNDING/ACCESS DECISIONS**
  For full details see funding body website
  Scottish Medicines Consortium (SMC) decisions
  ▶ Formoterol fumarate dihydrate/glycopyrronium/budesonide
  (*Trixeo Aerosphere®*) for the maintenance treatment in adults
  with moderate to severe chronic obstructive pulmonary
  disease who are not adequately treated by a combination of
  an inhaled corticosteroid and a long-acting beta$_2$-agonist or
  combination of a long-acting beta$_2$-agonist and a long-acting
  muscarinic antagonist (February 2021) SMC No. SMC2321
  Recommended with restrictions

- **MEDICINAL FORMS** There can be variation in the licensing of
  different medicines containing the same drug.
  Pressurised inhalation
  CAUTIONARY AND ADVISORY LABELS 8, 10
  ▶ Formoterol fumarate with glycopyrronium and budesonide (Non-
    proprietary)
    Formoterol fumarate dihydrate 5 microgram per 1 dose,
    Glycopyrronium (as Glycopyrronium bromide) 7.2 microgram per
    1 dose, Budesonide 160 microgram per 1 dose Trixeo Aerosphere
    5micrograms/dose / 7.2micrograms/dose / 160micrograms/dose
    pressurised inhaler | 120 dose PoM £44.50

3 | Respiratory system

Mometasone furoate

☞ 292

08-Oct-2024

● **INDICATIONS AND DOSE**

Prophylaxis of asthma

▶ BY INHALATION OF POWDER

▶ Child 12–17 years: Initially 400 micrograms once daily, to be inhaled in the evening, alternatively initially 200 micrograms twice daily; reduced to 200 micrograms once daily, to be inhaled in the evening, dose to be reduced if control maintained

▶ Adult: Initially 400 micrograms once daily, to be inhaled in the evening, alternatively initially 200 micrograms twice daily; reduced to 200 micrograms once daily, to be inhaled in the evening, dose to be reduced if control maintained

Prophylaxis of severe asthma

▶ BY INHALATION OF POWDER

▶ Child 12–17 years: Initially 400 micrograms twice daily, reduce to the lowest effective dose when control achieved

▶ Adult: Initially 400 micrograms twice daily, reduce to the lowest effective dose when control achieved

● INTERACTIONS → Appendix 1: corticosteroids

● **SIDE-EFFECTS**

▶ **Common or very common** Candida infection

● **PRESCRIBING AND DISPENSING INFORMATION** For choice of therapy, see Asthma, acute p. 274 and Asthma, chronic p. 271.

● **PATIENT AND CARER ADVICE** Patients or carers should be given advice on how to administer mometasone by inhaler. Medicines for Children leaflet: Mometasone furoate inhaler for asthma prevention (prophylaxis) www.medicinesforchildren.org. uk/medicines/mometasone-furoate-inhaler-for-asthma-prevention-prophylaxis/

● **NATIONAL FUNDING/ACCESS DECISIONS**

For full details see funding body website

Scottish Medicines Consortium (SMC) decisions

▶ Mometasone furoate (*Asmanex® Twisthaler®*) for asthma (November 2003) SMC No. 79/03 Recommended with restrictions

● **MEDICINAL FORMS** There can be variation in the licensing of different medicines containing the same drug.

Inhalation powder

CAUTIONARY AND ADVISORY LABELS 8, 10

▶ Asmanex Twisthaler (Organon Pharma (UK) Ltd)

Mometasone furoate 200 microgram per 1 dose Asmanex 200micrograms/dose Twisthaler | 30 dose PoM £15.70 DT = £15.70 | 60 dose PoM £23.54 DT = £23.54

Mometasone furoate 400 microgram per 1 dose Asmanex 400micrograms/dose Twisthaler | 30 dose PoM £21.78 DT = £21.78 | 60 dose PoM £36.05 DT = £36.05

☞ 285

Mometasone furoate with glycopyrronium bromide and indacaterol

19-Jul-2022

The properties listed below are those particular to the combination only. For the properties of the components please consider, mometasone furoate above, glycopyrronium bromide p. 281.

● **INDICATIONS AND DOSE**

Prophylaxis of asthma

▶ BY INHALATION OF POWDER

▶ Adult: 1 inhalation once daily

● **INTERACTIONS** → Appendix 1: beta₂ agonists · corticosteroids · glycopyrronium

● **SIDE-EFFECTS**

▶ **Common or very common** Asthma exacerbated · cough · cystitis · dysphonia · fever · gastrointestinal disorders · hypersensitivity · increased risk of infection · muscle complaints · odynophagia · oropharyngeal complaints · pain · skin reactions · tension headache · throat complaints

▶ **Uncommon** Cataract · dry mouth · dysuria · eye pruritus · genital pruritus

● **PREGNANCY** EvGr Use only if potential benefit outweighs risk—limited information available. Ⓜ

● **BREAST FEEDING** EvGr Avoid—present in milk in *animal* studies. Ⓜ

● **HEPATIC IMPAIRMENT** EvGr Avoid in severe impairment unless potential benefit outweighs risk (limited information available). Ⓜ

● **RENAL IMPAIRMENT** EvGr Use with caution in severe impairment or end-stage renal disease—limited information available. Ⓜ

● **PATIENT AND CARER ADVICE** EvGr Patients and carers should be given advice on appropriate inhaler technique and reminded that the capsules are not for oral administration. Ⓜ

● **NATIONAL FUNDING/ACCESS DECISIONS**

For full details see funding body website

Scottish Medicines Consortium (SMC) decisions

▶ Indacaterol/glycopyrronium/mometasone furoate (*Enerzair Breezhaler®*) for the maintenance treatment of asthma in adult patients not adequately controlled with a maintenance combination of a long-acting beta₂-agonist and a high dose of an inhaled corticosteroid, who experienced one or more asthma exacerbations in the previous year (May 2021) SMC No. SMC2355 Recommended

All Wales Medicines Strategy Group (AWMSG) decisions

▶ Indacaterol/glycopyrronium/mometasone (*Enerzair Breezhaler®*) for the maintenance treatment of asthma in adult patients not adequately controlled with a maintenance combination of a long-acting beta₂-agonist and a high dose of an inhaled corticosteroid, who experienced one or more asthma exacerbations in the previous year (May 2021) AWMSG No. 3141 Recommended

● **MEDICINAL FORMS** There can be variation in the licensing of different medicines containing the same drug.

Inhalation powder

▶ Enerzair Breezhaler (Novartis Pharmaceuticals UK Ltd)

Glycopyrronium (as Glycopyrronium bromide) 46 microgram per 1 dose, Indacaterol (as Indacaterol acetate) 114 microgram per 1 dose, Mometasone furoate 136 microgram per 1 dose Enerzair Breezhaler 114micrograms/dose / 46micrograms/dose / 136micrograms/dose inhalation powder capsules with device | 30 capsule PoM £44.50

ENZYME INHIBITORS

Human alpha₁-proteinase inhibitor

05-Oct-2021

● **DRUG ACTION** Human alpha₁-proteinase inhibitor is a normal plasma constituent; it inhibits neutrophil elastase (an enzyme released in response to inflammation) in the lungs.

● **INDICATIONS AND DOSE**

Progression of emphysema in patients with severe alpha₁-proteinase inhibitor deficiency, despite optimal treatment with other standard therapies (specialist use only)

▶ BY INTRAVENOUS INFUSION

▶ Adult: 60 mg/kg once weekly

- **CONTRA-INDICATIONS** IgA deficiency with confirmed antibodies against IgA—increased risk of severe hypersensitivity reactions
- **CAUTIONS** Consider vaccination against hepatitis A and hepatitis B · hypersensitivity reactions · IgA deficiency (without known antibodies to IgA)—increased risk of hypersensitivity reactions

  CAUTIONS, FURTHER INFORMATION
  ▸ Hypersensitivity reactions Hypersensitivity reactions may occur, even in patients who have previously tolerated treatment. Manufacturer advises close monitoring, including vital signs, during the first infusions. If a reaction occurs, manufacturer advises to decrease the rate of infusion or discontinue treatment; if symptoms improve promptly after stopping, the infusion may be resumed at a slower infusion rate.

- **SIDE-EFFECTS**
  ▸ **Common or very common** Dizziness · headache · nausea
  ▸ **Uncommon** Asthenia · confusion · flushing · hypersensitivity · hypotension · sensation abnormal · skin reactions · syncope · tachycardia · throat oedema
  ▸ **Rare or very rare** Chest pain · chills · fever · hyperhidrosis
  ▸ **Frequency not known** Eye swelling · facial swelling · lip swelling · lymph node pain

- **PREGNANCY** Manufacturer advises caution—no information available.

- **BREAST FEEDING** Manufacturer advises avoid—no information available.

- **PRESCRIBING AND DISPENSING INFORMATION** Manufacturer advises to record the brand name and batch number after each administration (in case of transmission of infective agents).

- **PATIENT AND CARER ADVICE** Manufacturer advises patients receiving treatment at home should receive appropriate training regarding self-administration, and be informed of the signs of hypersensitivity reactions.
  Driving and skilled tasks Manufacturer advises patients and carers should be counselled on the effects on driving and performance of skilled tasks—increased risk of dizziness.

- **NATIONAL FUNDING/ACCESS DECISIONS**
  For full details see funding body website
  Scottish Medicines Consortium (SMC) decisions
  ▸ **Human alpha1-proteinase inhibitor (*Respreeza*®) for maintenance treatment, to slow the progression of emphysema in adults with documented severe alpha1-proteinase inhibitor (A1-PI) deficiency (August 2016)** SMC No. 1157/16 Not recommended
  All Wales Medicines Strategy Group (AWMSG) decisions
  ▸ **Human alpha1-proteinase inhibitor (*Respreeza*®) for maintenance treatment, to slow the progression of emphysema in adults with documented severe alpha1-proteinase inhibitor deficiency (March 2017)** AWMSG No. 47 Not recommended

- **MEDICINAL FORMS** There can be variation in the licensing of different medicines containing the same drug.
  Powder and solvent for solution for infusion
  ELECTROLYTES: May contain Sodium
  ▸ **Respreeza** (CSL Behring UK Ltd)
  Human alpha1-proteinase inhibitor 1 gram Respreeza 1000mg powder and solvent for solution for infusion vials | 1 vial [PoM] £220.00 (Hospital only)

IMMUNOSUPPRESSANTS › MONOCLONAL ANTIBODIES

Benralizumab
05-May-2021

- **DRUG ACTION** Benralizumab is a humanised monoclonal antibody that interferes with interleukin-5 receptor binding, thereby reducing the survival of eosinophils and basophils.

- **INDICATIONS AND DOSE**
  Severe eosinophilic asthma (specialist use only)
  ▸ BY SUBCUTANEOUS INJECTION
  ▸ Adult: Initially 30 mg every 4 weeks for the first 3 doses, then maintenance 30 mg every 8 weeks, to be administered into the thigh, abdomen or upper arm

  PHARMACOKINETICS
  ▸ The half-life of benralizumab is approx. 15 days.

- **CAUTIONS** Pre-existing helminth infection
  CAUTIONS, FURTHER INFORMATION
  ▸ Helminth infection Manufacturer advises to treat pre-existing helminth infections before starting benralizumab—if patient becomes infected during therapy and does not respond to anti-helminth treatment, discontinue benralizumab until infection is resolved.

- **SIDE-EFFECTS**
  ▸ **Common or very common** Fever · headache · hypersensitivity (may be delayed) · increased risk of infection · skin reactions
  ▸ **Frequency not known** Anaphylactic reaction

- **PREGNANCY** Manufacturer advises avoid unless potential benefit outweighs risk—limited data available.

- **BREAST FEEDING** Manufacturer advises avoid—no information available.

- **DIRECTIONS FOR ADMINISTRATION** Manufacturer advises to take the syringe out of the refrigerator at least 30 minutes before administration, and to avoid injecting into areas of the skin that are tender, bruised, erythematous, or hardened—consult product literature for further information.

- **PRESCRIBING AND DISPENSING INFORMATION** For choice of therapy, see Asthma, acute p. 274 and Asthma, chronic p. 271.

- **HANDLING AND STORAGE** Manufacturer advises store in a refrigerator (2–8°C) and protect from light.

- **PATIENT AND CARER ADVICE** Manufacturer advises patients and their carers should be instructed to seek medical advice if their asthma remains uncontrolled or if symptoms worsen after initiation of treatment.

- **NATIONAL FUNDING/ACCESS DECISIONS**
  For full details see funding body website
  NICE decisions
  ▸ **Benralizumab for treating severe eosinophilic asthma (updated September 2019)** NICE TA565 Recommended with restrictions
  Scottish Medicines Consortium (SMC) decisions
  ▸ **Benralizumab (*Fasenra*®) as add-on maintenance treatment in adult patients with severe eosinophilic asthma inadequately controlled despite high-dose inhaled corticosteroids plus long-acting beta-agonists (June 2019)** SMC No. SMC2155 Recommended with restrictions

- **MEDICINAL FORMS** There can be variation in the licensing of different medicines containing the same drug.
  Solution for injection
  ▸ **Fasenra** (AstraZeneca UK Ltd)
  Benralizumab 30 mg per 1 ml Fasenra 30mg/1ml solution for injection pre-filled pens | 1 pre-filled disposable injection [PoM] £1,955.00

Mepolizumab

05-May-2021

- **DRUG ACTION** Mepolizumab is a humanised anti-interleukin-5 (anti-IL-5) monoclonal antibody; it reduces the production and survival of eosinophils.

- **INDICATIONS AND DOSE**

Add on treatment for severe refractory eosinophilic asthma (under expert supervision)
  - ▸ BY SUBCUTANEOUS INJECTION
  - ▸ Adult: 100 mg every 4 weeks

- **CAUTIONS** Helminth infection

  CAUTIONS, FURTHER INFORMATION
  - ▸ Helminth infections Manufacturer advises pre-existing helminth infections should be treated before initiation of therapy; if patients become infected during treatment and do not respond to anti-helminth treatment, consider treatment interruption.

- **SIDE-EFFECTS**
  - ▸ **Common or very common** Abdominal pain upper · administration related reaction · back pain · fever · headache · hypersensitivity · increased risk of infection · nasal congestion · skin reactions
  - ▸ **Frequency not known** Angioedema

- **PREGNANCY** Manufacturer advises avoid unless potential benefit outweighs risk—limited data available.

- **BREAST FEEDING** Manufacturer advises avoid—present in milk in *animal* studies.

- **DIRECTIONS FOR ADMINISTRATION** Manufacturer advises injection is given into the thigh, abdomen, or upper arm. Patients may self-administer *Nucala*® pre-filled devices into the thigh or abdomen after appropriate training in preparation and administration.

- **PRESCRIBING AND DISPENSING INFORMATION** Mepolizumab is a biological medicine. Biological medicines must be prescribed and dispensed by brand name, see *Biological medicines* and *Biosimilar medicines*, under Guidance on prescribing p. 1; record the brand name and batch number after each administration.
  For choice of therapy, see Asthma, acute p. 274 and Asthma, chronic p. 271.

- **PATIENT AND CARER ADVICE** Patients and their carers should be advised to seek medical advice if their asthma remains uncontrolled or worsens after initiation of treatment.

- **NATIONAL FUNDING/ACCESS DECISIONS**
  For full details see funding body website
  NICE decisions
  - ▸ Mepolizumab for treating severe eosinophilic asthma (February 2021) NICE TA671 Recommended with restrictions
  Scottish Medicines Consortium (SMC) decisions
  - ▸ Mepolizumab (*Nucala*®) as an add-on treatment for severe refractory eosinophilic asthma in adult patients (June 2016) SMC No. 1149/16 Recommended with restrictions

- **MEDICINAL FORMS** There can be variation in the licensing of different medicines containing the same drug.
  Solution for injection
  EXCIPIENTS: May contain Edetic acid (edta), polysorbates
  - ▸ Nucala (GlaxoSmithKline UK Ltd)
    Mepolizumab 100 mg per 1 ml Nucala 100mg/1ml solution for injection pre-filled pens | 1 pre-filled disposable injection [PoM] £840.00
    Nucala 40mg/0.4ml solution for injection pre-filled syringes | 1 pre-filled disposable injection [PoM] £336.00 (Hospital only)
    Nucala 100mg/1ml solution for injection pre-filled syringes | 1 pre-filled disposable injection [PoM] £840.00

Omalizumab

17-May-2021

- **INDICATIONS AND DOSE**

Prophylaxis of severe persistent allergic asthma
  - ▸ BY SUBCUTANEOUS INJECTION
  - ▸ Adult: Dose according to immunoglobulin E concentration and body-weight (consult product literature)

Add-on therapy for chronic spontaneous urticaria in patients who have had an inadequate response to H₁ antihistamine treatment
  - ▸ BY SUBCUTANEOUS INJECTION
  - ▸ Adult: 300 mg every 4 weeks

- **CAUTIONS** Autoimmune disease · susceptibility to helminth infection—discontinue if infection does not respond to anthelmintic

- **SIDE-EFFECTS**
  - ▸ **Common or very common** Headache · skin reactions
  - ▸ **Uncommon** Cough · diarrhoea · dizziness · drowsiness · dyspepsia · fatigue · flushing · increased risk of infection · influenza like illness · limb swelling · nausea · paraesthesia · photosensitivity reaction · postural hypotension · respiratory disorders · syncope · weight increased
  - ▸ **Rare or very rare** Angioedema · hypersensitivity · systemic lupus erythematosus (SLE)
  - ▸ **Frequency not known** Alopecia · eosinophilic granulomatosis with polyangiitis · immune thrombocytopenic purpura · joint disorders · lymphadenopathy · myalgia

  SIDE-EFFECTS, FURTHER INFORMATION **Eosinophilic granulomatosis with polyangiitis (Churg-Strauss syndrome)** Churg-Strauss syndrome has occurred rarely in patients given omalizumab; the reaction is usually associated with the reduction of oral corticosteroid therapy. Churg-Strauss syndrome can present as eosinophilia, vasculitic rash, cardiac complications, worsening pulmonary symptoms, or peripheral neuropathy.
  Hypersensitivity reactions Hypersensitivity reactions can also occur immediately following treatment with omalizumab or sometimes more than 24 hours after the first injection.

- **PREGNANCY** Manufacturer advises avoid unless essential—crosses the placenta.

- **BREAST FEEDING** Manufacturer advises avoid—present in milk in *animal* studies.

- **HEPATIC IMPAIRMENT** Manufacturer advises caution (no information available).

- **RENAL IMPAIRMENT** Manufacturer advises caution—no information available.

- **PRESCRIBING AND DISPENSING INFORMATION** Omalizumab is a biological medicine. Biological medicines must be prescribed and dispensed by brand name, see *Biological medicines* and *Biosimilar medicines*, under Guidance on prescribing p. 1; record the brand name and batch number after each administration.
  - ▸ When used for Asthma For choice of therapy, see Asthma, acute p. 274 and Asthma, chronic p. 271.

- **NATIONAL FUNDING/ACCESS DECISIONS**
  For full details see funding body website
  NICE decisions
  - ▸ Omalizumab for severe persistent allergic asthma (April 2013) NICE TA278 Recommended
  - ▸ Omalizumab for previously treated chronic spontaneous urticaria (June 2015) NICE TA339 Recommended with restrictions
  Scottish Medicines Consortium (SMC) decisions
  - ▸ Omalizumab (*Xolair*®) as add-on therapy for the treatment of chronic spontaneous urticaria in adult and adolescent

(12 years and above) patients with inadequate response to H₁-antihistamine treatment (January 2015) SMC No. 1017/14 Recommended with restrictions

● **MEDICINAL FORMS** There can be variation in the licensing of different medicines containing the same drug.

Solution for injection

▸ Xolair (Novartis Pharmaceuticals UK Ltd)
Omalizumab 150 mg per 1 ml Xolair 300mg/2ml solution for injection pre-filled pens | 1 pre-filled disposable injection [PoM] £512.30 (Hospital only)
Xolair 150mg/1ml solution for injection pre-filled syringes | 1 pre-filled disposable injection [PoM] £256.15 DT = £256.15
Xolair 75mg/0.5ml solution for injection pre-filled pens | 1 pre-filled disposable injection [PoM] £128.07 (Hospital only)
Xolair 150mg/1ml solution for injection pre-filled pens | 1 pre-filled disposable injection [PoM] £256.15 (Hospital only)
Xolair 300mg/2ml solution for injection pre-filled syringes | 1 pre-filled disposable injection [PoM] £512.30 (Hospital only)
Xolair 75mg/0.5ml solution for injection pre-filled syringes | 1 pre-filled disposable injection [PoM] £128.07 DT = £128.07

Reslizumab
05-May-2021

● **DRUG ACTION** Reslizumab is a humanised monoclonal antibody that interferes with interleukin-5 receptor binding, thereby reducing the survival and activity of eosinophils.

● **INDICATIONS AND DOSE**

Severe eosinophilic asthma (adjunctive therapy when inadequately controlled by high-dose corticosteroids plus another standard treatment) (specialist use only)
▸ BY INTRAVENOUS INFUSION
▸ Adult: (consult product literature)

PHARMACOKINETICS
▸ The half-life of reslizumab is approx. 24 days.

● **CAUTIONS** Hypersensitivity reactions · pre-existing helminth infection

CAUTIONS, FURTHER INFORMATION
▸ Helminth infection Manufacturer advises to treat pre-existing helminth infections before starting reslizumab—consider temporarily discontinuing reslizumab if patient becomes infected during therapy and does not respond to anti-helminth treatment.
▸ Hypersensitivity reactions Serious hypersensitivity reactions, including life-threatening anaphylaxis, can occur and manufacturer advises to monitor closely during treatment and for at least 20 minutes after completion of infusion; in the event of a hypersensitivity reaction, treatment should be permanently discontinued.

● **SIDE-EFFECTS**
▸ **Uncommon** Anaphylactic reaction · myalgia
▸ **Frequency not known** Secondary malignancy

● **PREGNANCY** Manufacturer advises avoid—limited information available.

● **BREAST FEEDING** Manufacturer advises avoid during first few days after birth—risk of transfer of antibodies to infant cannot be excluded; present in milk in *animal* studies.

● **DIRECTIONS FOR ADMINISTRATION** For *intravenous infusion*, manufacturer advises give intermittently in Sodium Chloride 0.9%; administer over 20–50 minutes through an in-line 0.2 micron filter.

● **PRESCRIBING AND DISPENSING INFORMATION** Reslizumab is a biological medicine. Biological medicines must be prescribed and dispensed by brand name, see *Biological medicines* and *Biosimilar medicines*, under Guidance on prescribing p. 1; record the brand name and batch number after each administration.
For choice of therapy, see Asthma, acute p. 274 and Asthma, chronic p. 271.

● **HANDLING AND STORAGE** Manufacturer advises store in a refrigerator (2–8°C); consult product literature for storage conditions after preparation of infusion.

● **PATIENT AND CARER ADVICE** Manufacturer advises patients and their carers should be instructed to seek medical advice if their asthma remains uncontrolled or if symptoms worsen after initiation of treatment.

● **NATIONAL FUNDING/ACCESS DECISIONS**
For full details see funding body website

NICE decisions
▸ **Reslizumab for treating severe eosinophilic asthma (October 2017) NICE TA479** Recommended with restrictions

Scottish Medicines Consortium (SMC) decisions
▸ **Reslizumab (*Cinqaero*®) as add-on therapy in adult patients with severe eosinophilic asthma inadequately controlled despite high-dose inhaled corticosteroids plus another medicinal product for maintenance treatment (December 2017) SMC No. 1233/17** Not recommended

● **MEDICINAL FORMS** There can be variation in the licensing of different medicines containing the same drug.

Solution for infusion
EXCIPIENTS: May contain Sucrose

▸ Cinqaero (Teva UK Ltd)
Reslizumab 10 mg per 1 ml Cinqaero 100mg/10ml concentrate for solution for infusion vials | 1 vial [PoM] £499.99 (Hospital only)
Cinqaero 25mg/2.5ml concentrate for solution for infusion vials | 1 vial [PoM] £124.99 (Hospital only)

Tezepelumab
21-Aug-2023

● **DRUG ACTION** Tezepelumab is a monoclonal antibody that interferes with thymic stromal lymphopoietin (TSLP) binding, thereby reducing the production of inflammatory biomarkers and cytokines.

● **INDICATIONS AND DOSE**

Severe asthma [add-on maintenance therapy] (initiated by a specialist)
▸ BY SUBCUTANEOUS INJECTION
▸ Adult: 210 mg every 4 weeks

PHARMACOKINETICS
▸ The half-life of tezepelumab is approx. 26 days.

● **CAUTIONS** Helminth infections · serious infections
CAUTIONS, FURTHER INFORMATION
▸ Infections [EvGr] Pre-existing helminth infections and serious infections should be treated before starting tezepelumab. During tezepelumab therapy, if a helminth infection develops and does not respond to anti-helminth treatment, or a serious infection develops, discontinue tezepelumab until the infection is resolved. Ⓜ

● **INTERACTIONS** → Appendix 1: monoclonal antibodies

● **SIDE-EFFECTS**
▸ **Common or very common** Arthralgia · increased risk of infection · skin reactions
▸ **Frequency not known** Hypersensitivity

● **PREGNANCY** [EvGr] Avoid unless potential benefit outweighs risk—limited information available. Ⓜ

● **BREAST FEEDING** [EvGr] Avoid during first few days after birth—risk of transfer to infant cannot be excluded; present in milk in *animal* studies. Ⓜ

● **DIRECTIONS FOR ADMINISTRATION** [EvGr] Inject into the thigh or abdomen (except for the 5 cm around the navel), or upper arm (if not self-administered); rotate injection site and avoid skin that is tender, bruised, erythematous, or hardened. Ⓜ Patients may self-administer *Tezspire*® after appropriate training in preparation and administration.

● **PRESCRIBING AND DISPENSING INFORMATION** Tezepelumab is a biological medicine. Biological medicines must be prescribed and dispensed by brand name, see *Biological medicines* and *Biosimilar medicines*, under Guidance on prescribing p. 1; record the brand name and batch number after each administration.

For choice of therapy, see Asthma, acute p. 274 and Asthma, chronic p. 271.

● **HANDLING AND STORAGE** Store in a refrigerator (2–8°C) and protect from light; may be kept at room temperature (max. 25°C) for max. 30 days.

● **PATIENT AND CARER ADVICE** Patients and their carers should be instructed to seek medical advice if their asthma remains uncontrolled or worsens after initiation of treatment. Patients and their carers should be advised of the signs and symptoms of a cardiac event and to seek immediate medical attention if they occur.
Self-administration Patients or their carers should be given training in subcutaneous injection technique.

A patient leaflet and user manual should be provided.

● **NATIONAL FUNDING/ACCESS DECISIONS**
For full details see funding body website
NICE decisions
▶ **Tezepelumab for treating severe asthma (April 2023)**
NICE TA880 Recommended with restrictions
Scottish Medicines Consortium (SMC) decisions
▶ **Tezepelumab (*Tezspire*®) as add-on maintenance treatment in adults and adolescents 12 years and older with severe asthma who are inadequately controlled despite high dose inhaled corticosteroids plus another medicinal product for maintenance treatment (August 2023)** SMC No. SMC2541 Recommended with restrictions

● **MEDICINAL FORMS** There can be variation in the licensing of different medicines containing the same drug.
Solution for injection
EXCIPIENTS: May contain L-proline, polysorbates
▶ Tezspire (AstraZeneca UK Ltd) ▼
Tezepelumab 110 mg per 1 ml Tezspire 210mg/1.91ml solution for injection pre-filled pens | 1 pre-filled disposable injection PoM £1,265.00 (Hospital only)
Tezspire 210mg/1.91ml solution for injection pre-filled syringes | 1 pre-filled disposable injection PoM £1,265.00 (Hospital only)

LEUKOTRIENE RECEPTOR ANTAGONISTS

Montelukast

02-May-2024

● **INDICATIONS AND DOSE**
Prophylaxis of asthma
▶ BY MOUTH
▸ Child 6 months–5 years: 4 mg once daily, dose to be taken in the evening
▸ Child 6-14 years: 5 mg once daily, dose to be taken in the evening
▸ Child 15-17 years: 10 mg once daily, dose to be taken in the evening
▸ Adult: 10 mg once daily, dose to be taken in the evening

Symptomatic relief of seasonal allergic rhinitis in patients with asthma
▶ BY MOUTH
▸ Child 15-17 years: 10 mg once daily, dose to be taken in the evening
▸ Adult: 10 mg once daily, dose to be taken in the evening

IMPORTANT SAFETY INFORMATION
MHRA/CHM ADVICE: MONTELUKAST (*SINGULAIR*®): REMINDER OF THE RISK OF NEUROPSYCHIATRIC REACTIONS (SEPTEMBER 2019)
Healthcare professionals are advised to be alert for neuropsychiatric reactions, including speech impairment and obsessive-compulsive symptoms, in adults, adolescents, and children taking montelukast. Patients should be advised to read the list of neuropsychiatric reactions in the information leaflet and seek immediate medical attention if they occur.

For further details, see: www.gov.uk/drug-safety-update/montelukast-singulair-reminder-of-the-risk-of-neuropsychiatric-reactions.

MHRA/CHM ADVICE: MONTELUKAST: REMINDER OF THE RISK OF NEUROPSYCHIATRIC REACTIONS (APRIL 2024)
Following a review of the available evidence, warnings about the risk of neuropsychiatric reactions associated with montelukast have been strengthened and highlighted in product literature to increase awareness. Such reactions include new or worsening changes in mood, sleep, or behaviour (e.g. nightmares, aggression, anxiety, depression, or thoughts of self-injury), and have been reported in adults, adolescents, and children. In addition to advice issued in 2019, healthcare professionals are advised to discontinue montelukast in patients who develop new or worsening neuropsychiatric symptoms.

The MHRA has produced videos to support this advice—guidance for healthcare professionals is available at: www.youtube.com/watch?v=rpFog4QNf4k and guidance for patients, parents, and carers is available at: www.youtube.com/watch?v=e5hv96JGjtw.

For further details, see: www.gov.uk/drug-safety-update/montelukast-reminder-of-the-risk-of-neuropsychiatric-reactions.

● **INTERACTIONS** → Appendix 1: montelukast

● **SIDE-EFFECTS**
▶ **Common or very common** Diarrhoea · fever · gastrointestinal discomfort · headache · nausea · skin reactions · upper respiratory tract infection · vomiting
▶ **Uncommon** Akathisia · anxiety · arthralgia · asthenia · behaviour abnormal · depression · dizziness · drowsiness · dry mouth · haemorrhage · malaise · mood altered · muscle complaints · oedema · seizure · sensation abnormal · sleep disorders
▶ **Rare or very rare** Angioedema · concentration impaired · disorientation · eosinophilic granulomatosis with polyangiitis · erythema nodosum · hallucination · hepatic disorders · memory impairment · palpitations · psychiatric disorders · pulmonary eosinophilia · speech disorder · suicidal behaviours · tremor

SIDE-EFFECTS, FURTHER INFORMATION Eosinophilic granulomatosis with polyangiitis (Churg-Strauss syndrome) has occurred very rarely in association with the use of montelukast; in many of the reported cases the reaction followed the reduction or withdrawal of oral corticosteroid therapy. Prescribers should be alert to the development of eosinophilia, vasculitic rash, worsening pulmonary symptoms, cardiac complications, or peripheral neuropathy.

● **PREGNANCY** Manufacturer advises avoid unless essential. There is limited evidence for the safe use of montelukast during pregnancy; however, it can be taken as normal in women who have shown a significant improvement in asthma not achievable with other drugs before becoming pregnant.

● **BREAST FEEDING** Manufacturer advises avoid unless essential.

● **DIRECTIONS FOR ADMINISTRATION** Manufacturer advises granules may be swallowed or mixed with cold, soft food (not liquid) and taken immediately.

● **PRESCRIBING AND DISPENSING INFORMATION** Flavours of chewable tablet formulations may include cherry.
▶ When used for Asthma For choice of therapy, see Asthma, acute p. 274 and Asthma, chronic p. 271.

● **PATIENT AND CARER ADVICE**
Administration Patients or carers should be given advice on how to administer montelukast granules.
Risk of neuropsychiatric reactions Patients and carers should be advised to seek medical attention if changes in behaviour occur—see also *Important safety information*.
Medicines for Children leaflet: Montelukast for asthma
www.medicinesforchildren.org.uk/medicines/montelukast-for-asthma/

● **MEDICINAL FORMS** There can be variation in the licensing of different medicines containing the same drug.

Oral tablet
▸ Montelukast (Non-proprietary)
Montelukast (as Montelukast sodium) 10 mg Montelukast 10mg tablets | 28 tablet PoM £32.36 DT = £1.20
▸ Singulair (Organon Pharma (UK) Ltd)
Montelukast (as Montelukast sodium) 10 mg Singulair 10mg tablets | 28 tablet PoM £26.97 DT = £1.20

Oral granules
▸ Montelukast (Non-proprietary)
Montelukast (as Montelukast sodium) 4 mg Montelukast 4mg granules sachets sugar free | 28 sachet PoM £6.33–£10.00 DT = £6.67 SF
▸ Singulair (Organon Pharma (UK) Ltd)
Montelukast (as Montelukast sodium) 4 mg Singulair Paediatric 4mg granules sachets | 28 sachet PoM £25.69 DT = £6.67 SF

Chewable tablet
CAUTIONARY AND ADVISORY LABELS 23, 24
EXCIPIENTS: May contain Aspartame
▸ Montelukast (Non-proprietary)
Montelukast (as Montelukast sodium) 4 mg Montelukast 4mg chewable tablets sugar free | 28 tablet PoM £30.83 DT = £0.94 SF
Montelukast (as Montelukast sodium) 5 mg Montelukast 5mg chewable tablets sugar free | 28 tablet PoM £30.83 DT = £1.09 SF
▸ Singulair (Organon Pharma (UK) Ltd)
Montelukast (as Montelukast sodium) 4 mg Singulair Paediatric 4mg chewable tablets | 28 tablet PoM £25.69 DT = £0.94 SF
Montelukast (as Montelukast sodium) 5 mg Singulair Paediatric 5mg chewable tablets | 28 tablet PoM £25.69 DT = £1.09 SF

PHOSPHODIESTERASE TYPE-4 INHIBITORS

Roflumilast
14-Jul-2022

● **DRUG ACTION** Roflumilast is a phosphodiesterase type-4 inhibitor with anti-inflammatory properties.

● **INDICATIONS AND DOSE**

Adjunct to bronchodilators for the maintenance treatment of patients with severe chronic obstructive pulmonary disease associated with chronic bronchitis and a history of frequent exacerbations
▸ BY MOUTH
▸ Adult: Initially 250 micrograms once daily for 28 days, then maintenance 500 micrograms once daily

● **CONTRA-INDICATIONS** Cancer (except basal cell carcinoma) · concomitant treatment with immunosuppressive drugs (except short-term systemic corticosteroids) · history of depression associated with suicidal ideation or behaviour · moderate to severe cardiac failure · severe acute infectious disease · severe immunological disease

● **CAUTIONS** History of psychiatric illness (discontinue if new or worsening psychiatric symptoms occur) · latent infection (such as tuberculosis, viral hepatitis, herpes infection)

● **INTERACTIONS** → Appendix 1: phosphodiesterase type-4 inhibitors

● **SIDE-EFFECTS**
▸ **Common or very common** Appetite decreased · diarrhoea · gastrointestinal discomfort · headache · insomnia · nausea · weight decreased
▸ **Uncommon** Anxiety · asthenia · back pain · dizziness · gastrointestinal disorders · malaise · muscle complaints ·

muscle weakness · palpitations · skin reactions · tremor · vertigo · vomiting
▸ **Rare or very rare** Angioedema · constipation · depression · gynaecomastia · haematochezia · respiratory tract infection · suicidal behaviours · taste altered

● **CONCEPTION AND CONTRACEPTION** Women of child-bearing age should use effective contraception.

● **PREGNANCY** Manufacturer advises avoid—toxicity in *animal* studies.

● **BREAST FEEDING** Manufacturer advises avoid—present in milk in *animal* studies.

● **HEPATIC IMPAIRMENT** Manufacturer advises caution in mild impairment; avoid in moderate to severe impairment.

● **MONITORING REQUIREMENTS** Monitor body-weight.

● **PATIENT AND CARER ADVICE** Patients and carers should be instructed to report changes in behaviour or mood and any suicidal ideation. Patients should be advised to check their body-weight on a regular basis and seek medical advice in the event of an unexplained weight decrease.

● **NATIONAL FUNDING/ACCESS DECISIONS**
For full details see funding body website
NICE decisions
▸ **Roflumilast for treating chronic obstructive pulmonary disease (July 2017)** NICE TA461 Recommended with restrictions

Scottish Medicines Consortium (SMC) decisions
▸ **Roflumilast (*Daxas*®) for the maintenance treatment of severe chronic obstructive pulmonary disease (COPD) (forced expiratory volume in one second [FEV1]) post-bronchodilator less than 50% predicted) associated with chronic bronchitis in adult patients with a history of frequent exacerbations as add on to bronchodilator treatment (September 2017)** SMC No. 635/10 Not recommended

● **MEDICINAL FORMS** There can be variation in the licensing of different medicines containing the same drug.
Oral tablet
▸ Roflumilast (Non-proprietary)
Roflumilast 500 microgram Roflumilast 500microgram tablets | 30 tablet PoM £37.71 DT = £37.71
▸ Daxas (AstraZeneca UK Ltd)
Roflumilast 250 microgram Daxas 250microgram tablets | 28 tablet PoM £35.20 DT = £35.20
Roflumilast 500 microgram Daxas 500microgram tablets | 30 tablet PoM £37.71 DT = £37.71

SYMPATHOMIMETICS ❭ VASOCONSTRICTOR

Ephedrine hydrochloride
29-Mar-2022

● **INDICATIONS AND DOSE**

Reversal of hypotension from spinal or epidural anaesthesia
▸ BY SLOW INTRAVENOUS INJECTION
▸ Adult: 3–7.5 mg every 3–4 minutes (max. per dose 9 mg), adjusted according to response; maximum 30 mg per course

Reversible airways obstruction
▸ BY MOUTH
▸ Adult: 15–60 mg 3 times a day

Neuropathic oedema
▸ BY MOUTH
▸ Adult: 30–60 mg 3 times a day

● **UNLICENSED USE** Not licensed for neuropathic oedema.

● **CAUTIONS**

GENERAL CAUTIONS Diabetes mellitus · elderly · hypertension · hyperthyroidism · ischaemic heart disease · prostatic hypertrophy (risk of acute urinary retention)

SPECIFIC CAUTIONS
▶ With intravenous use Susceptibility to angle-closure glaucoma
● INTERACTIONS → Appendix 1: sympathomimetics, vasoconstrictor
● SIDE-EFFECTS
GENERAL SIDE-EFFECTS
▶ **Common or very common** Anxiety · headache · insomnia · nausea
▶ **Frequency not known** Tremor
SPECIFIC SIDE-EFFECTS
▶ **Common or very common**
▶ With intravenous use Arrhythmias · asthenia · confusion · depression · dyspnoea · hyperhidrosis · irritability · palpitations · vomiting
▶ **Rare or very rare**
▶ With intravenous use Acute urinary retention
▶ With oral use Myocardial infarction
▶ **Frequency not known**
▶ With intravenous use Acute angle closure glaucoma · angina pectoris · appetite decreased · cardiac arrest · dizziness · hypokalaemia · intracranial haemorrhage · psychotic disorder · pulmonary oedema
▶ With oral use Arrhythmias · circulation impaired · dry mouth · enuresis · hypertension · sedation
● PREGNANCY
▶ With oral use Manufacturer advises avoid.
▶ With intravenous use Increased fetal heart rate reported with parenteral ephedrine.
● BREAST FEEDING Present in milk; manufacturer advises avoid—irritability and disturbed sleep reported.
● RENAL IMPAIRMENT
▶ With oral use EvGr Use with caution. M
● LESS SUITABLE FOR PRESCRIBING
▶ With oral use Ephedrine tablets are less suitable and less safe for use as a bronchodilator than the selective beta₂ agonists.
● EXCEPTIONS TO LEGAL CATEGORY
▶ With oral use For exceptions relating to ephedrine tablets see *Medicines, Ethics and Practice*, London, Pharmaceutical Press (always consult latest edition).

● MEDICINAL FORMS There can be variation in the licensing of different medicines containing the same drug. Forms available from special-order manufacturers include: oral suspension, oral solution, solution for injection
Oral tablet
▶ Ephedrine hydrochloride (Non-proprietary)
Ephedrine hydrochloride 15 mg Ephedrine hydrochloride 15mg tablets | 28 tablet PoM £150.24 DT = £125.00
Ephedrine hydrochloride 30 mg Ephedrine hydrochloride 30mg tablets | 28 tablet PoM £227.68 DT = £180.00
Solution for injection
▶ Ephedrine hydrochloride (Non-proprietary)
Ephedrine hydrochloride 3 mg per 1 ml Ephedrine 30mg/10ml solution for injection ampoules | 10 ampoule PoM £124.09–£175.22
Ephedrine 30mg/10ml solution for injection pre-filled syringes | 1 pre-filled disposable injection PoM £9.50 DT = £9.50 | 10 pre-filled disposable injection PoM £95.00
Ephedrine hydrochloride 30 mg per 1 ml Ephedrine 30mg/1ml solution for injection ampoules | 10 ampoule PoM £172.76–£326.00

XANTHINES

Aminophylline

03-Aug-2023

● **INDICATIONS AND DOSE**
Severe acute asthma in patients not previously treated with theophylline
▶ BY SLOW INTRAVENOUS INJECTION
▶ Child: 5 mg/kg (max. per dose 500 mg), to be followed by intravenous infusion
▶ Adult: 250–500 mg (max. per dose 5 mg/kg), to be followed by intravenous infusion
Severe acute asthma
▶ BY INTRAVENOUS INFUSION
▶ Child 1 month-11 years: 1 mg/kg/hour, adjusted according to plasma-theophylline concentration
▶ Child 12-17 years: 500–700 micrograms/kg/hour, adjusted according to plasma-theophylline concentration
▶ Adult: 500–700 micrograms/kg/hour, adjusted according to plasma-theophylline concentration
▶ Elderly: 300 micrograms/kg/hour, adjusted according to plasma-theophylline concentration
Severe acute exacerbation of chronic obstructive pulmonary disease in patients not previously treated with theophylline
▶ BY SLOW INTRAVENOUS INJECTION
▶ Adult: 250–500 mg (max. per dose 5 mg/kg), to be followed by intravenous infusion
Severe acute exacerbation of chronic obstructive pulmonary disease
▶ BY INTRAVENOUS INFUSION
▶ Adult: 500–700 micrograms/kg/hour, adjusted according to plasma-theophylline concentration
▶ Elderly: 300 micrograms/kg/hour, adjusted according to plasma-theophylline concentration
DOSE ADJUSTMENTS DUE TO INTERACTIONS
▶ Dose adjustment may be necessary if smoking started or stopped during treatment.
DOSES AT EXTREMES OF BODY-WEIGHT
▶ To avoid excessive dosage in obese patients, dose should be calculated on the basis of ideal weight for height.
PHARMACOKINETICS
▶ Aminophylline is a stable mixture or combination of theophylline and ethylenediamine; the ethylenediamine confers greater solubility in water.
▶ Theophylline is metabolised in the liver. The plasma-theophylline concentration is increased in heart failure, hepatic impairment, and in viral infections. The plasma-theophylline concentration is decreased in smokers, and by alcohol consumption. Differences in the half-life of aminophylline are important because the toxic dose is close to the therapeutic dose.

● UNLICENSED USE Aminophylline injection not licensed for use in children under 6 months.
● CAUTIONS Arrhythmias following rapid intravenous injection · cardiac arrhythmias or other cardiac disease · elderly (increased plasma-theophylline concentration) · epilepsy · fever · hypertension · peptic ulcer · risk of hypokalaemia · thyroid disorder
● INTERACTIONS → Appendix 1: aminophylline
● SIDE-EFFECTS Abdominal pain · anxiety · arrhythmia (more common when given too rapidly by intravenous injection) · confusion · delirium · diarrhoea · dizziness · electrolyte imbalance · gastrointestinal haemorrhage · gastrooesophageal reflux disease · headache · hyperthermia · hyperventilation · hypotension (more common when given too rapidly by intravenous injection) ·

insomnia · mania · metabolic disorder · nausea · pain · palpitations · seizure (more common when given too rapidly by intravenous injection) · skin reactions · tachycardia (more common when given too rapidly by intravenous injection) · thirst · tremor · vertigo · visual impairment · vomiting

● SIDE-EFFECTS, FURTHER INFORMATION Potentially serious hypokalaemia may result from beta$_2$-agonist therapy. Particular caution is required in severe asthma, because this effect may be potentiated by concomitant treatment with theophylline and its derivatives, corticosteroids, and diuretics, and by hypoxia. Plasma-potassium concentration should therefore be monitored in severe asthma.

Overdose Theophylline and related drugs in overdose can cause vomiting (which may be severe and intractable), agitation, restlessness, dilated pupils, sinus tachycardia, and hyperglycaemia. More serious effects are haematemesis, convulsions, and supraventricular and ventricular arrhythmias. Severe hypokalaemia may develop rapidly.

For specific details on the management of poisoning, see *Theophylline*, under Emergency treatment of poisoning p. 1554.

● ALLERGY AND CROSS-SENSITIVITY Allergy to ethylenediamine can cause urticaria, erythema, and exfoliative dermatitis.

● PREGNANCY Neonatal irritability and apnoea have been reported. Theophylline can be taken as normal during pregnancy as it is particularly important that asthma should be well controlled during pregnancy.

● BREAST FEEDING Present in milk—irritability in infant reported. Theophylline can be taken as normal during breast-feeding.

● HEPATIC IMPAIRMENT Manufacturer advises caution (risk of reduced clearance).
Dose adjustments Manufacturer advises maintenance dose reduction—consult product literature.

● MONITORING REQUIREMENTS
▸ Aminophylline is monitored therapeutically in terms of plasma-theophylline concentrations; a blood sample should be taken 4–6 hours after starting treatment.
▸ Measurement of plasma-theophylline concentration may be helpful and is **essential** if a loading dose of intravenous aminophylline is to be given to patients who are already taking theophylline, because serious side-effects such as convulsions and arrhythmias can occasionally precede other symptoms of toxicity.
▸ In most individuals, a plasma-theophylline concentration of 10–20 mg/litre (55–110 micromol/litre) is required for satisfactory bronchodilation, although a lower plasma-theophylline concentration of 5–15 mg/litre may be effective. Adverse effects can occur within the range 10–20 mg/litre and both the frequency and severity increase at concentrations above 20 mg/litre.

● DIRECTIONS FOR ADMINISTRATION For *intravenous injection*, manufacturer advises give **very slowly** over at least 20 minutes (with close monitoring).
▸ In children For *intravenous infusion*, expert sources advise dilute to a concentration of 1 mg/mL with Glucose 5% *or* Sodium Chloride 0.9%.
▸ In adults For *intravenous infusion*, manufacturer advises give continuously in Glucose 5% *or* Sodium Chloride 0.9%.

● PRESCRIBING AND DISPENSING INFORMATION Patients taking oral theophylline should not normally receive a loading dose of intravenous aminophylline.
▸ When used for Asthma For choice of therapy, see Asthma, acute p. 274 and Asthma, chronic p. 271. Consider intravenous aminophylline for treatment of severe and life-threatening acute asthma only after consultation with senior medical staff.

● MEDICINAL FORMS There can be variation in the licensing of different medicines containing the same drug. Forms available from special-order manufacturers include: solution for infusion
Solution for injection
▸ Aminophylline (Non-proprietary)
   Aminophylline 25 mg per 1 ml Aminophylline 250mg/10ml solution for injection ampoules | 10 ampoule PoM £13.50–£15.00 DT = £15.00

Theophylline
15-Apr-2024

● INDICATIONS AND DOSE
UNIPHYLLIN CONTINUS ®
Chronic asthma
▸ BY MOUTH USING MODIFIED-RELEASE MEDICINES
▸ Child 2-11 years: 9 mg/kg every 12 hours (max. per dose 200 mg), dose may be increased in some children with chronic asthma; increased to 10–16 mg/kg every 12 hours (max. per dose 400 mg), may be appropriate to give larger evening or morning dose to achieve optimum therapeutic effect when symptoms most severe; in patients whose night or daytime symptoms persist despite other therapy, who are not currently receiving theophylline, total daily requirement may be added as single evening or morning dose
▸ Child 12-17 years: 200 mg every 12 hours, adjusted according to response to 400 mg every 12 hours, may be appropriate to give larger evening or morning dose to achieve optimum therapeutic effect when symptoms most severe; in patients whose night or daytime symptoms persist despite other therapy, who are not currently receiving theophylline, total daily requirement may be added as single evening or morning dose

Reversible airways obstruction | Severe acute asthma | Chronic asthma
▸ BY MOUTH USING MODIFIED-RELEASE MEDICINES
▸ Adult: 200 mg every 12 hours, adjusted according to response to 400 mg every 12 hours, may be appropriate to give larger evening or morning dose to achieve optimum therapeutic effect when symptoms most severe; in patients whose night or daytime symptoms persist despite other therapy, who are not currently receiving theophylline, total daily requirement may be added as single evening or morning dose

DOSE ADJUSTMENTS DUE TO INTERACTIONS
▸ Dose adjustment may be necessary if smoking started or stopped during treatment.

PHARMACOKINETICS
▸ Theophylline is metabolised in the liver. The plasma-theophylline concentration is increased in heart failure, hepatic impairment, and in viral infections. The plasma-theophylline concentration is decreased in smokers, and by alcohol consumption. Differences in the half-life of theophylline are important because the toxic dose is close to the therapeutic dose.

● CAUTIONS Cardiac arrhythmias or other cardiac disease · elderly (increased plasma-theophylline concentration) · epilepsy · fever · hypertension · peptic ulcer · risk of hypokalaemia · thyroid disorder
CAUTIONS, FURTHER INFORMATION
▸ Elderly Screening Tool of Older Persons' potentially inappropriate Prescriptions (STOPP) criteria to aid medication reviews (see Prescribing in the elderly p. 31 for information): potentially inappropriate as monotherapy for COPD (safer and more effective alternatives available; risk of adverse effects due to narrow therapeutic index).

● INTERACTIONS → Appendix 1: theophylline

● SIDE-EFFECTS Anxiety · arrhythmias · diarrhoea · dizziness · gastrointestinal discomfort · gastrooesophageal reflux disease · headache · hyperuricaemia · nausea · palpitations · seizure · skin reactions · sleep disorders · tremor · urinary disorders · vomiting

SIDE-EFFECTS, FURTHER INFORMATION Potentially serious hypokalaemia may result from beta$_2$-agonist therapy. Particular caution is required in severe asthma, because this effect may be potentiated by concomitant treatment with theophylline and its derivatives, corticosteroids, and diuretics, and by hypoxia. Plasma-potassium concentration should therefore be monitored in severe asthma.

Overdose Theophylline in overdose can cause vomiting (which may be severe and intractable), agitation, restlessness, dilated pupils, sinus tachycardia, and hyperglycaemia. More serious effects are haematemesis, convulsions, and supraventricular and ventricular arrhythmias. Severe hypokalaemia may develop rapidly.

For details on the management of poisoning, see Theophylline, under Emergency treatment of poisoning p. 1554.

● **PREGNANCY** Neonatal irritability and apnoea have been reported. Theophylline can be taken as normal during pregnancy as it is particularly important that asthma should be well controlled during pregnancy.

● **BREAST FEEDING** Present in milk—irritability in infant reported; modified-release preparations preferable. Theophylline can be taken as normal during breast-feeding.

● **HEPATIC IMPAIRMENT** Manufacturer advises caution (risk of increased exposure).
Dose adjustments Manufacturer advises consider dose reduction.

● **MONITORING REQUIREMENTS**
▶ In most individuals, a plasma-theophylline concentration of 10–20 mg/litre (55–110 micromol/litre) is required for satisfactory bronchodilation, although a lower plasma-theophylline concentration of 5–15 mg/litre may be effective. Adverse effects can occur within the range 10–20 mg/litre and both the frequency and severity increase at concentrations above 20 mg/litre.
▶ Plasma-theophylline concentration is measured 5 days after starting oral treatment and at least 3 days after any dose adjustment. A blood sample should usually be taken 4–6 hours after an oral dose of a modified-release preparation (sampling times may vary—consult local guidelines).

● **PRESCRIBING AND DISPENSING INFORMATION**
▶ When used for Asthma For choice of therapy, see Asthma, acute p. 274 and Asthma, chronic p. 271.

The rate of absorption from modified-release preparations can vary between brands. If a prescription for a modified-release oral theophylline preparation does not specify a brand name, the pharmacist should contact the prescriber and agree the brand to be dispensed. Additionally, it is essential that a patient discharged from hospital should be maintained on the brand on which that patient was stabilised as an in-patient.

● **MEDICINAL FORMS** There can be variation in the licensing of different medicines containing the same drug.
Modified-release tablet
CAUTIONARY AND ADVISORY LABELS 25
▶ Uniphyllin Continus (Ennogen Healthcare International Ltd)
Theophylline 200 mg Uniphyllin Continus 200mg tablets | 56 tablet [P] £29.80 DT = £29.80
Theophylline 300 mg Uniphyllin Continus 300mg tablets | 56 tablet [P] £29.80 DT = £29.80
Theophylline 400 mg Uniphyllin Continus 400mg tablets | 56 tablet [P] £29.80 DT = £29.80

Nebuliser solutions

● **HYPERTONIC SODIUM CHLORIDE SOLUTIONS**
MUCOCLEAR® 3%

● **INDICATIONS AND DOSE**

Mobilise lower respiratory tract secretions in mucous consolidation (e.g. cystic fibrosis) | Mild to moderate acute viral bronchiolitis in infants
▶ BY INHALATION OF NEBULISED SOLUTION
▶ Adult: 4 mL 2–4 times a day, temporary irritation, such as coughing, hoarseness, or reversible bronchoconstriction may occur; an inhaled bronchodilator can be used before treatment with hypertonic sodium chloride to reduce the risk of these adverse effects

MucoClear 3% inhalation solution 4ml ampoules (Pari Medical Ltd) **Sodium chloride 30 mg per 1 ml** 20 ampoule · NHS indicative price = £12.98 · Drug Tariff (Part IXa)60 ampoule · NHS indicative price = £27.00 · Drug Tariff (Part IXa)

MUCOCLEAR® 6%

● **INDICATIONS AND DOSE**

Mobilise lower respiratory tract secretions in mucous consolidation (e.g. cystic fibrosis)
▶ BY INHALATION OF NEBULISED SOLUTION
▶ Adult: 4 mL twice daily, temporary irritation, such as coughing, hoarseness, or reversible bronchoconstriction may occur; an inhaled bronchodilator can be used before treatment with hypertonic sodium chloride to reduce the risk of these adverse effects

MucoClear 6% inhalation solution 4ml ampoules (Pari Medical Ltd) **Sodium chloride 60 mg per 1 ml** 20 ampoule · NHS indicative price = £12.98 · Drug Tariff (Part IXa)60 ampoule · NHS indicative price = £27.00 · Drug Tariff (Part IXa)

NEBUSAL®

● **INDICATIONS AND DOSE**

Mobilise lower respiratory tract secretions in mucous consolidation (e.g. cystic fibrosis)
▶ BY INHALATION OF NEBULISED SOLUTION
▶ Adult: 4 mL up to twice daily, temporary irritation, such as coughing, hoarseness, or reversible bronchoconstriction may occur; an inhaled bronchodilator can be used before treatment with hypertonic sodium chloride to reduce the risk of these adverse effects

Nebusal 7% inhalation solution 4ml vials (Accord-UK Ltd) **Sodium chloride 70 mg per 1 ml** 60 vial · NHS indicative price = £27.00 · Drug Tariff (Part IXa)

PULMOCLEAR®

● **INDICATIONS AND DOSE**

Mobilise lower respiratory tract secretions and prevent drying of bronchial mucous.
▶ BY INHALATION OF NEBULISED SOLUTION
▶ Adult: (consult product literature)

PulmoClear 6% inhalation solution 4ml vials (TriOn Pharma Ltd) 60 vial · NHS indicative price = £16.59 · Drug Tariff (Part IXa)

PulmoClear 3% inhalation solution 4ml vials (TriOn Pharma Ltd) **Sodium chloride 30 mg per 1 ml** 60 vial · NHS indicative price = £16.47 · Drug Tariff (Part IXa)

PulmoClear 7% inhalation solution 4ml vials (TriOn Pharma Ltd) **Sodium chloride 70 mg per 1 ml** 60 vial · NHS indicative price = £16.59 · Drug Tariff (Part IXa)

RESP-EASE®

● **INDICATIONS AND DOSE**

Mobilise lower respiratory tract secretions and prevent drying of bronchial mucous.

▶ BY INHALATION OF NEBULISED SOLUTION

▸ Adult: (consult product literature)

Resp-Ease 3% inhalation solution 4ml ampoules (Venture Healthcare Ltd) **Sodium chloride 30 mg per 1 ml** 60 ampoule · NHS indicative price = £21.60 · Drug Tariff (Part IXa)

Resp-Ease 6% inhalation solution 4ml ampoules (Venture Healthcare Ltd) **Sodium chloride 60 mg per 1 ml** 60 ampoule · NHS indicative price = £21.60 · Drug Tariff (Part IXa)

Resp-Ease 7% inhalation solution 4ml vials (Venture Healthcare Ltd) **Sodium chloride 70 mg per 1 ml** 60 vial · NHS indicative price = £21.60 · Drug Tariff (Part IXa)

Peak flow meters: low range

● LOW RANGE PEAK FLOW METERS

MEDI® LOW RANGE

Range 40–420 litres/minute.
Compliant to standard EN ISO 23747:2007 except for scale range.

Medi peak flow meter low range (Medicareplus International Ltd)
1 device · NHS indicative price = £6.50 · Drug Tariff (Part IXa) price = £4.50

MINI-WRIGHT® LOW RANGE

Range 30–400 litres/minute.
Compliant to standard EN ISO 23747:2007 except for scale range.

Mini-Wright peak flow meter low range (Clement Clarke International Ltd)
1 device · NHS indicative price = £7.23 · Drug Tariff (Part IXa) price = £4.50

POCKETPEAK® LOW RANGE

Range 50–400 litres/minute.
Compliant to standard EN ISO 23747:2007 except for scale range.

nSpire Pocket Peak peak flow meter low range (nSpire Health Ltd)
1 device · NHS indicative price = £6.53 · Drug Tariff (Part IXa) price = £4.50

Peak flow meters: standard range

● STANDARD RANGE PEAK FLOW METERS

AIRZONE®

Range 60–720 litres/minute.
Conforms to standard EN ISO 23747:2007.

AirZone peak flow meter standard range (Clement Clarke International Ltd)
1 device · NHS indicative price = £4.76 · Drug Tariff (Part IXa) price = £4.25

MEDI® STANDARD RANGE

Range 60–800 litres/minute.
Conforms to standard EN ISO 23747:2007.

Medi peak flow meter standard range (Medicareplus International Ltd)
1 device · NHS indicative price = £4.50 · Drug Tariff (Part IXa) price = £4.25

MICROPEAK®

Range 60–900 litres/minute.
Conforms to standard EN ISO 23747:2007.

MicroPeak peak flow meter standard range (Micro Medical Ltd)
1 device · NHS indicative price = £6.50 · Drug Tariff (Part IXa) price = £4.25

MINI-WRIGHT® STANDARD RANGE

Range 60–800 litres/minute.
Conforms to standard EN ISO 23747:2007.

Mini-Wright peak flow meter standard range (Clement Clarke International Ltd)
1 device · NHS indicative price = £7.18 · Drug Tariff (Part IXa) price = £4.25

PIKO-1®

Range 15–999 litres/minute.
Conforms to standard EN ISO 23747:2007.

nSpire PiKo-1 peak flow meter standard range (nSpire Health Ltd)
1 device · NHS indicative price = £9.50 · Drug Tariff (Part IXa) price = £4.25

PINNACLE®

Range 60–900 litres/minute.
Conforms to standard EN ISO 23747:2007.

Fyne Dynamics Pinnacle peak flow meter standard range (Fyne Dynamics Ltd)
1 device · NHS indicative price = £6.50 · Drug Tariff (Part IXa) price = £4.25

POCKETPEAK® STANDARD RANGE

Range 60–800 litres/minute.
Conforms to standard EN ISO 23747:2007.

nSpire Pocket Peak peak flow meter standard range (nSpire Health Ltd)
1 device · NHS indicative price = £6.53 · Drug Tariff (Part IXa) price = £4.25

VITALOGRAPH®

Range 50–800 litres/minute.
Conforms to standard EN ISO 23747:2007.

Vitalograph peak flow meter standard range (Vitalograph Ltd)
1 device · NHS indicative price = £4.83 · Drug Tariff (Part IXa) price = £4.25

Spacers

● SPACERS

A2A SPACER®

For use with all pressurised (aerosol) inhalers.

A2A Spacer (Clement Clarke International Ltd)
1 device · NHS indicative price = £4.15 · Drug Tariff (Part IXa)

A2A Spacer with medium mask (Clement Clarke International Ltd)
1 device · NHS indicative price = £6.68 · Drug Tariff (Part IXa)

A2A Spacer with small mask (Clement Clarke International Ltd)
1 device · NHS indicative price = £6.68 · Drug Tariff (Part IXa)

ABLE SPACER®

Small-volume device. For use with all pressurised (aerosol) inhalers.

Able Spacer 2 (Clement Clarke International Ltd)
1 device · NHS indicative price = £4.39 · Drug Tariff (Part IXa)

Able Spacer 2 with medium mask (Clement Clarke International Ltd)
1 device · NHS indicative price = £7.16 · Drug Tariff (Part IXa)

Able Spacer 2 with small mask (Clement Clarke International Ltd)
1 device · NHS indicative price = £7.16 · Drug Tariff (Part IXa)

AEROCHAMBER PLUS®

Medium-volume device. For use with all pressurised (aerosol) inhalers.

AeroChamber Plus (Trudell Medical UK Ltd)
1 device · NHS indicative price = £5.21 · Drug Tariff (Part IXa)

AeroChamber Plus with adult mask (Trudell Medical UK Ltd)
1 device · NHS indicative price = £8.69 · Drug Tariff (Part IXa)

AeroChamber Plus with child mask (Trudell Medical UK Ltd)
1 device · NHS indicative price = £8.69 · Drug Tariff (Part IXa)

AeroChamber Plus with infant mask (Trudell Medical UK Ltd)
1 device · NHS indicative price = £8.69 · Drug Tariff (Part IXa)

BABYHALER®

For paediatric use with *Flixotide*®, and *Ventolin*® inhalers.

● PRESCRIBING AND DISPENSING INFORMATION

Not available for NHS prescription.

Babyhaler (GlaxoSmithKline UK Ltd)
1 device · No NHS indicative price available · Drug Tariff (Part IXa)

EASYCHAMBER® SPACER

For use with all pressurised (aerosol) inhalers.

EasyChamber Spacer (TriOn Pharma Ltd)
1 device · NHS indicative price = £3.98 · Drug Tariff (Part IXa)

EasyChamber Spacer with adult mask 6 years - adult (TriOn Pharma Ltd)
1 device · NHS indicative price = £6.59 · Drug Tariff (Part IXa)

EasyChamber Spacer with child mask 2-6 years (TriOn Pharma Ltd)
1 device · NHS indicative price = £6.55 · Drug Tariff (Part IXa)

EasyChamber Spacer with infant mask 0-24 months (TriOn Pharma Ltd)
1 device · NHS indicative price = £6.53 · Drug Tariff (Part IXa)

OPTICHAMBER ®
For use with all pressurised (aerosol) inhalers.

OptiChamber (Respironics (UK) Ltd)
1 device · NHS indicative price = £4.28 · Drug Tariff (Part IXa)

OPTICHAMBER ® **DIAMOND**
For use with all pressurised (aerosol) inhalers.

OptiChamber Diamond (Respironics (UK) Ltd)
1 device · NHS indicative price = £4.49 · Drug Tariff (Part IXa)

OptiChamber Diamond with large LiteTouch mask 5 years-adult (Respironics (UK) Ltd)
1 device · NHS indicative price = £7.49 · Drug Tariff (Part IXa)

OptiChamber Diamond with medium LiteTouch mask 1-5 years (Respironics (UK) Ltd)
1 device · NHS indicative price = £7.49 · Drug Tariff (Part IXa)

OptiChamber Diamond with small LiteTouch mask 0-18 months (Respironics (UK) Ltd)
1 device · NHS indicative price = £7.49 · Drug Tariff (Part IXa)

POCKET CHAMBER ®
Small volume device. For use with all pressurised (aerosol) inhalers.

Pocket Chamber (nSpire Health Ltd)
1 device · NHS indicative price = £4.18 · Drug Tariff (Part IXa)

Pocket Chamber with adult mask (nSpire Health Ltd)
1 device · NHS indicative price = £9.75 · Drug Tariff (Part IXa)

Pocket Chamber with child mask (nSpire Health Ltd)
1 device · NHS indicative price = £9.75 · Drug Tariff (Part IXa)

Pocket Chamber with infant mask (nSpire Health Ltd)
1 device · NHS indicative price = £9.75 · Drug Tariff (Part IXa)

Pocket Chamber with teenager mask (nSpire Health Ltd)
1 device · NHS indicative price = £9.75 · Drug Tariff (Part IXa)

SPACE CHAMBER PLUS ®
For use with all pressurised (aerosol) inhalers.

Space Chamber Plus (Medical Developments International Ltd)
1 device · NHS indicative price = £4.34 · Drug Tariff (Part IXa)

Space Chamber Plus with large mask (Medical Developments International Ltd)
1 device · NHS indicative price = £7.10 · Drug Tariff (Part IXa)

Space Chamber Plus with medium mask (Medical Developments International Ltd)
1 device · NHS indicative price = £7.10 · Drug Tariff (Part IXa)

Space Chamber Plus with small mask (Medical Developments International Ltd)
1 device · NHS indicative price = £7.10 · Drug Tariff (Part IXa)

VOLUMATIC ®
Large-volume device. For use with *Clenil Modulite*®, *Flixotide*®, *Seretide*®, *Serevent*®, and *Ventolin*® inhalers.

Volumatic (GlaxoSmithKline UK Ltd)
1 device · NHS indicative price = £3.88 · Drug Tariff (Part IXa)

Volumatic with paediatric mask (GlaxoSmithKline UK Ltd)
1 device · NHS indicative price = £6.83 · Drug Tariff (Part IXa)

VORTEX ®
Medium-volume device. For use with all pressurised (aerosol) inhalers.

2　Allergic conditions

Antihistamines, allergen immunotherapy and allergic emergencies

02-Aug-2022

Antihistamines

All antihistamines are of potential value in the treatment of nasal allergies, particularly seasonal allergic rhinitis (hayfever), and they may be of some value in vasomotor rhinitis. They reduce rhinorrhoea and sneezing but are usually less effective for nasal congestion. Antihistamines are used topically in the eye, in the nose, and on the skin.

Oral antihistamines are also of some value in preventing urticaria and are used to treat urticarial rashes, pruritus, and insect bites and stings; they are also used in drug allergies. Antihistamines may also be given in anaphylaxis following initial stabilisation of the patient, especially in patients with persistent cutaneous symptoms—for further information, see *Anaphylaxis*.

Antihistamines (including cinnarizine p. 499, cyclizine p. 492, and promethazine teoclate p. 500) may also have a role in nausea and vomiting. Buclizine is included as an anti-emetic in a preparation for migraine. Antihistamines may also have a role in occasional insomnia.

All older antihistamines cause sedation but alimemazine tartrate p. 322 and **promethazine** may be more sedating whereas chlorphenamine maleate p. 323 and cyclizine may be less so. This sedating activity is sometimes used to manage the pruritus associated with some allergies. There is little evidence that any one of the older, 'sedating' antihistamines is superior to another and patients vary widely in their response.

Non-sedating antihistamines such as acrivastine p. 318, bilastine p. 319, cetirizine hydrochloride p. 319, desloratadine p. 319 (an active metabolite of loratadine p. 321), fexofenadine hydrochloride p. 320 (an active metabolite of terfenadine), levocetirizine hydrochloride p. 320 (an isomer of cetirizine hydrochloride), loratadine and mizolastine p. 321 cause less sedation and psychomotor impairment than the older antihistamines because they penetrate the blood brain barrier only to a slight extent.

Considerations in the elderly

The use of first-generation antihistamines in elderly patients is potentially inappropriate (STOPP criteria) as safer, less toxic antihistamines are widely available.

For further information, see *STOPP/START criteria* in Prescribing in the elderly p. 31.

Allergen immunotherapy

Immunotherapy using allergen vaccines containing house dust mite, animal dander (cat or dog), or grass pollen extract p. 327 and tree pollen extract p. 329 can reduce symptoms of asthma and allergic rhinoconjunctivitis. Vaccines containing wasp venom extract p. 330 or bee venom extract p. 327 may be used to reduce the risk of severe anaphylaxis and systemic reactions in individuals with hypersensitivity to wasp and bee stings. An oral preparation of grass pollen extract is licensed for disease-modifying treatment of grass pollen-induced rhinitis and conjunctivitis, and an oral preparation of house dust mite extract p. 328 is licensed for disease-modifying treatment of house dust mite allergic rhinitis or asthma in certain patients. EvGr Desensitisation treatment with peanut protein p. 328 may be offered to patients with peanut allergy in childhood, and treatment can be continued into adulthood. Ⓐ Those requiring immunotherapy must be referred to a hospital specialist for accurate diagnosis, assessment, and treatment.

Omalizumab p. 308 is a monoclonal antibody that binds to immunoglobulin E (IgE). It is used as additional therapy in individuals with proven IgE-mediated sensitivity to inhaled allergens, whose severe persistent allergic asthma cannot be controlled adequately with high dose inhaled corticosteroid together with a long-acting beta₂ agonist. Omalizumab should be initiated by physicians in specialist centres experienced in the treatment of severe persistent asthma. Omalizumab is also indicated as add-on therapy for the treatment of chronic spontaneous urticaria in patients who have had an inadequate response to H_1 antihistamine treatment.

Anaphylaxis and allergic emergencies

Anaphylaxis

Anaphylaxis is a severe, life-threatening, generalised or systemic hypersensitivity reaction. It is characterised by rapidly developing airway and/or breathing and/or circulation problems, and is usually associated with skin and mucosal changes; prompt treatment is required.

The most common allergens that cause anaphylaxis include food (e.g. peanuts, sesame, tree nuts, soy, shellfish, and cow's milk—see Food allergy p. 77), drugs (e.g. antibacterials, aspirin and other NSAIDs, neuromuscular blocking drugs, chlorhexidine, contrast media, and vaccines), venom (e.g. insect stings), and latex. In the case of drugs, anaphylaxis is more likely after parenteral administration; resuscitation facilities must always be available for injections associated with special risk. Anaphylactic reactions may also be associated with *additives and excipients* in foods and medicines. Refined arachis (peanut) oil, which may be present in some medicinal products, is unlikely to cause an allergic reaction— nevertheless it is wise to check the full formula of preparations which may contain allergens.

Certain patients may be at higher risk of anaphylaxis, either because of an existing comorbidity (such as asthma) or because of an increased likelihood of repeated exposure to the same allergen (such as those with venom or food allergies).

Recommendations on the management of anaphylaxis reflect the *Resuscitation Council (UK)—Emergency treatment of anaphylaxis: Guidelines for healthcare providers (May* 2021*)* and *NICE—Anaphylaxis: assessment and referral after emergency treatment guidelines (CG134, updated August* 2020).

Initial treatment of anaphylaxis

Cardiopulmonary arrest may follow an anaphylactic reaction—start cardiopulmonary resuscitation (CPR) immediately. For guidance on CPR, see Life support algorithm (image) Inside back cover.

[EvGr] Immediately call for an ambulance or the resuscitation team and begin initial treatment for anaphylaxis.

Remove the trigger causing the anaphylactic reaction if possible (e.g. stopping the suspected drug or removing the stinger after an insect sting). Place the patient in a comfortable position taking into account their presenting signs and symptoms—lay the patient flat (with or without legs raised) to aid in the restoration of blood pressure, or in a semi-recumbent position for patients with airway and breathing problems (and no evidence of cardiovascular instability) to make breathing easier, or in the recovery position for unconscious patients who are breathing normally; pregnant females should lie on their left side to prevent aortocaval compression.

Intramuscular adrenaline/epinephrine p. 256 should be given as first line treatment for anaphylaxis. If there is doubt about the diagnosis, give intramuscular adrenaline/epinephrine and seek expert advice. Adrenaline/epinephrine provides physiological reversal of the immediate symptoms associated with hypersensitivity reactions. Assess response to treatment by monitoring vital signs (such as blood pressure, pulse, respiratory function, and level of consciousness) and auscultate for wheeze.

A repeat dose of intramuscular adrenaline/epinephrine should be given after a 5-minute interval if there is no improvement in the patient's condition. Patients who have no improvement in respiratory and/or cardiovascular problems despite 2 appropriate doses of intramuscular adrenaline/epinephrine, should have their care escalated quickly and managed as having refractory anaphylaxis. Ⓐ For further information, see *Refractory anaphylaxis*.

[EvGr] Nebulised adrenaline/epinephrine may be effective as an adjunct to treat upper airways obstruction caused by laryngeal oedema, but only after treatment with intramuscular adrenaline/epinephrine and not as an alternative.

High-flow oxygen should be given as soon as it is available.

Intravenous fluids should be given to patients with hypotension/shock, or if there is poor response to an initial dose of adrenaline/epinephrine.

Antihistamines are not recommended as part of the initial emergency treatment of anaphylaxis. Following stabilisation of the patient, a non-sedating oral antihistamine such as cetirizine hydrochloride p. 319 (in preference to chlorphenamine maleate) may be considered, especially in patients with persistent cutaneous symptoms (urticaria and/or angioedema). If oral administration is not possible, intramuscular or intravenous chlorphenamine maleate p. 323 can be given.

The routine use of corticosteroids for the emergency treatment of anaphylaxis is not recommended. Consider corticosteroids after initial resuscitation for refractory reactions or ongoing asthma/shock; corticosteroids must not be given preferentially to adrenaline/epinephrine p. 256. Corticosteroids should be given via the oral route where possible.

Inhaled bronchodilator therapy with salbutamol p. 287 and/or ipratropium bromide p. 281 may also be considered for patients with persisting respiratory problems, but should not be used as an alternative to further treatment with adrenaline/epinephrine. Ⓐ For guidance on the management of bronchospasm in severe asthma, see Asthma, acute p. 274.

For further guidance on the initial management of anaphylaxis, see Resuscitation Council (UK) guideline: **Emergency treatment of anaphylaxis** (available at: www.resus.org.uk/library/additional-guidance/guidance-anaphylaxis/emergency-treatment).

Refractory anaphylaxis

Refractory anaphylaxis is defined as anaphylaxis that requires ongoing treatment due to persisting respiratory and/or cardiovascular problems despite 2 appropriate doses of intramuscular adrenaline/epinephrine—[EvGr] seek early critical care support.

Patients should be treated with an intravenous adrenaline/epinephrine infusion. Intravenous adrenaline/epinephrine should only be given by experienced specialists and in a setting where patients can be carefully monitored. If an intravenous infusion cannot be administered safely (e.g. due to a patient being outside a hospital setting), continue to give intramuscular adrenaline/epinephrine at 5-minute intervals while life-threatening cardiovascular and/or respiratory features persist. Adrenaline/epinephrine therapy should be supported with intravenous fluid therapy. Ⓐ For further guidance on the use of intravenous adrenaline/epinephrine and other treatment options in refractory anaphylaxis (such as nebulised adrenaline/epinephrine, bronchodilators, vasopressors, corticosteroids, and glucagon (in patients on beta-blockers)), see Resuscitation Council (UK) guideline: **Emergency treatment of anaphylaxis** (available at: www.resus.org.uk/library/additional-guidance/guidance-anaphylaxis/emergency-treatment).

Discharge and follow-up

[EvGr] Prior to discharge from hospital, patients (or their family or carers) should be provided with 2 adrenaline/epinephrine auto-injectors, trained on their correct use, and advised to carry these with them at all times. The provision of adrenaline/epinephrine auto-injectors are appropriate for all patients who have had anaphylaxis, with the exception of those with a drug-induced reaction (unless future exposure to the trigger drug will be difficult to avoid). Patients who are provided with auto-injectors should have appropriate follow-up including contact with their general practitioner.

Patients and their family or carers should also be provided with information about anaphylaxis, the risk of a biphasic reaction (with clear instructions to return to hospital if symptoms return), avoidance of suspected triggers, and what to do if an anaphylactic reaction occurs. An emergency management or action plan should be provided, and referral to a specialist allergy clinic made. Ⓐ

Angioedema

Allergic angioedema

Angioedema can be caused by an allergic reaction. It involves the swelling of deeper tissues, most commonly in the eyelids and lips, and sometimes the tongue and throat. Allergic angioedema that occurs with life-threatening airway and/or breathing and/or circulatory problems should be managed as **anaphylaxis**. For further guidance, see *Anaphylaxis*.

Hereditary angioedema

The treatment of hereditary angioedema should be under specialist supervision. Unlike allergic angioedema, adrenaline/epinephrine, corticosteroids, and antihistamines should not be used for the treatment of acute attacks (including attacks involving laryngeal oedema) as they are ineffective and may delay appropriate treatment—intubation may be necessary. The administration of C1-esterase inhibitor p. 331, an endogenous complement blocker derived from human plasma, (in fresh frozen plasma or in partially purified form) can terminate acute attacks of *hereditary angioedema*; it can also be used for short-term prophylaxis before dental, medical, or surgical procedures. Conestat alfa p. 331 and icatibant p. 333 are licensed for the treatment of acute attacks of hereditary angioedema in adults with C1-esterase inhibitor deficiency.

Tranexamic acid p. 127 and danazol [unlicensed indication] are used for short-term and long-term prophylaxis of hereditary angioedema. Short-term prophylaxis with tranexamic acid or danazol is started several days before planned procedures (e.g. dental work) and continued for 2–5 days afterwards. Danazol should be avoided in children because of its androgenic effects.

Lanadelumab p. 332 or berotralstat p. 332 may be an option for the prevention of recurrent attacks of hereditary angioedema. For guidance on their use, see NICE pathway: **Immune system conditions** (available at: pathways.nice.org. uk/pathways/blood-and-immune-system-conditions).

Dose of intramuscular injection of adrenaline (epinephrine) for the emergency treatment of anaphylaxis by healthcare professionals

Age	Dose	Volume of adrenaline
Child up to 6 months	100-150 micrograms	0.1-0.15 mL 1 in 1000 (1 mg/mL) adrenaline[1]
Child 6 months– 5 years	150 micrograms	0.15 mL 1 in 1000 (1 mg/mL) adrenaline[2]
Child 6-11 years	300 micrograms	0.3 mL 1 in 1000 (1 mg/mL) adrenaline
Child 12-17 years	500 micrograms	0.5 mL 1 in 1000 (1 mg/mL) adrenaline[3]
Adult	500 micrograms	0.5 mL 1 in 1000 (1 mg/mL) adrenaline

Repeat dose after 5 minutes if no response. If life-threatening features persist, further doses can be given every 5 minutes until specialist critical care available.

1. Use suitable syringe for measuring small volume
2. Use suitable syringe for measuring small volume
3. 300 micrograms (0.3 mL) if child is small or prepubertal

ANTIHISTAMINES > NON-SEDATING

Acrivastine

23-Apr-2021

● **INDICATIONS AND DOSE**

Symptomatic relief of allergy such as hayfever, chronic idiopathic urticaria

▶ BY MOUTH

▸ Child 12-17 years: 8 mg 3 times a day

▸ Adult: 8 mg 3 times a day

● **CONTRA-INDICATIONS** Avoid in Acute porphyrias p. 1202 · elderly

● **INTERACTIONS** → Appendix 1: antihistamines, non-sedating

● **SIDE-EFFECTS**

▸ **Common or very common** Drowsiness · dry mouth

▸ **Frequency not known** Dizziness · rash

SIDE-EFFECTS, FURTHER INFORMATION Non-sedating antihistamines such as acrivastine cause less sedation and psychomotor impairment than the older antihistamines, but can still occur; sedation is generally minimal. This is because non-sedating antihistamines penetrate the blood brain barrier to a much lesser extent.

● **ALLERGY AND CROSS-SENSITIVITY** [EvGr] Contra-indicated if history of hypersensitivity to triprolidine. Ⓜ

● **PREGNANCY** Most manufacturers of antihistamines advise avoiding their use during pregnancy; however, there is no evidence of teratogenicity.

● **BREAST FEEDING** Most antihistamines are present in breast milk in varying amounts; although not known to be harmful, most manufacturers advise avoiding their use in mothers who are breast-feeding.

● **RENAL IMPAIRMENT** [EvGr] Avoid in severe impairment. Ⓜ

● **PATIENT AND CARER ADVICE**

Driving and skilled tasks Patients and their carers should be advised that drowsiness can occur and may affect performance of skilled tasks (e.g. cycling or driving).

● **MEDICINAL FORMS** There can be variation in the licensing of different medicines containing the same drug.

Oral capsule

▸ Acrivastine (Non-proprietary)

Acrivastine 8 mg Acrivastine 8mg capsules | 24 capsule Ⓟ £4.45-£7.90

▸ **Benadryl Allergy Relief** (McNeil Products Ltd)
Acrivastine 8 mg Benadryl Allergy Relief 8mg capsules |
48 capsule P £11.23

Bilastine
14-Dec-2020

● INDICATIONS AND DOSE

Symptomatic relief of allergic rhinoconjunctivitis and urticaria
▸ BY MOUTH
▸ Child 12-17 years: 20 mg once daily
▸ Adult: 20 mg once daily

● **CONTRA-INDICATIONS** Avoid in Acute porphyrias p. 1202

● **INTERACTIONS** → Appendix 1: antihistamines, non-sedating

● **SIDE-EFFECTS**
▸ **Common or very common** Drowsiness · headache
▸ **Uncommon** Anxiety · appetite increased · asthenia · bundle branch block · diarrhoea · dry mouth · dyspnoea · fever · gastritis · gastrointestinal discomfort · insomnia · nasal complaints · nausea · oral herpes · pre-existing condition improved · pruritus · QT interval prolongation · sinus arrhythmia · thirst · tinnitus · vertigo · weight increased

SIDE-EFFECTS, FURTHER INFORMATION Non-sedating antihistamines such as bilastine cause less sedation and psychomotor impairment than the older antihistamines, but can still occur; sedation is generally minimal. This is because non-sedating antihistamines penetrate the blood brain barrier to a much lesser extent.

● **PREGNANCY** Avoid—limited information available. Most manufacturers of antihistamines advise avoiding their use during pregnancy; however, there is no evidence of teratogenicity.

● **BREAST FEEDING** Avoid—no information available. Most antihistamines are present in breast milk in varying amounts; although not known to be harmful, most manufacturers advise avoiding their use in mothers who are breast-feeding.

● **DIRECTIONS FOR ADMINISTRATION** Manufacturer advises tablet should be taken 1 hour before or 2 hours after food or fruit juice.

● **PATIENT AND CARER ADVICE** Patients or carers should be given advice on how to administer bilastine tablets.
Driving and skilled tasks Patients and their carers should be advised that drowsiness can occur and may affect performance of skilled tasks (e.g. cycling or driving).

● **MEDICINAL FORMS** There can be variation in the licensing of different medicines containing the same drug.
Oral tablet
CAUTIONARY AND ADVISORY LABELS 23
▸ **Ilaxten** (A. Menarini Farmaceutica Internazionale SRL)
Bilastine 20 mg Ilaxten 20mg tablets | 30 tablet PoM £6.00 DT = £6.00

Cetirizine hydrochloride
10-Nov-2021

● INDICATIONS AND DOSE

Symptomatic relief of allergy such as hay fever, chronic idiopathic urticaria, atopic dermatitis
▸ BY MOUTH
▸ Child 2-5 years: 2.5 mg twice daily
▸ Child 6-11 years: 5 mg twice daily
▸ Child 12-17 years: 10 mg once daily
▸ Adult: 10 mg once daily

● **CAUTIONS** Epilepsy

● **INTERACTIONS** → Appendix 1: antihistamines, non-sedating

● **SIDE-EFFECTS**
▸ **Uncommon** Agitation · asthenia · diarrhoea · malaise · paraesthesia · skin reactions
▸ **Rare or very rare** Aggression · angioedema · confusion · depression · hallucination · hepatic function abnormal · insomnia · movement disorders · oculogyration · oedema · seizure · syncope · tachycardia · taste altered · thrombocytopenia · tic · tremor · urinary disorders · vision disorders · weight increased
▸ **Frequency not known** Abdominal pain · appetite increased · dizziness · drowsiness · dry mouth · headache · memory loss · nausea · pharyngitis · suicidal ideation · vertigo

SIDE-EFFECTS, FURTHER INFORMATION Non-sedating antihistamines such as cetirizine hydrochloride cause less sedation and psychomotor impairment than the older antihistamines, but can still occur; sedation is generally minimal. This is because non-sedating antihistamines penetrate the blood brain barrier to a much lesser extent.

● **PREGNANCY** Most manufacturers of antihistamines advise avoiding their use during pregnancy; however, there is no evidence of teratogenicity.

● **BREAST FEEDING** Most antihistamines are present in breast milk in varying amounts; although not known to be harmful, most manufacturers advise avoiding their use in mothers who are breast-feeding.

● **RENAL IMPAIRMENT**
▸ In adults Avoid if eGFR less than 10 mL/minute/1.73 m^2.
▸ In children Avoid if estimated glomerular filtration rate less than 10 mL/minute/1.73 m^2.
Dose adjustments
▸ In adults Use half normal dose if eGFR 30–50 mL/minute/1.73 m^2. Use half normal dose and reduce dose frequency to alternate days if eGFR 10–30 mL/minute/1.73 m^2.
▸ In children Use half normal dose if estimated glomerular filtration rate 30–50 mL/minute/1.73 m^2. Use half normal dose and reduce dose frequency to alternate days if estimated glomerular filtration rate 10–30 mL/minute/1.73 m^2.

● **PATIENT AND CARER ADVICE**
Medicines for Children leaflet: Cetirizine for hayfever
www.medicinesforchildren.org.uk/medicines/cetirizine-for-hayfever/
Driving and skilled tasks Patients and their carers should be advised that drowsiness can occur and may affect performance of skilled tasks (e.g. cycling or driving).

● **PROFESSION SPECIFIC INFORMATION**
Dental practitioners' formulary Cetirizine Tablets 10 mg may be prescribed.
Cetirizine Oral Solution 5 mg/5 mL may be prescribed.

● **MEDICINAL FORMS** There can be variation in the licensing of different medicines containing the same drug.
Oral tablet
▸ **Cetirizine hydrochloride** (Non-proprietary)
Cetirizine hydrochloride 10 mg Cetirizine 10mg tablets | 30 tablet PoM £0.79–£0.92 DT = £0.79
Oral solution
EXCIPIENTS: May contain Propylene glycol
▸ **Cetirizine hydrochloride** (Non-proprietary)
Cetirizine hydrochloride 1 mg per 1 ml Cetirizine 1mg/ml oral solution sugar free | 200 ml PoM £18.27 DT = £16.51 SF

Desloratadine
23-Apr-2021

● INDICATIONS AND DOSE

Symptomatic relief of allergy such as allergic rhinitis, urticaria, chronic idiopathic urticaria
▸ BY MOUTH
▸ Child 1-5 years: 1.25 mg once daily

continued →

- Child 6-11 years: 2.5 mg once daily
- Child 12-17 years: 5 mg once daily
- Adult: 5 mg once daily

PHARMACOKINETICS
- Desloratadine is a metabolite of loratadine.

- **INTERACTIONS** → Appendix 1: antihistamines, non-sedating

- **SIDE-EFFECTS**
- **Common or very common** Asthenia · dry mouth · headache
- **Rare or very rare** Akathisia · arrhythmias · diarrhoea · dizziness · drowsiness · gastrointestinal discomfort · hallucination · hepatic disorders · insomnia · myalgia · nausea · palpitations · seizure · vomiting
- **Frequency not known** Behaviour abnormal · photosensitivity reaction · QT interval prolongation

  SIDE-EFFECTS, FURTHER INFORMATION Non-sedating antihistamines such as desloratadine cause less sedation and psychomotor impairment than the older antihistamines, but can still occur; sedation is generally minimal. This is because non-sedating antihistamines penetrate the blood brain barrier to a much lesser extent.

- **ALLERGY AND CROSS-SENSITIVITY** EvGr Contra-indicated if history of hypersensitivity to loratadine. Ⓜ

- **PREGNANCY** Most manufacturers of antihistamines advise avoiding their use during pregnancy; however, there is no evidence of teratogenicity.

- **BREAST FEEDING** Most antihistamines are present in breast milk in varying amounts; although not known to be harmful, most manufacturers advise avoiding their use in mothers who are breast-feeding.

- **RENAL IMPAIRMENT** EvGr Use with caution in severe impairment. Ⓜ

- **PRESCRIBING AND DISPENSING INFORMATION** Flavours of oral liquid formulations may include bubblegum.

- **PATIENT AND CARER ADVICE**
  Driving and skilled tasks Patients and their carers should be advised that drowsiness can occur and may affect performance of skilled tasks (e.g. cycling or driving).

- **MEDICINAL FORMS** There can be variation in the licensing of different medicines containing the same drug.
  Oral tablet
  - **Desloratadine (Non-proprietary)**
    Desloratadine 5 mg Desloratadine 5mg tablets | 30 tablet PoM £6.60 DT = £2.68
  - **Neoclarityn** (Organon Pharma (UK) Ltd)
    Desloratadine 5 mg Neoclarityn 5mg tablets | 30 tablet PoM £6.77 DT = £2.68

  Oral solution
  EXCIPIENTS: May contain Propylene glycol, sorbitol
  - **Desloratadine (Non-proprietary)**
    Desloratadine 500 microgram per 1 ml Desloratadine 2.5mg/5ml oral solution sugar free | 150 ml PoM £8.12 DT = £10.15 SF
  - **Neoclarityn** (Organon Pharma (UK) Ltd)
    Desloratadine 500 microgram per 1 ml Neoclarityn 2.5mg/5ml oral solution | 100 ml PoM £6.77 SF | 150 ml PoM £10.15 DT = £10.15 SF

Fexofenadine hydrochloride
14-Dec-2020

- **INDICATIONS AND DOSE**

Symptomatic relief of seasonal allergic rhinitis
- BY MOUTH
- Child 6-11 years: 30 mg twice daily
- Child 12-17 years: 120 mg once daily
- Adult: 120 mg once daily

Symptomatic relief of chronic idiopathic urticaria
- BY MOUTH
- Child 12-17 years: 180 mg once daily

- Adult: 180 mg once daily

PHARMACOKINETICS
- Fexofenadine is a metabolite of terfenadine.

- **INTERACTIONS** → Appendix 1: antihistamines, non-sedating

- **SIDE-EFFECTS**
- **Common or very common** Dizziness · drowsiness · headache · nausea
- **Uncommon** Fatigue
- **Frequency not known** Diarrhoea · nervousness · palpitations · skin reactions · sleep disorders · tachycardia

  SIDE-EFFECTS, FURTHER INFORMATION Non-sedating antihistamines such as fexofenadine cause less sedation and psychomotor impairment than the older antihistamines, but can still occur; sedation is generally minimal. This is because non-sedating antihistamines penetrate the blood brain barrier to a much lesser extent.

- **PREGNANCY** Most manufacturers of antihistamines advise avoiding their use during pregnancy; however, there is no evidence of teratogenicity.

- **BREAST FEEDING** Most antihistamines are present in breast milk in varying amounts; although not known to be harmful, most manufacturers advise avoiding their use in mothers who are breast-feeding.

- **PATIENT AND CARER ADVICE**
  Driving and skilled tasks Patients and their carers should be advised that drowsiness can occur and may affect performance of skilled tasks (e.g. cycling or driving).

- **MEDICINAL FORMS** There can be variation in the licensing of different medicines containing the same drug. Forms available from special-order manufacturers include: oral suspension, oral solution
  Oral tablet
  CAUTIONARY AND ADVISORY LABELS 5
  - **Fexofenadine hydrochloride (Non-proprietary)**
    Fexofenadine hydrochloride 120 mg Fexofenadine 120mg tablets | 30 tablet PoM £7.15 DT = £1.02
    Fexofenadine hydrochloride 180 mg Fexofenadine 180mg tablets | 30 tablet PoM £9.65 DT = £1.48
  - **Telfast** (Opella Healthcare UK Ltd)
    Fexofenadine hydrochloride 30 mg Telfast 30mg tablets | 60 tablet PoM £5.46 DT = £5.46
    Fexofenadine hydrochloride 180 mg Telfast 180mg tablets | 30 tablet PoM £7.58 DT = £1.48

Levocetirizine hydrochloride
14-Dec-2020

- **INDICATIONS AND DOSE**

Symptomatic relief of allergy such as hay fever, urticaria
- BY MOUTH
- Child 6-17 years: 5 mg once daily
- Adult: 5 mg once daily

PHARMACOKINETICS
- Levocetirizine is an isomer of cetirizine.

- **CONTRA-INDICATIONS** Avoid in Acute porphyrias p. 1202

- **INTERACTIONS** → Appendix 1: antihistamines, non-sedating

- **SIDE-EFFECTS**
- **Common or very common** Asthenia · constipation (in children) · drowsiness · dry mouth
- **Uncommon** Abdominal pain
- **Frequency not known** Aggression · agitation · angioedema · appetite increased · arthralgia · depression · diarrhoea (very common in children) · dizziness · dyspnoea · hallucination · hepatitis · myalgia · nausea · oedema · palpitations · paraesthesia · seizure · skin reactions · sleep disorders (very common in children) · suicidal ideation · syncope ·

tachycardia · taste altered · tremor · urinary disorders · vertigo · vision disorders · vomiting · weight increased

SIDE-EFFECTS, FURTHER INFORMATION Non-sedating antihistamines such as levocetirizine cause less sedation and psychomotor impairment than the older antihistamines, but can still occur; sedation is generally minimal. This is because non-sedating antihistamines penetrate the blood brain barrier to a much lesser extent.

- **PREGNANCY** Most manufacturers of antihistamines advise avoiding their use during pregnancy; however, there is no evidence of teratogenicity.
- **BREAST FEEDING** Most antihistamines are present in breast milk in varying amounts; although not known to be harmful, most manufacturers advise avoiding their use in mothers who are breast-feeding.
- **RENAL IMPAIRMENT**
  - In adults Avoid if eGFR less than 10 mL/minute/1.73 m^2.
  - In children Avoid if estimated glomerular filtration rate less than 10 mL/minute/1.73 m^2.
    Dose adjustments
    - In adults 5 mg on alternate days if eGFR 30–50 mL/minute/1.73 m^2. 5 mg every 3 days if eGFR 10–30 mL/minute/1.73 m^2.
    - In children Reduce dose frequency to alternate days if estimated glomerular filtration rate 30–50 mL/minute/1.73 m^2. Reduce dose frequency to every 3 days if estimated glomerular filtration rate 10–30 mL/minute/1.73 m^2.
- **PATIENT AND CARER ADVICE**
  Driving and skilled tasks Patients and their carers should be advised that drowsiness can occur and may affect performance of skilled tasks (e.g. cycling or driving).

- **MEDICINAL FORMS** There can be variation in the licensing of different medicines containing the same drug.
  Oral tablet
  - Levocetirizine hydrochloride (Non-proprietary)
    Levocetirizine dihydrochloride 5 mg Levocetirizine 5mg tablets | 30 tablet [PoM] £4.66 DT = £4.36
  - Xyzal (UCB Pharma Ltd)
    Levocetirizine dihydrochloride 5 mg Xyzal 5mg tablets | 30 tablet [PoM] £4.39 DT = £4.36
  Oral solution
  - Xyzal (UCB Pharma Ltd)
    Levocetirizine dihydrochloride 500 microgram per 1 ml Xyzal 0.5mg/ml oral solution | 200 ml [PoM] £6.00 DT = £6.00 [SF]

Loratadine
10-Nov-2021

- **INDICATIONS AND DOSE**
  Symptomatic relief of allergy such as hay fever, chronic idiopathic urticaria
  - BY MOUTH
  - Child 2–11 years (body-weight up to 31 kg): 5 mg once daily
  - Child 2–11 years (body-weight 31 kg and above): 10 mg once daily
  - Child 12–17 years: 10 mg once daily
  - Adult: 10 mg once daily

- **INTERACTIONS** → Appendix 1: antihistamines, non-sedating

- **SIDE-EFFECTS**
  - **Common or very common** Drowsiness · nervousness (in children)
  - **Uncommon** Appetite increased · headache (very common in children) · insomnia
  - **Rare or very rare** Alopecia · angioedema · dizziness · dry mouth · fatigue (very common in children) · gastritis · hepatic function abnormal · nausea · palpitations · rash · seizure · tachycardia

SIDE-EFFECTS, FURTHER INFORMATION Non-sedating antihistamines such as loratadine cause less sedation and psychomotor impairment than the older antihistamines, but can still occur; sedation is generally minimal. This is because non-sedating antihistamines penetrate the blood brain barrier to a much lesser extent.

- **PREGNANCY** Most manufacturers of antihistamines advise avoiding their use during pregnancy; however, there is no evidence of teratogenicity.
- **BREAST FEEDING** Most antihistamines are present in breast milk in varying amounts; although not known to be harmful, most manufacturers advise avoiding their use in mothers who are breast-feeding.
- **HEPATIC IMPAIRMENT** Manufacturer advises caution in severe impairment (risk of increased exposure).
  Dose adjustments Manufacturer advises initial dose reduction to alternate days in severe impairment.
- **PATIENT AND CARER ADVICE**
  Medicines for Children leaflet: Loratadine for allergy symptoms www.medicinesforchildren.org.uk/medicines/loratadine-for-allergy-symptoms/
  Driving and skilled tasks Patients and their carers should be advised that drowsiness can occur and may affect performance of skilled tasks (e.g. cycling or driving).
- **PROFESSION SPECIFIC INFORMATION**
  Dental practitioners' formulary Loratadine 10 mg tablets may be prescribed.
  Loratadine syrup 5 mg/5 mL may be prescribed.

- **MEDICINAL FORMS** There can be variation in the licensing of different medicines containing the same drug.
  Oral tablet
  - Loratadine (Non-proprietary)
    Loratadine 10 mg Loratadine 10mg tablets | 30 tablet [PoM] [Ẋ] DT = £0.70
  Oral solution
  EXCIPIENTS: May contain Propylene glycol
  - Loratadine (Non-proprietary)
    Loratadine 1 mg per 1 ml Loratadine 5mg/5ml oral solution | 100 ml [PoM] £2.54 DT = £2.54
    Loratadine 5mg/5ml oral solution sugar free | 100 ml [P] £3.78 DT = £3.78 [SF]

Mizolastine
14-Dec-2020

- **INDICATIONS AND DOSE**
  Symptomatic relief of allergy such as hay fever, urticaria
  - BY MOUTH
  - Child 12–17 years: 10 mg once daily
  - Adult: 10 mg once daily

- **CONTRA-INDICATIONS** Cardiac disease · susceptibility to QT-interval prolongation

- **INTERACTIONS** → Appendix 1: antihistamines, non-sedating

- **SIDE-EFFECTS**
  - **Common or very common** Appetite increased · asthenia · diarrhoea · dizziness · drowsiness · dry mouth · gastrointestinal discomfort · headache · nausea · weight increased
  - **Uncommon** Anxiety · arrhythmias · arthralgia · depression · myalgia · palpitations
  - **Rare or very rare** Hypersensitivity
  - **Frequency not known** Asthma exacerbated · bronchospasm · QT interval prolongation

SIDE-EFFECTS, FURTHER INFORMATION Non-sedating antihistamines such as mizolastine cause less sedation and psychomotor impairment than the older antihistamines, but can still occur; sedation is generally minimal. This is because non-sedating antihistamines penetrate the blood brain barrier to a much lesser extent.

- PREGNANCY Most manufacturers of antihistamines advise avoiding their use during pregnancy; however, there is no evidence of teratogenicity.
- BREAST FEEDING Most antihistamines are present in breast milk in varying amounts; although not known to be harmful, most manufacturers advise avoiding their use in mothers who are breast-feeding.
- HEPATIC IMPAIRMENT Manufacturer advises avoid in significant impairment.
- PATIENT AND CARER ADVICE
Driving and skilled tasks Patients and their carers should be advised that drowsiness can occur and may affect performance of skilled tasks (e.g. cycling or driving).

- MEDICINAL FORMS No licensed medicines listed.

Rupatadine

29-Apr-2019

- DRUG ACTION Rupatadine is a second generation non-sedating antihistamine.

- INDICATIONS AND DOSE

Symptomatic relief of allergic rhinitis and urticaria
▸ BY MOUTH USING TABLETS
▸ Child 12-17 years: 10 mg once daily
▸ Adult: 10 mg once daily

- CAUTIONS Elderly—limited information available · history of QT-interval prolongation · predisposition to arrhythmia · uncorrected hypokalaemia
- INTERACTIONS → Appendix 1: antihistamines, non-sedating
- SIDE-EFFECTS
▸ **Common or very common** Asthenia · dizziness · drowsiness · dry mouth · headache
▸ **Uncommon** Appetite increased · arthralgia · back pain · concentration impaired · constipation · cough · diarrhoea · dry throat · eosinophilia (in children) · epistaxis · fever · gastrointestinal discomfort · increased risk of infection · irritability · malaise · myalgia · nasal dryness · nausea · neutropenia (in children) · night sweats (in children) · oropharyngeal pain · skin reactions · thirst · vomiting · weight increased
▸ **Rare or very rare** Palpitations · tachycardia
SIDE-EFFECTS, FURTHER INFORMATION Non-sedating antihistamines such as rupatadine cause less sedation and psychomotor impairment than the older antihistamines, but can still occur; sedation is generally minimal. This is because non-sedating antihistamines penetrate the blood brain barrier to a much lesser extent.
- PREGNANCY Most manufacturers of antihistamines advise avoiding their use during pregnancy; however, there is no evidence of teratogenicity.
- BREAST FEEDING Most antihistamines are present in breast milk in varying amounts; although not known to be harmful, most manufacturers advise avoiding their use in mothers who are breast-feeding.
- HEPATIC IMPAIRMENT Manufacturer advises avoid (no information available).
- RENAL IMPAIRMENT Manufacturer advises avoid—no information available.

- MEDICINAL FORMS There can be variation in the licensing of different medicines containing the same drug.
Oral tablet
▸ Rupatadine (Non-proprietary)
Rupatadine (as Rupatadine fumarate) 10 mg Rupatadine 10mg tablets | 30 tablet PoM £37.00–£75.82 DT = £75.82

ANTIHISTAMINES › SEDATING

Alimemazine tartrate

27-Jun-2023

(Trimeprazine tartrate)

- INDICATIONS AND DOSE

Urticaria | Pruritus
▸ BY MOUTH
▸ Child 2-4 years: 2.5 mg 3–4 times a day
▸ Child 5-11 years: 5 mg 3–4 times a day
▸ Child 12-17 years: 10 mg 2–3 times a day, in severe cases doses up to 100 mg per day have been used
▸ Adult: 10 mg 2–3 times a day, in severe cases doses up to 100 mg per day have been used
▸ Elderly: 10 mg 1–2 times a day

- CONTRA-INDICATIONS Epilepsy · hepatic dysfunction · history of narrow angle glaucoma · hypothyroidism · myasthenia gravis · Parkinson's disease · phaeochromocytoma · prostatic hypertrophy (in adults) · renal dysfunction
- CAUTIONS Cardiovascular diseases (due to tachycardia-inducing and hypotensive effects of phenothiazines) · elderly · exposure to sunlight should be avoided during treatment with high doses · pyloroduodenal obstruction · susceptibility to QT interval prolongation · urinary retention · volume depleted patients who are more susceptible to orthostatic hypotension
- INTERACTIONS → Appendix 1: antihistamines, sedating
- SIDE-EFFECTS Agitation · agranulocytosis · amenorrhoea · atrioventricular block · autonomic dysfunction · bile thrombus · consciousness impaired · drug fever · dry mouth · eosinophilia · erectile dysfunction · eye disorder · galactorrhoea · gynaecomastia · hepatic disorders · hyperprolactinaemia · hyperthermia · hypotension · insomnia · leucopenia (on prolonged high dose) · movement disorders · muscle rigidity · nasal congestion · neuroleptic malignant syndrome (discontinue—potentially fatal) · pallor · parkinsonism · photosensitivity reaction · postural hypotension (more common in the elderly or in volume depletion) · QT interval prolongation · respiratory depression · seizure · skin reactions · tardive dyskinesia (more common after long term high doses) · tremor · ventricular fibrillation (increased risk with hypokalaemia and cardiac disease) · ventricular tachycardia (increased risk with hypokalaemia and cardiac disease)
SIDE-EFFECTS, FURTHER INFORMATION Drowsiness may diminish after a few days.
Patients on high dosage may develop photosensitivity and should avoid exposure to direct sunlight.
Children and elderly patients are more susceptible to side-effects.
- PREGNANCY Most manufacturers of antihistamines advise avoiding their use during pregnancy; however, there is no evidence of teratogenicity. Use in the latter part of the third trimester may cause adverse effects in neonates such as irritability, paradoxical excitability, and tremor.
- BREAST FEEDING Most antihistamines are present in breast milk in varying amounts; although not known to be harmful, most manufacturers advise avoiding their use in mothers who are breast-feeding.
- HEPATIC IMPAIRMENT Manufacturer advises avoid—no information available.
- RENAL IMPAIRMENT EvGr Avoid. ⟨M⟩
- PATIENT AND CARER ADVICE
Driving and skilled tasks Drowsiness may affect performance of skilled tasks (e.g. cycling or driving); sedating effects enhanced by alcohol.

- **MEDICINAL FORMS** There can be variation in the licensing of different medicines containing the same drug. Forms available from special-order manufacturers include: oral solution

Oral tablet
CAUTIONARY AND ADVISORY LABELS 2
- **Alimemazine tartrate (Non-proprietary)**
  Alimemazine tartrate 10 mg Alimemazine 10mg tablets | 28 tablet [PoM] £106.10 DT = £48.80

Oral solution
CAUTIONARY AND ADVISORY LABELS 2
- **Alimemazine tartrate (Non-proprietary)**
  Alimemazine tartrate 1.5 mg per 1 ml Alimemazine 7.5mg/5ml oral solution | 100 ml [PoM] £179.55 DT = £135.00
  Alimemazine 7.5mg/5ml oral solution sugar free | 100 ml [PoM] £107.74-£168.00 DT = £168.00 [SF]
  Alimemazine tartrate 2 mg per 1 ml Alimemazine 10mg/5ml oral solution sugar free | 100 ml [PoM] £191.10 DT = £191.10 [SF]
  Alimemazine tartrate 6 mg per 1 ml Alimemazine 30mg/5ml oral solution sugar free | 100 ml [PoM] £146.10-£230.00 DT = £230.00 [SF]
  Alimemazine 30mg/5ml oral solution | 100 ml [PoM] £243.51 DT = £231.63
- **Alfresed** (Syri Ltd)
  Alimemazine tartrate 1.5 mg per 1 ml Alfresed 7.5mg/5ml syrup | 100 ml [PoM] £89.00 DT = £135.00
  Alimemazine tartrate 6 mg per 1 ml Alfresed 30mg/5ml syrup | 100 ml [PoM] £99.00 DT = £231.63
- **Itzenal** (Zentiva Pharma UK Ltd)
  Alimemazine tartrate 1.5 mg per 1 ml Itzenal 7.5mg/5ml oral solution sugar free | 100 ml [PoM] £89.00 DT = £168.00 [SF]
  Alimemazine tartrate 6 mg per 1 ml Itzenal 30mg/5ml oral solution sugar free | 100 ml [PoM] £99.00 DT = £230.00 [SF]

Chlorphenamine maleate   10-Oct-2023
(Chlorpheniramine maleate)

- **INDICATIONS AND DOSE**

Symptomatic relief of allergy such as hay fever, urticaria, food allergy, drug reactions | Relief of itch associated with chickenpox
- BY MOUTH
- Child 1-23 months: 1 mg twice daily
- Child 2-5 years: 1 mg every 4–6 hours
- Child 6-11 years: 2 mg every 4–6 hours
- Child 12-17 years: 4 mg every 4–6 hours
- Adult: 4 mg every 4–6 hours
- Elderly: 4 mg every 4–6 hours, consider maximum 12 mg per day due to risk of side-effects

Symptomatic relief of allergy such as hay fever, urticaria, food allergy, drug reactions
- BY INTRAMUSCULAR INJECTION, OR BY INTRAVENOUS INJECTION
- Child 1-5 months: 250 micrograms/kg for 1 dose (max. per dose 2.5 mg), to be repeated if necessary; maximum 4 doses per day
- Child 6 months-5 years: 2.5 mg for 1 dose, to be repeated if necessary; maximum 4 doses per day
- Child 6-11 years: 5 mg for 1 dose, to be repeated if necessary; maximum 4 doses per day
- Child 12-17 years: 10 mg for 1 dose, to be repeated if necessary; maximum 4 doses per day
- Adult: 10 mg for 1 dose, to be repeated if necessary; maximum 4 doses per day

Emergency treatment of anaphylactic reactions
- BY INTRAMUSCULAR INJECTION, OR BY INTRAVENOUS INJECTION
- Child 1-5 months: 250 micrograms/kg for 1 dose (max. per dose 2.5 mg), to be repeated if necessary; maximum 4 doses per day
- Child 6 months-5 years: 2.5 mg for 1 dose, to be repeated if necessary; maximum 4 doses per day

- Child 6-11 years: 5 mg for 1 dose, to be repeated if necessary; maximum 4 doses per day
- Child 12-17 years: 10 mg for 1 dose, to be repeated if necessary; maximum 4 doses per day
- Adult: 10 mg for 1 dose, to be repeated if necessary; maximum 4 doses per day

- **UNLICENSED USE** Expert sources advise that chlorphenamine may be used in children under 1 year of age for the treatment of allergies and of itch associated with chickenpox, but it is not licensed for this age group.

> **IMPORTANT SAFETY INFORMATION**
> **MHRA/CHM ADVICE: OVER-THE-COUNTER COUGH AND COLD MEDICINES FOR CHILDREN (APRIL 2009)**
> Children under 6 years should not be given over-the-counter cough and cold medicines containing chlorphenamine.

- **CAUTIONS** Epilepsy · prostatic hypertrophy (in adults) · pyloroduodenal obstruction · susceptibility to angle-closure glaucoma · urinary retention

- **INTERACTIONS** → Appendix 1: antihistamines, sedating

- **SIDE-EFFECTS**

GENERAL SIDE-EFFECTS
- **Common or very common** Concentration impaired · coordination abnormal · dizziness · dry mouth · fatigue · headache · nausea · vision blurred
- **Frequency not known** Agitation · appetite decreased · blood disorder · bronchial secretion viscosity increased · depression · diarrhoea · haemolytic anaemia · hypotension · irritability · muscle twitching · muscle weakness · nightmare · palpitations · photosensitivity reaction · skin reactions · tinnitus · urinary retention · vomiting

SPECIFIC SIDE-EFFECTS
- **Common or very common**
- With oral use Drowsiness
- **Frequency not known**
- With oral use Angioedema · arrhythmias · chest tightness · confusion · gastrointestinal discomfort · hepatic disorders
- With parenteral use Central nervous system stimulation · confusional psychosis (in adults) · dyspepsia · gastrointestinal disorder · hepatitis · sedation

SIDE-EFFECTS, FURTHER INFORMATION Children and elderly patients are more susceptible to side-effects.

- **PREGNANCY** Most manufacturers of antihistamines advise avoiding their use during pregnancy; however, there is no evidence of teratogenicity. Use in the latter part of the third trimester may cause adverse effects in neonates such as irritability, paradoxical excitability, and tremor.

- **BREAST FEEDING** Most antihistamines are present in breast milk in varying amounts; although not known to be harmful, most manufacturers advise avoiding their use in mothers who are breast-feeding.

- **HEPATIC IMPAIRMENT** Manufacturer advises caution.

- **DIRECTIONS FOR ADMINISTRATION** For *intravenous injection*, manufacturer advises give over 1 minute; if small dose required, dilute with Sodium Chloride 0.9%.

- **PATIENT AND CARER ADVICE**
  Medicines for Children leaflet: Chlorphenamine maleate for allergy www.medicinesforchildren.org.uk/medicines/chlorphenamine-maleate-for-allergy/
  Driving and skilled tasks Drowsiness may affect performance of skilled tasks (e.g. cycling or driving); sedating effects enhanced by alcohol.

- **PROFESSION SPECIFIC INFORMATION**
  Dental practitioners' formulary Chlorphenamine tablets may be prescribed.
    Chlorphenamine oral solution may be prescribed.

● **EXCEPTIONS TO LEGAL CATEGORY**
▸ With intramuscular use or intravenous use Prescription only medicine restriction does not apply to chlorphenamine injection where administration is for saving life in emergency.

● **MEDICINAL FORMS** There can be variation in the licensing of different medicines containing the same drug. Forms available from special-order manufacturers include: oral solution

Solution for injection
▸ **Chlorphenamine maleate (Non-proprietary)**
Chlorphenamine maleate 10 mg per 1 ml Chlorphenamine 10mg/1ml solution for injection ampoules | 5 ampoule PoM £22.50 DT = £25.49 (Hospital only) | 5 ampoule PoM £25.49 DT = £25.49

Oral tablet
CAUTIONARY AND ADVISORY LABELS 2
▸ **Chlorphenamine maleate (Non-proprietary)**
Chlorphenamine maleate 4 mg Chlorphenamine 4mg tablets | 28 tablet P £8.05 DT = £0.81
▸ **Allerief** (Crescent Pharma Ltd)
Chlorphenamine maleate 4 mg Allerief 4mg tablets | 28 tablet P £3.07 DT = £0.81
▸ **Hayleve** (Genesis Pharmaceuticals Ltd)
Chlorphenamine maleate 4 mg Hayleve 4mg tablets | 28 tablet P £2.47 DT = £0.81
▸ **Piriton** (Haleon UK Trading Ltd)
Chlorphenamine maleate 4 mg Piriton 4mg tablets | 500 tablet P £21.25
Piriton Allergy 4mg tablets | 30 tablet P £3.49 | 60 tablet P £5.59

Oral solution
CAUTIONARY AND ADVISORY LABELS 2
▸ **Chlorphenamine maleate (Non-proprietary)**
Chlorphenamine maleate 400 microgram per 1 ml Chlorphenamine 2mg/5ml oral solution sugar free | 150 ml P £7.99 DT = £7.99 SF
▸ **Allerief** (Crescent Pharma Ltd)
Chlorphenamine maleate 400 microgram per 1 ml Allerief 2mg/5ml oral solution | 150 ml P £2.21 DT = £7.99 SF
▸ **Piriton** (Haleon UK Trading Ltd)
Chlorphenamine maleate 400 microgram per 1 ml Piriton 2mg/5ml syrup | 150 ml P £3.91 DT = £3.91

Cyproheptadine hydrochloride 04-Sep-2020

● **INDICATIONS AND DOSE**
Symptomatic relief of allergy such as hay fever, urticaria | Pruritus
▸ BY MOUTH
▸ Adult: 4 mg 3 times a day, usual dose 4–20 mg daily; maximum 32 mg per day

● **CONTRA-INDICATIONS** Avoid in Acute porphyrias p. 1202
● **CAUTIONS** Epilepsy · prostatic hypertrophy · pyloroduodenal obstruction · susceptibility to angle-closure glaucoma · urinary retention
● **INTERACTIONS** → Appendix 1: antihistamines, sedating
● **SIDE-EFFECTS** Aggression · agranulocytosis · anxiety · appetite abnormal · arrhythmias · bronchial secretion viscosity increased · chest tightness · chills · confusion · constipation · coordination abnormal · diarrhoea · dizziness · drowsiness · dry mouth · dry throat · epigastric distress · epistaxis · fatigue · haemolytic anaemia · hallucination · headache · hepatic disorders · hyperhidrosis · hypotension · insomnia · labyrinthitis · leucopenia · menstruation irregular · mood altered · nasal complaints · nausea · neuritis · oedema · palpitations · paraesthesia · photosensitivity reaction · seizure · skin reactions · thrombocytopenia · tinnitus · tremor · urinary disorders · vertigo · vision disorders · vomiting · weight increased · wheezing
● **PREGNANCY** Most manufacturers of antihistamines advise avoiding their use during pregnancy; however, there is no evidence of teratogenicity. Use in the latter part of the

third trimester may cause adverse effects in neonates such as irritability, paradoxical excitability, and tremor.

● **BREAST FEEDING** Most antihistamines are present in breast milk in varying amounts; although not known to be harmful, most manufacturers advise avoiding their use in mothers who are breast-feeding.

● **PATIENT AND CARER ADVICE**
Driving and skilled tasks Drowsiness may affect performance of skilled tasks (e.g. driving); sedating effects enhanced by alcohol.

● **MEDICINAL FORMS** There can be variation in the licensing of different medicines containing the same drug. Forms available from special-order manufacturers include: oral suspension, oral solution

Oral tablet
CAUTIONARY AND ADVISORY LABELS 2
▸ **Periactin** (Teva UK Ltd)
Cyproheptadine hydrochloride 4 mg Periactin 4mg tablets | 30 tablet P £5.99 DT = £5.99

Hydroxyzine hydrochloride 27-Apr-2021

● **DRUG ACTION** Hydroxyzine is a sedating antihistamine which exerts its actions by antagonising the effects of histamine.

● **INDICATIONS AND DOSE**
Pruritus
▸ BY MOUTH
▸ Child 6 months–5 years: 5–15 mg daily in divided doses, dose adjusted according to weight; maximum 2 mg/kg per day
▸ Child 6–17 years (body-weight up to 40 kg): Initially 15–25 mg daily in divided doses, dose increased as necessary, adjusted according to weight; maximum 2 mg/kg per day
▸ Child 6–17 years (body-weight 40 kg and above): Initially 15–25 mg daily in divided doses, increased if necessary to 50–100 mg daily in divided doses, dose adjusted according to weight
▸ Adult: Initially 25 mg daily, dose to be taken at night; increased if necessary to 25 mg 3–4 times a day
▸ Elderly: Initially 25 mg daily, dose to be taken at night; increased if necessary to 25 mg twice daily

IMPORTANT SAFETY INFORMATION
MHRA/CHM ADVICE: RISK OF QT-INTERVAL PROLONGATION AND TORSADE DE POINTES (APRIL 2015)
Following concerns of heart rhythm abnormalities, the safety and efficacy of hydroxyzine has been reviewed by the European Medicines Agency. The review concludes that hydroxyzine is associated with a small risk of QT-interval prolongation and torsade de pointes; these events are most likely to occur in patients who have risk factors for QT prolongation, e.g. concomitant use of drugs that prolong the QT-interval, cardiovascular disease, family history of sudden cardiac death, significant electrolyte imbalance (low plasma-potassium or plasma-magnesium concentrations), or significant bradycardia. To minimise the risk of such adverse effects, the following dose restrictions have been made and new cautions and contra-indications added:
● Hydroxyzine is contra-indicated in patients with prolonged QT-interval or who have risk factors for QT-interval prolongation;
● Avoid use in the elderly due to increased susceptibility to the side-effects of hydroxyzine;
● Consider the risks of QT-interval prolongation and torsade de pointes before prescribing to patients taking drugs that lower heart rate or plasma-potassium concentration;

- In children with body-weight up to 40 kg, the maximum daily dose is 2 mg/kg;
- In adults, the maximum daily dose is 100 mg;
- In the elderly, the maximum daily dose is 50 mg (if use of hydroxyzine cannot be avoided);
- The lowest effective dose for the shortest period of time should be prescribed.

- **CONTRA-INDICATIONS** Acquired or congenital QT interval prolongation · predisposition to QT interval prolongation

  CONTRA-INDICATIONS, FURTHER INFORMATION
- ▶ QT interval prolongation Risk factors for QT interval prolongation include significant electrolyte imbalance, bradycardia, cardiovascular disease, and family history of sudden cardiac death.

- **CAUTIONS** Bladder outflow obstruction · breathing problems · cardiovascular disease · children · decreased gastrointestinal motility · dementia · elderly · epilepsy · hypertension · hyperthyroidism · myasthenia gravis · prostatic hypertrophy (in adults) · pyloroduodenal obstruction · stenosing peptic ulcer · susceptibility to angle-closure glaucoma · urinary retention

  CAUTIONS, FURTHER INFORMATION Elderly patients are particularly susceptible to side-effects; manufacturers advise avoid or reduce dose.

  Children have an increased susceptibility to side-effects, particularly CNS effects.

- **INTERACTIONS** → Appendix 1: antihistamines, sedating

- **SIDE-EFFECTS**
- ▶ **Rare or very rare** Severe cutaneous adverse reactions (SCARs) · skin reactions
- ▶ **Frequency not known** Agranulocytosis · alopecia · anticholinergic syndrome · anxiety · appetite decreased · arrhythmias · asthenia · blood disorder · bronchial secretion viscosity increased · chest tightness · chills · coma · concentration impaired · confusion · constipation · depression · diarrhoea · dizziness · drowsiness · dry mouth · dry throat · dyskinesia (on discontinuation) · epigastric pain · fever · flushing · gastrointestinal disorders · haemolytic anaemia · hallucination · headache · hepatic function abnormal · hyperhidrosis · hypotension · irritability · labyrinthitis · leucopenia · malaise · menstruation irregular · movement disorders · myalgia · nasal congestion · nausea · palpitations · paraesthesia · QT interval prolongation · respiratory disorders · respiratory tract dryness · seizure (with high doses) · sexual dysfunction · sleep disorders · speech slurred · taste bitter · thrombocytopenia · tinnitus · tremor (with high doses) · urinary disorders · vertigo · vision disorders · vomiting

  SIDE-EFFECTS, FURTHER INFORMATION Paradoxical stimulation may occur rarely, especially with high doses or in the elderly. Drowsiness may diminish after a few days of treatment.

- **ALLERGY AND CROSS-SENSITIVITY** Manufacturer advises hydroxyzine should be avoided in patients with previous hypersensitivity to cetirizine or other piperazine derivatives, and aminophylline.

- **PREGNANCY** Manufacturers advise avoid—toxicity in *animal* studies with higher doses. Use in the latter part of the third trimester may cause irritability, paradoxical excitability, and tremor in the neonate.

- **BREAST FEEDING** Manufacturer advises avoid—expected to be present in milk but effect unknown.

- **HEPATIC IMPAIRMENT** Manufacturer advises caution in mild to moderate impairment (increased risk of accumulation); avoid in severe impairment.
  Dose adjustments Manufacturer advises dose reduction of 33% in mild to moderate impairment.

- **RENAL IMPAIRMENT** [EvGr] Use with caution. ◈M◈

- **Dose adjustments** [EvGr] Reduce daily dose by half in moderate to severe renal impairment. ◈M◈

- **EFFECT ON LABORATORY TESTS** May interfere with methacholine test—manufacturer advises stop treatment 96 hours prior to test. May interfere with skin testing for allergy—manufacturer advises stop treatment one week prior to test.

- **PATIENT AND CARER ADVICE**
  Driving and skilled tasks Drowsiness may affect performance of skilled tasks (e.g. cycling or driving); sedating effects enhanced by alcohol.

- **MEDICINAL FORMS** There can be variation in the licensing of different medicines containing the same drug. Forms available from special-order manufacturers include: oral suspension, oral solution

  Oral tablet
  CAUTIONARY AND ADVISORY LABELS 2
- ▶ Hydroxyzine hydrochloride (Non-proprietary)
  Hydroxyzine hydrochloride 10 mg Hydroxyzine 10mg tablets | 84 tablet [PoM] £2.80 DT = £2.01
  Hydroxyzine hydrochloride 25 mg Hydroxyzine 25mg tablets | 28 tablet [PoM] £1.50 DT = £0.86

  Oral solution
  CAUTIONARY AND ADVISORY LABELS 2
  EXCIPIENTS: May contain Alcohol, sucrose

Ketotifen
14-Dec-2020

- **INDICATIONS AND DOSE**

  Allergic rhinitis
- ▶ BY MOUTH
- ▶ Child 3–17 years: 1 mg twice daily
- ▶ Adult: 1 mg twice daily, increased if necessary to 2 mg twice daily, to be taken with food

  Allergic rhinitis in readily sedated patients
- ▶ BY MOUTH
- ▶ Adult: Initially 0.5–1 mg once daily, dose to be taken at night

- **CONTRA-INDICATIONS** Avoid in Acute porphyrias p. 1202

- **CAUTIONS** Epilepsy · prostatic hypertrophy (in adults) · pyloroduodenal obstruction · susceptibility to angle-closure glaucoma · urinary retention

- **INTERACTIONS** → Appendix 1: antihistamines, sedating

- **SIDE-EFFECTS**
- ▶ **Common or very common** Anxiety · insomnia · irritability
- ▶ **Uncommon** Cystitis · dizziness · dry mouth · skin reactions
- ▶ **Rare or very rare** Hepatitis · sedation · seizure · Stevens-Johnson syndrome · weight increased

  SIDE-EFFECTS, FURTHER INFORMATION Drowsiness is a significant side-effect with most of the older antihistamines although paradoxical stimulation may occur rarely, especially with high doses or in children and the elderly. Drowsiness may diminish after a few days of treatment and is considerably less of a problem with the newer antihistamines.

- **PREGNANCY** Most manufacturers of antihistamines advise avoiding their use during pregnancy; however, there is no evidence of teratogenicity. Use in the latter part of the third trimester may cause adverse effects in neonates such as irritability, paradoxical excitability, and tremor.

- **BREAST FEEDING** Most antihistamines are present in breast milk in varying amounts; although not known to be harmful, most manufacturers advise avoiding their use in mothers who are breast-feeding.

- **PATIENT AND CARER ADVICE**
  Driving and skilled tasks Drowsiness may affect performance of skilled tasks (e.g. driving or cycling); sedating effects enhanced by alcohol.

● **NATIONAL FUNDING/ACCESS DECISIONS**
For full details see funding body website
All Wales Medicines Strategy Group (AWMSG) decisions
▶ Ketotifen (*Ketofall*®) for symptomatic treatment of seasonal allergic conjunctivitis (June 2020) AWMSG No. 3930 Recommended with restrictions

● **MEDICINAL FORMS** There can be variation in the licensing of different medicines containing the same drug. Forms available from special-order manufacturers include: oral solution

Oral tablet
CAUTIONARY AND ADVISORY LABELS 2, 21
▶ Zaditen (CD Pharma Srl)
Ketotifen (as Ketotifen fumarate) 1 mg Zaditen 1mg tablets | 60 tablet PoM £14.56 DT = £14.56

Oral solution
CAUTIONARY AND ADVISORY LABELS 2, 21
▶ Zaditen (CD Pharma Srl)
Ketotifen (as Ketotifen fumarate) 200 microgram per 1 ml Zaditen 1mg/5ml elixir | 300 ml PoM £17.25 DT = £17.25 SF

Promethazine hydrochloride
27-Jun-2023

● **INDICATIONS AND DOSE**

Symptomatic relief of allergy such as hay fever and urticaria | Insomnia associated with urticaria and pruritus
▶ BY MOUTH
▶ Child 2-4 years: 5 mg twice daily, alternatively 5–15 mg once daily, dose to be taken at night
▶ Child 5-9 years: 5–10 mg twice daily, alternatively 10–25 mg once daily, dose to be taken at night
▶ Child 10-17 years: 10–20 mg 2–3 times a day, alternatively 25 mg once daily, dose to be taken at night, increased if necessary to 25 mg twice daily
▶ Adult: 10–20 mg 2–3 times a day
▶ BY DEEP INTRAMUSCULAR INJECTION
▶ Adult: 25–50 mg (max. per dose 100 mg)

Emergency treatment of anaphylactic reactions
▶ BY SLOW INTRAVENOUS INJECTION
▶ Adult: 25–50 mg, to be administered as a solution containing 2.5 mg/mL in water for injections; maximum 100 mg per course

Sedation (short-term use)
▶ BY MOUTH
▶ Child 2-4 years: 15–20 mg
▶ Child 5-9 years: 20–25 mg
▶ Child 10-17 years: 25–50 mg
▶ Adult: 25–50 mg
▶ BY DEEP INTRAMUSCULAR INJECTION
▶ Adult: 25–50 mg

Nausea | Vomiting | Vertigo | Labyrinthine disorders | Motion sickness
▶ BY MOUTH
▶ Child 2-4 years: 5 mg, to be taken at bedtime on night before travel, repeat following morning if necessary
▶ Child 5-9 years: 10 mg, to be taken at bedtime on night before travel, repeat following morning if necessary
▶ Child 10-17 years: 20–25 mg, to be taken at bedtime on night before travel, repeat following morning if necessary
▶ Adult: 20–25 mg, to be taken at bedtime on night before travel, repeat following morning if necessary

IMPORTANT SAFETY INFORMATION
MHRA/CHM ADVICE: OVER-THE-COUNTER COUGH AND COLD MEDICINES FOR CHILDREN (APRIL 2009)
Children under 6 years should not be given over-the-counter cough and cold medicines containing promethazine.

● **CAUTIONS**

GENERAL CAUTIONS Epilepsy · prostatic hypertrophy (in adults) · pyloroduodenal obstruction · severe coronary artery disease · susceptibility to angle-closure glaucoma · susceptibility to QT interval prolongation · urinary retention

SPECIFIC CAUTIONS
▶ With intravenous use Avoid extravasation with intravenous injection

● **INTERACTIONS** → Appendix 1: antihistamines, sedating

● **SIDE-EFFECTS**

GENERAL SIDE-EFFECTS Arrhythmias · blood disorder · confusion · dizziness · drowsiness · dry mouth · headache · hypotension · jaundice · movement disorders · palpitations · photosensitivity reaction · QT interval prolongation · urinary retention · vision blurred

SPECIFIC SIDE-EFFECTS
▶ With oral use Agranulocytosis · angle closure glaucoma · anticholinergic syndrome · anxiety · insomnia · leucopenia · nasal congestion · nausea · rash · seizure · thrombocytopenia · tinnitus · tremor · vomiting
▶ With parenteral use Appetite decreased · epigastric discomfort · fatigue · haemolytic anaemia · hypersensitivity · muscle spasms · nightmare · restlessness · skin reactions

SIDE-EFFECTS, FURTHER INFORMATION Elderly patients are more susceptible to anticholinergic side-effects.

● **PREGNANCY** Most manufacturers of antihistamines advise avoiding their use during pregnancy; however, there is no evidence of teratogenicity. Use in the latter part of the third trimester may cause adverse effects in neonates such as irritability, paradoxical excitability, and tremor.

● **BREAST FEEDING** Most antihistamines are present in breast milk in varying amounts; although not known to be harmful, most manufacturers advise avoiding their use in mothers who are breast-feeding.

● **HEPATIC IMPAIRMENT** Manufacturer advises caution.

● **RENAL IMPAIRMENT** EvGr Use with caution. Ⓜ

● **PATIENT AND CARER ADVICE**
Driving and skilled tasks Drowsiness may affect the performance of skilled tasks (e.g. cycling or driving); sedating effects enhanced by alcohol.

● **PROFESSION SPECIFIC INFORMATION**
Dental practitioners' formulary Promethazine Hydrochloride Tablets 10 mg or 25 mg may be prescribed. Promethazine Hydrochloride Oral Solution (elixir) 5 mg/5 mL may be prescribed.

● **LESS SUITABLE FOR PRESCRIBING** Promethazine is less suitable for prescribing for sedation.

● **EXCEPTIONS TO LEGAL CATEGORY** Prescription only medicine restriction does not apply to promethazine hydrochloride injection where administration is for saving life in emergency.

● **MEDICINAL FORMS** There can be variation in the licensing of different medicines containing the same drug. Forms available from special-order manufacturers include: oral suspension, oral solution

Solution for injection
EXCIPIENTS: May contain Sulfites
▶ Phenergan (Opella Healthcare UK Ltd)
Promethazine hydrochloride 25 mg per 1 ml Phenergan 25mg/1ml solution for injection ampoules | 10 ampoule PoM £6.74 DT = £6.74

Oral tablet
CAUTIONARY AND ADVISORY LABELS 2
▶ Promethazine hydrochloride (Non-proprietary)
Promethazine hydrochloride 10 mg Promethazine hydrochloride 10mg tablets | 56 tablet PoM £5.12 DT = £4.23
Promethazine hydrochloride 25 mg Promethazine hydrochloride 25mg tablets | 56 tablet PoM £34.19 DT = £3.67

▶ **Sominex** (Dexcel-Pharma Ltd)
Promethazine hydrochloride 20 mg Sominex 20mg tablets |
8 tablet P £1.89 DT = £1.89 | 16 tablet P £2.69 DT = £2.69
Oral solution
CAUTIONARY AND ADVISORY LABELS 2
EXCIPIENTS: May contain Sulfites
ELECTROLYTES: May contain Sodium
▶ **Phenergan** (Opella Healthcare UK Ltd)
Promethazine hydrochloride 1 mg per 1 ml Phenergan 5mg/5ml
elixir | 100 ml P £4.08 DT = £4.08 SF

VACCINES > ALLERGEN-TYPE VACCINES

Bee venom extract
30-Sep-2024

● **INDICATIONS AND DOSE**
Hypersensitivity to bee venom (under expert supervision)
▶ BY SUBCUTANEOUS INJECTION
▶ Adult: (consult product literature)

IMPORTANT SAFETY INFORMATION
DESENSITISING VACCINES
In view of concerns about the safety of desensitising
vaccines, it is recommended that they are used by
specialists and only for licensed indications.
EvGr Desensitising vaccines should generally be
avoided or used with particular care in patients with
asthma. M

● **CONTRA-INDICATIONS** Consult product literature
● **CAUTIONS** Consult product literature
● **INTERACTIONS** → Appendix 1: bee venom extract
● **SIDE-EFFECTS** Consult product literature.
Hypersensitivity reactions Hypersensitivity reactions
to immunotherapy can be life-threatening.
Cardiopulmonary resuscitation must be immediately
available and patients need to be monitored for at least
30 minutes after administration. If symptoms or signs of
hypersensitivity develop (e.g. rash, urticaria,
bronchospasm, faintness), **even when mild**, the patient
should be observed until these have resolved completely.
● **PREGNANCY** EvGr Avoid initiating up-dosing treatment
(no information available). If pregnancy occurs during
maintenance treatment, *Alutard SQ Bee Venom*® may be
continued after the general condition of the patient is
evaluated, including reactions to previous injections. M
● **BREAST FEEDING** Specialist sources indicate probably
compatible (no information available). High molecular
weight makes excretion into milk unlikely and inactivation
in the gastrointestinal tract suggests limited absorption by
the infant.
● **DIRECTIONS FOR ADMINISTRATION** EvGr For *subcutaneous
injection (Alutard SQ Bee Venom*®), the vial must be turned
slowly upside down 10 to 20 times to make a homogenous
suspension before use. Administer slowly, either laterally
in the distal part of the upper arm or dorsally in the
proximal part of the forearm. M
● **PRESCRIBING AND DISPENSING INFORMATION** Each set of
allergen extracts usually contains vials for the
administration of graded amounts of allergen to patients
undergoing hyposensitisation. Maintenance sets
containing vials at the highest strength are also available.
Product literature must be consulted for details of
allergens, vial strengths, and administration.
● **HANDLING AND STORAGE** Store unopened vials in a
refrigerator (2–8°C) and protect from light. Once opened,
vials may be stored for a maximum of 6 months in a
refrigerator (2–8°C) when used for one individual patient.
● **PATIENT AND CARER ADVICE** Patients and carers should be
counselled to avoid physical exercise, hot baths, and

alcohol on the day of injection—potential amplification of
anaphylactic reaction. They should also be advised to seek
immediate medical attention if severe delayed systemic
reactions develop, and to inform their doctor before the
next injection of any local or systemic reactions that occur
subsequently.
Asthma Patients and carers should be advised to seek
immediate medical attention if their asthma deteriorates
suddenly during treatment.
Driving and skilled tasks Patients and carers should be
counselled on the effects on driving and performance of
skilled tasks—increased risk of dizziness or vertigo.
● **NATIONAL FUNDING/ACCESS DECISIONS**
For full details see funding body website
NICE decisions
▶ *Pharmalgen*® for the treatment of bee and wasp venom
allergy (February 2012) NICE TA246 Recommended with
restrictions

● **MEDICINAL FORMS** There can be variation in the licensing of
different medicines containing the same drug.
Suspension for injection
▶ **Alutard SQ Bee Venom** (ALK-Abello Ltd)
Bee venom 100 SQ-U per 1 ml Alutard SQ Bee Venom 500 SQ-U/5ml
suspension for injection vials | 1 vial PoM ℥ (Hospital only)
Bee venom 1000 SQ-U per 1 ml Alutard SQ Bee Venom 5,000 SQ-
U/5ml suspension for injection vials | 1 vial PoM ℥ (Hospital only)
Bee venom 10000 SQ-U per 1 ml Alutard SQ Bee Venom 50,000 SQ-
U/5ml suspension for injection vials | 1 vial PoM ℥ (Hospital only)
Bee venom 100000 SQ-U per 1 ml Alutard SQ Bee Venom
maintenance pack suspension for injection vials | 1 vial PoM £462.61
(Hospital only)

Grass pollen extract
17-Nov-2021

● **INDICATIONS AND DOSE**
**Treatment of seasonal allergic hay fever due to grass
pollen in patients who have failed to respond to anti-
allergy drugs**
▶ BY SUBCUTANEOUS INJECTION
▶ Adult: (consult product literature)

**Treatment of seasonal allergic hay fever due to grass
pollen in patients who have failed to respond to anti-
allergy drugs (initiated under specialist supervision)**
▶ BY MOUTH
▶ Adult: 1 tablet daily, treatment to be started at least
4 months before start of pollen season and continue for
up to 3 years

IMPORTANT SAFETY INFORMATION
DESENSITISING VACCINES
In view of concerns about the safety of desensitising
vaccines, it is recommended that they are used by
specialists and only for licensed indications.
EvGr Desensitising vaccines should generally be
avoided or used with particular care in patients with
asthma. M

● **CONTRA-INDICATIONS** Consult product literature
● **CAUTIONS** Consult product literature
● **INTERACTIONS** → Appendix 1: grass pollen extract
● **SIDE-EFFECTS** Consult product literature.
Hypersensitivity reactions Hypersensitivity reactions
to immunotherapy can be life-threatening.
Cardiopulmonary resuscitation must be immediately
available and patients need to be monitored for at least
30 minutes (oral) or 1 hour (subcutaneous) after
administration. If symptoms or signs of hypersensitivity
develop (e.g. rash, urticaria, bronchospasm, faintness),
even when mild, the patient should be observed until
these have resolved completely.

- PREGNANCY Should be avoided in pregnant women—consult product literature.
- MONITORING REQUIREMENTS The first dose of grass pollen extract (*Grazax®*) should be taken under medical supervision and the patient should be monitored for 20–30 minutes.
- DIRECTIONS FOR ADMINISTRATION Manufacturer advises oral lyophilisates should be placed under the tongue and allowed to disperse. Advise patient not to swallow for 1 minute, or eat or drink for 5 minutes after taking the tablet. The first should be taken under medical supervision and the patient should be monitored for 20–30 minutes.
- PRESCRIBING AND DISPENSING INFORMATION Each set of allergen extracts usually contains vials for the administration of graded amounts of allergen to patients undergoing hyposensitisation. Maintenance sets containing vials at the highest strength are also available. Product literature must be consulted for details of allergens, vial strengths, and administration.
- PATIENT AND CARER ADVICE Patients or carers should be given advice on how to administer oral lyophilisates.

- MEDICINAL FORMS There can be variation in the licensing of different medicines containing the same drug.
Form unstated
  - Pollinex Grasses + Rye (Allergy Therapeutics (UK) Ltd)
    Pollinex Grasses + Rye suspension for injection treatment and extension course vials | 4 vial [PoM] £450.00
Oral lyophilisate
  - Grazax (ALK-Abello Ltd)
    Timothy grass (Phleum pratense) pollen allergen extract 75000 SQ-T Grazax 75,000 SQ-T oral lyophilisates | 30 tablet [PoM] £80.12 DT = £80.12 [SF]

House dust mite extract
01-Apr-2025

- INDICATIONS AND DOSE
Moderate to severe house dust mite allergic rhinitis [in patients who have failed to respond to anti-allergy drugs] (initiated by a specialist)
  - BY MOUTH
  - Adult 18–65 years: 1 tablet daily for up to 18 months, consider discontinuation of treatment if no improvement during the first 12 months
House dust mite allergic asthma not controlled by inhaled corticosteroids [in patients with mild to severe house dust mite allergic rhinitis] (initiated by a specialist)
  - BY MOUTH
  - Adult 18–65 years: 1 tablet daily for up to 18 months, consider discontinuation of treatment if no improvement during the first 12 months

IMPORTANT SAFETY INFORMATION
DESENSITISING VACCINES
In view of concerns about the safety of desensitising vaccines, it is recommended that they are used by specialists and only for licensed indications.
[EvGr] Desensitising vaccines should generally be avoided or used with particular care in patients with asthma. [M]

- CONTRA-INDICATIONS Consult product literature
- CAUTIONS Consult product literature
- SIDE-EFFECTS Consult product literature.
  Hypersensitivity reactions Hypersensitivity reactions to immunotherapy can be life-threatening. Cardiopulmonary resuscitation must be immediately available and patients need to be monitored for at least 30 minutes after administration. If symptoms or signs of hypersensitivity develop (e.g. rash, urticaria,

bronchospasm, faintness), **even when mild**, the patient should be observed until these have resolved completely.

- PREGNANCY [EvGr] Avoid initiation during pregnancy—limited information available. If pregnancy occurs during treatment, *Acarizax®* may be continued after the general condition and lung function of the patient are evaluated, including reactions to previous doses–close supervision of patients with pre-existing asthma is recommended. [M]
- DIRECTIONS FOR ADMINISTRATION [EvGr] Oral lyophilisates should be placed under the tongue and allowed to disperse. Advise patient not to swallow for 1 minute, or eat or drink for 5 minutes after taking the tablet. The first dose should be taken under medical supervision and the patient should be monitored for at least 30 minutes. [M]
- PATIENT AND CARER ADVICE
Administration Patients or carers should be given advice on how to administer oral lyophilisates.
Asthma Patients or carers should be advised to seek immediate medical attention if their asthma deteriorates suddenly during treatment.
Eosinophilic oesophagitis Patients or carers should be advised to seek medical attention if severe or persistent gastro-oesophageal symptoms (such as dysphagia or dyspepsia) develop during treatment.
Missed doses If treatment is interrupted for more than 7 days, patients or carers should be advised to seek medical advice before resuming treatment.
- NATIONAL FUNDING/ACCESS DECISIONS
For full details see funding body website
NICE decisions
  - **12 SQ-HDM SLIT for treating allergic rhinitis and allergic asthma caused by house dust mites [in patients with allergic rhinitis] (March 2025)** NICE TA1045 Recommended
  - **12 SQ-HDM SLIT for treating allergic rhinitis and allergic asthma caused by house dust mites [in patients with allergic asthma] (March 2025)** NICE TA1045 Not recommended

- MEDICINAL FORMS There can be variation in the licensing of different medicines containing the same drug.
Oral lyophilisate
  - Acarizax (ALK-Abello Ltd)
    Acarizax 12 SQ-HDM oral lyophilisates | 30 tablet [PoM] £80.12 [SF]

Peanut protein
20-Oct-2022

- INDICATIONS AND DOSE
Peanut allergy [in conjunction with dietary restriction] (under expert supervision)
  - BY MOUTH
  - Adult: (consult product literature)

IMPORTANT SAFETY INFORMATION
DESENSITISING VACCINES
In view of concerns about the safety of desensitising vaccines, it is recommended that they are used by specialists and only for licensed indications.
[EvGr] Desensitising vaccines should generally be avoided or used with particular care in patients with asthma. [M]

- CONTRA-INDICATIONS Consult product literature
- CAUTIONS Consult product literature
- SIDE-EFFECTS Consult product literature.
  Hypersensitivity reactions Allergic reactions mostly occur during the first 2 hours after ingestion of the dose and are usually mild or moderate; however severe reactions including life-threatening anaphylaxis may occur. Severe reactions such as difficulty swallowing, difficulty breathing, vomiting, diarrhoea, or severe flushing or itching of the skin require immediate

treatment. Self-injectable adrenaline must be available to the patient at all times. Patients need to be monitored for at least 1 hour after the last dose.

Eosinophilic oesophagitis In patients who experience severe or persistent gastrointestinal symptoms, including dysphagia, gastroesophageal reflux, chest pain, or abdominal pain, the manufacturer advises treatment must be discontinued and a diagnosis of eosinophilic oesophagitis should be considered.

- PREGNANCY [EvGr] Avoid initiation during pregnancy—no information available. If pregnancy occurs during treatment, discontinue *Palforzia*® unless potential benefit outweighs risk of anaphylactic reaction to continuing treatment. [M]

- BREAST FEEDING [EvGr] Use with caution—no information available; peanut allergens present in milk after maternal consumption of peanuts. [M]

- PRESCRIBING AND DISPENSING INFORMATION *Palforzia*® is a biological medicine. Biological medicines must be prescribed and dispensed by brand name, see *Biological medicines* and *Biosimilar medicines*, under Guidance on prescribing p. 1; record the brand name and batch number after each administration.

  Palforzia® contains peanut protein as defatted powder of *Arachis hypogaea L.*, semen (peanuts) which desensitises patients with peanut allergy.

  The manufacturer of *Palforzia*® has provided a user manual for healthcare professionals.

- PATIENT AND CARER ADVICE Patients or carers should be instructed on the potential risk factors for systemic allergic reactions and how to recognise their signs and symptoms. Patients should be advised to carry self-injectable adrenaline at all times; if use is necessary, immediate medical care should be sought and treatment stopped until the patient has been assessed.

  A safety booklet for patients and caregivers, and a patient alert card should be provided.

  Driving and skilled tasks Patients and carers should be counselled on the effects on driving and performance of skilled tasks—exercise caution for 2 hours after a dose in case of allergic reaction.

- MEDICINAL FORMS There can be variation in the licensing of different medicines containing the same drug.

  Form unstated
  CAUTIONARY AND ADVISORY LABELS 21
  - Palforzia (Diagenics Ltd) ▼
  Palforzia Level 3 (12mg daily) 2 week up-dosing pack |
  48 capsule [PoM] £141.68 (Hospital only)
  Palforzia initial dose escalation pack | 13 capsule [PoM] £10.12 (Hospital only)
  Palforzia Level 7 (120mg daily) 2 week up-dosing pack |
  32 capsule [PoM] £141.68 (Hospital only)
  Palforzia Level 8 (160mg daily) 2 week up-dosing pack |
  64 capsule [PoM] £141.68 (Hospital only)
  Palforzia Level 10 (240mg daily) 2 week up-dosing pack |
  64 capsule [PoM] £141.68 (Hospital only)

  Oral powder
  CAUTIONARY AND ADVISORY LABELS 21
  - Palforzia (Diagenics Ltd) ▼
  Peanut protein (as defatted powder of Arachis hypogaea L., semen [peanuts]) 500 microgram Palforzia 0.5mg oral powder in capsules for opening | 2 capsule [PoM] [S] (Hospital only)
  Peanut protein (as defatted powder of Arachis hypogaea L., semen [peanuts]) 1 mg Palforzia Level 1 (3mg daily) 2 week up-dosing pack | 48 capsule [PoM] £141.68 (Hospital only)
  Palforzia Level 2 (6mg daily) 2 week up-dosing pack |
  96 capsule [PoM] £141.68 (Hospital only)
  Palforzia 1mg oral powder in capsules for opening |
  11 capsule [PoM] [S] (Hospital only)
  Peanut protein (as defatted powder of Arachis hypogaea L., semen [peanuts]) 10 mg Palforzia 10mg oral powder in capsules for opening | 16 capsule [PoM] [S] (Hospital only)

Peanut protein (as defatted powder of Arachis hypogaea L., semen [peanuts]) 20 mg Palforzia Level 4 (20mg daily) 2 week up-dosing pack | 16 capsule [PoM] £141.68 (Hospital only)
Palforzia 20mg oral powder in capsules for opening |
16 capsule [PoM] [S] (Hospital only)
Palforzia Level 5 (40mg daily) 2 week up-dosing pack |
32 capsule [PoM] £141.68 (Hospital only)
Palforzia Level 6 (80mg daily) 2 week up-dosing pack |
64 capsule [PoM] £141.68 (Hospital only)
Peanut protein (as defatted powder of Arachis hypogaea L., semen [peanuts]) 100 mg Palforzia Level 9 (200mg daily) 2 week up-dosing pack | 32 capsule [PoM] £141.68 (Hospital only)
Palforzia 100mg oral powder in capsules for opening |
16 capsule [PoM] [S] (Hospital only)
Peanut protein (as defatted powder of Arachis hypogaea L., semen [peanuts]) 300 mg Palforzia Level 11 (300mg daily) 2 week up-dosing pack | 15 sachet [PoM] £141.68 (Hospital only)
Palforzia maintenance pack 300mg oral powder sachets |
30 sachet [PoM] £303.60 (Hospital only)

Tree pollen extract

07-Oct-2024

- INDICATIONS AND DOSE

Treatment of seasonal allergic hay fever due to tree pollen in patients who have failed to respond to anti-allergy drugs (under expert supervision)
▸ BY SUBCUTANEOUS INJECTION
- Adult: (consult product literature)

Moderate-to-severe allergic rhinitis and/or conjunctivitis due to pollen from the birch homologous group (initiated by a specialist)
▸ BY SUBLINGUAL ADMINISTRATION USING ORAL LYOPHILISATE
- Adult: 1 tablet once daily, initiate treatment at least 16 weeks before expected start of the tree pollen season and continue throughout. Discontinue if no improvement observed within first year of treatment

> **IMPORTANT SAFETY INFORMATION**
> DESENSITISING VACCINES
> In view of concerns about the safety of desensitising vaccines, it is recommended that they are used by specialists and only for licensed indications.
>   [EvGr] Desensitising vaccines should generally be avoided or used with particular care in patients with asthma. [M]

- CONTRA-INDICATIONS Consult product literature
- CAUTIONS Consult product literature
- INTERACTIONS → Appendix 1: tree pollen extract
- SIDE-EFFECTS Consult product literature.

  Hypersensitivity reactions Hypersensitivity reactions to immunotherapy can be life-threatening. Cardiopulmonary resuscitation must be immediately available and patients need to be monitored for at least 30 minutes (oral) or 1 hour (subcutaneous) after administration. If symptoms or signs of hypersensitivity develop (e.g. rash, urticaria, bronchospasm, faintness), **even when mild**, the patient should be observed until these have resolved completely.

- PREGNANCY
▸ With subcutaneous use [EvGr] Avoid (no information available). [M]
▸ With sublingual use [EvGr] Avoid initiation during pregnancy (no information available). If pregnancy occurs during treatment, *Itulazax*® may be continued after the general condition and lung function of the patient are evaluated, including reactions to previous doses—close supervision of patients with pre-existing asthma is recommended. [M]

- BREAST FEEDING Specialist sources indicate probably compatible (no information available). High molecular weight makes excretion into milk unlikely and inactivation in the gastrointestinal tract suggests limited absorption by the infant.

- **DIRECTIONS FOR ADMINISTRATION** [EvGr] Oral lyophilisates should be placed under the tongue and allowed to disperse. Advise patient not to swallow for 1 minute, or eat or drink for 5 minutes afterwards. The first dose should be taken under medical supervision and the patient should be monitored for at least 30 minutes. Ⓜ

- **PRESCRIBING AND DISPENSING INFORMATION**
▸ With subcutaneous use Each set of allergen extracts usually contains vials for the administration of graded amounts of allergen to patients undergoing hyposensitisation. Maintenance sets containing vials at the highest strength are also available. Product literature must be consulted for details of allergens, vial strengths, and administration.

- **PATIENT AND CARER ADVICE**
Administration Patients or carers should be given advice on how to administer oral lyophilisates.
Asthma
▸ With sublingual use Patients or carers should be advised to seek immediate medical attention if their asthma deteriorates suddenly during treatment.
Eosinophilic oesophagitis
▸ With sublingual use Patients or carers should be advised to seek medical attention if severe or persistent gastro-oesophageal symptoms (such as dysphagia or dyspepsia) develop during treatment.
Missed doses
▸ With sublingual use If treatment is interrupted for more than 7 days, patients or carers should be advised to seek medical advice before resuming treatment.

- **MEDICINAL FORMS** There can be variation in the licensing of different medicines containing the same drug.
Form unstated
▸ Pollinex Trees (Allergy Therapeutics (UK) Ltd)
Pollinex Trees suspension for injection treatment and extension course vials | 4 vial [PoM] £450.00
Oral lyophilisate
CAUTIONARY AND ADVISORY LABELS 26
▸ Itulazax (ALK-Abello Ltd) ▼
Birch (Betula verrucosa) pollen allergen extract 12 SQ-Bet Itulazax 12 SQ-Bet oral lyophilisates | 30 tablet [PoM] £80.12 [SF]
Suspension for injection
▸ Pollinex Trees (Allergy Therapeutics (UK) Ltd)
Pollinex Trees No 3 suspension for injection 1ml vials | 1 vial [PoM] 🛇
Pollinex Trees No 2 suspension for injection 1ml vials | 1 vial [PoM] 🛇
Pollinex Trees No 1 suspension for injection 1ml vials | 1 vial [PoM] 🛇

Wasp venom extract

30-Sep-2024

- **INDICATIONS AND DOSE**
Hypersensitivity to wasp venom (under expert supervision)
▸ BY SUBCUTANEOUS INJECTION
▸ Adult: (consult product literature)

IMPORTANT SAFETY INFORMATION
DESENSITISING VACCINES
In view of concerns about the safety of desensitising vaccines, it is recommended that they are used by specialists and only for licensed indications.
[EvGr] Desensitising vaccines should generally be avoided or used with particular care in patients with asthma. Ⓜ

- **CONTRA-INDICATIONS** Consult product literature
- **CAUTIONS** Consult product literature
- **INTERACTIONS** → Appendix 1: wasp venom extract
- **SIDE-EFFECTS** Consult product literature.

Hypersensitivity reactions Hypersensitivity reactions to immunotherapy can be life-threatening. Cardiopulmonary resuscitation must be immediately available and patients need to be monitored for at least 30 minutes after administration. If symptoms or signs of hypersensitivity develop (e.g. rash, urticaria, bronchospasm, faintness), **even when mild**, the patient should be observed until these have resolved completely.

- **PREGNANCY** [EvGr] Avoid initiating up-dosing treatment (no information available). If pregnancy occurs during maintenance treatment, *Alutard SQ Wasp Venom*® may be continued after the general condition of the patient is evaluated, including reactions to previous injections. Ⓜ

- **BREAST FEEDING** Specialist sources indicate probably compatible (no information available). High molecular weight makes excretion into milk unlikely and inactivation in the gastrointestinal tract suggests limited absorption by the infant.

- **DIRECTIONS FOR ADMINISTRATION** [EvGr] For *subcutaneous injection (Alutard SQ Wasp Venom*®), the vial must be turned slowly upside down 10 to 20 times to make a homogenous suspension before use. Administer slowly, either laterally in the distal part of the upper arm or dorsally in the proximal part of the forearm. Ⓜ

- **PRESCRIBING AND DISPENSING INFORMATION** Each set of allergen extracts usually contains vials for the administration of graded amounts of allergen to patients undergoing hyposensitisation. Maintenance sets containing vials at the highest strength are also available. Product literature must be consulted for details of allergens, vial strengths, and administration.

- **HANDLING AND STORAGE** Store unopened vials in a refrigerator (2–8°C) and protect from light. Once opened, vials may be stored for a maximum of 6 months in a refrigerator (2–8°C) when used for one individual patient.

- **PATIENT AND CARER ADVICE** Patients and carers should be counselled to avoid physical exercise, hot baths, and alcohol on the day of injection—potential amplification of anaphylactic reaction. They should also be advised to seek immediate medical attention if severe delayed systemic reactions develop, and to inform their doctor before the next injection of any local or systemic reactions that occur subsequently.
Asthma Patients and carers should be advised to seek immediate medical attention if their asthma deteriorates suddenly during treatment.
Driving and skilled tasks Patients and carers should be counselled on the effects on driving and performance of skilled tasks—increased risk of dizziness or vertigo.

- **NATIONAL FUNDING/ACCESS DECISIONS**
For full details see funding body website
NICE decisions
▸ *Pharmalgen*® for bee and wasp venom allergy (February 2012) NICE TA246 Recommended with restrictions

- **MEDICINAL FORMS** There can be variation in the licensing of different medicines containing the same drug.
Suspension for injection
▸ Alutard SQ Wasp Venom (ALK-Abello Ltd)
Wasp venom 100 SQ-U per 1 ml Alutard SQ Wasp Venom 500 SQ-U/5ml suspension for injection vials | 1 vial [PoM] 🛇 (Hospital only)
Wasp venom 1000 SQ-U per 1 ml Alutard SQ Wasp Venom 5,000 SQ-U/5ml suspension for injection vials | 1 vial [PoM] 🛇 (Hospital only)
Wasp venom 10000 SQ-U per 1 ml Alutard SQ Wasp Venom 50,000 SQ-U/5ml suspension for injection vials | 1 vial [PoM] 🛇 (Hospital only)
Wasp venom 100000 SQ-U per 1 ml Alutard SQ Wasp Venom maintenance pack suspension for injection vials | 1 vial [PoM] £462.61 (Hospital only)

2.1 Angioedema

DRUGS USED IN HEREDITARY ANGIOEDEMA ›
COMPLEMENT REGULATORY PROTEINS

C1-esterase inhibitor
30-Oct-2020

- **INDICATIONS AND DOSE**

BERINERT ®

Acute attacks of hereditary angioedema (under expert supervision)
- ▸ BY SLOW INTRAVENOUS INJECTION, OR BY INTRAVENOUS INFUSION
- ▸ Adult: 20 units/kg

Short-term prophylaxis of hereditary angioedema before dental, medical, or surgical procedures (under expert supervision)
- ▸ BY SLOW INTRAVENOUS INJECTION, OR BY INTRAVENOUS INFUSION
- ▸ Adult: 1000 units for 1 dose, to be administered less than 6 hours before procedure

CINRYZE ®

Acute attacks of hereditary angioedema (under expert supervision)
- ▸ BY SLOW INTRAVENOUS INJECTION
- ▸ Adult: 1000 units for 1 dose, dose may be repeated if necessary after 60 minutes (or sooner for patients experiencing laryngeal attacks or if treatment initiation is delayed)

Short-term prophylaxis of hereditary angioedema before dental, medical, or surgical procedures (under expert supervision)
- ▸ BY SLOW INTRAVENOUS INJECTION
- ▸ Adult: 1000 units for 1 dose, to be administered up to 24 hours before procedure

Long-term prophylaxis of severe, recurrent attacks of hereditary angioedema where acute treatment is inadequate, or when oral prophylaxis is inadequate or not tolerated (under expert supervision)
- ▸ BY SLOW INTRAVENOUS INJECTION
- ▸ Adult: 1000 units every 3–4 days, interval between doses to be adjusted according to response

- **CAUTIONS** Vaccination against hepatitis A and hepatitis B may be required

- **SIDE-EFFECTS**
- ▸ **Rare or very rare** Dizziness · dyspnoea · flushing · headache · hypersensitivity · hypertension · hypotension · nausea · tachycardia · thrombosis (with high doses) · urticaria

- **PREGNANCY** Manufacturer advises avoid unless essential.

- **PRESCRIBING AND DISPENSING INFORMATION** C1-esterase inhibitor is prepared from human plasma.

- **NATIONAL FUNDING/ACCESS DECISIONS**
  For full details see funding body website

  All Wales Medicines Strategy Group (AWMSG) decisions
  - ▸ C1 inhibitor (human) (*Cinryze*®) for the treatment and pre-procedure prevention of attacks of hereditary angioedema (HAE) in adults; routine prevention of angioedema attacks in adults with severe and recurrent attacks of HAE, where acute treatment is inadequate, or when oral prophylaxis is inadequate or not tolerated (October 2017) AWMSG No. 3295 Recommended

- **MEDICINAL FORMS** There can be variation in the licensing of different medicines containing the same drug.

  Powder and solvent for solution for injection
  ELECTROLYTES: May contain Sodium
  - ▸ Berinert P (CSL Behring UK Ltd)
    C1-esterase inhibitor human 500 unit Berinert 500unit powder and solvent for solution for injection vials | 1 vial [PoM] £670.00 DT = £670.00
    C1-esterase inhibitor human 1500 unit Berinert 1,500unit powder and solvent for solution for injection vials | 1 vial [PoM] £2,010.00 DT = £2,010.00
  - ▸ Cinryze (Takeda UK Ltd) ▼
    C1-esterase inhibitor human 500 unit Cinryze 500unit powder and solvent for solution for injection vials | 2 vial [PoM] £1,336.00

Conestat alfa
15-Jun-2021

- **INDICATIONS AND DOSE**

Acute attacks of hereditary angioedema in patients with C1-esterase inhibitor deficiency (under expert supervision)
- ▸ BY SLOW INTRAVENOUS INJECTION
- ▸ Adult (body-weight up to 84 kg): 50 units/kg for 1 dose, to be administered over 5 minutes, dose may be repeated if there has been an inadequate response after 120 minutes; maximum 2 doses per day
- ▸ Adult (body-weight 84 kg and above): 4200 units for 1 dose, to be administered over 5 minutes, dose may be repeated if there has been an inadequate response after 120 minutes; maximum 2 doses per day

- **CONTRA-INDICATIONS** Rabbit allergy

- **SIDE-EFFECTS**
- ▸ **Common or very common** Nausea
- ▸ **Uncommon** Abdominal discomfort · auricular swelling · diarrhoea · dizziness · headache · numbness · oral paraesthesia · throat irritation · urticaria · vertigo

- **ALLERGY AND CROSS-SENSITIVITY** [EvGr] Caution—possible risk of hypersensitivity reaction in presence of a clinical allergy to cows' milk. ⟨M⟩

- **PREGNANCY** Use only if potential benefit outweighs risk—toxicity in *animal* studies.

- **BREAST FEEDING** Use only if potential benefit outweighs risk—no information available.

- **PRESCRIBING AND DISPENSING INFORMATION** Conestat alfa is a biological medicine. Biological medicines must be prescribed and dispensed by brand name, see *Biological medicines* and *Biosimilar medicines*, under Guidance on prescribing p. 1; record the brand name and batch number after each administration.

- **PATIENT AND CARER ADVICE**
  Driving and skilled tasks Patients and carers should be counselled on the effects on driving and performance of skilled tasks—increased risk of headache, vertigo or dizziness.

- **NATIONAL FUNDING/ACCESS DECISIONS**
  For full details see funding body website

  Scottish Medicines Consortium (SMC) decisions
  - ▸ Conestat alfa (*Ruconest*®) for the treatment of acute angioedema attacks in adults and adolescents with hereditary angioedema (HAE) due to C1-esterase inhibitor deficiency (August 2018) SMC No. 745/11 Recommended

  All Wales Medicines Strategy Group (AWMSG) decisions
  - ▸ Conestat alfa (*Ruconest*®) for the treatment of acute angioedema attacks in adults, adolescents and children (aged 2 years and above) with hereditary angioedema (HAE) due to C1-esterase inhibitor deficiency (May 2021) AWMSG No. 4519 Recommended

- **MEDICINAL FORMS** There can be variation in the licensing of different medicines containing the same drug.
  Powder and solvent for solution for injection
  ELECTROLYTES: May contain Sodium
  ▶ Ruconest (Pharming Group N.V.)
    Conestat alfa 2100 unit Ruconest 2,100unit powder and solvent for solution for injection vials | 1 vial [PoM] £715.00 (Hospital only)

DRUGS USED IN HEREDITARY ANGIOEDEMA ›
KALLIKREIN INHIBITORS

Berotralstat

01-Apr-2022

- **DRUG ACTION** Berotralstat is a plasma kallikrein inhibitor, which limits the production of bradykinin, a potent vasodilator associated with angioedema attacks.

- **INDICATIONS AND DOSE**

  Prevention of recurrent attacks of hereditary angioedema
  ▶ BY MOUTH
  ▶ Adult (body-weight 40 kg and above): 150 mg once daily, dose to be taken with food

- **CONTRA-INDICATIONS** Body-weight less than 40 kg · not a treatment for acute attacks of angioedema—initiate individualised treatment for breakthrough attacks

- **CAUTIONS** Risk factors for QT prolongation
  CAUTIONS, FURTHER INFORMATION
  ▶ QT prolongation [EvGr] If treatment with berotralstat is unavoidable, monitoring is recommended—consult product literature. ⓜ

- **INTERACTIONS** → Appendix 1: berotralstat

- **SIDE-EFFECTS**
  ▶ **Common or very common** Diarrhoea · gastrointestinal discomfort · gastrointestinal disorders · headaches · rash · vomiting

- **CONCEPTION AND CONTRACEPTION** [EvGr] Females of childbearing potential should use effective contraception during and for at least 1 month after last treatment. Efficacy of desogestrel-containing contraceptives may be reduced—consult product literature. ⓜ

- **PREGNANCY** [EvGr] Avoid—limited information available. ⓜ

- **BREAST FEEDING** [EvGr] Avoid—present in milk in *animal* studies. ⓜ

- **HEPATIC IMPAIRMENT** [EvGr] Avoid in moderate or severe impairment (risk of increased exposure). ⓜ

- **RENAL IMPAIRMENT** [EvGr] Avoid in severe impairment (increased risk of prolonged QT); if treatment is unavoidable, monitoring is required—consult product literature. ⓜ

- **PATIENT AND CARER ADVICE**
  Missed doses If a dose is missed or not taken at the usual time, the missed dose should be taken as soon as possible on the same day. The next dose should be taken at the usual time.

- **NATIONAL FUNDING/ACCESS DECISIONS**
  For full details see funding body website
  NICE decisions
  ▶ Berotralstat for preventing recurrent attacks of hereditary angioedema (October 2021) NICE TA738 Recommended with restrictions

  Scottish Medicines Consortium (SMC) decisions
  ▶ Berotralstat (*Orladeyo* ®) for the routine prevention of recurrent attacks of hereditary angioedema (HAE) in adult and adolescent patients aged 12 years and older (March 2022) SMC No. SMC2405 Recommended with restrictions

- **MEDICINAL FORMS** There can be variation in the licensing of different medicines containing the same drug.
  Oral capsule
  CAUTIONARY AND ADVISORY LABELS 21
  EXCIPIENTS: May contain Gelatin
  ▶ Orladeyo (BioCryst Ireland Ltd) ▼
    Berotralstat (as Berotralstat dihydrochloride) 150 mg Orladeyo 150mg capsules | 28 capsule [PoM] £10,205.00 (Hospital only)

Lanadelumab

09-Nov-2020

- **DRUG ACTION** Lanadelumab is a humanised monoclonal antibody which inhibits plasma kallikrein activity, thereby limiting the production of bradykinin, a potent vasodilator associated with angioedema attacks in patients with hereditary angioedema.

- **INDICATIONS AND DOSE**

  Prevention of recurrent attacks of hereditary angioedema (initiated under specialist supervision)
  ▶ BY SUBCUTANEOUS INJECTION
  ▶ Adult: 300 mg every 2 weeks, reduced to 300 mg every 4 weeks, in those stable and attack free—consult product literature

- **CONTRA-INDICATIONS** Not a treatment for acute attacks of angioedema—initiate individualised treatment for breakthrough attacks

- **SIDE-EFFECTS**
  ▶ **Common or very common** Dizziness · hypersensitivity · myalgia · oral disorders · skin reactions

- **PREGNANCY** Manufacturer advises preferable to avoid—limited or no information available; *animal* studies do not indicate toxicity.

- **BREAST FEEDING** Manufacturer advises avoid during first few days after birth—possible risk from transfer of antibodies to infant. After this time, use during breast-feeding only if clinically needed.

- **EFFECT ON LABORATORY TESTS** Manufacturer advises may increase activated partial thromboplastin time (aPTT) due to an interaction with the aPTT assay—consult product literature.

- **DIRECTIONS FOR ADMINISTRATION** Manufacturer advises to withdraw dose from the vial into a syringe with an 18 gauge needle and inject, using a suitable gauge needle, into the abdomen, thigh, or upper outer arm within 2 hours—consult product literature for further information. *Takhzyro* ® may be self-administered or administered by a carer after appropriate training in subcutaneous injection technique.

- **PRESCRIBING AND DISPENSING INFORMATION**
  Lanadelumab is a biological medicine. Biological medicines must be prescribed and dispensed by brand name, see *Biological medicines* and *Biosimilar medicines*, under Guidance on prescribing p. 1; manufacturer advises to record the brand name and batch number after each administration.

- **HANDLING AND STORAGE** Manufacturer advises store in a refrigerator (2–8°C) and protect from light—consult product literature for further information regarding storage outside refrigerator.

- **PATIENT AND CARER ADVICE**
  Self-administration Manufacturer advises patients and their carers should be given training in subcutaneous injection technique if appropriate.
  Missed doses Manufacturer advises if a dose is missed, it should be taken as soon as possible ensuring at least 10 days between doses.

- **NATIONAL FUNDING/ACCESS DECISIONS**
  For full details see funding body website
  NICE decisions
  ▶ Lanadelumab for preventing recurrent attacks of hereditary angioedema (October 2019) NICE TA606 Recommended with restrictions
  Scottish Medicines Consortium (SMC) decisions
  ▶ Lanadelumab (*Takhzyro*®) for routine prevention of recurrent attacks of hereditary angioedema (HAE) in patients aged 12 years and older (December 2019) SMC No. SMC2206 Recommended with restrictions

- **MEDICINAL FORMS** There can be variation in the licensing of different medicines containing the same drug.
  Solution for injection
  EXCIPIENTS: May contain Polysorbates
  ▶ Takhzyro (Takeda UK Ltd)
    Lanadelumab 150 mg per 1 ml Takhzyro 150mg/1ml solution for injection pre-filled syringes | 1 pre-filled disposable injection [PoM] £12,420.00 (Hospital only)
    Takhzyro 300mg/2ml solution for injection pre-filled syringes | 1 pre-filled disposable injection [PoM] £12,420.00 (Hospital only)

DRUGS USED IN HEREDITARY ANGIOEDEMA ›
SELECTIVE BRADYKININ B$_2$ ANTAGONISTS

Icatibant
22-Oct-2020

- **INDICATIONS AND DOSE**
  Acute attacks of hereditary angioedema in patients with C1-esterase inhibitor deficiency
  ▶ BY SUBCUTANEOUS INJECTION
  ▶ Adult: 30 mg for 1 dose, then 30 mg after 6 hours if required, then 30 mg after 6 hours if required; maximum 3 doses per day

- **CAUTIONS** Ischaemic heart disease · stroke
- **INTERACTIONS** → Appendix 1: icatibant
- **SIDE-EFFECTS**
  ▶ **Common or very common** Dizziness · fever · headache · nausea · skin reactions
- **PREGNANCY** Manufacturer advises use only if potential benefit outweighs risk—toxicity in *animal* studies.
- **BREAST FEEDING** Manufacturer advises avoid for 12 hours after administration.
- **NATIONAL FUNDING/ACCESS DECISIONS**
  For full details see funding body website
  Scottish Medicines Consortium (SMC) decisions
  ▶ Icatibant (*Firazyr*®) for the symptomatic treatment of acute attacks of hereditary angioedema (HAE) in adults (type I and II HAE) (March 2012) SMC No. 476/08 Recommended
  All Wales Medicines Strategy Group (AWMSG) decisions
  ▶ Icatibant acetate (*Firazyr*®) for the symptomatic treatment of acute attacks of hereditary angioedema (HAE) in adults, adolescents and children aged 2 years and older, with C1 esterase-inhibitor deficiency (June 2018) AWMSG No. 3293 Recommended

- **MEDICINAL FORMS** There can be variation in the licensing of different medicines containing the same drug.
  Solution for injection
  ▶ Icatibant (Non-proprietary)
    Icatibant (as Icatibant acetate) 10 mg per 1 ml Icatibant 30mg/3ml solution for injection pre-filled syringes | 1 pre-filled disposable injection [PoM] £1,395.00 | 1 pre-filled disposable injection [PoM] £837.00-£1,395.00 (Hospital only) | 3 pre-filled disposable injection [PoM] £4,185.00 (Hospital only)
  ▶ Firazyr (Takeda UK Ltd)
    Icatibant (as Icatibant acetate) 10 mg per 1 ml Firazyr 30mg/3ml solution for injection pre-filled syringes | 1 pre-filled disposable injection [PoM] £1,395.00 (Hospital only)

3   Conditions affecting sputum viscosity

MUCOLYTICS

Acetylcysteine
01-Aug-2024

- **INDICATIONS AND DOSE**
  NACSYS® EFFERVESCENT TABLETS
  Reduction of sputum viscosity
  ▶ BY MOUTH
  ▶ Adult: 600 mg once daily

- **CAUTIONS** Asthma · history of peptic ulceration
- **INTERACTIONS** → Appendix 1: acetylcysteine
- **SIDE-EFFECTS**
  ▶ **Uncommon** Diarrhoea · fever · gastrointestinal discomfort · headache · hypotension · nausea · stomatitis · tinnitus · vomiting
  ▶ **Rare or very rare** Haemorrhage
  ▶ **Frequency not known** Face oedema

- **MEDICINAL FORMS** There can be variation in the licensing of different medicines containing the same drug.
  Effervescent tablet
  CAUTIONARY AND ADVISORY LABELS 13
  ELECTROLYTES: May contain Sodium
  ▶ NACSYS (Alturix Ltd)
    Acetylcysteine 600 mg NACSYS 600mg effervescent tablets | 30 tablet [PoM] £5.50 DT = £5.50 [SF]

Carbocisteine
02-Jan-2024

- **INDICATIONS AND DOSE**
  Reduction of sputum viscosity
  ▶ BY MOUTH
  ▶ Adult: Initially 2.25 g daily in 3 divided doses, then reduced to 1.5 g daily in 2–4 divided doses, dose to be reduced as condition improves

- **CONTRA-INDICATIONS** Active peptic ulceration
- **CAUTIONS** History of peptic ulceration (may disrupt the gastric mucosal barrier)
- **SIDE-EFFECTS** Gastrointestinal haemorrhage · skin reactions · Stevens-Johnson syndrome · vomiting
- **PREGNANCY** Manufacturer advises avoid in first trimester.
- **BREAST FEEDING** No information available.
- **PRESCRIBING AND DISPENSING INFORMATION** Flavours of oral liquid formulations may include cherry, raspberry, cinnamon, or rum.

- **MEDICINAL FORMS** There can be variation in the licensing of different medicines containing the same drug.
  Oral solution
  ▶ Carbocisteine (Non-proprietary)
    Carbocisteine 50 mg per 1 ml Carbocisteine 250mg/5ml oral solution sugar free | 300 ml [PoM] £9.49 DT = £8.39 [SF]
    Carbocisteine 250mg/5ml oral solution | 300 ml [PoM] £7.55 DT = £5.48
    Carbocisteine 75 mg per 1 ml Carbocisteine 750mg/10ml oral solution 10ml sachets sugar free | 15 sachet [PoM] £3.85 DT = £5.54 [SF]
    Carbocisteine 150 mg per 1 ml Carbocisteine 750mg/5ml oral solution sugar free | 100 ml [PoM] £19.23 [SF] | 200 ml [PoM] £37.42 DT = £37.42 [SF]
  ▶ Mucodyne (Sanofi)
    Carbocisteine 50 mg per 1 ml Mucodyne 250mg/5ml syrup | 300 ml [PoM] £8.39 DT = £5.48

Oral capsule

▸ Carbocisteine (Non-proprietary)
Carbocisteine 375 mg Carbocisteine 375mg capsules |
120 capsule [PoM] £18.98 DT = £2.69
Carbocisteine 750 mg Carbocisteine 750mg capsules |
60 capsule [PoM] £30.36 DT = £18.98

Erdosteine

23-Jul-2021

● **INDICATIONS AND DOSE**

Symptomatic treatment of acute exacerbations of chronic bronchitis

▸ BY MOUTH
▸ Adult: 300 mg twice daily for up to 10 days

● **CAUTIONS** History of peptic ulceration (may disrupt the gastric mucosal barrier)

● **SIDE-EFFECTS**
▸ **Common or very common** Epigastric pain · taste altered
▸ **Uncommon** Allergic dermatitis · angioedema · common cold · diarrhoea · dyspnoea · headache · nausea · vomiting

● **PREGNANCY** Manufacturer advises avoid—no information available.

● **BREAST FEEDING** Manufacturer advises avoid—no information available.

● **HEPATIC IMPAIRMENT** Manufacturer advises caution in mild to moderate hepatic failure; avoid in severe hepatic failure.
Dose adjustments Manufacturer advises max. 300 mg daily in mild to moderate hepatic failure.

● **RENAL IMPAIRMENT** [EvGr] Avoid if creatinine clearance less than 25 mL/minute (no information available). Ⓜ See p. 21.

● **NATIONAL FUNDING/ACCESS DECISIONS**
For full details see funding body website
Scottish Medicines Consortium (SMC) decisions
▸ Erdosteine (*Erdotin*®) for chronic bronchitis in adults (November 2007) SMC No. 415/07 Not recommended

● **MEDICINAL FORMS** There can be variation in the licensing of different medicines containing the same drug.
Oral capsule
▸ Erdotin (Galen Ltd)
Erdosteine 300 mg Erdotin 300mg capsules | 20 capsule [PoM]
£5.00 DT = £5.00

3.1 Cystic fibrosis

Cystic fibrosis

07-Aug-2024

Description of condition

Cystic fibrosis is a genetic disorder affecting the lungs, pancreas, liver, intestine, and reproductive organs. The main clinical signs are pulmonary disease, with recurrent infections and the production of copious viscous sputum, and malabsorption due to pancreatic insufficiency. Other complications include hepatobiliary disease, osteoporosis, cystic fibrosis-related diabetes, and distal intestinal obstruction syndrome.

Aims of treatment

The aim of treatment includes preventing and managing lung infections, loosening and removing thick, sticky mucus from the lungs, preventing or treating intestinal obstruction, and providing sufficient nutrition and hydration.

Lung function is a key predictor of life expectancy in people with cystic fibrosis and optimising lung function is a major aim of care.

Non-drug treatment

Specialist physiotherapists should assess patients with cystic fibrosis and provide advice on airway clearance, nebuliser use, musculoskeletal disorders, physical activity, and urinary incontinence. The importance of airway clearance techniques should be discussed with patients and their parents or carers and appropriate training provided. Patients should be advised that regular exercise improves both lung function and overall fitness.

Drug treatment

Treatment for cystic fibrosis lung disease is based on the prevention of lung infection and the maintenance of lung function. [EvGr] In patients with cystic fibrosis, who have clinical evidence of lung disease, the frequency of routine review should be based on their clinical condition, but adults should be reviewed at least every 3 months. More frequent review is required immediately after diagnosis. Ⓐ

Cystic fibrosis transmembrane conductance regulator (CFTR) modulators
[EvGr] CFTR modulators can be used for the treatment of cystic fibrosis in certain patients (specialist use). Ⓐ

Mucolytics
[EvGr] Patients with cystic fibrosis who have evidence of lung disease should be offered a mucolytic. Dornase alfa p. 335 is the first choice mucolytic. If there is an inadequate response, dornase alfa p. 335 and hypertonic sodium chloride p. 314, or hypertonic sodium chloride p. 314 alone should be considered.

Mannitol dry powder for inhalation p. 338 is recommended as an option when dornase alfa p. 335 is unsuitable (because of ineligibility, intolerance, or inadequate response), when lung function is rapidly declining, and if other osmotic drugs are not considered appropriate (see mannitol p. 338 National funding/access decisions). Ⓐ

Pulmonary infection
Staphylococcus aureus
[EvGr] Patients who are not taking prophylaxis and have a new *Staphylococcus aureus* infection can be given an oral anti-*Staph. aureus* antibacterial, if they are clinically well. If they are clinically unwell and have pulmonary disease, oral or intravenous (depending on infection severity) broad-spectrum antibacterials with activity against *Staph. aureus* should be given (consult local protocol).

A long-term antibacterial should be considered to suppress **chronic** *Staph. aureus* respiratory infections in patients whose pulmonary disease is stable. In patients with chronic *Staph. aureus* respiratory infections who become clinically unwell with pulmonary disease, oral or intravenous (depending on infection severity) broad-spectrum antibacterials with activity against *Staph. aureus* should be given. In those patients with new evidence of **meticillin-resistant** *Staphylococcus aureus* (MRSA) respiratory infection (with or without pulmonary exacerbation), specialist microbiological advice should be sought.

Antibacterials should not be routinely used to suppress chronic MRSA in patients with stable pulmonary disease.

If a patient with cystic fibrosis and chronic MRSA respiratory infection becomes unwell with a pulmonary exacerbation or shows a decline in pulmonary function, specialist microbiological advice should be sought. Ⓐ

Pseudomonas aeruginosa
[EvGr] If a patient with cystic fibrosis develops a new *Pseudomonas aeruginosa* infection, eradication therapy with a course of oral antibacterial should be started (by intravenous injection, if they are clinically unwell), in combination with an inhaled antibacterial. An extended course of oral and inhaled antibacterial should follow (consult local protocol).

If eradication therapy is not successful, sustained treatment with an inhaled antibacterial should be offered. Nebulised colistimethate sodium p. 645 should be considered as first-line treatment (but see also colistimethate sodium by dry powder inhalation p. 645 National funding/access decisions).

In patients with **chronic** *Ps. aeruginosa* infection (when treatment has not eradicated the infection) who become clinically unwell with pulmonary exacerbations, an oral antibacterial or a combination of two intravenous antibacterial drugs of different classes (depending on infection severity) should be used. Changing antibacterial regimens should be considered to treat exacerbations (consult local protocol).

Nebulised aztreonam p. 626, nebulised tobramycin p. 598, or tobramycin dry powder for inhalation p. 598 (see tobramycin p. 598 National funding/access decisions) should be considered for those who are deteriorating despite regular inhaled colistimethate sodium p. 645. Ⓐ

Burkholderia cepacia complex
EvGr Patients who develop a new *Burkholderia cepacia* complex infection, should be given eradication therapy with a combination of intravenous antibacterial drugs (specialist microbiological advice should be sought on the choice of antibacterials). Ⓐ There is no evidence to support using antibacterials to suppress **chronic** *Burkholderia cepacia* complex infection in patients with cystic fibrosis who have stable pulmonary status.

EvGr Specialist microbiological advice should be sought for patients with chronic *Burkholderia cepacia* complex infection (when treatment has not eradicated the infection) and who become clinically unwell with a pulmonary disease exacerbation.

An inhaled antibacterial should be considered for those who have chronic *Burkholderia cepacia* complex infection and declining pulmonary status; treatment should be stopped if there is no observed benefit. Ⓐ

Haemophilus influenzae
EvGr *Haemophilus influenzae* infection in the absence of clinical evidence of pulmonary infection should be treated with an appropriate oral antibacterial drug. In those who are unwell with clinical evidence of pulmonary infection, an appropriate antibacterial should be given by mouth or intravenously depending on the severity of the illness (consult local protocol). Ⓐ

Non-tuberculous mycobacteria
EvGr Non-tuberculous mycobacterial eradication therapy should be considered for patients with cystic fibrosis who are clinically unwell and whose pulmonary disease has not responded to other recommended treatments. Specialist microbiological advice should be sought on the choice of antibacterial and on the duration of treatment. Ⓐ

Aspergillus fumigatus complex
EvGr Treatment with an antifungal drug should only be considered to suppress **chronic** *Aspergillus fumigatus* complex respiratory infection in patients with declining pulmonary status. Specialist microbiological advice should be sought on the choice of antifungal drug. Ⓐ

Unidentified infections
EvGr An oral or intravenous (depending on the exacerbation severity) broad-spectrum antibacterial should be used for patients who have a pulmonary disease exacerbation and no clear cause. If a causative pathogen is identified, an appropriate treatment should be selected (consult local protocol). Ⓐ

Immunomodulatory drugs
EvGr Long-term treatment with azithromycin p. 620 [unlicensed indication], at an immunomodulatory dose, should be offered to patients with deteriorating lung function or repeated pulmonary exacerbations. In those patients with continued deterioration in lung function or

continuing pulmonary exacerbations, long-term azithromycin p. 620 should be discontinued and the use of an oral corticosteroid considered. Ⓐ

Nutrition and exocrine pancreatic insufficiency
EvGr The cystic fibrosis specialist dietitian should offer advice on optimal nutrition.

Pancreatin p. 76 should be offered to patients with exocrine pancreatic insufficiency. Dose should be adjusted as needed to minimise any symptoms or signs of malabsorption (see Exocrine pancreatic insufficiency p. 75). An acid-suppressing drug, such as an H_2 receptor antagonist or a proton pump inhibitor [unlicensed indications] can be considered for patients who have persistent symptoms or signs of malabsorption.

A short-term trial of an appetite stimulant (for example up to 3 months) [unlicensed indication] can be considered in adult patients if attempts to increase calorie intake are not effective. Ⓐ

Distal intestinal obstruction syndrome
EvGr Oral or intravenous fluids should be offered to ensure adequate hydration for patients with distal intestinal obstruction syndrome. Meglumine amidotrizoate with sodium amidotrizoate solution (orally or via an enteral tube) should be considered as first-line treatment for distal intestinal obstruction syndrome. An iso-osmotic polyethylene glycol and electrolyte solution (macrogols) (orally or via an enteral tube) can be considered as a second-line treatment. Surgery is a last resort, if prolonged treatment with a polyethylene glycol solution is not effective. Suspected distal intestinal obstruction syndrome should be managed in a specialist cystic fibrosis centre. Ⓐ

Liver disease
EvGr If liver function blood tests are abnormal in patients with cystic fibrosis, ursodeoxycholic acid p. 100 [unlicensed indication] can be given until liver function is restored. Ⓐ

Bone mineral density
EvGr Patients should be monitored for cystic fibrosis-related low bone mineral density. Ⓐ

Cystic fibrosis-related diabetes
EvGr Patients should be monitored for cystic fibrosis-related diabetes. Ⓐ

Useful Resources
Cystic fibrosis: diagnosis and management. National Institute for Health and Care Excellence. NICE guideline 78. October 2017
www.nice.org.uk/guidance/NG78

MUCOLYTICS

Dornase alfa
17-Aug-2020

(Phosphorylated glycosylated recombinant human deoxyribonuclease 1 (rhDNase))

● **DRUG ACTION** Dornase alfa is a genetically engineered version of a naturally occurring human enzyme which cleaves extracellular deoxyribonucleic acid (DNA).

● **INDICATIONS AND DOSE**

Management of cystic fibrosis patients with a forced vital capacity (FVC) of greater than 40% of predicted to improve pulmonary function
▸ BY INHALATION OF NEBULISED SOLUTION
▸ Adult: 2500 units once daily, administered by jet nebuliser, patients over 21 years may benefit from twice daily dosage

DOSE EQUIVALENCE AND CONVERSION
▸ Dornase alfa 1000 units is equivalent to 1 mg.

- **SIDE-EFFECTS** Chest pain · conjunctivitis · dyspepsia · dysphonia · dyspnoea · fever · increased risk of infection · skin reactions
- **PREGNANCY** No evidence of teratogenicity; manufacturer advises use only if potential benefit outweighs risk.
- **BREAST FEEDING** Amount probably too small to be harmful—manufacturer advises caution.
- **DIRECTIONS FOR ADMINISTRATION** Dornase alfa is administered undiluted by inhalation using a jet nebuliser; ultrasonic nebulisers are unsuitable. Expert sources advise usually once daily at least 1 hour before physiotherapy.

- **MEDICINAL FORMS** There can be variation in the licensing of different medicines containing the same drug.
Nebuliser liquid
  - ▸ Pulmozyme (Roche Products Ltd)
  Dornase alfa 1 mg per 1 ml Pulmozyme 2.5mg nebuliser liquid 2.5ml ampoules | 30 ampoule [PoM] £496.43 DT = £496.43

Ivacaftor
06-Aug-2024

- **DRUG ACTION** Ivacaftor is a cystic fibrosis transmembrane conductance regulator (CFTR) protein potentiator that increases chloride transport in the abnormal CFTR protein.

- **INDICATIONS AND DOSE**
Cystic fibrosis (specialist use only)
  - ▸ BY MOUTH USING GRANULES
  - ▸ Adult: Use tablets
Cystic fibrosis (specialist use only)
  - ▸ BY MOUTH USING TABLETS
  - ▸ Adult: 150 mg every 12 hours
DOSE ADJUSTMENTS DUE TO INTERACTIONS
  - ▸ [EvGr] *For tablets,* reduce dose to 150 mg twice a week with concurrent use of potent CYP3A4 inhibitors; the evening dose of ivacaftor should not be taken.
  - ▸ *For tablets,* reduce dose to 150 mg once daily with concurrent use of moderate CYP3A4 inhibitors; the evening dose of ivacaftor should not be taken. Ⓜ

IMPORTANT SAFETY INFORMATION
MHRA/CHM ADVICE: IVACAFTOR, TEZACAFTOR, ELEXACAFTOR (*KAFTRIO*®) IN COMBINATION WITH IVACAFTOR (*KALYDECO*®): RISK OF SERIOUS LIVER INJURY; UPDATED ADVICE ON LIVER FUNCTION TESTING (FEBRUARY 2022)
A European review of safety data identified a case of liver failure requiring transplantation in an adult patient, with pre-existing cirrhosis and portal hypertension, taking ivacaftor/tezacaftor/elexacaftor (*Kaftrio*®) in combination with ivacaftor (*Kalydeco*®). Other cases of serious liver injury, characterised by elevations in alanine aminotransferase (ALT), aspartate aminotransferase (AST), and total bilirubin, were also identified in 2 adult patients, with no history of liver disease, taking this combination.
  Healthcare professionals are advised to:
- measure total bilirubin levels in addition to ALT and AST levels before initiating treatment, every 3 months during the first year of treatment, and annually thereafter; more frequent monitoring should be considered in patients with a history of liver disease or transaminase elevations;
- use with caution and close monitoring in patients with advanced pre-existing liver disease, and only if the benefits outweigh the risks;
- promptly evaluate and measure liver function in patients who report symptoms that may indicate liver injury;
- discontinue treatment if significant elevation of liver enzymes occurs (see *Side-effects*), or signs and symptoms of liver injury develop; once liver abnormalities have resolved, consider the benefits and risks before resuming treatment.
Patients and carers should be counselled to seek immediate medical advice if signs of liver problems develop.

- **CAUTIONS** Organ transplantation (no information available)
- **INTERACTIONS** → Appendix 1: ivacaftor
- **SIDE-EFFECTS**
  - ▸ **Common or very common** Breast abnormalities · diarrhoea · dizziness · ear discomfort · flatulence · gastrointestinal discomfort · headache · hypoglycaemia · increased risk of infection · nasal complaints · nausea · oropharyngeal pain · ototoxicity · respiratory disorders · skin reactions · throat erythema · tympanic membrane hyperaemia
  - ▸ **Uncommon** Gynaecomastia
  - ▸ **Frequency not known** Hepatic disorders
  SIDE-EFFECTS, FURTHER INFORMATION Manufacturer advises interrupt treatment if transaminase levels more than 5 times the upper limit of normal *or* transaminase levels more than 3 times the upper limit of normal **and** blood bilirubin more than twice the upper limit of normal—consult product literature.
- **PREGNANCY** Manufacturer advises avoid—limited information available.
- **BREAST FEEDING** Manufacturer advises avoid—present in milk in *animal* studies.
- **HEPATIC IMPAIRMENT** [EvGr] Avoid unless benefit outweighs risk in severe impairment (risk of increased exposure–serious liver injury reported). Ⓜ
  Dose adjustments [EvGr] *For tablets,* reduce dose to 150 mg once daily in moderate impairment; in severe impairment reduce starting dose to 150 mg on alternate days or less frequently, adjust dosing interval according to clinical response and tolerability. The evening dose of ivacaftor should not be taken. Ⓜ
- **RENAL IMPAIRMENT** Manufacturer advises caution in severe impairment or end-stage renal disease—limited information available.
- **MONITORING REQUIREMENTS** [EvGr] Monitor liver function before treatment, every 3 months during the first year of treatment, then annually thereafter (more frequent monitoring should be considered in patients with a history of liver disease or transaminase elevations). Ⓜ
- **DIRECTIONS FOR ADMINISTRATION** [EvGr] *Tablets* should be taken with fat-containing food. Ⓜ
- **PRESCRIBING AND DISPENSING INFORMATION** Ivacaftor should be prescribed by a physician experienced in the treatment of cystic fibrosis.
- **PATIENT AND CARER ADVICE**
  Missed doses [EvGr] If a dose is more than 6 hours late, the missed dose should not be taken and the next dose should be taken at the normal time. Ⓜ
  Driving and skilled tasks [EvGr] Patients and their carers should be counselled on the effects on driving and skilled tasks—increased risk of dizziness. Ⓜ
- **NATIONAL FUNDING/ACCESS DECISIONS**
  For full details see funding body website
  Scottish Medicines Consortium (SMC) decisions
  - ▸ **Ivacaftor (*Kalydeco*®) for the treatment of patients with cystic fibrosis (CF) aged 18 years and older who have an R117H mutation in the CF transmembrane conductance regulator (CFTR) gene (December 2016) SMC No. 1193/16 Not recommended**

- **MEDICINAL FORMS** There can be variation in the licensing of different medicines containing the same drug.

Oral tablet

CAUTIONARY AND ADVISORY LABELS 25

▸ Kalydeco (Vertex Pharmaceuticals (Europe) Ltd)
  Ivacaftor 75 mg Kalydeco 75mg tablets | 28 tablet [PoM] £7,000.00 (Hospital only)
  Ivacaftor 150 mg Kalydeco 150mg tablets | 28 tablet [PoM] £7,000.00 (Hospital only) | 56 tablet [PoM] £14,000.00 (Hospital only)

Ivacaftor with tezacaftor and elexacaftor

13-Aug-2024

The properties listed below are those particular to the combination only. For the properties of the components please consider, ivacaftor p. 336, tezacaftor with ivacaftor p. 339.

- **INDICATIONS AND DOSE**

Cystic fibrosis (in combination with ivacaftor) [using tablets containing 75/50/100 mg ivacaftor/tezacaftor/elexacaftor] (specialist use only)

▸ BY MOUTH

▸ Adult: 2 tablets, to be taken in the morning and, *Ivacaftor* 150 mg to be taken in the evening (about 12 hours apart)

DOSE ADJUSTMENTS DUE TO INTERACTIONS

▸ [EvGr] With concurrent use of potent CYP3A4 inhibitors, reduce dose to 2 *tablets* twice a week, taken approximately 3–4 days apart; the evening dose of ivacaftor should not be taken.

▸ With concurrent use of moderate CYP3A4 inhibitors, reduce dose to 2 *tablets* every other morning, with ivacaftor taken in the mornings alternate to ivacaftor/tezacaftor/elexacaftor; the evening dose of ivacaftor should not be taken. ⟨M⟩

IMPORTANT SAFETY INFORMATION

MHRA/CHM ADVICE: IVACAFTOR, TEZACAFTOR, ELEXACAFTOR (*KAFTRIO*®) IN COMBINATION WITH IVACAFTOR (*KALYDECO*®): RISK OF SERIOUS LIVER INJURY; UPDATED ADVICE ON LIVER FUNCTION TESTING (FEBRUARY 2022)

A European review of safety data identified a case of liver failure requiring transplantation in an adult patient, with pre-existing cirrhosis and portal hypertension, taking ivacaftor/tezacaftor/elexacaftor (*Kaftrio*®) in combination with ivacaftor (*Kalydeco*®). Other cases of serious liver injury, characterised by elevations in alanine aminotransferase (ALT), aspartate aminotransferase (AST), and total bilirubin, were also identified in 2 adult patients, with no history of liver disease, taking this combination.

Healthcare professionals are advised to:

- measure total bilirubin levels in addition to ALT and AST levels before initiating treatment, every 3 months during the first year of treatment, and annually thereafter; more frequent monitoring should be considered in patients with a history of liver disease or transaminase elevations;
- use with caution and close monitoring in patients with advanced pre-existing liver disease, and only if the benefits outweigh the risks;
- promptly evaluate and measure liver function in patients who report symptoms that may indicate liver injury;
- discontinue treatment if significant elevation of liver enzymes occurs (see *Side-effects* of ivacaftor p. 336), or signs and symptoms of liver injury develop; once liver abnormalities have resolved, consider the benefits and risks before resuming treatment.

Patients and carers should be counselled to seek immediate medical advice if signs of liver problems develop.

- **INTERACTIONS** → Appendix 1: elexacaftor · ivacaftor · tezacaftor

- **SIDE-EFFECTS**

▸ **Common or very common** Breast abnormalities · diarrhoea · dizziness · ear discomfort · flatulence · gastrointestinal discomfort · headache · hypoglycaemia · increased risk of infection · nasal complaints · nausea · oropharyngeal pain · ototoxicity · respiratory disorders · skin reactions · throat erythema · tympanic membrane hyperaemia

▸ **Uncommon** Gynaecomastia

▸ **Frequency not known** Anxiety · concentration impaired · depressed mood · liver injury · memory impairment · mood altered · sleep disorder

SIDE-EFFECTS, FURTHER INFORMATION Manufacturer advises interrupt treatment if transaminase levels more than 5 times the upper limit of normal *or* transaminase levels more than 3 times the upper limit of normal **and** blood bilirubin more than twice the upper limit of normal—consult product literature.

- **HEPATIC IMPAIRMENT** [EvGr] Avoid in severe impairment; use with caution only if benefit outweighs risk in moderate impairment (risk of increased exposure–serious liver injury reported). ⟨M⟩
  Dose adjustments [EvGr] In moderate impairment, alternate dose between 1 and 2 *tablets* in the mornings, and omit evening dose of ivacaftor. ⟨M⟩

- **DIRECTIONS FOR ADMINISTRATION** [EvGr] *Tablets* should be taken with fat-containing food. ⟨M⟩

- **PATIENT AND CARER ADVICE**
  Missed doses Manufacturer advises if the morning dose is more than 6 hours late, the missed dose should be taken and the evening dose of ivacaftor omitted; the next morning dose should be taken at the normal time. If the evening dose of ivacaftor is more than 6 hours late, the missed dose should **not** be taken and the next morning dose should be taken at the normal time.

- **NATIONAL FUNDING/ACCESS DECISIONS**
  For full details see funding body website

NICE decisions

▸ Ivacaftor-tezacaftor-elexacaftor, tezacaftor-ivacaftor and lumacaftor-ivacaftor for treating cystic fibrosis (July 2024) NICE TA988 Recommended

Scottish Medicines Consortium (SMC) decisions

▸ Ivacaftor with tezacaftor and elexacaftor (*Kaftrio*®) in combination with ivacaftor for the treatment of cystic fibrosis in patients aged 2 years and older who have at least one F508del mutation in the cystic fibrosis transmembrane conductance regulator gene (July 2024) SMC No. SMC2713 Recommended

---

- **MEDICINAL FORMS** There can be variation in the licensing of different medicines containing the same drug.

Oral tablet

CAUTIONARY AND ADVISORY LABELS 25

▸ Kaftrio (Vertex Pharmaceuticals (Europe) Ltd) ▼
  Tezacaftor 25 mg, Ivacaftor 37.5 mg, Elexacaftor 50 mg Kaftrio 37.5mg/25mg/50mg tablets | 56 tablet [PoM] £8,346.30 (Hospital only)
  Tezacaftor 50 mg, Ivacaftor 75 mg, Elexacaftor 100 mg Kaftrio 75mg/50mg/100mg tablets | 56 tablet [PoM] £8,346.30 (Hospital only)

Lumacaftor with ivacaftor

12-Aug-2024

The properties listed below are those particular to the combination only. For the properties of the components please consider, ivacaftor p. 336.

● **INDICATIONS AND DOSE**

Cystic fibrosis (specialist use only)

▶ BY MOUTH USING TABLETS

▶ Adult: 400/250 mg every 12 hours

DOSE ADJUSTMENTS DUE TO INTERACTIONS

▶ [EvGr] Reduce initial dose to 200/125 mg once daily for the first week in those already taking a potent CYP3A4 inhibitor. Ⓜ

DOSE EQUIVALENCE AND CONVERSION

▶ Dose expressed as *x/y* mg of lumacaftor/ivacaftor.

● **CAUTIONS** Forced expiratory volume in 1 second (FEV$_1$) less than 40% of the predicted normal value—additional monitoring recommended at initiation of treatment · pulmonary exacerbation—no information available

● **INTERACTIONS** → Appendix 1: ivacaftor · lumacaftor

● **SIDE-EFFECTS**

▶ **Common or very common** Breast abnormalities · diarrhoea · dizziness · dyspnoea · ear discomfort · flatulence · gastrointestinal discomfort · headache · increased risk of infection · menstrual cycle irregularities · nasal complaints · nausea · oropharyngeal pain · ototoxicity · productive cough · rash · respiratory disorders · sputum increased · throat erythema · tympanic membrane hyperaemia · vomiting

▶ **Uncommon** Gynaecomastia · hepatic encephalopathy · hepatitis cholestatic · hypertension

SIDE-EFFECTS, FURTHER INFORMATION Manufacturer advises interrupt treatment if transaminase levels more than 5 times the upper limit of normal *or* transaminase levels more than 3 times the upper limit of normal **and** blood bilirubin more than twice the upper limit of normal—consult product literature.

● **HEPATIC IMPAIRMENT** [EvGr] Use with caution only if benefit outweighs risk in severe impairment (risk of increased exposure—serious liver injury reported). Ⓜ **Dose adjustments** [EvGr] Reduce evening dose to 200/125 mg in moderate impairment; in severe impairment, reduce dose to 200/125 mg every 12 hours or less frequently. Ⓜ

● **PRE-TREATMENT SCREENING** If the patient's genotype is unknown, a validated genotyping method should be performed to confirm the presence of the F508del mutation on both alleles of the CFTR gene before starting treatment.

● **MONITORING REQUIREMENTS** Manufacturer advises monitor blood pressure periodically during treatment.

● **EFFECT ON LABORATORY TESTS** False positive urine screening tests for tetrahydrocannabinol have been reported—manufacturer advises consider alternative confirmatory method.

● **DIRECTIONS FOR ADMINISTRATION** Manufacturer advises *tablets* should be taken with fat-containing food.

● **PATIENT AND CARER ADVICE**

Missed doses If a dose is more than 6 hours late, the missed dose should not be taken and the next dose should be taken at the normal time.

● **NATIONAL FUNDING/ACCESS DECISIONS**

For full details see funding body website

NICE decisions

▶ Ivacaftor–tezacaftor–elexacaftor, tezacaftor–ivacaftor and lumacaftor–ivacaftor for treating cystic fibrosis (July 2024) NICE TA988 Recommended

Scottish Medicines Consortium (SMC) decisions

▶ Lumacaftor with ivacaftor (*Orkambi*®) for the treatment of cystic fibrosis in patients aged 1 year and older who are homozygous for the F508del mutation in the cystic fibrosis transmembrane conductance regulator gene (July 2024) SMC No. SMC2712 Recommended

● **MEDICINAL FORMS** There can be variation in the licensing of different medicines containing the same drug.

Oral tablet

CAUTIONARY AND ADVISORY LABELS 25
EXCIPIENTS: May contain Propylene glycol

▶ Orkambi (Vertex Pharmaceuticals (Europe) Ltd)
Lumacaftor 100 mg, Ivacaftor 125 mg Orkambi 100mg/125mg tablets | 112 tablet [PoM] £8,000.00 (Hospital only)
Ivacaftor 125 mg, Lumacaftor 200 mg Orkambi 200mg/125mg tablets | 112 tablet [PoM] £8,000.00 (Hospital only)

Mannitol

15-Oct-2021

● **INDICATIONS AND DOSE**

Treatment of cystic fibrosis as an add-on therapy to standard care

▶ BY INHALATION OF POWDER

▶ Adult: Maintenance 400 mg twice daily, an initiation dose assessment must be carried out under medical supervision, for details of the initiation dose regimen, consult product literature

● **CONTRA-INDICATIONS** Bronchial hyperresponsiveness to inhaled mannitol · impaired lung function (forced expiratory volume in 1 second < 30% of predicted) · non-CF bronchiectasis

● **CAUTIONS** Asthma · haemoptysis

● **INTERACTIONS** → Appendix 1: mannitol

● **SIDE-EFFECTS**

▶ **Common or very common** Chest discomfort · condition aggravated · cough · haemoptysis · headache · respiratory disorders · throat complaints · vomiting

▶ **Uncommon** Abdominal pain upper · appetite decreased · asthma · burping · cold sweat · cystic fibrosis related diabetes · dehydration · diarrhoea · dizziness · dysphonia · dyspnoea · ear pain · fatigue · fever · gastrointestinal disorders · hypoxia · increased risk of infection · influenza like illness · insomnia · joint disorders · malaise · morbid thoughts · nausea · odynophagia · oral disorders · pain · rhinorrhoea · skin reactions · sputum discolouration · urinary incontinence

● **PREGNANCY** Manufacturer advises avoid.

● **BREAST FEEDING** Manufacturer advises avoid.

● **PRE-TREATMENT SCREENING** Patients must be assessed for bronchial hyperresponsiveness to inhaled mannitol before starting the therapeutic dose regimen; an initiation dose assessment must be carried out under medical supervision—for details of the initiation dose regimen, consult product literature.

● **DIRECTIONS FOR ADMINISTRATION** [EvGr] The dose should be administered 5–15 minutes after a bronchodilator and before physiotherapy; the second daily dose should be taken 2–3 hours before bedtime. Ⓜ

● **PATIENT AND CARER ADVICE** Patients or carers should be given advice on how to administer mannitol inhalation powder.

● **NATIONAL FUNDING/ACCESS DECISIONS**

For full details see funding body website

NICE decisions

▶ Mannitol dry powder for inhalation for treating cystic fibrosis (November 2012) NICE TA266 Recommended

3

Respiratory system

Scottish Medicines Consortium (SMC) decisions

▶ Mannitol (*Bronchitol*®) for the treatment of cystic fibrosis (CF) in adults aged 18 years and above as an add-on therapy to best standard of care (December 2013) SMC No. 837/13 Recommended with restrictions

● MEDICINAL FORMS There can be variation in the licensing of different medicines containing the same drug.

Inhalation powder

▶ Mannitol (Non-proprietary)

Mannitol 5 mg Osmohale 5mg inhalation powder capsules | 1 capsule [PoM] [x] (Hospital only)

Mannitol 10 mg Osmohale 10mg inhalation powder capsules | 1 capsule [PoM] [x] (Hospital only)

Mannitol 20 mg Osmohale 20mg inhalation powder capsules | 1 capsule [PoM] [x] (Hospital only)

Mannitol 40 mg Osmohale 40mg inhalation powder capsules | 15 capsule [PoM] [x] (Hospital only)

▶ Bronchitol (Chapper Healthcare)

Mannitol 40 mg Bronchitol 40mg inhalation powder capsules with two devices | 280 capsule [PoM] £231.66 DT = £231.66 Bronchitol 40mg inhalation powder capsules with device | 10 capsule [PoM] £8.27 (Hospital only)

Tezacaftor with ivacaftor
01-Aug-2024

The properties listed below are those particular to the combination only. For the properties of the components please consider, ivacaftor p. 336.

● INDICATIONS AND DOSE

Cystic fibrosis (in combination with ivacaftor) (specialist use only)

▶ BY MOUTH

▶ Adult: 100/150 mg, to be taken in the morning and, *Ivacaftor* 150 mg to be taken in the evening (about 12 hours apart)

DOSE ADJUSTMENTS DUE TO INTERACTIONS

▶ [EvGr] With concurrent use of potent CYP3A4 inhibitors, reduce dose to 100/150 mg tezacaftor/ivacaftor twice a week, taken approximately 3–4 days apart; the evening dose of ivacaftor should not be taken.

▶ With concurrent use of moderate CYP3A4 inhibitors, reduce dose to 100/150 mg tezacaftor/ivacaftor every other morning, with ivacaftor 150 mg taken in the mornings alternate to tezacaftor/ivacaftor; the evening dose of ivacaftor should not be taken. ⟨M⟩

DOSE EQUIVALENCE AND CONVERSION

▶ Combination dose expressed as *x/y* mg of tezacaftor/ivacaftor.

● INTERACTIONS → Appendix 1: ivacaftor · tezacaftor

● SIDE-EFFECTS

▶ **Common or very common** Abdominal pain · breast abnormalities · diarrhoea · dizziness · ear discomfort · headache · increased risk of infection · nasal congestion · nausea · oropharyngeal pain · ototoxicity · rash · sinus congestion · throat erythema · tympanic membrane hyperaemia

▶ **Uncommon** Gynaecomastia

▶ **Frequency not known** Hepatic function abnormal

SIDE-EFFECTS, FURTHER INFORMATION Manufacturer advises interrupt treatment if transaminase levels more than 5 times the upper limit of normal *or* transaminase levels more than 3 times the upper limit of normal **and** blood bilirubin more than twice the upper limit of normal—consult product literature.

● HEPATIC IMPAIRMENT [EvGr] Use with caution only if benefit outweighs risk in severe impairment (risk of increased exposure–serious liver injury reported). ⟨M⟩

Dose adjustments [EvGr] Omit evening dose of ivacaftor in moderate or severe impairment; in severe impairment, tezacaftor/ivacaftor should be taken once daily or less

frequently, adjust dosing interval according to clinical response and tolerability. ⟨M⟩

● DIRECTIONS FOR ADMINISTRATION [EvGr] Doses should be taken with fat-containing food. ⟨M⟩

● PATIENT AND CARER ADVICE

Missed doses Manufacturer advises if a dose is more than 6 hours late, the missed dose should not be taken and the next dose should be taken at the normal time.

● NATIONAL FUNDING/ACCESS DECISIONS

For full details see funding body website

NICE decisions

▶ Ivacaftor-tezacaftor-elexacaftor, tezacaftor-ivacaftor and lumacaftor-ivacaftor for treating cystic fibrosis (July 2024) NICE TA988 Recommended

Scottish Medicines Consortium (SMC) decisions

▶ Tezacaftor with ivacaftor (*Symkevi*®) in combination with ivacaftor for the treatment of patients with cystic fibrosis aged 6 years and older who are homozygous for the F508del mutation or who are heterozygous for the F508del mutation and have one of the following mutations in the cystic fibrosis transmembrane conductance regulator gene: P67L, R117C, L206W, R352Q, A455E, D579G, 711+3A→G, S945L, S977F, R1070W, D1152H, 2789+5G→A, 3272-26A→G, and 3849 +10kbC→T (July 2024) SMC No. SMC2711 Recommended

---

● MEDICINAL FORMS There can be variation in the licensing of different medicines containing the same drug.

Oral tablet

CAUTIONARY AND ADVISORY LABELS 25

▶ Symkevi (Vertex Pharmaceuticals (Europe) Ltd)

Tezacaftor 50 mg, Ivacaftor 75 mg Symkevi 50mg/75mg tablets | 28 tablet [PoM] £6,293.91 (Hospital only)

Tezacaftor 100 mg, Ivacaftor 150 mg Symkevi 100mg/150mg tablets | 28 tablet [PoM] £6,293.91 (Hospital only)

---

4   Cough and congestion

Aromatic inhalations, cough preparations and systemic nasal decongestants
03-May-2024

Aromatic inhalations in adults

Inhalations containing volatile substances such as eucalyptus oil are traditionally used and although the vapour may contain little of the additive it encourages deliberate inspiration of warm moist air which is often comforting in bronchitis; boiling water should not be used owing to the risk of scalding. In practice, inhalations are also used for the relief of nasal obstruction in acute rhinitis or sinusitis.

Cough preparations in adults

Cough suppressants

Cough may be a symptom of an underlying disorder, such as asthma, gastro-oesophageal reflux disease, or rhinitis, which should be addressed before prescribing cough suppressants. Cough may be a side-effect of another drug, such as an ACE inhibitor, or it can be associated with smoking or environmental pollutants. Cough can also have a significant habit component. When there is no identifiable cause, cough suppressants may be useful, for example if sleep is disturbed. They may cause sputum retention and this may be harmful in patients with chronic bronchitis and bronchiectasis.

There is some evidence to suggest that codeine phosphate p. 517 provides no benefit for symptoms of acute cough. Codeine phosphate is also constipating and can cause dependence; **dextromethorphan** has fewer side-effects.

Sedating antihistamines are used as the cough suppressant component of many compound cough preparations on sale to the public; all tend to cause drowsiness which may reflect their main mode of action.

MHRA/CHM advice: Pholcodine-containing cough and cold medicines: withdrawal from UK market as a precautionary measure (March 2023)

Following a review of cumulative safety information, the MHRA has found that pholcodine use in the 12 months preceding anaesthesia was significantly associated with an increased risk of peri-anaesthetic anaphylaxis to neuromuscular blocking agents (NMBAs). Although the absolute risk is very small, pholcodine-containing preparations are being withdrawn because their benefits do not outweigh this risk.

Healthcare professionals are advised to ask patients scheduled to receive general anaesthesia with NMBAs if they have taken pholcodine, particularly in the past 12 months. Patients or carers should be advised of this risk, and that there is no increased risk of allergic reactions, including anaphylaxis, with other allergens following pholcodine use.

Palliative care

Diamorphine hydrochloride p. 518 and methadone hydrochloride p. 570 have been used to control distressing cough in terminal lung cancer although morphine p. 525 is now preferred. In other circumstances they are contra-indicated because they induce sputum retention and ventilatory failure as well as causing opioid dependence. Methadone hydrochloride linctus should be avoided because it has a long duration of action and tends to accumulate.

Demulcent and expectorant cough preparations
Demulcent cough preparations contain soothing substances such as syrup or glycerol and some patients believe that such preparations relieve a dry irritating cough. Preparations such as **simple linctus** have the advantage of being harmless and inexpensive; **paediatric simple linctus** is particularly useful in children.

Expectorants are claimed to promote expulsion of bronchial secretions, but there is no evidence that any drug can specifically facilitate expectoration.

[EvGr] An over-the-counter cough medicine containing the expectorant guaifenesin may be used for acute cough; there is some evidence to suggest it may reduce symptoms. (A)

Compound preparations are on sale to the public for the treatment of cough and colds but should not be used in children under 6 years; the rationale for some is dubious. Care should be taken to give the correct dose and to not use more than one preparation at a time.

Nasal decongestants, systemic

Nasal decongestants for administration by mouth may not be as effective as preparations for local application but they do not give rise to rebound nasal congestion on withdrawal. Pseudoephedrine hydrochloride p. 1367 is available over the counter; it has few sympathomimetic effects but is only recommended for short-term use.

Aromatic inhalations in children

The use of strong aromatic decongestants (applied as rubs or to pillows) is not advised for infants under the age of 3 months. Carers of young infants in whom nasal obstruction with mucus is a problem can readily be taught appropriate techniques of suction aspiration but sodium chloride 0.9% given as nasal drops is preferred; administration before feeds may ease feeding difficulties caused by nasal congestion.

Cough preparations in children

The use of over-the-counter cough suppressants containing codeine phosphate should be avoided in children under 12 years and in children of any age known to be CYP2D6 ultra-rapid metabolisers. Cough suppressants containing similar opioid analgesics such as dextromethorphan are not generally recommended in children and should be avoided in children under 6 years.

Pholcodine-containing cough and cold preparations are not recommended and are being withdrawn due to safety concerns (see *MHRA/CHM advice* in *Cough preparations in adults*, above).

MHRA/CHM advice: Over-the-counter cough and cold medicines for children (March 2008 and February 2009)
Children under 6 years should not be given over-the-counter cough and cold medicines containing the following ingredients:

- brompheniramine, chlorphenamine maleate p. 323, diphenhydramine, doxylamine, promethazine, or triprolidine (antihistamines);
- dextromethorphan (cough suppressant);
- guaifenesin or ipecacuanha (expectorants);
- phenylephrine hydrochloride, pseudoephedrine hydrochloride, ephedrine hydrochloride p. 311, oxymetazoline, or xylometazoline hydrochloride p. 1368 (decongestants).

Over-the-counter cough and cold medicines can be considered for children aged 6–12 years after basic principles of best care have been tried, but treatment should be restricted to five days or less. Children should not be given more than 1 cough or cold preparation at a time because different brands may contain the same active ingredient; care should be taken to give the correct dose.

COUGH AND COLD PREPARATIONS

Citric acid

17-Jul-2024

- **DRUG ACTION** Formulated as simple linctus

- **INDICATIONS AND DOSE**

Cough
▶ BY MOUTH
▸ Adult: 5 mL 3–4 times a day, this dose is for Simple Linctus, BP (2.5%)

- **PRESCRIBING AND DISPENSING INFORMATION** Flavours of oral liquid formulations may include anise.
  When prepared extemporaneously, the BP states Simple Linctus, BP consists of citric acid monohydrate 2.5%, in a suitable vehicle with an anise flavour.

- **MEDICINAL FORMS** There can be variation in the licensing of different medicines containing the same drug.

Oral solution
▸ Citric acid (Non-proprietary)
  Citric acid monohydrate 6.25 mg per 1 ml Care Simple linctus paediatric sugar free | 200 ml [GSL] £1.75 DT = £1.75 [SF]
  Bell's Children's Cough Relief | 200 ml [GSL] £1.27 DT = £2.26
  Simple linctus paediatric | 200 ml [GSL] £1.52–£2.26 DT = £2.26
  Citric acid monohydrate 25 mg per 1 ml Simple linctus sugar free | 200 ml [GSL] £2.62 DT = £2.62 [SF] | 2000 ml [GSL] £23.00–£26.20 [SF]
  Simple linctus | 200 ml [GSL] £1.27–£1.49 DT = £1.49

MENTHOL AND DERIVATIVES

Eucalyptus with menthol

18-Mar-2020

- **INDICATIONS AND DOSE**

Aromatic inhalation for relief of nasal congestion
▶ BY INHALATION
▸ Adult: Add one teaspoonful to a pint of hot, **not** boiling, water and inhale the vapour; repeat after 4 hours if necessary

- **PRESCRIBING AND DISPENSING INFORMATION** When prepared extemporaneously, the BP states Menthol and Eucalyptus Inhalation, BP 1980 consists of racementhol or levomenthol 2 g, eucalyptus oil 10 mL, light magnesium carbonate 7 g, water to 100 mL.

- **PROFESSION SPECIFIC INFORMATION**
Dental practitioners' formulary Menthol and Eucalyptus Inhalation BP, 1980 may be prescribed.

- **MEDICINAL FORMS** No licensed medicines listed.

5   Interstitial lung disease

Other drugs used for Interstitial lung disease Nintedanib, p. 1120

ANTIFIBROTICS

Pirfenidone

28-Jul-2021

- **DRUG ACTION** The exact mechanism of action of pirfenidone is not yet understood, but it is believed to slow down the progression of idiopathic pulmonary fibrosis by exerting both antifibrotic and anti-inflammatory properties.

- **INDICATIONS AND DOSE**

Treatment of mild to moderate idiopathic pulmonary fibrosis (initiated under specialist supervision)
- BY MOUTH
- Adult: Initially 267 mg 3 times a day for 7 days, then increased to 534 mg 3 times a day for 7 days, then increased to 801 mg 3 times a day

DOSE ADJUSTMENTS DUE TO INTERACTIONS
- Caution with concomitant use with ciprofloxacin— reduce dose of pirfenidone to 534 mg three times daily with high-dose ciprofloxacin (750 mg twice daily).

IMPORTANT SAFETY INFORMATION
MHRA/CHM ADVICE: PIRFENIDONE (*ESBRIET*®): RISK OF SERIOUS LIVER INJURY; UPDATED ADVICE ON LIVER FUNCTION TESTING (NOVEMBER 2020)

A European review of safety data identified severe, sometimes fatal, cases of drug-induced liver injury (including liver failure) associated with pirfenidone therapy. Healthcare professionals are advised to monitor liver function and counsel patients to seek immediate medical attention if they experience signs and symptoms of liver injury; prompt clinical evaluation and measurement of liver function should be performed in those affected—see *Monitoring requirements*. Patients also taking inhibitors of cytochrome P450 isoenzymes involved in the metabolism of pirfenidone should be closely monitored for toxicity.

- **CAUTIONS**
- Photosensitivity Manufacturer advises avoid exposure to direct sunlight—if photosensitivity reaction or rash occurs, dose adjustment or treatment interruption may be required (consult product literature).
- Treatment interruption If treatment is interrupted for 14 consecutive days or more, the initial 2 week titration regimen should be repeated; if treatment is interrupted for less than 14 consecutive days, the dose can be resumed at the previous daily dose without titration.

- **INTERACTIONS** → Appendix 1: pirfenidone

- **SIDE-EFFECTS**
- **Common or very common** Appetite decreased · arthralgia · asthenia · constipation · diarrhoea · dizziness · drowsiness · gastrointestinal discomfort · gastrointestinal disorders · headache · hot flush · increased risk of infection · insomnia · musculoskeletal chest pain · myalgia · nausea ·

photosensitivity reaction · productive cough · skin reactions · sunburn · taste altered · vomiting · weight decreased
- **Uncommon** Agranulocytosis · angioedema · hepatic disorders · hyponatraemia
- **Frequency not known** Severe cutaneous adverse reactions (SCARs)

SIDE-EFFECTS, FURTHER INFORMATION Gastrointestinal side-effects may require dose reduction or treatment interruption—consult product literature.

- **PREGNANCY** Manufacturer advises avoid—no information available.

- **BREAST FEEDING** Manufacturer advises avoid—no information available.

- **HEPATIC IMPAIRMENT** Manufacturer advises caution in mild to moderate impairment (risk of increased exposure); avoid in severe impairment (no information available).

- **RENAL IMPAIRMENT** EvGr Caution if creatinine clearance 30–50 mL/minute; avoid if creatinine clearance less than 30 mL/minute. Ⓜ See p. 21.

- **MONITORING REQUIREMENTS**
- Manufacturer advises monitor for weight loss.
- Manufacturer advises monitor liver function (ALT, AST, and bilirubin) before starting treatment, then at monthly intervals for the first 6 months, and then every 3 months thereafter; review if abnormal liver function tests—dose reduction, treatment interruption or discontinuation may be required (consult product literature).

- **PATIENT AND CARER ADVICE**
Driving and skilled tasks Dizziness or malaise may affect performance of skilled tasks (e.g. driving).

- **NATIONAL FUNDING/ACCESS DECISIONS**
For full details see funding body website
NICE decisions
- Pirfenidone for treating idiopathic pulmonary fibrosis (February 2018) NICE TA504 Recommended with restrictions
Scottish Medicines Consortium (SMC) decisions
- Pirfenidone (*Esbriet*®) in adults for the treatment of mild to moderate idiopathic pulmonary fibrosis (IPF) (August 2013) SMC No. 835/13 Recommended with restrictions

---

- **MEDICINAL FORMS** There can be variation in the licensing of different medicines containing the same drug.
Oral tablet
CAUTIONARY AND ADVISORY LABELS 11, 21, 25
- Pirfenidone (Non-proprietary)
Pirfenidone 267 mg Pirfenidone 267mg tablets | 63 tablet PoM £371.00-£451.73 (Hospital only) | 63 tablet PoM £426.63-£501.92 | 252 tablet PoM £1,505.78-£1,806.93 (Hospital only) | 252 tablet PoM £1,706.55-£2,007.70
Pirfenidone 801 mg Pirfenidone 801mg tablets | 84 tablet PoM £1,706.55-£2,007.70 | 84 tablet PoM £1,500.00-£1,806.93 (Hospital only)
- Esbriet (Roche Products Ltd)
Pirfenidone 267 mg Esbriet 267mg tablets | 63 tablet PoM £501.92 (Hospital only) | 252 tablet PoM £2,007.70 (Hospital only)
Pirfenidone 801 mg Esbriet 801mg tablets | 84 tablet PoM £2,007.70 (Hospital only)

6 Respiratory depression, respiratory distress syndrome and apnoea

Respiratory stimulants

Overview

Respiratory stimulants (analeptic drugs) have a limited place in the treatment of ventilatory failure in patients with chronic obstructive pulmonary disease. They are effective only when given by intravenous injection or infusion and have a short duration of action. Their use has largely been replaced by ventilatory support including nasal intermittent positive pressure ventilation. However, occasionally when ventilatory support is contra-indicated and in patients with hypercapnic respiratory failure who are becoming drowsy or comatose, respiratory stimulants in the short term may arouse patients sufficiently to co-operate and clear their secretions.

Respiratory stimulants can also be harmful in respiratory failure since they stimulate non-respiratory as well as respiratory muscles. They should only be given under **expert supervision** in hospital and must be combined with active physiotherapy. There is at present no oral respiratory stimulant available for long-term use in chronic respiratory failure.

RESPIRATORY STIMULANTS

Doxapram hydrochloride

22-Nov-2018

● **INDICATIONS AND DOSE**

Postoperative respiratory depression

▸ INITIALLY BY INTRAVENOUS INJECTION

▸ Adult: Initially 1–1.5 mg/kg, to be administered over at least 30 seconds, repeated if necessary after intervals of one hour, alternatively (by intravenous infusion) 2–3 mg/minute, adjusted according to response

Acute respiratory failure

▸ BY INTRAVENOUS INFUSION

▸ Adult: 1.5–4 mg/minute, adjusted according to response, to be given concurrently with oxygen and whenever possible monitor with frequent measurement of blood gas tensions

● CONTRA-INDICATIONS Cerebral oedema · cerebrovascular accident · coronary artery disease · epilepsy and other convulsive disorders · hyperthyroidism · physical obstruction of respiratory tract · severe hypertension · status asthmaticus

● CAUTIONS Give with beta$_2$ agonist in bronchoconstriction · give with oxygen in severe irreversible airways obstruction or severely decreased lung compliance (because of increased work load of breathing) · hypertension · impaired cardiac reserve · phaeochromocytoma

● INTERACTIONS → Appendix 1: doxapram

● SIDE-EFFECTS Arrhythmias · chest discomfort · confusion · cough · dizziness · dyspnoea · fever · flushing · hallucination · headache · hyperhidrosis · movement disorders · nausea · neuromuscular dysfunction · oral disorders · perineal warmth · reflexes abnormal · respiratory disorders · seizure · urinary disorders · vomiting

● PREGNANCY No evidence of harm, but manufacturer advises avoid unless benefit outweighs risk.

● HEPATIC IMPAIRMENT Manufacturer advises use with caution.

● MONITORING REQUIREMENTS Frequent arterial blood gas and pH measurements are necessary during treatment to ensure correct dosage.

● MEDICINAL FORMS There can be variation in the licensing of different medicines containing the same drug.

Solution for injection

▸ Doxapram hydrochloride (Non-proprietary)
Doxapram hydrochloride 20 mg per 1 ml Doxapram 100mg/5ml solution for injection ampoules | 5 ampoule PoM £110.00 (Hospital only) | 5 ampoule PoM £126.50

Chapter 4
Nervous system

CONTENTS

1 Dementia

Dementia

14-Sep-2018

Description of condition

Dementia is a progressive clinical syndrome characterised by a range of cognitive and behavioural symptoms that can include memory loss, problems with reasoning and communication, a change in personality, and a reduced ability to carry out daily activities such as washing or dressing. Alzheimer's disease is the most common type of dementia; other common types of dementia include vascular dementia (due to cerebrovascular disease), dementia with Lewy bodies, mixed dementia, and frontotemporal dementia.

Aims of treatment

The aim of treatment is to promote independence, maintain function, and manage symptoms of dementia.

Non-drug treatment

[EvGr] Patients with all types of *mild-to-moderate* dementia presenting with **cognitive symptoms** should be given the opportunity to participate in a structured group cognitive stimulation programme. Group reminiscence therapy (use of life stories to improve psychological well-being), and cognitive rehabilitation or occupational therapy to support daily functional ability, should also be considered. [A]

Management of cognitive symptoms

[EvGr] Some commonly prescribed drugs are associated with increased antimuscarinic (anticholinergic) burden, and therefore cognitive impairment; their use should be minimised. [A] Drugs with antimuscarinic effects include some antidepressants (e.g. amitriptyline hydrochloride p. 431, paroxetine p. 425), antihistamines (e.g. chlorphenamine maleate p. 323, promethazine hydrochloride p. 326), antipsychotics (e.g. olanzapine p. 459, quetiapine p. 462), and urinary antispasmodics (e.g. solifenacin succinate p. 899, tolterodine tartrate p. 900).

Alzheimer's disease

[EvGr] In newly diagnosed patients, drug treatment should only be initiated under the advice of a specialist clinician experienced in the management of Alzheimer's disease.

In patients with *mild-to-moderate* Alzheimer's disease, monotherapy with donepezil hydrochloride p. 345, galantamine p. 346, or rivastigmine p. 347 (acetylcholinesterase inhibitors) are first-line treatment options. If acetylcholinesterase inhibitors are not tolerated or contra-indicated, memantine hydrochloride p. 349 is a suitable alternative in patients with *moderate* Alzheimer's disease. Memantine hydrochloride is the drug of choice in patients with *severe* Alzheimer's disease.

In patients already receiving an acetylcholinesterase inhibitor to treat Alzheimer's disease, the addition of memantine hydrochloride should be considered if they develop *moderate* or *severe* disease; in this case, memantine hydrochloride can be initiated in primary care without advice from a specialist clinician. [A]

In patients with moderate Alzheimer's disease, discontinuing acetylcholinesterase inhibitor treatment can cause a substantial worsening in cognitive function; [EvGr] treatment discontinuation should not be based on disease severity alone. [A]

Non-Alzheimer's dementia

[EvGr] Donepezil hydrochloride [unlicensed indication] or rivastigmine [unlicensed indication] should be given to patients with *mild-to-moderate* dementia with Lewy bodies; galantamine [unlicensed indication] can be considered only if treatment with both donepezil hydrochloride or rivastigmine is not tolerated. Donepezil hydrochloride [unlicensed indication] or rivastigmine [unlicensed indication] can also be considered in patients with *severe* dementia with Lewy bodies. Memantine hydrochloride [unlicensed indication] can be considered as an alternative in patients with dementia with Lewy bodies in whom acetylcholinesterase inhibitors are contra-indicated or not tolerated.

Acetylcholinesterase inhibitors [unlicensed indication] or memantine hydrochloride [unlicensed indication] should only be considered in patients with vascular dementia if they have suspected co-morbid Alzheimer's disease, Parkinson's disease dementia, or dementia with Lewy bodies.

Acetylcholinesterase inhibitors and memantine hydrochloride are **not** recommended in patients with frontotemporal dementia or cognitive impairment caused by multiple sclerosis. Ⓐ

For management of Parkinson's disease dementia see Parkinson's disease p. 470.

Management of non-cognitive symptoms

Agitation, aggression, distress and psychosis

EvGr Patients with dementia should be offered psychosocial and environmental interventions such as counselling and management of pain and delirium to reduce distress.

Antipsychotic drugs should only be offered to patients with dementia if they are either at risk of harming themselves or others, or experiencing agitation, hallucinations or delusions that are causing them severe distress. Ⓐ The CHM/MHRA has reported (2009) an increased risk of stroke and a small increased risk of death when antipsychotic drugs are used in elderly patients with dementia. The balance of risks and benefits should be carefully assessed, including any previous history of stroke or transient ischaemic attack and any risk factors for cerebrovascular disease such as hypertension, diabetes, smoking, and atrial fibrillation.

EvGr Antipsychotic drugs should be used at the lowest effective dose and for the shortest time possible, with a regular review at least every 6 weeks. Ⓐ

In patients who have dementia with Lewy bodies or Parkinson's disease dementia, antipsychotic drugs can worsen the motor features of the condition, and in some cases cause severe antipsychotic sensitivity reactions. See also management of psychotic symptoms in Parkinson's disease p. 470.

Depression and anxiety

EvGr Psychological treatments (e.g. cognitive behavioural therapy (CBT), multisensory stimulation, relaxation, or animal-assisted therapies) should be considered for patients with *mild-to-moderate* dementia who have mild to moderate depression or anxiety; antidepressants should be reserved for pre-existing severe mental health problems. Ⓐ

Sleep disturbances

EvGr Patients should be offered non-drug treatment approaches to manage sleep problems and insomnia, including sleep hygiene education, exposure to daylight, and increasing exercise and activity. Ⓐ

Useful Resources

Dementia: assessment, management and support for people living with dementia and their carers. National Institute for Health and Care Excellence. NICE guideline 97. June 2018.
www.nice.org.uk/guidance/ng97

> **Other drugs used for Dementia** Risperidone, p. 464

AMYLOID BETA-DIRECTED ANTIBODIES

Donanemab

03-Dec-2024

- **DRUG ACTION** Donanemab is a humanised monoclonal antibody which binds to insoluble N-terminal truncated form of amyloid beta (N3pG Aβ), thereby reducing amyloid plaques in the brain.

- **INDICATIONS AND DOSE**

Mild cognitive impairment or mild dementia in Alzheimer's disease [in apolipoprotein E ε 4 (ApoEε4) heterozygotes or non-carriers] (under expert supervision)
- ▸ BY INTRAVENOUS INFUSION
- ▸ Adult: Initially 700 mg every 4 weeks for the first 3 doses, for dose interruption or treatment

discontinuation due to side-effects—consult product literature, followed by 1.4 g every 4 weeks for up to a total of 18 months, for dose interruption or treatment discontinuation due to side-effects—consult product literature

- **CONTRA-INDICATIONS** MRI findings suggestive of cerebral amyloid angiopathy—consult product literature

- **CAUTIONS** Infusion-related reactions · risk factors for intracerebral haemorrhage

  CAUTIONS, FURTHER INFORMATION
  - ▸ Infusion-related reactions EvGr Infusion-related reactions can occur and donanemab should only be administered when appropriately trained staff are available; these reactions can be managed by reducing the rate or stopping the infusion and appropriate management initiated. Patients should be closely monitored for signs of infusion-related reactions during and for at least 30 minutes after completion of the infusion. Premedication may be considered for subsequent infusions. Ⓜ

- **INTERACTIONS** → Appendix 1: donanemab

- **SIDE-EFFECTS**
  - ▸ **Common or very common** Amyloid related imaging abnormalities · CNS haemorrhage · cortical superficial siderosis · headache · infusion related reaction · nausea · vomiting
  - ▸ **Uncommon** Hypersensitivity

- **PREGNANCY** EvGr Avoid (no information available). Ⓜ

- **BREAST FEEDING** EvGr Use only if potential benefit outweighs risk (no information available). Ⓜ

- **MONITORING REQUIREMENTS** EvGr Monitor for signs and symptoms of amyloid related imaging abnormalities (ARIA) during treatment—consult product literature. Ⓜ

- **DIRECTIONS FOR ADMINISTRATION** EvGr For *intravenous infusion* (*Kisunla*®), dilute requisite dose in Sodium Chloride 0.9% to a final concentration of 4–10 mg/mL (gently invert, do not shake); give over at least 30 minutes. Ⓜ

- **PRESCRIBING AND DISPENSING INFORMATION** Donanemab is a biological medicine. Biological medicines must be prescribed and dispensed by brand name, see *Biological medicines* and *Biosimilar medicines*, under Guidance on prescribing p. 1; record the brand name and batch number after each administration.

- **HANDLING AND STORAGE** Store in a refrigerator at 2–8°C and protect from light—consult product literature for further information regarding storage conditions outside refrigerator and after preparation of the infusion.

- **MEDICINAL FORMS** There can be variation in the licensing of different medicines containing the same drug.

Solution for infusion
EXCIPIENTS: May contain Polysorbates, sucrose
ELECTROLYTES: May contain Sodium
- ▸ **Kisunla** (Eli Lilly and Company Ltd) ▼
  Donanemab 17.5 mg per 1 ml Kisunla 350mg/20ml concentrate for solution for infusion vials | 1 vial PoM £613.60 (Hospital only)

Lecanemab

27-Feb-2025

- **DRUG ACTION** Lecanemab is a humanised monoclonal antibody which binds to amyloid beta (Aβ) aggregates, thereby reducing amyloid plaques in the brain.

● INDICATIONS AND DOSE

Mild cognitive impairment or mild dementia in Alzheimer's disease [in apolipoprotein E ε 4 (ApoEε4) heterozygotes or non-carriers] (under expert supervision)

▸ BY INTRAVENOUS INFUSION

▸ Adult: 10 mg/kg every 2 weeks, for dose interruption or treatment discontinuation due to side-effects—consult product literature

- **CONTRA-INDICATIONS** MRI findings suggestive of cerebral amyloid angiopathy—consult product literature

- **CAUTIONS** Infusion-related reactions · risk factors for intracerebral haemorrhage

  CAUTIONS, FURTHER INFORMATION
  ▸ Infusion-related reactions [EvGr] Infusion-related reactions can occur during or within 2.5 hours after completion of the infusion; these reactions can be managed by reducing the rate or stopping the infusion and appropriate management initiated. Pre-medication with antihistamines, paracetamol, NSAIDs, or corticosteroids may be considered for subsequent infusions. ⓜ

- **INTERACTIONS** → Appendix 1: lecanemab

- **SIDE-EFFECTS**
  ▸ **Common or very common** Amyloid related imaging abnormalities · atrial fibrillation · CNS haemorrhage · headache · hypersensitivity · infusion related reaction · skin reactions · superficial siderosis of central nervous system
  ▸ **Frequency not known** Fall

- **CONCEPTION AND CONTRACEPTION** [EvGr] Females of childbearing potential should use effective contraception during treatment and for up to 3 months after last treatment. ⓜ

- **PREGNANCY** [EvGr] Avoid unless potential benefit outweighs risk (no information available). ⓜ

- **BREAST FEEDING** [EvGr] Avoid (no information available). ⓜ

- **MONITORING REQUIREMENTS** [EvGr] Monitor for signs and symptoms of amyloid related imaging abnormalities (ARIA) during treatment, especially during the first 14 weeks—consult product literature. ⓜ

- **DIRECTIONS FOR ADMINISTRATION** [EvGr] For *intravenous infusion (Leqembi®)*, dilute requisite dose in 250 mL of Sodium Chloride 0.9% (gently invert, do not shake); give over approximately 1 hour through a low-protein binding 0.2 micron in-line filter. ⓜ

- **PRESCRIBING AND DISPENSING INFORMATION** Lecanemab is a biological medicine. Biological medicines must be prescribed and dispensed by brand name, see *Biological medicines* and *Biosimilar medicines*, under Guidance on prescribing p. 1; record the brand name and batch number after each administration.

  The manufacturer of *Leqembi®* has provided a *Guide for Healthcare Professionals*.

- **HANDLING AND STORAGE** Store in a refrigerator at 2–8°C and protect from light—consult product literature for storage conditions after dilution.

- **PATIENT AND CARER ADVICE**
  Patient alert card A patient alert card should be provided.

- **NATIONAL FUNDING/ACCESS DECISIONS**
  For full details see funding body website
  Scottish Medicines Consortium (SMC) decisions
  ▸ Lecanemab (*Leqembi®*) for the treatment of mild cognitive impairment and mild dementia due to Alzheimer's disease in adult patients that are apolipoprotein E ε 4 (ApoEε4) heterozygotes or non-carriers (February 2025) SMC No. SMC2700 Not recommended

- **MEDICINAL FORMS** There can be variation in the licensing of different medicines containing the same drug.
  Solution for infusion
  EXCIPIENTS: May contain Polysorbates
  ▸ **Leqembi** (Eisai Ltd) ▼
    Lecanemab 100 mg per 1 ml Leqembi 200mg/2ml concentrate for solution for infusion vials | 1 vial [PoM] £275.00 (Hospital only)
    Leqembi 500mg/5ml concentrate for solution for infusion vials | 1 vial [PoM] £545.00 (Hospital only)

ANTICHOLINESTERASES > CENTRALLY ACTING

Donepezil hydrochloride

15-Apr-2024

- **DRUG ACTION** Donepezil is a reversible inhibitor of acetylcholinesterase.

● INDICATIONS AND DOSE

Mild to moderate dementia in Alzheimer's disease

▸ BY MOUTH

▸ Adult: Initially 5 mg once daily for one month, then increased if necessary up to 10 mg daily, doses to be given at bedtime

- **CAUTIONS** Asthma · chronic obstructive pulmonary disease · sick sinus syndrome · supraventricular conduction abnormalities · susceptibility to peptic ulcers

  CAUTIONS, FURTHER INFORMATION
  ▸ Elderly For acetylcholinesterase inhibitors, Screening Tool of Older Persons' potentially inappropriate Prescriptions (STOPP) criteria to aid medication reviews (see Prescribing in the elderly p. 31 for information): potentially inappropriate in patients with a known history of persistent bradycardia (heart rate less than 60 beats per minute), heart block, recurrent unexplained syncope, or concurrent treatment with drugs that reduce heart rate (risk of cardiac conduction failure, syncope, and injury).

- **INTERACTIONS** → Appendix 1: anticholinesterases, centrally acting

- **SIDE-EFFECTS**
  ▸ **Common or very common** Aggression · agitation · appetite decreased · common cold · diarrhoea · dizziness · fatigue · gastrointestinal disorders · hallucination · headache · injury · muscle cramps · nausea · pain · skin reactions · sleep disorders · syncope · urinary incontinence · vomiting
  ▸ **Uncommon** Arrhythmias · gastrointestinal haemorrhage · hypersalivation · seizure
  ▸ **Rare or very rare** Cardiac conduction disorders · hepatic disorders · movement disorders · neuroleptic malignant syndrome (discontinue—potentially fatal) · rhabdomyolysis
  ▸ **Frequency not known** QT interval prolongation · sexual dysfunction

  SIDE-EFFECTS, FURTHER INFORMATION Dose should be started low and increased if tolerated and necessary.

- **HEPATIC IMPAIRMENT** Manufacturer advises caution (risk of increased exposure in mild to moderate impairment; no information available in severe impairment).
  Dose adjustments Manufacturer advises dose escalation should be performed according to individual tolerability in mild to moderate impairment.

- **DIRECTIONS FOR ADMINISTRATION** Manufacturer advises donepezil orodispersible tablet should be placed on the tongue, allowed to disperse, and swallowed.
- **PATIENT AND CARER ADVICE** Patient or carers should be given advice on how to administer donepezil hydrochloride orodispersible tablets.
- **NATIONAL FUNDING/ACCESS DECISIONS** For full details see funding body website

NICE decisions
▸ **Donepezil, galantamine, rivastigmine, and memantine for the treatment of Alzheimer's disease (updated June 2018)** NICE TA217 Recommended with restrictions

- **MEDICINAL FORMS** There can be variation in the licensing of different medicines containing the same drug. Forms available from special-order manufacturers include: oral suspension

Oral tablet
▸ **Donepezil hydrochloride (Non-proprietary)**
Donepezil hydrochloride 5 mg Donepezil 5mg tablets | 28 tablet PoM £71.82 DT = £1.14
Donepezil hydrochloride 10 mg Donepezil 10mg tablets | 28 tablet PoM £100.66 DT = £1.19
▸ **Aricept** (Eisai Ltd)
Donepezil hydrochloride 5 mg Aricept 5mg tablets | 28 tablet PoM £59.85 DT = £1.14
Donepezil hydrochloride 10 mg Aricept 10mg tablets | 28 tablet PoM £83.89 DT = £1.19

Oral solution
▸ **Donepezil hydrochloride (Non-proprietary)**
Donepezil hydrochloride 1 mg per 1 ml Donepezil 1mg/ml oral solution sugar free | 150 ml PoM £114.07 DT = £114.07 SF

Orodispersible tablet
▸ **Donepezil hydrochloride (Non-proprietary)**
Donepezil hydrochloride 5 mg Donepezil 5mg orodispersible tablets sugar free | 28 tablet PoM £50.87 DT = £45.87 SF
Donepezil hydrochloride 10 mg Donepezil 10mg orodispersible tablets sugar free | 28 tablet PoM £127.60 DT = £124.03 SF
▸ **Apozyl** (Novumgen Ltd)
Donepezil hydrochloride 5 mg Apozyl 5mg orodispersible tablets | 28 tablet PoM £19.21 DT = £45.87 SF
Donepezil hydrochloride 10 mg Apozyl 10mg orodispersible tablets | 28 tablet PoM £62.92 DT = £124.03 SF
▸ **Aricept Evess** (Eisai Ltd)
Donepezil hydrochloride 5 mg Aricept Evess 5mg orodispersible tablets | 28 tablet PoM £59.85 DT = £45.87 SF
Donepezil hydrochloride 10 mg Aricept Evess 10mg orodispersible tablets | 28 tablet PoM £83.89 DT = £124.03 SF

Galantamine

15-Apr-2024

- **DRUG ACTION** Galantamine is a reversible inhibitor of acetylcholinesterase and it also has nicotinic receptor agonist properties.

- **INDICATIONS AND DOSE**

Mild to moderately severe dementia in Alzheimer's disease
▸ BY MOUTH USING IMMEDIATE-RELEASE MEDICINES
▸ Adult: Initially 4 mg twice daily for 4 weeks, increased to 8 mg twice daily for at least 4 weeks; maintenance 8–12 mg twice daily
▸ BY MOUTH USING MODIFIED-RELEASE CAPSULES
▸ Adult: Initially 8 mg once daily for 4 weeks, increased to 16 mg once daily for at least 4 weeks; maintenance 16–24 mg daily

- **CAUTIONS** Avoid in gastro-intestinal obstruction · avoid in urinary outflow obstruction · avoid whilst recovering from bladder surgery · avoid whilst recovering from gastro-intestinal surgery · cardiac disease · chronic obstructive pulmonary disease · congestive heart failure · electrolyte disturbances · history of seizures · history of severe asthma · pulmonary infection · sick sinus syndrome ·

supraventricular conduction abnormalities · susceptibility to peptic ulcers · unstable angina

CAUTIONS, FURTHER INFORMATION
▸ Elderly For acetylcholinesterase inhibitors, Screening Tool of Older Persons' potentially inappropriate Prescriptions (STOPP) criteria to aid medication reviews (see Prescribing in the elderly p. 31 for information): potentially inappropriate in patients with a known history of persistent bradycardia (heart rate less than 60 beats per minute), heart block, recurrent unexplained syncope, or concurrent treatment with drugs that reduce heart rate (risk of cardiac conduction failure, syncope, and injury).

- **INTERACTIONS** → Appendix 1: anticholinesterases, centrally acting

- **SIDE-EFFECTS**
▸ **Common or very common** Appetite decreased · arrhythmias · asthenia · depression · diarrhoea · dizziness · drowsiness · fall · gastrointestinal discomfort · hallucinations · headache · hypertension · malaise · muscle spasms · nausea · skin reactions · syncope · tremor · vomiting · weight decreased
▸ **Uncommon** Atrioventricular block · dehydration · flushing · hyperhidrosis · hypersomnia · hypotension · muscle weakness · palpitations · paraesthesia · seizure · taste altered · tinnitus · vision blurred
▸ **Rare or very rare** Hepatitis · severe cutaneous adverse reactions (SCARs)

- **PREGNANCY** Use with caution—toxicity in *animal* studies.

- **BREAST FEEDING** Avoid—no information available.

- **HEPATIC IMPAIRMENT** Manufacturer advises caution in moderate impairment (risk of increased plasma concentrations); avoid in severe impairment (no information available).
Dose adjustments Manufacturer advises for *immediate-release* preparations in moderate impairment, initially 4 mg once daily (preferably in the morning) for at least 7 days, then 4 mg twice daily for at least 4 weeks; maximum 8 mg twice daily.
   Manufacturer advises for *modified-release* preparations in moderate impairment, initially 8 mg on alternate days (preferably in the morning) for 7 days, then 8 mg once daily for 4 weeks; maximum 16 mg daily.

- **RENAL IMPAIRMENT** EvGr Avoid if creatinine clearance less than 9 mL/minute (no information available). Ⓜ See p. 21.

- **PATIENT AND CARER ADVICE** Manufacturer recommends that patients are warned of the signs of serious skin reactions; they should be advised to stop taking galantamine immediately and seek medical advice if symptoms occur.

- **NATIONAL FUNDING/ACCESS DECISIONS** For full details see funding body website

NICE decisions
▸ **Donepezil, galantamine, rivastigmine, and memantine for the treatment of Alzheimer's disease (updated June 2018)** NICE TA217 Recommended with restrictions

- **MEDICINAL FORMS** There can be variation in the licensing of different medicines containing the same drug. Forms available from special-order manufacturers include: oral tablet

Oral tablet
CAUTIONARY AND ADVISORY LABELS 3, 21

Oral solution
CAUTIONARY AND ADVISORY LABELS 3, 21
▸ **Galantamine (Non-proprietary)**
Galantamine (as Galantamine hydrobromide) 4 mg per 1 ml Galantamine 20mg/5ml oral solution sugar free | 100 ml PoM £120.00 DT = £120.00 SF

- ▸ **Galzemic** (Zentiva Pharma UK Ltd)
  **Galantamine (as Galantamine hydrobromide) 4 mg per
  1 ml** Galzemic 4mg/ml oral solution | 100 ml [PoM] £90.00 DT =
  £120.00 [SF]
- ▸ **Reminyl** (Takeda UK Ltd)
  **Galantamine (as Galantamine hydrobromide) 4 mg per
  1 ml** Reminyl 4mg/ml oral solution | 100 ml [PoM] £120.00 DT =
  £120.00 [SF]

Modified-release capsule

CAUTIONARY AND ADVISORY LABELS 3, 21, 25

- ▸ **Galantamine** (Non-proprietary)
  Galantamine (as Galantamine hydrobromide) 8 mg Galantamine
  8mg modified-release capsules | 28 capsule [PoM] £52.91 DT = £51.88
  Galantamine (as Galantamine hydrobromide) 16 mg Galantamine
  16mg modified-release capsules | 28 capsule [PoM] £66.19 DT =
  £64.90
  Galantamine (as Galantamine hydrobromide) 24 mg Galantamine
  24mg modified-release capsules | 28 capsule [PoM] £81.39 DT =
  £79.80
- ▸ **Gaalin** (Milpharm Ltd)
  Galantamine (as Galantamine hydrobromide) 8 mg Gaalin 8mg
  modified-release capsules | 28 capsule [PoM] £51.88 DT = £51.88
  Galantamine (as Galantamine hydrobromide) 16 mg Gaalin 16mg
  modified-release capsules | 28 capsule [PoM] £64.90 DT = £64.90
  Galantamine (as Galantamine hydrobromide) 24 mg Gaalin 24mg
  modified-release capsules | 28 capsule [PoM] £79.80 DT = £79.80
- ▸ **Galantex XL** (Zentiva Pharma UK Ltd)
  Galantamine (as Galantamine hydrobromide) 8 mg Galzemic XL
  8mg capsules | 28 capsule [PoM] £19.03 DT = £51.88
  Galantamine (as Galantamine hydrobromide) 16 mg Galzemic XL
  16mg capsules | 28 capsule [PoM] £23.82 DT = £64.90
  Galantamine (as Galantamine hydrobromide) 24 mg Galzemic XL
  24mg capsules | 28 capsule [PoM] £29.30 DT = £79.80
- ▸ **Gatalin XL** (Aspire Pharma Ltd)
  Galantamine (as Galantamine hydrobromide) 8 mg Gatalin XL
  8mg capsules | 28 capsule [PoM] £25.94 DT = £51.88
  Galantamine (as Galantamine hydrobromide) 16 mg Gatalin XL
  16mg capsules | 28 capsule [PoM] £32.45 DT = £64.90
  Galantamine (as Galantamine hydrobromide) 24 mg Gatalin XL
  24mg capsules | 28 capsule [PoM] £39.90 DT = £79.80
- ▸ **Gazylan XL** (Teva UK Ltd)
  Galantamine (as Galantamine hydrobromide) 8 mg Gazylan XL
  8mg capsules | 28 capsule [PoM] £19.04 DT = £51.88
  Galantamine (as Galantamine hydrobromide) 16 mg Gazylan XL
  16mg capsules | 28 capsule [PoM] £23.83 DT = £64.90
  Galantamine (as Galantamine hydrobromide) 24 mg Gazylan XL
  24mg capsules | 28 capsule [PoM] £29.31 DT = £79.80
- ▸ **Lotprosin XL** (Accord-UK Ltd)
  Galantamine (as Galantamine hydrobromide) 8 mg Lotprosin XL
  8mg capsules | 28 capsule [PoM] £51.88 DT = £51.88
  Galantamine (as Galantamine hydrobromide) 16 mg Lotprosin XL
  16mg capsules | 28 capsule [PoM] £64.90 DT = £64.90
  Galantamine (as Galantamine hydrobromide) 24 mg Lotprosin XL
  24mg capsules | 28 capsule [PoM] £79.80 DT = £79.80
- ▸ **Luventa XL** (Fontus Health Ltd)
  Galantamine (as Galantamine hydrobromide) 8 mg Luventa XL
  8mg capsules | 28 capsule [PoM] £25.42 DT = £51.88
  Galantamine (as Galantamine hydrobromide) 16 mg Luventa XL
  16mg capsules | 28 capsule [PoM] £31.80 DT = £64.90
  Galantamine (as Galantamine hydrobromide) 24 mg Luventa XL
  24mg capsules | 28 capsule [PoM] £39.10 DT = £79.80
- ▸ **Reminyl XL** (Takeda UK Ltd)
  Galantamine (as Galantamine hydrobromide) 8 mg Reminyl XL
  8mg capsules | 28 capsule [PoM] £51.88 DT = £51.88
  Galantamine (as Galantamine hydrobromide) 16 mg Reminyl XL
  16mg capsules | 28 capsule [PoM] £64.90 DT = £64.90
  Galantamine (as Galantamine hydrobromide) 24 mg Reminyl XL
  24mg capsules | 28 capsule [PoM] £79.80 DT = £79.80

Rivastigmine

15-Apr-2024

- ● **DRUG ACTION** Rivastigmine is a reversible non-
  competitive inhibitor of acetylcholinesterases.

- ● **INDICATIONS AND DOSE**

Mild to moderate dementia in Alzheimer's disease
- ▸ BY MOUTH
- ▸ Adult: Initially 1.5 mg twice daily, increased in steps of
  1.5 mg twice daily, dose to be increased at intervals of
  at least 2 weeks according to response and tolerance;
  usual dose 3–6 mg twice daily (max. per dose 6 mg
  twice daily), if treatment interrupted for more than
  several days, retitrate from 1.5 mg twice daily
- ▸ BY TRANSDERMAL APPLICATION USING PATCHES
- ▸ Adult: Apply 4.6 mg/24 hours daily for at least 4 weeks,
  increased if tolerated to 9.5 mg/24 hours daily for a
  further 6 months, then increased if necessary to
  13.3 mg/24 hours daily, increase to 13.3 mg/24 hours
  patch if well tolerated and cognitive deterioration or
  functional decline demonstrated; use caution in
  patients with body-weight less than 50 kg, if treatment
  interrupted for more than 3 days, retitrate from
  4.6 mg/24 hours patch

Mild to moderate dementia in Parkinson's disease
- ▸ BY MOUTH
- ▸ Adult: Initially 1.5 mg twice daily, increased in steps of
  1.5 mg twice daily, dose to be increased at intervals of
  at least 2 weeks according to response and tolerance;
  usual dose 3–6 mg twice daily (max. per dose 6 mg
  twice daily), if treatment interrupted for more than
  several days, retitrate from 1.5 mg twice daily

DOSE EQUIVALENCE AND CONVERSION
- ▸ When switching from oral to transdermal therapy,
  patients taking 3–6 mg by mouth daily should initially
  switch to 4.6 mg/24 hours patch, then titrate as above.
  Patients taking 9 mg by mouth daily should switch to
  9.5 mg/24 hours patch if oral dose stable and well
  tolerated; if oral dose not stable or well tolerated,
  patients should switch to 4.6 mg/24 hours patch, then
  titrate as above. Patients taking 12 mg by mouth daily
  should switch to 9.5 mg/24 hours patch. The first patch
  should be applied on the day following the last oral
  dose.

ZEYZELF ® PATCHES

Mild to moderate dementia in Alzheimer's disease
- ▸ BY TRANSDERMAL APPLICATION USING PATCHES
- ▸ Adult: Apply 4.6 mg/24 hours twice weekly for at least
  4 weeks, increased if tolerated to 9.5 mg/24 hours twice
  weekly, if further dose increases are necessary after
  6 months of treatment with the 9.5 mg/24 hours twice
  weekly patch, switch to a higher strength daily patch. If
  treatment interrupted for more than 3 days, retitrate
  from 4.6 mg/24 hours twice weekly patch

DOSE EQUIVALENCE AND CONVERSION
- ▸ When switching from oral to *Zeyzelf*® transdermal
  therapy, patients taking 3–6 mg by mouth daily should
  initially switch to 4.6 mg/24 hours twice weekly patch,
  then titrate as above. Patients taking 9 mg by mouth
  daily should switch to 9.5 mg/24 hours twice weekly
  patch if oral dose stable and well tolerated; if oral dose
  not stable or well tolerated, patients should switch to
  4.6 mg/24 hours twice weekly patch, then titrate as
  above. Patients taking 12 mg by mouth daily should
  switch to 9.5 mg/24 hours twice weekly patch. The first
  patch should be applied on the day following the last
  oral dose.

IMPORTANT SAFETY INFORMATION
Daily application transdermal patches which are
available in strengths of 4.6 mg/24 hours,

9.5 mg/24 hours, and 13.3 mg/24 hours should **not** be confused with *Zeyzelf*® twice weekly application transdermal patches which are available in strengths of 4.6 mg/24 hours and 9.5 mg/24 hours.

● **CAUTIONS** Bladder outflow obstruction · conduction abnormalities · duodenal ulcers · gastric ulcers · history of asthma · history of chronic obstructive pulmonary disease · history of seizures · patients at risk of developing torsade de pointes · risk of fatal overdose with patch administration errors · sick sinus syndrome · susceptibility to ulcers

CAUTIONS, FURTHER INFORMATION

▸ Elderly For acetylcholinesterase inhibitors, Screening Tool of Older Persons' potentially inappropriate Prescriptions (STOPP) criteria to aid medication reviews (see Prescribing in the elderly p. 31 for information): potentially inappropriate in patients with a known history of persistent bradycardia (heart rate less than 60 beats per minute), heart block, recurrent unexplained syncope, or concurrent treatment with drugs that reduce heart rate (risk of cardiac conduction failure, syncope, and injury).

● **INTERACTIONS** → Appendix 1: anticholinesterases, centrally acting

● **SIDE-EFFECTS**

GENERAL SIDE-EFFECTS

▸ **Common or very common** Anxiety · appetite decreased · arrhythmias · asthenia · dehydration · depression · diarrhoea · dizziness · drowsiness · fall · gastrointestinal discomfort · headache · hypertension · movement disorders · nausea · skin reactions · syncope · tremor · urinary incontinence · urinary tract infection · vomiting · weight decreased

▸ **Uncommon** Aggression · atrioventricular block

▸ **Rare or very rare** Pancreatitis · seizure

▸ **Frequency not known** Hepatitis

SPECIFIC SIDE-EFFECTS

▸ **Common or very common**

▸ With oral use Confusion · gait abnormal · hallucinations · hyperhidrosis · hypersalivation · malaise · parkinsonism · sleep disorders

▸ With transdermal use Delirium · fever

▸ **Uncommon**

▸ With oral use Hypotension

▸ With transdermal use Gastric ulcer

▸ **Rare or very rare**

▸ With oral use Angina pectoris · gastrointestinal disorders · gastrointestinal haemorrhage

▸ **Frequency not known**

▸ With transdermal use Hallucination · nightmare

SIDE-EFFECTS, FURTHER INFORMATION Dose should be started low and increased according to response if tolerated.

Treatment should be interrupted if dehydration resulting from prolonged vomiting or diarrhoea occurs and withheld until resolution—retitrate dose if necessary.

Transdermal administration is less likely to cause side-effects.

● **HEPATIC IMPAIRMENT** Manufacturer advises caution (risk of increased exposure; no information available in severe impairment).
Dose adjustments Manufacturer advises cautious dose titration according to individual tolerability.

● **RENAL IMPAIRMENT**
Dose adjustments
▸ With oral use EvGr Titrate according to individual tolerability (risk of increased exposure). Ⓜ

● **MONITORING REQUIREMENTS** Monitor body-weight.

● **DIRECTIONS FOR ADMINISTRATION**

▸ With transdermal use Manufacturer advises apply patches to clean, dry, non-hairy, non-irritated skin on back, upper arm, or chest, removing after 24 hours and siting a replacement patch on a different area (avoid using the same area for 14 days).
ZEYZELF ® PATCHES Apply patches on fixed days to clean, dry, non-hairy, non-irritated skin on back, upper arm, or chest. Remove after 4 and 3 days respectively, and site replacement patch on a different area (avoid using the same area for 14 days).

● **PATIENT AND CARER ADVICE**

▸ With transdermal use Patients and carers should be given advice on patch administration, particularly to remove the previous patch before applying the new patch—consult product literature.

● **NATIONAL FUNDING/ACCESS DECISIONS**
For full details see funding body website
NICE decisions
▸ **Donepezil, galantamine, rivastigmine, and memantine for the treatment of Alzheimer's disease (updated June 2018)**
NICE TA217 Recommended with restrictions

● **MEDICINAL FORMS** There can be variation in the licensing of different medicines containing the same drug.
Oral solution
CAUTIONARY AND ADVISORY LABELS 21
▸ **Rivastigmine (Non-proprietary)**
Rivastigmine (as Rivastigmine hydrogen tartrate) 2 mg per 1 ml Rivastigmine 2mg/ml oral solution sugar free | 120 ml PoM £85.00 DT = £85.00 SF

Oral capsule
CAUTIONARY AND ADVISORY LABELS 21, 25
▸ **Rivastigmine (Non-proprietary)**
Rivastigmine (as Rivastigmine hydrogen tartrate)
1.5 mg Rivastigmine 1.5mg capsules | 28 capsule PoM £33.91 DT = £1.87 | 56 capsule PoM £3.82
Rivastigmine (as Rivastigmine hydrogen tartrate)
3 mg Rivastigmine 3mg capsules | 28 capsule PoM £33.91 DT = £2.35 | 56 capsule PoM £4.88
Rivastigmine (as Rivastigmine hydrogen tartrate)
4.5 mg Rivastigmine 4.5mg capsules | 28 capsule PoM £33.91 DT = £4.17
Rivastigmine (as Rivastigmine hydrogen tartrate)
6 mg Rivastigmine 6mg capsules | 28 capsule PoM £33.91 DT = £7.47 | 56 capsule PoM £56.53

Transdermal patch
▸ **Rivastigmine (Non-proprietary)**
Rivastigmine 4.6 mg per 24 hour Rivastigmine 4.6mg/24hours transdermal patches | 30 patch PoM £37.60 DT = £77.97
Rivastigmine 9.5 mg per 24 hour Rivastigmine 9.5mg/24hours transdermal patches | 30 patch PoM £37.60 DT = £19.97
Rivastigmine 13.3 mg per 24 hour Rivastigmine 13.3mg/24hours transdermal patches | 30 patch PoM £50.66 DT = £77.97
▸ **Almuriva** (Sandoz Ltd)
Rivastigmine 4.6 mg per 24 hour Almuriva 4.6mg/24hours transdermal patches | 30 patch PoM £77.97 DT = £77.97
Rivastigmine 9.5 mg per 24 hour Almuriva 9.5mg/24hours transdermal patches | 30 patch PoM £77.97 DT = £19.97
Rivastigmine 13.3 mg per 24 hour Almuriva 13.3mg/24hours transdermal patches | 30 patch PoM £77.97 DT = £77.97
▸ **Alzest** (Dr Reddy's Laboratories (UK) Ltd)
Rivastigmine 4.6 mg per 24 hour Alzest 4.6mg/24hours transdermal patches | 30 patch PoM £35.10 DT = £77.97
Rivastigmine 9.5 mg per 24 hour Alzest 9.5mg/24hours transdermal patches | 30 patch PoM £19.97 DT = £19.97
Rivastigmine 13.3 mg per 24 hour Alzest 13.3mg/24hours transdermal patches | 30 patch PoM £54.58 DT = £77.97
▸ **Exelon** (Novartis Pharmaceuticals UK Ltd)
Rivastigmine 4.6 mg per 24 hour Exelon 4.6mg/24hours transdermal patches | 30 patch PoM £77.97 DT = £77.97
Rivastigmine 9.5 mg per 24 hour Exelon 9.5mg/24hours transdermal patches | 30 patch PoM £77.97 DT = £19.97
Rivastigmine 13.3 mg per 24 hour Exelon 13.3mg/24hours transdermal patches | 30 patch PoM £77.97 DT = £77.97

▶ **Rivatev** (Teva UK Ltd)
Rivastigmine 13.3 mg per 24 hour Erastig 13.3mg/24hours transdermal patches | 30 patch [PoM] £73.90 DT = £77.97

▶ **Zeyzelf** (Luye Pharma Ltd)
Rivastigmine 4.6 mg per 24 hour Zeyzelf 4.6mg/24hours twice weekly transdermal patches | 8 patch [PoM] £35.09
Rivastigmine 9.5 mg per 24 hour Zeyzelf 9.5mg/24hours twice weekly transdermal patches | 8 patch [PoM] £35.09

DOPAMINERGIC DRUGS › NMDA RECEPTOR ANTAGONISTS

Memantine hydrochloride
09-Mar-2021

- **DRUG ACTION** Memantine is a glutamate receptor antagonist.

● **INDICATIONS AND DOSE**

Moderate to severe dementia in Alzheimer's disease
▶ BY MOUTH
▶ **Adult:** Initially 5 mg once daily, then increased in steps of 5 mg every week; usual maintenance 20 mg daily; maximum 20 mg per day

Oscillopsia in multiple sclerosis
▶ BY MOUTH
▶ **Adult:** Initially 10 mg daily, then increased to 40 mg daily, over 1 week; increased if necessary to 60 mg daily, over 1 week, on specialist advice only

- **UNLICENSED USE** [EvGr] Memantine hydrochloride is used for oscillopsia in multiple sclerosis, ⟨E⟩ but is not licensed for this indication.

- **CAUTIONS** Epilepsy · history of convulsions · risk factors for epilepsy

- **INTERACTIONS** → Appendix 1: memantine

- **SIDE-EFFECTS**
▶ **Common or very common** Balance impaired · constipation · dizziness · drowsiness · dyspnoea · headache · hypersensitivity · hypertension
▶ **Uncommon** Confusion · embolism and thrombosis · fatigue · fungal infection · hallucination · heart failure · vomiting
▶ **Rare or very rare** Seizure
▶ **Frequency not known** Hepatitis · pancreatitis · psychotic disorder

- **PREGNANCY** Manufacturer advises avoid unless essential—no information available.

- **BREAST FEEDING** Manufacturer advises avoid—no information available.

- **HEPATIC IMPAIRMENT** Manufacturer advises avoid in severe impairment—no information available.

- **RENAL IMPAIRMENT** Avoid if eGFR less than $5 \, mL/minute/1.73 \, m^2$.
Dose adjustments Reduce dose to 10 mg daily if eGFR $30–49 \, mL/minute/1.73 \, m^2$, if well tolerated after at least 7 days dose can be increased in steps to 20 mg daily; reduce dose to 10 mg daily if eGFR $5–29 \, mL/minute/1.73 \, m^2$.

- **DIRECTIONS FOR ADMINISTRATION** For *oral solution*, manufacturer advises solution should be dosed onto a spoon or into a glass of water.

- **NATIONAL FUNDING/ACCESS DECISIONS**
For full details see funding body website
NICE decisions
▶ **Donepezil, galantamine, rivastigmine, and memantine for the treatment of Alzheimer's disease (updated June 2018)**
NICE TA217 Recommended with restrictions

- **MEDICINAL FORMS** There can be variation in the licensing of different medicines containing the same drug.
Oral tablet
▶ **Memantine hydrochloride (Non-proprietary)**
Memantine hydrochloride 5 mg Memantine 5mg tablets | 7 tablet [PoM] [⅏]
Memantine hydrochloride 10 mg Memantine 10mg tablets | 28 tablet [PoM] £29.33 DT = £1.98
Memantine hydrochloride 15 mg Memantine 15mg tablets | 7 tablet [PoM] [⅏]
Memantine hydrochloride 20 mg Memantine 20mg tablets | 28 tablet [PoM] £58.66 DT = £2.94
▶ **Ebixa** (Lundbeck Ltd)
Memantine hydrochloride 5 mg Ebixa 5mg tablets | 7 tablet [PoM] [⅏]
Memantine hydrochloride 10 mg Ebixa 10mg tablets | 28 tablet [PoM] £34.50 DT = £1.98
Memantine hydrochloride 15 mg Ebixa 15mg tablets | 7 tablet [PoM] [⅏]
Memantine hydrochloride 20 mg Ebixa 20mg tablets | 28 tablet [PoM] £69.01 DT = £2.94
Oral solution
▶ **Memantine hydrochloride (Non-proprietary)**
Memantine hydrochloride 10 mg per 1 ml Memantine 10mg/ml oral solution sugar free | 50 ml [PoM] £54.00 DT = £12.87 [SF] | 100 ml [PoM] £13.93-£123.23 [SF]
▶ **Ebixa** (Lundbeck Ltd)
Memantine hydrochloride 10 mg per 1 ml Ebixa 5mg/0.5ml pump actuation oral solution | 50 ml [PoM] £61.61 DT = £12.87 [SF] | 100 ml [PoM] £123.23 [SF]
Form unstated
▶ **Memantine hydrochloride (Non-proprietary)**
Memantine 5mg/10mg/15mg/20mg tablets treatment initiation pack | 28 tablet [PoM] £80.00 DT = £43.13
▶ **Ebixa** (Lundbeck Ltd)
Ebixa tablets treatment initiation pack | 28 tablet [PoM] £43.13 DT = £43.13
▶ **Valios** (Dr Reddy's Laboratories (UK) Ltd)
Valios 5mg/10mg/15mg/20mg orodispersible tablets initiation pack | 28 tablet [PoM] £31.24 DT = £31.24 [SF]
Orodispersible tablet
EXCIPIENTS: May contain Aspartame
▶ **Valios** (Dr Reddy's Laboratories (UK) Ltd)
Memantine hydrochloride 5 mg Valios 5mg orodispersible tablets sugar free | 28 tablet [PoM] £12.50 DT = £12.50 [SF]
Memantine hydrochloride 10 mg Valios 10mg orodispersible tablets sugar free | 28 tablet [PoM] £24.99 DT = £24.99 [SF]
Memantine hydrochloride 15 mg Valios 15mg orodispersible tablets sugar free | 7 tablet [PoM] [⅏] [SF]
Memantine hydrochloride 20 mg Valios 20mg orodispersible tablets sugar free | 28 tablet [PoM] £49.98 DT = £49.98 [SF]

2 Epilepsy and other seizure disorders

Epilepsy
02-Oct-2024

Epilepsy control

The object of treatment is to prevent the occurrence of seizures by maintaining an effective dose of one or more antiepileptic drugs (antiseizure medications). Careful adjustment of doses is necessary, starting with low doses and increasing gradually until seizures are controlled or there are significant adverse effects.

When choosing an antiepileptic drug, the seizure type, epilepsy syndrome, need for treatment, risks and benefits of treatment with antiepileptic drugs (including their importance in reducing the risk of epilepsy-related death), and the patient's age, sex, comorbidities, concomitant medication, and personal circumstances (such as education, employment, and likelihood of pregnancy) should be taken into account.

The dosage frequency is often determined by the plasma-drug half-life, and should be kept as low as possible to encourage adherence with the prescribed regimen. Most antiepileptics, when used in the usual dosage, can be given twice daily. Lamotrigine p. 366, perampanel p. 371, phenobarbital p. 388, and phenytoin p. 372, which have long half-lives, can be given once daily at bedtime. However, with large doses, some antiepileptics may need to be given more frequently to avoid adverse effects associated with high peak plasma-drug concentration.

Management

[EvGr] When monotherapy with a first-line antiepileptic drug is unsuccessful (does not reduce or stop seizures, or if side-effects are intolerable), monotherapy with an alternative drug should be tried; the diagnosis should be checked before starting an alternative drug if the first drug showed lack of efficacy. The change from one antiepileptic drug to another should be cautious, slowly withdrawing the first drug only when the new regimen has been established. Combination (adjunctive) therapy with two or more antiepileptic drugs may be necessary, but the concurrent use of antiepileptic drugs increases the risk of adverse effects and drug interactions. If combination therapy does not reduce seizures, revert to the regimen (monotherapy or combination therapy) that provided the best balance between tolerability and efficacy. A single antiepileptic drug should be prescribed wherever possible. ⓐ

For guidance on when to refer patients to tertiary epilepsy services, see NICE guideline: **Epilepsies in children, young people and adults** (see *Useful resources*).

In light of prescribing data showing ongoing exposure to valproate in pregnancy, and of potential risks associated with valproate use in males, the MHRA has issued a National Patient Safety Alert. This outlines new regulatory measures for initiation of valproate in individuals (males or females) aged under 55 years, and continued use in females of childbearing potential. In addition to these measures, further advice has been issued around the use in males and the need to use effective contraception. For further information, see *Important safety information*, *Conception and contraception*, and *Pregnancy* in sodium valproate p. 378 and valproic acid p. 409.

The MHRA also advise that topiramate must not be used in females of childbearing potential unless the conditions of the Pregnancy Prevention Programme are met. Topiramate must not be used during pregnancy unless there is no other suitable alternative. For further information, see *Important safety information*, *Conception and contraception*, and *Pregnancy* in topiramate p. 384.

MHRA/CHM advice: Antiepileptics: risk of suicidal thoughts and behaviour (August 2008)

A Europe-wide review concluded that all antiepileptic drugs may be associated with a small increased risk of suicidal thoughts and behaviour; symptoms may occur as early as 1 week after starting treatment. The MHRA has recommended that patients and their carers should be advised to seek medical advice if any mood changes, distressing thoughts, or feelings about suicide or self-harming develop, and that the patient should be referred for appropriate treatment if necessary. Patients should also be advised not to stop or switch antiepileptic treatment and to seek advice from a healthcare professional if concerned.

MHRA/CHM advice: Antiepileptic drugs: updated advice on switching between different manufacturers' products (November 2017)

The CHM has reviewed spontaneous adverse reactions received by the MHRA and publications that reported potential harm arising from switching of antiepileptic drugs in patients previously stabilised on a branded product to a generic. The CHM concluded that reports of loss of seizure control and/or worsening of side-effects around the time of switching between products could be explained as chance associations, but that a causal role of switching could not be ruled out in all cases. The following guidance has been issued to help minimise risk:

- Different antiepileptic drugs vary considerably in their characteristics, which influences the risk of whether switching between different manufacturers' products of a particular drug may cause adverse effects or loss of seizure control;
- Antiepileptic drugs have been divided into three risk-based categories to help healthcare professionals decide whether it is necessary to maintain continuity of supply of a specific manufacturer's product. These categories are listed below;
- If it is felt desirable for a patient to be maintained on a specific manufacturer's product this should be prescribed either by specifying a brand name, or by using the generic drug name and name of the manufacturer (otherwise known as the Marketing Authorisation Holder);
- This advice relates only to antiepileptic drug use for treatment of epilepsy; it does not apply to their use in other indications (e.g. mood stabilisation, neuropathic pain);
- Please report on a Yellow Card any suspected adverse reactions to antiepileptic drugs;
- Dispensing pharmacists should ensure the continuity of supply of a particular product when the prescription specifies it. If the prescribed product is unavailable, it may be necessary to dispense a product from a different manufacturer to maintain continuity of treatment of that antiepileptic drug. Such cases should be discussed and agreed with both the prescriber and patient (or carer);
- Usual dispensing practice can be followed when a specific product is not stated.

Category 1
Carbamazepine p. 355, phenobarbital, phenytoin, primidone p. 389. For these drugs, doctors are advised to ensure that their patient is maintained on a specific manufacturer's product.

Category 2
Clobazam p. 390, clonazepam p. 391, eslicarbazepine acetate p. 359, lamotrigine, oxcarbazepine p. 370, perampanel, rufinamide p. 376, topiramate, valproate, zonisamide p. 387. For these drugs, the need for continued supply of a particular manufacturer's product should be based on clinical judgement and consultation with the patient and/or carer taking into account factors such as seizure frequency, treatment history, and potential implications to the patient of having a breakthrough seizure. Non-clinical factors as for Category 3 drugs should also be considered.

Category 3
Brivaracetam p. 354, ethosuximide p. 360, gabapentin p. 362, lacosamide p. 364, levetiracetam p. 368, pregabalin p. 374, tiagabine p. 383, vigabatrin p. 385. For these drugs, it is usually unnecessary to ensure that patients are maintained on a specific manufacturer's product as therapeutic equivalence can be assumed, however, other factors are important when considering whether switching is appropriate. Differences between alternative products (e.g. product name, packaging, appearance, and taste) may be perceived negatively by patients and/or carers, and may lead to dissatisfaction, anxiety, confusion, dosing errors, and reduced adherence. In addition, difficulties for patients with co-morbid autism, mental health problems, or learning disability should also be considered.

Antiepileptic hypersensitivity syndrome

Antiepileptic hypersensitivity syndrome is a rare but potentially fatal syndrome associated with some antiepileptic drugs (**carbamazepine, lacosamide, lamotrigine, oxcarbazepine, phenobarbital, phenytoin,**

primidone, and **rufinamide**); rarely cross-sensitivity occurs between some of these antiepileptic drugs. Some other antiepileptics (**eslicarbazepine, stiripentol**, and **zonisamide**) have a theoretical risk. The symptoms usually start between 1 and 8 weeks of exposure; fever, rash, and lymphadenopathy are most commonly seen. Other systemic signs include liver dysfunction, haematological, renal, and pulmonary abnormalities, vasculitis, and multi-organ failure. If signs or symptoms of hypersensitivity syndrome occur, the drug should be withdrawn immediately, the patient must not be re-exposed, and expert advice should be sought.

Withdrawal

[EvGr] The decision to withdraw antiepileptic drugs from a seizure-free patient may be considered after the patient has been seizure-free for at least two years, depending on their individual circumstances. An assessment to determine the risk of seizure recurrence if antiepileptic drugs are discontinued should be carried out. If there is any doubt or concern, the assessment should be done by an epilepsy specialist. (A) Even in patients who have been seizure-free for several years, there is a significant risk of seizure recurrence on drug withdrawal.

[EvGr] In patients receiving several antiepileptic drugs, only one drug should be withdrawn at a time. Avoid abrupt withdrawal, particularly of barbiturates and benzodiazepines, because this can precipitate severe rebound seizures. Reduction in dosage should be gradual and for most drugs, this would usually be over at least three months. In the case of barbiturates and benzodiazepines, withdrawal of the drug would typically be over a longer period to reduce the risk of drug-related withdrawal symptoms.

If seizures recur during or after discontinuation of an antiepileptic drug, the last dose reduction should be reversed and guidance sought from an epilepsy specialist. (A)

Driving

If a driver has a seizure (of any type) they must stop driving immediately and inform the Driver and Vehicle Licensing Agency (DVLA).

Patients who have had a first unprovoked epileptic seizure or a single isolated seizure must not drive for 6 months; driving may then be resumed, provided the patient has been assessed by a specialist as fit to drive and investigations do not suggest a risk of further seizures.

Patients with established epilepsy may drive a motor vehicle provided they are not a danger to the public and are compliant with treatment and follow up. To continue driving, these patients must be seizure-free for at least one year (or have a pattern of seizures established for one year where there is no influence on their level of consciousness or the ability to act); also, they must not have a history of unprovoked seizures.

Note: additional criteria apply for drivers of large goods or passenger carrying vehicles—consult DVLA guidance.

Patients who have had a *seizure while asleep* are not permitted to drive for one year from the date of each seizure, unless:

- a history or pattern of sleep seizures occurring **only** ever while asleep has been established over the course of at least one year from the date of the first sleep seizure; or
- an established pattern of purely asleep seizures can be demonstrated over the course of three years if the patient has previously had seizures whilst awake (or awake and asleep).

The DVLA recommends that patients should not drive during medication changes or withdrawal of antiepileptic drugs, and for 6 months after their last dose. If a seizure occurs due to a prescribed change or withdrawal of epilepsy treatment, the patient will have their driving license revoked for 1 year; relicensing may be considered earlier if treatment

has been reinstated for 6 months and no further seizures have occurred.

Pregnancy

There is an increased risk of teratogenicity associated with the use of antiepileptic drugs (especially if used during the first trimester and particularly if the patient is taking two or more antiepileptic drugs).

In light of prescribing data showing ongoing exposure to valproate in pregnancy, the MHRA has issued a National Patient Safety Alert. This outlines new regulatory measures for initiation of valproate in individuals aged under 55 years, and continued use in females of childbearing potential. In addition to these measures, further advice has been issued around the use in males and the need to use effective contraception. For further information, see *Important safety information, Conception and contraception*, and *Pregnancy* in sodium valproate p. 378 and valproic acid p. 409.

The MHRA also advise that topiramate must not be used in females of childbearing potential unless the conditions of the Pregnancy Prevention Programme are met. Topiramate must not be used during pregnancy unless there is no other suitable alternative. For further information, see *Important safety information, Conception and contraception*, and *Pregnancy* in topiramate p. 384.

MHRA/CHM advice: Antiepileptic drugs in pregnancy: updated advice following comprehensive safety review (January 2021)
Valproate, in particular, is highly teratogenic and evidence supports that use in pregnancy leads to congenital malformations (approximately 10% risk) and neurodevelopmental disorders (approximately 30–40% risk). Prescribers are reminded that valproate must **not** be used in females of childbearing potential unless the conditions of the Pregnancy Prevention Programme are met and alternative treatments are ineffective or not tolerated. Valproate must not be used during pregnancy unless there is no other suitable alternative. For further information, see sodium valproate and valproic acid.

In the context of the known harms associated with valproate, the CHM initiated a safety review on the use of other key antiepileptic drugs in pregnancy for the risk of major congenital malformations, neurodevelopmental disorders or delay, and other effects on the child. Safety data for carbamazepine, gabapentin, lamotrigine, levetiracetam, oxcarbazepine, phenobarbital, phenytoin, pregabalin, topiramate, and zonisamide were reviewed. Much of the evidence base related to epilepsy, and as such, the review focused on the risks and decisions for epilepsy treatment.

The review confirmed that lamotrigine and levetiracetam are the safer of the drugs reviewed; large studies of pregnancies exposed to lamotrigine or levetiracetam monotherapy did not suggest an increased risk of major congenital malformations (at usual maintenance doses). Data for neurodevelopmental outcomes were more limited; available studies did not suggest an increased risk of neurodevelopmental disorders or delay associated with *in-utero* exposure to either lamotrigine or levetiracetam, however the data were inadequate to completely rule out the possibility of an increased risk. Lamotrigine and levetiracetam were not associated with an increased risk of fetal loss, intra-uterine growth restriction, or preterm birth.

For carbamazepine, phenobarbital, phenytoin, and topiramate, the data showed that use during pregnancy was associated with an increased risk of major congenital malformations; the risk for carbamazepine, phenobarbital, and topiramate was shown to be dose dependent. There is the possibility of adverse effects on neurodevelopment associated with the use of phenobarbital and phenytoin, and an increased risk of intra-uterine growth restriction with phenobarbital, topiramate, and zonisamide. The available data for carbamazepine did not suggest an increased risk of neurodevelopmental disorders or delay associated with in-utero exposure; however, the data were inadequate to completely rule out the possibility of an increased risk. For information on other antiepileptic drugs, see *Pregnancy* in the individual drug monographs.

Specialists should discuss the risks associated with antiepileptic drugs and untreated epilepsy during pregnancy with female patients when initiating treatment and during annual reviews; a safety information leaflet is available to aid discussion. Treatment should be reviewed according to the patient's clinical condition and circumstance. Female patients should be advised not to stop their antiepileptic treatment without discussing this with their doctor, and to seek urgent medical advice if they are on antiepileptic drugs and think they could be pregnant. Those who are planning a pregnancy should be urgently referred to a specialist for advice on antiepileptic treatment and offered folic acid.

With any antiepileptic drug used during pregnancy, monotherapy and use of the lowest effective dose are recommended where possible. Plasma concentrations of antiepileptic drugs (particularly lamotrigine and phenytoin) can be affected by physiological changes during pregnancy and post-partum. Prescribers should consult product literature and relevant clinical guidance for dosing and monitoring recommendations. For further information, also see *Monitoring in Pregnancy* in individual drug monographs.

Other considerations
Prescribers should also carefully consider the choice of antiepileptic therapy in pre-pubescent girls who may later become pregnant. Females of childbearing potential who take antiepileptic drugs should be given advice about the need for a highly effective contraception method to avoid unplanned pregnancy—for further information, see *Contraception in patients taking medication with teratogenic potential* in Contraceptives, hormonal p. 912. Some antiepileptic drugs can reduce the efficacy of hormonal contraceptives, and the efficacy of some antiepileptics may be affected by hormonal contraceptives.

Once an unplanned pregnancy is discovered, specialist advice should be sought; the risk of harm to the mother and fetus from convulsive seizures outweighs the risk of continued therapy. The likelihood of a female who is taking antiepileptic drugs having a baby with no malformations is at least 90%, and it is important that female patients do not stop taking essential treatment because of concern over harm to the fetus. To reduce the risk of neural tube defects, folate supplementation is advised throughout the first trimester.

Female patients who have seizures in the second half of pregnancy should be assessed for eclampsia before any change is made to antiepileptic treatment. Status epilepticus should be treated according to the standard protocol. Routine injection of vitamin K at birth minimises the risk of neonatal haemorrhage associated with antiepileptics. Withdrawal effects in the newborn may occur with some antiepileptic drugs.

Epilepsy and Pregnancy Register
All pregnant females with epilepsy, whether taking medication or not, should be encouraged to notify the UK Epilepsy and Pregnancy Register (available at: www.epilepsyandpregnancy.co.uk).

Breast-feeding
Females taking antiepileptic monotherapy should generally be encouraged to breast-feed; if a female is on combination therapy or if there are other risk factors, such as premature birth, close monitoring is recommended. Patients and their family should be made aware of signs of toxicity in the infant and advised to seek medical advice if these occur.

All infants should be monitored for sedation, feeding difficulties, adequate weight gain, and developmental milestones. Infants should also be monitored for adverse effects associated with the antiepileptic drug particularly with newer antiepileptics, if the antiepileptic is readily transferred into breast-milk causing high infant serum-drug concentrations (e.g. ethosuximide, lamotrigine, primidone, and zonisamide), or if slower metabolism in the infant causes drugs to accumulate (e.g. phenobarbital and lamotrigine). Serum-drug concentration monitoring should be undertaken in breast-fed infants if suspected adverse reactions develop; if toxicity develops it may be necessary to introduce formula feeds to limit the infant's drug exposure, or to wean the infant off breast-milk altogether.

Primidone, phenobarbital, and the benzodiazepines are associated with an established risk of drowsiness in breast-fed babies and caution is required.

Withdrawal effects may occur in infants if a mother suddenly stops breast-feeding, particularly if she is taking phenobarbital, primidone, or lamotrigine.

Focal seizures with or without secondary generalisation

Focal seizures with or without secondary generalisation is also referred to as focal seizures with or without evolution to bilateral tonic-clonic seizures.

[EvGr] Consider lamotrigine p. 366 or levetiracetam p. 368 as first-line options for treating focal seizures. If monotherapy with either lamotrigine or levetiracetam is unsuccessful, the other of these options should be considered. If monotherapy with these drugs is unsuccessful, consider carbamazepine p. 355, oxcarbazepine p. 370, or zonisamide p. 387 as second-line monotherapy options. Lacosamide p. 364 should be considered as third-line monotherapy.

If monotherapy is unsuccessful, adjunctive treatment should be considered. First-line options for adjunctive treatment include carbamazepine, lacosamide, lamotrigine, levetiracetam, oxcarbazepine, topiramate p. 384, or zonisamide. Second-line options include brivaracetam p. 354, cenobamate p. 358, eslicarbazepine acetate p. 359, perampanel p. 371, pregabalin p. 374, or sodium valproate p. 378 (in males, and females unable to have children). Third-line options include phenobarbital p. 388, phenytoin p. 372, tiagabine p. 383, or vigabatrin p. 385. (A)

Generalised seizures

Tonic-clonic seizures
[EvGr] Offer sodium valproate as first-line monotherapy for generalised tonic-clonic seizures in males, and females unable to have children. If treatment with sodium valproate is unsuccessful, consider lamotrigine or levetiracetam [unlicensed use] as alternative second-line options. If monotherapy with either lamotrigine or levetiracetam is unsuccessful, the other of these options should be tried.

For females who are able to have children, offer lamotrigine p. 366 or levetiracetam p. 368 [unlicensed use] as first-line monotherapy. If monotherapy with either lamotrigine or levetiracetam is unsuccessful, the other of these options should be tried.

If monotherapy is unsuccessful, adjunctive treatment should be considered. First-line options for adjunctive treatment include clobazam p. 390, lamotrigine, levetiracetam, perampanel p. 371, sodium valproate p. 378 (in males, and females unable to have children), or topiramate p. 384. Second-line options include brivaracetam p. 354 [unlicensed use], lacosamide p. 364, phenobarbital p. 388, primidone p. 389, or zonisamide p. 387 [unlicensed use]. (A)

Patients with absence or myoclonic seizures may have their seizures exacerbated if treated with carbamazepine, gabapentin, lamotrigine, oxcarbazepine, phenytoin, pregabalin, tiagabine, or vigabatrin.

Absence seizures
[EvGr] Offer ethosuximide p. 360 as first-line treatment for absence seizures. If treatment with ethosuximide is unsuccessful, consider sodium valproate as second-line monotherapy or adjunctive treatment for males, and females

unable to have children. If treatment with sodium valproate is unsuitable or unsuccessful, lamotrigine or levetiracetam [unlicensed use] should be considered as third-line monotherapy or adjunctive treatment. If treatment with either lamotrigine or levetiracetam is unsuccessful, the other of these options should be considered. Ⓐ

Patients with absence seizures may have their seizures exacerbated if treated with carbamazepine, gabapentin, oxcarbazepine, phenobarbital, phenytoin, pregabalin, tiagabine, or vigabatrin.

Myoclonic seizures

Myoclonic seizures (myoclonic jerks) occur in a variety of syndromes, and response to treatment varies considerably.

EvGr Offer sodium valproate as first-line treatment for myoclonic seizures in males, and females unable to have children. If treatment with sodium valproate is unsuccessful, levetiracetam should be offered as second-line monotherapy or adjunctive treatment.

For females who are able to have children, offer levetiracetam [unlicensed use] as first-line monotherapy.

If treatment with levetiracetam is unsuccessful, consider monotherapy or adjunctive treatment (for all patients) with brivaracetam [unlicensed use], clobazam, clonazepam p. 391, lamotrigine, phenobarbital, piracetam p. 468, topiramate [unlicensed use], or zonisamide [unlicensed use].

In patients with myoclonic seizures, the use of carbamazepine, gabapentin, oxcarbazepine, phenytoin, pregabalin, tiagabine, or vigabatrin is not recommended because they may exacerbate seizures. Ⓐ Lamotrigine may also occasionally exacerbate myoclonic seizures.

Atonic or tonic seizures

Atonic or tonic seizures are usually seen in childhood, in specific epilepsy syndromes, or associated with cerebral damage or learning disabilities. They may respond poorly to the traditional drugs.

EvGr Offer sodium valproate as first-line treatment for atonic or tonic seizures in males, and females unable to have children. If treatment with sodium valproate is unsuccessful, lamotrigine should be offered as second-line monotherapy or adjunctive treatment.

For females who are able to have children, offer lamotrigine as first-line monotherapy.

If treatment with lamotrigine is unsuccessful, consider monotherapy or adjunctive treatment (for all patients) with clobazam, rufinamide p. 376 [unlicensed use], or topiramate [unlicensed use].

If all other treatments are unsuccessful, consider felbamate [unlicensed] as adjunctive treatment under the supervision of a neurologist with expertise in epilepsy. Ⓐ

Patients with atonic or tonic seizures may have their seizures exacerbated if treated with carbamazepine, gabapentin, oxcarbazepine, pregabalin, tiagabine, or vigabatrin.

Epilepsy syndromes

Some drugs are licensed for use in particular epilepsy syndromes. The epilepsy syndromes are specific types of epilepsy that are characterised according to a number of features including seizure type, age of onset, and EEG characteristics. Patients with an epilepsy syndrome that is likely to be drug-resistant (failure of adequate trials of two antiepileptic drugs (whether as monotherapy or in combination) to achieve sustained seizure freedom) should be referred to a tertiary epilepsy service. For further guidance on epilepsy syndromes, see NICE guideline: **Epilepsies in children, young people and adults** (see *Useful resources*).

Dravet syndrome

EvGr A neurologist with expertise in epilepsy should be involved in decisions regarding the treatment of Dravet syndrome.

Sodium valproate should be considered as first-line treatment for all patients with Dravet syndrome, including females, because of the severity of the syndrome and the lack of evidence for other effective first-line options. If sodium valproate is started or continued in females who are able to have children, ensure that the potential risks and benefits of treatment are discussed, and that the likelihood of pregnancy is considered and a pregnancy prevention programme put in place, if appropriate.

If monotherapy with sodium valproate is unsuccessful, consider triple therapy with clobazam and stiripentol p. 382 as first-line adjunctive therapy.

If triple therapy with sodium valproate, clobazam, and stiripentol is unsuccessful, cannabidiol p. 355 with clobazam may be considered as second-line adjunctive treatment in certain patients.

Fenfluramine p. 361 may also be considered as adjunctive treatment to other antiepileptic drugs in certain patients.

Under the supervision of a neurologist with expertise in epilepsy, further adjunctive treatment options include topiramate [unlicensed use] or levetiracetam [unlicensed use]; or if all other treatments are unsuccessful, potassium bromide [unlicensed] may be considered. Ⓐ

Patients with Dravet syndrome may have their seizures exacerbated if treated with carbamazepine, gabapentin, lacosamide, lamotrigine, oxcarbazepine, phenobarbital, pregabalin, tiagabine, or vigabatrin.

Lennox-Gastaut syndrome

EvGr A neurologist with expertise in epilepsy should be involved in decisions regarding the treatment of Lennox-Gastaut syndrome.

Sodium valproate should be considered as first-line treatment for all patients with Lennox-Gastaut syndrome, including females, because of the severity of the syndrome and the lack of evidence for other effective first-line options. If sodium valproate is started or continued in females who are able to have children, ensure that the potential risks and benefits of treatment are discussed, and that the likelihood of pregnancy is considered and a pregnancy prevention programme put in place, if appropriate.

If monotherapy with sodium valproate is unsuccessful, consider lamotrigine as second-line monotherapy or adjunctive treatment. Third-line adjunctive treatment options include cannabidiol with clobazam in certain patients, or clobazam, rufinamide, or topiramate.

Felbamate [unlicensed] may be considered as adjunctive therapy under the supervision of a neurologist with expertise in epilepsy when all other treatment options are unsuccessful. Ⓐ

Patients with Lennox-Gastaut syndrome may have their seizures exacerbated if treated with carbamazepine, gabapentin, lacosamide, lamotrigine, oxcarbazepine, phenobarbital, pregabalin, tiagabine, or vigabatrin.

Repeated or cluster seizures, prolonged seizures, and status epilepticus

Repeated or cluster seizures (typically 3 or more self-terminating seizures in 24 hours), prolonged convulsive seizures (a seizure that continues for more than 2 minutes longer than the patient's usual seizure), and convulsive status epilepticus (a seizure that lasts 5 minutes or longer, or recurrent seizures without recovery in between) should be managed as a medical emergency.

For further guidance on the management of convulsive status epilepticus, see Status epilepticus p. 392, and for a quick reference resource with doses of benzodiazepines for use in convulsive status epilepticus, see *Seizures* in Medical emergencies in the community p. 2028.

Repeated or cluster seizures, or prolonged seizures

EvGr The patient's individualised emergency management plan should be followed, if immediately available. If an individualised emergency management plan is not available, treatment with a benzodiazepine (such as clobazam p. 390 or midazolam p. 394) should be urgently considered for patients with repeated or cluster seizures, or prolonged convulsive seizures. For convulsive seizures that last 5 minutes or longer, or recurrent seizures without recovery in between, follow the recommendations for convulsive status epilepticus, see Status epilepticus p. 392.

If there is concern that repeated or cluster seizures, or prolonged seizures (convulsive or non-convulsive) may recur, an emergency management plan should be agreed with the patient if they do not have one already.

Expert guidance should be sought if the patient has further episodes of repeated or cluster seizures. Ⓐ

Febrile convulsions

Brief febrile convulsions need no specific treatment; antipyretic medication (e.g. paracetamol p. 507), is commonly used to reduce fever and prevent further convulsions but evidence to support this practice is lacking. *Prolonged febrile convulsions* (those lasting 5 minutes or longer), or *recurrent febrile convulsions* without recovery must be treated actively as for convulsive status epilepticus, see Status epilepticus p. 392. Long-term anticonvulsant prophylaxis for febrile convulsions is rarely indicated.

Useful resources

Epilepsies in children, young people and adults. National Institute for Health and Care Excellence. NICE guideline 217. April 2022.
www.nice.org.uk/guidance/ng217

> **Other drugs used for Epilepsy and other seizure disorders** Acetazolamide, p. 1343 · Magnesium sulfate, p. 1193

ANTIEPILEPTICS

Brivaracetam

04-Aug-2022

● **INDICATIONS AND DOSE**

Adjunctive therapy of focal seizures with or without secondary generalisation
▸ BY MOUTH, OR BY INTRAVENOUS INJECTION, OR BY INTRAVENOUS INFUSION
▸ Adult: Initially 25–50 mg twice daily, adjusted according to response; usual maintenance 25–100 mg twice daily (max. per dose 100 mg twice daily)

IMPORTANT SAFETY INFORMATION
MHRA/CHM ADVICE: ANTIEPILEPTICS: RISK OF SUICIDAL THOUGHTS AND BEHAVIOUR (AUGUST 2008)
See Epilepsy p. 349.

MHRA/CHM ADVICE: ANTIEPILEPTIC DRUGS: UPDATED ADVICE ON SWITCHING BETWEEN DIFFERENT MANUFACTURERS' PRODUCTS (NOVEMBER 2017)
See Epilepsy p. 349.

MHRA/CHM ADVICE: ANTIEPILEPTIC DRUGS IN PREGNANCY: UPDATED ADVICE FOLLOWING COMPREHENSIVE SAFETY REVIEW (JANUARY 2021)
See Epilepsy p. 349.

● INTERACTIONS → Appendix 1: antiepileptics

● SIDE-EFFECTS
▸ **Common or very common** Anxiety · appetite decreased · constipation · cough · depression · dizziness · drowsiness · fatigue · increased risk of infection · insomnia · irritability · nausea · vertigo · vomiting
▸ **Uncommon** Behaviour abnormal · neutropenia · psychotic disorder

▸ **Frequency not known** Severe cutaneous adverse reactions (SCARs) · suicidal behaviours

● **PREGNANCY** Manufacturer advises avoid unless potential benefit outweighs risk—limited information available. See also *Pregnancy* in Epilepsy p. 349.

● **BREAST FEEDING** Manufacturer advises avoid—present in milk in *animal* studies.

● **HEPATIC IMPAIRMENT** EvGr Caution (risk of increased exposure). Ⓜ
Dose adjustments EvGr Initial dose of 25 mg twice daily; max. maintenance dose of 75 mg twice daily (limited information available). Ⓜ

● **TREATMENT CESSATION** EvGr Avoid abrupt withdrawal—reduce daily dose in steps of 50 mg at weekly intervals, then reduce to 20 mg daily for a final week. Ⓜ

● **DIRECTIONS FOR ADMINISTRATION**
▸ With intravenous use For intermittent *intravenous infusion*, manufacturer advises dilute in Glucose 5% *or* Sodium Chloride 0.9% *or* Lactated Ringer's solution; give over 15 minutes.
▸ With oral use Manufacturer advises oral solution can be diluted in water or juice shortly before swallowing.

● **PRESCRIBING AND DISPENSING INFORMATION**
Manufacturer advises if switching between oral therapy and intravenous therapy (for those temporarily unable to take oral medication), the total daily dose and the frequency of administration should be maintained.

● **PATIENT AND CARER ADVICE**
Missed doses Manufacturer advises if one or more doses are missed, a single dose should be taken as soon as possible and the next dose should be taken at the usual time.
Driving and skilled tasks Manufacturer advises patients and carers should be cautioned on the effects on driving and performance of skilled tasks—increased risk of dizziness.

● **NATIONAL FUNDING/ACCESS DECISIONS**
For full details see funding body website
Scottish Medicines Consortium (SMC) decisions
▸ Brivaracetam (*Briviact*®) as adjunctive therapy in the treatment of partial-onset seizures with or without secondary generalisation in adult and adolescent patients from 16 years of age with epilepsy (July 2016) SMC No. 1160/16 Recommended with restrictions

All Wales Medicines Strategy Group (AWMSG) decisions
▸ Brivaracetam (*Briviact*®) as adjunctive therapy in the treatment of partial-onset seizures with or without secondary generalisation in patients from 2 years of age with epilepsy (July 2022) AWMSG No. 4614 Recommended with restrictions

● **MEDICINAL FORMS** There can be variation in the licensing of different medicines containing the same drug.
Solution for injection
CAUTIONARY AND ADVISORY LABELS 2
ELECTROLYTES: May contain Sodium
▸ Briviact (UCB Pharma Ltd)
Brivaracetam 10 mg per 1 ml Briviact 50mg/5ml solution for injection vials | 10 vial PoM £222.75
Oral tablet
CAUTIONARY AND ADVISORY LABELS 2, 8, 25
▸ Briviact (UCB Pharma Ltd)
Brivaracetam 10 mg Briviact 10mg tablets | 14 tablet PoM £34.64 DT = £34.64
Brivaracetam 25 mg Briviact 25mg tablets | 56 tablet PoM £129.64 DT = £129.64
Brivaracetam 50 mg Briviact 50mg tablets | 56 tablet PoM £129.64 DT = £129.64
Brivaracetam 75 mg Briviact 75mg tablets | 56 tablet PoM £129.64 DT = £129.64
Brivaracetam 100 mg Briviact 100mg tablets | 56 tablet PoM £129.64 DT = £129.64

Oral solution

CAUTIONARY AND ADVISORY LABELS 2, 8
EXCIPIENTS: May contain Sorbitol
ELECTROLYTES: May contain Sodium

▸ Briviact (UCB Pharma Ltd)
Brivaracetam 10 mg per 1 ml Briviact 10mg/ml oral solution |
300 ml [PoM] £115.83 DT = £115.83 [SF]

Cannabidiol
21-Mar-2023

● **INDICATIONS AND DOSE**

**Seizures associated with Lennox-Gastaut syndrome
[adjunctive treatment with clobazam] (specialist use
only) | Seizures associated with Dravet syndrome
[adjunctive treatment with clobazam] (specialist use
only)**

▸ BY MOUTH
▸ Adult: Initially 2.5 mg/kg twice daily for 1 week, then
increased to 5 mg/kg twice daily, then increased in
steps of 2.5 mg/kg twice daily if required, dose to be
adjusted according to response at weekly intervals,
food may affect absorption (take at the same time with
respect to food); maximum 20 mg/kg per day

**Seizures associated with tuberous sclerosis complex
[adjunctive treatment] (specialist use only)**

▸ BY MOUTH
▸ Adult: Initially 2.5 mg/kg twice daily for 1 week, then
increased to 5 mg/kg twice daily, then increased in
steps of 2.5 mg/kg twice daily if required, dose to be
adjusted according to response at weekly intervals,
food may affect absorption (take at the same time with
respect to food); maximum 25 mg/kg per day

> **IMPORTANT SAFETY INFORMATION**
>
> MHRA/CHM ADVICE: ANTIEPILEPTICS: RISK OF SUICIDAL
> THOUGHTS AND BEHAVIOUR (AUGUST 2008)
> See Epilepsy p. 349.
>
> MHRA/CHM ADVICE: ANTIEPILEPTIC DRUGS: UPDATED ADVICE ON
> SWITCHING BETWEEN DIFFERENT MANUFACTURERS' PRODUCTS
> (NOVEMBER 2017)
> See Epilepsy p. 349.
>
> MHRA/CHM ADVICE: ANTIEPILEPTIC DRUGS IN PREGNANCY:
> UPDATED ADVICE FOLLOWING COMPREHENSIVE SAFETY REVIEW
> (JANUARY 2021)
> See Epilepsy p. 349.

● **CAUTIONS** Elderly

● **INTERACTIONS** → Appendix 1: cannabidiol

● **SIDE-EFFECTS**
▸ **Common or very common** Aggression · appetite decreased ·
cough · diarrhoea · drowsiness · fatigue · fever · increased
risk of infection · irritability · nausea · rash · seizure ·
vomiting · weight decreased
▸ **Frequency not known** Anaemia · suicidal behaviours

● **PREGNANCY** Manufacturer advises avoid unless potential
benefit outweighs risk—toxicity in *animal* studies. See also
Pregnancy in Epilepsy p. 349.

● **BREAST FEEDING** Manufacturer advises avoid—limited
information available.

● **HEPATIC IMPAIRMENT** Manufacturer advises caution in
moderate to severe impairment (risk of increased
exposure).
Dose adjustments Manufacturer advises dose reduction in
moderate to severe impairment—consult product
literature.

● **MONITORING REQUIREMENTS** Manufacturer advises
monitor liver function at baseline, at 1 month, 3 months,
and 6 months of treatment, then periodically thereafter;
more frequent monitoring is recommended in patients
with raised baseline ALT or AST or taking valproate.

Restart monitoring schedule if dose increased above
10 mg/kg/day. If transaminase or bilirubin levels increase
significantly or symptoms of hepatic dysfunction occur,
treatment should be withheld or permanently
discontinued based on severity—consult product
literature.

● **TREATMENT CESSATION** Manufacturer advises avoid abrupt
withdrawal—withdraw treatment gradually.

● **DIRECTIONS FOR ADMINISTRATION** For administration
advice via nasogastric or gastrostomy tube—consult
product literature.

● **PATIENT AND CARER ADVICE** Oral solution should be
discarded 12 weeks after first opening.
Missed doses If doses are missed for more than 7 days,
dose titration should be re-started.
Driving and skilled tasks Patients and carers should be
counselled on the effects on driving and performance of
skilled tasks—increased risk of somnolence and sedation.
Effects of alcohol increased.

For information on 2015 legislation regarding driving
whilst taking certain controlled drugs, including cannabis,
see Drugs and driving under Guidance on prescribing p. 1.

● **NATIONAL FUNDING/ACCESS DECISIONS**
For full details see funding body website

NICE decisions

▸ **Cannabidiol with clobazam for treating seizures associated
with Dravet syndrome (December 2019)** NICE TA614
Recommended with restrictions
▸ **Cannabidiol with clobazam for treating seizures associated
with Lennox-Gastaut syndrome (December 2019)** NICE TA615
Recommended with restrictions
▸ **Cannabidiol for treating seizures caused by tuberous sclerosis
complex (March 2023)** NICE TA873 Recommended with
restrictions

Scottish Medicines Consortium (SMC) decisions

▸ Cannabidiol (*Epidyolex*®) as adjunctive therapy of seizures
associated with Dravet syndrome (DS) in conjunction with
clobazam, for patients 2 years of age and older (September
2020) SMC No. SMC2262 Recommended
▸ Cannabidiol (*Epidyolex*®) as adjunctive therapy of seizures
associated with Lennox-Gastaut syndrome (LGS) in
conjunction with clobazam, for patients 2 years of age and
older (September 2020) SMC No. SMC2263 Recommended
▸ Cannabidiol (*Epidyolex*®) as adjunctive therapy of seizures
associated with tuberous sclerosis complex (TSC) for patients
2 years of age and older (February 2022) SMC No. SMC2402
Recommended

● **MEDICINAL FORMS** There can be variation in the licensing of
different medicines containing the same drug. Forms available
from special-order manufacturers include: oral solution

Oral solution

CAUTIONARY AND ADVISORY LABELS 2, 8
EXCIPIENTS: May contain Benzyl alcohol, ethanol, sesame oil

▸ Epidyolex (Jazz Pharmaceuticals Operations UK Ltd)
Cannabidiol 100 mg per 1 ml Epidyolex 100mg/ml oral solution |
100 ml [PoM] £850.29 DT = £850.29 [CD5] [SF]

Carbamazepine
16-Jul-2024

● **INDICATIONS AND DOSE**

**Focal and secondary generalised tonic-clonic seizures |
Primary generalised tonic-clonic seizures**

▸ BY MOUTH USING IMMEDIATE-RELEASE MEDICINES
▸ Adult: Initially 100–200 mg 1–2 times a day, increased
in steps of 100–200 mg every 2 weeks; usual dose
0.8–1.2 g daily in divided doses; increased if necessary
up to 1.6–2 g daily in divided doses
▸ Elderly: Reduce initial dose

continued →

▸ BY RECTUM

▸ Adult: Up to 1 g daily in 4 divided doses for up to 7 days, for short-term use when oral therapy temporarily not possible

Trigeminal neuralgia

▸ BY MOUTH USING IMMEDIATE-RELEASE MEDICINES

▸ Adult: Initially 100 mg 1–2 times a day, some patients may require higher initial dose, increase gradually according to response; usual dose 200 mg 3–4 times a day, increased if necessary up to 1.6 g daily

Prophylaxis of bipolar disorder unresponsive to lithium

▸ BY MOUTH USING IMMEDIATE-RELEASE MEDICINES

▸ Adult: Initially 400 mg daily in divided doses, increased until symptoms controlled; usual dose 400–600 mg daily; maximum 1.6 g per day

Adjunct in acute alcohol withdrawal

▸ BY MOUTH USING IMMEDIATE-RELEASE MEDICINES

▸ Adult: Initially 800 mg daily in divided doses, then reduced to 200 mg daily for usual treatment duration of 7–10 days, dose to be reduced gradually over 5 days

Diabetic neuropathy

▸ BY MOUTH USING IMMEDIATE-RELEASE MEDICINES

▸ Adult: Initially 100 mg 1–2 times a day, increased gradually according to response; usual dose 200 mg 3–4 times a day, increased if necessary up to 1.6 g daily

Focal and generalised tonic-clonic seizures

▸ BY MOUTH USING IMMEDIATE-RELEASE MEDICINES

▸ Child 1 month-11 years: Initially 5 mg/kg once daily, dose to be taken at night, alternatively initially 2.5 mg/kg twice daily, then increased in steps of 2.5–5 mg/kg every 3–7 days as required; maintenance 5 mg/kg 2–3 times a day, increased if necessary up to 20 mg/kg daily

▸ Child 12-17 years: Initially 100–200 mg 1–2 times a day, then increased to 200–400 mg 2–3 times a day, increased if necessary up to 1.8 g daily, dose should be increased slowly

DOSE EQUIVALENCE AND CONVERSION

▸ Suppositories of 125 mg may be considered to be approximately equivalent in therapeutic effect to tablets of 100 mg but final adjustment should always depend on clinical response (plasma concentration monitoring recommended).

CARBAGEN ® SR

Focal and secondary generalised tonic-clonic seizures | Primary generalised tonic-clonic seizures

▸ BY MOUTH

▸ Adult: Initially 100–400 mg daily in 1–2 divided doses, increased in steps of 100–200 mg every 2 weeks, dose should be increased slowly; usual dose 0.8–1.2 g daily in 1–2 divided doses, increased if necessary up to 1.6–2 g daily in 1–2 divided doses

▸ Elderly: Reduce initial dose

Trigeminal neuralgia

▸ BY MOUTH

▸ Adult: Initially 100–200 mg daily in 1–2 divided doses, some patients may require higher initial dose, increase gradually according to response; usual dose 600–800 mg daily in 1–2 divided doses, increased if necessary up to 1.6 g daily in 1–2 divided doses

Prophylaxis of bipolar disorder unresponsive to lithium

▸ BY MOUTH

▸ Adult: Initially 400 mg daily in 1–2 divided doses, increased until symptoms controlled; usual dose 400–600 mg daily in 1–2 divided doses; maximum 1.6 g per day

Focal and generalised tonic-clonic seizures | Prophylaxis of bipolar disorder

▸ BY MOUTH

▸ Child 5-11 years: Initially 5 mg/kg daily in 1–2 divided doses, then increased in steps of 2.5–5 mg/kg every 3–7 days as required, dose should be increased slowly; maintenance 10–15 mg/kg daily in 1–2 divided doses, increased if necessary up to 20 mg/kg daily in 1–2 divided doses

▸ Child 12-17 years: Initially 100–400 mg daily in 1–2 divided doses, then increased to 400–1200 mg daily in 1–2 divided doses, increased if necessary up to 1.8 g daily in 1–2 divided doses, dose should be increased slowly

TEGRETOL ® PROLONGED RELEASE

Focal and secondary generalised tonic-clonic seizures | Primary generalised tonic-clonic seizures

▸ BY MOUTH

▸ Adult: Initially 100–400 mg daily in 2 divided doses, increased in steps of 100–200 mg every 2 weeks, dose should be increased slowly; usual dose 0.8–1.2 g daily in 2 divided doses, increased if necessary up to 1.6–2 g daily in 2 divided doses

▸ Elderly: Reduce initial dose

Focal and generalised tonic-clonic seizures | Prophylaxis of bipolar disorder

▸ BY MOUTH

▸ Child 5-11 years: Initially 5 mg/kg daily in 2 divided doses, then increased in steps of 2.5–5 mg/kg every 3–7 days as required; maintenance 10–15 mg/kg daily in 2 divided doses, increased if necessary up to 20 mg/kg daily in 2 divided doses

▸ Child 12-17 years: Initially 100–400 mg daily in 2 divided doses, dose should be increased slowly; maintenance 400–1200 mg daily in 2 divided doses, increased if necessary up to 1.8 g daily in 2 divided doses

Trigeminal neuralgia

▸ BY MOUTH

▸ Adult: Initially 100–200 mg daily in 2 divided doses, some patients may require higher initial dose. After initial dose, increase according to response; usual dose 600–800 mg daily in 2 divided doses, increased if necessary up to 1.6 g daily in 2 divided doses, dose should be increased slowly

Prophylaxis of bipolar disorder unresponsive to lithium

▸ BY MOUTH

▸ Adult: Initially 400 mg daily in 2 divided doses, increased until symptoms controlled; usual dose 400–600 mg daily in 2 divided doses; maximum 1.6 g per day

● UNLICENSED USE

▸ In children Not licensed for use in prophylaxis of bipolar disorder.

▸ In adults Not licensed for use in acute alcohol withdrawal. Use in diabetic neuropathy is an unlicensed indication.

IMPORTANT SAFETY INFORMATION

MHRA/CHM ADVICE: TEGRETOL ® 100 MG/5 ML LIQUID (CARBAMAZEPINE): TEMPORARY STOCK-OUT AND UPDATE TO POSOLOGY (REDUCTION OF MAXIMUM DAILY DOSE) (APRIL 2024)

Tegretol ® 100 mg/5 mL liquid/oral suspension will imminently be out of stock due to manufacturing constraints associated with the excipient sorbitol, therefore the maximum dose of *Tegretol* ® liquid has been reduced to 1200 mg per day. Patients that require *Tegretol* ® liquid should be switched to alternative oral formulations of *Tegretol* ®, such as immediate-release or prolonged-release tablets, where possible. If this is not feasible, other antiepileptic medicines should be considered. Patients requiring more than the maximum daily dose of *Tegretol*® liquid should be permanently switched to an appropriate alternative. For treatment guidelines and advice on switching antiepileptic medicines, see Epilepsy p. 349.

MHRA/CHM ADVICE: ANTIEPILEPTICS: RISK OF SUICIDAL THOUGHTS AND BEHAVIOUR (AUGUST 2008)
See Epilepsy p. 349.

MHRA/CHM ADVICE: ANTIEPILEPTIC DRUGS: UPDATED ADVICE ON SWITCHING BETWEEN DIFFERENT MANUFACTURERS' PRODUCTS (NOVEMBER 2017)
See Epilepsy p. 349 and see also *Prescribing and dispensing information*.

MHRA/CHM ADVICE: ANTIEPILEPTIC DRUGS IN PREGNANCY: UPDATED ADVICE FOLLOWING COMPREHENSIVE SAFETY REVIEW (JANUARY 2021)
See Epilepsy p. 349.

● CONTRA-INDICATIONS Acute porphyrias p. 1202 · AV conduction abnormalities (unless paced) · history of bone-marrow depression

● CAUTIONS Cardiac disease · history of haematological reactions to other drugs · presence of HLA-B*1502 or HLA-A*3101 allele · seizures (may be exacerbated) · skin reactions · susceptibility to angle-closure glaucoma

CAUTIONS, FURTHER INFORMATION MHRA advises consider vitamin D supplementation in patients who are immobilised for long periods or who have inadequate sun exposure or dietary intake of calcium.

▸ Blood, hepatic, or skin disorders [EvGr] Carbamazepine should be withdrawn immediately in cases of aggravated liver dysfunction or acute liver disease. Leucopenia that is severe, progressive, or associated with clinical symptoms requires withdrawal (if necessary under cover of a suitable alternative). ⟨M⟩

▸ HLA allele [EvGr] The presence of HLA-B*1502 allele, particularly in individuals of Han Chinese or Thai origin, is strongly associated with an increased risk of Stevens-Johnson syndrome—see also *Pre-treatment screening*.

  The presence of HLA-A*3101 allele, particularly in individuals of European or Japanese origin, is associated with an increased risk of cutaneous adverse reactions but there are insufficient data to support pre-treatment screening. Consider use if potential benefit outweighs risk. ⟨M⟩

▸ Seizure exacerbation [EvGr] Carbamazepine may exacerbate seizures in patients with absence or myoclonic seizures (including juvenile myoclonic epilepsy), tonic or atonic seizures, Dravet syndrome, Lennox-Gastaut syndrome, and myoclonic-atonic seizures. ⟨A⟩

● INTERACTIONS → Appendix 1: antiepileptics

● SIDE-EFFECTS

▸ **Common or very common** Dizziness · drowsiness · dry mouth · eosinophilia · fatigue · fluid imbalance · gastrointestinal discomfort · headache · hyponatraemia · leucopenia · movement disorders · nausea · oedema · skin reactions · thrombocytopenia · vision disorders · vomiting · weight increased

▸ **Uncommon** Constipation · diarrhoea · eye disorders · tic · tremor

▸ **Rare or very rare** Aggression · agranulocytosis · albuminuria · alopecia · anaemia · angioedema · anxiety · appetite decreased · arrhythmias · arthralgia · azotaemia · bone disorders · bone marrow disorders · cardiac conduction disorders · circulatory collapse · confusion · congestive heart failure · conjunctivitis · coronary artery disease aggravated · depression · dyspnoea · embolism and thrombosis · erythema nodosum · fever · folate deficiency · galactorrhoea · gynaecomastia · haematuria · haemolytic anaemia · hallucinations · hearing impairment · hepatic disorders · hirsutism · hyperacusia · hyperhidrosis · hypersensitivity · hypertension ·

hypogammaglobulinaemia · hypotension · lens opacity · leucocytosis · lymphadenopathy · meningitis aseptic · muscle complaints · muscle weakness · nephritis tubulointerstitial · nervous system disorder · neuroleptic malignant syndrome (discontinue—potentially fatal) · oral disorders · pancreatitis · paraesthesia · paresis · peripheral neuropathy · photosensitivity reaction · pneumonia · pneumonitis · pseudolymphoma · psychosis · red blood cell abnormalities · renal impairment · severe cutaneous adverse reactions (SCARs) · sexual dysfunction · speech impairment · spermatogenesis abnormal · syncope · systemic lupus erythematosus (SLE) · taste altered · tinnitus · urinary disorders · vanishing bile duct syndrome · vasculitis

▸ **Frequency not known** Bone fracture · colitis · human herpesvirus 6 infection reactivation · memory loss · nail loss · suicidal behaviours

SIDE-EFFECTS, FURTHER INFORMATION Some side-effects (such as headache, ataxia, drowsiness, nausea, vomiting, blurring of vision, dizziness and allergic skin reactions) are dose-related, and may be dose-limiting. These side-effects are more common at the start of treatment and in the elderly.

Overdose For details on the management of poisoning, see Active elimination techniques, under Emergency treatment of poisoning p. 1554.

● ALLERGY AND CROSS-SENSITIVITY Antiepileptic hypersensitivity syndrome associated with carbamazepine. See under Epilepsy p. 349 for more information. [EvGr] Caution—cross-sensitivity reported with oxcarbazepine, phenytoin, primidone, and phenobarbital. ⟨M⟩

● PREGNANCY An increased risk of major congenital malformations has been seen with carbamazepine, see *Pregnancy* in Epilepsy p. 349 for further details.
Monitoring [EvGr] Plasma-drug concentration should be monitored and may be maintained on the lower side of the therapeutic range provided seizure control is maintained. ⟨M⟩

● BREAST FEEDING Amount probably too small to be harmful.
Monitoring Monitor infant for possible adverse reactions.

● HEPATIC IMPAIRMENT Manufacturer advises caution and close monitoring—no information available.

● RENAL IMPAIRMENT [EvGr] Use with caution. ⟨M⟩

● PRE-TREATMENT SCREENING [EvGr] Test for HLA-B*1502 allele in individuals of Han Chinese or Thai origin, and consider testing in other at-risk Asian populations such as individuals of Filipino or Malaysian origin (avoid unless no alternative). ⟨M⟩

● MONITORING REQUIREMENTS
▸ Plasma concentration for optimum response 4–12 mg/litre (20–50 micromol/litre) measured after 1–2 weeks.
▸ Manufacturer recommends blood counts and hepatic and renal function tests (but evidence of practical value uncertain).

● TREATMENT CESSATION When stopping treatment with carbamazepine for bipolar disorder, reduce the dose gradually over a period of at least 4 weeks.

● DIRECTIONS FOR ADMINISTRATION
▸ In children Expert sources advise oral liquid has been used rectally—should be retained for at least 2 hours (but may have laxative effect).

TEGRETOL® PROLONGED RELEASE Manufacturer advises *Tegretol*® *Prolonged Release* tablets can be halved but should not be chewed.

● PRESCRIBING AND DISPENSING INFORMATION
Switching between formulations Different formulations of oral preparations may vary in bioavailability. Patients being treated for epilepsy should be maintained on a specific manufacturer's product.
  Patients requiring *Tegretol*® 100 mg/5 mL liquid should

Nervous system　**4**

be switched to an appropriate alternative—see *Important safety information*.

- **PATIENT AND CARER ADVICE**
Blood, hepatic, or skin disorders Patients or their carers should be told how to recognise signs of blood, liver, or skin disorders, and advised to seek immediate medical attention if symptoms such as fever, rash, mouth ulcers, bruising, or bleeding develop.
Medicines for Children leaflet: Carbamazepine (oral) for preventing seizures www.medicinesforchildren.org.uk/medicines/carbamazepine-oral-for-preventing-seizures/

- **PROFESSION SPECIFIC INFORMATION**
Dental practitioners' formulary Carbamazepine Tablets may be prescribed.

- **MEDICINAL FORMS** There can be variation in the licensing of different medicines containing the same drug. Forms available from special-order manufacturers include: oral suspension, oral solution

Oral tablet
CAUTIONARY AND ADVISORY LABELS 3, 8
▸ Carbamazepine (Non-proprietary)
   Carbamazepine 100 mg Carbamazepine 100mg tablets | 84 tablet [PoM] £3.30 DT = £2.07
   Carbamazepine 200 mg Carbamazepine 200mg tablets | 84 tablet [PoM] £5.50 DT = £3.83
   Carbamazepine 400 mg Carbamazepine 400mg tablets | 56 tablet [PoM] £7.00 DT = £5.02
▸ Tegretol (Novartis Pharmaceuticals UK Ltd)
   Carbamazepine 100 mg Tegretol 100mg tablets | 84 tablet [PoM] £2.07 DT = £2.07
   Carbamazepine 200 mg Tegretol 200mg tablets | 84 tablet [PoM] £3.83 DT = £3.83
   Carbamazepine 400 mg Tegretol 400mg tablets | 56 tablet [PoM] £5.02 DT = £5.02

Modified-release tablet
CAUTIONARY AND ADVISORY LABELS 3, 8, 25
▸ Curatil Prolonged Release (Tillomed Laboratories Ltd)
   Carbamazepine 200 mg Curatil Prolonged Release 200mg tablets | 56 tablet [PoM] £3.83 DT = £5.20 (Hospital only)
▸ Tegretol Retard (Novartis Pharmaceuticals UK Ltd)
   Carbamazepine 200 mg Tegretol Prolonged Release 200mg tablets | 56 tablet [PoM] £5.20 DT = £5.20
   Carbamazepine 400 mg Tegretol Prolonged Release 400mg tablets | 56 tablet [PoM] £10.24 DT = £10.24

Suppository
CAUTIONARY AND ADVISORY LABELS 3, 8
▸ Carbamazepine (Non-proprietary)
   Carbamazepine 125 mg Carbamazepine 125mg suppositories | 5 suppository [PoM] £123.60 DT = £123.60
   Carbamazepine 250 mg Carbamazepine 250mg suppositories | 5 suppository [PoM] £177.22 DT = £177.22

Oral suspension
CAUTIONARY AND ADVISORY LABELS 3, 8
▸ Carbamazepine (Non-proprietary)
   Carbamazepine 20 mg per 1 ml Carbamazepine 100mg/5ml oral suspension sugar free | 300 ml [PoM] £26.38 DT = £13.95 [SF]
▸ Tegretol (Novartis Pharmaceuticals UK Ltd)
   Carbamazepine 20 mg per 1 ml Tegretol 100mg/5ml liquid | 300 ml [PoM] £6.12 DT = £13.95 [SF]

Oral solution
CAUTIONARY AND ADVISORY LABELS 3, 8

Cenobamate

01-Mar-2022

- **INDICATIONS AND DOSE**

Adjunctive treatment of focal seizures with or without secondary generalisation
▸ BY MOUTH
▸ Adult: Initially 12.5 mg once daily for 2 weeks, followed by 25 mg once daily for a further 2 weeks, then 50 mg once daily for a further 2 weeks, then increased in steps of 50 mg every 2 weeks, according to response; 200 mg

once daily is the usual target dose; increased if necessary up to 400 mg once daily

> **IMPORTANT SAFETY INFORMATION**
> MHRA/CHM ADVICE: ANTIEPILEPTICS: RISK OF SUICIDAL THOUGHTS AND BEHAVIOUR (AUGUST 2008)
> See Epilepsy p. 349.
>
> MHRA/CHM ADVICE: ANTIEPILEPTIC DRUGS: UPDATED ADVICE ON SWITCHING BETWEEN DIFFERENT MANUFACTURERS' PRODUCTS (NOVEMBER 2017)
> See Epilepsy p. 349 and see also *Prescribing and dispensing information*.
>
> MHRA/CHM ADVICE: ANTIEPILEPTIC DRUGS IN PREGNANCY: UPDATED ADVICE FOLLOWING COMPREHENSIVE SAFETY REVIEW (JANUARY 2021)
> See Epilepsy p. 349.

- **CONTRA-INDICATIONS** Familial short QT syndrome
- **CAUTIONS** Elderly
- **INTERACTIONS** → Appendix 1: cenobamate
- **SIDE-EFFECTS**
▸ **Common or very common** Confusion · constipation · diarrhoea · dizziness · drowsiness · dry mouth · fatigue · gait abnormal · headache · hepatic function abnormal · hypersomnia · irritability · memory impairment · movement disorders · nausea · nystagmus · skin reactions · speech impairment · vertigo · vision disorders · vomiting
▸ **Uncommon** Suicidal behaviours
▸ **Rare or very rare** Drug reaction with eosinophilia and systemic symptoms (DRESS)
- **CONCEPTION AND CONTRACEPTION** [EvGr] Women of childbearing potential should use effective contraception during treatment and for 4 weeks after last dose. [M]
- **PREGNANCY** [EvGr] Avoid unless potential benefit outweighs risk—toxicity in *animal* studies. [M] See also *Pregnancy* in Epilepsy p. 349.
- **BREAST FEEDING** [EvGr] Avoid—present in milk in *animal* studies. [M]
- **HEPATIC IMPAIRMENT** [EvGr] Caution in mild or moderate impairment (increased exposure in chronic hepatic disease); avoid in severe impairment (no information available). [M]
  Dose adjustments [EvGr] Consider up to 50% reduction in target dose; max. dose of 200 mg daily in mild or moderate impairment. [M]
- **RENAL IMPAIRMENT** [EvGr] Caution; avoid in end-stage renal disease or haemodialysis patients (no information available). [M]
  Dose adjustments [EvGr] Consider reduction of target dose in mild or moderate (creatinine clearance 30 to less than 90 mL/minute) or severe (creatinine clearance less than 30 mL/minute) impairment; max. dose of 300 mg daily. [M] See p. 21.
- **TREATMENT CESSATION** [EvGr] Avoid abrupt withdrawal—withdraw treatment gradually over at least 2 weeks. [M]
- **PATIENT AND CARER ADVICE**
Drug reaction with eosinophilia and systemic symptoms (DRESS syndrome) Patients and carers should be told how to recognise signs of DRESS syndrome, and advised to seek immediate medical attention if symptoms such as fever, rash, or lymphadenopathy develop.
Driving and skilled tasks Patients and carers should be counselled on the effects on driving and performance of skilled tasks—increased risk of somnolence, dizziness, fatigue, impaired vision, and other CNS-related effects.

● **NATIONAL FUNDING/ACCESS DECISIONS**
For full details see funding body website
NICE decisions
▶ Cenobamate for treating focal onset seizures in epilepsy
(December 2021) NICE TA753 Recommended with restrictions
Scottish Medicines Consortium (SMC) decisions
▶ Cenobamate (*Ontozry*®) for the adjunctive treatment of focal
onset seizures with or without secondary generalisation in
adult patients with epilepsy (February 2022) SMC No. SMC2408
Recommended with restrictions

● **MEDICINAL FORMS** There can be variation in the licensing of
different medicines containing the same drug.
Oral tablet
CAUTIONARY AND ADVISORY LABELS 2, 8
▶ Ontozry (Angelini Pharma UK-I Ltd) ▼
Cenobamate 12.5 mg Ontozry 12.5mg tablets | 14 tablet [PoM] 🅔
Cenobamate 25 mg Ontozry 25mg tablets | 14 tablet [PoM] 🅔
Cenobamate 50 mg Ontozry 50mg tablets | 14 tablet [PoM] £85.54
DT = £85.54 | 28 tablet [PoM] £91.00 DT = £91.00
Cenobamate 100 mg Ontozry 100mg tablets | 14 tablet [PoM]
£87.36 DT = £87.36 | 28 tablet [PoM] £136.50 DT = £136.50
Cenobamate 150 mg Ontozry 150mg tablets | 14 tablet [PoM]
£89.18 DT = £89.18 | 28 tablet [PoM] £182.00 DT = £182.00
Cenobamate 200 mg Ontozry 200mg tablets | 14 tablet [PoM]
£91.00 DT = £91.00 | 28 tablet [PoM] £182.00 DT = £182.00

Eslicarbazepine acetate
17-Oct-2022

● **INDICATIONS AND DOSE**
**Monotherapy of focal seizures with or without secondary
generalisation**
▶ BY MOUTH
▶ Adult: Initially 400 mg once daily for 1–2 weeks, then
increased to 800 mg once daily, then increased if
necessary to 1.2 g once daily (max. per dose 1.6 g)
▶ Elderly: Initially 400 mg once daily for 1–2 weeks, then
increased to 800 mg once daily (max. per dose 1.2 g)

**Adjunctive therapy of focal seizures with or without
secondary generalisation**
▶ BY MOUTH
▶ Adult: Initially 400 mg once daily for 1–2 weeks, then
increased to 800 mg once daily (max. per dose 1.2 g)

IMPORTANT SAFETY INFORMATION
MHRA/CHM ADVICE: ANTIEPILEPTICS: RISK OF SUICIDAL
THOUGHTS AND BEHAVIOUR (AUGUST 2008)
See Epilepsy p. 349.

MHRA/CHM ADVICE: ANTIEPILEPTIC DRUGS: UPDATED ADVICE ON
SWITCHING BETWEEN DIFFERENT MANUFACTURERS' PRODUCTS
(NOVEMBER 2017)
See Epilepsy p. 349 and see also *Prescribing and
dispensing information*.

MHRA/CHM ADVICE: ANTIEPILEPTIC DRUGS IN PREGNANCY:
UPDATED ADVICE FOLLOWING COMPREHENSIVE SAFETY REVIEW
(JANUARY 2021)
See Epilepsy p. 349.

● **CONTRA-INDICATIONS** Second- or third-degree AV block
● **CAUTIONS** Hyponatraemia · PR-interval prolongation ·
presence of HLA-B*1502 or HLA-A*3101 allele

CAUTIONS, FURTHER INFORMATION
▶ HLA allele [EvGr] The presence of HLA-B*1502 allele,
particularly in individuals of Han Chinese or Thai origin, is
strongly associated with an increased risk of
carbamazepine-induced Stevens-Johnson syndrome; this
may also occur with eslicarbazepine acetate, a
structurally-related antiepileptic—see also *Pre-treatment
screening*.
The presence of HLA-A*3101 allele, particularly in
individuals of European or Japanese origin, is associated

with an increased risk of carbamazepine-induced
cutaneous adverse reactions. This may also occur with
eslicarbazepine acetate, a structurally-related
antiepileptic, but there are insufficient data to support
pre-treatment screening. Consider use if potential benefit
outweighs risk. ⟨M⟩

● **INTERACTIONS** → Appendix 1: antiepileptics
● **SIDE-EFFECTS**
▶ **Common or very common** Appetite decreased · asthenia ·
concentration impaired · diarrhoea · dizziness · drowsiness
· electrolyte imbalance · gait abnormal · headaches ·
movement disorders · nausea · skin reactions · sleep
disorders · tremor · vertigo · vision disorders · vomiting ·
weight changes
▶ **Uncommon** Alopecia · altered smell sensation · anaemia ·
anxiety · bone metabolism disorder · bradycardia ·
cerebellar syndrome · chest pain · chills · confusion ·
constipation · crying · dehydration · depression · dry mouth
· eye disorders · flushing · gastritis · gastrointestinal
discomfort · haemorrhage · hearing impairment ·
hyperhidrosis · hypertension · hypotension ·
hypothyroidism · increased risk of infection · liver disorder
· malaise · memory impairment · mood altered · muscle
weakness · myalgia · pain in extremity · palpitations ·
peripheral coldness · peripheral neuropathy · peripheral
oedema · psychomotor retardation · psychotic disorder ·
sensation abnormal · speech impairment · tinnitus ·
toothache
▶ **Frequency not known** Angioedema · inappropriate
antidiuretic hormone secretion like-syndrome · leucopenia
· pancreatitis · severe cutaneous adverse reactions (SCARs)
· suicidal behaviours · thrombocytopenia

● **ALLERGY AND CROSS-SENSITIVITY** Antiepileptic
hypersensitivity syndrome theoretically associated with
eslicarbazepine. See under Epilepsy p. 349 for more
information.

● **PREGNANCY** [EvGr] Caution—reproductive toxicity in
animal studies. ⟨M⟩ See also *Pregnancy* in Epilepsy p. 349.

● **BREAST FEEDING** Manufacturer advises avoid—present in
milk in *animal* studies.

● **HEPATIC IMPAIRMENT** Manufacturer advises caution in
mild to moderate impairment—limited information; avoid
in severe impairment—no information available.

● **RENAL IMPAIRMENT** Manufacturer advises avoid if
creatinine clearance less than 30 mL/minute.
Dose adjustments See p. 21.
Manufacturer advises reduce initial dose to 200 mg once
daily or 400 mg every other day for 2 weeks, then increase
to 400 mg once daily if creatinine clearance
30–60 mL/minute. The dose may be further increased
based on individual response.

● **PRE-TREATMENT SCREENING** [EvGr] Test for HLA-B*1502
allele in individuals of Han Chinese or Thai origin, and
consider testing in other at-risk Asian populations such as
individuals of Filipino or Malaysian origin (consider use if
potential benefit outweighs risk). ⟨M⟩

● **MONITORING REQUIREMENTS** Monitor plasma-sodium
concentration in patients at risk of hyponatraemia and
discontinue treatment if hyponatraemia occurs.

● **PRESCRIBING AND DISPENSING INFORMATION**
Switching between formulations Care should be taken when
switching between oral formulations. The need for
continued supply of a particular manufacturer's product
should be based on clinical judgement and consultation
with the patient or their carer, taking into account factors
such as seizure frequency and treatment history.

● **PATIENT AND CARER ADVICE**
Driving and skilled tasks Manufacturer advises patients and
carers should be cautioned on the effects on driving and

performance of skilled tasks—increased risk of dizziness, somnolence and visual disorders.

- **NATIONAL FUNDING/ACCESS DECISIONS**
  For full details see funding body website
  Scottish Medicines Consortium (SMC) decisions
  ▶ Eslicarbazepine acetate (*Zebinix*®) for the treatment of adjunctive therapy in adults with partial-onset seizures with or without secondary generalisation (November 2010) SMC No. 592/09 Recommended with restrictions
  All Wales Medicines Strategy Group (AWMSG) decisions
  ▶ Eslicarbazepine acetate (*Zebinix*®) as adjunctive therapy in adults, adolescents and children aged above six years, with partial-onset seizures with or without secondary generalisation (June 2019) AWMSG No. 1214 Recommended with restrictions

- **MEDICINAL FORMS** There can be variation in the licensing of different medicines containing the same drug.
  Oral tablet
  CAUTIONARY AND ADVISORY LABELS 8
  ▶ **Eslicarbazepine acetate (Non-proprietary)**
    Eslicarbazepine acetate 200 mg Eslicarbazepine 200mg tablets | 60 tablet PoM £68.00 DT = £68.00
    Eslicarbazepine acetate 800 mg Eslicarbazepine 800mg tablets | 30 tablet PoM £135.99 DT = £55.75
  ▶ **Arupsan** (Accord-UK Ltd)
    Eslicarbazepine acetate 200 mg Arupsan 200mg tablets | 60 tablet PoM £68.00 DT = £68.00
    Eslicarbazepine acetate 800 mg Arupsan 800mg tablets | 30 tablet PoM £109.28 DT = £55.75
  ▶ **Zebinix** (BIAL Pharma UK Ltd)
    Eslicarbazepine acetate 200 mg Zebinix 200mg tablets | 60 tablet PoM £68.00 DT = £68.00
    Eslicarbazepine acetate 800 mg Zebinix 800mg tablets | 30 tablet PoM £136.00 DT = £55.75
  Oral suspension
  CAUTIONARY AND ADVISORY LABELS 8
  ▶ **Zebinix** (BIAL Pharma UK Ltd)
    Eslicarbazepine acetate 50 mg per 1 ml Zebinix 50mg/1ml oral suspension | 200 ml PoM £56.67 DT = £56.67 SF

Ethosuximide

26-Oct-2021

- **INDICATIONS AND DOSE**

  Absence seizures | Atypical absence seizures (adjunct) | Myoclonic seizures
  ▶ BY MOUTH
  ▶ Child 1 month–5 years: Initially 5 mg/kg twice daily (max. per dose 125 mg), dose to be increased every 5–7 days; maintenance 10–20 mg/kg twice daily (max. per dose 500 mg), total daily dose may rarely be given in 3 divided doses
  ▶ Child 6–17 years: Initially 250 mg twice daily, then increased in steps of 250 mg every 5–7 days; usual dose 500–750 mg twice daily, increased if necessary up to 1 g twice daily
  ▶ Adult: Initially 500 mg daily in 2 divided doses, then increased in steps of 250 mg every 5–7 days; usual dose 1–1.5 g daily in 2 divided doses, increased if necessary up to 2 g daily

IMPORTANT SAFETY INFORMATION

MHRA/CHM ADVICE: ANTIEPILEPTICS: RISK OF SUICIDAL THOUGHTS AND BEHAVIOUR (AUGUST 2008)
See Epilepsy p. 349.

MHRA/CHM ADVICE: ANTIEPILEPTIC DRUGS: UPDATED ADVICE ON SWITCHING BETWEEN DIFFERENT MANUFACTURERS' PRODUCTS (NOVEMBER 2017)
See Epilepsy p. 349.

MHRA/CHM ADVICE: ANTIEPILEPTIC DRUGS IN PREGNANCY: UPDATED ADVICE FOLLOWING COMPREHENSIVE SAFETY REVIEW (JANUARY 2021)
See Epilepsy p. 349.

- **CAUTIONS** Avoid in Acute porphyrias p. 1202
- **INTERACTIONS** → Appendix 1: antiepileptics
- **SIDE-EFFECTS**
  ▶ **Common or very common** Appetite decreased · dizziness · drowsiness · gastrointestinal discomfort · gastrointestinal disorder · headache · movement disorders · nausea · skin reactions · vomiting
  ▶ **Uncommon** Aggression · agranulocytosis · bone marrow disorders · concentration impaired · depression · diarrhoea · eosinophilia · fatigue · haemorrhage · hiccups · leucopenia · lupus erythematosus · mood altered · myopia · oral disorders · psychotic disorder · severe cutaneous adverse reactions (SCARs) · sleep disorders · suicidal behaviours · weight decreased
  ▶ **Frequency not known** Generalised tonic-clonic seizure · libido increased · thrombocytopenia

  SIDE-EFFECTS, FURTHER INFORMATION Blood counts required if features of fever, sore throat, mouth ulcers, bruising or bleeding.

- **PREGNANCY** See also *Pregnancy* in Epilepsy p. 349.
  Monitoring EvGr Plasma-drug concentration should be regularly monitored during pregnancy; lowest effective dose must not be exceeded. M
- **BREAST FEEDING** Present in milk. Hyperexcitability and sedation reported.
- **HEPATIC IMPAIRMENT** Use with caution.
- **RENAL IMPAIRMENT** EvGr Use with caution—monitor drug concentration. M
- **PATIENT AND CARER ADVICE**
  Blood disorders Patients or their carers should be told how to recognise signs of blood disorders, and advised to seek immediate medical attention if symptoms such as fever, mouth ulcers, bruising, or bleeding develop.

- **MEDICINAL FORMS** There can be variation in the licensing of different medicines containing the same drug.
  Oral solution
  CAUTIONARY AND ADVISORY LABELS 8
  ▶ **Ethosuximide (Non-proprietary)**
    Ethosuximide 50 mg per 1 ml Ethosuximide 250mg/5ml syrup | 200 ml PoM £173.00 DT = £147.96
    Ethosuximide 250mg/5ml oral solution sugar free | 125 ml PoM £108.13 DT = £108.13 SF | 200 ml PoM £1,730.00 DT = £173.00 SF | 250 ml PoM £216.25 DT = £216.25 SF
  ▶ **Emeside** (Fontus Health Ltd)
    Ethosuximide 50 mg per 1 ml Emeside 250mg/5ml syrup | 200 ml PoM £91.43 DT = £147.96
  Oral capsule
  CAUTIONARY AND ADVISORY LABELS 8
  ▶ **Ethosuximide (Non-proprietary)**
    Ethosuximide 250 mg Ethosuximide 250mg capsules | 56 capsule PoM £210.68 DT = £76.20
  ▶ **Emeside** (Fontus Health Ltd)
    Ethosuximide 250 mg Emeside 250mg capsules | 56 capsule PoM £88.50 DT = £76.20
  ▶ **Epesri** (Strides Pharma UK Ltd)
    Ethosuximide 250 mg Epesri 250mg capsules | 56 capsule PoM £100.41 DT = £76.20

Fenfluramine

09-Nov-2023

- **DRUG ACTION** Fenfluramine is a serotonin-releasing agent that stimulates multiple 5-HT receptor subtypes; this action on serotonin receptors in the brain may contribute to its anti-seizure activity.

- **INDICATIONS AND DOSE**

Adjunctive therapy of seizures associated with Dravet syndrome (specialist use only)
- ► BY MOUTH
- ► Adult: Initially 0.1 mg/kg twice daily for 1 week, then increased if necessary to 0.2 mg/kg twice daily for 1 week, adjusted according to response; maintenance 0.35 mg/kg twice daily, for patients requiring more rapid titration, the dose may be increased every 4 days; maximum 26 mg per day

DOSE ADJUSTMENTS DUE TO INTERACTIONS
- ► When used with stiripentol, a lower maintenance dose of 0.2 mg/kg twice daily is recommended; maximum 17 mg per day.

IMPORTANT SAFETY INFORMATION

MHRA/CHM ADVICE: ANTIEPILEPTICS: RISK OF SUICIDAL THOUGHTS AND BEHAVIOUR (AUGUST 2008)
See Epilepsy p. 349.

MHRA/CHM ADVICE: ANTIEPILEPTIC DRUGS: UPDATED ADVICE ON SWITCHING BETWEEN DIFFERENT MANUFACTURERS' PRODUCTS (NOVEMBER 2017)
See Epilepsy p. 349.

MHRA/CHM ADVICE: ANTIEPILEPTIC DRUGS IN PREGNANCY: UPDATED ADVICE FOLLOWING COMPREHENSIVE SAFETY REVIEW (JANUARY 2021)
See Epilepsy p. 349.

- **CONTRA-INDICATIONS** Pulmonary arterial hypertension · valvular heart disease (aortic or mitral)

- **CAUTIONS** History of anorexia nervosa · history of bulimia nervosa

- **INTERACTIONS** → Appendix 1: fenfluramine

- **SIDE-EFFECTS**
- ► **Common or very common** Agitation · appetite decreased · asthenia · ataxia · behaviour abnormal · constipation · diarrhoea · drowsiness · fall · fever · hypersalivation · increased risk of infection · insomnia · mood altered · muscle tone decreased · status epilepticus · tremor · vomiting · weight decreased
- ► **Frequency not known** Angle closure glaucoma · mydriasis · pulmonary arterial hypertension · suicidal behaviours

- **PREGNANCY** [EvGr] Avoid—limited information available. Ⓜ See also *Pregnancy* in Epilepsy p. 349.

- **BREAST FEEDING** [EvGr] Avoid—present in milk in *animal* studies. Ⓜ

- **HEPATIC IMPAIRMENT** [EvGr] Avoid in moderate or severe impairment (no information available). Ⓜ

- **MONITORING REQUIREMENTS**
- ► [EvGr] An echocardiogram should be performed before starting treatment, then every 6 months for the first 2 years, and annually thereafter; if pathological valvular changes or pulmonary arterial hypertension develop, a follow-up echocardiogram should be performed at an earlier timeframe—consult product literature.
- ► Monitor body-weight during treatment. Ⓜ

- **PRESCRIBING AND DISPENSING INFORMATION** *Fintepla*® should be prescribed and dispensed according to the controlled access programme.
  The manufacturer has provided a *Prescriber Guide*.

- **PATIENT AND CARER ADVICE** The manufacturer of *Fintepla*® has provided a *Patient and Caregiver Guide*.

- **NATIONAL FUNDING/ACCESS DECISIONS**
For full details see funding body website
NICE decisions
- ► **Fenfluramine for treating seizures associated with Dravet syndrome (July 2022)** NICE TA808 Recommended with restrictions

Scottish Medicines Consortium (SMC) decisions
- ► **Fenfluramine (*Fintepla*®) for the treatment of seizures associated with Dravet syndrome as an add-on therapy to other antiepileptic medicines for patients 2 years of age and older (October 2023)** SMC No. SMC2569 Recommended

---

- **MEDICINAL FORMS** There can be variation in the licensing of different medicines containing the same drug.
Oral solution
CAUTIONARY AND ADVISORY LABELS 2, 8
EXCIPIENTS: May contain Glucose, hydroxybenzoates (parabens)
- ► **Fintepla** (UCB Pharma Ltd) ▼
  Fenfluramine (as Fenfluramine hydrochloride) 2.2 mg per 1 ml Fintepla 2.2mg/ml oral solution | 120 ml [PoM] £1,802.88 (Hospital only) [SF] | 360 ml [PoM] £5,408.65 (Hospital only) [SF]

Fosphenytoin sodium

10-May-2021

- **DRUG ACTION** Fosphenytoin is a pro-drug of phenytoin.

- **INDICATIONS AND DOSE**

Status epilepticus
- ► BY INTRAVENOUS INFUSION
- ► Adult: Initially 20 mg(PE)/kg, dose to be administered at a rate of 100–150 mg(PE)/minute, then 4–5 mg(PE)/kg daily in 1–2 divided doses, dose to be administered at a rate of 50–100 mg(PE)/minute, dose to be adjusted according to response and trough plasma-phenytoin concentration
- ► Elderly: Consider 10–25% reduction in dose or infusion rate

Prophylaxis or treatment of seizures associated with neurosurgery or head injury
- ► BY INTRAMUSCULAR INJECTION, OR BY INTRAVENOUS INFUSION
- ► Adult: Initially 10–15 mg(PE)/kg, intravenous infusion to be administered at a rate of 50–100 mg(PE)/minute, then 4–5 mg(PE)/kg daily in 1–2 divided doses, intravenous infusion to be administered at a rate of 50–100 mg(PE)/minute, dose to be adjusted according to response and trough plasma-phenytoin concentration
- ► Elderly: Consider 10–25% reduction in dose or infusion rate

Temporary substitution for oral phenytoin
- ► BY INTRAMUSCULAR INJECTION, OR BY INTRAVENOUS INFUSION
- ► Adult: Same dose and same dosing frequency as oral phenytoin therapy, intravenous infusion to be administered at a rate of 50–100 mg(PE)/minute
- ► Elderly: Consider 10–25% reduction in dose or infusion rate

DOSE EQUIVALENCE AND CONVERSION
- ► Doses are expressed as phenytoin sodium equivalent (PE); fosphenytoin sodium 1.5 mg ≡ phenytoin sodium 1 mg.

- **UNLICENSED USE** Fosphenytoin sodium doses in BNF may differ from those in product literature.

IMPORTANT SAFETY INFORMATION

MHRA/CHM ADVICE: ANTIEPILEPTICS: RISK OF SUICIDAL THOUGHTS AND BEHAVIOUR (AUGUST 2008)
See Epilepsy p. 349.

MHRA/CHM ADVICE: ANTIEPILEPTIC DRUGS: UPDATED ADVICE ON SWITCHING BETWEEN DIFFERENT MANUFACTURERS' PRODUCTS (NOVEMBER 2017)
See Epilepsy p. 349.

MHRA/CHM ADVICE: ANTIEPILEPTIC DRUGS IN PREGNANCY: UPDATED ADVICE FOLLOWING COMPREHENSIVE SAFETY REVIEW (JANUARY 2021)
See Epilepsy p. 349.

- **CONTRA-INDICATIONS** Acute porphyrias p. 1202 · second-degree heart block · sino-atrial block · sinus bradycardia · Stokes-Adams syndrome · third-degree heart block

- **CAUTIONS** Heart failure · hypotension · injection solutions alkaline (irritant to tissues) · respiratory depression · resuscitation facilities must be available

- **INTERACTIONS** → Appendix 1: antiepileptics

- **SIDE-EFFECTS**
- ▸ **Common or very common** Asthenia · chills · dizziness · drowsiness · dry mouth · dysarthria · euphoric mood · headache · hypotension · movement disorders · nausea · nystagmus · sensation abnormal · skin reactions · stupor · taste altered · tinnitus · tremor · vasodilation · vertigo · vision disorders · vomiting
- ▸ **Uncommon** Cardiac arrest · confusion · hearing impairment · muscle complaints · muscle weakness · nervousness · oral disorders · reflexes abnormal · severe cutaneous adverse reactions (SCARs) · systemic lupus erythematosus (SLE) · thinking abnormal
- ▸ **Frequency not known** Acute psychosis · agranulocytosis · appetite disorder · atrial conduction depression (more common if injection too rapid) · atrioventricular block · bone disorders · bone fracture · bone marrow disorders · bradycardia · cardiotoxicity · cerebrovascular insufficiency · circulatory collapse (more common if injection too rapid) · coarsening of the facial features · constipation · delirium · Dupuytren's contracture · encephalopathy · granulocytopenia · groin tingling · hair changes · hepatic disorders · hyperglycaemia · hypersensitivity · insomnia · leucopenia · lymphadenopathy · nephritis tubulointerstitial · Peyronie's disease · pneumonitis · polyarteritis nodosa · polyarthritis · purple glove syndrome · respiratory disorders · sensory peripheral polyneuropathy · suicidal behaviours · thrombocytopenia · tonic seizure · ventricular conduction depression (more common if injection too rapid) · ventricular fibrillation (more common if injection too rapid)

SIDE-EFFECTS, FURTHER INFORMATION Fosphenytoin has been associated with severe cardiovascular reactions including asystole, ventricular fibrillation, and cardiac arrest. Hypotension, bradycardia, and heart block have also been reported. The following are recommended: monitor heart rate, blood pressure, and respiratory function for duration of infusion; observe patient for at least 30 minutes after infusion; if hypotension occurs, reduce infusion rate or discontinue; reduce dose or infusion rate in elderly, and in renal or hepatic impairment.

- **ALLERGY AND CROSS-SENSITIVITY** Cross-sensitivity reported with carbamazepine.

- **PREGNANCY** An increased risk of major congenital malformations and possibility of adverse effects on neurodevelopment have been seen with phenytoin, see *Pregnancy* in Epilepsy p. 349.
Monitoring Changes in plasma-protein binding make interpretation of plasma-phenytoin concentrations difficult—monitor unbound fraction.
EvGr Doses should be adjusted on the basis of plasma-drug concentration monitoring—phenytoin pharmacokinetics altered during pregnancy. Ⓜ

- **BREAST FEEDING** Small amounts present in milk, but not known to be harmful.

- **HEPATIC IMPAIRMENT** Manufacturer advises caution—monitor free plasma-phenytoin concentration (rather than total plasma-phenytoin concentration) in hepatic impairment or hypoalbuminaemia and in hyperbilirubinaemia.
Dose adjustments Manufacturer advises consider a 10–25% reduction in dose or infusion rate (except in the treatment of status epilepticus) in hepatic impairment or hypoalbuminaemia.

- **RENAL IMPAIRMENT** EvGr Caution—monitor free plasma-phenytoin concentration (rather than total plasma-phenytoin concentration) in renal impairment or hypoalbuminaemia. Ⓜ
Dose adjustments EvGr Consider a 10–25% reduction in dose or infusion rate (except in the treatment of status epilepticus) in renal impairment or hypoalbuminaemia. Ⓜ

- **PRE-TREATMENT SCREENING** HLA-B* 1502 allele in individuals of Han Chinese or Thai origin—avoid unless essential (increased risk of Stevens-Johnson syndrome).

- **MONITORING REQUIREMENTS**
- ▸ Manufacturer recommends blood counts (but evidence of practical value uncertain).
- ▸ With intravenous use Monitor heart rate, blood pressure, ECG, and respiratory function for during infusion.

- **DIRECTIONS FOR ADMINISTRATION** For *intermittent intravenous infusion* (*Pro-Epanutin*®), manufacturer advises give *in* Glucose 5% *or* Sodium Chloride 0.9%; dilute to a concentration of 1.5–25 mg (phenytoin sodium equivalent (PE))/mL.

- **PRESCRIBING AND DISPENSING INFORMATION** Prescriptions for fosphenytoin sodium should state the dose in terms of phenytoin sodium equivalent (PE); fosphenytoin sodium 1.5 mg ≡ phenytoin sodium 1 mg.

- **MEDICINAL FORMS** There can be variation in the licensing of different medicines containing the same drug.
Solution for injection
ELECTROLYTES: May contain Phosphate
- ▸ **Pro-Epanutin** (Pfizer Ltd)
Fosphenytoin sodium 75 mg per 1 ml Pro-Epanutin 750mg/10ml concentrate for solution for injection vials │ 10 vial PoM £400.00 (Hospital only)

Gabapentin

17-Oct-2022

- **INDICATIONS AND DOSE**

Adjunctive treatment of focal seizures with or without secondary generalisation
- ▸ BY MOUTH
- ▸ Child 6-11 years: 10 mg/kg once daily (max. per dose 300 mg) on day 1, then 10 mg/kg twice daily (max. per dose 300 mg) on day 2, then 10 mg/kg 3 times a day (max. per dose 300 mg) on day 3; usual dose 25–35 mg/kg daily in 3 divided doses, some children may not tolerate daily increments; longer intervals (up to weekly) may be more appropriate, daily dose maximum to be given in 3 divided doses; maximum 70 mg/kg per day
- ▸ Child 12-17 years: Initially 300 mg once daily on day 1, then 300 mg twice daily on day 2, then 300 mg 3 times a day on day 3, alternatively initially 300 mg 3 times a day on day 1, then increased in steps of 300 mg every 2–3 days in 3 divided doses, adjusted according to response; usual dose 0.9–3.6 g daily in 3 divided doses (max. per dose 1.6 g 3 times a day), some children may not tolerate daily increments; longer intervals (up to weekly) may be more appropriate
- ▸ Adult: Initially 300 mg once daily on day 1, then 300 mg twice daily on day 2, then 300 mg 3 times a day on day 3, alternatively initially 300 mg 3 times a day on day 1, then increased in steps of 300 mg every 2–3 days in 3 divided doses, adjusted according to response;

usual dose 0.9–3.6 g daily in 3 divided doses (max. per dose 1.6 g 3 times a day)

Monotherapy for focal seizures with or without secondary generalisation
▸ BY MOUTH
▸ Child 12-17 years: Initially 300 mg once daily on day 1, then 300 mg twice daily on day 2, then 300 mg 3 times a day on day 3, alternatively initially 300 mg 3 times a day on day 1, then increased in steps of 300 mg every 2–3 days in 3 divided doses, adjusted according to response; usual dose 0.9–3.6 g daily in 3 divided doses (max. per dose 1.6 g 3 times a day), some children may not tolerate daily increments; longer intervals (up to weekly) may be more appropriate
▸ Adult: Initially 300 mg once daily on day 1, then 300 mg twice daily on day 2, then 300 mg 3 times a day on day 3, alternatively initially 300 mg 3 times a day on day 1, then increased in steps of 300 mg every 2–3 days in 3 divided doses, adjusted according to response; usual dose 0.9–3.6 g daily in 3 divided doses (max. per dose 1.6 g 3 times a day)

Peripheral neuropathic pain
▸ BY MOUTH
▸ Adult: Initially 300 mg once daily on day 1, then 300 mg twice daily on day 2, then 300 mg 3 times a day on day 3, alternatively initially 300 mg 3 times a day on day 1, then increased in steps of 300 mg every 2–3 days in 3 divided doses, adjusted according to response; maximum 3.6 g per day

Menopausal symptoms, particularly hot flushes, in women with breast cancer
▸ BY MOUTH
▸ Adult: 300 mg 3 times a day, initial dose should be lower and titrated up over three days

Oscillopsia in multiple sclerosis
▸ BY MOUTH
▸ Adult: Initially 300 mg once daily, then increased in steps of 300 mg, every 4–7 days, adjusted according to response; usual maximum 900 mg 3 times a day

Spasticity in multiple sclerosis
▸ BY MOUTH
▸ Adult: Initially 300 mg once daily for 1–2 weeks, then 300 mg twice daily for 1–2 weeks, then 300 mg 3 times a day for 1–2 weeks, alternatively initially 100 mg 3 times a day, then increased in steps of 100 mg 3 times a day, every 1–2 weeks, adjusted according to response; usual maximum 900 mg 3 times a day

Muscular symptoms in motor neurone disease
▸ BY MOUTH
▸ Adult: Initially 300 mg once daily for 1–2 weeks, then 300 mg twice daily for 1–2 weeks, then 300 mg 3 times a day for 1–2 weeks, adjusted according to response; usual maximum 900 mg 3 times a day

● **UNLICENSED USE** Not licensed at doses over 50 mg/kg daily in children under 12 years.
  EvGr Gabapentin is used for the treatment of menopausal symptoms, Ⓐ but is not licensed for this indication. EvGr Gabapentin is used for oscillopsia in multiple sclerosis, Ⓔ but is not licensed for this indication. EvGr Gabapentin is used for spasticity in multiple sclerosis, Ⓔ but is not licensed for this indication. EvGr Gabapentin is used for muscular symptoms in motor neurone disease, Ⓔ but is not licensed for this indication.

IMPORTANT SAFETY INFORMATION
The levels of propylene glycol, acesulfame K and saccharin sodium may exceed the recommended WHO daily intake limits if high doses of gabapentin oral solution (Rosemont brand) are given to adolescents or adults with low body-weight (39–50 kg)—consult product literature.

MHRA/CHM ADVICE: ANTIEPILEPTICS: RISK OF SUICIDAL THOUGHTS AND BEHAVIOUR (AUGUST 2008)
See Epilepsy p. 349.

MHRA/CHM ADVICE: GABAPENTIN (_NEURONTIN_®): RISK OF SEVERE RESPIRATORY DEPRESSION (OCTOBER 2017)
Gabapentin has been associated with a rare risk of severe respiratory depression even without concomitant opioid medicines. Patients with compromised respiratory function, respiratory or neurological disease, renal impairment, concomitant use of central nervous system (CNS) depressants, and elderly people might be at higher risk of experiencing severe respiratory depression and dose adjustments may be necessary in these patients.

MHRA/CHM ADVICE: ANTIEPILEPTIC DRUGS: UPDATED ADVICE ON SWITCHING BETWEEN DIFFERENT MANUFACTURERS' PRODUCTS (NOVEMBER 2017)
See Epilepsy p. 349.

MHRA/CHM ADVICE: GABAPENTIN (_NEURONTIN_®) AND RISK OF ABUSE AND DEPENDENCE: NEW SCHEDULING REQUIREMENTS FROM 1 APRIL (APRIL 2019)
Following concerns about abuse, gabapentin has been reclassified as a Class C controlled substance and is now a Schedule 3 drug, but is exempt from safe custody requirements. Healthcare professionals should evaluate patients carefully for a history of drug abuse before prescribing gabapentin, and observe patients for signs of abuse and dependence. Patients should be informed of the potentially fatal risks of interactions between gabapentin and alcohol, and with other medicines that cause CNS depression, particularly opioids.

MHRA/CHM ADVICE: ANTIEPILEPTIC DRUGS IN PREGNANCY: UPDATED ADVICE FOLLOWING COMPREHENSIVE SAFETY REVIEW (JANUARY 2021)
See Epilepsy p. 349.

● **CAUTIONS** Diabetes mellitus · elderly · high doses of oral solution in adolescents and adults with low body-weight · history of substance abuse · respiratory depression, see _Important safety information_ · seizures (may be exacerbated)
CAUTIONS, FURTHER INFORMATION
▸ Seizure exacerbation EvGr Gabapentin may exacerbate seizures in patients with absence or myoclonic seizures (including juvenile myoclonic epilepsy), tonic or atonic seizures, Dravet syndrome, Lennox-Gastaut syndrome, and myoclonic-atonic seizures. Ⓐ

● **INTERACTIONS** → Appendix 1: antiepileptics

● **SIDE-EFFECTS**
▸ **Common or very common** Anxiety · appetite abnormal · arthralgia · asthenia · behaviour abnormal · confusion · constipation · cough · depression · diarrhoea · dizziness · drowsiness · dry mouth · dry throat · dysarthria · dyspnoea · emotional lability · fever · flatulence · gait abnormal · gastrointestinal discomfort · headache · hypertension · increased risk of infection · insomnia · leucopenia · malaise · memory loss · movement disorders · muscle complaints · nausea · nystagmus · oedema · pain · reflexes abnormal · sensation abnormal · sexual dysfunction · skin reactions · thinking abnormal · tooth disorder · tremor · vasodilation · vertigo · visual impairment · vomiting · weight increased
▸ **Uncommon** Cognitive impairment · dysphagia · hyperglycaemia · palpitations
▸ **Rare or very rare** Hypoglycaemia · loss of consciousness · respiratory depression
▸ **Frequency not known** Acute kidney injury · alopecia · angioedema · breast enlargement · chest pain · drug use disorders · gynaecomastia · hallucination · hepatic disorders · hyponatraemia · pancreatitis · rhabdomyolysis · severe cutaneous adverse reactions (SCARs) · suicidal

behaviours · thrombocytopenia · tinnitus · urinary incontinence · withdrawal syndrome

- **PREGNANCY** Manufacturer advises avoid unless benefit outweighs risk — toxicity reported. See also *Pregnancy* in Epilepsy p. 349.
- **BREAST FEEDING** Present in milk—manufacturer advises use only if potential benefit outweighs risk. See also *Breast-feeding* in Epilepsy p. 349.
- **RENAL IMPAIRMENT**
  Dose adjustments See p. 21.
  ▶ In adults Manufacturer advises reduce dose to 600–1800 mg daily in 3 divided doses if creatinine clearance 50–79 mL/minute. Manufacturer advises reduce dose to 300–900 mg daily in 3 divided doses if creatinine clearance 30–49 mL/minute. Manufacturer advises reduce dose to 150–600 mg daily in 3 divided doses if creatinine clearance 15–29 mL/minute (150 mg daily dose to be given as 300 mg in 3 divided doses on alternate days). Manufacturer advises reduce dose to 150–300 mg daily in 3 divided doses if creatinine clearance is less than 15 mL/minute (150 mg daily dose to be given as 300 mg in 3 divided doses on alternate days)—further dose reductions may be required in proportion to creatinine clearance, consult product literature.
  ▶ In children Manufacturer advises reduce dose if creatinine clearance less than 80 mL/minute (consult product literature).
- **MONITORING REQUIREMENTS** Monitor for signs of gabapentin abuse.
- **EFFECT ON LABORATORY TESTS** False positive readings with some urinary protein tests.
- **DIRECTIONS FOR ADMINISTRATION** Expert sources advise capsules can be opened but the bitter taste is difficult to mask.
- **PATIENT AND CARER ADVICE**
  Medicines for Children leaflet: Gabapentin for neuropathic pain www.medicinesforchildren.org.uk/medicines/gabapentin-for-neuropathic-pain/
  Medicines for Children leaflet: Gabapentin for preventing seizures www.medicinesforchildren.org.uk/medicines/gabapentin-for-preventing-seizures/
  Patient leaflet NHS England has produced a patient leaflet with information on the reclassification of gabapentin.

- **MEDICINAL FORMS** There can be variation in the licensing of different medicines containing the same drug. Forms available from special-order manufacturers include: oral suspension, oral solution

Oral tablet
CAUTIONARY AND ADVISORY LABELS 3, 5, 8, 25
▶ Gabapentin (Non-proprietary)
  Gabapentin 600 mg Gabapentin 600mg tablets | 100 tablet PoM £52.76 DT = £5.42 CD3
  Gabapentin 800 mg Gabapentin 800mg tablets | 100 tablet PoM £78.00 DT = £14.69 CD3
▶ Neurontin (Viatris UK Healthcare Ltd)
  Gabapentin 600 mg Neurontin 600mg tablets | 100 tablet PoM £84.80 DT = £5.42 CD3
  Gabapentin 800 mg Neurontin 800mg tablets | 100 tablet PoM £98.13 DT = £14.69 CD3

Oral capsule
CAUTIONARY AND ADVISORY LABELS 3, 5, 8, 25
▶ Gabapentin (Non-proprietary)
  Gabapentin 100 mg Gabapentin 100mg capsules | 100 capsule PoM £18.29 DT = £1.53 CD3
  Gabapentin 300 mg Gabapentin 300mg capsules | 100 capsule PoM £42.40 DT = £2.26 CD3
  Gabapentin 400 mg Gabapentin 400mg capsules | 100 capsule PoM £49.06 DT = £2.93 CD3
▶ Neurontin (Viatris UK Healthcare Ltd)
  Gabapentin 100 mg Neurontin 100mg capsules | 100 capsule PoM £18.29 DT = £1.53 CD3
  Gabapentin 300 mg Neurontin 300mg capsules | 100 capsule PoM £42.40 DT = £2.26 CD3
  Gabapentin 400 mg Neurontin 400mg capsules | 100 capsule PoM £49.06 DT = £2.93 CD3

Oral solution
CAUTIONARY AND ADVISORY LABELS 3, 5, 8
EXCIPIENTS: May contain Propylene glycol
ELECTROLYTES: May contain Potassium, sodium
▶ Gabapentin (Non-proprietary)
  Gabapentin 50 mg per 1 ml Neurontin 250mg/5ml oral solution | 470 ml PoM ⚠ CD3
  Gabapentin 50mg/ml oral solution sugar free | 150 ml PoM £67.29 DT = £18.98 Schedule 3 (CD No Register Exempt Safe Custody) SF

Lacosamide

11-Nov-2022

- **INDICATIONS AND DOSE**

Monotherapy of focal seizures with or without secondary generalisation
▶ BY MOUTH, OR BY INTRAVENOUS INFUSION
▶ Child (body-weight 50 kg and above): Initially 50 mg twice daily, then increased to 100 mg twice daily after 1 week, alternatively initially 100 mg twice daily; increased in steps of 50 mg twice daily (max. per dose 300 mg twice daily) if necessary and if tolerated, dose to be increased at weekly intervals
▶ Child 2–17 years (body-weight 10–39 kg): Initially 1 mg/kg twice daily, then increased to 2 mg/kg twice daily after 1 week; increased in steps of 1 mg/kg twice daily (max. per dose 6 mg/kg twice daily) if necessary and if tolerated, dose to be increased at weekly intervals
▶ Child 2–17 years (body-weight 40–49 kg): Initially 1 mg/kg twice daily, then increased to 2 mg/kg twice daily after 1 week; increased in steps of 1 mg/kg twice daily (max. per dose 5 mg/kg twice daily) if necessary and if tolerated, dose to be increased at weekly intervals
▶ Adult: Initially 50 mg twice daily, then increased to 100 mg twice daily after 1 week, alternatively initially 100 mg twice daily; increased in steps of 50 mg twice daily (max. per dose 300 mg twice daily) if necessary and if tolerated, dose to be increased at weekly intervals

Monotherapy of focal seizures with or without secondary generalisation (alternative loading dose regimen when it is necessary to rapidly attain therapeutic plasma concentrations) (under close medical supervision)
▶ BY MOUTH, OR BY INTRAVENOUS INFUSION
▶ Child (body-weight 50 kg and above): Loading dose 200 mg, followed by 100 mg twice daily, to be given 12 hours after initial dose; increased in steps of 50 mg twice daily (max. per dose 300 mg twice daily) if necessary and if tolerated, dose to be increased at weekly intervals
▶ Adult: Loading dose 200 mg, followed by 100 mg twice daily, to be given 12 hours after initial dose; increased in steps of 50 mg twice daily (max. per dose 300 mg twice daily) if necessary and if tolerated, dose to be increased at weekly intervals

Adjunctive treatment of focal seizures with or without secondary generalisation
▶ BY MOUTH, OR BY INTRAVENOUS INFUSION
▶ Child (body-weight 50 kg and above): Initially 50 mg twice daily, then increased to 100 mg twice daily after 1 week; increased in steps of 50 mg twice daily (max. per dose 200 mg twice daily) if necessary and if tolerated, dose to be increased at weekly intervals
▶ Child 2–17 years (body-weight 10–19 kg): Initially 1 mg/kg twice daily, then increased to 2 mg/kg twice daily after 1 week; increased in steps of 1 mg/kg twice daily (max. per dose 6 mg/kg twice daily) if necessary and if tolerated, dose to be increased at weekly intervals
▶ Child 2–17 years (body-weight 20–29 kg): Initially 1 mg/kg twice daily, then increased to 2 mg/kg twice daily after

1 week; increased in steps of 1 mg/kg twice daily (max. per dose 5 mg/kg twice daily) if necessary and if tolerated, dose to be increased at weekly intervals

▸ Child 2-17 years (body-weight 30–49 kg): Initially 1 mg/kg twice daily, then increased to 2 mg/kg twice daily after 1 week; increased in steps of 1 mg/kg twice daily (max. per dose 4 mg/kg twice daily) if necessary and if tolerated, dose to be increased at weekly intervals

▸ Adult: Initially 50 mg twice daily, then increased to 100 mg twice daily after 1 week; increased in steps of 50 mg twice daily (max. per dose 200 mg twice daily) if necessary and if tolerated, dose to be increased at weekly intervals

Adjunctive treatment of primary generalised tonic-clonic seizures

▸ BY MOUTH, OR BY INTRAVENOUS INFUSION

▸ Child (body-weight 50 kg and above): Initially 50 mg twice daily, then increased to 100 mg twice daily after 1 week; increased in steps of 50 mg twice daily (max. per dose 200 mg twice daily) if necessary and if tolerated, dose to be increased at weekly intervals

▸ Child 4-17 years (body-weight 10–19 kg): Initially 1 mg/kg twice daily, then increased to 2 mg/kg twice daily after 1 week; increased in steps of 1 mg/kg twice daily (max. per dose 6 mg/kg twice daily) if necessary and if tolerated, dose to be increased at weekly intervals

▸ Child 4-17 years (body-weight 20–29 kg): Initially 1 mg/kg twice daily, then increased to 2 mg/kg twice daily after 1 week; increased in steps of 1 mg/kg twice daily (max. per dose 5 mg/kg twice daily) if necessary and if tolerated, dose to be increased at weekly intervals

▸ Child 4-17 years (body-weight 30–49 kg): Initially 1 mg/kg twice daily, then increased to 2 mg/kg twice daily after 1 week; increased in steps of 1 mg/kg twice daily (max. per dose 4 mg/kg twice daily) if necessary and if tolerated, dose to be increased at weekly intervals

▸ Adult: Initially 50 mg twice daily, then increased to 100 mg twice daily after 1 week; increased in steps of 50 mg twice daily (max. per dose 200 mg twice daily) if necessary and if tolerated, dose to be increased at weekly intervals

Adjunctive treatment of focal seizures with or without secondary generalisation (alternative loading dose regimen when it is necessary to rapidly attain therapeutic plasma concentrations) (under close medical supervision) | Adjunctive treatment of primary generalised tonic-clonic seizures (alternative loading dose regimen when it is necessary to rapidly attain therapeutic plasma concentrations) (under close medical supervision)

▸ BY MOUTH, OR BY INTRAVENOUS INFUSION

▸ Child (body-weight 50 kg and above): Loading dose 200 mg, followed by 100 mg twice daily, to be given 12 hours after initial dose; increased in steps of 50 mg twice daily (max. per dose 200 mg twice daily) if necessary and if tolerated, dose to be increased at weekly intervals

▸ Adult: Loading dose 200 mg, followed by 100 mg twice daily, to be given 12 hours after initial dose; increased in steps of 50 mg twice daily (max. per dose 200 mg twice daily) if necessary and if tolerated, dose to be increased at weekly intervals

IMPORTANT SAFETY INFORMATION

MHRA/CHM ADVICE: ANTIEPILEPTICS: RISK OF SUICIDAL THOUGHTS AND BEHAVIOUR (AUGUST 2008)
See Epilepsy p. 349.

MHRA/CHM ADVICE: ANTIEPILEPTIC DRUGS: UPDATED ADVICE ON SWITCHING BETWEEN DIFFERENT MANUFACTURERS' PRODUCTS (NOVEMBER 2017)
See Epilepsy p. 349.

MHRA/CHM ADVICE: ANTIEPILEPTIC DRUGS IN PREGNANCY: UPDATED ADVICE FOLLOWING COMPREHENSIVE SAFETY REVIEW (JANUARY 2021)
See Epilepsy p. 349.

● **CONTRA-INDICATIONS** Second- or third-degree AV block

● **CAUTIONS** Conduction problems · elderly · risk of PR-interval prolongation · seizures (may be exacerbated) · severe cardiac disease

CAUTIONS, FURTHER INFORMATION

▸ Seizure exacerbation [EvGr] Lacosamide may exacerbate seizures in patients with Dravet syndrome and Lennox-Gastaut syndrome. Ⓐ

● **INTERACTIONS** → Appendix 1: antiepileptics

● **SIDE-EFFECTS**

▸ **Common or very common** Asthenia · cognitive disorder · concentration impaired · confusion · constipation · depression · diarrhoea · dizziness · drowsiness · dry mouth · dysarthria · dyspepsia · feeling drunk · flatulence · gait abnormal · headache · insomnia · memory impairment · mood altered · movement disorders · muscle spasms · myoclonic seizure · nausea · nystagmus · sensation abnormal · skin reactions · tinnitus · tremor · vertigo · vision disorders · vomiting

▸ **Uncommon** Agitation · angioedema · arrhythmias · atrioventricular block · behaviour abnormal · hallucination · psychotic disorder · suicidal behaviours · syncope

▸ **Frequency not known** Agranulocytosis · appetite decreased (in children) · fever (in children) · increased risk of infection (in children) · severe cutaneous adverse reactions (SCARs)

● **ALLERGY AND CROSS-SENSITIVITY** Antiepileptic hypersensitivity syndrome associated with lacosamide. See under Epilepsy p. 349 for more information.

● **PREGNANCY** [EvGr] Avoid unless potential benefit outweighs risk—embryotoxic in *animal* studies. Ⓜ See also *Pregnancy* in Epilepsy p. 349.

● **BREAST FEEDING** Specialist sources indicate use with caution only if no suitable alternative—present in milk; monitor infant neurodevelopment and monitor infant for adverse effects.

● **HEPATIC IMPAIRMENT** Manufacturer advises caution (risk of increased exposure), particularly in severe impairment (no information available).
Dose adjustments Manufacturer advises consider dose reduction—consult product literature.

● **RENAL IMPAIRMENT**
Dose adjustments [EvGr] Dose reduction may be required (consult product literature). Ⓜ

● **DIRECTIONS FOR ADMINISTRATION** For *intermittent intravenous infusion*, manufacturer advises give undiluted or dilute with Glucose 5% *or* Sodium Chloride 0.9% *or* Lactated Ringer's Solution; give over 15–60 minutes—give doses greater than 200 mg over at least 30 minutes.

● **PRESCRIBING AND DISPENSING INFORMATION** Flavours of syrup may include strawberry.

● **PATIENT AND CARER ADVICE** Patients and carers should be counselled on the symptoms of cardiac arrhythmia and advised to seek immediate medical advice if these occur.
Medicines for Children leaflet: Lacosamide for preventing seizures www.medicinesforchildren.org.uk/medicines/lacosamide-for-preventing-seizures/
Missed doses If a dose is more than 6 hours late, the missed dose should not be taken and the next dose should be taken at the normal time.
Driving and skilled tasks Patients and carers should be counselled on the effects on driving and performance of skilled tasks—increased risk of dizziness and blurred vision.

- **NATIONAL FUNDING/ACCESS DECISIONS**
For full details see funding body website
Scottish Medicines Consortium (SMC) decisions
▸ Lacosamide (*Vimpat*®) as adjunctive therapy in the treatment of partial-onset seizures with or without secondary generalisation in patients with epilepsy aged 16 years or older (February 2009) SMC No. 532/09 Recommended with restrictions
▸ Lacosamide (*Vimpat*®) as adjunctive therapy in the treatment of partial-onset seizures with or without secondary generalisation in adolescents and children from 4 years of age with epilepsy (February 2018) SMC No. 1301/18 Recommended with restrictions

All Wales Medicines Strategy Group (AWMSG) decisions
▸ Lacosamide (*Vimpat*®) as adjunctive therapy in the treatment of partial-onset seizures with or without secondary generalisation in children from 2 years of age up to 15 years of age with epilepsy (October 2022) AWMSG No. 4698 Recommended

- **MEDICINAL FORMS** There can be variation in the licensing of different medicines containing the same drug.
Solution for infusion
ELECTROLYTES: May contain Sodium
▸ **Lacosamide (Non-proprietary)**
Lacosamide 10 mg per 1 ml Lacosamide 200mg/20ml solution for infusion vials | 1 vial [PoM] £29.70 DT = £29.70 (Hospital only)
▸ **Vimpat** (UCB Pharma Ltd)
Lacosamide 10 mg per 1 ml Vimpat 200mg/20ml solution for infusion vials | 1 vial [PoM] £29.70 DT = £29.70

Oral tablet
CAUTIONARY AND ADVISORY LABELS 8
▸ **Lacosamide (Non-proprietary)**
Lacosamide 50 mg Lacosamide 50mg tablets | 14 tablet [PoM] £10.81 DT = £1.37
Lacosamide 100 mg Lacosamide 100mg tablets | 14 tablet [PoM] £1.38–£21.62 | 56 tablet [PoM] £86.50 DT = £4.91
Lacosamide 150 mg Lacosamide 150mg tablets | 14 tablet [PoM] £32.44 DT = £32.44 | 56 tablet [PoM] £129.74 DT = £129.74
Lacosamide 200 mg Lacosamide 200mg tablets | 56 tablet [PoM] £168.66 DT = £7.50
▸ **Vimpat** (UCB Pharma Ltd)
Lacosamide 50 mg Vimpat 50mg tablets | 14 tablet [PoM] £10.81 DT = £1.37
Lacosamide 100 mg Vimpat 100mg tablets | 14 tablet [PoM] £21.62 | 56 tablet [PoM] £86.50 DT = £4.91
Lacosamide 150 mg Vimpat 150mg tablets | 14 tablet [PoM] £32.44 DT = £32.44 | 56 tablet [PoM] £129.74 DT = £129.74
Lacosamide 200 mg Vimpat 200mg tablets | 56 tablet [PoM] £144.16 DT = £7.50

Oral solution
CAUTIONARY AND ADVISORY LABELS 8
EXCIPIENTS: May contain Aspartame, propylene glycol
ELECTROLYTES: May contain Sodium
▸ **Lacosamide (Non-proprietary)**
Lacosamide 10 mg per 1 ml Lacosamide 10mg/ml oral solution sugar free | 200 ml [PoM] £25.70–£29.70 DT = £25.74 [SF]
▸ **Vimpat** (UCB Pharma Ltd)
Lacosamide 10 mg per 1 ml Vimpat 10mg/ml syrup | 200 ml [PoM] £25.74 DT = £25.74 [SF]

Lamotrigine

17-Oct-2022

- **INDICATIONS AND DOSE**

Monotherapy of focal seizures | Monotherapy of primary and secondary generalised tonic-clonic seizures | Monotherapy of seizures associated with Lennox-Gastaut syndrome
▸ BY MOUTH
▸ Child 12-17 years: Initially 25 mg once daily for 14 days, then increased to 50 mg once daily for further 14 days, then increased in steps of up to 100 mg every 7–14 days; maintenance 100–200 mg daily in 1–2 divided doses; increased if necessary up to 500 mg

daily, dose titration should be repeated if restarting after interval of more than 5 days
▸ Adult: Initially 25 mg once daily for 14 days, then increased to 50 mg once daily for further 14 days, then increased in steps of up to 100 mg every 7–14 days; maintenance 100–200 mg daily in 1–2 divided doses; increased if necessary up to 500 mg daily, dose titration should be repeated if restarting after interval of more than 5 days

Adjunctive therapy of focal seizures with valproate | Adjunctive therapy of primary and secondary generalised tonic-clonic seizures with valproate | Adjunctive therapy of seizures associated with Lennox-Gastaut syndrome with valproate
▸ BY MOUTH
▸ Child 2-11 years (body-weight up to 13 kg): Initially 2 mg once daily on alternate days for first 14 days, then 300 micrograms/kg once daily for further 14 days, then increased in steps of up to 300 micrograms/kg every 7–14 days; maintenance 1–5 mg/kg daily in 1–2 divided doses, dose titration should be repeated if restarting after interval of more than 5 days; maximum 200 mg per day
▸ Child 2-11 years (body-weight 13 kg and above): Initially 150 micrograms/kg once daily for 14 days, then 300 micrograms/kg once daily for further 14 days, then increased in steps of up to 300 micrograms/kg every 7–14 days; maintenance 1–5 mg/kg daily in 1–2 divided doses, dose titration should be repeated if restarting after interval of more than 5 days; maximum 200 mg per day
▸ Child 12-17 years: Initially 25 mg once daily on alternate days for 14 days, then 25 mg once daily for further 14 days, then increased in steps of up to 50 mg every 7–14 days; maintenance 100–200 mg daily in 1–2 divided doses, dose titration should be repeated if restarting after interval of more than 5 days
▸ Adult: Initially 25 mg once daily on alternate days for 14 days, then 25 mg once daily for further 14 days, then increased in steps of up to 50 mg every 7–14 days; maintenance 100–200 mg daily in 1–2 divided doses, dose titration should be repeated if restarting after interval of more than 5 days

Adjunctive therapy of focal seizures (with enzyme inducing drugs) without valproate | Adjunctive therapy of primary and secondary generalised tonic-clonic seizures (with enzyme inducing drugs) without valproate | Adjunctive therapy of seizures associated with Lennox-Gastaut syndromes (with enzyme inducing drugs) without valproate
▸ BY MOUTH
▸ Child 2-11 years: Initially 300 micrograms/kg twice daily for 14 days, then 600 micrograms/kg twice daily for further 14 days, then increased in steps of up to 1.2 mg/kg every 7–14 days; maintenance 5–15 mg/kg daily in 1–2 divided doses, dose titration should be repeated if restarting after interval of more than 5 days; maximum 400 mg per day
▸ Child 12-17 years: Initially 50 mg once daily for 14 days, then 50 mg twice daily for further 14 days, then increased in steps of up to 100 mg every 7–14 days; maintenance 200–400 mg daily in 2 divided doses, increased if necessary up to 700 mg daily, dose titration should be repeated if restarting after interval of more than 5 days
▸ Adult: Initially 50 mg once daily for 14 days, then 50 mg twice daily for further 14 days, then increased in steps of up to 100 mg every 7–14 days; maintenance 200–400 mg daily in 2 divided doses, increased if necessary up to 700 mg daily, dose titration should be repeated if restarting after interval of more than 5 days

Adjunctive therapy of focal seizures (without enzyme inducing drugs) without valproate | Adjunctive therapy of primary and secondary generalised tonic-clonic seizures (without enzyme inducing drugs) without valproate | Adjunctive therapy of seizures associated with Lennox-Gastaut syndromes (without enzyme inducing drugs) without valproate

▶ BY MOUTH
▶ Child 2-11 years: Initially 300 micrograms/kg daily in 1–2 divided doses for 14 days, then 600 micrograms/kg daily in 1–2 divided doses for further 14 days, then increased in steps of up to 600 micrograms/kg every 7–14 days; maintenance 1–10 mg/kg daily in 1–2 divided doses, dose titration should be repeated if restarting after interval of more than 5 days; maximum 200 mg per day
▶ Child 12-17 years: Initially 25 mg once daily for 14 days, then increased to 50 mg once daily for further 14 days, then increased in steps of up to 100 mg every 7–14 days; maintenance 100–200 mg daily in 1–2 divided doses, dose titration should be repeated if restarting after interval of more than 5 days
▶ Adult: Initially 25 mg once daily for 14 days, then increased to 50 mg once daily for further 14 days, then increased in steps of up to 100 mg every 7–14 days; maintenance 100–200 mg daily in 1–2 divided doses, dose titration should be repeated if restarting after interval of more than 5 days

Monotherapy or adjunctive therapy of bipolar disorder (without enzyme inducing drugs) without valproate

▶ BY MOUTH
▶ Adult: Initially 25 mg once daily for 14 days, then 50 mg daily in 1–2 divided doses for further 14 days, then 100 mg daily in 1–2 divided doses for further 7 days; maintenance 200 mg daily in 1–2 divided doses, patients stabilised on lamotrigine for bipolar disorder may require dose adjustments if other drugs are added to or withdrawn from their treatment regimens—consult product literature, dose titration should be repeated if restarting after interval of more than 5 days; maximum 400 mg per day

Adjunctive therapy of bipolar disorder with valproate

▶ BY MOUTH
▶ Adult: Initially 25 mg once daily on alternate days for 14 days, then 25 mg once daily for further 14 days, then 50 mg daily in 1–2 divided doses for further 7 days; maintenance 100 mg daily in 1–2 divided doses, patients stabilised on lamotrigine for bipolar disorder may require dose adjustments if other drugs are added to or withdrawn from their treatment regimens—consult product literature, dose titration should be repeated if restarting after interval of more than 5 days; maximum 200 mg per day

Adjunctive therapy of bipolar disorder (with enzyme inducing drugs) without valproate

▶ BY MOUTH
▶ Adult: Initially 50 mg once daily for 14 days, then 50 mg twice daily for further 14 days, then increased to 100 mg twice daily for further 7 days, then increased to 150 mg twice daily for further 7 days; maintenance 200 mg twice daily, patients stabilised on lamotrigine for bipolar disorder may require dose adjustments if other drugs are added to or withdrawn from their treatment regimens—consult product literature, dose titration should be repeated if restarting after interval of more than 5 days

IMPORTANT SAFETY INFORMATION

MHRA/CHM ADVICE: ANTIEPILEPTICS: RISK OF SUICIDAL THOUGHTS AND BEHAVIOUR (AUGUST 2008)
See Epilepsy p. 349.

MHRA/CHM ADVICE: ANTIEPILEPTIC DRUGS: UPDATED ADVICE ON SWITCHING BETWEEN DIFFERENT MANUFACTURERS' PRODUCTS (NOVEMBER 2017)
See Epilepsy p. 349 and see also *Prescribing and dispensing information*.

MHRA/CHM ADVICE: ANTIEPILEPTIC DRUGS IN PREGNANCY: UPDATED ADVICE FOLLOWING COMPREHENSIVE SAFETY REVIEW (JANUARY 2021)
See Epilepsy p. 349.

● **CAUTIONS** Brugada syndrome · Parkinson's disease (may be exacerbated) · seizures (may be exacerbated)

CAUTIONS, FURTHER INFORMATION
▶ Seizure exacerbation [EvGr] Lamotrigine may exacerbate seizures in patients with myoclonic seizures (including juvenile myoclonic epilepsy), Dravet syndrome, and Lennox-Gastaut syndrome. ⟨A⟩

● **INTERACTIONS** → Appendix 1: antiepileptics

● **SIDE-EFFECTS**
▶ **Common or very common** Aggression · agitation · arthralgia · diarrhoea · dizziness · drowsiness · dry mouth · fatigue · headache · irritability · nausea · pain · rash · sleep disorders · tremor · vomiting
▶ **Uncommon** Alopecia · movement disorders · vision disorders
▶ **Rare or very rare** Confusion · conjunctivitis · disseminated intravascular coagulation · face oedema · fever · haemophagocytic lymphohistiocytosis · hallucination · hepatic disorders · lupus-like syndrome · lymphadenopathy · meningitis aseptic · multi organ failure · nystagmus · seizure · severe cutaneous adverse reactions (SCARs) · tic
▶ **Frequency not known** Suicidal behaviours

SIDE-EFFECTS, FURTHER INFORMATION Serious skin reactions including Stevens-Johnson syndrome and toxic epidermal necrolysis have developed (especially in children); most rashes occur in the first 8 weeks. Rash is sometimes associated with hypersensitivity syndrome and is more common in patients with history of allergy or rash from other antiepileptic drugs. Consider withdrawal if rash or signs of hypersensitivity syndrome develop. Factors associated with increased risk of serious skin reactions include concomitant use of valproate, initial lamotrigine dosing higher than recommended, and more rapid dose escalation than recommended.

● **ALLERGY AND CROSS-SENSITIVITY** Antiepileptic hypersensitivity syndrome associated with lamotrigine. See under Epilepsy p. 349 for more information.

● **PREGNANCY** See also *Pregnancy* in Epilepsy p. 349. **Monitoring** [EvGr] Plasma-drug concentration should be monitored before, during, and after pregnancy, including shortly after birth, and doses adjusted according to response—plasma levels alter during pregnancy and may increase rapidly after birth. ⟨M⟩

● **BREAST FEEDING** Present in milk, but limited data suggest no harmful effect on infant.

● **HEPATIC IMPAIRMENT** Manufacturer advises caution in moderate to severe impairment. **Dose adjustments** Manufacturer advises dose reduction of approx. 50% in moderate impairment, and approx. 75% in severe impairment; adjust according to response.

● **RENAL IMPAIRMENT** [EvGr] Caution in renal failure; metabolite may accumulate. ⟨M⟩ **Dose adjustments** [EvGr] Consider reducing maintenance dose in significant impairment. ⟨M⟩

● **TREATMENT CESSATION** Avoid abrupt withdrawal (taper off over 2 weeks or longer) unless serious skin reaction occurs.

● **PRESCRIBING AND DISPENSING INFORMATION** Patients being treated for epilepsy may need to be maintained on a specific manufacturer's branded or generic lamotrigine product.

Switching between formulations Care should be taken when switching between oral formulations in the treatment of epilepsy. The need for continued supply of a particular manufacturer's product should be based on clinical judgement and consultation with the patient or their carer, taking into account factors such as seizure frequency and treatment history.

● **PATIENT AND CARER ADVICE**

Skin reactions Warn patients and carers to see their doctor immediately if rash or signs or symptoms of hypersensitivity syndrome develop.

Blood disorders Patients and their carers should be alert for symptoms and signs suggestive of bone-marrow failure, such as anaemia, bruising, or infection. Aplastic anaemia, bone-marrow depression, and pancytopenia have been associated rarely with lamotrigine.

Medicines for Children leaflet: Lamotrigine for preventing seizures www.medicinesforchildren.org.uk/medicines/lamotrigine-for-preventing-seizures/

● **MEDICINAL FORMS** There can be variation in the licensing of different medicines containing the same drug. Forms available from special-order manufacturers include: oral suspension, oral solution

Dispersible tablet

CAUTIONARY AND ADVISORY LABELS 8, 13

▸ Lamotrigine (Non-proprietary)

Lamotrigine 5 mg Lamotrigine 5mg dispersible tablets sugar free | 28 tablet [PoM] £16.00 DT = £13.18 [SF]

Lamotrigine 25 mg Lamotrigine 25mg dispersible tablets sugar free | 56 tablet [PoM] £20.00 DT = £14.69 [SF]

Lamotrigine 100 mg Lamotrigine 100mg dispersible tablets sugar free | 56 tablet [PoM] £58.68 DT = £14.63 [SF]

▸ Lamictal (GlaxoSmithKline UK Ltd)

Lamotrigine 2 mg Lamictal 2mg dispersible tablets | 30 tablet [PoM] £18.81 DT = £18.81 [SF]

Lamotrigine 5 mg Lamictal 5mg dispersible tablets | 30 tablet [PoM] £10.05 [SF]

Lamotrigine 25 mg Lamictal 25mg dispersible tablets | 56 tablet [PoM] £23.53 DT = £14.69 [SF]

Lamotrigine 100 mg Lamictal 100mg dispersible tablets | 56 tablet [PoM] £69.04 DT = £14.63 [SF]

Oral tablet

CAUTIONARY AND ADVISORY LABELS 8

▸ Lamotrigine (Non-proprietary)

Lamotrigine 25 mg Lamotrigine 25mg tablets | 56 tablet [PoM] £2.77 DT = £1.66

Lamotrigine 50 mg Lamotrigine 50mg tablets | 56 tablet [PoM] £3.73 DT = £2.19

Lamotrigine 100 mg Lamotrigine 100mg tablets | 56 tablet [PoM] £5.39 DT = £2.86

Lamotrigine 200 mg Lamotrigine 200mg tablets | 56 tablet [PoM] £9.63 DT = £4.34

▸ Lamictal (GlaxoSmithKline UK Ltd)

Lamotrigine 25 mg Lamictal 25mg tablets | 56 tablet [PoM] £23.53 DT = £1.66

Lamotrigine 50 mg Lamictal 50mg tablets | 56 tablet [PoM] £40.02 DT = £2.19

Lamotrigine 100 mg Lamictal 100mg tablets | 56 tablet [PoM] £69.04 DT = £2.86

Lamotrigine 200 mg Lamictal 200mg tablets | 56 tablet [PoM] £117.35 DT = £4.34

Oral suspension

▸ Lamotrigine (Non-proprietary)

Lamotrigine 10 mg per 1 ml Lamotrigine 10mg/ml oral suspension sugar free | 300 ml [PoM] £43.87 DT = £43.87 [SF]

Levetiracetam

30-Nov-2023

● **INDICATIONS AND DOSE**

Monotherapy of focal seizures with or without secondary generalisation

▸ BY MOUTH, OR BY INTRAVENOUS INFUSION

▸ Child 16-17 years: Initially 250 mg once daily for 1 week, then increased to 250 mg twice daily, dose then increased in steps of 250 mg twice daily every 2 weeks up to maximum 1.5 g twice daily, to be adjusted according to response

▸ Adult: Initially 250 mg once daily for 1–2 weeks, then increased to 250 mg twice daily, dose then increased in steps of 250 mg twice daily every 2 weeks up to maximum 1.5 g twice daily, to be adjusted according to response

Adjunctive therapy of focal seizures with or without secondary generalisation

▸ BY MOUTH

▸ Child 1-5 months: Initially 7 mg/kg once daily, dose then increased in steps of up to 7 mg/kg twice daily every 2 weeks up to maximum 21 mg/kg twice daily

▸ Child 6 months-17 years (body-weight up to 50 kg): Initially 10 mg/kg once daily, dose then increased in steps of up to 10 mg/kg twice daily every 2 weeks up to maximum 30 mg/kg twice daily

▸ Child 12-17 years (body-weight 50 kg and above): Initially 250 mg twice daily, dose then increased in steps of 500 mg twice daily every 2–4 weeks up to maximum 1.5 g twice daily

▸ Adult: Initially 250 mg twice daily, dose then increased in steps of 500 mg twice daily every 2–4 weeks up to maximum 1.5 g twice daily

▸ BY INTRAVENOUS INFUSION

▸ Child 4-17 years (body-weight up to 50 kg): Initially 10 mg/kg once daily, dose then increased in steps of up to 10 mg/kg twice daily every 2 weeks up to maximum 30 mg/kg twice daily

▸ Child 12-17 years (body-weight 50 kg and above): Initially 250 mg twice daily, dose then increased in steps of 500 mg twice daily every 2 weeks up to maximum 1.5 g twice daily

▸ Adult: Initially 250 mg twice daily, dose then increased in steps of 500 mg twice daily every 2–4 weeks up to maximum 1.5 g twice daily

Adjunctive therapy of myoclonic seizures and tonic-clonic seizures

▸ BY MOUTH, OR BY INTRAVENOUS INFUSION

▸ Child 12-17 years (body-weight up to 50 kg): Initially 10 mg/kg once daily, dose then increased in steps of up to 10 mg/kg twice daily every 2 weeks up to maximum 30 mg/kg twice daily

▸ Child 12-17 years (body-weight 50 kg and above): Initially 250 mg twice daily, dose then increased in steps of 500 mg twice daily every 2 weeks up to maximum 1.5 g twice daily

▸ Adult: Initially 250 mg twice daily, dose then increased in steps of 500 mg twice daily every 2–4 weeks up to maximum 1.5 g twice daily

Convulsive status epilepticus (administered on expert advice)

▸ BY INTRAVENOUS INFUSION

▸ Child: 40 mg/kg for 1 dose (max. per dose 3 g), consult local protocols

● **UNLICENSED USE** [EvGr] Initial dosing recommendations for levetiracetam ⓔ in BNF Publications differ from product licence.

▸ With intravenous use in children [EvGr] Levetiracetam is used for the treatment of convulsive status epilepticus, Ⓐ but is not licensed for this indication.

▶ With oral use in children EvGr *Granules* and *granules for oral solution* are not licensed for use in children aged under 6 years, for initial treatment in children with body-weight less than 25 kg, or for the administration of doses below 250 mg— *oral solution* should be used. ◈M◈

> **IMPORTANT SAFETY INFORMATION**
> **MHRA/CHM ADVICE: ANTIEPILEPTICS: RISK OF SUICIDAL THOUGHTS AND BEHAVIOUR (AUGUST 2008)**
> See Epilepsy p. 349.
>
> **MHRA/CHM ADVICE: ANTIEPILEPTIC DRUGS: UPDATED ADVICE ON SWITCHING BETWEEN DIFFERENT MANUFACTURERS' PRODUCTS (NOVEMBER 2017)**
> See Epilepsy p. 349.
>
> **MHRA/CHM ADVICE: ANTIEPILEPTIC DRUGS IN PREGNANCY: UPDATED ADVICE FOLLOWING COMPREHENSIVE SAFETY REVIEW (JANUARY 2021)**
> See Epilepsy p. 349.

● **CAUTIONS** Risk factors for QT interval prolongation

● **INTERACTIONS** → Appendix 1: antiepileptics

● **SIDE-EFFECTS**

▶ **Common or very common** Anxiety · appetite decreased · asthenia · behaviour abnormal · cough · depression · diarrhoea · dizziness · drowsiness · gastrointestinal discomfort · headache · increased risk of infection · insomnia · mood altered · movement disorders · nausea · skin reactions · tremor · vertigo · vomiting

▶ **Uncommon** Alopecia · concentration impaired · confusion · hallucination · leucopenia · memory impairment · muscle weakness · myalgia · paraesthesia · psychotic disorder · suicidal behaviours · thrombocytopenia · vision disorders · weight changes

▶ **Rare or very rare** Acute kidney injury · agranulocytosis · bone marrow disorders · delirium · encephalopathy · gait abnormal · hepatic disorders · hyponatraemia · neutropenia · pancreatitis · personality disorder · QT interval prolongation · rhabdomyolysis · seizures exacerbated · severe cutaneous adverse reactions (SCARs) · thinking abnormal

▶ **Frequency not known** Neuroleptic malignant syndrome (discontinue—potentially fatal)

● **PREGNANCY** See also *Pregnancy* in Epilepsy p. 349.
Monitoring EvGr Clinical response should be monitored during pregnancy—plasma concentrations decrease during pregnancy (by up to 60% in the third trimester). ◈M◈

● **BREAST FEEDING** Present in milk—manufacturer advises avoid.

● **HEPATIC IMPAIRMENT** Manufacturer advises caution in severe impairment.
Dose adjustments Manufacturer advises maintenance dose reduction of 50% in severe impairment if creatinine clearance is less than 60 mL/minute/1.73 m^2—consult product literature.

● **RENAL IMPAIRMENT**
Dose adjustments
> ▶ In children Reduce dose if estimated glomerular filtration rate less than 80 mL/minute/1.73 m^2 (consult product literature).
> ▶ In adults Maximum 2 g daily if eGFR 50–80 mL/minute/1.73 m^2. Maximum 1.5 g daily if eGFR 30–50 mL/minute/1.73 m^2. Maximum 1 g daily if eGFR less than 30 mL/minute/1.73 m^2.

● **DIRECTIONS FOR ADMINISTRATION**

▶ With intravenous use for Focal seizures or Myoclonic seizures or Tonic-clonic seizures EvGr Dilute calculated dose with at least 100 mL Glucose 5% or Sodium Chloride 0.9%; give over 15 minutes. ◈M◈

▶ With intravenous use for Convulsive status epilepticus in children EvGr Dilute calculated dose with Glucose 5% or

Sodium Chloride 0.9% to a concentration of 50 mg/mL and give over 5 minutes. ◈A◈

▶ With oral use For administration of *oral solution*, manufacturer advises dose may be diluted in a glass of water.

● **PRESCRIBING AND DISPENSING INFORMATION** If switching between oral therapy and intravenous therapy (for those temporarily unable to take oral medication), the intravenous dose should be the same as the established oral dose.

● **PATIENT AND CARER ADVICE** Patients and caregivers should be advised to seek medical advice if signs of depression or suicidal ideation emerge. Patients should consult their doctor immediately if seizures worsen. Medicines for Children leaflet: Levetiracetam for preventing seizures www.medicinesforchildren.org.uk/medicines/levetiracetam-for-preventing-seizures/
Driving and skilled tasks Patients and carers should be cautioned on the effects on driving and performance of skilled tasks—increased risk of somnolence or other CNS side-effects.

● **MEDICINAL FORMS** There can be variation in the licensing of different medicines containing the same drug. Forms available from special-order manufacturers include: oral solution

Oral tablet
CAUTIONARY AND ADVISORY LABELS 3, 8
▶ **Levetiracetam (Non-proprietary)**
Levetiracetam 250 mg Levetiracetam 250mg tablets | 60 tablet PoM £25.25 DT = £1.98
Levetiracetam 500 mg Levetiracetam 500mg tablets | 60 tablet PoM £46.25 DT = £5.54 | 200 tablet PoM £17.70
Levetiracetam 750 mg Levetiracetam 750mg tablets | 60 tablet PoM £81.25 DT = £3.70
Levetiracetam 1 gram Levetiracetam 1g tablets | 60 tablet PoM £92.25 DT = £5.02
▶ **Keppra** (UCB Pharma Ltd)
Levetiracetam 250 mg Keppra 250mg tablets | 60 tablet PoM £28.01 DT = £1.98
Levetiracetam 500 mg Keppra 500mg tablets | 60 tablet PoM £49.32 DT = £5.54
Levetiracetam 750 mg Keppra 750mg tablets | 60 tablet PoM £84.02 DT = £3.70
Levetiracetam 1 gram Keppra 1g tablets | 60 tablet PoM £95.34 DT = £5.02

Solution for infusion
ELECTROLYTES: May contain Sodium
▶ **Levetiracetam (Non-proprietary)**
Levetiracetam 100 mg per 1 ml Levetiracetam 500mg/5ml concentrate for solution for infusion vials | 10 vial PoM £127.50 DT = £127.31 (Hospital only)
▶ **Desitrend** (Desitin Pharma Ltd)
Levetiracetam 100 mg per 1 ml Desitrend 500mg/5ml concentrate for solution for infusion ampoules | 10 ampoule PoM £127.31 DT = £127.31
▶ **Keppra** (UCB Pharma Ltd)
Levetiracetam 100 mg per 1 ml Keppra 500mg/5ml concentrate for solution for infusion vials | 10 vial PoM £127.31 DT = £127.31 (Hospital only)

Oral solution
CAUTIONARY AND ADVISORY LABELS 3, 8
▶ **Levetiracetam (Non-proprietary)**
Levetiracetam 100 mg per 1 ml Levetiracetam 100mg/ml oral solution sugar free | 150 ml PoM £26.40 SF | 300 ml PoM £66.95 DT = £5.55 SF
▶ **Eltam** (Medley Pharma Ltd)
Levetiracetam 100 mg per 1 ml Eltam 100mg/ml oral solution | 150 ml PoM £23.30 SF | 300 ml PoM £48.95 DT = £5.55 SF
▶ **Keppra** (UCB Pharma Ltd)
Levetiracetam 100 mg per 1 ml Keppra 100mg/ml oral solution | 150 ml PoM £33.48 SF | 300 ml PoM £66.95 DT = £5.55 SF

Granules for oral solution
CAUTIONARY AND ADVISORY LABELS 3, 8
▶ **Levetiracetam (Non-proprietary)**
Levetiracetam 250 mg Levetiracetam 250mg granules for oral solution sachets sugar free | 60 sachet PoM £22.41-£39.22 SF

Levetiracetam 500 mg Levetiracetam 500mg granules for oral solution sachets sugar free | 60 sachet [PoM] £39.46-£69.06 [SF]
Levetiracetam 750 mg Levetiracetam 750mg granules for oral solution sachets sugar free | 60 sachet [PoM] £57.87-£111.41 [SF]
Levetiracetam 1 gram Levetiracetam 1g granules for oral solution sachets sugar free | 60 sachet [PoM] £76.27-£133.48 [SF]
Levetiracetam 1.5 gram Levetiracetam 1.5g granules for oral solution sachets sugar free | 60 sachet [PoM] £110.73-£193.78 [SF]

Oral granules
CAUTIONARY AND ADVISORY LABELS 3, 8
▸ Desitrend (Desitin Pharma Ltd)
Levetiracetam 250 mg Desitrend 250mg granules sachets | 60 sachet [PoM] £22.41 DT = £22.41 [SF]
Levetiracetam 500 mg Desitrend 500mg granules sachets | 60 sachet [PoM] £39.46 DT = £39.46 [SF]
Levetiracetam 1 gram Desitrend 1000mg granules sachets | 60 sachet [PoM] £76.27 DT = £76.27 [SF]

Oxcarbazepine

17-Oct-2022

● **INDICATIONS AND DOSE**

Monotherapy for the treatment of focal seizures with or without secondary generalised tonic-clonic seizures
▸ BY MOUTH
▸ Child 6–17 years: Initially 4–5 mg/kg twice daily (max. per dose 300 mg), then increased in steps of up to 5 mg/kg twice daily, adjusted according to response, dose to be adjusted at weekly intervals; maximum 46 mg/kg per day
▸ Adult: Initially 300 mg twice daily, then increased in steps of up to 600 mg daily, adjusted according to response, dose to be adjusted at weekly intervals; usual dose 0.6–2.4 g daily in divided doses

Adjunctive therapy for the treatment of focal seizures with or without secondary generalised tonic-clonic seizures
▸ BY MOUTH
▸ Child 6–17 years: Initially 4–5 mg/kg twice daily (max. per dose 300 mg), then increased in steps of up to 5 mg/kg twice daily, adjusted according to response, dose to be adjusted at weekly intervals; maintenance 15 mg/kg twice daily; maximum 46 mg/kg per day
▸ Adult: Initially 300 mg twice daily, then increased in steps of up to 600 mg daily, adjusted according to response, dose to be adjusted at weekly intervals; usual dose 0.6–2.4 g daily in divided doses

Treatment of primary generalised tonic-clonic seizures
▸ BY MOUTH
▸ Adult: Initially 300 mg twice daily, then increased in steps of up to 600 mg daily, adjusted according to response, dose to be increased at weekly intervals; usual dose 0.6–2.4 g daily in divided doses

DOSE ADJUSTMENTS DUE TO INTERACTIONS
▸ In adjunctive therapy, the dose of concomitant antiepileptics may need to be reduced when using high doses of oxcarbazepine.

● **UNLICENSED USE** Not licensed for the treatment of primary generalised tonic-clonic seizures.

IMPORTANT SAFETY INFORMATION

MHRA/CHM ADVICE: ANTIEPILEPTICS: RISK OF SUICIDAL THOUGHTS AND BEHAVIOUR (AUGUST 2008)
See Epilepsy p. 349.

MHRA/CHM ADVICE: ANTIEPILEPTIC DRUGS: UPDATED ADVICE ON SWITCHING BETWEEN DIFFERENT MANUFACTURERS' PRODUCTS (NOVEMBER 2017)
See Epilepsy p. 349 and see also *Prescribing and dispensing information*.

MHRA/CHM ADVICE: ANTIEPILEPTIC DRUGS IN PREGNANCY: UPDATED ADVICE FOLLOWING COMPREHENSIVE SAFETY REVIEW (JANUARY 2021)
See Epilepsy p. 349.

● **CAUTIONS** Avoid in Acute porphyrias p. 1202 · cardiac conduction disorders · heart failure · hyponatraemia · presence of HLA-B*1502 or HLA-A*3101 allele · seizures (may be exacerbated)

CAUTIONS, FURTHER INFORMATION
▸ HLA allele [EvGr] The presence of HLA-B*1502 allele, particularly in individuals of Han Chinese or Thai origin, is strongly associated with an increased risk of carbamazepine-induced Stevens-Johnson syndrome; this may also occur with oxcarbazepine, a structurally-related antiepileptic—see also *Pre-treatment screening*.
  The presence of HLA-A*3101 allele, particularly in individuals of European or Japanese origin, is associated with an increased risk of carbamazepine-induced cutaneous adverse reactions. This may also occur with oxcarbazepine, a structurally-related antiepileptic, but there are insufficient data to support pre-treatment screening. Consider use if potential benefit outweighs risk. [M]
▸ Seizure exacerbation [EvGr] Oxcarbazepine may exacerbate seizures in patients with absence or myoclonic seizures (including juvenile myoclonic epilepsy), tonic or atonic seizures, Dravet syndrome, Lennox-Gastaut syndrome, and myoclonic-atonic seizures. [A]

● **INTERACTIONS** → Appendix 1: antiepileptics

● **SIDE-EFFECTS**
▸ **Common or very common** Abdominal pain · agitation · alopecia · asthenia · ataxia · concentration impaired · confusion · constipation · depression · diarrhoea · dizziness · drowsiness · emotional lability · headache · hyponatraemia · memory loss · nausea · nystagmus · skin reactions · speech impairment · tremor · vertigo · vision disorders · vomiting · weight increased
▸ **Uncommon** Hypertension · hypothyroidism · leucopenia
▸ **Rare or very rare** Agranulocytosis · angioedema · arrhythmia · atrioventricular block · bone disorders · bone fracture · bone marrow disorders · hepatitis · inappropriate antidiuretic hormone secretion like-syndrome · neutropenia · pancreatitis · severe cutaneous adverse reactions (SCARs) · systemic lupus erythematosus (SLE) · thrombocytopenia
▸ **Frequency not known** Suicidal behaviours

● **ALLERGY AND CROSS-SENSITIVITY** Caution in patients with hypersensitivity to carbamazepine. Antiepileptic hypersensitivity syndrome associated with oxcarbazepine. See under Epilepsy p. 349 for more information.

● **PREGNANCY** See also *Pregnancy* in Epilepsy p. 349.
Monitoring [EvGr] Clinical response should be monitored carefully during pregnancy, and plasma concentration monitoring of the active metabolite should be considered during and after pregnancy (if doses were increased during pregnancy)—plasma levels of the active metabolite may gradually decrease during pregnancy. [M]

● **BREAST FEEDING** Amount probably too small to be harmful but manufacturer advises avoid.

● **HEPATIC IMPAIRMENT** Manufacturer advises caution in severe impairment (no information available).

● **RENAL IMPAIRMENT**
Dose adjustments [EvGr] Halve initial dose if creatinine clearance less than 30 mL/minute; increase according to response at intervals of at least 1 week. [M] See p. 21.

● **PRE-TREATMENT SCREENING** [EvGr] Test for HLA-B*1502 allele in individuals of Han Chinese or Thai origin, and consider testing in other at-risk Asian populations such as individuals of Filipino or Malaysian origin (consider use if potential benefit outweighs risk). ⟨M⟩

- **MONITORING REQUIREMENTS**
- ▶ Monitor plasma-sodium concentration in patients at risk of hyponatraemia.
- ▶ Monitor body-weight in patients with heart failure.

- **PRESCRIBING AND DISPENSING INFORMATION** Patients may need to be maintained on a specific manufacturer's branded or generic oxcarbazepine product.
Switching between formulations Care should be taken when switching between oral formulations. The need for continued supply of a particular manufacturer's product should be based on clinical judgement and consultation with the patient or their carer, taking into account factors such as seizure frequency and treatment history.

- **PATIENT AND CARER ADVICE**
Blood, hepatic, or skin disorders Patients or their carers should be told how to recognise signs of blood, liver, or skin disorders, and advised to seek immediate medical attention if symptoms such as lethargy, confusion, muscular twitching, fever, rash, blistering, mouth ulcers, bruising, or bleeding develop.
Medicines for Children: Oxcarbazepine for preventing seizures
www.medicinesforchildren.org.uk/medicines/oxcarbazepine-for-preventing-seizures/

- **MEDICINAL FORMS** There can be variation in the licensing of different medicines containing the same drug. Forms available from special-order manufacturers include: oral suspension

Oral tablet
CAUTIONARY AND ADVISORY LABELS 3, 8
- ▶ Oxcarbazepine (Non-proprietary)
  Oxcarbazepine 150 mg Oxcarbazepine 150mg tablets | 50 tablet PoM £20.11 DT = £20.11
  Oxcarbazepine 300 mg Oxcarbazepine 300mg tablets | 50 tablet PoM £24.48 DT = £12.45
  Oxcarbazepine 600 mg Oxcarbazepine 600mg tablets | 50 tablet PoM £56.48 DT = £53.36
- ▶ Trileptal (Novartis Pharmaceuticals UK Ltd)
  Oxcarbazepine 150 mg Trileptal 150mg tablets | 50 tablet PoM £12.24 DT = £20.11
  Oxcarbazepine 300 mg Trileptal 300mg tablets | 50 tablet PoM £24.48 DT = £12.45
  Oxcarbazepine 600 mg Trileptal 600mg tablets | 50 tablet PoM £48.96 DT = £53.36

Oral suspension
CAUTIONARY AND ADVISORY LABELS 3, 8
EXCIPIENTS: May contain Propylene glycol
- ▶ Trileptal (Novartis Pharmaceuticals UK Ltd)
  Oxcarbazepine 60 mg per 1 ml Trileptal 60mg/ml oral suspension | 250 ml PoM £48.96 DT = £48.96 SF

Perampanel
22-Jun-2021

- **INDICATIONS AND DOSE**
Adjunctive treatment of focal seizures with or without secondary generalised seizures
- ▶ BY MOUTH
- ▶ Child 4-11 years (body-weight up to 20 kg): Initially 1 mg once daily, dose to be taken before bedtime, then increased, if tolerated, in steps of 1 mg at intervals of at least every 2 weeks, adjusted according to response; maintenance 2–4 mg once daily, then increased, if tolerated, in steps of 0.5 mg at intervals of at least every 2 weeks, adjusted according to response; maximum 6 mg per day
- ▶ Child 4-11 years (body-weight 20-29 kg): Initially 1 mg once daily, dose to be taken before bedtime, then increased, if tolerated, in steps of 1 mg at intervals of at least every 2 weeks, adjusted according to response; maintenance 4–6 mg once daily; maximum 8 mg per day

- ▶ Child 4-11 years (body-weight 30 kg and above): Initially 2 mg once daily, dose to be taken before bedtime, then increased, if tolerated, in steps of 2 mg at intervals of at least every 2 weeks, adjusted according to response; maintenance 4–8 mg once daily; maximum 12 mg per day
- ▶ Child 12-17 years: Initially 2 mg once daily, dose to be taken before bedtime, then increased, if tolerated, in steps of 2 mg at intervals of at least every 2 weeks, adjusted according to response; maintenance 4–8 mg once daily; maximum 12 mg per day
- ▶ Adult: Initially 2 mg once daily, dose to be taken before bedtime, then increased, if tolerated, in steps of 2 mg at intervals of at least every 2 weeks, adjusted according to response; maintenance 4–8 mg once daily; maximum 12 mg per day

Adjunctive treatment of primary generalised tonic-clonic seizures
- ▶ BY MOUTH
- ▶ Child 7-11 years (body-weight up to 20 kg): Initially 1 mg once daily, dose to be taken before bedtime, then increased, if tolerated, in steps of 1 mg at intervals of at least every 2 weeks, adjusted according to response; maintenance 2–4 mg once daily, then increased, if tolerated, in steps of 0.5 mg at intervals of at least every 2 weeks, adjusted according to response; maximum 6 mg per day
- ▶ Child 7-11 years (body-weight 20-29 kg): Initially 1 mg once daily, dose to be taken before bedtime, then increased in steps of 1 mg at intervals of at least every 2 weeks, adjusted according to response; maintenance 4–6 mg once daily; maximum 8 mg per day
- ▶ Child 7-11 years (body-weight 30 kg and above): Initially 2 mg once daily, dose to be taken before bedtime, then increased, if tolerated, in steps of 2 mg at intervals of at least every 2 weeks, adjusted according to response; maintenance 4–8 mg once daily; maximum 12 mg per day
- ▶ Child 12-17 years: Initially 2 mg once daily, dose to be taken before bedtime, then increased, if tolerated, in steps of 2 mg at intervals of at least every 2 weeks, adjusted according to response, maintenance up to 8 mg once daily; maximum 12 mg per day
- ▶ Adult: Initially 2 mg once daily, dose to be taken before bedtime, then increased, if tolerated, in steps of 2 mg at intervals of at least every 2 weeks, adjusted according to response, maintenance up to 8 mg once daily; maximum 12 mg per day

DOSE ADJUSTMENTS DUE TO INTERACTIONS
- ▶ Titrate at intervals of at least 1 week with concomitant carbamazepine, fosphenytoin, oxcarbazepine, or phenytoin.

IMPORTANT SAFETY INFORMATION
MHRA/CHM ADVICE: ANTIEPILEPTICS: RISK OF SUICIDAL THOUGHTS AND BEHAVIOUR (AUGUST 2008)
See Epilepsy p. 349.

MHRA/CHM ADVICE: ANTIEPILEPTIC DRUGS: UPDATED ADVICE ON SWITCHING BETWEEN DIFFERENT MANUFACTURERS' PRODUCTS (NOVEMBER 2017)
See Epilepsy p. 349 and see also *Prescribing and dispensing information.*

MHRA/CHM ADVICE: ANTIEPILEPTIC DRUGS IN PREGNANCY: UPDATED ADVICE FOLLOWING COMPREHENSIVE SAFETY REVIEW (JANUARY 2021)
See Epilepsy p. 349.

- **INTERACTIONS** → Appendix 1: antiepileptics
- **SIDE-EFFECTS**
- ▶ **Common or very common** Anxiety · appetite abnormal · back pain · behaviour abnormal · confusion · dizziness ·

drowsiness · dysarthria · fatigue · gait abnormal · irritability · movement disorders · nausea · vertigo · vision disorders · weight increased
- **Uncommon** Suicidal behaviours
- **Frequency not known** Homicidal ideation · severe cutaneous adverse reactions (SCARs)
- **PREGNANCY** [EvGr] Avoid—embryotoxic in *animal* studies. Ⓜ See also *Pregnancy* in Epilepsy p. 349.
- **BREAST FEEDING** Avoid—present in milk in *animal* studies.
- **HEPATIC IMPAIRMENT** [EvGr] Caution in mild to moderate impairment; avoid in severe impairment. Ⓜ
  Dose adjustments [EvGr] Maximum 8 mg per day in mild to moderate impairment. Ⓜ
- **RENAL IMPAIRMENT** [EvGr] Avoid in moderate or severe impairment. Ⓜ
- **PRESCRIBING AND DISPENSING INFORMATION**
  Switching between formulations Care should be taken when switching between oral formulations. The need for continued supply of a particular manufacturer's product should be based on clinical judgement and consultation with the patient or their carer, taking into account factors such as seizure frequency and treatment history.
  Patients may need to be maintained on a specific manufacturer's branded or generic perampanel product.
- **PATIENT AND CARER ADVICE**
  Driving and skilled tasks Manufacturer advises patients and carers should be cautioned on the effects on driving and performance of skilled tasks—increased risk of dizziness and drowsiness.
- **NATIONAL FUNDING/ACCESS DECISIONS**
  For full details see funding body website
  Scottish Medicines Consortium (SMC) decisions
- Perampanel (*Fycompa*®) for the adjunctive treatment of partial-onset seizures with or without secondary generalised seizures in patients with epilepsy aged 12 years and older (December 2012) SMC No. 819/12 Recommended with restrictions
- Perampanel oral suspension (*Fycompa*®) for the adjunctive treatment of partial-onset seizures with or without secondary generalised seizures in patients with epilepsy aged 12 years and older (August 2019) SMC No. SMC2172 Recommended with restrictions
  All Wales Medicines Strategy Group (AWMSG) decisions
- Perampanel (*Fycompa*®) for the adjunctive treatment of partial-onset seizures with or without secondary generalised seizures in patients from 4 years of age up to 12 years of age (May 2021) AWMSG No. 4770 Recommended with restrictions

- **MEDICINAL FORMS** There can be variation in the licensing of different medicines containing the same drug. Forms available from special-order manufacturers include: oral suspension

Oral tablet
CAUTIONARY AND ADVISORY LABELS 3, 8, 25
- Fycompa (Eisai Ltd)
  Perampanel 2 mg Fycompa 2mg tablets | 7 tablet [PoM] £35.00 DT = £35.00 | 28 tablet [PoM] £140.00 DT = £140.00
  Perampanel 4 mg Fycompa 4mg tablets | 28 tablet [PoM] £140.00 DT = £140.00
  Perampanel 6 mg Fycompa 6mg tablets | 28 tablet [PoM] £140.00 DT = £140.00
  Perampanel 8 mg Fycompa 8mg tablets | 28 tablet [PoM] £140.00 DT = £140.00
  Perampanel 10 mg Fycompa 10mg tablets | 28 tablet [PoM] £140.00 DT = £140.00
  Perampanel 12 mg Fycompa 12mg tablets | 28 tablet [PoM] £140.00 DT = £140.00

Oral suspension
CAUTIONARY AND ADVISORY LABELS 3, 8
EXCIPIENTS: May contain Sorbitol
- Fycompa (Eisai Ltd)
  Perampanel 500 microgram per 1 ml Fycompa 0.5mg/ml oral suspension | 340 ml [PoM] £127.50 DT = £127.50 [SF]

Phenytoin

18-Oct-2022

- **INDICATIONS AND DOSE**

Tonic-clonic seizures | Focal seizures
- BY MOUTH
- Child 1 month–11 years: Initially 1.5–2.5 mg/kg twice daily (max. per dose 150 mg), then adjusted according to response to 2.5–5 mg/kg twice daily (max. per dose 150 mg), dose also adjusted according to plasma-phenytoin concentration, increased if necessary up to 7.5 mg/kg twice daily (max. per dose 150 mg)
- Child 12–17 years: Initially 75–150 mg twice daily, then adjusted according to response to 150–200 mg twice daily, dose also adjusted according to plasma-phenytoin concentration, increased if necessary up to 300 mg twice daily

Tonic-clonic seizures | Focal seizures | Prevention and treatment of seizures during or following neurosurgery or severe head injury
- BY MOUTH
- Adult: Initially 3–4 mg/kg daily, alternatively 150–300 mg once daily, alternatively 150–300 mg daily in 2 divided doses; usual maintenance 200–500 mg daily, to be taken preferably with or after food, dose to be increased gradually as necessary (with plasma-phenytoin concentration monitoring), exceptionally, higher doses may be used

Prevention and treatment of seizures during or following neurosurgery or severe head injury
- BY MOUTH
- Child: Initially 2.5 mg/kg twice daily, then adjusted according to response to 4–8 mg/kg daily, dose also adjusted according to plasma-phenytoin concentration; maximum 300 mg per day

Status epilepticus | Acute symptomatic seizures associated with head trauma or neurosurgery
- INITIALLY BY SLOW INTRAVENOUS INJECTION, OR BY INTRAVENOUS INFUSION
- Child 1 month–11 years: Loading dose 20 mg/kg for 1 dose, then (by slow intravenous injection or by intravenous infusion) 2.5–5 mg/kg twice daily
- Child 12–17 years: Loading dose 20 mg/kg for 1 dose, then (by intravenous infusion or by slow intravenous injection) up to 100 mg 3–4 times a day
- Adult: Loading dose 20 mg/kg for 1 dose (max. per dose 2 g), then (by intravenous infusion or by slow intravenous injection or by mouth) maintenance 100 mg every 6–8 hours, dose to be adjusted according to plasma-concentration monitoring

DOSE EQUIVALENCE AND CONVERSION
- Preparations containing phenytoin sodium are **not** bioequivalent to those containing phenytoin base (such as *Epanutin Infatabs*® and *Epanutin*® suspension); 100 mg of phenytoin sodium is approximately equivalent in therapeutic effect to 92 mg phenytoin base. The dose is the same for all phenytoin products when initiating therapy. However, if switching between these products the difference in phenytoin content may be clinically significant. Care is needed when making changes between formulations and plasma-phenytoin concentration monitoring is recommended.

PHARMACOKINETICS
- Phenytoin has a narrow therapeutic index and the relationship between dose and plasma-drug concentration is non-linear; small dosage increases in some patients may produce large increases in plasma-drug concentration with acute toxic side-effects. Similarly, a few missed doses or a small change in drug absorption may result in a marked change in plasma-

drug concentration. Monitoring of plasma-drug concentration improves dosage adjustment.

● **UNLICENSED USE**
▸ With oral use Licensed for use in children (age range not specified by manufacturer).
▸ With intravenous use Phenytoin doses in BNF publications may differ from those in product literature.

IMPORTANT SAFETY INFORMATION

MHRA/CHM ADVICE: ANTIEPILEPTICS: RISK OF SUICIDAL THOUGHTS AND BEHAVIOUR (AUGUST 2008)
See Epilepsy p. 349.

NHS IMPROVEMENT PATIENT SAFETY ALERT: RISK OF DEATH AND SEVERE HARM FROM ERROR WITH INJECTABLE PHENYTOIN (NOVEMBER 2016)
Use of injectable phenytoin is error-prone throughout the prescribing, preparation, administration and monitoring processes; all relevant staff should be made aware of appropriate guidance on the safe use of injectable phenytoin to reduce the risk of error.

MHRA/CHM ADVICE: ANTIEPILEPTIC DRUGS: UPDATED ADVICE ON SWITCHING BETWEEN DIFFERENT MANUFACTURERS' PRODUCTS (NOVEMBER 2017)
See Epilepsy p. 349 and see also *Prescribing and dispensing information*.

MHRA/CHM ADVICE: ANTIEPILEPTIC DRUGS IN PREGNANCY: UPDATED ADVICE FOLLOWING COMPREHENSIVE SAFETY REVIEW (JANUARY 2021)
See Epilepsy p. 349.

● **CONTRA-INDICATIONS**
GENERAL CONTRA-INDICATIONS Acute porphyrias p. 1202
SPECIFIC CONTRA-INDICATIONS
▸ With intravenous use Second- and third-degree heart block · sino-atrial block · sinus bradycardia · Stokes-Adams syndrome

● **CAUTIONS**
GENERAL CAUTIONS Enteral feeding (interrupt feeding for 2 hours before and after dose; more frequent monitoring may be necessary) · presence of HLA-B*1502 allele · seizures (may be exacerbated)
SPECIFIC CAUTIONS
▸ With intravenous use Heart failure · hypotension · injection solutions alkaline (irritant to tissues) · respiratory depression · resuscitation facilities must be available
CAUTIONS, FURTHER INFORMATION MHRA advises consider vitamin D supplementation in patients who are immobilised for long periods or who have inadequate sun exposure or dietary intake of calcium.
  EvGr Intramuscular phenytoin should not be used (absorption is slow and erratic). M
▸ HLA allele EvGr Limited evidence suggests that the presence of HLA-B*1502 allele, particularly in individuals of Han Chinese or Thai origin, may be associated with an increased risk of Stevens-Johnson syndrome. Consider use if potential benefit outweighs risk. M
▸ Seizure exacerbation EvGr Phenytoin may exacerbate seizures in patients with absence or myoclonic seizures (including juvenile myoclonic epilepsy), and myoclonic-atonic seizures. A

● **INTERACTIONS** → Appendix 1: antiepileptics

● **SIDE-EFFECTS**
GENERAL SIDE-EFFECTS Agranulocytosis · bone disorders · bone fracture · bone marrow disorders · cerebrovascular insufficiency · coarsening of the facial features · confusion · constipation · dizziness · drowsiness · Dupuytren's contracture · dysarthria · eosinophilia · fever · gingival hyperplasia (maintain good oral hygiene) · granulocytopenia · hair changes · headache · hepatic disorders · hypersensitivity · insomnia · joint disorders · leucopenia · lip swelling · lymphatic abnormalities · macrocytosis · megaloblastic anaemia · movement disorders · muscle twitching · nausea · neoplasms · nephritis tubulointerstitial · nervousness · nystagmus · paraesthesia · Peyronie's disease · pneumonitis · polyarteritis nodosa · pseudolymphoma · sensory peripheral polyneuropathy · severe cutaneous adverse reactions (SCARs) · skin reactions · suicidal behaviours · systemic lupus erythematosus (SLE) · taste altered · thrombocytopenia · tremor · vertigo · vomiting
SPECIFIC SIDE-EFFECTS
▸ With oral use Electrolyte imbalance · vitamin D deficiency
▸ With parenteral use Arrhythmias · atrial conduction depression (more common if injection too rapid) · cardiac arrest · extravasation necrosis · hypotension · injection site necrosis · purple glove syndrome · respiratory arrest (more common if injection too rapid) · respiratory disorder · tonic seizure (more common if injection too rapid) · ventricular conduction depression (more common if injection too rapid) · ventricular fibrillation (more common if injection too rapid)

SIDE-EFFECTS, FURTHER INFORMATION **Rash** Discontinue; if mild re-introduce cautiously but discontinue immediately if recurrence.
  Bradycardia and hypotension With intravenous use; reduce rate of administration if bradycardia or hypotension occurs.
Overdose Symptoms of phenytoin toxicity include nystagmus, diplopia, slurred speech, ataxia, confusion, and hyperglycaemia.

● **ALLERGY AND CROSS-SENSITIVITY** Cross-sensitivity reported with carbamazepine. Antiepileptic hypersensitivity syndrome associated with phenytoin. See under Epilepsy p. 349 for more information.

● **PREGNANCY** An increased risk of major congenital malformations and possibility of adverse effects on neurodevelopment have been seen with phenytoin, see *Pregnancy* in Epilepsy p. 349.
Monitoring Changes in plasma-protein binding make interpretation of plasma-phenytoin concentrations difficult—monitor unbound fraction.
  EvGr Doses should be adjusted on the basis of plasma-drug concentration monitoring—phenytoin pharmacokinetics altered during pregnancy. M

● **BREAST FEEDING** Small amounts present in milk, but not known to be harmful.

● **HEPATIC IMPAIRMENT** Manufacturer advises caution (increased risk of accumulation and toxicity due to decreased protein binding in hepatic impairment, hypoalbuminaemia, or hyperbilirubinaemia).
Dose adjustments
▸ With oral use Manufacturer advises consider dose reduction.
▸ With intravenous use Manufacturer advises consider maintenance dose reduction.

● **MONITORING REQUIREMENTS**
▸ In adults The usual total plasma-phenytoin concentration for optimum response is 10–20 mg/litre (or 40–80 micromol/litre). In pregnancy, the elderly, and certain disease states where protein binding may be reduced, careful interpretation of total plasma-phenytoin concentration is necessary; it may be more appropriate to measure free plasma-phenytoin concentration.
▸ In children Therapeutic plasma-phenytoin concentrations reduced in first 3 months of life because of reduced protein binding. Trough plasma concentration for optimum response: neonate–3 months, 6–15 mg/litre (25–60 micromol/litre); child 3 months–18 years, 10–20 mg/litre (40–80 micromol/litre).
▸ Blood counts Manufacturer recommends blood counts (but

evidence of practical value uncertain).

▶ With intravenous use Monitor ECG and blood pressure.

● DIRECTIONS FOR ADMINISTRATION Manufacturer advises each injection or infusion should be preceded and followed by an injection of Sodium Chloride 0.9% through the same needle or catheter to avoid local venous irritation.

▶ With intravenous use in children EvGr For *intravenous injection*, give into a large vein at a rate not exceeding 1 mg/kg/minute (max. 50 mg/minute). ⒹManufacturer advises for *intravenous infusion*, dilute to a concentration not exceeding 10 mg/mL with Sodium Chloride 0.9% and give into a large vein through an in-line filter (0.22–0.50 micron). EvGr Give at a rate not exceeding 1 mg/kg/minute (max. 50 mg/minute). ⒹComplete administration within 1 hour of preparation.

▶ With intravenous use in adults Manufacturer advises for *intravenous injection*, give into a large vein at a rate not exceeding 50 mg/minute; rate of 25 mg/minute or lower may be more appropriate in some patients (including the elderly and those with heart disease). Manufacturer advises for *intravenous infusion*, dilute in 50–100 mL Sodium Chloride 0.9% (final concentration not to exceed 10 mg/mL) and give into a large vein through an in-line filter (0.22–0.50 micron) at a rate not exceeding 50 mg/minute; rate of 25 mg/minute or lower may be more appropriate in some patients (including the elderly and those with heart disease). Complete administration within 1 hour of preparation.

● PRESCRIBING AND DISPENSING INFORMATION
Switching between formulations Different formulations of oral preparations may vary in bioavailability. Patients being treated for epilepsy should be maintained on a specific manufacturer's product.

● PATIENT AND CARER ADVICE
Blood or skin disorders Patients or their carers should be told how to recognise signs of blood or skin disorders, and advised to seek immediate medical attention if symptoms such as fever, rash, mouth ulcers, bruising, or bleeding develop. Leucopenia that is severe, progressive, or associated with clinical symptoms requires withdrawal (if necessary under cover of a suitable alternative).
Medicines for Children leaflet: Phenytoin for preventing seizures www.medicinesforchildren.org.uk/medicines/phenytoin-for-preventing-seizures/

● MEDICINAL FORMS There can be variation in the licensing of different medicines containing the same drug. Forms available from special-order manufacturers include: chewable tablet, oral suspension, oral solution

Oral tablet
CAUTIONARY AND ADVISORY LABELS 8
▶ Phenytoin (Non-proprietary)
Phenytoin sodium 100 mg Phenytoin sodium 100mg tablets | 28 tablet PoM £12.26 DT = £10.18

Solution for injection
EXCIPIENTS: May contain Alcohol, propylene glycol
ELECTROLYTES: May contain Sodium
▶ Phenytoin (Non-proprietary)
Phenytoin sodium 50 mg per 1 ml Phenytoin sodium 250mg/5ml solution for injection ampoules | 5 ampoule PoM £24.40 (Hospital only) | 10 ampoule PoM £34.00 (Hospital only)
▶ Epanutin (Viatris UK Healthcare Ltd)
Phenytoin sodium 50 mg per 1 ml Epanutin Ready-Mixed Parenteral 250mg/5ml solution for injection ampoules | 10 ampoule PoM £48.79 (Hospital only)

Oral suspension
CAUTIONARY AND ADVISORY LABELS 8
▶ Phenytoin (Non-proprietary)
Phenytoin 6 mg per 1 ml Dilantin-30 suspension | 250 ml PoM Ⓢ
▶ Epanutin (Viatris UK Healthcare Ltd)
Phenytoin 6 mg per 1 ml Epanutin 30mg/5ml oral suspension | 500 ml PoM £4.27 DT = £4.27

Oral capsule
CAUTIONARY AND ADVISORY LABELS 8
▶ Phenytoin (Non-proprietary)
Phenytoin sodium 25 mg Phenytoin sodium 25mg capsules | 28 capsule PoM £7.24 DT = £13.14
Phenytoin sodium 50 mg Phenytoin sodium 50mg capsules | 28 capsule PoM £7.07 DT = £7.07
Phenytoin sodium 100 mg Phenytoin sodium 100mg capsules | 84 capsule PoM £9.56 DT = £10.33
Phenytoin sodium 300 mg Phenytoin sodium 300mg capsules | 28 capsule PoM £9.11 DT = £16.55

Chewable tablet
CAUTIONARY AND ADVISORY LABELS 8, 24
▶ Phenytoin (Non-proprietary)
Phenytoin 50 mg Dilantin Infatabs 50mg chewable tablets | 100 tablet PoM Ⓢ
▶ Epanutin (Viatris UK Healthcare Ltd)
Phenytoin 50 mg Epanutin Infatabs 50mg chewable tablets | 200 tablet PoM £13.18 DT = £13.18

Pregabalin

17-Oct-2022

● INDICATIONS AND DOSE
Peripheral and central neuropathic pain
▶ BY MOUTH
▶ Adult: Initially 150 mg daily in 2–3 divided doses, then increased if necessary to 300 mg daily in 2–3 divided doses, dose to be increased after 3–7 days, then increased if necessary up to 600 mg daily in 2–3 divided doses, dose to be increased after 7 days

Adjunctive therapy for focal seizures with or without secondary generalisation
▶ BY MOUTH
▶ Adult: Initially 25 mg twice daily, then increased in steps of 50 mg daily, dose to be increased at 7 day intervals, increased to 300 mg daily in 2–3 divided doses for 7 days, then increased if necessary up to 600 mg daily in 2–3 divided doses

Generalised anxiety disorder
▶ BY MOUTH
▶ Adult: Initially 150 mg daily in 2–3 divided doses, then increased in steps of 150 mg daily if required, dose to be increased at 7 day intervals, increased if necessary up to 600 mg daily in 2–3 divided doses

● UNLICENSED USE Pregabalin doses in BNF may differ from those in product literature.

IMPORTANT SAFETY INFORMATION
MHRA/CHM ADVICE: ANTIEPILEPTICS: RISK OF SUICIDAL THOUGHTS AND BEHAVIOUR (AUGUST 2008)
See Epilepsy p. 349.

MHRA/CHM ADVICE: ANTIEPILEPTIC DRUGS: UPDATED ADVICE ON SWITCHING BETWEEN DIFFERENT MANUFACTURERS' PRODUCTS (NOVEMBER 2017)
See Epilepsy p. 349.

MHRA/CHM ADVICE: PREGABALIN (*LYRICA*®) AND RISK OF ABUSE AND DEPENDENCE: NEW SCHEDULING REQUIREMENTS FROM 1 APRIL (APRIL 2019)
Following concerns about abuse, pregabalin has been reclassified as a Class C controlled substance and is now a Schedule 3 drug, but is exempt from safe custody requirements. Healthcare professionals should evaluate patients carefully for a history of drug abuse before prescribing pregabalin, and observe patients for signs of abuse and dependence. Patients should be informed of the potentially fatal risks of interactions between pregabalin and alcohol, and with other medicines that cause CNS depression, particularly opioids.

MHRA/CHM ADVICE: ANTIEPILEPTIC DRUGS IN PREGNANCY: UPDATED ADVICE FOLLOWING COMPREHENSIVE SAFETY REVIEW (JANUARY 2021)
See Epilepsy p. 349.

MHRA/CHM ADVICE: PREGABALIN (*LYRICA*®): FINDINGS OF SAFETY STUDY ON RISKS DURING PREGNANCY (APRIL 2022)
MHRA and European reviews of a Nordic population-based cohort study have concluded that pregabalin use for all authorised indications during the first trimester of pregnancy may cause a slightly increased risk of major congenital malformations in the unborn child, when compared with patients taking lamotrigine, duloxetine or no antiepileptic drug.

Healthcare professionals are advised to:
- counsel patients taking pregabalin on the potential risks to an unborn baby and the need to use effective contraception during treatment;
- avoid use of pregabalin during pregnancy unless clearly necessary and the benefits outweigh the risks—in such cases, use the lowest effective dose;
- advise patients taking pregabalin that are planning to, or become pregnant, to discuss their treatment with their prescriber.

MHRA/CHM ADVICE: PREGABALIN (*LYRICA*®): REPORTS OF SEVERE RESPIRATORY DEPRESSION (FEBRUARY 2021)
A European review of pregabalin safety data identified worldwide reports of severe respiratory depression, in some cases without concomitant opioid treatment. Healthcare professionals are advised to consider whether adjustments in dose or dosing regimen are necessary in patients at higher risk of respiratory depression, including those:
- with compromised respiratory function, respiratory or neurological disease, or renal impairment;
- taking other CNS depressants (including opioid-containing medicines);
- aged older than 65 years.

Patients should be advised to seek medical help if they experience any trouble breathing or shallow breathing; a noticeable change in breathing may be associated with sleepiness.

- **CAUTIONS** Conditions that may precipitate encephalopathy · elderly · history of substance abuse · respiratory depression · seizures (may be exacerbated) · severe congestive heart failure

CAUTIONS, FURTHER INFORMATION
▸ Respiratory depression [EvGr] Patients with compromised respiratory function, respiratory or neurological disease, renal impairment, concomitant use of central nervous system (CNS) depressants, and the elderly might be at higher risk of experiencing severe respiratory depression and dose adjustments may be necessary in these patients. ⟨M⟩

▸ Seizure exacerbation [EvGr] Pregabalin may exacerbate seizures in patients with absence or myoclonic seizures (including juvenile myoclonic epilepsy), tonic or atonic seizures, Dravet syndrome, Lennox-Gastaut syndrome, and myoclonic-atonic seizures. ⟨A⟩

- **INTERACTIONS** → Appendix 1: antiepileptics

- **SIDE-EFFECTS**
▸ **Common or very common** Abdominal distension · appetite abnormal · asthenia · cervical spasm · concentration impaired · confusion · constipation · diarrhoea · dizziness · drowsiness · dry mouth · feeling abnormal · gait abnormal · gastrointestinal disorders · headache · increased risk of infection · joint disorders · memory loss · mood altered · movement disorders · muscle complaints · nausea · oedema · pain · sensation abnormal · sexual dysfunction · sleep disorders · speech impairment · vertigo · vision disorders · vomiting · weight changes
▸ **Uncommon** Aggression · anxiety · arrhythmias · atrioventricular block · breast abnormalities · chest tightness · chills · consciousness impaired · cough · depression · dry eye · dyspnoea · epistaxis · eye discomfort ·

eye disorders · eye inflammation · fever · hallucination · hyperacusia · hypertension · hypoglycaemia · hypotension · malaise · menstrual cycle irregularities · nasal complaints · neutropenia · oral disorders · peripheral coldness · psychiatric disorders · reflexes decreased · skin reactions · snoring · sweat changes · syncope · taste loss · thirst · urinary disorders · vasodilation
▸ **Rare or very rare** Altered smell sensation · ascites · dysgraphia · dysphagia · gynaecomastia · hepatic disorders · pancreatitis · pulmonary oedema · QT interval prolongation · renal impairment · rhabdomyolysis · Stevens-Johnson syndrome · suicidal behaviours · throat tightness
▸ **Frequency not known** Drug use disorders · encephalopathy · respiratory depression · withdrawal syndrome

- **PREGNANCY** [EvGr] Avoid unless benefit clearly outweighs potential risk—use in the first trimester of pregnancy is associated with a slightly increased risk of major birth defects in the unborn child. ⟨M⟩ See also *Pregnancy* in Epilepsy p. 349 and *Important safety information*.

- **BREAST FEEDING** See *Breast-feeding* in Epilepsy p. 349.

- **RENAL IMPAIRMENT**
Dose adjustments [EvGr] Initially 75 mg daily and maximum 300 mg daily in 2–3 divided doses if creatinine clearance 30–60 mL/minute.
Initially 25–50 mg daily and maximum 150 mg daily in 1–2 divided doses if creatinine clearance 15–30 mL/minute.
Initially 25 mg once daily and maximum 75 mg once daily if creatinine clearance less than 15 mL/minute. ⟨M⟩ See p. 21.

- **MONITORING REQUIREMENTS** Monitor for signs of pregabalin abuse.

- **TREATMENT CESSATION** Avoid abrupt withdrawal (taper over at least 1 week).

- **PRESCRIBING AND DISPENSING INFORMATION** Flavours of oral liquid formulations may include strawberry.

- **PATIENT AND CARER ADVICE**
Patient leaflet NHS England has produced a patient leaflet with information on the reclassification of pregabalin.
The MHRA has produced a patient leaflet regarding risks in pregnancy: www.gov.uk/government/publications/pregabalin-and-risks-in-pregnancy.
Driving and skilled tasks Patients and carers should be counselled on the effects on driving and performance of skilled tasks—increased risk of dizziness or vision disorders.

- **NATIONAL FUNDING/ACCESS DECISIONS**
For full details see funding body website
Scottish Medicines Consortium (SMC) decisions
▸ **Pregabalin (*Lyrica*®) for central neuropathic pain in adults (August 2007)** SMC No. 389/07 Not recommended
▸ **Pregabalin oral solution (*Lyrica*®) for the treatment of peripheral and central neuropathic pain in adults, and as adjunctive therapy in adults with partial seizures with or without secondary generalization (June 2012)** SMC No. 765/12 Recommended with restrictions

- **MEDICINAL FORMS** There can be variation in the licensing of different medicines containing the same drug. Forms available from special-order manufacturers include: oral suspension, oral solution
Oral tablet
CAUTIONARY AND ADVISORY LABELS 3, 8
▸ Pregabalin (Non-proprietary)
Pregabalin 25 mg Pregabalin 25mg tablets | 56 tablet [PoM] £7.61 DT = £7.61 [CD3]
Pregabalin 50 mg Pregabalin 50mg tablets | 84 tablet [PoM] £7.83 DT = £7.83 [CD3]
Pregabalin 75 mg Pregabalin 75mg tablets | 56 tablet [PoM] £7.99 DT = £7.99 [CD3]

Pregabalin 100 mg Pregabalin 100mg tablets | 84 tablet [PoM]
£10.80 DT = £10.80 [CD3]

Pregabalin 150 mg Pregabalin 150mg tablets | 56 tablet [PoM]
£10.56 DT = £10.56 [CD3]

Pregabalin 200 mg Pregabalin 200mg tablets | 84 tablet [PoM]
£13.25 DT = £13.25 [CD3]

Pregabalin 225 mg Pregabalin 225mg tablets | 56 tablet [PoM]
£6.39 DT = £6.39 [CD3]

Pregabalin 300 mg Pregabalin 300mg tablets | 56 tablet [PoM]
£13.28 DT = £13.28 [CD3]

Oral capsule

CAUTIONARY AND ADVISORY LABELS 3, 8

▶ **Pregabalin (Non-proprietary)**
Pregabalin 25 mg Pregabalin 25mg capsules | 56 capsule [PoM]
£64.40 DT = £1.30 [CD3] | 84 capsule [PoM] £1.95–£86.94 [CD3]
Pregabalin 50 mg Pregabalin 50mg capsules | 56 capsule [PoM]
£54.74–£64.40 [CD3] | 84 capsule [PoM] £96.60 DT = £4.75 [CD3]
Pregabalin 75 mg Pregabalin 75mg capsules | 56 capsule [PoM]
£64.40 DT = £1.30 [CD3]
Pregabalin 100 mg Pregabalin 100mg capsules | 84 capsule [PoM]
£96.60 DT = £2.14 [CD3]
Pregabalin 150 mg Pregabalin 150mg capsules | 56 capsule [PoM]
£64.40 DT = £2.11 [CD3]
Pregabalin 200 mg Pregabalin 200mg capsules | 84 capsule [PoM]
£96.60 DT = £3.40 [CD3]
Pregabalin 225 mg Pregabalin 225mg capsules | 56 capsule [PoM]
£64.40 DT = £2.26 [CD3]
Pregabalin 300 mg Pregabalin 300mg capsules | 56 capsule [PoM]
£64.40 DT = £2.41 [CD3]

▶ **Alzain** (Dr Reddy's Laboratories (UK) Ltd)
Pregabalin 25 mg Alzain 25mg capsules | 56 capsule [PoM] £4.99 DT
= £1.30 [CD3]
Pregabalin 50 mg Alzain 50mg capsules | 56 capsule [PoM]
£5.99 [CD3] | 84 capsule [PoM] £6.99 DT = £4.75 [CD3]
Pregabalin 75 mg Alzain 75mg capsules | 56 capsule [PoM] £5.99 DT
= £1.30 [CD3]
Pregabalin 100 mg Alzain 100mg capsules | 84 capsule [PoM] £6.99
DT = £2.14 [CD3]
Pregabalin 150 mg Alzain 150mg capsules | 56 capsule [PoM] £6.99
DT = £2.11 [CD3]
Pregabalin 200 mg Alzain 200mg capsules | 84 capsule [PoM] £8.99
DT = £3.40 [CD3]
Pregabalin 225 mg Alzain 225mg capsules | 56 capsule [PoM] £7.99
DT = £2.26 [CD3]
Pregabalin 300 mg Alzain 300mg capsules | 56 capsule [PoM] £8.99
DT = £2.41 [CD3]

▶ **Axalid** (Kent Pharma (UK) Ltd)
Pregabalin 25 mg Axalid 25mg capsules | 56 capsule [PoM] £19.95
DT = £1.30 [CD3]
Pregabalin 50 mg Axalid 50mg capsules | 56 capsule [PoM]
£19.95 [CD3]
Pregabalin 75 mg Axalid 75mg capsules | 56 capsule [PoM] £19.95
DT = £1.30 [CD3]
Pregabalin 100 mg Axalid 100mg capsules | 56 capsule [PoM]
£19.95 [CD3]
Pregabalin 150 mg Axalid 150mg capsules | 56 capsule [PoM]
£19.95 DT = £2.11 [CD3]
Pregabalin 200 mg Axalid 200mg capsules | 56 capsule [PoM]
£19.95 [CD3]
Pregabalin 225 mg Axalid 225mg capsules | 56 capsule [PoM]
£19.95 DT = £2.26 [CD3]
Pregabalin 300 mg Axalid 300mg capsules | 56 capsule [PoM]
£19.95 DT = £2.41 [CD3]

▶ **Lyrica** (Viatris UK Healthcare Ltd)
Pregabalin 25 mg Lyrica 25mg capsules | 56 capsule [PoM] £64.40
DT = £1.30 [CD3] | 84 capsule [PoM] £96.60 [CD3]
Pregabalin 50 mg Lyrica 50mg capsules | 84 capsule [PoM] £96.60
DT = £4.75 [CD3]
Pregabalin 75 mg Lyrica 75mg capsules | 56 capsule [PoM] £64.40
DT = £1.30 [CD3]
Pregabalin 100 mg Lyrica 100mg capsules | 84 capsule [PoM]
£96.60 DT = £2.14 [CD3]
Pregabalin 150 mg Lyrica 150mg capsules | 56 capsule [PoM]
£64.40 DT = £2.11 [CD3]
Pregabalin 200 mg Lyrica 200mg capsules | 84 capsule [PoM]
£96.60 DT = £3.40 [CD3]
Pregabalin 225 mg Lyrica 225mg capsules | 56 capsule [PoM]
£64.40 DT = £2.26 [CD3]
Pregabalin 300 mg Lyrica 300mg capsules | 56 capsule [PoM]
£64.40 DT = £2.41 [CD3]

Oral solution

CAUTIONARY AND ADVISORY LABELS 3, 8

▶ **Pregabalin (Non-proprietary)**
Pregabalin 20 mg per 1 ml Pregabalin 20mg/ml oral solution sugar
free | 473 ml [PoM] £99.48 DT = £32.67 Schedule 3 (CD No Register
Exempt Safe Custody) [SF] | 500 ml [PoM] £54.29–£105.16 Schedule
3 (CD No Register Exempt Safe Custody) [SF]

▶ **Lyrica** (Viatris UK Healthcare Ltd)
Pregabalin 20 mg per 1 ml Lyrica 20mg/ml oral solution |
473 ml [PoM] £99.48 DT = £32.67 Schedule 3 (CD No Register Exempt
Safe Custody) [SF]

Rufinamide

11-Nov-2021

● INDICATIONS AND DOSE

**Adjunctive treatment of seizures in Lennox-Gastaut
syndrome without valproate (initiated by a specialist)**

▶ BY MOUTH

▶ Child 1–3 years: Initially 5 mg/kg twice daily, then
increased in steps of up to 5 mg/kg twice daily (max.
per dose 22.5 mg/kg twice daily), adjusted according to
response, dose to be increased at intervals of not less
than 3 days to the target dose (maximum dose), each
dose should be given to the nearest 0.5 mL

▶ Child 4–17 years (body-weight up to 30 kg): Initially
100 mg twice daily, then increased in steps of 100 mg
twice daily (max. per dose 500 mg twice daily), adjusted
according to response, dose to be increased at intervals
of not less than 3 days

▶ Child 4–17 years (body-weight 30–50 kg): Initially 200 mg
twice daily, then increased in steps of 200 mg twice
daily (max. per dose 900 mg twice daily), adjusted
according to response, dose to be increased at intervals
of not less than 2 days

▶ Child 4–17 years (body-weight 50.1–70 kg): Initially 200 mg
twice daily, then increased in steps of 200 mg twice
daily (max. per dose 1.2 g twice daily), adjusted
according to response, dose to be increased at intervals
of not less than 2 days

▶ Child 4–17 years (body-weight 70.1 kg and above): Initially
200 mg twice daily, then increased in steps of 200 mg
twice daily (max. per dose 1.6 g twice daily), adjusted
according to response, dose to be increased at intervals
of not less than 2 days

▶ Adult (body-weight 30–50 kg): Initially 200 mg twice
daily, then increased in steps of 200 mg twice daily
(max. per dose 900 mg twice daily), adjusted according
to response, dose to be increased at intervals of not less
than 2 days

▶ Adult (body-weight 50.1–70 kg): Initially 200 mg twice
daily, then increased in steps of 200 mg twice daily
(max. per dose 1.2 g twice daily), adjusted according to
response, dose to be increased at intervals of not less
than 2 days

▶ Adult (body-weight 70.1 kg and above): Initially 200 mg
twice daily, then increased in steps of 200 mg
twice daily (max. per dose 1.6 g twice daily), adjusted
according to response, dose to be increased at intervals
of not less than 2 days

**Adjunctive treatment of seizures in Lennox-Gastaut
syndrome with valproate (initiated by a specialist)**

▶ BY MOUTH

▶ Child 1–3 years: Initially 5 mg/kg twice daily, then
increased in steps of up to 5 mg/kg twice daily (max.
per dose 15 mg/kg twice daily), adjusted according to
response, dose to be increased at intervals of not less
than 3 days to the target dose (maximum dose), each
dose should be given to the nearest 0.5 mL

▶ Child 4–17 years (body-weight up to 30 kg): Initially
100 mg twice daily, then increased in steps of 100 mg
twice daily (max. per dose 300 mg twice daily), adjusted

according to response, dose to be increased at intervals of not less than 2 days
- Child 4-17 years (body-weight 30-50 kg): Initially 200 mg twice daily, then increased in steps of 200 mg twice daily (max. per dose 600 mg twice daily), adjusted according to response, dose to be increased at intervals of not less than 2 days
- Child 4-17 years (body-weight 50.1-70 kg): Initially 200 mg twice daily, then increased in steps of 200 mg twice daily (max. per dose 800 mg twice daily), adjusted according to response, dose to be increased at intervals of not less than 2 days
- Child 4-17 years (body-weight 70.1 kg and above): Initially 200 mg twice daily, then increased in steps of 200 mg twice daily (max. per dose 1.1 g twice daily), adjusted according to response, dose to be increased at intervals of not less than 2 days
- Adult (body-weight 30-50 kg): Initially 200 mg twice daily, then increased in steps of 200 mg twice daily (max. per dose 600 mg twice daily), adjusted according to response, dose to be increased at intervals of not less than 2 days
- Adult (body-weight 50.1-70 kg): Initially 200 mg twice daily, then increased in steps of 200 mg twice daily (max. per dose 800 mg twice daily), adjusted according to response, dose to be increased at intervals of not less than 2 days
- Adult (body-weight 70.1 kg and above): Initially 200 mg twice daily, then increased in steps of 200 mg twice daily (max. per dose 1.1 g twice daily), adjusted according to response, dose to be increased at intervals of not less than 2 days

---

IMPORTANT SAFETY INFORMATION

MHRA/CHM ADVICE: ANTIEPILEPTICS: RISK OF SUICIDAL THOUGHTS AND BEHAVIOUR (AUGUST 2008)
See Epilepsy p. 349.

MHRA/CHM ADVICE: ANTIEPILEPTIC DRUGS: UPDATED ADVICE ON SWITCHING BETWEEN DIFFERENT MANUFACTURERS' PRODUCTS (NOVEMBER 2017)
See Epilepsy p. 349 and see also *Prescribing and dispensing information*.

MHRA/CHM ADVICE: ANTIEPILEPTIC DRUGS IN PREGNANCY: UPDATED ADVICE FOLLOWING COMPREHENSIVE SAFETY REVIEW (JANUARY 2021)
See Epilepsy p. 349.

- **CAUTIONS** Patients at risk of further shortening of QTc interval
- **INTERACTIONS** → Appendix 1: antiepileptics
- **SIDE-EFFECTS**
- **Common or very common** Anxiety · appetite decreased · back pain · constipation · diarrhoea · dizziness · drowsiness · eating disorder · epistaxis · fatigue · gait abnormal · gastrointestinal discomfort · headache · increased risk of infection · insomnia · movement disorders · nausea · nystagmus · oligomenorrhoea · seizures · skin reactions · tremor · vertigo · vision disorders · vomiting · weight decreased
- **Uncommon** Hypersensitivity
- **Frequency not known** Suicidal behaviours
- **ALLERGY AND CROSS-SENSITIVITY** Antiepileptic hypersensitivity syndrome associated with rufinamide. See under Epilepsy p. 349 for more information.
- **PREGNANCY** Manufacturer advises avoid unless essential—toxicity in *animal* studies. See also *Pregnancy* in Epilepsy p. 349.
- **BREAST FEEDING** Manufacturer advises avoid—no information available.

- **HEPATIC IMPAIRMENT** Manufacturer advises caution in mild to moderate impairment; avoid in severe impairment (no information available).
Dose adjustments Manufacturer advises cautious dose titration in mild to moderate impairment.
- **DIRECTIONS FOR ADMINISTRATION** Manufacturer advises tablets may be crushed and given in half a glass of water.
- **PRESCRIBING AND DISPENSING INFORMATION**
Switching between formulations Care should be taken when switching between oral formulations. The need for continued supply of a particular manufacturer's product should be based on clinical judgement and consultation with the patient or their carer, taking into account factors such as seizure frequency and treatment history.
　Patients may need to be maintained on a specific manufacturer's branded or generic rufinamide product.
- **PATIENT AND CARER ADVICE** Counselling on antiepileptic hypersensitivity syndrome is advised.
Medicines for Children leaflet: Rufinamide for preventing seizures www.medicinesforchildren.org.uk/medicines/rufinamide-for-preventing-seizures/
Driving and skilled tasks Manufacturer advises patients and carers should be cautioned on the effects on driving and performance of skilled tasks—increased risk of dizziness, somnolence and blurred vision.
- **NATIONAL FUNDING/ACCESS DECISIONS**
For full details see funding body website
Scottish Medicines Consortium (SMC) decisions
- **Rufinamide (*Inovelon*®) as adjunctive therapy in the treatment of seizures associated with Lennox-Gastaut syndrome in patients four years and older (November 2008)** SMC No. 416/07 Recommended with restrictions
- **Rufinamide 40 mg/mL oral suspension (*Inovelon*®) as adjunctive therapy in the treatment of seizures associated with Lennox-Gastaut syndrome (LGS) in patients 4 years of age or older (July 2012)** SMC No. 795/12 Recommended with restrictions
- **Rufinamide (*Inovelon*®) as adjunctive therapy in the treatment of seizures associated with Lennox-Gastaut syndrome in patients aged 1 year up to 4 years (April 2019)** SMC No. SMC2146 Recommended with restrictions
All Wales Medicines Strategy Group (AWMSG) decisions
- **Rufinamide 40 mg/mL oral suspension (*Inovelon*®) as adjunctive therapy in the treatment of seizures associated with Lennox-Gastaut syndrome in patients 1 year of age and older (June 2019)** AWMSG No. 991 Recommended with restrictions

---

- **MEDICINAL FORMS** There can be variation in the licensing of different medicines containing the same drug.
Oral tablet
CAUTIONARY AND ADVISORY LABELS 8, 21
- Inovelon (Eisai Ltd)
　Rufinamide 100 mg Inovelon 100mg tablets | 10 tablet [PoM] £5.15 DT = £5.15
　Rufinamide 200 mg Inovelon 200mg tablets | 60 tablet [PoM] £61.77 DT = £61.77
　Rufinamide 400 mg Inovelon 400mg tablets | 60 tablet [PoM] £102.96 DT = £102.96
Oral suspension
CAUTIONARY AND ADVISORY LABELS 8, 21
EXCIPIENTS: May contain Propylene glycol
- Inovelon (Eisai Ltd)
　Rufinamide 40 mg per 1 ml Inovelon 40mg/ml oral suspension | 460 ml [PoM] £94.71 DT = £94.71 [SF]

Sodium valproate

(Valproate sodium)

25-Feb-2025

- **INDICATIONS AND DOSE**

All forms of epilepsy

▶ BY MOUTH USING IMMEDIATE-RELEASE MEDICINES

▸ Child 1 month–11 years: Initially 10–15 mg/kg daily in 1–2 divided doses (max. per dose 600 mg); maintenance 25–30 mg/kg daily in 2 divided doses, doses up to 60 mg/kg daily in 2 divided doses may be used in infantile spasms; monitor clinical chemistry and haematological parameters if dose exceeds 40 mg/kg daily

▸ Child 12-17 years: Initially 600 mg daily in 1–2 divided doses, increased in steps of 150–300 mg every 3 days; maintenance 1–2 g daily in 2 divided doses; maximum 2.5 g per day

▸ Adult: Initially 600 mg daily in 1–2 divided doses, then increased in steps of 150–300 mg every 3 days; maintenance 1–2 g daily, alternatively maintenance 20–30 mg/kg daily; maximum 2.5 g per day

Initiation of valproate treatment

▶ INITIALLY BY INTRAVENOUS INJECTION

▸ Adult: Initially 10 mg/kg, (usually 400–800 mg), followed by (by intravenous infusion or by intravenous injection) up to 2.5 g daily in 2–4 divided doses, alternatively (by continuous intravenous infusion) up to 2.5 g daily; (by intravenous injection or by intravenous infusion or by continuous intravenous infusion) usual dose 1–2 g daily, alternatively (by intravenous injection or by intravenous infusion or by continuous intravenous infusion) usual dose 20–30 mg/kg daily, intravenous injection to be administered over 3–5 minutes

Continuation of valproate treatment

▶ BY INTRAVENOUS INJECTION, OR BY INTRAVENOUS INFUSION, OR BY CONTINUOUS INTRAVENOUS INFUSION

▸ Adult: If switching from oral therapy to intravenous therapy give the same dose as current oral daily dose, give over 3–5 minutes by intravenous injection or in 2–4 divided doses by intravenous infusion

Migraine prophylaxis

▶ BY MOUTH USING IMMEDIATE-RELEASE MEDICINES

▸ Adult: Initially 200 mg twice daily, then increased if necessary to 1.2–1.5 g daily in divided doses

EPILIM CHRONOSPHERE ®

All forms of epilepsy

▶ BY MOUTH

▸ Adult: Total daily dose to be given in 1–2 divided doses (consult product literature)

EPILIM CHRONO ®

All forms of epilepsy

▶ BY MOUTH

▸ Adult: Total daily dose to be given in 1–2 divided doses (consult product literature)

EPISENTA ® CAPSULES

All forms of epilepsy

▶ BY MOUTH

▸ Adult: Total daily dose to be given in 1–2 divided doses (consult product literature)

Mania

▶ BY MOUTH

▸ Adult: Initially 750 mg daily in 1–2 divided doses, adjusted according to response, usual dose 1–2 g daily in 1–2 divided doses, doses greater than 45 mg/kg daily require careful monitoring

EPISENTA ® GRANULES

All forms of epilepsy

▶ BY MOUTH

▸ Adult: Total daily dose to be given in 1–2 divided doses (consult product literature)

Mania

▶ BY MOUTH

▸ Adult: Initially 750 mg daily in 1–2 divided doses, adjusted according to response, usual dose 1–2 g daily in 1–2 divided doses, doses greater than 45 mg/kg daily require careful monitoring

EPIVAL ®

All forms of epilepsy

▶ BY MOUTH

▸ Adult: Total daily dose to be given in 1–2 divided doses (consult product literature)

- **UNLICENSED USE** Not licensed for migraine prophylaxis.

IMPORTANT SAFETY INFORMATION

MHRA/CHM ADVICE: ANTIEPILEPTICS: RISK OF SUICIDAL THOUGHTS AND BEHAVIOUR (AUGUST 2008)

See Epilepsy p. 349.

MHRA/CHM ADVICE: ANTIEPILEPTIC DRUGS: UPDATED ADVICE ON SWITCHING BETWEEN DIFFERENT MANUFACTURERS' PRODUCTS (NOVEMBER 2017)

See Epilepsy p. 349 and see also *Prescribing and dispensing information*.

MHRA/CHM ADVICE: VALPROATE MEDICINES: CONTRA-INDICATED IN WOMEN AND GIRLS OF CHILDBEARING POTENTIAL UNLESS CONDITIONS OF PREGNANCY PREVENTION PROGRAMME ARE MET (APRIL 2018)

Valproate is highly teratogenic and evidence supports that use in pregnancy leads to neurodevelopmental disorders (approx. 30–40% risk) and congenital malformations (approx. 10% risk).

Valproate must not be used in women and girls of childbearing potential unless the conditions of the Pregnancy Prevention Programme are met (see *Conception and contraception*) and only if other treatments are ineffective or not tolerated, as judged by an experienced specialist.

Use of valproate in pregnancy is contra-indicated for migraine prophylaxis [unlicensed] and bipolar disorder; it must only be considered for epilepsy if there is no suitable alternative treatment (see *Pregnancy*).

Women and girls (and their carers) must be fully informed of the risks and the need to avoid exposure to valproate medicines in pregnancy; supporting materials have been provided to use in the implementation of the Pregnancy Prevention Programme (see *Prescribing and dispensing Information*). The MHRA advises that:

- GPs must recall all women and girls who may be of childbearing potential, provide the Patient Guide, check they have been reviewed by a specialist in the last year and are on highly effective contraception;
- Specialists must book in review appointments at least annually with women and girls under the Pregnancy Prevention Programme, re-evaluate treatment as necessary, explain clearly the conditions as outlined in the supporting materials and complete and sign the Risk Acknowledgement Form—copies of the form must be given to the patient or carer and sent to their GP;
- Pharmacists must ensure valproate medicines are dispensed in whole packs whenever possible—all packs dispensed to women and girls of childbearing potential should have a warning label either on the carton or via a sticker. They must also discuss risks in pregnancy with female patients each time valproate medicines are dispensed, ensure they have the Patient Guide and have seen their GP or specialist to discuss their treatment and the need for contraception.

MHRA/CHM ADVICE: VALPROATE MEDICINES: ARE YOU ACTING IN COMPLIANCE WITH THE PREGNANCY PREVENTION MEASURES? (DECEMBER 2018)

The MHRA advises that all healthcare professionals must continue to identify and review all female patients on valproate, including when used outside licensed indications (off-label use) and provide them with the patient information materials every time they attend appointments or receive their medicines.

Guidance for psychiatrists on the withdrawal of, and alternatives to, valproate in women of childbearing potential who have a psychiatric illness is available from the Royal College of Psychiatrists.

MHRA/CHM ADVICE: VALPROATE MEDICINES AND SERIOUS HARMS IN PREGNANCY: NEW ANNUAL RISK ACKNOWLEDGEMENT FORM AND CLINICAL GUIDANCE FROM PROFESSIONAL BODIES TO SUPPORT COMPLIANCE WITH THE PREGNANCY PREVENTION PROGRAMME (APRIL 2019)

The Annual Risk Acknowledgement Form has been updated and should be used for all future reviews of female patients on valproate. Specialists should comply with guidance given on the form if they consider the patient is not at risk of pregnancy, including the need for review in case her risk status changes.

Guidance has been published to support healthcare professionals with the use of valproate. These include a summary by NICE of their guidance and safety advice, pan-college guidance by national healthcare bodies, and paediatric guidance by the British Paediatric Neurology Association and the Royal College of Paediatrics and Child Health.

MHRA/CHM ADVICE (UPDATED JANUARY 2020): VALPROATE PREGNANCY PREVENTION PROGRAMME

The Guide for Healthcare Professionals has been updated and should be used for all future reviews of female patients on valproate medicines, in conjunction with other supporting materials (see *Prescribing and dispensing Information*).

MHRA/CHM ADVICE (UPDATED MAY 2020): VALPROATE PREGNANCY PREVENTION PROGRAMME: TEMPORARY ADVICE FOR MANAGEMENT DURING CORONAVIRUS (COVID-19)

The MHRA has issued temporary guidance for female patients on valproate during the coronavirus (COVID-19) pandemic to support adherence to the Pregnancy Prevention Programme, particularly for those who are shielding due to other health conditions, and should be followed until further notice.

MHRA/CHM ADVICE: ANTIEPILEPTIC DRUGS IN PREGNANCY: UPDATED ADVICE FOLLOWING COMPREHENSIVE SAFETY REVIEW (JANUARY 2021)

See Epilepsy p. 349.

MHRA/CHM ADVICE: VALPROATE: REMINDER OF CURRENT PREGNANCY PREVENTION PROGRAMME REQUIREMENTS; INFORMATION ON NEW SAFETY MEASURES TO BE INTRODUCED IN THE COMING MONTHS (DECEMBER 2022)

In light of data showing ongoing exposure to valproate in pregnancy and evolving information about the potential risks of valproate in other patients, healthcare professionals are reminded of the risks in pregnancy and requirements of the existing Pregnancy Prevention Programme, and are also advised of the potential risk of infertility in male patients. The CHM has recommended regulatory actions to strengthen safety measures for valproate which will be introduced over the coming months. In the meantime, healthcare professionals are advised that patients currently taking valproate should continue to do so unless recommended to stop by a specialist. All other suitable treatment options should be considered and findings from the safety review of antiepileptic drugs in pregnancy consulted before initiating valproate treatment in female patients aged under 55 years (see Epilepsy p. 349). Two specialists are required to independently consider and document that there is no other effective or tolerated treatment before prescribing valproate for male or female patients aged under 55 years.

MHRA/CHM ADVICE: VALPROATE: RE-ANALYSIS OF STUDY ON RISKS IN CHILDREN OF MEN TAKING VALPROATE (AUGUST 2023)

The MHRA continues to review all emerging data on valproate medicines, including findings from a retrospective observational study which suggested an increased risk of neurodevelopmental disorders in children of men who took valproate, when compared with those of men who took lamotrigine or levetiracetam, in the 3 months before conception. However, errors have been identified in the study and the MHRA has determined that a full re-analysis is required before conclusions can be made. In the meantime, healthcare professionals are reminded that the use of valproate in females of childbearing potential should be in accordance with the Pregnancy Prevention Programme, and that all patients currently taking valproate should continue to do so unless advised to stop by a specialist. Patients should continue to be informed of the risks of valproate in pregnancy.

MHRA/CHM ADVICE: FULL PACK DISPENSING OF VALPROATE-CONTAINING MEDICINES (OCTOBER 2023)

Valproate medicines have been dispensed to patients in alternative packaging because the prescribed amount was different to that of the manufacturer's original full pack. This resulted in patients not always receiving all the risk materials about the use of these medicines in pregnancy. Pharmacists are advised that all patients (male and female) must receive their valproate medicines in the manufacturer's original full pack (i.e. original pack dispensing) and the amount dispensed must be as close as possible to the amount stated on the prescription (NHS or private). Rarely, exceptions to this requirement can be made on an individual patient basis, provided a risk assessment is carried out on the need to dispense repackaged valproate medicines (e.g. in a monitored dosage system), whereby a patient information leaflet must be supplied.

NATIONAL PATIENT SAFETY ALERT: VALPROATE: ORGANISATIONS TO PREPARE FOR NEW REGULATORY MEASURES FOR OVERSIGHT OF PRESCRIBING TO NEW PATIENTS AND EXISTING FEMALE PATIENTS (NOVEMBER 2023)

Following a comprehensive review of safety data, and advice from the CHM and an expert group, the MHRA requests that organisations put a plan in place to implement the following new regulatory measures for valproate medicines:

- valproate must not be started in new patients (male or female) aged under 55 years, unless two specialists independently consider and document that there is no other effective or tolerated treatment, or there are compelling reasons why the reproductive risks do not apply;
- at the next annual specialist review, females of childbearing potential should be reviewed using a revised valproate Risk Acknowledgement Form, which will include the need for a second specialist signature if the patient is to continue with valproate; subsequent annual reviews with one specialist should be carried out unless the patient's situation changes.

These measures are in response to data showing ongoing exposure to valproate in pregnancy and evolving information about the potential risk of impaired fertility in male patients on valproate.

Current safety measures continue to apply, including the Pregnancy Prevention Programme for females of childbearing potential on valproate. All patients currently taking valproate should continue to do so unless advised to stop by a specialist. General practice and pharmacy teams should discuss the current warnings, upcoming measures, and new educational materials with patients.

MHRA/CHM ADVICE: VALPROATE (*DYZANTIL*®, *EPILIM*®, *EPILIM CHRONO*® OR *CHRONOSPHERE*®, *EPISENTA*®, AND *EPIVAL*®): NEW SAFETY AND EDUCATIONAL MATERIALS TO SUPPORT REGULATORY MEASURES IN MEN AND WOMEN UNDER 55 YEARS OF AGE (JANUARY 2024)

Healthcare professionals are advised to review, and integrate into their clinical practice, the updated safety and educational materials that support the new regulatory measures as outlined in the National Patient Safety Alert, above (see also *Prescribing and dispensing information*). General practice and pharmacy teams should continue to prescribe and dispense valproate according to current safety measures. If required, patients should be referred to a specialist to discuss treatment options. Patients on valproate medicines should be fully informed of the potential risks and counselled on treatment options at initial prescribing and at all subsequent reviews.

Healthcare professionals should advise patients to:
- not stop taking valproate medicines without advice from a specialist as their epilepsy or bipolar disorder may worsen;
- attend any offered appointments to discuss their treatment plan and to talk to a healthcare professional if they have any concerns;
- consult the new Patient Guide and Patient Information Leaflet for information on the risks of valproate.

MHRA/CHM ADVICE: VALPROATE USE IN MEN: AS A PRECAUTION, MEN AND THEIR PARTNERS SHOULD USE EFFECTIVE CONTRACEPTION (SEPTEMBER 2024)

The MHRA has reviewed findings from a retrospective observational study (see advice issued in August 2023, above) that suggest a potential increased risk of neurodevelopmental disorders in children born to men taking valproate medicines in the 3 months before conception; however, causality is unconfirmed. In addition to current safety measures, healthcare professionals should advise male patients (of any age) who may father a child:
- about this risk at treatment initiation or at the next treatment review, irrespective of indication and also after intravenous valproate;
- to use effective contraception (i.e. condoms plus contraception used by their female partner) during and for 3 months after valproate treatment;
- to refrain from donating sperm during and for 3 months after valproate treatment.

Healthcare professionals are also advised that:
- male patients who are planning a family in the next year should be referred to a specialist to discuss alternative treatment;
- female partners of male patients taking valproate medicines who are pregnant or planning a pregnancy (including those undergoing IVF) should be referred for prenatal counselling.

MHRA/CHM ADVICE: VALPROATE (*DYZANTIL*®, *EPILIM*®, *EPILIM CHRONO*® OR *CHRONOSPHERE*®, *EPISENTA*®, AND *EPIVAL*®): REVIEW BY TWO SPECIALISTS IS REQUIRED FOR INITIATING VALPROATE BUT NOT FOR MALE PATIENTS ALREADY TAKING VALPROATE (FEBRUARY 2025)

Healthcare professionals are reminded that the current safety measure advising all patients under 55 years of age to be reviewed by two specialists before initiating valproate remains in place, however, the CHM has advised that this will not be required for male patients who are already taking valproate. Healthcare professionals are also reminded that all previously issued safety measures continue to apply.

The CHM has produced infographics to clarify the situations where review by two specialists may be required.

For female patients under 55 years of age, see: assets.publishing.service.gov.uk/media/67adf28c6e6c8d18118acd69/250213_MHRA_Valproate_Infographic_Female_under_55_CC_V7.pdf.

For male patients under 55 years of age, see: assets.publishing.service.gov.uk/media/67adf2aa6e6c8d18118acd6a/250213_MHRA_Valproate_Infographic_Male_under_55_CC_V7.pdf.

For male and female patients aged 55 years or older, see: assets.publishing.service.gov.uk/media/67adf2c62c594609b38acd71/250213_MHRA_Valproate_Infographic_55_or_older_CC_V7.pdf.

For further information and resources, including a list of who may qualify as a specialist, see the MHRA Valproate Safety Measures information page, available at: www.gov.uk/government/collections/valproate-safety-measures.

● **CONTRA-INDICATIONS** Acute porphyrias p. 1202 · known or suspected mitochondrial disorders (higher rate of acute liver failure and liver-related deaths) · personal or family history of severe hepatic dysfunction · urea cycle disorders (risk of hyperammonaemia)

● **CAUTIONS** Systemic lupus erythematosus

CAUTIONS, FURTHER INFORMATION The MHRA advises consider vitamin D supplementation in patients that are immobilised for long periods or who have inadequate sun exposure or dietary intake of calcium.

▸ Liver toxicity Liver dysfunction (including fatal hepatic failure) has occurred in association with valproate (especially in children under 3 years and in those with metabolic or degenerative disorders, organic brain disease or severe seizure disorders associated with mental retardation) usually in first 6 months and usually involving multiple antiepileptic therapy. EvGr Raised liver enzymes during valproate treatment are usually transient but patients should be reassessed clinically and liver function (including prothrombin time) monitored until return to normal—discontinue if abnormally prolonged prothrombin time (particularly in association with other relevant abnormalities). Ⓜ

● **INTERACTIONS** → Appendix 1: antiepileptics

● **SIDE-EFFECTS**

GENERAL SIDE-EFFECTS

▸ **Common or very common** Abdominal pain · agitation · alopecia (regrowth may be curly) · anaemia · behaviour abnormal · concentration impaired · confusion · deafness · diarrhoea · drowsiness · haemorrhage · hallucination · headache · hepatic disorders · hypersensitivity · hyponatraemia · memory loss · menstrual cycle irregularities · movement disorders · nail disorder · nausea · nystagmus · oral disorders · seizures · stupor · thrombocytopenia · tremor · urinary disorders · vomiting · weight increased

▸ **Uncommon** Androgenetic alopecia · angioedema · bone disorders · bone fracture · bone marrow disorders · coma · encephalopathy · hair changes · hypothermia · leucopenia · pancreatitis · paraesthesia · parkinsonism · peripheral oedema · pleural effusion · renal failure · SIADH · skin reactions · vasculitis · virilism

▸ **Rare or very rare** Agranulocytosis · cerebral atrophy · cognitive disorder · dementia · diplopia · gynaecomastia · hyperammonaemia · hypothyroidism · infertility male · learning disability · myelodysplastic syndrome · nephritis tubulointerstitial · obesity · polycystic ovaries · red blood cell abnormalities · rhabdomyolysis · severe cutaneous adverse reactions (SCARs) · systemic lupus erythematosus (SLE) · urine abnormalities

▶ **Frequency not known** Alertness increased · suicidal behaviours

SPECIFIC SIDE-EFFECTS
▶ **Common or very common**
▶ With intravenous use Dizziness

SIDE-EFFECTS, FURTHER INFORMATION **Hepatic dysfunction** Withdraw treatment immediately if persistent vomiting and abdominal pain, anorexia, jaundice, oedema, malaise, drowsiness, or loss of seizure control.

Pancreatitis Discontinue treatment if symptoms of pancreatitis develop.

● CONCEPTION AND CONTRACEPTION The MHRA advises that all women and girls of childbearing potential being treated with valproate medicines must be supported on a Pregnancy Prevention Programme—pregnancy should be excluded before treatment initiation. Highly effective contraception must be used during treatment i.e. at least 1, preferably highly effective user-independent contraceptive method (such as an intra-uterine device or implant), or 2 complementary forms including a barrier method. The MHRA advises that all male patients being treated with valproate medicines and who may father children should use effective contraception (i.e. condoms plus contraception used by their female partner) during and for 3 months after treatment. The MHRA advises that male patients taking valproate medicines should be informed of the risk of infertility, and of data showing testicular toxicity in *animal* studies.

● PREGNANCY For *migraine prophylaxis* [unlicensed] and *bipolar disorder*, the MHRA advises that valproate medicines must not be used. For *epilepsy*, the MHRA advises valproate must not be used unless two specialists independently consider and document that there is no other effective or tolerated treatment (see also *Important safety information*). If valproate is to be used, the lowest effective dose should be prescribed in divided doses to be taken throughout the day; modified-release preparations may be preferable to avoid high peak plasma-valproate concentrations. There is no dose threshold considered to be without any risk, however, the risk of birth defects and neurodevelopmental disorders is greater at higher doses. EvGr Specialist prenatal monitoring should be instigated when valproate has been taken in pregnancy. Ⓜ Neonatal bleeding (related to hypofibrinaemia) reported. Neonatal hepatotoxicity also reported. See also *Pregnancy* in Epilepsy p. 349.

● BREAST FEEDING Present in milk—risk of haematological disorders in breast-fed newborns and infants.

● HEPATIC IMPAIRMENT Manufacturer advises avoid.

● RENAL IMPAIRMENT
Dose adjustments EvGr Consider dose reduction. Ⓜ

● MONITORING REQUIREMENTS
▶ Plasma-valproate concentrations are not a useful index of efficacy, therefore routine monitoring is unhelpful.
▶ Monitor liver function before therapy and during first 6 months especially in patients most at risk.
▶ Measure full blood count and ensure no undue potential for bleeding before starting and before surgery.

● EFFECT ON LABORATORY TESTS False-positive urine tests for ketones.

● TREATMENT CESSATION EvGr Avoid abrupt withdrawal; if treatment with valproate is stopped, reduce the dose gradually over at least 4 weeks. Ⓐ

● DIRECTIONS FOR ADMINISTRATION Manufacturer advises for *intravenous injection*, give over 3–5 minutes. For *intravenous infusion*, dilute with Glucose 5% *or* Sodium Chloride 0.9%. Reconstitute *Epilim* ® with solvent provided then dilute with infusion fluid if required. Displacement value may be significant, consult local guidelines.

EPILIM CHRONOSPHERE ® Manufacturer advises granules may be mixed with soft food or drink that is cold or at room temperature, and swallowed immediately without chewing.

EPILIM ® SYRUP Manufacturer advises may be diluted, preferably in Syrup BP; use within 14 days.

EPISENTA ® CAPSULES Manufacturer advises contents of capsule may be mixed with soft food or drink that is cold or at room temperature and swallowed immediately without chewing.

EPISENTA ® GRANULES Manufacturer advises granules may be mixed with soft food or drink that is cold or at room temperature and swallowed immediately without chewing.

EPIVAL ® Manufacturer advises tablets may be halved but not crushed or chewed.

● PRESCRIBING AND DISPENSING INFORMATION The Pregnancy Prevention Programme is supported by the following safety and educational materials: *Patient Guide, Guide for Healthcare Professionals, Annual Risk Acknowledgement Form for Female Patients, Risk Acknowledgement Form for Male Patients Starting Valproate, Patient Card, Pharmacy Poster,* and *Warning Stickers.*

In addition, the MHRA advises that pharmacists must dispense valproate medicines in the manufacturer's original full pack.

See the MHRA Valproate Safety Measures information page, available at: www.gov.uk/government/collections/valproate-safety-measures.

The Royal Pharmaceutical Society has also produced a safe supply algorithm, available at: www.rpharms.com/safesupplyvalproate.

Switching between formulations Care should be taken when switching between oral formulations in the treatment of *epilepsy*. The need for continued supply of a particular manufacturer's product should be based on clinical judgement and consultation with the patient or their carer, taking into account factors such as seizure frequency and treatment history.

Patients being treated for epilepsy may need to be maintained on a specific manufacturer's branded or generic oral sodium valproate product.

EPILIM CHRONOSPHERE ® Prescribe dose to the nearest whole 50-mg sachet.

● PATIENT AND CARER ADVICE The MHRA advises that patients should **not** stop taking valproate without first discussing it with a specialist. Female patients or their carers should be advised to immediately contact their GP for an urgent referral to a specialist in case of suspected pregnancy. Female partners of male patients taking valproate medicines should be referred for prenatal counselling if pregnancy is suspected.

Blood or hepatic disorders Patients or their carers should be told how to recognise signs and symptoms of blood or liver disorders and advised to seek immediate medical attention if symptoms develop.

Pancreatitis Patients or their carers should be told how to recognise signs and symptoms of pancreatitis and advised to seek immediate medical attention if symptoms such as abdominal pain, nausea, or vomiting develop.

Patient guide A patient guide must be provided.

Pregnancy Prevention Programme Pharmacists must ensure that female patients have a patient card—see also *Important safety information*.

Decision aid NHS England has produced a patient decision aid for females of childbearing potential who are considering or are taking valproate medicines for epilepsy, available at: www.england.nhs.uk/publication/decision-support-tool-is-valproate-the-right-epilepsy-treatment-for-me/.

Medicines for Children leaflet: Sodium valproate for preventing seizures www.medicinesforchildren.org.uk/medicines/sodium-valproate-for-preventing-seizures/

4

Nervous system

EPILIM CHRONOSPHERE ® Patients and carers should be counselled on the administration of granules.

EPISENTA ® **CAPSULES** Patients and carers should be counselled on the administration of capsules.

EPISENTA ® **GRANULES** Patients and carers should be counselled on the administration of granules.

● **MEDICINAL FORMS** There can be variation in the licensing of different medicines containing the same drug. Forms available from special-order manufacturers include: oral suspension, oral solution

Oral tablet

CAUTIONARY AND ADVISORY LABELS 8, 10, 21

▸ Epilim (Sanofi) ▼
Sodium valproate 100 mg Epilim 100mg crushable tablets | 30 tablet PoM £1.68 DT = £1.68

Modified-release tablet

CAUTIONARY AND ADVISORY LABELS 8, 10, 21, 25

▸ Dyzantil (Aspire Pharma Ltd)
Sodium valproate 200 mg Dyzantil 200mg modified-release tablets | 30 tablet PoM £2.45 DT = £3.50
Sodium valproate 300 mg Dyzantil 300mg modified-release tablets | 30 tablet PoM £3.67 DT = £5.24
Sodium valproate 500 mg Dyzantil 500mg modified-release tablets | 30 tablet PoM £6.11 DT = £8.73

▸ Epilim Chrono (Sanofi) ▼
Sodium valproate 200 mg Epilim Chrono 200 tablets | 30 tablet PoM £3.50 DT = £3.50
Sodium valproate 300 mg Epilim Chrono 300 tablets | 30 tablet PoM £5.24 DT = £5.24
Sodium valproate 500 mg Epilim Chrono 500 tablets | 30 tablet PoM £8.73 DT = £8.73

▸ Epival CR (G.L. Pharma UK Ltd) ▼
Sodium valproate 300 mg Epival CR 300mg tablets | 30 tablet PoM £3.40 DT = £5.24
Sodium valproate 500 mg Epival CR 500mg tablets | 30 tablet PoM £5.67 DT = £8.73

Gastro-resistant tablet

CAUTIONARY AND ADVISORY LABELS 5, 8, 10, 25

▸ Sodium valproate (non-proprietary) ▼
Sodium valproate 200 mg Sodium valproate 200mg gastro-resistant tablets | 30 tablet PoM £2.51–£3.80 DT = £2.67
Sodium valproate 500 mg Sodium valproate 500mg gastro-resistant tablets | 30 tablet PoM £5.90–£30.00 DT = £5.95

▸ Epilim (Sanofi) ▼
Sodium valproate 200 mg Epilim 200 gastro-resistant tablets | 30 tablet PoM £1.99 DT = £2.67
Sodium valproate 500 mg Epilim 500 gastro-resistant tablets | 30 tablet PoM £5.78 DT = £5.95

Powder and solvent for solution for injection

▸ Sodium valproate (non-proprietary) ▼
Sodium valproate 400 mg Sodium valproate 400mg powder and solvent for solution for injection vials | 4 vial PoM £53.28 (Hospital only)

▸ Epilim (Sanofi) ▼
Sodium valproate 400 mg Epilim Intravenous 400mg powder and solvent for solution for injection vials | 1 vial PoM £13.32 DT = £13.32

Solution for injection

▸ Sodium valproate (non-proprietary) ▼
Sodium valproate 100 mg per 1 ml Sodium valproate 400mg/4ml solution for injection ampoules | 5 ampoule PoM £57.90 DT = £57.90
Sodium valproate 400mg/4ml solution for injection vials | 5 vial PoM £60.00 (Hospital only)
Sodium valproate 300mg/3ml solution for injection vials | 5 vial PoM £60.00 (Hospital only)

▸ Episenta (Desitin Pharma Ltd) ▼
Sodium valproate 100 mg per 1 ml Episenta 300mg/3ml solution for injection ampoules | 5 ampoule PoM £35.00 DT = £35.00

Modified-release capsule

CAUTIONARY AND ADVISORY LABELS 8, 10, 21, 25

▸ Episenta (Desitin Pharma Ltd) ▼
Sodium valproate 150 mg Episenta 150mg modified-release capsules | 30 capsule PoM £2.76 DT = £2.76
Sodium valproate 300 mg Episenta 300mg modified-release capsules | 30 capsule PoM £4.56 DT = £4.56

Oral solution

CAUTIONARY AND ADVISORY LABELS 8, 10, 21

▸ Sodium valproate (non-proprietary) ▼
Sodium valproate 40 mg per 1 ml Sodium valproate 200mg/5ml oral solution sugar free | 300 ml PoM £7.29–£15.00 DT = £14.40 SF
Sodium valproate 200 mg per 1 ml Depakin 200mg/ml oral solution | 40 ml PoM Ⓧ

▸ Epilim (Sanofi) ▼
Sodium valproate 40 mg per 1 ml Epilim 200mg/5ml liquid | 300 ml PoM £7.78 DT = £14.40 SF
Epilim 200mg/5ml syrup | 300 ml PoM £9.33 DT = £9.33

Modified-release granules

CAUTIONARY AND ADVISORY LABELS 8, 10, 21, 25

▸ Epilim Chronosphere MR (Sanofi) ▼
Sodium valproate 50 mg Epilim Chronosphere MR 50mg granules sachets | 30 sachet PoM £30.00 DT = £30.00 SF
Sodium valproate 100 mg Epilim Chronosphere MR 100mg granules sachets | 30 sachet PoM £30.00 DT = £30.00 SF
Sodium valproate 250 mg Epilim Chronosphere MR 250mg granules sachets | 30 sachet PoM £30.00 DT = £30.00 SF
Sodium valproate 500 mg Epilim Chronosphere MR 500mg granules sachets | 30 sachet PoM £30.00 DT = £30.00 SF
Sodium valproate 750 mg Epilim Chronosphere MR 750mg granules sachets | 30 sachet PoM £30.00 DT = £30.00 SF
Sodium valproate 1 gram Epilim Chronosphere MR 1000mg granules sachets | 30 sachet PoM £30.00 DT = £30.00 SF

▸ Episenta (Desitin Pharma Ltd) ▼
Sodium valproate 500 mg Episenta 500mg modified-release granules sachets | 30 sachet PoM £6.30 DT = £30.00 SF
Sodium valproate 1 gram Episenta 1000mg modified-release granules sachets | 30 sachet PoM £12.30 DT = £30.00 SF

Stiripentol

16-Aug-2023

● **INDICATIONS AND DOSE**

Adjunctive therapy of refractory generalised tonic-clonic seizures in patients with severe myoclonic epilepsy in infancy (Dravet syndrome) in combination with clobazam and valproate (under expert supervision)

▸ BY MOUTH

▸ Adult: Doses of up to 50 mg/kg daily in 2–3 divided doses should be continued for as long as efficacy is observed

DOSE EQUIVALENCE AND CONVERSION

▸ Stiripentol capsules and oral powder sachets are **not** bioequivalent. If a switch of formulation is required, manufacturer advises this is done under clinical supervision in case of intolerance.

IMPORTANT SAFETY INFORMATION

MHRA/CHM ADVICE: ANTIEPILEPTICS: RISK OF SUICIDAL THOUGHTS AND BEHAVIOUR (AUGUST 2008)
See Epilepsy p. 349.

MHRA/CHM ADVICE: ANTIEPILEPTIC DRUGS: UPDATED ADVICE ON SWITCHING BETWEEN DIFFERENT MANUFACTURERS' PRODUCTS (NOVEMBER 2017)
See Epilepsy p. 349.

MHRA/CHM ADVICE: ANTIEPILEPTIC DRUGS IN PREGNANCY: UPDATED ADVICE FOLLOWING COMPREHENSIVE SAFETY REVIEW (JANUARY 2021)
See Epilepsy p. 349.

● **CONTRA-INDICATIONS** History of psychosis in the form of episodes of delirium

● **INTERACTIONS** → Appendix 1: antiepileptics

● **SIDE-EFFECTS**

▸ **Common or very common** Agitation · appetite decreased · behaviour abnormal · drowsiness · irritability · movement disorders · muscle tone decreased · nausea · neutropenia · sleep disorders · vomiting · weight decreased

▸ **Uncommon** Diplopia · fatigue · photosensitivity reaction · skin reactions

▸ **Rare or very rare** Thrombocytopenia

- ▸ **Frequency not known** Suicidal behaviours
- ● **ALLERGY AND CROSS-SENSITIVITY** Antiepileptic hypersensitivity syndrome theoretically associated with stiripentol. See under Epilepsy p. 349 for more information.
- ● **PREGNANCY** See also *Pregnancy* in Epilepsy p. 349.
- ● **BREAST FEEDING** Present in milk in *animal* studies.
- ● **HEPATIC IMPAIRMENT** Manufacturer advises avoid (no information available).
- ● **RENAL IMPAIRMENT** [EvGr] Avoid—no information available. ⟨M⟩
- ● **MONITORING REQUIREMENTS** Perform full blood count and liver function tests prior to initiating treatment and every 6 months thereafter.
- ● **NATIONAL FUNDING/ACCESS DECISIONS**
  For full details see funding body website
  Scottish Medicines Consortium (SMC) decisions
- ▸ Stiripentol (*Diacomit*®) for use in conjunction with clobazam and valproate as adjunctive therapy of refractory generalised tonic-clonic seizures in patients with severe myoclonic epilepsy in infancy (SMEI; Dravet's syndrome) whose seizures are not adequately controlled with clobazam and valproate (September 2017) SMC No. 524/08 Recommended
  All Wales Medicines Strategy Group (AWMSG) decisions
- ▸ Stiripentol (*Diacomit*®) for use in conjunction with clobazam and valproate as adjunctive therapy of refractory generalized tonic-clonic seizures in patients with severe myoclonic epilepsy in infancy (SMEI; Dravet syndrome) whose seizures are not adequately controlled with clobazam and valproate (November 2017) AWMSG No. 3468 Recommended

- ● **MEDICINAL FORMS** There can be variation in the licensing of different medicines containing the same drug.
  Oral capsule
  CAUTIONARY AND ADVISORY LABELS 1, 8, 21
  - ▸ **Diacomit** (Alan Pharmaceuticals)
    Stiripentol 250 mg Diacomit 250mg capsules | 60 capsule [PoM] £284.00 DT = £284.00
    Stiripentol 500 mg Diacomit 500mg capsules | 60 capsule [PoM] £493.00 DT = £493.00
  Powder for oral suspension
  CAUTIONARY AND ADVISORY LABELS 1, 8, 13, 21
  EXCIPIENTS: May contain Aspartame
  - ▸ **Diacomit** (Alan Pharmaceuticals)
    Stiripentol 250 mg Diacomit 250mg oral powder sachets | 60 sachet [PoM] £284.00 DT = £284.00
    Stiripentol 500 mg Diacomit 500mg oral powder sachets | 60 sachet [PoM] £493.00 DT = £493.00

Tiagabine
17-Oct-2022

- ● **INDICATIONS AND DOSE**
  Adjunctive treatment for focal seizures with or without secondary generalisation that are not satisfactorily controlled by other antiepileptics (with enzyme-inducing drugs)
  - ▸ BY MOUTH
  - ▸ **Child 12-17 years:** Initially 5–10 mg daily in 1–2 divided doses, then increased in steps of 5–10 mg/24 hours every week; maintenance 30–45 mg daily in 2–3 divided doses
  - ▸ **Adult:** Initially 5–10 mg daily in 1–2 divided doses, then increased in steps of 5–10 mg/24 hours every week; maintenance 30–45 mg daily in 2–3 divided doses

  Adjunctive treatment for focal seizures with or without secondary generalisation that are not satisfactorily controlled by other antiepileptics (without enzyme-inducing drugs)
  - ▸ BY MOUTH
  - ▸ **Child 12-17 years:** Initially 5–10 mg daily in 1–2 divided doses, then increased in steps of 5–10 mg/24 hours every week; maintenance 15–30 mg daily in 2–3 divided doses
  - ▸ **Adult:** Initially 5–10 mg daily in 1–2 divided doses, then increased in steps of 5–10 mg/24 hours every week; maintenance 15–30 mg daily in 2–3 divided doses

> **IMPORTANT SAFETY INFORMATION**
> MHRA/CHM ADVICE: ANTIEPILEPTICS: RISK OF SUICIDAL THOUGHTS AND BEHAVIOUR (AUGUST 2008)
> See Epilepsy p. 349.
>
> MHRA/CHM ADVICE: ANTIEPILEPTIC DRUGS: UPDATED ADVICE ON SWITCHING BETWEEN DIFFERENT MANUFACTURERS' PRODUCTS (NOVEMBER 2017)
> See Epilepsy p. 349.
>
> MHRA/CHM ADVICE: ANTIEPILEPTIC DRUGS IN PREGNANCY: UPDATED ADVICE FOLLOWING COMPREHENSIVE SAFETY REVIEW (JANUARY 2021)
> See Epilepsy p. 349.

- ● **CAUTIONS** Avoid in Acute porphyrias p. 1202 · seizures (may be exacerbated)
  CAUTIONS, FURTHER INFORMATION
  - ▸ Seizure exacerbation [EvGr] Tiagabine may exacerbate seizures in patients with absence or myoclonic seizures (including juvenile myoclonic epilepsy), tonic or atonic seizures, Dravet syndrome, and Lennox-Gastaut syndrome. ⟨A⟩
- ● **INTERACTIONS** → Appendix 1: antiepileptics
- ● **SIDE-EFFECTS**
  - ▸ **Common or very common** Abdominal pain · behaviour abnormal · concentration impaired · depression · diarrhoea · dizziness · emotional lability · fatigue · gait abnormal · insomnia · nausea · nervousness · speech disorder · tremor · vision disorders · vomiting
  - ▸ **Uncommon** Drowsiness · psychosis · skin reactions
  - ▸ **Rare or very rare** Delusions · hallucination
  - ▸ **Frequency not known** Suicidal behaviours
- ● **PREGNANCY** [EvGr] Avoid unless potential benefit outweighs risk—toxicity in *animal* studies. ⟨M⟩ See also *Pregnancy* in Epilepsy p. 349.
- ● **HEPATIC IMPAIRMENT** Manufacturer advises caution in mild to moderate impairment (risk of increased exposure); avoid in severe impairment.
  Dose adjustments Manufacturer advises dose reduction and/or longer dose interval with careful titration in mild to moderate impairment.
- ● **PATIENT AND CARER ADVICE**
  Medicines for Children leaflet: Tiagabine for epilepsy
  www.medicinesforchildren.org.uk/medicines/tiagabine-for-epilepsy/
  Driving and skilled tasks May impair performance of skilled tasks (e.g. driving).

- ● **MEDICINAL FORMS** There can be variation in the licensing of different medicines containing the same drug. Forms available from special-order manufacturers include: oral suspension
  Oral tablet
  CAUTIONARY AND ADVISORY LABELS 21
  - ▸ **Gabitril** (Teva UK Ltd)
    Tiagabine (as Tiagabine hydrochloride monohydrate)
    5 mg Gabitril 5mg tablets | 100 tablet [PoM] £52.04 DT = £52.04
    Tiagabine (as Tiagabine hydrochloride monohydrate)
    10 mg Gabitril 10mg tablets | 100 tablet [PoM] £104.09 DT = £104.09

Tiagabine (as Tiagabine hydrochloride monohydrate)
15 mg Gabitril 15mg tablets | 100 tablet [PoM] £156.13 DT = £156.13

Topiramate

18-Sep-2024

● **INDICATIONS AND DOSE**

Monotherapy of generalised tonic-clonic seizures or focal seizures with or without secondary generalisation

▸ BY MOUTH

▸ Child 6-17 years: Initially 0.5–1 mg/kg once daily (max. per dose 25 mg) for 1 week, dose to be taken at night, then increased in steps of 250–500 micrograms/kg twice daily, dose to be increased by a maximum of 25 mg twice daily at intervals of 1–2 weeks; usual dose 50 mg twice daily (max. per dose 7.5 mg/kg twice daily), if child cannot tolerate titration regimens recommended above then smaller steps or longer interval between steps may be used; maximum 500 mg per day

▸ Adult: Initially 25 mg once daily for 1 week, dose to be taken at night, then increased in steps of 25–50 mg every 1–2 weeks, dose to be taken in 2 divided doses; usual dose 100–200 mg daily in 2 divided doses, adjusted according to response, doses of 1 g daily have been used in refractory epilepsy; maximum 500 mg per day

Adjunctive treatment of generalised tonic-clonic seizures or focal seizures with or without secondary generalisation | Adjunctive treatment for seizures associated with Lennox-Gastaut syndrome

▸ BY MOUTH

▸ Child 2-17 years: Initially 1–3 mg/kg once daily (max. per dose 25 mg) for 1 week, dose to be taken at night, then increased in steps of 0.5–1.5 mg/kg twice daily, dose to be increased by a maximum of 25 mg twice daily at intervals of 1–2 weeks; usual dose 2.5–4.5 mg/kg twice daily (max. per dose 7.5 mg/kg twice daily), if child cannot tolerate recommended titration regimen then smaller steps or longer interval between steps may be used; maximum 400 mg per day

▸ Adult: Initially 25–50 mg once daily for 1 week, dose to be taken at night, then increased in steps of 25–50 mg every 1–2 weeks, dose to be taken in 2 divided doses; usual dose 200–400 mg daily in 2 divided doses; maximum 400 mg per day

Migraine prophylaxis

▸ BY MOUTH

▸ Adult: Initially 25 mg once daily for 1 week, dose to be taken at night, then increased in steps of 25 mg every week; usual dose 50–100 mg daily in 2 divided doses; maximum 200 mg per day

IMPORTANT SAFETY INFORMATION

MHRA/CHM ADVICE: ANTIEPILEPTICS: RISK OF SUICIDAL THOUGHTS AND BEHAVIOUR (AUGUST 2008)
See Epilepsy p. 349.

MHRA/CHM ADVICE: ANTIEPILEPTIC DRUGS: UPDATED ADVICE ON SWITCHING BETWEEN DIFFERENT MANUFACTURERS' PRODUCTS (NOVEMBER 2017)
See Epilepsy p. 349 and see also *Prescribing and dispensing information*.

MHRA/CHM ADVICE: ANTIEPILEPTIC DRUGS IN PREGNANCY: UPDATED ADVICE FOLLOWING COMPREHENSIVE SAFETY REVIEW (JANUARY 2021)
See Epilepsy p. 349.

MHRA/CHM ADVICE: TOPIRAMATE (*TOPAMAX®*): START OF SAFETY REVIEW TRIGGERED BY A STUDY REPORTING AN INCREASED RISK OF NEURODEVELOPMENTAL DISABILITIES IN CHILDREN WITH PRENATAL EXPOSURE (JULY 2022)
The MHRA has started a new safety review of topiramate following a large observational study that found a dose-dependent association between prenatal exposure and an increased risk of autism spectrum disorders, intellectual disability, and neurodevelopmental disorders in children. Healthcare professionals are reminded that topiramate must be prescribed according to current guidance. In addition, females of childbearing potential or their carers should be counselled on the importance of avoiding pregnancy due to these emerging risks, as well as the established risks associated with topiramate use in pregnancy.

MHRA/CHM ADVICE: TOPIRAMATE (*TOPAMAX®*): INTRODUCTION OF NEW SAFETY MEASURES, INCLUDING A PREGNANCY PREVENTION PROGRAMME (JUNE 2024)
Following the safety review above, the MHRA concluded that the use of topiramate during pregnancy is associated with significant harm to the unborn child, including a higher risk of congenital malformations and low birth-weight, and a potential increased risk of intellectual disability, autism spectrum disorders, and ADHD.

Topiramate must not be used in females of childbearing potential unless the conditions of the Pregnancy Prevention Programme are met (see *Conception and contraception*). Use of topiramate in pregnancy is contra-indicated for migraine prophylaxis, and it must only be considered for epilepsy if there is no suitable alternative treatment (see *Pregnancy*).

Female patients (and their carers) must be fully informed of the risks associated with the use of topiramate during pregnancy; supporting materials have been provided to use in the implementation of the Pregnancy Prevention Programme (see *Prescribing and dispensing information*). The MHRA advises that:

● Prescribers must identify all new and existing females of childbearing potential on topiramate, explain clearly the conditions of the Pregnancy Prevention Programme, provide the Patient Guide, and complete and sign the Risk Awareness Form (at treatment initiation and at each annual review)—copies of the form must be given to the patient or carer and, if necessary, sent to their GP;

● Pharmacists must ensure topiramate is dispensed in whole packs whenever possible—all packs dispensed to females of childbearing potential should have a warning symbol either on the carton or via a sticker. They must also provide the Patient Card and check if the patient is using highly effective contraception, if they are not, patients should be advised to contact their GP for a follow-up appointment.

● **CAUTIONS** Avoid in Acute porphyrias p. 1202 · risk of metabolic acidosis · risk of nephrolithiasis—ensure adequate hydration (especially in strenuous activity or warm environment)

● **INTERACTIONS** → Appendix 1: antiepileptics

● **SIDE-EFFECTS**

▸ **Common or very common** Alopecia · anaemia · anxiety · appetite abnormal · asthenia · behaviour abnormal · cognitive impairment · concentration impaired · confusion · constipation · cough · depression · diarrhoea · dizziness · drowsiness · dry mouth · dyspnoea · ear discomfort · eye disorders · feeling abnormal · fever (in children) · gait abnormal · gastrointestinal discomfort · gastrointestinal disorders · haemorrhage · hypersensitivity · joint disorders · malaise · memory loss · mood altered · movement disorders · muscle complaints · muscle weakness · nasal complaints · nasopharyngitis · nausea · oral disorders · pain · seizures · sensation abnormal · skin reactions · sleep disorders · speech impairment · taste altered · tinnitus · tremor · urinary disorders · urolithiases · vertigo (in children) · vision disorders · vomiting (in children) · weight changes

▶ **Uncommon** Abnormal sensation in eye · anhidrosis · arrhythmias · aura · cerebellar syndrome · consciousness impaired · crying · drooling · dry eye · dysgraphia · dysphonia · eosinophilia (in children) · facial swelling · hallucinations · hearing impairment · hyperthermia (in children) · hypokalaemia · hypotension · influenza like illness · learning disability (in children) · leucopenia · lymphadenopathy · metabolic acidosis · musculoskeletal stiffness · palpitations · pancreatitis · paranasal sinus hypersecretion · peripheral coldness · peripheral neuropathy · polydipsia · psychotic disorder · renal pain · sexual dysfunction · smell altered · suicidal behaviours · syncope · thinking abnormal · thirst · thrombocytopenia · vasodilation

▶ **Rare or very rare** Eye inflammation · face oedema · glaucoma · hepatic disorders · limb discomfort · neutropenia · Raynaud's phenomenon · renal tubular acidosis · severe cutaneous adverse reactions (SCARs) · unresponsive to stimuli

SIDE-EFFECTS, FURTHER INFORMATION Topiramate has been associated with acute myopia with secondary angle-closure glaucoma, typically occurring within 1 month of starting treatment. Choroidal effusions resulting in anterior displacement of the lens and iris have also been reported. If raised intra-ocular pressure occurs: seek specialist ophthalmological advice; use appropriate measures to reduce intra-ocular pressure and stop topiramate as rapidly as feasible.

● **CONCEPTION AND CONTRACEPTION** The MHRA advises that all females of childbearing potential being treated with topiramate must follow the requirements of the Pregnancy Prevention Programme—pregnancy should be excluded before treatment initiation. Highly effective contraception must be used during and for at least 4 weeks after stopping treatment.

● **PREGNANCY** For *migraine prophylaxis*, the MHRA advises that topiramate must not be used. For *epilepsy*, the MHRA advises that topiramate must not be used unless there is no suitable alternative treatment; in such cases, patients must be counselled about the risks (see *Important safety information*). EvGr If used during pregnancy, careful prenatal monitoring should be performed. Ⓜ See also *Pregnancy* in Epilepsy p. 349.

● **BREAST FEEDING** Manufacturer advises avoid—present in milk.

● **HEPATIC IMPAIRMENT** Manufacturer advises caution (risk of decreased clearance).

● **RENAL IMPAIRMENT** EvGr Use with caution. Ⓜ
Dose adjustments EvGr Half usual starting and maintenance dose if creatinine clearance 70 mL/minute or less (reduced clearance and longer time to steady-state plasma concentration). Ⓜ See p. 21.

● **DIRECTIONS FOR ADMINISTRATION**
TOPAMAX ® CAPSULES Manufacturer advises swallow whole or sprinkle contents of capsule on soft food and swallow immediately without chewing.

● **PRESCRIBING AND DISPENSING INFORMATION** The Pregnancy Prevention Programme is supported by the following safety and educational materials: *Patient Guide, Guide for Healthcare Professionals, Risk Awareness Form, Patient Card*, and *Warning Stickers*.

  In addition, the MHRA advises that pharmacists must dispense topiramate in whole packs—see also *Important safety information*.
Switching between formulations Care should be taken when switching between oral formulations in the treatment of epilepsy. The need for continued supply of a particular manufacturer's product should be based on clinical judgement and consultation with the patient or their carer, taking into account factors such as seizure frequency and treatment history.

Patients being treated for epilepsy may need to be maintained on a specific manufacturer's branded or generic topiramate product.

● **PATIENT AND CARER ADVICE**
Pregnancy Prevention Programme A patient card and patient guide must be provided to females of childbearing potential—see also *Important safety information*.
Medicines for Children leaflet: Topiramate for preventing seizures www.medicinesforchildren.org.uk/medicines/topiramate-for-preventing-seizures/
Driving and skilled tasks Patients and carers should be counselled on the effects on driving and performance of skilled tasks—increased risk of dizziness and visual disturbances.

TOPAMAX ® CAPSULES Patients or carers should be given advice on how to administer *Topamax ® Sprinkle* capsules.

● **MEDICINAL FORMS** There can be variation in the licensing of different medicines containing the same drug. Forms available from special-order manufacturers include: oral suspension, oral solution

Oral tablet
CAUTIONARY AND ADVISORY LABELS 2, 8
▶ Topiramate (non-proprietary) ▼
  Topiramate 25 mg Topiramate 25mg tablets | 60 tablet PoM £16.40 DT = £1.68
  Topiramate 50 mg Topiramate 50mg tablets | 60 tablet PoM £26.94 DT = £2.40
  Topiramate 100 mg Topiramate 100mg tablets | 60 tablet PoM £48.25 DT = £2.97
  Topiramate 200 mg Topiramate 200mg tablets | 60 tablet PoM £93.70 DT = £7.89
▶ Topamax (Janssen-Cilag Ltd) ▼
  Topiramate 25 mg Topamax 25mg tablets | 60 tablet PoM £19.29 DT = £1.68
  Topiramate 50 mg Topamax 50mg tablets | 60 tablet PoM £31.69 DT = £2.40
  Topiramate 100 mg Topamax 100mg tablets | 60 tablet PoM £56.76 DT = £2.97
  Topiramate 200 mg Topamax 200mg tablets | 60 tablet PoM £110.23 DT = £7.89

Oral solution
▶ Topiramate (non-proprietary) ▼
  Topiramate 20 mg per 1 ml Topiramate 20mg/ml oral solution sugar free | 150 ml PoM £165.00-£320.00 SF | 280 ml PoM £330.72-£594.00 SF

Oral suspension
CAUTIONARY AND ADVISORY LABELS 2, 8
▶ Topiramate (non-proprietary) ▼
  Topiramate 10 mg per 1 ml Topiramate 50mg/5ml oral suspension sugar free | 150 ml PoM £186.00-£228.96 DT = £228.96 SF
  Topiramate 20 mg per 1 ml Topiramate 100mg/5ml oral suspension sugar free | 280 ml PoM £330.72 DT = £330.72 SF

Oral capsule
CAUTIONARY AND ADVISORY LABELS 2, 8
▶ Topamax (Janssen-Cilag Ltd) ▼
  Topiramate 15 mg Topamax 15mg sprinkle capsules | 60 capsule PoM £14.79 DT = £14.79
  Topiramate 25 mg Topamax 25mg sprinkle capsules | 60 capsule PoM £22.18 DT = £22.18
  Topiramate 50 mg Topamax 50mg sprinkle capsules | 60 capsule PoM £36.45 DT = £36.45

Vigabatrin

19-Mar-2024

● **INDICATIONS AND DOSE**

Adjunctive treatment of focal seizures with or without secondary generalisation not satisfactorily controlled with other antiepileptics (under expert supervision)
▶ BY MOUTH
▶ Child 1-23 months: Initially 15–20 mg/kg twice daily (max. per dose 250 mg), to be increased over 2–3 weeks to usual maintenance dose, usual maintenance 30–40 mg/kg twice daily (max. per dose 75 mg/kg)

continued →

▶ Child 2-11 years: Initially 15–20 mg/kg twice daily (max. per dose 250 mg), to be increased over 2–3 weeks to usual maintenance dose, usual maintenance 30–40 mg/kg twice daily (max. per dose 1.5 g)

▶ Child 12-17 years: Initially 250 mg twice daily, to be increased over 2–3 weeks to usual maintenance dose, usual maintenance 1–1.5 g twice daily

▶ Adult: Initially 1 g once daily, alternatively initially 1 g daily in 2 divided doses, then increased in steps of 500 mg every week, adjusted according to response; usual dose 2–3 g daily; maximum 3 g per day

▶ BY RECTUM

▶ Child 1-23 months: Initially 15–20 mg/kg twice daily (max. per dose 250 mg), to be increased over 2–3 weeks to usual maintenance dose, usual maintenance 30–40 mg/kg twice daily (max. per dose 75 mg/kg)

▶ Child 2-11 years: Initially 15–20 mg/kg twice daily (max. per dose 250 mg), to be increased over 2–3 weeks to usual maintenance dose, usual maintenance 30–40 mg/kg twice daily (max. per dose 1.5 g)

▶ Child 12-17 years: Initially 250 mg twice daily, to be increased over 2–3 weeks to usual maintenance dose, usual maintenance 1–1.5 g twice daily

● UNLICENSED USE Granules not licensed for rectal use. Tablets not licensed to be crushed and dispersed in liquid. Vigabatrin doses in BNF Publications may differ from those in product literature.

IMPORTANT SAFETY INFORMATION

MHRA/CHM ADVICE: ANTIEPILEPTICS: RISK OF SUICIDAL THOUGHTS AND BEHAVIOUR (AUGUST 2008)

See Epilepsy p. 349.

MHRA/CHM ADVICE: ANTIEPILEPTIC DRUGS: UPDATED ADVICE ON SWITCHING BETWEEN DIFFERENT MANUFACTURERS' PRODUCTS (NOVEMBER 2017)

See Epilepsy p. 349.

MHRA/CHM ADVICE: ANTIEPILEPTIC DRUGS IN PREGNANCY: UPDATED ADVICE FOLLOWING COMPREHENSIVE SAFETY REVIEW (JANUARY 2021)

See Epilepsy p. 349.

● CONTRA-INDICATIONS Visual field defects

● CAUTIONS Elderly · history of behavioural problems · history of depression · history of psychosis · seizures (may be exacerbated)

CAUTIONS, FURTHER INFORMATION

▶ Seizure exacerbation EvGr Vigabatrin may exacerbate seizures in patients with absence or myoclonic seizures (including juvenile myoclonic epilepsy), tonic or atonic seizures, Dravet syndrome, Lennox-Gastaut syndrome, and myoclonic-atonic seizures. Ⓐ

▶ Visual field defects Vigabatrin is associated with visual field defects. The onset of symptoms varies from 1 month to several years after starting. In most cases, visual field defects have persisted despite discontinuation, and further deterioration after discontinuation cannot be excluded. EvGr Visual field testing should be carried out before treatment and at 6-month intervals. Patients and their carers should be warned to report any new visual symptoms that develop and those with symptoms should be referred for an urgent ophthalmological opinion. Gradual withdrawal of vigabatrin should be considered. Ⓜ

● INTERACTIONS → Appendix 1: antiepileptics

● SIDE-EFFECTS

GENERAL SIDE-EFFECTS

▶ Rare or very rare Suicidal behaviours

SPECIFIC SIDE-EFFECTS

▶ Common or very common

▶ With oral use Abdominal pain · alopecia · anaemia · anxiety · arthralgia · behaviour abnormal · concentration impaired · depression · dizziness · drowsiness · eye disorders · fatigue · headache · insomnia · memory loss · mood altered · nausea · oedema · paraesthesia · speech disorder · thinking abnormal · tremor · vision disorders · vomiting · weight increased

▶ Uncommon

▶ With oral use Movement disorders · psychotic disorder · seizure (patients with myoclonic seizures at greater risk) · skin reactions

▶ Rare or very rare

▶ With oral use Angioedema · encephalopathy · hallucination · hepatitis · optic neuritis

▶ Frequency not known

▶ With oral use Intramyelinic oedema (particularly in infants) · muscle tone increased

SIDE-EFFECTS, FURTHER INFORMATION **Encephalopathic symptoms** Encephalopathic symptoms including marked sedation, stupor, and confusion with non-specific slow wave EEG can occur rarely -reduce dose or withdraw.

Visual field defects About one-third of patients treated with vigabatrin have suffered visual field defects; counselling and careful monitoring for this side-effect are required.

● PREGNANCY EvGr Avoid unless essential—toxicity in *animal* studies. Ⓜ See also *Pregnancy* in Epilepsy p. 349.

● BREAST FEEDING Present in milk—manufacturer advises avoid.

● RENAL IMPAIRMENT

Dose adjustments EvGr Consider reduced dose or increased dose interval if creatinine clearance less than 60 mL/minute. Ⓜ See p. 21.

● MONITORING REQUIREMENTS

▶ Closely monitor neurological function.

● DIRECTIONS FOR ADMINISTRATION

▶ With oral use EvGr The contents of a sachet of granules should be dissolved in at least 100 mL of water, fruit juice, or milk immediately before taking. Ⓜ Expert sources advise film-coated tablets may be crushed and dispersed in liquid.

▶ With oral use in children EvGr Soluble tablets should be dissolved in a small volume of water (approximately 5 or 10 mL) before administration. Ⓜ

▶ With rectal use Expert sources advise contents of a sachet of granules should be dissolved in a small amount of water and administered rectally.

● PATIENT AND CARER ADVICE Patients and their carers should be warned to report any new visual symptoms that develop.

Medicines for Children leaflet: Vigabatrin for preventing seizures www.medicinesforchildren.org.uk/medicines/vigabatrin-for-preventing-seizures/

Driving and skilled tasks Patients and carers should be cautioned on the effects on driving and performance of skilled or hazardous tasks—increased risk of visual field defects.

● NATIONAL FUNDING/ACCESS DECISIONS

For full details see funding body website

Scottish Medicines Consortium (SMC) decisions

▶ Vigabatrin (*Kigabeq*®) for children from 1 month to less than 7 years of age: as monotherapy for the treatment of infantile spasms (West's syndrome); in combination with other antiepileptic medicinal products for patients with resistant partial epilepsy (focal onset seizures) with or without secondary generalisation, where all other appropriate medicinal product combinations have proved inadequate or have not been tolerated (June 2021) SMC No. SMC2352 Recommended with restrictions

● **MEDICINAL FORMS** There can be variation in the licensing of different medicines containing the same drug. Forms available from special-order manufacturers include: oral solution

Oral tablet

CAUTIONARY AND ADVISORY LABELS 3, 8

▸ Sabril (Sanofi)
Vigabatrin 500 mg Sabril 500mg tablets | 100 tablet [PoM] £44.41 DT = £44.41

Granules for oral solution

CAUTIONARY AND ADVISORY LABELS 3, 8, 13

▸ Sabril (Sanofi)
Vigabatrin 500 mg Sabril 500mg granules for oral solution sachets | 50 sachet [PoM] £24.60 DT = £24.60 [SF]

Zonisamide   11-Nov-2021

● **INDICATIONS AND DOSE**

Monotherapy for treatment of focal seizures with or without secondary generalisation in adults with newly diagnosed epilepsy

▸ BY MOUTH

▸ Adult: Initially 100 mg once daily for 2 weeks, then increased in steps of 100 mg every 2 weeks, usual maintenance dose 300 mg once daily; maximum 500 mg per day

Adjunctive treatment for refractory focal seizures with or without secondary generalisation

▸ BY MOUTH

▸ Child 6-17 years (body-weight 20-54 kg): Initially 1 mg/kg once daily for 7 days, then increased in steps of 1 mg/kg every 7 days, usual maintenance 6–8 mg/kg once daily (max. per dose 500 mg once daily), dose to be increased at 2-week intervals in patients who are **not** receiving concomitant carbamazepine, phenytoin, phenobarbital or other potent inducers of cytochrome P450 enzyme CYP3A4

▸ Child 6-17 years (body-weight 55 kg and above): Initially 1 mg/kg once daily for 7 days, then increased in steps of 1 mg/kg every 7 days, usual maintenance 300–500 mg once daily, dose to be increased at 2-week intervals in patients who are **not** receiving concomitant carbamazepine, phenytoin, phenobarbital or other potent inducers of cytochrome P450 enzyme CYP3A4

▸ Adult: Initially 50 mg daily in 2 divided doses for 7 days, then increased to 100 mg daily in 2 divided doses, then increased in steps of 100 mg every 7 days, usual maintenance 300–500 mg daily in 1–2 divided doses, dose to be increased at 2-week intervals in patients who are **not** receiving concomitant carbamazepine, phenytoin, phenobarbital or other potent inducers of cytochrome P450 enzyme CYP3A4

IMPORTANT SAFETY INFORMATION

MHRA/CHM ADVICE: ANTIEPILEPTICS: RISK OF SUICIDAL THOUGHTS AND BEHAVIOUR (AUGUST 2008)

See Epilepsy p. 349.

MHRA/CHM ADVICE: ANTIEPILEPTIC DRUGS: UPDATED ADVICE ON SWITCHING BETWEEN DIFFERENT MANUFACTURERS' PRODUCTS (NOVEMBER 2017)

See Epilepsy p. 349 and see also *Prescribing and dispensing information*.

MHRA/CHM ADVICE: ANTIEPILEPTIC DRUGS IN PREGNANCY: UPDATED ADVICE FOLLOWING COMPREHENSIVE SAFETY REVIEW (JANUARY 2021)

See Epilepsy p. 349.

● **CAUTIONS** Elderly · history of eye disorders · low body-weight or poor appetite—monitor weight throughout treatment (fatal cases of weight loss reported in children) · metabolic acidosis—monitor serum bicarbonate concentration in children and those with other risk factors (consider dose reduction or discontinuation if metabolic acidosis develops) · risk factors for renal stone formation (particularly predisposition to nephrolithiasis)

CAUTIONS, FURTHER INFORMATION [EvGr] Avoid overheating and ensure adequate hydration especially in children, during strenuous activity or if in warm environment (fatal cases of heat stroke reported in children). ⓜ

● **INTERACTIONS** → Appendix 1: antiepileptics

● **SIDE-EFFECTS**

▸ **Common or very common** Alopecia · anxiety · appetite decreased · ataxia · bradyphrenia · concentration impaired · confusion · constipation · depression · diarrhoea · dizziness · drowsiness · fatigue · fever · gastrointestinal discomfort · hypersensitivity · influenza like illness · insomnia · memory loss · mood altered · nausea · nystagmus · paraesthesia · peripheral oedema · psychosis · rash (consider discontinuation) · skin reactions · speech disorder · tremor · urolithiases · vision disorders · vomiting · weight decreased

▸ **Uncommon** Behaviour abnormal · gallbladder disorders · hallucination · hypokalaemia · increased risk of infection · leucopenia · respiratory disorder · seizures · suicidal behaviours · thrombocytopenia

▸ **Rare or very rare** Agranulocytosis · alveolitis allergic · angle closure glaucoma · anhidrosis · bone marrow disorders · coma · dyspnoea · eye pain · heat stroke · hepatocellular injury · hydronephrosis · leucocytosis · lymphadenopathy · metabolic acidosis · myasthenic syndrome · neuroleptic malignant syndrome · pancreatitis · renal failure · renal tubular acidosis · rhabdomyolysis · severe cutaneous adverse reactions (SCARs) · urine abnormal

▸ **Frequency not known** Sudden unexplained death in epilepsy

● **ALLERGY AND CROSS-SENSITIVITY** Contra-indicated in sulfonamide hypersensitivity.
Antiepileptic hypersensitivity syndrome theoretically associated with zonisamide. See under Epilepsy p. 349 for more information.

● **CONCEPTION AND CONTRACEPTION** Manufacturer advises women of childbearing potential should use effective contraception during treatment and for one month after last dose—avoid in women of childbearing potential not using effective contraception unless clearly necessary and the potential benefit outweighs risk; patients should be fully informed of the risks related to the use of zonisamide during pregnancy.

● **PREGNANCY** An increased risk of intra-uterine growth restriction has been seen with zonisamide, see *Pregnancy* in Epilepsy p. 349.

● **BREAST FEEDING** Manufacturer advises avoid for 4 weeks after last dose.

● **HEPATIC IMPAIRMENT** Avoid in severe impairment.
Dose adjustments Initially increase dose at 2-week intervals if mild or moderate impairment.

● **RENAL IMPAIRMENT**
Dose adjustments Initially increase dose at 2-week intervals; discontinue if renal function deteriorates.

● **TREATMENT CESSATION** Avoid abrupt withdrawal (consult product literature for recommended withdrawal regimens in children).

● **PRESCRIBING AND DISPENSING INFORMATION**
Switching between formulations Care should be taken when switching between oral formulations. The need for continued supply of a particular manufacturer's product should be based on clinical judgement and consultation with the patient or their carer, taking into account factors

4
Nervous system

such as seizure frequency and treatment history.

Patients may need to be maintained on a specific manufacturer's branded or generic zonisamide product.

- **PATIENT AND CARER ADVICE** Children and their carers should be made aware of how to prevent and recognise overheating and dehydration.
Medicines for Children leaflet: Zonisamide for preventing seizures www.medicinesforchildren.org.uk/medicines/zonisamide-for-preventing-seizures/

- **NATIONAL FUNDING/ACCESS DECISIONS**
For full details see funding body website
Scottish Medicines Consortium (SMC) decisions
- Zonisamide (*Zonegran®*) as adjunctive therapy in the treatment of partial seizures, with or without secondary generalisation, in adolescents, and children aged 6 years and above (March 2014) SMC No. 949/14 Recommended with restrictions

- **MEDICINAL FORMS** There can be variation in the licensing of different medicines containing the same drug. Forms available from special-order manufacturers include: oral suspension, oral solution

Oral suspension
CAUTIONARY AND ADVISORY LABELS 3, 8, 10
- Zonisamide (Non-proprietary)
  Zonisamide 20 mg per 1 ml Zonisamide 20mg/ml oral suspension sugar free | 150 ml [PoM] £109.14 [SF]
- Desizon (Desitin Pharma Ltd)
  Zonisamide 20 mg per 1 ml Desizon 20mg/ml oral suspension | 250 ml [PoM] £181.90 DT = £181.90

Oral capsule
CAUTIONARY AND ADVISORY LABELS 3, 8, 10
- Zonisamide (Non-proprietary)
  Zonisamide 25 mg Zonisamide 25mg capsules | 14 capsule [PoM] £15.18 DT = £9.86
  Zonisamide 50 mg Zonisamide 50mg capsules | 56 capsule [PoM] £47.04 DT = £11.08
  Zonisamide 100 mg Zonisamide 100mg capsules | 56 capsule [PoM] £62.72 DT = £12.59
- Zonegran (Advanz Pharma)
  Zonisamide 25 mg Zonegran 25mg capsules | 14 capsule [PoM] £8.82 DT = £9.86
  Zonisamide 50 mg Zonegran 50mg capsules | 56 capsule [PoM] £47.04 DT = £11.08
  Zonisamide 100 mg Zonegran 100mg capsules | 56 capsule [PoM] £62.72 DT = £12.59

ANTIEPILEPTICS > BARBITURATES

Phenobarbital

17-Oct-2022

(Phenobarbitone)

- **INDICATIONS AND DOSE**

All forms of epilepsy except typical absence seizures
- BY MOUTH
- Adult: 60–180 mg once daily, dose to be taken at night

Status epilepticus
- BY INTRAVENOUS INJECTION
- Adult: 10 mg/kg (max. per dose 1 g)
- BY SLOW INTRAVENOUS INJECTION

- Neonate: Initially 20 mg/kg, then 2.5–5 mg/kg 1–2 times a day.

- Child 1 month-11 years: Initially 20 mg/kg, then 2.5–5 mg/kg 1–2 times a day
- Child 12-17 years: Initially 20 mg/kg (max. per dose 1 g), then 300 mg twice daily

IMPORTANT SAFETY INFORMATION
MHRA/CHM ADVICE: ANTIEPILEPTICS: RISK OF SUICIDAL THOUGHTS AND BEHAVIOUR (AUGUST 2008)
See Epilepsy p. 349.

MHRA/CHM ADVICE: ANTIEPILEPTIC DRUGS: UPDATED ADVICE ON SWITCHING BETWEEN DIFFERENT MANUFACTURERS' PRODUCTS (NOVEMBER 2017)
See Epilepsy p. 349 and see also *Prescribing and dispensing information*.

MHRA/CHM ADVICE: ANTIEPILEPTIC DRUGS IN PREGNANCY: UPDATED ADVICE FOLLOWING COMPREHENSIVE SAFETY REVIEW (JANUARY 2021)
See Epilepsy p. 349.

- **CAUTIONS** Avoid in Acute porphyrias p. 1202 · children · debilitated · elderly · history of alcohol abuse · history of drug abuse · respiratory depression (avoid if severe) · seizures (may be exacerbated)

CAUTIONS, FURTHER INFORMATION MHRA advises consider vitamin D supplementation in patients who are immobilised for long periods or who have inadequate sun exposure or dietary intake of calcium.
- Seizure exacerbation [EvGr] Phenobarbital may exacerbate seizures in patients with absence seizures, Dravet syndrome, and Lennox-Gastaut syndrome. Ⓐ

- **INTERACTIONS** → Appendix 1: antiepileptics

- **SIDE-EFFECTS**

GENERAL SIDE-EFFECTS Agranulocytosis · anticonvulsant hypersensitivity syndrome · behaviour abnormal · bone disorders · bone fracture · cognitive impairment · confusion · depression · drowsiness · folate deficiency · hepatic disorders · memory loss · movement disorders · nystagmus · respiratory depression · severe cutaneous adverse reactions (SCARs) · skin reactions · suicidal behaviours

SPECIFIC SIDE-EFFECTS
- With oral use Anxiety · hallucination · hypotension · megaloblastic anaemia · thrombocytopenia
- With parenteral use Agitation · anaemia · aplastic anaemia · Dupuytren's contracture · hypocalcaemia · irritability

Overdose For details on the management of poisoning, see Active elimination techniques, under Emergency treatment of poisoning p. 1554.

- **ALLERGY AND CROSS-SENSITIVITY** Cross-sensitivity reported with carbamazepine. Antiepileptic hypersensitivity syndrome associated with phenobarbital. See under Epilepsy p. 349 for more information.

- **PREGNANCY** An increased risk of major congenital malformations and intra-uterine growth restriction, and possibility of adverse effects on neurodevelopment have been seen with phenobarbital, see *Pregnancy* in Epilepsy p. 349 for further details.

- **BREAST FEEDING** Avoid if possible; drowsiness may occur.

- **HEPATIC IMPAIRMENT** Manufacturer advises caution in mild to moderate impairment; avoid in severe impairment.

- **RENAL IMPAIRMENT** [EvGr] Use with caution in mild to moderate impairment; avoid in severe impairment. Ⓜ

- **MONITORING REQUIREMENTS**
- Plasma-phenobarbital concentration for optimum response is 15–40 mg/litre (60–180 micromol/litre); however, monitoring the plasma-drug concentration is less useful than with other drugs because tolerance occurs.

- **TREATMENT CESSATION** Avoid abrupt withdrawal (dependence with prolonged use).

- **DIRECTIONS FOR ADMINISTRATION** For administration by *mouth*, tablets may be crushed.
- In adults EvGr For *intravenous injection*, dilute injection solution 1 in 10 with Water for Injections; ⟨M⟩ give at a rate not more than 100 mg/minute.
- In children EvGr For *intravenous injection*, dilute injection solution 1 in 10 with Water for Injections; ⟨M⟩ give at a rate not more than 1 mg/kg/minute.
- **PRESCRIBING AND DISPENSING INFORMATION** Switching between formulations Different formulations of oral preparations may vary in bioavailability. Patients should be maintained on a specific manufacturer's product.
- **PATIENT AND CARER ADVICE** Medicines for Children leaflet: Phenobarbital for preventing seizures www.medicinesforchildren.org.uk/medicines/phenobarbital-for-preventing-seizures/

- **MEDICINAL FORMS** There can be variation in the licensing of different medicines containing the same drug. Forms available from special-order manufacturers include: oral tablet, oral capsule, oral suspension, oral solution

Oral tablet
CAUTIONARY AND ADVISORY LABELS 2, 8
- **Phenobarbital (Non-proprietary)**
  Phenobarbital 15 mg Phenobarbital 15mg tablets | 28 tablet PoM £24.95 DT = £7.64 CD3
  Phenobarbital 30 mg Phenobarbital 30mg tablets | 28 tablet PoM £0.81 DT = £0.81 CD3
  Phenobarbital 60 mg Phenobarbital 60mg tablets | 28 tablet PoM £7.99 DT = £2.41 CD3

Solution for injection
EXCIPIENTS: May contain Propylene glycol
- **Phenobarbital (Non-proprietary)**
  Phenobarbital sodium 30 mg per 1 ml Phenobarbital 30mg/1ml solution for injection ampoules | 10 ampoule PoM £158.84-£171.45 DT = £158.84 CD3
  Phenobarbital sodium 60 mg per 1 ml Phenobarbital 60mg/1ml solution for injection ampoules | 10 ampoule PoM £138.52-£185.86 DT = £167.61 CD3
  Phenobarbital sodium 200 mg per 1 ml Phenobarbital 200mg/1ml solution for injection ampoules | 10 ampoule PoM £112.94-£140.71 DT = £136.61 CD3

Oral solution
CAUTIONARY AND ADVISORY LABELS 2, 8
EXCIPIENTS: May contain Alcohol
- **Phenobarbital (Non-proprietary)**
  Phenobarbital 3 mg per 1 ml Phenobarbital 15mg/5ml elixir | 500 ml PoM £83.00 DT = £83.00 CD3

Primidone
11-Aug-2022

- **DRUG ACTION** Primidone is partially converted to phenobarbital, but is also considered to have some antiepileptic action in its own right.

- **INDICATIONS AND DOSE**

All forms of epilepsy except typical absence seizures
- BY MOUTH
- Child 1 month–1 year: Initially 125 mg daily, dose to be taken at bedtime, then increased in steps of 125 mg every 3 days, adjusted according to response; maintenance 125–250 mg twice daily
- Child 2–4 years: Initially 125 mg once daily, dose to be taken at bedtime, then increased in steps of 125 mg every 3 days, adjusted according to response; maintenance 250–375 mg twice daily
- Child 5–8 years: Initially 125 mg once daily, dose to be taken at bedtime, then increased in steps of 125 mg every 3 days, adjusted according to response; maintenance 375–500 mg twice daily
- Child 9–17 years: Initially 125 mg once daily, dose to be taken at bedtime, then increased in steps of 125 mg every 3 days, increased to 250 mg twice daily, then increased in steps of 250 mg every 3 days (max. per dose 750 mg twice daily), adjusted according to response
- Adult: Initially 125 mg once daily, dose to be taken at bedtime, then increased in steps of 125 mg every 3 days, increased to 500 mg daily in 2 divided doses, then increased in steps of 250 mg every 3 days, adjusted according to response; maintenance 0.75–1.5 g daily in 2 divided doses

Essential tremor
- BY MOUTH
- Adult: Initially 50 mg daily, then adjusted according to response to up to 750 mg daily, dose to be increased over 2–3 weeks

---

IMPORTANT SAFETY INFORMATION

MHRA/CHM ADVICE: ANTIEPILEPTICS: RISK OF SUICIDAL THOUGHTS AND BEHAVIOUR (AUGUST 2008)
See Epilepsy p. 349.

MHRA/CHM ADVICE: ANTIEPILEPTIC DRUGS: UPDATED ADVICE ON SWITCHING BETWEEN DIFFERENT MANUFACTURERS' PRODUCTS (NOVEMBER 2017)
See Epilepsy p. 349 and see also *Prescribing and dispensing information.*

MHRA/CHM ADVICE: ANTIEPILEPTIC DRUGS IN PREGNANCY: UPDATED ADVICE FOLLOWING COMPREHENSIVE SAFETY REVIEW (JANUARY 2021)
See Epilepsy p. 349.

- **CAUTIONS** Avoid in Acute porphyrias p. 1202 · children · debilitated · elderly · history of alcohol abuse · history of drug abuse · respiratory depression (consider dose reduction)

  CAUTIONS, FURTHER INFORMATION MHRA advises consider vitamin D supplementation in patients who are immobilised for long periods or who have inadequate sun exposure or dietary intake of calcium.

- **INTERACTIONS** → Appendix 1: antiepileptics
- **SIDE-EFFECTS**
  - **Common or very common** Apathy · movement disorders · nausea · nystagmus · visual impairment
  - **Uncommon** Dizziness · headache · hypersensitivity · skin reactions · vomiting
  - **Rare or very rare** Arthralgia · bone disorders · Dupuytren's contracture · leucopenia · lymphadenopathy · megaloblastic anaemia (may be treated with folic acid) · psychotic disorder · severe cutaneous adverse reactions (SCARs) · systemic lupus erythematosus (SLE) · thrombocytopenia
  - **Frequency not known** Bone fracture · confusion · drowsiness · hallucination · suicidal behaviours
- **ALLERGY AND CROSS-SENSITIVITY** Cross-sensitivity reported with carbamazepine. Antiepileptic hypersensitivity syndrome associated with primidone. See under Epilepsy p. 349 for more information.
- **PREGNANCY** EvGr Caution—increased risk of congenital malformations following exposure during pregnancy. ⟨M⟩ See also *Pregnancy* in Epilepsy p. 349.
- **HEPATIC IMPAIRMENT** Manufacturer advises caution. **Dose adjustments** Manufacturer advises consider dose reduction.
- **RENAL IMPAIRMENT** EvGr Use with caution. ⟨M⟩ **Dose adjustments** EvGr Consider dose reduction. ⟨M⟩
- **MONITORING REQUIREMENTS**
  - Monitor plasma concentrations of derived phenobarbital; plasma concentration for optimum response is 15–40 mg/litre (60–180 micromol/litre).
- **TREATMENT CESSATION** Avoid abrupt withdrawal (dependence with prolonged use).

● **PRESCRIBING AND DISPENSING INFORMATION**
Switching between formulations Different formulations of oral
preparations may vary in bioavailability. Patients being
treated for epilepsy should be maintained on a specific
manufacturer's product.

● **MEDICINAL FORMS** There can be variation in the licensing of
different medicines containing the same drug. Forms available
from special-order manufacturers include: oral capsule, oral
suspension

Oral tablet
CAUTIONARY AND ADVISORY LABELS 2, 8
▸ **Primidone (Non-proprietary)**
  Primidone 50 mg Primidone 50mg tablets | 100 tablet [PoM]
  £163.82 DT = £118.71
  Primidone 125 mg Primidone 125mg tablets | 50 tablet [PoM]
  £65.00 DT = £65.00
  Primidone 250 mg Primidone 250mg tablets | 100 tablet [PoM]
  £145.00 DT = £75.49
▸ **Enodama** (Desitin Pharma Ltd)
  Primidone 50 mg Enodama 50mg tablets | 100 tablet [PoM] £90.00
  DT = £118.71

Oral suspension
▸ **Primidone (Non-proprietary)**
  Primidone 25 mg per 1 ml Liskantin Saft 125mg/5ml oral
  suspension | 250 ml [PoM] [Ⓢ] (Hospital only)

HYPNOTICS, SEDATIVES AND ANXIOLYTICS ⟩ BENZODIAZEPINES

⌑ 397

Clobazam

26-Oct-2021

● **INDICATIONS AND DOSE**

Adjunct in epilepsy
▸ BY MOUTH
▸ Child 6-17 years: Initially 5 mg daily, dose to be
  increased if necessary at intervals of 5 days,
  maintenance 0.3–1 mg/kg daily, daily doses of up to
  30 mg may be given as a single dose at bedtime, higher
  doses should be divided; maximum 60 mg per day
▸ Adult: 20–30 mg daily, then increased if necessary up
  to 60 mg daily

Anxiety (short-term use)
▸ BY MOUTH
▸ Adult: 20–30 mg daily in divided doses, alternatively
  20–30 mg once daily, dose to be taken at bedtime;
  increased if necessary up to 60 mg daily in divided
  doses, dose only increased in severe anxiety (in
  hospital patients), for debilitated patients, use elderly
  dose
▸ Elderly: 10–20 mg daily

IMPORTANT SAFETY INFORMATION

SAFE PRACTICE
Clobazam has been confused with clonazepam; care
must be taken to ensure the correct drug is prescribed
and dispensed.

MHRA/CHM ADVICE: ANTIEPILEPTICS: RISK OF SUICIDAL
THOUGHTS AND BEHAVIOUR (AUGUST 2008)
See Epilepsy p. 349.

MHRA/CHM ADVICE: ANTIEPILEPTIC DRUGS: UPDATED ADVICE ON
SWITCHING BETWEEN DIFFERENT MANUFACTURERS' PRODUCTS
(NOVEMBER 2017)
See Epilepsy p. 349 and see also *Prescribing and
dispensing information.*

MHRA/CHM ADVICE: ANTIEPILEPTIC DRUGS IN PREGNANCY:
UPDATED ADVICE FOLLOWING COMPREHENSIVE SAFETY REVIEW
(JANUARY 2021)
See Epilepsy p. 349.

● **CONTRA-INDICATIONS** Respiratory depression

● **CAUTIONS** Muscle weakness · organic brain changes

CAUTIONS, FURTHER INFORMATION The effectiveness of
clobazam may decrease significantly after weeks or
months of continuous therapy.

● **INTERACTIONS** → Appendix 1: benzodiazepines

● **SIDE-EFFECTS** Appetite decreased · consciousness
impaired · constipation · drug abuse · dry mouth · fall · gait
unsteady · libido loss · movement disorders · muscle
spasms · nystagmus · psychotic disorder · respiratory
disorder · severe cutaneous adverse reactions (SCARs) ·
skin reactions · speech impairment · suicidal behaviours ·
weight increased

● **PREGNANCY** See *Pregnancy* in Epilepsy p. 349.

● **BREAST FEEDING** Benzodiazepines are present in milk, and
should be avoided if possible during breast-feeding.
Monitoring All infants should be monitored for sedation,
feeding difficulties, adequate weight gain, and
developmental milestones.

● **MONITORING REQUIREMENTS**
▸ In children Routine measurement of plasma concentrations
  of antiepileptic drugs is not usually justified, because the
  target concentration ranges are arbitrary and often vary
  between individuals. However, plasma drug
  concentrations may be measured in children with
  worsening seizures, status epilepticus, suspected
  noncompliance, or suspected toxicity. Similarly,
  haematological and biochemical monitoring should not be
  undertaken unless clinically indicated.

● **PRESCRIBING AND DISPENSING INFORMATION**
Switching between formulations Care should be taken when
switching between oral formulations in the treatment of
epilepsy. The need for continued supply of a particular
manufacturer's product should be based on clinical
judgement and consultation with the patient or their
carer, taking into account factors such as seizure
frequency and treatment history.
  Patients being treated for epilepsy may need to be
maintained on a specific manufacturer's branded or
generic clobazam product.

● **PATIENT AND CARER ADVICE**
Medicines for Children leaflet: Clobazam for preventing seizures
www.medicinesforchildren.org.uk/medicines/clobazam-for-
preventing-seizures/

● **NATIONAL FUNDING/ACCESS DECISIONS**
NHS restrictions Clobazam is not prescribable in NHS
primary care except for the treatment of epilepsy; endorse
prescription 'SLS'.

● **MEDICINAL FORMS** There can be variation in the licensing of
different medicines containing the same drug. Forms available
from special-order manufacturers include: oral capsule, oral
suspension

Oral tablet
CAUTIONARY AND ADVISORY LABELS 2, 8
▸ **Clobazam (Non-proprietary)**
  Clobazam 10 mg Clobazam 10mg tablets | 30 tablet [PoM] £6.51 DT
  = £3.62 [CD4-1]
  Clobazam 20 mg Clobazam 20mg tablets | 30 tablet [PoM] £9.75-
  £15.60 DT = £9.75 [CD4-1]
▸ **Frisium** (Atnahs Pharma UK Ltd)
  Clobazam 10 mg Frisium 10mg tablets | 30 tablet [PoM] £2.51 DT =
  £3.62 [CD4-1]

Oral suspension
CAUTIONARY AND ADVISORY LABELS 2, 8
EXCIPIENTS: May contain Hydroxybenzoates (parabens), polysorbates,
propylene glycol
▸ **Clobazam (Non-proprietary)**
  Clobazam 1 mg per 1 ml Clobazam 5mg/5ml oral suspension sugar
  free | 150 ml [PoM] £90.00 DT = £49.35 [CD4-1] [SF] | 250 ml [PoM]
  £131.23-£231.28 [CD4-1] [SF]
  Clobazam 2 mg per 1 ml Clobazam 10mg/5ml oral suspension sugar
  free | 150 ml [PoM] £95.00 DT = £39.92 [CD4-1] [SF] | 250 ml [PoM]
  £131.98-£233.24 [CD4-1] [SF]

▶ **Perizam** (Rosemont Pharmaceuticals Ltd)
Clobazam 1 mg per 1 ml Perizam 1mg/ml oral suspension | 150 ml [PoM] £90.00 DT = £49.35 [CD4-1] [SF]
Clobazam 2 mg per 1 ml Perizam 2mg/ml oral suspension | 150 ml [PoM] £95.00 DT = £39.92 [CD4-1] [SF]

▶ **Zacco** (Syri Ltd)
Clobazam 1 mg per 1 ml Zacco 5mg/5ml oral suspension | 150 ml [PoM] £50.00 DT = £49.35 [CD4-1] [SF]
Clobazam 2 mg per 1 ml Zacco 10mg/5ml oral suspension | 150 ml [PoM] £55.00 DT = £39.92 [CD4-1] [SF]

⏷ 397

Clonazepam

26-Oct-2021

● **INDICATIONS AND DOSE**

All forms of epilepsy

▶ BY MOUTH
▶ Child 1-11 months: Initially 250 micrograms once daily for 4 nights, dose to be increased over 2–4 weeks, usual dose 0.5–1 mg daily, dose to be taken at night; may be given in 3 divided doses if necessary
▶ Child 1-4 years: Initially 250 micrograms once daily for 4 nights, dose to be increased over 2–4 weeks, usual dose 1–3 mg daily, dose to be taken at night; may be given in 3 divided doses if necessary
▶ Child 5-11 years: Initially 500 micrograms once daily for 4 nights, dose to be increased over 2–4 weeks, usual dose 3–6 mg daily, dose to be taken at night; may be given in 3 divided doses if necessary
▶ Child 12-17 years: Initially 1 mg once daily for 4 nights, dose to be increased over 2–4 weeks, usual dose 4–8 mg daily, dose usually taken at night; may be given in 3–4 divided doses if necessary

All forms of epilepsy | Myoclonus

▶ BY MOUTH
▶ Adult: Initially 1 mg once daily for 4 nights, dose to be increased over 2–4 weeks, usual dose 4–8 mg daily, adjusted according to response, dose usually taken at night; may be given in 3–4 divided doses if necessary
▶ Elderly: Initially 500 micrograms once daily for 4 nights, dose to be increased over 2–4 weeks, usual dose 4–8 mg daily, adjusted according to response, dose usually taken at night; may be given in 3–4 divided doses if necessary

Panic disorders (with or without agoraphobia) resistant to antidepressant therapy

▶ BY MOUTH
▶ Adult: 1–2 mg daily

● **UNLICENSED USE** Clonazepam doses in BNF Publications may differ from those in product literature. Use for panic disorders (with or without agoraphobia) resistant to antidepressant therapy is an unlicensed indication.

IMPORTANT SAFETY INFORMATION

SAFE PRACTICE
Clonazepam has been confused with clobazam; care must be taken to ensure the correct drug is prescribed and dispensed.

MHRA/CHM ADVICE: ANTIEPILEPTICS: RISK OF SUICIDAL THOUGHTS AND BEHAVIOUR (AUGUST 2008)
See Epilepsy p. 349.

MHRA/CHM ADVICE: ANTIEPILEPTIC DRUGS: UPDATED ADVICE ON SWITCHING BETWEEN DIFFERENT MANUFACTURERS' PRODUCTS (NOVEMBER 2017)
See Epilepsy p. 349 and see also *Prescribing and dispensing information*.

MHRA/CHM ADVICE: ANTIEPILEPTIC DRUGS IN PREGNANCY: UPDATED ADVICE FOLLOWING COMPREHENSIVE SAFETY REVIEW (JANUARY 2021)
See Epilepsy p. 349.

● **CONTRA-INDICATIONS** Coma · current alcohol abuse · current drug abuse · respiratory depression

● **CAUTIONS** Acute porphyrias p. 1202 · airways obstruction · brain damage · cerebellar ataxia · depression · spinal ataxia · suicidal ideation

CAUTIONS, FURTHER INFORMATION The effectiveness of clonazepam may decrease significantly after weeks or months of continuous therapy.

● **INTERACTIONS** → Appendix 1: benzodiazepines

● **SIDE-EFFECTS**
▶ **Common or very common** Nystagmus
▶ **Frequency not known** Alopecia · bronchial secretion increased (in children) · cardiac arrest · concentration impaired · drooling (in children) · epigastric discomfort · gastrointestinal disorder · heart failure · hypersalivation (in children) · incomplete precocious puberty (in children) · increased risk of fall (in adults) · increased risk of fracture (in adults) · movement disorders · muscle tone decreased · psychotic disorder · seizure presentation change · sexual dysfunction · skin reactions · speech impairment · suicidal behaviours · urinary incontinence

● **PREGNANCY** See *Pregnancy* in Epilepsy p. 349.

● **BREAST FEEDING** Present in milk, and should be avoided if possible during breast-feeding.
Monitoring All infants should be monitored for sedation, feeding difficulties, adequate weight gain, and developmental milestones.

● **MONITORING REQUIREMENTS**
▶ In children Routine measurement of plasma concentrations of antiepileptic drugs is not usually justified, because the target concentration ranges are arbitrary and often vary between individuals. However, plasma drug concentrations may be measured in children with worsening seizures, status epilepticus, suspected noncompliance, or suspected toxicity. Similarly, haematological and biochemical monitoring should not be undertaken unless clinically indicated.

● **PRESCRIBING AND DISPENSING INFORMATION** The RCPCH and NPPG recommend that, when a liquid special of clonazepam is required, the following strength is used: 2 mg/5 mL.
Switching between formulations Care should be taken when switching between oral formulations in the treatment of epilepsy. The need for continued supply of a particular manufacturer's product should be based on clinical judgement and consultation with the patient or their carer, taking into account factors such as seizure frequency and treatment history.
  Patients being treated for epilepsy may need to be maintained on a specific manufacturer's branded or generic oral clonazepam product.

● **PATIENT AND CARER ADVICE**
Medicines for Children leaflet: Clonazepam for preventing seizures www.medicinesforchildren.org.uk/medicines/clonazepam-for-preventing-seizures/

● **MEDICINAL FORMS** There can be variation in the licensing of different medicines containing the same drug. Forms available from special-order manufacturers include: orodispersible tablet, oral suspension, oral solution

Oral tablet
CAUTIONARY AND ADVISORY LABELS 2, 8
▶ Clonazepam (Non-proprietary)
Clonazepam 500 microgram Clonazepam 500microgram tablets | 100 tablet [PoM] £32.27 DT = £17.28 [CD4-1]
Clonazepam 1 mg Clonazepam 1mg tablets | 100 tablet [PoM] £41.95–£73.40 DT = £41.95 [CD4-1]
Clonazepam 2 mg Clonazepam 2mg tablets | 100 tablet [PoM] £34.99 DT = £10.07 [CD4-1]

Oral solution

CAUTIONARY AND ADVISORY LABELS 2, 8
EXCIPIENTS: May contain Ethanol

▸ **Clonazepam (Non-proprietary)**
Clonazepam 100 microgram per 1 ml Clonazepam 500micrograms/5ml oral solution sugar free | 150 ml [PoM] £69.50 DT = £57.34 [CD4-1] [SF]
Clonazepam 400 microgram per 1 ml Clonazepam 2mg/5ml oral solution sugar free | 150 ml [PoM] £90.30 DT = £83.93 [CD4-1] [SF]

2.1 Status epilepticus

Status epilepticus

23-May-2024

Description of condition

Status epilepticus, defined as a seizure that lasts 5 minutes or longer, or recurrent seizures without recovery in between, should be managed as a medical emergency to prevent neurological injury and death. Status epilepticus may be convulsive or non-convulsive. Non-convulsive status epilepticus can be difficult to detect and its management requires specialist advice.

Causes of status epilepticus include poorly-controlled epilepsy (therapy non-adherence or withdrawal), eclampsia, metabolic abnormalities, alcohol or drug withdrawal, infection such as CNS infections, a tumour, airway obstruction, hypoxia, and shock.

Aims of treatment

The aim of treatment is to stop the seizure as soon as possible. After 5 minutes, seizures are unlikely to stop without medical intervention, and seizures become harder to stop the longer they last.

Convulsive status epilepticus

For a quick reference resource with doses of benzodiazepines for the management of convulsive status epilepticus, see *Seizures* in Medical emergencies in the community p. 2028.

The immediate management of convulsive status epilepticus includes securing the patient's airway, giving oxygen, and monitoring cardiac and respiratory function. Underlying causes should be managed appropriately. In patients with established epilepsy, obtaining serum-antiepileptic concentrations can determine if non-adherence is a cause, and may inform treatment doses.

[EvGr] The individualised emergency management plan of patients with epilepsy, if immediately available, should be followed. Where such a plan is unavailable or in those with other underlying causes, patients in the community should immediately be given buccal midazolam p. 394 [unlicensed] or rectal diazepam p. 398. If intravenous access and resuscitation facilities are immediately available, intravenous lorazepam p. 393 should be given.

Where there is no response to the first benzodiazepine dose, emergency services should be called if in the community or expert advice sought if in hospital. The patient's individualised emergency management plan, if immediately available, should continue to be followed; otherwise, a second benzodiazepine dose should be given if the seizure has not stopped within 5-10 minutes of the first dose.

If there is no response to two benzodiazepine doses, levetiracetam p. 368 [unlicensed use], phenytoin p. 372, or sodium valproate p. 378 may be given as second-line treatment, taking into account that levetiracetam may be quicker to give and has fewer side-effects. If there is no response, an alternative second-line treatment option should be considered under expert advice. Phenobarbital p. 388 may also be considered if these options are not effective or suitable.

If second-line treatment options are unsuccessful, consider general anaesthesia as third-line treatment under expert advice.

If there is concern that convulsive status epilepticus may recur, an emergency management plan should be agreed with the patient if they do not have one already. [A]

Useful Resources

Epilepsies in children, young people and adults. National Institute for Health and Care Excellence. NICE guideline 217. April 2022.
www.nice.org.uk/guidance/ng217

> **Other drugs used for Status epilepticus** Fosphenytoin sodium, p. 361

ANTIEPILEPTICS > BARBITURATES

Thiopental sodium

10-May-2021

(Thiopentone sodium)

● **INDICATIONS AND DOSE**

Status epilepticus (only if other measures fail)

▸ BY SLOW INTRAVENOUS INJECTION
▸ Adult: 75–125 mg for 1 dose, to be administered as a 2.5% (25 mg/mL) solution

Induction of anaesthesia

▸ BY SLOW INTRAVENOUS INJECTION
▸ Adult: Initially 100–150 mg, to be administered over 10–15 seconds usually as a 2.5% (25 mg/mL) solution, followed by 100–150 mg after 0.5–1 minute if required, dose to be given in fit and premedicated adults; debilitated patients or adults over 65 years may require a lower dose or increased administration time, alternatively initially up to 4 mg/kg (max. per dose 500 mg)

Anaesthesia of short duration

▸ BY SLOW INTRAVENOUS INJECTION
▸ Adult: Initially 100–150 mg, to be administered over 10–15 seconds usually as a 2.5% (25 mg/mL) solution, followed by 100–150 mg after 0.5–1 minute if required, dose to be given in fit and premedicated adults; debilitated patients or adults over 65 years may require a lower dose or increased administration time, alternatively initially up to 4 mg/kg (max. per dose 500 mg)

Reduction of raised intracranial pressure if ventilation controlled

▸ BY SLOW INTRAVENOUS INJECTION
▸ Adult: 1.5–3 mg/kg, repeated if necessary

> **IMPORTANT SAFETY INFORMATION**
> Thiopental sodium should only be administered by, or under the direct supervision of, personnel experienced in its use, with adequate training in anaesthesia and airway management, and when resuscitation equipment is available.

● **CONTRA-INDICATIONS** Acute porphyrias p. 1202 · myotonic dystrophy

● **CAUTIONS** Acute circulatory failure (shock) · avoid intra-arterial injection · cardiovascular disease · elderly · hypovolaemia · reconstituted solution is highly alkaline (extravasation causes tissue necrosis and severe pain) · respiratory diseases (avoid in acute asthma)

● **INTERACTIONS** → Appendix 1: thiopental

● **SIDE-EFFECTS**
▸ **Common or very common** Arrhythmia · myocardial contractility decreased

▸ **Frequency not known** Appetite decreased · circulatory collapse · cough · electrolyte imbalance · extravasation necrosis · hypotension · respiratory disorders · skin eruption · sneezing

● PREGNANCY May depress neonatal respiration when used during delivery.

● BREAST FEEDING Breast-feeding can be resumed as soon as mother has recovered sufficiently from anaesthesia.

● HEPATIC IMPAIRMENT Manufacturer advises caution.
Dose adjustments Manufacturer advises dose reduction.

● RENAL IMPAIRMENT [EvGr] Caution in severe impairment. ⟨M⟩

● PATIENT AND CARER ADVICE
Driving and skilled tasks Patients given sedatives and analgesics during minor outpatient procedures should be very carefully warned about the risk of driving or undertaking skilled tasks afterwards. For a short general anaesthetic the risk extends to **at least 24 hours** after administration. Responsible persons should be available to take patients home. The dangers of taking **alcohol** should also be emphasised.

● MEDICINAL FORMS There can be variation in the licensing of different medicines containing the same drug. Forms available from special-order manufacturers include: solution for injection

Powder for solution for injection

▸ Thiopental sodium (Non-proprietary)
Thiopental sodium 500 mg Thiopental 500mg powder for solution for injection vials | 10 vial [PoM] £57.60 | 10 vial [PoM] £69.00 (Hospital only)

HYPNOTICS, SEDATIVES AND ANXIOLYTICS › BENZODIAZEPINES

[⚑ 397]

Lorazepam

11-Aug-2022

● **INDICATIONS AND DOSE**
Short-term use in anxiety
▸ BY MOUTH
▸ Adult: 1–4 mg daily in divided doses
▸ Elderly: 0.5–2 mg daily in divided doses
Short-term use in anxiety [for debilitated patients]
▸ BY MOUTH
▸ Adult: 0.5–2 mg daily in divided doses
Short-term use in insomnia associated with anxiety
▸ BY MOUTH
▸ Adult: 1–2 mg once daily, to be taken at bedtime
Acute panic attacks
▸ BY SLOW INTRAVENOUS INJECTION
▸ Adult: 25–30 micrograms/kg every 6 hours as required, usual dose 1.5–2.5 mg every 6 hours as required
▸ BY INTRAMUSCULAR INJECTION
▸ Adult: 25–30 micrograms/kg every 6 hours as required, usual dose 1.5–2.5 mg every 6 hours as required, only use intramuscular route when oral and intravenous routes not possible
Conscious sedation for procedures
▸ BY MOUTH
▸ Adult: 2–3 mg for 1 dose, to be taken the night before operation and 2–4 mg for 1 dose, to be taken 1–2 hours before operation
▸ BY SLOW INTRAVENOUS INJECTION
▸ Adult: 50 micrograms/kg for 1 dose, to be administered 30–45 minutes before operation
▸ BY INTRAMUSCULAR INJECTION
▸ Adult: 50 micrograms/kg for 1 dose, to be administered 60–90 minutes before operation

Premedication
▸ BY MOUTH
▸ Adult: 2–3 mg for 1 dose, to be taken the night before operation and 2–4 mg for 1 dose, to be taken 1–2 hours before operation
▸ BY SLOW INTRAVENOUS INJECTION
▸ Adult: 50 micrograms/kg for 1 dose, to be administered 30–45 minutes before operation
▸ BY INTRAMUSCULAR INJECTION
▸ Adult: 50 micrograms/kg for 1 dose, to be administered 60–90 minutes before operation

Status epilepticus | Febrile convulsions | Convulsions caused by poisoning
▸ BY SLOW INTRAVENOUS INJECTION
▸ Child 1 month-11 years: 100 micrograms/kg for 1 dose (max. per dose 4 mg), then 100 micrograms/kg for 1 dose (max. per dose 4 mg), to be given 5–10 minutes after first dose if required
▸ Child 12-17 years: 4 mg for 1 dose, then 4 mg for 1 dose, to be given 5–10 minutes after first dose if required
▸ Adult: 4 mg for 1 dose, then 4 mg for 1 dose, to be given 5–10 minutes after first dose if required

● UNLICENSED USE
▸ In children Not licensed for use in febrile convulsions. Not licensed for use in convulsions caused by poisoning.

> **IMPORTANT SAFETY INFORMATION**
> ANAESTHESIA
> Benzodiazepines should only be administered for anaesthesia by, or under the direct supervision of, personnel experienced in their use, with adequate training in anaesthesia and airway management.

● CONTRA-INDICATIONS CNS depression · compromised airway · respiratory depression

● CAUTIONS Muscle weakness · organic brain changes · parenteral administration
CAUTIONS, FURTHER INFORMATION
▸ Paradoxical effects A paradoxical increase in hostility and aggression may be reported by patients taking benzodiazepines. The effects range from talkativeness and excitement to aggressive and antisocial acts. Adjustment of the dose (up or down) sometimes attenuates the impulses. Increased anxiety and perceptual disorders are other paradoxical effects.
▸ Special precautions for parenteral administration When given parenterally, facilities for managing respiratory depression with mechanical ventilation must be available. Close observation required until full recovery from sedation.

● INTERACTIONS → Appendix 1: benzodiazepines

● SIDE-EFFECTS
GENERAL SIDE-EFFECTS
▸ **Common or very common** Apnoea · asthenia · coma · disinhibition · extrapyramidal symptoms · hypothermia · memory loss · speech slurred
▸ **Uncommon** Allergic dermatitis · constipation · sexual dysfunction
▸ **Rare or very rare** Agranulocytosis · hyponatraemia · pancytopenia · SIADH · thrombocytopenia
▸ **Frequency not known** Suicidal behaviours
SPECIFIC SIDE-EFFECTS
▸ **Common or very common**
▸ With parenteral use Vertigo
▸ **Rare or very rare**
▸ With oral use Saliva altered
▸ **Frequency not known**
▸ With oral use Psychosis
▸ With parenteral use Leucopenia

● BREAST FEEDING Benzodiazepines are present in milk, and should be avoided if possible during breast-feeding.

4

Nervous system

- **DIRECTIONS FOR ADMINISTRATION**
- In children For *intravenous injection*, dilute with an equal volume of Sodium Chloride 0.9% (for neonates, dilute injection solution to a concentration of 100 micrograms/mL). Give into a large vein over 3–5 minutes; max. rate 50 micrograms/kg over 3 minutes.
- In adults For *intramuscular injection*, solution for injection should be diluted with an equal volume of water for injections or sodium chloride 0.9% (but only use when oral and intravenous routes not possible). For *slow intravenous injection*, solution for injection should preferably be diluted with an equal volume of water for injections or sodium chloride 0.9%. Give into a large vein.

- **PATIENT AND CARER ADVICE**
Driving and skilled tasks Patients given sedatives and analgesics during minor outpatient procedures should be very carefully warned about the risks of undertaking skilled tasks (e.g. driving) afterwards. For intravenous benzodiazepines the risk extends to **at least 24 hours** after administration. Responsible persons should be available to take patients home afterwards. The dangers of taking **alcohol** should be emphasised.

- **MEDICINAL FORMS** There can be variation in the licensing of different medicines containing the same drug. Forms available from special-order manufacturers include: oral suspension, oral solution, solution for injection

Solution for injection
EXCIPIENTS: May contain Benzyl alcohol, propylene glycol
- Lorazepam (Non-proprietary)
   Lorazepam 2 mg per 1 ml Lorazepam 2mg/1ml solution for injection Carpuject cartridges | 10 cartridge PoM ⚠ (Hospital only) CD4-1
   Lorazepam 2mg/1ml solution for injection vials |
   10 vial PoM ⚠ CD4-1
   Lorazepam 4 mg per 1 ml Ativan 4mg/1ml solution for injection vials | 25 vial PoM ⚠ (Hospital only) CD4-1
   Lorazepam 4mg/1ml solution for injection ampoules |
   10 ampoule PoM £150.00 DT = £150.00 CD4-1

Oral tablet
CAUTIONARY AND ADVISORY LABELS 2
EXCIPIENTS: May contain Tartrazine
- Lorazepam (Non-proprietary)
   Lorazepam 250 microgram Lorazepam 250microgram tablets | 28 tablet PoM £32.20–£56.00 DT = £32.20 CD4-1
   Lorazepam 500 microgram Lorazepam 500microgram tablets | 28 tablet PoM £24.50 DT = £16.74 CD4-1
   Lorazepam 1 mg Lorazepam 1mg tablets | 28 tablet PoM £28.00 DT = £2.43 CD4-1
   Lorazepam 2.5 mg Lorazepam 2.5mg tablets | 28 tablet PoM £11.43 DT = £3.31 CD4-1

Oral solution
CAUTIONARY AND ADVISORY LABELS 2
EXCIPIENTS: May contain Ethanol
- Lorazepam (Non-proprietary)
   Lorazepam 1 mg per 1 ml Lorazepam 1mg/ml oral solution sugar free | 150 ml PoM £126.83–£181.63 DT = £181.63 CD4-1 SF

► 397

Midazolam

10-Jul-2024

- **INDICATIONS AND DOSE**

Status epilepticus | Febrile convulsions
- BY BUCCAL ADMINISTRATION
- Child 1–2 months: 300 micrograms/kg for 1 dose (max. per dose 2.5 mg), then 300 micrograms/kg for 1 dose (max. per dose 2.5 mg), to be given 5–10 minutes after first dose if required
- Child 3–11 months: 2.5 mg for 1 dose, then 2.5 mg for 1 dose, to be given 5–10 minutes seizer first dose if required
- Child 1–4 years: 5 mg for 1 dose, then 5 mg for 1 dose, to be given 5–10 minutes after first dose if required
- Child 5–9 years: 7.5 mg for 1 dose, then 7.5 mg for 1 dose, to be given 5–10 minutes after first dose if required

- Child 10–17 years: 10 mg for 1 dose, then 10 mg for 1 dose, to be given 5–10 minutes after first dose if required
- Adult: 10 mg for 1 dose, then 10 mg for 1 dose, to be given 5–10 minutes after first dose if required

Conscious sedation for procedures
- BY SLOW INTRAVENOUS INJECTION
- Adult: Initially 2–2.5 mg for 1 dose, to be administered 5–10 minutes before procedure at a rate of approximately 2 mg/minute, dose increased in steps of 1 mg if required, usual total dose is 3.5–5 mg; maximum 7.5 mg per course
- Elderly: Initially 0.5–1 mg for 1 dose, to be administered 5–10 minutes before procedure at a rate of approximately 2 mg/minute, dose increased in steps of 0.5–1 mg if required; maximum 3.5 mg per course

Sedative in combined anaesthesia
- INITIALLY BY INTRAVENOUS INJECTION
- Adult: 30–100 micrograms/kg, repeated if necessary, alternatively (by continuous intravenous infusion) 30–100 micrograms/kg/hour
- Elderly: Lower doses needed

Premedication
- BY DEEP INTRAMUSCULAR INJECTION
- Adult: 70–100 micrograms/kg for 1 dose, to be administered 20–60 minutes before induction
- Elderly: 25–50 micrograms/kg for 1 dose, to be administered 20–60 minutes before induction
- BY INTRAVENOUS INJECTION
- Adult: 1–2 mg for 1 dose, to be administered 5–30 minutes before procedure, dose can be repeated if necessary
- Elderly: 0.5 mg for 1 dose, to be administered 5–30 minutes before procedure, dose can be repeated if necessary, repeat dose slowly as required

Premedication [for debilitated patients]
- BY DEEP INTRAMUSCULAR INJECTION
- Adult: 25–50 micrograms/kg for 1 dose, to be administered 20–60 minutes before induction
- BY INTRAVENOUS INJECTION
- Adult: 0.5 mg for 1 dose, to be administered 5–30 minutes before procedure, dose can be repeated if necessary, repeat dose slowly as required

Induction of anaesthesia (but rarely used)
- BY SLOW INTRAVENOUS INJECTION
- Adult: 150–200 micrograms/kg daily in divided doses (max. per dose 5 mg), dose to be given at intervals of 2 minutes, maximum total dose 600 micrograms/kg
- Elderly: 50–150 micrograms/kg daily in divided doses (max. per dose 5 mg), dose to be given at intervals of 2 minutes, maximum total dose 600 micrograms/kg

Induction of anaesthesia (but rarely used) [for debilitated patients]
- BY SLOW INTRAVENOUS INJECTION
- Adult: 50–150 micrograms/kg daily in divided doses (max. per dose 5 mg), dose to be given at intervals of 2 minutes, maximum total dose 600 micrograms/kg

Sedation of patient receiving intensive care
- INITIALLY BY SLOW INTRAVENOUS INJECTION
- Adult: Initially 30–300 micrograms/kg, dose to be given in steps of 1–2.5 mg every 2 minutes, then (by slow intravenous injection or by continuous intravenous infusion) 30–200 micrograms/kg/hour, reduce dose (or reduce or omit initial dose) in hypovolaemia, vasoconstriction, or hypothermia, lower doses may be adequate if opioid analgesic also used

Agitation in palliative care for the imminently dying [initial titration]
▶ BY SUBCUTANEOUS INJECTION, OR BY SLOW INTRAVENOUS INJECTION
▶ Adult: 2.5–5 mg every 1 hour as required, usual max. 60 mg per day, doses higher than usual max. occasionally used on expert advice, increased if necessary up to 10 mg every 1 hour as required, usual max. 60 mg per day, doses higher than usual max. occasionally used on expert advice

Agitation in palliative care for the imminently dying [maintenance dose after initial titration]
▶ BY CONTINUOUS SUBCUTANEOUS INFUSION, OR BY CONTINUOUS INTRAVENOUS INFUSION
▶ Adult: 10–60 mg/24 hours, higher doses occasionally used on expert advice

Convulsions in palliative care for the imminently dying [prophylaxis or maintenance dose after acute treatment]
▶ BY CONTINUOUS SUBCUTANEOUS INFUSION
▶ Adult: 20–30 mg/24 hours

● **UNLICENSED USE** Unlicensed oromucosal formulations are also available and may have different doses—refer to product literature. Oromucosal solution not licensed for use in children under 3 months. Oromucosal solution not licensed for use in adults over 18 years. Specialist sources support use in palliative care, but it is not licensed for these indications.

IMPORTANT SAFETY INFORMATION
ANAESTHESIA
Benzodiazepines should only be administered for anaesthesia by, or under the direct supervision of, personnel experienced in their use, with adequate training in anaesthesia and airway management.

NHS NEVER EVENT: MIS-SELECTION OF HIGH-STRENGTH MIDAZOLAM DURING CONSCIOUS SEDATION (JANUARY 2018).
In clinical areas performing conscious sedation, high-strength preparations (5 mg/mL in 2 mL and 10 mL ampoules, or 2 mg/mL in 5 mL ampoules) should **not** be selected in place of the 1 mg/mL preparation.
  The areas where high-strength midazolam is used should be restricted to those performing general anaesthesia, intensive care, palliative care, or areas where its use has been formally risk-assessed in the organisation. In these situations the higher strength may be more appropriate to administer the prescribed dose.
  It is advised that flumazenil is available when midazolam is used, to reverse the effects if necessary.

● **CONTRA-INDICATIONS** CNS depression · compromised airway · severe respiratory depression

● **CAUTIONS** Cardiac disease · children (particularly if cardiovascular impairment) · debilitated patients (reduce dose) (in children) · hypothermia · hypovolaemia (risk of severe hypotension) · risk of airways obstruction and hypoventilation in children under 6 months (monitor respiratory rate and oxygen saturation) · vasoconstriction
CAUTIONS, FURTHER INFORMATION
▶ Recovery when used for sedation Midazolam has a fast onset of action, recovery is faster than for other benzodiazepines such as diazepam, but may be significantly longer in the elderly, in patients with a low cardiac output, or after repeated dosing.

● **INTERACTIONS** → Appendix 1: benzodiazepines

● **SIDE-EFFECTS**
GENERAL SIDE-EFFECTS
▶ **Common or very common** Level of consciousness decreased · vomiting
▶ **Uncommon** Skin reactions

▶ **Rare or very rare** Apnoea · bradycardia · cardiac arrest · constipation · dry mouth · dyspnoea · hiccups · movement disorders · physical assault · respiratory disorders · vasodilation
▶ **Frequency not known** Appetite increased · disinhibition (severe; with sedative and peri-operative use) (in children) · fall · gastrointestinal disorder · saliva altered · urinary incontinence · vertigo
SPECIFIC SIDE-EFFECTS
▶ **Frequency not known**
▶ With buccal use Thrombosis
▶ With parenteral use Angioedema · drug abuse · drug withdrawal seizure · embolism and thrombosis
SIDE-EFFECTS, FURTHER INFORMATION Higher doses are associated with prolonged sedation and risk of hypoventilation. The co-administration of midazolam with other sedative, hypnotic, or CNS-depressant drugs results in increased sedation. Midazolam accumulates in adipose tissue, which can significantly prolong sedation, especially in patients with obesity, hepatic impairment or renal impairment.

Overdose There have been reports of overdosage when high strength midazolam has been used for conscious sedation. The use of high-strength midazolam (5mg/mL in 2mL and 10mL ampoules, or 2mg/mL in 5mL ampoules) should be restricted to general anaesthesia, intensive care, palliative care, or other situations where the risk has been assessed. It is advised that flumazenil is available when midazolam is used, to reverse the effects if necessary.

● **BREAST FEEDING** Small amount present in milk—avoid breast-feeding for 24 hours after administration (although amount probably too small to be harmful after single doses).

● **HEPATIC IMPAIRMENT** For *parenteral preparations* manufacturer advises caution in all degrees of impairment. **Dose adjustments** For *parenteral preparations* manufacturer advises consider dose reduction in all degrees of impairment.

● **RENAL IMPAIRMENT** Manufacturer advises use with caution in chronic renal failure.

● **DIRECTIONS FOR ADMINISTRATION** For *intravenous infusion* (*Hypnovel*®), give continuously in Glucose 5% or Sodium chloride 0.9%.
  For *buccal* administration, give the full dose slowly over 4–5 seconds into one buccal cavity (space between the gum and the cheek). Alternatively, give half the dose over 2–3 seconds into one side of the mouth, and then the other half into the other side of the mouth.

● **PRESCRIBING AND DISPENSING INFORMATION**
Palliative care For further information on the use of midazolam in palliative care, see www.medicinescomplete. com/#/content/palliative/benzodiazepines-and-z-drugs.

● **PATIENT AND CARER ADVICE** Patients or carers should be given advice on how and when to administer midazolam oromucosal solution.
  Patients given sedatives and analgesics during minor outpatient procedures should be very carefully warned about the risks of undertaking skilled tasks (e.g. driving) afterwards. For intravenous benzodiazepines the risk extends to **at least 24 hours** after administration. Responsible persons should be available to take patients home afterwards. The dangers of taking **alcohol** should be emphasised.
Medicines for Children leaflet: Midazolam for stopping seizures www.medicinesforchildren.org.uk/medicines/midazolam-for-stopping-seizures/

- **NATIONAL FUNDING/ACCESS DECISIONS**
For full details see funding body website
Scottish Medicines Consortium (SMC) decisions
▶ Midazolam oromucosal solution (*Epistatus*®) for the treatment of prolonged, acute, convulsive seizures in children and adolescents aged 10 to less than 18 years (November 2017) SMC No. 1279/17 Recommended

- **MEDICINAL FORMS** There can be variation in the licensing of different medicines containing the same drug. Forms available from special-order manufacturers include: oromucosal solution, solution for injection, infusion, solution for infusion

Solution for injection
▶ **Midazolam (Non-proprietary)**
Midazolam (as Midazolam hydrochloride) 1 mg per 1 ml Midazolam 5mg/5ml solution for injection ampoules | 10 ampoule [PoM] £13.59–£16.89 DT = £13.59 [CD3]
Midazolam 5mg/5ml solution for injection pre-filled syringes | 1 pre-filled disposable injection [PoM] £11.53 (Hospital only) [CD3]
Midazolam 2mg/2ml solution for injection ampoules | 10 ampoule [PoM] £9.30 DT = £9.30 [CD3]
Midazolam (as Midazolam hydrochloride) 2 mg per 1 ml Midazolam 10mg/5ml solution for injection ampoules | 10 ampoule [PoM] £6.75–£9.80 DT = £9.80 [CD3]
Midazolam (as Midazolam hydrochloride) 5 mg per 1 ml Midazolam 50mg/10ml solution for injection ampoules | 10 ampoule [PoM] £7.26 DT = £33.00 (Hospital only) [CD3] | 10 ampoule [PoM] £33.00–£33.77 DT = £33.00 [CD3]
Midazolam 15mg/3ml solution for injection ampoules | 10 ampoule [PoM] £7.26 (Hospital only) [CD3]
Midazolam 10mg/2ml solution for injection ampoules | 10 ampoule [PoM] £5.11–£8.94 DT = £5.43 [CD3]
▶ **Hypnovel** (Neon Healthcare Ltd)
Midazolam (as Midazolam hydrochloride) 5 mg per 1 ml Hypnovel 10mg/2ml solution for injection ampoules | 10 ampoule [PoM] £7.11 DT = £5.43 [CD3]

Solution for infusion
▶ **Midazolam (Non-proprietary)**
Midazolam (as Midazolam hydrochloride) 1 mg per 1 ml Midazolam 50mg/50ml solution for infusion vials | 1 vial [PoM] £9.56–£13.20 [CD3]
Midazolam (as Midazolam hydrochloride) 2 mg per 1 ml Midazolam 100mg/50ml solution for infusion vials | 1 vial [PoM] £14.85 (Hospital only) [CD3] | 1 vial [PoM] £9.96 [CD3]

Oromucosal solution
CAUTIONARY AND ADVISORY LABELS 2
EXCIPIENTS: May contain Ethanol
▶ **Midazolam (Non-proprietary)**
Midazolam (as Midazolam hydrochloride) 5 mg per 1 ml Midazolam 10mg/2ml oromucosal solution pre-filled oral syringes sugar free | 4 unit dose [PoM] £91.00–£91.50 DT = £91.50 Schedule 3 (CD No Register Exempt Safe Custody) [SF]
Midazolam 5mg/1ml oromucosal solution pre-filled oral syringes sugar free | 4 unit dose [PoM] £85.00–£85.50 DT = £85.50 Schedule 3 (CD No Register Exempt Safe Custody) [SF]
Midazolam 2.5mg/0.5ml oromucosal solution pre-filled oral syringes sugar free | 4 unit dose [PoM] £81.00–£82.00 DT = £82.00 Schedule 3 (CD No Register Exempt Safe Custody) [SF]
Midazolam 7.5mg/1.5ml oromucosal solution pre-filled oral syringes sugar free | 4 unit dose [PoM] £88.00–£89.00 DT = £89.00 Schedule 3 (CD No Register Exempt Safe Custody) [SF]
▶ **Buccolam** (Neuraxpharm UK Ltd)
Midazolam (as Midazolam hydrochloride) 5 mg per 1 ml Buccolam 7.5mg/1.5ml oromucosal solution pre-filled oral syringes | 4 unit dose [PoM] £89.00 DT = £89.00 Schedule 3 (CD No Register Exempt Safe Custody) [SF]
Buccolam 10mg/2ml oromucosal solution pre-filled oral syringes | 4 unit dose [PoM] £91.50 DT = £91.50 Schedule 3 (CD No Register Exempt Safe Custody) [SF]
Buccolam 5mg/1ml oromucosal solution pre-filled oral syringes | 4 unit dose [PoM] £85.50 DT = £85.50 Schedule 3 (CD No Register Exempt Safe Custody) [SF]
Buccolam 2.5mg/0.5ml oromucosal solution pre-filled oral syringes | 4 unit dose [PoM] £82.00 DT = £82.00 Schedule 3 (CD No Register Exempt Safe Custody) [SF]
▶ **Epistatus** (SERB)
Midazolam (as Midazolam maleate) 10 mg per 1 ml Epistatus 5mg/0.5ml oromucosal solution pre-filled oral syringes | 1 unit dose [PoM] £43.75 DT = £43.75 Schedule 3 (CD No Register Exempt Safe Custody) [SF]

Epistatus 10mg/1ml oromucosal solution pre-filled oral syringes | 1 unit dose [PoM] £45.76 DT = £45.76 Schedule 3 (CD No Register Exempt Safe Custody) [SF]
Epistatus 2.5mg/0.25ml oromucosal solution pre-filled oral syringes | 1 unit dose [PoM] £43.75 DT = £43.75 Schedule 3 (CD No Register Exempt Safe Custody) [SF]
Epistatus 7.5mg/0.75ml oromucosal solution pre-filled oral syringes | 1 unit dose [PoM] £43.75 DT = £43.75 Schedule 3 (CD No Register Exempt Safe Custody) [SF]

3 Mental health disorders

3.1 Anxiety

> **Other drugs used for Anxiety** Duloxetine, p. 426 · Escitalopram, p. 423 · Lorazepam, p. 393 · Moclobemide, p. 420 · Paroxetine, p. 425 · Pericyazine, p. 447 · Pregabalin, p. 374 · Trazodone hydrochloride, p. 429 · Trifluoperazine, p. 450 · Venlafaxine, p. 427

ANTIDEPRESSANTS › SEROTONIN RECEPTOR AGONISTS

Buspirone hydrochloride

07-Jan-2021

- **INDICATIONS AND DOSE**
Anxiety (short-term use)
▶ BY MOUTH
▶ Adult: 5 mg 2–3 times a day, increased if necessary up to 45 mg daily, dose to be increased at intervals of 2–3 days; usual dose 15–30 mg daily in divided doses
DOSE ADJUSTMENTS DUE TO INTERACTIONS
▶ Manufacturer advises reduce dose to 2.5 mg twice daily with concurrent use of potent inhibitors of CYP3A4.

- **CONTRA-INDICATIONS** Epilepsy

- **CAUTIONS** Angle-closure glaucoma · does not alleviate symptoms of benzodiazepine withdrawal · myasthenia gravis
CAUTIONS, FURTHER INFORMATION Manufacturer advises a patient taking a benzodiazepine still needs to have the benzodiazepine withdrawn gradually; it is advisable to do this before starting buspirone.

- **INTERACTIONS** → Appendix 1: buspirone

- **SIDE-EFFECTS**
▶ **Common or very common** Abdominal pain · anger · anxiety · chest pain · cold sweat · concentration impaired · confusion · constipation · depression · diarrhoea · dizziness · drowsiness · dry mouth · fatigue · headache · laryngeal pain · movement disorders · musculoskeletal pain · nasal congestion · nausea · paraesthesia · skin reactions · sleep disorders · tachycardia · tinnitus · tremor · vision disorders · vomiting
▶ **Rare or very rare** Depersonalisation · emotional lability · galactorrhoea · hallucination · memory loss · parkinsonism · psychotic disorder · seizure · serotonin syndrome · syncope · urinary retention

- **PREGNANCY** Avoid.

- **BREAST FEEDING** Avoid.

- **HEPATIC IMPAIRMENT** Manufacturer advises caution; avoid in severe hepatic failure.
Dose adjustments Manufacturer advises titrate individual dose carefully in cirrhosis—consult product literature.

- **RENAL IMPAIRMENT** Avoid if eGFR less than 20 mL/minute/1.73 m^2.
Dose adjustments Reduce dose.

- **PATIENT AND CARER ADVICE**
Driving and skilled tasks May affect performance of skilled tasks (e.g. driving); effects of alcohol may be enhanced.

- **MEDICINAL FORMS** There can be variation in the licensing of different medicines containing the same drug. Forms available from special-order manufacturers include: oral suspension, oral solution

  Oral tablet
  ▸ Buspirone hydrochloride (Non-proprietary)
  Buspirone hydrochloride 5 mg Buspirone 5mg tablets | 30 tablet [PoM] £13.30 DT = £3.56
  Buspirone hydrochloride 7.5 mg Buspirone 7.5mg tablets | 30 tablet [PoM] £15.00 DT = £15.00
  Buspirone hydrochloride 10 mg Buspirone 10mg tablets | 30 tablet [PoM] £28.50 DT = £4.32
  Buspirone hydrochloride 15 mg Buspirone 15mg tablets | 30 tablet [PoM] £23.33-£37.32 DT = £23.33

HYPNOTICS, SEDATIVES AND ANXIOLYTICS ›
BENZODIAZEPINES

Benzodiazepines

> **IMPORTANT SAFETY INFORMATION**
>
> MHRA/CHM ADVICE: BENZODIAZEPINES AND OPIOIDS: REMINDER OF RISK OF POTENTIALLY FATAL RESPIRATORY DEPRESSION (MARCH 2020)
>
> The MHRA reminds healthcare professionals that benzodiazepines and benzodiazepine-like drugs co-prescribed with opioids can produce additive CNS depressant effects, thereby increasing the risk of sedation, respiratory depression, coma, and death. Healthcare professionals are advised to only co-prescribe if there is no alternative and, if necessary, the lowest possible doses should be given for the shortest duration. Patients should be closely monitored for signs of respiratory depression at initiation of treatment and when there is any change in prescribing, such as dose adjustments or new interactions. If methadone is co-prescribed with a benzodiazepine or benzodiazepine-like drug, the respiratory depressant effect of methadone may be delayed; patients should be monitored for at least 2 weeks after initiation or changes in prescribing. Patients should be informed of the signs and symptoms of respiratory depression and sedation, and advised to seek urgent medical attention should these occur.

- **CONTRA-INDICATIONS** Acute pulmonary insufficiency · marked neuromuscular respiratory weakness · not for use alone to treat chronic psychosis (in adults) · not for use alone to treat depression (or anxiety associated with depression) (in adults) · obsessional states · phobic states · sleep apnoea syndrome · unstable myasthenia gravis

- **CAUTIONS** Avoid prolonged use (and abrupt withdrawal thereafter) · debilitated patients (reduce dose) (in adults) · elderly (reduce dose) · history of alcohol dependence or abuse · history of drug dependence or abuse · myasthenia gravis · personality disorder (within the fearful group— dependent, avoidant, obsessive-compulsive) may increase risk of dependence · respiratory disease

  CAUTIONS, FURTHER INFORMATION
  ▸ Paradoxical effects A paradoxical increase in hostility and aggression may be reported by patients taking benzodiazepines. The effects range from talkativeness and excitement to aggressive and antisocial acts. Adjustment of the dose (up or down) sometimes attenuates the impulses. Increased anxiety and perceptual disorders are other paradoxical effects.
  ▸ Elderly Screening Tool of Older Persons' potentially inappropriate Prescriptions (STOPP) criteria to aid medication reviews (see Prescribing in the elderly p. 31 for information). Potentially inappropriate:
    - for a duration of 4 weeks or longer (no indication for longer treatment; risk of adverse events; all benzodiazepines should be withdrawn gradually if taken

for more than 2 weeks as there is a risk of causing a benzodiazepine withdrawal syndrome if stopped abruptly)
    - with acute or chronic respiratory failure i.e. $PaO_2 < 8\,kPa$ with or without $PaCO_2 > 6.5\,kPa$ (risk of exacerbation of respiratory failure)
    - in patients prone to falls (sedative, may cause reduced sensorium and impair balance)

- **SIDE-EFFECTS**
  ▸ **Common or very common** Alertness decreased · anxiety · ataxia (more common in elderly) · confusion (more common in elderly) · depression · dizziness · drowsiness · dysarthria · fatigue · headache · hypotension · mood altered · muscle weakness · nausea · respiratory depression (particularly with high dose and intravenous use—facilities for its treatment are essential) · sleep disorders · tremor · vision disorders · withdrawal syndrome
  ▸ **Uncommon** Agitation (more common in children and elderly) · anterograde amnesia · behaviour abnormal · hallucination · libido disorder · rash
  ▸ **Rare or very rare** Aggression (more common in children and elderly) · blood disorder · delusions · jaundice · paradoxical drug reaction · restlessness (with sedative and peri-operative use) · urinary retention
  ▸ **Frequency not known** Drug dependence

  Overdose Benzodiazepines taken alone cause drowsiness, ataxia, dysarthria, nystagmus, and occasionally respiratory depression, and coma. For details on the management of poisoning, see Benzodiazepines, under Emergency treatment of poisoning p. 1554.

- **PREGNANCY** Risk of neonatal withdrawal symptoms when used during pregnancy. Avoid regular use and use only if there is a clear indication such as seizure control. High doses administered during late pregnancy or labour may cause neonatal hypothermia, hypotonia, and respiratory depression.

- **HEPATIC IMPAIRMENT** In general, manufacturers advise caution in mild to moderate impairment; avoid in severe impairment. Benzodiazepines with a shorter half-life are considered safer.
  Dose adjustments In general, manufacturers advise dose reduction in mild to moderate impairment, adjust dose according to response.

- **RENAL IMPAIRMENT** In general, manufacturers advise caution (risk of increased cerebral sensitivity to benzodiazepines).
  Dose adjustments In general, manufacturers advise to consider dose reduction.

- **PATIENT AND CARER ADVICE**
  Driving and skilled tasks May cause drowsiness, impair judgement and increase reaction time, and so affect ability to drive or perform skilled tasks; effects of alcohol increased. Moreover the hangover effects of a night dose may impair performance on the following day.

  For information on 2015 legislation regarding driving whilst taking certain controlled drugs, including benzodiazepines, see *Drugs and driving* under Guidance on prescribing p. 1.

☞ above

Alprazolam
14-Oct-2021

- **INDICATIONS AND DOSE**

  Short-term use in anxiety
  ▸ **BY MOUTH**
  ▸ **Adult:** 250–500 micrograms 3 times a day, increased if necessary up to 3 mg daily, for debilitated patients, use elderly dose
  ▸ **Elderly:** 250 micrograms 2–3 times a day, increased if necessary up to 3 mg daily

- **CONTRA-INDICATIONS** Respiratory depression
- **CAUTIONS** Muscle weakness · organic brain changes
- **INTERACTIONS** → Appendix 1: benzodiazepines
- **SIDE-EFFECTS**
  - ▶ **Common or very common** Appetite decreased · concentration impaired · constipation · dermatitis · dry mouth · memory loss · movement disorders · sexual dysfunction · weight changes
  - ▶ **Uncommon** Menstruation irregular · urinary incontinence
  - ▶ **Frequency not known** Angioedema · autonomic dysfunction · gastrointestinal disorder · hepatic disorders · hyperprolactinaemia · peripheral oedema · photosensitivity reaction · psychosis · suicide · thinking abnormal
- **BREAST FEEDING** Benzodiazepines are present in milk, and should be avoided if possible during breast-feeding.
- **NATIONAL FUNDING/ACCESS DECISIONS**
  NHS restrictions Alprazolam tablets are not prescribable in NHS primary care.

- **MEDICINAL FORMS** There can be variation in the licensing of different medicines containing the same drug.
  Oral tablet
  CAUTIONARY AND ADVISORY LABELS 2
  - ▶ **Xanax** (Viatris UK Healthcare Ltd)
    Alprazolam 250 microgram Xanax 250microgram tablets | 60 tablet [PoM] £3.18 [CD4-1]
    Alprazolam 500 microgram Xanax 500microgram tablets | 60 tablet [PoM] £6.09 [CD4-1]

▶ 397

Chlordiazepoxide hydrochloride

14-Oct-2021

- **INDICATIONS AND DOSE**
  Short-term use in anxiety
  - ▶ BY MOUTH
    - ▶ Adult: 10 mg 3 times a day, increased if necessary to 60–100 mg daily in divided doses, for debilitated patients, use elderly dose
    - ▶ Elderly: 5 mg 3 times a day, increased if necessary to 30–50 mg daily in divided doses

  Treatment of alcohol withdrawal in moderate dependence
  - ▶ BY MOUTH
    - ▶ Adult: 10–30 mg 4 times a day, dose to be gradually reduced over 5–7 days, consult local protocols for titration regimens

  Treatment of alcohol withdrawal in severe dependence
  - ▶ BY MOUTH
    - ▶ Adult: 10–50 mg 4 times a day and 10–40 mg as required for the first 2 days, dose to be gradually reduced over 7–10 days, consult local protocols for titration regimens; maximum 250 mg per day

- **CONTRA-INDICATIONS** Chronic psychosis · respiratory depression
- **CAUTIONS** Muscle weakness · organic brain changes
- **INTERACTIONS** → Appendix 1: benzodiazepines
- **SIDE-EFFECTS**
  - ▶ **Common or very common** Movement disorders
  - ▶ **Rare or very rare** Abdominal distress · agranulocytosis · bone marrow disorders · erectile dysfunction · leucopenia · menstrual disorder · skin eruption · thrombocytopenia · urinary incontinence · vertigo
  - ▶ **Frequency not known** Appetite increased · gait abnormal · increased risk of fall · level of consciousness decreased · memory loss · psychosis · saliva altered · suicidal behaviours
- **BREAST FEEDING** Benzodiazepines are present in milk, and should be avoided if possible during breast-feeding.

- **HEPATIC IMPAIRMENT**
  Dose adjustments Manufacturer advises dose reduction to max. 50% of the usual dose in mild to moderate impairment.
- **RENAL IMPAIRMENT**
  Dose adjustments Manufacturer advises dose reduction to max. 50% of the usual dose.
- **NATIONAL FUNDING/ACCESS DECISIONS**
  NHS restrictions *Librium*® is not prescribable in NHS primary care.

- **MEDICINAL FORMS** There can be variation in the licensing of different medicines containing the same drug. Forms available from special-order manufacturers include: oral suspension, oral solution
  Oral capsule
  CAUTIONARY AND ADVISORY LABELS 2
  - ▶ **Chlordiazepoxide hydrochloride (Non-proprietary)**
    Chlordiazepoxide hydrochloride 5 mg Chlordiazepoxide 5mg capsules | 100 capsule [PoM] £20.00 DT = £6.12 [CD4-1]
    Chlordiazepoxide hydrochloride 10 mg Chlordiazepoxide 10mg capsules | 100 capsule [PoM] £25.00 DT = £7.19 [CD4-1]
  - ▶ **Librium** (Viatris UK Healthcare Ltd)
    Chlordiazepoxide hydrochloride 5 mg Librium 5mg capsules | 100 capsule [PoM] £5.38 DT = £6.12 [CD4-1]
    Chlordiazepoxide hydrochloride 10 mg Librium 10mg capsules | 100 capsule [PoM] £7.46 DT = £7.19 [CD4-1]

▶ 397

Diazepam

16-Apr-2024

- **INDICATIONS AND DOSE**
  Muscle spasm of varied aetiology
  - ▶ BY MOUTH
    - ▶ Adult: 2–15 mg daily in divided doses, then increased if necessary to 60 mg daily, adjusted according to response, dose only increased in spastic conditions

  Acute muscle spasm
  - ▶ BY INTRAMUSCULAR INJECTION, OR BY SLOW INTRAVENOUS INJECTION
    - ▶ Adult: 10 mg for 1 dose, then 10 mg for 1 dose, to be administered 4 hours after first dose if required

  Tetanus
  - ▶ BY INTRAVENOUS INJECTION
    - ▶ Child: 100–300 micrograms/kg every 1–4 hours
    - ▶ Adult: 100–300 micrograms/kg every 1–4 hours
  - ▶ BY CONTINUOUS INTRAVENOUS INFUSION
    - ▶ Child: 3–10 mg/kg/24 hours, dose to be adjusted according to response
    - ▶ Adult: 3–10 mg/kg/24 hours, dose to be adjusted according to response
  - ▶ BY NASODUODENAL TUBE
    - ▶ Child: 3–10 mg/kg, dose to be given over 24 hours, dose to be adjusted according to response
    - ▶ Adult: 3–10 mg/kg, dose to be given over 24 hours, dose to be adjusted according to response

  Muscle spasm in cerebral spasticity or in postoperative skeletal muscle spasm
  - ▶ BY MOUTH
    - ▶ Child 1-11 months: Initially 250 micrograms/kg twice daily
    - ▶ Child 1-4 years: Initially 2.5 mg twice daily
    - ▶ Child 5-11 years: Initially 5 mg twice daily
    - ▶ Child 12-17 years: Initially 10 mg twice daily, dose can be increased if necessary up to maximum 40 mg per day

  Anxiety
  - ▶ BY MOUTH
    - ▶ Adult: 2 mg 3 times a day, dose can be increased if necessary to 15–30 mg daily in divided doses
    - ▶ Elderly: 1 mg 3 times a day, dose can be increased if necessary to 7.5–15 mg daily in divided doses

Anxiety [for debilitated patients]
▶ BY MOUTH
▸ Adult: 1 mg 3 times a day, dose can be increased if necessary to 7.5–15 mg daily in divided doses

Insomnia associated with anxiety
▶ BY MOUTH
▸ Adult: 5–15 mg once daily, to be taken at bedtime

Severe acute anxiety | Control of acute panic attacks | Acute alcohol withdrawal
▶ BY INTRAMUSCULAR INJECTION, OR BY SLOW INTRAVENOUS INJECTION
▸ Adult: 10 mg for 1 dose, then 10 mg for 1 dose, to be administered 4 hours after first dose if required

Acute drug-induced dystonic reactions
▶ BY INTRAVENOUS INJECTION
▸ Adult: 5–10 mg for 1 dose, then 5–10 mg, to be administered at least 10 minutes after previous dose as required

Acute anxiety and agitation
▶ BY RECTUM
▸ Adult: 500 micrograms/kg for 1 dose, then 500 micrograms/kg, to be given 12 hours after previous dose as required
▸ Elderly: 250 micrograms/kg for 1 dose, then 250 micrograms/kg, to be given 12 hours after previous dose as required

Premedication
▶ BY MOUTH
▸ Adult: 5–10 mg for 1 dose, to be given 1–2 hours before procedure
▸ Elderly: 2.5–5 mg for 1 dose, to be given 1–2 hours before procedure
▶ BY INTRAVENOUS INJECTION
▸ Adult: 100–200 micrograms/kg for 1 dose, to be administered immediately before procedure
▸ Elderly: 100 micrograms/kg for 1 dose, to be administered immediately before procedure

Premedication [for debilitated patients]
▶ BY MOUTH
▸ Adult: 2.5–5 mg for 1 dose, to be given 1–2 hours before procedure
▶ BY INTRAVENOUS INJECTION
▸ Adult: 100 micrograms/kg for 1 dose, to be administered immediately before procedure

Sedation in dental procedures carried out in hospital
▶ BY MOUTH
▸ Adult: Up to 20 mg for 1 dose, to be given 1–2 hours before procedure

Conscious sedation for procedures, and in conjunction with local anaesthesia
▶ BY MOUTH
▸ Adult: 5–10 mg for 1 dose, to be given 1–2 hours before procedure
▸ Elderly: 2.5–5 mg for 1 dose, to be given 1–2 hours before procedure

Conscious sedation for procedures, and in conjunction with local anaesthesia [for debilitated patients]
▶ BY MOUTH
▸ Adult: 2.5–5 mg for 1 dose, to be given 1–2 hours before procedure

Sedative cover for minor surgical and medical procedures
▶ BY INTRAVENOUS INJECTION
▸ Adult: 10–20 mg for 1 dose, to be administered immediately before procedure

Status epilepticus | Febrile convulsions | Convulsions due to poisoning
▶ BY INTRAVENOUS INJECTION
▸ Neonate: 300–400 micrograms/kg for 1 dose, then 300–400 micrograms/kg for 1 dose, to be administered 10 minutes after first dose if required.
▸ Child 1 month-11 years: 300–400 micrograms/kg for 1 dose (max. per dose 10 mg), then 300–400 micrograms/kg for 1 dose (max. per dose 10 mg), to be administered 10 minutes after first dose if required
▸ Child 12-17 years: 10 mg for 1 dose, then 10 mg for 1 dose, to be administered 10 minutes after first dose if required
▸ Adult: 10 mg for 1 dose, then 10 mg for 1 dose, to be administered 10 minutes after first dose if required
▶ BY RECTUM
▸ Neonate: 1.25–2.5 mg for 1 dose, then 1.25–2.5 mg for 1 dose, to be administered 5–10 minutes after first dose if required.
▸ Child 1 month-1 year: 5 mg for 1 dose, then 5 mg for 1 dose, to be administered 5–10 minutes after first dose if required
▸ Child 2-11 years: 5–10 mg for 1 dose, then 5–10 mg for 1 dose, to be administered 5–10 minutes after first dose if required
▸ Child 12-17 years: 10–20 mg for 1 dose, then 10–20 mg for 1 dose, to be administered 5–10 minutes after first dose if required
▸ Adult: 10–20 mg for 1 dose, then 10–20 mg for 1 dose, to be administered 5–10 minutes after first dose if required
▸ Elderly: 10 mg for 1 dose, then 10 mg for 1 dose, to be administered 5–10 minutes after first dose if required

Life-threatening acute drug-induced dystonic reactions
▶ BY INTRAVENOUS INJECTION
▸ Child 1 month-11 years: 100 micrograms/kg, dose can be repeated if necessary
▸ Child 12-17 years: 5–10 mg, dose can be repeated if necessary

Dyspnoea associated with anxiety in palliative care
▶ BY MOUTH
▸ Adult: 5–10 mg daily

Pain of muscle spasm in palliative care
▶ BY MOUTH
▸ Adult: 5–10 mg daily

● UNLICENSED USE
▸ With rectal use in children *Diazepam Desitin*®, *Diazepam Rectubes*®, and *Stesolid Rectal Tubes*® not licensed for use in children under 1 year.

> IMPORTANT SAFETY INFORMATION
> ANAESTHESIA
> Benzodiazepines should only be administered for anaesthesia by, or under the direct supervision of, personnel experienced in their use, with adequate training in anaesthesia and airway management.

● CONTRA-INDICATIONS Avoid injections containing benzyl alcohol in neonates · chronic psychosis (in adults) · CNS depression · compromised airway · hyperkinesis · respiratory depression

● CAUTIONS
GENERAL CAUTIONS Muscle weakness · organic brain changes · parenteral administration (close observation required until full recovery from sedation)
SPECIFIC CAUTIONS
▸ With intravenous use High risk of venous thrombophlebitis with intravenous use (reduced by using an emulsion formulation)
CAUTIONS, FURTHER INFORMATION
▸ Special precautions for intravenous injection When given intravenously facilities for reversing respiratory

depression with mechanical ventilation must be immediately available.

- **INTERACTIONS** → Appendix 1: benzodiazepines
- **SIDE-EFFECTS**
  GENERAL SIDE-EFFECTS
  ▸ **Common or very common** Appetite abnormal · concentration impaired · gastrointestinal disorder · movement disorders · muscle spasms · palpitations · sensory disorder · vomiting
  ▸ **Uncommon** Constipation · diarrhoea · hypersalivation · speech slurred
  ▸ **Rare or very rare** Bradycardia · bronchial secretion increased · cardiac arrest · dry mouth · gynaecomastia · heart failure · leucopenia · loss of consciousness · memory loss · respiratory arrest · sexual dysfunction · syncope · urinary incontinence · vertigo
  ▸ **Frequency not known** Apnoea · nystagmus
  SPECIFIC SIDE-EFFECTS
  ▸ **Uncommon**
  ▸ With intravenous or oral or rectal use Skin reactions
  ▸ **Rare or very rare**
  ▸ With intravenous or oral use Psychiatric disorder · psychosis
  ▸ With rectal use Psychosis
  ▸ **Frequency not known**
  ▸ With intramuscular use Chest pain · embolism and thrombosis · fall · increased risk of dementia · psychiatric disorders · soft tissue necrosis · urticaria
- **PREGNANCY** Women who have seizures in the second half of pregnancy should be assessed for eclampsia before any change is made to antiepileptic treatment. Status epilepticus should be treated according to the standard protocol.
  Epilepsy and Pregnancy Register All pregnant women with epilepsy, whether taking medication or not, should be encouraged to notify the UK Epilepsy and Pregnancy Register (Tel: 0800 389 1248).
- **BREAST FEEDING** Present in milk, and should be avoided if possible during breast-feeding.
- **DIRECTIONS FOR ADMINISTRATION**
  ▸ With intravenous use Diazepam is adsorbed by plastics of infusion bags and giving sets. Expert sources advise emulsion formulation preferred for intravenous use.
  ▸ In children EvGr For *continuous intravenous infusion* (emulsion) (*Diazemuls ®*), dilute to a concentration of max. 400 micrograms/mL with Glucose 5% or 10%; max. 6 hours between addition and completion of infusion. For *continuous intravenous infusion* (solution) (*Diazepam, Hameln*), dilute to a concentration of max. 80 micrograms/mL with Glucose 5% or Sodium Chloride 0.9%. ⟨M⟩
  ▸ For Status epilepticus or Febrile convulsions or Convulsions due to poisoning or Life-threatening acute drug-induced dystonic reactions in children EvGr For *intravenous injection*, give over 3–5 minutes. ⟨M⟩
  ▸ In adults EvGr For *intravenous injection*, administer into a large vein at a rate of no more than 5 mg/minute. For *intravenous infusion* (solution) (*Diazepam, Hameln*), give continuously *in* Glucose 5% or Sodium Chloride 0.9%. Dilute to a concentration of not more than 40 mg in 500 mL. For *intravenous infusion* (emulsion) (*Diazemuls ®*), give continuously *in* Glucose 5% or 10%. May be diluted to a max. concentration of 200 mg in 500 mL; max. 6 hours between addition and completion of administration. May be given *via* drip tubing *in* Glucose 5% or 10% or Sodium Chloride 0.9%. ⟨M⟩
  ▸ With intramuscular use or intravenous use in adults EvGr Solution for injection should not be diluted, except for intravenous infusion. ⟨M⟩
  ▸ With intramuscular use EvGr Only use intramuscular route when oral and intravenous routes not possible. ⟨M⟩

- **PRESCRIBING AND DISPENSING INFORMATION**
  Palliative care For further information on the use of diazepam in palliative care, see www.medicinescomplete. com/#/content/palliative/benzodiazepines-and-z-drugs.
- **PATIENT AND CARER ADVICE** Patients or carers should be given advice on how and when to administer rectal diazepam. Patients given sedatives and analgesics during minor outpatient procedures should be very carefully warned about the risks of undertaking skilled tasks (e.g. driving) afterwards. For intravenous benzodiazepines the risk extends to **at least 24 hours** after administration. Responsible persons should be available to take patients home afterwards. The dangers of taking **alcohol** should be emphasised.
  Medicines for Children leaflet: Diazepam (rectal) for stopping seizures www.medicinesforchildren.org.uk/medicines/ diazepam-rectal-for-stopping-seizures/
  Medicines for Children leaflet: Diazepam for muscle spasm www.medicinesforchildren.org.uk/medicines/diazepam-for- muscle-spasm/
- **PROFESSION SPECIFIC INFORMATION**
  Dental practitioners' formulary Diazepam Tablets may be prescribed.
  Diazepam Oral Solution 2 mg/5 mL may be prescribed.

- **MEDICINAL FORMS** There can be variation in the licensing of different medicines containing the same drug. Forms available from special-order manufacturers include: oral suspension, oral solution, suppository
  Oral tablet
  CAUTIONARY AND ADVISORY LABELS 2
  ▸ Diazepam (Non-proprietary)
    Diazepam 2 mg Diazepam 2mg tablets | 28 tablet PoM £0.79 DT = £0.65 CD4–1
    Diazepam 5 mg Diazepam 5mg tablets | 28 tablet PoM £0.81 DT = £0.67 CD4–1
    Diazepam 10 mg Diazepam 10mg tablets | 28 tablet PoM £0.87 DT = £0.75 CD4–1
  Solution for injection
  EXCIPIENTS: May contain Benzyl alcohol, ethanol, propylene glycol
  ▸ Diazepam (Non-proprietary)
    Diazepam 5 mg per 1 ml Diazepam 10mg/2ml solution for injection ampoules | 10 ampoule PoM £9.75–£31.00 DT = £31.00 CD4–1
  Oral suspension
  CAUTIONARY AND ADVISORY LABELS 2
  EXCIPIENTS: May contain Ethanol, hydroxybenzoates (parabens), potassium sorbate, sucrose
  Oral solution
  CAUTIONARY AND ADVISORY LABELS 2
  EXCIPIENTS: May contain Hydroxybenzoates (parabens), propylene glycol, sorbic acid, sorbitol
  ▸ Diazepam (Non-proprietary)
    Diazepam 400 microgram per 1 ml Diazepam 2mg/5ml oral solution sugar free | 100 ml PoM £95.00 DT = £95.00 CD4–1 SF
  Enema
  CAUTIONARY AND ADVISORY LABELS 2
  EXCIPIENTS: May contain Benzyl alcohol, ethanol, propylene glycol
  ▸ Diazepam (Non-proprietary)
    Diazepam 2 mg per 1 ml Diazepam 5mg/2.5ml rectal solution tube | 5 tube PoM £5.85 DT = £5.85 CD4–1
    Diazepam 4 mg per 1 ml Diazepam 10mg/2.5ml rectal solution tube | 5 tube PoM £8.78 DT = £8.78 CD4–1

⟨F 397⟩

Oxazepam

14-Oct-2021

- **INDICATIONS AND DOSE**
  Anxiety (short-term use)
  ▸ BY MOUTH
  ▸ Adult: 15–30 mg 3–4 times a day, for debilitated patients, use elderly dose
  ▸ Elderly: 10–20 mg 3–4 times a day

Insomnia associated with anxiety
▶ BY MOUTH
▶ Adult: 15–25 mg once daily (max. per dose 50 mg), dose to be taken at bedtime

- **CONTRA-INDICATIONS** Chronic psychosis · respiratory depression

- **CAUTIONS** Muscle weakness · organic brain changes

  CAUTIONS, FURTHER INFORMATION
  ▶ Paradoxical effects A paradoxical increase in hostility and aggression may be reported by patients taking benzodiazepines. The effects range from talkativeness and excitement to aggressive and antisocial acts. Adjustment of the dose (up or down) sometimes attenuates the impulses. Increased anxiety and perceptual disorders are other paradoxical effects.

- **INTERACTIONS** → Appendix 1: benzodiazepines

- **SIDE-EFFECTS** Fever · gastrointestinal disorder · leucopenia · memory loss · oedema · psychosis · saliva altered · speech slurred · suicidal ideation · syncope · urinary incontinence · urticaria · vertigo

- **BREAST FEEDING** Benzodiazepines are present in milk, and should be avoided if possible during breast-feeding.

- **MEDICINAL FORMS** There can be variation in the licensing of different medicines containing the same drug. Forms available from special-order manufacturers include: oral suspension

  Oral tablet
  CAUTIONARY AND ADVISORY LABELS 2
  ▶ Oxazepam (Non-proprietary)
  Oxazepam 10 mg Oxazepam 10mg tablets | 28 tablet [PoM] £13.73 DT = £4.04 [CD4-1]
  Oxazepam 15 mg Oxazepam 15mg tablets | 28 tablet [PoM] £13.44 DT = £2.93 [CD4-1]

3.2 Attention deficit hyperactivity disorder

Attention deficit hyperactivity disorder

04-Aug-2018

Description of condition

Attention deficit hyperactivity disorder (ADHD) is a behavioural disorder characterised by hyperactivity, impulsivity and inattention, which can lead to functional impairment such as psychological, social, educational or occupational difficulties. While these symptoms tend to co-exist, some patients are predominantly hyperactive and impulsive, while others are principally inattentive. Symptoms typically appear in children aged 3–7 years, but may not be recognised until after 7 years of age, especially if hyperactivity is not present. ADHD is more commonly diagnosed in males than in females.

ADHD is usually a persisting disorder and some children continue to have symptoms throughout adolescence and into adulthood, where inattentive symptoms tend to persist, and hyperactive-impulsive symptoms tend to recede over time. ADHD is also associated with an increased risk of disorders such as oppositional defiant disorder (ODD), conduct disorder, and possibly mood disorders such as depression, mania, and anxiety, as well as substance misuse.

Aims of treatment

The aims of treatment are to reduce functional impairment, severity of symptoms, and to improve quality of life.

Non-drug treatment

[EvGr] Patients should be advised about the importance of a balanced diet, good nutrition and regular exercise. [A]

Environmental modifications are changes made to the physical environment that can help reduce the impact of ADHD symptoms on a person's day-to-day life. [EvGr] The modifications should be specific to the person's circumstances, and may involve changes to seating arrangements, lighting and noise, reducing distractions, optimising work or education by having shorter periods of focus with movement breaks, and reinforcing verbal requests with written instructions. These changes should form part of the discussion at the time of diagnosis of ADHD and be trialled and reviewed for effectiveness before drug treatment is started.

ADHD focused psychological interventions which may involve elements of, or a complete course of cognitive behavioural therapy (CBT) may be effective in patients who have refused drug treatment, have difficulty with adherence, are intolerant of, or unresponsive to drug treatment. In patients who have benefited from drug treatment, but whose symptoms are still causing significant impairment in at least one area of function (such as interpersonal relationships, education and occupational attainment, and risk awareness), consider a combination of non-drug treatment with drug treatment. [A]

Drug treatment

[EvGr] Drug treatment should be initiated by a specialist trained in the diagnosis and management of ADHD. Following dose stabilisation, continuation and monitoring of drug treatment can be undertaken by the patient's general practitioner under a shared care arrangement. Treatment should be started in patients with ADHD whose symptoms are still causing significant impairment in at least one area of function, despite environmental modifications. Patients with ADHD and anxiety disorder, tic disorder, or autism spectrum disorder should be offered the same treatment options as other patients with ADHD.

Lisdexamfetamine mesilate p. 406 or methylphenidate hydrochloride p. 403 are recommended as first-line treatment. If symptoms have not improved following a 6-week trial of either drug, switching to the alternative first-line treatment should be considered. Dexamfetamine sulfate p. 405 [unlicensed] can be tried if the patient is having a beneficial response to lisdexamfetamine mesilate but cannot tolerate its longer duration of effect.

Modified-release preparations of stimulants are preferred because of their pharmacokinetic profile, convenience, improved adherence, reduced risk of drug diversion (drugs being forwarded to others for non-prescription use or misuse), and the lack of need to be taken to work. Immediate-release preparations can be given when more flexible dosing regimens are required, or during initial dose titration. A combination of modified-release and immediate-release preparations taken at different times of the day can be used to extend the duration of effect. The magnitude, duration of effect, and side-effects of stimulants vary between patients.

In patients who are intolerant to both methylphenidate hydrochloride p. 403 and lisdexamfetamine mesilate, or who have not responded to separate 6-week trials of both drugs, treatment with the non-stimulant atomoxetine p. 402 can be considered.

Advice from, or referral to a tertiary specialist ADHD service should be considered if the patient is unresponsive to one or more stimulant drugs (e.g. methylphenidate hydrochloride p. 403 and lisdexamfetamine mesilate) and atomoxetine p. 402. A specialist service should also be consulted for advice before starting treatment with guanfacine p. 407 [unlicensed], or an atypical antipsychotic in addition to stimulants in patients with ADHD and co-existing pervasive aggression, rages or irritability. If sustained orthostatic hypotension or fainting episodes occur with guanfacine p. 407 treatment, the dose should be reduced or an alternative treatment offered. ⒜

Other treatment options such as bupropion hydrochloride p. 566, modafinil p. 559, tricyclic antidepressants, and venlafaxine p. 427 [all unlicensed] have been used in the management of ADHD, but due to limited evidence their use is not recommended without specialist advice.

[EvGr] Patients should be monitored for effectiveness of medication and side-effects, as well as changes in sleep pattern, sexual dysfunction (associated with atomoxetine below), and stimulant diversion or misuse. If the patient develops new, or has worsening of existing seizures, review drug treatment and stop any drug that might be contributing to the seizures; treatment can be cautiously reintroduced if it is unlikely to be the cause. Monitor patients for the development of tics associated with stimulant use. If tics are stimulant related, consider a dose reduction, stopping treatment, or changing to a non-stimulant drug. If there is worsening of behaviour, consider adjusting drug treatment and reviewing the diagnosis.

Treatment should be reviewed by a specialist at least once a year and trials of treatment-free periods, or dose reductions considered where appropriate. ⒜

Useful Resources

Attention deficit hyperactivity disorder: diagnosis and management. National Institute for Health and Care Excellence. Clinical guideline 87. March 2018. www.nice.org.uk/guidance/ng87

CNS STIMULANTS > CENTRALLY ACTING SYMPATHOMIMETICS

Atomoxetine

26-Oct-2021

● **INDICATIONS AND DOSE**

Attention deficit hyperactivity disorder (initiated by a specialist)

▶ BY MOUTH

▸ Child 6–17 years (body-weight up to 70 kg): Initially 500 micrograms/kg daily for 7 days, dose is increased according to response; maintenance 1.2 mg/kg daily, total daily dose may be given either as a single dose in the morning or in 2 divided doses with last dose no later than early evening, high daily doses to be given under the direction of a specialist; maximum 1.8 mg/kg per day; maximum 120 mg per day

▸ Child 6–17 years (body-weight 70 kg and above): Initially 40 mg daily for 7 days, dose is increased according to response; maintenance 80 mg daily, total daily dose may be given either as a single dose in the morning or in 2 divided doses with last dose no later than early evening, high daily doses to be given under the direction of a specialist; maximum 120 mg per day

▸ Adult (body-weight up to 70 kg): Initially 500 micrograms/kg daily for 7 days, dose is increased according to response; maintenance 1.2 mg/kg daily, total daily dose may be given either as a single dose in the morning or in 2 divided doses with last dose no later than early evening, high daily doses to be given under the direction of a specialist; maximum 1.8 mg/kg per day; maximum 120 mg per day

▸ Adult (body-weight 70 kg and above): Initially 40 mg daily for 7 days, dose is increased according to response; maintenance 80–100 mg daily, total daily dose may be given either as a single dose in the morning or in 2 divided doses with last dose no later than early evening, high daily doses to be given under the direction of a specialist; maximum 120 mg per day

● **UNLICENSED USE** Atomoxetine doses in BNF may differ from those in product literature.

▸ In children Doses above 100 mg daily not licensed.

▸ In adults Dose maximum of 120 mg not licensed.

● **CONTRA-INDICATIONS** Phaeochromocytoma · severe cardiovascular disease · severe cerebrovascular disease

● **CAUTIONS** Aggressive behaviour · cardiovascular disease · cerebrovascular disease · emotional lability · history of seizures · hostility · hypertension · mania · psychosis · QT-interval prolongation · structural cardiac abnormalities · susceptibility to angle-closure glaucoma · tachycardia

● **INTERACTIONS** → Appendix 1: atomoxetine

● **SIDE-EFFECTS**

▸ **Common or very common** Anxiety · appetite decreased · arrhythmias (uncommon in children) · asthenia · chills (in adults) · constipation · depression · dizziness · drowsiness · dry mouth (in adults) · feeling jittery (in adults) · flatulence (in adults) · gastrointestinal discomfort · genital pain (rare in children) · headaches · hyperhidrosis (uncommon in children) · menstrual cycle irregularities (in adults) · mood altered · mydriasis (in children) · nausea · palpitations (uncommon in children) · prostatitis (in adults) · sensation abnormal (uncommon in children) · sexual dysfunction (rare in children) · skin reactions · sleep disorders · taste altered (in adults) · thirst (in adults) · tremor (uncommon in children) · urinary disorders (rare in children) · vasodilation (in adults) · vomiting · weight decreased

▸ **Uncommon** Behaviour abnormal · chest pain (very common in children) · dyspnoea · feeling cold (in adults) · hypersensitivity · muscle spasms (in adults) · peripheral coldness (in adults) · QT interval prolongation · suicidal behaviour · syncope · tic (very common in children) · vision blurred

▸ **Rare or very rare** Hallucination (uncommon in children) · hepatic disorders · psychosis (uncommon in children) · Raynaud's phenomenon · seizure (uncommon in children)

▸ **Frequency not known** Sudden cardiac death

● **PREGNANCY** Manufacturer advises avoid unless potential benefit outweighs risk.

● **BREAST FEEDING** Avoid-present in milk in *animal* studies.

● **HEPATIC IMPAIRMENT**

Dose adjustments Manufacturer advises halve dose in moderate impairment and quarter dose in severe impairment.

● **MONITORING REQUIREMENTS**

▸ Monitor for appearance or worsening of anxiety, depression or tics.

▸ Pulse, blood pressure, psychiatric symptoms, appetite, weight and height should be recorded at initiation of therapy, following each dose adjustment, and at least every 6 months thereafter.

● **PATIENT AND CARER ADVICE**

Suicidal ideation Following reports of suicidal thoughts and behaviour, patients and their carers should be informed about the risk and told to report clinical worsening, suicidal thoughts or behaviour, irritability, agitation, or depression.

Hepatic impairment Following rare reports of hepatic disorders, patients and carers should be advised of the risk and be told how to recognise symptoms; prompt medical attention should be sought in case of abdominal pain, unexplained nausea, malaise, darkening of the urine, or jaundice.

Medicines for Children leaflet: Atomoxetine for ADHD www.medicinesforchildren.org.uk/medicines/atomoxetine-for-adhd/

● NATIONAL FUNDING/ACCESS DECISIONS
For full details see funding body website
Scottish Medicines Consortium (SMC) decisions
▸ **Atomoxetine oral solution (*Strattera*®) for treatment of attention-deficit/hyperactivity disorder (ADHD) in children of 6 years and older, in adolescents and in adults as part of a comprehensive treatment programme (December 2015)** SMC No. 1107/15 Recommended with restrictions

● MEDICINAL FORMS There can be variation in the licensing of different medicines containing the same drug. Forms available from special-order manufacturers include: oral suspension, oral solution

Oral solution
CAUTIONARY AND ADVISORY LABELS 3
▸ Strattera (Eli Lilly and Company Ltd)
Atomoxetine (as Atomoxetine hydrochloride) 4 mg per 1 ml Strattera 4mg/1ml oral solution | 300 ml [PoM] £85.00 DT = £85.00 [SF]

Oral capsule
CAUTIONARY AND ADVISORY LABELS 3, 25
▸ Atomoxetine (Non-proprietary)
Atomoxetine (as Atomoxetine hydrochloride) 10 mg Atomoxetine 10mg capsules | 7 capsule [PoM] £9.12 | 28 capsule [PoM] £53.09 DT = £44.71
Atomoxetine (as Atomoxetine hydrochloride) 18 mg Atomoxetine 18mg capsules | 7 capsule [PoM] £9.12 | 28 capsule [PoM] £53.09 DT = £41.25
Atomoxetine (as Atomoxetine hydrochloride) 25 mg Atomoxetine 25mg capsules | 7 capsule [PoM] £9.18 | 28 capsule [PoM] £53.49 DT = £42.25
Atomoxetine (as Atomoxetine hydrochloride) 40 mg Atomoxetine 40mg capsules | 7 capsule [PoM] £9.15 | 28 capsule [PoM] £53.09 DT = £44.21
Atomoxetine (as Atomoxetine hydrochloride) 60 mg Atomoxetine 60mg capsules | 28 capsule [PoM] £53.67 DT = £43.16
Atomoxetine (as Atomoxetine hydrochloride) 80 mg Atomoxetine 80mg capsules | 28 capsule [PoM] £70.79 DT = £46.03
Atomoxetine (as Atomoxetine hydrochloride) 100 mg Atomoxetine 100mg capsules | 28 capsule [PoM] £70.79 DT = £43.46

Methylphenidate hydrochloride　07-Oct-2022

● **INDICATIONS AND DOSE**
Attention deficit hyperactivity disorder (initiated under specialist supervision)
▸ BY MOUTH USING IMMEDIATE-RELEASE MEDICINES
▸ Child 6-17 years: Initially 5 mg 1–2 times a day, increased in steps of 5–10 mg daily if required, at weekly intervals, increased if necessary up to 60 mg daily in 2–3 divided doses, increased if necessary up to 2.1 mg/kg daily in 2–3 divided doses, the licensed maximum dose is 60 mg daily in 2–3 doses, higher dose (up to a maximum of 90 mg daily) under the direction of a specialist, discontinue if no response after 1 month, if effect wears off in evening (with rebound hyperactivity) a dose at bedtime may be appropriate (establish need with trial bedtime dose). Treatment may be started using a modified-release preparation
▸ Adult: Initially 5 mg 2–3 times a day, dose is increased if necessary at weekly intervals according to response, increased if necessary up to 100 mg daily in 2–3 divided doses, if effect wears off in evening (with rebound hyperactivity) a dose at bedtime may be appropriate (establish need with trial bedtime dose). Treatment may be started using a modified-release preparation

Narcolepsy
▸ BY MOUTH USING IMMEDIATE-RELEASE MEDICINES
▸ Adult: 10–60 mg daily in divided doses; usual dose 20–30 mg daily in divided doses, dose to be taken before meals

DOSE EQUIVALENCE AND CONVERSION
▸ When switching from *immediate-release* preparations to *modified-release* preparations—consult product literature.

CONCERTA® XL
Attention deficit hyperactivity disorder
▸ BY MOUTH
▸ Child 6-17 years: Initially 18 mg once daily, dose to be taken in the morning, increased in steps of 18 mg every week, adjusted according to response; increased if necessary up to 2.1 mg/kg daily, licensed max. dose is 54 mg once daily, to be increased to higher dose only under direction of specialist; discontinue if no response after 1 month; maximum 108 mg per day
▸ Adult: Initially 18 mg once daily, dose to be taken in the morning; adjusted at weekly intervals according to response; maximum 108 mg per day

DOSE EQUIVALENCE AND CONVERSION
▸ Total daily dose of 15 mg of standard-release formulation is considered equivalent to *Concerta*® XL 18 mg once daily.

DELMOSART® PROLONGED-RELEASE TABLET
Attention deficit hyperactivity disorder (under expert supervision)
▸ BY MOUTH
▸ Child 6-17 years: Initially 18 mg once daily, dose to be taken in the morning, then increased in steps of 18 mg every week if required, discontinue if no response after 1 month; maximum 54 mg per day
▸ Adult: Initially 18 mg once daily, dose to be taken in the morning, then increased in steps of 18 mg every week if required, discontinue if no response after 1 month; maximum 54 mg per day

DOSE EQUIVALENCE AND CONVERSION
▸ Total daily dose of 15 mg of standard-release formulation is considered equivalent to *Delmosart*® 18 mg once daily.

EQUASYM® XL
Attention deficit hyperactivity disorder
▸ BY MOUTH
▸ Child 6-17 years: Initially 10 mg once daily, dose to be taken in the morning before breakfast; increased gradually at weekly intervals if necessary; increased if necessary up to 2.1 mg/kg daily, licensed max. dose is 60 mg daily, to be increased to higher dose only under direction of specialist; discontinue if no response after 1 month; maximum 90 mg per day
▸ Adult: Initially 10 mg once daily, dose to be taken in the morning before breakfast; increased gradually at weekly intervals if necessary; maximum 100 mg per day

MEDIKINET® XL
Attention deficit hyperactivity disorder
▸ BY MOUTH
▸ Child 6-17 years: Initially 10 mg once daily, dose to be taken in the morning with breakfast; adjusted at weekly intervals according to response; increased if necessary up to 2.1 mg/kg daily, licensed max. dose is 60 mg daily, to be increased to higher dose only under direction of specialist; discontinue if no response after 1 month; maximum 90 mg per day
▸ Adult: Initially 10 mg once daily, dose to be taken in the morning with breakfast; adjusted at weekly intervals according to response; maximum 100 mg per day

continued →

XAGGITIN ® XL

Attention deficit hyperactivity disorder (under expert supervision)
▶ BY MOUTH
▶ Child 6-17 years: Initially 18 mg once daily, dose to be taken in the morning, increased in steps of 18 mg every week, adjusted according to response, discontinue if no response after 1 month; maximum 54 mg per day
▶ Adult: Initially 18 mg once daily, dose to be taken in the morning, increased in steps of 18 mg every week, adjusted according to response, discontinue if no response after 1 month; maximum 54 mg per day

DOSE EQUIVALENCE AND CONVERSION
▶ Total daily dose of 15 mg of standard-release formulation is considered equivalent to *Xaggitin* ® XL 18 mg once daily.

● UNLICENSED USE Doses over 60 mg daily not licensed; doses of *Concerta* ® *XL* over 54 mg daily not licensed. Not licensed for use in narcolepsy. Not licensed for use in adults for attention deficit hyperactivity disorder.

IMPORTANT SAFETY INFORMATION

MHRA/CHM ADVICE: METHYLPHENIDATE LONG-ACTING (MODIFIED-RELEASE) PREPARATIONS: CAUTION IF SWITCHING BETWEEN PRODUCTS DUE TO DIFFERENCES IN FORMULATIONS (SEPTEMBER 2022)

All long-acting preparations of methylphenidate contain an immediate-release component and a modified-release component. The biphasic-release profiles of different preparations are not all equivalent and contain different proportions of immediate-release and modified-release components. The MHRA has advised caution when switching between such preparations, due to differences in dosing frequency, administration with food, amount and timing of the modified-release component, and overall clinical effect.

Healthcare professionals are advised to:
● follow the specific dosage recommendations for each preparation;
● discuss the reasons for switching with patients or their carers, including any possible changes in symptoms and side-effects;
● take patient preferences into account when considering a switch;
● provide counselling on administration of the new preparation, especially with regards to food;
● follow current clinical guidance on prescribing by brand name, or by manufacturer name if generic;
● avoid frequent switching between different preparations.

● CONTRA-INDICATIONS Anorexia nervosa · arrhythmias · cardiomyopathy · cardiovascular disease · cerebrovascular disorders · heart failure · hyperthyroidism · mania · phaeochromocytoma · psychosis · severe depression · severe hypertension · structural cardiac abnormalities · suicidal tendencies · uncontrolled bipolar disorder · vasculitis

● CAUTIONS Agitation · alcohol dependence · anxiety · drug dependence · epilepsy (discontinue if increased seizure frequency) · family history of Tourette syndrome · susceptibility to angle-closure glaucoma · tics

CONCERTA ® XL Dysphagia (dose form not appropriate) · restricted gastro-intestinal lumen (dose form not appropriate)

DELMOSART ® PROLONGED-RELEASE TABLET Dysphagia (dose form not appropriate) · restricted gastro-intestinal lumen (dose form not appropriate)

XAGGITIN ® XL Dysphagia (dose form not appropriate)

● INTERACTIONS → Appendix 1: methylphenidate

● SIDE-EFFECTS
▶ **Common or very common** Aggression (or hostility) · alopecia · anxiety · appetite decreased · arrhythmias · arthralgia · asthenia · behaviour abnormal · cough · depression · diarrhoea · dizziness · drowsiness · dry mouth · feeling jittery · fever · gastrointestinal discomfort · growth retardation (in children) · headaches · hyperhidrosis · hypertension · increased risk of infection · laryngeal pain · mood altered · movement disorders · muscle complaints · nausea · oropharyngeal pain · palpitations · paraesthesia · sexual dysfunction · skin reactions · sleep disorders · thirst · tic · toothache (in adults) · vertigo · vision disorders · vomiting · weight decreased
▶ **Uncommon** Angioedema · chest discomfort · constipation · dry eye · dyspnoea · haematuria · hallucinations · hot flush · psychotic disorder · speech impairment · suicidal behaviours · tremor · urinary disorders
▶ **Rare or very rare** Anaemia · angina pectoris · cardiac arrest · cerebrovascular insufficiency · confusion · gynaecomastia · hepatic coma · hepatic disorders · hyperfocus · leucopenia · mydriasis · myocardial infarction · neuroleptic malignant syndrome (discontinue—potentially fatal) · peripheral coldness · Raynaud's phenomenon · seizures · sudden cardiac death · thinking abnormal · thrombocytopenia
▶ **Frequency not known** Delusions · drug dependence · hyperpyrexia · intracranial haemorrhage · pancytopenia · trismus (in adults) · vasculitis

● PREGNANCY Limited experience—avoid unless potential benefit outweighs risk.

● BREAST FEEDING Limited information available—avoid.

● MONITORING REQUIREMENTS
▶ Monitor for psychiatric disorders.
▶ Pulse, blood pressure, psychiatric symptoms, appetite, weight and height should be recorded at initiation of therapy, following each dose adjustment, and at least every 6 months thereafter.

● TREATMENT CESSATION Avoid abrupt withdrawal.

● DIRECTIONS FOR ADMINISTRATION

EQUASYM ® XL Manufacturer advises contents of capsule can be sprinkled on a tablespoon of apple sauce (then swallowed immediately without chewing).

MEDIKINET ® XL Manufacturer advises contents of capsule can be sprinkled on a tablespoon of apple sauce or yoghurt (then swallowed immediately without chewing).

● PRESCRIBING AND DISPENSING INFORMATION Different versions of modified-release preparations may not have the same clinical effect. To avoid confusion between these different formulations of methylphenidate, prescribers should specify the brand or manufacturer name, if generic, to be dispensed—see also *Important safety information*.

CONCERTA ® XL Consists of an immediate-release component (22% of the dose) and a modified-release component (78% of the dose).

EQUASYM ® XL Consists of an immediate-release component (30% of the dose) and a modified-release component (70% of the dose).

MEDIKINET ® XL Consists of an immediate-release component (50% of the dose) and a modified-release component (50% of the dose).

● PATIENT AND CARER ADVICE
Medicines for Children leaflet: Methylphenidate for ADHD
www.medicinesforchildren.org.uk/medicines/methylphenidate-for-adhd/

Driving and skilled tasks Prescribers and other healthcare professionals should advise patients if treatment is likely to affect their ability to perform skilled tasks (e.g. driving). This applies especially to drugs with sedative effects; patients should be warned that these effects are increased by alcohol. General information about a patient's fitness to drive is available from the Driver and Vehicle Licensing

Agency at www.gov.uk/government/organisations/driver-and-vehicle-licensing-agency.

2015 legislation regarding driving whilst taking certain drugs, may also apply to methylphenidate, see *Drugs and driving* under Guidance on prescribing p. 1.

CONCERTA ® XL Tablet membrane may pass through gastro-intestinal tract unchanged.

DELMOSART ® PROLONGED-RELEASE TABLET Manufacturer advises tablet membrane may pass through gastro-intestinal tract unchanged.

- **MEDICINAL FORMS** There can be variation in the licensing of different medicines containing the same drug. Forms available from special-order manufacturers include: oral suspension, oral solution

Oral tablet
- ▸ Methylphenidate hydrochloride (Non-proprietary)
  Methylphenidate hydrochloride 5 mg Methylphenidate 5mg tablets | 30 tablet PoM £4.84 DT = £3.03 CD2
  Methylphenidate hydrochloride 10 mg Methylphenidate 10mg tablets | 30 tablet PoM £10.00 DT = £3.47 CD2
  Methylphenidate hydrochloride 20 mg Methylphenidate 20mg tablets | 30 tablet PoM £16.38 DT = £10.92 CD2
- ▸ Medikinet (Medice UK Ltd)
  Methylphenidate hydrochloride 5 mg Medikinet 5mg tablets | 30 tablet PoM £3.03 DT = £3.03 CD2
  Methylphenidate hydrochloride 10 mg Medikinet 10mg tablets | 30 tablet PoM £5.49 DT = £3.47 CD2
  Methylphenidate hydrochloride 20 mg Medikinet 20mg tablets | 30 tablet PoM £10.92 DT = £10.92 CD2
- ▸ Ritalin (InfectoPharm Ltd)
  Methylphenidate hydrochloride 10 mg Ritalin 10mg tablets | 30 tablet PoM £6.68 DT = £3.47 CD2
- ▸ Tranquilyn (Genesis Pharmaceuticals Ltd)
  Methylphenidate hydrochloride 5 mg Tranquilyn 5mg tablets | 30 tablet PoM £3.03 DT = £3.03 CD2
  Methylphenidate hydrochloride 10 mg Tranquilyn 10mg tablets | 30 tablet PoM £5.49 DT = £3.47 CD2
  Methylphenidate hydrochloride 20 mg Tranquilyn 20mg tablets | 30 tablet PoM £10.92 DT = £10.92 CD2

Modified-release tablet
CAUTIONARY AND ADVISORY LABELS 25
- ▸ Concerta XL (Janssen-Cilag Ltd)
  Methylphenidate hydrochloride 18 mg Concerta XL 18mg tablets | 30 tablet PoM £31.19 DT = £31.19 CD2
  Methylphenidate hydrochloride 27 mg Concerta XL 27mg tablets | 30 tablet PoM £36.81 DT = £36.81 CD2
  Methylphenidate hydrochloride 36 mg Concerta XL 36mg tablets | 30 tablet PoM £42.45 DT = £42.45 CD2
  Methylphenidate hydrochloride 54 mg Concerta XL 54mg tablets | 30 tablet PoM £73.62 DT = £36.80 CD2
- ▸ Delmosart (Accord-UK Ltd)
  Methylphenidate hydrochloride 18 mg Delmosart 18mg modified-release tablets | 30 tablet PoM £15.57 DT = £31.19 CD2
  Methylphenidate hydrochloride 27 mg Delmosart 27mg modified-release tablets | 30 tablet PoM £18.39 DT = £36.81 CD2
  Methylphenidate hydrochloride 36 mg Delmosart 36mg modified-release tablets | 30 tablet PoM £21.21 DT = £42.45 CD2
  Methylphenidate hydrochloride 54 mg Delmosart 54mg modified-release tablets | 30 tablet PoM £36.79 DT = £36.80 CD2
- ▸ Xaggitin XL (Ethypharm UK Ltd)
  Methylphenidate hydrochloride 18 mg Xaggitin XL 18mg tablets | 30 tablet PoM £15.58 DT = £31.19 CD2
  Methylphenidate hydrochloride 27 mg Xaggitin XL 27mg tablets | 30 tablet PoM £18.40 DT = £36.81 CD2
  Methylphenidate hydrochloride 36 mg Xaggitin XL 36mg tablets | 30 tablet PoM £21.22 DT = £42.45 CD2
  Methylphenidate hydrochloride 54 mg Xaggitin XL 54mg tablets | 30 tablet PoM £36.80 DT = £36.80 CD2

Modified-release capsule
CAUTIONARY AND ADVISORY LABELS 25
- ▸ Equasym XL (Takeda UK Ltd)
  Methylphenidate hydrochloride 10 mg Equasym XL 10mg capsules | 30 capsule PoM £25.00 DT = £25.00 CD2
  Methylphenidate hydrochloride 20 mg Equasym XL 20mg capsules | 30 capsule PoM £30.00 DT = £30.00 CD2
  Methylphenidate hydrochloride 30 mg Equasym XL 30mg capsules | 30 capsule PoM £35.00 DT = £35.00 CD2
- ▸ Medikinet XL (Medice UK Ltd) ▼
  Methylphenidate hydrochloride 5 mg Medikinet XL 5mg capsules | 30 capsule PoM £24.04 DT = £24.04 CD2
  Methylphenidate hydrochloride 10 mg Medikinet XL 10mg capsules | 30 capsule PoM £24.04 DT = £25.00 CD2
  Methylphenidate hydrochloride 20 mg Medikinet XL 20mg capsules | 30 capsule PoM £28.86 DT = £30.00 CD2
  Methylphenidate hydrochloride 30 mg Medikinet XL 30mg capsules | 30 capsule PoM £33.66 DT = £35.00 CD2
  Methylphenidate hydrochloride 40 mg Medikinet XL 40mg capsules | 30 capsule PoM £57.72 DT = £57.72 CD2
  Methylphenidate hydrochloride 50 mg Medikinet XL 50mg capsules | 30 capsule PoM £62.52 DT = £62.52 CD2
  Methylphenidate hydrochloride 60 mg Medikinet XL 60mg capsules | 30 capsule PoM £67.32 DT = £67.32 CD2

Oral solution
- ▸ Methylphenidate hydrochloride (Non-proprietary)
  Methylphenidate hydrochloride 2 mg per 1 ml Methylphenidate 2mg/ml oral solution sugar free | 150 ml PoM £85.00 DT = £85.00 CD2 SF

CNS STIMULANTS > CENTRALLY ACTING SYMPATHOMIMETICS > AMFETAMINES

Dexamfetamine sulfate
09-May-2024
(Dexamphetamine sulphate)

- **INDICATIONS AND DOSE**

Narcolepsy
- ▸ BY MOUTH
- ▸ Adult: Initially 10 mg daily in divided doses, increased in steps of 10 mg every week, maintenance dose to be given in 2–4 divided doses; maximum 60 mg per day
- ▸ Elderly: Initially 5 mg daily in divided doses, increased in steps of 5 mg every week, maintenance dose to be given in 2–4 divided doses; maximum 60 mg per day

Refractory attention deficit hyperactivity disorder (initiated under specialist supervision)
- ▸ BY MOUTH
- ▸ Child 6-17 years: Initially 2.5 mg 2–3 times a day, increased in steps of 5 mg once weekly if required, usual maximum 1 mg/kg daily, up to 20 mg daily (40 mg daily has been required in some children); maintenance dose to be given in 2–4 divided doses
- ▸ Adult: Initially 5 mg twice daily, dose is increased at weekly intervals according to response, maintenance dose to be given in 2–4 divided doses; maximum 60 mg per day

- **UNLICENSED USE** Not licensed for use in adults for refractory attention deficit hyperactivity disorder.

- **CONTRA-INDICATIONS** Advanced arteriosclerosis · anorexia · arrhythmias (life-threatening) · cardiomyopathies · cardiovascular disease · cerebrovascular disorders · heart failure · history of alcohol abuse · history of drug abuse · hyperexcitability · hyperthyroidism · moderate hypertension · psychiatric disorders · psychosis · severe hypertension · structural cardiac abnormalities · suicidal tendencies

  CONTRA-INDICATIONS, FURTHER INFORMATION
- ▸ Psychiatric disorders Psychiatric disorders include severe depression, schizophrenia, borderline personality disorder and uncontrolled bipolar disorder. Co-morbidity with psychiatric disorders is common in attention deficit hyperactivity disorder. Manufacturer advises if new psychiatric symptoms develop or exacerbation of psychiatric disorders occurs, continue use only if benefits outweigh risks.

- **CAUTIONS** History of epilepsy (discontinue if seizures occur) · mild hypertension · susceptibility to angle-closure glaucoma · tics · Tourette syndrome

CAUTIONS, FURTHER INFORMATION

▸ Tics and Tourette syndrome Discontinue use if tics occur.
▸ Growth restriction in children Monitor height and weight as growth restriction may occur during prolonged therapy (drug-free periods may allow catch-up in growth but withdraw slowly to avoid inducing depression or renewed hyperactivity).

● INTERACTIONS → Appendix 1: amfetamines

● SIDE-EFFECTS

▸ **Common or very common** Abdominal pain · anxiety · appetite decreased · arrhythmias · arthralgia · behaviour abnormal · depression · dry mouth · headache · mood altered · movement disorders · muscle cramps · nausea · palpitations · poor weight gain · sleep disorders · vertigo · vomiting · weight decreased
▸ **Rare or very rare** Anaemia · angina pectoris · cardiac arrest · central nervous system vasculitis · cerebrovascular insufficiency · fatigue · growth retardation · hallucination · hepatic coma · hepatic function abnormal · intracranial haemorrhage · leucopenia · mydriasis · psychosis · seizure · skin reactions · suicidal behaviours · thrombocytopenia · tic (in those at risk) · vision disorders
▸ **Frequency not known** Acidosis · alopecia · cardiomyopathy · chest pain · circulatory collapse · colitis ischaemic · concentration impaired · confusion · diarrhoea · dizziness · drug dependence · hyperhidrosis · hypermetabolism · hyperpyrexia · kidney injury · myocardial infarction · neuroleptic malignant syndrome (discontinue—potentially fatal) · obsessive-compulsive disorder · reflexes increased · rhabdomyolysis · sexual dysfunction · sudden death · taste altered · tremor

Overdose Amfetamines cause wakefulness, excessive activity, paranoia, hallucinations, and hypertension followed by exhaustion, convulsions, hyperthermia, and coma. See Stimulants under Emergency treatment of poisoning p. 1554.

● PREGNANCY Avoid (retrospective evidence of uncertain significance suggesting possible embryotoxicity).

● BREAST FEEDING Significant amount in milk—avoid.

● RENAL IMPAIRMENT EvGr Use with caution (no information available). ⟨M⟩

● MONITORING REQUIREMENTS

▸ Monitor growth in children.
▸ Monitor for aggressive behaviour or hostility during initial treatment.
▸ Pulse, blood pressure, psychiatric symptoms, appetite, weight and height should be recorded at initiation of therapy, following each dose adjustment, and at least every 6 months thereafter.

● TREATMENT CESSATION Avoid abrupt withdrawal.

● DIRECTIONS FOR ADMINISTRATION

▸ In children Manufacturer advises tablets can be halved.

● PRESCRIBING AND DISPENSING INFORMATION Data on safety and efficacy of long-term use not complete.

● PATIENT AND CARER ADVICE

Driving and skilled tasks Prescribers and other healthcare professionals should advise patients if treatment is likely to affect their ability to perform skilled tasks (e.g. driving). This applies especially to drugs with sedative effects; patients should be warned that these effects are increased by alcohol.

For information on 2015 legislation regarding driving whilst taking certain controlled drugs, including amfetamines, see *Drugs and driving* under Guidance on prescribing p. 1.

● MEDICINAL FORMS There can be variation in the licensing of different medicines containing the same drug. Forms available from special-order manufacturers include: modified-release capsule, oral suspension, oral solution

Oral tablet

▸ Dexamfetamine sulfate (Non-proprietary)
  Dexamfetamine sulfate 5 mg Dexamfetamine 5mg tablets | 28 tablet PoM £33.13 DT = £20.65 CD2
▸ Amfexa (Medice UK Ltd)
  Dexamfetamine sulfate 5 mg Amfexa 5mg tablets | 30 tablet PoM £19.89 CD2
  Dexamfetamine sulfate 10 mg Amfexa 10mg tablets | 30 tablet PoM £39.78 DT = £39.78 CD2
  Dexamfetamine sulfate 20 mg Amfexa 20mg tablets | 30 tablet PoM £79.56 DT = £79.56 CD2

Oral solution

▸ Dexamfetamine sulfate (Non-proprietary)
  Dexamfetamine sulfate 1 mg per 1 ml Dexamfetamine 5mg/5ml oral solution sugar free | 150 ml PoM £178.50 DT = £178.50 CD2 SF

Modified-release capsule

▸ Dexamfetamine sulfate (Non-proprietary)
  Dexamfetamine sulfate 5 mg Dexedrine 5mg Spansules | 100 capsule PoM ⚠ CD2
  Dexamfetamine sulfate 10 mg Dexedrine 10mg Spansules | 100 capsule PoM ⚠ CD2
▸ Dexedrine Spansules (Imported (United States))
  Dexamfetamine sulfate 15 mg Dexedrine 15mg Spansules | 100 capsule PoM ⚠ CD2

Lisdexamfetamine mesilate
29-Oct-2020

● DRUG ACTION Lisdexamfetamine is a prodrug of dexamfetamine.

● **INDICATIONS AND DOSE**

Attention deficit hyperactivity disorder (initiated by a specialist)

▸ BY MOUTH

▸ Child 6-17 years: Initially 30 mg once daily, alternatively initially 20 mg once daily, increased in steps of 10–20 mg every week if required, dose to be taken in the morning, discontinue if response insufficient after 1 month; maximum 70 mg per day
▸ Adult: Initially 30 mg once daily, increased in steps of 20 mg every week if required, dose to be taken in the morning, discontinue if response insufficient after 1 month; maximum 70 mg per day

● CONTRA-INDICATIONS Advanced arteriosclerosis · agitated states · hyperthyroidism · moderate hypertension · severe hypertension · symptomatic cardiovascular disease

● CAUTIONS Bipolar disorder · history of cardiovascular disease · history of substance abuse · may lower seizure threshold (discontinue if seizures occur) · psychotic disorders · susceptibility to angle-closure glaucoma · tics · Tourette syndrome

CAUTIONS, FURTHER INFORMATION

▸ Cardiovascular disease Manufacturer advises caution in patients with underlying conditions that might be compromised by increases in blood pressure or heart rate; see also *Contra-indications*.

● INTERACTIONS → Appendix 1: amfetamines

● SIDE-EFFECTS

▸ **Common or very common** Abdominal pain upper · anxiety · appetite decreased · behaviour abnormal · constipation · diarrhoea · dizziness · dry mouth · dyspnoea · fatigue · feeling jittery · headache · hyperhidrosis (uncommon in children) · insomnia · mood altered · movement disorders (uncommon in children) · nausea · palpitations · sexual dysfunction (uncommon in children) · tachycardia · tremor · weight decreased

► **Uncommon** Depression (very common in children) · drowsiness (very common in children) · fever (very common in children) · logorrhea · psychiatric disorders (very common in children) · skin reactions (very common in children) · taste altered · vision blurred · vomiting (very common in children)

► **Frequency not known** Angioedema · cardiomyopathy (uncommon in children) · drug dependence · hallucination (uncommon in children) · hepatitis allergic · mydriasis (uncommon in children) · psychotic disorder · Raynaud's phenomenon (uncommon in children) · seizure · Stevens-Johnson syndrome

Overdose Amfetamines cause wakefulness, excessive activity, paranoia, hallucinations, and hypertension followed by exhaustion, convulsions, hyperthermia, and coma. See Stimulants under Emergency treatment of poisoning p. 1554.

● **PREGNANCY** Manufacturer advises use only if potential benefit outweighs risk.

● **BREAST FEEDING** Manufacturer advises avoid—present in human milk.

● **RENAL IMPAIRMENT**
Dose adjustments Manufacturer advises max. dose 50 mg daily in severe impairment.

● **MONITORING REQUIREMENTS**
► Manufacturer advises monitor for aggressive behaviour or hostility during initial treatment.
► Manufacturer advises monitor pulse, blood pressure, and for psychiatric symptoms before treatment initiation, following each dose adjustment, and at least every 6 months thereafter. Monitor weight in adults before treatment initiation and during treatment; in children, height and weight should be recorded before treatment initiation, and height, weight and appetite monitored at least every 6 months during treatment.

● **TREATMENT CESSATION** Avoid abrupt withdrawal.

● **DIRECTIONS FOR ADMINISTRATION** Manufacturer advises swallow whole or mix contents of capsule with soft food such as yoghurt or in a glass of water or orange juice; contents should be dispersed completely and consumed immediately.

● **PATIENT AND CARER ADVICE** Patients and carers should be counselled on the administration of capsules.
Driving and skilled tasks Prescribers and other healthcare professionals should advise patients if treatment is likely to affect their ability to perform skilled tasks (e.g. driving). This applies especially to drugs with sedative effects; patients should be warned that these effects are increased by alcohol. General information about a patient's fitness to drive is available from the Driver and Vehicle Licensing Agency at www.gov.uk/government/organisations/driver-and-vehicle-licensing-agency.

For information on 2015 legislation regarding driving whilst taking certain controlled drugs, including amfetamines, see *Drugs and driving* under Guidance on prescribing p. 1.

● **NATIONAL FUNDING/ACCESS DECISIONS**
For full details see funding body website
Scottish Medicines Consortium (SMC) decisions
► Lisdexamfetamine dimesylate (*Elvanse*®) for use as part of a comprehensive treatment programme for attention deficit/hyperactivity disorder (ADHD) in children aged 6 years of age and over when response to previous methylphenidate treatment is considered clinically inadequate (May 2013) SMC No. 863/13 Recommended
► Lisdexamfetamine dimesylate (*Elvanse Adult*®) for use as part of a comprehensive treatment programme for attention deficit/hyperactivity disorder (ADHD) in adults (September 2015) SMC No. 1079/15 Recommended

All Wales Medicines Strategy Group (AWMSG) decisions
► Lisdexamfetamine dimesylate (*Elvanse*®) for use as part of a treatment programme for attention deficit/hyperactivity disorder (ADHD) in children aged 6 years and over when response to previous methylphenidate treatment is considered clinically inadequate. Treatment must be under the supervision of a specialist in childhood and/or adolescent behavioural disorders (December 2013) AWMSG No. 188 Recommended
► Lisdexamfetamine dimesylate (*Elvanse Adult*®) for use as part of a comprehensive treatment programme for attention deficit/hyperactivity disorder (ADHD) in adults (October 2015) AWMSG No. 2534 Recommended

● **MEDICINAL FORMS** There can be variation in the licensing of different medicines containing the same drug.
Oral capsule
CAUTIONARY AND ADVISORY LABELS 3
► **Elvanse** (Takeda UK Ltd)
Lisdexamfetamine dimesylate 20 mg Elvanse Adult 20mg capsules | 28 capsule [PoM] £54.62 DT = £54.62 [CD2]
Elvanse 20mg capsules | 28 capsule [PoM] £54.62 DT = £54.62 [CD2]
Lisdexamfetamine dimesylate 30 mg Elvanse Adult 30mg capsules | 28 capsule [PoM] £58.24 DT = £58.24 [CD2]
Elvanse 30mg capsules | 28 capsule [PoM] £58.24 DT = £58.24 [CD2]
Lisdexamfetamine dimesylate 40 mg Elvanse 40mg capsules | 28 capsule [PoM] £62.82 DT = £62.82 [CD2]
Lisdexamfetamine dimesylate 50 mg Elvanse Adult 50mg capsules | 28 capsule [PoM] £68.60 DT = £68.60 [CD2]
Elvanse 50mg capsules | 28 capsule [PoM] £68.60 DT = £68.60 [CD2]
Lisdexamfetamine dimesylate 60 mg Elvanse 60mg capsules | 28 capsule [PoM] £75.18 DT = £75.18 [CD2]
Elvanse Adult 60mg capsules | 28 capsule [PoM] £75.18 DT = £75.18 [CD2]
Lisdexamfetamine dimesylate 70 mg Elvanse 70mg capsules | 28 capsule [PoM] £83.16 DT = £83.16 [CD2]
Elvanse Adult 70mg capsules | 28 capsule [PoM] £83.16 DT = £83.16 [CD2]

SYMPATHOMIMETICS 〉 ALPHA$_2$-ADRENOCEPTOR AGONISTS

Guanfacine
24-Apr-2024

● **INDICATIONS AND DOSE**
Attention deficit hyperactivity disorder in children for whom stimulants are not suitable, not tolerated or ineffective (initiated under specialist supervision)
► BY MOUTH
► Child 6-12 years (body-weight 25 kg and above): Initially 1 mg once daily; adjusted in steps of 1 mg every week if necessary and if tolerated; maintenance 0.05–0.12 mg/kg once daily (max. per dose 4 mg), for optimal weight-adjusted dose titrations, consult product literature
► Child 13-17 years (body-weight 34-41.4 kg): Initially 1 mg once daily; adjusted in steps of 1 mg every week if necessary and if tolerated; maintenance 0.05–0.12 mg/kg once daily (max. per dose 4 mg), for optimal weight-adjusted dose titrations, consult product literature
► Child 13-17 years (body-weight 41.5-49.4 kg): Initially 1 mg once daily; adjusted in steps of 1 mg every week if necessary and if tolerated; maintenance 0.05–0.12 mg/kg once daily (max. per dose 5 mg), for optimal weight-adjusted dose titrations, consult product literature
► Child 13-17 years (body-weight 49.5-58.4 kg): Initially 1 mg once daily; adjusted in steps of 1 mg every week if necessary and if tolerated; maintenance 0.05–0.12 mg/kg once daily (max. per dose 6 mg), for optimal weight-adjusted dose titrations, consult product literature

continued →

Nervous system

4

▸ Child 13–17 years (body-weight 58.5 kg and above): Initially 1 mg once daily; adjusted in steps of 1 mg every week if necessary and if tolerated; maintenance 0.05–0.12 mg/kg once daily (max. per dose 7 mg), for optimal weight-adjusted dose titrations, consult product literature

DOSE ADJUSTMENTS DUE TO INTERACTIONS
▸ EvGr Reduce dose by half with concurrent use of moderate and potent inhibitors of CYP3A4 and ciprofloxacin; further titrate dose if needed.
▸ Consider increasing dose by 1 mg per week, up to max. 7 mg daily if needed, with concurrent use of potent inducers of CYP3A4. M

● **CAUTIONS** Bradycardia (risk of torsade de pointes) · heart block (risk of torsade de pointes) · history of cardiovascular disease · history of QT-interval prolongation · hypokalaemia (risk of torsade de pointes)

● **INTERACTIONS** → Appendix 1: guanfacine

● **SIDE-EFFECTS**
▸ **Common or very common** Anxiety · appetite decreased · arrhythmias · asthenia · constipation · depression · diarrhoea · dizziness · drowsiness · dry mouth · gastrointestinal discomfort · headache · hypotension · mood altered · nausea · skin reactions · sleep disorders · urinary disorders · vomiting · weight increased
▸ **Uncommon** Asthma · atrioventricular block · chest pain · hallucination · loss of consciousness · pallor · seizure · syncope
▸ **Rare or very rare** Hypertension · hypertensive encephalopathy · malaise
▸ **Frequency not known** Erectile dysfunction

SIDE-EFFECTS, FURTHER INFORMATION Somnolence and sedation may occur, predominantly during the first 2–3 weeks of treatment and with dose increases; manufacturer advises to consider dose reduction or discontinuation of treatment if symptoms are clinically significant or persistent.

Overdose Features may include hypotension, initial hypertension, bradycardia, lethargy, and respiratory depression. Manufacturer advises that patients who develop lethargy should be observed for development of more serious toxicity for up to 24 hours.

● **CONCEPTION AND CONTRACEPTION** Manufacturer recommends effective contraception in females of childbearing potential.

● **PREGNANCY** Manufacturer advises avoid—toxicity in *animal* studies.

● **BREAST FEEDING** Manufacturer advises avoid—present in milk in *animal* studies.

● **HEPATIC IMPAIRMENT** Manufacturer advises caution (pharmacokinetics have not been assessed in paediatric patients with hepatic impairment).
Dose adjustments Manufacturer advises consider dose reduction.

● **RENAL IMPAIRMENT**
Dose adjustments EvGr Dose reduction may be required in severe impairment and end-stage renal disease (no information available in children with renal impairment). M

● **MONITORING REQUIREMENTS**
▸ Manufacturer advises to conduct a baseline evaluation to identify patients at risk of somnolence, sedation, hypotension, bradycardia, QT-prolongation, and arrhythmia; this should include assessment of cardiovascular status. Monitor for signs of these adverse effects weekly during dose titration and then every 3 months during the first year of treatment, and every 6 months thereafter. Monitor BMI prior to treatment and then every 3 months for the first year of treatment, and

every 6 months thereafter. More frequent monitoring is advised following dose adjustments.
▸ Monitor blood pressure and pulse during dose downward titration and following discontinuation of treatment.

● **TREATMENT CESSATION** Manufacturer advises avoid abrupt withdrawal; consider dose tapering to minimise potential withdrawal effects.

● **DIRECTIONS FOR ADMINISTRATION** Manufacturer advises avoid administration with high fat meals (may increase absorption).

● **PATIENT AND CARER ADVICE** Patients or carers should be counselled on administration of guanfacine modified-release tablets.
Missed doses Manufacturer advises that patients and carers should inform their prescriber if more than one dose is missed; consider dose re-titration.
Driving and skilled tasks Manufacturer advises patients and carers should be counselled about the effects on driving and performance of skilled tasks—increased risk of dizziness and syncope.

● **MEDICINAL FORMS** There can be variation in the licensing of different medicines containing the same drug.
Modified-release tablet
CAUTIONARY AND ADVISORY LABELS 2, 25
▸ Intuniv (Takeda UK Ltd) ▼
Guanfacine (as Guanfacine hydrochloride) 1 mg Intuniv 1mg modified-release tablets | 28 tablet PoM £56.00 DT = £56.00
Guanfacine (as Guanfacine hydrochloride) 2 mg Intuniv 2mg modified-release tablets | 28 tablet PoM £58.52 DT = £58.52
Guanfacine (as Guanfacine hydrochloride) 3 mg Intuniv 3mg modified-release tablets | 28 tablet PoM £65.52 DT = £65.52
Guanfacine (as Guanfacine hydrochloride) 4 mg Intuniv 4mg modified-release tablets | 28 tablet PoM £76.16 DT = £76.16

3.3 Bipolar disorder and mania

Mania and hypomania

02-Oct-2024

Overview

Antimanic drugs are used in bipolar disorder to manage acute episodes of mania or hypomania, and to prevent recurrence. Patients with suspected bipolar disorder should be referred to a specialist mental health service and treatment should be initiated on specialist advice.

EvGr An antidepressant drug may also be required for the treatment of co-existing bipolar depression, but should be avoided in patients with rapid-cycling bipolar disorder, a recent history of mania or hypomania, or with rapid mood fluctuations. Consider stopping the antidepressant drug if the patient develops mania or hypomania. A

Antipsychotic drugs

EvGr Antipsychotic drugs (such as haloperidol p. 445, olanzapine p. 459, quetiapine p. 462, and risperidone p. 464) are used in the treatment of acute episodes of mania or hypomania; if the response to antipsychotic drugs is inadequate, lithium or valproate may be added. In patients already taking prophylactic treatment with lithium or valproate, if there is no improvement despite optimising the dose of lithium or valproate, an antipsychotic drug can be added to treat the acute episode of mania or hypomania. An antipsychotic drug may also be used concomitantly with lithium or valproate in the initial treatment of severe acute episodes of mania. A Valproate is highly teratogenic; for information on regulatory measures issued by the MHRA/CHM to ensure appropriate and safe use, see *valproate* below.

Asenapine p. 413, a second-generation antipsychotic drug, is licensed for the treatment of moderate to severe manic episodes associated with bipolar disorder.

Olanzapine can be used for the long-term management of bipolar disorder; it is licensed for the prevention of recurrence in patients whose manic episode has responded to olanzapine therapy.

EvGr When discontinuing antipsychotic drugs, the dose should be reduced gradually over at least 4 weeks to minimise the risk of recurrence. A

Benzodiazepines

EvGr Use of benzodiazepines (such as lorazepam) may be helpful in the initial stages of treatment for behavioural disturbance or agitation. A Benzodiazepines should not be used for long periods because of the risk of dependence.

Lithium

EvGr Lithium salts (lithium carbonate p. 414 and lithium citrate p. 415) are used for the treatment of acute episodes of mania or hypomania in bipolar disorder. Lithium is also used for the long-term management of bipolar disorder to prevent recurrence of acute episodes. A

The decision to give prophylactic lithium must be based on careful consideration of the likelihood of recurrence in the individual patient, and the benefit of treatment weighed against the risks. The full prophylactic effect of lithium may not occur for six to twelve months after the initiation of therapy.

Valproate

EvGr Valproate (valproic acid below (as the semisodium salt) and sodium valproate p. 378) is used for the treatment of manic episodes associated with bipolar disorder if lithium is not tolerated or contra-indicated. Valproate is also used for the long-term management of bipolar disorder to prevent recurrence of acute episodes, in combination with lithium if treatment with lithium alone is ineffective, or as monotherapy if lithium is not tolerated or contra-indicated. A

Safety measures around the use of valproate have been revised, and the MHRA/CHM has issued a National Patient Safety Alert. This outlines new regulatory measures for initiation of valproate in individuals (males or females) aged under 55 years, and continued use in females of childbearing potential. Due to the high teratogenic risk associated with valproate, it must not be used in females of childbearing potential unless the conditions of the Pregnancy Prevention Programme are met and alternative treatments are ineffective or not tolerated. Valproate must not be used during pregnancy in patients with bipolar disorder. In addition to these measures, further advice has been issued around the use in males and the need to use effective contraception. For further information, see *Important safety information*, *Conception and contraception*, and *Pregnancy* in valproic acid and sodium valproate.

Carbamazepine

Carbamazepine p. 355 is licensed for the long-term management of bipolar disorder, to prevent recurrence of acute episodes in patients unresponsive to lithium therapy.

Other drugs used for Bipolar disorder and mania
Chlorpromazine hydrochloride, p. 443 · Lamotrigine, p. 366 · Paliperidone, p. 461 · Prochlorperazine, p. 448 · Zuclopenthixol acetate, p. 451

ANTIEPILEPTICS

Valproic acid   25-Feb-2025

● **INDICATIONS AND DOSE**

Treatment of manic episodes associated with bipolar disorder
▶ BY MOUTH
▸ Adult: Initially 750 mg daily in 2–3 divided doses, then increased to 1–2 g daily, adjusted according to response, doses greater than 45 mg/kg daily require careful monitoring

Migraine prophylaxis
▶ BY MOUTH
▸ Adult: Initially 250 mg twice daily, then increased if necessary to 1 g daily in divided doses

DOSE EQUIVALENCE AND CONVERSION
▸ Semisodium valproate comprises equimolar amounts of sodium valproate and valproic acid.

CONVULEX ®

Epilepsy
▶ BY MOUTH
▸ Adult: Initially 600 mg daily in 2–4 divided doses, increased in steps of 150–300 mg every 3 days; usual maintenance 1–2 g daily in 2–4 divided doses, max. 2.5 g daily in 2–4 divided doses

DOSE EQUIVALENCE AND CONVERSION
▸ *Convulex* ® has a 1:1 dose relationship with products containing sodium valproate, but nevertheless care is needed if switching or making changes.

● **UNLICENSED USE** Not licensed for migraine prophylaxis.

IMPORTANT SAFETY INFORMATION

MHRA/CHM ADVICE: ANTIEPILEPTICS: RISK OF SUICIDAL THOUGHTS AND BEHAVIOUR (AUGUST 2008)
See Epilepsy p. 349.

MHRA/CHM ADVICE: ANTIEPILEPTIC DRUGS: UPDATED ADVICE ON SWITCHING BETWEEN DIFFERENT MANUFACTURERS' PRODUCTS (NOVEMBER 2017)
See Epilepsy p. 349 and see also *Prescribing and dispensing information.*

MHRA/CHM ADVICE: VALPROATE MEDICINES: CONTRA-INDICATED IN WOMEN AND GIRLS OF CHILDBEARING POTENTIAL UNLESS CONDITIONS OF PREGNANCY PREVENTION PROGRAMME ARE MET (APRIL 2018)
Valproate is highly teratogenic and evidence supports that use in pregnancy leads to neurodevelopmental disorders (approx. 30–40% risk) and congenital malformations (approx. 10% risk).

Valproate must not be used in women and girls of childbearing potential unless the conditions of the Pregnancy Prevention Programme are met (see *Conception and contraception*) and only if other treatments are ineffective or not tolerated, as judged by an experienced specialist.

Use of valproate in pregnancy is contra-indicated for migraine prophylaxis [unlicensed] and bipolar disorder; it must only be considered for epilepsy if there is no suitable alternative treatment (see *Pregnancy*).

Women and girls (and their carers) must be fully informed of the risks and the need to avoid exposure to valproate medicines in pregnancy; supporting materials have been provided to use in the implementation of the Pregnancy Prevention Programme (see *Prescribing and dispensing information*). The MHRA advises that:
● GPs must recall all women and girls who may be of childbearing potential, provide the Patient Guide, check they have been reviewed by a specialist in the last year and are on highly effective contraception;

- Specialists must book in review appointments at least annually with women and girls under the Pregnancy Prevention Programme, re-evaluate treatment as necessary, explain clearly the conditions as outlined in the supporting materials and complete and sign the Risk Acknowledgement Form—copies of the form must be given to the patient or carer and sent to their GP;
- Pharmacists must ensure valproate medicines are dispensed in whole packs whenever possible—all packs dispensed to women and girls of childbearing potential should have a warning label either on the carton or via a sticker. They must also discuss risks in pregnancy with female patients each time valproate medicines are dispensed, ensure they have the Patient Guide and have seen their GP or specialist to discuss their treatment and the need for contraception.

MHRA/CHM ADVICE: VALPROATE MEDICINES: ARE YOU ACTING IN COMPLIANCE WITH THE PREGNANCY PREVENTION MEASURES? (DECEMBER 2018)

The MHRA advises that all healthcare professionals must continue to identify and review all female patients on valproate, including when used outside licensed indications (off-label use) and provide them with the patient information materials every time they attend appointments or receive their medicines.

Guidance for psychiatrists on the withdrawal of, and alternatives to, valproate in women of childbearing potential who have a psychiatric illness is available from the Royal College of Psychiatrists.

MHRA/CHM ADVICE: VALPROATE MEDICINES AND SERIOUS HARMS IN PREGNANCY: NEW ANNUAL RISK ACKNOWLEDGEMENT FORM AND CLINICAL GUIDANCE FROM PROFESSIONAL BODIES TO SUPPORT COMPLIANCE WITH THE PREGNANCY PREVENTION PROGRAMME (APRIL 2019)

The Annual Risk Acknowledgement Form has been updated and should be used for all future reviews of female patients on valproate. Specialists should comply with guidance given on the form if they consider the patient is not at risk of pregnancy, including the need for review in case her risk status changes.

Guidance has been published to support healthcare professionals with the use of valproate. These include a summary by NICE of their guidance and safety advice, pan-college guidance by national healthcare bodies, and paediatric guidance by the British Paediatric Neurology Association and the Royal College of Paediatrics and Child Health.

MHRA/CHM ADVICE (UPDATED JANUARY 2020): VALPROATE PREGNANCY PREVENTION PROGRAMME

The Guide for Healthcare Professionals has been updated and should be used for all future reviews of female patients on valproate medicines, in conjunction with other supporting materials (see *Prescribing and dispensing Information*).

MHRA/CHM ADVICE (UPDATED MAY 2020): VALPROATE PREGNANCY PREVENTION PROGRAMME: TEMPORARY ADVICE FOR MANAGEMENT DURING CORONAVIRUS (COVID-19)

The MHRA has issued temporary guidance for female patients on valproate during the coronavirus (COVID-19) pandemic to support adherence to the Pregnancy Prevention Programme, particularly for those who are shielding due to other health conditions, and should be followed until further notice.

MHRA/CHM ADVICE: ANTIEPILEPTIC DRUGS IN PREGNANCY: UPDATED ADVICE FOLLOWING COMPREHENSIVE SAFETY REVIEW (JANUARY 2021)

See Epilepsy p. 349.

MHRA/CHM ADVICE: VALPROATE: REMINDER OF CURRENT PREGNANCY PREVENTION PROGRAMME REQUIREMENTS; INFORMATION ON NEW SAFETY MEASURES TO BE INTRODUCED IN THE COMING MONTHS (DECEMBER 2022)

In light of data showing ongoing exposure to valproate in pregnancy and evolving information about the potential risks of valproate in other patients, healthcare professionals are reminded of the risks in pregnancy and requirements of the existing Pregnancy Prevention Programme, and are also advised of the potential risk of infertility in male patients. The CHM has recommended regulatory actions to strengthen safety measures for valproate which will be introduced over the coming months. In the meantime, healthcare professionals are advised that patients currently taking valproate should continue to do so unless recommended to stop by a specialist. All other suitable treatment options should be considered and findings from the safety review of antiepileptic drugs in pregnancy consulted before initiating valproate treatment in female patients aged under 55 years (see Epilepsy p. 349). Two specialists are required to independently consider and document that there is no other effective or tolerated treatment before prescribing valproate for male or female patients aged under 55 years.

MHRA/CHM ADVICE: VALPROATE: RE-ANALYSIS OF STUDY ON RISKS IN CHILDREN OF MEN TAKING VALPROATE (AUGUST 2023)

The MHRA continues to review all emerging data on valproate medicines, including findings from a retrospective observational study which suggested an increased risk of neurodevelopmental disorders in children of men who took valproate, when compared with those of men who took lamotrigine or levetiracetam, in the 3 months before conception. However, errors have been identified in the study and the MHRA has determined that a full re-analysis is required before conclusions can be made. In the meantime, healthcare professionals are reminded that the use of valproate in females of childbearing potential should be in accordance with the Pregnancy Prevention Programme, and that all patients currently taking valproate should continue to do so unless advised to stop by a specialist. Patients should continue to be informed of the risks of valproate in pregnancy.

MHRA/CHM ADVICE: FULL PACK DISPENSING OF VALPROATE-CONTAINING MEDICINES (OCTOBER 2023)

Valproate medicines have been dispensed to patients in alternative packaging because the prescribed amount was different to that of the manufacturer's original full pack. This resulted in patients not always receiving all the risk materials about the use of these medicines in pregnancy. Pharmacists are advised that all patients (male and female) must receive their valproate medicines in the manufacturer's original full pack (i.e. original pack dispensing) and the amount dispensed must be as close as possible to the amount stated on the prescription (NHS or private). Rarely, exceptions to this requirement can be made on an individual patient basis, provided a risk assessment is carried out on the need to dispense repackaged valproate medicines (e.g. in a monitored dosage system), whereby a patient information leaflet must be supplied.

NATIONAL PATIENT SAFETY ALERT: VALPROATE: ORGANISATIONS TO PREPARE FOR NEW REGULATORY MEASURES FOR OVERSIGHT OF PRESCRIBING TO NEW PATIENTS AND EXISTING FEMALE PATIENTS (NOVEMBER 2023)

Following a comprehensive review of safety data, and advice from the CHM and an expert group, the MHRA requests that organisations put a plan in place to implement the following new regulatory measures for valproate medicines:

- valproate must not be started in new patients (male or female) aged under 55 years, unless two specialists independently consider and document that there is no other effective or tolerated treatment, or there are compelling reasons why the reproductive risks do not apply;

- at the next annual specialist review, females of childbearing potential should be reviewed using a revised valproate Risk Acknowledgement Form, which will include the need for a second specialist signature if the patient is to continue with valproate; subsequent annual reviews with one specialist should be carried out unless the patient's situation changes.

These measures are in response to data showing ongoing exposure to valproate in pregnancy and evolving information about the potential risk of impaired fertility in male patients on valproate.

Current safety measures continue to apply, including the Pregnancy Prevention Programme for females of childbearing potential on valproate. All patients currently taking valproate should continue to do so unless advised to stop by a specialist. General practice and pharmacy teams should discuss the current warnings, upcoming measures, and new educational materials with patients.

MHRA/CHM ADVICE: VALPROATE (*BELVO®*, *CONVULEX®*, *DEPAKOTE®*, AND *SYONELL®*): NEW SAFETY AND EDUCATIONAL MATERIALS TO SUPPORT REGULATORY MEASURES IN MEN AND WOMEN UNDER 55 YEARS OF AGE (JANUARY 2024)

Healthcare professionals are advised to review, and integrate into their clinical practice, the updated safety and educational materials that support the new regulatory measures as outlined in the National Patient Safety Alert, above (see also *Prescribing and dispensing information*). General practice and pharmacy teams should continue to prescribe and dispense valproate according to current safety measures. If required, patients should be referred to a specialist to discuss treatment options. Patients on valproate medicines should be fully informed of the potential risks and counselled on treatment options at initial prescribing and at all subsequent reviews.

Healthcare professionals should advise patients to:

- not stop taking valproate medicines without advice from a specialist as their epilepsy or bipolar disorder may worsen;
- attend any offered appointments to discuss their treatment plan and to talk to a healthcare professional if they have any concerns;
- consult the new Patient Guide and Patient Information Leaflet for information on the risks of valproate.

MHRA/CHM ADVICE: VALPROATE USE IN MEN: AS A PRECAUTION, MEN AND THEIR PARTNERS SHOULD USE EFFECTIVE CONTRACEPTION (SEPTEMBER 2024)

The MHRA has reviewed findings from a retrospective observational study (see advice issued in August 2023, above) that suggest a potential increased risk of neurodevelopmental disorders in children born to men taking valproate medicines in the 3 months before conception; however, causality is unconfirmed. In addition to current safety measures, healthcare professionals should advise male patients (of any age) who may father a child:

- about this risk at treatment initiation or at the next treatment review, irrespective of indication and also after intravenous valproate;
- to use effective contraception (i.e. condoms plus contraception used by their female partner) during and for 3 months after valproate treatment;
- to refrain from donating sperm during and for 3 months after valproate treatment.

Healthcare professionals are also advised that:

- male patients who are planning a family in the next year should be referred to a specialist to discuss alternative treatment;
- female partners of male patients taking valproate medicines who are pregnant or planning a pregnancy (including those undergoing IVF) should be referred for prenatal counselling.

MHRA/CHM ADVICE: VALPROATE (*BELVO®*, *CONVULEX®*, *DEPAKOTE®*, AND *SYONELL®*): REVIEW BY TWO SPECIALISTS IS REQUIRED FOR INITIATING VALPROATE BUT NOT FOR MALE PATIENTS ALREADY TAKING VALPROATE (FEBRUARY 2025)

Healthcare professionals are reminded that the current safety measure advising all patients under 55 years of age to be reviewed by two specialists before initiating valproate remains in place, however, the CHM has advised that this will not be required for male patients who are already taking valproate. Healthcare professionals are also reminded that all previously issued safety measures continue to apply.

The CHM has produced infographics to clarify the situations where review by two specialists may be required.

For female patients under 55 years of age, see: assets. publishing.service.gov.uk/media/ 67adf28c6e6c8d18118acd69/250213_MHRA_Valproate_ Infographic_Female_under_55_CC_V7.pdf.

For male patients under 55 years of age, see: assets. publishing.service.gov.uk/media/ 67adf2aa6e6c8d18118acd6a/250213_MHRA_Valproate_ Infographic_Male_under_55_CC_V7.pdf.

For male and female patients aged 55 years and older, see: assets.publishing.service.gov.uk/media/ 67adf2c62c594609b38acd71/250213_MHRA_Valproate_ Infographic_55_or_older_CC_V7.pdf.

For further information and resources, including a list of who may qualify as a specialist, see the MHRA Valproate Safety Measures information page, available at: www.gov.uk/government/collections/valproate-safety-measures.

- ● **CONTRA-INDICATIONS** Acute porphyrias p. 1202 · known or suspected mitochondrial disorders (higher rate of acute liver failure and liver-related deaths) · personal or family history of severe hepatic dysfunction · urea cycle disorders (risk of hyperammonaemia)

- ● **CAUTIONS** Systemic lupus erythematosus

  CAUTIONS, FURTHER INFORMATION

  ▸ Liver toxicity Liver dysfunction (including fatal hepatic failure) has occurred in association with valproate (especially in children under 3 years and in those with metabolic or degenerative disorders, organic brain disease or severe seizure disorders associated with mental retardation) usually in first 6 months and usually involving multiple antiepileptic therapy. EvGr Raised liver enzymes during valproate treatment are usually transient but patients should be reassessed clinically and liver function (including prothrombin time) monitored until return to normal—discontinue if abnormally prolonged prothrombin time (particularly in association with other relevant abnormalities). Ⓜ

  The MHRA advises consider vitamin D supplementation in patients who are immobilised for long periods or who have inadequate sun exposure or dietary intake of calcium.

- ● **INTERACTIONS** → Appendix 1: antiepileptics

- ● **SIDE-EFFECTS**

  ▸ **Common or very common** Abdominal pain · agitation · alopecia · anaemia · behaviour abnormal · concentration impaired · confusion · diarrhoea · drowsiness · haemorrhage · hallucination · headache · hearing loss · hepatic disorders · hypersensitivity · hyponatraemia · memory impairment · menstrual cycle irregularities · movement disorders · nail disorder · nausea · nystagmus · oral disorders · seizures · stupor · thrombocytopenia · tremor · urinary disorders · vomiting · weight increased

  ▸ **Uncommon** Angioedema · bone disorders · bone fracture · bone marrow disorders · coma · encephalopathy · eosinophilic pleural effusion · hair changes ·

hyperandrogenism · hypothermia · leucopenia · pancreatitis · paraesthesia · parkinsonism · peripheral oedema · renal failure · SIADH · skin reactions · vasculitis · virilism
▶ **Rare or very rare** Agranulocytosis · cerebral atrophy · cognitive disorder · dementia · diplopia · hyperammonaemia · hypothyroidism · infertility male · learning disability · myelodysplastic syndrome · nephritis tubulointerstitial · obesity · polycystic ovarian syndrome · red blood cell abnormalities · rhabdomyolysis · severe cutaneous adverse reactions (SCARs) · systemic lupus erythematosus (SLE)
▶ **Frequency not known** Gynaecomastia · hypocarnitinaemia · suicidal behaviours

SIDE-EFFECTS, FURTHER INFORMATION **Hepatic dysfunction** Withdraw treatment immediately if persistent vomiting and abdominal pain, anorexia, jaundice, oedema, malaise, drowsiness, or loss of seizure control.

Pancreatitis Discontinue treatment if symptoms of pancreatitis develop.

● CONCEPTION AND CONTRACEPTION The MHRA advises that all women and girls of childbearing potential being treated with valproate medicines must be supported on a Pregnancy Prevention Programme—pregnancy should be excluded before treatment initiation. Highly effective contraception must be used during treatment i.e. at least 1, preferably highly effective user-independent contraceptive method (such as an intra-uterine device or implant), or 2 complementary forms including a barrier method. The MHRA advises that all male patients being treated with valproate medicines and who may father children should use effective contraception (i.e. condoms plus contraception used by their female partner) during and for 3 months after treatment. The MHRA advises that male patients taking valproate medicines should be informed of the risk of infertility, and of data showing testicular toxicity in *animal* studies.

● PREGNANCY For *migraine prophylaxis* [unlicensed] and *bipolar disorder*, the MHRA advises that valproate medicines must not be used. For *epilepsy*, the MHRA advises valproate must not be used unless two specialists independently consider and document that there is no other effective or tolerated treatment (see also *Important safety information*). If valproate is to be used, the lowest effective dose should be prescribed in divided doses to be taken throughout the day; modified-release preparations may be preferable to avoid high peak plasma-valproate concentrations. There is no dose threshold considered to be without any risk, however, the risk of birth defects and neurodevelopmental disorders is greater at higher doses. EvGr Specialist prenatal monitoring should be instigated when valproate has been taken in pregnancy. Ⓜ Neonatal bleeding (related to hypofibrinaemia). Neonatal hepatotoxicity also reported. See also *Pregnancy* in Epilepsy p. 349.

● BREAST FEEDING Present in milk—risk of haematological disorders in breast-fed newborns and infants.

● HEPATIC IMPAIRMENT Manufacturer advises avoid.

● RENAL IMPAIRMENT
Dose adjustments EvGr Consider dose reduction. Ⓜ

● MONITORING REQUIREMENTS
▶ Monitor closely if dose greater than 45 mg/kg daily.
▶ Monitor liver function before therapy and during first 6 months especially in patients most at risk.
▶ Measure full blood count and ensure no undue potential for bleeding before starting and before surgery.

● EFFECT ON LABORATORY TESTS False-positive urine tests for ketones.

● TREATMENT CESSATION EvGr In bipolar disorder, avoid abrupt withdrawal; if treatment with valproate is stopped, reduce the dose gradually over at least 4 weeks. Ⓐ

● PRESCRIBING AND DISPENSING INFORMATION The Pregnancy Prevention Programme is supported by the following safety and educational materials: *Patient Guide*, *Guide for Healthcare Professionals*, *Annual Risk Acknowledgement Form for Female Patients*, *Risk Acknowledgement Form for Male Patients Starting Valproate*, *Patient Card*, *Pharmacy Poster*, and *Warning Stickers*.

In addition, the MHRA advises that pharmacists must dispense valproate medicines in the manufacturer's original full pack.

See the MHRA Valproate Safety Measures information page, available at: www.gov.uk/government/collections/valproate-safety-measures.

The Royal Pharmaceutical Society has also produced a safe supply algorithm, available at: www.rpharms.com/safesupplyvalproate.

CONVULEX ® Patients being treated for epilepsy may need to be maintained on a specific manufacturer's branded or generic oral valproic acid product.

● PATIENT AND CARER ADVICE The MHRA advises that patients should **not** stop taking valproate without first discussing it with a specialist. Female patients or their carers should be advised to immediately contact their GP for an urgent referral to a specialist in case of suspected pregnancy. Female partners of male patients taking valproate medicines should be referred for prenatal counselling if pregnancy is suspected.
Blood or hepatic disorders Patients or their carers should be told how to recognise signs and symptoms of blood or liver disorders and advised to seek immediate medical attention if symptoms develop.
Pancreatitis Patients or their carers should be told how to recognise signs and symptoms of pancreatitis and advised to seek immediate medical attention if symptoms such as abdominal pain, nausea, or vomiting develop.
Patient guide A patient guide must be provided.
Pregnancy Prevention Programme Pharmacists must ensure that female patients have a patient card—see also *Important safety information*.
Decision aid NHS England has produced a patient decision aid for females of childbearing potential who are considering or are taking valproate medicines for epilepsy, available at: www.england.nhs.uk/publication/decision-support-tool-is-valproate-the-right-epilepsy-treatment-for-me/.

● MEDICINAL FORMS There can be variation in the licensing of different medicines containing the same drug. Forms available from special-order manufacturers include: oral suspension, oral solution

Gastro-resistant capsule
CAUTIONARY AND ADVISORY LABELS 8, 10, 21, 25
▶ **Valproic acid (Non-proprietary)**
Valproic acid (as Valproate semisodium) 125 mg Depakote 125mg sprinkle gastro-resistant capsules | 100 capsule PoM ⓧ
▶ **Convulex** (G.L. Pharma UK Ltd) ▼
Valproic acid 150 mg Convulex 150mg gastro-resistant capsules | 30 capsule PoM £2.80 DT = £2.80
Valproic acid 300 mg Convulex 300mg gastro-resistant capsules | 30 capsule PoM £5.60 DT = £5.60
Valproic acid 500 mg Convulex 500mg gastro-resistant capsules | 30 capsule PoM £7.38 DT = £7.38

Gastro-resistant tablet
CAUTIONARY AND ADVISORY LABELS 10, 21, 25
▶ **Belvo** (Consilient Health Ltd)
Valproic acid (as Valproate semisodium) 250 mg Belvo 250mg gastro-resistant tablets | 30 tablet PoM £5.69 DT = £5.69
Valproic acid (as Valproate semisodium) 500 mg Belvo 500mg gastro-resistant tablets | 30 tablet PoM £11.37 DT = £11.37
▶ **Depakote** (Sanofi) ▼
Valproic acid (as Valproate semisodium) 250 mg Depakote 250mg gastro-resistant tablets | 30 tablet PoM £5.69 DT = £5.69

Valproic acid (as Valproate semisodium) **500 mg** Depakote 500mg gastro-resistant tablets | 30 tablet [PoM] £11.37 DT = £11.37
▸ **Syonell** (Lupin Healthcare (UK) Ltd)
Valproic acid (as Valproate semisodium) **250 mg** Syonell 250mg gastro-resistant tablets | 30 tablet [PoM] £4.55 DT = £5.69
Valproic acid (as Valproate semisodium) **500 mg** Syonell 500mg gastro-resistant tablets | 30 tablet [PoM] £9.10 DT = £11.37

ANTIPSYCHOTICS ⟩ SECOND-GENERATION

▸ 442

Asenapine
19-Jul-2021

● **INDICATIONS AND DOSE**

Moderate to severe manic episodes associated with bipolar disorder, as monotherapy or combination therapy
▸ BY SUBLINGUAL ADMINISTRATION
▸ Adult: 5 mg twice daily, increased if necessary to 10 mg twice daily, adjusted according to response

● **CAUTIONS** Dementia with Lewy bodies

● **INTERACTIONS** → Appendix 1: antipsychotics, second generation

● **SIDE-EFFECTS**
▸ **Common or very common** Anxiety · appetite increased · nausea · oral disorders · taste altered
▸ **Uncommon** Bundle branch block · dysarthria · dysphagia · sexual dysfunction · syncope
▸ **Rare or very rare** Accommodation disorder · pulmonary embolism · rhabdomyolysis

● **PREGNANCY** Use only if potential benefit outweighs risk— toxicity in *animal* studies.

● **BREAST FEEDING** Manufacturer advises discontinue breast-feeding—present in milk in *animal* studies.

● **HEPATIC IMPAIRMENT** Manufacturer advises caution in moderate impairment; avoid in severe impairment (risk of increased exposure).

● **RENAL IMPAIRMENT** [EvGr] Use with caution if creatinine clearance less than 15 mL/minute (no information available), Ⓜ see p. 21.

● **DIRECTIONS FOR ADMINISTRATION** Manufacturer advises *sublingual tablets* should be placed under the tongue and allowed to dissolve completely. Patients should be advised not to consume food or drink for at least 10 minutes after administration. When used as combination therapy, asenapine sublingual tablets should be administered last.

● **PATIENT AND CARER ADVICE** Patient or carer should be given advice on how to administer asenapine sublingual tablets.

● **MEDICINAL FORMS** There can be variation in the licensing of different medicines containing the same drug.
Sublingual tablet
CAUTIONARY AND ADVISORY LABELS 2, 26
▸ **Sycrest** (Organon Pharma (UK) Ltd)
Asenapine (as Asenapine maleate) 5 mg Sycrest 5mg sublingual tablets | 60 tablet [PoM] £102.60 DT = £102.60 [SF]
Asenapine (as Asenapine maleate) 10 mg Sycrest 10mg sublingual tablets | 60 tablet [PoM] £102.60 DT = £102.60 [SF]

LITHIUM SALTS

Lithium salts
03-May-2023

● **CONTRA-INDICATIONS** Addison's disease · cardiac disease associated with rhythm disorder · cardiac insufficiency · dehydration · family history of Brugada syndrome · low sodium diets · personal history of Brugada syndrome · untreated hypothyroidism

● **CAUTIONS** Avoid abrupt withdrawal · cardiac disease · concurrent ECT (may lower seizure threshold) · diuretic treatment (risk of toxicity) · elderly (reduce dose) · epilepsy (may lower seizure threshold) · myasthenia gravis · psoriasis (risk of exacerbation) · QT interval prolongation · review dose as necessary in diarrhoea · review dose as necessary in intercurrent infection (especially if sweating profusely) · review dose as necessary in vomiting · surgery

● **SIDE-EFFECTS**
▸ **Common or very common** Electrolyte imbalance
▸ **Rare or very rare** Nephrotic syndrome
▸ **Frequency not known** Abdominal discomfort · alopecia · angioedema · appetite decreased · arrhythmias · atrioventricular block · cardiomyopathy · cerebellar syndrome · circulatory collapse · coma · confusion · consciousness impaired · delirium · diarrhoea · dizziness · drug reaction with eosinophilia and systemic symptoms (DRESS) · dry mouth · encephalopathy · feeling dazed · folliculitis · gastritis · goitre · hyperglycaemia · hyperparathyroidism · hypersalivation · hypotension · hypothyroidism · idiopathic intracranial hypertension · leucocytosis · memory impairment · movement disorders · muscle weakness · myasthenia gravis · nausea · neoplasms · nephrogenic diabetes insipidus · neuroleptic malignant syndrome (discontinue—potentially fatal) · nystagmus · parathyroid hyperplasia · peripheral neuropathy · peripheral oedema · polydipsia · polyuria · QT interval prolongation · reflexes abnormal · renal disorders · renal impairment · rhabdomyolysis · seizure · serotonin syndrome · sexual dysfunction · skin reactions · skin ulcer · speech impairment · taste altered · thyrotoxicosis · tremor · vertigo · vision disorders · vomiting · weight increased

SIDE-EFFECTS, FURTHER INFORMATION **Overdose** Signs of intoxication require withdrawal of treatment and include increasing gastro-intestinal disturbances (vomiting, diarrhoea), visual disturbances, polyuria, muscle weakness, fine tremor increasing to coarse tremor, CNS disturbances (confusion and drowsiness increasing to lack of coordination, restlessness, stupor); abnormal reflexes, myoclonus, incontinence, hypernatraemia. With severe overdosage seizures, cardiac arrhythmias (including sino-atrial block, bradycardia and first-degree heart block), blood pressure changes, circulatory failure, renal failure, coma and sudden death reported.
For details on the management of poisoning, see Lithium, under Emergency treatment of poisoning p. 1554.

● **CONCEPTION AND CONTRACEPTION** Manufacturer advises effective contraception during treatment for women of child bearing potential.

● **PREGNANCY** Avoid if possible, particularly in the first trimester (risk of teratogenicity, including cardiac abnormalities). Close monitoring of serum-lithium concentration advised in pregnancy (risk of toxicity in neonate).
Dose adjustments Dose requirements increased during the second and third trimesters (but on delivery return abruptly to normal).

● **BREAST FEEDING** Present in milk and risk of toxicity in infant—avoid.

● **RENAL IMPAIRMENT** See p. 21. [EvGr] Caution in mild to moderate impairment; avoid in severe impairment. Ⓜ

● **MONITORING REQUIREMENTS**
▸ Serum concentrations Lithium salts have a narrow therapeutic/toxic ratio and should therefore not be prescribed unless facilities for monitoring serum-lithium concentrations are available.
[EvGr] Samples should be taken 12 hours post dose; for twice-daily dosing, morning dose to be withheld until sample taken. Ⓔ[EvGr] Serum-lithium concentrations should be monitored 1 week after treatment initiation, and 1 week after each dose (or formulation) change, and then weekly until concentrations are stable. Ⓐ
[EvGr]   An initial serum-lithium concentration between

0.6–0.8 mmol/litre is recommended for the treatment and prophylaxis of bipolar disorder in lithium-naïve patients, and between 0.4–0.6 mmol/litre for the treatment and prophylaxis of recurrent major depressive disorder (unipolar depression). Where the effect of lithium is sub-optimal, specialists may advise increasing the dose to obtain a serum concentration of 0.8–1 mmol/litre in bipolar disorder and 0.6–0.8 mmol/litre in unipolar depression. A lower initial serum-lithium concentration of 0.4–0.6 mmol/litre is recommended for patients aged 65 years and older, adjusted according to response on specialist advice. (E)

[EvGr] When serum-lithium concentrations are stable, monitor every 3 months for the first year, and every 6 months thereafter. Serum-lithium concentrations should be monitored every 3 months if patients: are 65 years and older; are taking drugs that interact with lithium; are at risk of impaired renal or thyroid function, have raised calcium levels, or other complications; have poor symptom control or poor adherence; or whose last serum-lithium concentration was 0.8 mmol/litre or higher. (A)[EvGr] Additional monitoring is required if a patient develops significant intercurrent disease, if there is a significant change in a patient's sodium or fluid intake, or if signs of lithium toxicity occur. (M)

▶ [EvGr] Before treatment initiation, assess body-weight or BMI, renal and thyroid function, urea and electrolytes (including calcium levels), and a full blood count. An ECG is recommended in patients with cardiovascular disease or risk factors for it.

▶ Body-weight or BMI, renal and thyroid function, and urea and electrolytes (including calcium levels) should be monitored at least every 6 months during treatment, and more often if there is evidence of impaired renal or thyroid function, raised calcium levels, or an increase in mood symptoms that might be related to impaired thyroid function or altered calcium levels. Specialists may recommend regular monitoring of cardiac function for some patients. (E)

● **TREATMENT CESSATION** [EvGr] If lithium is to be discontinued, the dose should be reduced gradually over a period of at least 4 weeks (preferably over a period of up to 3 months). Patients should be monitored closely for early signs of mania or depression during dose reduction and for 3 months after discontinuation of lithium. (A)

● **PATIENT AND CARER ADVICE** Patients and carers should be advised to report signs and symptoms of lithium toxicity, hypothyroidism, renal dysfunction (including polyuria and polydipsia), and benign intracranial hypertension (persistent headache and visual disturbance); medical attention should be sought if any of these occur. Patients and carers should also be counselled on the signs of relapse. Maintain adequate fluid intake and avoid dietary changes which reduce or increase sodium intake. Patients and carers should be made aware of the risk of dehydration due to factors such as excessive alcohol intake, hot climates, and vomiting or diarrhoea. Medical attention should be sought if dehydration occurs.

Lithium treatment packs A lithium treatment pack should be given to patients on initiation of treatment with lithium. The pack consists of a patient information booklet, lithium alert card, and a record book for tracking serum-lithium concentration. Packs may be purchased from

3M
0845 610 1112

NHS trusts can order supplies from cmswebshop.corp. xerox.com/NHS/Login.aspx.
Driving and skilled tasks May impair performance of skilled tasks (e.g. driving, operating machinery).

▶ 413

Lithium carbonate

10-Sep-2024

● **INDICATIONS AND DOSE**

Treatment and prophylaxis of mania (initiated by a specialist) | Treatment and prophylaxis of bipolar disorder (initiated by a specialist) | Treatment and prophylaxis of recurrent major depressive disorder [unipolar depression] (initiated by a specialist) | Treatment and prophylaxis of aggressive or self-harming behaviour (initiated by a specialist)

▶ BY MOUTH

▶ Adult: Initially 200–600 mg once daily, to be taken at night, dose adjusted according to serum-lithium concentration

▶ Elderly: Initially 100–250 mg once daily, to be taken at night, dose adjusted according to serum-lithium concentration

DOSE EQUIVALENCE AND CONVERSION

▶ There is no clinically significant difference between the pharmacokinetics of *Priadel*® and *Camcolit*® modified-release tablets; however, other preparations may not be bioequivalent. Lithium should be prescribed by brand name and formulation (tablets and liquids are not interchangeable)—changing the preparation or formulation requires the same monitoring of serum-lithium concentration as initiation of lithium.

● **UNLICENSED USE** [EvGr] Lithium carbonate is used in the doses provided in the BNF for the treatment and prophylaxis of mania, bipolar disorder, recurrent major depressive disorder (unipolar depression), and aggressive or self-harming behaviour (E), but these may differ from those licensed.

● **INTERACTIONS** → Appendix 1: lithium

● **SIDE-EFFECTS** Cardiac arrest · hyperthyroidism · parkinsonism

● **MEDICINAL FORMS** There can be variation in the licensing of different medicines containing the same drug. Forms available from special-order manufacturers include: oral suspension

Oral tablet
CAUTIONARY AND ADVISORY LABELS 10
▶ Lithium carbonate (Non-proprietary)
Lithium carbonate 250 mg Lithium carbonate 250mg tablets | 100 tablet [PoM] £95.70–£155.64 DT = £176.53

Modified-release tablet
CAUTIONARY AND ADVISORY LABELS 10, 25
▶ Camcolit (Essential Pharma Ltd)
Lithium carbonate 400 mg Camcolit 400 modified-release tablets | 100 tablet [PoM] £48.18 DT = £18.60
▶ Liskonum (Teofarma S.r.l.)
Lithium carbonate 450 mg Liskonum 450mg modified-release tablets | 60 tablet [PoM] £11.84 DT = £11.84
▶ Priadel (lithium carbonate) (Essential Pharma Ltd)
Lithium carbonate 200 mg Priadel 200mg modified-release tablets | 100 tablet [PoM] £16.42 DT = £16.42
Lithium carbonate 400 mg Priadel 400mg modified-release tablets | 100 tablet [PoM] £18.60 DT = £18.60

Lithium citrate

F 413

10-Sep-2024

- **INDICATIONS AND DOSE**

LI-LIQUID ®

Treatment and prophylaxis of mania (initiated by a specialist) | Treatment and prophylaxis of bipolar disorder (initiated by a specialist) | Treatment and prophylaxis of recurrent major depressive disorder [unipolar depression] (initiated by a specialist) | Treatment and prophylaxis of aggressive or self-harming behaviour (initiated by a specialist)

▸ BY MOUTH

▸ Adult: Initially 0.509–1.527 g daily in 1–2 divided doses, dose adjusted according to serum-lithium concentration

▸ Elderly: Initially 254.5–631.2 mg daily in 1–2 divided doses, dose adjusted according to serum-lithium concentration

DOSE EQUIVALENCE AND CONVERSION

▸ *Li-Liquid* ® containing lithium citrate 509 mg in 5 mL is equivalent to lithium carbonate 200 mg; *Li-Liquid* ® containing lithium citrate 1.018 g in 5 mL is equivalent to lithium carbonate 400 mg.

▸ **Preparations may vary widely in bioavailability;** lithium should be prescribed by brand name and formulation (tablets and liquids are not interchangeable)—changing the preparation or formulation requires the same monitoring of serum-lithium concentration as initiation of lithium.

PRIADEL ® LIQUID

Treatment and prophylaxis of mania (initiated by a specialist) | Treatment and prophylaxis of bipolar disorder (initiated by a specialist) | Treatment and prophylaxis of recurrent major depressive disorder [unipolar depression] (initiated by a specialist) | Treatment and prophylaxis of aggressive or self-harming behaviour (initiated by a specialist)

▸ BY MOUTH

▸ Adult: Initially 0.52–1.56 g daily in 1–2 divided doses, dose adjusted according to serum-lithium concentration

▸ Elderly: Initially 260–645 mg daily in 1–2 divided doses, dose adjusted according to serum-lithium concentration

DOSE EQUIVALENCE AND CONVERSION

▸ *Priadel* ® liquid containing lithium citrate 520 mg in 5 mL is equivalent to lithium carbonate 204 mg.

▸ **Preparations may vary widely in bioavailability;** lithium should be prescribed by brand name and formulation (tablets and liquids are not interchangeable)—changing the preparation or formulation requires the same monitoring of serum-lithium concentration as initiation of lithium.

- **UNLICENSED USE** EvGr Lithium citrate is used in the doses provided in the BNF for the treatment and prophylaxis of mania, bipolar disorder, recurrent major depressive disorder (unipolar depression), and aggressive or self-harming behaviour Ⓔ, but these may differ from those licensed.

- **INTERACTIONS** → Appendix 1: lithium

- **SIDE-EFFECTS** Thirst

- **MEDICINAL FORMS** There can be variation in the licensing of different medicines containing the same drug.

Oral solution

CAUTIONARY AND ADVISORY LABELS 10

▸ Li-Liquid (Rosemont Pharmaceuticals Ltd)
Lithium citrate 101.8 mg per 1 ml Li-Liquid 509mg/5ml oral solution | 150 ml [PoM] £5.79 DT = £5.79

Lithium citrate 203.6 mg per 1 ml Li-Liquid 1.018g/5ml oral solution | 150 ml [PoM] £17.49 DT = £17.49

▸ Priadel (lithium citrate) (Essential Pharma Ltd)
Lithium citrate 104 mg per 1 ml Priadel 520mg/5ml liquid | 150 ml [PoM] £12.11 DT = £12.11 [SF]

3.4 Depression

Depression

05-Aug-2022

Description of condition

Depression is a common condition characterised by low mood, loss of interest or pleasure in most activities, and a range of associated emotional, cognitive, physical, and behavioural symptoms (such as sleep and appetite disturbance, lack of concentration, low self-confidence, agitation, guilt or self-blame, and suicidal thoughts or acts). It is one of the leading causes of disability and can have a major detrimental effect on an individual's life.

Risk factors for depression include a personal or family history of depressive illness, history of other mental health conditions, other chronic comorbidities, female sex, recent childbirth, older age, and psychosocial issues (such as relationship problems, bereavement, unemployment, poverty, or homelessness).

Depression severity depends on the intensity, frequency and duration of symptoms, and their impact on daily functioning. This can be classified as subthreshold, mild, moderate, or severe.

Patients classified as having chronic depressive symptoms include those who for at least 2 years, either continually meet the criteria for diagnosis of a major depressive episode, or have persistent subthreshold symptoms, or persistent low mood (with or without concurrent episodes of major depression).

Recurrence rates of depression are high and increase with each depressive episode.

Aims of treatment

Treatment aims to improve the patient's mood and quality of life, and to reduce the risk of relapse or recurrence.

Management

Patients with depression should be assessed for the risk of suicide, comorbid conditions associated with depression (such as anxiety, Dementia p. 343, personality disorders, or psychotic symptoms), and any other risk factors. For further guidance, see NICE guideline: **Depression in adults: treatment and management** (see *Useful resources*).

Lifestyle changes such as regular physical activity, eating a healthy diet, not over-using alcohol, and getting enough sleep should be encouraged, as these may help to improve the patient's sense of well-being.

EvGr The choice of treatment for depression should be based on the patient's clinical needs, their preference, and response to any previous treatment. Initial treatment options that may be offered include the use of an antidepressant and/or psychological and psychosocial treatment (guided self-help, cognitive behavioural therapy (CBT), behavioural activation (BA), group physical activity provided by a trained healthcare professional, group mindfulness and meditation, interpersonal psychotherapy (IPT), counselling, or short-term psychodynamic psychotherapy (STPP)). Any of these treatment options can be used first line, with patients made aware of any waiting times for particular treatments. Ⓐ For further guidance on treatment options, see *Subthreshold or mild depression*, *Moderate or severe depression*, and *Chronic depressive symptoms*.

Patients with moderate or severe depression or chronic

depressive symptoms should be referred to specialist mental health services if they have not benefited from previous treatments, and they either have multiple complicating problems or significant co-existing conditions.

For patients who are assessed to be at risk of suicide, toxicity in overdose should be taken into account if drug treatment is prescribed and referral to specialist mental health services considered; EvGr withholding treatment for depression on the basis of the patient's suicide risk is not recommended. Ⓐ

All patients receiving treatment should be monitored for suicidal ideation, particularly in the early weeks of treatment, and for treatment concordance. Patients and their family/carers should be advised to be vigilant for worsening behavioural symptoms (such as mood changes), especially during high-risk periods such as times of increased stress or when starting or changing treatment, and to seek help from a healthcare professional if concerned.

For all patients, response to treatment should be reviewed 2 to 4 weeks after initiation. Patients on antidepressants should usually be reviewed within 2 weeks of initiation; however, those who are thought to be at risk of suicide or who are aged 18 to 25 years, should be reviewed 1 week after starting treatment (or increasing the dose), with ongoing reviews repeated as often as necessary but within 4 weeks. Patients should be informed that the effects of antidepressant treatment are usually seen within 4 weeks of initiation and that treatment is usually continued for at least 6 months. Thereafter, ongoing reviews should continue according to the patients' needs.

Patients taking antidepressants should also be advised about the risk of withdrawal symptoms if they abruptly stop, miss doses, or do not take a full dose. Discontinuation of an antidepressant usually involves a step-wise dose reduction, with smaller reductions considered as the dose becomes lower; more rapid withdrawal may be appropriate in some circumstances. Successful withdrawal of an antidepressant drug may take weeks or months to complete.

For further information on prescribing or discontinuing antidepressants, and the management of withdrawal symptoms, see Antidepressant drugs p. 417, *Treatment cessation* in drug monographs, and NICE guidelines: **Depression in adults: treatment and management** (see *Useful resources*) and **Medicines associated with dependence or withdrawal symptoms: safe prescribing and withdrawal management for adults** (available at: www.nice.org.uk/guidance/ng215).

Pregnancy and breast-feeding

The management of depression during pregnancy and the postnatal period should take into account the potential risks and benefits of treatments (including that of stopping or changing treatment), the patient's preference, and the possible risks from untreated depression, on the female and the fetus or baby. Before starting any treatment, discuss the higher threshold for intervention with drug treatment because of the changing risk-benefit ratio, and the likely benefits of psychological treatment. Specialist advice, preferably from a specialist in perinatal mental health, should be sought if there is uncertainty about the risks associated with specific drug treatments.

For further guidance on the management of depression in pregnancy and breast-feeding, see NICE guideline: **Antenatal and postnatal mental health: clinical management and service guidance** (available at: www.nice.org.uk/guidance/cg192) and Clinical Knowledge Summary (CKS): **Depression - antenatal and postnatal** (available at: cks.nice.org.uk/topics/depression-antenatal-postnatal/).

Subthreshold or mild depression

EvGr For patients with a new episode of subthreshold or mild depression, psychological and psychosocial therapy (such as guided self-help, CBT, or BA) should be considered as first-line treatment options.

Antidepressants should not be offered routinely, unless it is the patient's preference. Where this is the case, an SSRI such as citalopram p. 422, escitalopram p. 423, sertraline p. 425, fluoxetine p. 424, fluvoxamine maleate p. 424, or paroxetine p. 425 should be offered as appropriate. Ⓐ

For patients who decide against treatment, offer active monitoring with the option to reconsider treatment at any time, and arrange a further assessment (usually within 2 to 4 weeks).

EvGr St John's wort (Hypericum perforatum) is a herbal remedy that may improve subthreshold or mild depression; however its use is not recommended for the treatment of depression because of potentially serious interactions with other drugs, variation in potency between different preparations, and the uncertainty about appropriate doses to be used. Ⓐ

For guidance on alternative treatment options for patients who have limited or no response to first-line treatment, see *Further treatment*.

Moderate or severe depression

EvGr For patients with a new episode of moderate or severe depression, combination therapy with an antidepressant and individual CBT should ideally be offered as first-line treatment; however, monotherapy with an antidepressant or a psychological treatment (such as individual CBT, BA or problem solving) may also be offered as a first-line option. SSRIs should be considered as the first choice of antidepressant treatment as they are well tolerated and have a good safety profile. Other antidepressant options include serotonin and noradrenaline reuptake inhibitors (SNRIs) such as duloxetine p. 426 and venlafaxine p. 427, or an antidepressant based on the patient's previous treatment history such as a tricyclic antidepressant (TCA). Ⓐ Note that TCAs are associated with the greatest risk in overdose, although lofepramine p. 436 has the best safety profile.

Electroconvulsive therapy (ECT) for the treatment of severe depression should be considered if a rapid response is needed, or if based on the patient's previous experience, it is their preference over other treatments.

For guidance on alternative treatment options for patients who have limited or no response to first-line treatment, see *Further treatment*.

Further treatment

For patients who have not responded after 4 weeks of antidepressant treatment, or after 4 to 6 weeks of psychological therapy or combined antidepressant and psychological therapy, assess for treatment adherence and consider other factors or health conditions that may explain why the treatment is not working.

EvGr For patients with limited or no response to psychological monotherapy, consider switching to an alternative psychological treatment, adding in an SSRI, or switching to an SSRI alone.

If there has been limited or no response to antidepressant monotherapy, consider the addition of a group exercise intervention; switching to a psychological therapy; increasing the antidepressant dose; switching to a different antidepressant in the same class or different class; or changing to a combination of psychological therapy and an antidepressant.

For patients with limited or no response to treatment with a combination of psychological therapy and an antidepressant, consider switching to another psychological therapy; increasing the antidepressant dose; switching to another antidepressant drug in the same class or different class; or adding in another medication.

Vortioxetine p. 439 may be considered as a treatment option for patients with limited or no response to at least two antidepressant drugs.

Referral to a specialist mental health setting or seeking specialist advice should be considered when switching to an antidepressant from a different class such as a TCA or MAOI; when adding in an additional antidepressant from a different class; when combining an antidepressant with either a second-generation antipsychotic, lithium carbonate p. 414, or lithium citrate p. 415; or when combining antidepressant drugs with ECT, lamotrigine p. 366 [unlicensed use], or liothyronine sodium p. 891 [unlicensed use].

ECT, transcranial magnetic stimulation, and implanted vagus nerve stimulation may also be considered as treatment options for certain patients with depression. ◇A◇

Relapse prevention

Continuation of treatment following full or partial remission may reduce the risk of relapse, this should be discussed with the patient and a shared decision made whether to continue or to stop treatment.

[EvGr] For patients in remission following psychological treatment alone, but who are at a higher risk of relapse, consider continuing psychological therapy.

For patients on antidepressant monotherapy who are in remission but at higher risk of relapse, consider continuing the antidepressant, combining the antidepressant with a course of psychological therapy (such as group CBT or mindfulness-based cognitive therapy (MBCT)), or switching to a course of psychological therapy alone.

For patients in remission following combination treatment with an antidepressant and psychological therapy who are at higher risk of relapse, consider continuing one or both treatments. ◇A◇

The risk of relapse should be reassessed on completion of psychological therapy, and at least every 6 months for those who continue on antidepressant treatment.

Chronic depressive symptoms

Some patients presenting with chronic depressive symptoms may not have sought treatment for their depression previously. [EvGr] For patients with symptoms that significantly impair functioning, treatment options include monotherapy with either CBT or drug treatment with an SSRI, SNRI, or a TCA; or combination therapy with CBT and either an SSRI or a TCA. Note that TCAs are associated with the greatest risk in overdose, although lofepramine has a better safety profile. ◇A◇

For patients who do not respond to SSRIs or SNRIs, consider alternative drug treatments in specialist settings or on specialist advice (alternatives include TCAs, moclobemide p. 420, irreversible MAOIs, or amisulpride p. 453 [unlicensed use]).

For further guidance on alternative treatment options for patients who have limited or no response to treatment, or for guidance on treatment options for patients who have had, or are still receiving treatment for depression and present with chronic depressive symptoms, see *Further treatment*.

Useful Resources

Depression in adults: treatment and management. National Institute for Health and Care Excellence. NICE guideline 222. June 2022.
www.nice.org.uk/guidance/ng222

Antidepressant drugs
05-Aug-2022

Overview
Choice
The major classes of antidepressant drugs include the tricyclic and related antidepressants, the selective serotonin re-uptake inhibitors (SSRIs), and the monoamine oxidase

inhibitors (MAOIs). A number of antidepressant drugs cannot be accommodated easily into this classification.

There is little to choose between the different classes of antidepressant drugs in terms of efficacy, so choice should be based on the individual patient's requirements, including the presence of concomitant disease, existing therapy, suicide risk, and previous response to antidepressant therapy. During the first few weeks of treatment, there is an increased potential for agitation, anxiety, and suicidal ideation.

SSRIs are better tolerated and are safer in overdose than other classes of antidepressants. In patients with unstable angina or who have had a recent myocardial infarction, sertraline p. 425 has been shown to be safe.

Tricyclic antidepressants have similar efficacy to SSRIs but are more likely to be discontinued because of side-effects; toxicity in overdosage is also a problem. SSRIs are less sedating and have fewer antimuscarinic and cardiotoxic effects than tricyclic antidepressants.

MAOIs have dangerous interactions with some foods and drugs, and should be reserved for use by specialists.

Management
For guidance on the management of depression, see Depression p. 415.

Patients should be reviewed every 1–2 weeks at the start of antidepressant treatment. Treatment should be continued for at least 4 weeks (6 weeks in the elderly) before considering whether to switch antidepressant due to lack of efficacy. In cases of partial response, continue for a further 2–4 weeks (elderly patients may take longer to respond).

Following remission, antidepressant treatment should be continued at the same dose for at least 6 months (about 12 months in the elderly), or for at least 12 months in patients receiving treatment for generalised anxiety disorder (as the likelihood of relapse is high).

For guidance on the prescribing of antidepressant drugs, and management of withdrawal, see NICE guideline: **Medicines associated with dependence or withdrawal symptoms: safe prescribing and withdrawal management for adults** (available at: www.nice.org.uk/guidance/ng215).

Hyponatraemia and antidepressant therapy
Hyponatraemia (usually in the elderly and possibly due to inappropriate secretion of antidiuretic hormone) has been associated with all types of antidepressants; however, it has been reported more frequently with SSRIs than with other antidepressants. Hyponatraemia should be considered in all patients who develop drowsiness, confusion, or convulsions while taking an antidepressant.

Suicidal behaviour and antidepressant therapy
The use of antidepressants has been linked with suicidal thoughts and behaviour; children, young adults, and patients with a history of suicidal behaviour are particularly at risk. Where necessary patients should be monitored for suicidal behaviour, self-harm, or hostility, particularly at the beginning of treatment or if the dose is changed.

Serotonin syndrome
Serotonin syndrome or serotonin toxicity is a relatively uncommon adverse drug reaction caused by excessive central and peripheral serotonergic activity. Onset of symptoms, which range from mild to life-threatening, can occur within hours or days following the initiation, dose escalation, or overdose of a serotonergic drug, the addition of a new serotonergic drug, or the replacement of one serotonergic drug by another without allowing a long enough washout period in-between, particularly when the first drug is an irreversible MAOI or a drug with a long half-life. Severe toxicity, which is a medical emergency, usually occurs with a combination of serotonergic drugs, one of which is generally an MAOI.

The characteristic symptoms of serotonin syndrome fall

into 3 main areas, although features from each group may not be seen in all patients—neuromuscular hyperactivity (such as tremor, hyperreflexia, clonus, myoclonus, rigidity), autonomic dysfunction (tachycardia, blood pressure changes, hyperthermia, diaphoresis, shivering, diarrhoea), and altered mental state (agitation, confusion, mania).

Treatment consists of withdrawal of the serotonergic medication and supportive care; specialist advice should be sought.

Anxiety disorders and obsessive-compulsive disorder

Management of acute anxiety generally involves the use of a benzodiazepine or buspirone hydrochloride p. 396. For chronic anxiety (of longer than 4 weeks' duration) it may be appropriate to use an antidepressant. Combined therapy with a benzodiazepine may be required until the antidepressant takes effect. Patients with *generalised anxiety disorder*, a form of chronic anxiety, should be offered psychological treatment before initiating an antidepressant. If drug treatment is needed, an SSRI such as escitalopram p. 423, paroxetine p. 425, or sertraline [unlicensed], can be used. Duloxetine p. 426 and venlafaxine p. 427 (serotonin and noradrenaline reuptake inhibitors (SNRIs)) are also recommended for the treatment of generalised anxiety disorder; if the patient cannot tolerate SSRIs or SNRIs (or if treatment has failed to control symptoms), pregabalin p. 374 can be considered.

Panic disorder is treated with SSRIs; clomipramine hydrochloride [unlicensed] or imipramine hydrochloride [unlicensed] can be used second-line. Venlafaxine, an SNRI, is also licensed for panic disorder.

Obsessive-compulsive disorder, post-traumatic stress disorder, and phobic states such as *social anxiety disorder* are treated with SSRIs. Clomipramine hydrochloride p. 432 can be used second-line for obsessive-compulsive disorder. Moclobemide p. 420 is licensed for the treatment of social anxiety disorder.

Tricyclic and related antidepressant drugs

Choice

Tricyclic and related antidepressants block the re-uptake of both serotonin and noradrenaline, although to different extents. For example, clomipramine hydrochloride is more selective for serotonergic transmission, and imipramine hydrochloride p. 435 is more selective for noradrenergic transmission. Tricyclic and related antidepressant drugs can be roughly divided into those with additional sedative properties and those that are less sedating. Agitated and anxious patients tend to respond best to the sedative compounds, whereas withdrawn and apathetic patients will often obtain most benefit from the less sedating ones. Those with **sedative** properties include amitriptyline hydrochloride p. 431, clomipramine hydrochloride, dosulepin hydrochloride p. 433, doxepin p. 434, mianserin hydrochloride p. 430, trazodone hydrochloride p. 429, and trimipramine p. 438. Those with **less sedative** properties include imipramine hydrochloride, lofepramine p. 436, and nortriptyline p. 437.

Tricyclic and related antidepressants also have varying degrees of antimuscarinic side-effects and cardiotoxicity in overdosage, which may be important in individual patients. Lofepramine has a lower incidence of side-effects and is less dangerous in overdosage but is infrequently associated with hepatic toxicity. Imipramine hydrochloride is also well established, but has more marked antimuscarinic side-effects than other tricyclic and related antidepressants. Amitriptyline hydrochloride and dosulepin hydrochloride are effective but they are particularly dangerous in overdosage; dosulepin hydrochloride should be initiated by a specialist.

Dosage

About 10 to 20% of patients fail to respond to tricyclic and related antidepressant drugs and inadequate dosage may account for some of these failures. It is important to use doses that are sufficiently high for effective treatment but not so high as to cause toxic effects. Low doses should be used for initial treatment in the **elderly**. In most patients the long half-life of tricyclic antidepressant drugs allows **once-daily** administration, usually at night; the use of modified-release preparations is therefore unnecessary.

Some tricyclic antidepressants are used in the management of *panic* and other *anxiety disorders*. Some tricyclic antidepressants may also have a role in some forms of *neuralgia* and in *nocturnal enuresis* in children.

Children and adolescents

Studies have shown that tricyclic antidepressants are not effective for treating depression in children.

Considerations in the elderly

The use of tricyclic antidepressants in elderly patients is potentially inappropriate (STOPP criteria):

- if prescribed in those with dementia, narrow angle glaucoma, cardiac conduction abnormalities, prostatism, or history of urinary retention (risk of worsening these conditions);
- if initiated as first-line antidepressant treatment (higher risk of adverse drug reactions than with SSRIs or SNRIs).

For further information, see *STOPP/START criteria* in Prescribing in the elderly p. 31.

Monoamine-oxidase inhibitors

Monoamine-oxidase inhibitors are used much less frequently than tricyclic and related antidepressants, or SSRIs and related antidepressants because of the dangers of dietary and drug interactions and the fact that it is easier to prescribe MAOIs when tricyclic antidepressants have been unsuccessful than vice versa.

Tranylcypromine p. 420 has a greater stimulant action than phenelzine p. 420 or isocarboxazid p. 420 and is more likely to cause a hypertensive crisis. Isocarboxazid and phenelzine are more likely to cause hepatotoxicity than tranylcypromine.

Moclobemide p. 420 should be reserved as a second line treatment.

Phobic patients and depressed patients with atypical, hypochondriacal, or hysterical features are said to respond best to MAOIs. However, MAOIs should be tried in any patients who are refractory to treatment with other antidepressants as there is occasionally a dramatic response. Response to treatment may be delayed for 3 weeks or more and may take an additional 1 or 2 weeks to become maximal.

Interactions

Other antidepressants should not be started for 2 weeks after treatment with MAOIs has been stopped (3 weeks if starting clomipramine or imipramine). Conversely, an MAOI should not be started until:

- at least 2 weeks after a previous MAOI has been stopped (then started at a reduced dose)
- at least 7–14 days after a tricyclic or related antidepressant (3 weeks in the case of clomipramine or imipramine) has been stopped
- at least a week after an SSRI or related antidepressant (at least 5 weeks in the case of fluoxetine) has been stopped

Other antidepressant drugs

The thioxanthene flupentixol p. 444 (*Fluanxol®*) has antidepressant properties when given by mouth in low doses. Flupentixol is also used for the treatment of psychoses.

Other drugs used for Depression Quetiapine, p. 462

ANTIDEPRESSANTS › MELATONIN RECEPTOR AGONISTS

Agomelatine

07-May-2021

- **DRUG ACTION** A melatonin receptor agonist and a selective serotonin-receptor antagonist; it does not affect the uptake of serotonin, noradrenaline, or dopamine.

- **INDICATIONS AND DOSE**

Major depression
▸ BY MOUTH
▸ Adult: 25 mg once daily, to be taken at bedtime, increased if necessary to 50 mg once daily, to be taken at bedtime, increased dose may be used after 2 weeks of initial treatment

- **CAUTIONS** Alcoholism · bipolar disorder · diabetes · elderly with dementia (safety and efficacy not established) · excessive alcohol consumption · hypomania · mania · non-alcoholic fatty liver disease · obesity · patients 75 years of age or older (safety and efficacy not established)

- **INTERACTIONS** → Appendix 1: agomelatine

- **SIDE-EFFECTS**
▸ **Common or very common** Abdominal pain · anxiety · back pain · constipation · diarrhoea · dizziness · drowsiness · fatigue · headaches · nausea · sleep disorders · vomiting · weight changes
▸ **Uncommon** Aggression · confusion · hyperhidrosis · mood altered · movement disorders · paraesthesia · skin reactions · suicidal behaviours · tinnitus · vision blurred
▸ **Rare or very rare** Angioedema · face oedema · hallucination · hepatic disorders · urinary retention

SIDE-EFFECTS, FURTHER INFORMATION The use of antidepressants has been linked with suicidal thoughts and behaviour; children, young adults, and patients with a history of suicidal behaviour are particularly at risk. Where necessary patients should be monitored for suicidal behaviour, self-harm, or hostility, particularly at the beginning of treatment or if the dose is changed.

- **PREGNANCY** Manufacturer advises avoid.

- **BREAST FEEDING** Avoid—present in milk in *animal* studies.

- **HEPATIC IMPAIRMENT** Manufacturer advises caution if transaminases are elevated; avoid in hepatic impairment or if transaminases exceed 3 times the upper limit of normal.

- **RENAL IMPAIRMENT** [EvGr] Caution in moderate to severe impairment. ⓜ

- **MONITORING REQUIREMENTS** Test liver function before treatment and after 3, 6, 12 and 24 weeks of treatment, and then regularly thereafter when clinically indicated (restart monitoring schedule if dose increased); discontinue if serum transaminases exceed 3 times the upper limit of reference range or symptoms of liver disorder.

- **PATIENT AND CARER ADVICE**
Hepatotoxicity Patients should be told how to recognise signs of liver disorder, and advised to seek immediate medical attention if symptoms such as dark urine, light coloured stools, jaundice, bruising, fatigue, abdominal pain, or pruritus develop.

Patients should be given a booklet with more information on the risk of hepatic side-effects.

- **MEDICINAL FORMS** There can be variation in the licensing of different medicines containing the same drug.

Oral tablet
▸ Agomelatine (Non-proprietary)
Agomelatine 25 mg Agomelatine 25mg tablets | 28 tablet [PoM] £30.00 DT = £17.22

▸ Valdoxan (Servier Laboratories Ltd)
Agomelatine 25 mg Valdoxan 25mg tablets | 28 tablet [PoM] £30.00 DT = £17.22

ANTIDEPRESSANTS › MONOAMINE-OXIDASE INHIBITORS

Monoamine-oxidase inhibitors 

- **DRUG ACTION** MAOIs inhibit monoamine oxidase, thereby causing an accumulation of amine neurotransmitters.

- **CONTRA-INDICATIONS** Cerebrovascular disease · not indicated in manic phase · phaeochromocytoma · severe cardiovascular disease

- **CAUTIONS** Acute porphyrias p. 1202 · avoid in agitated patients · blood disorders · cardiovascular disease · concurrent electroconvulsive therapy · diabetes mellitus · elderly (great caution) · epilepsy · severe hypertensive reactions to certain drugs and foods · surgery

- **SIDE-EFFECTS** Akathisia · anxiety · appetite increased · arrhythmia · asthenia · behaviour abnormal · blood disorder · confusion · constipation · dizziness · drowsiness · dry mouth · dysuria · hallucination · headache · hyperhidrosis · insomnia · jaundice · nausea · paraesthesia · peripheral neuritis · postural hypotension (more common in elderly) · reflexes increased · skin reactions · suicidal behaviours · tremor · vision blurred · vomiting · weight increased

SIDE-EFFECTS, FURTHER INFORMATION Risk of postural hypotension and hypertensive responses. Discontinue if palpitations or frequent headaches occur.

- **PREGNANCY** Increased risk of neonatal malformations—manufacturer advises avoid unless there are compelling reasons.

- **HEPATIC IMPAIRMENT** In general, manufacturers advise avoid.

- **MONITORING REQUIREMENTS** Monitor blood pressure (risk of postural hypotension and hypertensive responses).

- **TREATMENT CESSATION**
Withdrawal If possible avoid abrupt withdrawal.
MAOIs are associated with withdrawal symptoms on cessation of therapy. Symptoms include agitation, irritability, ataxia, movement disorders, insomnia, drowsiness, vivid dreams, cognitive impairment, and slowed speech. Withdrawal symptoms occasionally experienced when discontinuing MAOIs include hallucinations and paranoid delusions. If possible MAOIs should be withdrawn slowly.

Withdrawal effects may occur within 5 days of stopping treatment with antidepressant drugs; they are usually mild and self-limiting, but in some cases may be severe. The risk of withdrawal symptoms is increased if the antidepressant is stopped suddenly after regular administration for 8 weeks or more. The dose should preferably be reduced gradually over about 4 weeks, or longer if withdrawal symptoms emerge (6 months in patients who have been on long-term maintenance treatment).

- **PATIENT AND CARER ADVICE** Patients should be advised to eat only fresh foods and avoid food that is suspected of being stale or 'going off'. This is especially important with meat, fish, poultry or offal; game should be avoided. The danger of interaction persists for up to 2 weeks after treatment with MAOIs is discontinued. Patients should also be advised to avoid alcoholic drinks or de-alcoholised (low alcohol) drinks.
Driving and skilled tasks Drowsiness may affect performance of skilled tasks (e.g. driving).

4

Nervous system

ANTIDEPRESSANTS > MONOAMINE-OXIDASE A AND B INHIBITORS, IRREVERSIBLE

⌐ 419

Isocarboxazid
07-May-2021

● **INDICATIONS AND DOSE**

Depressive illness

▸ BY MOUTH

▸ Adult: Initially 30 mg daily until improvement occurs, initial dose may be given in single or divided doses, dose may be increased if necessary after 4 weeks, increased if necessary up to 60 mg daily for 4–6 weeks, dose to be increased under close supervision only, then reduced to 10–20 mg daily, usual maintenance dose, but up to 40 mg daily may be required

▸ Elderly: 5–10 mg daily

● INTERACTIONS → Appendix 1: MAOIs, irreversible

● SIDE-EFFECTS Granulocytopenia · peripheral oedema · sexual dysfunction

● BREAST FEEDING Avoid.

● RENAL IMPAIRMENT EvGr Use with caution. Ⓜ

● LESS SUITABLE FOR PRESCRIBING Less suitable for prescribing.

● MEDICINAL FORMS There can be variation in the licensing of different medicines containing the same drug. Forms available from special-order manufacturers include: oral suspension

Oral tablet

CAUTIONARY AND ADVISORY LABELS 3, 10

▸ Isocarboxazid (Non-proprietary)

Isocarboxazid 10 mg Isocarboxazid 10mg tablets | 56 tablet PoM £249.10–£302.10 DT = £287.71

⌐ 419

Phenelzine
21-May-2020

● **INDICATIONS AND DOSE**

Depressive illness

▸ BY MOUTH

▸ Adult: Initially 15 mg 3 times a day, response is usually seen within first week; dose may be increased if necessary after 2 weeks if response is not evident, increased if necessary to 15 mg 4 times a day, doses up to 30 mg three times a day may be used in hospital patients; response may not become apparent for up to 4 weeks; once satisfactory response has been achieved, reduce dose gradually to lowest suitable maintenance dose (15 mg on alternate days may be adequate)

● INTERACTIONS → Appendix 1: MAOIs, irreversible

● SIDE-EFFECTS

▸ **Rare or very rare** Neuroleptic malignant syndrome (discontinue—potentially fatal)

▸ **Frequency not known** Cardiovascular insufficiency · delirium · electrolyte imbalance · fatal progressive hepatocellular necrosis · feeling jittery · fever · gastrointestinal disorder · glaucoma · hypermetabolism · hypertensive crisis · impaired driving ability · intracranial haemorrhage · lupus-like syndrome · malaise · mood altered · movement disorders · muscle tone increased · muscle twitching · nystagmus · oedema · respiratory disorders · schizophrenia · seizure · sexual dysfunction · shock-like coma · speech repetitive

● BREAST FEEDING Avoid—no information available.

● LESS SUITABLE FOR PRESCRIBING Less suitable for prescribing.

● MEDICINAL FORMS There can be variation in the licensing of different medicines containing the same drug.

Oral tablet

CAUTIONARY AND ADVISORY LABELS 3, 10

▸ Nardil (Neon Healthcare Ltd)

Phenelzine (as Phenelzine sulfate) 15 mg Nardil 15mg tablets | 100 tablet PoM £120.00 DT = £120.00

⌐ 419

Tranylcypromine
22-May-2020

● **INDICATIONS AND DOSE**

Depressive illness

▸ BY MOUTH

▸ Adult: Initially 10 mg twice daily, dose to be taken at a time no later than 3 p.m, dose may be increased if necessary after 1 week, increased if necessary to 30 mg daily in divided doses, 10 mg to be taken in the morning and 20 mg to be taken in the afternoon, doses above 30 mg daily under close supervision only; maintenance 10 mg daily

● CONTRA-INDICATIONS History of hepatic disease · hyperthyroidism

● INTERACTIONS → Appendix 1: MAOIs, irreversible

● SIDE-EFFECTS

▸ **Rare or very rare** Hepatocellular injury

▸ **Frequency not known** Chest pain · diarrhoea · drug dependence · extrasystole · flushing · hypertension · hypomania · mydriasis · pain · pallor · photophobia · sleep disorder · throbbing headache

● BREAST FEEDING Present in milk in *animal* studies.

● LESS SUITABLE FOR PRESCRIBING Less suitable for prescribing.

● MEDICINAL FORMS There can be variation in the licensing of different medicines containing the same drug.

Oral tablet

CAUTIONARY AND ADVISORY LABELS 3, 10

▸ Tranylcypromine (Non-proprietary)

Tranylcypromine (as Tranylcypromine sulfate) 10 mg Tranylcypromine 10mg tablets | 28 tablet PoM £500.00 DT = £485.00

ANTIDEPRESSANTS > MONOAMINE-OXIDASE A INHIBITORS, REVERSIBLE

Moclobemide
08-Nov-2020

● DRUG ACTION Moclobemide is reported to act by reversible inhibition of monoamine oxidase type A (it is therefore termed a RIMA).

● **INDICATIONS AND DOSE**

Depressive illness

▸ BY MOUTH

▸ Adult: Initially 300 mg daily in divided doses, adjusted according to response; usual dose 150–600 mg daily, dose to be taken after food

Social anxiety disorder

▸ BY MOUTH

▸ Adult: Initially 300 mg daily for 3 days, then increased to 600 mg daily in 2 divided doses continued for 8–12 weeks to assess efficacy

DOSE ADJUSTMENTS DUE TO INTERACTIONS

▸ Manufacturer advises reduce dose to half or one-third of the usual dose with concurrent use of cimetidine.

● CONTRA-INDICATIONS Acute confusional states · phaeochromocytoma

- **CAUTIONS** Avoid in agitated or excited patients (or give with sedative for up to 2–3 weeks) · may provoke manic episodes in bipolar disorders · thyrotoxicosis
- **INTERACTIONS** → Appendix 1: moclobemide
- **SIDE-EFFECTS**
▶ **Common or very common** Anxiety · constipation · diarrhoea · dizziness · dry mouth · headache · hypotension · irritability · nausea · paraesthesia · skin reactions · sleep disorder · vomiting
▶ **Uncommon** Asthenia · confusion · flushing · oedema · suicidal behaviours · taste altered · visual impairment
▶ **Rare or very rare** Appetite decreased · delusions · hyponatraemia · serotonin syndrome
- **PREGNANCY** Safety in pregnancy has not been established—manufacturer advises avoid unless there are compelling reasons.
- **BREAST FEEDING** Amount too small to be harmful, but patient information leaflet advises avoid.
- **HEPATIC IMPAIRMENT** Manufacturer advises caution in severe impairment (risk of decreased metabolism). **Dose adjustments** Manufacturer advises dose reduction to half or one-third of the daily dose in severe impairment.
- **TREATMENT CESSATION** Withdrawal effects may occur within 5 days of stopping treatment with antidepressant drugs; they are usually mild and self-limiting, but in some cases may be severe. The risk of withdrawal symptoms is increased if the antidepressant is stopped suddenly after regular administration for 8 weeks or more. The dose should preferably be reduced gradually over about 4 weeks, or longer if withdrawal symptoms emerge (6 months in patients who have been on long-term maintenance treatment).
- **PATIENT AND CARER ADVICE** Moclobemide is claimed to cause less potentiation of the pressor effect of tyramine than the traditional (irreversible) MAOIs, but patients should avoid consuming large amounts of tyramine-rich food (such as mature cheese, yeast extracts and fermented soya bean products).

- **MEDICINAL FORMS** There can be variation in the licensing of different medicines containing the same drug. Forms available from special-order manufacturers include: oral suspension

Oral tablet
CAUTIONARY AND ADVISORY LABELS 10, 21
▶ Moclobemide (Non-proprietary)
Moclobemide 150 mg Moclobemide 150mg tablets | 30 tablet PoM £15.86 DT = £9.33
Moclobemide 300 mg Moclobemide 300mg tablets | 30 tablet PoM £22.30 DT = £13.99
▶ Manerix (Viatris UK Healthcare Ltd)
Moclobemide 150 mg Manerix 150mg tablets | 30 tablet PoM £9.33 DT = £9.33
Moclobemide 300 mg Manerix 300mg tablets | 30 tablet PoM £13.99 DT = £13.99

ANTIDEPRESSANTS 〉 NORADRENALINE REUPTAKE INHIBITORS

Reboxetine
13-Jun-2021

- **DRUG ACTION** Reboxetine is a selective inhibitor of noradrenaline re-uptake.

- **INDICATIONS AND DOSE**
Major depression
▶ BY MOUTH
▶ Adult 18-65 years: 4 mg twice daily for 3–4 weeks, then increased if necessary to 10 mg daily in divided doses; maximum 12 mg per day

- **CAUTIONS** Bipolar disorder · history of cardiovascular disease · history of epilepsy · prostatic hypertrophy ·

susceptibility to angle-closure glaucoma · urinary retention

- **INTERACTIONS** → Appendix 1: reboxetine
- **SIDE-EFFECTS**
▶ **Common or very common** Accommodation disorder · akathisia · anxiety · appetite decreased · chills · constipation · dizziness · dry mouth · headache · hyperhidrosis · hypertension · hypotension · insomnia · nausea · palpitations · paraesthesia · sexual dysfunction · skin reactions · tachycardia · taste altered · urinary disorders · urinary tract infection · vasodilation · vomiting
▶ **Uncommon** Mydriasis · vertigo
▶ **Rare or very rare** Glaucoma
▶ **Frequency not known** Aggression · hallucination · hyponatraemia · irritability · peripheral coldness · potassium depletion (long term use) · Raynaud's phenomenon · suicidal behaviours · testicular pain
- **PREGNANCY** Use only if potential benefit outweighs risk—limited information available.
- **BREAST FEEDING** Small amount present in milk—use only if potential benefit outweighs risk.
- **HEPATIC IMPAIRMENT** Manufacturer advises caution (risk of increased exposure). **Dose adjustments** Manufacturer advises initial dose reduction to 2 mg twice daily, increased according to tolerance.
- **RENAL IMPAIRMENT**
Dose adjustments EvGr Initial dose 2 mg twice daily, increased according to tolerance. 
- **TREATMENT CESSATION** Caution— avoid abrupt withdrawal.
- **PATIENT AND CARER ADVICE**
Driving and skilled tasks Counselling advised.

- **MEDICINAL FORMS** There can be variation in the licensing of different medicines containing the same drug.
Oral tablet
▶ Edronax (Pfizer Ltd)
Reboxetine (as Reboxetine mesilate) 4 mg Edronax 4mg tablets | 60 tablet PoM £18.91 DT = £18.91

ANTIDEPRESSANTS 〉 SELECTIVE SEROTONIN RE-UPTAKE INHIBITORS

Selective serotonin re-uptake inhibitors

- **DRUG ACTION** Selectively inhibit the re-uptake of serotonin (5-hydroxytryptamine, 5-HT).

> **IMPORTANT SAFETY INFORMATION**
> MHRA/CHM ADVICE: SSRI/SNRI ANTIDEPRESSANT MEDICINES: SMALL INCREASED RISK OF POSTPARTUM HAEMORRHAGE WHEN USED IN THE MONTH BEFORE DELIVERY (JANUARY 2021)
> SSRIs are known to increase the risk of bleeding due to their effect on platelet function. Observational data suggest that the use of SSRIs in the last month before delivery may increase the risk of postpartum haemorrhage. Healthcare professionals should continue to consider the benefits and risks of antidepressant use during pregnancy, and the risks of untreated depression in pregnancy.
>
> Healthcare professionals should also consider this finding in the context of individual patient risk factors for bleeding or thrombotic events. Anticoagulant medication in women at high risk of thrombotic events should not be stopped but healthcare professionals should be aware of the risk identified.

- **CONTRA-INDICATIONS** Poorly controlled epilepsy · SSRIs should not be used if the patient enters a manic phase

- **CAUTIONS** Cardiac disease · concurrent electroconvulsive therapy · diabetes mellitus · epilepsy (discontinue if convulsions develop) · history of bleeding disorders (especially gastro-intestinal bleeding) · history of mania · susceptibility to angle-closure glaucoma

  CAUTIONS, FURTHER INFORMATION
  ► Elderly Screening Tool of Older Persons' potentially inappropriate Prescriptions (STOPP) criteria to aid medication reviews (see Prescribing in the elderly p. 31 for information): potentially inappropriate with current or recent significant hyponatraemia i.e. serum sodium less than 130 mmol/L (risk of exacerbating or precipitating hyponatraemia).

- **SIDE-EFFECTS**
  ► **Common or very common** Anxiety · appetite abnormal · arrhythmias · arthralgia · asthenia · concentration impaired · confusion · constipation · depersonalisation · diarrhoea · dizziness · drowsiness · dry mouth · fever · gastrointestinal discomfort · haemorrhage · headache · hyperhidrosis · malaise · memory loss · menstrual cycle irregularities · myalgia · mydriasis · nausea (dose-related) · palpitations · paraesthesia · QT interval prolongation · sexual dysfunction · skin reactions · sleep disorders · taste altered · tinnitus · tremor · urinary disorders · visual impairment · vomiting · weight changes · yawning
  ► **Uncommon** Alopecia · angioedema · behaviour abnormal · hallucination · leucopenia · mania · movement disorders · photosensitivity reaction · postural hypotension · seizure · suicidal behaviours · syncope
  ► **Rare or very rare** Galactorrhoea · hepatitis · hyperprolactinaemia · hyponatraemia · serotonin syndrome · severe cutaneous adverse reactions (SCARs) · SIADH · thrombocytopenia
  ► **Frequency not known** Increased risk of fracture · withdrawal syndrome

  SIDE-EFFECTS, FURTHER INFORMATION Symptoms of sexual dysfunction may persist after treatment has stopped.

  Overdose Symptoms of poisoning by selective serotonin re-uptake inhibitors include nausea, vomiting, agitation, tremor, nystagmus, drowsiness, and sinus tachycardia; convulsions may occur. Rarely, severe poisoning results in the serotonin syndrome, with marked neuropsychiatric effects, neuromuscular hyperactivity, and autonomic instability; hyperthermia, rhabdomyolysis, renal failure, and coagulopathies may develop.

  For details on the management of poisoning, see Selective serotonin re-uptake inhibitors, under Emergency treatment of poisoning p. 1554.

- **PREGNANCY** Specialist sources indicate SSRIs may be suitable for use in pregnancy, but the risks and benefits of use must be considered, and the lowest effective dose should be used. The available data regarding malformation risk for all SSRIs are conflicting and confounded, and a causal association between the use of SSRIs in pregnancy, and spontaneous miscarriage, preterm delivery, low birth weight, and adverse effects on infant neurodevelopment remains unconfirmed. Published data on first trimester use of fluoxetine and paroxetine are contradictory. Some studies suggest a small increased risk of cardiovascular malformations with the use of fluoxetine, and congenital malformations (particularly cardiovascular) with the use of paroxetine, however other studies do not support an association. There may be a small increased risk of persistent pulmonary hypertension in the newborn with the use of SSRIs beyond 20 weeks' gestation, and use in the later stages of pregnancy may result in neonatal withdrawal syndrome—neonates should be monitored for associated central nervous system, motor, respiratory, and gastro-intestinal symptoms. There may also be a small increased risk of postpartum haemorrhage when used in the month before delivery (see *Important safety information*).

- **BREAST FEEDING** Specialist sources indicate that sertraline and paroxetine are the SSRIs of choice in breast-feeding based on passage into milk, half-life, and published evidence of safety. However, all SSRIs can be used in breast-feeding with caution, and since there are risks with switching an SSRI, it may be more clinically appropriate to continue treatment with an SSRI that has been effective, or restart treatment with an SSRI that has previously been effective. With all SSRIs, infants should be monitored for drowsiness, poor feeding, adequate weight gain, gastro-intestinal disturbances, irritability, and restlessness.

- **HEPATIC IMPAIRMENT** In general, manufacturers advise caution (prolonged half-life).

- **TREATMENT CESSATION** Gastro-intestinal disturbances, headache, anxiety, dizziness, paraesthesia, electric shock sensation in the head, neck, and spine, tinnitus, sleep disturbances, fatigue, influenza-like symptoms, and sweating are the most common features of abrupt withdrawal of an SSRI or marked reduction of the dose; palpitation and visual disturbances can occur less commonly. The dose should be tapered over at least a few weeks to avoid these effects. For some patients, it may be necessary to withdraw treatment over a longer period; consider obtaining specialist advice if symptoms persist.

  Withdrawal effects may occur within 5 days of stopping treatment with antidepressant drugs; they are usually mild and self-limiting, but in some cases may be severe. The risk of withdrawal symptoms is increased if the antidepressant is stopped suddenly after regular administration for 8 weeks or more.

- **PATIENT AND CARER ADVICE**
  Driving and skilled tasks May also impair performance of skilled tasks (e.g. driving, operating machinery).

◄ 421

Citalopram

01-May-2023

- **INDICATIONS AND DOSE**

  Depressive illness
  ► BY MOUTH USING TABLETS
  ► Adult: 20 mg once daily, increased in steps of 20 mg daily if required, dose to be increased at intervals of 3–4 weeks; maximum 40 mg per day
  ► Elderly: 10–20 mg once daily; maximum 20 mg per day
  ► BY MOUTH USING ORAL DROPS
  ► Adult: 16 mg once daily, increased in steps of 16 mg daily if required, dose to be increased at intervals of 3–4 weeks; maximum 32 mg per day
  ► Elderly: 8–16 mg daily; maximum 16 mg per day

  Panic disorder
  ► BY MOUTH USING TABLETS
  ► Adult: Initially 10 mg daily, increased in steps of 10 mg daily if required, dose to be increased gradually; usual dose 20–30 mg daily; maximum 40 mg per day
  ► Elderly: Initially 10 mg daily, increased in steps of 10 mg daily if required, dose to be increased gradually; maximum 20 mg per day
  ► BY MOUTH USING ORAL DROPS
  ► Adult: Initially 8 mg once daily, increased in steps of 8 mg if required, dose to be increased gradually; usual dose 16–24 mg daily; maximum 32 mg per day
  ► Elderly: Initially 8 mg once daily, increased in steps of 8 mg if required, dose to be increased gradually; maximum 16 mg per day

  DOSE EQUIVALENCE AND CONVERSION
  ► 4 oral drops (8 mg) is equivalent in therapeutic effect to 10 mg tablet.

- **CONTRA-INDICATIONS** QT-interval prolongation

- **CAUTIONS** Susceptibility to QT-interval prolongation
- **INTERACTIONS** → Appendix 1: SSRIs
- **SIDE-EFFECTS**
  ▶ **Common or very common** Acute angle closure glaucoma · apathy · flatulence · hypersalivation · migraine · rhinitis
  ▶ **Uncommon** Oedema
  ▶ **Rare or very rare** Cough · generalised tonic-clonic seizure
  ▶ **Frequency not known** Hypokalaemia
- **BREAST FEEDING** Specialist sources indicate use with caution. Present in milk in small to moderate amounts; long half-life increases risk of accumulation in the infant.
- **HEPATIC IMPAIRMENT**
  Dose adjustments For *tablets* manufacturer advises initial dose of 10 mg daily for the first two weeks in mild to moderate impairment—dose may be increased to max. 20 mg daily; use with extra caution and careful dose titration in severe impairment.

  For *oral drops* manufacturer advises initial dose of 8 mg daily for the first two weeks in mild to moderate impairment—dose may be increased to max. 16 mg daily; use with extra caution and careful dose titration in severe impairment.
- **RENAL IMPAIRMENT** [EvGr] Use with caution; no information available for creatinine clearance less than 20 mL/minute. ⟨M⟩ See p. 21.
- **TREATMENT CESSATION** The dose should preferably be reduced gradually over about 4 weeks, or longer if withdrawal symptoms emerge (6 months in patients who have been on long-term maintenance treatment).
- **DIRECTIONS FOR ADMINISTRATION** Manufacturer advises *Cipramil*® oral drops should be mixed with water, orange juice, or apple juice before taking.
- **PATIENT AND CARER ADVICE** Counselling on administration of oral drops is advised.
  Driving and skilled tasks Patients should be advised of the effects of citalopram on driving and skilled tasks.

- **MEDICINAL FORMS** There can be variation in the licensing of different medicines containing the same drug.
  Oral tablet
  ▶ **Citalopram (Non-proprietary)**
  Citalopram (as Citalopram hydrobromide) 10 mg Citalopram 10mg tablets | 28 tablet [PoM] £0.18 DT = £0.70 (Hospital only) | 28 tablet [PoM] £1.20 DT = £0.70 | 250 tablet [PoM] £5.65-£7.06
  Citalopram (as Citalopram hydrobromide) 20 mg Citalopram 20mg tablets | 28 tablet [PoM] £0.20 DT = £0.73 (Hospital only) | 28 tablet [PoM] £7.16 DT = £0.73 | 250 tablet [PoM] £7.03-£8.79
  Citalopram (as Citalopram hydrobromide) 40 mg Citalopram 40mg tablets | 28 tablet [PoM] £0.30 DT = £1.07 (Hospital only) | 28 tablet [PoM] £1.85 DT = £1.07
  ▶ **Cipramil** (Lundbeck Ltd)
  Citalopram (as Citalopram hydrobromide) 20 mg Cipramil 20mg tablets | 28 tablet [PoM] £8.95 DT = £0.73
  Oral drops
  EXCIPIENTS: May contain Alcohol
  ▶ **Citalopram (Non-proprietary)**
  Citalopram (as Citalopram hydrochloride) 40 mg per 1 ml Citalopram 40mg/ml oral drops sugar free | 15 ml [PoM] £14.09 DT = £10.81 [SF]
  ▶ **Cipramil** (Lundbeck Ltd)
  Citalopram (as Citalopram hydrochloride) 40 mg per 1 ml Cipramil 40mg/ml drops | 15 ml [PoM] £10.08 DT = £10.81 [SF]

Escitalopram   [F 421]   01-May-2023

- **DRUG ACTION** Escitalopram is the active enantiomer of citalopram.

- **INDICATIONS AND DOSE**
  Depressive illness | Generalised anxiety disorder | Obsessive-compulsive disorder
  ▶ BY MOUTH
  ▶ **Adult:** 10 mg once daily; increased if necessary up to 20 mg once daily
  ▶ **Elderly:** Initially 5 mg once daily; increased if necessary to 10 mg once daily

  Panic disorder
  ▶ BY MOUTH
  ▶ **Adult:** Initially 5 mg once daily for 7 days, then increased to 10 mg once daily; increased if necessary up to 20 mg once daily
  ▶ **Elderly:** Initially 5 mg once daily; increased if necessary to 10 mg once daily

  Social anxiety disorder
  ▶ BY MOUTH
  ▶ **Adult:** Initially 10 mg once daily for 2–4 weeks, dose to be adjusted after 2–4 weeks of treatment; usual maintenance 5–20 mg once daily

  DOSE EQUIVALENCE AND CONVERSION
  ▶ 1 drop of oral solution contains 1 mg of escitalopram.

- **CONTRA-INDICATIONS** QT-interval prolongation
- **CAUTIONS** Susceptibility to QT-interval prolongation
- **INTERACTIONS** → Appendix 1: SSRIs
- **SIDE-EFFECTS**
  ▶ **Common or very common** Sinusitis
  ▶ **Uncommon** Oedema
- **BREAST FEEDING** Specialist sources indicate use with caution. Present in milk in small amounts; long half-life increases risk of accumulation in the infant.
- **HEPATIC IMPAIRMENT**
  Dose adjustments Manufacturer advises initially 5 mg once daily for 2 weeks in mild to moderate impairment, thereafter increased to 10 mg once daily according to response; titrate dose with extra caution in severe impairment.
- **RENAL IMPAIRMENT** [EvGr] Use with caution if creatinine clearance less than 30 mL/minute, ⟨M⟩ see p. 21.
- **TREATMENT CESSATION** The dose should preferably be reduced gradually over about 4 weeks, or longer if withdrawal symptoms emerge (6 months in patients who have been on long-term maintenance treatment).
- **DIRECTIONS FOR ADMINISTRATION** Manufacturer advises oral drops can be mixed with water, orange juice, or apple juice before taking.
- **PATIENT AND CARER ADVICE** Counselling on administration of oral drops advised.
  Driving and skilled tasks Patients should be counselled about the effects on driving.

- **MEDICINAL FORMS** There can be variation in the licensing of different medicines containing the same drug.
  Oral tablet
  ▶ **Escitalopram (Non-proprietary)**
  Escitalopram (as Escitalopram oxalate) 5 mg Escitalopram 5mg tablets | 28 tablet [PoM] £10.76 DT = £2.34
  Escitalopram (as Escitalopram oxalate) 10 mg Escitalopram 10mg tablets | 28 tablet [PoM] £17.89 DT = £1.29
  Escitalopram (as Escitalopram oxalate) 20 mg Escitalopram 20mg tablets | 28 tablet [PoM] £30.24 DT = £1.44
  ▶ **Cipralex** (Lundbeck Ltd)
  Escitalopram (as Escitalopram oxalate) 5 mg Cipralex 5mg tablets | 28 tablet [PoM] £8.97 DT = £2.34

Escitalopram (as Escitalopram oxalate) 10 mg Cipralex 10mg tablets | 28 tablet [PoM] £14.91 DT = £1.29
Escitalopram (as Escitalopram oxalate) 20 mg Cipralex 20mg tablets | 28 tablet [PoM] £25.20 DT = £1.44

Oral drops
▸ Cipralex (Lundbeck Ltd)
Escitalopram (as Escitalopram oxalate) 20 mg per 1 ml Cipralex 20mg/ml oral drops | 15 ml [PoM] £20.16 DT = £20.16 [SF]

⟁ 421

Fluoxetine

01-May-2023

● **INDICATIONS AND DOSE**

Major depression
▸ BY MOUTH
▸ Adult: Initially 20 mg once daily, daily dose may be administered as a divided dose, increased if necessary up to 60 mg once daily, daily dose may be administered as a divided dose; dose may be increased after 3–4 weeks of initial dose, and at appropriate intervals thereafter
▸ Elderly: Initially 20 mg once daily, daily dose may be administered as a divided dose, increased if necessary up to 40 mg once daily, daily dose may be administered as a divided dose; dose may be increased after 3–4 weeks of initial dose, and at appropriate intervals thereafter, usual maximum dose is 40 mg per day but doses up to 60 mg per day can be used

Bulimia nervosa
▸ BY MOUTH
▸ Adult: 60 mg once daily, daily dose may be administered as a divided dose
▸ Elderly: Up to 40 mg once daily, daily dose may be administered as a divided dose; usual maximum dose is 40 mg per day but doses up to 60 mg per day can be used

Obsessive-compulsive disorder
▸ BY MOUTH
▸ Adult: 20 mg once daily, daily dose may be administered as a divided dose, increased if necessary up to 60 mg once daily, daily dose may be administered as a divided dose, dose to be increased gradually, review treatment if inadequate response after 10 weeks
▸ Elderly: 20 mg once daily, daily dose may be administered as a divided dose, increased if necessary up to 40 mg once daily, daily dose may be administered as a divided dose, dose to be increased gradually; usual maximum dose is 40 mg per day but doses up to 60 mg per day can be used, review treatment if inadequate response after 10 weeks

Menopausal symptoms, particularly hot flushes, in women with breast cancer (except those taking tamoxifen)
▸ BY MOUTH
▸ Adult: 20 mg once daily

PHARMACOKINETICS
▸ Consider the long half-life of fluoxetine when adjusting dosage (or in overdosage).

● **UNLICENSED USE** [EvGr] Fluoxetine is used for menopausal symptoms, Ⓑ but it is not licensed for this indication.
● **INTERACTIONS** → Appendix 1: SSRIs
● **SIDE-EFFECTS**
▸ **Common or very common** Chills · feeling abnormal · postmenopausal haemorrhage · uterine disorder · vasodilation · vision blurred
▸ **Uncommon** Cold sweat · dysphagia · dyspnoea · hypotension · mood altered · muscle twitching · self-injurious behaviour · temperature sensation altered · thinking abnormal
▸ **Rare or very rare** Atelectasis · buccoglossal syndrome · interstitial lung disease · neutropenia · oesophageal pain · pharyngitis · serum sickness · speech disorder · vasculitis

● **BREAST FEEDING** Specialist sources indicate use with caution. Present in milk in moderate to significant amounts; very long half-life increases risk of accumulation in the infant.

● **HEPATIC IMPAIRMENT**
Dose adjustments Manufacturer advises dose reduction or increasing dose interval.

● **DIRECTIONS FOR ADMINISTRATION** Manufacturer advises dispersible tablets can be dispersed in water for administration or swallowed whole with plenty of water.

● **PATIENT AND CARER ADVICE** Patients and carers should be counselled on the administration of dispersible tablets.
Driving and skilled tasks Patients should be counselled about the effects on driving and skilled tasks.

● **MEDICINAL FORMS** There can be variation in the licensing of different medicines containing the same drug. Forms available from special-order manufacturers include: oral suspension, oral solution

Oral tablet
▸ Fluoxetine (Non-proprietary)
Fluoxetine (as Fluoxetine hydrochloride) 10 mg Fluoxetine 10mg tablets | 30 tablet [PoM] £61.73-£104.98 DT = £61.73

Dispersible tablet
CAUTIONARY AND ADVISORY LABELS 10
▸ Olena (Advanz Pharma)
Fluoxetine (as Fluoxetine hydrochloride) 20 mg Olena 20mg dispersible tablets | 28 tablet [PoM] £3.44 DT = £3.44 [SF]

Oral capsule
▸ Fluoxetine (Non-proprietary)
Fluoxetine (as Fluoxetine hydrochloride) 10 mg Fluoxetine 10mg capsules | 30 capsule [PoM] £53.60 DT = £5.27
Fluoxetine (as Fluoxetine hydrochloride) 20 mg Fluoxetine 20mg capsules | 30 capsule [PoM] £1.90 DT = £0.78
Fluoxetine (as Fluoxetine hydrochloride) 30 mg Fluoxetine 30mg capsules | 30 capsule [PoM] £9.99 DT = £2.82
Fluoxetine (as Fluoxetine hydrochloride) 40 mg Fluoxetine 40mg capsules | 30 capsule [PoM] £4.50 DT = £1.98
Fluoxetine (as Fluoxetine hydrochloride) 60 mg Fluoxetine 60mg capsules | 30 capsule [PoM] £54.36 DT = £1.74

Oral solution
▸ Fluoxetine (Non-proprietary)
Fluoxetine (as Fluoxetine hydrochloride) 4 mg per 1 ml Fluoxetine 20mg/5ml oral solution | 70 ml [PoM] £20.00 DT = £5.91
Fluoxetine 20mg/5ml oral solution sugar free | 70 ml [PoM] £12.95 DT = £12.95 [SF]
▸ Prozep (Rosemont Pharmaceuticals Ltd)
Fluoxetine (as Fluoxetine hydrochloride) 4 mg per 1 ml Prozep 20mg/5ml oral solution | 70 ml [PoM] £12.95 DT = £12.95 [SF]

⟁ 421

Fluvoxamine maleate

01-May-2023

● **INDICATIONS AND DOSE**

Depressive illness
▸ BY MOUTH
▸ Adult: Initially 50–100 mg daily, dose to be taken in the evening, dose to be increased gradually, increased if necessary up to 300 mg daily, doses over 150 mg daily are given in divided doses; maintenance 100 mg daily

Obsessive-compulsive disorder
▸ BY MOUTH
▸ Adult: Initially 50 mg daily, dose to be taken in the evening, dose is increased gradually if necessary after several weeks, increased if necessary up to 300 mg daily; maintenance 100–300 mg daily, doses over 150 mg daily are given in divided doses, if no improvement in obsessive-compulsive disorder within 10 weeks, treatment should be reconsidered

● **INTERACTIONS** → Appendix 1: SSRIs
● **SIDE-EFFECTS**
▸ **Rare or very rare** Hepatic function abnormal (discontinue)

▶ **Frequency not known** Glaucoma · neuroleptic malignant-like syndrome (discontinue—potentially fatal) · withdrawal syndrome neonatal

● **BREAST FEEDING** Specialist sources indicate use with caution. Present in milk in small amounts; long half-life increases risk of accumulation in the infant.

● **HEPATIC IMPAIRMENT**
Dose adjustments Manufacturer advises low initial dose.

● **RENAL IMPAIRMENT**
Dose adjustments [EvGr] Start with a low dose. ⟨M⟩

● **TREATMENT CESSATION** The dose should preferably be reduced gradually over about 4 weeks, or longer if withdrawal symptoms emerge (6 months in patients who have been on long-term maintenance treatment).

● **PATIENT AND CARER ADVICE**
Driving and skilled tasks Patients should be counselled about the effects on driving and skilled tasks.

● **MEDICINAL FORMS** There can be variation in the licensing of different medicines containing the same drug. Forms available from special-order manufacturers include: oral suspension
Oral tablet
▶ Faverin (Viatris UK Healthcare Ltd)
Fluvoxamine maleate 50 mg Faverin 50mg tablets |
60 tablet [PoM] £17.10 DT = £17.10
Fluvoxamine maleate 100 mg Faverin 100mg tablets |
30 tablet [PoM] £17.10 DT = £17.10

F 421

Paroxetine

25-May-2023

● **INDICATIONS AND DOSE**
Major depression | Social anxiety disorder | Post-traumatic stress disorder | Generalised anxiety disorder
▶ BY MOUTH
▶ Adult: 20 mg daily, dose to be taken in the morning, no evidence of greater efficacy at higher doses; maximum 50 mg per day
▶ Elderly: 20 mg daily, dose to be taken in the morning, no evidence of greater efficacy at higher doses; maximum 40 mg per day

Obsessive-compulsive disorder
▶ BY MOUTH
▶ Adult: Initially 20 mg daily, dose to be taken in the morning, increased in steps of 10 mg, dose to be increased gradually, increased to 40 mg daily, no evidence of greater efficacy at higher doses; maximum 60 mg per day
▶ Elderly: Initially 20 mg daily, dose to be taken in the morning, increased in steps of 10 mg, dose to be increased gradually; maximum 40 mg per day

Panic disorder
▶ BY MOUTH
▶ Adult: Initially 10 mg daily, dose to be taken in the morning, increased in steps of 10 mg, dose to be increased gradually, increased to 40 mg daily, no evidence of greater efficacy at higher doses; maximum 60 mg per day
▶ Elderly: Initially 10 mg daily, dose to be taken in the morning, increased in steps of 10 mg, dose to be increased gradually; maximum 40 mg per day

Menopausal symptoms, particularly hot flushes, in women with breast cancer (except those taking tamoxifen).
▶ BY MOUTH
▶ Adult: 10 mg once daily

● **UNLICENSED USE** [EvGr] Paroxetine is used for menopausal symptoms, ⟨B⟩ but it is not licensed for this indication.

● **CAUTIONS** Achlorhydria · high gastric pH

CAUTIONS, FURTHER INFORMATION
▶ Achlorhydria or high gastric pH Causes reduced absorption of the oral suspension.

● **INTERACTIONS** → Appendix 1: SSRIs

● **SIDE-EFFECTS**
▶ **Common or very common** Vision blurred
▶ **Uncommon** Diabetic control impaired
▶ **Rare or very rare** Acute glaucoma · hepatic disorders · peripheral oedema
▶ **Frequency not known** Colitis microscopic

● **BREAST FEEDING** Specialist sources indicate can be used. Present in milk in small amounts; long half-life increases risk of accumulation in the infant.

● **HEPATIC IMPAIRMENT**
Dose adjustments Manufacturer advises dose at the lower end of the range.

● **RENAL IMPAIRMENT** [EvGr] Use with caution if creatinine clearance less than 30 mL/minute, ⟨M⟩ see p. 21.

● **TREATMENT CESSATION** Associated with a higher risk of withdrawal reactions. The dose should preferably be reduced gradually over about 4 weeks, or longer if withdrawal symptoms emerge (6 months in patients who have been on long-term maintenance treatment).

● **PATIENT AND CARER ADVICE**
Driving and skilled tasks Patients should be counselled about the effect on driving.

● **MEDICINAL FORMS** There can be variation in the licensing of different medicines containing the same drug. Forms available from special-order manufacturers include: oral suspension, oral solution
Oral tablet
CAUTIONARY AND ADVISORY LABELS 21
▶ Paroxetine (Non-proprietary)
Paroxetine (as Paroxetine hydrochloride) 10 mg Paroxetine 10mg tablets | 28 tablet [PoM] £17.03 DT = £1.15
Paroxetine (as Paroxetine hydrochloride) 20 mg Paroxetine 20mg tablets | 30 tablet [PoM] £12.18 DT = £1.19
Paroxetine (as Paroxetine hydrochloride) 30 mg Paroxetine 30mg tablets | 30 tablet [PoM] £21.39 DT = £1.41
Paroxetine (as Paroxetine hydrochloride) 40 mg Paroxetine 40mg tablets | 28 tablet [PoM] £17.03 | 30 tablet [PoM] £17.03 DT = £8.11
▶ Seroxat (GlaxoSmithKline UK Ltd)
Paroxetine (as Paroxetine hydrochloride) 10 mg Seroxat 10mg tablets | 28 tablet [PoM] £14.21 DT = £1.15
Paroxetine (as Paroxetine hydrochloride) 30 mg Seroxat 30mg tablets | 30 tablet [PoM] £26.74 DT = £1.41
Oral suspension
CAUTIONARY AND ADVISORY LABELS 5, 21

F 421

Sertraline

18-Aug-2023

● **INDICATIONS AND DOSE**
Depressive illness
▶ BY MOUTH
▶ Adult: Initially 50 mg once daily, then increased in steps of 50 mg at intervals of at least 1 week if required; maintenance 50 mg once daily; maximum 200 mg per day

Obsessive-compulsive disorder
▶ BY MOUTH
▶ Adult: Initially 50 mg once daily, then increased in steps of 50 mg at intervals of at least 1 week if required; maximum 200 mg per day

Panic disorder | Post-traumatic stress disorder | Social anxiety disorder
▶ BY MOUTH
▶ Adult: Initially 25 mg once daily for 1 week, then increased to 50 mg once daily, then increased in steps of 50 mg at intervals of at least 1 week if required, increase only if response is partial and if drug is tolerated; maximum 200 mg per day

- **INTERACTIONS** → Appendix 1: SSRIs
- **SIDE-EFFECTS**
- ▸ **Common or very common** Chest pain · depression · gastrointestinal disorders · increased risk of infection · neuromuscular dysfunction · vasodilation
- ▸ **Uncommon** Back pain · burping · chills · cold sweat · dysphagia · dyspnoea · ear pain · euphoric mood · hypertension · hypothyroidism · migraine · muscle complaints · muscle weakness · oedema · oral disorders · osteoarthritis · periorbital oedema · respiratory disorders · sensation abnormal · speech disorder · thinking abnormal · thirst
- ▸ **Rare or very rare** Balanoposthitis · bone disorder · cardiac disorder · coma · conversion disorder · diabetes mellitus · drug dependence · dysphonia · eye disorders · gait abnormal · genital discharge · glaucoma · hair texture abnormal · hepatic disorders · hiccups · hypercholesterolaemia · hypoglycaemia · injury · lymphadenopathy · myocardial infarction · neoplasms · neuroleptic malignant syndrome · oliguria · peripheral ischaemia · psychotic disorder · rhabdomyolysis · vasodilation procedure · vision disorders · vulvovaginal atrophy
- ▸ **Frequency not known** Cerebrovascular insufficiency · gynaecomastia · hyperglycaemia · interstitial lung disease · pancreatitis
- **BREAST FEEDING** Specialist sources indicate can be used. Present in milk in small amounts; long half-life increases risk of accumulation in the infant.
- **HEPATIC IMPAIRMENT** Manufacturer advises avoid in severe impairment (no information available). **Dose adjustments** Manufacturer advises dose reduction or increasing dose interval in mild to moderate impairment.
- **TREATMENT CESSATION** The dose should preferably be reduced gradually over about 4 weeks, or longer if withdrawal symptoms emerge (6 months in patients who have been on long-term maintenance treatment).
- **DIRECTIONS FOR ADMINISTRATION** EvGr Sertraline *concentrate for oral solution* must be diluted before use; the requisite dose is diluted with approximately 120 mL (one glass) of water, ginger ale, lemon/lime soda, lemonade, or orange juice only and taken immediately. Ⓜ
- **PATIENT AND CARER ADVICE** Patients or carers should be given advice on how to administer sertraline concentrate for oral solution. **Driving and skilled tasks** Patients should be counselled on the effects on driving and skilled tasks.

- **MEDICINAL FORMS** There can be variation in the licensing of different medicines containing the same drug. Forms available from special-order manufacturers include: oral tablet, oral suspension

Oral tablet

- ▸ Sertraline (Non-proprietary)
  Sertraline (as Sertraline hydrochloride) 25 mg Sertraline 25mg tablets | 28 tablet PoM £20.28 DT = £11.05
  Sertraline (as Sertraline hydrochloride) 50 mg Sertraline 50mg tablets | 28 tablet PoM £17.82 DT = £0.90 | 250 tablet PoM £9.10 | 500 tablet PoM £46.36–£270.48
  Sertraline (as Sertraline hydrochloride) 100 mg Sertraline 100mg tablets | 28 tablet PoM £29.16 DT = £1.09 | 250 tablet PoM £10.97 | 500 tablet PoM £36.29–£442.61
  Sertraline (as Sertraline hydrochloride) 150 mg Sertraline 150mg tablets | 30 tablet PoM £14.85–£25.76 DT = £14.85
  Sertraline (as Sertraline hydrochloride) 200 mg Sertraline 200mg tablets | 30 tablet PoM £19.80–£37.22 DT = £19.80
- ▸ Contulen (HFA Healthcare Ltd)
  Sertraline (as Sertraline hydrochloride) 50 mg Contulen 50mg tablets | 28 tablet PoM £17.82 DT = £0.90
  Sertraline (as Sertraline hydrochloride) 100 mg Contulen 100mg tablets | 28 tablet PoM £29.16 DT = £1.09
- ▸ Lustral (Viatris UK Healthcare Ltd)
  Sertraline (as Sertraline hydrochloride) 50 mg Lustral 50mg tablets | 28 tablet PoM £17.82 DT = £0.90

Sertraline (as Sertraline hydrochloride) 100 mg Lustral 100mg tablets | 28 tablet PoM £29.16 DT = £1.09

Oral suspension

- ▸ Sertraline (Non-proprietary)
  Sertraline (as Sertraline hydrochloride) 10 mg per 1 ml Sertraline 50mg/5ml oral suspension sugar free | 150 ml PoM £201.80–£363.24 SF

Concentrate for oral solution

CAUTIONARY AND ADVISORY LABELS 13
EXCIPIENTS: May contain Alcohol, butylated hydroxytoluene

- ▸ Sertraline (Non-proprietary)
  Sertraline (as Sertraline hydrochloride) 20 mg per 1 ml Sertraline 100mg/5ml concentrate for oral solution sugar free | 60 ml PoM £52.63–£54.00 SF

ANTIDEPRESSANTS › SEROTONIN AND NORADRENALINE RE-UPTAKE INHIBITORS

Duloxetine

08-Nov-2023

- **DRUG ACTION** Inhibits the re-uptake of serotonin and noradrenaline.

- **INDICATIONS AND DOSE**

Major depressive disorder
- ▸ BY MOUTH
- ▸ Adult: 60 mg once daily, dose can be increased if necessary up to a maximum of 120 mg per day in patients who are responding to treatment and have a history of repeated episodes of major depression

Generalised anxiety disorder
- ▸ BY MOUTH
- ▸ Adult: Initially 30 mg once daily, usual maintenance 60 mg once daily, dose can be increased if necessary up to a maximum of 120 mg per day

Diabetic neuropathy
- ▸ BY MOUTH
- ▸ Adult: 60 mg once daily, discontinue if inadequate response after 2 months; review treatment at least every 3 months; dose can be increased if necessary up to a maximum of 120 mg daily in divided doses

Moderate to severe stress urinary incontinence
- ▸ BY MOUTH
- ▸ Adult (female): 40 mg twice daily, patient should be assessed for benefit and tolerability after 2–4 weeks, alternatively initially 20 mg twice daily for 2 weeks, this can minimise side-effects, then increased to 40 mg twice daily, patient should be assessed for benefit and tolerability after 2–4 weeks.

IMPORTANT SAFETY INFORMATION

SNRI ANTIDEPRESSANT MEDICINES: SMALL INCREASED RISK OF POSTPARTUM HAEMORRHAGE WHEN USED IN THE MONTH BEFORE DELIVERY

Serotonin and noradrenaline re-uptake inhibitors (SNRIs) are known to increase the risk of bleeding due to their effect on platelet function. Observational data suggest that the use of SNRIs in the last month before delivery may increase the risk of postpartum haemorrhage. Healthcare professionals should continue to consider the benefits and risks of antidepressant use during pregnancy, and the risks of untreated depression in pregnancy.

Healthcare professionals should also consider this finding in the context of individual patient risk factors for bleeding or thrombotic events. Anticoagulant medication in women at high risk of thrombotic events should not be stopped but healthcare professionals should be aware of the risk identified.

- **CAUTIONS** Bleeding disorders · cardiac disease · elderly · history of mania · history of seizures · hypertension (avoid if uncontrolled) · raised intra-ocular pressure · susceptibility to angle-closure glaucoma

● INTERACTIONS → Appendix 1: SNRIs

● SIDE-EFFECTS

▶ **Common or very common** Anxiety · appetite decreased · constipation · diarrhoea · dizziness · drowsiness · dry mouth · fall · fatigue · flushing · gastrointestinal discomfort · gastrointestinal disorders · headache · muscle complaints · nausea · pain · palpitations · paraesthesia · sexual dysfunction · skin reactions · sleep disorders · sweat changes · tinnitus · tremor · urinary disorders · vision disorders · vomiting · weight changes · yawning

▶ **Uncommon** Apathy · arrhythmias · behaviour abnormal · burping · chills · concentration impaired · disorientation · dysphagia · ear pain · feeling abnormal · gait abnormal · haemorrhage · hepatic disorders · hyperglycaemia · increased risk of infection · malaise · menstrual disorder · movement disorders · mydriasis · peripheral coldness · photosensitivity reaction · postural hypotension · suicidal behaviours · syncope · taste altered · temperature sensation altered · testicular pain · thirst · throat tightness · vertigo

▶ **Rare or very rare** Angioedema · cutaneous vasculitis · dehydration · galactorrhoea · glaucoma · hallucination · hyperprolactinaemia · hypertensive crisis · hyponatraemia · hypothyroidism · interstitial lung disease · mania · menopausal symptoms · oral disorders · pneumonia eosinophilic · seizure · serotonin syndrome · SIADH · Stevens-Johnson syndrome · urine odour abnormal

▶ **Frequency not known** Stress cardiomyopathy

SIDE-EFFECTS, FURTHER INFORMATION Symptoms of sexual dysfunction may persist after treatment has stopped.

● PREGNANCY Toxicity in *animal* studies—avoid in patients with stress urinary incontinence; in other conditions use only if potential benefit outweighs risk. Risk of neonatal withdrawal symptoms if used near term.

● BREAST FEEDING Present in milk—manufacturer advises avoid.

● HEPATIC IMPAIRMENT Manufacturer advises avoid.

● RENAL IMPAIRMENT [EvGr] Avoid if creatinine clearance less than 30 mL/minute, ⟨M⟩ see p. 21.

● TREATMENT CESSATION Nausea, vomiting, headache, anxiety, dizziness, paraesthesia, sleep disturbances, and tremor are the most common features of abrupt withdrawal or marked reduction of the dose; dose should be reduced over at least 1–2 weeks.

● PATIENT AND CARER ADVICE
Driving and skilled tasks Patients and carers should be counselled on the effects on driving and performance of skilled tasks—increased risk of dizziness.

● NATIONAL FUNDING/ACCESS DECISIONS
CYMBALTA ® For full details see funding body website
Scottish Medicines Consortium (SMC) decisions
▶ **Duloxetine (*Cymbalta*®) for diabetic peripheral neuropathic pain in adults (September 2006)** SMC No. 285/06 Recommended with restrictions

● MEDICINAL FORMS There can be variation in the licensing of different medicines containing the same drug.
Gastro-resistant capsule
CAUTIONARY AND ADVISORY LABELS 2
▶ **Duloxetine (Non-proprietary)**
Duloxetine (as Duloxetine hydrochloride) 20 mg Duloxetine 20mg gastro-resistant capsules | 28 capsule [PoM] £22.18 DT = £6.09
Duloxetine (as Duloxetine hydrochloride) 30 mg Duloxetine 30mg gastro-resistant capsules | 28 capsule [PoM] £26.88 DT = £1.36
Duloxetine (as Duloxetine hydrochloride) 40 mg Duloxetine 40mg gastro-resistant capsules | 56 capsule [PoM] £44.35 DT = £6.64
Duloxetine (as Duloxetine hydrochloride) 60 mg Duloxetine 60mg gastro-resistant capsules | 28 capsule [PoM] £33.26 DT = £1.72

Duloxetine (as Duloxetine hydrochloride) 90 mg Duloxetine 90mg gastro-resistant capsules | 28 capsule [PoM] £30.72 DT = £28.42
Duloxetine (as Duloxetine hydrochloride) 120 mg Duloxetine 120mg gastro-resistant capsules | 28 capsule [PoM] £37.32 DT = £33.82
▶ **Cymbalta** (Eli Lilly and Company Ltd)
Duloxetine (as Duloxetine hydrochloride) 30 mg Cymbalta 30mg gastro-resistant capsules | 28 capsule [PoM] £22.40 DT = £1.36
Duloxetine (as Duloxetine hydrochloride) 60 mg Cymbalta 60mg gastro-resistant capsules | 28 capsule [PoM] £27.72 DT = £1.72
▶ **Depalta** (GlucoRx Ltd)
Duloxetine (as Duloxetine hydrochloride) 30 mg Depalta 30mg gastro-resistant capsules | 28 capsule [PoM] £2.95 DT = £1.36
Duloxetine (as Duloxetine hydrochloride) 60 mg Depalta 60mg gastro-resistant capsules | 28 capsule [PoM] £4.25 DT = £1.72
▶ **Duciltia** (Pharmathen S.A.)
Duloxetine (as Duloxetine hydrochloride) 30 mg Duciltia 30mg gastro-resistant capsules | 28 capsule [PoM] £22.40 DT = £1.36
Duloxetine (as Duloxetine hydrochloride) 60 mg Duciltia 60mg gastro-resistant capsules | 28 capsule [PoM] £27.72 DT = £1.72
▶ **Yentreve** (Eli Lilly and Company Ltd)
Duloxetine (as Duloxetine hydrochloride) 20 mg Yentreve 20mg gastro-resistant capsules | 28 capsule [PoM] £18.48 DT = £6.09
Duloxetine (as Duloxetine hydrochloride) 40 mg Yentreve 40mg gastro-resistant capsules | 56 capsule [PoM] £36.96 DT = £6.64

Venlafaxine

12-Apr-2023

● DRUG ACTION A serotonin and noradrenaline re-uptake inhibitor.

● INDICATIONS AND DOSE
Major depression
▶ BY MOUTH USING IMMEDIATE-RELEASE MEDICINES
▶ Adult: 75 mg daily in 2 divided doses, then increased if necessary up to 375 mg daily in 2 divided doses, dose to be increased if necessary at intervals of at least 2 weeks, faster dose titration may be necessary in some patients
▶ BY MOUTH USING MODIFIED-RELEASE MEDICINES
▶ Adult: 75 mg once daily, increased if necessary up to 375 mg once daily, dose to be increased if necessary at intervals of at least 2 weeks, faster dose titration may be necessary in some patients

Generalised anxiety disorder
▶ BY MOUTH USING MODIFIED-RELEASE MEDICINES
▶ Adult: 75 mg once daily, increased if necessary up to 225 mg once daily, dose to be increased at intervals of at least 2 weeks

Social anxiety disorder
▶ BY MOUTH USING MODIFIED-RELEASE MEDICINES
▶ Adult: 75 mg once daily, there is no evidence of greater efficacy at higher doses, increased if necessary up to 225 mg once daily, dose to be increased if necessary at intervals of at least 2 weeks

Panic disorder
▶ BY MOUTH USING MODIFIED-RELEASE MEDICINES
▶ Adult: Initially 37.5 mg once daily for 7 days, increased to 75 mg once daily, increased if necessary up to 225 mg once daily, dose to be increased at intervals of at least 2 weeks

Menopausal symptoms, particularly hot flushes, in women with breast cancer
▶ BY MOUTH USING MODIFIED-RELEASE MEDICINES
▶ Adult: 37.5 mg once daily for one week, then increased if necessary to 75 mg once daily

- **UNLICENSED USE** [EvGr] Venlafaxine is used for menopausal symptoms, ⚖ but it is not licensed for this indication.

IMPORTANT SAFETY INFORMATION

MHRA/CHM ADVICE: SSRI/SNRI ANTIDEPRESSANT MEDICINES: SMALL INCREASED RISK OF POSTPARTUM HAEMORRHAGE WHEN USED IN THE MONTH BEFORE DELIVERY (JANUARY 2021)

Serotonin and noradrenaline re-uptake inhibitors (SNRIs) are known to increase the risk of bleeding due to their effect on platelet function. Observational data suggest that the use of SNRIs in the last month before delivery may increase the risk of postpartum haemorrhage. Healthcare professionals should continue to consider the benefits and risks of antidepressant use during pregnancy, and the risks of untreated depression in pregnancy.

Healthcare professionals should also consider this finding in the context of individual patient risk factors for bleeding or thrombotic events. Anticoagulant medication in women at high risk of thrombotic events should not be stopped but healthcare professionals should be aware of the risk identified.

- **CONTRA-INDICATIONS** Uncontrolled hypertension

- **CAUTIONS** Conditions associated with high risk of cardiac arrhythmia · diabetes · heart disease (monitor blood pressure) · history of bleeding disorders · history of epilepsy · history or family history of mania · susceptibility to angle-closure glaucoma

- **INTERACTIONS** → Appendix 1: SNRIs

- **SIDE-EFFECTS**
  - **Common or very common** Anxiety · appetite decreased · arrhythmias · asthenia · chills · confusion · constipation · depersonalisation · diarrhoea · dizziness · dry mouth · dyspnoea · headache · hot flush · hypertension · menstrual cycle irregularities · movement disorders · muscle tone increased · mydriasis · nausea · palpitations · paraesthesia · sedation · sexual dysfunction · skin reactions · sleep disorders · sweat changes · taste altered · tinnitus · tremor · urinary disorders · vision disorders · vomiting · weight changes · yawning
  - **Uncommon** Alopecia · angioedema · apathy · behaviour abnormal · derealisation · haemorrhage · hallucination · hypotension · mood altered · photosensitivity reaction · syncope
  - **Rare or very rare** Agranulocytosis · angle closure glaucoma · bone marrow disorders · delirium · hepatitis · hyponatraemia · interstitial lung disease · neuroleptic malignant syndrome · neutropenia · pancreatitis · pulmonary eosinophilia · QT interval prolongation · rhabdomyolysis · seizure · serotonin syndrome · severe cutaneous adverse reactions (SCARs) · SIADH · thrombocytopenia
  - **Frequency not known** Suicidal behaviours · vertigo · withdrawal syndrome

  SIDE-EFFECTS, FURTHER INFORMATION Symptoms of sexual dysfunction may persist after treatment has stopped.

- **PREGNANCY** Avoid unless potential benefit outweighs risk—toxicity in *animal* studies. Risk of withdrawal effects in neonate.

- **BREAST FEEDING** Present in milk—avoid.

- **HEPATIC IMPAIRMENT** Manufacturer advises caution (inter-individual variability in clearance; limited information available in severe impairment).
  Dose adjustments Manufacturer advises consider dose reduction of 50% in mild to moderate impairment and of more than 50% in severe impairment.

- **RENAL IMPAIRMENT** [EvGr] Use with caution (inter-individual variability in clearance). Ⓜ
  Dose adjustments [EvGr] Use half normal dose if eGFR less than 30 mL/minute/1.73 m^2; Ⓜ see p. 21.

- **TREATMENT CESSATION** Associated with a higher risk of withdrawal effects compared with other antidepressants.
  Gastro-intestinal disturbances, headache, anxiety, dizziness, paraesthesia, tremor, sleep disturbances, and sweating are most common features of withdrawal if treatment stopped abruptly or if dose reduced markedly; dose should be reduced over several weeks.

- **PATIENT AND CARER ADVICE**
  Driving and skilled tasks May affect performance of skilled tasks (e.g. driving).

- **MEDICINAL FORMS** There can be variation in the licensing of different medicines containing the same drug. Forms available from special-order manufacturers include: oral suspension, oral solution

Oral tablet

CAUTIONARY AND ADVISORY LABELS 2, 21

▸ Venlafaxine (Non-proprietary)
  Venlafaxine (as Venlafaxine hydrochloride) 37.5 mg Venlafaxine 37.5mg tablets | 56 tablet [PoM] £3.58 DT = £1.86
  Venlafaxine (as Venlafaxine hydrochloride) 75 mg Venlafaxine 75mg tablets | 56 tablet [PoM] £9.81 DT = £4.63

Modified-release tablet

CAUTIONARY AND ADVISORY LABELS 2, 21, 25

▸ Venlafaxine (Non-proprietary)
  Venlafaxine (as Venlafaxine hydrochloride) 37.5 mg Venlafaxine 37.5mg modified-release tablets | 30 tablet [PoM] £7.30–£9.90 DT = £7.30
  Venlafaxine (as Venlafaxine hydrochloride) 75 mg Venlafaxine 75mg modified-release tablets | 30 tablet [PoM] £2.91 DT = £2.91
  Venlafaxine (as Venlafaxine hydrochloride) 150 mg Venlafaxine 150mg modified-release tablets | 28 tablet [PoM] £3.99–£18.70 | 30 tablet [PoM] £4.14 DT = £4.27
  Venlafaxine (as Venlafaxine hydrochloride) 225 mg Venlafaxine 225mg modified-release tablets | 30 tablet [PoM] £25.12–£33.60 DT = £33.60
  Venlafaxine (as Venlafaxine hydrochloride) 300 mg Venlafaxine 300mg modified-release tablets | 30 tablet [PoM] £41.25–£77.56 DT = £41.25

▸ Sunveniz XL (Sun Pharma UK Ltd)
  Venlafaxine (as Venlafaxine hydrochloride) 75 mg Sunveniz XL 75mg tablets | 30 tablet [PoM] £11.14 DT = £2.91
  Venlafaxine (as Venlafaxine hydrochloride) 150 mg Sunveniz XL 150mg tablets | 30 tablet [PoM] £18.64 DT = £4.27

▸ Venladex XL (Dexcel-Pharma Ltd)
  Venlafaxine (as Venlafaxine hydrochloride) 75 mg Venladex XL 75mg tablets | 28 tablet [PoM] £11.20
  Venlafaxine (as Venlafaxine hydrochloride) 150 mg Venladex XL 150mg tablets | 28 tablet [PoM] £18.70
  Venlafaxine (as Venlafaxine hydrochloride) 225 mg Venladex XL 225mg tablets | 28 tablet [PoM] £31.36

▸ ViePax XL (Dexcel-Pharma Ltd)
  Venlafaxine (as Venlafaxine hydrochloride) 75 mg ViePax XL 75mg tablets | 28 tablet [PoM] £2.60
  Venlafaxine (as Venlafaxine hydrochloride) 150 mg ViePax XL 150mg tablets | 28 tablet [PoM] £3.90

Modified-release capsule

CAUTIONARY AND ADVISORY LABELS 2, 21, 25

▸ Venlafaxine (Non-proprietary)
  Venlafaxine (as Venlafaxine hydrochloride) 37.5 mg Venlafaxine 37.5mg modified-release capsules | 28 capsule [PoM] £5.25–£10.73 DT = £5.25
  Venlafaxine (as Venlafaxine hydrochloride) 75 mg Venlafaxine 75mg modified-release capsules | 28 capsule [PoM] £3.29–£22.94 DT = £2.71
  Venlafaxine (as Venlafaxine hydrochloride) 150 mg Venlafaxine 150mg modified-release capsules | 28 capsule [PoM] £4.72–£38.26 DT = £9.95
  Venlafaxine (as Venlafaxine hydrochloride) 225 mg Venlafaxine 225mg modified-release capsules | 28 capsule [PoM] £28.97 DT = £12.80 | 30 capsule [PoM] £27.69

▸ Efexor XL (Viatris UK Healthcare Ltd)
  Venlafaxine (as Venlafaxine hydrochloride) 75 mg Efexor XL 75mg capsules | 28 capsule [PoM] £22.08 DT = £2.71
  Venlafaxine (as Venlafaxine hydrochloride) 150 mg Efexor XL 150mg capsules | 28 capsule [PoM] £36.81 DT = £9.95
  Venlafaxine (as Venlafaxine hydrochloride) 225 mg Efexor XL 225mg capsules | 28 capsule [PoM] £47.11 DT = £12.80

▶ **Majoven XL** (Bristol Laboratories Ltd)
Venlafaxine (as Venlafaxine hydrochloride) 37.5 mg Majoven XL
37.5mg capsules | 28 capsule [PoM] £5.25 DT = £5.25
Venlafaxine (as Venlafaxine hydrochloride) 75 mg Majoven XL
75mg capsules | 28 capsule [PoM] £22.08 DT = £2.71
Venlafaxine (as Venlafaxine hydrochloride) 150 mg Majoven XL
150mg capsules | 28 capsule [PoM] £36.81 DT = £9.95

▶ **Politid XL** (Accord-UK Ltd)
Venlafaxine (as Venlafaxine hydrochloride) 75 mg Politid XL 75mg
capsules | 28 capsule [PoM] £23.41 DT = £2.71

▶ **Venaxx XL** (Advanz Pharma)
Venlafaxine (as Venlafaxine hydrochloride) 75 mg Venaxx XL
75mg capsules | 28 capsule [PoM] £10.40 DT = £2.71
Venlafaxine (as Venlafaxine hydrochloride) 150 mg Venaxx XL
150mg capsules | 28 capsule [PoM] £17.40 DT = £9.95

▶ **Vencarm XL** (Aspire Pharma Ltd)
Venlafaxine (as Venlafaxine hydrochloride) 37.5 mg Vencarm XL
37.5mg capsules | 28 capsule [PoM] £3.30 DT = £5.25
Venlafaxine (as Venlafaxine hydrochloride) 75 mg Vencarm XL
75mg capsules | 28 capsule [PoM] £2.59 DT = £2.71
Venlafaxine (as Venlafaxine hydrochloride) 150 mg Vencarm XL
150mg capsules | 28 capsule [PoM] £3.89 DT = £9.95
Venlafaxine (as Venlafaxine hydrochloride) 225 mg Vencarm XL
225mg capsules | 28 capsule [PoM] £9.90 DT = £12.80

▶ **Venlablue XL** (Zentiva Pharma UK Ltd)
Venlafaxine (as Venlafaxine hydrochloride) 37.5 mg Venlablue XL
37.5mg capsules | 28 capsule [PoM] £5.25 DT = £5.25
Venlafaxine (as Venlafaxine hydrochloride) 75 mg Venlablue XL
75mg capsules | 28 capsule [PoM] £6.95 DT = £2.71
Venlafaxine (as Venlafaxine hydrochloride) 150 mg Venlablue XL
150mg capsules | 28 capsule [PoM] £9.95 DT = £9.95

▶ **Venlasov XL** (Sovereign Medical Ltd)
Venlafaxine (as Venlafaxine hydrochloride) 75 mg Venlasov XL
75mg capsules | 28 capsule [PoM] £3.13 DT = £2.71
Venlafaxine (as Venlafaxine hydrochloride) 150 mg Venlasov XL
150mg capsules | 28 capsule [PoM] £4.72 DT = £9.95

▶ **Vensir XL** (Morningside Healthcare Ltd)
Venlafaxine (as Venlafaxine hydrochloride) 75 mg Vensir XL 75mg
capsules | 28 capsule [PoM] £6.95 DT = £2.71
Venlafaxine (as Venlafaxine hydrochloride) 150 mg Vensir XL
150mg capsules | 28 capsule [PoM] £9.95 DT = £9.95
Venlafaxine (as Venlafaxine hydrochloride) 225 mg Vensir XL
225mg capsules | 28 capsule [PoM] £29.55 DT = £12.80

▶ **Venzip XL** (Milpharm Ltd)
Venlafaxine (as Venlafaxine hydrochloride) 75 mg Venzip XL
75mg capsules | 28 capsule [PoM] £22.08 DT = £2.71
Venlafaxine (as Venlafaxine hydrochloride) 150 mg Venzip XL
150mg capsules | 28 capsule [PoM] £36.81 DT = £9.95

Oral solution
CAUTIONARY AND ADVISORY LABELS 2, 21
EXCIPIENTS: May contain Hydroxybenzoates (parabens)
▶ **Venlafaxine (Non-proprietary)**
Venlafaxine (as Venlafaxine hydrochloride) 7.5 mg per
1 ml Venlafaxine 37.5mg/5ml oral solution sugar free | 150 ml [PoM]
£186.90 DT = £186.90 [SF]
Venlafaxine (as Venlafaxine hydrochloride) 15 mg per
1 ml Venlafaxine 75mg/5ml oral solution sugar free | 150 ml [PoM]
£244.65 DT = £244.65 [SF]

ANTIDEPRESSANTS > SEROTONIN UPTAKE INHIBITORS

Trazodone hydrochloride   25-May-2021

● **INDICATIONS AND DOSE**

Depressive illness (particularly where sedation is required)
▶ BY MOUTH
▶ Adult: Initially 150 mg daily in divided doses, dose to
be taken after food, alternatively initially 150 mg once
daily, dose to be taken at bedtime, increased if
necessary to 300 mg daily; increased if necessary to
600 mg daily in divided doses, higher dose for use in
hospital patients only
▶ Elderly: Initially 100 mg daily in divided doses, dose to
be taken after food, alternatively initially 100 mg once
daily, dose to be taken at bedtime, increased if
necessary to 300 mg daily; increased if necessary to
600 mg daily in divided doses, higher dose for use in
hospital patients only

Anxiety
▶ BY MOUTH
▶ Adult: 75 mg daily, increased if necessary to 300 mg
daily

● **CONTRA-INDICATIONS** During the manic phase of bipolar
disorder · immediate recovery period after myocardial
infarction

● **CAUTIONS** Arrhythmias · cardiovascular disease · chronic
constipation · epilepsy · history of bipolar disorder · history
of psychosis · hyperthyroidism (risk of arrhythmias) ·
increased intra-ocular pressure · patients with a significant
risk of suicide · prostatic hypertrophy · susceptibility to
angle-closure glaucoma · urinary retention

CAUTIONS, FURTHER INFORMATION Manufacturer advises
treatment should be stopped if the patient enters a manic
phase.
 Elderly patients are particularly susceptible to many of
the side-effects of tricyclic antidepressants; manufacturer
advises low initial doses should be used, with close
monitoring, particularly for psychiatric and cardiac side-
effects.

● **INTERACTIONS** → Appendix 1: trazodone

● **SIDE-EFFECTS** Aggression · agranulocytosis · alertness
decreased · anaemia · anxiety · aphasia · appetite abnormal
· arrhythmias · arthralgia · asthenia · blood disorder · chest
pain · confusion · constipation · delirium · delusions ·
diarrhoea · dizziness · drowsiness · dry mouth · dyspnoea ·
eosinophilia · fever · gastroenteritis · gastrointestinal
discomfort · hallucination · headache · hepatic disorders ·
hyperhidrosis · hypersalivation · hypertension ·
hyponatraemia · influenza like illness · jaundice
(discontinue) · leucopenia · libido decreased · mania ·
memory loss · movement disorders · myalgia · nasal
congestion · nausea · neuroleptic malignant syndrome
(discontinue—potentially fatal) · oedema · pain ·
palpitations · paraesthesia · paralytic ileus · postural
hypotension · priapism (discontinue) · QT interval
prolongation · seizure · serotonin syndrome · SIADH · skin
reactions · sleep disorders · suicidal behaviours · syncope ·
taste altered · thrombocytopenia · tremor · urinary disorder
· vertigo · vision blurred · vomiting · weight decreased ·
withdrawal syndrome

SIDE-EFFECTS, FURTHER INFORMATION The risk of side-
effects is reduced by titrating slowly to the minimum
effective dose (every 2–3 days). Consider using a lower
starting dose in elderly patients.

Overdose The tricyclic-related antidepressant drugs may
be associated with a lower risk of cardiotoxicity in
overdosage.
 Tricyclic and related antidepressants cause dry mouth,
coma of varying degree, hypotension, hypothermia,
hyperreflexia, extensor plantar responses, convulsions,
respiratory failure, cardiac conduction defects, and
arrhythmias. Dilated pupils and urinary retention also
occur. For details on the management of poisoning see
Tricyclic and related antidepressants under Emergency
treatment of poisoning p. 1554.

● **PREGNANCY** Avoid during first trimester—limited
information available. Monitor infant for signs of
withdrawal if used until delivery.

● **BREAST FEEDING** The amount secreted into breast milk is
too small to be harmful.

● **HEPATIC IMPAIRMENT** Manufacturer advises caution,
particularly in severe impairment (increased risk of side-
effects).

- **RENAL IMPAIRMENT** [EvGr] Use with caution, particularly in severe impairment. [M]

- **TREATMENT CESSATION** Withdrawal effects may occur within 5 days of stopping treatment with antidepressant drugs; they are usually mild and self-limiting, but in some cases may be severe. The risk of withdrawal symptoms is increased if the antidepressant is stopped suddenly after regular administration for 8 weeks or more. The dose should preferably be reduced gradually over about 4 weeks, or longer if withdrawal symptoms emerge (6 months in patients who have been on long-term maintenance treatment). If possible tricyclic and related antidepressants should be withdrawn slowly.

- **PRESCRIBING AND DISPENSING INFORMATION** Limited quantities of tricyclic antidepressants should be prescribed at any one time because their cardiovascular and epileptogenic effects are dangerous in overdosage.

- **PATIENT AND CARER ADVICE**
Driving and skilled tasks Drowsiness may affect the performance of skilled tasks (e.g. driving).
   Effects of alcohol enhanced.

- **MEDICINAL FORMS** There can be variation in the licensing of different medicines containing the same drug. Forms available from special-order manufacturers include: oral suspension, oral solution

Oral tablet
CAUTIONARY AND ADVISORY LABELS 2, 21
▸ Trazodone hydrochloride (Non-proprietary)
   Trazodone hydrochloride 50 mg Trazodone 50mg tablets |
   84 tablet [PoM] £23.43–£38.66 DT = £23.43
   Trazodone hydrochloride 100 mg Trazodone 100mg tablets |
   56 tablet [PoM] £26.75–£44.14 DT = £26.75
   Trazodone hydrochloride 150 mg Trazodone 150mg tablets |
   28 tablet [PoM] £34.00 DT = £1.98

Oral solution
CAUTIONARY AND ADVISORY LABELS 2, 21
▸ Trazodone hydrochloride (Non-proprietary)
   Trazodone hydrochloride 10 mg per 1 ml Trazodone 50mg/5ml
   oral solution sugar free | 120 ml [PoM] £180.00 DT = £7.17 [SF]
   Trazodone hydrochloride 20 mg per 1 ml Trazodone 100mg/5ml
   oral solution sugar free | 120 ml [PoM] £155.00–£315.92 DT =
   £315.92 [SF]

Oral capsule
CAUTIONARY AND ADVISORY LABELS 2, 21
▸ Trazodone hydrochloride (Non-proprietary)
   Trazodone hydrochloride 50 mg Trazodone 50mg capsules |
   84 capsule [PoM] £35.00 DT = £2.05
   Trazodone hydrochloride 100 mg Trazodone 100mg capsules |
   56 capsule [PoM] £41.00 DT = £1.98

ANTIDEPRESSANTS > TETRACYCLIC ANTIDEPRESSANTS

Mianserin hydrochloride
14-Dec-2021

- **INDICATIONS AND DOSE**

Depressive illness (particularly where sedation is required)
▸ BY MOUTH
▸ Adult: Initially 30–40 mg daily in divided doses, alternatively initially 30–40 mg once daily, dose to be taken at bedtime, increase dose gradually as necessary; usual dose 30–90 mg
▸ Elderly: Initially 30 mg daily in divided doses, alternatively initially 30 mg once daily, dose to be taken at bedtime, increase dose gradually as necessary; usual dose 30–90 mg

- **CONTRA-INDICATIONS** Acute porphyrias p. 1202 · during the manic phase of bipolar disorder

- **CAUTIONS** Arrhythmias · cardiovascular disease · diabetes · elderly · epilepsy · heart block · history of bipolar disorder · history of psychosis · immediate recovery period after

myocardial infarction · increased intra-ocular pressure · patients with a significant risk of suicide · phaeochromocytoma (risk of arrhythmias) · prostatic hypertrophy · susceptibility to angle-closure glaucoma

CAUTIONS, FURTHER INFORMATION Manufacturer advises treatment should be stopped if the patient enters a manic phase.

- **INTERACTIONS** → Appendix 1: mianserin

- **SIDE-EFFECTS** Agranulocytosis · arthritis · bone marrow disorders · breast abnormalities · dizziness · granulocytopenia · gynaecomastia · hepatic disorders · hyperhidrosis · hyponatraemia · joint disorders · lactation in absence of pregnancy · leucopenia · mood altered · neuromuscular irritability · oedema · paranoid delusions · postural hypotension · psychosis · rash · seizure · sexual dysfunction · suicidal behaviours · tremor · withdrawal syndrome

SIDE-EFFECTS, FURTHER INFORMATION The risk of side-effects is reduced by titrating slowly to the minimum effective dose (every 2–3 days). Consider using a lower starting dose in elderly patients.

Overdose The tricyclic-related antidepressant drugs may be associated with a lower risk of cardiotoxicity in overdosage.
   Tricyclic and related antidepressants cause dry mouth, coma of varying degree, hypotension, hypothermia, hyperreflexia, extensor plantar responses, convulsions, respiratory failure, cardiac conduction defects, and arrhythmias. Dilated pupils and urinary retention also occur. For details on the management of poisoning see Tricyclic and related antidepressants under Emergency treatment of poisoning p. 1554.

- **PREGNANCY** Avoid.

- **BREAST FEEDING** The amount secreted into breast milk is too small to be harmful.

- **HEPATIC IMPAIRMENT** Manufacturer advises caution; avoid in severe impairment.

- **RENAL IMPAIRMENT** [EvGr] Use with caution. [M]

- **MONITORING REQUIREMENTS** A full **blood count** is recommended every 4 weeks during the first 3 months of treatment; clinical monitoring should continue subsequently and treatment should be stopped and a full blood count obtained if *fever, sore throat, stomatitis,* or other signs of infection develop.

- **TREATMENT CESSATION** Withdrawal effects may occur within 5 days of stopping treatment with antidepressant drugs; they are usually mild and self-limiting, but in some cases may be severe. The risk of withdrawal symptoms is increased if the antidepressant is stopped suddenly after regular administration for 8 weeks or more. The dose should preferably be reduced gradually over about 4 weeks, or longer if withdrawal symptoms emerge (6 months in patients who have been on long-term maintenance treatment). If possible tricyclic and related antidepressants should be withdrawn slowly.

- **PRESCRIBING AND DISPENSING INFORMATION** Limited quantities of tricyclic antidepressants should be prescribed at any one time because their cardiovascular and epileptogenic effects are dangerous in overdosage.

- **PATIENT AND CARER ADVICE**
Driving and skilled tasks Drowsiness may affect the performance of skilled tasks (e.g. driving).
   Effects of alcohol enhanced.

- **MEDICINAL FORMS** There can be variation in the licensing of different medicines containing the same drug. Forms available from special-order manufacturers include: oral suspension, oral solution

Oral tablet
CAUTIONARY AND ADVISORY LABELS 2, 25
▸ **Mianserin hydrochloride (Non-proprietary)**
  Mianserin hydrochloride 10 mg Mianserin 10mg tablets | 28 tablet [PoM] £19.56–£21.00 DT = £19.56
  Mianserin hydrochloride 30 mg Mianserin 30mg tablets | 28 tablet [PoM] £52.00 DT = £47.75

Mirtazapine
12-Apr-2023

- **DRUG ACTION** Mirtazapine is a presynaptic alpha$_2$-adrenoreceptor antagonist which increases central noradrenergic and serotonergic neurotransmission.

- **INDICATIONS AND DOSE**

Major depression
▸ BY MOUTH
▸ Adult: Initially 15–30 mg once daily for 2–4 weeks, dose to be taken at bedtime, then adjusted according to response to up to 45 mg once daily, dose to be taken at bedtime, alternatively up to 45 mg daily in 2 divided doses

- **CAUTIONS** Cardiac disorders · diabetes mellitus · elderly · history of mania (discontinue if patient entering manic phase) · history of seizures · history of urinary retention · hypotension · psychoses (may aggravate psychotic symptoms) · susceptibility to angle-closure glaucoma

- **INTERACTIONS** → Appendix 1: mirtazapine

- **SIDE-EFFECTS**
▸ **Common or very common** Anxiety · appetite increased · arthralgia · back pain · confusion · constipation · diarrhoea · dizziness · drowsiness · dry mouth · fatigue · headache (on discontinuation) · myalgia · nausea · oedema · postural hypotension · sleep disorders · tremor · vomiting · weight increased
▸ **Uncommon** Hallucination · mania · movement disorders · oral disorders · syncope
▸ **Rare or very rare** Aggression · pancreatitis
▸ **Frequency not known** Agranulocytosis · arrhythmias · bone marrow disorders · dysarthria · eosinophilia · granulocytopenia · hyponatraemia · jaundice (discontinue) · QT interval prolongation · rhabdomyolysis · seizure · serotonin syndrome · severe cutaneous adverse reactions (SCARs) · SIADH · skin reactions · sudden death · suicidal behaviours · thrombocytopenia · urinary retention · withdrawal syndrome

- **PREGNANCY** Use with caution—limited experience; monitor neonate for withdrawal effects.

- **BREAST FEEDING** Present in milk; use only if potential benefit outweighs risk.

- **HEPATIC IMPAIRMENT** Manufacturer advises caution (risk of increased plasma concentration, no information available in severe impairment).

- **RENAL IMPAIRMENT** Clearance reduced by 30% if creatinine clearance less than 40 mL/minute; clearance reduced by 50% if creatinine clearance less than 10 mL/minute. See p. 21.

- **TREATMENT CESSATION** Nausea, vomiting, dizziness, agitation, anxiety, and headache are most common features of withdrawal if treatment stopped abruptly or if dose reduced markedly; dose should be reduced over several weeks.

- **DIRECTIONS FOR ADMINISTRATION** Orodispersible tablet should be placed on the tongue, allowed to disperse and swallowed.

- **PATIENT AND CARER ADVICE** Counselling on administration of orodispersible tablet advised.
Blood Disorders Patients should be advised to report any fever, sore throat, stomatitis or other signs of infection during treatment. Blood count should be performed and the drug stopped immediately if blood dyscrasia suspected.

- **MEDICINAL FORMS** There can be variation in the licensing of different medicines containing the same drug. Forms available from special-order manufacturers include: oral capsule, oral suspension, oral solution

Oral tablet
CAUTIONARY AND ADVISORY LABELS 2, 25
▸ **Mirtazapine (Non-proprietary)**
  Mirtazapine 15 mg Mirtazapine 15mg tablets | 28 tablet [PoM] £3.95 DT = £0.98
  Mirtazapine 30 mg Mirtazapine 30mg tablets | 28 tablet [PoM] £4.50 DT = £1.14
  Mirtazapine 45 mg Mirtazapine 45mg tablets | 28 tablet [PoM] £4.95 DT = £1.40

Oral solution
CAUTIONARY AND ADVISORY LABELS 2
▸ **Mirtazapine (Non-proprietary)**
  Mirtazapine 15 mg per 1 ml Mirtazapine 15mg/ml oral solution sugar free | 66 ml [PoM] £137.59 DT = £137.59 [SF]

Orodispersible tablet
CAUTIONARY AND ADVISORY LABELS 2
EXCIPIENTS: May contain Aspartame
▸ **Mirtazapine (Non-proprietary)**
  Mirtazapine 15 mg Mirtazapine 15mg orodispersible tablets | 30 tablet [PoM] £3.95 DT = £1.79
  Mirtazapine 30 mg Mirtazapine 30mg orodispersible tablets | 30 tablet [PoM] £4.50 DT = £1.79
  Mirtazapine 45 mg Mirtazapine 45mg orodispersible tablets | 30 tablet [PoM] £4.95 DT = £2.00

ANTIDEPRESSANTS › TRICYCLIC ANTIDEPRESSANTS

Amitriptyline hydrochloride
20-Oct-2020

- **INDICATIONS AND DOSE**

Abdominal pain or discomfort (in patients who have not responded to laxatives, loperamide, or antispasmodics)
▸ BY MOUTH
▸ Adult: Initially 5–10 mg daily, to be taken at night; increased in steps of 10 mg at least every 2 weeks as required; maximum 30 mg per day

Major depressive disorder [not recommended—increased risk of fatality in overdose]
▸ BY MOUTH
▸ Adult: Initially 50 mg daily in 2 divided doses, then increased in steps of 25 mg once daily on alternate days if required, maximum 150 mg daily in 2 divided doses
▸ Elderly: Initially 10–25 mg daily, increased if necessary up to 100–150 mg daily in 2 divided doses, dose increases dependent on individual patient response and tolerability—doses above 100 mg should be used with caution

Major depressive disorder in patients with cardiovascular disease [not recommended—increased risk of fatality in overdose]
▸ BY MOUTH
▸ Adult: Initially 10–25 mg daily, increased if necessary up to 100–150 mg daily in 2 divided doses, dose increases dependent on individual patient response and tolerability—doses above 100 mg should be used with caution

Neuropathic pain | Migraine prophylaxis | Chronic tension-type headache prophylaxis
▸ BY MOUTH
▸ Adult: Initially 10–25 mg daily, dose to be taken in the evening, then increased, if tolerated, in   continued →

steps of 10–25 mg every 3–7 days in 1–2 divided doses; usual dose 25–75 mg daily, dose to be taken in the evening, doses above 100 mg should be used with caution (doses above 75 mg should be used with caution in the elderly and in patients with cardiovascular disease); maximum per dose 75 mg

Emotional lability in multiple sclerosis

▶ BY MOUTH

▸ Adult: Initially 10–25 mg daily; increased, if tolerated, in steps of 10–25 mg every 1–7 days; maximum 75 mg per day

- **UNLICENSED USE** Not licensed for use in abdominal pain or discomfort in patients who have not responded to laxatives, loperamide, or antispasmodics. EvGr Amitriptyline hydrochloride is used for emotional lability in multiple sclerosis, Ⓔ but is not licensed for this indication.

- **CONTRA-INDICATIONS** Arrhythmias · during manic phase of bipolar disorder · heart block · immediate recovery period after myocardial infarction

- **CAUTIONS** Cardiovascular disease · chronic constipation · diabetes · epilepsy · history of bipolar disorder · history of psychosis · hyperthyroidism (risk of arrhythmias) · increased intra-ocular pressure · patients with a significant risk of suicide · phaeochromocytoma (risk of arrhythmias) · prostatic hypertrophy · pyloric stenosis · susceptibility to angle-closure glaucoma · urinary retention

  CAUTIONS, FURTHER INFORMATION EvGr Treatment should be stopped if the patient enters a manic phase. Ⓜ
  Elderly patients are particularly susceptible to many of the side-effects of tricyclic antidepressants; EvGr low initial doses should be used, with close monitoring, particularly for psychiatric and cardiac side-effects. Ⓜ

- **INTERACTIONS** → Appendix 1: tricyclic antidepressants

- **SIDE-EFFECTS**
▸ **Common or very common** Accommodation disorder · anxiety · arrhythmias · behaviour abnormal · cardiac conduction disorders · concentration impaired · confusion · constipation · dizziness · drowsiness · dry mouth · fatigue · headache · hyperhidrosis · hyponatraemia · hypotension · movement disorders · mydriasis · nasal congestion · nausea · palpitations · paraesthesia · QT interval prolongation · sexual dysfunction · speech impairment · taste altered · thirst · tremor · urinary disorders · weight changes
▸ **Uncommon** Circulatory collapse · diarrhoea · face oedema · galactorrhoea · heart failure aggravated · hepatic disorders · hypertension · mood altered · oral disorders · seizure · skin reactions · sleep disorders · tinnitus · vomiting
▸ **Rare or very rare** Acute glaucoma · agranulocytosis · alopecia · appetite decreased · bone marrow depression · cardiomyopathy · delirium · eosinophilia · fever · gynaecomastia · hallucination · interstitial lung disease · leucopenia · paralytic ileus · photosensitivity reaction · polyneuropathy · pulmonary eosinophilia · suicidal behaviours · thrombocytopenia
▸ **Frequency not known** Angioedema · anticholinergic syndrome · dry eye · hypersensitivity myocarditis · hyperthermia · increased risk of fracture · severe cutaneous adverse reactions (SCARs)

  SIDE-EFFECTS, FURTHER INFORMATION The risk of side-effects is reduced by titrating slowly to the minimum effective dose (every 2–3 days). Consider using a lower starting dose in elderly patients.

  Overdose Overdosage with amitriptyline is associated with a relatively high rate of fatality. Symptoms of overdosage may include dry mouth, coma of varying degree, hypotension, hypothermia, hyperreflexia, extensor plantar responses, convulsions, respiratory failure, cardiac conduction defects, and arrhythmias. Dilated pupils and urinary retention also occur. For details on the management of poisoning, see Tricyclic and related antidepressants, under Emergency treatment of poisoning p. 1554.

- **PREGNANCY** Use only if potential benefit outweighs risk.

- **BREAST FEEDING** The amount secreted into breast milk is too small to be harmful.

- **HEPATIC IMPAIRMENT** Manufacturer advises use with caution in mild-to-moderate impairment; avoid in severe impairment.

- **TREATMENT CESSATION** Withdrawal effects may occur within 5 days of stopping treatment with antidepressant drugs; they are usually mild and self-limiting, but in some cases may be severe. The risk of withdrawal symptoms is increased if the antidepressant is stopped suddenly after regular administration for 8 weeks or more. The dose should preferably be reduced gradually over about 4 weeks, or longer if withdrawal symptoms emerge (6 months in patients who have been on long-term maintenance treatment). If possible tricyclic and related antidepressants should be withdrawn slowly.

- **PRESCRIBING AND DISPENSING INFORMATION** Limited quantities of tricyclic antidepressants should be prescribed at any one time because their cardiovascular and epileptogenic effects are dangerous in overdosage.

- **PATIENT AND CARER ADVICE**
  Driving and skilled tasks Drowsiness may affect the performance of skilled tasks (e.g. driving).
  Effects of alcohol enhanced.

- **LESS SUITABLE FOR PRESCRIBING** Amitriptyline hydrochloride is less suitable for prescribing, see Tricyclic and related antidepressant drugs in Antidepressant drugs p. 417.

- **MEDICINAL FORMS** There can be variation in the licensing of different medicines containing the same drug. Forms available from special-order manufacturers include: oral suspension, oral solution

Oral tablet
CAUTIONARY AND ADVISORY LABELS 2
▶ Amitriptyline hydrochloride (Non-proprietary)
  Amitriptyline hydrochloride 10 mg Amitriptyline 10mg tablets | 28 tablet PoM £0.79 DT = £0.61
  Amitriptyline hydrochloride 25 mg Amitriptyline 25mg tablets | 28 tablet PoM £0.89 DT = £0.64
  Amitriptyline hydrochloride 50 mg Amitriptyline 50mg tablets | 28 tablet PoM £1.08 DT = £0.79

Oral solution
CAUTIONARY AND ADVISORY LABELS 2
▶ Amitriptyline hydrochloride (Non-proprietary)
  Amitriptyline hydrochloride 2 mg per 1 ml Amitriptyline 10mg/5ml oral solution sugar free | 150 ml PoM £122.76 DT = £55.86 SF
  Amitriptyline hydrochloride 5 mg per 1 ml Amitriptyline 25mg/5ml oral solution sugar free | 150 ml PoM £18.00 DT = £14.22 SF
  Amitriptyline hydrochloride 10 mg per 1 ml Amitriptyline 50mg/5ml oral solution sugar free | 150 ml PoM £24.00 DT = £15.08 SF

Clomipramine hydrochloride

16-Feb-2021

- **INDICATIONS AND DOSE**

Depressive illness
▶ BY MOUTH
▸ Adult: Initially 10 mg daily, then increased if necessary to 30–150 mg daily in divided doses, dose to be increased gradually, alternatively increased if necessary to 30–150 mg once daily, dose to be taken at bedtime; maximum 250 mg per day
▸ Elderly: Initially 10 mg daily, then increased to 30–75 mg daily, dose to be increased carefully over approximately 10 days

Phobic and obsessional states
▶ BY MOUTH
▸ Adult: Initially 25 mg daily, then increased to 100–150 mg daily, dose to be increased gradually over 2 weeks; maximum 250 mg per day
▸ Elderly: Initially 10 mg daily, then increased to 100–150 mg daily, dose to be increased gradually over 2 weeks; maximum 250 mg per day

Adjunctive treatment of cataplexy associated with narcolepsy
▶ BY MOUTH
▸ Adult: Initially 10 mg daily, dose to be gradually increased until satisfactory response; increased if necessary to 10–75 mg daily

- **CONTRA-INDICATIONS** Acute porphyrias p. 1202 · arrhythmias · during the manic phase of bipolar disorder · heart block · immediate recovery period after myocardial infarction

- **CAUTIONS** Cardiovascular disease · chronic constipation · epilepsy · history of bipolar disorder · history of psychosis · hyperthyroidism (risk of arrhythmias) · increased intra-ocular pressure · patients with a significant risk of suicide · phaeochromocytoma (risk of arrhythmias) · prostatic hypertrophy · risk factors for QT interval prolongation—correct hypokalaemia before initiating treatment · susceptibility to angle-closure glaucoma · urinary retention

  CAUTIONS, FURTHER INFORMATION [EvGr] Treatment should be stopped or dose reduced if the patient enters a manic phase. ⟨M⟩

  Elderly patients are particularly susceptible to many of the side-effects of tricyclic antidepressants; [EvGr] low initial doses should be used, with close monitoring, particularly for psychiatric and cardiac side-effects. ⟨M⟩

- **INTERACTIONS** → Appendix 1: tricyclic antidepressants

- **SIDE-EFFECTS**
▸ **Common or very common** Aggression · anxiety · arrhythmias · breast enlargement · concentration impaired · confusion · constipation · delirium · depersonalisation · depression exacerbated · diarrhoea · dizziness · drowsiness · dry mouth · fatigue · galactorrhoea · gastrointestinal disorder · hallucination · headache · hot flush · hyperhidrosis · hypotension · memory loss · mood altered · movement disorders · muscle tone increased · muscle weakness · mydriasis · nausea · palpitations · paraesthesia · photosensitivity reaction · sexual dysfunction · skin reactions · sleep disorders · speech disorder · taste altered · tinnitus · tremor · urinary disorders · vision disorders · vomiting · weight increased · yawning
▸ **Uncommon** Psychosis · seizure
▸ **Rare or very rare** Agranulocytosis · alopecia · cardiac conduction disorders · eosinophilia · glaucoma · hepatic disorders · hyperpyrexia · interstitial lung disease · leucopenia · neuroleptic malignant syndrome (discontinue—potentially fatal) · oedema · QT interval prolongation · SIADH · thrombocytopenia · vaginal haemorrhage
▸ **Frequency not known** Increased risk of fracture · rhabdomyolysis · serotonin syndrome · suicidal behaviours · withdrawal syndrome

  SIDE-EFFECTS, FURTHER INFORMATION The patient should be encouraged to persist with treatment as some tolerance to these side-effects seems to develop.

  The risk of side-effects is reduced by titrating slowly to the minimum effective dose (every 2–3 days). Consider using a lower starting dose in elderly patients.

  Overdose Tricyclic and related antidepressants cause dry mouth, coma of varying degree, hypotension, hypothermia, hyperreflexia, extensor plantar responses, convulsions, respiratory failure, cardiac conduction defects, and arrhythmias. Dilated pupils and urinary retention also occur. For details on the management of poisoning see Tricyclic and related antidepressants under Emergency treatment of poisoning p. 1554.

- **PREGNANCY** Neonatal withdrawal symptoms reported if used during third trimester.

- **BREAST FEEDING** The amount secreted into breast milk is too small to be harmful.

- **HEPATIC IMPAIRMENT** Manufacturer advises caution; avoid in severe impairment (risk of hypertensive crisis).

- **MONITORING REQUIREMENTS** Manufacturer advises monitor cardiac and hepatic function during long-term use.

- **TREATMENT CESSATION** Withdrawal effects may occur within 5 days of stopping treatment with antidepressant drugs; they are usually mild and self-limiting, but in some cases may be severe. The risk of withdrawal symptoms is increased if the antidepressant is stopped suddenly after regular administration for 8 weeks or more. The dose should preferably be reduced gradually over about 4 weeks, or longer if withdrawal symptoms emerge (6 months in patients who have been on long-term maintenance treatment). If possible tricyclic and related antidepressants should be withdrawn slowly.

- **PRESCRIBING AND DISPENSING INFORMATION** Limited quantities of tricyclic antidepressants should be prescribed at any one time because their cardiovascular and epileptogenic effects are dangerous in overdosage.

- **PATIENT AND CARER ADVICE**
  Driving and skilled tasks Drowsiness may affect the performance of skilled tasks (e.g. driving).
  Effects of alcohol enhanced.

- **MEDICINAL FORMS** There can be variation in the licensing of different medicines containing the same drug. Forms available from special-order manufacturers include: modified-release tablet, oral suspension, oral solution
  Oral capsule
  CAUTIONARY AND ADVISORY LABELS 2
▸ **Clomipramine hydrochloride (Non-proprietary)**
  Clomipramine hydrochloride 10 mg Clomipramine 10mg capsules | 28 capsule [PoM] £6.72 DT = £3.93
  Clomipramine hydrochloride 25 mg Clomipramine 25mg capsules | 28 capsule [PoM] £9.36 DT = £4.67
  Clomipramine hydrochloride 50 mg Clomipramine 50mg capsules | 28 capsule [PoM] £13.34 DT = £7.65

Dosulepin hydrochloride
07-Jan-2021

(Dothiepin hydrochloride)

- **INDICATIONS AND DOSE**

Depressive illness, particularly where sedation is required (not recommended—increased risk of fatality in overdose) (initiated by a specialist)
▶ BY MOUTH
▸ Adult: Initially 75 mg daily in divided doses, alternatively initially 75 mg once daily, dose to be taken at bedtime, increased if necessary to 150 mg daily, doses to be increased gradually; up to 225 mg daily in some circumstances (e.g. hospital use)
▸ Elderly: Initially 50–75 mg daily in divided doses, alternatively initially 50–75 mg once daily, dose to be taken at bedtime, increased if necessary to 75–150 mg daily, doses to be increased gradually; up to 225 mg daily in some circumstances (e.g. hospital use)

- **CONTRA-INDICATIONS** Acute porphyrias p. 1202 · arrhythmias · during the manic phase of bipolar disorder · heart block · immediate recovery period after myocardial infarction

- **CAUTIONS** Cardiovascular disease · chronic constipation · diabetes · epilepsy · history of bipolar disorder · history of psychosis · hyperthyroidism (risk of arrhythmias) · increased intra-ocular pressure · patients with a significant risk of suicide · phaeochromocytoma (risk of arrhythmias) · prostatic hypertrophy · susceptibility to angle-closure glaucoma · urinary retention

  CAUTIONS, FURTHER INFORMATION EvGr Treatment should be stopped if the patient enters a manic phase. ⓜ

  Elderly patients are particularly susceptible to many of the side-effects of tricyclic antidepressants; EvGr low initial doses should be used, with close monitoring, particularly for psychiatric and cardiac side-effects. ⓜ

- **INTERACTIONS** → Appendix 1: tricyclic antidepressants

- **SIDE-EFFECTS** Accommodation disorder · agranulocytosis · alveolitis · anticholinergic syndrome · appetite abnormal · arrhythmias · asthenia · bone marrow depression · cardiac conduction disorder · confusion · constipation · dizziness · drowsiness · dry mouth · endocrine disorder · eosinophilia · epigastric discomfort · galactorrhoea · gynaecomastia · hepatic disorders · hyperhidrosis · hypertension · hyponatraemia · hypotension · increased risk of fracture · leucopenia · mood altered · movement disorders · nausea · nervousness · paranoid delusions · photosensitivity reaction · psychosis · seizures · sexual dysfunction · SIADH · skin reactions · speech disorder · suicidal behaviours · testicular hypertrophy · thrombocytopenia · tremor · urinary hesitation · vomiting · weight changes · withdrawal syndrome

  SIDE-EFFECTS, FURTHER INFORMATION The risk of side-effects are reduced by titrating slowly to the minimum effective dose (every 2–3 days). Consider using a lower starting dose in elderly patients.

  Overdose Overdosage with dosulepin is associated with a relatively high rate of fatality.

  Tricyclic and related antidepressants cause dry mouth, coma of varying degree, hypotension, hypothermia, hyperreflexia, extensor plantar responses, convulsions, respiratory failure, cardiac conduction defects, and arrhythmias. Dilated pupils and urinary retention also occur. For details on the management of poisoning see Tricyclic and related antidepressants under Emergency treatment of poisoning.

- **PREGNANCY** Use only if potential benefit outweighs risk.

- **BREAST FEEDING** The amount secreted into breast milk is too small to be harmful.

- **HEPATIC IMPAIRMENT** Manufacturer advises caution in mild to moderate impairment; avoid in severe impairment.

- **TREATMENT CESSATION** Withdrawal effects may occur within 5 days of stopping treatment with antidepressant drugs; they are usually mild and self-limiting, but in some cases may be severe. The risk of withdrawal symptoms is increased if the antidepressant is stopped suddenly after regular administration for 8 weeks or more. The dose should preferably be reduced gradually over about 4 weeks, or longer if withdrawal symptoms emerge. (6 months in patients who have been on long-term maintenance treatment). If possible tricyclic and related antidepressants should be withdrawn slowly.

- **PRESCRIBING AND DISPENSING INFORMATION** Limited quantities of tricyclic antidepressants should be prescribed at any one time because their cardiovascular and epileptogenic effects are dangerous in overdosage.

  A maximum prescription equivalent to 2 weeks' supply of 75 mg daily should be considered in patients with increased risk factors for suicide at initiation of treatment, during any dose adjustment, and until improvement occurs.

- **PATIENT AND CARER ADVICE**
  Driving and skilled tasks Drowsiness may affect the performance of skilled tasks (e.g. driving).
  Effects of alcohol enhanced.

- **LESS SUITABLE FOR PRESCRIBING** Dosulepin hydrochloride is less suitable for prescribing, see Tricyclic and related antidepressant drugs in Antidepressant drugs p. 417.

- **MEDICINAL FORMS** There can be variation in the licensing of different medicines containing the same drug. Forms available from special-order manufacturers include: oral suspension, oral solution

Oral tablet
CAUTIONARY AND ADVISORY LABELS 2
- ▸ **Dosulepin hydrochloride (Non-proprietary)**
  Dosulepin hydrochloride 75 mg Dosulepin 75mg tablets |
  28 tablet PoM £7.97 DT = £7.97
- ▸ **Prothiaden** (Teofarma S.r.l.)
  Dosulepin hydrochloride 75 mg Prothiaden 75mg tablets |
  28 tablet PoM £2.97 DT = £7.97

Oral capsule
CAUTIONARY AND ADVISORY LABELS 2
- ▸ **Dosulepin hydrochloride (Non-proprietary)**
  Dosulepin hydrochloride 25 mg Dosulepin 25mg capsules |
  28 capsule PoM £7.06 DT = £6.48
- ▸ **Prothiaden** (Teofarma S.r.l.)
  Dosulepin hydrochloride 25 mg Prothiaden 25mg capsules |
  28 capsule PoM £1.70 DT = £6.48

Doxepin
20-Apr-2021

- **INDICATIONS AND DOSE**

  Depressive illness (particularly where sedation is required)
  ▸ BY MOUTH
  ▸ Adult: Initially 75 mg daily in divided doses, alternatively 75 mg once daily, adjusted according to response, dose to taken at bedtime; maintenance 25–300 mg daily, doses above 100 mg given in 3 divided doses
  ▸ Elderly: Start with lower doses and adjust according to response

- **CONTRA-INDICATIONS** Acute porphyrias p. 1202 · during manic phase of bipolar disorder

- **CAUTIONS** Arrhythmias · cardiovascular disease · chronic constipation · diabetes · epilepsy · heart block · history of bipolar disorder · history of psychosis · hyperthyroidism (risk of arrhythmias) · immediate recovery period after myocardial infarction · increased intra-ocular pressure · patients with significant risk of suicide · phaeochromocytoma (risk of arrhythmias) · prostatic hypertrophy · susceptibility to angle-closure glaucoma · urinary retention

  CAUTIONS, FURTHER INFORMATION Treatment should be stopped if the patient enters a manic phase.
  ▸ Elderly Elderly patients are particularly susceptible to many of the side-effects of tricyclic antidepressants; low initial doses should be used, with close monitoring, particularly for psychiatric and cardiac side-effects.

- **INTERACTIONS** → Appendix 1: tricyclic antidepressants

- **SIDE-EFFECTS** Agitation · agranulocytosis · alopecia · anticholinergic syndrome · appetite decreased · asthenia · asthma exacerbated · bone marrow depression · breast enlargement · cardiovascular effects · chills · confusion · constipation · diarrhoea · dizziness · drowsiness · dry mouth · dyspepsia · eosinophilia · face oedema · flushing · galactorrhoea · gynaecomastia · haemolytic anaemia · hallucination · headache · hyperhidrosis · hyperpyrexia · increased risk of fracture · jaundice · leucopenia · mania · movement disorders · nausea · oral ulceration · paranoid delusions · photosensitivity reaction · postural hypotension · psychosis · seizure · sensation abnormal · sexual dysfunction · SIADH · skin reactions · sleep disorders · suicidal behaviours · tachycardia · taste altered · testicular swelling · thrombocytopenia · tinnitus · tremor · urinary retention · vision blurred · vomiting · weight increased

SIDE-EFFECTS, FURTHER INFORMATION The risk of side-effects is reduced by titrating slowly to the minimum effective dose (every 2–3 days). Consider using a lower starting dose in elderly patients.

Overdose Tricyclic and related antidepressants cause dry mouth, coma of varying degree, hypotension, hypothermia, hyperreflexia, extensor plantar responses, convulsions, respiratory failure, cardiac conduction defects, and arrhythmias. Dilated pupils and urinary retention also occur. For details on the management of poisoning see Tricyclic and related antidepressants under Emergency treatment of poisoning p. 1554.

● PREGNANCY Use with caution—limited information available.

● BREAST FEEDING The amount secreted into breast milk is too small to be harmful. Accumulation of metabolite may cause sedation and respiratory depression in neonate.

● HEPATIC IMPAIRMENT Manufacturer advises caution in mild to moderate impairment; avoid in severe impairment.
Dose adjustments Manufacturer advises consider dose reduction in mild to moderate impairment.

● RENAL IMPAIRMENT [EvGr] Use with caution. ◈M◈
Dose adjustments [EvGr] Consider dose reduction. ◈M◈

● TREATMENT CESSATION Withdrawal effects may occur within 5 days of stopping treatment with antidepressant drugs; they are usually mild and self-limiting, but in some cases may be severe. The risk of withdrawal symptoms is increased if the antidepressant is stopped suddenly after regular administration for 8 weeks or more. The dose should preferably be reduced gradually over about 4 weeks, or longer if withdrawal symptoms emerge (6 months in patients who have been on long-term maintenance treatment). If possible tricyclic and related antidepressants should be withdrawn slowly.

● PRESCRIBING AND DISPENSING INFORMATION Limited quantities of tricyclic antidepressants should be prescribed at any one time because their cardiovascular and epileptogenic effects are dangerous in overdosage.

● PATIENT AND CARER ADVICE
Driving and skilled tasks Drowsiness may affect performance of skilled tasks (e.g. driving).
Effects of alcohol enhanced.

● MEDICINAL FORMS There can be variation in the licensing of different medicines containing the same drug. Forms available from special-order manufacturers include: oral suspension, oral solution

Oral capsule
CAUTIONARY AND ADVISORY LABELS 2
▶ Doxepin (Non-proprietary)
　Doxepin (as Doxepin hydrochloride) 10 mg Doxepin 10mg capsules
　| 28 capsule [PoM] £81.50-£146.70 DT = £81.50
　Doxepin (as Doxepin hydrochloride) 25 mg Doxepin 25mg capsules
　| 28 capsule [PoM] £97.00 DT = £30.16
　Doxepin (as Doxepin hydrochloride) 50 mg Doxepin 50mg capsules
　| 28 capsule [PoM] £154.00 DT = £34.38

Imipramine hydrochloride　　　10-Nov-2021

● **INDICATIONS AND DOSE**
Depressive illness
▶ BY MOUTH
▶ Adult: Initially up to 75 mg daily in divided doses, then increased to 150–200 mg daily, up to 150 mg may be given as a single dose at bedtime, dose to be increased gradually
▶ Elderly: Initially 10 mg daily, increased to 30–50 mg daily, dose to be increased gradually

Depressive illness in hospital patients
▶ BY MOUTH
▶ Adult: Initially up to 75 mg daily in divided doses, dose to be increased gradually, increased to up to 300 mg daily in divided doses

Nocturnal enuresis
▶ BY MOUTH
▶ Child 6-7 years: 25 mg once daily, to be taken at bedtime, initial period of treatment (including gradual withdrawal) 3 months—full physical examination before further course
▶ Child 8-10 years: 25–50 mg once daily, to be taken at bedtime, initial period of treatment (including gradual withdrawal) 3 months—full physical examination before further course
▶ Child 11-17 years: 50–75 mg once daily, to be taken at bedtime, initial period of treatment (including gradual withdrawal) 3 months—full physical examination before further course

● CONTRA-INDICATIONS Acute porphyrias p. 1202 · arrhythmia · during the manic phase of bipolar disorder · heart block · immediate recovery period after myocardial infarction

● CAUTIONS Cardiovascular disease · chronic constipation · diabetes · epilepsy · history of bipolar disorder · history of psychosis · hyperthyroidism (risk of arrhythmias) · increased intra-ocular pressure · patients with a significant risk of suicide · phaeochromocytoma (risk of arrhythmias) · prostatic hypertrophy (in adults) · susceptibility to angle-closure glaucoma · urinary retention

CAUTIONS, FURTHER INFORMATION [EvGr] Treatment should be stopped if the patient enters a manic phase. ◈M◈
　Elderly patients are particularly susceptible to many of the side-effects of tricyclic antidepressants; [EvGr] low initial doses should be used, with close monitoring, particularly for psychiatric and cardiac side-effects. ◈M◈

● INTERACTIONS → Appendix 1: tricyclic antidepressants

● SIDE-EFFECTS
▶ **Common or very common** Anxiety · appetite decreased · arrhythmias · asthenia · cardiac conduction disorders · confusion · delirium · depression · dizziness · drowsiness · epilepsy · hallucination · headache · hepatic disorders · hypotension · mood altered · nausea · palpitations · paraesthesia · sexual dysfunction · skin reactions · sleep disorder · tremor · vomiting · weight changes
▶ **Uncommon** Psychosis
▶ **Rare or very rare** Aggression · agranulocytosis · alopecia · bone marrow depression · enlarged mammary gland · eosinophilia · fever · galactorrhoea · gastrointestinal disorders · glaucoma · heart failure · interstitial lung disease · leucopenia · movement disorders · mydriasis · oedema · oral disorders · peripheral vasospastic reaction · photosensitivity reaction · SIADH · speech disorder · thrombocytopenia
▶ **Frequency not known** Anticholinergic syndrome · cardiovascular effects · drug fever · hyponatraemia · increased risk of fracture · neurological effects · paranoid delusions exacerbated · psychiatric disorder · suicidal

behaviours · tinnitus · urinary disorder · withdrawal syndrome

SIDE-EFFECTS, FURTHER INFORMATION The risk of side-effects is reduced by titrating slowly to the minimum effective dose (every 2–3 days). Consider using a lower starting dose in elderly patients.

Overdose Tricyclic and related antidepressants cause dry mouth, coma of varying degree, hypotension, hypothermia, hyperreflexia, extensor plantar responses, convulsions, respiratory failure, cardiac conduction defects, and arrhythmias. Dilated pupils and urinary retention also occur. For details on the management of poisoning see Tricyclic and related antidepressants under Emergency treatment of poisoning p. 1554.

● PREGNANCY Colic, tachycardia, dyspnoea, irritability, muscle spasms, respiratory depression and withdrawal symptoms reported in neonates when used in the third trimester.

● BREAST FEEDING The amount secreted into breast milk is too small to be harmful.

● HEPATIC IMPAIRMENT Manufacturer advises caution in mild to moderate impairment; avoid in severe impairment.

● RENAL IMPAIRMENT EvGr Caution in severe impairment. M

● TREATMENT CESSATION Withdrawal effects may occur within 5 days of stopping treatment with antidepressant drugs; they are usually mild and self-limiting, but in some cases may be severe. The risk of withdrawal symptoms is increased if the antidepressant is stopped suddenly after regular administration for 8 weeks or more. The dose should preferably be reduced gradually over about 4 weeks, or longer if withdrawal symptoms emerge (6 months in patients who have been on long-term maintenance treatment). If possible tricyclic antidepressants should be withdrawn slowly.

● PRESCRIBING AND DISPENSING INFORMATION Limited quantities of tricyclic antidepressants should be prescribed at any one time because their cardiovascular and epileptogenic effects are dangerous in overdosage.

● PATIENT AND CARER ADVICE
Medicines for Children leaflet: Imipramine for various conditions www.medicinesforchildren.org.uk/medicines/imipramine/
Driving and skilled tasks Drowsiness may affect the performance of skilled tasks (e.g. driving).
Effects of alcohol enhanced.

● MEDICINAL FORMS There can be variation in the licensing of different medicines containing the same drug. Forms available from special-order manufacturers include: oral suspension, oral solution

Oral tablet
CAUTIONARY AND ADVISORY LABELS 2
► Imipramine hydrochloride (Non-proprietary)
Imipramine hydrochloride 10 mg Imipramine 10mg tablets | 28 tablet PoM £5.20 DT = £1.19
Imipramine hydrochloride 25 mg Imipramine 25mg tablets | 28 tablet PoM £5.42 DT = £0.97
Oral solution
CAUTIONARY AND ADVISORY LABELS 2
► Imipramine hydrochloride (Non-proprietary)
Imipramine hydrochloride 5 mg per 1 ml Imipramine 25mg/5ml oral solution sugar free | 150 ml PoM £250.00 DT = £250.00 SF

Lofepramine

21-Apr-2021

● **INDICATIONS AND DOSE**

Depressive illness
► BY MOUTH
► Adult: 140–210 mg daily in divided doses
► Elderly: May respond to lower doses

● CONTRA-INDICATIONS Acute porphyrias p. 1202 · arrhythmias · during the manic phase of bipolar disorder · heart block · immediate recovery period after myocardial infarction

● CAUTIONS Cardiovascular disease · chronic constipation · diabetes · epilepsy · history of bipolar disorder · history of psychosis · hyperthyroidism (risk of arrhythmias) · increased intra-ocular pressure · patients with a significant risk of suicide · phaeochromocytoma (risk of arrhythmias) · prostatic hypertrophy · susceptibility to angle-closure glaucoma · urinary retention

CAUTIONS, FURTHER INFORMATION EvGr Treatment should be stopped if the patient enters a manic phase. M

Elderly patients are particularly susceptible to many of the side-effects of tricyclic antidepressants; EvGr low initial doses should be used, with close monitoring, particularly for psychiatric and cardiac side-effects M.

● INTERACTIONS → Appendix 1: tricyclic antidepressants

● SIDE-EFFECTS Accommodation disorder · agitation · agranulocytosis · arrhythmias · bone marrow disorders · cardiac conduction disorder · confusion · constipation · coordination abnormal · dizziness · drowsiness · dry mouth · eosinophilia · face oedema · galactorrhoea · glaucoma · granulocytopenia · gynaecomastia · hallucination · headache · heart failure aggravated · hepatic disorders · hyperhidrosis (on discontinuation) · hyponatraemia · hypotension · increased risk of fracture · leucopenia · malaise · mood altered · mucositis · nausea · paraesthesia · paranoid delusions · photosensitivity reaction · psychosis · respiratory depression · seizure · sexual dysfunction · SIADH · skin haemorrhage · skin reactions · sleep disorder · suicidal behaviours · taste altered · testicular disorders · thrombocytopenia · tinnitus · tremor · urinary disorders · vomiting · withdrawal syndrome

SIDE-EFFECTS, FURTHER INFORMATION The risk of side-effects is reduced by titrating slowly to the minimum effective dose (every 2–3 days). Consider using a lower starting dose in elderly patients.

Overdose Tricyclic and related antidepressants cause dry mouth, coma of varying degree, hypotension, hypothermia, hyperreflexia, extensor plantar responses, convulsions, respiratory failure, cardiac conduction defects, and arrhythmias. Dilated pupils and urinary retention also occur. Lofepramine is associated with the lowest risk of fatality in overdosage, in comparison with other tricyclic antidepressant drugs. For details on the management of poisoning see Tricyclic and related antidepressants under Emergency treatment of poisoning p. 1554.

● PREGNANCY Neonatal withdrawal symptoms and respiratory depression reported if used during third trimester.

● BREAST FEEDING The amount secreted into breast milk is too small to be harmful.

● HEPATIC IMPAIRMENT Manufacturer advises caution in mild to moderate impairment; avoid in severe impairment.

● RENAL IMPAIRMENT EvGr Use with caution in mild to moderate impairment; avoid in severe impairment. M

● TREATMENT CESSATION Withdrawal effects may occur within 5 days of stopping treatment with antidepressant drugs; they are usually mild and self-limiting, but in some cases may be severe. The risk of withdrawal symptoms is increased if the antidepressant is stopped suddenly after regular administration for 8 weeks or more. The dose should preferably be reduced gradually over about 4 weeks, or longer if withdrawal symptoms emerge (6 months in patients who have been on long-term maintenance treatment). If possible tricyclic and related antidepressants should be withdrawn slowly.

- **PRESCRIBING AND DISPENSING INFORMATION** Limited quantities of tricyclic antidepressants should be prescribed at any one time because their cardiovascular and epileptogenic effects are dangerous in overdosage.

- **PATIENT AND CARER ADVICE**
Driving and skilled tasks Drowsiness may affect the performance of skilled tasks (e.g. driving).
Effects of alcohol enhanced.

- **MEDICINAL FORMS** There can be variation in the licensing of different medicines containing the same drug. Forms available from special-order manufacturers include: oral suspension, oral solution

Oral tablet
CAUTIONARY AND ADVISORY LABELS 2
- ▸ Lofepramine (Non-proprietary)
  Lofepramine (as Lofepramine hydrochloride) 70 mg Lofepramine 70mg tablets | 56 tablet [PoM] £50.00 DT = £24.89

Oral suspension
CAUTIONARY AND ADVISORY LABELS 2
- ▸ Lofepramine (Non-proprietary)
  Lofepramine (as Lofepramine hydrochloride) 14 mg per 1 ml Lofepramine 70mg/5ml oral suspension sugar free | 150 ml [PoM] £140.07 DT = £140.07 [SF]

Nortriptyline

07-Nov-2020

- **INDICATIONS AND DOSE**

Depressive illness
- ▸ BY MOUTH
- ▸ Adult: To be initiated at a low dose, then increased if necessary to 75–100 mg daily in divided doses, alternatively increased if necessary to 75–100 mg once daily; maximum 150 mg per day
- ▸ Elderly: To be initiated at a low dose, then increased if necessary to 30–50 mg daily in divided doses

Neuropathic pain
- ▸ BY MOUTH
- ▸ Adult: Initially 10 mg once daily, to be taken at night, increased if necessary to 75 mg daily, dose to be increased gradually; higher doses to be given under specialist supervision

- **UNLICENSED USE** Not licensed for use in neuropathic pain.

- **CONTRA-INDICATIONS** Arrhythmias · during the manic phase of bipolar disorder · heart block · immediate recovery period after myocardial infarction

- **CAUTIONS** Cardiovascular disease · chronic constipation · diabetes · epilepsy · history of bipolar disorder · history of psychosis · hyperthyroidism (risk of arrhythmias) · increased intra-ocular pressure · patients with a significant risk of suicide · phaeochromocytoma (risk of arrhythmias) · prostatic hypertrophy · susceptibility to angle-closure glaucoma · urinary retention

  CAUTIONS, FURTHER INFORMATION [EvGr] Treatment should be stopped if the patient enters a manic phase. ⟨M⟩
  Elderly patients are particularly susceptible to many of the side-effects of tricyclic antidepressants; [EvGr] low initial doses should be used, with close monitoring, particularly for psychiatric and cardiac side-effects. ⟨M⟩

- **INTERACTIONS** → Appendix 1: tricyclic antidepressants

- **SIDE-EFFECTS** Agranulocytosis · alopecia · anxiety · appetite decreased · arrhythmias · asthenia · atrioventricular block · bone marrow disorders · breast enlargement · confusion · constipation · delusions · diarrhoea · dizziness · drowsiness · drug cross-reactivity · drug fever · dry mouth · eosinophilia · fever · flushing · galactorrhoea · gastrointestinal discomfort · gynaecomastia · hallucination · headache · hepatic disorders · hyperhidrosis · hypertension · hypomania · hypotension · increased risk of fracture · increased risk of

infection · malaise · movement disorders · mydriasis · myocardial infarction · nausea · oedema · oral disorders · palpitations · paralytic ileus · peripheral neuropathy · photosensitivity reaction · psychosis exacerbated · seizure · sensation abnormal · sexual dysfunction · SIADH · skin reactions · sleep disorders · stroke · suicidal behaviours · taste altered · testicular swelling · thrombocytopenia · tinnitus · tremor · urinary disorders · urinary tract dilation · vision disorders · vomiting · weight changes

SIDE-EFFECTS, FURTHER INFORMATION The risk of side-effects is reduced by titrating slowly to the minimum effective dose (every 2–3 days). Consider using a lower starting dose in elderly patients.

Overdose Tricyclic and related antidepressants cause dry mouth, coma of varying degree, hypotension, hypothermia, hyperreflexia, extensor plantar responses, convulsions, respiratory failure, cardiac conduction defects, and arrhythmias. Dilated pupils and urinary retention also occur. For details on the management of poisoning see Tricyclic and related antidepressants under Emergency treatment of poisoning p. 1554.

- **PREGNANCY** Use only if potential benefit outweighs risk.

- **BREAST FEEDING** The amount secreted into breast milk is too small to be harmful.

- **HEPATIC IMPAIRMENT** Manufacturer advises avoid in severe impairment.

- **MONITORING REQUIREMENTS**
- ▸ Manufacturer advises plasma-nortriptyline concentration monitoring if dose above 100 mg daily, but evidence of practical value uncertain.

- **TREATMENT CESSATION** Withdrawal effects may occur within 5 days of stopping treatment with antidepressant drugs; they are usually mild and self-limiting, but in some cases may be severe. The risk of withdrawal symptoms is increased if the antidepressant is stopped suddenly after regular administration for 8 weeks or more. The dose should preferably be reduced gradually over about 4 weeks, or longer if withdrawal symptoms emerge (6 months in patients who have been on long-term maintenance treatment). If possible tricyclic and related antidepressants should be withdrawn slowly.

- **PRESCRIBING AND DISPENSING INFORMATION** Limited quantities of tricyclic antidepressants should be prescribed at any one time because their cardiovascular and epileptogenic effects are dangerous in overdosage.

- **PATIENT AND CARER ADVICE** Drowsiness may affect the performance of skilled tasks (e.g. driving). Effects of alcohol enhanced.

- **MEDICINAL FORMS** There can be variation in the licensing of different medicines containing the same drug. Forms available from special-order manufacturers include: oral suspension, oral solution

Oral tablet
CAUTIONARY AND ADVISORY LABELS 2
- ▸ Nortriptyline (Non-proprietary)
  Nortriptyline (as Nortriptyline hydrochloride) 10 mg Nortriptyline 10mg tablets | 28 tablet [PoM] £2.14 | 84 tablet [PoM] £6.42 | 100 tablet [PoM] £33.41 DT = £4.03
  Nortriptyline (as Nortriptyline hydrochloride) 25 mg Nortriptyline 25mg tablets | 28 tablet [PoM] £2.46 | 30 tablet [PoM] £12.43 | 84 tablet [PoM] £7.38 | 100 tablet [PoM] £35.22 DT = £2.00
  Nortriptyline (as Nortriptyline hydrochloride) 50 mg Nortriptyline 50mg tablets | 30 tablet [PoM] £84.50 DT = £27.61

Trimipramine

15-Nov-2020

● INDICATIONS AND DOSE

Depressive illness (particularly where sedation required)
▸ BY MOUTH
▸ **Adult:** Initially 50–75 mg daily in divided doses, alternatively initially 50–75 mg once daily, dose to be taken at bedtime, increased if necessary to 150–300 mg daily
▸ **Elderly:** Initially 10–25 mg 3 times a day, maintenance 75–150 mg daily

● CONTRA-INDICATIONS Acute porphyrias p. 1202 · arrhythmias · during the manic phase of bipolar disorder · heart block · immediate recovery period after myocardial infarction

● CAUTIONS Cardiovascular disease · chronic constipation · diabetes · epilepsy · history of bipolar disorder · history of psychosis · hyperthyroidism (risk of arrhythmias) · increased intra-ocular pressure · patients with a significant risk of suicide · phaeochromocytoma (risk of arrhythmias) · prostatic hypertrophy · susceptibility to angle-closure glaucoma · urinary retention

CAUTIONS, FURTHER INFORMATION EvGr Treatment should be stopped if the patient enters a manic phase. Ⓜ
   Elderly patients are particularly susceptible to many of the side-effects of tricyclic antidepressants; EvGr low initial doses should be used, with close monitoring, particularly for psychiatric and cardiac side-effects. Ⓜ

● INTERACTIONS → Appendix 1: tricyclic antidepressants

● SIDE-EFFECTS Accommodation disorder · agitation · agranulocytosis · anticholinergic syndrome · arrhythmias · bone marrow depression · constipation · drowsiness · dry mouth · hyperglycaemia · hyperhidrosis · hypotension · increased risk of fracture · jaundice cholestatic · mood altered · paranoid delusions · peripheral neuropathy · rash · respiratory depression · seizure · sexual dysfunction · suicidal behaviours · tremor · urinary hesitation · withdrawal syndrome

SIDE-EFFECTS, FURTHER INFORMATION The risk of side-effects is reduced by titrating slowly to the minimum effective dose (every 2–3 days). Consider using a lower starting dose in elderly patients.

Overdose Tricyclic and related antidepressants cause dry mouth, coma of varying degree, hypotension, hypothermia, hyperreflexia, extensor plantar responses, convulsions, respiratory failure, cardiac conduction defects, and arrhythmias. Dilated pupils and urinary retention also occur. For details on the management of poisoning see Tricyclic and related antidepressants under Emergency treatment of poisoning p. 1554.

● PREGNANCY Use only if potential benefit outweighs risk.

● BREAST FEEDING The amount secreted into breast milk is too small to be harmful.

● HEPATIC IMPAIRMENT Manufacturer advises avoid in severe impairment.

● TREATMENT CESSATION Withdrawal effects may occur within 5 days of stopping treatment with antidepressant drugs; they are usually mild and self-limiting, but in some cases may be severe. The risk of withdrawal symptoms is increased if the antidepressant is stopped suddenly after regular administration for 8 weeks or more. The dose should preferably be reduced gradually over about 4 weeks, or longer if withdrawal symptoms emerge (6 months in patients who have been on long-term maintenance treatment). If possible tricyclic and related antidepressants should be withdrawn slowly.

● PRESCRIBING AND DISPENSING INFORMATION Limited quantities of tricyclic antidepressants should be prescribed at any one time because their cardiovascular and epileptogenic effects are dangerous in overdosage.

● PATIENT AND CARER ADVICE
Driving and skilled tasks Drowsiness may affect the performance of skilled tasks (e.g. driving).
   Effects of alcohol enhanced.

● MEDICINAL FORMS There can be variation in the licensing of different medicines containing the same drug. Forms available from special-order manufacturers include: oral suspension, oral solution

Oral tablet
CAUTIONARY AND ADVISORY LABELS 2
▸ **Trimipramine (Non-proprietary)**
   Trimipramine (as Trimipramine maleate) 10 mg Trimipramine 10mg tablets | 28 tablet PoM £197.18 DT = £197.18
   Trimipramine (as Trimipramine maleate) 25 mg Trimipramine 25mg tablets | 28 tablet PoM £205.44 DT = £205.44
Oral capsule
CAUTIONARY AND ADVISORY LABELS 2
▸ **Trimipramine (Non-proprietary)**
   Trimipramine (as Trimipramine maleate) 50 mg Trimipramine 50mg capsules | 28 capsule PoM £190.00 DT = £25.61

ANTIDEPRESSANTS ⟩ OTHER

Tryptophan

04-Oct-2017

(L-Tryptophan)

● DRUG ACTION Tryptophan is an essential dietary amino acid, and is a precursor of serotonin; it re-establishes the inhibitory action of serotonin on the amygdaloid nuclei, thereby reducing feelings of anxiety and depression.

● INDICATIONS AND DOSE

Treatment-resistant depression (used alone or as adjunct to other antidepressant drugs) (initiated under direction of hospital consultant)
▸ BY MOUTH
▸ **Adult:** 1 g 3 times a day; maximum 6 g per day

● CONTRA-INDICATIONS History of eosinophilia myalgia syndrome following use of tryptophan

● INTERACTIONS → Appendix 1: tryptophan

● SIDE-EFFECTS Asthenia · dizziness · drowsiness · eosinophilia myalgia syndrome · headache · myalgia · myopathy · nausea · oedema · suicidal behaviours

SIDE-EFFECTS, FURTHER INFORMATION If patients experience any symptoms of eosinophilia myalgia syndrome (EMS), manufacturer advises to withhold treatment until possibility of EMS is excluded.

● PREGNANCY Manufacturer advises caution—no information available.

● BREAST FEEDING Manufacturer advises avoid—no information available.

● MONITORING REQUIREMENTS Manufacturer advises close monitoring for signs of suicidal thoughts, particularly in patients at high risk and during early treatment and dose changes.

● PATIENT AND CARER ADVICE Manufacturer advises patients and carers should be advised to seek medical advice immediately if any clinical worsening, suicidal thoughts, or unusual behaviour develops.
Driving and skilled tasks Manufacturer advises patients should be counselled on the effects on driving and performance of skilled tasks—increased risk of drowsiness.

- **MEDICINAL FORMS** There can be variation in the licensing of different medicines containing the same drug. Forms available from special-order manufacturers include: oral capsule

Oral capsule
- ▶ **Optimax** (Esteve Pharmaceuticals Ltd)
  Tryptophan 500 mg Optimax 500mg capsules | 84 capsule [PoM] £45.82 DT = £45.82

Vortioxetine
22-Apr-2021

- **DRUG ACTION** Vortioxetine inhibits the re-uptake of serotonin (5-HT) and is an antagonist at 5-HT$_3$ and an agonist at 5-HT$_{1A}$ receptors. This multimodal activity appears to be associated with antidepressant and anxiolytic-like effects.

● INDICATIONS AND DOSE

Major depression
- ▶ BY MOUTH
- ▶ Adult: Initially 10 mg once daily; adjusted according to response to 5–20 mg once daily
- ▶ Elderly: Initially 5 mg once daily; increased if necessary up to 20 mg once daily

IMPORTANT SAFETY INFORMATION

MHRA/CHM ADVICE: SSRI/SNRI ANTIDEPRESSANT MEDICINES: SMALL INCREASED RISK OF POSTPARTUM HAEMORRHAGE WHEN USED IN THE MONTH BEFORE DELIVERY (JANUARY 2021)

Selective serotonin re-uptake inhibitors (SSRIs) and serotonin and noradrenaline re-uptake inhibitors (SNRIs) are known to increase the risk of bleeding due to their effect on platelet function. Observational data suggest that the use of SSRIs and SNRIs in the last month before delivery may increase the risk of postpartum haemorrhage. This risk might also apply to vortioxetine. Healthcare professionals should continue to consider the benefits and risks of antidepressant use during pregnancy, and the risks of untreated depression in pregnancy.

Healthcare professionals should also consider this finding in the context of individual patient risk factors for bleeding or thrombotic events. Anticoagulant medication in women at high risk of thrombotic events should not be stopped but healthcare professionals should be aware of the risk identified.

- **CAUTIONS** Bleeding disorders · cirrhosis of the liver (risk of hyponatraemia) · elderly (risk of hyponatraemia) · history of mania (discontinue if patient entering manic phase) · history of seizures · susceptibility to angle-closure glaucoma · unstable epilepsy

  CAUTIONS, FURTHER INFORMATION
- ▶ **Seizures** Manufacturer advises discontinue treatment in patients who develop seizures or if there is an increase in seizure frequency.
- ▶ **Elderly** Manufacturer advises caution when treating elderly patients with doses over 10 mg daily—limited information.
- **INTERACTIONS** → Appendix 1: vortioxetine
- **SIDE-EFFECTS**
- ▶ **Common or very common** Abnormal dreams · constipation · diarrhoea · dizziness · nausea · skin reactions · vomiting
- ▶ **Uncommon** Flushing · night sweats
- ▶ **Frequency not known** Angioedema · haemorrhage · hyponatraemia · neuroleptic malignant syndrome (discontinue immediately) · serotonin syndrome (discontinue immediately)
- **PREGNANCY** Manufacturer advises avoid unless potential benefit outweighs risk—toxicity in *animal* studies. If used during the later stages of pregnancy, there is a risk of neonatal withdrawal symptoms and persistent pulmonary hypertension in the newborn.

- **BREAST FEEDING** Manufacturer advises avoid—present in milk in *animal* studies.
- **HEPATIC IMPAIRMENT** Manufacturer advises caution in severe impairment (no information available).
- **RENAL IMPAIRMENT** [EvGr] Use with caution (limited information available). ⓜ
- **TREATMENT CESSATION** Manufacturer advises treatment can be stopped abruptly, without need for gradual dose reduction.
- **PATIENT AND CARER ADVICE**
  Driving and skilled tasks Manufacturer advises patients and carers should be counselled on the effects on driving and performance of skilled tasks, especially when starting treatment or changing the dose.
- **NATIONAL FUNDING/ACCESS DECISIONS**
  For full details see funding body website
  NICE decisions
- ▶ **Vortioxetine for treating major depressive episodes (November 2015)** NICE TA367 Recommended with restrictions

- **MEDICINAL FORMS** There can be variation in the licensing of different medicines containing the same drug.
  Oral tablet
- ▶ **Brintellix** (Lundbeck Ltd)
  Vortioxetine (as Vortioxetine hydrobromide) 5 mg Brintellix 5mg tablets | 28 tablet [PoM] £27.72 DT = £27.72
  Vortioxetine (as Vortioxetine hydrobromide) 10 mg Brintellix 10mg tablets | 28 tablet [PoM] £27.72 DT = £27.72
  Vortioxetine (as Vortioxetine hydrobromide) 20 mg Brintellix 20mg tablets | 28 tablet [PoM] £27.72 DT = £27.72

3.5 Inappropriate sexual behaviour

ANTIPSYCHOTICS ⟩ FIRST-GENERATION

▶ 442

Benperidol
21-Oct-2021

- **● INDICATIONS AND DOSE**

  Control of deviant antisocial sexual behaviour
- ▶ BY MOUTH
- ▶ Adult: 0.25–1.5 mg daily in divided doses, adjusted according to response, for debilitated patients, use elderly dose
- ▶ Elderly: Initially 0.125–0.75 mg daily in divided doses, adjusted according to response

- **CONTRA-INDICATIONS** CNS depression · comatose states · phaeochromocytoma
- **CAUTIONS** Risk factors for stroke
- **INTERACTIONS** → Appendix 1: benperidol
- **SIDE-EFFECTS** Appetite decreased · blood disorder · cardiac arrest · depression · dyspepsia · embolism and thrombosis · headache · hepatic disorders · hyperhidrosis · hypertension · nausea · oculogyric crisis · oedema · oligomenorrhoea · paradoxical drug reaction · pruritus · psychiatric disorder · temperature regulation disorders · weight change
- **PREGNANCY** Extrapyramidal effects and withdrawal syndrome have been reported occasionally in the neonate when antipsychotic drugs are taken during the third trimester of pregnancy. Following maternal use of antipsychotic drugs in the third trimester, neonates should be monitored for symptoms including agitation, hypertonia, hypotonia, tremor, drowsiness, feeding problems, and respiratory distress.
- **BREAST FEEDING** There is limited information available on the short- and long-term effects of antipsychotic drugs on the breast-fed infant. *Animal* studies indicate possible

adverse effects of antipsychotic medicines on the developing nervous system. Chronic treatment with antipsychotic drugs whilst breast-feeding should be avoided unless absolutely necessary.

- **HEPATIC IMPAIRMENT** Manufacturer advises caution.
- **RENAL IMPAIRMENT** EvGr Caution in renal failure. M
- **MONITORING REQUIREMENTS** Manufacturer advises regular blood counts and liver function tests during long-term treatment.
- **PRESCRIBING AND DISPENSING INFORMATION** The proprietary name *Benquil*® has been used for benperidol tablets.
- **MEDICINAL FORMS** There can be variation in the licensing of different medicines containing the same drug. Forms available from special-order manufacturers include: oral suspension

Oral tablet

CAUTIONARY AND ADVISORY LABELS 2

▸ Anquil (Neon Healthcare Ltd)
  Benperidol 250 microgram Anquil 250microgram tablets |
  112 tablet PoM £200.32

3.6 Psychoses and schizophrenia

Psychoses and related disorders

15-Feb-2021

Overview

Antipsychotic drugs, formerly called 'major tranquillisers', are also known as neuroleptics. They have varying effects and properties; these include sedative, anxiolytic, antimanic, mood stabilising, and antidepressant properties. Antipsychotic drugs are used for a number of mental health disorders, mainly schizophrenia and bipolar disorder (sometimes called manic depression), but may also be used in severe or difficult to treat anxiety or depression.

Schizophrenia

Schizophrenia is the most common psychotic disorder. The symptoms of psychosis and schizophrenia are usually divided into 'positive symptoms' such as hallucinations and delusions, and 'negative symptoms' such as emotional apathy and social withdrawal. Each patient will have a unique combination of symptoms and experiences. Typically, patients experience a prodromal period characterised by some deterioration in personal functioning and emergence of negative symptoms. This is followed by an acute phase marked by positive symptoms, which may resolve or reduce following treatment, but in some cases negative symptoms can remain and interfere with daily functioning.

The initial aim of treatment is to reduce acute phase symptoms and return the patient to their baseline level of functioning. Many patients who have one episode of schizophrenia will go on to have further episodes and generally require maintenance treatment with antipsychotic drugs to prevent relapses.

Antipsychotic drugs are effective in the treatment of acute schizophrenic episodes; they are more effective at alleviating positive symptoms than negative symptoms.

EvGr An oral antipsychotic drug in combination with psychological therapy should be offered to patients with schizophrenia. The choice of drug depends on factors such as the potential to cause extrapyramidal symptoms (including akathisia), cardiovascular adverse effects, metabolic adverse effects (including weight gain and diabetes), hormonal adverse effects (including increase in prolactin concentration), and patient and carer preference. Treatment with an antipsychotic drug should be considered an explicit individual therapeutic trial; doses should be started low and slowly titrated up to the minimum effective dose according to patient response and tolerability. Patients should receive an antipsychotic drug at an optimum dose for 4–6 weeks before it is deemed ineffective. A

Prescribing more than one antipsychotic drug at a time should be avoided except in exceptional circumstances (e.g. clozapine p. 457 augmentation or when changing medication during titration) because of the increased risk of adverse effects such as extrapyramidal symptoms, QT-interval prolongation, and sudden cardiac death. EvGr It is important to record the reasons for continuing, changing, and stopping treatment, and the effects of such changes, including side-effects experienced.

Clozapine should be offered if schizophrenia is not controlled despite the sequential use of at least 2 different antipsychotic drugs (one of which should be a second-generation antipsychotic drug), each for an adequate duration. If symptoms do not respond adequately to an optimised dose of clozapine, consider other causes of non-response (e.g. adherence to therapy, concurrent use of other drugs), review diagnosis, and check plasma-clozapine concentration before adding a second antipsychotic drug to augment clozapine; allow 8–10 weeks' treatment to assess response. A EvGr Patients must be registered with a clozapine patient monitoring service. M

EvGr Long-acting depot injectable antipsychotic drugs can be considered for patients with psychosis and schizophrenia where it is a clinical priority to avoid non-adherence. A

Antipsychotic drugs

First-generation antipsychotic drugs

The first-generation antipsychotic drugs (also known as typical or conventional) act predominantly by blocking dopamine D_2 receptors in the brain. They are more likely to cause a range of side-effects, particularly acute extrapyramidal symptoms and hyperprolactinaemia.

First-generation antipsychotics include the **phenothiazine** derivatives (chlorpromazine hydrochloride p. 443, fluphenazine decanoate, levomepromazine p. 502, pericyazine p. 447, prochlorperazine p. 448, promazine hydrochloride p. 468, and trifluoperazine p. 450), the **butyrophenones** (benperidol p. 439 and haloperidol p. 445), the **thioxanthenes** (flupentixol p. 444 and zuclopenthixol p. 450), the **diphenylbutylpiperidines** (pimozide p. 448) and the **substituted benzamides** (sulpiride p. 449).

Second-generation antipsychotic drugs

The second-generation antipsychotic drugs (also referred to as atypical) act on a range of receptors in comparison to first-generation antipsychotic drugs and are generally associated with a lower risk for acute extrapyramidal symptoms and tardive dyskinesia; the extent varies between individual drugs. However, second-generation antipsychotic drugs are associated with several other important adverse effects, such as weight gain and glucose intolerance.

Second-generation antipsychotics include amisulpride p. 453, aripiprazole p. 454, asenapine p. 413, cariprazine p. 456, clozapine, lurasidone hydrochloride p. 458, olanzapine p. 459, paliperidone p. 461, quetiapine p. 462, and risperidone p. 464.

Prescribing high-dose antipsychotic drugs

A *high-dose* antipsychotic is defined as a total daily dose of a single antipsychotic drug which exceeds the maximum licensed dose with respect to the age of the patient and the indication being treated, and a total daily dose of two or more antipsychotic drugs which exceeds the maximum licensed dose using the percentage method.

For further information and advice on prescribing high-dose antipsychotic medication, see The Royal College of Psychiatrists consensus statement available at www.rcpsych.ac.uk/.

There is no robust evidence that high doses of antipsychotic drug treatment is any more effective than standard doses for the treatment of schizophrenia. The majority of adverse effects associated with antipsychotic treatment are dose-related and there is clear evidence for a greater side-effect burden with high-dose antipsychotic drug use. Antipsychotic polypharmacy and 'when required' antipsychotic drug treatment are strongly associated with high-dose prescribing.

Important: When prescribing an antipsychotic drug for administration in an emergency situation (e.g. for rapid tranquillisation), the aim of treatment is to calm and sedate the patient without inducing sleep. EvGr The initial prescription should be written as a single dose, and not repeated until the effects of the initial dose has been reviewed. Oral and intramuscular drugs should be prescribed separately. The patient must be monitored for side-effects and vital signs at least every hour until there are no further concerns about their physical health status. Monitor the patient every 15 minutes if a high-dose antipsychotic drug has been given. A

Prescribing for the elderly

EvGr The balance of risk and benefit should be considered and discussed with the patient or carers before prescribing antipsychotic drugs for elderly patients. A In elderly patients with dementia, the use of antipsychotic drugs are associated with a small increased risk of mortality and an increased risk of stroke or transient ischaemic attack (see Dementia p. 343). Furthermore, elderly patients are particularly susceptible to postural hypotension.

It is recommended that:

- EvGr Antipsychotic drugs should not be used in elderly patients with dementia, unless they are at risk of harming themselves or others, or experiencing agitation, hallucinations or delusions that are causing them severe distress.
- The lowest effective dose should be used for the shortest period of time.
- Treatment should be reviewed regularly; at least every 6 weeks (earlier for in-patients). A

Prescribing of antipsychotic drugs in patients with learning disabilities

EvGr In patients with learning disabilities who are taking antipsychotic drugs and not experiencing psychotic symptoms, the following considerations should be taken into account:

- a reduction in dose or the discontinuation of long-term antipsychotic treatment;
- review of the patient's condition after dose reduction or discontinuation of an antipsychotic drug;
- referral to a psychiatrist experienced in working with patients who have learning disabilities and mental health problems;
- annual documentation of the reasons for continuing a prescription if the antipsychotic drug is not reduced in dose or discontinued. A

Side-effects and choice of antipsychotic drug

There is little difference in efficacy between each of the antipsychotic drugs (other than clozapine p. 457), and response and tolerability to each antipsychotic drug varies. EvGr There is no first-line antipsychotic drug that is suitable for all patients and the properties of individual antipsychotic drugs should be considered and discussed with the patient or carers when prescribing. A

Both first-generation and second-generation antipsychotic drugs are associated with side-effects that are common and contribute significantly to non-adherence and treatment discontinuation.

Extrapyramidal symptoms

Extrapyramidal symptoms are dose-related and are most likely to occur with high doses of high-potency first-generation antipsychotic drugs such as the piperazine phenothiazines (fluphenazine decanoate and trifluoperazine p. 450), the butyrophenones (benperidol p. 439 and haloperidol p. 445), and the first-generation depot preparations. They are less common with some second-generation antipsychotics which have a lower liability for both acute and late onset extrapyramidal symptoms; particularly clozapine, olanzapine p. 459, quetiapine p. 462, and aripiprazole p. 454. Extrapyramidal symptoms cannot be predicted accurately because they depend on the dose, the class of antipsychotic drug, and on individual susceptibility.

Extrapyramidal symptoms consist of:

- *parkinsonian symptoms* (including bradykinesia, tremor), which may occur more commonly in elderly females or those with pre-existing neurological damage such as stroke, and may appear gradually;
- *dystonia* (uncontrolled muscle spasm in any part of the body), which occurs more commonly in young males; acute dystonia can appear within hours of starting antipsychotics;
- *akathisia* (restlessness), which characteristically occurs within hours to weeks of starting antipsychotic treatment or on dose increase and may be mistaken for psychotic agitation;
- *tardive dyskinesia* (abnormal involuntary movements of lips, tongue, face, and jaw), which can develop on long-term or high-dose therapy, or even after discontinuation; in some patients it can be irreversible.

EvGr When *parkinsonian* symptoms are identified, treatment should be reviewed with the aim of reducing exposure to high-dose and high-potency antipsychotic drugs. Although antimuscarinic drugs can relieve symptom burden, they should not be routinely prescribed for prophylaxis with antipsychotic drugs. A

Tardive dyskinesia is the most serious manifestation of late-onset extrapyramidal symptoms for which there is no satisfactory treatment; it occurs more commonly in elderly females. EvGr Antipsychotic treatment should be carefully and regularly reviewed; any changes to dose or drug should be made gradually, over weeks or months, to minimise the risk of withdrawal tardive dyskinesia. A However, some manufacturers suggest that drug withdrawal at the earliest signs of tardive dyskinesia (fine vermicular movements of the tongue) may halt its full development.

Hyperprolactinaemia

Most antipsychotic drugs, both first- and second-generation, increase prolactin concentration to some extent because dopamine inhibits prolactin release. Aripiprazole reduces prolactin concentration in a dose-dependent manner because it is a dopamine-receptor partial agonist. Risperidone p. 464, amisulpride p. 453, sulpiride p. 449, and first-generation antipsychotic drugs are most likely to cause symptomatic hyperprolactinaemia. Hyperprolactinaemia is very rare with aripiprazole, asenapine p. 413, cariprazine p. 456, clozapine, and quetiapine treatment.

The clinical symptoms of hyperprolactinaemia include sexual dysfunction, reduced bone mineral density, menstrual disturbances, breast enlargement, galactorrhoea, and a possible increased risk of breast cancer.

Sexual dysfunction

Sexual dysfunction is reported as a side-effect of all antipsychotic medication; physical illness, psychiatric illness, and substance misuse are contributing factors. Antipsychotic-induced sexual dysfunction is caused by more than one mechanism. Reduced dopamine transmission and hyperprolactinaemia decrease libido; antimuscarinic effects can cause disorders of arousal; and alpha$_1$-adrenoceptor antagonists are associated with erection and ejaculation problems in men. Risperidone, haloperidol, and olanzapine have a higher prevalence to cause sexual dysfunction. The antipsychotic drugs with the lowest risk of sexual dysfunction are aripiprazole and quetiapine.

Expert sources advise to consider dose reduction or discontinuation (where appropriate), or switching medication if sexual dysfunction is thought to be antipsychotic-induced.

Cardiovascular side-effects

Antipsychotic drugs are associated with cardiovascular side-effects such as tachycardia, arrhythmias, and hypotension. QT-interval prolongation is a particular concern with pimozide p. 448. Overall risk is probably dose-related but there is also a higher probability of QT-interval prolongation in patients using any intravenous antipsychotic drug, or any antipsychotic drug or combination of antipsychotic drugs with doses exceeding the recommended maximum.

Antipsychotic drugs with a low tendency to prolong QT interval include aripiprazole, asenapine p. 413, clozapine, flupentixol p. 444, fluphenazine decanoate, loxapine p. 447, olanzapine, paliperidone p. 461, prochlorperazine p. 448, risperidone, and sulpiride.

Hypotension

Postural hypotension is a common cardiac side-effect of antipsychotic drugs, usually presenting acutely during the initial dose titration; however, it can also be a chronic problem. Postural hypotension can lead to syncope and dangerous falls related injuries, especially in the elderly. The second-generation antipsychotics most likely to cause postural hypotension are clozapine and quetiapine. Slow dose titration is commonly used to minimise postural hypotension.

Hyperglycaemia and diabetes

Schizophrenia is associated with insulin resistance and diabetes; the risk of diabetes is probably increased in all patients with schizophrenia who take antipsychotic drugs. Some evidence suggests first-generation antipsychotic drugs are less likely to cause diabetes than second-generation antipsychotic drugs, and of the first-generation antipsychotic drugs, fluphenazine decanoate and haloperidol have the lowest risk. Amisulpride and aripiprazole have the lowest risk of diabetes of the second-generation antipsychotic drugs.

Weight gain

All antipsychotic drugs may cause weight gain, but the risk and extent varies. Clozapine and olanzapine commonly cause weight gain. Amisulpride, asenapine p. 413, aripiprazole, cariprazine p. 456, haloperidol, lurasidone hydrochloride p. 458, sulpiride, and trifluoperazine are least likely to cause weight gain.

Neuroleptic malignant syndrome

Neuroleptic malignant syndrome (hyperthermia, fluctuating level of consciousness, muscle rigidity, and autonomic dysfunction with fever, tachycardia, labile blood pressure, and sweating) is a rare but potentially fatal side-effect of all antipsychotic drugs.

Expert sources advise discontinuation of the antipsychotic drug is essential for at least 5 days, preferably longer. The signs and symptoms of neuroleptic malignant syndrome should be allowed to resolve completely. Bromocriptine and dantrolene have been used for treatment.

Monitoring

[EvGr] Weight should be measured at the start of therapy with antipsychotic drugs, then weekly for the first 6 weeks, then at 12 weeks, at 1 year, and then yearly.

Fasting blood glucose, HbA$_{1c}$, and blood lipid concentrations should be measured at baseline, at 12 weeks, at 1 year, and then yearly. Prolactin concentrations should also be measured at baseline.

Before initiating antipsychotic drugs, an ECG may be required, particularly if physical examination identifies cardiovascular risk factors (e.g. high blood pressure), if there is a personal history of cardiovascular disease, or if the patient is being admitted as an inpatient.

Blood pressure monitoring is advised before starting therapy, at 12 weeks, at 1 year and then yearly during treatment and dose titration of antipsychotic drugs. (A)

Expert sources advise to monitor full blood count, urea and electrolytes, and liver function tests at the start of therapy with antipsychotic drugs, and then yearly thereafter.

MHRA/CHM advice: Clozapine and other antipsychotics

The MHRA/CHM have released important safety information regarding antipsychotics and monitoring blood concentrations for toxicity. For further information, see *Important safety information* in the amisulpride p. 453, aripiprazole p. 454, clozapine p. 457, olanzapine p. 459, olanzapine embonate p. 466, quetiapine p. 462, risperidone p. 464, and sulpiride p. 449 monographs.

Antipsychotic depot injections

[EvGr] Long-acting depot injections can be considered for patients with psychosis or schizophrenia who prefer such treatment after an acute episode or where avoiding non-adherence to antipsychotic medication is a clinical priority.
(A) First-generation antipsychotic depot injections may give rise to a higher incidence of adverse-effects such as extrapyramidal reactions. Extrapyramidal reactions occur less frequently with second-generation antipsychotic depot preparations, such as aripiprazole, paliperidone p. 461, risperidone and olanzapine embonate.

There are very few differences in efficacy between individual first-generation antipsychotic depot injections; zuclopenthixol decanoate p. 453 may be more effective in preventing relapses than other first-generation antipsychotic depot preparations.

Individual responses to antipsychotic drugs are variable. Expert sources advise in order to achieve optimum effect, dosage and dosage interval must be titrated according to the patient's response.

ANTIPSYCHOTICS

Antipsychotic drugs

- **CAUTIONS** Blood dyscrasias · cardiovascular disease · conditions predisposing to seizures · depression · diabetes (may raise blood glucose) · epilepsy · history of jaundice · myasthenia gravis · Parkinson's disease (may be exacerbated) (in adults) · photosensitisation (may occur with higher dosages) · prostatic hypertrophy (in adults) · severe respiratory disease · susceptibility to angle-closure glaucoma

CAUTIONS, FURTHER INFORMATION

- ▸ Cardiovascular disease An ECG may be required, particularly if physical examination identifies cardiovascular risk factors, personal history of cardiovascular disease, or if the patient is being admitted as an inpatient.
- ▸ Elderly Screening Tool of Older Persons' potentially inappropriate Prescriptions (STOPP) criteria to aid medication reviews (see Prescribing in the elderly p. 31 for information). Potentially inappropriate:
  - for all antipsychotics (other than quetiapine and clozapine) in patients with parkinsonism or Lewy Body Disease (risk of severe extrapyramidal symptoms)
  - in behavioural and psychological symptoms of dementia (BPSD), unless symptoms are severe and other non-pharmacological treatments have failed (increased risk of stroke)
  - for use as a hypnotic, unless sleep disorder is due to psychosis or dementia (risk of confusion, hypotension, extrapyramidal side-effects, and falls)
  - in patients prone to falls (may cause gait dyspraxia, parkinsonism)

- if prescribed a **phenothiazine** (other than prochlorperazine for nausea, vomiting, or vertigo; chlorpromazine for relief of persistent hiccups; levomepromazine as an antiemetic in palliative care) as first-line treatment (sedative, significant antimuscarinic (anticholinergic) toxicity in older people, and safer and more efficacious alternatives exist)
- if prescribed an antipsychotic drug with **moderate or marked antimuscarinic effects** (e.g. chlorpromazine, clozapine, flupentixol, fluphenazine, pipothiazine, promazine, and zuclopenthixol) in patients with a history of prostatism or urinary retention (high risk of urinary retention)

- **SIDE-EFFECTS**
▶ **Common or very common** Agitation · amenorrhoea · arrhythmias · constipation · dizziness · drowsiness · dry mouth · erectile dysfunction · fatigue · galactorrhoea · gynaecomastia · hyperglycaemia · hyperprolactinaemia · hypersalivation · hypotension (dose-related) · insomnia · leucopenia · movement disorders · muscle rigidity · neutropenia · parkinsonism · postural hypotension (dose-related) · QT interval prolongation · rash · seizure · tremor · urinary retention · vomiting · weight increased
▶ **Uncommon** Agranulocytosis · confusion · neuroleptic malignant syndrome (discontinue—potentially fatal)
▶ **Rare or very rare** Sudden death · withdrawal syndrome neonatal

SIDE-EFFECTS, FURTHER INFORMATION For depot antipsychotics—side-effects may persist until the drug has been cleared from its depot site.

Overdose Phenothiazines cause less depression of consciousness and respiration than other sedatives. Hypotension, hypothermia, sinus tachycardia, and arrhythmias may complicate poisoning. For details on the management of poisoning see Antipsychotics under Emergency treatment of poisoning p. 1554.

- **PREGNANCY** Extrapyramidal effects and withdrawal syndrome have been reported occasionally in the neonate when antipsychotic drugs are taken during the third trimester of pregnancy. Following maternal use of antipsychotic drugs in the third trimester, neonates should be monitored for symptoms including agitation, hypertonia, hypotonia, tremor, drowsiness, feeding problems, and respiratory distress.

- **BREAST FEEDING** There is limited information available on the short- and long-term effects of antipsychotic drugs on the breast-fed infant. *Animal studies* indicate possible adverse effects of antipsychotic medicines on the developing nervous system. Chronic treatment with antipsychotic drugs whilst breast-feeding should be avoided unless absolutely necessary. Phenothiazine derivatives are sometimes used in breast-feeding women for short-term treatment of nausea and vomiting.

- **MONITORING REQUIREMENTS**
▶ It is advisable to monitor prolactin concentration at the start of therapy, at 6 months, and then yearly. Patients taking antipsychotic drugs not normally associated with symptomatic hyperprolactinaemia should be considered for prolactin monitoring if they show symptoms of hyperprolactinaemia (such as breast enlargement and galactorrhoea).
▶ Patients with schizophrenia should have physical health monitoring (including cardiovascular disease risk assessment) at least once per year.
▶ In children Regular clinical monitoring of endocrine function should be considered when children are taking an antipsychotic drug known to increase prolactin levels; this includes measuring weight and height, assessing sexual maturation, and monitoring menstrual function.

- **TREATMENT CESSATION** There is a high risk of relapse if medication is stopped after 1–2 years. Withdrawal of antipsychotic drugs after long-term therapy should always be gradual and closely monitored to avoid the risk of acute withdrawal syndromes or rapid relapse. Patients should be monitored for 2 years after withdrawal of antipsychotic medication for signs and symptoms of relapse.

- **PRESCRIBING AND DISPENSING INFORMATION** Patient decision aid Antipsychotic medicines for treating agitation, aggression and distress in people living with dementia. National Institute for Health and Care Excellence. June 2018. www.nice.org.uk/about/what-we-do/our-programmes/nice-guidance/nice-guidelines/shared-decision-making

- **PATIENT AND CARER ADVICE** As photosensitisation may occur with higher dosages, patients should avoid direct sunlight.
Driving and skilled tasks Drowsiness may affect performance of skilled tasks (e.g. driving or operating machinery), especially at start of treatment; effects of alcohol are enhanced.

ANTIPSYCHOTICS > FIRST-GENERATION

◀ 442

Chlorpromazine hydrochloride   27-Jun-2023

- **INDICATIONS AND DOSE**

Schizophrenia and other psychoses | Mania | Short-term adjunctive management of severe anxiety | Psychomotor agitation, excitement, and violent or dangerously impulsive behaviour
▶ BY MOUTH
▶ Adult: Initially 25 mg 3 times a day, adjusted according to response, alternatively initially 75 mg once daily, adjusted according to response, dose to be taken at night; maintenance 75–300 mg daily, increased if necessary up to 1 g daily, this dose may be required in psychoses; use a third to half adult dose in the elderly or debilitated patients
▶ BY RECTUM
▶ Adult: 100 mg every 6–8 hours, dose expressed as chlorpromazine base

Intractable hiccup
▶ BY MOUTH
▶ Adult: 25–50 mg 3–4 times a day

Relief of acute symptoms of psychoses (under expert supervision)
▶ BY DEEP INTRAMUSCULAR INJECTION
▶ Adult: 25–50 mg every 6–8 hours

Nausea and vomiting in palliative care (where other drugs have failed or are not available)
▶ BY MOUTH
▶ Child 1–5 years: 500 micrograms/kg every 4–6 hours; maximum 40 mg per day
▶ Child 6–11 years: 500 micrograms/kg every 4–6 hours; maximum 75 mg per day
▶ Child 12–17 years: 10–25 mg every 4–6 hours
▶ Adult: 10–25 mg every 4–6 hours
▶ BY DEEP INTRAMUSCULAR INJECTION
▶ Child 1–5 years: 500 micrograms/kg every 6–8 hours; maximum 40 mg per day
▶ Child 6–11 years: 500 micrograms/kg every 6–8 hours; maximum 75 mg per day
▶ Child 12–17 years: Initially 25 mg, then 25–50 mg every 3–4 hours until vomiting stops
▶ Adult: Initially 25 mg, then 25–50 mg every 3–4 hours until vomiting stops
▶ BY RECTUM
▶ Adult: 100 mg every 6–8 hours

DOSE EQUIVALENCE AND CONVERSION
▶ For equivalent therapeutic effect 100 mg chlorpromazine base given *rectally* as a   continued →

suppository ≡ 20–25 mg chlorpromazine hydrochloride *by intramuscular injection* ≡ 40–50 mg of chlorpromazine base or hydrochloride given *by mouth*.

- **UNLICENSED USE** Rectal route is not licensed.
- **CONTRA-INDICATIONS** CNS depression · comatose states · hypothyroidism · phaeochromocytoma
- **CAUTIONS** Susceptibility to QT interval prolongation
- **INTERACTIONS** → Appendix 1: phenothiazines
- **SIDE-EFFECTS**
  GENERAL SIDE-EFFECTS
  ▸ **Common or very common** Anxiety · glucose tolerance impaired · mood altered · muscle tone increased
  ▸ **Frequency not known** Accommodation disorder · angioedema · atrioventricular block · cardiac arrest · embolism and thrombosis · eye deposit · eye disorders · gastrointestinal disorders · hepatic disorders · hypertriglyceridaemia · hyponatraemia · photosensitivity reaction · respiratory disorders · sexual dysfunction · SIADH · skin reactions · systemic lupus erythematosus (SLE) · temperature regulation disorder · trismus
  SPECIFIC SIDE-EFFECTS
  ▸ With intramuscular use Nasal congestion
  SIDE-EFFECTS, FURTHER INFORMATION Acute dystonic reactions may occur; children are particularly susceptible.
- **HEPATIC IMPAIRMENT** Manufacturer advises caution in severe hepatic failure (increased risk of accumulation).
- **RENAL IMPAIRMENT** EvGr Caution in severe renal failure (risk of accumulation). (M)
- **MONITORING REQUIREMENTS**
  ▸ With intramuscular use Patients should remain supine, with blood pressure monitoring for 30 minutes after intramuscular injection.
- **PRESCRIBING AND DISPENSING INFORMATION**
  Palliative care For further information on the use of chlorpromazine hydrochloride in palliative care, see www.medicinescomplete.com/#/content/palliative/antipsychotics.
- **HANDLING AND STORAGE** Owing to the risk of contact sensitisation, pharmacists, nurses, and other health workers should avoid direct contact with chlorpromazine; tablets should not be crushed and solutions should be handled with care.

- **MEDICINAL FORMS** There can be variation in the licensing of different medicines containing the same drug. Forms available from special-order manufacturers include: oral capsule, oral suspension, oral solution, suppository

Oral tablet
CAUTIONARY AND ADVISORY LABELS 2, 11
  ▸ **Chlorpromazine hydrochloride (Non-proprietary)**
  Chlorpromazine hydrochloride 10 mg Chlorpromazine 10mg tablets | 28 tablet PoM £10.85–£18.98 DT = £10.85
  Chlorpromazine hydrochloride 25 mg Chlorpromazine 25mg tablets | 28 tablet PoM £37.13 DT = £20.79
  Chlorpromazine hydrochloride 50 mg Chlorpromazine 50mg tablets | 28 tablet PoM £37.50 DT = £20.75
  Chlorpromazine hydrochloride 100 mg Chlorpromazine 100mg tablets | 28 tablet PoM £39.99 DT = £36.90

Suppository
CAUTIONARY AND ADVISORY LABELS 2, 11

Oral solution
CAUTIONARY AND ADVISORY LABELS 2, 11
  ▸ **Chlorpromazine hydrochloride (Non-proprietary)**
  Chlorpromazine hydrochloride 5 mg per 1 ml Chlorpromazine 25mg/5ml syrup | 150 ml PoM £6.00 DT = £6.00
  Chlorpromazine 25mg/5ml oral solution sugar free | 150 ml PoM £6.80 DT = £7.02 SF
  Chlorpromazine 25mg/5ml oral solution | 150 ml PoM £6.00 DT = £6.00
  Chlorpromazine hydrochloride 20 mg per 1 ml Chlorpromazine 100mg/5ml oral solution | 150 ml PoM £35.68 DT = £35.68

⚑ 442

Flupentixol

21-Oct-2021

(Flupenthixol)

- **INDICATIONS AND DOSE**

Schizophrenia and other psychoses, particularly with apathy and withdrawal but not mania or psychomotor hyperactivity
▸ BY MOUTH
▸ Adult: Initially 3–9 mg twice daily, adjusted according to response, for debilitated patients, use elderly dose; maximum 18 mg per day
▸ Elderly: Initially 0.75–4.5 mg twice daily, adjusted according to response

Depressive illness
▸ BY MOUTH
▸ Adult: Initially 1 mg once daily, dose to be taken in the morning, increased if necessary to 2 mg after 1 week, doses above 2 mg to be given in divided doses, last dose to be taken before 4 pm; discontinue if no response after 1 week at maximum dosage; maximum 3 mg per day
▸ Elderly: Initially 500 micrograms daily, dose to be taken in the morning, then increased if necessary to 1 mg after 1 week, doses above 1 mg to be given in divided doses, last dose to be taken before 4 pm; discontinue if no response after 1 week at maximum dosage; maximum 1.5 mg per day

- **CONTRA-INDICATIONS** Circulatory collapse · CNS depression · comatose states · excitable patients · impaired consciousness · overactive patients
- **CAUTIONS** Cardiac disorders · cardiovascular disease · cerebral arteriosclerosis · elderly · hyperthyroidism · hypothyroidism · parkinsonism · phaeochromocytoma · QT-interval prolongation · senile confusional states
- **INTERACTIONS** → Appendix 1: flupentixol
- **SIDE-EFFECTS**
  ▸ **Common or very common** Appetite abnormal · asthenia · concentration impaired · depression · diarrhoea · dyspnoea · gastrointestinal discomfort · headache · hyperhidrosis · myalgia · nervousness · palpitations · sexual dysfunction · skin reactions · urinary disorder · vision disorders
  ▸ **Uncommon** Flatulence · hot flush · nausea · oculogyration · photosensitivity reaction · speech disorder
  ▸ **Rare or very rare** Glucose tolerance impaired · jaundice · thrombocytopenia
  ▸ **Frequency not known** Suicidal behaviours · venous thromboembolism
- **PREGNANCY** Avoid unless potential benefit outweighs risk.
- **BREAST FEEDING** Present in breast milk—avoid.
- **HEPATIC IMPAIRMENT** Manufacturer advises caution—monitor serum drug concentration.
- **RENAL IMPAIRMENT** EvGr Caution in renal failure (increased risk of cerebral sensitivity). (M)
- **PATIENT AND CARER ADVICE** Although drowsiness may occur, can also have an alerting effect so should not be taken in the evening.

- **MEDICINAL FORMS** There can be variation in the licensing of different medicines containing the same drug. Forms available from special-order manufacturers include: oral suspension, oral solution

Oral tablet
CAUTIONARY AND ADVISORY LABELS 2
  ▸ **Depixol** (Lundbeck Ltd)
  Flupentixol (as Flupentixol dihydrochloride) 3 mg Depixol 3mg tablets | 100 tablet PoM £13.92 DT = £13.92

▶ Fluanxol (Lundbeck Ltd)
Flupentixol (as Flupentixol dihydrochloride)
500 microgram Fluanxol 500microgram tablets | 60 tablet PoM
£2.88 DT = £2.88
Flupentixol (as Flupentixol dihydrochloride) 1 mg Fluanxol 1mg
tablets | 60 tablet PoM £4.86 DT = £4.86

◀ 442

Haloperidol

10-Jul-2024

● **INDICATIONS AND DOSE**

Prophylaxis of postoperative nausea and vomiting [in patients at moderate to high risk and when alternatives ineffective or not tolerated]
▶ BY INTRAMUSCULAR INJECTION
▸ Adult: 1–2 mg, to be given at induction or 30 minutes before the end of anaesthesia
▸ Elderly: 500 micrograms, to be given at induction or 30 minutes before the end of anaesthesia

Combination treatment of postoperative nausea and vomiting [when alternatives ineffective or not tolerated]
▶ BY INTRAMUSCULAR INJECTION
▸ Adult: 1–2 mg
▸ Elderly: 500 micrograms

Schizophrenia and schizoaffective disorder
▶ BY MOUTH
▸ Adult: 2–10 mg daily in 1–2 divided doses; usual dose 2–4 mg daily, in first-episode schizophrenia, up to 10 mg daily, in multiple-episode schizophrenia, dose adjusted according to response at intervals of 1–7 days. Individual benefit-risk should be assessed when considering doses above 10 mg daily; maximum 20 mg per day
▸ Elderly: Initially, use half the lowest adult dose, then adjust gradually according to response up to maximum 5 mg daily, doses above 5 mg daily should only be considered in patients who have tolerated higher doses and after reassessment of the individual benefit-risk

Acute delirium [when non-pharmacological treatments ineffective]
▶ BY MOUTH
▸ Adult: 1–10 mg daily in 1–3 divided doses, treatment should be started at the lowest possible dose and adjusted in increments at 2–4 hourly intervals if required; maximum 10 mg per day
▸ Elderly: Initially, use half the lowest adult dose, then adjust gradually according to response up to maximum 5 mg daily, doses above 5 mg daily should only be considered in patients who have tolerated higher doses and after reassessment of the individual benefit-risk
▶ BY INTRAMUSCULAR INJECTION
▸ Adult: 1–10 mg, treatment should be started at the lowest possible dose and adjusted in increments at 2–4 hourly intervals if required; maximum 10 mg per day
▸ Elderly: Initially 500 micrograms, dose adjusted gradually according to response up to maximum 5 mg daily, doses above 5 mg daily should only be considered in patients who have tolerated higher doses and after reassessment of the individual benefit-risk

Moderate to severe manic episodes associated with bipolar I disorder
▶ BY MOUTH
▸ Adult: 2–10 mg daily in 1–2 divided doses, dose adjusted according to response at intervals of 1–3 days. Individual benefit-risk should be assessed when considering doses above 10 mg daily; continued use should be evaluated early in treatment; maximum 15 mg per day
▸ Elderly: Initially, use half the lowest adult dose, then adjust gradually according to response up to maximum

5 mg daily, doses above 5 mg daily should only be considered in patients who have tolerated higher doses and after reassessment of the individual benefit-risk; continued use should be evaluated early in treatment

Acute psychomotor agitation associated with psychotic disorder or manic episodes of bipolar I disorder
▶ BY MOUTH
▸ Adult: 5–10 mg, dose may be repeated after 12 hours if necessary; continued use should be evaluated early in treatment; maximum 20 mg per day
▸ Elderly: Initially 2.5 mg, dose may be repeated after 12 hours if necessary up to maximum 5 mg daily, doses above 5 mg daily should only be considered in patients who have tolerated higher doses and after reassessment of the individual benefit-risk; continued use should be evaluated early in treatment

Rapid control of severe acute psychomotor agitation associated with psychotic disorder or manic episodes of bipolar I disorder [when oral therapy is not appropriate]
▶ BY INTRAMUSCULAR INJECTION
▸ Adult: 5 mg, dose may be repeated hourly if required— in the majority of patients, doses of up to 15 mg daily are usually sufficient; continued use should be evaluated early in treatment; maximum 20 mg per day
▸ Elderly: 2.5 mg, dose may be repeated hourly if required up to maximum 5 mg daily, doses above 5 mg daily should only be considered in patients who have tolerated higher doses and after reassessment of the individual benefit-risk; continued use should be evaluated early in treatment

Persistent aggression and psychotic symptoms in moderate to severe Alzheimer's dementia and vascular dementia [when non-pharmacological treatments ineffective and there is a risk of harm to self or others]
▶ BY MOUTH
▸ Adult: 0.5–5 mg daily in 1–2 divided doses, dose adjusted according to response at intervals of 1–3 days. Reassess treatment after no more than 6 weeks
▸ Elderly: Initially 500 micrograms daily, dose adjusted gradually according to response up to maximum 5 mg daily. Reassess treatment after no more than 6 weeks, doses above 5 mg daily should only be considered in patients who have tolerated higher doses and after reassessment of the individual benefit-risk

Severe tic disorders, including Tourette's syndrome [when educational, psychological and other pharmacological treatments ineffective]
▶ BY MOUTH
▸ Adult: 0.5–5 mg daily in 1–2 divided doses, dose adjusted according to response at intervals of 1–7 days. Reassess treatment every 6–12 months
▸ Elderly: Initially, use half the lowest adult dose, then adjust gradually according to response up to maximum 5 mg daily. Reassess treatment every 6–12 months, doses above 5 mg daily should only be considered in patients who have tolerated higher doses and after reassessment of the individual benefit-risk

Mild to moderate chorea in Huntington's disease [when alternatives ineffective or not tolerated]
▶ BY MOUTH
▸ Adult: 2–10 mg daily in 1–2 divided doses, dose adjusted according to response at intervals of 1–3 days
▸ Elderly: Initially, use half the lowest adult dose, then adjust gradually according to response up to maximum 5 mg daily, doses above 5 mg daily should only be considered in patients who have tolerated higher doses and after reassessment of the individual benefit-risk

continued →

Mild to moderate chorea in Huntington's disease [when alternatives ineffective or not tolerated and oral therapy inappropriate]
▶ BY INTRAMUSCULAR INJECTION
▶ Adult: 2–5 mg, dose may be repeated hourly if required; maximum 10 mg per day
▶ Elderly: Initially 1 mg, dose may be repeated hourly if required up to maximum 5 mg daily, doses above 5 mg daily should only be considered in patients who have tolerated higher doses and after reassessment of the individual benefit-risk

Nausea and vomiting in palliative care
▶ BY MOUTH, OR BY SUBCUTANEOUS INJECTION
▶ Adult: 0.5–1.5 mg once daily, dose to be given at bedtime and 0.5–1.5 mg every 2 hours as required, max. 10 mg per day in total taking into account regular and as required dosing
▶ INITIALLY BY CONTINUOUS SUBCUTANEOUS INFUSION
▶ Adult: 0.5–1.5 mg/24 hours and (by subcutaneous injection) 0.5–1.5 mg every 2 hours as required, max. 10 mg per day in total taking into account regular and as required dosing

Agitation or delirium in palliative care [regular dosing]
▶ BY MOUTH, OR BY SUBCUTANEOUS INJECTION
▶ Adult: 0.5 mg once daily, dose to be given at bedtime, dose to be adjusted if necessary in 0.5–1 mg increments up to max. 10 mg per day in total taking into account regular and as required dosing
▶ BY CONTINUOUS SUBCUTANEOUS INFUSION
▶ Adult: 0.5 mg/24 hours, dose to be adjusted if necessary in 0.5–1 mg increments up to max. 10 mg per day in total taking into account regular and as required dosing

Agitation or delirium in palliative care [regular dosing for patients in severe distress and/or immediate danger to self or others]
▶ BY MOUTH, OR BY SUBCUTANEOUS INJECTION
▶ Adult: 1.5–3 mg once daily, dose to be given at bedtime, dose to be adjusted if necessary in 0.5–1 mg increments up to max. 10 mg per day in total taking into account regular and as required dosing

Agitation or delirium in palliative care [as required dosing]
▶ BY MOUTH, OR BY SUBCUTANEOUS INJECTION
▶ Adult: 0.5 mg every 2 hours as required, max. 10 mg per day in total taking into account regular and as required dosing

Agitation in palliative care for the imminently dying [initial titration]
▶ BY SUBCUTANEOUS INJECTION
▶ Adult: 1.5–5 mg every 1 hour as required, usual max. 10 mg per day, doses higher than usual max. occasionally used on expert advice
▶ Elderly: 0.5–2.5 mg every 1 hour as required, usual max. 10 mg per day, doses higher than usual max. occasionally used on expert advice

Agitation in palliative care for the imminently dying [maintenance dose after initial titration]
▶ BY CONTINUOUS SUBCUTANEOUS INFUSION
▶ Adult: 2.5–10 mg/24 hours, higher doses occasionally used on expert advice

● **UNLICENSED USE** Not licensed for use in palliative care.

IMPORTANT SAFETY INFORMATION
▶ With intramuscular use or subcutaneous use
When prescribing, dispensing or administering, check that this injection is the correct preparation—this preparation is usually used in hospital for the rapid control of an *acute episode* and should **not** be confused with depot preparations of haloperidol decanoate which

are usually used in the community or clinics for *maintenance* treatment.

MHRA/CHM ADVICE: HALOPERIDOL (*HALDOL* ®): REMINDER OF RISKS WHEN USED IN ELDERLY PATIENTS FOR THE ACUTE TREATMENT OF DELIRIUM (DECEMBER 2021)
The MHRA reminds healthcare professionals that elderly patients are at an increased risk of adverse neurological and cardiac effects, and special caution is required when using haloperidol for the acute treatment of delirium in frail, elderly patients. Haloperidol should only be considered when non-pharmacological interventions are ineffective and no contra-indications are present (e.g. Parkinson's disease and dementia with Lewy bodies). Before initiating treatment, a baseline ECG and correction of any electrolyte disturbances is recommended; cardiac and electrolyte monitoring should be repeated during treatment. Monitor patients for any extrapyramidal adverse effects e.g. acute dystonia, parkinsonism, tardive dyskinesia, akathisia, hypersalivation, and dysphagia.
The lowest possible dose for the shortest possible time should be used, and any dose increase should be gradual and reviewed frequently.

● **CONTRA-INDICATIONS** CNS depression · comatose states · congenital long QT syndrome · dementia with Lewy bodies · history of torsade de pointes · history of ventricular arrhythmia · Parkinson's disease · progressive supranuclear palsy · QTc-interval prolongation · recent acute myocardial infarction · uncompensated heart failure · uncorrected hypokalaemia

● **CAUTIONS**

GENERAL CAUTIONS Bradycardia · electrolyte disturbances (correct before treatment initiation) · family history of QTc-interval prolongation · history of heavy alcohol exposure · hyperthyroidism · hypotension (including orthostatic hypotension) · prolactin-dependent tumours · prolactinaemia · risk factors for stroke

SPECIFIC CAUTIONS
▶ When used for Acute delirium [when non-pharmacological treatments ineffective] Frail, elderly patients

● **INTERACTIONS** → Appendix 1: haloperidol

● **SIDE-EFFECTS**

GENERAL SIDE-EFFECTS
▶ **Common or very common** Depression · eye disorders · headache · nausea · neuromuscular dysfunction · psychotic disorder · vision disorders · weight decreased
▶ **Uncommon** Breast abnormalities · dyspnoea · gait abnormal · hepatic disorders · hyperhidrosis · menstrual cycle irregularities · muscle complaints · musculoskeletal stiffness · oedema · photosensitivity reaction · restlessness · sexual dysfunction · skin reactions · temperature regulation disorders
▶ **Rare or very rare** Hypoglycaemia · respiratory disorders · SIADH · trismus
▶ **Frequency not known** Hypersensitivity vasculitis · pancytopenia · rhabdomyolysis · thrombocytopenia

SPECIFIC SIDE-EFFECTS
▶ With oral use Angioedema
▶ With parenteral use Hypertension · severe cutaneous adverse reactions (SCARs)

SIDE-EFFECTS, FURTHER INFORMATION Haloperidol is a less sedating antipsychotic.

● **PREGNANCY** Manufacturer advises it is preferable to avoid—moderate amount of data indicate no malformative or fetal/neonatal toxicity, however there are isolated case reports of birth defects following fetal exposure, mostly in combination with other drugs; reproductive toxicity shown in *animal* studies.

● **HEPATIC IMPAIRMENT** Manufacturer advises caution.

Dose adjustments Manufacturer advises halve initial dose and then adjust if necessary with smaller increments and at longer intervals.

- **RENAL IMPAIRMENT** Manufacturer advises use with caution.

  Dose adjustments Manufacturer advises consider lower initial dose in severe impairment and then adjust if necessary with smaller increments and at longer intervals.

- **MONITORING REQUIREMENTS**
- ► Manufacturer advises monitor electrolytes before treatment initiation and periodically during treatment.
- ► EvGr A baseline ECG is recommended before treatment initiation and the need for further ECGs during treatment must be assessed on an individual basis. ECG monitoring is recommended up to 6 hours after administration of *intramuscular* doses for prophylaxis or treatment of postoperative nausea and vomiting. Continuous ECG monitoring is recommended for repeated *intramuscular* doses. M EvGr However, serial ECG monitoring may be used in psychiatric settings where continuous ECG monitoring is not available—if an ECG cannot be performed (for example, in rapid control of severe acute psychomotor agitation), or if one has not been done recently, *intramuscular* haloperidol should be avoided. E

- **DIRECTIONS FOR ADMINISTRATION** For *continuous subcutaneous infusion* dilute with a suitable volume of Water for Injections.

- **PRESCRIBING AND DISPENSING INFORMATION**

  Palliative care For further information on the use of haloperidol in palliative care, see www.medicinescomplete. com/#/content/palliative/haloperidol.

- **MEDICINAL FORMS** There can be variation in the licensing of different medicines containing the same drug. Forms available from special-order manufacturers include: oral suspension, oral solution

Solution for injection
- ► **Haloperidol (Non-proprietary)**
  Haloperidol 5 mg per 1 ml Haloperidol 5mg/1ml solution for injection ampoules | 5 ampoule PoM £16.50 | 10 ampoule PoM £69.00 DT = £67.35

Oral tablet
CAUTIONARY AND ADVISORY LABELS 2
- ► **Haloperidol (Non-proprietary)**
  Haloperidol 500 microgram Haloperidol 500microgram tablets | 28 tablet PoM £473.86 DT = £475.50
  Haloperidol 1.5 mg Haloperidol 1.5mg tablets | 28 tablet PoM £9.00 DT = £8.07
  Haloperidol 5 mg Haloperidol 5mg tablets | 28 tablet PoM £13.20 DT = £7.94
  Haloperidol 10 mg Haloperidol 10mg tablets | 28 tablet PoM £22.01 DT = £21.21

Oral solution
CAUTIONARY AND ADVISORY LABELS 2
- ► **Haloperidol (Non-proprietary)**
  Haloperidol 1 mg per 1 ml Haloperidol 5mg/5ml oral solution sugar free | 100 ml PoM £19.50 DT = £19.38 SF
  Haloperidol 2 mg per 1 ml Haloperidol 10mg/5ml oral solution sugar free | 100 ml PoM £46.75 DT = £8.01 SF
- ► **Haldol** (Essential Pharma Ltd)
  Haloperidol 2 mg per 1 ml Haldol 2mg/ml oral solution | 100 ml PoM £4.45 DT = £8.01 SF
- ► **Halkid** (Syri Ltd)
  Haloperidol 200 microgram per 1 ml Halkid 200micrograms/ml oral solution | 100 ml PoM £89.90 DT = £89.90 SF

► 442

Loxapine
25-Apr-2017

- **DRUG ACTION** Loxapine is a dopamine D_2 and serotonin 5-HT_{2A} receptor antagonist. It also binds to noradrenergic, histaminergic, and cholinergic receptors.

- **INDICATIONS AND DOSE**

  Rapid control of mild-to-moderate agitation in patients with schizophrenia or bipolar disorder (specialist supervision in hospital)
  - ► BY INHALATION
  - ► Adult: 9.1 mg as a single dose, followed by 9.1 mg after 2 hours if required, alternatively 4.5 mg as a single dose, followed by 4.5 mg after 2 hours if required, lower dose may be given if more appropriate or if the higher dose not previously tolerated

- **CONTRA-INDICATIONS** Acute respiratory symptoms · asthma · cardiovascular disease · cerebrovascular disease · chronic obstructive pulmonary disease · dehydration—risk of hypotension · elderly patients (especially those with dementia-related psychosis) · hypovolaemia—risk of hypotension

- **CAUTIONS** Bronchodilator treatment should be available for treatment of possible severe respiratory side-effects (bronchospasm) · history of extrapyramidal symptoms · risk factors for hypoventilation

- **INTERACTIONS** → Appendix 1: loxapine

- **SIDE-EFFECTS**
- ► **Common or very common** Taste altered · throat irritation
- ► **Uncommon** Bronchospasm · oculogyration · restlessness
- ► **Frequency not known** Dry eye · hypertension · syncope · vision blurred

- **PREGNANCY** Manufacturer advises use only if potential benefit outweighs risk.

- **BREAST FEEDING** Manufacturer advises to avoid for 48 hours after dose (express and discard milk produced during this time)—present in milk in *animal* studies.

- **MONITORING REQUIREMENTS** Manufacturer advises to observe patient during the first hour after each dose for signs and symptoms of bronchospasm.

- **DIRECTIONS FOR ADMINISTRATION** Manufacturer advises remove pull-tab and wait for green light to turn on (product must be used within 15 minutes of pulling tab); instruct patient to inhale through mouthpiece and then hold breath briefly. When green light turns off, this indicates the dose has been delivered.

- **PRESCRIBING AND DISPENSING INFORMATION** Educational risk minimisation materials are available for health care professionals.

  Adasuve® 4.5 mg inhalation powder may be difficult to obtain.

- **MEDICINAL FORMS** No licensed medicines listed.

► 442

Pericyazine
27-Jun-2023
(Periciazine)

- **INDICATIONS AND DOSE**

  Schizophrenia | Psychoses
  - ► BY MOUTH
  - ► Adult: Initially 75 mg daily in divided doses, then increased in steps of 25 mg every week, adjusted according to response; maximum 300 mg per day
  - ► Elderly: Initially 15–30 mg daily in divided doses, then increased in steps of 25 mg every week, adjusted according to response; maximum 300 mg per day

continued →

Short-term adjunctive management of severe anxiety, psychomotor agitation, and violent or dangerously impulsive behaviour

▶ BY MOUTH

▶ Adult: Initially 15–30 mg daily in 2 divided doses, adjusted according to response, larger dose to be taken at bedtime

▶ Elderly: Initially 5–10 mg daily in 2 divided doses, adjusted according to response, larger dose to be taken at bedtime

● CONTRA-INDICATIONS CNS depression · comatose states · phaeochromocytoma

● CAUTIONS Hypothyroidism · susceptibility to QT interval prolongation

● INTERACTIONS → Appendix 1: phenothiazines

● SIDE-EFFECTS Atrioventricular block · cardiac arrest · consciousness impaired · contact dermatitis · glucose tolerance impaired · hepatic disorders · hyperthermia · nasal congestion · priapism · respiratory depression

● HEPATIC IMPAIRMENT Can precipitate coma; phenothiazines are hepatotoxic.

● RENAL IMPAIRMENT EvGr Use with caution (risk of accumulation). Ⓜ

● MEDICINAL FORMS There can be variation in the licensing of different medicines containing the same drug. Forms available from special-order manufacturers include: oral suspension, oral solution

Oral tablet

CAUTIONARY AND ADVISORY LABELS 2

▶ Pericyazine (Non-proprietary)
Pericyazine 2.5 mg Pericyazine 2.5mg tablets | 84 tablet [PoM] £52.81 DT = £52.81
Pericyazine 10 mg Pericyazine 10mg tablets | 84 tablet [PoM] £132.39 DT = £132.39

Oral solution

CAUTIONARY AND ADVISORY LABELS 2

▶ Pericyazine (Non-proprietary)
Pericyazine 2 mg per 1 ml Pericyazine 10mg/5ml oral solution | 100 ml [PoM] £82.80 DT = £82.80

⬥ 442

Pimozide

28-Oct-2021

● INDICATIONS AND DOSE

Schizophrenia

▶ BY MOUTH

▶ Adult: Initially 2 mg daily, adjusted according to response, then increased in steps of 2–4 mg at intervals of not less than 1 week; usual dose 2–20 mg daily

▶ Elderly: Initially 1 mg daily, adjusted according to response, increased in steps of 2–4 mg at intervals of not less than 1 week; usual dose 2–20 mg daily

Monosymptomatic hypochondriacal psychosis | Paranoid psychosis

▶ BY MOUTH

▶ Adult: Initially 4 mg daily, adjusted according to response, then increased in steps of 2–4 mg at intervals of not less than 1 week; maximum 16 mg per day

▶ Elderly: Initially 2 mg daily, adjusted according to response, increased in steps of 2–4 mg at intervals of not less than 1 week; maximum 16 mg per day

● CONTRA-INDICATIONS CNS depression · comatose states · history of arrhythmias · history or family history of congenital QT prolongation · phaeochromocytoma

● INTERACTIONS → Appendix 1: pimozide

● SIDE-EFFECTS

▶ **Common or very common** Appetite decreased · depression · headache · hyperhidrosis · restlessness · sebaceous gland overactivity · urinary disorders · vision blurred

▶ **Uncommon** Dysarthria · face oedema · muscle spasms · oculogyric crisis · skin reactions

▶ **Frequency not known** Cardiac arrest · embolism and thrombosis · generalised tonic-clonic seizure · glycosuria · hyponatraemia · libido decreased · neck stiffness · temperature regulation disorders

● HEPATIC IMPAIRMENT Manufacturer advises caution.

● RENAL IMPAIRMENT EvGr Caution in renal failure. Ⓜ

● MONITORING REQUIREMENTS

▶ ECG monitoring Following reports of sudden unexplained death, an ECG is recommended before treatment. It is also recommended that patients taking pimozide should have an annual ECG (if the QT interval is prolonged, treatment should be reviewed and either withdrawn or dose reduced under close supervision) and that pimozide should not be given with other antipsychotic drugs (including depot preparations), tricyclic antidepressants or other drugs which prolong the QT interval, such as certain antimalarials, antiarrhythmic drugs and certain antihistamines and should not be given with drugs which cause electrolyte disturbances (especially diuretics).

● MEDICINAL FORMS There can be variation in the licensing of different medicines containing the same drug. Forms available from special-order manufacturers include: oral suspension

Oral tablet

CAUTIONARY AND ADVISORY LABELS 2

▶ Pimozide (Non-proprietary)
Pimozide 1 mg Orap 1mg tablets | 100 tablet [PoM] Ⓢ (Hospital only)

▶ Orap (Eumedica Pharma Ltd)
Pimozide 4 mg Orap 4mg tablets | 100 tablet [PoM] £40.31 DT = £40.31

⬥ 442

Prochlorperazine

15-Apr-2024

● INDICATIONS AND DOSE

Schizophrenia and other psychoses | Mania

▶ BY MOUTH

▶ Adult: 12.5 mg twice daily for 7 days, dose to be adjusted at intervals of 4–7 days according to response; usual dose 75–100 mg per day

▶ BY DEEP INTRAMUSCULAR INJECTION

▶ Adult: 12.5–25 mg 2–3 times a day

Short-term adjunctive management of severe anxiety

▶ BY MOUTH

▶ Adult: 15–20 mg daily in divided doses; maximum 40 mg per day

Nausea and vomiting, acute attack

▶ BY MOUTH

▶ Adult: Initially 20 mg for 1 dose, then 10 mg for 1 dose, to be given 2 hours after first dose

▶ BY DEEP INTRAMUSCULAR INJECTION

▶ Adult: 12.5 mg as required, to be followed if necessary after 6 hours by an oral dose

Nausea and vomiting, prevention

▶ BY MOUTH

▶ Adult: 5–10 mg 2–3 times a day

▶ BY DEEP INTRAMUSCULAR INJECTION

▶ Adult: 12.5 mg as required, to be followed if necessary after 6 hours by an oral dose

Prevention and treatment of nausea and vomiting

▶ BY MOUTH

▶ Child 1–11 years (body-weight 10 kg and above): 250 micrograms/kg 2–3 times a day

▶ Child 12–17 years: 5–10 mg up to 3 times a day as required

▶ BY INTRAMUSCULAR INJECTION

▶ Child 2–4 years: 1.25–2.5 mg up to 3 times a day as required

▸ Child 5-11 years: 5–6.25 mg up to 3 times a day as required
▸ Child 12-17 years: 12.5 mg up to 3 times a day as required

Labyrinthine disorders
▸ BY MOUTH
▸ Adult: 5 mg 3 times a day, dose can be increased gradually to 30 mg daily in divided doses if necessary, then reduced to 5–10 mg per day after several weeks

Nausea and vomiting in previously diagnosed migraine
▸ BY BUCCAL ADMINISTRATION
▸ Child 12-17 years: 3–6 mg twice daily
▸ Adult: 3–6 mg twice daily

Acute migraine
▸ BY MOUTH
▸ Adult: 10 mg for 1 dose, to be taken as soon as migraine symptoms develop

DOSE EQUIVALENCE AND CONVERSION
▸ Doses are expressed as prochlorperazine maleate or mesilate; 1 mg prochlorperazine maleate ≡ 1 mg prochlorperazine mesilate.

● UNLICENSED USE [EvGr] Prochlorperazine is used for the treatment of acute migraine, ⓐ but is not licensed for this indication.
  Injection not licensed for use in children. *Buccastem M*® tablets not licensed for use in children.

● CONTRA-INDICATIONS Avoid oral route in child under 10 kg · CNS depression · comatose states · phaeochromocytoma

● CAUTIONS

GENERAL CAUTIONS Elderly · hypotension (more likely after intramuscular injection) · susceptibility to QT interval prolongation

SPECIFIC CAUTIONS
▸ With systemic use Hypothyroidism (in adults)

CAUTIONS, FURTHER INFORMATION
▸ Elderly Screening Tool of Older Persons' potentially inappropriate Prescriptions (STOPP) criteria to aid medication reviews (see Prescribing in the elderly p. 31 for information): potentially inappropriate in patients with parkinsonism (risk of exacerbating parkinsonian symptoms).

● INTERACTIONS → Appendix 1: phenothiazines

● SIDE-EFFECTS

GENERAL SIDE-EFFECTS
▸ **Rare or very rare** Glucose tolerance impaired · hyponatraemia · SIADH
▸ **Frequency not known** Photosensitivity reaction

SPECIFIC SIDE-EFFECTS
▸ **Rare or very rare**
▸ With buccal use Blood disorder · hepatic disorders
▸ **Frequency not known**
▸ With buccal use Embolism and thrombosis · oral disorders · skin eruption
▸ With intramuscular use Atrioventricular block · cardiac arrest · eye disorders · jaundice · nasal congestion · respiratory depression · skin reactions
▸ With oral use Atrioventricular block · autonomic dysfunction · cardiac arrest · consciousness impaired · hyperthermia · jaundice · nasal congestion · oculogyric crisis · respiratory depression · skin reactions

SIDE-EFFECTS, FURTHER INFORMATION Acute dystonias are more common with potent first-generation antipsychotics. The risk is increased in men, young adults, children, antipsychotic-naïve patients, rapid dose escalation, and abrupt treatment discontinuation.

● HEPATIC IMPAIRMENT Manufacturer advises avoid.

● RENAL IMPAIRMENT
Dose adjustments Start with small doses in severe renal impairment because of increased cerebral sensitivity.

● DIRECTIONS FOR ADMINISTRATION Manufacturer advises buccal tablets are placed high between upper lip and gum and left to dissolve.

● PATIENT AND CARER ADVICE Patients or carers should be given advice on how to administer prochlorperazine buccal tablets.

● MEDICINAL FORMS There can be variation in the licensing of different medicines containing the same drug.

Solution for injection
▸ Stemetil (Sanofi)
  Prochlorperazine mesilate 12.5 mg per 1 ml Stemetil 12.5mg/1ml solution for injection ampoules | 10 ampoule [PoM] £5.23 DT = £5.23

Oral tablet
CAUTIONARY AND ADVISORY LABELS 2
▸ Prochlorperazine (Non-proprietary)
  Prochlorperazine maleate 5 mg Prochlorperazine 5mg tablets | 28 tablet [PoM] £3.00 DT = £1.32 | 84 tablet [PoM] £3.96-£7.80
▸ Stemetil (Sanofi)
  Prochlorperazine maleate 5 mg Stemetil 5mg tablets | 28 tablet [PoM] £1.98 DT = £1.32 | 84 tablet [PoM] £5.94

Buccal tablet
CAUTIONARY AND ADVISORY LABELS 2
▸ Prochlorperazine (Non-proprietary)
  Prochlorperazine maleate 3 mg Prochlorperazine 3mg buccal tablets | 8 tablet [PoM] £3.25 | 50 tablet [PoM] £22.99 DT = £8.05

F 442

Sulpiride
21-Oct-2021

● **INDICATIONS AND DOSE**

Schizophrenia with predominantly negative symptoms
▸ BY MOUTH
▸ Adult: 200–400 mg twice daily; maximum 800 mg per day
▸ Elderly: Lower initial dose to be given, increased gradually according to response

Schizophrenia with mainly positive symptoms
▸ BY MOUTH
▸ Adult: 200–400 mg twice daily; maximum 2.4 g per day
▸ Elderly: Lower initial dose to be given, increased gradually according to response

IMPORTANT SAFETY INFORMATION
MHRA/CHM ADVICE: CLOZAPINE AND OTHER ANTIPSYCHOTICS: MONITORING BLOOD CONCENTRATIONS FOR TOXICITY (AUGUST 2020)
Following fatal cases involving toxicity of clozapine and other antipsychotic medicines, the MHRA advises that monitoring blood concentration of sulpiride may be helpful in certain circumstances, such as patients presenting symptoms suggestive of toxicity, or when concomitant medicines may interact to increase blood concentration of sulpiride.

● CONTRA-INDICATIONS CNS depression · comatose states · phaeochromocytoma

● CAUTIONS Aggressive patients (even low doses may aggravate symptoms) · agitated patients (even low doses may aggravate symptoms) · excited patients (even low doses may aggravate symptoms)

● INTERACTIONS → Appendix 1: sulpiride

● SIDE-EFFECTS
▸ **Common or very common** Breast abnormalities
▸ **Uncommon** Muscle tone increased · orgasm abnormal
▸ **Rare or very rare** Oculogyric crisis
▸ **Frequency not known** Cardiac arrest · dyspnoea · embolism and thrombosis · hyponatraemia · SIADH · trismus · urticaria

- **RENAL IMPAIRMENT**
Dose adjustments [EvGr] Reduce dose or increase dose interval; increase in small steps. ◈

- **MONITORING REQUIREMENTS** Sulpiride does not affect blood pressure to the same extent as other antipsychotic drugs and so blood pressure monitoring is not mandatory for this drug.

- **PRESCRIBING AND DISPENSING INFORMATION** Flavours of oral liquid formulations may include lemon and aniseed.

- **MEDICINAL FORMS** There can be variation in the licensing of different medicines containing the same drug. Forms available from special-order manufacturers include: oral suspension, oral solution

Oral tablet
CAUTIONARY AND ADVISORY LABELS 2
- ▶ **Sulpiride (Non-proprietary)**
Sulpiride 200 mg Sulpiride 200mg tablets | 30 tablet [PoM] £12.20 DT = £3.06
Sulpiride 400 mg Sulpiride 400mg tablets | 30 tablet [PoM] £23.50 DT = £11.90

Oral solution
CAUTIONARY AND ADVISORY LABELS 2
- ▶ **Sulpiride (Non-proprietary)**
Sulpiride 40 mg per 1 ml Sulpiride 200mg/5ml oral solution sugar free | 150 ml [PoM] £93.64 DT = £93.64 [SF]

☞ 442

Trifluoperazine

27-Jun-2023

- **INDICATIONS AND DOSE**

Schizophrenia and other psychoses | Short-term adjunctive management of psychomotor agitation, excitement, and violent or dangerously impulsive behaviour
▶ BY MOUTH
▶ Adult: Initially 5 mg twice daily, daily dose may be increased by 5 mg after 1 week. If necessary, dose may be further increased in steps of 5 mg at intervals of 3 days. When satisfactory control has been achieved, reduce gradually until an effective maintenance level has been established
▶ Elderly: Initially up to 2.5 mg twice daily, daily dose may be increased by 5 mg after 1 week. If necessary, dose may be further increased in steps of 5 mg at intervals of 3 days. When satisfactory control has been achieved, reduce gradually until an effective maintenance level has been established

Short-term adjunctive management of severe anxiety
▶ BY MOUTH
▶ Adult: 2–4 mg daily in divided doses, increased if necessary to 6 mg daily
▶ Elderly: Up to 2 mg daily in divided doses, increased if necessary to 6 mg daily

Severe nausea and vomiting
▶ BY MOUTH
▶ Adult: 2–4 mg daily in divided doses; maximum 6 mg per day

- **CONTRA-INDICATIONS** CNS depression · comatose states · phaeochromocytoma

- **CAUTIONS** Susceptibility to QT interval prolongation

- **INTERACTIONS** → Appendix 1: phenothiazines

- **SIDE-EFFECTS** Alertness decreased · anxiety · appetite decreased · blood disorder · cardiac arrest · embolism and thrombosis · hyperpyrexia · jaundice cholestatic · lens opacity · muscle weakness · oedema · pancytopenia · photosensitivity reaction · skin reactions · thrombocytopenia · urinary hesitation · vision blurred · withdrawal syndrome

SIDE-EFFECTS, FURTHER INFORMATION Extrapyramidal symptoms are more frequent at doses exceeding 6 mg

daily. Acute dystonias are more common with potent first generation antipsychotics. The risk is increased in men, young adults, children, antipsychotic-naïve patients, rapid dose escalation, and abrupt treatment discontinuation.

- **HEPATIC IMPAIRMENT** Manufacturer advises avoid.

- **MONITORING REQUIREMENTS** Trifluoperazine does not affect blood pressure to the same extent as other antipsychotic drugs and so blood pressure monitoring is not mandatory for this drug.

- **MEDICINAL FORMS** There can be variation in the licensing of different medicines containing the same drug.

Oral tablet
CAUTIONARY AND ADVISORY LABELS 2
- ▶ **Trifluoperazine (Non-proprietary)**
Trifluoperazine (as Trifluoperazine hydrochloride)
1 mg Trifluoperazine 1mg tablets | 112 tablet [PoM] £47.30–£99.80 DT = £59.12
Trifluoperazine (as Trifluoperazine hydrochloride)
5 mg Trifluoperazine 5mg tablets | 112 tablet [PoM] £107.91–£165.00 DT = £134.89

Oral solution
CAUTIONARY AND ADVISORY LABELS 2
- ▶ **Trifluoperazine (Non-proprietary)**
Trifluoperazine (as Trifluoperazine hydrochloride)
200 microgram per 1 ml Trifluoperazine 1mg/5ml oral solution sugar free | 200 ml [PoM] £136.88 DT = £136.88 [SF]
Trifluoperazine (as Trifluoperazine hydrochloride) 1 mg per 1 ml Trifluoperazine 5mg/5ml oral solution sugar free | 150 ml [PoM] £83.98 DT = £76.87 [SF]

☞ 442

Zuclopenthixol

21-Oct-2021

- **INDICATIONS AND DOSE**

Schizophrenia and other psychoses
▶ BY MOUTH
▶ Adult: Initially 20–30 mg daily in divided doses, increased if necessary up to 150 mg daily; usual maintenance 20–50 mg daily (max. per dose 40 mg), for debilitated patients, use elderly dose
▶ Elderly: Initially 5–15 mg daily in divided doses, increased if necessary up to 150 mg daily; usual maintenance 20–50 mg daily (max. per dose 40 mg)

- **CONTRA-INDICATIONS** Apathetic states · CNS depression · comatose states · phaeochromocytoma · withdrawn states

- **CAUTIONS** Hyperthyroidism · hypothyroidism

- **INTERACTIONS** → Appendix 1: zuclopenthixol

- **SIDE-EFFECTS** Anxiety · appetite abnormal · asthenia · concentration impaired · depression · diarrhoea · dyspnoea · eye disorders · fever · flatulence · gait abnormal · gastrointestinal discomfort · glucose tolerance impaired · headaches · hepatic disorders · hot flush · hyperacusia · hyperhidrosis · hyperlipidaemia · hypothermia · malaise · memory loss · myalgia · nasal congestion · nausea · neuromuscular dysfunction · pain · palpitations · paraesthesia · photosensitivity reaction · reflexes increased · seborrhoea · sexual dysfunction · skin reactions · sleep disorders · speech disorder · syncope · thirst · thrombocytopenia · tinnitus · urinary disorders · venous thromboembolism · vertigo · vision disorders · vulvovaginal dryness · weight decreased · withdrawal syndrome

- **HEPATIC IMPAIRMENT** Manufacturer advises caution—monitor serum drug concentration.
Dose adjustments Manufacturer advises dose reduction of half the recommended dose.

- **RENAL IMPAIRMENT** [EvGr] Caution in renal failure. ◈
Dose adjustments [EvGr] Use half normal dose in renal failure. ◈

- **MEDICINAL FORMS** There can be variation in the licensing of different medicines containing the same drug.

Oral tablet

CAUTIONARY AND ADVISORY LABELS 2

▸ **Clopixol** (Lundbeck Ltd)

Zuclopenthixol (as Zuclopenthixol dihydrochloride) 2 mg Clopixol 2mg tablets | 100 tablet [PoM] £3.14 DT = £3.14

Zuclopenthixol (as Zuclopenthixol dihydrochloride) **10 mg** Clopixol 10mg tablets | 100 tablet [PoM] £8.06 DT = £8.06

Zuclopenthixol (as Zuclopenthixol dihydrochloride) **25 mg** Clopixol 25mg tablets | 100 tablet [PoM] £16.13 DT = £16.13

Oral drops

▸ **Zuclopenthixol** (Non-proprietary)

Zuclopenthixol (as Zuclopenthixol dihydrochloride) 20 mg per 1 ml Ciatyl-Z 20mg/ml oral drops | 30 ml [PoM] [🄴] (Hospital only)

⚑ 442

Zuclopenthixol acetate

21-Oct-2021

- **INDICATIONS AND DOSE**

Short-term management of acute psychosis | Short-term management of mania | Short-term management of exacerbation of chronic psychosis

▸ BY DEEP INTRAMUSCULAR INJECTION

▸ Adult: 50–150 mg, then 50–150 mg after 2–3 days if required, (1 additional dose may be needed 1–2 days after the first injection); maximum cumulative dose 400 mg in 2 weeks and maximum 4 injections; maximum duration of treatment 2 weeks—if maintenance treatment necessary change to an oral antipsychotic 2–3 days after last injection, or to a longer acting antipsychotic depot injection given concomitantly with last injection of zuclopenthixol acetate; to be administered into the gluteal muscle or lateral thigh

▸ Elderly: 50–100 mg, then 50–100 mg after 2–3 days if required, (1 additional dose may be needed 1–2 days after the first injection); maximum cumulative dose 400 mg in 2 weeks and maximum 4 injections; maximum duration of treatment 2 weeks—if maintenance treatment necessary change to an oral antipsychotic 2–3 days after last injection, or to a longer acting antipsychotic depot injection given concomitantly with last injection of zuclopenthixol acetate; to be administered into the gluteal muscle or lateral thigh

> **IMPORTANT SAFETY INFORMATION**
>
> When prescribing, dispensing, or administering, check that this is the correct preparation—this preparation is usually used in hospital for an *acute episode* and should **not** be confused with depot preparations which are usually used in the community or clinics for *maintenance* treatment.
>
> **SAFE PRACTICE**
>
> Zuclopenthixol acetate has been confused with zuclopenthixol decanoate; care must be taken to ensure the correct drug is prescribed and dispensed.

- **CONTRA-INDICATIONS** CNS depression · comatose states · phaeochromocytoma

- **CAUTIONS** Hyperthyroidism · hypothyroidism

- **INTERACTIONS** → Appendix 1: zuclopenthixol

- **SIDE-EFFECTS** Anxiety · appetite abnormal · asthenia · concentration impaired · depression · diarrhoea · dyspnoea · eye disorders · fever · flatulence · gait abnormal · gastrointestinal discomfort · glucose tolerance impaired · headaches · hepatic disorders · hot flush · hyperacusia · hyperhidrosis · hyperlipidaemia · hypothermia (dose-related) · malaise · memory loss · myalgia · nasal congestion · nausea · neuromuscular dysfunction · pain ·

palpitations · paraesthesia · photosensitivity reaction · reflexes increased · seborrhoea · sexual dysfunction · skin reactions · sleep disorders · speech disorder · syncope · thirst · thrombocytopenia · tinnitus · urinary disorders · venous thromboembolism · vertigo · vision disorders · vulvovaginal dryness · weight decreased · withdrawal syndrome

- **HEPATIC IMPAIRMENT** Manufacturer advises caution—monitor serum drug concentration.

  Dose adjustments Manufacturer advises dose reduction to half the recommended dose.

- **RENAL IMPAIRMENT** [EvGr] Caution in renal failure. ⟨M⟩

  Dose adjustments [EvGr] Use half normal dose in renal failure. ⟨M⟩

- **MEDICINAL FORMS** There can be variation in the licensing of different medicines containing the same drug.

Solution for injection

▸ **Clopixol Acuphase** (Lundbeck Ltd)

Zuclopenthixol acetate 50 mg per 1 ml Clopixol Acuphase 50mg/1ml solution for injection ampoules | 5 ampoule [PoM] £24.21 DT = £24.21 (Hospital only)

ANTIPSYCHOTICS › FIRST-GENERATION (DEPOT INJECTIONS)

⚑ 442

Flupentixol decanoate

21-Oct-2021

(Flupenthixol Decanoate)

- **INDICATIONS AND DOSE**

Maintenance in schizophrenia and other psychoses

▸ BY DEEP INTRAMUSCULAR INJECTION

▸ Adult: Test dose 20 mg, dose to be injected into the upper outer buttock or lateral thigh, then 20–40 mg after at least 7 days, then 20–40 mg every 2–4 weeks, adjusted according to response, usual maintenance dose 50 mg every 4 weeks to 300 mg every 2 weeks; maximum 400 mg per week

▸ Elderly: Dose is initially quarter to half adult dose

- **CONTRA-INDICATIONS** Children · CNS depression · comatose states · excitable patients · overactive patients

- **CAUTIONS** An alternative antipsychotic may be necessary if symptoms such as aggression or agitation appear · hyperthyroidism · hypothyroidism · phaeochromocytoma · when transferring from oral to depot therapy, the dose by mouth should be reduced gradually

- **INTERACTIONS** → Appendix 1: flupentixol

- **SIDE-EFFECTS**

▸ **Common or very common** Appetite abnormal · asthenia · concentration impaired · depression · diarrhoea · dyspnoea · gastrointestinal discomfort · headache · hyperhidrosis · myalgia · nervousness · palpitations · sexual dysfunction · skin reactions · urinary disorder · vision disorders

▸ **Uncommon** Flatulence · hot flush · nausea · oculogyration · photosensitivity reaction · speech disorder

▸ **Rare or very rare** Glucose tolerance impaired · jaundice · thrombocytopenia

▸ **Frequency not known** Suicidal behaviours · venous thromboembolism

  SIDE-EFFECTS, FURTHER INFORMATION Side-effects may persist until the drug has been cleared from its depot site.

- **HEPATIC IMPAIRMENT** Manufacturer advises caution—monitor serum drug concentration.

  Dose adjustments Manufacturer advises initiate at low dose orally to check for tolerability before switching to depot formulation.

- **RENAL IMPAIRMENT** [EvGr] Caution in renal failure (increased risk of cerebral sensitivity). ⟨M⟩

- **MONITORING REQUIREMENTS** Treatment requires careful monitoring for optimum effect.
- **DIRECTIONS FOR ADMINISTRATION** In general, manufacturers advise not more than 2–3 mL of oily injection should be administered at any one site (consult product literature). Use correct injection technique (including use of z-track technique) and rotate injection sites. When initiating therapy with sustained-release preparations of conventional antipsychotics, expert sources advise patients should first be given a small test-dose as undesirable side-effects are prolonged.

- **MEDICINAL FORMS** There can be variation in the licensing of different medicines containing the same drug.

Solution for injection

▸ **Depixol** (Lundbeck Ltd)
Flupentixol decanoate 20 mg per 1 ml Depixol 40mg/2ml solution for injection ampoules | 10 ampoule [PoM] £25.39 DT = £25.39
Depixol 20mg/1ml solution for injection ampoules | 10 ampoule [PoM] £15.17 DT = £15.17
Flupentixol decanoate 100 mg per 1 ml Depixol Conc 100mg/1ml solution for injection ampoules | 10 ampoule [PoM] £62.51 DT = £62.51
Flupentixol decanoate 200 mg per 1 ml Depixol Low Volume 200mg/1ml solution for injection ampoules | 5 ampoule [PoM] £97.59 DT = £97.59

▸ **Psytixol** (Viatris UK Healthcare Ltd)
Flupentixol decanoate 20 mg per 1 ml Psytixol 40mg/2ml solution for injection ampoules | 10 ampoule [PoM] £25.38 DT = £25.39
Psytixol 20mg/1ml solution for injection ampoules | 10 ampoule [PoM] £15.16 DT = £15.17
Flupentixol decanoate 100 mg per 1 ml Psytixol 50mg/0.5ml solution for injection ampoules | 10 ampoule [PoM] £34.12 DT = £34.12
Psytixol 100mg/1ml solution for injection ampoules | 10 ampoule [PoM] £62.50 DT = £62.51
Flupentixol decanoate 200 mg per 1 ml Psytixol 200mg/1ml solution for injection ampoules | 5 ampoule [PoM] £97.58 DT = £97.59

▶ 442

Haloperidol decanoate

05-Oct-2021

- **INDICATIONS AND DOSE**

Maintenance in schizophrenia and schizoaffective disorder [in patients currently stabilised on oral haloperidol]

▸ BY DEEP INTRAMUSCULAR INJECTION
▸ Adult: Initially 25–150 mg every 4 weeks, initial dose should be based on previous daily dose of oral haloperidol (10–15 times the daily dose of oral haloperidol is recommended), adjusted in steps of up to 50 mg every 4 weeks if required, adjustment of the dosing interval may be required, depending on individual patient response; usual maintenance 50–200 mg every 4 weeks (max. per dose 300 mg every 4 weeks), dose to be administered into gluteal muscle, the individual benefit-risk should be assessed when considering doses above 200 mg every 4 weeks, if supplementation with oral haloperidol is required, the combined total dose of haloperidol from both formulations must not exceed the corresponding maximum oral haloperidol dose of 20 mg per day
▸ Elderly: Initially 12.5–25 mg every 4 weeks, increased if necessary to 25–75 mg every 4 weeks, adjustment of the dosing interval may be required, depending on individual patient response, dose to be administered into gluteal muscle, doses above 75 mg every 4 weeks should only be considered in patients who have tolerated higher doses and after reassessment of the individual benefit-risk, if supplementation with oral haloperidol is required, the combined total dose of haloperidol from both formulations must not exceed the corresponding maximum oral haloperidol dose of 5 mg per day, or the previously administered oral

haloperidol dose in patients who have received long-term treatment with oral haloperidol

DOSE EQUIVALENCE AND CONVERSION
▸ A range of equivalent doses is quoted in the literature; the consensus is that 2 mg per day of *oral* haloperidol is approximately equivalent to 15 mg per week of haloperidol decanoate *depot injection*.

> **IMPORTANT SAFETY INFORMATION**
> When prescribing, dispensing or administering, check that this is the correct preparation—this preparation is used for *maintenance* treatment and should **not** be used for the rapid control of an *acute episode*.

- **CONTRA-INDICATIONS** CNS depression · comatose states · congenital long QT syndrome · dementia with Lewy bodies · history of torsade de pointes · history of ventricular arrhythmia · Parkinson's disease · progressive supranuclear palsy · QT-interval prolongation · recent acute myocardial infarction · uncompensated heart failure · uncorrected hypokalaemia
- **CAUTIONS** Bradycardia · electrolyte disturbances (correct before treatment initiation) · family history of QTc-interval prolongation · history of heavy alcohol exposure · hyperthyroidism · hypotension (including orthostatic hypotension) · prolactin-dependent tumours · prolactinaemia · risk factors for stroke · when transferring from oral to depot therapy, the dose by mouth should be reduced gradually
- **INTERACTIONS** → Appendix 1: haloperidol
- **SIDE-EFFECTS**
▸ **Common or very common** Depression · sexual dysfunction
▸ **Uncommon** Eye disorders · headache · neuromuscular dysfunction · vision disorders
▸ **Frequency not known** Angioedema · breast abnormalities · cardiac arrest · dyspnoea · gait abnormal · hepatic disorders · hyperhidrosis · hypersensitivity vasculitis · hypoglycaemia · menstrual cycle irregularities · muscle complaints · musculoskeletal stiffness · nausea · oedema · pancytopenia · photosensitivity reaction · psychotic disorder · respiratory disorders · restlessness · rhabdomyolysis · SIADH · skin reactions · temperature regulation disorders · thrombocytopenia · trismus · weight decreased

SIDE-EFFECTS, FURTHER INFORMATION Haloperidol is a less sedating antipsychotic.

- **PREGNANCY** Manufacturer advises it is preferable to avoid—moderate amount of data indicate no malformative or fetal/neonatal toxicity, however there are isolated case reports of birth defects following fetal exposure, mostly in combination with other drugs; reproductive toxicity shown in *animal* studies.
- **HEPATIC IMPAIRMENT** Manufacturer advises caution.
Dose adjustments Manufacturer advises halve initial dose and then adjust if necessary with smaller increments and at longer intervals.
- **RENAL IMPAIRMENT** Manufacturer advises use with caution.
Dose adjustments Manufacturer advises consider lower initial dose in severe impairment and then adjust if necessary with smaller increments and at longer intervals.
- **MONITORING REQUIREMENTS**
▸ Manufacturer advises perform ECG before treatment initiation and assess need for further ECGs during treatment on an individual basis.
▸ Manufacturer advises monitor electrolytes before treatment initiation and periodically during treatment.
- **DIRECTIONS FOR ADMINISTRATION** In general, manufacturers advise not more than 2–3 mL of oily injection should be administered at any one site. Use

correct injection technique (including use of z-track technique) and rotate of injection sites. When initiating therapy with sustained-release preparations of conventional antipsychotics, expert sources advise patients should first be given a small test-dose as undesirable side-effects are prolonged.

- **MEDICINAL FORMS** There can be variation in the licensing of different medicines containing the same drug.
  Solution for injection
  EXCIPIENTS: May contain Benzyl alcohol, sesame oil
  ▸ **Haldol decanoate** (Essential Pharma Ltd)
  Haloperidol (as Haloperidol decanoate) 50 mg per 1 ml Haldol Decanoate 50mg/1ml solution for injection ampoules | 5 ampoule [PoM] £19.06 DT = £19.06
  Haloperidol (as Haloperidol decanoate) 100 mg per 1 ml Haldol Decanoate 100mg/1ml solution for injection ampoules | 5 ampoule [PoM] £25.26 DT = £25.26

⚑ 442   Zuclopenthixol decanoate

21-Oct-2021

- **INDICATIONS AND DOSE**

Maintenance in schizophrenia and paranoid psychoses
  ▸ BY DEEP INTRAMUSCULAR INJECTION
  ▸ Adult: Test dose 100 mg, dose to be administered into the upper outer buttock or lateral thigh, followed by 200–500 mg after at least 7 days, then 200–500 mg every 1–4 weeks, adjusted according to response, higher doses of more than 500mg can be used; do not exceed 600 mg weekly
  ▸ Elderly: A quarter to half usual starting dose to be used

> **IMPORTANT SAFETY INFORMATION**
>
> When prescribing, dispensing, or administering, check that this is the correct preparation—this preparation is used for *maintenance* treatment and should **not** be used for the short-term management of an *acute episode*.
>
> **SAFE PRACTICE**
> Zuclopenthixol decanoate has been confused with zuclopenthixol acetate; care must be taken to ensure the correct drug is prescribed and dispensed.

- **CONTRA-INDICATIONS** CNS depression · comatose states · phaeochromocytoma
- **CAUTIONS** Hyperthyroidism · hypothyroidism · QT interval prolongation · when transferring from oral to depot therapy, the dose by mouth should be reduced gradually
- **INTERACTIONS** → Appendix 1: zuclopenthixol
- **SIDE-EFFECTS** Anxiety · appetite abnormal · asthenia · concentration impaired · depression · diarrhoea · dyspnoea · eye disorders · fever · flatulence · gait abnormal · gastrointestinal discomfort · glucose tolerance impaired · headaches · hepatic disorders · hot flush · hyperacusia · hyperhidrosis · hyperlipidaemia · hypothermia · malaise · memory loss · myalgia · nasal congestion · nausea · neuromuscular dysfunction · pain · palpitations · paraesthesia · photosensitivity reaction · reflexes increased · seborrhoea · sexual dysfunction · skin reactions · sleep disorders · speech disorder · syncope · thirst · thrombocytopenia · tinnitus · urinary disorders · venous thromboembolism · vertigo · vision disorders · vulvovaginal dryness · weight decreased · withdrawal syndrome
  SIDE-EFFECTS, FURTHER INFORMATION Side-effects may persist until the drug has been cleared from its depot site.
- **HEPATIC IMPAIRMENT** Manufacturer advises caution— monitor serum drug concentration.
  Dose adjustments Manufacturer advises dose reduction to half the recommended dose.
- **RENAL IMPAIRMENT** [EvGr] Caution in renal failure. ⟨M⟩

Dose adjustments [EvGr] Use half normal dose in renal failure. ⟨M⟩

- **MONITORING REQUIREMENTS** Treatment requires careful monitoring for optimum effect.
- **DIRECTIONS FOR ADMINISTRATION** In general, manufacturers advise not more than 2–3 mL of oily injection should be administered at any one site (consult product literature). Use correct injection technique (including use of z-track technique) and rotate injection sites. When initiating therapy with sustained-release preparations of conventional antipsychotics, expert sources advise patients should first be given a small test-dose as undesirable side-effects are prolonged.

- **MEDICINAL FORMS** There can be variation in the licensing of different medicines containing the same drug.
  Solution for injection
  ▸ **Clopixol** (Lundbeck Ltd)
  Zuclopenthixol decanoate 200 mg per 1 ml Clopixol 200mg/1ml solution for injection ampoules | 10 ampoule [PoM] £31.51 DT = £31.51
  Zuclopenthixol decanoate 500 mg per 1 ml Clopixol Conc 500mg/1ml solution for injection ampoules | 5 ampoule [PoM] £37.18 DT = £37.18

ANTIPSYCHOTICS › SECOND-GENERATION

⚑ 442   Amisulpride

06-Jul-2021

- **DRUG ACTION** Amisulpride is a selective dopamine receptor antagonist with high affinity for mesolimbic D_2 and D_3 receptors.

- **INDICATIONS AND DOSE**

Acute psychotic episode in schizophrenia
  ▸ BY MOUTH
  ▸ Adult: 400–800 mg daily in 2 divided doses, adjusted according to response; maximum 1.2 g per day

Schizophrenia with predominantly negative symptoms
  ▸ BY MOUTH
  ▸ Adult: 50–300 mg daily

> **IMPORTANT SAFETY INFORMATION**
>
> MHRA/CHM ADVICE: CLOZAPINE AND OTHER ANTIPSYCHOTICS: MONITORING BLOOD CONCENTRATIONS FOR TOXICITY (AUGUST 2020)
>
> Following fatal cases involving toxicity of clozapine and other antipsychotic medicines, the MHRA advises that monitoring blood concentration of amisulpride may be helpful in certain circumstances, such as patients presenting symptoms suggestive of toxicity, or when concomitant medicines may interact to increase blood concentration of amisulpride.

- **CONTRA-INDICATIONS** CNS depression · comatose states · phaeochromocytoma · prolactin-dependent tumours
- **INTERACTIONS** → Appendix 1: antipsychotics, second generation
- **SIDE-EFFECTS**
  ▸ **Common or very common** Anxiety · breast pain · nausea · oculogyric crisis · orgasm abnormal · trismus · vision blurred
  ▸ **Uncommon** Bone disorders · dyslipidaemia · hepatic disorders · nasal congestion · pneumonia aspiration
  ▸ **Rare or very rare** Angioedema · embolism and thrombosis · hyponatraemia · neoplasms · SIADH · urticaria
  ▸ **Frequency not known** Photosensitivity reaction
- **PREGNANCY** Avoid.
- **BREAST FEEDING** Avoid—no information available.

- RENAL IMPAIRMENT Manufacturer advises caution if creatinine clearance less than 10 mL/minute (no information available).
  Dose adjustments See p. 21.
    Manufacturer advises halve dose if creatinine clearance 30–60 mL/minute.
    Manufacturer advises use one-third dose if creatinine clearance 10–30 mL/minute.
- MONITORING REQUIREMENTS Amisulpride does not affect blood pressure to the same extent as other antipsychotic drugs and so blood pressure monitoring is not mandatory for this drug.
- PRESCRIBING AND DISPENSING INFORMATION Flavours of oral liquid formulations may include caramel.

- MEDICINAL FORMS There can be variation in the licensing of different medicines containing the same drug. Forms available from special-order manufacturers include: oral suspension, oral solution

Oral tablet
CAUTIONARY AND ADVISORY LABELS 2
- Amisulpride (Non-proprietary)
  Amisulpride 50 mg Amisulpride 50mg tablets | 60 tablet PoM
  £13.09 DT = £8.80
  Amisulpride 100 mg Amisulpride 100mg tablets | 60 tablet PoM
  £20.30 DT = £10.91
  Amisulpride 200 mg Amisulpride 200mg tablets | 60 tablet PoM
  £33.93 DT = £21.14
  Amisulpride 400 mg Amisulpride 400mg tablets | 60 tablet PoM
  £84.09 DT = £83.76

Oral solution
CAUTIONARY AND ADVISORY LABELS 2
- Amisulpride (Non-proprietary)
  Amisulpride 100 mg per 1 ml Amisulpride 100mg/ml oral solution sugar free | 60 ml PoM £88.75 DT = £88.75 SF

F 442

Aripiprazole

08-Apr-2025

- DRUG ACTION Aripiprazole is a dopamine D_2 partial agonist with weak $5\text{-}HT_{1a}$ partial agonism and $5\text{-}HT_{2A}$ receptor antagonism.

● INDICATIONS AND DOSE

Schizophrenia
- BY MOUTH
- Adult: 10–15 mg once daily; usual dose 15 mg once daily (max. per dose 30 mg once daily)

Treatment and recurrence prevention of mania
- BY MOUTH
- Adult: 15 mg once daily, increased if necessary up to 30 mg once daily

Rapid control of agitation and disturbed behaviour in schizophrenia and mania
- BY INTRAMUSCULAR INJECTION USING IMMEDIATE-RELEASE MEDICINES
- Adult: Initially 5.25–15 mg for 1 dose, alternatively usual dose 9.75 mg for 1 dose, followed by 5.25–15 mg after 2 hours if required, maximum 3 injections daily; maximum daily combined oral and parenteral dose 30 mg

Maintenance of schizophrenia in patients stabilised with oral aripiprazole who are CYP2D6 poor metabolisers [using once-monthly intramuscular depot injection]
- BY DEEP INTRAMUSCULAR INJECTION USING DEPOT INJECTION
- Adult: 300 mg every month, minimum of 26 days between injections, treatment with prescribed daily dose of oral aripiprazole should be continued for 14 consecutive days after the first injection, for dose adjustment due to side-effects and for advice on missed doses—consult product literature, alternatively initially 600 mg for 1 dose, to be administered as 2 consecutive 300 mg injections, along with a single

previously prescribed dose of oral aripiprazole, then maintenance 300 mg every month, minimum of 26 days between injections, for dose adjustment due to side-effects and for advice on missed doses—consult product literature

Maintenance of schizophrenia in patients stabilised with oral aripiprazole [using once-monthly intramuscular depot injection]
- BY DEEP INTRAMUSCULAR INJECTION USING DEPOT INJECTION
- Adult: 400 mg every month, minimum of 26 days between injections, treatment with 10–20 mg oral aripiprazole daily should be continued for 14 consecutive days after the first injection, for dose adjustment due to side-effects and for advice on missed doses—consult product literature, alternatively initially 800 mg for 1 dose, to be administered as 2 consecutive 400 mg injections, along with a single dose of 20 mg oral aripiprazole, then maintenance 400 mg every month, minimum of 26 days between injections, for dose adjustment due to side-effects and for advice on missed doses—consult product literature

DOSE ADJUSTMENTS DUE TO INTERACTIONS
- With oral use Manufacturer advises double the dose with concurrent use of potent inducers of CYP3A4. Manufacturer advises reduce dose by half with concurrent use of potent inhibitors of CYP3A4 or CYP2D6.
- With intramuscular use For dose adjustments of immediate-release and depot intramuscular injections, including *Abilify Maintena*®, due to concurrent use of interacting drugs—consult product literature.

ABILIFY MAINTENA®
Maintenance of schizophrenia in patients stabilised with oral aripiprazole who are CYP2D6 poor metabolisers [using a two-month intramuscular depot injection]
- BY DEEP INTRAMUSCULAR INJECTION USING DEPOT INJECTION
- Adult: 720 mg every 2 months, keep 56 days between injections (may be given up to 2 weeks before or 2 weeks after scheduled dose), treatment with prescribed daily dose of oral aripiprazole should be continued for 14 consecutive days after the first injection, for dose adjustments due to side-effects and for advice on missed doses—consult product literature, alternatively initially 1.02 g for 1 dose, to be administered consecutively using one 720 mg aripiprazole two-month intramuscular depot injection and one 300 mg aripiprazole once-monthly intramuscular depot injection, along with a single dose of 20 mg oral aripiprazole, then maintenance 720 mg every 2 months, keep 56 days between injections (may be given up to 2 weeks before or 2 weeks after scheduled dose), for dose adjustments due to side-effects and for advice on missed doses—consult product literature

Maintenance of schizophrenia in patients stabilised with aripiprazole once-monthly intramuscular depot injection who are CYP2D6 poor metabolisers [using a two-month intramuscular depot injection]
- BY DEEP INTRAMUSCULAR INJECTION USING DEPOT INJECTION
- Adult: 720 mg every 2 months, keep 56 days between injections (may be given up to 2 weeks before or 2 weeks after scheduled dose), initial dose to be given a minimum of 26 days after previous 300 mg aripiprazole once-monthly intramuscular depot injection, for dose adjustments due to side-effects and for advice on missed doses—consult product literature

Maintenance of schizophrenia in patients stabilised with oral aripiprazole [using a two-month intramuscular depot injection]
▸ BY DEEP INTRAMUSCULAR INJECTION USING DEPOT INJECTION
▸ Adult: 960 mg every 2 months, keep 56 days between injections (may be given up to 2 weeks before or 2 weeks after scheduled dose), treatment with 10–20 mg oral aripiprazole daily should be continued for 14 consecutive days after the first injection, for dose adjustments due to side-effects and for advice on missed doses—consult product literature, alternatively initially 1.36 g for 1 dose, to be administered consecutively using one 960 mg aripiprazole two-month intramuscular depot injection and one 400 mg aripiprazole once-monthly intramuscular depot injection, along with a single dose of 20 mg oral aripiprazole, then maintenance 960 mg every 2 months, keep 56 days between injections (may be given up to 2 weeks before or 2 weeks after scheduled dose), for dose adjustments due to side-effects and for advice on missed doses—consult product literature

Maintenance of schizophrenia in patients stabilised with aripiprazole once-monthly intramuscular depot injection [using a two-month intramuscular depot injection]
▸ BY DEEP INTRAMUSCULAR INJECTION USING DEPOT INJECTION
▸ Adult: 960 mg every 2 months, keep 56 days between injections (may be given up to 2 weeks before or 2 weeks after scheduled dose), initial dose to be given a minimum of 26 days after previous 400 mg aripiprazole once-monthly intramuscular depot injection, for dose adjustments due to side-effects and for advice on missed doses—consult product literature

IMPORTANT SAFETY INFORMATION
When prescribing, dispensing, or administering, check that the correct preparation is used—the preparation usually used in hospital for the rapid control of an *acute episode* (solution for injection containing aripiprazole 7.5 mg/mL) should **not** be confused with depot preparations administered once-monthly (powder and solvent for prolonged-release suspension for injection containing aripiprazole 300 mg or 400 mg) or every two-months (prolonged-release suspension for injection containing aripiprazole 720 mg or 960 mg), which are usually used in the community or clinics for *maintenance treatment*.

MHRA/CHM ADVICE: CLOZAPINE AND OTHER ANTIPSYCHOTICS: MONITORING BLOOD CONCENTRATIONS FOR TOXICITY (AUGUST 2020)
Following fatal cases involving toxicity of clozapine and other antipsychotic medicines, the MHRA advises that monitoring blood concentration of aripiprazole may be helpful in certain circumstances, such as patients presenting symptoms suggestive of toxicity, or when concomitant medicines may interact to increase blood concentration of aripiprazole.

MHRA/CHM ADVICE: ARIPIPRAZOLE (*ABILIFY*® AND GENERIC BRANDS): RISK OF PATHOLOGICAL GAMBLING (DECEMBER 2023)
There has been an increase in reports, via the Yellow Card Scheme, of gambling disorder and pathological gambling associated with aripiprazole in patients with and without a history of such disorders; the majority were reported to resolve upon dose reduction or treatment discontinuation. In addition, concerns have been raised with the MHRA about a lack of awareness of this issue, especially when gambling is a recognised common risk factor linked to suicide. Healthcare professionals are advised to counsel patients and their carers about this risk and to be alert for the development of new or increased urges to gamble and other impulse control symptoms, such as excessive eating or spending, or hypersexuality. The prescriber should consider reducing the dose or stopping the drug if these symptoms occur.

● CAUTIONS Cerebrovascular disease · elderly (reduce initial dose) · risk of aspiration pneumonia
● INTERACTIONS → Appendix 1: antipsychotics, second generation
● SIDE-EFFECTS

GENERAL SIDE-EFFECTS
▸ **Common or very common** Anxiety · appetite abnormal · diabetes mellitus · gastrointestinal discomfort · headache · musculoskeletal stiffness · nausea · vision disorders · weight decreased
▸ **Uncommon** Alopecia · depression · diarrhoea · hiccups · hypertension · sexual dysfunction · suicidal behaviours · thrombocytopenia
▸ **Frequency not known** Cardiac arrest · diabetic hyperosmolar coma · diabetic ketoacidosis · dysphagia · embolism and thrombosis · generalised tonic-clonic seizure · hepatic disorders · hyperhidrosis · hyponatraemia · laryngospasm · oropharyngeal spasm · pancreatitis · pathological gambling · peripheral oedema · photosensitivity reaction · pneumonia aspiration · rhabdomyolysis · serotonin syndrome · speech disorder · syncope · temperature regulation disorder · urinary incontinence

SPECIFIC SIDE-EFFECTS
▸ **Uncommon**
▸ With intramuscular use Altered smell sensation · anaemia · asthenia · behaviour abnormal · breast tenderness · chest discomfort · cough · drooling · dyslipidaemia · eye pain · fever · gait abnormal · gastrointestinal disorders · glycosuria · hyperinsulinaemia · joint disorders · muscle complaints · muscle tone increased · nephrolithiasis · oculogyric crisis · pain · skin reactions · sleep disorder · taste altered · thirst · vulvovaginal dryness
▸ **Frequency not known**
▸ With intramuscular use Binge eating · drug reaction with eosinophilia and systemic symptoms (DRESS) · poriomania · psychiatric disorders
▸ With oral use Aggression · chest pain · myalgia
● PREGNANCY Use only if potential benefit outweighs risk.
● BREAST FEEDING Manufacturer advises avoid—present in milk.
● HEPATIC IMPAIRMENT Manufacturer advises caution in severe impairment (oral treatment preferred to intramuscular administration; limited information available).
● MONITORING REQUIREMENTS
▸ Aripiprazole does not affect blood pressure to the same extent as other antipsychotic drugs and so blood pressure monitoring is not mandatory for this drug.
▸ With intramuscular use Treatment requires careful monitoring for optimum effect.
● DIRECTIONS FOR ADMINISTRATION
▸ With oral use Orodispersible tablets should be placed on the tongue and allowed to dissolve, or be dispersed in water and swallowed.
▸ With intramuscular use Use correct injection technique (including the use of z-track technique) and rotate injection sites. EvGr Inject *once-monthly depot preparations* slowly into the gluteal or deltoid muscle. For initiating treatment with 2 injections Ⓜ—consult product literature. EvGr Inject *two-month depot preparations* slowly into the gluteal muscle. For initiating treatment with 2 injections (a once-monthly depot injection and a two-month depot injection) Ⓜ—consult product literature.

- **PRESCRIBING AND DISPENSING INFORMATION**
▶ With intramuscular use A user manual for depot injections has been provided for healthcare professionals.

- **PATIENT AND CARER ADVICE** Patients or carers should be given advice on how to administer aripiprazole orodispersible tablets.

- **NATIONAL FUNDING/ACCESS DECISIONS**
For full details see funding body website

Scottish Medicines Consortium (SMC) decisions
▶ Aripiprazole prolonged-release suspension for injection (*Abilify Maintena*®) for maintenance treatment of schizophrenia in adult patients stabilised with oral aripiprazole (May 2014) SMC No. 962/14 Recommended

- **MEDICINAL FORMS** There can be variation in the licensing of different medicines containing the same drug. Forms available from special-order manufacturers include: oral solution

Oral tablet
CAUTIONARY AND ADVISORY LABELS 2
▶ Aripiprazole (Non-proprietary)
Aripiprazole 1 mg Aripiprazole 1mg tablets | 28 tablet PoM £29.50–£53.10
Aripiprazole 2.5 mg Aripiprazole 2.5mg tablets | 28 tablet PoM £29.50–£53.10
Aripiprazole 5 mg Aripiprazole 5mg tablets | 28 tablet PoM £115.25 DT = £1.63
Aripiprazole 10 mg Aripiprazole 10mg tablets | 28 tablet PoM £115.25 DT = £1.65
Aripiprazole 15 mg Aripiprazole 15mg tablets | 28 tablet PoM £115.25 DT = £1.77
Aripiprazole 30 mg Aripiprazole 30mg tablets | 28 tablet PoM £230.50 DT = £4.98
▶ Abilify (Otsuka Pharmaceuticals (U.K.) Ltd)
Aripiprazole 5 mg Abilify 5mg tablets | 28 tablet PoM £96.04 DT = £1.63
Aripiprazole 10 mg Abilify 10mg tablets | 28 tablet PoM £96.04 DT = £1.65
Aripiprazole 15 mg Abilify 15mg tablets | 28 tablet PoM £96.04 DT = £1.77
Aripiprazole 30 mg Abilify 30mg tablets | 28 tablet PoM £192.08 DT = £4.98
▶ Arpoya (Torrent Pharma (UK) Ltd)
Aripiprazole 5 mg Arpoya 5mg tablets | 28 tablet PoM £1.90 DT = £1.63
Aripiprazole 10 mg Arpoya 10mg tablets | 28 tablet PoM £1.94 DT = £1.65
Aripiprazole 15 mg Arpoya 15mg tablets | 28 tablet PoM £2.43 DT = £1.77

Solution for injection
EXCIPIENTS: May contain Sulfobutylether beta cyclodextrin sodium
▶ Abilify (Otsuka Pharmaceuticals (U.K.) Ltd)
Aripiprazole 7.5 mg per 1 ml Abilify 9.75mg/1.3ml solution for injection vials | 1 vial PoM £3.43 DT = £3.43

Oral solution
CAUTIONARY AND ADVISORY LABELS 2
EXCIPIENTS: May contain Disodium edetate, hydroxybenzoates (parabens), propylene glycol, sucrose
▶ Aripiprazole (Non-proprietary)
Aripiprazole 1 mg per 1 ml Aripiprazole 1mg/ml oral solution sugar free | 150 ml PoM £101.20 DT = £101.20 SF
Aripiprazole 1mg/ml oral solution | 150 ml PoM £101.22 DT = £22.22
▶ Abilify (Otsuka Pharmaceuticals (U.K.) Ltd)
Aripiprazole 1 mg per 1 ml Abilify 1mg/ml oral solution | 150 ml PoM £102.90 DT = £22.22

Powder and solvent for prolonged-release suspension for inj
▶ Aripiprazole (Non-proprietary)
Aripiprazole 400 mg Aripiprazole 400mg powder and solvent for prolonged-release suspension for injection vials | 1 vial PoM £220.41 DT = £220.41
Aripiprazole 400mg powder and solvent for prolonged-release suspension for injection pre-filled syringes | 1 pre-filled disposable injection PoM £220.41 DT = £220.41

Prolonged-release suspension for injection
▶ Abilify Maintena (Otsuka Pharmaceuticals (U.K.) Ltd)
Aripiprazole 300 mg per 1 ml Abilify Maintena 720mg/2.4ml prolonged-release suspension for injection pre-filled syringes | 1 pre-filled disposable injection PoM £440.00
Abilify Maintena 960mg/3.2ml prolonged-release suspension for injection pre-filled syringes | 1 pre-filled disposable injection PoM £440.00 DT = £440.00

Orodispersible tablet
CAUTIONARY AND ADVISORY LABELS 2
EXCIPIENTS: May contain Aspartame
▶ Aripiprazole (Non-proprietary)
Aripiprazole 10 mg Aripiprazole 10mg orodispersible tablets sugar free | 28 tablet PoM £79.27 DT = £24.70 SF
Aripiprazole 15 mg Aripiprazole 15mg orodispersible tablets sugar free | 28 tablet PoM £79.27 DT = £20.31 SF
▶ Abilify (Otsuka Pharmaceuticals (U.K.) Ltd)
Aripiprazole 10 mg Abilify 10mg orodispersible tablets | 28 tablet PoM £96.04 DT = £24.70 SF
Aripiprazole 15 mg Abilify 15mg orodispersible tablets | 28 tablet PoM £96.04 DT = £20.31 SF
▶ Elozar (Novumgen Ltd)
Aripiprazole 10 mg Elozar 10mg orodispersible tablets | 28 tablet PoM £15.67 DT = £24.70 SF
Aripiprazole 15 mg Elozar 15mg orodispersible tablets | 28 tablet PoM £17.67 DT = £20.31 SF

F 442

Cariprazine

27-May-2022

- **INDICATIONS AND DOSE**
Schizophrenia
▶ BY MOUTH
▶ Adult: 1.5 mg once daily, increased in steps of 1.5 mg if required; maximum 6 mg per day

- **INTERACTIONS** → Appendix 1: antipsychotics, second generation

- **SIDE-EFFECTS**
▶ **Common or very common** Anxiety · appetite abnormal · bradyphrenia · drooling · dyslipidaemia · eye disorders · gait abnormal · hypertension · joint stiffness · muscle tightness · musculoskeletal stiffness · nausea · oral disorders · pain · reflexes abnormal · sleep disorders · speech impairment · teeth grinding · vision disorders
▶ **Uncommon** Anaemia · cardiac conduction disorder · delirium · depression · diabetes mellitus · dysaesthesia · eosinophilia · eye irritation · gastrooesophageal reflux disease · grimacing · hiccups · pruritus · sexual dysfunction · suicidal behaviour · thirst · urinary disorders · vertigo
▶ **Rare or very rare** Cataract · dysphagia · hypothyroidism · memory loss · rhabdomyolysis
▶ **Frequency not known** Hepatitis toxic

- **CONCEPTION AND CONTRACEPTION** Manufacturer advises highly effective contraception in women of childbearing potential during treatment and for at least 10 weeks after the last dose; addition of barrier method recommended in women using systemically-acting hormonal contraceptives.

- **PREGNANCY** Manufacturer advises avoid—toxicity in *animal* studies.

- **BREAST FEEDING** Manufacturer advises avoid—present in milk in *animal* studies.

- **HEPATIC IMPAIRMENT** Manufacturer advises avoid in severe impairment (no information available).

- **RENAL IMPAIRMENT** Manufacturer advises avoid in severe impairment (no information available).

- **NATIONAL FUNDING/ACCESS DECISIONS**
For full details see funding body website

Scottish Medicines Consortium (SMC) decisions
▶ Cariprazine (*Reagila*®) for the treatment of schizophrenia in adult patients (May 2019) SMC No. SMC2137 Recommended with restrictions

All Wales Medicines Strategy Group (AWMSG) decisions
▶ Cariprazine (*Reagila*®) for the treatment of schizophrenia in adult patients (May 2022) AWMSG No. 5032 Recommended with restrictions

● **MEDICINAL FORMS** There can be variation in the licensing of different medicines containing the same drug.

Oral capsule
▶ Reagila (Recordati Pharmaceuticals Ltd)
Cariprazine (as Cariprazine hydrochloride) **1.5 mg** Reagila 1.5mg capsules | 28 capsule [PoM] £80.36 DT = £80.36
Cariprazine (as Cariprazine hydrochloride) **3 mg** Reagila 3mg capsules | 28 capsule [PoM] £80.36 DT = £80.36
Cariprazine (as Cariprazine hydrochloride) **4.5 mg** Reagila 4.5mg capsules | 28 capsule [PoM] £80.36 DT = £80.36
Cariprazine (as Cariprazine hydrochloride) **6 mg** Reagila 6mg capsules | 28 capsule [PoM] £80.36 DT = £80.36

▶ 442

Clozapine
04-May-2021

● **DRUG ACTION** Clozapine is a dopamine D_1, dopamine D_2, 5-HT$_{2A}$, alpha$_1$-adrenoceptor, and muscarinic-receptor antagonist.

● **INDICATIONS AND DOSE**

Schizophrenia in patients unresponsive to, or intolerant of, conventional antipsychotic drugs
▶ BY MOUTH
▶ Adult 18–59 years: 12.5 mg 1–2 times a day for day 1, then 25–50 mg for day 2, then increased, if tolerated, in steps of 25–50 mg daily, dose to be increased gradually over 14–21 days, increased to up to 300 mg daily in divided doses, larger dose to be taken at night, up to 200 mg daily may be taken as a single dose at bedtime; increased in steps of 50–100 mg 1–2 times a week if required, it is preferable to increase once a week; usual dose 200–450 mg daily, max. 900 mg per day, if restarting after interval of more than 48 hours, 12.5 mg once or twice on first day (but may be feasible to increase more quickly than on initiation)—extreme caution if previous respiratory or cardiac arrest with initial dosing
▶ Adult 60 years and over: 12.5 mg once daily for day 1, then increased to 25–37.5 mg for day 2, then increased, if tolerated, in steps of up to 25 mg daily, dose to be increased gradually over 14–21 days, increased to up to 300 mg daily in divided doses, larger dose at to be taken night, up to 200 mg daily may be taken as a single dose at bedtime; increased in steps of 50–100 mg 1–2 times a week if required, it is preferable to increase once a week; usual dose 200–450 mg daily, max. 900 mg per day, if restarting after interval of more than 48 hours, 12.5 mg once or twice on first day (but may be feasible to increase more quickly than on initiation)—extreme caution if previous respiratory or cardiac arrest with initial dosing

Psychosis in Parkinson's disease
▶ BY MOUTH
▶ Adult: 12.5 mg once daily, dose to be taken at bedtime, then increased in steps of 12.5 mg up to twice weekly, adjusted according to response; usual dose 25–37.5 mg once daily, dose to be taken at bedtime; increased in steps of 12.5 mg once weekly, this applies only in exceptional cases, increased if necessary up to 100 mg daily in 1–2 divided doses; Usual maximum 50 mg/24 hours

IMPORTANT SAFETY INFORMATION
MHRA/CHM ADVICE: CLOZAPINE: REMINDER OF POTENTIALLY FATAL RISK OF INTESTINAL OBSTRUCTION, FAECAL IMPACTION, AND PARALYTIC ILEUS (OCTOBER 2017)
Clozapine has been associated with varying degrees of impairment of intestinal peristalsis—see Cautions and Contra-indications for further information. Patients and their carers should be advised to seek immediate medical advice before taking the next dose of clozapine if constipation develops.

MHRA/CHM ADVICE: CLOZAPINE AND OTHER ANTIPSYCHOTICS: MONITORING BLOOD CONCENTRATIONS FOR TOXICITY (AUGUST 2020)
Following fatal cases involving toxicity of clozapine and other antipsychotic medicines, the MHRA recommends monitoring blood concentration of clozapine for toxicity in certain clinical situations such as when:
● a patient stops smoking or switches to an e-cigarette;
● concomitant medicines may interact to increase blood clozapine levels;
● a patient has pneumonia or other serious infection;
● reduced clozapine metabolism is suspected;
● toxicity is suspected.
Clozapine blood concentration monitoring should be carried out in addition to the required blood tests to manage the risk of agranulocytosis.

● **CONTRA-INDICATIONS** Alcoholic and toxic psychoses · bone-marrow disorders · coma · drug intoxication · history of agranulocytosis · history of circulatory collapse · history of neutropenia · paralytic ileus · severe cardiac disorders (e.g. myocarditis) · severe CNS depression · uncontrolled epilepsy

● **CAUTIONS** Age over 60 years · prostatic hypertrophy · susceptibility to angle-closure glaucoma · taper off other antipsychotics before starting

CAUTIONS, FURTHER INFORMATION
▶ Agranulocytosis Neutropenia and potentially fatal agranulocytosis reported. Leucocyte and differential blood counts must be normal before starting; monitor counts every week for 18 weeks then at least every 2 weeks and if clozapine continued and blood count stable after 1 year at least every 4 weeks (and 4 weeks after discontinuation); if leucocyte count below 3000/mm^3 or if absolute neutrophil count below 1500/mm^3 discontinue permanently and refer to haematologist. Patients who have a low white blood cell count because of benign ethnic neutropenia may be started on clozapine with the agreement of a haematologist. Avoid drugs which depress leucopoiesis; patients should report immediately symptoms of infection, especially influenza-like illness.
▶ Myocarditis and cardiomyopathy Fatal myocarditis (most commonly in first 2 months) and cardiomyopathy reported.
● Perform physical examination and take full medical history before starting
● Specialist examination required if cardiac abnormalities or history of heart disease found—clozapine initiated only in absence of severe heart disease and if benefit outweighs risk
● Persistent tachycardia especially in first 2 months should prompt observation for other indicators for myocarditis or cardiomyopathy
● If myocarditis or cardiomyopathy suspected clozapine should be stopped and patient evaluated urgently by cardiologist
● Discontinue permanently in clozapine-induced myocarditis or cardiomyopathy
▶ Intestinal obstruction Impairment of intestinal peristalsis, including constipation, intestinal obstruction, faecal impaction, and paralytic ileus, (including fatal cases) reported. Clozapine should be used with caution in patients receiving drugs that may cause constipation (e.g. antimuscarinic drugs) or in those with a history of colonic disease or lower abdominal surgery. It is essential that constipation is recognised and actively treated.

● **INTERACTIONS** → Appendix 1: antipsychotics, second generation

- **SIDE-EFFECTS**
- ▶ **Common or very common** Appetite decreased · eosinophilia · fever · headache · hypertension · leucocytosis · nausea · speech impairment · sweating abnormal · syncope · temperature regulation disorders · urinary disorders · vision blurred
- ▶ **Uncommon** Fall
- ▶ **Rare or very rare** Anaemia · cardiac arrest · cardiac inflammation · cardiomyopathy · circulatory collapse · delirium · diabetes mellitus · diabetic hyperosmolar coma · dyslipidaemia · dysphagia · embolism and thrombosis · gastrointestinal disorders · glucose tolerance impaired · hepatic disorders · increased risk of infection · intestinal obstruction (including fatal cases) · ketoacidosis · nephritis tubulointerstitial · obesity · obsessive-compulsive disorder · pancreatitis · parotid gland enlargement · pericardial effusion · respiratory disorders · restlessness · sexual dysfunction · skin reactions · sleep apnoea · thrombocytopenia · thrombocytosis
- ▶ **Frequency not known** Angina pectoris · angioedema · chest pain · cholinergic syndrome · diarrhoea · gastrointestinal discomfort · hypersensitivity vasculitis · mitral valve incompetence · muscle complaints · muscle weakness · myocardial infarction · nasal congestion · palpitations · polyserositis · pseudophaeochromocytoma · renal failure · rhabdomyolysis · sepsis · systemic lupus erythematosus (SLE)

SIDE-EFFECTS, FURTHER INFORMATION Hypersalivation associated with clozapine therapy can be treated with hyoscine hydrobromide [unlicensed indication], provided that the patient is not at particular risk from the additive antimuscarinic side-effects of hyoscine and clozapine.

- **PREGNANCY** Use with caution.
- **BREAST FEEDING** Avoid.
- **HEPATIC IMPAIRMENT** Manufacturer advises caution— monitor liver function (discontinue if liver enzymes are greater than 3 times the upper limit of normal or jaundice occurs); avoid in symptomatic or progressive impairment and in hepatic failure.
- **RENAL IMPAIRMENT** EvGr Avoid in severe impairment. Ⓜ
- **MONITORING REQUIREMENTS**
- ▶ Monitor leucocyte and differential blood counts. Clozapine requires differential white blood cell monitoring weekly for 18 weeks, then fortnightly for up to one year, and then monthly as part of the clozapine patient monitoring service.
- ▶ Blood clozapine concentration should be monitored in certain clinical situations—consult product literature.
- ▶ Close medical supervision during initiation (risk of collapse because of hypotension and convulsions).
- ▶ Blood lipids and weight should be measured at baseline, at 3 months (weight should be measured at frequent intervals during the first 3 months), and then yearly with antipsychotics. Patients taking clozapine require more frequent monitoring of these parameters: every 3 months for the first year, then yearly.
- ▶ Fasting blood glucose should be measured at baseline, at 4–6 months, and then yearly. Patients taking clozapine should have fasting blood glucose tested at baseline, after one months' treatment, then every 4–6 months.
- ▶ Patient, prescriber, and supplying pharmacist must be registered with the appropriate Patient Monitoring Service—it takes several days to do this.
- **TREATMENT CESSATION** On planned withdrawal reduce dose over 1–2 weeks to avoid risk of rebound psychosis. If abrupt withdrawal necessary observe patient carefully.
- **DIRECTIONS FOR ADMINISTRATION** Manufacturer advises shake oral suspension well for 90 seconds when dispensing or if visibly settled and stand for 24 hours before use; otherwise shake well for 10 seconds before use. May be

diluted with water. Orodispersible tablets should be placed on the tongue, allowed to dissolve and swallowed.

- **PRESCRIBING AND DISPENSING INFORMATION** Clozapine has been used for psychosis in Parkinson's disease in children aged 16 years and over.
- **PATIENT AND CARER ADVICE** Patients or carers should be given advice on how to administer clozapine oral suspension and orodispersible tablets.

- **MEDICINAL FORMS** There can be variation in the licensing of different medicines containing the same drug. Forms available from special-order manufacturers include: oral suspension, oral solution

Oral tablet

CAUTIONARY AND ADVISORY LABELS 2, 10

- ▶ **Clozapine** (Non-proprietary)
  Clozapine 25 mg Clozapine 25mg tablets | 28 tablet [PoM] £3.02 (Hospital only) | 84 tablet [PoM] £8.40 DT = £16.64 (Hospital only) | 100 tablet [PoM] £10.00 (Hospital only)
  Clozapine 100 mg Clozapine 100mg tablets | 28 tablet [PoM] £12.07 (Hospital only) | 84 tablet [PoM] £33.60 DT = £66.53 (Hospital only) | 100 tablet [PoM] £39.00 (Hospital only)
- ▶ **Clozaril** (Viatris UK Healthcare Ltd)
  Clozapine 25 mg Clozaril 25mg tablets | 28 tablet [PoM] £3.02 (Hospital only) | 84 tablet [PoM] £8.40 DT = £16.64 (Hospital only) | 100 tablet [PoM] £10.00 (Hospital only)
  Clozapine 100 mg Clozaril 100mg tablets | 28 tablet [PoM] £12.07 (Hospital only) | 84 tablet [PoM] £33.60 DT = £66.53 (Hospital only) | 100 tablet [PoM] £39.00 (Hospital only)
- ▶ **Denzapine** (Britannia Pharmaceuticals Ltd)
  Clozapine 25 mg Denzapine 25mg tablets | 84 tablet [PoM] £16.64 DT = £16.64 | 100 tablet [PoM] £19.80
  Clozapine 50 mg Denzapine 50mg tablets | 100 tablet [PoM] £39.60 DT = £39.60
  Clozapine 100 mg Denzapine 100mg tablets | 84 tablet [PoM] £66.53 DT = £66.53 | 100 tablet [PoM] £79.20
  Clozapine 200 mg Denzapine 200mg tablets | 100 tablet [PoM] £158.40 DT = £158.40
- ▶ **Zaponex** (Leyden Delta B.V.)
  Clozapine 25 mg Zaponex 25mg tablets | 84 tablet [PoM] £8.28 DT = £16.64 | 500 tablet [PoM] £48.39
  Clozapine 100 mg Zaponex 100mg tablets | 84 tablet [PoM] £33.88 DT = £66.53 | 500 tablet [PoM] £196.43

Oral suspension

CAUTIONARY AND ADVISORY LABELS 2, 10

- ▶ **Denzapine** (Britannia Pharmaceuticals Ltd)
  Clozapine 50 mg per 1 ml Denzapine 50mg/ml oral suspension | 100 ml [PoM] £77.73 DT = £77.73 [SF]

Orodispersible tablet

CAUTIONARY AND ADVISORY LABELS 2, 10
EXCIPIENTS: May contain Aspartame

- ▶ **Zaponex** (Leyden Delta B.V.)
  Clozapine 12.5 mg Zaponex 12.5mg orodispersible tablets | 28 tablet [PoM] £2.77 DT = £2.77 [SF]
  Clozapine 25 mg Zaponex 25mg orodispersible tablets | 28 tablet [PoM] £5.55 DT = £5.55 [SF]
  Clozapine 50 mg Zaponex 50mg orodispersible tablets | 28 tablet [PoM] £11.09 DT = £11.09 [SF]
  Clozapine 100 mg Zaponex 100mg orodispersible tablets | 28 tablet [PoM] £22.18 DT = £22.18 [SF]
  Clozapine 200 mg Zaponex 200mg orodispersible tablets | 28 tablet [PoM] £44.35 DT = £44.35 [SF]

F 442

Lurasidone hydrochloride

08-Jul-2021

- **DRUG ACTION** Lurasidone is a dopamine D_2, $5\text{-}HT_{2A}$, $5\text{-}HT_7$, alpha$_{2A}$- and alpha$_{2C}$- adrenoceptor antagonist, and is a partial agonist at $5\text{-}HT_{1a}$ receptors.

- **INDICATIONS AND DOSE**

Schizophrenia

- ▶ BY MOUTH
- ▶ Adult: Initially 37 mg once daily, increased if necessary up to 148 mg once daily, for advice on restarting treatment following interruption—consult product literature

Schizophrenia [when given with moderate CYP3A4 inhibitors (e.g. diltiazem, erythromycin, fluconazole, and verapamil)]
▶ BY MOUTH
▶ Adult: Initially 18.5 mg once daily (max. per dose 74 mg once daily)

● **CAUTIONS** High doses in elderly · susceptibility to QT-interval prolongation

● **INTERACTIONS** → Appendix 1: antipsychotics, second generation

● **SIDE-EFFECTS**
▶ **Common or very common** Anxiety · drooling · gastrointestinal discomfort · hypersensitivity · musculoskeletal stiffness · nausea · oculogyric crisis · pain · pruritus · psychiatric disorders · sleep disorders · tongue spasm
▶ **Uncommon** Appetite decreased · dysarthria · dysuria · gait abnormal · gastrointestinal disorders · hot flush · hyperhidrosis · hypertension · hyponatraemia · joint stiffness · myalgia · nasopharyngitis · vision blurred
▶ **Rare or very rare** Angioedema · eosinophilia · rhabdomyolysis
▶ **Frequency not known** Anaemia · angina pectoris · atrioventricular block · breast abnormalities · diarrhoea · dysmenorrhoea · dysphagia · renal failure · Stevens-Johnson syndrome · suicidal behaviour · vertigo

● **PREGNANCY** EvGr Use only if potential benefit outweighs risk—limited information available. M

● **BREAST FEEDING** EvGr Use only if potential benefit outweighs risk—present in milk in *animal* studies. M

● **HEPATIC IMPAIRMENT** Manufacturer advises caution in moderate to severe impairment (risk of increased exposure).
Dose adjustments Manufacturer advises initially 18.5 mg once daily in moderate to severe impairment, increased if necessary up to 74 mg once daily in moderate impairment, or up to max. 37 mg once daily in severe impairment.

● **RENAL IMPAIRMENT** EvGr Use only if potential benefit outweighs risk if creatinine clearance less than 15 mL/minute. M
Dose adjustments EvGr Initially 18.5 mg once daily, up to max. 74 mg once daily if creatinine clearance less than 50 mL/minute, M see p. 21.

● **NATIONAL FUNDING/ACCESS DECISIONS**
For full details see funding body website
All Wales Medicines Strategy Group (AWMSG) decisions
▶ Lurasidone (*Latuda*®) for the treatment of schizophrenia in adults and adolescents aged 13 years and over (March 2021) AWMSG No. 4394 Recommended

● **MEDICINAL FORMS** There can be variation in the licensing of different medicines containing the same drug.
Oral tablet
CAUTIONARY AND ADVISORY LABELS 2, 21, 25
▶ Lurasidone hydrochloride (Non-proprietary)
Lurasidone (as Lurasidone hydrochloride) **18.5 mg** Lurasidone 18.5mg tablets | 28 tablet PoM £79.99 DT = £80.00
Lurasidone (as Lurasidone hydrochloride) **37 mg** Lurasidone 37mg tablets | 28 tablet PoM £79.99 DT = £80.00
Lurasidone (as Lurasidone hydrochloride) **74 mg** Lurasidone 74mg tablets | 28 tablet PoM £79.99 DT = £80.00
▶ Latuda (CNX Therapeutics Ltd)
Lurasidone (as Lurasidone hydrochloride) **18.5 mg** Latuda 18.5mg tablets | 28 tablet PoM £80.00 DT = £80.00
Lurasidone (as Lurasidone hydrochloride) **37 mg** Latuda 37mg tablets | 28 tablet PoM £80.00 DT = £80.00
Lurasidone (as Lurasidone hydrochloride) **74 mg** Latuda 74mg tablets | 28 tablet PoM £80.00 DT = £80.00

⚑ 442

Olanzapine

25-Sep-2024

● **DRUG ACTION** Olanzapine is a dopamine D_1, D_2, D_4, 5-HT_2, histamine-1-, and muscarinic-receptor antagonist.

● **INDICATIONS AND DOSE**
Schizophrenia | Combination therapy for mania
▶ BY MOUTH
▶ Adult: 10 mg daily, adjusted according to response, usual dose 5–20 mg daily, doses greater than 10 mg daily only after reassessment, when one or more factors present that might result in slower metabolism (e.g. females, elderly, non-smoker) consider lower initial dose and more gradual dose increase; maximum 20 mg per day

Preventing recurrence in bipolar disorder
▶ BY MOUTH
▶ Adult: 10 mg daily, adjusted according to response, usual dose 5–20 mg daily, doses greater than 10 mg daily only after reassessment, when one or more factors present that might result in slower metabolism (e.g. females, elderly, non-smoker) consider lower initial dose and more gradual dose increase; maximum 20 mg per day

Monotherapy for mania
▶ BY MOUTH
▶ Adult: 15 mg daily, adjusted according to response, usual dose 5–20 mg daily, doses greater than 15 mg daily only after reassessment, when one or more factors present that might result in slower metabolism (e.g. females, elderly, non-smoker) consider lower initial dose and more gradual dose increase; maximum 20 mg per day

Control of agitation and disturbed behaviour in schizophrenia or mania
▶ BY INTRAMUSCULAR INJECTION
▶ Adult: Initially 5–10 mg for 1 dose; usual dose 10 mg for 1 dose, followed by 5–10 mg after 2 hours if required, maximum 3 injections daily for 3 days; maximum daily combined oral and parenteral dose 20 mg, when one or more factors present that might result in slower metabolism (e.g. females, elderly, non-smoker) consider lower initial dose and more gradual dose increase
▶ Elderly: Initially 2.5–5 mg, followed by 2.5–5 mg after 2 hours if required, maximum 3 injections daily for 3 days; maximum daily combined oral and parenteral dose 20 mg, when one or more factors present that might result in slower metabolism (e.g. females, elderly, non-smoker) consider lower initial dose and more gradual dose increase

---

IMPORTANT SAFETY INFORMATION
MHRA/CHM ADVICE: CLOZAPINE AND OTHER ANTIPSYCHOTICS: MONITORING BLOOD CONCENTRATIONS FOR TOXICITY (AUGUST 2020)
Following fatal cases involving toxicity of clozapine and other antipsychotic medicines, the MHRA advises that monitoring blood concentration of olanzapine may be helpful in certain circumstances, such as patients presenting symptoms suggestive of toxicity, or when concomitant medicines may interact to increase blood concentration of olanzapine.

● **CONTRA-INDICATIONS**
▶ With intramuscular use Acute myocardial infarction · bradycardia · recent heart surgery · severe hypotension · sick sinus syndrome · unstable angina

● **CAUTIONS** Bone-marrow depression · hypereosinophilic disorders · low leucocyte count · low neutrophil count · myeloproliferative disease · paralytic ileus
CAUTIONS, FURTHER INFORMATION
▸ CNS and respiratory depression
▸ With intramuscular use Blood pressure, pulse and respiratory rate should be monitored for at least 4 hours after intramuscular injection, particularly in those also receiving a benzodiazepine or another antipsychotic (leave at least one hour between administration of olanzapine intramuscular injection and parenteral benzodiazepines).

● **INTERACTIONS** → Appendix 1: antipsychotics, second generation

● **SIDE-EFFECTS**
GENERAL SIDE-EFFECTS
▸ **Common or very common** Anticholinergic syndrome · appetite increased · arthralgia · asthenia · eosinophilia · fever · glycosuria · oedema · sexual dysfunction
▸ **Uncommon** Abdominal distension · alopecia · breast enlargement · diabetes mellitus · embolism and thrombosis · epistaxis · memory loss · oculogyration · photosensitivity reaction · urinary disorders
▸ **Rare or very rare** Hepatic disorders · hypothermia · pancreatitis · rhabdomyolysis · thrombocytopenia
SPECIFIC SIDE-EFFECTS
▸ **Common or very common**
▸ With oral use Hypersomnia
▸ **Uncommon**
▸ With intramuscular use Respiratory disorders · speech impairment
▸ With oral use Diabetic coma · dysarthria · ketoacidosis
▸ **Rare or very rare**
▸ With intramuscular use Withdrawal syndrome
▸ **Frequency not known**
▸ With intramuscular use Cerebrovascular adverse events · drug reaction with eosinophilia and systemic symptoms (DRESS) · erythema · fall · gait abnormal · hallucinations · pneumonia

● **PREGNANCY** Use only if potential benefit outweighs risk; neonatal lethargy, tremor, and hypertonia reported when used in third trimester.

● **BREAST FEEDING** Avoid—present in milk.

● **HEPATIC IMPAIRMENT** Manufacturer advises caution.
Dose adjustments ⟨EvGr⟩ Consider initial dose of 5 mg and cautious titration. ⟨M⟩

● **RENAL IMPAIRMENT**
Dose adjustments ⟨EvGr⟩ Consider initial dose of 5 mg. ⟨M⟩

● **MONITORING REQUIREMENTS**
▸ Blood lipids and weight should be measured at baseline, at 3 months (weight should be measured at frequent intervals during the first 3 months), and then yearly with antipsychotic drugs. Patients taking olanzapine require more frequent monitoring of these parameters: every 3 months for the first year, then yearly.
▸ Fasting blood glucose should be measured at baseline, at 4–6 months, and then yearly. Patients taking olanzapine should have fasting blood glucose tested at baseline, after one months' treatment, then every 4–6 months.

● **DIRECTIONS FOR ADMINISTRATION** Manufacturer advises olanzapine orodispersible tablet may be placed on the tongue and allowed to dissolve, or dispersed in water, orange juice, apple juice, milk, or coffee.

● **PRESCRIBING AND DISPENSING INFORMATION**
▸ With intramuscular use When prescribing, dispensing, or administering, check that this injection is the correct preparation—this preparation is usually used in hospital for the rapid control of an *acute episode* and should **not** be confused with depot preparations which are usually used in the community or clinics for *maintenance* treatment.

● **PATIENT AND CARER ADVICE** Patients or carers should be given advice on how to administer orodispersible tablets.

● **MEDICINAL FORMS** There can be variation in the licensing of different medicines containing the same drug. Forms available from special-order manufacturers include: oral suspension, oral solution

Oral tablet
CAUTIONARY AND ADVISORY LABELS 2
▸ **Olanzapine (Non-proprietary)**
Olanzapine 2.5 mg Olanzapine 2.5mg tablets | 28 tablet [PoM] £22.28 DT = £1.17
Olanzapine 5 mg Olanzapine 5mg tablets | 28 tablet [PoM] £44.57 DT = £1.81
Olanzapine 7.5 mg Olanzapine 7.5mg tablets | 28 tablet [PoM] £2.14 DT = £1.34 | 56 tablet [PoM] £2.50–£133.72
Olanzapine 10 mg Olanzapine 10mg tablets | 28 tablet [PoM] £89.15 DT = £2.29
Olanzapine 15 mg Olanzapine 15mg tablets | 28 tablet [PoM] £121.56 DT = £2.29
Olanzapine 20 mg Olanzapine 20mg tablets | 28 tablet [PoM] £162.07 DT = £2.39
▸ **Zyprexa** (Neon Healthcare Ltd)
Olanzapine 2.5 mg Zyprexa 2.5mg tablets | 28 tablet [PoM] £21.85 DT = £1.17
Olanzapine 5 mg Zyprexa 5mg tablets | 28 tablet [PoM] £43.70 DT = £1.81
Olanzapine 7.5 mg Zyprexa 7.5mg tablets | 56 tablet [PoM] £131.10
Olanzapine 10 mg Zyprexa 10mg tablets | 28 tablet [PoM] £87.40 DT = £2.29
Olanzapine 15 mg Zyprexa 15mg tablets | 28 tablet [PoM] £119.18 DT = £2.29
Olanzapine 20 mg Zyprexa 20mg tablets | 28 tablet [PoM] £158.90 DT = £2.39

Powder for solution for injection
EXCIPIENTS: May contain Maltose
▸ **Ceyxa** (Nordic Pharma Ltd)
Olanzapine 10 mg Ceyxa 10mg powder for solution for injection vials | 1 vial [PoM] £35.95 (Hospital only)
▸ **Xyquila** (Eramol (UK) Ltd)
Olanzapine 10 mg Xyquila 10mg powder for solution for injection vials | 1 vial [PoM] £24.50 (Hospital only)

Oral lyophilisate
▸ **Zyprexa** (Neon Healthcare Ltd)
Olanzapine 5 mg Zyprexa 5mg Velotabs | 28 tablet [PoM] £48.07 DT = £48.07 [SF]
Olanzapine 10 mg Zyprexa 10mg Velotabs | 28 tablet [PoM] £87.40 DT = £87.40 [SF]
Olanzapine 15 mg Zyprexa 15mg Velotabs | 28 tablet [PoM] £131.10 DT = £131.10 [SF]
Olanzapine 20 mg Zyprexa 20mg Velotabs | 28 tablet [PoM] £174.79 DT = £174.79 [SF]

Orodispersible tablet
CAUTIONARY AND ADVISORY LABELS 2
EXCIPIENTS: May contain Aspartame
▸ **Olanzapine (Non-proprietary)**
Olanzapine 5 mg Olanzapine 5mg orodispersible tablets sugar free | 28 tablet [PoM] £5.13–£49.02 DT = £5.13 [SF]
Olanzapine 5mg orodispersible tablets | 28 tablet [PoM] £30.00 DT = £6.31
Olanzapine 10 mg Olanzapine 10mg orodispersible tablets | 28 tablet [PoM] £50.00 DT = £9.12
Olanzapine 10mg orodispersible tablets sugar free | 28 tablet [PoM] £7.05–£89.04 DT = £7.05 [SF]
Olanzapine 15 mg Olanzapine 15mg orodispersible tablets sugar free | 28 tablet [PoM] £8.73–£133.72 DT = £8.73 [SF]
Olanzapine 20 mg Olanzapine 20mg orodispersible tablets sugar free | 28 tablet [PoM] £11.34–£178.28 DT = £11.34 [SF]
Olanzapine 20mg orodispersible tablets | 28 tablet [PoM] £80.00 DT = £13.38

Paliperidone

`F 442`

27-Apr-2023

- **DRUG ACTION** Paliperidone is a metabolite of risperidone.

- **INDICATIONS AND DOSE**

Schizophrenia | Psychotic or manic symptoms of schizoaffective disorder

- ▶ BY MOUTH
- ▶ Adult: 6 mg once daily, dose to be taken in the morning, then adjusted in steps of 3 mg if required, dose to be adjusted over at least 5 days; usual dose 3–12 mg daily

Schizophrenia [in patients stabilised on oral paliperidone or oral risperidone] | Schizophrenia [in patients previously responsive to oral paliperidone or risperidone]

- ▶ BY DEEP INTRAMUSCULAR INJECTION
- ▶ Adult: 150 mg for 1 dose on day 1, followed by 100 mg for 1 dose on day 8, then maintenance 75 mg once a month, alternatively maintenance 25–150 mg once a month, dose to be adjusted according to response, for maintenance doses required to achieve similar previous steady-state levels of paliperidone or risperidone—consult product literature, for advice on missed doses—consult product literature

Schizophrenia [in patients stabilised on intramuscular risperidone]

- ▶ BY DEEP INTRAMUSCULAR INJECTION
- ▶ Adult: 25–150 mg once a month, dose to be adjusted according to response, starting dose is based on previous intramuscular risperidone and should be initiated in place of the next scheduled dose—consult product literature, for advice on missed doses—consult product literature

BYANNLI ® PRE-FILLED SYRINGES

Schizophrenia [in patients stabilised on once- or three-monthly intramuscular paliperidone]

- ▶ BY DEEP INTRAMUSCULAR INJECTION
- ▶ Adult: 700–1000 mg every 6 months, dose to be adjusted according to response, starting dose is based on previous once- or three-monthly intramuscular paliperidone and should be initiated in place of the next scheduled dose—consult product literature, for advice on missed doses—consult product literature

TREVICTA ® PRE-FILLED SYRINGES

Schizophrenia [in patients stabilised on once-monthly intramuscular paliperidone]

- ▶ BY DEEP INTRAMUSCULAR INJECTION
- ▶ Adult: 175–525 mg every 3 months, dose to be adjusted according to response, starting dose is based on previous once-monthly intramuscular paliperidone and should be initiated in place of the next scheduled dose—consult product literature, for advice on missed doses—consult product literature

- **CAUTIONS**

GENERAL CAUTIONS Cataract surgery (risk of intraoperative floppy iris syndrome) · dementia with Lewy bodies · elderly patients with dementia · elderly patients with risk factors for stroke · predisposition to gastro-intestinal obstruction · prolactin-dependent tumours

SPECIFIC CAUTIONS

- ▶ With intramuscular use When transferring from oral to depot therapy, the dose by mouth should be reduced gradually

- **INTERACTIONS** → Appendix 1: antipsychotics, second generation

- **SIDE-EFFECTS**

GENERAL SIDE-EFFECTS

- ▶ **Common or very common** Anxiety · appetite abnormal · asthenia · cardiac conduction disorders · cough · depression · diarrhoea · drooling · eye disorders · facial spasm · fever · gastrointestinal discomfort · glabellar reflex abnormal · headache · hypertension · increased risk of infection · joint disorders · laryngeal pain · mood altered · muscle complaints · muscle contracture · musculoskeletal stiffness · nasal congestion · nausea · neuromuscular dysfunction · oral disorders · oropharyngeal spasm · pain · respiratory disorders · skin reactions · vision disorders · weight decreased

- ▶ **Uncommon** Alopecia · anaemia · breast abnormalities · chest discomfort · chills · concentration impaired · conjunctivitis · cystitis · diabetes mellitus · dry eye · dysarthria · dysphagia · dyspnoea · ear pain · epistaxis · fall · gait abnormal · gastrointestinal disorders · generalised tonic-clonic seizure · hypoglycaemia · induration · malaise · menstrual cycle irregularities · muscle weakness · oedema · palpitations · sensation abnormal · sexual dysfunction · sleep disorders · syncope · taste altered · thirst · thrombocytopenia · tinnitus · urinary disorders · vertigo

- ▶ **Rare or very rare** Angioedema · cerebrovascular insufficiency · coma · consciousness impaired · dandruff · diabetic ketoacidosis · dysphonia · embolism and thrombosis · flushing · glaucoma · hypothermia · ischaemia · jaundice · pancreatitis · polydipsia · posture abnormal · rhabdomyolysis · SIADH · sleep apnoea · vaginal discharge · water intoxication · withdrawal syndrome

- ▶ **Frequency not known** Severe cutaneous adverse reactions (SCARs)

SPECIFIC SIDE-EFFECTS

- ▶ **Common or very common**
- ▶ With intramuscular use Cervical spasm · tetany
- ▶ **Rare or very rare**
- ▶ With intramuscular use Catatonia · unresponsive to stimuli
- ▶ **Frequency not known**
- ▶ With intramuscular use Injection site necrosis

- **PREGNANCY** EvGr Use only if potential benefit outweighs risk (toxicity in *animal* studies). Ⓜ
- ▶ With oral use EvGr If discontinuation during pregnancy is necessary, withdraw gradually. Ⓜ

BYANNLI ® PRE-FILLED SYRINGES EvGr Consider long-acting nature of formulation (paliperidone may be detected in plasma up to 4 years after single dose). Ⓜ

TREVICTA ® PRE-FILLED SYRINGES EvGr Consider long-acting nature of formulation (paliperidone may be detected in plasma up to 18 months after single dose). Ⓜ

- **BREAST FEEDING** EvGr Avoid (present in milk). Ⓜ

BYANNLI ® PRE-FILLED SYRINGES EvGr Consider long-acting nature of formulation (paliperidone may be detected in plasma up to 4 years after single dose). Ⓜ

TREVICTA ® PRE-FILLED SYRINGES EvGr Consider long-acting nature of formulation (paliperidone may be detected in plasma up to 18 months after single dose). Ⓜ

- **HEPATIC IMPAIRMENT** EvGr Caution in severe impairment (no information available). Ⓜ

- **RENAL IMPAIRMENT** See p. 21.
- ▶ With oral use EvGr Avoid if creatinine clearance less than 10 mL/minute. Ⓜ
- ▶ With intramuscular use EvGr Avoid if creatinine clearance less than 50 mL/minute. Ⓜ

Dose adjustments

- ▶ With oral use EvGr Reduce initial dose to 3 mg once daily if creatinine clearance 50–79 mL/minute (max. 6 mg once daily). Reduce initial dose to 3 mg on alternate days if creatinine clearance 10–49 mL/minute (max. 3 mg once daily). Ⓜ

▶ With intramuscular use [EvGr] For once-monthly formulations, reduce initial dose to 100 mg on day 1 then 75 mg on day 8 if creatinine clearance 50–79 mL/minute; recommended maintenance dose 50 mg (range 25–100 mg) once a month if creatinine clearance 50–79 mL/minute. Ⓜ

BYANNLI ® PRE-FILLED SYRINGES Dose adjustments [EvGr] Max. dose 700 mg every 6 months if creatinine clearance 50-80 mL/minute. Ⓜ

● MONITORING REQUIREMENTS
▶ With intramuscular use Treatment requires careful monitoring for optimum effect.

● DIRECTIONS FOR ADMINISTRATION
▶ With intramuscular use Use correct injection technique (including the use of z-track technique) and rotate injection sites. For once-monthly formulations, inject initial doses (days 1 and 8) slowly into the deltoid muscle; maintenance doses may be injected slowly into the deltoid or gluteal muscle.
▶ With oral use Always take tablets with breakfast or always take on an empty stomach.

BYANNLI ® PRE-FILLED SYRINGES Inject slowly into the gluteal muscle.

TREVICTA ® PRE-FILLED SYRINGES Inject slowly into the deltoid or gluteal muscle.

● PRESCRIBING AND DISPENSING INFORMATION The 25 mg pre-filled syringes for once-monthly dosing may be difficult to obtain.

● PATIENT AND CARER ADVICE Patients or carers should be given advice on how to administer tablets.

● NATIONAL FUNDING/ACCESS DECISIONS

TREVICTA ® PRE-FILLED SYRINGES For full details see funding body website

Scottish Medicines Consortium (SMC) decisions
▶ Paliperidone palmitate (*Trevicta* ®), a three-monthly injection, is indicated for the maintenance treatment of schizophrenia in adult patients who are clinically stable on one-monthly paliperidone palmitate injectable product (September 2016) SMC No. 1181/16 Recommended

● MEDICINAL FORMS There can be variation in the licensing of different medicines containing the same drug.
Prolonged-release suspension for injection
EXCIPIENTS: May contain Polysorbates
▶ **Paliperidone (Non-proprietary)**
Paliperidone (as Paliperidone palmitate) 100 mg per 1 ml Paliperidone 50mg/0.5ml prolonged-release suspension for injection pre-filled syringes | 1 pre-filled disposable injection [PoM] £147.14-£294.28 DT = £183.92
Paliperidone 75mg/0.75ml prolonged-release suspension for injection pre-filled syringes | 1 pre-filled disposable injection [PoM] £195.92-£391.84 DT = £244.90 | 1 pre-filled disposable injection [PoM] £220.41 DT = £244.90 (Hospital only)
Paliperidone 100mg/1ml prolonged-release suspension for injection pre-filled syringes | 1 pre-filled disposable injection [PoM] £251.26-£502.52 DT = £314.07 | 1 pre-filled disposable injection [PoM] £282.66 DT = £314.07 (Hospital only)
Paliperidone 150mg/1.5ml prolonged-release suspension for injection pre-filled syringes | 1 pre-filled disposable injection [PoM] £314.07-£628.14 DT = £392.59 | 1 pre-filled disposable injection [PoM] £353.33 DT = £392.59 (Hospital only)
▶ **Byannli** (Janssen-Cilag Ltd)
Paliperidone (as Paliperidone palmitate) 200 mg per 1 ml Byannli 1000mg/5ml prolonged-release suspension for injection pre-filled syringes | 1 pre-filled disposable injection [PoM] £2,355.54 (Hospital only)
Byannli 700mg/3.5ml prolonged-release suspension for injection pre-filled syringes | 1 pre-filled disposable injection [PoM] £1,884.42 (Hospital only)
▶ **Trevicta** (Janssen-Cilag Ltd)
Paliperidone (as Paliperidone palmitate) 200 mg per 1 ml Trevicta 175mg/0.875ml prolonged-release suspension for injection pre-filled syringes | 1 pre-filled disposable injection [PoM] £551.76 DT = £551.76

Trevicta 263mg/1.315ml prolonged-release suspension for injection pre-filled syringes | 1 pre-filled disposable injection [PoM] £734.70 DT = £734.70
Trevicta 350mg/1.75ml prolonged-release suspension for injection pre-filled syringes | 1 pre-filled disposable injection [PoM] £942.21 DT = £942.21
Trevicta 525mg/2.625ml prolonged-release suspension for injection pre-filled syringes | 1 pre-filled disposable injection [PoM] £1,177.77 DT = £1,177.77
▶ **Xeplion** (Janssen-Cilag Ltd)
Paliperidone (as Paliperidone palmitate) 100 mg per 1 ml Xeplion 100mg/1ml prolonged-release suspension for injection pre-filled syringes | 1 pre-filled disposable injection [PoM] £314.07 DT = £314.07
Xeplion 150mg/1.5ml prolonged-release suspension for injection pre-filled syringes | 1 pre-filled disposable injection [PoM] £392.59 DT = £392.59
Xeplion 50mg/0.5ml prolonged-release suspension for injection pre-filled syringes | 1 pre-filled disposable injection [PoM] £183.92 DT = £183.92
Xeplion 75mg/0.75ml prolonged-release suspension for injection pre-filled syringes | 1 pre-filled disposable injection [PoM] £244.90 DT = £244.90

Modified-release tablet
CAUTIONARY AND ADVISORY LABELS 2, 25
▶ **Invega** (Janssen-Cilag Ltd)
Paliperidone 3 mg Invega 3mg modified-release tablets | 28 tablet [PoM] £97.28 DT = £97.28
Paliperidone 6 mg Invega 6mg modified-release tablets | 28 tablet [PoM] £97.28 DT = £97.28
Paliperidone 9 mg Invega 9mg modified-release tablets | 28 tablet [PoM] £145.92 DT = £145.92

☛ 442

Quetiapine

22-Aug-2022

● DRUG ACTION Quetiapine is a dopamine D_1, dopamine D_2, 5-HT_2, alpha$_1$-adrenoceptor, and histamine-1 receptor antagonist.

● INDICATIONS AND DOSE
Schizophrenia
▶ BY MOUTH USING IMMEDIATE-RELEASE MEDICINES
▶ Adult: 25 mg twice daily for day 1, then 50 mg twice daily for day 2, then 100 mg twice daily for day 3, then 150 mg twice daily for day 4, then, adjusted according to response, usual dose 300–450 mg daily in 2 divided doses, the rate of dose titration may need to be slower and the daily dose lower in elderly patients; maximum 750 mg per day
▶ BY MOUTH USING MODIFIED-RELEASE MEDICINES
▶ Adult: 300 mg once daily for day 1, then 600 mg once daily for day 2, then, adjusted according to response, usual dose 600 mg once daily, maximum dose under specialist supervision; maximum 800 mg per day
▶ Elderly: Initially 50 mg once daily, adjusted according to response. adjusted in steps of 50 mg daily

Treatment of mania in bipolar disorder
▶ BY MOUTH USING IMMEDIATE-RELEASE MEDICINES
▶ Adult: 50 mg twice daily for day 1, then 100 mg twice daily for day 2, then 150 mg twice daily for day 3, then 200 mg twice daily for day 4, then adjusted in steps of up to 200 mg daily, adjusted according to response, usual dose 400–800 mg daily in 2 divided doses, the rate of dose titration may need to be slower and the daily dose lower in elderly patients; maximum 800 mg per day
▶ BY MOUTH USING MODIFIED-RELEASE MEDICINES
▶ Adult: 300 mg once daily for day 1, then 600 mg once daily for day 2, then, adjusted according to response, usual dose 400–800 mg once daily
▶ Elderly: Initially 50 mg once daily, adjusted according to response. adjusted in steps of 50 mg daily

Treatment of depression in bipolar disorder
▶ BY MOUTH USING IMMEDIATE-RELEASE MEDICINES
▶ Adult: 50 mg once daily for day 1, dose to be taken at bedtime, then 100 mg once daily for day 2, then 200 mg once daily for day 3, then 300 mg once daily for day 4, then, adjusted according to response; usual dose 300 mg once daily, the rate of dose titration may need to be slower and the daily dose lower in elderly patients; maximum 600 mg per day
▶ BY MOUTH USING MODIFIED-RELEASE MEDICINES
▶ Adult: 50 mg once daily for day 1, dose to be taken at bedtime, then 100 mg once daily for day 2, then 200 mg once daily for day 3, then 300 mg once daily for day 4, then, adjusted according to response; usual dose 300 mg once daily; maximum 600 mg per day

Prevention of mania and depression in bipolar disorder
▶ BY MOUTH USING IMMEDIATE-RELEASE MEDICINES
▶ Adult: Continue at the dose effective for treatment of bipolar disorder and adjust to lowest effective dose; usual dose 300–800 mg daily in 2 divided doses
▶ BY MOUTH USING MODIFIED-RELEASE MEDICINES
▶ Adult: Continue at the dose effective for treatment of bipolar disorder and adjust to lowest effective dose; usual dose 300–800 mg once daily

Adjunctive treatment of major depression
▶ BY MOUTH USING MODIFIED-RELEASE MEDICINES
▶ Adult: 50 mg once daily for 2 days, dose to be taken at bedtime, then 150 mg once daily for 2 days, then, adjusted according to response, usual dose 150–300 mg once daily
▶ Elderly: Initially 50 mg once daily for 3 days, then increased if necessary to 100 mg once daily for 4 days, then adjusted in steps of 50 mg, adjusted according to response, usual dose 50–300 mg once daily, dose of 300 mg should not be reached before day 22 of treatment

DOSE EQUIVALENCE AND CONVERSION
▶ Patients can be switched from immediate-release to modified-release tablets at the equivalent daily dose; to maintain clinical response, dose titration may be required.

IMPORTANT SAFETY INFORMATION

MHRA/CHM ADVICE: CLOZAPINE AND OTHER ANTIPSYCHOTICS: MONITORING BLOOD CONCENTRATIONS FOR TOXICITY (AUGUST 2020)

Following fatal cases involving toxicity of clozapine and other antipsychotic medicines, the MHRA advises that monitoring blood concentration of quetiapine may be helpful in certain circumstances, such as patients presenting symptoms suggestive of toxicity, or when concomitant medicines may interact to increase blood concentration of quetiapine.

● **CAUTIONS** Cerebrovascular disease · elderly · history or risk factors for sleep apnoea · patients at risk of aspiration pneumonia · treatment of depression in patients under 25 years (increased risk of suicide)

● **INTERACTIONS** → Appendix 1: antipsychotics, second generation

● **SIDE-EFFECTS**
▶ **Common or very common** Appetite increased · asthenia · dysarthria · dyspepsia · dyspnoea · fever · headache · irritability · palpitations · peripheral oedema · rhinitis · sleep disorders · suicidal behaviours · syncope · vision blurred · withdrawal syndrome
▶ **Uncommon** Anaemia · diabetes mellitus · dysphagia · hyponatraemia · hypothyroidism · sexual dysfunction · skin reactions · thrombocytopenia
▶ **Rare or very rare** Angioedema · breast swelling · gastrointestinal disorders · hepatic disorders · hypothermia ·

menstrual disorder · metabolic syndrome · pancreatitis · rhabdomyolysis · severe cutaneous adverse reactions (SCARs) · SIADH · venous thromboembolism
▶ **Frequency not known** Sleep apnoea

● **PREGNANCY** Use only if potential benefit outweighs risk.

● **BREAST FEEDING** Manufacturer advises avoid.

● **HEPATIC IMPAIRMENT** Manufacturer advises caution (risk of increased plasma concentrations).
Dose adjustments Manufacturer advises for *immediate-release tablets*, initially 25 mg daily, increased daily in steps of 25–50 mg.
Manufacturer advises for *modified-release tablets*, initially 50 mg daily, increased daily in steps of 50 mg.

● **MEDICINAL FORMS** There can be variation in the licensing of different medicines containing the same drug. Forms available from special-order manufacturers include: oral suspension, oral solution, oral powder

Oral tablet
CAUTIONARY AND ADVISORY LABELS 2
▶ **Quetiapine (Non-proprietary)**
Quetiapine (as Quetiapine fumarate) 25 mg Quetiapine 25mg tablets | 30 tablet [PoM] £24.30 | 60 tablet [PoM] £40.59 DT = £1.84
Quetiapine (as Quetiapine fumarate) 50 mg Quetiapine 50mg tablets | 60 tablet [PoM] £10.32-£12.50 DT = £12.50
Quetiapine (as Quetiapine fumarate) 100 mg Quetiapine 100mg tablets | 60 tablet [PoM] £135.72 DT = £9.41
Quetiapine (as Quetiapine fumarate) 150 mg Quetiapine 150mg tablets | 60 tablet [PoM] £135.72 DT = £10.47
Quetiapine (as Quetiapine fumarate) 200 mg Quetiapine 200mg tablets | 60 tablet [PoM] £159.72 DT = £14.82
Quetiapine (as Quetiapine fumarate) 300 mg Quetiapine 300mg tablets | 60 tablet [PoM] £204.00 DT = £9.85
Quetiapine (as Quetiapine fumarate) 400 mg Quetiapine 400mg tablets | 60 tablet [PoM] £25.00-£41.26 DT = £25.00
▶ **Seroquel** (Luye Pharma Ltd)
Quetiapine (as Quetiapine fumarate) 25 mg Seroquel 25mg tablets | 60 tablet [PoM] £48.60 DT = £1.84
Quetiapine (as Quetiapine fumarate) 100 mg Seroquel 100mg tablets | 60 tablet [PoM] £135.72 DT = £9.41
Quetiapine (as Quetiapine fumarate) 200 mg Seroquel 200mg tablets | 60 tablet [PoM] £135.72 DT = £14.82
Quetiapine (as Quetiapine fumarate) 300 mg Seroquel 300mg tablets | 60 tablet [PoM] £204.00 DT = £9.85

Modified-release tablet
CAUTIONARY AND ADVISORY LABELS 2, 23, 25
▶ **Quetiapine (Non-proprietary)**
Quetiapine (as Quetiapine fumarate) 50 mg Quetiapine 50mg modified-release tablets | 60 tablet [PoM] £64.28 DT = £67.66
Quetiapine (as Quetiapine fumarate) 150 mg Quetiapine 150mg modified-release tablets | 60 tablet [PoM] £107.45 DT = £113.10
Quetiapine (as Quetiapine fumarate) 200 mg Quetiapine 200mg modified-release tablets | 60 tablet [PoM] £107.45 DT = £113.10
Quetiapine (as Quetiapine fumarate) 300 mg Quetiapine 300mg modified-release tablets | 60 tablet [PoM] £161.50 DT = £170.00
Quetiapine (as Quetiapine fumarate) 400 mg Quetiapine 400mg modified-release tablets | 60 tablet [PoM] £214.89 DT = £226.20
▶ **Atrolak XL** (Accord-UK Ltd)
Quetiapine (as Quetiapine fumarate) 50 mg Atrolak XL 50mg tablets | 60 tablet [PoM] £67.65 DT = £67.66
Quetiapine (as Quetiapine fumarate) 150 mg Atrolak XL 150mg tablets | 60 tablet [PoM] £107.45 DT = £113.10
Quetiapine (as Quetiapine fumarate) 200 mg Atrolak XL 200mg tablets | 60 tablet [PoM] £113.09 DT = £113.10
Quetiapine (as Quetiapine fumarate) 300 mg Atrolak XL 300mg tablets | 60 tablet [PoM] £169.99 DT = £170.00
Quetiapine (as Quetiapine fumarate) 400 mg Atrolak XL 400mg tablets | 60 tablet [PoM] £226.19 DT = £226.20
▶ **Biquelle XL** (Aspire Pharma Ltd)
Quetiapine (as Quetiapine fumarate) 50 mg Biquelle XL 50mg tablets | 30 tablet [PoM] £14.73 | 60 tablet [PoM] £29.45 DT = £67.66
Quetiapine (as Quetiapine fumarate) 150 mg Biquelle XL 150mg tablets | 30 tablet [PoM] £24.73 | 60 tablet [PoM] £49.45 DT = £113.10
Quetiapine (as Quetiapine fumarate) 200 mg Biquelle XL 200mg tablets | 30 tablet [PoM] £24.73 | 60 tablet [PoM] £49.45 DT = £113.10

Quetiapine (as Quetiapine fumarate) 300 mg Biquelle XL 300mg tablets | 30 tablet [PoM] £37.23 | 60 tablet [PoM] £74.45 DT = £170.00

Quetiapine (as Quetiapine fumarate) 400 mg Biquelle XL 400mg tablets | 30 tablet [PoM] £49.48 | 60 tablet [PoM] £98.95 DT = £226.20

Quetiapine (as Quetiapine fumarate) 600 mg Biquelle XL 600mg tablets | 30 tablet [PoM] £70.73 DT = £70.73

▶ **Brancico XL** (Zentiva Pharma UK Ltd)

Quetiapine (as Quetiapine fumarate) 50 mg Brancico XL 50mg tablets | 60 tablet [PoM] £8.99 DT = £67.66

Quetiapine (as Quetiapine fumarate) 150 mg Brancico XL 150mg tablets | 60 tablet [PoM] £19.49 DT = £113.10

Quetiapine (as Quetiapine fumarate) 200 mg Brancico XL 200mg tablets | 60 tablet [PoM] £19.49 DT = £113.10

Quetiapine (as Quetiapine fumarate) 300 mg Brancico XL 300mg tablets | 60 tablet [PoM] £33.74 DT = £170.00

Quetiapine (as Quetiapine fumarate) 400 mg Brancico XL 400mg tablets | 60 tablet [PoM] £44.99 DT = £226.20

▶ **Mintreleq XL** (Aristo Pharma Ltd)

Quetiapine (as Quetiapine fumarate) 50 mg Mintreleq XL 50mg tablets | 60 tablet [PoM] £14.99 DT = £67.66

Quetiapine (as Quetiapine fumarate) 150 mg Mintreleq XL 150mg tablets | 60 tablet [PoM] £29.99 DT = £113.10

Quetiapine (as Quetiapine fumarate) 200 mg Mintreleq XL 200mg tablets | 60 tablet [PoM] £29.99 DT = £113.10

Quetiapine (as Quetiapine fumarate) 300 mg Mintreleq XL 300mg tablets | 60 tablet [PoM] £49.99 DT = £170.00

Quetiapine (as Quetiapine fumarate) 400 mg Mintreleq XL 400mg tablets | 60 tablet [PoM] £64.99 DT = £226.20

▶ **Seroquel XL** (Luye Pharma Ltd)

Quetiapine (as Quetiapine fumarate) 50 mg Seroquel XL 50mg tablets | 60 tablet [PoM] £67.66 DT = £67.66

Quetiapine (as Quetiapine fumarate) 150 mg Seroquel XL 150mg tablets | 60 tablet [PoM] £113.10 DT = £113.10

Quetiapine (as Quetiapine fumarate) 200 mg Seroquel XL 200mg tablets | 60 tablet [PoM] £113.10 DT = £113.10

Quetiapine (as Quetiapine fumarate) 300 mg Seroquel XL 300mg tablets | 60 tablet [PoM] £170.00 DT = £170.00

Quetiapine (as Quetiapine fumarate) 400 mg Seroquel XL 400mg tablets | 60 tablet [PoM] £226.20 DT = £226.20

▶ **Sondate XL** (Teva UK Ltd)

Quetiapine (as Quetiapine fumarate) 50 mg Sondate XL 50mg tablets | 60 tablet [PoM] £11.99 DT = £67.66

Quetiapine (as Quetiapine fumarate) 150 mg Sondate XL 150mg tablets | 60 tablet [PoM] £25.99 DT = £113.10

Quetiapine (as Quetiapine fumarate) 200 mg Sondate XL 200mg tablets | 60 tablet [PoM] £25.99 DT = £113.10

Quetiapine (as Quetiapine fumarate) 300 mg Sondate XL 300mg tablets | 60 tablet [PoM] £44.99 DT = £170.00

Quetiapine (as Quetiapine fumarate) 400 mg Sondate XL 400mg tablets | 60 tablet [PoM] £59.99 DT = £226.20

▶ **Zaluron XL** (Fontus Health Ltd)

Quetiapine (as Quetiapine fumarate) 50 mg Zaluron XL 50mg tablets | 60 tablet [PoM] £27.96 DT = £67.66

Quetiapine (as Quetiapine fumarate) 150 mg Zaluron XL 150mg tablets | 60 tablet [PoM] £46.96 DT = £113.10

Quetiapine (as Quetiapine fumarate) 200 mg Zaluron XL 200mg tablets | 60 tablet [PoM] £46.96 DT = £113.10

Quetiapine (as Quetiapine fumarate) 300 mg Zaluron XL 300mg tablets | 60 tablet [PoM] £70.71 DT = £170.00

Quetiapine (as Quetiapine fumarate) 400 mg Zaluron XL 400mg tablets | 60 tablet [PoM] £93.98 DT = £226.20

Oral suspension

CAUTIONARY AND ADVISORY LABELS 2

▶ **Quetiapine (Non-proprietary)**

Quetiapine (as Quetiapine fumarate) 20 mg per 1 ml Quetiapine 20mg/ml oral suspension sugar free | 150 ml [PoM] £208.95 DT = £208.95 [SF]

⚑ 442

Risperidone

21-Jan-2025

● **DRUG ACTION** Risperidone is a dopamine D_2, 5-HT_{2A}, alpha$_1$-adrenoceptor, and histamine-1 receptor antagonist.

● INDICATIONS AND DOSE

Acute and chronic psychosis

▶ BY MOUTH

▶ **Adult:** 2 mg daily in 1–2 divided doses for day 1, then 4 mg daily in 1–2 divided doses for day 2, slower titration is appropriate in some patients, usual dose 4–6 mg daily, doses above 10 mg daily only if benefit considered to outweigh risk; maximum 16 mg per day

▶ **Elderly:** Initially 500 micrograms twice daily, then increased in steps of 500 micrograms twice daily, increased to 1–2 mg twice daily

Mania

▶ BY MOUTH

▶ **Adult:** Initially 2 mg once daily, then increased in steps of 1 mg daily if required; usual dose 1–6 mg daily

▶ **Elderly:** Initially 500 micrograms twice daily, then increased in steps of 500 micrograms twice daily, increased to 1–2 mg twice daily

Short-term treatment (up to 6 weeks) of persistent aggression in patients with moderate to severe Alzheimer's dementia unresponsive to non-pharmacological interventions and when there is a risk of harm to self or others

▶ BY MOUTH

▶ **Adult:** Initially 250 micrograms twice daily, then increased in steps of 250 micrograms twice a day on alternate days, adjusted according to response; usual dose 500 micrograms twice daily (max. per dose 1 mg twice daily)

OKEDI ® PRE-FILLED SYRINGES

Schizophrenia [in patients stabilised on oral risperidone 3 mg daily]

▶ BY DEEP INTRAMUSCULAR INJECTION

▶ **Adult:** Initially 75 mg every 28 days, treatment to be initiated about 24 hours after the last oral risperidone dose. Before treatment initiation risperidone-naïve patients should be titrated with oral risperidone for at least 14 days; patients stabilised on other oral antipsychotics, but with previous response to risperidone, should be titrated with oral risperidone for at least 6 days. Those stabilised on oral risperidone may be switched without titration; increased if necessary up to 100 mg every 28 days, dose to be adjusted at intervals of 28 days; usual maintenance 75 mg every 28 days, dose may be given up to 3 days before the 28-day time point

Schizophrenia [in patients stabilised on oral risperidone 4 mg daily or more]

▶ BY DEEP INTRAMUSCULAR INJECTION

▶ **Adult:** Initially 100 mg every 28 days, treatment to be initiated about 24 hours after the last oral risperidone dose. Before treatment initiation risperidone-naïve patients should be titrated with oral risperidone for at least 14 days; patients stabilised on other oral antipsychotics, but with previous response to risperidone, should be titrated with oral risperidone for at least 6 days. Those stabilised on oral risperidone may be switched without titration, dose to be adjusted as necessary at intervals of 28 days; usual maintenance 75 mg every 28 days, dose may be given up to 3 days before the 28-day time point

Schizophrenia [in patients switching from intramuscular risperidone 37.5 mg every 2 weeks]
▶ BY DEEP INTRAMUSCULAR INJECTION
▶ Adult: 75 mg every 28 days, treatment to be initiated 2 weeks after the last bi-weekly injection, dose may be given up to 3 days before the 28-day time point

Schizophrenia [in patients switching from intramuscular risperidone 50 mg every 2 weeks]
▶ BY DEEP INTRAMUSCULAR INJECTION
▶ Adult: 100 mg every 28 days, treatment to be initiated 2 weeks after the last bi-weekly injection, dose may be given up to 3 days before the 28-day time point

RISPERDAL CONSTA® INJECTION

Schizophrenia [in patients stabilised on oral antipsychotics e.g. risperidone up to 4 mg daily for 2 weeks or more]
▶ BY DEEP INTRAMUSCULAR INJECTION
▶ Adult: Initially 25 mg every 2 weeks, oral antipsychotics should be continued during the first 3 weeks of treatment; increased if necessary up to 37.5–50 mg every 2 weeks, dose to be increased at intervals of at least 4 weeks; usual maintenance 25 mg every 2 weeks

Schizophrenia [in patients stabilised on oral antipsychotics e.g. risperidone over 4 mg daily]
▶ BY DEEP INTRAMUSCULAR INJECTION
▶ Adult: Initially 37.5 mg every 2 weeks, oral antipsychotics should be continued during the first 3 weeks of treatment; increased if necessary up to 50 mg every 2 weeks, dose to be increased at intervals of at least 4 weeks

---

IMPORTANT SAFETY INFORMATION

SAFE PRACTICE
Risperidone has been confused with ropinirole; care must be taken to ensure the correct drug is prescribed and dispensed.

MHRA/CHM ADVICE: CLOZAPINE AND OTHER ANTIPSYCHOTICS: MONITORING BLOOD CONCENTRATIONS FOR TOXICITY (AUGUST 2020)
Following fatal cases involving toxicity of clozapine and other antipsychotic medicines, the MHRA advises that monitoring blood concentration of risperidone may be helpful in certain circumstances, such as patients presenting symptoms suggestive of toxicity, or when concomitant medicines may interact to increase blood concentration of risperidone.

● CAUTIONS Avoid in Acute porphyrias p. 1202 · cataract surgery (risk of intra-operative floppy iris syndrome) · dehydration · dementia with Lewy bodies · prolactin-dependent tumours

● INTERACTIONS → Appendix 1: antipsychotics, second generation

● SIDE-EFFECTS
▶ **Common or very common** Anaemia · anxiety · appetite abnormal · asthenia · chest discomfort · conjunctivitis · cough · depression · diarrhoea · dyspnoea · epistaxis · fall · fever · gastrointestinal discomfort · headache · hypertension · increased risk of infection · joint disorders · laryngeal pain · muscle spasms · nasal congestion · nausea · oedema · oral disorders · pain · sexual dysfunction · skin reactions · sleep disorders · urinary disorders · vision disorders · weight decreased
▶ **Uncommon** Alopecia · breast abnormalities · cardiac conduction disorders · cerebrovascular insufficiency · chills · coma · concentration impaired · consciousness impaired · cystitis · diabetes mellitus · dry eye · dysarthria · dysphagia · dysphonia · ear pain · eye disorders · feeling abnormal · flushing · gait abnormal · gastrointestinal disorders ·

induration · malaise · menstrual cycle irregularities · mood altered · muscle weakness · palpitations · polydipsia · posture abnormal · procedural pain · respiratory disorders · sensation abnormal · syncope · taste altered · thirst · thrombocytopenia · tinnitus · vaginal discharge · vertigo
▶ **Rare or very rare** Angioedema · catatonia · dandruff · diabetic ketoacidosis · embolism and thrombosis · eyelid crusting · glaucoma · hypoglycaemia · hypothermia · jaundice · pancreatitis · peripheral coldness · rhabdomyolysis · SIADH · sleep apnoea · water intoxication · withdrawal syndrome
▶ **Frequency not known** Cardiac arrest · severe cutaneous adverse reactions (SCARs)

● PREGNANCY Use only if potential benefit outweighs risk.

● BREAST FEEDING Use only if potential benefit outweighs risk—small amount present in milk.

● HEPATIC IMPAIRMENT [EvGr] Caution. ◈M◈
Dose adjustments
▶ With oral use [EvGr] Dose reduction to half the usual dose, and slower dose titration. ◈M◈

OKEDI® PRE-FILLED SYRINGES [EvGr] Caution (no information available)—increased risk of exposure. ◈M◈
Dose adjustments [EvGr] Careful titration with oral risperidone, by halving initial doses and slowing titration, is recommended; if an oral dose of at least 3 mg daily is tolerated, treatment with 75 mg as a deep intramuscular depot injection may be initiated. ◈M◈

RISPERDAL CONSTA® INJECTION [EvGr] Caution (no information available). ◈M◈
Dose adjustments [EvGr] If an oral dose of at least 2 mg daily is tolerated, 25 mg as a deep intramuscular depot injection can be given every 2 weeks. ◈M◈

● RENAL IMPAIRMENT [EvGr] Caution. ◈M◈
Dose adjustments
▶ With oral use [EvGr] Initial and subsequent doses should be halved, with slower dose titration. ◈M◈

OKEDI® PRE-FILLED SYRINGES [EvGr] Avoid in moderate to severe impairment (no information available). ◈M◈

RISPERDAL CONSTA® INJECTION [EvGr] Caution (no information available). ◈M◈
Dose adjustments [EvGr] If an oral dose of at least 2 mg daily is tolerated, 25 mg as a deep intramuscular depot injection can be given every 2 weeks. ◈M◈

● MONITORING REQUIREMENTS
▶ With intramuscular use Treatment requires careful monitoring for optimum effect.

● DIRECTIONS FOR ADMINISTRATION
▶ With oral use Orodispersible tablets should be placed on the tongue, allowed to dissolve and swallowed. Manufacturer advises oral liquid may be diluted with any non-alcoholic drink, except tea.
▶ With intramuscular use Use correct injection technique (including the use of z-track technique) and rotate injection sites.

OKEDI® PRE-FILLED SYRINGES [EvGr] Inject into the deltoid or gluteal muscle. ◈M◈

RISPERDAL CONSTA® INJECTION [EvGr] Inject into the deltoid or gluteal muscle. ◈M◈

● HANDLING AND STORAGE

RISPERDAL CONSTA® INJECTION Store in a refrigerator (2–8°C) and protect from light; may be stored at room temperature (below 25°C) for up to 7 days—consult product literature about storage after reconstitution.

● PATIENT AND CARER ADVICE Patients or carers should be given advice on how to administer risperidone orodispersible tablets and oral liquid (counselling on use of dose syringe advised).

- **MEDICINAL FORMS** There can be variation in the licensing of different medicines containing the same drug. Forms available from special-order manufacturers include: oral solution

Oral tablet

CAUTIONARY AND ADVISORY LABELS 2

▸ **Risperidone (Non-proprietary)**
Risperidone 250 microgram Risperidone 250microgram tablets | 20 tablet [PoM] £38.00–£56.00
Risperidone 500 microgram Risperidone 500microgram tablets | 20 tablet [PoM] £6.18 DT = £1.92
Risperidone 1 mg Risperidone 1mg tablets | 20 tablet [PoM] £10.16 DT = £0.90 | 60 tablet [PoM] £2.64–£14.93
Risperidone 2 mg Risperidone 2mg tablets | 60 tablet [PoM] £60.10 DT = £1.77
Risperidone 3 mg Risperidone 3mg tablets | 60 tablet [PoM] £88.38 DT = £1.87
Risperidone 4 mg Risperidone 4mg tablets | 60 tablet [PoM] £116.67 DT = £2.10
Risperidone 6 mg Risperidone 6mg tablets | 28 tablet [PoM] £82.50 DT = £14.91

Oral solution

CAUTIONARY AND ADVISORY LABELS 2

▸ **Risperidone (Non-proprietary)**
Risperidone 1 mg per 1 ml Risperidone 1mg/ml oral solution sugar free | 100 ml [PoM] £9.46 DT = £3.41 [SF]

Powder and solvent for prolonged-release suspension for inj

EXCIPIENTS: May contain Polysorbates

▸ **Okedi** (ROVI Biotech Ltd)
Risperidone 75 mg Okedi 75mg powder and solvent for prolonged-release suspension for injection pre-filled syringes | 1 pre-filled disposable injection [PoM] £222.64 (Hospital only)
Risperidone 100 mg Okedi 100mg powder and solvent for prolonged-release suspension for injection pre-filled syringes | 1 pre-filled disposable injection [PoM] £285.52 (Hospital only)

▸ **Risperdal Consta** (Janssen-Cilag Ltd)
Risperidone 25 mg Risperdal Consta 25mg powder and solvent for prolonged-release suspension for injection vials | 1 vial [PoM] £79.69 DT = £79.69
Risperidone 37.5 mg Risperdal Consta 37.5mg powder and solvent for prolonged-release suspension for injection vials | 1 vial [PoM] £111.32 DT = £111.32
Risperidone 50 mg Risperdal Consta 50mg powder and solvent for prolonged-release suspension for injection vials | 1 vial [PoM] £142.76 DT = £142.76

Orodispersible tablet

CAUTIONARY AND ADVISORY LABELS 2

EXCIPIENTS: May contain Aspartame

▸ **Risperidone (Non-proprietary)**
Risperidone 500 microgram Risperidone 500microgram orodispersible tablets sugar free | 28 tablet [PoM] £7.82–£23.03 DT = £5.03 [SF]
Risperidone 1 mg Risperidone 1mg orodispersible tablets sugar free | 28 tablet [PoM] £25.31 DT = £16.38 [SF]
Risperidone 2 mg Risperidone 2mg orodispersible tablets sugar free | 28 tablet [PoM] £45.82 DT = £45.82 [SF]
Risperidone 3 mg Risperidone 3mg orodispersible tablets sugar free | 28 tablet [PoM] £43.48 DT = £43.48 [SF]
Risperidone 4 mg Risperidone 4mg orodispersible tablets sugar free | 28 tablet [PoM] £56.02 DT = £56.02 [SF]

ANTIPSYCHOTICS > SECOND-GENERATION (DEPOT INJECTIONS)

▶ 442

Olanzapine embonate

21-Mar-2023

(Olanzapine pamoate)

● **INDICATIONS AND DOSE**

Maintenance in schizophrenia in patients tolerant to olanzapine by mouth (patients taking 10 mg oral olanzapine daily)

▸ BY DEEP INTRAMUSCULAR INJECTION
▸ Adult 18-75 years: Initially 210 mg every 2 weeks, alternatively initially 405 mg every 4 weeks, then maintenance 150 mg every 2 weeks, alternatively maintenance 300 mg every 4 weeks, maintenance dose to be started after 2 months of initial treatment, dose to be administered into the gluteal muscle, consult product literature if supplementation with oral olanzapine required

Maintenance in schizophrenia in patients tolerant to olanzapine by mouth (patients taking 15 mg oral olanzapine daily)

▸ BY DEEP INTRAMUSCULAR INJECTION
▸ Adult 18-75 years: Initially 300 mg every 2 weeks, then maintenance 210 mg every 2 weeks, alternatively maintenance 405 mg every 4 weeks, maintenance dose to be started after 2 months of initial treatment, dose to be administered into the gluteal muscle, consult product literature if supplementation with oral olanzapine required

Maintenance in schizophrenia in patients tolerant to olanzapine by mouth (patients taking 20 mg oral olanzapine daily)

▸ BY DEEP INTRAMUSCULAR INJECTION
▸ Adult: Initially 300 mg every 2 weeks, then maintenance 300 mg every 2 weeks (max. per dose 300 mg every 2 weeks), adjusted according to response, dose to be administered into the gluteal muscle, consult product literature if supplementation with oral olanzapine required

IMPORTANT SAFETY INFORMATION

When prescribing, dispensing or administering, check that this is the correct preparation—this preparation is used for *maintenance* treatment and should **not** be used for the rapid control of an *acute* episode.

MHRA/CHM ADVICE: CLOZAPINE AND OTHER ANTIPSYCHOTICS: MONITORING BLOOD CONCENTRATIONS FOR TOXICITY (AUGUST 2020)

Following fatal cases involving toxicity of clozapine and other antipsychotic medicines, the MHRA advises that monitoring blood concentration of olanzapine may be helpful in certain circumstances, such as patients presenting symptoms suggestive of toxicity, or when concomitant medicines may interact to increase blood concentration of olanzapine.

● **CAUTIONS** Bone-marrow depression · hypereosinophilic disorders · low leucocyte count · low neutrophil count · myeloproliferative disease · paralytic ileus · when transferring from oral to depot therapy, the dose by mouth should be reduced gradually

● **INTERACTIONS** → Appendix 1: antipsychotics, second generation

● **SIDE-EFFECTS**
▸ **Common or very common** Anticholinergic syndrome · appetite increased · arthralgia · asthenia · eosinophilia · fever · glycosuria · oedema · sexual dysfunction
▸ **Uncommon** Abdominal distension · alopecia · breast enlargement · diabetes mellitus · diabetic coma · dysarthria · embolism and thrombosis · epistaxis · ketoacidosis · memory loss · oculogyration · photosensitivity reaction · urinary disorders
▸ **Rare or very rare** Drug reaction with eosinophilia and systemic symptoms (DRESS) · hepatic disorders · hypothermia · pancreatitis · rhabdomyolysis · thrombocytopenia
▸ **Frequency not known** Erythema · gait abnormal · increased risk of fall · pneumonia · visual hallucinations

SIDE-EFFECTS, FURTHER INFORMATION Side-effects may persist until the drug has been cleared from its depot site.

Overdose Post-injection reactions have been reported leading to signs and symptoms of overdose.

- **PREGNANCY** Use only if potential benefit outweighs risk; neonatal lethargy, tremor, and hypertonia reported when used in third trimester.
- **BREAST FEEDING** Avoid—present in milk.
- **HEPATIC IMPAIRMENT** Manufacturer advises caution. **Dose adjustments** Manufacturer advises consider initial dose of 150 mg every 4 weeks.
- **RENAL IMPAIRMENT**
  Dose adjustments [EvGr] Consider initial dose of 150 mg every 4 weeks. ⟨M⟩
- **MONITORING REQUIREMENTS**
  ▸ Observe patient for at least 3 hours after injection.
  ▸ Treatment requires careful monitoring for optimum effect.
  ▸ Blood lipids and weight should be measured at baseline, at 3 months (weight should be measured at frequent intervals during the first 3 months), and then yearly with antipsychotic drugs. Patients taking olanzapine require more frequent monitoring of these parameters: every 3 months for the first year, then yearly.
  ▸ Fasting blood glucose should be measured at baseline, at 4–6 months, and then yearly. Patients taking olanzapine should have fasting blood glucose tested at baseline, after one months' treatment, then every 4–6 months.
- **DIRECTIONS FOR ADMINISTRATION** Use correct injection technique (including use of z-track technique) and rotate injection sites.

- **MEDICINAL FORMS** There can be variation in the licensing of different medicines containing the same drug.
  Powder and solvent for prolonged-release suspension for inj
  ▸ Zypadhera (Neon Healthcare Ltd)
  Olanzapine (as Olanzapine embonate monohydrate)
  210 mg Zypadhera 210mg powder and solvent for prolonged-release suspension for injection vials | 1 vial [PoM] £142.76
  Olanzapine (as Olanzapine embonate monohydrate)
  300 mg Zypadhera 300mg powder and solvent for prolonged-release suspension for injection vials | 1 vial [PoM] £222.64
  Olanzapine (as Olanzapine embonate monohydrate)
  405 mg Zypadhera 405mg powder and solvent for prolonged-release suspension for injection vials | 1 vial [PoM] £285.52

4　Movement disorders

Cerebral palsy and spasticity　05-Apr-2019

Overview

Cerebral palsy is a group of permanent, non-progressive abnormalities of the developing fetal or neonatal brain that lead to movement and posture disorders, causing activity limitation and functional impact. There can be accompanying clinical and developmental comorbidities. These include disturbances of sensation, perception, cognition, communication and behaviour, epilepsy, and secondary musculoskeletal problems (such as muscle contracture and abnormal torsion). Cerebral palsy is not curable and the comorbidities can impact on many areas of participation and quality of life, particularly eating, drinking, comfort, and sleep.

There are an increasing number of adults now living with cerebral palsy. These patients have a wide range of abilities — from full independence in everyday life to requiring 24 hour care and attention. It is therefore important that patients and their family and carers are provided with information about the network of general and specialised adult services available, to ensure their changing needs are met. The management of adults with cerebral palsy is a continuation from childhood under the care of specialists. For guidance on the management of patients with cerebral palsy, see *Cerebral Palsy and Spasticity* in BNF for Children.

Useful Resources

Cerebral palsy in under 25s: assessment and management. National Institute for Health and Care Excellence. Clinical guideline 62. January 2017.
www.nice.org.uk/guidance/ng62
　Spasticity in under 19s: management. National Institute for Health and Care Excellence. Clinical guideline 145. July 2012 (updated November 2016).
www.nice.org.uk/guidance/cg145
　Cerebral Palsy in adults. National Institute for Health and Care Excellence. Clinical guideline 119. January 2019.
www.nice.org.uk/guidance/ng119

Motor neurone disease　13-Nov-2020

Description of condition

Motor neurone disease is a neurodegenerative condition affecting the brain and spinal cord. Degeneration of motor neurones leads to progressive muscle weakness; resulting symptoms include muscle cramps, wasting and stiffness, loss of dexterity, reduced respiratory function and cognitive dysfunction. The most common form is amyotrophic lateral sclerosis.
　[EvGr] Patients suspected of having developed motor neurone disease should be referred to a neurologist without delay. ⟨A⟩

Aims of treatment

As there is no cure, treatment focuses on maintaining functional ability and managing symptoms.

Non-drug treatment

Non-drug treatment includes nutrition, psychosocial support, physiotherapy, exercise programmes and use of special equipment or mobility aids.

Management of symptoms

Muscular symptoms

[EvGr] Quinine p. 713 [unlicensed indication] is recommended as first line treatment for muscle cramps. If quinine is ineffective, not tolerated or contra-indicated, baclofen p. 1289 [unlicensed indication] should be considered as second line treatment. Subsequent treatment options include tizanidine p. 1291 [unlicensed indication], dantrolene sodium p. 1541 [unlicensed indication] or gabapentin p. 362 [unlicensed indication].
　Symptoms of muscle stiffness, spasticity or increased tone can be managed with baclofen, tizanidine, dantrolene sodium or gabapentin [unlicensed indication]. Treatment of severe spasticity may require specialist referral. ⟨A⟩
　The MHRA/CHM have released important safety information on the use of antiepileptic drugs and the risk of suicidal thoughts and behaviour. For further information, see Epilepsy p. 349.

Saliva problems

[EvGr] A trial of an antimuscarinic drug [unlicensed indication] can be considered for excessive drooling of saliva. Glycopyrronium bromide p. 281 is recommended in patients who have cognitive impairment as it has fewer central nervous system side-effects. If initial treatment is ineffective, not tolerated or contra-indicated, referral for specialist administration of botulinum toxin type A p. 469 may be required.
　Humidification, nebulisers and carbocisteine p. 333 can be used to treat patients with thick, tenacious saliva. ⟨A⟩

Respiratory symptoms

[EvGr] Reversible causes of worsening respiratory impairment (such as respiratory tract infections or secretion problems) should be treated before considering other options.

Patients experiencing breathlessness can be treated with opioids [unlicensed indication], or benzodiazepines [unlicensed indication] if the patient's symptoms are exacerbated by anxiety. Non-invasive ventilation should be considered in patients with respiratory impairment. ◈

Amyotrophic lateral sclerosis

Riluzole p. 1282 is licensed for use in patients with amyotrophic lateral sclerosis to extend life or to extend the time to mechanical ventilation—see *National funding/access decisions* under riluzole.

Useful Resources

Motor neurone disease: assessment and management. National Institute for Health and Care Excellence. Clinical guideline NG42. February 2016.
www.nice.org.uk/guidance/ng42

4.1 Dystonias and other involuntary movements

Essential tremor, chorea, tics, and related disorders

14-Sep-2020

Drugs used in essential tremor, chorea, tics, and related disorders

Tetrabenazine p. 469 is mainly used to control movement disorders in Huntington's chorea and related disorders. Tetrabenazine can also be prescribed for the treatment of tardive dyskinesia if switching or withdrawing the causative antipsychotic drug is not effective. It acts by depleting nerve endings of dopamine. It is effective in only a proportion of patients and its use may be limited by the development of depression.

Haloperidol p. 445 [unlicensed indication], olanzapine p. 459 [unlicensed indication], risperidone p. 464 [unlicensed indication], and quetiapine p. 462 [unlicensed indication], can also be used to suppress chorea in Huntington's disease.

Haloperidol can also improve motor tics and symptoms of Tourette syndrome and related choreas. Other treatments for Tourette syndrome include pimozide p. 448 [unlicensed indication] (**important**: ECG monitoring required), clonidine hydrochloride p. 172 [unlicensed indication], and sulpiride p. 449 [unlicensed indication]. Trihexyphenidyl hydrochloride p. 473 in high dosage can also improve some movement disorders; it is sometimes necessary to build the dose up over many weeks. Chlorpromazine hydrochloride p. 443 and haloperidol are used to relieve intractable hiccup.

Propranolol hydrochloride p. 178 or another beta-adrenoceptor blocking drug may be useful in treating essential tremor or tremors associated with anxiety or thyrotoxicosis.

Primidone p. 389 in some cases provides relief from benign essential tremor; the dose is increased slowly to reduce side-effects.

Piracetam below is used as an adjunctive treatment for myoclonus of cortical origin. After an acute episode, attempts should be made every 6 months to decrease or discontinue treatment.

Riluzole p. 1282 is used to extend life in patients with motor neurone disease who have amyotrophic lateral sclerosis.

Torsion dystonia and other involuntary movements

Treatment with botulinum toxin type A p. 469 can be considered after an acquired non-progressive brain injury if rapid-onset spasticity causes postural or functional difficulties.

> **Other drugs used for Dystonias and other involuntary movements** Diazepam, p. 398 · Orphenadrine hydrochloride, p. 472 · Pericyazine, p. 447 · Pramipexole, p. 485 · Procyclidine hydrochloride, p. 472 · Ropinirole, p. 487 · Rotigotine, p. 488 · Trifluoperazine, p. 450

ANTIPSYCHOTICS > FIRST-GENERATION

◤ 442

Promazine hydrochloride

27-Jun-2023

● **INDICATIONS AND DOSE**

Short-term adjunctive management of psychomotor agitation
▸ BY MOUTH
▸ Adult: 100–200 mg 4 times a day

Agitation and restlessness in elderly
▸ BY MOUTH
▸ Elderly: 25–50 mg 4 times a day

● **CONTRA-INDICATIONS** CNS depression · comatose states · phaeochromocytoma

● **CAUTIONS** Cerebral arteriosclerosis · susceptibility to QT interval prolongation

● **INTERACTIONS** → Appendix 1: phenothiazines

● **SIDE-EFFECTS** Apathy · autonomic dysfunction · cardiac arrest · cardiovascular effects · consciousness impaired · corneal opacity · epilepsy · eye discolouration · gastrointestinal disorder · glaucoma · haemolytic anaemia · headache · hepatic disorders · hyperpyrexia · hypersensitivity · hyperthermia (dose-related) · hypothermia (dose-related) · lens opacity · menstrual disorder · nasal congestion · photosensitivity reaction · skin reactions · urinary hesitation · vision blurred · withdrawal syndrome

● **HEPATIC IMPAIRMENT** Manufacturer advises caution.

● **RENAL IMPAIRMENT** EvGr Use with caution. Ⓜ

● **LESS SUITABLE FOR PRESCRIBING** Promazine hydrochloride is less suitable for prescribing.

● **MEDICINAL FORMS** There can be variation in the licensing of different medicines containing the same drug. Forms available from special-order manufacturers include: oral suspension, oral solution

Oral tablet
CAUTIONARY AND ADVISORY LABELS 2
▸ **Promazine hydrochloride (Non-proprietary)**
   Promazine hydrochloride 25 mg Promazine 25mg tablets | 100 tablet PoM £90.64 DT = £90.64
   Promazine hydrochloride 50 mg Promazine 50mg tablets | 100 tablet PoM £132.76 DT = £132.76
Oral solution
CAUTIONARY AND ADVISORY LABELS 2
▸ **Promazine hydrochloride (Non-proprietary)**
   Promazine hydrochloride 5 mg per 1 ml Promazine 25mg/5ml syrup | 150 ml PoM £60.19 DT = £60.19
   Promazine 25mg/5ml oral solution | 150 ml PoM £60.19 DT = £60.19
   Promazine hydrochloride 10 mg per 1 ml Promazine 50mg/5ml syrup | 150 ml PoM £75.36 DT = £75.36
   Promazine 50mg/5ml oral solution | 150 ml PoM £51.11–£75.36 DT = £75.36

CNS STIMULANTS

Piracetam

20-Aug-2021

● **INDICATIONS AND DOSE**

Adjunctive treatment of cortical myoclonus
▸ BY MOUTH
▸ Adult: Initially 7.2 g daily in 2–3 divided doses, then increased in steps of 4.8 g every 3–4 days, adjusted according to response, subsequently, attempts should

be made to reduce dose of concurrent therapy; maximum 24 g per day

- **CONTRA-INDICATIONS** Cerebral haemorrhage · Huntington's chorea
- **CAUTIONS** Gastric ulcer · history of haemorrhagic stroke · increased risk of bleeding · major surgery · underlying disorders of haemostasis
- **SIDE-EFFECTS**
  ▸ **Common or very common** Anxiety · movement disorders · weight increased
  ▸ **Uncommon** Asthenia · depression · drowsiness
  ▸ **Frequency not known** Angioedema · confusion · diarrhoea · epilepsy exacerbated · gastrointestinal discomfort · haemorrhagic disorder · hallucination · headache · insomnia · nausea · skin reactions · vertigo · vomiting
- **PREGNANCY** Avoid.
- **BREAST FEEDING** Avoid.
- **HEPATIC IMPAIRMENT** Manufacturer advises caution in combined hepatic and renal impairment.
  Dose adjustments Manufacturer advises dose reduction in combined hepatic and renal impairment.
- **RENAL IMPAIRMENT** EvGr Avoid if creatinine clearance less than 20 mL/minute. ◈M◈
  Dose adjustments EvGr Use two-thirds of normal dose in 2 or 3 divided doses if creatinine clearance 50–80 mL/minute.
  Use one-third of normal dose in 2 divided doses if creatinine clearance 30–50 mL/minute.
  Use one-sixth of normal dose as a single dose if creatinine clearance 20–30 mL/minute. ◈M◈
  See p. 21.
- **TREATMENT CESSATION** Avoid abrupt withdrawal.
- **DIRECTIONS FOR ADMINISTRATION** Manufacturer advises follow the oral solution with a glass of water (or soft drink) to reduce bitter taste.
- **PRESCRIBING AND DISPENSING INFORMATION** Piracetam has been used in children 16 years and over as adjunctive treatment for cortical myoclonus.
- **MEDICINAL FORMS** There can be variation in the licensing of different medicines containing the same drug.
  Oral tablet
  CAUTIONARY AND ADVISORY LABELS 3
  ▸ **Nootropil** (UCB Pharma Ltd)
  Piracetam 800 mg Nootropil 800mg tablets | 90 tablet PoM
  £11.75 DT = £11.75
  Piracetam 1.2 gram Nootropil 1200mg tablets | 60 tablet PoM
  £10.97 DT = £10.97

MONOAMINE DEPLETING DRUGS

| Tetrabenazine
15-Jun-2021

- **INDICATIONS AND DOSE**
  Movement disorders due to Huntington's chorea, hemiballismus, senile chorea, and related neurological conditions
  ▸ BY MOUTH
  ▸ Adult: Initially 25 mg 3 times a day, then increased, if tolerated, in steps of 25 mg every 3–4 days; maximum 200 mg per day
  ▸ Elderly: Lower initial dose may be necessary

  Moderate to severe tardive dyskinesia
  ▸ BY MOUTH
  ▸ Adult: Initially 12.5 mg daily, dose to be gradually increased according to response

- **CONTRA-INDICATIONS** Depression · parkinsonism · phaeochromocytoma · prolactin-dependent tumours
- **CAUTIONS** Susceptibility to QT-interval prolongation

- **INTERACTIONS** → Appendix 1: tetrabenazine
- **SIDE-EFFECTS**
  ▸ **Common or very common** Anxiety · confusion · constipation · depression · diarrhoea · drowsiness · hypotension · insomnia · nausea · parkinsonism · vomiting
  ▸ **Uncommon** Consciousness impaired · hyperthermia
  ▸ **Rare or very rare** Neuroleptic malignant syndrome (discontinue—potentially fatal) · skeletal muscle damage
  ▸ **Frequency not known** Bradycardia · dizziness · dry mouth · epigastric pain · suicidal behaviours
- **PREGNANCY** Avoid unless essential—toxicity in *animal* studies.
- **BREAST FEEDING** Avoid.
- **HEPATIC IMPAIRMENT** Manufacturer advises caution (increased risk of exposure), particularly in severe impairment (no information available).
  Dose adjustments Manufacturer advises initial dose reduction of 50% and slower dose titration in mild to moderate impairment.
- **RENAL IMPAIRMENT** EvGr Use with caution (no information available). ◈M◈
- **TREATMENT CESSATION** Avoid abrupt withdrawal.
- **PATIENT AND CARER ADVICE**
  Driving and skilled tasks May affect performance of skilled tasks (e.g. driving).

- **MEDICINAL FORMS** There can be variation in the licensing of different medicines containing the same drug. Forms available from special-order manufacturers include: oral suspension
  Oral tablet
  CAUTIONARY AND ADVISORY LABELS 2
  ▸ **Tetrabenazine (Non-proprietary)**
  Tetrabenazine 25 mg Tetrabenazine 25mg tablets | 112 tablet PoM £183.15 DT = £161.97
  ▸ **Xenazine** (Alliance Pharmaceuticals Ltd)
  Tetrabenazine 25 mg Xenazine 25 tablets | 112 tablet PoM £100.00 DT = £161.97

MUSCLE RELAXANTS > PERIPHERALLY ACTING > NEUROTOXINS (BOTULINUM TOXINS)

| Botulinum toxin type A
12-Apr-2022

- **INDICATIONS AND DOSE**
  Hand and wrist disability due to upper limb spasticity associated with stroke (specialist use only) | Foot and ankle disability due to lower limb spasticity associated with stroke (specialist use only) | Blepharospasm (specialist use only) | Hemifacial spasm (specialist use only) | Spasmodic torticollis (specialist use only) | Severe hyperhidrosis of the axillae (specialist use only) | Prophylaxis of headaches in chronic migraine (specialist use only) | Temporary improvement of moderate to severe upper facial lines in adults under 65 years (specialist use only) | Management of bladder dysfunctions (specialist use only) | Chronic sialorrhoea [due to neurological disorders] (specialist use only)
  ▸ BY SUBCUTANEOUS INJECTION, OR BY INTRADERMAL INJECTION, OR BY INTRAMUSCULAR INJECTION, OR BY LOCAL INFILTRATION
  ▸ Adult: (consult product literature)

  DOSE EQUIVALENCE AND CONVERSION
  ▸ **Important**: information is specific to each individual preparation.

- **CONTRA-INDICATIONS** Acute urinary retention (specific to use in bladder disorders only) · catheterisation difficulties (specific to use in bladder disorders only) · infection at injection site · presence of bladder calculi (specific to use in bladder disorders only) · urinary tract infection (specific to use in bladder disorders only)

- **CAUTIONS**
  GENERAL CAUTIONS Atrophy in target muscle · chronic respiratory disorder · elderly · excessive weakness in target muscle · history of aspiration · history of dysphagia · inflammation in target muscle · neurological disorders · neuromuscular disorders · off-label use (fatal adverse events reported)
  SPECIFIC CAUTIONS
  ‣ When used for Blepharospasm or hemifacial spasm Risk of angle-closure glaucoma
  CAUTIONS, FURTHER INFORMATION Neuromuscular or neurological disorders can lead to increased sensitivity and exaggerated muscle weakness including dysphagia and respiratory compromise.
  ‣ Blepharospasm or hemifacial spasm When used for blepharospasm and hemifacial spasm, reduced blinking can lead to corneal exposure, persistent epithelial defect and corneal ulceration (especially in those with VIIth nerve disorders)— EvGr careful testing of corneal sensation in previously operated eyes, avoidance of injection in lower lid area to avoid ectropion, and vigorous treatment of epithelial defect needed. Ⓜ

- **INTERACTIONS** → Appendix 1: botulinum toxins

- **SIDE-EFFECTS**
  ‣ **Common or very common** Alopecia · asthenia · autonomic dysreflexia · bladder diverticulum · brow ptosis · constipation · dizziness · drowsiness · dry eye · dry mouth · dysphagia (most common after injection into sternocleidomastoid muscle and salivary gland) · ecchymosis (minimised by applying gentle pressure at injection site immediately after injection) · eye discomfort · eye disorders · eye inflammation · facial paresis · fall · fever · gait abnormal · haematuria · headaches · hot flush · increased risk of infection · influenza like illness · insomnia · joint disorders · leukocyturia · malaise · muscle complaints · muscle weakness · musculoskeletal stiffness · nausea · oedema · pain · sensation abnormal · skin reactions · subcutaneous nodule · urinary disorders · vision disorders
  ‣ **Uncommon** Anxiety · coordination abnormal · depression · dysphonia · dyspnoea · facial paralysis · memory loss · oral paraesthesia · photosensitivity reaction · postural hypotension · speech impairment · taste altered · vertigo
  ‣ **Frequency not known** Abdominal pain · angioedema · angle closure glaucoma · appetite decreased · arrhythmia · diarrhoea · hearing impairment · hypersensitivity · myocardial infarction · myopathy · nerve disorders · neuromuscular dysfunction · pneumonia aspiration (potentially fatal) · respiratory disorders · seizure · syncope · tinnitus · vomiting

- **CONCEPTION AND CONTRACEPTION** Avoid in women of child-bearing age unless using effective contraception.

- **PREGNANCY** Avoid unless essential—toxicity in *animal* studies (manufacturer of *Botox*® advise avoid).

- **BREAST FEEDING** Low risk of systemic absorption but avoid unless essential.

- **PRESCRIBING AND DISPENSING INFORMATION** Preparations are not interchangeable.

- **PATIENT AND CARER ADVICE** Patients and carers should be warned of the signs and symptoms of toxin spread, such as muscle weakness and breathing difficulties; they should be advised to seek immediate medical attention if swallowing, speech or breathing difficulties occur.

- **NATIONAL FUNDING/ACCESS DECISIONS**
  For full details see funding body website
  NICE decisions
  ‣ Botulinum toxin type A for the prevention of headaches in adults with chronic migraine (June 2012) NICE TA260 Recommended with restrictions

‣ Xeomin® (botulinum neurotoxin type A) for treating chronic sialorrhoea (October 2019) NICE TA605 Recommended
Scottish Medicines Consortium (SMC) decisions
‣ Botulinum toxin type A (*Botox*®) for the management of bladder dysfunctions in adult patients who are not adequately managed with anticholinergics: overactive bladder with symptoms of urinary incontinence, urgency and frequency (July 2014) SMC No. 931/13 Recommended with restrictions
‣ Botulinum toxin A (*Botox*®) for the prophylaxis of headaches in adults with chronic migraine (headaches on at least 15 days per month of which at least 8 days are with migraine) (February 2017) SMC No. 692/11 Recommended with restrictions
‣ Clostridium botulinum neurotoxin type A (*Xeomin*®) for adult patients with chronic sialorrhoea due to neurological conditions (November 2019) SMC No. SMC2212 Recommended

- **MEDICINAL FORMS** There can be variation in the licensing of different medicines containing the same drug.
  Powder for solution for injection
  ‣ **Azzalure** (Galderma (UK) Ltd)
    Botulinum toxin type A 125 unit Azzalure 125unit powder for solution for injection vials | 2 vial PoM £126.99
  ‣ **Bocouture** (Merz Aesthetics UK Ltd)
    Botulinum toxin type A 50 unit Bocouture 50unit powder for solution for injection vials | 1 vial PoM 🅧
    Botulinum toxin type A 100 unit Bocouture 100unit powder for solution for injection vials | 1 vial PoM 🅧
  ‣ **Botox** (AbbVie Ltd)
    Botulinum toxin type A 50 unit Botox 50unit powder for solution for injection vials | 1 vial PoM £77.50 (Hospital only)
    Botulinum toxin type A 100 unit Botox 100unit powder for solution for injection vials | 1 vial PoM £138.20 (Hospital only)
    Botulinum toxin type A 200 unit Botox 200unit powder for solution for injection vials | 1 vial PoM £276.40 (Hospital only)
  ‣ **Dysport** (Ipsen Ltd)
    Botulinum toxin type A 300 unit Dysport 300unit powder for solution for injection vials | 1 vial PoM £92.40
    Botulinum toxin type A 500 unit Dysport 500unit powder for solution for injection vials | 2 vial PoM £308.00
  ‣ **Letybo** (Croma-Pharma GmbH)
    Botulinum toxin type A 50 unit Letybo 50unit powder for solution for injection vials | 1 vial PoM £65.00 | 2 vial PoM £120.00 | 6 vial PoM £350.00
  ‣ **Xeomin** (Merz Pharma UK Ltd)
    Botulinum toxin type A 50 unit Xeomin 50unit powder for solution for injection vials | 1 vial PoM £72.00
    Botulinum toxin type A 100 unit Xeomin 100unit powder for solution for injection vials | 1 vial PoM £129.90
    Botulinum toxin type A 200 unit Xeomin 200unit powder for solution for injection vials | 1 vial PoM £259.80 (Hospital only)

4.2 Parkinson's disease

Parkinson's disease   29-May-2024

Description of condition

Parkinson's disease is a progressive neurodegenerative condition resulting from the death of dopaminergic cells of the substantia nigra in the brain.

Patients with Parkinson's disease classically present with motor-symptoms including hypokinesia, bradykinesia, rigidity, rest tremor, and postural instability.

Non-motor symptoms include dementia, depression, sleep disturbances, bladder and bowel dysfunction, speech and language changes, swallowing problems and weight loss.

EvGr Patients with suspected Parkinson's disease should be referred to a specialist and reviewed every 6 to 12 months. When Parkinson's disease diagnosis is confirmed, patients should be advised to inform the DVLA and their car insurer. Ⓐ

Aims of treatment

Parkinson's disease is an incurable progressive condition, and the aim of treatment is to control the symptoms and to improve the patient's quality of life.

Non-drug treatment

[EvGr] Parkinson's disease patients should be offered physiotherapy if balance or motor function problems are present, speech and language therapy if they develop communication, swallowing or saliva problems, and occupational therapy if they experience difficulties with their daily activities. Dietitian referral should be considered. ⟨A⟩

Drug treatment

Drug management of motor symptoms in Parkinson's disease
First-line treatment

[EvGr] In early stages of Parkinson's disease, patients whose motor symptoms decrease their quality of life should be offered *levodopa* combined with *carbidopa* (co-careldopa p. 476) or *benserazide* (co-beneldopa p. 475).

Parkinson's disease patients whose motor symptoms *do not* affect their quality of life, could be prescribed a choice of *levodopa*, *non-ergot-derived dopamine-receptor agonists* (pramipexole p. 485, ropinirole p. 487 or rotigotine p. 488) or *monoamine-oxidase-B inhibitors* (rasagiline p. 489 or selegiline hydrochloride p. 490).

Before starting antiparkinsonian treatment, the patient's individual circumstances, including symptoms, comorbidities and preferences, should be discussed together with the potential benefits and harms from the different drugs available.

Patients and their carers should be informed about the risk of adverse reactions from antiparkinsonian drugs, including psychotic symptoms, excessive sleepiness and sudden onset of sleep with dopamine-receptor agonists, and impulse control disorders with all dopaminergic therapy (especially *dopamine-receptor agonists*). For further information *see Impulse control disorders*. ⟨A⟩

Levodopa treatment is associated with motor complications, including response fluctuations and dyskinesias. Response fluctuations are characterised by large variations in motor performance, with normal function during the 'on' period, and weakness and restricted mobility during the 'off' period. 'End-of-dose' deterioration with progressively shorter duration of benefit can also occur. Modified-release preparations may help with 'end-of-dose' deterioration or nocturnal immobility.

The overall improvement in motor performance is more noticeable with *levodopa* than with *dopamine-receptor agonists*, and motor complications are less likely to occur with *dopamine-receptor agonists* when used alone long-term. Conversely, excessive sleepiness, hallucinations, and impulse control disorders are more likely to occur with *dopamine-receptor agonists* than with *levodopa*.

[EvGr] To avoid the potential for acute akinesia or neuroleptic malignant syndrome, antiparkinsonian drug concentrations should not be allowed to fall suddenly due to poor absorption or abrupt withdrawal. ⟨A⟩

Adjuvant therapy

[EvGr] If a patient with Parkinson's disease develops dyskinesia or motor fluctuations, specialist advice should be sought before modifying antiparkinsonian drug therapy.

Patients who develop dyskinesia or motor fluctuations despite optimal *levodopa* therapy should be offered a choice of *non-ergotic dopamine-receptor agonists* (pramipexole, ropinirole, rotigotine), *monoamine oxidase B inhibitors* (rasagiline or selegiline hydrochloride) or COMT inhibitors (entacapone p. 474 or tolcapone p. 475) as an adjunct to *levodopa*.

An *ergot-derived dopamine-receptor agonist* (bromocriptine p. 482, cabergoline p. 484 or pergolide) should **only** be considered as an adjunct to *levodopa* if symptoms are not

adequately controlled with a *non-ergot-derived dopamine-receptor agonist*.

If dyskinesia is not adequately managed by modifying existing therapy, amantadine hydrochloride p. 480 should be considered. ⟨A⟩

Drug management of non-motor symptoms in Parkinson's disease

Daytime sleepiness and sudden onset of sleep

[EvGr] Patients who experience daytime sleepiness or sudden onset of sleep, should have their Parkinson's drug treatment adjusted under specialist medical guidance. If reversible pharmacological and physical causes have been excluded, modafinil p. 559 should be considered to treat excessive daytime sleepiness, and treatment should be reviewed at least every 12 months.

Patients with Parkinson's disease who have daytime sleepiness or sudden onset of sleep should be advised not to drive, to inform the DVLA about their symptoms, and to think about any occupational hazards. ⟨A⟩

Nocturnal akinesia

[EvGr] When treating nocturnal akinesia in patients with Parkinson's disease, *levodopa* or oral *dopamine-receptor agonists* should be considered as first-line options and rotigotine p. 488 as second-line (if both *levodopa* or oral *dopamine-receptor agonists* are ineffective). ⟨A⟩

Postural hypotension

[EvGr] Patients with Parkinson's disease who develop postural hypotension should have their drug treatment reviewed to address any pharmacological cause. If drug therapy is required, midodrine hydrochloride p. 217 should be considered as the first option and fludrocortisone acetate p. 787 [unlicensed indication] as an alternative. ⟨A⟩

Depression

See Depression p. 415.

Psychotic symptoms

[EvGr] Hallucinations and delusions need not be treated if they are well tolerated. Otherwise, the dosage of any antiparkinsonism drugs that might have triggered hallucinations or delusions should be reduced, taking into account the severity of symptoms and possible withdrawal effects. Specialist advice should be sought before modifying drug treatment.

In Parkinson's disease patients with no cognitive impairment, quetiapine p. 462 [unlicensed indication] can be considered to treat hallucinations and delusions. If standard treatment is not effective, clozapine p. 457 should be offered to treat hallucinations and delusions in patients with Parkinson's disease. ⟨A⟩ It is important to acknowledge that other antipsychotic medicines (such as phenothiazines and butyrophenones) can worsen the motor features of Parkinson's disease.

Rapid eye movement sleep behaviour disorder

[EvGr] Clonazepam p. 391 [unlicensed indication] or melatonin p. 555 [unlicensed indication] should be considered to treat rapid eye movement sleep behaviour disorder in Parkinson's patients once possible pharmacological causes have been addressed. ⟨A⟩

Drooling of saliva

[EvGr] Drug treatment for drooling of saliva in patients with Parkinson's disease should only be considered if non-drug treatment such as speech and language therapy is not available or is ineffective.

Glycopyrronium bromide p. 281 [unlicensed indication] should be considered as first-line treatment and botulinum toxin type A p. 469 as second-line.

Other antimuscarinic drugs, should only be considered if the risk of cognitive adverse effects is thought to be minimal; topical preparations, such as *atropine* [unlicensed indication], should be used if possible to reduce the risk of adverse events. Ⓐ

Parkinson's disease dementia

[EvGr] An acetylcholinesterase inhibitor should be offered to patients with mild-to-moderate Parkinson's disease dementia and considered for patients with severe Parkinson's disease dementia [unlicensed indications apart from rivastigmine capsules and oral solution p. 347 for the treatment of mild-to-moderate dementia in patients with Parkinson's disease]. If acetylcholinesterase inhibitors are not tolerated or contra-indicated, memantine hydrochloride p. 349 [unlicensed indication] should be considered. Ⓐ For further information *see* Dementia p. 343

Advanced Parkinson's disease

[EvGr] Patients with advanced Parkinson's disease can be offered apomorphine hydrochloride p. 481 as intermittent injections or continuous subcutaneous infusions. Ⓐ To control nausea and vomiting associated with *apomorphine*, the manufacturers recommend that administration of domperidone p. 494 [unlicensed in those weighing less than 35 kg] will usually need to be started two days before *apomorphine* therapy, and then discontinued as soon as possible. To reduce the risk of serious arrhythmia due to QT prolongation associated to the concomitant use of domperidone p. 494 and apomorphine hydrochloride p. 481, the MHRA/CHM recommend an assessment of cardiac risk factors and ECG monitoring and to ensure that the benefits outweighs the risks when initiating treatment.

[EvGr] Deep brain stimulation should *only* be considered for patients with advanced Parkinson's disease whose symptoms are *not* adequately controlled by best drug therapy.

Intestinal gel containing co-careldopa p. 476 or continuous subcutaneous infusion of foslevodopa with foscarbidopa p. 478 may be used to treat advanced levodopa-responsive Parkinson's disease with severe motor fluctuations and hyperkinesia or dyskinesia, if the use of *apomorphine* or deep brain stimulation is not possible or fails to control symptoms. Ⓐ

Impulse control disorders

Impulse control disorders (compulsive gambling, hypersexuality, binge eating, or obsessive shopping) can develop in a person with Parkinson's disease who is on any dopaminergic therapy at any stage in the disease course particularly if the patient has a history of previous impulsive behaviours, alcohol consumption, or smoking. [EvGr] Patients should be informed about the different types of impulse control disorders and that dopamine-receptor agonist therapy may be reduced or stopped if problematic impulse control disorders develop.

When managing impulse control disorders, dopamine-receptor agonist doses should be reduced gradually and patients should be monitored for symptoms of dopamine agonist withdrawal. Specialist cognitive behavioural therapy should be offered if modifying dopaminergic therapy is not effective. Ⓐ

Useful Resources

Parkinson's disease in adults. National Institute for Health and Care Excellence. NICE guideline 71. July 2017.
www.nice.org.uk/guidance/NG71

ANTIMUSCARINICS

Orphenadrine hydrochloride
27-Apr-2021

- **DRUG ACTION** Orphenadrine exerts its antiparkinsonian action by reducing the effects of the relative central cholinergic excess that occurs as a result of dopamine deficiency.

- **INDICATIONS AND DOSE**

Parkinsonism | Drug-induced extrapyramidal symptoms (but not tardive dyskinesia)
- ▶ BY MOUTH
- ▶ Adult: Initially 150 mg daily in divided doses, then increased in steps of 50 mg every 2–3 days, adjusted according to response; usual dose 150–300 mg daily in divided doses; maximum 400 mg per day
- ▶ Elderly: Preferably dose at lower end of range

- **CONTRA-INDICATIONS** Acute porphyrias p. 1202 · gastro-intestinal obstruction

- **CAUTIONS** Cardiovascular disease · elderly · hypertension · in patients susceptible to angle-closure glaucoma · liable to abuse · prostatic hypertrophy · psychotic disorders · pyrexia

- **INTERACTIONS** → Appendix 1: orphenadrine

- **SIDE-EFFECTS**
- ▶ **Common or very common** Accommodation disorder · anxiety · dizziness · dry mouth · gastrointestinal disorder · nausea
- ▶ **Uncommon** Confusion · constipation · coordination abnormal · euphoric mood · hallucination · insomnia · sedation · seizure · tachycardia · urinary retention
- ▶ **Rare or very rare** Memory loss

- **PREGNANCY** Caution.

- **BREAST FEEDING** Caution.

- **HEPATIC IMPAIRMENT** Manufacturer advises caution.

- **RENAL IMPAIRMENT** [EvGr] Use with caution. Ⓜ

- **TREATMENT CESSATION** Avoid abrupt withdrawal in patients taking long-term treatment.

- **PATIENT AND CARER ADVICE**
Driving and skilled tasks May affect performance of skilled tasks (e.g. driving).

- **MEDICINAL FORMS** There can be variation in the licensing of different medicines containing the same drug. Forms available from special-order manufacturers include: oral solution
Oral solution
- ▶ Orphenadrine hydrochloride (Non-proprietary)
  Orphenadrine hydrochloride 10 mg per 1 ml Orphenadrine 50mg/5ml oral solution sugar free | 150 ml [PoM] £139.59 DT = £139.59 [SF]

Procyclidine hydrochloride
25-Aug-2022

- **DRUG ACTION** Procyclidine exerts its antiparkinsonian action by reducing the effects of the relative central cholinergic excess that occurs as a result of dopamine deficiency.

- **INDICATIONS AND DOSE**
Parkinsonism
- ▶ BY MOUTH
- ▶ Adult: 2.5 mg 3 times a day, then increased in steps of 2.5–5 mg daily as required, dose to be increased at 2–3 day intervals, usual maintenance 15–30 mg daily in 2–4 divided doses, maximum daily dose only to be used in exceptional circumstances; maximum 60 mg per day
- ▶ Elderly: Lower end of range preferable

Drug-induced extrapyramidal symptoms (but not tardive dyskinesia)
▶ BY MOUTH
▶ Adult: 2.5 mg 3 times a day, then increased in steps of 2.5 mg daily as required, usual maintenance 10–30 mg daily in 2–3 divided doses
▶ Elderly: Lower end of range preferable

Acute dystonia
▶ BY INTRAMUSCULAR INJECTION, OR BY INTRAVENOUS INJECTION
▶ Adult: 5–10 mg, occasionally, more than 10 mg, dose usually effective in 5–10 minutes but may need 30 minutes for relief
▶ Elderly: Lower end of range preferable

● **CONTRA-INDICATIONS** Gastro-intestinal obstruction

● **CAUTIONS** Cardiovascular disease · elderly · hypertension · liable to abuse · prostatic hypertrophy · psychotic disorders · pyrexia · those susceptible to angle-closure glaucoma

● **INTERACTIONS** → Appendix 1: procyclidine

● **SIDE-EFFECTS**
▶ **Common or very common** Constipation · dry mouth · urinary retention · vision blurred
▶ **Uncommon** Anxiety · cognitive impairment · confusion · dizziness · gingivitis · hallucination · memory loss · nausea · rash · vomiting
▶ **Rare or very rare** Psychotic disorder

● **PREGNANCY** Use only if potential benefit outweighs risk.

● **BREAST FEEDING** No information available.

● **HEPATIC IMPAIRMENT** Manufacturer advises caution.

● **RENAL IMPAIRMENT** EvGr Use with caution. Ⓜ

● **TREATMENT CESSATION** Avoid abrupt withdrawal in patients taking long-term treatment.

● **PATIENT AND CARER ADVICE**
Driving and skilled tasks May affect performance of skilled tasks (e.g. driving).

● **MEDICINAL FORMS** There can be variation in the licensing of different medicines containing the same drug. Forms available from special-order manufacturers include: oral suspension, oral solution

Solution for injection
▶ Procyclidine hydrochloride (Non-proprietary)
Procyclidine hydrochloride 5 mg per 1 ml Procyclidine 10mg/2ml solution for injection ampoules | 5 ampoule PoM £72.50-£105.00 DT = £72.50

Oral tablet
▶ Procyclidine hydrochloride (Non-proprietary)
Procyclidine hydrochloride 5 mg Procyclidine 5mg tablets | 28 tablet PoM £2.52 DT = £1.26 | 100 tablet PoM £4.50-£8.94 | 500 tablet PoM £22.50-£44.63
▶ Kemadrin (Aspen Pharma Trading Ltd)
Procyclidine hydrochloride 5 mg Kemadrin 5mg tablets | 100 tablet PoM £4.72 | 500 tablet PoM £23.62

Oral solution
▶ Procyclidine hydrochloride (Non-proprietary)
Procyclidine hydrochloride 500 microgram per 1 ml Procyclidine 2.5mg/5ml oral solution sugar free | 150 ml PoM £47.30 DT = £47.30 SF
Procyclidine hydrochloride 1 mg per 1 ml Procyclidine 5mg/5ml oral solution sugar free | 150 ml PoM £70.04 DT = £70.04 SF

Trihexyphenidyl hydrochloride   27-Apr-2021
(Benzhexol hydrochloride)

● **DRUG ACTION** Trihexyphenidyl exerts its effects by reducing the effects of the relative central cholinergic excess that occurs as a result of dopamine deficiency.

● **INDICATIONS AND DOSE**

Parkinson's disease (if used in combination with co-careldopa or co-beneldopa)
▶ BY MOUTH
▶ Adult: Maintenance 2–6 mg daily in divided doses, use not recommended because of toxicity in the elderly and the risk of aggravating dementia

Parkinsonism | Drug-induced extrapyramidal symptoms (but not tardive dyskinesia)
▶ BY MOUTH
▶ Adult: 1 mg daily, then increased in steps of 2 mg every 3–5 days, adjusted according to response; maintenance 5–15 mg daily in 3–4 divided doses, not recommended for use in Parkinson's disease because of toxicity in the elderly and the risk of aggravating dementia; maximum 20 mg per day
▶ Elderly: Lower end of range preferable, not recommended for use in Parkinson's disease because of toxicity in the elderly and the risk of aggravating dementia

● **CONTRA-INDICATIONS** Myasthenia gravis

● **CAUTIONS** Cardiovascular disease · elderly · gastro-intestinal obstruction · hypertension · liable to abuse · prostatic hypertrophy · psychotic disorders · pyrexia · those susceptible to angle-closure glaucoma

● **INTERACTIONS** → Appendix 1: trihexyphenidyl

● **SIDE-EFFECTS** Anxiety · bronchial secretion decreased · confusion · constipation · delusions · dizziness · dry mouth · dysphagia · euphoric mood · fever · flushing · hallucination · insomnia · memory loss · myasthenia gravis aggravated · mydriasis · nausea · skin reactions · tachycardia · thirst · urinary disorders · vision disorders · vomiting

● **PREGNANCY** Use only if potential benefit outweighs risk.

● **BREAST FEEDING** Avoid.

● **HEPATIC IMPAIRMENT** Manufacturer advises caution.

● **RENAL IMPAIRMENT** EvGr Use with caution. Ⓜ

● **TREATMENT CESSATION** Avoid abrupt withdrawal in patients taking long-term treatment.

● **DIRECTIONS FOR ADMINISTRATION** Manufacturer advises tablets should be taken with or after food.

● **PATIENT AND CARER ADVICE**
Driving and skilled tasks May affect performance of skilled tasks (e.g. driving).

● **MEDICINAL FORMS** There can be variation in the licensing of different medicines containing the same drug. Forms available from special-order manufacturers include: oral suspension, oral solution

Oral tablet
▶ Trihexyphenidyl hydrochloride (Non-proprietary)
Trihexyphenidyl hydrochloride 2 mg Trihexyphenidyl 2mg tablets | 84 tablet PoM £50.00 DT = £3.10
Trihexyphenidyl hydrochloride 5 mg Trihexyphenidyl 5mg tablets | 84 tablet PoM £50.00 DT = £8.14

Oral solution
EXCIPIENTS: May contain Propylene glycol
▶ Trihexyphenidyl hydrochloride (Non-proprietary)
Trihexyphenidyl hydrochloride 1 mg per 1 ml Trihexyphenidyl 5mg/5ml oral solution | 200 ml PoM £108.44 DT = £108.44
Trihexyphenidyl 5mg/5ml syrup | 200 ml PoM £108.44 DT = £108.44

DOPAMINERGIC DRUGS > CATECHOL-O-METHYLTRANSFERASE INHIBITORS

Entacapone
15-Apr-2024

- **DRUG ACTION** Entacapone prevents the peripheral breakdown of levodopa, by inhibiting catechol-*O*-methyltransferase, allowing more levodopa to reach the brain.

- **INDICATIONS AND DOSE**

  Adjunct to co-beneldopa or co-careldopa in Parkinson's disease with 'end-of-dose' motor fluctuations (under expert supervision)
  ▸ BY MOUTH
  ▸ Adult: 200 mg, dose to be given with each dose of levodopa with dopa-decarboxylase inhibitor; maximum 2 g per day

- **CONTRA-INDICATIONS** History of neuroleptic malignant syndrome · history of non-traumatic rhabdomyolysis · phaeochromocytoma

- **CAUTIONS** Concurrent levodopa dose may need to be reduced by about 10–30% · ischaemic heart disease

- **INTERACTIONS** → Appendix 1: entacapone

- **SIDE-EFFECTS**
  ▸ **Common or very common** Abdominal pain · confusion · constipation · diarrhoea · dizziness · dry mouth · fall · fatigue · hallucination · hyperhidrosis · ischaemic heart disease · movement disorders · nausea · sleep disorders · urine discolouration · vomiting
  ▸ **Uncommon** Myocardial infarction
  ▸ **Rare or very rare** Agitation · appetite decreased · skin reactions · weight decreased
  ▸ **Frequency not known** Colitis · drowsiness · hair colour changes · hepatic disorders · impulse-control disorder · nail discolouration · neuroleptic malignant syndrome · rhabdomyolysis · sudden onset of sleep

- **PREGNANCY** Avoid—no information available.

- **BREAST FEEDING** Avoid—present in milk in *animal* studies.

- **HEPATIC IMPAIRMENT** Manufacturer advises avoid.

- **TREATMENT CESSATION** Avoid abrupt withdrawal.

- **PATIENT AND CARER ADVICE** Patient counselling is advised (may colour urine reddish-brown, concomitant iron-containing products).
  Driving and skilled tasks
  Sudden onset of sleep Excessive daytime sleepiness and sudden onset of sleep can occur with entacapone.

  Patients starting treatment should be warned of the risk and of the need to exercise caution when driving or operating machinery. Those who have experienced excessive sedation or sudden onset of sleep should refrain from driving or operating machines until these effects have stopped occurring.

  Management of excessive daytime sleepiness should focus on the identification of an underlying cause, such as depression or concomitant medication. Patients should be counselled on improving sleep behaviour.

- **MEDICINAL FORMS** There can be variation in the licensing of different medicines containing the same drug. Forms available from special-order manufacturers include: oral suspension, oral solution

  Oral tablet
  CAUTIONARY AND ADVISORY LABELS 14
  ▸ Entacapone (Non-proprietary)
    Entacapone 200 mg Entacapone 200mg tablets | 30 tablet [PoM] £14.65 DT = £7.03 | 100 tablet [PoM] £23.43–£48.83

▸ Comtess (Orion Pharma (UK) Ltd)
  Entacapone 200 mg Comtess 200mg tablets | 30 tablet [PoM] £17.24 DT = £7.03 | 100 tablet [PoM] £57.45

Combinations available: *Levodopa with carbidopa and entacapone,* p. 479

Opicapone
28-May-2024

- **DRUG ACTION** Opicapone prevents the peripheral breakdown of levodopa, by inhibiting catechol-*O*-methyltransferase, allowing more levodopa to reach the brain.

- **INDICATIONS AND DOSE**

  Adjunct to co-beneldopa or co-careldopa in Parkinson's disease with 'end-of-dose' motor fluctuations (under expert supervision)
  ▸ BY MOUTH
  ▸ Adult: 50 mg once daily, dose to be taken at bedtime, at least one hour before or after levodopa combinations

- **CONTRA-INDICATIONS** Catecholamine-secreting neoplasms · history of neuroleptic malignant syndrome · history of non-traumatic rhabdomyolysis · paraganglioma · phaeochromocytoma

- **CAUTIONS** Concurrent levodopa dose may need to be reduced · elderly over 85 years (limited information available)

- **INTERACTIONS** → Appendix 1: opicapone

- **SIDE-EFFECTS**
  ▸ **Common or very common** Constipation · dizziness · drowsiness · dry mouth · hallucinations · headache · hypotension · movement disorders · muscle complaints · sleep disorders · vomiting
  ▸ **Uncommon** Anxiety · appetite decreased · depression · dry eye · dyspnoea · ear congestion · gastrointestinal discomfort · hypertension · hypertriglyceridaemia · musculoskeletal stiffness · nocturia · pain in extremity · palpitations · syncope · taste altered · urine discolouration · weight decreased

  SIDE-EFFECTS, FURTHER INFORMATION Manufacturer advises consider liver function tests in patients who experience progressive anorexia, asthenia and weight decrease within a relatively short period of time.

- **PREGNANCY** Manufacturer advises avoid—limited information available.

- **BREAST FEEDING** Manufacturer advises avoid—no information available.

- **HEPATIC IMPAIRMENT** Manufacturer advises caution in moderate impairment (risk of increased exposure); avoid in severe impairment (no information available).
  Dose adjustments Manufacturer advises consider dose reduction in moderate impairment.

- **NATIONAL FUNDING/ACCESS DECISIONS**
  For full details see funding body website
  Scottish Medicines Consortium (SMC) decisions
  ▸ Opicapone (*Ongentys*®) as adjunctive therapy to preparations of levodopa/dopa-decarboxylase inhibitors in adult patients with Parkinson's disease and end-of-dose motor fluctuations who cannot be stabilised on those combinations (January 2022) SMC No. SMC2430 Recommended
  All Wales Medicines Strategy Group (AWMSG) decisions
  ▸ Opicapone (*Ongentys*®) as adjunctive therapy to preparations of levodopa/dopa-decarboxylase inhibitors in adult patients with Parkinson's disease and end-of-dose motor fluctuations who cannot be stabilised on those combinations (May 2024) AWMSG No. 5285 Recommended

- **MEDICINAL FORMS** There can be variation in the licensing of different medicines containing the same drug.

  Oral capsule
  - ▸ Ongentys (BIAL Pharma UK Ltd)

    Opicapone 50 mg Ongentys 50mg capsules | 30 capsule [PoM] £59.00 DT = £59.00

Tolcapone

04-Aug-2021

- **DRUG ACTION** Tolcapone prevents the peripheral breakdown of levodopa, by inhibiting catechol-*O*-methyltransferase, allowing more levodopa to reach the brain.

- ● **INDICATIONS AND DOSE**

  Adjunct to co-beneldopa or co-careldopa in Parkinson's disease with 'end-of-dose' motor fluctuations if another inhibitor of peripheral catechol-O-methyltransferase inappropriate (under expert supervision)
  - ▸ BY MOUTH
  - ▸ Adult: 100 mg 3 times a day (max. per dose 200 mg 3 times a day) continuing beyond 3 weeks **only** if substantial improvement, leave 6 hours between each dose; first daily dose should be taken at the same time as levodopa with dopa-decarboxylase inhibitor, dose maximum only in exceptional circumstances

- **CONTRA-INDICATIONS** Phaeochromocytoma · previous history of hyperthermia · previous history of neuroleptic malignant syndrome · previous history of rhabdomyolysis · severe dyskinesia

- **CAUTIONS** Most patients receiving more than 600 mg levodopa daily require reduction of levodopa dose by about 30%

  CAUTIONS, FURTHER INFORMATION
  - ▸ Hepatotoxicity Potentially life-threatening hepatotoxicity including fulminant hepatitis reported rarely, usually in women and during the first 6 months, but late-onset liver injury also reported; discontinue if abnormal liver function tests or symptoms of liver disorder; do not re-introduce tolcapone once discontinued.

- **INTERACTIONS** → Appendix 1: tolcapone

- **SIDE-EFFECTS**
  - ▸ **Common or very common** Appetite decreased · chest pain · confusion · constipation · diarrhoea · dizziness · drowsiness · dry mouth · gastrointestinal discomfort · hallucination · headache · hyperhidrosis · influenza like illness · movement disorders · nausea · postural hypotension · sleep disorders · syncope · upper respiratory tract infection · urine discolouration · vomiting
  - ▸ **Uncommon** Hepatocellular injury
  - ▸ **Rare or very rare** Eating disorders · neuroleptic malignant syndrome (reported on dose reduction or withdrawal) · pathological gambling · psychiatric disorders · sexual dysfunction

- **PREGNANCY** Toxicity in *animal* studies—use only if potential benefit outweighs risk.

- **BREAST FEEDING** Avoid—present in milk in *animal* studies.

- **HEPATIC IMPAIRMENT** Manufacturer advises avoid.

- **RENAL IMPAIRMENT** [EvGr] Caution if creatinine clearance less than 30 mL/minute. ⟨M⟩ See p. 21.

- **MONITORING REQUIREMENTS** Test liver function before treatment, and monitor every 2 weeks for first year, every 4 weeks for next 6 months and then every 8 weeks thereafter (restart monitoring schedule if dose increased).

- **TREATMENT CESSATION** Avoid abrupt withdrawal.

- **PATIENT AND CARER ADVICE** Patients should be told how to recognise signs of liver disorder and advised to seek immediate medical attention if symptoms such as

anorexia, nausea, vomiting, fatigue, abdominal pain, dark urine, or pruritus develop.

- **MEDICINAL FORMS** There can be variation in the licensing of different medicines containing the same drug.

  Oral tablet

  CAUTIONARY AND ADVISORY LABELS 14, 25
  - ▸ Tasmar (Viatris UK Healthcare Ltd)

    Tolcapone 100 mg Tasmar 100mg tablets | 100 tablet [PoM] £95.20 DT = £95.20

DOPAMINERGIC DRUGS › DOPAMINE PRECURSORS

Co-beneldopa

06-Nov-2024

- ● **INDICATIONS AND DOSE**

  Parkinson's disease
  - ▸ BY MOUTH USING IMMEDIATE-RELEASE MEDICINES
  - ▸ Adult: Initially 50 mg 3–4 times a day, then increased in steps of 100 mg daily, dose to be increased once or twice weekly according to response; maintenance 400–800 mg daily in divided doses
  - ▸ Elderly: Initially 50 mg 1–2 times a day, then increased in steps of 50 mg daily, dose to be increased every 3–4 days according to response

  Parkinson's disease (in advanced disease)
  - ▸ BY MOUTH USING IMMEDIATE-RELEASE MEDICINES
  - ▸ Adult: Initially 100 mg 3 times a day, then increased in steps of 100 mg daily, dose to be increased once or twice weekly according to response; maintenance 400–800 mg daily in divided doses

  Parkinson's disease (patients not taking levodopa/dopa-decarboxylase inhibitor therapy)
  - ▸ BY MOUTH USING MODIFIED-RELEASE MEDICINES
  - ▸ Adult: Initially 1 capsule 3 times a day; maximum 6 capsules per day

  Parkinson's disease (patients transferring from immediate-release levodopa/dopa-decarboxylase inhibitor preparations)
  - ▸ BY MOUTH USING MODIFIED-RELEASE MEDICINES
  - ▸ Adult: Initially 1 capsule substituted for every 100 mg of levodopa and given at same dosage frequency, increased every 2–3 days according to response; average increase of 50% needed over previous levodopa dose and titration may take up to 4 weeks, supplementary dose of immediate-release *Madopar*® may be needed with first morning dose; if response still poor to total daily dose of *Madopar*® CR plus *Madopar*® corresponding to 1.2 g levodopa—consider alternative therapy.

  DOSE EQUIVALENCE AND CONVERSION
  - ▸ Dose is expressed as levodopa.

> **IMPORTANT SAFETY INFORMATION**
>
> IMPULSE CONTROL DISORDERS
>
> Treatment with levodopa is associated with impulse control disorders, including pathological gambling, binge eating, and hypersexuality. Patients and their carers should be informed about the risk of impulse control disorders. See Parkinson's disease p. 470.

- **CONTRA-INDICATIONS** Angle-closure glaucoma · suspicious undiagnosed skin lesions or history of skin melanoma (risk of activation)

- **CAUTIONS** Cushing's syndrome · diabetes mellitus · endocrine disorders · history of convulsions · history of myocardial infarction with residual arrhythmia · history of peptic ulcer · hyperthyroidism · open-angle glaucoma (monitor intra-ocular pressure) · osteomalacia · phaeochromocytoma · psychiatric illness (avoid if severe

4

Nervous system

and discontinue if deterioration) · severe cardiovascular disease · severe pulmonary disease

- **INTERACTIONS** → Appendix 1: levodopa
- **SIDE-EFFECTS**
  - ▸ **Common or very common** Anxiety · appetite decreased · arrhythmia · depression · diarrhoea · hallucination · movement disorders · nausea · parkinsonism · postural hypotension · sleep disorder · taste altered · vomiting
  - ▸ **Rare or very rare** Leucopenia
  - ▸ **Frequency not known** Aggression · agranulocytosis · compulsions · confusion · delusions · dopamine dysregulation syndrome · drowsiness · eating disorders · euphoric mood · flushing · gastrointestinal haemorrhage · haemolytic anaemia · hyperhidrosis · oral disorders · pancytopenia · pathological gambling · psychosis · sexual dysfunction · skin reactions · sudden onset of sleep (can occur without warning) · thrombocytopenia · tongue discolouration · tooth discolouration · urine discolouration
- **PREGNANCY** Caution in pregnancy—toxicity has occurred in *animal* studies.
- **BREAST FEEDING** May suppress lactation; present in milk—avoid.
- **HEPATIC IMPAIRMENT** Manufacturer advises caution in mild to moderate impairment; avoid in decompensated hepatic function.
- **RENAL IMPAIRMENT** Use with caution.
- **EFFECT ON LABORATORY TESTS** False positive tests for urinary ketones have been reported.
- **TREATMENT CESSATION** Avoid abrupt withdrawal (risk of neuroleptic malignant syndrome and rhabdomyolysis).
- **DIRECTIONS FOR ADMINISTRATION** EvGr Dispersible tablets can be dispersed in water or orange squash (not orange juice).

  Dispersible tablets, capsules, and modified-release capsules should be taken 30 minutes before or 1 hour after meals.

  If undesirable gastrointestinal effects occur, this may be controlled by taking doses with a low-protein snack or liquid. ⓜ

- **PRESCRIBING AND DISPENSING INFORMATION** Co-beneldopa is a mixture of benserazide hydrochloride and levodopa in mass proportions corresponding to 1 part of benserazide and 4 parts of levodopa.

  When transferring patients from another levodopa/dopa-decarboxylase inhibitor preparation, the previous preparation should be discontinued 12 hours before (although interval can be shorter).

  When switching from modified-release levodopa to dispersible co-beneldopa, reduce dose by approximately 30%.

  When administered as an adjunct to other antiparkinsonian drugs, once therapeutic effect apparent, the other drugs may be reduced or withdrawn.

- **PATIENT AND CARER ADVICE** Patients or carers should be given advice on how to administer co-beneldopa preparations.

  Dopamine dysregulation syndrome Manufacturer advises patients and their carers should be informed of the risk of developing dopamine dysregulation syndrome; addiction-like symptoms should be reported.

  Driving and skilled tasks

  Sudden onset of sleep Excessive daytime sleepiness and sudden onset of sleep can occur with co-beneldopa.

  Patients starting treatment should be warned of the risk and of the need to exercise caution when driving or operating machinery. Those who have experienced excessive sedation or sudden onset of sleep should refrain from driving or operating machines until these effects have stopped occurring.

Management of excessive daytime sleepiness should focus on the identification of an underlying cause, such as depression or concomitant medication. Patients should be counselled on improving sleep behaviour.

- **MEDICINAL FORMS** There can be variation in the licensing of different medicines containing the same drug. Forms available from special-order manufacturers include: oral suspension, oral solution

Dispersible tablet

CAUTIONARY AND ADVISORY LABELS 10, 14

▸ **Madopar** (Roche Products Ltd)

Benserazide (as Benserazide hydrochloride) 12.5 mg, Levodopa 50 mg Madopar 50mg/12.5mg dispersible tablets | 100 tablet PoM £5.90 DT = £5.90 SF

Benserazide (as Benserazide hydrochloride) 25 mg, Levodopa 100 mg Madopar 100mg/25mg dispersible tablets | 100 tablet PoM £10.45 DT = £10.45 SF

Modified-release capsule

CAUTIONARY AND ADVISORY LABELS 5, 10, 14, 25

▸ **Madopar CR** (Roche Products Ltd)

Benserazide (as Benserazide hydrochloride) 25 mg, Levodopa 100 mg Madopar CR capsules | 100 capsule PoM £12.77 DT = £12.77

Oral capsule

CAUTIONARY AND ADVISORY LABELS 10, 14

▸ **Co-beneldopa (Non-proprietary)**

Benserazide (as Benserazide hydrochloride) 12.5 mg, Levodopa 50 mg Co-beneldopa 12.5mg/50mg capsules | 100 capsule PoM £7.21 DT = £7.21

▸ **Madopar** (Roche Products Ltd)

Benserazide (as Benserazide hydrochloride) 12.5 mg, Levodopa 50 mg Madopar 50mg/12.5mg capsules | 100 capsule PoM £4.96 DT = £7.21

Benserazide (as Benserazide hydrochloride) 25 mg, Levodopa 100 mg Madopar 100mg/25mg capsules | 100 capsule PoM £6.91 DT = £6.91

Benserazide (as Benserazide hydrochloride) 50 mg, Levodopa 200 mg Madopar 200mg/50mg capsules | 100 capsule PoM £11.78 DT = £11.78

Co-careldopa

06-Nov-2024

- **INDICATIONS AND DOSE**

Parkinson's disease

▸ BY MOUTH

▸ Adult: Initially 25/100 mg 3 times a day, then increased in steps of 12.5/50 mg once daily or on alternate days, alternatively increased in steps of 25/100 mg once daily or on alternate days, dose to be adjusted according to response; dose increased until 800 mg levodopa (with 200 mg carbidopa) daily in divided doses is reached, then maintenance up to 200/2000 mg daily in divided doses, adjusted according to response, when co-careldopa is used, the total daily dose of carbidopa should be at least 70 mg. A lower dose may not achieve full inhibition of extracerebral dopa-decarboxylase, with a resultant increase in side-effects

Parkinson's disease—alternative regimen

▸ BY MOUTH

▸ Adult: Initially 12.5/50 mg 3–4 times a day, alternatively initially 10/100 mg 3–4 times a day, then increased in steps of 12.5/50 mg once daily or on alternate days, adjusted according to response, alternatively increased in steps of 10/100 mg once daily or on alternate days, adjusted according to response, dose increased until 800 mg levodopa (with up to 200 mg carbidopa) daily in divided doses is reached, then maintenance up to 200/2000 mg daily in divided doses, adjusted according to response, when co-careldopa is used, the total daily dose of carbidopa should be at least 70 mg. A lower dose may not achieve full inhibition of extracerebral dopa-decarboxylase, with a resultant increase in side-effects

DOSE EQUIVALENCE AND CONVERSION
- The proportions are expressed in the form x/y where x and y are the strengths in milligrams of carbidopa and levodopa respectively.
- 2 tablets *Sinemet* ® 12.5 mg/50 mg is equivalent to 1 tablet *Sinemet* ® Plus 25 mg/100 mg.

CARAMET ® CR

Parkinson's disease (patients not receiving levodopa/dopa-decarboxylase inhibitor preparations, expressed as levodopa)
- BY MOUTH USING MODIFIED-RELEASE TABLETS
- Adult: Initially 100–200 mg twice daily, dose to be given at least 6 hours apart; dose adjusted according to response at intervals of at least 2 days

Parkinson's disease (patients transferring from immediate-release levodopa/dopa-decarboxylase inhibitor preparations)
- BY MOUTH USING MODIFIED-RELEASE TABLETS
- Adult: Discontinue previous preparation at least 12 hours before first dose of *Caramet* ® CR; substitute *Caramet* ® CR to provide a similar amount of levodopa daily and extend dosing interval by 30–50%; dose then adjusted according to response at intervals of at least 2 days.

DUODOPA ®

Severe Parkinson's disease inadequately controlled by other preparations
- Adult: Administered as intestinal gel, for use with enteral tube (consult product literature)

HALF SINEMET ® CR

Parkinson's disease (for fine adjustment of Sinemet ® CR dose)
- BY MOUTH
- Adult: (consult product literature)

SINEMET ® CR

Parkinson's disease (patients not receiving levodopa/dopa-decarboxylase inhibitor therapy)
- BY MOUTH
- Adult: Initially 1 tablet twice daily, both dose and interval then adjusted according to response at intervals of not less than 3 days

Parkinson's disease (patients transferring from immediate-release levodopa/dopa-decarboxylase inhibitor preparations)
- BY MOUTH
- Adult: 1 tablet twice daily, dose can be substituted for a daily dose of levodopa 300–400 mg in immediate-release *Sinemet* ® tablets (substitute *Sinemet* ® CR to provide approximately 10% more levodopa per day and extend dosing interval by 30–50%); dose and interval then adjusted according to response at intervals of not less than 3 days.

> **IMPORTANT SAFETY INFORMATION**
> IMPULSE CONTROL DISORDERS
> Treatment with levodopa is associated with impulse control disorders, including pathological gambling, binge eating, and hypersexuality. Patients and their carers should be informed about the risk of impulse control disorders. See Parkinson's disease p. 470.

- **CONTRA-INDICATIONS** Angle-closure glaucoma · suspicious undiagnosed skin lesions or history of skin melanoma (risk of activation)
- **CAUTIONS** Acute stroke · Cushing's syndrome · diabetes mellitus · endocrine disorders · history of convulsions · history of myocardial infarction with residual arrhythmia ·

history of peptic ulcer · hyperthyroidism · open-angle glaucoma (monitor intra-ocular pressure) · osteomalacia · phaeochromocytoma · psychiatric illness (avoid if severe and discontinue if deterioration) · severe cardiovascular disease · severe pulmonary disease

- **INTERACTIONS** → Appendix 1: carbidopa · levodopa
- **SIDE-EFFECTS**
- **Rare or very rare** Drowsiness · seizure · sudden onset of sleep (can occur without warning)
- **Frequency not known** Agranulocytosis · alertness decreased · alopecia · anaemia · angioedema · anxiety · appetite decreased · asthenia · cardiac disorder · chest pain · compulsions · confusion · constipation · delusions · dementia · depression · diarrhoea · dizziness · dopamine dysregulation syndrome · dry mouth · dyskinesia (may be dose-limiting) · dysphagia · dyspnoea · eating disorders · euphoric mood · eye disorders · fall · focal tremor · gait abnormal · gastrointestinal discomfort · gastrointestinal disorders · gastrointestinal haemorrhage · haemolytic anaemia · hallucination · headache · Henoch-Schönlein purpura · hiccups · hoarseness · Horner's syndrome exacerbated · hypertension · hypotension · leucopenia · malaise · malignant melanoma · movement disorders · muscle complaints · nausea · neuroleptic malignant syndrome (on abrupt discontinuation) · oedema · on and off phenomenon · oral disorders · palpitations · pathological gambling · postural disorders · psychotic disorder · respiration abnormal · sensation abnormal · sexual dysfunction · skin reactions · sleep disorders · suicidal ideation · sweat changes · syncope · taste bitter · teeth grinding · thrombocytopenia · trismus · urinary disorders · urine dark · vasodilation · vision disorders · vomiting · weight changes

SIDE-EFFECTS, FURTHER INFORMATION Also available as an intestinal gel—for specific side-effects consult product literature.

- **PREGNANCY** Use with caution—toxicity has occurred in *animal* studies.
- **BREAST FEEDING** May suppress lactation; present in milk—avoid.
- **HEPATIC IMPAIRMENT** Manufacturer advises use with caution in hepatic disease.
- **RENAL IMPAIRMENT** EvGr Use with caution. ⓜ
- **MONITORING REQUIREMENTS**
- With intestinal use: Evaluate patients for history, signs, or known risk factors for polyneuropathy before initiating treatment, and periodically thereafter.
- **EFFECT ON LABORATORY TESTS** False positive tests for urinary ketones have been reported.
- **TREATMENT CESSATION** Avoid abrupt withdrawal (risk of neuroleptic malignant syndrome and rhabdomyolysis).
- **PRESCRIBING AND DISPENSING INFORMATION** Co-careldopa is a mixture of carbidopa and levodopa; the proportions are expressed in the form x/y where x and y are the strengths in milligrams of carbidopa and levodopa respectively.

  When transferring patients from another levodopa/dopa-decarboxylase inhibitor preparation, the previous preparation should be discontinued at least 12 hours before.

  Co-careldopa 25/100 provides an adequate dose of carbidopa when low doses of levodopa are needed.
- **PATIENT AND CARER ADVICE** Manufacturer advises patients and their carers should be informed of the risk of developing dopamine dysregulation syndrome; addiction-like symptoms should be reported.
  Driving and skilled tasks
  Sudden onset of sleep Excessive daytime sleepiness and

sudden onset of sleep can occur with co-careldopa.

Patients starting treatment should be warned of the risk and of the need to exercise caution when driving or operating machinery. Those who have experienced excessive sedation or sudden onset of sleep should refrain from driving or operating machines until these effects have stopped occurring.

Management of excessive daytime sleepiness should focus on the identification of an underlying cause, such as depression or concomitant medication. Patients should be counselled on improving sleep behaviour.

● NATIONAL FUNDING/ACCESS DECISIONS

DUODOPA ® For full details see funding body website

Scottish Medicines Consortium (SMC) decisions

► Co-careldopa (*Duodopa* ®) for the treatment of advanced levodopa-responsive Parkinson's disease with severe motor fluctuations and hyper-/dyskinesia when available combinations of Parkinson medicinal products have not given satisfactory results (June 2016) SMC No. 316/06 Recommended with restrictions

All Wales Medicines Strategy Group (AWMSG) decisions

► Levodopa-carbidopa intestinal gel (*Duodopa* ®) for the treatment of advanced levodopa-responsive Parkinson's disease with severe motor fluctuations and hyper-/dyskinesia when available combinations of Parkinson medicinal products have not given satisfactory results and patients are not eligible for deep brain stimulation (March 2018) AWMSG No. 3397 Recommended with restrictions

● MEDICINAL FORMS There can be variation in the licensing of different medicines containing the same drug. Forms available from special-order manufacturers include: oral suspension, oral solution

Oral tablet

CAUTIONARY AND ADVISORY LABELS 10, 14

► Co-careldopa (Non-proprietary)

Carbidopa (as Carbidopa monohydrate) 12.5 mg, Levodopa 50 mg Co-careldopa 12.5mg/50mg tablets | 90 tablet PoM £19.31 DT = £3.88 | 100 tablet PoM £4.19–£5.40

Carbidopa (as Carbidopa monohydrate) 25 mg, Levodopa 100 mg Co-careldopa 25mg/100mg tablets | 100 tablet PoM £13.50 DT = £5.07

Carbidopa (as Carbidopa monohydrate) 10 mg, Levodopa 100 mg Co-careldopa 10mg/100mg tablets | 100 tablet PoM £14.00 DT = £14.00

Carbidopa (as Carbidopa monohydrate) 25 mg, Levodopa 250 mg Co-careldopa 25mg/250mg tablets | 100 tablet PoM £35.00 DT = £35.00

► Sinemet 110 (Organon Pharma (UK) Ltd)

Carbidopa (as Carbidopa monohydrate) 10 mg, Levodopa 100 mg Sinemet 10mg/100mg tablets | 100 tablet PoM £7.30 DT = £14.00

► Sinemet 275 (Organon Pharma (UK) Ltd)

Carbidopa (as Carbidopa monohydrate) 25 mg, Levodopa 250 mg Sinemet 25mg/250mg tablets | 100 tablet PoM £18.29 DT = £35.00

► Sinemet 62.5 (Organon Pharma (UK) Ltd)

Carbidopa (as Carbidopa monohydrate) 12.5 mg, Levodopa 50 mg Sinemet 12.5mg/50mg tablets | 90 tablet PoM £6.28 DT = £3.88

► Sinemet Plus (Organon Pharma (UK) Ltd)

Carbidopa (as Carbidopa monohydrate) 25 mg, Levodopa 100 mg Sinemet Plus 25mg/100mg tablets | 100 tablet PoM £12.88 DT = £5.07

Modified-release tablet

CAUTIONARY AND ADVISORY LABELS 10, 14, 25

► Caramet CR (Teva UK Ltd)

Carbidopa (as Carbidopa monohydrate) 25 mg, Levodopa 100 mg Caramet 25mg/100mg CR tablets | 60 tablet PoM £11.47 DT = £11.60

► Half Sinemet CR (Organon Pharma (UK) Ltd)

Carbidopa (as Carbidopa monohydrate) 25 mg, Levodopa 100 mg Half Sinemet CR 25mg/100mg tablets | 60 tablet PoM £11.60 DT = £11.60

► Lecado (Sandoz Ltd)

Carbidopa (as Carbidopa monohydrate) 25 mg, Levodopa 100 mg Lecado 100mg/25mg modified-release tablets | 60 tablet PoM £9.86 DT = £11.60

Carbidopa (as Carbidopa monohydrate) 50 mg, Levodopa 200 mg Lecado 200mg/50mg modified-release tablets | 60 tablet PoM £9.86 DT = £11.60

► Sinemet CR (Organon Pharma (UK) Ltd)

Carbidopa (as Carbidopa monohydrate) 50 mg, Levodopa 200 mg Sinemet CR 50mg/200mg tablets | 60 tablet PoM £11.60 DT = £11.60

Intestinal gel

CAUTIONARY AND ADVISORY LABELS 10, 14

► Duodopa (AbbVie Ltd)

Carbidopa monohydrate 5 mg per 1 ml, Levodopa 20 mg per 1 ml Duodopa intestinal gel 100ml cassette | 7 cassette PoM £539.00

Foslevodopa with foscarbidopa   28-May-2024

● DRUG ACTION Foslevodopa and foscarbidopa are prodrugs of levodopa and carbidopa, respectively.

● INDICATIONS AND DOSE

Severe Parkinson's disease inadequately controlled by other preparations

► BY CONTINUOUS SUBCUTANEOUS INFUSION

► Adult: Initial dose and starting infusion rate are based on levodopa equivalents calculated from the patients levodopa-containing medications, dose and rate are then adjusted according to response to a maximum daily foslevodopa dose of 6 g (25 mL), consult product literature for further information, including instructions on how to convert from different levodopa formulations to levodopa equivalents, how to determine the infusion volume and rate, and the loading dose

DOSE EQUIVALENCE AND CONVERSION

► Each mL of *Produodopa* ® solution for infusion contains 240 mg foslevodopa and 12 mg foscarbidopa.

IMPORTANT SAFETY INFORMATION

IMPULSE CONTROL DISORDERS

Treatment with levodopa is associated with impulse control disorders, including pathological gambling, binge eating, and hypersexuality. Patients and their carers should be informed about the risk of impulse control disorders. See Parkinson's disease p. 470.

● CONTRA-INDICATIONS Acute stroke · angle-closure glaucoma · Cushing's syndrome · hyperthyroidism · phaeochromocytoma · severe cardiac arrhythmia · severe heart failure · suspicious undiagnosed skin lesions or history of skin melanoma (risk of activation)

● CAUTIONS Asthma · endocrine disorders · history of convulsions · history of myocardial infarction with residual arrhythmia · history of peptic ulcer disease · low-salt diet (*Produodopa* ® is high in sodium) · open-angle glaucoma · psychiatric illness or history of psychosis · severe cardiovascular disease · severe pulmonary disease

● INTERACTIONS → Appendix 1: foslevodopa

● SIDE-EFFECTS

► Common or very common Abdominal pain · anxiety · appetite decreased · asthenia · cognitive disorder · confusion · constipation · delusions · depression · diarrhoea · dizziness · drowsiness · dry mouth · dyspnoea · fall · hallucinations · headache · hypertension · hypotension · impulse-control disorder · insomnia · malaise · movement disorders · muscle spasms · nausea · nerve disorders · on and off phenomenon · paranoia · peripheral oedema · psychotic disorder · sensation abnormal · skin reactions ·

suicidal ideation · syncope · urinary disorders · vomiting · weight decreased

▸ **Uncommon** Dopamine dysregulation syndrome · palpitations

● **PREGNANCY** [EvGr] Avoid unless potential benefit outweighs risk (no information available for foslevodopa or foscarbidopa; levodopa and carbidopa have shown toxicity in *animal* studies). ⟨M⟩

● **BREAST FEEDING** [EvGr] Discontinue breast-feeding (no information available for foslevodopa or foscarbidopa; levodopa and carbidopa may be present in milk, and levodopa may suppress lactation). ⟨M⟩

● **HEPATIC IMPAIRMENT** [EvGr] Caution (no information available). ⟨M⟩

● **RENAL IMPAIRMENT** [EvGr] Caution (no information available). ⟨M⟩

● **MONITORING REQUIREMENTS**
▸ [EvGr] Before starting treatment, evaluate patients for history or signs of polyneuropathy, and periodically thereafter.
▸ During treatment, monitor for mental changes including depression with suicidal thoughts, hallucinations, and impulse control disorders (review treatment if symptoms develop).
▸ With prolonged treatment, hepatic, haematological, renal, and cardiovascular monitoring is advisable.
▸ Examine skin regularly for melanoma. ⟨M⟩

● **EFFECT ON LABORATORY TESTS** False positive tests for urinary ketones have been reported.

● **TREATMENT CESSATION** [EvGr] Avoid abrupt withdrawal (risk of neuroleptic malignant syndrome and rhabdomyolysis). ⟨M⟩

● **DIRECTIONS FOR ADMINISTRATION** Take vial out of the refrigerator and allow to reach room temperature before administration using the *Vyafuser*® infusion pump— consult product literature. Patients and carers may administer *Produodopa*® after appropriate training in subcutaneous infusion technique.

● **HANDLING AND STORAGE** Store in a refrigerator (2–8°C). Once removed from refrigerator, may be stored at room temperature (up to a maximum 30°C) for a single period of up to 28 days. Once the content of a vial is transferred into the syringe, the contents of the syringe should be administered within 24 hours.

● **PATIENT AND CARER ADVICE** Patients and their carers should be informed of the risk of developing dopamine dysregulation syndrome or impulse control disorders; addiction-like symptoms should be reported.
Patient guide Patients and carers should be given a *Patient Guide*.
Driving and skilled tasks Patients and carers should be cautioned on the effects on driving and performance of skilled tasks—increased risk of dizziness/orthostatic hypotension, and sudden onset of sleep (see below).
Sudden onset of sleep Excessive daytime sleepiness and sudden onset of sleep can occur with *Produodopa*®.

Patients starting treatment should be warned of the risk and of the need to exercise caution when driving or operating machinery. Those who have experienced excessive sedation or sudden onset of sleep should refrain from driving or operating machines until these effects have resolved.

Management of excessive daytime sleepiness should focus on the identification of an underlying cause, such as depression or concomitant medication. Patients should be counselled on improving sleep behaviour.

● **NATIONAL FUNDING/ACCESS DECISIONS**
For full details see funding body website
NICE decisions
▸ **Foslevodopa-foscarbidopa for treating advanced Parkinson's with motor symptoms (November 2023)** NICE TA934 Recommended with restrictions

Scottish Medicines Consortium (SMC) decisions
▸ **Foslevodopa-foscarbidopa (*Produodopa*®) for the treatment of advanced levodopa-responsive Parkinson's disease with severe motor fluctuations and hyperkinesia or dyskinesia when available combinations of Parkinson medicinal products have not given satisfactory results (March 2024)** SMC No. SMC2574 Recommended with restrictions

● **MEDICINAL FORMS** There can be variation in the licensing of different medicines containing the same drug.
Solution for infusion
CAUTIONARY AND ADVISORY LABELS 10
ELECTROLYTES: May contain Sodium
▸ **Produodopa** (AbbVie Ltd)
Foscarbidopa 12 mg per 1 ml, Foslevodopa 240 mg per 1 ml Produodopa 2.4g/10ml / 120mg/10ml solution for infusion vials | 7 vial [PoM] £592.90 (Hospital only)

Levodopa with carbidopa and entacapone

30-Dec-2024

The properties listed below are those particular to the combination only. For the properties of the components please consider, co-careldopa p. 476, entacapone p. 474.

● **INDICATIONS AND DOSE**

LECIGON ® 20/5/20

Severe Parkinson's disease inadequately controlled by other preparations
▸ Adult: Administered as intestinal gel using a pump for continuous delivery directly into the duodenum or upper jejunum, initial morning and continuous maintenance doses are based on previous levodopa dose regimen, then adjusted according to response to a maximum daily levodopa dose of 2 g (100 mL). Consult product literature for further information

DOSE EQUIVALENCE AND CONVERSION
▸ Each mL of *Lecigon*® intestinal gel contains 20 mg levodopa, 5 mg carbidopa, and 20 mg entacapone.

STALEVO ® 100/25/200

Parkinson's disease and end-of-dose motor fluctuations not adequately controlled with levodopa and dopa-decarboxylase inhibitor treatment
▸ BY MOUTH
▸ Adult: 1 tablet for each dose; maximum 10 tablets per day

STALEVO ® 125/31.25/200

Parkinson's disease and end-of-dose motor fluctuations not adequately controlled with levodopa and dopa-decarboxylase inhibitor treatment
▸ BY MOUTH
▸ Adult: 1 tablet for each dose; maximum 10 tablets per day

STALEVO ® 150/37.5/200

Parkinson's disease and end-of-dose motor fluctuations not adequately controlled with levodopa and dopa-decarboxylase inhibitor treatment
▸ BY MOUTH
▸ Adult: 1 tablet for each dose; maximum 10 tablets per day

continued →

Nervous system

4

STALEVO ® 175/43.75/200

Parkinson's disease and end-of-dose motor fluctuations not adequately controlled with levodopa and dopa-decarboxylase inhibitor treatment

▶ BY MOUTH
▶ Adult: 1 tablet for each dose; maximum 8 tablets per day

STALEVO ® 200/50/200

Parkinson's disease and end-of-dose motor fluctuations not adequately controlled with levodopa and dopa-decarboxylase inhibitor treatment

▶ BY MOUTH
▶ Adult: 1 tablet for each dose; maximum 7 tablets per day

STALEVO ® 50/12.5/200

Parkinson's disease and end-of-dose motor fluctuations not adequately controlled with levodopa and dopa-decarboxylase inhibitor treatment

▶ BY MOUTH
▶ Adult: 1 tablet for each dose; maximum 10 tablets per day

STALEVO ® 75/18.75/200

Parkinson's disease and end-of-dose motor fluctuations not adequately controlled with levodopa and dopa-decarboxylase inhibitor treatment

▶ BY MOUTH
▶ Adult: 1 tablet for each dose; maximum 10 tablets per day

● **INTERACTIONS** → Appendix 1: carbidopa · entacapone · levodopa

● **HEPATIC IMPAIRMENT** EvGr Caution in mild to moderate impairment (risk of increased exposure to entacapone); avoid in severe impairment. Ⓜ

● **PRESCRIBING AND DISPENSING INFORMATION**
▶ With intestinal use The manufacturer of *Lecigon* ® has provided *Risk minimisation materials* for healthcare professionals.
▶ With oral use Patients receiving standard-release co-careldopa or co-beneldopa alone, initiate *Stalevo* ® at a dose that provides similar (or slightly lower) amount of levodopa. Patients with dyskinesia or receiving more than 800 mg levodopa daily, introduce entacapone before transferring to *Stalevo* ® (levodopa dose may need to be reduced by 10–30% initially). Patients receiving entacapone and standard-release co-careldopa or co-beneldopa, initiate *Stalevo* ® at a dose that provides similar (or slightly higher) amount of levodopa.

● **HANDLING AND STORAGE**
▶ With intestinal use For *Lecigon* ®, store in a refrigerator (2–8°C) and protect from light. Cartridge may be used for up to 24 hours once removed from the refrigerator—consult product literature.

● **PATIENT AND CARER ADVICE**
Driving and skilled tasks
Sudden onset of sleep Excessive daytime sleepiness and sudden onset of sleep can occur with carbidopa with entacapone and levodopa.

Patients starting treatment with these drugs should be warned of the risk and of the need to exercise caution when driving or operating machinery. Those who have experienced excessive sedation or sudden onset of sleep should refrain from driving or operating machines until these effects have stopped occurring.

Management of excessive daytime sleepiness should focus on the identification of an underlying cause, such as depression or concomitant medication. Patients should be counselled on improving sleep behaviour.

● **NATIONAL FUNDING/ACCESS DECISIONS**
For full details see funding body website
Scottish Medicines Consortium (SMC) decisions
▶ Levodopa/carbidopa/entacapone (*Lecigon* ®) for the treatment of advanced Parkinson's disease with severe motor fluctuations and hyperkinesia or dyskinesia when available oral combinations of Parkinson medicinal products have not given satisfactory results (December 2024) SMC No. SMC2507 Not recommended

All Wales Medicines Strategy Group (AWMSG) decisions
▶ Levodopa/carbidopa/entacapone (*Lecigon* ®) for the treatment of advanced Parkinson's disease with severe motor fluctuations and hyperkinesia or dyskinesia when available oral combinations of Parkinson medicinal products have not given satisfactory results (April 2023) AWMSG No. 4871 Recommended with restrictions

● **MEDICINAL FORMS** There can be variation in the licensing of different medicines containing the same drug.
Oral tablet
CAUTIONARY AND ADVISORY LABELS 10, 14 (urine reddish-brown)
▶ Stalevo (Orion Pharma (UK) Ltd)
  Carbidopa 25 mg, Levodopa 100 mg, Entacapone 200 mg Stalevo 100mg/25mg/200mg tablets | 30 tablet [PoM] £20.79 DT = £20.79 | 100 tablet [PoM] £69.31 DT = £69.31
  Carbidopa 18.75 mg, Levodopa 75 mg, Entacapone 200 mg Stalevo 75mg/18.75mg/200mg tablets | 30 tablet [PoM] £20.79 DT = £20.79 | 100 tablet [PoM] £69.31 DT = £69.31
  Carbidopa 37.5 mg, Levodopa 150 mg, Entacapone 200 mg Stalevo 150mg/37.5mg/200mg tablets | 30 tablet [PoM] £20.79 DT = £20.79 | 100 tablet [PoM] £69.31 DT = £69.31
  Carbidopa 12.5 mg, Levodopa 50 mg, Entacapone 200 mg Stalevo 50mg/12.5mg/200mg tablets | 30 tablet [PoM] £20.79 DT = £20.79 | 100 tablet [PoM] £69.31 DT = £69.31
  Carbidopa 31.25 mg, Levodopa 125 mg, Entacapone 200 mg Stalevo 125mg/31.25mg/200mg tablets | 30 tablet [PoM] £20.79 DT = £20.79 | 100 tablet [PoM] £69.31 DT = £69.31
  Carbidopa 43.75 mg, Levodopa 175 mg, Entacapone 200 mg Stalevo 175mg/43.75mg/200mg tablets | 30 tablet [PoM] £20.79 DT = £20.79 | 100 tablet [PoM] £69.31 DT = £69.31
  Carbidopa 50 mg, Entacapone 200 mg, Levodopa 200 mg Stalevo 200mg/50mg/200mg tablets | 30 tablet [PoM] £20.79 DT = £20.79 | 100 tablet [PoM] £69.31 DT = £69.31
Intestinal gel
CAUTIONARY AND ADVISORY LABELS 10, 14 (urine reddish-brown)
ELECTROLYTES: May contain Sodium
▶ Lecigon (Britannia Pharmaceuticals Ltd)
  Carbidopa monohydrate 5 mg per 1 ml, Entacapone 20 mg per 1 ml, Levodopa 20 mg per 1 ml Lecigon 20mg/ml + 5mg/ml + 20mg/ml intestinal gel 47ml cartridges | 7 cartridge [PoM] £532.06 (Hospital only)

DOPAMINERGIC DRUGS › DOPAMINE RECEPTOR AGONISTS

Amantadine hydrochloride

05-Jan-2024

● **DRUG ACTION** Amantadine is a weak dopamine agonist with modest antiparkinsonian effects.

● **INDICATIONS AND DOSE**
Parkinson's disease
▶ BY MOUTH
▶ Adult: 100 mg daily for 1 week, then increased to 100 mg twice daily, usually administered in conjunction with other treatment. Some patients may require higher doses; maximum 400 mg per day
▶ Elderly: 100 mg daily, adjusted according to response

Post-herpetic neuralgia
▶ BY MOUTH
▶ Adult: 100 mg twice daily for 14 days (continued for another 14 days if necessary)

Treatment of influenza A (but not recommended)
▸ BY MOUTH
▸ Adult: 100 mg daily 4–5 days

Prophylaxis of influenza A (but not recommended)
▸ BY MOUTH
▸ Adult: 100 mg daily usually for 6 weeks or with influenza vaccination for 2–3 weeks after vaccination

Fatigue in multiple sclerosis (initiated by a specialist)
▸ BY MOUTH
▸ Adult: 100 mg daily for 1 week, dose to be taken in the morning, then increased to 100 mg twice daily; maximum 400 mg per day

● UNLICENSED USE [EvGr] Amantadine is used for fatigue in multiple sclerosis, ⟨E⟩ but is not licensed for this indication.

IMPORTANT SAFETY INFORMATION
IMPULSE CONTROL DISORDERS
Treatment with dopaminergic drugs is associated with impulse control disorders, including pathological gambling, binge eating, and hypersexuality. Patients and their carers should be informed about the risk of impulse control disorders. See Parkinson's disease p. 470.

● CONTRA-INDICATIONS Epilepsy · history of gastric ulceration

● CAUTIONS Confused or hallucinatory states · congestive heart disease (may exacerbate oedema) · elderly · tolerance to the effects of amantadine may develop in Parkinson's disease

● INTERACTIONS → Appendix 1: dopamine receptor agonists

● SIDE-EFFECTS
▸ **Common or very common** Anxiety · appetite decreased · concentration impaired · confusion · constipation · depression · dizziness · dry mouth · hallucination · headache · hyperhidrosis · lethargy · mood altered · movement disorders · myalgia · nausea · palpitations · peripheral oedema · postural hypotension · skin reactions · sleep disorders · speech slurred · vision disorders · vomiting
▸ **Uncommon** Psychosis · seizure · tremor
▸ **Rare or very rare** Cardiovascular insufficiency · diarrhoea · eye disorders · eye inflammation · heart failure · leucopenia · neuroleptic malignant syndrome · photosensitivity reaction · urinary disorders
▸ **Frequency not known** Delirium

● PREGNANCY Avoid; toxicity in *animal* studies.

● BREAST FEEDING Avoid; present in milk; toxicity in infant reported.

● HEPATIC IMPAIRMENT Manufacturer advises use with caution in liver disorders.

● RENAL IMPAIRMENT [EvGr] Avoid if creatinine clearance less than 15 mL/minute. ⟨M⟩ See p. 21.
Dose adjustments [EvGr] Reduce dose (consult product literature). ⟨M⟩

● TREATMENT CESSATION Avoid abrupt withdrawal in Parkinson's disease.

● PATIENT AND CARER ADVICE
Driving and skilled tasks May affect performance of skilled tasks (e.g. driving).

● NATIONAL FUNDING/ACCESS DECISIONS
For full details see funding body website

NICE decisions
▸ Oseltamivir, amantadine (review) and zanamivir for the prophylaxis of influenza (September 2008) NICE TA158 Not recommended
▸ Amantadine, oseltamivir and zanamivir for the treatment of influenza (February 2009) NICE TA168 Not recommended

● MEDICINAL FORMS There can be variation in the licensing of different medicines containing the same drug. Forms available from special-order manufacturers include: oral tablet

Oral solution
▸ Amantadine hydrochloride (Non-proprietary)
Amantadine hydrochloride 10 mg per 1 ml Amantadine 50mg/5ml oral solution sugar free | 150 ml [PoM] £140.00 DT = £140.00 [SF]
▸ Trilasym (Fontus Health Ltd)
Amantadine hydrochloride 10 mg per 1 ml Trilasym 50mg/5ml oral solution | 150 ml [PoM] £99.99 DT = £140.00 [SF]

Oral capsule
▸ Amantadine hydrochloride (Non-proprietary)
Amantadine hydrochloride 100 mg Amantadine 100mg capsules | 14 capsule [PoM] £3.68-£10.25 | 56 capsule [PoM] £41.00 DT = £16.73

Apomorphine hydrochloride
28-May-2021

● **INDICATIONS AND DOSE**
Refractory motor fluctuations in Parkinson's disease ('off' episodes) inadequately controlled by co-beneldopa or co-careldopa or other dopaminergics (for capable and motivated patients) (under expert supervision)
▸ BY SUBCUTANEOUS INJECTION
▸ Adult: Initially 1 mg, dose to be administered at the first sign of 'off' episode, then 2 mg after 30 minutes, dose to be given if inadequate or no response following initial dose, thereafter increase dose at minimum 40-minute intervals until satisfactory response obtained, this determines threshold dose; usual dose 3–30 mg daily in divided doses (max. per dose 10 mg), subcutaneous infusion may be preferable in those requiring division of injections into more than 10 doses; maximum 100 mg per day

Refractory motor fluctuations in Parkinson's disease ('off' episodes) inadequately controlled by co-beneldopa or co-careldopa or other dopaminergics (in patients requiring division into more than 10 injections daily) (under expert supervision)
▸ BY CONTINUOUS SUBCUTANEOUS INFUSION
▸ Adult: Initially 1 mg/hour, adjusted according to response, then increased in steps of up to 500 micrograms/hour, dose to be increased at intervals not more often than every 4 hours; usual dose 1–4 mg/hour, alternatively usual dose 15–60 micrograms/kg/hour, change infusion site every 12 hours and give during waking hours only (tolerance may occur unless there is a 4-hour treatment-free period at night—24-hour infusions not recommended unless severe night time symptoms); intermittent bolus doses may be needed; maximum 100 mg per day

---

IMPORTANT SAFETY INFORMATION
IMPULSE CONTROL DISORDERS
Treatment with dopamine-receptor agonists are associated with impulse control disorders, including pathological gambling, binge eating, and hypersexuality. Patients and their carers should be informed about the risk of impulse control disorders. Ergot- and non-ergot-derived dopamine-receptor agonists do not differ in their propensity to cause impulse control disorders, so switching between dopamine-receptor agonists will not control these side-effects. See Parkinson's disease p. 470.

● CONTRA-INDICATIONS Avoid if 'on' response to levodopa marred by severe dyskinesia or dystonia · dementia · psychosis · respiratory depression

● CAUTIONS Cardiovascular disease · history of postural hypotension (special care on initiation) · neuropsychiatric conditions · pulmonary disease · susceptibility to QT-interval prolongation

- **INTERACTIONS** → Appendix 1: dopamine receptor agonists
- **SIDE-EFFECTS**
  ▶ **Common or very common** Confusion · dizziness · drowsiness · hallucinations · nausea · psychiatric disorders · subcutaneous nodule · vomiting · yawning
  ▶ **Uncommon** Dyskinesia (may require discontinuation) · dyspnoea · haemolytic anaemia · injection site necrosis · postural hypotension · skin reactions · sudden onset of sleep · thrombocytopenia
  ▶ **Rare or very rare** Bronchospasm · eosinophilia · hypersensitivity
  ▶ **Frequency not known** Aggression · agitation · dopamine dysregulation syndrome · eating disorders · pathological gambling · peripheral oedema · sexual dysfunction · syncope
- **ALLERGY AND CROSS-SENSITIVITY** EvGr Contra-indicated if history of hypersensitivity to opioids. ⟨E⟩
- **PREGNANCY** Avoid unless clearly necessary.
- **BREAST FEEDING** No information available; may suppress lactation.
- **HEPATIC IMPAIRMENT** Manufacturer advises avoid in hepatic insufficiency.
- **RENAL IMPAIRMENT** EvGr Use with caution. ⟨M⟩
- **MONITORING REQUIREMENTS**
  ▶ Monitor hepatic, haemopoietic, renal, and cardiovascular function.
  ▶ *With concomitant levodopa* test initially and every 6 months for haemolytic anaemia and thrombocytopenia (development calls for specialist haematological care with dose reduction and possible discontinuation).
- **TREATMENT CESSATION** Antiparkinsonian drug therapy should never be stopped abruptly as this carries a small risk of neuroleptic malignant syndrome.
- **PATIENT AND CARER ADVICE** Manufacturer advises patients and their carers should be informed of the risk of developing dopamine dysregulation syndrome; addiction-like symptoms should be reported.
  Driving and skilled tasks
  Sudden onset of sleep Excessive daytime sleepiness and sudden onset of sleep can occur with dopamine-receptor agonists.

  Patients starting treatment with these drugs should be warned of the risk and of the need to exercise caution when driving or operating machinery. Those who have experienced excessive sedation or sudden onset of sleep should refrain from driving or operating machines until these effects have stopped occurring.

  Management of excessive daytime sleepiness should focus on the identification of an underlying cause, such as depression or concomitant medication. Patients should be counselled on improving sleep behaviour.
  Drugs and driving Prescribers and other healthcare professionals should advise patients if treatment is likely to affect their ability to perform skilled tasks (e.g. driving). This applies especially to drugs with sedative effects; patients should be warned that these effects are increased by alcohol. General information about a patient's fitness to drive is available from the Driver and Vehicle Licensing Agency at www.gov.uk/government/organisations/driver-and-vehicle-licensing-agency.

  2015 legislation regarding driving whilst taking certain drugs, may also apply to apomorphine, see *Drugs and driving* under Guidance on prescribing p. 1.
  Hypotensive reactions Hypotensive reactions can occur in some patients taking dopamine-receptor agonists; these can be particularly problematic during the first few days of treatment and care should be exercised when driving or operating machinery.

- **MEDICINAL FORMS** There can be variation in the licensing of different medicines containing the same drug. Forms available from special-order manufacturers include: solution for injection, solution for infusion

Solution for injection
CAUTIONARY AND ADVISORY LABELS 10
EXCIPIENTS: May contain Sulfites
  ▶ **APO-go** (Britannia Pharmaceuticals Ltd)
    Apomorphine hydrochloride 10 mg per 1 ml APO-go 50mg/5ml solution for injection ampoules | 5 ampoule PoM £73.11 DT = £73.11
  ▶ **APO-go Pen** (Britannia Pharmaceuticals Ltd)
    Apomorphine hydrochloride 10 mg per 1 ml APO-go PEN 30mg/3ml solution for injection | 5 pre-filled disposable injection PoM £123.91 DT = £123.91
  ▶ **Dacepton** (EVER Pharma UK Ltd)
    Apomorphine hydrochloride hemihydrate 10 mg per 1 ml Dacepton 30mg/3ml solution for injection cartridges | 5 cartridge PoM £123.00 DT = £123.00

Solution for infusion
CAUTIONARY AND ADVISORY LABELS 10
EXCIPIENTS: May contain Sulfites
  ▶ **APO-go PFS** (Britannia Pharmaceuticals Ltd)
    Apomorphine hydrochloride 5 mg per 1 ml APO-go PFS 50mg/10ml solution for infusion pre-filled syringes | 5 pre-filled disposable injection PoM £73.11 DT = £73.11
  ▶ **APO-go POD** (Britannia Pharmaceuticals Ltd)
    Apomorphine hydrochloride hemihydrate 5 mg per 1 ml APO-go POD 100mg/20ml solution for infusion cartridges | 5 cartridge PoM £146.22
  ▶ **Dacepton** (EVER Pharma UK Ltd)
    Apomorphine hydrochloride hemihydrate 5 mg per 1 ml Dacepton 100mg/20ml solution for infusion vials | 5 vial PoM £145.00 DT = £145.00

Bromocriptine
06-Nov-2024

- **DRUG ACTION** Bromocriptine is a stimulant of dopamine receptors in the brain; it also inhibits release of prolactin by the pituitary.

- **INDICATIONS AND DOSE**

Prevention of lactation
  ▶ BY MOUTH
  ▶ Adult: Initially 2.5 mg daily for 1 day, then 2.5 mg twice daily for 14 days

Suppression of lactation
  ▶ BY MOUTH
  ▶ Adult: Initially 2.5 mg daily for 2–3 days, then 2.5 mg twice daily for 14 days

Hypogonadism | Galactorrhoea | Infertility
  ▶ BY MOUTH
  ▶ Adult: Initially 1–1.25 mg daily, dose to be taken at bedtime, increase dose gradually; usual dose 7.5 mg daily in divided doses, increased if necessary up to 30 mg daily, usual dose in infertility without hyperprolactinaemia is 2.5 mg twice daily

Acromegaly
  ▶ BY MOUTH
  ▶ Adult: Initially 1–1.25 mg daily, dose to be taken at bedtime, then increased to 5 mg every 6 hours, increase dose gradually

Prolactinoma
  ▶ BY MOUTH
  ▶ Adult: Initially 1–1.25 mg daily, dose to be taken at bedtime, then increased to 5 mg every 6 hours, increase dose gradually. Occasionally patients may require up to 30 mg daily

Parkinson's disease
  ▶ BY MOUTH
  ▶ Adult: Initially 1–1.25 mg daily for 1 week, dose to be taken at night, then 2–2.5 mg daily for 1 week, dose to be taken at night, then 2.5 mg twice daily for 1 week, then 2.5 mg 3 times a day for 1 week, then increased in

steps of 2.5 mg every 3–14 days, adjusted according to response; maintenance 10–30 mg daily

---

IMPORTANT SAFETY INFORMATION

FIBROTIC AND SEROSAL REACTIONS

Bromocriptine, particularly with long-term and high-dose treatment, has been associated with pulmonary, pleural, retroperitoneal, and pericardial fibrosis (the latter often manifests as cardiac failure), pleural and pericardial effusions, and constrictive pericarditis. Baseline investigations and regular monitoring for signs and symptoms of these reactions should be undertaken and treatment stopped if they are suspected. See also *Contra-indications* and *Monitoring requirements*.

IMPULSE CONTROL DISORDERS

Treatment with dopamine-receptor agonists is associated with impulse control disorders, including pathological gambling, binge eating, and hypersexuality. Patients and their carers should be informed about the risk of impulse control disorders. Ergot- and non-ergot-derived dopamine-receptor agonists do not differ in their propensity to cause impulse control disorders, so switching between dopamine-receptor agonists will not control these side-effects. See Parkinson's disease p. 470.

MHRA/CHM ADVICE: BROMOCRIPTINE: MONITOR BLOOD PRESSURE WHEN PRESCRIBING BROMOCRIPTINE FOR PREVENTION OR INHIBITION OF POST-PARTUM PHYSIOLOGICAL LACTATION (OCTOBER 2024)

The MHRA conducted a safety review following a Yellow Card report, and issued the following advice to remind healthcare professionals that bromocriptine should only be used for prevention or suppression of postpartum lactation where medically indicated, in cases such as intrapartum loss, neonatal death, or a mother with HIV infection. It should not be used in women with postpartum hypertension, or for routine suppression of lactation, or for relieving symptoms of postpartum breast pain and engorgement. Serious side-effects have been reported; blood pressure should be carefully monitored, especially during the first days of treatment and with any subsequent dose increases. See *Contra-indications* for further information.

- **CONTRA-INDICATIONS** Cardiac valvulopathy (exclude before long-term treatment) · hypertension in postpartum women or in puerperium · hypertensive disorders of pregnancy (e.g. pre-eclampsia, eclampsia, or pregnancy-induced hypertension) · uncontrolled hypertension

  ##### CONTRA-INDICATIONS, FURTHER INFORMATION
  ▸ Use in prevention or suppression of lactation or other non-life threatening indications EvGr Avoid in these indications for patients with a history of severe cardiovascular conditions, including coronary artery disease, or symptoms (or history) of severe psychiatric disorders. Very rarely hypertension, myocardial infarction, seizures or stroke (both sometimes preceded by severe headache or visual disturbances), and psychiatric disorders have been reported in postpartum women given bromocriptine for lactation suppression—caution with drugs that affect blood pressure and avoid other ergot alkaloids. Discontinue immediately if hypertension, suggestive chest pain, severe progressive or unremitting headache, or signs of CNS toxicity develop. ⟨M⟩

- **CAUTIONS** Cardiovascular disease · history of peptic ulcer (particularly in acromegalic patients) · history of serious mental disorders (especially psychotic disorders) · Raynaud's syndrome

  ##### CAUTIONS, FURTHER INFORMATION
  ▸ Hyperprolactinemic patients In hyperprolactinaemic patients, the source of the hyperprolactinaemia should be

established (i.e. exclude pituitary tumour before treatment).

- **INTERACTIONS** → Appendix 1: dopamine receptor agonists

- **SIDE-EFFECTS**
  ▸ **Common or very common** Constipation · drowsiness · headache · nasal congestion · nausea
  ▸ **Uncommon** Allergic dermatitis · alopecia · confusion · dizziness · dry mouth · fatigue · hallucination · hypotension · leg cramps · movement disorders · vomiting
  ▸ **Rare or very rare** Abdominal pain · arrhythmias · cardiac valvulopathy · diarrhoea · dyspnoea · gastrointestinal disorders · gastrointestinal haemorrhage · insomnia · neuroleptic malignant-like syndrome · pallor · paraesthesia · pericardial effusion · pericarditis · peripheral oedema · psychotic disorder · pulmonary fibrosis · respiratory disorders · sudden onset of sleep (can occur without warning) · tinnitus · vision disorders
  ▸ **Frequency not known** Eating disorders · hypertension · myocardial infarction · pathological gambling · psychiatric disorders · seizure · sexual dysfunction · stroke

  ##### SIDE-EFFECTS, FURTHER INFORMATION Treatment should be withdrawn if gastro-intestinal bleeding occurs.

- **ALLERGY AND CROSS-SENSITIVITY** EvGr Bromocriptine should not be used in patients with hypersensitivity to ergot alkaloids. ⟨M⟩

- **CONCEPTION AND CONTRACEPTION** Caution—provide contraceptive advice if appropriate (oral contraceptives may increase prolactin concentration).

- **BREAST FEEDING** Suppresses lactation; avoid breast feeding for about 5 days if lactation prevention fails.

- **HEPATIC IMPAIRMENT**
  Dose adjustments Manufacturer advises dose adjustment may be necessary—risk of increased plasma concentration.

- **MONITORING REQUIREMENTS**
  ▸ Specialist evaluation—monitor for pituitary enlargement, particularly during pregnancy; monitor visual field to detect secondary field loss in macroprolactinoma.
  ▸ EvGr Monitor blood pressure for a few days after starting treatment ⟨M⟩ and following dosage increase.
  ▸ EvGr Baseline chest X-rays/lung function tests, serum creatinine, and inflammatory markers (such as erythrocyte sedimentation rate) should be obtained before starting treatment. Monitor for fibrotic or serosal inflammatory changes during treatment (manifesting as dyspnoea, persistent cough, chest pain, cardiac failure, back pain, lower limb oedema, or renal impairment) and discontinue treatment if these are suspected. ⟨M⟩

- **TREATMENT CESSATION** Antiparkinsonian drug therapy should never be stopped abruptly as this carries a small risk of neuroleptic malignant syndrome.

- **PATIENT AND CARER ADVICE** Patients and their carers should be informed about the signs and symptoms of impulse control disorders.
  Driving and skilled tasks
  Sudden onset of sleep Excessive daytime sleepiness and sudden onset of sleep can occur with dopamine-receptor agonists.

  Patients starting treatment with these drugs should be warned of the risk and of the need to exercise caution when driving or operating machinery. Those who have experienced excessive sedation or sudden onset of sleep should refrain from driving or operating machines until these effects have stopped occurring.

  Management of excessive daytime sleepiness should focus on the identification of an underlying cause, such as depression or concomitant medication. Patients should be counselled on improving sleep behaviour.
  Hypotensive reactions Hypotensive reactions can occur in some patients taking dopamine-receptor agonists; these can be particularly problematic during the first few days of

treatment and care should be exercised when driving or operating machinery.

- ● MEDICINAL FORMS There can be variation in the licensing of different medicines containing the same drug. Forms available from special-order manufacturers include: oral suspension
Oral tablet
CAUTIONARY AND ADVISORY LABELS 10, 21
▸ Bromocriptine (Non-proprietary)
Bromocriptine (as Bromocriptine mesilate) 2.5 mg Bromocriptine 2.5mg tablets | 30 tablet [PoM] £70.99 DT = £57.81

▌Cabergoline

06-Nov-2024

- ● DRUG ACTION Cabergoline is a stimulant of dopamine receptors in the brain and it also inhibits release of prolactin by the pituitary.

- ● INDICATIONS AND DOSE
Prevention of lactation
▸ BY MOUTH
▸ Adult: 1 mg, to be taken as a single dose on the first day postpartum

Suppression of established lactation
▸ BY MOUTH
▸ Adult: 250 micrograms every 12 hours for 2 days

Hyperprolactinaemic disorders
▸ BY MOUTH
▸ Adult: Initially 500 micrograms once weekly, dose may be taken as a single dose or as 2 divided doses on separate days, then increased in steps of 500 micrograms every month until optimal therapeutic response reached, increase dose following monthly monitoring of serum prolactin levels; usual dose 0.25–2 mg once weekly, usually 1 mg weekly; reduce initial dose and increase more gradually if patient intolerant, doses over 1 mg weekly to be given as divided dose; maximum 4.5 mg per week

Alone or as adjunct to co-beneldopa or co-careldopa in Parkinson's disease where dopamine-receptor agonists other than ergot derivative not appropriate
▸ BY MOUTH
▸ Adult: Initially 1 mg daily, then increased in steps of 0.5–1 mg every 7–14 days, concurrent dose of levodopa may be decreased gradually while dose of cabergoline is increased; maximum 3 mg per day

IMPORTANT SAFETY INFORMATION
FIBROTIC REACTIONS
Cabergoline has been associated with pulmonary, retroperitoneal, and pericardial fibrotic reactions.
   Manufacturer advises exclude cardiac valvulopathy with echocardiography before starting treatment with these ergot derivatives for Parkinson's disease or chronic endocrine disorders (excludes suppression of lactation); it may also be appropriate to measure the erythrocyte sedimentation rate and serum creatinine and to obtain a chest X-ray. Patients should be monitored for dyspnoea, persistent cough, chest pain, cardiac failure, and abdominal pain or tenderness. If long-term treatment is expected, then lung-function tests may also be helpful. Patients taking cabergoline should be regularly monitored for cardiac fibrosis by echocardiography (within 3–6 months of initiating treatment and subsequently at 6–12 month intervals).

IMPULSE CONTROL DISORDERS
Treatment with dopamine-receptor agonists are associated with impulse control disorders, including pathological gambling, binge eating, and hypersexuality. Patients and their carers should be informed about the risk of impulse control disorders. Ergot- and non-ergot-

derived dopamine-receptor agonists do not differ in their propensity to cause impulse control disorders, so switching between dopamine-receptor agonists will not control these side-effects. See Parkinson's disease p. 470.

PREVENTION OR SUPPRESSION OF LACTATION
Healthcare professionals are reminded that cabergoline should not be used in women with postpartum hypertension. Serious side-effects have been reported; blood pressure should be carefully monitored, especially during the first days of treatment and with any subsequent dose increases. See *Contra-indications* for further information.

- ● CONTRA-INDICATIONS Cardiac valvulopathy—exclude before treatment (does not apply to suppression of lactation) · eclampsia · history of pericardial fibrotic disorders · history of puerperal psychosis · history of pulmonary fibrotic disorders · history of retroperitoneal fibrotic disorders · hypertension in postpartum women · pre-eclampsia · uncontrolled hypertension

CONTRA-INDICATIONS, FURTHER INFORMATION
▸ Use in prevention or suppression of lactation [EvGr] Hypertension, myocardial infarction, seizures or stroke (both sometimes preceded by severe headache or visual disturbances), and psychiatric disorders have been reported in postpartum women given cabergoline for lactation suppression—caution with drugs that affect blood pressure and avoid other ergot alkaloids. Discontinue immediately if hypertension, suggestive chest pain, severe progressive or unremitting headache, or signs of CNS toxicity develop. ⟨M⟩

- ● CAUTIONS Cardiovascular disease · history of peptic ulcer · history of serious mental disorders (especially psychotic disorders) · Raynaud's syndrome

CAUTIONS, FURTHER INFORMATION
▸ Hyperprolactinemic patients In hyperprolactinaemic patients, the source of the hyperprolactinaemia should be established (i.e. exclude pituitary tumour before treatment).

- ● INTERACTIONS → Appendix 1: dopamine receptor agonists
- ● SIDE-EFFECTS
▸ **Common or very common** Asthenia · breast pain · cardiac valve disorders · confusion · constipation · depression · dizziness · drowsiness · dyspnoea · gastritis · gastrointestinal discomfort · hallucination · headache · hot flush · hypotension · movement disorders · nausea · oedema · pericardial effusion · pericarditis · sexual dysfunction · sleep disorder · vertigo · vomiting
▸ **Uncommon** Alopecia · delusions · digital vasospasm · epistaxis · erythromelalgia · fibrosis · hepatic function abnormal · leg cramps · palpitations · paraesthesia · psychotic disorder · pulmonary fibrosis · rash · respiratory disorders · syncope · vision disorders
▸ **Frequency not known** Aggression · angina pectoris · chest pain · hypertension · myocardial infarction · pathological gambling · psychiatric disorder · seizure · stroke · sudden onset of sleep (can occur without warning) · tremor

- ● ALLERGY AND CROSS-SENSITIVITY [EvGr] Cabergoline should not be used in patients with hypersensitivity to ergot alkaloids. ⟨M⟩

- ● CONCEPTION AND CONTRACEPTION Exclude pregnancy before starting and perform monthly pregnancy tests during the amenorrhoeic period. Caution—advise non-hormonal contraception if pregnancy not desired. Discontinue 1 month before intended conception (ovulatory cycles persist for 6 months).

- ● PREGNANCY Discontinue if pregnancy occurs during treatment (specialist advice needed).

- **BREAST FEEDING** Suppresses lactation; avoid breast-feeding if lactation prevention fails.
- **HEPATIC IMPAIRMENT** Manufacturer advises caution in severe impairment (risk of increased exposure). **Dose adjustments** Manufacturer advises consider dose reduction in severe impairment.
- **MONITORING REQUIREMENTS**
  ‣ Monitor for fibrotic disease.
  ‣ Monitor blood pressure for a few days after starting treatment and following dosage increase.
- **TREATMENT CESSATION** Antiparkinsonian drug therapy should never be stopped abruptly as this carries a small risk of neuroleptic malignant syndrome.
- **PRESCRIBING AND DISPENSING INFORMATION** Dispense in original container (contains desiccant).
- **PATIENT AND CARER ADVICE**
  Driving and skilled tasks
  Sudden onset of sleep Excessive daytime sleepiness and sudden onset of sleep can occur with dopamine-receptor agonists.

  Patients starting treatment with these drugs should be warned of the risk and of the need to exercise caution when driving or operating machinery. Those who have experienced excessive sedation or sudden onset of sleep should refrain from driving or operating machines until these effects have stopped occurring.

  Management of excessive daytime sleepiness should focus on the identification of an underlying cause, such as depression or concomitant medication. Patients should be counselled on improving sleep behaviour.
  Hypotensive reactions Hypotensive reactions can occur in some patients taking dopamine-receptor agonists; these can be particularly problematic during the first few days of treatment and care should be exercised when driving or operating machinery.

- **MEDICINAL FORMS** There can be variation in the licensing of different medicines containing the same drug.

  Oral tablet
  CAUTIONARY AND ADVISORY LABELS 10, 21
  ‣ **Cabergoline (Non-proprietary)**
    Cabergoline 500 microgram Cabergoline 500microgram tablets | 8 tablet PoM £28.54 DT = £15.16
    Cabergoline 1 mg Cabergoline 1mg tablets | 20 tablet PoM £72.00 DT = £60.75
    Cabergoline 2 mg Cabergoline 2mg tablets | 20 tablet PoM £112.13 DT = £112.13
  ‣ **Cabaser** (Pfizer Ltd)
    Cabergoline 1 mg Cabaser 1mg tablets | 20 tablet PoM £83.00 DT = £60.75
    Cabergoline 2 mg Cabaser 2mg tablets | 20 tablet PoM £83.00 DT = £112.13
  ‣ **Dostinex** (Pfizer Ltd)
    Cabergoline 500 microgram Dostinex 500microgram tablets | 8 tablet PoM £30.04 DT = £15.16

Pramipexole

29-Jul-2021

- **INDICATIONS AND DOSE**

  Parkinson's disease, used alone or as an adjunct to co-beneldopa or co-careldopa
  ‣ BY MOUTH USING IMMEDIATE-RELEASE MEDICINES
  ‣ Adult: Initially 88 micrograms 3 times a day, if tolerated dose to be increased by doubling dose every 5–7 days, increased to 350 micrograms 3 times a day, then increased in steps of 180 micrograms 3 times a day if required, dose to be increased at weekly intervals, during dose titration and maintenance, levodopa dose may be reduced, maximum daily dose to be given in 3 divided doses; maximum 3.3 mg per day

‣ BY MOUTH USING MODIFIED-RELEASE MEDICINES
‣ Adult: Initially 260 micrograms once daily, dose to be increased by doubling dose every 5–7 days, increased to 1.05 mg once daily, then increased in steps of 520 micrograms every week if required, during dose titration and maintenance, levodopa dose may be reduced according to response; maximum 3.15 mg per day

Moderate to severe restless legs syndrome
‣ BY MOUTH USING IMMEDIATE-RELEASE MEDICINES
‣ Adult: Initially 88 micrograms once daily, dose to be taken 2–3 hours before bedtime, dose to be increased by doubling dose every 4–7 days if necessary, repeat dose titration if restarting treatment after an interval of more than a few days; maximum 540 micrograms per day

DOSE EQUIVALENCE AND CONVERSION
‣ Doses and strengths are stated in terms of pramipexole (base).
‣ Equivalent strengths of pramipexole (base) in terms of pramipexole dihydrochloride monohydrate (salt) for immediate-release preparations are as follows:
‣ 88 micrograms base ≡ 125 micrograms salt;
‣ 180 micrograms base ≡ 250 micrograms salt;
‣ 350 micrograms base ≡ 500 micrograms salt;
‣ 700 micrograms base ≡ 1 mg salt.
‣ Equivalent strengths of pramipexole (base) in terms of pramipexole dihydrochloride monohydrate (salt) for modified-release preparations are as follows:
‣ 260 micrograms base ≡ 375 micrograms salt;
‣ 520 micrograms base ≡ 750 micrograms salt;
‣ 1.05 mg base ≡ 1.5 mg salt;
‣ 1.57 mg base ≡ 2.25 mg salt;
‣ 2.1 mg base ≡ 3 mg salt;
‣ 2.62 mg base ≡ 3.75 mg salt;
‣ 3.15 mg base ≡ 4.5 mg salt.

> **IMPORTANT SAFETY INFORMATION**
> IMPULSE CONTROL DISORDERS
> Treatment with dopamine-receptor agonists is associated with impulse control disorders, including pathological gambling, binge eating, and hypersexuality. Patients and their carers should be informed about the risk of impulse control disorders. Ergot- and non-ergot-derived dopamine-receptor agonists do not differ in their propensity to cause impulse control disorders, so switching between dopamine-receptor agonists will not control these side-effects. See Parkinson's disease p. 470

- **CAUTIONS** Psychotic disorders · risk of visual disorders (ophthalmological testing recommended) · severe cardiovascular disease
- **INTERACTIONS** → Appendix 1: dopamine receptor agonists
- **SIDE-EFFECTS**
  ‣ **Common or very common** Appetite abnormal · behaviour abnormal · confusion · constipation · dizziness · drowsiness · fatigue · hallucination · headache · hypotension · movement disorders · nausea · peripheral oedema · psychiatric disorders · sleep disorders · vision disorders · vomiting · weight changes
  ‣ **Uncommon** Anxiety · binge eating · delirium · delusions · dyspnoea · heart failure · hiccups · mania · memory loss · pathological gambling · pneumonia · sexual dysfunction · SIADH · skin reactions · sudden onset of sleep (can occur without warning) · syncope
  ‣ **Frequency not known** Depression · dopamine agonist withdrawal syndrome · generalised pain · sweating abnormal
- **PREGNANCY** Use only if potential benefit outweighs risk—no information available.

- **BREAST FEEDING** May suppress lactation; avoid—present in milk in *animal* studies.
- **RENAL IMPAIRMENT** EvGr For *immediate-release* tablets in restless legs syndrome, use with caution if creatinine clearance less than 20 mL/minute (no information available). For *modified-release* tablets, avoid if creatinine clearance less than 30 mL/minute (no information available). ⓜ

  Dose adjustments EvGr For *immediate-release* tablets in Parkinson's disease, initially 88 micrograms twice daily (max. 1.57 mg daily in 2 divided doses) if creatinine clearance 20–50 mL/minute; initially 88 micrograms once daily (max. 1.1 mg once daily) if creatinine clearance less than 20 mL/minute. If renal function declines during treatment, reduce dose by the same percentage as the decline in creatinine clearance.

  For *modified-release* tablets, initially 260 micrograms on alternate days if creatinine clearance 30–50 mL/minute, increased to 260 micrograms once daily after 1 week, further increased if necessary by 260 micrograms daily at weekly intervals to max. 1.57 mg daily. ⓜ
  See p. 21.

- **MONITORING REQUIREMENTS** Risk of postural hypotension (especially on initiation)—monitor blood pressure.

- **TREATMENT CESSATION** Antiparkinsonian drug therapy should never be stopped abruptly as this carries a small risk of neuroleptic malignant syndrome.

- **PATIENT AND CARER ADVICE**
  Driving and skilled tasks
  Sudden onset of sleep Excessive daytime sleepiness and sudden onset of sleep can occur with dopamine-receptor agonists.

  Patients starting treatment with these drugs should be warned of the risk and of the need to exercise caution when driving or operating machinery. Those who have experienced excessive sedation or sudden onset of sleep should refrain from driving or operating machines until these effects have stopped occurring.

  Management of excessive daytime sleepiness should focus on the identification of an underlying cause, such as depression or concomitant medication. Patients should be counselled on improving sleep behaviour.
  Hypotensive reactions Hypotensive reactions can occur in some patients taking dopamine-receptor agonists; these can be particularly problematic during the first few days of treatment and care should be exercised when driving or operating machinery.

- **MEDICINAL FORMS** There can be variation in the licensing of different medicines containing the same drug.

Oral tablet
CAUTIONARY AND ADVISORY LABELS 10
▸ **Pramipexole (Non-proprietary)**
  Pramipexole (as Pramipexole dihydrochloride monohydrate)
  88 microgram Pramipexole 88microgram tablets | 30 tablet PoM £9.55 DT = £1.60
  Pramipexole (as Pramipexole dihydrochloride monohydrate)
  180 microgram Pramipexole 180microgram tablets | 30 tablet PoM £17.19 DT = £4.43
  Pramipexole (as Pramipexole dihydrochloride monohydrate)
  350 microgram Pramipexole 350microgram tablets | 30 tablet PoM £38.96 DT = £12.31
  Pramipexole (as Pramipexole dihydrochloride monohydrate)
  700 microgram Pramipexole 700microgram tablets | 30 tablet PoM £68.76 DT = £7.56 | 100 tablet PoM £9.33
▸ **Mirapexin** (Boehringer Ingelheim Ltd)
  Pramipexole (as Pramipexole dihydrochloride monohydrate)
  88 microgram Mirapexin 0.088mg tablets | 30 tablet PoM £11.24 DT = £1.60
  Pramipexole (as Pramipexole dihydrochloride monohydrate)
  180 microgram Mirapexin 0.18mg tablets | 30 tablet PoM £22.49 DT = £4.43

Pramipexole (as Pramipexole dihydrochloride monohydrate)
350 microgram Mirapexin 0.35mg tablets | 30 tablet PoM £44.97 DT = £12.31
Pramipexole (as Pramipexole dihydrochloride monohydrate)
700 microgram Mirapexin 0.7mg tablets | 30 tablet PoM £89.94 DT = £7.56

Modified-release tablet
CAUTIONARY AND ADVISORY LABELS 10, 25
▸ **Pramipexole (Non-proprietary)**
  Pramipexole (as Pramipexole dihydrochloride monohydrate)
  260 microgram Pramipexole 260microgram modified-release tablets | 30 tablet PoM £30.87 DT = £7.91
  Pramipexole (as Pramipexole dihydrochloride monohydrate)
  520 microgram Pramipexole 520microgram modified-release tablets | 30 tablet PoM £61.73 DT = £13.78
  Pramipexole (as Pramipexole dihydrochloride monohydrate)
  1.05 mg Pramipexole 1.05mg modified-release tablets | 30 tablet PoM £123.46 DT = £20.21
  Pramipexole (as Pramipexole dihydrochloride monohydrate)
  1.57 mg Pramipexole 1.57mg modified-release tablets | 30 tablet PoM £172.01-£192.24 DT = £191.11
  Pramipexole (as Pramipexole dihydrochloride monohydrate)
  2.1 mg Pramipexole 2.1mg modified-release tablets | 30 tablet PoM £246.91 DT = £245.47
  Pramipexole (as Pramipexole dihydrochloride monohydrate)
  2.62 mg Pramipexole 2.62mg modified-release tablets | 30 tablet PoM £404.72 DT = £404.72
  Pramipexole (as Pramipexole dihydrochloride monohydrate)
  3.15 mg Pramipexole 3.15mg modified-release tablets | 30 tablet PoM £467.84 DT = £467.84
▸ **Mirapexin** (Boehringer Ingelheim Ltd)
  Pramipexole (as Pramipexole dihydrochloride monohydrate)
  260 microgram Mirapexin 0.26mg modified-release tablets | 30 tablet PoM £32.49 DT = £7.91
  Pramipexole (as Pramipexole dihydrochloride monohydrate)
  520 microgram Mirapexin 0.52mg modified-release tablets | 30 tablet PoM £64.98 DT = £13.78
  Pramipexole (as Pramipexole dihydrochloride monohydrate)
  1.05 mg Mirapexin 1.05mg modified-release tablets | 30 tablet PoM £129.96 DT = £20.21
  Pramipexole (as Pramipexole dihydrochloride monohydrate)
  1.57 mg Mirapexin 1.57mg modified-release tablets | 30 tablet PoM £202.36 DT = £191.11
  Pramipexole (as Pramipexole dihydrochloride monohydrate)
  2.1 mg Mirapexin 2.1mg modified-release tablets | 30 tablet PoM £259.91 DT = £245.47
  Pramipexole (as Pramipexole dihydrochloride monohydrate)
  2.62 mg Mirapexin 2.62mg modified-release tablets | 30 tablet PoM £337.27 DT = £404.72
  Pramipexole (as Pramipexole dihydrochloride monohydrate)
  3.15 mg Mirapexin 3.15mg modified-release tablets | 30 tablet PoM £389.87 DT = £467.84
▸ **Pipexus** (Ethypharm UK Ltd)
  Pramipexole (as Pramipexole dihydrochloride monohydrate)
  260 microgram Pipexus 0.26mg modified-release tablets | 30 tablet PoM £16.25 DT = £7.91
  Pramipexole (as Pramipexole dihydrochloride monohydrate)
  520 microgram Pipexus 0.52mg modified-release tablets | 30 tablet PoM £32.49 DT = £13.78
  Pramipexole (as Pramipexole dihydrochloride monohydrate)
  1.05 mg Pipexus 1.05mg modified-release tablets | 30 tablet PoM £64.98 DT = £20.21
  Pramipexole (as Pramipexole dihydrochloride monohydrate)
  1.57 mg Pipexus 1.57mg modified-release tablets | 30 tablet PoM £101.18 DT = £191.11
  Pramipexole (as Pramipexole dihydrochloride monohydrate)
  2.1 mg Pipexus 2.1mg modified-release tablets | 30 tablet PoM £129.96 DT = £245.47
  Pramipexole (as Pramipexole dihydrochloride monohydrate)
  2.62 mg Pipexus 2.62mg modified-release tablets | 30 tablet PoM £168.64 DT = £404.72
  Pramipexole (as Pramipexole dihydrochloride monohydrate)
  3.15 mg Pipexus 3.15mg modified-release tablets | 30 tablet PoM £194.94 DT = £467.84

Ropinirole

04-Aug-2021

● **INDICATIONS AND DOSE**

Parkinson's disease, either used alone or as adjunct to co-beneldopa or co-careldopa

▸ BY MOUTH USING IMMEDIATE-RELEASE MEDICINES
▸ Adult: Initially 750 micrograms daily in 3 divided doses, then increased in steps of 750 micrograms daily, dose to be increased at weekly intervals, increased to 3 mg daily in 3 divided doses, then increased in steps of 1.5–3 mg daily, adjusted according to response, dose to be increased at weekly intervals; usual dose 9–16 mg daily in 3 divided doses, higher doses may be required if used with levodopa, when administered as adjunct to levodopa, concurrent dose of levodopa may be reduced by approx. 20%, daily maximum dose to be given in 3 divided doses; maximum 24 mg per day

▸ BY MOUTH USING MODIFIED-RELEASE MEDICINES
▸ Adult: Initially 2 mg once daily for 1 week, then 4 mg once daily, increased in steps of 2 mg at intervals of at least 1 week, adjusted according to response, increased to up to 8 mg once daily, dose to be increased further if still no response; increased in steps of 2–4 mg at intervals of at least 2 weeks if required, consider slower titration in patients over 75 years, when administered as adjunct to levodopa, concurrent dose of levodopa may gradually be reduced by approx. 30%; maximum 24 mg per day

Parkinson's disease in patients transferring from ropinirole immediate-release tablets

▸ BY MOUTH USING MODIFIED-RELEASE MEDICINES
▸ Adult: Initially ropinirole modified-release once daily substituted for total daily dose equivalent of ropinirole immediate-release tablets; if control not maintained after switching, titrate dose as above

Moderate to severe restless legs syndrome

▸ BY MOUTH USING IMMEDIATE-RELEASE MEDICINES
▸ Adult: Initially 250 micrograms once daily for 2 days, increased if tolerated to 500 micrograms once daily for 5 days, then increased if tolerated to 1 mg once daily for 7 days, then increased in steps of 500 micrograms daily, adjusted according to response, dose to be increased at weekly intervals; usual dose 2 mg once daily, doses to be taken at night; maximum 4 mg per day

● **UNLICENSED USE** Doses in the BNF may differ from those in product literature.

> **IMPORTANT SAFETY INFORMATION**
>
> **SAFE PRACTICE**
> Ropinirole has been confused with risperidone; care must be taken to ensure the correct drug is prescribed and dispensed.
>
> **IMPULSE CONTROL DISORDERS**
> Treatment with dopamine-receptor agonists is associated with impulse control disorders, including pathological gambling, binge eating, and hypersexuality. Patients and their carers should be informed about the risk of impulse control disorders. Ergot- and non-ergot-derived dopamine-receptor agonists do not differ in their propensity to cause impulse control disorders, so switching between dopamine-receptor agonists will not control these side-effects. See Parkinson's disease p. 470

● **CAUTIONS** Elderly · major psychotic disorders · severe cardiovascular disease (risk of hypotension—monitor blood pressure)

● **INTERACTIONS** → Appendix 1: dopamine receptor agonists

● **SIDE-EFFECTS**

▸ **Common or very common** Confusion · dizziness · drowsiness · early morning awakening · fatigue · gastrointestinal discomfort · hallucination · movement disorders · nausea · nervousness · peripheral oedema · syncope · vertigo · vomiting

▸ **Uncommon** Hypotension · sexual dysfunction · sudden onset of sleep

▸ **Rare or very rare** Hepatic reaction

▸ **Frequency not known** Behaviour abnormal · compulsions · delirium · delusions · dopamine dysregulation syndrome · eating disorders · pathological gambling · psychotic disorder

● **PREGNANCY** Avoid unless potential benefit outweighs risk—toxicity in *animal* studies.

● **BREAST FEEDING** May suppress lactation—avoid.

● **HEPATIC IMPAIRMENT**

▸ When used for Parkinson's disease Manufacturer advises avoid (no information available).

▸ When used for Restless legs syndrome Manufacturer advises caution in moderate impairment; avoid in severe impairment.

● **RENAL IMPAIRMENT** EvGr Avoid if creatinine clearance less than 30 mL/minute (no information available). Ⓜ See p. 21.

● **TREATMENT CESSATION** Antiparkinsonian drug therapy should never be stopped abruptly as this carries a small risk of neuroleptic malignant syndrome.

● **PATIENT AND CARER ADVICE** Manufacturer advises patients and their carers should be informed of the risk of developing dopamine dysregulation syndrome; addiction-like symptoms should be reported.

Missed doses

▸ When used for Parkinson's disease Manufacturer advises if treatment is interrupted for one day or more, re-initiation by dose titration should be considered—consult product literature.

▸ When used for Moderate to severe restless legs syndrome Manufacturer advises if treatment is interrupted for more than a few days, re-initiation by dose titration is recommended.

Driving and skilled tasks

Sudden onset of sleep Excessive daytime sleepiness and sudden onset of sleep can occur with dopamine-receptor agonists.

Patients starting treatment with these drugs should be warned of the risk and of the need to exercise caution when driving or operating machinery. Those who have experienced excessive sedation or sudden onset of sleep should refrain from driving or operating machines until these effects have stopped occurring.

Management of excessive daytime sleepiness should focus on the identification of an underlying cause, such as depression or concomitant medication. Patients should be counselled on improving sleep behaviour.

Hypotensive reactions Hypotensive reactions can occur in some patients taking dopamine-receptor agonists; these can be particularly problematic during the first few days of treatment and care should be exercised when driving or operating machinery.

● **NATIONAL FUNDING/ACCESS DECISIONS**

For full details see funding body website

Scottish Medicines Consortium (SMC) decisions

▸ **Ropinirole tablets (*Adartrel*®) for the treatment of moderate to severe idiopathic restless legs syndrome (July 2006)** SMC No. 165/05 Recommended with restrictions

▸ **Ropinirole (*Requip XL*®) for the treatment of idiopathic Parkinson's Disease (September 2008)** SMC No. 491/08 Recommended

- **MEDICINAL FORMS** There can be variation in the licensing of different medicines containing the same drug. Forms available from special-order manufacturers include: oral suspension, oral solution

Oral tablet

CAUTIONARY AND ADVISORY LABELS 10, 21

▸ **Ropinirole (Non-proprietary)**
Ropinirole (as Ropinirole hydrochloride)
250 microgram Ropinirole 250microgram tablets | 12 tablet PoM £10.61 DT = £7.08
Ropinirole (as Ropinirole hydrochloride)
500 microgram Ropinirole 500microgram tablets | 28 tablet PoM £16.00 DT = £10.52
Ropinirole (as Ropinirole hydrochloride) 1 mg Ropinirole 1mg tablets | 84 tablet PoM £53.75 DT = £26.04
Ropinirole (as Ropinirole hydrochloride) 2 mg Ropinirole 2mg tablets | 28 tablet PoM £31.60 DT = £21.54 | 84 tablet PoM £59.13–£97.80
Ropinirole (as Ropinirole hydrochloride) 5 mg Ropinirole 5mg tablets | 84 tablet PoM £242.80 DT = £195.92

▸ **Adartrel** (GlaxoSmithKline UK Ltd)
Ropinirole (as Ropinirole hydrochloride) 250 microgram Adartrel 250microgram tablets | 12 tablet PoM £3.94 DT = £7.08
Ropinirole (as Ropinirole hydrochloride) 500 microgram Adartrel 500microgram tablets | 28 tablet PoM £15.75 DT = £10.52
Ropinirole (as Ropinirole hydrochloride) 2 mg Adartrel 2mg tablets | 28 tablet PoM £31.51 DT = £21.54

▸ **ReQuip** (GlaxoSmithKline UK Ltd)
Ropinirole (as Ropinirole hydrochloride) 250 microgram ReQuip 250microgram tablets | 21 tablet PoM £5.70
Ropinirole (as Ropinirole hydrochloride) 1 mg ReQuip 1mg tablets | 84 tablet PoM £56.71 DT = £26.04
Ropinirole (as Ropinirole hydrochloride) 2 mg ReQuip 2mg tablets | 84 tablet PoM £113.44
Ropinirole (as Ropinirole hydrochloride) 5 mg ReQuip 5mg tablets | 84 tablet PoM £195.92 DT = £195.92

Modified-release tablet

CAUTIONARY AND ADVISORY LABELS 10, 25

▸ **Ropinirole (Non-proprietary)**
Ropinirole (as Ropinirole hydrochloride) 2 mg Ropinirole 2mg modified-release tablets | 28 tablet PoM £12.78 DT = £12.54
Ropinirole (as Ropinirole hydrochloride) 4 mg Ropinirole 4mg modified-release tablets | 28 tablet PoM £25.58 DT = £25.09
Ropinirole (as Ropinirole hydrochloride) 8 mg Ropinirole 8mg modified-release tablets | 28 tablet PoM £42.95 DT = £42.11

▸ **Eppinix XL** (Ethypharm UK Ltd)
Ropinirole (as Ropinirole hydrochloride) 2 mg Ipinnia XL 2mg tablets | 28 tablet PoM £5.64 DT = £12.54
Ropinirole (as Ropinirole hydrochloride) 3 mg Ipinnia XL 3mg tablets | 28 tablet PoM £8.46 DT = £8.46
Ropinirole (as Ropinirole hydrochloride) 4 mg Ipinnia XL 4mg tablets | 28 tablet PoM £11.29 DT = £25.09
Ropinirole (as Ropinirole hydrochloride) 6 mg Ipinnia XL 6mg tablets | 28 tablet PoM £15.32 DT = £15.32
Ropinirole (as Ropinirole hydrochloride) 8 mg Ipinnia XL 8mg tablets | 28 tablet PoM £18.95 DT = £42.11

▸ **Raponer XL** (Accord-UK Ltd)
Ropinirole (as Ropinirole hydrochloride) 2 mg Raponer XL 2mg tablets | 28 tablet PoM £12.54 DT = £12.54
Ropinirole (as Ropinirole hydrochloride) 4 mg Raponer XL 4mg tablets | 28 tablet PoM £25.09 DT = £25.09
Ropinirole (as Ropinirole hydrochloride) 8 mg Raponer XL 8mg tablets | 28 tablet PoM £42.11 DT = £42.11

▸ **ReQuip XL** (GlaxoSmithKline UK Ltd)
Ropinirole (as Ropinirole hydrochloride) 2 mg ReQuip XL 2mg tablets | 28 tablet PoM £12.54 DT = £12.54
Ropinirole (as Ropinirole hydrochloride) 4 mg ReQuip XL 4mg tablets | 28 tablet PoM £25.09 DT = £25.09
Ropinirole (as Ropinirole hydrochloride) 8 mg ReQuip XL 8mg tablets | 28 tablet PoM £42.11 DT = £42.11

▸ **Repinex XL** (Aspire Pharma Ltd)
Ropinirole (as Ropinirole hydrochloride) 2 mg Repinex XL 2mg tablets | 28 tablet PoM £6.20 DT = £12.54
Ropinirole (as Ropinirole hydrochloride) 4 mg Repinex XL 4mg tablets | 28 tablet PoM £12.50 DT = £25.09
Ropinirole (as Ropinirole hydrochloride) 8 mg Repinex XL 8mg tablets | 28 tablet PoM £21.00 DT = £42.11

▸ **Ropiqual XL** (Milpharm Ltd)
Ropinirole (as Ropinirole hydrochloride) 2 mg Ropiqual XL 2mg tablets | 28 tablet PoM £12.54 DT = £12.54
Ropinirole (as Ropinirole hydrochloride) 4 mg Ropiqual XL 4mg tablets | 28 tablet PoM £25.09 DT = £25.09
Ropinirole (as Ropinirole hydrochloride) 8 mg Ropiqual XL 8mg tablets | 28 tablet PoM £42.11 DT = £42.11

Rotigotine

09-Mar-2021

- **INDICATIONS AND DOSE**

Monotherapy in Parkinson's disease
▸ BY TRANSDERMAL APPLICATION USING PATCHES
▸ Adult: Initially 2 mg/24 hours, then increased in steps of 2 mg/24 hours every week if required; maximum 8 mg/24 hours per day

Adjunctive therapy with co-beneldopa or co-careldopa in Parkinson's disease
▸ BY TRANSDERMAL APPLICATION USING PATCHES
▸ Adult: Initially 4 mg/24 hours, then increased in steps of 2 mg/24 hours every week if required; maximum 16 mg/24 hours per day

Moderate to severe restless legs syndrome
▸ BY TRANSDERMAL APPLICATION USING PATCHES
▸ Adult: Initially 1 mg/24 hours, then increased in steps of 1 mg/24 hours every week if required; maximum 3 mg/24 hours per day

IMPORTANT SAFETY INFORMATION
IMPULSE CONTROL DISORDERS
Treatment with dopamine-receptor agonists is associated with impulse control disorders, including pathological gambling, binge eating, and hypersexuality. Patients and their carers should be informed about the risk of impulse control disorders. Ergot- and non-ergot-derived dopamine-receptor agonists do not differ in their propensity to cause impulse control disorders, so switching between dopamine-receptor agonists will not control these side-effects. See Parkinson's disease p. 470

- **CAUTIONS** Avoid exposure of patch to heat · remove patch (aluminium-containing) before magnetic resonance imaging or cardioversion

- **INTERACTIONS** → Appendix 1: dopamine receptor agonists

- **SIDE-EFFECTS**
▸ **Common or very common** Asthenia · behaviour abnormal · constipation · dizziness · drowsiness · dry mouth · dyskinesia · eating disorders · fall · gastrointestinal discomfort · hallucinations · headache · hiccups · hyperhidrosis · hypertension · hypotension · loss of consciousness · malaise · nausea · palpitations · pathological gambling · perception altered · peripheral oedema · psychiatric disorders · skin reactions · sleep disorders · sudden onset of sleep (can occur without warning) · syncope · vertigo · vomiting · weight changes
▸ **Uncommon** Agitation · angioedema · arrhythmias · confusion · sexual dysfunction · vision disorders
▸ **Rare or very rare** Delirium · delusions · irritability · psychotic disorder · seizure
▸ **Frequency not known** Dopamine dysregulation syndrome · rhabdomyolysis

- **PREGNANCY** Avoid—no information available.

- **BREAST FEEDING** May suppress lactation; avoid—present in milk in *animal* studies.

- **HEPATIC IMPAIRMENT** Manufacturer advises caution in severe impairment (no information available).
Dose adjustments Manufacturer advises consider dose reduction in severe impairment.

- **MONITORING REQUIREMENTS** Ophthalmic testing recommended.

- **TREATMENT CESSATION** Antiparkinsonian drug therapy should never be stopped abruptly as this carries a small risk of neuroleptic malignant syndrome.
- **DIRECTIONS FOR ADMINISTRATION** Manufacturer advises apply patch to clean, dry, intact, healthy and non-irritated skin on torso, thigh, hip, shoulder or upper arm by pressing the patch firmly against the skin for about 30 seconds. Patches should be removed after 24 hours and the replacement patch applied on a different area (avoid using the same area for 14 days)—consult product literature for further information.
- **PATIENT AND CARER ADVICE** Manufacturer advises patients and their carers should be informed of the risk of developing dopamine dysregulation syndrome; addiction-like symptoms should be reported.

Driving and skilled tasks

Sudden onset of sleep Excessive daytime sleepiness and sudden onset of sleep can occur with dopamine-receptor agonists.

Patients starting treatment with these drugs should be warned of the risk and of the need to exercise caution when driving or operating machinery. Those who have experienced excessive sedation or sudden onset of sleep should refrain from driving or operating machines until these effects have stopped occurring.

Management of excessive daytime sleepiness should focus on the identification of an underlying cause, such as depression or concomitant medication. Patients should be counselled on improving sleep behaviour.

Hypotensive reactions Hypotensive reactions can occur in some patients taking dopamine-receptor agonists; these can be particularly problematic during the first few days of treatment and care should be exercised when driving or operating machinery.

- **NATIONAL FUNDING/ACCESS DECISIONS**
  For full details see funding body website

  Scottish Medicines Consortium (SMC) decisions
  ▸ Rotigotine (*Neupro*®) for advanced-stage idiopathic Parkinson's disease (August 2007) SMC No. 392/07 Recommended with restrictions
  ▸ Rotigotine (*Neupro*®) for early-stage Parkinson's disease (July 2007) SMC No. 289/06 Recommended
  ▸ Rotigotine (*Neupro*®) for Restless Legs Syndrome (RLS) (August 2009) SMC No. 548/09 Recommended with restrictions

- **MEDICINAL FORMS** There can be variation in the licensing of different medicines containing the same drug.

  Transdermal patch
  CAUTIONARY AND ADVISORY LABELS 10
  ▸ Rotigotine (Non-proprietary)
    Rotigotine 1 mg per 24 hour Rotigotine 1mg/24hours transdermal patches | 28 patch PoM £77.24 DT = £77.24
    Rotigotine 2 mg per 24 hour Rotigotine 2mg/24hours transdermal patches | 28 patch PoM £81.10 DT = £81.10
    Rotigotine 3 mg per 24 hour Rotigotine 3mg/24hours transdermal patches | 28 patch PoM £102.35 DT = £102.35
    Rotigotine 4 mg per 24 hour Rotigotine 4mg/24hours transdermal patches | 28 patch PoM £123.60 DT = £123.60
    Rotigotine 6 mg per 24 hour Rotigotine 6mg/24hours transdermal patches | 28 patch PoM £149.93 DT = £149.93
    Rotigotine 8 mg per 24 hour Rotigotine 8mg/24hours transdermal patches | 28 patch PoM £149.93 DT = £149.93
  ▸ Neupro (UCB Pharma Ltd)
    Rotigotine 1 mg per 24 hour Neupro 1mg/24hours transdermal patches | 28 patch PoM £77.24 DT = £77.24
    Rotigotine 2 mg per 24 hour Neupro 2mg/24hours transdermal patches | 28 patch PoM £81.10 DT = £81.10
    Rotigotine 3 mg per 24 hour Neupro 3mg/24hours transdermal patches | 28 patch PoM £102.35 DT = £102.35
    Rotigotine 4 mg per 24 hour Neupro 4mg/24hours transdermal patches | 28 patch PoM £123.60 DT = £123.60
    Rotigotine 6 mg per 24 hour Neupro 6mg/24hours transdermal patches | 28 patch PoM £149.93 DT = £149.93

Rotigotine 8 mg per 24 hour Neupro 8mg/24hours transdermal patches | 28 patch PoM £149.93 DT = £149.93

DOPAMINERGIC DRUGS ❭ MONOAMINE-OXIDASE B INHIBITORS

Rasagiline
15-Apr-2024

- **DRUG ACTION** Rasagiline is a monoamine-oxidase B inhibitor.

- **INDICATIONS AND DOSE**

  Parkinson's disease, used alone or as adjunct to co-beneldopa or co-careldopa for 'end-of-dose' fluctuations
  ▸ BY MOUTH
  ▸ Adult: 1 mg daily

- **INTERACTIONS** → Appendix 1: MAO-B inhibitors

- **SIDE-EFFECTS**
  ▸ **Common or very common** Abdominal pain · abnormal dreams · angina pectoris · arthralgia · arthritis · conjunctivitis · depression · dermatitis · dry mouth · fall · fever · flatulence · hallucination · headache · increased risk of infection · leucopenia · malaise · nausea · neoplasms · pain · postural hypotension · urinary urgency · vertigo · vomiting · weight decreased
  ▸ **Uncommon** Appetite decreased · confusion
  ▸ **Frequency not known** Dopamine dysregulation syndrome · drowsiness · eating disorders · pathological gambling · psychiatric disorders · sexual dysfunction · sudden onset of sleep

- **PREGNANCY** Manufacturer advises avoid—no information available.

- **BREAST FEEDING** Use with caution—may suppress lactation.

- **HEPATIC IMPAIRMENT** Manufacturer advises caution in mild impairment; avoid in moderate to severe impairment (risk of increased exposure).

- **TREATMENT CESSATION** Avoid abrupt withdrawal.

- **PATIENT AND CARER ADVICE**

  Driving and skilled tasks

  Sudden onset of sleep Excessive daytime sleepiness and sudden onset of sleep can occur with rasagiline.

  Patients starting treatment should be warned of the risk and of the need to exercise caution when driving or operating machinery. Those who have experienced excessive sedation or sudden onset of sleep should refrain from driving or operating machines until these effects have stopped occurring.

  Management of excessive daytime sleepiness should focus on the identification of an underlying cause, such as depression or concomitant medication. Patients should be counselled on improving sleep behaviour.

- **MEDICINAL FORMS** There can be variation in the licensing of different medicines containing the same drug. Forms available from special-order manufacturers include: oral suspension, oral solution

  Oral tablet
  ▸ Rasagiline (Non-proprietary)
    Rasagiline 1 mg Rasagiline 1mg tablets | 28 tablet PoM £70.72 DT = £4.02
  ▸ Azilect (Teva UK Ltd)
    Rasagiline 1 mg Azilect 1mg tablets | 28 tablet PoM £70.72 DT = £4.02

4

Nervous system

Safinamide

26-Jun-2019

- **DRUG ACTION** Safinamide is a monoamine-oxidase B inhibitor.

- **INDICATIONS AND DOSE**

Parkinson's disease, as an adjunct to levodopa alone or in combination with other antiparkinsonian drugs, for mid- to late-stage fluctuations
  - ▶ BY MOUTH
  - ▶ Adult: 50 mg once daily, increased if necessary to 100 mg once daily

- **CONTRA-INDICATIONS** Active retinopathy · albinism · family history of hereditary retinal disease · retinal degeneration · uveitis

- **CAUTIONS** Hypertension (may raise blood pressure) · may exacerbate pre-existing dyskinesia (requiring levodopa dose reduction)

- **INTERACTIONS** → Appendix 1: MAO-B inhibitors

- **SIDE-EFFECTS**
- ▶ **Common or very common** Cataract · dizziness · drowsiness · headache · hypotension · injury · nausea · sleep disorders
- ▶ **Uncommon** Anaemia · anxiety · appetite abnormal · arrhythmias · asthenia · cognitive disorder · confusion · constipation · cough · decreased leucocytes · depression · diarrhoea · dry mouth · dysarthria · dyslipidaemia · dyspnoea · emotional lability · eye disorders · eye inflammation · gastrointestinal discomfort · gastrointestinal disorders · glaucoma · hallucination · hyperglycaemia · hypertension · increased risk of infection · joint disorders · movement disorders · muscle complaints · muscle weakness · neoplasms · oral disorders · pain · palpitations · peripheral oedema · photosensitivity reaction · psychotic disorder · QT interval prolongation · red blood cell abnormality · rhinorrhoea · sensation abnormal · sensation of pressure · sexual dysfunction · skin reactions · sweat changes · syncope · temperature sensation altered · urinary disorders · varicose veins · vertigo · vision disorders · vomiting · weight changes
- ▶ **Rare or very rare** Alopecia · arterial spasm · atherosclerosis · benign prostatic hyperplasia · breast abnormalities · bronchospasm · cachexia · concentration impaired · delirium · diabetic retinopathy · dysphonia · eosinophilia · eye pain · fat embolism · fever · gambling · haemorrhage · hyperbilirubinaemia · hyperkalaemia · illusion · malaise · myocardial infarction · oropharyngeal complaints · osteoarthritis · paranoia · psychiatric disorders · pyuria · reflexes decreased · suicidal ideation · taste altered

- **PREGNANCY** Manufacturer advises avoid—toxicity in *animal* studies.

- **BREAST FEEDING** Manufacturer advises avoid—present in milk in *animal* studies.

- **HEPATIC IMPAIRMENT** Manufacturer advises caution in moderate impairment (risk of increased exposure); avoid in severe impairment.
Dose adjustments Manufacturer advises max. daily dose should not exceed 50 mg daily in moderate impairment.

- **MEDICINAL FORMS** There can be variation in the licensing of different medicines containing the same drug.

Oral tablet
- ▶ Xadago (Zambon UK Ltd)
  Safinamide (as Safinamide methansulfonate) 50 mg Xadago 50mg tablets | 30 tablet [PoM] £69.00 DT = £69.00
  Safinamide (as Safinamide methansulfonate) 100 mg Xadago 100mg tablets | 30 tablet [PoM] £69.00 DT = £69.00

Selegiline hydrochloride

28-May-2021

- **DRUG ACTION** Selegiline is a monoamine-oxidase B inhibitor.

- **INDICATIONS AND DOSE**

Parkinson's disease, used alone or as adjunct to co-beneldopa or co-careldopa to reduce 'end of dose' deterioration | Symptomatic parkinsonism
  - ▶ BY MOUTH USING IMMEDIATE-RELEASE MEDICINES
  - ▶ Adult: Initially 5 mg once daily for 2–4 weeks, then increased if tolerated to 10 mg daily, dose to be taken in the morning
  - ▶ BY MOUTH USING ORAL LYOPHILISATE
  - ▶ Adult: 1.25 mg once daily, dose to be taken before breakfast

DOSE EQUIVALENCE AND CONVERSION
  - ▶ 1.25-mg oral lyophilisate is equivalent to 10-mg tablet.
  - ▶ Patients receiving 10 mg conventional selegiline hydrochloride tablets can be switched to oral lyophilisates (*Zelapar*®) 1.25 mg.

- **CONTRA-INDICATIONS** Active duodenal ulceration · active gastric ulceration · avoid or use with great caution in postural hypotension (when used in combination with levodopa)

- **CAUTIONS** Angina · arrhythmias · duodenal ulceration · gastric ulceration · history of hepatic dysfunction · patients predisposed to confusion and psychosis · psychosis · uncontrolled hypertension

- **INTERACTIONS** → Appendix 1: MAO-B inhibitors

- **SIDE-EFFECTS**
- ▶ **Common or very common** Arrhythmias · arthralgia · back pain · confusion · constipation · depression · diarrhoea · dizziness · dry mouth · fall · fatigue · hallucination · headache · hyperhidrosis · hypertension · hypotension · movement disorders · muscle cramps · nasal congestion · nausea · oral disorders · sleep disorders · throat pain · tremor · vertigo
- ▶ **Uncommon** Alopecia · angina pectoris · anxiety · appetite decreased · chest pain · dyspnoea · leucopenia · mood altered · myopathy · palpitations · peripheral oedema · pharyngitis · psychosis · skin eruption · thrombocytopenia · urinary disorders · vision blurred
- ▶ **Frequency not known** Hypersexuality

SIDE-EFFECTS, FURTHER INFORMATION Side-effects of levodopa may be increased—concurrent levodopa dosage can be reduced by 10–30% in steps of 10% every 3–4 days.

- **PREGNANCY** Avoid—no information available.

- **BREAST FEEDING** Avoid—no information available.

- **HEPATIC IMPAIRMENT** Manufacturer advises caution in severe impairment.

- **RENAL IMPAIRMENT** [EvGr] Use with caution in severe impairment. Ⓜ

- **TREATMENT CESSATION** Avoid abrupt withdrawal.

- **DIRECTIONS FOR ADMINISTRATION** Oral lyophilisates should be placed on the tongue and allowed to dissolve. Advise patient not to drink, rinse, or wash mouth out for 5 minutes after taking the tablet.

- **PATIENT AND CARER ADVICE** Patients or carers should be advised on how to administer selegiline hydrochloride oral lyophilisates.
Driving and skilled tasks Prescribers and other healthcare professionals should advise patients if treatment is likely to affect their ability to perform skilled tasks (e.g. driving). This applies especially to drugs with sedative effects; patients should be warned that these effects are increased by alcohol. General information about a patient's fitness to drive is available from the Driver and Vehicle Licensing Agency at www.dvla.gov.uk.

2015 legislation regarding driving whilst taking certain drugs, may also apply to selegiline, see *Drugs and driving* under Guidance on prescribing p. 1.

● **MEDICINAL FORMS** There can be variation in the licensing of different medicines containing the same drug. Forms available from special-order manufacturers include: oral solution

Oral tablet

▸ Eldepryl (Orion Pharma (UK) Ltd)
  Selegiline hydrochloride 5 mg Eldepryl 5mg tablets |
  100 tablet [PoM] £16.52 DT = £16.52
  Selegiline hydrochloride 10 mg Eldepryl 10mg tablets |
  100 tablet [PoM] £32.23 DT = £32.23

5   Nausea and labyrinth disorders

Nausea and labyrinth disorders

01-Oct-2021

Drug treatment

Antiemetics are generally only prescribed when the cause of vomiting is known because otherwise, they may delay diagnosis, particularly in children. If antiemetic drug treatment is indicated, the drug is chosen according to the aetiology of vomiting.

Antihistamines (e.g. cinnarizine p. 499, cyclizine p. 492, promethazine hydrochloride p. 326, promethazine teoclate p. 500) are effective against nausea and vomiting resulting from many underlying conditions. The duration of action and incidence of adverse effects, such as drowsiness and antimuscarinic effects, differ between antihistamines.

The phenothiazines (e.g. chlorpromazine hydrochloride p. 443, prochlorperazine p. 448, trifluoperazine p. 450) are dopamine antagonists and act centrally by blocking the chemoreceptor trigger zone. Severe dystonic reactions sometimes occur with phenothiazines, especially in children. [EvGr] Prochlorperazine can be used for chemotherapy-induced and radiation-induced nausea and vomiting. ⟨A⟩ It is less sedating and available as a buccal tablet, which can be useful in patients with persistent vomiting or with severe nausea.

[EvGr] Other antipsychotic drugs including haloperidol p. 445 [unlicensed use] and levomepromazine p. 502 are used for the relief of nausea and vomiting in palliative care. ⟨A⟩ For information on the use of antiemetics in palliative care, see Prescribing in palliative care p. 26.

Metoclopramide hydrochloride p. 494 is an effective antiemetic and its activity closely resembles that of the phenothiazines. Metoclopramide hydrochloride also acts directly on the gastric smooth muscle stimulating gastric emptying and it may be superior to the phenothiazines for emesis associated with gastro-intestinal and biliary disease.

Domperidone p. 494 acts at the chemoreceptor trigger zone. It has the advantage over metoclopramide hydrochloride and the phenothiazines of being less likely to cause central effects, such as sedation and dystonic reactions, because it does not readily cross the blood-brain barrier. [EvGr] In Parkinson's disease, low-dose domperidone can be used to treat nausea caused by dopaminergic drugs.

The 5HT$_3$-receptor antagonists, granisetron p. 496, ondansetron p. 497, and palonosetron p. 498, are used in the management of nausea and vomiting in patients receiving cytotoxics. ⟨A⟩ A combination of palonosetron with netupitant p. 499, a neurokinin 1-receptor antagonist, is also available.

[EvGr] Dexamethasone has antiemetic effects and is used in the management of chemotherapy-induced nausea and vomiting. It can be used alone or in combination with other antiemetics such as a 5HT$_3$-receptor antagonist.

The neurokinin 1-receptor antagonists, aprepitant p. 495 and fosaprepitant p. 496, are used to prevent nausea and vomiting associated with chemotherapy. They are usually given in combination with dexamethasone and a 5HT$_3$-receptor antagonist. ⟨A⟩ For further information on the prevention of nausea and vomiting caused by chemotherapy, see Cytotoxic drugs p. 1027.

Nabilone p. 493 is a synthetic cannabinoid with antiemetic properties. [EvGr] It can be considered as an add-on treatment for chemotherapy-induced nausea and vomiting unresponsive to optimised conventional antiemetics. ⟨A⟩

Nausea and vomiting during pregnancy

Nausea and vomiting in the first trimester of pregnancy is common and will usually resolve spontaneously within 16 to 20 weeks. [EvGr] For women who have nausea and vomiting, offer appropriate self-care advice (such as rest, oral hydration and dietary changes), and inform them about other available support (e.g. self-help information and support groups) and when to seek urgent medical advice. Take into consideration that a number of interventions may have already been tried. Antiemetics should be considered for women with persistent symptoms where self-care measures have been ineffective. If a non-pharmacological option is preferred, ginger may be helpful for mild to moderate nausea.

For women who choose pharmacological treatment, offer an antiemetic considering the advantages and disadvantages of each option, as well as patient preference, and their experience with treatments in previous pregnancies. Although few drug options are specifically licensed for nausea and vomiting associated with pregnancy, their use is established practice. Antiemetic options include: chlorpromazine hydrochloride, cyclizine, doxylamine with pyridoxine p. 493, metoclopramide hydrochloride, prochlorperazine, promethazine hydrochloride p. 326, promethazine teoclate p. 500, and ondansetron. For further information on antiemetic options, see NICE guideline: **Antenatal care** (available at: www.nice.org.uk/guidance/ng201). Assess the response to treatment after 24 hours; if the response is inadequate, switch to an antiemetic from a different therapeutic class. Reassess after 24 hours and if symptoms have not settled, specialist opinion should be sought. For women who have moderate to severe nausea and vomiting, consider intravenous fluids and adjunctive treatment with acupressure.

Hyperemesis gravidarum is a more serious condition, which requires regular antiemetic therapy, intravenous fluid and electrolyte replacement, and sometimes nutritional support. For women with severe or persistent hyperemesis gravidarum, antiemetics given by the parenteral or rectal routes may be more suitable than the oral route. Supplementation with thiamine p. 1238 must be considered in order to reduce the risk of Wernicke's encephalopathy. ⟨A⟩

Postoperative nausea and vomiting

The incidence of postoperative nausea and vomiting depends on many factors including the anaesthetic used, and the type and duration of surgery. Other risk factors include female sex, younger age, non-smokers, a history of postoperative nausea and vomiting or motion sickness, and intraoperative and postoperative use of opioids. Therapy to prevent postoperative nausea and vomiting should be based on the assessed risk of postoperative nausea and vomiting in each patient. [EvGr] A combination of two or more antiemetic drugs that have different mechanisms of action is often indicated in those with risk factors for postoperative nausea and vomiting. When a prophylactic antiemetic drug has failed, postoperative nausea and vomiting should be treated with an antiemetic drug from a different therapeutic class.

Drugs used include 5HT$_3$-receptor antagonists (e.g. granisetron, ondansetron), dexamethasone, droperidol p. 502 and haloperidol p. 445. Ⓐ Cyclizine is licensed for the prevention and treatment of postoperative nausea and vomiting caused by opioids and general anaesthetics. Prochlorperazine is licensed for the prevention and treatment of nausea and vomiting.

Motion sickness

Antiemetics should be given to prevent motion sickness rather than after nausea or vomiting develop. Hyoscine hydrobromide p. 501 is licensed to prevent motion sickness symptoms such as nausea, vomiting, and vertigo. Antihistamine drugs may also be effective; the less sedating antihistamines include cinnarizine and cyclizine, and the more sedating antihistamines include promethazine hydrochloride p. 326 and promethazine teoclate p. 500. Domperidone, metoclopramide hydrochloride, 5HT$_3$-receptor antagonists, and the phenothiazines (except promethazine—an antihistamine phenothiazine) are **ineffective** in motion sickness.

Ménière's disease

Patients presenting with symptoms of Ménière's disease should be referred to an ear, nose, and throat specialist to confirm the diagnosis.

[EvGr] Antihistamines (e.g. cinnarizine, cyclizine, promethazine teoclate p. 500) and phenothiazines (e.g. prochlorperazine) are used to help alleviate nausea, vomiting, and vertigo in acute attacks of Ménière's disease. Buccal prochlorperazine, or deep intramuscular injections of prochlorperazine or cyclizine, can be used to rapidly relieve nausea and vomiting in severe acute attacks.

Betahistine dihydrochloride p. 503 is an analogue of histamine. It can be trialled to reduce the frequency and severity of hearing loss, tinnitus, and vertigo in patients with recurrent attacks of Ménière's disease. Ⓐ

Nausea and vomiting associated with migraine

For information on the use of antiemetics in migraine attacks, see Migraine p. 536.

ANTIEMETICS AND ANTINAUSEANTS ›
ANTIHISTAMINES

| Cyclizine

27-Oct-2023

● **INDICATIONS AND DOSE**

Nausea | Vomiting | Vertigo | Labyrinthine disorders
▸ BY MOUTH, OR BY INTRAVENOUS INJECTION, OR BY INTRAMUSCULAR INJECTION
▸ Adult: 50 mg up to 3 times a day

Motion sickness
▸ BY MOUTH
▸ Adult: 50 mg up to 3 times a day, take 1–2 hours before departure
▸ BY INTRAVENOUS INJECTION, OR BY INTRAMUSCULAR INJECTION
▸ Adult: 50 mg up to 3 times a day

Nausea and vomiting of known cause | Nausea and vomiting associated with vestibular disorders
▸ BY MOUTH, OR BY INTRAVENOUS INJECTION
▸ Child 1 month-5 years: 0.5–1 mg/kg up to 3 times a day (max. per dose 25 mg), for motion sickness, take 1–2 hours before departure
▸ Child 6-11 years: 25 mg up to 3 times a day, for motion sickness, take 1–2 hours before departure
▸ Child 12-17 years: 50 mg up to 3 times a day, for motion sickness, take 1–2 hours before departure

▸ BY RECTUM
▸ Child 2-5 years: 12.5 mg up to 3 times a day
▸ Child 6-11 years: 25 mg up to 3 times a day
▸ Child 12-17 years: 50 mg up to 3 times a day
▸ BY CONTINUOUS INTRAVENOUS INFUSION, OR BY CONTINUOUS SUBCUTANEOUS INFUSION
▸ Child 1-23 months: 3 mg/kg/24 hours
▸ Child 2-5 years: 50 mg/24 hours
▸ Child 6-11 years: 75 mg/24 hours
▸ Child 12-17 years: 150 mg/24 hours

Nausea and vomiting in palliative care
▸ BY CONTINUOUS SUBCUTANEOUS INFUSION
▸ Child 1-23 months: 3 mg/kg/24 hours
▸ Child 2-5 years: 50 mg/24 hours
▸ Child 6-11 years: 75 mg/24 hours
▸ Child 12-17 years: 150 mg/24 hours
▸ Adult: 150 mg/24 hours
▸ BY MOUTH
▸ Child 1 month-5 years: 0.5–1 mg/kg up to 3 times a day (max. per dose 25 mg)
▸ Child 6-11 years: 25 mg up to 3 times a day
▸ Child 12-17 years: 50 mg up to 3 times a day
▸ Adult: 50 mg up to 3 times a day
▸ BY INTRAVENOUS INJECTION
▸ Child 1 month-5 years: 0.5–1 mg/kg up to 3 times a day (max. per dose 25 mg)
▸ Child 6-11 years: 25 mg up to 3 times a day
▸ Child 12-17 years: 50 mg up to 3 times a day
▸ BY CONTINUOUS INTRAVENOUS INFUSION
▸ Child 1-23 months: 3 mg/kg/24 hours
▸ Child 2-5 years: 50 mg/24 hours
▸ Child 6-11 years: 75 mg/24 hours
▸ Child 12-17 years: 150 mg/24 hours
▸ BY RECTUM
▸ Child 2-5 years: 12.5 mg up to 3 times a day
▸ Child 6-11 years: 25 mg up to 3 times a day
▸ Child 12-17 years: 50 mg up to 3 times a day

● UNLICENSED USE Tablets not licensed for use in children under 6 years. Injection not licensed for use in children.

● CAUTIONS Epilepsy · glaucoma (in children) · may counteract haemodynamic benefits of opioids · neuromuscular disorders—increased risk of transient paralysis with intravenous use · prostatic hypertrophy (in adults) · pyloroduodenal obstruction · severe heart failure—may cause fall in cardiac output and associated increase in heart rate, mean arterial pressure and pulmonary wedge pressure · susceptibility to angle-closure glaucoma (in adults) · urinary retention

● INTERACTIONS → Appendix 1: antihistamines, sedating

● SIDE-EFFECTS

GENERAL SIDE-EFFECTS
▸ **Rare or very rare** Agitation (more common at high doses) · angle closure glaucoma · depression
▸ **Frequency not known** Abdominal pain · agranulocytosis · angioedema · anxiety · apnoea · appetite decreased · arrhythmias · asthenia · bronchospasm · constipation · diarrhoea · disorientation · dizziness · drowsiness · dry mouth · dry throat · euphoric mood · haemolytic anaemia · hallucinations · headache · hepatic disorders · hypertension · hypotension · increased gastric reflux · insomnia · leucopenia · movement disorders · muscle complaints · nasal dryness · nausea · oculogyric crisis · palpitations · paraesthesia · photosensitivity reaction · seizure · skin reactions · speech disorder · thrombocytopenia · tinnitus · tremor · urinary retention · vision blurred · vomiting

SPECIFIC SIDE-EFFECTS
▸ With oral use Level of consciousness decreased

▶ **With parenteral use** Chills · consciousness impaired · injection site necrosis · pain · paralysis · sensation of pressure · thrombophlebitis

● **PREGNANCY** Manufacturer advises avoid; however, there is no evidence of teratogenicity. The use of sedating antihistamines in the latter part of the third trimester may cause adverse effects in neonates such as irritability, paradoxical excitability, and tremor.

● **BREAST FEEDING** No information available. Most antihistamines are present in breast milk in varying amounts; although not known to be harmful, most manufacturers advise avoiding their use in mothers who are breast-feeding.

● **HEPATIC IMPAIRMENT** Manufacturer advises caution.

● **DIRECTIONS FOR ADMINISTRATION** For administration *by mouth*, tablets may be crushed.

▶ **In children** For *intravenous injection*, give over 3–5 minutes. Mixing and compatibility for the use of syringe drivers in palliative care Cyclizine may precipitate at concentrations above 10 mg/mL or in the presence of Sodium Chloride 0.9% *or* as the concentration of diamorphine relative to cyclizine increases; mixtures of diamorphine and cyclizine are also likely to precipitate after 24 hours.

● **PRESCRIBING AND DISPENSING INFORMATION**

Palliative care For further information on the use of cyclizine in palliative care, see www.medicinescomplete. com/#/content/palliative/antihistaminic-antimuscarinic-anti-emetics.

● **PATIENT AND CARER ADVICE**

Driving and skilled tasks Drowsiness may affect performance of skilled tasks (e.g. cycling, driving); effects of alcohol enhanced.

● **MEDICINAL FORMS** There can be variation in the licensing of different medicines containing the same drug. Forms available from special-order manufacturers include: oral suspension, oral solution, suppository

Oral tablet
CAUTIONARY AND ADVISORY LABELS 2
▶ Cyclizine (Non-proprietary)
Cyclizine hydrochloride 50 mg Cyclizine 50mg tablets | 30 tablet P £1.82–£5.00 | 100 tablet P £16.60 DT = £4.39
Solution for injection
▶ Cyclizine (Non-proprietary)
Cyclizine lactate 50 mg per 1 ml Cyclizine 50mg/1ml solution for injection ampoules | 5 ampoule PoM £6.80–£16.25 DT = £3.54 | 10 ampoule PoM £10.28–£35.00

Doxylamine with pyridoxine   13-Aug-2020

● **DRUG ACTION** Doxylamine is a first-generation antihistamine which selectively binds H_1 receptors in the brain; pyridoxine (vitamin B_6) is a water-soluble vitamin.

● **INDICATIONS AND DOSE**

Nausea and vomiting in pregnancy
▶ BY MOUTH
▶ Adult: 20/20 mg once daily for 2 days, to be taken at bedtime; increased if necessary to 10/10 mg, to be taken in the morning and 20/20 mg, to be taken at bedtime; increased if necessary to 10/10 mg, to be taken in the morning, 10/10 mg, to be taken mid-afternoon and 20/20 mg, to be taken at bedtime; maximum 40/40 mg per day

DOSE EQUIVALENCE AND CONVERSION
▶ Dose expressed as *x/y* mg of doxylamine/pyridoxine.

● **CAUTIONS** Asthma · bladder neck obstruction · increased intra-ocular pressure · narrow angle glaucoma · pyloroduodenal obstruction · stenosing peptic ulcer

● **INTERACTIONS** → Appendix 1: antihistamines, sedating

● **SIDE-EFFECTS**
▶ **Common or very common** Dizziness · drowsiness · dry mouth · fatigue
▶ **Frequency not known** Akathisia · anxiety · chest discomfort · constipation · diarrhoea · disorientation · dyspnoea · gastrointestinal discomfort · headaches · hyperhidrosis · irritability · malaise · palpitations · paraesthesia · skin reactions · sleep disorders · tachycardia · urinary disorders · vertigo · vision disorders

● **PATIENT AND CARER ADVICE**
Driving and skilled tasks Manufacturer advises patients and carers should be counselled on the effects on driving and performance of skilled tasks—increased risk of somnolence and dizziness.

● **NATIONAL FUNDING/ACCESS DECISIONS**
For full details see funding body website
Scottish Medicines Consortium (SMC) decisions
▶ Doxylamine succinate and pyridoxine hydrochloride (*Xonvea*®) for the treatment of nausea and vomiting of pregnancy in women who do not respond to conservative management (May 2019) SMC No. SMC2140 Not recommended
All Wales Medicines Strategy Group (AWMSG) decisions
▶ Doxylamine succinate/pyridoxine hydrochloride (*Xonvea*®) for the treatment of nausea and vomiting of pregnancy in those patients who do not respond to conservative management (June 2019) AWMSG No. 2170 Not recommended

● **MEDICINAL FORMS** There can be variation in the licensing of different medicines containing the same drug.
Gastro-resistant tablet
CAUTIONARY AND ADVISORY LABELS 2, 23, 25
▶ Xonvea (Exeltis UK Ltd)
Doxylamine succinate 10 mg, Pyridoxine hydrochloride 10 mg Xonvea 10mg/10mg gastro-resistant tablets | 20 tablet PoM £28.50 DT = £28.50

ANTIEMETICS AND ANTINAUSEANTS ›
CANNABINOIDS

Nabilone   21-Jan-2020

● **INDICATIONS AND DOSE**

Nausea and vomiting caused by cytotoxic chemotherapy, unresponsive to conventional antiemetics (preferably in hospital setting) (under close medical supervision)
▶ BY MOUTH
▶ Adult: Initially 1 mg twice daily, increased if necessary to 2 mg twice daily throughout each cycle of cytotoxic therapy and, if necessary, for 48 hours after the last dose of each cycle, the first dose should be taken the night before initiation of cytotoxic treatment and the second dose 1–3 hours before the first dose of cytotoxic drug, daily dose maximum should be given in 3 divided doses; maximum 6 mg per day

● **CAUTIONS** Adverse effects on mental state can persist for 48–72 hours after stopping · elderly · heart disease · history of psychiatric disorder · hypertension

● **INTERACTIONS** → Appendix 1: nabilone

● **SIDE-EFFECTS** Abdominal pain · appetite decreased · concentration impaired · confusion · depression · dizziness · drowsiness · drug use disorders · dry mouth · euphoric mood · feeling of relaxation · hallucination · headache · hypotension · movement disorders · nausea · psychosis · sleep disorder · tachycardia · tremor · vertigo · visual impairment

SIDE-EFFECTS, FURTHER INFORMATION Drowsiness and dizziness occur frequently with standard doses.

● **PREGNANCY** Avoid unless essential.

● **BREAST FEEDING** Avoid—no information available.

- **HEPATIC IMPAIRMENT** Manufacturer advises avoid in severe impairment (primarily biliary excretion).
- **PATIENT AND CARER ADVICE**
Behavioural effects Patients should be made aware of possible changes of mood and other adverse behavioural effects.
Driving and skilled tasks Drowsiness may affect performance of skilled tasks (e.g. driving).
Effects of alcohol enhanced.
For information on 2015 legislation regarding driving whilst taking certain controlled drugs, including nabilone, see *Drugs and driving* under Guidance on prescribing p. 1.

- **MEDICINAL FORMS** There can be variation in the licensing of different medicines containing the same drug. Forms available from special-order manufacturers include: oral capsule
Oral capsule
CAUTIONARY AND ADVISORY LABELS 2
▸ **Nabilone (Non-proprietary)**
Nabilone 250 microgram Nabilone 250microgram capsules | 20 capsule [PoM] £172.50 DT = £172.50 [CD2]
Nabilone 1 mg Nabilone 1mg capsules | 20 capsule [PoM] £225.40 DT = £225.40 [CD2]

ANTIEMETICS AND ANTINAUSEANTS ›
DOPAMINE RECEPTOR ANTAGONISTS

| Domperidone
11-Nov-2021

- **INDICATIONS AND DOSE**
Relief of nausea and vomiting
▸ BY MOUTH
▸ Child 12-17 years (body-weight 35 kg and above): 10 mg up to 3 times a day for a usual maximum of 1 week
▸ Adult (body-weight 35 kg and above): 10 mg up to 3 times a day for a usual maximum of 1 week

Gastro-intestinal pain in palliative care
▸ BY MOUTH
▸ Adult: 10 mg 3 times a day, to be taken before meals

IMPORTANT SAFETY INFORMATION
MHRA/CHM ADVICE (UPDATED DECEMBER 2019): DOMPERIDONE FOR NAUSEA AND VOMITING: LACK OF EFFICACY IN CHILDREN; REMINDER OF CONTRA-INDICATIONS IN ADULTS AND ADOLESCENTS
Domperidone is no longer indicated for the relief of nausea and vomiting in children aged under 12 years or those weighing less than 35 kg. A European review concluded that domperidone is not as effective in this population as previously thought and alternative treatments should be considered. Healthcare professionals are advised to adhere to the licensed dose and to use the lowest effective dose for the shortest possible duration (max. treatment duration should not usually exceed 1 week).
Healthcare professionals are also reminded of the existing contra-indications for use of domperidone (see *Contra-indications*, *Hepatic impairment*, and *Interactions*).

- **CONTRA-INDICATIONS** Cardiac disease · conditions where cardiac conduction is, or could be, impaired · gastro-intestinal haemorrhage · gastro-intestinal mechanical obstruction · gastro-intestinal mechanical perforation · if increased gastro-intestinal motility harmful · prolactinoma
- **CAUTIONS** Patients over 60 years—increased risk of ventricular arrhythmia
- **INTERACTIONS** → Appendix 1: domperidone
- **SIDE-EFFECTS**
▸ **Common or very common** Dry mouth
▸ **Uncommon** Anxiety · asthenia · breast abnormalities · diarrhoea · drowsiness · headache · lactation disorders · libido loss

▸ **Frequency not known** Arrhythmias · depression · gynaecomastia · menstrual cycle irregularities · movement disorders · oculogyric crisis · QT interval prolongation · seizure · sudden cardiac death · urinary retention
- **PREGNANCY** Use only if potential benefit outweighs risk.
- **BREAST FEEDING** Amount too small to be harmful.
- **HEPATIC IMPAIRMENT** Manufacturer advises avoid in moderate to severe impairment.
- **RENAL IMPAIRMENT**
Dose adjustments [EvGr] For repeated doses, consider dose reduction and reduce frequency of administration (consult product literature). [M]
- **PRESCRIBING AND DISPENSING INFORMATION**
Palliative care For further information on the use of domperidone in palliative care, see www.medicinescomplete.com/#/content/palliative/domperidone.
- **PATIENT AND CARER ADVICE**
Arrhythmia Patients and their carers should be told how to recognise signs of arrhythmia and advised to seek medical attention if symptoms such as palpitation or syncope develop.

- **MEDICINAL FORMS** There can be variation in the licensing of different medicines containing the same drug. Forms available from special-order manufacturers include: oral suspension
Oral tablet
CAUTIONARY AND ADVISORY LABELS 22
▸ **Domperidone (Non-proprietary)**
Domperidone (as Domperidone maleate) 10 mg Domperidone 10mg tablets | 30 tablet [PoM] £2.17 DT = £0.84 | 100 tablet [PoM] £7.23 DT = £2.80
Oral suspension
CAUTIONARY AND ADVISORY LABELS 22
▸ **Domperidone (Non-proprietary)**
Domperidone 1 mg per 1 ml Domperidone 1mg/ml oral suspension sugar free | 200 ml [PoM] £49.32 DT = £49.32 [SF]

| Metoclopramide hydrochloride
24-Feb-2025

- **INDICATIONS AND DOSE**
Symptomatic treatment of nausea and vomiting including that associated with acute migraine | Prevention of delayed (but not acute) chemotherapy-induced nausea and vomiting | Prevention of radiotherapy-induced nausea and vomiting | Prevention of postoperative nausea and vomiting
▸ BY MOUTH, OR BY INTRAMUSCULAR INJECTION, OR BY SLOW INTRAVENOUS INJECTION
▸ Adult (body-weight up to 60 kg): Up to 500 micrograms/kg daily in 3 divided doses for a maximum of 5 days
▸ Adult (body-weight 60 kg and above): 10 mg up to 3 times a day for a maximum of 5 days

Hiccup in palliative care
▸ BY MOUTH, OR BY INTRAMUSCULAR INJECTION, OR BY SUBCUTANEOUS INJECTION
▸ Adult: 10 mg every 6–8 hours

Nausea and vomiting in palliative care
▸ BY MOUTH
▸ Adult: 10 mg 3 times a day
▸ BY CONTINUOUS SUBCUTANEOUS INFUSION
▸ Adult: 30–100 mg/24 hours

Acute migraine
▸ BY MOUTH, OR BY SLOW INTRAVENOUS INJECTION, OR BY INTRAMUSCULAR INJECTION
▸ Adult: 10 mg for 1 dose, to be administered as soon as migraine symptoms develop

- **UNLICENSED USE** Metoclopramide may be used as detailed below, although these situations are considered unlicensed:

- EvGr hiccup, and nausea and vomiting in palliative care; D

- EvGr Acute migraine. A

> **IMPORTANT SAFETY INFORMATION**
> **MHRA/CHM ADVICE—METOCLOPRAMIDE: RISK OF NEUROLOGICAL ADVERSE EFFECTS—RESTRICTED DOSE AND DURATION OF USE (AUGUST 2013)**
> The benefits and risks of metoclopramide have been reviewed by the European Medicines Agency's Committee on Medicinal Products for Human Use, which concluded that the risk of neurological effects such as extrapyramidal disorders and tardive dyskinesia outweigh the benefits in long-term or high-dose treatment. To help minimise the risk of potentially serious neurological adverse effects, the following restrictions to indications, dose, and duration of use have been made:
> - In adults aged over 18 years, metoclopramide should only be used for prevention of postoperative nausea and vomiting, radiotherapy-induced nausea and vomiting, delayed (but not acute) chemotherapy-induced nausea and vomiting, and symptomatic treatment of nausea and vomiting, including that associated with acute migraine (where it may also be used to improve absorption of oral analgesics);
> - Metoclopramide should only be prescribed for short-term use (up to 5 days);
> - Usual recommended dose is 10 mg, repeated up to 3 times daily;
> - Intravenous doses should be administered as a slow bolus over at least 3 minutes;
> - Oral liquid formulations should be given via an appropriately designed, graduated oral syringe to ensure dose accuracy.
> This advice does not apply to the unlicensed use of metoclopramide in palliative care.

- **CONTRA-INDICATIONS** 3–4 days after gastrointestinal surgery · epilepsy · gastro-intestinal haemorrhage · gastro-intestinal obstruction · gastro-intestinal perforation · phaeochromocytoma

- **CAUTIONS** Asthma · atopic allergy · bradycardia · cardiac conduction disturbances · children · elderly · may mask underlying disorders such as cerebral irritation · Parkinson's disease · uncorrected electrolyte imbalance · young adults

  CAUTIONS, FURTHER INFORMATION
  ▸ Elderly Screening Tool of Older Persons' potentially inappropriate Prescriptions (STOPP) criteria to aid medication reviews (see Prescribing in the elderly p. 31 for information): potentially inappropriate in patients with parkinsonism (risk of exacerbating parkinsonian symptoms).

- **INTERACTIONS** → Appendix 1: metoclopramide

- **SIDE-EFFECTS**

  GENERAL SIDE-EFFECTS
  ▸ **Common or very common** Asthenia · depression · diarrhoea · drowsiness · hypotension · menstrual cycle irregularities · movement disorders · parkinsonism
  ▸ **Uncommon** Arrhythmias · hallucination · hyperprolactinaemia · level of consciousness decreased
  ▸ **Rare or very rare** Confusion · galactorrhoea · seizure
  ▸ **Frequency not known** Atrioventricular block · blood disorders · cardiac arrest · gynaecomastia · hypertension · neuroleptic malignant syndrome (discontinue—potentially fatal) · QT interval prolongation · shock · syncope · tremor

  SPECIFIC SIDE-EFFECTS
  ▸ With parenteral use Anxiety · dizziness · dyspnoea · oedema · skin reactions · visual impairment

SIDE-EFFECTS, FURTHER INFORMATION Metoclopramide can induce acute dystonic reactions involving facial and skeletal muscle spasms and oculogyric crises. These dystonic effects are more common in the young (especially girls and young women) and the very old; they usually occur shortly after starting treatment with metoclopramide and subside within 24 hours of stopping it. Injection of an antiparkinsonian drug such as procyclidine will abort dystonic attacks.

- **PREGNANCY** Not known to be harmful.

- **BREAST FEEDING** Small amount present in milk; avoid.

- **HEPATIC IMPAIRMENT** Manufacturer advises caution in severe impairment (risk of accumulation).
  Dose adjustments Manufacturer advises dose reduction of 50% in severe impairment.

- **RENAL IMPAIRMENT**
  Dose adjustments EvGr Reduce daily dose by 75% in end-stage renal disease.
  Reduce dose by 50% in moderate to severe impairment. M

- **DIRECTIONS FOR ADMINISTRATION** Manufacturer advises oral liquid preparation to be given via a graduated oral dosing syringe.
  EvGr For *intravenous injection*, give over at least 3 minutes. M

- **PRESCRIBING AND DISPENSING INFORMATION**
  Palliative care For further information on the use of metoclopramide hydrochloride in palliative care, see www.medicinescomplete.com/#/content/palliative/metoclopramide.

- **PATIENT AND CARER ADVICE** Counselling on use of pipette advised with oral solution.

- **MEDICINAL FORMS** There can be variation in the licensing of different medicines containing the same drug. Forms available from special-order manufacturers include: oral solution

  Solution for injection
  ▸ **Metoclopramide hydrochloride (Non-proprietary)**
  Metoclopramide hydrochloride 5 mg per 1 ml Metoclopramide 10mg/2ml solution for injection ampoules | 5 ampoule PoM £1.31-£5.34 | 10 ampoule PoM £0.49-£4.84 DT = £5.43 (Hospital only) | 10 ampoule PoM £4.84 DT = £5.43

  Oral tablet
  ▸ **Metoclopramide hydrochloride (Non-proprietary)**
  Metoclopramide hydrochloride 5 mg Metoclopramide 5mg tablets | 28 tablet PoM £3.75-£6.00 DT = £3.75
  Metoclopramide hydrochloride 10 mg Metoclopramide 10mg tablets | 28 tablet PoM £3.75 DT = £0.83
  ▸ **Maxolon** (Advanz Pharma)
  Metoclopramide hydrochloride 10 mg Maxolon 10mg tablets | 84 tablet PoM £5.24

  Oral solution
  ▸ **Metoclopramide hydrochloride (Non-proprietary)**
  Metoclopramide hydrochloride 1 mg per 1 ml Metoclopramide 5mg/5ml oral solution sugar free | 150 ml PoM £19.77 DT = £9.05 SF

ANTIEMETICS AND ANTINAUSEANTS ⟩
NEUROKININ-1 RECEPTOR ANTAGONISTS

Aprepitant
11-Sep-2018

- **INDICATIONS AND DOSE**

  Adjunct treatment to prevent nausea and vomiting associated with moderately and highly emetogenic chemotherapy
  ▸ BY MOUTH
  ▸ Adult: Initially 125 mg, dose to be taken 1 hour before chemotherapy, then 80 mg once daily for 2 days, consult product literature for dose of concomitant dexamethasone and 5HT$_3$-antagonist

- **CONTRA-INDICATIONS** Acute porphyrias p. 1202
- **INTERACTIONS** → Appendix 1: neurokinin-1 receptor antagonists
- **SIDE-EFFECTS**
  - ▸ **Common or very common** Appetite decreased · asthenia · constipation · gastrointestinal discomfort · headache · hiccups
  - ▸ **Uncommon** Anaemia · anxiety · burping · dizziness · drowsiness · dry mouth · febrile neutropenia · gastrointestinal disorders · hot flush · malaise · nausea · palpitations · skin reactions · urinary disorders · vomiting
  - ▸ **Rare or very rare** Bradycardia · cardiovascular disorder · chest discomfort · cognitive disorder · conjunctivitis · cough · disorientation · euphoric mood · gait abnormal · hyperhidrosis · increased risk of infection · muscle spasms · muscle weakness · oedema · oropharyngeal pain · photosensitivity reaction · polydipsia · seborrhoea · severe cutaneous adverse reactions (SCARs) · sneezing · stomatitis · taste altered · throat irritation · tinnitus · weight decreased
  - ▸ **Frequency not known** Dysarthria · dyspnoea · insomnia · miosis · sensation abnormal · visual acuity decreased · wheezing
- **CONCEPTION AND CONTRACEPTION** Manufacturer advises effectiveness of hormonal contraceptives may be reduced—alternative non-hormonal methods of contraception necessary during treatment and for 2 months after stopping aprepitant.
- **PREGNANCY** Manufacturer advises avoid unless clearly necessary—no information available.
- **BREAST FEEDING** Manufacturer advises avoid—present in milk in *animal* studies.
- **HEPATIC IMPAIRMENT** Manufacturer advises caution in moderate to severe impairment—limited information available.

- **MEDICINAL FORMS** There can be variation in the licensing of different medicines containing the same drug. Forms available from special-order manufacturers include: oral suspension

Oral capsule
  - ▸ Aprepitant (Non-proprietary)
    Aprepitant 80 mg Aprepitant 80mg capsules | 2 capsule [PoM] £31.61 DT = £31.61 | 2 capsule [PoM] £31.61 DT = £31.61 (Hospital only)
    Aprepitant 125 mg Aprepitant 125mg capsules | 5 capsule [PoM] £79.03 DT = £79.03 | 5 capsule [PoM] £79.03 DT = £79.03 (Hospital only)
  - ▸ Emend (Merck Sharp & Dohme (UK) Ltd)
    Aprepitant 80 mg Emend 80mg capsules | 2 capsule [PoM] [S] DT = £31.61
    Aprepitant 125 mg Emend 125mg capsules | 1 capsule [PoM] [S]

Fosaprepitant

02-Nov-2020

- **DRUG ACTION** Fosaprepitant is a prodrug of aprepitant.

- **INDICATIONS AND DOSE**

Adjunct to dexamethasone and a 5HT$_3$-receptor antagonist in preventing nausea and vomiting associated with moderately and highly emetogenic chemotherapy
  - ▸ BY INTRAVENOUS INFUSION
  - ▸ Adult: 150 mg, dose to be administered over 20–30 minutes and given 30 minutes before chemotherapy on day 1 of cycle only, consult product literature for dose of concomitant corticosteroid and 5HT$_3$-receptor antagonist

- **CONTRA-INDICATIONS** Acute porphyrias p. 1202
- **INTERACTIONS** → Appendix 1: neurokinin-1 receptor antagonists

- **SIDE-EFFECTS**
  - ▸ **Common or very common** Appetite decreased · asthenia · constipation · gastrointestinal discomfort · headache · hiccups
  - ▸ **Uncommon** Anaemia · anxiety · burping · dizziness · drowsiness · dry mouth · febrile neutropenia · flushing · gastrointestinal disorders · malaise · nausea · palpitations · skin reactions · thrombophlebitis · urinary disorders · vomiting
  - ▸ **Rare or very rare** Bradycardia · cardiovascular disorder · chest discomfort · cognitive disorder · conjunctivitis · cough · disorientation · euphoric mood · gait abnormal · hyperhidrosis · increased risk of infection · muscle spasms · muscle weakness · oedema · oropharyngeal pain · photosensitivity reaction · polydipsia · seborrhoea · severe cutaneous adverse reactions (SCARs) · sneezing · stomatitis · taste altered · throat irritation · tinnitus · weight decreased
  - ▸ **Frequency not known** Dysarthria · dyspnoea · insomnia · miosis · sensation abnormal · visual acuity decreased · wheezing
- **CONCEPTION AND CONTRACEPTION** Effectiveness of hormonal contraceptives reduced—effective non-hormonal methods of contraception necessary during treatment and for 2 months after stopping fosaprepitant.
- **PREGNANCY** Avoid unless potential benefit outweighs risk—no information available.
- **BREAST FEEDING** Avoid—present in milk in *animal* studies.
- **HEPATIC IMPAIRMENT** Manufacturer advises caution in moderate to severe impairment—limited information available.
- **DIRECTIONS FOR ADMINISTRATION** For *intravenous infusion* (*Ivemend*®), manufacturer advises give intermittently *in* Sodium Chloride 0.9%; reconstitute each 150 mg vial with 5 mL Sodium Chloride 0.9% gently without shaking to avoid foaming, then dilute in 145 mL infusion fluid; give over 20–30 minutes.
- **NATIONAL FUNDING/ACCESS DECISIONS**
  For full details see funding body website
  Scottish Medicines Consortium (SMC) decisions
  - ▸ Fosaprepitant (*Ivemend*®) for the prevention of acute and delayed nausea and vomiting associated with highly emetogenic cisplatin based cancer chemotherapy in adults (March 2011) SMC No. 678/11 Recommended

- **MEDICINAL FORMS** There can be variation in the licensing of different medicines containing the same drug.
  Powder for solution for infusion
  - ▸ Ivemend (Merck Sharp & Dohme (UK) Ltd)
    Fosaprepitant (as Fosaprepitant dimeglumine) 150 mg Ivemend 150mg powder for solution for infusion vials | 1 vial [PoM] £47.42

ANTIEMETICS AND ANTINAUSEANTS ›
SEROTONIN (5HT3) RECEPTOR ANTAGONISTS

Granisetron

16-Jul-2020

- **DRUG ACTION** Granisetron is a specific 5HT$_3$-receptor antagonist which blocks 5HT$_3$ receptors in the gastro-intestinal tract and in the CNS.

- **INDICATIONS AND DOSE**

Nausea and vomiting induced by cytotoxic chemotherapy for planned duration of 3–5 days where oral antiemetics cannot be used
  - ▸ BY TRANSDERMAL APPLICATION USING PATCHES
  - ▸ Adult: Apply 3.1 mg/24 hours, apply patch to clean, dry, non-irritated, non-hairy skin on upper arm (or abdomen if upper arm cannot be used) 24–48 hours before treatment, patch may be worn for up to 7 days;

remove at least 24 hours after completing chemotherapy

Prevention of postoperative nausea and vomiting
▶ BY INTRAVENOUS INJECTION
▶ Adult: 1 mg, to be administered before induction of anaesthesia, dose to be diluted to 5 mL and given over 30 seconds

Treatment of postoperative nausea and vomiting
▶ BY INTRAVENOUS INJECTION
▶ Adult: 1 mg, dose to be diluted to 5 mL and given over 30 seconds; maximum 3 mg per day

Management of nausea and vomiting induced by cytotoxic chemotherapy or radiotherapy
▶ BY MOUTH
▶ Adult: 1–2 mg, to be taken within 1 hour before start of treatment, then 2 mg daily in 1–2 divided doses for up to 1 week following treatment, when intravenous route also used, maximum combined total dose 9 mg in 24 hours
▶ BY INTRAVENOUS INJECTION, OR BY INTRAVENOUS INFUSION
▶ Adult: 10–40 micrograms/kg (max. per dose 3 mg), to be given 5 minutes before start of treatment, dose may be repeated if necessary, further maintenance doses must not be given less than 10 minutes apart, for intravenous injection, each 1 mg granisetron diluted to 5 mL and given over not less than 30 seconds, for intravenous infusion, to be given over 5 minutes; maximum 9 mg per day

● CAUTIONS Subacute intestinal obstruction · susceptibility to QT-interval prolongation (including electrolyte disturbances)

● INTERACTIONS → Appendix 1: 5-HT3-receptor antagonists

● SIDE-EFFECTS
GENERAL SIDE-EFFECTS
▶ Common or very common Constipation · headache
SPECIFIC SIDE-EFFECTS
▶ Common or very common
▶ With intravenous or oral use Diarrhoea · insomnia
▶ Uncommon
▶ With intravenous or oral use Extrapyramidal symptoms · QT interval prolongation · serotonin syndrome
▶ With transdermal use Appetite decreased · arthralgia · dry mouth · flushing · generalised oedema · vertigo
▶ Rare or very rare
▶ With transdermal use Dystonia

● PREGNANCY Manufacturer advises avoid.

● BREAST FEEDING Avoid—no information available.

● HEPATIC IMPAIRMENT Manufacturer advises caution.

● DIRECTIONS FOR ADMINISTRATION For *intravenous infusion*, manufacturer advises give intermittently in Glucose 5% or Sodium Chloride 0.9%; dilute up to 3 mL in 20–50 mL infusion fluid; give over 5 minutes.

● PATIENT AND CARER ADVICE
▶ With transdermal use Patients should be advised not to expose the site of the patch to sunlight during use and for 10 days after removal.

● MEDICINAL FORMS There can be variation in the licensing of different medicines containing the same drug.

Solution for injection
▶ Granisetron (Non-proprietary)
Granisetron (as Granisetron hydrochloride) 1 mg per 1 ml Granisetron 3mg/3ml concentrate for solution for injection ampoules | 10 ampoule [PoM] £72.00 DT = £72.00
Granisetron 1mg/1ml concentrate for solution for injection ampoules | 10 ampoule [PoM] £24.20 DT = £24.20

Oral tablet
▶ Granisetron (Non-proprietary)
Granisetron (as Granisetron hydrochloride) 1 mg Granisetron 1mg tablets | 10 tablet [PoM] £51.20 DT = £41.91

▶ Kytril (Atnahs Pharma UK Ltd)
Granisetron (as Granisetron hydrochloride) 1 mg Kytril 1mg tablets | 10 tablet [PoM] £52.39 DT = £41.91

Transdermal patch
▶ Sancuso (Kyowa Kirin International UK NewCo Ltd)
Granisetron 3.1 mg per 24 hour Sancuso 3.1mg/24hours transdermal patches | 1 patch [PoM] £56.00 DT = £56.00

Ondansetron

12-Feb-2024

● DRUG ACTION Ondansetron is a specific 5HT$_3$-receptor antagonist which blocks 5HT$_3$ receptors in the gastro-intestinal tract and in the CNS.

● INDICATIONS AND DOSE

Moderately emetogenic chemotherapy or radiotherapy
▶ BY MOUTH
▶ Adult: Initially 8 mg for 1 dose, dose to be taken 1–2 hours before treatment, then 8 mg every 12 hours for up to 5 days
▶ INITIALLY BY INTRAMUSCULAR INJECTION, OR BY SLOW INTRAVENOUS INJECTION
▶ Adult: Initially 8 mg for 1 dose, dose to be administered immediately before treatment, then (by mouth) 8 mg every 12 hours for up to 5 days
▶ INITIALLY BY INTRAMUSCULAR INJECTION, OR BY INTRAVENOUS INFUSION
▶ Elderly: Initially 8 mg for 1 dose, dose to be administered immediately before treatment, then (by mouth) 8 mg every 12 hours for up to 5 days

Severely emetogenic chemotherapy (consult product literature for dose of concomitant corticosteroid)
▶ BY MOUTH
▶ Adult: 24 mg for 1 dose, dose to be taken 1–2 hours before treatment, then 8 mg every 12 hours for up to 5 days
▶ INITIALLY BY INTRAMUSCULAR INJECTION, OR BY SLOW INTRAVENOUS INJECTION
▶ Adult: Initially 8 mg for 1 dose, dose to be administered immediately before treatment, followed by (by intramuscular injection or by slow intravenous injection) 8 mg every 4 hours if required for 2 doses, alternatively (by continuous intravenous infusion) 1 mg/hour for up to 24 hours, then (by mouth) 8 mg every 12 hours for up to 5 days
▶ INITIALLY BY INTRAMUSCULAR INJECTION
▶ Adult 65-74 years: Initially 8 mg for 1 dose, dose to be administered immediately before treatment, followed by (by intramuscular injection) 8 mg every 4 hours if required for 2 doses, alternatively (by continuous intravenous infusion) 1 mg/hour for up to 24 hours, then (by mouth) 8 mg every 12 hours for up to 5 days
▶ INITIALLY BY INTRAVENOUS INFUSION
▶ Adult: Initially 16 mg for 1 dose, dose to be administered immediately before treatment, followed by (by intramuscular injection or by slow intravenous injection) 8 mg every 4 hours if required for 2 doses, then (by mouth) 8 mg every 12 hours for up to 5 days
▶ Adult 65-74 years: Initially 8–16 mg for 1 dose, dose to be administered immediately before treatment, followed by (by intramuscular injection or by intravenous infusion) 8 mg every 4 hours if required for 2 doses, then (by mouth) 8 mg every 12 hours for up to 5 days
▶ Adult 75 years and over: Initially 8 mg for 1 dose, dose to be administered immediately before treatment, followed by (by intravenous infusion) 8 mg every 4 hours if required for 2 doses, then (by mouth) 8 mg every 12 hours for up to 5 days

continued →

4
Nervous system

Prevention of postoperative nausea and vomiting
▶ INITIALLY BY MOUTH
▶ Adult: 16 mg for 1 dose, dose to be taken 1 hour before anaesthesia, alternatively (by intramuscular injection or by slow intravenous injection) 4 mg for 1 dose, dose to be administered at induction of anaesthesia

Treatment of postoperative nausea and vomiting
▶ BY INTRAMUSCULAR INJECTION, OR BY SLOW INTRAVENOUS INJECTION
▶ Adult: 4 mg for 1 dose

IMPORTANT SAFETY INFORMATION

MHRA/CHM ADVICE: ONDANSETRON: SMALL INCREASED RISK OF ORAL CLEFTS FOLLOWING USE IN THE FIRST 12 WEEKS OF PREGNANCY (JANUARY 2020)

Epidemiological studies have identified a small increased risk of cleft lip and/or cleft palate in babies born to women who used oral ondansetron during the first trimester of pregnancy. Healthcare professionals are advised that if there is a clinical need for ondansetron in pregnancy, patients should be counselled on the potential benefits and risks, and the final decision made jointly.

● **CONTRA-INDICATIONS** Congenital long QT syndrome

● **CAUTIONS** Adenotonsillar surgery · subacute intestinal obstruction · susceptibility to QT-interval prolongation (including electrolyte disturbances)

● **INTERACTIONS** → Appendix 1: 5-HT3-receptor antagonists

● **SIDE-EFFECTS**
GENERAL SIDE-EFFECTS
▶ **Common or very common** Constipation · feeling hot · headache · sensation abnormal
▶ **Uncommon** Arrhythmias · chest pain · hiccups · hypotension · movement disorders · oculogyric crisis · seizure
▶ **Rare or very rare** Dizziness · QT interval prolongation · vision disorders
▶ **Frequency not known** Myocardial ischaemia
SPECIFIC SIDE-EFFECTS
▶ **Rare or very rare**
▶ With oral use Skin toxicity · toxic epidermal necrolysis
▶ With parenteral use Abdominal pain · bullous dermatitis · depression · diarrhoea · severe cutaneous adverse reactions (SCARs)

● **PREGNANCY** Manufacturer advises avoid in first trimester—small increased risk of congenital abnormalities such as orofacial clefts, see *Important safety information*.

● **BREAST FEEDING** Present in milk in *animal* studies—avoid.

● **HEPATIC IMPAIRMENT** Manufacturer advises caution in moderate to severe impairment (decreased clearance). **Dose adjustments** Manufacturer advises maximum 8 mg daily in moderate to severe impairment.

● **DIRECTIONS FOR ADMINISTRATION** For *intravenous infusion* (*Zofran*®), give continuously or intermittently in Glucose 5% *or* Glucose 5% with Potassium Chloride 0.3% *or* Sodium Chloride 0.9% *or* Sodium Chloride 0.9% with Potassium Chloride 0.3% *or* Mannitol 10% *or* Ringers Solution; for intermittent infusion, dilute the required dose in 50–100 mL of infusion fluid and give over at least 15 minutes.
  Orodispersible films and lyophylisates should be placed on the tongue, allowed to disperse and swallowed.

● **PRESCRIBING AND DISPENSING INFORMATION** Flavours of oral liquid formulations may include strawberry.

● **PATIENT AND CARER ADVICE** Patients or carers should be given advice on how to administer orodispersible films and lyophilisates.

● **MEDICINAL FORMS** There can be variation in the licensing of different medicines containing the same drug. Forms available from special-order manufacturers include: oral suspension, oral solution

Oral tablet
▶ Ondansetron (Non-proprietary)
  Ondansetron (as Ondansetron hydrochloride dihydrate)
  4 mg Ondansetron 4mg tablets | 10 tablet PoM £11.70 DT = £1.94 | 30 tablet PoM £4.23-£86.33
  Ondansetron (as Ondansetron hydrochloride dihydrate)
  8 mg Ondansetron 8mg tablets | 10 tablet PoM £57.55 DT = £5.72

Solution for injection
▶ Ondansetron (Non-proprietary)
  Ondansetron (as Ondansetron hydrochloride dihydrate) 2 mg per 1 ml Ondansetron 8mg/4ml solution for injection ampoules | 5 ampoule PoM £38.37-£61.60 (Hospital only) | 5 ampoule PoM £28.00-£70.14 | 10 ampoule PoM £7.80
  Ondansetron 4mg/2ml solution for injection pre-filled syringes | 1 pre-filled disposable injection PoM £29.97 (Hospital only)
  Ondansetron 8mg/4ml solution for injection pre-filled syringes | 1 pre-filled disposable injection PoM £59.95 (Hospital only)
  Ondansetron 4mg/2ml solution for injection ampoules | 5 ampoule PoM £28.47-£29.70 (Hospital only) | 5 ampoule PoM £14.00-£36.00 | 10 ampoule PoM £20.00 DT = £20.00
▶ Zofran (Novartis Pharmaceuticals UK Ltd)
  Ondansetron (as Ondansetron hydrochloride dihydrate) 2 mg per 1 ml Zofran 4mg/2ml solution for injection ampoules | 10 ampoule PoM £59.94 DT = £20.00
  Zofran 8mg/4ml solution for injection ampoules | 8 ampoule PoM £95.92

Oral solution
▶ Ondansetron (Non-proprietary)
  Ondansetron (as Ondansetron hydrochloride) 800 microgram per 1 ml Ondansetron 4mg/5ml oral solution sugar free | 50 ml PoM £38.37 DT = £14.08 SF
  Ondansetron (as Ondansetron hydrochloride) 1.6 mg per 1 ml Ondansetron 8mg/5ml oral solution sugar free | 100 ml PoM £130.46 DT = £130.46 SF

Orodispersible film
▶ Setofilm (Norgine Pharmaceuticals Ltd)
  Ondansetron 4 mg Setofilm 4mg orodispersible films | 10 film PoM £28.50 DT = £28.50 SF
  Ondansetron 8 mg Setofilm 8mg orodispersible films | 10 film PoM £57.00 DT = £57.00 SF

Orodispersible tablet
▶ Ondansetron (Non-proprietary)
  Ondansetron 4 mg Ondansetron 4mg orodispersible tablets | 10 tablet PoM £35.97 DT = £15.09
  Ondansetron 8 mg Ondansetron 8mg orodispersible tablets | 10 tablet PoM £71.94 DT = £71.94

Palonosetron

22-Jan-2020

● **DRUG ACTION** Palonosetron is a specific 5HT$_3$-receptor antagonist which blocks 5HT$_3$ receptors in the gastro-intestinal tract and in the CNS.

● **INDICATIONS AND DOSE**

Moderately emetogenic chemotherapy
▶ INITIALLY BY MOUTH
▶ Adult: 500 micrograms, dose to be taken 1 hour before treatment, alternatively (by intravenous injection) 250 micrograms for 1 dose, dose to be administered over 30 seconds, 30 minutes before treatment

Severely emetogenic chemotherapy
▶ BY INTRAVENOUS INJECTION
▶ Adult: 250 micrograms for 1 dose, dose to be administered over 30 seconds, 30 minutes before treatment

● **CAUTIONS** History of constipation · intestinal obstruction · susceptibility to QT-interval prolongation (including electrolyte disturbances)

● **INTERACTIONS** → Appendix 1: 5-HT3-receptor antagonists

● **SIDE-EFFECTS**

GENERAL SIDE-EFFECTS

▸ **Common or very common** Constipation · headache

SPECIFIC SIDE-EFFECTS

▸ **Common or very common**
▸ With intravenous use Diarrhoea · dizziness · electrolyte imbalance · metabolic disorder
▸ **Uncommon**
▸ With intravenous use Amblyopia · anxiety · appetite decreased · arrhythmias · arthralgia · asthenia · drowsiness · dry mouth · dyspepsia · euphoric mood · eye irritation · feeling hot · fever · flatulence · glycosuria · hiccups · hyperbilirubinaemia · hyperglycaemia · hypertension · hypotension · influenza like illness · motion sickness · myocardial ischaemia · paraesthesia · peripheral neuropathy · QT interval prolongation · skin reactions · sleep disorders · tinnitus · urinary retention · vasodilation · vein discolouration
▸ With oral use Atrioventricular block · dyspnoea · eye swelling · insomnia · myalgia
▸ **Rare or very rare**
▸ With intravenous use Shock

● **PREGNANCY** Avoid—no information available.

● **BREAST FEEDING** Avoid—no information available.

● **PATIENT AND CARER ADVICE**

Driving and skilled tasks Dizziness or drowsiness may affect performance of skilled tasks (e.g. driving).

● **MEDICINAL FORMS** There can be variation in the licensing of different medicines containing the same drug.

Solution for injection

▸ Palonosetron (Non-proprietary)
    Palonosetron (as Palonosetron hydrochloride) 50 microgram per 1 ml Palonosetron 250micrograms/5ml solution for injection vials | 1 vial PoM £53.10–£800.00 (Hospital only) | 1 vial PoM £53.10 | 10 vial PoM £860.50
▸ Aloxi (Chugai Pharma UK Ltd)
    Palonosetron (as Palonosetron hydrochloride) 50 microgram per 1 ml Aloxi 250micrograms/5ml solution for injection vials | 1 vial PoM £55.89

Palonosetron with netupitant   12-Nov-2020

The properties listed below are those particular to the combination only. For the properties of the components please consider, palonosetron p. 498.

● **INDICATIONS AND DOSE**

Moderately emetogenic chemotherapy | Highly emetogenic cisplatin-based chemotherapy

▸ BY MOUTH
▸ Adult: 1 capsule, to be taken approximately 1 hour before the start of each chemotherapy cycle

● **CAUTIONS** Patients over 75 years

● **INTERACTIONS** → Appendix 1: 5-HT3-receptor antagonists · neurokinin-1 receptor antagonists

● **SIDE-EFFECTS**

▸ **Common or very common** Asthenia · constipation · headache
▸ **Uncommon** Alopecia · cardiac conduction disorders · cardiomyopathy · diarrhoea · dizziness · flatulence · gastrointestinal discomfort · hiccups · hypertension · increased leucocytes · neutropenia · QT interval prolongation · sleep disorders · urticaria · vertigo
▸ **Rare or very rare** Acute psychosis · arrhythmias · conjunctivitis · cystitis · dysphagia · feeling hot · hypokalaemia · hypotension · leucopenia · mitral valve incompetence · mood altered · myocardial ischaemia · numbness · pain · tongue coated · vision blurred

● **CONCEPTION AND CONTRACEPTION** Manufacturer recommends exclude pregnancy before treatment in females of childbearing age; ensure effective contraception during treatment and for one month after treatment.

● **PREGNANCY** Manufacturer advises avoid—toxicity in *animal* studies.

● **BREAST FEEDING** Manufacturer advises avoid during treatment and for 1 month after last dose—no information available.

● **HEPATIC IMPAIRMENT** Manufacturer advises caution in severe impairment (risk of increased exposure, limited information available).

● **NATIONAL FUNDING/ACCESS DECISIONS**

For full details see funding body website

Scottish Medicines Consortium (SMC) decisions

▸ Palonosetron with netupitant (*Akynzeo*®) in adults for the prevention of acute and delayed nausea and vomiting associated with highly emetogenic cisplatin-based cancer chemotherapy and moderately emetogenic cancer chemotherapy (January 2016) SMC No. 1109/15 Recommended with restrictions

● **MEDICINAL FORMS** There can be variation in the licensing of different medicines containing the same drug.

Oral capsule

CAUTIONARY AND ADVISORY LABELS 25

▸ Akynzeo (Chugai Pharma UK Ltd)
    Palonosetron (as Palonosetron hydrochloride) 500 microgram, Netupitant 300 mg Akynzeo 300mg/0.5mg capsules | 1 capsule PoM £69.00 (Hospital only)

ANTIHISTAMINES › SEDATING ANTIHISTAMINES

Cinnarizine   27-Apr-2021

● **INDICATIONS AND DOSE**

Relief of symptoms of vestibular disorders, such as vertigo, tinnitus, nausea, and vomiting in Ménière's disease

▸ BY MOUTH
▸ Child 5–11 years: 15 mg 3 times a day
▸ Child 12–17 years: 30 mg 3 times a day
▸ Adult: 30 mg 3 times a day

Motion sickness

▸ BY MOUTH
▸ Child 5–11 years: Initially 15 mg, dose to be taken 2 hours before travel, then 7.5 mg every 8 hours if required, dose to be taken during journey
▸ Child 12–17 years: Initially 30 mg, dose to be taken 2 hours before travel, then 15 mg every 8 hours if required, dose to be taken during journey
▸ Adult: Initially 30 mg, dose to be taken 2 hours before travel, then 15 mg every 8 hours if required, dose to be taken during journey

● **CONTRA-INDICATIONS** Avoid in Acute porphyrias p. 1202

● **CAUTIONS** Epilepsy · glaucoma (in children) · Parkinson's disease (in adults) · prostatic hypertrophy (in adults) · pyloroduodenal obstruction · susceptibility to angle-closure glaucoma (in adults) · urinary retention

● **INTERACTIONS** → Appendix 1: antihistamines, sedating

● **SIDE-EFFECTS**

▸ **Common or very common** Drowsiness · gastrointestinal discomfort · nausea · weight increased
▸ **Uncommon** Fatigue · hyperhidrosis · vomiting
▸ **Frequency not known** Dry mouth · gastrointestinal disorder · headache · jaundice cholestatic · movement disorders · muscle rigidity · parkinsonism · skin reactions · subacute cutaneous lupus erythematosus · tremor

● **PREGNANCY** Manufacturer advises avoid; however, there is no evidence of teratogenicity. The use of sedating antihistamines in the latter part of the third trimester may cause adverse effects in neonates such as irritability, paradoxical excitability, and tremor.

- **BREAST FEEDING** Most antihistamines are present in breast milk in varying amounts; although not known to be harmful, most manufacturers advise avoiding their use in mothers who are breast-feeding.
- **HEPATIC IMPAIRMENT** Manufacturer advises caution in hepatic insufficiency—no information available.
- **RENAL IMPAIRMENT** [EvGr] Use with caution (no information available). ⟨M⟩
- **PATIENT AND CARER ADVICE**
  Driving and skilled tasks Drowsiness may affect performance of skilled tasks (e.g. cycling, driving); sedating effects enhanced by alcohol.

- **MEDICINAL FORMS** There can be variation in the licensing of different medicines containing the same drug. Forms available from special-order manufacturers include: oral suspension
  Oral tablet
  CAUTIONARY AND ADVISORY LABELS 2
  - Cinnarizine (Non-proprietary)
    Cinnarizine 15 mg Cinnarizine 15mg tablets | 84 tablet [P] £6.88 DT = £4.12
  - Stugeron (Johnson & Johnson Ltd)
    Cinnarizine 15 mg Stugeron 15mg tablets | 15 tablet [P] £3.30

Cinnarizine with dimenhydrinate

10-Sep-2020

The properties listed below are those particular to the combination only. For the properties of the components please consider, cinnarizine p. 499.

- **INDICATIONS AND DOSE**

Vertigo
- BY MOUTH
- Adult: 1 tablet 3 times a day

- **INTERACTIONS** → Appendix 1: antihistamines, sedating · dimenhydrinate

- **MEDICINAL FORMS** There can be variation in the licensing of different medicines containing the same drug.
  Oral tablet
  CAUTIONARY AND ADVISORY LABELS 2, 21
  - Cinnarizine with dimenhydrinate (Non-proprietary)
    Cinnarizine 20 mg, Dimenhydrinate 40 mg Cinnarizine 20mg / Dimenhydrinate 40mg tablets | 100 tablet [PoM] £23.00-£24.00 DT = £24.00
  - Arlevert (Hennig Arzneimittel GmbH & Co. KG)
    Cinnarizine 20 mg, Dimenhydrinate 40 mg Arlevert tablets | 100 tablet [PoM] £24.00 DT = £24.00

Promethazine teoclate

27-Jun-2023

- **INDICATIONS AND DOSE**

Nausea | Vomiting | Labyrinthine disorders
- BY MOUTH
- Child 5-9 years: 12.5–37.5 mg daily
- Child 10-17 years: 25–75 mg daily; maximum 100 mg per day
- Adult: 25–75 mg daily; maximum 100 mg per day

Motion sickness prevention
- BY MOUTH
- Child 5-9 years: 12.5 mg once daily, dose to be taken at bedtime on night before travel or 1–2 hours before travel
- Child 10-17 years: 25 mg once daily, dose to be taken at bedtime on night before travel or 1–2 hours before travel

- Adult: 25 mg once daily, dose to be taken at bedtime on night before travel or 1–2 hours before travel

Motion sickness treatment
- BY MOUTH
- Child 5-9 years: Initially 12.5 mg, dose to be taken at onset of motion sickness, then 12.5 mg for a further two doses, doses to be taken at bedtime, starting on the evening of onset
- Child 10-17 years: Initially 25 mg, dose to be taken at onset of motion sickness, then 25 mg for a further two doses, doses to be taken at bedtime, starting on the evening of onset
- Adult: Initially 25 mg, dose to be taken at onset of motion sickness, then 25 mg for a further two doses, doses to be taken at bedtime, starting on the evening of onset

> **IMPORTANT SAFETY INFORMATION**
> MHRA/CHM ADVICE: OVER-THE-COUNTER COUGH AND COLD MEDICINES FOR CHILDREN (APRIL 2009)
> Children under 6 years should not be given over-the-counter cough and cold medicines containing promethazine.

- **CAUTIONS** Asthma · bronchiectasis · bronchitis · epilepsy · prostatic hypertrophy (in adults) · pyloroduodenal obstruction · Reye's syndrome · severe coronary artery disease · susceptibility to angle-closure glaucoma · susceptibility to QT interval prolongation · urinary retention

- **INTERACTIONS** → Appendix 1: antihistamines, sedating

- **SIDE-EFFECTS** Anticholinergic syndrome · anxiety · appetite decreased · arrhythmia · blood disorder · bronchial secretion viscosity increased · confusion · dizziness · drowsiness · dry mouth · epigastric discomfort · fatigue · haemolytic anaemia · headache · hypotension · jaundice · movement disorders · muscle spasms · nightmare · palpitations · photosensitivity reaction · urinary retention · vision blurred

  SIDE-EFFECTS, FURTHER INFORMATION Elderly patients are more susceptible to anticholinergic side-effects. In children paradoxical stimulation may occur, especially with high doses.

- **PREGNANCY** Most manufacturers of antihistamines advise avoiding their use during pregnancy; however, there is no evidence of teratogenicity. Use in the latter part of the third trimester may cause adverse effects in neonates such as irritability, paradoxical excitability, and tremor.

- **BREAST FEEDING** Most antihistamines are present in breast milk in varying amounts; although not known to be harmful, most manufacturers advise avoiding their use in mothers who are breast-feeding.

- **HEPATIC IMPAIRMENT** Manufacturer advises caution.

- **RENAL IMPAIRMENT** [EvGr] Use with caution. ⟨M⟩

- **PATIENT AND CARER ADVICE**
  Driving and skilled tasks Drowsiness may affect performance of skilled tasks (e.g. cycling or driving); sedating effects enhanced by alcohol.

- **MEDICINAL FORMS** There can be variation in the licensing of different medicines containing the same drug.
  Oral tablet
  CAUTIONARY AND ADVISORY LABELS 2
  - Promethazine teoclate (Non-proprietary)
    Promethazine teoclate 25 mg Promethazine teoclate 25mg tablets | 28 tablet [PoM] [Σ] DT = £4.65

ANTIMUSCARINICS

F 896

Hyoscine hydrobromide

16-Jan-2024

(Scopolamine hydrobromide)

● **INDICATIONS AND DOSE**

Motion sickness

▶ BY MOUTH

▸ Child 4-9 years: 75–150 micrograms, dose to be taken up to 30 minutes before the start of journey, then 75–150 micrograms every 6 hours if required; maximum 450 micrograms per day

▸ Child 10-17 years: 150–300 micrograms, dose to be taken up to 30 minutes before the start of journey, then 150–300 micrograms every 6 hours if required; maximum 900 micrograms per day

▸ Adult: 150–300 micrograms, dose to be taken up to 30 minutes before the start of journey, then 150–300 micrograms every 6 hours if required; maximum 900 micrograms per day

▶ BY TRANSDERMAL APPLICATION

▸ Child 10-17 years: Apply 1 patch, apply behind ear 5–6 hours before journey, then apply 1 patch after 72 hours if required, remove old patch and site replacement patch behind the other ear

▸ Adult: Apply 1 patch, apply behind ear 5–6 hours before journey, then apply 1 patch after 72 hours if required, remove old patch and site replacement patch behind the other ear

Hypersalivation associated with clozapine therapy

▶ BY MOUTH

▸ Adult: 300 micrograms up to 3 times a day; maximum 900 micrograms per day

Excessive respiratory secretion in palliative care

▶ BY SUBCUTANEOUS INJECTION

▸ Adult: 400 micrograms every 4 hours as required, hourly use is occasionally necessary, particularly in excessive respiratory secretions

▶ BY CONTINUOUS SUBCUTANEOUS INFUSION

▸ Adult: 1.2–2 mg/24 hours

Bowel colic in palliative care

▶ BY SUBCUTANEOUS INJECTION

▸ Adult: 400 micrograms every 4 hours as required, hourly use is occasionally necessary

▶ BY SUBCUTANEOUS INFUSION

▸ Adult: 1.2–2 mg/24 hours

Bowel colic pain in palliative care

▶ BY MOUTH USING SUBLINGUAL TABLETS

▸ Adult: 300 micrograms 3 times a day, as *Kwells*®.

Premedication

▶ BY SUBCUTANEOUS INJECTION, OR BY INTRAMUSCULAR INJECTION

▸ Adult: 200–600 micrograms, to be administered 30–60 minutes before induction of anaesthesia

● **UNLICENSED USE** Not licensed for hypersalivation associated with clozapine therapy.

IMPORTANT SAFETY INFORMATION

Antimuscarinic drugs used for premedication to general anaesthesia should only be administered by, or under the direct supervision of, personnel experienced in their use.

MHRA/CHM ADVICE: HYOSCINE HYDROBROMIDE PATCHES (*SCOPODERM*® 1.5 MG PATCH OR *SCOPODERM*® TTS PATCH): RISK OF ANTICHOLINERGIC SIDE EFFECTS, INCLUDING HYPERTHERMIA (JULY 2023)

There has been a small number of reports of serious and life-threatening anticholinergic side-effects associated with the use of hyoscine hydrobromide patches, including a fatality from hyperthermia in a child, particularly with unlicensed use. These side-effects (which include hyperthermia, urinary retention, delirium, hallucinations, seizures, respiratory paralysis, and coma) may persist for 24 hours or longer after patch removal as the drug in the skin continues to enter the bloodstream. Healthcare professionals are reminded to:

● be alert for potential signs and symptoms of anticholinergic side-effects, particularly with unlicensed use, and to manage promptly if they occur;

● be aware that children and the elderly are more susceptible to anticholinergic toxicity;

● counsel patients and their carers to seek immediate medical attention and remove the patch if signs and symptoms of serious anticholinergic side-effects occur; immediate action should also be taken to reduce body heat if a high temperature develops.

● **CAUTIONS** Epilepsy

CAUTIONS, FURTHER INFORMATION

▸ Anticholinergic syndrome

▸ With systemic use in adults In some patients, especially the elderly, hyoscine may cause the central anticholinergic syndrome (excitement, ataxia, hallucinations, behavioural abnormalities, and drowsiness).

▸ With systemic use in children In some children hyoscine may cause the central anticholinergic syndrome (excitement, ataxia, hallucinations, behavioural abnormalities, and drowsiness).

● **INTERACTIONS** → Appendix 1: hyoscine

● **SIDE-EFFECTS**

▸ **Common or very common**

▸ With transdermal use Eye disorders · eyelid irritation

▸ **Rare or very rare**

▸ With transdermal use Concentration impaired · glaucoma · hallucinations · memory impairment · restlessness

▸ **Frequency not known**

▸ With oral use Asthma · cardiovascular disorders · central nervous system stimulation · gastrointestinal disorder · hallucination · hypersensitivity · hyperthermia · hypohidrosis · mydriasis · oedema · respiratory tract reaction · restlessness · seizure

▸ With parenteral use Agitation · angle closure glaucoma · arrhythmias · delirium · dysphagia · dyspnoea · epilepsy exacerbated · hallucination · hypersensitivity · idiosyncratic drug reaction · loss of consciousness · mydriasis · neuroleptic malignant syndrome (discontinue—potentially fatal) · psychotic disorder · thirst

▸ With transdermal use Balance impaired · coma · delirium · hyperthermia · respiratory paralysis · seizure

SIDE-EFFECTS, FURTHER INFORMATION Since systemic absorption can follow transdermal use, also consider the side-effects of systemic antimuscarinics.

● **PREGNANCY** Use only if potential benefit outweighs risk. Injection may depress neonatal respiration.

● **BREAST FEEDING** Amount too small to be harmful.

● **HEPATIC IMPAIRMENT** Manufacturer advises caution.

● **RENAL IMPAIRMENT** EvGr Use with caution. Ⓜ

● **DIRECTIONS FOR ADMINISTRATION**

▸ With transdermal use in children Expert sources advise *patch* applied to hairless area of skin behind ear; if less than whole patch required **either** cut with scissors along full thickness ensuring membrane is not peeled away **or** cover portion to prevent contact with skin.

▸ With oral use in children For administration by *mouth*, expert sources advise injection solution may be given orally.

● **PRESCRIBING AND DISPENSING INFORMATION**

Palliative care For further information on the use of hyoscine hydrobromide in palliative care, see www.medicinescomplete.com/#/content/palliative/hyoscine-hydrobromide.

● **PATIENT AND CARER ADVICE**
▶ With transdermal use Explain accompanying instructions to patient and in particular emphasise advice to wash hands after handling and to wash application site after removing, and to use one patch at a time.
Driving and skilled tasks
▶ With transdermal use Drowsiness may persist for up to 24 hours or longer after removal of patch; effects of alcohol enhanced.

● **MEDICINAL FORMS** There can be variation in the licensing of different medicines containing the same drug. Forms available from special-order manufacturers include: oral suspension, oral solution
Oral tablet
CAUTIONARY AND ADVISORY LABELS 2
▶ Kwells (Dexcel-Pharma Ltd)
Hyoscine hydrobromide 150 microgram Kwells Kids 150microgram tablets | 12 tablet P £2.50 DT = £2.50
Hyoscine hydrobromide 300 microgram Kwells 300microgram tablets | 12 tablet P £2.50 DT = £2.50
▶ Travel Calm (The Boots Company Plc)
Hyoscine hydrobromide 300 microgram Travel Calm 300microgram tablets | 12 tablet P Ⓢ DT = £2.50
Solution for injection
▶ Hyoscine hydrobromide (Non-proprietary)
Hyoscine hydrobromide 400 microgram per 1 ml Hyoscine hydrobromide 400micrograms/1ml solution for injection ampoules | 10 ampoule PoM £53.49 DT = £38.73
Hyoscine hydrobromide 600 microgram per 1 ml Hyoscine hydrobromide 600micrograms/1ml solution for injection ampoules | 10 ampoule PoM £179.42–£266.00 DT = £179.42
Transdermal patch
CAUTIONARY AND ADVISORY LABELS 19
▶ Scopoderm (Baxter Healthcare Ltd)
Hyoscine 1 mg per 72 hour Scopoderm 1.5mg patches | 2 patch P £12.87 DT = £12.87

ANTIPSYCHOTICS > FIRST-GENERATION

ᴳ 442

Droperidol
04-May-2021

● **DRUG ACTION** Droperidol is a butyrophenone, structurally related to haloperidol, which blocks dopamine receptors in the chemoreceptor trigger zone.

● **INDICATIONS AND DOSE**
Prevention and treatment of postoperative nausea and vomiting
▶ BY INTRAVENOUS INJECTION
▶ Adult: 0.625–1.25 mg, dose to be given 30 minutes before end of surgery, then 0.625–1.25 mg every 6 hours as required
▶ Elderly: 625 micrograms, dose to be given 30 minutes before end of surgery, then 625 micrograms every 6 hours as required

Prevention of nausea and vomiting caused by opioid analgesics in postoperative patient-controlled analgesia (PCA)
▶ BY INTRAVENOUS INJECTION
▶ Adult: 15–50 micrograms of droperidol for every 1 mg of morphine in PCA, reduce dose in elderly; maximum 5 mg per day

● **CONTRA-INDICATIONS** Bradycardia · comatose states · hypokalaemia · hypomagnesaemia · phaeochromocytoma · QT-interval prolongation

● **CAUTIONS** Chronic obstructive pulmonary disease · CNS depression · electrolyte disturbances · history of alcohol abuse · respiratory failure

● **INTERACTIONS** → Appendix 1: droperidol

● **SIDE-EFFECTS**
▶ **Uncommon** Anxiety · oculogyration
▶ **Rare or very rare** Blood disorder · cardiac arrest · dysphoria
▶ **Frequency not known** Coma · epilepsy · hallucination · oligomenorrhoea · respiratory disorders · SIADH · syncope

● **BREAST FEEDING** Limited information available—avoid repeated administration.

● **HEPATIC IMPAIRMENT** Manufacturer advises caution.
Dose adjustments
▶ When used for Prevention and treatment of postoperative nausea and vomiting Manufacturer advises maximum 625 micrograms repeated every 6 hours as required.
▶ When used for Prevention of nausea and vomiting caused by opioid analgesics in postoperative patient-controlled analgesia Manufacturer advises dose reduction (no information available).

● **RENAL IMPAIRMENT**
Dose adjustments
▶ When used for Prevention and treatment of postoperative nausea and vomiting EvGr Maximum 625 micrograms repeated every 6 hours as required. Ⓜ
▶ When used for Prevention of nausea and vomiting caused by opioid analgesics in postoperative patient-controlled analgesia EvGr Reduce dose (no information available). Ⓜ

● **MONITORING REQUIREMENTS** Continuous pulse oximetry required if risk of ventricular arrhythmia—continue for 30 minutes following administration.

● **MEDICINAL FORMS** There can be variation in the licensing of different medicines containing the same drug.
Solution for injection
▶ Droperidol (Non-proprietary)
Droperidol 2.5 mg per 1 ml Droperidol 2.5mg/1ml solution for injection vials | 10 vial PoM £39.40 (Hospital only)
Droperidol 2.5mg/1ml solution for injection ampoules | 10 ampoule PoM £80.00 (Hospital only)

ᴳ 442

Levomepromazine
29-Nov-2023
(Methotrimeprazine)

● **INDICATIONS AND DOSE**
Pain in palliative care (reserved for distressed patients with severe pain unresponsive to other measures)
▶ BY CONTINUOUS SUBCUTANEOUS INFUSION, OR BY INTRAMUSCULAR INJECTION, OR BY INTRAVENOUS INJECTION
▶ Adult: Seek specialist advice

Agitation in palliative care for the imminently dying [initial titration]
▶ BY SUBCUTANEOUS INJECTION
▶ Adult: 12.5–25 mg every 1 hour as required, dose to be adjusted according to response; maximum 200 mg per day
▶ Elderly: 6.25–12.5 mg every 1 hour as required, dose to be adjusted according to response; maximum 200 mg per day

Agitation in palliative care for the imminently dying [maintenance dose after initial titration]
▶ BY CONTINUOUS SUBCUTANEOUS INFUSION
▶ Adult: 12.5–200 mg/24 hours

Nausea and vomiting in palliative care [regular dosing]
▶ BY MOUTH, OR BY SUBCUTANEOUS INJECTION
▶ Adult: 6–6.25 mg once daily, dose to be given at bedtime, if necessary, dose to be progressively increased every 4–5 days up to max. 25 mg per day in total taking into account regular and as required dosing
▶ BY CONTINUOUS SUBCUTANEOUS INFUSION
▶ Adult: 6.25 mg/24 hours, if necessary, dose to be progressively increased every 4–5 days up to max.

25 mg per day in total taking into account regular and as required dosing

Nausea and vomiting in palliative care [as required dosing]
▶ BY MOUTH, OR BY SUBCUTANEOUS INJECTION
▸ Adult: 6–6.25 mg every 2 hours as required, max. 25 mg per day in total taking into account regular and as required dosing

Schizophrenia (bed patients)
▶ BY MOUTH
▸ Adult: Initially 100–200 mg daily in 3 divided doses, increased if necessary to 1 g daily

Schizophrenia
▶ BY MOUTH
▸ Adult: Initially 25–50 mg daily in divided doses, dose can be increased as necessary

● UNLICENSED USE Specialist sources support use as detailed below in the doses provided in the BNF, but these may differ from those licensed:
  ● agitation in palliative care for the imminently dying;
  ● nausea and vomiting in palliative care.

● CONTRA-INDICATIONS CNS depression · comatose states · phaeochromocytoma

● CAUTIONS Patients receiving large initial doses should remain supine · susceptibility to QT interval prolongation
  CAUTIONS, FURTHER INFORMATION Risk of postural hypotension; not recommended for ambulant patients over 50 years unless risk of hypotensive reaction assessed.

● INTERACTIONS → Appendix 1: phenothiazines

● SIDE-EFFECTS
▸ **Common or very common** Asthenia · heat stroke
▸ **Uncommon** Embolism and thrombosis
▸ **Rare or very rare** Cardiac arrest · hepatic disorders
▸ **Frequency not known** Allergic dermatitis · delirium · gastrointestinal disorders · glucose tolerance impaired · hyponatraemia · photosensitivity reaction · priapism · SIADH

● HEPATIC IMPAIRMENT Manufacturer advises consider avoiding.

● DIRECTIONS FOR ADMINISTRATION For *continuous subcutaneous infusion* dilute with a suitable volume of Sodium Chloride 0.9%.
▸ With oral use for Nausea and vomiting in palliative care A 25 mg tablet can be quartered to achieve a 6.25 mg dose.

● PRESCRIBING AND DISPENSING INFORMATION
  Palliative care For further information on the use of levomepromazine in palliative care, see www.medicinescomplete.com/#/content/palliative/levomepromazine.

● MEDICINAL FORMS There can be variation in the licensing of different medicines containing the same drug. Forms available from special-order manufacturers include: oral tablet, oral suspension, oral solution

Oral tablet
CAUTIONARY AND ADVISORY LABELS 2
▸ Levomepromazine (Non-proprietary)
  Levomepromazine maleate 6 mg Levomepromazine 6mg tablets | 28 tablet PoM £247.20 DT = £247.20
  Levomepromazine maleate 25 mg Levomepromazine 25mg tablets | 84 tablet PoM £20.26-£34.22 DT = £34.22
  Levomepromazine maleate 50 mg Levomepromazine 50mg tablets | 84 tablet PoM £34.00 DT = £34.00
  Levomepromazine maleate 100 mg Levomepromazine 100mg tablets | 28 tablet PoM ℞ (Hospital only)
  Nozinan 100mg tablets | 100 tablet PoM ℞ (Hospital only)
▸ Levorol (Galvany Pharma Ltd)
  Levomepromazine maleate 6.25 mg Levorol 6.25mg tablets | 28 tablet PoM £181.00 DT = £181.00

▸ Nozinan (Neuraxpharm UK Ltd)
  Levomepromazine maleate 25 mg Nozinan 25mg tablets | 84 tablet PoM £20.26 DT = £34.22
Solution for injection
▸ Levomepromazine (Non-proprietary)
  Levomepromazine hydrochloride 25 mg per 1 ml Levomepromazine 25mg/1ml solution for injection ampoules | 10 ampoule PoM £20.13 DT = £20.13
▸ Nozinan (Neuraxpharm UK Ltd)
  Levomepromazine hydrochloride 25 mg per 1 ml Nozinan 25mg/1ml solution for injection ampoules | 10 ampoule PoM £20.13 DT = £20.13
Oral solution
▸ Levorol (Galvany Pharma Ltd)
  Levomepromazine (as Levomepromazine hydrochloride) 5 mg per 1 ml Levorol 5mg/ml oral solution | 100 ml PoM £175.00 DT = £175.00 SF

5.1   Ménière's disease

HISTAMINE ANALOGUES

Betahistine dihydrochloride
23-Nov-2020

● **INDICATIONS AND DOSE**
Vertigo, tinnitus and hearing loss associated with Ménière's disease
▶ BY MOUTH
▸ Adult: Initially 16 mg 3 times a day, dose preferably taken with food; maintenance 24–48 mg daily

● CONTRA-INDICATIONS Phaeochromocytoma
● CAUTIONS Asthma · history of peptic ulcer
● INTERACTIONS → Appendix 1: betahistine
● SIDE-EFFECTS
▸ **Common or very common** Gastrointestinal discomfort · headache · nausea
▸ **Frequency not known** Allergic dermatitis · vomiting

● PREGNANCY Avoid unless clearly necessary—no information available.

● BREAST FEEDING Use only if potential benefit outweighs risk—no information available.

● MEDICINAL FORMS There can be variation in the licensing of different medicines containing the same drug. Forms available from special-order manufacturers include: oral suspension, oral solution

Oral tablet
CAUTIONARY AND ADVISORY LABELS 21
▸ Betahistine dihydrochloride (Non-proprietary)
  Betahistine dihydrochloride 8 mg Betahistine 8mg tablets | 84 tablet PoM £10.50 DT = £1.81 | 120 tablet PoM £1.48-£13.50
  Betahistine dihydrochloride 16 mg Betahistine 16mg tablets | 84 tablet PoM £17.19 DT = £2.37
  Betahistine dihydrochloride 24 mg Betahistine 24mg tablets | 60 tablet PoM £5.71-£9.00 | 84 tablet PoM £8.00 DT = £8.00
▸ Serc (Viatris UK Healthcare Ltd)
  Betahistine dihydrochloride 8 mg Serc 8mg tablets | 120 tablet PoM £9.04
  Betahistine dihydrochloride 16 mg Serc 16mg tablets | 84 tablet PoM £12.65 DT = £2.37

6   Pain

Pain, chronic
23-Sep-2023

Overview

Pain is described as an unpleasant sensory and emotional experience associated with, or resembling that associated with, actual or potential tissue damage. Physiologically, it can be described as **neuropathic, nociceptive** or **nociplastic**, and be classified as either **acute** or **chronic**, and **primary** or **secondary** in nature. Nociceptive pain generally responds to treatment with conventional analgesics, whereas neuropathic and nociplastic pain respond poorly to conventional analgesics and can be difficult to treat.

Chronic pain is defined as pain that has been present for more than 12 weeks (beyond the expected time of wound healing). It is a complex phenomenon and can have a considerable impact on quality of life, resulting in significant suffering and disability (which are particularly prominent in presentations of chronic primary pain).

Chronic **primary** pain is defined as pain that has no clear underlying condition, or where the pain (or its impact) appears to be out of proportion to any observable injury or disease. Types of chronic primary pain include complex regional pain syndrome, fibromyalgia (chronic widespread pain), primary headache and orofacial pain, primary visceral, and primary musculoskeletal pain. **Secondary** pain however, is caused by an underlying condition (such as endometriosis, osteoarthritis, rheumatoid arthritis, and ulcerative colitis) and can be organised into 6 pain categories: cancer-related, neuropathic, post-surgical or post-traumatic, secondary headache or orofacial, secondary musculoskeletal, and secondary visceral. Chronic primary and secondary pain can coexist.

EvGr **Depression** is a common comorbidity in those with chronic pain; individuals should be monitored and treated for depression as appropriate. Optimising antidepressant therapy should be considered in individuals with moderate depression and chronic pain. ⒶFor information on the treatment of depression, see Depression p. 415.

Aims of treatment

Treatment aims to reduce pain and the impact of chronic pain on quality of life, mood, and function.

Management of chronic pain

A wide range of both pharmacological and non-pharmacological management strategies are available for chronic pain. Where possible, treatment options should be guided by any known underlying chronic pain condition(s). For guidance on the management of pain in specific conditions, see Diverticular disease and diverticulitis p. 39, Endometriosis p. 867, Irritable bowel syndrome p. 52, Low back pain and sciatica p. 1291, Migraine p. 536, Neuropathic pain p. 547, Osteoarthritis p. 1249, Rheumatoid arthritis p. 1249, Spondyloarthritis p. 1250, and Ulcerative colitis p. 41. For guidance on the management of pain in palliative care, see Prescribing in palliative care p. 26.

Consider specialist referral when non-specialist management is failing, the pain is poorly controlled, the patient is experiencing significant distress, and/or where a specialist intervention is being considered.

Non-drug treatment

EvGr Exercise and exercise therapies, regardless of their form, are recommended in the management of chronic pain; strategies to improve adherence (such as supervised exercise sessions) should be implemented.

Transcutaneous electrical nerve stimulation (TENS), either high or low frequency, may be considered for the relief of chronic pain.

Referral to a pain management programme and psychologically-based interventions such as cognitive behavioural therapy, biofeedback, and progressive relaxation should be considered for patients with chronic pain; brief education (consisting of examination, information, reassurance, and advice to stay active) should be given to all patients.

The use of self-management resources (safe, low-technology, community-based, and affordable programmes) should be considered to complement other therapies in the treatment of chronic pain. ⒶFor information on self-management resources, see SIGN clinical guideline: **Management of chronic pain** (see *Useful resources*).

Drug treatment

A variety of analgesics are used in the treatment of chronic pain and can be divided into **non-opioid**, **opioid**, and **adjuvant** analgesics.

Individual responses to analgesia vary considerably, both in terms of efficacy and side-effects; even with the same chronic pain syndrome, the underlying pain mechanisms may differ between individuals. This provides challenges with assessment and management in routine clinical practice. EvGr If an individual either fails to tolerate, or has an inadequate response to a drug, then it is worthwhile considering a different agent from the same class. Ⓐ

Individuals using analgesics to manage chronic pain should be reviewed at least annually, with review frequency increased if there are any changes to their medication, underlying pain syndrome or comorbidities.

For comparative information on analgesic options, see Analgesics p. 505.

Non-opioid analgesics

Non-opioid analgesics include paracetamol p. 507 and NSAIDs (in both oral and topical forms). For information on the use of NSAIDs, see Non-steroidal anti-inflammatory drugs p. 1292.

Compound preparations

EvGr The use of single-ingredient analgesics is preferred to allow for independent titration of each drug; however, fixed dose combination analgesics (except those with low-dose opioids) may be considered for those with stable chronic pain. Ⓐ

Opioid analgesics

Opioid analgesics can be divided into those used for mild-to-moderate pain (such as codeine phosphate p. 517) and those used for moderate-to-severe pain (such as morphine p. 525 or oxycodone hydrochloride p. 528).

EvGr Opioids should only be considered in carefully selected individuals for the short- to medium-term treatment of chronic non-malignant pain, when other therapies have been insufficient; the benefits should outweigh the risks of serious harms (such as addiction, overdose, and death). With continuous longer-term use of opioids, tolerance and dependence compromise both safety and efficacy. Prescribers should have knowledge of opioid pharmacology, and be competent and experienced in the use of strong opioids.

When starting treatment with an opioid there should be an agreement between the prescriber and patient about the expected outcomes—with advanced agreement on the reduction and cessation of the opioid if these are not met. Opioids should be reviewed at least annually but more frequently if required; consideration should be given to a gradual reduction of the opioid to the lowest effective dose or complete cessation. Pain specialist advice or review should be sought for individuals taking doses >90 mg/day morphine equivalent. Ⓐ

There is a rationale for switching between opioids if the initial choice is ineffective or if side-effects are unacceptable. EvGr Caution should be used with dose comparisons and switching due to limited evidence for the accuracy of dose equivalence tables and considerable variation between individuals. ⒶFor more information on opioid dose conversions or equivalents, see Prescribing in palliative care p. 26. Resources for the prescribing of opioids have been produced by the Faculty of Pain Medicine in partnership with PHE, and are available at: fpm.ac.uk/opioids-aware.

Adjuvant analgesics

Adjuvant analgesics include drugs such as antidepressants, antiepileptics, benzodiazepines and other muscle relaxants, bone-modulating drugs, corticosteroids, and topical capsaicin, lidocaine, and rubefacients.

In addition to the use of some antidepressants in certain types of chronic secondary pain, EvGr the use of an antidepressant [unlicensed], either amitriptyline, citalopram, duloxetine, fluoxetine, paroxetine, or sertraline to manage chronic primary pain may be considered. A

Useful Resources

Chronic pain (primary and secondary) in over 16s: assessment of all chronic pain and management of chronic primary pain. National Institute for Health and Care Excellence. NICE guideline 193. April 2021.
www.nice.org.uk/guidance/ng193

Management of chronic pain. Scottish Intercollegiate Guidelines Network. SIGN guideline 136. August 2019.
www.sign.ac.uk/our-guidelines/management-of-chronic-pain/

Analgesics

06-Dec-2023

Pain relief

The non-opioid drugs, paracetamol p. 507 and aspirin p. 142 (and other NSAIDs), are particularly suitable for pain in musculoskeletal conditions, whereas the opioid analgesics are more suitable for moderate to severe pain, particularly of visceral origin.

Pain in sickle-cell disease

The pain of mild sickle-cell crises is managed with paracetamol, a NSAID, codeine phosphate p. 517, or dihydrocodeine tartrate p. 518. Severe crises may require the use of morphine p. 525 or diamorphine hydrochloride p. 518; concomitant use of a NSAID may potentiate analgesia and allow lower doses of the opioid to be used. Pethidine hydrochloride p. 531 should be avoided if possible because accumulation of a neurotoxic metabolite can precipitate seizures; the relatively short half-life of pethidine hydrochloride necessitates frequent injections.

Dental and orofacial pain

Analgesics should be used judiciously in dental care as a **temporary** measure until the cause of the pain has been dealt with.

Dental pain of inflammatory origin, such as that associated with pulpitis, apical infection, localised osteitis or pericoronitis is usually best managed by treating the infection, providing drainage, restorative procedures, and other local measures. Analgesics provide temporary relief of pain (usually for about 1 to 7 days) until the causative factors have been brought under control. In the case of pulpitis, intra-osseous infection or abscess, reliance on analgesics alone is usually inappropriate.

Similarly the pain and discomfort associated with acute problems of the oral mucosa (e.g. acute herpetic gingivostomatitis, erythema multiforme) may be relieved by benzydamine hydrochloride mouthwash or spray p. 1380 until the cause of the mucosal disorder has been dealt with. However, where a patient is febrile, the antipyretic action of paracetamol or ibuprofen p. 1302 is often helpful.

The *choice* of an analgesic for dental purposes should be based on its suitability for the patient. Most dental pain is relieved effectively by non-steroidal anti-inflammatory drugs (NSAIDs). NSAIDs that are used for dental pain include ibuprofen, diclofenac sodium p. 1297, and aspirin. Paracetamol has analgesic and antipyretic effects but no anti-inflammatory effect.

Opioid analgesics such as dihydrocodeine tartrate act on the central nervous system and are traditionally used for *moderate to severe pain*. However, opioid analgesics are relatively ineffective in dental pain and their side-effects can be unpleasant. Paracetamol, ibuprofen, or aspirin are adequate for most cases of dental pain and an opioid is rarely required.

Combining a non-opioid with an opioid analgesic can provide greater relief of pain than either analgesic given alone. However, this applies only when an adequate dose of each analgesic is used. Most combination analgesic preparations have not been shown to provide greater relief of pain than an adequate dose of the non-opioid component given alone. Moreover, combination preparations have the disadvantage of an increased number of side-effects.

Any analgesic given before a dental procedure should have a low risk of increasing postoperative bleeding. In the case of pain after the dental procedure, taking an analgesic before the effect of the local anaesthetic has worn off can improve control. Postoperative analgesia with ibuprofen or aspirin is usually continued for about 24 to 72 hours.

Temporomandibular dysfunction can be related to anxiety in some patients who may clench or grind their teeth (bruxism) during the day or night. The muscle spasm (which appears to be the main source of pain) may be treated empirically with an overlay appliance which provides a free sliding occlusion and may also interfere with grinding. In addition, diazepam p. 398, which has muscle relaxant as well as anxiolytic properties, may be helpful but it should only be prescribed on a short-term basis during the acute phase. Analgesics such as aspirin or ibuprofen may also be required.

Dysmenorrhoea

Use of an oral contraceptive prevents the pain of dysmenorrhoea which is generally associated with ovulatory cycles. If treatment is necessary paracetamol or a NSAID will generally provide adequate relief of pain. The vomiting and severe pain associated with dysmenorrhoea in women with endometriosis may call for an antiemetic (in addition to an analgesic). Antispasmodics (such as alverine citrate p. 97) have been advocated for dysmenorrhoea but the antispasmodic action does not generally provide significant relief.

Non-opioid analgesics and compound analgesic preparations

Aspirin is indicated for headache, transient musculoskeletal pain, dysmenorrhoea, and pyrexia. In inflammatory conditions, most physicians prefer anti-inflammatory treatment with another NSAID which may be better tolerated and more convenient for the patient. Aspirin is used increasingly for its antiplatelet properties. Aspirin tablets or dispersible aspirin tablets are adequate for most purposes as they act rapidly.

Gastric irritation may be a problem; it is minimised by taking the dose after food. Enteric-coated preparations are available, but have a slow onset of action and are therefore unsuitable for single-dose analgesic use (though their prolonged action may be useful for night pain).

Aspirin interacts significantly with a number of other drugs and its interaction with warfarin sodium p. 165 is a **special hazard**.

Paracetamol is similar in efficacy to aspirin, but has no demonstrable anti-inflammatory activity; it is less irritant to the stomach and for that reason is now generally preferred to aspirin, particularly in the elderly. **Overdosage** with paracetamol is particularly dangerous as it may cause hepatic damage which is sometimes not apparent for 4 to 6 days.

Nefopam hydrochloride p. 509 may have a place in the relief of persistent pain unresponsive to other non-opioid analgesics. It causes little or no respiratory depression, but sympathomimetic and antimuscarinic side-effects may be troublesome.

Non-steroidal anti-inflammatory analgesics (NSAIDs) are particularly useful for the treatment of patients with chronic disease accompanied by pain and inflammation. Some of them are also used in the short-term treatment of mild to moderate pain including transient musculoskeletal pain but paracetamol is now often preferred, particularly in the elderly. They are also suitable for the relief of pain in *dysmenorrhoea* and to treat pain caused by *secondary bone tumours*, many of which produce lysis of bone and release prostaglandins. Selective inhibitors of cyclo-oxygenase-2 may be used in preference to non-selective NSAIDs for patients at high risk of developing serious gastro-intestinal side-effects. Several NSAIDs are also used for postoperative analgesia.

A non-opioid analgesic administered by intrathecal infusion (**ziconotide**) is licensed for the treatment of chronic severe pain; ziconotide can be used by a hospital specialist as an adjunct to opioid analgesics.

Compound analgesic preparations

Compound analgesic preparations that contain a simple analgesic (such as aspirin p. 142 or paracetamol p. 507) with an opioid component reduce the scope for effective titration of the individual components in the management of pain of varying intensity.

Compound analgesic preparations containing paracetamol or aspirin with a *low dose* of an opioid analgesic (e.g. 8 mg of codeine phosphate p. 517 per compound tablet) are commonly used, but the advantages have not been substantiated. The low dose of the opioid may be enough to cause opioid side-effects (in particular, constipation) and can complicate the treatment of **overdosage** yet may not provide significant additional relief of pain.

A *full dose* of the opioid component (e.g. 60 mg codeine phosphate) in compound analgesic preparations effectively augments the analgesic activity but is associated with the full range of opioid side-effects (including nausea, vomiting, severe constipation, drowsiness, respiratory depression, and risk of dependence on long-term administration). **Important**: the elderly are particularly susceptible to opioid side-effects and should receive lower doses.

In general, when assessing pain, it is necessary to weigh up carefully whether there is a need for a non-opioid and an opioid analgesic to be taken simultaneously.

Caffeine is a weak stimulant that is often included, in small doses, in analgesic preparations. It is claimed that the addition of caffeine may enhance the analgesic effect, but the alerting effect, mild habit-forming effect and possible provocation of headache may not always be desirable. Moreover, in excessive dosage or on withdrawal caffeine may itself induce headache.

Co-proxamol tablets (dextropropoxyphene in combination with paracetamol) are no longer licensed because of safety concerns, particularly toxicity in overdose. Co-proxamol tablets [unlicensed] may still be prescribed for patients who find it difficult to change, because alternatives are not effective or suitable.

Opioid analgesics and dependence

Opioid analgesics are usually used to relieve moderate to severe pain particularly of visceral origin. Repeated administration may cause dependence and tolerance, but this is no deterrent in the control of pain in terminal illness. Regular use of a potent opioid may be appropriate for certain cases of chronic non-malignant pain.

For general guidance on the use of opioid analgesics in chronic pain, see Pain, chronic p. 503.

Strong opioids

Morphine p. 525 remains the most valuable opioid analgesic for severe pain although it frequently causes nausea and vomiting. It is the standard against which other opioid analgesics are compared. In addition to relief of pain, morphine also confers a state of euphoria and mental detachment.

Morphine is the opioid of choice for the oral treatment of *severe pain in palliative care*. It is given regularly every 4 hours (or every 12 or 24 hours as modified-release preparations).

Buprenorphine p. 511 has both opioid agonist and antagonist properties and may precipitate withdrawal symptoms, including pain, in patients dependent on other opioids. It has abuse potential and may itself cause dependence. It has a much longer duration of action than morphine and sublingually is an effective analgesic for 6 to 8 hours. Unlike most opioid analgesics, the effects of buprenorphine are only partially reversed by naloxone hydrochloride p. 1564.

Dipipanone hydrochloride used alone is less sedating than morphine but the only preparation available contains an antiemetic and is therefore not suitable for regular regimens in palliative care.

Diamorphine hydrochloride p. 518 (heroin) is a powerful opioid analgesic. It may cause less nausea and hypotension than morphine. In *palliative care* the greater solubility of diamorphine hydrochloride allows effective doses to be injected in smaller volumes and this is important in the emaciated patient.

Alfentanil p. 1537, fentanyl p. 520 and remifentanil p. 1538 are used by injection for intra-operative analgesia; fentanyl is available in a transdermal drug delivery system as a self-adhesive patch which is changed every 72 hours.

Methadone hydrochloride p. 570 is less sedating than morphine and acts for longer periods. In prolonged use, methadone hydrochloride should not be administered more often than twice daily to avoid the risk of accumulation and opioid overdosage. Methadone hydrochloride may be used instead of morphine in the occasional patient who experiences excitation (or exacerbation of pain) with morphine.

Oxycodone hydrochloride p. 528 has an efficacy and side-effect profile similar to that of morphine. It is commonly used as a second-line drug if morphine is not tolerated or does not control the pain.

Papaveretum is rarely used; morphine is easier to prescribe and less prone to error with regard to the strength and dose.

Pentazocine p. 531 has both agonist and antagonist properties and precipitates withdrawal symptoms, including pain in patients dependent on other opioids. By injection it is more potent than dihydrocodeine tartrate p. 518 or codeine phosphate, but hallucinations and thought disturbances may occur. It is not recommended and, in particular, should be avoided after myocardial infarction as it may increase pulmonary and aortic blood pressure as well as cardiac work.

Pethidine hydrochloride p. 531 produces prompt but short-lasting analgesia; it is less constipating than morphine, but even in high doses is a less potent analgesic. It is not suitable for severe continuing pain. It is used for analgesia in labour; however, other opioids, such as morphine or diamorphine hydrochloride, are often preferred for obstetric pain. Remifentanil patient-controlled analgesia (PCA) can also be used for pain relief during labour and birth [unlicensed use]—consult hospital protocols.

Tapentadol p. 533 produces analgesia by two mechanisms. It is an opioid-receptor agonist and it also inhibits noradrenaline reuptake. Nausea, vomiting, and constipation are less likely to occur with tapentadol than with other strong opioid analgesics.

Tramadol hydrochloride p. 534 produces analgesia by two mechanisms: an opioid effect and an enhancement of serotonergic and adrenergic pathways. It has fewer of the typical opioid side-effects (notably, less respiratory depression, less constipation and less addiction potential); psychiatric reactions have been reported.

Weak opioids

Codeine phosphate can be used for the relief of mild to moderate pain where other painkillers such as paracetamol or ibuprofen p. 1302 have proved ineffective.

Dihydrocodeine tartrate has an analgesic efficacy similar to that of codeine phosphate. Higher doses may provide some additional pain relief but this may be at the cost of more nausea and vomiting.

Meptazinol p. 525 is claimed to have a low incidence of repiratory depression. It has a reported length of action of 2 to 7 hours with onset within 15 minutes.

Postoperative analgesia

EvGr Offer a multimodal approach using a combination of analgesics from different classes to manage postoperative pain. ⓐ For further information on postoperative analgesia, see Peri-operative analgesia p. 1532. The use of intra-operative opioids affects the prescribing of postoperative analgesics. A postoperative opioid analgesic should be given with care since it may potentiate any residual respiratory depression.

Morphine p. 525 is used most widely. Tramadol hydrochloride p. 534 is not as effective in severe pain as other opioid analgesics. Buprenorphine p. 511 may antagonise the analgesic effect of previously administered opioids and is generally not recommended. Pethidine hydrochloride p. 531 is generally not recommended for postoperative pain because it is metabolised to norpethidine which may accumulate, particularly in renal impairment; norpethidine stimulates the central nervous system and may cause convulsions.

Opioids are also given epidurally [unlicensed route] in the postoperative period but are associated with side-effects such as pruritus, urinary retention, nausea and vomiting; respiratory depression can be delayed, particularly with morphine.

Patient-controlled analgesia (PCA) can be used to relieve postoperative pain—consult individual hospital protocols.

Pain management and opioid dependence

Although caution is necessary, patients who are dependent on opioids or have a history of drug dependence may be treated with opioid analgesics when there is a clinical need. Treatment with opioid analgesics in this patient group should normally be carried out with the advice of specialists. However, doctors do not require a special licence to prescribe opioid analgesics to patients with opioid dependence for relief of pain due to organic disease or injury.

> **Other drugs used for Pain** Diclofenac potassium, p. 1296 · Levomepromazine, p. 502 · Mefenamic acid, p. 1308

ANAESTHETICS, GENERAL ⟩ VOLATILE LIQUID ANAESTHETICS

Methoxyflurane

22-Jan-2019

● **INDICATIONS AND DOSE**

Moderate-to-severe pain associated with trauma (under close medical supervision)

▸ BY INHALATION

▸ Adult: 3–6 mL as required, avoid administration on consecutive days; administer using inhaler device; maximum 15 mL per week

> **IMPORTANT SAFETY INFORMATION**
> Manufacturer advises methoxyflurane should only be self-administered under the supervision of personnel experienced in its use, using a hand-held *Penthrox*® inhaler device.

● **CONTRA-INDICATIONS** Cardiovascular disease · history of liver damage associated with use of methoxyflurane or other halogenated anaesthetics · impaired consciousness · respiratory depression · susceptibility to malignant hyperthermia

● **CAUTIONS** Elderly—increased risk of hypotension · repeated administration more than once every 3 months—increased risk of hepatic injury · risk factors for hepatic impairment · risk factors for renal impairment

● **INTERACTIONS** → Appendix 1: volatile halogenated anaesthetics

● **SIDE-EFFECTS**

▸ **Common or very common** Dizziness · drowsiness · dry mouth · headache · nausea

▸ **Uncommon** Anxiety · appetite increased · chills · concentration impaired · cough · depression · fatigue · feeling abnormal · flushing · hyperhidrosis · hypertension · hypotension · memory loss · mood altered · oral disorders · paraesthesia · peripheral neuropathy · speech impairment · taste altered · vision disorders · vomiting

▸ **Frequency not known** Choking · confusion · consciousness impaired · dissociation · hepatic disorders · hypoxia · nephrotoxicity (with high doses) · nystagmus · renal failure

● **ALLERGY AND CROSS-SENSITIVITY** Contra-indicated in patients with hypersensitivity to fluorinated anaesthetics.

● **PREGNANCY** Manufacturer advises use with caution—limited information available.

● **BREAST FEEDING** Manufacturer advises use with caution—limited information available.

● **HEPATIC IMPAIRMENT** Manufacturer advises caution (risk of increased exposure).

● **RENAL IMPAIRMENT** Manufacturer advises avoid.

● **PRESCRIBING AND DISPENSING INFORMATION** The manufacturer of *Penthrox*® has provided an *Administration Checklist* and an *Administration Guide* for healthcare professionals.

● **HANDLING AND STORAGE** Manufacturer advises exposure of healthcare professionals to methoxyflurane should be minimised—risk of serious side-effects.

● **PATIENT AND CARER ADVICE** Manufacturer advises that patients should be given advice on appropriate inhaler technique.

A patient alert card should be provided.

Driving and skilled tasks Manufacturer advises patients and carers should be counselled on the effects on driving and performance of skilled tasks—increased risk of dizziness and drowsiness.

● **MEDICINAL FORMS** There can be variation in the licensing of different medicines containing the same drug.

Inhalation vapour liquid

EXCIPIENTS: May contain Butylated hydroxytoluene

▸ Penthrox (Galen Ltd)

Methoxyflurane 999 mg per 1 gram Penthrox inhalation vapour liquid 3ml bottles with device | 1 bottle PoM £18.46

ANALGESICS ⟩ NON-OPIOID

Paracetamol

19-Apr-2024

(Acetaminophen)

● **INDICATIONS AND DOSE**

Mild to moderate pain | Pyrexia

▸ BY MOUTH

▸ Adult: 0.5–1 g, every 4–6 hours; maximum 4 g per day

▸ BY INTRAVENOUS INFUSION

▸ Adult (body-weight up to 51 kg): 15 mg/kg, every 4–6 hours, dose to be administered over 15 minutes; maximum 60 mg/kg per day

continued →

4

Nervous system

▸ Adult (body-weight 51 kg and above): 1 g, every 4–6 hours, dose to be administered over 15 minutes; maximum 4 g per day
▸ BY RECTUM
▸ Adult: 0.5–1 g, every 4–6 hours; maximum 4 g per day

Mild to moderate pain in patients with risk factors for hepatotoxicity | Pyrexia in patients with risk factors for hepatotoxicity
▸ BY INTRAVENOUS INFUSION
▸ Adult (body-weight up to 51 kg): 15 mg/kg, every 4–6 hours, dose to be administered over 15 minutes; maximum 60 mg/kg per day
▸ Adult (body-weight 51 kg and above): 1 g, every 4–6 hours, dose to be administered over 15 minutes; maximum 3 g per day

Pain | Pyrexia with discomfort
▸ BY MOUTH
▸ Child 3–5 months: 60 mg, every 4–6 hours; maximum 4 doses per day
▸ Child 6–23 months: 120 mg, every 4–6 hours; maximum 4 doses per day
▸ Child 2–3 years: 180 mg, every 4–6 hours; maximum 4 doses per day
▸ Child 4–5 years: 240 mg, every 4–6 hours; maximum 4 doses per day
▸ Child 6–7 years: 240–250 mg, every 4–6 hours; maximum 4 doses per day
▸ Child 8–9 years: 360–375 mg, every 4–6 hours; maximum 4 doses per day
▸ Child 10–11 years: 480–500 mg, every 4–6 hours; maximum 4 doses per day
▸ Child 12–15 years: 480–750 mg, every 4–6 hours; maximum 4 doses per day
▸ Child 16–17 years: 0.5–1 g, every 4–6 hours; maximum 4 doses per day
▸ BY RECTUM
▸ Child 3–11 months: 60–125 mg every 4–6 hours as required, maximum 4 doses per day
▸ Child 1–4 years: 125–250 mg every 4–6 hours as required, maximum 4 doses per day
▸ Child 5–11 years: 250–500 mg every 4–6 hours as required, maximum 4 doses per day
▸ Child 12–17 years: 500 mg every 4–6 hours

Post-immunisation pyrexia in infants
▸ BY MOUTH
▸ Child 2–3 months: 60 mg for 1 dose, then 60 mg for 1 dose, to be given 4–6 hours after first dose if required
▸ Child 4 months: 60 mg for 1 dose, then 60 mg, to be given 4–6 hours after previous dose; maximum 4 doses per day

Acute migraine
▸ BY MOUTH
▸ Adult: 1 g for 1 dose, to be taken as soon as migraine symptoms develop

● **UNLICENSED USE** Paracetamol oral suspension 500 mg/5 mL not licensed for use in children under 16 years.

IMPORTANT SAFETY INFORMATION
HEALTH SERVICES SAFETY INVESTIGATIONS BODY (HSSIB) PATIENT SAFETY INVESTIGATIONS: UNINTENTIONAL OVERDOSE OF PARACETAMOL IN ADULTS WITH LOW BODYWEIGHT (FEBRUARY 2022)
A review of oral paracetamol prescriptions for adult inpatients with low body-weight (less than 50 kg) identified multiple incidents of overdose, including one death. To minimise the risk of harm, the HSSIB has issued advice: www.hssib.org.uk/patient-safety-investigations/unintentional-overdose-of-paracetamol-in-adults-with-low-bodyweight/.

● **CAUTIONS** Before administering, check when paracetamol last administered and cumulative paracetamol dose over previous 24 hours · body-weight under 50 kg · chronic alcohol consumption · chronic dehydration · chronic malnutrition · long-term use (especially in those who are malnourished)

CAUTIONS, FURTHER INFORMATION [EvGr] Some patients may be at increased risk of experiencing toxicity at therapeutic doses, particularly those with a body-weight under 50 kg and those with risk factors for hepatotoxicity. Clinical judgement should be used to adjust the dose of oral and intravenous paracetamol in these patients.
   Co-administration of enzyme-inducing antiepileptic medications may increase toxicity; doses should be reduced. (E)

● **INTERACTIONS** → Appendix 1: paracetamol

● **SIDE-EFFECTS**

GENERAL SIDE-EFFECTS
▸ **Rare or very rare** Thrombocytopenia

SPECIFIC SIDE-EFFECTS
▸ **Common or very common**
▸ With rectal use Anorectal erythema
▸ **Rare or very rare**
▸ With intravenous use Hypersensitivity · hypotension · leucopenia · malaise · neutropenia
▸ With rectal use Angioedema · liver injury · severe cutaneous adverse reactions (SCARs) · skin reactions
▸ **Frequency not known**
▸ With intravenous use Flushing · skin reactions · tachycardia
▸ With oral use Agranulocytosis · bronchospasm · hepatic function abnormal · rash · severe cutaneous adverse reactions (SCARs)
▸ With rectal use Agranulocytosis · blood disorder

Overdose Liver damage and less frequently renal damage can occur following overdose.
   Nausea and vomiting, the only early features of poisoning, usually settle within 24 hours. Persistence beyond this time, often associated with the onset of right subcostal pain and tenderness, usually indicates development of hepatic necrosis.
   For specific details on the management of poisoning, see Paracetamol, under Emergency treatment of poisoning p. 1554.

● **PREGNANCY** Not known to be harmful.

● **BREAST FEEDING** Amount too small to be harmful.

● **HEPATIC IMPAIRMENT** Manufacturer advises caution (increased risk of toxicity).

● **RENAL IMPAIRMENT** [EvGr] Caution in severe impairment (consult product literature). (M)
Dose adjustments
▸ With intravenous use [EvGr] Increase infusion dose interval to at least every 6 hours if creatinine clearance 30 mL/minute or less. (M) See p. 21.

● **DIRECTIONS FOR ADMINISTRATION** For *intravenous infusion* (*Perfalgan®*), manufacturer advises give in Glucose 5% *or* Sodium Chloride 0.9%; dilute to a concentration of not less than 1 mg/mL and use within an hour; may also be given undiluted.

● **PRESCRIBING AND DISPENSING INFORMATION** BP directs that when Paediatric Paracetamol Oral Suspension or Paediatric Paracetamol Mixture is prescribed Paracetamol Oral Suspension 120 mg/5 mL should be dispensed.

● **PATIENT AND CARER ADVICE**
Medicines for Children leaflet: Paracetamol for mild-to-moderate pain www.medicinesforchildren.org.uk/medicines/paracetamol/

● **PROFESSION SPECIFIC INFORMATION**
Dental practitioners' formulary Paracetamol Tablets may be prescribed.

Paracetamol Soluble Tablets 500 mg may be prescribed.
Paracetamol Oral Suspension may be prescribed.

- **EXCEPTIONS TO LEGAL CATEGORY** Paracetamol capsules or tablets can be sold to the public provided packs contain no more than 32 capsules or tablets; pharmacists can sell multiple packs up to a total quantity of 100 capsules or tablets in justifiable circumstances.

- **MEDICINAL FORMS** There can be variation in the licensing of different medicines containing the same drug. Forms available from special-order manufacturers include: oral suspension, oral solution, oral powder, suppository

Oral tablet
CAUTIONARY AND ADVISORY LABELS 29(500 mg tablets in adults), 30

▸ **Paracetamol (Non-proprietary)**
Paracetamol 500 mg Paracetamol 500mg caplets | 32 tablet [PoM] £0.90 DT = £0.67 | 100 tablet [PoM] £2.50 DT = £2.09
Paracetamol 500mg tablets | 32 tablet [PoM] [⅀] DT = £0.67 | 100 tablet [PoM] £3.30 DT = £2.09 | 1000 tablet [PoM] £20.90–£31.60
Paracetamol 1 gram Paracetamol 1g tablets | 100 tablet [PoM] £9.20 DT = £9.20

Suppository
CAUTIONARY AND ADVISORY LABELS 30

▸ **Paracetamol (Non-proprietary)**
Paracetamol 80 mg Paracetamol 80mg suppositories | 10 suppository [P] £10.00 DT = £10.00
Paracetamol 120 mg Paracetamol 120mg suppositories | 10 suppository [P] £38.72 DT = £23.01
Paracetamol 125 mg Paracetamol 125mg suppositories | 10 suppository [P] £12.07–£15.00 DT = £13.80
Paracetamol 240 mg Paracetamol 240mg suppositories | 10 suppository [P] £62.31 DT = £62.31
Paracetamol 250 mg Paracetamol 250mg suppositories | 10 suppository [P] £15.00–£27.60 DT = £27.60
Paracetamol 500 mg Paracetamol 500mg suppositories | 10 suppository [P] £41.27 DT = £41.27
Paracetamol 1 gram Paracetamol 1g suppositories | 10 suppository [P] £59.50–£60.00 DT = £59.50

▸ **Alvedon** (Esteve Pharmaceuticals Ltd)
Paracetamol 60 mg Alvedon 60mg suppositories | 10 suppository [P] £11.95
Paracetamol 125 mg Alvedon 125mg suppositories | 10 suppository [P] £13.80 DT = £13.80
Paracetamol 250 mg Alvedon 250mg suppositories | 10 suppository [P] £27.60 DT = £27.60

Oral suspension
CAUTIONARY AND ADVISORY LABELS 30

▸ **Paracetamol (Non-proprietary)**
Paracetamol 24 mg per 1 ml Paracetamol 120mg/5ml oral suspension paediatric | 100 ml [P] £3.69–£6.28
Paracetamol 120mg/5ml oral suspension paediatric sugar free | 100 ml [P] £3.01 DT = £2.71 [SF] | 200 ml [P] £4.84–£6.02 [SF] | 500 ml [P] £13.55–£18.90 [SF]
Paracetamol 50 mg per 1 ml Paracetamol 250mg/5ml oral suspension | 100 ml [P] £6.40 DT = £3.77 | 200 ml [P] £2.35 | 500 ml [P] £18.85–£31.70
Paracetamol 250mg/5ml oral suspension sugar free | 100 ml [P] £2.42–£4.47 [SF] | 200 ml [P] £12.00 DT = £9.17 [SF] | 500 ml [P] £13.83–£17.00 [SF] | 1000 ml [P] £42.40 [SF]
Paracetamol 100 mg per 1 ml Paracetamol 500mg/5ml oral suspension sugar free | 150 ml [PoM] £93.02 DT = £55.70 [SF]

▸ **Calpol** (McNeil Products Ltd)
Paracetamol 24 mg per 1 ml Calpol Infant Original 120mg/5ml oral suspension | 200 ml [P] £4.73
Calpol Infant 120mg/5ml oral suspension 5ml sachets sugar free | 12 sachet [GSL] £3.04 DT = £3.04 [SF] | 20 sachet [GSL] £4.85 DT = £4.85 [SF]
Calpol Infant 120mg/5ml oral suspension sugar free | 200 ml [P] £4.73 [SF]
Paracetamol 50 mg per 1 ml Calpol Six Plus 250mg/5ml oral suspension 5ml sachets sugar free | 12 sachet [GSL] £3.67 DT = £3.67 [SF]
Calpol Six Plus 250mg/5ml oral suspension sugar free | 100 ml [P] £3.42 [SF] | 200 ml [P] £5.60 DT = £9.17 [SF]

Effervescent tablet
CAUTIONARY AND ADVISORY LABELS 13, 29(500 mg tablets in adults), 30

▸ **Paracetamol (Non-proprietary)**
Paracetamol 500 mg Paracetamol 500mg soluble tablets | 100 tablet [PoM] [⅀] DT = £17.60
Paracetamol 500mg effervescent tablets | 60 tablet [PoM] £3.68–£8.10 | 100 tablet [PoM] £5.10–£11.58 DT = £4.56

▸ **Altridexamol** (TriOn Pharma Ltd)
Paracetamol 1 gram Altridexamol 1000mg effervescent tablets | 50 tablet [PoM] £7.89 DT = £7.89 [SF]

Oral capsule
CAUTIONARY AND ADVISORY LABELS 29(500 mg capsules in adults), 30

▸ **Paracetamol (Non-proprietary)**
Paracetamol 500 mg Paracetamol 500mg capsules | 100 capsule [PoM] £3.19 DT = £3.09

Solution for infusion

▸ **Paracetamol (Non-proprietary)**
Paracetamol 10 mg per 1 ml Paracetamol 500mg/50ml solution for infusion bottles | 10 bottle [PoM] £14.30 (Hospital only)
Paracetamol 500mg/50ml solution for infusion vials | 10 vial [PoM] £26.40
Paracetamol 1g/100ml solution for infusion bottles | 10 bottle [PoM] £12.45–£15.62 (Hospital only)
Paracetamol 1g/100ml solution for infusion vials | 10 vial [PoM] £132.00 (Hospital only)
Paracetamol 100mg/10ml solution for infusion ampoules | 20 ampoule [PoM] £101.00 (Hospital only)

Oral solution
CAUTIONARY AND ADVISORY LABELS 30

▸ **Paracetamol (Non-proprietary)**
Paracetamol 24 mg per 1 ml Paracetamol 120mg/5ml oral solution paediatric sugar free | 500 ml [P] [⅀] [SF]
Paracetamol 100 mg per 1 ml Paracetamol 500mg/5ml oral solution sugar free | 200 ml [PoM] £18.00 DT = £18.00 [SF]

Orodispersible tablet
CAUTIONARY AND ADVISORY LABELS 30

▸ **Calpol Fastmelts** (McNeil Products Ltd)
Paracetamol 250 mg Calpol Six Plus Fastmelts 250mg tablets | 24 tablet [P] £5.33 DT = £5.33 [SF]

Combinations available: *Co-codamol,* p. 515 · *Dihydrocodeine with paracetamol,* p. 519 · *Tramadol with paracetamol,* p. 536

ANALGESICS ❭ NON-OPIOID, CENTRALLY ACTING

Nefopam hydrochloride
23-Apr-2021

- **INDICATIONS AND DOSE**

Moderate pain
▸ BY MOUTH
▸ Adult: Initially 60 mg 3 times a day, adjusted according to response; usual dose 30–90 mg 3 times a day
▸ Elderly: Initially 30 mg 3 times a day, adjusted according to response; usual dose 30–90 mg 3 times a day

- **CONTRA-INDICATIONS** Convulsive disorders · not indicated for myocardial infarction

- **CAUTIONS** Angle-closure glaucoma · elderly · urinary retention

- **INTERACTIONS** → Appendix 1: nefopam

- **SIDE-EFFECTS**
▸ **Uncommon** Coma · drowsiness · headache · hyperhidrosis · insomnia · tachycardia · vision blurred · vomiting
▸ **Rare or very rare** Urine discolouration
▸ **Frequency not known** Abdominal pain · angioedema · confusion · diarrhoea · dizziness · dry mouth · gastrointestinal disorder · hallucination · hypotension · nausea · nervousness · palpitations · paraesthesia · seizure · syncope · tremor · urinary retention

- **PREGNANCY** No information available—avoid unless no safer treatment.

- **HEPATIC IMPAIRMENT** Manufacturer advises caution.

- **RENAL IMPAIRMENT** [EvGr] Use with caution. (M)
Dose adjustments [EvGr] Reduce daily dose in end-stage renal disease. (M)

- **MEDICINAL FORMS** There can be variation in the licensing of different medicines containing the same drug. Forms available from special-order manufacturers include: oral suspension

Oral tablet
CAUTIONARY AND ADVISORY LABELS 2, 14
▸ **Nefopam hydrochloride (Non-proprietary)**
Nefopam hydrochloride 30 mg Nefopam 30mg tablets |
30 tablet [PoM] £1.89–£4.97 | 90 tablet [PoM] £68.73 DT = £3.87
Nefopam hydrochloride 60 mg Nefopam 60mg tablets |
60 tablet [PoM] £19.90 DT = £19.90

ANALGESICS › NON-STEROIDAL ANTI-INFLAMMATORY DRUGS

Aspirin with codeine
14-Jul-2020

The properties listed below are those particular to the combination only. For the properties of the components please consider, aspirin p. 142, codeine phosphate p. 517.

● INDICATIONS AND DOSE

Mild to moderate pain | Pyrexia
▸ BY MOUTH
▸ Adult: 1–2 tablets every 4–6 hours as required; maximum 8 tablets per day

- **INTERACTIONS** → Appendix 1: aspirin · opioids
- **PRESCRIBING AND DISPENSING INFORMATION** When co-codaprin tablets or dispersible tablets are prescribed and no strength is stated, tablets or dispersible tablets, respectively, containing codeine phosphate 8 mg and aspirin 400 mg should be dispensed.
- **LESS SUITABLE FOR PRESCRIBING** Aspirin with codeine is less suitable for prescribing.
- **EXCEPTIONS TO LEGAL CATEGORY** Aspirin with codeine can be sold to the public provided packs contain no more than 32 capsules or tablets; pharmacists can sell multiple packs up to a total quantity of 100 capsules or tablets in justifiable circumstances.
- **MEDICINAL FORMS** No licensed medicines listed.

ANALGESICS › OPIOIDS

Opioids 

> **IMPORTANT SAFETY INFORMATION**
> **MHRA/CHM ADVICE: BENZODIAZEPINES AND OPIOIDS: REMINDER OF RISK OF POTENTIALLY FATAL RESPIRATORY DEPRESSION (MARCH 2020)**
> The MHRA reminds healthcare professionals that opioids co-prescribed with benzodiazepines and benzodiazepine-like drugs can produce additive CNS depressant effects, thereby increasing the risk of sedation, respiratory depression, coma, and death. Healthcare professionals are advised to only co-prescribe if there is no alternative and, if necessary, the lowest possible doses should be given for the shortest duration. Patients should be closely monitored for signs of respiratory depression at initiation of treatment and when there is any change in prescribing, such as dose adjustments or new interactions. If methadone is co-prescribed with a benzodiazepine or benzodiazepine-like drug, the respiratory depressant effect of methadone may be delayed; patients should be monitored for at least 2 weeks after initiation or changes in prescribing. Patients should be informed of the signs and symptoms of respiratory depression and sedation, and advised to seek urgent medical attention should these occur.

> **MHRA/CHM ADVICE: OPIOIDS: RISK OF DEPENDENCE AND ADDICTION (SEPTEMBER 2020)**
> New safety recommendations have been issued following a review of the risks of dependence and addiction associated with prolonged use (longer than 3 months) of opioids for non-malignant pain.
> Healthcare professionals are advised to:
> - discuss with patients that prolonged use of opioids, even at therapeutic doses, may lead to dependence and addiction;
> - agree a treatment strategy and plan for end of treatment with the patient before starting opioids;
> - counsel patients and their carers on the risks of tolerance and potentially fatal unintentional overdose, as well as signs and symptoms of overdose;
> - provide regular monitoring and support to patients at increased risk, such as those with current or history of substance use disorder (including alcohol misuse) or mental health disorders;
> - taper dosage slowly at the end of treatment to reduce the risk of withdrawal effects associated with abrupt discontinuation (tapering high doses may take weeks or months);
> - consider hyperalgesia in patients on long-term opioid treatment who present with increased pain sensitivity;
> - consult product literature for the latest advice and warnings for opioid use during pregnancy (see also *Pregnancy*).
>
> The MHRA has also issued a safety leaflet for patients— see *Patient and carer advice*.

> **MHRA/CHM ADVICE: PROLONGED-RELEASE OPIOIDS: REMOVAL OF INDICATION FOR RELIEF OF POST-OPERATIVE PAIN (MARCH 2025)**
> Following a safety review by the MHRA and advice from the CHM, treatment of postoperative pain will be removed from the licensed indications of modified-release morphine and modified-release oxycodone due to the potential for harm and increased risk of persistent postoperative opioid use (PPOU) and opioid-induced ventilatory impairment (OIVI). Modified-release opioids provide relief from chronic severe pain and should not be used for acute pain relief after surgery; transdermal patches are also not recommended for such use. Modified-release opioids are associated with PPOU, defined as continued opioid use beyond 90 days after surgery, and OIVI, a serious form of respiratory depression that causes central respiratory depression, sedation, and upper airway obstruction.
> Before surgery, healthcare professionals should discuss with the patient:
> - the risks of PPOU and dependence, and potential risk of addiction and withdrawal reactions;
> - the risk of OIVI, especially in those with underlying respiratory conditions;
> - that postoperative pain is normally short-lived and should only require short-term treatment with immediate-release opioids;
> - pain management strategies involving immediate-release opioids and multimodal analgesia, and plan for end of treatment.
>
> Healthcare professionals should review the treatment, before and after surgery, of patients whose pain is managed with opioids pre-operatively, in line with Consensus Best Practice Guidelines (available at: www.cpoc.org.uk/sites/cpoc/files/documents/2021-03/surgery-and-opioids-2021.pdf).
> At discharge from hospital, healthcare professionals should:
> - only prescribe and supply a sufficient amount of immediate-release opioids for acute postoperative pain relief to minimise the risk of PPOU, dependence,

stockpiling of unused opioids, and potential for diversion;
- communicate the pain management plan with primary care practice taking over care in the community and document in the patient's clinical notes.

Healthcare professionals should advise patients to:
- talk to their doctor about pain management and ongoing needs if they are already on modified-release opioids before surgery, as the risk of respiratory depression and PPOU is higher;
- dial 999 if they notice new or increased trouble with breathing;
- contact their doctor if they feel unable to stop taking opioids as originally planned.

Patients or their carer who are concerned about using more opioids than prescribed should also be counselled to seek advice from the NHS website (available at: www.nhs.uk/live-well/pain/how-to-get-nhs-help-for-your-pain/), or in Northern Ireland, the Health and Social Care website (available at: online.hscni.net/our-work/pharmacy-and-medicines-management/patient-initiatives/long-term-pain/).

- **CONTRA-INDICATIONS** Acute respiratory depression · comatose patients · head injury (opioid analgesics interfere with pupillary responses vital for neurological assessment) · raised intracranial pressure (opioid analgesics interfere with pupillary responses vital for neurological assessment) · risk of paralytic ileus

- **CAUTIONS** Adrenocortical insufficiency (reduced dose is recommended) · asthma (avoid during an acute attack) · central sleep apnoea · convulsive disorders · current or history of mental health disorder · current or history of substance use disorder · debilitated patients (reduced dose is recommended) (in adults) · diseases of the biliary tract · elderly (reduced dose is recommended) · hypotension · hypothyroidism (reduced dose is recommended) · impaired respiratory function (avoid in chronic obstructive pulmonary disease) · inflammatory bowel disorders · myasthenia gravis · obstructive bowel disorders · prostatic hypertrophy (in adults) · shock · urethral stenosis

  CAUTIONS, FURTHER INFORMATION
  ▸ Dependence and addiction Prolonged use of opioid analgesics may lead to drug dependence and addiction, even at therapeutic doses. There is an increased risk in individuals with current or history of substance use disorder or mental health disorders. See also *Important safety information*.
  ▸ Central sleep apnoea Opioids cause a dose-dependent increased risk of central sleep apnoea, Ⓔⱽᴳʳ consider total opioid dose reduction. Ⓜ
  ▸ Palliative care Ⓔⱽᴳʳ In the control of pain in terminal illness, the cautions listed should not necessarily be a deterrent to the use of opioid analgesics. Ⓜ
  ▸ Elderly Screening Tool of Older Persons' potentially inappropriate Prescriptions (STOPP) criteria to aid medication reviews (see Prescribing in the elderly p. 31 for information). Potentially inappropriate:
    - if prescribed a **strong, oral,** or **transdermal** opioid (i.e. morphine, oxycodone, fentanyl, buprenorphine, diamorphine, methadone, tramadol, pethidine, pentazocine) as first-line therapy for mild pain (WHO analgesic ladder not observed)
    - if used regularly without concomitant laxative (risk of severe constipation)
    - if prescribed a **long-acting (modified-release)** opioid without a **short-acting (immediate-release)** opioid for breakthrough pain (risk of persistence of severe pain)

- **SIDE-EFFECTS**
  ▸ **Common or very common** Arrhythmias · confusion · constipation · dizziness · drowsiness · dry mouth · euphoric mood · flushing · hallucination · headache · hyperhidrosis ·

hypotension (with high doses) · miosis · nausea (more common on initiation) · palpitations · respiratory depression (with high doses) · skin reactions · urinary retention · vertigo · visual impairment · vomiting (more common on initiation) · withdrawal syndrome
▸ **Uncommon** Drug dependence · dysphoria · seizure

  SIDE-EFFECTS, FURTHER INFORMATION **Respiratory depression** Respiratory depression is a major concern with opioid analgesics and it may be treated by artificial ventilation or be reversed by naloxone.

  Dependence, addiction, and withdrawal Long term use of opioids in non-malignant pain (longer than 3 months) carries an increased risk of dependence and addiction, even at therapeutic doses. At the end of treatment the dosage should be tapered slowly to reduce the risk of withdrawal effects; tapering from a high dose may take weeks or months. See also *Important safety information*.

  Overdose Opioids (narcotic analgesics) cause coma, respiratory depression, and pinpoint pupils. For details on the management of poisoning, see Opioids, under Emergency treatment of poisoning p. 1554 and consider the specific antidote, naloxone hydrochloride.

- **PREGNANCY** Respiratory depression and withdrawal symptoms can occur in the neonate if opioid analgesics are used during delivery; also gastric stasis and inhalation pneumonia has been reported in the mother if opioid analgesics are used during labour.

- **TREATMENT CESSATION** Avoid abrupt withdrawal after long-term treatment; they should be withdrawn gradually to avoid abstinence symptoms.

- **PRESCRIBING AND DISPENSING INFORMATION** The *Faculty of Pain Medicine* has produced resources for healthcare professionals around opioid prescribing: www.fpm.ac.uk/faculty-of-pain-medicine/opioids-aware

- **PATIENT AND CARER ADVICE**
  MHRA safety leaflet: Opioid medicines and the risk of addiction www.gov.uk/guidance/opioid-medicines-and-the-risk-of-addiction

  Driving and skilled tasks Drowsiness may affect performance of skilled tasks (e.g. driving); effects of alcohol enhanced. Driving at the start of therapy with opioid analgesics, and following dose changes, should be avoided.

  For information on 2015 legislation regarding driving whilst taking certain controlled drugs, including opioids, see *Drugs and driving* under Guidance on prescribing p. 1.

⊩ 510

Buprenorphine

15-Feb-2024

- **DRUG ACTION** Buprenorphine is an opioid-receptor partial agonist (it has opioid agonist and antagonist properties).

- **INDICATIONS AND DOSE**
  Moderate to severe pain
  ▸ BY SUBLINGUAL ADMINISTRATION
  ▸ Child (body-weight 16-25 kg): 100 micrograms every 6–8 hours
  ▸ Child (body-weight 25-37.5 kg): 100–200 micrograms every 6–8 hours
  ▸ Child (body-weight 37.5-50 kg): 200–300 micrograms every 6–8 hours
  ▸ Child (body-weight 50 kg and above): 200–400 micrograms every 6–8 hours
  ▸ Adult: 200–400 micrograms every 6–8 hours
  ▸ BY INTRAMUSCULAR INJECTION, OR BY SLOW INTRAVENOUS INJECTION
  ▸ Child 6 months-11 years: 3–6 micrograms/kg every 6–8 hours (max. per dose 9 micrograms/kg)
  ▸ Child 12-17 years: 300–600 micrograms every 6–8 hours

continued →

▸ Adult: 300–600 micrograms every 6–8 hours

Premedication

▸ BY SUBLINGUAL ADMINISTRATION
▸ Adult: 400 micrograms
▸ BY INTRAMUSCULAR INJECTION
▸ Adult: 300 micrograms

Intra-operative analgesia

▸ BY SLOW INTRAVENOUS INJECTION
▸ Adult: 300–450 micrograms

Adjunct in the treatment of opioid dependence (under expert supervision)

▸ BY SUBLINGUAL ADMINISTRATION USING SUBLINGUAL TABLETS
▸ Adult: Initially 0.8–4 mg for 1 dose on the first day, adjusted in steps of 2–4 mg daily if required; usual dose 12–24 mg daily, for further information about switching from methadone to sublingual buprenorphine, consult product literature; maximum 32 mg per day
▸ BY MOUTH USING ORAL LYOPHILISATE
▸ Adult: Initially 2 mg daily, followed by 2–4 mg if required on day one, adjusted in steps of 2–6 mg daily if required, for adjustment of dosing interval following stabilisation or for further information about switching from methadone to buprenorphine, consult product literature; maximum 18 mg per day

Moderate to severe chronic pain unresponsive to non-opioid analgesics in opioid-naïve patients (administered on expert advice)

▸ BY TRANSDERMAL APPLICATION USING PATCHES
▸ Adult: Initially 5 micrograms/hour, using the 7-day patches, *Bunov*®, *Bupramyl*®, *Butec*®, *BuTrans*®, *Panitaz*®, *Rebrikel*®, *Reletrans*®, or *Sevodyne*®. If necessary, dose should be adjusted at intervals of at least 3 days. Maximum 2 patches can be used at any one time, applied at same time to avoid confusion. For chronic non-cancer pain, usual maximum one 20 microgram/hour patch, seek specialist advice if further dose increases required. For further information including morphine equivalent doses and the management of breakthrough pain, see Opioid analgesics in Prescribing in palliative care p. 26.

Moderate to severe chronic cancer pain in patients currently treated with an opioid analgesic (administered on expert advice) | Severe chronic non-cancer pain in patients currently treated with an opioid analgesic (administered on expert advice)

▸ BY TRANSDERMAL APPLICATION USING PATCHES
▸ Adult: Initial dose should be based on previous 24-hour opioid requirement. If necessary, dose should be adjusted when the next patch is due. Maximum 2 patches can be used at any one time, applied at the same time to avoid confusion. For chronic non-cancer pain, usual maximum one 35 microgram/hour patch, seek specialist advice if further dose increases required. For further information including conversion from long-term oral morphine to transdermal buprenorphine, and for the management of breakthrough pain, see Opioid analgesics, in Prescribing in palliative care p. 26.

PHARMACOKINETICS

▸ With transdermal use For 7-day patches (*Bunov*®, *Bupramyl*®, *Butec*®, *BuTrans*®, *Panitaz*®, *Rebrikel*®, *Reletrans*®, *Sevodyne*®): analgesic effect should be evaluated after the system has been worn for at least 3 days to allow for gradual increase in plasma-buprenorphine concentration. It takes approximately 12 hours for the plasma-buprenorphine concentration to decrease by 50% after patch is removed. For 4-day patches (*Bupeaze*®, *Carlosafine*®, *Relevtec*®, *Transtec*®): analgesic effect should be evaluated after the system has been worn

for at least 1 day to allow for gradual increase in plasma-buprenorphine concentration. It takes approximately 30 hours for the plasma-buprenorphine concentration to decrease by 50% after patch is removed. For 3-day patches (*Hapoctasin*®): analgesic effect should be evaluated after the system has been worn for at least 1 day to allow for gradual increase in plasma-buprenorphine concentration. It takes approximately 25 hours for the plasma-buprenorphine concentration to decrease by 50% after patch is removed.

BUVIDAL®

Adjunct in the treatment of opioid dependence (under expert supervision)

▸ BY SUBCUTANEOUS INJECTION
▸ Adult: (consult product literature)

PHARMACOKINETICS

▸ *Buvidal*® injections are available in formulations that can be given weekly or monthly depending on the strength of the injection.
▸ Weekly *Buvidal*® (8 mg, 16 mg, 24 mg, and 32 mg injections) has a terminal half-life ranging from 3 to 5 days.
▸ Monthly *Buvidal*® (64 mg, 96 mg, 128 mg, and 160 mg injections) has a terminal half-life ranging from 19 to 25 days.

SIXMO®

Adjunct in the treatment of opioid dependence [in clinically stable patients who require no more than 8 mg per day of sublingual buprenorphine] (under expert supervision)

▸ BY SUBCUTANEOUS IMPLANTATION
▸ Adult 18–65 years: 296.8 mg, dose consists of 4 implants (each containing 74.2 mg) to be left in place for 6 months, sublingual buprenorphine should be discontinued 12 to 24 hours prior to insertion, for supplemental sublingual buprenorphine, treatment discontinuation, and re-treatment—consult product literature

● UNLICENSED USE [EvGr] Buprenorphine transdermal patches are used in the doses provided in the BNF for chronic pain, ⟨E⟩ but these may differ from those licensed. Sublingual tablets not licensed for use in children under 6 years.

> IMPORTANT SAFETY INFORMATION
> Do not confuse the formulations of transdermal patches which are available in various strengths as 7-day, 4-day and 3-day patches; prescription by brand name is recommended. See *Prescribing and dispensing information.*

● CONTRA-INDICATIONS
SIXMO® Contra-indications for magnetic resonance imaging (MRI) · history of keloid or hypertrophic scar formation

● CAUTIONS
GENERAL CAUTIONS Impaired consciousness
SPECIFIC CAUTIONS
▸ With transdermal use Fever or external heat · other opioids should not be administered within 24 hours of patch removal (long duration of action)
▸ When used for Adjunct in the treatment of opioid dependence Hepatitis B infection · hepatitis C infection · pre-existing liver enzyme abnormalities
CAUTIONS, FURTHER INFORMATION
▸ Fever or external heat
▸ With transdermal use Manufacturer advises monitor patients using patches for increased side-effects if fever present (increased absorption possible); avoid exposing

application site to external heat (may also increase absorption).

BUVIDAL[®] Susceptibility to QT-interval prolongation

SIXMO[®] History of connective tissue disease · history of recurrent meticillin-resistant *Staphylococcus aureus* infection

● **INTERACTIONS** → Appendix 1: opioids

● **SIDE-EFFECTS**

GENERAL SIDE-EFFECTS

▶ **Common or very common** Anxiety · depression · diarrhoea · tremor

SPECIFIC SIDE-EFFECTS

▶ **Common or very common**

▶ When used by implant Appetite abnormal · asthenia · chills · gastrointestinal discomfort · hot flush · increased risk of infection · malaise · pain · procedural pain · sleep disorders

▶ With parenteral use Appetite decreased (in adults) · arthralgia (in adults) · asthenia (in adults) · asthma (in adults) · behaviour abnormal (in adults) · chest pain (in adults) · chills (in adults) · cough (in adults) · dysmenorrhoea (in adults) · dyspnoea (in adults) · eye disorders (in adults) · fever (in adults) · gastrointestinal discomfort (in adults) · gastrointestinal disorders (in adults) · hypersensitivity · increased risk of infection (in adults) · insomnia (in adults) · lymphadenopathy (in adults) · malaise (in adults) · migraine (in adults) · muscle complaints (in adults) · muscle tone increased (in adults) · pain (in adults) · paraesthesia (in adults) · peripheral oedema (in adults) · speech disorder (in adults) · syncope (in adults) · thinking abnormal (in adults) · vasodilation (in adults) · withdrawal syndrome neonatal · yawning (in adults)

▶ With sublingual use Fatigue · sleep disorders

▶ With transdermal use Appetite decreased · asthenia · dyspnoea · gastrointestinal discomfort · muscle weakness · oedema · sleep disorders

▶ **Uncommon**

▶ When used by implant Cold sweat · dehydration · device complications · dysmenorrhoea · eye disorders · feeling cold · fever · flatulence · haematochezia · irritability · joint disorders · level of consciousness decreased · limb discomfort · lymphadenopathy · migraine · muscle spasms · neutropenia · oedema · post procedural complication · sensation abnormal · sexual dysfunction · swelling · thinking abnormal · urinary disorders · vision blurred · weight changes · yawning

▶ With parenteral use Procedural dizziness (in adults)

▶ With sublingual use Apnoea · appetite decreased · atrioventricular block · coma · conjunctivitis · coordination abnormal · cyanosis · depersonalisation · diplopia · dyspepsia · dyspnoea · hypertension · pallor · paraesthesia · psychosis · speech slurred · tinnitus · urinary disorder

▶ With transdermal use Aggression · chest pain · chills · circulatory collapse · concentration impaired · cough · dry eye · fever · gastrointestinal disorders · hiccups · hypertension · injury · memory loss · migraine · mood altered · movement disorders · muscle complaints · respiratory disorders · sensation abnormal · sexual dysfunction · speech impairment · syncope · taste altered · tinnitus · urinary disorders · vision blurred · weight decreased

▶ **Rare or very rare**

▶ With sublingual use Angioedema · bronchospasm

▶ With transdermal use Angina pectoris · asthma exacerbated · dehydration · dysphagia · ear pain · eyelid oedema · increased risk of infection · influenza like illness · muscle contractions involuntary · psychotic disorder · vasodilation

▶ **Frequency not known**

▶ When used by implant Hepatic disorders · hepatic encephalopathy

▶ With parenteral use Angioedema · bronchospasm · death (in adults) · hepatic disorders · hepatic encephalopathy (in adults) · psychotic disorder · vision blurred

▶ With sublingual use Cerebrospinal fluid pressure increased · circulation impaired · haemorrhagic diathesis · hepatic disorders · oral disorders · syncope

▶ With transdermal use Biliary colic · depersonalisation · withdrawal syndrome neonatal

Overdose The effects of buprenorphine are only partially reversed by naloxone.

● **PREGNANCY**

SIXMO[®] [EvGr] Avoid—inappropriate due to inflexible dosing of preparation. (M)

● **BREAST FEEDING** Present in low levels in breast milk. **Monitoring** Neonates should be monitored for drowsiness, adequate weight gain, and developmental milestones.

● **HEPATIC IMPAIRMENT** Manufacturer advises caution; avoid in severe impairment (limited information available).

For *transdermal patch*, manufacturer advises consider avoiding in severe impairment.

Dose adjustments For *oral lyophilisate*, manufacturer advises initial dose reduction in mild to moderate impairment.

● **RENAL IMPAIRMENT** Some manufacturers advise caution in severe impairment (risk of increased and prolonged effects; consult product literature).

Dose adjustments For *sublingual tablets*, some manufacturers advise dose reduction may be required in severe impairment (consult product literature).

● **PRE-TREATMENT SCREENING** Documentation of viral hepatitis status is recommended before commencing therapy for opioid dependence.

● **MONITORING REQUIREMENTS**

▶ Monitor liver function; when used in opioid dependence baseline liver function test is recommended before commencing therapy, and regular liver function tests should be performed throughout treatment.

▶ [EvGr] For *subcutaneous implant*, monitor for signs of infection and problems with wound healing 1 week after insertion and regularly thereafter. (M)

● **DIRECTIONS FOR ADMINISTRATION**

▶ In children Manufacturer advises *sublingual tablets* may be halved.

▶ In adults Manufacturer advises *oral lyophilisates* should be placed on the tongue and allowed to dissolve. Patients should be advised not to swallow for 2 minutes and not to consume food or drink for at least 5 minutes after administration.

▶ With transdermal use [EvGr] Apply 7-day patches to dry, non-irritated, non-hairy skin on upper torso or upper arm. Site replacement patch on a different area. Avoid applying to the same area for at least 3 weeks.

Apply 3-day or 4-day patches to dry, non-irritated, non-hairy skin on upper torso. Site replacement patch on a different area. Avoid applying to the same area for at least 7 days. (M)

● **PRESCRIBING AND DISPENSING INFORMATION**

▶ With transdermal use Transdermal buprenorphine patches are not suitable for acute pain or in those patients whose analgesic requirements are changing rapidly because the long time to steady state prevents rapid titration of the dose. Transdermal patches are available in strengths of 5, 10, 15 and 20 micrograms/hour as 7-day formulations; and 35, 52.5 and 70 micrograms/hour as 4-day or 3-day formulations. Prescribers and dispensers must ensure that the correct preparation is prescribed and dispensed; prescription by brand name is recommended to reduce the risk of confusion and errors. Preparations that should be applied up to every 3 days (72 hours) include *Hapoctasin*[®]. Preparations that should be applied up to every 4 days

(96 hours) include *Bupeaze* ®, *Carlosafine* ®, *Relevtec* ®, and *Transtec* ®. Preparations that should be applied up to every 7 days include *Bunov* ®, *Bupramyl* ®, *Butec* ®, *BuTrans* ®, *Panitaz* ®, *Rebrikel* ®, *Reletrans* ®, and *Sevodyne* ®.

▸ With oral use in adults *Espranor* ® oral lyophilisate has different bioavailability to other buprenorphine products and is not interchangeable with them—consult product literature before switching between products.

SIXMO ® Patients previously treated with sublingual buprenorphine, or sublingual buprenorphine with naloxone, must be on stable daily buprenorphine doses of 2 to 8 mg for at least 30 days before switching to *Sixmo* ® subcutaneous implant. Educational risk minimisation materials for *Sixmo* ® subcutaneous implant are available for healthcare professionals.

● **PATIENT AND CARER ADVICE** Patients or carers should be given advice on how to administer buprenorphine products.

For *subcutaneous implant*, patients and carers should be advised to seek immediate medical attention if spontaneous expulsion of the implant occurs and to store it in a closed glass jar away from others.

Alert card For *subcutaneous implant*, a patient alert card should be provided.

Driving and skilled tasks For *subcutaneous implant*, patients and carers should be counselled on the risk of somnolence lasting for up to 1 week after insertion.

● **NATIONAL FUNDING/ACCESS DECISIONS** For full details see funding body website

NICE decisions

▸ Methadone and buprenorphine for the management of opioid dependence (January 2007) NICE TA114 Recommended

Scottish Medicines Consortium (SMC) decisions

▸ Buprenorphine transdermal patches (*Butec* ®) for the treatment of chronic non-malignant pain of moderate intensity when an opioid is necessary for obtaining adequate analgesia in adults (January 2017) SMC No. 1213/17 Recommended with restrictions

▸ Buprenorphine oral lyophilisate (*Espranor* ®) as substitution treatment for opioid drug dependence, within a framework of medical, social and psychological treatment (June 2017) SMC No. 1245/17 Recommended with restrictions

▸ Buprenorphine (*Buvidal* ®) for the treatment of opioid dependence within a framework of medical, social and psychological treatment (August 2019) SMC No. SMC2169 Recommended with restrictions

▸ Buprenorphine implant (*Sixmo* ®) as substitution treatment for opioid dependence in clinically stable adult patients who require no more than 8 mg/day of sublingual buprenorphine, within a framework of medical, social and psychological treatment (December 2021) SMC No. SMC2372 Recommended

All Wales Medicines Strategy Group (AWMSG) decisions

▸ Buprenorphine (*Buvidal* ®) for the treatment of opioid dependence within a framework of medical, social and psychological treatment (September 2019) AWMSG No. 3977 Recommended

▸ Buprenorphine implant (*Sixmo* ®) as substitution treatment for opioid dependence in clinically stable adult patients who require no more than 8 mg/day of sublingual buprenorphine, within a framework of medical, social and psychological treatment (February 2022) AWMSG No. 4262 Not recommended

● **MEDICINAL FORMS** There can be variation in the licensing of different medicines containing the same drug.

Prolonged-release subcutaneous implant

▸ Sixmo (Accord-UK Ltd) ▼
Buprenorphine (as Buprenorphine hydrochloride) 74.2 mg Sixmo 74.2mg implant | 4 device PoM £1,438.20 CD3

Sublingual tablet

CAUTIONARY AND ADVISORY LABELS 2, 26

▸ **Buprenorphine (Non-proprietary)**
Buprenorphine (as Buprenorphine hydrochloride) 400 microgram Buprenorphine 400microgram sublingual tablets sugar free | 7 tablet PoM £1.60 DT = £1.36 CD3 SF
Buprenorphine (as Buprenorphine hydrochloride) 2 mg Buprenorphine 2mg sublingual tablets sugar free | 7 tablet PoM £5.38 DT = £1.35 CD3 SF
Buprenorphine (as Buprenorphine hydrochloride) 8 mg Buprenorphine 8mg sublingual tablets sugar free | 7 tablet PoM £16.15 DT = £3.13 CD3 SF

▸ **Prefibin** (Sandoz Ltd)
Buprenorphine (as Buprenorphine hydrochloride) 400 microgram Prefibin 0.4mg sublingual tablets | 7 tablet PoM £1.60 DT = £1.36 CD3 SF
Buprenorphine (as Buprenorphine hydrochloride) 2 mg Prefibin 2mg sublingual tablets | 7 tablet PoM £5.38 DT = £1.35 CD3 SF
Buprenorphine (as Buprenorphine hydrochloride) 8 mg Prefibin 8mg sublingual tablets | 7 tablet PoM £16.15 DT = £3.13 CD3 SF

▸ **Subutex** (Indivior UK Ltd)
Buprenorphine (as Buprenorphine hydrochloride) 400 microgram Subutex 0.4mg sublingual tablets | 7 tablet PoM £1.36 DT = £1.36 CD3 SF
Buprenorphine (as Buprenorphine hydrochloride) 2 mg Subutex 2mg sublingual tablets | 7 tablet PoM £4.45 DT = £1.35 CD3 SF
Buprenorphine (as Buprenorphine hydrochloride) 8 mg Subutex 8mg sublingual tablets | 7 tablet PoM £13.34 DT = £3.13 CD3 SF

▸ **Temgesic** (Eumedica Pharma Ltd)
Buprenorphine (as Buprenorphine hydrochloride) 200 microgram Temgesic 200microgram sublingual tablets | 50 tablet PoM £5.04 DT = £5.04 CD3 SF
Buprenorphine (as Buprenorphine hydrochloride) 400 microgram Temgesic 400microgram sublingual tablets | 50 tablet PoM £10.07 DT = £10.07 CD3 SF

▸ **Tephine** (Sandoz Ltd)
Buprenorphine (as Buprenorphine hydrochloride) 200 microgram Tephine 200microgram sublingual tablets | 50 tablet PoM £4.27 DT = £5.04 CD3 SF
Buprenorphine (as Buprenorphine hydrochloride) 400 microgram Tephine 400microgram sublingual tablets | 50 tablet PoM £8.54 DT = £10.07 CD3 SF

Transdermal patch

CAUTIONARY AND ADVISORY LABELS 2

▸ **BuTrans** (Napp Pharmaceuticals Ltd)
Buprenorphine 5 microgram per 1 hour BuTrans 5micrograms/hour transdermal patches | 4 patch PoM £17.60 DT = £17.60 CD3
Buprenorphine 10 microgram per 1 hour BuTrans 10micrograms/hour transdermal patches | 4 patch PoM £31.55 DT = £31.55 CD3
Buprenorphine 15 microgram per 1 hour BuTrans 15micrograms/hour transdermal patches | 4 patch PoM £49.15 DT = £49.15 CD3
Buprenorphine 20 microgram per 1 hour BuTrans 20micrograms/hour transdermal patches | 4 patch PoM £57.46 DT = £57.46 CD3

▸ **Bunov** (Glenmark Pharmaceuticals Europe Ltd)
Buprenorphine 5 microgram per 1 hour Bunov 5micrograms/hour transdermal patches | 4 patch PoM £5.54 DT = £17.60 CD3
Buprenorphine 10 microgram per 1 hour Bunov 10micrograms/hour transdermal patches | 4 patch PoM £9.94 DT = £31.55 CD3
Buprenorphine 20 microgram per 1 hour Bunov 20micrograms/hour transdermal patches | 4 patch PoM £18.10 DT = £57.46 CD3

▸ **Bupeaze** (Dr Reddy's Laboratories (UK) Ltd)
Buprenorphine 35 microgram per 1 hour Bupeaze 35micrograms/hour transdermal patches | 4 patch PoM £9.47 DT = £15.80 CD3
Buprenorphine 52.5 microgram per 1 hour Bupeaze 52.5micrograms/hour transdermal patches | 4 patch PoM £13.99 DT = £23.71 CD3
Buprenorphine 70 microgram per 1 hour Bupeaze 70micrograms/hour transdermal patches | 4 patch PoM £17.99 DT = £31.60 CD3

▸ **Butec** (Qdem Pharmaceuticals Ltd)
Buprenorphine 5 microgram per 1 hour Butec 5micrograms/hour transdermal patches | 4 patch PoM £7.92 DT = £17.60 CD3

Buprenorphine 10 microgram per 1 hour Butec
10micrograms/hour transdermal patches | 4 patch [PoM] £14.20 DT =
£31.55 [CD3]

Buprenorphine 15 microgram per 1 hour Butec
15micrograms/hour transdermal patches | 4 patch [PoM] £22.12 DT =
£49.15 [CD3]

Buprenorphine 20 microgram per 1 hour Butec
20micrograms/hour transdermal patches | 4 patch [PoM] £25.86 DT =
£57.46 [CD3]

▶ **Carlosafine** (Glenmark Pharmaceuticals Europe Ltd)

Buprenorphine 35 microgram per 1 hour Carlosafine
35micrograms/hour transdermal patches | 4 patch [PoM] £9.48 DT =
£15.80 [CD3]

Buprenorphine 52.5 microgram per 1 hour Carlosafine
52.5micrograms/hour transdermal patches | 4 patch [PoM] £14.23 DT
= £23.71 [CD3]

Buprenorphine 70 microgram per 1 hour Carlosafine
70micrograms/hour transdermal patches | 4 patch [PoM] £18.96 DT =
£31.60 [CD3]

▶ **Hapoctasin** (Accord-UK Ltd)

Buprenorphine 35 microgram per 1 hour Hapoctasin
35micrograms/hour transdermal patches | 4 patch [PoM] £9.48 DT =
£15.80 [CD3]

Buprenorphine 52.5 microgram per 1 hour Hapoctasin
52.5micrograms/hour transdermal patches | 4 patch [PoM] £14.23 DT
= £23.71 [CD3]

Buprenorphine 70 microgram per 1 hour Hapoctasin
70micrograms/hour transdermal patches | 4 patch [PoM] £18.96 DT =
£31.60 [CD3]

▶ **Panitaz** (Dr Reddy's Laboratories (UK) Ltd)

Buprenorphine 10 microgram per 1 hour Panitaz
10micrograms/hour transdermal patches | 4 patch [PoM] £12.62 DT =
£31.55 [CD3]

Buprenorphine 20 microgram per 1 hour Panitaz
20micrograms/hour transdermal patches | 4 patch [PoM] £22.98 DT =
£57.46 [CD3]

▶ **Rebrikel** (Zentiva Pharma UK Ltd)

Buprenorphine 5 microgram per 1 hour Rebrikel
5micrograms/hour transdermal patches | 4 patch [PoM] £5.25 DT =
£17.60 [CD3]

Buprenorphine 10 microgram per 1 hour Rebrikel
10micrograms/hour transdermal patches | 4 patch [PoM] £9.43 DT =
£31.55 [CD3]

Buprenorphine 20 microgram per 1 hour Rebrikel
20micrograms/hour transdermal patches | 4 patch [PoM] £17.19 DT =
£57.46 [CD3]

▶ **Reletrans** (Sandoz Ltd)

Buprenorphine 5 microgram per 1 hour Reletrans
5micrograms/hour transdermal patches | 4 patch [PoM] £6.34 DT =
£17.60 [CD3]

Buprenorphine 10 microgram per 1 hour Reletrans
10micrograms/hour transdermal patches | 4 patch [PoM] £11.36 DT =
£31.55 [CD3]

Buprenorphine 15 microgram per 1 hour Reletrans
15micrograms/hour transdermal patches | 4 patch [PoM] £17.70 DT =
£49.15 [CD3]

Buprenorphine 20 microgram per 1 hour Reletrans
20micrograms/hour transdermal patches | 4 patch [PoM] £20.06 DT =
£57.46 [CD3]

Buprenorphine 25 microgram per 1 hour Reletrans
25microgram/hour transdermal patches | 4 patch [PoM] £31.70 DT =
£31.70 [CD3]

Buprenorphine 30 microgram per 1 hour Reletrans
30micrograms/hour transdermal patches | 4 patch [PoM] £38.04 DT =
£38.04 [CD3]

Buprenorphine 40 microgram per 1 hour Reletrans
40micrograms/hour transdermal patches | 4 patch [PoM] £50.72 DT =
£50.72 [CD3]

▶ **Relevtec** (Sandoz Ltd)

Buprenorphine 35 microgram per 1 hour Relevtec
35micrograms/hour transdermal patches | 4 patch [PoM] £11.06 DT =
£15.80 [CD3]

Buprenorphine 52.5 microgram per 1 hour Relevtec
52.5micrograms/hour transdermal patches | 4 patch [PoM] £16.60 DT
= £23.71 [CD3]

Buprenorphine 70 microgram per 1 hour Relevtec
70micrograms/hour transdermal patches | 4 patch [PoM] £22.12 DT =
£31.60 [CD3]

▶ **Sevodyne** (Aspire Pharma Ltd)

Buprenorphine 5 microgram per 1 hour Sevodyne
5micrograms/hour transdermal patches | 4 patch [PoM] £5.53 DT =
£17.60 [CD3]

Buprenorphine 10 microgram per 1 hour Sevodyne
10micrograms/hour transdermal patches | 4 patch [PoM] £9.93 DT =
£31.55 [CD3]

Buprenorphine 15 microgram per 1 hour Sevodyne
15micrograms/hour transdermal patches | 4 patch [PoM] £15.48 DT =
£49.15 [CD3]

Buprenorphine 20 microgram per 1 hour Sevodyne
20micrograms/hour transdermal patches | 4 patch [PoM] £18.09 DT =
£57.46 [CD3]

▶ **Transtec** (Grunenthal Ltd)

Buprenorphine 35 microgram per 1 hour Transtec
35micrograms/hour transdermal patches | 4 patch [PoM] £15.80 DT =
£15.80 [CD3]

Buprenorphine 52.5 microgram per 1 hour Transtec
52.5micrograms/hour transdermal patches | 4 patch [PoM] £23.71 DT
= £23.71 [CD3]

Buprenorphine 70 microgram per 1 hour Transtec
70micrograms/hour transdermal patches | 4 patch [PoM] £31.60 DT =
£31.60 [CD3]

Oral lyophilisate

CAUTIONARY AND ADVISORY LABELS 2
EXCIPIENTS: May contain Aspartame, gelatin

▶ **Espranor** (Martindale Pharmaceuticals Ltd)

Buprenorphine (as Buprenorphine hydrochloride) 2 mg Espranor
2mg oral lyophilisates | 28 tablet [PoM] £25.40 DT = £25.40 [CD3] [SF]

Buprenorphine (as Buprenorphine hydrochloride) 8 mg Espranor
8mg oral lyophilisates | 28 tablet [PoM] £76.20 DT = £76.20 [CD3] [SF]

Prolonged-release solution for injection

▶ **Buvidal** (Camurus AB)

Buprenorphine 50 mg per 1 ml Buvidal 16mg/0.32ml prolonged-
release solution for injection pre-filled syringes | 1 pre-filled
disposable injection [PoM] £55.93 DT = £55.93 [CD3]
Buvidal 8mg/0.16ml prolonged-release solution for injection pre-filled
syringes | 1 pre-filled disposable injection [PoM] £55.93 DT =
£55.93 [CD3]
Buvidal 24mg/0.48ml prolonged-release solution for injection pre-
filled syringes | 1 pre-filled disposable injection [PoM] £55.93 DT =
£55.93 [CD3]
Buvidal 32mg/0.64ml prolonged-release solution for injection pre-
filled syringes | 1 pre-filled disposable injection [PoM] £55.93 DT =
£55.93 [CD3]

Buprenorphine 355.56 mg per 1 ml Buvidal 96mg/0.27ml
prolonged-release solution for injection pre-filled syringes | 1 pre-
filled disposable injection [PoM] £239.70 DT = £239.70 [CD3]
Buvidal 160mg/0.45ml prolonged-release solution for injection pre-
filled syringes | 1 pre-filled disposable injection [PoM] £239.70 DT =
£239.70 [CD3]
Buvidal 64mg/0.18ml prolonged-release solution for injection pre-
filled syringes | 1 pre-filled disposable injection [PoM] £239.70 DT =
£239.70 [CD3]
Buvidal 128mg/0.36ml prolonged-release solution for injection pre-
filled syringes | 1 pre-filled disposable injection [PoM] £239.70 DT =
£239.70 [CD3]

▶ 510

Co-codamol

13-Nov-2020

The properties listed below are those particular to the
combination only. For the properties of the components
please consider, paracetamol p. 507.

● **INDICATIONS AND DOSE**

**Moderate pain [using co-codamol 8/500 preparations
only]**

▶ BY MOUTH USING TABLETS, OR BY MOUTH USING
EFFERVESCENT TABLETS

▶ Adult: 1–2 tablets every 4–6 hours as required;
maximum 8 tablets per day

▶ BY MOUTH USING CAPSULES

▶ Adult: 1–2 capsules every 4–6 hours as required;
maximum 8 capsules per day   continued →

Moderate pain [using co-codamol 15/500 preparations only]

▶ BY MOUTH USING TABLETS, OR BY MOUTH USING EFFERVESCENT TABLETS
▸ Adult: 1–2 tablets every 4–6 hours as required; maximum 8 tablets per day
▶ BY MOUTH USING CAPSULES
▸ Adult: 1–2 capsules every 4–6 hours as required; maximum 8 capsules per day

Moderate to severe pain [using co-codamol 30/500 preparations only]

▶ BY MOUTH USING TABLETS, OR BY MOUTH USING EFFERVESCENT TABLETS
▸ Adult: 1–2 tablets every 4–6 hours as required; maximum 8 tablets per day
▶ BY MOUTH USING CAPSULES
▸ Adult: 1–2 capsules every 4–6 hours as required; maximum 8 capsules per day
▶ BY MOUTH USING ORAL SOLUTION
▸ Adult: 5–10 mL every 4–6 hours as required; maximum 40 mL per day

KAPAKE ® 15/500

Mild to moderate pain

▶ BY MOUTH
▸ Adult: 2 tablets every 4–6 hours as required; maximum 8 tablets per day

SOLPADOL ® CAPLETS

Severe pain

▶ BY MOUTH
▸ Adult: 2 tablets every 4–6 hours as required; maximum 8 tablets per day

SOLPADOL ® CAPSULES

Severe pain

▶ BY MOUTH
▸ Adult: 2 capsules every 4–6 hours as required; maximum 8 capsules per day

SOLPADOL ® EFFERVESCENT TABLETS

Severe pain

▶ BY MOUTH USING EFFERVESCENT TABLETS
▸ Adult: 2 tablets every 4–6 hours as required, tablets to be dispersed in water; maximum 8 tablets per day

● CONTRA-INDICATIONS Acute ulcerative colitis · antibiotic-associated colitis · conditions where abdominal distention develops · conditions where inhibition of peristalsis should be avoided · known ultra-rapid codeine metabolisers

● CAUTIONS Acute abdomen · alcohol dependence · avoid abrupt withdrawal after long-term treatment · cardiac arrhythmias · chronic alcoholism · chronic dehydration · chronic malnutrition · not recommended for adolescents aged 12–18 years with breathing problems

CAUTIONS, FURTHER INFORMATION
▸ Variation in metabolism The capacity to metabolise codeine to morphine can vary considerably between individuals; there is a marked increase in morphine toxicity in patients who are ultra-rapid codeine metabolisers (CYP2D6 ultra-rapid metabolisers) and a reduced therapeutic effect in poor codeine metabolisers.

● INTERACTIONS → Appendix 1: opioids · paracetamol

● SIDE-EFFECTS Abdominal pain · addiction · agranulocytosis · blood disorder · irritability · pancreatitis · restlessness · severe cutaneous adverse reactions (SCARs) · thrombocytopenia

Overdose Liver damage (and less frequently renal damage) following overdosage with paracetamol.

● BREAST FEEDING Manufacturer advises avoid (recommendation also supported by MHRA and specialist sources). Present in milk and mothers vary considerably in their capacity to metabolise codeine; risk of opioid toxicity in infant.

● HEPATIC IMPAIRMENT Manufacturer advises caution in mild to moderate impairment; avoid in severe impairment. **Dose adjustments** Manufacturer advises consider dose reduction in mild to moderate impairment.

● RENAL IMPAIRMENT Reduce dose or avoid codeine; increased and prolonged effect; increased cerebral sensitivity.

● PRESCRIBING AND DISPENSING INFORMATION Co-codamol is a mixture of codeine phosphate and paracetamol; the proportions are expressed in the form x/y, where x and y are the strengths in milligrams of codeine phosphate and paracetamol respectively.

When co-codamol tablets, dispersible (or effervescent) tablets, or capsules are prescribed and **no strength is stated**, tablets, dispersible (or effervescent) tablets, or capsules, respectively, containing codeine phosphate 8 mg and paracetamol 500 mg should be dispensed.

The Drug Tariff allows tablets of co-codamol labelled 'dispersible' to be dispensed against an order for 'effervescent' and *vice versa*.

● LESS SUITABLE FOR PRESCRIBING Co-codamol is less suitable for prescribing.

● EXCEPTIONS TO LEGAL CATEGORY Co-codamol 8/500 can be sold to the public in certain circumstances; for exemptions see *Medicines, Ethics and Practice*, London, Pharmaceutical Press (always consult latest edition).

● MEDICINAL FORMS There can be variation in the licensing of different medicines containing the same drug. Forms available from special-order manufacturers include: oral suspension, oral solution

Oral tablet
CAUTIONARY AND ADVISORY LABELS 2(does not apply to the 8/500 tablet), 29, 30
▶ Co-codamol (Non-proprietary)
Codeine phosphate 8 mg, Paracetamol 500 mg Co-codamol 8mg/500mg tablets | 100 tablet PoM £3.75 DT = £3.03 CD5
Codeine phosphate 15 mg, Paracetamol 500 mg Co-codamol 15mg/500mg tablets | 100 tablet PoM £15.00 DT = £3.42 CD5
Codeine phosphate 30 mg, Paracetamol 500 mg Co-codamol 30mg/500mg caplets | 100 tablet PoM £3.90 DT = £3.47 CD5
Co-codamol 30mg/500mg tablets | 30 tablet PoM £1.53 DT = £1.04 CD5 | 100 tablet PoM £7.53 DT = £3.47 CD5
▶ Codipar (Advanz Pharma)
Codeine phosphate 15 mg, Paracetamol 500 mg Codipar 15mg/500mg tablets | 100 tablet PoM £8.25 DT = £3.42 CD5
▶ Emcozin (GlucoRx Ltd)
Codeine phosphate 30 mg, Paracetamol 500 mg Emcozin 30mg/500mg tablets | 100 tablet PoM £2.94 DT = £3.47 CD5
▶ Migraleve Yellow (McNeil Products Ltd)
Codeine phosphate 8 mg, Paracetamol 500 mg Migraleve Yellow tablets | 16 tablet PoM ⚠ CD5
▶ Solpadeine Max (Omega Pharma Ltd)
Codeine phosphate 12.8 mg, Paracetamol 500 mg Solpadeine Max 12.8mg/500mg tablets | 24 tablet P £5.04 CD5
▶ Solpadol (Phoenix Labs Ltd)
Codeine phosphate 30 mg, Paracetamol 500 mg Solpadol 30mg/500mg caplets | 100 tablet PoM £6.74 DT = £3.47 CD5
▶ Zapain (Advanz Pharma)
Codeine phosphate 30 mg, Paracetamol 500 mg Zapain 30mg/500mg tablets | 50 tablet PoM £1.56 CD5 | 100 tablet PoM £3.11 DT = £3.47 CD5

Effervescent tablet
CAUTIONARY AND ADVISORY LABELS 2(does not apply to the 8/500 tablet), 13, 29, 30
EXCIPIENTS: May contain Aspartame
ELECTROLYTES: May contain Sodium
▶ Co-codamol (Non-proprietary)
Codeine phosphate 8 mg, Paracetamol 500 mg Co-codamol 8mg/500mg effervescent tablets sugar free | 100 tablet PoM £10.25 DT = £10.25 CD5 SF
Co-codamol 8mg/500mg effervescent tablets | 100 tablet PoM £8.75 DT = £7.28 CD5

Codeine phosphate 15 mg, Paracetamol 500 mg Co-codamol 15mg/500mg effervescent tablets sugar free | 100 tablet [PoM] £8.25–£13.20 DT = £8.25 [CD5] [SF]

Codeine phosphate 30 mg, Paracetamol 500 mg Co-codamol 30mg/500mg effervescent tablets | 32 tablet [PoM] £5.40 DT = £2.32 [CD5] | 100 tablet [PoM] £19.20 DT = £7.25 [CD5] Co-codamol 30mg/500mg effervescent tablets sugar free | 100 tablet [PoM] £8.90 [CD5] [SF]

▸ **Solpadol** (Phoenix Labs Ltd)
Codeine phosphate 30 mg, Paracetamol 500 mg Solpadol 30mg/500mg effervescent tablets | 100 tablet [PoM] £8.90 DT = £7.25 [CD5]

Oral capsule
CAUTIONARY AND ADVISORY LABELS 2(does not apply to the 8/500 capsule), 29, 30
EXCIPIENTS: May contain Sulfites

▸ **Co-codamol (Non-proprietary)**
Codeine phosphate 8 mg, Paracetamol 500 mg Co-codamol 8mg/500mg capsules | 32 capsule [PoM] £11.38 DT = £12.03 [CD5] | 100 capsule [PoM] £51.56 DT = £37.59 [CD5]

Codeine phosphate 30 mg, Paracetamol 500 mg Co-codamol 30mg/500mg capsules | 100 capsule [PoM] £8.72 DT = £5.54 [CD5]

▸ **Codipar** (Advanz Pharma)
Codeine phosphate 15 mg, Paracetamol 500 mg Codipar 15mg/500mg capsules | 100 capsule [PoM] £7.25 DT = £7.25 [CD5]

▸ **Tylex** (UCB Pharma Ltd)
Codeine phosphate 30 mg, Paracetamol 500 mg Tylex 30mg/500mg capsules | 100 capsule [PoM] £7.93 DT = £5.54 [CD5]

▸ **Zapain** (Advanz Pharma)
Codeine phosphate 30 mg, Paracetamol 500 mg Zapain 30mg/500mg capsules | 50 capsule [PoM] £1.93 [CD5] | 100 capsule [PoM] £3.85 DT = £5.54 [CD5]

◤ 510

Codeine phosphate
28-Mar-2024

- **INDICATIONS AND DOSE**

Diarrhoea
▸ BY MOUTH
- Child 12–17 years: 15–60 mg 3–4 times a day
- Adult: 15–60 mg 3–4 times a day

Short-term treatment of acute moderate pain
▸ BY MOUTH
- Child 12–17 years: 30–60 mg every 6 hours as required for maximum 3 days
- Adult: 30–60 mg every 6 hours as required for maximum 3 days

Dry or painful cough
▸ BY MOUTH
- Adult: 15–30 mg 3–4 times a day, dose to be given using linctus

---

IMPORTANT SAFETY INFORMATION

MHRA/CHM ADVICE (JULY 2013) CODEINE FOR ANALGESIA: RESTRICTED USE IN CHILDREN DUE TO REPORTS OF MORPHINE TOXICITY

Codeine should only be used to relieve acute moderate pain in children older than 12 years and only if it cannot be relieved by other painkillers such as paracetamol or ibuprofen alone. A significant risk of serious and life-threatening adverse reactions has been identified in children with obstructive sleep apnoea who received codeine after tonsillectomy or adenoidectomy:

- in children aged 12–18 years, the maximum daily dose of codeine should not exceed 240 mg. Doses may be taken up to four times a day at intervals of no less than 6 hours. The lowest effective dose should be used and duration of treatment should be limited to 3 days
- codeine is contra-indicated in all children (under 18 years) who undergo the removal of tonsils or adenoids for the treatment of obstructive sleep apnoea
- codeine is not recommended for use in children whose breathing may be compromised, including those with neuromuscular disorders, severe cardiac or respiratory conditions, respiratory infections, multiple trauma or extensive surgical procedures
- codeine is contra-indicated in patients of any age who are known to be ultra-rapid metabolisers of codeine (CYP2D6 ultra-rapid metabolisers)
- codeine should not be used in breast-feeding mothers because it can pass to the baby through breast milk
- parents and carers should be advised on how to recognise signs and symptoms of morphine toxicity, and to stop treatment and seek medical attention if signs or symptoms of toxicity occur (including reduced consciousness, lack of appetite, somnolence, constipation, respiratory depression, 'pin-point' pupils, nausea, vomiting)

MHRA/CHM ADVICE (APRIL 2015) CODEINE FOR COUGH AND COLD: RESTRICTED USE IN CHILDREN

Do not use codeine in children under 12 years as it is associated with a risk of respiratory side effects. Codeine is not recommended for adolescents (12–18 years) who have problems with breathing. When prescribing or dispensing codeine-containing medicines for cough and cold, consider that codeine is contra-indicated in:
- children younger than 12 years old
- patients of any age known to be CYP2D6 ultra-rapid metabolisers
- breastfeeding mothers

MHRA/CHM ADVICE: CODEINE LINCTUS (CODEINE ORAL SOLUTIONS): RECLASSIFICATION TO PRESCRIPTION-ONLY MEDICINE (FEBRUARY 2024)

Following the results of a public consultation, codeine linctus has been reclassified as a prescription-only medicine (POM) due to the risk of dependence, addiction, and overdose. Healthcare professionals are reminded that codeine linctus is only authorised for the treatment of dry cough, and only considered to be effective for chronic coughs lasting over 8 weeks.

- **CONTRA-INDICATIONS** Acute ulcerative colitis · antibiotic-associated colitis · children under 18 years who undergo the removal of tonsils or adenoids for the treatment of obstructive sleep apnoea · conditions where abdominal distension develops · conditions where inhibition of peristalsis should be avoided · known ultra-rapid codeine metabolisers

- **CAUTIONS** Acute abdomen · cardiac arrhythmias · gallstones · not recommended for adolescents aged 12–18 years with breathing problems

  CAUTIONS, FURTHER INFORMATION
  ▸ Variation in metabolism The capacity to metabolise codeine to morphine can vary considerably between individuals; there is a marked increase in morphine toxicity in patients who are ultra-rapid codeine metabolisers (CYP2D6 ultra-rapid metabolisers) and a reduced therapeutic effect in poor codeine metabolisers.

- **INTERACTIONS** → Appendix 1: opioids

- **SIDE-EFFECTS** Abdominal cramps · addiction · appetite decreased · biliary spasm · depression · dyskinesia · dyspnoea · face oedema · fatigue · fever · hyperglycaemia · hypersensitivity · hypothermia · intracranial pressure increased · lymphadenopathy · malaise · mood altered · muscle rigidity (with high doses) · nightmare · pancreatitis · restlessness · sexual dysfunction · splenomegaly · ureteral spasm · urinary disorders · vision disorders

- **BREAST FEEDING** Manufacturer advises avoid (recommendation also supported by MHRA and specialist sources). Present in milk and mothers vary considerably in their capacity to metabolise codeine; risk of opioid toxicity in infant.

- **HEPATIC IMPAIRMENT** [EvGr] Caution in mild to moderate

Nervous system   **4**

impairment; avoid in severe impairment. ⟨M⟩
Dose adjustments [EvGr] Reduce dose in mild to moderate impairment. ⟨M⟩

- **RENAL IMPAIRMENT** Avoid use or reduce dose; opioid effects increased and prolonged and increased cerebral sensitivity occurs.

- **PRESCRIBING AND DISPENSING INFORMATION** BP directs that when Diabetic Codeine Linctus is prescribed, Codeine Linctus formulated with a vehicle appropriate for administration to diabetics, whether or not labelled 'Diabetic Codeine Linctus', shall be dispensed or supplied.

- **PATIENT AND CARER ADVICE**
Medicines for Children leaflet: Codeine phosphate for pain
www.medicinesforchildren.org.uk/medicines/codeine-phosphate-for-pain/

- **MEDICINAL FORMS** There can be variation in the licensing of different medicines containing the same drug. Forms available from special-order manufacturers include: oral suspension, oral solution

Oral tablet
CAUTIONARY AND ADVISORY LABELS 2
▸ **Codeine phosphate (Non-proprietary)**
Codeine phosphate 15 mg Codeine 15mg tablets | 28 tablet [PoM] £0.94 DT = £0.94 [CD5] | 100 tablet [PoM] £3.36 DT = £3.36 [CD5]
Codeine phosphate 30 mg Codeine 30mg tablets | 28 tablet [PoM] £1.34 DT = £1.16 [CD5] | 100 tablet [PoM] £6.40 DT = £4.14 [CD5]
Codeine phosphate 60 mg Codeine 60mg tablets | 28 tablet [PoM] £2.54 DT = £2.40 [CD5]

Oral solution
CAUTIONARY AND ADVISORY LABELS 2
▸ **Codeine phosphate (Non-proprietary)**
Codeine phosphate 3 mg per 1 ml Codeine 15mg/5ml linctus sugar free | 200 ml [PoM] £21.96 DT = £5.31 [CD5] [SF] | 2000 ml [PoM] £39.80 [CD5] [SF]
Codeine 15mg/5ml linctus | 200 ml [PoM] £19.50–£31.20 DT = £2.40 [CD5]
Codeine phosphate 5 mg per 1 ml Codeine 25mg/5ml oral solution | 500 ml [PoM] £6.64 DT = £6.64 [CD5]
▸ **Galcodine** (Thornton & Ross Ltd)
Codeine phosphate 3 mg per 1 ml Galcodine 15mg/5ml linctus | 2000 ml [PoM] £9.90 [CD5] [SF]

Combinations available: *Aspirin with codeine*, p. 510

�F 510

Diamorphine hydrochloride
13-Nov-2020
(Heroin hydrochloride)

- **INDICATIONS AND DOSE**

Acute pain
▸ BY INTRAMUSCULAR INJECTION, OR BY SUBCUTANEOUS INJECTION
▸ Adult: 5 mg every 4 hours if required
▸ BY SLOW INTRAVENOUS INJECTION
▸ Adult: 1.25–2.5 mg every 4 hours if required

Acute pain (heavier, well-muscled patients)
▸ BY INTRAMUSCULAR INJECTION, OR BY SUBCUTANEOUS INJECTION
▸ Adult: Up to 10 mg every 4 hours if required
▸ BY SLOW INTRAVENOUS INJECTION
▸ Adult: 2.5–5 mg every 4 hours if required

Chronic pain not currently treated with a strong opioid analgesic
▸ BY SUBCUTANEOUS INJECTION, OR BY INTRAMUSCULAR INJECTION
▸ Adult: Initially 2.5–5 mg every 4 hours, adjusted according to response
▸ BY SUBCUTANEOUS INFUSION
▸ Adult: Initially 5–10 mg, adjusted according to response, dose to be administered over 24 hours

Acute pulmonary oedema
▸ BY SLOW INTRAVENOUS INJECTION
▸ Adult: 2.5–5 mg, dose to be administered at a rate of 1 mg/minute

Myocardial infarction
▸ BY SLOW INTRAVENOUS INJECTION
▸ Adult: 5 mg, followed by 2.5–5 mg if required, dose to be administered at a rate of 1–2 mg/minute
▸ Elderly: 2.5 mg, followed by 1.25–2.5 mg if required, dose to be administered at a rate of 1–2 mg/minute

Myocardial infarction (frail patients)
▸ BY SLOW INTRAVENOUS INJECTION
▸ Adult: 2.5 mg, followed by 1.25–2.5 mg if required, dose to be administered at a rate of 1–2 mg/minute

- **CONTRA-INDICATIONS** Delayed gastric emptying · phaeochromocytoma

- **CAUTIONS** CNS depression · severe cor pulmonale · severe diarrhoea · toxic psychosis

- **INTERACTIONS** → Appendix 1: opioids

- **SIDE-EFFECTS** Biliary spasm · circulatory depression · intracranial pressure increased · mood altered

- **BREAST FEEDING** Therapeutic doses unlikely to affect infant; withdrawal symptoms in infants of dependent mothers; breast-feeding not best method of treating dependence in offspring.

- **HEPATIC IMPAIRMENT** Manufacturer advises caution.
Dose adjustments Manufacturer advises dose reduction.

- **RENAL IMPAIRMENT** Avoid use or reduce dose; opioid effects increased and prolonged; increased cerebral sensitivity.

- **MEDICINAL FORMS** There can be variation in the licensing of different medicines containing the same drug. Forms available from special-order manufacturers include: solution for injection, powder for solution for injection

Powder for solution for injection
▸ **Diamorphine hydrochloride (Non-proprietary)**
Diamorphine hydrochloride 5 mg Diamorphine 5mg powder for solution for injection ampoules | 5 ampoule [PoM] £12.80 DT = £12.80 [CD2]
Diamorphine hydrochloride 10 mg Diamorphine 10mg powder for solution for injection ampoules | 5 ampoule [PoM] £16.56 [CD2]
Diamorphine hydrochloride 30 mg Diamorphine 30mg powder for solution for injection ampoules | 5 ampoule [PoM] £16.52 DT = £16.52 [CD2]
Diamorphine hydrochloride 100 mg Diamorphine 100mg powder for solution for injection ampoules | 5 ampoule [PoM] £42.39 DT = £42.39 [CD2]

�F 510

Dihydrocodeine tartrate
16-Feb-2021

- **INDICATIONS AND DOSE**

Moderate to severe pain
▸ BY MOUTH USING IMMEDIATE-RELEASE MEDICINES
▸ Child 4–11 years: 0.5–1 mg/kg every 4–6 hours (max. per dose 30 mg)
▸ Child 12–17 years: 30 mg every 4–6 hours
▸ Adult: 30 mg every 4–6 hours as required
▸ BY DEEP SUBCUTANEOUS INJECTION, OR BY INTRAMUSCULAR INJECTION
▸ Adult: Up to 50 mg every 4–6 hours as required

Chronic severe pain
▸ BY MOUTH USING MODIFIED-RELEASE MEDICINES
▸ Child 12–17 years: 60–120 mg every 12 hours
▸ Adult: 60–120 mg every 12 hours

DF118 FORTE ®
Severe pain
▸ BY MOUTH
▸ Child 12-17 years: 40–80 mg 3 times a day
▸ Adult: 40–80 mg 3 times a day

- **CAUTIONS** Pancreatitis · severe cor pulmonale
- **INTERACTIONS** → Appendix 1: opioids
- **SIDE-EFFECTS**
  GENERAL SIDE-EFFECTS Dysuria · mood altered
  SPECIFIC SIDE-EFFECTS
- ► With oral use Biliary spasm · bronchospasm · hypothermia · sexual dysfunction · ureteral spasm
- **BREAST FEEDING** Specialist sources indicate caution—use the lowest effective dose for the shortest possible duration; monitor infant for adverse effects, including sedation, breathing difficulties, constipation, difficulty feeding and poor weight gain.
- **HEPATIC IMPAIRMENT** Manufacturer advises caution; consider avoiding.
  Dose adjustments Manufacturer advises dose reduction, if used.
- **RENAL IMPAIRMENT** Avoid use or reduce dose; opioid effects increased and prolonged and increased cerebral sensitivity occurs.
- **PROFESSION SPECIFIC INFORMATION**
  Dental practitioners' formulary Dihydrocodeine tablets 30 mg may be prescribed.

- **MEDICINAL FORMS** There can be variation in the licensing of different medicines containing the same drug. Forms available from special-order manufacturers include: oral suspension, oral solution

Oral tablet
CAUTIONARY AND ADVISORY LABELS 2
► Dihydrocodeine tartrate (Non-proprietary)
  Dihydrocodeine tartrate 30 mg Dihydrocodeine 30mg tablets | 28 tablet [PoM] £3.00 DT = £2.08 [CD5] | 30 tablet [PoM] £2.23–£3.50 [CD5] | 84 tablet [PoM] £6.62 [CD5] | 100 tablet [PoM] £10.20 DT = £7.43 [CD5] | 112 tablet [PoM] £8.84 [CD5]

Oral solution
CAUTIONARY AND ADVISORY LABELS 2

Modified-release tablet
CAUTIONARY AND ADVISORY LABELS 2, 25
► Dihydrocodeine tartrate (Non-proprietary)
  Dihydrocodeine tartrate 60 mg Dihydrocodeine 60mg modified-release tablets | 56 tablet [PoM] £5.20 DT = £5.20 [CD5]
  Dihydrocodeine tartrate 90 mg Dihydrocodeine 90mg modified-release tablets | 56 tablet [PoM] £8.66 DT = £8.66 [CD5]
  Dihydrocodeine tartrate 120 mg Dihydrocodeine 120mg modified-release tablets | 56 tablet [PoM] £10.95 DT = £10.95 [CD5]

▶ 510

Dihydrocodeine with paracetamol

26-Jan-2023

The properties listed below are those particular to the combination only. For the properties of the components please consider, paracetamol p. 507.

- **INDICATIONS AND DOSE**

Mild to moderate pain [using 10/500 preparations only]
► BY MOUTH
► Adult: 1–2 tablets every 4–6 hours as required, to be given using 10/500 mg strength tablet; maximum 8 tablets per day

Severe pain [using 20/500 preparations only]
► BY MOUTH
► Adult: 1–2 tablets every 4–6 hours as required, to be given using 20/500 mg strength tablet; maximum 8 tablets per day

Severe pain [using 30/500 preparations only]
► BY MOUTH
► Adult: 1–2 tablets every 4–6 hours as required, to be given using 30/500 mg strength tablet; maximum 8 tablets per day

DOSE EQUIVALENCE AND CONVERSION
► Tablets contain a mixture of dihydrocodeine tartrate and paracetamol; the proportions are expressed in the form x/y, where x and y are the strengths in milligrams of dihydrocodeine and paracetamol respectively.

IMPORTANT SAFETY INFORMATION
MHRA/CHM ADVICE: DIHYDROCODEINE WITH PARACETAMOL (CO-DYDRAMOL): PRESCRIBE AND DISPENSE BY STRENGTH TO MINIMISE RISK OF MEDICATION ERROR (JANUARY 2018)
The MHRA has advised that dihydrocodeine with paracetamol preparations are prescribed and dispensed by strength to minimise dispensing errors and the risk of accidental opioid overdose—see Prescribing and dispensing information.

- **CAUTIONS** Alcohol dependence · before administering, check when paracetamol last administered and cumulative paracetamol dose over previous 24 hours · chronic alcoholism · chronic dehydration · chronic malnutrition · pancreatitis · severe cor pulmonale
- **INTERACTIONS** → Appendix 1: opioids · paracetamol
- **SIDE-EFFECTS** Abdominal pain · blood disorder · leucopenia · malaise · neutropenia · pancreatitis · paraesthesia · paralytic ileus · severe cutaneous adverse reactions (SCARs) · thrombocytopenia
  Overdose Liver damage (and less frequently renal damage) following overdosage with paracetamol.
- **BREAST FEEDING** Specialist sources indicate caution—use the lowest effective dose for the shortest possible duration; monitor infant for adverse effects, including sedation, breathing difficulties, constipation, difficulty feeding and poor weight gain.
- **HEPATIC IMPAIRMENT** Manufacturer advises consider avoiding in mild to moderate impairment; avoid in severe impairment.
  Dose adjustments Manufacturer advises dose reduction in mild to moderate impairment, if used.
- **RENAL IMPAIRMENT** Reduce dose or avoid dihydrocodeine; increased and prolonged effect; increased cerebral sensitivity.
- **PRESCRIBING AND DISPENSING INFORMATION** The MHRA advises when prescribing dihydrocodeine with paracetamol, the tablet strength and dose must be clearly indicated; when dispensing dihydrocodeine with paracetamol, ensure the prescribed strength is supplied—contact the prescriber if in doubt.
  The BP defines *Co-dydramol* Tablets as containing dihydrocodeine tartrate 10 mg and paracetamol 500 mg.
- **LESS SUITABLE FOR PRESCRIBING** Dihydrocodeine with paracetamol is less suitable for prescribing.

- **MEDICINAL FORMS** There can be variation in the licensing of different medicines containing the same drug. Forms available from special-order manufacturers include: oral suspension, oral solution

Oral tablet
CAUTIONARY AND ADVISORY LABELS 2, 29, 30
► Dihydrocodeine with paracetamol (Non-proprietary)
  Dihydrocodeine tartrate 10 mg, Paracetamol 500 mg Co-dydramol 10mg/500mg tablets | 30 tablet [PoM] £2.56 DT = £1.17 [CD5] | 100 tablet [PoM] £9.45 DT = £3.90 [CD5]
  Dihydrocodeine tartrate 20 mg, Paracetamol 500 mg Co-dydramol 20mg/500mg tablets | 56 tablet [PoM] [⚡] DT = £5.87 [CD5] | 112 tablet [PoM] [⚡] DT = £11.13 [CD5]
  Dihydrocodeine tartrate 30 mg, Paracetamol 500 mg Co-dydramol 30mg/500mg tablets | 56 tablet [PoM] [⚡] DT = £6.82 [CD5]
► Remedeine (Crescent Pharma Ltd)
  Dihydrocodeine tartrate 20 mg, Paracetamol 500 mg Remedeine tablets | 56 tablet [PoM] £5.87 DT = £5.87 [CD5] | 112 tablet [PoM] £11.13 DT = £11.13 [CD5]

Dihydrocodeine tartrate 30 mg, Paracetamol 500 mg Remedeine
Forte tablets | 56 tablet [PoM] £6.82 DT = £6.82 [CD5]

F 510

Dipipanone hydrochloride with cyclizine

10-May-2021

● **INDICATIONS AND DOSE**

Acute pain

▶ BY MOUTH

▶ Adult: Initially 1 tablet every 6 hours, then increased if necessary up to 3 tablets every 6 hours, dose to be increased gradually

● CAUTIONS Diabetes mellitus · palliative care (not recommended) · phaeochromocytoma

● INTERACTIONS → Appendix 1: antihistamines, sedating · opioids

● SIDE-EFFECTS Agranulocytosis · anxiety · biliary spasm · consciousness impaired · dry throat · dysuria · hallucinations · hepatic disorders · insomnia · intracranial pressure increased · mood altered · movement disorders · muscle complaints · nasal dryness · psychosis · renal spasm · speech disorder · tremor · vision blurred

● BREAST FEEDING No information available.

● HEPATIC IMPAIRMENT Manufacturer advises caution in mild to moderate impairment; avoid in severe impairment.
Dose adjustments Manufacturer advises dose reduction in mild to moderate impairment; adjust according to response.

● RENAL IMPAIRMENT [EvGr] Avoid in severe impairment. ⓜ
Dose adjustments [EvGr] Reduce dose in mild to moderate impairment (risk of increased and prolonged effects). ⓜ

● MEDICINAL FORMS There can be variation in the licensing of different medicines containing the same drug.

Oral tablet

▶ Dipipanone hydrochloride with cyclizine (Non-proprietary)
Dipipanone hydrochloride 10 mg, Cyclizine hydrochloride 30 mg Dipipanone 10mg / Cyclizine 30mg tablets | 50 tablet [PoM] £440.65 DT = £440.65 [CD2]

F 510

Fentanyl

04-May-2023

● **INDICATIONS AND DOSE**

Chronic severe pain currently treated with a weak opioid analgesic (administered on expert advice)

▶ BY TRANSDERMAL APPLICATION

▶ Adult: Initially 12 micrograms/hour every 72 hours, when starting, evaluation of the analgesic effect should not be made before the system has been worn for 24 hours (to allow for the gradual increase in plasma-fentanyl concentration)—previous analgesic therapy should be phased out gradually from time of first patch application, dose should be adjusted at 72 hour intervals in steps of 12–25 micrograms/hour if necessary. After a dose increase, the system should be worn through two 72-hour applications before any further increase in dose, more than one patch may be used at a time (but applied at the same time to avoid confusion)—consider additional or alternative analgesic therapy if dose required exceeds 300 micrograms/hour (important: it takes 20 hours or more for the plasma-fentanyl concentration to decrease by 50%—replacement opioid therapy should be initiated at a low dose and increased gradually). For further information including opioid dose conversion and the management of breakthrough pain, see *Opioid analgesics* under Prescribing in palliative care p. 26.

Chronic severe pain currently treated with a strong opioid analgesic (administered on expert advice)

▶ BY TRANSDERMAL APPLICATION

▶ Adult: Initial dose based on previous 24-hour opioid requirement—consult product literature, for evaluating analgesic efficacy and dose increments, see under *Chronic severe pain currently treated with a weak opioid analgesic*, for conversion from long term oral morphine to transdermal fentanyl, see *Opioid analgesics* under Prescribing in palliative care p. 26.

Spontaneous respiration: analgesia and enhancement of anaesthesia, during operation

▶ BY SLOW INTRAVENOUS INJECTION

▶ Adult: Initially 50–100 micrograms (max. per dose 200 micrograms), dose maximum on specialist advice, then 25–50 micrograms as required

▶ BY INTRAVENOUS INFUSION

▶ Adult: 3–4.8 micrograms/kg/hour, adjusted according to response

Assisted ventilation: analgesia and enhancement of anaesthesia during operation

▶ BY SLOW INTRAVENOUS INJECTION

▶ Adult: Initially 300–3500 micrograms, then 100–200 micrograms as required

▶ BY INTRAVENOUS INFUSION

▶ Adult: Initially 10 micrograms/kg, dose to be given over 10 minutes, then 6 micrograms/kg/hour, adjusted according to response, may require up to 180 micrograms/kg/hour during cardiac surgery

Assisted ventilation: analgesia and respiratory depression in intensive care

▶ BY SLOW INTRAVENOUS INJECTION

▶ Adult: Initially 300–3500 micrograms, then 100–200 micrograms as required

▶ BY INTRAVENOUS INFUSION

▶ Adult: Initially 10 micrograms/kg, dose to be given over 10 minutes, then 6 micrograms/kg/hour, adjusted according to response, may require up to 180 micrograms/kg/hour during cardiac surgery

Breakthrough pain in patients receiving opioid therapy for chronic cancer pain (administered on expert advice)

▶ BY BUCCAL ADMINISTRATION USING LOZENGES

▶ Adult: Initially 200 micrograms, dose to be given over 15 minutes, then 200 micrograms after 15 minutes if required, no more than 2 dose units for each pain episode; if adequate pain relief not achieved with 1 dose unit for consecutive breakthrough pain episodes, increase the strength of the dose unit until adequate pain relief achieved with 4 lozenges or less daily, if more than 4 episodes of breakthrough pain each day, adjust background analgesia

▶ BY BUCCAL ADMINISTRATION USING BUCCAL FILMS

▶ Adult: Initially 200 micrograms, adjusted according to response, consult product literature for information on dose adjustments, maximum 1.2 mg per episode of breakthrough pain; leave at least 4 hours between treatment of episodes of breakthrough pain, if more than 4 episodes of breakthrough pain each day occur on more than 4 consecutive days, adjust background analgesia

DOSE EQUIVALENCE AND CONVERSION

▶ Fentanyl films are **not bioequivalent** to other fentanyl preparations.

▶ Fentanyl preparations for the treatment of breakthrough pain are not interchangeable; if patients are switched from another fentanyl-containing preparation, a new dose titration is required.

4

Nervous system

DOSES AT EXTREMES OF BODY-WEIGHT

▶ To avoid excessive dosage in obese patients, weight-based doses may need to be calculated on the basis of ideal bodyweight.

ABSTRAL ®

Breakthrough pain in patients receiving opioid therapy for chronic cancer pain (administered on expert advice)

▶ BY MOUTH USING SUBLINGUAL TABLETS

▶ Adult: Initially 100 micrograms, then 100 micrograms after 15–30 minutes if required, dose to be adjusted according to response—consult product literature, no more than 2 dose units 15–30 minutes apart, for each pain episode; max. 800 micrograms per episode of breakthrough pain; leave at least 2 hours between treatment of episodes of breakthrough pain, if more than 4 episodes of breakthrough pain each day, adjust background analgesia

EFFENTORA ®

Breakthrough pain in patients receiving opioid therapy for chronic cancer pain (administered on expert advice)

▶ BY MOUTH USING BUCCAL TABLET

▶ Adult: Initially 100 micrograms, then 100 micrograms after 30 minutes if required, dose to be adjusted according to response—consult product literature, no more than 2 dose units for each pain episode; max. 800 micrograms per episode of breakthrough pain; leave at least 4 hours between treatment of episodes of breakthrough pain during titration

INSTANYL ®

Breakthrough pain in patients receiving opioid therapy for chronic cancer pain (administered on expert advice)

▶ BY INTRANASAL ADMINISTRATION

▶ Adult: Initially 50 micrograms, dose to be administered into one nostril, then 50 micrograms after 10 minutes if required, dose to be adjusted according to response, maximum 2 sprays for each pain episode and minimum 4 hours between treatment of each pain episode, if more than 4 breakthrough pain episodes daily, adjust background analgesia

PECFENT ®

Breakthrough pain in patients receiving opioid therapy for chronic cancer pain (administered on expert advice)

▶ BY INTRANASAL ADMINISTRATION

▶ Adult: Initially 100 micrograms, adjusted according to response, dose to be administered into one nostril only, maximum 2 sprays for each pain episode and minimum 4 hours between treatment of each pain episode, if more than 4 breakthrough pain episodes daily, adjust background analgesia

---

IMPORTANT SAFETY INFORMATION

MHRA/CHM ADVICE: TRANSDERMAL FENTANYL PATCHES: LIFE-THREATENING AND FATAL OPIOID TOXICITY FROM ACCIDENTAL EXPOSURE, PARTICULARLY IN CHILDREN (OCTOBER 2018)

Accidental exposure to transdermal fentanyl can occur if a patch is swallowed or transferred to another individual. Always fully inform patients and their carers about directions for safe use of fentanyl patches, including the importance of:

● not exceeding the prescribed dose;
● following the correct frequency of patch application, avoiding touching the adhesive side of patches, and washing hands after application;
● not cutting patches and avoiding exposure of patches to heat including via hot water;
● ensuring that old patches are removed before applying a new one;
● following instructions for safe storage and properly disposing of used patches or those which are not needed.

Patients and carers should be advised to seek immediate medical attention if overdose is suspected—see *Side-effects* and *Patient and carer advice* for further information.

MHRA/CHM ADVICE: TRANSDERMAL FENTANYL PATCHES FOR NON-CANCER PAIN: DO NOT USE IN OPIOID-NAÏVE PATIENTS (SEPTEMBER 2020)

A review noted that serious harm, including fatalities, has been reported with the use of fentanyl patches in both opioid-naïve and opioid-tolerant patients. There is considerable risk of respiratory depression with the use of fentanyl, especially in opioid-naïve patients, and significant risk with too rapid an escalation of dose, even in long-term opioid-tolerant patients.

The MHRA advises healthcare professionals that the use of fentanyl transdermal patches is contra-indicated in opioid-naïve patients; other analgesics and other opioids for non-malignant pain should be used before prescribing fentanyl patches. Patients and their carers should be reminded about the directions for safe use of fentanyl patches (see above).

● **CONTRA-INDICATIONS**
▶ With transdermal use Opioid-naïve patients

● **CAUTIONS**

GENERAL CAUTIONS Bradyarrhythmias · cerebral tumour · diabetes mellitus (with *Actiq* ® and *Cynril* ® lozenges) · impaired consciousness

SPECIFIC CAUTIONS
▶ With buccal use Mucositis—absorption from oral preparations may be increased, caution during dose titration

CAUTIONS, FURTHER INFORMATION
▶ With transdermal use EvGr Transdermal fentanyl patches are not suitable for acute pain or in those patients whose analgesic requirements are changing rapidly because the long time to steady state prevents rapid titration of the dose. ◈M◈
▶ With intravenous use EvGr Repeated intra-operative doses should be given with care since the resulting respiratory depression can persist postoperatively and occasionally it may become apparent for the first time postoperatively when monitoring of the patient might be less intensive. ◈M◈

● **INTERACTIONS** → Appendix 1: opioids

● **SIDE-EFFECTS**
▶ **Common or very common**
▶ With parenteral use Apnoea · hypertension · movement disorders · muscle rigidity · post procedural complications · respiratory disorders · vascular pain
▶ With sublingual use Asthenia · dyspnoea · oral disorders
▶ With transdermal use Anxiety · appetite decreased · asthenia · depression · diarrhoea · dyspnoea · gastrointestinal discomfort · hypertension · insomnia · malaise · muscle complaints · peripheral oedema · sensation abnormal · temperature sensation altered · tremor
▶ **Uncommon**
▶ With parenteral use Airway complication of anaesthesia · chills · hiccups · hypothermia
▶ With sublingual use Altered smell sensation · anxiety · appetite decreased · bruising tendency · concentration impaired · depression · emotional lability · erectile dysfunction · gastrointestinal discomfort · impaired gastric emptying · joint disorders · malaise · memory loss · musculoskeletal stiffness · night sweats · numbness · oropharyngeal pain · overdose · paranoia · psychiatric disorder · sleep disorders · taste altered · throat tightness · tremor · vision blurred
▶ With transdermal use Consciousness impaired · cyanosis · fever · gastrointestinal disorders · influenza like illness ·

memory loss · respiratory disorders · seizures · sexual dysfunction · vision blurred
▸ **Rare or very rare**
▸ With transdermal use Apnoea
▸ **Frequency not known**
▸ With buccal use Adrenal insufficiency · androgen deficiency · anxiety · appetite decreased · asthenia · coma · depersonalisation · depression · diarrhoea · dyspnoea · emotional lability · fever · gait abnormal · gastrointestinal discomfort · gastrointestinal disorders · gingival haemorrhage · gingivitis · injury · loss of consciousness · malaise · myoclonus · oral disorders · peripheral oedema · sensation abnormal · sleep disorders · speech slurred · taste altered · thinking abnormal · throat oedema · vasodilation · vision disorders · weight decreased · withdrawal syndrome neonatal
▸ With intranasal use Diarrhoea · epistaxis · fatigue · fever · hot flush · insomnia · malaise · motion sickness · myoclonus · nasal complaints · peripheral oedema · sensation abnormal · stomatitis · taste altered · throat irritation
▸ With parenteral use Biliary spasm · cardiac arrest · cough · hyperalgesia · loss of consciousness
▸ With sublingual use Addiction · consciousness impaired · diarrhoea · fall · fever · hot flush · peripheral oedema · withdrawal syndrome neonatal
▸ With transdermal use Myoclonus · withdrawal syndrome neonatal

SIDE-EFFECTS, FURTHER INFORMATION **Muscle rigidity** Intravenous administration of fentanyl can cause muscle rigidity, which may involve the thoracic muscles. Manufacturer advises administration by slow intravenous injection to avoid; higher doses may require premedication with benzodiazepines and muscle relaxants.

Transdermal use Monitor patients using patches for increased side-effects if fever is present (increased absorption possible); avoid exposing application site to external heat, for example a hot bath or sauna (may also increase absorption).

● **BREAST FEEDING**
▸ With buccal use or intranasal use or sublingual use Manufacturer advises avoid during treatment and for 5 days after last administration—present in milk.
▸ With intravenous use Manufacturer advises avoid during treatment and for 24 hours after last administration—present in milk.
▸ With transdermal use Manufacturer advises avoid during treatment and for 72 hours after removal of patch—present in milk.

● **HEPATIC IMPAIRMENT** Manufacturer advises caution (risk of accumulation).
Dose adjustments Manufacturer advises cautious dose titration.

● **RENAL IMPAIRMENT** Manufacturer advises caution (risk of increased and prolonged effects).
Dose adjustments
▸ With intravenous use Manufacturer advises consider dose reduction.

● **DIRECTIONS FOR ADMINISTRATION**
▸ With transdermal use EvGr For *patches*, apply to dry, non-irritated, non-irradiated, non-hairy skin on torso or upper arm, removing after 72 hours and siting replacement patch on a different area (avoid using the same area for several days). Ⓜ
▸ With intravenous use EvGr For *intravenous infusion*, give continuously or intermittently in Glucose 5% or Sodium Chloride 0.9%. Ⓜ
▸ With buccal use EvGr For *buccal* films, moisten mouth, place film on inner lining of cheek (pink side to cheek), hold for at least 5 seconds until it sticks, and leave to dissolve (15–30 minutes); if more than 1 film required do not overlap, but use another area of the mouth. Avoid liquids for 5 minutes after application; avoid food until the film has dissolved. Ⓜ
▸ With buccal use EvGr Patients should be advised to place the lozenge in the mouth against the cheek and move it around the mouth using the applicator; each lozenge should be sucked over a 15 minute period. In patients with a dry mouth, water may be used to moisten the buccal mucosa. Patients with diabetes should be advised each lozenge contains approximately 2 g glucose. Ⓜ

EFFENTORA ® Place tablet between cheek and gum and leave to dissolve; if more than 1 tablet required, place second tablet on the other side of the mouth; tablet may alternatively be placed under the tongue (sublingually).

INSTANYL ® Patient should sit or stand during administration.

● **PRESCRIBING AND DISPENSING INFORMATION** Prescriptions for fentanyl patches can be written to show the strength in terms of the release rate and it is acceptable to write *'Fentanyl 25 patches'* to prescribe patches that release fentanyl 25 micrograms per hour. The dosage should be expressed in terms of the interval between applying a patch and replacing it with a new one, e.g. *'one patch to be applied every 72 hours'*. The total quantity of patches to be supplied should be written in words and figures.

● **PATIENT AND CARER ADVICE**
▸ With transdermal use Patients and carers should be informed about safe use, including correct administration and disposal, strict adherence to dosage instructions, and the symptoms and signs of opioid overdosage. Patches should be removed immediately in case of breathing difficulties, marked drowsiness, confusion, dizziness, or impaired speech, and patients and carers should seek prompt medical attention.
▸ With buccal use Patients or carers should be given advice on how to administer fentanyl buccal films or fentanyl lozenges.
▸ With intranasal use Patients or carers should be given advice on how to administer fentanyl nasal spray.

ABSTRAL ® Patients should be advised not to eat or drink until the tablet is completely dissolved.
In patients with a dry mouth, the buccal mucosa may be moistened with water before administration of tablet.

EFFENTORA ® Patients or carers should be given advice on how to administer *Effentora*® buccal tablets.
Patients should be advised not to eat or drink until the tablet is completely dissolved; after 30 minutes, if any remnants remain, they may be swallowed with a glass of water. Patients with a dry mouth should be advised to drink water to moisten the buccal mucosa before administration of the tablets; if appropriate effervescence does not occur, a switch of therapy may be advised.

INSTANYL ® Avoid concomitant use of other nasal preparations.
Patients or carers should be given advice on how to administer *Instanyl*® spray.

PECFENT ® Avoid concomitant use of other nasal preparations.
Patients or carers should be given advice on how to administer *PecFent*® spray.

● **NATIONAL FUNDING/ACCESS DECISIONS**
ABSTRAL ® For full details see funding body website
Scottish Medicines Consortium (SMC) decisions
▸ **Fentanyl sublingual tablets (*Abstral*®) for the management of breakthrough pain in adult patients using opioid therapy for chronic cancer pain (February 2009)** SMC No. 534/09 Recommended with restrictions

EFFENTORA ® For full details see funding body website
Scottish Medicines Consortium (SMC) decisions
▸ Fentanyl buccal tablets (*Effentora*®) for breakthrough pain in adults with cancer (February 2009) SMC No. 510/08 Recommended with restrictions

INSTANYL ® For full details see funding body website
Scottish Medicines Consortium (SMC) decisions
▸ Fentanyl nasal spray (*Instanyl*®) for the management of breakthrough pain in adults already receiving maintenance opioid therapy for chronic cancer pain (November 2009) SMC No. 579/09 Recommended with restrictions

PECFENT ® For full details see funding body website
Scottish Medicines Consortium (SMC) decisions
▸ Fentanyl pectin nasal spray (*PecFent*®) for the management of breakthrough pain in adults who are already receiving maintenance opioid therapy for chronic cancer pain (January 2011) SMC No. 663/10 Recommended with restrictions

● MEDICINAL FORMS There can be variation in the licensing of different medicines containing the same drug. Forms available from special-order manufacturers include: solution for injection, infusion, solution for infusion

Solution for injection
▸ **Fentanyl (Non-proprietary)**
Fentanyl (as Fentanyl citrate) 50 microgram per 1 ml Fentanyl 100micrograms/2ml solution for injection ampoules | 10 ampoule PoM £14.33 DT = £16.24 (Hospital only) CD2 | 10 ampoule PoM £11.50-£16.24 DT = £16.24 CD2 Fentanyl 500micrograms/10ml solution for injection ampoules | 10 ampoule PoM £14.50-£18.30 CD2 | 10 ampoule PoM £14.50 (Hospital only) CD2
▸ **Sublimaze** (Piramal Critical Care Ltd)
Fentanyl (as Fentanyl citrate) 50 microgram per 1 ml Sublimaze 500micrograms/10ml solution for injection ampoules | 5 ampoule PoM £6.53 DT = £6.53 CD2

Spray
CAUTIONARY AND ADVISORY LABELS 2
▸ **PecFent** (Kyowa Kirin International UK NewCo Ltd)
Fentanyl (as Fentanyl citrate) 100 microgram per 1 dose PecFent 100micrograms/dose nasal spray | 8 dose PoM £36.48 DT = £36.48 CD2 | 32 dose PoM £145.92 DT = £145.92 CD2
Fentanyl (as Fentanyl citrate) 400 microgram per 1 dose PecFent 400micrograms/dose nasal spray | 8 dose PoM £36.48 DT = £36.48 CD2 | 32 dose PoM £145.92 DT = £145.92 CD2

Buccal tablet
CAUTIONARY AND ADVISORY LABELS 2
ELECTROLYTES: May contain Sodium
▸ **Effentora** (Teva UK Ltd)
Fentanyl (as Fentanyl citrate) 100 microgram Effentora 100microgram buccal tablets | 28 tablet PoM £139.72 DT = £139.72 CD2 SF
Fentanyl (as Fentanyl citrate) 800 microgram Effentora 800microgram buccal tablets | 4 tablet PoM £19.96 CD2 SF | 28 tablet PoM £139.72 DT = £139.72 CD2 SF

Solution for infusion
▸ **Fentanyl (Non-proprietary)**
Fentanyl (as Fentanyl citrate) 50 microgram per 1 ml Fentanyl 2.5mg/50ml solution for infusion vials | 1 vial PoM £9.80 (Hospital only) CD2

Sublingual tablet
CAUTIONARY AND ADVISORY LABELS 2, 26
▸ **Abstral** (Kyowa Kirin International UK NewCo Ltd)
Fentanyl (as Fentanyl citrate) 100 microgram Abstral 100microgram sublingual tablets | 10 tablet PoM £49.99 DT = £49.99 CD2 SF | 30 tablet PoM £149.70 CD2 SF
Fentanyl (as Fentanyl citrate) 200 microgram Abstral 200microgram sublingual tablets | 10 tablet PoM £49.99 DT = £49.99 CD2 SF | 30 tablet PoM £149.70 CD2 SF
Fentanyl (as Fentanyl citrate) 300 microgram Abstral 300microgram sublingual tablets | 10 tablet PoM £49.99 DT = £49.99 CD2 SF | 30 tablet PoM £149.70 CD2 SF
Fentanyl (as Fentanyl citrate) 400 microgram Abstral 400microgram sublingual tablets | 10 tablet PoM £49.99 DT = £49.99 CD2 SF | 30 tablet PoM £149.70 CD2 SF
Fentanyl (as Fentanyl citrate) 600 microgram Abstral 600microgram sublingual tablets | 30 tablet PoM £149.70 DT = £149.70 CD2 SF

Fentanyl (as Fentanyl citrate) 800 microgram Abstral 800microgram sublingual tablets | 30 tablet PoM £149.70 DT = £149.70 CD2 SF
▸ **Fenhuma** (Glenmark Pharmaceuticals Europe Ltd)
Fentanyl (as Fentanyl citrate) 100 microgram Fenhuma 100microgram sublingual tablets | 10 tablet PoM £37.49 DT = £49.99 CD2 SF | 30 tablet PoM £112.28 CD2 SF
Fentanyl (as Fentanyl citrate) 200 microgram Fenhuma 200microgram sublingual tablets | 10 tablet PoM £37.49 DT = £49.99 CD2 SF | 30 tablet PoM £112.28 CD2 SF
Fentanyl (as Fentanyl citrate) 300 microgram Fenhuma 300microgram sublingual tablets | 10 tablet PoM £37.49 DT = £49.99 CD2 SF | 30 tablet PoM £112.28 CD2 SF
Fentanyl (as Fentanyl citrate) 400 microgram Fenhuma 400microgram sublingual tablets | 10 tablet PoM £37.49 DT = £49.99 CD2 SF | 30 tablet PoM £112.28 CD2 SF
Fentanyl (as Fentanyl citrate) 600 microgram Fenhuma 600microgram sublingual tablets | 30 tablet PoM £112.28 DT = £149.70 CD2 SF
Fentanyl (as Fentanyl citrate) 800 microgram Fenhuma 800microgram sublingual tablets | 30 tablet PoM £112.28 DT = £149.70 CD2 SF
▸ **Iremia** (Kent Pharma (UK) Ltd)
Fentanyl (as Fentanyl citrate) 67 microgram Iremia 67microgram sublingual tablets | 4 tablet PoM £14.00 CD2 SF
Fentanyl (as Fentanyl citrate) 133 microgram Iremia 133microgram sublingual tablets | 4 tablet PoM £14.00 CD2 SF
Fentanyl (as Fentanyl citrate) 267 microgram Iremia 267microgram sublingual tablets | 4 tablet PoM £14.00 CD2 SF
Fentanyl (as Fentanyl citrate) 400 microgram Iremia 400microgram sublingual tablets | 4 tablet PoM £14.00 CD2 SF
Fentanyl (as Fentanyl citrate) 533 microgram Iremia 533microgram sublingual tablets | 4 tablet PoM £14.00 CD2 SF
Fentanyl (as Fentanyl citrate) 800 microgram Iremia 800microgram sublingual tablets | 4 tablet PoM £14.00 CD2 SF

Transdermal patch
CAUTIONARY AND ADVISORY LABELS 2
▸ **Durogesic DTrans** (Janssen-Cilag Ltd)
Fentanyl 12 microgram per 1 hour Durogesic DTrans 12micrograms/hour transdermal patches | 5 patch PoM £12.59 DT = £12.59 CD2
Fentanyl 25 microgram per 1 hour Durogesic DTrans 25micrograms/hour transdermal patches | 5 patch PoM £17.99 DT = £17.99 CD2
Fentanyl 50 microgram per 1 hour Durogesic DTrans 50micrograms/hour transdermal patches | 5 patch PoM £33.66 DT = £33.66 CD2
Fentanyl 75 microgram per 1 hour Durogesic DTrans 75micrograms/hour transdermal patches | 5 patch PoM £46.99 DT = £46.99 CD2
Fentanyl 100 microgram per 1 hour Durogesic DTrans 100micrograms/hour transdermal patches | 5 patch PoM £57.86 DT = £57.86 CD2
▸ **Fencino** (Luye Pharma Ltd)
Fentanyl 12 microgram per 1 hour Fencino 12micrograms/hour transdermal patches | 5 patch PoM £8.46 DT = £12.59 CD2
Fentanyl 25 microgram per 1 hour Fencino 25micrograms/hour transdermal patches | 5 patch PoM £12.10 DT = £17.99 CD2
Fentanyl 50 microgram per 1 hour Fencino 50micrograms/hour transdermal patches | 5 patch PoM £22.62 DT = £33.66 CD2
Fentanyl 75 microgram per 1 hour Fencino 75micrograms/hour transdermal patches | 5 patch PoM £31.54 DT = £46.99 CD2
Fentanyl 100 microgram per 1 hour Fencino 100micrograms/hour transdermal patches | 5 patch PoM £38.88 DT = £57.86 CD2
▸ **Fenylat** (Luye Pharma Ltd)
Fentanyl 12 microgram per 1 hour Fenylat 12micrograms/hour transdermal patches | 5 patch PoM £8.46 DT = £12.59 CD2
Fentanyl 25 microgram per 1 hour Fenylat 25micrograms/hour transdermal patches | 5 patch PoM £12.10 DT = £17.99 CD2
Fentanyl 50 microgram per 1 hour Fenylat 50micrograms/hour transdermal patches | 5 patch PoM £22.62 DT = £33.66 CD2
Fentanyl 75 microgram per 1 hour Fenylat 75micrograms/hour transdermal patches | 5 patch PoM £31.54 DT = £46.99 CD2
Fentanyl 100 microgram per 1 hour Fenylat 100micrograms/hour transdermal patches | 5 patch PoM £38.88 DT = £57.86 CD2
▸ **Matrifen** (Teva UK Ltd)
Fentanyl 12 microgram per 1 hour Matrifen 12micrograms/hour transdermal patches | 5 patch PoM £7.52 DT = £12.59 CD2
Fentanyl 25 microgram per 1 hour Matrifen 25micrograms/hour transdermal patches | 5 patch PoM £10.76 DT = £17.99 CD2

Nervous system

4

Fentanyl 50 microgram per 1 hour Matrifen 50micrograms/hour transdermal patches | 5 patch [PoM] £20.12 DT = £33.66 [CD2]

Fentanyl 75 microgram per 1 hour Matrifen 75micrograms/hour transdermal patches | 5 patch [PoM] £28.06 DT = £46.99 [CD2]

Fentanyl 100 microgram per 1 hour Matrifen 100micrograms/hour transdermal patches | 5 patch [PoM] £34.59 DT = £57.86 [CD2]

▸ **Mezolar Matrix** (Sandoz Ltd)

Fentanyl 12 microgram per 1 hour Mezolar Matrix 12micrograms/hour transdermal patches | 5 patch [PoM] £7.53 DT = £12.59 [CD2]

Fentanyl 25 microgram per 1 hour Mezolar Matrix 25micrograms/hour transdermal patches | 5 patch [PoM] £10.77 DT = £17.99 [CD2]

Fentanyl 37.5 microgram per 1 hour Mezolar Matrix 37.5microgram/hour transdermal patches | 5 patch [PoM] £15.46 DT = £15.46 [CD2]

Fentanyl 50 microgram per 1 hour Mezolar Matrix 50micrograms/hour transdermal patches | 5 patch [PoM] £20.13 DT = £33.66 [CD2]

Fentanyl 75 microgram per 1 hour Mezolar Matrix 75micrograms/hour transdermal patches | 5 patch [PoM] £28.07 DT = £46.99 [CD2]

Fentanyl 100 microgram per 1 hour Mezolar Matrix 100micrograms/hour transdermal patches | 5 patch [PoM] £34.60 DT = £57.86 [CD2]

▸ **Opiodur** (Zentiva Pharma UK Ltd)

Fentanyl 12 microgram per 1 hour Opiodur 12micrograms/hour transdermal patches | 5 patch [PoM] £5.64 DT = £12.59 [CD2]

Fentanyl 25 microgram per 1 hour Opiodur 25micrograms/hour transdermal patches | 5 patch [PoM] £8.07 DT = £17.99 [CD2]

Fentanyl 50 microgram per 1 hour Opiodur 50micrograms/hour transdermal patches | 5 patch [PoM] £15.09 DT = £33.66 [CD2]

Fentanyl 75 microgram per 1 hour Opiodur 75micrograms/hour transdermal patches | 5 patch [PoM] £21.05 DT = £46.99 [CD2]

Fentanyl 100 microgram per 1 hour Opiodur 100micrograms/hour transdermal patches | 5 patch [PoM] £25.94 DT = £57.86 [CD2]

▸ **Victanyl** (Accord-UK Ltd)

Fentanyl 12 microgram per 1 hour Victanyl 12micrograms/hour transdermal patches | 5 patch [PoM] £12.58 DT = £12.59 [CD2]

Fentanyl 25 microgram per 1 hour Victanyl 25micrograms/hour transdermal patches | 5 patch [PoM] £25.89 DT = £17.99 [CD2]

Fentanyl 50 microgram per 1 hour Victanyl 50micrograms/hour transdermal patches | 5 patch [PoM] £48.36 DT = £33.66 [CD2]

Fentanyl 75 microgram per 1 hour Victanyl 75micrograms/hour transdermal patches | 5 patch [PoM] £67.41 DT = £46.99 [CD2]

Fentanyl 100 microgram per 1 hour Victanyl 100micrograms/hour transdermal patches | 5 patch [PoM] £83.09 DT = £57.86 [CD2]

▸ **Yemex** (Sandoz Ltd)

Fentanyl 12 microgram per 1 hour Yemex 12micrograms/hour transdermal patches | 5 patch [PoM] £12.59 DT = £12.59 [CD2]

Fentanyl 25 microgram per 1 hour Yemex 25micrograms/hour transdermal patches | 5 patch [PoM] £17.99 DT = £17.99 [CD2]

Fentanyl 50 microgram per 1 hour Yemex 50micrograms/hour transdermal patches | 5 patch [PoM] £33.66 DT = £33.66 [CD2]

Fentanyl 75 microgram per 1 hour Yemex 75micrograms/hour transdermal patches | 5 patch [PoM] £46.99 DT = £46.99 [CD2]

Fentanyl 100 microgram per 1 hour Yemex 100micrograms/hour transdermal patches | 5 patch [PoM] £57.86 DT = £57.86 [CD2]

Lozenge

CAUTIONARY AND ADVISORY LABELS 2
EXCIPIENTS: May contain Propylene glycol

▸ **Actiq** (Teva UK Ltd)

Fentanyl (as Fentanyl citrate) 200 microgram Actiq 200microgram lozenges with integral oromucosal applicator | 3 lozenge [PoM] £21.05 DT = £21.05 [CD2] | 30 lozenge [PoM] £210.41 DT = £210.41 [CD2]

Fentanyl (as Fentanyl citrate) 400 microgram Actiq 400microgram lozenges with integral oromucosal applicator | 30 lozenge [PoM] £210.41 DT = £210.41 [CD2]

Fentanyl (as Fentanyl citrate) 600 microgram Actiq 600microgram lozenges with integral oromucosal applicator | 3 lozenge [PoM] £21.05 DT = £21.05 [CD2] | 30 lozenge [PoM] £210.41 DT = £210.41 [CD2]

Fentanyl (as Fentanyl citrate) 800 microgram Actiq 800microgram lozenges with integral oromucosal applicator | 3 lozenge [PoM] £21.05 DT = £21.05 [CD2] | 30 lozenge [PoM] £210.41 DT = £210.41 [CD2]

Fentanyl (as Fentanyl citrate) 1.2 mg Actiq 1.2mg lozenges with integral oromucosal applicator | 30 lozenge [PoM] £210.41 DT = £210.41 [CD2]

Fentanyl (as Fentanyl citrate) 1.6 mg Actiq 1.6mg lozenges with integral oromucosal applicator | 30 lozenge [PoM] £210.41 DT = £210.41 [CD2]

▸ **Cynril** (Fontus Health Ltd)

Fentanyl (as Fentanyl citrate) 200 microgram Cynril 200microgram lozenges with integral oromucosal applicator | 3 lozenge [PoM] £16.80 DT = £21.05 [CD2]

Fentanyl (as Fentanyl citrate) 400 microgram Cynril 400microgram lozenges with integral oromucosal applicator | 3 lozenge [PoM] £16.80 DT = £21.05 [CD2]

Fentanyl (as Fentanyl citrate) 600 microgram Cynril 600microgram lozenges with integral oromucosal applicator | 3 lozenge [PoM] £16.80 DT = £21.05 [CD2]

Fentanyl (as Fentanyl citrate) 800 microgram Cynril 800microgram lozenges with integral oromucosal applicator | 3 lozenge [PoM] £16.80 DT = £21.05 [CD2]

Fentanyl (as Fentanyl citrate) 1.2 mg Cynril 1.2mg lozenges with integral oromucosal applicator | 3 lozenge [PoM] £16.80 DT = £16.80 [CD2]

Fentanyl (as Fentanyl citrate) 1.6 mg Cynril 1.6mg lozenges with integral oromucosal applicator | 3 lozenge [PoM] £16.80 DT = £16.80 [CD2]

▶ 510

Hydromorphone hydrochloride

11-May-2021

● **INDICATIONS AND DOSE**

Severe pain in cancer

▸ BY MOUTH USING IMMEDIATE-RELEASE MEDICINES
▸ **Child 12-17 years:** 1.3 mg every 4 hours, dose to be increased if necessary according to severity of pain
▸ **Adult:** 1.3 mg every 4 hours, dose to be increased if necessary according to severity of pain
▸ BY MOUTH USING MODIFIED-RELEASE MEDICINES
▸ **Child 12-17 years:** 4 mg every 12 hours, dose to be increased if necessary according to severity of pain
▸ **Adult:** 4 mg every 12 hours, dose to be increased if necessary according to severity of pain

● **CONTRA-INDICATIONS** Acute abdomen

● **CAUTIONS** Pancreatitis · toxic psychosis

● **INTERACTIONS** → Appendix 1: opioids

● **SIDE-EFFECTS**

▸ **Common or very common** Abdominal pain · anxiety · appetite decreased · asthenia · sleep disorders
▸ **Uncommon** Depression · diarrhoea · dyspnoea · erectile dysfunction · malaise · movement disorders · paraesthesia · peripheral oedema · taste altered · tremor
▸ **Frequency not known** Hyperalgesia · paralytic ileus · withdrawal syndrome neonatal

● **BREAST FEEDING** Avoid—no information available.

● **HEPATIC IMPAIRMENT** Manufacturer advises avoid.

● **RENAL IMPAIRMENT** [EvGr] Use with caution. [M]
Dose adjustments [EvGr] Consider dose reduction (risk of increased and prolonged effects). [M]

● **DIRECTIONS FOR ADMINISTRATION** For *immediate-release* capsules, manufacturer advises swallow whole capsule or sprinkle contents on soft food. For *modified-release* capsules, manufacturer advises swallow whole or open capsule and sprinkle contents on soft cold food (swallow the pellets within the capsule whole; do not crush or chew).

● **PATIENT AND CARER ADVICE** Patients or carers should be given advice on how to administer hydromorphone hydrochloride capsules and modified-release capsules.

● **MEDICINAL FORMS** There can be variation in the licensing of different medicines containing the same drug. Forms available from special-order manufacturers include: oral solution

Modified-release capsule

CAUTIONARY AND ADVISORY LABELS 2

▸ **Palladone SR** (Napp Pharmaceuticals Ltd)

Hydromorphone hydrochloride 2 mg Palladone SR 2mg capsules | 56 capsule [PoM] £20.98 DT = £20.98 [CD2]

Hydromorphone hydrochloride 4 mg Palladone SR 4mg capsules |
56 capsule [PoM] £28.75 DT = £28.75 [CD2]
Hydromorphone hydrochloride 8 mg Palladone SR 8mg capsules |
56 capsule [PoM] £56.08 DT = £56.08 [CD2]

Oral capsule
CAUTIONARY AND ADVISORY LABELS 2
▸ Palladone (Napp Pharmaceuticals Ltd)
   Hydromorphone hydrochloride 1.3 mg Palladone 1.3mg capsules
| 56 capsule [PoM] £8.82 DT = £8.82 [CD2]

▸ 510

Meptazinol

11-May-2021

● **INDICATIONS AND DOSE**

Moderate to severe pain, including post-operative pain and renal colic
▸ BY MOUTH
  ▸ Adult: 200 mg every 3–6 hours as required
▸ BY INTRAMUSCULAR INJECTION
  ▸ Adult: 75–100 mg every 2–4 hours if required
▸ BY SLOW INTRAVENOUS INJECTION
  ▸ Adult: 50–100 mg every 2–4 hours if required

Obstetric analgesia
▸ BY INTRAMUSCULAR INJECTION
  ▸ Adult: 2 mg/kg, usual dose 100–150 mg

● **CONTRA-INDICATIONS** Myocardial infarction ·
phaeochromocytoma

● **INTERACTIONS** → Appendix 1: opioids

● **SIDE-EFFECTS**
▸ **Common or very common** Diarrhoea · gastrointestinal
discomfort
  Overdose Effects only partially reversed by naloxone.

● **BREAST FEEDING** Use only if potential benefit outweighs
risk.

● **HEPATIC IMPAIRMENT** Manufacturer advises caution.
Dose adjustments Manufacturer advises dose reduction.

● **RENAL IMPAIRMENT**
Dose adjustments [EvGr] Reduce dose in moderate to severe
impairment (risk of increased and prolonged effects;
increased cerebral sensitivity). ⟨M⟩

● **MEDICINAL FORMS** There can be variation in the licensing of
different medicines containing the same drug.
Oral tablet
CAUTIONARY AND ADVISORY LABELS 2
▸ Meptid (Almirall Ltd)
  Meptazinol (as Meptazinol hydrochloride) 200 mg Meptid 200mg
tablets | 112 tablet [PoM] £22.11 DT = £22.11

▸ 510

Morphine

03-Apr-2024

● **INDICATIONS AND DOSE**

Pain
▸ BY SUBCUTANEOUS INJECTION
  ▸ Child 1–5 months: Initially 100–200 micrograms/kg
every 6 hours, dose to be adjusted according to
response
  ▸ Child 6 months–1 year: Initially 100–200 micrograms/kg
every 4 hours, dose to be adjusted according to
response
  ▸ Child 2–11 years: Initially 200 micrograms/kg every
4 hours (max. per dose 10 mg), dose to be adjusted
according to response
  ▸ Child 12–17 years: Initially 2.5–10 mg every 4 hours,
dose to be adjusted according to response
▸ INITIALLY BY INTRAVENOUS INJECTION
  ▸ Child 1–5 months: 100 micrograms/kg every 6 hours, to
be administered over at least 5 minutes, dose to be
adjusted according to response, alternatively (by
intravenous injection) initially 100 micrograms/kg for

1 dose, to be administered over at least 5 minutes,
followed by (by continuous intravenous infusion)
10–30 micrograms/kg/hour, dose to be adjusted
according to response
  ▸ Child 6 months–11 years: 100 micrograms/kg every
4 hours, to be administered over at least 5 minutes,
dose to be adjusted according to response,
alternatively (by intravenous injection) initially
100 micrograms/kg for 1 dose, to be administered over
at least 5 minutes, followed by (by continuous
intravenous infusion) 20–30 micrograms/kg/hour, dose
to be adjusted according to response
  ▸ Child 12–17 years: 5 mg every 4 hours, to be
administered over at least 5 minutes, dose to be
adjusted according to response, alternatively (by
intravenous injection) initially 5 mg for 1 dose, to be
administered over at least 5 minutes, followed by (by
continuous intravenous infusion)
20–30 micrograms/kg/hour, dose to be adjusted
according to response
▸ BY MOUTH USING IMMEDIATE-RELEASE MEDICINES, OR BY
RECTUM
  ▸ Child 1–2 months: Initially 50–100 micrograms/kg every
4 hours, dose to be adjusted according to response
  ▸ Child 3–5 months: 100–150 micrograms/kg every
4 hours, dose to be adjusted according to response
  ▸ Child 6–11 months: 200 micrograms/kg every 4 hours,
dose to be adjusted according to response
  ▸ Child 1 year: Initially 200–300 micrograms/kg every
4 hours, dose to be adjusted according to response
  ▸ Child 2–11 years: Initially 200–300 micrograms/kg every
4 hours (max. per dose 10 mg), dose to be adjusted
according to response
  ▸ Child 12–17 years: Initially 5–10 mg every 4 hours, dose
to be adjusted according to response

Acute pain
▸ BY MOUTH USING IMMEDIATE-RELEASE MEDICINES, OR BY
INTRAMUSCULAR INJECTION
  ▸ Adult: Initially 10 mg every 4 hours, use reduced dose
5 mg every 4 hours in frail patients, dose to be adjusted
according to response, dose can be given more
frequently during titration
  ▸ Elderly: Initially 5 mg every 4 hours, dose to be
adjusted according to response, dose can be given more
frequently during titration
▸ BY SUBCUTANEOUS INJECTION
  ▸ Adult: Initially 10 mg every 4 hours, use reduced dose
5 mg every 4 hours in frail patients, dose to be adjusted
according to response, subcutaneous injection not
suitable for oedematous patients, dose can be given
more frequently during titration
  ▸ Elderly: Initially 5 mg every 4 hours, dose to be
adjusted according to response, subcutaneous
injection not suitable for oedematous patients, dose
can be given more frequently during titration
▸ BY SLOW INTRAVENOUS INJECTION
  ▸ Adult: Initially 5 mg every 4 hours, use reduced dose in
frail and elderly patients, dose to be adjusted according
to response, dose can be adjusted more frequently
during titration

Chronic pain
▸ BY MOUTH USING IMMEDIATE-RELEASE MEDICINES, OR BY
INTRAMUSCULAR INJECTION
  ▸ Adult: Initially 5–10 mg every 4 hours, dose to be
adjusted according to response
▸ BY SUBCUTANEOUS INJECTION
  ▸ Adult: Initially 5–10 mg every 4 hours, dose to be
adjusted according to response, subcutaneous
injection not suitable for oedematous patients

continued →

▶ BY RECTUM
▸ Adult: Initially 15–30 mg every 4 hours, dose to be adjusted according to response

Pain [with modified-release 12-hourly preparations]
▶ BY MOUTH USING MODIFIED-RELEASE MEDICINES
▸ Adult: Every 12 hours, dose adjusted according to daily morphine requirements, dosage requirements should be reviewed if the brand is altered

Pain [with modified-release 24-hourly preparations]
▶ BY MOUTH USING MODIFIED-RELEASE MEDICINES
▸ Adult: Every 24 hours, dose adjusted according to daily morphine requirements, dosage requirements should be reviewed if the brand is altered

Pain in palliative care [starting dose for opioid-naïve patients]
▶ BY MOUTH
▸ Adult: Initially 20–30 mg daily in divided doses, using immediate-release preparation 4-hourly or a 12-hourly modified-release preparation, for management of breakthrough pain and advice on dose titration, see *Opioid analgesics* under Prescribing in palliative care p. 26.

Pain in palliative care [starting dose for patients being switched from a regular weak opioid]
▶ BY MOUTH
▸ Adult: Initially 40–60 mg daily in divided doses, using immediate-release preparation 4-hourly or a 12-hourly modified-release preparation, for management of breakthrough pain and advice on dose titration, see *Opioid analgesics* under Prescribing in palliative care p. 26, use dose for elderly in frail patients.
▸ Elderly: Initially 20–30 mg daily in divided doses, using immediate-release preparation 4-hourly or a 12-hourly modified-release preparation, for management of breakthrough pain and advice on dose titration, see *Opioid analgesics* under Prescribing in palliative care p. 26.

Pain in palliative care [starting dose for strong opioid-naïve patients]
▶ BY CONTINUOUS SUBCUTANEOUS INFUSION
▸ Adult: Initially 20 mg/24 hours, for management of breakthrough pain and advice on dose titration, see *Opioid analgesics* under Prescribing in palliative care p. 26, use dose for elderly in frail patients.
▸ Elderly: Initially 10 mg/24 hours, for management of breakthrough pain and advice on dose titration, see *Opioid analgesics* under Prescribing in palliative care p. 26.

Cough in palliative care [starting dose for opioid-naïve patients]
▶ BY MOUTH USING IMMEDIATE-RELEASE MEDICINES
▸ Adult: 2.5–5 mg every 4–6 hours, if necessary, increase dose until cough relieved or until unacceptable side-effects occur
▶ BY MOUTH USING MODIFIED-RELEASE MEDICINES
▸ Adult: 5–10 mg every 12 hours, if necessary, increase dose until cough relieved or until unacceptable side-effects occur

Breathlessness at rest in palliative care [starting dose for opioid-naïve patients]
▶ BY MOUTH USING IMMEDIATE-RELEASE MEDICINES
▸ Adult: Initially 500 micrograms every 12 hours for 48 hours, then increased to 500 micrograms every 6 hours for 48 hours, then increased to 1 mg every 4 hours for 1 week, then increased to 2 mg every 4 hours for 1 week, then increased to 3 mg every 4 hours for 1 week, then increased to 5 mg every 4 hours, if necessary, continue to adjust dose each week by 30-50%; usual maximum 30 mg per day

▶ BY MOUTH USING MODIFIED-RELEASE MEDICINES
▸ Adult: Initially 5 mg every 12 hours, if necessary, daily dose to be increased in steps of 10 mg at weekly intervals; usual maximum 30 mg per day

Premedication
▶ BY SUBCUTANEOUS INJECTION, OR BY INTRAMUSCULAR INJECTION
▸ Adult: Up to 10 mg, dose to be administered 60–90 minutes before operation

Patient controlled analgesia (PCA)
▶ BY INTRAVENOUS INFUSION
▸ Adult: (consult local protocol)

Myocardial infarction
▶ BY SLOW INTRAVENOUS INJECTION
▸ Adult: 5–10 mg for 1 dose, to be administered at a rate of 1–2 mg/minute, dose can be repeated if required, use reduced dose 2.5–5 mg in frail patients
▸ Elderly: 2.5–5 mg for 1 dose, to be administered at a rate of 1–2 mg/minute, dose can be repeated if required

Acute pulmonary oedema
▶ BY SLOW INTRAVENOUS INJECTION
▸ Adult: 5–10 mg for 1 dose, to be administered at a rate of 2 mg/minute, use reduced dose 2.5–5 mg in frail patients
▸ Elderly: 2.5–5 mg for 1 dose, to be administered at a rate of 2 mg/minute

DOSE EQUIVALENCE AND CONVERSION
▸ The doses stated refer equally to morphine hydrochloride and sulfate.

● UNLICENSED USE
▸ With oral use in adults [EvGr] Morphine is used in the treatment of cough and breathlessness at rest in palliative care, ⓓ but is not licensed for these indications.
▸ With oral use in children *Oramorph* ® solution and *MXL* ® capsules not licensed for use in children aged under 1 year. *Sevredol* ® tablets not licensed for use in children under 3 years. *MST Continus* ® preparations licensed to treat children with cancer pain (age-range not specified by manufacturer). *Actimorph* ® orodispersible tablets not licensed for use in children under 6 months.
▸ With rectal use Suppositories are not licensed for use.

IMPORTANT SAFETY INFORMATION
Do not confuse *modified-release* 12-hourly preparations with 24-hourly preparations, see *Prescribing and dispensing information.*
▸ In children
Different strengths of *oral solution*, such as 10 mg/5 mL and 20 mg/mL, are available. In addition, a 100 micrograms/mL oral solution is available as an unlicensed 'specials' product that is used in and supplied from secondary care settings. Care should be taken to ensure that the correct strength of oral solution is prescribed and dispensed, and the dose stated as both quantity and volume.

HEALTH SERVICES SAFETY INVESTIGATIONS BODY (HSSIB) PATIENT SAFETY INVESTIGATIONS: UNINTENTIONAL OVERDOSE OF MORPHINE SULFATE ORAL SOLUTION (APRIL 2022)
A review of an unintentional overdose of morphine sulfate 10 mg/5 mL *oral solution* identified that it may have contributed to a patient's death. The patient had not seen the dispensing label on the outer carton, and mistakenly thought the strength on the bottle was the prescribed dose. To minimise the risk of harm, the HSSIB has issued advice: www.hssib.org.uk/patient-safety-investigations/unintentional-overdose-of-morphine-sulfate-oral-solution/.

● CONTRA-INDICATIONS Acute abdomen · delayed gastric emptying · heart failure secondary to chronic lung disease · phaeochromocytoma

- **CAUTIONS** Cardiac arrhythmias · pancreatitis · severe cor pulmonale
- **INTERACTIONS** → Appendix 1: opioids
- **SIDE-EFFECTS**
▶ **Common or very common**
▶ With oral use Appetite decreased · asthenia · gastrointestinal discomfort · insomnia · malaise · neuromuscular dysfunction
▶ **Uncommon**
▶ With oral use Agitation · bronchospasm · ileus · mood altered · myoclonus · peripheral oedema · pulmonary oedema · sensation abnormal · syncope · taste altered
▶ **Frequency not known**
▶ With oral use Amenorrhoea · biliary pain · cough decreased · hyperalgesia · hypertension · pancreatitis exacerbated · sexual dysfunction · sleep apnoea · thinking abnormal · ureteral spasm · withdrawal syndrome neonatal
▶ With parenteral use Alertness decreased · bile duct disorders · mood altered · myoclonus · sexual dysfunction · ureteral spasm · urinary disorders · vision disorders
- **BREAST FEEDING** Therapeutic doses unlikely to affect infant.
- **HEPATIC IMPAIRMENT** Manufacturer advises caution. Avoid *oral preparations* in acute impairment; for *injectable preparations*—consult product literature.
  Dose adjustments Manufacturer advises consider dose reduction—consult product literature.
- **RENAL IMPAIRMENT** Avoid use or reduce dose; opioid effects increased and prolonged; increased cerebral sensitivity.
- **MONITORING REQUIREMENTS** Possible association between acute chest syndrome in patients with sickle cell disease treated with morphine during a vaso-occlusive crisis—manufacturer advises close monitoring for acute chest syndrome symptoms during treatment.
- **DIRECTIONS FOR ADMINISTRATION**
▶ In adults For *continuous subcutaneous infusion*, dilute with Water for Injections, Sodium Chloride 0.9%, or Glucose 5%.
▶ In children For *continuous intravenous infusion*, dilute with Glucose 5% or 10% or Sodium Chloride 0.9%.
▶ With oral use For *modified release capsules*—swallow whole or open capsule and sprinkle contents on soft food. EvGr For *orodispersible tablets*— place on the tongue, allow to disperse and swallow. Alternatively, tablets can be placed in a spoon and dispersed in a small amount of water before administration. ◈M◈
- **PRESCRIBING AND DISPENSING INFORMATION**
  Prescriptions must specify the 'form'.
▶ With oral use Modified-release preparations are available as 12-hourly or 24-hourly formulations; prescribers must ensure that the correct preparation is prescribed. Preparations that should be given 12-hourly include *MST Continus®*, *Morphgesic® SR*, and *Zomorph®*. Preparations that should be given 24-hourly include *MXL®*.
▶ With oral use in children Oral solutions are available in different strengths; prescribers must ensure that the correct preparation is prescribed—see *Important safety information* for details.
▶ With rectal use Both the strength of the suppositories and the morphine salt contained in them must be specified by the prescriber.
▶ When used for Breathlessness at rest in palliative care [starting dose for opioid-naïve patients] When a stable dose has been maintained for 2 weeks using immediate-release medicines, consider switching to a modified-release preparation.
  Palliative care For further information on the use of morphine in palliative care, see www.medicinescomplete. com/#/content/palliative/morphine.

- **PATIENT AND CARER ADVICE** Patients or carers should be given advice on how to administer morphine modified-release capsules and orodispersible tablets.
  Medicines for Children leaflet: Morphine for pain
  www.medicinesforchildren.org.uk/medicines/morphine-for-pain/
- **EXCEPTIONS TO LEGAL CATEGORY**
  Morphine Oral Solutions Prescription-only medicines or schedule 2 controlled drug. The proportion of morphine hydrochloride may be altered when specified by the prescriber; if above 13 mg per 5 mL the solution becomes a schedule 2 controlled drug. It is usual to adjust the strength so that the dose volume is 5 or 10 mL.
  Oral solutions of morphine can be prescribed by writing the formula:
  Morphine hydrochloride 5 mg
  Chloroform water to 5 mL

- **MEDICINAL FORMS** There can be variation in the licensing of different medicines containing the same drug. Forms available from special-order manufacturers include: oral capsule, oral solution, solution for injection, infusion, solution for infusion

Oral tablet
CAUTIONARY AND ADVISORY LABELS 2
▶ **Sevredol** (Napp Pharmaceuticals Ltd)
  Morphine sulfate 10 mg Sevredol 10mg tablets | 56 tablet PoM £5.31 DT = £5.31 CD2
  Morphine sulfate 20 mg Sevredol 20mg tablets | 56 tablet PoM £10.61 DT = £10.61 CD2
  Morphine sulfate 50 mg Sevredol 50mg tablets | 56 tablet PoM £28.02 DT = £28.02 CD2

Modified-release tablet
CAUTIONARY AND ADVISORY LABELS 2, 25
▶ **MST Continus** (Napp Pharmaceuticals Ltd)
  Morphine sulfate 5 mg MST Continus 5mg tablets | 60 tablet PoM £3.29 DT = £3.29 CD2
  Morphine sulfate 10 mg MST Continus 10mg tablets | 60 tablet PoM £5.20 DT = £5.20 CD2
  Morphine sulfate 15 mg MST Continus 15mg tablets | 60 tablet PoM £9.10 DT = £9.10 CD2
  Morphine sulfate 30 mg MST Continus 30mg tablets | 60 tablet PoM £12.47 DT = £12.47 CD2
  Morphine sulfate 60 mg MST Continus 60mg tablets | 60 tablet PoM £24.32 DT = £24.32 CD2
  Morphine sulfate 100 mg MST Continus 100mg tablets | 60 tablet PoM £38.50 DT = £38.50 CD2
  Morphine sulfate 200 mg MST Continus 200mg tablets | 60 tablet PoM £81.34 DT = £81.34 CD2
▶ **Morphgesic SR** (Advanz Pharma)
  Morphine sulfate 10 mg Morphgesic SR 10mg tablets | 60 tablet PoM £3.85 DT = £5.20 CD2
  Morphine sulfate 30 mg Morphgesic SR 30mg tablets | 60 tablet PoM £9.24 DT = £12.47 CD2
  Morphine sulfate 60 mg Morphgesic SR 60mg tablets | 60 tablet PoM £18.04 DT = £24.32 CD2
  Morphine sulfate 100 mg Morphgesic SR 100mg tablets | 60 tablet PoM £28.54 DT = £38.50 CD2

Solution for injection
▶ **Morphine (Non-proprietary)**
  Morphine sulfate 1 mg per 1 ml Morphine sulfate 5mg/5ml solution for injection ampoules | 10 ampoule PoM £78.80 DT = £78.80 CD2
  Morphine sulfate 1mg/1ml solution for injection ampoules | 10 ampoule PoM £62.30 (Hospital only) CD2
  Morphine sulfate 10mg/10ml solution for injection ampoules | 10 ampoule PoM £15.00–£82.50 DT = £17.50 CD2
  Morphine sulfate 10 mg per 1 ml Morphine sulfate 10mg/1ml solution for injection ampoules | 10 ampoule PoM £5.80–£19.27 DT = £2.81 CD2 | 10 ampoule PoM £14.72 DT = £2.81 (Hospital only) CD2
  Morphine sulfate 15 mg per 1 ml Morphine sulfate 15mg/1ml solution for injection ampoules | 10 ampoule PoM £10.74 DT = £12.17 (Hospital only) CD2 | 10 ampoule PoM £12.17 DT = £12.17 CD2
  Morphine sulfate 20 mg per 1 ml Morphine sulfate 20mg/1ml solution for injection ampoules | 10 ampoule PoM £254.73–£411.20 DT = £254.73 CD2
  Morphine sulfate 30 mg per 1 ml Morphine sulfate 30mg/1ml solution for injection ampoules | 10 ampoule PoM £15.79 DT =

£48.44 (Hospital only) [CD2] | 10 ampoule [PoM] £48.44 DT = £48.44 [CD2]
Morphine sulfate 60mg/2ml solution for injection ampoules | 5 ampoule [PoM] £12.00 DT = £12.00 [CD2]

Modified-release capsule
CAUTIONARY AND ADVISORY LABELS 2
- **MXL** (Napp Pharmaceuticals Ltd)
  Morphine sulfate 30 mg MXL 30mg capsules | 28 capsule [PoM] £10.91 [CD2]
  Morphine sulfate 60 mg MXL 60mg capsules | 28 capsule [PoM] £14.95 [CD2]
  Morphine sulfate 90 mg MXL 90mg capsules | 28 capsule [PoM] £22.04 DT = £22.04 [CD2]
  Morphine sulfate 120 mg MXL 120mg capsules | 28 capsule [PoM] £29.15 DT = £29.15 [CD2]
  Morphine sulfate 150 mg MXL 150mg capsules | 28 capsule [PoM] £36.43 DT = £36.43 [CD2]
  Morphine sulfate 200 mg MXL 200mg capsules | 28 capsule [PoM] £46.15 [CD2]
- **Zomorph** (Ethypharm UK Ltd)
  Morphine sulfate 10 mg Zomorph 10mg modified-release capsules | 60 capsule [PoM] £3.47 DT = £3.47 [CD2]
  Morphine sulfate 30 mg Zomorph 30mg modified-release capsules | 60 capsule [PoM] £8.30 DT = £8.30 [CD2]
  Morphine sulfate 60 mg Zomorph 60mg modified-release capsules | 60 capsule [PoM] £16.20 DT = £16.20 [CD2]
  Morphine sulfate 100 mg Zomorph 100mg modified-release capsules | 60 capsule [PoM] £21.80 DT = £21.80 [CD2]
  Morphine sulfate 200 mg Zomorph 200mg modified-release capsules | 60 capsule [PoM] £43.60 DT = £43.60 [CD2]

Solution for infusion
- **Morphine (Non-proprietary)**
  Morphine sulfate 1 mg per 1 ml Morphine sulfate 50mg/50ml solution for infusion vials | 1 vial [PoM] £5.78-£8.00 [CD2] | 10 vial [PoM] £73.20 [CD2]
  Morphine sulfate 2 mg per 1 ml Morphine sulfate 100mg/50ml solution for infusion vials | 1 vial [PoM] £6.48-£10.00 [CD2] | 10 vial [PoM] £119.40 [CD2]

Oral solution
CAUTIONARY AND ADVISORY LABELS 2
- **Morphine (Non-proprietary)**
  Morphine sulfate 2 mg per 1 ml Morphine sulfate 10mg/5ml oral solution | 100 ml [PoM] £2.76-£3.00 [CD5] | 300 ml [PoM] £9.00 DT = £8.33 [CD5] | 500 ml [PoM] £13.80-£14.15 [CD5]
- **Oramorph** (Glenwood GmbH)
  Morphine sulfate 2 mg per 1 ml Oramorph 10mg/5ml oral solution | 100 ml [PoM] £1.89 [CD5] | 300 ml [PoM] £5.45 DT = £8.33 [CD5] | 500 ml [PoM] £8.50 [CD5]
  Morphine sulfate 20 mg per 1 ml Oramorph 20mg/ml concentrated oral solution | 120 ml [PoM] £19.50 DT = £19.50 [CD2] [SF]

Orodispersible tablet
CAUTIONARY AND ADVISORY LABELS 2
- **Actimorph** (Ethypharm UK Ltd)
  Morphine sulfate 1 mg Actimorph 1mg orodispersible tablets | 56 tablet [PoM] £2.00 DT = £2.00 [CD2] [SF]
  Morphine sulfate 2.5 mg Actimorph 2.5mg orodispersible tablets | 56 tablet [PoM] £2.50 DT = £2.50 [CD2] [SF]
  Morphine sulfate 5 mg Actimorph 5mg orodispersible tablets | 56 tablet [PoM] £3.50 DT = £3.50 [CD2] [SF]
  Morphine sulfate 10 mg Actimorph 10mg orodispersible tablets | 56 tablet [PoM] £4.75 DT = £4.75 [CD2] [SF]
  Morphine sulfate 20 mg Actimorph 20mg orodispersible tablets | 56 tablet [PoM] £9.50 DT = £9.50 [CD2] [SF]
  Morphine sulfate 30 mg Actimorph 30mg orodispersible tablets | 56 tablet [PoM] £13.00 DT = £13.00 [CD2] [SF]

Infusion
- **Sendolor** (Eurocept International bv)
  Morphine hydrochloride 1 mg per 1 ml Sendolor 100mg/100ml infusion bags | 1 bag [PoM] £23.13 (Hospital only) [CD2]

► 510

Oxycodone hydrochloride
10-Apr-2025

● **INDICATIONS AND DOSE**

Postoperative pain
- ► BY MOUTH USING IMMEDIATE-RELEASE MEDICINES
- ► Adult: Initially 5 mg every 4–6 hours, dose to be increased if necessary according to severity of pain,

some patients may require higher doses than the maximum daily dose; maximum 400 mg per day
- ► BY SLOW INTRAVENOUS INJECTION
- ► Adult: 1–10 mg every 4 hours as required
- ► BY INTRAVENOUS INFUSION
- ► Adult: Initially 2 mg/hour, adjusted according to response
- ► BY SUBCUTANEOUS INJECTION
- ► Adult: Initially 5 mg every 4 hours as required
- ► BY SUBCUTANEOUS INFUSION
- ► Adult: Initially 7.5 mg/24 hours, adjusted according to response

Patient controlled analgesia (PCA)
- ► BY INTRAVENOUS INFUSION
- ► Adult: (consult local protocol)

Severe pain
- ► BY MOUTH USING IMMEDIATE-RELEASE MEDICINES
- ► Adult: Initially 5 mg every 4–6 hours, dose to be increased if necessary according to severity of pain, some patients may require higher doses than the maximum daily dose; maximum 400 mg per day
- ► BY MOUTH USING MODIFIED-RELEASE MEDICINES
- ► Adult: Initially 10 mg every 12 hours (max. per dose 200 mg every 12 hours), dose to be increased if necessary according to severity of pain, some patients might require higher doses than the maximum daily dose, use 12-hourly modified-release preparations for this dose; see *Prescribing and dispensing information*
- ► BY SLOW INTRAVENOUS INJECTION
- ► Adult: 1–10 mg every 4 hours as required
- ► BY INTRAVENOUS INFUSION
- ► Adult: Initially 2 mg/hour, adjusted according to response
- ► BY SUBCUTANEOUS INJECTION
- ► Adult: Initially 5 mg every 4 hours as required
- ► BY SUBCUTANEOUS INFUSION
- ► Adult: Initially 7.5 mg/24 hours, adjusted according to response

Moderate to severe pain in palliative care [starting dose for strong opioid-naïve patients] (administered on expert advice)
- ► BY MOUTH USING IMMEDIATE-RELEASE MEDICINES
- ► Adult: Initially 5 mg every 4–6 hours, for management of breakthrough pain and advice on dose titration, see *Opioid analgesics* under Prescribing in palliative care p. 26, use dose for elderly in frail patients.
- ► Elderly: Initially 2.5 mg every 4–6 hours, for management of breakthrough pain and advice on dose titration, see *Opioid analgesics* under Prescribing in palliative care p. 26.
- ► BY MOUTH USING MODIFIED-RELEASE MEDICINES
- ► Adult: Initially 10 mg every 12 hours, use 12-hourly modified-release preparations for this dose; see *Prescribing and dispensing information*, for management of breakthrough pain and advice on dose titration, see *Opioid analgesics* under Prescribing in palliative care p. 26, use dose for elderly in frail patients.
- ► Elderly: Initially 5 mg every 12 hours, use 12-hourly modified-release preparations for this dose; see *Prescribing and dispensing information*, for management of breakthrough pain and advice on dose titration, see *Opioid analgesics* under Prescribing in palliative care p. 26.
- ► BY CONTINUOUS SUBCUTANEOUS INFUSION
- ► Adult: Initially 7.5 mg/24 hours, for management of breakthrough pain and advice on dose titration, see *Opioid analgesics* under Prescribing in palliative care p. 26.

DOSE EQUIVALENCE AND CONVERSION
- ► When switching between formulations in patients already receiving oxycodone, 2 mg oral oxycodone is

approximately equivalent to 1 mg parenteral oxycodone.

ONEXILA XL®

Severe pain
▶ BY MOUTH
▶ **Adult:** Initially 10 mg every 24 hours, dose to be increased if necessary according to severity of pain, some patients may require higher doses than the maximum daily dose; maximum 400 mg per day

> **IMPORTANT SAFETY INFORMATION**
> Do not confuse modified-release 12-hourly preparations with 24-hourly preparations, see *Prescribing and dispensing information*.

- **CONTRA-INDICATIONS** Acute abdomen · chronic constipation · cor pulmonale · delayed gastric emptying
- **CAUTIONS** Pancreatitis · toxic psychosis
- **INTERACTIONS** → Appendix 1: opioids
- **SIDE-EFFECTS**
  GENERAL SIDE-EFFECTS
  ▶ **Common or very common** Anxiety · bronchospasm · depression · diarrhoea · dyspnoea · gastrointestinal discomfort · hiccups · mood altered · tremor
  ▶ **Uncommon** Biliary colic · burping · chills · dehydration · dysphagia · gastrointestinal disorders · malaise · memory loss · neuromuscular dysfunction · oedema · sensation abnormal · sexual dysfunction · speech disorder · syncope · taste altered · thirst · vasodilation
  ▶ **Frequency not known** Aggression · amenorrhoea · cholestasis
  SPECIFIC SIDE-EFFECTS
  ▶ **Common or very common**
  ▶ With oral use Appetite abnormal · asthenic conditions · cognitive impairment · insomnia · movement disorders · perception altered · psychiatric disorders · urinary frequency increased
  ▶ With parenteral use Appetite decreased · asthenia · cough decreased · sleep disorders · thinking abnormal
  ▶ **Uncommon**
  ▶ With oral use Chest pain · cough · hyperacusia · increased risk of infection · injury · lacrimation disorder · migraine · oral disorders · pain · SIADH · voice alteration
  ▶ With parenteral use Fever · hypogonadism · ureteral spasm
  ▶ **Rare or very rare**
  ▶ With oral use Haemorrhage · lymphadenopathy · muscle spasms · photosensitivity reaction · tooth discolouration · weight changes
  ▶ **Frequency not known**
  ▶ With parenteral use Dental caries · hyperalgesia · withdrawal syndrome neonatal
- **BREAST FEEDING** Present in milk—avoid.
- **HEPATIC IMPAIRMENT** [EvGr] Caution in mild impairment; avoid in moderate to severe impairment ⟨M⟩.
  Dose adjustments [EvGr] Initial dose reduction of 50% in mild impairment; adjust according to response. ⟨M⟩
- **RENAL IMPAIRMENT** [EvGr] Caution (risk of increased and prolonged effects). ⟨M⟩
  Dose adjustments [EvGr] Initial dose reduction of 50%; adjust according to response. ⟨M⟩
- **DIRECTIONS FOR ADMINISTRATION** For intravenous infusion (*Oxynorm*®), manufacturer advises give continuously *or* intermittently in Glucose 5% or Sodium Chloride 0.9%; dilute to a concentration of 1 mg/mL.
- **PRESCRIBING AND DISPENSING INFORMATION** Modified-release preparations are available as 12-hourly or 24-hourly formulations. Preparations that should be given 12-hourly include *Abtard*®, *Carexil*®, *Ixyldone*®, *Leveraxo*®, *Longtec*®, *Oxeltra*®, *OxyContin*®, *Oxypro*®, *Oxylan*®,

Reltebon®, and *Renocontin*®. Preparations that should be given 24-hourly include *Onexila*® XL.

Palliative care For further information on the use of oxycodone in palliative care, see www.medicinescomplete.com/#/content/palliative/oxycodone.

- **NATIONAL FUNDING/ACCESS DECISIONS**
  For full details see funding body website
  Scottish Medicines Consortium (SMC) decisions
  ▶ Oxycodone injection (*OxyNorm*®) for the treatment of moderate to severe pain in patients with cancer (October 2004) SMC No. 125/04 Recommended with restrictions
  ▶ Oxycodone 5 mg, 10 mg, 20 mg, 40 mg and 80 mg prolonged release tablets (*OxyContin*®) for the treatment of severe non-malignant pain requiring a strong opioid (September 2005) SMC No. 197/05 Recommended with restrictions
  ▶ Oxycodone hydrochloride 50 mg/mL injection (*OxyNorm*®) for the treatment of moderate to severe pain in patients with cancer (November 2010) SMC No. 648/10 Recommended with restrictions

- **MEDICINAL FORMS** There can be variation in the licensing of different medicines containing the same drug. Forms available from special-order manufacturers include: oral solution, solution for infusion

Oral tablet
CAUTIONARY AND ADVISORY LABELS 2
EXCIPIENTS: May contain Lecithin
▶ Oxyact (G.L. Pharma UK Ltd)
Oxycodone hydrochloride 5 mg Oxyact 5mg tablets | 20 tablet [PoM] £1.95 [CD2] | 56 tablet [PoM] £5.15 DT = £5.15 [CD2]
Oxycodone hydrochloride 10 mg Oxyact 10mg tablets | 56 tablet [PoM] £10.29 DT = £10.29 [CD2]
Oxycodone hydrochloride 20 mg Oxyact 20mg tablets | 56 tablet [PoM] £20.57 DT = £20.57 [CD2]

Modified-release tablet
CAUTIONARY AND ADVISORY LABELS 2, 25
▶ Ixyldone (Morningside Healthcare Ltd)
Oxycodone hydrochloride 5 mg Ixyldone 5mg modified-release tablets | 28 tablet [PoM] £2.96 DT = £12.52 [CD2]
Oxycodone hydrochloride 10 mg Ixyldone 10mg modified-release tablets | 56 tablet [PoM] £5.94 DT = £25.04 [CD2]
Oxycodone hydrochloride 15 mg Ixyldone 15mg modified-release tablets | 56 tablet [PoM] £9.05 DT = £38.12 [CD2]
Oxycodone hydrochloride 20 mg Ixyldone 20mg modified-release tablets | 56 tablet [PoM] £11.88 DT = £50.08 [CD2]
Oxycodone hydrochloride 30 mg Ixyldone 30mg modified-release tablets | 56 tablet [PoM] £18.10 DT = £76.23 [CD2]
Oxycodone hydrochloride 40 mg Ixyldone 40mg modified-release tablets | 56 tablet [PoM] £23.79 DT = £100.19 [CD2]
Oxycodone hydrochloride 60 mg Ixyldone 60mg modified-release tablets | 56 tablet [PoM] £36.19 DT = £152.49 [CD2]
Oxycodone hydrochloride 80 mg Ixyldone 80mg modified-release tablets | 56 tablet [PoM] £47.58 DT = £200.39 [CD2]
▶ Longtec (Qdem Pharmaceuticals Ltd)
Oxycodone hydrochloride 5 mg Longtec 5mg modified-release tablets | 28 tablet [PoM] £4.69 DT = £12.52 [CD2]
Oxycodone hydrochloride 10 mg Longtec 10mg modified-release tablets | 56 tablet [PoM] £9.39 DT = £25.04 [CD2]
Oxycodone hydrochloride 15 mg Longtec 15mg modified-release tablets | 56 tablet [PoM] £14.30 DT = £38.12 [CD2]
Oxycodone hydrochloride 20 mg Longtec 20mg modified-release tablets | 56 tablet [PoM] £18.78 DT = £50.08 [CD2]
Oxycodone hydrochloride 30 mg Longtec 30mg modified-release tablets | 56 tablet [PoM] £28.58 DT = £76.23 [CD2]
Oxycodone hydrochloride 40 mg Longtec 40mg modified-release tablets | 56 tablet [PoM] £37.57 DT = £100.19 [CD2]
Oxycodone hydrochloride 60 mg Longtec 60mg modified-release tablets | 56 tablet [PoM] £57.18 DT = £152.49 [CD2]
Oxycodone hydrochloride 80 mg Longtec 80mg modified-release tablets | 56 tablet [PoM] £75.14 DT = £200.39 [CD2]
Oxycodone hydrochloride 120 mg Longtec 120mg modified-release tablets | 56 tablet [PoM] £114.38 DT = £305.02 [CD2]
▶ Oxeltra (Wockhardt UK Ltd)
Oxycodone hydrochloride 5 mg Oxeltra 5mg modified-release tablets | 28 tablet [PoM] £3.13 DT = £12.52 [CD2]
Oxycodone hydrochloride 10 mg Oxeltra 10mg modified-release tablets | 56 tablet [PoM] £6.26 DT = £25.04 [CD2]

Oxycodone hydrochloride 15 mg Oxeltra 15mg modified-release tablets | 56 tablet [PoM] £9.53 DT = £38.12 [CD2]
Oxycodone hydrochloride 20 mg Oxeltra 20mg modified-release tablets | 56 tablet [PoM] £12.52 DT = £50.08 [CD2]
Oxycodone hydrochloride 30 mg Oxeltra 30mg modified-release tablets | 56 tablet [PoM] £19.06 DT = £76.23 [CD2]
Oxycodone hydrochloride 40 mg Oxeltra 40mg modified-release tablets | 56 tablet [PoM] £25.05 DT = £100.19 [CD2]
Oxycodone hydrochloride 60 mg Oxeltra 60mg modified-release tablets | 56 tablet [PoM] £38.12 DT = £152.49 [CD2]
Oxycodone hydrochloride 80 mg Oxeltra 80mg modified-release tablets | 56 tablet [PoM] £50.10 DT = £200.39 [CD2]

▸ **OxyContin** (Napp Pharmaceuticals Ltd)
Oxycodone hydrochloride 5 mg OxyContin 5mg modified-release tablets | 28 tablet [PoM] £12.52 DT = £12.52 [CD2]
Oxycodone hydrochloride 10 mg OxyContin 10mg modified-release tablets | 56 tablet [PoM] £25.04 DT = £25.04 [CD2]
Oxycodone hydrochloride 15 mg OxyContin 15mg modified-release tablets | 56 tablet [PoM] £38.12 DT = £38.12 [CD2]
Oxycodone hydrochloride 20 mg OxyContin 20mg modified-release tablets | 56 tablet [PoM] £50.08 DT = £50.08 [CD2]
Oxycodone hydrochloride 30 mg OxyContin 30mg modified-release tablets | 56 tablet [PoM] £76.23 DT = £76.23 [CD2]
Oxycodone hydrochloride 40 mg OxyContin 40mg modified-release tablets | 56 tablet [PoM] £100.19 DT = £100.19 [CD2]
Oxycodone hydrochloride 60 mg OxyContin 60mg modified-release tablets | 56 tablet [PoM] £152.49 DT = £152.49 [CD2]
Oxycodone hydrochloride 80 mg OxyContin 80mg modified-release tablets | 56 tablet [PoM] £200.39 DT = £200.39 [CD2]

▸ **Oxylan** (G.L. Pharma UK Ltd)
Oxycodone hydrochloride 5 mg Oxylan 5mg prolonged-release tablets | 14 tablet [PoM] £1.95 [CD2] | 28 tablet [PoM] £2.66 DT = £12.52 [CD2]
Oxycodone hydrochloride 10 mg Oxylan 10mg prolonged-release tablets | 14 tablet [PoM] £1.95 [CD2] | 56 tablet [PoM] £5.32 DT = £25.04 [CD2]
Oxycodone hydrochloride 15 mg Oxylan 15mg prolonged-release tablets | 56 tablet [PoM] £7.82 DT = £38.12 [CD2]
Oxycodone hydrochloride 20 mg Oxylan 20mg prolonged-release tablets | 56 tablet [PoM] £9.84 DT = £50.08 [CD2]
Oxycodone hydrochloride 30 mg Oxylan 30mg prolonged-release tablets | 56 tablet [PoM] £16.18 DT = £76.23 [CD2]
Oxycodone hydrochloride 40 mg Oxylan 40mg prolonged-release tablets | 56 tablet [PoM] £21.17 DT = £100.19 [CD2]
Oxycodone hydrochloride 60 mg Oxylan 60mg prolonged-release tablets | 56 tablet [PoM] £32.43 DT = £152.49 [CD2]
Oxycodone hydrochloride 80 mg Oxylan 80mg prolonged-release tablets | 56 tablet [PoM] £42.62 DT = £200.39 [CD2]

▸ **Oxypro** (Ridge Pharma Ltd)
Oxycodone hydrochloride 5 mg Oxypro 5mg modified-release tablets | 28 tablet [PoM] £3.13 DT = £12.52 [CD2]
Oxycodone hydrochloride 10 mg Oxypro 10mg modified-release tablets | 56 tablet [PoM] £6.26 DT = £25.04 [CD2]
Oxycodone hydrochloride 15 mg Oxypro 15mg modified-release tablets | 56 tablet [PoM] £9.53 DT = £38.12 [CD2]
Oxycodone hydrochloride 20 mg Oxypro 20mg modified-release tablets | 56 tablet [PoM] £12.52 DT = £50.08 [CD2]
Oxycodone hydrochloride 30 mg Oxypro 30mg modified-release tablets | 56 tablet [PoM] £19.06 DT = £76.23 [CD2]
Oxycodone hydrochloride 40 mg Oxypro 40mg modified-release tablets | 56 tablet [PoM] £25.05 DT = £100.19 [CD2]
Oxycodone hydrochloride 60 mg Oxypro 60mg modified-release tablets | 56 tablet [PoM] £38.12 DT = £152.49 [CD2]
Oxycodone hydrochloride 80 mg Oxypro 80mg modified-release tablets | 56 tablet [PoM] £50.10 DT = £200.39 [CD2]

▸ **Reltebon** (Accord-UK Ltd)
Oxycodone hydrochloride 5 mg Reltebon 5mg modified-release tablets | 28 tablet [PoM] £6.26 DT = £12.52 [CD2]
Oxycodone hydrochloride 10 mg Reltebon 10mg modified-release tablets | 56 tablet [PoM] £12.52 DT = £25.04 [CD2]
Oxycodone hydrochloride 15 mg Reltebon 15mg modified-release tablets | 56 tablet [PoM] £19.06 DT = £38.12 [CD2]
Oxycodone hydrochloride 20 mg Reltebon 20mg modified-release tablets | 56 tablet [PoM] £25.04 DT = £50.08 [CD2]
Oxycodone hydrochloride 30 mg Reltebon 30mg modified-release tablets | 56 tablet [PoM] £38.11 DT = £76.23 [CD2]
Oxycodone hydrochloride 40 mg Reltebon 40mg modified-release tablets | 56 tablet [PoM] £50.09 DT = £100.19 [CD2]
Oxycodone hydrochloride 60 mg Reltebon 60mg modified-release tablets | 56 tablet [PoM] £76.24 DT = £152.49 [CD2]

Oxycodone hydrochloride 80 mg Reltebon 80mg modified-release tablets | 56 tablet [PoM] £100.19 DT = £200.39 [CD2]

Solution for injection

▸ **Oxycodone hydrochloride (Non-proprietary)**
Oxycodone hydrochloride 10 mg per 1 ml Oxycodone 20mg/2ml solution for injection ampoules | 5 ampoule [PoM] £15.00–£16.00 DT = £16.00 [CD2]
Oxycodone 10mg/1ml solution for injection ampoules | 5 ampoule [PoM] £7.50–£13.32 DT = £13.32 [CD2]
Oxycodone hydrochloride 50 mg per 1 ml Oxycodone 50mg/1ml solution for injection ampoules | 5 ampoule [PoM] [Ⓢ] DT = £70.10 (Hospital only) [CD2] | 5 ampoule [PoM] £67.50–£70.10 DT = £70.10 [CD2]

▸ **OxyNorm** (Napp Pharmaceuticals Ltd)
Oxycodone hydrochloride 10 mg per 1 ml OxyNorm 10mg/1ml solution for injection ampoules | 5 ampoule [PoM] £8.00 DT = £13.32 [CD2]
OxyNorm 20mg/2ml solution for injection ampoules | 5 ampoule [PoM] £16.00 DT = £16.00 [CD2]
Oxycodone hydrochloride 50 mg per 1 ml OxyNorm 50mg/1ml solution for injection ampoules | 5 ampoule [PoM] £70.10 DT = £70.10 [CD2]

▸ **Shortec** (Qdem Pharmaceuticals Ltd)
Oxycodone hydrochloride 10 mg per 1 ml Shortec 10mg/1ml solution for injection ampoules | 5 ampoule [PoM] £6.80 DT = £13.32 [CD2]
Shortec 20mg/2ml solution for injection ampoules | 5 ampoule [PoM] £13.60 DT = £16.00 [CD2]
Oxycodone hydrochloride 50 mg per 1 ml Shortec 50mg/1ml solution for injection ampoules | 5 ampoule [PoM] £59.59 DT = £70.10 [CD2]

Oral capsule
CAUTIONARY AND ADVISORY LABELS 2

▸ **Oxycodone hydrochloride (Non-proprietary)**
Oxycodone hydrochloride 5 mg Oxycodone 5mg capsules | 56 capsule [PoM] £6.17 DT = £11.43 [CD2]
Oxycodone hydrochloride 10 mg Oxycodone 10mg capsules | 56 capsule [PoM] £12.35 DT = £22.86 [CD2]
Oxycodone hydrochloride 20 mg Oxycodone 20mg capsules | 56 capsule [PoM] £24.69 DT = £45.71 [CD2]

▸ **Lynlor** (Accord-UK Ltd)
Oxycodone hydrochloride 5 mg Lynlor 5mg capsules | 56 capsule [PoM] £6.86 DT = £11.43 [CD2]
Oxycodone hydrochloride 10 mg Lynlor 10mg capsules | 56 capsule [PoM] £13.72 DT = £22.86 [CD2]
Oxycodone hydrochloride 20 mg Lynlor 20mg capsules | 56 capsule [PoM] £27.43 DT = £45.71 [CD2]

▸ **OxyNorm** (Napp Pharmaceuticals Ltd)
Oxycodone hydrochloride 5 mg OxyNorm 5mg capsules | 56 capsule [PoM] £11.43 DT = £11.43 [CD2]
Oxycodone hydrochloride 10 mg OxyNorm 10mg capsules | 56 capsule [PoM] £22.86 DT = £22.86 [CD2]
Oxycodone hydrochloride 20 mg OxyNorm 20mg capsules | 56 capsule [PoM] £45.71 DT = £45.71 [CD2]

▸ **Shortec** (Qdem Pharmaceuticals Ltd)
Oxycodone hydrochloride 5 mg Shortec 5mg capsules | 56 capsule [PoM] £6.86 DT = £11.43 [CD2]
Oxycodone hydrochloride 10 mg Shortec 10mg capsules | 56 capsule [PoM] £13.72 DT = £22.86 [CD2]
Oxycodone hydrochloride 20 mg Shortec 20mg capsules | 56 capsule [PoM] £27.43 DT = £45.71 [CD2]

Oral solution
CAUTIONARY AND ADVISORY LABELS 2

▸ **Oxycodone hydrochloride (Non-proprietary)**
Oxycodone hydrochloride 1 mg per 1 ml Oxycodone 5mg/5ml oral solution sugar free | 250 ml [PoM] £9.71–£10.40 DT = £7.62 [CD2] [SF]
Oxycodone hydrochloride 10 mg per 1 ml Oxycodone 10mg/ml oral solution sugar free | 120 ml [PoM] £46.43–£46.63 DT = £46.63 [CD2] [SF]

▸ **OxyNorm** (Napp Pharmaceuticals Ltd)
Oxycodone hydrochloride 1 mg per 1 ml OxyNorm liquid 1mg/ml oral solution | 250 ml [PoM] £9.71 DT = £7.62 [CD2] [SF]
Oxycodone hydrochloride 10 mg per 1 ml OxyNorm 10mg/ml concentrate oral solution | 120 ml [PoM] £46.63 DT = £46.63 [CD2] [SF]

Oxycodone with naloxone

The properties listed below are those particular to the combination only. For the properties of the components please consider, oxycodone hydrochloride p. 528, naloxone hydrochloride p. 1564.

● INDICATIONS AND DOSE

Severe pain requiring opioid analgesia in patients not currently treated with opioid analgesics
▸ BY MOUTH
▸ Adult: Initially 10/5 mg every 12 hours (max. per dose 40/20 mg every 12 hours), dose to be increased according to response; patients already receiving opioid analgesics can start with a higher dose

Second-line treatment of symptomatic severe to very severe idiopathic restless legs syndrome after failure of dopaminergic therapy
▸ BY MOUTH
▸ Adult: Initially 5/2.5 mg every 12 hours, adjusted weekly according to response, usual dose 10/5 mg every 12 hours; maximum 60/30 mg per day

DOSE EQUIVALENCE AND CONVERSION
▸ Dose quantities are expressed in the form x/y where x and y are the strengths in milligrams of oxycodone and naloxone respectively.

● INTERACTIONS → Appendix 1: opioids

● MEDICINAL FORMS There can be variation in the licensing of different medicines containing the same drug. Forms available from special-order manufacturers include: oral suspension

Modified-release tablet
CAUTIONARY AND ADVISORY LABELS 2, 25
▸ Myloxifin (Ridge Pharma Ltd)
Naloxone hydrochloride 2.5 mg, Oxycodone hydrochloride 5 mg Myloxifin 5mg/2.5mg modified-release tablets | 28 tablet [PoM] £15.07 DT = £21.16 [CD2]
Naloxone hydrochloride 5 mg, Oxycodone hydrochloride 10 mg Myloxifin 10mg/5mg modified-release tablets | 56 tablet [PoM] £30.14 DT = £42.32 [CD2]
Naloxone hydrochloride 10 mg, Oxycodone hydrochloride 20 mg Myloxifin 20mg/10mg modified-release tablets | 56 tablet [PoM] £60.28 DT = £84.62 [CD2]
Naloxone hydrochloride 20 mg, Oxycodone hydrochloride 40 mg Myloxifin 40mg/20mg modified-release tablets | 56 tablet [PoM] £120.60 DT = £169.28 [CD2]
▸ Sofonac (G.L. Pharma UK Ltd)
Naloxone hydrochloride 2.5 mg, Oxycodone hydrochloride 5 mg Sofonac 5mg/2.5mg modified-release tablets | 28 tablet [PoM] £8.46 DT = £21.16 [CD2]
Naloxone hydrochloride 5 mg, Oxycodone hydrochloride 10 mg Sofonac 10mg/5mg modified-release tablets | 56 tablet [PoM] £16.93 DT = £42.32 [CD2]
Naloxone hydrochloride 10 mg, Oxycodone hydrochloride 20 mg Sofonac 20mg/10mg modified-release tablets | 56 tablet [PoM] £33.85 DT = £84.62 [CD2]
Naloxone hydrochloride 20 mg, Oxycodone hydrochloride 40 mg Sofonac 40mg/20mg modified-release tablets | 56 tablet [PoM] £67.71 DT = £169.28 [CD2]
▸ Targinact (Napp Pharmaceuticals Ltd)
Naloxone hydrochloride 2.5 mg, Oxycodone hydrochloride 5 mg Targinact 5mg/2.5mg modified-release tablets | 28 tablet [PoM] £21.16 DT = £21.16 [CD2]
Naloxone hydrochloride 5 mg, Oxycodone hydrochloride 10 mg Targinact 10mg/5mg modified-release tablets | 56 tablet [PoM] £42.32 DT = £42.32 [CD2]
Naloxone hydrochloride 10 mg, Oxycodone hydrochloride 20 mg Targinact 20mg/10mg modified-release tablets | 56 tablet [PoM] £84.62 DT = £84.62 [CD2]
Naloxone hydrochloride 20 mg, Oxycodone hydrochloride 40 mg Targinact 40mg/20mg modified-release tablets | 56 tablet [PoM] £169.28 DT = £169.28 [CD2]

F 510

Pentazocine

24-Sep-2021

● INDICATIONS AND DOSE

Moderate to severe pain
▸ BY MOUTH
▸ Adult: 50 mg every 3–4 hours, dose to be taken preferably after food, usual dose 25–100 mg every 3–4 hours; maximum 600 mg per day

Moderate pain
▸ BY SUBCUTANEOUS INJECTION, OR BY INTRAMUSCULAR INJECTION, OR BY INTRAVENOUS INJECTION
▸ Adult: 30 mg every 3–4 hours as required; maximum 360 mg per day

Severe pain
▸ BY SUBCUTANEOUS INJECTION, OR BY INTRAMUSCULAR INJECTION, OR BY INTRAVENOUS INJECTION
▸ Adult: 45–60 mg every 3–4 hours as required; maximum 360 mg per day

● CONTRA-INDICATIONS Acute porphyrias p. 1202 · heart failure secondary to chronic lung disease · patients dependent on opioids (can precipitate withdrawal)

● CAUTIONS Arterial hypertension · cardiac arrhythmias · myocardial infarction · pancreatitis · phaeochromocytoma · pulmonary hypertension

● INTERACTIONS → Appendix 1: opioids

● SIDE-EFFECTS Biliary spasm · blood disorder · chills · circulatory depression · face oedema · facial plethora · generalised tonic-clonic seizure · hypertension · hypothermia · intracranial pressure increased · mood altered · myalgia · paraesthesia · sexual dysfunction · sleep disorders · syncope · toxic epidermal necrolysis · tremor · ureteral spasm

Overdose Effects only partially reversed by naloxone.

● BREAST FEEDING Use with caution—limited information available.

● HEPATIC IMPAIRMENT [EvGr] Caution in severe impairment (risk of increased bioavailability). ⓜ
Dose adjustments [EvGr] Reduce dose in severe impairment. ⓜ

● RENAL IMPAIRMENT [EvGr] Use with caution in severe impairment. ⓜ
Dose adjustments [EvGr] Reduce dose in severe impairment (risk of increased and prolonged effects). ⓜ

● LESS SUITABLE FOR PRESCRIBING Pentazocine is less suitable for prescribing.

● MEDICINAL FORMS There can be variation in the licensing of different medicines containing the same drug.
Oral tablet
CAUTIONARY AND ADVISORY LABELS 2, 21
▸ Pentazocine (Non-proprietary)
Pentazocine hydrochloride 25 mg Pentazocine 25mg tablets | 28 tablet [PoM] £27.39 DT = £27.39 [CD3]
Oral capsule
CAUTIONARY AND ADVISORY LABELS 2, 21
▸ Pentazocine (Non-proprietary)
Pentazocine hydrochloride 50 mg Pentazocine 50mg capsules | 28 capsule [PoM] £28.50 DT = £28.50 [CD3]

F 510

Pethidine hydrochloride

01-Jun-2021

(Meperidine)

● INDICATIONS AND DOSE

Acute pain
▸ BY MOUTH
▸ Adult: 50–150 mg every 4 hours

continued →

▶ BY SUBCUTANEOUS INJECTION, OR BY INTRAMUSCULAR INJECTION
▸ Adult: 25–100 mg, then 25–100 mg after 4 hours, for debilitated patients use dose described for elderly patients
▸ Elderly: Initially 25 mg, then 25–100 mg after 4 hours
▶ BY SLOW INTRAVENOUS INJECTION
▸ Adult: 25–50 mg, then 25–50 mg after 4 hours, for debilitated patients use dose described for elderly patients
▸ Elderly: Initially 25 mg, then 25–50 mg after 4 hours

Obstetric analgesia
▶ BY SUBCUTANEOUS INJECTION, OR BY INTRAMUSCULAR INJECTION
▸ Adult: 50–100 mg, then 50–100 mg after 1–3 hours if required; maximum 400 mg per day

Premedication
▶ BY INTRAMUSCULAR INJECTION
▸ Adult: 25–100 mg, dose to be given 1 hour before operation, for debilitated patients use dose described for elderly patients
▸ Elderly: 25 mg, dose to be given 1 hour before operation

Postoperative pain
▶ BY SUBCUTANEOUS INJECTION, OR BY INTRAMUSCULAR INJECTION
▸ Adult: 25–100 mg every 2–3 hours if required, for debilitated patients use dose described for elderly patients
▸ Elderly: Initially 25 mg every 2–3 hours if required

● CONTRA-INDICATIONS Phaeochromocytoma

● CAUTIONS Accumulation of metabolites may result in toxicity · cardiac arrhythmias · not suitable for severe continuing pain · severe cor pulmonale

● INTERACTIONS → Appendix 1: opioids

● SIDE-EFFECTS

GENERAL SIDE-EFFECTS Biliary spasm · dysuria · hypothermia

SPECIFIC SIDE-EFFECTS
▸ With oral use Agitation · mood altered · muscle rigidity · sexual dysfunction · ureteral spasm
▸ With parenteral use Anxiety · asthenia · coordination abnormal · delirium · syncope · tremor
Overdose Convulsions reported in overdosage.

● BREAST FEEDING Present in milk but not known to be harmful.

● HEPATIC IMPAIRMENT Manufacturer advises caution in mild to moderate impairment; avoid in severe impairment.
Dose adjustments Manufacturer advises dose reduction in mild to moderate impairment.

● RENAL IMPAIRMENT [EvGr] Caution in mild to moderate impairment; avoid in severe impairment (risk of increased and prolonged effects). Ⓜ
Dose adjustments [EvGr] Reduce dose in mild to moderate impairment. Ⓜ

● MEDICINAL FORMS There can be variation in the licensing of different medicines containing the same drug. Forms available from special-order manufacturers include: oral capsule, oral solution, solution for injection

Oral tablet
CAUTIONARY AND ADVISORY LABELS 2
▸ Pethidine hydrochloride (Non-proprietary)
Pethidine hydrochloride 50 mg Pethidine 50mg tablets | 50 tablet [PoM] £58.58-£68.50 [CD2]

Solution for injection
▸ Pethidine hydrochloride (Non-proprietary)
Pethidine hydrochloride 50 mg per 1 ml Pethidine 50mg/1ml solution for injection ampoules | 10 ampoule [PoM] £5.11-£6.00 DT = £5.11 [CD2]

Pethidine 100mg/2ml solution for injection ampoules | 10 ampoule [PoM] £4.66-£6.50 DT = £4.66 [CD2]

▶ 510

Sufentanil

03-Jul-2024

● DRUG ACTION Sufentanil is a potent, highly selective μ-opioid receptor agonist.

● INDICATIONS AND DOSE

Acute moderate to severe pain
▶ BY SUBLINGUAL ADMINISTRATION
▸ Adult (under close medical supervision): 30 micrograms every 1 hour as required for a maximum duration of 48 hours

● CAUTIONS Acute pancreatitis · brain tumour · history of bradyarrhythmias (increased risk of bradycardia) · increased susceptibility to cerebral effects of CO_2 retention (including increased intracranial pressure and impaired consciousness)

● INTERACTIONS → Appendix 1: opioids

● SIDE-EFFECTS
▸ **Common or very common** Anaemia · anxiety · electrolyte imbalance · fever · gastrointestinal discomfort · gastrointestinal disorders · hypersensitivity · hypertension · hypoproteinaemia · hypoxia · insomnia · laryngeal pain · leucocytosis · muscle complaints · post procedural complications
▸ **Uncommon** Angina pectoris · apathy · apnoea · asthenia · burping · chest discomfort · chills · conjunctivitis · diabetes mellitus · diarrhoea · epistaxis · eye pain · feeling hot · headaches · hiccups · hyperbilirubinaemia · hyperglycaemia · hyperlipidaemia · hypovolaemia · increased risk of infection · lipoma · local swelling · memory impairment · movement disorders · oral hypoaesthesia · pain · procedural complications · psychiatric disorders · pulmonary embolism · pulmonary oedema · reflexes increased · renal impairment · respiratory disorders · sensation abnormal · thrombocytopenia · tremor · urinary hesitation · urinary tract pain
▸ **Frequency not known** Coma

● PREGNANCY [EvGr] Avoid (toxicity in *animal* studies). Ⓜ

● BREAST FEEDING Specialist sources indicate safer alternatives may be preferable if breast-feeding a neonate or preterm infant (no information available).

● HEPATIC IMPAIRMENT [EvGr] Caution in moderate to severe impairment (risk of prolonged effects; limited information available). Ⓜ

● RENAL IMPAIRMENT [EvGr] Caution in severe impairment (risk of prolonged effects; limited information available). Ⓜ

● DIRECTIONS FOR ADMINISTRATION Sublingual tablets should be placed under the tongue and allowed to dissolve. Patients should avoid eating or drinking, and minimise talking for 10 minutes after each dose. Doses should be administered by a healthcare professional, using the single dose applicator.

● PRESCRIBING AND DISPENSING INFORMATION The manufacturer of *Dzuveo®* has provided an *Information Guide Intended to Healthcare Professionals*.

● HANDLING AND STORAGE Protect from light.

● MEDICINAL FORMS There can be variation in the licensing of different medicines containing the same drug.
Sublingual tablet
CAUTIONARY AND ADVISORY LABELS 2, 26
▸ Dzuveo (Aguettant Ltd)
Sufentanil (as Sufentanil citrate) 30 microgram Dzuveo 30microgram sublingual tablets | 5 tablet [PoM] £60.00 (Hospital only) [CD2] [SF]

Tapentadol

▶ 510   01-Sep-2022

● INDICATIONS AND DOSE

Moderate to severe acute pain which can be managed only with opioid analgesics

▶ BY MOUTH USING IMMEDIATE-RELEASE MEDICINES
▶ Adult: Initially 50 mg every 4–6 hours, adjusted according to response, on the first day of treatment, an additional dose of 50 mg may be taken 1 hour after the initial dose; maximum 700 mg in the first 24 hours; maximum 600 mg per day

Severe chronic pain which can be managed only with opioid analgesics

▶ BY MOUTH USING MODIFIED-RELEASE MEDICINES
▶ Adult: Initially 50 mg every 12 hours, adjusted according to response; maximum 500 mg per day

---

IMPORTANT SAFETY INFORMATION

MHRA/CHM ADVICE: TAPENTADOL (*PALEXIA*®): RISK OF SEIZURES AND REPORTS OF SEROTONIN SYNDROME WHEN CO-ADMINISTERED WITH OTHER MEDICINES (JANUARY 2019)

Tapentadol can induce seizures and should be prescribed with caution in patients with a history of seizure disorders or epilepsy. Seizure risk may be increased in patients taking other medicines that lower seizure threshold, for example, antidepressants such as selective serotonin reuptake inhibitors (SSRIs), serotonin-noradrenaline reuptake inhibitors (SNRIs), tricyclic antidepressants, and antipsychotics.

Serotonin syndrome has been reported when tapentadol is used in combination with serotonergic antidepressants—withdrawal of the serotonergic medicine, together with supportive symptomatic care, usually brings about a rapid improvement in serotonin syndrome.

● INTERACTIONS → Appendix 1: opioids

● SIDE-EFFECTS
▶ **Common or very common** Anxiety · appetite decreased · asthenia · concentration impaired · depressed mood · diarrhoea · dyspnoea · feeling of body temperature change · gastrointestinal discomfort · mucosal dryness · muscle contractions involuntary · muscle spasms · oedema · sleep disorders · tremor
▶ **Uncommon** Cognitive impairment · dysarthria · feeling abnormal · irritability · level of consciousness decreased · memory impairment · movement disorders · perception altered · sensation abnormal · sexual dysfunction · syncope · urinary disorders · weight decreased
▶ **Rare or very rare** Impaired gastric emptying

● BREAST FEEDING Avoid—no information available.

● HEPATIC IMPAIRMENT EvGr Caution in moderate impairment; avoid in severe impairment (no information available). Ⓜ
Dose adjustments EvGr Reduce initial daily dose in moderate impairment. For *immediate-release tablets*, initiate at 50 mg up to every 8 hours; for *oral solution*, initiate at 25 mg up to every 8 hours; for *modified-release preparations*, initiate at 50 mg up to once every 24 hours. Ⓜ

● RENAL IMPAIRMENT Manufacturer advises avoid in severe impairment (no information available).

● DIRECTIONS FOR ADMINISTRATION EvGr Modified-release capsules may be swallowed whole with water. Alternatively, capsules may be opened and the contents sprinkled onto approximately 1 tablespoon of cold, soft food (e.g. apple sauce), and swallowed immediately without chewing. Ⓜ

● NATIONAL FUNDING/ACCESS DECISIONS
For full details see funding body website
Scottish Medicines Consortium (SMC) decisions
▶ Tapentadol (*Palexia SR*®) for the management of severe chronic pain in adults (June 2011) SMC No. 654/10 Recommended with restrictions

● MEDICINAL FORMS There can be variation in the licensing of different medicines containing the same drug.

Oral tablet

CAUTIONARY AND ADVISORY LABELS 2
▶ Palexia (Grunenthal Ltd)
Tapentadol (as Tapentadol hydrochloride) 50 mg Palexia 50mg tablets | 28 tablet PoM £12.46 DT = £12.46 CD2 | 56 tablet PoM £24.91 CD2
Tapentadol (as Tapentadol hydrochloride) 75 mg Palexia 75mg tablets | 28 tablet PoM £18.68 DT = £18.68 CD2 | 56 tablet PoM £37.37 DT = £37.37 CD2

Oral solution

CAUTIONARY AND ADVISORY LABELS 2
EXCIPIENTS: May contain Propylene glycol
▶ Palexia (Grunenthal Ltd)
Tapentadol (as Tapentadol hydrochloride) 20 mg per 1 ml Palexia 20mg/ml oral solution | 100 ml PoM £17.80 DT = £17.80 CD2 SF

Modified-release tablet

CAUTIONARY AND ADVISORY LABELS 2, 25
▶ Tapentadol (Non-proprietary)
Tapentadol 50 mg Tapentadol 50mg modified-release tablets | 28 tablet PoM £14.21 DT = £12.46 CD2 | 56 tablet PoM £28.39 DT = £24.91 CD2
Tapentadol 100 mg Tapentadol 100mg modified-release tablets | 56 tablet PoM £56.80 DT = £49.82 CD2
Tapentadol 150 mg Tapentadol 150mg modified-release tablets | 56 tablet PoM £85.20 DT = £74.73 CD2
Tapentadol 200 mg Tapentadol 200mg modified-release tablets | 56 tablet PoM £113.59 DT = £99.64 CD2
Tapentadol 250 mg Tapentadol 250mg modified-release tablets | 56 tablet PoM £124.55 DT = £124.55 CD2
▶ Ationdo SR (Grunenthal Ltd)
Tapentadol 25 mg Ationdo SR 25mg tablets | 56 tablet PoM £8.72 DT = £8.72 CD2
Tapentadol 50 mg Ationdo SR 50mg tablets | 56 tablet PoM £14.94 DT = £24.91 CD2
Tapentadol 100 mg Ationdo SR 100mg tablets | 56 tablet PoM £29.88 DT = £49.82 CD2
Tapentadol 150 mg Ationdo SR 150mg tablets | 56 tablet PoM £44.83 DT = £74.73 CD2
Tapentadol 200 mg Ationdo SR 200mg tablets | 56 tablet PoM £59.77 DT = £99.64 CD2
Tapentadol 250 mg Ationdo SR 250mg tablets | 56 tablet PoM £74.72 DT = £124.55 CD2
▶ Lupaxis (Dr Reddy's Laboratories (UK) Ltd)
Tapentadol 50 mg Lupaxis 50mg prolonged-release tablets | 28 tablet PoM £12.46 DT = £12.46 CD2 | 56 tablet PoM £24.91 DT = £24.91 CD2
Tapentadol 100 mg Lupaxis 100mg prolonged-release tablets | 56 tablet PoM £49.82 DT = £49.82 CD2
Tapentadol 150 mg Lupaxis 150mg prolonged-release tablets | 56 tablet PoM £74.73 DT = £74.73 CD2
Tapentadol 200 mg Lupaxis 200mg prolonged-release tablets | 56 tablet PoM £99.64 DT = £99.64 CD2
Tapentadol 250 mg Lupaxis 250mg prolonged-release tablets | 56 tablet PoM £124.55 DT = £124.55 CD2
▶ Palexia SR (Grunenthal Ltd)
Tapentadol 50 mg Palexia SR 50mg tablets | 28 tablet PoM £12.46 DT = £12.46 CD2 | 56 tablet PoM £24.91 DT = £24.91 CD2
Tapentadol 100 mg Palexia SR 100mg tablets | 56 tablet PoM £49.82 DT = £49.82 CD2
Tapentadol 150 mg Palexia SR 150mg tablets | 56 tablet PoM £74.73 DT = £74.73 CD2
Tapentadol 200 mg Palexia SR 200mg tablets | 56 tablet PoM £99.64 DT = £99.64 CD2
Tapentadol 250 mg Palexia SR 250mg tablets | 56 tablet PoM £124.55 DT = £124.55 CD2
▶ Tadomon (G.L. Pharma UK Ltd)
Tapentadol 25 mg Tadomon 25mg prolonged-release tablets | 56 tablet PoM £6.23 DT = £8.72 CD2

Tapentadol 50 mg Tadomon 50mg prolonged-release tablets | 28 tablet [PoM] £6.23 DT = £12.46 [CD2] | 56 tablet [PoM] £12.46 DT = £24.91 [CD2]

Tapentadol 100 mg Tadomon 100mg prolonged-release tablets | 56 tablet [PoM] £24.91 DT = £49.82 [CD2]

Tapentadol 150 mg Tadomon 150mg prolonged-release tablets | 56 tablet [PoM] £37.37 DT = £74.73 [CD2]

Tapentadol 200 mg Tadomon 200mg prolonged-release tablets | 56 tablet [PoM] £49.82 DT = £99.64 [CD2]

Tapentadol 250 mg Tadomon 250mg prolonged-release tablets | 56 tablet [PoM] £62.28 DT = £124.55 [CD2]

▸ **Vecicom** (Celix Pharma Ltd)

Tapentadol 50 mg Vecicom 50mg prolonged-release tablets | 28 tablet [PoM] £8.72 DT = £12.46 [CD2] | 56 tablet [PoM] £17.44 DT = £24.91 [CD2]

Tapentadol 100 mg Vecicom 100mg prolonged-release tablets | 56 tablet [PoM] £34.87 DT = £49.82 [CD2]

Tapentadol 150 mg Vecicom 150mg prolonged-release tablets | 56 tablet [PoM] £52.31 DT = £74.73 [CD2]

Tapentadol 200 mg Vecicom 200mg prolonged-release tablets | 56 tablet [PoM] £69.96 DT = £99.64 [CD2]

Tapentadol 250 mg Vecicom 250mg prolonged-release tablets | 56 tablet [PoM] £87.19 DT = £124.55 [CD2]

Modified-release capsule

CAUTIONARY AND ADVISORY LABELS 2
EXCIPIENTS: May contain Gelatin

▸ **Tapimio** (Neuraxpharm UK Ltd)

Tapentadol (as Tapentadol phosphate) 50 mg Tapimio 50mg modified-release capsules | 28 capsule [PoM] £10.59 DT = £10.59 [CD2] | 56 capsule [PoM] £21.17 DT = £21.17 [CD2]

Tapentadol (as Tapentadol phosphate) 100 mg Tapimio 100mg modified-release capsules | 56 capsule [PoM] £42.35 DT = £42.35 [CD2]

Tapentadol (as Tapentadol phosphate) 150 mg Tapimio 150mg modified-release capsules | 56 capsule [PoM] £63.52 DT = £63.52 [CD2]

Tapentadol (as Tapentadol phosphate) 200 mg Tapimio 200mg modified-release capsules | 56 capsule [PoM] £84.69 DT = £84.69 [CD2]

Tapentadol (as Tapentadol phosphate) 250 mg Tapimio 250mg modified-release capsules | 56 capsule [PoM] £105.87 DT = £105.87 [CD2]

⚑ 510

Tramadol hydrochloride

25-Aug-2022

● **INDICATIONS AND DOSE**

Moderate to severe pain

▸ BY INTRAMUSCULAR INJECTION, OR BY INTRAVENOUS INJECTION, OR BY INTRAVENOUS INFUSION, OR BY SUBCUTANEOUS INJECTION

▸ Adult: 50–100 mg every 4–6 hours, intravenous injection to be given over 2–3 minutes; Usual maximum 400 mg/24 hours

Moderate to severe acute pain

▸ BY MOUTH USING IMMEDIATE-RELEASE MEDICINES

▸ Child 12–17 years: Initially 100 mg, then 50–100 mg every 4–6 hours; Usual maximum 400 mg/24 hours

▸ Adult: Initially 100 mg, then 50–100 mg every 4–6 hours; Usual maximum 400 mg/24 hours

Moderate to severe chronic pain

▸ BY MOUTH USING IMMEDIATE-RELEASE MEDICINES

▸ Child 12–17 years: Initially 50 mg, then, adjusted according to response; Usual maximum 400 mg/24 hours

▸ Adult: Initially 50 mg, then, adjusted according to response; Usual maximum 400 mg/24 hours

Postoperative pain

▸ BY INTRAVENOUS INJECTION, OR BY INTRAMUSCULAR INJECTION, OR BY INTRAVENOUS INFUSION, OR BY SUBCUTANEOUS INJECTION

▸ Adult: Initially 100 mg, then 50 mg every 10–20 minutes if required up to total maximum 250 mg (including initial dose) in first hour, then 50–100 mg every 4–6 hours, intravenous injection to be given over 2–3 minutes; Usual maximum 400 mg/24 hours

Moderate to severe pain (with modified-release 12-hourly preparations)

▸ BY MOUTH USING MODIFIED-RELEASE MEDICINES

▸ Child 12–17 years: 50–100 mg twice daily, increased if necessary to 150–200 mg twice daily, doses exceeding the usual maximum not generally required; Usual maximum 400 mg/24 hours

▸ Adult: 50–100 mg twice daily, increased if necessary to 150–200 mg twice daily, doses exceeding the usual maximum not generally required; Usual maximum 400 mg/24 hours

Moderate to severe pain (with modified-release 24-hourly preparations)

▸ BY MOUTH USING MODIFIED-RELEASE MEDICINES

▸ Child 12–17 years: Initially 100–150 mg once daily, increased if necessary up to 400 mg once daily; Usual maximum 400 mg/24 hours

▸ Adult: Initially 100–150 mg once daily, increased if necessary up to 400 mg once daily; Usual maximum 400 mg/24 hours

> **IMPORTANT SAFETY INFORMATION**
> Do not confuse modified-release 12-hourly preparations with 24-hourly preparations, see *Prescribing and dispensing information.*

● **CONTRA-INDICATIONS** Acute intoxication with alcohol · acute intoxication with analgesics · acute intoxication with hypnotics · acute intoxication with opioids · compromised respiratory function (in children) · not suitable for narcotic withdrawal treatment · uncontrolled epilepsy

● **CAUTIONS** Excessive bronchial secretions · history of epilepsy—use tramadol only if compelling reasons · impaired consciousness · not suitable as a substitute in opioid-dependent patients · postoperative use (in children) · susceptibility to seizures—use tramadol only if compelling reasons · variation in metabolism

CAUTIONS, FURTHER INFORMATION

▸ Variation in metabolism The capacity to metabolise tramadol can vary considerably between individuals; there is a risk of developing side-effects of opioid toxicity in patients who are ultra-rapid tramadol metabolisers (CYP2D6 ultra-rapid metabolisers) and the therapeutic effect may be reduced in poor tramadol metabolisers.

▸ Postoperative use Manufacturer advises extreme caution when used for postoperative pain relief in children—reports of rare, but life threatening adverse events after tonsillectomy and/or adenoidectomy for obstructive sleep apnoea; if used, monitor closely for symptoms of opioid toxicity.

● **INTERACTIONS** → Appendix 1: opioids

● **SIDE-EFFECTS**

GENERAL SIDE-EFFECTS

▸ **Common or very common** Fatigue

▸ **Rare or very rare** Dyspnoea · epileptiform seizure · respiratory disorders · vision blurred

▸ **Frequency not known** Asthma exacerbated · hypoglycaemia

SPECIFIC SIDE-EFFECTS

▸ **Uncommon**

▸ With parenteral use Circulatory collapse · gastrointestinal discomfort

▸ **Rare or very rare**

▸ With parenteral use Angioedema · appetite change · behaviour abnormal · cognitive disorder · dysuria · hypersensitivity · mood altered · movement disorders · muscle weakness · perception disorders · psychiatric disorder · sensation abnormal · sleep disorders

► **Frequency not known**
► With oral use Blood disorder · drug abuse · hiccups · hypertension · hyponatraemia · nightmare · paraesthesia · serotonin syndrome · syncope · urinary disorder

● **PREGNANCY** Embryotoxic in *animal* studies— manufacturers advise avoid.

● **BREAST FEEDING** Amount probably too small to be harmful, but manufacturer advises avoid.

● **HEPATIC IMPAIRMENT** Manufacturers advise caution (risk of delayed elimination); some *oral preparations* should be avoided in severe impairment—consult product literature. **Dose adjustments** Manufacturers advise consider increasing dosage interval.

● **RENAL IMPAIRMENT** Avoid use or reduce dose; opioid effects increased and prolonged and increased cerebral sensitivity occurs. Caution (avoid for *oral drops*) in severe impairment.

● **TREATMENT CESSATION** Manufacturer advises consider tapering the dose gradually to prevent withdrawal symptoms.

● **DIRECTIONS FOR ADMINISTRATION** Manufacturer advises tramadol hydrochloride *orodispersible tablets* should be sucked and then swallowed. May also be dispersed in water. Manufacturers advise some tramadol hydrochloride modified-release capsule preparations may be opened and the contents swallowed immediately without chewing— check individual preparations.
   For *intravenous infusion*, manufacturer advises dilute in Glucose 5% or Sodium Chloride 0.9%.

● **PRESCRIBING AND DISPENSING INFORMATION** Modified-release preparations are available as 12-hourly or 24-hourly formulations. Non-proprietary preparations of modified-release tramadol may be available as either 12-hourly or 24-hourly formulations; prescribers and dispensers must ensure that the correct formulation is prescribed and dispensed. Branded preparations that should be given 12-hourly include *Brimisol*® *PR, Marol*®, *Maxitram*® *SR, Tilodol*® *SR, Tramquel*® *SR, Tramulief*® *SR, Zamadol*® *SR,* and *Zydol SR*®. Preparations that should be given 24-hourly include *Tradorec XL*®, *Zamadol*® *24hr,* and *Zydol XL*®.

● **PATIENT AND CARER ADVICE** Patients or carers should be given advice on how to administer tramadol hydrochloride orodispersible tablets.
   Medicines for Children leaflet: Tramadol for pain
   www.medicinesforchildren.org.uk/medicines/tramadol-for-pain/

● **MEDICINAL FORMS** There can be variation in the licensing of different medicines containing the same drug. Forms available from special-order manufacturers include: oral suspension

Modified-release tablet
CAUTIONARY AND ADVISORY LABELS 2, 25
► **Tramadol hydrochloride (Non-proprietary)**
   Tramadol hydrochloride 100 mg Tramadol 100mg modified-release tablets | 60 tablet [PoM] £20.66 [CD3]
   Tramadol hydrochloride 150 mg Tramadol 150mg modified-release tablets | 60 tablet [PoM] £27.94 [CD3]
   Tramadol hydrochloride 200 mg Tramadol 200mg modified-release tablets | 60 tablet [PoM] £43.20 [CD3]
► **Brimisol PR** (Bristol Laboratories Ltd)
   Tramadol hydrochloride 100 mg Brimisol PR 100mg tablets | 60 tablet [PoM] [℥] [CD3]
   Tramadol hydrochloride 200 mg Brimisol PR 200mg tablets | 60 tablet [PoM] £36.00 [CD3]
► **Marol** (Teva UK Ltd)
   Tramadol hydrochloride 100 mg Marol 100mg modified-release tablets | 60 tablet [PoM] £6.94 [CD3]
   Tramadol hydrochloride 150 mg Marol 150mg modified-release tablets | 60 tablet [PoM] £10.39 [CD3]
   Tramadol hydrochloride 200 mg Marol 200mg modified-release tablets | 60 tablet [PoM] £14.19 [CD3]
► **Tilodol SR** (Sandoz Ltd)
   Tramadol hydrochloride 100 mg Tilodol SR 100mg tablets | 60 tablet [PoM] £15.52 [CD3]
   Tramadol hydrochloride 150 mg Tilodol SR 150mg tablets | 60 tablet [PoM] £23.28 [CD3]
   Tramadol hydrochloride 200 mg Tilodol SR 200mg tablets | 60 tablet [PoM] £31.04 [CD3]
► **Tramulief SR** (Advanz Pharma)
   Tramadol hydrochloride 100 mg Tramulief SR 100mg tablets | 60 tablet [PoM] £6.98 [CD3]
   Tramadol hydrochloride 150 mg Tramulief SR 150mg tablets | 60 tablet [PoM] £10.48 [CD3]
   Tramadol hydrochloride 200 mg Tramulief SR 200mg tablets | 60 tablet [PoM] £14.28 [CD3]
► **Zydol SR** (Grunenthal Ltd)
   Tramadol hydrochloride 50 mg Zydol SR 50mg tablets | 60 tablet [PoM] £4.60 DT = £4.60 [CD3]
   Tramadol hydrochloride 100 mg Zydol SR 100mg tablets | 60 tablet [PoM] £17.22 [CD3]
   Tramadol hydrochloride 150 mg Zydol SR 150mg tablets | 60 tablet [PoM] £25.83 [CD3]
   Tramadol hydrochloride 200 mg Zydol SR 200mg tablets | 60 tablet [PoM] £34.40 [CD3]
► **Zydol XL** (Grunenthal Ltd)
   Tramadol hydrochloride 400 mg Zydol XL 400mg tablets | 30 tablet [PoM] £32.47 [CD3]

Soluble tablet
CAUTIONARY AND ADVISORY LABELS 2, 13
► **Zydol** (Grunenthal Ltd)
   Tramadol hydrochloride 50 mg Zydol 50mg soluble tablets | 20 tablet [PoM] £2.79 Schedule 3 (CD No Register Exempt Safe Custody) [SF] | 100 tablet [PoM] £13.33 DT = £13.33 Schedule 3 (CD No Register Exempt Safe Custody) [SF]

Solution for injection
► **Tramadol hydrochloride (Non-proprietary)**
   Tramadol hydrochloride 50 mg per 1 ml Tramadol 100mg/2ml solution for injection ampoules | 5 ampoule [PoM] £4.00 DT = £4.00 (Hospital only) [CD3] | 10 ampoule [PoM] £11.00 [CD3]
► **Zydol** (Grunenthal Ltd)
   Tramadol hydrochloride 50 mg per 1 ml Zydol 100mg/2ml solution for injection ampoules | 5 ampoule [PoM] £4.00 DT = £4.00 [CD3]

Modified-release capsule
CAUTIONARY AND ADVISORY LABELS 2, 25
► **Tramadol hydrochloride (Non-proprietary)**
   Tramadol hydrochloride 50 mg Tramadol 50mg modified-release capsules | 60 capsule [PoM] £7.24 DT = £7.24 [CD3]
   Tramadol hydrochloride 100 mg Tramadol 100mg modified-release capsules | 60 capsule [PoM] £14.47 DT = £14.47 [CD3]
   Tramadol hydrochloride 150 mg Tramadol 150mg modified-release capsules | 60 capsule [PoM] £21.71 DT = £21.71 [CD3]
   Tramadol hydrochloride 200 mg Tramadol 200mg modified-release capsules | 60 capsule [PoM] £28.93 DT = £28.93 [CD3]
► **Maxitram SR** (Chiesi Ltd)
   Tramadol hydrochloride 50 mg Maxitram SR 50mg capsules | 60 capsule [PoM] £4.55 DT = £7.24 [CD3]
   Tramadol hydrochloride 100 mg Maxitram SR 100mg capsules | 60 capsule [PoM] £12.14 DT = £14.47 [CD3]
   Tramadol hydrochloride 150 mg Maxitram SR 150mg capsules | 60 capsule [PoM] £18.21 DT = £21.71 [CD3]
   Tramadol hydrochloride 200 mg Maxitram SR 200mg capsules | 60 capsule [PoM] £24.28 DT = £28.93 [CD3]
► **Zamadol SR** (Viatris UK Healthcare Ltd)
   Tramadol hydrochloride 50 mg Zamadol SR 50mg capsules | 60 capsule [PoM] £7.24 DT = £7.24 [CD3]
   Tramadol hydrochloride 100 mg Zamadol SR 100mg capsules | 60 capsule [PoM] £14.47 DT = £14.47 [CD3]
   Tramadol hydrochloride 150 mg Zamadol SR 150mg capsules | 60 capsule [PoM] £21.71 DT = £21.71 [CD3]
   Tramadol hydrochloride 200 mg Zamadol SR 200mg capsules | 60 capsule [PoM] £28.93 DT = £28.93 [CD3]

Oral capsule
CAUTIONARY AND ADVISORY LABELS 2
► **Tramadol hydrochloride (Non-proprietary)**
   Tramadol hydrochloride 50 mg Tramadol 50mg capsules | 30 capsule [PoM] £2.50 DT = £0.68 [CD3] | 100 capsule [PoM] £7.63 DT = £2.27 [CD3]
► **Zamadol** (Viatris UK Healthcare Ltd)
   Tramadol hydrochloride 50 mg Zamadol 50mg capsules | 100 capsule [PoM] £8.00 DT = £2.27 [CD3]

▸ **Zydol** (Grunenthal Ltd)
Tramadol hydrochloride 50 mg Zydol 50mg capsules |
100 capsule PoM £7.63 DT = £2.27 CD3

Orodispersible tablet
CAUTIONARY AND ADVISORY LABELS 2
▸ **Zamadol Melt** (Viatris UK Healthcare Ltd)
Tramadol hydrochloride 50 mg Zamadol Melt 50mg tablets |
60 tablet PoM £7.12 DT = £7.12 Schedule 3 (CD No Register Exempt
Safe Custody) SF

Tramadol with dexketoprofen
24-Apr-2018

The properties listed below are those particular to the
combination only. For the properties of the components
please consider, tramadol hydrochloride p. 534,
dexketoprofen p. 1295.

● **INDICATIONS AND DOSE**
Moderate to severe acute pain
▸ BY MOUTH
▸ Adult: 75/25 mg every 8 hours as required for up to
5 days
▸ Elderly: 75/25 mg every 8 hours as required for up to
5 days; Usual maximum 150/50 mg/24 hours
DOSE EQUIVALENCE AND CONVERSION
▸ Dose expressed as x/y mg of tramadol/dexketoprofen.

● INTERACTIONS → Appendix 1: NSAIDs · opioids

● MEDICINAL FORMS There can be variation in the licensing of
different medicines containing the same drug.
Oral tablet
CAUTIONARY AND ADVISORY LABELS 2, 22
▸ **Skudexa** (A. Menarini Farmaceutica Internazionale SRL)
Dexketoprofen 25 mg, Tramadol hydrochloride 75 mg Skudexa
75mg/25mg tablets | 10 tablet PoM £3.68 CD3 | 20 tablet PoM
£5.52 DT = £5.52 CD3

Tramadol with paracetamol
22-Feb-2018

The properties listed below are those particular to the
combination only. For the properties of the components
please consider, paracetamol p. 507, tramadol hydrochloride
p. 534.

● **INDICATIONS AND DOSE**
Moderate to severe pain
▸ BY MOUTH
▸ Child 12-17 years: 75/650 mg every 6 hours as required
▸ Adult: 75/650 mg every 6 hours as required
DOSE EQUIVALENCE AND CONVERSION
▸ The proportions are expressed in the form x/y, where x
and y are the strengths in milligrams of tramadol and
paracetamol respectively.

● INTERACTIONS → Appendix 1: opioids · paracetamol

● MEDICINAL FORMS There can be variation in the licensing of
different medicines containing the same drug.
Oral tablet
CAUTIONARY AND ADVISORY LABELS 2, 25, 29, 30
▸ **Tramadol with paracetamol (Non-proprietary)**
Tramadol hydrochloride 37.5 mg, Paracetamol 325 mg Tramadol
37.5mg / Paracetamol 325mg tablets | 60 tablet PoM £12.95 DT =
£12.95 CD3
▸ **Tramacet** (Grunenthal Ltd)
Tramadol hydrochloride 37.5 mg, Paracetamol 325 mg Tramacet
37.5mg/325mg tablets | 60 tablet PoM £9.68 DT = £12.95 CD3
Effervescent tablet
CAUTIONARY AND ADVISORY LABELS 2, 13, 29, 30
ELECTROLYTES: May contain Sodium
▸ **Tramacet** (Grunenthal Ltd)
Tramadol hydrochloride 37.5 mg, Paracetamol 325 mg Tramacet
37.5mg/325mg effervescent tablets | 60 tablet PoM £9.68 DT =
£9.68 Schedule 3 (CD No Register Exempt Safe Custody) SF

6.1 Headache

Cluster headache and other trigeminal autonomic cephalalgias

06-Jul-2023

Management
Cluster headache rarely responds to standard analgesics.
Sumatriptan p. 545 given by subcutaneous injection is the
drug of choice for the *treatment* of cluster headache. If an
injection is unsuitable, sumatriptan nasal spray or
zolmitriptan nasal spray p. 546 [both unlicensed use] may be
used. Alternatively, 100% oxygen at a rate of
10−15 litres/minute for 10−20 minutes is useful in aborting
an attack.

Prophylaxis of cluster headache is considered if the attacks
are frequent, last over 3 weeks, or if they cannot be treated
effectively. Verapamil hydrochloride p. 191 or lithium [both
unlicensed use] are used for prophylaxis.

Prednisolone p. 791 can be used for short-term
prophylaxis of episodic cluster headache [unlicensed use]
either as monotherapy, or in combination with verapamil
hydrochloride during verapamil titration.

The other trigeminal autonomic cephalalgias, paroxysmal
hemicrania (sensitive to indometacin p. 1305), and short-
lasting unilateral neuralgiform headache attacks with
conjunctival injection and tearing, are seen rarely and are
best managed by a specialist.

> **Other drugs used for Headache** Clonidine hydrochloride,
> p. 172 · Pizotifen, p. 540

6.1a Migraine

Migraine
02-Oct-2024

Description of condition
Migraine is a common type of primary headache disorder. It
occurs more commonly in females than in males, and is
characterised by recurrent attacks of typically moderate to
severe headaches that usually last between 4−72 hours. The
headache is usually unilateral, pulsating, aggravated by
routine physical activity, and may be severe enough to
impact or prevent daily activities. It is frequently
accompanied by nausea and vomiting, photophobia and
phonophobia, or both. Migraine is subdivided into migraine
with or *without* aura, and is defined as either episodic or
chronic.

Migraine *with* aura consists of visual symptoms (zigzag or
flickering lights, spots, lines, or loss of vision), sensory
symptoms (pins and needles, or numbness), or dysphasia,
which usually precede the onset of headache. Symptoms
usually develop gradually and resolve within 1 hour.

Episodic migraine is defined as headache which occurs on
less than 15 days per month, and can be further subdivided
into low frequency (1−9 days per month) and high frequency
(10−14 days per month). Chronic migraine is defined as
headache which occurs on at least 15 days per month and
has the characteristics of a migraine headache on at least
8 days per month for greater than 3 months.

In some females, the drop in oestrogen levels just before
menstruation is a trigger for migraine, with symptoms
generally occurring from two days before the start of
bleeding up until three days after.

Medication-overuse headache is a complication of
migraine; the frequent use of acute treatment for migraine

increases the frequency and intensity of headache, and can become the cause of the headache.

Aims of treatment

Treatment of acute migraine aims to stop the attack, or to significantly reduce the severity of the headache and other associated symptoms. Preventative treatment aims to reduce the frequency, severity and duration of migraine attacks, and development of medication-overuse headache.

Lifestyle advice

EvGr Patients should be encouraged to eat regular meals, and to maintain adequate hydration, sleep and exercise. A Other potential triggers include stress, relaxation after stress, some foods and drinks, and bright lights. EvGr Known triggers should be avoided; keeping a headache diary may be useful to identify potential triggers and should be continued for a minimum of 8 weeks. A

Acute migraine treatment

EvGr The choice of treatment for acute migraine should be guided by the patient's preference, response to previous treatment, the severity and frequency of headache attacks, other associated symptoms, and co-morbidities. Treatment should ideally be restricted to 2 days per week and patients should be advised of the risk of developing medication-overuse headache.

Monotherapy, with either aspirin p. 142, ibuprofen p. 1302, or a $5HT_1$-receptor agonist ('triptan') is recommended as first-line treatment and should be taken as soon as the patient knows that they are developing a migraine (start of headache phase).

In patients who experience aura with their migraine, it is recommended that $5HT_1$-receptor agonists are taken at the start of the headache and not at the start of the aura (unless the aura and headache start at the same time).

Based on its clinical efficacy and safety profile, sumatriptan p. 545 is the $5HT_1$-receptor agonist of choice. A Alternative $5HT_1$-receptor agonists include almotriptan p. 543, eletriptan p. 543, frovatriptan p. 544, naratriptan p. 544, rizatriptan p. 545, and zolmitriptan p. 546. EvGr In patients who do not respond to one $5HT_1$-receptor agonist, a different $5HT_1$-receptor agonist should be tried as response can be variable between patients. Subcutaneous sumatriptan p. 545 or nasal zolmitriptan p. 546 can be given to patients who present with early vomiting or who have severe migraine attacks. A

EvGr Other NSAIDs that may be used for the treatment of acute migraine include, naproxen p. 1310 [unlicensed indication], tolfenamic acid p. 539, and diclofenac potassium p. 1296. In patients presenting with severe nausea and vomiting, diclofenac sodium suppositories p. 1297 [unlicensed indication] may be an option. Mefenamic acid p. 1308 [unlicensed indication] can also be used for menstrual migraine in females already using it for other indications such as dysmenorrhea, or menorrhagia. E

EvGr Treatment with paracetamol p. 507 can be considered in patients who are unable to take other acute treatment options.

In patients who fail to respond to monotherapy, combination therapy with sumatriptan p. 545 and naproxen p. 1310 can be given.

For patients in whom at least two $5HT_1$-receptor agonists have been ineffective, or for patients where they are unsuitable and who have failed to respond to NSAIDs and paracetamol, rimegepant p. 542 can be considered.

In addition to their use as antiemetics, metoclopramide hydrochloride p. 494 [unlicensed indication] or prochlorperazine p. 448 [unlicensed indication] can also be given as a single dose at the onset of migraine symptoms for the treatment of headache. They can be given orally or by injection, depending on the severity of the patients' symptoms and the setting. A

Antiemetics

EvGr Metoclopramide hydrochloride p. 494 or prochlorperazine p. 448 can be given orally or by injection to relieve nausea or vomiting. Metoclopramide hydrochloride should not be used regularly due to the risk of extrapyramidal side effects. A

EvGr Domperidone p. 494 [unlicensed in those weighing less than 35 kg] may be used as an alternative antiemetic. E

Preventative migraine treatment

EvGr The decision to start prophylactic treatment should be based on the impact of the migraine on the patient's quality of life. The choice of treatment depends on factors such as patient preference, drug interactions, and other co-morbidities. Treatment should be started at a low dose and gradually increased to the maximum effective and tolerated dose.

Propranolol hydrochloride p. 178 is recommended as first-line preventative treatment in patients with episodic or chronic migraine. A EvGr For patients in whom propranolol is unsuitable, other beta-blockers that can be considered are metoprolol tartrate p. 182, atenolol p. 180 [unlicensed indication], nadolol p. 177, and timolol maleate p. 179. Bisoprolol fumarate p. 180 [unlicensed indication] may also be considered, especially in patients already taking it for cardiac reasons under the advice of their cardiologist. E

EvGr If a beta-blocker is unsuitable in patients with episodic or chronic migraine, topiramate p. 384 can be given. A However, the MHRA has advised that topiramate must not be used in females of childbearing potential unless the conditions of the Pregnancy Prevention Programme are met; it must not be used during pregnancy for migraine prophylaxis. For further information, see *Important safety information, Conception and contraception*, and *Pregnancy* in topiramate.

EvGr Amitriptyline hydrochloride p. 431 is effective for migraine prophylaxis and should be considered for patients with episodic or chronic migraine. A less sedative tricyclic antidepressant can be used if amitriptyline hydrochloride is not tolerated.

Candesartan cilexetil p. 202 [unlicensed use] can be considered in patients with episodic or chronic migraine, although there is limited evidence to support its use. However, it should be avoided in pregnancy; A for further information, see *Conception and contraception* and *Pregnancy* in candesartan cilexetil.

EvGr Sodium valproate p. 378 [unlicensed use] can be considered as an option in patients aged 55 years and over with episodic or chronic migraine. A The MHRA has advised that sodium valproate must not be used in females of childbearing potential unless the conditions of the Pregnancy Prevention Programme are met and alternative treatments are ineffective or not tolerated; it must not be used during pregnancy for migraine prophylaxis. In light of prescribing data showing ongoing exposure to valproate in pregnancy, and also of potential risks associated with valproate use in males, the MHRA/CHM has released new regulatory measures around its use in individuals (males or females) aged under 55 years. In addition to these measures, further advice has been issued about the use in males and the need to use effective contraception. For further information, see *Important safety information, Conception and contraception*, and *Pregnancy* for sodium valproate p. 378.

EvGr Flunarizine [unlicensed] can also be considered in patients with episodic or chronic migraine (avoid in pregnancy, specialist use only). Pizotifen p. 540 is used but evidence to recommend its use is limited.

Preventative treatment should be tried for at least 3 months at the maximum tolerated dose, before deciding whether or not it is effective. ⟨A⟩ A good response to treatment is defined as a 50% reduction in the severity and frequency of migraine attacks. [EvGr] A review of ongoing prophylaxis should be considered after 6–12 months; treatment can be gradually withdrawn in many patients. Patients should be referred to a neurology or specialist headache clinic if trials with 3 or more drugs have been unsuccessful.

An oral calcitonin gene-related peptide (CGRP) inhibitor, such as atogepant p. 540 or rimegepant p. 542, can be used for the prophylaxis of migraine in patients in whom at least 3 prophylactic treatments have been ineffective. Rimegepant is an option for patients with episodic migraine who have at least 4 migraine attacks per month, and atogepant is an option for patients with either episodic or chronic migraine who have at least 4 migraine days per month. Parenteral CGRP inhibitors may be used for the prophylaxis of either episodic or chronic migraine (specialist use).

Botulinum toxin type A p. 469 (specialist use) is recommended for prophylaxis of chronic migraine where medication-overuse has been addressed and where 3 or more oral prophylactic treatments have failed. ⟨A⟩

Menstrual migraine prophylaxis

[EvGr] Frovatriptan p. 544 [unlicensed indication] can be given instead of, or in addition to, standard prophylactic treatment in females with perimenstrual migraine. It is given from 2 days before until 3 days after menstruation starts. Zolmitriptan p. 546 [unlicensed indication] or naratriptan p. 544 [unlicensed indication] are suitable alternatives to frovatriptan p. 544. In order for treatment to be effective, the patient's menstrual cycle must be regular.

Females with menstrual-related migraine who are using $5HT_1$-receptor agonists for both perimenstrual prophylaxis and at other times in the month should be advised of the increased risk of developing medication-overuse headache. ⟨A⟩

Medication-overuse headache

[EvGr] Medication overuse should be addressed in patients overusing acute treatments such as $5HT_1$-receptor agonists, combination analgesics, ergots, or opioids for migraine. ⟨A⟩ Withdrawing the overused medication can reduce the frequency and intensity of headaches but is often associated with transient worsening. Not all patients overusing acute treatment will develop medication-overuse headache; in some patients, continued headaches may be a sign of poorly treated migraine.

Useful Resources

Pharmacological management of migraine. Scottish Intercollegiate Guidelines Network. A national clinical guideline 155. February 2018 (updated March 2023). www.sign.ac.uk/our-guidelines/pharmacological-management-of-migraine/

> **Other drugs used for Migraine** Clonidine hydrochloride, p. 172 · Valproic acid, p. 409

Paracetamol with isometheptene

11-Nov-2019

The properties listed below are those particular to the combination only. For the properties of the components please consider, paracetamol p. 507.

- **INDICATIONS AND DOSE**

Treatment of acute attacks of migraine
- ▶ BY MOUTH
- ▶ Adult: 2 capsules, dose to be taken at onset of attack, followed by 1 capsule every 1 hour if required, maximum of 5 capsules in 12 hours

- **CONTRA-INDICATIONS** Acute porphyrias p. 1202 · glaucoma · severe cardiovascular disease · severe hypertension
- **INTERACTIONS** → Appendix 1: paracetamol · sympathomimetics, vasoconstrictor
- **PATIENT AND CARER ADVICE** Patient counselling is advised (dosage).
- **LESS SUITABLE FOR PRESCRIBING** Isometheptene with paracetamol is less suitable for prescribing (more effective treatments available).
- **MEDICINAL FORMS** There can be variation in the licensing of different medicines containing the same drug.

Oral capsule
CAUTIONARY AND ADVISORY LABELS 30
- ▶ Midrid (DHP Healthcare Ltd)
  Isometheptene mucate 65 mg, Paracetamol 325 mg Midrid 325mg/65mg capsules | 15 capsule Ⓟ £4.81 DT = £4.81

Aspirin with metoclopramide

14-Jul-2020

The properties listed below are those particular to the combination only. For the properties of the components please consider, aspirin p. 142, metoclopramide hydrochloride p. 494.

- **INDICATIONS AND DOSE**

Acute migraine
- ▶ BY MOUTH
- ▶ Adult: 1 sachet, sachet to be mixed in water, and dose to be taken at the start of the attack, then 1 sachet after 2 hours if required; maximum 3 sachets per day

> **IMPORTANT SAFETY INFORMATION**
> Metoclopramide can cause **severe extrapyramidal effects**, particularly in children and young adults.

- **CAUTIONS** Treatment should not exceed 3 months due to risk of tardive dyskinesia
- **INTERACTIONS** → Appendix 1: aspirin · metoclopramide
- **PRESCRIBING AND DISPENSING INFORMATION** Flavours of oral powder formulations may include lemon.
- **MEDICINAL FORMS** No licensed medicines listed.

Tolfenamic acid
01-Aug-2023

- **INDICATIONS AND DOSE**

Treatment of acute migraine
▶ BY MOUTH
▶ Adult: 200 mg, dose to be taken at onset, then 200 mg after 1–2 hours if required

> **IMPORTANT SAFETY INFORMATION**
> MHRA/CHM ADVICE: NSAIDS: POTENTIAL RISKS FOLLOWING PROLONGED USE AFTER 20 WEEKS OF PREGNANCY (JUNE 2023)
> See Non-steroidal anti-inflammatory drugs p. 1292.

- **CONTRA-INDICATIONS** Active gastro-intestinal bleeding · active gastro-intestinal ulceration · history of gastro-intestinal bleeding related to previous NSAID therapy · history of gastro-intestinal haemorrhage (two or more distinct episodes) · history of gastro-intestinal perforation related to previous NSAID therapy · history of recurrent gastro-intestinal ulceration (two or more distinct episodes) · severe heart failure

- **CAUTIONS** Allergic disorders · cardiac impairment (NSAIDs may impair renal function) · cerebrovascular disease · coagulation defects · connective-tissue disorders · dehydration (risk of renal impairment) · elderly (risk of serious side-effects and fatalities) · heart failure · history of gastro-intestinal disorders (e.g. ulcerative colitis, Crohn's disease) · ischaemic heart disease · may mask symptoms of infection · peripheral arterial disease · risk factors for cardiovascular events · uncontrolled hypertension

- **INTERACTIONS** → Appendix 1: NSAIDs

- **SIDE-EFFECTS** Agranulocytosis · angioedema · aplastic anaemia · asthma · confusion · constipation · Crohn's disease aggravated · depression · diarrhoea · dizziness · drowsiness · dyspnoea · dysuria (most common in men) · euphoric mood · fatigue · fertility decreased female · gastrointestinal discomfort · gastrointestinal disorders · haemolytic anaemia · haemorrhage · hallucination · headache · heart failure · hepatic disorders · hypersensitivity · hypertension · increased risk of arterial thromboembolism · malaise · meningitis aseptic (patients with connective-tissue disorders such as systemic lupus erythematosus may be especially susceptible) · nausea · nephritis tubulointerstitial · nephropathy · neutropenia · oedema · optic neuritis · oral ulceration · pancreatitis · paraesthesia · photosensitivity reaction · renal failure (more common in patients with pre-existing renal impairment) · respiratory disorders · severe cutaneous adverse reactions (SCARs) · skin reactions · thrombocytopenia · tinnitus · tremor · vertigo · visual impairment · vomiting

- **SIDE-EFFECTS, FURTHER INFORMATION** For information about cardiovascular and gastrointestinal side-effects, and a possible exacerbation of symptoms in asthma, see Non-steroidal anti-inflammatory drugs. p. 1292

- **ALLERGY AND CROSS-SENSITIVITY** EvGr Contra-indicated in patients with a history of hypersensitivity to aspirin or any other NSAID—which includes those in whom attacks of asthma, angioedema, urticaria or rhinitis have been precipitated by aspirin or any other NSAID. Ⓜ

- **CONCEPTION AND CONTRACEPTION** EvGr Caution—long-term use of some NSAIDs is associated with reduced female fertility, which is reversible on stopping treatment. Ⓜ

- **PREGNANCY** Avoid use in first and second trimesters unless essential; the MHRA advises additional antenatal monitoring may be required if treatment is considered necessary by a doctor from week 20 of pregnancy onwards. Avoid use in third trimester. See *NSAIDs in Pregnancy* in Non-steroidal anti-inflammatory drugs p. 1292 for further details.

- **BREAST FEEDING** Amount too small to be harmful. Use with caution during breast-feeding.

- **HEPATIC IMPAIRMENT** Manufacturer advises caution in mild to moderate impairment; avoid in severe impairment.

- **RENAL IMPAIRMENT** In general, for *NSAIDs* the MHRA advises to avoid where possible; if necessary, use with caution (risk of fluid retention and further renal impairment, including renal failure).

- **MEDICINAL FORMS** There can be variation in the licensing of different medicines containing the same drug.

Oral tablet
CAUTIONARY AND ADVISORY LABELS 21
▶ Tolfenamic acid (Non-proprietary)
Tolfenamic acid 200 mg Tolfenamic acid 200mg tablets | 10 tablet PoM £27.08 DT = £27.08

ANTIHISTAMINES › SEDATING ANTIHISTAMINES

Paracetamol with buclizine hydrochloride and codeine phosphate
22-Nov-2019

The properties listed below are those particular to the combination only. For the properties of the components please consider, paracetamol p. 507, codeine phosphate p. 517.

- **INDICATIONS AND DOSE**

MIGRALEVE ®

Acute migraine
▶ BY MOUTH
▶ Child 12-15 years: Initially 1 tablet, (pink tablet) to be taken at onset of attack, or if it is imminent, followed by 1 tablet every 4 hours if required, (yellow tablet) to be taken following initial dose; maximum 1 pink and 3 yellow tablets in 24 hours
▶ Child 16-17 years: Initially 2 tablets, (pink tablets) to be taken at onset of attack or if it is imminent, followed by 2 tablets every 4 hours if required, (yellow tablets) to be taken following initial dose; maximum 2 pink and 6 yellow tablets in 24 hours
▶ Adult: Initially 2 tablets, (pink tablets) to be taken at onset of attack or if it is imminent, followed by 2 tablets every 4 hours if required, (yellow tablets) to be taken following initial dose; maximum 2 pink and 6 yellow tablets in 24 hours

- **INTERACTIONS** → Appendix 1: antihistamines, sedating · opioids · paracetamol

- **PRESCRIBING AND DISPENSING INFORMATION** See co-codamol p. 515 for *Migraleve* ® Yellow preparations.

- **LESS SUITABLE FOR PRESCRIBING**

MIGRALEVE ® *Migraleve* ® is less suitable for prescribing.

- **MEDICINAL FORMS** There can be variation in the licensing of different medicines containing the same drug.

Oral tablet
CAUTIONARY AND ADVISORY LABELS 2, 17, 30
▶ Migraleve Pink (McNeil Products Ltd)
Buclizine hydrochloride 6.25 mg, Codeine phosphate 8 mg, Paracetamol 500 mg Migraleve Pink tablets | 12 tablet P £5.00 CD5 | 24 tablet P £7.95 CD5

Pizotifen

21-May-2024

- **INDICATIONS AND DOSE**

Prevention of vascular headache | Prevention of classical migraine | Prevention of common migraine | Prevention of cluster headache
- BY MOUTH
- Adult: Initially 500 micrograms once daily, then increased to 1.5 mg once daily, dose to be increased gradually and taken at night, alternatively increased to 1.5 mg daily in 3 divided doses, doses to be increased gradually; increased if necessary up to 4.5 mg daily (max. per dose 3 mg)

Prophylaxis of migraine
- BY MOUTH
- Child 5-17 years: Initially 500 micrograms once daily, dose to be taken at night, then increased if necessary up to 1.5 mg daily in divided doses, dose to be increased gradually, max. single dose (at night) 1 mg

- **CONTRA-INDICATIONS** Acute porphyrias p. 1202
- **CAUTIONS** Avoid abrupt withdrawal · history of epilepsy · susceptibility to angle-closure glaucoma · urinary retention
- **INTERACTIONS** → Appendix 1: antihistamines, sedating
- **SIDE-EFFECTS**
- **Common or very common** Appetite increased · dizziness · drowsiness · dry mouth · fatigue · nausea · weight increased
- **Uncommon** Constipation
- **Rare or very rare** Aggression · anxiety · arthralgia · central nervous system stimulation · depression · hallucination · muscle complaints · paraesthesia · seizure · skin reactions · sleep disorders
- **Frequency not known** Hepatic disorders
- **PREGNANCY** Avoid unless potential benefit outweighs risk.
- **BREAST FEEDING** Amount probably too small to be harmful, but manufacturer advises avoid.
- **HEPATIC IMPAIRMENT** Manufacturer advises caution. **Dose adjustments** Manufacturer advises consider dose reduction.
- **RENAL IMPAIRMENT** EvGr Use with caution. M **Dose adjustments** EvGr Consider dose reduction. M
- **PATIENT AND CARER ADVICE** Medicines for Children leaflet: Pizotifen for migraine headaches www.medicinesforchildren.org.uk/medicines/pizotifen-for-migraine-headaches/
Driving and skilled tasks Drowsiness may affect performance of skilled tasks (e.g. driving); effects of alcohol enhanced.

- **MEDICINAL FORMS** There can be variation in the licensing of different medicines containing the same drug. Forms available from special-order manufacturers include: oral solution
Oral tablet
CAUTIONARY AND ADVISORY LABELS 2
- Pizotifen (Non-proprietary)
Pizotifen (as Pizotifen hydrogen malate)
500 microgram Pizotifen 500microgram tablets | 28 tablet PoM £3.00 DT = £1.37
Pizotifen (as Pizotifen hydrogen malate) 1.5 mg Pizotifen 1.5mg tablets | 28 tablet PoM £4.60 DT = £1.77

CALCITONIN GENE-RELATED PEPTIDE INHIBITORS

Atogepant

08-Jul-2024

- **DRUG ACTION** Atogepant is a calcitonin gene-related peptide (CGRP) receptor antagonist which inhibits the function of CGRP, thereby preventing migraine attacks.

- **INDICATIONS AND DOSE**

Prophylaxis of episodic or chronic migraine [in patients who have at least 4 migraine days per month]
- BY MOUTH
- Adult: 60 mg once daily
DOSE ADJUSTMENTS DUE TO INTERACTIONS
- EvGr Reduce dose to 10 mg once daily with concurrent use of potent CYP3A4 inhibitors, OATP inhibitors, or telmisartan. M

- **INTERACTIONS** → Appendix 1: atogepant
- **SIDE-EFFECTS**
- **Common or very common** Appetite decreased · constipation · drowsiness · fatigue · nausea · weight decreased
- **PREGNANCY** EvGr Avoid (toxicity in *animal* studies). M
- **BREAST FEEDING** EvGr Avoid (present in milk in *animal* studies). M
- **HEPATIC IMPAIRMENT** EvGr Avoid in severe impairment (risk of increased exposure). M
- **RENAL IMPAIRMENT**
Dose adjustments EvGr Reduce dose to 10 mg once daily if creatinine clearance less than 30 mL/minute. M See p. 21.
- **PATIENT AND CARER ADVICE**
Driving and skilled tasks Patients and carers should be counselled on the effects on driving and performance of skilled tasks—increased risk of somnolence.
- **NATIONAL FUNDING/ACCESS DECISIONS** For full details see funding body website
NICE decisions
- **Atogepant for preventing migraine (May 2024)** NICE TA973 Recommended with restrictions
Scottish Medicines Consortium (SMC) decisions
- Atogepant (*Aquipta*®) for the prophylaxis of migraine in adults who have at least four migraine days per month (October 2023) SMC No. SMC2599 Recommended with restrictions

- **MEDICINAL FORMS** There can be variation in the licensing of different medicines containing the same drug.
Oral tablet
- Aquipta (AbbVie Ltd) ▼
Atogepant 10 mg Aquipta 10mg tablets | 28 tablet PoM £182.16 DT = £182.16
Atogepant 60 mg Aquipta 60mg tablets | 28 tablet PoM £182.16 DT = £182.16

Eptinezumab

04-Apr-2023

- **DRUG ACTION** Eptinezumab is a human monoclonal antibody that binds to the calcitonin gene-related peptide (CGRP) ligand, inhibiting the function of CGRP at its receptor, and thereby preventing migraine attacks.

- **INDICATIONS AND DOSE**

Prophylaxis of migraine [in patients who have at least 4 migraine days per month] (initiated by a specialist)
- BY INTRAVENOUS INFUSION
- Adult: 100 mg every 12 weeks; increased if necessary to 300 mg every 12 weeks, assess need for dose escalation within first 12 weeks; increased dose to be given on the

next scheduled date. Review treatment 6 months after initiation

● **SIDE-EFFECTS**
▸ **Common or very common** Fatigue · hypersensitivity · nasopharyngitis
● **PREGNANCY** [EvGr] Avoid—limited information available. ⟨M⟩
● **BREAST FEEDING** [EvGr] Avoid during first few days after birth—possible risk from transfer of antibodies to infant. After this time, use during breast-feeding only if clinically needed. ⟨M⟩
● **DIRECTIONS FOR ADMINISTRATION** [EvGr] For *intravenous infusion*, dilute requisite dose with 100 mL of Sodium Chloride 0.9%; give over about 30 minutes through an in-line or add-on filter (0.2 or 0.22 micron). ⟨M⟩
● **PRESCRIBING AND DISPENSING INFORMATION** Eptinezumab is a biological medicine. Biological medicines must be prescribed and dispensed by brand name, see *Biological medicines* and *Biosimilar medicines*, under Guidance on prescribing p. 1; record the brand name and batch number after each administration.
● **HANDLING AND STORAGE** Store in a refrigerator (2-8°C) and protect from light—consult product literature for storage conditions after preparation of the infusion.
● **NATIONAL FUNDING/ACCESS DECISIONS** For full details see funding body website
  NICE decisions
▸ **Eptinezumab for preventing migraine (March 2023)** NICE TA871 Recommended with restrictions
  Scottish Medicines Consortium (SMC) decisions
▸ **Eptinezumab (*Vyepti*®) for the prophylaxis of migraine in adults who have at least 4 migraine days per month (February 2023)** SMC No. SMC2547 Recommended with restrictions

● **MEDICINAL FORMS** There can be variation in the licensing of different medicines containing the same drug.
  Solution for infusion
  EXCIPIENTS: May contain Polysorbates, sorbitol
▸ **Vyepti** (Lundbeck Ltd) ▼
  Eptinezumab 100 mg per 1 ml Vyepti 100mg/1ml concentrate for solution for infusion vials | 1 vial [PoM] £1,350.00 (Hospital only)

Erenumab
30-Mar-2021

● **DRUG ACTION** Erenumab is a human monoclonal antibody that binds to the calcitonin gene-related peptide (CGRP) receptor, inhibiting the function of CGRP, and thereby preventing migraine attacks.

● **INDICATIONS AND DOSE**

  Prophylaxis of migraine (in patients who have at least 4 migraine days per month) (initiated by a specialist)
▸ BY SUBCUTANEOUS INJECTION
▸ Adult: 70 mg every 4 weeks; increased if necessary to 140 mg every 4 weeks, consider discontinuing if no response after 3 months of treatment

● **INTERACTIONS** → Appendix 1: erenumab
● **SIDE-EFFECTS**
▸ **Common or very common** Angioedema · constipation · hypersensitivity · muscle spasms · oedema · skin reactions · swelling
▸ **Frequency not known** Alopecia · oral disorders
● **PREGNANCY** Manufacturer advises avoid—limited information available.
● **BREAST FEEDING** Manufacturer advises avoid during first few days after birth—possible risk from transfer of antibodies to infant. After this time, use during breast-feeding only if clinically needed.

● **DIRECTIONS FOR ADMINISTRATION** Manufacturer advises injection into the abdomen, thigh, or upper arm (if not self-administered). Patients may self-administer *Aimovig*® after appropriate training in subcutaneous injection technique.
● **PRESCRIBING AND DISPENSING INFORMATION** Erenumab is a biological medicine. Biological medicines must be prescribed and dispensed by brand name, see *Biological medicines* and *Biosimilar medicines*, under Guidance on prescribing p. 1; manufacturer advises to record the brand name and batch number after each administration.
● **HANDLING AND STORAGE** Manufacturer advises store in a refrigerator (2-8°C) and protect from light—consult product literature for further information regarding storage outside refrigerator.
● **PATIENT AND CARER ADVICE** Self-administration Manufacturer advises that patients and their carers should be given training in subcutaneous injection technique if appropriate.
● **NATIONAL FUNDING/ACCESS DECISIONS** For full details see funding body website
  NICE decisions
▸ **Erenumab for preventing migraine (March 2021)** NICE TA682 Recommended with restrictions
  Scottish Medicines Consortium (SMC) decisions
▸ **Erenumab (*Aimovig*®) for the prophylaxis of migraine in adults who have at least 4 migraine days per month (April 2019)** SMC No. SMC2134 Recommended with restrictions

● **MEDICINAL FORMS** There can be variation in the licensing of different medicines containing the same drug.
  Solution for injection
  EXCIPIENTS: May contain Polysorbates, sucrose
▸ **Aimovig** (Novartis Pharmaceuticals UK Ltd)
  Erenumab 70 mg per 1 ml Aimovig 70mg/1ml solution for injection pre-filled pens | 1 pre-filled disposable injection [PoM] £386.50 DT = £386.50
  Erenumab 140 mg per 1 ml Aimovig 140mg/1ml solution for injection pre-filled pens | 1 pre-filled disposable injection [PoM] £386.50 (Hospital only)

Fremanezumab
01-Mar-2022

● **DRUG ACTION** Fremanezumab is a humanised monoclonal antibody that binds to the calcitonin gene-related peptide (CGRP) ligand, inhibiting the function of CGRP at its receptor, and thereby preventing migraine attacks.

● **INDICATIONS AND DOSE**

  Prophylaxis of migraine [in patients who have at least 4 migraine days per month] (initiated by a specialist)
▸ BY SUBCUTANEOUS INJECTION
▸ Adult: 225 mg once a month, alternatively 675 mg every 3 months, review treatment within first 3 months and regularly thereafter

● **CAUTIONS** Major cardiovascular disease (no information available)
● **SIDE-EFFECTS** Hypersensitivity
● **PREGNANCY** Manufacturer advises avoid—limited information available.
● **BREAST FEEDING** Manufacturer advises avoid during first few days after birth—possible risk from transfer of antibodies to infant. After this time, use during breast-feeding only if clinically needed.
● **DIRECTIONS FOR ADMINISTRATION** Manufacturer advises injection into the abdomen, thigh or upper arm. Patients may self-administer *Ajovy*® after appropriate training in subcutaneous injection technique.
● **PRESCRIBING AND DISPENSING INFORMATION** Fremanezumab is a biological medicine. Biological

medicines must be prescribed and dispensed by brand name, see *Biological medicines* and *Biosimilar medicines*, under Guidance on prescribing p. 1; manufacturer advises to record the brand name and batch number after each administration.

- **HANDLING AND STORAGE** Manufacturer advises store in a refrigerator (2–8°C) and protect from light—consult product literature for further information regarding storage outside refrigerator.
- **PATIENT AND CARER ADVICE**
Self-administration Manufacturer advises patients and their carers should be given training in subcutaneous injection technique if appropriate.
- **NATIONAL FUNDING/ACCESS DECISIONS**
For full details see funding body website
NICE decisions
▸ Fremanezumab for preventing migraine (February 2022) NICE TA764 Recommended with restrictions
Scottish Medicines Consortium (SMC) decisions
▸ Fremanezumab (*Ajovy*®) for the prophylaxis of migraine in adults who have at least four migraine days per month (January 2020) SMC No. SMC2226 Recommended with restrictions

- **MEDICINAL FORMS** There can be variation in the licensing of different medicines containing the same drug.
Solution for injection
EXCIPIENTS: May contain Edetic acid (edta), polysorbates, sucrose
▸ **Ajovy** (Teva UK Ltd)
Fremanezumab 150 mg per 1 ml Ajovy 225mg/1.5ml solution for injection pre-filled syringes | 1 pre-filled disposable injection PoM £450.00
Ajovy 225mg/1.5ml solution for injection pre-filled pens | 1 pre-filled disposable injection PoM £450.00 | 3 pre-filled disposable injection PoM £1,350.00

Galcanezumab
04-May-2021

- **DRUG ACTION** Galcanezumab is a humanised monoclonal antibody that binds to the calcitonin gene-related peptide (CGRP) ligand, inhibiting the function of CGRP at its receptor, and thereby preventing migraine attacks.

- **INDICATIONS AND DOSE**
Prophylaxis of migraine [in patients who have at least 4 migraine days per month] (initiated by a specialist)
▸ BY SUBCUTANEOUS INJECTION
▸ Adult: Loading dose 240 mg for 1 dose, then maintenance 120 mg once a month, maintenance dosing to start 1 month after loading dose. Review treatment 3 months after initiation

- **SIDE-EFFECTS**
▸ **Common or very common** Constipation · skin reactions · vertigo
▸ **Rare or very rare** Anaphylactic reaction · angioedema
- **PREGNANCY** Manufacturer advises avoid—limited information available.
- **BREAST FEEDING** Manufacturer advises avoid during first few days after birth—possible risk from transfer of antibodies to infant. After this time, use during breast-feeding only if clinically needed.
- **DIRECTIONS FOR ADMINISTRATION** Manufacturer advises injection into the abdomen, thigh, back of the upper arm, or the gluteal region. Patients may self-administer *Emgality*® after appropriate training in subcutaneous injection technique.
- **PRESCRIBING AND DISPENSING INFORMATION** Galcanezumab is a biological medicine. Biological medicines must be prescribed and dispensed by brand name, see *Biological medicines* and *Biosimilar medicines*,

under Guidance on prescribing p. 1; manufacturer advises to record the brand name and batch number after each administration.

- **HANDLING AND STORAGE** Manufacturer advises store in a refrigerator (2–8°C) and protect from light—consult product literature for further information regarding storage outside refrigerator.
- **PATIENT AND CARER ADVICE**
Self-administration Manufacturer advises patients and their carers should be given training in subcutaneous injection technique if appropriate.
Driving and skilled tasks Manufacturer advises patients and their carers should be counselled on the effects on driving and performance of skilled tasks—increased risk of vertigo.
- **NATIONAL FUNDING/ACCESS DECISIONS**
For full details see funding body website
NICE decisions
▸ Galcanezumab for preventing migraine (November 2020) NICE TA659 Recommended with restrictions
Scottish Medicines Consortium (SMC) decisions
▸ Galcanezumab (*Emgality*®) for the prophylaxis of migraine in adults who have at least 4 migraine days per month (April 2021) SMC No. SMC2313 Recommended with restrictions

- **MEDICINAL FORMS** There can be variation in the licensing of different medicines containing the same drug.
Solution for injection
EXCIPIENTS: May contain Polysorbates
▸ **Emgality** (Organon Pharma (UK) Ltd)
Galcanezumab 120 mg per 1 ml Emgality 120mg/1ml solution for injection pre-filled pens | 1 pre-filled disposable injection PoM £450.00 DT = £450.00

Rimegepant
08-Jul-2024

- **DRUG ACTION** Rimegepant is a calcitonin gene-related peptide (CGRP) receptor antagonist which inhibits the function of CGRP, thereby preventing migraine attacks.

- **INDICATIONS AND DOSE**
Treatment of acute migraine
▸ BY MOUTH
▸ Adult: 75 mg once daily if required
Prophylaxis of episodic migraine [in patients who have at least 4 migraine attacks per month]
▸ BY MOUTH
▸ Adult: 75 mg once daily on alternate days

- **INTERACTIONS** → Appendix 1: rimegepant
- **SIDE-EFFECTS**
▸ **Common or very common** Nausea
▸ **Uncommon** Hypersensitivity

SIDE-EFFECTS, FURTHER INFORMATION Hypersensitivity reactions, including dyspnoea and rash, can occur days after administration. If a hypersensitivity reaction occurs, rimegepant should be discontinued.
- **PREGNANCY** EvGr Avoid—limited information available. Ⓜ
- **BREAST FEEDING** Specialist sources indicate present in milk but amount probably too small to be harmful. Consider an alternative drug if breast-feeding a neonate (pre or full-term)—limited information available.
- **HEPATIC IMPAIRMENT** EvGr Avoid in severe impairment (increased risk of exposure). Ⓜ
- **RENAL IMPAIRMENT** EvGr Caution in severe impairment (increased risk of exposure). Ⓜ
- **DIRECTIONS FOR ADMINISTRATION** Rimegepant oral lyophilisates should be placed on or under the tongue and allowed to dissolve.

- **PATIENT AND CARER ADVICE** Patients or their carers should be given advice on how to administer rimegepant oral lyophilisates.

- **NATIONAL FUNDING/ACCESS DECISIONS**
For full details see funding body website
NICE decisions
▶ Rimegepant for preventing migraine (July 2023) NICE TA906
Recommended with restrictions
▶ Rimegepant for treating migraine (October 2023) NICE TA919
Recommended with restrictions
Scottish Medicines Consortium (SMC) decisions
▶ Rimegepant (*Vydura*®) for the acute treatment of migraine with or without aura in adults (May 2023) SMC No. SMC2521
Recommended with restrictions
▶ Rimegepant (*Vydura*®) for the preventive treatment of episodic migraine in adults who have at least 4 migraine attacks per month (September 2023) SMC No. SMC2603
Recommended with restrictions

- **MEDICINAL FORMS** There can be variation in the licensing of different medicines containing the same drug.
Oral lyophilisate
EXCIPIENTS: May contain Gelatin
▶ Vydura (Pfizer Ltd) ▼
Rimegepant (as Rimegepant sulfate) 75 mg Vydura 75mg oral lyophilisates | 2 tablet [PoM] £25.80 DT = £25.80 [SF] | 8 tablet [PoM] £103.20 DT = £103.20 [SF]

TRIPTANS

Almotriptan
03-Aug-2021

- **INDICATIONS AND DOSE**
Treatment of acute migraine
▶ BY MOUTH
▶ Adult: 12.5 mg, dose to be taken as soon as possible after onset, followed by 12.5 mg after 2 hours if required, dose to be taken only if migraine recurs (patient not responding to initial dose should not take second dose for same attack); maximum 25 mg per day

- **UNLICENSED USE** Not licensed for use in elderly.

- **CONTRA-INDICATIONS** Coronary vasospasm · ischaemic heart disease · peripheral vascular disease · previous cerebrovascular accident · previous myocardial infarction · previous transient ischaemic attack · Prinzmetal's angina · severe hypertension · uncontrolled hypertension

- **CAUTIONS** Conditions which predispose to coronary artery disease · elderly

- **INTERACTIONS** → Appendix 1: triptans

- **SIDE-EFFECTS**
▶ **Common or very common** Asthenia · dizziness · drowsiness · nausea · vomiting
▶ **Uncommon** Bone pain · chest pain · diarrhoea · dry mouth · dyspepsia · headache · myalgia · palpitations · paraesthesia · throat tightness · tinnitus
▶ **Rare or very rare** Coronary vasospasm · myocardial infarction · tachycardia
▶ **Frequency not known** Intestinal ischaemia · seizure · vision disorders

SIDE-EFFECTS, FURTHER INFORMATION Discontinue if symptoms of heat, heaviness, pressure or tightness (including throat and chest) occur.

- **ALLERGY AND CROSS-SENSITIVITY** [EvGr] Caution in patients with sensitivity to sulfonamides. ⟨M⟩

- **PREGNANCY** There is limited experience of using 5HT$_1$-receptor agonists during pregnancy; manufacturers advise that they should be avoided unless the potential benefit outweighs the risk.

- **BREAST FEEDING** Present in milk in *animal* studies—withhold breast-feeding for 24 hours.

- **HEPATIC IMPAIRMENT** Manufacturer advises caution in mild to moderate impairment; avoid in severe impairment—no information available.

- **RENAL IMPAIRMENT**
Dose adjustments [EvGr] Max. 12.5 mg in 24 hours if creatinine clearance less than 30 mL/minute. ⟨M⟩ See p. 21.

- **MEDICINAL FORMS** There can be variation in the licensing of different medicines containing the same drug.
Oral tablet
CAUTIONARY AND ADVISORY LABELS 3
▶ Almotriptan (Non-proprietary)
Almotriptan (as Almotriptan hydrogen malate)
12.5 mg Almotriptan 12.5mg tablets | 3 tablet [PoM] £9.07 DT = £7.14 | 6 tablet [PoM] £18.14 DT = £14.28 | 9 tablet [PoM] £27.20 DT = £21.42

Eletriptan
03-Aug-2021

- **INDICATIONS AND DOSE**
Treatment of acute migraine
▶ BY MOUTH
▶ Adult: 40 mg, followed by 40 mg after 2 hours if required, dose to be taken only if migraine recurs (patient not responding to initial dose should not take second dose for same attack); increased if necessary to 80 mg, dose to be taken for subsequent attacks if 40 mg dose inadequate; maximum 80 mg per day

- **UNLICENSED USE** Not licensed for use in elderly.

- **CONTRA-INDICATIONS** Arrhythmias · coronary vasospasm · heart failure · ischaemic heart disease · peripheral vascular disease · previous cerebrovascular accident · previous myocardial infarction · previous transient ischaemic attack · Prinzmetal's angina · severe hypertension · uncontrolled hypertension

- **CAUTIONS** Conditions which predispose to coronary artery disease · elderly

- **INTERACTIONS** → Appendix 1: triptans

- **SIDE-EFFECTS**
▶ **Common or very common** Arrhythmias · asthenia · chest discomfort · chills · dizziness · drowsiness · dry mouth · feeling hot · flushing · gastrointestinal discomfort · headache · hyperhidrosis · increased risk of infection · muscle complaints · muscle tone increased · muscle weakness · nausea · pain · palpitations · sensation abnormal · throat tightness · vertigo
▶ **Uncommon** Agitation · appetite decreased · arthralgia · arthritis · confusion · depersonalisation · depression · diarrhoea · dyspnoea · ear pain · eye pain · insomnia · lacrimation disorder · malaise · mood altered · movement disorders · oedema · oral disorders · peripheral vascular disease · respiratory disorder · skin reactions · speech disorder · stupor · taste altered · thinking abnormal · thirst · tinnitus · tremor · urinary disorders · urinary tract disorder · vision disorders · yawning
▶ **Rare or very rare** Asthma · breast pain · burping · conjunctivitis · constipation · gastrointestinal disorders · hyperbilirubinaemia · lymphadenopathy · menorrhagia · myopathy · shock · voice alteration
▶ **Frequency not known** Coronary vasospasm · hypertension · myocardial infarction · myocardial ischaemia · serotonin syndrome · stroke · syncope · vomiting

SIDE-EFFECTS, FURTHER INFORMATION Discontinue if symptoms of heat, heaviness, pressure or tightness (including throat and chest) occur.

- **PREGNANCY** There is limited experience of using 5HT$_1$-receptor agonists during pregnancy; manufacturers advise that they should be avoided unless the potential benefit outweighs the risk.

- **BREAST FEEDING** Present in milk—avoid breast-feeding for 24 hours.
- **HEPATIC IMPAIRMENT** Manufacturer advises avoid in severe impairment.
- **RENAL IMPAIRMENT** [EvGr] Avoid if creatinine clearance less than 30 mL/minute, [M] see p. 21.
  Dose adjustments [EvGr] Reduce initial dose to 20 mg (maximum 40 mg in 24 hours) in mild to moderate impairment. [M]

- **MEDICINAL FORMS** There can be variation in the licensing of different medicines containing the same drug.
  Oral tablet
  CAUTIONARY AND ADVISORY LABELS 3
  ▸ Eletriptan (Non-proprietary)
  Eletriptan (as Eletriptan hydrobromide) 20 mg Eletriptan 20mg tablets | 6 tablet [PoM] £21.38-£32.00 DT = £22.50
  Eletriptan (as Eletriptan hydrobromide) 40 mg Eletriptan 40mg tablets | 6 tablet [PoM] £21.38-£22.50 DT = £22.50
  ▸ Relpax (Viatris UK Healthcare Ltd)
  Eletriptan (as Eletriptan hydrobromide) 20 mg Relpax 20mg tablets | 6 tablet [PoM] £22.50 DT = £22.50
  Eletriptan (as Eletriptan hydrobromide) 40 mg Relpax 40mg tablets | 6 tablet [PoM] £22.50 DT = £22.50

Frovatriptan

04-Mar-2020

- **INDICATIONS AND DOSE**
  Treatment of acute migraine
  ▸ BY MOUTH
  ▸ Adult: 2.5 mg, dose to be taken as soon as possible after onset, followed by 2.5 mg after 2 hours if required, dose to be taken only if migraine recurs (patient not responding to initial dose should not take second dose for same attack); maximum 5 mg per day

  Menstrual migraine prophylaxis
  ▸ BY MOUTH
  ▸ Adult: 2.5 mg twice daily, to be taken from 2 days before until 3 days after bleeding starts

- **UNLICENSED USE** Not licensed for use in elderly.
  [EvGr] Frovatriptan may be used for menstrual migraine prophylaxis, [A] but it is not licensed for this indication.
- **CONTRA-INDICATIONS** Coronary vasospasm · ischaemic heart disease · peripheral vascular disease · previous cerebrovascular accident · previous myocardial infarction · previous transient ischaemic attack · Prinzmetal's angina · severe hypertension · uncontrolled hypertension
- **CAUTIONS** Conditions which predispose to coronary artery disease · elderly
- **INTERACTIONS** → Appendix 1: triptans
- **SIDE-EFFECTS**
- ▸ **Common or very common** Asthenia · chest discomfort · dizziness · drowsiness · dry mouth · flushing · gastrointestinal discomfort · headache · hyperhidrosis · nausea · sensation abnormal · throat complaints · vision disorders
- ▸ **Uncommon** Anxiety · arrhythmias · arthralgia · concentration impaired · confusion · dehydration · depression · diarrhoea · dysphagia · ear discomfort · eye discomfort · gastrointestinal disorders · hypertension · increased risk of infection · malaise · musculoskeletal stiffness · neuromuscular dysfunction · pain · palpitations · peripheral coldness · psychiatric disorders · skin reactions · sleep disorders · taste altered · temperature sensation altered · thirst · tinnitus · tremor · urinary disorders · vertigo
- ▸ **Rare or very rare** Breast tenderness · burping · constipation · ear disorder · epistaxis · fever · hiccups · hyperacusia · hypoglycaemia · irritable bowel syndrome · lymphadenopathy · memory loss · movement disorder ·

oesophageal spasm · oral disorders · piloerection · reflexes decreased · renal pain · respiratory disorders · self mutilation
- ▸ **Frequency not known** Angioedema · coronary vasospasm · hypersensitivity · myocardial infarction

  SIDE-EFFECTS, FURTHER INFORMATION Discontinue if symptoms of heat, heaviness, pressure or tightness (including throat and chest) occur.
- **PREGNANCY** There is limited experience of using 5HT$_1$-receptor agonists during pregnancy; manufacturers advise that they should be avoided unless the potential benefit outweighs the risk.
- **BREAST FEEDING** Present in milk in *animal* studies—withhold breast-feeding for 24 hours.
- **HEPATIC IMPAIRMENT** Manufacturer advises avoid in severe impairment—no information available.

- **MEDICINAL FORMS** There can be variation in the licensing of different medicines containing the same drug.
  Oral tablet
  CAUTIONARY AND ADVISORY LABELS 3
  ▸ Frovatriptan (Non-proprietary)
  Frovatriptan (as Frovatriptan succinate monohydrate) 2.5 mg Frovatriptan 2.5mg tablets | 6 tablet [PoM] £18.13 DT = £12.32
  ▸ Migard (A. Menarini Farmaceutica Internazionale SRL)
  Frovatriptan (as Frovatriptan succinate monohydrate) 2.5 mg Migard 2.5mg tablets | 6 tablet [PoM] £16.67 DT = £12.32
  ▸ Mylatrip (Viatris UK Healthcare Ltd)
  Frovatriptan (as Frovatriptan succinate monohydrate) 2.5 mg Mylatrip 2.5mg tablets | 6 tablet [PoM] £16.50 DT = £12.32

Naratriptan

03-Aug-2021

- **INDICATIONS AND DOSE**
  Treatment of acute migraine
  ▸ BY MOUTH
  ▸ Adult: 2.5 mg, followed by 2.5 mg after at least 4 hours if required, to be taken only if migraine recurs (patient not responding to initial dose should not take second dose for same attack); maximum 5 mg per day

  Menstrual migraine prophylaxis
  ▸ BY MOUTH
  ▸ Adult: 2.5 mg twice daily, to be taken from 2 days before until 3 days after bleeding starts

- **UNLICENSED USE** [EvGr] Naratriptan is used for menstrual migraine prophylaxis, [A] but is not licensed for this indication. Not licensed for use in elderly.
- **CONTRA-INDICATIONS** Coronary vasospasm · ischaemic heart disease · moderate or severe hypertension · peripheral vascular disease · previous cerebrovascular accident · previous myocardial infarction · previous transient ischaemic attack · Prinzmetal's angina · uncontrolled hypertension
- **CAUTIONS** Conditions which predispose to coronary artery disease · elderly
- **INTERACTIONS** → Appendix 1: triptans
- **SIDE-EFFECTS**
- ▸ **Common or very common** Dizziness · drowsiness · fatigue · feeling hot · malaise · nausea · paraesthesia · vomiting
- ▸ **Uncommon** Arrhythmias · feeling abnormal · pain · palpitations · visual impairment
- ▸ **Rare or very rare** Angina pectoris · colitis ischaemic · coronary vasospasm · face oedema · myocardial infarction · peripheral vascular disease · skin reactions

  SIDE-EFFECTS, FURTHER INFORMATION Discontinue if symptoms of heat, heaviness, pressure or tightness (including throat and chest) occur.

- **ALLERGY AND CROSS-SENSITIVITY** [EvGr] Caution in patients with sensitivity to sulfonamides. [M]
- **PREGNANCY** There is limited experience of using $5HT_1$-receptor agonists during pregnancy; manufacturers advise that they should be avoided unless the potential benefit outweighs the risk.
- **BREAST FEEDING** Withhold breast-feeding for 24 hours.
- **HEPATIC IMPAIRMENT** Manufacturer advises caution in mild to moderate impairment (risk of decreased clearance); avoid in severe impairment.
  Dose adjustments Manufacturer advises maximum 2.5 mg in 24 hours in mild to moderate impairment.
- **RENAL IMPAIRMENT** [EvGr] Caution; avoid if creatinine clearance less than 15 mL/minute. [M] See p. 21.
  Dose adjustments [EvGr] Max. 2.5 mg in 24 hours. [M]
- **PATIENT AND CARER ADVICE**
  Driving and skilled tasks Drowsiness may affect performance of skilled tasks (e.g. driving).

- **MEDICINAL FORMS** There can be variation in the licensing of different medicines containing the same drug.
  Oral tablet
  CAUTIONARY AND ADVISORY LABELS 3
  - ▸ Naratriptan (Non-proprietary)
    Naratriptan (as Naratriptan hydrochloride) 2.5 mg Naratriptan 2.5mg tablets | 6 tablet [PoM] £24.55 DT = £1.46 | 12 tablet [PoM] £2.92–£8.68 DT = £2.92
  - ▸ Naramig (GlaxoSmithKline UK Ltd)
    Naratriptan (as Naratriptan hydrochloride) 2.5 mg Naramig 2.5mg tablets | 6 tablet [PoM] £24.55 DT = £1.46

Rizatriptan
24-May-2021

- **INDICATIONS AND DOSE**
Treatment of acute migraine
  - ▸ BY MOUTH
  - ▸ Adult: 10 mg, dose to be taken as soon as possible after onset, followed by 10 mg after 2 hours if required, dose to be taken only if migraine recurs (patient not responding to initial dose should not take second dose for same attack); maximum 20 mg per day

DOSE ADJUSTMENTS DUE TO INTERACTIONS
  - ▸ Manufacturer advises reduce dose to 5 mg with concurrent use of propranolol.

- **UNLICENSED USE** Not licensed for use in elderly.
- **CONTRA-INDICATIONS** Coronary vasospasm · ischaemic heart disease · peripheral vascular disease · previous cerebrovascular accident · previous myocardial infarction · previous transient ischaemic attack · Prinzmetal's angina · severe hypertension · uncontrolled hypertension
- **CAUTIONS** Conditions which predispose to coronary artery disease · elderly
- **INTERACTIONS** → Appendix 1: triptans
- **SIDE-EFFECTS**
- ▸ **Common or very common** Alertness decreased · asthenia · diarrhoea · dizziness · drowsiness · dry mouth · dyspepsia · feeling abnormal · headache · insomnia · musculoskeletal stiffness · nausea · pain · palpitations · sensation abnormal · throat complaints · vasodilation · vomiting
- ▸ **Uncommon** Angioedema · arrhythmias · ataxia · disorientation · dyspnoea · face oedema · hyperhidrosis · hypertension · muscle weakness · myalgia · nervousness · skin reactions · syncope · taste altered · thirst · tongue swelling · tremor · vertigo · vision blurred
- ▸ **Rare or very rare** Hypersensitivity · stroke · wheezing
- ▸ **Frequency not known** Colitis ischaemic · myocardial infarction · myocardial ischaemia · peripheral vascular disease · seizure · serotonin syndrome · toxic epidermal necrolysis

SIDE-EFFECTS, FURTHER INFORMATION Discontinue if symptoms of heat, heaviness, pressure or tightness (including throat and chest) occur.

- **PREGNANCY** There is limited experience of using $5HT_1$-receptor agonists during pregnancy; manufacturers advise that they should be avoided unless the potential benefit outweighs the risk.
- **BREAST FEEDING** Present in milk in *animal* studies—withhold breast-feeding for 24 hours.
- **HEPATIC IMPAIRMENT** Manufacturer advises caution in mild to moderate impairment; avoid in severe impairment (no information available).
  Dose adjustments Manufacturer advises dose reduction to 5 mg in mild to moderate impairment.
- **RENAL IMPAIRMENT** [EvGr] Avoid in severe impairment. [M]
  Dose adjustments [EvGr] Reduce dose to 5 mg in mild to moderate impairment. [M]
- **DIRECTIONS FOR ADMINISTRATION** Rizatriptan orodispersible tablets should be placed on the tongue, allowed to disperse and swallowed. Rizatriptan oral lyophilisates should be placed on the tongue and allowed to dissolve.
- **PATIENT AND CARER ADVICE** Patients or carers should be given advice on how to administer rizatriptan orodispersible tablets and oral lyophilisates.
  Driving and skilled tasks Drowsiness may affect performance of skilled tasks (e.g. driving).

- **MEDICINAL FORMS** There can be variation in the licensing of different medicines containing the same drug.
  Oral tablet
  CAUTIONARY AND ADVISORY LABELS 3
  - ▸ Rizatriptan (Non-proprietary)
    Rizatriptan (as Rizatriptan benzoate) 5 mg Rizatriptan 5mg tablets | 3 tablet [PoM] £13.37 | 6 tablet [PoM] £29.60 DT = £28.26
    Rizatriptan (as Rizatriptan benzoate) 10 mg Rizatriptan 10mg tablets | 3 tablet [PoM] £8.26–£15.60 DT = £9.65 | 6 tablet [PoM] £16.52–£31.20
  - ▸ Maxalt (Organon Pharma (UK) Ltd)
    Rizatriptan (as Rizatriptan benzoate) 5 mg Maxalt 5mg tablets | 6 tablet [PoM] £26.74 DT = £28.26
    Rizatriptan (as Rizatriptan benzoate) 10 mg Maxalt 10mg tablets | 3 tablet [PoM] £13.37 DT = £9.65 | 6 tablet [PoM] £26.74
  Orodispersible tablet
  CAUTIONARY AND ADVISORY LABELS 3
  EXCIPIENTS: May contain Aspartame
  - ▸ Rizatriptan (Non-proprietary)
    Rizatriptan (as Rizatriptan benzoate) 5 mg Rizatriptan 5mg orodispersible tablets sugar free | 6 tablet [PoM] £18.98 [SF] | 12 tablet [PoM] £26.98–£37.96 [SF]
    Rizatriptan (as Rizatriptan benzoate) 10 mg Rizatriptan 10mg orodispersible tablets sugar free | 3 tablet [PoM] £13.37 DT = £4.87 [SF] | 6 tablet [PoM] £3.87–£26.74 [SF]
  Oral lyophilisate
  CAUTIONARY AND ADVISORY LABELS 3
  EXCIPIENTS: May contain Aspartame
  - ▸ Maxalt Melt (Organon Pharma (UK) Ltd)
    Rizatriptan (as Rizatriptan benzoate) 10 mg Maxalt Melt 10mg oral lyophilisates | 3 tablet [PoM] £13.37 DT = £13.37 [SF] | 6 tablet [PoM] £26.74 DT = £26.74 [SF] | 12 tablet [PoM] £53.48 DT = £53.48 [SF]

Sumatriptan
24-May-2021

- **INDICATIONS AND DOSE**
Treatment of acute migraine
  - ▸ BY MOUTH
  - ▸ Adult: Initially 50–100 mg for 1 dose, followed by 50–100 mg after at least 2 hours if required, to be taken only if migraine recurs (patient not responding to initial dose should not take second dose for same attack); maximum 300 mg per day continued →

▶ BY SUBCUTANEOUS INJECTION
▶ **Adult 18–65 years:** Initially 3–6 mg for 1 dose, followed by 3–6 mg after at least 1 hour if required, to be taken only if migraine recurs (patient not responding to initial dose should not take second dose for same attack), dose to be administered using an auto-injector; not for intravenous injection which may cause coronary vasospasm and angina; maximum 12 mg per day
▶ BY INTRANASAL ADMINISTRATION
▶ **Adult 18–65 years:** Initially 10–20 mg, to be administered into one nostril, followed by 10–20 mg after at least 2 hours if required, to be taken only if migraine recurs (patient not responding to initial dose should not take second dose for same attack); maximum 40 mg per day

Treatment of acute cluster headache
▶ BY SUBCUTANEOUS INJECTION
▶ **Adult:** Initially 6 mg for 1 dose, followed by 6 mg after at least 1 hour if required, to be taken only if headache recurs (patient not responding to initial dose should not take second dose for same attack), dose to be administered using an auto-injector; not for intravenous injection which may cause coronary vasospasm and angina; maximum 12 mg per day
▶ BY INTRANASAL ADMINISTRATION
▶ **Adult 18-65 years:** Initially 10–20 mg, dose to be administered into one nostril, followed by 10–20 mg after at least 2 hours if required, to be taken only if headache recurs (patient not responding to initial dose should not take second dose for same attack); maximum 40 mg per day

● **UNLICENSED USE** Not licensed for use in elderly.

● **CONTRA-INDICATIONS** Coronary vasospasm · ischaemic heart disease · mild uncontrolled hypertension · moderate and severe hypertension · peripheral vascular disease · previous cerebrovascular accident · previous myocardial infarction · previous transient ischaemic attack · Prinzmetal's angina

● **CAUTIONS** Conditions which predispose to coronary artery disease · elderly · history of seizures · mild, controlled hypertension · risk factors for seizures

● **INTERACTIONS** → Appendix 1: triptans

● **SIDE-EFFECTS**
GENERAL SIDE-EFFECTS
▶ **Common or very common** Asthenia · dizziness · drowsiness · dyspnoea · feeling abnormal · flushing · myalgia · nausea · pain · sensation abnormal · skin reactions · temperature sensation altered · vomiting
▶ **Rare or very rare** Hypersensitivity
▶ **Frequency not known** Angina pectoris · anxiety · arrhythmias · arthralgia · colitis ischaemic · coronary vasospasm · diarrhoea · dystonia · hyperhidrosis · hypotension · myocardial infarction · nystagmus · palpitations · Raynaud's phenomenon · seizure · tremor · vision disorders
SPECIFIC SIDE-EFFECTS
▶ **Common or very common**
▶ With intranasal use Epistaxis · nasal irritation · taste altered · throat irritation
▶ With subcutaneous use Haemorrhage · swelling
SIDE-EFFECTS, FURTHER INFORMATION Discontinue if symptoms of heat, heaviness, pressure or tightness (including throat and chest) occur.

● **ALLERGY AND CROSS-SENSITIVITY** EvGr Caution in patients with sensitivity to sulfonamides. M

● **PREGNANCY** There is limited experience of using 5HT$_1$-receptor agonists during pregnancy; manufacturers advise that they should be avoided unless the potential benefit outweighs the risk.

● **BREAST FEEDING** Present in milk but amount probably too small to be harmful; withhold breast-feeding for 12 hours after treatment.

● **HEPATIC IMPAIRMENT** Manufacturer advises caution (reduced pre-systemic clearance increases exposure); avoid in severe impairment (no information available).
Dose adjustments
▶ With oral use Manufacturer advises consider dose reduction to 25–50 mg in mild to moderate impairment.

● **RENAL IMPAIRMENT** EvGr Use with caution. M

● **PATIENT AND CARER ADVICE**
Driving and skilled tasks Drowsiness may affect performance of skilled tasks (e.g. driving).

● **EXCEPTIONS TO LEGAL CATEGORY** Sumatriptan 50 mg tablets can be sold to the public to treat previously diagnosed migraine; max. daily dose 100 mg.

● **MEDICINAL FORMS** There can be variation in the licensing of different medicines containing the same drug.

Solution for injection
CAUTIONARY AND ADVISORY LABELS 3, 10
▶ Sumatriptan (Non-proprietary)
Sumatriptan (as Sumatriptan succinate) 6 mg per 1 ml Sumatriptan 3mg/0.5ml solution for injection pre-filled pens | 2 pre-filled disposable injection PoM £39.50 DT = £39.50
Sumatriptan (as Sumatriptan succinate) 12 mg per 1 ml Sumatriptan 6mg/0.5ml solution for injection pre-filled pens | 2 pre-filled disposable injection PoM £62.11 DT = £62.11
▶ Imigran Subject (GlaxoSmithKline UK Ltd)
Sumatriptan (as Sumatriptan succinate) 12 mg per 1 ml Imigran Subject 6mg/0.5ml solution for injection syringe refill pack | 2 pre-filled disposable injection PoM £48.49 DT = £48.49
Imigran Subject 6mg/0.5ml solution for injection pre-filled syringes with device | 2 pre-filled disposable injection PoM £50.96 DT = £50.96

Oral tablet
CAUTIONARY AND ADVISORY LABELS 3, 10
▶ Sumatriptan (Non-proprietary)
Sumatriptan (as Sumatriptan succinate) 50 mg Sumatriptan 50mg tablets | 6 tablet PoM £24.85 DT = £0.88
Sumatriptan (as Sumatriptan succinate) 100 mg Sumatriptan 100mg tablets | 6 tablet PoM £41.18 DT = £1.17
▶ Imigran (GlaxoSmithKline UK Ltd)
Sumatriptan (as Sumatriptan succinate) 50 mg Imigran Radis 50mg tablets | 6 tablet PoM £23.90 DT = £0.88
Imigran 50mg tablets | 6 tablet PoM £31.85 DT = £0.88
Sumatriptan (as Sumatriptan succinate) 100 mg Imigran 100mg tablets | 6 tablet PoM £51.48 DT = £1.17
Imigran Radis 100mg tablets | 6 tablet PoM £42.90 DT = £1.17

Spray
CAUTIONARY AND ADVISORY LABELS 3, 10
▶ Imigran (GlaxoSmithKline UK Ltd)
Sumatriptan 100 mg per 1 ml Imigran 10mg nasal spray | 2 unit dose PoM £14.16 DT = £14.16
Sumatriptan 200 mg per 1 ml Imigran 20mg nasal spray | 2 unit dose PoM £14.16 | 6 unit dose PoM £42.47 DT = £42.47

Zolmitriptan

03-Sep-2020

● **INDICATIONS AND DOSE**
Treatment of acute migraine
▶ BY MOUTH
▶ **Adult:** 2.5 mg, followed by 2.5 mg after at least 2 hours if required, dose to be taken only if migraine recurs, then increased if necessary to 5 mg, dose to be taken only for subsequent attacks in patients not achieving satisfactory relief with 2.5 mg dose; maximum 10 mg per day
▶ BY INTRANASAL ADMINISTRATION
▶ **Adult:** 5 mg, dose to be administered as soon as possible after onset into one nostril only, followed by

5 mg after at least 2 hours if required, dose to be administered only if migraine recurs; maximum 10 mg per day

Treatment of acute cluster headache
▸ BY INTRANASAL ADMINISTRATION
▸ Adult: 5 mg, dose to be administered as soon as possible after onset into one nostril only, followed by 5 mg after at least 2 hours if required, dose to be administered only if migraine recurs; maximum 10 mg per day

Menstrual migraine prophylaxis
▸ BY MOUTH
▸ Adult: 2.5 mg 3 times a day, to be taken from 2 days before until 3 days after bleeding starts

DOSE ADJUSTMENTS DUE TO INTERACTIONS
▸ Manufacturer advises max. dose 5 mg in 24 hours with concurrent use of moderate and potent inhibitors of CYP1A2, cimetidine and moclobemide.

DOSE EQUIVALENCE AND CONVERSION
▸ 1 spray of *Zomig*® nasal spray = 5 mg zolmitriptan.

● UNLICENSED USE [EvGr] Zolmitriptan is used for menstrual migraine prophylaxis, ⒶA but is not licensed for this indication. Not licensed for use in elderly. Not licensed for treatment of cluster headaches.

● CONTRA-INDICATIONS Arrhythmias associated with accessory cardiac conduction pathways · coronary vasospasm · ischaemic heart disease · moderate to severe hypertension · peripheral vascular disease · previous cerebrovascular accident · previous myocardial infarction · Prinzmetal's angina · transient ischaemic attack · uncontrolled hypertension · Wolff-Parkinson-White syndrome

● CAUTIONS Conditions which predispose to coronary artery disease · elderly

● INTERACTIONS → Appendix 1: triptans

● SIDE-EFFECTS
GENERAL SIDE-EFFECTS
▸ **Common or very common** Abdominal pain · asthenia · chest discomfort · dizziness · drowsiness · dry mouth · dysphagia · feeling hot · headache · limb discomfort · muscle weakness · nausea · pain · palpitations · sensation abnormal · vomiting
▸ **Uncommon** Tachycardia · urinary disorders
▸ **Rare or very rare** Angina pectoris · angioedema · coronary vasospasm · gastrointestinal disorders · gastrointestinal infarction · hypersensitivity · myocardial infarction · splenic infarction · urticaria
SPECIFIC SIDE-EFFECTS
▸ **Common or very common**
▸ With intranasal use Feeling abnormal · haemorrhage · myalgia · nasal discomfort · taste altered · throat pain
▸ With oral use Muscle complaints · sensation of pressure · throat complaints
▸ **Rare or very rare**
▸ With oral use Diarrhoea

SIDE-EFFECTS, FURTHER INFORMATION Discontinue if symptoms of heat, heaviness, pressure or tightness (including throat and chest) occur.

● PREGNANCY There is limited experience of using 5HT₁-receptor agonists during pregnancy; manufacturers advise that they should be avoided unless the potential benefit outweighs the risk.

● BREAST FEEDING Use with caution—present in milk in *animal* studies.

● HEPATIC IMPAIRMENT Manufacturer advises caution in moderate to severe impairment (risk of increased exposure).
Dose adjustments Manufacturer advises maximum 5 mg in 24 hours in moderate to severe impairment.

● DIRECTIONS FOR ADMINISTRATION Zolmitriptan orodispersible tablets should be placed on the tongue, allowed to disperse and swallowed.

● PATIENT AND CARER ADVICE Patients or carers should be given advice on how to administer zolmitriptan orodispersible tablets.

● MEDICINAL FORMS There can be variation in the licensing of different medicines containing the same drug.
Oral tablet
▸ Zolmitriptan (Non-proprietary)
Zolmitriptan 2.5 mg Zolmitriptan 2.5mg tablets | 6 tablet [PoM] £24.00 DT = £29.50 | 12 tablet [PoM] £58.99 DT = £58.99
Zolmitriptan 5 mg Zolmitriptan 5mg tablets | 6 tablet [PoM] £36.00-£64.70 DT = £36.00 | 12 tablet [PoM] £72.00
▸ Zomig (Grunenthal Ltd)
Zolmitriptan 2.5 mg Zomig 2.5mg tablets | 6 tablet [PoM] £23.94 DT = £29.50
Spray
▸ Zolmitriptan (Non-proprietary)
Zolmitriptan 50 mg per 1 ml Zolmitriptan 5mg/0.1ml nasal spray unit dose | 6 unit dose [PoM] £36.50 DT = £36.50
▸ Zomig (Grunenthal Ltd)
Zolmitriptan 50 mg per 1 ml Zomig 5mg/0.1ml nasal spray 0.1ml unit dose | 6 unit dose [PoM] £36.50 DT = £36.50
Orodispersible tablet
EXCIPIENTS: May contain Aspartame
▸ Zolmitriptan (Non-proprietary)
Zolmitriptan 2.5 mg Zolmitriptan 2.5mg orodispersible tablets sugar free | 6 tablet [PoM] £22.79 DT = £10.53 [SF]
Zolmitriptan 5 mg Zolmitriptan 5mg orodispersible tablets sugar free | 6 tablet [PoM] £36.00 DT = £14.13 [SF]
▸ Zomig Rapimelt (Grunenthal Ltd)
Zolmitriptan 2.5 mg Zomig Rapimelt 2.5mg orodispersible tablets | 6 tablet [PoM] £23.99 DT = £10.53 [SF]
Zolmitriptan 5 mg Zomig Rapimelt 5mg orodispersible tablets | 6 tablet [PoM] £23.94 DT = £14.13 [SF]

6.2 Neuropathic pain

Neuropathic pain

06-Oct-2020

MHRA/CHM important safety information

When using antiepileptics for the management of neuropathic pain, see Epilepsy p. 349 for information on the use of antiepileptic drugs and the risk of suicidal thoughts and behaviour.

For information on the use of opioids and risk of dependence and addiction, see *Important safety information* in individual drug monographs.

Overview and management

Neuropathic pain, which occurs as a result of damage to neural tissue, includes *phantom limb pain, compression neuropathies, peripheral neuropathies* (e.g. due to Diabetic complications p. 802, chronic excessive alcohol intake, HIV infection p. 735, chemotherapy, idiopathic neuropathy), *trauma, central pain* (e.g. pain following stroke, spinal cord injury, and syringomyelia), and *postherpetic neuralgia* (peripheral nerve damage following acute herpes zoster infection (shingles)). The pain may occur in an area of sensory deficit and is sometimes accompanied by pain that is evoked by a non-noxious stimulus (allodynia).

Trigeminal neuralgia is also caused by dysfunction of neural tissue, but its management is distinct from other forms of neuropathic pain.

Neuropathic pain is generally managed with a **tricyclic antidepressant** or with certain **antiepileptic drugs**. Amitriptyline hydrochloride p. 431 and pregabalin p. 374 are effective treatments for neuropathic pain. Amitriptyline hydrochloride and pregabalin can be used in combination if the patient has an inadequate response to either drug at the maximum tolerated dose.

Nortriptyline p. 437 [unlicensed indication] may be better tolerated than amitriptyline hydrochloride.

Gabapentin p. 362 is also effective for the treatment of neuropathic pain.

Neuropathic pain may respond to **opioid analgesics**. There is evidence of efficacy for tramadol hydrochloride p. 534, morphine p. 525, and oxycodone hydrochloride p. 528; however, treatment with morphine or oxycodone hydrochloride should be initiated only under specialist supervision. Tramadol hydrochloride can be prescribed when other treatments have been unsuccessful, while the patient is waiting for assessment by a specialist.

Patients with localised pain who are unable to take oral medicines may benefit from **topical local anaesthetic preparations**, such as lidocaine hydrochloride medicated plasters p. 117, while awaiting specialist review.

Capsaicin below is licensed for neuropathic pain (but the intense burning sensation during initial treatment may limit use). Capsaicin 0.075% cream is licensed for the symptomatic relief of *postherpetic neuralgia*. A self-adhesive patch containing capsaicin 8% is licensed for the treatment of peripheral neuropathic pain. It should be used under specialist supervision.

A corticosteroid may help to relieve pressure in compression neuropathy and thereby reduce pain.

Neuromodulation by spinal cord stimulation may be of benefit in some patients. Many patients with chronic neuropathic pain require multidisciplinary management, including physiotherapy and psychological support.

Trigeminal neuralgia

Surgery may be the treatment of choice in many patients; a neurological assessment will identify those who stand to benefit. Carbamazepine p. 355 taken during the acute stages of trigeminal neuralgia, reduces the frequency and severity of attacks. It is very effective for the severe pain associated with trigeminal neuralgia and (less commonly) glossopharyngeal neuralgia. Blood counts and electrolytes should be monitored when high doses are given. Small doses should be used initially to reduce the incidence of side-effects e.g. dizziness. Some cases respond to phenytoin p. 372; the drug may be given by intravenous infusion (possibly as fosphenytoin sodium p. 361) in a crisis (specialist use only).

Chronic facial pain

Chronic oral and facial pain including *persistent idiopathic facial pain* (also termed 'atypical facial pain') and *temporomandibular dysfunction* (previously termed temporomandibular joint pain dysfunction syndrome) may call for prolonged use of analgesics or for other drugs. **Tricyclic antidepressants** may be useful for facial pain [unlicensed indication], but are not on the Dental Practitioners' List. Disorders of this type require specialist referral and psychological support to accompany drug treatment. Patients on long-term therapy need to be monitored both for progress and for side-effects.

> **Other drugs used for Neuropathic pain** Amantadine hydrochloride, p. 480

ANALGESICS > PLANT ALKALOIDS

| Capsaicin

09-Nov-2020

- **INDICATIONS AND DOSE**

Localised neuropathic pain
▸ TO THE SKIN USING CREAM
▸ Adult: Apply 3–4 times a day, using 0.075% strength; apply sparingly, not more often than every 4 hours

AXSAIN ®

Post-herpetic neuralgia
▸ TO THE SKIN
▸ Adult: Apply 3–4 times a day, apply sparingly; **important; after** lesions have healed, not more often than every 4 hours

Painful diabetic neuropathy (under expert supervision)
▸ TO THE SKIN
▸ Adult: Apply 3–4 times a day for 8 weeks then review, apply sparingly, not more often than every 4 hours

QUTENZA ®

Peripheral neuropathic pain (under the supervision of a physician)
▸ BY TRANSDERMAL APPLICATION USING PATCHES
▸ Adult: (consult product literature)

ZACIN ®

Symptomatic relief in osteoarthritis
▸ TO THE SKIN
▸ Adult: Apply 4 times a day, apply sparingly, not more often than every 4 hours

- **UNLICENSED USE** [EvGr] Capsaicin is used in the treatment of localised neuropathic pain, [E] but is not licensed for this indication.

- **CAUTIONS**

GENERAL CAUTIONS Avoid contact with broken skin · avoid contact with inflamed skin

SPECIFIC CAUTIONS
▸ With topical use Avoid contact with eyes · avoid hot shower or bath just before or after application (burning sensation enhanced) · avoid inhalation of vapours · not to be used under tight bandages
▸ With transdermal use Avoid contact with the face, scalp or in proximity to mucous membranes · avoid holding near eyes or mucous membranes · diabetes · history of cardiovascular disease · uncontrolled hypertension

CAUTIONS, FURTHER INFORMATION
▸ Diabetes
▸ With transdermal use [EvGr] Particular attention should be given to diabetic patients with coronary artery disease, hypertension, or cardiovascular autonomic neuropathy. [M]

- **SIDE-EFFECTS**

GENERAL SIDE-EFFECTS
▸ **Uncommon** Cough

SPECIFIC SIDE-EFFECTS
▸ **Common or very common**
▸ With transdermal use Sensation abnormal
▸ **Uncommon**
▸ With transdermal use Atrioventricular block · eye irritation · muscle spasms · nausea · palpitations · peripheral oedema · skin reactions · tachycardia · taste altered · throat irritation
▸ **Rare or very rare**
▸ With topical use Sneezing · watering eye
▸ **Frequency not known**
▸ With topical use Asthma exacerbated · dyspnoea · skin burning sensation (particularly if too much used or if administered more than 4 times daily) · skin irritation

- **MONITORING REQUIREMENTS**
▸ With transdermal use Monitor blood pressure during treatment procedure.

- **HANDLING AND STORAGE**
▸ With topical use Wash hands immediately after use (or wash hands 30 minutes after application if hands treated).
▸ With transdermal use Nitrile gloves to be worn while handling patches and cleaning treatment areas (latex gloves do not provide adequate protection).

● **NATIONAL FUNDING/ACCESS DECISIONS**
For full details see funding body website
Scottish Medicines Consortium (SMC) decisions
▶ Capsaicin (*Qutenza*®) for the treatment of peripheral
neuropathic pain in non-diabetic adults either alone or in
combination with other medicinal products for pain (October
2014) SMC No. 673/11 Recommended with restrictions

● **MEDICINAL FORMS** There can be variation in the licensing of
different medicines containing the same drug. Forms available
from special-order manufacturers include: cutaneous cream
Cutaneous patch
EXCIPIENTS: May contain Butylated hydroxyanisole
▶ Qutenza (Grunenthal Ltd)
Capsaicin 179 mg Qutenza 179mg cutaneous patches |
1 patch [PoM] £210.00 DT = £210.00
Cutaneous cream
EXCIPIENTS: May contain Benzyl alcohol, cetostearyl alcohol (including
cetyl and stearyl alcohol)
▶ Capsaicin (Non-proprietary)
Capsaicin 250 microgram per 1 gram Capsaicin 0.025% cream |
1 gram [PoM] [S]
Capsaicin 750 microgram per 1 gram Capsaicin 0.075% cream |
1 gram [PoM] [S]

7 Sleep disorders

7.1 Insomnia

Hypnotics and anxiolytics

04-Mar-2021

Overview

Most anxiolytics ('sedatives') will induce sleep when given at
night and most hypnotics will sedate when given during the
day. Prescribing of these drugs is widespread but
dependence (both physical and psychological) and tolerance
occur. This may lead to difficulty in withdrawing the drug
after the patient has been taking it regularly for more than a
few weeks. Hypnotics and anxiolytics should therefore be
reserved for short courses to alleviate acute conditions after
causal factors have been established.

Benzodiazepines are the most commonly used anxiolytics
and hypnotics; they act at benzodiazepine receptors which
are associated with gamma-aminobutyric acid (GABA)
receptors. Older drugs such as meprobamate and
barbiturates are **not** recommended—they have more side-
effects and interactions than benzodiazepines and are much
more dangerous in overdosage.

Benzodiazepine indications

● Benzodiazepines are indicated for the short-term relief
(two to four weeks only) of anxiety that is severe,
disabling, or causing the patient unacceptable distress,
occurring alone or in association with insomnia or short-
term psychosomatic, organic, or psychotic illness.
● The use of benzodiazepines to treat short-term 'mild'
anxiety is inappropriate.
● Benzodiazepines should be used to treat insomnia only
when it is severe, disabling, or causing the patient extreme
distress.

Dependence and withdrawal

Withdrawal of a benzodiazepine should be gradual because
abrupt withdrawal may produce confusion, toxic psychosis,
convulsions, or a condition resembling delirium tremens.

The benzodiazepine withdrawal syndrome may develop at
any time up to 3 weeks after stopping a long-acting
benzodiazepine, but may occur within a day in the case of a
short-acting one. It is characterised by insomnia, anxiety,
loss of appetite and of body-weight, tremor, perspiration,
tinnitus, and perceptual disturbances. Some symptoms may

be similar to the original complaint and encourage further
prescribing; some symptoms may continue for weeks or
months after stopping benzodiazepines.

Benzodiazepine withdrawal should be flexible and carried
out at a reduction rate that is tolerable for the patient. The
rate should depend on the initial dose of benzodiazepine,
duration of use, and the patient's clinical response. Short-
term users of benzodiazepines (2–4 weeks only) can usually
taper off within 2–4 weeks. However, long-term users should
be withdrawn over a much longer period of several months
or more.

A suggested protocol for withdrawal for prescribed long-
term benzodiazepine patients is as follows:

● Transfer patient stepwise, one dose at a time over about a
week, to an equivalent daily dose of diazepam preferably
taken at night.
● Reduce diazepam dose, usually by 1–2 mg every 2–
4 weeks (in patients taking high doses of benzodiazepines,
initially it may be appropriate to reduce the dose by up to
one-tenth every 1–2 weeks). If uncomfortable withdrawal
symptoms occur, maintain this dose until symptoms
lessen.
● Reduce diazepam dose further, if necessary in smaller
steps; steps of 500 micrograms may be appropriate towards
the end of withdrawal. Then stop completely.
● For long-term patients, the period needed for complete
withdrawal may vary from several months to a year or
more.

Approximate equivalent doses, diazepam 5 mg
   ≡ alprazolam 250 micrograms
   ≡ clobazam 10 mg
   ≡ clonazepam 250 micrograms
   ≡ flurazepam 7.5–15 mg
   ≡ chlordiazepoxide 12.5 mg
   ≡ loprazolam 0.5–1 mg
   ≡ lorazepam 500 micrograms
   ≡ lormetazepam 0.5–1 mg
   ≡ nitrazepam 5 mg
   ≡ oxazepam 10 mg
   ≡ temazepam 10 mg

Withdrawal symptoms for long-term users usually resolve
within 6–18 months of the last dose. Some patients will
recover more quickly, others may take longer. The addition
of beta-blockers, antidepressants and antipsychotics should
be **avoided** where possible.

Counselling can be of considerable help both during and
after the taper.

Hypnotics

Before a hypnotic is prescribed the cause of the insomnia
should be established and, where possible, underlying
factors should be treated. However, it should be noted that
some patients have unrealistic sleep expectations, and
others understate their alcohol consumption which is often
the cause of the insomnia. Short-acting hypnotics are
preferable in patients with sleep onset insomnia, when
sedation the following day is undesirable, or when
prescribing for elderly patients. Long-acting hypnotics are
indicated in patients with poor sleep maintenance (e.g. early
morning waking) that causes daytime effects, when an
anxiolytic effect is needed during the day, or when sedation
the following day is acceptable.

Transient insomnia may occur in those who normally sleep
well and may be due to extraneous factors such as noise,
shift work, and jet lag. If a hypnotic is indicated one that is
rapidly eliminated should be chosen, and only one or two
doses should be given.

Short-term insomnia is usually related to an emotional
problem or serious medical illness. It may last for a few
weeks and may recur; a hypnotic can be useful but should
not be given for more than three weeks (preferably only one

week). Intermittent use is desirable with omission of some doses. A short-acting drug is usually appropriate.

Chronic insomnia is rarely benefited by hypnotics and is sometimes due to mild dependence caused by injudicious prescribing of hypnotics. Psychiatric disorders such as anxiety, depression, and abuse of drugs and alcohol are common causes. Sleep disturbance is very common in depressive illness and early wakening is often a useful pointer. The underlying psychiatric complaint should be treated, adapting the drug regimen to alleviate insomnia. For example, clomipramine hydrochloride p. 432 or mirtazapine p. 431 prescribed for depression will also help to promote sleep if taken at night. Other causes of insomnia include daytime cat-napping and physical causes such as pain, pruritus, and dyspnoea.

Hypnotics should **not** be prescribed indiscriminately and routine prescribing is undesirable. They should be reserved for short courses in the acutely distressed. Tolerance to their effects develops within 3 to 14 days of continuous use and long-term efficacy cannot be assured. A major drawback of long-term use is that withdrawal can cause rebound insomnia and a withdrawal syndrome.

Where prolonged administration is unavoidable hypnotics should be discontinued as soon as feasible and the patient warned that sleep may be disturbed for a few days before normal rhythm is re-established; broken sleep with vivid dreams may persist for several weeks.

Elderly
Benzodiazepines and the Z–drugs should be avoided in the elderly, because the elderly are at greater risk of becoming ataxic and confused, leading to falls and injury.

Dental patients
Some anxious patients may benefit from the use of hypnotics during dental procedures such as temazepam p. 552 or diazepam p. 398. Temazepam is preferred when it is important to minimise any residual effect the following day.

Benzodiazepines
Benzodiazepines used as hypnotics include nitrazepam p. 552 and flurazepam p. 551 which have a prolonged action and may give rise to residual effects on the following day; repeated doses tend to be cumulative.

Loprazolam p. 551, lormetazepam p. 551, and temazepam act for a shorter time and they have little or no hangover effect. Withdrawal phenomena are more common with the short-acting benzodiazepines.

If insomnia is associated with daytime anxiety then the use of a long-acting benzodiazepine anxiolytic such as diazepam given as a single dose at night may effectively treat both symptoms.

Zolpidem, and zopiclone
Zolpidem tartrate p. 556 and zopiclone p. 557 are non-benzodiazepine hypnotics (sometimes referred to as Z-drugs), but they act at the benzodiazepine receptor. They are not licensed for long-term use; dependence has been reported in a small number of patients. Both zolpidem tartrate and zopiclone have a short duration of action.

Chloral and derivatives
There is no convincing evidence that they are particularly useful in the elderly and their role as hypnotics is now very limited.

Clomethiazole
Clomethiazole p. 553 may be a useful hypnotic for elderly patients because of its freedom from hangover but, as with all hypnotics, routine administration is undesirable and dependence occurs.

Antihistamines
Some **antihistamines** such as promethazine hydrochloride p. 326 are on sale to the public for occasional insomnia; their prolonged duration of action can often cause drowsiness the following day. The sedative effect of antihistamines may diminish after a few days of continued treatment; antihistamines are associated with headache, psychomotor impairment and antimuscarinic effects.

Alcohol
Alcohol is a poor hypnotic because the diuretic action interferes with sleep during the latter part of the night. Alcohol also disturbs sleep patterns, and so can worsen sleep disorders.

Melatonin
Melatonin p. 555 is a pineal hormone; it is licensed for the short-term treatment of insomnia in adults over 55 years; and for the short-term treatment of jet-lag in adults.

Anxiolytics

Benzodiazepine anxiolytics can be effective in alleviating anxiety states. Although these drugs are sometimes prescribed for stress-related symptoms, unhappiness, or minor physical disease, their use in such conditions is inappropriate. Benzodiazepine anxiolytics should not be used as sole treatment for chronic anxiety, and they are not appropriate for treating depression or chronic psychosis. In bereavement, psychological adjustment may be inhibited by benzodiazepines.

Anxiolytic benzodiazepine treatment should be limited to the lowest possible dose for the shortest possible time. Dependence is particularly likely in patients with a history of alcohol or drug abuse and in patients with marked personality disorders.

Some antidepressant drugs are licensed for use in anxiety and related disorders. Some antipsychotic drugs, in low doses, are also sometimes used in severe anxiety for their sedative action, but long-term use should be avoided because of the risk of adverse effects. The use of antihistamines (e.g. hydroxyzine hydrochloride p. 324) for their sedative effect in anxiety is not appropriate.

Beta-adrenoceptor blocking drugs do not affect psychological symptoms of anxiety, such as worry, tension, and fear, but they do reduce autonomic symptoms, such as palpitation and tremor; they do not reduce non-autonomic symptoms, such as muscle tension. Beta-blockers are therefore indicated for patients with predominantly somatic symptoms; this, in turn, may prevent the onset of worry and fear.

Benzodiazepines
Benzodiazepines (diazepam, alprazolam p. 397, chlordiazepoxide hydrochloride p. 398, clobazam p. 390, lorazepam p. 393, and oxazepam p. 400) are indicated for the *short-term relief of severe anxiety*; long-term use should be avoided. Shorter-acting compounds may be preferred in patients with hepatic impairment but they carry a greater risk of withdrawal symptoms.

In *panic disorders* (with or without agoraphobia) resistant to antidepressant therapy, a benzodiazepine may be used; alternatively, a benzodiazepine may be used as short-term adjunctive therapy at the start of antidepressant treatment to prevent the initial worsening of symptoms.

Diazepam or lorazepam are very occasionally administered intravenously for the *control of panic attacks*. This route is the most rapid but the procedure is not without risk and should be used only when alternative measures have failed. The intramuscular route has no advantage over the oral route.

Buspirone
Buspirone hydrochloride p. 396 is thought to act at specific serotonin ($5HT_{1A}$) receptors. Response to treatment may take up to 2 weeks. It does not alleviate the symptoms of benzodiazepine withdrawal. Therefore a patient taking a benzodiazepine still needs to have the benzodiazepine withdrawn gradually; it is advisable to do this before starting buspirone hydrochloride. The dependence and abuse potential of buspirone hydrochloride is low; it is, however,

licensed for short-term use only (but specialists occasionally use it for several months).

Meprobamate

Meprobamate is **less effective** than the benzodiazepines, more hazardous in overdosage, and can also induce dependence. It is **not** recommended.

Barbiturates

The intermediate-acting **barbiturates** have a place only in the treatment of severe intractable insomnia in patients **already taking** barbiturates; they should be **avoided** in the elderly. Intermediate-acting barbiturate preparations containing amobarbital sodium, butobarbital, and secobarbital sodium are available on a named patient basis.

The long-acting barbiturate phenobarbital is still sometimes of value in epilepsy but its use as a sedative is unjustified.

The very short-acting barbiturate thiopental sodium p. 392 is used in anaesthesia.

Increased hostility and aggression after barbiturates and alcohol usually indicates intoxication.

HYPNOTICS, SEDATIVES AND ANXIOLYTICS › BENZODIAZEPINES

Flurazepam

F 397   14-Oct-2021

● **INDICATIONS AND DOSE**

Insomnia (short-term use)

▶ BY MOUTH

▸ Adult: 15–30 mg once daily, dose to be taken at bedtime, for debilitated patients, use elderly dose
▸ Elderly: 15 mg once daily, dose to be taken at bedtime

● **CONTRA-INDICATIONS** Respiratory depression

● **CAUTIONS** Acute porphyrias p. 1202 · hypoalbuminaemia · muscle weakness

CAUTIONS, FURTHER INFORMATION

▸ Paradoxical effects A paradoxical increase in hostility and aggression may be reported by patients taking benzodiazepines. The effects range from talkativeness and excitement to aggressive and antisocial acts. Adjustment of the dose (up or down) sometimes attenuates the impulses. Increased anxiety and perceptual disorders are other paradoxical effects.

● **INTERACTIONS** → Appendix 1: benzodiazepines

● **SIDE-EFFECTS**

▸ **Common or very common** Taste altered
▸ **Rare or very rare** Abdominal discomfort · skin eruption · vertigo
▸ **Frequency not known** Agranulocytosis · extrapyramidal symptoms · leucopenia · pancytopenia · psychotic disorder · suicidal behaviours · thrombocytopenia

● **BREAST FEEDING** Benzodiazepines are present in milk, and should be avoided if possible during breast-feeding.

● **HEPATIC IMPAIRMENT**

Dose adjustments Manufacturer advises dose of 15 mg in mild to moderate impairment.

● **NATIONAL FUNDING/ACCESS DECISIONS**

NHS restrictions Flurazepam capsules are not prescribable in NHS primary care.

● **MEDICINAL FORMS** There can be variation in the licensing of different medicines containing the same drug.

Oral capsule

CAUTIONARY AND ADVISORY LABELS 19

▸ Dalmane (Viatris UK Healthcare Ltd)
Flurazepam (as Flurazepam hydrochloride) **15 mg** Dalmane 15mg capsules | 30 capsule [PoM] £6.73 [CD4–1]
Flurazepam (as Flurazepam hydrochloride) **30 mg** Dalmane 30mg capsules | 30 capsule [PoM] £8.63 [CD4–1]

Loprazolam

F 397   14-Oct-2021

● **INDICATIONS AND DOSE**

Insomnia (short-term use)

▶ BY MOUTH

▸ Adult: 1 mg once daily, then increased to 1.5–2 mg once daily if required, dose to be taken at bedtime, for debilitated patients, use elderly dose
▸ Elderly: 0.5–1 mg once daily, dose to be taken at bedtime

● **CONTRA-INDICATIONS** Respiratory depression

● **CAUTIONS** Acute porphyrias p. 1202 · hypoalbuminaemia · muscle weakness

CAUTIONS, FURTHER INFORMATION

▸ Paradoxical effects A paradoxical increase in hostility and aggression may be reported by patients taking benzodiazepines. The effects range from talkativeness and excitement to aggressive and antisocial acts. Adjustment of the dose (up or down) sometimes attenuates the impulses. Increased anxiety and perceptual disorders are other paradoxical effects.

● **INTERACTIONS** → Appendix 1: benzodiazepines

● **SIDE-EFFECTS** Adjustment disorder · cognitive disorder · gastrointestinal disorder · muscle tone decreased · speech disorder · suicidal ideation

● **BREAST FEEDING** Benzodiazepines are present in milk, and should be avoided if possible during breast-feeding.

● **MEDICINAL FORMS** There can be variation in the licensing of different medicines containing the same drug.

Oral tablet

CAUTIONARY AND ADVISORY LABELS 19

▸ Loprazolam (Non-proprietary)
Loprazolam (as Loprazolam mesilate) 1 mg Loprazolam 1mg tablets | 28 tablet [PoM] £36.00 DT = £27.95 [CD4–1]

Lormetazepam

F 397   14-Oct-2021

● **INDICATIONS AND DOSE**

Insomnia (short-term use)

▶ BY MOUTH

▸ Adult: 0.5–1.5 mg once daily, dose to be taken at bedtime, for debilitated patients, use elderly dose
▸ Elderly: 500 micrograms once daily, dose to be taken at bedtime

● **CONTRA-INDICATIONS** Not for use alone to treat insomnia associated with depression · respiratory depression

● **CAUTIONS** Acute porphyrias p. 1202 · hypoalbuminaemia · muscle weakness

CAUTIONS, FURTHER INFORMATION

▸ Paradoxical effects A paradoxical increase in hostility and aggression may be reported by patients taking benzodiazepines. The effects range from talkativeness and excitement to aggressive and antisocial acts. Adjustment of the dose (up or down) sometimes attenuates the impulses. Increased anxiety and perceptual disorders are other paradoxical effects.

● **INTERACTIONS** → Appendix 1: benzodiazepines

● **SIDE-EFFECTS**

▸ **Common or very common** Asthenia
▸ **Rare or very rare** Agranulocytosis · allergic dermatitis · apnoea · appetite change · coma · constipation · disinhibition · extrapyramidal symptoms · hyponatraemia · hypothermia · leucopenia · memory loss · obstructive pulmonary disease exacerbated · pancytopenia · saliva altered · sexual dysfunction · SIADH · speech slurred · thrombocytopenia

► **Frequency not known** Psychosis · suicidal behaviours
● BREAST FEEDING Benzodiazepines are present in milk, and should be avoided if possible during breast-feeding.

● MEDICINAL FORMS There can be variation in the licensing of different medicines containing the same drug. Forms available from special-order manufacturers include: oral suspension
Oral tablet
CAUTIONARY AND ADVISORY LABELS 19
► Lormetazepam (Non-proprietary)
Lormetazepam 500 microgram Lormetazepam 500microgram tablets | 30 tablet [PoM] £18.94 DT = £8.58 [CD4-1]
Lormetazepam 1 mg Lormetazepam 1mg tablets | 30 tablet [PoM] £9.17 DT = £8.10 [CD4-1]

⚑ 397

Nitrazepam
14-Oct-2021

● **INDICATIONS AND DOSE**
Insomnia (short-term use)
► BY MOUTH
► Adult: 5–10 mg daily, dose to be taken at bedtime, for debilitated patients, use elderly dose
► Elderly: 2.5–5 mg daily, dose to be taken at bedtime

● CONTRA-INDICATIONS Chronic psychosis · respiratory depression
● CAUTIONS Acute porphyrias p. 1202 · hypoalbuminaemia · muscle weakness
CAUTIONS, FURTHER INFORMATION
► Paradoxical effects A paradoxical increase in hostility and aggression may be reported by patients taking benzodiazepines. The effects range from talkativeness and excitement to aggressive and antisocial acts. Adjustment of the dose (up or down) sometimes attenuates the impulses. Increased anxiety and perceptual disorders are other paradoxical effects.

● INTERACTIONS → Appendix 1: benzodiazepines
● **SIDE-EFFECTS**
► **Common or very common** Movement disorders
► **Uncommon** Concentration impaired
► **Rare or very rare** Abdominal distress · muscle cramps · psychiatric disorder · skin reactions · Stevens-Johnson syndrome · vertigo
► **Frequency not known** Drug abuse

● BREAST FEEDING Benzodiazepines are present in milk, and should be avoided if possible during breast-feeding.

● MEDICINAL FORMS There can be variation in the licensing of different medicines containing the same drug. Forms available from special-order manufacturers include: oral suspension
Oral tablet
CAUTIONARY AND ADVISORY LABELS 19
► Nitrazepam (Non-proprietary)
Nitrazepam 5 mg Nitrazepam 5mg tablets | 28 tablet [PoM] £5.00 DT = £1.71 [CD4-1]
► Mogadon (Viatris UK Healthcare Ltd)
Nitrazepam 5 mg Mogadon 5mg tablets | 30 tablet [PoM] £5.76 [CD4-1]
Oral suspension
CAUTIONARY AND ADVISORY LABELS 19
► Nitrazepam (Non-proprietary)
Nitrazepam 500 microgram per 1 ml Nitrazepam 2.5mg/5ml oral suspension | 70 ml [PoM] £159.60 DT = £159.60 [CD4-1]

⚑ 397

Temazepam
14-Oct-2021

● **INDICATIONS AND DOSE**
Insomnia (short-term use)
► BY MOUTH
► Adult: 10–20 mg once daily, alternatively 30–40 mg once daily, higher dose range only to be administered

in exceptional circumstances, dose to be taken at bedtime, for debilitated patients, use elderly dose
► Elderly: 10 mg once daily, alternatively 20 mg once daily, higher dose only to be administered in exceptional circumstances, dose to be taken at bedtime
Conscious sedation for dental procedures
► BY MOUTH
► Adult: 15–30 mg, to be administered 30–60 minutes before procedure
Premedication before surgery or investigatory procedures
► BY MOUTH
► Adult: 10–20 mg, to be taken 1–2 hours before procedure, alternatively 30 mg, to be taken 1–2 hours before procedure, higher alternate dose only administered in exceptional circumstances
► Elderly: 10 mg, to be taken 1–2 hours before procedure, alternatively 20 mg, to be taken 1–2 hours before procedure, higher alternate dose only administered in exceptional circumstances

● UNLICENSED USE Temazepam doses in BNF may differ from those in product literature.
Not licensed for conscious sedation for dental procedures.
● CONTRA-INDICATIONS Chronic psychosis · CNS depression · compromised airway · respiratory depression
● CAUTIONS Hypoalbuminaemia · muscle weakness · organic brain changes
CAUTIONS, FURTHER INFORMATION
► Paradoxical effects A paradoxical increase in hostility and aggression may be reported by patients taking benzodiazepines. The effects range from talkativeness and excitement to aggressive and antisocial acts. Adjustment of the dose (up or down) sometimes attenuates the impulses. Increased anxiety and perceptual disorders are other paradoxical effects.

● INTERACTIONS → Appendix 1: benzodiazepines
● SIDE-EFFECTS Drug abuse · dry mouth · gastrointestinal disorder · hypersalivation · psychosis · speech slurred · urinary incontinence
● BREAST FEEDING Benzodiazepines are present in milk, and should be avoided if possible during breast-feeding.
● HEPATIC IMPAIRMENT
Dose adjustments
► When used for Insomnia Manufacturer advises initiate at 5 mg once daily, increase to 10 mg or 20 mg once daily in extreme cases. Dose to be taken at bedtime.
● RENAL IMPAIRMENT
Dose adjustments
► When used for Insomnia Manufacturer advises initiate at 5 mg once daily, increase to 10 mg or 20 mg once daily in extreme cases. Dose to be taken at bedtime.
● PATIENT AND CARER ADVICE
Driving and skilled tasks Patients given sedatives and analgesics during minor outpatient procedures should be very carefully warned about the risks of undertaking skilled tasks (e.g. driving) afterwards. Responsible persons should be available to take patients home afterwards. The dangers of taking **alcohol** should be emphasised.
● PROFESSION SPECIFIC INFORMATION
Dental practitioners' formulary Temazepam tablets and oral solution may be prescribed.

- **MEDICINAL FORMS** There can be variation in the licensing of different medicines containing the same drug. Forms available from special-order manufacturers include: oral suspension, oral solution

Oral tablet
CAUTIONARY AND ADVISORY LABELS 19
▸ **Temazepam (Non-proprietary)**
Temazepam 10 mg Temazepam 10mg tablets | 28 tablet [PoM] £44.50 DT = £26.34 [CD3]
Temazepam 20 mg Temazepam 20mg tablets | 28 tablet [PoM] £31.25 DT = £26.53 [CD3]

Oral solution
CAUTIONARY AND ADVISORY LABELS 19
▸ **Temazepam (Non-proprietary)**
Temazepam 2 mg per 1 ml Temazepam 10mg/5ml oral solution sugar free | 300 ml [PoM] £167.55 DT = £167.55 [CD3] [SF]

HYPNOTICS, SEDATIVES AND ANXIOLYTICS ›
NON-BENZODIAZEPINE HYPNOTICS AND SEDATIVES

Chloral hydrate
27-Apr-2023

- **INDICATIONS AND DOSE**

Severe insomnia [short-term use when insomnia is interfering with daily life and other therapies have failed]
▸ BY MOUTH USING ORAL SOLUTION
▸ Adult: 430–860 mg once daily (max. per dose 2 g) for a maximum of 2 weeks, dose to be taken with water or milk at bedtime, repeat courses are not recommended and can only be administered after reassessment by a specialist

Severe insomnia, using cloral betaine 707 mg ($\equiv$ 414 mg chloral hydrate) tablets [short-term use when insomnia is interfering with daily life and other therapies have failed]
▸ BY MOUTH USING TABLETS
▸ Adult: 1–2 tablets once daily for a maximum of 2 weeks, dose to be taken with water or milk at bedtime, repeat courses are not recommended and can only be administered after reassessment by a specialist, alternatively 414–828 mg once daily for a maximum of 2 weeks, dose to be taken with water or milk at bedtime, repeat courses are not recommended and can only be administered after reassessment by a specialist; maximum 4 tablets per day; maximum 2 g per day

- **CONTRA-INDICATIONS** Acute porphyrias p. 1202 · gastritis · severe cardiac disease
- **CAUTIONS** Avoid contact with mucous membranes · avoid contact with skin · avoid prolonged use (and abrupt withdrawal thereafter) · reduce dose in frail elderly
- **INTERACTIONS** → Appendix 1: chloral hydrate
- **SIDE-EFFECTS** Agitation · allergic dermatitis · ataxia · confusion · delirium (more common on abrupt discontinuation) · drug use disorders · gastrointestinal discomfort · gastrointestinal disorders · headache · injury · ketonuria · kidney injury
- **PREGNANCY** Avoid.
- **BREAST FEEDING** Risk of sedation in infant—avoid.
- **HEPATIC IMPAIRMENT** Manufacturer advises avoid in marked impairment.
Dose adjustments Manufacturer advises consider dose reduction in the elderly with hepatic impairment.
- **RENAL IMPAIRMENT** [EvGr] Caution in mild to moderate impairment; avoid in severe impairment. [M]
Dose adjustments [EvGr] Dose adjustment may be necessary in mild to moderate impairment. [M]

- **DIRECTIONS FOR ADMINISTRATION** For administration *by mouth*, expert sources advise dilute liquid with plenty of water or juice to mask unpleasant taste.
- **PRESCRIBING AND DISPENSING INFORMATION** Flavours of oral liquid formulations may include black currant.
- **PATIENT AND CARER ADVICE**
Driving and skilled tasks Drowsiness may persist the next day and affect performance of skilled tasks (e.g. driving); effects of alcohol enhanced.
- **LESS SUITABLE FOR PRESCRIBING** Chloral hydrate is less suitable for prescribing in insomnia.
- **MEDICINAL FORMS** There can be variation in the licensing of different medicines containing the same drug. Forms available from special-order manufacturers include: oral solution

Oral solution
CAUTIONARY AND ADVISORY LABELS 1(paediatric solution only), 19 (solution other than paediatric only), 27
EXCIPIENTS: May contain Glucose, propylene glycol
▸ **Chloral hydrate (Non-proprietary)**
Chloral hydrate 28.66 mg per 1 ml Chloral hydrate 143.3mg/5ml oral solution BP | 150 ml [PoM] £244.25 DT = £244.25
Chloral hydrate 100 mg per 1 ml Chloral hydrate 500mg/5ml oral solution | 150 ml [PoM] £244.25 DT = £244.25

Clomethiazole
15-Nov-2021
(Chlormethiazole)

- **INDICATIONS AND DOSE**

Severe insomnia (short-term use)
▸ BY MOUTH USING CAPSULES
▸ Elderly: 192–384 mg once daily, dose to be taken at bedtime
▸ BY MOUTH USING ORAL SOLUTION
▸ Elderly: 5–10 mL once daily, dose to be taken at bedtime

Restlessness and agitation
▸ BY MOUTH USING CAPSULES
▸ Elderly: 192 mg 3 times a day
▸ BY MOUTH USING ORAL SOLUTION
▸ Elderly: 5 mL 3 times a day

Alcohol withdrawal
▸ BY MOUTH USING CAPSULES
▸ Adult: Initially 2–4 capsules, to be repeated if necessary after some hours. 9–12 capsules daily in 3–4 divided doses on day 1 (first 24 hours), then 6–8 capsules daily in 3–4 divided doses on day 2, then 4–6 capsules daily in 3–4 divided doses on day 3, dose then to be gradually reduced over days 4–6, total duration of treatment for no more than 9 days
▸ BY MOUTH USING ORAL SOLUTION
▸ Adult: Initially 10–20 mL, to be repeated if necessary after some hours, then 45–60 mL daily in 3–4 divided doses on day 1 (first 24 hours), then 30–40 mL daily in 3–4 divided doses on day 2, then 20–30 mL daily in 3–4 divided doses on day 3, dose then to be gradually reduced over days 4–6, total duration of treatment for no more than 9 days

- **CONTRA-INDICATIONS** Acute pulmonary insufficiency · alcohol-dependent patients who continue to drink
- **CAUTIONS** Avoid prolonged use (and abrupt withdrawal thereafter) · cardiac disease (confusional state may indicate hypoxia) · chronic pulmonary insufficiency · elderly · excessive sedation may occur (particularly with higher doses) · history of drug abuse · marked personality disorder · respiratory disease (confusional state may indicate hypoxia) · sleep apnoea syndrome
- **INTERACTIONS** → Appendix 1: clomethiazole

- **SIDE-EFFECTS** Agitation · bronchial secretion increased · confusion · conjunctival irritation · drug dependence · excessive sedation · gastrointestinal disorder · hangover · nasal complaints · skin reactions · upper airway secretion increased
- **PREGNANCY** Avoid if possible—especially during the first and third trimesters.
- **BREAST FEEDING** Use only if benefit outweighs risk—present in breast milk but effects unknown.
- **HEPATIC IMPAIRMENT** Manufacturer advises caution in moderate to severe impairment (risk of increased exposure).
  Dose adjustments Manufacturer advises consider dose reduction in moderate hepatic disorders associated with alcoholism.
- **RENAL IMPAIRMENT** [EvGr] Use with caution. (M) Increased cerebral sensitivity.
- **PATIENT AND CARER ADVICE**
  Driving and skilled tasks Drowsiness may persist the next day and affect performance of skilled tasks (e.g. driving); effects of alcohol enhanced.

- **MEDICINAL FORMS** There can be variation in the licensing of different medicines containing the same drug.
  Oral solution
  CAUTIONARY AND ADVISORY LABELS 19
  EXCIPIENTS: May contain Alcohol
  ▸ **Clomethiazole (Non-proprietary)**
  Clomethiazole (as Clomethiazole edisilate) 31.5 mg per 1 ml Clomethiazole 31.5mg/ml oral solution sugar free | 300 ml [PoM] £31.50 DT = £31.50 [SF]
  Oral capsule
  CAUTIONARY AND ADVISORY LABELS 19
  ▸ **Clomethiazole (Non-proprietary)**
  Clomethiazole 192 mg Clomethiazole 192mg capsules | 60 capsule [PoM] £34.44 DT = £34.44

▌ Daridorexant

03-May-2024

- **DRUG ACTION** Daridorexant is an orexin OX_1- and OX_2-receptor antagonist that blocks the action of orexin neuropeptides, thereby decreasing wakefulness.

- **INDICATIONS AND DOSE**

  Insomnia [short-term use when symptoms present for at least 3 months]
  ▸ BY MOUTH
  ▸ Adult: 50 mg once daily, dose to be taken within 30 minutes before bedtime, alternatively 25 mg once daily, dose to be taken within 30 minutes before bedtime, lower dose may be more appropriate for some patients

  DOSE ADJUSTMENTS DUE TO INTERACTIONS
  ▸ [EvGr] Give a dose of 25 mg once daily with concurrent use of moderate CYP3A4 inhibitors, ciclosporin, or ciprofloxacin. (M)

- **CONTRA-INDICATIONS** Narcolepsy
- **CAUTIONS** Depression (worsening of symptoms including suicidal ideation) · elderly (limited information available in patients older than 75 years) · psychiatric illness (suicidal ideation reported in those with pre-existing disorders)
- **INTERACTIONS** → Appendix 1: daridorexant
- **SIDE-EFFECTS**
  ▸ **Common or very common** Dizziness · fatigue · headache · nausea
  ▸ **Uncommon** Hallucinations · sleep paralysis
- **PREGNANCY** [EvGr] Avoid unless essential (limited information available). (M)
- **BREAST FEEDING** Specialist sources indicate use with caution and monitor breast-fed infant for sedation, poor

feeding, and poor weight gain (amount in milk likely to be small as daridorexant is about 99.7% bound to plasma proteins). Consider an alternative drug, particularly if breast-feeding a neonate (pre- or full-term). No information on human lactation is available.

- **HEPATIC IMPAIRMENT** [EvGr] Avoid in severe impairment (no information available). (M)
  Dose adjustments [EvGr] Lower dose of 25 mg once daily is recommended in moderate impairment (risk of increased exposure). (M)
- **DIRECTIONS FOR ADMINISTRATION** Tablets may be taken with or without food; however, administration soon after a large meal may reduce the effect on sleep onset.
- **PRESCRIBING AND DISPENSING INFORMATION** [EvGr] Treatment duration should be as short as possible; the need for continued treatment should be assessed within 3 months of starting daridorexant and periodically thereafter. (M)
- **PATIENT AND CARER ADVICE** Patients or their carers should be counselled on the administration of daridorexant.
  Driving and skilled tasks Drowsiness may persist the next day, especially in the first few days of treatment—leave about 9 hours between taking daridorexant and performing skilled tasks (e.g. driving or operating machinery); effects of alcohol and other CNS depressants enhanced.
- **NATIONAL FUNDING/ACCESS DECISIONS**
  For full details see funding body website
  NICE decisions
  ▸ **Daridorexant for treating long-term insomnia (October 2023)** NICE TA922 Recommended with restrictions
  Scottish Medicines Consortium (SMC) decisions
  ▸ **Daridorexant (*Quviviq*®) for the treatment of adult patients with insomnia characterised by symptoms present for at least 3 months and considerable impact on daytime functioning (April 2024)** SMC No. SMC2611 Recommended with restrictions

- **MEDICINAL FORMS** There can be variation in the licensing of different medicines containing the same drug.
  Oral tablet
  CAUTIONARY AND ADVISORY LABELS 19
  ▸ **Quviviq** (Idorsia Pharmaceuticals UK Ltd) ▼
  Daridorexant (as Daridorexant hydrochloride) 25 mg Quviviq 25mg tablets | 30 tablet [PoM] £42.00 DT = £42.00
  Daridorexant (as Daridorexant hydrochloride) 50 mg Quviviq 50mg tablets | 30 tablet [PoM] £42.00 DT = £42.00

▌ Eszopiclone

04-Mar-2025

- **DRUG ACTION** Eszopiclone is an isomer of zopiclone.

- **INDICATIONS AND DOSE**

  Insomnia [short-term use]
  ▸ BY MOUTH
  ▸ Adult: 1 mg once daily for up to 4 weeks, dose to be taken at bedtime, dose may be increased if necessary to 2 or 3 mg once daily (usual max. total treatment duration 4 weeks), in certain cases (e.g. chronic insomnia) it may be necessary to extend treatment for up to a max. of 6 months
  ▸ Elderly: 1 mg once daily for up to 4 weeks, dose to be taken at bedtime, dose may be increased if necessary to 2 mg once daily (usual max. total treatment duration 4 weeks)

  DOSE ADJUSTMENTS DUE TO INTERACTIONS
  ▸ [EvGr] In adults 18–64 years, max. dose 2 mg once daily with concurrent use of potent CYP3A4 inhibitors. (M)

- **CONTRA-INDICATIONS** Myasthenia gravis · previous complex sleep-related behaviours associated with hypnotics · respiratory failure · severe sleep apnoea syndrome

- **CAUTIONS** Chronic pulmonary insufficiency (increased risk of respiratory depression) · depression · elderly · history of alcohol abuse · history of drug abuse · prolonged use (monitor regularly for signs of dependence) · psychiatric illness

CAUTIONS, FURTHER INFORMATION

▸ Elderly For hypnotic Z-drugs, Screening Tool of Older Persons' potentially inappropriate Prescriptions (STOPP) criteria to aid medication reviews (see Prescribing in the elderly p. 31 for information): potentially innapropriate in elderly (may cause protracted daytime sedation and/or ataxia).

- **INTERACTIONS** → Appendix 1: eszopiclone

- **SIDE-EFFECTS**

▸ **Common or very common** Anxiety · asthenia · depression · diarrhoea · dizziness · dry mouth · gastrointestinal discomfort · headaches · increased risk of infection · memory impairment · muscle complaints · nausea · pain · skin reactions · sleep disorders · taste altered · thinking abnormal · vision blurred · vomiting

▸ **Uncommon** Albuminuria · anaemia · appetite abnormal · breast pain · colitis · confusion · dry eye · dyspnoea · ear pain · eosinophilia · fever · gait abnormal · hallucination · hiccups · hyperhidrosis · hypertension · hyperthyroidism · hypokalaemia · joint disorder · leucopenia · menstrual cycle irregularities · mood altered · movement disorders · muscle weakness · nephrolithiasis · oral disorders · paraesthesia · peripheral oedema · photosensitivity reaction · renal pain · sexual dysfunction · stupor · syncope · thirst · tinnitus · tremor · urinary disorders · vertigo · weight changes

▸ **Rare or very rare** Pruritus (common in elderly)

▸ **Frequency not known** Altered smell sensation · drug dependence · withdrawal syndrome

- **PREGNANCY** [EvGr] Avoid (eszopiclone has shown toxicity in *animal* studies; *zopiclone* increases risk of neonatal withdrawal symptoms, and use during late pregnancy or labour may cause neonatal hypothermia, hypotonia, and respiratory depression). ⟨M⟩

- **BREAST FEEDING** [EvGr] Avoid (no information available for eszopiclone; *zopiclone* is present in milk). ⟨M⟩

- **HEPATIC IMPAIRMENT** [EvGr] Avoid in severe impairment (may precipitate encephalopathy). ⟨M⟩

- **RENAL IMPAIRMENT** [EvGr] Caution in severe impairment. ⟨M⟩
  Dose adjustments [EvGr] Max. dose 2 mg once daily in severe impairment. ⟨M⟩

- **PATIENT AND CARER ADVICE**
  Driving and skilled tasks Drowsiness may persist the next day and increased risk of dizziness or blurred vision may affect performance of skilled tasks (e.g. driving, or operating machinery); effects of alcohol and other CNS depressants enhanced.

- **MEDICINAL FORMS** There can be variation in the licensing of different medicines containing the same drug.

  Oral tablet
  CAUTIONARY AND ADVISORY LABELS 19

  ▸ Lunivia (Axunio Pharma GmbH)
    Eszopiclone 1 mg Lunivia 1mg tablets | 30 tablet [PoM] £3.99 [CD4–1]
    Eszopiclone 2 mg Lunivia 2mg tablets | 30 tablet [PoM] £3.99 [CD4–1]
    Eszopiclone 3 mg Lunivia 3mg tablets | 30 tablet [PoM] £3.99 [CD4–1]

Melatonin

14-Dec-2022

- **INDICATIONS AND DOSE**

Insomnia [short-term use]

▸ BY MOUTH USING MODIFIED-RELEASE TABLETS

▸ Adult 55 years and over: 2 mg once daily for up to 13 weeks, dose to be taken 1–2 hours before bedtime

Jet lag [short-term use]

▸ BY MOUTH USING IMMEDIATE-RELEASE MEDICINES

▸ Adult: 3 mg once daily for up to 5 days, the first dose should be taken at the habitual bedtime after arrival at destination. Doses should not be taken before 8 p.m. or after 4 a.m, dose may be increased to 5 or 6 mg once daily if necessary, or reduced to 1 or 2 mg once daily if sufficient. Maximum of 16 treatment courses per year

Insomnia in patients with learning disabilities and behaviour that challenges [where sleep hygiene measures have been insufficient] (initiated under specialist supervision)

▸ BY MOUTH USING MODIFIED-RELEASE TABLETS

▸ Adult: Initially 2 mg once daily, dose to be taken 30–60 minutes before bedtime, increased if necessary to 4–6 mg once daily, dose to be taken 30–60 minutes before bedtime, dose can be increased if necessary up to maximum 10 mg per day

DOSE EQUIVALENCE AND CONVERSION

▸ Caution is advised when switching between *immediate-release* formulations as the peak plasma-melatonin concentration may be higher with the oral solution than with tablets.

PHARMACOKINETICS

▸ The intake of food with *immediate-release* formulations may increase the bioavailability of melatonin—see *Directions for administration*.

- **UNLICENSED USE** [EvGr] Melatonin is used for insomnia in patients with learning disabilities and behaviour that challenges, ⟨E⟩ but is not licensed for this indication.

- **CAUTIONS** Autoimmune disease · susceptibility to seizures (risk of increased seizure frequency)

CAUTIONS, FURTHER INFORMATION

▸ Autoimmune disease [EvGr] Avoid—limited information available in patients with autoimmune disease; exacerbation reported occasionally. ⟨M⟩

- **INTERACTIONS** → Appendix 1: melatonin

- **SIDE-EFFECTS**

▸ **Common or very common** Arthralgia · increased risk of infection · pain

▸ **Uncommon** Anxiety · asthenia · chest pain · dizziness · drowsiness · dry mouth · gastrointestinal discomfort · headaches · hyperbilirubinaemia · hypertension · menopausal symptoms · mood altered · movement disorders · nausea · night sweats · oral disorders · skin reactions · sleep disorders · urine abnormalities · weight increased

▸ **Rare or very rare** Aggression · angina pectoris · arthritis · concentration impaired · crying · depression · disorientation · electrolyte imbalance · excessive tearing · gastrointestinal disorders · haematuria · hot flush · hypertriglyceridaemia · leucopenia · memory loss · muscle complaints · nail disorder · palpitations · paraesthesia · partial complex seizure · prostatitis · sexual dysfunction · syncope · thirst · thrombocytopenia · urinary disorders · vertigo · vision disorders · vomiting

▸ **Frequency not known** Angioedema · galactorrhoea · hyperglycaemia

- **PREGNANCY** No information available—avoid.

- **BREAST FEEDING** Present in milk—avoid.

- **HEPATIC IMPAIRMENT** [EvGr] For *modified-release tablets*, avoid (risk of decreased clearance; limited information available). For *immediate-release formulations*, avoid in moderate or severe impairment (risk of decreased clearance; limited information available). ◈M◈

● **RENAL IMPAIRMENT** EvGr For *modified-release tablets*, caution (no information available). For *immediate-release formulations*, caution (increased risk of exposure; limited information available); avoid in severe impairment. ◈M◈

● **DIRECTIONS FOR ADMINISTRATION** EvGr Modified-release tablets should be taken with or after food. Licensed immediate-release formulations should be taken on an empty stomach, 2 hours before or 2 hours after food (ideally at least 3 hours after food in those with significantly impaired glucose tolerance or diabetes)— intake with carbohydrate-rich meals may impair blood glucose control. The immediate-release tablet *Adaflex®* may be crushed and mixed with water immediately before administration. ◈M◈

● **PRESCRIBING AND DISPENSING INFORMATION** Licensed doses differ between preparations—further information can be found in the product literature for the individual preparations. Melatonin is available as a modified-release tablet (*Circadin®* and *Slenyto®*) and also as immediate-release formulations, including a tablet (*Adaflex®*, *Ceyesto®*, and *Syncrodin®*), hard capsule, and oral solution. *Circadin®* is licensed for the short-term treatment of primary insomnia in adults aged 55 years and over, and some immediate-release formulations, such as *Adaflex®*, *Ceyesto®*, and *Syncrodin®*, are licensed for the short-term treatment of jet lag in adults. *Adaflex®*, *Ceyesto®*, and *Slenyto®* are used for the treatment of insomnia associated with behavioural disorders in children and adolescents. Unlicensed preparations are also available, however, there is variability in clinical effect of unlicensed formulations.

● **PATIENT AND CARER ADVICE** Patients or their carers should be counselled on the administration of melatonin.

● **MEDICINAL FORMS** There can be variation in the licensing of different medicines containing the same drug. Forms available from special-order manufacturers include: oral tablet, modified-release tablet, oral capsule, oral solution

Oral tablet
CAUTIONARY AND ADVISORY LABELS 2
▸ **Melatonin (Non-proprietary)**
Melatonin 500 microgram VesPro Melatonin 500microgram tablets | 1000 tablet PoM 🔾
Melatonin 1 mg Melatonin 1mg tablets | 90 tablet PoM 🔾
Melatonin 3 mg Melatonin 3mg tablets | 30 tablet PoM £19.81 DT = £16.92
Melatonin 5 mg Melatonin Extra Strength 5mg tablets | 60 tablet PoM 🔾
Melatonin 5mg tablets | 30 tablet PoM £10.89 DT = £10.89
▸ **Adaflex** (AGB-Pharma)
Melatonin 1 mg Adaflex 1mg tablets | 30 tablet PoM £10.89 DT = £10.89
Melatonin 2 mg Adaflex 2mg tablets | 30 tablet PoM £10.89 DT = £10.89
Melatonin 3 mg Adaflex 3mg tablets | 30 tablet PoM £10.89 DT = £16.92
Melatonin 4 mg Adaflex 4mg tablets | 30 tablet PoM £10.89 DT = £10.89
Melatonin 5 mg Adaflex 5mg tablets | 30 tablet PoM £10.89 DT = £10.89
▸ **Ceyesto** (Alturix Ltd)
Melatonin 3 mg Ceyesto 3mg tablets | 30 tablet PoM £10.99 DT = £16.92
▸ **Syncrodin** (Pharma Nord (UK) Ltd)
Melatonin 3 mg Syncrodin 3mg tablets | 30 tablet PoM £14.95 DT = £16.92

Modified-release tablet
CAUTIONARY AND ADVISORY LABELS 2, 21, 25
▸ **Melatonin (Non-proprietary)**
Melatonin 2 mg Melatonin 2mg modified-release tablets | 30 tablet PoM £15.39 DT = £2.71
Melatonin 3 mg Melatonin 3mg modified-release tablets | 120 tablet PoM 🔾

▸ **Circadin** (Flynn Pharma Ltd)
Melatonin 2 mg Circadin 2mg modified-release tablets | 30 tablet PoM £15.39 DT = £2.71
▸ **Slenyto** (Flynn Pharma Ltd)
Melatonin 1 mg Slenyto 1mg modified-release tablets | 60 tablet PoM £32.96 DT = £32.96
Melatonin 5 mg Slenyto 5mg modified-release tablets | 30 tablet PoM £82.40 DT = £82.40

Oral capsule
CAUTIONARY AND ADVISORY LABELS 2
▸ **Melatonin (Non-proprietary)**
Melatonin 500 microgram Melatonin 500microgram capsules | 200 capsule PoM 🔾
Melatonin 1 mg Melatonin 1mg capsules | 60 capsule PoM 🔾
Melatonin 2 mg Melatonin 2mg capsules | 30 capsule PoM £103.50 DT = £57.50
Icenia Melatonin 2mg capsules | 60 capsule PoM 🔾
Melatonin 2.5 mg Melatonin 2.5mg capsules | 60 capsule PoM 🔾 DT = £149.94
Melatonin 3 mg Icenia Melatonin 3mg capsules | 60 capsule PoM 🔾 Melatonin 3mg capsules | 30 capsule PoM £62.50–£113.00 DT = £62.50
Melatonin 5 mg Icenia Melatonin 5mg capsules | 60 capsule PoM 🔾 Melatonin 5mg capsules | 30 capsule PoM £105.00–£189.00 DT = £105.00
Melatonin 10 mg Melatonin 10mg capsules | 60 capsule PoM 🔾
Melatonin 20 mg S.Gard 20mg capsules | 60 capsule PoM 🔾

Oral solution
CAUTIONARY AND ADVISORY LABELS 2
EXCIPIENTS: May contain Propylene glycol, sorbitol
▸ **Melatonin (Non-proprietary)**
Melatonin 1 mg per 1 ml Melatonin 1mg/ml oral solution sugar free | 50 ml PoM £6.85–£7.53 SF | 60 ml PoM £19.77–£60.00 SF | 100 ml PoM £19.80–£86.67 SF | 150 ml PoM £22.59–£130.00 DT = £18.76 SF
Melatonin 2 mg per 1 ml Melatonin 2mg/ml oral solution sugar free | 25 ml PoM £55.00–£60.00 DT = £60.00 SF
▸ **Ceyesto** (Alturix Ltd)
Melatonin 1 mg per 1 ml Ceyesto 1mg/ml oral solution | 100 ml PoM £17.10 SF | 150 ml PoM £25.65 DT = £18.76 SF

Zolpidem tartrate
15-Apr-2024

● **INDICATIONS AND DOSE**
Insomnia (short-term use)
▸ BY MOUTH
▸ **Adult:** 10 mg daily for up to 4 weeks, dose to be taken at bedtime, for debilitated patients, use elderly dose
▸ **Elderly:** 5 mg daily for up to 4 weeks, dose to be taken at bedtime

● **CONTRA-INDICATIONS** Acute respiratory depression · marked neuromuscular respiratory weakness · myasthenia gravis · obstructive sleep apnoea · psychotic illness · severe respiratory depression

● **CAUTIONS** Avoid prolonged use (and abrupt withdrawal thereafter) · depression · elderly · history of alcohol abuse · history of drug abuse · muscle weakness

CAUTIONS, FURTHER INFORMATION
▸ **Elderly** For hypnotic Z-drugs, Screening Tool of Older Persons' potentially inappropriate Prescriptions (STOPP) criteria to aid medication reviews (see Prescribing in the elderly p. 31 for information): potentially inappropriate in elderly (may cause protracted daytime sedation and/or ataxia).

● **INTERACTIONS** → Appendix 1: zolpidem

● **SIDE-EFFECTS**
▸ **Common or very common** Abdominal pain · anterograde amnesia · anxiety · back pain · diarrhoea · dizziness · fatigue · hallucination · headache · increased risk of infection · nausea · sleep disorders · vomiting
▸ **Uncommon** Confusion · diplopia · irritability
▸ **Frequency not known** Angioedema · behaviour abnormal · concentration impaired · delusions · depression · drug

dependence · fall · gait abnormal · hepatic disorders · hyperhidrosis · level of consciousness decreased · libido disorder · muscle weakness · psychosis · respiratory depression · skin reactions · speech disorder · withdrawal syndrome

- **PREGNANCY** Avoid regular use (risk of neonatal withdrawal symptoms); high doses during late pregnancy or labour may cause neonatal hypothermia, hypotonia, and respiratory depression.
- **BREAST FEEDING** Small amounts present in milk—avoid.
- **HEPATIC IMPAIRMENT** Manufacturer advises caution in mild to moderate impairment (risk of decreased clearance); avoid in severe impairment.
  Dose adjustments Manufacturer advises initial dose reduction to 5 mg daily in mild to moderate impairment.
- **RENAL IMPAIRMENT** [EvGr] Use with caution. ⟨M⟩
- **PATIENT AND CARER ADVICE**
  Driving and skilled tasks Drowsiness may persist the next day—leave at least 8 hours between taking zolpidem and performing skilled tasks (e.g. driving, or operating machinery); effects of alcohol and other CNS depressants enhanced.
- **NATIONAL FUNDING/ACCESS DECISIONS**
  For full details see funding body website
  NICE decisions
- ▸ **Guidance on the use of zaleplon, zolpidem, and zopiclone for the short-term management of insomnia (April 2004)**
  NICE TA77 Recommended

- **MEDICINAL FORMS** There can be variation in the licensing of different medicines containing the same drug.
  Oral tablet
  CAUTIONARY AND ADVISORY LABELS 19
  - ▸ **Zolpidem tartrate (Non-proprietary)**
    Zolpidem tartrate 5 mg Zolpidem 5mg tablets | 28 tablet [PoM]
    £3.08 DT = £1.65 [CD4–1]
    Zolpidem tartrate 10 mg Zolpidem 10mg tablets | 28 tablet [PoM]
    £4.48 DT = £1.23 [CD4–1]

| Zopiclone

04-Mar-2025

- **INDICATIONS AND DOSE**
  Insomnia (short-term use)
  - ▸ BY MOUTH
  - ▸ Adult: 7.5 mg once daily for up to 4 weeks, dose to be taken at bedtime
  - ▸ Elderly: Initially 3.75 mg once daily for up to 4 weeks, dose to be taken at bedtime, dose may be increased if necessary to 7.5 mg once daily

  Insomnia (short-term use) in patients with chronic pulmonary insufficiency
  - ▸ BY MOUTH
  - ▸ Adult: Initially 3.75 mg once daily for up to 4 weeks, dose to be taken at bedtime, dose may be increased if necessary to 7.5 mg once daily

- **CONTRA-INDICATIONS** Marked neuromuscular respiratory weakness · myasthenia gravis · previous complex sleep-related behaviours associated with hypnotics · respiratory failure · severe sleep apnoea syndrome
- **CAUTIONS** Avoid prolonged use (risk of tolerance and withdrawal symptoms) · chronic pulmonary insufficiency (increased risk of respiratory depression) · depression · elderly · history of alcohol abuse · history of drug abuse · muscle weakness · psychiatric illness

  CAUTIONS, FURTHER INFORMATION
  - ▸ Elderly For hypnotic Z-drugs, Screening Tool of Older Persons' potentially inappropriate Prescriptions (STOPP) criteria to aid medication reviews (see Prescribing in the elderly p. 31 for information): potentially innapropriate in

elderly (may cause protracted daytime sedation and/or ataxia).

- **INTERACTIONS** → Appendix 1: zopiclone
- **SIDE-EFFECTS**
  - ▸ **Common or very common** Dry mouth · taste bitter
  - ▸ **Uncommon** Anxiety · dizziness · fatigue · headache · nausea · sleep disorders · vomiting
  - ▸ **Rare or very rare** Behaviour abnormal · confusion · dyspnoea · fall · hallucination · irritability · libido disorder · memory impairment · skin reactions
  - ▸ **Frequency not known** Cognitive disorder · concentration impaired · delusions · depressed mood · diplopia · drug dependence · dyspepsia · movement disorders · muscle weakness · paraesthesia · respiratory depression · speech disorder · withdrawal syndrome
- **PREGNANCY** Not recommended (risk of neonatal withdrawal symptoms). Use during late pregnancy or labour may cause neonatal hypothermia, hypotonia, and respiratory depression.
- **BREAST FEEDING** Present in milk—avoid.
- **HEPATIC IMPAIRMENT** Manufacturer advises caution in mild to moderate impairment; avoid in severe impairment (risk of decreased elimination).
  Dose adjustments Manufacturer advises dose reduction to 3.75 mg in mild to moderate impairment, dose can be increased with caution if necessary.
- **RENAL IMPAIRMENT**
  Dose adjustments [EvGr] Start with reduced dose of 3.75 mg. ⟨M⟩
- **PATIENT AND CARER ADVICE**
  Driving and skilled tasks Drowsiness may persist the next day and affect performance of skilled tasks (e.g. driving); effects of alcohol enhanced.
- **NATIONAL FUNDING/ACCESS DECISIONS**
  For full details see funding body website
  NICE decisions
- ▸ **Guidance on the use of zaleplon, zolpidem and zopiclone for the short-term management of insomnia (April 2004)**
  NICE TA77 Recommended

- **MEDICINAL FORMS** There can be variation in the licensing of different medicines containing the same drug. Forms available from special-order manufacturers include: oral suspension, oral solution
  Oral tablet
  CAUTIONARY AND ADVISORY LABELS 19, 25
  - ▸ **Zopiclone (Non-proprietary)**
    Zopiclone 3.75 mg Zopiclone 3.75mg tablets | 28 tablet [PoM] £1.24 DT = £1.07 [CD4–1]
    Zopiclone 7.5 mg Zopiclone 7.5mg tablets | 28 tablet [PoM] £1.24 DT = £1.07 [CD4–1]
  - ▸ **Zimovane** (Sanofi)
    Zopiclone 3.75 mg Zimovane LS 3.75mg tablets | 14 tablet [PoM] £0.82 [CD4–1]
    Zopiclone 7.5 mg Zimovane 7.5mg tablets | 14 tablet [PoM] £1.63 [CD4–1]

7.2   Narcolepsy

> **Other drugs used for Narcolepsy** Dexamfetamine sulfate, p. 405 · Methylphenidate hydrochloride, p. 403

Nervous system

4

CENTRAL NERVOUS SYSTEM DEPRESSANTS

Sodium oxybate

14-Oct-2021

- **DRUG ACTION** A central nervous system depressant.

- **INDICATIONS AND DOSE**

Narcolepsy with cataplexy (under expert supervision)
- BY MOUTH
- Adult: Initially 2.25 g daily, dose to be taken on retiring and 2.25 g after 2.5–4 hours, then increased in steps of 1.5 g daily in 2 divided doses, dose adjusted according to response at intervals of 1–2 weeks; dose titration should be repeated if restarting after interval of more than 14 days, maximum 9 g daily in 2 divided doses

DOSE ADJUSTMENTS DUE TO INTERACTIONS
- Manufacturer advises reduce dose by 20 % with concurrent use of sodium valproate or valproic acid.

- **CONTRA-INDICATIONS** Major depression · succinic semi-aldehyde dehydrogenase deficiency

- **CAUTIONS** Body mass index of 40 kg/m^2 or greater (higher risk of sleep apnoea) · elderly · epilepsy · heart failure (high sodium content) · history of depression · history of drug abuse · hypertension (high sodium content) · respiratory disorders · risk of discontinuation effects including rebound cataplexy and withdrawal symptoms

- **INTERACTIONS** → Appendix 1: sodium oxybate

- **SIDE-EFFECTS**
- **Common or very common** Abdominal pain upper · anxiety · appetite abnormal · arthralgia · asthenia · back pain · concentration impaired · confusion · depression · diarrhoea · dizziness · dyspnoea · fall · feeling drunk · headache · hyperhidrosis · hypertension · increased risk of infection · movement disorders · muscle spasms · nasal congestion · nausea · palpitations · peripheral oedema · sedation · sensation abnormal · skin reactions · sleep disorders · sleep paralysis · snoring · taste altered · tremor · urinary disorders · vertigo · vision blurred · vomiting · weight decreased
- **Uncommon** Behaviour abnormal · faecal incontinence · hallucination · memory loss · psychosis · suicidal behaviours · thinking abnormal
- **Frequency not known** Angioedema · dehydration · delusions · dry mouth · homicidal ideation · loss of consciousness · mood altered · respiratory depression · seizure · sleep apnoea

- **PREGNANCY** Avoid.

- **HEPATIC IMPAIRMENT** Manufacturer advises caution (risk of increased exposure).
  Dose adjustments Manufacturer advises initial dose reduction of 50%.

- **RENAL IMPAIRMENT** EvGr Consider reducing sodium intake (contains 0.18 g Na$^+$ per gram of sodium oxybate). Ⓜ

- **DIRECTIONS FOR ADMINISTRATION** Manufacturer advises dilute each dose with 60 mL water; prepare both doses before retiring. Observe the same time interval (2–3 hours) each night between the last meal and the first dose.

- **PATIENT AND CARER ADVICE** Patients or carers should be given advice on how to administer sodium oxybate oral solution.
  Driving and skilled tasks Leave at least 6 hours between taking sodium oxybate and performing skilled tasks (e.g. driving or operating machinery); effects of alcohol and other CNS depressants enhanced.

- **MEDICINAL FORMS** There can be variation in the licensing of different medicines containing the same drug.
  Oral solution
  CAUTIONARY AND ADVISORY LABELS 13, 19
  ELECTROLYTES: May contain Sodium
  - **Sodium oxybate (Non-proprietary)**
    Sodium oxybate 500 mg per 1 ml Sodium oxybate 500mg/ml oral solution sugar free | 180 ml PoM £357.00–£360.00 DT = £360.00 (Hospital only) CD2 SF
  - **Xyrem** (UCB Pharma Ltd)
    Sodium oxybate 500 mg per 1 ml Xyrem 500mg/ml oral solution | 180 ml PoM £360.00 DT = £360.00 (Hospital only) CD2 SF

CNS STIMULANTS

Pitolisant

28-May-2019

- **DRUG ACTION** Pitolisant is a histamine H$_3$-receptor antagonist which enhances the activity of brain histaminergic neurons.

- **INDICATIONS AND DOSE**

Narcolepsy with or without cataplexy (initiated by a specialist)
- BY MOUTH
- Adult: Initially 9 mg once daily for 1 week, then increased if necessary to 18 mg once daily for 1 week, then increased if necessary to 36 mg once daily, dose to be taken in the morning with breakfast, dose can be decreased (down to 4.5 mg per day) or increased (up to 36 mg per day) according to response and tolerance

- **CAUTIONS** Acid-related gastric disorders · epilepsy · history of psychiatric disorders · severe anorexia · severe obesity

- **INTERACTIONS** → Appendix 1: pitolisant

- **SIDE-EFFECTS**
- **Common or very common** Anxiety · asthenia · depression · dizziness · gastrointestinal discomfort · headaches · mood altered · nausea · sleep disorders · tremor · vertigo · vomiting
- **Uncommon** Appetite abnormal · arrhythmias · arthralgia · blepharospasm · chest pain · concentration impaired · constipation · diarrhoea · drowsiness · dry mouth · epilepsy · feeling abnormal · fluid retention · gastrointestinal disorders · hallucinations · hot flush · hypertension · hypotension · malaise · metrorrhagia · movement disorders · muscle complaints · muscle weakness · oedema · on and off phenomenon · oral paraesthesia · pain · paraesthesia · QT interval prolongation · sexual dysfunction · skin reactions · suicidal ideation · sweat changes · tinnitus · urinary frequency increased · visual acuity decreased · weight decreased (review treatment if significant) · weight increased (review treatment if significant) · yawning
- **Rare or very rare** Behaviour abnormal · cognitive impairment · confusion · loss of consciousness · memory impairment · obsessive thoughts · photosensitivity reaction · sense of oppression · swallowing difficulty

- **CONCEPTION AND CONTRACEPTION** Manufacturer advises effective contraception in women of childbearing potential for at least 21 days after treatment discontinuation—pitolisant may reduce the effectiveness of hormonal contraceptives.

- **PREGNANCY** Manufacturer advises avoid unless potential benefit outweighs risk—toxicity in *animal* studies.

- **BREAST FEEDING** Manufacturer advises avoid—present in milk in *animal* studies.

- **HEPATIC IMPAIRMENT** Manufacturer advises caution in moderate impairment; avoid in severe impairment.
  Dose adjustments Manufacturer advises consider dose increase two weeks after initiation in moderate impairment; maximum daily dose of 18 mg.

● **RENAL IMPAIRMENT**
Dose adjustments Manufacturer advises use with caution; maximum daily dose should not exceed 18 mg.

● **MEDICINAL FORMS** There can be variation in the licensing of different medicines containing the same drug.
Oral tablet
▸ Wakix (Bioprojet UK Ltd) ▼
  Pitolisant (as Pitolisant hydrochloride) **4.5 mg** Wakix 4.5mg tablets | 30 tablet PoM £310.00 DT = £310.00
  Pitolisant (as Pitolisant hydrochloride) **18 mg** Wakix 18mg tablets | 30 tablet PoM £310.00 DT = £310.00

CNS STIMULANTS › CENTRALLY ACTING SYMPATHOMIMETICS

Modafinil
11-May-2021

● **INDICATIONS AND DOSE**
Excessive sleepiness associated with narcolepsy with or without cataplexy
▸ BY MOUTH
▸ Adult: Initially 200 mg daily in 2 divided doses, dose to be taken in the morning and at noon, alternatively initially 200 mg once daily, dose to be taken in the morning, adjusted according to response to 200–400 mg daily in 2 divided doses, alternatively adjusted according to response to 200–400 mg once daily
▸ Elderly: Initially 100 mg daily

IMPORTANT SAFETY INFORMATION
MHRA/CHM ADVICE (UPDATED NOVEMBER 2020): MODAFINIL (*PROVIGIL*®): INCREASED RISK OF CONGENITAL MALFORMATIONS IF USED DURING PREGNANCY
A European review and other safety data found that use of modafinil during pregnancy potentially increases the risk of congenital malformations such as heart defects, hypospadias, and orofacial clefts. Healthcare professionals are advised that modafinil should not be used during pregnancy; alternative treatment options should be considered, including behaviour modifying measures, sleep hygiene, and scheduled daytime naps. Modafinil may also reduce the effectiveness of some hormonal contraceptives, including oral contraceptives, therefore alternative or additional methods of contraception are required—see also *Interactions*. Females of childbearing potential should be advised on the use of contraception (see *Conception and contraception*) and informed of the risk of congenital malformations.

● **CONTRA-INDICATIONS** Arrhythmia · history of clinically significant signs of CNS stimulant-induced mitral valve prolapse (including ischaemic ECG changes, chest pain and arrhythmias) · history of cor pulmonale · history of left ventricular hypertrophy · moderate to severe uncontrolled hypertension

● **CAUTIONS** History of alcohol abuse · history of depression · history of drug abuse · history of mania · history of psychosis · possibility of dependence

● **INTERACTIONS** → Appendix 1: modafinil

● **SIDE-EFFECTS**
▸ **Common or very common** Anxiety · appetite abnormal · arrhythmias · asthenia · chest pain · confusion · constipation · depression · diarrhoea · dizziness · drowsiness · dry mouth · gastrointestinal discomfort · headaches · mood altered · nausea · palpitations · sensation abnormal · sleep disorders · thinking abnormal · vasodilation · vision disorders
▸ **Uncommon** Allergic rhinitis · arthralgia · asthma · behaviour abnormal · central nervous system stimulation ·

cough aggravated · diabetes mellitus · dry eye · dysphagia · dyspnoea · eosinophilia · epistaxis · gastrointestinal disorders · hypercholesterolaemia · hyperglycaemia · hyperhidrosis · hypertension · hypotension · increased risk of infection · leucopenia · libido decreased · memory loss · menstrual disorder · movement disorders · muscle complaints · muscle tone increased · muscle weakness · oral disorders · pain · peripheral oedema · psychiatric disorders · skin reactions · speech disorder · suicidal behaviours · taste altered · thirst · tremor · urinary frequency increased · urine abnormal · vertigo · vomiting · weight changes
▸ **Rare or very rare** Hallucination · psychosis
▸ **Frequency not known** Angioedema · delusions · fever · hypersensitivity · lymphadenopathy · severe cutaneous adverse reactions (SCARs)

SIDE-EFFECTS, FURTHER INFORMATION Discontinue treatment if rash develops. Discontinue treatment if psychiatric symptoms develop.

● **CONCEPTION AND CONTRACEPTION** The MHRA advises females of childbearing potential should use effective contraception during treatment and for 2 months after last treatment—see also *Important safety information*.

● **PREGNANCY** Manufacturer advises avoid—increased risk of congenital malformations (see also *Important safety information*).

● **BREAST FEEDING** Avoid—present in milk in *animal* studies.

● **HEPATIC IMPAIRMENT** Manufacturer advises caution in severe impairment (risk of increased plasma concentrations).
Dose adjustments Manufacturer advises dose reduction of 50% in severe impairment.

● **RENAL IMPAIRMENT** EvGr Use with caution—limited information available. ⟨M⟩

● **PRE-TREATMENT SCREENING** ECG required before initiation.

● **MONITORING REQUIREMENTS** Monitor blood pressure and heart rate in hypertensive patients.

● **MEDICINAL FORMS** There can be variation in the licensing of different medicines containing the same drug. Forms available from special-order manufacturers include: oral suspension, oral solution
Oral tablet
▸ Modafinil (Non-proprietary)
  Modafinil **100 mg** Modafinil 100mg tablets | 30 tablet PoM £5.18 DT = £1.95
  Modafinil **200 mg** Modafinil 200mg tablets | 30 tablet PoM £9.12 DT = £8.26
▸ Provigil (Teva UK Ltd)
  Modafinil **100 mg** Provigil 100mg tablets | 30 tablet PoM £52.60 DT = £1.95

Solriamfetol
03-Aug-2022

● **DRUG ACTION** Solriamfetol increases the levels of dopamine and noradrenaline in the brain by inhibiting re-uptake, thereby improving wakefulness.

● **INDICATIONS AND DOSE**
Excessive sleepiness associated with narcolepsy [with or without cataplexy] (initiated by a specialist)
▸ BY MOUTH
▸ Adult: 75 mg once daily, increased if necessary up to 150 mg once daily, dose to be taken upon awakening and not within 9 hours of bedtime, dose to be increased by doubling the dose after at least 3 days, according to response, in patients with severe symptoms, a starting dose of 150 mg once daily may be considered; maximum 150 mg per day

continued →

Excessive sleepiness associated with obstructive sleep apnoea (initiated by a specialist)
▸ BY MOUTH
▸ Adult: 37.5 mg once daily, increased if necessary up to 150 mg once daily, dose to be taken upon awakening and not within 9 hours of bedtime, dose to be increased by doubling the dose at intervals of at least 3 days, according to response; maximum 150 mg per day

● CONTRA-INDICATIONS Cardiac arrhythmias · hypertension (uncontrolled) · myocardial infarction (within the past year) · unstable angina pectoris

● CAUTIONS Elderly (limited information available—consider lower doses and close monitoring) · history of alcohol abuse · history of stimulant abuse · history of, or concurrent, psychosis or bipolar disorder (risk of exacerbation of psychiatric symptoms) · increased intra-ocular pressure (risk of mydriasis) · patients at risk of angle-closure glaucoma (risk of mydriasis) · patients at risk of major cardiovascular events

● INTERACTIONS → Appendix 1: solriamfetol

● SIDE-EFFECTS
▸ **Common or very common** Abdominal pain · anxiety · appetite decreased · chest discomfort · constipation · cough · diarrhoea · dizziness · dry mouth · feeling jittery · headache · hyperhidrosis · insomnia · irritability · nausea · palpitations · teeth grinding · vomiting
▸ **Uncommon** Concentration impaired · dyspnoea · hypertension · tachycardia · thirst · tremor · weight decreased
▸ **Frequency not known** Mydriasis

● CONCEPTION AND CONTRACEPTION Manufacturer advises females of childbearing potential or their male partners should use effective contraception during treatment.

● PREGNANCY Manufacturer advises avoid—toxicity in *animal* studies.

● BREAST FEEDING Specialist sources indicate use with caution—limited information available. Monitor breast-fed infants for adverse reactions such as agitation, insomnia, poor feeding, and reduced weight gain.

● RENAL IMPAIRMENT Manufacturer advises caution in moderate to severe impairment—increased risk of elevations in blood pressure and heart rate; avoid in end-stage renal disease.
Dose adjustments Manufacturer advises a starting dose of 37.5 mg once daily, increased if necessary after 5 days to a maximum of 75 mg once daily, in moderate impairment; a dose of 37.5 mg once daily should not be exceeded in severe impairment.

● MONITORING REQUIREMENTS Manufacturer advises assess blood pressure and heart rate before initiation and monitor periodically during treatment, including after dose increases; pre-existing hypertension should be controlled before starting treatment.

● PATIENT AND CARER ADVICE
Driving and skilled tasks Manufacturer advises patients and carers should be counselled on the effects on driving and performance of skilled tasks—increased risk of dizziness and attention disturbances.

Patients should be frequently reassessed, and if appropriate, advised to avoid driving or any other potentially dangerous activity, especially at the start of treatment or when a dose is changed. Patients with abnormal levels of sleepiness should be advised that their level of wakefulness may not return to normal.

● NATIONAL FUNDING/ACCESS DECISIONS
For full details see funding body website
NICE decisions
▸ Solriamfetol for treating excessive daytime sleepiness caused by narcolepsy (January 2022) NICE TA758 Recommended with restrictions
▸ Solriamfetol for treating excessive daytime sleepiness caused by obstructive sleep apnoea (March 2022) NICE TA777 Not recommended
Scottish Medicines Consortium (SMC) decisions
▸ Solriamfetol (*Sunosi*®) to improve wakefulness and reduce excessive daytime sleepiness (EDS) in adult patients with obstructive sleep apnoea (OSA) whose EDS has not been satisfactorily treated by primary OSA therapy, such as continuous positive airway pressure (CPAP) (March 2022) SMC No. SMC2419 Not recommended
▸ Solriamfetol (*Sunosi*®) to improve wakefulness and reduce excessive daytime sleepiness (EDS) in adult patients with narcolepsy (with or without cataplexy) (July 2022) SMC No. SMC2439 Recommended with restrictions

● MEDICINAL FORMS There can be variation in the licensing of different medicines containing the same drug.
Oral tablet
▸ Sunosi (Atnahs Pharma UK Ltd) ▼
Solriamfetol (as Solriamfetol hydrochloride) 75 mg Sunosi 75mg tablets | 28 tablet [PoM] £177.52 (Hospital only)
Solriamfetol (as Solriamfetol hydrochloride) 150 mg Sunosi 150mg tablets | 28 tablet [PoM] £248.64 (Hospital only)

8 Substance dependence

Substance dependence

17-May-2022

Guidance on treatment of drug misuse

The UK health departments have produced guidance on the treatment of drug misuse in the UK. *Drug Misuse and Dependence: UK Guidelines on Clinical Management* (2017) is available at www.gov.uk/government/publications/drug-misuse-and-dependence-uk-guidelines-on-clinical-management.

Alcohol dependence

See Alcohol dependence p. 562.

Nicotine dependence

See Smoking cessation p. 565.

Opioid dependence

The management of opioid dependence requires medical, social, and psychological treatment; access to a multidisciplinary team is recommended. Treatment for opioid dependence should be initiated under the supervision of an appropriately qualified prescriber.

Untreated heroin dependence shows early withdrawal symptoms within 8 hours, with peak symptoms at 36–72 hours; symptoms subside substantially after 5 days. Methadone hydrochloride p. 570 or buprenorphine p. 511 withdrawal occurs later, with longer-lasting symptoms.

Opioid substitution therapy

Methadone hydrochloride and buprenorphine are used as substitution therapy in opioid dependence. Substitute medication should be commenced with a short period of stabilisation, followed by either a withdrawal regimen or by maintenance treatment. Maintenance treatment enables patients to achieve stability, reduces drug use and crime, and improves health; it should be regularly reviewed to ensure the patient continues to derive benefit. The prescriber should monitor for signs of toxicity, and the patient should be told to be aware of warning signs of toxicity on initiation and during titration.

A withdrawal regimen after stabilisation with methadone hydrochloride or buprenorphine should be attempted only after careful consideration. Enforced withdrawal is ineffective for sustained abstinence, and it increases the risk of patients relapsing and subsequently overdosing because of loss of tolerance. Complete withdrawal from opioids usually takes up to 4 weeks in an inpatient or residential setting, and up to 12 weeks in a community setting. If abstinence is not achieved, illicit drug use is resumed, or the patient cannot tolerate withdrawal, the withdrawal regimen should be stopped and maintenance therapy should be resumed at the optimal dose. Following successful withdrawal treatment, further support and monitoring to maintain abstinence should be provided for a period of at least 6 months.

Missed doses
Patients who miss 3 days or more of their regular prescribed dose of opioid maintenance therapy are at risk of overdose because of loss of tolerance. Consider reducing the dose in these patients.

If the patient misses 5 or more days of treatment, an assessment of illicit drug use is also recommended before restarting substitution therapy; this is particularly important for patients taking buprenorphine because of the risk of precipitated withdrawal.

Buprenorphine
Buprenorphine is preferred by some patients because it is less sedating than methadone hydrochloride; for this reason it may be more suitable for employed patients or those undertaking other skilled tasks such as driving. Buprenorphine is safer than methadone hydrochloride when used in conjunction with other sedating drugs, and has fewer drug interactions. Dose reductions may be easier than with methadone hydrochloride because the withdrawal symptoms are milder, and patients generally require fewer adjunctive medications; there is also a lower risk of overdose. Buprenorphine can be given on alternate days in higher doses and it requires a shorter drug-free period than methadone hydrochloride before induction with naltrexone hydrochloride p. 564 for prevention of relapse.

Patients dependent on high doses of opioids may be at increased risk of precipitated withdrawal. Precipitated withdrawal can occur in any patient if buprenorphine is administered when other opioid agonist drugs are in circulation. Precipitated opioid withdrawal, if it occurs, starts within 1–3 hours of the first buprenorphine dose and peaks at around 6 hours. Non-opioid adjunctive therapy, such as lofexidine hydrochloride p. 572, may be required if symptoms are severe.

To reduce the risk of precipitated withdrawal, the first dose of buprenorphine should be given when the patient is exhibiting signs of withdrawal, or 6–12 hours after the last use of heroin (or other short-acting opioid), or 24–48 hours after the last dose of methadone hydrochloride. It is possible to titrate the dose of buprenorphine within one week—more rapidly than with methadone hydrochloride therapy—but care is still needed to avoid toxicity or precipitated withdrawal; dividing the dose on the first day may be useful.

A combination preparation containing buprenorphine with naloxone p. 571 can be prescribed for patients when there is a risk of dose diversion for parenteral administration; the naloxone hydrochloride p. 1564 component precipitates withdrawal if the preparation is injected, but it has little effect when the preparation is taken sublingually.

Where there is a risk of diversion of opioid substitution medicines, or difficulties with adherence to daily supervised opioid substitution medication, buprenorphine prolonged-release injection may be an option.

Methadone
Methadone hydrochloride, a long-acting opioid agonist, is usually administered in a single daily dose as methadone hydrochloride oral solution 1 mg/mL. Patients with a long history of opioid misuse, those who typically abuse a variety of sedative drugs and alcohol, and those who experience increased anxiety during withdrawal of opioids may prefer methadone hydrochloride to buprenorphine because it has a more pronounced sedative effect.

Methadone hydrochloride is initiated at least 8 hours after the last heroin dose, provided that there is objective evidence of withdrawal symptoms. A supplementary dose on the first day may be considered if there is evidence of persistent opioid withdrawal symptoms. Because of the long half-life, plasma concentrations progressively rise during initial treatment even if the patient remains on the same daily dose (it takes 3–10 days for plasma concentrations to reach steady-state in patients on a stable dose); a dose tolerated on the first day of treatment may become a toxic dose on the third day as cumulative toxicity develops. Thus, titration to the optimal dose in methadone hydrochloride maintenance treatment may take several weeks.

Opioid substitution during pregnancy
Acute withdrawal of opioids should be avoided in pregnancy because it can cause fetal death. Opioid substitution therapy is recommended during pregnancy because it carries a lower risk to the fetus than continued use of illicit drugs. If a woman who is stabilised on methadone hydrochloride or buprenorphine for treatment of opioid dependence becomes pregnant, therapy should be continued [buprenorphine is not licensed for use in pregnancy]. Many pregnant patients choose a withdrawal regimen, but withdrawal during the first trimester should be avoided because it is associated with an increased risk of spontaneous miscarriage. Withdrawal of methadone hydrochloride or buprenorphine should be undertaken gradually during the second trimester, with dose reductions made every 3–5 days. If illicit drug use occurs, the patient should be re-stabilised at the optimal maintenance dose and consideration should be given to stopping the withdrawal regimen.

Further withdrawal of methadone hydrochloride p. 570 or buprenorphine p. 511 in the third trimester is not recommended because maternal withdrawal, even if mild, is associated with fetal distress, stillbirth, and the risk of neonatal mortality. Drug metabolism can be increased in the third trimester; it may be necessary to either increase the dose of methadone hydrochloride or change to twice-daily consumption (or a combination of both strategies) to prevent withdrawal symptoms from developing.

The neonate should be monitored for respiratory depression and signs of withdrawal if the mother is prescribed high doses of opioid substitute.

Signs of neonatal withdrawal from opioids usually develop 24–72 hours after delivery but symptoms may be delayed for up to 14 days, so monitoring may be required for several weeks. Symptoms include a high-pitched cry, rapid breathing, hungry but ineffective suckling, and excessive wakefulness; severe, but rare symptoms include hypertonicity and convulsions.

Opioid substitution during breastfeeding
Doses of methadone and buprenorphine should be kept as low as possible in breast-feeding mothers. Increased sleepiness, breathing difficulties, or limpness in breast-fed babies of mothers taking opioid substitutes should be reported urgently to a healthcare professional.

Adjunctive therapy and symptomatic treatment
Adjunctive therapy may be required for the management of opioid withdrawal symptoms. Loperamide hydrochloride p. 74 may be used for the control of diarrhoea; mebeverine hydrochloride p. 98 for controlling stomach cramps; paracetamol p. 507 and **non-steroidal anti-inflammatory drugs** for muscular pains and headaches; metoclopramide

4
Nervous system

hydrochloride p. 494 or prochlorperazine p. 448 may be useful for nausea or vomiting. Topical **rubefacients** can be helpful for relieving muscle pain associated with methadone hydrochloride withdrawal. If a patient is suffering from insomnia, short-acting **benzodiazepines** or zopiclone p. 557 may be prescribed, but because of the potential for abuse, prescriptions should be limited to a short course of a few days only. If anxiety or agitation is severe, specialist advice should be sought.

Lofexidine

Lofexidine hydrochloride p. 572 may alleviate some of the physical symptoms of opioid withdrawal by attenuating the increase in adrenergic neurotransmission that occurs during opioid withdrawal. Lofexidine hydrochloride can be prescribed as an adjuvant to opioid substitution therapy, initiated either at the same time as the opioid substitute or during withdrawal of the opioid substitute. Alternatively, lofexidine hydrochloride may be prescribed instead of an opioid substitute in patients who have mild or uncertain dependence (including young people), and those with a short history of illicit drug use.

Opioid-receptor antagonists

Patients dependant on opioids can be given a supply of naloxone hydrochloride p. 1564 to be used in case of accidental overdose.

Naltrexone hydrochloride p. 564 precipitates withdrawal symptoms in opioid-dependent subjects. Because the effects of opioid-receptor agonists are blocked by naltrexone hydrochloride, it is prescribed as an aid to prevent relapse in formerly opioid-dependent patients.

Opioid dependence in children

In younger patients (under 18 years), the harmful effects of drug misuse are more often related to acute intoxication than to dependence, so substitution therapy is usually inappropriate. Maintenance treatment with opioid substitution therapy is therefore controversial in young people; however, it may be useful for the older adolescent who has a history of opioid use to undergo a period of stabilisation with buprenorphine or methadone hydrochloride before starting a withdrawal regimen.

8.1 Alcohol dependence

Alcohol dependence

14-Sep-2020

Description of condition

Alcohol dependence is a cluster of behavioural, cognitive and physiological factors that typically include a strong desire to drink alcohol, tolerance to its effects, and difficulties controlling its use. Someone who is alcohol-dependent may persist in drinking, despite harmful consequences, such as physical or mental health problems.

In severely dependent patients who have been drinking excessively for a prolonged period of time, an abrupt reduction in alcohol intake may result in the development of an alcohol withdrawal syndrome, which, in the absence of medical management, can lead to seizures, delirium tremens, and death.

Assisted alcohol withdrawal

EvGr Patients with mild alcohol dependence usually do not need assisted alcohol withdrawal. Patients with moderate dependence can generally be treated in a community setting unless they are at high risk of developing alcohol withdrawal seizures or delirium tremens; individuals with severe dependence should undergo withdrawal in an inpatient setting. Patients with decompensated liver disease should be treated under specialist supervision.

A long-acting benzodiazepine, such as chlordiazepoxide hydrochloride p. 398 or diazepam p. 398, is recommended to attenuate alcohol withdrawal symptoms; local clinical protocols should be followed.

In primary care, *fixed-dose reducing regimens* are used. This involves using a standard, initial dose (determined by the severity of alcohol dependence or level of alcohol consumption), followed by dose reduction to zero, usually over 7–10 days. In inpatient or residential settings, a *fixed-dose regimen* or a *symptom-triggered regimen* can be used. A symptom-triggered approach involves tailoring the drug regimen according to the severity of withdrawal and any complications in an individual patient; adequate monitoring facilities should be available. The patient should be monitored on a regular basis and treatment only continued as long as there are withdrawal symptoms.

Carbamazepine p. 355 [unlicensed indication] can be used as an alternative treatment in acute alcohol withdrawal. The MHRA/CHM have released important safety information on the use of antiepileptic drugs and the risk of suicidal thoughts and behaviour. For further information, see Epilepsy p. 349.

EvGr Clomethiazole p. 553 may be considered as an alternative to a benzodiazepine or carbamazepine p. 355. It should only be used in an inpatient setting and should not be prescribed if the patient is liable to continue drinking alcohol. **Note:** Alcohol combined with clomethiazole p. 553, particularly in patients with cirrhosis, can lead to fatal respiratory depression even with short-term use.

EvGr When managing withdrawal from **co-existing** benzodiazepine and alcohol dependence, the dose of benzodiazepine used for withdrawal should be increased. The initial daily dose is calculated, based on the requirements for alcohol withdrawal plus the equivalent regularly used daily dose of benzodiazepine. A single benzodiazepine (chlordiazepoxide hydrochloride p. 398 or diazepam p. 398) should be used rather than multiple benzodiazepines. Inpatient withdrawal regimens should last for 2–3 weeks or longer, depending on the severity of benzodiazepine dependence. When withdrawal is managed in the community, or where there is a high level of benzodiazepine dependence, or both, the regimen should last for a minimum of 3 weeks (according to the patient's symptoms).

If alcohol withdrawal seizures occur, a fast-acting benzodiazepine (such as lorazepam p. 393 [unlicensed indication]) should be prescribed to reduce the likelihood of further seizures. If alcohol withdrawal seizures develop in a person during treatment for acute alcohol withdrawal, review their withdrawal drug regimen.

Delirium tremens

EvGr Delirium tremens is a medical emergency that requires specialist inpatient care. In patients with delirium tremens (characterised by agitation, confusion, paranoia, and visual and auditory hallucinations), oral lorazepam p. 393 should be used as first-line treatment. If symptoms persist or oral medication is declined, parenteral lorazepam p. 393 [unlicensed], or haloperidol p. 445 [unlicensed] can be given as adjunctive therapy. If delirium tremens develops during treatment for acute alcohol withdrawal, the withdrawal drug regimen should also be reviewed.

Alcohol dependence

EvGr In harmful drinkers or patients with mild alcohol dependence, a psychological intervention (such as cognitive behavioural therapy) should be offered. In those who have not responded to psychological interventions alone or who have specifically requested a pharmacological treatment, acamprosate calcium p. 563 or oral naltrexone hydrochloride p. 564 can be used in combination with a psychological intervention.

Acamprosate calcium below or oral naltrexone hydrochloride p. 564 in combination with a psychological intervention are recommended for relapse prevention in patients with moderate and severe alcohol dependence, to start after successful assisted withdrawal. Disulfiram below is an alternative for patients in whom acamprosate calcium below and oral naltrexone hydrochloride p. 564 are not suitable, or if the patient prefers disulfiram below and understands the risks of taking the drug.

Nalmefene p. 564 is recommended for the reduction of alcohol consumption in patients with alcohol dependence who have a high drinking risk level, without physical withdrawal symptoms, and who do not require immediate detoxification (see *National funding/access decisions* for nalmefene p. 564).

Patients with severe alcohol-related hepatitis with a discriminant function of 32 or more can be given corticosteroids but only after any active infection or gastro-intestinal bleeding is treated, any renal impairment is controlled, and following discussion of the potential benefits and risks of treatment. Corticosteroid treatment has been shown to improve survival in the short term (1 month) but not over a longer term (3 months to 1 year). It has also been shown to increase the risk of serious infections within the first 3 months of starting treatment.

Patients with chronic alcohol-related pancreatitis should be offered nutritional support; those who have symptoms of steatorrhoea or who have poor nutritional status due to Exocrine pancreatic insufficiency p. 75 should be prescribed pancreatic enzyme supplements; supplements are not indicated when pain is the only symptom. Ⓐ

Wernicke's encephalopathy

EvGr Patients with alcohol dependence are at risk of developing Wernicke's encephalopathy; patients at high risk are those who are malnourished, at risk of malnourishment, or have decompensated liver disease. Parenteral thiamine p. 1238, followed by oral thiamine p. 1238, should be given to patients with suspected Wernicke's encephalopathy, those who are malnourished or at risk of malnourishment, those who have decompensated liver disease or who are attending hospital for acute treatment. Prophylactic oral thiamine p. 1238 should also be given to harmful or dependent drinkers if they are in acute withdrawal, or before and during assisted alcohol withdrawal. Ⓐ Parenteral thiamine is available as part of a vitamin B substances with ascorbic acid p. 1238 preparation.

Useful Resources

Alcohol-use disorders: diagnosis, assessment and management of harmful drinking and alcohol dependence. National Institute for Health and Care Excellence. Clinical guideline 115. February 2011.
www.nice.org.uk/guidance/cg115

Alcohol-use disorders: diagnosis and management of physical complications. National Institute for Health and Care Excellence. Clinical guideline 100. June 2010 (updated April 2017).
www.nice.org.uk/guidance/cg100

ALDEHYDE DEHYDROGENASE INHIBITORS

Disulfiram
15-Jun-2021

- **INDICATIONS AND DOSE**

Adjunct in the treatment of alcohol dependence (under expert supervision)
▶ BY MOUTH
▶ Adult: 200 mg daily, increased if necessary up to 500 mg daily

- **UNLICENSED USE** Disulfiram doses in BNF may differ from those in product literature.

- **CONTRA-INDICATIONS** Cardiac failure · coronary artery disease · history of cerebrovascular accident · hypertension · psychosis · severe personality disorder · suicide risk

- **CAUTIONS** Alcohol challenge **not** recommended on routine basis (if considered essential—specialist units only with resuscitation facilities) · avoid in Acute porphyrias p. 1202 · diabetes mellitus · epilepsy · respiratory disease

- **INTERACTIONS** → Appendix 1: disulfiram

- **SIDE-EFFECTS** Allergic dermatitis · breath odour · depression · drowsiness · encephalopathy · fatigue · hepatocellular injury · libido decreased · mania · nausea · nerve disorders · paranoia · psychotic disorder · vomiting

- **PREGNANCY** High concentrations of acetaldehyde which occur in presence of alcohol may be teratogenic; avoid in first trimester.

- **BREAST FEEDING** Avoid—no information available.

- **HEPATIC IMPAIRMENT** Manufacturer advises caution.

- **RENAL IMPAIRMENT** EvGr Use with caution. Ⓜ

- **PRE-TREATMENT SCREENING** Before initiating disulfiram, prescribers should evaluate the patient's suitability for treatment, because some patient factors, for example memory impairment or social circumstances, make compliance to treatment or abstinence from alcohol difficult.

- **MONITORING REQUIREMENTS** During treatment with disulfiram, patients should be monitored at least every 2 weeks for the first 2 months, then each month for the following 4 months, and at least every 6 months thereafter.

- **PATIENT AND CARER ADVICE** Manufacturer advises patients and their carers should be counselled on the disulfiram-alcohol reaction—reactions may occur following exposure to small amounts of alcohol found in perfume, aerosol sprays, or low alcohol and "non-alcohol" beers and wines; symptoms may be severe and life-threatening and can include nausea, flushing, palpitations, arrhythmias, hypotension, respiratory depression, and coma. EvGr Patients and their carers should be counselled on the signs of hepatotoxicity—patients should discontinue treatment and seek immediate medical attention if they feel unwell or symptoms such as fever or jaundice develop. Ⓐ

- **MEDICINAL FORMS** There can be variation in the licensing of different medicines containing the same drug.

Oral tablet
CAUTIONARY AND ADVISORY LABELS 2
▶ Disulfiram (Non-proprietary)
Disulfiram 200 mg Disulfiram 200mg tablets | 50 tablet PoM £228.21 DT = £210.55
Disulfiram 250 mg Antabuse 250mg tablets | 100 tablet PoM Ⓢ (Hospital only)
Disulfiram 500 mg Esperal 500mg tablets | 20 tablet PoM Ⓢ

GAMMA-AMINOBUTYRIC ACID ANALOGUES AND DERIVATIVES

Acamprosate calcium
24-Jun-2021

- **INDICATIONS AND DOSE**

Maintenance of abstinence in alcohol-dependent patients
▶ BY MOUTH
▶ Adult 18–65 years (body-weight up to 60 kg): 666 mg once daily, to be taken at breakfast and 333 mg twice daily, to be taken at midday and at night
▶ Adult 18–65 years (body-weight 60 kg and above): 666 mg 3 times a day

- **CAUTIONS** Continued alcohol abuse (risk of treatment failure)

4 Nervous system

- **SIDE-EFFECTS**
▶ **Common or very common** Abdominal pain · diarrhoea · flatulence · nausea · sexual dysfunction · skin reactions · vomiting
- **PREGNANCY** Manufacturer advises avoid unless potential benefit outweighs risk.
- **BREAST FEEDING** Avoid.
- **HEPATIC IMPAIRMENT** Manufacturer advises caution in severe hepatic failure—no information available.
- **RENAL IMPAIRMENT** EvGr Avoid in renal impairment if serum-creatinine greater than 120 micromol/litre. ⟨M⟩
- **PRESCRIBING AND DISPENSING INFORMATION** Acamprosate calcium has been used for the maintenance of abstinence in alcohol dependence in children aged 16 years and over.

- **MEDICINAL FORMS** There can be variation in the licensing of different medicines containing the same drug.
Gastro-resistant tablet
CAUTIONARY AND ADVISORY LABELS 5, 21, 25
ELECTROLYTES: May contain Calcium
  ▶ **Acamprosate calcium (Non-proprietary)**
  Acamprosate calcium 333 mg Acamprosate 333mg gastro-resistant tablets | 168 tablet PoM £39.20 DT = £23.99
  ▶ **Campral EC** (Merck Serono Ltd)
  Acamprosate calcium 333 mg Campral EC 333mg tablets | 168 tablet PoM £28.80 DT = £23.99

OPIOID RECEPTOR ANTAGONISTS

Nalmefene

20-May-2021

- **INDICATIONS AND DOSE**
Reduction of alcohol consumption in patients with alcohol dependence who have a high drinking risk level without physical withdrawal symptoms, and who do not require immediate detoxification
▶ BY MOUTH
  ▶ Adult: 18 mg daily if required, taken on each day there is a risk of drinking alcohol, preferably taken 1–2 hours before the anticipated time of drinking, if a dose has not been taken before drinking alcohol, 1 dose should be taken as soon as possible; maximum 18 mg per day

- **CONTRA-INDICATIONS** Recent history of acute alcohol withdrawal syndrome · recent or current opioid use
- **CAUTIONS** Continued treatment for more than 1 year · history of seizure disorders (including alcohol withdrawal seizures) · psychiatric illness
- **INTERACTIONS** → Appendix 1: nalmefene
- **SIDE-EFFECTS**
▶ **Common or very common** Appetite decreased · asthenia · concentration impaired · confusion · diarrhoea · dizziness · drowsiness · dry mouth · feeling abnormal · headache · hyperhidrosis · libido decreased · malaise · muscle spasms · nausea · palpitations · restlessness · sensation abnormal · sleep disorders · tachycardia · tremor · vomiting · weight decreased
▶ **Frequency not known** Dissociation · hallucinations
- **PREGNANCY** Manufacturer advises avoid—toxicity in *animal* studies.
- **BREAST FEEDING** Manufacturer advises avoid—present in milk in *animal* studies.
- **HEPATIC IMPAIRMENT** Manufacturer advises caution in mild to moderate impairment (risk of increased exposure); avoid in severe impairment (no information available).
- **RENAL IMPAIRMENT** EvGr Use with caution in mild to moderate impairment; avoid in severe impairment. ⟨M⟩
- **PRE-TREATMENT SCREENING** Before initiating treatment, prescribers should evaluate the patient's clinical status, alcohol dependence, and level of alcohol consumption.

Nalmefene should only be prescribed for patients who continue to have a high drinking risk level two weeks after the initial assessment.
- **MONITORING REQUIREMENTS** During treatment, patients should be monitored regularly and the need for continued treatment assessed.
- **NATIONAL FUNDING/ACCESS DECISIONS**
For full details see funding body website
NICE decisions
▶ **Nalmefene for reducing alcohol consumption in people with alcohol dependence (November 2014)** NICE TA325 Recommended with restrictions

- **MEDICINAL FORMS** There can be variation in the licensing of different medicines containing the same drug.
Oral tablet
CAUTIONARY AND ADVISORY LABELS 25
  ▶ **Selincro** (Lundbeck Ltd)
  Nalmefene (as Nalmefene hydrochloride) 18 mg Selincro 18mg tablets | 28 tablet PoM £84.84 DT = £84.84

Naltrexone hydrochloride

25-Feb-2025

- **DRUG ACTION** Naltrexone is an opioid-receptor antagonist.

- **INDICATIONS AND DOSE**
Adjunct to prevent relapse in formerly opioid-dependent patients (who have remained opioid-free for at least 7–10 days) (initiated under specialist supervision)
▶ BY MOUTH
  ▶ Adult: Initially 25 mg daily, then increased to 50 mg daily, total weekly dose may be divided and given on 3 days of the week for improved compliance (e.g. 100 mg on Monday and Wednesday, and 150 mg on Friday); maximum 350 mg per week

Adjunct to prevent relapse in formerly alcohol-dependent patients (initiated under specialist supervision)
▶ BY MOUTH
  ▶ Adult: 25 mg once daily on the first day, then increased if tolerated to 50 mg daily

Gambling-related harm (under expert supervision)
▶ BY MOUTH
  ▶ Adult: Initially 25 mg once daily for 3 days, then increased if tolerated to 50 mg once daily for 4–6 months, higher doses up to a max. of 150 mg daily may be given where clinically indicated

- **UNLICENSED USE** Naltrexone may be used as detailed below, although these situations are considered unlicensed:
  • initial dose of 25 mg once daily as adjunct to prevent relapse in formerly alcohol-dependent patients
  • EvGr Gambling-related harm ⟨A⟩
- **CONTRA-INDICATIONS** Patients currently dependent on opioids
- **CAUTIONS** Concomitant use of opioids
CAUTIONS, FURTHER INFORMATION
  ▶ Concomitant use of opioids Concomitant use of opioids should be avoided but increased dose of opioid analgesic may be required for pain—manufacturer advises to monitor for opioid intoxication.
- **INTERACTIONS** → Appendix 1: naltrexone
- **SIDE-EFFECTS**
▶ **Common or very common** Abdominal pain · anxiety · appetite abnormal · arthralgia · asthenia · chest pain · chills · constipation · diarrhoea · dizziness · eye disorders · headache · hyperhidrosis · mood altered · myalgia · nausea · palpitations · sexual dysfunction · skin reactions · sleep disorders · tachycardia · thirst · vomiting

▶ **Uncommon** Alopecia · confusion · cough · depression · drowsiness · dry mouth · dysphonia · dyspnoea · ear discomfort · eye discomfort · eye swelling · feeling hot · fever · flatulence · flushing · hallucination · hepatic disorders · lymphadenopathy · nasal complaints · oropharyngeal pain · pain · paranoia · peripheral coldness · seborrhoea · sinus disorder · sputum increased · tinnitus · tremor · ulcer · urinary disorders · vertigo · vision disorders · weight changes · yawning

▶ **Rare or very rare** Immune thrombocytopenic purpura · rhabdomyolysis · suicidal behaviours

▶ **Frequency not known** Withdrawal syndrome

● PREGNANCY Use only if benefit outweighs risk.

● BREAST FEEDING Avoid—potential toxicity.

● HEPATIC IMPAIRMENT Manufacturer advises caution in mild to moderate impairment; avoid in severe or acute impairment, acute hepatitis, or hepatic failure.
Dose adjustments Manufacturer advises consider dose adjustment in mild to moderate impairment.

● RENAL IMPAIRMENT [EvGr] Caution in mild to moderate impairment; avoid in severe impairment. Ⓜ
Dose adjustments [EvGr] Consider dose adjustment in mild to moderate impairment. Ⓜ

● PRE-TREATMENT SCREENING Test for opioid dependence with naloxone before treatment.

● MONITORING REQUIREMENTS Liver function tests needed before and during treatment.

● PATIENT AND CARER ADVICE Patients should be warned that an attempt to overcome the blockade of opioid receptors by overdosing could result in acute opioid intoxication.

● NATIONAL FUNDING/ACCESS DECISIONS
For full details see funding body website
NICE decisions
▶ **Naltrexone for the management of opioid dependence (January 2007) NICE TA115** Recommended

● MEDICINAL FORMS There can be variation in the licensing of different medicines containing the same drug. Forms available from special-order manufacturers include: oral capsule, oral suspension, oral solution
Oral tablet
▶ Naltrexone hydrochloride (Non-proprietary)
Naltrexone hydrochloride 50 mg Naltrexone 50mg tablets |
28 tablet [PoM] £23.00-£110.00 DT = £102.28
▶ Adepend (AOP Orphan Ltd)
Naltrexone hydrochloride 50 mg Adepend 50mg tablets |
28 tablet [PoM] £47.43 DT = £102.28

8.2 Nicotine dependence

Smoking cessation

08-Mar-2025

Overview

Smoking tobacco is the main cause of preventable illness and premature death in the UK. It is linked to a number of diseases such as cancer (primarily lung cancer), chronic obstructive pulmonary disease, and cardiovascular disease, and can lead to complications during pregnancy. Smoking cessation reduces the risk of developing or worsening of smoking-related illnesses, and the benefits begin as soon as an individual stops smoking.

Smoking cessation may be associated with temporary withdrawal symptoms caused by nicotine dependence, making it difficult for people to stop. These symptoms include nicotine cravings, irritability, depression, restlessness, poor concentration, light-headedness, sleep disturbances, and increased appetite. Weight gain is a concern for many people who stop smoking, however it is less likely to occur when drug treatment is used to aid smoking cessation.

Alternative forms of tobacco (smokeless tobacco) that are placed in the nose or mouth and not burned, are also associated with significant health risks such as oropharyngeal cancers, cardiovascular disease, and periodontal disease. As with smoking cessation, smokeless tobacco cessation reduces the risk of tobacco-related health problems, but may cause withdrawal symptoms.

Management

[EvGr] Individuals who use smokeless tobacco should be advised to stop, and be offered referral to local specialist tobacco cessation services for interventions and support. Ⓐ For further guidance on smokeless tobacco cessation, see NICE guideline: **Tobacco: preventing uptake, promoting quitting and treating dependence** (see *Useful resources*).
[EvGr] Individuals who smoke tobacco should be advised to stop smoking and be offered interventions and support to facilitate smoking cessation. They should also be advised that stopping in one step ('stop in one go') offers the best chance of lasting success, and that a combination of drug treatment and behavioural support is likely to be the most effective approach. The 'stop in one go' approach is when an individual makes a commitment to stop smoking on or before a particular date (the quit date), rather than by gradually reducing their smoking. Individuals who are unwilling, or not ready, to stop smoking in one go may benefit from a 'harm reduction approach' that includes cutting down before stopping smoking, reducing smoking (without intending to stop), or temporarily not smoking. Although existing evidence is not clear about the health benefits of smoking reduction, it may mean individuals are more likely to stop smoking altogether in the future.

Individuals who wish to stop or reduce their harm from smoking should be referred to local stop-smoking services, if appropriate, where they will be provided with advice, drug treatment, and behavioural support options such as individual counselling or group meetings. Attendance at Allen Carr's Easyway in-person group seminar may be offered as an alternative intervention. Individuals who decline referral to local stop-smoking services should be referred to a suitable healthcare professional who can also offer stop-smoking interventions.

Follow-up appointments should be offered to individuals attempting to stop smoking and those reducing their harm. Individuals who do not achieve their quitting or harm-reduction goals, should be encouraged to try again and the various intervention options available should be discussed. Ⓐ

Drug treatment

For guidance on smoking cessation during pregnancy, see *Pregnancy*.
[EvGr] Nicotine replacement therapy (NRT) p. 567, nicotine-receptor partial agonists (cytisinicline p. 567 or varenicline p. 570), and bupropion hydrochloride p. 566, are effective drug treatments to aid smoking cessation and should be offered alongside behavioural support. The choice of drug treatment should take into consideration the individual's likely adherence, preferences, and previous experience of smoking-cessation aids, as well as contra-indications and side-effects of each preparation. Cytisinicline, varenicline, or a combination of long-acting NRT (transdermal patch) and short-acting NRT (lozenges, gum, sublingual tablets, inhalator, nasal spray and oral spray), are the most effective treatment options and thus the preferred choices. If these options are not appropriate, bupropion hydrochloride or single therapy NRT should be considered instead. Ⓐ

Nicotine transdermal patches are generally applied for 16 hours, with the patch removed overnight; if individuals experience strong nicotine cravings upon waking, a 24-hour

Nervous system

4

patch can be used instead. Short-acting nicotine preparations are used whenever the urge to smoke occurs or to prevent cravings; there is no evidence that one form of NRT is more effective than another. [EvGr] The use of NRT combined with cytisinicline, varenicline, or bupropion hydrochloride is not recommended, and bupropion hydrochloride should not be prescribed with either cytisinicline or varenicline.

A quit date should be agreed when drug treatment is prescribed for smoking cessation, and treatment should be available before the individual stops smoking. For those who have successfully stopped smoking, offer the opportunity for a further course of varenicline, NRT, or bupropion hydrochloride [unlicensed] to prevent a relapse to smoking.

Individuals who are unwilling or not ready to stop smoking may also benefit from the use of NRT as part of a 'harm reduction approach', because the amount of nicotine in NRT is much lower and the way these products deliver nicotine makes them less addictive than smoking tobacco. These individuals should be advised that NRT will make it easier to reduce how much they smoke and improve their chance of stopping smoking in the long-term. NRT can be used for as long as needed to help prevent a return to previous levels of smoking. ⟨A⟩

E-cigarettes

E-cigarettes deliver nicotine without the toxins found in tobacco. Nicotine containing e-cigarettes have been shown to be of similar effectiveness to other cessation options such as varenicline or long-acting and short-acting NRT. It is likely that e-cigarettes are substantially less harmful to health than tobacco smoking and can help some individuals to stop smoking, but long-term effects are still largely unknown. [EvGr] People who wish to use e-cigarettes should be advised that although these products are not licensed drugs, they are regulated by the Tobacco and Related Products Regulations 2016. ⟨A⟩ The MHRA advises healthcare professionals to document e-cigarette use when taking a medical history, inform patients to be vigilant for suspected adverse reactions after use, and ensure that any suspected adverse reactions or safety concerns are reported to the Yellow Card scheme. In the UK, sale of e-cigarettes is prohibited in children under 18 years of age.

Pregnancy

[EvGr] Pregnant females should always be advised to stop smoking completely, and be informed about the risks to the unborn child of smoking during pregnancy and the harmful effects of exposure to second-hand smoke for both mother and baby. All pregnant females who smoke or have stopped smoking in the last 2 weeks should be referred to local stop-smoking services, and ongoing intensive support should be offered during and following pregnancy. For pregnant females who are reluctant or unable to attend stop-smoking services, consider alternative options such as home visits, and providing details for telephone quitlines or online stop-smoking support. Smoking cessation should also be encouraged for all members of the household.

Nicotine replacement therapy (NRT) p. 567 should be considered along with behavioural support at the earliest opportunity in pregnancy. Pregnant females should be advised that compared to smoking tobacco, using NRT has much lower risks and is less addictive because of the much lower amount of nicotine in NRT and the way these products deliver nicotine. NRT may be continued after pregnancy, if needed, to prevent a relapse to smoking. ⟨A⟩

Concomitant drugs

Polycyclic aromatic hydrocarbons found in tobacco smoke increase the metabolism of some drugs by inducing hepatic enzymes, often requiring an increase in dose. Information about drugs interacting with tobacco smoke can be found under *Interactions* of the relevant drug monograph.

Useful Resources

Tobacco: preventing uptake, promoting quitting and treating dependence. National Institute for Health and Care Excellence guideline NG209. November 2021, updated February 2025.
www.nice.org.uk/guidance/ng209

National Centre for Smoking Cessation and Training.
www.ncsct.co.uk

ANTIDEPRESSANTS › SEROTONIN AND NORADRENALINE RE-UPTAKE INHIBITORS

Bupropion hydrochloride
(Amfebutamone hydrochloride)

21-Apr-2021

● INDICATIONS AND DOSE

To aid smoking cessation in combination with motivational support in nicotine-dependent patients

► BY MOUTH

► Adult: Initially 150 mg daily for 6 days, then 150 mg twice daily (max. per dose 150 mg), minimum 8 hours between doses; period of treatment 7–9 weeks, start treatment 1–2 weeks before target stop date, discontinue if abstinence not achieved at 7 weeks, consider maximum 150 mg daily in patients with risk factors for seizures; maximum 300 mg per day

► Elderly: 150 mg daily for 7–9 weeks, start treatment 1–2 weeks before target stop date, discontinue if abstinence not achieved at 7 weeks; maximum 150 mg per day

IMPORTANT SAFETY INFORMATION

MHRA/CHM ADVICE: BUPROPION (*ZYBAN*®): RISK OF SEROTONIN SYNDROME WITH USE WITH OTHER SEROTONERGIC DRUGS (NOVEMBER 2020)

Cases of serotonin syndrome have been reported in patients taking bupropion with other serotonergic drugs, such as selective serotonin re-uptake inhibitors (SSRIs) and serotonin and noradrenaline re-uptake inhibitors (SNRIs); some cases were associated with an overdose of bupropion.

The MHRA reminds healthcare professionals not to exceed the recommended dose when prescribing bupropion with other serotonergic drugs; patients should be counselled on the milder symptoms of serotonin syndrome and advised to seek medical attention should these occur, particularly during treatment initiation and dose increases. They should also be advised to never exceed the prescribed dose of bupropion, and encouraged to read the patient information leaflet for information on side-effects. If serotonin syndrome is suspected, a dose reduction or discontinuation of bupropion, depending on the severity of the symptoms, should be considered.

● **CONTRA-INDICATIONS** Acute alcohol withdrawal · acute benzodiazepine withdrawal · bipolar disorder · CNS tumour · eating disorders · history of seizures · severe hepatic cirrhosis

● **CAUTIONS** Alcohol abuse · diabetes · elderly · history of head trauma · predisposition to seizures (prescribe only if benefit clearly outweighs risk)

● **INTERACTIONS** → Appendix 1: bupropion

● **SIDE-EFFECTS**

► **Common or very common** Abdominal pain · anxiety · concentration impaired · constipation · dizziness · dry mouth · fever · gastrointestinal disorder · headache · hyperhidrosis · hypersensitivity · insomnia (reduced by avoiding dose at bedtime) · nausea · skin reactions · taste altered · tremor · vomiting

► **Uncommon** Appetite decreased · asthenia · chest pain · confusion · tachycardia · tinnitus · vasodilation · visual impairment

► **Rare or very rare** Angioedema · arthralgia · behaviour abnormal · bronchospasm · delusions · depersonalisation · dyspnoea · hallucination · hepatic disorders · irritability · memory loss · movement disorders · muscle complaints · palpitations · paraesthesia · parkinsonism · postural hypotension · seizure · sleep disorders · Stevens-Johnson syndrome · syncope · urinary disorders

► **Frequency not known** Anaemia · hyponatraemia · leucopenia · psychosis · suicidal behaviours · thrombocytopenia

● **PREGNANCY** Avoid—no information available.

● **BREAST FEEDING** Present in milk—avoid.

● **HEPATIC IMPAIRMENT** Manufacturer advises use with caution—monitor closely for adverse effects; avoid in severe cirrhosis.
Dose adjustments Manufacturer advises reduce dose to 150 mg daily in mild to moderate impairment.

● **RENAL IMPAIRMENT** [EvGr] Use with caution. ⟨M⟩
Dose adjustments [EvGr] Reduce dose to 150 mg daily. ⟨M⟩

● **MONITORING REQUIREMENTS** Manufacturer advises monitor blood pressure before and during treatment.

● **PATIENT AND CARER ADVICE** Manufacturer advises patients and carers should be instructed to report any clinical worsening of depression, suicidal behaviour or thoughts and unusual changes in behaviour.
Driving and skilled tasks Manufacturer advises patients and carers should be counselled on the effects on driving and performance of skilled tasks—increased risk of dizziness and light-headedness.

● **MEDICINAL FORMS** There can be variation in the licensing of different medicines containing the same drug.
Modified-release tablet
CAUTIONARY AND ADVISORY LABELS 25
► Zyban (GlaxoSmithKline UK Ltd)
Bupropion hydrochloride 150 mg Zyban 150mg modified-release tablets | 60 tablet [PoM] £41.76 DT = £41.76

NICOTINIC RECEPTOR AGONISTS

Cytisinicline
05-Aug-2024

(Cytisine)

● **DRUG ACTION** Cytisinicline (cytisine), a plant alkaloid that resembles nicotine, is a nicotine-receptor partial agonist.

● **INDICATIONS AND DOSE**
To aid smoking cessation
► BY MOUTH
► Adult 18-65 years: Initially 1.5 mg every 2 hours from day 1 to 3, maximum 9 mg per day, then reduced to 1.5 mg every 2.5 hours from day 4 to 12, maximum 7.5 mg per day, smoking should be stopped no later than day 5, then reduced to 1.5 mg every 3 hours from day 13 to 16, maximum 6 mg per day, then reduced to 1.5 mg every 5 hours from day 17 to 20, maximum 4.5 mg per day, then reduced to 1.5–3 mg per day from day 21 to 25

● **CONTRA-INDICATIONS** Arrhythmias · recent myocardial infarction · recent stroke · unstable angina

● **CAUTIONS** Cardiovascular disease · diabetes · gastric and duodenal ulcer · gastro-oesophageal reflux disease · history of psychiatric illness (may exacerbate underlying illness including depression) · hyperthyroidism · peripheral vascular disease · phaeochromocytoma · schizophrenia

● **INTERACTIONS** → Appendix 1: cytisinicline

● **SIDE-EFFECTS**
► **Common or very common** Anxiety · appetite change · concentration impaired · constipation · diarrhoea · dizziness · drowsiness · dry mouth · fatigue · gastrointestinal discomfort · headaches · hypertension · malaise · mood altered · myalgia · nausea · oral disorders · skin reactions · sleep disorders · tachycardia · taste altered · vomiting · weight increased

► **Uncommon** Dyspnoea · excessive tearing · hyperhidrosis · libido decreased · sputum increased

● **CONCEPTION AND CONTRACEPTION** [EvGr] Females of childbearing potential should use highly effective contraception during treatment; additional barrier method recommended in females using hormonal contraceptives— effect on hormonal contraception unknown. ⟨M⟩

● **PREGNANCY** [EvGr] Avoid (limited information available). ⟨M⟩

● **BREAST FEEDING** [EvGr] Avoid (no information available). ⟨M⟩

● **PRESCRIBING AND DISPENSING INFORMATION** Discontinue if treatment fails and consider resuming after 2 to 3 months.

● **NATIONAL FUNDING/ACCESS DECISIONS**
For full details see funding body website
All Wales Medicines Strategy Group (AWMSG) decisions
► Cytisinicline (cytisine) for smoking cessation and reduction of nicotine cravings in smokers willing to stop smoking (July 2024) AWMSG No. 3708 Recommended

● **MEDICINAL FORMS** There can be variation in the licensing of different medicines containing the same drug.
Oral tablet
► Cytisinicline (Non-proprietary)
Cytisinicline 1.5 mg Cytisine 1.5mg tablets | 100 tablet [PoM] £115.00 DT = £115.00

Nicotine
17-Mar-2022

● **INDICATIONS AND DOSE**
Nicotine replacement therapy in individuals who smoke fewer than 20 cigarettes each day
► BY MOUTH USING CHEWING GUM
► Adult: 2 mg as required, chew 1 piece of gum when the urge to smoke occurs or to prevent cravings, if attempting smoking cessation, treatment should continue for 3 months before reducing the dose
► BY SUBLINGUAL ADMINISTRATION USING SUBLINGUAL TABLETS
► Adult: 1 tablet every 1 hour, increased to 2 tablets every 1 hour if required, if attempting smoking cessation, treatment should continue for up to 3 months before reducing the dose; maximum 40 tablets per day

Nicotine replacement therapy in individuals who smoke more than 20 cigarettes each day or who require more than 15 pieces of 2-mg strength gum each day
► BY MOUTH USING CHEWING GUM
► Adult: 4 mg as required, chew 1 piece of gum when the urge to smoke occurs or to prevent cravings, individuals should not exceed 15 pieces of 4-mg strength gum daily, if attempting smoking cessation, treatment should continue for 3 months before reducing the dose

Nicotine replacement therapy in individuals who smoke more than 20 cigarettes each day
► BY SUBLINGUAL ADMINISTRATION USING SUBLINGUAL TABLETS
► Adult: 2 tablets every 1 hour, if attempting smoking cessation, treatment should continue for up to 3 months before reducing the dose; maximum 40 tablets per day
continued →

4 — Nervous system

Nicotine replacement therapy
▶ BY INHALATION USING INHALATOR
▶ **Adult:** As required, the cartridges can be used when the urge to smoke occurs or to prevent cravings, individuals should not exceed 12 cartridges of the 10-mg strength daily, or 6 cartridges of the 15-mg strength daily
▶ BY MOUTH USING LOZENGES
▶ **Adult:** 1 lozenge every 1–2 hours as required, one lozenge should be used when the urge to smoke occurs, individuals who smoke less than 20 cigarettes each day should usually use the lower-strength lozenges; individuals who smoke more than 20 cigarettes each day and those who fail to stop smoking with the low-strength lozenges should use the higher-strength lozenges; If attempting smoking cessation, treatment should continue for 6–12 weeks before attempting a reduction in dose; maximum 15 lozenges per day
▶ BY MOUTH USING OROMUCOSAL SPRAY
▶ **Adult:** 1–2 sprays as required, individuals can spray in the mouth when the urge to smoke occurs or to prevent cravings, individuals should not exceed 2 sprays per episode (up to 4 sprays every hour); maximum 64 sprays per day
▶ BY INTRANASAL ADMINISTRATION USING NASAL SPRAY
▶ **Adult:** 1 spray as required, individuals can spray into each nostril when the urge to smoke occurs, up to twice every hour for 16 hours daily, if attempting smoking cessation, treatment should continue for 8 weeks before reducing the dose; maximum 64 sprays per day
▶ BY TRANSDERMAL APPLICATION USING PATCHES
▶ **Adult:** Individuals who smoke more than 10 cigarettes daily should apply a high-strength patch daily for 6–8 weeks, followed by the medium-strength patch for 2 weeks, and then the low-strength patch for the final 2 weeks; individuals who smoke fewer than 10 cigarettes daily can usually start with the medium-strength patch for 6–8 weeks, followed by the low-strength patch for 2–4 weeks; a slower titration schedule can be used in individuals who are not ready to quit but want to reduce cigarette consumption before a quit attempt; if abstinence is not achieved, or if withdrawal symptoms are experienced, the strength of the patch used should be maintained or increased until the patient is stabilised; individuals using the high-strength patch who experience excessive side-effects, that do not resolve within a few days, should change to a medium-strength patch for the remainder of the initial period and then use the low-strength patch for 2–4 weeks

● CAUTIONS

GENERAL CAUTIONS Diabetes mellitus—blood-glucose concentration should be monitored closely when initiating treatment · haemodynamically unstable patients hospitalised with cerebrovascular accident · haemodynamically unstable patients hospitalised with myocardial infarction · haemodynamically unstable patients hospitalised with severe arrhythmias · phaeochromocytoma · uncontrolled hyperthyroidism

SPECIFIC CAUTIONS
▶ When used by inhalation Bronchospastic disease · chronic throat disease · obstructive lung disease
▶ With intranasal use Bronchial asthma (may exacerbate)
▶ With oral use Gastritis (can be aggravated by swallowed nicotine) · *gum* may also stick to and damage dentures · oesophagitis (can be aggravated by swallowed nicotine) · peptic ulcers (can be aggravated by swallowed nicotine)
▶ With transdermal use *Patches* should not be placed on broken skin · patients with skin disorders

CAUTIONS, FURTHER INFORMATION Most warnings for nicotine replacement therapy also apply to continued cigarette smoking, but the risk of continued smoking outweighs any risks of using nicotine preparations.

Specific cautions for individual preparations are usually related to the local effect of nicotine.

● SIDE-EFFECTS

GENERAL SIDE-EFFECTS
▶ **Common or very common** Dizziness · headache · hyperhidrosis · nausea · palpitations · skin reactions · vomiting
▶ **Uncommon** Flushing

SPECIFIC SIDE-EFFECTS
▶ **Common or very common**
▶ When used by inhalation Asthenia · cough · dry mouth · flatulence · gastrointestinal discomfort · hiccups · hypersensitivity · nasal complaints · oral disorders · taste altered · throat complaints
▶ With intranasal use Chest discomfort · cough · dyspnoea · epistaxis · nasal complaints · paraesthesia · throat irritation
▶ With oral use Anxiety · appetite abnormal · burping · diarrhoea · dyspepsia (may be caused by swallowed nicotine) · gastrointestinal disorders · hiccups · increased risk of infection · mood altered · oral disorders · sleep disorders
▶ With sublingual use Asthenia · cough · dry mouth · flatulence · gastrointestinal discomfort · hiccups · hypersensitivity · oral disorders · rhinitis · taste altered · throat complaints
▶ **Uncommon**
▶ When used by inhalation Abnormal dreams · arrhythmias · bronchospasm · burping · chest discomfort · dysphonia · dyspnoea · hypertension · malaise
▶ With intranasal use Abnormal dreams · asthenia · hypertension · malaise
▶ With oral use Anger · asthma exacerbated · cough · dyspepsia aggravated · dysphagia · haemorrhage · laryngospasm · nasal complaints · nocturia · numbness · overdose · pain · palpitations exacerbated · peripheral oedema · tachycardia · taste altered · throat complaints · vascular disorders
▶ With sublingual use Abnormal dreams · arrhythmias · bronchospasm · burping · chest discomfort · dysphonia · dyspnoea · hypertension · malaise · nasal complaints
▶ With transdermal use Arrhythmias · asthenia · chest discomfort · dyspnoea · hypertension · malaise · myalgia · paraesthesia
▶ **Rare or very rare**
▶ When used by inhalation Dysphagia
▶ With intranasal use Arrhythmias
▶ With oral use Coagulation disorder · platelet disorder
▶ With sublingual use Dysphagia
▶ With transdermal use Abdominal discomfort · angioedema · pain in extremity
▶ **Frequency not known**
▶ When used by inhalation Angioedema · excessive tearing · vision blurred
▶ With intranasal use Abdominal discomfort · angioedema · excessive tearing · oropharyngeal complaints
▶ With sublingual use Excessive tearing · muscle tightness · vision blurred

SIDE-EFFECTS, FURTHER INFORMATION Some systemic effects occur on initiation of therapy, particularly if the patient is using high-strength preparations; however, the patient may confuse side-effects of the nicotine-replacement preparation with nicotine withdrawal symptoms. Common symptoms of nicotine withdrawal include malaise, headache, dizziness, sleep disturbance, coughing, influenza–like symptoms, depression, irritability, increased appetite, weight gain, restlessness, anxiety, drowsiness, aphthous ulcers, decreased heart rate, and impaired concentration.

● PREGNANCY EvGr The use of nicotine replacement therapy is preferable to the continuation of smoking.

Nicotine replacement therapy should be considered alongside behavioural support, at the earliest opportunity in pregnancy and continued after pregnancy if needed. If patches are used, they should be removed before bed. ⓐ See also *Pregnancy* in Smoking cessation p. 565.

- **BREAST FEEDING** Nicotine is present in milk; however, the amount to which the infant is exposed is small and less hazardous than second-hand smoke. Intermittent therapy is preferred.

- **HEPATIC IMPAIRMENT** Manufacturer advises caution in moderate to severe impairment (risk of decreased clearance).

- **RENAL IMPAIRMENT** EvGr Use with caution in severe renal impairment. ⓜ

- **DIRECTIONS FOR ADMINISTRATION** EvGr Acidic beverages, such as coffee or fruit juice, may decrease the absorption of nicotine through the buccal mucosa and should be avoided for 15 minutes before the use of oral nicotine replacement therapy. ⓜ
Administration by transdermal patch Patches should be applied on waking to dry, non-hairy skin on the hip, trunk, or upper arm and held in position for 10–20 seconds to ensure adhesion; place next patch on a different area and avoid using the same site for several days.
Administration by nasal spray EvGr Initially 1 spray should be used in both nostrils but when withdrawing from therapy, the dose can be gradually reduced to 1 spray in 1 nostril. ⓜ
Administration by oral spray The oral spray should be released into the mouth, holding the spray as close to the mouth as possible and avoiding the lips. The patient should not inhale while spraying and avoid swallowing for a few seconds after use. If using the oral spray for the first time, or if unit not used for 2 or more days, prime the unit before administration.
Administration by sublingual tablet Each tablet should be placed under the tongue and allowed to dissolve.
Administration by lozenge Slowly allow each lozenge to dissolve in the mouth; periodically move the lozenge from one side of the mouth to the other. Lozenges last for 10–30 minutes, depending on their size.
Administration by inhalation Insert the cartridge into the device and draw in air through the mouthpiece; each session can last for approximately 5 minutes. The amount of nicotine from 1 puff of the cartridge is less than that from a cigarette, therefore it is necessary to inhale more often than when smoking a cigarette. A single 15 mg cartridge lasts for approximately 40 minutes of intense use.
Administration by medicated chewing gum Chew the gum until the taste becomes strong, then rest it between the cheek and gum; when the taste starts to fade, repeat this process. One piece of gum lasts for approximately 30 minutes.

- **PRESCRIBING AND DISPENSING INFORMATION** Flavours of chewing gum and lozenges may include mint, freshfruit, freshmint, icy white, or cherry.

- **PATIENT AND CARER ADVICE** Patient or carers should be given advice on how to administer nicotine chewing gum, inhalators, lozenges, sublingual tablets, oral spray, nasal spray and patches.

- **MEDICINAL FORMS** There can be variation in the licensing of different medicines containing the same drug.

Spray
EXCIPIENTS: May contain Ethanol
- ▶ **Nicorette** (McNeil Products Ltd)
Nicotine 500 microgram per 1 dose Nicorette 500micrograms/dose nasal spray | 10 ml GSL £21.05 DT = £21.05
- ▶ **Nicorette QuickMist** (McNeil Products Ltd)
Nicotine 1 mg per 1 dose Nicorette QuickMist SmartTrack 1mg/dose mouthspray | 13.2 ml GSL £15.05 DT = £14.97 SF | 26.4 ml GSL £23.92 SF

Nicorette QuickMist 1mg/dose mouthspray freshmint | 13.2 ml GSL £14.97 DT = £14.97 SF | 26.4 ml GSL £23.29 SF
Nicorette QuickMist 1mg/dose mouthspray cool berry | 13.2 ml GSL £14.97 DT = £14.97 SF | 26.4 ml GSL £23.29 SF

Inhalation vapour impregnated plug
- ▶ **Nicorette** (McNeil Products Ltd)
Nicotine 15 mg Nicorette 15mg Inhalator | 4 cartridge GSL £6.43 DT = £6.43 | 20 cartridge GSL £22.64 DT = £22.64 | 36 cartridge GSL £35.66 DT = £35.66

Sublingual tablet
CAUTIONARY AND ADVISORY LABELS 26
- ▶ **Nicorette Microtab** (McNeil Products Ltd)
Nicotine (as Nicotine cyclodextrin complex) 2 mg Nicorette Microtab 2mg sublingual tablets | 100 tablet GSL £19.14 DT = £19.14 SF

Transdermal patch
- ▶ **NiQuitin** (Omega Pharma Ltd)
Nicotine 7 mg per 24 hour NiQuitin 7mg patches | 7 patch GSL £11.48 DT = £10.49
Nicotine 14 mg per 24 hour NiQuitin 14mg patches | 7 patch GSL £11.48 DT = £10.82
Nicotine 21 mg per 24 hour NiQuitin 21mg patches | 7 patch GSL £11.48 DT = £9.97
- ▶ **NiQuitin Clear** (Omega Pharma Ltd)
Nicotine 7 mg per 24 hour NiQuitin Clear 7mg patches | 7 patch GSL £11.48 DT = £10.49
Nicotine 14 mg per 24 hour NiQuitin Clear 14mg patches | 7 patch GSL £11.48 DT = £10.82 | 14 patch GSL £18.79
Nicotine 21 mg per 24 hour NiQuitin Clear 21mg patches | 7 patch GSL £11.48 DT = £9.97 | 14 patch GSL £18.79
NiQuitin Pre-Quit Clear 21mg patches | 7 patch GSL £11.48 DT = £9.97
- ▶ **Nicorette invisi** (McNeil Products Ltd)
Nicotine 10 mg per 16 hour Nicorette invisi 10mg/16hours patches | 7 patch GSL £11.40 DT = £11.40
Nicotine 15 mg per 16 hour Nicorette invisi 15mg/16hours patches | 7 patch GSL £11.43 DT = £11.43
Nicotine 25 mg per 16 hour Nicorette invisi 25mg/16hours patches | 7 patch GSL £11.40 DT = £11.40 | 14 patch GSL £18.72
- ▶ **Nicotinell TTS** (Haleon UK Trading Ltd)
Nicotine 7 mg per 24 hour Nicotinell TTS 10 patches | 7 patch GSL £10.49 DT = £10.49
Nicotine 14 mg per 24 hour Nicotinell TTS 20 patches | 7 patch GSL £10.82 DT = £10.82
Nicotine 21 mg per 24 hour Nicotinell TTS 30 patches | 7 patch GSL £11.48 DT = £9.97 | 21 patch GSL £28.20

Medicated chewing-gum
- ▶ **Nicorette** (McNeil Products Ltd)
Nicotine 2 mg Nicorette Freshmint 2mg medicated chewing gum | 30 piece GSL £4.80 SF | 105 piece GSL £11.89 DT = £11.89 SF | 210 piece GSL £19.34 SF
Nicorette Fruitfusion 2mg medicated chewing gum | 30 piece GSL £4.89 SF | 105 piece GSL £11.89 DT = £11.89 SF
Nicorette Original 2mg medicated chewing gum | 105 piece GSL £11.89 DT = £11.89 SF | 210 piece GSL £19.34 DT = £19.34 SF
Nicotine 4 mg Nicorette Fruitfusion 4mg medicated chewing gum | 105 piece GSL £14.55 DT = £14.55 SF
Nicorette Original 4mg medicated chewing gum | 105 piece GSL £14.55 DT = £14.55 SF | 210 piece GSL £23.93 DT = £23.93 SF
Nicorette Freshmint 4mg medicated chewing gum | 105 piece GSL £14.55 DT = £14.55 SF | 210 piece GSL £23.93 DT = £23.93 SF
- ▶ **Nicorette Icy White** (McNeil Products Ltd)
Nicotine 2 mg Nicorette Icy White 2mg medicated chewing gum | 30 piece GSL £4.80 SF | 105 piece GSL £11.89 DT = £11.89 SF | 210 piece GSL £19.34 DT = £19.34 SF
Nicotine 4 mg Nicorette Icy White 4mg medicated chewing gum | 105 piece GSL £14.55 DT = £14.55 SF
- ▶ **Nicotinell** (Haleon UK Trading Ltd)
Nicotine 2 mg Nicotinell Mint 2mg medicated chewing gum | 96 piece GSL £10.93 DT = £10.93 SF | 204 piece GSL £20.71 SF
Nicotinell Fruit 2mg medicated chewing gum | 96 piece GSL £10.93 DT = £10.93 SF | 204 piece GSL £20.71 SF
Nicotine 4 mg Nicotinell Mint 4mg medicated chewing gum | 96 piece GSL £13.57 DT = £13.57 SF
Nicotinell Fruit 4mg medicated chewing gum | 96 piece GSL £13.57 DT = £13.57 SF

Nervous system

4

Lozenge
EXCIPIENTS: May contain Aspartame
ELECTROLYTES: May contain Sodium
▸ **Nicotine (Non-proprietary)**
   Nicotine 4 mg Nicorette Fruit 4mg lozenges | 160 lozenge GSL
   £21.70 SF

Varenicline

05-Aug-2021

● **DRUG ACTION** Varenicline is a selective nicotine-receptor
partial agonist.

● **INDICATIONS AND DOSE**

To aid smoking cessation
▸ BY MOUTH
▸ Adult: Initially 500 micrograms once daily for 3 days,
   increased to 500 micrograms twice daily for 4 days,
   then 1 mg twice daily for 11 weeks; reduced if not
   tolerated to 500 micrograms twice daily, usually to be
   started 1–2 weeks before target stop date but can be
   started up to a maximum of 5 weeks before target stop
   date, 12-week course can be repeated in abstinent
   individuals to reduce risk of relapse

● **CAUTIONS** Conditions that may lower seizure threshold ·
history of cardiovascular disease · history of psychiatric
illness (may exacerbate underlying illness including
depression) · predisposition to seizures

● **SIDE-EFFECTS**
▸ **Common or very common** Appetite abnormal · asthenia ·
chest discomfort · constipation · diarrhoea · dizziness ·
drowsiness · dry mouth · gastrointestinal discomfort ·
gastrointestinal disorders · headache · joint disorders ·
muscle complaints · nausea · oral disorders · pain · skin
reactions · sleep disorders · vomiting · weight increased
▸ **Uncommon** Allergic rhinitis · anxiety · arrhythmias ·
behaviour abnormal · burping · conjunctivitis · depression ·
eye pain · fever · fungal infection · haemorrhage ·
hallucination · hot flush · hyperglycaemia · influenza like
illness · malaise · menorrhagia · mood swings · numbness ·
palpitations · seizure · sexual dysfunction · suicidal
ideation · sweat changes · thinking abnormal · tinnitus ·
tremor · urinary disorders
▸ **Rare or very rare** Angioedema · bradyphrenia ·
coordination abnormal · costochondritis · cyst · diabetes
mellitus · dysarthria · eye disorders · feeling cold ·
glycosuria · muscle tone increased · polydipsia · psychosis ·
scleral discolouration · severe cutaneous adverse reactions
(SCARs) · snoring · vaginal discharge · vision disorders
▸ **Frequency not known** Loss of consciousness

● **PREGNANCY** Avoid—toxicity in *animal* studies.

● **BREAST FEEDING** Avoid—present in milk in *animal* studies.

● **RENAL IMPAIRMENT**
Dose adjustments EvGr If creatinine clearance less than
30 mL/minute, initial dose 500 micrograms once daily,
increased after 3 days to 1 mg once daily. Ⓜ See p. 21.

● **TREATMENT CESSATION** Risk of relapse, irritability,
depression, and insomnia on discontinuation; consider
dose tapering on completion of 12-week course.

● **PATIENT AND CARER ADVICE**
Driving and skilled tasks Manufacturer advises patients and
carers should be cautioned on the effects on driving and
performance of skilled tasks—increased risk of dizziness,
somnolence, and transient loss of consciousness.

● **NATIONAL FUNDING/ACCESS DECISIONS**
For full details see funding body website
NICE decisions
▸ **Varenicline for smoking cessation (July 2007)** NICE TA123
Recommended

● **MEDICINAL FORMS** There can be variation in the licensing of
different medicines containing the same drug.
Oral tablet
CAUTIONARY AND ADVISORY LABELS 3
▸ **Varenicline (Non-proprietary)**
   Varenicline (as Varenicline tartrate) 500 microgram Varenicline
   500microgram tablets | 28 tablet PoM £23.21-£42.92 |
   56 tablet PoM £46.40-£76.00
   Varenicline (as Varenicline tartrate) 1 mg Varenicline 1mg tablets
   | 28 tablet PoM £23.20-£38.00 | 56 tablet PoM £46.40-£76.60
Form unstated
▸ **Varenicline (Non-proprietary)**
   Varenicline 1mg tablets and Varenicline 500microgram tablets |
   25 tablet PoM £23.20-£38.00 | 53 tablet PoM £56.50-£81.18

8.3 Opioid dependence

Other drugs used for Opioid dependence Buprenorphine,
p. 511 · Naltrexone hydrochloride, p. 564

ANALGESICS › OPIOIDS

◄ 510

Methadone hydrochloride

23-Sep-2024

● **INDICATIONS AND DOSE**

Severe pain
▸ BY MOUTH, OR BY SUBCUTANEOUS INJECTION, OR BY
   INTRAMUSCULAR INJECTION
▸ Adult: 5–10 mg every 6–8 hours, adjusted according to
   response, on prolonged use not to be given more
   frequently than every 12 hours

Adjunct in treatment of opioid dependence
▸ BY MOUTH USING ORAL SOLUTION
▸ Adult: Initially 10–30 mg daily, increased in steps of
   5–10 mg daily if required until no signs of withdrawal
   nor evidence of intoxication, dose to be increased in
   the first week, then increased every few days as
   necessary up to usual dose, maximum weekly dose
   increase of 30 mg; usual dose 60–120 mg daily

**Adjunct in treatment of opioid dependence if tolerance
low or not known**
▸ BY MOUTH USING ORAL SOLUTION
▸ Adult: Initially 10–20 mg daily, increased in steps of
   5–10 mg daily if required until no signs of withdrawal
   nor evidence of intoxication, dose to be increased in
   the first week, then increased every few days as
   necessary up to usual dose, maximum weekly dose
   increase of 30 mg; usual dose 60–120 mg daily

**Adjunct in treatment of opioid dependence if tolerance
high (under expert supervision)**
▸ BY MOUTH USING ORAL SOLUTION
▸ Adult: Initially up to 40 mg daily, increased in steps of
   5–10 mg daily if required until no signs of withdrawal
   nor evidence of intoxication, dose to be increased in
   the first week, then increased every few days as
   necessary up to usual dose, maximum weekly dose
   increase of 30 mg; usual dose 60–120 mg daily

Cough in palliative care
▸ INITIALLY BY MOUTH USING LINCTUS
▸ Adult: 1–2 mg every 4–6 hours, (by mouth) reduced to
   1–2 mg twice daily, use twice daily frequency if
   prolonged use

DOSE EQUIVALENCE AND CONVERSION
▸ See buprenorphine p. 511 for dose adjustments in
   opioid substitution therapy, for patients taking
   methadone who want to switch to buprenorphine.

- **UNLICENSED USE** Methadone hydrochloride doses for opioid dependence in the BNF may differ from those in the product literature.

> **IMPORTANT SAFETY INFORMATION**
> Many preparations of Methadone oral solution are licensed for opioid drug addiction only but some are also licensed for analgesia in severe pain.

- **CONTRA-INDICATIONS** Phaeochromocytoma
- **CAUTIONS** Risk factors for QT-interval prolongation
  CAUTIONS, FURTHER INFORMATION
  ► QT-interval prolongation [EvGr] ECG monitoring recommended in patients with the following risk factors for QT-interval prolongation while taking methadone: history of cardiac conduction abnormalities, family history of sudden death, heart or liver disease, electrolyte abnormalities, or concomitant treatment with drugs that can prolong QT interval; patients requiring more than 100 mg daily should also be monitored. Ⓜ

- **INTERACTIONS** → Appendix 1: opioids
- **SIDE-EFFECTS**

  GENERAL SIDE-EFFECTS Asthma exacerbated · dry eye · dysuria · hyperprolactinaemia · hypothermia · menstrual cycle irregularities · mood altered · nasal dryness · QT interval prolongation

  SPECIFIC SIDE-EFFECTS
  ► With oral use Galactorrhoea · intracranial pressure increased
  ► With parenteral use Biliary spasm · muscle rigidity · oedema · restlessness · sexual dysfunction · sleep disorder · ureteral spasm · withdrawal syndrome neonatal

  SIDE-EFFECTS, FURTHER INFORMATION Methadone is a long-acting opioid therefore effects may be cumulative.

  Methadone, even in low doses is a special hazard for children; non-dependent adults are also at risk of toxicity; dependent adults are at risk if tolerance is incorrectly assessed during induction.

  Overdose Methadone has a very long duration of action; patients may need to be monitored for long periods following large overdoses.

- **BREAST FEEDING** Withdrawal symptoms in infant; breast-feeding permissible during maintenance but dose should be as low as possible and infant monitored to avoid sedation (high doses of methadone carry an increased risk of sedation and respiratory depression in the neonate).

- **HEPATIC IMPAIRMENT** Manufacturer advises caution; consider avoiding in severe impairment (risk of increased exposure).
  Dose adjustments Manufacturer advises consider dose reduction.

- **RENAL IMPAIRMENT** Avoid use or reduce dose; opioid effects increased and prolonged and increased cerebral sensitivity occurs.

- **TREATMENT CESSATION** Avoid abrupt withdrawal.

- **PRESCRIBING AND DISPENSING INFORMATION** Flavours of oral liquid formulations may include tolu.

  Palliative care For further information on the use of methadone in palliative care, see www.medicinescomplete. com/#/content/palliative/methadone

  METHADOSE ® The final strength of the methadone mixture to be dispensed to the patient must be specified on the prescription.

  Important—care is required in prescribing and dispensing the **correct strength** since any confusion could lead to an overdose; this preparation should be dispensed only **after dilution** as appropriate with *Methadose* ® Diluent (life of diluted solution 3 months) and is for drug dependent persons.

- **NATIONAL FUNDING/ACCESS DECISIONS**
  For full details see funding body website
  NICE decisions
  ► **Methadone and buprenorphine for the management of opioid dependence (January 2007)** NICE TA114 Recommended

- **LESS SUITABLE FOR PRESCRIBING** Methadone linctus is less suitable for prescribing for cough in terminal disease (has a tendency to accumulate).

- **MEDICINAL FORMS** There can be variation in the licensing of different medicines containing the same drug. Forms available from special-order manufacturers include: oral tablet, oral capsule, oral suspension, oral solution, solution for injection

  Oral tablet
  CAUTIONARY AND ADVISORY LABELS 2
  ► **Methadone hydrochloride (Non-proprietary)**
    Methadone hydrochloride 5 mg Methadone 5mg tablets | 50 tablet [PoM] £17.33-£32.58 DT = £17.33 [CD2]

  Solution for injection
  ► **Methadone hydrochloride (Non-proprietary)**
    Methadone hydrochloride 10 mg per 1 ml Methadone 10mg/1ml solution for injection ampoules | 10 ampoule [PoM] £8.47-£13.54 DT = £8.47 [CD2]
    Methadone hydrochloride 50 mg per 1 ml Methadone 50mg/1ml solution for injection ampoules | 10 ampoule [PoM] £19.67-£31.46 DT = £19.67 [CD2]

  Oral solution
  CAUTIONARY AND ADVISORY LABELS 2
  ► **Methadone hydrochloride (Non-proprietary)**
    Methadone hydrochloride 1 mg per 1 ml Methadone 1mg/ml oral solution | 100 ml [PoM] £0.92-£1.20 DT = £0.92 [CD2] | 500 ml [PoM] £4.30-£5.40 DT = £4.60 [CD2] | 2500 ml [PoM] £23.00-£32.10 [CD2] Methadone 1mg/ml oral solution sugar free | 50 ml [PoM] £1.00 [CD2] [SF] | 100 ml [PoM] £1.20 DT = £0.92 [CD2] [SF] | 500 ml [PoM] £4.30-£6.00 DT = £4.60 [CD2] [SF] | 2500 ml [PoM] £23.00-£32.10 [CD2] [SF]
  ► **Methadose** (Rosemont Pharmaceuticals Ltd)
    Methadone hydrochloride 10 mg per 1 ml Methadose 10mg/ml oral solution concentrate | 150 ml [PoM] £12.01 DT = £12.01 [CD2] [SF] | 500 ml [PoM] £30.75 [CD2] [SF]
    Methadone hydrochloride 20 mg per 1 ml Methadose 20mg/ml oral solution concentrate | 150 ml [PoM] £24.02 DT = £24.02 [CD2] [SF]
  ► **Metharose** (Rosemont Pharmaceuticals Ltd)
    Methadone hydrochloride 1 mg per 1 ml Metharose 1mg/ml oral solution sugar free | 500 ml [PoM] £6.82 DT = £4.60 [CD2] [SF]
  ► **Physeptone** (Martindale Pharmaceuticals Ltd)
    Methadone hydrochloride 1 mg per 1 ml Physeptone 1mg/ml mixture | 100 ml [PoM] £1.27 DT = £0.92 [CD2] | 500 ml [PoM] £6.42 DT = £4.60 [CD2] | 2500 ml [PoM] £32.10 [CD2] Physeptone 1mg/ml oral solution sugar free | 100 ml [PoM] £1.27 DT = £0.92 [CD2] [SF] | 500 ml [PoM] £6.42 DT = £4.60 [CD2] [SF] | 2500 ml [PoM] £32.10 [CD2] [SF]

OPIOID RECEPTOR ANTAGONISTS

Buprenorphine with naloxone 18-Nov-2022

The properties listed below are those particular to the combination only. For the properties of the components please consider, buprenorphine p. 511, naloxone hydrochloride p. 1564.

- **INDICATIONS AND DOSE**

  Adjunct in the treatment of opioid dependence (dose expressed as buprenorphine) (under expert supervision)
  ► BY SUBLINGUAL ADMINISTRATION
  ► Adult: Initially 4 mg once daily, dose may be repeated up to twice on day 1 depending on the individual patient's requirement, then maintenance, dose adjusted according to response, total weekly dose may be divided and given on alternate days or 3 times weekly—consult product literature, for maintenance treatment, *Suboxone* ® sublingual film may alternatively be administered buccally; maximum 24 mg per day.

continued →

DOSE EQUIVALENCE AND CONVERSION

▶ [EvGr] *Suboxone*® sublingual tablets and sublingual film are **not** bioequivalent. If a switch of formulation is required, patients should be monitored for symptoms of overdose or withdrawal—consult product literature. Ⓜ

ZUBSOLV ®

Adjunct in the treatment of opioid dependence (dose expressed as buprenorphine) (under expert supervision)

▶ BY SUBLINGUAL ADMINISTRATION

▶ Adult 18-65 years: Initially 1.4–2.9 mg once daily, an additional 1.4 mg or 2.9 mg may be taken on day 1 depending on the individual patient's requirement, then maintenance, dose adjusted according to response, total weekly dose may be divided and given on alternate days or 3 times weekly—consult product literature; maximum 17.2 mg per day

DOSE EQUIVALENCE AND CONVERSION

▶ [EvGr] *Zubsolv*® is **not** interchangeable with other buprenorphine products on a milligram-for-milligram basis due to differences in bioavailability. Patients should not be switched between products. Ⓜ

● **INTERACTIONS** → Appendix 1: opioids

● **DIRECTIONS FOR ADMINISTRATION** [EvGr] For *Suboxone*® sublingual films, up to 2 films may be used at the same time if required to make up the prescribed dose, placed on opposite sides of the mouth. A third film may be administered if required once the first 2 films have dissolved Ⓜ.

● **NATIONAL FUNDING/ACCESS DECISIONS**
For full details see funding body website
Scottish Medicines Consortium (SMC) decisions

▶ Buprenorphine/naloxone (*Suboxone*®) as substitution treatment for opioid drug dependence (March 2007) SMC No. 355/07 Recommended with restrictions

▶ Buprenorphine/naloxone (*Suboxone*®) sublingual film as substitution treatment for opioid drug dependence (February 2021) SMC No. SMC2316 Recommended with restrictions

▶ Buprenorphine/naloxone (*Zubsolv*®) as substitution treatment for opioid drug dependence (November 2022) SMC No. SMC2123 Recommended with restrictions

All Wales Medicines Strategy Group (AWMSG) decisions

▶ Buprenorphine/naloxone (*Suboxone*®) sublingual film as substitution treatment for opioid drug dependence (April 2021) AWMSG No. 4590 Recommended with restrictions

● **MEDICINAL FORMS** There can be variation in the licensing of different medicines containing the same drug.

Sublingual tablet
CAUTIONARY AND ADVISORY LABELS 2, 26

▶ **Suboxone** (Indivior UK Ltd)
Naloxone (as Naloxone hydrochloride dihydrate) 500 microgram, Buprenorphine (as Buprenorphine hydrochloride) 2 mg Suboxone 2mg/500microgram sublingual tablets | 28 tablet [PoM] £25.40 DT = £25.40 [CD3] [SF]
Naloxone (as Naloxone hydrochloride dihydrate) 2 mg, Buprenorphine (as Buprenorphine hydrochloride) 8 mg Suboxone 8mg/2mg sublingual tablets | 28 tablet [PoM] £76.19 DT = £76.19 [CD3] [SF]
Naloxone (as Naloxone hydrochloride dihydrate) 4 mg, Buprenorphine (as Buprenorphine hydrochloride) 16 mg Suboxone 16mg/4mg sublingual tablets | 28 tablet [PoM] £152.38 DT = £152.38 [CD3] [SF]

▶ **Zubsolv** (Accord-UK Ltd)
Naloxone (as Naloxone hydrochloride dihydrate) 360 microgram, Buprenorphine (as Buprenorphine hydrochloride) 1.4 mg Zubsolv 1.4mg/0.36mg sublingual tablets | 28 tablet [PoM] £25.40 DT = £25.40 [CD3] [SF]
Naloxone (as Naloxone hydrochloride dihydrate) 710 microgram, Buprenorphine (as Buprenorphine hydrochloride) 2.9 mg Zubsolv 2.9mg/0.71mg sublingual tablets | 28 tablet [PoM] £38.77 DT = £38.77 [CD3] [SF]
Naloxone (as Naloxone hydrochloride dihydrate) 1.4 mg, Buprenorphine (as Buprenorphine hydrochloride) 5.7 mg Zubsolv 5.7mg/1.4mg sublingual tablets | 28 tablet [PoM] £76.19 DT = £76.19 [CD3] [SF]
Naloxone (as Naloxone hydrochloride dihydrate) 2.1 mg, Buprenorphine (as Buprenorphine hydrochloride) 8.6 mg Zubsolv 8.6mg/2.1mg sublingual tablets | 28 tablet [PoM] £118.08 DT = £118.08 [CD3] [SF]
Naloxone (as Naloxone hydrochloride dihydrate) 2.9 mg, Buprenorphine (as Buprenorphine hydrochloride) 11.4 mg Zubsolv 11.4mg/2.9mg sublingual tablets | 28 tablet [PoM] £152.38 DT = £152.38 [CD3] [SF]

SYMPATHOMIMETICS > ALPHA$_2$-ADRENOCEPTOR AGONISTS

Lofexidine hydrochloride
03-Apr-2020

● **DRUG ACTION** Lofexidine is an alpha$_2$-adrenergic agonist.

● **INDICATIONS AND DOSE**
Management of symptoms of opioid withdrawal

▶ BY MOUTH

▶ Adult: Initially 800 micrograms daily in divided doses, increased in steps of 400–800 micrograms daily (max. per dose 800 micrograms) as required recommended duration of treatment 7–10 days if no opioid use (but longer may be required); maximum 2.4 mg per day

● **CAUTIONS** Bradycardia · cerebrovascular disease · depression · hypotension (monitor pulse rate and blood pressure) · metabolic disturbances · recent myocardial infarction · risk factors for QT interval prolongation · severe coronary insufficiency

● **INTERACTIONS** → Appendix 1: lofexidine

● **SIDE-EFFECTS**

▶ **Common or very common** Bradycardia · dizziness · drowsiness · hypotension · mucosal dryness

▶ **Frequency not known** QT interval prolongation

● **PREGNANCY** Use only if benefit outweighs risk—no information available.

● **BREAST FEEDING** Use only if benefit outweighs risk—no information available.

● **RENAL IMPAIRMENT** Caution in chronic impairment.

● **MONITORING REQUIREMENTS** Monitoring of blood pressure and pulse rate is recommended on initiation, for at least 72 hours or until a stable dose is achieved, and on discontinuation.

● **TREATMENT CESSATION** Treatment should be withdrawn gradually over 2–4 days (or longer) to reduce the risk of rebound hypertension and associated symptoms.

● **PRESCRIBING AND DISPENSING INFORMATION** Lofexidine has been used in children over 12 years in the management of symptoms of opioid withdrawal.
Available from specialist importing companies.

● **PATIENT AND CARER ADVICE** The patient should take part of the dose at bedtime to offset insomnia associated with opioid withdrawal.

● **MEDICINAL FORMS** No licensed medicines listed.

Chapter 5
Infection

CONTENTS

1 Amoebic infection

> **Other drugs used for Amoebic infection** Metronidazole, p. 628

ANTIPROTOZOALS

Mepacrine hydrochloride   01-Jul-2020

- **INDICATIONS AND DOSE**

Giardiasis
▶ BY MOUTH
▶ Adult: 100 mg every 8 hours for 5–7 days

- **UNLICENSED USE** Not licensed for use in giardiasis.
- **CAUTIONS** Avoid in psoriasis · elderly · history of psychosis
- **INTERACTIONS** → Appendix 1: mepacrine
- **SIDE-EFFECTS** Aplastic anaemia (long term use) · central nervous system stimulation (with high doses) · corneal deposits · dermatosis (long term use) · dizziness · exfoliative dermatitis (severe; long term use) · gastrointestinal disorder · headache · hepatitis (long term use) · nail discolouration · nausea (with high doses) · oral discolouration · skin discolouration (long term use) · toxic psychosis (transient; with high doses) · urine discolouration (long term use) · visual impairment · vomiting (with high doses)
- **HEPATIC IMPAIRMENT** Use with caution.

- **MEDICINAL FORMS** There can be variation in the licensing of different medicines containing the same drug. Forms available from special-order manufacturers include: oral tablet

Oral tablet
CAUTIONARY AND ADVISORY LABELS 4, 9, 14, 21

2 Bacterial infection

Antibacterials, principles of therapy

15-Jan-2025

Antibacterial drug choice

Before selecting an antibacterial the clinician must first consider three factors— the patient, the known or likely causative organism, and the risk of bacterial resistance with repeated courses.

Factors related to the patient which must be considered include history of allergy, renal and hepatic function, susceptibility to infection (i.e. whether immunocompromised), ability to tolerate drugs by mouth, severity of illness, risk of complications, ethnic origin, age, whether taking other medication and, if female, whether pregnant, breast-feeding or taking an oral contraceptive.

The known or likely organism and its antibacterial sensitivity, in association with the factors above, will provide one or more antibacterial option. EvGr In patients receiving antibacterial prophylaxis, an antibacterial from a different class should be used. Ⓐ

Some patients may be at higher risk of treatment failure. They include those who have had repeated antibacterial courses, a previous or current culture with resistant bacteria, or those at higher risk of developing complications.

Antibacterials, considerations before starting therapy

The following precepts should be considered before starting:
- Viral infections should not be treated with antibacterials. However, antibacterials may be used to treat secondary bacterial infection (e.g. bacterial pneumonia secondary to influenza);
- Samples should be taken for culture and sensitivity testing as appropriate; '**blind**' antibacterial prescribing for unexplained pyrexia usually leads to further difficulty in establishing the diagnosis;
- Knowledge of **prevalent organisms** and their current sensitivity is of great help in choosing an antibacterial

before bacteriological confirmation is available. Generally, narrow-spectrum antibacterials are preferred to broad-spectrum antibacterials unless there is a clear clinical indication (e.g. life-threatening sepsis);

- The **dose** of an antibacterial varies according to a number of factors including age, weight, hepatic function, renal function, and severity of infection. The prescribing of the so-called 'standard' dose in serious infections may result in failure of treatment or even death of the patient; therefore it is important to prescribe a dose appropriate to the condition. An inadequate dose may also increase the likelihood of antibacterial resistance. On the other hand, for an antibacterial with a narrow margin between the toxic and therapeutic dose (e.g. an aminoglycoside) it is also important to avoid an excessive dose and the concentration of the drug in the plasma may need to be monitored;
- The **route** of administration of an antibacterial often depends on the severity of the infection. Life-threatening infections require intravenous therapy. Antibacterials that are well absorbed may be given by mouth even for some serious infections. Parenteral administration is also appropriate when the oral route cannot be used (e.g. because of vomiting) or if absorption is inadequate. Whenever possible, painful intramuscular injections should be avoided in children;
- **Duration** of therapy depends on the nature of the infection and the response to treatment. Courses should not be unduly prolonged because they encourage resistance, they may lead to side-effects and they are costly. However, in certain infections such as tuberculosis or osteomyelitis it may be necessary to treat for prolonged periods. The prescription for an antibacterial should specify the duration of treatment or the date when treatment is to be reviewed.

For further guidance on the appropriate and effective use of antibacterials, see Antimicrobial stewardship p. 18.

Advice to be given to patients and their family and/or carers

If an antibacterial is given, advise patients about directions for correct use and possible side-effects using verbal and written information.

If an antibacterial is **not** given, advise patients about an antibacterial not being needed currently—discuss alternative options as appropriate, such as self-care with over-the-counter preparations, back-up (delayed) prescribing, or other non-pharmacological interventions.

Patients should be advised to seek medical help if symptoms worsen rapidly or significantly at any time, if symptoms do not start to improve within an agreed time, if problems arise as a result of treatment, or if the patient becomes systemically very unwell.

For further information on advice for patients and their family and/or carers when deciding if antibacterial treatment is necessary, see *Advice for patients and their family and/or carers* in Antimicrobial stewardship p. 18.

Antibacterials, considerations during therapy

[EvGr] Review choice of antibacterial if susceptibility results indicate bacterial resistance and symptoms are not improving—consult local microbiologist as needed. ⬩ If no bacterium is cultured, the antibacterial can be continued or stopped on clinical grounds.

[EvGr] Review intravenous antibacterials within 48 hours and consider stepping down to oral antibacterials where possible. ⬩

Superinfection

In general, broad-spectrum antibacterial drugs such as the cephalosporins are more likely to be associated with adverse reactions related to the selection of resistant organisms e.g.

fungal infections or *antibiotic-associated colitis* (pseudomembranous colitis); other problems associated with superinfection include vaginitis and pruritus ani.

Notifiable diseases

In England, registered medical practitioners must report a suspected case of a notifiable disease listed below, or any other suspected infectious disease that may present a significant risk to human health as soon as possible. Urgent cases must be reported to the local health protection team by telephone within 24 hours, and all other cases reported using the online notification service within 3 days. For further information on reporting notifiable diseases, including the online service, see: **www.gov.uk/guidance/notifiable-diseases-and-how-to-report-them**.

Anthrax	Mpox (monkeypox)
Botulism	Mumps
Brucellosis	Paratyphoid fever
Cholera	Plague
COVID-19	Poliomyelitis (acute)
Diarrhoea (infectious bloody)	Rabies
Diphtheria	Rubella
Encephalitis (acute)	Severe acute respiratory
Food poisoning	syndrome (SARS)
Haemolytic uraemic syndrome	Scarlet fever
(HUS)	Smallpox
Haemorrhagic fever (viral)	Streptococcal disease (Group A,
Hepatitis (acute infectious)	invasive)
Legionnaires' disease	Tetanus
Leprosy	Tuberculosis
Malaria	Typhoid fever
Measles	Typhus
Meningitis (acute)	Whooping cough
Meningococcal septicaemia	Yellow fever

In Wales, information on notifiable diseases is available from Public Health Wales (**publichealthwales.nhs.wales/services-and-teams/aware-health-protection-team/**).

In Northern Ireland, information on notifiable diseases is available from the Public Health Agency (**www.niinfectioncontrolmanual.net/notifiable-diseases/**).

In Scotland, information on notifiable diseases is available from Public Health Scotland (**publichealthscotland.scot/our-areas-of-work/health-protection/notifiable-diseases-health-risk-states-and-infections/overview/**).

Antibacterials, use for prophylaxis

18-Aug-2024

Rheumatic fever: prevention of recurrence

- Phenoxymethylpenicillin p. 634 *or* sulfadiazine p. 654.

Invasive group A streptococcal infection: prevention of secondary cases

- Phenoxymethylpenicillin.
- Patients who are penicillin allergic: azithromycin p. 620 [unlicensed use], *or* clarithromycin p. 621 [unlicensed use], *or* erythromycin p. 624 (in pregnancy or within 28 days of giving birth).

The local health protection team should be contacted for advice on who should receive chemoprophylaxis. For further information, see UKHSA guidance: **UK guidelines for the management of contacts of invasive group A streptococcus (iGAS) infection in community settings** (see *Useful resources*).

Meningococcal disease: prevention of secondary cases

Neisseria meningitidis (meningococcus) can cause invasive meningococcal disease (IMD), including meningitis and septicaemia, albeit rarely. The aim of antibacterial prophylaxis is to eliminate asymptomatic carriage of *Neisseria meningitidis* from close contacts of the index case (including those with conjunctivitis), thereby reducing onward transmission and secondary cases.

Advice regarding the management of close contacts of a case of meningococcal disease should be sought from the local health protection team.

The following recommendations on antibacterial prophylaxis reflect advice from UKHSA **Guidance for public health management of meningococcal disease in the UK** (see *Useful resources*):

- Irrespective of vaccination status, antibacterial prophylaxis should be offered as soon as possible (ideally within 24 hours) after the diagnosis of the index case, to individuals who have had:
  ▸ Prolonged close contact with the index case (including conjunctivitis cases) in a household type setting during the 7 days before onset of illness.
  ▸ Sexual or other intimate contact during the 7 days before onset of illness.
  ▸ Transient close contact with the index case only if they have been directly exposed to large particle droplets or secretions from the respiratory tract of a case around the time of admission to hospital.

The health protection team will lead on contact tracing and advise on the need for antibacterial prophylaxis for individuals who do not clearly fall into these categories.

Index cases treated with cephalosporins (such as ceftriaxone or cefotaxime) do not require antibacterial prophylaxis. If the index case (including conjunctivitis cases) is treated with any other antibacterial drug, antibacterial prophylaxis should be offered when the individual is able to take oral medication, and ideally before discharge from hospital.

Vaccination against *Neisseria meningitidis* should also be considered for the index case and close contacts following a case of IMD. For information on vaccination, see Meningococcal vaccines p. 1486 and UKHSA: **Guidance for public health management of meningococcal disease in the UK** (see *Useful resources*).

Choice of antibacterial prophylaxis

- *First line*:
▸ Ciprofloxacin p. 648;
▸ Alternative if ciprofloxacin unsuitable, or if recent travel to the Middle East or Asia: rifampicin p. 674.
- *In pregnancy*:
▸ Ciprofloxacin, ceftriaxone p. 609 [unlicensed use], *or* azithromycin [unlicensed use].

Haemophilus influenzae type b infection: prevention of secondary disease

Haemophilus influenzae type b (Hib) can cause severe life-threatening disease in healthy individuals. With invasive Hib disease, the index case has a small, but significant risk of secondary Hib infection, particularly within 6 months of the first episode. Close contacts of the index case (mainly in a household, or a pre-school or primary school setting) are also at increased risk of developing invasive Hib disease, especially within the first week of the index case becoming ill. Antibacterial prophylaxis aims to reduce the risk of secondary disease in the index case and among close contacts by eliminating asymptomatic pharyngeal carriage of Hib.

The following recommendations on antibacterial prophylaxis reflect advice from Public Health England's (PHE) guidance: **Revised recommendations for the prevention of secondary *Haemophilus influenzae* type b (Hib) disease** (see *Useful resources*).

For confirmed or probable cases of invasive Hib disease in all children aged under 10 years, and in individuals of any age who have a vulnerable individual (any individual who is immunosuppressed or has asplenia, or any child aged under 10 years old) in their household, antibacterial prophylaxis should be given prior to hospital discharge.

All household contacts of a confirmed or probable index case should be given antibacterial prophylaxis if there is a vulnerable individual in the household.

For a pre-school or primary school setting that has an outbreak (2 or more cases of invasive Hib disease within 120 days), antibacterial prophylaxis is recommended for all room contacts, including staff.

For a pre-school or primary school setting where the levels of contact are similar to those in a household (e.g. a small number of children attending the same child-minder for several hours each day), antibacterial prophylaxis for the close contact group should be considered.

For all eligible contacts, antibacterial prophylaxis should be offered up to 4 weeks after illness onset in the index case.

In addition to antibacterial prophylaxis, vaccination with a Hib-containing vaccine should be considered following a case of invasive Hib disease. For information on vaccination, see *Post-exposure management of invasive Haemophilus influenzae type b disease* in Haemophilus influenzae type b conjugate vaccine p. 1479.

Choice of antibacterial prophylaxis

- *First line*:
▸ Rifampicin;
▸ Alternative if rifampicin unsuitable: ceftriaxone [unlicensed] (based on limited evidence), *or* oral ciprofloxacin [unlicensed] *or* azithromycin [unlicensed] (however effectiveness in healthy individuals has not been determined).

Diphtheria: prevention of secondary cases

The risk of infection with diphtheria is directly related to the closeness and duration of contact with diphtheria cases or asymptomatic carriers. Antibacterial prophylaxis aims to reduce the risk of secondary disease by treating incubating disease in recently exposed contacts and eliminating asymptomatic carriage of diphtheria.

Management of close contacts of confirmed or probable diphtheria cases or asymptomatic carriers is led by the local health protection teams.

The following recommendations on antibacterial prophylaxis reflect advice from UKHSA guidance: **Public health control and management of diphtheria in England** (see *Useful resources*).

Close contacts of a confirmed or probable case or asymptomatic carrier of diphtheria should be investigated immediately, kept under surveillance, and be given antibacterial prophylaxis. Close contacts include individuals who have contact with a case or known carrier in a household type of setting, or through kissing or sexual contact, or who have been exposed to respiratory droplets or an undressed wound of a cutaneous case where splash or droplet contamination has occurred (such as healthcare workers).

In addition to antibacterial prophylaxis, vaccination with a diphtheria-containing vaccine should be considered. For information on vaccination, see *Post-exposure management* in Diphtheria vaccine p. 1477.

Choice of antibacterial prophylaxis

- *First line*:
▸ Azithromycin p. 620 [unlicensed use], *or* clarithromycin p. 621 [unlicensed use], *or* erythromycin p. 624 (in pregnancy);

▸ Alternative if more easily administered: benzathine benzylpenicillin p. 632 [unlicensed use].

Pertussis: prevention of secondary cases

Pertussis is highly contagious and can spread rapidly from person-to-person through contact with infectious respiratory particles. Prolonged and close contact with an index case during their early catarrhal phase is typically required for significant risk of pertussis transmission to arise, but the index case can remain infectious for up to 21 days following the onset of coughing.

The following recommendations on antibacterial prophylaxis reflect advice from UKHSA: **Guidance on the management of cases of pertussis in England during the re-emergence of pertussis in 2024** (see *Useful resources*).

In households, healthcare and relevant community settings, antibacterial prophylaxis should be offered to close contacts of the index case if the onset of coughing in the index case was within the preceding 14 days, and the close contact is in a priority group for public health action. Group 1 priority group includes individuals at increased risk of severe complications from pertussis ('vulnerable'). Group 2 priority group includes individuals who are at increased risk of transmitting pertussis to a 'vulnerable' individual in group 1, and who have not received a pertussis-containing vaccine more than one week and less than 5 years ago.

For further information on priority groups for public health action and definitions of close contacts, see UKHSA: **Guidance on the management of cases of pertussis in England during the re-emergence of pertussis in 2024** (see *Useful resources*).

Choice of antibacterial prophylaxis

- *First line*:
▸ Azithromycin [unlicensed use], clarithromycin, *or* erythromycin;
▸ Alternative if macrolides contra-indicated or not tolerated: co-trimoxazole p. 652 [unlicensed use].
- *In pregnancy*:
▸ Erythromycin is the preferred macrolide, with azithromycin [unlicensed use] second line, and clarithromycin third line.

Pneumococcal infection in asplenia or in patients with sickle-cell disease, antibacterial prophylaxis

- Phenoxymethylpenicillin p. 634.
- If penicillin-allergic, erythromycin.

Antibacterial prophylaxis is not fully reliable. Antibacterial prophylaxis may be discontinued in children over 5 years of age with sickle-cell disease who have received pneumococcal immunisation and who do not have a history of severe pneumococcal infection.

Tuberculosis antibacterial prophylaxis in susceptible close contacts or those who have become tuberculin positive

See *Close contacts* and *Treatment of latent tuberculosis* under Tuberculosis p. 670.

Human and animal bites, antibacterial prophylaxis

See *Human and animal bites* in Skin infections, antibacterial therapy p. 589.

Early-onset neonatal infection, antibacterial prophylaxis

For guidance on antibacterials that can be offered to females during labour to prevent early-onset neonatal infection, see NICE guideline: **Neonatal infection** (see *Useful resources*).

Gastro-intestinal procedures, antibacterial prophylaxis

Operations on stomach or oesophagus

- Single dose of i/v gentamicin p. 596 *or* i/v cefuroxime p. 606 *or* i/v co-amoxiclav p. 638 (additional intra-operative or postoperative doses may be given for prolonged procedures or if there is major blood loss).

Intravenous antibacterial prophylaxis should be given up to 30 minutes before the procedure.

Add i/v teicoplanin p. 616 (*or* vancomycin p. 617) if high risk of meticillin-resistant *Staphylococcus aureus*.

Open biliary surgery

- Single dose of i/v cefuroxime + i/v metronidazole p. 628 *or* i/v gentamicin + i/v metronidazole *or* i/v co-amoxiclav alone (additional intra-operative or postoperative doses may be given for prolonged procedures or if there is major blood loss).

Intravenous antibacterial prophylaxis should be given up to 30 minutes before the procedure.

Where i/v metronidazole is suggested, it may alternatively be given by suppository but to allow adequate absorption, it should be given 2 hours before surgery.

Add i/v teicoplanin (*or* vancomycin) if high risk of meticillin-resistant *Staphylococcus aureus*.

Resections of colon and rectum for carcinoma, and resections in inflammatory bowel disease, and appendicectomy

- Single dose of i/v gentamicin + i/v metronidazole *or* i/v cefuroxime + i/v metronidazole *or* i/v co-amoxiclav alone (additional intra-operative or postoperative doses may be given for prolonged procedures or if there is major blood loss).

Intravenous antibacterial prophylaxis should be given up to 30 minutes before the procedure.

Where i/v metronidazole is suggested, it may alternatively be given by suppository but to allow adequate absorption, it should be given 2 hours before surgery.

Add i/v teicoplanin (*or* vancomycin) if high risk of meticillin-resistant *Staphylococcus aureus*.

Endoscopic retrograde cholangiopancreatography

- Single dose of i/v gentamicin *or* oral *or* i/v ciprofloxacin p. 648.

Intravenous antibacterial prophylaxis should be given up to 30 minutes before the procedure.

Prophylaxis recommended if pancreatic pseudocyst, immunocompromised, history of liver transplantation, or risk of incomplete biliary drainage. For biliary complications following liver transplantation, add i/v amoxicillin p. 635 or i/v teicoplanin (*or* vancomycin).

Percutaneous endoscopic gastrostomy or jejunostomy

- Single dose of i/v co-amoxiclav *or* i/v cefuroxime.

Intravenous antibacterial prophylaxis should be given up to 30 minutes before the procedure.

Use single dose of i/v teicoplanin (*or* vancomycin) if history of allergy to penicillins or cephalosporins, or if high risk of meticillin-resistant *Staphylococcus aureus*.

Orthopaedic surgery, antibacterial prophylaxis

Joint replacement including hip and knee

- Single dose of i/v cefuroxime alone *or* i/v flucloxacillin p. 643 + i/v gentamicin (additional intra-operative or postoperative doses may be given for prolonged procedures or if there is major blood loss).

Intravenous antibacterial prophylaxis should be given up to 30 minutes before the procedure.

If history of allergy to penicillins or to cephalosporins or if high risk of meticillin-resistant *Staphylococcus aureus*, use single dose of i/v teicoplanin (*or* vancomycin) + i/v gentamicin (additional intra-operative or postoperative doses may be given for prolonged procedures or if there is major blood loss).

Closed fractures

- Single dose of i/v cefuroxime *or* i/v flucloxacillin (additional intra-operative or postoperative doses may be given for prolonged procedures or if there is major blood loss).

Intravenous antibacterial prophylaxis should be given up to 30 minutes before the procedure.

If history of allergy to penicillins or to cephalosporins or if high risk of meticillin-resistant *Staphylococcus aureus*, use single dose of i/v teicoplanin (*or* vancomycin) (additional intra-operative or postoperative doses may be given for prolonged procedures or if there is major blood loss).

Open fractures

- Use i/v co-amoxiclav alone *or* i/v cefuroxime + i/v metronidazole (*or* i/v clindamycin p. 618 alone if history of allergy to penicillins or to cephalosporins).

Add i/v teicoplanin (*or* vancomycin) if high risk of meticillin-resistant *Staphylococcus aureus*. Start prophylaxis within 3 hours of injury and continue until soft tissue closure (max. 72 hours).

At first debridement also use a single dose of i/v cefuroxime p. 606 + i/v metronidazole p. 628 + i/v gentamicin p. 596 *or* i/v co-amoxiclav p. 638 + i/v gentamicin (*or* i/v clindamycin p. 618 + i/v gentamicin if history of allergy to penicillins or to cephalosporins).

At time of skeletal stabilisation and definitive soft tissue closure use a single dose of i/v gentamicin + i/v teicoplanin p. 616 (*or* vancomycin p. 617) (intravenous antibacterial prophylaxis should be given up to 30 minutes before the procedure).

High lower-limb amputation

- Use i/v co-amoxiclav alone *or* i/v cefuroxime + i/v metronidazole.

Intravenous antibacterial prophylaxis should be given up to 30 minutes before the procedure.

Continue antibacterial prophylaxis for at least 2 doses after procedure (max. duration of prophylaxis 5 days). If history of allergy to penicillin or to cephalosporins, or if high risk of meticillin-resistant *Staphylococcus aureus*, use i/v teicoplanin (*or* vancomycin) + i/v gentamicin + i/v metronidazole.

Where i/v metronidazole is suggested, it may alternatively be given by suppository but to allow adequate absorption, it should be given 2 hours before surgery.

Urological procedures, antibacterial prophylaxis

Transrectal prostate biopsy

- Single dose of oral ciprofloxacin p. 648 + oral metronidazole *or* i/v gentamicin + i/v metronidazole (additional intra-operative or postoperative doses may be given for prolonged procedures or if there is major blood loss).

Intravenous antibacterial prophylaxis should be given up to 30 minutes before the procedure.

Use single dose of i/v gentamicin + i/v metronidazole if high risk of meticillin-resistant *Staphylococcus aureus* (additional intra-operative or postoperative doses of antibacterial may be given for prolonged procedures or if there is major blood loss).

Where i/v metronidazole is suggested, it may alternatively be given by suppository but to allow adequate absorption, it should be given 2 hours before surgery.

Transurethral resection of prostate

- Single dose of oral ciprofloxacin *or* i/v gentamicin *or* i/v cefuroxime (additional intra-operative or postoperative doses may be given for prolonged procedures or if there is major blood loss).

Intravenous antibacterial prophylaxis should be given up to 30 minutes before the procedure.

Use single dose of i/v gentamicin if high risk of meticillin-resistant *Staphylococcus aureus* (additional intra-operative or postoperative doses may be given for prolonged procedures or if there is major blood loss).

Preterm prelabour rupture of membranes (P-PROM): prevention of intra-uterine infection

- [EvGr] Erythromycin p. 624. [A]
- Alternative if oral erythromycin is contra-indicated or unsuitable: [EvGr] consider an oral penicillin for up to 10 days or until established labour, whichever is sooner. [A]

For further guidance on P-PROM, see NICE guideline: **Preterm labour and birth** (see *Useful resources*).

Assisted vaginal birth (ventouse or forceps), antibacterial prophylaxis

- [EvGr] Single dose of i/v co-amoxiclav given within 6 hours after cord clamping.
- If penicillin allergic, use a locally agreed alternative. [A]

For further guidance on assisted vaginal birth, see NICE guideline: **Intrapartum care** (see *Useful resources*).

Obstetric and gynaecological surgery, antibacterial prophylaxis

Caesarean section

- Single dose of i/v cefuroxime (additional intra-operative or postoperative doses may be given for prolonged procedures or if there is major blood loss).

Intravenous antibacterial prophylaxis should be given up to 30 minutes before the procedure.

Substitute i/v clindamycin if history of allergy to penicillins or cephalosporins. Add i/v teicoplanin (*or* vancomycin) if high risk of meticillin-resistant *Staphylococcus aureus*.

Hysterectomy

- Single dose of i/v cefuroxime + i/v metronidazole *or* i/v gentamicin + i/v metronidazole *or* i/v co-amoxiclav alone (additional intra-operative or postoperative doses may be given for prolonged procedures or if there is major blood loss).

Intravenous antibacterial prophylaxis should be given up to 30 minutes before the procedure.

Use single dose of i/v gentamicin + i/v metronidazole or add i/v teicoplanin (*or* vancomycin) to other regimens if high risk of meticillin-resistant *Staphylococcus aureus* (additional intra-operative or postoperative doses may be given for prolonged procedures or if there is major blood loss).

Where i/v metronidazole is suggested, it may alternatively be given by suppository but to allow adequate absorption, it should be given 2 hours before surgery.

Termination of pregnancy

- Single dose of oral metronidazole (additional intra-operative or postoperative doses may be given for prolonged procedures or if there is major blood loss).

If genital chlamydial infection cannot be ruled out, give doxycycline p. 655 postoperatively.

Cardiology procedures, antibacterial prophylaxis

Cardiac pacemaker insertion

- Single dose of i/v cefuroxime alone *or* i/v flucloxacillin p. 643 + i/v gentamicin *or* i/v teicoplanin (*or* vancomycin) + i/v gentamicin (additional intra-operative or postoperative doses may be given for prolonged procedures or if there is major blood loss).

Intravenous antibacterial prophylaxis should be given up to 30 minutes before the procedure.

Use single dose of i/v teicoplanin (*or* vancomycin) + i/v cefuroxime *or* i/v teicoplanin (*or* vancomycin) + i/v gentamicin if high risk of meticillin-resistant *Staphylococcus aureus* (additional intra-operative or postoperative doses may be given for prolonged procedures or if there is major blood loss).

Vascular surgery, antibacterial prophylaxis

Reconstructive arterial surgery of abdomen, pelvis or legs

- Single dose of i/v cefuroxime alone *or* i/v flucloxacillin + i/v gentamicin (additional intra-operative or postoperative doses may be given for prolonged procedures or if there is major blood loss).

Intravenous antibacterial prophylaxis should be given up to 30 minutes before the procedure.

Add i/v metronidazole for patients at risk from anaerobic infections including those with diabetes, gangrene, or undergoing amputation. Use single dose of i/v teicoplanin (*or* vancomycin) + i/v gentamicin if history of allergy to penicillins or cephalosporins, or if high risk of meticillin-resistant *Staphylococcus aureus* (additional intra-operative or postoperative doses may be given for prolonged procedures or if there is major blood loss).

Infective endocarditis, antibacterial prophylaxis

NICE guidance: Antimicrobial prophylaxis against infective endocarditis in adults and children undergoing interventional procedures (March 2008, updated 2016)

- Chlorhexidine mouthwash is **not** recommended for the prevention of infective endocarditis in at risk patients undergoing dental procedures.

Antibacterial prophylaxis is **not** *routinely* recommended for the prevention of infective endocarditis in patients undergoing the following procedures:

- dental;
- upper and lower respiratory tract (including ear, nose, and throat procedures and bronchoscopy);
- genito-urinary tract (including urological, gynaecological, and obstetric procedures);
- upper and lower gastro-intestinal tract.

Whilst these procedures can cause bacteraemia, there is no clear association with the development of infective endocarditis. Prophylaxis may expose patients to the adverse effects of antimicrobials when the evidence of benefit has not been proven.

Any infection in patients at risk of endocarditis should be investigated promptly and treated appropriately to reduce the risk of endocarditis.

If patients at risk of endocarditis are undergoing a gastro-intestinal or genito-urinary tract procedure at a site where infection is suspected, they should receive appropriate antibacterial therapy that includes cover against organisms that cause infective endocarditis.

Patients at risk of infective endocarditis should be:

- advised to maintain good oral hygiene;
- told how to recognise signs of infective endocarditis, and advised when to seek expert advice.

Patients at risk of infective endocarditis include those with valve replacement, acquired valvular heart disease with stenosis or regurgitation, structural congenital heart disease (including surgically corrected or palliated structural conditions, but excluding isolated atrial septal defect, fully repaired ventricular septal defect, fully repaired patent ductus arteriosus, and closure devices considered to be endothelialised), hypertrophic cardiomyopathy, or a previous episode of infective endocarditis.

Dermatological procedures

Advice of a Working Party of the British Society for Antimicrobial Chemotherapy is that patients who undergo dermatological procedures do not require antibacterial prophylaxis against endocarditis.

The British Association of Dermatologists Therapy Guidelines and Audit Subcommittee advise that such dermatological procedures include skin biopsies and excision of moles or of malignant lesions.

Joint prostheses and dental treatment, antibacterial prophylaxis

Advice of a Working Party of the British Society for Antimicrobial Chemotherapy is that patients with prosthetic joint implants (including total hip replacements) do not require antibiotic prophylaxis for dental treatment. The Working Party considers that it is unacceptable to expose patients to the adverse effects of antibiotics when there is no evidence that such prophylaxis is of any benefit, but that those who develop any intercurrent infection require prompt treatment with antibiotics to which the infecting organisms are sensitive.

The Working Party has commented that joint infections have rarely been shown to follow dental procedures and are even more rarely caused by oral streptococci.

Immunosuppression and indwelling intraperitoneal catheters

Advice of a Working Party of the British Society for Antimicrobial Chemotherapy is that patients who are immunosuppressed (including transplant patients) and patients with indwelling intraperitoneal catheters do not require antibiotic prophylaxis for dental treatment provided there is no other indication for prophylaxis.

The Working Party has commented that there is little evidence that dental treatment is followed by infection in immunosuppressed and immunodeficient patients nor is there evidence that dental treatment is followed by infection in patients with indwelling intraperitoneal catheters.

Useful Resources

Intrapartum care. National Institute for Health and Care Excellence. NICE guideline 235. September 2023.
www.nice.org.uk/guidance/ng235

Neonatal infection: antibiotics for prevention and treatment. National Institute for Health and Care Excellence. NICE guideline 195. April 2021.
www.nice.org.uk/guidance/ng195

Preterm labour and birth. National Institute for Health and Care Excellence. NICE guideline 25. November 2015 (updated June 2022).
www.nice.org.uk/guidance/ng25

UK guidelines for the management of contacts of invasive group A streptococcus (iGAS) infection in community settings. UK Health Security Agency. March 2023.
www.gov.uk/government/publications/invasive-group-a-streptococcal-disease-managing-community-contacts

Revised recommendations for the prevention of secondary *Haemophilus influenzae* type b (Hib) disease. Public Health England. 2009 (updated July 2013).
www.gov.uk/government/publications/haemophilus-influenzae-type-b-hib-revised-recommendations-for-the-prevention-of-secondary-cases

Public health control and management of diphtheria in England. UK Health Security Agency. November 2023.
www.gov.uk/government/publications/diphtheria-public-health-control-and-management-in-england-and-wales

Guidance for public health management of meningococcal disease in the UK. UK Health Security Agency. 2018, updated September 2024.
www.gov.uk/government/publications/meningococcal-disease-guidance-on-public-health-management

Guidance on the management of cases of pertussis in England during the re-emergence of pertussis in 2024. UK

Health Security Agency. February 2024, updated August 2024.

www.gov.uk/government/publications/pertussis-guidelines-for-public-health-management

Sepsis

15-Jan-2025

Overview

Sepsis is a clinical syndrome caused by activation of the body's immune and coagulation systems due to infection. It is defined as life-threatening organ dysfunction caused by a dysregulated host response to an infection. Septic shock is a subset of sepsis, which describes circulatory, cellular, and metabolic abnormalities, with raised serum lactate and persistent hypotension despite fluid replacement; it carries a greater risk of mortality than sepsis alone. Signs and symptoms of sepsis can be very non-specific and variable. The risk of sepsis should be considered in anyone presenting with possible infection; early recognition and prompt treatment is essential in improving outcomes in patients who are deteriorating and at risk of organ dysfunction and death.

Initial management of suspected or confirmed sepsis

For additional guidance on the management of meningococcal septicaemia, including **choice of antibacterial therapy**, see Central nervous system infections, antibacterial therapy p. 580.

EvGr In patients with suspected or confirmed sepsis, a systematic approach should be used to assess their risk of severe illness or death, and of deterioration due to sepsis. The risk should be re-evaluated at regular intervals depending on sepsis severity (alongside other clinical parameters), or if there is a deterioration or unexpected change in the patient's condition. ⒶFor information on assessing the risk of severe illness or death using criteria for risk stratification *or* the National Early Warning Score 2 (NEWS2) as appropriate (alongside other considerations), and for guidance on urgent transfer to hospital, monitoring and escalation of care, see NICE guideline: **Suspected sepsis: recognition, diagnosis and early management** (see *Useful resources*).

EvGr Neutropenic sepsis should be suspected in unwell patients who have received systemic anticancer treatment in the last 30 days, or who have received or are receiving immunosuppressant treatment for reasons unrelated to cancer. ⒶFor guidance on the management of neutropenic sepsis, see NICE CG151: **Neutropenic sepsis: prevention and management in people with cancer** (available at: www.nice.org.uk/guidance/cg151).

Initial treatment of suspected or confirmed sepsis includes the use of intravenous antibacterials, fluid resuscitation, inotropes/vasopressors, and oxygen, as clinically indicated.

Pre-hospital antibacterial therapy

EvGr For patients in remote or rural locations with suspected sepsis and high-risk criteria for severe illness or death, antibacterial treatment should be given prior to hospital transfer according to local policy/guidance if the combined transfer and handover time to the emergency department is likely to be longer than 1 hour. Ⓐ

Antibacterial therapy in hospital

EvGr Microbiological and blood samples should be taken before administering antibacterial treatment.

Patients who require empirical antibacterial treatment for suspected sepsis but who have no confirmed diagnosis, should be given broad-spectrum intravenous antibacterial treatment according to local guidelines. A thorough clinical examination should be carried out to identify sources of infection. If there is a clear source of infection, treat in line with local antimicrobial guidance for that condition.

The time-frame during which antibacterials should be administered depends on assessment of the patient's risk of severe illness or death from sepsis. For patients assessed as high-risk of severe illness or death, antibacterial treatment should be administered within 1 hour of severity assessment (if not already given prior to hospital transfer).

The purpose of deferring antibacterial administration in non-high risk sepsis is to allow time to gather information for a more specific diagnosis, and therefore targeted treatment. Once a decision is made to give antibacterials, administration should not be delayed. ⒶFor guidance on timing of antibacterials for patients not assessed as high-risk, see NICE guideline: **Suspected sepsis: recognition, diagnosis and early management** (see *Useful resources*).

EvGr When the source of infection is confirmed or microbiological results are available, the choice of antibacterial should be reviewed, and where appropriate changed to a narrower-spectrum agent. Ⓐ

Intravenous fluids and inotropes/vasopressors

EvGr The need for intravenous fluids should be assessed without delay, taking into consideration the patient's lactate concentration, systolic blood pressure, and their risk of severe illness or death. If fluid resuscitation is indicated, a crystalloid with a sodium content in the range of 130–154 mmol/litre should be used, with a bolus of 500 mL given over less than 15 minutes (within 1 hour of identifying that they are at high risk). A second bolus may be given if there is no improvement. For guidance on sodium content of crystalloids, see Fluids and electrolytes p. 1175. Human albumin solution (4–5 %) should be considered for fluid resuscitation only in patients with septic shock. Where appropriate, patients should also be assessed by a critical care specialist for inotropic or vasopressor support. ⒶFor further guidance, see NICE guideline: **Suspected sepsis: recognition, diagnosis and early management** (see *Useful resources*).

Oxygen

EvGr Oxygen should be given if required to achieve a target saturation of 94–98 %, or 88–92 % for those at risk of hypercapnic respiratory failure. Ⓐ

Useful Resources

Suspected sepsis: recognition, diagnosis and early management. National Institute for Health and Care Excellence. NICE guideline 51. July 2016, updated March 2024.

www.nice.org.uk/guidance/ng51

Cardiovascular system infections, antibacterial therapy

Endocarditis: initial 'blind' therapy

- *Native valve endocarditis*, amoxicillin p. 635 (*or* ampicillin p. 637)
- ▸ Consider adding low-dose gentamicin p. 596
- ▸ *If penicillin-allergic, or if meticillin-resistant Staphylococcus aureus* suspected, or if severe sepsis, use vancomycin p. 617 + low-dose gentamicin
- ▸ If severe sepsis with risk factors for Gram-negative infection, use vancomycin + meropenem p. 601
- *If prosthetic valve endocarditis*, vancomycin + rifampicin p. 674 + low-dose gentamicin

Endocarditis (native valve) caused by staphylococci

- Flucloxacillin p. 643

5
Infection

▶ *Suggested duration of treatment* 4 weeks (at least 6 weeks if secondary lung abscess or osteomyelitis also present)

● *If penicillin-allergic or if meticillin-resistant Staphylococcus aureus*, vancomycin + rifampicin

▶ *Suggested duration of treatment* 4 weeks (at least 6 weeks if secondary lung abscess or osteomyelitis also present)

Endocarditis (prosthetic valve) caused by staphylococci

● Flucloxacillin + rifampicin + low-dose gentamicin

▶ *Suggested duration of treatment* at least 6 weeks; review need to continue gentamicin at 2 weeks—seek specialist advice if gentamicin considered necessary beyond 2 weeks

● *If penicillin-allergic or if meticillin-resistant Staphylococcus aureus*, vancomycin + rifampicin + low-dose gentamicin

▶ *Suggested duration of treatment* at least 6 weeks; review need to continue gentamicin at 2 weeks—seek specialist advice if gentamicin considered necessary beyond 2 weeks

Endocarditis caused by fully-sensitive streptococci

● Benzylpenicillin sodium p. 633

▶ *Suggested duration of treatment* 4–6 weeks (6 weeks for prosthetic valve endocarditis)

● *If penicillin-allergic*, vancomycin (*or* teicoplanin p. 616) + low-dose gentamicin

▶ *Suggested duration of treatment* 4–6 weeks (stop gentamicin after 2 weeks)

Endocarditis caused by less-sensitive streptococci

● Benzylpenicillin sodium + low-dose gentamicin

▶ *Suggested duration of treatment* 4–6 weeks (6 weeks for prosthetic valve endocarditis); review need to continue gentamicin at 2 weeks—seek specialist advice if gentamicin considered necessary beyond 2 weeks; stop gentamicin at 2 weeks if micro-organisms moderately sensitive to penicillin

● *If penicillin-allergic or highly penicillin-resistant*, vancomycin (*or* teicoplanin) + low-dose gentamicin

▶ *Suggested duration of treatment* 4–6 weeks (6 weeks for prosthetic valve endocarditis); review need to continue gentamicin at 2 weeks—seek specialist advice if gentamicin considered necessary beyond 2 weeks; stop gentamicin at 2 weeks if micro-organisms moderately sensitive to penicillin

Endocarditis caused by enterococci

● Amoxicillin (*or* ampicillin) + low dose gentamicin *or* benzylpenicillin sodium + low-dose gentamicin

▶ *Suggested duration of treatment* 4–6 weeks (6 weeks for prosthetic valve endocarditis); review need to continue gentamicin at 2 weeks—seek specialist advice if gentamicin considered necessary beyond 2 weeks

● *If penicillin-allergic or penicillin-resistant*, vancomycin (*or* teicoplanin) + low-dose gentamicin

▶ *Suggested duration of treatment* 4–6 weeks (6 weeks for prosthetic valve endocarditis); review need to continue gentamicin at 2 weeks—seek specialist advice if gentamicin considered necessary beyond 2 weeks

● If gentamicin resistant, amoxicillin (*or* ampicillin)

▶ Add streptomycin p. 598 (if susceptible) for 2 weeks

▶ *Suggested duration of treatment* at least 6 weeks

Endocarditis caused by *Haemophilus*, *Actinobacillus*, *Cardiobacterium*, *Eikenella*, and *Kingella* species ('HACEK' micro-organisms)

● Amoxicillin (*or* ampicillin) + low-dose gentamicin

▶ *Suggested duration of treatment* 4 weeks (6 weeks for prosthetic valve endocarditis); stop gentamicin after 2 weeks

● *If amoxicillin-resistant*, ceftriaxone p. 609 (*or* cefotaxime p. 608) + low-dose gentamicin

▶ *Suggested duration of treatment* 4 weeks (6 weeks for prosthetic valve endocarditis); stop gentamicin after 2 weeks

Central nervous system infections, antibacterial therapy

03-Jun-2024

Meningitis and meningococcal disease

Meningitis involves inflammation of the membranes covering the brain and spinal cord (meninges)—causes can be infective (bacterial, viral, or fungal) or non-infective (certain cancers, autoimmune disorders, injury, or drugs). The most common causative organisms of acute bacterial meningitis are *Neisseria meningitidis* (meningococcus), *Streptococcus pneumoniae* (pneumococcus), and *Haemophilus influenzae* type b (Hib). *Listeria monocytogenes* is a rare cause of meningitis, usually affecting adults aged over 60 years, very young children, and those with other risk factors including pregnancy, cancer, kidney or liver disease, diabetes, alcohol misuse, and immunosuppression. Meningococcal disease refers to invasive infection caused by *N. meningitidis*, which can result in meningococcal meningitis, meningococcal septicaemia, or more commonly, a combination of both.

EvGr Bacterial meningitis and meningococcal disease are medical emergencies that require prompt recognition and treatment. Bacterial meningitis should be strongly suspected in patients with all the symptoms in the 'red flag' combination (fever, headache, neck stiffness, and altered level of consciousness or cognition), however, bacterial meningitis can still be strongly suspected even in the absence of some of these symptoms. Meningococcal disease should be strongly suspected in patients with a non-blanching petechial or purpuric rash with or without the 'red flag' symptoms of meningitis, however, the absence of a rash does not rule out meningococcal disease. Ⓐ For further guidance on the recognition of bacterial meningitis and meningococcal disease, see NICE guideline: **Meningitis (bacterial) and meningococcal disease: recognition, diagnosis and management** (see *Useful resources*).

Acute bacterial meningitis and meningococcal septicaemia are notifiable diseases in the UK. For further information, see *Notifiable diseases* in Antibacterials, principles of therapy p. 573.

Management

EvGr Patients with suspected bacterial meningitis or meningococcal disease should be transferred to hospital as an emergency.

Patients with strongly suspected meningococcal disease should be given intravenous or intramuscular antibacterials as soon as possible outside of hospital, unless this will delay transfer to hospital. Patients with strongly suspected bacterial meningitis should be given intravenous or intramuscular antibacterials if there is likely to be a clinically significant delay in transfer to hospital.

Advice from an infection specialist should be obtained for all cases of bacterial meningitis, particularly for individuals who have recently travelled outside of the UK and may be at risk of antimicrobial resistance, and for those who are colonised with cephalosporin-resistant *Enterobacterales*.

For suspected bacterial meningitis and meningococcal disease, antibacterials should be started within 1 hour of the patient arriving at hospital if an appropriate first dose has not already been given in the community. Microbiological samples should be taken prior to starting treatment in hospital if it is safe to do so and will not cause a clinically significant delay. Empirical antibacterial therapy for suspected bacterial meningitis should be continued until investigation results suggest that an alternative treatment is required. Ⓐ

For further guidance on the investigation of bacterial meningitis and meningococcal disease, treatment of bacterial meningitis once the causative organism is known, and the management of complications and long-term effects, see NICE guideline: **Meningitis (bacterial) and meningococcal disease: recognition, diagnosis and management** (see *Useful resources*).

Choice of antibacterial therapy for bacterial meningitis and meningococcal disease (in individuals aged 1 month and older)

Emergency treatment of strongly suspected bacterial meningitis or meningococcal disease prior to transfer to hospital

- EvGr Ceftriaxone p. 609 or benzylpenicillin sodium p. 633.
- Do not give antibacterials outside of hospital if the patient has a severe allergy to a beta-lactam antibacterial. Ⓐ

Empirical antibacterial therapy for suspected bacterial meningitis in hospital

- EvGr *First line (including patients with non-severe allergy to a beta-lactam antibacterial)* : ceftriaxone. If ceftriaxone is contra-indicated for reasons other than allergy, cefotaxime p. 608 may be used.
- ▶ *Alternative in patients with severe allergy to a beta-lactam antibacterial* : consider chloramphenicol p. 660 and seek advice from an infection specialist. Ⓐ

Patients with risk factors for L. monocytogenes:

- EvGr *First line*: amoxicillin p. 635 in addition to ceftriaxone (or cefotaxime).
- ▶ *Alternative in those with non-severe allergy to a beta-lactam antibacterial* : consider co-trimoxazole p. 652 [unlicensed use] in addition to ceftriaxone (or cefotaxime), and seek advice from an infection specialist.
- ▶ *Alternative in those with severe allergy to a beta-lactam antibacterial*: consider co-trimoxazole [unlicensed use] and chloramphenicol, and seek advice from an infection specialist. Ⓐ

Antibacterial therapy for meningococcal disease in hospital

- EvGr *First line (including patients with non-severe allergy to a beta-lactam antibacterial)* : ceftriaxone.
- *Alternative in patients with severe allergy to a beta-lactam antibacterial* : consider chloramphenicol and seek advice from an infection specialist. Ⓐ

Corticosteroids

Corticosteroids for bacterial meningitis

For some causes of bacterial meningitis, there is evidence that corticosteroids may reduce mortality in adults, and reduce hearing impairment in both adults and children.

EvGr For patients aged 3 months and older with strongly suspected or confirmed bacterial meningitis, give dexamethasone p. 786.

For infants aged between 28 days and 3 months with strongly suspected or confirmed bacterial meningitis, seek advice on giving dexamethasone from an infection specialist.

The first dose of dexamethasone should be given with or before the first dose of antibacterial treatment if possible, however, antibacterial treatment should not be delayed to administer dexamethasone. If antibacterial treatment was started less than 12 hours ago, dexamethasone should be given as soon as possible. Otherwise, seek advice from an infection specialist to decide whether dexamethasone is still likely to provide benefit.

If *S. pneumoniae* or *H. influenzae* type b are found to be the cause, continue dexamethasone. For all other causative organisms, stop dexamethasone treatment. If no causative organism is found, seek advice from an infection specialist on whether to continue dexamethasone. Ⓐ

Corticosteroids for meningococcal disease

EvGr Corticosteroids are not routinely recommended for patients with meningococcal disease, however, low-dose replacement corticosteroids can be considered for those with meningococcal septic shock unresponsive to high-dose vasoactive agents. Ⓐ

Prevention of secondary cases

EvGr The local health protection team should be contacted as soon as a case of meningococcal disease is suspected to undertake a public health assessment and to consider antibacterial chemoprophylaxis of cases and close contacts. Ⓐ For further information on the prevention of secondary cases of meningococcal disease or invasive *H. influenzae* type b infection, see Antibacterials, use for prophylaxis p. 574. For guidance on the public health management of meningococcal disease in the UK, see UKHSA guideline: **Guidance for public health management of meningococcal disease in the UK** (see *Useful resources*).

Useful Resources

Guidance for public health management of meningococcal disease in the UK. UK Health Security Agency. 2018, updated November 2024.
www.gov.uk/government/publications/meningococcal-disease-guidance-on-public-health-management

Meningitis (bacterial) and meningococcal disease: recognition, diagnosis and management. National Institute for Health and Care Excellence. NICE guideline 240. March 2024.
www.nice.org.uk/guidance/ng240

Diabetic foot infections, antibacterial therapy
14-Nov-2024

Diabetic foot infection

Diabetic foot infection is defined as any type of skin, soft tissue or bone infection below the ankle in patients with diabetes. It includes cellulitis, paronychia, abscesses, myositis, tendonitis, necrotising fasciitis, osteomyelitis, and septic arthritis. It is defined clinically by the presence of at least 2 of the following: local swelling or induration, erythema, local tenderness or pain, local warmth, or purulent discharge.

For guidance on classification of infection severity, see NICE guideline: **Diabetic foot problems** (see *Useful resources*).

Treatment

EvGr Refer patients immediately to acute services and inform the multidisciplinary foot care service if they have a limb-threatening or life-threatening problem, such as ulceration with fever or any signs of sepsis, ulceration with limb ischaemia, or gangrene.

Antibacterial treatment should be started as soon as possible if diabetic foot infection is suspected. Samples (such as soft tissue, bone sample, or deep swab) should be taken for microbiological testing before, or as close as possible to, the start of antibacterial treatment.

Offer an antibacterial taking into account the severity of infection, risk of complications, previous microbiological results, recent antibacterial use, and patient preferences. Ⓐ

For other considerations such as switching from intravenous to oral antibacterials, and for advice to be given to patients, see Antibacterials, principles of therapy p. 573.

Infection 5

Reassessment

[EvGr] Reassess if symptoms worsen rapidly or significantly at any time, do not start to improve within 1–2 days of starting antibacterial treatment, or the patient becomes systemically very unwell or has severe pain out of proportion to the infection. Take into account other diagnoses (such as pressure sores, gout, or non-infected ulcers), signs and symptoms of a more serious illness (such as limb ischaemia, osteomyelitis, necrotising fasciitis, or sepsis), and previous antibacterial use.

Review the choice of antibacterial when microbiological results are available and change according to the results, using a narrower-spectrum antibacterial if appropriate. (A)

Choice of antibacterial therapy

[EvGr] Treatment should be based on clinical assessment, infection severity, suspected micro-organism, and be guided by microbiological results when available. Treatment duration should be based on the severity of infection, and clinical assessment of response to treatment. Review the need for continued antibacterials regularly.

Offer oral antibacterials to patients who are able to take oral treatment and the severity of their condition does not require intravenous treatment. (A)

Mild infection

- **Oral** *first line* :
- ▶ [EvGr] Flucloxacillin p. 643.
- ▶ Alternative in penicillin allergy or flucloxacillin unsuitable: clarithromycin p. 621, doxycycline p. 655, or erythromycin p. 624 (in pregnancy). (A)

Moderate or severe infection

[EvGr] Treatment duration is based on clinical assessment; minimum of 7 days and up to 6 weeks for osteomyelitis (use oral antibacterials for prolonged treatment). In severe infection, intravenous antibacterials should be given for at least 48 hours (until stabilised). (A)

- **Oral** or **Intravenous** *first line* :
- ▶ [EvGr] Flucloxacillin **with** or **without** intravenous gentamicin p. 596 **and/or** metronidazole p. 628, *or* co-amoxiclav p. 638 **with** or **without** intravenous gentamicin p. 596, *or* intravenous ceftriaxone p. 609 **with** metronidazole p. 628.
- ▶ Alternative in penicillin allergy: co-trimoxazole p. 652 [unlicensed] **with** or **without** intravenous gentamicin p. 596 **and/or** metronidazole p. 628.
- ▶ Additional antibacterial choices if *Pseudomonas aeruginosa* suspected or confirmed: intravenous piperacillin with tazobactam p. 631, *or* clindamycin p. 618 **with** ciprofloxacin p. 648 **and/or** intravenous gentamicin p. 596. Ciprofloxacin should only be used if other antibacterials are inappropriate.
- ▶ If meticillin-resistant *Staphylococcus aureus* (MRSA) confirmed or suspected **add** intravenous vancomycin p. 617, or intravenous teicoplanin p. 616, or linezolid p. 664 (specialist use only if vancomycin or teicoplanin cannot be used).
- ▶ Other antibacterials may be appropriate based on microbiological results and specialist advice. (A)

Useful Resources

Diabetic foot problems: prevention and management. National Institute for Health and Care Excellence. NICE guideline 19. August 2015, updated September 2024. www.nice.org.uk/guidance/ng19

Ear infections, antibacterial therapy

03-May-2022

Otitis externa

Otitis externa is inflammation of the external ear canal; it can be triggered by a bacterial infection caused by *Pseudomonas aeruginosa* or *Staphylococcus aureus*. For further information, including use of topical treatments, see *Otitis externa* in Ear p. 1357. Oral antibacterials are rarely indicated but if they are required, consider seeking specialist advice.

Choice of antibacterial therapy
If pseudomonas suspected

- [EvGr] Ciprofloxacin p. 648 (*or* an aminoglycoside). (E)

No penicillin allergy

- [EvGr] Flucloxacillin p. 643. (E)

Penicillin allergy or intolerance

- [EvGr] Clarithromycin p. 621 (*or* azithromycin p. 620 *or* erythromycin p. 624). (E)

Otitis media

Acute otitis media is inflammation in the middle ear associated with effusion and accompanied by an ear infection. Acute otitis media is commonly seen in children and is generally caused by viruses (respiratory syncytial virus, rhinovirus, adenovirus, influenza virus, and parainfluenza virus) or bacteria (*Haemophilus influenzae, Streptococcus pneumoniae, Streptococcus pyogenes*, and *Moraxella catarrhalis*); both virus and bacteria often co-exist. For further information, see *Acute otitis media* in Ear p. 1357.

Choice of antibacterial therapy in children
No penicillin allergy

- *First line*: [EvGr] amoxicillin p. 635. (A)
- *Second line* (worsening symptoms despite 2 to 3 days of antibacterial treatment): [EvGr] co-amoxiclav p. 638. (A)

Penicillin allergy or intolerance

- *First line*: [EvGr] clarithromycin p. 621 or erythromycin p. 624 (in pregnancy). (A)
- *Second line* (worsening symptoms despite 2 to 3 days of antibacterial treatment): [EvGr] Consult local microbiologist. (A)

Eye infections, antibacterial therapy

Conjunctivitis (purulent)

- Chloramphenicol eye drops p. 1335.

Gastro-intestinal system infections, antibacterial therapy

14-Nov-2024

Gastro-enteritis

Frequently self-limiting and may not be bacterial.

- Antibacterial not usually indicated.

Campylobacter enteritis

Frequently self-limiting; treat if immunocompromised or if severe infection.

- Clarithromycin p. 621 (*or* azithromycin p. 620 *or* erythromycin p. 624)
- *Alternative*, ciprofloxacin p. 648
- ▶ Strains with decreased sensitivity to ciprofloxacin isolated frequently

Diverticulitis, acute

Acute diverticulitis is a condition where diverticula (small pouches protruding from the walls of the large intestine) suddenly become inflamed or infected. Complicated acute diverticulitis refers to diverticulitis associated with complications such as abscess, bowel perforation and peritonitis, fistula, intestinal obstruction, haemorrhage, or sepsis. For further information on acute diverticulitis including the non-antibacterial management, see Diverticular disease and diverticulitis p. 39.

Treatment

[EvGr] For patients with acute diverticulitis who are systemically well, consider a watchful waiting and a no antibacterial prescribing strategy. Advise patients to re-present if symptoms persist or worsen.

For patients who are systemically unwell, immunosuppressed, or have significant comorbidities, an antibacterial prescribing strategy should be offered.

Oral antibacterials should be offered to patients who are systemically unwell but do not meet the referral criteria for suspected complicated acute diverticulitis.

Patients with persistent or worsening symptoms should be reassessed in primary care and considered for referral to hospital for further assessment.

Patients with suspected complicated acute diverticulitis and uncontrolled abdominal pain should be referred for same-day hospital assessment.

Patients admitted to hospital with suspected or confirmed complicated acute diverticulitis should be treated with intravenous antibacterials. ⒶFor guidance on the management of suspected sepsis, see NICE guideline **Sepsis** at: www.nice.org.uk/guidance/ng51.

For other considerations such as switching from intravenous to oral antibacterials, and for advice to be given to patients, see Antibacterials, principles of therapy p. 573.

[EvGr] Antibacterial prophylaxis is not recommended to prevent recurrent acute diverticulitis. Ⓐ

Choice of antibacterial therapy

[EvGr] Patients unable to take oral treatment should be referred to hospital. Ⓐ

Suspected or confirmed uncomplicated acute diverticulitis

- *Oral first line* :

▸ [EvGr] Co-amoxiclav p. 638.

▸ Alternative in penicillin allergy or co-amoxiclav unsuitable: cefalexin p. 603 (caution in penicillin allergy) **with** metronidazole p. 628, *or* trimethoprim p. 665 **with** metronidazole p. 628, *or* ciprofloxacin p. 648 (only if other antibacterials are inappropriate, and if switching from intravenous route under specialist advice) **with** metronidazole p. 628. Ⓐ

Suspected or confirmed complicated acute diverticulitis

- *Intravenous first line* :

▸ [EvGr] Co-amoxiclav, *or* cefuroxime p. 606 **with** metronidazole p. 628, *or* amoxicillin p. 635 **with** gentamicin p. 596 **and** metronidazole p. 628.

▸ Alternative only in penicillin and cephalosporins allergy: ciprofloxacin p. 648 **with** metronidazole p. 628.

▸ For alternative antibacterials consult local microbiologist. Ⓐ

Salmonella (non-typhoid)

Treat invasive or severe infection. Do not treat less severe infection unless there is a risk of developing invasive infection (e.g. immunocompromised patients, those with haemoglobinopathy, or children under 6 months of age).

- Ciprofloxacin *or* cefotaxime p. 608

Shigellosis

Antibacterial not indicated for mild cases.

- Ciprofloxacin *or* azithromycin
- *Alternatives if micro-organism sensitive*, amoxicillin p. 635 *or* trimethoprim p. 665

Typhoid fever

Infections from Middle-East, South Asia, and South-East Asia may be multiple-antibacterial-resistant and sensitivity should be tested.

- Cefotaxime (*or* ceftriaxone p. 609)
- ▸ Azithromycin may be an alternative in mild or moderate disease caused by multiple-antibacterial-resistant organisms.
- *Alternative if micro-organism sensitive*, ciprofloxacin

Clostridioides difficile infection

Clostridioides difficile (*C. difficile*) infection occurs when normal gut microbiota are suppressed, allowing levels of toxin producing strains of *C. difficile* to flourish. The toxin damages the lining of the colon and causes diarrhoea. Infection can be mild, moderate, severe, or life-threatening; complications include pseudomembranous colitis, toxic megacolon, colonic perforation, sepsis, and death.

C. difficile infection is most common in patients who are currently taking or have recently taken antibacterials. Clindamycin, cephalosporins (especially third and fourth generation), fluoroquinolones, and broad-spectrum penicillins have been frequently associated with *C. difficile* infection. Infection risk increases with longer duration of antibacterial treatment, concurrent use of multiple antibacterials, or multiple antibacterial courses. Other risk factors for *C. difficile* infection include current use of acid suppressing drugs (such as proton pump inhibitors), age over 65 years, prolonged hospitalisation, underlying comorbidity, exposure to other people with the infection, and previous history of *C. difficile* infection(s).

For guidance on classification of *C. difficile* infection severity and non-antibacterial management options (such as faecal microbiota transplant for patients with recurrent episodes of *C. difficile* infection), see NICE guideline: **Clostridioides difficile infection** (see *Useful resources*). For guidance on diagnosis, infection control, and the management of life-threatening disease, see UK Health Security Agency (UKHSA) collection: **Clostridioides difficile: guidance, data and analysis** (available at: www.gov.uk/government/collections/clostridium-difficile-guidance-data-and-analysis).

Treatment

[EvGr] Offer an antibacterial to patients with suspected or confirmed *C. difficile* infection. Consider seeking prompt specialist advice before starting treatment.

Antibacterials are not recommended for preventing *C. difficile* infection. ⒶFor other considerations such as advice to be given to patients, and if appropriate their family or carers, see Antibacterials, principles of therapy p. 573.

[EvGr] Urgent referral to hospital and specialist advice should be sought for patients with life-threatening infection.

Refer patients with suspected or confirmed *C. difficile* infection to hospital if they are severely unwell, or their signs or symptoms worsen rapidly or significantly at any time.

Consider referral to hospital for patients with a high risk of complications or recurrence due to individual factors such as age, frailty, or comorbidities. Ⓐ

Reassessment

[EvGr] Reassess if signs or symptoms worsen rapidly or significantly at any time, or do not improve as expected.

Consider stopping antibacterial therapy if subsequent stool sample tests do not confirm *C. difficile* infection.

Clinical judgement should be used to determine if antibacterial treatment is ineffective (not usually possible until day 7 as diarrhoea may take 1–2 weeks to resolve). Ⓐ

Choice of antibacterial therapy

EvGr For patients who cannot take oral medicines, seek specialist advice about other enteral routes (such as nasogastric tube or rectal catheter). Ⓐ

First episode of mild, moderate, or severe C. difficile infection

- *Oral first line* :
  ‣ EvGr Vancomycin p. 617. Ⓐ
- *Oral second line* :
  ‣ EvGr Fidaxomicin p. 661. Ⓐ
- If first and second line antibacterials are ineffective: EvGr Seek specialist advice. Ⓐ

Further episode of C. difficile infection

- *Oral first line* for infection within 12 weeks of symptom resolution (relapse):
  ‣ EvGr Fidaxomicin p. 661. Ⓐ
- *Oral first line* for infection more than 12 weeks after symptom resolution (recurrence):
  ‣ EvGr Vancomycin p. 617 or fidaxomicin p. 661. Ⓐ

Life-threatening C. difficile infection

- EvGr Specialist may offer oral vancomycin p. 617 **with** intravenous metronidazole p. 628. Ⓐ

Biliary-tract infection

- Ciprofloxacin *or* gentamicin p. 596 *or* a cephalosporin

Peritonitis

- A cephalosporin + metronidazole *or* gentamicin + metronidazole *or* gentamicin + clindamycin p. 618 *or* piperacillin with tazobactam p. 631 alone

Peritonitis: peritoneal dialysis-associated

- Vancomycin p. 617 (*or* teicoplanin p. 616) + ceftazidime p. 608 added to dialysis fluid *or* vancomycin added to dialysis fluid + ciprofloxacin by mouth
  ‣ *Suggested duration of treatment* 14 days or longer

Useful Resources

Diverticular disease: diagnosis and management. National Institute for Health and Care Excellence. NICE guideline 147. November 2019, updated September 2024. www.nice.org.uk/guidance/ng147

Clostridioides difficile infection: antimicrobial prescribing. National Institute for Health and Care Excellence. NICE guideline 199. July 2021. www.nice.org.uk/guidance/ng199

Genital system infections, antibacterial therapy
                                                    12-Jun-2023

Bacterial vaginosis

- Oral metronidazole p. 628
  ‣ *Suggested duration of treatment* 5–7 days (or high-dose metronidazole as a single dose)
- *Alternatively*, topical metronidazole for 5 days *or* topical clindamycin p. 957 for 7 days

Uncomplicated genital chlamydial infection and uncomplicated non-gonococcal urethritis (non-specific urethritis)

EvGr Contact tracing recommended. Ⓐ

- *First line*: EvGr doxycycline p. 655 Ⓐ
- *Alternative if tetracycline allergy or unsuitable*: EvGr azithromycin p. 620. Ⓐ

For other treatment options and further guidance on the management of chlamydial infections and non-gonococcal urethritis, see the British Association for Sexual Health and HIV guidelines: **UK national guideline for the management of infection with *Chlamydia trachomatis*** and **UK national guideline on the management of non-gonococcal urethritis** (see *Useful resources*).

Gonorrhoea: uncomplicated

EvGr Prior to treating gonococcal infection obtain cultures from all potentially exposed sites for antimicrobial susceptibility testing. Contact tracing and test of cure following treatment are recommended. For sexual contacts presenting within 14 days of exposure, epidemiological treatment should be considered, whereas for contacts presenting after 14 days of exposure, treatment is only recommended following a positive test. Sexual intercourse should be avoided until 7 days after patients and their partner(s) have completed treatment. Ⓐ

- *First line*:
  ‣ EvGr If antimicrobial susceptibility unknown: ceftriaxone p. 609
  ‣ If micro-organism is sensitive to ciprofloxacin: ciprofloxacin p. 648 Ⓐ
- *Alternatives due to allergy, needle phobia or contra-indications*:
  ‣ EvGr Gentamicin p. 596 **plus** azithromycin
  ‣ If parenteral administration is not possible: cefixime p. 608 [unlicensed use] **plus** azithromycin
  ‣ In non-pharyngeal infections: spectinomycin [unlicensed] **plus** azithromycin
  ‣ If unable to take standard therapy: azithromycin Ⓐ

For guidance on the management of other types of gonococcal infections, see the British Association for Sexual Health and HIV guideline: **National guideline for the management of infection with *Neisseria gonorrhoeae*** (see *Useful resources*).

Pelvic inflammatory disease

Contact tracing recommended.

- Doxycycline + metronidazole + single-dose of i/m ceftriaxone *or* ofloxacin p. 652 + metronidazole
  ‣ *Suggested duration of treatment* 14 days (except i/m ceftriaxone).
  ‣ In severely ill patients initial treatment with doxycycline + i/v ceftriaxone + i/v metronidazole, then switch to oral treatment with doxycycline + metronidazole to complete 14 days' treatment

Syphilis

EvGr Contact tracing recommended. Ⓐ

Early syphilis (primary, secondary, and early latent–less than 2 years since infection) and late latent syphilis (more than 2 years since infection)

- *First line*: EvGr benzathine benzylpenicillin p. 632 Ⓐ
- *Alternatives include*: EvGr Doxycycline Ⓐ

Asymptomatic contacts of patients with infectious syphilis

- *First line*: EvGr Benzathine benzylpenicillin Ⓐ
- *Alternatives include*: EvGr Doxycycline Ⓐ

For guidance on other treatment options and further information on the management of syphilis, including in pregnancy, and in symptomatic late disease, see the British Association for Sexual Health and HIV guideline: **UK national guidelines on the management of syphilis** (see *Useful resources*).

Useful Resources

UK national guideline on the management of non-gonococcal urethritis. British Association for Sexual Health and HIV. 2015, updated December 2018. www.bashh.org/guidelines

UK national guideline for the management of infection with *Chlamydia trachomatis*. British Association for Sexual Health and HIV. 2015, updated September 2018.
www.bashh.org/guidelines

National guideline for the management of infection with *Neisseria gonorrhoeae*. British Association for Sexual Health and HIV. 2018, updated March 2020.
www.bashh.org/guidelines

UK national guidelines on the management of syphilis. British Association for Sexual Health and HIV. 2015, updated July 2019.
www.bashh.org/guidelines

Musculoskeletal system infections, antibacterial therapy

Osteomyelitis

For management of osteomyelitis below the ankle in individuals with diabetes mellitus, see Diabetic foot infections, antibacterial therapy p. 581.

Seek specialist advice if chronic infection or prostheses present.

- Flucloxacillin p. 643
- ▸ Consider adding fusidic acid p. 663 or rifampicin p. 674 for initial 2 weeks.
- ▸ *Suggested duration of treatment* 6 weeks for acute infection
- *If penicillin-allergic*, clindamycin p. 618
- ▸ Consider adding fusidic acid or rifampicin for initial 2 weeks.
- ▸ *Suggested duration of treatment* 6 weeks for acute infection
- *If meticillin-resistant Staphylococcus aureus suspected*, vancomycin p. 617 (*or* teicoplanin p. 616)
- ▸ Consider adding fusidic acid or rifampicin for initial 2 weeks.
- ▸ *Suggested duration of treatment* 6 weeks for acute infection

Septic arthritis

For management of septic arthritis below the ankle in individuals with diabetes mellitus, see Diabetic foot infections, antibacterial therapy p. 581.

Seek specialist advice if prostheses present.

- Flucloxacillin
- ▸ *Suggested duration of treatment* 4–6 weeks (longer if infection complicated).
- *If penicillin-allergic*, clindamycin
- ▸ *Suggested duration of treatment* 4–6 weeks (longer if infection complicated).
- *If meticillin-resistant Staphylococcus aureus suspected*, vancomycin (*or* teicoplanin)
- ▸ *Suggested duration of treatment* 4–6 weeks (longer if infection complicated).
- *If gonococcal arthritis or Gram-negative infection suspected*, cefotaxime p. 608 (*or* ceftriaxone p. 609)
- ▸ *Suggested duration of treatment* 4–6 weeks (longer if infection complicated; treat gonococcal infection for 2 weeks).

Nose infections, antibacterial therapy

31-Oct-2017

Sinusitis (acute)

Acute sinusitis is generally triggered by a viral infection, although occasionally it may become complicated by a bacterial infection caused by *Streptococcus pneumoniae*, *Haemophylus influenzae*, *Moraxella catarrhalis*, or *Staphylococcus aureus*. For further information *see* Sinusitis (acute) p. 1368.

Treatment

EvGr Antibacterial therapy should *only* be offered to patients with acute sinusitis who are systemically very unwell, have signs and symptoms of a more serious illness, those who are at high-risk of complications due to pre-existing comorbidities, or whenever bacterial sinusitis is suspected.

Patients presenting with symptoms for around 10 days or more with no improvement may be prescribed a back-up antibiotic prescription, which can be used if symptoms do not improve within 7 days or if they worsen significantly at any time. Ⓐ For further information *see*, Sinusitis (acute) p. 1368.

Choice of antibacterial therapy
No penicillin allergy

- *First line*:
- ▸ EvGr Non-life threatening symptoms: phenoxymethylpenicillin p. 634.
- ▸ Systemically very unwell, signs and symptoms of a more serious illness, or at high-risk of complications: co-amoxiclav p. 638. Ⓐ
- *Second line* (worsening symptoms despite 2 or 3 days of antibiotic treatment):
- ▸ EvGr Non-life threatening symptoms: co-amoxiclav.
- ▸ Systemically very unwell, signs and symptoms of a more serious illness or at high-risk of complications: consult local microbiologist. Ⓐ

Penicillin allergy or intolerance

- *First line*: EvGr doxycycline p. 655 or clarithromycin p. 621 (erythromycin p. 624 in pregnancy). Ⓐ
- *Second line* (worsening symptoms despite 2 or 3 days of antibiotic treatment): EvGr Consult local microbiologist. Ⓐ

Useful Resources

Sinusitis (acute): antimicrobial prescribing. National Institute for Health and Care Excellence. NICE guideline 79. October 2017.
www.nice.org.uk/guidance/ng79

Oral bacterial infections

07-Oct-2021

Antibacterial drugs

Antibacterial drugs should only be prescribed for the *treatment* of oral infections on the basis of defined need. They may be used in conjunction with (but not as an alternative to) other appropriate measures, such as providing drainage or extracting a tooth.

The 'blind' prescribing of an antibacterial for unexplained pyrexia, cervical lymphadenopathy, or facial swelling can lead to difficulty in establishing the diagnosis. In severe oral infections, a sample should always be taken for bacteriology.

Oral infections which may require antibacterial treatment include acute periapical or periodontal abscess, cellulitis, acutely created oral-antral communication (and acute sinusitis), severe pericoronitis, localised osteitis, acute necrotising ulcerative gingivitis, and destructive forms of chronic periodontal disease. Most of these infections are readily resolved by the early establishment of drainage and removal of the cause (typically an infected necrotic pulp). Antibacterials may be required if treatment has to be delayed, in immunocompromised patients, or in those with conditions such as diabetes or Paget's disease. Certain rarer infections including bacterial sialadenitis, osteomyelitis, actinomycosis, and infections involving fascial spaces such as Ludwig's angina, require antibiotics and specialist hospital care.

Antibacterial drugs may also be useful after dental surgery in some cases of spreading infection. Infection may spread to involve local lymph nodes, to fascial spaces (where it can cause airway obstruction), or into the bloodstream (where it can lead to cavernous sinus thrombosis and other serious complications). Extension of an infection can also lead to maxillary sinusitis; osteomyelitis is a complication, which usually arises when host resistance is reduced.

If the oral infection fails to respond to antibacterial treatment within 48 hours the antibacterial should be changed, preferably on the basis of bacteriological investigation. Failure to respond may also suggest an incorrect diagnosis, lack of essential additional measures (such as drainage), poor host resistance, or poor patient compliance.

Combination of a penicillin (or a macrolide) with metronidazole p. 628 may sometimes be helpful for the treatment of severe oral infections or oral infections that have not responded to initial antibacterial treatment.

For information on antibacterials used for the treatment of pericoronitis, acute necrotising ulcerative gingivitis, dental abscess, and sore throat, see Oropharyngeal infections, antibacterial therapy p. 1383.

Penicillins

Phenoxymethylpenicillin p. 634 is effective for dentoalveolar abscess.

Broad-spectrum penicillins

Amoxicillin p. 635 is as effective as phenoxymethylpenicillin but is better absorbed; however, it may encourage emergence of resistant organisms.

Like phenoxymethylpenicillin, amoxicillin is ineffective against bacteria that produce beta-lactamases.

Amoxicillin may be useful for short course oral regimens.

Co-amoxiclav p. 638 is active against beta-lactamase-producing bacteria that are resistant to amoxicillin. Co-amoxiclav may be used for severe dental infection with spreading cellulitis or dental infection not responding to first-line antibacterial treatment.

Cephalosporins

The cephalosporins offer little advantage over the penicillins in dental infections, often being less active against anaerobes. Infections due to oral streptococci (often termed viridans streptococci) which become resistant to penicillin are usually also resistant to cephalosporins. This is of importance in the case of patients who have had rheumatic fever and are on long-term penicillin therapy. Cefalexin p. 603 and cefradine p. 605 have been used in the treatment of oral infections.

Tetracyclines

In adults, tetracyclines can be effective against oral anaerobes but the development of resistance (especially by oral streptococci) has reduced their usefulness for the treatment of acute oral infections; they may still have a role in the treatment of destructive (refractory) forms of periodontal disease on specialist advice. Doxycycline p. 655 has a longer duration of action than tetracycline p. 659 or oxytetracycline p. 658 and need only be given once daily; it is reported to be more active against anaerobes than some other tetracyclines.

Macrolides

The macrolides are an alternative for oral infections in penicillin-allergic patients or where a beta-lactamase producing organism is involved. However, many organisms are now resistant to macrolides or rapidly develop resistance; their use should therefore be limited to short courses.

Clindamycin

Clindamycin p. 618 should not be used routinely for the treatment of oral infections because it may be no more effective than penicillins against anaerobes and there may be cross-resistance with erythromycin-resistant bacteria.

Metronidazole

Metronidazole is an alternative to a penicillin for the treatment of many oral infections where the patient is allergic to penicillin or the infection is due to beta-lactamase-producing anaerobes.

Respiratory system infections, antibacterial therapy

14-Nov-2024

Epiglottitis (*Haemophilus influenzae*)

- Cefotaxime p. 608 (*or* ceftriaxone p. 609)
- *If history of immediate hypersensitivity reaction to penicillin or to cephalosporins*, chloramphenicol p. 660

Bronchiectasis (non-cystic fibrosis), acute exacerbation

Bronchiectasis is a persistent or progressive condition caused by chronic inflammatory damage to the airways and is characterised by thick-walled, dilated bronchi. Signs and symptoms may range from intermittent expectoration and infection, to chronic cough, persistent daily production of sputum, bacterial colonisation, and recurrent infections. An acute exacerbation is defined as sustained deterioration of the patient's signs and symptoms from their baseline, and presents with worsening local symptoms, with or without increased wheeze, breathlessness or haemoptysis and may be accompanied by fever or pleurisy.

Treatment

[EvGr] Obtain a sputum sample and send for culture and susceptibility testing. Antibacterial therapy should be given to all patients with an acute exacerbation. (A)

For patients receiving prophylactic antibacterial therapy, switching from intravenous to oral antibacterials, and for advice to be given to patients, see Antibacterials, principles of therapy p. 573.

[EvGr] Refer patients to hospital if they have signs or symptoms suggestive of a more serious illness such as cardiorespiratory failure or sepsis. (A)

Reassessment

[EvGr] Reassess if symptoms worsen rapidly or significantly at any time and consider:

- Other diagnoses such as pneumonia, or signs and symptoms of a more serious illness such as cardiorespiratory failure, or sepsis;
- Previous antibacterial use that may have led to resistance.

Review choice of antibacterial if susceptibility results indicate bacterial resistance and symptoms are not improving—consult local microbiologist as needed. (A)

Choice of antibacterial therapy

[EvGr] The recommended total duration of treatment is 7–14 days.

Treatment should be guided by the most recent sputum culture and susceptibility results when available.

Seek specialist advice for patients whose symptoms are not improving with repeated courses, or who are resistant to, or cannot take oral antibacterials. (A)

- *Oral first line* :
  ▸ [EvGr] Amoxicillin p. 635, clarithromycin p. 621, or doxycycline p. 655.
  ▸ Alternative if at high risk of treatment failure (repeated courses of antibacterials, previous culture with resistant or

atypical bacteria, or high risk of complications): co-amoxiclav p. 638, or levofloxacin p. 650 (only if co-amoxiclav is inappropriate, and under specialist advice). Ⓐ

- **Intravenous** *first line* (severely unwell or unable to take oral treatment):
- ▸ EvGr Co-amoxiclav, piperacillin with tazobactam p. 631, or levofloxacin (only if co-amoxiclav and piperacillin with tazobactam are inappropriate, and under specialist advice). Ⓐ

Antibacterial prophylaxis

EvGr For patients with repeated acute exacerbations, a trial of antibacterial prophylaxis may be given on specialist advice only. Ⓐ

Chronic obstructive pulmonary disease, acute exacerbation

An acute exacerbation of chronic obstructive pulmonary disease (COPD) is a sustained worsening of symptoms from the patient's usual stable state, that is beyond the usual day to day variations. Many exacerbations are not caused by bacterial infections, but instead can be triggered by other factors such as smoking or viral infections.

For the non-antibacterial management of acute exacerbations of COPD, see Chronic obstructive pulmonary disease p. 276.

Treatment

EvGr Consider antibacterial treatment taking into account:

- The severity of symptoms, sputum colour changes and increases in volume and thickness;
- The need for hospital admission;
- Previous exacerbations and hospital admission history, and risk of developing complications. Ⓐ

For other considerations such as in patients receiving prophylactic antibacterial therapy, switching from intravenous to oral antibacterials, and for advice to be given to patients, see Antibacterials, principles of therapy p. 573.

EvGr Refer patients to hospital if they have signs or symptoms suggestive of a more serious illness such as cardiorespiratory failure or sepsis. Ⓐ

Reassessment

EvGr Reassess if symptoms worsen rapidly or significantly at any time and consider:

- Other diagnoses such as pneumonia, or signs and symptoms of a more serious illness such as cardiorespiratory failure, or sepsis;
- Previous antibacterial use that may have led to resistance.

Send a sputum sample for testing if there is no improvement after antibacterial therapy and this has not already been done.

Review choice of antibacterial if susceptibility results indicate bacterial resistance and symptoms are not improving—consult local microbiologist as needed. Ⓐ

Choice of antibacterial therapy

EvGr The recommended total duration of treatment is 5 days.

Treatment should be guided by the most recent sputum culture and susceptibility results when available.

Seek specialist advice for patients whose symptoms are not improving with repeated courses, or who are resistant to, or cannot take oral antibacterials. Ⓐ

- **Oral** *first line* :
- ▸ EvGr Amoxicillin, clarithromycin, or doxycycline.
- ▸ Alternative if at high risk of treatment failure (repeated courses of antibacterials, previous culture with resistant or atypical bacteria, or high risk of complications): co-amoxiclav, co-trimoxazole p. 652, or levofloxacin (only if co-amoxiclav and co-trimoxazole are inappropriate, and under specialist advice). Ⓐ

- **Oral** *second line* (if no improvement after at least 2 to 3 days):
- ▸ EvGr Use a first line antibacterial from a different class to the antibacterial used previously.
- ▸ Alternative if at high risk of treatment failure: co-amoxiclav, co-trimoxazole, or levofloxacin (only if co-amoxiclav and co-trimoxazole are inappropriate, and under specialist advice). Ⓐ
- **Intravenous** *first line* (severely unwell or unable to take oral treatment):
- ▸ EvGr Amoxicillin, co-amoxiclav, clarithromycin, co-trimoxazole, or piperacillin with tazobactam. Ⓐ
- **Intravenous** *second line* : EvGr Choice should be made in consultation with a local microbiologist. Ⓐ

Cough, acute

Acute cough is usually self-limiting and often resolves within 3–4 weeks without antibacterials. It is most commonly caused by a viral upper respiratory tract infection, but can have other infective causes such as acute bronchitis or pneumonia, or non-infective causes such as interstitial lung disease or gastro-oesophageal reflux disease.

Treatment

EvGr Patients should be advised that an acute cough is usually self-limiting and to manage their symptoms using self-care treatments. These include honey and over-the-counter cough medicines containing expectorants or cough suppressants, however there is limited evidence to support the use of such products. For more information, see Aromatic inhalations, cough preparations and systemic nasal decongestants p. 339.

Patients with an acute cough who are systemically very unwell should be offered immediate antibacterial treatment.

Do not routinely offer an antibacterial to treat an acute cough associated with an upper respiratory tract infection or acute bronchitis in patients who are not systemically very unwell or at higher risk of complications. Ⓐ

Patients with a pre-existing co-morbidity, young children who were born prematurely, and patients aged over 65 years of age and the presence of certain criteria (hospitalisation in the previous year, type 1 or 2 diabetes, history of congestive heart failure, or currently taking oral corticosteroids) are considered to be at a higher risk of complications if they present with an acute cough. EvGr Immediate or back-up antibacterial treatment should be considered in these patients based on the face-to-face clinical examination. If back-up treatment is given, advise patients to start treatment if symptoms worsen rapidly or significantly at any time. Ⓐ

For general advice to give to patients, see Antibacterials, principles of therapy p. 573.

EvGr Seek specialist advice, or refer patients with an acute cough to hospital if they have signs or symptoms of a more serious illness or condition. Ⓐ

Reassessment

EvGr Reassess if symptoms worsen rapidly or significantly taking into account alternative diagnoses, signs or symptoms suggestive of a more serious condition, and previous antibacterial use which may have led to resistant bacteria. Ⓐ

Choice of antibacterial therapy

EvGr The recommended duration of oral treatment is 5 days. Ⓐ

- **First line**
- ▸ EvGr Doxycycline p. 655.
- ▸ Alternative *first line* choices: amoxicillin p. 635, clarithromycin p. 621, or erythromycin p. 624. Ⓐ
- Choice during pregnancy:
- ▸ EvGr Amoxicillin or erythromycin. Ⓐ

5

Infection

Pneumonia, community-acquired

Pneumonia is an acute infection of the lung parenchyma that presents with symptoms such as cough, chest pain, dyspnoea, and fever. It is classified as community-acquired if acquired outside of hospital or in a nursing home.

For recommendations on the management of suspected or confirmed pneumonia secondary to COVID-19 infection, see NICE rapid guideline: **Managing COVID-19** (available at: www.nice.org.uk/guidance/ng191). For further information on COVID-19, see COVID-19 p. 714.

Treatment

EvGr Offer an antibacterial taking into account the severity assessment, risk of complications, local antimicrobial resistance and surveillance data, recent antibacterial use, and recent microbiological results. A For severity assessment and guidance on monitoring, see NICE guideline on pneumonia in adults (see *Useful resources*).

EvGr Antibacterial treatment should be started as soon as possible and within 4 hours of establishing a diagnosis (within 1 hour if the patient has suspected sepsis and meets any of the high risk criteria for this — see NICE guideline on sepsis at: www.nice.org.uk/guidance/ng51).

Refer patients to hospital as recommended in the NICE guideline on pneumonia in adults, or if they have signs or symptoms suggestive of a more serious illness (such as cardiorespiratory failure or sepsis).

In patients with moderate or high-severity community-acquired pneumonia, obtain blood and sputum cultures and consider performing pneumococcal and legionella urinary antigen tests.

Do not routinely offer a glucocorticoid to patients with community-acquired pneumonia unless they have other conditions for which glucocorticoid treatment is indicated. A

For other considerations such as switching from intravenous to oral antibacterials, and for advice to be given to patients, see Antibacterials, principles of therapy p. 573.

Reassessment

EvGr Reassess if signs or symptoms do not improve or worsen rapidly or significantly, and consider other possible non-bacterial causes such as influenza.

If a sample has been sent for microbiological testing, review the choice of antibacterial and consider changing according to the results, using a narrower-spectrum antibacterial if appropriate.

Send a sample (such as sputum sample) for testing if there is no improvement after antibacterial therapy and this has not already been done.

Refer patients to hospital if symptoms do not improve as expected with antibacterial treatment. A

Choice of antibacterial therapy

EvGr Treatment should be based on severity assessment using clinical judgement and CRB65 or CURB65, suspected micro-organism, and in moderate and high-severity community-acquired pneumonia microbiological results when available.

Offer oral antibacterials to patients who are able to take oral treatment and the severity of their condition does not require intravenous treatment.

Consider referral to hospital or seeking specialist advice if bacteria are resistant to oral antibacterials or patients cannot take oral treatment. A

Low severity

- **Oral** *first line* :
  - ▸ EvGr Amoxicillin.
  - ▸ Alternative in penicillin allergy or amoxicillin unsuitable (e.g. atypical pathogens suspected): clarithromycin, doxycycline, or erythromycin (in pregnancy). A

Moderate severity

- **Oral** *first line* :
  - ▸ EvGr Amoxicillin.
  - ▸ If atypical pathogens suspected: amoxicillin **with** clarithromycin **or** erythromycin (in pregnancy).
  - ▸ Alternative in penicillin allergy: clarithromycin, or doxycycline. A

High severity

- **Oral** *or* **Intravenous** *first line* :
  - ▸ EvGr Co-amoxiclav p. 638 **with** clarithromycin **or** oral erythromycin (in pregnancy).
  - ▸ Alternative in penicillin allergy: levofloxacin p. 650 (consult local microbiologist if fluoroquinolone not appropriate). A

Pneumonia, hospital-acquired

Pneumonia is an acute infection of the lung parenchyma that presents with symptoms such as cough, chest pain, dyspnoea, and fever. It is classified as hospital-acquired when it develops 48 hours or more after hospital admission.

For recommendations on the management of suspected or confirmed pneumonia secondary to COVID-19 infection, see NICE rapid guideline: **Managing COVID-19** (available at: www.nice.org.uk/guidance/ng191). For further information on COVID-19, see COVID-19 p. 714.

Treatment

EvGr In patients with signs or symptoms of pneumonia starting within 48 hours of hospital admission, follow recommendations for patients with community-acquired pneumonia.

Offer an antibacterial taking into account:

- The severity of signs or symptoms;
- The number of days in hospital before onset of symptoms;
- The risk of complications;
- Local hospital and ward-based antimicrobial resistance data;
- Recent antibacterial use;
- Recent microbiological test results;
- Recent contact with health or social care settings;
- Risk of adverse effects such as *Clostridioides difficile* infection.

Antibacterial treatment should be started as soon as possible and within 4 hours of establishing a diagnosis (within 1 hour if the patient has suspected sepsis and meets any of the high risk criteria for this — see NICE guideline on sepsis at: www.nice.org.uk/guidance/ng51).

A sample (for example, sputum sample, nasopharyngeal swab, or tracheal aspirate) should be taken for microbiological testing. A

For other considerations such as switching from intravenous to oral antibacterials, and for advice to be given to patients, see Antibacterials, principles of therapy p. 573.

Reassessment

EvGr Reassess if symptoms do not improve or worsen rapidly or significantly.

When microbiological results are available, review choice of antibacterial and change treatment according to the results, using a narrower-spectrum antibacterial if appropriate.

Seek advice from a microbiologist if symptoms do not improve as expected with treatment, or multidrug-resistant bacteria are present. A

Choice of antibacterial therapy

EvGr For patients with non-severe signs or symptoms and not at higher risk of resistance, treatment should be guided by microbiological results when available. For patients with severe signs or symptoms or at higher risk of resistance, treatment should be based on specialist microbiological advice and local resistance data.

Higher risk of resistance includes signs or symptoms starting more than 5 days after hospital admission, relevant comorbidity, recent use of broad-spectrum antibacterials, colonisation with multidrug-resistant bacteria, and recent contact with a health or social care setting before the current admission.

In patients with signs or symptoms of pneumonia starting within 3 to 5 days of hospital admission who are not at higher risk of resistance, consider following the recommendations for community-acquired pneumonia for choice of antibacterial treatment. Ⓐ

Non-severe signs or symptoms and not at higher risk of resistance

- **Oral** *first line* :
  ▸ EvGr Co-amoxiclav p. 638.
  ▸ Alternative in penicillin allergy or co-amoxiclav unsuitable (based on specialist microbiological advice and local resistance data): doxycycline p. 655, cefalexin p. 603 (caution in penicillin allergy), co-trimoxazole p. 652 [unlicensed use], or levofloxacin p. 650 [unlicensed use] (only if other antibacterials are inappropriate, and if switching from intravenous levofloxacin under specialist advice). Ⓐ

Severe signs or symptoms or at higher risk of resistance

- **Intravenous** *first line* :
  ▸ EvGr Piperacillin with tazobactam p. 631, ceftazidime p. 608, ceftazidime with avibactam p. 612, ceftriaxone p. 609, cefuroxime p. 606, meropenem p. 601, or levofloxacin [unlicensed use] (only if other first-line antibacterials are inappropriate).
  ▸ If meticillin-resistant *Staphylococcus aureus* confirmed or suspected **add** vancomycin p. 617, or teicoplanin p. 616, or linezolid p. 664 (under specialist advice only if vancomycin cannot be used). Ⓐ

Useful resources

Bronchiectasis (non-cystic fibrosis), acute exacerbation: antimicrobial prescribing. National Institute for Health and Care Excellence. NICE guideline 117. December 2018, updated September 2024.
www.nice.org.uk/guidance/ng117

Chronic obstructive pulmonary disease (acute exacerbation): antimicrobial prescribing. National Institute for Health and Care Excellence. NICE guideline 114, updated September 2024.
www.nice.org.uk/guidance/ng114

Cough (acute): antimicrobial prescribing. National Institute for Health and Care Excellence. NICE guideline 120. February 2019.
www.nice.org.uk/guidance/ng120

Pneumonia in adults: diagnosis and management. National Institute for Health and Care Excellence. Clinical guideline 191. December 2014, updated October 2023.
www.nice.org.uk/guidance/cg191

Pneumonia (community-acquired): antimicrobial prescribing. National Institute for Health and Care Excellence. NICE guideline 138. September 2019, updated September 2024.
www.nice.org.uk/guidance/ng138

Pneumonia (hospital-acquired): antimicrobial prescribing. National Institute for Health and Care Excellence. NICE guideline 139. September 2019, updated September 2024.
www.nice.org.uk/guidance/ng139

Skin infections, antibacterial therapy

06-May-2021

Impetigo

Impetigo is a contagious, superficial bacterial infection of the skin that affects all age groups, but it is more common in young children. Transmission occurs directly through close contact with an infected individual or indirectly via contaminated objects such as toys, clothing, or towels.

Impetigo can develop as a primary infection or as a secondary complication of pre-existing skin conditions such as eczema, scabies, or chickenpox. The two main clinical forms are non-bullous impetigo (most common form) and bullous impetigo. Non-bullous impetigo is characterised by thin-walled vesicles or pustules that rupture quickly, forming a golden-brown crust, while bullous impetigo is characterised by the presence of fluid-filled vesicles and blisters that rupture, leaving a thin, flat, yellow-brown crust.

Initial treatment

EvGr Patients, and if appropriate their family or carers, should be advised on good hygiene measures to reduce the spread of impetigo to other body areas and to other people.

In patients with **localised non-bullous impetigo** who are not systemically unwell or at high risk of complications, consider hydrogen peroxide 1% cream p. 1453; if unsuitable (e.g. if impetigo is around the eyes), offer a topical antibacterial.

In patients with **widespread non-bullous impetigo** who are not systemically unwell or at high risk of complications, offer a topical **or** oral antibacterial. Take into account that both routes of administration are effective; any previous use of topical antibacterials that could have led to resistance; and the preferences of the patient and, their family or carers (if appropriate), including the practicalities of administration (particularly to large areas).

In patients with **non-bullous impetigo** who are systemically unwell or at high risk of complications and in all patients with **bullous impetigo**, offer an oral antibacterial.

Combination treatment with a topical and oral antibacterial is not recommended. Ⓐ

For other considerations such as advice to be given to patients, and if appropriate their family or carers, see Antibacterials, principles of therapy p. 573.

EvGr Refer patients to hospital if they have any signs or symptoms suggestive of a more serious condition or illness, or if they have widespread impetigo and are immunocompromised.

Consider referral to hospital or seeking specialist advice for patients who are systemically unwell, have a higher risk of complications, or if impetigo is difficult to treat (such as bullous impetigo (particularly in children aged under 1 year) or frequently recurrent impetigo). Ⓐ

Reassessment and further treatment

EvGr Reassess if symptoms worsen rapidly or significantly at any time, or do not improve after completion of the treatment course. Take into consideration other possible diagnoses (such as herpes simplex infection), signs or symptoms suggesting a more serious illness or condition (such as cellulitis), and previous antibacterial use that might have led to resistance.

For patients whose impetigo is worsening or has not improved after treatment with hydrogen peroxide 1% cream, offer a topical antibacterial if the infection remains localised, or a topical **or** oral antibacterial if infection has become widespread.

Offer an oral antibacterial to patients whose impetigo is worsening or has not improved after completing a course of topical antibacterial.

For patients whose impetigo is worsening or has not improved after completing a course of topical or oral antibacterials, consider sending a skin swab for microbiological testing.

For patients with impetigo that recurs frequently, send a skin swab for microbiological testing and consider taking a nasal swab and starting treatment for decolonisation (using topical treatments and personal hygiene measures).

If a skin swab has been sent for microbiological testing, review the choice of antibacterial and change according to the results if symptoms are not improving, using a narrower-spectrum antibacterial if possible. Ⓐ

5

Infection

Choice of antibacterial therapy

[EvGr] Treatment should be based on infection severity and number of lesions, suspected micro-organism, local antibacterial resistance data, and be guided by microbiological results if available. ◬

- **Topical** *first line* if hydrogen peroxide unsuitable or ineffective:
  - ▸ [EvGr] fusidic acid p. 663.
  - ▸ Alternative if fusidic acid resistance suspected or confirmed: mupirocin p. 1399. ◬
- **Oral** *first line* :
  - ▸ [EvGr] Flucloxacillin p. 643.
  - ▸ Alternative if penicillin allergy or flucloxacillin unsuitable: clarithromycin p. 621 or erythromycin p. 624 (in pregnancy). ◬
- If meticillin-resistant *Staphylococcus aureus* (MRSA) infection suspected or confirmed: [EvGr] Consult local microbiologist. ◬

Cellulitis and erysipelas

Cellulitis and erysipelas are infections of the subcutaneous tissues, which usually result from contamination of a break in the skin. Both conditions are characterised by acute localised inflammation and oedema. Lesions are more superficial in erysipelas and have a well-defined, raised margin.

For management of an infected leg ulcer, see *Leg Ulcer*, and for infection below the ankle in patients with diabetes, see Diabetic foot infections, antibacterial therapy p. 581.

Treatment

[EvGr] Consider taking a swab for microbiological testing **only** if the skin is broken and there is risk of infection by an uncommon pathogen (for example, after a penetrating injury, exposure to water-born organisms, or an infection acquired outside the UK).

Drawing around the extent of the infection to monitor progress before initiating antibacterial treatment can also be considered, taking into account that redness may be less visible on darker skin tones.

Offer an antibacterial taking into account the severity of symptoms, site of infection, risk of uncommon pathogens, previous microbiological results from a swab, and the patient's meticillin-resistant *Staphylococcus aureus* (MRSA) status if known. ◬

For other considerations such as in patients receiving prophylactic antibacterial therapy, switching from intravenous to oral antibacterials, and for advice to be given to patients, see Antibacterials, principles of therapy p. 573.

[EvGr] Manage any underlying condition that may predispose to cellulitis or erysipelas, such as diabetes mellitus, venous insufficiency, eczema, and oedema.

Refer patients to hospital if they have signs or symptoms suggestive of a more serious illness, such as orbital cellulitis, osteomyelitis, septic arthritis, necrotising fasciitis, or sepsis.

Consider referral to hospital or seeking specialist advice for patients who have lymphangitis, are severely unwell, are unable to take oral antibacterials, have infection near the eyes or nose, or that could be caused by an uncommon pathogen. ◬

Reassessment

[EvGr] Reassess if symptoms worsen rapidly or significantly at any time, do not improve within 2–3 days of starting an antibacterial, or the patient becomes systemically very unwell, has severe pain out of proportion to the infection, or has redness or swelling spreading beyond the initial presentation (taking into account that some initial spreading may occur). Take into consideration other possible diagnoses (such as an inflammatory reaction to an insect bite or deep vein thrombosis), any underlying condition that may predispose to cellulitis or erysipelas, signs or symptoms suggesting a more serious illness, results from

microbiological tests, and previous antibacterial use that might have led to resistance.

Consider taking a swab for testing if the skin is broken and this has not already been done.

If a swab has been sent for microbiological testing, review the choice of antibacterial and change according to the results if signs or symptoms are not improving, using a narrower-spectrum antibacterial if possible.

Consider referral to hospital or seeking specialist advice if the infection has spread and is not responding to oral antibacterials. ◬

Choice of antibacterial therapy

[EvGr] Treatment should be based on clinical assessment, infection severity, suspected micro-organism, and site of infection.

Offer oral antibacterials to patients who are able to take oral treatment and the severity of their condition does not require intravenous treatment.

Consider referral to hospital or seeking specialist advice if bacteria are resistant to oral antibacterials, patients cannot take oral treatment, or have infection near the eyes or nose. ◬

First choice antibacterials

- **Oral** or **Intravenous** *first line* :
  - ▸ [EvGr] Flucloxacillin p. 643.
  - ▸ Alternative in penicillin allergy or flucloxacillin unsuitable: clarithromycin p. 621, oral erythromycin p. 624 (in pregnancy), or oral doxycycline p. 655. ◬
- **Oral** or **Intravenous** *first line if infection near the eyes or nose* :
  - ▸ [EvGr] Co-amoxiclav p. 638.
  - ▸ Alternative in penicillin allergy or co-amoxiclav unsuitable: clarithromycin **with** metronidazole p. 628. ◬

Alternative choice antibacterials for severe infection

- **Oral** or **Intravenous**:
  - ▸ [EvGr] Co-amoxiclav, clindamycin p. 618, intravenous cefuroxime p. 606, or intravenous ceftriaxone p. 609 (ambulatory care only).
  - ▸ If meticillin-resistant *Staphylococcus aureus* confirmed or suspected, **add** intravenous vancomycin p. 617, intravenous teicoplanin p. 616, or linezolid p. 664 (specialist use only if vancomycin or teicoplanin cannot be used).
  - ▸ For ambulatory care, and in MRSA confirmed or suspected infections, other antibacterials may be appropriate based on microbiological results and specialist advice. ◬

Antibacterial prophylaxis

[EvGr] For patients who have been treated in hospital, or under specialist advice, for at least 2 separate episodes of cellulitis or erysipelas in the previous 12 months, a trial of antibacterial prophylaxis may be considered by a specialist.

If cellulitis or erysipelas recurs, stop or change the prophylactic antibacterial to an alternative once the acute infection has been treated.

Review antibacterial prophylaxis at least every 6 months, assessing the success of therapy and discussing continuing, stopping or changing prophylaxis taking into account the patient's preference for antibacterial use and the risk of antibacterial resistance. ◬

Leg Ulcer

Leg ulcers usually develop on the lower leg, between the shin and the ankle, and take more than 4–6 weeks to heal. Although the majority of leg ulcers may be colonised with bacteria, this does not necessarily mean that the wound is infected. Signs and symptoms of an infected leg ulcer include redness (may be less visible on darker skin tones) or swelling spreading beyond the ulcer, localised warmth, increased pain, or fever.

Treatment

[EvGr] Any underlying condition that may cause a leg ulcer, such as venous insufficiency and oedema should be managed to promote healing.

Taking a sample for microbiological testing at initial presentation with a leg ulcer is not recommended, even if the ulcer may be infected.

Offer an antibacterial to patients who have signs or symptoms of infection taking into account the severity of signs or symptoms, risk of developing complications, and previous antibacterial use. ⟨A⟩

For other considerations such as switching from intravenous to oral antibacterials and for advice to be given to patients, see Antibacterials, principles of therapy p. 573.

[EvGr] Refer patients to hospital if they have signs or symptoms suggestive of a more serious condition or illness, such as sepsis, necrotising fasciitis, or osteomyelitis.

Consider referral to hospital or seeking specialist advice for patients with an infected leg ulcer who are unable to take oral treatment, have lymphangitis, or are at a higher risk of complications due to comorbidities (such as diabetes or immunosuppression). ⟨A⟩

Reassessment

[EvGr] Reassess if signs or symptoms worsen rapidly or significantly at any time, do not improve within 2–3 days, or the patient becomes systemically unwell or has severe pain out of proportion to the infection. Take into consideration previous antibacterial use that might have led to resistance, and be aware that full resolution of an infected leg ulcer is not expected until after the antibacterial course is completed.

Consider taking a sample from the leg ulcer (after cleaning) for microbiological testing if signs or symptoms of infection are worsening or have not improved as expected. Review the choice of antibacterial(s) and change according to the results if signs or symptoms are not improving, using a narrower-spectrum antibacterial if possible.

Consider referral to hospital or seeking specialist advice if patients have a spreading infection that is not responding to oral antibacterials. ⟨A⟩

Choice of antibacterial therapy

[EvGr] Treatment should be based on clinical assessment, infection severity, suspected micro-organism, and be guided by microbiological results if available.

Offer oral antibacterials to patients who are able to take oral treatment and the severity of their condition does not require intravenous treatment. ⟨A⟩

Non-severely unwell patients

- **Oral** *first line* :
  - ▸ [EvGr] Flucloxacillin.
  - ▸ Alternative in penicillin allergy or flucloxacillin unsuitable: doxycycline, clarithromycin, or erythromycin (in pregnancy). ⟨A⟩
- **Oral** *second line* (guided by microbiological results when available):
  - ▸ [EvGr] Co-amoxiclav.
  - ▸ Alternative in penicillin allergy: co-trimoxazole p. 652 [unlicensed]. ⟨A⟩

Severely unwell patients

- **Oral** or **Intravenous** *first line* (guided by microbiological results if available):
  - ▸ [EvGr] Intravenous flucloxacillin **with** or **without** intravenous gentamicin p. 596 **and/or** metronidazole, *or* intravenous co-amoxiclav **with** or **without** intravenous gentamicin.
  - ▸ Alternative in penicillin allergy: intravenous co-trimoxazole [unlicensed] **with** or **without** intravenous gentamicin **and/or** metronidazole. ⟨A⟩
- **Oral** or **Intravenous** *second line* (guided by microbiological results when available or following specialist advice):

- ▸ [EvGr] Intravenous piperacillin with tazobactam p. 631, *or* intravenous ceftriaxone **with** or **without** metronidazole. ⟨A⟩

Antibacterials to be added if meticillin-resistant Staphylococcus aureus (MRSA) infection suspected or confirmed

- **Oral** or **Intravenous** (in addition to antibacterials listed above):
  - ▸ [EvGr] Intravenous vancomycin, intravenous teicoplanin, or linezolid (specialist use only if vancomycin or teicoplanin cannot be used). ⟨A⟩

Insect bites and stings

Redness, itchiness, or pain and swelling after an insect sting or bite (including bites from spiders and ticks) is often caused by a localised inflammatory or allergic reaction rather than an infection, especially when there is a rapid onset. Rarely, symptoms may last for up to 10 days.

For the management of patients with a known or suspected tick bite, see Lyme disease p. 669. [EvGr] Consider referral or seeking specialist advice for patients with fever or persistent lesions after an insect bite or sting from outside the UK, as this may indicate a more serious illness such as rickettsial infection or malaria.

Antibacterials are not recommended for an insect bite or sting unless the patient has signs or symptoms of an infection. For the management of patients with a suspected infection, see *Cellulitis and erysipelas*. ⟨A⟩

Human and animal bites

Human and animal bites that cause a break in the skin are an infection risk. Contributing factors of infection include the species causing the bite, type and location of the wound, and the patient's individual risk factors (such as comorbidities, and age (with the elderly being at higher risk of infection)).

For guidance on the management of insect bites, see *Insects bites and stings*.

Management

[EvGr] Patients with a human or an animal bite should be assessed for their risk of tetanus, rabies, or a blood-borne viral infection (such as HIV, and hepatitis B and C), and should be managed accordingly. ⟨A⟩ For guidance on the management of tetanus- and rabies-prone wounds, see Tetanus vaccine p. 1493 or Rabies vaccine p. 1490.

[EvGr] The patient's wound should be cleaned by irrigation and debrided as necessary.

For bites from wild or exotic animals (including birds and non-traditional pets), advice should be sought from a microbiologist as the spectrum of bacteria involved may be different and there may be a risk of other serious non-bacterial infections. Consider seeking advice for bites from unfamiliar domestic animals (including farm animals).

Refer patients to hospital if they have signs or symptoms suggesting a more serious illness or condition (such as severe cellulitis, abscess, osteomyelitis, septic arthritis, necrotising fasciitis, or sepsis), or a penetrating wound involving the arteries, joints, nerves, muscles, tendons, bones or the central nervous system.

Consider referral to hospital or seeking specialist advice for patients who have lymphangitis, are systemically unwell, have a bite in an area of poor circulation, are at risk of a serious wound infection due to comorbidities, or are unable to take oral antibacterials. ⟨A⟩

For considerations such as switching from intravenous to oral antibacterials, and for advice to be given to patients, see Antibacterials, principles of therapy p. 573.

Prophylaxis for an uninfected bite

[EvGr] Offer antibacterial prophylaxis to patients with a:

- cat or human bite that has broken the skin and drawn blood; or
- dog or other traditional pet bite (excluding cat bites) that has broken the skin and drawn blood if it:

- has penetrated bone, joint, tendon or vascular structures;
- is deep, a puncture or crush wound, or has caused significant tissue damage; or
- is visibly contaminated (for example if there is dirt or a tooth in the wound).

Consider antibacterial prophylaxis in a patient with:

- a cat bite that has broken the skin but **not** drawn blood and the wound could be deep; or
- a human bite that has broken the skin but **not** drawn blood, *or* a dog or other traditional pet bite (excluding cat bites) that has broken the skin and drawn blood, if it:

- involves a high-risk area (such as the hands, feet, face, genitals, skin overlying cartilaginous structures, or an area of poor circulation), or
- is in an individual at risk of a serious wound infection because of a comorbidity (such as diabetes, immunosuppression, asplenia, or decompensated liver disease).

Consider referral to hospital or seeking specialist advice for patients who develop an infection despite taking antibacterial prophylaxis. ⒶⒶ

Treatment for an infected bite
[EvGr] To guide treatment for wounds that have a purulent or non-purulent discharge, a swab should be taken for microbiological testing.

Antibacterial therapy should be offered to patients if there are signs or symptoms of infection (such as increased pain, inflammation, fever, discharge, or an unpleasant smell). ⒶⒶ

Reassessment
[EvGr] Reassess the patient's wound if either:

- signs or symptoms of infection develop, worsen rapidly or significantly at any time, or do not improve within 1–2 days of starting an antibacterial; or
- the patient becomes systemically unwell or has severe pain out of proportion to the infection.

If a skin swab has been sent for microbiological testing, review the choice of antibacterial and change according to the results if needed, using a narrower-spectrum antibacterial if possible.

Consider referral or seeking specialist advice if the infected wound is not responding to oral antibacterial therapy. ⒶⒶ

Choice of antibacterial for prophylaxis and treatment
[EvGr] For bites from a human, cat, dog, or other traditional pet, offer oral antibacterials to patients who are able to take medication orally and the severity of their condition does not require intravenous antibacterials. ⒶⒶ

- *Oral* first line :
- [EvGr] Co-amoxiclav p. 638.
- Alternative in penicillin allergy or co-amoxiclav unsuitable: doxycycline p. 655 **with** metronidazole p. 628; seek specialist advice in pregnancy. ⒶⒶ

- *Intravenous* first line :
- [EvGr] Co-amoxiclav.
- Alternative in penicillin allergy or co-amoxiclav unsuitable: cefuroxime p. 606 *or* ceftriaxone p. 609, **with** metronidazole; seek specialist advice if a cephalosporin is not appropriate. ⒶⒶ

Secondary bacterial infection of common skin conditions

Common skin conditions that cause breaks in the skin are an infection risk, as bacteria that live on the skin may infiltrate the damaged area. The most commonly infected skin conditions are chickenpox, eczema, psoriasis, scabies, and shingles. For guidance on the management of underlying skin conditions and non-antibacterial treatment, see Eczema p. 1405, Herpesvirus infections p. 727, Psoriasis p. 1406, and Skin infections p. 1395.

[EvGr] For secondary bacterial infections of common skin conditions other than eczema (such as chickenpox, psoriasis, scabies, and shingles) there is no evidence available for antibacterial use—seek specialist advice if needed. ⒶⒶ

The following recommendations cover the management of patients with secondary bacterial skin infection of **eczema**. Signs and symptoms of secondary bacterial infection of eczema can include weeping, pustules, crusts, no response to treatment, rapidly worsening eczema, fever, and malaise. Even if weeping and crusts are present, not all eczema flares are caused by a bacterial infection.

Treatment of secondary bacterial skin infection of eczema
[EvGr] Taking a routine skin swab for microbiological testing at initial presentation is not recommended as eczema is often colonised with bacteria but may not be clinically infected.

In patients who are not systemically unwell, an antibacterial is not routinely recommended. Take into account the evidence of limited benefit of antibacterials when used in addition to topical corticosteroids, risk of antimicrobial resistance with repeated courses, extent and severity of signs or symptoms, and risk of developing complications (higher in individuals with underlying conditions such as immunosuppression).

If an antibacterial is offered to patients who are not systemically unwell, the choice between a topical or oral antibacterial should take into account the preferences of the patient (and their family/carers), previous use of topical antibacterials as resistance can develop rapidly with extended or repeated use, practicalities of administration (particularly to large areas), and the extent and severity of signs or symptoms. A topical antibacterial may be more appropriate for a localised infection that is not severe, whereas, an oral antibacterial may be more appropriate if the infection is widespread or severe.

Offer an oral antibacterial to patients who are systemically unwell (such as with a fever or malaise).

Underlying eczema and flares should be managed with emollients and topical corticosteroids regardless of whether antibacterials are offered (see Eczema p. 1405). ⒶⒶ

For other considerations such as advice to be given to patients, see Antibacterials, principles of therapy p. 573.

[EvGr] Refer patients to hospital if they have signs or symptoms suggestive of a more serious illness, such as necrotising fasciitis or sepsis. For patients with signs and symptoms of cellulitis, see *Cellulitis and erysipelas*.

Consider referral to hospital or seeking specialist advice for patients who are systemically unwell or at high risk of complications, or have infections that recur often. ⒶⒶ

Reassessment
[EvGr] Reassess if symptoms worsen rapidly or significantly at any time, do not improve after completion of an antibacterial course, the patient becomes systemically unwell, or has pain out of proportion to the infection. Take into consideration other possible diagnoses (such as eczema herpeticum), signs or symptoms suggesting a more serious illness, and previous antibacterial use that might have led to resistance.

For patients whose infection is worsening or has not improved as expected, consider sending a skin swab for microbiological testing.

For patients with secondary bacterial infection of eczema that recurs frequently, send a skin swab for microbiological testing and consider taking a nasal swab and starting treatment for decolonisation.

If a skin swab has been sent for microbiological testing, review the choice of antibacterial and change according to the results if symptoms are not improving, using a narrower-spectrum antibacterial if possible.

Consider referral to hospital or seeking specialist advice if the infection has spread and is not responding to oral antibacterials. ⒶⒶ

Choice of antibacterial therapy

[EvGr] Treatment should be based on infection severity, suspected micro-organism, local antibacterial resistance data, and be guided by microbiological results if available. Ⓐ

- *Topical* first line :
▸ [EvGr] Fusidic acid p. 663.
▸ If fusidic acid unsuitable or ineffective: offer an oral antibacterial. Ⓐ
- *Oral* first line :
▸ [EvGr] Flucloxacillin p. 643.
▸ Alternative if penicillin allergy or flucloxacillin unsuitable: clarithromycin p. 621 or erythromycin p. 624 (in pregnancy). Ⓐ
- If meticillin-resistant *Staphylococcus aureus* (MRSA) infection suspected or confirmed: [EvGr] Consult a local microbiologist. Ⓐ

Mastitis during breast-feeding

Treat if severe, if systemically unwell, if nipple fissure present, if symptoms do not improve after 12–24 hours of effective milk removal, or if culture indicates infection. Continue breast-feeding or expressing milk during treatment.

- Flucloxacillin
▸ *Suggested duration of treatment* 10–14 days.
- *If penicillin-allergic*, erythromycin
▸ *Suggested duration of treatment* 10–14 days.

Useful Resources

Cellulitis and erysipelas: antimicrobial prescribing. National Institute for Health and Care Excellence. NICE guideline 141. September 2019.
www.nice.org.uk/guidance/ng141

Human and animal bites: antimicrobial prescribing. National Institute for Health and Care Excellence. NICE guideline 184. November 2020.
www.nice.org.uk/guidance/ng184

Impetigo: antimicrobial prescribing. National Institute for Health and Care Excellence. NICE guideline 153. February 2020.
www.nice.org.uk/guidance/ng153

Insect bites and stings: antimicrobial prescribing. National Institute for Health and Care Excellence. NICE guideline 182. September 2020.
www.nice.org.uk/guidance/ng182

Leg ulcer infection: antimicrobial prescribing. National Institute for Health and Care Excellence. NICE guideline 152. February 2020.
www.nice.org.uk/guidance/ng152

Secondary bacterial infection of eczema and other common skin conditions: antimicrobial prescribing. National Institute for Health and Care Excellence. NICE guideline 190. March 2021.
www.nice.org.uk/guidance/ng190

> **Other drugs used for Bacterial infection** Rifabutin, p. 673

ANTIBACTERIALS > AMINOGLYCOSIDES

Aminoglycosides   15-May-2024

Overview

These include amikacin p. 594, gentamicin p. 596, neomycin sulfate p. 597, streptomycin p. 598, and tobramycin p. 598. All are bactericidal and active against some Gram-positive and many Gram-negative organisms. Amikacin, gentamicin, and tobramycin are also active against *Pseudomonas aeruginosa*; streptomycin is active against *Mycobacterium tuberculosis* and is now almost entirely reserved for tuberculosis.

The aminoglycosides are not absorbed from the gut (although there is a risk of absorption in inflammatory bowel disease and liver failure) and must therefore be given by injection for systemic infections.

Gentamicin is the aminoglycoside of choice in the UK and is used widely for the treatment of serious infections. It has a broad spectrum but is inactive against anaerobes and has poor activity against haemolytic streptococci and pneumococci. When used for the 'blind' therapy of undiagnosed serious infections it is usually given in conjunction with a penicillin or metronidazole p. 628 (or both). Gentamicin is used together with another antibiotic for the treatment of endocarditis. Streptomycin may be used as an alternative in gentamicin-resistant enterococcal endocarditis.

Loading and maintenance doses of gentamicin may be calculated on the basis of the patient's weight and renal function (e.g. using a nomogram); adjustments are then made according to serum-gentamicin concentrations. High doses are occasionally indicated for serious infections, especially in the neonate or in the immunocompromised patient. Whenever possible treatment should not exceed 7 days.

Amikacin is more stable than gentamicin to enzyme inactivation. Amikacin is used in the treatment of serious infections caused by gentamicin-resistant Gram-negative bacilli.

Tobramycin has similar activity to gentamicin but is more active against *Pseudomonas aeruginosa*. Tobramycin can also be administered by nebuliser or by inhalation of powder on a cyclical basis (28 days of tobramycin followed by a 28-day tobramycin-free interval) for the treatment of chronic pulmonary *Pseudomonas aeruginosa* infection in cystic fibrosis; however, resistance may develop and some patients do not respond to treatment.

Neomycin sulfate is too toxic for parenteral administration and can only be used for infections of the skin or mucous membranes or to reduce the bacterial population of the colon prior to bowel surgery or in hepatic failure. Oral administration may lead to malabsorption. Small amounts of neomycin sulfate may be absorbed from the gut in patients with hepatic failure and, as these patients may also be uraemic, cumulation may occur with resultant ototoxicity.

Once daily dosage

Once daily administration of aminoglycosides is more convenient, provides adequate serum concentrations, and in many cases has largely superseded *multiple-daily dose regimens* (given in 2–3 divided doses during the 24 hours). Local guidelines on dosage and serum concentrations should be consulted. A once-daily, high-dose regimen of an aminoglycoside should be avoided in patients with endocarditis due to Gram-positive bacteria, HACEK endocarditis, burns of more than 20% of the total body surface area, or creatinine clearance less than 20 mL/minute. There is insufficient evidence to recommend a once daily, high-dose regimen of an aminoglycoside in pregnancy.

Serum concentrations

Serum concentration monitoring avoids both excessive and subtherapeutic concentrations thus preventing toxicity and ensuring efficacy. Serum-aminoglycoside concentrations should be monitored in patients receiving parenteral aminoglycosides and **must** be determined in the elderly, in obesity, and in cystic fibrosis, or if high doses are being given, or if there is renal impairment.

Aminoglycosides (by injection)

> **IMPORTANT SAFETY INFORMATION**
>
> **MHRA/CHM ADVICE: AMINOGLYCOSIDES (GENTAMICIN, AMIKACIN, TOBRAMYCIN, AND NEOMYCIN): INCREASED RISK OF DEAFNESS IN PATIENTS WITH MITOCHONDRIAL MUTATIONS (JANUARY 2021)**
>
> The use of aminoglycosides is associated with rare cases of ototoxicity. A safety review found an increased risk of deafness in patients with mitochondrial mutations (particularly the m.1555A>G mutation), including cases where the patient's aminoglycoside serum levels were within the recommended range. Nevertheless, these mitochondrial mutations are considered rare and penetrance is uncertain.
>
> Healthcare professionals are advised to consider the need for aminoglycoside treatment versus alternative options in patients with susceptible mutations. The need for genetic testing especially in those requiring recurrent or long-term treatment with aminoglycosides should also be considered, however, urgent treatment should not be delayed. To minimise the risks of adverse effects, continuous monitoring of renal and auditory function, as well as hepatic and laboratory parameters, is recommended for all patients. Those with known mitochondrial mutations or a family history of ototoxicity are advised to inform their doctor or pharmacist before using an aminoglycoside.

- **CONTRA-INDICATIONS** Myasthenia gravis (aminoglycosides may impair neuromuscular transmission)
- **CAUTIONS** Auditory disorder · care must be taken with dosage (the main side-effects of the aminoglycosides are dose-related) · conditions characterised by muscular weakness (aminoglycosides may impair neuromuscular transmission) · if possible, dehydration should be corrected before starting an aminoglycoside · vestibular disorder · whenever possible, parenteral treatment should not exceed 7 days
- **SIDE-EFFECTS**
  - **Common or very common** Aphonia · appetite decreased · bronchospasm · chest discomfort · cough · deafness · diarrhoea · dizziness · dysphonia · fever · haemoptysis · headache · increased risk of infection · nausea · oropharyngeal pain · renal impairment · skin reactions · taste altered · tinnitus · vomiting
  - **Rare or very rare** Anaemia · azotaemia · eosinophilia · hearing loss (sometimes irreversible) · hypomagnesaemia · paraesthesia
  - **Frequency not known** Confusion · lethargy · leucopenia · muscle weakness · nephrotoxicity · peripheral neuropathy · thrombocytopenia · vertigo

  SIDE-EFFECTS, FURTHER INFORMATION Ototoxicity and nephrotoxicity are important side-effects to consider with aminoglycoside therapy. Nephrotoxicity occurs most commonly in patients with renal impairment, who may require reduced doses; monitoring is particularly important in the elderly.
- **PREGNANCY** There is a risk of auditory or vestibular nerve damage in the infant when aminoglycosides are used in the second and third trimesters of pregnancy. The risk is greatest with streptomycin. The risk is probably very small with gentamicin and tobramycin, but their use should be avoided unless essential.
  Monitoring If given during pregnancy, serum-aminoglycoside concentration monitoring is essential.
- **RENAL IMPAIRMENT** EvGr Aminoglycosides are primarily renally excreted and accumulation can occur in renal impairment (increased risk of ototoxicity and nephrotoxicity)—serum-aminoglycoside concentrations **must** be frequently monitored in patients with renal impairment. ⓜ

Dose adjustments EvGr Reduce dose and/or increase the dose interval according to impairment (consult product literature). ⓜ

- **MONITORING REQUIREMENTS**
  - Serum concentrations Serum concentration monitoring avoids both excessive and subtherapeutic concentrations thus preventing toxicity and ensuring efficacy. Serum-aminoglycoside concentrations should be measured in all patients receiving parenteral aminoglycosides and **must** be determined in obesity, if high doses are being given and in cystic fibrosis.
  - In adults Serum aminoglycoside concentrations **must** be determined in the elderly. In patients with normal renal function, aminoglycoside concentrations should be measured after 3 or 4 doses of a multiple daily dose regimen and after a dose change. For multiple daily dose regimens, blood samples should be taken approximately 1 hour after intramuscular or intravenous administration ('peak' concentration) and also just before the next dose ('trough' concentration). If the pre-dose ('trough') concentration is high, the interval between doses must be increased. If the post-dose ('peak') concentration is high, the dose must be decreased. For once daily dose regimens, consult local guidelines on serum concentration monitoring.
  - In children In children with normal renal function, aminoglycoside concentrations should be measured after 3 or 4 doses of a multiple daily dose regimen. Blood samples should be taken just before the next dose is administered ('trough' concentration). If the pre-dose ('trough') concentration is high, the interval between doses must be increased. For multiple daily dose regimens, blood samples should also be taken approximately 1 hour after intramuscular or intravenous administration ('peak' concentration). If the post-dose ('peak') concentration is high, the dose must be decreased.
  - Renal function should be assessed before starting an aminoglycoside and during treatment.
  - Auditory and vestibular function should also be monitored during treatment.

⬗ above

Amikacin

13-May-2024

- **INDICATIONS AND DOSE**

Serious Gram-negative infections resistant to gentamicin (multiple daily dose regimen)
- BY INTRAMUSCULAR INJECTION, OR BY SLOW INTRAVENOUS INJECTION, OR BY INTRAVENOUS INFUSION
- Adult: 15 mg/kg daily in 2 divided doses, increased to 22.5 mg/kg daily in 3 divided doses for up to 10 days, higher dose to be used in severe infections; maximum 1.5 g per day; maximum 15 g per course

Serious Gram-negative infections resistant to gentamicin (once daily dose regimen)
- BY INTRAVENOUS INFUSION
- Adult: Initially 15 mg/kg once daily (max. per dose 1.5 g once daily), dose to be adjusted according to serum-amikacin concentration; maximum 15 g per course

Acute prostatitis (once daily dose regimen)
- BY INTRAVENOUS INFUSION, OR BY SLOW INTRAVENOUS INJECTION
- Adult: Initially 15 mg/kg once daily (max. per dose 1.5 g once daily), dose to be adjusted according to serum-amikacin concentration; maximum 15 g per course

Acute pyelonephritis (once daily dose regimen) | Urinary tract infection (catheter-associated, once daily dose regimen)
▸ BY INTRAVENOUS INFUSION, OR BY SLOW INTRAVENOUS INJECTION
▸ Adult: Initially 15 mg/kg once daily (max. per dose 1.5 g once daily), dose to be adjusted according to serum-amikacin concentration; maximum 15 g per course

DOSES AT EXTREMES OF BODY-WEIGHT
▸ To avoid excessive dosage in obese patients, use ideal weight for height to calculate dose and monitor serum-amikacin concentration closely

ARIKAYCE ® LIPOSOMAL NEBULISER DISPERSION

Non-tuberculous mycobacterial lung infections caused by *Mycobacterium avium* complex in patients without cystic fibrosis [in combination with other drugs] (specialist use only)
▸ BY INHALATION OF NEBULISED SUSPENSION
▸ Adult: 590 mg once daily for 12 months after negative sputum cultures, or for up to 6 months if negative sputum cultures not confirmed; treatment should not exceed 18 months

DOSE EQUIVALENCE AND CONVERSION
▸ For *Arikayce®*: one vial contains amikacin sulfate equivalent to 590 mg amikacin in a liposomal formulation; the mean dose delivered to the lungs when nebulised is approximately 312 mg amikacin.

IMPORTANT SAFETY INFORMATION

MHRA/CHM ADVICE: LIPOSOMAL AND LIPID-COMPLEX FORMULATIONS: NAME CHANGE TO REDUCE MEDICATION ERRORS (JULY 2020)
Serious harm and fatal overdoses have occurred following confusion between liposomal, pegylated-liposomal, lipid-complex, and conventional formulations of the same drug substance. Medicines with these formulations will explicitly include 'liposomal', 'pegylated-liposomal', or 'lipid-complex' within their name to reduce the risk of potentially fatal medication errors.

The MHRA reminds healthcare professionals that liposomal, pegylated-liposomal, lipid-complex, and conventional formulations containing the same drug substance are **not** interchangeable. Healthcare professionals are advised to make a clear distinction between formulations when prescribing, dispensing, administering, and communicating about them. The product name and dose should be verified before administration and the maximum dose should not be exceeded.

● CONTRA-INDICATIONS
▸ When used by inhalation Myasthenia gravis (aminoglycosides may impair neuromuscular transmission)

● CAUTIONS
▸ When used by inhalation History of reactive airway disease, asthma, or bronchospasm (pre-treat with a short-acting bronchodilator) · known or suspected neuromuscular disorders · underlying pulmonary disease (discontinue if signs of exacerbation occur)

● INTERACTIONS → Appendix 1: aminoglycosides

● SIDE-EFFECTS

GENERAL SIDE-EFFECTS
▸ Common or very common Arthralgia · balance impaired

SPECIFIC SIDE-EFFECTS
▸ Common or very common
▸ When used by inhalation Dry mouth · dyspnoea · fatigue · interstitial lung disease · myalgia · respiratory disorders · sputum increased · throat irritation · weight decreased

▸ Uncommon
▸ When used by inhalation Anxiety
▸ Rare or very rare
▸ With parenteral use Albuminuria · hearing impairment · hypotension · muscle twitching · tremor
▸ Frequency not known
▸ When used by inhalation Hypersensitivity · neuromuscular disorders · ototoxicity
▸ With parenteral use Apnoea · neuromuscular blockade · paralysis

SIDE-EFFECTS, FURTHER INFORMATION Since systemic absorption can follow inhaled use, also consider the side-effects of systemic aminoglycosides.

● PREGNANCY
ARIKAYCE ® LIPOSOMAL NEBULISER DISPERSION [EvGr] Avoid—no information available. Ⓜ

● BREAST FEEDING
ARIKAYCE ® LIPOSOMAL NEBULISER DISPERSION [EvGr] Avoid—no information available. Ⓜ

● RENAL IMPAIRMENT
▸ When used by inhalation [EvGr] Avoid in severe impairment (no information available). Ⓜ

● PRE-TREATMENT SCREENING NHS England commissions genetic testing under the *National genomic test directory* indication: R65 - Aminoglycoside exposure posing risk to hearing. The testing criteria is significant exposure to aminoglycosides posing risk of ototoxicity. This testing is relevant to individuals with a predisposition to gram-negative infections or with hearing loss who have been exposed to aminoglycosides. For further information, see www.england.nhs.uk/publication/national-genomic-test-directories/.

● MONITORING REQUIREMENTS
▸ With intravenous use *Multiple daily dose regimen*: one-hour ('peak') serum concentration should not exceed 30 mg/litre; pre-dose ('trough') concentration should be less than 10 mg/litre. *Once daily dose regimen*: pre-dose ('trough') concentration should be less than 5 mg/litre.
▸ When used by inhalation [EvGr] Auditory and vestibular function, and renal function should be monitored during treatment. Ⓜ

● DIRECTIONS FOR ADMINISTRATION For *intravenous infusion* (*Amikin®*); manufacturer advises dilute in Glucose 5% *or* Sodium Chloride 0.9%. To be given over 30–60 minutes.

● PRESCRIBING AND DISPENSING INFORMATION
Amikacin is available as both *conventional* and *liposomal* formulations. These different formulations vary in their licensed indications, pharmacokinetics, dosage and administration, and are **not** interchangeable.
▸ With intravenous use Once daily dose regimen not to be used for endocarditis, febrile neutropenia, or meningitis. Consult local guidelines.

● PATIENT AND CARER ADVICE
ARIKAYCE ® LIPOSOMAL NEBULISER DISPERSION Patients and carers should be given advice on how to administer doses using the *Lamira®* nebuliser system.
Driving and skilled tasks Patients and carers should be cautioned on the effects on driving and performance of skilled tasks—increased risk of dizziness and vestibular disturbances.

● NATIONAL FUNDING/ACCESS DECISIONS
For full details see funding body website

Scottish Medicines Consortium (SMC) decisions
▸ Amikacin liposomal nebuliser dispersion (*Arikayce®*) for the treatment of non-tuberculous mycobacterial lung infections caused by *Mycobacterium avium* complex in adults with limited treatment options who do not have cystic fibrosis (December 2021) SMC No. SMC2432 Recommended

All Wales Medicines Strategy Group (AWMSG) decisions

- Amikacin liposomal nebuliser dispersion (*Arikayce*®) for the treatment of non-tuberculous mycobacterial lung infections caused by *Mycobacterium avium* complex in adults with limited treatment options who do not have cystic fibrosis (September 2021) AWMSG No. 2140 Recommended

● **MEDICINAL FORMS** There can be variation in the licensing of different medicines containing the same drug. Forms available from special-order manufacturers include: solution for injection

Solution for injection

- Amikacin (Non-proprietary)
  Amikacin (as Amikacin sulfate) 250 mg per 1 ml Amikacin 500mg/2ml solution for injection ampoules | 5 ampoule [PoM] £60.00 (Hospital only)
  Amikacin 500mg/2ml solution for injection vials | 5 vial [PoM] £40.00–£60.00 (Hospital only) | 5 vial [PoM] £60.00
- Amikin (Vianex S.A.)
  Amikacin (as Amikacin sulfate) 50 mg per 1 ml Amikin 100mg/2ml solution for injection vials | 5 vial [PoM] £10.33 (Hospital only)

Nebuliser dispersion

- Arikayce (Insmed Ltd)
  Amikacin liposomal 590 mg Arikayce liposomal 590mg nebuliser dispersion vials with Lamira Nebuliser Handset | 28 vial [PoM] £9,513.00 (Hospital only)

F 594

Gentamicin

10-Feb-2025

● **INDICATIONS AND DOSE**

Moderate diabetic foot infection | Severe diabetic foot infection | Acute diverticulitis [in combination with amoxicillin and metronidazole] | Leg ulcer infection [in combination with other drugs]

▶ BY INTRAVENOUS INFUSION

- Adult: Initially 5–7 mg/kg once daily, subsequent doses adjusted according to serum-gentamicin concentration

Gram-positive bacterial endocarditis or HACEK endocarditis (in combination with other antibacterials)

▶ BY INTRAMUSCULAR INJECTION, OR BY SLOW INTRAVENOUS INJECTION, OR BY INTRAVENOUS INFUSION

- Adult: 1 mg/kg every 12 hours, intravenous injection to be administered over at least 3 minutes, to be given in a multiple daily dose regimen

Septicaemia | Meningitis and other CNS infections | Biliary-tract infection | Endocarditis | Pneumonia in hospital patients | Adjunct in listerial meningitis | Prostatitis

▶ BY INTRAVENOUS INFUSION, OR BY SLOW INTRAVENOUS INJECTION, OR BY INTRAMUSCULAR INJECTION

- Adult: 3–5 mg/kg daily in 3 divided doses, to be given in a multiple daily dose regimen, divided doses to be given every 8 hours, intravenous injection to be administered over at least 3 minutes

▶ BY INTRAVENOUS INFUSION

- Adult: Initially 5–7 mg/kg, subsequent doses adjusted according to serum-gentamicin concentration, to be given in a once daily dose regimen

CNS infections (administered on expert advice)

▶ BY INTRATHECAL INJECTION

- Adult: 1 mg daily, increased if necessary to 5 mg daily, seek specialist advice

Surgical prophylaxis

▶ BY SLOW INTRAVENOUS INJECTION

- Adult: 1.5 mg/kg, intravenous injection to be administered over at least 3 minutes, administer dose up to 30 minutes before the procedure, dose may be repeated every 8 hours for high-risk procedures; up to 3 further doses may be given

Surgical prophylaxis in joint replacement surgery

▶ BY INTRAVENOUS INFUSION

- Adult: 5 mg/kg for 1 dose, administer dose up to 30 minutes before the procedure

Acute pyelonephritis (once daily dose regimen) | Urinary tract infection (catheter-associated, once daily dose regimen)

▶ BY INTRAVENOUS INFUSION

- Adult: Initially 5–7 mg/kg once daily, subsequent doses adjusted according to serum-gentamicin concentration

Uncomplicated gonorrhoea [anogenital and pharyngeal infection—in combination with azithromycin]

▶ BY INTRAMUSCULAR INJECTION

- Adult: 240 mg for 1 dose

DOSES AT EXTREMES OF BODY-WEIGHT

- With intramuscular use or intravenous use To avoid excessive dosage in obese patients, use ideal weight for height to calculate parenteral dose and monitor serum-gentamicin concentration closely.

● **UNLICENSED USE** Gentamicin doses in BNF Publications may differ from those in product literature.

[EvGr] Gentamicin is used in the doses provided in BNF Publications for the treatment of uncomplicated gonorrhoea, ⟨A⟩ but these are not licensed.

IMPORTANT SAFETY INFORMATION

MHRA/CHM ADVICE: POTENTIAL FOR HISTAMINE-RELATED ADVERSE DRUG REACTIONS WITH SOME BATCHES (NOVEMBER 2017)

Following reports that some batches of gentamicin sulphate active pharmaceutical ingredient (API) used to manufacture gentamicin may contain higher than expected levels of histamine, which is a residual from the manufacturing process, the MHRA advise to monitor patients for signs of histamine-related adverse reactions; particular caution is required in patients taking concomitant drugs known to cause histamine release, in children, and in patients with severe renal impairment.

● **INTERACTIONS** → Appendix 1: aminoglycosides

● **SIDE-EFFECTS**

- **Rare or very rare** Fanconi syndrome acquired
- **Frequency not known** Antibiotic associated colitis · blood disorder · central neuropathy · depression · encephalopathy · hallucination · hepatic function abnormal · neurotoxicity · pseudomembranous enterocolitis · seizure · severe cutaneous adverse reactions (SCARs) · stomatitis · vestibular damage

● **PRE-TREATMENT SCREENING** NHS England commissions genetic testing under the *National genomic test directory* indication: R65 - Aminoglycoside exposure posing risk to hearing. The testing criteria is significant exposure to aminoglycosides posing risk of ototoxicity. This testing is relevant to individuals with a predisposition to gram-negative infections or with hearing loss who have been exposed to aminoglycosides. For further information, see www.england.nhs.uk/publication/national-genomic-test-directories/.

● **MONITORING REQUIREMENTS**

- With intramuscular use or intravenous use For multiple daily dose regimen, one-hour ('peak') serum concentration should be 5–10 mg/litre; pre-dose ('trough') concentration should be less than 2 mg/litre. For multiple daily dose regimen in endocarditis, one-hour ('peak') serum concentration should be 3–5 mg/litre; pre-dose ('trough') concentration should be less than 1 mg/litre. Serum-gentamicin concentration should be measured after 3 or 4 doses, then at least every 3 days and after a dose change (more frequently in renal impairment).

▸ **With intravenous use** For once-daily dose regimen, consult local guidelines on monitoring serum-gentamicin concentration.

● **DIRECTIONS FOR ADMINISTRATION** For *intrathecal* injection, use preservative-free intrathecal preparations only.

　　EvGr For *intravenous infusion*, give intermittently *or* via drip tubing in Glucose 5% or Sodium Chloride 0.9%. Suggested volume for intermittent infusion 50–100 mL given over 20–30 minutes (given over 60 minutes for once daily dose regimen). Ⓜ

● **PRESCRIBING AND DISPENSING INFORMATION** For choice of antibacterial therapy, see Antibacterials, use for prophylaxis p. 574, Cardiovascular system infections, antibacterial therapy p. 579, Central nervous system infections, antibacterial therapy p. 580, Diabetic foot infections, antibacterial therapy p. 581, Gastro-intestinal system infections, antibacterial therapy p. 582, Genital system infections, antibacterial therapy p. 584, Respiratory system infections, antibacterial therapy p. 586, Skin infections, antibacterial therapy p. 589, Urinary-tract infections p. 681.

▸ **With intravenous use** Local guidelines may vary in the dosing advice provided for once daily administration.

▸ **With intrathecal use** Only preservative-free intrathecal preparation should be used.

● **MEDICINAL FORMS** There can be variation in the licensing of different medicines containing the same drug. Forms available from special-order manufacturers include: solution for injection, infusion

Solution for injection

▸ Gentamicin (Non-proprietary)
　Gentamicin (as Gentamicin sulfate) 5 mg per 1 ml Gentamicin Intrathecal 5mg/1ml solution for injection ampoules | 5 ampoule PoM £36.28 (Hospital only)
　Gentamicin (as Gentamicin sulfate) 10 mg per 1 ml Gentamicin 20mg/2ml solution for injection ampoules | 5 ampoule PoM £12.95 DT = £11.25
　Gentamicin Paediatric 20mg/2ml solution for injection vials | 5 vial PoM £11.25
　Gentamicin (as Gentamicin sulfate) 40 mg per 1 ml Gentamicin 80mg/2ml solution for injection ampoules | 5 ampoule PoM £6.88 DT = £6.88 | 5 ampoule PoM £6.88 DT = £6.88 (Hospital only) | 10 ampoule PoM £12.00 | 10 ampoule PoM £13.76 (Hospital only)

▸ Cidomycin (Advanz Pharma)
　Gentamicin (as Gentamicin sulfate) 40 mg per 1 ml Cidomycin 80mg/2ml solution for injection vials | 5 vial PoM £6.88 DT = £6.88 (Hospital only)
　Cidomycin 80mg/2ml solution for injection ampoules | 5 ampoule PoM £6.88 DT = £6.88

Infusion

▸ Gentamicin (Non-proprietary)
　Gentamicin (as Gentamicin sulfate) 1 mg per 1 ml Gentamicin 80mg/80ml infusion polyethylene bottles | 20 bottle PoM £54.78 (Hospital only)
　Gentamicin (as Gentamicin sulfate) 3 mg per 1 ml Gentamicin 360mg/120ml infusion polyethylene bottles | 20 bottle PoM £237.05 (Hospital only)
　Gentamicin 240mg/80ml infusion polyethylene bottles | 20 bottle PoM £166.98 (Hospital only)

| Neomycin sulfate　　　　　　　　　　29-Mar-2023

● **INDICATIONS AND DOSE**

Bowel sterilisation before surgery
▸ BY MOUTH
▸ Adult: 1 g every 1 hour for 4 hours, then 1 g every 4 hours for 2–3 days

Hepatic coma
▸ BY MOUTH
▸ Adult: Up to 4 g daily in divided doses usually for 5–7 days

---

IMPORTANT SAFETY INFORMATION

MHRA/CHM ADVICE: AMINOGLYCOSIDES (GENTAMICIN, AMIKACIN, TOBRAMYCIN, AND NEOMYCIN): INCREASED RISK OF DEAFNESS IN PATIENTS WITH MITOCHONDRIAL MUTATIONS (JANUARY 2021)
The use of aminoglycosides is associated with rare cases of ototoxicity. A safety review found an increased risk of deafness in patients with mitochondrial mutations (particularly the m.1555A>G mutation), including cases where the patient's aminoglycoside serum levels were within the recommended range. Nevertheless, these mitochondrial mutations are considered rare and penetrance is uncertain.

Healthcare professionals are advised to consider the need for aminoglycoside treatment versus alternative options in patients with susceptible mutations. The need for genetic testing especially in those requiring recurrent or long-term treatment with aminoglycosides should also be considered, however, urgent treatment should not be delayed. To minimise the risks of adverse effects, continuous monitoring of renal and auditory function, as well as hepatic and laboratory parameters, is recommended for all patients. Those with known mitochondrial mutations or a family history of ototoxicity are advised to inform their doctor or pharmacist before using an aminoglycoside.

● **CONTRA-INDICATIONS** Intestinal obstruction · myasthenia gravis (aminoglycosides may impair neuromuscular transmission)

● **CAUTIONS** Avoid prolonged use

　CAUTIONS, FURTHER INFORMATION Although neomycin is associated with the same cautions as other aminoglycosides it is generally considered too toxic for systemic use.

● **INTERACTIONS** → Appendix 1: neomycin

● **SIDE-EFFECTS** Blood disorder · confusion · diarrhoea · drug cross-reactivity · electrolyte imbalance · gastrointestinal disorders · haemolytic anaemia · nausea · nephrotoxicity · nystagmus · oral disorders · ototoxicity · paraesthesia · superinfection · vomiting

　SIDE-EFFECTS, FURTHER INFORMATION Although neomycin is associated with the same side effects as other aminoglycosides, it is poorly absorbed after oral administration.

● **PREGNANCY** There is a risk of auditory or vestibular nerve damage in the infant when aminoglycosides are used in the second and third trimesters of pregnancy.

● **HEPATIC IMPAIRMENT** Manufacturer advises caution (increased risk of ototoxicity and nephrotoxicity).

● **RENAL IMPAIRMENT** Avoid–risk of ototoxicity and nephrotoxicity.

● **PRE-TREATMENT SCREENING** NHS England commissions genetic testing under the *National genomic test directory* indication: R65 - Aminoglycoside exposure posing risk to hearing. The testing criteria is significant exposure to aminoglycosides posing risk of ototoxicity. This testing is relevant to individuals with a predisposition to gram-negative infections or with hearing loss who have been exposed to aminoglycosides. For further information, see www.england.nhs.uk/publication/national-genomic-test-directories/.

● **MONITORING REQUIREMENTS**
▸ Renal function should be assessed before starting an aminoglycoside and during treatment.

5

Infection

▸ Auditory and vestibular function should also be monitored during treatment.

● MEDICINAL FORMS There can be variation in the licensing of different medicines containing the same drug. Forms available from special-order manufacturers include: oral solution

Oral solution
▸ Neomycin sulfate (Non-proprietary)
   Neomycin sulfate 25 mg per 1 ml Neo-Fradin 125mg/5ml oral solution | 480 ml PoM ⟨Ⅹ⟩ (Hospital only)

▶ 594

Streptomycin

29-Mar-2023

● INDICATIONS AND DOSE

Tuberculosis, resistant to other treatment, in combination with other drugs
▸ BY DEEP INTRAMUSCULAR INJECTION
▸ Adult: 15 mg/kg daily (max. per dose 1 g), reduce dose in those under 50 kg and those over 40 years

Adjunct to doxycycline in brucellosis (administered on expert advice)
▸ BY DEEP INTRAMUSCULAR INJECTION
▸ Adult: (consult local protocol)

Enterococcal endocarditis
▸ Adult: (consult local protocol)

● UNLICENSED USE Use in tuberculosis is an unlicensed indication.

> IMPORTANT SAFETY INFORMATION
> Side-effects increase after a cumulative dose of 100 g, which should only be exceeded in exceptional circumstances.

● INTERACTIONS → Appendix 1: aminoglycosides

● SIDE-EFFECTS Amblyopia · angioedema · Clostridioides difficile colitis · haemolytic anaemia · ototoxicity · pancytopenia

● PRE-TREATMENT SCREENING NHS England commissions genetic testing under the *National genomic test directory* indication: R65 - Aminoglycoside exposure posing risk to hearing. The testing criteria is significant exposure to aminoglycosides posing risk of ototoxicity. This testing is relevant to individuals with a predisposition to gram-negative infections or with hearing loss who have been exposed to aminoglycosides. For further information, see www.england.nhs.uk/publication/national-genomic-test-directories/.

● MONITORING REQUIREMENTS
▸ One-hour ('peak') concentration should be 15–40 mg/litre; pre-dose ('trough') concentration should be less than 5 mg/litre (less than 1 mg/litre in renal impairment or in those over 50 years).

● MEDICINAL FORMS Forms available from special-order manufacturers include: powder for solution for injection

▶ 594

Tobramycin

13-May-2024

● INDICATIONS AND DOSE

Septicaemia | Meningitis and other CNS infections | Biliary-tract infection | Acute pyelonephritis or prostatitis | Pneumonia in hospital patients
▸ BY INTRAMUSCULAR INJECTION, OR BY SLOW INTRAVENOUS INJECTION, OR BY INTRAVENOUS INFUSION
▸ Adult: 3 mg/kg daily in 3 divided doses; increased if necessary up to 5 mg/kg daily in 3–4 divided doses, increased dose used in severe infection; dose to be reduced back to 3 mg/kg daily as soon as clinically indicated

Urinary-tract infection
▸ BY INTRAMUSCULAR INJECTION
▸ Adult: 2–3 mg/kg for 1 dose

Chronic *Pseudomonas aeruginosa* infection in patients with cystic fibrosis
▸ BY INHALATION OF NEBULISED SOLUTION
▸ Adult: 300 mg every 12 hours for 28 days, subsequent courses repeated after 28-day interval without tobramycin nebuliser solution
▸ BY INHALATION OF POWDER
▸ Adult: 112 mg every 12 hours for 28 days, subsequent courses repeated after 28-day interval without tobramycin inhalation powder

DOSES AT EXTREMES OF BODY-WEIGHT
▸ With intramuscular use or intravenous use To avoid excessive dosage in obese patients, use ideal weight for height to calculate parenteral dose and monitor serum-tobramycin concentration closely.

VANTOBRA ® NEBULISER SOLUTION

Chronic pulmonary *Pseudomonas aeruginosa* infection in patients with cystic fibrosis
▸ BY INHALATION OF NEBULISED SOLUTION
▸ Adult: 170 mg every 12 hours for 28 days, subsequent courses repeated after 28-day interval without tobramycin nebuliser solution

● CAUTIONS
▸ When used by inhalation Auditory disorder · conditions characterised by muscular weakness (may impair neuromuscular transmission) · history of prolonged previous or concomitant intravenous aminoglycosides (increased risk of ototoxicity) · renal impairment (limited information available) · severe haemoptysis (risk of further haemorrhage) · vestibular disorder

● INTERACTIONS → Appendix 1: aminoglycosides

● SIDE-EFFECTS
▸ **Common or very common**
▸ When used by inhalation Malaise · respiratory disorder · sputum discolouration
▸ **Rare or very rare**
▸ When used by inhalation Abdominal pain · asthenia · asthma · drowsiness · ear disorder · ear pain · epistaxis · hypoxia · lymphadenopathy · oral ulceration · pain
▸ **Frequency not known**
▸ With parenteral use Granulocytopenia · leucocytosis · nerve disorders · urine abnormalities

SIDE-EFFECTS, FURTHER INFORMATION Manufacturer advises to monitor serum-tobramycin concentration in patients with known or suspected signs of auditory dysfunction; if ototoxicity develops — discontinue treatment until serum concentration falls below 2 mg/litre.

   With inhaled use Since systemic absorption can follow inhaled use, also consider the side-effects of systemic aminoglycosides.

● RENAL IMPAIRMENT
▸ When used by inhalation EvGr Monitor serum-tobramycin concentration; if nephrotoxicity develops—discontinue treatment until serum concentration falls below 2 mg/litre. ⟨M⟩

● PRE-TREATMENT SCREENING NHS England commissions genetic testing under the *National genomic test directory* indication: R65 - Aminoglycoside exposure posing risk to hearing. The testing criteria is significant exposure to aminoglycosides posing risk of ototoxicity. This testing is relevant to individuals with a predisposition to gram-negative infections or with hearing loss who have been exposed to aminoglycosides. For further information, see www.england.nhs.uk/publication/national-genomic-test-directories/.

- **MONITORING REQUIREMENTS**
  - With intramuscular use or intravenous use One-hour ('peak') serum concentration should not exceed 10 mg/litre; pre-dose ('trough') concentration should be less than 2 mg/litre.
  - When used by inhalation Measure lung function before and after initial dose of tobramycin and monitor for bronchospasm; if bronchospasm occurs in a patient not using a bronchodilator, repeat test using bronchodilator. Manufacturer advises monitor renal function before treatment and then annually.
- **DIRECTIONS FOR ADMINISTRATION**
  - With intravenous use For *intravenous infusion*, manufacturer advises give intermittently or via drip tubing in Glucose 5% or Sodium Chloride 0.9%. For adult intermittent infusion suggested volume 50–100 mL given over 20–60 minutes.
  - When used by inhalation Manufacturer advises other inhaled drugs should be administered before tobramycin.
- **PATIENT AND CARER ADVICE** Patient counselling is advised for Tobramycin dry powder for inhalation (administration).

  VANTOBRA ® NEBULISER SOLUTION

  Missed doses Manufacturer advises if a dose is more than 6 hours late, the missed dose should not be taken and the next dose should be taken at the normal time.
- **NATIONAL FUNDING/ACCESS DECISIONS**
  For full details see funding body website

  NICE decisions
  - Tobramycin by dry powder inhalation for pseudomonal lung infection in cystic fibrosis (March 2013) NICE TA276 Recommended with restrictions

- **MEDICINAL FORMS** There can be variation in the licensing of different medicines containing the same drug.

  Solution for injection
  - **Tobramycin (Non-proprietary)**
    Tobramycin 40 mg per 1 ml Tobramycin 80mg/2ml solution for injection vials | 1 vial [PoM] £5.37 DT = £5.37 | 5 vial [PoM] £20.80 DT = £20.80
    Tobramycin 240mg/6ml solution for injection vials | 1 vial [PoM] £19.20 DT = £19.20

  Inhalation powder
  - **Tobi Podhaler** (Viatris UK Healthcare Ltd)
    Tobramycin 28 mg Tobi Podhaler 28mg inhalation powder capsules with device | 224 capsule [PoM] £1,790.00 DT = £1,790.00

  Nebuliser liquid
  - **Tobramycin (Non-proprietary)**
    Tobramycin 60 mg per 1 ml Tobramycin 300mg/5ml nebuliser liquid ampoules | 56 ampoule [PoM] £719.00–£1,187.00 DT = £1,187.00 | 56 ampoule [PoM] £1,075.79 DT = £1,187.00 (Hospital only)
  - **Bramitob** (Chiesi Ltd)
    Tobramycin 75 mg per 1 ml Bramitob 300mg/4ml nebuliser solution 4ml ampoules | 56 ampoule [PoM] £1,187.00 DT = £1,187.00
  - **Munuza** (Aristo Pharma Ltd)
    Tobramycin 60 mg per 1 ml Munuza 300mg/5ml nebuliser solution 5ml ampoules | 56 ampoule [PoM] £779.99 DT = £1,187.00
  - **TOBI** (Viatris UK Healthcare Ltd)
    Tobramycin 60 mg per 1 ml Tobi 300mg/5ml nebuliser solution 5ml ampoules | 56 ampoule [PoM] £1,305.92 DT = £1,187.00
  - **Tymbrineb** (Teva UK Ltd)
    Tobramycin 60 mg per 1 ml Tymbrineb 300mg/5ml nebuliser solution 5ml ampoules | 56 ampoule [PoM] £780.00 DT = £1,187.00
  - **Vantobra** (Pari Medical Ltd)
    Tobramycin 100 mg per 1 ml Vantobra 170mg/1.7ml nebuliser solution 1.7ml ampoules | 56 ampoule [PoM] £950.00

Carbapenems
29-Sep-2021

Overview

The carbapenems are beta-lactam antibacterials with a broad-spectrum of activity which includes many Gram-positive and Gram-negative bacteria, and anaerobes; imipenem (imipenem with cilastatin p. 600) and meropenem p. 601 have activity against *Pseudomonas aeruginosa* but emerging acquired resistance can be a problem. The carbapenems are not active against meticillin-resistant *Staphylococcus aureus* (MRSA) and *Enterococcus faecium*.

Imipenem (imipenem with cilastatin) and meropenem are used for the treatment of severe and complicated infections including hospital-acquired pneumonia, intra-abdominal infections, skin and soft-tissue infections, and urinary-tract infections.

Ertapenem below is licensed for treating abdominal and gynaecological infections and for community-acquired pneumonia, but it is not active against atypical respiratory pathogens and its activity against penicillin-resistant pneumococci is unknown. It is also licensed for treating foot infections of the skin and soft tissue in patients with diabetes. Unlike the other carbapenems, ertapenem is not active against *Pseudomonas* or against *Acinetobacter* spp.

Imipenem is partially inactivated in the kidney by enzymatic activity and is therefore administered in combination with cilastatin (imipenem with cilastatin), a specific enzyme inhibitor, which blocks its renal metabolism. Meropenem and ertapenem are stable to the renal enzyme which inactivates imipenem and therefore can be given without cilastatin.

Side-effects of imipenem with cilastatin are similar to those of other beta-lactam antibiotics. Meropenem has less seizure-inducing potential and can be used to treat central nervous system infection.

Ertapenem
25-Oct-2021

- **INDICATIONS AND DOSE**

  Abdominal infections | Acute gynaecological infections | Community-acquired pneumonia
  - BY INTRAVENOUS INFUSION
  - Adult: 1 g once daily

  Diabetic foot infections of the skin and soft-tissue
  - BY INTRAVENOUS INFUSION
  - Adult: 1 g once daily

  Surgical prophylaxis, colorectal surgery
  - BY INTRAVENOUS INFUSION
  - Adult: 1 g for 1 dose, dose to be completed within 1 hour before surgery

- **CAUTIONS** CNS disorders—risk of seizures · elderly
- **INTERACTIONS** → Appendix 1: carbapenems
- **SIDE-EFFECTS**
  - **Common or very common** Diarrhoea · headache · nausea · skin reactions · thrombophlebitis · vomiting
  - **Uncommon** Appetite decreased · arrhythmias · asthenia · confusion · constipation · dizziness · drowsiness · dry mouth · gastrointestinal discomfort · gastrointestinal disorders · hypotension · increased risk of infection · insomnia · oedema · pseudomembranous enterocolitis · seizure · swelling · taste altered · throat discomfort
  - **Rare or very rare** Anxiety · cholecystitis · depression · dysphagia · eye disorder · haemorrhage · hepatic disorders · hypersensitivity · hypoglycaemia · malaise · muscle cramps · nasal congestion · neutropenia · renal impairment · shoulder pain · syncope · thrombocytopenia · tremor

▶ **Frequency not known** Aggression · antibiotic associated colitis · delirium · drug reaction with eosinophilia and systemic symptoms (DRESS) · gait abnormal · hallucination · level of consciousness decreased · movement disorders · muscle weakness · psychiatric disorder · tooth discolouration

● ALLERGY AND CROSS-SENSITIVITY [EvGr] Avoid if history of **immediate hypersensitivity** reaction to beta-lactam antibacterials.

   Use with caution in patients with sensitivity to beta-lactam antibacterials. Ⓜ

● PREGNANCY Manufacturer advises avoid unless potential benefit outweighs risk.

● BREAST FEEDING Present in milk—manufacturer advises avoid.

● RENAL IMPAIRMENT
Dose adjustments Risk of seizures; max. 500 mg daily if eGFR less than 30 mL/minute/1.73 m^2.

● DIRECTIONS FOR ADMINISTRATION For *intravenous infusion* (*Invanz*®), manufacturer advises give intermittently *in* Sodium Chloride 0.9%. Reconstitute 1 g with 10 mL Water for Injections *or* Sodium Chloride 0.9%; dilute requisite dose in infusion fluid to a final concentration not exceeding 20 mg/mL; give over 30 minutes; incompatible with glucose solutions.

● PRESCRIBING AND DISPENSING INFORMATION For choice of antibacterial therapy, see Antibacterials, use for prophylaxis p. 574, Diabetic foot infections, antibacterial therapy p. 581, Gastro-intestinal system infections, antibacterial therapy p. 582, Respiratory system infections, antibacterial therapy p. 586.

● MEDICINAL FORMS There can be variation in the licensing of different medicines containing the same drug.
Powder for solution for infusion
ELECTROLYTES: May contain Sodium
▶ Ertapenem (Non-proprietary)
   Ertapenem (as Ertapenem sodium) 1 gram Ertapenem 1g powder for concentrate for solution for infusion vials | 1 vial [PoM] £36.00 DT = £31.65 (Hospital only) | 10 vial [PoM] £316.50 | 10 vial [PoM] £315.00-£316.50 (Hospital only)
▶ Invanz (Merck Sharp & Dohme (UK) Ltd)
   Ertapenem (as Ertapenem sodium) 1 gram Invanz 1g powder for solution for infusion vials | 1 vial [PoM] £31.65 DT = £31.65 (Hospital only)

Imipenem with cilastatin
24-Nov-2020

● INDICATIONS AND DOSE
Aerobic and anaerobic Gram-positive and Gram-negative infections (not indicated for CNS infections) | Hospital-acquired septicaemia
▶ BY INTRAVENOUS INFUSION
▶ Adult: 500 mg every 6 hours, alternatively 1 g every 8 hours
Infection caused by *Pseudomonas* or other less sensitive organisms | Empirical treatment of infection in febrile patients with neutropenia | Life-threatening infection
▶ BY INTRAVENOUS INFUSION
▶ Adult: 1 g every 6 hours
DOSE EQUIVALENCE AND CONVERSION
▶ Dose expressed in terms of imipenem.

● CAUTIONS CNS disorders · epilepsy
● INTERACTIONS → Appendix 1: carbapenems
● SIDE-EFFECTS
▶ **Common or very common** Diarrhoea · eosinophilia · nausea · skin reactions · thrombophlebitis · vomiting
▶ **Uncommon** Bone marrow disorders · confusion · dizziness · drowsiness · hallucination · hypotension · leucopenia ·

movement disorders · psychiatric disorder · seizure · thrombocytopenia · thrombocytosis
▶ **Rare or very rare** Agranulocytosis · anaphylactic reaction · angioedema · chest discomfort · colitis haemorrhagic · cyanosis · dyspnoea · encephalopathy · flushing · focal tremor · gastrointestinal discomfort · haemolytic anaemia · headache · hearing loss · hepatic disorders · hyperhidrosis · hyperventilation · increased risk of infection · myasthenia gravis aggravated · oral disorders · palpitations · paraesthesia · polyarthralgia · polyuria · pseudomembranous enterocolitis · renal impairment · severe cutaneous adverse reactions (SCARs) · spinal pain · tachycardia · taste altered · tinnitus · tongue discolouration · tooth discolouration · urine discolouration · vertigo
▶ **Frequency not known** Agitation · antibiotic associated colitis

● ALLERGY AND CROSS-SENSITIVITY [EvGr] Avoid if history of **immediate hypersensitivity** reaction to beta-lactam antibacterials.

   Use with caution in patients with sensitivity to beta-lactam antibacterials. Ⓜ

● PREGNANCY Manufacturer advises avoid unless potential benefit outweighs risk (toxicity in *animal* studies).

● BREAST FEEDING [EvGr] Specialist sources indicate suitable for use in breast-feeding. Ⓓ

● RENAL IMPAIRMENT Manufacturer advises caution if creatinine clearance less than 90 mL/minute.
Dose adjustments Manufacturer advises reduce dose if creatinine clearance less than 90 mL/minute (risk of CNS side-effects)—consult product literature. See p. 21.

● EFFECT ON LABORATORY TESTS Positive Coombs' test.

● DIRECTIONS FOR ADMINISTRATION For *intravenous infusion*, manufacturer advises dilute to a concentration of 5 mg (as imipenem)/mL in Sodium Chloride 0.9%; give up to 500 mg (as imipenem) over 20–30 minutes, give dose greater than 500 mg (as imipenem) over 40–60 minutes.

● MEDICINAL FORMS There can be variation in the licensing of different medicines containing the same drug.
Powder for solution for infusion
ELECTROLYTES: May contain Sodium
▶ Imipenem with cilastatin (Non-proprietary)
   Cilastatin (as Cilastatin sodium) 500 mg, Imipenem (as Imipenem monohydrate) 500 mg Imipenem 500mg / Cilastatin 500mg powder for solution for infusion vials | 10 vial [PoM] £170.10

Imipenem with cilastatin and relebactam
21-Sep-2020

The properties listed below are those particular to the combination only. For the properties of the components please consider, imipenem with cilastatin above.

● INDICATIONS AND DOSE
Aerobic Gram-negative infections [in patients with limited treatment options] (administered on expert advice)
▶ BY INTRAVENOUS INFUSION
▶ Adult: 500 mg every 6 hours, duration should be tailored to site of infection—consult product literature
DOSE EQUIVALENCE AND CONVERSION
▶ Dose expressed in terms of imipenem.

● CAUTIONS Neutropenia (consider alternative treatment options) · severe infections (consider alternative treatment options) · supra-normal creatinine clearance
CAUTIONS, FURTHER INFORMATION
▶ Supra-normal creatinine clearance Manufacturer advises the usual dose may not be sufficient to treat patients with creatinine clearance 150 mL/minute or more, and alternative treatment options should be considered.

- **INTERACTIONS** → Appendix 1: carbapenems
- **RENAL IMPAIRMENT** Manufacturer advises caution if creatinine clearance less than 90 mL/minute.
  Dose adjustments Manufacturer advises reduce dose if creatinine clearance less than 90 mL/minute—consult product literature. See p. 21.
- **DIRECTIONS FOR ADMINISTRATION** Manufacturer advises for *intravenous infusion*, dilute to a concentration of 5 mg (as imipenem)/mL with Sodium Chloride 0.9% (preferably) *or* Glucose 5%; give intermittently over 30 minutes. For a list of compatible infusion bags and infusion sets—consult product literature.

- **MEDICINAL FORMS** There can be variation in the licensing of different medicines containing the same drug.
  Powder for solution for infusion
  ELECTROLYTES: May contain Sodium
  ▸ **Recarbrio** (Merck Sharp & Dohme (UK) Ltd) ▼
    Relebactam (as Relebactam monohydrate) 250 mg, Cilastatin (as Cilastatin sodium) 500 mg, Imipenem (as Imipenem monohydrate) 500 mg Recarbrio 500mg/500mg/250mg powder for solution for infusion vials | 25 vial [PoM] £3,838.75 (Hospital only)

Meropenem

18-Aug-2021

- ● **INDICATIONS AND DOSE**

Aerobic and anaerobic Gram-positive and Gram-negative infections | Hospital-acquired septicaemia
▸ BY INTRAVENOUS INFUSION, OR BY INTRAVENOUS INJECTION
▸ Adult: 0.5–1 g every 8 hours

Exacerbations of chronic lower respiratory-tract infection in cystic fibrosis
▸ BY INTRAVENOUS INFUSION, OR BY INTRAVENOUS INJECTION
▸ Adult: 2 g every 8 hours

Meningitis
▸ BY INTRAVENOUS INFUSION, OR BY INTRAVENOUS INJECTION
▸ Adult: 2 g every 8 hours

Endocarditis (in combination with another antibacterial)
▸ BY INTRAVENOUS INFUSION, OR BY INTRAVENOUS INJECTION
▸ Adult: 2 g every 8 hours

- **UNLICENSED USE** Not licensed for use in endocarditis.
- **INTERACTIONS** → Appendix 1: carbapenems
- **SIDE-EFFECTS**
▸ **Common or very common** Abdominal pain · diarrhoea · headache · inflammation · nausea · pain · skin reactions · thrombocytosis · vomiting
▸ **Uncommon** Agranulocytosis · antibiotic associated colitis · eosinophilia · haemolytic anaemia · increased risk of infection · leucopenia · neutropenia · paraesthesia · severe cutaneous adverse reactions (SCARs) · thrombocytopenia · thrombophlebitis
▸ **Rare or very rare** Seizure
▸ **Frequency not known** Pseudomembranous enterocolitis

- **ALLERGY AND CROSS-SENSITIVITY** [EvGr] Avoid if history of **immediate hypersensitivity** reaction to beta-lactam antibacterials.
  Use with caution in patients with sensitivity to beta-lactam antibacterials. ⟨M⟩
- **PREGNANCY** Use only if potential benefit outweighs risk— no information available.
- **BREAST FEEDING** Unlikely to be absorbed (however, manufacturer advises avoid).
- **RENAL IMPAIRMENT**
  Dose adjustments See p. 21.
  [EvGr] Use normal dose every 12 hours if creatinine clearance 26–50 mL/minute.
  Use half normal dose every 12 hours if creatinine clearance 10–25 mL/minute.

Use half normal dose every 24 hours if creatinine clearance less than 10 mL/minute. ⟨M⟩
- **MONITORING REQUIREMENTS** Manufacturer advises monitor liver function—risk of hepatotoxicity.
- **EFFECT ON LABORATORY TESTS** Positive Coombs' test.
- **DIRECTIONS FOR ADMINISTRATION** Manufacturer advises *intravenous injection* to be administered over 5 minutes.
  For *intravenous infusion* (*Meronem®*), manufacturer advises give intermittently in Glucose 5% *or* Sodium Chloride 0.9%. Dilute dose in infusion fluid to a final concentration of 1–20 mg/mL; give over 15–30 minutes.

- **MEDICINAL FORMS** There can be variation in the licensing of different medicines containing the same drug.
  Powder for solution for injection
  ELECTROLYTES: May contain Sodium
  ▸ **Meropenem** (Non-proprietary)
    Meropenem (as Meropenem trihydrate) 500 mg Meropenem 500mg powder for solution for injection vials | 10 vial [PoM] £121.80 DT = £117.70 (Hospital only)
    Meropenem (as Meropenem trihydrate) 1 gram Meropenem 1g powder for solution for injection vials | 10 vial [PoM] £243.60 DT = £235.40 (Hospital only)
    Meropenem (as Meropenem trihydrate) 2 gram Meropenem 2g powder for solution for injection vials | 10 vial [PoM] £190.00 (Hospital only)
  ▸ **Meronem** (Pfizer Ltd)
    Meropenem (as Meropenem trihydrate) 500 mg Meronem 500mg powder for solution for injection vials | 10 vial [PoM] £103.14 DT = £117.70 (Hospital only)
    Meropenem (as Meropenem trihydrate) 1 gram Meronem 1g powder for solution for injection vials | 10 vial [PoM] £206.28 DT = £235.40 (Hospital only)

Meropenem with vaborbactam

15-Jul-2022

The properties listed below are those particular to the combination only. For the properties of the components please consider, meropenem above.

- ● **INDICATIONS AND DOSE**

Complicated urinary-tract infection [including pyelonephritis] | Complicated intra-abdominal infection
▸ BY INTRAVENOUS INFUSION
▸ Adult: 2/2 g every 8 hours for 5–10 days; may be continued for up to 14 days

Hospital-acquired pneumonia | Ventilator-associated pneumonia
▸ BY INTRAVENOUS INFUSION
▸ Adult: 2/2 g every 8 hours for 7–14 days

Bacteraemia [occurring in association with or suspected to be associated with the licensed indications]
▸ BY INTRAVENOUS INFUSION
▸ Adult: 2/2 g every 8 hours, duration should be tailored to site of infection

Aerobic Gram-negative infections [in patients with limited treatment options] (administered on expert advice)
▸ BY INTRAVENOUS INFUSION
▸ Adult: 2/2 g every 8 hours, duration should be tailored to site of infection

DOSE EQUIVALENCE AND CONVERSION
▸ Dose expressed as *x/y* g of meropenem/vaborbactam.

- **INTERACTIONS** → Appendix 1: carbapenems · vaborbactam
- **SIDE-EFFECTS**
▸ **Common or very common** Diarrhoea · electrolyte imbalance · headache · hypoglycaemia · hypotension · nausea · thrombocytosis · vomiting
▸ **Uncommon** Appetite decreased · bronchospasm · chest discomfort · Clostridioides difficile colitis · dizziness · eosinophilia · gastrointestinal discomfort · hallucination · hyperglycaemia · increased risk of infection · infusion related reaction · insomnia · lethargy · leucopenia ·

neutropenia · pain · paraesthesia · renal impairment · skin reactions · thrombocytopenia · tremor · urinary incontinence · vascular pain

▸ **Rare or very rare** Seizure

▸ **Frequency not known** Agranulocytosis · angioedema · delirium · haemolytic anaemia · severe cutaneous adverse reactions (SCARs)

● PREGNANCY Manufacturer advises avoid—no or limited information available.

● BREAST FEEDING Manufacturer advises discontinue breast-feeding.

● RENAL IMPAIRMENT [EvGr] Caution if creatinine clearance 39 mL/minute or less. ⓜ

Dose adjustments See p. 21.

[EvGr] Reduce dose to 1/1 g every 8 hours if creatinine clearance 20–39 mL/minute.

Reduce dose to 1/1 g every 12 hours if creatinine clearance 10–19 mL/minute.

Reduce dose to 0.5/0.5 g every 12 hours if creatinine clearance less than 10 mL/minute. ⓜ

● DIRECTIONS FOR ADMINISTRATION [EvGr] For *continuous intravenous infusion*, reconstitute each 1/1 g vial to produce a 0.05/0.05 g/mL solution with 20 mL Sodium Chloride 0.9%. Dilute reconstituted solution to a final volume of 250 mL with Sodium Chloride 0.9%; give over 3 hours. ⓜ

● PATIENT AND CARER ADVICE

Driving and skilled tasks Manufacturer advises patients and carers should be counselled on the effects on driving and performance of skilled tasks—increased risk of dizziness, lethargy, and paraesthesia.

● NATIONAL FUNDING/ACCESS DECISIONS

For full details see funding body website

Scottish Medicines Consortium (SMC) decisions

▸ Meropenem/vaborbactam (*Vaborem*®) for the treatment of: complicated urinary tract infection; complicated intra-abdominal infection; hospital-acquired pneumonia; bacteraemia that occurs in association with, or is suspected to be associated with any of these infections; infections due to aerobic Gram-negative organisms in adults with limited treatment options (October 2020) SMC No. SMC2278 Recommended with restrictions

All Wales Medicines Strategy Group (AWMSG) decisions

▸ Meropenem/vaborbactam (*Vaborem*®) for the treatment of: complicated urinary tract infection; complicated intra-abdominal infection; hospital-acquired pneumonia; bacteraemia that occurs in association with, or is suspected to be associated with any of these infections; infections due to aerobic Gram-negative organisms in adults with limited treatment options (October 2020) AWMSG No. 2760 Recommended with restrictions

● MEDICINAL FORMS There can be variation in the licensing of different medicines containing the same drug.

Powder for solution for infusion

ELECTROLYTES: May contain Sodium

▸ Vaborem (A. Menarini Farmaceutica Internazionale SRL) Meropenem (as Meropenem trihydrate) 1 gram, Vaborbactam 1 gram Vaborem 1g/1g powder for concentrate for solution for infusion vials | 6 vial [PoM] £334.00 (Hospital only)

ANTIBACTERIALS > CEPHALOSPORINS

Cephalosporins

03-Feb-2021

Overview

The cephalosporins are broad-spectrum antibiotics which are used for the treatment of septicaemia, pneumonia, meningitis, biliary-tract infections, peritonitis, and urinary-tract infections. The pharmacology of the cephalosporins is similar to that of the penicillins, excretion being principally renal. Cephalosporins penetrate the cerebrospinal fluid poorly unless the meninges are inflamed; cefotaxime p. 608 and ceftriaxone p. 609 are suitable cephalosporins for infections of the CNS (e.g meningitis).

The principal side-effect of the cephalosporins is hypersensitivity. Cross-reactivity between penicillins and first and early second-generation cephalosporins has been reported to occur in up to 10%, and for third-generation cephalosporins in 2–3%, of penicillin-allergic patients. If a cephalosporin is essential in patients with a history of immediate hypersensitivity to penicillin, because a suitable alternative antibacterial is not available, then cefixime p. 608, cefotaxime, ceftazidime p. 608, ceftriaxone, or cefuroxime p. 606 can be used with caution; cefaclor p. 605, cefadroxil p. 603, cefalexin p. 603, cefradine p. 605, and ceftaroline fosamil p. 614 should be avoided.

The orally active 'first generation' cephalosporins, cefalexin, cefradine, and cefadroxil and the 'second generation' cephalosporin, cefaclor, have a similar antimicrobial spectrum. They are useful for urinary-tract infections, respiratory-tract infections, otitis media, and skin and soft-tissue infections. Cefaclor has good activity against *H. influenzae*. Cefadroxil has a long duration of action and can be given twice daily; it has poor activity against *H. influenzae*. **Cefuroxime axetil**, an ester of the 'second generation' cephalosporin cefuroxime, has the same antibacterial spectrum as the parent compound; it is poorly absorbed and needs to be given with food to maximise absorption.

Cefixime is an orally active 'third generation' cephalosporin. It has a longer duration of action than the other cephalosporins that are active by mouth. It is only licensed for acute infections.

Cefuroxime is a 'second generation' cephalosporin that is less susceptible than the earlier cephalosporins to inactivation by beta-lactamases. It is, therefore, active against certain bacteria which are resistant to the other drugs and has greater activity against *Haemophilus influenzae*.

Cefotaxime, ceftazidime and ceftriaxone are 'third generation' cephalosporins with greater activity than the 'second generation' cephalosporins against certain Gram-negative bacteria. However, they are less active than cefuroxime against Gram-positive bacteria, most notably *Staphylococcus aureus*. Their broad antibacterial spectrum may encourage superinfection with resistant bacteria or fungi.

Ceftazidime has good activity against pseudomonas. It is also active against other Gram-negative bacteria.

Ceftriaxone has a longer half-life and therefore needs to be given only once daily. Indications include serious infections such as septicaemia, pneumonia, and meningitis. The calcium salt of ceftriaxone forms a precipitate in the gall bladder which may rarely cause symptoms but these usually resolve when the antibiotic is stopped.

Ceftaroline fosamil is a 'fifth generation' cephalosporin with bactericidal activity similar to cefotaxime; however, ceftaroline fosamil has an extended spectrum of activity against Gram-positive bacteria that includes meticillin-resistant *Staphylococcus aureus* and multi-drug resistant *Streptococcus pneumoniae*. Ceftaroline fosamil is licensed for the treatment of community-acquired pneumonia and complicated skin and soft-tissue infections, but there is no experience of its use in pneumonia caused by meticillin-resistant *S. aureus*.

Cefiderocol p. 614, a siderophore cephalosporin, is used for treating infections due to Gram-negative aerobic organisms in individuals who have limited treatment options, particularly when other antimicrobial agents have failed.

Cephalosporins 

- **DRUG ACTION** Cephalosporins are antibacterials that attach to penicillin binding proteins to interrupt cell wall biosynthesis, leading to bacterial cell lysis and death.

- **SIDE-EFFECTS**
- ▸ **Common or very common** Abdominal pain · diarrhoea · dizziness · eosinophilia · headache · leucopenia · nausea · neutropenia · pseudomembranous enterocolitis · skin reactions · thrombocytopenia · vomiting
- ▸ **Uncommon** Anaphylactic reaction · angioedema
- ▸ **Rare or very rare** Agranulocytosis · haemolytic anaemia · nephritis tubulointerstitial (reversible) · severe cutaneous adverse reactions (SCARs)

- **ALLERGY AND CROSS-SENSITIVITY** [EvGr] Contra-indicated in patients with cephalosporin hypersensitivity. Ⓜ
- ▸ Cross-sensitivity with other beta-lactam antibacterials Cross-reactivity between penicillins and first and early second-generation cephalosporins has been reported to occur in up to 10%, and for third-generation cephalosporins in 2–3%, of penicillin-allergic patients. [EvGr] Patients with a history of **immediate hypersensitivity** to penicillin and other beta-lactams should not receive a cephalosporin. Cephalosporins should be used with caution in patients with sensitivity to penicillin and other beta-lactams. Ⓜ

- **EFFECT ON LABORATORY TESTS** False positive urinary glucose (if tested for reducing substances). False positive Coombs' test.

ANTIBACTERIALS › CEPHALOSPORINS, FIRST-GENERATION

⚑ above

Cefadroxil

- **INDICATIONS AND DOSE**

Susceptible infections due to sensitive Gram-positive and Gram-negative bacteria
- ▸ BY MOUTH
- ▸ Child 6-17 years (body-weight up to 40 kg): 0.5 g twice daily
- ▸ Child 6-17 years (body-weight 40 kg and above): 0.5–1 g twice daily
- ▸ Adult: 0.5–1 g twice daily

Skin infections | Soft-tissue infections | Uncomplicated urinary-tract infections
- ▸ BY MOUTH
- ▸ Child 6-17 years (body-weight 40 kg and above): 1 g once daily
- ▸ Adult: 1 g daily

- **INTERACTIONS** → Appendix 1: cephalosporins

- **SIDE-EFFECTS**
- ▸ **Common or very common** Dyspepsia · glossitis
- ▸ **Uncommon** Increased risk of infection
- ▸ **Rare or very rare** Arthralgia · drug fever · fatigue · hepatic disorders · insomnia · nervousness · serum sickness-like reaction

- **PREGNANCY** Not known to be harmful.

- **BREAST FEEDING** Present in milk in low concentration, but appropriate to use.

- **RENAL IMPAIRMENT**
  Dose adjustments
  - ▸ In adults 1 g initially, then 500 mg every 12 hours if eGFR 26–50 mL/minute/1.73 m^2. 1 g initially, then 500 mg every 24 hours if eGFR 11–26 mL/minute/1.73 m^2. 1 g initially, then 500 mg every 36 hours if eGFR less than 11 mL/minute/1.73 m^2.
    - ▸ In children Reduce dose if estimated glomerular filtration rate less than 50 mL/minute/1.73 m^2.

- **MEDICINAL FORMS** There can be variation in the licensing of different medicines containing the same drug.
  Oral capsule
  CAUTIONARY AND ADVISORY LABELS 9
  - ▸ Cefadroxil (Non-proprietary)
    Cefadroxil (as Cefadroxil monohydrate) 500 mg Cefadroxil 500mg capsules | 20 capsule [PoM] £22.38 DT = £22.38

⚑ above

Cefalexin

(Cephalexin)

26-Oct-2021

- **INDICATIONS AND DOSE**

Susceptible infections due to sensitive Gram-positive and Gram-negative bacteria
- ▸ BY MOUTH
- ▸ Child 1-11 months: 12.5 mg/kg twice daily, alternatively 125 mg twice daily
- ▸ Child 1-4 years: 12.5 mg/kg twice daily, alternatively 125 mg 3 times a day
- ▸ Child 5-11 years: 12.5 mg/kg twice daily, alternatively 250 mg 3 times a day
- ▸ Child 12-17 years: 500 mg 2–3 times a day
- ▸ Adult: 250 mg every 6 hours, alternatively 500 mg every 8–12 hours; increased to 1–1.5 g every 6–8 hours, increased dose used in severe infections

Serious susceptible infections due to sensitive Gram-positive and Gram-negative bacteria
- ▸ BY MOUTH
- ▸ Child 1 month-11 years: 25 mg/kg 2–4 times a day (max. per dose 1 g)
- ▸ Child 12-17 years: 1–1.5 g 3–4 times a day

Hospital-acquired pneumonia | Acute diverticulitis [in combination with metronidazole]
- ▸ BY MOUTH
- ▸ Adult: 500 mg 2–3 times a day for 5 days then review, alternatively 1–1.5 g 3–4 times a day for 5 days then review, increased dose used in severe infection

Prophylaxis of recurrent urinary-tract infection
- ▸ BY MOUTH
- ▸ Child 3 months-15 years: 12.5 mg/kg once daily (max. per dose 125 mg), dose to be taken at night
- ▸ Child 16-17 years: 125 mg once daily, dose to be taken at night, alternatively 500 mg for 1 dose, dose to be taken following exposure to a trigger
- ▸ Adult: 125 mg once daily, dose to be taken at night, alternatively 500 mg for 1 dose, dose to be taken following exposure to a trigger

Acute pyelonephritis | Urinary-tract infection (catheter-associated)
- ▸ BY MOUTH
- ▸ Child 3-11 months: 125 mg twice daily for 7 to 10 days, alternatively 12.5 mg/kg twice daily for 7 to 10 days, alternatively 25 mg/kg 2–4 times a day (max. per dose 1 g) for 7 to 10 days, increased dose used in severe infections
- ▸ Child 1-4 years: 125 mg 3 times a day for 7 to 10 days, alternatively 12.5 mg/kg twice daily for 7 to 10 days, alternatively 25 mg/kg 2–4 times a day (max. per dose 1 g) for 7 to 10 days, increased dose used in severe infections
- ▸ Child 5-11 years: 250 mg 3 times a day for 7 to 10 days, alternatively 12.5 mg/kg twice daily for 7 to 10 days, alternatively 25 mg/kg 2–4 times a day (max. per dose 1 g) for 7 to 10 days, increased dose used in severe infections
- ▸ Child 12-17 years: 500 mg 2–3 times a day for 7 to 10 days, alternatively 1–1.5 g 3–4 times a day for 7 to 10 days, increased dose used in severe infections

continued →

▶ Adult: 500 mg 2–3 times a day for 7 to 10 days, alternatively 1–1.5 g 3–4 times a day for 7 to 10 days, increased dose used in severe infections

Lower urinary-tract infection in pregnancy
▶ BY MOUTH
▶ Child 12-17 years: 500 mg twice daily for 7 days
▶ Adult: 500 mg twice daily for 7 days

Lower urinary-tract infection
▶ BY MOUTH
▶ Child 3-11 months: 12.5 mg/kg twice daily for 3 days, alternatively 125 mg twice daily for 3 days
▶ Child 1-4 years: 12.5 mg/kg twice daily for 3 days, alternatively 125 mg 3 times a day for 3 days
▶ Child 5-11 years: 12.5 mg/kg twice daily for 3 days, alternatively 250 mg 3 times a day for 3 days
▶ Child 12-15 years: 500 mg twice daily for 3 days

● **UNLICENSED USE** [EvGr] Cefalexin is used for prophylaxis of recurrent urinary-tract infection, Ⓐ but is not licensed for this indication.

● **INTERACTIONS** → Appendix 1: cephalosporins

● **SIDE-EFFECTS** Agitation · arthritis · confusion · fatigue · gastrointestinal discomfort · genital pruritus · hallucination · hepatitis (transient) · hypersensitivity · increased risk of infection · jaundice cholestatic (transient) · joint disorders · vaginal discharge

● **PREGNANCY** Not known to be harmful.

● **BREAST FEEDING** Present in milk in low concentration, but appropriate to use.

● **RENAL IMPAIRMENT**
Dose adjustments
▶ In adults Max. 3 g daily if eGFR 40–50 mL/minute/1.73 m^2. Max. 1.5 g daily if eGFR 10–40 mL/minute/1.73 m^2. Max. 750 mg daily if eGFR less than 10 mL/minute/1.73 m^2.
▶ In children Reduce dose in moderate impairment.

● **PRESCRIBING AND DISPENSING INFORMATION** For choice of antibacterial therapy, see Gastro-intestinal system infections, antibacterial therapy p. 582, Respiratory system infections, antibacterial therapy p. 586, Urinary-tract infections p. 681.

● **PATIENT AND CARER ADVICE**
Medicines for Children leaflet: Cefalexin for bacterial infections www.medicinesforchildren.org.uk/medicines/cefalexin-for-bacterial-infections/

● **PROFESSION SPECIFIC INFORMATION**
Dental practitioners' formulary Cefalexin Capsules may be prescribed.
Cefalexin Tablets may be prescribed.
Cefalexin Oral Suspension may be prescribed.

● **MEDICINAL FORMS** There can be variation in the licensing of different medicines containing the same drug.
Oral tablet
CAUTIONARY AND ADVISORY LABELS 9
▶ Cefalexin (Non-proprietary)
Cefalexin 250 mg Cefalexin 250mg tablets | 28 tablet [PoM] £4.40 DT = £2.48
Cefalexin 500 mg Cefalexin 500mg tablets | 21 tablet [PoM] £4.60 DT = £2.63
Oral suspension
CAUTIONARY AND ADVISORY LABELS 9
▶ Cefalexin (Non-proprietary)
Cefalexin 25 mg per 1 ml Cefalexin 125mg/5ml oral suspension sugar free | 100 ml [PoM] £2.92-£5.50 DT = £2.92 [SF]
Cefalexin 125mg/5ml oral suspension | 100 ml [PoM] £3.70 DT = £5.12
Cefalexin 50 mg per 1 ml Cefalexin 250mg/5ml oral suspension sugar free | 100 ml [PoM] £3.38-£6.10 DT = £3.38 [SF]
Cefalexin 250mg/5ml oral suspension | 100 ml [PoM] £4.11 DT = £5.64

Oral capsule
CAUTIONARY AND ADVISORY LABELS 9
▶ Cefalexin (Non-proprietary)
Cefalexin 250 mg Cefalexin 250mg capsules | 28 capsule [PoM] £3.30 DT = £2.37
Cefalexin 500 mg Cefalexin 500mg capsules | 21 capsule [PoM] £4.80 DT = £2.53

⟨F 603

Cefazolin
25-Aug-2020

● **INDICATIONS AND DOSE**
Surgical prophylaxis
▶ BY SLOW INTRAVENOUS INJECTION, OR BY INTRAVENOUS INFUSION, OR BY DEEP INTRAMUSCULAR INJECTION
▶ Adult: 1 g, to be administered 30–60 minutes before surgery, then 0.5–1 g if required, during surgery (in procedures lasting 2 hours or more)

Skin infection | Soft tissue infection | Bone infection | Joint infection
▶ BY SLOW INTRAVENOUS INJECTION, OR BY INTRAVENOUS INFUSION, OR BY DEEP INTRAMUSCULAR INJECTION
▶ Adult: 1–2 g daily in 2–3 divided doses, for sensitive bacteria; increased to 3–4 g daily in 3–4 divided doses, for moderately-sensitive bacteria; increased if necessary up to 6 g daily in 3–4 divided doses, for severe infections, single doses greater than 1 g should be given by intravenous infusion

● **INTERACTIONS** → Appendix 1: cephalosporins

● **SIDE-EFFECTS**
▶ **Common or very common** Appetite decreased
▶ **Uncommon** Drug fever · interstitial lung disease · oral candidiasis (particularly in long term use) · seizure (in renal impairment) · thrombophlebitis
▶ **Rare or very rare** Akathisia · anaemia · anal pruritus · anxiety · asthenia · bone marrow disorders · chest pain · coagulation disorder · colour vision change · confusion · cough · drowsiness · dyspnoea · epileptogenic activity · face oedema · genital pruritus · hepatitis (transient) · hot flush · hyperglycaemia · hypersensitivity · hypoglycaemia · increased leucocytes · increased risk of infection · jaundice cholestatic (transient) · lymphopenia · malaise · nephropathy · proteinuria · respiratory disorders · sleep disorders · tongue swelling · vertigo

SIDE-EFFECTS, FURTHER INFORMATION Blood disorders including: leucopenia, granulocytopenia, thrombocytopenia, lymphopenia, eosinophillia and increased leucocytes are reversible.

● **PREGNANCY** Manufacturer advises avoid unless essential—limited data available but not known to harmful in *animal* studies. [EvGr] Specialist sources indicate suitable for use in pregnancy. Ⓓ

● **BREAST FEEDING** Present in milk in low concentration, but appropriate to use.

● **RENAL IMPAIRMENT** See p. 21. Manufacturer advises caution if creatinine clearance 54 mL/minute or less, or serum creatinine 1.6 mg/dL or above (increased risk of convulsions).
Dose adjustments Manufacturer advises dose reduction in impairment—consult product literature.

● **DIRECTIONS FOR ADMINISTRATION** Displacement value may be significant when reconstituting injection, consult local guidelines or product literature.
For *intravenous injection*, manufacturer advises reconstitute with Water for Injection *or* Glucose 5 or 10% *or* Sodium Chloride 0.9%; give over 3 to 5 minutes—consult product literature.
For intermittent *intravenous infusion*, manufacturer advises dilute reconstituted solution with Water for Injection *or* Glucose 5% *or* Sodium Chloride 0.9% *or*

Compound Sodium Lactate *or* Ringer's Solution; give over 30 to 60 minutes—consult product literature.

For *intramuscular injection*, manufacturer advises reconstitute with Water for Injection *or* Glucose 10% *or* Sodium Chloride 0.9% *or* Lidocaine Hydrochloride 0.5%; give as a deep *intramuscular injection*—consult product literature.

- **PRESCRIBING AND DISPENSING INFORMATION** For choice of antibacterial therapy, see Antibacterials, use for prophylaxis p. 574, Skin infections, antibacterial therapy p. 589, Musculoskeletal system infections, antibacterial therapy p. 585.

- **MEDICINAL FORMS** There can be variation in the licensing of different medicines containing the same drug.

Powder for solution for injection
ELECTROLYTES: May contain Sodium

- **Cefazolin (Non-proprietary)**
  Cefazolin (as Cefazolin sodium) 1 gram Cefazolin 1g powder for solution for injection vials | 10 vial [PoM] £161.83
  Cefazolin (as Cefazolin sodium) 2 gram Cefazolin 2g powder for solution for injection vials | 10 vial [PoM] £183.90

Cefradine
(Cephradine)
22-Jul-2021　　▶ 603

- **INDICATIONS AND DOSE**

Susceptible infections due to sensitive Gram-positive and Gram-negative bacteria | Surgical prophylaxis
▶ BY MOUTH
- Child 7-11 years: 25–50 mg/kg daily in 2–4 divided doses
- Child 12-17 years: 250–500 mg 4 times a day, alternatively 0.5–1 g twice daily; increased if necessary up to 1 g 4 times a day, increased dose may be used in severe infections
- Adult: 250–500 mg 4 times a day, alternatively 0.5–1 g twice daily; increased if necessary up to 1 g 4 times a day, increased dose may be used in severe infections

- **INTERACTIONS** → Appendix 1: cephalosporins

- **SIDE-EFFECTS**
▶ **Rare or very rare** Antibiotic associated colitis
▶ **Frequency not known** Akathisia · aplastic anaemia · arthralgia · blood disorder · chest tightness · confusion · gastrointestinal discomfort · glossitis · hepatitis (transient) · hypersensitivity · increased risk of infection · jaundice cholestatic · muscle tone increased · nervousness · oedema · sleep disorder

- **PREGNANCY** Not known to be harmful.

- **BREAST FEEDING** Present in milk in low concentration, but appropriate to use.

- **RENAL IMPAIRMENT**
Dose adjustments See p. 21.
▶ In adults [EvGr] Use half normal dose if creatinine clearance 5–20 mL/minute. Use one-quarter normal dose if creatinine clearance less than 5 mL/minute. ◈M◈
▶ In children [EvGr] Reduce dose if creatinine clearance less than 20 mL/minute. ◈M◈

- **PROFESSION SPECIFIC INFORMATION**
Dental practitioners' formulary Cefradine Capsules may be prescribed.

- **MEDICINAL FORMS** There can be variation in the licensing of different medicines containing the same drug.

Oral capsule
CAUTIONARY AND ADVISORY LABELS 9

- **Cefradine (Non-proprietary)**
  Cefradine 250 mg Cefradine 250mg capsules | 20 capsule [PoM] £19.60 DT = £19.34
  Cefradine 500 mg Cefradine 500mg capsules | 20 capsule [PoM] £24.80 DT = £12.50

ANTIBACTERIALS ⟩ CEPHALOSPORINS, SECOND-GENERATION

▶ 603

Cefaclor
12-Apr-2021

- **INDICATIONS AND DOSE**

Susceptible infections due to sensitive Gram-positive and Gram-negative bacteria
▶ BY MOUTH USING IMMEDIATE-RELEASE MEDICINES
- Child 1-11 months: 20 mg/kg daily in 3 divided doses, alternatively 62.5 mg 3 times a day
- Child 1-4 years: 20 mg/kg daily in 3 divided doses, alternatively 125 mg 3 times a day
- Child 5-11 years: 20 mg/kg daily in 3 divided doses, usual max. 1 g daily, alternatively 250 mg 3 times a day
- Child 12-17 years: 250 mg 3 times a day; maximum 4 g per day
- Adult: 250 mg 3 times a day; maximum 4 g per day
▶ BY MOUTH USING MODIFIED-RELEASE MEDICINES
- Child 12-17 years: 375 mg every 12 hours, dose to be taken with food
- Adult: 375 mg every 12 hours, dose to be taken with food

Severe susceptible infections due to sensitive Gram-positive and Gram-negative bacteria
▶ BY MOUTH USING IMMEDIATE-RELEASE MEDICINES
- Child 1-11 months: 40 mg/kg daily in 3 divided doses, usual max. 1 g daily, alternatively 125 mg 3 times a day
- Child 1-4 years: 40 mg/kg daily in 3 divided doses, usual max. 1 g daily, alternatively 250 mg 3 times a day
- Child 5-11 years: 40 mg/kg daily in 3 divided doses, usual max. 1 g daily
- Child 12-17 years: 500 mg 3 times a day; maximum 4 g per day
- Adult: 500 mg 3 times a day; maximum 4 g per day

Pneumonia
▶ BY MOUTH USING MODIFIED-RELEASE MEDICINES
- Child 12-17 years: 750 mg every 12 hours, dose to be taken with food
- Adult: 750 mg every 12 hours, dose to be taken with food

Lower urinary-tract infections
▶ BY MOUTH USING MODIFIED-RELEASE MEDICINES
- Child 12-17 years: 375 mg every 12 hours, dose to be taken with food
- Adult: 375 mg every 12 hours, dose to be taken with food

Asymptomatic carriage of *Haemophilus influenzae* or mild exacerbations in cystic fibrosis
▶ BY MOUTH USING IMMEDIATE-RELEASE MEDICINES
- Child 1-11 months: 125 mg every 8 hours
- Child 1-6 years: 250 mg 3 times a day
- Child 7-17 years: 500 mg 3 times a day

- **INTERACTIONS** → Appendix 1: cephalosporins

- **SIDE-EFFECTS** Akathisia · anxiety · aplastic anaemia · arthralgia · arthritis · asthenia · colitis · confusion · drowsiness · dyspnoea · fever · genital pruritus · hallucination · hepatitis (transient) · hypersensitivity · increased risk of infection · insomnia · jaundice cholestatic (transient) · lymphadenopathy · lymphocytosis · muscle tone increased · oedema · paraesthesia · proteinuria · syncope · vasodilation

SIDE-EFFECTS, FURTHER INFORMATION Cefaclor is associated with protracted skin reactions, especially in children.

- **PREGNANCY** Not known to be harmful.

- **BREAST FEEDING** Present in milk in low concentration, but appropriate to use.

- **RENAL IMPAIRMENT** [EvGr] Use with caution. ◈M◈

- **MEDICINAL FORMS** There can be variation in the licensing of different medicines containing the same drug.

Oral suspension
CAUTIONARY AND ADVISORY LABELS 9

▸ Cefaclor (Non-proprietary)
  Cefaclor (as Cefaclor monohydrate) 50 mg per 1 ml Cefaclor 250mg/5ml oral suspension | 100 ml PoM £8.26 DT = £8.26

▸ Distaclor (Flynn Pharma Ltd)
  Cefaclor (as Cefaclor monohydrate) 25 mg per 1 ml Distaclor 125mg/5ml oral suspension | 100 ml PoM £4.13 DT = £4.13
  Cefaclor (as Cefaclor monohydrate) 50 mg per 1 ml Distaclor 250mg/5ml oral suspension | 100 ml PoM £8.26 DT = £8.26

Modified-release tablet
CAUTIONARY AND ADVISORY LABELS 9, 21, 25

▸ Cefaclor (Non-proprietary)
  Cefaclor (as Cefaclor monohydrate) 375 mg Cefaclor 375mg modified-release tablets | 14 tablet PoM £9.10 DT = £9.10

▸ Distaclor MR (Flynn Pharma Ltd)
  Cefaclor (as Cefaclor monohydrate) 375 mg Distaclor MR 375mg tablets | 14 tablet PoM £9.10 DT = £9.10

Oral capsule
CAUTIONARY AND ADVISORY LABELS 9

▸ Cefaclor (Non-proprietary)
  Cefaclor (as Cefaclor monohydrate) 500 mg Cefaclor 500mg capsules | 21 capsule PoM £7.50 DT = £7.50

▸ Distaclor (Flynn Pharma Ltd)
  Cefaclor (as Cefaclor monohydrate) 500 mg Distaclor 500mg capsules | 21 capsule PoM £7.50 DT = £7.50

F 603

Cefoxitin

21-Aug-2019

- **INDICATIONS AND DOSE**

Complicated urinary tract infection | Pyelonephritis
▸ BY SLOW INTRAVENOUS INJECTION
▸ Adult: 2 g every 4–6 hours; maximum 12 g per day

- **INTERACTIONS** → Appendix 1: cephalosporins

- **SIDE-EFFECTS** Anaemia · bone marrow failure · encephalopathy · fever · hypersensitivity · local reaction · myasthenia gravis aggravated · overgrowth of nonsusceptible organisms · renal impairment · thrombophlebitis

- **PREGNANCY** Manufacturer advises not known to be harmful.

- **BREAST FEEDING** EvGr Specialist sources indicate present in milk in low concentrations, but appropriate to use. ◇

- **RENAL IMPAIRMENT**
  Dose adjustments Manufacturer advises increase dosing interval to every 8-12 hours if creatinine clearance 30-50 mL/minute, or every 12-24 hours if creatinine clearance 10-29 mL/minute. Consult product literature if creatinine clearance less than 10 mL/minute. See p. 21.

- **DIRECTIONS FOR ADMINISTRATION** For *slow intravenous injection*, reconstitute with 10 mL Water for Injections; give over 3 to 5 minutes.

- **MEDICINAL FORMS** There can be variation in the licensing of different medicines containing the same drug. Forms available from special-order manufacturers include: powder for solution for injection

Powder for solution for injection
ELECTROLYTES: May contain Sodium

▸ Cefoxitin (Non-proprietary)
  Cefoxitin (as Cefoxitin sodium) 1 gram Cefoxitin 1g powder for solution for injection vials | 10 vial PoM ▣
  Cefoxitin (as Cefoxitin sodium) 2 gram Cefoxitin 2g powder for solution for injection vials | 10 vial PoM ▣

▸ Renoxitin (Renascience Pharma Ltd)
  Cefoxitin (as Cefoxitin sodium) 1 gram Renoxitin 1g powder for solution for injection vials | 10 vial PoM £163.80 (Hospital only)
  Cefoxitin (as Cefoxitin sodium) 2 gram Renoxitin 2g powder for solution for injection vials | 10 vial PoM £282.45 (Hospital only)

F 603

Cefuroxime

07-Apr-2022

- **INDICATIONS AND DOSE**

Susceptible infections due to Gram-positive and Gram-negative bacteria
▸ BY MOUTH
▸ Child 3 months–1 year: 10 mg/kg twice daily (max. per dose 125 mg)
▸ Child 2-11 years: 15 mg/kg twice daily (max. per dose 250 mg)
▸ Child 12-17 years: 250 mg twice daily, dose may be doubled in severe lower respiratory-tract infections or if pneumonia is suspected
▸ Adult: 250 mg twice daily, dose may be doubled in severe lower respiratory-tract infections or if pneumonia is suspected
▸ BY INTRAVENOUS INFUSION, OR BY INTRAVENOUS INJECTION, OR BY INTRAMUSCULAR INJECTION
▸ Child: 20 mg/kg every 8 hours (max. per dose 750 mg); increased to 50–60 mg/kg every 6–8 hours (max. per dose 1.5 g), increased dose used for severe infection and cystic fibrosis
▸ Adult: 750 mg every 6–8 hours; increased if necessary up to 1.5 g every 6–8 hours, increased dose used for severe infections

Hospital-acquired pneumonia
▸ BY INTRAVENOUS INJECTION, OR BY INTRAVENOUS INFUSION
▸ Adult: 750 mg every 8 hours; increased if necessary to 750 mg every 6 hours, increased dose used for severe infections, alternatively 1.5 g every 6–8 hours, increased dose used for severe infections

Cellulitis | Erysipelas
▸ BY INTRAVENOUS INJECTION, OR BY INTRAVENOUS INFUSION
▸ Child: 20 mg/kg every 8 hours (max. per dose 750 mg); increased if necessary up to 50–60 mg/kg every 6–8 hours (max. per dose 1.5 g)
▸ Adult: 750 mg every 6–8 hours; increased if necessary up to 1.5 g every 6–8 hours

Prophylaxis of infection from human bites [in combination with other drugs] | Prophylaxis of infection from animal bites [in combination with other drugs] | Treatment of infection from human bites [in combination with other drugs] | Treatment of infection from animal bites [in combination with other drugs]
▸ BY INTRAVENOUS INFUSION, OR BY INTRAVENOUS INJECTION
▸ Adult: 750 mg every 8 hours; increased if necessary to 750 mg every 6 hours, increased dose used for severe infections, alternatively 1.5 g every 6–8 hours, increased dose used for severe infections

Acute diverticulitis [in combination with metronidazole]
▸ BY INTRAVENOUS INJECTION, OR BY INTRAVENOUS INFUSION
▸ Adult: 750 mg every 6–8 hours; increased if necessary up to 1.5 g every 6–8 hours, use increased dose in severe infection

Lyme disease
▸ BY MOUTH
▸ Child 3 months–11 years: 15 mg/kg twice daily (max. per dose 500 mg) for 14–21 days (for 28 days in Lyme arthritis)
▸ Child 12-17 years: 500 mg twice daily for 14–21 days (for 28 days in Lyme arthritis)
▸ Adult: 500 mg twice daily for 14–21 days (for 28 days in Lyme arthritis)

Surgical prophylaxis
▸ INITIALLY BY INTRAVENOUS INJECTION
▸ Adult: 1.5 g for 1 dose, to be administered up to 30 minutes before the procedure, then (by intravenous injection or by intramuscular injection) 750 mg every

8 hours if required for up to 3 doses (in high risk procedures)

Open fractures, prophylaxis
► BY INTRAVENOUS INFUSION, OR BY INTRAVENOUS INJECTION
► Adult: 1.5 g every 8 hours until soft tissue closure (maximum duration 72 hours)

Acute prostatitis
► BY INTRAVENOUS INFUSION, OR BY INTRAVENOUS INJECTION
► Adult: 1.5 g every 6–8 hours

Urinary-tract infection (lower)
► BY MOUTH
► Child (body-weight up to 40 kg): 15 mg/kg twice daily (max. per dose 250 mg)
► Child (body-weight 40 kg and above): 250 mg twice daily
► Adult: 250 mg twice daily

Urinary tract infection (catheter-associated)
► BY INTRAVENOUS INFUSION, OR BY INTRAVENOUS INJECTION
► Child 3 months-15 years: 20 mg/kg every 8 hours (max. per dose 750 mg); increased to 50–60 mg/kg every 6–8 hours (max. per dose 1.5 g), increased dose used for severe infection
► Child 16-17 years: 0.75–1.5 g every 6–8 hours
► Adult: 0.75–1.5 g every 6–8 hours

Acute pyelonephritis
► BY MOUTH
► Child (body-weight up to 40 kg): 15 mg/kg twice daily (max. per dose 250 mg)
► Child (body-weight 40 kg and above): 250 mg twice daily
► Adult: 250 mg twice daily
► BY INTRAVENOUS INFUSION, OR BY INTRAVENOUS INJECTION
► Child 3 months-15 years: 20 mg/kg every 8 hours (max. per dose 750 mg); increased to 50–60 mg/kg every 6–8 hours (max. per dose 1.5 g), increased dose used for severe infection
► Child 16-17 years: 0.75–1.5 g every 6–8 hours
► Adult: 0.75–1.5 g every 6–8 hours

● **UNLICENSED USE**
► In adults EvGr Cefuroxime is used for the treatment of hospital-acquired pneumonia, Ⓐ but is not licensed for this indication.
► In children EvGr Cefuroxime is used for the treatment of cellulitis, Ⓐ but the dose increase is not licensed for this indication. EvGr Cefuroxime is used for the treatment of erysipelas, Ⓐ but the dose increase is not licensed for this indication.
► With oral use in children Not licensed for treatment of Lyme disease in children under 12 years.
► With oral use Duration of treatment in Lyme disease is unlicensed.

● **INTERACTIONS** → Appendix 1: cephalosporins

● **SIDE-EFFECTS**
► **Common or very common**
► With oral use Increased risk of infection
► **Uncommon**
► With parenteral use Gastrointestinal disorder
► **Frequency not known**
► With oral use Drug fever · hepatic disorders · Jarisch-Herxheimer reaction · serum sickness
► With parenteral use Cutaneous vasculitis · drug fever · increased risk of infection

● **PREGNANCY** Not known to be harmful.

● **BREAST FEEDING** Present in milk in low concentration, but appropriate to use.

● **RENAL IMPAIRMENT**
Dose adjustments
► With intravenous use in adults Use parenteral dose of 750 mg twice daily if eGFR 10–20 mL/minute/1.73 m^2. Use parenteral dose of 750 mg once daily if eGFR less than 10 mL/minute/1.73 m^2.

► In children Reduce parenteral dose if estimated glomerular filtration rate less than 20 mL/minute/1.73 m^2.

● **DIRECTIONS FOR ADMINISTRATION**
► With intramuscular use or intravenous use Manufacturer advises single doses over 750 mg should be administered by the intravenous route only.
► With intravenous use in children Displacement value may be significant when reconstituting injection, consult local guidelines. For *intermittent intravenous infusion*, manufacturer advises dilute reconstituted solution further in Glucose 5% *or* Sodium Chloride 0.9%; give over 30–60 minutes.
► With intravenous use in adults For *intravenous infusion* (*Zinacef*®), manufacturer advises give intermittently or via drip tubing in Glucose 5% *or* Sodium Chloride 0.9%. Dissolve initially in Water for Injections (at least 2 mL for each 250 mg, 15 mL for 1.5 g); suggested volume 50–100 mL given over 30–60 minutes.

● **PRESCRIBING AND DISPENSING INFORMATION** For choice of antibacterial therapy, see Antibacterials, use for prophylaxis p. 574, Gastro-intestinal system infections, antibacterial therapy p. 582, Lyme disease p. 669, Respiratory system infections, antibacterial therapy p. 586, Skin infections, antibacterial therapy p. 589, Urinary-tract infections p. 681.

● **MEDICINAL FORMS** There can be variation in the licensing of different medicines containing the same drug. Forms available from special-order manufacturers include: solution for injection, infusion

Oral tablet
CAUTIONARY AND ADVISORY LABELS 9, 21, 25
► Cefuroxime (Non-proprietary)
Cefuroxime (as Cefuroxime axetil) 250 mg Cefuroxime 250mg tablets | 14 tablet PoM £25.98 DT = £9.11

Powder for solution for injection
ELECTROLYTES: May contain Sodium
► Cefuroxime (Non-proprietary)
Cefuroxime (as Cefuroxime sodium) 50 mg Cefuroxime 50mg powder for solution for injection vials | 10 vial PoM £49.95 (Hospital only)
Cefuroxime (as Cefuroxime sodium) 250 mg Cefuroxime 250mg powder for solution for injection vials | 10 vial PoM £9.25 (Hospital only)
Cefuroxime (as Cefuroxime sodium) 750 mg Cefuroxime 750mg powder for solution for injection vials | 10 vial PoM £25.20 | 10 vial PoM £23.40-£34.10 (Hospital only)
Cefuroxime (as Cefuroxime sodium) 1.5 gram Cefuroxime 1.5g powder for solution for injection vials | 10 vial PoM £50.50 | 10 vial PoM £47.00-£69.20 (Hospital only)
► Zinacef (Sandoz Ltd)
Cefuroxime (as Cefuroxime sodium) 250 mg Zinacef 250mg powder for solution for injection vials | 5 vial PoM £4.70 (Hospital only)
Cefuroxime (as Cefuroxime sodium) 750 mg Zinacef 750mg powder for solution for injection vials | 5 vial PoM £11.72 (Hospital only)
Cefuroxime (as Cefuroxime sodium) 1.5 gram Zinacef 1.5g powder for solution for injection vials | 1 vial PoM £4.70 (Hospital only)

Oral suspension
CAUTIONARY AND ADVISORY LABELS 9, 21
EXCIPIENTS: May contain Aspartame, sucrose
► Zinnat (Sandoz Ltd)
Cefuroxime (as Cefuroxime axetil) 25 mg per 1 ml Zinnat 125mg/5ml oral suspension | 70 ml PoM £5.20 DT = £5.20

ANTIBACTERIALS › CEPHALOSPORINS, THIRD-GENERATION

⚑ 603

Cefixime

26-Jul-2023

● **INDICATIONS AND DOSE**

Acute infections due to sensitive Gram-positive and Gram-negative bacteria
▶ BY MOUTH
▸ Child 6–11 months: 75 mg daily
▸ Child 1–4 years: 100 mg daily
▸ Child 5–9 years: 200 mg daily
▸ Child 10–17 years: 200–400 mg daily, alternatively 100–200 mg twice daily
▸ Adult: 200–400 mg daily in 1–2 divided doses

Uncomplicated gonorrhoea [anogenital and pharyngeal infection—in combination with azithromycin]
▶ BY MOUTH
▸ Adult: 400 mg for 1 dose

Disseminated gonococcal infection [when sensitivity confirmed]
▶ BY MOUTH
▸ Adult: 400 mg twice daily, following intravenous antibacterial treatment, starting 24–48 hours after symptoms improve, to give 7 days treatment in total

● UNLICENSED USE [EvGr] Cefixime is used for the treatment of uncomplicated gonorrhoea and disseminated gonococcal infection, ⟨A⟩ but is not licensed for these indications.

● INTERACTIONS → Appendix 1: cephalosporins

● SIDE-EFFECTS Acute kidney injury · arthralgia · drug fever · dyspepsia · dyspnoea · face oedema · flatulence · genital pruritus · hypereosinophilia · jaundice · serum sickness-like reaction · thrombocytosis · vulvovaginal infection

● PREGNANCY Not known to be harmful.

● BREAST FEEDING Manufacturer advises avoid unless essential—no information available.

● RENAL IMPAIRMENT [EvGr] Caution in severe impairment. ⟨M⟩
Dose adjustments See p. 21.
▸ In adults [EvGr] Reduce dose if creatinine clearance less than 20 mL/minute (max. 200 mg once daily). ⟨M⟩
▸ In children [EvGr] Reduce dose if creatinine clearance less than 20 mL/minute (should not exceed 200 mg once daily). ⟨M⟩

● PRESCRIBING AND DISPENSING INFORMATION For choice of antibacterial therapy, see Genital system infections, antibacterial therapy p. 584.

● MEDICINAL FORMS There can be variation in the licensing of different medicines containing the same drug.
Oral tablet
CAUTIONARY AND ADVISORY LABELS 9
▸ Suprax (Advanz Pharma)
Cefixime 200 mg Suprax 200mg tablets | 7 tablet [PoM] £13.23 DT = £13.23

⚑ 603

Cefotaxime

24-Jul-2024

● **INDICATIONS AND DOSE**

Uncomplicated gonorrhoea
▶ BY INTRAMUSCULAR INJECTION
▸ Adult: 500–1000 mg for 1 dose

Disseminated gonococcal infection
▶ BY INTRAVENOUS INJECTION, OR BY INTRAVENOUS INFUSION
▸ Adult: 1 g every 8 hours for 7 days, may be switched 24–48 hours after symptoms improve to a suitable oral antibacterial

Infections due to sensitive Gram-positive and Gram-negative bacteria | Surgical prophylaxis | Haemophilus epiglottitis
▶ BY INTRAMUSCULAR INJECTION, OR BY INTRAVENOUS INJECTION, OR BY INTRAVENOUS INFUSION
▸ Adult: 1 g every 12 hours

Severe susceptible infections due to sensitive Gram-positive and Gram-negative bacteria | Meningitis
▶ BY INTRAVENOUS INJECTION, OR BY INTRAVENOUS INFUSION
▸ Adult: 8 g daily in 4 divided doses, increased if necessary to 12 g daily in 3–4 divided doses

● UNLICENSED USE [EvGr] Cefotaxime is used in the doses provided in BNF Publications for the treatment of disseminated gonococcal infection, ⟨A⟩ but these are not licensed.

● INTERACTIONS → Appendix 1: cephalosporins

● SIDE-EFFECTS
▶ **Uncommon** Drug fever · Jarisch-Herxheimer reaction · renal impairment · seizure
▶ **Frequency not known** Arrhythmia (following rapid injection) · bronchospasm · encephalopathy · fungal infection · hepatic disorders

● PREGNANCY Not known to be harmful.

● BREAST FEEDING Present in milk in low concentration, but appropriate to use.

● RENAL IMPAIRMENT
Dose adjustments See p. 21.
[EvGr] If eGFR less than 5 mL/minute/1.73 m^2, initial dose of 1 g then use half normal dose. ⟨M⟩

● DIRECTIONS FOR ADMINISTRATION
▸ With intramuscular use For *intramuscular injection*, doses over 1 g should be divided between more than one site.
▸ With intravenous use For *intravenous infusion*, manufacturer advises give reconstituted solution intermittently *in* Glucose 5% *or* Sodium Chloride 0.9%. Suggested volume 40–100 mL given over 20–60 minutes; incompatible with alkaline solutions.

● PRESCRIBING AND DISPENSING INFORMATION For choice of antibacterial therapy, see Central nervous system infections, antibacterial therapy p. 580, Genital system infections, antibacterial therapy p. 584, Respiratory system infections, antibacterial therapy p. 586.

● MEDICINAL FORMS There can be variation in the licensing of different medicines containing the same drug.
Powder for solution for injection
▸ Cefotaxime (Non-proprietary)
Cefotaxime (as Cefotaxime sodium) 500 mg Cefotaxime 500mg powder for solution for injection vials | 10 vial [PoM] £21.00-£30.00 (Hospital only)
Cefotaxime (as Cefotaxime sodium) 1 gram Cefotaxime 1g powder for solution for injection vials | 10 vial [PoM] £35.00 | 10 vial [PoM] £35.00-£42.00 (Hospital only)
Cefotaxime (as Cefotaxime sodium) 2 gram Cefotaxime 2g powder for solution for injection vials | 10 vial [PoM] £55.00-£56.25 (Hospital only)

⚑ 603

Ceftazidime

29-Nov-2021

● **INDICATIONS AND DOSE**

Prophylaxis for transurethral resection of prostate
▶ BY INTRAVENOUS INJECTION, OR BY INTRAVENOUS INFUSION, OR BY DEEP INTRAMUSCULAR INJECTION
▸ Adult: 1 g for 1 dose, dose to be administered up to 30 minutes before procedure, dose may be repeated if necessary when catheter removed

Pseudomonal lung infection in cystic fibrosis

▸ BY INTRAVENOUS INFUSION, OR BY INTRAVENOUS INJECTION, OR BY DEEP INTRAMUSCULAR INJECTION

▸ Adult: 100–150 mg/kg daily in 3 divided doses (max. per dose 3 g)

Complicated urinary-tract infection

▸ BY INTRAVENOUS INJECTION, OR BY INTRAVENOUS INFUSION, OR BY DEEP INTRAMUSCULAR INJECTION

▸ Adult: 1–2 g every 8–12 hours

Septicaemia | Hospital-acquired pneumonia

▸ BY INTRAVENOUS INFUSION, OR BY INTRAVENOUS INJECTION

▸ Adult: 2 g every 8 hours

Febrile neutropenia

▸ BY INTRAVENOUS INFUSION, OR BY INTRAVENOUS INJECTION

▸ Adult: 2 g every 8 hours

Meningitis

▸ BY INTRAVENOUS INFUSION, OR BY INTRAVENOUS INJECTION

▸ Adult: 2 g every 8 hours

Susceptible infections due to sensitive Gram-positive and Gram-negative bacteria

▸ BY INTRAVENOUS INFUSION, OR BY INTRAVENOUS INJECTION, OR BY DEEP INTRAMUSCULAR INJECTION

▸ Adult: 1–2 g every 8 hours

● INTERACTIONS → Appendix 1: cephalosporins

● SIDE-EFFECTS

▸ **Common or very common** Thrombocytosis · thrombophlebitis

▸ **Uncommon** Antibiotic associated colitis · increased risk of infection

▸ **Rare or very rare** Acute kidney injury

▸ **Frequency not known** Coma · encephalopathy · jaundice · lymphocytosis · myoclonus · neurological effects · paraesthesia · seizure · taste altered · tremor

● PREGNANCY Not known to be harmful.

● BREAST FEEDING Present in milk in low concentration, but appropriate to use.

● HEPATIC IMPAIRMENT Manufacturer advises caution in severe impairment (no information available).

● RENAL IMPAIRMENT [EvGr] Use with caution. ⟨M⟩
Dose adjustments [EvGr] Reduce dose if creatinine clearance 50 mL/minute or less—consult product literature. ⟨M⟩ See p. 21.

● DIRECTIONS FOR ADMINISTRATION Intramuscular administration used when intravenous administration not possible; single doses over 1 g by intravenous route only.

For *intravenous infusion* give intermittently *or via* drip tubing *in* Glucose 5% or 10% *or* Sodium Chloride 0.9%. Dissolve 2 g initially in 10 mL (3 g in 15 mL) infusion fluid, dilute further up to a concentration of 40 mg/mL. Give over up to 30 minutes.

● MEDICINAL FORMS There can be variation in the licensing of different medicines containing the same drug. Forms available from special-order manufacturers include: infusion, solution for infusion

Powder for solution for injection

ELECTROLYTES: May contain Sodium

▸ Ceftazidime (Non-proprietary)

Ceftazidime (as Ceftazidime pentahydrate) **500 mg** Ceftazidime 500mg powder for solution for injection vials | 1 vial [PoM] £4.25–£6.42 (Hospital only)

Ceftazidime (as Ceftazidime pentahydrate) **1 gram** Ceftazidime 1g powder for solution for injection vials | 1 vial [PoM] £12.42 (Hospital only) | 10 vial [PoM] £13.90-£103.90 (Hospital only)

Ceftazidime (as Ceftazidime pentahydrate) **2 gram** Ceftazidime 2g powder for solution for injection vials | 1 vial [PoM] £26.16 (Hospital only) | 10 vial [PoM] £27.70-£218.80 (Hospital only)

Combinations available: *Ceftazidime with avibactam,* p. 612

F 603

Ceftriaxone

24-Jul-2024

● INDICATIONS AND DOSE

Community-acquired pneumonia | Intra-abdominal infections | Complicated urinary-tract infections | Acute exacerbations of chronic obstructive pulmonary disease

▸ BY INTRAVENOUS INFUSION, OR BY INTRAVENOUS INJECTION, OR BY DEEP INTRAMUSCULAR INJECTION

▸ Adult: 1–2 g once daily, 2 g dose to be used for severe cases

Hospital-acquired pneumonia

▸ BY INTRAVENOUS INFUSION, OR BY INTRAVENOUS INJECTION, OR BY DEEP INTRAMUSCULAR INJECTION

▸ Adult: 2 g once daily

Cellulitis | Erysipelas | Moderate diabetic foot infection | Severe diabetic foot infection | Leg ulcer infection

▸ BY INTRAVENOUS INJECTION, OR BY INTRAVENOUS INFUSION

▸ Adult: 2 g once daily

Prophylaxis of infection from human bites [in combination with other drugs] | Prophylaxis of infection from animal bites [in combination with other drugs] | Treatment of infection from human bites [in combination with other drugs] | Treatment of infection from animal bites [in combination with other drugs]

▸ BY INTRAVENOUS INJECTION, OR BY INTRAVENOUS INFUSION

▸ Adult: 2 g once daily

Complicated skin and soft tissue infections | Infections of bones and joints

▸ BY INTRAVENOUS INFUSION, OR BY INTRAVENOUS INJECTION, OR BY DEEP INTRAMUSCULAR INJECTION

▸ Adult: 2 g once daily

Suspected bacterial infection in neutropenic patients

▸ BY INTRAVENOUS INFUSION, OR BY INTRAVENOUS INJECTION

▸ Adult: 2–4 g once daily, doses at the higher end of the recommended range used in severe cases

▸ BY DEEP INTRAMUSCULAR INJECTION

▸ Adult: 2 g once daily, increased if necessary up to 4 g daily in 2 divided doses, doses at the higher end of the recommended range used in severe cases

Suspected meningococcal disease [pre-hospital treatment] | Suspected bacterial meningitis [pre-hospital treatment where there is likely to be a clinically significant delay in transfer to hospital]

▸ BY DEEP INTRAMUSCULAR INJECTION

▸ Child 1 month: 250 mg for 1 dose, administer prior to urgent transfer to hospital unless this will delay transfer. The actual dose given should be communicated to the receiving hospital, where the child's weight should be obtained as soon as possible and the remainder of the dose given if necessary (see dosing for *Bacterial meningitis* and *Meningococcal disease*)

▸ Child 2-11 months: 500 mg for 1 dose, administer prior to urgent transfer to hospital unless this will delay transfer. The actual dose given should be communicated to the receiving hospital, where the child's weight should be obtained as soon as possible and the remainder of the dose given if necessary (see dosing for *Bacterial meningitis* and *Meningococcal disease*)

▸ Child 1-4 years: 1 g for 1 dose, administer prior to urgent transfer to hospital unless this will delay transfer. The actual dose given should be communicated to the receiving hospital, where the child's weight should be obtained as soon as possible and the remainder of the dose given if necessary (see dosing for *Bacterial meningitis* and *Meningococcal disease*)

continued →

▸ Child 5-8 years: 1.5 g for 1 dose, administer prior to urgent transfer to hospital unless this will delay transfer. The actual dose given should be communicated to the receiving hospital, where the child's weight should be obtained as soon as possible and the remainder of the dose given if necessary (see dosing for *Bacterial meningitis* and *Meningococcal disease*)

▸ Child 9-11 years: 2 g for 1 dose, administer prior to urgent transfer to hospital unless this will delay transfer. The actual dose given should be communicated to the receiving hospital, where the child's weight should be obtained as soon as possible and the remainder of the dose given if necessary (see dosing for *Bacterial meningitis* and *Meningococcal disease*)

▸ BY INTRAVENOUS INJECTION, OR BY DEEP INTRAMUSCULAR INJECTION

▸ Child 12-17 years: 2 g for 1 dose, administer prior to urgent transfer to hospital unless this will delay transfer

▸ Adult: 2 g for 1 dose, administer prior to urgent transfer to hospital unless this will delay transfer

Bacterial meningitis | Meningococcal disease

▸ BY INTRAVENOUS INFUSION, OR BY INTRAVENOUS INJECTION

▸ Adult: 2 g every 12 hours, alternatively 4 g once daily

▸ BY INTRAVENOUS INFUSION

▸ Child 1 month-11 years (body-weight up to 50 kg): 100 mg/kg once daily (max. per dose 4 g), if the *total* daily dose exceeds 2 g consider giving in 2 divided doses

▸ Child 9-11 years (body-weight 50 kg and above): 2 g every 12 hours, alternatively 4 g once daily

▸ Child 12-17 years: 2 g every 12 hours, alternatively 4 g once daily

▸ BY INTRAVENOUS INJECTION

▸ Child 9-11 years (body-weight 50 kg and above): 2 g every 12 hours, alternatively 4 g once daily, doses of 50 mg/kg or more should be given by intravenous infusion

▸ Child 12-17 years: 2 g every 12 hours, alternatively 4 g once daily

Bacterial endocarditis

▸ BY INTRAVENOUS INFUSION, OR BY INTRAVENOUS INJECTION

▸ Adult: 2-4 g once daily, doses at the higher end of the recommended range used in severe cases

▸ BY INTRAVENOUS INFUSION

▸ Child 1 month-11 years (body-weight up to 50 kg): 100 mg/kg once daily (max. per dose 4 g)

▸ Child 9-11 years (body-weight 50 kg and above): 2-4 g once daily, doses at the higher end of the recommended range used in severe cases

▸ Child 12-17 years: 2-4 g once daily, doses at the higher end of the recommended range used in severe cases

▸ BY INTRAVENOUS INJECTION

▸ Child 9-11 years (body-weight 50 kg and above): 2-4 g once daily, doses at the higher end of the recommended range used in severe cases; doses of 50 mg/kg or more should be given by infusion

▸ Child 12-17 years: 2-4 g once daily, doses at the higher end of the recommended range used in severe cases

▸ BY DEEP INTRAMUSCULAR INJECTION

▸ Child 1 month-11 years (body-weight up to 50 kg): 100 mg/kg daily; maximum 4 g per day

▸ Child 9-11 years (body-weight 50 kg and above): 2 g once daily, increased if necessary up to 4 g daily in 2 divided doses, doses at the higher end of the recommended range used in severe cases

▸ Child 12-17 years: 2 g once daily, increased if necessary up to 4 g daily in 2 divided doses, doses at the higher end of the recommended range used in severe cases

▸ Adult: 2 g once daily, increased if necessary up to 4 g daily in 2 divided doses, doses at the higher end of the recommended range used in severe cases

Surgical prophylaxis

▸ BY INTRAVENOUS INFUSION, OR BY INTRAVENOUS INJECTION, OR BY DEEP INTRAMUSCULAR INJECTION

▸ Adult: 2 g for 1 dose, dose to be administered 30-90 minutes before procedure

Pelvic inflammatory disease

▸ BY DEEP INTRAMUSCULAR INJECTION

▸ Child 12-17 years (body-weight 45 kg and above): 1 g for 1 dose

▸ Adult: 1 g for 1 dose

Uncomplicated gonorrhoea

▸ BY DEEP INTRAMUSCULAR INJECTION

▸ Child 12-17 years (body-weight 45 kg and above): 1 g for 1 dose

▸ Adult: 1 g for 1 dose

Gonococcal conjunctivitis

▸ BY DEEP INTRAMUSCULAR INJECTION

▸ Adult: 1 g for 1 dose

Gonococcal epididymo-orchitis

▸ BY DEEP INTRAMUSCULAR INJECTION

▸ Adult: 1 g for 1 dose, to be followed by an additional antibacterial course to treat epididymo-orchitis

Disseminated gonococcal infection

▸ BY DEEP INTRAMUSCULAR INJECTION, OR BY INTRAVENOUS INFUSION, OR BY INTRAVENOUS INJECTION

▸ Adult: 1 g every 24 hours for 7 days, may be switched 24-48 hours after symptoms improve to a suitable oral antibacterial

Syphilis

▸ BY INTRAVENOUS INFUSION, OR BY INTRAVENOUS INJECTION, OR BY DEEP INTRAMUSCULAR INJECTION

▸ Adult: 0.5-1 g once daily for 10-14 days, dose increased to 2 g once daily for neurosyphilis

Lyme disease [affecting central nervous system]

▸ BY INTRAVENOUS INFUSION, OR BY INTRAVENOUS INJECTION

▸ Adult: 2 g twice daily for 21 days, alternatively 4 g once daily for 21 days

Lyme arthritis | Acrodermatitis chronica atrophicans

▸ BY INTRAVENOUS INFUSION, OR BY INTRAVENOUS INJECTION

▸ Adult: 2 g once daily for 28 days

Lyme carditis

▸ BY INTRAVENOUS INFUSION, OR BY INTRAVENOUS INJECTION

▸ Adult: 2 g once daily for 21 days

Prevention of secondary case of meningococcal meningitis

▸ BY DEEP INTRAMUSCULAR INJECTION

▸ Adult: 250 mg for 1 dose

Prevention of secondary case of *Haemophilus influenzae* type b disease

▸ BY DEEP INTRAMUSCULAR INJECTION, OR BY INTRAVENOUS INJECTION, OR BY INTRAVENOUS INFUSION

▸ Adult: 1 g once daily for 2 days

Acute otitis media

▸ BY DEEP INTRAMUSCULAR INJECTION

▸ Adult: 1-2 g for 1 dose, dose can be given for 3 days if severely ill or previous therapy failed

Acute prostatitis

▸ BY SLOW INTRAVENOUS INJECTION, OR BY INTRAVENOUS INFUSION

▸ Adult: 2 g once daily

● UNLICENSED USE [EvGr] Not licensed for prophylaxis of *Haemophilus influenzae* type b disease. ⟨E⟩ Not licensed for prophylaxis of meningococcal meningitis. [EvGr] Ceftriaxone is used for the treatment of pelvic inflammatory disease, ⟨A⟩ but is not licensed for this indication. [EvGr] Ceftriaxone is used in the doses provided in BNF Publications for the treatment of uncomplicated gonorrhoea, gonococcal epididymo-orchitis, gonococcal conjunctivitis and disseminated gonococcal infection, ⟨A⟩ but these are not licensed. EvGr Ceftriaxone is used for Lyme disease affecting the central nervous system, ⟨A⟩ but the dose is not licensed for this indication.

- **CAUTIONS**

GENERAL CAUTIONS History of hypercalciuria · history of kidney stones

SPECIFIC CAUTIONS

▸ With intravenous use Concomitant treatment with intravenous calcium (including total parenteral nutrition containing calcium)

- **INTERACTIONS** → Appendix 1: cephalosporins
- **SIDE-EFFECTS**

▸ **Uncommon** Anaemia · coagulation disorder · fungal infection

▸ **Rare or very rare** Bronchospasm · glycosuria · haematuria · oedema

▸ **Frequency not known** Antibiotic associated colitis · cholelithiasis · hypersensitivity · nephrolithiasis · oral disorders · pancreatitis · seizure · vertigo

SIDE-EFFECTS, FURTHER INFORMATION Precipitates of calcium ceftriaxone can occur in the gall bladder and urine (particularly in very young, dehydrated or those who are immobilised)—consider discontinuation if symptomatic.

- **PREGNANCY** Manufacturer advises use only if benefit outweighs risk—limited data available but not known to be harmful in *animal* studies. EvGr Specialist sources indicate suitable for use in pregnancy. ⟨D⟩
- **BREAST FEEDING** EvGr Specialist sources advise ceftriaxone is compatible with breastfeeding—present in milk in low concentration but limited effects to breast-fed infant. ⟨D⟩
- **HEPATIC IMPAIRMENT** Manufacturer advises caution in severe impairment (no information available).
- **RENAL IMPAIRMENT**

Dose adjustments See p. 21.

Manufacturer advises a dose reduction may be required in severe renal impairment in combination with hepatic impairment (limited information available)—monitor for efficacy.

▸ In adults Manufacturer advises max. 2 g daily if creatinine clearance less than 10 mL/minute.

▸ In children Expert sources advise max. 50 mg/kg daily or max. 2 g daily if estimated glomerular filtration rate less than 10 mL/minute/1.73 m^2.

- **MONITORING REQUIREMENTS** Manufacturer advises to monitor full blood count regularly during prolonged treatment.
- **DIRECTIONS FOR ADMINISTRATION**

▸ With intravenous use in children EvGr For doses greater than 2 g daily, consider giving in two divided doses. ⟨M⟩ Displacement value may be significant, consult local guidelines. EvGr For *intravenous infusion* (preferred route), dilute reconstituted solution with Glucose 5% *or* Sodium Chloride 0.9%; give over at least 30 minutes. ⟨M⟩ Not to be given simultaneously with parenteral nutrition or infusion fluids containing calcium, even by different infusion lines; may be infused sequentially with infusion fluids containing calcium if infusion lines at different sites are used, or if the infusion lines are replaced or thoroughly flushed between infusions with Sodium Chloride 0.9% to avoid precipitation—consult product literature. EvGr For *intravenous injection*, give over 5 minutes. ⟨M⟩ Local policies may advise that doses of 50 mg/kg can be given by intravenous injection over 5 minutes to children under 12 years, although this is not licensed.

▸ With intramuscular use in children EvGr The maximum single intramuscular dose is 2 g. Doses over 1 g should be divided between more than one site. Doses greater than 2 g must be given in two divided doses 12 hours apart or by intravenous administration. For *intramuscular injection*, may be mixed with 1% Lidocaine Hydrochloride Injection to reduce pain at intramuscular injection site. Intramuscular injection should only be considered when the intravenous route is not possible or less appropriate. ⟨M⟩ If administered by intramuscular injection, the lower end of the dose range should be used for the shortest time possible; volume depends on the age and size of the child. Displacement value may be significant, consult local guidelines.

▸ With intravenous use in adults EvGr For doses greater than 2 g daily, consider giving in two divided doses. For *intravenous infusion* (preferred route), give intermittently *or via* drip tubing *in* Glucose 5% or 10% *or* Sodium Chloride 0.9%. Reconstitute 2-g vial with 40 mL infusion fluid. Give by intermittent infusion over at least 30 minutes. ⟨M⟩ Not to be given simultaneously with total parenteral nutrition or infusion fluids containing calcium, even by different infusion lines. May be infused sequentially with infusion fluids containing calcium if infusion lines at different sites are used, or if the infusion lines are replaced or thoroughly flushed between infusions with Sodium Chloride 0.9% to avoid precipitation—consult product literature. EvGr For *intravenous injection*, give over 5 minutes. ⟨M⟩

▸ With intramuscular use in adults EvGr The maximum single intramuscular dose is 2 g. Doses over 1 g should be divided between more than one site. Doses greater than 2 g must be given in two divided doses 12 hours apart or by intravenous administration. For *intramuscular injection*, may be mixed with 1% Lidocaine Hydrochloride Injection to reduce pain at intramuscular injection site. ⟨M⟩ Displacement value may be significant, consult local guidelines.

- **PRESCRIBING AND DISPENSING INFORMATION** For choice of antibacterial therapy, see Antibacterials, use for prophylaxis p. 574, Cardiovascular system infections, antibacterial therapy p. 579, Central nervous system infections, antibacterial therapy p. 580, Diabetic foot infections, antibacterial therapy p. 581, Gastro-intestinal system infections, antibacterial therapy p. 582, Genital system infections, antibacterial therapy p. 584, Lyme disease p. 669, Musculoskeletal system infections, antibacterial therapy p. 585, Respiratory system infections, antibacterial therapy p. 586, Skin infections, antibacterial therapy p. 589, Urinary-tract infections p. 681.

- **MEDICINAL FORMS** There can be variation in the licensing of different medicines containing the same drug. Forms available from special-order manufacturers include: infusion

Powder for solution for injection

ELECTROLYTES: May contain Sodium

▸ Ceftriaxone (Non-proprietary)

Ceftriaxone (as Ceftriaxone sodium) 250 mg Ceftriaxone 250mg powder for solution for injection vials | 1 vial PoM £2.30 DT = £2.40 (Hospital only) | 10 vial PoM £24.00 (Hospital only)

Ceftriaxone (as Ceftriaxone sodium) 1 gram Ceftriaxone 1g powder for solution for injection vials | 1 vial PoM £6.50 DT = £9.58 | 5 vial PoM £45.00 (Hospital only) | 10 vial PoM £60.00-£95.80 | 10 vial PoM £86.22-£95.80 (Hospital only)

Ceftriaxone (as Ceftriaxone sodium) 2 gram Ceftriaxone 2g powder for solution for injection vials | 1 vial PoM £18.30 DT = £19.18 (Hospital only) | 10 vial PoM £191.80 (Hospital only) Ceftriaxone 2g powder for solution for infusion vials | 10 vial PoM ⊠ (Hospital only)

▸ Rocephin (Roche Products Ltd)

Ceftriaxone (as Ceftriaxone sodium) 250 mg Rocephin 250mg powder for solution for injection vials | 1 vial PoM £2.40 DT = £2.40 (Hospital only)

Ceftriaxone (as Ceftriaxone sodium) 1 gram Rocephin 1g powder for solution for injection vials | 1 vial PoM £9.58 DT = £9.58 (Hospital only)

Ceftriaxone (as Ceftriaxone sodium) 2 gram Rocephin 2g powder for solution for injection vials | 1 vial [PoM] £19.18 DT = £19.18 (Hospital only)

ANTIBACTERIALS > CEPHALOSPORINS, THIRD-GENERATION WITH BETA-LACTAMASE INHIBITOR

⚑ 603

Ceftazidime with avibactam

06-Nov-2020

The properties listed below are those particular to the combination only. For the properties of the components please consider, ceftazidime p. 608.

● **INDICATIONS AND DOSE**

Complicated intra-abdominal infection
▸ BY INTRAVENOUS INFUSION
▸ Adult: 2/0.5 g every 8 hours for 5–14 days

Complicated urinary tract infection, including pyelonephritis
▸ BY INTRAVENOUS INFUSION
▸ Adult: 2/0.5 g every 8 hours for 5–10 days

Hospital-acquired pneumonia, including ventilator-associated pneumonia
▸ BY INTRAVENOUS INFUSION
▸ Adult: 2/0.5 g every 8 hours for 7–14 days

Infections due to Gram-negative bacteria with limited treatment options
▸ BY INTRAVENOUS INFUSION
▸ Adult: 2/0.5 g every 8 hours, duration of treatment guided by infection severity, pathogen, and response

DOSE EQUIVALENCE AND CONVERSION
▸ Dose expressed as *x*/*y* g ceftazidime/avibactam

● INTERACTIONS → Appendix 1: cephalosporins

● SIDE-EFFECTS
▸ **Common or very common** Increased risk of infection · thrombocytosis
▸ **Uncommon** Acute kidney injury · Clostridioides difficile colitis · lymphocytosis · paraesthesia · taste altered
▸ **Frequency not known** Jaundice

● PREGNANCY Manufacturer advises avoid unless potential benefit outweighs risk—toxicity in *animal* studies.

● BREAST FEEDING Manufacturer advises avoid—presence of avibactam in milk unknown.

● RENAL IMPAIRMENT [EvGr] Use with caution. Ⓜ
Dose adjustments [EvGr] Reduce dose if creatinine clearance 50 mL/minute or less—consult product literature. Ⓜ See p. 21.

● DIRECTIONS FOR ADMINISTRATION Manufacturer advises for *intravenous infusion* (*Zavicefta*®) give in Glucose 5%, *or* Sodium Chloride 0.9%, *or* Sodium Chloride 0.45% with Glucose 2.5% combination *or* Lactated Ringer's solution. Reconstitute each 2 g/0.5 g vial with 10 mL water for injections; dilute requisite dose in an appropriate infusion bag and give over 120 minutes.

● PATIENT AND CARER ADVICE
Driving and skilled tasks Manufacturer advises patients and carers should be counselled on the effects on driving and performance of skilled tasks—risk of dizziness.

● MEDICINAL FORMS There can be variation in the licensing of different medicines containing the same drug.
Powder for solution for infusion
ELECTROLYTES: May contain Sodium
▸ Zavicefta (Pfizer Ltd)
Avibactam (as Avibactam sodium) 500 mg, Ceftazidime (as Ceftazidime pentahydrate) 2 gram Zavicefta 2g/0.5g powder for concentrate for solution for infusion vials | 10 vial [PoM] £857.00 (Hospital only)

⚑ 603

Ceftolozane with tazobactam

31-Aug-2020

● **INDICATIONS AND DOSE**

Complicated intra-abdominal infection
▸ BY INTRAVENOUS INFUSION
▸ Adult: 1/0.5 g every 8 hours for 4–14 days

Complicated urinary tract infection | Acute pyelonephritis
▸ BY INTRAVENOUS INFUSION
▸ Adult: 1/0.5 g every 8 hours for 7 days

Hospital-acquired pneumonia | Ventilator-associated pneumonia
▸ BY INTRAVENOUS INFUSION
▸ Adult: 2/1 g every 8 hours for 8–14 days

DOSE EQUIVALENCE AND CONVERSION
▸ Dose expressed as x/y g where x and y are ceftolozane and tazobactam respectively.

● INTERACTIONS → Appendix 1: cephalosporins

● SIDE-EFFECTS
▸ **Common or very common** Anxiety · Clostridioides difficile colitis · constipation · electrolyte imbalance · hypotension · insomnia · thrombocytosis
▸ **Uncommon** Anaemia · angina pectoris · arrhythmias · dyspnoea · gastrointestinal discomfort · gastrointestinal disorders · hyperglycaemia · increased risk of infection · ischaemic stroke · renal impairment · venous thrombosis
▸ **Frequency not known** Antibiotic associated colitis

● PREGNANCY Manufacturer advises to use only if potential benefit outweighs risk—toxicity in *animal* studies with tazobactam.

● BREAST FEEDING Manufacturer advises avoid—no information available.

● RENAL IMPAIRMENT Manufacturer advises monitor for changes in renal function.
Dose adjustments See p. 21.
▸ When used for Complicated intra-abdominal infection or Complicated urinary tract infection or Acute pyelonephritis Manufacturer advises reduce dose to 500/250 mg every 8 hours if creatinine clearance 30–50 mL/minute and 250/125 mg every 8 hours if creatinine clearance 15–29 mL/minute.
▸ When used for Hospital-acquired pneumonia or Ventilator-associated pneumonia Manufacturer advises reduce dose to 1/0.5 g every 8 hours if creatinine clearance 30–50 mL/minute and 500/250 mg every 8 hours if creatinine clearance 15–29 mL/minute.

● DIRECTIONS FOR ADMINISTRATION For *intravenous infusion* (*Zerbaxa*®), give intermittently in Glucose 5% or Sodium Chloride 0.9%; reconstitute initially each vial with 10 mL Water for Injections or Sodium Chloride 0.9% to give a final volume of 11.4 mL; dilute requisite dose in 100 mL of Glucose 5% or Sodium Chloride 0.9%; give over 1 hour.

● HANDLING AND STORAGE Manufacturer advises store in a refrigerator at 2°C–8°C.

● PATIENT AND CARER ADVICE
Driving and skilled tasks Manufacturer advises ceftolozane with tazobactam may influence driving and performance of skilled tasks—increased risk of dizziness.

● NATIONAL FUNDING/ACCESS DECISIONS
For full details see funding body website
Scottish Medicines Consortium (SMC) decisions
▸ Ceftolozane with tazobactam (*Zerbaxa*®) for the treatment of the following infections in adults: complicated intra-abdominal infections, acute pyelonephritis, and complicated urinary tract infections (May 2016) SMC No. 1146/16 Not recommended

- **MEDICINAL FORMS** There can be variation in the licensing of different medicines containing the same drug.
  Powder for solution for infusion
  ELECTROLYTES: May contain Sodium
  ▸ Zerbaxa (Merck Sharp & Dohme (UK) Ltd)
    Tazobactam (as Tazobactam sodium) 500 mg, Ceftolozane (as Ceftolozane sulfate) 1 gram Zerbaxa 1g/0.5g powder for concentrate for solution for infusion vials | 10 vial [PoM] £670.30 (Hospital only)

ANTIBACTERIALS › CEPHALOSPORINS, OTHER

▸ 603

Cefepime
19-Aug-2020

- **INDICATIONS AND DOSE**

  Infections due to sensitive Gram-positive and Gram-negative bacteria
  ▸ BY INTRAVENOUS INJECTION, OR BY INTRAVENOUS INFUSION, OR BY INTRAMUSCULAR INJECTION
  ▸ Adult (body-weight up to 41 kg): 50 mg/kg every 12 hours (max. per dose 2 g), increased if necessary to 50 mg/kg every 8 hours (max. per dose 2 g), increased dose used for severe infections, intravenous route preferred in severe infections

  Mild to moderate urinary tract infections
  ▸ BY INTRAVENOUS INJECTION, OR BY INTRAVENOUS INFUSION, OR BY INTRAMUSCULAR INJECTION
  ▸ Adult (body-weight 41 kg and above): 0.5–1 g every 12 hours

  Mild to moderate infections due to sensitive Gram-positive and Gram-negative bacteria
  ▸ BY INTRAVENOUS INJECTION, OR BY INTRAVENOUS INFUSION, OR BY INTRAMUSCULAR INJECTION
  ▸ Adult (body-weight 41 kg and above): 1 g every 12 hours

  Severe infections due to sensitive Gram-positive and Gram-negative bacteria
  ▸ BY INTRAVENOUS INJECTION, OR BY INTRAVENOUS INFUSION
  ▸ Adult (body-weight 41 kg and above): 2 g every 12 hours, increased if necessary to 2 g every 8 hours, increased dose used for very severe infections

- **INTERACTIONS** → Appendix 1: cephalosporins

- **SIDE-EFFECTS**
  ▸ **Common or very common** Anaemia
  ▸ **Uncommon** Gastrointestinal disorders · increased risk of infection
  ▸ **Rare or very rare** Constipation · dyspnoea · genital pruritus · paraesthesia · seizure · taste altered · vasodilation
  ▸ **Frequency not known** Anaphylactic shock · antibiotic associated colitis · aplastic anaemia · Clostridioides difficile colitis · coma · confusion · consciousness impaired · encephalopathy · haemorrhage · hallucination · myoclonus · nephrotoxicity · renal failure

- **PREGNANCY** Manufacturer advises caution—no data available but not known to be harmful in *animal* studies.

- **BREAST FEEDING** Manufacturer advises caution—present in milk in very low quantities.

- **RENAL IMPAIRMENT** Manufacturer advises use with caution.
  Dose adjustments Manufacturer advises reduce dose—consult product literature.

- **DIRECTIONS FOR ADMINISTRATION** After reconstitution the solution is yellow to yellow-brown. Displacement value may be significant when reconstituting injection, consult local guidelines. For *intravenous infusion*, manufacturer advises reconstitute with 50 mL Glucose 5% or 10% *or* Sodium Chloride 0.9%; give over 30 minutes. For *intravenous injection*, manufacturer advises reconstitute with 10 mL Glucose 5% or 10% *or* Sodium Chloride 0.9%.

For *intramuscular injection*, manufacturer advises reconstitute with 3 mL Water for Injection.

- **NATIONAL FUNDING/ACCESS DECISIONS**
  For full details see funding body website
  All Wales Medicines Strategy Group (AWMSG) decisions
  ▸ Cefepime (*Renapime*®) for resistant pseudomonas infections (November 2019) AWMSG No. 4129 Recommended with restrictions

- **MEDICINAL FORMS** There can be variation in the licensing of different medicines containing the same drug.
  Powder for solution for injection
  ▸ Renapime (Renascience Pharma Ltd)
    Cefepime (as Cefepime dihydrochloride monohydrate)
    1 gram Renapime 1g powder for solution for injection vials | 10 vial [PoM] £70.00
    Cefepime (as Cefepime dihydrochloride monohydrate)
    2 gram Renapime 2g powder for solution for injection vials | 10 vial [PoM] £110.00

▸ 603

Cefepime with enmetazobactam
01-Jul-2024

The properties listed below are those particular to the combination only. For the properties of the components please consider, cefepime above.

- **INDICATIONS AND DOSE**

  Complicated urinary tract infection [including pyelonephritis] | Hospital-acquired pneumonia [including ventilator-associated pneumonia]
  ▸ BY INTRAVENOUS INFUSION
  ▸ Adult: 2.5 g every 8 hours for 7–10 days; may be continued for up to 14 days, treatment up to 14 days may be required if bacteraemia occurs in association with, or suspected to be associated with these indications

  DOSE EQUIVALENCE AND CONVERSION
  ▸ *Exblifep*® contains 2 g cefepime and 0.5 g enmetazobactam. Doses in BNF Publications are expressed as the total of both drug strengths.

- **CAUTIONS** History of allergic diathesis · history of asthma · supra-normal creatinine clearance
  CAUTIONS, FURTHER INFORMATION
  ▸ Supra-normal creatinine clearance [EvGr] Prolong duration of infusion to 4 hours if creatinine clearance greater than 150 mL/minute. ⟨M⟩

- **INTERACTIONS** → Appendix 1: cephalosporins

- **SIDE-EFFECTS**
  ▸ **Uncommon** Clostridioides difficile colitis · colitis · vulvovaginal infection
  ▸ **Rare or very rare** Constipation · taste altered · vulvovaginal pruritus
  ▸ **Frequency not known** Hypersensitivity

- **PREGNANCY** [EvGr] Use only if potential benefit outweighs risk (toxicity in *animal* studies with enmetazobactam). ⟨M⟩

- **BREAST FEEDING** [EvGr] Avoid (present in milk in *animal* studies and limited data suggests present in human milk). ⟨M⟩

- **RENAL IMPAIRMENT**
  Dose adjustments [EvGr] Reduce dose in moderate to severe impairment—consult product literature. ⟨M⟩

- **DIRECTIONS FOR ADMINISTRATION** After reconstitution the solution can develop a yellow to amber colour. [EvGr] For *intermittent intravenous infusion (Exblifep*®), give in Glucose 5% *or* Sodium Chloride 0.9% *or* Sodium Chloride 0.45% with Glucose 2.5%. Reconstitute each vial with 10 mL infusion fluid withdrawn from an appropriate 250 mL infusion bag, mix the vial gently to dissolve, then dilute requisite dose in the remaining infusion fluid—consult product literature. ⟨M⟩

▶ When used for Complicated urinary tract infection [including pyelonephritis] [EvGr] Give over 2 hours. ⟨M⟩

▶ When used for Hospital-acquired pneumonia [including ventilator-associated pneumonia] [EvGr] Give over 4 hours. ⟨M⟩

● HANDLING AND STORAGE Store in a refrigerator (2–8°C) and protect from light—consult product literature for storage after reconstitution and dilution.

● MEDICINAL FORMS There can be variation in the licensing of different medicines containing the same drug.

Powder for solution for infusion

▶ Exblifep (Advanz Pharma) ▼

Enmetazobactam 500 mg, Cefepime (as Cefepime dihydrochloride monohydrate) 2 gram Exblifep 2g/0.5g powder for concentrate for solution for infusion vials | 10 vial [PoM] £814.15

Cefiderocol

02-Oct-2020

● INDICATIONS AND DOSE

Aerobic Gram-negative infections [in patients with limited treatment options] (administered on expert advice)

▶ BY INTRAVENOUS INFUSION

▶ Adult: 2 g every 8 hours, duration should be tailored to site of infection—consult product literature

● CAUTIONS Seizure disorders · supra-normal creatinine clearance

CAUTIONS, FURTHER INFORMATION

▶ Supra-normal creatinine clearance Manufacturer advises to increase frequency of infusion to 2 g every 6 hours in patients with creatinine clearance of 120 mL/minute or more.

● INTERACTIONS → Appendix 1: cephalosporins

● SIDE-EFFECTS

▶ **Common or very common** Clostridioides difficile colitis · cough · hepatic function abnormal · increased risk of infection

● PREGNANCY Manufacturer advises avoid—limited data available but not known to be harmful in *animal* studies.

● BREAST FEEDING Manufacturer advises avoid—not known if present in human milk. A specialist source confirms lack of information in human lactation, but states acceptable to use (cephalosporins generally not expected to cause adverse effects in breastfed infants).

● RENAL IMPAIRMENT Manufacturer advises use with caution if creatinine clearance less than 60 mL/minute. **Dose adjustments** Manufacturer advises reduce dose if creatinine clearance less than 60 mL/minute—consult product literature. See p. 21.

● MONITORING REQUIREMENTS Manufacturer advises monitor renal function regularly—dose adjustment may be required.

● EFFECT ON LABORATORY TESTS Manufacturer advises may cause false-positive urine tests for protein, ketones, or occult blood.

● DIRECTIONS FOR ADMINISTRATION Manufacturer advises for *intravenous infusion*, give intermittently in Glucose 5% *or* Sodium Chloride 0.9%. Dilute reconstituted solution to 100 mL with infusion fluid; give over 3 hours.

● HANDLING AND STORAGE Store in a refrigerator (2–8°C)—consult product literature for storage after reconstitution and dilution. Protect from light.

● MEDICINAL FORMS There can be variation in the licensing of different medicines containing the same drug.

Powder for solution for infusion

ELECTROLYTES: May contain Sodium

▶ Fetcroja (Shionogi BV) ▼

Cefiderocol (as Cefiderocol sulfate tosylate) 1 gram Fetcroja 1g powder for concentrate for solution for infusion vials | 10 vial [PoM] £1,319.00 (Hospital only)

Ceftaroline fosamil

04-Nov-2020

● INDICATIONS AND DOSE

Community-acquired pneumonia

▶ BY INTRAVENOUS INFUSION

▶ Adult: 600 mg every 12 hours for 5–7 days

Complicated skin infections | Complicated soft-tissue infections

▶ BY INTRAVENOUS INFUSION

▶ Adult: 600 mg every 12 hours for 5–14 days, for high dose regimen consult product literature

● CAUTIONS Seizure disorders

● INTERACTIONS → Appendix 1: cephalosporins

● SIDE-EFFECTS

▶ **Uncommon** Anaemia · Clostridioides difficile colitis · hypersensitivity

▶ **Frequency not known** Antibiotic associated colitis

● PREGNANCY Manufacturer advises avoid unless essential—limited information; *animal* studies do not indicate toxicity.

● BREAST FEEDING Manufacturer advises avoid—no information available.

● RENAL IMPAIRMENT
Dose adjustments Manufacturer advises reduce dose if creatinine clearance less than 51 mL/minute—consult product literature. See p. 21.

● DIRECTIONS FOR ADMINISTRATION For *intravenous infusion*, give intermittently *in* Glucose 5% *or* Sodium Chloride 0.9%. Dilute reconstituted solution to 50, 100, or 250 mL with infusion fluid; give over 5 to 60 minutes. Consult product literature for administration of high-dose regimen.

● NATIONAL FUNDING/ACCESS DECISIONS
For full details see funding body website

Scottish Medicines Consortium (SMC) decisions

▶ Ceftaroline fosamil (*Zinforo*®) for the treatment of complicated skin and soft tissue infections (cSSTIs) (January 2013) SMC No. 830/12 Recommended with restrictions

● MEDICINAL FORMS There can be variation in the licensing of different medicines containing the same drug.

Powder for solution for infusion

▶ Zinforo (Pfizer Ltd)

Ceftaroline fosamil (as Ceftaroline fosamil acetic acid solvate monohydrate) 600 mg Zinforo 600mg powder for concentrate for solution for infusion vials | 10 vial [PoM] £375.00 (Hospital only)

Ceftobiprole

28-Apr-2021

● INDICATIONS AND DOSE

Hospital-acquired pneumonia (excluding ventilator-associated pneumonia) | Community-acquired pneumonia

▶ BY INTRAVENOUS INFUSION

▶ Adult: 500 mg every 8 hours

● CAUTIONS Pre-existing seizure disorder—increased risk of seizures · supra-normal creatinine clearance

CAUTIONS, FURTHER INFORMATION

▸ **Supra-normal creatinine clearance** Manufacturer advises to measure baseline renal function and increase duration of infusion if creatinine clearance greater than 150 mL/minute.

● INTERACTIONS → Appendix 1: cephalosporins

● SIDE-EFFECTS

▸ **Common or very common** Drowsiness · dyspepsia · electrolyte imbalance · hypersensitivity · increased risk of infection · taste altered

▸ **Uncommon** Anaemia · anxiety · asthma · Clostridioides difficile colitis · dyspnoea · laryngeal pain · muscle spasms · peripheral oedema · renal failure · sleep disorders · thrombocytosis

▸ **Frequency not known** Antibiotic associated colitis · seizure

● PREGNANCY Manufacturer advises avoid unless essential—no information available.

● BREAST FEEDING Manufacturer advises avoid—present in milk in *animal* studies.

● RENAL IMPAIRMENT EvGr Use with caution in severe impairment (risk of increased exposure, limited information available). ⟨M⟩
Dose adjustments EvGr Reduce dose to 500 mg every 12 hours in moderate impairment, and 250 mg every 12 hours in severe impairment. ⟨M⟩

● DIRECTIONS FOR ADMINISTRATION Manufacturer advises for *intravenous infusion* (*Zevtera*®), give intermittently in Glucose 5%, or Sodium Chloride 0.9%, or Lactated Ringer's solution; reconstitute each 500 mg with 10 mL Water for injections or Glucose 5%; dilute in 250 mL infusion fluid and give over 2 hours (increased to 4 hours if creatinine clearance greater than 150 mL/minute). Do not mix with calcium-containing solutions (except Lactated Ringer's solution) in the same intravenous line—precipitation may occur.

● HANDLING AND STORAGE Manufacturer advises store in a refrigerator (2–8°C)—consult product literature for storage after reconstitution and dilution.

● PATIENT AND CARER ADVICE
Driving and skilled tasks Manufacturer advises patients and carers should be counselled on the effects on driving and performance of skilled tasks—increased risk of dizziness.

● MEDICINAL FORMS There can be variation in the licensing of different medicines containing the same drug.
Powder for solution for infusion
ELECTROLYTES: May contain Sodium
▸ Zevtera (Advanz Pharma)
Ceftobiprole (as Ceftobiprole medocaril sodium) 500 mg Zevtera 500mg powder for concentrate for solution for infusion vials | 10 vial PoM £396.30 (Hospital only)

ANTIBACTERIALS › GLYCOPEPTIDE ANTIBACTERIALS

Dalbavancin
11-Aug-2021

● DRUG ACTION Dalbavancin is a glycopeptide antibacterial; it has bactericidal activity against Gram-positive bacteria including various staphylococci. However, there are reports of *Staphylococcus aureus* with reduced susceptibility to glycopeptides and increasing reports of glycopeptide-resistant enterococci.

● INDICATIONS AND DOSE
Acute bacterial skin and skin structure infections
▸ BY INTRAVENOUS INFUSION
▸ Adult: 1500 mg for 1 dose, alternatively 1000 mg, then 500 mg after 1 week

● SIDE-EFFECTS
▸ **Common or very common** Diarrhoea · headache · nausea

▸ **Uncommon** Anaemia · appetite decreased · Clostridioides difficile colitis · constipation · cough · dizziness · eosinophilia · flushing · gastrointestinal discomfort · increased risk of infection · infusion related reaction · insomnia · leucopenia · neutropenia · skin reactions · taste altered · thrombocytosis · vomiting · vulvovaginal pruritus

▸ **Rare or very rare** Bronchospasm

▸ **Frequency not known** Ototoxicity

● ALLERGY AND CROSS-SENSITIVITY Manufacturer advises use with caution in patients with other glycopeptide sensitivity.

● PREGNANCY Manufacturer advises avoid unless essential—toxicity in *animal* studies.

● BREAST FEEDING Manufacturer advises avoid—present in milk in *animal* studies.

● HEPATIC IMPAIRMENT Manufacturer advises caution in moderate to severe impairment (no information available).

● RENAL IMPAIRMENT
Dose adjustments Manufacturer advises reduce dose to 1000 mg as a single infusion *or* reduce dose to 750 mg followed one week later by 375 mg if creatinine clearance less than 30 mL/minute. See p. 21.

● DIRECTIONS FOR ADMINISTRATION Manufacturer advises for *intravenous infusion* (*Xydalba*®), reconstitute each 500 mg vial to produce a 20 mg/mL solution with 25 mL Water for Injections. Dilute reconstituted solution to a concentration of 1–5 mg/mL with Glucose 5%; give intermittently over 30 minutes (avoid rapid infusion—risk of 'red man' syndrome).

● NATIONAL FUNDING/ACCESS DECISIONS
For full details see funding body website
Scottish Medicines Consortium (SMC) decisions
▸ **Dalbavancin (*Xydalba*®) for the treatment of acute bacterial skin and skin structure infections (ABSSSI) in adults (January 2017)** SMC No. 1105/15 Recommended with restrictions
All Wales Medicines Strategy Group (AWMSG) decisions
▸ **Dalbavancin (*Xydalba*®) for the treatment of acute bacterial skin and skin structure infections (ABSSSI) in adults (July 2018)** AWMSG No. 2001 Recommended with restrictions

● MEDICINAL FORMS There can be variation in the licensing of different medicines containing the same drug.
Powder for solution for infusion
▸ Xydalba (Advanz Pharma)
Dalbavancin (as Dalbavancin hydrochloride) 500 mg Xydalba 500mg powder for concentrate for solution for infusion vials | 1 vial PoM £558.70 (Hospital only)

Oritavancin
14-Jun-2022

● DRUG ACTION Oritavancin is a glycopeptide antibacterial; it has bactericidal activity against Gram-positive bacteria including various staphylococci. However, there are reports of *Staphylococcus aureus* with reduced susceptibility to glycopeptides and increasing reports of glycopeptide-resistant enterococci.

● INDICATIONS AND DOSE
Acute bacterial skin and skin structure infections
▸ BY INTRAVENOUS INFUSION
▸ Adult: 1.2 g for 1 dose

● CONTRA-INDICATIONS Concomitant use with unfractionated heparin

CONTRA-INDICATIONS, FURTHER INFORMATION
▸ Concomitant use with unfractionated heparin EvGr Use of intravenous unfractionated heparin is contra-indicated for 120 hours after oritavancin administration—activated partial thromboplastin time test results may remain falsely elevated for up to 120 hours after oritavancin administration. ⟨M⟩

- **INTERACTIONS** → Appendix 1: oritavancin
- **SIDE-EFFECTS**
  ‣ **Common or very common** Abscess · anaemia · constipation · diarrhoea · dizziness · headache · increased risk of infection · limb abscess · myalgia · nausea · peripheral oedema · skin reactions · tachycardia · vomiting
  ‣ **Uncommon** Abdominal pain · angioedema · chest discomfort · dyspnoea · eosinophilia · fever · flushing · hypersensitivity · hypersensitivity vasculitis · hyperuricaemia · hypoglycaemia · respiratory disorders · tenosynovitis · thrombocytopenia
  ‣ **Rare or very rare** Chills · hypoxia · pain · tremor · vancomycin-like infusion reaction
  ‣ **Frequency not known** Antibiotic associated colitis · infusion related reaction · pseudomembranous enterocolitis
- **ALLERGY AND CROSS-SENSITIVITY** [EvGr] Use with caution in patients with history of glycopeptide sensitivity—monitor closely during and after infusion. Ⓜ
- **PREGNANCY** [EvGr] Avoid unless potential benefit outweighs risk—no information available. Ⓜ
- **BREAST FEEDING** [EvGr] Avoid—present in milk in *animal* studies. Ⓜ
- **EFFECT ON LABORATORY TESTS** [EvGr] Oritavancin may interfere with certain laboratory coagulation tests—consult product literature. Ⓜ
- **DIRECTIONS FOR ADMINISTRATION** [EvGr] For *intravenous infusion* (*Tenkasi ®*), reconstitute each 400 mg vial with 40 mL Water for Injection to produce a 10 mg/mL solution. Dilute reconstituted solution to a concentration of 1.2 mg/mL with Glucose 5%; give over 3 hours. Ⓜ
- **PATIENT AND CARER ADVICE**
  Driving and skilled tasks Patients and carers should be counselled on the effects on driving and performance of skilled tasks—increased risk of dizziness.
- **NATIONAL FUNDING/ACCESS DECISIONS**
  For full details see funding body website
  Scottish Medicines Consortium (SMC) decisions
  ‣ Oritavancin (*Tenkasi ®*) for the treatment of acute bacterial skin and skin structure infections in adults (May 2022) SMC No. SMC2285 Recommended with restrictions

- **MEDICINAL FORMS** There can be variation in the licensing of different medicines containing the same drug.
  Powder for solution for infusion
  ‣ Tenkasi (A. Menarini Farmaceutica Internazionale SRL)
    Oritavancin (as Oritavancin diphosphate) 400 mg Tenkasi 400mg powder for concentrate for solution for infusion vials | 3 vial [PoM] £1,500.00 (Hospital only)

Teicoplanin

25-Oct-2021

- **DRUG ACTION** The glycopeptide antibiotic teicoplanin has bactericidal activity against aerobic and anaerobic Gram-positive bacteria including multi-resistant staphylococci. However, there are reports of *Staphylococcus aureus* with reduced susceptibility to glycopeptides and increasing reports of glycopeptide-resistant enterococci. Teicoplanin is similar to vancomycin, but has a significantly longer duration of action, allowing once daily administration after the loading dose.

- **INDICATIONS AND DOSE**
  Clostridioides difficile **infection**
  ‣ BY MOUTH
  ‣ Adult: 100–200 mg twice daily for 7–14 days

Moderate diabetic foot infection | Severe diabetic foot infection | Leg ulcer infection
‣ BY INTRAVENOUS INJECTION, OR BY INTRAVENOUS INFUSION
‣ Adult: Initially 6 mg/kg every 12 hours for 3 doses, then 6 mg/kg once daily

Cellulitis | Erysipelas
‣ BY INTRAVENOUS INJECTION, OR BY INTRAVENOUS INFUSION
‣ Adult: Initially 6 mg/kg every 12 hours for 3 doses, then 6 mg/kg once daily

Serious infections caused by Gram-positive bacteria (e.g. complicated skin and soft-tissue infections, pneumonia, complicated urinary tract infections)
‣ BY INTRAVENOUS INJECTION, OR BY INTRAVENOUS INFUSION, OR BY INTRAMUSCULAR INJECTION
‣ Adult: Initially 6 mg/kg every 12 hours for 3 doses, then 6 mg/kg once daily

Streptococcal or enterococcal endocarditis (in combination with another antibacterial) | Bone and joint infections
‣ INITIALLY BY INTRAVENOUS INJECTION, OR BY INTRAVENOUS INFUSION
‣ Adult: 12 mg/kg every 12 hours for 3–5 doses, then (by intravenous injection or by intravenous infusion or by intramuscular injection) 12 mg/kg once daily

Surgical prophylaxis
‣ BY INTRAVENOUS INJECTION
‣ Adult: 400 mg for 1 dose, to be administered up to 30 minutes before the procedure

Surgical prophylaxis in open fractures
‣ BY INTRAVENOUS INFUSION
‣ Adult: 800 mg for 1 dose, to be administered up to 30 minutes before skeletal stabilisation and definitive soft-tissue closure

Peritonitis associated with peritoneal dialysis (added to dialysis fluid)
‣ BY INTRAPERITONEAL INFUSION
‣ Adult: (consult local protocol)

PHARMACOKINETICS
‣ Teicoplanin should **not** be given by mouth for systemic infections because it is not absorbed significantly.

- **UNLICENSED USE** Not licensed for surgical prophylaxis.
- **INTERACTIONS** → Appendix 1: teicoplanin
- **SIDE-EFFECTS**
  ‣ **Common or very common** Fever · pain · skin reactions
  ‣ **Uncommon** Bronchospasm · diarrhoea · dizziness · eosinophilia · headache · hearing impairment · hypersensitivity · leucopenia · nausea · ototoxicity · thrombocytopenia · vomiting
  ‣ **Rare or very rare** Abscess
  ‣ **Frequency not known** Agranulocytosis · angioedema · chills · neutropenia · overgrowth of nonsusceptible organisms · renal impairment · seizure · severe cutaneous adverse reactions (SCARs) · thrombophlebitis

  SIDE-EFFECTS, FURTHER INFORMATION Teicoplanin is associated with a lower incidence of nephrotoxicity than vancomycin.

- **ALLERGY AND CROSS-SENSITIVITY** [EvGr] Caution if history of vancomycin sensitivity. Ⓜ
- **PREGNANCY** Manufacturer advises use only if potential benefit outweighs risk.
- **BREAST FEEDING** No information available.
- **RENAL IMPAIRMENT**
  Dose adjustments Use normal dose regimen on days 1–4, then use normal maintenance dose every 48 hours if eGFR 30–80 mL/minute/1.73 m^2 and use normal maintenance dose every 72 hours if eGFR less than 30 mL/minute/1.73 m^2.

Monitoring Monitor renal and auditory function during prolonged treatment in renal impairment.

- **MONITORING REQUIREMENTS**
- ▸ With intramuscular use or intravenous use Manufacturer advises monitor serum-teicoplanin trough concentration at steady state after completion of loading dose and during maintenance treatment—consult product literature.
- ▸ Blood counts and liver and kidney function tests required.
- ▸ Manufacturer advises monitoring for adverse reactions when doses of 12 mg/kg twice daily are administered.

- **DIRECTIONS FOR ADMINISTRATION**
- ▸ With intravenous use For intravenous infusion (*Targocid®*), manufacturer advises give intermittently in Glucose 5% *or* Sodium Chloride 0.9%; reconstitute initially with Water for Injections provided; infuse over 30 minutes. Continuous infusion not usually recommended.
- ▸ With oral use Manufacturer advises injection can be used to prepare solution for oral administration.

- **PRESCRIBING AND DISPENSING INFORMATION** For choice of antibacterial therapy, see Antibacterials, use for prophylaxis p. 574, Cardiovascular system infections, antibacterial therapy p. 579, Diabetic foot infections, antibacterial therapy p. 581, Gastro-intestinal system infections, antibacterial therapy p. 582, Musculoskeletal system infections, antibacterial therapy p. 585, Respiratory system infections, antibacterial therapy p. 586, Skin infections, antibacterial therapy p. 589, Urinary-tract infections p. 681.

- **MEDICINAL FORMS** There can be variation in the licensing of different medicines containing the same drug. Forms available from special-order manufacturers include: solution for injection

Powder and solvent for solution for injection
ELECTROLYTES: May contain Sodium
- ▸ **Teicoplanin (Non-proprietary)**
  Teicoplanin 200 mg Teicoplanin 200mg powder and solvent for solution for injection vials | 1 vial [PoM] £5.04 DT = £3.93 (Hospital only) | 1 vial [PoM] £5.34 DT = £3.93
  Teicoplanin 400 mg Teicoplanin 400mg powder and solvent for solution for injection vials | 1 vial [PoM] £8.58 DT = £7.32 (Hospital only) | 1 vial [PoM] £9.08 DT = £7.32
- ▸ **Targocid** (Sanofi)
  Teicoplanin 200 mg Targocid 200mg powder and solvent for solution for injection vials | 1 vial [PoM] £3.93 DT = £3.93
  Teicoplanin 400 mg Targocid 400mg powder and solvent for solution for injection vials | 1 vial [PoM] £7.32 DT = £7.32

Vancomycin

10-Feb-2025

- **DRUG ACTION** The glycopeptide antibiotic vancomycin has bactericidal activity against aerobic and anaerobic Gram-positive bacteria including multi-resistant staphylococci. However, there are reports of *Staphylococcus aureus* with reduced susceptibility to glycopeptides. There are increasing reports of glycopeptide-resistant enterococci. Penetration into cerebrospinal fluid is poor.

- **INDICATIONS AND DOSE**

Clostridioides difficile infection
- ▸ BY MOUTH
- ▸ Adult: 125 mg every 6 hours for 10 days; increased if necessary to 500 mg every 6 hours for 10 days, increased dose to be used if life-threatening or refractory infection

Moderate diabetic foot infection | Severe diabetic foot infection | Leg ulcer infection
- ▸ BY INTRAVENOUS INFUSION
- ▸ Adult: 15–20 mg/kg every 8–12 hours (max. per dose 2 g), dose to be adjusted according to plasma-concentration monitoring

Cellulitis | Erysipelas
- ▸ BY INTRAVENOUS INFUSION
- ▸ Adult: 15–20 mg/kg every 8–12 hours (max. per dose 2 g), dose to be adjusted according to plasma-concentration monitoring

Complicated skin and soft tissue infections | Bone infections | Joint infections | Community-acquired pneumonia | Hospital-acquired pneumonia [including ventilator-associated pneumonia] | Infective endocarditis | Acute bacterial meningitis | Bacteraemia [occurring in association with or suspected to be associated with the licensed indications]
- ▸ BY INTRAVENOUS INFUSION
- ▸ Adult: 15–20 mg/kg every 8–12 hours (max. per dose 2 g), dose to be adjusted according to plasma-concentration monitoring, duration should be tailored to type and severity of infection and the individual clinical response—consult product literature for further information, in seriously ill patients, a loading dose of 25–30 mg/kg (usual max. 2 g) can be used to facilitate rapid attainment of the target trough serum-vancomycin concentration

Perioperative prophylaxis of bacterial endocarditis [in patients at high risk of developing bacterial endocarditis when undergoing major surgical procedures]
- ▸ BY INTRAVENOUS INFUSION
- ▸ Adult: 15 mg/kg for 1 dose, to be given prior to induction of anaesthesia, a second dose may be required depending on duration of surgery

Surgical prophylaxis (when high risk of MRSA)
- ▸ BY INTRAVENOUS INFUSION
- ▸ Adult: 1 g for 1 dose

Peritonitis associated with peritoneal dialysis
- ▸ BY INTRAPERITONEAL ADMINISTRATION
- ▸ Adult: (consult local protocol)

PHARMACOKINETICS
- ▸ Vancomycin should **not** be given by mouth for systemic infections because it is not absorbed significantly.

- **UNLICENSED USE** Vancomycin doses in BNF Publications may differ from those in product literature. Use of vancomycin (added to dialysis fluid) for the treatment of peritonitis associated with peritoneal dialysis is an unlicensed route.

- **CONTRA-INDICATIONS**
- ▸ With intravenous use Previous hearing loss

- **CAUTIONS**
- ▸ With oral use Systemic absorption may be enhanced in patients with inflammatory disorders of the intestinal mucosa or with *Clostridioides difficile*-induced pseudomembranous colitis (increased risk of adverse reactions)

- **INTERACTIONS** → Appendix 1: vancomycin

- **SIDE-EFFECTS**

  GENERAL SIDE-EFFECTS Agranulocytosis · dizziness · drug fever · eosinophilia · hypersensitivity · nausea · nephritis tubulointerstitial · neutropenia (more common after 1 week or cumulative dose of 25g) · renal failure · severe cutaneous adverse reactions (SCARs) · skin reactions · thrombocytopenia · tinnitus (discontinue) · vasculitis · vertigo

  SPECIFIC SIDE-EFFECTS
  - ▸ Common or very common
  - ▸ With intravenous use Vancomycin infusion reaction
  - ▸ Rare or very rare
  - ▸ With intravenous use Pseudomembranous enterocolitis
  - ▸ Frequency not known
  - ▸ With intravenous use Back pain · bradycardia · cardiac arrest (on rapid intravenous injection) · cardiogenic shock (on rapid intravenous injection) · chest pain · diarrhoea ·

dyspnoea · hearing loss · hypotension · muscle complaints · wheezing

SIDE-EFFECTS, FURTHER INFORMATION Vancomycin is associated with a higher incidence of nephrotoxicity than teicoplanin.

● ALLERGY AND CROSS-SENSITIVITY [EvGr] Caution if teicoplanin sensitivity. ⓜ

● PREGNANCY Manufacturer advises use only if potential benefit outweighs risk.
Monitoring Plasma-vancomycin concentration monitoring essential to reduce risk of fetal toxicity.

● BREAST FEEDING Present in milk—significant absorption following oral administration unlikely.

● RENAL IMPAIRMENT Manufacturer advises serial monitoring of renal function.

▸ With intravenous use Manufacturer advises use with caution—increased risk of toxic effects with prolonged high blood concentration.
Dose adjustments

  ▸ With oral use Manufacturer advises dose adjustment is unlikely to be required unless substantial oral absorption occurs in inflammatory disorders of the intestinal mucosa or with *Clostridioides difficile*-induced pseudomembranous colitis, see *Monitoring*.

  ▸ With intravenous use Manufacturer advises initial dose must not be reduced—consult product literature.

● MONITORING REQUIREMENTS

▸ With intravenous use Manufacturer advises initial doses should be based on body-weight; subsequent dose adjustments should be based on serum-vancomycin concentrations to achieve targeted therapeutic concentrations. All patients require serum-vancomycin measurement (on the second day of treatment, immediately before the next dose if renal function normal, earlier if renal impairment—consult product literature). Frequency of monitoring depends on the clinical situation and response to treatment; regular monitoring indicated in high-dose therapy and longer-term use, particularly in patients with impaired renal function, impaired hearing, or concurrent use of nephrotoxic or ototoxic drugs. Manufacturer advises pre-dose ('trough') concentration should normally be 10–20 mg/litre depending on the site of infection and the susceptibility of the pathogen; trough concentration of 15–20 mg/litre is usually recommended to cover susceptible pathogens with MIC greater than or equal to 1 mg/litre—consult product literature.

   Manufacturer advises periodic testing of auditory function. Manufacturer advises monitor blood counts, urinalysis, hepatic and renal function periodically in all patients; monitor leucocyte count regularly in patients receiving long-term vancomycin or if given concurrently with other drugs that may cause neutropenia or agranulocytosis.

   Manufacturer advises monitor vestibular and auditory function during and after treatment in the elderly; avoid concurrent or sequential use of other ototoxic drugs.

▸ With oral use Manufacturer advises monitoring serum-vancomycin concentration in inflammatory intestinal disorders.

   Manufacturer advises serial tests of auditory function may be helpful to minimise the risk of ototoxicity in patients with an underlying hearing loss, or who are receiving concomitant therapy with other ototoxic drugs.

● DIRECTIONS FOR ADMINISTRATION

▸ With intravenous use Avoid rapid infusion (risk of anaphylactoid reactions) and rotate infusion sites.

   For *intravenous infusion*, give intermittently in Glucose 5% or Sodium chloride 0.9%; reconstitute each 500 mg with 10 mL water for injections and dilute with infusion fluid to a concentration of up to 5 mg/mL (10 mg/mL in fluid restriction but increased risk of infusion-related

effects); give over at least 60 minutes (rate not to exceed 10 mg/minute for doses over 500 mg); use continuous infusion only if intermittent not feasible.

▸ With oral use Injection can be used to prepare solution for oral administration—consult product literature.

● PRESCRIBING AND DISPENSING INFORMATION For choice of antibacterial therapy, see Antibacterials, use for prophylaxis p. 574, Cardiovascular system infections, antibacterial therapy p. 579, Central nervous system infections, antibacterial therapy p. 580, Diabetic foot infections, antibacterial therapy p. 581, Gastro-intestinal system infections, antibacterial therapy p. 582, Musculoskeletal system infections, antibacterial therapy p. 585, Respiratory system infections, antibacterial therapy p. 586, Skin infections, antibacterial therapy p. 589.

● MEDICINAL FORMS There can be variation in the licensing of different medicines containing the same drug. Forms available from special-order manufacturers include: oral suspension, oral solution, solution for injection, infusion

Oral capsule

CAUTIONARY AND ADVISORY LABELS 9

▸ Vancomycin (Non-proprietary)
  Vancomycin (as Vancomycin hydrochloride) 125 mg Vancomycin 125mg capsules | 28 capsule [PoM] £150.60 DT = £127.32
  Vancomycin (as Vancomycin hydrochloride) 250 mg Vancomycin 250mg capsules | 28 capsule [PoM] £131.75 DT = £131.74

Powder for solution for infusion

▸ Vancomycin (Non-proprietary)
  Vancomycin (as Vancomycin hydrochloride) 500 mg Vancomycin 500mg powder for solution for infusion vials | 5 vial [PoM] [℞] (Hospital only)
  Vancomycin 500mg powder for concentrate for solution for infusion vials | 1 vial [PoM] £10.05 | 1 vial [PoM] £5.49–£14.47 (Hospital only) | 5 vial [PoM] £50.25 | 10 vial [PoM] £62.50–£100.05 (Hospital only) | 10 vial [PoM] £100.05
  Vancomycin (as Vancomycin hydrochloride) 1 gram Vancomycin 1g powder for solution for infusion vials | 5 vial [PoM] [℞] (Hospital only)
  Vancomycin 1g powder for concentrate for solution for infusion vials | 1 vial [PoM] £17.25 | 1 vial [PoM] £11.25 (Hospital only) | 5 vial [PoM] £86.25 | 10 vial [PoM] £125.00–£172.50 (Hospital only) | 10 vial [PoM] £172.50

ANTIBACTERIALS ⟩ LINCOSAMIDES

▌Clindamycin
22-Mar-2024

● DRUG ACTION Clindamycin is active against Gram-positive cocci, including streptococci and penicillin-resistant staphylococci, and also against many anaerobes, especially *Bacteroides fragilis*. It is well concentrated in bone and excreted in bile and urine.

● INDICATIONS AND DOSE

Staphylococcal bone and joint infections such as osteomyelitis | Peritonitis | Intra-abdominal sepsis | Meticillin-resistant *Staphylococcus aureus* (MRSA) in bronchiectasis, bone and joint infections, and skin and soft-tissue infections

▸ BY MOUTH

▸ Child: 3–6 mg/kg 4 times a day (max. per dose 450 mg)

▸ Adult: 150–300 mg every 6 hours; increased if necessary up to 450 mg every 6 hours, increased dose used in severe infection

▸ BY INTRAMUSCULAR INJECTION, OR BY INTRAVENOUS INFUSION

▸ Adult: 0.6–2.7 g daily in 2–4 divided doses, dose can be increased if necessary up to 4.8 g daily in 4 divided doses in life-threatening infection; single doses above 600 mg to be administered by intravenous infusion only, single doses by intravenous infusion not to exceed 1.2 g

Moderate diabetic foot infection | Severe diabetic foot infection
▸ BY MOUTH
▸ Adult: 150–300 mg every 6 hours; increased if necessary up to 450 mg every 6 hours
▸ BY INTRAVENOUS INFUSION
▸ Adult: 0.6–2.7 g daily in 2–4 divided doses (max. per dose 1.2 g); increased if necessary up to 4.8 g daily in 4 divided doses, increased dose used in life-threatening infection, single doses not to exceed 1.2 g

Cellulitis | Erysipelas
▸ BY MOUTH
▸ Child: 3–6 mg/kg 4 times a day (max. per dose 450 mg) for 7 days then review
▸ Adult: 150–300 mg every 6 hours for 7 days then review, alternatively 450 mg every 6 hours for 7 days then review
▸ BY INTRAVENOUS INFUSION
▸ Adult: 0.6–2.7 g daily in 2–4 divided doses (max. per dose 1.2 g); increased if necessary up to 4.8 g daily in 4 divided doses, increased dose used in life-threatening infection, single doses not to exceed 1.2 g

Treatment of mild to moderate pneumocystis pneumonia (in combination with primaquine)
▸ BY MOUTH
▸ Adult: 600 mg every 8 hours

Treatment of falciparum malaria (to be given with or following quinine)
▸ BY MOUTH
▸ Child: 7–13 mg/kg every 8 hours (max. per dose 450 mg) for 7 days
▸ Adult: 450 mg every 8 hours for 7 days

● UNLICENSED USE Not licensed for treatment of mild to moderate pneumocystis infection.
 Not licensed for treatment of falciparum malaria.
● CONTRA-INDICATIONS Diarrhoeal states
● CAUTIONS Avoid in Acute porphyrias p. 1202
● INTERACTIONS → Appendix 1: clindamycin
● SIDE-EFFECTS
 GENERAL SIDE-EFFECTS
▸ **Common or very common** Abdominal pain · diarrhoea (discontinue) · pseudomembranous enterocolitis · skin reactions
▸ **Uncommon** Nausea · vomiting
▸ **Frequency not known** Agranulocytosis · Clostridioides difficile colitis · eosinophilia · jaundice · leucopenia · neutropenia · severe cutaneous adverse reactions (SCARs) · taste altered · thrombocytopenia
 SPECIFIC SIDE-EFFECTS
▸ **Frequency not known**
▸ With oral use Angioedema · gastrointestinal disorders · vulvovaginal infection
▸ With parenteral use Cardiac arrest · colitis · hypotension · increased risk of infection · thrombophlebitis

 SIDE-EFFECTS, FURTHER INFORMATION Clindamycin has been associated with antibiotic-associated colitis, which may be fatal. Although antibiotic-associated colitis can occur with most antibacterials, it occurs more frequently with clindamycin. If *C. difficile* infection is suspected or confirmed, discontinue the antibiotic if appropriate. Seek specialist advice if the antibiotic cannot be stopped and the diarrhoea is severe.

● PREGNANCY Manufacturer advises not known to be harmful in the second and third trimesters; use with caution in the first trimester—limited data.
● BREAST FEEDING EvGr Specialist sources indicate use with caution—present in milk. Monitor infant for effects on the gastrointestinal flora such as diarrhoea, candidiasis, or rarely, blood in the stool indicating possible antibiotic-associated colitis. ⓓ

● MONITORING REQUIREMENTS Monitor liver and renal function if treatment exceeds 10 days.
▸ In children Monitor liver and renal function in neonates and infants.
● DIRECTIONS FOR ADMINISTRATION Avoid rapid intravenous administration. For *intravenous infusion* (*Dalacin® C Phosphate*), manufacturer advises give continuously *or* intermittently in Glucose 5% *or* Sodium Chloride 0.9%; dilute to not more than 18 mg/mL and give over 10–60 minutes at a rate not exceeding 30 mg/minute (1.2 g over at least 60 minutes; higher doses by continuous infusion).
● PRESCRIBING AND DISPENSING INFORMATION For choice of antibacterial therapy, see Diabetic foot infections, antibacterial therapy p. 581, Gastro-intestinal system infections, antibacterial therapy p. 582, Malaria, treatment p. 708, Musculoskeletal system infections, antibacterial therapy p. 585, Pneumocystis pneumonia p. 697, Respiratory system infections, antibacterial therapy p. 586, Skin infections, antibacterial therapy p. 589.
● PATIENT AND CARER ADVICE Patients and their carers should be advised to discontinue and contact a doctor immediately if severe, prolonged or bloody diarrhoea develops.
▸ With oral use Capsules should be swallowed with a glass of water.
● PROFESSION SPECIFIC INFORMATION

 Dental practitioners' formulary Clindamycin capsules may be prescribed.

● MEDICINAL FORMS There can be variation in the licensing of different medicines containing the same drug. Forms available from special-order manufacturers include: oral suspension, oral solution

Solution for injection
EXCIPIENTS: May contain Benzyl alcohol
▸ Clindamycin (Non-proprietary)
 Clindamycin (as Clindamycin phosphate) 150 mg per 1 ml Clindamycin 600mg/4ml solution for injection ampoules | 5 ampoule [PoM] £61.75 (Hospital only) | 10 ampoule [PoM] £100.00 (Hospital only)
 Clindamycin 300mg/2ml solution for injection ampoules | 5 ampoule [PoM] £31.01 (Hospital only) | 10 ampoule [PoM] £55.00 (Hospital only)
▸ Dalacin C (Pfizer Ltd)
 Clindamycin (as Clindamycin phosphate) 150 mg per 1 ml Dalacin C Phosphate 300mg/2ml solution for injection ampoules | 5 ampoule [PoM] £31.01 (Hospital only)
 Dalacin C Phosphate 600mg/4ml solution for injection ampoules | 5 ampoule [PoM] £61.75 (Hospital only)

Oral capsule
CAUTIONARY AND ADVISORY LABELS 9, 27
▸ Clindamycin (Non-proprietary)
 Clindamycin (as Clindamycin hydrochloride) 75 mg Clindamycin 75mg capsules | 24 capsule [PoM] £7.45 DT = £7.45
 Clindamycin (as Clindamycin hydrochloride) 150 mg Clindamycin 150mg capsules | 24 capsule [PoM] £13.72 DT = £2.56 | 100 capsule [PoM] £10.00-£55.08
 Clindamycin (as Clindamycin hydrochloride) 300 mg Clindamycin 300mg capsules | 30 capsule [PoM] £42.00 DT = £13.30
▸ Dalacin C (Pfizer Ltd)
 Clindamycin (as Clindamycin hydrochloride) 75 mg Dalacin C 75mg capsules | 24 capsule [PoM] £7.45 DT = £7.45
 Clindamycin (as Clindamycin hydrochloride) 150 mg Dalacin C 150mg capsules | 24 capsule [PoM] £13.72 DT = £2.56 | 100 capsule [PoM] £55.08

Macrolides

10-Aug-2023

Overview

The macrolides have an antibacterial spectrum that is similar but not identical to that of penicillin; they are thus an alternative in penicillin-allergic patients. They are active against many-penicillin-resistant staphylococci, but some are now also resistant to the macrolides.

Indications for the macrolides include campylobacter enteritis, respiratory infections (including pneumonia, whooping cough, Legionella, chlamydia, and mycoplasma infection), and skin infections.

Erythromycin p. 624 may be used in the treatment of early syphilis, and uncomplicated genital chlamydial infection. Erythromycin has poor activity against *Haemophilus influenzae*. Erythromycin causes nausea, vomiting, and diarrhoea in some patients; in mild to moderate infections this can be avoided by giving a lower dose, but if a more serious infection, such as Legionella pneumonia, is suspected higher doses are needed.

Azithromycin below is a macrolide with slightly less activity than erythromycin against Gram-positive bacteria, but enhanced activity against some Gram-negative organisms including *H. influenzae*. Plasma concentrations are very low, but tissue concentrations are much higher. It has a long tissue half-life and once daily dosage is recommended. Azithromycin is also used in the treatment of uncomplicated genital chlamydial infection, non-gonococcal urethritis, uncomplicated gonorrhoea, typhoid [unlicensed indication], trachoma [unlicensed indication], and Lyme disease [unlicensed indication].

Clarithromycin p. 621 is an erythromycin derivative with slightly greater activity than the parent compound. Tissue concentrations are higher than with erythromycin. Clarithromycin is also used in regimens for *Helicobacter pylori* eradication.

Spiramycin is also a macrolide which is used for the treatment of toxoplasmosis.

Macrolides

- **CAUTIONS**
- With intravenous use or oral use Electrolyte disturbances (predisposition to QT interval prolongation) · may aggravate myasthenia gravis · predisposition to QT interval prolongation

- **SIDE-EFFECTS**
- **Common or very common** Appetite decreased · diarrhoea · dizziness · gastrointestinal discomfort · gastrointestinal disorders · headache · hearing impairment · insomnia · nausea · pancreatitis · paraesthesia · skin reactions · taste altered · vasodilation · vision disorders · vomiting
- **Uncommon** Angioedema · anxiety · arrhythmias · candida infection · chest pain · constipation · drowsiness · eosinophilia · hepatic disorders · leucopenia · neutropenia · palpitations · QT interval prolongation · severe cutaneous adverse reactions (SCARs) · tinnitus · vertigo
- **Rare or very rare** Infantile hypertrophic pyloric stenosis (in children) · myasthenia gravis · nephritis tubulointerstitial · pseudomembranous enterocolitis
- **Frequency not known** Clostridioides difficile colitis · hallucination · hypotension · seizure · smell altered · thrombocytopenia · tongue discolouration

- **PATIENT AND CARER ADVICE**
- In children Parents and carers should be advised to seek medical attention if vomiting or irritability with feeding occurs, due to the risk of infantile hypertrophic pyloric stenosis.

Azithromycin

04-Dec-2023

above

- **INDICATIONS AND DOSE**

Mild diphtheria [confirmed or probable]
- BY MOUTH
- Child 6 months–11 years: 12 mg/kg once daily (max. per dose 500 mg) for 7–10 days
- Child 12–17 years: 500 mg once daily for 7–10 days
- Adult: 500 mg once daily for 7–10 days

Prevention of secondary case of diphtheria
- BY MOUTH
- Child 6 months–11 years: 12 mg/kg once daily (max. per dose 500 mg) for 6 days
- Child 12–17 years: 500 mg once daily for 6 days
- Adult: 500 mg once daily for 6 days

Prevention of secondary case of invasive group A streptococcal infection in patients who are allergic to penicillin
- BY MOUTH
- Child 6 months–11 years: 12 mg/kg once daily (max. per dose 500 mg) for 5 days
- Child 12–17 years: 500 mg once daily for 5 days
- Adult: 500 mg once daily for 5 days

Respiratory-tract infections, otitis media, skin and soft-tissue infections
- BY MOUTH
- Child 6 months–17 years (body-weight up to 15 kg): 10 mg/kg once daily for 3 days
- Child 6 months–17 years (body-weight 15–25 kg): 10 mg/kg once daily for 3 days, alternatively 200 mg once daily for 3 days
- Child 6 months–17 years (body-weight 26–35 kg): 10 mg/kg once daily for 3 days, alternatively 300 mg once daily for 3 days
- Child 6 months–17 years (body-weight 36–45 kg): 10 mg/kg once daily for 3 days, alternatively 400 mg once daily for 3 days
- Child 6 months–17 years (body-weight 46 kg and above): 500 mg once daily for 3 days
- Adult: 500 mg once daily for 3 days, alternatively initially 500 mg once daily for 1 day, then 250 mg once daily for 4 days

Uncomplicated genital chlamydia | Uncomplicated non-gonococcal urethritis
- BY MOUTH
- Child 12–17 years (body-weight 45 kg and above): 1 g once daily for 1 day, then 500 mg once daily for 2 days
- Adult: 1 g once daily for 1 day, then 500 mg once daily for 2 days

Uncomplicated gonorrhoea
- BY MOUTH
- Adult: 2 g for 1 dose

Lyme disease [erythema migrans and/or non-focal symptoms]
- BY MOUTH
- Adult: 500 mg once daily for 17 days

Mild to moderate typhoid due to multiple-antibacterial resistant organisms
- BY MOUTH
- Adult: 500 mg once daily for 7 days

Community-acquired pneumonia, low to moderate severity
- BY MOUTH
- Adult: 500 mg once daily for 3 days, alternatively initially 500 mg once daily for 1 day, then 250 mg once daily for 4 days

Community-acquired pneumonia, high severity

▶ INITIALLY BY INTRAVENOUS INFUSION
▶ Adult: Initially 500 mg once daily for at least 2 days, then (by mouth) 500 mg once daily for a total treatment duration of 7–10 days

Antibacterial prophylaxis for insertion of intra-uterine device

▶ BY MOUTH
▶ Adult: 1 g for 1 dose

● **UNLICENSED USE** UKHSA advises azithromycin may be used as detailed below, although these situations are considered outside the scope of its licence:
  ● treatment and prevention of diphtheria;
  ● prevention of secondary cases of invasive group A streptococcal infection.
▶ In children Azithromycin may be used as detailed below, although these situations are considered outside the scope of its licence:
  ● EvGr dose for uncomplicated genital chlamydia;
  ● uncomplicated non-gonococcal urethritis. ⟨A⟩
▶ In adults Azithromycin may be used as detailed below, although these situations are considered outside the scope of its licence:
  ● EvGr dose for uncomplicated genital chlamydia;
  ● uncomplicated non-gonococcal urethritis;
  ● Lyme disease; ⟨A⟩
  ● mild to moderate typhoid due to multiple-antibacterial resistant organisms;
  ● community-acquired pneumonia (high severity) when oral treatment continues for more than 3 days.

● **INTERACTIONS** → Appendix 1: macrolides

● **SIDE-EFFECTS**

GENERAL SIDE-EFFECTS
▶ **Uncommon** Numbness · oedema · photosensitivity reaction
▶ **Frequency not known** Acute kidney injury · aggression · akathisia · haemolytic anaemia · syncope

SPECIFIC SIDE-EFFECTS
▶ **Common or very common**
▶ With oral use Arthralgia

● **PREGNANCY** Manufacturers advise use only if adequate alternatives not available.

● **BREAST FEEDING** Present in milk; use only if no suitable alternatives.

● **HEPATIC IMPAIRMENT** Manufacturer advises caution; consider avoiding in severe impairment (no information available).

● **RENAL IMPAIRMENT** See p. 21.
▶ In adults EvGr Use with caution if eGFR less than 10 mL/minute/1.73 m^2. ⓜ
▶ In children EvGr Use with caution if estimated glomerular filtration rate less than 10 mL/minute/1.73 m^2. ⓜ

● **DIRECTIONS FOR ADMINISTRATION** For *intravenous infusion* (*Zedbac*®), manufacturer advises give intermittently *in* Glucose 5% *or* Sodium Chloride 0.9%. Reconstitute 500 mg with 4.8 mL Water for Injections to produce a 100 mg/mL solution, then dilute 5 mL of solution with infusion fluid to a final concentration of 1 or 2 mg/mL; give the 1 mg/mL solution over 3 hours *or* give the 2 mg/mL solution over 1 hour.

● **PRESCRIBING AND DISPENSING INFORMATION** For choice of antibacterial therapy, see Antibacterials, use for prophylaxis p. 574, Ear infections, antibacterial therapy p. 582, Genital system infections, antibacterial therapy p. 584, Lyme disease p. 669, Respiratory system infections, antibacterial therapy p. 586, Skin infections, antibacterial therapy p. 589.

● **PATIENT AND CARER ADVICE**
Medicines for Children leaflet: Azithromycin for bacterial infection
www.medicinesforchildren.org.uk/medicines/azithromycin-for-bacterial-infection/

● **PROFESSION SPECIFIC INFORMATION**
Dental practitioners' formulary Azithromycin Capsules may be prescribed.
　Azithromycin Tablets may be prescribed.
　Azithromycin Oral Suspension 200 mg/5 mL may be prescribed.

● **MEDICINAL FORMS** There can be variation in the licensing of different medicines containing the same drug. Forms available from special-order manufacturers include: oral suspension

Oral tablet
CAUTIONARY AND ADVISORY LABELS 5, 9
▶ Azithromycin (Non-proprietary)
　Azithromycin 250 mg Azithromycin 250mg tablets | 4 tablet [PoM] £1.49 DT = £0.92 | 6 tablet [PoM] £1.38-£3.16
　Azithromycin 500 mg Azithromycin 500mg tablets | 3 tablet [PoM] £1.29 DT = £0.95

Oral suspension
CAUTIONARY AND ADVISORY LABELS 5, 9
▶ Azithromycin (Non-proprietary)
　Azithromycin 40 mg per 1 ml Azithromycin 200mg/5ml oral suspension | 15 ml [PoM] £6.18 DT = £4.06 | 30 ml [PoM] £19.88 DT = £11.04
▶ Zithromax (Pfizer Ltd)
　Azithromycin 40 mg per 1 ml Zithromax 200mg/5ml oral suspension | 15 ml [PoM] £4.06 DT = £4.06 | 22.5 ml [PoM] £6.10 DT = £6.10 | 30 ml [PoM] £11.04 DT = £11.04

Oral capsule
CAUTIONARY AND ADVISORY LABELS 5, 9, 23
▶ Azithromycin (Non-proprietary)
　Azithromycin (as Azithromycin dihydrate) 250 mg Azithromycin 250mg capsules | 4 capsule [PoM] £2.11-£3.58 | 6 capsule [PoM] £4.97 DT = £2.26
▶ Zithromax (Pfizer Ltd)
　Azithromycin (as Azithromycin dihydrate) 250 mg Zithromax 250mg capsules | 4 capsule [PoM] £7.16 | 6 capsule [PoM] £10.74 DT = £2.26

Powder for solution for infusion
ELECTROLYTES: May contain Sodium
▶ Azithromycin (Non-proprietary)
　Azithromycin (as Azithromycin dihydrate) 500 mg Azithromycin 500mg powder for concentrate for solution for infusion vials | 1 vial [PoM] £9.50 (Hospital only)
▶ Zedbac (Aspire Pharma Ltd)
　Azithromycin (as Azithromycin dihydrate) 500 mg Zedbac 500mg powder for solution for infusion vials | 1 vial [PoM] £9.50 (Hospital only)

F 620

Clarithromycin

10-Nov-2023

● **INDICATIONS AND DOSE**

Mild diabetic foot infection

▶ BY MOUTH USING IMMEDIATE-RELEASE MEDICINES
▶ Adult: 500 mg twice daily for 7 days then review

Leg ulcer infection

▶ BY MOUTH USING IMMEDIATE-RELEASE MEDICINES
▶ Adult: 500 mg twice daily for 7 days

Cellulitis | Erysipelas

▶ BY MOUTH USING IMMEDIATE-RELEASE MEDICINES
▶ Child 1 month–11 years (body-weight up to 8 kg): 7.5 mg/kg twice daily for 5–7 days then review (review after 7 days if infection near the eyes or nose)
▶ Child 1 month–11 years (body-weight 8-11 kg): 62.5 mg twice daily for 5–7 days then review (review after 7 days if infection near the eyes or nose)
▶ Child 1 month–11 years (body-weight 12-19 kg): 125 mg twice daily for 5–7 days then review (review after 7 days if infection near the eyes or nose)　　continued →

- Child 1 month-11 years (body-weight 20-29 kg): 187.5 mg twice daily for 5–7 days then review (review after 7 days if infection near the eyes or nose)
- Child 1 month-11 years (body-weight 30-40 kg): 250 mg twice daily for 5–7 days then review (review after 7 days if infection near the eyes or nose)
- Child 12-17 years: 250–500 mg twice daily for 5–7 days then review (review after 7 days if infection near the eyes or nose)
- Adult: 500 mg twice daily for 5–7 days then review (review after 7 days if infection near the eyes or nose)
▶ BY INTRAVENOUS INFUSION
- Adult: 500 mg every 12 hours

Impetigo | Secondary bacterial infection of eczema
▶ BY MOUTH USING IMMEDIATE-RELEASE MEDICINES
- Child 1 month-11 years (body-weight up to 8 kg): 7.5 mg/kg twice daily for 5–7 days
- Child 1 month-11 years (body-weight 8-11 kg): 62.5 mg twice daily for 5–7 days
- Child 1 month-11 years (body-weight 12-19 kg): 125 mg twice daily for 5–7 days
- Child 1 month-11 years (body-weight 20-29 kg): 187.5 mg twice daily for 5–7 days
- Child 1 month-11 years (body-weight 30-40 kg): 250 mg twice daily for 5–7 days
- Child 12-17 years: 250 mg twice daily for 5–7 days, alternatively 500 mg twice daily for 5–7 days, increased dose used in severe infections
- Adult: 250 mg twice daily for 5–7 days, alternatively 500 mg twice daily for 5–7 days, increased dose used in severe infections

Community-acquired pneumonia
▶ BY MOUTH USING IMMEDIATE-RELEASE MEDICINES
- Child 1 month-11 years (body-weight up to 8 kg): 7.5 mg/kg twice daily for 5 days
- Child 1 month-11 years (body-weight 8-11 kg): 62.5 mg twice daily for 5 days
- Child 1 month-11 years (body-weight 12-19 kg): 125 mg twice daily for 5 days
- Child 1 month-11 years (body-weight 20-29 kg): 187.5 mg twice daily for 5 days
- Child 1 month-11 years (body-weight 30-40 kg): 250 mg twice daily for 5 days
- Child 12-17 years: 250–500 mg twice daily for 5 days
- Adult: 500 mg twice daily for 5 days
▶ BY INTRAVENOUS INFUSION
- Adult: 500 mg every 12 hours

Hospital-acquired pneumonia
▶ BY MOUTH USING IMMEDIATE-RELEASE MEDICINES
- Child 1 month-11 years (body-weight up to 8 kg): 7.5 mg/kg twice daily for 5 days then review
- Child 1 month-11 years (body-weight 8-11 kg): 62.5 mg twice daily for 5 days then review
- Child 1 month-11 years (body-weight 12-19 kg): 125 mg twice daily for 5 days then review
- Child 1 month-11 years (body-weight 20-29 kg): 187.5 mg twice daily for 5 days then review
- Child 1 month-11 years (body-weight 30-40 kg): 250 mg twice daily for 5 days then review
- Child 12-17 years: 500 mg twice daily for 5 days then review

Respiratory-tract infections | Mild to moderate skin and soft-tissue infections
▶ BY MOUTH USING IMMEDIATE-RELEASE MEDICINES
- Child 1 month-11 years (body-weight up to 8 kg): 7.5 mg/kg twice daily
- Child 1 month-11 years (body-weight 8-11 kg): 62.5 mg twice daily
- Child 1 month-11 years (body-weight 12-19 kg): 125 mg twice daily

- Child 1 month-11 years (body-weight 20-29 kg): 187.5 mg twice daily
- Child 1 month-11 years (body-weight 30-40 kg): 250 mg twice daily
- Child 12-17 years: 250 mg twice daily usually for 7–14 days, alternatively 500 mg twice daily usually for 7–14 days, increased dose used if required in severe infections
- Adult: 250 mg twice daily usually for 7–14 days, alternatively 500 mg twice daily usually for 7–14 days, increased dose used if required in severe infections
▶ BY MOUTH USING MODIFIED-RELEASE MEDICINES
- Child 12-17 years: 500 mg once daily usually for 7–14 days, alternatively 1 g once daily usually for 7–14 days, increased dose used if required in severe infections
- Adult: 500 mg once daily usually for 7–14 days, alternatively 1 g once daily usually for 7–14 days, increased dose used if required in severe infections
▶ BY INTRAVENOUS INFUSION
- Adult: 500 mg every 12 hours maximum duration 5 days, switch to oral route when appropriate, to be administered into a large proximal vein

Acute exacerbation of chronic obstructive pulmonary disease
▶ BY MOUTH USING IMMEDIATE-RELEASE MEDICINES
- Adult: 500 mg twice daily for 5 days
▶ BY INTRAVENOUS INFUSION
- Adult: 500 mg every 12 hours, to be administered into a large proximal vein

Acute exacerbation of bronchiectasis
▶ BY MOUTH USING IMMEDIATE-RELEASE MEDICINES
- Child 1 month-11 years (body-weight up to 8 kg): 7.5 mg/kg twice daily for 7–14 days
- Child 1 month-11 years (body-weight 8-11 kg): 62.5 mg twice daily for 7–14 days
- Child 1 month-11 years (body-weight 12-19 kg): 125 mg twice daily for 7–14 days
- Child 1 month-11 years (body-weight 20-29 kg): 187.5 mg twice daily for 7–14 days
- Child 1 month-11 years (body-weight 30-40 kg): 250 mg twice daily for 7–14 days
- Child 12-17 years: 250–500 mg twice daily for 7–14 days
- Adult: 500 mg twice daily for 7–14 days

Acute cough [if systemically very unwell or at higher risk of complications] | Acute sore throat
▶ BY MOUTH USING IMMEDIATE-RELEASE MEDICINES
- Child 1 month-11 years (body-weight up to 8 kg): 7.5 mg/kg twice daily for 5 days (10 days for scarlet fever)
- Child 1 month-11 years (body-weight 8-11 kg): 62.5 mg twice daily for 5 days (10 days for scarlet fever)
- Child 1 month-11 years (body-weight 12-19 kg): 125 mg twice daily for 5 days (10 days for scarlet fever)
- Child 1 month-11 years (body-weight 20-29 kg): 187.5 mg twice daily for 5 days (10 days for scarlet fever)
- Child 1 month-11 years (body-weight 30-40 kg): 250 mg twice daily for 5 days (10 days for scarlet fever)
- Child 12-17 years: 250–500 mg twice daily for 5 days (10 days for scarlet fever)
- Adult: 250–500 mg twice daily for 5 days

Prevention of secondary case of invasive group A streptococcal infection
▶ BY MOUTH USING IMMEDIATE-RELEASE MEDICINES
- Neonate: 7.5 mg/kg twice daily for 10 days.

- Child 1 month-11 years (body-weight up to 8 kg): 7.5 mg/kg twice daily for 10 days
- Child 1 month-11 years (body-weight 8-11 kg): 62.5 mg twice daily for 10 days
- Child 1 month-11 years (body-weight 12-19 kg): 125 mg twice daily for 10 days

> Child 1 month–11 years (body-weight 20–29 kg): 187.5 mg twice daily for 10 days
> Child 1 month–11 years (body-weight 30–40 kg): 250 mg twice daily for 10 days
> Child 12–17 years: 250–500 mg twice daily for 10 days
> Adult: 250–500 mg twice daily for 10 days

Acute otitis media
▸ BY MOUTH USING IMMEDIATE-RELEASE MEDICINES
> Child 1 month–11 years (body-weight up to 8 kg): 7.5 mg/kg twice daily for 5–7 days
> Child 1 month–11 years (body-weight 8–11 kg): 62.5 mg twice daily for 5–7 days
> Child 1 month–11 years (body-weight 12–19 kg): 125 mg twice daily for 5–7 days
> Child 1 month–11 years (body-weight 20–29 kg): 187.5 mg twice daily for 5–7 days
> Child 1 month–11 years (body-weight 30–40 kg): 250 mg twice daily for 5–7 days
> Child 12–17 years: 250–500 mg twice daily for 5–7 days
> Adult: 250 mg twice daily usually for 7–14 days, alternatively 500 mg twice daily usually for 7–14 days, increased dose used if required in severe infections
▸ BY INTRAVENOUS INFUSION
> Adult: 500 mg every 12 hours maximum duration 5 days, switch to oral route when appropriate, to be administered into a large proximal vein

Mild diphtheria [confirmed or probable]
▸ BY MOUTH USING IMMEDIATE-RELEASE MEDICINES
> Child 1 month–11 years: 7.5 mg/kg twice daily (max. per dose 500 mg) for 14 days
> Child 12–17 years: 500 mg twice daily for 14 days
> Adult: 500 mg twice daily for 14 days

Prevention of secondary case of diphtheria
▸ BY MOUTH USING IMMEDIATE-RELEASE MEDICINES
> Child 1 month–11 years: 7.5 mg/kg twice daily (max. per dose 500 mg) for 7 days
> Child 12–17 years: 500 mg twice daily for 7 days
> Adult: 500 mg twice daily for 7 days

Prevention of pertussis
▸ BY MOUTH USING IMMEDIATE-RELEASE MEDICINES
> Child 1 month–11 years (body-weight up to 8 kg): 7.5 mg/kg twice daily for 7 days
> Child 1 month–11 years (body-weight 8–11 kg): 62.5 mg twice daily for 7 days
> Child 1 month–11 years (body-weight 12–19 kg): 125 mg twice daily for 7 days
> Child 1 month–11 years (body-weight 20–29 kg): 187.5 mg twice daily for 7 days
> Child 1 month–11 years (body-weight 30–40 kg): 250 mg twice daily for 7 days
> Child 12–17 years: 500 mg twice daily for 7 days
> Adult: 500 mg twice daily for 7 days

***Helicobacter pylori* eradication [in combination with other drugs]**
▸ BY MOUTH USING IMMEDIATE-RELEASE MEDICINES
> Adult: 500 mg twice daily for 7 days for first- and second-line eradication therapy; 10 days for third-line eradication therapy

Acute sinusitis
▸ BY MOUTH USING IMMEDIATE-RELEASE MEDICINES
> Child 1 month–11 years (body-weight up to 8 kg): 7.5 mg/kg twice daily for 5 days
> Child 1 month–11 years (body-weight 8–11 kg): 62.5 mg twice daily for 5 days
> Child 1 month–11 years (body-weight 12–19 kg): 125 mg twice daily for 5 days
> Child 1 month–11 years (body-weight 20–29 kg): 187.5 mg twice daily for 5 days
> Child 1 month–11 years (body-weight 30–40 kg): 250 mg twice daily for 5 days

> Child 12–17 years: 250 mg twice daily for 5 days, alternatively 500 mg twice daily for 5 days
> Adult: 500 mg twice daily for 5 days

● **UNLICENSED USE** UKHSA advises clarithromycin may be used as detailed below, although these situations are considered unlicensed:
  ● prevention of secondary cases of invasive group A streptococcal infection;
  ● treatment and prevention of diphtheria.
  EvGr Duration of treatment for acute sinusitis differs from product literature and adheres to national guidelines. Ⓐ
▸ In children EvGr Duration of treatment for acute otitis media differs from product literature and adheres to national guidelines. Ⓐ Tablets not licensed for use in children under 12 years; oral suspension not licensed for use in infants under 6 months.
▸ In adults EvGr Combination regimens and durations for *Helicobacter pylori* eradication may differ from product literature but adhere to national guidelines. Ⓐ

● **INTERACTIONS** → Appendix 1: macrolides

● **SIDE-EFFECTS**
  GENERAL SIDE-EFFECTS
▸ **Uncommon** Burping · dry mouth · haemorrhage · muscle complaints · oral disorders · thrombocytosis · tremor
▸ **Frequency not known** Abnormal dreams · agranulocytosis · depersonalisation · depression · mania · myopathy · psychotic disorder · renal failure · tooth discolouration · urine discolouration
  SPECIFIC SIDE-EFFECTS
▸ **Uncommon**
▸ With oral use Increased risk of infection
▸ With parenteral use Cardiac arrest · dyskinesia · loss of consciousness · pulmonary embolism
▸ **Frequency not known**
▸ With oral use Disorientation

● **PREGNANCY** Manufacturer advises avoid, particularly in the first trimester, unless potential benefit outweighs risk.

● **BREAST FEEDING** Manufacturer advises avoid unless potential benefit outweighs risk—present in milk.

● **HEPATIC IMPAIRMENT** Manufacturer advises caution; avoid in severe failure if renal impairment also present.

● **RENAL IMPAIRMENT** EvGr Avoid if severe hepatic impairment also present. For *modified-release* preparations, avoid if creatinine clearance less than 30 mL/minute. Ⓜ
  Dose adjustments EvGr For *immediate-release* preparations, use half normal dose if creatinine clearance less than 30 mL/minute, max. duration 14 days.
    For *modified-release* preparations, use half normal dose if creatinine clearance 30–60 mL/minute. Ⓜ
    See p. 21.

● **DIRECTIONS FOR ADMINISTRATION** For *intravenous infusion* (*Klaricid*® *I.V.*), manufacturer advises give intermittently in Glucose 5% *or* Sodium Chloride 0.9%; dissolve initially in Water for Injections (500 mg in 10 mL) then dilute to a concentration of 2 mg/mL; give over 60 minutes.

● **PRESCRIBING AND DISPENSING INFORMATION** For choice of antibacterial therapy, see Antibacterials, use for prophylaxis p. 574, Diabetic foot infections, antibacterial therapy p. 581, Ear infections, antibacterial therapy p. 582, Helicobacter pylori infection p. 93, Nose infections, antibacterial therapy p. 585, Oropharyngeal infections, antibacterial therapy p. 1383, Respiratory system infections, antibacterial therapy p. 586, Skin infections, antibacterial therapy p. 589.

● **PATIENT AND CARER ADVICE**
  Medicines for Children leaflet: Clarithromycin for bacterial infections www.medicinesforchildren.org.uk/medicines/clarithromycin-for-bacterial-infections/

- PROFESSION SPECIFIC INFORMATION

Dental practitioners' formulary Clarithromycin Tablets may be prescribed.

Clarithromycin Oral Suspension may be prescribed.

- MEDICINAL FORMS There can be variation in the licensing of different medicines containing the same drug. Forms available from special-order manufacturers include: infusion

Oral tablet

CAUTIONARY AND ADVISORY LABELS 9

- Clarithromycin (Non-proprietary)

Clarithromycin 250 mg Clarithromycin 250mg tablets | 14 tablet [PoM] £5.51 DT = £2.00

Clarithromycin 500 mg Clarithromycin 500mg tablets | 14 tablet [PoM] £11.96 DT = £3.78

Modified-release tablet

CAUTIONARY AND ADVISORY LABELS 9, 21, 25

- Xetinin XL (Morningside Healthcare Ltd)

Clarithromycin 500 mg Xetinin XL 500mg tablets | 7 tablet [PoM] £6.72 DT = £6.72 | 14 tablet [PoM] £13.23 DT = £13.23

Oral suspension

CAUTIONARY AND ADVISORY LABELS 9

- Clarithromycin (Non-proprietary)

Clarithromycin 25 mg per 1 ml Clarithromycin 125mg/5ml oral suspension | 70 ml [PoM] £10.42 DT = £5.05

Clarithromycin 50 mg per 1 ml Clarithromycin 250mg/5ml oral suspension | 70 ml [PoM] £21.02 DT = £9.48

Powder for solution for infusion

ELECTROLYTES: May contain Sodium

- Clarithromycin (Non-proprietary)

Clarithromycin 500 mg Clarithromycin 500mg powder for solution for infusion vials | 1 vial [PoM] £11.25 (Hospital only)

Clarithromycin 500mg powder for concentrate for solution for infusion vials | 1 vial [PoM] £11.15 (Hospital only) | 10 vial [PoM] £111.50 | 10 vial [PoM] £112.50 (Hospital only)

F 620

Erythromycin

04-Dec-2024

- INDICATIONS AND DOSE

Susceptible infections in patients with penicillin hypersensitivity (e.g. respiratory-tract infections (including Legionella infection), skin and oral infections, and campylobacter enteritis)

▸ BY MOUTH

▸ Child 1–23 months: 125 mg 4 times a day, alternatively 250 mg twice daily, increased to 250 mg 4 times a day, increased dose may be used in severe infections

▸ Child 2–7 years: 250 mg 4 times a day, alternatively 500 mg twice daily, increased to 500 mg 4 times a day, increased dose may be used in severe infections

▸ Child 8-17 years: 250–500 mg 4 times a day, alternatively 500–1000 mg twice daily, increased to 500–1000 mg 4 times a day, increased dose may be used in severe infections

▸ Adult: 250–500 mg 4 times a day, alternatively 500–1000 mg twice daily, increased to 500–1000 mg 4 times a day, increased dose may be used in severe infections

▸ BY INTRAVENOUS INFUSION

▸ Child: 12.5 mg/kg every 6 hours (max. per dose 1 g)

▸ Adult: 6.25 mg/kg every 6 hours (max. per dose 500 mg), for mild infections when oral treatment not possible, increased to 12.5 mg/kg every 6 hours (max. per dose 1 g), increased dose may be used in severe infections

Impetigo | Secondary bacterial infection of eczema

▸ BY MOUTH

▸ Child 8-17 years: 250–500 mg 4 times a day for 5–7 days

▸ Adult: 250–500 mg 4 times a day for 5–7 days

Cellulitis | Erysipelas

▸ BY MOUTH

▸ Child 8-17 years: 250–500 mg 4 times a day for 5–7 days then review

▸ Adult: 500 mg 4 times a day for 5–7 days then review

Prevention of recurrent cellulitis (specialist use only) | Prevention of recurrent erysipelas (specialist use only)

▸ BY MOUTH

▸ Adult: 250 mg twice daily

Mild diabetic foot infection

▸ BY MOUTH

▸ Adult: 500 mg 4 times a day for 7 days then review

Leg ulcer infection

▸ BY MOUTH

▸ Adult: 500 mg 4 times a day for 7 days

Community-acquired pneumonia

▸ BY MOUTH

▸ Child 8-17 years: 250–500 mg 4 times a day for 5 days

▸ Adult: 500 mg 4 times a day for 5 days

Acute cough [if systemically very unwell or at higher risk of complications]

▸ BY MOUTH

▸ Child 1-23 months: 125 mg 4 times a day for 5 days, alternatively 250 mg twice daily for 5 days

▸ Child 2-7 years: 250 mg 4 times a day for 5 days, alternatively 500 mg twice daily for 5 days

▸ Child 8-17 years: 250–500 mg 4 times a day for 5 days, alternatively 500–1000 mg twice daily for 5 days

▸ Adult: 250–500 mg 4 times a day for 5 days, alternatively 500–1000 mg twice daily for 5 days

Acute sore throat

▸ BY MOUTH

▸ Child 8-17 years: 250–500 mg 4 times a day for 5 days, alternatively 500–1000 mg twice daily for 5 days

▸ Adult: 250–500 mg 4 times a day for 5 days, alternatively 500–1000 mg twice daily for 5 days

Acute otitis media

▸ BY MOUTH

▸ Child 8-17 years: 250–500 mg 4 times a day for 5–7 days, alternatively 500–1000 mg twice daily for 5–7 days

Early syphilis

▸ BY MOUTH

▸ Adult: 500 mg 4 times a day for 14 days

Uncomplicated genital chlamydia

▸ BY MOUTH

▸ Adult: 500 mg twice daily for 14 days

Chronic prostatitis

▸ BY MOUTH

▸ Adult: 250–500 mg 4 times a day, total daily dose may alternatively be given in two divided doses, dose may be increased to 4 g daily in divided doses in severe infections

▸ BY INTRAVENOUS INFUSION

▸ Adult: 6.25 mg/kg every 6 hours (max. per dose 500 mg), for mild infections when oral treatment is not possible, increased to 12.5 mg/kg every 6 hours (max. per dose 1 g), increased dose may be used in severe infections

Prevention and treatment of pertussis

▸ BY MOUTH

▸ Child 1-23 months: 125 mg 4 times a day, alternatively 250 mg twice daily, increased to 250 mg 4 times a day, increased dose may be used in severe infections

▸ Child 2-7 years: 250 mg 4 times a day, alternatively 500 mg twice daily, increased to 500 mg 4 times a day, increased dose may be used in severe infections

▸ Child 8-17 years: 250–500 mg 4 times a day, alternatively 500–1000 mg twice daily, increased to

500–1000 mg 4 times a day, increased dose may be used in severe infections
▸ Adult: (consult local protocol)

Mild diphtheria [confirmed or probable]
▸ BY MOUTH
▸ Child 1 month–11 years: 10–15 mg/kg 4 times a day (max. per dose 500 mg) for 14 days, alternatively 20–30 mg/kg twice daily (max. per dose 1 g) for 14 days
▸ Child 12–17 years: 500 mg 4 times a day for 14 days, alternatively 1 g twice daily for 14 days
▸ Adult: 500 mg 4 times a day for 14 days, alternatively 1 g twice daily for 14 days

Prevention of secondary case of diphtheria
▸ BY MOUTH
▸ Child 1 month–11 years: 10–15 mg/kg 4 times a day (max. per dose 500 mg) for 7 days, alternatively 20–30 mg/kg twice daily (max. per dose 1 g) for 7 days
▸ Child 12–17 years: 500 mg 4 times a day for 7 days, alternatively 1 g twice daily for 7 days
▸ Adult: 500 mg 4 times a day for 7 days, alternatively 1 g twice daily for 7 days

Prevention of secondary case of invasive group A streptococcal infection [penicillin-allergic patients who are pregnant or within 28 days of delivery]
▸ BY MOUTH
▸ Child 8–17 years: 250–500 mg every 6 hours for 10 days
▸ Adult: 250–500 mg every 6 hours for 10 days

Prevention of pneumococcal infection in asplenia or in patients with sickle-cell disease (if penicillin-allergic)
▸ BY MOUTH
▸ Adult: 500 mg twice daily, antibiotic prophylaxis is not fully reliable. It may be discontinued in those with sickle-cell disease who have received pneumococcal immunisation and who do not have a history of severe pneumococcal infection

Rosacea
▸ BY MOUTH
▸ Adult: 500 mg twice daily courses usually last 6–12 weeks and are repeated intermittently

Acne
▸ BY MOUTH
▸ Adult: 500 mg twice daily

Gastro-intestinal stasis
▸ BY MOUTH
▸ Adult: 250–500 mg 3 times a day for up to 4 weeks, to be taken before food
▸ BY INTRAVENOUS INFUSION
▸ Adult: 3 mg/kg 3 times a day

Prophylaxis of intra-uterine infection [in preterm prelabour rupture of membranes]
▸ BY MOUTH
▸ Adult: 250 mg 4 times a day for up to 10 days or until established labour, whichever is sooner

● UNLICENSED USE EvGr Duration of treatment for acute otitis media differs from product literature and adheres to national guidelines. Ⓐ
   UKHSA advises erythromycin is used in the doses provided in BNF Publications for the treatment and prevention of diphtheria, but these may differ from those licensed.
   EvGr Erythromycin is used for the prevention of recurrent cellulitis, Ⓐ but the dose is not licensed for this indication.
   EvGr Erythromycin is used for the prevention of recurrent erysipelas, Ⓐ but the dose is not licensed for this indication.
   EvGr Erythromycin may be used for gastro-intestinal stasis, Ⓔ but it is not licensed for this indication.
   EvGr Erythromycin is used for the prophylaxis of intra-uterine infection in women with preterm prelabour

rupture of membranes, Ⓐ but is not licensed for this indication.

IMPORTANT SAFETY INFORMATION

MHRA/CHM ADVICE: ERYTHROMYCIN: CAUTION REQUIRED DUE TO CARDIAC RISKS (QT INTERVAL PROLONGATION); DRUG INTERACTION WITH RIVAROXABAN (DECEMBER 2020)
A European review of safety data highlighted an increased risk of cardiotoxicity (i.e. QT interval prolongation) associated with erythromycin. Healthcare professionals are advised that erythromycin should not be given to patients with a history of QT interval prolongation or ventricular arrhythmia (including torsade de pointes), or those with electrolyte disturbances. The benefit-risk balance of treatment should be assessed in patients at increased risk of a cardiac event; caution is required in those with cardiac disease or heart failure, conduction disturbances or clinically relevant bradycardia, or if taking concomitant medicines associated with QT interval prolongation. Patients and carers should be directed to the patient information leaflet and advised to seek medical attention if signs or symptoms of a cardiac event develop. A potential drug interaction between rivaroxaban and erythromycin resulting in an increased risk of bleeding has also been identified—consult product literature.

MHRA/CHM ADVICE: ERYTHROMYCIN: UPDATE ON KNOWN RISK OF INFANTILE HYPERTROPHIC PYLORIC STENOSIS (DECEMBER 2020)
A European review of safety data suggested an overall two- to three-fold increase in the risk of infantile hypertrophic pyloric stenosis after exposure to erythromycin during infancy, in general, and found the risk to be highest in the first 14 days after birth. Healthcare professionals are advised to assess the benefit-risk balance of erythromycin therapy in infants. Parents and carers should be advised to seek medical attention if vomiting or irritability with feeding occurs in infants during treatment.

● CAUTIONS Avoid in Acute porphyrias p. 1202
● INTERACTIONS → Appendix 1: macrolides
● SIDE-EFFECTS
GENERAL SIDE-EFFECTS
▸ **Rare or very rare** Hearing loss (can occur after large doses)
SPECIFIC SIDE-EFFECTS
▸ With oral use Cerebral impairment
▸ With parenteral use Atrioventricular block
● PREGNANCY EvGr Use only if potential benefit outweighs risk Ⓜ (recommendation also supported by specialist sources).
▸ When used for Early syphilis EvGr Avoid (drug may not reach fetus in adequate concentration to prevent congenital syphilis). Ⓐ
● BREAST FEEDING Only small amounts in milk—not known to be harmful.
● HEPATIC IMPAIRMENT Manufacturer advises caution.
● RENAL IMPAIRMENT
Dose adjustments Some manufacturers advise consider dose reduction in moderate to severe impairment (ototoxicity) (consult product literature).
● DIRECTIONS FOR ADMINISTRATION
▸ With intravenous use in children Dilute reconstituted solution further in Glucose 5% (neutralised with Sodium Bicarbonate) or Sodium Chloride 0.9% to a concentration of 1–5 mg/mL; give over 20–60 minutes. Concentration of up to 10 mg/mL may be used in fluid-restriction if administered via a central venous catheter.
▸ With intravenous use in adults For *intravenous infusion* (as

lactobionate), give intermittently *in* Glucose 5% (neutralised with Sodium Bicarbonate) *or* Sodium Chloride 0.9%; dissolve initially in Water for Injections (1 g in 20 mL) then dilute to a concentration of 1–5 mg/mL; give over 20–60 minutes.

- **PRESCRIBING AND DISPENSING INFORMATION** For choice of antibacterial therapy, see Antibacterials, use for prophylaxis p. 574, Diabetic foot infections, antibacterial therapy p. 581, Ear infections, antibacterial therapy p. 582, Gastro-intestinal system infections, antibacterial therapy p. 582, Genital system infections, antibacterial therapy p. 584, Oropharyngeal infections, antibacterial therapy p. 1383, Respiratory system infections, antibacterial therapy p. 586, Skin infections, antibacterial therapy p. 589.

- **PATIENT AND CARER ADVICE**
Medicines for Children leaflet: Erythromycin for bacterial infections www.medicinesforchildren.org.uk/medicines/erythromycin-for-bacterial-infections/

- **PROFESSION SPECIFIC INFORMATION**

Dental practitioners' formulary Erythromycin tablets e/c may be prescribed.
Erythromycin ethyl succinate oral suspension may be prescribed.
Erythromycin stearate tablets may be prescribed.
Erythromycin ethyl succinate tablets may be prescribed.

- **MEDICINAL FORMS** There can be variation in the licensing of different medicines containing the same drug.

Oral tablet
CAUTIONARY AND ADVISORY LABELS 9
- Erythromycin (Non-proprietary)
Erythromycin (as Erythromycin stearate) 250 mg Erythromycin stearate 250mg tablets | 100 tablet PoM ⓧ DT = £18.20
Erythromycin (as Erythromycin ethyl succinate) 500 mg Erythromycin ethyl succinate 500mg tablets | 28 tablet PoM £15.95 DT = £15.95
Erythromycin (as Erythromycin stearate) 500 mg Erythromycin stearate 500mg tablets | 100 tablet PoM ⓧ DT = £36.40
- Erythrocin (Advanz Pharma)
Erythromycin (as Erythromycin stearate) 250 mg Erythrocin 250 tablets | 100 tablet PoM £18.20 DT = £18.20
Erythromycin (as Erythromycin stearate) 500 mg Erythrocin 500 tablets | 100 tablet PoM £36.40 DT = £36.40

Gastro-resistant tablet
CAUTIONARY AND ADVISORY LABELS 5, 9, 25
- Erythromycin (Non-proprietary)
Erythromycin 250 mg Erythromycin 250mg gastro-resistant tablets | 28 tablet PoM £12.31 DT = £3.54

Oral suspension
CAUTIONARY AND ADVISORY LABELS 9
- Erythromycin (Non-proprietary)
Erythromycin (as Erythromycin ethyl succinate) 25 mg per 1 ml Erythromycin ethyl succinate 125mg/5ml oral suspension | 100 ml PoM £8.20 DT = £7.07
Erythromycin ethyl succinate 125mg/5ml oral suspension sugar free | 100 ml PoM £8.20 DT = £6.92 SF
Erythromycin (as Erythromycin ethyl succinate) 50 mg per 1 ml Erythromycin ethyl succinate 250mg/5ml oral suspension | 100 ml PoM £13.80 DT = £12.40
Erythromycin ethyl succinate 250mg/5ml oral suspension sugar free | 100 ml PoM £13.80 DT = £12.42 SF
Erythromycin (as Erythromycin ethyl succinate) 100 mg per 1 ml Erythromycin ethyl succinate 500mg/5ml oral suspension | 100 ml PoM £23.46

Powder for solution for infusion
- Erythromycin (Non-proprietary)
Erythromycin (as Erythromycin lactobionate)
1 gram Erythromycin 1g powder for solution for infusion vials | 1 vial PoM £22.00-£22.92 (Hospital only)

ANTIBACTERIALS ﹥ MONOBACTAMS

Aztreonam

04-Nov-2024

- **DRUG ACTION** Aztreonam is a monocyclic beta-lactam ('monobactam') antibiotic with an antibacterial spectrum limited to Gram-negative aerobic bacteria including *Pseudomonas aeruginosa, Neisseria meningitidis*, and *Haemophilus influenzae*; it should not be used alone for 'blind' treatment since it is not active against Gram-positive organisms. Aztreonam is also effective against *Neisseria gonorrhoeae* (but not against concurrent chlamydial infection).

- **INDICATIONS AND DOSE**

Gram-negative infections including *Pseudomonas aeruginosa, Haemophilus influenzae,* and *Neisseria meningitidis*
- BY DEEP INTRAMUSCULAR INJECTION, OR BY INTRAVENOUS INFUSION, OR BY INTRAVENOUS INJECTION
- Adult: 1 g every 8 hours, alternatively 2 g every 12 hours, single doses over 1 g intravenous route only

Severe gram-negative infections including *Pseudomonas aeruginosa, Haemophilus influenzae, Neisseria meningitidis,* and lung infections in cystic fibrosis
- BY INTRAVENOUS INFUSION, OR BY INTRAVENOUS INJECTION
- Adult: 2 g every 6–8 hours

Gonorrhoea | Cystitis
- BY INTRAMUSCULAR INJECTION
- Adult: 1 g for 1 single dose

Urinary-tract infections
- BY DEEP INTRAMUSCULAR INJECTION, OR BY INTRAVENOUS INFUSION, OR BY INTRAVENOUS INJECTION
- Adult: 0.5–1 g every 8–12 hours

Chronic pulmonary *Pseudomonas aeruginosa* infection in patients with cystic fibrosis
- BY INHALATION OF NEBULISED SOLUTION
- Adult: 75 mg 3 times a day for 28 days, doses to be administered at least 4 hours apart, subsequent courses repeated after 28-day interval without aztreonam nebuliser solution

- **CAUTIONS**
- When used by inhalation Haemoptysis— risk of further haemorrhage

- **SIDE-EFFECTS**

GENERAL SIDE-EFFECTS
- **Common or very common** Dyspnoea · respiratory disorders

SPECIFIC SIDE-EFFECTS
- **Common or very common**
- When used by inhalation Cough · haemoptysis · joint disorders · laryngeal pain · nasal complaints · rash
- **Rare or very rare**
- With parenteral use Anaemia · asthenia · breast tenderness · chest pain · confusion · diplopia · dizziness · eosinophilia · haemorrhage · headache · hepatic disorders · hypotension · insomnia · leucocytosis · myalgia · nasal congestion · neutropenia · oral disorders · pancytopenia · paraesthesia · pseudomembranous enterocolitis · seizure · thrombocytopenia · thrombocytosis · tinnitus · vertigo · vulvovaginal candidiasis
- **Frequency not known**
- With parenteral use Abdominal pain · angioedema · Clostridioides difficile colitis · diarrhoea · nausea · skin reactions · taste altered · toxic epidermal necrolysis · vomiting

- **ALLERGY AND CROSS-SENSITIVITY** EvGr Contra-indicated in aztreonam hypersensitivity.
Use with caution in patients with hypersensitivity to other beta-lactam antibiotics (although aztreonam may be

less likely than other beta-lactams to cause hypersensitivity in penicillin-sensitive patients). ⟨M⟩

● **PREGNANCY**
▸ With systemic use No information available; manufacturer of injection advises avoid.
▸ When used by inhalation No information available; manufacturer of powder for nebuliser solution advises avoid unless essential.

● **BREAST FEEDING** Amount in milk probably too small to be harmful.

● **HEPATIC IMPAIRMENT**
▸ With systemic use Manufacturer advises caution in chronic impairment with cirrhosis.
  Dose adjustments
  ▸ With systemic use Manufacturer advises dose reduction of 20—25% for long term treatment of patients with chronic impairment with cirrhosis, especially in alcoholic cirrhosis and concomitant renal impairment.

● **RENAL IMPAIRMENT**
  Dose adjustments
  ▸ With systemic use If eGFR 10–30 mL/minute/1.73 m^2, usual initial dose of injection, then half normal dose. If eGFR less than 10 mL/minute/1.73 m^2, usual initial dose of injection, then one-quarter normal dose.

● **MONITORING REQUIREMENTS**
▸ When used by inhalation Measure lung function before and after initial dose of aztreonam and monitor for bronchospasm.

● **EFFECT ON LABORATORY TESTS**
▸ With systemic use False positive Coombs' test.

● **DIRECTIONS FOR ADMINISTRATION**
▸ With intravenous use For *intravenous injection*, manufacturer advises give over 3–5 minutes. For *intravenous infusion* (*Azactam*®), manufacturer advises give intermittently *in* Glucose 5% *or* Sodium Chloride 0.9%. Dissolve initially in Water for Injections (1 g per 3 mL) then dilute to a concentration of less than 20 mg/mL; to be given over 20–60 minutes.
▸ When used by inhalation Manufacturer advises other inhaled drugs should be administered before aztreonam; a bronchodilator should be administered before each dose.

● **NATIONAL FUNDING/ACCESS DECISIONS**
  For full details see funding body website
  Scottish Medicines Consortium (SMC) decisions
▸ Aztreonam lysine (*Cayston*®) for suppressive therapy of chronic pulmonary infections due to *Pseudomonas aeruginosa* in patients with cystic fibrosis aged six years and older (January 2015) SMC No. 753/12 Recommended with restrictions

● **MEDICINAL FORMS** There can be variation in the licensing of different medicines containing the same drug.
  Powder and solvent for nebuliser solution
  ▸ Cayston (Gilead Sciences Ltd)
    Aztreonam (as Aztreonam lysine) **75 mg** Cayston 75mg powder and solvent for nebuliser solution vials with Altera Nebuliser Handset | 84 vial PoM £2,181.53 DT = £2,181.53
  Powder for solution for injection
  ▸ Azactam (Bristol-Myers Squibb Pharmaceuticals Ltd)
    Aztreonam **1 gram** Azactam 1g powder for solution for injection vials | 1 vial PoM £9.40 (Hospital only)
    Aztreonam **2 gram** Azactam 2g powder for solution for injection vials | 1 vial PoM £18.82 (Hospital only)

Aztreonam with avibactam　　　　04-Nov-2024

The properties listed below are those particular to the combination only. For the properties of the components please consider, aztreonam p. 626.

● **INDICATIONS AND DOSE**
Complicated urinary-tract infection [including pyelonephritis] | Complicated intra-abdominal infection
▸ BY INTRAVENOUS INFUSION
▸ Adult: Loading dose 2/0.67 g for 1 dose, then maintenance 1.5/0.5 g every 6 hours for 5–10 days in total, maintenance dose to be started 6 hours after initial loading dose

Hospital-acquired pneumonia [including ventilator-associated pneumonia]
▸ BY INTRAVENOUS INFUSION
▸ Adult: Loading dose 2/0.67 g for 1 dose, then maintenance 1.5/0.5 g every 6 hours for 7–14 days in total, maintenance dose to be started 6 hours after initial loading dose

Aerobic Gram-negative infections [in patients with limited treatment options] (administered on expert advice)
▸ BY INTRAVENOUS INFUSION
▸ Adult: Loading dose 2/0.67 g for 1 dose, then maintenance 1.5/0.5 g every 6 hours, duration should be tailored to site of infection and may continue for up to 14 days in total, maintenance dose to be started 6 hours after initial loading dose

DOSE EQUIVALENCE AND CONVERSION
▸ Dose expressed as *x/y* g of aztreonam/avibactam.

● **SIDE-EFFECTS**
▸ **Common or very common** Abdominal pain · anaemia · confusion · diarrhoea · dizziness · fever · nausea · skin reactions · thrombocytopenia · thrombocytosis · thrombophlebitis · vomiting
▸ **Uncommon** Angioedema · asthenia · chest discomfort · Clostridioides difficile colitis · encephalopathy · extrasystole · flushing · haemorrhage · headache · hyperhidrosis · hypotension · insomnia · leucocytosis · oral disorders · respiratory disorders · taste altered · toxic epidermal necrolysis
▸ **Rare or very rare** Breast tenderness · diplopia · dyspnoea · hepatic disorders · increased risk of infection · malaise · myalgia · nasal complaints · neutropenia · pancytopenia · paraesthesia · pseudomembranous enterocolitis · seizure · tinnitus · vertigo

● **PREGNANCY** EvGr Avoid unless potential benefit outweighs risk (toxicity in *animal* studies with avibactam). ⟨M⟩

● **BREAST FEEDING** EvGr Avoid (presence of avibactam in milk unknown). ⟨M⟩

● **RENAL IMPAIRMENT** EvGr Avoid if creatinine clearance 15 mL/minute or less (consult product literature for information on use in patients on renal replacement therapy). ⟨M⟩
  Dose adjustments See p. 21.
    EvGr Reduce maintenance dose to 0.75/0.25 g every 6 hours if creatinine clearance 31–50 mL/minute.
    Reduce loading dose to 1.35/0.45 g and maintenance dose to 0.675/0.225 g every 8 hours if creatinine clearance 16–30 mL/minute. ⟨M⟩

● **DIRECTIONS FOR ADMINISTRATION** For *intravenous infusion*, reconstitute each 1.5/0.5 g vial with 10 mL Water for Injections. Dilute requisite volume of reconstituted solution to a final concentration of 1.5/0.5–40/13.3 mg/mL in Glucose 5% *or* Sodium Chloride 0.9%; give over 3 hours.

● **HANDLING AND STORAGE** Store in a refrigerator (2–8°C) and protect from light—consult product literature about storage after dilution.

● **PATIENT AND CARER ADVICE**
Driving and skilled tasks Patients and carers should be
counselled on the effects on driving and performance of
skilled tasks—increased risk of dizziness.

● **MEDICINAL FORMS** There can be variation in the licensing of
different medicines containing the same drug.
Powder for solution for infusion
ELECTROLYTES: May contain Sodium
▸ **Emblaveo** (Pfizer Ltd)
Avibactam (as Avibactam sodium) 500 mg, Aztreonam
1.5 gram Emblaveo 1.5g/0.5g powder for concentrate for solution for
infusion vials | 10 vial [PoM] £1,500.00 (Hospital only)

ANTIBACTERIALS > NITROIMIDAZOLE DERIVATIVES

Metronidazole

10-Nov-2021

● **DRUG ACTION** Metronidazole is an antimicrobial drug with
high activity against anaerobic bacteria and protozoa.

● **INDICATIONS AND DOSE**
Anaerobic infections
▸ BY MOUTH
▸ Child 1 month: 7.5 mg/kg every 12 hours usually treated
for 7 days
▸ Child 2 months-11 years: 7.5 mg/kg every 8 hours (max.
per dose 400 mg) usually treated for 7 days
▸ Child 12-17 years: 400 mg every 8 hours usually treated
for 7 days
▸ Adult: 400 mg every 8 hours usually treated for 7 days,
alternatively 500 mg every 8 hours usually treated for
7 days
▸ BY RECTUM
▸ Child 1-11 months: 125 mg 3 times a day for 3 days, then
125 mg twice daily for usual total treatment duration of
7 days
▸ Child 1-4 years: 250 mg 3 times a day for 3 days, then
250 mg twice daily for usual total treatment duration of
7 days
▸ Child 5-9 years: 500 mg 3 times a day for 3 days, then
500 mg twice daily for usual total treatment duration of
7 days
▸ Child 10-17 years: 1 g 3 times a day for 3 days, then 1 g
twice daily for usual total treatment duration of 7 days
▸ Adult: 1 g 3 times a day for 3 days, then 1 g twice daily
for usual total treatment duration of 7 days
▸ BY INTRAVENOUS INFUSION
▸ Adult: 500 mg every 8 hours usually treated for 7 days
(for 10 days in *Clostridioides difficile* infection)

**Moderate diabetic foot infection | Severe diabetic foot
infection | Leg ulcer infection [in combination with other
drugs]**
▸ BY MOUTH
▸ Adult: 400 mg every 8 hours
▸ BY INTRAVENOUS INFUSION
▸ Adult: 500 mg every 8 hours

Cellulitis | Erysipelas
▸ BY MOUTH
▸ Child 1 month: 7.5 mg/kg every 12 hours for 7 days then
review
▸ Child 2 months-11 years: 7.5 mg/kg every 8 hours (max.
per dose 400 mg) for 7 days then review
▸ Child 12-17 years: 400 mg every 8 hours for 7 days then
review
▸ Adult: 400 mg every 8 hours for 7 days then review
▸ BY INTRAVENOUS INFUSION
▸ Adult: 500 mg every 8 hours

**Prophylaxis of infection from human bites [in
combination with other drugs] | Prophylaxis of infection
from animal bites [in combination with other drugs]**
▸ BY MOUTH
▸ Child 12-17 years: 400 mg 3 times a day for 3 days
▸ Adult: 400 mg 3 times a day for 3 days
▸ BY INTRAVENOUS INFUSION
▸ Child 1 month: Loading dose 15 mg/kg for 1 dose, then
7.5 mg/kg every 8 hours
▸ Child 2 months-17 years: 7.5 mg/kg every 8 hours (max.
per dose 500 mg)
▸ Adult: 500 mg every 8 hours

**Treatment of infection from human bites [in combination
with other drugs] | Treatment of infection from animal
bites [in combination with other drugs]**
▸ BY MOUTH
▸ Child 12-17 years: 400 mg 3 times a day for 5–7 days
▸ Adult: 400 mg 3 times a day for 5–7 days
▸ BY INTRAVENOUS INFUSION
▸ Child 1 month: Loading dose 15 mg/kg for 1 dose, then
7.5 mg/kg every 8 hours
▸ Child 2 months-17 years: 7.5 mg/kg every 8 hours (max.
per dose 500 mg)
▸ Adult: 500 mg every 8 hours

***Helicobacter pylori* eradication [in combination with other
drugs]**
▸ BY MOUTH
▸ Adult: 400 mg twice daily for 7 days for first- and
second-line eradication therapy; 10 days for third-line
eradication therapy

Fistulating Crohn's disease
▸ BY MOUTH
▸ Adult: 10–20 mg/kg daily in divided doses, usual dose
400–500 mg 3 times a day usually given for 1 month
but no longer than 3 months because of concerns about
peripheral neuropathy

Acute diverticulitis [in combination with other drugs]
▸ BY MOUTH
▸ Adult: 400 mg 3 times a day for 5 days then review
▸ BY INTRAVENOUS INFUSION
▸ Adult: 500 mg every 8 hours

Pressure sores
▸ BY MOUTH
▸ Adult: 400 mg every 8 hours for 7 days

**Bacterial vaginosis (notably *Gardnerella vaginalis*
infection)**
▸ BY MOUTH
▸ Adult: 400–500 mg twice daily for 5–7 days,
alternatively 2 g for 1 dose

Bacterial vaginosis
▸ BY VAGINA USING VAGINAL GEL
▸ Adult: 1 applicatorful once daily for 5 days, dose to be
administered at night

DOSE EQUIVALENCE AND CONVERSION
▸ 1 applicatorful of vaginal gel delivers a 5 g dose of
metronidazole 0.75%.

Pelvic inflammatory disease
▸ BY MOUTH
▸ Child 12-17 years: 400 mg twice daily for 14 days
▸ Adult: 400 mg twice daily for 14 days

Acute ulcerative gingivitis
▸ BY MOUTH
▸ Child 1-2 years: 50 mg every 8 hours for 3 days
▸ Child 3-6 years: 100 mg every 12 hours for 3 days
▸ Child 7-9 years: 100 mg every 8 hours for 3 days
▸ Child 10-17 years: 200–250 mg every 8 hours for 3 days
▸ Adult: 400 mg every 8 hours for 3 days

Acute oral infections
▸ BY MOUTH
▸ Child 1-2 years: 50 mg every 8 hours for 3–7 days
▸ Child 3-6 years: 100 mg every 12 hours for 3–7 days
▸ Child 7-9 years: 100 mg every 8 hours for 3–7 days
▸ Child 10-17 years: 200–250 mg every 8 hours for 3–7 days
▸ Adult: 400 mg every 8 hours for 3–7 days

Surgical prophylaxis
▸ BY MOUTH
▸ Adult: 400–500 mg for 1 dose, to be administered 2 hours before surgery, then 400–500 mg every 8 hours if required for up to 3 doses (in high-risk procedures)
▸ BY RECTUM
▸ Adult: 1 g for 1 dose, to be administered 2 hours before surgery, then 1 g every 8 hours if required for up to 3 doses (in high-risk procedures)
▸ BY INTRAVENOUS INFUSION
▸ Adult: 500 mg for 1 dose, to be administered up to 30 minutes before the procedure, to be used if rectal administration inappropriate, then 500 mg every 8 hours if required for up to 3 doses (in high-risk procedures)

Invasive intestinal amoebiasis
▸ BY MOUTH
▸ Child 1-2 years: 200 mg 3 times a day for 5 days
▸ Child 3-6 years: 200 mg 4 times a day for 5 days
▸ Child 7-9 years: 400 mg 3 times a day for 5 days
▸ Child 10-17 years: 800 mg 3 times a day for 5 days
▸ Adult: 800 mg 3 times a day for 5 days

Extra-intestinal amoebiasis (including liver abscess)
▸ BY MOUTH
▸ Child 1-2 years: 200 mg 3 times a day for 5–10 days
▸ Child 3-6 years: 200 mg 4 times a day for 5–10 days
▸ Child 7-9 years: 400 mg 3 times a day for 5–10 days
▸ Child 10-17 years: 800 mg 3 times a day for 5–10 days
▸ Adult: 800 mg 3 times a day for 5–10 days

Urogenital trichomoniasis
▸ BY MOUTH
▸ Child 1-2 years: 50 mg 3 times a day for 7 days
▸ Child 3-6 years: 100 mg twice daily for 7 days
▸ Child 7-9 years: 100 mg 3 times a day for 7 days
▸ Child 10-17 years: 200 mg 3 times a day for 7 days, alternatively 400–500 mg twice daily for 5–7 days, alternatively 2 g for 1 dose
▸ Adult: 200 mg 3 times a day for 7 days, alternatively 400–500 mg twice daily for 5–7 days, alternatively 2 g for 1 dose

Giardiasis
▸ BY MOUTH
▸ Child 1-2 years: 500 mg once daily for 3 days
▸ Child 3-6 years: 600–800 mg once daily for 3 days
▸ Child 7-9 years: 1 g once daily for 3 days
▸ Child 10-17 years: 2 g once daily for 3 days, alternatively 400 mg 3 times a day for 5 days, alternatively 500 mg twice daily for 7–10 days
▸ Adult: 2 g once daily for 3 days, alternatively 400 mg 3 times a day for 5 days, alternatively 500 mg twice daily for 7–10 days

Established case of tetanus
▸ BY INTRAVENOUS INFUSION
▸ Adult: (consult product literature)

● UNLICENSED USE
▸ With systemic use in adults Metronidazole doses in the BNF may differ from those in product literature.
EvGr Combination regimens and durations for *Helicobacter pylori* eradication may differ from product literature but adhere to national guidelines. Ⓐ

● CAUTIONS
▸ With vaginal use Not recommended during menstruation · some systemic absorption may occur with vaginal gel

● INTERACTIONS → Appendix 1: metronidazole

● SIDE-EFFECTS
▸ **Common or very common**
▸ With systemic use Dry mouth · myalgia · nausea · oral disorders · taste metallic · vomiting
▸ With vaginal use Pelvic discomfort · vulvovaginal candidiasis · vulvovaginal disorders
▸ **Uncommon**
▸ With systemic use Asthenia · headache · leucopenia (with long term or intensive therapy)
▸ With vaginal use Menstrual cycle irregularities · vaginal haemorrhage
▸ **Rare or very rare**
▸ With systemic use Agranulocytosis · angioedema · appetite decreased · ataxia · cerebellar syndrome · confusion · diarrhoea · dizziness · drowsiness · encephalopathy · epigastric pain · epileptiform seizure (with long term or intensive therapy) · flushing · hallucination · hepatic disorders · meningitis aseptic · mucositis · nerve disorders · neutropenia · pancreatitis · pancytopenia · peripheral neuropathy (with long term or intensive therapy) · psychotic disorder · seizure · severe cutaneous adverse reactions (SCARs) · skin reactions · thrombocytopenia · urine dark · vision disorders
▸ **Frequency not known**
▸ With systemic use Depressed mood · gastrointestinal disorder · hearing impairment · taste altered · tinnitus · vertigo

● PREGNANCY
▸ With systemic use Manufacturer advises avoidance of high-dose regimens; use only if potential benefit outweighs risk.

● BREAST FEEDING
▸ With systemic use Significant amount in milk; manufacturer advises avoid large single doses though otherwise compatible; may give milk a bitter taste.

● HEPATIC IMPAIRMENT
▸ With oral use or rectal use Manufacturer advises caution in hepatic encephalopathy (risk of decreased clearance).
▸ With intravenous use Manufacturer advises caution in severe impairment (risk of decreased clearance).
Dose adjustments
▸ With oral use or rectal use Manufacturer advises dose reduction to one-third of the daily dose in hepatic encephalopathy (dose may be given once daily).
▸ With intravenous use Manufacturer advises consider dose reduction in severe impairment.

● MONITORING REQUIREMENTS
▸ With systemic use Clinical and laboratory monitoring advised if treatment exceeds 10 days.

● DIRECTIONS FOR ADMINISTRATION EvGr For *intravenous infusion*, give over 20–60 minutes. Ⓜ

● PRESCRIBING AND DISPENSING INFORMATION For choice of antibacterial therapy, see Antibacterials, use for prophylaxis p. 574, Antiprotozoal drugs p. 702, Diabetic foot infections, antibacterial therapy p. 581, Gastro-intestinal system infections, antibacterial therapy p. 582, Genital system infections, antibacterial therapy p. 584, Helicobacter pylori infection p. 93, Oropharyngeal infections, antibacterial therapy p. 1383, Skin infections, antibacterial therapy p. 589.

Metronidazole is well absorbed orally and the intravenous route is normally reserved for severe infections. Metronidazole by the rectal route is an effective alternative to the intravenous route when oral administration is not possible.

- **PATIENT AND CARER ADVICE**

Medicines for Children leaflet: Metronidazole for bacterial infections www.medicinesforchildren.org.uk/medicines/metronidazole-for-bacterial-infections/

- **PROFESSION SPECIFIC INFORMATION**

Dental practitioners' formulary Metronidazole Tablets may be prescribed.

Metronidazole Oral Suspension may be prescribed.

- **MEDICINAL FORMS** There can be variation in the licensing of different medicines containing the same drug. Forms available from special-order manufacturers include: oral suspension, oral solution, suppository

Oral tablet

CAUTIONARY AND ADVISORY LABELS 4, 9, 21, 25, 27

▸ Metronidazole (Non-proprietary)

Metronidazole 200 mg Metronidazole 200mg tablets |
21 tablet [PoM] £4.00 DT = £0.85
Metronidazole 400 mg Metronidazole 400mg tablets |
21 tablet [PoM] £12.00 DT = £0.97
Metronidazole 500 mg Metronidazole 500mg tablets |
21 tablet [PoM] £42.95 DT = £18.69

▸ Flagyl (Purple Orchid Health Ltd)

Metronidazole 400 mg Flagyl 400mg tablets | 14 tablet [PoM]
£6.34

Suppository

CAUTIONARY AND ADVISORY LABELS 4, 9

▸ Flagyl (Purple Orchid Health Ltd)

Metronidazole 500 mg Flagyl 500mg suppositories |
10 suppository [PoM] £15.18 DT = £15.18
Metronidazole 1 gram Flagyl 1g suppositories |
10 suppository [PoM] £23.06 DT = £23.06

Oral suspension

CAUTIONARY AND ADVISORY LABELS 4, 9

▸ Metronidazole (Non-proprietary)

**Metronidazole (as Metronidazole benzoate) 40 mg per
1 ml** Metronidazole 200mg/5ml oral suspension | 100 ml [PoM]
£70.52 DT = £61.48

Vaginal gel

EXCIPIENTS: May contain Disodium edetate, hydroxybenzoates (parabens), propylene glycol

▸ Zidoval (Viatris UK Healthcare Ltd)

Metronidazole 7.5 mg per 1 gram Zidoval 0.75% vaginal gel |
40 gram [PoM] £4.31 DT = £4.31

Infusion

ELECTROLYTES: May contain Sodium

▸ Metronidazole (Non-proprietary)

Metronidazole 5 mg per 1 ml Metronidazole 500mg/100ml infusion
100ml Viaflo bags | 60 bag [PoM] £288.60 (Hospital only)

ANTIBACTERIALS > PENICILLINS

Penicillins

14-Jul-2021

Benzylpenicillin and phenoxymethylpenicillin

Benzylpenicillin sodium p. 633 (Penicillin G) remains an important and useful antibiotic but is inactivated by bacterial beta-lactamases. It is effective for many streptococcal (including pneumococcal), gonococcal, and meningococcal infections and also for anthrax, diphtheria, tetanus, gas-gangrene, and leptospirosis. Pneumococci, meningococci, and gonococci which have decreased sensitivity to penicillin have been isolated; benzylpenicillin sodium is no longer the drug of first choice for pneumococcal meningitis. Benzylpenicillin is inactivated by gastric acid and absorption from the gastro-intestinal tract is low; therefore it must be given by injection.

Benzathine benzylpenicillin p. 632 is used for the treatment of early syphilis and late latent syphilis; it is given by intramuscular injection.

Phenoxymethylpenicillin p. 634 (Penicillin V) has a similar antibacterial spectrum to benzylpenicillin sodium, but is less active. It is gastric acid-stable, so is suitable for oral administration. It should not be used for serious infections because absorption can be unpredictable and plasma concentrations variable. It is indicated principally for respiratory-tract infections in children, for streptococcal tonsillitis, and for continuing treatment after one or more injections of benzylpenicillin sodium when clinical response has begun. It should not be used for meningococcal or gonococcal infections. Phenoxymethylpenicillin is used for prophylaxis against streptococcal infections following rheumatic fever and against pneumococcal infections following splenectomy or in sickle-cell disease.

Penicillinase-resistant penicillins

Most staphylococci are now resistant to benzylpenicillin because they produce penicillinases. Flucloxacillin p. 643, however, is not inactivated by these enzymes and is thus effective in infections caused by penicillin-resistant staphylococci, which is the sole indication for its use. Flucloxacillin is acid-stable and can, therefore, be given by mouth as well as by injection. Flucloxacillin is well absorbed from the gut.

Temocillin p. 644 is active against Gram-negative bacteria and is stable against a wide range of beta-lactamases. It should be reserved for the treatment of infections caused by beta-lactamase-producing strains of Gram-negative bacteria, including those resistant to third-generation cephalosporins. Temocillin is not active against *Pseudomonas aeruginosa* or *Acinetobacter* spp.

Broad-spectrum penicillins

Ampicillin p. 637 is active against certain Gram-positive and Gram-negative organisms but is inactivated by penicillinases including those produced by *Staphylococcus aureus* and by common Gram-negative bacilli such as *Escherichia coli*. Almost all staphylococci, approx. 60% of *E. coli* strains and approx. 20% of *Haemophilus influenzae* strains are now resistant. The likelihood of resistance should therefore be considered before using ampicillin for the 'blind' treatment of infections; in particular, it should not be used for hospital patients without checking sensitivity.

Ampicillin is well excreted in the bile and urine. It is principally indicated for the treatment of exacerbations of chronic bronchitis and middle ear infections, both of which may be due to *Streptococcus pneumoniae* and *H. influenzae*, and for urinary-tract infections.

Ampicillin can be given by mouth but less than half the dose is absorbed, and absorption is further decreased by the presence of food in the gut.

Maculopapular rashes commonly occur with ampicillin (and amoxicillin p. 635) but are not usually related to true penicillin allergy. They almost always occur in patients with glandular fever; broad-spectrum penicillins should not therefore be used for 'blind' treatment of a sore throat. The risk of rash is also increased in patients with acute or chronic lymphocytic leukaemia or in cytomegalovirus infection.

Amoxicillin is a derivative of ampicillin and has a similar antibacterial spectrum. It is better absorbed than ampicillin when given by mouth, producing higher plasma and tissue concentrations; unlike ampicillin, absorption is not affected by the presence of food in the stomach. Amoxicillin is also used for the treatment of Lyme disease.

Co-amoxiclav p. 638 consists of amoxicillin with the betalactamase inhibitor clavulanic acid. Clavulanic acid itself has no significant antibacterial activity but, by inactivating beta-lactamases, it makes the combination active against beta-lactamase-producing bacteria that are resistant to amoxicillin. These include resistant strains of *Staph. aureus*, *E. coli*, and *H. influenzae*, as well as many *Bacteroides* and *Klebsiella* spp. Co-amoxiclav should be reserved for infections likely, or known, to be caused by amoxicillin-resistant beta-lactamase-producing strains.

A combination of ampicillin with flucloxacillin (as co-fluampicil p. 637) is available to treat infections involving either streptococci or staphylococci.

Antipseudomonal penicillins

Piperacillin, a ureidopenicillin, is only available in combination with the beta-lactamase inhibitor tazobactam. **Ticarcillin**, a carboxypenicillin, is only available in combination with the beta-lactamase inhibitor clavulanic acid. Both preparations have a broad spectrum of activity against a range of Gram-positive and Gram-negative bacteria, and anaerobes. Piperacillin with tazobactam below has activity against a wider range of Gram-negative organisms than ticarcillin with clavulanic acid and it is more active against *Pseudomonas aeruginosa*. These antibacterials are not active against MRSA. They are used in the treatment of septicaemia, hospital-acquired pneumonia, and complicated infections involving the urinary tract, skin and soft tissues, or intra-abdomen. For severe pseudomonas infections these antipseudomonal penicillins can be given with an aminoglycoside (e.g. gentamicin p. 596) since they have a synergistic effect.

Mecillinams

Pivmecillinam hydrochloride p. 642 has significant activity against many Gram-negative bacteria including *Escherichia coli*, klebsiella, enterobacter, and salmonellae. It is not active against *Pseudomonas aeruginosa* or enterococci. Pivmecillinam hydrochloride is hydrolysed to mecillinam, which is the active drug.

Penicillins

- **DRUG ACTION** The penicillins are bactericidal and act by interfering with bacterial cell wall synthesis. They diffuse well into body tissues and fluids, but penetration into the cerebrospinal fluid is poor except when the meninges are inflamed. They are excreted in the urine in therapeutic concentrations.

- **CAUTIONS** History of allergy

- **SIDE-EFFECTS**
- **Common or very common** Diarrhoea · hypersensitivity · nausea · skin reactions · thrombocytopenia · vomiting
- **Uncommon** Arthralgia · leucopenia
- **Rare or very rare** Agranulocytosis · angioedema · haemolytic anaemia · hepatic disorders · nephritis tubulointerstitial · neutropenia · pseudomembranous enterocolitis · seizure · severe cutaneous adverse reactions (SCARs)

  SIDE-EFFECTS, FURTHER INFORMATION Diarrhoea frequently occurs during oral penicillin therapy. It is most common with broad-spectrum penicillins, which can cause antibiotic-associated colitis.

- **ALLERGY AND CROSS-SENSITIVITY** The most important side-effect of the penicillins is hypersensitivity which causes rashes and anaphylaxis and can be fatal. Allergic reactions to penicillins occur in 1–10% of exposed individuals; anaphylactic reactions occur in fewer than 0.05% of treated patients. Patients with a history of atopic allergy (e.g. asthma, eczema, hay fever) are at a higher risk of anaphylactic reactions to penicillins. Individuals with a history of anaphylaxis, urticaria, or rash immediately after penicillin administration are at risk of immediate hypersensitivity to a penicillin; these individuals should not receive a penicillin. Individuals with a history of a minor rash (i.e. non-confluent, non-pruritic rash restricted to a small area of the body) or a rash that occurs more than 72 hours after penicillin administration are probably not allergic to penicillin and in these individuals a penicillin should not be withheld unnecessarily for serious infections; the possibility of an allergic reaction should,

however, be borne in mind. Other beta-lactam antibiotics (including cephalosporins) can be used in these patients.

Patients who are allergic to one penicillin will be allergic to all because the hypersensitivity is related to the basic penicillin structure. Patients with a history of immediate hypersensitivity to penicillins may also react to the cephalosporins and other beta-lactam antibiotics, they should not receive these antibiotics. If a penicillin (or another beta-lactam antibiotic) is essential in an individual with immediate hypersensitivity to penicillin then specialist advice should be sought on hypersensitivity testing or using a beta-lactam antibiotic with a different structure to the penicillin that caused the hypersensitivity.

ANTIBACTERIALS › PENICILLINS, ANTIPSEUDOMONAL WITH BETA-LACTAMASE INHIBITOR

◤ above

Piperacillin with tazobactam
10-Feb-2025

- **INDICATIONS AND DOSE**

  Hospital-acquired pneumonia | Septicaemia | Complicated infections involving the urinary-tract | Complicated infections involving the skin | Complicated infections involving the soft-tissues | Acute exacerbation of chronic obstructive pulmonary disease | Acute exacerbation of bronchiectasis | Moderate diabetic foot infection | Severe diabetic foot infection | Leg ulcer infection
  - ▸ BY INTRAVENOUS INFUSION
  - ▸ Adult: 4.5 g every 8 hours; increased if necessary to 4.5 g every 6 hours, increased frequency may be used for severe infections

  Infections in neutropenic patients
  - ▸ BY INTRAVENOUS INFUSION
  - ▸ Adult: 4.5 g every 6 hours

  DOSE EQUIVALENCE AND CONVERSION
  - ▸ Doses are expressed as piperacillin with tazobactam: the total of piperacillin and tazobactam components (both as sodium salts) in a ratio of 8:1.
  - ▸ Piperacillin with tazobactam 4.5 g consists of piperacillin 4 g and tazobactam 500 mg; piperacillin with tazobactam 2.25 g consists of piperacillin 2 g and tazobactam 250 mg.

- **UNLICENSED USE** [EvGr] Piperacillin with tazobactam is used for the treatment of acute exacerbation of chronic obstructive pulmonary disease, Ⓐ but is not licensed for this indication.

  [EvGr] Piperacillin with tazobactam is used for the treatment of acute exacerbation of bronchiectasis, Ⓐ but is not licensed for this indication.

- **CAUTIONS** High doses may lead to hypernatraemia (owing to sodium content of preparations)

- **INTERACTIONS** → Appendix 1: penicillins

- **SIDE-EFFECTS**
- **Common or very common** Anaemia · candida infection · constipation · gastrointestinal discomfort · headache · insomnia
- **Uncommon** Flushing · hypokalaemia · hypotension · myalgia · thrombophlebitis
- **Rare or very rare** Epistaxis · stomatitis
- **Frequency not known** Eosinophilia · pancytopenia · pneumonia eosinophilic · renal failure · thrombocytosis

- **PREGNANCY** Manufacturers advise use only if potential benefit outweighs risk.

- **BREAST FEEDING** Trace amount in milk, but appropriate to use.

5

Infection

- RENAL IMPAIRMENT

  Dose adjustments See p. 21.

  [EvGr] Max. 4.5 g every 8 hours if creatinine clearance 20–40 mL/minute.

  Max. 4.5 g every 12 hours if creatinine clearance less than 20 mL/minute. ◆M◆

- EFFECT ON LABORATORY TESTS False-positive urinary glucose (if tested for reducing substances).

- DIRECTIONS FOR ADMINISTRATION For *intravenous infusion*, give intermittently in Glucose 5% or Sodium chloride 0.9%. Reconstitute initially (2.25 g in 10 mL, 4.5 g in 20 mL) with water for injections, or glucose 5% (*Tazocin*® brand only), or sodium chloride 0.9%, then dilute to 50–150 mL with infusion fluid; give over 30 minutes.

- PRESCRIBING AND DISPENSING INFORMATION For choice of antibacterial therapy, see Diabetic foot infections, antibacterial therapy p. 581, Respiratory system infections, antibacterial therapy p. 586, Skin infections, antibacterial therapy p. 589, Urinary-tract infections p. 681.

- MEDICINAL FORMS There can be variation in the licensing of different medicines containing the same drug. Forms available from special-order manufacturers include: infusion, powder for solution for infusion

  Powder for solution for infusion

  ELECTROLYTES: May contain Sodium

  - Piperacillin with tazobactam (Non-proprietary)

    Tazobactam (as Tazobactam sodium) 250 mg, Piperacillin (as Piperacillin sodium) 2 gram Piperacillin 2g / Tazobactam 250mg powder for solution for infusion vials | 1 vial [PoM] £7.85 (Hospital only) | 10 vial [PoM] £7.65–£108.90 (Hospital only)

    Tazobactam (as Tazobactam sodium) 500 mg, Piperacillin (as Piperacillin sodium) 4 gram Piperacillin 4g / Tazobactam 500mg powder for solution for infusion vials | 1 vial [PoM] £15.75–£19.97 (Hospital only) | 10 vial [PoM] £48.00–£223.90 (Hospital only)

  - Tazocin (Pfizer Ltd)

    Tazobactam (as Tazobactam sodium) 250 mg, Piperacillin (as Piperacillin sodium) 2 gram Tazocin 2g/0.25g powder for solution for infusion vials | 1 vial [PoM] £7.65 (Hospital only)

    Tazobactam (as Tazobactam sodium) 500 mg, Piperacillin (as Piperacillin sodium) 4 gram Tazocin 4g/0.5g powder for solution for infusion vials | 1 vial [PoM] £15.17 (Hospital only)

ANTIBACTERIALS > PENICILLINS, BETA-LACTAMASE SENSITIVE

◀ 631

Benzathine benzylpenicillin

10-Nov-2023

(Benzathine penicillin G)

- INDICATIONS AND DOSE

  Erysipelas | Yaws | Pinta | Prevention of secondary case of diphtheria

  ▸ BY DEEP INTRAMUSCULAR INJECTION

  ▸ Adult: 1.2 million units for 1 dose, outer quadrant of the gluteus maximus or Hochstetter's ventrogluteal field is the preferred site of injection

  Early syphilis [primary, secondary, and early latent—less than 2 years since infection] | Asymptomatic contacts of patients with infectious syphilis

  ▸ BY DEEP INTRAMUSCULAR INJECTION

  ▸ Adult: 2.4 million units for 1 dose, outer quadrant of the gluteus maximus or Hochstetter's ventrogluteal field is the preferred site of injection, in the third trimester of pregnancy (week 28 onwards) the dose should be repeated after 7 days

  Late latent syphilis [more than 2 years since infection]

  ▸ BY DEEP INTRAMUSCULAR INJECTION

  ▸ Adult: 2.4 million units once weekly for 3 weeks, outer quadrant of the gluteus maximus or Hochstetter's ventrogluteal field is the preferred site of injection

  Prophylaxis of rheumatic fever [without cardiac involvement] | Prophylaxis of poststreptococcal glomerulonephritis [without cardiac involvement] | Prophylaxis of erysipelas [without cardiac involvement]

  ▸ BY DEEP INTRAMUSCULAR INJECTION

  ▸ Adult: 1.2 million units every 3–4 weeks for at least 5 years or up to 21 years of age (whichever is longer), outer quadrant of the gluteus maximus or Hochstetter's ventrogluteal field is the preferred site of injection

  Prophylaxis of rheumatic fever [transient cardiac involvement] | Prophylaxis of poststreptococcal glomerulonephritis [transient cardiac involvement] | Prophylaxis of erysipelas [transient cardiac involvement]

  ▸ BY DEEP INTRAMUSCULAR INJECTION

  ▸ Adult: 1.2 million units every 3–4 weeks for at least 10 years or up to 21 years of age (whichever is longer), outer quadrant of the gluteus maximus or Hochstetter's ventrogluteal field is the preferred site of injection

  Prophylaxis of rheumatic fever [persistent cardiac involvement] | Prophylaxis of poststreptococcal glomerulonephritis [persistent cardiac involvement] | Prophylaxis of erysipelas [persistent cardiac involvement]

  ▸ BY DEEP INTRAMUSCULAR INJECTION

  ▸ Adult: 1.2 million units every 3–4 weeks for at least 10 years or up to 40 years of age (whichever is longer); life-long prophylaxis may be necessary, outer quadrant of the gluteus maximus or Hochstetter's ventrogluteal field is the preferred site of injection

- UNLICENSED USE UKHSA advises benzathine benzylpenicillin is used for the prevention of diphtheria, but is not licensed for this indication.

> IMPORTANT SAFETY INFORMATION
>
> When prescribing, dispensing, or administering, check that this is the correct preparation—benzathine benzylpenicillin is a long-acting form of benzylpenicillin and is **not** interchangeable with benzylpenicillin sodium.
>
> SAFE PRACTICE
>
> Benzathine benzylpenicillin has been confused with benzylpenicillin sodium; care must be taken to ensure the correct drug is prescribed and dispensed.

- INTERACTIONS → Appendix 1: penicillins

- SIDE-EFFECTS

  ▸ **Common or very common** Increased risk of infection

  ▸ **Uncommon** Oral disorders

  ▸ **Rare or very rare** Nephropathy

  ▸ **Frequency not known** Antibiotic associated colitis · encephalopathy · Hoigne's syndrome · Jarisch-Herxheimer reaction

- ALLERGY AND CROSS-SENSITIVITY Contra-indicated in patients allergic to peanuts or soya (contains phospholipids from soya lecithin).

- PREGNANCY Manufacturer advises not known to be harmful.

- BREAST FEEDING Manufacturer advises present in milk in small amounts but not known to be harmful. Monitor infant for effects on the gastrointestinal flora; discontinue breast feeding if diarrhoea, candidiasis or rash in the infant occur.

- **HEPATIC IMPAIRMENT** Manufacturer advises caution in impairment (possible risk of delayed metabolism and excretion in severe impairment).
- **RENAL IMPAIRMENT** Manufacturer advises caution in impairment (possible risk of delayed metabolism and excretion in severe impairment).
  Dose adjustments Manufacturer advises reduce daily dose by 25% and give as a single dose if creatinine clearance 15–59 mL/minute; reduce daily dose by 50–80% and give in 2–3 divided doses if creatinine clearance less than 15 mL/minute (maximum 1–3 million units per day). See p. 21.
- **MONITORING REQUIREMENTS**
- ▶ Manufacturer advises observe the patient for hypersensitivity reactions for at least 30 minutes after the injection.
- ▶ Manufacturer advises monitor renal, hepatic and haematopoietic function periodically in patients on long-term treatment.
- **EFFECT ON LABORATORY TESTS** False-positive direct Coombs' test. False-positive urinary glucose. False-positive urobilinogen. False-positive urinary protein using precipitation techniques, the Folin-Ciocalteu-Lowry method, or the biuret method. False-positive urinary amino acids using the ninhydrin method. Increased levels of urinary 17-ketosteriods using the Zimmermann reaction.
- **DIRECTIONS FOR ADMINISTRATION** For *deep intramuscular injection*, manufacturer advises reconstitute with Water for Injections and inject slowly with low pressure. No more than 5 mL should be administered per injection site and do not administer into tissues with reduced perfusion. Avoid rubbing the injection site after the injection.
- **PRESCRIBING AND DISPENSING INFORMATION** For choice of antibacterial therapy, see Antibacterials, use for prophylaxis p. 574, Genital system infections, antibacterial therapy p. 584.

- **MEDICINAL FORMS** There can be variation in the licensing of different medicines containing the same drug.
  Powder and solvent for suspension for injection
  EXCIPIENTS: May contain Lecithin, polysorbates
  - ▶ Benzathine benzylpenicillin (Non-proprietary)
    Benzathine benzylpenicillin 1.2 mega unit Extencilline 1.2million unit powder and solvent for suspension for injection vials | 50 vial [PoM] [⅀] (Hospital only)
    Benzathine benzylpenicillin 2.4 mega unit Benzetacil 2.4million unit powder and solvent for suspension for injection vials | 1 vial [PoM] [⅀] (Hospital only)
    Retarpen 2.4million unit powder and solvent for suspension for injection vials | 50 vial [PoM] [⅀] (Hospital only)
    Benzathine benzylpenicillin 600000 unit Extencilline 600,000units powder and solvent for suspension for injection vials | 50 vial [PoM] [⅀] (Hospital only)

▶ **631**

Benzylpenicillin sodium

10-Feb-2025

(Penicillin G)

- **INDICATIONS AND DOSE**

Mild to moderate susceptible infections | Throat infections | Otitis media | Pneumonia | Cellulitis
- ▶ BY INTRAMUSCULAR INJECTION
- ▶ Adult: 0.6–1.2 g every 6 hours
- ▶ BY SLOW INTRAVENOUS INJECTION, OR BY INTRAVENOUS INFUSION
- ▶ Adult: 0.6–1.2 g every 6 hours, dose may be increased if necessary in more serious infections (consult product literature)

Endocarditis (in combination with other antibacterial if necessary)
- ▶ BY SLOW INTRAVENOUS INJECTION, OR BY INTRAVENOUS INFUSION
- ▶ Adult: 1.2 g every 4 hours, increased if necessary to 2.4 g every 4 hours, dose may be increased in infections such as enterococcal endocarditis

Anthrax (in combination with other antibacterials)
- ▶ BY SLOW INTRAVENOUS INJECTION, OR BY INTRAVENOUS INFUSION
- ▶ Adult: 2.4 g every 4 hours

Intrapartum prophylaxis against group B streptococcal infection
- ▶ BY SLOW INTRAVENOUS INJECTION, OR BY INTRAVENOUS INFUSION
- ▶ Adult: Initially 3 g for 1 dose, then 1.5 g every 4 hours until delivery

Meningitis | Meningococcal disease
- ▶ BY SLOW INTRAVENOUS INJECTION, OR BY INTRAVENOUS INFUSION
- ▶ Adult: 2.4 g every 4 hours
- ▶ BY INTRAVENOUS INFUSION
- ▶ Neonate up to 7 days: 50 mg/kg every 12 hours.
- ▶ Neonate 7 days to 28 days: 50 mg/kg every 8 hours.
- ▶ Child: 50 mg/kg every 4–6 hours (max. per dose 2.4 g)

Suspected meningococcal disease [pre-hospital treatment]
- ▶ BY INTRAVENOUS INJECTION, OR BY INTRAMUSCULAR INJECTION
- ▶ Neonate: 300 mg for 1 dose, administer prior to urgent transfer to hospital unless this will delay transfer.
- ▶ Child 1-11 months: 300 mg for 1 dose, administer prior to urgent transfer to hospital unless this will delay transfer
- ▶ Child 1-9 years: 600 mg for 1 dose, administer prior to urgent transfer to hospital unless this will delay transfer
- ▶ Child 10-17 years: 1.2 g for 1 dose, administer prior to urgent transfer to hospital unless this will delay transfer
- ▶ Adult: 1.2 g for 1 dose, administer prior to urgent transfer to hospital unless this will delay transfer

Suspected bacterial meningitis [pre-hospital treatment where there is likely to be a clinically significant delay in transfer to hospital]
- ▶ BY INTRAVENOUS INJECTION, OR BY INTRAMUSCULAR INJECTION
- ▶ Child 1-11 months: 300 mg for 1 dose, administer prior to transfer to hospital
- ▶ Child 1-9 years: 600 mg for 1 dose, administer prior to transfer to hospital
- ▶ Child 10-17 years: 1.2 g for 1 dose, administer prior to transfer to hospital
- ▶ Adult: 1.2 g for 1 dose, administer prior to transfer to hospital

Severe diphtheria [confirmed or probable] (in combination with a macrolide)
- ▶ BY SLOW INTRAVENOUS INJECTION, OR BY INTRAVENOUS INFUSION
- ▶ Adult: 1.2–2.4 g every 6 hours for 14 days

- **UNLICENSED USE** UKHSA advises benzylpenicillin sodium is used in the doses provided in BNF Publications for the

treatment of diphtheria, but these may differ from those licensed.
▸ In adults Benzylpenicillin sodium doses in the BNF may differ from those in product literature.

> **IMPORTANT SAFETY INFORMATION**
>
> Intrathecal injection of benzylpenicillin sodium is **not** recommended.
>
> When prescribing, dispensing, or administering, check that this is the correct preparation—benzylpenicillin sodium is a short-acting form of benzylpenicillin and is **not** interchangeable with benzathine benzylpenicillin.
>
> **SAFE PRACTICE**
>
> Benzylpenicillin sodium has been confused with benzathine benzylpenicillin; care must be taken to ensure the correct drug is prescribed and dispensed.

● CAUTIONS Accumulation of sodium from injection can occur with high doses

● INTERACTIONS → Appendix 1: penicillins

● SIDE-EFFECTS
▸ **Common or very common** Fever · Jarisch-Herxheimer reaction
▸ **Rare or very rare** Neurotoxicity
▸ **Frequency not known** Coma

● PREGNANCY Not known to be harmful.

● BREAST FEEDING Trace amounts in milk, but appropriate to use.

● RENAL IMPAIRMENT Accumulation of sodium from injection can occur in renal failure. High doses may cause neurotoxicity, including cerebral irritation, convulsions, or coma.
Dose adjustments
  ▸ In adults EvGr Reduce dose (consult product literature).
  Ⓜ
  ▸ In children Expert sources advise use normal dose every 8–12 hours if estimated glomerular filtration rate 10–50 mL/minute/1.73 m^2; use normal dose every 12 hours if estimated glomerular filtration rate less than 10 mL/minute/1.73 m^2. See p. 21.

● EFFECT ON LABORATORY TESTS False-positive urinary glucose (if tested for reducing substances).

● DIRECTIONS FOR ADMINISTRATION
▸ In children Intravenous route recommended in neonates and infants. For *intravenous infusion*, dilute with Glucose 5% *or* Sodium Chloride 0.9%; give over 15–30 minutes. Longer administration time is particularly important when using doses of 50 mg/kg (or greater) to avoid CNS toxicity.
▸ In adults For *intravenous infusion*, give intermittently *in* Glucose 5% *or* Sodium chloride 0.9%; suggested volume 100 mL given over 30–60 minutes. Continuous infusion not usually recommended.

● PRESCRIBING AND DISPENSING INFORMATION For choice of antibacterial therapy, see Anthrax p. 667, Antibacterials, use for prophylaxis p. 574, Cardiovascular system infections, antibacterial therapy p. 579, Central nervous system infections, antibacterial therapy p. 580, Respiratory system infections, antibacterial therapy p. 586, Skin infections, antibacterial therapy p. 589.

● MEDICINAL FORMS There can be variation in the licensing of different medicines containing the same drug. Forms available from special-order manufacturers include: infusion

Powder for solution for injection
ELECTROLYTES: May contain Sodium
  ▸ Benzylpenicillin sodium (Non-proprietary)
  Benzylpenicillin sodium 600 mg Benzylpenicillin sodium 600mg powder for solution for injection vials | 1 vial PoM £2.56 | 2 vial PoM £6.01 | 10 vial PoM £25.59 | 25 vial PoM £75.12
  Benzylpenicillin sodium 1.2 gram Benzylpenicillin sodium 1.2g powder for solution for injection vials | 25 vial PoM £109.49

⚑ 631

Phenoxymethylpenicillin
(Penicillin V)

11-Nov-2021

● INDICATIONS AND DOSE

Oral infections | Otitis media
▸ BY MOUTH
▸ Child 1–11 months: 62.5 mg 4 times a day, increased if necessary up to 12.5 mg/kg 4 times a day
▸ Child 1–5 years: 125 mg 4 times a day, increased if necessary up to 12.5 mg/kg 4 times a day
▸ Child 6–11 years: 250 mg 4 times a day, increased if necessary up to 12.5 mg/kg 4 times a day
▸ Child 12–17 years: 500 mg 4 times a day, increased if necessary up to 1 g 4 times a day
▸ Adult: 500 mg every 6 hours, increased if necessary up to 1 g every 6 hours

Acute sore throat
▸ BY MOUTH
▸ Child 1–11 months: 62.5 mg 4 times a day for 5–10 days, alternatively 125 mg twice daily for 5–10 days
▸ Child 1–5 years: 125 mg 4 times a day for 5–10 days, alternatively 250 mg twice daily for 5–10 days
▸ Child 6–11 years: 250 mg 4 times a day for 5–10 days, alternatively 500 mg twice daily for 5–10 days
▸ Child 12–17 years: 500 mg 4 times a day for 5–10 days, alternatively 1000 mg twice daily for 5–10 days
▸ Adult: 500 mg 4 times a day for 5–10 days, alternatively 1000 mg twice daily for 5–10 days

Prevention of recurrent cellulitis (specialist use only) | Prevention of recurrent erysipelas (specialist use only)
▸ BY MOUTH
▸ Adult: 250 mg twice daily

Prevention of recurrence of rheumatic fever
▸ BY MOUTH
▸ Child 1 month–5 years: 125 mg twice daily
▸ Child 6–17 years: 250 mg twice daily
▸ Adult: 250 mg twice daily

Prevention of secondary case of invasive group A streptococcal infection
▸ BY MOUTH
▸ Child 1–11 months: 62.5 mg every 6 hours for 10 days
▸ Child 1–5 years: 125 mg every 6 hours for 10 days
▸ Child 6–11 years: 250 mg every 6 hours for 10 days
▸ Child 12–17 years: 250–500 mg every 6 hours for 10 days
▸ Adult: 250–500 mg every 6 hours for 10 days

Prevention of pneumococcal infection in asplenia or in patients with sickle-cell disease
▸ BY MOUTH
▸ Child 1–11 months: 62.5 mg twice daily
▸ Child 1–4 years: 125 mg twice daily
▸ Child 5–17 years: 250 mg twice daily
▸ Adult: 250 mg twice daily

Acute sinusitis
▸ BY MOUTH
▸ Child 1–11 months: 62.5 mg 4 times a day for 5 days
▸ Child 1–5 years: 125 mg 4 times a day for 5 days
▸ Child 6–11 years: 250 mg 4 times a day for 5 days
▸ Child 12–17 years: 500 mg 4 times a day for 5 days
▸ Adult: 500 mg 4 times a day for 5 days

● UNLICENSED USE EvGr Duration of treatment for acute sinusitis adheres to national guidelines. Ⓐ See Sinusitis (acute) p. 1368 for further information.
  EvGr Phenoxymethylpenicillin is used for the prevention of recurrent cellulitis, Ⓐ but is not licensed for this indication.
  EvGr Phenoxymethylpenicillin is used for the prevention of recurrent erysipelas, Ⓐ but is not licensed for this indication.

Phenoxymethylpenicillin doses in BNF Publications may differ from product literature.

- **INTERACTIONS** → Appendix 1: penicillins
- **SIDE-EFFECTS** Circulatory collapse · coagulation disorder · eosinophilia · faeces soft · fever · increased risk of infection · neurotoxicity · oral disorders · paraesthesia
- **PREGNANCY** Not known to be harmful.
- **BREAST FEEDING** Trace amounts in milk, but appropriate to use.
- **EFFECT ON LABORATORY TESTS** False-positive urinary glucose (if tested for reducing substances).
- **PRESCRIBING AND DISPENSING INFORMATION** For choice of antibacterial therapy, see Antibacterials, use for prophylaxis p. 574, Nose infections, antibacterial therapy p. 585, Oral bacterial infections p. 585, Oropharyngeal infections, antibacterial therapy p. 1383, Skin infections, antibacterial therapy p. 589.
- **PATIENT AND CARER ADVICE**
  Medicines for Children leaflet: Penicillin V for bacterial infections www.medicinesforchildren.org.uk/medicines/penicillin-v-for-bacterial-infections/
  Medicines for Children leaflet: Penicillin V for prevention of pneumococcal infection www.medicinesforchildren.org.uk/medicines/penicillin-v-for-prevention-of-pneumococcal-infection/
- **PROFESSION SPECIFIC INFORMATION**
  Dental practitioners' formulary Phenoxymethylpenicillin Tablets may be prescribed.
  Phenoxymethylpenicillin Oral Solution may be prescribed.

- **MEDICINAL FORMS** There can be variation in the licensing of different medicines containing the same drug.
  Oral tablet
  CAUTIONARY AND ADVISORY LABELS 9, 23
  - Phenoxymethylpenicillin (Non-proprietary)
    Phenoxymethylpenicillin (as Phenoxymethylpenicillin potassium) 250 mg Phenoxymethylpenicillin 250mg tablets | 28 tablet [PoM] £5.00 DT = £1.07
    Phenoxymethylpenicillin (as Phenoxymethylpenicillin potassium) 500 mg Phenoxymethylpenicillin 500mg tablets | 20 tablet [PoM] £3.99

  Oral solution
  CAUTIONARY AND ADVISORY LABELS 9, 23
  - Phenoxymethylpenicillin (Non-proprietary)
    Phenoxymethylpenicillin (as Phenoxymethylpenicillin potassium) 25 mg per 1 ml Phenoxymethylpenicillin 125mg/5ml oral solution | 100 ml [PoM] £25.00 DT = £2.32
    Phenoxymethylpenicillin 125mg/5ml oral solution sugar free | 100 ml [PoM] £25.00 DT = £5.29 [SF]
    Phenoxymethylpenicillin (as Phenoxymethylpenicillin potassium) 50 mg per 1 ml Phenoxymethylpenicillin 250mg/5ml oral solution | 100 ml [PoM] £35.00 DT = £3.05
    Phenoxymethylpenicillin 250mg/5ml oral solution sugar free | 100 ml [PoM] £35.00 DT = £3.35 [SF]

ANTIBACTERIALS › PENICILLINS, BROAD-SPECTRUM

F 631

Amoxicillin
24-Jul-2024

(Amoxycillin)

- **INDICATIONS AND DOSE**
  Susceptible infections (e.g. sinusitis, salmonellosis, oral infections)
  ▸ BY MOUTH
  - Child 1-11 months: 125 mg 3 times a day, increased if necessary up to 30 mg/kg 3 times a day
  - Child 1-4 years: 250 mg 3 times a day, increased if necessary up to 30 mg/kg 3 times a day

- Child 5-11 years: 500 mg 3 times a day, increased if necessary up to 30 mg/kg 3 times a day (max. per dose 1 g)
- Child 12-17 years: 500 mg 3 times a day, increased if necessary up to 1 g 3 times a day, use increased dose in severe infections
- Adult: 500 mg every 8 hours, increased if necessary to 1 g every 8 hours, increased dose used in severe infections
▸ BY INTRAMUSCULAR INJECTION
- Adult: 500 mg every 8 hours
▸ BY INTRAVENOUS INJECTION, OR BY INTRAVENOUS INFUSION
- Adult: 500 mg every 8 hours, increased to 1 g every 6 hours, use increased dose in severe infections

Community-acquired pneumonia
▸ BY MOUTH
- Child 1-11 months: 125 mg 3 times a day for 5 days, increased if necessary up to 30 mg/kg 3 times a day
- Child 1-4 years: 250 mg 3 times a day for 5 days, increased if necessary up to 30 mg/kg 3 times a day
- Child 5-11 years: 500 mg 3 times a day for 5 days, increased if necessary up to 30 mg/kg 3 times a day (max. per dose 1 g)
- Child 12-17 years: 500 mg 3 times a day for 5 days, increased if necessary up to 1 g 3 times a day
- Adult: 500 mg 3 times a day for 5 days, increased if necessary to 1 g 3 times a day

Acute exacerbation of bronchiectasis
▸ BY MOUTH
- Child 1-11 months: 125 mg 3 times a day for 7–14 days
- Child 1-4 years: 250 mg 3 times a day for 7–14 days
- Child 5-17 years: 500 mg 3 times a day for 7–14 days
- Adult: 500 mg 3 times a day for 7–14 days

Acute exacerbation of chronic obstructive pulmonary disease
▸ BY MOUTH
- Adult: 500 mg 3 times a day for 5 days, increased if necessary to 1 g 3 times a day, increased dose used in severe infections
▸ BY INTRAVENOUS INJECTION, OR BY INTRAVENOUS INFUSION
- Adult: 500 mg every 8 hours, increased to 1 g every 6 hours, increased dose used in severe infections

Acute cough [if systemically very unwell or at higher risk of complications]
▸ BY MOUTH
- Child 1-11 months: 125 mg 3 times a day for 5 days
- Child 1-4 years: 250 mg 3 times a day for 5 days
- Child 5-17 years: 500 mg 3 times a day for 5 days
- Adult: 500 mg 3 times a day for 5 days

Acute otitis media
▸ BY MOUTH
- Child 1-11 months: 125 mg 3 times a day for 5–7 days
- Child 1-4 years: 250 mg 3 times a day for 5–7 days
- Child 5-17 years: 500 mg 3 times a day for 5–7 days

Lyme disease [erythema migrans and/or non-focal symptoms] | Lyme disease [affecting cranial nerves or peripheral nervous system]
▸ BY MOUTH
- Adult: 1 g 3 times a day for 21 days

Lyme arthritis | Acrodermatitis chronica atrophicans
▸ BY MOUTH
- Adult: 1 g 3 times a day for 28 days

Anthrax (treatment and post-exposure prophylaxis)
▸ BY MOUTH
- Adult: 500 mg 3 times a day

Dental abscess (short course)
▸ BY MOUTH
- Adult: 3 g for 1 dose, then 3 g for 1 dose, to be given 8 hours after the first dose   continued →

Infection

5

Listerial meningitis
▸ BY INTRAVENOUS INFUSION
▸ Adult: 2 g every 4 hours

Endocarditis (in combination with another antibiotic if necessary)
▸ BY INTRAVENOUS INFUSION
▸ Adult: 2 g every 4 hours

Helicobacter pylori eradication [in combination with other drugs]
▸ BY MOUTH
▸ Adult: 1 g twice daily for 7 days for first- and second-line eradication therapy; 10 days for third-line eradication therapy

Acute diverticulitis [in combination with gentamicin and metronidazole]
▸ BY INTRAVENOUS INJECTION, OR BY INTRAVENOUS INFUSION
▸ Adult: 500 mg every 8 hours; increased if necessary to 1 g every 6 hours, increased dose used in severe infections

Prophylaxis of recurrent urinary-tract infection
▸ BY MOUTH
▸ Adult: 250 mg once daily, dose to be taken at night, alternatively 500 mg for 1 dose, dose to be taken following exposure to a trigger

Lower urinary-tract infection in pregnancy
▸ BY MOUTH
▸ Adult: 500 mg 3 times a day for 7 days

Lower urinary-tract infection
▸ BY MOUTH
▸ Child 3–11 months: 125 mg 3 times a day for 3 days
▸ Child 1–4 years: 250 mg 3 times a day for 3 days
▸ Child 5–15 years: 500 mg 3 times a day for 3 days

Urinary-tract infections (short course)
▸ BY MOUTH
▸ Adult: 3 g for 1 dose, then 3 g for 1 dose, to be given 10–12 hours after the first dose

Asymptomatic bacteriuria in pregnancy
▸ BY MOUTH
▸ Adult: 250–500 mg 3 times a day, alternatively 750–1000 mg twice daily

Urinary-tract infection (catheter-associated)
▸ BY MOUTH
▸ Child 16–17 years: 500 mg 3 times a day for 7 days
▸ Adult: 500 mg 3 times a day for 7 days

● **UNLICENSED USE** Amoxicillin doses in BNF Publications may differ from those in product literature.

EvGr Duration of treatment for acute otitis media differs from product literature and adheres to national guidelines.

Amoxicillin is used for the treatment of acute exacerbation of bronchiectasis, A but is not licensed for this indication.

EvGr Amoxicillin is used for prophylaxis of recurrent urinary-tract infection, A but is not licensed for this indication.

EvGr Combination regimens and durations for *Helicobacter pylori* eradication may differ from product literature but adhere to national guidelines. A

● **CAUTIONS**

GENERAL CAUTIONS Acute lymphocytic leukaemia (increased risk of erythematous rashes) · chronic lymphocytic leukaemia (increased risk of erythematous rashes) · cytomegalovirus infection (increased risk of erythematous rashes) · glandular fever (erythematous rashes common) · maintain adequate hydration with high doses (particularly during parenteral therapy)

SPECIFIC CAUTIONS
▸ With intravenous use Accumulation of sodium can occur with high parenteral doses

● **INTERACTIONS** → Appendix 1: penicillins

● **SIDE-EFFECTS**

GENERAL SIDE-EFFECTS
▸ **Rare or very rare** Antibiotic associated colitis · colitis haemorrhagic · crystalluria · dizziness · hyperkinesia · hypersensitivity vasculitis · mucocutaneous candidiasis
▸ **Frequency not known** Enterocolitis · Jarisch-Herxheimer reaction

SPECIFIC SIDE-EFFECTS
▸ **Rare or very rare**
▸ With oral use Black hairy tongue

● **PREGNANCY** Not known to be harmful.

● **BREAST FEEDING** Trace amount in milk, but appropriate to use.

● **HEPATIC IMPAIRMENT** Manufacturer advises caution.

● **RENAL IMPAIRMENT** Increased risk of convulsions. Accumulation of sodium from injection can occur in patients with renal impairment. Risk of crystalluria with high doses (particularly during parenteral therapy).
Dose adjustments See p. 21.
▸ In adults EvGr Reduce dose if eGFR 30 mL/minute/1.73 m^2 or less (consult product literature). M
▸ In children EvGr Reduce dose if estimated glomerular filtration rate 30 mL/minute/1.73 m^2 or less (consult product literature). M

● **DIRECTIONS FOR ADMINISTRATION** For *intravenous infusion* (*Amoxil*®), give intermittently *in* Glucose 5% *or* Sodium chloride 0.9%. Reconstituted solutions diluted and given without delay; suggested volume 100 mL given over 30–60 minutes or *give via* drip tubing *in* Glucose 5% *or* Sodium chloride 0.9%; continuous infusion not usually recommended.

● **PRESCRIBING AND DISPENSING INFORMATION** For choice of antibacterial therapy, see Anthrax p. 667, Cardiovascular system infections, antibacterial therapy p. 579, Central nervous system infections, antibacterial therapy p. 580, Ear infections, antibacterial therapy p. 582, Gastro-intestinal system infections, antibacterial therapy p. 582, Helicobacter pylori infection p. 93, Lyme disease p. 669, Nose infections, antibacterial therapy p. 585, Oral bacterial infections p. 585, Oropharyngeal infections, antibacterial therapy p. 1383, Respiratory system infections, antibacterial therapy p. 586, Urinary-tract infections p. 681.

● **PATIENT AND CARER ADVICE** Patient counselling is advised for amoxicillin oral suspension (use of oral dosing syringe). Medicines for Children leaflet: Amoxicillin for bacterial infections www.medicinesforchildren.org.uk/medicines/amoxicillin-for-bacterial-infections/

● **PROFESSION SPECIFIC INFORMATION**

Dental practitioners' formulary Amoxicillin capsules may be prescribed.

Amoxicillin sachets may be prescribed as Amoxicillin Oral Powder.

Amoxicillin Oral Suspension may be prescribed.

● **MEDICINAL FORMS** There can be variation in the licensing of different medicines containing the same drug.

Powder for solution for injection
ELECTROLYTES: May contain Sodium
▸ Amoxicillin (Non-proprietary)
  Amoxicillin (as Amoxicillin sodium) 250 mg Amoxicillin 250mg powder for solution for injection vials | 10 vial PoM £7.50 | 10 vial PoM £7.50 (Hospital only)
  Amoxicillin (as Amoxicillin sodium) 500 mg Amoxicillin 500mg powder for solution for injection vials | 10 vial PoM £12.00 DT = £9.60 (Hospital only) | 10 vial PoM £9.60 DT = £9.60
  Amoxicillin (as Amoxicillin sodium) 1 gram Amoxicillin 1g powder for solution for injection vials | 1 vial PoM £1.92 DT = £1.92 | 10 vial PoM £16.50 (Hospital only)

Oral suspension

CAUTIONARY AND ADVISORY LABELS 9
EXCIPIENTS: May contain Sucrose

▸ Amoxicillin (Non-proprietary)

Amoxicillin (as Amoxicillin trihydrate) 25 mg per 1 ml Amoxicillin 125mg/5ml oral suspension sugar free | 100 ml [PoM] £25.00 DT = £1.23 [SF]
Amoxicillin 125mg/5ml oral suspension | 100 ml [PoM] £25.00 DT = £1.43

Amoxicillin (as Amoxicillin trihydrate) 50 mg per 1 ml Amoxicillin 250mg/5ml oral suspension sugar free | 100 ml [PoM] £35.00 DT = £1.65 [SF]
Amoxicillin 250mg/5ml oral suspension | 100 ml [PoM] £35.00 DT = £1.61

Amoxicillin (as Amoxicillin trihydrate) 100 mg per 1 ml Amoxicillin 500mg/5ml oral suspension sugar free | 100 ml [PoM] £5.75-£10.00 DT = £6.45 [SF]

Oral capsule

CAUTIONARY AND ADVISORY LABELS 9

▸ Amoxicillin (Non-proprietary)

Amoxicillin (as Amoxicillin trihydrate) 250 mg Amoxicillin 250mg capsules | 15 capsule [PoM] £5.00 DT = £0.75 | 21 capsule [PoM] £8.99 DT = £1.05 | 500 capsule [PoM] £28.00-£120.00

Amoxicillin (as Amoxicillin trihydrate) 500 mg Amoxicillin 500mg capsules | 15 capsule [PoM] £7.85 DT = £0.97 | 21 capsule [PoM] £15.00 DT = £1.36 | 100 capsule [PoM] £6.48-£75.00

Powder for oral suspension

CAUTIONARY AND ADVISORY LABELS 9, 13

▸ Amoxicillin (Non-proprietary)

Amoxicillin (as Amoxicillin trihydrate) 3 gram Amoxicillin 3g oral powder sachets sugar free | 2 sachet [PoM] £45.10 DT = £45.10 [SF]

Combinations available: *Co-amoxiclav,* p. 638

F 631

Ampicillin

24-Jul-2024

● **INDICATIONS AND DOSE**

Susceptible infections (including bronchitis, urinary-tract infections, otitis media, sinusitis, uncomplicated community-acquired pneumonia, salmonellosis)

▸ BY MOUTH

▸ Child 1-11 months: 125 mg 4 times a day, increased if necessary up to 30 mg/kg 4 times a day

▸ Child 1-4 years: 250 mg 4 times a day, increased if necessary up to 30 mg/kg 4 times a day

▸ Child 5-11 years: 500 mg 4 times a day, increased if necessary up to 30 mg/kg 4 times a day (max. per dose 1 g)

▸ Child 12-17 years: 500 mg 4 times a day, increased if necessary to 1 g 4 times a day, use increased dose in severe infection

▸ Adult: 0.5–1 g every 6 hours

▸ BY INTRAVENOUS INJECTION, OR BY INTRAVENOUS INFUSION

▸ Adult: 500 mg every 4–6 hours

▸ BY INTRAMUSCULAR INJECTION

▸ Adult: 500 mg every 4–6 hours

Endocarditis (in combination with another antibacterial if necessary)

▸ BY INTRAVENOUS INFUSION

▸ Adult: 2 g every 4 hours

Listerial meningitis

▸ BY INTRAVENOUS INFUSION

▸ Adult: 2 g every 4 hours

● **UNLICENSED USE** Ampicillin doses in BNF Publications may differ from those in product literature.

● **CAUTIONS**

GENERAL CAUTIONS Acute lymphocytic leukaemia (increased risk of erythematous rashes) · chronic lymphocytic leukaemia (increased risk of erythematous rashes) · cytomegalovirus infection (increased risk of erythematous rashes) · glandular fever (erythematous rashes common)

SPECIFIC CAUTIONS

▸ With intravenous use Accumulation of electrolytes contained in parenteral preparations can occur with high doses

● INTERACTIONS → Appendix 1: penicillins

● SIDE-EFFECTS Colitis haemorrhagic

● PREGNANCY Not known to be harmful.

● BREAST FEEDING Trace amounts in milk, but appropriate to use.

● RENAL IMPAIRMENT Rashes more common in renal impairment. Accumulation of sodium from injection can occur in patients with renal failure.
Dose adjustments [EvGr] Consider dose reduction or increase dose interval if creatinine clearance less than 10 mL/minute, ⟨M⟩ see p. 21.

● DIRECTIONS FOR ADMINISTRATION

▸ With oral use Administer at least 30 minutes before food.

▸ With intravenous use For *intravenous infusion*, give intermittently *in* Glucose 5% *or* Sodium Chloride 0.9%. Reconstituted solutions diluted and given without delay; suggested volume 100 mL given over 30–60 minutes *via* drip tubing *in* Glucose 5% *or* Sodium Chloride 0.9%. Continuous infusion not usually recommended.

● PATIENT AND CARER ADVICE
Medicines for Children leaflet: Ampicillin for infection
www.medicinesforchildren.org.uk/medicines/ampicillin-for-infection/

● MEDICINAL FORMS There can be variation in the licensing of different medicines containing the same drug.

Oral capsule

CAUTIONARY AND ADVISORY LABELS 9, 23

▸ Ampicillin (Non-proprietary)

Ampicillin 500 mg Ampicillin 500mg capsules | 28 capsule [PoM] £47.96 DT = £47.96

Powder for solution for injection

▸ Ampicillin (Non-proprietary)

Ampicillin (as Ampicillin sodium) 500 mg Ampicillin 500mg powder for solution for injection vials | 10 vial [PoM] £82.22

F 631

Co-fluampicil

06-Feb-2025

● **INDICATIONS AND DOSE**

Mixed infections involving beta-lactamase-producing staphylococci

▸ BY MOUTH

▸ Child 10-17 years: 250/250 mg every 6 hours

▸ Adult: 250/250 mg every 6 hours

Severe mixed infections involving beta-lactamase-producing staphylococci

▸ BY MOUTH

▸ Child 10-17 years: 500/500 mg every 6 hours

▸ Adult: 500/500 mg every 6 hours

> **IMPORTANT SAFETY INFORMATION**
>
> HEPATIC DISORDERS
>
> Cholestatic jaundice and hepatitis may occur very rarely, up to two months after treatment with flucloxacillin has been stopped. Administration for more than 2 weeks and increasing age are risk factors. Manufacturer advises:
> - flucloxacillin should not be used in patients with a history of hepatic dysfunction associated with flucloxacillin;
> - flucloxacillin should be used with caution in patients with hepatic impairment;
> - careful enquiry should be made about hypersensitivity reactions to beta-lactam antibacterials.

● CAUTIONS Acute lymphocytic leukaemia (increased risk of erythematous rashes) · chronic lymphocytic leukaemia (increased risk of erythematous rashes) · cytomegalovirus infection (increased risk of erythematous rashes) · glandular fever (erythematous rashes common)

- **INTERACTIONS** → Appendix 1: penicillins
- **SIDE-EFFECTS** Bronchospasm · coma · dyspnoea · electrolyte imbalance · eosinophilia · erythema nodosum · gastrointestinal disorder · hallucination · Jarisch-Herxheimer reaction · myalgia · purpura non-thrombocytopenic · vasculitis
- **PREGNANCY** Not known to be harmful.
- **BREAST FEEDING** Trace amount in milk, but appropriate to use.
- **HEPATIC IMPAIRMENT** Manufacturer advises caution.
- **RENAL IMPAIRMENT**
  Dose adjustments EvGr Reduce dose or frequency if creatinine clearance less than 10 mL/minute, Ⓜ see p. 21.
- **EFFECT ON LABORATORY TESTS** False-positive urinary glucose (if tested for reducing substances).
- **PRESCRIBING AND DISPENSING INFORMATION** Dose expressed as a combination of equal parts by mass of flucloxacillin and ampicillin.

- **MEDICINAL FORMS** No licensed medicines listed.

ANTIBACTERIALS > PENICILLINS, BROAD-SPECTRUM WITH BETA-LACTAMASE INHIBITOR

⚑ 631

Co-amoxiclav

12-Aug-2024

- **INDICATIONS AND DOSE**

Infections due to beta-lactamase-producing strains (where amoxicillin alone not appropriate) [doses for 375 mg (250/125 mg) or 625 mg (500/125 mg) tablets]
▸ BY MOUTH USING TABLETS
▸ Child 12-17 years: 375 mg 3 times a day, alternatively 625 mg 3 times a day
▸ Adult: 375 mg 3 times a day, alternatively 625 mg 3 times a day

Infections due to beta-lactamase-producing strains (where amoxicillin alone not appropriate) [doses for 1 g (875/125 mg) tablets]
▸ BY MOUTH USING TABLETS
▸ Child 6-17 years (body-weight 25-39 kg): 1 g twice daily
▸ Child 6-17 years (body-weight 40 kg and above): 1 g twice daily, alternatively 1 g 3 times a day
▸ Adult: 1 g twice daily, alternatively 1 g 3 times a day

Infections due to beta-lactamase-producing strains (where amoxicillin alone not appropriate) [doses for 125/31 mg per 5 mL suspension]
▸ BY MOUTH USING ORAL SUSPENSION
▸ Child 1-11 months: 0.25 mL/kilogram 3 times a day, dose doubled if necessary
▸ Child 1-5 years: 0.25 mL/kilogram 3 times a day, dose doubled if necessary, alternatively 5 mL 3 times a day, dose doubled if necessary

Infections due to beta-lactamase-producing strains (where amoxicillin alone not appropriate) [doses for 250/62 mg per 5 mL suspension]
▸ BY MOUTH USING ORAL SUSPENSION
▸ Child 6-11 years: 0.15 mL/kilogram 3 times a day, dose doubled if necessary, alternatively 5 mL 3 times a day, dose doubled if necessary

Infections due to beta-lactamase-producing strains (where amoxicillin alone not appropriate) [doses for 400/57 mg per 5 mL suspension]
▸ BY MOUTH USING ORAL SUSPENSION
▸ Child 2-23 months: 0.15 mL/kilogram twice daily, dose doubled if necessary

▸ Child 2-6 years (body-weight 13-21 kg): 2.5 mL twice daily, dose doubled if necessary
▸ Child 7-12 years (body-weight 22-40 kg): 5 mL twice daily, dose doubled if necessary
▸ Child 12-17 years (body-weight 41 kg and above): 10 mL twice daily, alternatively 10 mL 3 times a day
▸ Adult: 10 mL twice daily, alternatively 10 mL 3 times a day

Infections due to beta-lactamase-producing strains (where amoxicillin alone not appropriate) [doses for 600 mg (500/100 mg) or 1.2 g (1000/200 mg) injection]
▸ BY INTRAVENOUS INJECTION, OR BY INTRAVENOUS INFUSION
▸ Adult: 1.2 g every 8 hours

Infections due to beta-lactamase-producing strains (where amoxicillin alone not appropriate) [doses for 2.2 g (2000/200 mg) injection]
▸ BY INTRAVENOUS INFUSION
▸ Adult: 1.1 g every 8 hours, alternatively 2.2 g every 12 hours, increased if necessary to 2.2 g every 8 hours

Acute diverticulitis [doses for 625 mg (500/125 mg) tablets]
▸ BY MOUTH USING TABLETS
▸ Adult: 625 mg 3 times a day for 5 days then review

Acute diverticulitis [doses for 600 mg (500/100 mg) or 1.2 g (1000/200 mg) injection]
▸ BY INTRAVENOUS INJECTION, OR BY INTRAVENOUS INFUSION
▸ Adult: 1.2 g every 8 hours

Moderate or severe diabetic foot infection [doses for 625 mg (500/125 mg) tablets]
▸ BY MOUTH USING TABLETS
▸ Adult: 625 mg 3 times a day

Moderate or severe diabetic foot infection [doses for 600 mg (500/100 mg) or 1.2 g (1000/200 mg) injection]
▸ BY INTRAVENOUS INJECTION, OR BY INTRAVENOUS INFUSION
▸ Adult: 1.2 g every 8 hours

Leg ulcer infection [doses for 625 mg (500/125 mg) tablets]
▸ BY MOUTH USING TABLETS
▸ Adult: 625 mg 3 times a day for 7 days

Leg ulcer infection [doses for 600 mg (500/100 mg) or 1.2 g (1000/200 mg) injection]
▸ BY INTRAVENOUS INJECTION, OR BY INTRAVENOUS INFUSION
▸ Adult: 1.2 g every 8 hours

Cellulitis [doses for 375 mg (250/125 mg) or 625 mg (500/125 mg) tablets] | Erysipelas [doses for 375 mg (250/125 mg) or 625 mg (500/125 mg) tablets]
▸ BY MOUTH USING TABLETS
▸ Child 12-17 years: 375 mg 3 times a day for 5–7 days then review (review after 7 days in severe infection or if infection near the eyes or nose), alternatively 625 mg 3 times a day for 5–7 days then review (review after 7 days in severe infection or if infection near the eyes or nose)
▸ Adult: 625 mg 3 times a day for 7 days then review

Cellulitis [doses for 125/31 mg per 5 mL suspension] | Erysipelas [doses for 125/31 mg per 5 mL suspension]
▸ BY MOUTH USING ORAL SUSPENSION
▸ Child 1-11 months: 0.25 mL/kilogram 3 times a day for 5–7 days then review (review after 7 days in severe infection or if infection near the eyes or nose), dose doubled if necessary
▸ Child 1-5 years: 0.25 mL/kilogram 3 times a day for 5–7 days then review (review after 7 days in severe infection or if infection near the eyes or nose), dose doubled if necessary, alternatively 5 mL 3 times a day for 5–7 days then review (review after 7 days in severe infection or if infection near the eyes or nose), dose doubled if necessary

Cellulitis [doses for 250/62 mg per 5 mL suspension] | Erysipelas [doses for 250/62 mg per 5 mL suspension]
- ▸ BY MOUTH USING ORAL SUSPENSION
- ▸ Child 6-11 years: 0.15 mL/kilogram 3 times a day for 5–7 days then review (review after 7 days in severe infection or if infection near the eyes or nose), dose doubled if necessary, alternatively 5 mL 3 times a day for 5–7 days then review (review after 7 days in severe infection or if infection near the eyes or nose), dose doubled if necessary

Cellulitis [doses for 600 mg (500/100 mg) or 1.2 g (1000/200 mg) injection] | Erysipelas [doses for 600 mg (500/100 mg) or 1.2 g (1000/200 mg) injection]
- ▸ BY INTRAVENOUS INJECTION, OR BY INTRAVENOUS INFUSION
- ▸ Adult: 1.2 g every 8 hours

Prophylaxis of infection from human bites [doses for 375 mg (250/125 mg) or 625 mg (500/125 mg) tablets] | Prophylaxis of infection from animal bites [doses for 375 mg (250/125 mg) or 625 mg (500/125 mg) tablets]
- ▸ BY MOUTH USING TABLETS
- ▸ Child 12-17 years: 375 mg 3 times a day for 3 days, alternatively 625 mg 3 times a day for 3 days
- ▸ Adult: 375 mg 3 times a day for 3 days, alternatively 625 mg 3 times a day for 3 days

Prophylaxis of infection from human bites [doses for 125/31 mg per 5 mL suspension] | Prophylaxis of infection from animal bites [doses for 125/31 mg per 5 mL suspension]
- ▸ BY MOUTH USING ORAL SUSPENSION
- ▸ Child 1-11 months: 0.25 mL/kilogram 3 times a day for 3 days
- ▸ Child 1-5 years: 0.25 mL/kilogram 3 times a day for 3 days, alternatively 5 mL 3 times a day for 3 days

Prophylaxis of infection from human bites [doses for 250/62 mg per 5 mL suspension] | Prophylaxis of infection from animal bites [doses for 250/62 mg per 5 mL suspension]
- ▸ BY MOUTH USING ORAL SUSPENSION
- ▸ Child 6-11 years: 0.15 mL/kilogram 3 times a day for 3 days, alternatively 5 mL 3 times a day for 3 days

Prophylaxis of infection from human bites [doses for 600 mg (500/100 mg) or 1.2 g (1000/200 mg) injection] | Prophylaxis of infection from animal bites [doses for 600 mg (500/100 mg) or 1.2 g (1000/200 mg) injection]
- ▸ BY INTRAVENOUS INJECTION, OR BY INTRAVENOUS INFUSION
- ▸ Adult: 1.2 g every 8 hours

Treatment of infection from human bites [doses for 375 mg (250/125 mg) or 625 mg (500/125 mg) tablets] | Treatment of infection from animal bites [doses for 375 mg (250/125 mg) or 625 mg (500/125 mg) tablets]
- ▸ BY MOUTH USING TABLETS
- ▸ Child 12-17 years: 375 mg 3 times a day for 5–7 days, alternatively 625 mg 3 times a day for 5–7 days
- ▸ Adult: 375 mg 3 times a day for 5–7 days, alternatively 625 mg 3 times a day for 5–7 days

Treatment of infection from human bites [doses for 125/31 mg per 5 mL suspension] | Treatment of infection from animal bites [doses for 125/31 mg per 5 mL suspension]
- ▸ BY MOUTH USING ORAL SUSPENSION
- ▸ Child 1-11 months: 0.25 mL/kilogram 3 times a day for 5–7 days
- ▸ Child 1-5 years: 0.25 mL/kilogram 3 times a day for 5–7 days, alternatively 5 mL 3 times a day for 5–7 days

Treatment of infection from human bites [doses for 250/62 mg per 5 mL suspension] | Treatment of infection from animal bites [doses for 250/62 mg per 5 mL suspension]
- ▸ BY MOUTH USING ORAL SUSPENSION
- ▸ Child 6-11 years: 0.15 mL/kilogram 3 times a day for 5–7 days, alternatively 5 mL 3 times a day for 5–7 days

Treatment of infection from human bites [doses for 600 mg (500/100 mg) or 1.2 g (1000/200 mg) injection] | Treatment of infection from animal bites [doses for 600 mg (500/100 mg) or 1.2 g (1000/200 mg) injection]
- ▸ BY INTRAVENOUS INJECTION, OR BY INTRAVENOUS INFUSION
- ▸ Adult: 1.2 g every 8 hours

Severe dental infection with spreading cellulitis [doses for 375 mg (250/125 mg) tablets] | Dental infection not responding to first-line antibacterial [doses for 375 mg (250/125 mg) tablets]
- ▸ BY MOUTH USING TABLETS
- ▸ Child 12-17 years: 375 mg 3 times a day for 5 days
- ▸ Adult: 375 mg 3 times a day for 5 days

Surgical prophylaxis [doses for 600 mg (500/100 mg) or 1.2 g (1000/200 mg) injection]
- ▸ BY INTRAVENOUS INJECTION, OR BY INTRAVENOUS INFUSION
- ▸ Adult: 1.2 g for 1 dose, to be administered up to 30 minutes before the procedure, then 1.2 g every 8 hours for up to 3 further doses in high risk procedures

Surgical prophylaxis [doses for 2.2 g (2000/200 mg) injection]
- ▸ BY INTRAVENOUS INFUSION
- ▸ Adult: 1.1–2.2 g for 1 dose, to be administered up to 30 minutes before the procedure, then 1.1 g every 8 hours for up to 3 further doses in high risk procedures

Community-acquired pneumonia [doses for 625 mg (500/125 mg) tablets]
- ▸ BY MOUTH USING TABLETS
- ▸ Child 12-17 years: 625 mg 3 times a day for 5 days
- ▸ Adult: 625 mg 3 times a day for 5 days

Community-acquired pneumonia [doses for 125/31 mg per 5 mL suspension]
- ▸ BY MOUTH USING ORAL SUSPENSION
- ▸ Child 1-11 months: 0.5 mL/kilogram 3 times a day for 5 days
- ▸ Child 1-5 years: 0.5 mL/kilogram 3 times a day for 5 days, alternatively 10 mL 3 times a day for 5 days

Community-acquired pneumonia [doses for 250/62 mg per 5 mL suspension]
- ▸ BY MOUTH USING ORAL SUSPENSION
- ▸ Child 6-11 years: 0.3 mL/kilogram 3 times a day for 5 days, alternatively 10 mL 3 times a day for 5 days

Community-acquired pneumonia [doses for 600 mg (500/100 mg) or 1.2 g (1000/200 mg) injection]
- ▸ BY INTRAVENOUS INJECTION, OR BY INTRAVENOUS INFUSION
- ▸ Adult: 1.2 g every 8 hours

Hospital-acquired pneumonia [doses for 625 mg (500/125 mg) tablets]
- ▸ BY MOUTH USING TABLETS
- ▸ Child 12-17 years: 625 mg 3 times a day for 5 days then review
- ▸ Adult: 625 mg 3 times a day for 5 days then review

Hospital-acquired pneumonia [doses for 125/31 mg per 5 mL suspension]
- ▸ BY MOUTH USING ORAL SUSPENSION
- ▸ Child 1-11 months: 0.5 mL/kilogram 3 times a day for 5 days then review
- ▸ Child 1-5 years: 0.5 mL/kilogram 3 times a day for 5 days then review, alternatively 10 mL 3 times a day for 5 days then review

continued →

Hospital-acquired pneumonia [doses for 250/62 mg per 5 mL suspension]
▸ BY MOUTH USING ORAL SUSPENSION
▸ Child 6-11 years: 0.3 mL/kilogram 3 times a day for 5 days then review, alternatively 10 mL 3 times a day for 5 days then review

Acute exacerbation of bronchiectasis [doses for 375 mg (250/125 mg) or 625 mg (500/125 mg) tablets]
▸ BY MOUTH USING TABLETS
▸ Child 12-17 years: 375 mg 3 times a day for 7–14 days, alternatively 625 mg 3 times a day for 7–14 days
▸ Adult: 625 mg 3 times a day for 7–14 days

Acute exacerbation of bronchiectasis [doses for 125/31 mg per 5 mL suspension]
▸ BY MOUTH USING ORAL SUSPENSION
▸ Child 1-11 months: 0.25 mL/kilogram 3 times a day for 7–14 days
▸ Child 1-5 years: 0.25 mL/kilogram 3 times a day for 7–14 days, alternatively 5 mL 3 times a day for 7–14 days

Acute exacerbation of bronchiectasis [doses for 250/62 mg per 5 mL suspension]
▸ BY MOUTH USING ORAL SUSPENSION
▸ Child 6-11 years: 0.15 mL/kilogram 3 times a day for 7–14 days, alternatively 5 mL 3 times a day for 7–14 days

Acute exacerbation of bronchiectasis [doses for 600 mg (500/100 mg) or 1.2 g (1000/200 mg) injection]
▸ BY INTRAVENOUS INJECTION, OR BY INTRAVENOUS INFUSION
▸ Adult: 1.2 g every 8 hours

Acute exacerbation of chronic obstructive pulmonary disease [doses for 625 mg (500/125 mg) tablets]
▸ BY MOUTH USING TABLETS
▸ Adult: 625 mg 3 times a day for 5 days

Acute exacerbation of chronic obstructive pulmonary disease [doses for 600 mg (500/100 mg) or 1.2 g (1000/200 mg) injection]
▸ BY INTRAVENOUS INJECTION, OR BY INTRAVENOUS INFUSION
▸ Adult: 1.2 g every 8 hours

Acute sinusitis [doses for 375 mg (250/125 mg) or 625 mg (500/125 mg) tablets]
▸ BY MOUTH USING TABLETS
▸ Child 12-17 years: 375 mg 3 times a day for 5 days, alternatively 625 mg 3 times a day for 5 days
▸ Adult: 625 mg 3 times a day for 5 days

Acute sinusitis [doses for 125/31 mg per 5 mL suspension]
▸ BY MOUTH USING ORAL SUSPENSION
▸ Child 1-11 months: 0.25 mL/kilogram 3 times a day for 5 days
▸ Child 1-5 years: 0.25 mL/kilogram 3 times a day for 5 days, alternatively 5 mL 3 times a day for 5 days

Acute sinusitis [doses for 250/62 mg per 5 mL suspension]
▸ BY MOUTH USING ORAL SUSPENSION
▸ Child 6-11 years: 0.15 mL/kilogram 3 times a day for 5 days, alternatively 5 mL 3 times a day for 5 days

Acute otitis media [doses for 375 mg (250/125 mg) or 625 mg (500/125 mg) tablets]
▸ BY MOUTH USING TABLETS
▸ Child 12-17 years: 375 mg 3 times a day for 5–7 days, alternatively 625 mg 3 times a day for 5–7 days

Acute otitis media [doses for 125/31 mg per 5 mL suspension]
▸ BY MOUTH USING ORAL SUSPENSION
▸ Child 1-11 months: 0.25 mL/kilogram 3 times a day for 5–7 days
▸ Child 1-5 years: 0.25 mL/kilogram 3 times a day for 5–7 days, alternatively 5 mL 3 times a day for 5–7 days

Acute otitis media [doses for 250/62 mg per 5 mL suspension]
▸ BY MOUTH USING ORAL SUSPENSION
▸ Child 6-11 years: 0.15 mL/kilogram 3 times a day for 5–7 days, alternatively 5 mL 3 times a day for 5–7 days

Acute pyelonephritis [doses for 375 mg (250/125 mg) or 625 mg (500/125 mg) tablets] | Urinary-tract infection (catheter-associated) [doses for 375 mg (250/125 mg) or 625 mg (500/125 mg) tablets]
▸ BY MOUTH USING TABLETS
▸ Child 12-15 years: 375 mg 3 times a day for 7–10 days, alternatively 625 mg 3 times a day for 7–10 days
▸ Child 16-17 years: 625 mg 3 times a day for 7–10 days
▸ Adult: 625 mg 3 times a day for 7–10 days

Acute pyelonephritis [doses for 125/31 mg per 5 mL suspension] | Urinary-tract infection (catheter-associated) [doses for 125/31 mg per 5 mL suspension]
▸ BY MOUTH USING ORAL SUSPENSION
▸ Child 3-11 months: 0.25 mL/kilogram 3 times a day for 7–10 days, dose doubled if necessary
▸ Child 1-5 years: 0.25 mL/kilogram 3 times a day for 7–10 days, dose doubled if necessary, alternatively 5 mL 3 times a day for 7–10 days, dose doubled if necessary

Acute pyelonephritis [doses for 250/62 mg per 5 mL suspension] | Urinary-tract infection (catheter-associated) [doses for 250/62 mg per 5 mL suspension]
▸ BY MOUTH USING ORAL SUSPENSION
▸ Child 6-11 years: 0.15 mL/kilogram 3 times a day for 7–10 days, dose doubled if necessary, alternatively 5 mL 3 times a day for 7–10 days, dose doubled if necessary

Acute pyelonephritis [doses for 600 mg (500/100 mg) or 1.2 g (1000/200 mg) injection] | Urinary-tract infection (catheter-associated) [doses for 600 mg (500/100 mg) or 1.2 g (1000/200 mg) injection]
▸ BY INTRAVENOUS INJECTION, OR BY INTRAVENOUS INFUSION
▸ Adult: 1.2 g every 8 hours

DOSE EQUIVALENCE AND CONVERSION
▸ Doses are expressed as co-amoxiclav: the total of amoxicillin (as the trihydrate or as the sodium salt) and clavulanic acid (as potassium clavulanate) components.
▸ Co-amoxiclav preparations contain different ratios of amoxicillin and clavulanic acid to enable appropriate dosing of amoxicillin without exceeding the maximum daily dose of clavulanic acid.
▸ For *tablets*, co-amoxiclav 375 mg consists of amoxicillin 250 mg and clavulanic acid 125 mg (2:1); co-amoxiclav 625 mg consists of amoxicillin 500 mg and clavulanic acid 125 mg (4:1); co-amoxiclav 1 g consists of amoxicillin 875 mg and clavulanic acid 125 mg (7:1).
▸ For *oral suspension*, co-amoxiclav 125/31 mg per 5 mL consists of amoxicillin 125 mg and clavulanic acid 31 mg per 5 mL (4:1); co-amoxiclav 250/62 mg per 5 mL consists of amoxicillin 250 mg and clavulanic acid 62 mg per 5 mL (4:1); co-amoxiclav 400/57 mg per 5 mL consists of amoxicillin 400 mg and clavulanic acid 57 mg per 5 mL (7:1).
▸ For *injection*, co-amoxiclav 600 mg consists of amoxicillin 500 mg and clavulanic acid 100 mg (5:1); co-amoxiclav 1.2 g consists of amoxicillin 1 g and clavulanic acid 200 mg (5:1); co-amoxiclav 2.2 g consists of amoxicillin 2 g and clavulanic acid 200 mg (10:1).

● **UNLICENSED USE** Co-amoxiclav may be used as detailed below, although these situations are considered unlicensed:
  ● EvGr treatment of acute exacerbation of bronchiectasis

- treatment of hospital-acquired pneumonia
- duration of treatment for acute sinusitis
- duration of treatment for acute otitis media

Co-amoxiclav is used for the treatment of acute diverticulitis (A), but is not licensed orally for this indication.

> **IMPORTANT SAFETY INFORMATION**
> Co-amoxiclav preparations contain different ratios of amoxicillin and clavulanic acid to enable appropriate dosing of amoxicillin without exceeding the maximum daily dose of clavulanic acid.

- **CONTRA-INDICATIONS** History of co-amoxiclav-associated jaundice or hepatic dysfunction · history of penicillin-associated jaundice or hepatic dysfunction

- **CAUTIONS**
  GENERAL CAUTIONS Acute lymphocytic leukaemia (increased risk of erythematous rashes) · chronic lymphocytic leukaemia (increased risk of erythematous rashes) · cytomegalovirus infection (increased risk of erythematous rashes) · glandular fever (erythematous rashes common) · maintain adequate hydration with high doses (particularly during parental therapy)
  SPECIFIC CAUTIONS
  ▸ With intravenous use Accumulation of electrolytes contained in parenteral preparations can occur with high doses

- **INTERACTIONS** → Appendix 1: penicillins

- **SIDE-EFFECTS**
  GENERAL SIDE-EFFECTS
  ▸ **Common or very common** Increased risk of infection
  ▸ **Uncommon** Dizziness · dyspepsia · headache
  ▸ **Frequency not known** Acute kidney injury · antibiotic associated colitis · colitis haemorrhagic · crystalluria · enterocolitis · hypersensitivity vasculitis · Kounis syndrome · meningitis aseptic · pancreatitis acute
  SPECIFIC SIDE-EFFECTS
  ▸ With oral use Akathisia · black hairy tongue
  SIDE-EFFECTS, FURTHER INFORMATION Hepatic events have been reported mostly in males and elderly patients and may be associated with prolonged treatment.
     Signs and symptoms usually occur during or shortly after treatment but in some cases may occur several weeks after discontinuation.

- **PREGNANCY** Specialist sources indicate not known to be harmful. Avoid in preterm prelabour rupture of the membranes (PPROM)—possible increased risk of necrotising enterocolitis in the neonate.

- **BREAST FEEDING** Trace amount in milk, but appropriate to use.

- **HEPATIC IMPAIRMENT** Manufacturer advises caution.
  Monitoring Monitor liver function in liver disease.

- **RENAL IMPAIRMENT** Risk of crystalluria with high doses (particularly during parenteral therapy).
  ▸ With intravenous use Accumulation of electrolytes contained in parenteral preparations can occur in patients with renal failure.
  Dose adjustments See p. 21.
  ▸ With oral use in adults [EvGr] *Co-amoxiclav 375 mg (250/125 mg) tablets or 625 mg (500/125 mg) tablets*: if creatinine clearance 10–30 mL/minute, 375 mg twice daily or 625 mg twice daily; if creatinine clearance less than 10 mL/minute, 375 mg once daily or 625 mg once daily. *Co-amoxiclav 1 g (875/125 mg) tablets or 400/57 mg per 5 mL suspension*: avoid if creatinine clearance less than 30 mL/minute. (M)
  ▸ With intravenous use in adults [EvGr] *Co-amoxiclav 600 mg (500/100 mg) injection or 1.2 g (1000/200 mg) injection* : if creatinine clearance 10–30 mL/minute, 1.2 g initially, then

600 mg every 12 hours; if creatinine clearance less than 10 mL/minute, 1.2 g initially, then 600 mg every 24 hours. *Co-amoxiclav 2.2 g (2000/200 mg) injection*: avoid if creatinine clearance less than 30 mL/minute. Except when used for Surgical prophylaxis: if creatinine clearance less than 30 mL/minute, 1.1–2.2 g for 1 dose only. (M)
  ▸ With oral use in children *Co-amoxiclav 375 mg (250/125 mg) tablets, 625 mg (500/125 mg) tablets, 125/31 mg per 5 mL suspension, or 250/62 mg per 5 mL suspension* : use normal dose every 12 hours if estimated glomerular filtration rate 10–30 mL/minute/1.73 m². Use the normal dose recommended for mild or moderate infections every 12 hours if estimated glomerular filtration rate less than 10 mL/minute/1.73 m². [EvGr] *Co-amoxiclav 1 g (875/125 mg) tablets or 400/57 mg per 5 mL suspension*: avoid if creatinine clearance less than 30 mL/minute. (M)
  ▸ With intravenous use in children *Co-amoxiclav 600 mg (500/100 mg) injection or 1.2 g (1000/200 mg) injection* : use normal initial dose and then use half normal dose every 12 hours if estimated glomerular filtration rate 10–30 mL/minute/1.73 m²; use normal initial dose and then use half normal dose every 24 hours if estimated glomerular filtration rate less than 10 mL/minute/1.73 m². [EvGr] *Co-amoxiclav 2.2 g (2000/200 mg) injection*: avoid if creatinine clearance less than 30 mL/minute. (M)

- **DIRECTIONS FOR ADMINISTRATION**
  ▸ In children For *intermittent intravenous infusion using 600 mg (500/100 mg) or 1.2 g (1000/200 mg) injection*, dilute reconstituted solution to a concentration of 10 mg/mL with Sodium Chloride 0.9%; give over 30–40 minutes. For *intermittent intravenous infusion using 2.2 g (2000/200 mg) injection*, reconstitute 2.2 g initially with 20 mL Water for Injections, then dilute with at least 100 mL Sodium Chloride 0.9%; give over 30–40 minutes. For *intravenous injection using 600 mg (500/100 mg) or 1.2 g (1000/200 mg) injection*, administer over 3–4 minutes.
  ▸ In adults For *intermittent intravenous infusion using 600 mg (500/100 mg) injection*, reconstitute 600 mg initially with 10 mL Water for Injections, then dilute with 50 mL Sodium Chloride 0.9%; give over 30–40 minutes. For *intermittent intravenous infusion using 1.2 g (1000/200 mg) injection*, reconstitute 1.2 g initially with 20 mL Water for Injections, then dilute with 100 mL Sodium Chloride 0.9%; give over 30–40 minutes. For *intermittent intravenous infusion using 2.2 g (2000/200 mg) injection*, reconstitute 2.2 g initially with 20 mL Water for Injections, then dilute with at least 100 mL Sodium Chloride 0.9%; give over 30–40 minutes. For *intravenous injection using 600 mg (500/100 mg) or 1.2 g (1000/200 mg) injection*, administer over 3–4 minutes directly into a vein or via drip tubing.

- **PRESCRIBING AND DISPENSING INFORMATION** For choice of antibacterial therapy, see Antibacterials, principles of therapy p. 573, Antibacterials, use for prophylaxis p. 574, Diabetic foot infections, antibacterial therapy p. 581, Ear infections, antibacterial therapy p. 582, Gastro-intestinal system infections, antibacterial therapy p. 582, Nose infections, antibacterial therapy p. 585, Respiratory system infections, antibacterial therapy p. 586, Skin infections, antibacterial therapy p. 589, Urinary-tract infections p. 681.

- **PATIENT AND CARER ADVICE**
  Medicines for Children leaflet: Co-amoxiclav for bacterial infections www.medicinesforchildren.org.uk/medicines/co-amoxiclav-for-bacterial-infections/

- **PROFESSION SPECIFIC INFORMATION**
  Dental practitioners' formulary Co-amoxiclav 375 mg (250/125 mg) Tablets may be prescribed.
     Co-amoxiclav 125/31 mg per 5 mL Suspension may be prescribed.
     Co-amoxiclav 250/62 mg per 5 mL Suspension may be prescribed.

5

Infection

● **MEDICINAL FORMS** There can be variation in the licensing of
different medicines containing the same drug. Forms available
from special-order manufacturers include: infusion

Oral tablet
CAUTIONARY AND ADVISORY LABELS 9
▶ Co-amoxiclav (Non-proprietary)
   Clavulanic acid (as Potassium clavulanate) 125 mg, Amoxicillin
   (as Amoxicillin trihydrate) 250 mg Co-amoxiclav 250mg/125mg
   tablets | 21 tablet [PoM] £6.00 DT = £2.92
   Clavulanic acid (as Potassium clavulanate) 125 mg, Amoxicillin
   (as Amoxicillin trihydrate) 500 mg Co-amoxiclav 500mg/125mg
   tablets | 15 tablet [PoM] £4.96-£6.84 | 21 tablet [PoM] £12.00 DT =
   £2.73
   Clavulanic acid (as Potassium clavulanate) 125 mg, Amoxicillin
   (as Amoxicillin trihydrate) 875 mg Co-amoxiclav 875mg/125mg
   tablets | 14 tablet [PoM] £5.99 DT = £5.99
▶ Augmentin (GlaxoSmithKline UK Ltd)
   Clavulanic acid (as Potassium clavulanate) 125 mg, Amoxicillin
   (as Amoxicillin trihydrate) 250 mg Augmentin 375mg tablets |
   21 tablet [PoM] £5.03 DT = £2.92
   Clavulanic acid (as Potassium clavulanate) 125 mg, Amoxicillin
   (as Amoxicillin trihydrate) 500 mg Augmentin 625mg tablets |
   21 tablet [PoM] £9.60 DT = £2.73

Powder for solution for injection
ELECTROLYTES: May contain Potassium, sodium
▶ Co-amoxiclav (Non-proprietary)
   Clavulanic acid (as Potassium clavulanate) 100 mg, Amoxicillin
   (as Amoxicillin sodium) 500 mg Co-amoxiclav 500mg/100mg
   powder for solution for injection vials | 10 vial [PoM] £10.60-£14.90
   (Hospital only)
   Clavulanic acid (as Potassium clavulanate) 200 mg, Amoxicillin
   (as Amoxicillin sodium) 1000 mg Co-amoxiclav 1000mg/200mg
   powder for solution for injection vials | 10 vial [PoM] £27.50-£50.00
   (Hospital only)

Oral suspension
CAUTIONARY AND ADVISORY LABELS 9
EXCIPIENTS: May contain Aspartame
▶ Co-amoxiclav (Non-proprietary)
   Clavulanic acid (as Potassium clavulanate) 6.25 mg per 1 ml,
   Amoxicillin (as Amoxicillin trihydrate) 25 mg per 1 ml Co-
   amoxiclav 125mg/31mg/5ml oral suspension | 100 ml [PoM] £8.14 DT
   = £3.54
   Clavulanic acid (as Potassium clavulanate) 12.5 mg per 1 ml,
   Amoxicillin (as Amoxicillin trihydrate) 50 mg per 1 ml Co-
   amoxiclav 250mg/62mg/5ml oral suspension | 100 ml [PoM] £9.52 DT
   = £3.60
   Co-amoxiclav 250mg/62mg/5ml oral suspension sugar free |
   100 ml [PoM] £4.50 DT = £4.50 [SF]
   Clavulanic acid (as Potassium clavulanate) 11.4 mg per 1 ml,
   Amoxicillin (as Amoxicillin trihydrate) 80 mg per 1 ml Co-
   amoxiclav 400mg/57mg/5ml oral suspension | 35 ml [PoM] £4.13 DT
   = £4.13 | 70 ml [PoM] £5.79 DT = £5.79
   Co-amoxiclav 400mg/57mg/5ml oral suspension sugar free |
   70 ml [PoM] £6.97 DT = £6.97 [SF]
▶ Augmentin (GlaxoSmithKline UK Ltd)
   Clavulanic acid (as Potassium clavulanate) 6.25 mg per 1 ml,
   Amoxicillin (as Amoxicillin trihydrate) 25 mg per 1 ml Augmentin
   125/31 oral suspension | 100 ml [PoM] £3.54 DT = £3.54
   Clavulanic acid (as Potassium clavulanate) 12.5 mg per 1 ml,
   Amoxicillin (as Amoxicillin trihydrate) 50 mg per 1 ml Augmentin
   250/62 oral suspension | 100 ml [PoM] £3.60 DT = £3.60
▶ Augmentin-Duo (GlaxoSmithKline UK Ltd)
   Clavulanic acid (as Potassium clavulanate) 11.4 mg per 1 ml,
   Amoxicillin (as Amoxicillin trihydrate) 80 mg per 1 ml Augmentin-
   Duo 400/57 oral suspension | 35 ml [PoM] £4.13 DT = £4.13 |
   70 ml [PoM] £5.79 DT = £5.79

Powder for solution for infusion
ELECTROLYTES: May contain Potassium, sodium
▶ Co-amoxiclav (Non-proprietary)
   Clavulanic acid (as Potassium clavulanate) 200 mg, Amoxicillin
   (as Amoxicillin sodium) 2000 mg Co-amoxiclav 2000mg/200mg
   powder for solution for infusion vials | 10 vial [PoM] £55.00 (Hospital
   only)

**ANTIBACTERIALS > PENICILLINS,
MECILLINAM-TYPE**

F 631

Pivmecillinam hydrochloride   29-Jun-2023

● **INDICATIONS AND DOSE**
Acute uncomplicated cystitis
▶ BY MOUTH
▶ Child (body-weight 40 kg and above): Initially 400 mg for
  1 dose, then 200 mg every 8 hours for 8 tablets (total of
  10 tablets per course)
▶ Adult (body-weight 40 kg and above): Initially 400 mg for
  1 dose, then 200 mg every 8 hours for 8 tablets (total of
  10 tablets per course)

Chronic or recurrent bacteriuria
▶ BY MOUTH
▶ Child (body-weight 40 kg and above): 400 mg every
  6–8 hours
▶ Adult (body-weight 40 kg and above): 400 mg every
  6–8 hours

Urinary-tract infections
▶ BY MOUTH
▶ Child (body-weight up to 40 kg): 5–10 mg/kg every
  6 hours, alternatively 20–40 mg/kg daily in 3 divided
  doses

● **UNLICENSED USE** Not licensed for use in children under
3 months.

● **CONTRA-INDICATIONS** Carnitine deficiency · gastrointestinal obstruction · oesophageal strictures

● **CAUTIONS** Avoid in Acute porphyrias p. 1202

● **INTERACTIONS** → Appendix 1: penicillins

● **SIDE-EFFECTS**
▶ **Common or very common** Vulvovaginal fungal infection
▶ **Uncommon** Clostridioides difficile colitis · dizziness ·
  fatigue · gastrointestinal discomfort · gastrointestinal
  disorders · headache · oral ulceration · vertigo

● **PREGNANCY** Not known to be harmful, but manufacturer
advises avoid.

● **BREAST FEEDING** Trace amount in milk, but appropriate to
use.

● **MONITORING REQUIREMENTS** Liver and renal function
tests required in long-term use.

● **EFFECT ON LABORATORY TESTS** False positive urinary
glucose (if tested for reducing substances). False positive
newborn screening results for isovaleric acidaemia may
occur in neonates born to mothers receiving
pivmecillinam during late pregnancy.

● **DIRECTIONS FOR ADMINISTRATION** Manufacturer advises
tablets should be swallowed whole with plenty of fluid
during meals while sitting or standing.

● **PATIENT AND CARER ADVICE** Patient counselling is advised
on administration of pivmecillinam hydrochloride tablets
(posture).

● **MEDICINAL FORMS** There can be variation in the licensing of
different medicines containing the same drug.

Oral tablet
CAUTIONARY AND ADVISORY LABELS 9, 21, 27
▶ Pivmecillinam hydrochloride (Non-proprietary)
   Pivmecillinam hydrochloride 200 mg Pivmecillinam 200mg tablets
   | 10 tablet [PoM] £9.00 DT = £5.40
▶ Selexid (Karo Healthcare UK Ltd)
   Pivmecillinam hydrochloride 200 mg Selexid 200mg tablets |
   10 tablet [PoM] £5.40 DT = £5.40 | 18 tablet [PoM] £9.72

ANTIBACTERIALS 〉 PENICILLINS,
PENICILLINASE-RESISTANT

F 631

Flucloxacillin
29-Nov-2021

- **INDICATIONS AND DOSE**

Infections due to beta-lactamase-producing staphylococci including otitis externa | Adjunct in pneumonia
▶ BY MOUTH
- Child 1 month-1 year: 62.5–125 mg 4 times a day
- Child 2-9 years: 125–250 mg 4 times a day
- Child 10-17 years: 250–500 mg 4 times a day
- Adult: 250–500 mg 4 times a day
▶ BY INTRAMUSCULAR INJECTION
- Adult: 250–500 mg every 6 hours
▶ BY SLOW INTRAVENOUS INJECTION, OR BY INTRAVENOUS INFUSION
- Adult: 0.25–2 g every 6 hours

Impetigo
▶ BY MOUTH
- Child 1 month-1 year: 62.5–125 mg 4 times a day for 5–7 days
- Child 2-9 years: 125–250 mg 4 times a day for 5–7 days
- Child 10-17 years: 250–500 mg 4 times a day for 5–7 days
- Adult: 500 mg 4 times a day for 5–7 days
▶ BY INTRAMUSCULAR INJECTION
- Adult: 250–500 mg every 6 hours
▶ BY SLOW INTRAVENOUS INJECTION, OR BY INTRAVENOUS INFUSION
- Adult: 0.25–2 g every 6 hours

Cellulitis | Erysipelas
▶ BY MOUTH
- Child 1 month-1 year: 62.5–125 mg 4 times a day for 5–7 days then review
- Child 2-9 years: 125–250 mg 4 times a day for 5–7 days then review
- Child 10-17 years: 250–500 mg 4 times a day for 5–7 days then review
- Adult: 0.5–1 g 4 times a day for 5–7 days then review
▶ BY SLOW INTRAVENOUS INJECTION, OR BY INTRAVENOUS INFUSION
- Adult: 1–2 g every 6 hours

Secondary bacterial infection of eczema
▶ BY MOUTH
- Child 1 month-1 year: 62.5–125 mg 4 times a day for 5–7 days
- Child 2-9 years: 125–250 mg 4 times a day for 5–7 days
- Child 10-17 years: 250–500 mg 4 times a day for 5–7 days
- Adult: 500 mg 4 times a day for 5–7 days

Mild diabetic foot infection
▶ BY MOUTH
- Adult: 0.5–1 g 4 times a day for 7 days then review

Moderate diabetic foot infection | Severe diabetic foot infection
▶ BY MOUTH
- Adult: 1 g 4 times a day
▶ BY SLOW INTRAVENOUS INJECTION, OR BY INTRAVENOUS INFUSION
- Adult: 1–2 g every 6 hours

Leg ulcer infection
▶ BY MOUTH
- Adult: 0.5–1 g 4 times a day for 7 days
▶ BY SLOW INTRAVENOUS INJECTION, OR BY INTRAVENOUS INFUSION
- Adult: 1–2 g every 6 hours

Endocarditis (in combination with other antibacterial if necessary)
▶ BY SLOW INTRAVENOUS INJECTION, OR BY INTRAVENOUS INFUSION
- Adult (body-weight up to 85 kg): 8 g daily in 4 divided doses
- Adult (body-weight 85 kg and above): 12 g daily in 6 divided doses

Osteomyelitis
▶ BY SLOW INTRAVENOUS INJECTION, OR BY INTRAVENOUS INFUSION
- Adult: Up to 8 g daily in 3–4 divided doses

Surgical prophylaxis
▶ INITIALLY BY SLOW INTRAVENOUS INJECTION, OR BY INTRAVENOUS INFUSION
- Adult: 1–2 g for 1 dose, to be administered up to 30 minutes before the procedure, then (by mouth or by intramuscular injection or by slow intravenous injection or by intravenous infusion) 500 mg every 6 hours for up to 4 further doses if required in high risk procedures

Staphylococcal lung infection in cystic fibrosis
▶ BY MOUTH
- Child (body-weight up to 40 kg): 25 mg/kg 4 times a day, alternatively 100 mg/kg daily in 3 divided doses
- Child (body-weight 40 kg and above): 1 g 4 times a day, alternatively 4 g daily in 3 divided doses

Prevention of *Staphylococcus aureus* lung infection in cystic fibrosis—primary prevention
▶ BY MOUTH
- Child 1 month-3 years: 125 mg twice daily

Prevention of *Staphylococcus aureus* lung infection in cystic fibrosis—secondary prevention
▶ BY MOUTH
- Child: 50 mg/kg twice daily (max. per dose 1 g)

- UNLICENSED USE Flucloxacillin doses in BNF Publications may differ from those in product literature.

> **IMPORTANT SAFETY INFORMATION**
> HEPATIC DISORDERS
> Cholestatic jaundice and hepatitis may occur very rarely, up to two months after treatment with flucloxacillin has been stopped. Administration for more than 2 weeks and increasing age are risk factors. Manufacturer advises:
> - flucloxacillin should not be used in patients with a history of hepatic dysfunction associated with flucloxacillin
> - flucloxacillin should be used with caution in patients with hepatic impairment
> - careful enquiry should be made about hypersensitivity reactions to beta-lactam antibacterials

- CAUTIONS
▶ With intravenous use Accumulation of electrolytes can occur with high doses
- INTERACTIONS → Appendix 1: penicillins
- SIDE-EFFECTS
GENERAL SIDE-EFFECTS
▶ **Rare or very rare** Fever · myalgia
SPECIFIC SIDE-EFFECTS
▶ **Common or very common**
▶ With oral use Gastrointestinal disorders
▶ **Rare or very rare**
▶ With oral use Eosinophilia
▶ **Frequency not known**
▶ With oral use Hypokalaemia · oesophageal disorder · oral pain · oropharyngeal pain · throat irritation
▶ With parenteral use Bronchospasm · coma · dyspnoea · electrolyte imbalance · erythema nodosum · hallucination ·

Jarisch-Herxheimer reaction · nephropathy · neurotoxicity · oral candidiasis · platelet dysfunction · purpura non-thrombocytopenic · vasculitis

SIDE-EFFECTS, FURTHER INFORMATION Potentially life-threatening hypokalaemia can occur, especially in high doses. This can be resistant to potassium supplementation. Regular monitoring of serum potassium levels is recommended when using higher doses of flucloxacillin.

● **PREGNANCY** Not known to be harmful.

● **BREAST FEEDING** Trace amounts in milk, but appropriate to use.

● **HEPATIC IMPAIRMENT** Manufacturer advises caution; including in those with risk factors for hepatic reactions.

● **RENAL IMPAIRMENT** Accumulation of sodium from injection can occur in patients with renal failure.
▸ With intravenous use High doses may cause nephrotoxicity or neurotoxicity.
  Dose adjustments See p. 21.
  ▸ In adults EvGr Reduce dose or increase dose interval if creatinine clearance less than 10 mL/minute (consult product literature). Ⓜ
  ▸ In children Expert sources advise use normal dose every 8 hours if estimated glomerular filtration rate less than 10 mL/minute/1.73 m^2.

● **EFFECT ON LABORATORY TESTS** False-positive urinary glucose (if tested for reducing substances).

● **DIRECTIONS FOR ADMINISTRATION** For *intravenous infusion*, give intermittently *in* Glucose 5% *or* Sodium Chloride 0.9%; suggested volume 100 mL given over 30–60 minutes. *Via* drip tubing *in* Glucose 5% *or* Sodium Chloride 0.9%; continuous infusion not usually recommended.

● **PRESCRIBING AND DISPENSING INFORMATION** For choice of antibacterial therapy, see Antibacterials, use for prophylaxis p. 574, Cardiovascular system infections, antibacterial therapy p. 579, Diabetic foot infections, antibacterial therapy p. 581, Ear infections, antibacterial therapy p. 582, Musculoskeletal system infections, antibacterial therapy p. 585, Respiratory system infections, antibacterial therapy p. 586, Skin infections, antibacterial therapy p. 589.

● **PATIENT AND CARER ADVICE**
Medicines for Children leaflet: Flucloxacillin for bacterial infections
www.medicinesforchildren.org.uk/medicines/flucloxacillin-for-bacterial-infections/

● **MEDICINAL FORMS** There can be variation in the licensing of different medicines containing the same drug. Forms available from special-order manufacturers include: infusion

Oral solution
CAUTIONARY AND ADVISORY LABELS 9, 23
▸ Flucloxacillin (Non-proprietary)
  Flucloxacillin (as Flucloxacillin sodium) 25 mg per 1 ml Flucloxacillin 125mg/5ml oral solution | 100 ml PoM £20.83 DT = £2.38
  Flucloxacillin 125mg/5ml oral solution sugar free | 100 ml PoM £8.50 DT = £4.14 SF
  Flucloxacillin (as Flucloxacillin sodium) 50 mg per 1 ml Flucloxacillin 250mg/5ml oral solution sugar free | 100 ml PoM £12.50 DT = £5.93 SF
  Flucloxacillin 250mg/5ml oral solution | 100 ml PoM £47.10 DT = £2.72

Oral capsule
CAUTIONARY AND ADVISORY LABELS 9, 23
▸ Flucloxacillin (Non-proprietary)
  Flucloxacillin (as Flucloxacillin sodium) 250 mg Flucloxacillin 250mg capsules | 28 capsule PoM £5.00 DT = £1.41 | 100 capsule PoM £6.85-£19.00
  Flucloxacillin (as Flucloxacillin sodium) 500 mg Flucloxacillin 500mg capsules | 28 capsule PoM £10.50 DT = £2.38 | 100 capsule PoM £7.89-£37.50

Powder for solution for injection
▸ Flucloxacillin (Non-proprietary)
  Flucloxacillin (as Flucloxacillin sodium) 250 mg Flucloxacillin 250mg powder for solution for injection vials | 10 vial PoM £8.60-£178.00 DT = £8.60 (Hospital only)
  Flucloxacillin (as Flucloxacillin sodium) 500 mg Flucloxacillin 500mg powder for solution for injection vials | 10 vial PoM £17.20-£359.00 DT = £17.20 (Hospital only)
  Flucloxacillin (as Flucloxacillin sodium) 1 gram Flucloxacillin 1g powder for solution for injection vials | 10 vial PoM £34.50-£712.00 DT = £34.50 (Hospital only)
  Flucloxacillin (as Flucloxacillin sodium) 2 gram Flucloxacillin 2g powder for solution for injection vials | 1 vial PoM £6.00 (Hospital only)

Combinations available: *Co-fluampicil,* p. 637

◤ 631

Temocillin

22-May-2020

● **INDICATIONS AND DOSE**

Septicaemia | Urinary-tract infections | Lower respiratory-tract infections caused by susceptible Gram-negative bacteria
▸ BY INTRAMUSCULAR INJECTION, OR BY SLOW INTRAVENOUS INJECTION, OR BY INTRAVENOUS INFUSION
▸ Adult: 2 g every 12 hours, alternatively 2 g every 8 hours, higher daily dose to be used in critically ill patients
▸ BY CONTINUOUS INTRAVENOUS INFUSION
▸ Adult: (consult product literature)

● **CAUTIONS** Accumulation of sodium from injection can occur with high doses

● **INTERACTIONS** → Appendix 1: penicillins

● **SIDE-EFFECTS** Fever · myalgia · nervous system disorder · thrombophlebitis

● **PREGNANCY** Not known to be harmful.

● **BREAST FEEDING** Trace amounts in milk.

● **RENAL IMPAIRMENT** Accumulation of sodium from injection can occur in patients with renal failure.
  Dose adjustments Manufacturer advises reduce usual dose to 1 g every 12 hours if creatinine clearance 30–60 mL/minute; reduce usual dose to 1 g every 24 hours if creatinine clearance 10–30 mL/minute; reduce usual dose to 1 g every 48 hours *or* 500 mg every 24 hours if creatinine clearance less than 10 mL/minute; no information available to recommend dose adjustments with higher daily dose for use in critically ill patients. See p. 21.

● **EFFECT ON LABORATORY TESTS** False-positive urinary glucose (if tested for reducing substances).

● **DIRECTIONS FOR ADMINISTRATION** Manufacturer advises for *intramuscular injection*, reconstitute 1 g with 2 mL Water for Injections *or* Sodium Chloride 0.9% (*or* 0.5 or 1% lidocaine solution, if pain is experienced at injection site). Manufacturer advises for *slow intravenous injection*, reconstitute 1 g with 10 mL Water for Injections *or* Sodium Chloride 0.9%; give over 3–4 minutes. Manufacturer advises for *intermittent intravenous infusion*, give in Glucose 5% or 10% *or* Sodium Chloride 0.9% *or* Ringer's Solution *or* Lactated Ringer's Solution. Reconstitute 1 g with 10 mL Water for Injections *or* infusion fluid, then dilute in up to 150 mL infusion fluid; give over 30–40 minutes. For *continuous intravenous infusion*, consult product literature.

● **MEDICINAL FORMS** There can be variation in the licensing of different medicines containing the same drug.
Powder for solution for injection
ELECTROLYTES: May contain Sodium
▸ Negaban (Eumedica Pharma Ltd)
  Temocillin (as Temocillin sodium) 1 gram Negaban 1g powder for solution for injection vials | 1 vial PoM £25.45 DT = £25.45 (Hospital only)

ANTIBACTERIALS > POLYMYXINS

Colistimethate sodium
26-Feb-2024

(Colistin sulfomethate sodium)

- **DRUG ACTION** The polymyxin antibiotic, colistimethate sodium (colistin sulfomethate sodium), is active against Gram-negative organisms including *Pseudomonas aeruginosa*, *Acinetobacter baumanii*, and *Klebsiella pneumoniae*. It is not absorbed by mouth and thus needs to be given by injection for a systemic effect.

- **INDICATIONS AND DOSE**

Serious infections due to selected aerobic Gram-negative bacteria in patients with limited treatment options
  - BY INTRAVENOUS INFUSION
  - Adult: 9 million units daily in 2–3 divided doses, an initial loading dose of 9 million units should be used in those who are critically ill, loading and maintenance doses of up to 12 million units may be required in some cases, however clinical experience is limited and safety has not been established—consult product literature for details

Management of chronic pulmonary infections due to *Pseudomonas aeruginosa* in patients with cystic fibrosis
  - BY INHALATION OF NEBULISED SOLUTION
  - Child 2-17 years: 1–2 million units 2–3 times a day, for specific advice on administration using nebulisers— consult product literature; maximum 6 million units per day
  - Adult: 1–2 million units 2–3 times a day, for specific advice on administration using nebulisers—consult product literature; maximum 6 million units per day
  - BY INHALATION OF POWDER
  - Adult: 1.66 million units twice daily

- **CONTRA-INDICATIONS** Myasthenia gravis

- **CAUTIONS**
  - When used by inhalation Severe haemoptysis—risk of further haemorrhage

- **INTERACTIONS** → Appendix 1: colistimethate

- **SIDE-EFFECTS**
  - **Common or very common**
  - When used by inhalation Arthralgia · asthenia · asthma · balance impaired · chest discomfort · cough · dysphonia · dyspnoea · fever · haemorrhage · headache · lower respiratory tract infection · nausea · respiratory disorders · taste altered · throat complaints · tinnitus · vomiting
  - **Uncommon**
  - When used by inhalation Anxiety · appetite decreased · diarrhoea · drowsiness · ear congestion · flatulence · oral disorders · proteinuria · seizure · sputum purulent · thirst · weight change
  - **Rare or very rare**
  - With parenteral use Confusion · nephrotoxicity · presyncope · psychosis · speech slurred · visual impairment
  - **Frequency not known**
  - With parenteral use Apnoea · neurological effects · neurotoxicity · renal disorder · sensory disorder

  SIDE-EFFECTS, FURTHER INFORMATION Neurotoxicity and nephrotoxicity are dose-related.

- **PREGNANCY**
  - When used by inhalation Clinical use suggests probably safe.
  - With intravenous use Manufacturer advises use only if potential benefit outweighs risk.

- **BREAST FEEDING** Present in milk but poorly absorbed from gut; manufacturers advise avoid (or use only if potential benefit outweighs risk).

- **HEPATIC IMPAIRMENT**
  - With intravenous use Manufacturer advises caution (no information available).
- **RENAL IMPAIRMENT**
  - When used by inhalation Manufacturer advises caution.
  Dose adjustments
  - With intravenous use in adults Manufacturer advises reduce maintenance dose if creatinine clearance less than 50 mL/minute—consult product literature.
  Monitoring
  - With intravenous use In renal impairment, monitor plasma colistimethate sodium concentration during parenteral treatment—consult product literature. Recommended 'peak' plasma colistimethate sodium concentration (approx. 1 hour after intravenous injection or infusion) 5–15 mg/litre; pre-dose ('trough') concentration 2–6 mg/litre.

- **MONITORING REQUIREMENTS**
  - With intravenous use Monitor renal function.
  - When used by inhalation Measure lung function before and after initial dose of colistimethate sodium and monitor for bronchospasm; if bronchospasm occurs in a patient not using a bronchodilator, repeat test using a bronchodilator before the dose of colistimethate sodium.

- **DIRECTIONS FOR ADMINISTRATION**
  - When used by inhalation Manufacturer advises if other treatments are being administered, they should be taken in the order recommended by the physician. For *nebulisation*, consult product literature for information on reconstitution and dilution.
  - With intravenous use For *intravenous infusion*, manufacturer advises following reconstitution, dilute requisite dose, usually with 50 mL Sodium Chloride 0.9%; give over 30–60 minutes. Patients fitted with a totally implantable venous access device may tolerate an injection. For *slow intravenous injection* into a totally implantable venous access device, dilute to a concentration of 200 000 units/mL with Sodium Chloride 0.9%; give over at least 5 minutes.

- **PRESCRIBING AND DISPENSING INFORMATION**
  Colistimethate sodium is included in some preparations for topical application.

- **PATIENT AND CARER ADVICE**
  - When used by inhalation Patient should be advised to rinse mouth with water after each dose of dry powder inhalation. Patients or carers should be given advice on how to administer colistimethate sodium; first dose should be given under medical supervision.
  Driving and skilled tasks Manufacturer advises patients and carers should be counselled on the effects on driving and performance of skilled tasks—increased risk of dizziness, confusion and visual disturbances.

- **NATIONAL FUNDING/ACCESS DECISIONS**
  For full details see funding body website

  NICE decisions
  - Colistimethate sodium and tobramycin dry powders for inhalation for treating pseudomonas lung infection in cystic fibrosis (March 2013) NICE TA276 Recommended with restrictions

- **MEDICINAL FORMS** There can be variation in the licensing of different medicines containing the same drug.
  Inhalation powder
  - Colobreathe (Essential Pharma Ltd)
    Colistimethate sodium 1662500 unit Colobreathe 1,662,500unit inhalation powder capsules | 56 capsule [PoM] £968.80 DT = £968.80
  Powder for nebuliser solution
  - Colicym (Kent Pharma (UK) Ltd)
    Colistimethate sodium 1000000 unit Colicym 1million unit powder for nebuliser solution unit dose vials | 1 unit dose [PoM] £6.80 (Hospital only) | 10 unit dose [PoM] £68.00 (Hospital only) | 30 unit dose [PoM] £204.00 DT = £204.00 (Hospital only)

Powder for solution for injection
ELECTROLYTES: May contain Sodium
▶ **Colomycin** (Teva UK Ltd)
Colistimethate sodium 1000000 unit Colomycin 1million unit powder for solution for injection vials | 10 vial [PoM] £18.00 DT = £18.00 (Hospital only)
Colistimethate sodium 2000000 unit Colomycin 2million unit powder for solution for injection vials | 10 vial [PoM] £32.40 DT = £32.40

ANTIBACTERIALS > QUINOLONES

Quinolones

09-Feb-2021

MHRA/CHM advice: Systemic and inhaled fluoroquinolones

The MHRA and CHM have released important safety information regarding the use of systemic and inhaled fluoroquinolones. For restrictions and precautions, see *Important safety information* for all quinolones: ciprofloxacin p. 648, delafloxacin p. 649, levofloxacin p. 650, moxifloxacin p. 651, and ofloxacin p. 652.

Overview

In the UK, only fluoroquinolones are available; the recommendations below therefore refer to the use of fluoroquinolones.

Ciprofloxacin is active against both Gram-positive and Gram-negative bacteria. It is particularly active against Gram-negative bacteria, including *Salmonella*, *Shigella*, *Campylobacter*, *Neisseria*, and *Pseudomonas*. Ciprofloxacin has only moderate activity against Gram-positive bacteria such as *Streptococcus pneumoniae* and *Enterococcus faecalis*; it should not be used for pneumococcal pneumonia. It is active against *Chlamydia* and some mycobacteria. Most anaerobic organisms are not susceptible. Ciprofloxacin can be used for respiratory tract infections (but not for pneumococcal pneumonia), infections of the gastro-intestinal system (including typhoid fever), bone and joint infections, gonorrhoea and septicaemia caused by sensitive organisms.

Ofloxacin is licensed for urinary-tract infections, lower respiratory-tract infections, gonorrhoea, and non-gonococcal urethritis and cervicitis.

Levofloxacin is active against Gram-positive and Gram-negative organisms. It has greater activity against *Pneumococci* than ciprofloxacin.

Many *Staphylococci* are resistant to quinolones and their use should be avoided in MRSA infections.

Moxifloxacin is active against Gram-positive and Gram-negative organisms. It has greater activity against Gram-positive organisms, including *Pneumococci*, than ciprofloxacin. Moxifloxacin is not active against *Pseudomonas aeruginosa* or meticillin-resistant *Staphylococcus aureus* (MRSA).

Delafloxacin is active against Gram-positive (including MSRA) and Gram-negative organisms. It may be used for treating acute bacterial skin and skin structure infections (ABSSSI) in individuals when the use of standard treatments is considered inappropriate.

Quinolones

IMPORTANT SAFETY INFORMATION
The CSM has warned that quinolones may induce **convulsions** in patients with or without a history of convulsions; taking NSAIDs at the same time may also induce them.

TENDON DAMAGE
Tendon damage (including rupture) has been reported rarely in patients receiving quinolones. Tendon rupture

may occur within 48 hours of starting treatment; cases have also been reported several months after stopping a quinolone. Healthcare professionals are reminded that:
- quinolones are contra-indicated in patients with a history of tendon disorders related to quinolone use;
- patients over 60 years of age are more prone to tendon damage;
- the risk of tendon damage is increased by the concomitant use of corticosteroids;
- if tendinitis is suspected, the quinolone should be discontinued immediately.

MHRA/CHM ADVICE: SYSTEMIC AND INHALED FLUOROQUINOLONES: SMALL INCREASED RISK OF AORTIC ANEURYSM AND DISSECTION; ADVICE FOR PRESCRIBING IN HIGH-RISK PATIENTS (NOVEMBER 2018)
The MHRA advises that benefit-risk should be assessed and other therapeutic options considered before using fluoroquinolones in patients at risk of aortic aneurysm and dissection. Factors that increase the risk of aortic aneurysm and dissection include:
- family history of aneurysm disease;
- pre-existing aortic aneurysm and/or aortic dissection;
- other risk factors or conditions predisposing to aortic aneurysm and dissection (e.g. Marfan syndrome, vascular Ehlers-Danlos syndrome, Takayasu arteritis, giant cell arteritis, Behçet's disease, hypertension, and known atherosclerosis).

Patients (particularly the elderly and those at risk) and their carers should be informed about rare events of aortic aneurysm and dissection, and advised to seek immediate medical attention if sudden-onset severe abdominal, chest, or back pain develops.

MHRA/CHM ADVICE: FLUOROQUINOLONE ANTIBIOTICS: NEW RESTRICTIONS AND PRECAUTIONS FOR USE DUE TO VERY RARE REPORTS OF DISABLING AND POTENTIALLY LONG-LASTING OR IRREVERSIBLE SIDE EFFECTS (MARCH 2019)
Disabling, long-lasting, or potentially irreversible adverse reactions affecting musculoskeletal and nervous systems have been reported very rarely with fluoroquinolone antibiotics. Healthcare professionals are advised to inform patients to stop treatment at the first signs of a serious adverse reaction, such as tendinitis or tendon rupture, muscle pain, muscle weakness, joint pain, joint swelling, peripheral neuropathy, and CNS effects, and to contact their doctor immediately. Fluoroquinolones should not be prescribed for non-severe or self-limiting infections, or non-bacterial conditions. Unless other commonly recommended antibiotics are inappropriate, fluoroquinolones should not be prescribed for some mild to moderate infections, such as acute exacerbation of chronic bronchitis and chronic obstructive pulmonary disease, and ciprofloxacin or levofloxacin should not be prescribed for uncomplicated cystitis. Fluoroquinolones should be avoided in patients who have previously had serious adverse reactions. Use of fluoroquinolones with corticosteroids should also be avoided as it may exacerbate fluoroquinolone-induced tendinitis and tendon rupture. Fluoroquinolones should be prescribed with caution in patients older than 60 years and in patients with renal impairment or solid-organ transplants as they are at a higher risk of tendon injury.

MHRA/CHM ADVICE: SYSTEMIC AND INHALED FLUOROQUINOLONES: SMALL RISK OF HEART VALVE REGURGITATION; CONSIDER OTHER THERAPEUTIC OPTIONS FIRST IN PATIENTS AT RISK (DECEMBER 2020)
A European review of worldwide data found an increased risk of heart valve regurgitation associated with systemic and inhaled fluoroquinolones. A case-control study suggested a two-fold increased relative risk with current oral fluoroquinolone use compared with amoxicillin or azithromycin use. Healthcare professionals are advised that fluoroquinolones are authorised for use in serious,

life-threatening bacterial infections, and should only be used after careful benefit-risk assessment and consideration of other therapeutic options in patients with the following risk factors:
- congenital or pre-existing heart valve disease;
- connective tissue disorders (e.g. Marfan syndrome or Ehlers-Danlos syndrome);
- other risk factors or conditions predisposing to heart valve regurgitation (e.g. hypertension, Turner's syndrome, Behçet's disease, rheumatoid arthritis, and infective endocarditis).

Patients should be advised to seek immediate medical attention if they experience a rapid onset of shortness of breath (especially when lying down flat in bed), swelling of the ankles, feet, or abdomen, or new-onset heart palpitations.

MHRA/CHM ADVICE: FLUOROQUINOLONE ANTIBIOTICS: REMINDER OF THE RISK OF DISABLING AND POTENTIALLY LONG-LASTING OR IRREVERSIBLE SIDE EFFECTS (AUGUST 2023)

The risk of disabling and potentially long-lasting or irreversible adverse reactions affecting different, sometimes multiple, body systems resulted in the introduction of restrictions and precautions for fluoroquinolone antibiotics in 2019. However, a study of prescribing data has found no evidence that these measures changed fluoroquinolone prescribing patterns in primary care, and the MHRA has continued to receive reports of such reactions. Healthcare professionals are reminded to be alert to this risk and to continue to follow the advice issued in 2019 (see above).

MHRA/CHM ADVICE: FLUOROQUINOLONE ANTIBIOTICS: SUICIDAL THOUGHTS AND BEHAVIOUR (SEPTEMBER 2023)

Fluoroquinolones can cause psychiatric side-effects, including depression and psychosis, even after the first dose. In rare cases, these can lead to thoughts or attempts of suicide, and have been associated with the completed suicide of a patient without a history of psychiatric disorders. Fluoroquinolones can also worsen existing psychiatric symptoms and treatment should be stopped immediately if such side-effects, including new or worsening depression or psychosis, occur. Healthcare professionals are advised to counsel patients or their carers to:
- inform their healthcare professional if they are prescribed a fluoroquinolone and have pre-existing depression or psychosis;
- be alert to any changes in mood or behaviour, even after treatment has stopped for some time, and to inform friends and family about the risk and signs of psychiatric side-effects associated with fluoroquinolones—medical advice should be sought if these occur;
- stop taking the fluoroquinolone and seek immediate medical advice if suicidal thoughts or behaviour develop.

MHRA/CHM ADVICE: FLUOROQUINOLONE ANTIBIOTICS: MUST NOW ONLY BE PRESCRIBED WHEN OTHER COMMONLY RECOMMENDED ANTIBIOTICS ARE INAPPROPRIATE (JANUARY 2024)

Following a review of the effectiveness of current measures to reduce the identified risk of disabling and potentially long-lasting or irreversible adverse reactions, the MHRA has further restricted the use of fluoroquinolones. These adverse reactions, which may affect multiple body systems including musculoskeletal, nervous, psychiatric and sensory systems, have been reported in patients irrespective of their age and potential risk factors, and may last for months or years; the updated reporting incidence suggested a minimum frequency of between 1 and 10 per 10 000 patients. In addition to advice issued in 2019 and 2023 (see above), healthcare professionals are advised that

fluoroquinolones should only be used when other commonly recommended antibiotics are inappropriate i.e. in situations where:
- there is resistance to other first-line antibiotics recommended for the infection;
- other first-line antibiotics are contra-indicated in an individual patient;
- other first-line antibiotics have caused side-effects that required treatment to be stopped;
- treatment with other first-line antibiotics has failed.

Patients should be advised to stop fluoroquinolone treatment at the first sign of a serious musculoskeletal, neurological or psychiatric side effect and to contact their doctor immediately (see *Patient and carer advice*).

● **CONTRA-INDICATIONS**
▸ With intravenous use or oral use or when used by inhalation History of tendon disorders related to quinolone use

● **CAUTIONS**
▸ With intravenous use or oral use or when used by inhalation Can prolong the QT interval · conditions that predispose to seizures · diabetes (may affect blood glucose) · exposure to excessive sunlight and UV radiation should be avoided during treatment and for 48 hours after stopping treatment · G6PD deficiency · history of epilepsy · myasthenia gravis (risk of exacerbation) · psychiatric disorders
▸ With intravenous use or oral use Children or adolescents (arthropathy has developed in weight-bearing joints in young *animals*)

CAUTIONS, FURTHER INFORMATION
▸ With intravenous use or oral use in children Quinolones cause arthropathy in the weight-bearing joints of immature *animals* and are therefore generally not recommended in children and growing adolescents. However, the significance of this effect in humans is uncertain and in some specific circumstances use of ciprofloxacin may be justified in children.

● **SIDE-EFFECTS**
▸ **Common or very common** Appetite decreased · arthralgia · asthenia · constipation · diarrhoea · dizziness · dyspnoea · eye discomfort · eye disorders · fever · fungal infection · gastrointestinal discomfort · headache · myalgia · nausea · QT interval prolongation · skin reactions · sleep disorders · taste altered · tinnitus · vision disorders · vomiting
▸ **Uncommon** Altered smell sensation · anaemia · anxiety · arrhythmias · chest pain · confusion · cough · depression · drowsiness · dry eye · eosinophilia · eye inflammation · flatulence · hallucination · hearing impairment · hepatic disorders · hyperglycaemia · hyperhidrosis · hypersensitivity · hypoglycaemia · hypotension · leucopenia · muscle weakness · neutropenia · pain · palpitations · peripheral neuropathy (sometimes irreversible) · pseudomembranous enterocolitis · renal impairment · seizure · sensation abnormal · stomatitis · tendon disorders · thrombocytopenia · tremor · vertigo
▸ **Rare or very rare** Agranulocytosis · angioedema · arthritis · coordination abnormal · gait abnormal · haemolytic anaemia · hypoglycaemic coma · idiopathic intracranial hypertension · memory impairment · myasthenia gravis aggravated · pancreatitis · pancytopenia · photosensitivity reaction · polyneuropathy · psychotic disorder · severe cutaneous adverse reactions (SCARs) · suicidal behaviours · syncope · vasculitis
▸ **Frequency not known** Heart valve incompetence · increased risk of aortic aneurysm (more common in elderly) · increased risk of aortic dissection (more common in elderly) · rhabdomyolysis

SIDE-EFFECTS, FURTHER INFORMATION The drug should be discontinued if neurological, psychiatric, tendon disorders or hypersensitivity reactions (including severe rash) occur.

For more information regarding the safety of fluoroquinolones, please see Important Safety Information.

- **ALLERGY AND CROSS-SENSITIVITY** [EvGr] Use of quinolones contra-indicated in quinolone hypersensitivity. Ⓜ
- **PREGNANCY**
‣ With intravenous use or oral use or when used by inhalation Avoid in pregnancy—shown to cause arthropathy in *animal* studies; safer alternatives are available.
- **PATIENT AND CARER ADVICE**
‣ With systemic use or when used by inhalation Patients and their carers should be advised to stop fluoroquinolone treatment at the first signs of a serious musculoskeletal, neurological or psychiatric side effect and to contact their doctor immediately. The MHRA has produced a patient advice sheet on fluoroquinolones and serious adverse reactions affecting tendons, muscles, joints, and nerves, which should be provided to patients and their carers: assets.publishing.service.gov.uk/media/65aa9125c69eea0010883840/FQ_Patient_Information_Sheet_-_TO_PUBLISH.pdf.

⌐ 646

Ciprofloxacin
24-Jul-2024

- **INDICATIONS AND DOSE**

Moderate diabetic foot infection | Severe diabetic foot infection
‣ BY MOUTH
‣ Adult: 500 mg twice daily
‣ BY INTRAVENOUS INFUSION
‣ Adult: 400 mg every 8–12 hours, to be given over 60 minutes

Fistulating Crohn's disease
‣ BY MOUTH
‣ Adult: 500 mg twice daily

Acute diverticulitis [in combination with metronidazole] (administered on expert advice)
‣ BY MOUTH
‣ Adult: 500 mg twice daily for 5 days then review
‣ BY INTRAVENOUS INFUSION
‣ Adult: 400 mg every 8–12 hours, to be given over 60 minutes

Respiratory-tract infections
‣ BY MOUTH
‣ Adult: 500–750 mg twice daily
‣ BY INTRAVENOUS INFUSION
‣ Adult: 400 mg every 8–12 hours, to be given over 60 minutes

Pseudomonal lower respiratory-tract infection in cystic fibrosis
‣ BY MOUTH
‣ Adult: 750 mg twice daily

Urinary-tract infections
‣ BY MOUTH
‣ Adult: 250–750 mg twice daily
‣ BY INTRAVENOUS INFUSION
‣ Adult: 400 mg every 8–12 hours, to be given over 60 minutes

Acute prostatitis
‣ BY MOUTH
‣ Adult: 500 mg twice daily for 14 days then carry out a clinical assessment to decide whether to continue for a further 14 days
‣ BY INTRAVENOUS INFUSION
‣ Adult: 400 mg every 8–12 hours

Uncomplicated gonorrhoea [anogenital and pharyngeal infection, when sensitivity confirmed]
‣ BY MOUTH
‣ Adult: 500 mg for 1 dose

Disseminated gonococcal infection [when sensitivity confirmed]
‣ BY INTRAVENOUS INFUSION
‣ Adult: 500 mg every 12 hours for 7 days, may be switched 24–48 hours after symptoms improve to a suitable oral antibacterial
‣ BY MOUTH
‣ Adult: 500 mg twice daily, to be used following intravenous antibacterial treatment, starting 24–48 hours after symptoms improve, to give 7 days treatment in total

Most other infections
‣ BY MOUTH
‣ Adult: 500 mg twice daily; increased to 750 mg twice daily, increased dose used in severe or deep-seated infection
‣ BY INTRAVENOUS INFUSION
‣ Adult: 400 mg every 8–12 hours, to be given over 60 minutes

Surgical prophylaxis
‣ BY MOUTH
‣ Adult: 750 mg for 1 dose, to be taken 60 minutes before procedure

Anthrax (treatment and post-exposure prophylaxis)
‣ BY MOUTH
‣ Adult: 500 mg twice daily
‣ BY INTRAVENOUS INFUSION
‣ Adult: 400 mg every 12 hours, to be given over 60 minutes

Prevention of secondary case of meningococcal disease
‣ BY MOUTH
‣ Child 1-11 months: 30 mg/kg for 1 dose (max. per dose 125 mg)
‣ Child 1-4 years: 125 mg for 1 dose
‣ Child 5-11 years: 250 mg for 1 dose
‣ Child 12-17 years: 500 mg for 1 dose
‣ Adult: 500 mg for 1 dose

Acute pyelonephritis | Urinary tract infection (catheter-associated)
‣ BY MOUTH
‣ Adult: 500 mg twice daily for 7 days
‣ BY INTRAVENOUS INFUSION
‣ Adult: 400 mg every 8–12 hours

- **UNLICENSED USE** [EvGr] Ciprofloxacin is used for the treatment of disseminated gonococcal infection, Ⓐ but is not licensed for this indication.
‣ In children UKHSA advises that ciprofloxacin is used for the prevention of secondary case of meningococcal disease, but it is not licensed for this indication. Not licensed for use in children under 1 year of age.

- **CAUTIONS** Acute myocardial infarction (risk factor for QT interval prolongation) · avoid excessive alkalinity of urine (risk of crystalluria) · bradycardia (risk factor for QT interval prolongation) · congenital long QT syndrome (risk factor for QT interval prolongation) · electrolyte disturbances (risk factor for QT interval prolongation) · ensure adequate fluid intake (risk of crystalluria) · heart failure with reduced left ventricular ejection fraction (risk factor for QT interval prolongation) · history of symptomatic arrhythmias (risk factor for QT interval prolongation)

- **INTERACTIONS** → Appendix 1: quinolones

- **SIDE-EFFECTS**
‣ **Common or very common** Arthropathy (in children)
‣ **Uncommon** Akathisia · fungal superinfection · oedema · thrombocytosis · vasodilation
‣ **Rare or very rare** Antibiotic associated colitis · asthma · bone marrow depression · crystalluria · erythema nodosum · haematuria · intracranial pressure increased · leucocytosis · migraine · muscle cramps · muscle tone increased ·

nephritis tubulointerstitial · olfactory nerve disorder ·
status epilepticus
▶ **Frequency not known** Mood altered · self-injurious
behaviour
● PREGNANCY UKHSA advises a single dose of ciprofloxacin
may be used for prevention of secondary case of
meningococcal disease.
● BREAST FEEDING Amount too small to be harmful but
manufacturer advises avoid.
● RENAL IMPAIRMENT
Dose adjustments
▶ With oral use in adults Give 250–500 mg every 12 hours if
eGFR 30–60 mL/minute/1.73 m^2 (every 24 hours if eGFR
less than 30 mL/minute/1.73 m^2).
▶ With intravenous use in adults Give (200 mg over
30 minutes), 200–400 mg every 12 hours if eGFR
30–60 mL/minute/1.73m^2 (every 24 hours if eGFR less than
30 mL/minute/1.73 m^2).
▶ In children Reduce dose if estimated glomerular filtration
rate less than 30 mL/minute/1.73 m^2—consult product
literature.
● PRESCRIBING AND DISPENSING INFORMATION For choice
of antibacterial therapy, see Antibacterials, use for
prophylaxis p. 574, Anthrax p. 667, Diabetic foot
infections, antibacterial therapy p. 581, Gastro-intestinal
system infections, antibacterial therapy p. 582, Genital
system infections, antibacterial therapy p. 584,
Respiratory system infections, antibacterial therapy
p. 586, Urinary-tract infections p. 681.
● PATIENT AND CARER ADVICE Granules present in the oral
suspension should not be chewed.
Medicines for Children leaflet: Ciprofloxacin for bacterial infection
www.medicinesforchildren.org.uk/medicines/ciprofloxacin-for-
bacterial-infection/
Driving and skilled tasks May impair performance of skilled
tasks (e.g. driving); effects enhanced by alcohol.

● MEDICINAL FORMS There can be variation in the licensing of
different medicines containing the same drug. Forms available
from special-order manufacturers include: oral suspension
Oral tablet
CAUTIONARY AND ADVISORY LABELS 7, 9, 25
▶ Ciprofloxacin (Non-proprietary)
Ciprofloxacin (as Ciprofloxacin hydrochloride)
100 mg Ciprofloxacin 100mg tablets | 20 tablet [PoM] £48.00 DT =
£48.00
Ciprofloxacin (as Ciprofloxacin hydrochloride)
250 mg Ciprofloxacin 250mg tablets | 10 tablet [PoM] £1.17 DT =
£0.63 | 20 tablet [PoM] £1.23-£2.34
Ciprofloxacin (as Ciprofloxacin hydrochloride)
500 mg Ciprofloxacin 500mg tablets | 10 tablet [PoM] £1.57 DT =
£0.95 | 20 tablet [PoM] £1.70-£3.14
Ciprofloxacin (as Ciprofloxacin hydrochloride)
750 mg Ciprofloxacin 750mg tablets | 10 tablet [PoM] £8.00 DT =
£3.40
Oral suspension
CAUTIONARY AND ADVISORY LABELS 7, 9
▶ Ciproxin (Bayer Plc)
Ciprofloxacin 50 mg per 1 ml Ciproxin 250mg/5ml oral suspension
| 100 ml [PoM] £21.29 DT = £21.29
Solution for infusion
ELECTROLYTES: May contain Sodium
▶ Ciprofloxacin (Non-proprietary)
Ciprofloxacin (as Ciprofloxacin lactate) 2 mg per
1 ml Ciprofloxacin 400mg/200ml solution for infusion bottles |
10 bottle [PoM] £217.60-£260.10 (Hospital only)
Ciprofloxacin 200mg/100ml solution for infusion bottles |
10 bottle [PoM] £160.40-£171.10 (Hospital only)
Infusion
▶ Ciprofloxacin (Non-proprietary)
Ciprofloxacin (as Ciprofloxacin lactate) 2 mg per
1 ml Ciprofloxacin 400mg/200ml infusion bags | 10 bag [PoM]
£228.46 (Hospital only)

F 646

Delafloxacin
02-Aug-2022

● INDICATIONS AND DOSE
Acute bacterial skin and skin structure infections
▶ BY INTRAVENOUS INFUSION
▶ Adult: 300 mg every 12 hours for 5–14 days, to be given
over 60 minutes, switch from intravenous to oral route
when clinically appropriate
▶ BY MOUTH
▶ Adult: 450 mg twice daily for 5–14 days

● INTERACTIONS → Appendix 1: quinolones
● SIDE-EFFECTS
▶ **Common or very common** Hypertransaminasaemia
▶ **Uncommon** Alopecia · auditory hallucinations · chills · dry
mouth · dry throat · flushing · gastrointestinal disorders ·
haematuria · hypertension · increased risk of infection ·
local swelling · muscle spasms · myositis · oral disorders ·
peripheral oedema · seasonal allergy · sweat changes ·
wound complications
▶ **Rare or very rare** Paranoia
▶ **Frequency not known** Intracranial pressure increased · toxic
psychosis
● CONCEPTION AND CONTRACEPTION Manufacturer advises
females of childbearing potential should use effective
contraception during treatment.
● BREAST FEEDING Manufacturer advises avoid—present in
milk in *animal* studies.
● RENAL IMPAIRMENT [EvGr] Avoid in end-stage renal
disease. ⓜ
▶ With intravenous use [EvGr] Monitor serum creatinine in
patients with moderate to severe renal impairment as
intravenous vehicle may accumulate—if serum creatinine
increases, consider switching to oral formulation (no dose
adjustment required). ⓜ
▶ With oral use [EvGr] Caution in severe renal impairment—
monitor renal function. ⓜ
Dose adjustments
▶ With intravenous use [EvGr] Reduce dose to 200 mg every
12 hours if creatinine clearance is less than 30 mL/min;
alternatively, consider switching to oral formulation (no
dose adjustment required). ⓜ See p. 21.
● DIRECTIONS FOR ADMINISTRATION For *continuous*
intravenous infusion, manufacturer advises reconstitute
each 300 mg vial to produce a 25 mg/mL solution with
10.5 mL Glucose 5% *or* Sodium Chloride 0.9%, then dilute
required dose in 250 mL Glucose 5% *or* Sodium Chloride
0.9%; give over 60 minutes.
● PRESCRIBING AND DISPENSING INFORMATION For choice
of antibacterial therapy, see Skin infections, antibacterial
therapy p. 589.
● HANDLING AND STORAGE
▶ With intravenous use Consult product literature for storage
after reconstitution or dilution.
▶ With oral use Manufacturer advises protect from light.
● PATIENT AND CARER ADVICE
Driving and skilled tasks May impair performance of skilled
tasks (e.g. driving).
● NATIONAL FUNDING/ACCESS DECISIONS
For full details see funding body website

Scottish Medicines Consortium (SMC) decisions
▶ **Delafloxacin (*Quofenix*®) for the treatment of acute bacterial**
skin and skin structure infections in adults when it is
considered inappropriate to use other antibacterial agents
that are commonly recommended for the initial treatment of
these infections (July 2022) SMC No. SMC2453 Recommended
with restrictions

- **MEDICINAL FORMS** There can be variation in the licensing of different medicines containing the same drug.

Oral tablet

ELECTROLYTES: May contain Sodium

- Quofenix (A. Menarini Farmaceutica Internazionale SRL)
  Delafloxacin (as Delafloxacin meglumine) 450 mg Quofenix 450mg tablets | 10 tablet [PoM] £615.00 (Hospital only)

Powder for solution for infusion

EXCIPIENTS: May contain Disodium edetate, sulfobutylether beta cyclodextrin sodium

ELECTROLYTES: May contain Sodium

- Quofenix (A. Menarini Farmaceutica Internazionale SRL)
  Delafloxacin (as Delafloxacin meglumine) 300 mg Quofenix 300mg powder for concentrate for solution for infusion vials | 10 vial [PoM] £615.00 (Hospital only)

⚑ 646

Levofloxacin

15-Jul-2021

- **INDICATIONS AND DOSE**

Acute sinusitis

- BY MOUTH
- Adult: 500 mg once daily for 10–14 days

Acute exacerbation of chronic obstructive pulmonary disease

- BY MOUTH
- Adult: 500 mg once daily for 5 days

Acute exacerbation of bronchiectasis

- BY MOUTH
- Adult: 500 mg 1–2 times a day for 7–14 days
- BY INTRAVENOUS INFUSION
- Adult: 500 mg 1–2 times a day, to be given over at least 60 minutes

Community-acquired pneumonia

- BY MOUTH
- Adult: 500 mg twice daily for 5 days
- BY INTRAVENOUS INFUSION
- Adult: 500 mg twice daily for 5 days, to be given over at least 60 minutes

Hospital-acquired pneumonia (administered on expert advice)

- BY MOUTH
- Adult: 500 mg 1–2 times a day for 5 days then review
- BY INTRAVENOUS INFUSION
- Adult: 500 mg 1–2 times a day, to be given over at least 60 minutes, use twice daily if severe infection

Urinary-tract infections

- BY MOUTH
- Adult: 500 mg once daily for 7–14 days

Complicated urinary-tract infections

- BY INTRAVENOUS INFUSION
- Adult: 500 mg once daily, to be given over at least 60 minutes

Prostatitis (initiated under specialist supervision)

- BY MOUTH
- Adult: 500 mg once daily for 14 or 28 days based on clinical assessment
- BY INTRAVENOUS INFUSION
- Adult: 500 mg once daily, to be given over at least 60 minutes

Complicated skin infections | Complicated soft-tissue infections

- BY MOUTH
- Adult: 500 mg 1–2 times a day for 7–14 days
- BY INTRAVENOUS INFUSION
- Adult: 500 mg 1–2 times a day, to be given over at least 60 minutes

Inhalation of anthrax (treatment and post-exposure prophylaxis)

- BY MOUTH
- Adult: 500 mg once daily for 8 weeks

- BY INTRAVENOUS INFUSION
- Adult: 500 mg once daily, to be given over at least 60 minutes

Chronic pulmonary infections due to *Pseudomonas aeruginosa* in cystic fibrosis

- BY INHALATION OF NEBULISED SOLUTION
- Adult: 240 mg twice daily for 28 days, subsequent courses repeated after 28-day interval without levofloxacin nebuliser solution

***Helicobacter pylori* eradication [in combination with other drugs (see Helicobacter pylori infection p. 93)]**

- BY MOUTH
- Adult: 250 mg twice daily for 7 days for second-line eradication therapy; 10 days for third-line eradication therapy

- **UNLICENSED USE** Levofloxacin may be used as detailed below, although these situations are considered unlicensed:
  - [EvGr] treatment of acute exacerbation of bronchiectasis
  - treatment of hospital-acquired pneumonia
  - duration of treatment for acute exacerbation of chronic obstructive pulmonary disease
  - duration of treatment for community-acquired pneumonia
  - eradication of *Helicobacter pylori* Ⓐ

- **CAUTIONS** Risk factors for QT interval prolongation (e.g. electrolyte disturbances, acute myocardial infarction, heart failure with reduced left ventricular ejection fraction, bradycardia, congenital long QT syndrome, history of symptomatic arrhythmias)

- **INTERACTIONS** → Appendix 1: quinolones

- **SIDE-EFFECTS**
- **Common or very common**
- When used by inhalation Bronchial secretion changes · dysphonia · haemoptysis · increased risk of infection · respiratory disorders · weight decreased
- **Uncommon**
- When used by inhalation Costochondritis · hyperbilirubinaemia · joint stiffness
- With intravenous or oral use Increased risk of infection
- **Rare or very rare**
- With intravenous or oral use Nephritis tubulointerstitial · paranoia · SIADH
- **Frequency not known**
- With intravenous or oral use Alveolitis allergic · anosmia · bronchospasm · cardiac arrest · diarrhoea haemorrhagic · ligament rupture · movement disorders · muscle rupture · self-endangering behaviour

SIDE-EFFECTS, FURTHER INFORMATION Systemic side-effects may occur with nebulised levofloxacin.

Bronchospasm Manufacturer advises if acute symptomatic bronchospasm occurs after receiving nebulised levofloxacin, patients may benefit from the use of a short-acting inhaled bronchodilator at least 15 minutes to 4 hours prior to subsequent doses.

- **BREAST FEEDING** Manufacturer advises avoid.

- **RENAL IMPAIRMENT**
  Dose adjustments See p. 21.
  - With intravenous use or oral use [EvGr] Usual initial dose, then use half normal dose if creatinine clearance 20–50 mL/minute; consult product literature if creatinine clearance less than 20 mL/minute. Ⓜ
  - When used by inhalation [EvGr] Avoid if creatinine clearance less than 20 mL/minute. Ⓜ

- **PATIENT AND CARER ADVICE**
- When used by inhalation Manufacturer advises patients and carers should be given advice on how to administer levofloxacin.

Missed doses
‣ When used by inhalation Manufacturer advises if a dose is more than 4 hours late, the missed dose should not be taken and the next dose should be taken at the normal time.
Driving and skilled tasks May impair performance of skilled tasks (e.g. driving).

● NATIONAL FUNDING/ACCESS DECISIONS
For full details see funding body website
Scottish Medicines Consortium (SMC) decisions
‣ Levofloxacin (*Quinsair®*) for the management of chronic pulmonary infections due to *Pseudomonas aeruginosa* in adult patients with cystic fibrosis (August 2016)
SMC No. 1162/16 Recommended with restrictions
All Wales Medicines Strategy Group (AWMSG) decisions
‣ Levofloxacin (*Quinsair®*) for use as third-line therapy in patients who do not respond to, or are intolerant of, second-line treatment with tobramycin for the management of chronic pulmonary infections due to *Pseudomonas aeruginosa* in adult patients with cystic fibrosis (November 2016)
AWMSG No. 1012 Recommended with restrictions

● MEDICINAL FORMS There can be variation in the licensing of different medicines containing the same drug.
Oral tablet
CAUTIONARY AND ADVISORY LABELS 6, 9, 25
‣ Levofloxacin (Non-proprietary)
  Levofloxacin (as Levofloxacin hemihydrate) 250 mg Levofloxacin 250mg tablets | 5 tablet PoM £7.23 | 10 tablet PoM £14.45 DT = £11.09
  Levofloxacin (as Levofloxacin hemihydrate) 500 mg Levofloxacin 500mg tablets | 5 tablet PoM £12.93 DT = £3.60 | 10 tablet PoM £24.62 DT = £7.21
Solution for infusion
ELECTROLYTES: May contain Sodium
‣ Levofloxacin (Non-proprietary)
  Levofloxacin (as Levofloxacin hemihydrate) 5 mg per 1 ml Levofloxacin 500mg/100ml solution for infusion vials | 1 vial PoM £25.00 (Hospital only)
  Levofloxacin 500mg/100ml solution for infusion bottles | 10 bottle PoM £356.50
Nebuliser liquid
‣ Quinsair (Chiesi Ltd)
  Levofloxacin (as Levofloxacin hemihydrate) 100 mg per 1 ml Quinsair 240mg nebuliser solution ampoules | 56 ampoule PoM £2,181.53 DT = £2,181.53 (Hospital only)
Infusion
‣ Levofloxacin (Non-proprietary)
  Levofloxacin (as Levofloxacin hemihydrate) 5 mg per 1 ml Levofloxacin 500mg/100ml infusion bags | 10 bag PoM £220.00-£250.00 (Hospital only)

⌐ 646

Moxifloxacin

17-Apr-2020

● **INDICATIONS AND DOSE**
Sinusitis
‣ BY MOUTH
‣ Adult: 400 mg once daily for 7 days
Community-acquired pneumonia
‣ BY MOUTH
‣ Adult: 400 mg once daily for 7–14 days
‣ BY INTRAVENOUS INFUSION
‣ Adult: 400 mg once daily for 7–14 days, to be given over 60 minutes
Exacerbations of chronic bronchitis
‣ BY MOUTH
‣ Adult: 400 mg once daily for 5–10 days
Mild to moderate pelvic inflammatory disease
‣ BY MOUTH
‣ Adult: 400 mg once daily for 14 days

Complicated skin and soft-tissue infections which have failed to respond to other antibacterials or for patients who cannot be treated with other antibacterials
‣ BY MOUTH
‣ Adult: 400 mg once daily for 7–21 days
‣ BY INTRAVENOUS INFUSION
‣ Adult: 400 mg once daily for 7–21 days, to be given over 60 minutes

● CONTRA-INDICATIONS Acute myocardial infarction (risk factor for QT interval prolongation) · bradycardia (risk factor for QT interval prolongation) · congenital long QT syndrome (risk factor for QT interval prolongation) · electrolyte disturbances (risk factor for QT interval prolongation) · heart failure with reduced left ventricular ejection fraction (risk factor for QT interval prolongation) · history of symptomatic arrhythmias (risk factor for QT interval prolongation)

● INTERACTIONS → Appendix 1: quinolones

● SIDE-EFFECTS
GENERAL SIDE-EFFECTS
‣ **Common or very common** Increased risk of infection
‣ **Uncommon** Akathisia · angina pectoris · antibiotic associated colitis · asthma · dehydration · gastritis · hyperlipidaemia · malaise · oedema · pelvic pain · thrombocytosis · vasodilation
‣ **Rare or very rare** Cardiac arrest · concentration impaired · depersonalisation · dysphagia · emotional lability · generalised tonic-clonic seizure · hypertension · hyperuricaemia · muscle complaints · respiratory disorders · self-injurious behaviour · speech disorder
‣ **Frequency not known** Clostridioides difficile colitis
SPECIFIC SIDE-EFFECTS
‣ **Rare or very rare**
‣ With intravenous use Smell disorders
‣ With oral use Anosmia

● BREAST FEEDING Manufacturer advises avoid—present in milk in *animal* studies.

● HEPATIC IMPAIRMENT Manufacturer advises avoid in severe impairment or increased transaminases (5 times upper limit of normal).

● PATIENT AND CARER ADVICE
Driving and skilled tasks May impair performance of skilled tasks (e.g. driving).

● MEDICINAL FORMS There can be variation in the licensing of different medicines containing the same drug.
Oral tablet
CAUTIONARY AND ADVISORY LABELS 6, 9
‣ Moxifloxacin (Non-proprietary)
  Moxifloxacin (as Moxifloxacin hydrochloride) 400 mg Moxifloxacin 400mg tablets | 5 tablet PoM £11.19 DT = £10.99
Solution for infusion
ELECTROLYTES: May contain Sodium
‣ Moxifloxacin (Non-proprietary)
  Moxifloxacin (as Moxifloxacin hydrochloride) 1.6 mg per 1 ml Moxifloxacin 400mg/250ml solution for infusion bottles | 10 bottle PoM £399.50-£463.90 (Hospital only)
Infusion
‣ Moxifloxacin (Non-proprietary)
  Moxifloxacin (as Moxifloxacin hydrochloride) 1.6 mg per 1 ml Avelox I.V. 400mg/250ml infusion bags | 1 bag PoM ⓢ

▶ 646

Ofloxacin

03-May-2024

● **INDICATIONS AND DOSE**

Urinary-tract infections
▶ BY MOUTH
▸ Adult: 200–400 mg daily for 3 days, preferably taken in the morning

Complicated urinary-tract infections | Acute pyelonephritis | Lower respiratory-tract infections
▶ BY MOUTH
▸ Adult: 400 mg daily, preferably taken in the morning, increased if necessary to 400 mg twice daily for 7–10 days, dose increased for severe or complicated infections
▶ BY INTRAVENOUS INFUSION
▸ Adult: 200 mg twice daily, increased if necessary to 400 mg twice daily, dose increased for severe or complicated infections, to be given over at least 30 minutes for each 200 mg

Prostatitis
▶ BY MOUTH
▸ Adult: 200 mg twice daily for 14 or 28 days based on clinical assessment

Complicated skin and soft-tissue infections
▶ BY MOUTH
▸ Adult: 400 mg twice daily for 7–10 days
▶ BY INTRAVENOUS INFUSION
▸ Adult: 400 mg twice daily, to be given over at least 30 minutes for each 200 mg

Uncomplicated gonorrhoea
▶ BY MOUTH
▸ Adult: 400 mg as a single dose

Disseminated gonococcal infection [when sensitivity confirmed]
▶ BY MOUTH
▸ Adult: 400 mg twice daily, following intravenous antibacterial treatment, starting 24–48 hours after symptoms improve, to give 7 days treatment in total

Uncomplicated genital chlamydial infection | Non-gonococcal urethritis and cervicitis
▶ BY MOUTH
▸ Adult: 400 mg daily for 7 days, dose may be taken as a single daily dose or in divided doses

Pelvic inflammatory disease
▶ BY MOUTH
▸ Adult: 400 mg twice daily for 14 days

● **UNLICENSED USE** EvGr Ofloxacin is used for the treatment of disseminated gonococcal infection, Ⓐ but is not licensed for this indication.

● **CAUTIONS** Acute myocardial infarction (risk factor for QT interval prolongation) · bradycardia (risk factor for QT interval prolongation) · congenital long QT syndrome (risk factor for QT interval prolongation) · electrolyte disturbances (risk factor for QT interval prolongation) · heart failure with reduced left ventricular ejection fraction (risk factor for QT interval prolongation) · history of symptomatic arrhythmias (risk factor for QT interval prolongation)

● **INTERACTIONS** → Appendix 1: quinolones

● **SIDE-EFFECTS**

GENERAL SIDE-EFFECTS
▶ **Uncommon** Increased risk of infection
▶ **Rare or very rare** Bronchospasm · enterocolitis · enterocolitis haemorrhagic · hot flush · movement disorders
▶ **Frequency not known** Alveolitis allergic · bone marrow failure · ligament rupture · muscle rupture · myopathy · nephritis acute interstitial · self-endangering behaviour

SPECIFIC SIDE-EFFECTS
▶ With oral use Delirium

● **BREAST FEEDING** Amount probably too small to be harmful but manufacturer advises avoid.

● **HEPATIC IMPAIRMENT** Manufacturer advises caution.
Dose adjustments Manufacturer advises maximum 400 mg daily in hepatic failure (risk of decreased elimination).

● **RENAL IMPAIRMENT**
Dose adjustments Usual initial dose, then use half normal dose if creatinine clearance 20–50 mL/minute; 100 mg every 24 hours if creatinine clearance less than 20 mL/minute. See p. 21.

● **PRESCRIBING AND DISPENSING INFORMATION** For choice of antibacterial therapy, see Genital system infections, antibacterial therapy p. 584, Respiratory system infections, antibacterial therapy p. 586, Skin infections, antibacterial therapy p. 589, Urinary-tract infections p. 681.

● **PATIENT AND CARER ADVICE**
Driving and skilled tasks May affect performance of skilled tasks (e.g. driving); effects enhanced by alcohol.

● **MEDICINAL FORMS** There can be variation in the licensing of different medicines containing the same drug. Forms available from special-order manufacturers include: oral suspension, oral solution

Oral tablet
CAUTIONARY AND ADVISORY LABELS 6, 9, 11
▶ Ofloxacin (Non-proprietary)
Ofloxacin 200 mg Ofloxacin 200mg tablets | 10 tablet PoM £12.34 DT = £12.21
Ofloxacin 400 mg Ofloxacin 400mg tablets | 5 tablet PoM £12.80 DT = £11.12 | 10 tablet PoM £21.73–£22.24

ANTIBACTERIALS > SULFONAMIDES

Co-trimoxazole

06-Feb-2023

● **DRUG ACTION** Sulfamethoxazole and trimethoprim are used in combination (as co-trimoxazole) because of their synergistic activity (the importance of the sulfonamides has decreased as a result of increasing bacterial resistance and their replacement by antibacterials which are generally more active and less toxic).

● **INDICATIONS AND DOSE**

Treatment of susceptible infections
▶ BY MOUTH
▸ Child 6 weeks–5 months: 120 mg twice daily, alternatively 24 mg/kg twice daily
▸ Child 6 months–5 years: 240 mg twice daily, alternatively 24 mg/kg twice daily
▸ Child 6–11 years: 480 mg twice daily, alternatively 24 mg/kg twice daily (max. per dose 960 mg)
▸ Child 12–17 years: 960 mg twice daily
▸ Adult: 960 mg twice daily
▶ BY INTRAVENOUS INFUSION
▸ Adult: 960 mg every 12 hours, increased to 1.44 g every 12 hours, increased dose used in severe infection

Moderate diabetic foot infection | Severe diabetic foot infection
▶ BY MOUTH
▸ Adult: 960 mg twice daily
▶ BY INTRAVENOUS INFUSION
▸ Adult: 960 mg every 12 hours, increased if necessary to 1.44 g every 12 hours

Leg ulcer infection
▶ BY MOUTH
▸ Adult: 960 mg twice daily for 7 days
▶ BY INTRAVENOUS INFUSION
▸ Adult: 960 mg every 12 hours, increased to 1.44 g every 12 hours, increased dose used in severe infection

5

Infection

Hospital-acquired pneumonia
▶ BY MOUTH
▶ Adult: 960 mg twice daily for 5 days then review

Acute exacerbation of chronic obstructive pulmonary disease
▶ BY MOUTH
▶ Adult: 960 mg twice daily for 5 days
▶ BY INTRAVENOUS INFUSION
▶ Adult: 960 mg every 12 hours, increased if necessary to 1.44 g every 12 hours, increased dose used in severe infection

Treatment of *Pneumocystis jirovecii* (*Pneumocystis carinii*) infections (undertaken where facilities for appropriate monitoring available—consult microbiologist and product literature)
▶ BY MOUTH, OR BY INTRAVENOUS INFUSION
▶ Child: 120 mg/kg daily in 2–4 divided doses for 14–21 days, oral route preferred for children
▶ Adult: 120 mg/kg daily in 2–4 divided doses for 14–21 days

Prophylaxis of *Pneumocystis jirovecii* (*Pneumocystis carinii*) infections
▶ BY MOUTH
▶ Child: 450 mg/m^2 twice daily (max. per dose 960 mg) for 3 days of the week (either consecutively or on alternate days), dose regimens may vary, consult local guidelines
▶ Adult: 960 mg once daily, dose reduced if not tolerated to 480 mg once daily, alternatively 960 mg once daily on alternate days, to be given on 3 days of the week, alternatively 960 mg twice a day on alternate days, to be given on 3 days of the week

Acute prostatitis (initiated under specialist supervision)
▶ BY MOUTH
▶ Adult: 960 mg twice daily for 14 or 28 days based on clinical assessment

DOSE EQUIVALENCE AND CONVERSION
▶ Doses are expressed as co-trimoxazole: the total of sulfamethoxazole (sulphamethoxazole) and trimethoprim components in a ratio of 5:1.
▶ Co-trimoxazole 480 mg consists of sulfamethoxazole 400 mg and trimethoprim 80 mg.

● UNLICENSED USE Co-trimoxazole may be used as detailed below, although these situations are considered unlicensed:
  ● treatment of *Burkholderia cepacia* infections in cystic fibrosis
  ● treatment of *Stenotrophomonas maltophilia* infections
  ● EvGr treatment of hospital-acquired pneumonia
  ● treatment of moderate diabetic foot infection
  ● treatment of severe diabetic foot infection
  ● treatment of leg ulcer infection A
Not licensed for use in children under 6 weeks.

IMPORTANT SAFETY INFORMATION

RESTRICTIONS ON THE USE OF CO-TRIMOXAZOLE

Co-trimoxazole is licensed for the prophylaxis and treatment of *Pneumocystis jirovecii* (*Pneumocystis carinii*) pneumonia and toxoplasmosis; it is also licensed for the treatment of nocardiosis. *Stenotrophomonas maltophilia* has demonstrated susceptibility to co-trimoxazole. It should only be considered for use in acute exacerbations of chronic bronchitis and infections of the urinary tract when there is bacteriological evidence of sensitivity to co-trimoxazole and good reason to prefer this combination to a single antibacterial; similarly it should only be used in acute otitis media in children when there is good reason to prefer it.

● CONTRA-INDICATIONS Acute porphyrias p. 1202

● CAUTIONS Asthma · avoid in blood disorders (unless under specialist supervision) · avoid in infants under 6 weeks (except for treatment or prophylaxis of pneumocystis pneumonia) because of the risk of kernicterus · elderly (increased risk of serious side-effects) · G6PD deficiency (risk of haemolytic anaemia) · maintain adequate fluid intake · predisposition to folate deficiency · predisposition to hyperkalaemia

● INTERACTIONS → Appendix 1: sulfonamides · trimethoprim

● SIDE-EFFECTS
▶ **Common or very common** Diarrhoea · electrolyte imbalance · fungal overgrowth · headache · nausea · skin reactions
▶ **Uncommon** Vomiting
▶ **Rare or very rare** Agranulocytosis · angioedema · aplastic anaemia · appetite decreased · arthralgia · ataxia · cough · depression · dizziness · dyspnoea · eosinophilia · fever · haemolysis · haemolytic anaemia · hallucination · hepatic disorders · hypoglycaemia · leucopenia · megaloblastic anaemia · meningitis aseptic · metabolic acidosis · methaemoglobinaemia · myalgia · myocarditis allergic · nephritis tubulointerstitial · neutropenia · oral disorders · pancreatitis · peripheral neuropathy · photosensitivity reaction · pseudomembranous enterocolitis · renal impairment · renal tubular acidosis · respiratory disorders · rhabdomyolysis · seizure · serum sickness · severe cutaneous adverse reactions (SCARs) · systemic lupus erythematosus (SLE) · thrombocytopenia · tinnitus · uveitis · vasculitis · vertigo
▶ **Frequency not known** Haemophagocytic lymphohistiocytosis · psychotic disorder

SIDE-EFFECTS, FURTHER INFORMATION Co-trimoxazole is associated with rare but serious side effects. Discontinue immediately if blood disorders (including leucopenia, thrombocytopenia, megaloblastic anaemia, eosinophilia, haemophagocytic lymphohistiocytosis) or rash/skin reactions (including Stevens-Johnson syndrome, toxic epidermal necrolysis, acute generalised exanthematous pustulosis, drug reaction with eosinophilia and systemic symptoms) develop.

● ALLERGY AND CROSS-SENSITIVITY EvGr Contra-indicated if previous hypersensitivity to trimethoprim, sulfonamides or co-trimoxazole. Contra-indicated if previous Stevens-Johnson syndrome (SJS), toxic epidermal necrolysis (TEN) or drug reaction with eosinophilia and systemic symptoms (DRESS) with the use of co-trimoxazole. Contra-indicated if previous drug-induced thrombocytopenia with trimethoprim, sulfonamides or co-trimoxazole. M

● PREGNANCY Teratogenic risk in first trimester (trimethoprim a folate antagonist). Neonatal haemolysis and methaemoglobinaemia in third trimester; fear of increased risk of kernicterus in neonates appears to be unfounded.

● BREAST FEEDING Small risk of kernicterus in jaundiced infants and of haemolysis in G6PD-deficient infants (due to sulfamethoxazole).

● HEPATIC IMPAIRMENT Manufacturer advises avoid in severe liver disease.

● RENAL IMPAIRMENT EvGr Avoid if creatinine clearance less than 15 mL/minute or in severe insufficiency where plasma-sulfamethoxazole concentration cannot be monitored. Monitor plasma-sulfamethoxazole concentrations (consult product literature). M
  Dose adjustments See p. 21.
  ▶ In adults EvGr Use half normal dose if creatinine clearance 15–30 mL/minute. M
  ▶ In children EvGr Use half normal dose if creatinine clearance 15–30 mL/minute (consult product literature). M

● MONITORING REQUIREMENTS
▶ EvGr Monitor serum potassium and sodium in patients at risk of hyperkalaemia or hyponatraemia.

5

Infection

▶ Monitor blood counts on prolonged treatment. ⟨M⟩
▶ In children Plasma concentration monitoring may be required with high doses; seek expert advice

● **DIRECTIONS FOR ADMINISTRATION**
▶ In children For intermittent *intravenous infusion,* manufacturer advises may be further diluted in Glucose 5% and 10% *or* Sodium Chloride 0.9%. Dilute contents of 1 ampoule (5 mL) to 125 mL, 2 ampoules (10 mL) to 250 mL or 3 ampoules (15 mL) to 500 mL; suggested duration of infusion 60–90 minutes (but may be adjusted according to fluid requirements); if fluid restriction necessary, 1 ampoule (5 mL) may be diluted with 75 mL Glucose 5% and the required dose infused over max. 60 minutes; check container for haze or precipitant during administration. Expert sources advise in severe fluid restriction may be given undiluted via a central venous line.
▶ In adults For *intravenous infusion,* manufacturer advises give intermittently *in* Glucose 5% or 10% *or* Sodium Chloride 0.9%. Dilute contents of 1 ampoule (5 mL) to 125 mL, 2 ampoules (10 mL) to 250 mL or 3 ampoules (15 mL) to 500 mL; suggested duration of infusion 60–90 minutes (but may be adjusted according to fluid requirements); if fluid restriction necessary, 1 ampoule (5 mL) may be diluted with 75 mL Glucose 5% and infused over max. 60 minutes.

● **PRESCRIBING AND DISPENSING INFORMATION** For choice of antibacterial therapy, see Diabetic foot infections, antibacterial therapy p. 581, Pneumocystis pneumonia p. 697, Respiratory system infections, antibacterial therapy p. 586, Skin infections, antibacterial therapy p. 589, Urinary-tract infections p. 681.

● **MEDICINAL FORMS** There can be variation in the licensing of different medicines containing the same drug.

Solution for infusion
EXCIPIENTS: May contain Alcohol, propylene glycol, sulfites
ELECTROLYTES: May contain Sodium
▶ Co-trimoxazole (Non-proprietary)
 Trimethoprim 16 mg per 1 ml, Sulfamethoxazole 80 mg per 1 ml Co-trimoxazole 80mg/400mg/5ml solution for infusion ampoules | 10 ampoule PoM £47.15 DT = £47.15

Oral tablet
CAUTIONARY AND ADVISORY LABELS 9
▶ Co-trimoxazole (Non-proprietary)
 Trimethoprim 80 mg, Sulfamethoxazole 400 mg Co-trimoxazole 80mg/400mg tablets | 28 tablet PoM £3.95 DT = £1.41 | 100 tablet PoM £8.36–£10.91
 Trimethoprim 160 mg, Sulfamethoxazole 800 mg Co-trimoxazole 160mg/800mg tablets | 50 tablet PoM £11.73 | 100 tablet PoM £30.52 DT = £18.68

Oral suspension
CAUTIONARY AND ADVISORY LABELS 9
▶ Co-trimoxazole (Non-proprietary)
 Trimethoprim 8 mg per 1 ml, Sulfamethoxazole 40 mg per 1 ml Co-trimoxazole 40mg/200mg/5ml oral suspension sugar free | 100 ml PoM £9.95 DT = £15.13 SF
 Trimethoprim 16 mg per 1 ml, Sulfamethoxazole 80 mg per 1 ml Co-trimoxazole 80mg/400mg/5ml oral suspension | 100 ml PoM £10.95–£21.16 DT = £21.16

Sulfadiazine

03-Nov-2021

(Sulphadiazine)

● **DRUG ACTION** Sulfadiazine is a short-acting sulphonamide with bacteriostatic activity against a broad spectrum of organisms. The importance of the sulfonamides has decreased as a result of increasing bacterial resistance and their replacement by antibacterials which are generally more active and less toxic.

● **INDICATIONS AND DOSE**
Prevention of rheumatic fever recurrence
▶ BY MOUTH
▶ Adult (body-weight up to 30 kg): 500 mg daily
▶ Adult (body-weight 30 kg and above): 1 g daily

IMPORTANT SAFETY INFORMATION
SAFE PRACTICE
Sulfadiazine has been confused with sulfasalazine; care must be taken to ensure the correct drug is prescribed and dispensed.

● **CONTRA-INDICATIONS** Acute porphyrias p. 1202
● **CAUTIONS** Asthma · avoid in blood disorders · elderly · G6PD deficiency (risk of haemolytic anaemia) · maintain adequate fluid intake · predisposition to folate deficiency
● **INTERACTIONS** → Appendix 1: sulfonamides
● **SIDE-EFFECTS**
▶ **Rare or very rare** Haemolytic anaemia
▶ **Frequency not known** Agranulocytosis · aplastic anaemia · appetite decreased · ataxia · back pain · blood disorders · cough · crystalluria · cyanosis · depression · diarrhoea · dizziness · drowsiness · dyspnoea · eosinophilia · erythema nodosum · fatigue · fever · haematuria · hallucination · headache · hepatic disorders · hypoglycaemia · hypoprothrombinaemia · hypothyroidism · idiopathic intracranial hypertension · idiopathic pulmonary fibrosis · insomnia · leucopenia · meningitis aseptic · myocarditis · nausea · nephritis tubulointerstitial · nephrotoxicity · nerve disorders · neurological effects · neutropenia · oral disorders · pancreatitis · photosensitivity reaction · pseudomembranous enterocolitis · psychosis · pulmonary eosinophilia · renal impairment · renal tubular necrosis · seizure · serum sickness-like reaction · severe cutaneous adverse reactions (SCARs) · skin reactions · systemic lupus erythematosus (SLE) · thrombocytopenia · tinnitus · vasculitis · vertigo · vomiting

SIDE-EFFECTS, FURTHER INFORMATION Discontinue immediately if blood disorders (including leucopenia, thrombocytopenia, megaloblastic anaemia, eosinophilia) or rash (including Stevens-Johnson syndrome, toxic epidermal necrolysis) develop.

● **PREGNANCY** Risk of neonatal haemolysis and methaemoglobinaemia in third trimester; fear of increased risk of kernicterus in neonates appears to be unfounded.
● **BREAST FEEDING** Small risk of kernicterus in jaundiced infants and of haemolysis in G6PD-deficient infants.
● **HEPATIC IMPAIRMENT** Manufacturer advises caution in mild to moderate impairment; avoid in severe impairment or jaundice.
● **RENAL IMPAIRMENT** EvGr Caution in mild to moderate impairment; avoid in severe impairment (risk of crystalluria). ⟨M⟩
 Dose adjustments EvGr Dose reduction may be necessary. ⟨M⟩
● **MONITORING REQUIREMENTS** Monitor blood counts on prolonged treatment.

- **MEDICINAL FORMS** There can be variation in the licensing of different medicines containing the same drug. Forms available from special-order manufacturers include: oral suspension

Oral tablet

CAUTIONARY AND ADVISORY LABELS 9, 27

▸ **Sulfadiazine (Non-proprietary)**
   Sulfadiazine 500 mg Sulfadiazine 500mg tablets | 56 tablet [PoM] £395.42–£606.02 DT = £395.42

ANTIBACTERIALS › TETRACYCLINES AND RELATED DRUGS

Tetracyclines

Overview

The tetracyclines are broad-spectrum antibiotics whose value has decreased owing to increasing bacterial resistance. They remain, however, the treatment of choice for infections caused by chlamydia (trachoma, psittacosis, salpingitis, urethritis, and lymphogranuloma venereum), rickettsia (including Q-fever), brucella (doxycycline below with either streptomycin p. 598 or rifampicin p. 674), and the spirochaete, *Borrelia burgdorferi* (See Lyme disease). They are also used in respiratory and genital mycoplasma infections, in acne, in destructive (refractory) periodontal disease, in exacerbations of chronic bronchitis (because of their activity against *Haemophilus influenzae*), and for leptospirosis in penicillin hypersensitivity (as an alternative to erythromycin p. 624).

Tetracyclines have a role in the management of meticillin-resistant *Staphylococcus aureus* (MRSA) infection.

Microbiologically, there is little to choose between the various tetracyclines, the only exception being minocycline p. 658 which has a broader spectrum; it is active against *Neisseria meningitidis* and has been used for meningococcal prophylaxis but is no longer recommended because of side-effects including dizziness and vertigo. Compared to other tetracyclines, minocycline is associated with a greater risk of lupus-erythematosus-like syndrome. Minocycline sometimes causes irreversible pigmentation.

Tetracyclines 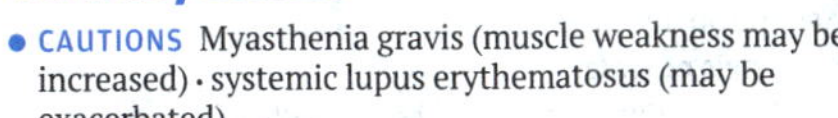

- **CAUTIONS** Myasthenia gravis (muscle weakness may be increased) · systemic lupus erythematosus (may be exacerbated)

- **SIDE-EFFECTS**
▸ **Common or very common** Angioedema · diarrhoea · headache · Henoch-Schönlein purpura · hypersensitivity · nausea · pericarditis · photosensitivity reaction · skin reactions · systemic lupus erythematosus exacerbated · vomiting
▸ **Uncommon** Dizziness · pancreatitis
▸ **Rare or very rare** Appetite decreased · discolouration of thyroid gland · dysphagia · eosinophilia · fontanelle bulging (in infants) · gastrointestinal disorders · glossitis · haemolytic anaemia · hepatic disorders · idiopathic intracranial hypertension · increased risk of infection · neutropenia · pseudomembranous enterocolitis · Stevens-Johnson syndrome · thrombocytopenia
▸ **Frequency not known** Tooth discolouration
   SIDE-EFFECTS, FURTHER INFORMATION Headache and visual disturbances may indicate benign intracranial hypertension (discontinue treatment if raised intracranial pressure develops).

- **PREGNANCY** Should **not** be given to pregnant women; effects on skeletal development have been documented in the first trimester in *animal* studies. Administration during the second or third trimester may cause discoloration of

the child's teeth, and maternal hepatotoxicity has been reported with large parenteral doses.

- **BREAST FEEDING** Should **not** be given to women who are breast-feeding (although absorption and therefore discoloration of teeth in the infant is probably usually prevented by chelation with calcium in milk).

- **HEPATIC IMPAIRMENT** In general, manufacturers advise caution.

▸ above

Demeclocycline hydrochloride   20-Jan-2022

- **INDICATIONS AND DOSE**

Susceptible infections (e.g. chlamydia, rickettsia and mycoplasma)
▸ BY MOUTH
▸ Adult: 150 mg 4 times a day, alternatively 300 mg twice daily

Treatment of hyponatraemia resulting from inappropriate secretion of antidiuretic hormone, if fluid restriction alone does not restore sodium concentration or is not tolerable
▸ BY MOUTH
▸ Adult: Initially 0.9–1.2 g daily in divided doses, maintenance 600–900 mg daily

- **CAUTIONS** Photosensitivity more common than with other tetracyclines

- **INTERACTIONS** → Appendix 1: tetracyclines

- **SIDE-EFFECTS**
▸ **Rare or very rare** Agranulocytosis · aplastic anaemia · hearing impairment · nephritis · severe cutaneous adverse reactions (SCARs)
▸ **Frequency not known** Intracranial pressure increased · muscle weakness · nephrogenic diabetes insipidus · stomatitis · vision disorders

- **HEPATIC IMPAIRMENT**
Dose adjustments Manufacturer advises maximum 1 g daily in divided doses.

- **RENAL IMPAIRMENT** [EvGr] Avoid unless potential benefit outweighs risk (risk of accumulation). ⓜ
Dose adjustments [EvGr] Reduce dose if use is essential. ⓜ

- **PATIENT AND CARER ADVICE** Patients should be advised to avoid exposure to sunlight or sun lamps.

- **MEDICINAL FORMS** There can be variation in the licensing of different medicines containing the same drug. Forms available from special-order manufacturers include: oral tablet, oral suspension, oral solution

Oral tablet
▸ **Demeclocycline hydrochloride (Non-proprietary)**
   Demeclocycline hydrochloride 150 mg Demeclocycline 150mg tablets | 100 tablet [PoM] 💊

Oral capsule
CAUTIONARY AND ADVISORY LABELS 7, 9, 11, 23
▸ **Demeclocycline hydrochloride (Non-proprietary)**
   Demeclocycline hydrochloride 150 mg Demeclocycline 150mg capsules | 28 capsule [PoM] £238.41–£381.46 DT = £238.41
   Demeclocycline hydrochloride 300 mg Ledermycin 300mg capsules | 16 capsule [PoM] 💊
   Demeclocycline 300mg capsules | 28 capsule [PoM] £452.98 DT = £452.98

▸ above

Doxycycline   18-Apr-2025

- **INDICATIONS AND DOSE**

Susceptible infections (e.g. chlamydia, rickettsia and mycoplasma)
▸ BY MOUTH USING IMMEDIATE-RELEASE MEDICINES
▸ Child 12–17 years: Initially 200 mg daily in 1–2 divided doses for 1 day, then 100 mg daily   continued →

▶ Adult: Initially 200 mg daily in 1–2 divided doses for 1 day, then 100 mg daily

Severe infections (including refractory urinary-tract infections)

▶ BY MOUTH USING IMMEDIATE-RELEASE MEDICINES
▶ Child 12–17 years: 200 mg daily
▶ Adult: 200 mg daily

Acute sinusitis | Acute cough [if systemically very unwell or at higher risk of complications] | Community-acquired pneumonia

▶ BY MOUTH USING IMMEDIATE-RELEASE MEDICINES
▶ Child 12–17 years: Initially 200 mg for 1 dose on first day, then 100 mg once daily for 5 days in total
▶ Adult: Initially 200 mg for 1 dose on first day, then 100 mg once daily for 5 days in total

Hospital-acquired pneumonia

▶ BY MOUTH USING IMMEDIATE-RELEASE MEDICINES
▶ Adult: Initially 200 mg for 1 dose on first day, then 100 mg once daily for 5 days in total then review

Acute exacerbation of bronchiectasis

▶ BY MOUTH USING IMMEDIATE-RELEASE MEDICINES
▶ Child 12–17 years: Initially 200 mg for 1 dose on first day, then 100 mg once daily for 7–14 days in total
▶ Adult: Initially 200 mg for 1 dose on first day, then 100 mg once daily for 7–14 days in total

Acute exacerbation of chronic obstructive pulmonary disease

▶ BY MOUTH USING IMMEDIATE-RELEASE MEDICINES
▶ Adult: Initially 200 mg for 1 dose on first day, then 100 mg once daily for 5 days in total, dose can be increased if necessary to 200 mg once daily in severe infections

Mild diabetic foot infection

▶ BY MOUTH USING IMMEDIATE-RELEASE MEDICINES
▶ Adult: Initially 200 mg for 1 dose on first day, then 100 mg once daily for 7 days in total then review, alternatively 200 mg once daily for 7 days in total then review

Cellulitis | Erysipelas

▶ BY MOUTH USING IMMEDIATE-RELEASE MEDICINES
▶ Adult: Initially 200 mg for 1 dose on first day, then 100 mg once daily for 5–7 days in total then review

Leg ulcer infection

▶ BY MOUTH USING IMMEDIATE-RELEASE MEDICINES
▶ Adult: Initially 200 mg for 1 dose on first day, then 100 mg once daily for 7 days in total, alternatively 200 mg once daily for 7 days in total

Prophylaxis of infection from human bites [in combination with other drugs] | Prophylaxis of infection from animal bites [in combination with other drugs]

▶ BY MOUTH USING IMMEDIATE-RELEASE MEDICINES
▶ Child 12–17 years: Initially 200 mg daily on first day, then 100–200 mg daily for 3 days in total
▶ Adult: Initially 200 mg daily on first day, then 100–200 mg daily for 3 days in total

Treatment of infection from human bites [in combination with other drugs] | Treatment of infection from animal bites [in combination with other drugs]

▶ BY MOUTH USING IMMEDIATE-RELEASE MEDICINES
▶ Child 12–17 years: Initially 200 mg daily on first day, then 100–200 mg daily for 5–7 days in total
▶ Adult: Initially 200 mg daily on first day, then 100–200 mg daily for 5–7 days in total

Acne vulgaris [adjunct to topical treatment]

▶ BY MOUTH USING IMMEDIATE-RELEASE MEDICINES
▶ Child 12–17 years: 100 mg once daily
▶ Adult: 100 mg once daily

Rosacea

▶ BY MOUTH USING IMMEDIATE-RELEASE MEDICINES
▶ Adult: 100 mg once daily

Papulopustular facial rosacea (without ocular involvement)

▶ BY MOUTH USING MODIFIED-RELEASE MEDICINES
▶ Adult: 40 mg once daily for 16 weeks, dose to be taken in the morning, consider discontinuing treatment if no response after 6 weeks

Early syphilis | Asymptomatic contacts of patients with infectious syphilis

▶ BY MOUTH USING IMMEDIATE-RELEASE MEDICINES
▶ Adult: 100 mg twice daily for 14 days

Late latent syphilis

▶ BY MOUTH USING IMMEDIATE-RELEASE MEDICINES
▶ Adult: 100 mg twice daily for 28 days

Neurosyphilis

▶ BY MOUTH USING IMMEDIATE-RELEASE MEDICINES
▶ Adult: 200 mg twice daily for 28 days

Uncomplicated genital chlamydia | Non-gonococcal urethritis

▶ BY MOUTH USING IMMEDIATE-RELEASE MEDICINES
▶ Child 12–17 years: 100 mg twice daily for 7 days
▶ Adult: 100 mg twice daily for 7 days

Pelvic inflammatory disease

▶ BY MOUTH USING IMMEDIATE-RELEASE MEDICINES
▶ Child 12–17 years: 100 mg twice daily for 14 days
▶ Adult: 100 mg twice daily for 14 days

Lyme disease [erythema migrans and/or non-focal symptoms] | Lyme disease [affecting cranial nerves or peripheral nervous system] | Lyme carditis

▶ BY MOUTH USING IMMEDIATE-RELEASE MEDICINES
▶ Adult: 200 mg daily in 1–2 divided doses for 21 days

Lyme disease [affecting central nervous system]

▶ BY MOUTH USING IMMEDIATE-RELEASE MEDICINES
▶ Adult: 400 mg daily in 1–2 divided doses for 21 days

Lyme arthritis | Acrodermatitis chronica atrophicans

▶ BY MOUTH USING IMMEDIATE-RELEASE MEDICINES
▶ Adult: 200 mg daily in 1–2 divided doses for 28 days

Anthrax (treatment or post-exposure prophylaxis)

▶ BY MOUTH USING IMMEDIATE-RELEASE MEDICINES
▶ Child 12–17 years: 100 mg twice daily
▶ Adult: 100 mg twice daily

Prophylaxis of malaria

▶ BY MOUTH USING IMMEDIATE-RELEASE MEDICINES
▶ Child 12–17 years (body-weight 25 kg and above): 100 mg once daily, to be started 1–2 days before entering endemic area and continued for 4 weeks after leaving
▶ Adult: 100 mg once daily, to be started 1–2 days before entering endemic area and continued for 4 weeks after leaving

Adjunct to quinine in treatment of *Plasmodium falciparum* malaria

▶ BY MOUTH USING IMMEDIATE-RELEASE MEDICINES
▶ Child 12–17 years: 200 mg daily for 7 days
▶ Adult: 200 mg daily for 7 days

Periodontitis (as an adjunct to gingival scaling and root planing)

▶ BY MOUTH USING IMMEDIATE-RELEASE MEDICINES
▶ Child 12–17 years: 20 mg twice daily for 3 months
▶ Adult: 20 mg twice daily for 3 months

Rocky Mountain spotted fever

▶ BY MOUTH USING DISPERSIBLE TABLETS
▶ Adult: 100 mg twice daily continue treatment for at least 3 days after fever subsides, minimum treatment duration is 5–7 days

- **UNLICENSED USE** Doxycycline may be used as detailed below, although these situations are considered outside the scope of its licence:
  - EvGr duration of treatment for acute sinusitis;
  - dose for treatment of acne vulgaris;
  - dose for treatment of early syphilis and late latent syphilis;
  - dose for treatment of asymptomatic contacts of patients with infectious syphilis;
  - Lyme disease ⟨A⟩;
  - treatment or post-exposure prophylaxis of anthrax;
  - malaria prophylaxis during pregnancy.

  Immediate-release doxycycline may be used for the treatment of rosacea, but it is not licensed for this indication.

- **CAUTIONS** Alcohol dependence

- **INTERACTIONS** → Appendix 1: tetracyclines

- **SIDE-EFFECTS**
- **Common or very common** Dyspnoea · hypotension · peripheral oedema · tachycardia
- **Uncommon** Gastrointestinal discomfort
- **Rare or very rare** Anxiety · arthralgia · Clostridioides difficile colitis · flushing · intracranial pressure increased with papilloedema · Jarisch-Herxheimer reaction · myalgia · photoonycholysis · severe cutaneous adverse reactions (SCARs) · skin hyperpigmentation (long term use) · stomatitis · tinnitus · vision disorders

- **PREGNANCY**
- When used for Prophylaxis of malaria UKHSA advises avoid—when travel to malarious areas is unavoidable and other regimens are unsuitable, doxycycline can be used if the entire course can be completed before 15 weeks' gestation. See also *Pregnancy* in Malaria, prophylaxis p. 702.

- **BREAST FEEDING**
- When used for Prophylaxis of malaria See *Breast-feeding* in Malaria, prophylaxis p. 702.

- **MONITORING REQUIREMENTS** When used for periodontitis, monitor for superficial fungal infection, particularly if predisposition to oral candidiasis.

- **DIRECTIONS FOR ADMINISTRATION** Manufacturer advises capsules and tablets should be swallowed whole with plenty of fluid, while sitting or standing.

- **PRESCRIBING AND DISPENSING INFORMATION** For choice of antibacterial therapy, see Anthrax p. 667, Diabetic foot infections, antibacterial therapy p. 581, Genital system infections, antibacterial therapy p. 584, Lyme disease p. 669, Malaria, prophylaxis p. 702, Malaria, treatment p. 708, Nose infections, antibacterial therapy p. 585, Respiratory system infections, antibacterial therapy p. 586, Skin infections, antibacterial therapy p. 589, Urinary-tract infections p. 681.

- **PATIENT AND CARER ADVICE** Counselling on administration advised.
  Photosensitivity Patients should be advised to avoid exposure to sunlight or sun lamps.

- **PROFESSION SPECIFIC INFORMATION**

  Dental practitioners' formulary Doxycycline Capsules 100 mg may be prescribed.
  Dispersible tablets may be prescribed as Dispersible Doxycycline Tablets.
  Tablets may be prescribed as Doxycycline Tablets 20 mg.

- **MEDICINAL FORMS** There can be variation in the licensing of different medicines containing the same drug. Forms available from special-order manufacturers include: oral suspension, oral solution

  Oral tablet
  CAUTIONARY AND ADVISORY LABELS 6, 11, 27
  - Periostat (Alliance Pharmaceuticals Ltd)
    Doxycycline (as Doxycycline hyclate) 20 mg Periostat 20mg tablets | 56 tablet [PoM] £17.30 DT = £17.30

Dispersible tablet
CAUTIONARY AND ADVISORY LABELS 6, 9, 11, 13
- Vibramycin-D (Pfizer Ltd)
  Doxycycline (as Doxycycline monohydrate) 100 mg Vibramycin-D 100mg dispersible tablets | 8 tablet [PoM] £4.91 DT = £4.91 [SF]

Modified-release capsule
CAUTIONARY AND ADVISORY LABELS 6, 11, 27
- Efracea (Galderma (UK) Ltd)
  Doxycycline (as Doxycycline monohydrate) 40 mg Efracea 40mg modified-release capsules | 14 capsule [PoM] £7.99 DT = £7.99

Oral capsule
CAUTIONARY AND ADVISORY LABELS 6, 9, 11, 27
- Doxycycline (Non-proprietary)
  Doxycycline (as Doxycycline hyclate) 50 mg Doxycycline 50mg capsules | 28 capsule [PoM] £2.00 DT = £1.68
  Doxycycline (as Doxycycline hyclate) 100 mg Doxycycline 100mg capsules | 6 capsule [PoM] £0.59-£1.00 | 8 capsule [PoM] £3.00 DT = £0.79 | 14 capsule [PoM] £5.25 | 50 capsule [PoM] £4.94-£19.00

F 655

Eravacycline
20-Jul-2022

- **INDICATIONS AND DOSE**

Complicated intra-abdominal infections
- BY INTRAVENOUS INFUSION
- Adult: 1 mg/kg every 12 hours for 4–14 days

DOSE ADJUSTMENTS DUE TO INTERACTIONS
- EvGr Increase dose to 1.5 mg/kg every 12 hours with concurrent use of potent CYP3A4 inducers or St John's wort. ⟨M⟩

- **INTERACTIONS** → Appendix 1: tetracyclines

- **SIDE-EFFECTS**
- **Common or very common** Thrombophlebitis
- **Uncommon** Hyperbilirubinaemia · hyperhidrosis

- **HEPATIC IMPAIRMENT** EvGr Caution in severe impairment (increased risk of exposure). ⟨M⟩

- **DIRECTIONS FOR ADMINISTRATION** EvGr For *intravenous infusion*, dilute reconstituted solution to a concentration of 0.3 mg/mL (range of 0.2 to 0.6 mg/mL) with Sodium Chloride 0.9%—consult product literature. Give over 1 hour. ⟨M⟩

- **HANDLING AND STORAGE** Store in a refrigerator (2–8°C) and protect from light—consult product literature about storage after dilution.

- **MEDICINAL FORMS** There can be variation in the licensing of different medicines containing the same drug.
  Powder for solution for infusion
  - Xerava (PAION Deutschland GmbH)
    Eravacycline 100 mg Xerava 100mg powder for concentrate for solution for infusion vials | 10 vial [PoM] £1,050.00 (Hospital only)

F 655

Lymecycline
20-Jan-2022

- **INDICATIONS AND DOSE**

Susceptible infections (e.g. chlamydia, rickettsia and mycoplasma)
- BY MOUTH
- Child 12-17 years: 408 mg twice daily, increased to 1.224–1.632 g daily, (in severe infection)
- Adult: 408 mg twice daily, increased to 1.224–1.632 g daily, (in severe infection)

Acne vulgaris [adjunct to topical treatment]
- BY MOUTH
- Child 12-17 years: 408 mg once daily
- Adult: 408 mg once daily

- **CONTRA-INDICATIONS** Children under 8 years (deposition in growing bone and teeth, by binding to calcium, causes staining and occasionally dental hypoplasia)

- **INTERACTIONS** → Appendix 1: tetracyclines

- **SIDE-EFFECTS**
- ▶ **Common or very common** Gastrointestinal discomfort
- ▶ **Frequency not known** Visual impairment
- **RENAL IMPAIRMENT** [EvGr] Caution; avoid in overt renal insufficiency. [M]

- **MEDICINAL FORMS** There can be variation in the licensing of different medicines containing the same drug.
  Oral capsule
  CAUTIONARY AND ADVISORY LABELS 6, 9
  - ▶ Lymecycline (Non-proprietary)
    Lymecycline 408 mg Lymecycline 408mg capsules | 28 capsule [PoM] £5.99 DT = £4.01 | 56 capsule [PoM] £15.00 DT = £8.02
  - ▶ Tetralysal (Galderma (UK) Ltd)
    Lymecycline 408 mg Tetralysal 300 capsules | 28 capsule [PoM] £6.95 DT = £4.01 | 56 capsule [PoM] £11.53 DT = £8.02

☞ 655

Minocycline
10-Feb-2022

- **INDICATIONS AND DOSE**

Susceptible infections (e.g. chlamydia, rickettsia and mycoplasma)
- ▶ BY MOUTH USING IMMEDIATE-RELEASE MEDICINES
- ▶ Child 12–17 years: 100 mg twice daily
- ▶ Adult: 100 mg twice daily

Acne
- ▶ BY MOUTH USING IMMEDIATE-RELEASE MEDICINES
- ▶ Child 12–17 years: 100 mg once daily, alternatively 50 mg twice daily
- ▶ Adult: 100 mg once daily, alternatively 50 mg twice daily
- ▶ BY MOUTH USING MODIFIED-RELEASE MEDICINES
- ▶ Child 12–17 years: 100 mg daily
- ▶ Adult: 100 mg daily

Prophylaxis of asymptomatic meningococcal carrier state (but no longer recommended)
- ▶ BY MOUTH USING IMMEDIATE-RELEASE MEDICINES
- ▶ Adult: 100 mg twice daily for 5 days, minocycline treatment is usually followed by administration of rifampicin

- **CONTRA-INDICATIONS** Children under 12 years (deposition in growing bone and teeth, by binding to calcium, causes staining and occasionally dental hypoplasia)
- **CAUTIONS** Systemic lupus erythematosus
- **INTERACTIONS** → Appendix 1: tetracyclines
- **SIDE-EFFECTS**
- ▶ **Rare or very rare** Acute kidney injury · hearing impairment · respiratory disorders · tinnitus
- ▶ **Frequency not known** Alopecia · arthralgia · ataxia · breast secretion · conjunctival discolouration · drug reaction with eosinophilia and systemic symptoms (DRESS) · dyspepsia · hyperbilirubinaemia · hyperhidrosis · oral discolouration · polyarteritis nodosa · sensation abnormal · tear discolouration · tongue discolouration · vertigo
- **RENAL IMPAIRMENT** [EvGr] Caution in severe impairment (risk of accumulation). [M]
  Dose adjustments [EvGr] Dose reduction may be required in severe impairment. [M]
- **MONITORING REQUIREMENTS** If treatment continued for longer than 6 months, monitor every 3 months for hepatotoxicity, pigmentation and for systemic lupus erythematosus—discontinue if these develop or if pre-existing systemic lupus erythematosus worsens.
- **DIRECTIONS FOR ADMINISTRATION** Manufacturer advises tablets or capsules should be swallowed whole with plenty of fluid while sitting or standing.
- **PATIENT AND CARER ADVICE** Counselling on administration advised (posture).

- **LESS SUITABLE FOR PRESCRIBING** Less suitable for prescribing (compared with other tetracyclines, minocycline is associated with a greater risk of lupus-erythematosus-like syndrome; it sometimes causes irreversible pigmentation).

- **MEDICINAL FORMS** There can be variation in the licensing of different medicines containing the same drug. Forms available from special-order manufacturers include: oral suspension, oral solution
  Oral tablet
  CAUTIONARY AND ADVISORY LABELS 6, 9
  - ▶ Minocycline (Non-proprietary)
    Minocycline (as Minocycline hydrochloride) 50 mg Minocycline 50mg tablets | 28 tablet [PoM] £10.00 DT = £6.18
    Minocycline (as Minocycline hydrochloride) 100 mg Minocycline 100mg tablets | 28 tablet [PoM] £13.50
  Modified-release capsule
  CAUTIONARY AND ADVISORY LABELS 6, 25
  - ▶ Acnamino MR (Dexcel-Pharma Ltd)
    Minocycline (as Minocycline hydrochloride) 100 mg Acnamino MR 100mg capsules | 56 capsule [PoM] £21.14 DT = £20.08
  - ▶ Minocin MR (Viatris UK Healthcare Ltd)
    Minocycline (as Minocycline hydrochloride) 100 mg Minocin MR 100mg capsules | 56 capsule [PoM] £20.08 DT = £20.08

☞ 655

Oxytetracycline
20-Jan-2022

- **INDICATIONS AND DOSE**

Susceptible infections (e.g. chlamydia, rickettsia and mycoplasma)
- ▶ BY MOUTH
- ▶ Child 12–17 years: 250–500 mg 4 times a day
- ▶ Adult: 250–500 mg 4 times a day

Rosacea
- ▶ BY MOUTH
- ▶ Adult: 500 mg twice daily usually for 6–12 weeks (course may be repeated intermittently)

Acne
- ▶ BY MOUTH
- ▶ Adult: 500 mg twice daily

- **CONTRA-INDICATIONS** Children under 12 years (deposition in growing bone and teeth, by binding to calcium, causes staining and occasionally dental hypoplasia)
- **INTERACTIONS** → Appendix 1: tetracyclines
- **SIDE-EFFECTS** Gastrointestinal discomfort · renal impairment
- **HEPATIC IMPAIRMENT**
  Dose adjustments Manufacturer advises avoid in high doses.
- **RENAL IMPAIRMENT** [EvGr] Avoid unless potential benefit outweighs risk (risk of accumulation). [M]
  Dose adjustments [EvGr] Reduce dose and/or increase dosing interval if use is essential. [M]
- **PROFESSION SPECIFIC INFORMATION**
  Dental practitioners' formulary Oxytetracycline Tablets may be prescribed.

- **MEDICINAL FORMS** There can be variation in the licensing of different medicines containing the same drug. Forms available from special-order manufacturers include: oral suspension
  Oral tablet
  CAUTIONARY AND ADVISORY LABELS 7, 9, 23
  - ▶ Oxytetracycline (Non-proprietary)
    Oxytetracycline (as Oxytetracycline dihydrate) 250 mg Oxytetracycline 250mg tablets | 28 tablet [PoM] £40.80 DT = £10.84

⬆ 655

Tetracycline

26-Jul-2023

- **INDICATIONS AND DOSE**

Susceptible infections (e.g. chlamydia, rickettsia, mycoplasma)
▸ BY MOUTH
▸ Child 12–17 years: 250 mg 4 times a day, increased if necessary to 500 mg 3–4 times a day, increased dose used in severe infections
▸ Adult: 250 mg 4 times a day, increased if necessary to 500 mg 3–4 times a day, increased dose used in severe infections

Rosacea
▸ BY MOUTH
▸ Adult: 500 mg twice daily usually for 6–12 weeks (course may be repeated intermittently)

Acne
▸ BY MOUTH
▸ Adult: 500 mg twice daily

Diabetic diarrhoea in autonomic neuropathy
▸ BY MOUTH
▸ Adult: 250 mg for 2 or 3 doses

Non-gonococcal urethritis
▸ BY MOUTH
▸ Adult: 500 mg 4 times a day for 7–14 days (21 days if failure or relapse after first course)

***Helicobacter pylori* eradication [in combination with other drugs (see Helicobacter pylori infection p. 93)]**
▸ BY MOUTH
▸ Adult: 500 mg 4 times a day for 7 days for first- and second-line eradication therapy; 10 days for third-line eradication therapy

- **UNLICENSED USE** Not licensed for treatment of diabetic diarrhoea in *autonomic neuropathy*. EvGr Tetracycline is used for the eradication of *Helicobacter pylori*, Ⓐ but is not licensed for this indication.

- **CONTRA-INDICATIONS** Children under 12 years (deposition in growing bone and teeth, by binding to calcium, causes staining and occasionally dental hypoplasia)

- **INTERACTIONS** → Appendix 1: tetracyclines

- **SIDE-EFFECTS**
▸ **Rare or very rare** Agranulocytosis · aplastic anaemia · nephritis · renal impairment
▸ **Frequency not known** Gastrointestinal discomfort · stomatitis · toxic epidermal necrolysis

- **HEPATIC IMPAIRMENT**
Dose adjustments Manufacturer advises avoid in high doses.

- **RENAL IMPAIRMENT** EvGr Avoid unless potential benefit outweighs risk (risk of accumulation). Ⓜ
Dose adjustments EvGr Reduce dose and/or increase dosing interval if use is essential. Ⓜ

- **DIRECTIONS FOR ADMINISTRATION** Manufacturer advises tablets should be swallowed whole with plenty of fluid while sitting or standing.

- **PRESCRIBING AND DISPENSING INFORMATION** For choice of antibacterial therapy, see Genital system infections, antibacterial therapy p. 584.

- **PATIENT AND CARER ADVICE** Counselling on administration advised.

- **PROFESSION SPECIFIC INFORMATION**
Dental practitioners' formulary Tetracycline Tablets may be prescribed.

- **MEDICINAL FORMS** There can be variation in the licensing of different medicines containing the same drug. Forms available from special-order manufacturers include: oral capsule, oral solution

Oral tablet
CAUTIONARY AND ADVISORY LABELS 7, 9, 23
▸ Tetracycline (Non-proprietary)
 Tetracycline hydrochloride 250 mg Tetracycline 250mg tablets | 28 tablet [PoM] £32.00 DT = £27.12

Tigecycline

02-Dec-2020

- **DRUG ACTION** Tigecycline is a glycylcycline antibacterial structurally related to the tetracyclines. Tigecycline is active against Gram-positive and Gram-negative bacteria, including tetracycline-resistant organisms, and some anaerobes. It is also active against meticillin-resistant *Staphylococcus aureus* and vancomycin-resistant enterococci, but *Pseudomonas aeruginosa* and many strains of *Proteus* spp. are resistant to tigecycline.

- **INDICATIONS AND DOSE**

Complicated skin and soft tissue infections (when other antibiotics are not suitable) | Complicated intra-abdominal infections (when other antibiotics are not suitable)
▸ BY INTRAVENOUS INFUSION
▸ Adult: Initially 100 mg for 1 dose, followed by 50 mg every 12 hours for 5–14 days

- **CONTRA-INDICATIONS** Diabetic foot infections

- **CAUTIONS** Cholestasis

- **INTERACTIONS** → Appendix 1: tigecycline

- **SIDE-EFFECTS**
▸ **Common or very common** Abscess · appetite decreased · diarrhoea · dizziness · gastrointestinal discomfort · headache · healing impaired · hyperbilirubinaemia · hypoglycaemia · hypoproteinaemia · increased risk of infection · nausea · sepsis · skin reactions · vomiting
▸ **Uncommon** Hepatic disorders · pancreatitis · thrombocytopenia · thrombophlebitis
▸ **Frequency not known** Acidosis · azotaemia · hyperphosphataemia · hypofibrinogenaemia · idiopathic intracranial hypertension · photosensitivity reaction · pseudomembranous enterocolitis · severe cutaneous adverse reactions (SCARs) · tooth discolouration

SIDE-EFFECTS, FURTHER INFORMATION Side-effects similar to those of the tetracyclines can potentially occur.

- **ALLERGY AND CROSS-SENSITIVITY** EvGr Contra-indicated in patients hypersensitive to tetracyclines. Ⓜ

- **PREGNANCY** Tetracyclines should **not** be given to pregnant women; effects on skeletal development have been documented in the first trimester in *animal* studies. Administration during the second or third trimester may cause discoloration of the child's teeth, and maternal hepatotoxicity has been reported with large parenteral doses.

- **BREAST FEEDING** Manufacturer advises avoid—present in milk in *animal* studies.

- **HEPATIC IMPAIRMENT** Manufacturer advises caution in severe impairment.
Dose adjustments Manufacturer advises dose reduction to 25 mg every 12 hours following the loading dose in severe impairment.

- **DIRECTIONS FOR ADMINISTRATION** For *intravenous infusion* (*Tygacil*®), give intermittently *in* Glucose 5% *or* Sodium Chloride 0.9%. Reconstitute each vial with 5.3 mL infusion fluid to produce a 10 mg/mL solution; dilute requisite dose in 100 mL infusion fluid; give over 30–60 minutes.

- **PATIENT AND CARER ADVICE**
Driving and skilled tasks Manufacturer advises patients and carers should be cautioned on the effects on driving and performance of skilled tasks—increased risk of dizziness.

- **MEDICINAL FORMS** There can be variation in the licensing of different medicines containing the same drug.
Powder for solution for infusion
  - ▸ Tigecycline (Non-proprietary)
  Tigecycline 50 mg Tigecycline 50mg powder for solution for infusion vials | 10 vial [PoM] £290.79–£323.10 (Hospital only)
  - ▸ Tygacil (Pfizer Ltd)
  Tigecycline 50 mg Tygacil 50mg powder for solution for infusion vials | 10 vial [PoM] £323.10 (Hospital only)

ANTIBACTERIALS › OTHER

Chloramphenicol

24-Jul-2024

- **DRUG ACTION** Chloramphenicol is a potent broad-spectrum antibiotic.

- **INDICATIONS AND DOSE**

Life threatening infections particularly those caused by *Haemophilus influenzae*|Typhoid fever
  - ▸ BY MOUTH, OR BY INTRAVENOUS INJECTION, OR BY INTRAVENOUS INFUSION
  - ▸ Adult: 12.5 mg/kg every 6 hours, in exceptional cases dose can be doubled for severe infections such as septicaemia and meningitis, providing high doses reduced as soon as clinically indicated

- **CONTRA-INDICATIONS** Acute porphyrias p. 1202
- **CAUTIONS** Avoid repeated courses and prolonged treatment
- **INTERACTIONS** → Appendix 1: chloramphenicol
- **SIDE-EFFECTS**
  - ▸ **Rare or very rare**
  - ▸ With parenteral use Aplastic anaemia (reversible or irreversible, with reports of resulting leukaemia)
  - ▸ **Frequency not known**
  - ▸ With oral use Bone marrow disorders · circulatory collapse · diarrhoea · enterocolitis · nausea · optic neuritis · oral disorders · ototoxicity · vomiting
  - ▸ With parenteral use Agranulocytosis · bone marrow disorders · depression · diarrhoea · dry mouth · fungal superinfection · headache · nausea · nerve disorders · thrombocytopenic purpura · urticaria · vision disorders · vomiting

  SIDE-EFFECTS, FURTHER INFORMATION Associated with serious haematological side-effects when given systemically and should therefore be reserved for the treatment of life-threatening infections.

- **PREGNANCY** Manufacturer advises avoid; neonatal 'grey-baby syndrome' if used in third trimester.
- **BREAST FEEDING** Manufacturer advises avoid; use another antibiotic; may cause bone-marrow toxicity in infant; concentration in milk usually insufficient to cause 'grey syndrome'.
- **HEPATIC IMPAIRMENT** Manufacturer advises caution (increased risk of bone-marrow depression)—monitor plasma-chloramphenicol concentration.
  Dose adjustments Manufacturer advises consider dose reduction.
- **RENAL IMPAIRMENT** [EvGr] Caution (increased risk of bone-marrow depression)—monitor plasma-chloramphenicol concentration. ⟨M⟩
  Dose adjustments [EvGr] Consider dose reduction. ⟨M⟩
- **MONITORING REQUIREMENTS**
  - ▸ Plasma concentration monitoring preferred in the elderly.
  - ▸ Recommended peak plasma concentration (approx. 2 hours after administration by mouth, intravenous injection or infusion) 10–25 mg/litre; pre-dose ('trough') concentration should not exceed 15 mg/litre.
  - ▸ Blood counts required before and periodically during treatment.

- **DIRECTIONS FOR ADMINISTRATION** [EvGr] For *intravenous infusion*, give intermittently or via drip tubing in Glucose 5% *or* Sodium Chloride 0.9%. ⟨M⟩

- **PRESCRIBING AND DISPENSING INFORMATION** For choice of antibacterial therapy, see Central nervous system infections, antibacterial therapy p. 580.

- **MEDICINAL FORMS** There can be variation in the licensing of different medicines containing the same drug.
Powder for solution for injection
ELECTROLYTES: May contain Sodium
  - ▸ Chloramphenicol (Non-proprietary)
  Chloramphenicol (as Chloramphenicol sodium succinate)
  1 gram Chloramphenicol 1g powder for solution for injection vials | 1 vial [PoM] £15.00–£88.00 (Hospital only) | 1 vial [PoM] £92.34–£92.40

Oral capsule
  - ▸ Chloramphenicol (Non-proprietary)
  Chloramphenicol 250 mg Chloramphenicol 250mg capsules | 60 capsule [PoM] £377.00 DT = £377.00

Daptomycin

18-Aug-2021

- **DRUG ACTION** Daptomycin is a lipopeptide antibacterial with a spectrum of activity similar to vancomycin but its efficacy against enterococci has not been established. It needs to be given with other antibacterials for mixed infections involving Gram-negative bacteria and some anaerobes.

- **INDICATIONS AND DOSE**

Complicated skin and soft-tissue infections caused by Gram-positive bacteria
  - ▸ BY INTRAVENOUS INFUSION
  - ▸ Child 12-23 months: 10 mg/kg once daily for up to 14 days, alternatively 12 mg/kg once daily, higher dose only if associated with *Staphylococcus aureus* bacteraemia—duration of treatment in accordance with risk of complications in individual patients
  - ▸ Child 2-6 years: 9 mg/kg once daily for up to 14 days, alternatively 12 mg/kg once daily, higher dose only if associated with *Staphylococcus aureus* bacteraemia—duration of treatment in accordance with risk of complications in individual patients
  - ▸ Child 7-11 years: 7 mg/kg once daily for up to 14 days, alternatively 9 mg/kg once daily, higher dose only if associated with *Staphylococcus aureus* bacteraemia—duration of treatment in accordance with risk of complications in individual patients
  - ▸ Child 12-17 years: 5 mg/kg once daily for up to 14 days, alternatively 7 mg/kg once daily, higher dose only if associated with *Staphylococcus aureus* bacteraemia—duration of treatment in accordance with risk of complications in individual patients

Complicated skin and soft-tissue infections caused by Gram-positive bacteria
  - ▸ BY SLOW INTRAVENOUS INJECTION, OR BY INTRAVENOUS INFUSION
  - ▸ Adult: 4 mg/kg once daily for 7–14 days or longer if necessary, alternatively 6 mg/kg once daily, higher dose only if associated with *Staphylococcus aureus* bacteraemia—duration of treatment may need to be longer than 14 days in accordance with risk of complications in individual patients

Right-sided infective endocarditis caused by
Staphylococcus aureus **(administered on expert advice)**
▸ BY SLOW INTRAVENOUS INJECTION, OR BY INTRAVENOUS
  INFUSION
▸ Adult: 6 mg/kg once daily, duration of treatment in
  accordance with official recommendations

● CAUTIONS Obesity (limited information on safety and
efficacy)

● INTERACTIONS → Appendix 1: daptomycin

● SIDE-EFFECTS
▸ **Common or very common** Anaemia · anxiety · asthenia ·
  constipation · diarrhoea · dizziness · fever · flatulence ·
  gastrointestinal discomfort · headache · hypertension ·
  hypotension · increased risk of infection · insomnia ·
  nausea · pain · skin reactions · vomiting
▸ **Uncommon** Appetite decreased · arrhythmias · arthralgia ·
  electrolyte imbalance · eosinophilia · flushing · glossitis ·
  hyperglycaemia · muscle weakness · myalgia · myopathy ·
  paraesthesia · renal impairment · taste altered ·
  thrombocytosis · tremor · vertigo
▸ **Rare or very rare** Jaundice
▸ **Frequency not known** Acute generalised exanthematous
  pustulosis (AGEP) · chills · Clostridioides difficile colitis ·
  cough · infusion related reaction · peripheral neuropathy ·
  respiratory disorders · syncope

SIDE-EFFECTS, FURTHER INFORMATION If unexplained
muscle pain, tenderness, weakness, or cramps develop
during treatment, measure creatine kinase every 2 days;
discontinue if unexplained muscular symptoms and
creatine elevated markedly.

● PREGNANCY Manufacturer advises use only if potential
benefit outweighs risk—no information available.

● BREAST FEEDING Present in milk in small amounts, but
absorption from gastrointestinal tract negligible.

● HEPATIC IMPAIRMENT Manufacturer advises caution in
severe impairment—no information available.

● RENAL IMPAIRMENT
▸ In children Manufacturer advises the dosage regimen has
  not been established—use with caution and monitor renal
  function regularly.
▸ In adults Manufacturer advises use only when potential
  benefit outweighs risk—higher risk of developing
  myopathy; monitor renal function regularly.
  Dose adjustments
  ▸ In adults Manufacturer advises use normal dose every
    48 hours if creatinine clearance less than 30 mL/minute.
    See p. 21.

● MONITORING REQUIREMENTS
▸ Manufacturer advises monitor plasma creatine
  phosphokinase (CPK) before treatment and then at least
  weekly during treatment; monitor CPK more frequently in
  patients at higher risk of developing myopathy, including
  those with renal impairment, taking other drugs
  associated with myopathy, or if CPK elevated more than
  5 times upper limit of normal before treatment.
▸ Manufacturer advises monitor renal function regularly
  during concomitant administration of potentially
  nephrotoxic drugs.

● EFFECT ON LABORATORY TESTS Interference with assay for
prothrombin time and INR—take blood sample
immediately before daptomycin dose.

● DIRECTIONS FOR ADMINISTRATION
▸ In children For *intravenous infusion*, manufacturer advises
  give intermittently in Sodium Chloride 0.9%; reconstitute
  with Sodium Chloride 0.9% (350 mg in 7 mL, 500 mg in
  10 mL); gently rotate vial without shaking; allow to stand
  for at least 10 minutes then rotate gently to dissolve;
  dilute requisite dose in 50 mL infusion fluid and give over

60 minutes for children aged 1–6 years and over
30 minutes for children aged 7–17 years.
▸ In adults For *intravenous infusion*, manufacturer advises
  give intermittently in Sodium Chloride 0.9%; reconstitute
  with Sodium Chloride 0.9% (350 mg in 7 mL, 500 mg in
  10 mL); gently rotate vial without shaking; allow to stand
  for at least 10 minutes then rotate gently to dissolve;
  dilute requisite dose in 50 mL infusion fluid and give over
  30 minutes. For *intravenous injection*, give over 2 minutes.

● HANDLING AND STORAGE Manufacturer advises store in a
refrigerator (2–8 °C)—consult product literature for
further information regarding storage after reconstitution
and dilution.

● NATIONAL FUNDING/ACCESS DECISIONS
For full details see funding body website
Scottish Medicines Consortium (SMC) decisions
▸ **Daptomycin (***Cubicin***®) for complicated skin and soft tissue
  infections in adults (April 2006)** SMC No. 248/06
  Recommended with restrictions
▸ **Daptomycin (***Cubicin***®) for the treatment of** *Staphylococcus*
  aureus **bacteraemia (SAB) when associated with right-sided
  infective endocarditis or with complicated skin and soft-tissue
  infection in adults (March 2008)** SMC No. 449/08
  Recommended with restrictions

● MEDICINAL FORMS There can be variation in the licensing of
different medicines containing the same drug.
Powder for solution for infusion
▸ Daptomycin (Non-proprietary)
  Daptomycin 350 mg Daptomycin 350mg powder for solution for
  infusion vials | 1 vial [PoM] £60.00-£62.00 (Hospital only) |
  1 vial [PoM] £60.00-£62.00
  Daptomycin 500 mg Daptomycin 500mg powder for solution for
  infusion vials | 1 vial [PoM] £88.00-£88.57 (Hospital only) |
  1 vial [PoM] £88.00-£88.57
▸ Cubicin (Merck Sharp & Dohme (UK) Ltd)
  Daptomycin 350 mg Cubicin 350mg powder for concentrate for
  solution for infusion vials | 1 vial [PoM] £62.00 (Hospital only)
  Daptomycin 500 mg Cubicin 500mg powder for concentrate for
  solution for infusion vials | 1 vial [PoM] £88.57 (Hospital only)

Fidaxomicin   16-Aug-2023

● DRUG ACTION Fidaxomicin is a macrocyclic antibacterial
that is poorly absorbed from the gastro-intestinal tract,
and, therefore, it should not be used to treat systemic
infections.

● **INDICATIONS AND DOSE**
***Clostridioides difficile* infection**
▸ BY MOUTH
▸ Adult: 200 mg every 12 hours for 10 days
***Clostridioides difficile* infection [extended-pulsed dosing]**
▸ BY MOUTH USING TABLETS
▸ Adult: Initially 200 mg every 12 hours on days 1–5,
  then 200 mg once daily on alternate days on days 7–25

● INTERACTIONS → Appendix 1: fidaxomicin

● SIDE-EFFECTS
▸ **Common or very common** Constipation · nausea · vomiting
▸ **Uncommon** Abdominal distension · appetite decreased ·
  dizziness · dry mouth · flatulence · headache · skin
  reactions · taste altered

● ALLERGY AND CROSS-SENSITIVITY [EvGr] Use with caution
in macrolide hypersensitivity. Ⓜ

● PREGNANCY Manufacturer advises avoid—no information
available.

● BREAST FEEDING Manufacturer advises avoid—no
information available.

● HEPATIC IMPAIRMENT Manufacturer advises caution in
moderate to severe impairment—limited information
available.

- **RENAL IMPAIRMENT** EvGr Caution in severe impairment (limited information available). Ⓜ
- **DIRECTIONS FOR ADMINISTRATION** Fidaxomicin oral suspension can be administered via an enteral feeding tube—consult product literature.
- **PATIENT AND CARER ADVICE** Patient or carer counselling is advised for fidaxomicin oral suspension.
- **NATIONAL FUNDING/ACCESS DECISIONS** For full details see funding body website

Scottish Medicines Consortium (SMC) decisions
- Fidaxomicin (*Dificlir*®) for the treatment of *Clostridium difficile* infections (CDI) also known as *C. Difficile*-associated diarrhoea (CDAD) (July 2012) SMC No. 791/12 Recommended with restrictions

- **MEDICINAL FORMS** There can be variation in the licensing of different medicines containing the same drug.

Oral tablet
CAUTIONARY AND ADVISORY LABELS 9, 25
EXCIPIENTS: May contain Lecithin
- Fidaxomicin (Non-proprietary)
Fidaxomicin 200 mg Fidaxomicin 200mg tablets | 20 tablet PoM £1,350.00 DT = £1,350.00

Oral suspension
CAUTIONARY AND ADVISORY LABELS 9
- Fidaxomicin (Non-proprietary)
Fidaxomicin 40 mg per 1 ml Fidaxomicin 40mg/ml oral suspension sugar free | 110 ml PoM £1,350.00 DT = £1,350.00 SF

Fosfomycin

28-Jul-2021

- **DRUG ACTION** Fosfomycin, a phosphonic acid antibacterial, is active against a range of Gram-positive and Gram-negative bacteria including *Staphylococcus aureus* and Enterobacteriaceae.

- **INDICATIONS AND DOSE**

Acute uncomplicated lower urinary-tract infections
- BY MOUTH USING GRANULES
- Adult: 3 g for 1 dose

Prophylaxis of urinary-tract infections in transurethral surgical procedures
- BY MOUTH USING GRANULES
- Adult: 3 g, to be given 3 hours before surgery. Dose may be repeated once, 24 hours after surgery

Osteomyelitis when first-line treatments are inappropriate or ineffective | Hospital-acquired lower respiratory-tract infections when first-line treatments are inappropriate or ineffective
- BY INTRAVENOUS INFUSION
- Adult: 12–24 g daily in 2–3 divided doses (max. per dose 8 g), use the high-dose regimen in severe infection suspected or known to be caused by less sensitive organisms

Complicated urinary-tract infections when first-line treatment ineffective or inappropriate
- BY INTRAVENOUS INFUSION
- Adult: 12–16 g daily in 2–3 divided doses (max. per dose 8 g)

Bacterial meningitis when first-line treatment ineffective or inappropriate
- BY INTRAVENOUS INFUSION
- Adult: 16–24 g daily in 3–4 divided doses (max. per dose 8 g), use the high-dose regimen in severe infection suspected or known to be caused by less sensitive organisms

- **CAUTIONS**
- With intravenous use Cardiac insufficiency · elderly (high doses) · hyperaldosteronism · hypernatraemia · hypertension · pulmonary oedema

- **SIDE-EFFECTS**
GENERAL SIDE-EFFECTS
- **Common or very common** Abdominal pain · diarrhoea · headache · nausea · vomiting
- **Uncommon** Skin reactions
- **Frequency not known** Antibiotic associated colitis · Clostridioides difficile colitis · pseudomembranous enterocolitis

SPECIFIC SIDE-EFFECTS
- **Common or very common**
- With oral use Dizziness · vulvovaginal infection
- **Uncommon**
- With parenteral use Appetite decreased · dyspnoea · electrolyte imbalance · fatigue · oedema · taste altered · vertigo
- **Rare or very rare**
- With parenteral use Bone marrow disorders · eosinophilia · hepatic disorders · visual impairment
- **Frequency not known**
- With parenteral use Agranulocytosis · asthmatic attack · confusion · leucopenia · neutropenia · tachycardia · thrombocytopenia

- **PREGNANCY** Manufacturer advises use only if potential benefit outweighs risk.
- **BREAST FEEDING** Manufacturer advises use only if potential benefit outweighs risk—present in milk.
- **RENAL IMPAIRMENT** See p. 21.
- With oral use EvGr Avoid if creatinine clearance less than 10 mL/minute. Ⓜ
- With intravenous use EvGr Caution if creatinine clearance 40–80 mL/minute; consult product literature if creatinine clearance less than 40 mL/minute. Ⓜ
- **MONITORING REQUIREMENTS**
- With intravenous use Monitor electrolytes and fluid balance.
- **DIRECTIONS FOR ADMINISTRATION**
- With intravenous use For *intravenous infusion* (*Fomicyt*®), manufacturer advises give intermittently *in* Glucose 5% *or* 10% *or* Water for Injections; reconstitute each 2-g or 4-g vial with 20 mL and 8-g vial with 40 mL infusion fluid; dilute reconstituted solution to a concentration of 40 mg/mL; give 2 g over 15 minutes.
- With oral use Manufacturer advises granules should be taken on an empty stomach (about 2–3 hours before or after a meal), preferably before bedtime and after emptying the bladder. The granules should be dissolved into a glass of water and taken immediately.
- **PRESCRIBING AND DISPENSING INFORMATION** Doses expressed as fosfomycin base.
- **NATIONAL FUNDING/ACCESS DECISIONS** For full details see funding body website

Scottish Medicines Consortium (SMC) decisions
- Fosfomycin (*Fomicyt*®) for the treatment of the following infections in adults and children including neonates: acute osteomyelitis; complicated urinary tract infections; nosocomial lower respiratory tract infections; bacterial meningitis; bacteraemia that occurs in association with, or is suspected to be associated with, any of the infections listed above (March 2015) SMC No. 1033/15 Recommended with restrictions
- Fosfomycin trometamol (*Monuril*®) for the treatment of acute lower uncomplicated urinary tract infections, caused by pathogens sensitive to fosfomycin in adult and adolescent female, and for prophylaxis in diagnostic and surgical transurethral procedures (September 2016) SMC No. 1163/16 Recommended

- **MEDICINAL FORMS** There can be variation in the licensing of different medicines containing the same drug.

Granules for oral solution
CAUTIONARY AND ADVISORY LABELS 9, 13, 23
EXCIPIENTS: May contain Sucrose
- ▶ **Fosfomycin (Non-proprietary)**
  Fosfomycin (as Fosfomycin trometamol) 3 gram Fosfomycin 3g granules for oral solution sachets | 1 sachet PoM £4.86-£7.90 DT = £4.86
  - ▶ Monuril (Zambon UK Ltd)
  Fosfomycin (as Fosfomycin trometamol) 3 gram Monuril 3g granules for oral solution sachets | 1 sachet PoM £4.86 DT = £4.86

Powder for solution for infusion
ELECTROLYTES: May contain Sodium
- ▶ **Fosfomycin (Non-proprietary)**
  Fosfomycin (as Fosfomycin sodium) 5 gram Infectofos 5g powder for solution for infusion vials | 10 vial PoM ⓧ (Hospital only)
  - ▶ Fomicyt (InfectoPharm Ltd)
  Fosfomycin (as Fosfomycin sodium) 2 gram Fomicyt 2g powder for solution for infusion vials | 10 vial PoM £160.03 (Hospital only)
  Fosfomycin (as Fosfomycin sodium) 4 gram Fomicyt 4g powder for solution for infusion vials | 10 vial PoM £320.06 (Hospital only)

Fusidic acid
05-Oct-2021

- **DRUG ACTION** Fusidic acid and its salts are narrow-spectrum antibiotics used for staphylococcal infections.

- **INDICATIONS AND DOSE**

Staphylococcal skin infection
- ▶ TO THE SKIN
- ▶ Child: Apply 3–4 times a day usually for 7 days
- ▶ Adult: Apply 3–4 times a day
- ▶ BY MOUTH USING TABLETS
- ▶ Child 12-17 years: 250 mg every 12 hours for 5-10 days, dose expressed as sodium fusidate
- ▶ Adult: 250 mg every 12 hours for 5-10 days, dose expressed as sodium fusidate

Non-bullous impetigo [in patients who are not systemically unwell or at high risk of complications] | Secondary bacterial infection of eczema [for localised infections only]
- ▶ TO THE SKIN
- ▶ Child: Apply 3 times a day for 5–7 days
- ▶ Adult: Apply 3 times a day for 5–7 days

Penicillin-resistant staphylococcal infection including osteomyelitis | Staphylococcal endocarditis in combination with other antibacterials
- ▶ BY MOUTH USING ORAL SUSPENSION
- ▶ Child 1-11 months: 15 mg/kg 3 times a day
- ▶ Child 1-4 years: 250 mg 3 times a day
- ▶ Child 5-11 years: 500 mg 3 times a day
- ▶ Child 12-17 years: 750 mg 3 times a day
- ▶ Adult: 750 mg 3 times a day
- ▶ BY MOUTH USING TABLETS
- ▶ Child 12-17 years: 500 mg every 8 hours, dose expressed as sodium fusidate, increased to 1 g every 8 hours, dose expressed as sodium fusidate, increased dose used for severe infections
- ▶ Adult: 500 mg every 8 hours, dose expressed as sodium fusidate, increased to 1 g every 8 hours, dose expressed as sodium fusidate, increased dose used for severe infections

Staphylococcal infections due to susceptible organisms
- ▶ BY INTRAVENOUS INFUSION
- ▶ Child (body-weight up to 50 kg): 6–7 mg/kg 3 times a day, dose expressed as sodium fusidate
- ▶ Child (body-weight 50 kg and above): 500 mg 3 times a day, dose expressed as sodium fusidate
- ▶ Adult (body-weight up to 50 kg): 6–7 mg/kg 3 times a day, dose expressed as sodium fusidate

- ▶ Adult (body-weight 50 kg and above): 500 mg 3 times a day, dose expressed as sodium fusidate

DOSE EQUIVALENCE AND CONVERSION
- ▶ With oral use
- ▶ Fusidic acid is incompletely absorbed and doses recommended for suspension are proportionately higher than those for sodium fusidate tablets.

- **CAUTIONS**
- ▶ With systemic use Impaired transport and metabolism of bilirubin
- ▶ With topical use Avoid contact of cream or ointment with eyes

CAUTIONS, FURTHER INFORMATION
- ▶ Avoiding resistance
- ▶ With topical use To avoid the development of resistance, fusidic acid should not be used for longer than 10 days and local microbiology advice should be sought before using it in hospital.

- **INTERACTIONS** → Appendix 1: fusidate

- **SIDE-EFFECTS**
  GENERAL SIDE-EFFECTS
- ▶ **Uncommon** Skin reactions
  SPECIFIC SIDE-EFFECTS
- ▶ **Common or very common**
- ▶ With intravenous use Thrombophlebitis · vascular pain (reduced if given via central vein)
- ▶ With oral use Diarrhoea · gastrointestinal discomfort · nausea · vomiting
- ▶ With systemic use Dizziness · drowsiness · hepatic disorders · hyperbilirubinaemia
- ▶ **Uncommon**
- ▶ With oral use Rash pustular
- ▶ With systemic use Appetite decreased · asthenia · headache · malaise · rhabdomyolysis
- ▶ **Rare or very rare**
- ▶ With topical use Angioedema · conjunctivitis
- ▶ **Frequency not known**
- ▶ With systemic use Agranulocytosis · anaemia · leucopenia · neutropenia · pancytopenia · renal failure · thrombocytopenia

  SIDE-EFFECTS, FURTHER INFORMATION Elevated liver enzymes, hyperbilirubinaemia and jaundice can occur with systemic use—these effects are usually reversible following withdrawal of therapy.

- **PREGNANCY**
- ▶ With systemic use Not known to be harmful; manufacturer advises use only if potential benefit outweighs risk.

- **BREAST FEEDING**
- ▶ With systemic use Present in milk—manufacturer advises caution.

- **HEPATIC IMPAIRMENT**
- ▶ With systemic use Manufacturer advises caution.

- **MONITORING REQUIREMENTS**
- ▶ With systemic use Manufacturer advises monitor liver function with high doses or on prolonged therapy; monitoring also advised for patients with biliary tract obstruction, those taking potentially hepatotoxic medication, or those taking concurrent medication with a similar excretion pathway.

- **DIRECTIONS FOR ADMINISTRATION** Manufacturer advises *for intravenous infusion*, give intermittently in Sodium Chloride 0.9% or Glucose 5%; reconstitute each vial with 10 mL buffer solution, then add contents of vial to 500 mL infusion fluid to give a solution containing approximately 1 mg/mL. Give requisite dose via a central line over 2 hours (give over at least 6 hours if administered via a large peripheral vein).

- **PRESCRIBING AND DISPENSING INFORMATION** For choice of antibacterial therapy, see Cardiovascular system infections, antibacterial therapy p. 579, Musculoskeletal system infections, antibacterial therapy p. 585, Skin infections, antibacterial therapy p. 589.

- **PROFESSION SPECIFIC INFORMATION**

Dental practitioners' formulary May be prescribed as Sodium Fusidate ointment.

- **MEDICINAL FORMS** There can be variation in the licensing of different medicines containing the same drug. Forms available from special-order manufacturers include: oral suspension

Oral tablet

CAUTIONARY AND ADVISORY LABELS 9

- ▸ **Fusidic acid (Non-proprietary)**
  Sodium fusidate 250 mg Sodium fusidate 250mg tablets | 1 tablet [PoM] [℞]
- ▸ **Fucidin** (LEO Pharma)
  Sodium fusidate 250 mg Fucidin 250mg tablets | 100 tablet [PoM] £54.99 DT = £54.99

Cutaneous ointment

EXCIPIENTS: May contain Cetostearyl alcohol (including cetyl and stearyl alcohol), woolfat and related substances (including lanolin)

- ▸ **Fucidin** (LEO Pharma)
  Sodium fusidate 20 mg per 1 gram Fucidin 20mg/g ointment | 15 gram [PoM] £2.68 DT = £2.68 | 30 gram [PoM] £4.55 DT = £4.55

Oral suspension

CAUTIONARY AND ADVISORY LABELS 9

- ▸ **Fucidin** (LEO Pharma)
  Fusidic acid 50 mg per 1 ml Fucidin 250mg/5ml oral suspension | 90 ml [PoM] £12.11 DT = £12.11

Cutaneous cream

EXCIPIENTS: May contain Butylated hydroxyanisole, cetostearyl alcohol (including cetyl and stearyl alcohol)

- ▸ **Fusidic acid (Non-proprietary)**
  Fusidic acid 20 mg per 1 gram Fusidic acid 2% cream | 15 gram [PoM] £3.20 DT = £1.92 | 30 gram [PoM] £7.00 DT = £3.59
- ▸ **Fucidin** (LEO Pharma)
  Fusidic acid 20 mg per 1 gram Fucidin 20mg/g cream | 15 gram [PoM] £1.92 DT = £1.92 | 30 gram [PoM] £3.59 DT = £3.59

Powder and solvent for solution for infusion

ELECTROLYTES: May contain Sodium

- ▸ **Fusidic acid (Non-proprietary)**
  Sodium fusidate 500 mg Sodium fusidate 500mg powder and solvent for solution for infusion vials | 1 vial [PoM] £21.95 DT = £21.95

Linezolid

19-Jul-2021

- **DRUG ACTION** Linezolid, an oxazolidinone antibacterial, is active against Gram-positive bacteria including meticillin-resistant *Staphylococcus aureus* (MRSA), and glycopeptide-resistant enterococci. Resistance to linezolid can develop with prolonged treatment or if the dose is less than that recommended. Linezolid is **not** active against common Gram-negative organisms; it must be given in combination with other antibacterials for mixed infections that also involve Gram-negative organisms.

- **INDICATIONS AND DOSE**

Pneumonia (when other antibacterials e.g. a glycopetide, such as vancomycin, cannot be used) (initiated under specialist supervision) | Complicated skin and soft-tissue infections caused by Gram-positive bacteria, when other antibacterials cannot be used (initiated under specialist supervision)

- ▸ BY MOUTH
- ▸ Adult: 600 mg every 12 hours usually for 10–14 days (maximum duration of treatment 28 days)
- ▸ BY INTRAVENOUS INFUSION
- ▸ Adult: 600 mg every 12 hours

Cellulitis (specialist use only) | Erysipelas (specialist use only)

- ▸ BY MOUTH, OR BY INTRAVENOUS INFUSION
- ▸ Adult: 600 mg every 12 hours

Moderate diabetic foot infection (specialist use only) | Severe diabetic foot infection (specialist use only) | Leg ulcer infection (specialist use only)

- ▸ BY MOUTH, OR BY INTRAVENOUS INFUSION
- ▸ Adult: 600 mg every 12 hours

IMPORTANT SAFETY INFORMATION

CHM ADVICE (OPTIC NEUROPATHY)

Severe optic neuropathy may occur rarely, particularly if linezolid is used for longer than 28 days. The CHM recommends that:

- patients should be warned to report symptoms of visual impairment (including blurred vision, visual field defect, changes in visual acuity and colour vision) immediately;
- patients experiencing new visual symptoms (regardless of treatment duration) should be evaluated promptly, and referred to an ophthalmologist if necessary;
- visual function should be monitored regularly if treatment is required for longer than 28 days.

BLOOD DISORDERS

Haematopoietic disorders (including thrombocytopenia, anaemia, leucopenia, and pancytopenia) have been reported in patients receiving linezolid. It is recommended that full blood counts are monitored weekly. Close monitoring is recommended in patients who:

- receive treatment for more than 10–14 days;
- have pre-existing myelosuppression;
- are receiving drugs that may have adverse effects on haemoglobin, blood counts, or platelet function;
- have severe renal impairment.

If significant myelosuppression occurs, treatment should be stopped unless it is considered essential, in which case intensive monitoring of blood counts and appropriate management should be implemented.

- **CAUTIONS** Acute confusional states · bipolar depression · carcinoid tumour · elderly (increased risk of blood disorders) · history of seizures · phaeochromocytoma · schizophrenia · thyrotoxicosis · uncontrolled hypertension

CAUTIONS, FURTHER INFORMATION

- ▸ Close observation Unless close observation and blood pressure monitoring possible, linezolid should be avoided in uncontrolled hypertension, phaeochromocytoma, carcinoid tumour, thyrotoxicosis, bipolar depression, schizophrenia, or acute confusional states.

- **INTERACTIONS** → Appendix 1: linezolid

- **SIDE-EFFECTS**

- ▸ **Common or very common** Anaemia · constipation · diarrhoea · dizziness · gastrointestinal discomfort · headache · hypertension · increased risk of infection · insomnia · localised pain · nausea · skin reactions · taste altered · thrombocytopenia · vomiting
- ▸ **Uncommon** Angioedema · antibiotic associated colitis · arrhythmias · bone marrow disorders · chills · dry mouth · eosinophilia · fatigue · gastritis · hyperhidrosis · hyponatraemia · leucopenia · nerve disorders · neutropenia · oral disorders · pancreatitis · polyuria · pseudomembranous enterocolitis · renal failure · seizure · sensation abnormal · thirst · thrombophlebitis · tinnitus · tongue discolouration · transient ischaemic attack · vision disorders · vulvovaginal disorder
- ▸ **Rare or very rare** Hypersensitivity vasculitis · lactic acidosis · rhabdomyolysis · severe cutaneous adverse reactions (SCARs) · tooth discolouration
- ▸ **Frequency not known** Alopecia · Clostridioides difficile colitis · serotonin syndrome · SIADH

- **PREGNANCY** Manufacturer advises use only if potential benefit outweighs risk—no information available.
- **BREAST FEEDING** Manufacturer advises avoid—present in milk in *animal* studies.
- **HEPATIC IMPAIRMENT** Manufacturer advises caution in severe impairment (no information available).
- **RENAL IMPAIRMENT** EvGr Use with caution if creatinine clearance less than 30 mL/minute (metabolites may accumulate), ⟨M⟩ see p. 21.
- **MONITORING REQUIREMENTS** Monitor full blood count (including platelet count) weekly.
- **DIRECTIONS FOR ADMINISTRATION**
- ▸ With intravenous use Manufacturer advises infusion to be administered over 30–120 minutes.
- **PRESCRIBING AND DISPENSING INFORMATION** For choice of antibacterial therapy, see Diabetic foot infections, antibacterial therapy p. 581, Respiratory system infections, antibacterial therapy p. 586, Skin infections, antibacterial therapy p. 589.
- **PATIENT AND CARER ADVICE** Patients should be advised to read the patient information leaflet given with linezolid.

- **MEDICINAL FORMS** There can be variation in the licensing of different medicines containing the same drug.

Infusion
EXCIPIENTS: May contain Glucose
ELECTROLYTES: May contain Sodium
- ▸ Linezolid (Non-proprietary)
  Linezolid 2 mg per 1 ml Linezolid 600mg/300ml infusion bags | 10 bag [PoM] £445.00-£706.30 (Hospital only)
- ▸ Zyvox (Pfizer Ltd)
  Linezolid 2 mg per 1 ml Zyvox 600mg/300ml infusion bags | 10 bag [PoM] £445.00 (Hospital only)

Oral tablet
CAUTIONARY AND ADVISORY LABELS 9, 10
- ▸ Linezolid (Non-proprietary)
  Linezolid 600 mg Linezolid 600mg tablets | 10 tablet [PoM] £239.16-£392.77 (Hospital only) | 10 tablet [PoM] £327.24-£445.00
- ▸ Zyvox (Pfizer Ltd)
  Linezolid 600 mg Zyvox 600mg tablets | 10 tablet [PoM] £445.00

Oral suspension
CAUTIONARY AND ADVISORY LABELS 9, 10
EXCIPIENTS: May contain Aspartame
- ▸ Zyvox (Pfizer Ltd)
  Linezolid 20 mg per 1 ml Zyvox 100mg/5ml granules for oral suspension | 150 ml [PoM] £222.50 DT = £222.50

Tedizolid

16-Nov-2020

- **DRUG ACTION** Tedizolid is an oxazolidinone antibacterial, which inhibits bacterial protein synthesis.

- **INDICATIONS AND DOSE**

Treatment of acute bacterial skin and skin structure infections
- ▸ BY INTRAVENOUS INFUSION, OR BY MOUTH
- ▸ Adult: 200 mg once daily for 6 days, patients should be switched from the intravenous to the oral route when clinically appropriate

- **CAUTIONS** Neutropenia—limited clinical experience · patients aged 75 years and over—limited clinical experience
- **INTERACTIONS** → Appendix 1: tedizolid
- **SIDE-EFFECTS**
  GENERAL SIDE-EFFECTS
- ▸ **Common or very common** Diarrhoea · dizziness · fatigue · headache · nausea · skin reactions · vomiting
- ▸ **Uncommon** Abscess · alopecia · anxiety · arthralgia · bradycardia · chills · Clostridioides difficile colitis · constipation · cough · dehydration · diabetic control impaired · drowsiness · dry mouth · fever · gastrointestinal

discomfort · gastrointestinal disorders · haematochezia · hyperhidrosis · hyperkalaemia · increased risk of infection · irritability · limb discomfort · lymphadenopathy · muscle spasms · nasal dryness · pain · peripheral oedema · pulmonary congestion · sensation abnormal · sleep disorders · taste altered · tremor · urine odour abnormal · vasodilation · vision blurred · vitreous floater · vulvovaginal pruritus
SPECIFIC SIDE-EFFECTS
- ▸ **Uncommon**
- ▸ With intravenous use Infusion related reaction
- **CONCEPTION AND CONTRACEPTION** Manufacturer recommends effective contraception in women of childbearing potential; an additional method of contraception is advised in women taking hormonal contraceptives—effectiveness may be reduced.
- **PREGNANCY** Manufacturer advises avoid—fetal developmental toxicity in *animal* studies.
- **BREAST FEEDING** Manufacturer advises avoid—present in milk in *animal* studies.
- **DIRECTIONS FOR ADMINISTRATION** For *intravenous infusion* (*Sivextro*®), manufacturer advises give intermittently in Sodium Chloride 0.9%; reconstitute each 200 mg vial with 4 mL Water for Injections, then dilute reconstituted solution in 250 mL Sodium Chloride 0.9%; give over approx. 1 hour.
- **PATIENT AND CARER ADVICE**
  Optic neuropathy Although neuropathy (peripheral and optic) has not been reported in patients treated with tedizolid, manufacturer advises patients and carers are warned to report symptoms of visual impairment (including blurred vision, visual field defect, changes in visual acuity and colour vision) immediately; patients should be evaluated promptly, and referred to an ophthalmologist if necessary.
  Missed doses Manufacturer advises that if a dose is more than 16 hours late, the missed dose should not be taken and the next dose should be taken at the normal time.
  Driving and skilled tasks Patients and carers should be counselled on the effects on driving and skilled tasks—increased risk of dizziness and fatigue.
- **NATIONAL FUNDING/ACCESS DECISIONS**
  For full details see funding body website

  Scottish Medicines Consortium (SMC) decisions
- ▸ **Tedizolid (*Sivextro*®) for the treatment of acute bacterial skin and skin structure infections in adults (August 2015)** SMC No. 1080/15 Recommended with restrictions

---

- **MEDICINAL FORMS** There can be variation in the licensing of different medicines containing the same drug.

Oral tablet
- ▸ Sivextro (Merck Sharp & Dohme (UK) Ltd)
  Tedizolid phosphate 200 mg Sivextro 200mg tablets | 6 tablet [PoM] £862.00

Powder for solution for infusion
- ▸ Sivextro (Merck Sharp & Dohme (UK) Ltd)
  Tedizolid phosphate 200 mg Sivextro 200mg powder for concentrate for solution for infusion vials | 6 vial [PoM] £862.00

Trimethoprim

11-Nov-2021

- **INDICATIONS AND DOSE**

Respiratory-tract infections
- ▸ BY MOUTH
- ▸ Child 4–5 weeks: 4 mg/kg twice daily (max. per dose 200 mg)
- ▸ Child 6 weeks–5 months: 4 mg/kg twice daily (max. per dose 200 mg), alternatively 25 mg twice daily
- ▸ Child 6 months–5 years: 4 mg/kg twice daily (max. per dose 200 mg), alternatively 50 mg twice daily

continued →

▸ Child 6–11 years: 4 mg/kg twice daily (max. per dose 200 mg), alternatively 100 mg twice daily
▸ Child 12–17 years: 200 mg twice daily
▸ Adult: 200 mg twice daily

Prophylaxis of recurrent urinary-tract infection
▸ BY MOUTH
▸ Child 4–5 weeks: 2 mg/kg once daily, dose to be taken at night
▸ Child 6 weeks–5 months: 2 mg/kg once daily, dose to be taken at night, alternatively 12.5 mg once daily, dose to be taken at night
▸ Child 6 months–5 years: 2 mg/kg once daily (max. per dose 100 mg), dose to be taken at night, alternatively 25 mg once daily, dose to be taken at night
▸ Child 6–11 years: 2 mg/kg once daily (max. per dose 100 mg), dose to be taken at night, alternatively 50 mg once daily, dose to be taken at night
▸ Child 12–15 years: 100 mg once daily, dose to be taken at night
▸ Child 16–17 years: 100 mg once daily, dose to be taken at night, alternatively 200 mg for 1 dose, dose to be taken following exposure to a trigger
▸ Adult: 100 mg once daily, dose to be taken at night, alternatively 200 mg for 1 dose, dose to be taken following exposure to a trigger

Treatment of mild to moderate *Pneumocystis jirovecii* (*Pneumocystis carinii*) pneumonia in patients who cannot tolerate co-trimoxazole (in combination with dapsone)
▸ BY MOUTH
▸ Child: 5 mg/kg every 6–8 hours
▸ Adult: 5 mg/kg every 6–8 hours

Acne resistant to other antibacterials
▸ BY MOUTH
▸ Adult: 300 mg twice daily

Shigellosis | Invasive salmonella infection
▸ BY MOUTH
▸ Adult: (consult product literature)

Acute diverticulitis [in combination with metronidazole]
▸ BY MOUTH
▸ Adult: 200 mg twice daily for 5 days then review

Acute prostatitis
▸ BY MOUTH
▸ Adult: 200 mg twice daily for 14 or 28 days based on clinical assessment

Acute pyelonephritis
▸ BY MOUTH
▸ Child 16–17 years: 200 mg twice daily for 14 days
▸ Adult: 200 mg twice daily for 14 days

Urinary-tract infection (catheter-associated)
▸ BY MOUTH
▸ Child 3–5 months: 4 mg/kg twice daily (max. per dose 200 mg) for 7–10 days, alternatively 25 mg twice daily for 7–10 days
▸ Child 6 months–5 years: 4 mg/kg twice daily (max. per dose 200 mg) for 7–10 days, alternatively 50 mg twice daily for 7–10 days
▸ Child 6–11 years: 4 mg/kg twice daily (max. per dose 200 mg) for 7–10 days, alternatively 100 mg twice daily for 7–10 days
▸ Child 12–15 years: 200 mg twice daily for 7–10 days
▸ Child 16–17 years: 200 mg twice daily for 7 days (14 days if upper urinary-tract symptoms are present)
▸ Adult: 200 mg twice daily for 7 days (14 days if upper urinary-tract symptoms are present)

Lower urinary-tract infection
▸ BY MOUTH
▸ Child 4–5 weeks: 4 mg/kg twice daily (max. per dose 200 mg)

▸ Child 6 weeks–2 months: 4 mg/kg twice daily (max. per dose 200 mg), alternatively 25 mg twice daily
▸ Child 3–5 months: 4 mg/kg twice daily (max. per dose 200 mg) for 3 days, alternatively 25 mg twice daily for 3 days
▸ Child 6 months–5 years: 4 mg/kg twice daily (max. per dose 200 mg) for 3 days, alternatively 50 mg twice daily for 3 days
▸ Child 6–11 years: 4 mg/kg twice daily (max. per dose 200 mg) for 3 days, alternatively 100 mg twice daily for 3 days
▸ Child 12–15 years: 200 mg twice daily for 3 days
▸ Child 16–17 years: 200 mg twice daily for 3 days (7 days in males)
▸ Adult: 200 mg twice daily for 3 days (7 days in males)

● UNLICENSED USE [EvGr] Trimethoprim can be given as a single dose for the prophylaxis of recurrent urinary-tract infection following exposure to a trigger, ⒶＡ but this dosing regimen is not licensed. Not licensed for treatment of pneumocystis pneumonia.
▸ In children Not licensed for use in children under 6 months for the prophylaxis of recurrent urinary-tract infection.
▸ In children Not licensed for use in children under 6 weeks.
▸ In adults Not licensed for treatment of acne resistant to other antibacterials.

● CONTRA-INDICATIONS Blood dyscrasias

● CAUTIONS Acute porphyrias p. 1202 · elderly · predisposition to folate deficiency

● INTERACTIONS → Appendix 1: trimethoprim

● SIDE-EFFECTS
▸ **Common or very common** Diarrhoea · electrolyte imbalance · fungal overgrowth · headache · nausea · skin reactions · vomiting
▸ **Rare or very rare** Agranulocytosis · angioedema · anxiety · appetite decreased · arthralgia · behaviour abnormal · bone marrow disorders · confusion · constipation · cough · depression · dizziness · dyspnoea · eosinophilia · erythema nodosum · fever · haemolysis · haemolytic anaemia · haemorrhage · hallucination · hepatic disorders · hypoglycaemia · lethargy · leucopenia · meningitis aseptic · movement disorders · myalgia · neutropenia · oral disorders · pancreatitis · paraesthesia · peripheral neuritis · photosensitivity reaction · pseudomembranous enterocolitis · renal impairment · seizure · severe cutaneous adverse reactions (SCARs) · sleep disorders · syncope · systemic lupus erythematosus (SLE) · thrombocytopenia · tinnitus · tremor · uveitis · vasculitis · vertigo · wheezing
▸ **Frequency not known** Gastrointestinal disorder · megaloblastic anaemia · methaemoglobinaemia

● PREGNANCY Teratogenic risk in first trimester (folate antagonist). Manufacturers advise avoid during pregnancy.

● BREAST FEEDING Present in milk—short-term use not known to be harmful.

● RENAL IMPAIRMENT Manufacturer advises caution in impairment.
Dose adjustments
▸ In adults Manufacturer advises dose reduction to half normal dose after 3 days if eGFR 15–30 mL/minute/1.73 m^2. Manufacturer advises dose reduction to half normal dose if eGFR less than 15 mL/minute/1.73 m^2.
▸ In children Manufacturer advises dose reduction to half normal dose after 3 days if estimated glomerular filtration rate 15–30 mL/minute/1.73 m^2. Manufacturer advises dose reduction to half normal dose if estimated glomerular filtration rate less than 15 mL/minute/1.73 m^2.

● MONITORING REQUIREMENTS
▸ Manufacturer advises monitor blood counts with long-term use and in those with, or at risk of, folate deficiency.

- Manufacturer advises monitor serum electrolytes in patients at risk of developing hyperkalaemia, and consider monitoring in other patients, particularly with long-term use.
- Manufacturer advises consider monitoring renal function, particularly with long-term use.
- Manufacturer advises monitoring of plasma-trimethoprim concentration may be considered with long-term use and under specialist advice.

● **PRESCRIBING AND DISPENSING INFORMATION** For choice of antibacterial therapy, see Gastro-intestinal system infections, antibacterial therapy p. 582, Pneumocystis pneumonia p. 697, Respiratory system infections, antibacterial therapy p. 586, Urinary-tract infections p. 681.

● **PATIENT AND CARER ADVICE**
Blood disorders On long-term treatment, patients and their carers should be told how to recognise signs of blood disorders and advised to seek immediate medical attention if symptoms such as fever, sore throat, rash, mouth ulcers, purpura, bruising or bleeding develop.
Medicines for Children leaflet: Trimethoprim for bacterial infections www.medicinesforchildren.org.uk/medicines/trimethoprim-for-bacterial-infections/

● **MEDICINAL FORMS** There can be variation in the licensing of different medicines containing the same drug. Forms available from special-order manufacturers include: oral suspension, oral solution
Oral tablet
CAUTIONARY AND ADVISORY LABELS 9
- Trimethoprim (Non-proprietary)
  Trimethoprim 100 mg Trimethoprim 100mg tablets | 28 tablet [PoM] £2.00 DT = £0.81
  Trimethoprim 200 mg Trimethoprim 200mg tablets | 6 tablet [PoM] £2.15 DT = £0.63 | 14 tablet [PoM] £10.00 DT = £1.47
Oral suspension
CAUTIONARY AND ADVISORY LABELS 9
- Trimethoprim (Non-proprietary)
  Trimethoprim 10 mg per 1 ml Trimethoprim 50mg/5ml oral suspension sugar free | 100 ml [PoM] £14.00 DT = £3.38 [SF]

Combinations available: *Co-trimoxazole,* p. 652

ANTIMYCOBACTERIALS > RIFAMYCINS

| Rifaximin

02-Dec-2020

● **DRUG ACTION** Rifaximin is a rifamycin that is poorly absorbed from the gastro-intestinal tract, and, therefore, should not be used to treat systemic infections.

● **INDICATIONS AND DOSE**
Travellers' diarrhoea that is not associated with fever, bloody diarrhoea, blood or leucocytes in the stool, or 8 or more unformed stools in the previous 24 hours
- BY MOUTH
- Adult: 200 mg every 8 hours for 3 days
Reduction in recurrence of hepatic encephalopathy
- BY MOUTH
- Adult: 550 mg twice daily

● **CONTRA-INDICATIONS** Intestinal obstruction

● **INTERACTIONS** → Appendix 1: rifaximin

● **SIDE-EFFECTS**
- **Common or very common** Arthralgia · ascites · constipation · depression · dizziness · dyspnoea · gastrointestinal discomfort · gastrointestinal disorders · headaches · muscle complaints · nausea · oedema · skin reactions · vomiting
- **Uncommon** Anaemia · anxiety · appetite decreased · asthenia · balance impaired · concentration impaired · confusion · cough · diplopia · drowsiness · dry lips · dry mouth · dry throat · ear pain · fall · haematuria · hot flush · hyperhidrosis · hyperkalaemia · increased risk of infection ·

lymphocytosis · memory loss · muscle weakness · nasal complaints · neutropenia · oropharyngeal pain · pain · palpitations · polymenorrhoea · respiratory disorders · seizure · sensation abnormal · sleep disorders · sunburn · taste altered · urinary disorders · urine abnormalities · vertigo
- **Rare or very rare** Hypertension · hypotension
- **Frequency not known** Angioedema · syncope · thrombocytopenia · urine discolouration

● **ALLERGY AND CROSS-SENSITIVITY** [EvGr] Contra-indicated if history of rifamycin hypersensitivity. ◈

● **PREGNANCY** Manufacturer advises avoid—toxicity in *animal* studies.

● **BREAST FEEDING** Unlikely to be present in milk in significant amounts, but manufacturer advises avoid.

● **HEPATIC IMPAIRMENT**
- When used for Hepatic encephalopathy Manufacturer advises caution in severe impairment (risk of increased exposure).

● **PRESCRIBING AND DISPENSING INFORMATION** Not recommended for diarrhoea associated with invasive organisms such as *Campylobacter* and *Shigella*.

● **NATIONAL FUNDING/ACCESS DECISIONS**
For full details see funding body website
NICE decisions
- Rifaximin for preventing episodes of overt hepatic encephalopathy (March 2015) NICE TA337 Recommended

● **MEDICINAL FORMS** There can be variation in the licensing of different medicines containing the same drug. Forms available from special-order manufacturers include: oral suspension
Oral tablet
CAUTIONARY AND ADVISORY LABELS 9(Xifaxanta ® brand only), 14
- Rifaximin (Non-proprietary)
  Rifaximin 550 mg Rifaximin 550mg tablets | 56 tablet [PoM] £259.23 DT = £259.23 | 98 tablet [PoM] £453.65
- Targaxan (Norgine Pharmaceuticals Ltd)
  Rifaximin 550 mg Targaxan 550mg tablets | 98 tablet [PoM] £453.65
- Xifaxanta (Norgine Pharmaceuticals Ltd)
  Rifaximin 200 mg Xifaxanta 200mg tablets | 9 tablet [PoM] £15.15 DT = £15.15
Oral suspension
- Rifaximin (Non-proprietary)
  Rifaximin 20 mg per 1 ml Normix 100mg/5ml granules for oral suspension | 100 ml [PoM] [℞]

2.1 Anthrax

Anthrax

03-Apr-2021

Treatment and post-exposure prophylaxis

Anthrax is a notifiable disease in the UK. For further information, see *Notifiable diseases* in Antibacterials, principles of therapy p. 573. If anthrax infection is suspected, discuss with an infectious disease specialist and arrange urgent consultation. For community level outbreaks, specialist advice should be sought from Public Health England (tel. 020 8200 4400) or, in Scotland, Health Protection Scotland (tel. 0141 300 1191).

Inhalation or *gastro-intestinal anthrax* should be treated initially with either ciprofloxacin p. 648 or, in patients over 12 years, doxycycline p. 655 [unlicensed use] and combined with one or two other antibacterials (such as benzylpenicillin sodium p. 633, clindamycin, rifampicin, and vancomycin). Alternatively, the combination of amoxicillin p. 635 and imipenem with cilastatin, or meropenem and chloramphenicol may be given.

Cutaneous anthrax should be treated with either oral ciprofloxacin [unlicensed use] or, in patients over 12 years, doxycycline [unlicensed use] for 7 days; treatment should be switched to amoxicillin if the infecting strain is susceptible.

Oral ciprofloxacin, doxycycline [unlicensed use], or amoxicillin may be given for *post-exposure prophylaxis*. Antibacterial prophylaxis should continue for up to 60 days, however a shorter period may be recommended. Vaccination against anthrax may be considered in selected cases. For further information, see Anthrax vaccine p. 1474.

Useful resources

Recommendations reflect Chemical, biological, radiological and nuclear incidents: clinical management and health protection. Second Edition. Public Health England. May 2018.

www.gov.uk/government/publications/chemical-biological-radiological-and-nuclear-incidents-recognise-and-respond

Chapter 13, Anthrax, in *Immunisation against infectious disease*- 'The Green Book'. Public Health England. February 2017.

www.gov.uk/government/publications/anthrax-the-green-book-chapter-13

2.2 Leprosy

Leprosy

Management

Advice from a member of the Panel of Leprosy Opinion is essential for the treatment of leprosy (Hansen's disease). Details can be obtained from the Hospital for Tropical Diseases, London (telephone (020) 3456 7890).

The World Health Organization has made recommendations to overcome the problem of dapsone below resistance and to prevent the emergence of resistance to other antileprotic drugs. Drugs recommended are dapsone, rifampicin p. 674, and clofazimine below. Other drugs with significant activity against *Mycobacterium leprae* include ofloxacin p. 652, minocycline p. 658 and clarithromycin p. 621, but none of these are as active as rifampicin; at present they should be reserved as second-line drugs for leprosy.

A three-drug regimen is recommended for *multibacillary leprosy* (lepromatous, borderline-lepromatous, and borderline leprosy) and a two-drug regimen for *paucibacillary leprosy* (borderline-tuberculoid, tuberculoid, and indeterminate).

Multibacillary leprosy should be treated with a combination of rifampicin, dapsone and clofazimine for at least 2 years. Treatment should be continued unchanged during both type I (reversal) or type II (erythema nodosum leprosum) reactions. During reversal reactions neuritic pain or weakness can herald the rapid onset of permanent nerve damage. Treatment with prednisolone p. 791 should be instituted at once. Mild type II reactions may respond to aspirin. Severe type II reactions may require corticosteroids; thalidomide p. 1092 [unlicensed] is also useful in patients who have become corticosteroid dependent, but it should be used only under **specialist supervision**. Thalidomide is teratogenic and, therefore, contra-indicated in pregnancy; it must **not** be given to women of child-bearing potential unless they comply with a pregnancy prevention programme. Increased doses of clofazimine are also useful.

Paucibacillary leprosy should be treated with rifampicin and dapsone for 6 months. If treatment is interrupted the regimen should be recommenced where it was left off to complete the full course.

Neither the multibacillary nor the paucibacillary antileprosy regimen is sufficient to treat tuberculosis.

Clofazimine

11-May-2021

● **INDICATIONS AND DOSE**

Multibacillary leprosy in combination with rifampicin and dapsone (3-drug regimen) (administered on expert advice)

▶ BY MOUTH

▶ Adult: 300 mg once a month, to be administered under supervision and 50 mg daily, to be self-administered, alternatively 300 mg once a month, to be administered under supervision and 100 mg once daily on alternate days, to be self-administered

Lepromatous lepra reactions (administered on expert advice)

▶ BY MOUTH

▶ Adult: 300 mg daily for max. 3 months

Severe type II (erythema nodosum leprosum) reactions (administered on expert advice)

▶ BY MOUTH

▶ Adult: 100 mg 3 times a day for one month, subsequent dose reductions are required, may take 4–6 weeks to attain full effect

● **CAUTIONS** Avoid if persistent abdominal pain and diarrhoea · may discolour soft contact lenses

● **INTERACTIONS** → Appendix 1: clofazimine

● **SIDE-EFFECTS** Abdominal pain · appetite decreased · dry eye · eye discolouration · fatigue · gastrointestinal disorders · hair colour changes (reversible) · headache · lymphadenopathy · nausea · photosensitivity reaction · red discolouration of body fluids · skin discolouration (including areas exposed to light) · skin reactions · splenic infarction · urine discolouration · visual impairment · vomiting (hospitalise if persistent) · weight decreased

● **PREGNANCY** Use with caution.

● **BREAST FEEDING** May alter colour of milk; skin discoloration of infant.

● **HEPATIC IMPAIRMENT** Use with caution.

● **RENAL IMPAIRMENT** EvGr Use with caution in severe impairment. Ⓜ

● **MEDICINAL FORMS** There can be variation in the licensing of different medicines containing the same drug. Forms available from special-order manufacturers include: oral capsule

Oral capsule

CAUTIONARY AND ADVISORY LABELS 8, 14, 21

▶ Clofazimine (Non-proprietary)

Clofazimine 50 mg Lamprene 50mg capsules | 100 capsule PoM Ⓢ

Dapsone

05-May-2020

● **INDICATIONS AND DOSE**

Multibacillary leprosy in combination with rifampicin and clofazimine (3-drug regimen) | Paucibacillary leprosy in combination with rifampicin (2-drug regimen)

▶ BY MOUTH

▶ Adult (body-weight up to 35 kg): 50 mg daily, alternatively 1–2 mg/kg daily, may be self-administered

▶ Adult (body-weight 35 kg and above): 100 mg daily, may be self-administered

Dermatitis herpetiformis

▶ BY MOUTH

▶ Adult: (consult product literature or local protocols)

Treatment of mild to moderate *Pneumocystis jirovecii* (*Pneumocystis carinii*) pneumonia (in combination with trimethoprim)
▶ BY MOUTH
▶ Adult: 100 mg once daily

Prophylaxis of *Pneumocystis jirovecii* (*Pneumocystis carinii*) pneumonia
▶ BY MOUTH
▶ Adult: 100 mg daily

● UNLICENSED USE Not licensed for treatment of pneumocystis (*P. jirovecii*) pneumonia.

● CAUTIONS Anaemia (treat severe anaemia before starting) · avoid in Acute porphyrias p. 1202 · cardiac disease · G6PD deficiency · pulmonary disease · susceptibility to haemolysis

● INTERACTIONS → Appendix 1: dapsone

● SIDE-EFFECTS Agranulocytosis · appetite decreased · haemolysis · haemolytic anaemia · headache · hepatic disorders · hypoalbuminaemia · insomnia · lepra reaction · methaemoglobinaemia · motor loss · nausea · peripheral neuropathy · photosensitivity reaction · psychosis · severe cutaneous adverse reactions (SCARs) · skin reactions · tachycardia · vomiting

SIDE-EFFECTS, FURTHER INFORMATION Side-effects are dose-related. If dapsone syndrome occurs (rash with fever and eosinophilia)—discontinue immediately (may progress to exfoliative dermatitis, hepatitis, hypoalbuminaemia, psychosis and death).

● PREGNANCY Folic acid p. 1161 (higher dose) should be given to mother throughout pregnancy; neonatal haemolysis and methaemoglobinaemia reported in third trimester.

● BREAST FEEDING Haemolytic anaemia; although significant amount in milk, risk to infant very small unless infant is G6PD deficient.

● PATIENT AND CARER ADVICE
Blood disorders On long-term treatment, patients and their carers should be told how to recognise signs of blood disorders and advised to seek immediate medical attention if symptoms such as fever, sore throat, rash, mouth ulcers, purpura, bruising or bleeding develop.

● MEDICINAL FORMS There can be variation in the licensing of different medicines containing the same drug. Forms available from special-order manufacturers include: oral suspension, oral solution
Oral tablet
CAUTIONARY AND ADVISORY LABELS 8
▶ Dapsone (Non-proprietary)
Dapsone 50 mg Dapsone 50mg tablets | 28 tablet PoM £32.00 DT = £6.18
Dapsone 100 mg Dapsone 100mg tablets | 28 tablet PoM £95.00 DT = £13.80

2.3 Lyme disease

Lyme disease

14-Nov-2018

Description of condition

Lyme disease, also known as Lyme borreliosis, is an infection caused by bacteria called *Borrelia burgdorferi*. It is transmitted to humans by the bite of an infected tick. Ticks are mainly found in grassy and wooded areas including urban gardens and parks. Most tick bites do not cause Lyme disease, and the prompt and correct removal of the tick reduces the risk of infection.

Lyme disease usually presents with a characteristic erythema migrans rash. This usually becomes visible 1–4 weeks after a tick bite, but can appear from 3 days to 3 months, and last for several weeks. It may be accompanied by non-focal (non-organ related) symptoms, such as fever, swollen glands, malaise, fatigue, neck pain or stiffness, joint or muscle pain, headache, cognitive impairment, or paraesthesia.

Other signs and symptoms of Lyme disease may also appear months or years after the initial infection and are typically characterised by focal symptoms (relating to at least 1 organ system). These include neurological (affecting cranial nerves, peripheral and central nervous systems), joint (Lyme arthritis), cardiac (Lyme carditis), or skin (acrodermatitis chronica atrophicans) manifestations.

Drug treatment

EvGr Patients diagnosed with Lyme disease should be given treatment with an antibacterial drug; the choice of drug should be based on presenting symptoms. In patients who present with focal symptoms, a discussion with, or referral to, a specialist should be considered but should not delay treatment.

In patients presenting with *erythema migrans rash with or without non-focal symptoms*, oral doxycycline p. 655 [unlicensed indication] is recommended as first-line treatment. If doxycycline p. 655 cannot be given, oral amoxicillin p. 635 should be used as an alternative. Oral azithromycin p. 620 [unlicensed indication] should be given if both doxycycline p. 655 and amoxicillin p. 635 are unsuitable.

In patients presenting with focal symptoms of *cranial nerve or peripheral nervous system* involvement, oral doxycycline p. 655 [unlicensed indication] is recommended as first-line treatment. If doxycycline p. 655 cannot be given, oral amoxicillin p. 635 should be used as an alternative.

In patients presenting with symptoms of *central nervous system* involvement, intravenous ceftriaxone p. 609 is recommended as first-line treatment. Oral doxycycline p. 655 [unlicensed indication] should be used as an alternative if ceftriaxone p. 609 cannot be given, or when switching to oral antibacterial treatment.

In patients with symptoms of *Lyme arthritis or acrodermatitis chronica atrophicans*, oral doxycycline p. 655 [unlicensed indication] is recommended as first-line treatment. If doxycycline p. 655 cannot be given, oral amoxicillin p. 635 should be used as an alternative. Intravenous ceftriaxone p. 609 should be given if both doxycycline p. 655 and amoxicillin p. 635 are unsuitable.

In patients with symptoms of *Lyme carditis who are haemodynamically stable*, oral doxycycline p. 655 [unlicensed indication] is recommended as first-line treatment. If doxycycline p. 655 cannot be given, intravenous ceftriaxone p. 609 should be used as an alternative.

In patients with symptoms of *Lyme carditis who are haemodynamically unstable*, intravenous ceftriaxone p. 609 is recommended. Oral doxycycline p. 655 [unlicensed indication] should be given when switching to oral antibacterial treatment. Ⓐ

Ongoing symptom management

EvGr If symptoms continue to persist or worsen after antibacterial treatment, patients should be assessed for possible alternative causes, re-infection with Lyme disease, treatment failure or non-adherence to previous antibacterial treatment, or progression to organ damage caused by Lyme disease (such as nerve palsy).

A second course of antibacterial treatment should be given to patients presenting with signs and symptoms of re-infection. In patients presenting with ongoing symptoms due to possible treatment failure, treatment with an alternative antibacterial drug should be considered. A third course of antibacterial treatment is not recommended, and further management should be discussed with a national reference laboratory or suitable specialist depending on symptoms (for example, a rheumatologist or neurologist). Ⓐ

Useful Resources

Lyme disease. National Institute for Health and Care Excellence. NICE guideline 95. April 2018. www.nice.org.uk/guidance/ng95

'Be tick aware'–Toolkit for raising awareness of the potential risk posed by ticks and tick-borne disease in England. Public Health England. March 2018. www.gov.uk/government/publications/tick-bite-risks-and-prevention-of-lyme-disease

2.4 Meticillin-resistant Staphylococcus aureus

MRSA

15-Jan-2025

Management

Meticillin-resistant *Staphylococcus aureus* (MRSA) are strains of *Staphylococcus aureus* that are resistant to a number of commonly used antibacterials including beta-lactam antibacterials (e.g. meticillin [now discontinued] and flucloxacillin). As with *Staph. aureus* colonisation, MRSA may colonise the skin, gut, or nose without displaying signs or symptoms of infection. Infection with MRSA can be difficult to manage; management includes appropriate infection control measures, adherence to local policies, and treatment guided by the sensitivity of the infecting strain. Consult a microbiologist or the local infection control team where appropriate.

EvGr Oral doxycycline p. 655, trimethoprim p. 665, ciprofloxacin p. 648, or co-trimoxazole p. 652 can be considered for lower *urinary-tract infections* caused by MRSA according to susceptibility. A **glycopeptide** can be considered for complicated urinary-tract infections. Ⓐ

For information on the management of MRSA-associated *skin and soft-tissue infections, hospital-acquired pneumonia, endocarditis, osteomyelitis*, and *septic arthritis*, see the corresponding treatment summary: Skin infections, antibacterial therapy p. 589, Respiratory system infections, antibacterial therapy p. 586, Cardiovascular system infections, antibacterial therapy p. 579, and Musculoskeletal system infections, antibacterial therapy p. 585.

For information on MRSA eradication of the nasal carriage, see Nose p. 1366.

2.5 Tuberculosis

Tuberculosis

18-Mar-2025

Overview

Tuberculosis is a curable infectious disease caused by bacteria of the *Mycobacterium tuberculosis* complex (*M. tuberculosis, M. africanum, M. bovis* or *M. microti*) and is spread by breathing in infected respiratory droplets from a person with infectious tuberculosis. The most common form of tuberculosis infection is in the lungs (**pulmonary**) but infection can also spread and develop in other parts of the body (**extrapulmonary**).

The initial infection with tuberculosis clears in the majority of individuals. However, in some cases the bacteria may become dormant and remain in the body with no symptoms (**latent** tuberculosis) or progress to being symptomatic (**active** tuberculosis) over the following weeks or months. In individuals with latent tuberculosis only a small proportion will develop active tuberculosis.

Many cases of tuberculosis can be prevented by public health measures and when clinical disease does occur most individuals can be cured if treated properly with the correct dose, combination and duration of treatment. Drug-resistant strains of tuberculosis are much harder to treat and significantly increase an individual's risk of long-term complications or death.

Treatment phases, overview

The standard treatment of active tuberculosis is completed in two phases—an **initial phase** using four drugs and a **continuation phase** using two drugs, in fully sensitive cases. EvGr The management of tuberculosis should be under specialist care by clinicians with training in, and experience of, the specialised care of individuals with tuberculosis. This tuberculosis service should include specialised nurses and health visitors. Ⓐ

Within the UK there are two regimens recommended for the treatment of tuberculosis: **unsupervised** or **supervised**. The choice of either regimen is dependent on a risk assessment to identify if an individual needs enhanced case management.

EvGr In all phases of treatment for tuberculosis, fixed-dose combination tablets should be used, and a daily dosing schedule should be offered in active pulmonary tuberculosis and considered as first choice in active extrapulmonary tuberculosis. Ⓐ

Initial phase

EvGr As standard treatment for individuals with active tuberculosis, offer rifampicin p. 674, ethambutol hydrochloride p. 678, pyrazinamide p. 680 and isoniazid p. 679 (with pyridoxine hydrochloride p. 1237) in the initial phase of therapy; modified according to drug susceptibility testing; and continued for 2 months.

Treatment should be started without waiting for culture results if clinical signs and symptoms are consistent with a tuberculosis diagnosis; consider completing the standard treatment even if subsequent culture results are negative. Ⓐ

Continuation phase

EvGr After the initial phase, offer standard continuation treatment with rifampicin and isoniazid (with pyridoxine hydrochloride) for a further 4 months in individuals with active tuberculosis without central nervous system involvement. Longer treatment for 10 months should be offered in individuals with active tuberculosis of the central nervous system, with or without spinal involvement.

Treatment should be modified according to drug susceptibility testing. Ⓐ

Unsupervised treatment

The unsupervised treatment regimen is for individuals who are likely to take antituberculosis drugs reliably and willingly without supervision.

Supervised treatment

For individuals requiring supervised treatment (directly observed therapy, DOT), this is offered as part of enhanced case management. EvGr Daily supervised treatment is the preferred option wherever feasible. A 3 times weekly dosing schedule can be considered in individuals with tuberculosis if they require enhanced case management and daily directly observed therapy is not available. Antituberculosis treatment dosing regimens of fewer than 3 times a week are not recommended.

Directly observed therapy should be offered to individuals who:
- have a current risk or history of non-adherence;
- have previously been treated for tuberculosis;
- have a history of homelessness, drug or alcohol misuse;

- are in prison or a young offender institution, or have been in the past 5 years;
- have a major psychiatric, memory or cognitive disorder;
- are in denial of the tuberculosis diagnosis;
- have multi-drug resistant tuberculosis;
- request directly observed therapy after discussion with the clinical team;
- are too ill to self-administer treatment. 

Individuals with comorbidities or coexisting conditions, including the immunocompromised

[EvGr] Individuals with comorbidities or coexisting conditions (such as HIV, severe liver disease, chronic kidney disease, diabetes, eye disease or vision impairment, a history of alcohol or substance misuse, or who are pregnant or breastfeeding) should be managed by a specialist multidisciplinary team with experience in managing tuberculosis and the comorbidity or coexisting condition.

For individuals who are HIV-positive with active TB, treatment with the standard regimen should not routinely exceed 6 months, unless the tuberculosis has central nervous system involvement, in which case treatment should not routinely extend beyond 12 months.

Care should be taken to avoid drug interactions when co-prescribing antiretroviral and antituberculosis drugs. For further information on the management of tuberculosis in HIV infection, see British HIV Association guideline: **Management of tuberculosis in adults living with HIV** (available at www.bhiva.org/guidelines).

Extrapulmonary tuberculosis

Central nervous system tuberculosis

[EvGr] Individuals with central nervous system tuberculosis should be offered standard treatment with **initial phase** drugs for 2 months (see *Initial phase* for specific drugs). After completion of the initial treatment phase, standard treatment with **continuation phase** drugs should then be offered (see *Continuation phase* for specific drugs); and continued for a further 10 months. Treatment for tuberculous meningitis should be offered if clinical signs and other laboratory findings are consistent with the diagnosis, even if a rapid diagnostic test is negative.

An initial high dose of *dexamethasone* or *prednisolone* should be offered at the same time as antituberculosis treatment, then slowly withdrawn over 4–8 weeks. For additional information on corticosteroid use, see NICE clinical guideline: **Tuberculosis** (see *Useful resources*).

[EvGr] Referral for surgery should only be considered in individuals who have raised intracranial pressure; or have spinal TB with spinal instability or evidence of spinal cord compression.

Pericardial tuberculosis

[EvGr] An initial high dose of oral *prednisolone* should be offered to individuals with active pericardial tuberculosis, at the same time as antituberculosis treatment, then slowly withdrawn over 2–3 weeks. For additional information on corticosteroid use, see NICE clinical guideline: **Tuberculosis** (see *Useful resources*).

Latent tuberculosis

Some individuals with latent tuberculosis are at increased risk of developing active tuberculosis (such as individuals who are HIV-positive, diabetic, injecting drug users, or receiving treatment with an anti-tumor necrosis factor alpha inhibitor). [EvGr] If for any reason these individuals do not have treatment for latent tuberculosis, they should be informed of the risks and symptoms of active tuberculosis.

Close contacts

[EvGr] Anyone aged under 65 years who is a close contact (prolonged, frequent or intense contact, for example household contacts or partners) of a person with pulmonary or laryngeal tuberculosis should be tested for latent tuberculosis. Drug treatment should be offered to all individuals aged under 65 years with evidence of latent tuberculosis, if the close contact has *suspected infectious* or *confirmed active* pulmonary or laryngeal drug-sensitive tuberculosis.

Immunocompromised

[EvGr] Individuals who are anticipated to be, or who are currently immunocompromised, should have a risk assessment carried out to establish whether tuberculosis testing should be offered. Take into account the severity and duration of their immunocompromise and any risk factors for tuberculosis (such as country of birth or recent contact with an index case with suspected infectious or confirmed pulmonary or laryngeal tuberculosis).

Individuals who are severely immunocompromised (such as those with HIV and a CD4 count of less than 200 cells/mm^3, or who have had a solid organ or allogeneic stem cell transplant) should be tested for latent tuberculosis using an appropriate method. Individuals who test positive should then be assessed for active disease, and if negative, offered treatment for latent tuberculosis. For further information on tuberculosis testing methods, see NICE clinical guideline: **Tuberculosis** (see *Useful resources*).

Healthcare workers

[EvGr] Any new NHS employees who are new entrants from a high incidence country should be offered appropriate testing for latent tuberculosis. Those who are not new entrants from a high incidence country, but who will be in contact with patients or clinical materials should be offered appropriate testing for latent tuberculosis if prior BCG vaccination cannot be verified. For further information on tuberculosis testing methods, see NICE clinical guideline: **Tuberculosis** (see *Useful resources*) and Bacillus Calmette-Guérin vaccine p. 1474.

[EvGr] Those who test positive should then be assessed for active disease, and if negative, offered treatment for latent tuberculosis.

For healthcare workers who are immunocompromised, follow standard advice for testing and treatment (see *Immunocompromised* above).

Treatment of latent tuberculosis

[EvGr] For individuals aged below 65 years, including those with HIV where treatment for latent tuberculosis is indicated, offer drug treatment with either 3 months of isoniazid (with pyridoxine hydrochloride p. 1237) and rifampicin or 6 months of isoniazid (with pyridoxine hydrochloride).

The choice of regimen is dependent on clinical factors, including age, risk of hepatotoxicity and possible drug interactions. [EvGr] Testing for HIV, hepatitis B and hepatitis C should be offered before starting antituberculosis treatment as this may affect choice of therapy.

Individuals aged 35 to 65 years should only be offered treatment if hepatotoxicity is not a concern.

For individuals aged under 35 years offer treatment with 3 months of isoniazid (with pyridoxine hydrochloride) and rifampicin if hepatotoxicity is a concern after an assessment of both liver function (including transaminase levels) and risk factors.

For individuals where interactions with rifamycins are a concern (for example, in people with HIV or who those have had a transplant), offer treatment with 6 months of isoniazid (with pyridoxine hydrochloride).

Individuals with severe liver disease should be treated under the care of a specialist team. Careful monitoring of liver function is necessary in individuals with non-severe liver disease, abnormal liver function, or who misuse alcohol or drugs.

Infection

Recommended dosage for standard unsupervised 6-month treatment

Rifampicin with isoniazid and pyrazinamide	Adult: ▸ body-weight up to 40 kg 3 tablets daily for 2 months (initial phase), use *Rifater*® Tablets, preferably taken before breakfast ; ▸ body-weight 40–49 kg 4 tablets daily for 2 months (initial phase), use *Rifater*® Tablets, preferably taken before breakfast ; ▸ body-weight 50–64 kg 5 tablets daily for 2 months (initial phase), use *Rifater*® Tablets, preferably taken before breakfast ; ▸ body-weight 65 kg and above 6 tablets daily for 2 months (initial phase), use *Rifater*® Tablets, preferably taken before breakfast
Ethambutol hydrochloride	Adult: 15 mg/kg once daily for 2 months (initial phase)
Rifampicin with isoniazid	Adult: ▸ body-weight up to 50 kg 450/300 mg daily for 4 months (continuation phase after 2-month initial phase), use *Rifinah*®150/100 Tablets, preferably taken before breakfast ; ▸ body-weight 50 kg and above 600/300 mg daily for 4 months (continuation phase after 2-month initial phase), use *Rifinah*®300/150 Tablets, preferably taken before breakfast

or (if combination preparations not appropriate):

Isoniazid	Child: 10 mg/kg once daily (max. per dose 300 mg) for 6 months (initial and continuation phases) Adult: 300 mg daily for 6 months (initial and continuation phases)
Rifampicin	Child: ▸ body-weight up to 50 kg 15 mg/kg once daily for 6 months (initial and continuation phases); maximum 450 mg per day ; ▸ body-weight 50 kg and above 15 mg/kg once daily for 6 months (initial and continuation phases); maximum 600 mg per day Adult: ▸ body-weight up to 50 kg 450 mg once daily for 6 months (initial and continuation phases) ; ▸ body-weight 50 kg and above 600 mg once daily for 6 months (initial and continuation phases)
Pyrazinamide	Child: ▸ body-weight up to 50 kg 35 mg/kg once daily for 2 months (initial phase); maximum 1.5 g per day ; ▸ body-weight 50 kg and above 35 mg/kg once daily for 2 months (initial phase); maximum 2 g per day Adult: ▸ body-weight up to 50 kg 1.5 g once daily for 2 months (initial phase); ▸ body-weight 50 kg and above 2 g once daily for 2 months (initial phase)
Ethambutol hydrochloride	Child: 20 mg/kg once daily for 2 months (initial phase) Adult: 15 mg/kg once daily for 2 months (initial phase)

In general, doses should be rounded up to facilitate administration of suitable volumes of liquid or an appropriate strength of tablet. The exception is ethambutol hydrochloride due to the risk of toxicity. Doses may also need to be recalculated to allow for weight gain in younger children. The fixed-dose combination preparations (*Rifater*®, *Rifinah*®) are unlicensed for use in children. Consideration may be given to use of these preparations in older children, provided the respective dose of each drug is appropriate for the weight of the child.

Recommended dosage for intermittent supervised 6-month treatment

Isoniazid	Child: 15 mg/kg 3 times a week (max. per dose 900 mg) for 6 months (initial and continuation phases) Adult: 15 mg/kg 3 times a week (max. per dose 900 mg) for 6 months (initial and continuation phases)
Rifampicin	Child: 15 mg/kg 3 times a week (max. per dose 900 mg) for 6 months (initial and continuation phases) Adult: 600–900 mg 3 times a week for 6 months (initial and continuation phases)
Pyrazinamide	Child: ▸ body-weight up to 50 kg 50 mg/kg 3 times a week (max. per dose 2 g 3 times a week) for 2 months (initial phase) ; ▸ body-weight 50 kg and above 50 mg/kg 3 times a week (max. per dose 2.5 g 3 times a week) for 2 months (initial phase) Adult: ▸ body-weight up to 50 kg 2 g 3 times a week for 2 months (initial phase); ▸ body-weight 50 kg and above 2.5 g 3 times a week for 2 months (initial phase)
Ethambutol hydrochloride	Child: 30 mg/kg 3 times a week for 2 months (initial phase) Adult: 30 mg/kg 3 times a week for 2 months (initial phase)

In general, doses should be rounded up to facilitate administration of suitable volumes of liquid or an appropriate strength of tablet. The exception is ethambutol hydrochloride due to the risk of toxicity. Doses may also need to be recalculated to allow for weight gain in younger children. The fixed-dose combination preparations (*Rifater*®, *Rifinah*®) are unlicensed for use in children. Consideration may be given to use of these preparations in older children, provided the respective dose of each drug is appropriate for the weight of the child.

For advice on immunisation against tuberculosis, see Bacillus Calmette-Guérin vaccine p. 1474.

Treatment failure

Major causes of treatment failure include incorrect prescribing by the clinician and inadequate compliance by the infected individual. [EvGr] All individuals diagnosed with tuberculosis should have an allocated case manager to help with the development of a health and social care plan, supervision of treatment, and support with the completion of treatment. Multidisciplinary tuberculosis teams should implement strategies (such as random urine tests, pill counts, home visits, health education counselling, and language appropriate reminder services) to help with adherence to, and successful completion of treatment. (A)

Treatment interruptions

A break in antituberculosis treatment of at least 2 weeks (during the initial phase) or missing more than 20% of prescribed doses is classified as treatment interruption. Re-establishing treatment appropriately following interruptions is key to ensuring treatment success without relapse, drug resistance or further adverse events. [EvGr] If an adverse reaction recurs upon re-introducing a particular drug, do not give that drug in future regimens and consider extending the total regimen accordingly. (A)

Treatment interruptions due to drug-induced hepatotoxicity

[EvGr] Following treatment interruption due to drug-induced hepatotoxicty, all potential causes of hepatotoxicity should be investigated. Once aspartate or alanine transaminase levels fall below twice the upper limit of normal, bilirubin levels have returned to the normal range, and hepatotoxic symptoms have resolved, antituberculosis therapy should be sequentially re-introduced at previous full doses over a period of no more than 10 days. Start with ethambutol hydrochloride p. 678 and either isoniazid p. 679 (with pyridoxine hydrochloride) or rifampicin p. 674.

In individuals with severe or highly infectious tuberculosis who need to interrupt the standard regimen, consider continuing treatment with at least 2 drugs with low risk of hepatotoxicity, such as ethambutol hydrochloride and streptomycin p. 598 (with or without a fluoroquinolone antibiotic, such as levofloxacin p. 650 or moxifloxacin p. 651), with ongoing monitoring by a liver specialist. (A)

Treatment interruptions due to cutaneous reactions

[EvGr] If an individual with severe or highly infectious tuberculosis has a cutaneous reaction, consider continuing treatment with a combination of at least 2 drugs with low risk for causing cutaneous reactions, such as ethambutol hydrochloride and streptomycin, with monitoring by a dermatologist. (A)

Drug-resistant tuberculosis

[EvGr] Treatment of drug-resistant tuberculosis should be managed by a multidisciplinary team with experience in such cases, and where appropriate facilities for infection-control exist. (A) The risk of resistance is minimised by ensuring therapy is administered in the correct dose and combination for the prescribed duration.

Single drug-resistant tuberculosis

[EvGr] For single drug-resistance in individuals with tuberculosis with central nervous system involvement, refer to a specialist with experience in managing drug-resistant tuberculosis. (A) For those without central nervous system involvement, the following treatment regimens are recommended:

Resistance to isoniazid:

- [EvGr] First 2 months (initial phase): rifampicin, pyrazinamide p. 680 and ethambutol hydrochloride;
- Continue with (continuation phase): rifampicin and ethambutol hydrochloride for 7 months (up to 10 months for extensive disease). (A)

Resistance to pyrazinamide:

- [EvGr] First 2 months (initial phase): rifampicin, ethambutol hydrochloride and isoniazid (with pyridoxine hydrochloride);
- Continue with (continuation phase): rifampicin p. 674 and isoniazid p. 679 (with pyridoxine hydrochloride p. 1237) for 7 months. (A)

Resistance to ethambutol hydrochloride p. 678:

- [EvGr] First 2 months (initial phase): rifampicin, pyrazinamide p. 680 and isoniazid (with pyridoxine hydrochloride);
- Continue with (continuation phase): rifampicin and isoniazid (with pyridoxine hydrochloride) for 4 months. (A)

Resistance to rifampicin:

- [EvGr] Rifampicin-resistant tuberculosis should be managed in the same way as multi-drug resistant tuberculosis. (A)

Multi-drug resistant tuberculosis (MDR-TB)

[EvGr] Advice on the management of patients with MDR-TB (resistance to isoniazid and rifampicin, with or without any other resistance), should be sought from local specialist advisory services for MDR-TB and the **British Thoracic Society** MDR-TB Clinical Advice Service (see: www.brit-thoracic.org.uk/quality-improvement/bts-mdr-tb-clinical-advice-service/). Testing for resistance to second-line drugs is recommended and treatment should be modified according to susceptibility. (A) Treatment regimens are comprised of different combinations of drugs such as bedaquiline, clofazimine [unlicensed use], delamanid [unlicensed], levofloxacin [unlicensed use] or moxifloxacin [unlicensed use], linezolid [unlicensed use], pretomanid [unlicensed], and pyrazinamide.

Useful Resources

Tuberculosis. National Institute for Health and Care Excellence. NICE guideline NG33. September 2019, updated February 2024.
www.nice.org.uk/guidance/ng33

ANTIMYCOBACTERIALS > RIFAMYCINS

Rifabutin   30-May-2023

● **INDICATIONS AND DOSE**

Prophylaxis of *Mycobacterium avium* complex infections in immunosuppressed patients with low CD4 count

▶ BY MOUTH
▶ Adult: 300 mg once daily, also consult product literature

Treatment of non-tuberculous mycobacterial disease, in combination with other drugs

▶ BY MOUTH
▶ Adult: 450–600 mg once daily for up to 6 months after cultures negative

Treatment of pulmonary tuberculosis, in combination with other drugs

▶ BY MOUTH
▶ Adult: 150–450 mg once daily for at least 6 months

Helicobacter pylori **eradication [in combination with other drugs (see Helicobacter pylori infection p. 93)]**

▶ BY MOUTH
▶ Adult: 150 mg twice daily for 10 days for third-line eradication therapy

- **UNLICENSED USE** EvGr Rifabutin is used for the eradication of *Helicobacter pylori*, Ⓐ but is not licensed for this indication.
- **CAUTIONS** Acute porphyrias p. 1202 · discolours soft contact lenses
- **INTERACTIONS** → Appendix 1: rifamycins
- **SIDE-EFFECTS** Agranulocytosis · anaemia · arthralgia · bronchospasm · chest pain · corneal deposits · decreased leucocytes · dyspnoea · eosinophilia · fever · haemolysis · hepatic disorders · influenza like illness · myalgia · nausea · neutropenia · pancytopenia · skin reactions · thrombocytopenia · urine discolouration · uveitis (more common following high doses or concomitant use with drugs that increase plasma concentration) · vomiting
- **ALLERGY AND CROSS-SENSITIVITY** EvGr Contra-indicated in patients with rifamycin hypersensitivity. Ⓜ
- **CONCEPTION AND CONTRACEPTION**
  Important Rifabutin induces hepatic enzymes and the effectiveness of hormonal contraceptives is reduced; alternative family planning advice should be offered.
- **PREGNANCY** Manufacturer advises avoid—no information available.
- **BREAST FEEDING** Manufacturer advises avoid—no information available.
- **HEPATIC IMPAIRMENT** Manufacturer advises caution in severe impairment.
- **RENAL IMPAIRMENT**
  Dose adjustments See p. 21.
  Manufacturer advises use half normal dose if creatinine clearance less than 30 mL/minute.
- **MONITORING REQUIREMENTS**
  ▸ *Renal function* should be checked before treatment.
  ▸ *Hepatic function* should be checked before treatment. If there is no evidence of liver disease (and pre-treatment liver function is normal), further checks are only necessary if the patient develops fever, malaise, vomiting, jaundice or unexplained deterioration during treatment. However, hepatic function should be monitored on prolonged therapy.
  ▸ Blood counts should be monitored on prolonged therapy.
  ▸ Those with alcohol dependence should have frequent checks of hepatic function, particularly in the first 2 months. Blood counts should also be monitored in these patients.
- **PRESCRIBING AND DISPENSING INFORMATION** If treatment interruption occurs, re-introduce with low dosage and increase gradually.
- **PATIENT AND CARER ADVICE**
  Soft contact lenses Patients or their carers should be advised that rifabutin discolours soft contact lenses.
  Hepatic disorders Patients or their carers should be told how to recognise signs of liver disorder, and advised to discontinue treatment and seek immediate medical attention if symptoms such as persistent nausea, vomiting, malaise or jaundice develop.

- **MEDICINAL FORMS** There can be variation in the licensing of different medicines containing the same drug. Forms available from special-order manufacturers include: oral suspension, oral solution
  Oral capsule
  CAUTIONARY AND ADVISORY LABELS 8, 14
  ▸ Mycobutin (Pfizer Ltd)
  Rifabutin 150 mg Mycobutin 150mg capsules | 30 capsule [PoM] £90.38 DT = £90.38

Rifampicin

30-May-2023

- **INDICATIONS AND DOSE**

Brucellosis in combination with other antibacterials | Legionnaires disease in combination with other antibacterials | Serious staphylococcal infections in combination with other antibacterials
▸ BY MOUTH, OR BY INTRAVENOUS INFUSION
▸ Child 1-11 months: 5–10 mg/kg twice daily
▸ Child 1-17 years: 10 mg/kg twice daily (max. per dose 600 mg)
▸ Adult: 0.6–1.2 g daily in 2–4 divided doses

Endocarditis in combination with other drugs
▸ BY MOUTH, OR BY INTRAVENOUS INFUSION
▸ Adult: 0.6–1.2 g daily in 2–4 divided doses

Tuberculosis, in combination with other drugs (intermittent supervised 6-month treatment) (under expert supervision)
▸ BY MOUTH
▸ Child: 15 mg/kg 3 times a week (max. per dose 900 mg) for 6 months (initial and continuation phases)
▸ Adult: 600–900 mg 3 times a week for 6 months (initial and continuation phases)

Tuberculosis, in combination with other drugs (standard unsupervised 6-month treatment)
▸ BY MOUTH
▸ Child (body-weight up to 50 kg): 15 mg/kg once daily for 6 months (initial and continuation phases); maximum 450 mg per day
▸ Child (body-weight 50 kg and above): 15 mg/kg once daily for 6 months (initial and continuation phases); maximum 600 mg per day
▸ Adult (body-weight up to 50 kg): 450 mg once daily for 6 months (initial and continuation phases)
▸ Adult (body-weight 50 kg and above): 600 mg once daily for 6 months (initial and continuation phases)

Prevention of tuberculosis in susceptible close contacts or those who have become tuberculin positive, in combination with isoniazid
▸ BY MOUTH
▸ Child 1 month-11 years (body-weight up to 50 kg): 15 mg/kg daily for 3 months; maximum 450 mg per day
▸ Child 1 month-11 years (body-weight 50 kg and above): 15 mg/kg daily for 3 months; maximum 600 mg per day
▸ Child 12-17 years (body-weight up to 50 kg): 450 mg daily for 3 months
▸ Child 12-17 years (body-weight 50 kg and above): 600 mg daily for 3 months
▸ Adult (body-weight up to 50 kg): 450 mg daily for 3 months
▸ Adult (body-weight 50 kg and above): 600 mg daily for 3 months

Prevention of tuberculosis in susceptible close contacts or those who have become tuberculin positive, who are isoniazid-resistant
▸ BY MOUTH
▸ Child 1 month-11 years (body-weight up to 50 kg): 15 mg/kg daily for 6 months; maximum 450 mg per day
▸ Child 1 month-11 years (body-weight 50 kg and above): 15 mg/kg daily for 6 months; maximum 600 mg per day
▸ Child 12-17 years (body-weight up to 50 kg): 450 mg daily for 6 months
▸ Child 12-17 years (body-weight 50 kg and above): 600 mg daily for 6 months

Prevention of tuberculosis in susceptible close contacts or those who have become tuberculin positive, who are isoniazid-resistant and under 35 years
▸ BY MOUTH
▸ Adult 18-34 years (body-weight up to 50 kg): 450 mg daily for 6 months

> Adult 18–34 years (body-weight 50 kg and above): 600 mg daily for 6 months

Prevention of secondary case of *Haemophilus influenzae* type b disease
> BY MOUTH
> Child 1–2 months: 10 mg/kg once daily for 4 days
> Child 3 months–11 years: 20 mg/kg once daily (max. per dose 600 mg) for 4 days
> Child 12–17 years: 600 mg once daily for 4 days
> Adult: 600 mg once daily for 4 days

Prevention of secondary case of meningococcal meningitis
> BY MOUTH
> Child 1–11 months: 5 mg/kg every 12 hours for 2 days
> Child 1–11 years: 10 mg/kg every 12 hours (max. per dose 600 mg), for 2 days
> Child 12–17 years: 600 mg every 12 hours for 2 days
> Adult: 600 mg every 12 hours for 2 days

Multibacillary leprosy in combination with dapsone and clofazimine (3-drug regimen) | Paucibacillary leprosy in combination with dapsone (2-drug regimen)
> BY MOUTH
> Adult (body-weight up to 35 kg): 450 mg once a month, supervised administration
> Adult (body-weight 35 kg and above): 600 mg once a month, supervised administration

● **CONTRA-INDICATIONS** Acute porphyrias p. 1202 · jaundice
● **CAUTIONS** Discolours soft contact lenses
● **INTERACTIONS** → Appendix 1: rifamycins
● **SIDE-EFFECTS**
  GENERAL SIDE-EFFECTS
  > **Common or very common** Nausea · thrombocytopenia · vomiting
  > **Uncommon** Diarrhoea · leucopenia
  > **Frequency not known** Abdominal discomfort · acute kidney injury · adrenal insufficiency · agranulocytosis · appetite decreased · disseminated intravascular coagulation · dyspnoea · eosinophilia · eye disorders · flushing · gastrointestinal disorders · haemolytic anaemia · hepatitis · hypersensitivity · influenza · intracranial haemorrhage · menstrual disorder · muscle weakness · myopathy · oedema · pseudomembranous enterocolitis · red discolouration of body fluids · severe cutaneous adverse reactions (SCARs) · shock · skin reactions · sputum discolouration · sweat changes · urine discolouration · vasculitis · wheezing
  SPECIFIC SIDE-EFFECTS
  > With intravenous use Bone pain · hyperbilirubinaemia · psychotic disorder
  > With oral use Psychosis

  SIDE-EFFECTS, FURTHER INFORMATION Side-effects that mainly occur with intermittent therapy include influenza-like symptoms (with chills, fever, dizziness, bone pain), respiratory symptoms (including shortness of breath), collapse and shock, haemolytic anaemia, thrombocytopenic purpura, and acute renal failure.
  Discontinue if serious side-effects develop.

● **ALLERGY AND CROSS-SENSITIVITY** EvGr Contra-indicated in patients with rifamycin hypersensitivity. Ⓜ

● **CONCEPTION AND CONTRACEPTION**
  Important Effectiveness of hormonal contraceptives is reduced and alternative family planning advice should be offered.

● **PREGNANCY** Manufacturers advise very high doses teratogenic in *animal* studies in first trimester; risk of neonatal bleeding may be increased in third trimester.

● **BREAST FEEDING** Amount too small to be harmful.

● **HEPATIC IMPAIRMENT** Manufacturer advises caution— monitor liver function weekly for two weeks, then every two weeks for the next six weeks.

Dose adjustments Manufacturer advises maximum 8 mg/kg per day.

● **RENAL IMPAIRMENT**
> In children Use with caution if doses above 10 mg/kg daily.
> In adults Use with caution if dose above 600 mg daily.

● **MONITORING REQUIREMENTS**
> *Renal function* should be checked before treatment.
> *Hepatic function* should be checked before treatment. If there is no evidence of liver disease (and pre-treatment liver function is normal), further checks are only necessary if the patient develops fever, malaise, vomiting, jaundice or unexplained deterioration during treatment. However, liver function should be monitored on prolonged therapy.
> Blood counts should be monitored in patients on prolonged therapy.
> In adults Those with alcohol dependence should have frequent checks of hepatic function, particularly in the first 2 months. Blood counts should also be monitored in these patients.

● **DIRECTIONS FOR ADMINISTRATION**
> With intravenous use in adults For *intravenous infusion* (*Rifadin* ®), give intermittently *in* Glucose 5% *or* Sodium Chloride 0.9%; reconstitute with solvent provided then dilute with 500 mL infusion fluid; give over 2–3 hours.
> With intravenous use in children Displacement value may be significant, consult local reconstitution guidelines; reconstitute with solvent provided. Expert sources advise may be further diluted with Glucose 5% *or* Sodium Chloride 0.9% to a final concentration of 1.2 mg/mL; infuse over 2–3 hours.

● **PRESCRIBING AND DISPENSING INFORMATION** If treatment interruption occurs, re-introduce with low dosage and increase gradually.
  Flavours of syrup may include raspberry.
> With oral use in children In general, doses should be rounded up to facilitate administration of suitable volumes of liquid or an appropriate strength of tablet. Doses may also need to be recalculated to allow for weight gain in younger children.

● **PATIENT AND CARER ADVICE**
  Soft contact lenses Patients or their carers should be advised that rifampicin discolours soft contact lenses.
  Hepatic disorders Patients or their carers should be told how to recognise signs of liver disorder, and advised to discontinue treatment and seek immediate medical attention if symptoms such as persistent nausea, vomiting, malaise or jaundice develop.
  Medicines for Children leaflet: Rifampicin for meningococcal prophylaxis www.medicinesforchildren.org.uk/medicines/rifampicin-for-meningococcal-prophylaxis/
  Medicines for Children leaflet: Rifampicin for treatment of tuberculosis www.medicinesforchildren.org.uk/medicines/rifampicin-for-treatment-of-tuberculosis/

● **MEDICINAL FORMS** There can be variation in the licensing of different medicines containing the same drug. Forms available from special-order manufacturers include: oral suspension, oral solution

Powder and solvent for solution for injection
> Rifampicin (Non-proprietary)
  Rifampicin 300 mg RIFA parenteral 300mg powder and solvent for solution for injection vials | 1 vial PoM Ⓢ (Hospital only)

Oral suspension
CAUTIONARY AND ADVISORY LABELS 8, 14, 23
EXCIPIENTS: May contain Sucrose
> Rifadin (Sanofi)
  Rifampicin 20 mg per 1 ml Rifadin 100mg/5ml syrup | 120 ml PoM £4.27 DT = £4.27

Oral capsule
CAUTIONARY AND ADVISORY LABELS 8, 14, 23
> Rifampicin (Non-proprietary)
  Rifampicin 150 mg Rifampicin 150mg capsules | 100 capsule PoM £98.27 DT = £98.27

Rifampicin 300 mg Rifampicin 300mg capsules | 60 capsule [PoM] £56.74 | 100 capsule [PoM] £165.18 DT = £94.57
▸ **Rifadin** (Sanofi)
Rifampicin 150 mg Rifadin 150mg capsules | 100 capsule [PoM] £18.32 DT = £98.27
Rifampicin 300 mg Rifadin 300mg capsules | 100 capsule [PoM] £36.63 DT = £94.57
▸ **Rimactane** (Sandoz Ltd)
Rifampicin 300 mg Rimactane 300mg capsules | 60 capsule [PoM] £21.98

Powder and solvent for solution for infusion
ELECTROLYTES: May contain Sodium
▸ **Rifadin** (Sanofi)
Rifampicin 600 mg Rifadin 600mg powder and solvent for solution for infusion vials | 1 vial [PoM] £9.20

Rifampicin with ethambutol, isoniazid and pyrazinamide

14-May-2020

The properties listed below are those particular to the combination only. For the properties of the components please consider, rifampicin p. 674, ethambutol hydrochloride p. 678, isoniazid p. 679, pyrazinamide p. 680.

● **INDICATIONS AND DOSE**

Initial treatment of tuberculosis
▸ BY MOUTH
▸ Adult (body-weight 30-39 kg): 2 tablets daily for 2 months (initial phase)
▸ Adult (body-weight 40-54 kg): 3 tablets daily for 2 months (initial phase)
▸ Adult (body-weight 55-69 kg): 4 tablets daily for 2 months (initial phase)
▸ Adult (body-weight 70 kg and above): 5 tablets daily for 2 months (initial phase)

DOSE EQUIVALENCE AND CONVERSION
▸ Tablet quantities refer to the number of *Voractiv* ® Tablets which should be taken. Each *Voractiv* ® Tablet contains ethambutol hydrochloride 275 mg, isoniazid 75 mg, pyrazinamide 400 mg and rifampicin 150 mg.

● INTERACTIONS → Appendix 1: ethambutol · isoniazid · pyrazinamide · rifamycins

● MEDICINAL FORMS There can be variation in the licensing of different medicines containing the same drug.
Oral tablet
CAUTIONARY AND ADVISORY LABELS 8, 14, 22
▸ Voractiv (Genus Pharmaceuticals Ltd)
Isoniazid 75 mg, Rifampicin 150 mg, Ethambutol hydrochloride 275 mg, Pyrazinamide 400 mg Voractiv tablets | 60 tablet [PoM] £39.50

Rifampicin with isoniazid

10-Mar-2020

The properties listed below are those particular to the combination only. For the properties of the components please consider, rifampicin p. 674, isoniazid p. 679.

● **INDICATIONS AND DOSE**

Treatment of tuberculosis (continuation phase)
▸ BY MOUTH
▸ Adult (body-weight up to 50 kg): 450/300 mg daily for 4 months (continuation phase after 2-month initial phase), use *Rifinah* ® 150/100 Tablets, preferably taken before breakfast.
▸ Adult (body-weight 50 kg and above): 600/300 mg daily for 4 months (continuation phase after 2-month initial phase), use *Rifinah* ® 300/150 Tablets, preferably taken before breakfast.

DOSE EQUIVALENCE AND CONVERSION
▸ *Rifinah* ® Tablets contain rifampicin and isoniazid; the proportions are expressed in the form x/y where x and y are the strengths in milligrams of rifampicin and isoniazid respectively.
▸ Each *Rifinah* ® 150/100 Tablet contains rifampicin 150 mg and isoniazid 100 mg.
▸ Each *Rifinah* ® 300/150 Tablet contains rifampicin 300 mg and isoniazid 150 mg.

● INTERACTIONS → Appendix 1: isoniazid · rifamycins

● MEDICINAL FORMS There can be variation in the licensing of different medicines containing the same drug.
Oral tablet
CAUTIONARY AND ADVISORY LABELS 8, 14, 23
▸ Rifinah (Sanofi)
Isoniazid 100 mg, Rifampicin 150 mg Rifinah 150mg/100mg tablets | 84 tablet [PoM] £19.09 DT = £19.09
Isoniazid 150 mg, Rifampicin 300 mg Rifinah 300mg/150mg tablets | 56 tablet [PoM] £25.22 DT = £25.22

Rifampicin with isoniazid and pyrazinamide

The properties listed below are those particular to the combination only. For the properties of the components please consider, rifampicin p. 674, isoniazid p. 679, pyrazinamide p. 680.

● **INDICATIONS AND DOSE**

Initial unsupervised treatment of tuberculosis (in combination with ethambutol)
▸ BY MOUTH
▸ Adult (body-weight up to 40 kg): 3 tablets daily for 2 months (initial phase), use *Rifater* ® Tablets, preferably taken before breakfast.
▸ Adult (body-weight 40-49 kg): 4 tablets daily for 2 months (initial phase), use *Rifater* ® Tablets, preferably taken before breakfast.
▸ Adult (body-weight 50-64 kg): 5 tablets daily for 2 months (initial phase), use *Rifater* ® Tablets, preferably taken before breakfast.
▸ Adult (body-weight 65 kg and above): 6 tablets daily for 2 months (initial phase), use *Rifater* ® Tablets, preferably taken before breakfast.

DOSE EQUIVALENCE AND CONVERSION
▸ Tablet quantities refer to the number of *Rifater* ® Tablets which should be taken. Each *Rifater* ® Tablet contains isoniazid 50 mg, pyrazinamide 300 mg and rifampicin 120 mg.

● INTERACTIONS → Appendix 1: isoniazid · pyrazinamide · rifamycins

● MEDICINAL FORMS There can be variation in the licensing of different medicines containing the same drug.
Oral tablet
CAUTIONARY AND ADVISORY LABELS 8, 14, 22
▸ Rifater (Sanofi)
Isoniazid 50 mg, Rifampicin 120 mg, Pyrazinamide 300 mg Rifater tablets | 100 tablet [PoM] £26.34

ANTIMYCOBACTERIALS > OTHER

Aminosalicylic acid

12-May-2021

● **INDICATIONS AND DOSE**

Multiple-drug resistant tuberculosis, in combination with other drugs

▸ BY MOUTH
▸ Adult: 4 g every 8 hours for a usual treatment duration of 24 months

Desensitisation regimen

▸ BY MOUTH
▸ Adult: (consult product literature)

● **CAUTIONS** Peptic ulcer

● **SIDE-EFFECTS**

▸ **Common or very common** Diarrhoea · dizziness · gastrointestinal discomfort · gastrointestinal disorders · hypersensitivity · nausea · skin reactions · vestibular syndrome · vomiting

▸ **Uncommon** Appetite decreased

▸ **Rare or very rare** Agranulocytosis · anaemia · crystalluria · gastrointestinal haemorrhage · headache · hepatic disorders · hypoglycaemia · hypothyroidism · leucopenia · methaemoglobinaemia · peripheral neuropathy · taste metallic · tendon pain · thrombocytopenia · visual impairment · weight decreased

● **PREGNANCY** Manufacturer advises avoid unless essential—toxicity in *animal* studies (highest risk during first trimester).

● **BREAST FEEDING** Present in milk—manufacturer advises avoid.

● **HEPATIC IMPAIRMENT** Manufacturer advises use with caution.

● **RENAL IMPAIRMENT** EvGr Caution in mild to moderate impairment; avoid in severe impairment (accumulation of inactive metabolites). ⟨M⟩

● **MONITORING REQUIREMENTS**

▸ Monitor for hypersensitivity reaction during the first 3 months of treatment—for desensitisation dosing regimen consult product literature.

▸ Monitor liver function—discontinue immediately if signs or symptoms of hepatic toxicity (including rash, fever and gastrointestinal disturbance).

● **DIRECTIONS FOR ADMINISTRATION** Manufacturer advises disperse granules in orange or tomato juice and take immediately (granules will not dissolve, ensure all granules are swallowed). Granules can be sprinkled on apple sauce or yoghurt for administration.

● **PATIENT AND CARER ADVICE** Patients should be advised that the skeletons of the granules may be seen in the stools. Counselling advised on administration.

● **MEDICINAL FORMS** There can be variation in the licensing of different medicines containing the same drug.

Gastro-resistant granules

CAUTIONARY AND ADVISORY LABELS 9, 25

▸ Granupas (Eurocept International bv)
 Aminosalicylic acid 1 gram per 1 gram Granupas gastro-resistant granules 4g sachets | 30 sachet PoM £331.00 DT = £331.00 SF

Bedaquiline

04-Apr-2023

● **INDICATIONS AND DOSE**

Multiple-drug resistant pulmonary tuberculosis, in combination with other drugs (under expert supervision)

▸ BY MOUTH
▸ Adult: Initially 400 mg once daily for 2 weeks, then 200 mg 3 times a week for 22 weeks, intervals of at least 48 hours between each dose, continue appropriate combination therapy after bedaquiline

● **CONTRA-INDICATIONS** QTc interval more than 500 milliseconds (derived using Fridericia's formula) · ventricular arrhythmia

● **CAUTIONS** Hypothyroidism · QTc interval (derived using Fridericia's formula) 450–500 milliseconds · risk factors for QT interval prolongation (e.g. electrolyte disturbances, heart failure, history of symptomatic arrhythmias, bradycardia, congenital long QT syndrome)

● **INTERACTIONS** → Appendix 1: bedaquiline

● **SIDE-EFFECTS**

▸ **Common or very common** Arthralgia · diarrhoea · dizziness · headache · hepatic function abnormal · myalgia · nausea · QT interval prolongation · vomiting

 SIDE-EFFECTS, FURTHER INFORMATION If syncope occurs, obtain ECG to identify if QT interval prolongation present.

● **PREGNANCY** Manufacturer advises avoid unless potential benefit outweighs risk.

● **BREAST FEEDING** Manufacturer advises avoid—present in milk in *animal* studies.

● **HEPATIC IMPAIRMENT** Manufacturer advises caution in moderate impairment; avoid in severe impairment—no information available.

● **RENAL IMPAIRMENT** EvGr Caution if creatinine clearance less than 30 mL/minute, ⟨M⟩ see p. 21.

● **MONITORING REQUIREMENTS**

▸ Determine serum potassium, calcium, and magnesium before starting treatment (correct if abnormal)—remeasure if QT prolongation occurs during treatment.

▸ Obtain ECG before starting treatment, and then at least monthly during treatment or more frequently if concomitant use with other drugs known to prolong the QT interval.

▸ Monitor liver function before starting treatment and then at least monthly during treatment—discontinue treatment if severe abnormalities in liver function tests.

● **PATIENT AND CARER ADVICE**

Missed doses If a dose is missed during the first two weeks of treatment, the missed dose should not be taken and the next dose should be taken at the usual time; if a dose is missed during weeks 3–24 of treatment, the missed dose should be taken as soon as possible and then the usual regimen resumed.

Driving and skilled tasks Dizziness may affect performance of skilled tasks (e.g. driving).

● **NATIONAL FUNDING/ACCESS DECISIONS**

For full details see funding body website

All Wales Medicines Strategy Group (AWMSG) decisions

▸ Bedaquiline (*Sirturo*®) for use as part of an appropriate combination regimen for pulmonary multidrug-resistant tuberculosis (MDR-TB) in adult and paediatric patients (5 years to less than 18 years of age and weighing at least 15 kg) when an effective treatment regimen cannot otherwise be composed for reasons of resistance or tolerability (November 2022) AWMSG No. 4860 Recommended

● **MEDICINAL FORMS** There can be variation in the licensing of different medicines containing the same drug.

Oral tablet

CAUTIONARY AND ADVISORY LABELS 4, 8, 21

▸ Sirturo (Janssen-Cilag Ltd)
 Bedaquiline (as Bedaquiline fumarate) 20 mg Sirturo 20mg tablets | 60 tablet PoM £1,193.64 (Hospital only)
 Bedaquiline (as Bedaquiline fumarate) 100 mg Sirturo 100mg tablets | 24 tablet PoM £2,387.28 (Hospital only)

Cycloserine

- **INDICATIONS AND DOSE**

Tuberculosis resistant to first-line drugs, in combination with other drugs
- BY MOUTH
  - Adult: Initially 250 mg every 12 hours for 2 weeks, then increased if necessary up to 500 mg every 12 hours, dose to be increased according to blood concentration and response

PHARMACOKINETICS
- Cycloserine penetrates the CNS.

- **CONTRA-INDICATIONS** Alcohol dependence · depression · epilepsy · psychotic states · severe anxiety

- **INTERACTIONS** → Appendix 1: cycloserine

- **SIDE-EFFECTS** Behaviour abnormal · coma · confusion · congestive heart failure · drowsiness · dysarthria · headache · hyperirritability · megaloblastic anaemia · memory loss · neurological effects · paraesthesia · paresis · psychosis · rash · reflexes increased · seizures · suicidal ideation · tremor · vertigo

SIDE-EFFECTS, FURTHER INFORMATION **CNS toxicity** Discontinue or reduce dose if symptoms of CNS toxicity occur.
Rashes or allergic dermatitis Discontinue or reduce dose if rashes or allergic dermatitis develop.

- **PREGNANCY** Manufacturer advises use only if potential benefit outweighs risk—crosses the placenta.

- **BREAST FEEDING** Present in milk—amount too small to be harmful.

- **RENAL IMPAIRMENT**
Dose adjustments Increase interval between doses if creatinine clearance less than 50 mL/minute.
Monitoring Monitor blood-cycloserine concentration if creatinine clearance less than 50 mL/minute.

- **MONITORING REQUIREMENTS**
  - Blood concentration monitoring required especially in renal impairment or if dose exceeds 500 mg daily or if signs of toxicity; blood concentration should not exceed 30 mg/litre.
  - Monitor haematological, renal, and hepatic function.

- **MEDICINAL FORMS** There can be variation in the licensing of different medicines containing the same drug.

Oral capsule
CAUTIONARY AND ADVISORY LABELS 2, 8
- Cycloserine (Non-proprietary)
  Cycloserine 250 mg Cycloserine 250mg capsules |
  100 capsule PoM £442.89 DT = £442.89

Delamanid

10-May-2021

- **INDICATIONS AND DOSE**

Multiple-drug resistant pulmonary tuberculosis, in combination with other drugs
- BY MOUTH
  - Adult: 100 mg twice daily for 24 weeks, continue appropriate combination therapy after delamanid

- **CONTRA-INDICATIONS** QTc interval more than 500 milliseconds (derived using Fridericia's formula) · serum albumin less than 28 g/litre

- **CAUTIONS** Risk factors for QT interval prolongation (e.g. electrolyte disturbances, acute myocardial infarction, heart failure with reduced left ventricular ejection fraction, severe hypertension, left ventricular hypertrophy, bradycardia, congenital long QT syndrome, history of symptomatic arrhythmias)

- **INTERACTIONS** → Appendix 1: delamanid

- **SIDE-EFFECTS**
  - **Common or very common** Anxiety · appetite decreased · asthenia · chest pain · cough · depression · dyslipidaemia · dyspnoea · ear pain · electrolyte imbalance · gastrointestinal discomfort · haemoptysis · headache · hyperhidrosis · hypertension · hypotension · malaise · muscle weakness · nausea · oropharyngeal pain · osteochondrosis · pain · palpitations · peripheral neuropathy · photophobia · psychotic disorder · QT interval prolongation · reticulocytosis · sensation abnormal · skin reactions · sleep disorders · throat irritation · tinnitus · tremor · vomiting
  - **Uncommon** Aggression · atrioventricular block · balance impaired · dehydration · delusional disorder, persecutory type · dysphagia · extrasystole · hepatic function abnormal · increased risk of infection · lethargy · leucopenia · oral paraesthesia · psychiatric disorders · thrombocytopenia · urinary disorders

- **CONCEPTION AND CONTRACEPTION** Effective contraception required during treatment.

- **PREGNANCY** Manufacturer advises avoid—toxicity in *animal* studies.

- **BREAST FEEDING** Manufacturer advises avoid—present in milk in *animal* studies.

- **HEPATIC IMPAIRMENT** Manufacturer advises avoid in moderate to severe impairment.

- **RENAL IMPAIRMENT** Manufacturer advises avoid in severe impairment—no information available.

- **MONITORING REQUIREMENTS**
  - Monitor serum albumin and electrolytes before starting treatment and then during treatment—discontinue treatment if serum albumin less than 28 g/litre.
  - Obtain ECG before starting treatment and then monthly during treatment (more frequently if serum albumin 28–34 g/litre, or if concomitant use of potent CYP3A4 inhibitors, or if risk factors for QT interval prolongation, or if QTc interval 450–500 milliseconds in men or 470–500 milliseconds in women)—discontinue treatment if QTc interval more than 500 milliseconds (derived using Fridericia's formula).

- **HANDLING AND STORAGE** Dispense in original container (contains desiccant).

- **MEDICINAL FORMS** There can be variation in the licensing of different medicines containing the same drug.

Oral tablet
CAUTIONARY AND ADVISORY LABELS 8, 21
- Deltyba (Imported) ▼
  Delamanid 50 mg Deltyba 50mg tablets | 48 tablet PoM ⓧ

Ethambutol hydrochloride

26-Oct-2021

- **INDICATIONS AND DOSE**

Tuberculosis, in combination with other drugs (standard unsupervised 6-month treatment)
- BY MOUTH
  - Child: 20 mg/kg once daily for 2 months (initial phase)
  - Adult: 15 mg/kg once daily for 2 months (initial phase)

Tuberculosis, in combination with other drugs (intermittent supervised 6-month treatment) (under expert supervision)
- BY MOUTH
  - Child: 30 mg/kg 3 times a week for 2 months (initial phase)
  - Adult: 30 mg/kg 3 times a week for 2 months (initial phase)

- **CONTRA-INDICATIONS** Optic neuritis · poor vision

- **CAUTIONS** Elderly · young children

CAUTIONS, FURTHER INFORMATION

▶ **Understanding warnings** Patients who cannot understand warnings about visual side-effects should, if possible, be given an alternative drug. In particular, ethambutol should be used with caution in children until they are at least 5 years old and capable of reporting symptomatic visual changes accurately.

● **INTERACTIONS** → Appendix 1: ethambutol

● **SIDE-EFFECTS**

▶ **Common or very common** Hyperuricaemia · nerve disorders · visual impairment

▶ **Rare or very rare** Nephritis tubulointerstitial

▶ **Frequency not known** Alveolitis allergic · appetite decreased · asthenia · confusion · dizziness · eosinophilia · fever · flatulence · gastrointestinal discomfort · gout · hallucination · headache · jaundice · leucopenia · nausea · nephrotoxicity · neutropenia · photosensitive lichenoid eruption · sensation abnormal · severe cutaneous adverse reactions (SCARs) · skin reactions · taste metallic · thrombocytopenia · tremor · vomiting

SIDE-EFFECTS, FURTHER INFORMATION Ocular toxicity is more common where excessive dosage is used or if the patient's renal function is impaired. Early discontinuation of the drug is almost always followed by recovery of eyesight.

● **PREGNANCY** Not known to be harmful.

● **BREAST FEEDING** Amount too small to be harmful.

● **RENAL IMPAIRMENT** Risk of optic nerve damage. EvGr Should preferably be avoided in patients with renal impairment. ⟨M⟩
Dose adjustments EvGr If creatinine clearance less than 30 mL/minute, use 15–25 mg/kg (max. 2.5 g) 3 times a week—monitor plasma-ethambutol concentration. ⟨M⟩ See p. 21.

● **MONITORING REQUIREMENTS**

▶ 'Peak' concentration (2–2.5 hours after dose) should be 2–6 mg/litre (7–22 micromol/litre); 'trough' (pre-dose) concentration should be less than 1 mg/litre (4 micromol/litre).

▶ Renal function should be checked before treatment.

▶ Visual acuity should be tested by Snellen chart before treatment with ethambutol.

▶ In young children, routine ophthalmological monitoring recommended.

● **PRESCRIBING AND DISPENSING INFORMATION** The RCPCH and NPPG recommend that, when a liquid special of ethambutol is required, the following strength is used: 400 mg/5 mL.

● **PATIENT AND CARER ADVICE**
Ocular toxicity The earliest features of ocular toxicity are subjective and patients should be advised to discontinue therapy immediately if they develop deterioration in vision and promptly seek further advice.
Medicines for Children leaflet: Ethambutol for treatment of tuberculosis www.medicinesforchildren.org.uk/medicines/ethambutol-for-treatments-of-tuberculosis/

● **MEDICINAL FORMS** There can be variation in the licensing of different medicines containing the same drug. Forms available from special-order manufacturers include: oral suspension, oral solution

Oral tablet
CAUTIONARY AND ADVISORY LABELS 8
▶ Ethambutol hydrochloride (Non-proprietary)
   Ethambutol hydrochloride 100 mg Ethambutol 100mg tablets | 56 tablet PoM £40.00 DT = £40.00
   Ethambutol hydrochloride 400 mg Ethambutol 400mg tablets | 56 tablet PoM £85.48 DT = £50.00

Combinations available: *Rifampicin with ethambutol, isoniazid and pyrazinamide,* p. 676

Isoniazid
10-Nov-2021

● **INDICATIONS AND DOSE**

Tuberculosis, in combination with other drugs (standard unsupervised 6-month treatment)

▶ BY MOUTH, OR BY INTRAMUSCULAR INJECTION, OR BY INTRAVENOUS INJECTION

▶ Child: 10 mg/kg once daily (max. per dose 300 mg) for 6 months (initial and continuation phases)

▶ Adult: 300 mg daily for 6 months (initial and continuation phases)

Tuberculosis, in combination with other drugs (intermittent supervised 6-month treatment) (under expert supervision)

▶ BY MOUTH, OR BY INTRAMUSCULAR INJECTION, OR BY INTRAVENOUS INJECTION

▶ Child: 15 mg/kg 3 times a week (max. per dose 900 mg) for 6 months (initial and continuation phases)

▶ Adult: 15 mg/kg 3 times a week (max. per dose 900 mg) for 6 months (initial and continuation phases)

Prevention of tuberculosis in susceptible close contacts or those who have become tuberculin positive

▶ INITIALLY BY MOUTH, OR BY INTRAMUSCULAR INJECTION, OR BY INTRAVENOUS INJECTION

▶ Child 1 month–11 years: 10 mg/kg daily (max. per dose 300 mg) for 6 months, alternatively (by mouth) 10 mg/kg daily (max. per dose 300 mg) for 3 months, to be taken in combination with rifampicin

▶ Child 12–17 years: 300 mg daily for 6 months, alternatively (by mouth) 300 mg daily for 3 months, to be taken in combination with rifampicin

▶ Adult: 300 mg daily for 6 months, alternatively (by mouth) 300 mg daily for 3 months, to be taken in combination with rifampicin

● **CONTRA-INDICATIONS** Drug-induced liver disease

● **CAUTIONS** Acute porphyrias p. 1202 · alcohol dependence · diabetes mellitus · epilepsy · history of psychosis · HIV infection · malnutrition · slow acetylator status (increased risk of side-effects)

CAUTIONS, FURTHER INFORMATION

▶ Peripheral neuropathy Pyridoxine hydrochloride p. 1237 should be given prophylactically in all patients from the start of treatment. Peripheral neuropathy is more likely to occur where there are pre-existing risk factors such as diabetes, alcohol dependence, chronic renal failure, pregnancy, malnutrition and HIV infection.

● **INTERACTIONS** → Appendix 1: isoniazid

● **SIDE-EFFECTS**

GENERAL SIDE-EFFECTS

▶ **Uncommon** Hepatic disorders

▶ **Rare or very rare** Severe cutaneous adverse reactions (SCARs)

▶ **Frequency not known** Agranulocytosis · aplastic anaemia · fever · gynaecomastia · haemolytic anaemia · nerve disorders · seizure · vasculitis

SPECIFIC SIDE-EFFECTS

▶ With oral use Acidosis · constipation · deafness · dry mouth · dysuria · erythema multiforme · euphoric mood · gastrointestinal disorder · hypoglycaemia · interstitial lung disease · lupus erythematosus · nausea · nicotinic acid deficiency · pancreatitis acute · psychiatric disorder · psychotic disorder · tinnitus · vertigo · vomiting · withdrawal syndrome

▶ With parenteral use Alopecia · anaemia · eosinophilia · hyperglycaemia · lupus-like syndrome · optic atrophy · pancreatitis · pellagra · psychosis · skin reactions · thrombocytopenia

5
Infection

SIDE-EFFECTS, FURTHER INFORMATION Hepatitis more common in those aged over 35 years and those with a daily alcohol intake.

- **PREGNANCY** Not known to be harmful; prophylactic pyridoxine recommended.
- **BREAST FEEDING** Theoretical risk of convulsions and neuropathy; prophylactic pyridoxine advisable in mother. **Monitoring** In breast-feeding, monitor infant for possible toxicity.
- **HEPATIC IMPAIRMENT** Manufacturer advises caution (increased risk of hepatotoxicity). **Monitoring** In patients with pre-existing liver disease or hepatic impairment monitor liver function regularly and particularly frequently in the first 2 months.
- **RENAL IMPAIRMENT** EvGr Use with caution (risk of ototoxicity and peripheral neuropathy; prophylactic pyridoxine hydrochloride p. 1237 recommended). Ⓜ **Dose adjustments**
  - With intramuscular use or intravenous use EvGr Dose reduction may be required in severe impairment (consult product literature). Ⓜ
- **MONITORING REQUIREMENTS**
  - *Renal function* should be checked before treatment.
  - *Hepatic function* should be checked before treatment. If there is no evidence of liver disease (and pre-treatment liver function is normal), further checks are only necessary if the patient develops fever, malaise, vomiting, jaundice or unexplained deterioration during treatment.
  - In adults Those with alcohol dependence should have frequent checks of hepatic function, particularly in the first 2 months.
- **PRESCRIBING AND DISPENSING INFORMATION**
  - With oral use in children In general, doses should be rounded up to facilitate administration of suitable volumes of liquid or an appropriate strength of tablet. The RCPCH and NPPG recommend that, when a liquid special of isoniazid is required, the following strength is used: 50 mg/5 mL.
  - In children Doses may need to be recalculated to allow for weight gain in younger children.
- **PATIENT AND CARER ADVICE**
  Hepatic disorders Patients or their carers should be told how to recognise signs of liver disorder, and advised to discontinue treatment and seek immediate medical attention if symptoms such as persistent nausea, vomiting, malaise or jaundice develop.
  Medicines for Children leaflet: Isoniazid for latent tuberculosis www.medicinesforchildren.org.uk/medicines/isoniazid-for-latent-tuberculosis/
  Medicines for Children leaflet: Isoniazid for treatment of tuberculosis www.medicinesforchildren.org.uk/medicines/isoniazid-for-treatment-of-tuberculosis/
- **MEDICINAL FORMS** There can be variation in the licensing of different medicines containing the same drug. Forms available from special-order manufacturers include: oral suspension, oral solution, solution for injection

  Solution for injection
  - Isoniazid (Non-proprietary)
    Isoniazid 20 mg per 1 ml Tebesium-S 100mg/5ml solution for injection ampoules | 12 ampoule PoM Ⓢ (Hospital only)
    Isoniazid 60 mg per 1 ml Cemidon Intravenoso 300mg/5ml solution for injection ampoules | 5 ampoule PoM Ⓢ (Hospital only)

  Oral tablet
  CAUTIONARY AND ADVISORY LABELS 8, 22
  - Isoniazid (Non-proprietary)
    Isoniazid 50 mg Isoniazid 50mg tablets | 56 tablet PoM £23.81 DT = £23.81
    Isoniazid 100 mg Isoniazid 100mg tablets | 28 tablet PoM £75.11 DT = £75.11

Isoniazid 300 mg Isoniazid 300mg tablets | 30 tablet PoM Ⓢ (Hospital only)

Combinations available: *Rifampicin with ethambutol, isoniazid and pyrazinamide,* p. 676 · *Rifampicin with isoniazid,* p. 676 · *Rifampicin with isoniazid and pyrazinamide,* p. 676

Pyrazinamide
11-Nov-2021

- **INDICATIONS AND DOSE**

Tuberculosis, in combination with other drugs (standard unsupervised 6-month treatment)
  - BY MOUTH
  - Child (body-weight up to 50 kg): 35 mg/kg once daily for 2 months (initial phase); maximum 1.5 g per day
  - Child (body-weight 50 kg and above): 35 mg/kg once daily for 2 months (initial phase); maximum 2 g per day
  - Adult (body-weight up to 50 kg): 1.5 g once daily for 2 months (initial phase)
  - Adult (body-weight 50 kg and above): 2 g once daily for 2 months (initial phase)

Tuberculosis, in combination with other drugs (intermittent supervised 6-month treatment) (under expert supervision)
  - BY MOUTH
  - Child (body-weight up to 50 kg): 50 mg/kg 3 times a week (max. per dose 2 g 3 times a week) for 2 months (initial phase)
  - Child (body-weight 50 kg and above): 50 mg/kg 3 times a week (max. per dose 2.5 g 3 times a week) for 2 months (initial phase)
  - Adult (body-weight up to 50 kg): 2 g 3 times a week for 2 months (initial phase)
  - Adult (body-weight 50 kg and above): 2.5 g 3 times a week for 2 months (initial phase)

- **CONTRA-INDICATIONS** Acute attack of gout (in adults)
- **CAUTIONS** Diabetes · gout (in adults)
- **INTERACTIONS** → Appendix 1: pyrazinamide
- **SIDE-EFFECTS** Appetite decreased · arthralgia · dysuria · flushing · gout aggravated · hepatic disorders · malaise · nausea · peptic ulcer aggravated · photosensitivity reaction · sideroblastic anaemia · skin reactions · splenomegaly · vomiting
- **PREGNANCY** Manufacturer advises use only if potential benefit outweighs risk.
- **BREAST FEEDING** Amount too small to be harmful.
- **HEPATIC IMPAIRMENT** Manufacturer advises avoid in severe impairment, acute hepatic disease and for up to 6 months after occurrence of hepatitis (risk of increased exposure).
- **RENAL IMPAIRMENT**
  Dose adjustments
  - In adults 25–30 mg/kg 3 times a week if eGFR less than 30 mL/minute/1.73 m^2.
  - In children If estimated glomerular filtration rate less than 30 mL/minute/1.73 m^2, use 25–30 mg/kg 3 times a week.
  Monitoring Monitor for gout in renal impairment.
- **MONITORING REQUIREMENTS**
  - *Renal function* should be checked before treatment.
  - *Hepatic function* should be checked before treatment. If there is no evidence of liver disease (and pre-treatment liver function is normal), further checks are only necessary if the patient develops fever, malaise, vomiting, jaundice or unexplained deterioration during treatment.
  - In adults Those with alcohol dependence should have frequent checks of hepatic function, particularly in the first 2 months.

Infection

5

- **PRESCRIBING AND DISPENSING INFORMATION**
▶ **In children** In general, doses should be rounded up to facilitate administration of suitable volumes of liquid or an appropriate strength of tablet. Doses may also need to be recalculated to allow for weight gain in younger children. The RCPCH and NPPG recommend that, when a liquid special of pyrazinamide is required, the following strength is used: 500 mg/5 mL.

- **PATIENT AND CARER ADVICE**
Hepatic disorders Patients or their carers should be told how to recognise signs of liver disorder, and advised to discontinue treatment and seek immediate medical attention if symptoms such as persistent nausea, vomiting, malaise or jaundice develop.
Medicines for Children leaflet: Pyrazinamide for the treatment of tuberculosis www.medicinesforchildren.org.uk/medicines/pyrazinamide-for-the-treatment-of-tuberculosis/

- **MEDICINAL FORMS** There can be variation in the licensing of different medicines containing the same drug. Forms available from special-order manufacturers include: oral suspension, oral solution

Oral tablet
CAUTIONARY AND ADVISORY LABELS 8
▶ Pyrazinamide (Non-proprietary)
Pyrazinamide 500 mg Pyrazinamide 500mg tablets | 30 tablet PoM £31.35–£40.06 DT = £40.06
▶ Zinamide (Genus Pharmaceuticals Ltd)
Pyrazinamide 500 mg Zinamide 500mg tablets | 30 tablet PoM £31.35 DT = £40.06

Combinations available: *Rifampicin with ethambutol, isoniazid and pyrazinamide*, p. 676 · *Rifampicin with isoniazid and pyrazinamide*, p. 676

2.6 Urinary tract infections

Urinary-tract infections

02-Jan-2025

Description of condition

Urinary-tract infections (UTIs) are common infections that can affect any part of the urinary tract; the terms 'male' and 'female' refer to all patients with a male urinary tract, and female urinary tract, respectively. UTIs occur more frequently in females, and are usually independent of any risk factor. They are predominantly caused by bacteria from the gastrointestinal tract entering the urinary tract, with *Escherichia coli* being the most common cause. Infection due to *Candida albicans* is rare, but may occur in hospitalised patients who are immunocompromised or have an indwelling catheter.

Lower UTIs are associated with inflammation of the bladder (cystitis) and urethra (urethritis). The most common signs and symptoms of lower UTIs are dysuria, increased urinary frequency and urgency, urine that is strong smelling, cloudy or contains blood, and persistent lower abdominal pain. A complicated lower UTI is a lower UTI with an increased risk of a more serious outcome or treatment failure, for example in a patient with a structural or functional abnormality of the urinary tract, or an underlying disease.

In some patients infection can ascend the urinary tract and lead to an upper UTI. Upper UTIs affect the proximal part of the ureters (pyelitis) or the proximal part of the ureters and the kidneys (pyelonephritis), and can cause renal scarring, abscess or failure, and sepsis. Upper UTIs usually present with accompanying loin pain and fever.

In pregnant females, asymptomatic bacteriuria is a risk factor for pyelonephritis and premature labour. UTIs in pregnancy have been associated with developmental delay and cerebral palsy in the infant, as well as fetal death.

Insertion of a catheter into the urinary tract increases the risk of developing a UTI, and the longer the catheter is in place for, further increases the risk of bacteriuria.

UTIs are considered recurrent after at least two episodes within 6 months or three or more episodes within 12 months.

Acute prostatitis is an infection of the prostate gland and is usually caused by a UTI. It can occur spontaneously or after certain medical procedures and can last for several weeks. Common symptoms include sudden onset of fever, acute urinary retention or irritative voiding symptoms. Possible complications include prostatic abscess, bacteraemia, epididymitis, and pyelonephritis. Chronic prostatitis is a complication of acute prostatitis and is defined as at least 3 months of urogenital pain usually associated with lower urinary tract symptoms.

Aims of treatment

The aims of treatment are to relieve symptoms, treat the underlying infection, prevent systemic infection, and to reduce the risk of complications.

Non-drug treatment

EvGr Patients with a UTI should be advised to drink plenty of fluids to avoid dehydration, and to use self-care strategies to reduce the risk of recurrent infections. These include wiping from front to back after defaecation, not delaying urination, and not wearing occlusive underwear.

To reduce the risk of recurrent infections, some females (non-pregnant) with recurrent UTIs may wish to try cranberry products (evidence of benefit uncertain) or D-mannose. Patients should be advised to consider the sugar content of these products. There is no evidence to support the use of cranberry products for the treatment of UTIs. Ⓐ

Drug treatment

EvGr When prescribing antibacterial therapy the severity of symptoms, risk of developing complications, previous urine culture and susceptibility results, and previous antibacterial use should be taken into consideration.

With the exception of pregnant females, asymptomatic bacteriuria is not routinely treated with antibacterials. Ⓐ

For other considerations such as for patients receiving prophylactic antibacterial therapy, switching from *intravenous* to *oral* antibacterials, and for advice to give to patients, see Antibacterials, principles of therapy p. 573.

EvGr Reassess patients if symptoms worsen at any time, or do not start to improve within 48 hours of starting treatment.

Refer patients to hospital if they have any symptoms or signs suggestive of a more serious illness or condition.

Review choice of antibacterial when microbiological results are available, and change treatment as appropriate if susceptibility results indicate bacterial resistance.

Advise patients that paracetamol or ibuprofen can be used for pain relief. Where appropriate, codeine may be used in patients with acute pyelonephritis or prostatitis. Ⓐ

There is no evidence to support the use of alkalising agents for the treatment of UTIs.

Uncomplicated lower urinary-tract infection

For complicated lower UTI, see *pyelonephritis, acute* for antibacterial choices.

Non-pregnant females

EvGr Acute, uncomplicated lower UTIs in these individuals can be self-limiting and for some, delaying antibacterial treatment with a back-up prescription to see if symptoms will resolve, may be an option. Consider a back-up antibacterial prescription for use if symptoms worsen or do not improve within 48 hours **or** an immediate antibacterial prescription. Ⓐ

Choice of antibacterial therapy

- **Oral** *first line* :
  - EvGr Nitrofurantoin p. 684, or trimethoprim p. 665 (if low risk of resistance). A
- **Oral** *second line* (if no improvement after at least 48 hours, **or** first line not suitable):
  - EvGr Nitrofurantoin (if not used first line), fosfomycin p. 662, pivmecillinam hydrochloride p. 642, or amoxicillin p. 635 (high rate of resistance, so only use if culture susceptible). A

Males

EvGr An immediate antibacterial prescription should be given and a midstream urine sample obtained before treatment is taken and sent for culture and susceptibility testing. A

Choice of antibacterial therapy

- **Oral** *first line* :
  - EvGr Nitrofurantoin, or trimethoprim. A
- **Oral** *second line* (if no improvement after at least 48 hours, **or** first line not suitable):
  - Consider pyelonephritis or prostatitis. See *pyelonephritis, acute*, or *prostatitis, acute* below for guidance.

Pregnant females

EvGr An immediate antibacterial prescription should be given and a midstream urine sample obtained before treatment is taken and sent for culture and susceptibility testing. A

Choice of antibacterial therapy

- **Oral** *first line* :
  - EvGr Nitrofurantoin. A
- **Oral** *second line* (if no improvement after at least 48 hours, **or** first line not suitable):
  - EvGr Amoxicillin (only if culture susceptible), or cefalexin p. 603. A
- **Alternative** *second line* :
  - EvGr Consult local microbiologist. A
- **Asymptomatic bacteriuria**:
  - EvGr Amoxicillin, cefalexin, or nitrofurantoin. A

Prostatitis, acute

EvGr An immediate antibacterial prescription should be given and a midstream urine sample obtained before treatment is taken and sent for culture and susceptibility testing.

Refer patients to hospital if symptoms are not improving after 48 hours of treatment, or if they have any signs or symptoms suggestive of a more serious condition such as sepsis, acute urinary retention, or prostatic abscess. A

Choice of antibacterial therapy

See *Important safety information* in ciprofloxacin p. 648, ofloxacin p. 652 and levofloxacin p. 650 for information relating to serious and long-lasting adverse effects associated with fluoroquinolones.

- **Oral** *first line* :
  - EvGr Ciprofloxacin, or ofloxacin.
  - Alternative first line if a fluoroquinolone is not appropriate (seek specialist advice): trimethoprim p. 665. A
- **Oral** *second line* (on specialist advice):
  - EvGr Levofloxacin, or co-trimoxazole p. 652. A
- **Intravenous** *first line* (if severely unwell or unable to take oral treatment). EvGr Antibacterials may be combined if concerned about sepsis.
  - Amikacin p. 594, ceftriaxone p. 609, cefuroxime p. 606, ciprofloxacin, gentamicin p. 596, or levofloxacin. A
- **Intravenous** *second line* :
  - EvGr Consult local microbiologist. A

Pyelonephritis, acute

EvGr An immediate antibacterial prescription should be given and a midstream urine sample obtained before treatment is taken and sent for culture and susceptibility testing.

Consider referring or seeking specialist advice for patients with acute pyelonephritis who are significantly dehydrated or are unable to take oral fluids and medicines, are pregnant, or have a higher risk of developing complications. A

Males and non-pregnant females

Choice of antibacterial therapy

- **Oral** *first line* :
  - EvGr Cefalexin p. 603. If sensitivity known: co-amoxiclav p. 638, or trimethoprim. If other first line antibacterials are inappropriate, ciprofloxacin may be used. A
- **Intravenous** *first line* (if severely unwell or unable to take oral treatment). EvGr Antibacterials may be combined if concerned about susceptibility or sepsis.
  - Amikacin, ceftriaxone, cefuroxime, or gentamicin. Co-amoxiclav may be used if given in combination or sensitivity known. If other first line antibacterials are inappropriate, ciprofloxacin may be used. A
- **Intravenous** *second line* :
  - EvGr Consult local microbiologist. A

Pregnant females

Choice of antibacterial therapy

- **Oral** *first line* :
  - EvGr Cefalexin. A
- **Intravenous** *first line* (if severely unwell or unable to take oral treatment):
  - EvGr Cefuroxime. A
- **Second line** or combining antibacterials if concerned about susceptibility or sepsis:
  - EvGr Consult local microbiologist. A

Recurrent urinary-tract infection

EvGr For patients with recurrent UTIs, refer or seek specialist advice for males, pregnant females, patients with suspected cancer, those presenting with recurrent upper UTI, patients who have had gender reassignment surgery that involved structural alteration of the urethra, and those with recurrent lower UTI with an unknown cause. A

Non-pregnant females

When behavioural and personal hygiene measures alone are not effective or appropriate, consider these alternative options in the following order to prevent recurrent UTIs, if appropriate for the patient:

- EvGr In perimenopausal, menopausal, and postmenopausal females, consider vaginal estriol p. 960 or estradiol p. 959 [unlicensed indication]; treatment should be reviewed within 12 months. Systemic oestrogens (hormone replacement therapy) should not be given specifically to reduce the risk of recurrent UTIs;
- Consider single-dose antibacterial prophylaxis [unlicensed indication] when there has been exposure to an identifiable trigger;
- Methenamine hippurate p. 683 may be considered for prophylaxis of recurrent uncomplicated lower UTI. Specialist advice should be sought if considering use in non-pregnant females with recurrent upper UTI or complicated lower UTI (lack of evidence to inform when methenamine hippurate may be beneficial in these patients). Treatment should be reviewed within 6 months and then annually, or earlier if required;
- Daily antibacterial prophylaxis should be considered if there is no improvement with the above measures. A

Males and pregnant females

EvGr When behavioural and personal hygiene measures alone are not effective or appropriate, seek specialist advice if considering methenamine hippurate for prophylaxis of recurrent UTI (lack of evidence to inform when methenamine hippurate may be beneficial in these patients). Treatment should be reviewed within 6 months and then annually, or earlier if required. If methenamine hippurate is not effective, with specialist advice, consider daily antibacterial prophylaxis as an alternative. A

Choice of antibacterial therapy

- **Oral** *first line* :
- ▶ EvGr Trimethoprim, or nitrofurantoin p. 684. A
- **Oral** *second line* :
- ▶ EvGr Amoxicillin p. 635 [unlicensed indication], or cefalexin.

Advise patients about the risk of resistance with long-term antibacterial use, seeking medical help if symptoms of an acute UTI develop, and to return for review within 6 months.

Review the success and ongoing need for antibacterial prophylaxis at least every 6 months. If antibacterial prophylaxis is stopped, ensure the patient has rapid access to treatment if they develop an acute UTI. A

Catheter-associated urinary-tract infection

EvGr For people with a catheter-associated urinary-tract infection, consider removing or changing the catheter as soon as possible if it has been in place for longer than 7 days, without delaying antibacterial treatment. An immediate antibacterial prescription should be given and a urine sample obtained before treatment is taken and sent for culture and susceptibility testing.

Consider referring or seeking specialist advice for patients with a catheter-associated UTI who are significantly dehydrated or unable to take oral fluids and medicines, are pregnant, have a higher risk of developing complications, have recurrent catheter-associated UTIs, or have bacteria resistant to oral antibacterials. A

Males and non-pregnant females
Choice of antibacterial therapy

- **Oral** *first line* (if **no** upper UTI symptoms):
- ▶ EvGr Amoxicillin (only if culture susceptible), nitrofurantoin, or trimethoprim (if low risk of resistance). A
- **Oral** *second line* (if **no** upper UTI symptoms and first-line not suitable):
- ▶ EvGr Pivmecillinam hydrochloride p. 642. A
- **Oral** *first line* (upper UTI symptoms):
- ▶ EvGr Cefalexin, co-amoxiclav (if culture susceptible), or trimethoprim (if culture susceptible). If other first line antibacterials are inappropriate, ciprofloxacin may be used. A
- **Intravenous** *first line* (if severely unwell or unable to take oral treatment). EvGr Antibacterials may be combined if concerned about susceptibility or sepsis.
- ▶ Amikacin, ceftriaxone, cefuroxime, gentamicin, or co-amoxiclav (only in combination, unless culture results confirm susceptibility). If other first line antibacterials are inappropriate, ciprofloxacin may be used. A
- **Intravenous** *second line* :
- ▶ EvGr Consult local microbiologist. A

Pregnant females
Choice of antibacterial therapy

- **Oral** *first line* :
- ▶ EvGr Cefalexin. A
- **Intravenous** *first line* (if severely unwell or unable to take oral treatment):
- ▶ EvGr Cefuroxime. A
- *Second line or combining if concerned about susceptibility or sepsis*:
- ▶ EvGr Consult local microbiologist. A

Useful Resources

Urinary tract infection (lower): antimicrobial prescribing. National Institute for Health and Care Excellence. NICE Guideline NG109. October 2018.
www.nice.org.uk/guidance/ng109

Management of suspected bacterial lower urinary tract infection in adult women. Scottish Intercollegiate Guidelines Network. Clinical guideline 160. September 2020.
www.sign.ac.uk/our-guidelines/management-of-suspected-bacterial-lower-urinary-tract-infection-in-adult-women/

Prostatitis (acute): antimicrobial prescribing. National Institute for Health and Care Excellence. NICE guideline NG110. October 2018, updated September 2024.
www.nice.org.uk/guidance/ng110

Pyelonephritis (acute): antimicrobial prescribing. National Institute for Health and Care Excellence. NICE guideline NG111. October 2018, updated September 2024.
www.nice.org.uk/guidance/ng111

Urinary tract infection (recurrent): antimicrobial prescribing. National Institute for Health and Care Excellence. NICE guideline NG112. October 2018, updated December 2024.
www.nice.org.uk/guidance/ng112

Urinary tract infection (catheter-associated): antimicrobial prescribing. National Institute for Health and Care Excellence. NICE guideline NG113. November 2018, updated September 2024.
www.nice.org.uk/guidance/ng113

Patient decision aids: Urinary tract infection (lower) National Institute for Health and Care Excellence. November 2018, updated April 2022.
www.nice.org.uk/about/what-we-do/our-programmes/nice-guidance/nice-guidelines/shared-decision-making

ANTIBACTERIALS

Methenamine hippurate　　　　　29-Oct-2024

(Hexamine hippurate)

- **DRUG ACTION** Methenamine hippurate is a urinary antiseptic which requires an acidic urine for its action. It has decreased effect on urea-degrading bacteria e.g. *Pseudomonas* and some strains of *Proteus*; these organisms usually affect patients with complicated urinary tract infections.

- **INDICATIONS AND DOSE**

Prophylaxis of uncomplicated lower urinary-tract infection
- ▶ BY MOUTH
- ▶ Adult: 1 g twice daily, seek specialist advice if considering use for prophylaxis during pregnancy, in male patients, or for recurrent upper UTI or recurrent complicated lower UTI (lack of evidence to inform when methenamine hippurate may be beneficial in these patients)

Prophylaxis of uncomplicated lower urinary-tract infections in patients with a catheter
- ▶ BY MOUTH
- ▶ Adult: 1 g 2–3 times a day

- **UNLICENSED USE** Methenamine hippurate is considered unlicensed for the situations detailed below:
  - prophylaxis of recurrent upper UTI;
  - prophylaxis of recurrent complicated lower UTI.

- **CONTRA-INDICATIONS** Gout · metabolic acidosis · renal parenchymal infection · severe dehydration
- **INTERACTIONS** → Appendix 1: methenamine
- **SIDE-EFFECTS**
▶ **Uncommon** Gastrointestinal discomfort · nausea · skin reactions · vomiting
▶ **Frequency not known** Diarrhoea
- **PREGNANCY** Specialist sources indicate not known to be harmful, however limited human data available.
- **BREAST FEEDING** [EvGr] Amount too small to be harmful ⓜ (recommendation also supported by tertiary sources).
- **HEPATIC IMPAIRMENT** [EvGr] Avoid ⓜ (risk of accumulation of ammonia metabolite).
- **RENAL IMPAIRMENT** Risk of hippurate crystalluria. [EvGr] Avoid if creatinine clearance less than 10 mL/minute, ⓜ see p. 21.
- **EFFECT ON LABORATORY TESTS** False results for urinary steroids, catecholamines and 5-hydroxyindole acetic acid can occur.
- **PATIENT AND CARER ADVICE** Patients and their carers should be advised to avoid using over-the-counter urinary-tract infection relief sachets containing potassium citrate or sodium citrate that make urine less acidic as this may reduce the effectiveness of methenamine. Patients and their carers should be advised to seek medical help if symptoms of acute urinary-tract infection occur.
- **MEDICINAL FORMS** There can be variation in the licensing of different medicines containing the same drug.
Oral tablet
▶ **Methenamine hippurate (Non-proprietary)**
Methenamine hippurate 1 gram Methenamine hippurate 1g tablets | 60 tablet [PoM] £19.74–£29.00 DT = £16.60
▶ **Hiprex** (Viatris UK Healthcare Ltd)
Methenamine hippurate 1 gram Hiprex 1g tablets | 60 tablet [PoM] £19.74 DT = £16.60

Nitrofurantoin

10-Aug-2023

- **INDICATIONS AND DOSE**
Lower urinary-tract infections
▶ BY MOUTH USING IMMEDIATE-RELEASE MEDICINES
▶ Child 3 months–11 years: 750 micrograms/kg 4 times a day (max. per dose 50 mg) for 3 days
▶ Child 12–15 years: 50 mg 4 times a day for 3 days (7 days in pregnant women)
▶ Child 16–17 years: 50 mg 4 times a day for 3 days (7 days in males and pregnant women)
▶ Adult: 50 mg 4 times a day for 3 days (7 days in males and pregnant women)
▶ BY MOUTH USING MODIFIED-RELEASE MEDICINES
▶ Child 12–15 years: 100 mg twice daily for 3 days (7 days in pregnant women)
▶ Child 16–17 years: 100 mg twice daily for 3 days (7 days in males and pregnant women)
▶ Adult: 100 mg twice daily for 3 days (7 days in males and pregnant women)
Urinary-tract infections (catheter-associated)
▶ BY MOUTH USING IMMEDIATE-RELEASE MEDICINES
▶ Child 16–17 years: 50 mg 4 times a day for 7 days, to be used if modified-release preparations are unavailable
▶ Adult: 50 mg 4 times a day for 7 days, to be used if modified-release preparations are unavailable
▶ BY MOUTH USING MODIFIED-RELEASE MEDICINES
▶ Child 16–17 years: 100 mg twice daily for 7 days
▶ Adult: 100 mg twice daily for 7 days
Severe chronic recurrent urinary-tract infections
▶ BY MOUTH USING IMMEDIATE-RELEASE MEDICINES
▶ Child 12–17 years: 100 mg 4 times a day for 3–7 days

▶ Adult: 100 mg 4 times a day for 7 days
Prophylaxis of recurrent urinary-tract infection
▶ BY MOUTH USING IMMEDIATE-RELEASE MEDICINES
▶ Child 3 months–11 years: 1 mg/kg once daily, dose to be taken at night
▶ Child 12–15 years: 50–100 mg once daily, dose to be taken at night
▶ Child 16–17 years: 50–100 mg once daily, dose to be taken at night, alternatively 100 mg for 1 dose, dose to be taken following exposure to a trigger
▶ Adult: 50–100 mg once daily, dose to be taken at night, alternatively 100 mg for 1 dose, dose to be taken following exposure to a trigger
Genito-urinary surgical prophylaxis
▶ BY MOUTH USING MODIFIED-RELEASE MEDICINES
▶ Child 12–17 years: 100 mg twice daily on day of procedure and for 3 days after
▶ Adult: 100 mg twice daily on day of procedure and for 3 days after

- **UNLICENSED USE** [EvGr] Duration of treatment for lower urinary-tract infection differs from product literature and adheres to national guidelines. ⓐ See Urinary-tract infections p. 681 for further information. [EvGr] Nitrofurantoin can be given as a single dose for the prophylaxis of recurrent urinary tract infection following exposure to a trigger, ⓐ but this dosing regimen is not licensed. See Urinary-tract infections p. 681 for further information.

> **IMPORTANT SAFETY INFORMATION**
> MHRA/CHM ADVICE: NITROFURANTOIN: REMINDER OF THE RISKS OF PULMONARY AND HEPATIC ADVERSE DRUG REACTIONS (APRIL 2023)
> Following a report of fatality in a patient who developed acute pulmonary damage and respiratory failure after a 10-day course of nitrofurantoin for the treatment of urinary-tract infection, the MHRA reminds healthcare professionals to:
> - increase vigilance for acute pulmonary reactions in the first week of treatment;
> - closely monitor patients on long-term therapy for new or worsening respiratory symptoms, especially if elderly;
> - discontinue treatment immediately if new or worsening symptoms of pulmonary damage occur;
> - use caution when prescribing to patients with pulmonary disease which may mask the signs and symptoms of adverse reactions.
> In addition, following discussion with NHS England about the risks of hepatic adverse reactions, the MHRA reminds healthcare professionals to:
> - be vigilant for signs and symptoms of hepatic dysfunction, especially with long-term therapy, and periodically monitor for signs and changes in biochemical tests that would indicate hepatitis or liver injury;
> - use caution when prescribing to patients with hepatic dysfunction which may mask the signs and symptoms of adverse reactions.
> Patients and their carers should be counselled to seek immediate medical advice if symptoms of pulmonary or hepatic adverse reactions develop.

- **CONTRA-INDICATIONS** Acute porphyrias p. 1202 · G6PD deficiency · infants less than 3 months old
- **CAUTIONS** Anaemia · diabetes mellitus · electrolyte imbalance · folate deficiency · pulmonary disease · susceptibility to peripheral neuropathy · urine may be coloured yellow or brown · vitamin B deficiency
- **INTERACTIONS** → Appendix 1: nitrofurantoin

- **SIDE-EFFECTS** Agranulocytosis·alopecia·anaemia· angioedema·aplastic anaemia·appetite decreased· arthralgia·asthenia·chest pain·chills·chronic pulmonary reaction (more common in elderly)·circulatory collapse·confusion·cough·cyanosis·depression· diarrhoea·dizziness·drowsiness·dyspnoea·eosinophilia ·euphoric mood·fever·granulocytopenia·haemolytic anaemia·headache·hepatic disorders·idiopathic intracranial hypertension·increased risk of infection· interstitial pneumonitis (more common in elderly)· leucopenia·lupus-like syndrome·nausea·nerve disorders ·nystagmus·pancreatitis·psychotic disorder·pulmonary fibrosis (more common in elderly)·pulmonary hypersensitivity·pulmonary reaction (possible association with lupus erythematosus-like syndrome)·respiratory disorders·skin reactions·Stevens-Johnson syndrome· thrombocytopenia·urine discolouration·vertigo· vomiting

  SIDE-EFFECTS, FURTHER INFORMATION Discontinue treatment if otherwise unexplained haematological or neurological syndromes (such as peripheral neuropathy) occur.

  Hepatic reactions Hepatic reactions, including fatal cases, have been reported. Discontinue treatment immediately if hepatitis occurs.

  Pulmonary reactions Acute pulmonary reactions usually occur within the first week of treatment and are reversible with cessation of therapy. Chronic pulmonary reactions can develop insidiously. Discontinue treatment immediately if pulmonary reactions occur.

- **PREGNANCY** Avoid at term—may produce neonatal haemolysis.

- **BREAST FEEDING** Avoid; only small amounts in milk but enough to produce haemolysis in G6PD-deficient infants.

- **HEPATIC IMPAIRMENT** Manufacturer advises caution.

- **RENAL IMPAIRMENT** Risk of peripheral neuropathy; antibacterial efficacy depends on renal secretion of the drug into urinary tract.

  ▸ In adults Avoid if eGFR less than 45 mL/minute/1.73 m^2; may be used with caution if eGFR 30–44 mL/minute/1.73 m^2 as a short-course only (3 to 7 days), to treat uncomplicated lower urinary-tract infection caused by suspected or proven multidrug resistant bacteria and only if potential benefit outweighs risk.

  ▸ In children Avoid if estimated glomerular filtration rate less than 45 mL/minute/1.73 m^2; may be used with caution if estimated glomerular filtration rate 30–44 mL/minute/1.73 m^2 as a short-course only (3 to 7 days), to treat uncomplicated lower urinary-tract infection caused by suspected or proven multidrug resistant bacteria and only if potential benefit outweighs risk.

- **MONITORING REQUIREMENTS** On long-term therapy, monitor liver function and monitor for pulmonary symptoms, especially in the elderly (discontinue if deterioration in lung function).

- **EFFECT ON LABORATORY TESTS** False positive urinary glucose (if tested for reducing substances).

- **PATIENT AND CARER ADVICE** Patients and their carers should be advised to seek immediate medical attention if signs or symptoms of pulmonary, hepatic, haematological, or neurological adverse reactions develop.
  Medicines for Children leaflet: Nitrofurantoin for urinary tract infections www.medicinesforchildren.org.uk/medicines/ nitrofurantoin-for-urinary-tract-infections/
  Driving and skilled tasks Patients and carers should be counselled on the effects on driving and performance of skilled tasks—increased risk of dizziness and drowsiness.

- **MEDICINAL FORMS** There can be variation in the licensing of different medicines containing the same drug. Forms available from special-order manufacturers include: oral suspension, oral solution

  Oral tablet
  CAUTIONARY AND ADVISORY LABELS 9, 14, 21
  ▸ **Nitrofurantoin (Non-proprietary)**
    Nitrofurantoin 50 mg Nitrofurantoin 50mg tablets | 28 tablet [PoM] £31.33 DT = £5.70 | 100 tablet [PoM] £20.36-£111.89
    Nitrofurantoin 100 mg Nitrofurantoin 100mg tablets | 28 tablet [PoM] £12.58 DT = £5.99 | 100 tablet [PoM] £21.39-£22.14

  Oral suspension
  CAUTIONARY AND ADVISORY LABELS 9, 14, 21
  ▸ **Nitrofurantoin (Non-proprietary)**
    Nitrofurantoin 5 mg per 1 ml Nitrofurantoin 25mg/5ml oral suspension sugar free | 300 ml [PoM] £525.17 DT = £394.56 [SF]

  Modified-release capsule
  CAUTIONARY AND ADVISORY LABELS 9, 14, 21, 25
  ▸ **Nitrofurantoin (Non-proprietary)**
    Nitrofurantoin 100 mg Nitrofurantoin 100mg modified-release capsules | 14 capsule [PoM] £9.50 DT = £9.50

  Oral capsule
  CAUTIONARY AND ADVISORY LABELS 9, 14, 21
  ▸ **Nitrofurantoin (Non-proprietary)**
    Nitrofurantoin 50 mg Nitrofurantoin 50mg capsules | 30 capsule [PoM] £15.42 DT = £1.93
    Nitrofurantoin 100 mg Nitrofurantoin 100mg capsules | 30 capsule [PoM] £13.56 DT = £4.22

3   Fungal infection

Antifungals, systemic use   31-Jan-2025

Fungal infections

The systemic treatment of common fungal infections is outlined below; specialist treatment is required in most forms of systemic or disseminated fungal infections. Local treatment is suitable for a number of fungal infections (genital, bladder, eye, ear, oropharynx, and skin).

Aspergillosis

Aspergillosis most commonly affects the respiratory tract but in severely immunocompromised patients, invasive forms can affect the heart, brain, and skin. Voriconazole p. 695 is the treatment of choice for aspergillosis; liposomal amphotericin B p. 689 is an alternative first-line treatment when voriconazole cannot be used. Caspofungin p. 687, or itraconazole p. 692, can be used in patients who are refractory to, or intolerant of voriconazole and liposomal amphotericin B. Itraconazole is also used for the treatment of chronic pulmonary aspergillosis or as an adjunct in the treatment of allergic bronchopulmonary aspergillosis [unlicensed indication]. Posaconazole p. 694 is licensed for use in patients with invasive aspergillosis who are refractory to, or intolerant of itraconazole or amphotericin B.

Candidiasis

Many superficial candidal infections including infections of the skin are treated locally; widespread or intractable infection requires systemic antifungal treatment. Vaginal candidiasis may be treated with locally acting antifungals or with fluconazole p. 690 given by mouth; for resistant organisms in adults, itraconazole can be given by mouth.

Oropharyngeal candidiasis generally responds to topical therapy but oral therapy may be required in some cases; see Oropharyngeal fungal infections p. 1384 for further information.

For *invasive or disseminated candidiasis*, an **echinocandin** can be used. Fluconazole is an alternative for *Candida albicans* infection in clinically stable patients who have not received an azole antifungal recently. Amphotericin B is an alternative when an echinocandin or fluconazole cannot be used, however, amphotericin B should be considered for the initial treatment of CNS candidiasis. Voriconazole can be used for infections caused by fluconazole-resistant *Candida* spp. when oral therapy is required, or in patients intolerant of amphotericin B or an echinocandin. In refractory cases, flucytosine p. 696 can be used with intravenous amphotericin B.

Cryptococcosis

Cryptococcosis is uncommon but infection in the immunocompromised, especially in HIV-positive patients, can be life-threatening; cryptococcal meningitis is the most common form of fungal meningitis. The treatment of choice in cryptococcal meningitis is amphotericin B by intravenous infusion and flucytosine by intravenous infusion for 2 weeks, followed by fluconazole by mouth for 8 weeks or until cultures are negative. In cryptococcosis, fluconazole is sometimes given alone as an alternative in HIV-positive patients with mild, localised infections or in those who cannot tolerate amphotericin B. Following successful treatment, fluconazole can be used for prophylaxis against relapse until immunity recovers.

Histoplasmosis

Histoplasmosis is rare in temperate climates; it can be life-threatening, particularly in HIV-infected persons. Itraconazole can be used for the treatment of immunocompetent patients with indolent non-meningeal infection, including chronic pulmonary histoplasmosis. Amphotericin B by intravenous infusion is used for the initial treatment of fulminant or severe infections, followed by a course of itraconazole by mouth. Following successful treatment, itraconazole can be used for prophylaxis against relapse until immunity recovers.

Skin and nail infections

Mild localised fungal infections of the skin (including tinea corporis, tinea cruris, and tinea pedis) respond to topical therapy. Systemic therapy is appropriate if topical therapy fails, if many areas are affected, or if the site of infection is difficult to treat such as in infections of the nails (onychomycosis) and of the scalp (tinea capitis). Oral imidazole or triazole antifungals (particularly itraconazole) and terbinafine p. 1401 are used more frequently than griseofulvin p. 697 because they have a broader spectrum of activity and require a shorter duration of treatment.

Tinea capitis is treated systemically; additional topical application of an antifungal may reduce transmission. Griseofulvin is used for tinea capitis in adults and children; it is effective against infections caused by *Trichophyton tonsurans* and *Microsporum spp*. Terbinafine is used for tinea capitis caused by *T. tonsurans* [unlicensed indication]. The role of terbinafine in the management of *Microsporum* infections is uncertain.

Pityriasis versicolor may be treated with itraconazole by mouth if topical therapy is ineffective; fluconazole by mouth is an alternative. Oral terbinafine is **not** effective for pityriasis versicolor.

Antifungal treatment may not be necessary in asymptomatic patients with tinea infection of the nails. If treatment is necessary, a systemic antifungal is more effective than topical therapy. Terbinafine and itraconazole have largely replaced griseofulvin for the systemic treatment of *onychomycosis*, particularly of the toenail; terbinafine is considered to be the drug of choice. Itraconazole can be administered as intermittent 'pulse' therapy. Topical antifungals also have a role in the treatment of onychomycosis.

Immunocompromised patients

Immunocompromised patients are at particular risk of fungal infections and may receive antifungal drugs prophylactically; oral triazole antifungals are the drugs of choice for prophylaxis. Fluconazole is more reliably absorbed than itraconazole, but fluconazole is not effective against *Aspergillus* spp. Itraconazole is preferred in patients at risk of invasive aspergillosis. Posaconazole can be used for prophylaxis in patients who are undergoing haematopoietic stem cell transplantation or receiving chemotherapy for acute myeloid leukaemia or myelodysplastic syndrome. Micafungin p. 688 can be used for prophylaxis of candidiasis in patients undergoing haematopoietic stem cell transplantation when fluconazole, itraconazole or posaconazole cannot be used.

Amphotericin B by intravenous infusion or caspofungin is used for the empirical *treatment* of serious fungal infections; caspofungin is not effective against fungal infections of the CNS.

Triazole antifungals

Triazole antifungal drugs have a role in the prevention and systemic treatment of fungal infections.

Fluconazole is very well absorbed after oral administration. It also achieves good penetration into the cerebrospinal fluid to treat fungal meningitis. Fluconazole is excreted largely unchanged in the urine and can be used to treat candiduria.

Itraconazole is active against a wide range of dermatophytes. Itraconazole capsules require an acid environment in the stomach for optimal absorption. Itraconazole has been associated with liver damage and should be avoided or used with caution in patients with liver disease; fluconazole is less frequently associated with hepatotoxicity.

Posaconazole is licensed for the treatment of invasive fungal infections unresponsive to conventional treatment.

Voriconazole is a broad-spectrum antifungal drug which is licensed for use in life-threatening infections.

Imidazole antifungals

The imidazole antifungals include clotrimazole p. 958, econazole nitrate p. 958, ketoconazole p. 959, and tioconazole p. 1401. They are used for the local treatment of vaginal candidiasis and for dermatophyte infections. Miconazole p. 1384 can be used locally for oral infections; it is also effective in intestinal infections. Systemic absorption may follow use of miconazole oral gel and may result in significant drug interactions.

Polyene antifungals

The polyene antifungals include amphotericin B and nystatin p. 1385; neither drug is absorbed when given by mouth. Nystatin p. 1385 is used for oral, oropharyngeal, and perioral infections by local application in the mouth. Nystatin is also used for *Candida albicans* infection of the skin.

Amphotericin B p. 689 by intravenous infusion is used for the treatment of systemic fungal infections and is active against most fungi and yeasts. It is highly protein bound and penetrates poorly into body fluids and tissues. When given parenterally amphotericin B is toxic and side-effects are common. Lipid formulations of amphotericin B are significantly less toxic and are recommended when the conventional formulation of amphotericin B is contra-indicated because of toxicity, especially nephrotoxicity or when response to conventional amphotericin B is inadequate; lipid formulations are more expensive.

Echinocandin antifungals

The echinocandin antifungals include anidulafungin p. 687, caspofungin p. 687 and micafungin p. 688. They are only active against *Aspergillus* spp. and *Candida* spp.; however, anidulafungin and micafungin are not used for the treatment of aspergillosis. Echinocandins are not effective against fungal infections of the CNS.

Other antifungals

Flucytosine p. 696 is used with amphotericin B in a synergistic combination. Bone marrow depression can occur which limits its use, particularly in HIV-positive patients; weekly blood counts are necessary during prolonged therapy. Resistance to flucytosine can develop during therapy and sensitivity testing is essential before and during treatment. Flucytosine has a role in the treatment of systemic candidiasis and cryptococcal meningitis.

Griseofulvin p. 697 is effective for widespread or intractable dermatophyte infections but has been superseded by newer antifungals, particularly for nail infections. It is the drug of choice for trichophyton infections in children. Duration of therapy is dependent on the site of the infection and may extend to a number of months.

Terbinafine p. 1401 is the drug of choice for fungal nail infections and is also used for ringworm infections where oral treatment is considered appropriate.

ANTIFUNGALS > ECHINOCANDIN ANTIFUNGALS

Anidulafungin
24-Nov-2020

● **INDICATIONS AND DOSE**

Invasive candidiasis
▶ BY INTRAVENOUS INFUSION
▶ Adult: Initially 200 mg once daily for 1 day, then 100 mg once daily

● **INTERACTIONS** → Appendix 1: anidulafungin

● **SIDE-EFFECTS**
▶ **Common or very common** Bronchospasm · cholestasis · diarrhoea · dyspnoea · headache · hyperglycaemia · hypertension · hypokalaemia · hypotension · nausea · seizure · skin reactions · vomiting
▶ **Uncommon** Abdominal pain upper · coagulation disorder · vasodilation

● **PREGNANCY** Manufacturer advises avoid unless potential benefit outweighs risk—toxicity in *animal* studies.

● **BREAST FEEDING** Manufacturer advises avoid unless potential benefit outweighs risk—present in milk in *animal* studies.

● **DIRECTIONS FOR ADMINISTRATION** For *intravenous infusion* (*Ecalta*®), give intermittently *in* Glucose 5% *or* Sodium Chloride 0.9%. Reconstitute each 100 mg with 30 mL Water for Injections and allow up to 5 minutes for reconstitution; dilute dose in infusion fluid to a concentration of 770 micrograms/mL; give at a rate not exceeding 1.1 mg/minute.

● **MEDICINAL FORMS** There can be variation in the licensing of different medicines containing the same drug.
Powder for solution for infusion
▶ Anidulafungin (Non-proprietary)
Anidulafungin 100 mg Anidulafungin 100mg powder for concentrate for solution for infusion vials | 1 vial [PoM] £299.98-£299.99 (Hospital only)
▶ Ecalta (Pfizer Ltd)
Anidulafungin 100 mg Ecalta 100mg powder for concentrate for solution for infusion vials | 1 vial [PoM] £299.99 (Hospital only)

Caspofungin
07-Aug-2020

● **INDICATIONS AND DOSE**

Invasive aspergillosis | Invasive candidiasis | Empirical treatment of systemic fungal infections in patients with neutropenia
▶ BY INTRAVENOUS INFUSION
▶ Adult (body-weight up to 81 kg): Loading dose 70 mg once daily for 1 day, then maintenance 50 mg once daily
▶ Adult (body-weight 81 kg and above): 70 mg once daily

DOSE ADJUSTMENTS DUE TO INTERACTIONS
▶ Manufacturer advises increase dose to 70 mg daily with concurrent use of some enzyme inducers (such as carbamazepine, dexamethasone, phenytoin, and rifampicin); no dose adjustment required for patients already on 70 mg daily.

● **INTERACTIONS** → Appendix 1: caspofungin

● **SIDE-EFFECTS**
▶ **Common or very common** Arthralgia · diarrhoea · dyspnoea · electrolyte imbalance · fever · headache · hyperhidrosis · nausea · skin reactions · vomiting
▶ **Uncommon** Anaemia · anxiety · appetite decreased · arrhythmias · ascites · chest discomfort · coagulation disorder · congestive heart failure · constipation · cough · disorientation · dizziness · drowsiness · dry mouth · dysphagia · excessive tearing · eyelid oedema · fatigue · flatulence · fluid overload · flushing · gastrointestinal discomfort · haematuria · hepatic disorders · hyperbilirubinaemia · hyperglycaemia · hypertension · hypotension · hypoxia · induration · insomnia · laryngeal pain · leucopenia · malaise · metabolic acidosis · muscle weakness · myalgia · nasal congestion · oedema · pain · palpitations · renal impairment · respiratory disorders · sensation abnormal · taste altered · thrombocytopenia · thrombophlebitis · tremor · vision blurred
▶ **Frequency not known** Severe cutaneous adverse reactions (SCARs)

● **PREGNANCY** Manufacturer advises avoid unless essential—toxicity in *animal* studies.

● **BREAST FEEDING** Present in milk in *animal* studies—manufacturer advises avoid.

● **HEPATIC IMPAIRMENT** No information available for severe impairment.
Dose adjustments 70 mg on first day then 35 mg once daily in moderate impairment.

● **DIRECTIONS FOR ADMINISTRATION** For *intravenous infusion* (*Cancidas*®), manufacturer advises give intermittently *in* Sodium Chloride 0.9%. Allow vial to reach room temperature; initially reconstitute each vial with 10.5 mL Water for Injections, mixing gently to dissolve then dilute requisite dose in 250 mL infusion fluid (35- or 50-mg doses may be diluted in 100 ml infusion fluid if necessary); give over 60 minutes; incompatible with glucose solutions.

● **MEDICINAL FORMS** There can be variation in the licensing of different medicines containing the same drug.
Powder for solution for infusion
▶ Caspofungin (Non-proprietary)
Caspofungin (as Caspofungin acetate) 50 mg Caspofungin 50mg powder for concentrate for solution for infusion vials | 1 vial [PoM] £238.87 DT = £238.87 | 1 vial [PoM] £327.67 DT = £238.87 (Hospital only)
Caspofungin (as Caspofungin acetate) 70 mg Caspofungin 70mg powder for concentrate for solution for infusion vials | 1 vial [PoM] £337.59-£416.78 (Hospital only)

Micafungin

28-Apr-2021

- **INDICATIONS AND DOSE**

Invasive candidiasis
- ▶ BY INTRAVENOUS INFUSION
- ▶ Adult (body-weight up to 40 kg): 2 mg/kg once daily for at least 14 days; increased if necessary to 4 mg/kg once daily, increase dose if response inadequate
- ▶ Adult (body-weight 40 kg and above): 100 mg once daily for at least 14 days; increased if necessary to 200 mg once daily, increase dose if response inadequate

Oesophageal candidiasis
- ▶ BY INTRAVENOUS INFUSION
- ▶ Adult (body-weight up to 40 kg): 3 mg/kg once daily
- ▶ Adult (body-weight 40 kg and above): 150 mg once daily

Prophylaxis of candidiasis in patients undergoing bone-marrow transplantation or who are expected to become neutropenic for over 10 days
- ▶ BY INTRAVENOUS INFUSION
- ▶ Adult (body-weight up to 40 kg): 1 mg/kg once daily continue for at least 7 days after neutrophil count is in desirable range
- ▶ Adult (body-weight 40 kg and above): 50 mg once daily continue for at least 7 days after neutrophil count is in desirable range

- **INTERACTIONS** → Appendix 1: micafungin

- **SIDE-EFFECTS** Anaemia · anxiety · appetite decreased · arrhythmias · confusion · constipation · diarrhoea · disseminated intravascular coagulation · dizziness · drowsiness · dyspnoea · electrolyte imbalance · eosinophilia · flushing · gastrointestinal discomfort · haemolysis · haemolytic anaemia · headache · hepatic disorders · hepatic failure (potentially life-threatening) · hyperbilirubinaemia · hyperhidrosis · hypersensitivity · hypertension · hypoalbuminaemia · hypotension · insomnia · leucopenia · nausea · neutropenia · palpitations · pancytopenia · peripheral oedema · renal impairment · severe cutaneous adverse reactions (SCARs) · shock · skin reactions · taste altered · thrombocytopenia · tremor · vomiting

- **PREGNANCY** Manufacturer advises avoid unless essential—toxicity in *animal* studies.

- **BREAST FEEDING** Manufacturer advises use only if potential benefit outweighs risk—present in milk in *animal* studies.

- **HEPATIC IMPAIRMENT** Manufacturer advises caution in chronic impairment; avoid in severe impairment (limited information available).

- **RENAL IMPAIRMENT** [EvGr] Use with caution; renal function may deteriorate. ⟨M⟩

- **MONITORING REQUIREMENTS**
- ▶ Monitor renal function.
- ▶ Monitor liver function—discontinue if significant and persistent abnormalities in liver function tests develop.

- **DIRECTIONS FOR ADMINISTRATION** For *intravenous infusion* (*Mycamine* ®), manufacturer advises give intermittently in Glucose 5% or Sodium Chloride 0.9%. Reconstitute each vial with 5 mL infusion fluid; gently rotate vial, without shaking, to dissolve; dilute requisite dose with infusion fluid to 100 mL (final concentration of 0.5–2 mg/mL); protect infusion from light; give over 60 minutes.

- **MEDICINAL FORMS** There can be variation in the licensing of different medicines containing the same drug.

Powder for solution for infusion
- ▶ Micafungin (Non-proprietary)
  Micafungin (as Micafungin sodium) 50 mg Micafungin 50mg powder for concentrate for solution for infusion vials | 1 vial [PoM] £196.08 (Hospital only)

Micafungin (as Micafungin sodium) 100 mg Micafungin 100mg powder for concentrate for solution for infusion vials | 1 vial [PoM] £341.00 (Hospital only)
- ▶ Mycamine (Sandoz Ltd)
  Micafungin (as Micafungin sodium) 50 mg Mycamine 50mg powder for solution for infusion vials | 1 vial [PoM] £196.08
  Micafungin (as Micafungin sodium) 100 mg Mycamine 100mg powder for solution for infusion vials | 1 vial [PoM] £341.00

Rezafungin

21-Oct-2024

- **DRUG ACTION** Rezafungin is an echinocandin antifungal which selectively inhibits $1,3-\beta$-D glucan synthase, a key enzyme in fungal cell wall formation.

- **INDICATIONS AND DOSE**

Invasive candidiasis
- ▶ BY INTRAVENOUS INFUSION
- ▶ Adult: Loading dose 400 mg for 1 dose, then maintenance 200 mg every week, maintenance dose to be started 1 week after initial loading dose

- **SIDE-EFFECTS**
- ▶ **Common or very common** Abdominal pain · anaemia · constipation · diarrhoea · electrolyte imbalance · fever · hypotension · infusion related reaction · nausea · skin reactions · vomiting · wheezing
- ▶ **Uncommon** Phototoxicity · tremor

- **PREGNANCY** [EvGr] Avoid unless potential benefit outweighs risk (limited information available). ⟨M⟩

- **BREAST FEEDING** Specialist sources indicate probably compatible (no information available). High plasma-protein binding suggests limited excretion into milk and poor oral bioavailability suggests limited absorption by the infant.

- **DIRECTIONS FOR ADMINISTRATION** For *intravenous infusion* (*Rezzayo* ®), give in Sodium Chloride 0.45% or 0.9%, or Glucose 5%. Reconstitute each vial with 9.5 mL Water for Injections, mixing gently to dissolve, then dilute requisite dose in infusion fluid to 250 mL and give over approximately 60 minutes. Infusion time may be increased up to 180 minutes to manage any infusion-related reactions.
  Missed doses If a dose is administered more than 3 days late, the next dose should be administered after at least 4 days.
  If a dose is more than 2 weeks late, treatment should be restarted with the loading dose.

- **PATIENT AND CARER ADVICE**
  Photosensitivity Patients should be advised to avoid unprotected exposure to sunlight and other UV radiation during treatment and for 7 days after last treatment.

- **NATIONAL FUNDING/ACCESS DECISIONS**
  For full details see funding body website
  Scottish Medicines Consortium (SMC) decisions
- ▶ Rezafungin acetate (*Rezzayo* ®) for the treatment of invasive candidiasis in adults (October 2024) SMC No. SMC2659 Recommended with restrictions

- **MEDICINAL FORMS** There can be variation in the licensing of different medicines containing the same drug.
  Powder for solution for infusion
  EXCIPIENTS: May contain Polysorbates
- ▶ Rezafungin (non-proprietary) ▼
  Rezafungin (as Rezafungin acetate) 200 mg Rezzayo 200mg powder for concentrate for solution for infusion vials | 1 vial [PoM] £1,999.95 (Hospital only)

ANTIFUNGALS > POLYENE ANTIFUNGALS

Amphotericin B
(Amphotericin)
07-Feb-2025

- **INDICATIONS AND DOSE**

FUNGIZONE ®

Systemic fungal infections
- ▸ BY INTRAVENOUS INFUSION
- ▸ Adult: Test dose 1 mg, to be given over 20–30 minutes, then 250 micrograms/kg daily, gradually increased over 2–4 days, increased if tolerated to 1 mg/kg daily, max. (severe infection) 1.5 mg/kg daily or on alternate days. Prolonged treatment usually necessary; if interrupted for longer than 7 days recommence at 250 micrograms/kg daily and increase gradually

DOSE EQUIVALENCE AND CONVERSION
- ▸ *Fungizone®* is a conventional formulation; it is not interchangeable with other formulations of amphotericin B.

LIPOSOMAL AMPHOTERICIN B

Severe systemic or deep mycoses (including disseminated candidiasis and aspergillosis)
- ▸ BY INTRAVENOUS INFUSION
- ▸ Adult: 3–5 mg/kg once daily for a minimum of 14 days

Mucormycosis
- ▸ BY INTRAVENOUS INFUSION
- ▸ Adult: 5–10 mg/kg once daily, slow escalation of doses should be avoided

Suspected or confirmed fungal infection in febrile neutropenic patients unresponsive to broad-spectrum antibacterials and where investigations have failed to define a bacterial or viral cause
- ▸ BY INTRAVENOUS INFUSION
- ▸ Adult: 3–5 mg/kg once daily continue treatment until patient is afebrile for 3 consecutive days; treatment should not exceed 42 days

Visceral leishmaniasis (unresponsive to the antimonial alone) (under expert supervision)
- ▸ BY INTRAVENOUS INFUSION
- ▸ Adult: 1–3 mg/kg once daily for 10–21 days to a cumulative dose of 21–30 mg/kg, alternatively initially 3 mg/kg once daily for 5 consecutive days, followed by 3 mg/kg for 1 dose, to be given 6 days later

HIV-associated cryptococcal meningitis (adjunct to flucytosine and fluconazole)
- ▸ BY INTRAVENOUS INFUSION
- ▸ Adult: 10 mg/kg for 1 dose, to be administered on day 1 in combination with flucytosine and fluconazole— consult product literature

DOSE EQUIVALENCE AND CONVERSION
- ▸ Liposomal amphotericin B is **not** interchangeable with conventional formulations of amphotericin B, e.g. *Fungizone®*.

IMPORTANT SAFETY INFORMATION

MHRA/CHM ADVICE: LIPOSOMAL AND LIPID-COMPLEX FORMULATIONS: NAME CHANGE TO REDUCE MEDICATION ERRORS (JULY 2020)

Serious harm and fatal overdoses have occurred following confusion between liposomal, pegylated-liposomal, lipid-complex, and conventional formulations of the same drug substance. Medicines with these formulations will explicitly include 'liposomal', 'pegylated-liposomal', or 'lipid-complex' within their name to reduce the risk of potentially fatal medication errors.

The MHRA reminds healthcare professionals that liposomal, pegylated-liposomal, lipid-complex, and conventional formulations containing the same drug substance are **not** interchangeable. Healthcare professionals are advised to make a clear distinction between formulations when prescribing, dispensing, administering, and communicating about amphotericin B. The product name and dose should be verified before administration and the maximum dose should not be exceeded.

- **CAUTIONS** Infusion-related reactions

CAUTIONS, FURTHER INFORMATION
- ▸ Infusion-related reactions [EvGr] Infusion-related reactions can be managed by stopping the infusion and restarting at a slower rate (over at least 2 hours), or by administering antipyretics, antihistamines or hydrocortisone as premedication. ⟨M⟩

FUNGIZONE ® Avoid rapid infusion (risk of arrhythmia)

- **INTERACTIONS** → Appendix 1: amphotericin B

- **SIDE-EFFECTS**
- ▸ **Common or very common** Anaemia · appetite decreased · azotaemia · chills · diarrhoea · dyspnoea · electrolyte imbalance · fever · headache · hepatic function abnormal (discontinue) · hyposthenuria · hypotension · nausea · nephrocalcinosis · renal impairment · renal tubular acidosis · skin reactions · vomiting
- ▸ **Uncommon** Agranulocytosis · arrhythmias · bronchospasm · flushing · gastrointestinal discomfort · hepatic disorders · leucopenia · myalgia · peripheral neuropathy · thrombocytopenia
- ▸ **Rare or very rare** Alveolitis allergic · arthralgia · cardiac arrest · coagulation disorder · deafness · encephalopathy · eosinophilia · haemorrhage · heart failure · hypersensitivity · hypertension · malaise · nephrogenic diabetes insipidus · pain · pulmonary oedema non-cardiogenic · seizure · severe cutaneous adverse reactions (SCARs) · shock · tinnitus · vertigo · vision disorders · weight decreased

- **PREGNANCY** Specialist sources indicate can be used if potential benefit outweighs risk (crosses human placenta).

- **BREAST FEEDING** Specialist sources indicate no information available but probably compatible due to high molecular weight, high protein binding, and poor oral absorption.

- **RENAL IMPAIRMENT** [EvGr] Liposomal amphotericin B may be less nephrotoxic than conventional, non-liposomal amphotericin B (*Fungizone®*). ⟨M⟩

- **MONITORING REQUIREMENTS** [EvGr] Monitor hepatic function, renal function, serum electrolytes (especially magnesium and potassium concentration) and full blood count at least once weekly—consider dose reduction, treatment interruption, or discontinuation if there is clinically significant worsening of renal function or other clinical parameters. ⟨M⟩

- **EFFECT ON LABORATORY TESTS** Liposomal amphotericin B may cause false elevations of serum phosphate—consult product literature.

- **DIRECTIONS FOR ADMINISTRATION** The product name and dose should be verified before administration to ensure that the correct amphotericin B preparation is administered.

FUNGIZONE ® **Amphotericin B (as sodium deoxycholate complex)** [EvGr] Incompatible with Sodium Chloride solutions.

For *intravenous infusion*, reconstitute each vial with 10 mL Water for Injections, and shake immediately to produce a 5 mg/mL clear colloidal solution. Dilute further in Glucose 5% to a concentration of 100 micrograms/mL; the pH of Glucose 5% should not be below 4.2 (check each container—consult product literature if pH less than 4.2). Infuse the test dose over 20–30 minutes, and subsequent

5
Infection

doses over 2–6 hours; an in-line filter (pore size no less than 1 micron) may be used.

When starting treatment, patient should be carefully observed throughout administration of test dose and for a minimum of 30 minutes after. ◈

LIPOSOMAL AMPHOTERICIN B EvGr Incompatible with Sodium Chloride solutions.

For *intravenous infusion*, reconstitute each vial with 12 mL Water for Injections and shake vigorously for 30 seconds to produce a 4 mg/mL dispersion. Using the 5 micron filter provided, dilute requisite dose in Glucose 5%, 10% or 20% to a final concentration of 0.2–2 mg/mL. Infuse over 30–60 minutes; for doses greater than 5 mg/kg, or to prevent infusion-related reactions—infuse over 2 hours. An in-line filter (pore size no less than 1 micron) may be used. ◈

● HANDLING AND STORAGE

FUNGIZONE ® Store in a refrigerator (2–8°C) and protect from light. For storage conditions after reconstitution and dilution—consult product literature.

LIPOSOMAL AMPHOTERICIN B Store at room temperature (below 25°C). For storage conditions after reconstitution and dilution—consult product literature.

● MEDICINAL FORMS There can be variation in the licensing of different medicines containing the same drug.

Powder for dispersion for infusion

▸ Amphotericin b (Non-proprietary)

Amphotericin B liposomal 50 mg Amphotericin B liposomal 50mg powder for dispersion for infusion vials | 1 vial PoM £81.00 (Hospital only) | 10 vial PoM £800.00-£821.87 (Hospital only)

Powder for solution for infusion

▸ Fungizone (Neon Healthcare Ltd)

Amphotericin B 50 mg Fungizone 50mg powder for concentrate for solution for infusion vials | 1 vial PoM £16.21 DT = £16.21

ANTIFUNGALS ＞ TRIAZOLE ANTIFUNGALS

Fluconazole
15-Nov-2024

● INDICATIONS AND DOSE

Candidal balanitis

▶ BY MOUTH

▸ Adult: 150 mg for 1 dose

Vaginal candidiasis

▶ BY MOUTH

▸ Adult: 150 mg for 1 dose

Vulvovaginal candidiasis (recurrent)

▶ BY MOUTH

▸ Adult: Initially 150 mg every 72 hours for 3 doses, then 150 mg once weekly for 6 months

Oropharyngeal candidiasis | Oesophageal candidiasis

▶ BY MOUTH, OR BY INTRAVENOUS INFUSION

▸ Child 1 month-11 years: Initially 6 mg/kg for 1 dose (max. per dose 400 mg), to be given on first day, then 3 mg/kg once daily (max. per dose 200 mg), treatment continued according to response

Oropharyngeal candidiasis

▶ BY MOUTH, OR BY INTRAVENOUS INFUSION

▸ Child 12-17 years: Initially 6 mg/kg for 1 dose (max. per dose 400 mg), to be given on first day, then 3 mg/kg once daily (max. per dose 200 mg), treatment continued according to response, alternatively initially 200–400 mg for 1 dose, to be given on first day, then 100–200 mg once daily for 7–21 days (duration may be increased in severely immunocompromised patients)

▸ Adult: Initially 200–400 mg for 1 dose, to be given on first day, then 100–200 mg once daily for 7–21 days (duration may be increased in severely immunocompromised patients)

Oesophageal candidiasis

▶ BY MOUTH, OR BY INTRAVENOUS INFUSION

▸ Child 12-17 years: Initially 6 mg/kg for 1 dose (max. per dose 400 mg), to be given on first day, then 3 mg/kg once daily (max. per dose 200 mg), treatment continued according to response, alternatively initially 200–400 mg for 1 dose, to be given on first day, then 100–200 mg once daily for 14–30 days (duration may be increased in severely immunocompromised patients)

▸ Adult: Initially 200–400 mg for 1 dose, to be given on first day, then 100–200 mg once daily for 14–30 days (duration may be increased in severely immunocompromised patients)

Candiduria

▶ BY MOUTH, OR BY INTRAVENOUS INFUSION

▸ Adult: 200–400 mg once daily for 7–21 days (duration may be increased in severely immunocompromised patients)

Chronic atrophic candidiasis

▶ BY MOUTH, OR BY INTRAVENOUS INFUSION

▸ Adult: 50 mg once daily for 14 days

Chronic mucocutaneous candidiasis

▶ BY MOUTH, OR BY INTRAVENOUS INFUSION

▸ Adult: 50–100 mg once daily for up to 28 days (duration may be increased in severe infection or severely immunocompromised patients)

Pityriasis versicolor [Tinea versicolor]

▶ BY MOUTH

▸ Adult: 300–400 mg once weekly for 1–3 weeks, alternatively 50 mg once daily for 2–4 weeks

Tinea pedis

▶ BY MOUTH

▸ Adult: 150 mg once weekly for up to 6 weeks, alternatively 50 mg once daily for up to 6 weeks

Tinea corporis | Tinea cruris | Dermal candidiasis

▶ BY MOUTH

▸ Adult: 150 mg once weekly for 2–4 weeks, alternatively 50 mg once daily for 2–4 weeks

Fungal nail infection

▶ BY MOUTH

▸ Adult: 150 mg once weekly continued until infected nail is replaced (uninfected nail grows in)

Invasive candidal infections (including candidaemia and disseminated candidiasis)

▶ BY MOUTH, OR BY INTRAVENOUS INFUSION

▸ Child 1 month-11 years: 6–12 mg/kg once daily (max. per dose 400 mg), dose dependent on the severity of the infection, treatment continued according to response

▸ Child 12-17 years: 6–12 mg/kg once daily (max. per dose 400 mg), dose dependent on the severity of the infection, treatment continued according to response, alternatively initially 800 mg for 1 dose, to be given on first day, then 400 mg once daily, in candidaemia continue treatment for 2 weeks after first negative blood culture and resolution of signs and symptoms

▸ Adult: Initially 800 mg for 1 dose, to be given on first day, then 400 mg once daily, in candidaemia continue treatment for 2 weeks after first negative blood culture and resolution of signs and symptoms

Cryptococcal meningitis

▶ BY MOUTH, OR BY INTRAVENOUS INFUSION

▸ Child 1 month-11 years: 6–12 mg/kg once daily (max. per dose 400 mg), dose dependent on the severity of the infection, treatment continued according to response

▸ Child 12-17 years: 6–12 mg/kg once daily (max. per dose 400 mg), dose dependent on the severity of the infection, treatment continued according to response, alternatively initially 400 mg for 1 dose, to be given on first day, then 200–400 mg once daily, dose can be

increased to 800 mg once daily in life-threatening infections, treatment continued according to response, usually for at least 6–8 weeks
▸ Adult: Initially 400 mg for 1 dose, to be given on first day, then 200–400 mg once daily, dose can be increased to 800 mg once daily in life-threatening infections, treatment continued according to response, usually for at least 6–8 weeks

Coccidioidomycosis
▸ BY MOUTH, OR BY INTRAVENOUS INFUSION
▸ Adult: 200–400 mg once daily for 11–24 months or longer according to response, dose can be increased if necessary to 800 mg once daily for some infections and especially for meningeal disease

Prevention of candidal infections in patients with prolonged neutropenia
▸ BY MOUTH, OR BY INTRAVENOUS INFUSION
▸ Adult: 200–400 mg once daily, start treatment before anticipated onset of neutropenia and continue for 7 days after neutrophil count in desirable range, dose adjusted according to risk

Prevention of candidal infections in immunocompromised patients
▸ BY MOUTH, OR BY INTRAVENOUS INFUSION
▸ Child: 3–12 mg/kg once daily (max. per dose 400 mg), start treatment before anticipated onset of neutropenia and continue for 7 days after neutrophil count in desirable range, dose according to extent and duration of neutropenia

Prevention of relapse of oropharyngeal or oesophageal candidiasis in HIV-infected patients at high risk of recurrence
▸ BY MOUTH, OR BY INTRAVENOUS INFUSION
▸ Adult: 100–200 mg once daily, alternatively 200 mg 3 times a week

Prevention of relapse of cryptococcal meningitis in patients at high risk of recurrence
▸ BY MOUTH, OR BY INTRAVENOUS INFUSION
▸ Adult: 200 mg once daily

● **CONTRA-INDICATIONS** Acute porphyrias p. 1202
● **CAUTIONS** Susceptibility to QT interval prolongation
● **INTERACTIONS** → Appendix 1: antifungals, azoles
● **SIDE-EFFECTS**
  GENERAL SIDE-EFFECTS
▸ **Common or very common** Diarrhoea · gastrointestinal discomfort · headache · nausea · skin reactions · vomiting
▸ **Uncommon** Dizziness · flatulence · hepatic disorders · seizure · taste altered
▸ **Rare or very rare** Agranulocytosis · alopecia · dyslipidaemia · hypokalaemia · leucopenia · neutropenia · QT interval prolongation · severe cutaneous adverse reactions (SCARs) · thrombocytopenia · torsade de pointes
  SPECIFIC SIDE-EFFECTS
▸ **Uncommon**
▸ **With parenteral use** Anaemia · appetite decreased · asthenia · constipation · drowsiness · dry mouth · fever · hyperhidrosis · insomnia · malaise · myalgia · paraesthesia · vertigo
▸ **Rare or very rare**
▸ **With parenteral use** Angioedema · face oedema · tremor
▸ **Frequency not known**
▸ **With oral use** Cardio-respiratory distress · oedema
  SIDE-EFFECTS, FURTHER INFORMATION If rash occurs, discontinue treatment (or monitor closely if infection invasive or systemic); severe cutaneous reactions are more likely in patients with AIDS.
● **CONCEPTION AND CONTRACEPTION** [EvGr] After single dose treatment in females of childbearing potential, a washout period of 1 week is recommended before becoming

pregnant. For longer courses of treatment in females of childbearing potential, effective contraception should be considered during and for 1 week after treatment. ⟨M⟩
● **PREGNANCY** [EvGr] Avoid unless potential benefit outweighs risk (multiple congenital abnormalities reported with long-term high doses). ⟨M⟩
● **BREAST FEEDING** Present in milk but amount probably too small to be harmful.
● **HEPATIC IMPAIRMENT** Manufacturer advises caution—limited information available.
● **RENAL IMPAIRMENT** [EvGr] Use with caution. ⟨M⟩
  Dose adjustments [EvGr] Usual initial dose then halve subsequent doses if creatinine clearance less than 50 mL/minute (consult product literature). ⟨M⟩ See p. 21.
● **MONITORING REQUIREMENTS** Monitor liver function with high doses or extended courses—discontinue if signs or symptoms of hepatic disease (risk of hepatic necrosis).
● **DIRECTIONS FOR ADMINISTRATION**
▸ In children For *intravenous infusion*, give over 10–30 minutes; do not exceed an infusion rate of 5–10 mL/minute.
● **PRESCRIBING AND DISPENSING INFORMATION** Flavours of oral liquid formulations may include orange.
● **PATIENT AND CARER ADVICE**
  Medicines for Children leaflet: Fluconazole for yeast and fungal infections www.medicinesforchildren.org.uk/medicines/fluconazole-for-yeast-and-fungal-infections/
● **PROFESSION SPECIFIC INFORMATION**
  Dental practitioners' formulary Fluconazole Capsules 50 mg may be prescribed.
  Fluconazole Oral Suspension 50 mg/5 mL may be prescribed.
● **EXCEPTIONS TO LEGAL CATEGORY** Fluconazole capsules can be sold to the public for vaginal candidiasis and associated candidal balanitis in those aged 16–60 years, in a container or packaging containing not more than 150 mg and labelled to show a max. dose of 150 mg.

● **MEDICINAL FORMS** There can be variation in the licensing of different medicines containing the same drug.
  Solution for infusion
  ELECTROLYTES: May contain Sodium
▸ **Fluconazole (Non-proprietary)**
  Fluconazole 2 mg per 1 ml Fluconazole 50mg/25ml solution for infusion vials | 1 vial [PoM] £20.00
  Fluconazole 100mg/50ml solution for infusion vials | 5 vial [PoM] £12.60 (Hospital only)
  Fluconazole 200mg/100ml solution for infusion bottles | 10 bottle [PoM] £427.20 (Hospital only) | 10 bottle [PoM] £510.90 | 20 bottle [PoM] £750.00 (Hospital only)
  Oral suspension
  CAUTIONARY AND ADVISORY LABELS 9
▸ **Fluconazole (Non-proprietary)**
  Fluconazole 10 mg per 1 ml Fluconazole 50mg/5ml oral suspension | 35 ml [PoM] £29.90 DT = £29.03
▸ **Diflucan** (Pfizer Ltd)
  Fluconazole 10 mg per 1 ml Diflucan 50mg/5ml oral suspension | 35 ml [PoM] £16.61 DT = £29.03
  Fluconazole 40 mg per 1 ml Diflucan 200mg/5ml oral suspension | 35 ml [PoM] £66.42 DT = £66.42
  Oral capsule
  CAUTIONARY AND ADVISORY LABELS 9 (50 mg and 200 mg strengths only)
▸ **Fluconazole (Non-proprietary)**
  Fluconazole 50 mg Fluconazole 50mg capsules | 7 capsule [PoM] £1.43 DT = £0.86
  Fluconazole 150 mg Fluconazole 150mg capsules | 1 capsule [PoM] £8.50 DT = £0.69
  Fluconazole 200 mg Fluconazole 200mg capsules | 7 capsule [PoM] £6.02 DT = £3.95
▸ **Diflucan** (Pfizer Ltd)
  Fluconazole 50 mg Diflucan 50mg capsules | 7 capsule [PoM] £16.61 DT = £0.86

Fluconazole 150 mg Diflucan 150mg capsules | 1 capsule [PoM]
£7.12 DT = £0.69
Fluconazole 200 mg Diflucan 200mg capsules | 7 capsule [PoM]
£66.42 DT = £3.95

Isavuconazole

24-May-2022

- **DRUG ACTION** Isavuconazole (an active metabolite of isavuconazonium sulfate) is a triazole antifungal that blocks the synthesis of ergosterol, a key component of the fungal cell membrane.

- **INDICATIONS AND DOSE**

Invasive aspergillosis | Mucormycosis in patients for whom amphotericin B is inappropriate
- ▸ BY MOUTH, OR BY INTRAVENOUS INFUSION
- ▸ Adult: Loading dose 200 mg every 8 hours for 48 hours (6 administrations in total), then maintenance 200 mg once daily, maintenance dose to be started at least 12 hours after the last loading dose; long-term treatment should be reviewed after 6-months

DOSE EQUIVALENCE AND CONVERSION
- ▸ Doses expressed as isavuconazole, though preparations contain the prodrug isavuconazonium sulfate. There is a significant difference between equivalent doses; 100 mg of isavuconazole is equivalent to 186.3 mg of isavuconazonium sulfate.

- **CONTRA-INDICATIONS** Acute porphyrias p. 1202 · short QT syndrome
- **CAUTIONS** Elderly—limited information
- **INTERACTIONS** → Appendix 1: antifungals, azoles
- **SIDE-EFFECTS**
  GENERAL SIDE-EFFECTS
- ▸ **Common or very common** Appetite decreased · asthenia · chest pain · confusion · delirium · diarrhoea · drowsiness · dyspnoea · electrolyte imbalance · gastrointestinal discomfort · headache · hepatic disorders · hyperbilirubinaemia · nausea · renal failure · respiratory disorders · skin reactions · thrombophlebitis · vomiting
- ▸ **Uncommon** Alopecia · anaemia · arrhythmias · back pain · circulatory collapse · constipation · depression · dizziness · encephalopathy · haemorrhage · hypersensitivity · hypoalbuminaemia · hypoglycaemia · hypotension · insomnia · leucopenia · malaise · malnutrition · neutropenia · palpitations · pancytopenia · paraesthesia · peripheral neuropathy · peripheral oedema · seizures · syncope · taste altered · thrombocytopenia · vertigo
- ▸ **Frequency not known** Severe cutaneous adverse reactions (SCARs)
  SPECIFIC SIDE-EFFECTS
- ▸ With intravenous use Infusion related reaction
  SIDE-EFFECTS, FURTHER INFORMATION Infusion-related reactions have been reported, including hypotension, dyspnoea, dizziness, paraesthesia, nausea, and headache—manufacturer advises discontinue treatment if these reactions occur.

- **PREGNANCY** Manufacturer advises avoid unless severe or life-threatening infection—toxicity in *animal* studies.
- **BREAST FEEDING** Manufacturer advises avoid—present in milk in *animal* studies.
- **HEPATIC IMPAIRMENT** Manufacturer advises caution in severe impairment (no information available)—monitor for drug toxicity.
- **DIRECTIONS FOR ADMINISTRATION** For *intravenous infusion*, manufacturer advises reconstitute each 200 mg with 5 mL Water for Injection; dilute dose to concentration of 0.8 mg/mL with Glucose 5% or Sodium Chloride 0.9% and give via a 0.2–1.2 micron filter over at least 1 hour.

- **HANDLING AND STORAGE**
- ▸ With intravenous use Manufacturer advises store in a refrigerator (2–8°C)—consult product literature for storage after reconstitution or dilution.

- **PATIENT AND CARER ADVICE**
  Driving and skilled tasks Manufacturer advises patients and carers should be cautioned on the effects on driving and performance of skilled tasks—increased risk of confusion, syncope and dizziness.

- **NATIONAL FUNDING/ACCESS DECISIONS**
  For full details see funding body website
  All Wales Medicines Strategy Group (AWMSG) decisions
- ▸ Isavuconazole (*Cresemba* ®) for the treatment of invasive aspergillosis in adults and the treatment of mucormycosis in adult patients for whom amphotericin B is inappropriate (January 2017) AWMSG No. 2433 Recommended

- **MEDICINAL FORMS** There can be variation in the licensing of different medicines containing the same drug.
  Powder for solution for infusion
  CAUTIONARY AND ADVISORY LABELS 3
- ▸ Cresemba (Pfizer Ltd)
  Isavuconazole (as Isavuconazonium sulfate) 200 mg Cresemba 200mg powder for concentrate for solution for infusion vials | 1 vial [PoM] £297.84 (Hospital only)
  Oral capsule
  CAUTIONARY AND ADVISORY LABELS 3, 25
- ▸ Cresemba (Pfizer Ltd)
  Isavuconazole (as Isavuconazonium sulfate) 40 mg Cresemba 40mg capsules | 35 capsule [PoM] £599.28 (Hospital only)
  Isavuconazole (as Isavuconazonium sulfate) 100 mg Cresemba 100mg capsules | 14 capsule [PoM] £599.28 (Hospital only)

Itraconazole

04-Aug-2022

- **INDICATIONS AND DOSE**

Vulvovaginal candidiasis
- ▸ BY MOUTH
- ▸ Adult: 200 mg twice daily for 1 day

Vulvovaginal candidiasis (recurrent)
- ▸ BY MOUTH
- ▸ Adult: 50–100 mg daily for 6 months

Oral or oesophageal candidiasis that has not responded to fluconazole
- ▸ BY MOUTH USING ORAL SOLUTION
- ▸ Adult: 100–200 mg twice daily for 2 weeks, continue for another 2 weeks if no response; the higher dose should not be used for longer than 2 weeks if no signs of improvement

Oral or oesophageal candidiasis in HIV-positive or other immunocompromised patients
- ▸ BY MOUTH USING ORAL SOLUTION
- ▸ Adult: 200 mg daily in 1–2 divided doses for 1 week (continue for another week if no response)

Systemic candidiasis where other antifungal drugs inappropriate or ineffective
- ▸ BY MOUTH
- ▸ Adult: 100–200 mg once daily
- ▸ BY INTRAVENOUS INFUSION
- ▸ Adult: 200 mg every 12 hours for 2 days, then 200 mg once daily for max. 12 days

Systemic candidiasis (invasive or disseminated) where other antifungal drugs inappropriate or ineffective
- ▸ BY MOUTH
- ▸ Adult: 200 mg twice daily

Pityriasis versicolor
- ▸ BY MOUTH
- ▸ Adult: 200 mg once daily for 7 days

Tinea pedis | Tinea manuum
▶ BY MOUTH
▶ Adult: 100 mg once daily for 30 days, alternatively 200 mg twice daily for 7 days

Tinea corporis | Tinea cruris
▶ BY MOUTH
▶ Adult: 100 mg once daily for 15 days, alternatively 200 mg once daily for 7 days

Onychomycosis
▶ BY MOUTH
▶ Adult: 200 mg once daily for 3 months, alternatively 200 mg twice daily for 7 days, subsequent courses repeated after 21-day intervals; fingernails 2 courses, toenails 3 courses

Aspergillosis
▶ BY MOUTH
▶ Adult: 200 mg twice daily

Systemic aspergillosis where other antifungal drugs inappropriate or ineffective
▶ BY INTRAVENOUS INFUSION
▶ Adult: 200 mg every 12 hours for 2 days, then 200 mg once daily for max. 12 days

Histoplasmosis
▶ BY MOUTH
▶ Adult: 200 mg 3 times a day for 3 days, then 200 mg 1–2 times a day
▶ BY INTRAVENOUS INFUSION
▶ Adult: 200 mg every 12 hours for 2 days, then 200 mg once daily for max. 12 days

Systemic cryptococcosis including cryptococcal meningitis where other antifungal drugs inappropriate or ineffective
▶ BY MOUTH
▶ Adult: 200 mg once daily, increased to 200 mg twice daily, increased dose used in invasive or disseminated disease and in cryptococcal meningitis
▶ BY INTRAVENOUS INFUSION
▶ Adult: 200 mg every 12 hours for 2 days, then 200 mg once daily for max. 12 days

Maintenance in HIV-infected patients to prevent relapse of underlying fungal infection and prophylaxis in neutropenia when standard therapy inappropriate
▶ BY MOUTH
▶ Adult: 200 mg once daily, increased to 200 mg twice daily, increased dose used only if low plasma-itraconazole concentration

Prophylaxis of deep fungal infections (when standard therapy inappropriate) in patients with haematological malignancy or undergoing bone-marrow transplantation who are expected to become neutropenic
▶ BY MOUTH USING ORAL SOLUTION
▶ Adult: 5 mg/kg daily in 2 divided doses, to be started before transplantation or before chemotherapy (taking care to avoid interaction with cytotoxic drugs) and continued until neutrophil count recovers, safety and efficacy not established in elderly patients

DOSE ADJUSTMENTS DUE TO INTERACTIONS
▶ EvGr Max. dose 200 mg daily with concurrent use of cobicistat-boosted regimens. Ⓜ

● **UNLICENSED USE** Itraconazole doses in BNF may differ from those in product literature.
● **CONTRA-INDICATIONS** Acute porphyrias p. 1202
● **CAUTIONS** Active liver disease · elderly · history of hepatotoxicity with other drugs · susceptibility to congestive heart failure

CAUTIONS, FURTHER INFORMATION
▶ Susceptibility to congestive heart failure There have been reports of heart failure associated with itraconazole. Those at risk may include patients receiving higher daily doses

and longer courses, patients with cardiac disease, patients with chronic lung disease, and patients receiving treatment with calcium channel blockers. Manufacturer advises avoid in patients with ventricular dysfunction, such as history of congestive heart failure, unless the infection is serious.

● **INTERACTIONS** → Appendix 1: antifungals, azoles
● **SIDE-EFFECTS**
GENERAL SIDE-EFFECTS
▶ **Common or very common** Alopecia · constipation · diarrhoea · dyspnoea · gastrointestinal discomfort · headache · heart failure · hepatic disorders · hyperbilirubinaemia · nausea · oedema · pulmonary oedema · skin reactions · vision disorders · vomiting
▶ **Uncommon** Hearing loss · taste altered
▶ **Rare or very rare** Angioedema · hypersensitivity vasculitis · hypertriglyceridaemia · pancreatitis · photosensitivity reaction · severe cutaneous adverse reactions (SCARs)
▶ **Frequency not known** Peripheral neuropathy (discontinue)

SPECIFIC SIDE-EFFECTS
▶ **Common or very common**
▶ With intravenous use Chest pain · confusion · cough · dizziness · drowsiness · electrolyte imbalance · fatigue · gastrointestinal disorder · granulocytopenia · hyperglycaemia · hyperhidrosis · hypersensitivity · hypertension · hypotension · myalgia · pain · renal impairment · tachycardia · tremor · urinary incontinence
▶ **Uncommon**
▶ With intravenous use Dysphonia · numbness · thrombocytopenia
▶ With oral use Flatulence · increased risk of infection · menstrual disorder
▶ **Rare or very rare**
▶ With oral use Erectile dysfunction · leucopenia · sensation abnormal · serum sickness · tinnitus · urinary frequency increased

SIDE-EFFECTS, FURTHER INFORMATION
Potentially life-threatening hepatotoxicity reported very rarely — discontinue if signs of hepatitis develop.

● **CONCEPTION AND CONTRACEPTION** Ensure effective contraception during treatment and until the next menstrual period following end of treatment.
● **PREGNANCY** Manufacturer advises use only in life-threatening situations (toxicity at high doses in *animal* studies).
● **BREAST FEEDING** Small amounts present in milk—may accumulate; manufacturer advises avoid.
● **HEPATIC IMPAIRMENT** Manufacturer advises use only in serious or life-saving situations where potential benefit outweighs risk of hepatotoxicity.
● **RENAL IMPAIRMENT**
▶ With oral use Manufacturer advises caution (risk of congestive heart failure).
▶ With intravenous use Manufacturer advises caution in mild to moderate impairment (risk of congestive heart failure); avoid if creatinine clearance less than 30 mL/minute. See p. 21.
Dose adjustments
▶ With oral use Manufacturer advises dose adjustment may be considered (bioavailability possibly reduced).

● **MONITORING REQUIREMENTS**
▶ Absorption reduced in AIDS and neutropenia (monitor plasma-itraconazole concentration and increase dose if necessary).
▶ Monitor liver function if treatment continues for longer than one month, if receiving other hepatotoxic drugs, or if history of hepatotoxicity with other drugs.

● **DIRECTIONS FOR ADMINISTRATION**
▶ With intravenous use For *intravenous infusion* (*Sporanox* ®), manufacturer advises give intermittently in Sodium

5 Infection

Chloride 0.9%; dilute 250 mg in 50 mL infusion fluid and infuse only 60 mL through an in-line filter (0.2 micron) over 60 minutes.

▶ With oral use For *oral liquid*, manufacturer advises do not take with food; swish around mouth and swallow, do not rinse afterwards.

● PRESCRIBING AND DISPENSING INFORMATION Flavours of oral liquid formulations may include cherry.

● PATIENT AND CARER ADVICE Patients should be told how to recognise signs of liver disorder and advised to seek prompt medical attention if symptoms such as anorexia, nausea, vomiting, fatigue, abdominal pain or dark urine develop.

Patients or carers should be given advice on how to administer itraconazole oral liquid.

● MEDICINAL FORMS There can be variation in the licensing of different medicines containing the same drug. Forms available from special-order manufacturers include: oral suspension, oral solution

Solution for infusion
EXCIPIENTS: May contain Propylene glycol
▶ **Itraconazole (Non-proprietary)**
Itraconazole 10 mg per 1 ml Itraconazole 250mg/25ml solution for infusion ampoules and diluent | 1 ampoule [PoM] £87.55 (Hospital only)

Oral solution
CAUTIONARY AND ADVISORY LABELS 9, 23
▶ **Itraconazole (Non-proprietary)**
Itraconazole 10 mg per 1 ml Itraconazole 50mg/5ml oral solution sugar free | 150 ml [PoM] £58.34 DT = £48.08 [SF]

Oral suspension
CAUTIONARY AND ADVISORY LABELS 9, 23

Oral capsule
CAUTIONARY AND ADVISORY LABELS 5, 9, 21, 25
▶ **Itraconazole (Non-proprietary)**
Itraconazole 100 mg Itraconazole 100mg capsules | 15 capsule [PoM] £13.77 DT = £5.44 | 28 capsule [PoM] £10.15 | 60 capsule [PoM] £26.76–£55.10

| Posaconazole

04-Sep-2024

● **INDICATIONS AND DOSE**

Invasive aspergillosis either refractory to, or in patients intolerant of, itraconazole or amphotericin B | Fusariosis either refractory to, or in patients intolerant of, amphotericin B | Chromoblastomycosis and mycetoma either refractory to, or in patients intolerant of, itraconazole | Coccidioidomycosis either refractory to, or in patients intolerant of, amphotericin B, itraconazole, or fluconazole
▶ BY MOUTH USING ORAL SUSPENSION
▶ Adult: 400 mg twice daily, to be taken with food, alternatively 200 mg 4 times a day, if unable to tolerate food
▶ BY MOUTH USING TABLETS, OR BY INTRAVENOUS INFUSION
▶ Adult: Loading dose 300 mg twice daily on first day, then 300 mg once daily, switch from intravenous to oral route when appropriate

Oropharyngeal candidiasis (severe infection or in immunocompromised patients only)
▶ BY MOUTH USING ORAL SUSPENSION
▶ Adult: Loading dose 200 mg on first day, then 100 mg once daily for 13 days, dose to be taken with food

Prophylaxis of invasive fungal infections in patients at high risk and undergoing high-dose immunosuppressive therapy for haematopoietic stem cell transplantation or receiving chemotherapy for acute myeloid leukaemia or myelodysplastic syndrome and expected to develop prolonged neutropenia
▶ BY MOUTH USING ORAL SUSPENSION
▶ Adult: 200 mg 3 times a day, dose to be taken with food, for chemotherapy patients, start several days before the expected onset of neutropenia and continue for 7 days after neutrophil count rises above 500 cells/mm^3
▶ BY MOUTH USING TABLETS, OR BY INTRAVENOUS INFUSION
▶ Adult: Loading dose 300 mg twice daily on first day, then 300 mg once daily, for chemotherapy patients, start several days before the expected onset of neutropenia and continue for 7 days after neutrophil count rises above 500 cells/mm^3, switch from intravenous to oral route when appropriate

DOSE EQUIVALENCE AND CONVERSION
▶ Posaconazole oral suspension is **not** interchangeable with tablets on a milligram-for-milligram basis.

PHARMACOKINETICS
▶ Posaconazole oral suspension should be taken with food (preferably a high fat meal) or nutritional supplement to ensure adequate exposure for systemic effects. Where possible, tablets should be used in preference to suspension because tablets have a higher bioavailability.

> **IMPORTANT SAFETY INFORMATION**
> Posaconazole tablets and oral suspension are **not** bioequivalent and should not be used interchangeably, due to differences in dosing frequency, administration with regards to food, and the plasma-drug concentration achieved. Directly switching between these preparations can lead to incorrect dosing which may result in a lack of efficacy if underdosed, or serious side-effects if overdosed. Prescribers should specify the dosage form for posaconazole on every prescription, and pharmacists should ensure that the correct preparation is supplied.

● CONTRA-INDICATIONS Acute porphyrias p. 1202

● CAUTIONS Administration by intravenous infusion, particularly by peripheral catheter—increased risk of QTc interval prolongation · body-weight over 120 kg—risk of treatment failure possibly increased · body-weight under 60 kg—risk of side effects increased · bradycardia · cardiomyopathy · history of QTc interval prolongation · symptomatic arrhythmias

● INTERACTIONS → Appendix 1: antifungals, azoles

● SIDE-EFFECTS
▶ **Common or very common** Appetite decreased · asthenia · constipation · diarrhoea · dizziness · drowsiness · dry mouth · electrolyte imbalance · gastrointestinal discomfort · gastrointestinal disorders · headache · hypertension · nausea · neutropenia · sensation abnormal · skin reactions · taste altered · vomiting
▶ **Uncommon** Alopecia · anaemia · aphasia · arrhythmias · burping · chest discomfort · confusion · cough · embolism and thrombosis · eosinophilia · feeling jittery · haemorrhage · hepatic disorders · hiccups · hyperglycaemia · hypoglycaemia · hypotension · leucopenia · lymphadenopathy · malaise · menstrual disorder · mucositis · nasal congestion · oedema · oral disorders · pain · palpitations · pancreatitis · peripheral neuropathy · QT interval prolongation · renal impairment · respiratory disorders · seizure · sleep disorders · splenic infarction · thrombocytopenia · tremor · vasculitis · vision disorders
▶ **Rare or very rare** Adrenal insufficiency · breast pain · cardiac arrest · coagulation disorder · depression ·

encephalopathy · haemolytic uraemic syndrome · hearing impairment · heart failure · interstitial lung disease · myocardial infarction · nephritis tubulointerstitial · pancytopenia · psychotic disorder · pulmonary hypertension · renal tubular acidosis · Stevens-Johnson syndrome · stroke · sudden cardiac death · syncope

● **CONCEPTION AND CONTRACEPTION** Manufacturer recommends effective contraception during treatment.

● **PREGNANCY** Manufacturer advises avoid unless potential benefit outweighs risk; toxicity in *animal* studies.

● **BREAST FEEDING** Manufacturer advises avoid—present in milk in *animal* studies.

● **HEPATIC IMPAIRMENT** Manufacturer advises caution (risk of increased exposure, limited information available).

● **RENAL IMPAIRMENT** Manufacturer advises monitor efficacy in severe impairment—variable exposure expected.
▸ With intravenous use Manufacturer advises caution if creatinine clearance less than 50 mL/minute—intravenous vehicle may accumulate. See p. 21.

● **MONITORING REQUIREMENTS**
▸ Monitor electrolytes (including potassium, magnesium, and calcium) before and during therapy.
▸ Monitor liver function before and during therapy.

● **DIRECTIONS FOR ADMINISTRATION** Manufacturer advises for *intravenous infusion* (*Noxafil®*), give continuously in Glucose 5% *or* Sodium Chloride 0.9%; dilute requisite dose in infusion fluid to produce a final concentration of 1–2 mg/mL; give via a central venous catheter or peripherally inserted central catheter over approx. 90 minutes (can give a single dose via peripheral venous catheter if central access not established—dilute to a final concentration of 2 mg/mL and give over approx. 30 minutes).

● **PRESCRIBING AND DISPENSING INFORMATION** Flavours of oral liquid formulations may include cherry.

● **HANDLING AND STORAGE**
▸ With intravenous use Manufacturer advises store in a refrigerator (2–8 °C).

● **PATIENT AND CARER ADVICE**
Driving and skilled tasks Manufacturer advises patients and carers should be counselled on the effects on driving and performance of skilled tasks—increased risk of dizziness and somnolence.

● **MEDICINAL FORMS** There can be variation in the licensing of different medicines containing the same drug.

Solution for infusion
ELECTROLYTES: May contain Sodium
▸ Noxafil (Merck Sharp & Dohme (UK) Ltd)
Posaconazole 18 mg per 1 ml Noxafil 300mg/16.7ml concentrate for solution for infusion vials | 1 vial PoM £211.00 (Hospital only)

Oral suspension
CAUTIONARY AND ADVISORY LABELS 3, 9, 21
▸ Posaconazole (Non-proprietary)
Posaconazole 40 mg per 1 ml Posaconazole 40mg/ml oral suspension | 105 ml PoM £491.20-£491.50 DT = £491.20 | 105 ml PoM £491.20 DT = £491.20 (Hospital only)
▸ Noxafil (Merck Sharp & Dohme (UK) Ltd)
Posaconazole 40 mg per 1 ml Noxafil 40mg/ml oral suspension | 105 ml PoM £491.20 DT = £491.20 (Hospital only)

Gastro-resistant tablet
CAUTIONARY AND ADVISORY LABELS 3, 9, 25
▸ Posaconazole (Non-proprietary)
Posaconazole 100 mg Posaconazole 100mg gastro-resistant tablets | 24 tablet PoM £385.00-£590.00 DT = £596.96 | 24 tablet PoM £507.42-£596.96 DT = £596.96 (Hospital only) | 96 tablet PoM £1,150.00-£2,387.85 | 96 tablet PoM £2,029.67-£2,387.85 (Hospital only)
▸ Noxafil (Merck Sharp & Dohme (UK) Ltd)
Posaconazole 100 mg Noxafil 100mg gastro-resistant tablets | 24 tablet PoM £596.96 DT = £596.96 | 96 tablet PoM £2,387.85

Voriconazole
02-Aug-2021

● **INDICATIONS AND DOSE**

Invasive aspergillosis | Serious infections caused by *Scedosporium* spp., *Fusarium* spp., or invasive fluconazole-resistant *Candida* spp. (including *C. krusei*)
▸ BY MOUTH
▸ Adult (body-weight up to 40 kg): Initially 200 mg every 12 hours for 2 doses, then 100 mg every 12 hours, increased if necessary to 150 mg every 12 hours
▸ Adult (body-weight 40 kg and above): Initially 400 mg every 12 hours for 2 doses, then 200 mg every 12 hours, increased if necessary to 300 mg every 12 hours
▸ BY INTRAVENOUS INFUSION
▸ Adult: Initially 6 mg/kg every 12 hours for 2 doses, then 4 mg/kg every 12 hours; reduced if not tolerated to 3 mg/kg every 12 hours; for max. 6 months

DOSE ADJUSTMENTS DUE TO INTERACTIONS
▸ With intravenous use Manufacturer advises increase maintenance dose to 5 mg/kg every 12 hours with concurrent use of fosphenytoin, phenytoin or rifabutin.
▸ With oral use Manufacturer advises increase maintenance dose with concurrent use of fosphenytoin or phenytoin; 400 mg every 12 hours for patients of body-weight 40 kg and above; 200 mg every 12 hours for patients of body-weight less than 40 kg. Manufacturer advises if concurrent use of rifabutin is unavoidable, increase maintenance dose to 350 mg every 12 hours for patients of body-weight 40 kg and above; 200 mg every 12 hours for patients of body-weight less than 40 kg.

● **CONTRA-INDICATIONS** Acute porphyrias p. 1202

● **CAUTIONS** Avoid exposure to sunlight · bradycardia · cardiomyopathy · electrolyte disturbances · history of QT interval prolongation · patients at risk of pancreatitis · symptomatic arrhythmias

● **INTERACTIONS** → Appendix 1: antifungals, azoles

● **SIDE-EFFECTS**
GENERAL SIDE-EFFECTS
▸ **Common or very common** Acute kidney injury · agranulocytosis · alopecia · anaemia · anxiety · arrhythmias · asthenia · bone marrow disorders · chest pain · chills · confusion · constipation · depression · diarrhoea · dizziness · drowsiness · dyspnoea · electrolyte imbalance · eye disorders · eye inflammation · fever · gastrointestinal discomfort · haemorrhage · hallucination · headache · hepatic disorders · hypoglycaemia · hypotension · increased risk of infection · insomnia · leucopenia · muscle tone increased · nausea · neutropenia · oedema · oral disorders · pain · pulmonary oedema · respiratory disorders · seizure · sensation abnormal · skin reactions · syncope · tetany · thrombocytopenia · tremor · vision disorders · vomiting
▸ **Uncommon** Adrenal insufficiency · arthritis · brain oedema · duodenitis · encephalopathy · eosinophilia · gallbladder disorders · hearing impairment · hypothyroidism · influenza like illness · lymphadenopathy · lymphangitis · movement disorders · nephritis · nerve disorders · pancreatitis · parkinsonism · phototoxicity · proteinuria · pseudomembranous enterocolitis · QT interval prolongation · renal tubular necrosis · severe cutaneous adverse reactions (SCARs) · taste altered · thrombophlebitis · tinnitus · vertigo
▸ **Rare or very rare** Angioedema · cardiac conduction disorders · disseminated intravascular coagulation · hyperthyroidism
▸ **Frequency not known** Cutaneous lupus erythematosus · periostitis (more common in transplant patients) · squamous cell carcinoma (more common in presence of phototoxicity)

SPECIFIC SIDE-EFFECTS
▸ With intravenous use Infusion related reaction

SIDE-EFFECTS, FURTHER INFORMATION **Hepatotoxicity**
Hepatitis, cholestasis, and acute hepatic failure have been reported; risk of hepatotoxicity increased in patients with haematological malignancy. Consider treatment discontinuation if severe abnormalities in liver function tests.

   Phototoxicity Phototoxicity occurs uncommonly. If phototoxicity occurs, consider treatment discontinuation; if treatment is continued, monitor for pre-malignant skin lesions and squamous cell carcinoma, and discontinue treatment if they occur.

● CONCEPTION AND CONTRACEPTION Effective contraception required during treatment.

● PREGNANCY Toxicity in *animal* studies—manufacturer advises avoid unless potential benefit outweighs risk.

● BREAST FEEDING Manufacturer advises avoid—no information available.

● HEPATIC IMPAIRMENT Manufacturer advises caution, particularly in severe impairment (no information available).
   Dose adjustments Manufacturer advises use usual initial loading dose then halve maintenance dose in mild to moderate cirrhosis.

● RENAL IMPAIRMENT [EvGr] Intravenous vehicle may accumulate if creatinine clearance less than 50 mL/minute—use intravenous infusion only if potential benefit outweighs risk, and monitor renal function; alternatively, use tablets or oral suspension (no dose adjustment required). Ⓜ See p. 21.

● MONITORING REQUIREMENTS
▸ Monitor renal function.
▸ Monitor liver function before starting treatment, then at least weekly for 1 month, and then monthly during treatment.

● DIRECTIONS FOR ADMINISTRATION For *intravenous infusion*, manufacturer advises reconstitute each 200 mg with 19 mL Water for Injections *or* Sodium Chloride 0.9% to produce a 10 mg/mL solution; dilute dose to concentration of 0.5–5 mg/mL with Glucose 5% or Sodium Chloride 0.9% and give intermittently at a rate not exceeding 3 mg/kg/hour.

● PRESCRIBING AND DISPENSING INFORMATION Flavours of oral liquid formulations may include orange.

● PATIENT AND CARER ADVICE Patients and their carers should be told how to recognise symptoms of liver disorder, and advised to seek immediate medical attention if symptoms such as persistent nausea, vomiting, malaise or jaundice develop.
   Patients and their carers should be advised that patients should avoid exposure to direct sunlight, and to avoid the use of sunbeds. In sunlight, patients should cover sun-exposed areas of skin and use a sunscreen with a high sun protection factor. Patients should seek medical attention if they experience sunburn or a severe skin reaction following exposure to light or sun.
   Patients and their carers should be advised to keep the alert card with them at all times.

● MEDICINAL FORMS There can be variation in the licensing of different medicines containing the same drug.
Oral tablet
CAUTIONARY AND ADVISORY LABELS 9, 11, 23
▸ Voriconazole (Non-proprietary)
   Voriconazole 50 mg Voriconazole 50mg tablets | 28 tablet [PoM] £191.62–£275.68 DT = £275.68 | 28 tablet [PoM] £65.50 DT = £275.68 (Hospital only)
   Voriconazole 100 mg Voriconazole 100mg tablets | 28 tablet [PoM] £275.68 DT = £275.68

   Voriconazole 200 mg Voriconazole 200mg tablets | 28 tablet [PoM] £218.00 DT = £1,102.74 (Hospital only) | 28 tablet [PoM] £758.92–£1,102.74 DT = £1,102.74
▸ VFEND (Pfizer Ltd)
   Voriconazole 50 mg VFEND 50mg tablets | 28 tablet [PoM] £275.68 DT = £275.68
   Voriconazole 200 mg VFEND 200mg tablets | 28 tablet [PoM] £1,102.74 DT = £1,102.74
Oral suspension
CAUTIONARY AND ADVISORY LABELS 9, 11, 23
▸ VFEND (Pfizer Ltd)
   Voriconazole 40 mg per 1 ml VFEND 40mg/ml oral suspension | 70 ml [PoM] £551.37 DT = £551.37
Powder for solution for infusion
EXCIPIENTS: May contain Sulfobutylether beta cyclodextrin sodium
ELECTROLYTES: May contain Sodium
▸ Voriconazole (Non-proprietary)
   Voriconazole 200 mg Voriconazole 200mg powder for solution for infusion vials | 1 vial [PoM] £69.43–£77.14 (Hospital only)
▸ VFEND (Pfizer Ltd)
   Voriconazole 200 mg VFEND 200mg powder for solution for infusion vials | 1 vial [PoM] £77.14 (Hospital only)

ANTIFUNGALS › OTHER

Flucytosine

17-Nov-2020

● **INDICATIONS AND DOSE**
Systemic yeast and fungal infections | Adjunct to amphotericin B in severe systemic candidiasis and in other severe or long-standing infections
▸ BY INTRAVENOUS INFUSION
▸ Adult: Usual dose 200 mg/kg daily in 4 divided doses usually for not more than 7 days, alternatively 100–150 mg/kg daily in 4 divided doses, lower dose may be sufficient for extremely sensitive organisms
Cryptococcal meningitis (adjunct to amphotericin B)
▸ BY INTRAVENOUS INFUSION
▸ Adult: 100 mg/kg daily in 4 divided doses for 2 weeks

● UNLICENSED USE Use in cryptococcal meningitis for 2 weeks is an unlicensed duration.

IMPORTANT SAFETY INFORMATION
MHRA/CHM ADVICE: FLUCYTOSINE (ANCOTIL ®): NEW CONTRA-INDICATION IN PATIENTS WITH DPD DEFICIENCY (OCTOBER 2020)
Patients with partial or complete dihydropyrimidine dehydrogenase (DPD) deficiency are at increased risk of severe and fatal toxicity during treatment with fluoropyrimidines. Healthcare professionals are advised that pre-treatment testing for DPD deficiency is not required in order to avoid delay in antimycotic therapy with flucytosine. However, if drug toxicity is confirmed or suspected, testing of DPD activity and withdrawal of treatment should be considered. Flucytosine is contra-indicated in patients with known complete DPD deficiency.

● CONTRA-INDICATIONS Complete dihydropyrimidine dehydrogenase deficiency

● CAUTIONS Blood disorders · elderly · partial dihydropyrimidine dehydrogenase deficiency

● INTERACTIONS → Appendix 1: flucytosine

● SIDE-EFFECTS Agranulocytosis · aplastic anaemia · blood disorder · cardiotoxicity · confusion · diarrhoea · hallucination · headache · hepatic disorders · leucopenia · nausea · rash · sedation · seizure · thrombocytopenia · toxic epidermal necrolysis · ventricular dysfunction · vertigo · vomiting

● PREGNANCY Teratogenic in *animal* studies; manufacturer advises use only if potential benefit outweighs risk.

● BREAST FEEDING Manufacturer advises avoid.

- **RENAL IMPAIRMENT**
Dose adjustments Use 50 mg/kg every 12 hours if creatinine clearance 20–40 mL/minute; use 50 mg/kg every 24 hours if creatinine clearance 10–20 mL/minute; use initial dose of 50 mg/kg if creatinine clearance less than 10 mL/minute and then adjust dose according to plasma-flucytosine concentration.
Monitoring In renal impairment liver- and kidney-function tests and blood counts required weekly.

- **MONITORING REQUIREMENTS**
- For plasma concentration monitoring, blood should be taken shortly before starting the next infusion; plasma concentration for optimum response 25–50 mg/litre (200–400 micromol/litre)—should not be allowed to exceed 80 mg/litre (620 micromol/litre).
- Liver- and kidney-function tests and blood counts required (weekly in blood disorders).

- **DIRECTIONS FOR ADMINISTRATION** For *intravenous infusion*, manufacturer advises give over 20–40 minutes.

- **MEDICINAL FORMS** No licensed medicines listed.

Griseofulvin
16-Jan-2020

- **INDICATIONS AND DOSE**
Dermatophyte infections of the skin, scalp, hair and nails where topical therapy has failed or is inappropriate
  - BY MOUTH
  - Adult: 500 mg daily, increased if necessary to 1 g daily, for severe infections; reduce dose when response occurs, daily dose may be taken once daily or in divided doses

Tinea capitis caused by *Trichophyton tonsurans*
  - BY MOUTH
  - Adult: 1 g once daily, alternatively 1 g daily in divided doses

- **UNLICENSED USE** Griseofulvin doses in BNF may differ from those in product literature.

- **CONTRA-INDICATIONS** Acute porphyrias p. 1202 · systemic lupus erythematosus (risk of exacerbation)

- **INTERACTIONS** → Appendix 1: griseofulvin

- **SIDE-EFFECTS**
  - **Common or very common** Diarrhoea · epigastric discomfort · headache · nausea · vomiting
  - **Uncommon** Appetite decreased · confusion · coordination abnormal · dizziness · drowsiness · insomnia · irritability · peripheral neuropathy · photosensitivity reaction · skin reactions · taste altered · toxic epidermal necrolysis
  - **Rare or very rare** Anaemia · hepatic disorders · leucopenia · neutropenia · systemic lupus erythematosus (SLE)

- **CONCEPTION AND CONTRACEPTION** Effective contraception required during and for at least 1 month after administration to women (important: effectiveness of oral contraceptives may be reduced, additional contraceptive precautions e.g. barrier method, required). Men should avoid fathering a child during and for at least 6 months after administration

- **PREGNANCY** Avoid (fetotoxicity and teratogenicity in *animals*).

- **BREAST FEEDING** Avoid—no information available.

- **HEPATIC IMPAIRMENT** Manufacturer advises caution in mild to moderate impairment (risk of deterioration); avoid in severe impairment.

- **PATIENT AND CARER ADVICE**
Driving and skilled tasks May impair performance of skilled tasks (e.g. driving); effects of alcohol enhanced.

- **MEDICINAL FORMS** There can be variation in the licensing of different medicines containing the same drug. Forms available from special-order manufacturers include: oral suspension
Oral tablet
CAUTIONARY AND ADVISORY LABELS 9, 21
  - ▸ Griseofulvin (Non-proprietary)
    Griseofulvin 125 mg Griseofulvin 125mg tablets | 100 tablet [PoM] £121.80 DT = £121.80
    Griseofulvin 500 mg Griseofulvin 500mg tablets | 90 tablet [PoM] £102.44 | 100 tablet [PoM] £113.82 DT = £113.82

3.1   Pneumocystis pneumonia

Pneumocystis pneumonia
25-Mar-2024

Overview
Pneumonia caused by *Pneumocystis jirovecii* (*Pneumocystis carinii*) occurs in immunosuppressed patients; it is a common cause of pneumonia in AIDS. Pneumocystis pneumonia should generally be treated by those experienced in its management. Blood gas measurement is used to assess disease severity.

Treatment
Mild to moderate disease
Co-trimoxazole p. 652 in high dosage is the drug of choice for the treatment of mild to moderate pneumocystis pneumonia.

Atovaquone p. 698 is licensed for the treatment of mild to moderate pneumocystis infection in patients who cannot tolerate co-trimoxazole. A combination of dapsone p. 668 with trimethoprim p. 665 is given by mouth for the treatment of mild to moderate disease [unlicensed indication].

A combination of clindamycin p. 618 and primaquine p. 713 by mouth is used in the treatment of mild to moderate disease [unlicensed indication].

Severe disease
Co-trimoxazole in high dosage, given by mouth or by intravenous infusion, is the drug of choice for the treatment of severe pneumocystis pneumonia. Pentamidine isetionate p. 698 given by intravenous infusion is an alternative for patients who cannot tolerate co-trimoxazole, or who have not responded to it. Pentamidine isetionate is a potentially toxic drug that can cause severe hypotension during or immediately after infusion.

Corticosteroid treatment can be lifesaving in those with severe pneumocystis pneumonia.

Adjunctive therapy
In moderate to severe infections associated with HIV infection, prednisolone p. 791 is given by mouth for 5 days (alternatively, hydrocortisone p. 787 may be given parenterally); the dose is then reduced to complete 21 days of treatment. Corticosteroid treatment should ideally be started at the same time as the anti-pneumocystis therapy and certainly no later than 24–72 hours afterwards. The corticosteroid should be withdrawn before anti-pneumocystis treatment is complete.

Prophylaxis
Prophylaxis against pneumocystis pneumonia should be given to all patients with a history of the infection. Prophylaxis against pneumocystis pneumonia should also be considered for severely immunocompromised patients. Prophylaxis should continue until immunity recovers sufficiently. It should not be discontinued if the patient has oral candidiasis, continues to lose weight, or is receiving cytotoxic therapy or long-term immunosuppressant therapy.

Co-trimoxazole by mouth is the drug of choice for prophylaxis against pneumocystis pneumonia. It is given daily or on alternate days (3 times a week); the dose may be reduced to improve tolerance.

Inhaled pentamidine isetionate is better tolerated than parenteral pentamidine isetionate. Intermittent inhalation of pentamidine isetionate is used for prophylaxis against pneumocystis pneumonia in patients unable to tolerate co-trimoxazole. It is effective but patients may be prone to extrapulmonary infection. Alternatively, dapsone can be used. Atovaquone has also been used for prophylaxis [unlicensed indication].

ANTIPROTOZOALS

Atovaquone

09-Sep-2021

- **INDICATIONS AND DOSE**

Treatment of mild to moderate *Pneumocystis jirovecii* (*Pneumocystis carinii*) pneumonia in patients intolerant of co-trimoxazole
- ▸ BY MOUTH
- ▸ Adult: 750 mg twice daily for 21 days, dose to be taken with food, particularly high fat food

Prophylaxis against pneumocystis pneumonia
- ▸ BY MOUTH
- ▸ Adult: 750 mg twice daily

- **UNLICENSED USE** Not licensed for prophylaxis against pneumocystis pneumonia.
- **CAUTIONS** Elderly · initial diarrhoea and difficulty in taking with food may reduce absorption (and require alternative therapy) · other causes of pulmonary disease should be sought and treated
- **INTERACTIONS** → Appendix 1: antimalarials
- **SIDE-EFFECTS**
- ▸ **Common or very common** Anaemia · angioedema · bronchospasm · diarrhoea · headache · hypersensitivity · hyponatraemia · insomnia · nausea · neutropenia · skin reactions · throat tightness · vomiting
- ▸ **Frequency not known** Stevens-Johnson syndrome
- **PREGNANCY** Manufacturer advises avoid unless potential benefit outweighs risk—no information available.
- **BREAST FEEDING** Manufacturer advises avoid.
- **HEPATIC IMPAIRMENT** Manufacturer advises use with caution in significant impairment and monitor closely—no information available.
- **RENAL IMPAIRMENT** [EvGr] Caution in significant impairment (no information available). ⬦
- **PRESCRIBING AND DISPENSING INFORMATION** Flavours of oral liquid formulations may include tutti-frutti.

- **MEDICINAL FORMS** There can be variation in the licensing of different medicines containing the same drug.

Oral suspension
CAUTIONARY AND ADVISORY LABELS 21
- ▸ Atovaquone (Non-proprietary)
  Atovaquone 150 mg per 1 ml Atovaquone 750mg/5ml oral suspension sugar free | 250 ml [PoM] £470.60-£780.00 [SF]
- ▸ Wellvone (GlaxoSmithKline UK Ltd)
  Atovaquone 150 mg per 1 ml Wellvone 750mg/5ml oral suspension | 226 ml [PoM] £486.37 DT = £486.37 [SF]

Pentamidine isetionate

05-Oct-2021

- **INDICATIONS AND DOSE**

Treatment of *Pneumocystis jirovecii* (*Pneumocystis carinii*) pneumonia (specialist use only)
- ▸ BY INTRAVENOUS INFUSION
- ▸ Adult: 4 mg/kg once daily for at least 14 days

Prophylaxis of *Pneumocystis jirovecii* (*Pneumocystis carinii*) pneumonia (specialist use only)
- ▸ BY INHALATION OF NEBULISED SOLUTION
- ▸ Adult: 300 mg every 4 weeks, alternatively 150 mg every 2 weeks, using suitable equipment—consult product literature

Visceral leishmaniasis (specialist use only)
- ▸ BY DEEP INTRAMUSCULAR INJECTION
- ▸ Adult: 3–4 mg/kg once daily on alternate days, maximum total of 10 injections, course may be repeated if necessary

Cutaneous leishmaniasis (specialist use only)
- ▸ BY DEEP INTRAMUSCULAR INJECTION
- ▸ Adult: 3–4 mg/kg 1–2 times a week until condition resolves

Trypanosomiasis (specialist use only)
- ▸ BY DEEP INTRAMUSCULAR INJECTION, OR BY INTRAVENOUS INFUSION
- ▸ Adult: 4 mg/kg once daily or on alternate days for a total of 7–10 injections

- **UNLICENSED USE** Not licensed for primary prevention of *Pneumocystis jirovecii* (*Pneumocystis carinii*) pneumonia by inhalation of nebulised solution.
- **CAUTIONS** Anaemia · bradycardia · cardiac disease · history of ventricular arrhythmias · hyperglycaemia · hypertension · hypoglycaemia · hypokalaemia · hypomagnesaemia · hypotension · leucopenia · risk of severe hypotension following administration · thrombocytopenia
- **INTERACTIONS** → Appendix 1: pentamidine
- **SIDE-EFFECTS**
- **GENERAL SIDE-EFFECTS**
- ▸ **Common or very common** Dizziness · hypoglycaemia (can be severe and sometimes fatal) · hypotension (can be severe and sometimes fatal) · local reaction · nausea · rash · taste altered
- ▸ **Rare or very rare** QT interval prolongation
- ▸ **Frequency not known** Pancreatitis acute (can be severe and sometimes fatal)
- **SPECIFIC SIDE-EFFECTS**
- ▸ **Common or very common**
- ▸ When used by inhalation Cough · dyspnoea · respiratory disorders
- ▸ With parenteral use Acute kidney injury · anaemia · azotaemia · electrolyte imbalance · flushing · haematuria · hyperglycaemia · induration · leucopenia · localised pain · myopathy · syncope · thrombocytopenia · vomiting
- ▸ **Rare or very rare**
- ▸ With parenteral use Arrhythmia (can be severe and sometimes fatal) · pancreatitis (can be severe and sometimes fatal)
- ▸ **Frequency not known**
- ▸ When used by inhalation Angioedema · appetite decreased · bradycardia · fatigue · renal failure
- ▸ With parenteral use Arrhythmias · perioral hypoaesthesia · sensation abnormal · Stevens-Johnson syndrome
- **PREGNANCY** Manufacturer advises avoid unless essential.
- **BREAST FEEDING** Manufacturer advises avoid unless essential—no information available.
- **HEPATIC IMPAIRMENT** Manufacturer advises caution.
- **RENAL IMPAIRMENT** [EvGr] Use with caution. ⬦
  Dose adjustments [EvGr] Reduce intravenous dose for pneumocystis pneumonia if creatinine clearance less than 10 mL/minute: in *life-threatening infection*, use 4 mg/kg once daily for 7–10 days, then 4 mg/kg on alternate days to complete course of at least 14 doses; in *less severe infection*, use 4 mg/kg on alternate days for at least 14 doses. ⬦ See p. 21.

- **MONITORING REQUIREMENTS**
▶ Monitor blood pressure before starting treatment, during administration, and at regular intervals, until treatment concluded.
▶ Carry out laboratory monitoring according to product literature.

- **DIRECTIONS FOR ADMINISTRATION** Manufacturer advises patient should be lying down when receiving drug parenterally. Direct intravenous injection should be avoided whenever possible and **never** given rapidly; intramuscular injections should be deep and preferably given into the buttock. For *intravenous infusion*, manufacturer advises reconstitute 300 mg with 3–5 mL Water for Injections (displacement value may be significant), then dilute required dose with 50–250 mL Glucose 5% *or* Sodium Chloride 0.9%; give over at least 60 minutes.
　Powder for injection (dissolved in water for injection) may be used for nebulisation.

- **HANDLING AND STORAGE** Pentamidine isetionate is toxic and personnel should be adequately protected during handling and administration—consult product literature.

- **MEDICINAL FORMS** There can be variation in the licensing of different medicines containing the same drug.
  Powder for solution for injection
  ▶ **Pentamidine isetionate (Non-proprietary)**
  Pentamidine isetionate 300 mg Pentamidine 300mg powder for solution for injection vials | 5 vial [PoM] £158.86 DT = £158.86 (Hospital only)
  ▶ **Pentacarinat** (Sanofi)
  Pentamidine isetionate 300 mg Pentacarinat 300mg powder for solution for injection vials | 5 vial [PoM] £158.86 DT = £158.86

4　Helminth infection

Helminth infections

03-Jul-2024

Specialist centres

Advice on prophylaxis and treatment of helminth infections is available from the following specialist centres:

Birmingham	(0121) 424 0357
Scotland	Contact local Infectious Diseases Unit
Liverpool	(0151) 705 3100
London	0845 155 5000 (treatment)

Threadworms

Anthelmintics are effective in threadworm (pinworms, *Enterobius vermicularis*) infections, but their use needs to be combined with hygienic measures to break the cycle of auto-infection. All members of the family require treatment.

　Adult threadworms do not live for longer than 6 weeks and for development of fresh worms, ova must be swallowed and exposed to the action of digestive juices in the upper intestinal tract. Direct multiplication of worms does not take place in the large bowel. Adult female worms lay ova on the perianal skin which causes pruritus; scratching the area then leads to ova being transmitted on fingers to the mouth, often via food eaten with unwashed hands. Washing hands and scrubbing nails before each meal and after each visit to the toilet is essential. A bath taken immediately after rising will remove ova laid during the night.

　Mebendazole p. 701 is the drug of choice for treating threadworm infection in patients of all ages over 6 months. It is given as a single dose; as reinfection is very common, a second dose may be given after 2 weeks.

Ascaricides (common roundworm infections)

Mebendazole is effective against *Ascaris lumbricoides* and is generally considered to be the drug of choice.

　Levamisole p. 701 [unlicensed] (available from 'special-order' manufacturers or specialist importing companies) is an alternative when mebendazole cannot be used. It is very well tolerated.

Tapeworm infections

Taenicides

Niclosamide [unlicensed] (available from 'special-order' manufacturers or specialist importing companies) is the most widely used drug for tapeworm infections and side-effects are limited to occasional gastro-intestinal upset, lightheadedness, and pruritus; it is not effective against larval worms. Fears of developing cysticercosis in *Taenia solium* infections have proved unfounded. All the same, an antiemetic can be given before treatment and a laxative can be given 2 hours after niclosamide.

　Praziquantel p. 702 [unlicensed] (available from 'special-order' manufacturers or specialist importing companies) is as effective as niclosamide.

Hydatid disease

Cysts caused by *Echinococcus granulosus* grow slowly and asymptomatic patients do not always require treatment. Surgical treatment remains the method of choice in many situations. Albendazole p. 700 [unlicensed] (available from 'special-order' manufacturers or specialist importing companies) is used in conjunction with surgery to reduce the risk of recurrence or as primary treatment in inoperable cases. Alveolar echinococcosis due to *E. multilocularis* is usually fatal if untreated. Surgical removal with albendazole cover is the treatment of choice, but where effective surgery is impossible, repeated cycles of albendazole (for a year or more) may help. Careful monitoring of liver function is particularly important during drug treatment.

Hookworms

Hookworms (ancylostomiasis, necatoriasis) live in the upper small intestine and draw blood from the point of their attachment to their host. An iron-deficiency anaemia may occur and, if present, effective treatment of the infection requires not only expulsion of the worms but treatment of the anaemia.

　Mebendazole has a useful broad-spectrum activity, and is effective against hookworms. Albendazole [unlicensed] (available from 'special-order' manufacturers or specialist importing companies) is an alternative. Levamisole is also is also effective in children.

Schistosomicides (bilharziasis)

Adult *Schistosoma haematobium* worms live in the genito-urinary veins and adult *S. mansoni* in those of the colon and mesentery. *S. japonicum* is more widely distributed in veins of the alimentary tract and portal system.

　Praziquantel [unlicensed] is available from Merck Serono (*Cysticide®*) and is effective against all human schistosomes. No serious adverse effects have been reported. Of all the available schistosomicides, it has the most attractive combination of effectiveness, broad-spectrum activity, and low toxicity.

Filaricides

Diethylcarbamazine [unlicensed] (available from 'special-order' manufacturers or specialist importing companies) is effective against microfilariae and adults of *Loa loa*, *Wuchereria bancrofti*, and *Brugia malayi*. To minimise reactions, treatment in adults and children over 1 month, is commenced with a dose of diethylcarbamazine citrate on the first day and increased gradually over 3 days. Length of treatment varies according to infection type, and usually gives a radical cure for these infections. Close medical supervision is necessary particularly in the early phase of treatment.

In heavy infections there may be a febrile reaction, and in heavy *Loa loa* infection there is a small risk of encephalopathy. In such cases specialist advice should be sought, and treatment must be given under careful in-patient supervision and stopped at the first sign of cerebral involvement.

Ivermectin below [unlicensed] is very effective in *onchocerciasis* and it is now the drug of choice; reactions are usually slight. Diethylcarbamazine or suramin should no longer be used for *onchocerciasis* because of their toxicity.

Cutaneous larva migrans (creeping eruption)

Dog and cat hookworm larvae may enter human skin where they produce slowly extending itching tracks usually on the foot. Single tracks can be treated with topical tiabendazole (no commercial preparation available). Multiple infections respond to ivermectin, albendazole or **tiabendazole** (thiabendazole) by mouth [all unlicensed].

Strongyloidiasis

Adult *Strongyloides stercoralis* live in the gut and produce larvae which penetrate the gut wall and invade the tissues, setting up a cycle of auto-infection. Ivermectin is the treatment of choice for chronic *Strongyloides* infection in adults and children over 5 years. Albendazole [unlicensed] (available from 'special order' manufacturers or specialist importing companies) is an alternative given to adults and children over 2 years.

ANTHELMINTICS

Albendazole

03-Jun-2024

● **INDICATIONS AND DOSE**

Chronic *Strongyloides* infection
▸ BY MOUTH
▸ Adult: 400 mg twice daily for 3 days, dose may be repeated after 3 weeks if necessary

Hydatid disease, in conjunction with surgery to reduce the risk of recurrence or as primary treatment in inoperable cases
▸ BY MOUTH
▸ Adult: (consult product literature)

Hookworm infections
▸ BY MOUTH
▸ Adult: 400 mg for 1 dose

● **UNLICENSED USE** Albendazole is an unlicensed drug.

● **CAUTIONS** Pre-existing neurocysticercosis (may trigger neurological symptoms)

● **INTERACTIONS** → Appendix 1: albendazole

● **SIDE-EFFECTS**
▸ **Common or very common** Abdominal pain · alopecia (reversible) · dizziness · gastrointestinal disorder · hair thinning · headache · nausea · vomiting
▸ **Uncommon** Diarrhoea · hepatic disorders · leucopenia · skin reactions
▸ **Rare or very rare** Agranulocytosis · bone marrow disorders · bone pain · proteinuria · Stevens-Johnson syndrome

● **PREGNANCY** Specialist sources indicate low risk due to poor oral bioavailability but consider avoiding during first trimester.

● **BREAST FEEDING** Specialist sources indicate present in milk but amount is clinically insignificant; a single oral dose is compatible with breast-feeding.

● **HEPATIC IMPAIRMENT** EvGr Caution in pre-existing liver disease (no information available). Ⓜ

● **MEDICINAL FORMS** There can be variation in the licensing of different medicines containing the same drug. Forms available from special-order manufacturers include: oral tablet, chewable tablet, oral suspension

Oral tablet
CAUTIONARY AND ADVISORY LABELS 9
▸ Albendazole (Non-proprietary)
  Albendazole 400 mg Eskazole 400mg tablets | 60 tablet PoM Ⓢ

Chewable tablet
CAUTIONARY AND ADVISORY LABELS 9
EXCIPIENTS: May contain Propylene glycol
▸ Albendazole (Non-proprietary)
  Albendazole 200 mg Zentel 200mg chewable tablets | 6 tablet PoM Ⓢ (Hospital only)
  Albendazole 400 mg Zentel 400mg chewable tablets | 1 tablet PoM Ⓢ

Diethylcarbamazine

● **INDICATIONS AND DOSE**

***Wuchereria bancrofti* infections | *Brugia malayi* infections**
▸ BY MOUTH
▸ Adult: Initially 1 mg/kg daily on the first day, then increased to 6 mg/kg daily in divided doses, dose to be increased gradually over 3 days

***Loa loa* infections**
▸ BY MOUTH
▸ Adult: Initially 1 mg/kg daily on the first day, then increased to 6 mg/kg daily in divided doses, dose to be increased gradually over 3 days; maximum 9 mg/kg per day

● **UNLICENSED USE** Diethylcarbamazine is an unlicensed drug.

● **MEDICINAL FORMS** No licensed medicines listed.

Ivermectin

07-Jul-2024

● **INDICATIONS AND DOSE**

Onchocerciasis
▸ BY MOUTH
▸ Adult: 150 micrograms/kg for 1 dose, repeat at intervals of 6 to 12 months, depending on symptoms, must be given until the adult worms die out

Scabies
▸ BY MOUTH
▸ Adult: 200 micrograms/kg for 1 dose, recovery may take up to 4 weeks after treatment; only repeat the dose within 2 weeks if new specific lesions occur, or if a parasitologic examination is positive at this date

Hyperkeratotic (crusted or 'Norwegian') scabies
▸ BY MOUTH
▸ Adult: 200 micrograms/kg for 1 dose, a repeat dose within 8 to 15 days may be necessary for recovery

Gastrointestinal strongyloidiasis
▸ BY MOUTH
▸ Adult (body-weight 36–50 kg): 9 mg for 1 dose
▸ Adult (body-weight 51–65 kg): 12 mg for 1 dose
▸ Adult (body-weight 66–79 kg): 15 mg for 1 dose
▸ Adult (body-weight 80 kg and above): 18 mg for 1 dose

Microfilaraemia in patients with lymphatic filariasis due to *Wuchereria bancrofti* infection
▸ BY MOUTH
▸ Adult (body-weight 15 kg and above): 150–200 micrograms/kg for 1 dose, to be repeated every 6 months. Consult product literature for more information

● **UNLICENSED USE** Ivermectin is used for the treatment of *onchocerciasis*, but is not licensed for this indication.

- **INTERACTIONS** → Appendix 1: ivermectin
- **SIDE-EFFECTS**
- **Common or very common** Skin reactions
- **Frequency not known** Abdominal pain · abnormal sensation in eye · anaemia · appetite decreased · arthralgia · asthenia · asthma exacerbated · coma · confusion · constipation · diarrhoea · difficulty standing · difficulty walking · dizziness · drowsiness · dyspnoea · encephalopathy · eye erythema · eye inflammation · fever · gastrointestinal disorders · haemorrhage · headache · hepatic disorders · hyperbilirubinaemia · hypereosinophilia · leucopenia · lymphatic abnormalities · Mazzotti reaction · myalgia · nausea · oedema · pain · postural hypotension · psychiatric disorder · severe cutaneous adverse reactions (SCARs) · stupor · tachycardia · tremor · urinary incontinence · vertigo · vomiting
- **PREGNANCY** [EvGr] Use only if potential benefit outweighs risk—no adverse effects in limited human data (recommendation also supported by specialist sources). ◇M◇
- **BREAST FEEDING** Specialist sources indicate present in milk but amount probably too small to be harmful.
- **DIRECTIONS FOR ADMINISTRATION** [EvGr] Tablets can be crushed before swallowing. ◇M◇
- **PATIENT AND CARER ADVICE** Patients and carers should be advised to take ivermectin on an empty stomach; 2 hours before or 2 hours after food (effect of food on absorption is unknown).
- **MEDICINAL FORMS** There can be variation in the licensing of different medicines containing the same drug. Forms available from special-order manufacturers include: oral tablet

Oral tablet
- **Ivermectin (Non-proprietary)**
  Ivermectin 3 mg Ivermectin 3mg tablets | 4 tablet [PoM] £49.20–£60.00 DT = £57.75
  Stromectol 3mg tablets | 4 tablet [PoM] [X] DT = £57.75

Levamisole

10-Mar-2020

- **INDICATIONS AND DOSE**
Roundworm infections
- BY MOUTH
- Adult: 120–150 mg for 1 dose

- **UNLICENSED USE** Not licensed.
- **CONTRA-INDICATIONS** Blood disorders
- **CAUTIONS** Epilepsy · Sjögren's syndrome
- **INTERACTIONS** → Appendix 1: levamisole
- **SIDE-EFFECTS** Arthralgia (long term use) · blood disorder (long term use) · diarrhoea · dizziness · headache · influenza like illness (long term use) · insomnia (long term use) · myalgia (long term use) · nausea · rash (long term use) · seizure (long term use) · taste altered (long term use) · vasculitis (long term use) · vomiting
- **PREGNANCY** Embryotoxic in *animal* studies, avoid if possible.
- **BREAST FEEDING** No information available.
- **HEPATIC IMPAIRMENT**
  Dose adjustments Use with caution—dose adjustment may be necessary.

- **MEDICINAL FORMS** There can be variation in the licensing of different medicines containing the same drug. Forms available from special-order manufacturers include: oral tablet

Oral tablet
CAUTIONARY AND ADVISORY LABELS 4
- **Ergamisol** (Imported (Belgium))
  Levamisole (as Levamisole hydrochloride) 50 mg Ergamisol 50mg tablets | 20 tablet [PoM] [X]

Mebendazole

10-Nov-2021

- **INDICATIONS AND DOSE**
Threadworm infections
- BY MOUTH
- Child 6 months-17 years: 100 mg for 1 dose, if reinfection occurs, second dose may be needed after 2 weeks
- Adult: 100 mg for 1 dose, if reinfection occurs, second dose may be needed after 2 weeks

Whipworm infections | Hookworm infections
- BY MOUTH
- Child 1-17 years: 100 mg twice daily for 3 days
- Adult: 100 mg twice daily for 3 days

Roundworm infections
- BY MOUTH
- Child 1 year: 100 mg twice daily for 3 days
- Child 2-17 years: 100 mg twice daily for 3 days, alternatively 500 mg for 1 dose
- Adult: 100 mg twice daily for 3 days, alternatively 500 mg for 1 dose

Threadworm infections (dose approved for use by community practitioner nurse prescribers)
- BY MOUTH
- Child 2-17 years: 100 mg for 1 dose, if reinfection occurs, second dose may be needed after 2 weeks
- Adult: 100 mg for 1 dose, if reinfection occurs, second dose may be needed after 2 weeks

- **UNLICENSED USE** Not licensed for use as a single dose of 500 mg in roundworm infections.
  Not licensed for use in children under 2 years.
- **INTERACTIONS** → Appendix 1: mebendazole
- **SIDE-EFFECTS**
- **Common or very common** Gastrointestinal discomfort
- **Uncommon** Diarrhoea · flatulence
- **Rare or very rare** Alopecia · dizziness · hepatitis · neutropenia · seizure · severe cutaneous adverse reactions (SCARs) · skin reactions
- **PREGNANCY** Manufacturer advises avoid—toxicity in *animal* studies.
- **BREAST FEEDING** Amount present in milk too small to be harmful but manufacturer advises avoid.
- **PRESCRIBING AND DISPENSING INFORMATION** Flavours of oral liquid formulations may include banana.
- **PATIENT AND CARER ADVICE**
  Medicines for Children leaflet: Mebendazole for worm infections www.medicinesforchildren.org.uk/medicines/mebendazole-for-worm-infections/
- **EXCEPTIONS TO LEGAL CATEGORY** Mebendazole tablets can be sold to the public if supplied for oral use in the treatment of enterobiasis in adults and children over 2 years provided its container or package is labelled to show a max. single dose of 100 mg and it is supplied in a container or package containing not more than 800 mg.

- **MEDICINAL FORMS** There can be variation in the licensing of different medicines containing the same drug.
Oral suspension
- **Vermox** (Janssen-Cilag Ltd)
  Mebendazole 20 mg per 1 ml Vermox 100mg/5ml oral suspension | 30 ml [PoM] £1.55 DT = £1.55

Chewable tablet
- **Vermox** (Janssen-Cilag Ltd)
  Mebendazole 100 mg Vermox 100mg chewable tablets | 6 tablet [PoM] £1.34 DT = £1.34 [SF]

Praziquantel

- **INDICATIONS AND DOSE**

Tapeworm infections (*Taenia solium*)
▸ BY MOUTH
▸ Adult: 5–10 mg/kg for 1 dose, to be taken after a light breakfast

Tapeworm infections (*Hymenolepis nana*)
▸ BY MOUTH
▸ Adult: 25 mg/kg for 1 dose, to be taken after a light breakfast

***Schistosoma haematobium* worm infections | *Schistosoma mansoni* worm infections**
▸ BY MOUTH
▸ Adult: 20 mg/kg, followed by 20 mg/kg after 4–6 hours

***Schistosoma japonicum* worm infections**
▸ BY MOUTH
▸ Adult: 20 mg/kg 3 times a day for 1 day

- **UNLICENSED USE** Praziquantel is an unlicensed drug.

- **INTERACTIONS** → Appendix 1: praziquantel

- **MEDICINAL FORMS** There can be variation in the licensing of different medicines containing the same drug. Forms available from special-order manufacturers include: oral tablet

Oral tablet
▸ Praziquantel (Non-proprietary)
Praziquantel 150 mg Cesol 150mg tablets | 6 tablet PoM ⅀
Praziquantel 600 mg Biltricide 600mg tablets | 6 tablet PoM ⅀

5 Protozoal infection

Antiprotozoal drugs

31-Jan-2025

Amoebicides

Metronidazole p. 628 is the drug of choice for *acute invasive amoebic dysentery* since it is very effective against vegetative forms of *Entamoeba histolytica* in ulcers. Tinidazole is also effective. Metronidazole and tinidazole are also active against amoebae which may have migrated to the liver. Treatment with metronidazole (or tinidazole) is followed by a 10-day course of diloxanide furoate.

Diloxanide furoate is the drug of choice for asymptomatic patients with *E. histolytica* cysts in the faeces; metronidazole and tinidazole are relatively ineffective. Diloxanide furoate is relatively free from toxic effects and the usual course is of 10 days, given alone for chronic infections or following metronidazole or tinidazole treatment.

For *amoebic abscesses* of the liver metronidazole is effective; tinidazole is an alternative. Aspiration of the abscess is indicated where it is suspected that it may rupture or where there is no improvement after 72 hours of metronidazole; the aspiration may need to be repeated. Aspiration aids penetration of metronidazole and, for abscesses with more than 100 mL of pus, if carried out in conjunction with drug therapy, may reduce the period of disability.

Diloxanide furoate is not effective against hepatic amoebiasis, but a 10-day course should be given at the completion of metronidazole or tinidazole treatment to destroy any amoebae in the gut.

Trichomonacides

Metronidazole is the treatment of choice for *Trichomonas vaginalis* infection. Contact tracing is recommended and sexual contacts should be treated simultaneously. If metronidazole is ineffective, tinidazole may be tried.

Antigiardial drugs

Metronidazole is the treatment of choice for *Giardia lamblia* infections. Alternative treatments are tinidazole or mepacrine hydrochloride p. 573.

Leishmaniacides

Cutaneous leishmaniasis frequently heals spontaneously but if skin lesions are extensive or unsightly, treatment is indicated, as it is in visceral leishmaniasis (kala-azar). Leishmaniasis should be treated under specialist supervision.

Sodium stibogluconate, an organic pentavalent antimony compound, is used for visceral leishmaniasis. The dosage varies with different geographical regions and expert advice should be obtained. Some early non-inflamed lesions of cutaneous leishmaniasis can be treated with intralesional injections of sodium stibogluconate under specialist supervision.

Amphotericin B p. 689 is used with or after an antimony compound for visceral leishmaniasis unresponsive to the antimonial alone; side-effects may be reduced by using liposomal amphotericin B.

Pentamidine isetionate p. 698 has been used in antimony-resistant visceral leishmaniasis, but although the initial response is often good, the relapse rate is high; it is associated with serious side-effects. Other treatments include paromomycin [unlicensed] (available from 'special-order' manufacturers or specialist importing companies).

Trypanocides

The prophylaxis and treatment of trypanosomiasis is difficult and differs according to the strain of organism. Expert advice should therefore be obtained.

Toxoplasmosis

Most infections caused by *Toxoplasma gondii* are self-limiting, and treatment is not necessary. Exceptions are patients with eye involvement (toxoplasma choroidoretinitis), and those who are immunosuppressed. Toxoplasmic encephalitis is a common complication of AIDS. The treatment of choice is a combination of pyrimethamine p. 714 and sulfadiazine p. 654, given for several weeks (expert advice **essential**). Pyrimethamine is a folate antagonist, and adverse reactions to this combination are relatively common (folinic acid supplements and weekly blood counts needed). Alternative regimens use combinations of pyrimethamine with clindamycin p. 618 or clarithromycin p. 621 or azithromycin p. 620. Long-term secondary prophylaxis is required after treatment of toxoplasmosis in immunocompromised patients; prophylaxis should continue until immunity recovers.

If toxoplasmosis is acquired in pregnancy, transplacental infection may lead to severe disease in the fetus; specialist advice should be sought on management. Spiramycin [unlicensed] (available from 'special-order' manufacturers or specialist importing companies) may reduce the risk of transmission of maternal infection to the fetus.

5.1 Malaria

Malaria, prophylaxis

18-Apr-2025

Prophylaxis against malaria

The recommendations on prophylaxis reflect guidelines agreed by the UK Malaria Expert Advisory Group (UKMEAG), published in the UKHSA Guidelines for malaria prevention in travellers from the UK, 2024. The advice is aimed at residents of the UK who travel to malaria-endemic areas.

For specialist centres offering advice on specific malaria-related problems, see Malaria, treatment p. 708.

The choice of drug for a particular individual should take into account:

- risk of exposure to malaria
- extent of drug resistance
- efficacy of the recommended drugs
- side-effects of the drugs
- patient-related factors (e.g. age, pregnancy, renal or hepatic impairment, compliance with prophylactic regimen)

For guidance on risk assessment when advising on malaria prevention, see UKHSA: **Guidelines for malaria prevention in travellers from the UK** (see *Useful resources*).

Protection against bites

Prophylaxis is not absolute, and breakthrough infection can occur with any of the drugs recommended. Personal protection against being bitten is very important and is recommended even in malaria-free areas as a preventive measure against other insect vector-borne diseases. Mosquito bed nets impregnated with a pyrethroid insecticide (such as permethrin p. 1404) improve protection and should be used unless sleeping in a well screened room with mosquito netting on windows and doors, or a room with switched on functioning air conditioning that is also sufficiently well sealed, into which mosquitoes cannot enter. The use of plug-in vaporised insecticides are also useful. Long-sleeved clothing, long trousers, and socks also provide protection against bites; clothing may be sprayed or impregnated with an insecticide such as permethrin.

Insect repellents give protection against bites, but attention to the correct application of the product is required. They should only be applied to exposed areas of skin, although some preparations can be sprayed onto clothing. A repellent should still be applied to exposed skin even if clothing has been sprayed or impregnated.

Diethyltoluamide (DEET) is available in various preparations, including sprays and modified-release formulations. A 50% DEET-based insect repellent is recommended as the first choice; there is no further increase in duration of protection beyond a DEET concentration of 50%. DEET is safe and effective when applied to the skin of adults and children over 2 months of age. It can be used during pregnancy and breast-feeding, however, ingestion should be avoided and so breast-feeding mothers should wash their hands and breast tissue before handling infants. DEET can be sprayed onto clothing, but it may damage synthetic fibres. When sunscreen is also required, DEET should be applied after the sunscreen. DEET reduces the SPF of sunscreen, so a sunscreen of SPF 30–50 should be applied. For alternative options if DEET is not tolerated or is unavailable, see UKHSA: **Guidelines for malaria prevention in travellers from the UK** (see *Useful resources*).

Length of prophylaxis

Prophylaxis should generally be started before travel into an endemic area; 1 week before travel for chloroquine p. 710; 2–3 weeks before travel for mefloquine p. 712; and 1–2 days before travel for atovaquone with proguanil hydrochloride p. 710 or doxycycline p. 655. Prophylaxis should be continued for 4 weeks after leaving the area (except for atovaquone with proguanil hydrochloride prophylaxis which should be stopped 1 week after leaving). For extensive journeys across different regions, the traveller must be protected in all areas of risk.

In those requiring long-term prophylaxis, chloroquine may be used, however there is considerable concern over the protective efficacy of chloroquine in certain areas where it was previously useful. Mefloquine is licensed for use up to 1 year (although, if it is tolerated in the short term, there is no evidence of harm when it is used for up to 3 years). Doxycycline can be used for up to 2 years, and atovaquone

with proguanil hydrochloride for up to 1 year. Prophylaxis with mefloquine, doxycycline, or atovaquone with proguanil hydrochloride may be considered for longer durations if it is justified by the risk of exposure to malaria. Specialist advice may be sought for long-term prophylaxis.

Return from malarial region

It is important to consider that any illness that occurs within 1 year and especially within 3 months of return, might be malaria, even if all recommended precautions against malaria were taken. Travellers should be warned of this and told that if they develop any illness after their return they should see a doctor early, and specifically mention their risk of exposure to malaria.

Malaria is a notifiable disease in England, Northern Ireland, and Wales. For further information, see *Notifiable diseases* in Antibacterials, principles of therapy p. 573.

Epilepsy

Both chloroquine and mefloquine are unsuitable for malaria prophylaxis in individuals with a history of epilepsy. In these patients, doxycycline or atovaquone with proguanil hydrochloride may be used. However doxycycline may interact with some antiepileptics and its dose may need to be adjusted, see *interactions* information in the doxycycline drug monograph.

Asplenia

Individuals with asplenia (or those with severe splenic dysfunction) are at particular risk of severe malaria and should avoid travel to malarious areas where possible; if travel to malarious areas is unavoidable, rigorous precautions are required against contracting the disease.

Pregnancy

Travel to malarious areas should be avoided during pregnancy; if travel is unavoidable, pregnant individuals must be informed about the risks and benefits of effective prophylaxis. Chloroquine can be given during all trimesters of pregnancy, but is not appropriate for most areas because its effectiveness has declined due to drug resistance. If travelling to high-risk areas or there is resistance to other drugs, mefloquine may be considered during the second or third trimester of pregnancy. Mefloquine can be used in the first trimester with caution if the benefits outweigh the risks. Doxycycline is contra-indicated during pregnancy, however it can be used for malaria prophylaxis if other regimens are unsuitable and if the entire course of doxycycline can be completed before 15 weeks' gestation [unlicensed]. Atovaquone with proguanil hydrochloride should be avoided during pregnancy, however it can be considered during the second and third trimesters if there is no suitable alternative. Folic acid p. 1161 (dosed as a pregnancy at 'high-risk' of neural tube defects) should be given for the length of time that atovaquone with proguanil hydrochloride is used during pregnancy, and in those planning to become pregnant.

Breast-feeding

Chloroquine and mefloquine are considered safe for use during breast-feeding. Atovaquone with proguanil hydrochloride and doxycycline should generally be avoided but can be used if other antimalarial options are unsuitable.

Prophylaxis is required in breast-fed infants; although antimalarials are present in breast milk, the amounts are too low to give reliable protection.

Anticoagulants

Travellers taking warfarin sodium should begin chemoprophylaxis 2–3 weeks before departure and the INR should be stable before departure. It should be measured before starting chemoprophylaxis, 7 days after starting, and after completing the course. For prolonged stays, the INR should be checked at regular intervals. Some antimalarials may alter the anticoagulant effect of warfarin, see *Interactions* in individual drug monographs for information.

Key to recommended regimens for prophylaxis against malaria

Codes for regimens	Details of regimens for prophylaxis against malaria
-	No risk
1	Chemoprophylaxis not recommended, but avoid mosquito bites and consider malaria if fever presents
2	Chloroquine only
3	Chloroquine or atovaquone with proguanil hydrochloride or doxycycline or mefloquine
4	Atovaquone with proguanil hydrochloride or doxycycline or mefloquine
5	Atovaquone with proguanil hydrochloride or doxycycline

Specific recommendations

Country	Comments on risk of malaria and regional or seasonal variation	Codes for regimens
Afghanistan	Low risk below 2000 m from May–November	1
	Very low risk below 2000 m from December–April	1
Andaman and Nicobar Islands (India)	Low risk	1
Angola	High risk	4
Argentina	No risk	1
Azerbaijan	No risk	1
Bangladesh	High risk in Chittagong Hill Tract districts (but not Chittagong city)	4
	Very low risk in Chittagong city and other areas, except Chittagong Hill Tract districts	1
Belize	No risk	1
Benin	High risk	4
Bhutan	Low risk in southern belt districts, along border with India: Chukha, Geyleg-phug, Samchi, Samdrup Jonkhar, and Shemgang	1
	No risk in areas other than those above	-
Bolivia	Low risk in Amazon basin	1
	Low risk in rural areas below 2500 m (other than above)	1
	No risk above 2500 m	-
Botswana	High risk from November–June in northern half, including Okavango Delta area	4
	Low risk from July–October in northern half, including Okavango Delta area	1
	Very low risk in southern half	1
Brazil	Low risk in Amazon basin, including city of Manaus	1
	Very low risk in areas other than those above	1
	No risk in Iguaçu Falls	-
Brunei Darussalam	Very low risk	1
Burkina Faso	High risk	4
Burundi	High risk	4
Cambodia	Low risk. Mefloquine resistance widespread in western provinces bordering Thailand	1
	Very low risk in Angkor Wat and Lake Tonle Sap, including Siem Reap	1
	No risk in Phnom Penh	-
Cameroon	High risk	4
Cape Verde	No risk	1
Central African Republic	High risk	4
Chad	High risk	4
China	No risk	1
	No risk in Hong Kong	-
Colombia	Low risk in rural areas below 1600 m	1
	Very low risk above 1600 m and in Cartagena	1
Comoros	High risk	4
Congo	High risk	4
Costa Rica	Low risk in Limon province, but not city of Limon (Puerto Limon)	1
	Very low risk in areas other than those above	1

Country	Comments on risk of malaria and regional or seasonal variation	Codes for regimens
Cote d'Ivoire (Ivory Coast)	High risk	4
Democratic Republic of the Congo	High risk	4
Djibouti	High risk	4
Dominican Republic	Low risk	1
	No risk in cities of Santiago and Santo Domingo	-
East Timor (Timor-Leste)	Very low risk	1
Ecuador	Low risk in areas below 1500 m including coastal provinces and Amazon basin	1
	No risk in Galapagos islands or city of Guayaquil	-
Egypt	No risk	1
El Salvador	No risk	1
Equatorial Guinea	High risk	4
Eritrea	High risk below 2200 m	4
	No risk in Asmara or in areas above 2200 m	-
Eswatini	Risk present in the northern and eastern regions bordering Mozambique and South Africa, including all the Lubombo district and Big Bend, Mhlume, Simunye, and Tshaneni regions	4
	Very low risk in areas other than those above	1
Ethiopia	High risk below 2000 m	4
	No risk in Addis Ababa or in areas above 2000 m	-
French Guiana	Risk present (particularly in border areas)	4
	Low risk in city of Cayenne or Devil's Island (Ile du Diable)	1
Gabon	High risk	4
Gambia	High risk	4
Georgia	Very low risk from June–October in rural south east	1
	No risk from November–May in rural south east	-
Ghana	High risk	4
Guatemala	Low risk below 1500 m	1
	No risk in Guatemala City, Antigua, or Lake Atitlan, and in areas above 1500 m	-
Guinea	High risk	4
Guinea-Bissau	High risk	4
Guyana	Risk present in all interior regions	4
	Very low risk in Georgetown and coastal region	1
Haiti	Risk present	3
Honduras	Low risk below 1000 m and in Roatán and other Bay Islands	1
	No risk in San Pedro Sula and Tegucigalpa and areas above 1000 m	-
India	Risk present in states of Assam and Orissa, districts of East Godavari, Srikakulam, Vishakhapatnam, and Vizianagaram in the state of Andhra Pradesh, and districts of Balaghat, Dindori, Mandla, and Seoni in the state of Madhya Pradesh	4
	Low risk in areas other than those above or below (including Goa, Andaman and Nicobar islands)	1
	No risk in Lakshadweep islands	-
Indonesia	High risk in Irian Jaya (Papua)	4
	Low risk in Bali, Lombok, and islands of Java and Sumatra	1
	No risk in city of Jakarta	-
Indonesia (Borneo)	Low risk	1
Iran	Low risk from March–November in rural south eastern provinces and in north, along Azerbaijan border in Ardabil, and near Turkmenistan border in North Khorasan	1
	Very low risk in areas other than those above	1
Iraq	Very low risk from May–November in rural northern area below 1500 m	1
	No risk in areas other than those above	-
Kenya	High risk	4
	Very low risk in city of Nairobi and in the highlands above 2500 m	1

Key to recommended regimens for prophylaxis against malaria

Codes for regimens	Details of regimens for prophylaxis against malaria
-	No risk
1	Chemoprophylaxis not recommended, but avoid mosquito bites and consider malaria if fever presents
2	Chloroquine only
3	Chloroquine or atovaquone with proguanil hydrochloride or doxycycline or mefloquine
4	Atovaquone with proguanil hydrochloride or doxycycline or mefloquine
5	Atovaquone with proguanil hydrochloride or doxycycline

Specific recommendations

Country	Comments on risk of malaria and regional or seasonal variation	Codes for regimens
Lao People's Democratic Republic (Laos)	Low risk	1
	Very low risk in city of Vientiane	1
Liberia	High risk	4
Madagascar	High risk	4
Malawi	High risk	4
Malaysia	Low risk in mainland Malaysia	1
Malaysia (Borneo)	Low risk in inland areas of Sabah and in inland, forested areas of Sarawak	1
	Very low risk in areas other than those above, including coastal areas of Sabah and Sarawak	1
Mali	High risk	4
Mauritania	High risk all year in southern provinces, and from July–October in the northern provinces	4
	Low risk from November–June in the northern provinces	1
Mauritius	No risk	1
Mayotte	Low risk	1
Mexico	Very low risk	1
Mozambique	High risk	4
Myanmar	Risk present at altitudes below 1000 m and on the border area with Thailand	5
Namibia	High risk in regions of Caprivi Strip, Kavango, and Kunene river	4
	Very low risk in areas other than those above	1
Nepal	Low risk below 1500 m, including the Terai district	1
	No risk in city of Kathmandu and on typical Himalayan treks	-
Nicaragua	Low risk	1
	Very low risk in Managua	1
Niger	High risk	4
Nigeria	High risk	4
North Korea	Very low risk in some southern areas	1
Pakistan	Low risk below 2000 m	1
	Very low risk above 2000 m	1
Panama	Low risk east of Canal Zone	1
	Very low risk west of Canal Zone	1
	No risk in Panama City or Canal Zone itself	-
Papua New Guinea	High risk below 1800 m	4
	Very low risk above 1800 m	1
Peru	Low risk in Amazon basin along border with Brazil, particularly in Loreto province and in rural areas below 2000 m including the Amazon basin bordering Bolivia	1
	No risk in city of Lima and coastal region south of Chiclayo	-
Philippines	Low risk in rural areas below 600 m and on islands of Luzon, Mindanao, Mindoro, and Palawan	1
	No risk in cities or on islands of Boracay, Bohol, Catanduanes, Cebu, or Leyte	-

Country	Comments on risk of malaria and regional or seasonal variation	Codes for regimens
Rwanda	High risk	4
São Tomé and Principe	High risk	4
Saudi Arabia	Low risk in south-western provinces along border with Yemen, including below 2000 m in Asir province	1
	No risk in cities of Jeddah, Makkah (Mecca), Medina, Riyadh, and Ta'if, or above 2000 m in Asir province	-
Senegal	High risk	4
Sierra Leone	High risk	4
Singapore	No risk	1
Solomon Islands	High risk	4
Somalia	High risk	4
South Africa	Risk from September–May in low altitude areas of Mpumalanga and Limpopo, particularly those bordering Mozambique, Eswatini, and Zimbabwe, including Kruger National Park	4
	Low risk from September–May in north-east KwaZulu-Natal and in designated areas of Mpumalanga and Limpopo	1
	Very low risk all year in North West Province (adjacent to Molopo river) and Northern Cape Province (adjacent to Orange river); and from June–August in low altitude areas of Mpumalanga and Limpopo, particularly those bordering Mozambique, Eswatini, and Zimbabwe, including Kruger National Park	1
South Korea	Very low risk in northern areas, in Gangwon-do and Gyeonggi-do provinces, and Incheon city (towards Demilitarized Zone)	1
South Sudan	High risk	4
Sri Lanka	No risk	1
Sudan	Risk present in all areas including Khartoum	4
Suriname	Low risk	1
	No risk in city of Paramaribo	-
Syria	Very low risk in small, remote foci of El Hasakah; possibility of additional cases cannot be excluded as up-to-date data not available	1
Tajikistan	No risk	1
Tanzania	High risk below 1800 m; risk also present in Zanzibar	4
	No risk above 1800 m	-
Thailand	Mefloquine resistance present. Low risk in rural forested borders with Cambodia, Laos, and Myanmar	1
	Very low risk in areas other than those above, including Kanchanaburi (Kwai Bridge)	1
	No risk in cities of Bangkok, Chiang Mai, Chiang Rai, Koh Phangan, Koh Samui, and Pattaya	-
Togo	High risk	4
Turkey	Very low risk	1
Uganda	High risk	4
Uzbekistan	No risk	1
Vanuatu	Risk present	4
Venezuela	Risk present (particularly in the Amazonas, Bolívar, Delta Amacuro, and Sucre states)	4
	No risk in city of Caracas or on Margarita Island	1
Vietnam	Low risk in rural areas, and in southern provinces of Tay Ninh, Lam Dong, Dak Lak, Gia Lai, and Kon Tum	1
	No risk in large cities (including Ho Chi Minh City (Saigon) and Hanoi), the Red River delta, coastal areas north of Nha Trang, and Phu Quoc Island	1
Western Sahara	No risk	1
Yemen	Risk present below 2000 m	4
	Very low risk on Socrota Island	1
	No risk above 2000 m, including Sana'a city	1
Zambia	High risk	4
Zimbabwe	High risk all year in Zambezi valley, and from November–June in areas below 1200 m	4
	Low risk from July–October in areas below 1200 m	1
	Very low risk all year in Harare and Bulawayo	1

There is relatively limited experience of chemoprophylaxis in those travellers taking direct-acting oral anticoagulants (DOACs).

Other medical conditions

For additional information on malaria prophylaxis in patients with other medical conditions, see UKHSA: **Guidelines for malaria prevention in travellers from the UK** (see *Useful resources*). Patients already taking hydroxychloroquine sulfate p. 1253 for another indication, and for whom chloroquine would be an appropriate antimalarial, can remain on hydroxychloroquine sulfate.

Emergency standby treatment

Travellers on prophylaxis who are visiting remote, malarious areas should carry standby emergency treatment if they are likely to be more than 24 hours away from medical care. Standby emergency treatment should also be considered in long-term travellers living in or visiting remote, malarious areas that may be far from appropriate medical attention; this does not replace the need to consider prophylaxis. Self-medication should be avoided if medical help is accessible.

In order to use standby treatment appropriately, travellers should be provided with written instructions which include seeking urgent medical attention if fever (38°C or more) develops more than 7 days after arriving in a malarious area, and that self-treatment is indicated if medical help is not available within 24 hours of fever onset.

In view of the continuing emergence of resistant strains and of the different regimens required for different areas, expert advice should be sought on the best treatment course for an individual traveller. A drug used for chemoprophylaxis should not be considered for standby treatment for the same traveller due to concerns over drug resistance and to minimise drug toxicity.

Malaria prophylaxis, specific recommendations

Travellers planning journeys across continents can travel into areas that have different malaria prophylaxis recommendations. The choice of prophylaxis medication must reflect overall risk to ensure protection in all areas; it may be possible to change from one regimen to another. Those travelling to remote or little-visited areas may require expert advice. For further information, see *Recommended regimens for prophylaxis against malaria*, and UKHSA: **Guidelines for malaria prevention in travellers from the UK** (see *Useful resources*).

Some countries not listed in *Recommended regimens for prophylaxis against malaria* may experience occasional instances of malaria transmission. For further guidance, see the National Travel Health Network and Centre (nathnac.net/) or TRAVAX (www.travax.nhs.uk/).

Important

Settled immigrants (or long-term visitors) in the UK may be unaware that any immunity they may have acquired while living in malarious areas is lost rapidly after migration to the UK, or that any non-malarious areas where they lived previously may now be malarious.

Useful resources

UK Health Security Agency: Guidelines for malaria prevention in travellers from the UK. July 2024.

www.gov.uk/government/publications/malaria-prevention-guidelines-for-travellers-from-the-uk

---

Malaria, treatment
03-May-2024

Advice for healthcare professionals

A number of specialist centres are able to provide advice on specific problems.

UKHSA Malaria Reference Laboratory (prophylaxis) www.gov.uk/government/collections/malaria-reference-laboratory-mrl

National Travel Health Network and Centre (NaTHNaC) www.travelhealthpro.org.uk/

TRAVAX (Public Health Scotland) www.travax.nhs.uk (for registered users of the NHS Travax website only)

Hospital for Tropical Diseases (HTD) (treatment) www.uclh.nhs.uk/our-services/find-service/tropical-and-infectious-diseases/htd-guidelines

Liverpool School of Tropical Medicine (LSTM) (treatment) 0151 705 3100 Monday to Friday: 9 a.m.–5 p.m. and via Royal Liverpool Hospital switchboard at all other times 0151 706 2000 www.lstmed.ac.uk/

Birmingham Infectious Diseases and Tropical Medicine 0121 424 2358

Advice for travellers

Hospital for Tropical Diseases travel clinic www.uclh.nhs.uk/our-services/find-service/tropical-and-infectious-diseases/travel-clinic-services

Fitfortravel www.fitfortravel.nhs.uk/home

WHO advice on international travel and health www.who.int/travel-advice

National Travel Health Network and Centre (NaTHNaC) www.travelhealthpro.org.uk/

Treatment of malaria

Malaria is a notifiable disease in England, Northern Ireland, and Wales. For further information, see *Notifiable diseases* in Antibacterials, principles of therapy p. 573.

The recommendations on treatment reflect UK malaria treatment guidelines 2016, agreed by UK malaria specialists. They are aimed for residents of the UK and for use in a non-endemic setting.

Expert advice must be sought in all patients suspected to have malaria. If malaria is diagnosed in a returned traveller, other members of the family or travelling group should be advised that they may have shared the same exposure risk and they should seek medical attention if they develop symptoms.

If the infective species is **not known**, or if the infection is **mixed** and includes falciparum parasites, initial treatment should be as for *falciparum malaria*.

Falciparum malaria

Falciparum malaria is caused by *Plasmodium falciparum*. Patients with falciparum malaria should usually be admitted to hospital initially due to the risk of rapid deterioration even after starting treatment.

Artemisinin combination therapy is recommended for the treatment of uncomplicated *P. falciparum* malaria. Artemether with lumefantrine p. 709 is the drug of choice. Oral quinine p. 713 or atovaquone with proguanil hydrochloride p. 710 can be used if an artemisinin combination therapy is not available. Quinine is highly effective but poorly-tolerated in prolonged treatment and should be used in combination with an additional drug, usually oral doxycycline p. 655 (or clindamycin p. 618 [unlicensed] in pregnant women and young children).

Severe or complicated falciparum malaria should be managed in a high dependency unit or intensive care setting. Intravenous **artesunate** (available for 'named-patient' use from infectious disease units or specialist tropical disease centres) is indicated in all patients with severe or complicated falciparum malaria, or those at high-risk of developing severe disease (such as if more than 2% of red blood cells are parasitized), or if the patient is unable to take oral treatment. Following a minimum of 24 hours of intravenous **artesunate** treatment, and when the patient has improved and is able take oral treatment, a full course of artemisinin combination therapy should be given. A full course of oral quinine with doxycycline (or clindamycin [unlicensed]), or atovaquone with proguanil hydrochloride are suitable alternatives.

Treatment of severe or complicated falciparum malaria should not be delayed whilst obtaining artesunate. Quinine by intravenous infusion [unlicensed] should be given if artesunate is not immediately available; it should be continued until the patient can take oral quinine to complete a full course. Oral doxycycline (or clindamycin [unlicensed]) should also be given when the patient can swallow.

In most parts of the world, *P. falciparum* is now resistant to chloroquine p. 710 which should not therefore be used for treatment. Mefloquine p. 712 is also no longer recommended for treatment because of concerns about adverse effects and non-completion of courses.

Specialist advice should be sought when considering the use of pyrimethamine with sulfadoxine as an alternative drug in combination with quinine.

Pregnancy
Falciparum malaria in pregnancy carries a higher risk of severe disease; it requires prompt treatment by specialists in hospital and close observation. Uncomplicated falciparum malaria in the second and third trimesters of pregnancy should be treated with artemether with lumefantrine below. Quinine with clindamycin [unlicensed indication] can be used in all trimesters. Quinine can increase the risk of uterine contractions and hypoglycemia.

Severe or complicated falciparum malaria is associated with a high risk of fatality, pregnancy loss, and complications. Due to efficacy, treatment with intravenous artesunate in any trimester of pregnancy is preferred; intravenous quinine (with clindamycin) can be used as an alternative.

Non-falciparum malaria
Non-falciparum malaria is usually caused by *Plasmodium vivax* and less commonly by *P. ovale*, *P. malariae*, and *P. knowlesi*. *P. knowlesi* is present in the Asia-Pacific region.

Either an artemisinin combination therapy (such as artemether with lumefantrine below) or chloroquine can be used for the treatment of non-falciparum malaria. Chloroquine-resistant *P. vivax* has been reported in the Indonesian archipelago, the Malay Peninsula, including Myanmar, and eastward to Southern Vietnam. Chloroquine can still be used for treatment of non-falciparum malaria from these regions with appropriate follow-up, however artemisinin combination therapy may be preferred.

Chloroquine alone is adequate for *P. malariae* and *P. knowlesi* infections but in the case of *P. vivax* and *P. ovale*, a *radical cure* (to destroy parasites in the liver and thus prevent relapses) is required. For a radical cure, primaquine p. 713 [unlicensed] is given with chloroquine treatment; the dose is dependent on the infecting organism. Patients should be screened for G6PD deficiency before initiating primaquine treatment, as primaquine may cause haemolysis in G6PD deficient individuals.

Severe or complicated non-falciparum malaria should be treated with parenteral **artesunate** or quinine [unlicensed] as for treatment of severe or complicated falciparum malaria.

Pregnancy
Chloroquine can be given for non-falciparum malaria treatment throughout pregnancy. Artemisinin combination therapy can be used in the second and third trimesters, and quinine may be used in the first trimester if there is concern about chloroquine-resistant *P. vivax*. In the case of *P. vivax* or *P. ovale* however, the radical cure with primaquine should be **postponed** until the pregnancy (and breast-feeding) is over; instead weekly chloroquine prophylaxis should be continued until delivery or completion of breast-feeding.

Artemether with lumefantrine 09-Sep-2021

● **INDICATIONS AND DOSE**

Treatment of acute uncomplicated falciparum malaria | Treatment of chloroquine-resistant non-falciparum malaria

▶ BY MOUTH
▸ Adult (body-weight 35 kg and above): Initially 4 tablets, followed by 4 tablets for 5 doses each given at 8, 24, 36, 48 and 60 hours (total 24 tablets over 60 hours)

● **UNLICENSED USE** Use in treatment of non-falciparum malaria is an unlicensed indication.

● **CONTRA-INDICATIONS** Family history of congenital QT interval prolongation · family history of sudden death · history of arrhythmias · history of clinically relevant bradycardia · history of congestive heart failure accompanied by reduced left ventricular ejection fraction

● **CAUTIONS** Avoid in Acute porphyrias p. 1202 · electrolyte disturbances (correct before and during treatment)

● **INTERACTIONS** → Appendix 1: antimalarials

● **SIDE-EFFECTS**
▸ **Common or very common** Abdominal pain · appetite decreased · arthralgia · asthenia · cough · diarrhoea · dizziness · gait abnormal · headache · movement disorders · myalgia · nausea · palpitations · QT interval prolongation · sensation abnormal · skin reactions · sleep disorders · vomiting
▸ **Uncommon** Drowsiness
▸ **Frequency not known** Angioedema

● **PREGNANCY** Toxicity in *animal* studies with artemether. Manufacturer advises use only if potential benefit outweighs risk.

● **BREAST FEEDING** Manufacturer advises avoid breastfeeding for at least 1 week after last dose. Present in milk in *animal* studies.

● **HEPATIC IMPAIRMENT** Manufacturer advises caution in severe impairment (no information available)—monitor ECG and plasma potassium concentration.

● **RENAL IMPAIRMENT** EvGr Caution in severe impairment (limited information available)—monitor ECG and plasma potassium concentration. Ⓜ

● **MONITORING REQUIREMENTS** Monitor patients unable to take food (greater risk of recrudescence).

● **DIRECTIONS FOR ADMINISTRATION** Manufacturer advises tablets may be crushed just before administration.

● **PATIENT AND CARER ADVICE**
Driving and skilled tasks Dizziness may affect performance of skilled tasks (e.g. driving).

● **MEDICINAL FORMS** There can be variation in the licensing of different medicines containing the same drug.
Oral tablet
CAUTIONARY AND ADVISORY LABELS 21
▸ Riamet (Novartis Pharmaceuticals UK Ltd)
   Artemether 20 mg, Lumefantrine 120 mg Riamet tablets |
   24 tablet PoM £22.50 DT = £22.50

Atovaquone with proguanil hydrochloride

18-Apr-2025

● **INDICATIONS AND DOSE**

Prophylaxis of falciparum malaria, particularly where resistance to other antimalarial drugs suspected [using 250 mg/100 mg tablets]

▸ BY MOUTH
  ▸ Adult (body-weight 40 kg and above): 1 tablet once daily, to be started 1–2 days before entering endemic area and continued for 1 week after leaving

Prophylaxis of falciparum malaria, particularly where resistance to other antimalarial drugs suspected [using 62.5 mg/25 mg tablets]

▸ BY MOUTH
  ▸ Adult (body-weight 30-39 kg): 3 tablets once daily, to be started 1–2 days before entering endemic area and continued for 1 week after leaving

Treatment of acute uncomplicated falciparum malaria [using 250 mg/100 mg tablets] | Treatment of non-falciparum malaria [using 250 mg/100 mg tablets]

▸ BY MOUTH
  ▸ Adult: 4 tablets once daily for 3 days

DOSE EQUIVALENCE AND CONVERSION
  ▸ Each 250 mg/100 mg tablet contains 250 mg of atovaquone and 100 mg of proguanil hydrochloride.
  ▸ Each 62.5 mg/25 mg tablet contains 62.5 mg of atovaquone and 25 mg of proguanil hydrochloride.

● **UNLICENSED USE** Not licensed for treatment of non-falciparum malaria.

● **CAUTIONS** Diarrhoea or vomiting (reduced absorption of atovaquone) · efficacy not evaluated in cerebral or complicated malaria (including hyperparasitaemia, pulmonary oedema or renal failure)

● **INTERACTIONS** → Appendix 1: antimalarials

● **SIDE-EFFECTS**
  ▸ **Common or very common** Abdominal pain · appetite decreased · cough · depression · diarrhoea · dizziness · fever · headache · nausea · skin reactions · sleep disorders · vomiting
  ▸ **Uncommon** Alopecia · anxiety · blood disorder · hyponatraemia · oral disorders · palpitations
  ▸ **Frequency not known** Hallucination · hepatic disorders · photosensitivity reaction · seizure · Stevens-Johnson syndrome · tachycardia · vasculitis

● **PREGNANCY**
  ▸ When used for Prophylaxis of malaria UKHSA advises avoid but may be considered during second and third trimesters if no suitable alternative available. See also *Pregnancy* in Malaria, prophylaxis p. 702.
  ▸ When used for Treatment of malaria EvGr Use only if potential benefit outweighs risk. Ⓜ

● **BREAST FEEDING** Specialist sources indicate use only if no suitable alternative available.

● **RENAL IMPAIRMENT** EvGr Avoid for malaria prophylaxis (and if possible for malaria treatment) if creatinine clearance less than 30 mL/minute, Ⓜ see p. 21.

● **PATIENT AND CARER ADVICE** Warn travellers about **importance** of avoiding mosquito bites, **importance** of taking prophylaxis regularly, and **importance** of immediate visit to doctor if ill within 1 year and **especially** within 3 months of return.

● **NATIONAL FUNDING/ACCESS DECISIONS**

NHS restrictions Drugs for malaria prophylaxis are not prescribable in NHS primary care; health authorities may investigate circumstances under which antimalarials are prescribed.

● **MEDICINAL FORMS** There can be variation in the licensing of different medicines containing the same drug.

Oral tablet

CAUTIONARY AND ADVISORY LABELS 21

▸ **Atovaquone with proguanil hydrochloride (Non-proprietary)**
  Proguanil hydrochloride 25 mg, Atovaquone 62.5 mg Proguanil 25mg / Atovaquone 62.5mg tablets | 12 tablet [PoM] £6.26 DT = £6.26
  Proguanil hydrochloride 100 mg, Atovaquone 250 mg Proguanil 100mg / Atovaquone 250mg tablets | 12 tablet [PoM] £25.21 DT = £25.21

▸ **Malarone** (GlaxoSmithKline UK Ltd)
  Proguanil hydrochloride 25 mg, Atovaquone 62.5 mg Malarone Paediatric 62.5mg/25mg tablets | 12 tablet [PoM] £6.26 DT = £6.26
  Proguanil hydrochloride 100 mg, Atovaquone 250 mg Malarone 250mg/100mg tablets | 12 tablet [PoM] £25.21 DT = £25.21

Chloroquine

16-Apr-2025

● **INDICATIONS AND DOSE**

Active rheumatoid arthritis (administered on expert advice) | Systemic and discoid lupus erythematosus (administered on expert advice)

▸ BY MOUTH USING TABLETS
  ▸ Adult: 155 mg daily; maximum 2.5 mg/kg per day

Prophylaxis of malaria

▸ BY MOUTH USING SYRUP
  ▸ Child (body-weight up to 4.5 kg): 25 mg once weekly, started 1 week before entering endemic area and continued for 4 weeks after leaving
  ▸ Child (body-weight 4.5-7 kg): 50 mg once weekly, started 1 week before entering endemic area and continued for 4 weeks after leaving
  ▸ Child (body-weight 8-10 kg): 75 mg once weekly, started 1 week before entering endemic area and continued for 4 weeks after leaving
  ▸ Child (body-weight 11-14 kg): 100 mg once weekly, started 1 week before entering endemic area and continued for 4 weeks after leaving
  ▸ Child (body-weight 15-16.4 kg): 125 mg once weekly, started 1 week before entering endemic area and continued for 4 weeks after leaving
  ▸ Child (body-weight 16.5-24 kg): 150 mg once weekly, started 1 week before entering endemic area and continued for 4 weeks after leaving
  ▸ Child (body-weight 25-44 kg): 225 mg once weekly, started 1 week before entering endemic area and continued for 4 weeks after leaving
  ▸ Child (body-weight 45 kg and above): 300 mg once weekly, started 1 week before entering endemic area and continued for 4 weeks after leaving
  ▸ Adult (body-weight 45 kg and above): 300 mg once weekly, started 1 week before entering endemic area and continued for 4 weeks after leaving

▸ BY MOUTH USING TABLETS
  ▸ Child (body-weight up to 6 kg): 38.75 mg once weekly, started 1 week before entering endemic area and continued for 4 weeks after leaving
  ▸ Child (body-weight 6-9 kg): 77.5 mg once weekly, started 1 week before entering endemic area and continued for 4 weeks after leaving
  ▸ Child (body-weight 10-15 kg): 116.25 mg once weekly, started 1 week before entering endemic area and continued for 4 weeks after leaving
  ▸ Child (body-weight 16-24 kg): 155 mg once weekly, started 1 week before entering endemic area and continued for 4 weeks after leaving
  ▸ Child (body-weight 25-44 kg): 232.5 mg once weekly, started 1 week before entering endemic area and continued for 4 weeks after leaving

▸ Child (body-weight 45 kg and above): 310 mg once weekly, started 1 week before entering endemic area and continued for 4 weeks after leaving
▸ Adult (body-weight 25–44 kg): 232.5 mg once weekly, started 1 week before entering endemic area and continued for 4 weeks after leaving
▸ Adult (body-weight 45 kg and above): 310 mg once weekly, started 1 week before entering endemic area and continued for 4 weeks after leaving

Treatment of non-falciparum malaria
▸ BY MOUTH
▸ Child: Initially 10 mg/kg (max. per dose 620 mg), then 5 mg/kg after 6–8 hours (max. per dose 310 mg), then 5 mg/kg daily (max. per dose 310 mg) for 2 days
▸ Adult: Initially 620 mg, then 310 mg after 6–8 hours, then 310 mg daily for 2 days, approximate total cumulative dose of 25 mg/kg of base

***P. vivax* or *P. ovale* infection during pregnancy while radical cure is postponed**
▸ BY MOUTH
▸ Adult: 310 mg once weekly

DOSE EQUIVALENCE AND CONVERSION
▸ Doses expressed as chloroquine base.
▸ Each tablet contains 155 mg of chloroquine base (equivalent to 250 mg of chloroquine phosphate). Syrup contains 50 mg/5 mL of chloroquine base (equivalent to 80 mg/5 mL of chloroquine phosphate).

DOSES AT EXTREMES OF BODY-WEIGHT
▸ In adults In active rheumatoid arthritis and systemic and discoid lupus erythematosus, to avoid excessive dosage in obese patients, the daily maximum dose should be calculated on the basis of ideal body weight.

● UNLICENSED USE Chloroquine doses for the treatment and prophylaxis of malaria in BNF Publications may differ from those in product literature.

> IMPORTANT SAFETY INFORMATION
> ▸ In adults
> Ocular toxicity is unlikely if the dose of chloroquine phosphate does not exceed 4 mg/kg daily (equivalent to chloroquine base approx. 2.5 mg/kg daily).
>
> MHRA/CHM ADVICE: HYDROXYCHLOROQUINE, CHLOROQUINE: INCREASED RISK OF CARDIOVASCULAR EVENTS WHEN USED WITH MACROLIDE ANTIBIOTICS; REMINDER OF PSYCHIATRIC REACTIONS (FEBRUARY 2022)
> An observational study has shown that co-administration of azithromycin with hydroxychloroquine in patients with rheumatoid arthritis was associated with an increased risk of cardiovascular events (including angina or chest pain and heart failure) and mortality. Healthcare professionals are reminded to consider the benefits and risks of co-prescribing systemic macrolides with chloroquine because of its similar safety profile to hydroxychloroquine. If such use cannot be avoided, caution is recommended in patients with risk factors for cardiac events and they should be advised to seek urgent medical attention if any signs or symptoms develop.
>
> A European safety review has reported that psychiatric reactions associated with chloroquine (including rare cases of suicidal behaviour) typically occurred within the first month of treatment; events have been reported in patients with no history of psychiatric disorders. Healthcare professionals are reminded to be vigilant for psychiatric reactions, and counsel patients and carers to seek medical advice if any new or worsening mental health symptoms develop.

● CAUTIONS Acute porphyrias p. 1202 · diabetes (may lower blood glucose) · G6PD deficiency · long-term therapy (risk of retinopathy and cardiomyopathy) · may aggravate

myasthenia gravis · may exacerbate psoriasis · neurological disorders, especially epilepsy (may lower seizure threshold)—avoid for prophylaxis of malaria if history of epilepsy · severe gastro-intestinal disorders

● INTERACTIONS → Appendix 1: antimalarials

● SIDE-EFFECTS
▸ **Rare or very rare** Cardiomyopathy · hallucination · hepatitis
▸ **Frequency not known** Abdominal pain · agranulocytosis · alopecia · anxiety · atrioventricular block · behaviour abnormal · bone marrow disorders · concentration impaired · confusion · corneal deposits · delusions · depression · diarrhoea · eye disorders · gastrointestinal disorder · headache · hearing impairment · hypoglycaemia · hypotension · interstitial lung disease · mania · movement disorders · myopathy · nausea · neuromyopathy · neutropenia · photosensitivity reaction · psychiatric disorder · psychosis · QT interval prolongation · seizure · severe cutaneous adverse reactions (SCARs) · skin reactions · sleep disorders · suicidal behaviour · thrombocytopenia · tinnitus · tongue protrusion · vision disorders · vomiting

SIDE-EFFECTS, FURTHER INFORMATION Side-effects which occur at doses used in the prophylaxis or treatment of malaria are generally not serious.

Overdose Chloroquine is very toxic in overdosage; overdosage is extremely hazardous and difficult to treat. Urgent advice from the National Poisons Information Service is essential. Life-threatening features include arrhythmias (which can have a very rapid onset) and convulsions (which can be intractable).

● PREGNANCY
▸ When used for Rheumatic disease in adults EvGr May be continued during pregnancy—no increased risk of adverse fetal outcomes reported, but cannot be completely excluded (limited information available). E
▸ When used for Prophylaxis of malaria or Treatment of malaria UKHSA advises can be used during all trimesters. See also *Pregnancy* in Malaria, prophylaxis p. 702 and Malaria, treatment p. 708.

● BREAST FEEDING
▸ When used for Rheumatic disease in adults EvGr May be used with caution during breast-feeding (very limited information available). Present in milk in small amounts—very long plasma half-life increases risk of accumulation in the infant. Monitor infant for irritability, insomnia, vomiting, diarrhoea, poor feeding, adequate weight gain, and ocular and hearing effects. Avoid in infants with G6PD deficiency, hyperbilirubinaemia, or jaundice (risk of haemolytic anaemia and kernicterus). E
▸ When used for Prophylaxis of malaria EvGr Present in milk but amount probably too small to be harmful. M
▸ When used for Treatment of malaria PHE advises safe for use.

● HEPATIC IMPAIRMENT Manufacturer advises caution, particularly in cirrhosis.

● RENAL IMPAIRMENT Manufacturers advise caution.
  Dose adjustments Only partially excreted by the kidneys and reduction of the dose is not required for prophylaxis of malaria except in severe impairment.
  For rheumatoid arthritis and lupus erythematosus, reduce dose.

● MONITORING REQUIREMENTS
▸ In adults A review group convened by the Royal College of Ophthalmologists has updated guidelines on monitoring for chloroquine and hydroxychloroquine retinopathy (*Hydroxychloroquine and Chloroquine Retinopathy: Recommendations on Monitoring* 2020). Chloroquine appears to be more retinotoxic than hydroxychloroquine. Annual monitoring (including fundus autofluorescence and spectral domain optical coherence tomography) is

recommended in all patients who have taken chloroquine for longer than 1 year.
- In children Expert sources advise ophthalmic examination with long-term therapy.

- **PATIENT AND CARER ADVICE** Warn travellers going to malarious areas about **importance** of avoiding mosquito bites, **importance** of taking prophylaxis regularly, and **importance** of immediate visit to doctor if ill within 1 year and **especially** within 3 months of return.

- **NATIONAL FUNDING/ACCESS DECISIONS**
NHS restrictions Drugs for malaria prophylaxis are not prescribable in NHS primary care; health authorities may investigate circumstances under which antimalarials are prescribed.

- **EXCEPTIONS TO LEGAL CATEGORY** *Tablets* can be sold to the public provided it is licensed and labelled for the prophylaxis of malaria.

- **MEDICINAL FORMS** There can be variation in the licensing of different medicines containing the same drug. Forms available from special-order manufacturers include: oral solution

Oral tablet
CAUTIONARY AND ADVISORY LABELS 5
- Avloclor (Alliance Pharmaceuticals Ltd)
Chloroquine phosphate 250 mg Avloclor 250mg tablets | 20 tablet P £8.59 DT = £8.59

Oral solution
CAUTIONARY AND ADVISORY LABELS 5
- Malarivon (Wallace Manufacturing Chemists Ltd)
Chloroquine phosphate 16 mg per 1 ml Malarivon 80mg/5ml syrup | 75 ml PoM £30.00 DT = £30.00

Mefloquine

18-Apr-2025

- **INDICATIONS AND DOSE**

Treatment of malaria
- BY MOUTH
- Adult: (consult product literature)

Prophylaxis of malaria
- BY MOUTH
- Child (body-weight 5-15 kg): 62.5 mg once weekly, dose to be started 2–3 weeks before entering endemic area and continued for 4 weeks after leaving
- Child (body-weight 16-24 kg): 125 mg once weekly, dose to be started 2–3 weeks before entering endemic area and continued for 4 weeks after leaving
- Child (body-weight 25-44 kg): 187.5 mg once weekly, dose to be started 2–3 weeks before entering endemic area and continued for 4 weeks after leaving
- Child (body-weight 45 kg and above): 250 mg once weekly, dose to be started 2–3 weeks before entering endemic area and continued for 4 weeks after leaving
- Adult (body-weight 25-44 kg): 187.5 mg once weekly, dose to be started 2–3 weeks before entering endemic area and continued for 4 weeks after leaving
- Adult (body-weight 45 kg and above): 250 mg once weekly, dose to be started 2–3 weeks before entering endemic area and continued for 4 weeks after leaving

- **UNLICENSED USE** Mefloquine doses in BNF Publications may differ from those in product literature.
Not licensed for use in children under 5 kg body-weight and under 3 months.

- **CONTRA-INDICATIONS** Avoid for prophylaxis if history of psychiatric disorders (including depression) or convulsions · avoid for standby treatment if history of convulsions · history of blackwater fever

- **CAUTIONS** Cardiac conduction disorders · epilepsy (avoid for prophylaxis) · infants less than 3 months (limited experience) · not recommended in infants under 5 kg · traumatic brain injury

CAUTIONS, FURTHER INFORMATION
- Neuropsychiatric reactions Mefloquine is associated with potentially serious neuropsychiatric reactions. Abnormal dreams, insomnia, anxiety, and depression occur commonly. Psychosis, suicidal ideation, and suicide have also been reported. Psychiatric symptoms such as insomnia, nightmares, acute anxiety, depression, restlessness, or confusion should be regarded as potentially prodromal for a more serious event. Adverse reactions may occur and persist up to several months after discontinuation because mefloquine has a long half-life. For a prescribing checklist, and further information on side-effects, particularly neuropsychiatric side-effects, which may be associated with the use of mefloquine for malaria prophylaxis, see the *Guide for Healthcare Professionals* provided by the manufacturer.

- **INTERACTIONS** → Appendix 1: antimalarials

- **SIDE-EFFECTS**
- **Common or very common** Anxiety · depression · diarrhoea · dizziness · gastrointestinal discomfort · headache · nausea · skin reactions · sleep disorders · vision disorders · vomiting
- **Frequency not known** Acute kidney injury · agranulocytosis · alopecia · aplastic anaemia · appetite decreased · arrhythmias · arthralgia · asthenia · behaviour abnormal · cardiac conduction disorders · cataract · chest pain · chills · concentration impaired · confusion · cranial nerve paralysis · delusional disorder · depersonalisation · drowsiness · dyspnoea · encephalopathy · eye disorder · fever · flushing · gait abnormal · hallucination · hearing impairment · hepatic disorders · hyperacusia · hyperhidrosis · hypertension · hypotension · leucocytosis · leucopenia · malaise · memory loss · mood altered · movement disorders · muscle complaints · muscle weakness · nephritis · nerve disorders · oedema · palpitations · pancreatitis · paraesthesia · pneumonia · pneumonitis · psychosis · seizure · self-endangering behaviour · speech disorder · Stevens-Johnson syndrome · suicidal behaviours · syncope · thrombocytopenia · tinnitus · tremor · vertigo

- **ALLERGY AND CROSS-SENSITIVITY** EvGr Contra-indicated in patients with hypersensitivity to quinine. M

- **CONCEPTION AND CONTRACEPTION** Manufacturer advises adequate contraception during prophylaxis and for 3 months after stopping (teratogenicity in *animal* studies).

- **PREGNANCY**
- When used for Treatment of malaria EvGr Not known to be harmful, M but see also *Pregnancy* in Malaria, treatment p. 708.
- When used for Prophylaxis of malaria UKHSA advises that use may be considered if travelling to high-risk areas or there is resistance to other drugs. See also *Pregnancy* in Malaria, prophylaxis p. 702.

- **BREAST FEEDING** Specialist sources indicate present in milk but amount probably too small to be harmful.

- **HEPATIC IMPAIRMENT** Manufacturer advises avoid in severe impairment—elimination may be prolonged.

- **RENAL IMPAIRMENT** Manufacturer advises caution.

- **DIRECTIONS FOR ADMINISTRATION** Expert sources advise tablet may be crushed and mixed with food such as jam or honey just before administration.

- **PATIENT AND CARER ADVICE** Manufacturer advises that patients receiving mefloquine for malaria prophylaxis should be informed to discontinue its use if neuropsychiatric symptoms occur and seek immediate medical advice so that mefloquine can be replaced with an alternative antimalarial. Travellers should also be warned about **importance** of avoiding mosquito bites, **importance** of taking prophylaxis regularly, and **importance** of immediate visit to doctor if ill within 1 year and especially within 3 months of return.

A patient alert card should be provided.
Driving and skilled tasks Dizziness or a disturbed sense of
balance may affect performance of skilled tasks (e.g.
driving); effects may occur and persist up to several
months after stopping mefloquine.

- **NATIONAL FUNDING/ACCESS DECISIONS**
NHS restrictions Drugs for malaria prophylaxis are not
prescribable in NHS primary care; health authorities may
investigate circumstances under which antimalarials are
prescribed.

- **MEDICINAL FORMS** There can be variation in the licensing of
different medicines containing the same drug.
Oral tablet
CAUTIONARY AND ADVISORY LABELS 10, 21, 27
  ▸ Lariam (Neon Healthcare Ltd)
    Mefloquine (as Mefloquine hydrochloride) 250 mg Lariam 250mg
    tablets | 8 tablet [PoM] £14.53 DT = £14.53

Primaquine

02-Sep-2024

- **INDICATIONS AND DOSE**
**Adjunct in the treatment of non-falciparum malaria
caused by *Plasmodium vivax* infection**
  ▸ BY MOUTH
  ▸ Adult: 30 mg daily for 14 days
**Adjunct in the treatment of non-falciparum malaria
caused by *Plasmodium ovale* infection**
  ▸ BY MOUTH
  ▸ Adult: 15 mg daily for 14 days
**Adjunct in the treatment of non-falciparum malaria
caused by *Plasmodium vivax* infection in patients with
mild G6PD deficiency (administered on expert advice)** |
**Adjunct in the treatment of non-falciparum malaria
caused by *Plasmodium ovale* infection in patients with
mild G6PD deficiency (administered on expert advice)**
  ▸ BY MOUTH
  ▸ Adult: 45 mg once weekly for 8 weeks
**Treatment of mild to moderate pneumocystis infection (in
combination with clindamycin)**
  ▸ BY MOUTH
  ▸ Adult: 30 mg daily

- **UNLICENSED USE** Not licensed.
- **CAUTIONS** G6PD deficiency · systemic diseases associated
with granulocytopenia (e.g. rheumatoid arthritis, lupus
erythematosus)
- **INTERACTIONS** → Appendix 1: antimalarials
- **SIDE-EFFECTS** Arrhythmia · dizziness · gastrointestinal
discomfort · haemolytic anaemia (in G6PD deficiency) ·
leucopenia · methaemoglobinaemia (in NADH
methaemoglobin reductase deficiency) · nausea · QT
interval prolongation · skin reactions · vomiting
- **PREGNANCY** Risk of neonatal haemolysis and
methaemoglobinaemia in third trimester.
- **BREAST FEEDING** No information available; theoretical
risk of haemolysis in G6PD-deficient infants.
- **PRE-TREATMENT SCREENING** Before starting primaquine,
blood should be tested for glucose-6-phosphate
dehydrogenase (G6PD) activity since the drug can cause
haemolysis in G6PD-deficient patients. Specialist advice
should be obtained in G6PD deficiency.

- **MEDICINAL FORMS** There can be variation in the licensing of
different medicines containing the same drug. Forms available
from special-order manufacturers include: oral suspension
Oral tablet
  ▸ Primaquine (Non-proprietary)
    Primaquine (as Primaquine phosphate) 7.5 mg Primaquine 7.5mg
    tablets | 100 tablet [℞]

Primaquine (as Primaquine phosphate) 15 mg Primaquine 15mg
tablets | 100 tablet [PoM] [℞] (Hospital only)

Quinine

27-Jul-2020

- **INDICATIONS AND DOSE**
Nocturnal leg cramps
  ▸ BY MOUTH
  ▸ Adult: 200–300 mg once daily, to be taken at bedtime
Non-falciparum malaria
  ▸ BY INTRAVENOUS INFUSION
  ▸ Adult: 10 mg/kg every 8 hours (max. per dose 700 mg),
    infused over 4 hours, given if patient is unable to take
    oral therapy. Change to oral chloroquine as soon as the
    patient's condition permits, reduce dose to 5–7 mg/kg
    if parenteral treatment is required for more than
    48 hours
Falciparum malaria
  ▸ BY MOUTH
  ▸ Child: 10 mg/kg every 8 hours (max. per dose 600 mg)
    for 7 days, to be given together with or followed by
    either doxycycline (in children over 12 years), or
    clindamycin
  ▸ Adult: 600 mg every 8 hours for 5–7 days, to be given
    together with or followed by either doxycycline or
    clindamycin
  ▸ BY INTRAVENOUS INFUSION
  ▸ Adult: Loading dose 20 mg/kg (max. per dose 1.4 g),
    infused over 4 hours, the loading dose of 20 mg/kg
    should **not** be used if the patient has received quinine
    or mefloquine during the previous 12 hours, then
    maintenance 10 mg/kg every 8 hours (max. per dose
    700 mg) until patient can swallow tablets to complete
    the 7-day course, maintenance dose to be given
    8 hours after the start of the loading dose and infused
    over 4 hours, to be given together with or followed by
    either doxycycline or clindamycin, reduce maintenance
    dose to 5–7 mg/kg if parenteral treatment is required
    for more than 48 hours
Falciparum malaria (in intensive care unit)
  ▸ BY INTRAVENOUS INFUSION
  ▸ Adult: Loading dose 7 mg/kg, infused over 30 minutes,
    followed immediately by 10 mg/kg, infused over
    4 hours, then maintenance 10 mg/kg every 8 hours
    (max. per dose 700 mg) until patient can swallow
    tablets to complete the 7-day course, maintenance
    dose to be given 8 hours after the start of the loading
    dose and infused over 4 hours, to be given together
    with or followed by either doxycycline or clindamycin,
    reduce maintenance dose to 5–7 mg/kg if parenteral
    treatment is required for more than 48 hours

DOSE EQUIVALENCE AND CONVERSION
  ▸ When using quinine for malaria, doses are valid for
    quinine hydrochloride, dihydrochloride, and sulfate;
    they are **not valid** for quinine bisulfate which contains
    a correspondingly smaller amount of quinine.
  ▸ Quinine (anhydrous base) 100 mg = quinine bisulfate
    169 mg; quinine dihydrochloride 122 mg; quinine
    hydrochloride 122 mg; and quinine sulfate 121 mg.
    Quinine bisulfate 300 mg tablets are available but
    provide less quinine than 300 mg of the
    dihydrochloride, hydrochloride, or sulfate.

- **UNLICENSED USE** Injection not licensed.

IMPORTANT SAFETY INFORMATION
**MHRA/CHM ADVICE: REMINDER OF DOSE-DEPENDENT QT-
PROLONGING EFFECTS (NOVEMBER 2017)**
Quinine has been associated with dose-dependent QT-
interval-prolonging effects and should be used with

caution in patients with risk factors for QT prolongation or in those with atrioventricular block—see Cautions for further information.

- **CONTRA-INDICATIONS** Haemoglobinuria · myasthenia gravis · optic neuritis · tinnitus
- **CAUTIONS** Atrial fibrillation (monitor ECG during parenteral treatment) · cardiac disease (monitor ECG during parenteral treatment) · conduction defects (monitor ECG during parenteral treatment) · elderly (monitor ECG during parenteral treatment) · electrolyte disturbance · G6PD deficiency · heart block (monitor ECG during parenteral treatment)
- **INTERACTIONS** → Appendix 1: antimalarials
- **SIDE-EFFECTS** Abdominal pain · agitation · agranulocytosis · angioedema · asthma · atrioventricular conduction changes · bronchospasm · cardiotoxicity · cerebral impairment · coagulation disorders · coma · confusion · death · diarrhoea · dyspnoea · fever · flushing · gastrointestinal disorder · haemoglobinuria · haemolysis · haemolytic uraemic syndrome · headache · hearing impairment · hypersensitivity · loss of consciousness · muscle weakness · myasthenia gravis aggravated · nausea · ocular toxicity · oedema · pancytopenia · photosensitivity reaction · QT interval prolongation · renal impairment · skin reactions · thrombocytopenia · tinnitus · vertigo · vision disorders · vomiting

Overdose Quinine is very toxic in overdosage; life-threatening features include arrhythmias (which can have a very rapid onset) and convulsions (which can be intractable).

For details on the management of poisoning, see Emergency treatment of poisoning p. 1554.

- **PREGNANCY** High doses are teratogenic in *first trimester*, but in malaria benefit of treatment outweighs risk.
- **BREAST FEEDING** Present in milk but not known to be harmful.
- **HEPATIC IMPAIRMENT**
- With oral use Manufacturer advises caution (risk of prolonged half-life).
  Dose adjustments
  - With intravenous use For treatment of malaria in severe impairment, reduce parenteral maintenance dose to 5–7 mg/kg of quinine salt.
  - With oral use Manufacturer advises dose reduction or increased dose interval.
- **RENAL IMPAIRMENT**
  Dose adjustments
  - With intravenous use For treatment of malaria in severe impairment, reduce parenteral maintenance dose to 5–7 mg/kg of quinine salt.
- **MONITORING REQUIREMENTS**
- With intravenous use Monitor blood glucose and electrolyte concentration during parenteral treatment.
- In adults Patients taking quinine for nocturnal leg cramps should be monitored closely during the early stages for adverse effects as well as for benefit.
- **DIRECTIONS FOR ADMINISTRATION** For *intravenous infusion*, expert sources advise give continuously in Glucose 5% or Sodium Chloride 0.9%. To be given over 4 hours.
- **PRESCRIBING AND DISPENSING INFORMATION** Intravenous injection of quinine is so hazardous that it has been superseded by infusion.

- **MEDICINAL FORMS** There can be variation in the licensing of different medicines containing the same drug. Forms available from special-order manufacturers include: oral capsule, oral suspension, oral solution, solution for infusion

Oral tablet
- Quinine (Non-proprietary)
  Quinine sulfate 200 mg Quinine sulfate 200mg tablets | 28 tablet [PoM] £7.61 DT = £4.71
  Quinine bisulfate 300 mg Quinine bisulfate 300mg tablets | 28 tablet [PoM] £50.00 DT = £5.05
  Quinine sulfate 300 mg Quinine sulfate 300mg tablets | 28 tablet [PoM] £3.80 DT = £2.34

5.2 Toxoplasmosis

ANTIPROTOZOALS

Pyrimethamine

13-Jan-2022

- **INDICATIONS AND DOSE**

  Toxoplasmosis in pregnancy (in combination with sulfadiazine and folinic acid)
  - BY MOUTH
  - Adult: 50 mg once daily until delivery

- **CAUTIONS** History of seizures—avoid large loading doses · predisposition to folate deficiency
- **INTERACTIONS** → Appendix 1: antimalarials
- **SIDE-EFFECTS**
  - **Common or very common** Anaemia · diarrhoea · dizziness · headache · leucopenia · nausea · skin reactions · thrombocytopenia · vomiting
  - **Uncommon** Fever
  - **Rare or very rare** Abdominal pain · oral ulceration · pancytopenia · pneumonia eosinophilic · seizure
- **PREGNANCY** Theoretical teratogenic risk in *first trimester* (folate antagonist). Adequate folate supplements should be given to the mother.
- **BREAST FEEDING** Significant amount in milk—avoid administration of other folate antagonists to infant. Avoid breast-feeding during toxoplasmosis treatment.
- **HEPATIC IMPAIRMENT** Manufacturer advises caution (limited information available).
  Dose adjustments Manufacturer advises consider dose reduction.
- **RENAL IMPAIRMENT** Manufacturer advises caution.
- **MONITORING REQUIREMENTS** Blood counts required with prolonged treatment.

- **MEDICINAL FORMS** There can be variation in the licensing of different medicines containing the same drug. Forms available from special-order manufacturers include: oral suspension
Oral tablet
- Daraprim (GlaxoSmithKline UK Ltd)
  Pyrimethamine 25 mg Daraprim 25mg tablets | 30 tablet [PoM] £13.00 DT = £13.00

6 Viral infection

6.1 Coronavirus

COVID-19

17-Apr-2023

Description of condition

COVID-19 is the syndrome caused by a novel coronavirus, SARS-CoV-2, which was originally detected late 2019 in Wuhan, Hubei Province, China. SARS-CoV-2 is primarily transmitted between people through respiratory particles, direct human contact, and contact with contaminated surfaces. A person can be infected when respiratory particles are inhaled, or come into contact with the eyes, nose or mouth.

COVID-19 is predominantly a respiratory illness with a range of symptoms of varying severity. Common symptoms include fever, a new continuous cough, loss or change in sense of smell or taste, loss of appetite, nausea or vomiting, diarrhoea, shortness of breath, fatigue, muscle aches, headache, sore throat, and nasal congestion or rhinorrhoea. Atypical symptoms such as delirium and reduced mobility may present in elderly and immunocompromised individuals, often without a fever. COVID-19 infection varies in severity from asymptomatic or mild upper respiratory tract infection in some individuals, to severe pneumonia and critical disease in others. Patients with COVID-19 may deteriorate rapidly, and life-threatening complications include thromboembolic events, cardiac disease, acute kidney injury, sepsis, septic shock, and acute respiratory and multi-organ failure. Individuals who are older, male, from deprived areas, or from black, Asian and minority ethnic groups are at higher risk of severe disease and death. The risk also increases in pregnancy and in those with obesity, certain underlying co-morbidities, frailty, impaired immunity, or a reduced ability to cough and clear secretions.

After acute infection with COVID-19, individuals may experience prolonged symptoms that persist for more than 4 weeks (known as 'long COVID'). For guidance on the management of 'long COVID', see NICE, SIGN and the Royal College of General Practitioners (RCGP) COVID-19 rapid guideline: **Managing the long-term effects of COVID-19** (available at: www.nice.org.uk/guidance/ng188).

COVID-19 vaccination significantly reduces the risk of infection, hospitalisation, and death. However, fully vaccinated individuals can still become infected with SARS-CoV-2 and transmit the infection to other individuals. For information on vaccination against COVID-19, see COVID-19 vaccines p. 1476.

Management

COVID-19 is a notifiable disease in the UK. For further information, see *Notifiable diseases* in Antibacterials, principles of therapy p. 573.

For guidance on infection prevention and control, and sampling and diagnostics, see the UKHSA collection: **Coronavirus (COVID-19): guidance** (available at: www.gov.uk/government/collections/coronavirus-covid-19-list-of-guidance).

For guidance on the management of COVID-19, see NICE rapid guideline: **Managing COVID-19** (see *Useful resources*).

Drug treatment

Individuals with COVID-19 have an increased risk of venous thromboembolism (VTE). For guidance on the prophylaxis and management of VTE, see NICE rapid guideline: **Managing COVID-19** (see *Useful resources*) and SIGN rapid guideline: **Prevention and management of venous thromboembolism in patients with COVID-19** (available at: www.sign.ac.uk/our-guidelines/prevention-and-management-of-venous-thromboembolism-in-covid-19/).

Dexamethasone p. 786 should be offered to patients with COVID-19 who need supplemental oxygen, or who have a level of hypoxia that requires supplemental oxygen but are unable to have or tolerate it. If dexamethasone is unsuitable or unavailable, either hydrocortisone p. 787 or prednisolone p. 791 can be used.

Other treatment options for patients hospitalised due to COVID-19, or for symptomatic patients who are at high risk of progression to severe disease, include antivirals (such as remdesivir p. 718, molnupiravir p. 716, or nirmatrelvir with ritonavir p. 717); SARS-CoV-2 neutralising monoclonal antibodies (such as sotrovimab p. 716); interleukin-6 inhibitors (such as tocilizumab p. 1258); or a Janus kinase inhibitor (such as baricitinib p. 1262 [unlicensed use]). For further guidance on drug treatments for COVID-19, see NICE rapid guideline: **Managing COVID-19** (see *Useful resources*).

Antibacterials are not recommended for preventing or treating pneumonia if it is likely to be caused by SARS-CoV-2, another virus, or a fungal infection. Empirical antibacterials should be started if a secondary bacterial infection is suspected in patients with COVID-19. For guidance on the management of suspected or confirmed bacterial pneumonia, see Respiratory system infections, antibacterial therapy p. 586.

Antifungals should only be offered for treatment of COVID-19-associated pulmonary aspergillosis (CAPA) if diagnosis is confirmed, or CAPA is suspected and a multidisciplinary team or local protocols support starting treatment.

For guidance on the management of COVID-19 infection in pregnancy, including therapies that should be offered to pregnant or postpartum females with COVID-19, see Royal College of Obstetricians and Gynaecologists, Royal College of Midwives, Royal College of Paediatrics and Child Health, PHE and Public Health Scotland guidance: **Coronavirus (COVID-19) infection in pregnancy** (available at: www.rcog.org.uk/en/guidelines-research-services/guidelines/coronavirus-pregnancy/). Exposure to COVID-19 antivirals in pregnant females should be reported to the UK COVID-19 antivirals in pregnancy registry. For further information, see www.medicinesinpregnancy.org/COVID-19-Antivirals-Pregnancy-Registry/.

For information on the fetal and neonatal risks of exposure to COVID-19 treatments, see UK Teratology Information Service (UKTIS): **Medications used to treat COVID-19 in pregnancy** (available at: www.medicinesinpregnancy.org/bumps/monographs/MEDICATIONS-USED-TO-TREAT-COVID-19-IN-PREGNANCY/).

For breastfeeding advice on drugs that may be used for COVID-19, see UK Drugs in Lactation Advisory Service (UKDILAS) guidance on the Specialist Pharmacy Service website (available at: www.sps.nhs.uk/articles/breastfeeding-with-covid-19-infection/).

Management of COVID-19 symptoms

Patients with a cough should be encouraged to avoid lying on their backs, if possible, because this may make coughing less effective. Cough should be initially managed using simple non-drug measures (such as honey). For cough that is distressing in a patient with COVID-19, consider short-term use of a cough suppressant (such as codeine phosphate or morphine).

Patients with fever should be advised to drink fluids regularly to avoid dehydration, and to take antipyretics (such as paracetamol or ibuprofen) as appropriate (whilst both fever and other symptoms that antipyretics would help treat are present).

Reversible causes of breathlessness (such as pulmonary oedema, pulmonary embolism, chronic obstructive pulmonary disorder, and asthma) should be identified and treated accordingly. When other significant medical pathology has been excluded or further investigation is inappropriate, non-drug management (such as relaxation and breathing techniques, and changing body positioning) may help to manage breathlessness as part of supportive care. If hypoxia is the likely cause of breathlessness, consider a trial of oxygen therapy if appropriate.

Reversible causes of anxiety should be addressed by discussing the patient's concerns. Consider a trial of a benzodiazepine (such as lorazepam) to manage anxiety or agitation.

Reversible causes of delirium should be assessed—see NICE guideline: **Delirium: prevention, diagnosis and management** (available at: www.nice.org.uk/guidance/cg103).

For further guidance on the management of COVID-19 symptoms, and for information on end of life care, see NICE rapid guideline: **Managing COVID-19** (see *Useful resources*).

Useful Resources

COVID-19 rapid guideline: managing COVID-19. National Institute for Health and Care Excellence. NICE guideline 191. March 2023.
www.nice.org.uk/guidance/ng191

ANTIVIRALS › SARS-COV-2 NEUTRALISING MONOCLONAL ANTIBODIES

Sotrovimab
27-Mar-2024

● **DRUG ACTION** Sotrovimab is an engineered human immunoglobulin monoclonal antibody that binds to the spike protein receptor binding domain of SARS-CoV-2, which prevents the virus from entering human cells.

● **INDICATIONS AND DOSE**

COVID-19 in patients who do not require oxygen supplementation and are at an increased risk of severe COVID-19 infection [if nirmatrelvir with ritonavir inappropriate]
▶ BY INTRAVENOUS INFUSION
▸ Adult: 500 mg for 1 dose, to be initiated as soon as possible after diagnosis and within 5 days of symptom onset

● **SIDE-EFFECTS**
▶ **Common or very common** Bronchospasm · hypersensitivity · infusion related reaction · skin reactions

● **PREGNANCY** EvGr Use only if potential benefit outweighs risk—no information available. ◈

● **BREAST FEEDING** Specialist sources indicate use with caution—no information available. Large molecular weight suggests limited excretion into milk. Monitor breast-fed infants for adequate feeding and hypersensitivity reactions.

● **DIRECTIONS FOR ADMINISTRATION** EvGr For *intravenous infusion* (*Xevudy*®), dilute in 50 mL or 100 mL Glucose 5% *or* Sodium Chloride 0.9% and administer over 30 minutes through an in-line 0.2 micron filter. ◈

● **PRESCRIBING AND DISPENSING INFORMATION** Sotrovimab is a biological medicine. Biological medicines must be prescribed and dispensed by brand name, see *Biological medicines* and *Biosimilar medicines*, under Guidance on prescribing p. 1; record the brand name and batch number after each administration.

● **HANDLING AND STORAGE** Store in a refrigerator (2°C–8°C) and protect from light—consult product literature about storage after dilution.

● **NATIONAL FUNDING/ACCESS DECISIONS**
For full details see funding body website
NICE decisions
▶ Nirmatrelvir plus ritonavir, sotrovimab and tocilizumab for treating COVID-19 (updated March 2024) NICE TA878 Recommended with restrictions
Scottish Medicines Consortium (SMC) decisions
▶ Sotrovimab (*Xevudy*®) for the treatment of symptomatic adults and adolescents (aged 12 years and over and weighing at least 40 kg) with acute COVID-19 infection who do require oxygen supplementation and who are at increased risk of progressing to severe COVID infection (March 2023) SMC No. SMC2555 Recommended with restrictions

● **MEDICINAL FORMS** There can be variation in the licensing of different medicines containing the same drug.
Solution for infusion
EXCIPIENTS: May contain Polysorbates
▶ **Xevudy** (GlaxoSmithKline UK Ltd) ▼
Sotrovimab 62.5 mg per 1 ml Xevudy 500mg/8ml concentrate for solution for infusion vials | 1 vial PoM £2,209.00 (Hospital only)

ANTIVIRALS › OTHER

Molnupiravir
25-Apr-2025

● **DRUG ACTION** Molnupiravir (a prodrug) is a ribonucleoside analogue that increases the number of mutations in viral RNA thus preventing multiplication of the virus.

● **INDICATIONS AND DOSE**

COVID-19 in patients who do not require oxygen supplementation and are at an increased risk of severe COVID-19 infection
▶ BY MOUTH
▸ Adult: 800 mg twice daily for 5 days, treatment to be started as soon as possible after diagnosis and within 5 days of symptom onset

---

IMPORTANT SAFETY INFORMATION

MHRA/CHM ADVICE: COVID-19 ANTIVIRALS: REPORTING TO THE UK COVID-19 ANTIVIRALS PREGNANCY REGISTRY (FEBRUARY 2022)

The safety of COVID-19 antiviral treatment, such as molnupiravir, during pregnancy has not been established. The MHRA, in collaboration with the UK Teratology Information Service (UKTIS), is operating the UK COVID-19 Antivirals Pregnancy Registry to collect information about and enable follow-up of reported exposures to COVID-19 antivirals in pregnancy; it is also collecting information on the outcomes of pregnancies, where conception occurred during or shortly after paternal exposure to antiviral treatment.

Healthcare professionals in England, Scotland, and Wales (as well as patients and their partners) are advised to report exposure to molnupiravir during pregnancy or around the time of conception, or of partners on molnupiravir around the time of conception. Healthcare professionals in Northern Ireland cannot currently report on behalf of a pregnant female or their partner but should encourage them to self-report. Since exposure can occur in very early pregnancy before pregnancy is recognised, healthcare professionals are advised to report (or to encourage patients to self-report), even if some time has passed since the end of molnupiravir treatment.

An exposed pregnancy should be reported by telephone to UKTIS—for more information, see the UKTIS Registry website (available at: www.medicinesinpregnancy.org/bumps/COVID-19-Antivirals-Pregnancy-Registry/).

● **SIDE-EFFECTS**
▶ **Common or very common** Diarrhoea · dizziness · nausea
▶ **Uncommon** Headache · skin reactions · vomiting

● **CONCEPTION AND CONTRACEPTION** EvGr Females of childbearing potential should use effective contraception during treatment and for 4 days after last treatment. ◈

● **PREGNANCY** EvGr Avoid—toxicity in *animal* studies. ◈ See also *Important safety information*.

● **BREAST FEEDING** EvGr Avoid during treatment and for 4 days after last treatment—no information available. ◈

● **PATIENT AND CARER ADVICE**
Missed doses If a dose is more than 10 hours late, the missed dose should not be taken and the next dose should be taken at the normal time.

- **NATIONAL FUNDING/ACCESS DECISIONS**
  For full details see funding body website
  NICE decisions
  ▶ Molnupiravir for treating COVID-19 (April 2025) NICE TA1056
  Recommended with restrictions
  Scottish Medicines Consortium (SMC) decisions
  ▶ Molnupiravir (*Lagevrio*®) for the treatment of mild to moderate coronavirus disease 2019 (COVID-19) in adults with a positive SARS-COV-2 diagnostic test and who have at least one risk factor for developing severe illness (April 2025) SMC No. SMC2556 Recommended with restrictions

- **MEDICINAL FORMS** There can be variation in the licensing of different medicines containing the same drug.
  Oral capsule
  CAUTIONARY AND ADVISORY LABELS 9
  ▶ Lagevrio (Merck Sharp & Dohme (UK) Ltd) ▼
    Molnupiravir 200 mg Lagevrio 200mg capsules | 40 capsule [PoM] £590.00

Nirmatrelvir with ritonavir

27-Mar-2024

(PF-07321332 with ritonavir)

The properties listed below are those particular to the combination only. For the properties of the components please consider, ritonavir p. 756.

- **DRUG ACTION** Nirmatrelvir is a peptidomimetic inhibitor of coronavirus 3C-like protease which prevents multiplication of SARS-CoV-2. Ritonavir inhibits CYP3A-mediated metabolism of nirmatrelvir thereby increasing the plasma concentration of nirmatrelvir.

- **INDICATIONS AND DOSE**

  COVID-19 in patients who do not require oxygen supplementation and are at an increased risk of severe COVID-19 infection
  ▶ BY MOUTH
  ▶ Adult: 300 mg (two pink tablets) and 100 mg (one white tablet) twice daily for 5 days, to be initiated as soon as possible after SARS-CoV-2 positive result and within 5 days of symptom onset, for each dose, nirmatrelvir (pink tablets) and ritonavir (white tablet) to be taken together

IMPORTANT SAFETY INFORMATION

MHRA/CHM ADVICE: COVID-19 ANTIVIRALS: REPORTING TO THE UK COVID-19 ANTIVIRALS PREGNANCY REGISTRY (FEBRUARY 2022)

The safety of COVID-19 antiviral treatment, such as nirmatrelvir with ritonavir, during pregnancy has not been established. The MHRA, in collaboration with the UK Teratology Information Service (UKTIS), is operating the UK COVID-19 Antivirals Pregnancy Registry to collect information about and enable follow-up of reported exposures to COVID-19 antivirals in pregnancy; it is also collecting information on the outcomes of pregnancies, where conception occurred during or shortly after paternal exposure to antiviral treatment.

Healthcare professionals in England, Scotland, and Wales (as well as patients and their partners) are advised to report exposure to nirmatrelvir with ritonavir during pregnancy or around the time of conception, or of partners on nirmatrelvir with ritonavir around the time of conception. Healthcare professionals in Northern Ireland cannot currently report on behalf of a pregnant female or their partner but should encourage them to self-report. Since exposure can occur in very early pregnancy before pregnancy is recognised, healthcare professionals are advised to report (or to encourage patients to self-report), even if some time has passed since the end of nirmatrelvir with ritonavir treatment.

An exposed pregnancy should be reported by telephone to UKTIS–for more information, see the UKTIS Registry website (available at: www.medicinesinpregnancy.org/bumps/COVID-19-Antivirals-Pregnancy-Registry/).

MHRA/CHM ADVICE: NIRMATRELVIR WITH RITONAVIR (*PAXLOVID*®): BE ALERT TO THE RISK OF DRUG INTERACTIONS WITH RITONAVIR (NOVEMBER 2023)

There is a risk of harmful interactions with the ritonavir component of *Paxlovid*® due to its potent inhibition of CYP3A4. Healthcare professionals are advised to obtain a detailed patient history of current medicines (including over-the-counter preparations, herbal remedies, and illicit or recreational drug use) and to consult resources, including product literature, for known and potential interactions before prescribing *Paxlovid*®. Patients should be informed of this risk and advised not to change or stop taking any medicines without consulting a healthcare professional.

- **CAUTIONS** Hepatitis · liver enzyme abnormalities · pre-existing liver diseases · uncontrolled or undiagnosed HIV-1 infection

  CAUTIONS, FURTHER INFORMATION
  ▶ HIV-1 infection [EvGr] As nirmatrelvir is co-administered with ritonavir, there may be a risk of developing resistance to HIV protease inhibitors in patients with uncontrolled or undiagnosed HIV-1 infection. [M]

- **INTERACTIONS** → Appendix 1: HIV-protease inhibitors · nirmatrelvir

- **SIDE-EFFECTS**
  ▶ **Common or very common** Diarrhoea · taste altered · vomiting

- **CONCEPTION AND CONTRACEPTION** [EvGr] Effectiveness of combined hormonal contraceptives may be reduced; alternative contraceptive methods or an additional barrier method is recommended during treatment and until completion of one menstrual cycle after stopping treatment. [M]

- **PREGNANCY** [EvGr] Avoid. [M] See also *Important safety information*.

- **BREAST FEEDING** [EvGr] Avoid during treatment and for 7 days after last treatment. [M]

- **HEPATIC IMPAIRMENT** [EvGr] Avoid in severe impairment (no information available). [M]

- **RENAL IMPAIRMENT** [EvGr] Caution in moderate impairment; avoid in severe impairment (increased exposure). [M]
  Dose adjustments [EvGr] Reduce dose to 150 mg nirmatrelvir (one pink tablet) and 100 mg ritonavir (one white tablet) twice daily in moderate impairment. [M]

- **PATIENT AND CARER ADVICE**
  Missed doses If a dose is more than 8 hours late, the missed dose should not be taken and the next dose should be taken at the normal time.

- **NATIONAL FUNDING/ACCESS DECISIONS**
  For full details see funding body website
  NICE decisions
  ▶ Nirmatrelvir plus ritonavir, sotrovimab and tocilizumab for treating COVID-19 (updated March 2024) NICE TA878 Recommended with restrictions
  Scottish Medicines Consortium (SMC) decisions
  ▶ Nirmatrelvir and ritonavir (*Paxlovid*®) for the treatment of COVID-19 in adults who do not require supplemental oxygen and who are at increased risk for progression to severe COVID-19 (updated March 2024) SMC No. SMC2557 Recommended with restrictions

Infection

5

- **MEDICINAL FORMS** There can be variation in the licensing of different medicines containing the same drug.

Form unstated

CAUTIONARY AND ADVISORY LABELS 9

▸ Paxlovid (Pfizer Ltd) ▼

Paxlovid 150mg/100mg tablets | 30 tablet [PoM] [£] DT = £2.50

Remdesivir

28-May-2024

- **DRUG ACTION** Remdesivir is an RNA polymerase inhibitor that disrupts the production of viral RNA, preventing multiplication of SARS-CoV-2.

- **INDICATIONS AND DOSE**

COVID-19 in patients hospitalised with pneumonia and requiring low-flow supplemental oxygen (under close medical supervision)

▸ BY INTRAVENOUS INFUSION

▸ Adult: Loading dose 200 mg for 1 dose, then maintenance 100 mg once daily for up to 5 days in total, treatment should be initiated within 10 days of initial COVID-19 symptoms, consider stopping treatment if continuous deterioration despite 48 hours of mechanical ventilation, course may be repeated if readmitted with COVID-19—consult interim clinical commissioning policy for further details (see *Prescribing and dispensing information*)

COVID-19 in immunocompromised patients hospitalised with pneumonia (under close medical supervision)

▸ BY INTRAVENOUS INFUSION

▸ Adult: Loading dose 200 mg for 1 dose, then maintenance 100 mg once daily for up to 10 days in total following a multidisciplinary assessment, consider stopping treatment if continuous deterioration despite 48 hours of mechanical ventilation, course may be repeated if readmitted with COVID-19—consult interim clinical commissioning policy for further details (see *Prescribing and dispensing information*)

COVID-19 in patients who do not require oxygen supplementation and are at an increased risk of progression to severe COVID-19 infection (under close medical supervision)

▸ BY INTRAVENOUS INFUSION

▸ Adult: Loading dose 200 mg for 1 dose, then maintenance 100 mg once daily for 3 days in total, treatment should be initiated within 7 days of initial COVID-19 symptoms

- **UNLICENSED USE** [EvGr] Remdesivir is used in the doses provided in the BNF for the treatment of COVID-19, Ⓐ but these may differ from those licensed.

IMPORTANT SAFETY INFORMATION

MHRA/CHM ADVICE: COVID-19 ANTIVIRALS: REPORTING TO THE UK COVID-19 ANTIVIRALS PREGNANCY REGISTRY (FEBRUARY 2022)

The safety of COVID-19 antiviral treatment, such as remdesivir, during pregnancy has not been established. The MHRA, in collaboration with the UK Teratology Information Service (UKTIS), is operating the UK COVID-19 Antivirals Pregnancy Registry to collect information about and enable follow-up of reported exposures to COVID-19 antivirals in pregnancy; it is also collecting information on the outcomes of pregnancies, where conception occurred during or shortly after paternal exposure to antiviral treatment.

  Healthcare professionals in England, Scotland, and Wales (as well as patients and their partners) are advised to report exposure to remdesivir during pregnancy or around the time of conception, or of partners on remdesivir around the time of conception. Healthcare

professionals in Northern Ireland cannot currently report on behalf of a pregnant female or their partner but should encourage them to self-report. Since exposure can occur in very early pregnancy before pregnancy is recognised, healthcare professionals are advised to report (or to encourage patients to self-report), even if some time has passed since the end of remdesivir treatment.

  An exposed pregnancy should be reported by telephone to UKTIS—for more information, see the UKTIS Registry website (available at: www.medicinesinpregnancy.org/bumps/COVID-19-Antivirals-Pregnancy-Registry/).

- **INTERACTIONS** → Appendix 1: remdesivir
- **SIDE-EFFECTS**
▸ **Common or very common** Headache · nausea · rash
▸ **Rare or very rare** Hypersensitivity · infusion related reaction
▸ **Frequency not known** Sinus bradycardia

SIDE-EFFECTS, FURTHER INFORMATION Manufacturer advises slower infusion rates, with a maximum infusion time of up to 120 minutes, to prevent signs and symptoms of hypersensitivity. If significant hypersensitivity occurs, discontinue immediately.

- **CONCEPTION AND CONTRACEPTION** Manufacturer advises females of childbearing potential should use effective contraception during treatment.

- **PREGNANCY** [EvGr] Avoid unless potential benefit outweighs risk—no information available. Ⓜ See also *Important safety information*.

- **BREAST FEEDING** Specialist sources indicate use with caution—limited information. Minimal oral absorption expected, but monitor breast-fed infants for adverse reactions such as diarrhoea, rash, hypotension, liver and renal impairment (increased risk of accumulation due to long half-life).

- **HEPATIC IMPAIRMENT** Manufacturer advises caution (no information available)—treatment should not be started if ALT is ≥5 times the upper limit of normal. If ALT increases during treatment, remdesivir may need to be withheld, consult product literature for further information.

- **RENAL IMPAIRMENT** Manufacturer advises avoid if eGFR less than 30 mL/minute/1.73 m^2— *Veklury*® formulation excipient (sulfobutylether beta cyclodextrin sodium) may accumulate. See p. 21.

- **MONITORING REQUIREMENTS**
▸ Manufacturer advises monitor liver function at baseline and periodically during treatment as indicated.
▸ Manufacturer advises monitor eGFR at baseline and periodically during treatment as indicated—severe renal toxicity in *animal* studies.

- **DIRECTIONS FOR ADMINISTRATION** [EvGr] For *intravenous infusion*, reconstitute each vial with 19 mL Water for Injections, then dilute in Sodium Chloride 0.9%; give over 30–120 minutes. Ⓜ For further information on dilution and infusion rates—consult product literature.

- **PRESCRIBING AND DISPENSING INFORMATION** NHS England Interim Clinical Commissioning Policy: Remdesivir for patients hospitalised due to COVID-19 (adults and children 12 years and older) (available at: www.england.nhs.uk/coronavirus/documents/interim-clinical-commissioning-policy-remdesivir-for-patients-hospitalised-due-to-covid-19-adults-and-adolescents-12-years-and-older/).

- **NATIONAL FUNDING/ACCESS DECISIONS**
For full details see funding body website

NICE decisions
▸ **Remdesivir and tixagevimab plus cilgavimab for treating COVID-19 (May 2024)** NICE TA971 Recommended with restrictions

Scottish Medicines Consortium (SMC) decisions

▸ Remdesivir (*Veklury*®) for the treatment of COVID-19 in adults and paediatric patients (May 2024) SMC No. SMC2550 Recommended with restrictions

● **MEDICINAL FORMS** There can be variation in the licensing of different medicines containing the same drug.

Powder for solution for infusion

EXCIPIENTS: May contain Sulfobutylether beta cyclodextrin sodium

▸ **Veklury** (Gilead Sciences Ltd) ▼

Remdesivir 100 mg Veklury 100mg powder for concentrate for solution for infusion vials | 1 vial [PoM] £340.00 (Hospital only)

6.2 Hepatitis

Hepatitis   26-May-2021

Overview

Acute infectious hepatitis is a notifiable disease in the UK. For further information, see *Notifiable diseases* in Antibacterials, principles of therapy p. 573.

Treatment for viral hepatitis should be initiated by a specialist. The management of uncomplicated acute viral hepatitis usually involves symptomatic supportive care. Early treatment of acute hepatitis C may reduce the risk of chronic infection and progression of liver disease. Hepatitis B and hepatitis C viruses are major causes of chronic hepatitis. Active or passive immunisation against hepatitis A and B infections is available, see Hepatitis A vaccine p. 1480 and Hepatitis B vaccine p. 1481.

Chronic hepatitis B

Treatment of chronic hepatitis B infection should be initiated by a specialist.

[EvGr] Entecavir below, peginterferon alfa p. 721, tenofovir alafenamide p. 720, and tenofovir disoproxil p. 751 are options for the treatment of chronic hepatitis B infection.

Entecavir and tenofovir disoproxil can be used in patients with decompensated liver disease. (A)

Other drugs licensed for the treatment of chronic hepatitis B infection include adefovir dipivoxil p. 720 and lamivudine p. 750.

[EvGr] If drug-resistance emerges during treatment, consider switching to, or adding another antiviral drug to which the virus is sensitive; ensure the antiviral drug does not share cross-resistance. (A) Hepatitis B viruses with reduced susceptibility to lamivudine have emerged following extended therapy.

Duration of treatment is dependent on several factors including response (e.g. viral suppression, antigen loss, seroconversion), patient characteristics (e.g. liver disease), and treatment tolerability. [EvGr] Treatment is usually continued long-term in patients with decompensated liver disease. (A)

For information on the treatment of HIV and chronic hepatitis B co-infection, see HIV infection p. 735.

Chronic hepatitis C

Treatment of chronic hepatitis C infection should be initiated by a specialist. Before starting treatment, the genotype of the infecting hepatitis C virus should be determined and the viral load measured as this may affect the choice and duration of treatment. [EvGr] All patients with chronic hepatitis C infection should be assessed for treatment with direct-acting antiviral agents. (A)

Sofosbuvir p. 724 in combination with ribavirin (with or without peginterferon alfa), sofosbuvir with velpatasvir p. 725 (with or without ribavirin), sofosbuvir with velpatasvir and voxilaprevir p. 726, and glecaprevir with pibrentasvir

p. 726 are licensed for the treatment of chronic hepatitis C infection of all genotypes.

Ledipasvir with sofosbuvir p. 724 (with or without ribavirin) is licensed for the treatment of chronic hepatitis C infection of genotypes 1, 3, 4, 5, or 6.

Elbasvir with grazoprevir p. 721 (with or without ribavirin) is licensed for the treatment of chronic hepatitis C infection of genotypes 1 or 4.

Other drugs licensed for the treatment of chronic hepatitis C infection include ribavirin p. 722 in combination with peginterferon alfa, or peginterferon alfa as monotherapy if ribavirin is contra-indicated or not tolerated.

6.3 Hepatitis infections

6.3a Chronic hepatitis B

ANTIVIRALS ⟩ NUCLEOSIDE ANALOGUES

▎Entecavir   11-Aug-2021

● **INDICATIONS AND DOSE**

Chronic hepatitis B in patients with compensated liver disease (with evidence of viral replication, and histologically documented active liver inflammation or fibrosis) not previously treated with nucleoside analogues

▸ BY MOUTH

▸ Adult: 500 micrograms once daily

Chronic hepatitis B in patients with compensated liver disease (with evidence of viral replication, and histologically documented active liver inflammation or fibrosis) and lamivudine-resistance

▸ BY MOUTH

▸ Adult: 1 mg once daily, consider other treatment if inadequate response after 6 months

Chronic hepatitis B in patients with decompensated liver disease

▸ BY MOUTH

▸ Adult: 1 mg once daily

● **CAUTIONS** HIV infection—risk of HIV resistance in patients not receiving 'highly active antiretroviral therapy' · lamivudine-resistant chronic hepatitis B—risk of entecavir resistance

CAUTIONS, FURTHER INFORMATION Manufacturer advises review treatment and consider discontinuation if deterioration in liver function occurs (risk of lactic acidosis)—consult product literature.

● **SIDE-EFFECTS**

▸ **Common or very common** Diarrhoea · dizziness · drowsiness · dyspepsia · fatigue · headache · insomnia · nausea · vomiting

▸ **Uncommon** Alopecia · rash

▸ **Frequency not known** Lactic acidosis

● **CONCEPTION AND CONTRACEPTION** Effective contraception required during treatment.

● **PREGNANCY** Toxicity in *animal* studies—manufacturer advises use only if potential benefit outweighs risk.

● **BREAST FEEDING** Manufacturer advises avoid—present in milk in *animal* studies.

● **RENAL IMPAIRMENT**

Dose adjustments [EvGr] Reduce dose if creatinine clearance less than 50 mL/minute (consult product literature). (M) See p. 21.

- **MONITORING REQUIREMENTS** Monitor liver function tests every 3 months, and viral markers for hepatitis B every 3–6 months during treatment (continue monitoring for at least 1 year after discontinuation—recurrent hepatitis may occur on discontinuation).
- **DIRECTIONS FOR ADMINISTRATION** Manufacturer advises to be taken at least 2 hours before or 2 hours after food.
- **PRESCRIBING AND DISPENSING INFORMATION** Flavours of oral liquid formulations may include orange.
- **PATIENT AND CARER ADVICE** Patients or carers should be counselled on the administration of entecavir tablets and oral solution.
- **NATIONAL FUNDING/ACCESS DECISIONS**
  For full details see funding body website
  NICE decisions
- ▶ Entecavir for the treatment of chronic hepatitis B (August 2008) NICE TA153 Recommended

- **MEDICINAL FORMS** There can be variation in the licensing of different medicines containing the same drug.
  Oral tablet
  - ▶ Entecavir (Non-proprietary)
    Entecavir (as Entecavir monohydrate) 500 microgram Entecavir 500microgram tablets | 30 tablet [PoM] £363.26 DT = £363.26 | 30 tablet [PoM] £363.26 DT = £363.26 (Hospital only)
    Entecavir (as Entecavir monohydrate) 1 mg Entecavir 1mg tablets | 30 tablet [PoM] £363.26 DT = £363.26 | 30 tablet [PoM] £363.26 DT = £363.26 (Hospital only)
  - ▶ Baraclude (Bristol-Myers Squibb Pharmaceuticals Ltd)
    Entecavir (as Entecavir monohydrate) 500 microgram Baraclude 0.5mg tablets | 30 tablet [PoM] £363.26 DT = £363.26
    Entecavir (as Entecavir monohydrate) 1 mg Baraclude 1mg tablets | 30 tablet [PoM] £363.26 DT = £363.26
  Oral solution
  - ▶ Baraclude (Bristol-Myers Squibb Pharmaceuticals Ltd)
    Entecavir (as Entecavir monohydrate) 50 microgram per 1 ml Baraclude 0.05mg/ml oral solution | 210 ml [PoM] £423.80 DT = £423.80 [SF]

ANTIVIRALS > NUCLEOSIDE REVERSE TRANSCRIPTASE INHIBITORS

☞ 744

Tenofovir alafenamide
01-Dec-2020

- **INDICATIONS AND DOSE**
  Chronic hepatitis B (initiated by a specialist)
  - ▶ BY MOUTH
  - ▶ Adult: 25 mg once daily, for duration of treatment—consult product literature

- **CAUTIONS** Decompensated liver disease · HIV co-infection
- **INTERACTIONS** → Appendix 1: tenofovir alafenamide
- **SIDE-EFFECTS**
- ▶ **Common or very common** Abdominal distension · arthralgia
- ▶ **Frequency not known** Hepatitis aggravated (during or following treatment) · nephrotoxicity
- **BREAST FEEDING** Manufacturer advises avoid—present in milk in *animal* studies.
- **HEPATIC IMPAIRMENT** Manufacturer advises caution in decompensated hepatic disease (no information available).
- **PRE-TREATMENT SCREENING** Manufacturer advises HIV antibody testing should be offered to those with unknown HIV-1 status before initiation of treatment.
- **MONITORING REQUIREMENTS** Manufacturer advises monitor liver function tests at repeated intervals during treatment and for at least 6 months after last dose—recurrent hepatitis may occur on discontinuation.
- **PATIENT AND CARER ADVICE**
  Missed doses Manufacturer advises if a dose is more than 18 hours late, the missed dose should not be taken and the next dose should be taken at the normal time.

- **MEDICINAL FORMS** There can be variation in the licensing of different medicines containing the same drug.
  Oral tablet
  CAUTIONARY AND ADVISORY LABELS 21
  - ▶ Vemlidy (Gilead Sciences Ltd)
    Tenofovir alafenamide (as Tenofovir alafenamide fumarate) 25 mg Vemlidy 25mg tablets | 30 tablet [PoM] £325.73 (Hospital only)

ANTIVIRALS > NUCLEOTIDE ANALOGUES

Adefovir dipivoxil
18-Aug-2021

- **INDICATIONS AND DOSE**
  Chronic hepatitis B infection with either compensated liver disease with evidence of viral replication, and histologically documented active liver inflammation and fibrosis, when other treatment not appropriate or decompensated liver disease in combination with another antiviral for chronic hepatitis B that has no cross-resistance to adefovir
  - ▶ BY MOUTH
  - ▶ Adult: 10 mg once daily

- **CAUTIONS** Elderly
  CAUTIONS, FURTHER INFORMATION Manufacturer advises review treatment and consider discontinuation if deterioration in liver function occurs (risk of lactic acidosis)—consult product literature.
- **INTERACTIONS** → Appendix 1: adefovir
- **SIDE-EFFECTS**
- ▶ **Common or very common** Asthenia · diarrhoea · flatulence · gastrointestinal discomfort · headache · nausea · renal impairment · skin reactions · vomiting
- ▶ **Frequency not known** Bone fracture · bone pain · hypophosphataemia · myopathy · nephrotoxicity · osteomalacia · pancreatitis · proximal renal tubulopathy
- **CONCEPTION AND CONTRACEPTION** Effective contraception required during treatment.
- **PREGNANCY** Toxicity in *animal* studies—manufacturer advises use only if potential benefit outweighs risk.
- **BREAST FEEDING** Manufacturer advises avoid—no information available.
- **RENAL IMPAIRMENT** [EvGr] Caution if creatinine clearance less than 30 mL/minute (use only if potential benefit outweighs risk, limited information available); no information available if creatinine clearance less than 10 mL/minute. Ⓜ
  Dose adjustments [EvGr] 10 mg every 48 hours if creatinine clearance 30–50 mL/minute; 10 mg every 72 hours if creatinine clearance 10–30 mL/minute. Ⓜ See p. 21.
- **MONITORING REQUIREMENTS**
- ▶ Monitor liver function tests every 3 months, and viral markers for hepatitis B every 3–6 months during treatment (continue monitoring for at least 1 year after discontinuation—recurrent hepatitis may occur on discontinuation).
- ▶ Monitor renal function before treatment then every 3 months, more frequently in patients receiving nephrotoxic drugs.

- **MEDICINAL FORMS** No licensed medicines listed.

IMMUNOSTIMULANTS > INTERFERONS

Peginterferon alfa
15-Dec-2021

- **DRUG ACTION** Polyethylene glycol-conjugated ('pegylated') derivatives of interferon alfa (**peginterferon alfa-2a** and **peginterferon alfa-2b**) are available; pegylation increases the persistence of the interferon in the blood.

- **INDICATIONS AND DOSE**

PEGASYS®

Combined with ribavirin for chronic hepatitis C | Monotherapy for chronic hepatitis C if ribavirin not tolerated or contra-indicated | Monotherapy for chronic hepatitis B
- ▶ BY SUBCUTANEOUS INJECTION
- ▶ Adult: (consult product literature)

- **CONTRA-INDICATIONS** For contra-indications consult product literature.
- **CAUTIONS** For cautions consult product literature.
- **INTERACTIONS** → Appendix 1: interferons
- **SIDE-EFFECTS**
- ▶ **Common or very common** Alopecia · anaemia · anxiety · appetite abnormal · arrhythmias · arthralgia · arthritis · asthenia · ataxia · behaviour abnormal · breast pain · chest discomfort · chills · concentration impaired · confusion · constipation · cough · crying · dehydration · depression · diarrhoea · dizziness · drowsiness · dry eye · dry mouth · dysphagia · dysphonia · dyspnoea · ear pain · eye discomfort · eye disorders · eye inflammation · feeling abnormal · fever · gastrointestinal discomfort · gastrointestinal disorders · haemolytic anaemia · haemorrhage · hair texture abnormal · headaches · hearing impairment · hyperbilirubinaemia · hypertension · hyperthyroidism · hyperuricaemia · hypotension · hypothyroidism · increased risk of infection · influenza like illness · leucopenia · lymphadenopathy · malaise · memory loss · menstrual cycle irregularities · mood altered · muscle complaints · muscle tone increased · muscle weakness · nail disorder · nasal complaints · nausea · neutropenia · oedema · oral disorders · ovarian disorder · pain · palpitations · photosensitivity reaction · prostatitis · respiratory disorders · sensation abnormal · sepsis · sexual dysfunction · skin reactions · sleep disorders · sweat changes · syncope · taste altered · thirst · throat complaints · thrombocytopenia · tinnitus · tremor · urinary disorders · urine abnormal · vaginal disorder · vasodilation · vertigo · vision disorders · vomiting · weight decreased
- ▶ **Uncommon** Diabetes mellitus · hallucination · hypersensitivity · hypertriglyceridaemia · myocardial infarction · nerve disorders · pancreatitis · psychosis · sarcoidosis · suicidal behaviours · thyroiditis
- ▶ **Rare or very rare** Angioedema · bone marrow disorders · cardiac inflammation · cardiomyopathy · cerebral ischaemia · CNS haemorrhage · coma · congestive heart failure · diabetic ketoacidosis · embolism and thrombosis · encephalopathy · facial paralysis · injection site necrosis · interstitial lung disease · ischaemic heart disease · myopathy · renal failure · retinopathy · seizure (more common with high doses in the elderly) · severe cutaneous adverse reactions (SCARs) · systemic lupus erythematosus (SLE) · ulcerative colitis · vasculitis
- ▶ **Frequency not known** Homicidal ideation · pericardial effusion · peripheral ischaemia · pulmonary arterial hypertension · pulmonary fibrosis · pure red cell aplasia · solid organ transplant rejection · tongue discolouration

- **CONCEPTION AND CONTRACEPTION** Effective contraception required during treatment—consult product literature.

- **PREGNANCY** Manufacturers recommend avoid unless potential benefit outweighs risk (toxicity in *animal* studies).
- **BREAST FEEDING** Manufacturers advise avoid—no information available.
- **HEPATIC IMPAIRMENT** Manufacturer advises avoid in severe impairment and decompensated cirrhosis.
- **RENAL IMPAIRMENT**
Dose adjustments See p. 21.
  Manufacturer advises reduce dose if creatinine clearance less than 30 mL/minute (consult product literature).
- **MONITORING REQUIREMENTS** Monitoring of lipid concentration is recommended.
- **NATIONAL FUNDING/ACCESS DECISIONS**
For full details see funding body website
NICE decisions
- ▶ **Peginterferon alfa and ribavirin for the treatment of chronic hepatitis C (September 2010)** NICE TA200 Recommended with restrictions

- **MEDICINAL FORMS** There can be variation in the licensing of different medicines containing the same drug.
Solution for injection
EXCIPIENTS: May contain Benzyl alcohol
- ▶ **Pegasys** (pharmaand GmbH)
Interferon alfa-2a (as Peginterferon alfa-2a) 180 microgram per 1 ml Pegasys 90micrograms/0.5ml solution for injection pre-filled syringes | 1 pre-filled disposable injection PoM £76.51 (Hospital only)
Interferon alfa-2a (as Peginterferon alfa-2a) 270 microgram per 1 ml Pegasys 135micrograms/0.5ml solution for injection pre-filled syringes | 1 pre-filled disposable injection PoM £107.76 (Hospital only)
Interferon alfa-2a (as Peginterferon alfa-2a) 360 microgram per 1 ml Pegasys 180micrograms/0.5ml solution for injection pre-filled syringes | 4 pre-filled disposable injection PoM £497.60 (Hospital only)

6.3b Chronic hepatitis C

ANTIVIRALS > HCV INHIBITORS

Elbasvir with grazoprevir
16-Aug-2022

- **DRUG ACTION** Elbasvir is an HCV NS5A inhibitor and grazoprevir is an HCV NS3/4A protease inhibitor; they reduce viral load by inhibiting hepatitis C virus RNA replication.

- **INDICATIONS AND DOSE**

Chronic hepatitis C infection of genotypes 1 or 4 [with or without ribavirin] (initiated by a specialist)
- ▶ BY MOUTH
- ▶ Adult: 50/100 mg once daily for 12 weeks (may extend to 16 weeks in some circumstances—consult product literature)

DOSE EQUIVALENCE AND CONVERSION
- ▶ Dose expressed as *x/y* mg of elbasvir/grazoprevir.

IMPORTANT SAFETY INFORMATION
MHRA/CHM ADVICE: DIRECT-ACTING ANTIVIRALS TO TREAT CHRONIC HEPATITIS C: RISK OF INTERACTION WITH VITAMIN K ANTAGONISTS AND CHANGES IN INR (JANUARY 2017)
An EU-wide review has identified that changes in liver function, secondary to hepatitis C treatment with direct-acting antivirals, may affect the efficacy of vitamin K antagonists; the MHRA has advised that INR should be

Infection
5

monitored closely in patients receiving concomitant treatment.

MHRA/CHM ADVICE: DIRECT-ACTING ANTIVIRAL INTERFERON-FREE REGIMENS TO TREAT CHRONIC HEPATITIS C: RISK OF HEPATITIS B REACTIVATION (JANUARY 2017)

An EU-wide review has concluded that direct-acting antiviral interferon-free regimens for chronic hepatitis C can cause hepatitis B reactivation in patients co-infected with hepatitis B and C viruses; the MHRA recommends to screen patients for hepatitis B before starting treatment—patients infected with both hepatitis B and C viruses must be monitored and managed according to current clinical guidelines.

MHRA/CHM ADVICE: DIRECT-ACTING ANTIVIRALS FOR CHRONIC HEPATITIS C: RISK OF HYPOGLYCAEMIA IN PATIENTS WITH DIABETES (DECEMBER 2018)

Rapid reduction in hepatitis C viral load during direct-acting antiviral therapy for hepatitis C may improve glucose metabolism in patients with diabetes and result in symptomatic hypoglycaemia if diabetic treatment is continued at the same dose.

The MHRA advises healthcare professionals:
- to monitor glucose levels closely in patients with diabetes during direct-acting antiviral therapy for hepatitis C, especially within the first 3 months of treatment and modify diabetic medication or doses when necessary;
- to be vigilant for changes in glucose tolerance and advise patients of the risk of hypoglycaemia;
- to inform the healthcare professional in charge of the diabetic care of the patient when direct-acting antiviral therapy is initiated.

- **CAUTIONS** Hepatitis B co-infection · re-treatment following previous exposure to elbasvir with grazoprevir, or to drugs of the same classes (NS5A inhibitors or NS3/4A inhibitors other than telaprevir, simeprevir, boceprevir)—efficacy not demonstrated

- **INTERACTIONS** → Appendix 1: elbasvir · grazoprevir

- **SIDE-EFFECTS**
▶ **Common or very common** Alopecia · anxiety · appetite decreased · arthralgia · asthenia · constipation · depression · diarrhoea · dizziness · dry mouth · gastrointestinal discomfort · headache · insomnia · irritability · myalgia · nausea · pruritus · vomiting
▶ **Frequency not known** Anaemia · hepatitis B reactivation · transient ischaemic attack

- **PREGNANCY** Manufacturer advises use only if potential benefit outweighs risk.

- **BREAST FEEDING** Manufacturer advises avoid—present in milk in *animal* studies.

- **HEPATIC IMPAIRMENT** Manufacturer advises avoid in moderate to severe impairment.

- **MONITORING REQUIREMENTS** Manufacturer advises monitor liver function before treatment, at week 8 in all patients, at week 12 in patients receiving 16 weeks of treatment, and then as clinically indicated—consider discontinuing treatment if alanine aminotransferase (ALT) is greater than 10 times the upper limit of normal; discontinue treatment if ALT elevation is accompanied by signs or symptoms of hepatic impairment or inflammation.

- **PATIENT AND CARER ADVICE**
Hepatic effects Patients and their carers should consult a healthcare professional if signs and symptoms of hepatic dysfunction occur (including fatigue, weakness, lack of appetite, nausea and vomiting, jaundice or discoloured faeces).
Vomiting If vomiting occurs within 4 hours of a dose, an additional dose should be taken.

Missed doses If a dose is more than 16 hours late, the missed dose should not be taken and the next dose should be taken at the normal time.

- **NATIONAL FUNDING/ACCESS DECISIONS**
For full details see funding body website
NICE decisions
▶ **Elbasvir–grazoprevir for treating chronic hepatitis C (October 2016) NICE TA413** Recommended
Scottish Medicines Consortium (SMC) decisions
▶ **Elbasvir with grazoprevir (*Zepatier*®) for chronic hepatitis C (January 2017) SMC No. 1203/17** Recommended

- **MEDICINAL FORMS** There can be variation in the licensing of different medicines containing the same drug.
Oral tablet
CAUTIONARY AND ADVISORY LABELS 3
ELECTROLYTES: May contain Sodium
▶ **Zepatier** (Merck Sharp & Dohme (UK) Ltd)
Elbasvir 50 mg, Grazoprevir 100 mg Zepatier 50mg/100mg tablets
| 28 tablet [PoM] £12,166.67

ANTIVIRALS > NUCLEOSIDE ANALOGUES

Ribavirin

20-Nov-2020

(Tribavirin)

- **INDICATIONS AND DOSE**
Bronchiolitis
▶ BY INHALATION OF AEROSOL, OR BY INHALATION OF NEBULISED SOLUTION
▶ Child 1-23 months: Inhale a solution containing 20 mg/mL for 12–18 hours for at least 3 days, maximum of 7 days, to be administered via small particle aerosol generator

Life-threatening RSV, parainfluenza virus, and adenovirus infection in immunocompromised children (administered on expert advice)
▶ BY INTRAVENOUS INFUSION
▶ Child: 33 mg/kg for 1 dose, to be administered over 15 minutes, then 16 mg/kg every 6 hours for 4 days, then 8 mg/kg every 8 hours for 3 days

COPEGUS ® TABLETS

Chronic hepatitis C (in combination with direct acting antivirals, or interferon alfa 2a, or peginterferon alfa 2a with or without direct acting antivirals)
▶ BY MOUTH
▶ Adult (body-weight up to 75 kg): 400 mg, dose to be taken in the morning and 600 mg, dose to be taken in the evening
▶ Adult (body-weight 75 kg and above): 600 mg twice daily

Chronic hepatitis C (in combination with peginterferon alfa 2b with or without direct acting antivirals)
▶ BY MOUTH
▶ Adult (body-weight up to 65 kg): 400 mg twice daily
▶ Adult (body-weight 65-80 kg): 400 mg, to be taken in the morning and 600 mg, to be taken in the evening
▶ Adult (body-weight 81-105 kg): 600 mg twice daily
▶ Adult (body-weight 106 kg and above): 600 mg, to be taken in the morning and 800 mg, to be taken in the evening

Chronic hepatitis C genotype 2 or 3 (not previously treated), or patients infected with HIV and hepatitis C (in combination with peginterferon alfa)
▶ BY MOUTH
▶ Adult: Usual dose 400 mg twice daily

REBETOL ® CAPSULES

Chronic hepatitis C (in combination with interferon alfa 2b, or peginterferon alfa 2b with or without boceprevir)
▶ BY MOUTH
▶ Adult (body-weight up to 65 kg): 400 mg twice daily
▶ Adult (body-weight 65–80 kg): 400 mg, dose to be taken in the morning and 600 mg, dose to be taken in the evening
▶ Adult (body-weight 81–104 kg): 600 mg twice daily
▶ Adult (body-weight 105 kg and above): 600 mg, dose to be taken in the morning and 800 mg, dose to be taken in the evening

● UNLICENSED USE
▶ When used by inhalation Inhalation licensed for use in children (age range not specified by manufacturer).
▶ With intravenous use Intravenous preparation not licensed.

● CONTRA-INDICATIONS
▶ With systemic use Consult product literature for specific contra-indications when ribavirin used in combination with other medicinal products · haemoglobinopathies · severe cardiac disease (in adults) · severe, uncontrolled cardiac disease in children with chronic hepatitis C · unstable or uncontrolled cardiac disease in previous 6 months (in adults)

● CAUTIONS
▶ When used by inhalation Maintain standard supportive respiratory and fluid management therapy
▶ With systemic use Anaemia (haemoglobin concentration should be monitored during the treatment and corrective action taken) (in adults) · cardiac disease (assessment including ECG recommended before and during treatment—discontinue if deterioration) · consult product literature for specific cautions when ribavirin used in combination with other medicinal products · gout (in adults) · haemolysis (haemoglobin concentration should be monitored during the treatment and corrective action taken) (in adults) · patients with a transplant—risk of rejection · risk of growth retardation in children, the reversibility of which is uncertain—if possible, consider starting treatment after pubertal growth spurt · severe dental disorders (in adults) · severe ocular disorders (in adults) · severe periodontal disorders (in adults) · severe psychiatric effects (in adults)

● INTERACTIONS → Appendix 1: ribavirin

● SIDE-EFFECTS
▶ **Common or very common** Alopecia · anaemia · anxiety · appetite decreased · arrhythmias · arthralgia · arthritis · asthenia · behaviour abnormal · chest pain · chills · concentration impaired · constipation · cough · depression · diarrhoea · dizziness · drowsiness · dry mouth · dysphagia · dyspnoea · ear pain · eye disorders · eye inflammation · eye pain · fever · gastrointestinal discomfort · gastrointestinal disorders · haemorrhage · headaches · hyperthyroidism · hypotension · hypothyroidism · increased risk of infection · influenza like illness · lymphadenopathy · malaise · memory loss · mood altered · muscle complaints · muscle weakness · nasal congestion · nausea · neutropenia · oral disorders · pain · palpitations · peripheral oedema · photosensitivity reaction · respiratory disorders · sensation abnormal · sexual dysfunction · skin reactions · sleep disorders · sweat changes · syncope · taste altered · thirst · throat pain · thrombocytopenia · tinnitus · tremor · vasodilation · vertigo · vision disorders · vomiting · weight decreased
▶ **Uncommon** Dehydration · diabetes mellitus · hallucination · hearing loss · hepatic disorders · hypertension · nerve disorders · sarcoidosis · suicidal behaviours · thyroiditis
▶ **Rare or very rare** Angina pectoris · angioedema · bone marrow disorders · cardiac inflammation · cerebral ischaemia · cholangitis · coma · congestive heart failure ·

facial paralysis · hepatic failure (discontinue) · hypersensitivity · interstitial pneumonitis · intracranial haemorrhage · myocardial infarction · myopathy · pancreatitis · psychotic disorder · pulmonary embolism · retinopathy · seizure · severe cutaneous adverse reactions (SCARs) · systemic lupus erythematosus (SLE) · vasculitis
▶ **Frequency not known** Haemolytic anaemia · homicidal ideation · nephrotic syndrome · pure red cell aplasia · renal failure · solid organ transplant rejection · tongue discolouration · ulcerative colitis

SIDE-EFFECTS, FURTHER INFORMATION Side effects listed are reported when oral ribavirin is used in combination with peginterferon alfa or interferon alfa, consult product literature for details.

● CONCEPTION AND CONTRACEPTION
▶ With systemic use Exclude pregnancy before treatment in females of childbearing age. Effective contraception essential during treatment and for 4 months after treatment in females and for 7 months after treatment in males of childbearing age. Routine monthly pregnancy tests recommended. Condoms must be used if partner of male patient is pregnant (ribavirin excreted in semen).
▶ When used by inhalation Women planning pregnancy should avoid exposure to aerosol.

● PREGNANCY Avoid; teratogenicity in *animal* studies.
▶ When used by inhalation Pregnant women should avoid exposure to aerosol.

● BREAST FEEDING Avoid—no information available.

● RENAL IMPAIRMENT Plasma-ribavirin concentration increased.
▶ In adults Manufacturer advises avoid oral ribavirin unless essential if eGFR less than 50 mL/minute/1.73 m^2— monitor haemoglobin concentration closely.
▶ In children Manufacturer advises use intravenous preparation with caution if estimated glomerular filtration rate less than 30 mL/minute/1.73 m^2.

● MONITORING REQUIREMENTS
▶ When used by inhalation Monitor electrolytes closely. Monitor equipment for precipitation.
▶ With systemic use in adults Determine full blood count, platelets, electrolytes, glucose, serum creatinine, liver function tests and uric acid before starting treatment and then on weeks 2 and 4 of treatment, then as indicated clinically—adjust dose if adverse reactions or laboratory abnormalities develop (consult product literature).

● PRESCRIBING AND DISPENSING INFORMATION Flavours of oral liquid formulations may include bubble-gum.

● NATIONAL FUNDING/ACCESS DECISIONS
For full details see funding body website
NICE decisions
▶ **Peginterferon alfa and ribavirin for the treatment of chronic hepatitis C (September 2010)** NICE TA200 Recommended with restrictions

● LESS SUITABLE FOR PRESCRIBING Ribavirin inhalation is less suitable for prescribing.

● MEDICINAL FORMS There can be variation in the licensing of different medicines containing the same drug.
Oral tablet
CAUTIONARY AND ADVISORY LABELS 21
▶ Ribavirin (Non-proprietary)
   Ribavirin 200 mg Ribavirin 200mg tablets | 42 tablet PoM £92.50 | 112 tablet PoM £246.65 | 168 tablet PoM £369.98
Oral capsule
CAUTIONARY AND ADVISORY LABELS 21
▶ Ribavirin (Non-proprietary)
   Ribavirin 200 mg Ribavirin 200mg capsules | 84 capsule PoM £160.69 | 140 capsule PoM £267.81 | 168 capsule PoM £321.38

ANTIVIRALS > NUCLEOTIDE ANALOGUES

Ledipasvir with sofosbuvir
08-Mar-2023

The properties listed below are those particular to the combination only. For the properties of the components please consider, sofosbuvir below.

- **DRUG ACTION** Sofosbuvir is a nucleotide analogue inhibitor and ledipasvir is an HCV inhibitor; they reduce viral load by inhibiting hepatitis C virus RNA replication.

- **INDICATIONS AND DOSE**

Chronic hepatitis C infection (under expert supervision)
- BY MOUTH
- Adult: 90/400 mg once daily, for treatment duration—consult product literature

DOSE ADJUSTMENTS DUE TO INTERACTIONS
- Manufacturer advises reduce dose of concurrent H_2-receptor antagonist if above a dose comparable to famotidine 40 mg twice daily.
- Manufacturer advises reduce dose of concurrent proton pump inhibitor if above a dose comparable to omeprazole 20 mg; take at the same time as sofosbuvir with ledipasvir.

DOSE EQUIVALENCE AND CONVERSION
- Dose expressed as x/y mg ledipasvir/sofosbuvir.

- **CAUTIONS** Retreatment following treatment failure—efficacy not established

- **INTERACTIONS** → Appendix 1: ledipasvir · sofosbuvir

- **SIDE-EFFECTS**
- **Common or very common** Fatigue · headache · rash
- **Frequency not known** Angioedema · hepatitis B reactivation · Stevens-Johnson syndrome

- **DIRECTIONS FOR ADMINISTRATION** Granules may be swallowed or mixed with non-acidic soft food that is at or below room temperature, and swallowed within 30 minutes without chewing.

- **PRESCRIBING AND DISPENSING INFORMATION** Dispense tablets in original container (contains desiccant).

- **PATIENT AND CARER ADVICE** Patients or carers should be given advice on how to administer granules.
Vomiting If vomiting occurs within 5 hours of administration, an additional dose should be taken.
Missed doses If a dose is more than 18 hours late, the missed dose should not be taken and the next dose should be taken at the normal time.

- **NATIONAL FUNDING/ACCESS DECISIONS**
For full details see funding body website

NICE decisions
- **Ledipasvir–sofosbuvir for treating chronic hepatitis C (November 2015)** NICE TA363 Recommended with restrictions

Scottish Medicines Consortium (SMC) decisions
- **Ledipasvir with sofosbuvir (*Harvoni*®) for the treatment of chronic hepatitis C (CHC) in adults (March 2015)** SMC No. 1030/15 Recommended with restrictions
- **Ledipasvir with sofosbuvir (*Harvoni*®) for the treatment of genotype 3 chronic hepatitis C (CHC) in adults (September 2015)** SMC No. 1084/15 Recommended with restrictions

- **MEDICINAL FORMS** There can be variation in the licensing of different medicines containing the same drug.

Oral tablet
CAUTIONARY AND ADVISORY LABELS 25
- Harvoni (Gilead Sciences Ltd)
Ledipasvir 45 mg, Sofosbuvir 200 mg Harvoni 45mg/200mg tablets | 28 tablet PoM £12,993.33 (Hospital only)
Ledipasvir 90 mg, Sofosbuvir 400 mg Harvoni 90mg/400mg tablets | 28 tablet PoM £12,993.33 (Hospital only)

Oral granules
CAUTIONARY AND ADVISORY LABELS 25
- Harvoni (Gilead Sciences Ltd)
Ledipasvir 33.75 mg, Sofosbuvir 150 mg Harvoni 33.75mg/150mg granules sachets | 28 sachet PoM £12,993.33 (Hospital only) SF
Ledipasvir 45 mg, Sofosbuvir 200 mg Harvoni 45mg/200mg granules sachets | 28 sachet PoM £12,993.33 (Hospital only) SF

Sofosbuvir
22-Mar-2023

- **INDICATIONS AND DOSE**

Chronic hepatitis C infection (under expert supervision)
- BY MOUTH
- Adult: 400 mg once daily, for duration of treatment—consult product literature

IMPORTANT SAFETY INFORMATION

MHRA/CHM ADVICE: DIRECT-ACTING ANTIVIRALS TO TREAT CHRONIC HEPATITIS C: RISK OF INTERACTION WITH VITAMIN K ANTAGONISTS AND CHANGES IN INR (JANUARY 2017)
An EU-wide review has identified that changes in liver function, secondary to hepatitis C treatment with direct-acting antivirals, may affect the efficacy of vitamin K antagonists; the MHRA has advised that INR should be monitored closely in patients receiving concomitant treatment.

MHRA/CHM ADVICE: DIRECT-ACTING ANTIVIRAL INTERFERON-FREE REGIMENS TO TREAT CHRONIC HEPATITIS C: RISK OF HEPATITIS B REACTIVATION (JANUARY 2017)
An EU-wide review has concluded that direct-acting antiviral interferon-free regimens for chronic hepatitis C can cause hepatitis B reactivation in patients co-infected with hepatitis B and C viruses; the MHRA recommends to screen patients for hepatitis B before starting treatment—patients infected with both hepatitis B and C viruses must be monitored and managed according to current clinical guidelines.

MHRA/CHM ADVICE: DIRECT-ACTING ANTIVIRALS FOR CHRONIC HEPATITIS C: RISK OF HYPOGLYCAEMIA IN PATIENTS WITH DIABETES (DECEMBER 2018)
Rapid reduction in hepatitis C viral load during direct-acting antiviral therapy for hepatitis C may improve glucose metabolism in patients with diabetes and result in symptomatic hypoglycaemia if diabetic treatment is continued at the same dose.
The MHRA advises healthcare professionals:
- to monitor glucose levels closely in patients with diabetes during direct-acting antiviral therapy for hepatitis C, especially within the first 3 months of treatment and modify diabetic medication or doses when necessary;
- to be vigilant for changes in glucose tolerance and advise patients of the risk of hypoglycaemia;
- to inform the healthcare professional in charge of the diabetic care of the patient when direct-acting antiviral therapy is initiated.

- **INTERACTIONS** → Appendix 1: sofosbuvir

- **SIDE-EFFECTS**
- **Common or very common** Alopecia · anaemia · anxiety · appetite decreased · arthralgia · asthenia · chest pain · chills · concentration impaired · constipation · cough · depression · diarrhoea · dizziness · dry mouth · dyspnoea · fever · gastrointestinal discomfort · gastrooesophageal reflux disease · headaches · influenza like illness · insomnia · irritability · memory loss · muscle complaints · nasopharyngitis · nausea · neutropenia · pain · skin reactions · vision blurred · vomiting · weight decreased
- **Frequency not known** Hepatitis B reactivation · Stevens-Johnson syndrome

SIDE-EFFECTS, FURTHER INFORMATION Side-effects listed are reported when sofosbuvir is used in combination with ribavirin or with ribavirin and peginterferon alfa.

- **PREGNANCY** Manufacturer advises avoid—limited information available.

- **BREAST FEEDING** Manufacturer advises avoid—present in milk in *animal* studies.

- **RENAL IMPAIRMENT** See p. 21. [EvGr] Caution if eGFR less than 30 mL/minute/1.73 m^2 (accumulation may occur; limited information available). ⟨M⟩

- **DIRECTIONS FOR ADMINISTRATION** Granules may be swallowed or mixed with non-acidic soft food that is at or below room temperature, and swallowed within 30 minutes without chewing.

- **PATIENT AND CARER ADVICE** Patients or carers should be given advice on how to administer granules.
  Vomiting If vomiting occurs within 2 hours of administration, an additional dose should be taken.
  Missed doses If a dose is more than 18 hours late, the missed dose should not be taken and the next dose should be taken at the normal time.
  Driving and skilled tasks Patients and carers should be cautioned on the effects on driving and performance of skilled tasks—increased risk of dizziness, impaired concentration, and blurred vision.

- **NATIONAL FUNDING/ACCESS DECISIONS**
  For full details see funding body website
  NICE decisions
  ▸ Sofosbuvir for treating chronic hepatitis C [with peginterferon alfa and ribavirin for adults with genotype 1, 3, 4, 5, or 6; with ribavirin for adults with genotype 2 or 3] (February 2015) NICE TA330 Recommended with restrictions
  ▸ Sofosbuvir for treating chronic hepatitis C [with ribavirin for adults with genotype 1, 4, 5, or 6] (February 2015) NICE TA330 Not recommended
  Scottish Medicines Consortium (SMC) decisions
  ▸ Sofosbuvir (*Sovaldi*®) in combination with other medicinal products for the treatment of chronic hepatitis C (CHC) in adults (June 2014) SMC No. 964/14 Recommended with restrictions

- **MEDICINAL FORMS** There can be variation in the licensing of different medicines containing the same drug.
  Oral tablet
  CAUTIONARY AND ADVISORY LABELS 21, 25
  ▸ **Sovaldi** (Gilead Sciences Ltd)
  Sofosbuvir 200 mg Sovaldi 200mg tablets | 28 tablet [PoM] £11,660.98 (Hospital only)
  Sofosbuvir 400 mg Sovaldi 400mg tablets | 28 tablet [PoM] £11,660.98 (Hospital only)
  Oral granules
  CAUTIONARY AND ADVISORY LABELS 21, 25
  ▸ **Sovaldi** (Gilead Sciences Ltd)
  Sofosbuvir 150 mg Sovaldi 150mg granules sachets | 28 sachet [PoM] £11,660.98 (Hospital only) [SF]
  Sofosbuvir 200 mg Sovaldi 200mg granules sachets | 28 sachet [PoM] £11,660.98 (Hospital only) [SF]

Sofosbuvir with velpatasvir

22-Mar-2023

The properties listed below are those particular to the combination only. For the properties of the components please consider, sofosbuvir p. 724.

- **DRUG ACTION** Sofosbuvir is a nucleotide analogue inhibitor and velpatasvir is an HCV inhibitor; they reduce viral load by inhibiting hepatitis C virus RNA replication.

- **INDICATIONS AND DOSE**
  Chronic hepatitis C infection (under expert supervision)
  ▸ BY MOUTH
  ▸ Adult: 400/100 mg once daily for 12 weeks (may extend to 24 weeks in some circumstances—consult product literature)
  DOSE ADJUSTMENTS DUE TO INTERACTIONS
  ▸ Manufacturer advises reduce dose of concurrent H$_2$-receptor antagonist if above a dose comparable to famotidine 40 mg twice daily.
  ▸ Manufacturer advises reduce dose of concurrent proton pump inhibitor if above a dose comparable to omeprazole 20 mg; take 4 hours after sofosbuvir with velpatasvir.
  DOSE EQUIVALENCE AND CONVERSION
  ▸ Dose expressed as x/y mg sofosbuvir/velpatasvir.

- **INTERACTIONS** → Appendix 1: sofosbuvir · velpatasvir

- **SIDE-EFFECTS**
  ▸ **Common or very common** Rash
  ▸ **Uncommon** Angioedema
  ▸ **Frequency not known** Fatigue · headache · hepatitis B reactivation · nausea · Stevens-Johnson syndrome

- **DIRECTIONS FOR ADMINISTRATION** Granules may be swallowed or mixed with non-acidic soft food that is at or below room temperature, and swallowed within 15 minutes without chewing.

- **PATIENT AND CARER ADVICE** Patients or carers should be given advice on how to administer granules.
  Vomiting If vomiting occurs within 3 hours of administration, an additional dose should be taken.
  Missed doses If a dose is more than 18 hours late, the missed dose should not be taken and the next dose should be taken at the normal time.

- **NATIONAL FUNDING/ACCESS DECISIONS**
  For full details see funding body website
  NICE decisions
  ▸ Sofosbuvir–velpatasvir for treating chronic hepatitis C (January 2017) NICE TA430 Recommended
  Scottish Medicines Consortium (SMC) decisions
  ▸ Sofosbuvir with velpatasvir (*Epclusa*®) for the treatment of chronic hepatitis C virus (HCV) infection in adults [with genotype 3 chronic HCV infection] (November 2016) SMC No. 1195/16 Recommended with restrictions
  ▸ Sofosbuvir with velpatasvir (*Epclusa*®) for the treatment of chronic hepatitis C virus (HCV) infection in adults [with genotype 2, 5 or 6 chronic HCV infection, or decompensated cirrhosis, irrespective of chronic HCV genotype] (October 2017) SMC No. 1271/17 Recommended with restrictions
  ▸ Sofosbuvir with velpatasvir (*Epclusa*®) for the treatment of chronic hepatitis C virus (HCV) infection in adults [with genotype 1 or 4 chronic HCV infection] (April 2018) SMC No. 1271/17 Recommended with restrictions

- **MEDICINAL FORMS** There can be variation in the licensing of different medicines containing the same drug.
  Oral tablet
  CAUTIONARY AND ADVISORY LABELS 25
  ▸ **Epclusa** (Gilead Sciences Ltd)
  Velpatasvir 50 mg, Sofosbuvir 200 mg Epclusa 200mg/50mg tablets | 28 tablet [PoM] £12,993.33 (Hospital only)
  Velpatasvir 100 mg, Sofosbuvir 400 mg Epclusa 400mg/100mg tablets | 28 tablet [PoM] £12,993.33 (Hospital only)

Oral granules

CAUTIONARY AND ADVISORY LABELS 25

▶ **Epclusa** (Gilead Sciences Ltd)
Velpatasvir 37.5 mg, Sofosbuvir 150 mg Epclusa 150mg/37.5mg granules sachets | 28 sachet [PoM] £12,993.33 (Hospital only) [SF]
Velpatasvir 50 mg, Sofosbuvir 200 mg Epclusa 200mg/50mg granules sachets | 28 sachet [PoM] £12,993.33 (Hospital only) [SF]

Sofosbuvir with velpatasvir and voxilaprevir

10-Nov-2020

The properties listed below are those particular to the combination only. For the properties of the components please consider, sofosbuvir p. 724.

● **INDICATIONS AND DOSE**

Chronic hepatitis C infection (specialist use only)
▶ BY MOUTH
▶ **Adult:** 1 tablet once daily, for duration of treatment, consult product literature

DOSE ADJUSTMENTS DUE TO INTERACTIONS
▶ Manufacturer advises reduce dose of concurrent H$_2$-receptor antagonist if above a dose comparable to famotidine 40 mg twice daily.
▶ Manufacturer advises reduce dose of concurrent proton pump inhibitor if above a dose comparable to omeprazole 20 mg.

● **CAUTIONS** Hepatitis B co-infection

● **INTERACTIONS** → Appendix 1: sofosbuvir · velpatasvir · voxilaprevir

● **SIDE-EFFECTS**
▶ **Common or very common** Abdominal pain · appetite decreased · diarrhoea · headache · muscle complaints · nausea · rash · vomiting
▶ **Uncommon** Angioedema
▶ **Frequency not known** Hepatitis B reactivation · Stevens-Johnson syndrome

● **HEPATIC IMPAIRMENT** Manufacturer advises avoid in moderate to severe impairment.

● **PATIENT AND CARER ADVICE**
Vomiting Manufacturer advises if vomiting occurs within 4 hours of administration, an additional dose should be taken.

● **NATIONAL FUNDING/ACCESS DECISIONS**
For full details see funding body website
NICE decisions
▶ Sofosbuvir–velpatasvir–voxilaprevir for treating chronic hepatitis C (February 2018) NICE TA507 Recommended with restrictions

Scottish Medicines Consortium (SMC) decisions
▶ Sofosbuvir with velpatasvir and voxilaprevir (*Vosevi*®) for the treatment of chronic hepatitis C virus (HCV) infection in adults (April 2018) SMC No. 1317/18 Recommended with restrictions

● **MEDICINAL FORMS** There can be variation in the licensing of different medicines containing the same drug.
Oral tablet
CAUTIONARY AND ADVISORY LABELS 21, 25

▶ **Vosevi** (Gilead Sciences Ltd)
Velpatasvir 100 mg, Voxilaprevir 100 mg, Sofosbuvir 400 mg Vosevi 400mg/100mg/100mg tablets | 28 tablet [PoM] £14,942.33

Glecaprevir with pibrentasvir

08-Dec-2021

● **INDICATIONS AND DOSE**

Chronic hepatitis C (specialist use only)
▶ BY MOUTH
▶ **Adult:** 300/120 mg once daily, for duration of treatment, consult product literature

DOSE EQUIVALENCE AND CONVERSION
▶ Dose expressed as x/y mg glecaprevir/pibrentasvir.

IMPORTANT SAFETY INFORMATION
HEPATITIS B INFECTION
Cases of hepatitis B reactivation, sometimes fatal, have been reported in patients co-infected with hepatitis B and C viruses; manufacturer advises to assess patients for hepatitis B prior to initiation of therapy and manage according to current clinical guidelines.

MHRA/CHM ADVICE: DIRECT-ACTING ANTIVIRALS TO TREAT CHRONIC HEPATITIS C: RISK OF INTERACTION WITH VITAMIN K ANTAGONISTS AND CHANGES IN INR (JANUARY 2017)
An EU-wide review has identified that changes in liver function, secondary to hepatitis C treatment with direct-acting antivirals, may affect the efficacy of vitamin K antagonists; the MHRA has advised that INR should be monitored closely in patients receiving concomitant treatment.

MHRA/CHM ADVICE: DIRECT-ACTING ANTIVIRALS FOR CHRONIC HEPATITIS C: RISK OF HYPOGLYCAEMIA IN PATIENTS WITH DIABETES (DECEMBER 2018)
Rapid reduction in hepatitis C viral load during direct-acting antiviral therapy for hepatitis C may improve glucose metabolism in patients with diabetes and result in symptomatic hypoglycaemia if diabetic treatment is continued at the same dose.
The MHRA advises healthcare professionals:
● to monitor glucose levels closely in patients with diabetes during direct-acting antiviral therapy for hepatitis C, especially within the first 3 months of treatment and modify diabetic medication or doses when necessary;
● to be vigilant for changes in glucose tolerance and advise patients of the risk of hypoglycaemia;
● to inform the healthcare professional in charge of the diabetic care of the patient when direct-acting antiviral therapy is initiated.

● **CAUTIONS** Hepatitis B infection · post-liver transplant patients · re-treatment of patients with prior exposure to NS3/4A- or NS5A-inhibitors—efficacy not established

● **INTERACTIONS** → Appendix 1: glecaprevir · pibrentasvir

● **SIDE-EFFECTS**
▶ **Common or very common** Asthenia · diarrhoea · headache · nausea
▶ **Uncommon** Angioedema
▶ **Frequency not known** Hepatitis B reactivation · pruritus · transient ischaemic attack

● **PREGNANCY** Manufacturer advises avoid—limited information available.

● **BREAST FEEDING** Manufacturer advises avoid—present in milk in *animal* studies.

● **HEPATIC IMPAIRMENT** Manufacturer advises avoid in moderate to severe impairment (risk of increased exposure).

● **PATIENT AND CARER ADVICE**
Missed doses Manufacturer advises if a dose is more than 18 hours late, the missed dose should not be taken and the next dose should be taken at the normal time.

- **NATIONAL FUNDING/ACCESS DECISIONS**
  For full details see funding body website
  NICE decisions
  ▸ Glecaprevir–pibrentasvir for treating chronic hepatitis C (January 2018) NICE TA499 Recommended with restrictions
  Scottish Medicines Consortium (SMC) decisions
  ▸ Glecaprevir with pibrentasvir (*Maviret*®) for the treatment of chronic hepatitis C virus (HCV) infection in adults (November 2017) SMC No. 1278/17 Recommended

- **MEDICINAL FORMS** There can be variation in the licensing of different medicines containing the same drug.
  Oral tablet
  CAUTIONARY AND ADVISORY LABELS 21, 25
  ▸ **Glecaprevir with pibrentasvir (Non-proprietary)**
    Pibrentasvir 40 mg, Glecaprevir 100 mg Glecaprevir 100mg / Pibrentasvir 40mg tablets | 84 tablet [PoM] £12,993.66 (Hospital only)

6.3c Chronic hepatitis D

ANTIVIRALS

Bulevirtide
28-Jun-2023

- **DRUG ACTION** Bulevirtide is a sodium-bile acid co-transporter inhibitor which binds to sodium-taurocholate co-transporting polypeptide thereby blocking the entry of hepatitis B virus and hepatitis D virus into hepatocytes.

- **INDICATIONS AND DOSE**
  Chronic hepatitis D infection with compensated liver disease (initiated by a specialist)
  ▸ BY SUBCUTANEOUS INJECTION
  ▸ Adult: 2 mg every 24 hours, consider discontinuation of treatment if sustained hepatitis B surface antigen seroconversion after 6 months or loss of virological and biochemical response

- **CONTRA-INDICATIONS** Decompensated liver disease

- **CAUTIONS** Co-infection with hepatitis B, hepatitis C or HIV · hepatitis exacerbation upon discontinuation of treatment—monitor liver function and hepatitis B and hepatitis D viral load

- **INTERACTIONS** → Appendix 1: bulevirtide

- **SIDE-EFFECTS**
  ▸ **Common or very common** Arthralgia · dizziness · eosinophilia · fatigue · headache · influenza like illness · nausea · pruritus

- **PREGNANCY** [EvGr] Avoid—no information available. ⓜ

- **BREAST FEEDING** [EvGr] Avoid—no information available. ⓜ

- **RENAL IMPAIRMENT** [EvGr] Caution (increased risk of elevated bile salts). ⓜ

- **MONITORING REQUIREMENTS** [EvGr] Monitor renal function. ⓜ

- **DIRECTIONS FOR ADMINISTRATION** [EvGr] Usual sites for subcutaneous injection are the upper thigh or abdomen. ⓜ
  Patients may self-administer *Hepcludex*®, after appropriate training in subcutaneous injection technique.

- **HANDLING AND STORAGE** Store in a refrigerator (2-8°C) and protect from light—consult product literature for storage conditions after preparation of the injection.

- **PATIENT AND CARER ADVICE**
  Missed doses If a dose is more than 4 hours late, the missed dose should not be taken and the next dose should be taken at the normal time.
  Driving and skilled tasks Patients and carers should be counselled on the effects on driving and performance of skilled tasks—increased risk of dizziness.

- **NATIONAL FUNDING/ACCESS DECISIONS**
  For full details see funding body website
  NICE decisions
  ▸ Bulevirtide for treating chronic hepatitis D (June 2023) NICE TA896 Recommended with restrictions
  Scottish Medicines Consortium (SMC) decisions
  ▸ Bulevirtide (*Hepcludex*®) for the treatment of chronic hepatitis delta virus (HDV) infection in plasma (or serum) HDV-RNA positive adult patients with compensated liver disease (March 2023) SMC No. SMC2520 Recommended with restrictions

- **MEDICINAL FORMS** There can be variation in the licensing of different medicines containing the same drug.
  Powder for solution for injection
  ▸ **Hepcludex** (Gilead Sciences Ltd) ▼
    Bulevirtide (as Bulevirtide acetate) 2 mg Hepcludex 2mg powder for solution for injection vials | 30 vial [PoM] £6,500.00 (Hospital only)

6.4 Herpesvirus infections

Herpesvirus infections
30-Jan-2023

Herpes simplex infections

Herpes infection of the mouth and lips and in the eye is generally associated with herpes simplex virus serotype 1 (HSV-1); other areas of the skin may also be infected, especially in immunodeficiency. Genital infection is most often associated with HSV-2 and also HSV-1.

[EvGr] Topical antiviral treatment is not routinely recommended in immunocompetent individuals with uncomplicated infection of the lips (herpes labialis or cold sores) or herpetic gingivostomatitis. However, some patients may find application of a topical antiviral drug helpful when used from the onset of the prodromal phase. Oral paracetamol p. 507 and/or ibuprofen p. 1302 may be given to relieve pain and fever. Other preparations that may be considered for symptom relief include topical anaesthetics or analgesics, and mouthwashes. Oral antiviral treatment may be considered in patients with severe, frequent or persistent oral infection.

Primary or recurrent genital herpes simplex infection is treated with an antiviral drug given by mouth.

Individuals suspected of having ocular herpes simplex infection should be referred for urgent, same-day specialist referral; treatment should not be initiated whilst awaiting review. If same-day review is not possible, specialist advice should be sought, which may include topical antiviral treatment in primary care. Some optometrists with appropriate expertise and training can initiate topical antiviral treatment in certain suspected cases.

Refer or seek specialist advice for treatment of herpes simplex infection in pregnancy. Ⓐ

Varicella-zoster infections

Varicella (chickenpox) is an acute disease caused by the varicella-zoster virus. [EvGr] Specialist advice should be sought on the management of chickenpox in neonates due to the higher risk of severe disease and complications. Chickenpox in otherwise healthy children is usually self-limiting and complications are rare; antiviral treatment is not routinely recommended.

Chickenpox is more severe in adolescents (aged 14 years and over) and adults than in children; antiviral treatment started within 24 hours of the onset of rash may be considered, particularly for those with severe infection or at risk of complications. Specialist advice should be sought on the diagnosis and management of chickenpox in immunocompromised patients. Ⓐ

Pregnant females who develop severe chickenpox may be at risk of complications, especially varicella pneumonia. [EvGr] Immediate specialist advice should be sought for the treatment of chickenpox during pregnancy. ⒶⒶ

Herpes zoster (shingles) is a viral infection of an individual nerve and the skin surface affected by the nerve. The infection is caused by the reactivation of the varicella-zoster virus, the same virus that causes chickenpox. [EvGr] Oral antiviral treatment should be offered to patients with shingles who are immunocompromised, have non-truncal involvement (e.g. neck, limbs, perineum), or to those with moderate to severe pain or rash. Consider oral antiviral treatment for patients aged over 50 years to reduce the risk of post-herpetic neuralgia. Treatment with the antiviral should be started within 72 hours of the onset of rash. Immunocompromised patients with severe or widespread infection, or severely immunocompromised patients, or patients with shingles in the ophthalmic distribution of the trigeminal nerve, should be admitted to hospital or specialist advice should be sought. ⒶⒶ

Chronic pain which persists after the rash has healed (post-herpetic neuralgia) requires specific management. For further information, see Neuropathic pain p. 547.

The risk and incidence of varicella-zoster infections can be reduced through vaccination of selected individuals. For further information, see Varicella-zoster vaccines p. 1495.

Post-exposure prophylaxis

UKHSA recommends post-exposure prophylaxis to attenuate disease and reduce the risk of complications (such as pneumonitis) in individuals at increased risk of severe chickenpox, such as neonates (especially in the first 7 days of life), children aged under one year, pregnant females, and immunosuppressed individuals, who have had a significant exposure to varicella-zoster virus during the infectious period and who are susceptible to the virus.

Post-exposure prophylaxis with aciclovir p. 729 [unlicensed use] is recommended for at risk individuals, except for certain susceptible neonates and for individuals for whom antivirals are contra-indicated or otherwise unsuitable (e.g. if there are significant concerns about renal impairment or intestinal malabsorption), where varicella-zoster immunoglobulin p. 1469 (VZIG) is recommended instead. Prophylactic intravenous aciclovir [unlicensed use] should also be considered in addition to VZIG for neonates whose mothers develop chickenpox 4 days before and up to 2 days after delivery, as they are at the highest risk of fatal outcome despite VZIG prophylaxis. Valaciclovir p. 731 [unlicensed use] can be used as an alternative to aciclovir as appropriate. Individuals on long term aciclovir or valaciclovir prophylaxis may require their dose to be temporarily increased. For further information on risk assessment and post-exposure guidance for specific risk groups, see UKHSA guidance: **Guidelines on post exposure prophylaxis (PEP) for varicella or shingles** (available at: www.gov.uk/government/publications/post-exposure-prophylaxis-for-chickenpox-and-shingles).

Individuals who develop chickenpox despite post-exposure prophylaxis require treatment with an antiviral.

During outbreaks in nurseries and pre-school settings where chickenpox is co-circulating with group A streptococcus infections (such as scarlet fever), post-exposure prophylaxis with the chickenpox varicella-zoster vaccine p. 1518 may be given to certain non-immune individuals in these settings. For further guidance, see *Post-exposure management of varicella (chickenpox)* in Varicella-zoster vaccines p. 1495.

Drug choice for treatment

Aciclovir is active against herpesviruses but does not eradicate them. [EvGr] Uses of aciclovir include systemic treatment of varicella-zoster and the systemic and topical treatment of herpes simplex infections of the skin and mucous membranes. ⒶⒶ Aciclovir eye ointment is licensed for herpes simplex infections of the eye.

[EvGr] Famciclovir p. 730, a prodrug of penciclovir, is similar to aciclovir and may be used in the treatment of herpes zoster and genital herpes.

Valaciclovir is an ester of aciclovir, which may be used in the treatment of herpes zoster and herpes simplex infections of the skin and mucous membranes (including genital herpes); ⒶⒶ it is also licensed for preventing cytomegalovirus disease following solid organ transplantation.

Intravenous foscarnet sodium p. 734 is licensed for mucocutaneous herpes simplex virus infection unresponsive to aciclovir in immunocompromised patients. Oral inosine pranobex below is also licensed for mucocutaneous infections due to the herpes simplex virus.

Cytomegalovirus infection

Cytomegalovirus (CMV) is a member of the herpesvirus group. In immunocompetent patients, CMV infection is often asymptomatic and self-limiting therefore treatment is not always required. In immunocompromised patients, such as those with AIDS and transplant recipients, the infection manifests more severely causing diseases associated with greater morbidity and mortality.

Drugs licensed for use in the management of CMV disease include ganciclovir p. 732 (related to aciclovir), cidofovir p. 732, foscarnet sodium, letermovir p. 735, valaciclovir p. 731, and valganciclovir p. 733 (an ester of ganciclovir p. 732). There is a possibility of ganciclovir resistance in those who repeatedly have a poor treatment response or when viral excretion continues despite treatment.

ANTIVIRALS ⟩ INOSINE COMPLEXES

Inosine pranobex

27-Apr-2021

(Inosine acedoben dimepranol)

● **INDICATIONS AND DOSE**

Mucocutaneous herpes simplex
▶ BY MOUTH
▶ Adult: 1 g 4 times a day for 7–14 days

Adjunctive treatment of genital warts
▶ BY MOUTH
▶ Adult: 1 g 3 times a day for 14–28 days

Subacute sclerosing panencephalitis
▶ BY MOUTH
▶ Adult: 50–100 mg/kg daily in 6 divided doses

● **CAUTIONS** History of gout · history of hyperuricaemia · history of urolithiasis

● **SIDE-EFFECTS** Arthralgia · constipation · diarrhoea · drowsiness · epigastric discomfort · fatigue · headache · insomnia · malaise · nausea · nervousness · polyuria · skin reactions · vertigo · vomiting

● **PREGNANCY** Manufacturer advises avoid.

● **RENAL IMPAIRMENT** Manufacturer advises caution; metabolised to uric acid.

● **LESS SUITABLE FOR PRESCRIBING** Inosine pranobex is less suitable for prescribing.

● **MEDICINAL FORMS** There can be variation in the licensing of different medicines containing the same drug.

Oral tablet
CAUTIONARY AND ADVISORY LABELS 9
▶ **Imunovir** (Kora Healthcare)
Inosine acedoben dimepranol 500 mg Imunovir 500mg tablets | 100 tablet [PoM] £46.77 DT = £46.77

ANTIVIRALS > NUCLEOSIDE ANALOGUES

Aciclovir
(Acyclovir)

23-Sep-2022

● **INDICATIONS AND DOSE**

Herpes simplex, treatment (non-genital)
▶ BY MOUTH
▹ Adult: 200 mg 5 times a day usually for 5 days (longer if new lesions appear during treatment or if healing incomplete)

Herpes simplex, treatment (non-genital) in immunocompromised or if absorption impaired
▶ BY MOUTH
▹ Adult: 400 mg 5 times a day usually for 5 days (longer if new lesions appear during treatment or if healing incomplete)

Herpes simplex, treatment in encephalitis
▶ BY INTRAVENOUS INFUSION
▹ Adult: 10 mg/kg every 8 hours for at least 14 days (at least 21 days if also immunocompromised)—confirm cerebrospinal fluid negative for herpes simplex virus before stopping treatment

Herpes simplex, treatment in the immunocompromised
▶ BY INTRAVENOUS INFUSION
▹ Adult: 5 mg/kg every 8 hours usually for 5 days, alternatively 10 mg/kg every 8 hours usually for 5 days, higher dose to be used only if resistant organisms suspected

Herpes simplex, suppression
▶ BY MOUTH
▹ Adult: 400 mg twice daily, alternatively 200 mg 4 times a day; increased to 400 mg 3 times a day, dose may be increased if recurrences occur on standard suppressive therapy or for suppression of genital herpes during late pregnancy (from 36 weeks gestation)

Herpes simplex, prophylaxis in the immunocompromised
▶ BY MOUTH
▹ Adult: 200–400 mg 4 times a day
▶ BY INTRAVENOUS INFUSION
▹ Adult: 5 mg/kg every 8 hours

Post-exposure prophylaxis of varicella zoster infection
▶ BY MOUTH
▹ Adult: 800 mg 4 times a day for 7 days, start course on day 7 after exposure; if the patient presents after this, the course may be started up to day 14 after exposure

Varicella zoster (chickenpox), treatment | Herpes zoster (shingles), treatment
▶ BY MOUTH
▹ Adult: 800 mg 5 times a day for 7 days
▶ BY INTRAVENOUS INFUSION
▹ Adult: 5 mg/kg every 8 hours usually for 5 days

Varicella zoster (chickenpox), treatment in encephalitis | Herpes zoster (shingles), treatment in encephalitis
▶ BY INTRAVENOUS INFUSION
▹ Adult: 10 mg/kg every 8 hours given for 10–14 days, possibly longer if also immunocompromised or if severe infection

Varicella zoster (chickenpox), treatment in immunocompromised
▶ BY INTRAVENOUS INFUSION
▹ Adult: 10 mg/kg every 8 hours usually for 5 days

Herpes zoster (shingles), treatment in immunocompromised
▶ BY MOUTH
▹ Adult: 800 mg 5 times a day continued for 2 days after crusting of lesions
▶ BY INTRAVENOUS INFUSION
▹ Adult: 10 mg/kg every 8 hours usually for 5 days

Genital herpes simplex, treatment of first episode
▶ BY MOUTH
▹ Adult: 200 mg 5 times a day usually for 5 days (longer if new lesions appear during treatment or if healing incomplete), alternatively 400 mg 3 times a day usually for 5 days (longer if new lesions appear during treatment or if healing incomplete)

Genital herpes simplex, treatment of first episode, in immunocompromised or HIV-positive
▶ BY MOUTH
▹ Adult: 400 mg 5 times a day for 7–10 days (longer if new lesions appear during treatment or if healing incomplete)

Severe genital herpes simplex, treatment, initial infection
▶ BY INTRAVENOUS INFUSION
▹ Adult: 5 mg/kg every 8 hours usually for 5 days, alternatively 10 mg/kg every 8 hours usually for 5 days, higher dose to be used only if resistant organisms suspected

Genital herpes simplex, treatment of recurrent infection
▶ BY MOUTH
▹ Adult: 800 mg 3 times a day for 2 days, alternatively 200 mg 5 times a day for 5 days, alternatively 400 mg 3 times a day for 3–5 days

Genital herpes simplex, treatment of recurrent infection in immunocompromised or HIV-positive patients
▶ BY MOUTH
▹ Adult: 400 mg 3 times a day for 5–10 days

DOSES AT EXTREMES OF BODY-WEIGHT
▶ With intravenous use To avoid excessive dosage in obese patients, dose should be calculated on the basis of ideal body-weight for height.

● UNLICENSED USE UKHSA advises aciclovir is used for post-exposure prophylaxis of varicella zoster infection, but it is not licensed for this indication.
   Intravenous infusion not licensed for herpes zoster.
   Aciclovir doses in BNF Publications may differ from those in product literature.

● CAUTIONS Elderly (risk of neurological reactions) · maintain adequate hydration (especially with infusion or high doses)

● INTERACTIONS → Appendix 1: aciclovir

● SIDE-EFFECTS
GENERAL SIDE-EFFECTS
▶ **Common or very common** Abdominal pain · diarrhoea · dizziness · fatigue · fever · headache · nausea · photosensitivity reaction · skin reactions · vomiting
▶ **Uncommon** Anaemia · leucopenia · thrombocytopenia
▶ **Rare or very rare** Agitation · angioedema · ataxia · coma · confusion · drowsiness · dysarthria · dyspnoea · encephalopathy · hallucination · hepatic disorders · psychosis · renal impairment · renal pain · seizure · tremor
▶ **Frequency not known** Crystalluria

SPECIFIC SIDE-EFFECTS
▶ **Rare or very rare**
▹ With intravenous use Inflammation localised
▶ **Frequency not known**
▹ With oral use Alopecia

● PREGNANCY Not known to be harmful—manufacturers advise use only when potential benefit outweighs risk.

● BREAST FEEDING Significant amount in milk after systemic administration—not known to be harmful but manufacturer advises caution.

● RENAL IMPAIRMENT See p. 21. Risk of neurological reactions increased. Maintain adequate hydration (especially during renal impairment).
Dose adjustments Consider dose reduction.
▹ With intravenous use Use normal intravenous dose every 12 hours if eGFR 25–50 mL/minute/1.73 m^2 (every 24 hours

if eGFR 10–25 mL/minute/1.73 m^2). Consult product literature for intravenous dose if eGFR less than 10 mL/minute/1.73 m^2.

▸ With oral use For *herpes zoster*, use normal oral dose every 8 hours if eGFR 10–25 mL/minute/1.73 m^2 (every 12 hours if eGFR less than 10 mL/minute/1.73 m^2). For *herpes simplex*, use normal oral dose every 12 hours if eGFR less than 10 mL/minute/1.73 m^2.

● **DIRECTIONS FOR ADMINISTRATION** For *intravenous infusion* Zovirax IV®, *Aciclovir IV* (Genus), give intermittently *in* Sodium chloride 0.9% *or* Sodium chloride and glucose; initially reconstitute to 25 mg/mL in water for injection or sodium chloride 0.9% then dilute to not more than 5 mg/mL with the infusion fluid; to be given over 1 hour; alternatively, may be administered in a concentration of 25 mg/mL using a suitable infusion pump and given over 1 hour; for *Aciclovir IV* (Hospira) dilute to not more than 5 mg/mL with infusion fluid; give over 1 hour.

● **PRESCRIBING AND DISPENSING INFORMATION** Flavours of oral liquid preparations may include banana, or orange.

▸ With oral use for Herpes simplex, suppression Interrupt therapy every 6–12 months to reassess recurrence frequency—consider restarting after two or more recurrences.

● **PROFESSION SPECIFIC INFORMATION**

Dental practitioners' formulary Aciclovir Tablets 200 mg or 800 mg may be prescribed.

Aciclovir Oral Suspension 200 mg/5mL may be prescribed.

● **MEDICINAL FORMS** There can be variation in the licensing of different medicines containing the same drug.

Oral tablet

CAUTIONARY AND ADVISORY LABELS 9

▸ Aciclovir (Non-proprietary)

Aciclovir 200 mg Aciclovir 200mg tablets | 25 tablet [PoM] £2.28 DT = £1.16

Aciclovir 400 mg Aciclovir 400mg tablets | 56 tablet [PoM] £4.62 DT = £2.56

Aciclovir 800 mg Aciclovir 800mg tablets | 35 tablet [PoM] £8.40 DT = £3.44

Dispersible tablet

CAUTIONARY AND ADVISORY LABELS 9

▸ Aciclovir (Non-proprietary)

Aciclovir 200 mg Aciclovir 200mg dispersible tablets | 25 tablet [PoM] £1.60 DT = £1.50

Aciclovir 400 mg Aciclovir 400mg dispersible tablets | 56 tablet [PoM] £5.18 DT = £4.50

Aciclovir 800 mg Aciclovir 800mg dispersible tablets | 35 tablet [PoM] £6.61 DT = £5.72

▸ Zovirax (GlaxoSmithKline UK Ltd)

Aciclovir 200 mg Zovirax 200mg dispersible tablets | 25 tablet [PoM] £2.85 DT = £1.50

Oral suspension

CAUTIONARY AND ADVISORY LABELS 9

▸ Aciclovir (Non-proprietary)

Aciclovir 40 mg per 1 ml Aciclovir 200mg/5ml oral suspension sugar free | 125 ml [PoM] £34.81 DT = £34.81 [SF]

Aciclovir 80 mg per 1 ml Aciclovir 400mg/5ml oral suspension sugar free | 100 ml [PoM] £52.70 DT = £31.00 [SF]

▸ Zovirax (GlaxoSmithKline UK Ltd)

Aciclovir 40 mg per 1 ml Zovirax 200mg/5ml oral suspension | 125 ml [PoM] £29.56 DT = £34.81 [SF]

Aciclovir 80 mg per 1 ml Zovirax Double Strength 400mg/5ml oral suspension | 100 ml [PoM] £33.02 DT = £31.00 [SF]

Solution for infusion

ELECTROLYTES: May contain Sodium

▸ Aciclovir (Non-proprietary)

Aciclovir (as Aciclovir sodium) 25 mg per 1 ml Aciclovir 1g/40ml solution for infusion vials | 1 vial [PoM] £40.00 (Hospital only)
Aciclovir 250mg/10ml concentrate for solution for infusion vials | 5 vial [PoM] £50.00-£55.00 (Hospital only)
Aciclovir 500mg/20ml solution for infusion vials | 5 vial [PoM] £100.00 (Hospital only)
Aciclovir 500mg/20ml concentrate for solution for infusion vials | 5 vial [PoM] £110.00 (Hospital only)

Powder for solution for infusion

ELECTROLYTES: May contain Sodium

▸ Aciclovir (Non-proprietary)

Aciclovir (as Aciclovir sodium) 250 mg Aciclovir 250mg powder for solution for Infusion vials | 5 vial [PoM] £16.50 (Hospital only)
Aciclovir 250mg powder for solution for infusion vials | 5 vial [PoM] £49.30 (Hospital only) | 10 vial [PoM] £91.30 (Hospital only)
Aciclovir (as Aciclovir sodium) 500 mg Aciclovir 500mg powder for solution for infusion vials | 10 vial [PoM] £182.00 (Hospital only)

▸ Zovirax I.V. (GlaxoSmithKline UK Ltd)

Aciclovir (as Aciclovir sodium) 250 mg Zovirax I.V. 250mg powder for solution for infusion vials | 5 vial [PoM] £16.70 (Hospital only)
Aciclovir (as Aciclovir sodium) 500 mg Zovirax I.V. 500mg powder for solution for infusion vials | 5 vial [PoM] £17.00 (Hospital only)

Famciclovir

27-Apr-2021

● **INDICATIONS AND DOSE**

Herpes zoster infection, treatment

▸ BY MOUTH

▸ Adult: 500 mg 3 times a day for 7 days, alternatively 750 mg 1–2 times a day for 7 days

Herpes zoster infection, treatment in immunocompromised patients

▸ BY MOUTH

▸ Adult: 500 mg 3 times a day for 10 days, continue for 2 days after crusting of lesions

Genital herpes, suppression

▸ BY MOUTH

▸ Adult: 250 mg twice daily, therapy to be interrupted every 6–12 months to reassess recurrence frequency—consider restarting after two or more recurrences

Genital herpes, suppression in immunocompromised or HIV-positive patients

▸ BY MOUTH

▸ Adult: 500 mg twice daily, therapy to be interrupted every 6–12 months to reassess recurrence frequency—consider restarting after two or more recurrences

Genital herpes infection, treatment of first episode

▸ BY MOUTH

▸ Adult: 250 mg 3 times a day for 5 days or longer if new lesions appear during treatment or if healing incomplete

Genital herpes infection, treatment of first episode in immunocompromised or HIV-positive patients

▸ BY MOUTH

▸ Adult: 500 mg twice daily for 10 days

Genital herpes infection, treatment of recurrent infection

▸ BY MOUTH

▸ Adult: 125 mg twice daily for 5 days, alternatively 1 g twice daily for 1 day

Genital herpes infection, treatment of recurrent infections in immunocompromised or HIV-positive patients

▸ BY MOUTH

▸ Adult: 500 mg twice daily for 5–10 days

Herpes simplex infection (non-genital), treatment in immunocompromised patients

▸ BY MOUTH

▸ Adult: 500 mg twice daily for 7 days

● **UNLICENSED USE** Famciclovir doses in BNF may differ from those in product literature.

● **SIDE-EFFECTS**

▸ **Common or very common** Abdominal pain · diarrhoea · dizziness · headache · nausea · skin reactions · vomiting

▸ **Uncommon** Angioedema · confusion · drowsiness

▸ **Rare or very rare** Hallucination · jaundice cholestatic · palpitations · thrombocytopenia

● **PREGNANCY** Manufacturers advise avoid unless potential benefit outweighs risk.

- **BREAST FEEDING** No information available—present in milk in *animal* studies.
- **HEPATIC IMPAIRMENT** Manufacturer advises efficacy may be decreased in severe impairment (risk of impaired conversion to active metabolite, no information available).
- **RENAL IMPAIRMENT**
  Dose adjustments [EvGr] Reduce dose (consult product literature). ⟨M⟩
- **PRESCRIBING AND DISPENSING INFORMATION** Famciclovir is a pro-drug of penciclovir.

- **MEDICINAL FORMS** There can be variation in the licensing of different medicines containing the same drug. Forms available from special-order manufacturers include: oral tablet

Oral tablet
CAUTIONARY AND ADVISORY LABELS 9

- Famciclovir (Non-proprietary)
  Famciclovir 125 mg Famciclovir 125mg tablets | 10 tablet [PoM] £53.45 DT = £53.45
  Famciclovir 250 mg Famciclovir 250mg tablets | 15 tablet [PoM] £133.42-£148.25 DT = £148.25 | 21 tablet [PoM] £207.55 DT = £207.55 | 56 tablet [PoM] £498.11-£553.46 DT = £553.46
  Famciclovir 500 mg Famciclovir 500mg tablets | 14 tablet [PoM] £299.23 DT = £299.23
- Famvir (Phoenix Labs Ltd)
  Famciclovir 125 mg Famvir 125mg tablets | 10 tablet [PoM] £53.45 DT = £53.45
  Famciclovir 250 mg Famvir 250mg tablets | 15 tablet [PoM] £160.34 DT = £148.25
  Famciclovir 500 mg Famvir 500mg tablets | 14 tablet [PoM] £299.23 DT = £299.23 | 30 tablet [PoM] £641.21 DT = £641.21

Valaciclovir
23-Sep-2022

- **INDICATIONS AND DOSE**

Post-exposure prophylaxis of varicella zoster infection
- BY MOUTH
- Adult: 1000 mg 3 times a day for 7 days, start course on day 7 after exposure; if the patient presents after this, the course may be started up to day 14 after exposure

Herpes zoster infection, treatment
- BY MOUTH
- Adult: 1 g 3 times a day for 7 days

Herpes zoster infection, treatment in immunocompromised patients
- BY MOUTH
- Adult: 1 g 3 times a day for at least 7 days and continued for 2 days after crusting of lesions

Herpes simplex, treatment of first infective episode
- BY MOUTH
- Adult: 500 mg twice daily for 5 days (longer if new lesions appear during treatment or healing is incomplete)

Herpes simplex infections treatment of first episode in immunocompromised or HIV-positive patients
- BY MOUTH
- Adult: 1 g twice daily for 10 days

Herpes simplex, treatment of recurrent infections
- BY MOUTH
- Adult: 500 mg twice daily for 3–5 days

Treatment of recurrent herpes simplex infections in immunocompromised or HIV-positive patients
- BY MOUTH
- Adult: 1 g twice daily for 5–10 days

Herpes labialis treatment
- BY MOUTH
- Adult: Initially 2 g, then 2 g after 12 hours

Herpes simplex, suppression of infections
- BY MOUTH
- Adult: 500 mg daily in 1–2 divided doses, therapy to be interrupted every 6–12 months to reassess recurrence frequency—consider restarting after two or more recurrences

Herpes simplex, suppression of infections in immunocompromised or HIV-positive patients
- BY MOUTH
- Adult: 500 mg twice daily, therapy to be interrupted every 6–12 months to reassess recurrence frequency— consider restarting after two or more recurrences

Genital herpes, reduction of transmission (administered on expert advice)
- BY MOUTH
- Adult: 500 mg once daily, to be taken by the infected partner

Prevention of cytomegalovirus disease following solid organ transplantation when valganciclovir or ganciclovir cannot be used
- BY MOUTH
- Adult: 2 g 4 times a day usually for 90 days, preferably starting within 72 hours of transplantation

- **UNLICENSED USE** UKHSA advises valaciclovir is used for post-exposure prophylaxis of varicella zoster infection, but it is not licensed for this indication.
- **CAUTIONS** Elderly (risk of neurological reactions) · maintain adequate hydration (especially with high doses)
- **INTERACTIONS** → Appendix 1: valaciclovir
- **SIDE-EFFECTS**
- **Common or very common** Diarrhoea · dizziness · headache · nausea · photosensitivity reaction · skin reactions · vomiting
- **Uncommon** Abdominal discomfort · agitation · confusion · dyspnoea · haematuria · hallucination · leucopenia · level of consciousness decreased · renal pain · thrombocytopenia · tremor
- **Rare or very rare** Angioedema · ataxia · coma · delirium · dysarthria · encephalopathy · nephrolithiasis · psychosis · renal impairment · seizure
- **Frequency not known** Microangiopathic haemolytic anaemia

  SIDE-EFFECTS, FURTHER INFORMATION Neurological reactions more frequent with higher doses.
- **PREGNANCY** Not known to be harmful—manufacturers advise use only when potential benefit outweighs risk.
- **BREAST FEEDING** Significant amount in milk after systemic administration—not known to be harmful but manufacturer advises caution.
- **HEPATIC IMPAIRMENT** Manufacturer advises caution with doses of 4 g or more per day (no information available).
- **RENAL IMPAIRMENT** See p. 21. Maintain adequate hydration.
  Dose adjustments Consider dose reduction.
    For *herpes zoster*, 1 g every 12 hours if eGFR 30–50 mL/minute/1.73 m^2 (1 g every 24 hours if eGFR 10–30 mL/minute/1.73 m^2; 500 mg every 24 hours if eGFR less than 10 mL/minute/1.73 m^2).
    For *treatment of herpes simplex*, 500 mg (1 g in immunocompromised or HIV-positive patients) every 24 hours if eGFR less than 30 mL/minute/1.73 m^2.
    For *treatment of herpes labialis*, if eGFR 30–50 mL/minute/1.73 m^2, initially 1 g, then 1 g 12 hours after initial dose (if eGFR 10–30 mL/minute/1.73 m^2, initially 500 mg, then 500 mg 12 hours after initial dose; if

eGFR less than 10 mL/minute/1.73 m^2, 500 mg as a single dose).

For *suppression of herpes simplex*, 250 mg (500 mg in immunocompromised or HIV-positive patients) every 24 hours if eGFR less than 30 mL/minute/1.73 m^2.

For *reduction of genital herpes transmission*, 250 mg every 24 hours if eGFR less than 15 mL/minute/1.73 m^2.

Reduce dose according to eGFR for *cytomegalovirus prophylaxis* following solid organ transplantation (consult product literature).

- **PRESCRIBING AND DISPENSING INFORMATION** Valaciclovir is a pro-drug of aciclovir.

- **MEDICINAL FORMS** There can be variation in the licensing of different medicines containing the same drug. Forms available from special-order manufacturers include: oral suspension

Oral tablet

CAUTIONARY AND ADVISORY LABELS 9

▸ Valaciclovir (Non-proprietary)
  Valaciclovir (as Valaciclovir hydrochloride) 500 mg Valaciclovir 500mg tablets | 10 tablet [PoM] £20.58 DT = £11.85 | 42 tablet [PoM] £49.77-£86.29
  Valaciclovir (as Valaciclovir hydrochloride) 1 gram Valaciclovir 1g tablets | 10 tablet [PoM] £33.98 DT = £33.98 | 21 tablet [PoM] £71.36-£73.47
▸ Valtrex (GlaxoSmithKline UK Ltd)
  Valaciclovir (as Valaciclovir hydrochloride) 250 mg Valtrex 250mg tablets | 60 tablet [PoM] £123.28 DT = £123.28
  Valaciclovir (as Valaciclovir hydrochloride) 500 mg Valtrex 500mg tablets | 10 tablet [PoM] £20.59 DT = £11.85 | 42 tablet [PoM] £86.30

6.4a Cytomegalovirus infections

ANTIVIRALS ⟩ NUCLEOSIDE ANALOGUES

Cidofovir

20-Mar-2019

- **DRUG ACTION** Cidofovir is a selective inhibitor of human cytomegalovirus (HCMV) DNA polymerase which inhibits viral DNA synthesis and thereby suppresses HCMV replication.

- **INDICATIONS AND DOSE**

Cytomegalovirus retinitis in patients with AIDS (in combination with probenecid) (specialist use only)
▸ BY INTRAVENOUS INFUSION
▸ Adult: Initially 5 mg/kg once weekly for 2 weeks, then maintenance 5 mg/kg every 2 weeks, maintenance treatment to be started 2 weeks after completion of induction treatment

- **CONTRA-INDICATIONS** Concomitant administration with potentially nephrotoxic drugs—discontinue potentially nephrotoxic drugs at least 7 days before starting cidofovir · patients unable to receive probenecid

- **CAUTIONS** Diabetes mellitus (increased risk of ocular hypotony) · ensure concomitant use of probenecid and Sodium Chloride 0.9%

CAUTIONS, FURTHER INFORMATION
▸ Probenecid and Sodium Chloride 0.9% Manufacturer advises oral probenecid and intravenous Sodium Chloride 0.9% must be administered with each cidofovir dose to prevent nephrotoxicity (consult cidofovir product literature for information on probenecid dosing and recommendations on intravenous hydration); see *Prescribing and dispensing information* for details on obtaining probenecid.

- **INTERACTIONS** → Appendix 1: cidofovir

- **SIDE-EFFECTS**
▸ **Common or very common** Alopecia · asthenia · chills · diarrhoea · dyspnoea · eye inflammation · fever · headache ·

nausea · neutropenia · ocular hypotony · proteinuria · rash · renal failure · vomiting
▸ **Uncommon** Fanconi syndrome acquired
▸ **Frequency not known** Hearing impairment · nephrotoxicity · pancreatitis

SIDE-EFFECTS, FURTHER INFORMATION Manufacturer advises intravenous sodium chloride 0.9% prehydration and concomitant oral probenecid for prevention of nephrotoxicity; consider treatment interruption, or discontinuation if changes in renal function occur— consult product literature.

- **CONCEPTION AND CONTRACEPTION** Manufacturer advises ensure effective contraception during and after treatment in women; men should be advised to use barrier contraception during and for 3 months after treatment. Cidofovir may cause impaired fertility in males—reduced testes weight and hypospermia observed in *animal* studies.

- **PREGNANCY** Manufacturer advises avoid—toxicity in *animal* studies.

- **BREAST FEEDING** Manufacturer advises avoid (no information available).

- **HEPATIC IMPAIRMENT** Manufacturer advises caution (no information available).

- **RENAL IMPAIRMENT** Manufacturer advises avoid if creatinine clearance is less than or equal to 55 mL/minute or if proteinuria is greater than or equal to 100 mg/dL. See p. 21.

- **MONITORING REQUIREMENTS**
▸ Manufacturer advises monitor serum creatinine, urine protein levels, and white blood cell count before each cidofovir dose.
▸ Manufacturer advises regular eye examinations (increased risk of iritis, ocular hypotony, and uveitis).

- **DIRECTIONS FOR ADMINISTRATION** Manufacturer advises for *intravenous infusion*, dilute with 100 mL Sodium Chloride 0.9% and mix thoroughly; give at a constant rate over 1 hour via an infusion pump.

- **PRESCRIBING AND DISPENSING INFORMATION** Probenecid is available from 'special-order' manufacturers or specialist importing companies—in case of difficulties, the cidofovir manufacturer (Tillomed) advises contacting their local representative. See probenecid product literature for prescribing information for probenecid, including information on interactions.

- **HANDLING AND STORAGE**
Caution in handling Manufacturer advises cidofovir should be considered a potential carcinogen and must be handled with caution (consult product literature); if contact with skin or mucous membranes occurs, wash thoroughly with water.

- **MEDICINAL FORMS** There can be variation in the licensing of different medicines containing the same drug.
Solution for infusion
ELECTROLYTES: May contain Sodium
▸ Cidofovir (non-proprietary) ▼
  Cidofovir 75 mg per 1 ml Cidofovir 375mg/5ml concentrate for solution for infusion vials | 1 vial [PoM] £3,250.00

Ganciclovir

15-Dec-2020

- **INDICATIONS AND DOSE**

Prevention of cytomegalovirus disease [pre-emptive therapy in patients with drug-induced immunosuppression]
▸ BY INTRAVENOUS INFUSION
▸ Adult: Initially 5 mg/kg every 12 hours for 7–14 days, then maintenance 6 mg/kg once daily, on 5 days of the week, alternatively maintenance 5 mg/kg once daily

Prevention of cytomegalovirus disease [universal prophylaxis in patients with drug-induced immunosuppression]
▶ BY INTRAVENOUS INFUSION
▸ Adult: 6 mg/kg once daily, on 5 days of the week, alternatively 5 mg/kg once daily

Treatment of cytomegalovirus disease [in immunocompromised patients]
▶ BY INTRAVENOUS INFUSION
▸ Adult: Initially 5 mg/kg every 12 hours for 14–21 days, then maintenance 6 mg/kg once daily, on 5 days of the week, alternatively maintenance 5 mg/kg once daily, maintenance only for patients at risk of relapse; if disease progresses initial induction treatment may be repeated

- **CONTRA-INDICATIONS** Abnormally low haemoglobin count (consult product literature) · abnormally low neutrophil count (consult product literature) · abnormally low platelet count (consult product literature)

- **CAUTIONS** History of cytopenia · potential carcinogen (including long-term carcinogenicity) · potential teratogen (including long-term teratogenicity) · radiotherapy

- **INTERACTIONS** → Appendix 1: ganciclovir

- **SIDE-EFFECTS**
▸ **Common or very common** Anaemia · anxiety · appetite decreased · arthralgia · asthenia · bone marrow disorders · chest pain · chills · confusion · constipation · cough · depression · diarrhoea · dizziness · dysphagia · dyspnoea · ear pain · eye disorders · eye inflammation · eye pain · fever · flatulence · gastrointestinal discomfort · headache · hepatic function abnormal · increased risk of infection · insomnia · leucopenia · malaise · muscle complaints · nausea · neutropenia · night sweats · pain · peripheral neuropathy · renal impairment · seizure · sensation abnormal · sepsis · skin reactions · taste altered · thinking abnormal · thrombocytopenia · vomiting · weight decreased
▸ **Uncommon** Alopecia · arrhythmia · deafness · haematuria · hypotension · infertility male · oral ulceration · pancreatitis · psychotic disorder · tremor · visual impairment
▸ **Rare or very rare** Agranulocytosis · hallucination

- **ALLERGY AND CROSS-SENSITIVITY** [EvGr] Contra-indicated in patients hypersensitive to valganciclovir.
    Caution in patients hypersensitive to aciclovir, valaciclovir, or famciclovir. Ⓜ

- **CONCEPTION AND CONTRACEPTION** Manufacturer advises women of childbearing potential should use effective contraception during and for at least 30 days after treatment; men with partners of childbearing potential should be advised to use barrier contraception during and for at least 90 days after treatment. Ganciclovir may cause temporary or permanent inhibition of spermatogenesis—impaired fertility observed in *animal* studies.

- **PREGNANCY** Manufacturer advises avoid unless potential benefit outweighs risk—teratogenicity in *animal* studies.

- **BREAST FEEDING** Manufacturer advises avoid—present in milk in *animal* studies.

- **RENAL IMPAIRMENT**
    Dose adjustments Manufacturer advises reduce dose for patients receiving mg/kg dosing if creatinine clearance less than 70 mL/minute—consult product literature. See p. 21.

- **MONITORING REQUIREMENTS** Monitor full blood count closely (severe deterioration may require correction and possibly treatment interruption).

- **DIRECTIONS FOR ADMINISTRATION** Manufacturer advises, for *intravenous infusion*, give intermittently in Glucose 5% or Sodium Chloride 0.9%. Reconstitute with Water for Injections (500 mg/10 mL) then dilute requisite dose to a concentration of not more than 10 mg/mL with infusion fluid; give over 1 hour into a vein with adequate flow, preferably using a plastic cannula.

- **HANDLING AND STORAGE** Caution in handling Ganciclovir is a potential teratogen and carcinogen. Manufacturer advises avoid inhalation of the powder or direct contact of the powder or reconstituted solution with the skin or mucous membranes; if contact occurs, wash thoroughly with soap and water; rinse eyes thoroughly with plain water.

- **MEDICINAL FORMS** There can be variation in the licensing of different medicines containing the same drug.
    Powder for solution for infusion
    ELECTROLYTES: May contain Sodium
    ▸ Ganciclovir (Non-proprietary)
        Ganciclovir (as Ganciclovir sodium) 500 mg Ganciclovir 500mg powder for concentrate for solution for infusion vials | 5 vial [PoM] £145.00-£148.82 (Hospital only)
    ▸ Cymevene (Neon Healthcare Ltd)
        Ganciclovir (as Ganciclovir sodium) 500 mg Cymevene 500mg powder for concentrate for solution for infusion vials | 5 vial [PoM] £148.83 (Hospital only)

Valganciclovir
06-Aug-2021

- **INDICATIONS AND DOSE**
Cytomegalovirus retinitis [induction and maintenance treatment in patients with AIDS]
▶ BY MOUTH
▸ Adult: Initially 900 mg twice daily for 21 days, then maintenance 900 mg daily, induction regimen may be repeated if retinitis progresses

Prevention of cytomegalovirus disease [following solid organ transplantation from a cytomegalovirus positive donor]
▶ BY MOUTH
▸ Adult: 900 mg daily for 100 days (for 100–200 days following kidney transplantation), to be started within 10 days of transplantation

DOSE EQUIVALENCE AND CONVERSION
▸ Oral valganciclovir 900 mg twice daily is equivalent to intravenous ganciclovir 5 mg/kg twice daily.

- **CONTRA-INDICATIONS** Abnormally low haemoglobin count (consult product literature) · abnormally low neutrophil count (consult product literature) · abnormally low platelet count (consult product literature)

- **CAUTIONS** History of cytopenia · potential carcinogen (including long-term carcinogenicity) · potential teratogen (including long-term teratogenicity) · radiotherapy

- **INTERACTIONS** → Appendix 1: valganciclovir

- **SIDE-EFFECTS**
▸ **Common or very common** Anaemia · anxiety · appetite decreased · arthralgia · asthenia · bone marrow disorders · chest pain · confusion · constipation · cough · depression · diarrhoea · dizziness · dysphagia · dyspnoea · ear pain · eye disorders · eye inflammation · eye pain · flatulence · gastrointestinal discomfort · headache · hepatic function abnormal · increased risk of infection · insomnia · leucopenia · malaise · muscle complaints · nausea · neutropenia · night sweats · pain · peripheral neuropathy · renal impairment · seizure · sensation abnormal · sepsis · skin reactions · taste altered · thinking abnormal · thrombocytopenia · vomiting · weight decreased
▸ **Uncommon** Alopecia · arrhythmia · deafness · haematuria · hallucination · hypotension · infertility male · oral ulceration · pancreatitis · psychotic disorder · tremor · visual impairment

- **ALLERGY AND CROSS-SENSITIVITY** [EvGr] Contra-indicated in patients hypersensitive to ganciclovir.

Caution in patients hypersensitive to aciclovir, valaciclovir, or famciclovir. ⓜ

- **CONCEPTION AND CONTRACEPTION** Manufacturer advises women of childbearing potential should use effective contraception during and for at least 30 days after treatment; men with partners of childbearing potential should be advised to use barrier contraception during and for at least 90 days after treatment. *Ganciclovir* may cause temporary or permanent inhibition of spermatogenesis—impaired fertility observed in *animal* studies.

- **PREGNANCY** Manufacturer advises avoid unless potential benefit outweighs risk—teratogenicity observed with *ganciclovir* in *animal* studies.

- **BREAST FEEDING** Manufacturer advises avoid— *ganciclovir* present in milk in *animal* studies.

- **RENAL IMPAIRMENT**
Dose adjustments Manufacturer advises reduce dose if creatinine clearance less than 60 mL/minute—consult product literature. See p. 21.

- **MONITORING REQUIREMENTS** Monitor full blood count closely (severe deterioration may require correction and possibly treatment interruption).

- **PRESCRIBING AND DISPENSING INFORMATION**
Valganciclovir is a pro-drug of ganciclovir.
    Flavours of oral liquid formulations may include tutti-frutti.

- **HANDLING AND STORAGE** Manufacturer advises reconstituted powder for oral solution should be stored in a refrigerator (2–8°C) for up to 49 days.
Caution in handling Valganciclovir is a potential teratogen and carcinogen. Manufacturer advises caution when handling the powder, reconstituted solution, or broken tablets and avoid inhalation of powder; if contact with skin or mucous membranes occurs, wash thoroughly with soap and water; rinse eyes thoroughly with plain water.

- **MEDICINAL FORMS** There can be variation in the licensing of different medicines containing the same drug. Forms available from special-order manufacturers include: oral solution

Oral tablet
CAUTIONARY AND ADVISORY LABELS 21
▸ Valganciclovir (Non-proprietary)
Valganciclovir (as Valganciclovir hydrochloride)
450 mg Valganciclovir 450mg tablets | 60 tablet PoM £1,081.46 DT = £1,081.46
▸ Valcyte (Neon Healthcare Ltd)
Valganciclovir (as Valganciclovir hydrochloride) 450 mg Valcyte 450mg tablets | 60 tablet PoM £1,081.46 DT = £1,081.46

Oral solution
CAUTIONARY AND ADVISORY LABELS 21
▸ Valcyte (Neon Healthcare Ltd)
Valganciclovir (as Valganciclovir hydrochloride) 50 mg per 1 ml Valcyte 50mg/ml oral solution | 88 ml PoM £230.32 DT = £230.32 SF

ANTIVIRALS ⟩ OTHER

Foscarnet sodium

27-Apr-2021

- **INDICATIONS AND DOSE**
Cytomegalovirus disease
▸ BY INTRAVENOUS INFUSION
▸ Adult: Initially 60 mg/kg every 8 hours for 2–3 weeks, alternatively initially 90 mg/kg every 12 hours for 2–3 weeks, then maintenance 60 mg/kg daily, then increased if tolerated to 90–120 mg/kg daily, if disease progresses on maintenance dose, repeat induction regimen

- **UNLICENSED USE** Licensed for CMV retinitis in AIDS patients only. Foscarnet doses in BNF may differ from those in product literature.

- **CAUTIONS** Conditions where excess sodium should be avoided · ensure adequate hydration

- **INTERACTIONS** → Appendix 1: foscarnet

- **SIDE-EFFECTS**
▸ **Common or very common** Aggression · anaemia · anxiety · appetite decreased · arrhythmias · asthenia · chest pain · chills · confusion · constipation · coordination abnormal · dehydration · depression · diarrhoea · dizziness · electrolyte imbalance · fever · gastrointestinal discomfort · genital discomfort (due to high concentrations excreted in urine) · genital ulceration (due to high concentrations excreted in urine) · haemorrhage · headache · hepatic function abnormal · hypertension · hypotension · leucopenia · malaise · muscle contractions involuntary · myalgia · nausea (reduce infusion rate) · neutropenia · numbness · oedema · palpitations · pancreatitis · paraesthesia (reduce infusion rate) · peripheral neuropathy · proteinuria · renal impairment · seizure · sepsis · skin reactions · thrombocytopenia · thrombophlebitis · tremor · urinary disorders · vomiting
▸ **Uncommon** Acidosis · angioedema · glomerulonephritis · nephropathy · pancytopenia
▸ **Frequency not known** Anaphylactoid reaction · diabetes insipidus · muscle weakness · myopathy · oesophageal ulcer · QT interval prolongation · renal pain · renal tubular acidosis · severe cutaneous adverse reactions (SCARs)

- **CONCEPTION AND CONTRACEPTION** Men should avoid fathering a child during and for 6 months after treatment.

- **PREGNANCY** Manufacturer advises avoid.

- **BREAST FEEDING** Avoid—present in milk in *animal* studies.

- **RENAL IMPAIRMENT** Manufacturer advises caution.
Dose adjustments Manufacturer advises dose reduction (consult product literature).

- **MONITORING REQUIREMENTS**
▸ Monitor electrolytes, particularly calcium and magnesium.
▸ Monitor serum creatinine every second day during induction and every week during maintenance.

- **DIRECTIONS FOR ADMINISTRATION** For *intravenous infusion* (*Foscavir*®), manufacturer advises give intermittently *in* Glucose 5% or Sodium Chloride 0.9%; dilute to a concentration of 12 mg/mL for infusion into peripheral vein (undiluted solution *via* central venous line only); infuse over at least 1 hour (infuse doses greater than 60 mg/kg over 2 hours).

- **MEDICINAL FORMS** There can be variation in the licensing of different medicines containing the same drug.

Solution for infusion
ELECTROLYTES: May contain Sodium
▸ Foscarnet sodium (Non-proprietary)
Foscarnet sodium 24 mg per 1 ml Foscarnet sodium 6g/250ml solution for infusion bottles | 1 bottle PoM £199.00 (Hospital only)
▸ Foscavir (Clinigen Healthcare Ltd)
Foscarnet sodium 24 mg per 1 ml Foscavir 6g/250ml solution for infusion bottles | 1 bottle PoM £75.00 (Hospital only)

Letermovir
31-Aug-2020

- **DRUG ACTION** Letermovir is a cytomegalovirus DNA terminase complex inhibitor that interferes with cytomegalovirus genome formation and virion maturation.

- **INDICATIONS AND DOSE**

Prevention of cytomegalovirus reactivation and disease [in recipients of an allogeneic haematopoietic stem cell transplant who are seropositive for the human cytomegalovirus] (initiated by a specialist)
  - ▸ BY MOUTH
  - ▸ Adult: 480 mg once daily for 100 days post-transplant, start within 28 days post-transplant, treatment beyond 100 days may be considered in some patients—consult product literature

  DOSE ADJUSTMENTS DUE TO INTERACTIONS
  - ▸ Manufacturer advises reduce dose to 240 mg once daily with concurrent use of ciclosporin.

- **INTERACTIONS** → Appendix 1: letermovir

- **SIDE-EFFECTS**
- ▸ **Common or very common** Diarrhoea · nausea · vomiting
- ▸ **Uncommon** Abdominal pain · appetite decreased · fatigue · headache · muscle spasms · peripheral oedema · taste altered · vertigo

- **CONCEPTION AND CONTRACEPTION** The effect on human fertility is not known—impairment of fertility has been observed in *animal* studies.

- **PREGNANCY** Manufacturer advises avoid—toxicity in *animal* studies.

- **BREAST FEEDING** Manufacturer advises avoid—present in milk in *animal* studies.

- **HEPATIC IMPAIRMENT** Manufacturer advises avoid in moderate impairment in those with co-existing moderate or severe renal impairment, and in severe impairment (risk of increased exposure).

- **NATIONAL FUNDING/ACCESS DECISIONS**
  For full details see funding body website
  NICE decisions
  - ▸ Letermovir for preventing cytomegalovirus disease after a stem cell transplant (July 2019) NICE TA591 Recommended
  Scottish Medicines Consortium (SMC) decisions
  - ▸ Letermovir (*Prevymis*®) for prophylaxis of cytomegalovirus (CMV) reactivation and disease in adult CMV-seropositive recipients [R+] of an allogeneic haematopoietic stem cell transplant (March 2019) SMC No. 1338/18 Recommended

- **MEDICINAL FORMS** There can be variation in the licensing of different medicines containing the same drug.
  Oral tablet
  CAUTIONARY AND ADVISORY LABELS 25
  - ▸ **Prevymis** (Merck Sharp & Dohme (UK) Ltd)
    Letermovir 240 mg Prevymis 240mg tablets | 28 tablet [PoM] £3,723.16 (Hospital only)

Maribavir
24-Apr-2025

- **DRUG ACTION** Maribavir is a cytomegalovirus UL97 protein kinase inhibitor which works by interfering with ATP binding, thereby stopping the virus from multiplying and infecting cells.

- **INDICATIONS AND DOSE**

Cytomegalovirus disease [in recipients of haematopoietic stem cell transplant or solid organ transplant] (initiated by a specialist)
  - ▸ BY MOUTH
  - ▸ Adult: 400 mg twice daily for 8 weeks, duration may be adjusted if necessary

  DOSE ADJUSTMENTS DUE TO INTERACTIONS
  - ▸ EvGr If concurrent use with potent or moderate CYP3A4 inducers (except rifampicin and St John's Wort) is unavoidable, increase dose to 1200 mg twice daily. Ⓜ

- **INTERACTIONS** → Appendix 1: maribavir
- **SIDE-EFFECTS**
- ▸ **Common or very common** Abdominal pain upper · appetite decreased · diarrhoea · fatigue · headache · nausea · taste altered · vomiting · weight decreased
- **PREGNANCY** EvGr Avoid—toxicity in *animal* studies. Ⓜ
- **BREAST FEEDING** EvGr Discontinue breast-feeding. Ⓜ
- **HEPATIC IMPAIRMENT** EvGr Caution in severe impairment (no information available). Ⓜ
- **MONITORING REQUIREMENTS** EvGr Virologic failure can occur during and after treatment; monitor cytomegalovirus DNA levels and investigate for resistance mutations in patients who do not respond to treatment—discontinue treatment if resistance mutations detected. Ⓜ
- **DIRECTIONS FOR ADMINISTRATION** EvGr *Livtencity*® tablets may be taken whole or crushed. Crushed tablets may also be administered via a nasogastric or orogastric tube. Ⓜ
- **PATIENT AND CARER ADVICE** Patients or carers should be given advice on how to administer maribavir tablets.
  Missed doses If a dose is more than 9 hours late, the missed dose should not be taken and the next dose should be taken at the normal time.
- **NATIONAL FUNDING/ACCESS DECISIONS**
  For full details see funding body website
  NICE decisions
  - ▸ Maribavir for treating refractory cytomegalovirus infection after transplant (January 2023) NICE TA860 Recommended
  Scottish Medicines Consortium (SMC) decisions
  - ▸ Maribavir (*Livtencity*®) for the treatment of cytomegalovirus infection and/or disease that are refractory (with or without resistance) to one or more prior therapies, including ganciclovir, valganciclovir, cidofovir or foscarnet in adult patients who have undergone a haematopoietic stem cell transplant or solid organ transplant (October 2023) SMC No. SMC2576 Recommended

- **MEDICINAL FORMS** There can be variation in the licensing of different medicines containing the same drug.
  Oral tablet
  - ▸ **Livtencity** (Takeda UK Ltd) ▼
    Maribavir 200 mg Livtencity 200mg tablets | 56 tablet [PoM] £11,550.00 (Hospital only)

6.5 HIV infection

HIV infection
03-Jul-2023

Overview

The human immunodeficiency virus (HIV) is a retrovirus that causes immunodeficiency by infecting and destroying cells of the immune system, particularly the CD4 cells. Acquired immune deficiency syndrome (AIDS) occurs when the number of CD4 cells fall to below 200 cells/microlitre; opportunistic infections and malignancies (AIDS-defining illnesses) can develop. The prognosis of HIV and AIDS has greatly improved due to more effective and better tolerated antiretroviral therapy (ART). The greatest risk to excess mortality and morbidity is delayed HIV diagnosis and treatment.

Aims of treatment

Treatment aims to achieve an undetectable viral load, to preserve immune function, to reduce the mortality and morbidity associated with chronic HIV infection, and to reduce onward transmission of HIV, whilst minimising drug toxicity. Treatment with a combination of ART aims to improve the physical and psychological well-being of infected people.

Initiation of treatment

[EvGr] All patients with suspected or diagnosed HIV should be reviewed promptly by a HIV specialist.

All patients diagnosed as being HIV positive should be offered immediate treatment, irrespective of CD4 cell counts. (A) Commitment to, and strict adherence to treatment over many years is required. Low adherence can be associated with drug resistance, progression to AIDS, and death. The treatment regimen should take into account dosing convenience, potential drug interactions, clinical symptoms, and comorbidities.

[EvGr] Treatment of HIV infection in *treatment-naive* patients is initiated with a combination of two nucleoside reverse transcriptase inhibitors (NRTIs) as a backbone regimen plus *one* of the following as a third drug: an integrase inhibitor (INI), a non-nucleoside reverse transcriptase inhibitor (NNRTI), *or* a boosted protease inhibitor (PI).

The regimen of choice contains a backbone of emtricitabine p. 748 and either tenofovir disoproxil p. 751 or tenofovir alafenamide p. 720. An alternative backbone regimen is abacavir p. 744 and lamivudine p. 750. The third drug of choice is either atazanavir p. 753 or darunavir p. 753 both boosted with ritonavir p. 756, or dolutegravir p. 739, or elvitegravir p. 740 boosted with cobicistat p. 757, or raltegravir p. 740, or rilpivirine p. 743. Efavirenz p. 741 may be used as an alternative third drug.

Patients who require treatment for both HIV and chronic hepatitis B should be treated with antivirals active against both diseases as part of fully suppressive combination ART. Regimens of choice are tenofovir disoproxil and emtricitabine, or tenofovir alafenamide p. 720 and emtricitabine. (A) For further information see British HIV Association guidelines for the treatment of HIV-1-positive adults with antiretroviral therapy available at: www.bhiva. org/guidelines.

Switching therapy

[EvGr] Deterioration of the condition (including clinical, virological, and CD4 cell count changes) may require a change in therapy. The choice of an alternative regimen should be guided by factors such as the response to previous treatment, tolerability, drug-drug interactions and the possibility of drug resistance. (A) For further information see British HIV Association guidelines for the treatment of HIV-1-positive adults with antiretroviral therapy available at: www.bhiva.org/guidelines.

HIV infection in pregnancy

[EvGr] Management of HIV infection in pregnancy should focus on the well-being of the women living with HIV, by ensuring that their ART regimen maximally suppresses viral replication as early as possible (if possible before conception) in order to minimise vertical transmission of HIV. Information on the teratogenic potential of most antiretroviral drugs is limited, however, all pregnant women living with HIV who conceive whilst on effective ART should continue this treatment throughout their pregnancy. All other women should start ART during their pregnancy. The recommended regimen is a NRTI backbone of either tenofovir disoproxil or abacavir with either emtricitabine or lamivudine; the third drug should be efavirenz or atazanavir boosted with ritonavir. All treatment options require careful assessment by a specialist. (A) For further information, including alternative ART options, see British HIV Association guidelines for the management of HIV in pregnancy and postpartum available at: www.bhiva.org/guidelines.

[EvGr] Pregnancies in women with HIV and babies born to them should be reported prospectively to the National Study of HIV in Pregnancy and Childhood at: www.ucl.ac.uk/nshpc/ **and** to the Antiretroviral Pregnancy Registry at: www.apregistry.com. (A)

HIV infection and breast-feeding

[EvGr] Breast-feeding by HIV-positive mothers may cause HIV infection in the infant and should be avoided. (A) For further information see British HIV Association guidelines for the management of HIV in pregnancy and postpartum available at: www.bhiva.org/guidelines.

HIV infection, pre-exposure prophylaxis

The risk of acquiring HIV is increased in:
- men or transgender individuals who have unprotected anal intercourse with men;
- sexual partners of people who are HIV-positive with a detectable viral load; and
- HIV-negative heterosexual individuals who have unprotected intercourse with a HIV-positive person, and are likely to repeat this with the same person or another person with a similar status.

[EvGr] Emtricitabine with tenofovir disoproxil p. 749 may be appropriate for pre-exposure prophylaxis to reduce the risk of sexually acquired HIV-1 infection in combination with safer sex practices in adults at high risk. Tenofovir disoproxil alone is an alternative for HIV-negative heterosexual individuals when emtricitabine is contra-indicated. (A) For further information see British HIV Association and British Association for Sexual Health and HIV guidelines on the use of HIV pre-exposure prophylaxis (PrEP) available at: www.bhiva.org/guidelines.

HIV infection, post-exposure prophylaxis

The Department of Health advises prompt prophylaxis with antiretroviral drugs [unlicensed indication] may be appropriate following exposure to HIV-contaminated material. Immediate expert advice should be sought in such cases. National guidelines on post-exposure prophylaxis for healthcare workers have been developed (by the Chief Medical Officer's Expert Advisory Group on AIDS), www.gov. uk/government/publications/eaga-guidance-on-hiv-post-exposure-prophylaxis and local ones may also be available.

[EvGr] Prompt prophylaxis with antiretroviral drugs [unlicensed indication] may also be appropriate following potential sexual exposure to HIV where there is a significant risk of viral transmission. The recommended treatment for post-exposure prophylaxis is emtricitabine with tenofovir disoproxil plus raltegravir for 28 days. (A) For further information see British Association for Sexual Health and HIV guidelines for the use of HIV post-exposure prophylaxis following sexual exposure available at: www.bashh.org.

Drug treatment

Drugs that are licensed for the treatment of HIV/AIDS are listed below according to drug class.

Nucleoside reverse transcriptase inhibitors (NRTI or 'nucleoside analogue'): abacavir (ABC), emtricitabine (FTC), lamivudine (3TC), tenofovir alafenamide fumarate p. 720 (TAF), tenofovir disoproxil fumarate (TDF), and zidovudine p. 752 (AZT).

Non-nucleoside reverse transcriptase inhibitors (NNRTI): doravirine p. 741 (DOR), efavirenz (EFV), etravirine p. 742 (ETR), nevirapine p. 742 (NVP), and rilpivirine p. 743 (RPV).

Protease inhibitors (PI): atazanavir (ATZ), darunavir (DRV), fosamprenavir p. 755 (FOS-APV), lopinavir (LPV), ritonavir (RTV), and saquinavir (SQV).

CCR5 antagonists: maraviroc p. 756 (MVC).

Integrase inhibitors (INI): bictegravir (BIC), cabotegravir below (CAB), dolutegravir p. 739 (DTG), elvitegravir p. 740 (EVG), and raltegravir (RAL).

Fusion inhibitors: enfuvirtide below (T-20).

Attachment inhibitors: fostemsavir below (FTR).

Pharmacokinetic enhancers: cobicistat p. 757 (c), and low-dose ritonavir (r). They boost the concentrations of other antiretrovirals metabolised by CYP3A4.

ANTIVIRALS > HIV-ATTACHMENT INHIBITORS

Fostemsavir
16-Nov-2021

- **DRUG ACTION** Fostemsavir is a prodrug of temsavir which inhibits the attachment of HIV to the host cell.

- **INDICATIONS AND DOSE**

HIV infection in combination with other antiretroviral drugs for resistant infection
- ▸ BY MOUTH
- ▸ Adult: 600 mg twice daily

- **CAUTIONS** Risk factors for QT-interval prolongation

- **INTERACTIONS** → Appendix 1: fostemsavir

- **SIDE-EFFECTS**
- ▸ **Common or very common** Central nervous system immune reconstitution inflammatory response · diarrhoea · dizziness · drowsiness · fatigue · flatulence · gastrointestinal discomfort · headache · immune reconstitution inflammatory syndrome · insomnia · myalgia · nausea · skin reactions · taste altered · vomiting

- **PREGNANCY** [EvGr] Avoid—limited information available. Ⓜ

- **HEPATIC IMPAIRMENT** [EvGr] Caution in patients with chronic hepatitis B or C (increased risk of severe hepatic side-effects)—monitor liver function. Ⓜ

- **PATIENT AND CARER ADVICE**
Driving and skilled tasks Patients and carers should be cautioned on the effects on driving and performance of skilled tasks—increased risk of headache, dizziness, and somnolence.

- **MEDICINAL FORMS** There can be variation in the licensing of different medicines containing the same drug.
Modified-release tablet
CAUTIONARY AND ADVISORY LABELS 25
- ▸ Rukobia (ViiV Healthcare UK Ltd) ▼
Fostemsavir 600 mg Rukobia 600mg modified-release tablets | 60 tablet [PoM] £2,900.00

ANTIVIRALS > HIV-FUSION INHIBITORS

Enfuvirtide
04-Sep-2020

- **DRUG ACTION** Enfuvirtide inhibits the fusion of HIV to the host cell.

- **INDICATIONS AND DOSE**

HIV infection in combination with other antiretroviral drugs for resistant infection or for patients intolerant to other antiretroviral regimens
- ▸ BY SUBCUTANEOUS INJECTION
- ▸ Adult: 90 mg twice daily

- **INTERACTIONS** → Appendix 1: enfuvirtide

- **SIDE-EFFECTS**
- ▸ **Common or very common** Anxiety · appetite decreased · asthenia · concentration impaired · conjunctivitis · diabetes mellitus · gastrooesophageal reflux disease · haematuria ·

hypertriglyceridaemia · increased risk of infection · influenza like illness · irritability · lymphadenopathy · myalgia · nasal congestion · nephrolithiasis · nightmare · numbness · pancreatitis · peripheral neuropathy · skin papilloma · skin reactions · tremor · vertigo · weight decreased

- ▸ **Frequency not known** Diarrhoea · hypersensitivity · immune reconstitution inflammatory syndrome · nausea · osteonecrosis

SIDE-EFFECTS, FURTHER INFORMATION **Hypersensitivity** Hypersensitivity reactions including rash, fever, nausea, vomiting, chills, rigors, low blood pressure, respiratory distress, glomerulonephritis, and raised liver enzymes reported; discontinue immediately if any signs or symptoms of systemic hypersensitivity develop and do not rechallenge.

Osteonecrosis Osteonecrosis has been reported in patients with advanced HIV disease or following long-term exposure to combination antiretroviral therapy.

- **PREGNANCY** Manufacturer advises use only if potential benefit outweighs risk.

- **HEPATIC IMPAIRMENT** Manufacturer advises caution (no information available); increased risk of hepatic side effects in patients with chronic hepatitis B or C.

- **DIRECTIONS FOR ADMINISTRATION** For *subcutaneous injection*, manufacturer advises reconstitute with 1.1 mL Water for Injections and allow to stand (for up to 45 minutes) to dissolve; do **not** shake or invert vial.

- **PATIENT AND CARER ADVICE**
Hypersensitivity reactions Patients or carers should be told how to recognise signs of hypersensitivity, and advised to discontinue treatment and seek immediate medical attention if symptoms develop.

- **MEDICINAL FORMS** No licensed medicines listed.

ANTIVIRALS > HIV-INTEGRASE INHIBITORS

Cabotegravir
27-Feb-2025

- **DRUG ACTION** Cabotegravir is an inhibitor of HIV integrase.

- **INDICATIONS AND DOSE**
APRETUDE TABLETS ®
Pre-exposure prophylaxis of HIV-1 infection [oral lead-in therapy] (specialist use only)
- ▸ BY MOUTH
- ▸ Adult: 30 mg once daily for approximately 1 month (at least 28 days) then, if tolerated, switch to intramuscular treatment with cabotegravir at month 2, for oral dose recommendations if cabotegravir injection is missed—consult product literature

APRETUDE ® **INJECTION**
Pre-exposure prophylaxis of HIV-1 infection (specialist use only)
- ▸ BY INTRAMUSCULAR INJECTION
- ▸ Adult: Initially 600 mg every month for 2 doses, to be started on the last day of oral lead-in therapy with cabotegravir or within 3 days thereafter (if used), then maintenance 600 mg every 2 months, to be given 2 months after previous injection

VOCABRIA TABLETS ®
HIV-1 infection [oral lead-in therapy, in combination with rilpivirine] (specialist use only)
- ▸ BY MOUTH
- ▸ Adult: 30 mg once daily for approximately 1 month (at least 28 days) then, if tolerated, switch to intramuscular treatment with cabotegravir and rilpivirine at month 2, for oral dose

continued →

recommendations if cabotegravir injection and rilpivirine injection are missed—consult product literature

VOCABRIA® INJECTION

HIV-1 infection [in combination with rilpivirine prolonged-release injection] (specialist use only)
▶ BY INTRAMUSCULAR INJECTION
▶ Adult: Initially 600 mg for 1 dose, to be started on the last day of oral lead-in therapy with cabotegravir and rilpivirine (if used), or on the last day of current regimen, then maintenance 400 mg every month, to be given 1 month after initial injection, alternatively initially 600 mg every month for 2 doses, to be started on the last day of oral lead-in therapy with cabotegravir and rilpivirine (if used), or on the last day of current regimen, then maintenance 600 mg every 2 months, to be given 2 months after previous injection

DOSE EQUIVALENCE AND CONVERSION
▶ For dose recommendations if switching between maintenance injections given every month or every 2 months—consult product literature.

● CAUTIONS
▶ When used for HIV-1 infection [in combination with rilpivirine prolonged-release injection] Co-infection with hepatitis B or C · risk factors for virological failure
▶ When used for HIV-1 infection [oral lead-in therapy, in combination with rilpivirine] Co-infection with hepatitis B or C · risk factors for virological failure

CAUTIONS, FURTHER INFORMATION
▶ Risk factors for virological failure
▶ When used for HIV-1 infection [oral lead-in therapy, in combination with rilpivirine] or HIV-1 infection [in combination with rilpivirine prolonged-release injection] EvGr Use with caution in patients with HIV-1 subtype A6/A1 or BMI of 30 kg/m^2 or more, if treatment history uncertain and pre-treatment resistance analyses absent. M

● INTERACTIONS → Appendix 1: cabotegravir

● SIDE-EFFECTS

GENERAL SIDE-EFFECTS
▶ **Common or very common** Anxiety · asthenia · depression · diarrhoea · dizziness · feeling hot · fever · flatulence · gastrointestinal discomfort · headache · malaise · myalgia · nausea · skin reactions · sleep disorders · vomiting · weight increased
▶ **Uncommon** Angioedema · drowsiness · hepatotoxicity · suicidal behaviours

SPECIFIC SIDE-EFFECTS
▶ With intramuscular use Pancreatitis

● PREGNANCY
▶ With oral use EvGr Avoid unless potential benefit outweighs risk—no information available. M
▶ With intramuscular use EvGr Avoid unless potential benefit outweighs risk—may remain in systemic circulation for up to 12 months or longer after last prolonged-release injection. M

● BREAST FEEDING
▶ With oral use EvGr Avoid—present in milk in *animal* studies. M
▶ With intramuscular use EvGr Avoid—may be present in milk for up to 12 months or longer after last prolonged-release injection. M

● HEPATIC IMPAIRMENT EvGr Caution in severe impairment (no information available). M

● MONITORING REQUIREMENTS EvGr Monitor liver function—discontinue treatment if hepatotoxicity develops. M

● TREATMENT CESSATION
▶ With intramuscular use EvGr May remain in circulation for up to 12 months or longer. M With *Vocabria*®, start an

alternative regimen no later than 1 month after final monthly injection or 2 months after final 2-month injection. With *Apretude*®, start an alternative regimen no later than 2 months after final injection.

● DIRECTIONS FOR ADMINISTRATION For *intramuscular injection*, inject into the gluteal muscle. Injections may be given up to 7 days before or after the scheduled dose. If injections are missed—consult product literature. For *Vocabria*®, cabotegravir and rilpivirine injections must be administered into separate gluteal muscle sites.

● PRESCRIBING AND DISPENSING INFORMATION The manufacturer of *Apretude*® has provided a *Guide for Prescribers* and a *Checklist for Prescribers*.

● PATIENT AND CARER ADVICE Patients or carers should be given advice on how to administer cabotegravir tablets. Patient guide and reminder card An *Apretude*® guide, and reminder card for individuals at risk must be provided. **Missed doses** If an **oral** dose is more than 12 hours late, the missed dose should not be taken and the next dose should be taken at the normal time. If vomiting occurs within 4 hours of taking an **oral** dose, a replacement dose should be taken.
Driving and skilled tasks Patients and carers should be counselled on the effects on driving and performance of skilled tasks—increased risk of fatigue, dizziness and somnolence.

● NATIONAL FUNDING/ACCESS DECISIONS
For full details see funding body website
NICE decisions
▶ Cabotegravir with rilpivirine for treating HIV-1 (January 2022) NICE TA757 Recommended
Scottish Medicines Consortium (SMC) decisions
▶ Cabotegravir (*Vocabria*®) prolonged-release injection in combination with rilpivirine prolonged-release injection, for the treatment of HIV-1 infection in adults who are virologically suppressed (plasma HIV-1 RNA concentration less than 50 copies/mL) on a stable antiretroviral regimen without present or past evidence of viral resistance to, and no prior virological failure with agents of the NNRTI and INI class (October 2021) SMC No. SMC2376 Recommended
▶ Cabotegravir (*Apretude*®) in combination with safer sex practices for pre-exposure prophylaxis to reduce the risk of sexually acquired HIV-1 infection in high-risk adults and adolescents, weighing at least 35 kg (February 2025) SMC No. SMC2718 Recommended with restrictions

● MEDICINAL FORMS There can be variation in the licensing of different medicines containing the same drug.
Prolonged-release suspension for injection
EXCIPIENTS: May contain Polysorbates
▶ **Apretude** (ViiV Healthcare UK Ltd) ▼
  Cabotegravir 200 mg per 1 ml Apretude 600mg/3ml prolonged-release suspension for injection vials | 1 vial [PoM] £1,197.02 (Hospital only)
▶ **Vocabria** (ViiV Healthcare UK Ltd) ▼
  Cabotegravir 200 mg per 1 ml Vocabria 600mg/3ml prolonged-release suspension for injection vials | 1 vial [PoM] £1,197.02 (Hospital only)
Oral tablet
▶ **Apretude** (ViiV Healthcare UK Ltd) ▼
  Cabotegravir 30 mg Apretude 30mg tablets | 30 tablet [PoM] £638.57 (Hospital only)
▶ **Vocabria** (ViiV Healthcare UK Ltd) ▼
  Cabotegravir 30 mg Vocabria 30mg tablets | 30 tablet [PoM] £638.57 (Hospital only)

Dolutegravir

20-Jul-2023

- **DRUG ACTION** Dolutegravir is an inhibitor of HIV integrase.

- **INDICATIONS AND DOSE**

HIV infection without resistance to other inhibitors of HIV integrase [in combination with other antiretroviral drugs] (specialist use only)
- ▶ BY MOUTH USING TABLETS
- ▶ Adult: 50 mg once daily
- ▶ BY MOUTH USING DISPERSIBLE TABLETS
- ▶ Adult: 30 mg once daily

HIV infection in patients with resistance to other inhibitors of HIV integrase [in combination with other antiretroviral drugs] (specialist use only)
- ▶ BY MOUTH USING TABLETS
- ▶ Adult: 50 mg twice daily, dose to be taken with food
- ▶ BY MOUTH USING DISPERSIBLE TABLETS
- ▶ Adult: 30 mg twice daily, dose to be taken with food

HIV infection [in combination with other antiretroviral drugs (with concomitant carbamazepine, efavirenz, etravirine (without boosted protease inhibitors, but see also Interactions), fosphenytoin, phenobarbital, phenytoin, primidone, nevirapine, oxcarbazepine, St John's wort, or rifampicin)] (specialist use only)
- ▶ BY MOUTH USING TABLETS
- ▶ Adult: 50 mg twice daily, avoid concomitant use with these drugs if resistance to other inhibitors of HIV integrase suspected
- ▶ BY MOUTH USING DISPERSIBLE TABLETS
- ▶ Adult: 30 mg twice daily, avoid concomitant use with these drugs if resistance to other inhibitors of HIV integrase suspected

DOSE EQUIVALENCE AND CONVERSION
- ▶ *Tivicay*® film-coated tablets and *Tivicay*® dispersible tablets are **not** bioequivalent. Follow correct dosing recommendations for the dosage form when switching formulations.

IMPORTANT SAFETY INFORMATION

MHRA/CHM ADVICE: DOLUTEGRAVIR (*TIVICAY*®, *TRIUMEQ*®, *JULUCA*®): UPDATED ADVICE ON INCREASED RISK OF NEURAL TUBE DEFECTS (OCTOBER 2020)
The MHRA has updated its safety recommendations based on an ongoing European review evaluating cases of neural tube defects in babies born to mothers who became pregnant during dolutegravir treatment that found a smaller increased risk than previously thought, almost comparable to other HIV drugs.

Healthcare professionals are advised to counsel women of childbearing potential on the possible risk of neural tube defects with dolutegravir, including consideration of effective contraceptive measures. The benefits and risks of continuing treatment in women who are trying to become pregnant should be discussed with the patient. If pregnancy is confirmed in the first trimester during treatment, the benefits and risks of continuing dolutegravir versus switching to another antiretroviral regimen should also be discussed, considering the gestational age and the critical time period of neural tube defect development.

- **INTERACTIONS** → Appendix 1: dolutegravir

- **SIDE-EFFECTS**
- ▶ **Common or very common** Anxiety · depression · diarrhoea · dizziness · fatigue · flatulence · gastrointestinal discomfort · headache · nausea · skin reactions · sleep disorders · vomiting

- ▶ **Uncommon** Arthralgia · hepatic disorders · hypersensitivity · immune reconstitution inflammatory syndrome · myalgia · suicidal behaviours

SIDE-EFFECTS, FURTHER INFORMATION **Hypersensitivity** Hypersensitivity reactions (including severe rash, or rash accompanied by fever, malaise, arthralgia, myalgia, blistering, oral lesions, conjunctivitis, angioedema, eosinophilia, or raised liver enzymes) reported uncommonly. Discontinue immediately if any sign or symptoms of hypersensitivity reactions develop.

Osteonecrosis Osteonecrosis has been reported in patients with advanced HIV disease or following long-term exposure to combination antiretroviral therapy.

- **PREGNANCY** [EvGr] Specialist sources indicate dolutegravir may be considered from 6 weeks' gestation if expected benefit outweighs risk—see *Important Safety Information*. Higher dose folic acid is recommended due to increased risk of neural tube defects—see *Prevention of neural tube defects (in those in the high-risk group who wish to become pregnant or who are at risk of becoming pregnant)* in folic acid p. 1161. (A)

- **HEPATIC IMPAIRMENT** Manufacturer advises caution in severe impairment—no information available.

- **DIRECTIONS FOR ADMINISTRATION** [EvGr] *Tivicay*® dispersible tablets may be dispersed in water and given within 30 minutes, or swallowed whole one at a time. Do not chew, cut, or crush. (M)

- **PATIENT AND CARER ADVICE** Patients or carers should be given advice on how to administer dolutegravir film-coated tablets and dispersible tablets.
Missed doses If a dose is more than 20 hours late on the once-daily regimen (or more than 8 hours late on the twice-daily regimen), the missed dose should not be taken and the next dose should be taken at the normal time.
Driving and skilled tasks Patients and carers should be counselled on the effects on driving and performance of skilled tasks—increased risk of dizziness.

- **NATIONAL FUNDING/ACCESS DECISIONS**
For full details see funding body website

Scottish Medicines Consortium (SMC) decisions
- ▶ Dolutegravir (*Tivicay*®) for use in combination with other antiretroviral medicinal products for the treatment of Human Immunodeficiency Virus (HIV) infected adults (May 2014)
SMC No. 961/14 Recommended

All Wales Medicines Strategy Group (AWMSG) decisions
- ▶ Dolutegravir (*Tivicay*®) for the treatment of Human Immunodeficiency Virus (HIV) infected adults in combination with other anti-retroviral medicinal products (October 2017)
AWMSG No. 3373 Recommended
- ▶ Dolutegravir 5 mg dispersible tablets (*Tivicay*®) in combination with other anti-retroviral medicinal products for the treatment of Human Immunodeficiency Virus (HIV) infected adults, adolescents and children of at least 4 weeks of age or older and weighing at least 3 kg (September 2021)
AWMSG No. 4611 Recommended

- **MEDICINAL FORMS** There can be variation in the licensing of different medicines containing the same drug.

Dispersible tablet
- ▶ Tivicay (ViiV Healthcare UK Ltd)
  Dolutegravir (as Dolutegravir sodium) 5 mg Tivicay 5mg dispersible tablets | 60 tablet [PoM] £159.60 (Hospital only) [SF]

Oral tablet
- ▶ Tivicay (ViiV Healthcare UK Ltd)
  Dolutegravir (as Dolutegravir sodium) 50 mg Tivicay 50mg tablets | 30 tablet [PoM] £498.75 DT = £498.75 (Hospital only)

Combinations available: *Abacavir with dolutegravir and lamivudine*, p. 745 · *Lamivudine with dolutegravir*, p. 750

Dolutegravir with rilpivirine
19-Aug-2020

The properties listed below are those particular to the combination only. For the properties of the components please consider, dolutegravir p. 739, rilpivirine p. 743.

- **INDICATIONS AND DOSE**

HIV-1 infection (initiated by a specialist)
▸ BY MOUTH
▸ Adult: 50/25 mg once daily

DOSE EQUIVALENCE AND CONVERSION
▸ Dose expressed as x/y mg dolutegravir/rilpivirine.

- **INTERACTIONS** → Appendix 1: dolutegravir · NNRTIs
- **PATIENT AND CARER ADVICE**
Missed doses If a dose is more than 12 hours late, the missed dose should not be taken and the next dose should be taken at the normal time.
Driving and skilled tasks Manufacturer advises patients and carers should be counselled on the effects on driving and performance of skilled tasks—increased risk of dizziness and drowsiness.
- **NATIONAL FUNDING/ACCESS DECISIONS**
For full details see funding body website
Scottish Medicines Consortium (SMC) decisions
▸ Dolutegravir / rilpivirine film-coated tablet (*Juluca*®) for the treatment of human immunodeficiency virus type 1 (HIV-1) infection in adults who are virologically suppressed (HIV-1 RNA <50 copies/mL) on a stable antiretroviral regimen for at least six months with no history of virological failure and no known or suspected resistance to any non-nucleoside reverse transcriptase inhibitor (NNRTI) or integrase strand transfer inhibitor (INSTI) (September 2018) SMC No. SMC2091 Recommended

All Wales Medicines Strategy Group (AWMSG) decisions
▸ Dolutegravir / rilpivirine (*Juluca*®) for treatment of human immunodeficiency virus type 1 (HIV-1) infection in adults who are virologically suppressed (HIV-1 RNA <50 copies/mL) on stable antiretroviral regimen for at least six months with no history of virological failure and no known or suspected resistance to any non-nucleoside reverse transcriptase inhibitor or integrase inhibitor (December 2018) AWMSG No. 2850 Recommended

- **MEDICINAL FORMS** There can be variation in the licensing of different medicines containing the same drug.
Oral tablet
CAUTIONARY AND ADVISORY LABELS 21
▸ Juluca (ViiV Healthcare UK Ltd)
Rilpivirine (as Rilpivirine hydrochloride) 25 mg, Dolutegravir (as Dolutegravir sodium) 50 mg Juluca 50mg/25mg tablets | 30 tablet [PoM] £699.02 (Hospital only)

Elvitegravir
17-May-2019

- **DRUG ACTION** Elvitegravir is an inhibitor of HIV integrase, which is an enzyme required for viral replication.

- **INDICATIONS AND DOSE**

HIV infection without resistance to other inhibitors of HIV integrase, in combination with low-dose ritonavir and atazanavir or lopinavir
▸ BY MOUTH
▸ Adult: 85 mg once daily, take at the same time as a once daily ritonavir-boosted regimen or with the first dose of a twice daily ritonavir-boosted regimen

HIV infection without resistance to other inhibitors of HIV integrase, in combination with low-dose ritonavir and darunavir or fosamprenavir
▸ BY MOUTH
▸ Adult: 150 mg once daily, take with the first dose of a twice daily ritonavir-boosted regimen

- **CAUTIONS** Elderly—limited information available
- **INTERACTIONS** → Appendix 1: elvitegravir
- **SIDE-EFFECTS**
▸ **Common or very common** Diarrhoea · fatigue · headache · nausea · rash · vomiting
▸ **Uncommon** Depression · dizziness · drowsiness · flatulence · gastrointestinal discomfort · insomnia · paraesthesia · suicidal ideation (in patients with history of depression or psychiatric illness) · taste altered
▸ **Frequency not known** Hyperglycaemia · osteonecrosis · weight increased
- **CONCEPTION AND CONTRACEPTION** Manufacturer advises women of child-bearing potential should use effective contraception during treatment (if using a hormonal contraceptive, it must contain norgestimate as the progestogen and at least 30 micrograms ethinylestradiol).
- **PREGNANCY** Manufacturer advises avoid unless essential—limited data available.
- **PATIENT AND CARER ADVICE**
Missed doses Manufacturer advises if a dose is more than 18 hours late, the missed dose should not be taken and the next dose should be taken at the normal time. If vomiting occurs within 1 hour of taking a dose, a replacement dose should be taken.

- **MEDICINAL FORMS** No licensed medicines listed.

Combinations available: *Elvitegravir with cobicistat, emtricitabine and tenofovir alafenamide*, p. 746 · *Elvitegravir with cobicistat, emtricitabine and tenofovir disoproxil*, p. 747

Raltegravir
10-Nov-2020

- **DRUG ACTION** Raltegravir is an inhibitor of HIV integrase.

- **INDICATIONS AND DOSE**

HIV-1 infection (initiated by a specialist)
▸ BY MOUTH USING TABLETS
▸ Adult: 400 mg twice daily, alternatively 1200 mg once daily, once daily dosing for use in patients who are treatment naive or virologically suppressed on an initial regimen of 400 mg twice daily—use 600 mg tablets only

- **CAUTIONS** Psychiatric illness (may exacerbate underlying illness including depression) · risk factors for myopathy · risk factors for rhabdomyolysis
- **INTERACTIONS** → Appendix 1: raltegravir
- **SIDE-EFFECTS**
▸ **Common or very common** Akathisia · appetite abnormal · asthenia · behaviour abnormal · depression · diarrhoea · dizziness · fever · gastrointestinal discomfort · gastrointestinal disorders · headaches · nausea · skin reactions · sleep disorders · vertigo · vomiting
▸ **Uncommon** Alopecia · anaemia · anxiety · arrhythmias · arthralgia · arthritis · body fat disorder · burping · cachexia · chest discomfort · chills · cognitive disorder · concentration impaired · confusion · constipation · diabetes mellitus · drowsiness · dry mouth · dyslipidaemia · dysphonia · erectile dysfunction · feeling jittery · glossitis · gynaecomastia · haemorrhage · hepatic disorders · hot flush · hyperglycaemia · hypersensitivity · hypertension · immune reconstitution inflammatory syndrome · increased risk of infection · lipodystrophy · lymph node abscess · lymphatic abnormalities · malaise · memory loss · menopausal symptoms · mood altered · myalgia · myopathy · nasal congestion · nephritis · nephrolithiasis · nerve disorders · neutropenia · nocturia · odynophagia · oedema · osteopenia · pain · palpitations · pancreatitis acute · polydipsia · psychiatric disorder · renal cyst · renal impairment · sensation abnormal · severe cutaneous adverse reactions (SCARs) · skin papilloma · submandibular

mass · suicidal behaviours · sweat changes · taste altered · tendinitis · thrombocytopenia · tinnitus · tremor · visual impairment · weight increased

▶ **Frequency not known** Osteonecrosis

SIDE-EFFECTS, FURTHER INFORMATION Rash occurs commonly. Discontinue if severe rash or rash accompanied by fever, malaise, arthralgia, myalgia, blistering, mouth ulceration, conjunctivitis, angioedema, hepatitis, or eosinophilia.

● PREGNANCY Manufacturer advises avoid—toxicity in *animal* studies.

● HEPATIC IMPAIRMENT Manufacturer advises caution in severe impairment (no information available), and in patients with chronic hepatitis B or C (consider interrupting or discontinuing treatment if impairment worsens; increased risk of hepatic side-effects).

● PRESCRIBING AND DISPENSING INFORMATION Dispense raltegravir chewable tablets in original container (contains desiccant).

● NATIONAL FUNDING/ACCESS DECISIONS
For full details see funding body website

Scottish Medicines Consortium (SMC) decisions

▶ Raltegravir (*Isentress*®) for the treatment of HIV in adults **(May 2010)** SMC No. 613/10 Recommended with restrictions

▶ Raltegravir 600 mg film-coated tablets (*Isentress*®) in combination with other anti-retroviral medicinal products for the treatment of human immunodeficiency virus (HIV-1) infection in adults and paediatric patients weighing at least 40 kg **(November 2017)** SMC No. 1280/17 Recommended with restrictions

● MEDICINAL FORMS There can be variation in the licensing of different medicines containing the same drug.

Oral tablet
CAUTIONARY AND ADVISORY LABELS 25

▶ **Raltegravir (Non-proprietary)**
Raltegravir 600 mg Raltegravir 600mg tablets | 60 tablet [PoM] £249.85–£471.41

▶ **Isentress** (Merck Sharp & Dohme (UK) Ltd)
Raltegravir 400 mg Isentress 400mg tablets | 60 tablet [PoM] £471.41 (Hospital only)
Raltegravir 600 mg Isentress 600mg tablets | 60 tablet [PoM] £471.41 (Hospital only)

ANTIVIRALS > NON-NUCLEOSIDE REVERSE TRANSCRIPTASE INHIBITORS

Doravirine
18-Oct-2022

● **INDICATIONS AND DOSE**

HIV-1 infection in combination with other antiretroviral drugs (initiated by a specialist)
▶ BY MOUTH
▶ Adult: 100 mg once daily

DOSE ADJUSTMENTS DUE TO INTERACTIONS
▶ [EvGr] If concurrent use of moderate inducers of CYP3A4, modafinil, or telotristat ethyl is unavoidable, increase dose to 100 mg twice daily. If co-administered with rifabutin, a dose of 100 mg twice daily is recommended. ◈

● INTERACTIONS → Appendix 1: NNRTIs

● SIDE-EFFECTS
▶ **Common or very common** Asthenia · diarrhoea · dizziness · drowsiness · gastrointestinal discomfort · gastrointestinal disorders · headache · hepatocellular injury · nausea · skin reactions · sleep disorders · vomiting
▶ **Uncommon** Anxiety · arthralgia · concentration impaired · confusion · constipation · depression · electrolyte imbalance · hypertension · malaise · memory loss · mood altered · muscle tone increased · myalgia · paraesthesia · suicidal ideation

▶ **Rare or very rare** Acute kidney injury · adjustment disorder · aggression · chest pain · chills · dyspnoea · hallucination · pain · rash pustular · renal disorder · thirst · tonsillar hypertrophy · urolithiases

● PREGNANCY Manufacturer advises avoid—no information available.

● HEPATIC IMPAIRMENT Manufacturer advises caution in severe impairment (no information available).

● PATIENT AND CARER ADVICE
Missed doses If a dose is more than 12 hours late, the missed dose should not be taken and the next dose should be taken at the normal time.
Driving and skilled tasks Manufacturer advises patients and carers should be counselled on the effects on driving and performance of skilled tasks—increased risk of fatigue, dizziness, and somnolence.

● NATIONAL FUNDING/ACCESS DECISIONS
For full details see funding body website

Scottish Medicines Consortium (SMC) decisions

▶ Doravirine (*Pifeltro*®) in combination with other antiretroviral medicinal products, for the treatment of adults infected with human immunodeficiency virus-1 (HIV-1) without past or present evidence of resistance to the non-nucleoside reverse transcriptase inhibitor (NNRTI) class **(March 2021)** SMC No. SMC2332 Recommended

All Wales Medicines Strategy Group (AWMSG) decisions

▶ Doravirine (*Pifeltro*®) in combination with other antiretroviral medicinal products, for the treatment of adults infected with HIV-1 without past or present evidence of resistance to the NNRTI class **(September 2020)** AWMSG No. 3109 Recommended

● MEDICINAL FORMS There can be variation in the licensing of different medicines containing the same drug.
Oral tablet
CAUTIONARY AND ADVISORY LABELS 25, 3

▶ **Pifeltro** (Merck Sharp & Dohme (UK) Ltd)
Doravirine 100 mg Pifeltro 100mg tablets | 30 tablet [PoM] £471.41 (Hospital only)

Combinations available: *Lamivudine with tenofovir disoproxil and doravirine,* p. 751

Efavirenz
27-Apr-2021

● **INDICATIONS AND DOSE**

HIV infection in combination with other antiretroviral drugs
▶ BY MOUTH USING CAPSULES
▶ Adult: 600 mg once daily
▶ BY MOUTH USING TABLETS
▶ Adult: 600 mg once daily

● CAUTIONS Acute porphyrias p. 1202 · elderly · history of psychiatric disorders · history of seizures · risk of QT interval prolongation

● INTERACTIONS → Appendix 1: NNRTIs

● SIDE-EFFECTS
▶ **Common or very common** Abdominal pain · anxiety · concentration impaired · depression · diarrhoea · dizziness · drowsiness · dyslipidaemia · fatigue · headache · movement disorders · nausea · skin reactions · sleep disorders · vomiting
▶ **Uncommon** Behaviour abnormal · confusion · flushing · gynaecomastia · hallucination · hepatic disorders · memory loss · mood altered · pancreatitis · psychosis · seizure · Stevens-Johnson syndrome · suicidal behaviours · thinking abnormal · tinnitus · tremor · vertigo · vision blurred
▶ **Rare or very rare** Delusions · photosensitivity reaction
▶ **Frequency not known** Immune reconstitution inflammatory syndrome · osteonecrosis

SIDE-EFFECTS, FURTHER INFORMATION **Rash** Rash, usually in the first 2 weeks, is the most common side-effect; discontinue if severe rash with blistering, desquamation, mucosal involvement or fever; if rash mild or moderate, may continue without interruption—usually resolves within 1 month.

CNS effects Administration at bedtime especially in first 2–4 weeks reduces CNS effects.

Abnormal hepatic function Manufacturer advises interrupt or discontinue treatment if transaminases more than 5 times the upper limit of normal.

- **PREGNANCY** Reports of neural tube defects when used in first trimester.

- **HEPATIC IMPAIRMENT** Greater risk of hepatic side-effects in chronic hepatitis B or C. Manufacturer advises avoid in severe impairment (limited information available).

- **RENAL IMPAIRMENT** Manufacturer advises caution in severe renal failure—no information available.

- **MONITORING REQUIREMENTS** Monitor liver function if receiving other hepatotoxic drugs.

- **DIRECTIONS FOR ADMINISTRATION** Manufacturer advises for patients who cannot swallow capsules, the capsule may be opened and contents added to a small amount of food—consult product literature. No additional food should be consumed for up to 2 hours after administration of efavirenz.

- **PATIENT AND CARER ADVICE**
Psychiatric disorders Patients or their carers should be advised to seek immediate medical attention if symptoms such as severe depression, psychosis or suicidal ideation occur.

- **MEDICINAL FORMS** There can be variation in the licensing of different medicines containing the same drug.
Oral tablet
CAUTIONARY AND ADVISORY LABELS 23
▸ Efavirenz (Non-proprietary)
Efavirenz 600 mg Efavirenz 600mg tablets | 30 tablet PoM £25.25-£452.94 (Hospital only)

Combinations available: *Efavirenz with emtricitabine and tenofovir disoproxil*, p. 746

Etravirine
15-Oct-2021

- **INDICATIONS AND DOSE**
HIV infection in combination with other antiretroviral drugs (including a boosted protease inhibitor) in patients previously treated with antiretrovirals (initiated by a specialist)
  ▸ BY MOUTH
  ▸ Adult: 200 mg twice daily, to be taken after food

- **CONTRA-INDICATIONS** Acute porphyrias p. 1202
- **CAUTIONS** Elderly
- **INTERACTIONS** → Appendix 1: NNRTIs
- **SIDE-EFFECTS**
▸ **Common or very common** Anaemia · anxiety · appetite decreased · asthenia · constipation · diabetes mellitus · diarrhoea · drowsiness · dry mouth · dyslipidaemia · dyspnoea exertional · gastrointestinal discomfort · gastrointestinal disorders · headache · hyperglycaemia · hypersensitivity · hypertension · memory loss · myocardial infarction · nausea · peripheral neuropathy · renal failure · sensation abnormal · skin reactions · sleep disorders · stomatitis · sweat changes · thrombocytopenia · vision blurred · vomiting
▸ **Uncommon** Angina pectoris · angioedema · atrial fibrillation · bronchospasm · concentration impaired · confusion · gynaecomastia · haematemesis · hepatic

disorders · immune reconstitution inflammatory syndrome · pancreatitis · seizure · syncope · tremor · vertigo
▸ **Rare or very rare** Haemorrhagic stroke · severe cutaneous adverse reactions (SCARs) · Stevens-Johnson syndrome (especially in children and adolescents)
▸ **Frequency not known** Osteonecrosis

SIDE-EFFECTS, FURTHER INFORMATION **Hypersensitivity reactions** Rash, usually in the second week, is the most common side-effect and appears more frequently in females. Life-threatening hypersensitivity reactions reported usually during week 3–6 of treatment and characterised by rash, eosinophilia, and systemic symptoms (including fever, general malaise, myalgia, arthralgia, blistering, oral lesions, conjunctivitis, and hepatitis). Discontinue permanently if hypersensitivity reaction or severe rash develop. If rash mild or moderate (without signs of hypersensitivity reaction), may continue without interruption—usually resolves within 2 weeks.

- **HEPATIC IMPAIRMENT** Manufacturer advises caution in moderate impairment and in patients with hepatitis B or C (increased risk of hepatic side effects); avoid in severe impairment (no information available).

- **DIRECTIONS FOR ADMINISTRATION** Manufacturer advises patients with swallowing difficulties may disperse tablets in a glass of water just before administration.

- **PRESCRIBING AND DISPENSING INFORMATION** Dispense in original container (contains desiccant).

- **PATIENT AND CARER ADVICE**
Hypersensitivity reactions Patients or carers should be told how to recognise hypersensitivity reactions and advised to seek immediate medical attention if hypersensitivity reaction or severe rash develop.
Vomiting If vomiting occurs 4 hours after taking tablets, no additional dose should be taken and the next dose should be taken at the usual time.
Missed doses If a dose is more than 6 hours late, the missed dose should not be taken and the next dose should be taken at the normal time.

- **NATIONAL FUNDING/ACCESS DECISIONS**
For full details see funding body website
All Wales Medicines Strategy Group (AWMSG) decisions
▸ Etravirine (*Intelence*®) in combination with a boosted protease inhibitor and other antiretroviral medicinal products, for the treatment of human immunodeficiency virus type 1 (HIV-1) infection in antiretroviral treatment-experienced adults and in antiretroviral treatment-experienced paediatric patients from 2 years of age (September 2021) AWMSG No. 4506 Recommended

- **MEDICINAL FORMS** There can be variation in the licensing of different medicines containing the same drug.
Oral tablet
CAUTIONARY AND ADVISORY LABELS 21
▸ Intelence (Janssen-Cilag Ltd)
Etravirine 100 mg Intelence 100mg tablets | 120 tablet PoM £301.27 (Hospital only)
Etravirine 200 mg Intelence 200mg tablets | 60 tablet PoM £301.27 (Hospital only)

Nevirapine
27-Apr-2021

- **INDICATIONS AND DOSE**
HIV infection in combination with other antiretroviral drugs (initial dose)
  ▸ BY MOUTH USING IMMEDIATE-RELEASE MEDICINES
  ▸ Adult: Initially 200 mg once daily for first 14 days, initial dose titration using 'immediate-release' preparation should not exceed 28 days; if rash occurs and is not resolved within 28 days, alternative treatment should be sought. If treatment interrupted

for more than 7 days, restart using the lower dose of the 'immediate-release' preparation for the first 14 days as for new treatment

HIV infection in combination with other antiretroviral drugs (maintenance dose following initial dose titration if no rash present)
▶ BY MOUTH USING IMMEDIATE-RELEASE MEDICINES
▶ Adult: 200 mg twice daily
▶ BY MOUTH USING MODIFIED-RELEASE MEDICINES
▶ Adult: 400 mg once daily

● **CONTRA-INDICATIONS** Acute porphyrias p. 1202 · post-exposure prophylaxis

● **CAUTIONS** Females (at greater risk of hepatic side effects) · high CD4 cell count (at greater risk of hepatic side effects)
  CAUTIONS, FURTHER INFORMATION
▶ **Hepatic effects** Patients with chronic hepatitis B or C, high CD4 cell count, and women are at increased risk of hepatic side effects—if plasma HIV-1 RNA detectable, manufacturer advises avoid in women with CD4 cell count greater than 250 cells/mm^3 or in men with CD4 cell count greater than 400 cells/mm^3 unless potential benefit outweighs risk.

● **INTERACTIONS** → Appendix 1: NNRTIs

● **SIDE-EFFECTS**
▶ **Common or very common** Abdominal pain · angioedema · diarrhoea · fatigue · fever · headache · hepatic disorders · hypersensitivity · hypertransaminasaemia · nausea · skin reactions · vomiting
▶ **Uncommon** Anaemia · arthralgia · myalgia · severe cutaneous adverse reactions (SCARs)
▶ **Frequency not known** Eosinophilia · osteonecrosis · weight increased

  SIDE-EFFECTS, FURTHER INFORMATION **Hepatic effects**
  Potentially life-threatening hepatotoxicity including fatal fulminant hepatitis reported usually in first 6 weeks; discontinue permanently if abnormalities in liver function tests accompanied by hypersensitivity reaction (rash, fever, arthralgia, myalgia, lymphadenopathy, hepatitis, renal impairment, eosinophilia, granulocytopenia); suspend if severe abnormalities in liver function tests but no hypersensitivity reaction—discontinue permanently if significant liver function abnormalities recur; monitor patient closely if mild to moderate abnormalities in liver function tests with no hypersensitivity reaction.
  Rash Rash, usually in first 6 weeks, is most common side-effect; incidence reduced if introduced at low dose and dose increased gradually (after 14 days); Discontinue permanently if severe rash or if rash accompanied by blistering, oral lesions, conjunctivitis, facial oedema, general malaise or hypersensitivity reactions; if rash mild or moderate may continue without interruption but dose should not be increased until rash resolves.
  Osteonecrosis Osteonecrosis has been reported in patients with advanced HIV disease or following long-term exposure to combination antiretroviral therapy.

● **HEPATIC IMPAIRMENT** For *modified-release* preparations, manufacturer advises avoid (no information available). For *immediate-release* preparations, manufacturer advises caution in moderate impairment and chronic hepatitis (increased risk of hepatic side effects; consider interrupting or discontinuing treatment if hepatic function worsens); avoid in severe impairment (no information available).

● **RENAL IMPAIRMENT** Manufacturer advises avoid *modified-release* preparation—no information available.

● **MONITORING REQUIREMENTS**
▶ **Hepatic disease** Close monitoring of liver function required during first 18 weeks; monitor liver function before treatment then every 2 weeks for 2 months then after 1 month and then regularly.

▶ **Rash** Monitor closely for skin reactions during first 18 weeks.

● **PATIENT AND CARER ADVICE**
  Hypersensitivity reactions Patients or carers should be told how to recognise hypersensitivity reactions and advised to discontinue treatment and seek immediate medical attention if severe skin reaction, hypersensitivity reactions, or symptoms of hepatitis develop.
  Missed doses If a dose is more than 8 hours late with the 'immediate-release' preparation (or more than 12 hours late with the modified-release preparation), the missed dose should not be taken and the next dose should be taken at the usual time.

● **MEDICINAL FORMS** There can be variation in the licensing of different medicines containing the same drug.
  Oral tablet
▶ **Nevirapine (Non-proprietary)**
  Nevirapine 200 mg Nevirapine 200mg tablets | 60 tablet [PoM] £170.00 (Hospital only)
  Oral suspension
▶ **Viramune** (Boehringer Ingelheim Ltd)
  Nevirapine (as Nevirapine hemihydrate) 10 mg per 1 ml Viramune 50mg/5ml oral suspension | 240 ml [PoM] £50.40 (Hospital only)
  Modified-release tablet
  CAUTIONARY AND ADVISORY LABELS 25
▶ **Nevirapine (Non-proprietary)**
  Nevirapine 400 mg Nevirapine 400mg modified-release tablets | 30 tablet [PoM] £127.50 (Hospital only)

Rilpivirine
27-Feb-2025

● **INDICATIONS AND DOSE**
  HIV-1 infection [in combination with other antiretroviral drugs] (specialist use only)
▶ BY MOUTH USING FILM-COATED TABLETS
▶ Adult: 25 mg once daily, dose to be taken with food

  HIV-1 infection [oral lead-in therapy, in combination with cabotegravir] (specialist use only)
▶ BY MOUTH USING FILM-COATED TABLETS
▶ Adult: 25 mg once daily for approximately 1 month (at least 28 days) with food then, if tolerated, switch to intramuscular treatment with cabotegravir and rilpivirine at month 2, for oral dose recommendations if cabotegravir injection and rilpivirine injection are missed—consult product literature

  HIV-1 infection [in combination with cabotegravir prolonged-release injection] (specialist use only)
▶ BY INTRAMUSCULAR INJECTION
▶ Adult: Initially 900 mg for 1 dose, to be started on the last day of oral lead-in therapy with cabotegravir and rilpivirine (if used), or on the last day of current regimen, then maintenance 600 mg every month, to be given 1 month after initial injection, alternatively initially 900 mg every month for 2 doses, to be started on the last day of oral lead-in therapy with cabotegravir and rilpivirine (if used), or on the last day of current regimen, then maintenance 900 mg every 2 months, to be given 2 months after previous injection

  DOSE EQUIVALENCE AND CONVERSION
▶ For dose recommendations if switching between maintenance injections given every month or every 2 months—consult product literature.

● **CAUTIONS** Acute porphyrias p. 1202 · co-infection with hepatitis B or C · risk factors for virological failure
  CAUTIONS, FURTHER INFORMATION
▶ **Risk factors for virological failure** [EvGr] Use with caution in patients with HIV-1 subtype A6/A1 or BMI of 30 kg/m^2 or more, if treatment history uncertain and pre-treatment resistance analyses absent. ◆M◆

- **INTERACTIONS** → Appendix 1: NNRTIs
- **SIDE-EFFECTS**
  GENERAL SIDE-EFFECTS
- ▶ **Common or very common** Depression · dizziness · drowsiness · gastrointestinal discomfort · headache · nausea · sleep disorders · vomiting
  SPECIFIC SIDE-EFFECTS
- ▶ **Common or very common**
- ▶ With intramuscular use Anxiety · asthenia · diarrhoea · feeling hot · fever · flatulence · malaise · myalgia · skin reactions · weight increased
- ▶ With oral use Appetite decreased · dry mouth · fatigue · rash
- ▶ **Uncommon**
- ▶ With intramuscular use Hepatotoxicity
- ▶ With oral use Immune reconstitution inflammatory syndrome
- ▶ **Frequency not known**
- ▶ With intramuscular use Pancreatitis
- **PREGNANCY**
- ▶ With oral use [EvGr] Use only if potential benefit outweighs risk—no toxicity observed in *animal* studies. If used, monitoring of viral load is recommended. ⟨M⟩
- ▶ With intramuscular use [EvGr] Avoid unless potential benefit outweighs risk—no information available. May remain in systemic circulation for up to 4 years after last prolonged-release injection. If used, monitoring of viral load is recommended. ⟨M⟩
- **BREAST FEEDING**
- ▶ With oral use [EvGr] Avoid—present in milk in *animal* studies. ⟨M⟩
- ▶ With intramuscular use [EvGr] Avoid—may be present in milk for up to 4 years after last prolonged-release injection. ⟨M⟩
- **HEPATIC IMPAIRMENT** Manufacturer advises caution in moderate impairment (limited information available); avoid in severe impairment (no information available).
- **RENAL IMPAIRMENT** Manufacturer advises caution in severe impairment.
- **MONITORING REQUIREMENTS** [EvGr] Monitor liver function in patients with hepatitis C—limited information available. ⟨M⟩
- **TREATMENT CESSATION**
- ▶ With intramuscular use [EvGr] May remain in circulation for up to 4 years; start an alternative regimen no later than 1 month after monthly regimen or 2 months after 2-monthly regimen. ⟨M⟩
- **DIRECTIONS FOR ADMINISTRATION**
- ▶ With intramuscular use For *Rekambys*®, rilpivirine and cabotegravir injections must be administered into separate gluteal muscle sites. Maintenance injections may be given up to 7 days before or after the scheduled dose. If injections are missed—consult product literature.
- **HANDLING AND STORAGE** Store rilpivirine prolonged-release injection (*Rekambys*®) in a refrigerator (2°C to 8°C)—may be stored unopened at room temperature (below 25°C) for up to 6 hours before use.
- **PATIENT AND CARER ADVICE** Patients or carers should be given advice on how to administer rilpivirine tablets. **Missed doses** If an **oral** dose is more than 12 hours late, the missed dose should not be taken and the next dose should be taken at the normal time. If vomiting occurs within 4 hours of taking an **oral** dose, a replacement dose should be taken.
  Driving and skilled tasks Patients and carers should be counselled on the effects on driving and performance of skilled tasks—increased risk of fatigue, dizziness and somnolence.

- **NATIONAL FUNDING/ACCESS DECISIONS** For full details see funding body website
  NICE decisions
- ▶ **Cabotegravir with rilpivirine for treating HIV-1 (January 2022)** NICE TA757 Recommended

- **MEDICINAL FORMS** There can be variation in the licensing of different medicines containing the same drug.
  Prolonged-release suspension for injection
- ▶ Rekambys (ViiV Healthcare UK Ltd) ▼
  Rilpivirine 300 mg per 1 ml Rekambys 900mg/3ml prolonged-release suspension for injection vials | 1 vial [PoM] £440.47 (Hospital only)
  Oral tablet
  CAUTIONARY AND ADVISORY LABELS 3, 21, 25
- ▶ Edurant (Janssen-Cilag Ltd)
  Rilpivirine (as Rilpivirine hydrochloride) 25 mg Edurant 25mg tablets | 30 tablet [PoM] £200.27 (Hospital only)

Combinations available: *Dolutegravir with rilpivirine,* p. 740 · *Emtricitabine with rilpivirine and tenofovir alafenamide,* p. 748 · *Emtricitabine with rilpivirine and tenofovir disoproxil,* p. 749

ANTIVIRALS > NUCLEOSIDE REVERSE TRANSCRIPTASE INHIBITORS

Nucleoside reverse transcriptase inhibitors 

- **SIDE-EFFECTS**
- ▶ **Common or very common** Abdominal pain · anaemia (may require transfusion) · asthenia · diarrhoea · dizziness · fever · flatulence · headache · insomnia · nausea · neutropenia · skin reactions · vomiting
- ▶ **Uncommon** Angioedema · pancreatitis
- ▶ **Rare or very rare** Lactic acidosis
- ▶ **Frequency not known** Immune reconstitution inflammatory syndrome · osteonecrosis · weight increased

  SIDE-EFFECTS, FURTHER INFORMATION Osteonecrosis has been reported in patients with advanced HIV disease or following long-term exposure to combination antiretroviral therapy.

- **PREGNANCY**
  Monitoring Mitochondrial dysfunction has been reported in infants exposed to nucleoside reverse transcriptase inhibitors in utero; the main effects include haematological, metabolic, and neurological disorders; all infants whose mothers received nucleoside reverse transcriptase inhibitors during pregnancy should be monitored for relevant signs or symptoms.
- **HEPATIC IMPAIRMENT** In general, manufacturers advise caution in patients with chronic hepatitis B or C (increased risk of hepatic side-effects).

▶ above

Abacavir

28-Apr-2021

- **INDICATIONS AND DOSE**

  HIV infection in combination with other antiretroviral drugs
- ▶ BY MOUTH
- ▶ Adult: 600 mg daily in 1–2 divided doses

- **CAUTIONS** HIV load greater than 100 000 copies/mL · patients at high risk of cardiovascular disease
- **INTERACTIONS** → Appendix 1: NRTIs
- **SIDE-EFFECTS**
- ▶ **Common or very common** Appetite decreased · lethargy
- ▶ **Rare or very rare** Severe cutaneous adverse reactions (SCARs)
- ▶ **Frequency not known** Hypersensitivity

SIDE-EFFECTS, FURTHER INFORMATION Life-threatening hypersensitivity reactions have been reported-characterised by fever or rash and possibly nausea, vomiting, diarrhoea, abdominal pain, dyspnoea, cough, lethargy, malaise, headache, and myalgia; less frequently mouth ulceration, oedema, hypotension, sore throat, acute respiratory distress syndrome, anaphylaxis, paraesthesia, arthralgia, conjunctivitis, lymphadenopathy, lymphocytopenia and renal failure; rarely myolysis. Laboratory abnormalities may include raised liver function tests and creatine kinase; symptoms usually appear in the first 6 weeks, but may occur at any time. Discontinue immediately if any symptom of hypersensitivity develops and do not rechallenge (risk of more severe hypersensitivity reaction).

- **ALLERGY AND CROSS-SENSITIVITY** [EvGr] Caution—increased risk of hypersensitivity reaction in presence of HLA-B*5701 allele. ⟨M⟩
- **HEPATIC IMPAIRMENT** Manufacturer advises caution in mild impairment; consider avoiding in moderate to severe impairment (no information available).
- **RENAL IMPAIRMENT** Manufacturer advises avoid in end-stage renal disease.
- **PRE-TREATMENT SCREENING** Test for HLA-B*5701 allele before treatment or if restarting treatment and HLA-B*5701 status not known.
- **MONITORING REQUIREMENTS** Monitor for symptoms of hypersensitivity reaction every 2 weeks for 2 months.
- **PRESCRIBING AND DISPENSING INFORMATION** Flavours of oral liquid formulations may include banana, or strawberry.
- **PATIENT AND CARER ADVICE** Patients and their carers should be told the importance of regular dosing (intermittent therapy may increase the risk of sensitisation), how to recognise signs of hypersensitivity, and advised to seek immediate medical attention if symptoms develop or before re-starting treatment.

  Patients should be provided with an alert card and advised to keep it with them at all times.

- **MEDICINAL FORMS** There can be variation in the licensing of different medicines containing the same drug.
  Oral tablet
  - Abacavir (Non-proprietary)
    Abacavir (as Abacavir sulfate) 300 mg Abacavir 300mg tablets | 60 tablet [PoM] £177.60-£177.61 (Hospital only)
  - Ziagen (ViiV Healthcare UK Ltd)
    Abacavir (as Abacavir sulfate) 300 mg Ziagen 300mg tablets | 60 tablet [PoM] £208.95 (Hospital only)

  Oral solution
  EXCIPIENTS: May contain Propylene glycol
  - Ziagen (ViiV Healthcare UK Ltd)
    Abacavir (as Abacavir sulfate) 20 mg per 1 ml Ziagen 20mg/ml oral solution | 240 ml [PoM] £55.72 (Hospital only) [SF]

Abacavir with dolutegravir and lamivudine
28-Jul-2021

The properties listed below are those particular to the combination only. For the properties of the components please consider, abacavir p. 744, lamivudine p. 750, dolutegravir p. 739.

- **INDICATIONS AND DOSE**

  HIV infection
  - BY MOUTH
  - Adult (body-weight 40 kg and above): 1 tablet once daily

- **INTERACTIONS** → Appendix 1: dolutegravir · NRTIs

- **RENAL IMPAIRMENT** [EvGr] Avoid if creatinine clearance less than 50 mL/minute (consult product literature). ⟨M⟩ See p. 21.
- **PATIENT AND CARER ADVICE**
  Missed doses If a dose is more than 20 hours late, the missed dose should not be taken and the next dose should be taken at the normal time.

- **MEDICINAL FORMS** There can be variation in the licensing of different medicines containing the same drug.
  Oral tablet
  - Triumeq (ViiV Healthcare UK Ltd)
    Dolutegravir (as Dolutegravir sodium) 50 mg, Lamivudine 300 mg, Abacavir (as Abacavir sulfate) 600 mg Triumeq 50mg/600mg/300mg tablets | 30 tablet [PoM] £798.16 (Hospital only)

Abacavir with lamivudine
28-Jul-2021

The properties listed below are those particular to the combination only. For the properties of the components please consider, abacavir p. 744, lamivudine p. 750.

- **INDICATIONS AND DOSE**

  HIV infection in combination with other antiretrovirals
  - BY MOUTH
  - Adult (body-weight 40 kg and above): 1 tablet once daily

- **INTERACTIONS** → Appendix 1: NRTIs
- **RENAL IMPAIRMENT** [EvGr] Avoid if creatinine clearance less than 50 mL/minute (consult product literature). ⟨M⟩ See p. 21.

- **MEDICINAL FORMS** There can be variation in the licensing of different medicines containing the same drug.
  Oral tablet
  - Abacavir with lamivudine (Non-proprietary)
    Lamivudine 300 mg, Abacavir 600 mg Abacavir 600mg / Lamivudine 300mg tablets | 30 tablet [PoM] £299.41 DT = £352.25 (Hospital only)
  - Kivexa (ViiV Healthcare UK Ltd)
    Lamivudine 300 mg, Abacavir 600 mg Kivexa 600mg/300mg tablets | 30 tablet [PoM] £352.25 DT = £352.25 (Hospital only)

Abacavir with lamivudine and zidovudine
28-Jul-2021

The properties listed below are those particular to the combination only. For the properties of the components please consider, abacavir p. 744, lamivudine p. 750, zidovudine p. 752.

- **INDICATIONS AND DOSE**

  HIV infection (use only if patient is stabilised for 6–8 weeks on the individual components in the same proportions)
  - BY MOUTH
  - Adult: 1 tablet twice daily

- **INTERACTIONS** → Appendix 1: NRTIs
- **RENAL IMPAIRMENT** [EvGr] Avoid if creatinine clearance less than 50 mL/minute (consult product literature). ⟨M⟩ See p. 21.

- **MEDICINAL FORMS** No licensed medicines listed.

Bictegravir with emtricitabine and tenofovir alafenamide

05-Jul-2024

The properties listed below are those particular to the combination only. For the properties of the components please consider, emtricitabine p. 748, tenofovir alafenamide p. 720.

- **INDICATIONS AND DOSE**

HIV-1 infection [doses for 50/200/25 mg tablets] (initiated by a specialist)
▶ BY MOUTH
▶ Adult: 1 tablet once daily

DOSE EQUIVALENCE AND CONVERSION
▶ Tablet strength expressed as x/y/z mg representing bictegravir/emtricitabine/tenofovir alafenamide, respectively.

- **INTERACTIONS** → Appendix 1: bictegravir · tenofovir alafenamide

- **SIDE-EFFECTS**
▶ **Common or very common** Depression · diarrhoea · dizziness · fatigue · headache · nausea · sleep disorders
▶ **Uncommon** Anaemia · angioedema · anxiety · arthralgia · flatulence · gastrointestinal discomfort · hyperbilirubinaemia · skin reactions · suicidal behaviours · vomiting
▶ **Rare or very rare** Stevens-Johnson syndrome
▶ **Frequency not known** Osteonecrosis

- **PREGNANCY** EvGr Use only if potential benefit outweighs risk (limited information on bictegravir). Ⓜ

- **HEPATIC IMPAIRMENT** EvGr Avoid in severe impairment (no information available). Ⓜ

- **RENAL IMPAIRMENT** EvGr Avoid if creatinine clearance is less than 30 mL/minute (limited information available). Ⓜ See p. 21. EvGr Caution in patients weighing <35kg with any degree of renal impairment (no information available). Ⓜ

- **PRESCRIBING AND DISPENSING INFORMATION** Dispense in original container (contains desiccant).

- **PATIENT AND CARER ADVICE**
Vomiting If vomiting occurs within 1 hour of taking a dose, a replacement dose should be taken.
Missed doses If a dose is more than 18 hours late, the missed dose should not be taken and the next dose should be taken at the normal time.
Driving and skilled tasks Patients and carers should be counselled on the effects on driving and performance of skilled tasks—increased risk of dizziness.

- **NATIONAL FUNDING/ACCESS DECISIONS**
For full details see funding body website
Scottish Medicines Consortium (SMC) decisions
▶ Bictegravir-emtricitabine-tenofovir alafenamide (*Biktarvy*®) for the treatment of adults infected with HIV-1 without any known mutations associated with resistance to the individual components (September 2018) SMC No. SMC2093 Recommended
All Wales Medicines Strategy Group (AWMSG) decisions
▶ Bictegravir/emtricitabine/tenofovir alafenamide (*Biktarvy*®) for the treatment of adults infected with human immunodeficiency virus-1 (HIV-1) without present or past evidence of viral resistance to the integrase inhibitor class, emtricitabine or tenofovir (December 2018) AWMSG No. 3414 Recommended with restrictions

- **MEDICINAL FORMS** There can be variation in the licensing of different medicines containing the same drug.
Oral tablet
CAUTIONARY AND ADVISORY LABELS 25
▶ Biktarvy (Gilead Sciences Ltd)
Tenofovir alafenamide (as Tenofovir alafenamide fumarate) 15 mg, Bictegravir (as Bictegravir sodium) 30 mg, Emtricitabine 120 mg Biktarvy 30mg/120mg/15mg tablets | 30 tablet PoM £879.51 (Hospital only)
Tenofovir alafenamide (as Tenofovir alafenamide fumarate) 25 mg, Bictegravir (as Bictegravir sodium) 50 mg, Emtricitabine 200 mg Biktarvy 50mg/200mg/25mg tablets | 30 tablet PoM £879.51 (Hospital only)

Efavirenz with emtricitabine and tenofovir disoproxil

25-Jul-2021

The properties listed below are those particular to the combination only. For the properties of the components please consider, tenofovir disoproxil p. 751, efavirenz p. 741, emtricitabine p. 748.

- **INDICATIONS AND DOSE**

HIV infection stabilised on antiretroviral therapy for more than 3 months
▶ BY MOUTH
▶ Adult: 1 tablet once daily

- **INTERACTIONS** → Appendix 1: NNRTIs · tenofovir disoproxil

- **HEPATIC IMPAIRMENT** Manufacturer advises caution in mild impairment; avoid in moderate to severe impairment (increased risk of hepatic side-effects).

- **RENAL IMPAIRMENT** EvGr Avoid if creatinine clearance less than 50 mL/minute. Ⓜ See p. 21.

- **PATIENT AND CARER ADVICE**
Missed doses If a dose is more than 12 hours late, the missed dose should not be taken and the next dose should be taken at the normal time.

- **MEDICINAL FORMS** There can be variation in the licensing of different medicines containing the same drug.
Oral tablet
CAUTIONARY AND ADVISORY LABELS 23, 25
▶ Efavirenz with emtricitabine and tenofovir disoproxil (Non-proprietary)
Emtricitabine 200 mg, Tenofovir disoproxil 245 mg, Efavirenz 600 mg Efavirenz 600mg / Emtricitabine 200mg / Tenofovir disoproxil 245mg tablets | 30 tablet PoM £532.87 | 30 tablet PoM £175.00–£532.87 (Hospital only)

Elvitegravir with cobicistat, emtricitabine and tenofovir alafenamide

22-Oct-2020

The properties listed below are those particular to the combination only. For the properties of the components please consider, emtricitabine p. 748, elvitegravir p. 740, cobicistat p. 757, tenofovir alafenamide p. 720.

- **INDICATIONS AND DOSE**

HIV-1 infection (specialist use only)
▶ BY MOUTH
▶ Adult: 1 tablet once daily

IMPORTANT SAFETY INFORMATION
MHRA/CHM ADVICE: ELVITEGRAVIR BOOSTED WITH COBICISTAT: AVOID USE IN PREGNANCY DUE TO RISK OF TREATMENT FAILURE AND MATERNAL-TO-CHILD TRANSMISSION OF HIV-1 (APRIL 2019)
Pharmacokinetic data show mean exposure of elvitegravir boosted with cobicistat (available in

combination in *Genvoya*® and *Stribild*®) to be lower during the second and third trimesters of pregnancy than postpartum. Low elvitegravir exposure may be associated with an increased risk of treatment failure and an increased risk of HIV-1 transmission to the unborn child. For further information, see *Pregnancy*.

- **INTERACTIONS** → Appendix 1: cobicistat · elvitegravir · tenofovir alafenamide

- **SIDE-EFFECTS**
▸ **Common or very common** Abnormal dreams · diarrhoea · dizziness · fatigue · flatulence · gastrointestinal discomfort · headache · nausea · skin reactions · vomiting
▸ **Uncommon** Anaemia · depression · suicidal behaviours
▸ **Frequency not known** Nephrotoxicity · osteonecrosis · weight increased

- **CONCEPTION AND CONTRACEPTION** Manufacturer advises effective contraception in women of childbearing potential; if using a hormonal contraceptive, it must contain drospirenone or norgestimate as the progestogen and at least 30 micrograms ethinylestradiol.

- **PREGNANCY** Manufacturer advises not to be initiated during pregnancy due to low elvitegravir exposure; women who become pregnant during therapy should be switched to an alternative regimen.

- **HEPATIC IMPAIRMENT** Manufacturer advises caution (increased risk of hepatic side-effects); avoid in severe impairment (no information available).

- **RENAL IMPAIRMENT** Manufacturer advises avoid if creatinine clearance less than 30 mL/minute—limited information available. See p. 21.

- **PRESCRIBING AND DISPENSING INFORMATION** Dispense in original container—contains desiccant.

- **PATIENT AND CARER ADVICE**
Missed doses Manufacturer advises if a dose is more than 18 hours late, the missed dose should not be taken and the next dose should be taken at the normal time.
Driving and skilled tasks Manufacturer advises patients and carers should be counselled on the effects on driving and performance of skilled tasks—increased risk of dizziness.

- **NATIONAL FUNDING/ACCESS DECISIONS**
For full details see funding body website
Scottish Medicines Consortium (SMC) decisions
▸ Elvitegravir, cobicistat, emtricitabine, tenofovir alafenamide (*Genvoya*®) for the treatment of adults and adolescents (aged 12 years and older with body weight at least 35 kg) infected with human immunodeficiency virus-1 (HIV-1) without any known mutations associated with resistance to the integrase inhibitor class, emtricitabine or tenofovir (May 2016) SMC No. 1142/16 Recommended

All Wales Medicines Strategy Group (AWMSG) decisions
▸ Elvitegravir / cobicistat / emtricitabine / tenofovir alafenamide (*Genvoya*®) for the treatment of adults and adolescents (aged 12 years and older with body weight at least 35 kg) infected with human immunodeficiency virus-1 (HIV-1) without any known mutations associated with resistance to the integrase inhibitor class, emtricitabine or tenofovir (July 2016) AWMSG No. 2248 Recommended

- **MEDICINAL FORMS** There can be variation in the licensing of different medicines containing the same drug.
Oral tablet
CAUTIONARY AND ADVISORY LABELS 21
▸ Genvoya (Gilead Sciences Ltd)
Tenofovir alafenamide (as Tenofovir alafenamide fumarate) 6 mg, Cobicistat 90 mg, Elvitegravir 90 mg, Emtricitabine 120 mg Genvoya 90mg/90mg/120mg/6mg tablets | 30 tablet PoM £879.51 (Hospital only)
Tenofovir alafenamide (as Tenofovir alafenamide fumarate) 10 mg, Cobicistat 150 mg, Elvitegravir 150 mg, Emtricitabine

200 mg Genvoya 150mg/150mg/200mg/10mg tablets | 30 tablet PoM £879.51 (Hospital only)

Elvitegravir with cobicistat, emtricitabine and tenofovir disoproxil

26-Jul-2021

The properties listed below are those particular to the combination only. For the properties of the components please consider, tenofovir disoproxil p. 751, emtricitabine p. 748, cobicistat p. 757, elvitegravir p. 740.

- **INDICATIONS AND DOSE**
HIV infection
▸ BY MOUTH
▸ Adult: 1 tablet once daily

IMPORTANT SAFETY INFORMATION
MHRA/CHM ADVICE: ELVITEGRAVIR BOOSTED WITH COBICISTAT: AVOID USE IN PREGNANCY DUE TO RISK OF TREATMENT FAILURE AND MATERNAL-TO-CHILD TRANSMISSION OF HIV-1 (APRIL 2019)
Pharmacokinetic data show mean exposure of elvitegravir boosted with cobicistat (available in combination in *Genvoya*® and *Stribild*®) to be lower during the second and third trimesters of pregnancy than postpartum. Low elvitegravir exposure may be associated with an increased risk of treatment failure and an increased risk of HIV-1 transmission to the unborn child. For further information, see *Pregnancy*.

- **INTERACTIONS** → Appendix 1: cobicistat · elvitegravir · tenofovir disoproxil

- **SIDE-EFFECTS**
▸ **Common or very common** Appetite decreased · asthenia · constipation · diarrhoea · dizziness · electrolyte imbalance · flatulence · gastrointestinal discomfort · headache · hyperbilirubinaemia · hyperglycaemia · hypersensitivity · hypertriglyceridaemia · nausea · neutropenia · pain · rash pustular · skin reactions · sleep disorders · vomiting
▸ **Uncommon** Anaemia · angioedema · depression (in patients with history of depression or psychiatric illness) · muscle weakness · myopathy · pancreatitis · proteinuria · renal failure · renal tubular disorders · suicidal ideation (in patients with history of depression or psychiatric illness)
▸ **Rare or very rare** Acute tubular necrosis · hepatic disorders · lactic acidosis · nephritis · nephrogenic diabetes insipidus · osteomalacia
▸ **Frequency not known** Autoimmune disorder · Grave's disease · inflammation · osteonecrosis · weight increased

- **CONCEPTION AND CONTRACEPTION** Women of child-bearing potential should use effective contraception during treatment (if using a hormonal contraceptive, it must contain norgestimate as the progestogen and at least 30 micrograms ethinylestradiol).

- **PREGNANCY** Manufacturer advises not to be initiated during pregnancy due to low elvitegravir exposure; women who become pregnant during therapy should be switched to an alternative regimen.

- **HEPATIC IMPAIRMENT** Manufacturer advises caution (increased risk of hepatic side-effects); avoid in severe impairment (no information available).

- **RENAL IMPAIRMENT** EvGr If creatinine clearance less than 90 mL/minute, only *initiate Stribild*® if other treatments cannot be used (avoid *initiating Stribild*® if creatinine clearance less than 70 mL/minute). If creatinine clearance less than 70 mL/minute, only *continue Stribild*® if potential benefit outweighs risk (discontinue *Stribild*® if creatinine clearance less than 50 mL/minute). Ⓜ See p. 21.

- **MONITORING REQUIREMENTS** Test urine glucose before treatment, then every 4 weeks for 1 year and then every 3 months.
- **PRESCRIBING AND DISPENSING INFORMATION** Dispense in original container (contains desiccant).
- **PATIENT AND CARER ADVICE** Patients or carers should be given advice on how to administer *Stribild*®.
  Missed doses If a dose is more than 18 hours late, the missed dose should not be taken and the next dose should be taken at the normal time.

- **MEDICINAL FORMS** There can be variation in the licensing of different medicines containing the same drug.
  Oral tablet
  CAUTIONARY AND ADVISORY LABELS 21
  ▸ Stribild (Gilead Sciences Ltd)
    Cobicistat 150 mg, Elvitegravir 150 mg, Emtricitabine 200 mg, Tenofovir disoproxil 245 mg Stribild 150mg/150mg/200mg/245mg tablets | 30 tablet [PoM] £879.51 (Hospital only)

⚑ 744

Emtricitabine
26-Jul-2021

(FTC)

- **INDICATIONS AND DOSE**
  HIV infection in combination with other antiretroviral drugs
  ▸ BY MOUTH USING CAPSULES
  ▸ Adult: 200 mg once daily
  ▸ BY MOUTH USING ORAL SOLUTION
  ▸ Adult: 240 mg once daily
  DOSE EQUIVALENCE AND CONVERSION
  ▸ 240 mg oral solution ≡ 200 mg capsule; where appropriate the capsule may be used instead of the oral solution.

- **SIDE-EFFECTS**
  ▸ **Common or very common** Abnormal dreams · dyspepsia · hyperbilirubinaemia · hyperglycaemia · hypersensitivity · hypertriglyceridaemia · pain · rash pustular

- **HEPATIC IMPAIRMENT**
  Monitoring On discontinuation, monitor patients with hepatitis B (risk of exacerbation of hepatitis).

- **RENAL IMPAIRMENT**
  Dose adjustments See p. 21.
    Manufacturer advises reduce dose or increase dosage interval if creatinine clearance less than 30 mL/minute (consult product literature).

- **PRESCRIBING AND DISPENSING INFORMATION** Flavours of oral liquid formulations may include candy.

- **PATIENT AND CARER ADVICE**
  Missed doses If a dose is more than 12 hours late, the missed dose should not be taken and the next dose should be taken at the normal time.

- **MEDICINAL FORMS** There can be variation in the licensing of different medicines containing the same drug.
  Oral solution
  ELECTROLYTES: May contain Sodium
  ▸ Emtriva (Gilead Sciences Ltd)
    Emtricitabine 10 mg per 1 ml Emtriva 10mg/ml oral solution | 170 ml [PoM] £39.53 (Hospital only) [SF]
  Oral capsule
  ▸ Emtriva (Gilead Sciences Ltd)
    Emtricitabine 200 mg Emtriva 200mg capsules | 30 capsule [PoM] £138.98 (Hospital only)

  Combinations available: *Darunavir with cobicistat, emtricitabine and tenofovir alafenamide,* p. 755

Emtricitabine with rilpivirine and tenofovir alafenamide
21-Aug-2020

The properties listed below are those particular to the combination only. For the properties of the components please consider, emtricitabine above, rilpivirine p. 743, tenofovir alafenamide p. 720.

- **INDICATIONS AND DOSE**
  HIV infection in patients with plasma HIV-1 RNA concentration of 100 000 **copies/mL or less (specialist use only)**
  ▸ BY MOUTH
  ▸ Adult: 1 tablet once daily

- **INTERACTIONS** → Appendix 1: NNRTIs · tenofovir alafenamide
- **SIDE-EFFECTS**
  ▸ **Common or very common** Appetite decreased · depression · diarrhoea · dizziness · drowsiness · dry mouth · fatigue · flatulence · gastrointestinal discomfort · headache · nausea · skin reactions · sleep disorders · vomiting
  ▸ **Uncommon** Anaemia · angioedema · arthralgia · immune reconstitution inflammatory syndrome · severe cutaneous adverse reactions (SCARs)
  ▸ **Frequency not known** Conjunctivitis · eosinophilia · fever · osteonecrosis

  SIDE-EFFECTS, FURTHER INFORMATION Systemic symptoms reported with severe skin reactions include fever, blisters, conjunctivitis, angioedema, elevated liver function tests, and eosinophilia.

- **HEPATIC IMPAIRMENT** Manufacturer advises caution in moderate impairment (increased risk of hepatic side-effects); avoid in severe impairment (no information available).

- **RENAL IMPAIRMENT** Manufacturer advises avoid if creatinine clearance less than 30 mL/minute—no information available. See p. 21.

- **PATIENT AND CARER ADVICE**
  Vomiting Manufacturer advises if vomiting occurs within 4 hours of taking a dose, a replacement dose should be taken.
  Driving and skilled tasks Manufacturer advises patients and carers should be counselled on the effects on driving and performance of skilled tasks—increased risk of dizziness.

- **NATIONAL FUNDING/ACCESS DECISIONS**
  For full details see funding body website
  Scottish Medicines Consortium (SMC) decisions
  ▸ Emtricitabine/rilpivirine/tenofovir alafenamide (*Odefsey*®) for the treatment of HIV-1 without known mutations associated with resistance to the non nucleoside reverse transcriptase inhibitor class, tenofovir or emtricitabine, and with a viral load HIV-1 RNA of 100,000 copies/mL or less (October 2016) SMC No. 1189/16 Recommended
  All Wales Medicines Strategy Group (AWMSG) decisions
  ▸ Emtricitabine/rilpivirine/tenofovir alafenamide (*Odefsey*®) for the treatment of HIV-1 without known mutations associated with resistance to the non-nucleoside reverse transcriptase inhibitor class, tenofovir or emtricitabine, and with a viral load HIV-1 RNA of 100,000 copies/mL or less (November 2016) AWMSG No. 3031 Recommended

- **MEDICINAL FORMS** There can be variation in the licensing of different medicines containing the same drug.
  Oral tablet
  CAUTIONARY AND ADVISORY LABELS 3, 21
  ▸ Odefsey (Gilead Sciences Ltd)
    Rilpivirine (as Rilpivirine hydrochloride) 25 mg, Tenofovir alafenamide (as Tenofovir alafenamide fumarate) 25 mg, Emtricitabine 200 mg Odefsey 200mg/25mg/25mg tablets | 30 tablet [PoM] £525.95 (Hospital only)

Emtricitabine with rilpivirine and tenofovir disoproxil

25-Jul-2021

The properties listed below are those particular to the combination only. For the properties of the components please consider, tenofovir disoproxil p. 751, emtricitabine p. 748, rilpivirine p. 743.

- **INDICATIONS AND DOSE**

HIV infection in patients with plasma HIV-1 RNA concentration less than 100 000 copies/mL
  - ▶ BY MOUTH
  - ▶ Adult: 1 tablet once daily

- **INTERACTIONS** → Appendix 1: NNRTIs · tenofovir disoproxil

- **HEPATIC IMPAIRMENT** Manufacturer advises caution in moderate impairment (increased risk of hepatic side-effects); avoid in severe impairment (no information available).

- **RENAL IMPAIRMENT** EvGr Caution if creatinine clearance 50–80 mL/minute; avoid if creatinine clearance less than 50 mL/minute. M See p. 21.

- **PATIENT AND CARER ADVICE** Patients or carers should be given advice on how to administer *Eviplera*®.
  Missed doses If a dose is more than 12 hours late, the missed dose should not be taken and the next dose should be taken at the normal time.

- **MEDICINAL FORMS** There can be variation in the licensing of different medicines containing the same drug.
  Oral tablet
  CAUTIONARY AND ADVISORY LABELS 21, 25
  - ▶ Eviplera (Gilead Sciences Ltd)
    Rilpivirine (as Rilpivirine hydrochloride) 25 mg, Emtricitabine 200 mg, Tenofovir disoproxil 245 mg Eviplera 200mg/25mg/245mg tablets | 30 tablet PoM £525.95 (Hospital only)

Emtricitabine with tenofovir alafenamide

10-Mar-2025

The properties listed below are those particular to the combination only. For the properties of the components please consider, emtricitabine p. 748, tenofovir alafenamide p. 720.

- **INDICATIONS AND DOSE**

HIV-1 infection in combination with other antiretroviral drugs [doses for 200/10 mg or 200/25 mg tablets] (initiated by a specialist)
  - ▶ BY MOUTH
  - ▶ Adult: 1 tablet once daily, tablet strength is dependent on drug regimen—consult product literature

Pre-exposure prophylaxis of HIV-1 infection [doses for 200/25 mg tablets] (initiated by a specialist)
  - ▶ BY MOUTH
  - ▶ Adult (male): 1 tablet once daily.

DOSE EQUIVALENCE AND CONVERSION
  - ▶ Tablet strength expressed as *x*/*y* mg representing emtricitabine/tenofovir alafenamide, respectively.

- **INTERACTIONS** → Appendix 1: tenofovir alafenamide

- **SIDE-EFFECTS**
- ▶ **Common or very common** Abnormal dreams · diarrhoea · dizziness · fatigue · flatulence · gastrointestinal discomfort · headache · nausea · skin reactions · vomiting
- ▶ **Uncommon** Anaemia · angioedema · arthralgia
- ▶ **Frequency not known** Immune reconstitution inflammatory syndrome · nephrotoxicity · osteonecrosis

- **HEPATIC IMPAIRMENT** EvGr Caution (increased risk of hepatic side-effects). M

- **RENAL IMPAIRMENT** EvGr Avoid if creatinine clearance less than 30 mL/minute (limited information available). M See p. 21.

- **PATIENT AND CARER ADVICE**
  Missed doses If a dose is more than 18 hours late, the missed dose should not be taken and the next dose should be taken at the normal time.
  Driving and skilled tasks Patients and carers should be counselled on the effects on driving and performance of skilled tasks—increased risk of dizziness.

- **NATIONAL FUNDING/ACCESS DECISIONS**
  For full details see funding body website
  Scottish Medicines Consortium (SMC) decisions
  - ▶ Emtricitabine / tenofovir alafenamide (*Descovy*®) in combination with other antiretroviral agents for the treatment of adults and adolescents (aged 12 years and older with body weight at least 35 kg) infected with human immunodeficiency virus type 1 (August 2016) SMC No. 1169/16 Recommended

  All Wales Medicines Strategy Group (AWMSG) decisions
  - ▶ Emtricitabine / tenofovir alafenamide (*Descovy*®) for treatment of adults and adolescents (aged 12 years and older with body weight at least 35 kg) infected with human immunodeficiency virus type 1 (HIV 1) (October 2016) AWMSG No. 2771 Recommended
  - ▶ Emtricitabine / tenofovir alafenamide (*Descovy*®) for pre-exposure prophylaxis to reduce the risk of sexually acquired HIV-1 infection in at-risk men who have sex with men, including adolescents (with body weight at least 35 kg) (February 2025) AWMSG No. 2566 Recommended with restrictions

- **MEDICINAL FORMS** There can be variation in the licensing of different medicines containing the same drug.
  Oral tablet
  CAUTIONARY AND ADVISORY LABELS 25
  - ▶ Descovy (Gilead Sciences Ltd)
    Tenofovir alafenamide (as Tenofovir alafenamide fumarate) 25 mg, Emtricitabine 200 mg Descovy 200mg/25mg tablets | 30 tablet PoM £355.73 DT = £355.73 (Hospital only)
    Tenofovir alafenamide (as Tenofovir alafenamide fumarate) 10 mg, Emtricitabine 200 mg Descovy 200mg/10mg tablets | 30 tablet PoM £355.73 DT = £355.73 (Hospital only)

Emtricitabine with tenofovir disoproxil

12-Oct-2020

The properties listed below are those particular to the combination only. For the properties of the components please consider, tenofovir disoproxil p. 751, emtricitabine p. 748.

- **INDICATIONS AND DOSE**

HIV-1 infection (initiated by a specialist)
  - ▶ BY MOUTH
  - ▶ Adult: 200/245 mg once daily

Pre-exposure prophylaxis of HIV-1 infection (initiated by a specialist)
  - ▶ BY MOUTH
  - ▶ Adult: 200/245 mg once daily

DOSE EQUIVALENCE AND CONVERSION
  - ▶ Dose expressed as x/y mg emtricitabine/tenofovir disoproxil.

- **INTERACTIONS** → Appendix 1: tenofovir disoproxil

- **HEPATIC IMPAIRMENT** Manufacturer advises caution (increased risk of hepatic side-effects).

- **RENAL IMPAIRMENT**
  - ▶ When used for HIV-1 infection Manufacturer advises avoid in

severe impairment.
- When used for Pre-exposure prophylaxis of HIV-1 infection Manufacturer advises avoid if creatinine clearance less than 60 mL/minute. See p. 21.
  Dose adjustments
  - When used for HIV-1 infection Manufacturer advises use normal dose every 2 days in moderate impairment.
- **DIRECTIONS FOR ADMINISTRATION** Patients with swallowing difficulties may disperse tablet in half a glass of water, orange juice, or grape juice.
- **PATIENT AND CARER ADVICE** Patients or carers should be given advice on how to administer emtricitabine with tenofovir tablets.
  Missed doses If a dose is more than 12 hours late, the missed dose should not be taken and the next dose should be taken at the normal time.
- **NATIONAL FUNDING/ACCESS DECISIONS** For full details see funding body website
  Scottish Medicines Consortium (SMC) decisions
- Emtricitabine/tenofovir disoproxil (*Truvada*®) in combination with safer sex practices for pre-exposure prophylaxis to reduce the risk of sexually acquired HIV-1 infection in adults at high risk (April 2017) SMC No. 1225/17 Recommended
  All Wales Medicines Strategy Group (AWMSG) decisions
- Emtricitabine/tenofovir disoproxil in combination with safer sex practices for pre-exposure prophylaxis to reduce the risk of sexually acquired HIV-1 infection in adults at high risk (June 2020) AWMSG No. 4623 Recommended

- **MEDICINAL FORMS** There can be variation in the licensing of different medicines containing the same drug. Forms available from special-order manufacturers include: oral tablet
  Oral tablet
  CAUTIONARY AND ADVISORY LABELS 21
  - Emtricitabine with tenofovir disoproxil (Non-proprietary)
    Emtricitabine 200 mg, Tenofovir disoproxil 245 mg Emtricitabine 200mg / Tenofovir disoproxil 245mg tablets | 30 tablet PoM £355.73 DT = £355.73 (Hospital only) | 30 tablet PoM £302.37 DT = £355.73
  - Truvada (Gilead Sciences Ltd)
    Emtricitabine 200 mg, Tenofovir disoproxil 245 mg Truvada 200mg/245mg tablets | 30 tablet PoM £355.73 DT = £355.73 (Hospital only)

▶ 744

Lamivudine

25-Jul-2021

(3TC)

- **INDICATIONS AND DOSE**

EPIVIR ® ORAL SOLUTION

HIV infection in combination with other antiretroviral drugs
- BY MOUTH
- Adult: 150 mg every 12 hours, alternatively 300 mg once daily

EPIVIR ® TABLETS

HIV infection in combination with other antiretroviral drugs
- BY MOUTH
- Adult: 150 mg every 12 hours, alternatively 300 mg once daily

ZEFFIX ®

Chronic hepatitis B infection either with compensated liver disease (with evidence of viral replication and histology of active liver inflammation or fibrosis) when first-line treatments cannot be used, or (in combination with another antiviral drug without cross-resistance to lamivudine) with decompensated liver disease
- BY MOUTH
- Adult: 100 mg once daily, patients receiving lamivudine for concomitant HIV infection should

continue to receive lamivudine in a dose appropriate for HIV infection

- **CAUTIONS** Recurrent hepatitis in patients with chronic hepatitis B may occur on discontinuation of lamivudine
- **INTERACTIONS** → Appendix 1: NRTIs
- **SIDE-EFFECTS**
  - **Common or very common** Alopecia · arthralgia · cough · gastrointestinal discomfort · hepatic disorders · malaise · muscle complaints · myopathy · nasal disorder
  - **Uncommon** Thrombocytopenia
  - **Rare or very rare** Paraesthesia · peripheral neuropathy · pure red cell aplasia
  - **Frequency not known** Respiratory tract infection · throat complaints
- **BREAST FEEDING** Can be used with caution in women infected with chronic hepatitis B alone, providing that adequate measures are taken to prevent hepatitis B infection in infants.
- **RENAL IMPAIRMENT**
  Dose adjustments EvGr Reduce dose if creatinine clearance less than 50 mL/minute (consult product literature). ⬥ See p. 21.
- **MONITORING REQUIREMENTS** When treating chronic hepatitis B with lamivudine, monitor liver function tests every 3 months, and viral markers of hepatitis B every 3–6 months, more frequently in patients with advanced liver disease or following transplantation (monitoring to continue for at least 1 year after discontinuation— recurrent hepatitis may occur on discontinuation).
- **PRESCRIBING AND DISPENSING INFORMATION** Flavours of oral liquid formulations may include banana and strawberry.

- **MEDICINAL FORMS** There can be variation in the licensing of different medicines containing the same drug.
  Oral tablet
  - Epivir (ViiV Healthcare UK Ltd)
    Lamivudine 150 mg Epivir 150mg tablets | 60 tablet PoM £143.32 DT = £143.32 (Hospital only)
    Lamivudine 300 mg Epivir 300mg tablets | 30 tablet PoM £157.51 DT = £157.51 (Hospital only)
  - Zeffix (GlaxoSmithKline UK Ltd)
    Lamivudine 100 mg Zeffix 100mg tablets | 28 tablet PoM £78.09 DT = £78.09
  Oral solution
  EXCIPIENTS: May contain Sucrose
  - Epivir (ViiV Healthcare UK Ltd)
    Lamivudine 10 mg per 1 ml Epivir 50mg/5ml oral solution | 240 ml PoM £39.01 DT = £39.01 (Hospital only)

Lamivudine with dolutegravir

23-Oct-2020

The properties listed below are those particular to the combination only. For the properties of the components please consider, lamivudine above, dolutegravir p. 739.

- **INDICATIONS AND DOSE**

HIV-1 infection
- BY MOUTH
- Adult: 300/50 mg once daily

DOSE EQUIVALENCE AND CONVERSION
- Dose expressed as x/y mg lamivudine/dolutegravir.

- **INTERACTIONS** → Appendix 1: dolutegravir · NRTIs
- **RENAL IMPAIRMENT** Manufacturer advises avoid if creatinine clearance less than 50 mL/minute. See p. 21.
- **PATIENT AND CARER ADVICE**
  Missed doses Manufacturer advises if a dose is more than 20 hours late, the missed dose should not be taken and the next dose should be taken at the normal time.

- **NATIONAL FUNDING/ACCESS DECISIONS**
  For full details see funding body website
  Scottish Medicines Consortium (SMC) decisions
  ▸ Dolutegravir / lamivudine (*Dovato*®) for treatment of Human Immunodeficiency Virus type 1 (HIV-1) infection in adults and adolescents above 12 years of age weighing at least 40 kg, with no known or suspected resistance to the integrase inhibitor class, or lamivudine (September 2019) SMC No. SMC2205 Recommended
  All Wales Medicines Strategy Group (AWMSG) decisions
  ▸ Dolutegravir / lamivudine (*Dovato*®) for treatment of Human Immunodeficiency Virus type 1 (HIV-1) infection in adults and adolescents above 12 years of age weighing at least 40 kg, with no known or suspected resistance to the integrase inhibitor class, or lamivudine (February 2020) AWMSG No. 3659 Recommended

- **MEDICINAL FORMS** There can be variation in the licensing of different medicines containing the same drug.
  Oral tablet
  ▸ Dovato (ViiV Healthcare UK Ltd)
    Dolutegravir (as Dolutegravir sodium) 50 mg, Lamivudine 300 mg Dovato 50mg/300mg tablets | 30 tablet PoM £656.26

Lamivudine with tenofovir disoproxil and doravirine
30-Mar-2021

The properties listed below are those particular to the combination only. For the properties of the components please consider, lamivudine p. 750, tenofovir disoproxil below, doravirine p. 741.

- **INDICATIONS AND DOSE**
  HIV-1 infection (initiated by a specialist)
  ▸ BY MOUTH
  ▸ Adult: 1 tablet once daily

  DOSE ADJUSTMENTS DUE TO INTERACTIONS
  ▸ Manufacturer advises if concurrent use of moderate inducers of CYP3A4, dabrafenib, modafinil or telotristat ethyl is unavoidable, increase doravirine dose to 100 mg twice daily. Manufacturer advises increasing doravirine dose to 100 mg twice daily with rifabutin. The extra doravirine 100 mg dose should be taken approximately 12 hours after the dose of *Delstrigo*®.

- **INTERACTIONS** → Appendix 1: NNRTIs · NRTIs · tenofovir disoproxil

- **PREGNANCY** Manufacturer advises avoid.

- **HEPATIC IMPAIRMENT** Manufacturer advises caution in severe impairment—no information available.

- **RENAL IMPAIRMENT** Manufacturer advises avoid if creatinine clearance less than 50 mL/minute. See p. 21.

- **PATIENT AND CARER ADVICE**
  Missed doses If a dose is more than 12 hours late, the missed dose should not be taken and the next dose should be taken at the normal time.
  Driving and skilled tasks Manufacturer advises patients and carers should be counselled on the effects on driving and performance of skilled tasks—increased risk of fatigue, dizziness, and somnolence.

- **NATIONAL FUNDING/ACCESS DECISIONS**
  For full details see funding body website
  Scottish Medicines Consortium (SMC) decisions
  ▸ Doravirine / lamivudine / tenofovir disoproxil fumarate (*Delstrigo*®) for the treatment of adults infected with human immunodeficiency virus-1 (HIV-1) without past or present evidence of resistance to the non-nucleoside reverse transcriptase inhibitor (NNRTI) class, lamivudine, or tenofovir (March 2021) SMC No. SMC2333 Recommended

All Wales Medicines Strategy Group (AWMSG) decisions
▸ Doravirine / lamivudine / tenofovir disoproxil fumarate (*Delstrigo*®) for the treatment of adults infected with HIV-1 without past or present evidence of resistance to the NNRTI class, lamivudine, or tenofovir (September 2020) AWMSG No. 3648 Recommended

- **MEDICINAL FORMS** There can be variation in the licensing of different medicines containing the same drug.
  Oral tablet
  CAUTIONARY AND ADVISORY LABELS 25, 3
  ▸ Delstrigo (Merck Sharp & Dohme (UK) Ltd)
    Doravirine 100 mg, Tenofovir disoproxil 245 mg, Lamivudine 300 mg Delstrigo 100mg/300mg/245mg tablets | 30 tablet PoM £578.55 (Hospital only)

▸ 744
Tenofovir disoproxil
23-Aug-2021

- **INDICATIONS AND DOSE**
  HIV infection in combination with other antiretroviral drugs | Chronic hepatitis B infection with compensated liver disease (with evidence of viral replication, and histologically documented active liver inflammation or fibrosis) | Chronic hepatitis B infection with decompensated liver disease
  ▸ BY MOUTH
  ▸ Adult: 245 mg once daily

  DOSE EQUIVALENCE AND CONVERSION
  ▸ 7.5 scoops of granules contains approx. 245 mg tenofovir disoproxil (as fumarate).

- **INTERACTIONS** → Appendix 1: tenofovir disoproxil

- **SIDE-EFFECTS**
  ▸ **Common or very common** Abdominal distension
  ▸ **Uncommon** Proximal renal tubulopathy
  ▸ **Rare or very rare** Acute tubular necrosis · hepatic disorders · nephritis · nephrogenic diabetes insipidus · renal impairment

- **HEPATIC IMPAIRMENT** Manufacturer advises caution in decompensated hepatic disease (limited information available).

- **RENAL IMPAIRMENT**
  Dose adjustments EvGr *Granules*: 132 mg once daily if creatinine clearance 30–50 mL/minute; 66 mg once daily if creatinine clearance 20–30 mL/minute; 33 mg once daily if creatinine clearance 10–20 mL/minute (limited information available; consult product literature).
    Tablets: 245 mg every 2 days if creatinine clearance 30–50 mL/minute; 245 mg every 3–4 days if creatinine clearance 10–30 mL/minute (limited information available; consult product literature). ⓜ
    See p. 21.

- **MONITORING REQUIREMENTS**
  ▸ Test renal function and serum phosphate before treatment, then every 4 weeks (more frequently if at increased risk of renal impairment) for 1 year and then every 3 months, interrupt treatment if renal function deteriorates or serum phosphate decreases.
  ▸ When treating chronic hepatitis B with tenofovir, monitor liver function tests every 3 months and viral markers for hepatitis B every 3–6 months during treatment (continue monitoring for at least 1 year after discontinuation— recurrent hepatitis may occur on discontinuation).

- **DIRECTIONS FOR ADMINISTRATION** *Granules*: Manufacturer advises mix 1 scoop of granules with 1 tablespoon of soft food (e.g. yoghurt, apple sauce) and take immediately without chewing. Do **not** mix granules with liquids.

- **PATIENT AND CARER ADVICE** Patients or carers should be given advice on how to administer tenofovir granules.

Missed doses If a dose is more than 12 hours late, the missed dose should not be taken and the next dose should be taken at the normal time.

- NATIONAL FUNDING/ACCESS DECISIONS
  For full details see funding body website
  NICE decisions
  ▶ **Tenofovir disoproxil for the treatment of chronic hepatitis B (July 2009)** NICE TA173 Recommended

- MEDICINAL FORMS There can be variation in the licensing of different medicines containing the same drug.
  Oral tablet
  CAUTIONARY AND ADVISORY LABELS 21
  ▶ **Tenofovir disoproxil (Non-proprietary)**
    Tenofovir disoproxil 245 mg Tenofovir disoproxil 245mg tablets | 30 tablet [PoM] £28.39 | 30 tablet [PoM] £28.37–£204.39 (Hospital only)
  ▶ **Viread** (Gilead Sciences Ltd)
    Tenofovir disoproxil 123 mg Viread 123mg tablets | 30 tablet [PoM] £102.60 (Hospital only)
    Tenofovir disoproxil 163 mg Viread 163mg tablets | 30 tablet [PoM] £135.98 (Hospital only)
    Tenofovir disoproxil 204 mg Viread 204mg tablets | 30 tablet [PoM] £170.19 (Hospital only)
    Tenofovir disoproxil 245 mg Viread 245mg tablets | 30 tablet [PoM] £204.39 (Hospital only)
  Oral granules
  CAUTIONARY AND ADVISORY LABELS 21
  ▶ **Viread** (Gilead Sciences Ltd)
    Tenofovir disoproxil 33 mg per 1 gram Viread 33mg/g granules | 60 gram [PoM] £54.50 (Hospital only)

◖ 744

Zidovudine

02-Sep-2021

(Azidothymidine; AZT)

- INDICATIONS AND DOSE

HIV infection in combination with other antiretroviral drugs
▶ BY MOUTH
▶ Adult: 250–300 mg twice daily

Prevention of maternal-fetal HIV transmission
▶ BY MOUTH, OR BY INTRAVENOUS INFUSION
▶ Adult: Seek specialist advice (combination therapy preferred) (consult local protocol)

HIV infection in combination with other antiretroviral drugs in patients temporarily unable to take zidovudine by mouth
▶ BY INTRAVENOUS INFUSION
▶ Adult: 0.8–1 mg/kg every 4 hours usually for not more than 2 weeks, dose approximating to 1.2–1.5 mg/kg every 4 hours by mouth

- CONTRA-INDICATIONS Abnormally low haemoglobin concentration (consult product literature) · abnormally low neutrophil counts (consult product literature)

- CAUTIONS Elderly · lactic acidosis · risk of haematological toxicity particularly with high dose and advanced disease · vitamin B_{12} deficiency (increased risk of neutropenia)

  CAUTIONS, FURTHER INFORMATION
  ▶ Lactic acidosis Lactic acidosis associated with hepatomegaly and hepatic steatosis has been reported with zidovudine. Use with caution in patients with hepatomegaly, hepatitis, or other risk factors for liver disease and hepatic steatosis (including obesity and alcohol abuse). Manufacturer advises discontinue treatment if symptoms of hyperlactataemia, lactic acidosis, progressive hepatomegaly or rapid deterioration of liver function become apparent.

- INTERACTIONS → Appendix 1: NRTIs

- SIDE-EFFECTS
  ▶ **Common or very common** Leucopenia · malaise · myalgia

▶ **Uncommon** Bone marrow disorders · dyspnoea · generalised pain · myopathy · thrombocytopenia
▶ **Rare or very rare** Alertness decreased · anxiety · appetite decreased · cardiomyopathy · chest pain · chills · cough · depression · drowsiness · dyspepsia · gynaecomastia · hepatic disorders · hyperhidrosis · influenza like illness · nail discolouration · oral discolouration · paraesthesia · pure red cell aplasia · seizure · taste altered · urinary frequency increased
▶ **Frequency not known** Lipoatrophy

SIDE-EFFECTS, FURTHER INFORMATION **Anaemia and myelosuppression** If anaemia or myelosuppression occur, reduce dose or interrupt treatment according to product literature, or consider other treatment.
  Lipodystrophy syndrome Metabolic effects may occur with zidovudine; plasma lipids and blood glucose concentrations should be measured routinely.

- HEPATIC IMPAIRMENT Manufacturer advises caution in moderate to severe impairment (increased risk of accumulation).
  Dose adjustments Manufacturer advises consider dose reduction in moderate to severe impairment—consult product literature.

- RENAL IMPAIRMENT
  Dose adjustments See p. 21.
    [EvGr] Reduce oral dose to 100 mg 3–4 times daily (300–400 mg daily) or intravenous dose to 1 mg/kg 3–4 times daily if creatinine clearance is less than 10 mL/minute. ⟨M⟩

- MONITORING REQUIREMENTS Monitor full blood count after 4 weeks of treatment, then every 3 months.

- DIRECTIONS FOR ADMINISTRATION For *intermittent intravenous infusion*, manufacturer advises dilute to a concentration of 2 mg/mL or 4 mg/mL with Glucose 5% and give over 1 hour.

- PRESCRIBING AND DISPENSING INFORMATION The abbreviation AZT which is sometimes used for zidovudine has also been used for another drug.

- MEDICINAL FORMS There can be variation in the licensing of different medicines containing the same drug.
  Solution for infusion
  ▶ **Retrovir** (ViiV Healthcare UK Ltd)
    Zidovudine 10 mg per 1 ml Retrovir IV 200mg/20ml concentrate for solution for infusion vials | 5 vial [PoM] £52.48 (Hospital only)
  Oral solution
  ▶ **Retrovir** (ViiV Healthcare UK Ltd)
    Zidovudine 10 mg per 1 ml Retrovir 100mg/10ml oral solution | 200 ml [PoM] £20.91 (Hospital only) [SF]
  Oral capsule
  ▶ **Zidovudine (Non-proprietary)**
    Zidovudine 100 mg Zidovudine 100mg capsules | 60 capsule [PoM] £53.31 (Hospital only)
    Zidovudine 250 mg Zidovudine 250mg capsules | 60 capsule [PoM] £13.32 (Hospital only)
  ▶ **Retrovir** (ViiV Healthcare UK Ltd)
    Zidovudine 100 mg Retrovir 100mg capsules | 100 capsule [PoM] £104.54 (Hospital only)
    Zidovudine 250 mg Retrovir 250mg capsules | 40 capsule [PoM] £104.54 (Hospital only)

Zidovudine with lamivudine

29-Jul-2021

The properties listed below are those particular to the combination only. For the properties of the components please consider, zidovudine above, lamivudine p. 750.

- INDICATIONS AND DOSE

HIV infection in combination with other antiretroviral drugs
▶ BY MOUTH
▶ Adult: 1 tablet twice daily

- **INTERACTIONS** → Appendix 1: NRTIs
- **RENAL IMPAIRMENT** [EvGr] Avoid if creatinine clearance less than 50 mL/minute (consult product literature). ⟨M⟩ See p. 21.
- **DIRECTIONS FOR ADMINISTRATION**
  COMBIVIR® **TABLETS** Manufacturer advises tablets may be crushed and mixed with semi-solid food or liquid just before administration.

- **MEDICINAL FORMS** There can be variation in the licensing of different medicines containing the same drug.
  Oral tablet
  ► **Zidovudine with lamivudine (Non-proprietary)**
    Lamivudine 150 mg, Zidovudine 300 mg Zidovudine 300mg / Lamivudine 150mg tablets | 60 tablet [PoM] £240.10-£255.10 DT = £300.12 (Hospital only)
  ► **Combivir** (ViiV Healthcare UK Ltd)
    Lamivudine 150 mg, Zidovudine 300 mg Combivir 150mg/300mg tablets | 60 tablet [PoM] £300.12 DT = £300.12 (Hospital only)

ANTIVIRALS ❯ PROTEASE INHIBITORS, HIV

Protease inhibitors

- **CONTRA-INDICATIONS** Acute porphyrias p. 1202
- **CAUTIONS** Haemophilia (increased risk of bleeding)
- **SIDE-EFFECTS**
  ► **Common or very common** Angioedema · anxiety · appetite abnormal · arthralgia · asthenia · diabetes mellitus · diarrhoea · dizziness · dyslipidaemia · fever · gastrointestinal discomfort · gastrointestinal disorders · headache · hepatic disorders · hypersensitivity · hypertension · myalgia · nausea · oral ulceration · pancreatitis · peripheral neuropathy · seizure · skin reactions · sleep disorders · syncope · taste altered · urinary frequency increased · vomiting
  ► **Uncommon** Alopecia · dry mouth · immune reconstitution inflammatory syndrome · myocardial infarction · osteonecrosis · weight increased
  ► **Rare or very rare** Stevens-Johnson syndrome
- **HEPATIC IMPAIRMENT** In general, manufacturers advise use with caution in patients with chronic hepatitis B or C (increased risk of hepatic side-effects).

⏻ above

Atazanavir

26-Apr-2023

- **INDICATIONS AND DOSE**
  HIV infection, in combination with other antiretroviral drugs—with low-dose ritonavir (initiated by a specialist)
  ► BY MOUTH
  ‣ Adult: 300 mg once daily
  HIV infection, in combination with other antiretroviral drugs—with cobicistat (initiated by a specialist)
  ► BY MOUTH
  ‣ Adult: 300 mg once daily

- **CAUTIONS** Cardiac conduction disorders · electrolyte disturbances · predisposition to QT interval prolongation
- **INTERACTIONS** → Appendix 1: HIV-protease inhibitors
- **SIDE-EFFECTS**
  ► **Uncommon** Chest pain · chronic kidney disease · depression · disorientation · drowsiness · drug reaction with eosinophilia and systemic symptoms (DRESS) · dyspnoea · gallbladder disorders · gynaecomastia · haematuria · malaise · memory loss · myopathy · nephritis tubulointerstitial · nephrolithiasis · proteinuria · torsade de pointes
  ► **Rare or very rare** Gait abnormal · oedema · palpitations · QT interval prolongation · renal pain · vasodilation

- **SIDE-EFFECTS, FURTHER INFORMATION** Mild to moderate rash occurs commonly, usually within the first 3 weeks of therapy. Severe rash occurs less frequently and may be accompanied by systemic symptoms. Discontinue if severe rash develops.
- **PREGNANCY** [EvGr] Theoretical risk of hyperbilirubinaemia in neonate if used at term. ⟨M⟩ For use with cobicistat, see atazanavir with cobicistat below.
  Monitoring [EvGr] In pregnancy, monitor viral load and plasma-atazanavir concentration during second and third trimesters. Postpartum patients should be closely monitored for adverse reactions. ⟨M⟩
- **HEPATIC IMPAIRMENT** Manufacturer advises caution in mild impairment; avoid in moderate to severe impairment (no information available).
- **RENAL IMPAIRMENT** [EvGr] Avoid in patients undergoing haemodialysis (limited information available). ⟨M⟩
- **MEDICINAL FORMS** There can be variation in the licensing of different medicines containing the same drug.
  Oral capsule
  CAUTIONARY AND ADVISORY LABELS 5, 21
  ► Atazanavir (Non-proprietary)
    Atazanavir (as Atazanavir sulfate) 200 mg Atazanavir 200mg capsules | 60 capsule [PoM] £303.38 (Hospital only)
    Atazanavir (as Atazanavir sulfate) 300 mg Atazanavir 300mg capsules | 30 capsule [PoM] £257.87-£303.38 (Hospital only)

Atazanavir with cobicistat

15-Dec-2020

The properties listed below are those particular to the combination only. For the properties of the components please consider, atazanavir above, cobicistat p. 757.

- **INDICATIONS AND DOSE**
  HIV infection, in combination with other antiretroviral drugs (initiated by a specialist)
  ► BY MOUTH
  ‣ Adult: 300/150 mg once daily
  DOSE EQUIVALENCE AND CONVERSION
  ► Dose expressed as x/y mg of atazanavir/cobicistat.

- **INTERACTIONS** → Appendix 1: cobicistat · HIV-protease inhibitors
- **PREGNANCY** [EvGr] Not to be initiated during pregnancy due to low atazanavir exposure; women who become pregnant during therapy should be switched to an alternative regimen. Darunavir with ritonavir may be considered as an alternative. ⟨M⟩

- **MEDICINAL FORMS** No licensed medicines listed.

⏻ above

Darunavir

15-Dec-2020

- **INDICATIONS AND DOSE**
  HIV infection in combination with other antiretroviral drugs in patients previously treated with antiretroviral therapy—with low-dose ritonavir
  ► BY MOUTH
  ‣ Adult: 600 mg twice daily, alternatively 800 mg once daily, once daily dose only to be used if no resistance to darunavir, if plasma HIV-RNA concentration less than 100 000 copies/mL, and if CD4 cell count greater than 100 cells × 10^6/ litre
  HIV infection in combination with other antiretroviral drugs in patients previously treated with antiretroviral therapy—with cobicistat
  ► BY MOUTH
  ‣ Adult: 800 mg once daily, dose appropriate if no resistance to darunavir, if plasma HIV-RNA   continued →

concentration less than 100 000 copies/mL, and if CD4 cell count greater than 100 cells $\times 10^6$/litre

HIV infection in combination with other antiretroviral drugs in patients not previously treated with antiretroviral therapy—with low-dose ritonavir
▶ BY MOUTH
▶ Adult: 800 mg once daily

HIV infection in combination with other antiretroviral drugs in patients not previously treated with antiretroviral therapy—with cobicistat
▶ BY MOUTH
▶ Adult: 800 mg once daily

● INTERACTIONS → Appendix 1: HIV-protease inhibitors

● SIDE-EFFECTS

▶ **Uncommon** Anaemia · angina pectoris · arrhythmias · burping · chest pain · concentration impaired · confusion · constipation · cough · depression · drowsiness · dry eye · dyspnoea · eye erythema · feeling hot · flushing · gout · gynaecomastia · haemorrhage · herpes simplex · hyperglycaemia · hypothyroidism · leucopenia · malaise · memory loss · mood altered · muscle spasms · muscle weakness · nail discolouration · nephrolithiasis · neutropenia · oral disorders · osteoporosis · pain · peripheral oedema · polydipsia · QT interval prolongation · renal impairment · sensation abnormal · sexual dysfunction · sweat changes · throat irritation · thrombocytopenia · urinary disorders · urine abnormalities · vertigo

▶ **Rare or very rare** Arthritis · chills · feeling abnormal · joint stiffness · musculoskeletal stiffness · palpitations · rhinorrhoea · severe cutaneous adverse reactions (SCARs) · visual impairment

SIDE-EFFECTS, FURTHER INFORMATION Mild to moderate rash occurs commonly, usually within the first 4 weeks of therapy and resolves without stopping treatment. Severe skin rash (including Stevens-Johnson syndrome and toxic epidermal necrolysis) occurs less frequently and may be accompanied by fever, malaise, arthralgia, myalgia, oral lesions, conjunctivitis, hepatitis, or eosinophilia; treatment should be stopped if this develops.

● ALLERGY AND CROSS-SENSITIVITY [EvGr] Use with caution in patients with sulfonamide sensitivity. [M]

● PREGNANCY Manufacturer advises use only if potential benefit outweighs risk; if required, use the twice daily dose regimen. For use with cobicistat, see darunavir with cobicistat below or darunavir with cobicistat, emtricitabine and tenofovir alafenamide p. 755.

● HEPATIC IMPAIRMENT Manufacturer advises caution in mild to moderate impairment; avoid in severe impairment (no information available).

● MONITORING REQUIREMENTS Monitor liver function before and during treatment.

● PRESCRIBING AND DISPENSING INFORMATION Flavours of oral liquid formulations may include strawberry.

● PATIENT AND CARER ADVICE
Vomiting [EvGr] If vomiting occurs more than 4 hours after a dose is taken, the missed dose should not be taken and the next dose should be taken at the normal time. [M]
Missed doses [EvGr] If a dose is more than 6 hours late on the twice-daily regimen (or more than 12 hours late on the once-daily regimen), the missed dose should not be taken and the next dose should be taken at the normal time. [M]

● MEDICINAL FORMS There can be variation in the licensing of different medicines containing the same drug.
Oral tablet
CAUTIONARY AND ADVISORY LABELS 21
▶ **Darunavir (Non-proprietary)**
Darunavir 400 mg Darunavir 400mg tablets | 60 tablet [PoM] £297.80 (Hospital only)

Darunavir 600 mg Darunavir 600mg tablets | 60 tablet [PoM] £400.00–£446.70 (Hospital only)
Darunavir 800 mg Darunavir 800mg tablets | 30 tablet [PoM] £297.80 DT = £268.00 (Hospital only)
▶ **Prezista** (Janssen-Cilag Ltd)
Darunavir 800 mg Prezista 800mg tablets | 30 tablet [PoM] £297.80 DT = £268.00 (Hospital only)
Oral suspension
CAUTIONARY AND ADVISORY LABELS 21
▶ **Prezista** (Janssen-Cilag Ltd)
Darunavir (as Darunavir ethanolate) 100 mg per 1 ml Prezista 100mg/ml oral suspension | 200 ml [PoM] £248.17 (Hospital only) [SF]

Darunavir with cobicistat
09-Dec-2020

The properties listed below are those particular to the combination only. For the properties of the components please consider, cobicistat p. 757, darunavir p. 753.

● INDICATIONS AND DOSE

HIV infection, in combination with other antiretroviral drugs (initiated by a specialist)
▶ BY MOUTH
▶ Adult: 800/150 mg once daily

DOSE EQUIVALENCE AND CONVERSION
▶ Dose expressed as x/y mg of darunavir/cobicistat.

IMPORTANT SAFETY INFORMATION
MHRA/CHM ADVICE: DARUNAVIR BOOSTED WITH COBICISTAT: AVOID USE IN PREGNANCY DUE TO RISK OF TREATMENT FAILURE AND MATERNAL-TO-CHILD TRANSMISSION OF HIV-1 (JULY 2018)
Pharmacokinetic data show mean exposure of darunavir boosted with cobicistat (available in combination in *Rezolsta*® and *Symtuza*®) to be lower during the second and third trimesters of pregnancy than during 6–12 weeks postpartum. Low darunavir exposure may be associated with an increased risk of treatment failure and an increased risk of HIV-1 transmission to the unborn child. For further information, see *Pregnancy*.

● CONTRA-INDICATIONS Treatment-experienced patients with 1 or more darunavir resistance-associated mutations, plasma HIV-RNA concentration of 100 000 copies/mL or greater, or CD4 count less than 100 cells $\times 10^6$/litre

● CAUTIONS Elderly

● INTERACTIONS → Appendix 1: cobicistat · HIV-protease inhibitors

● PREGNANCY Manufacturer advises not to be initiated during pregnancy due to low darunavir exposure; women who become pregnant during therapy should be switched to an alternative regimen. Darunavir with ritonavir may be considered as an alternative.

● NATIONAL FUNDING/ACCESS DECISIONS
For full details see funding body website
Scottish Medicines Consortium (SMC) decisions
▶ Darunavir/cobicistat (*Rezolsta*®) in combination with other antiretroviral medicinal products for the treatment of human immunodeficiency virus-1 (HIV-1) infection in adults aged 18 years or older. Genotypic testing should guide its use (August 2015) SMC No. 1081/15 Recommended

All Wales Medicines Strategy Group (AWMSG) decisions
▶ Darunavir with cobicistat (*Rezolsta*®) in combination with other antiretroviral medicinal products for the treatment of human immunodeficiency virus-1 (HIV-1) infection in adults and adolescents (aged 12 years and older with body weight at least 40 kg) (November 2020) AWMSG No. 3779 Recommended

● **MEDICINAL FORMS** There can be variation in the licensing of different medicines containing the same drug.

Oral tablet

CAUTIONARY AND ADVISORY LABELS 21

► Rezolsta (Janssen-Cilag Ltd)
Cobicistat 150 mg, Darunavir (as Darunavir ethanolate) **800 mg** Rezolsta 800mg/150mg tablets | 30 tablet PoM £317.24 (Hospital only)

Darunavir with cobicistat, emtricitabine and tenofovir alafenamide

10-Aug-2021

The properties listed below are those particular to the combination only. For the properties of the components please consider, darunavir p. 753, cobicistat p. 757, emtricitabine p. 748, tenofovir alafenamide p. 720.

● **INDICATIONS AND DOSE**

HIV infection (initiated by a specialist)

► BY MOUTH

► Adult: 1 tablet once daily

IMPORTANT SAFETY INFORMATION

MHRA/CHM ADVICE: DARUNAVIR BOOSTED WITH COBICISTAT: AVOID USE IN PREGNANCY DUE TO RISK OF TREATMENT FAILURE AND MATERNAL-TO-CHILD TRANSMISSION OF HIV-1 (JULY 2018)

Pharmacokinetic data show mean exposure of darunavir boosted with cobicistat (available in combination in *Rezolsta*® and *Symtuza*®) to be lower during the second and third trimesters of pregnancy than during 6–12 weeks postpartum. Low darunavir exposure may be associated with an increased risk of treatment failure and an increased risk of HIV-1 transmission to the unborn child. For further information, see *Pregnancy*.

● **INTERACTIONS** → Appendix 1: cobicistat · HIV-protease inhibitors · tenofovir alafenamide

● **PREGNANCY** Manufacturer advises not to be initiated during pregnancy due to low darunavir exposure; women who become pregnant during therapy should be switched to an alternative regimen.

● **RENAL IMPAIRMENT** EvGr Avoid if creatinine clearance less than 30 mL/minute (no information available). Ⓜ See p. 21.

● **PATIENT AND CARER ADVICE**
Driving and skilled tasks Manufacturer advises patients and carers should be counselled on the effects on driving and performance of skilled tasks—increased risk of dizziness.

● **NATIONAL FUNDING/ACCESS DECISIONS**
For full details see funding body website

Scottish Medicines Consortium (SMC) decisions

► Darunavir, cobicistat, emtricitabine, tenofovir alafenamide (*Symtuza*®) for the treatment of human immunodeficiency virus type 1 (HIV-1) infection in adults and adolescents (aged 12 years and older with body weight at least 40 kg) (January 2018) SMC No. 1290/18 Recommended

All Wales Medicines Strategy Group (AWMSG) decisions

► Darunavir / cobicistat / emtricitabine / tenofovir alafenamide (*Symtuza*®) for the treatment of human immunodeficiency virus type 1 (HIV-1) infection in adults and adolescents (aged 12 years and older with body weight at least 40 kg) (March 2018) AWMSG No. 2418 Recommended

● **MEDICINAL FORMS** There can be variation in the licensing of different medicines containing the same drug.

Oral tablet

CAUTIONARY AND ADVISORY LABELS 21

► Symtuza (Janssen-Cilag Ltd)
Tenofovir alafenamide (as Tenofovir alafenamide fumarate) **10 mg, Cobicistat 150 mg, Emtricitabine 200 mg, Darunavir (as Darunavir ethanolate) 800 mg** Symtuza 800mg/150mg/200mg/10mg tablets | 30 tablet PoM £672.97 (Hospital only)

◄ 753

Fosamprenavir

03-Aug-2020

● **DRUG ACTION** Fosamprenavir is a pro-drug of amprenavir.

● **INDICATIONS AND DOSE**

HIV infection in combination with other antiretroviral drugs—with low-dose ritonavir

► BY MOUTH

► Adult: 700 mg twice daily

DOSE EQUIVALENCE AND CONVERSION

► 700 mg fosamprenavir is equivalent to approximately 600 mg amprenavir.

● **INTERACTIONS** → Appendix 1: HIV-protease inhibitors

● **SIDE-EFFECTS**

► **Common or very common** Oral paraesthesia

SIDE-EFFECTS, FURTHER INFORMATION Rash may occur, usually in the second week of therapy; discontinue permanently if severe rash with systemic or allergic symptoms or, mucosal involvement; if rash mild or moderate, may continue without interruption—usually resolves and may respond to antihistamines.

● **PREGNANCY** Toxicity in *animal* studies; manufacturer advises use only if potential benefit outweighs risk.

● **HEPATIC IMPAIRMENT** Manufacturer advises caution.
Dose adjustments Manufacturer advises dose reduction to 450 mg twice daily in moderate impairment and 300 mg twice daily in severe impairment.

● **DIRECTIONS FOR ADMINISTRATION** Manufacturer advises in adults, oral suspension should be taken on an empty stomach.

● **PRESCRIBING AND DISPENSING INFORMATION** Flavours of oral liquid formulations may include grape, bubblegum, or peppermint.

● **PATIENT AND CARER ADVICE** Patients or carers should be given advice on how to administer fosamprenavir oral suspension.

● **MEDICINAL FORMS** No licensed medicines listed.

◄ 753

Lopinavir with ritonavir

21-Dec-2021

● **INDICATIONS AND DOSE**

HIV infection in combination with other antiretroviral drugs

► BY MOUTH USING TABLETS

► Adult: 400/100 mg twice daily, alternatively 800/200 mg once daily, once daily dose to be used only in adults with a HIV strain that has less than 3 mutations to protease inhibitors

► BY MOUTH USING ORAL SOLUTION

► Adult: 5 mL twice daily

DOSE EQUIVALENCE AND CONVERSION

► Oral solution contains 400 mg lopinavir, 100 mg ritonavir/5 mL (or 80 mg lopinavir, 20 mg ritonavir/mL).

● **CAUTIONS** Cardiac conduction disorders · pancreatitis · patients at high risk of cardiovascular disease · structural heart disease

- **INTERACTIONS** → Appendix 1: HIV-protease inhibitors
- **SIDE-EFFECTS**
  ▸ **Common or very common** Anaemia · increased risk of infection · leucopenia · lymphadenopathy · menstrual cycle irregularities · migraine · muscle spasms · muscle weakness · myopathy · neutropenia · night sweats · pain · sexual dysfunction
  ▸ **Uncommon** Atherosclerosis · atrioventricular block · cholangitis · constipation · deep vein thrombosis · haemorrhage · hyperbilirubinaemia · hypogonadism · nephritis · stomatitis · stroke · tinnitus · tremor · tricuspid valve incompetence · vasculitis · vertigo · visual impairment

  SIDE-EFFECTS, FURTHER INFORMATION Signs and symptoms suggestive of pancreatitis (including raised serum lipase) should be evaluated—discontinue if pancreatitis diagnosed.

- **PREGNANCY** For *tablets*, manufacturer advises only use if potential benefit outweighs risk—toxicity in *animal* studies (recommendation also supported by specialist sources). Avoid *oral solution* due to high alcohol and propylene glycol content.
- **HEPATIC IMPAIRMENT** For *oral solution*, manufacturer advises avoid due to propylene glycol content (risk of toxicity). For *tablets*, manufacturer advises avoid in severe impairment (no information available).
- **RENAL IMPAIRMENT** EvGr Avoid *oral solution* due to high propylene glycol content. Ⓜ
- **MONITORING REQUIREMENTS**
  ▸ Manufacturer advises monitor liver function before and during treatment.
  ▸ For *oral solution*, manufacturer advises monitor for signs of alcohol and propylene glycol toxicity (particularly in infants).
- **PRESCRIBING AND DISPENSING INFORMATION** For *oral solution*, manufacturer advises high alcohol (42 % v/v) and propylene glycol content—consider total amounts from all medicines that are to be given to infants in order to avoid toxicity; caution in patients for which consumption may be harmful.
- **PATIENT AND CARER ADVICE** Oral solution tastes bitter.
- **NATIONAL FUNDING/ACCESS DECISIONS** For full details see funding body website
  Scottish Medicines Consortium (SMC) decisions
  ▸ Lopinavir 200 mg, ritonavir 50 mg tablet (*Kaletra*®) for the treatment of HIV-1 infected adults and children above the age of 2 years in combination with other antiretroviral agents (November 2006) SMC No. 326/06 Recommended

- **MEDICINAL FORMS** There can be variation in the licensing of different medicines containing the same drug.
  Oral tablet
  CAUTIONARY AND ADVISORY LABELS 25
  ▸ **Lopinavir with ritonavir (Non-proprietary)**
    Ritonavir 50 mg, Lopinavir 200 mg Lopinavir 200mg / Ritonavir 50mg tablets | 120 tablet PoM £242.60-£285.40 (Hospital only)
  ▸ **Kaletra** (AbbVie Ltd)
    Ritonavir 25 mg, Lopinavir 100 mg Kaletra 100mg/25mg tablets | 60 tablet PoM £76.85 (Hospital only)
    Ritonavir 50 mg, Lopinavir 200 mg Kaletra 200mg/50mg tablets | 120 tablet PoM £285.41 (Hospital only)
  Oral solution
  CAUTIONARY AND ADVISORY LABELS 21
  EXCIPIENTS: May contain Alcohol, propylene glycol
  ▸ **Kaletra** (AbbVie Ltd)
    Ritonavir 20 mg per 1 ml, Lopinavir 80 mg per 1 ml Kaletra 80mg/20mg/1ml oral solution | 120 ml PoM £122.96 (Hospital only) | 300 ml PoM £307.39 (Hospital only)

Ritonavir

F 753

20-Jul-2023

- **INDICATIONS AND DOSE**

HIV infection in combination with other antiretroviral drugs (high-dose ritonavir)
  ▸ BY MOUTH
  ▸ Adult: Initially 300 mg every 12 hours for 3 days, increased in steps of 100 mg every 12 hours over not longer than 14 days; increased to 600 mg every 12 hours

Low-dose booster to increase effect of other protease inhibitors
  ▸ BY MOUTH
  ▸ Adult: 100–200 mg 1–2 times a day

- **CAUTIONS** Cardiac conduction disorders · pancreatitis · structural heart disease
- **INTERACTIONS** → Appendix 1: HIV-protease inhibitors
- **SIDE-EFFECTS**
  ▸ **Common or very common** Back pain · concentration impaired · confusion · cough · dehydration · feeling hot · flushing · gastrointestinal haemorrhage · gout · hypotension · menorrhagia · myopathy · oedema · oral paraesthesia · oropharyngeal pain · paraesthesia · peripheral coldness · pharyngitis · renal impairment · thrombocytopenia · vision blurred
  ▸ **Rare or very rare** Hyperglycaemia · toxic epidermal necrolysis

  SIDE-EFFECTS, FURTHER INFORMATION Signs and symptoms suggestive of pancreatitis (including raised serum lipase) should be evaluated — discontinue if pancreatitis diagnosed.

- **PREGNANCY**
  Dose adjustments Only use low-dose booster to increase the effect of other protease inhibitors.
- **HEPATIC IMPAIRMENT** When used as a *low-dose booster*, manufacturer advises caution in severe impairment; avoid in decompensated liver disease. When used in *high-doses*, manufacturer advises avoid in severe impairment.
  Dose adjustments Manufacturer advises consult product literature of co-administered protease inhibitor.
- **PATIENT AND CARER ADVICE**
  Driving and skilled tasks Patients and carers should be counselled on the effects on driving and performance of skilled tasks— increased risk of dizziness.

- **MEDICINAL FORMS** There can be variation in the licensing of different medicines containing the same drug.
  Oral tablet
  CAUTIONARY AND ADVISORY LABELS 21, 25
  ▸ **Ritonavir (Non-proprietary)**
    Ritonavir 100 mg Ritonavir 100mg tablets | 30 tablet PoM £16.52-£19.44 (Hospital only)
  ▸ **Norvir** (AbbVie Ltd)
    Ritonavir 100 mg Norvir 100mg tablets | 30 tablet PoM £19.44 (Hospital only)

ANTIVIRALS > OTHER

Maraviroc

31-Aug-2020

- **DRUG ACTION** Maraviroc is an antagonist of the CCR5 chemokine receptor.

- **INDICATIONS AND DOSE**

CCR5-tropic HIV infection in combination with other antiretroviral drugs in patients previously treated with antiretrovirals
  ▸ BY MOUTH
  ▸ Adult: 300 mg twice daily

- **CAUTIONS** Cardiovascular disease
- **INTERACTIONS** → Appendix 1: maraviroc
- **SIDE-EFFECTS**
▶ **Common or very common** Abdominal pain · anaemia · appetite decreased · asthenia · depression · diarrhoea · flatulence · headache · insomnia · nausea · rash
▶ **Uncommon** Hyperbilirubinaemia · increased risk of infection · myopathy · postural hypotension · proteinuria · renal failure · seizure
▶ **Rare or very rare** Angina pectoris · granulocytopenia · hepatic disorders · metastases · neoplasms · pancytopenia · severe cutaneous adverse reactions (SCARs)
▶ **Frequency not known** Fever · hypersensitivity · immune reconstitution inflammatory syndrome · organ dysfunction · osteonecrosis

SIDE-EFFECTS, FURTHER INFORMATION **Osteonecrosis** Osteonecrosis has been reported in patients with advanced HIV disease or following long-term exposure to combination antiretroviral therapy.

Hepatotoxicity Manufacturer advises consider discontinuation if signs or symptoms of acute hepatitis, or increased liver transaminases with systemic symptoms of hypersensitivity occur.

- **PREGNANCY** Manufacturer advises use only if potential benefit outweighs risk—toxicity in *animal* studies.
- **HEPATIC IMPAIRMENT** Manufacturer advises caution in impairment and in patients with chronic hepatitis (increased risk of hepatic side-effects; limited information available).
- **RENAL IMPAIRMENT** If eGFR less than 80 mL/minute/1.73 m^2, consult product literature.
- **NATIONAL FUNDING/ACCESS DECISIONS** For full details see funding body website
Scottish Medicines Consortium (SMC) decisions
▶ **Maraviroc (*Celsentri*®) for treatment-experienced adult patients infected with only CCR5-tropic HIV-1 detectable (October 2008)** SMC No. 458/08 Not recommended

- **MEDICINAL FORMS** There can be variation in the licensing of different medicines containing the same drug.
Oral tablet
▶ **Maraviroc (Non-proprietary)**
Maraviroc 150 mg Maraviroc 150mg tablets | 60 tablet [PoM] £467.23 (Hospital only)
Maraviroc 300 mg Maraviroc 300mg tablets | 60 tablet [PoM] £467.23 DT = £519.14 (Hospital only)
▶ **Celsentri** (ViiV Healthcare UK Ltd)
Maraviroc 150 mg Celsentri 150mg tablets | 60 tablet [PoM] £519.14 (Hospital only)
Maraviroc 300 mg Celsentri 300mg tablets | 60 tablet [PoM] £519.14 DT = £519.14 (Hospital only)

PHARMACOKINETIC ENHANCERS

Cobicistat
06-Aug-2021

- **INDICATIONS AND DOSE**
Pharmacokinetic enhancer used to increase the effect of atazanavir or darunavir
▶ BY MOUTH
▶ Adult: 150 mg once daily

- **INTERACTIONS** → Appendix 1: cobicistat
- **PREGNANCY** [EvGr] Not to be initiated during pregnancy. ⓂFor use with atazanavir, see atazanavir with cobicistat p. 753. For use with darunavir, see darunavir with cobicistat p. 754 or darunavir with cobicistat, emtricitabine and tenofovir alafenamide p. 755. For use with elvitegravir, see elvitegravir with cobicistat, emtricitabine and tenofovir disoproxil p. 747 or elvitegravir with cobicistat, emtricitabine and tenofovir alafenamide p. 746.

- **HEPATIC IMPAIRMENT** Manufacturer advises avoid in severe impairment—no information available.
- **RENAL IMPAIRMENT** [EvGr] No dose adjustment required; inhibits tubular secretion of creatinine; when any co-administered drug requires dose adjustment based on renal function, avoid initiating cobicistat if creatinine clearance less than 70 mL/minute. Ⓜ See p. 21.
- **PRESCRIBING AND DISPENSING INFORMATION** Dispense in original container (contains desiccant).
- **PATIENT AND CARER ADVICE**
Missed doses If a dose is more than 12 hours late, the missed dose should not be taken and the next dose should be taken at the normal time.

- **MEDICINAL FORMS** There can be variation in the licensing of different medicines containing the same drug.
Oral tablet
CAUTIONARY AND ADVISORY LABELS 21
▶ **Tybost** (Gilead Sciences Ltd)
Cobicistat 150 mg Tybost 150mg tablets | 30 tablet [PoM] £21.38 (Hospital only)

Combinations available: *Atazanavir with cobicistat*, p. 753 · *Darunavir with cobicistat*, p. 754 · *Darunavir with cobicistat, emtricitabine and tenofovir alafenamide*, p. 755 · *Elvitegravir with cobicistat, emtricitabine and tenofovir alafenamide*, p. 746 · *Elvitegravir with cobicistat, emtricitabine and tenofovir disoproxil*, p. 747

6.6 Influenza

Influenza
26-Jun-2024

Description of condition

Influenza is a highly infectious, acute respiratory infection caused by influenza viruses, of which there are three types (A, B, and C). Influenza A is more virulent and occurs more frequently; influenza B presents a milder course of disease but still has the potential to cause outbreaks; and influenza C causes mild or asymptomatic disease, similar to the common cold. Types A and B can be further categorised into subtypes depending on their principle H and N antigens. Transmission occurs via droplets, aerosols, or direct contact with respiratory secretions from an infected person, and the usual incubation period is 1–3 days.

Symptoms usually appear suddenly and may include chills, fever, headache, extreme fatigue, and myalgia. Dry cough, sore throat and nasal congestion may also be present. Complications are usually respiratory in nature and may include bronchitis, secondary bacterial pneumonia, or otitis media (in children); non-respiratory complications are rarer, and may be cardiac or neurological in nature.

Although influenza is usually self-limiting with recovery occurring within 2–7 days, it can be severe in some patients. Influenza is classified as uncomplicated or complicated, with the latter described as either requiring hospitalisation, having signs or symptoms of a lower respiratory-tract infection, central nervous system involvement, or exacerbation of an underlying condition. The risk of more serious illness is greater for those in at-risk groups, such as children aged under 6 months; pregnant females (including females up to 2 weeks post-partum); adults aged over 65 years; patients with long-term conditions such as respiratory, renal, hepatic, neurological or cardiac disease, diabetes mellitus, or morbid obesity (BMI $\geq$ 40 kg/m^2); or those with severe immunosuppression.

For further information on at-risk groups, see **UKHSA guidance on use of antiviral agents for the treatment and prophylaxis of seasonal influenza** (see *Useful resources*).

Other types of influenza include pandemic influenza, avian influenza, and swine influenza. For information and guidance on their management, see www.gov.uk/guidance/pandemic-flu, www.gov.uk/government/publications/avian-influenza-guidance-and-algorithms-for-managing-incidents-in-birds, and www.gov.uk/guidance/swine-influenza.

Aims of treatment

The management of influenza aims to reduce the duration and severity of illness, reduce the risk of complications, and to prevent infection.

Management

The antivirals oseltamivir p. 759 and zanamivir p. 760 are used for both treatment and post-exposure prophylaxis of influenza, although there is evidence that some strains of influenza are more likely to develop resistance to oseltamivir. In general, the risk of developing oseltamivir resistance is considered to be greater for influenza A(H1N1) pdm09 compared to other strains (such as influenza A(H3N2) and influenza B), with the risk of resistance being higher in patients who are severely immunosuppressed. Specialist advice regarding the management of influenza for individual patients can be obtained from local infection specialists where required. Additional advice can also be obtained from UKHSA's regional public health virologist and Respiratory Virus Unit. A consultant microbiologist or virologist can be consulted for advice on the resistance risk of individual influenza subtypes, and information on the dominant circulating strain can be found in UKHSA's weekly influenza reports at: www.gov.uk/government/collections/weekly-national-flu-reports.

Amantadine hydrochloride is not recommended for the treatment or post-exposure prophylaxis of influenza A.

Treatment of suspected or confirmed influenza

Where treatment with oseltamivir is indicated, it should be started as soon as possible, ideally within 48 hours of symptom onset. There is evidence to suggest that the risk of mortality may be reduced even if treatment is started up to 5 days after symptom onset; treatment initiation beyond 48 hours of onset is unlicensed and clinical judgement should be used. Where treatment with inhaled zanamivir is indicated, it should also be started as soon as possible, ideally within 48 hours (36 hours in children) of symptom onset; treatment initiation beyond this time is unlicensed and clinical judgement should be used. Where treatment with intravenous zanamivir is indicated, it should be commenced as soon as possible and within 6 days of symptom onset.

Uncomplicated influenza

Patients with uncomplicated influenza are usually managed in the community or accident and emergency departments. All patients should be advised about the symptoms of complicated influenza and to seek medical attention if their condition worsens.

For patients who are otherwise healthy (excluding pregnant females), no antiviral treatment is usually needed. For those considered to be at serious risk of developing complications, offer oseltamivir.

For patients in an at-risk group (including pregnant females but excluding those who are severely immunosuppressed), offer oseltamivir—do not wait for laboratory test results to treat. For pregnant females who meet additional criteria for requiring zanamivir first-line, treatment should be discussed with a local infection specialist. For further information, see **UKHSA guidance on use of antiviral agents for the treatment and prophylaxis of seasonal influenza** (see *Useful resources*).

For severely immunosuppressed patients, consider the subtype of influenza causing the infection, or if not yet known, take into account the current dominant circulating strain. Offer oseltamivir first-line unless the strain has a

higher risk for oseltamivir resistance, in which case inhaled zanamivir should be offered. For patients unable to use inhaled zanamivir due to underlying severe respiratory disease or inability to use the device (including children under 5 years), offer oseltamivir and assess response to therapy.

For patients with suspected or confirmed oseltamivir resistant influenza, offer inhaled zanamivir. For patients unable to use inhaled zanamivir, consider intravenous zanamivir [unlicensed indication].

Complicated influenza

All patients should be tested and treated, often in hospital—do not wait for laboratory test results to treat. For patients who are not severely immunosuppressed, oseltamivir should be offered first-line. If there is a risk of reduced gastrointestinal absorption, or if initial oseltamivir treatment is unsuccessful, offer inhaled zanamivir. For pregnant females who meet additional criteria for requiring zanamivir first-line, treatment should be discussed with a local infection specialist. For further information, see **UKHSA guidance on use of antiviral agents for the treatment and prophylaxis of seasonal influenza** (see *Useful resources*).

For severely immunosuppressed patients, consider the dominant circulating strain of influenza to guide treatment. Offer oseltamivir first-line unless the strain has a higher risk for developing oseltamivir resistance, in which case inhaled zanamivir should be offered.

For patients with suspected or confirmed oseltamivir resistant influenza, offer inhaled zanamivir.

For patients unable to use inhaled zanamivir, or for those with severe complicated illness such as multi-organ failure, consider intravenous zanamivir p. 760.

Post-exposure prophylaxis

Contacts in an at-risk group who are not adequately protected through vaccination (either due to infection by a different circulating strain or exposure within 14 days post-vaccination), should be offered prophylaxis following exposure to a person in the same household or residential setting with influenza-like illness (when influenza is circulating). Certain populations that are susceptible to localised outbreaks (such as those in care homes, prisons or detention centres), may be considered for antiviral prophylaxis regardless of vaccination status. For information on prophylaxis in these settings, refer to individual guidelines available at: www.gov.uk/government/collections/seasonal-influenza-guidance-data-and-analysis.

Prophylaxis should be started as soon as possible following exposure—ideally within 48 hours for oseltamivir p. 759 and 36 hours for inhaled zanamivir. Initiation beyond these times is unlicensed and specialist advice should be sought.

For patients in an at-risk group (including pregnant females but excluding severely immunosuppressed patients and children aged under 5 years), offer oseltamivir first-line regardless of the risk for resistance of the circulating or index case strain. For pregnant females who meet additional criteria for requiring zanamivir first-line, treatment should be discussed with a local infection specialist. For patients exposed to a strain with suspected or confirmed oseltamivir resistance, offer inhaled zanamivir.

For severely immunosuppressed patients (excluding children aged under 5 years), offer oseltamivir if the risk for oseltamivir resistance is low. However, if the risk for oseltamivir resistance is high, suspected or confirmed, offer inhaled zanamivir. For patients at higher risk of oseltamivir resistance who are unable to use inhaled zanamivir (due to underlying severe respiratory disease or inability to use the device), offer oseltamivir and advise patients to seek immediate medical attention if symptoms develop subsequently. For patients exposed to suspected or confirmed oseltamivir resistant influenza who are unable to use inhaled zanamivir, specialist advice should be sought and patients monitored closely for influenza-like illness, with arrangements made for prompt treatment if symptoms develop.

For children aged under 5 years in an at-risk group (including severely immunosuppressed children), offer oseltamivir first-line regardless of the risk of resistance for the circulating or index case strain. However, if the child is exposed to suspected or confirmed oseltamivir resistant influenza, monitor closely for influenza-like illness and promptly commence treatment if symptoms develop (see *Treatment of suspected or confirmed influenza*); seek specialist advise if the child is severely immunosuppressed.

Specialist advice is available through local health protection teams and public health virologists.

For further information, see **UKHSA guidance on use of antiviral agents for the treatment and prophylaxis of seasonal influenza** (see *Useful resources*).

For information on vaccination against influenza, see Influenza vaccine p. 1484.

Useful Resources

Recommendations reflect Guidance on use of antiviral agents for the treatment and prophylaxis of seasonal influenza. UK Health Security Agency. November 2021.
www.gov.uk/government/publications/influenza-treatment-and-prophylaxis-using-anti-viral-agents

> **Other drugs used for Influenza** Amantadine hydrochloride, p. 480

ANTIVIRALS > INFLUENZA > CAP-DEPENDENT ENDONUCLEASE INHIBITORS

Baloxavir marboxil
12-Jan-2022

- **DRUG ACTION** Baloxavir marboxil (a pro-drug of baloxavir) reduces replication of influenza A and B viruses by inhibiting viral cap-dependent endonuclease.

- **INDICATIONS AND DOSE**

Post-exposure prophylaxis of influenza
▸ BY MOUTH
▸ Child 12–17 years (body-weight up to 79 kg): 40 mg for 1 dose, to be taken as soon as possible within 48 hours following exposure
▸ Child 12–17 years (body-weight 80 kg and above): 80 mg for 1 dose, to be taken as soon as possible within 48 hours following exposure
▸ Adult (body-weight up to 79 kg): 40 mg for 1 dose, to be taken as soon as possible within 48 hours following exposure
▸ Adult (body-weight 80 kg and above): 80 mg for 1 dose, to be taken as soon as possible within 48 hours following exposure

Treatment of influenza
▸ BY MOUTH
▸ Child 12–17 years (body-weight up to 79 kg): 40 mg for 1 dose, to be taken as soon as possible within 48 hours of symptom onset
▸ Child 12–17 years (body-weight 80 kg and above): 80 mg for 1 dose, to be taken as soon as possible within 48 hours of symptom onset
▸ Adult (body-weight up to 79 kg): 40 mg for 1 dose, to be taken as soon as possible within 48 hours of symptom onset
▸ Adult (body-weight 80 kg and above): 80 mg for 1 dose, to be taken as soon as possible within 48 hours of symptom onset

- **INTERACTIONS** → Appendix 1: baloxavir marboxil
- **SIDE-EFFECTS**
▸ **Uncommon** Urticaria

▸ **Frequency not known** Angioedema
- **PREGNANCY** EvGr Avoid—limited information available. ⓜ
- **BREAST FEEDING** EvGr Avoid—present in milk in *animal* studies. ⓜ

- **MEDICINAL FORMS** There can be variation in the licensing of different medicines containing the same drug.
Oral tablet
▸ Baloxavir marboxil (non-proprietary) ▼
Baloxavir marboxil 20 mg Xofluza 20mg tablets | 2 tablet PoM ⓧ (Hospital only)
▸ Xofluza (Roche Products Ltd) ▼
Baloxavir marboxil 40 mg Xofluza 40mg tablets | 1 tablet PoM £100.00
Baloxavir marboxil 80 mg Xofluza 80mg tablets | 1 tablet PoM £100.00

ANTIVIRALS > INFLUENZA > NEURAMINIDASE INHIBITORS

Oseltamivir
02-Jul-2024

- **DRUG ACTION** Reduces replication of influenza A and B viruses by inhibiting viral neuraminidase.

- **INDICATIONS AND DOSE**

Prevention of influenza
▸ BY MOUTH
▸ Child 1–11 months: 3 mg/kg once daily (max. per dose 30 mg) for 10 days for post-exposure prophylaxis
▸ Child 1–12 years (body-weight up to 16 kg): 30 mg once daily for 10 days for post-exposure prophylaxis; for up to 6 weeks (or up to 12 weeks if immunocompromised) during an epidemic
▸ Child 1–12 years (body-weight 16–23 kg): 45 mg once daily for 10 days for post-exposure prophylaxis; for up to 6 weeks (or up to 12 weeks if immunocompromised) during an epidemic
▸ Child 1–12 years (body-weight 24–40 kg): 60 mg once daily for 10 days for post-exposure prophylaxis; for up to 6 weeks (or up to 12 weeks if immunocompromised) during an epidemic
▸ Child 1–12 years (body-weight 41 kg and above): 75 mg once daily for 10 days for post-exposure prophylaxis; for up to 6 weeks (or up to 12 weeks if immunocompromised) during an epidemic
▸ Child 13–17 years (body-weight up to 41 kg): 60 mg once daily for 10 days for post-exposure prophylaxis; for up to 6 weeks (or up to 12 weeks if immunocompromised) during an epidemic
▸ Child 13–17 years (body-weight 41 kg and above): 75 mg once daily for 10 days for post-exposure prophylaxis; for up to 6 weeks (or up to 12 weeks if immunocompromised) during an epidemic
▸ Adult (body-weight up to 41 kg): 60 mg once daily for 10 days for post-exposure prophylaxis; for up to 6 weeks (or up to 12 weeks if immunocompromised) during an epidemic
▸ Adult (body-weight 41 kg and above): 75 mg once daily for 10 days for post-exposure prophylaxis; for up to 6 weeks (or up to 12 weeks if immunocompromised) during an epidemic

Treatment of influenza
▸ BY MOUTH
▸ Child 1–11 months: 3 mg/kg twice daily (max. per dose 30 mg) for 5 days (10 days if immunocompromised)
▸ Child 1–12 years (body-weight 10–15 kg): 30 mg twice daily for 5 days (10 days if immunocompromised)
▸ Child 1–12 years (body-weight 16–23 kg): 45 mg twice daily for 5 days (10 days if immunocompromised)   continued →

- ▸ Child 1-12 years (body-weight 24–40 kg): 60 mg twice daily for 5 days (10 days if immunocompromised)
- ▸ Child 1-12 years (body-weight 41 kg and above): 75 mg twice daily for 5 days (10 days if immunocompromised)
- ▸ Child 13-17 years (body-weight up to 41 kg): 60 mg twice daily for 5 days (10 days if immunocompromised)
- ▸ Child 13-17 years (body-weight 41 kg and above): 75 mg twice daily for 5 days (10 days if immunocompromised)
- ▸ Adult (body-weight up to 41 kg): 60 mg twice daily for 5 days (10 days if immunocompromised)
- ▸ Adult (body-weight 41 kg and above): 75 mg twice daily for 5 days (10 days if immunocompromised)

- ● **UNLICENSED USE** Public Health England advises oseltamivir is used in the doses provided in BNF Publications for the prevention of influenza in children 1–12 years of age weighing less than 10 kg, but these are not licensed.
- ● **INTERACTIONS** → Appendix 1: oseltamivir
- ● **SIDE-EFFECTS**
- ▸ **Common or very common** Dizziness · gastrointestinal discomfort · herpes simplex · nausea · sleep disorders · vertigo · vomiting
- ▸ **Uncommon** Arrhythmia · consciousness impaired (in adults) · seizure · skin reactions
- ▸ **Rare or very rare** Angioedema · anxiety · behaviour abnormal · confusion · delirium · delusions · haemorrhage · hallucination · hepatic disorders · self-injurious behaviour · severe cutaneous adverse reactions (SCARs) · thrombocytopenia · visual impairment
- ● **PREGNANCY** Although safety data are limited, oseltamivir can be used in women who are pregnant when the potential benefit outweighs the risk (e.g. during a pandemic).
- ● **BREAST FEEDING** Although safety data are limited, oseltamivir can be used in women who are breast-feeding when the potential benefit outweighs the risk (e.g. during a pandemic). Oseltamivir is the preferred drug in women who are breast-feeding.
- ● **RENAL IMPAIRMENT**
- ▸ In adults Avoid for *treatment* and *prevention* if eGFR less than 10 mL/minute/1.73 m^2.
- ▸ In children Avoid for *treatment* and *prevention* if estimated glomerular filtration rate less than 10 mL/minute/1.73 m^2.
  Dose adjustments
  - ▸ In adults For *treatment*, use 30 mg twice daily if eGFR 30–60 mL/minute/1.73 m^2 (30 mg once daily if eGFR 10–30 mL/minute/1.73 m^2). For *prevention*, use 30 mg once daily if eGFR 30–60 mL/minute/1.73 m^2 (30 mg every 48 hours if eGFR 10–30 mL/minute/1.73 m^2).
  - ▸ In children For *treatment*, use 40% of normal dose twice daily if estimated glomerular filtration rate 30–60 mL/minute/1.73 m^2 (40% of normal dose once daily if estimated glomerular filtration rate 10–30 mL/minute/1.73 m^2). For *prevention*, use 40% of normal dose once daily if estimated glomerular filtration rate 30–60 mL/minute/1.73 m^2 (40% of normal dose every 48 hours if estimated glomerular filtration rate 10–30 mL/minute/1.73 m^2).
- ● **DIRECTIONS FOR ADMINISTRATION** If suspension not available, manufacturer advises capsules can be opened and the contents mixed with a small amount of sweetened food, such as sugar water or chocolate syrup, just before administration.
- ● **PRESCRIBING AND DISPENSING INFORMATION** Flavours of oral liquid formulations may include tutti-frutti.
  Public Health England advises that oseltamivir oral suspension should be reserved for children under the age of 1 year. Children over 1 year of age, adults with swallowing difficulties, and those receiving nasogastric

oseltamivir, should use capsules which can be opened and mixed into an appropriate sugary liquid.

- ● **PATIENT AND CARER ADVICE**
  Medicines for Children leaflet: Oseltamivir for influenza (flu) www.medicinesforchildren.org.uk/medicines/oseltamivir-for-influenza-flu/
- ● **NATIONAL FUNDING/ACCESS DECISIONS**
  For full details see funding body website
  NICE decisions
- ▸ **Oseltamivir, zanamivir, and amantadine for prophylaxis of influenza (September 2008)** NICE TA158 Recommended with restrictions
- ▸ **Oseltamivir, zanamivir, and amantadine for treatment of influenza (February 2009)** NICE TA168 Recommended with restrictions
  NHS restrictions *Tamiflu*® is not prescribable in NHS primary care except for the treatment and prophylaxis of influenza as indicated in the NICE guidance; endorse prescription 'SLS'.

- ● **MEDICINAL FORMS** There can be variation in the licensing of different medicines containing the same drug. Forms available from special-order manufacturers include: oral suspension, oral solution

Oral solution
CAUTIONARY AND ADVISORY LABELS 9
Oral suspension
CAUTIONARY AND ADVISORY LABELS 9
EXCIPIENTS: May contain Sorbitol
- ▸ Tamiflu (Roche Products Ltd)
  Oseltamivir (as Oseltamivir phosphate) 6 mg per 1 ml Tamiflu 6mg/ml oral suspension | 50 ml [PoM] £10.27 DT = £10.27 [SF]

Oral capsule
CAUTIONARY AND ADVISORY LABELS 9
- ▸ Oseltamivir (Non-proprietary)
  Oseltamivir (as Oseltamivir phosphate) 30 mg Oseltamivir 30mg capsules | 10 capsule [PoM] £6.50 DT = £7.71
- ▸ Ebilfumin (Teva UK Ltd)
  Oseltamivir (as Oseltamivir phosphate) 75 mg Ebilfumin 75mg capsules | 10 capsule [PoM] £14.64 DT = £15.41
- ▸ Tamiflu (Roche Products Ltd)
  Oseltamivir (as Oseltamivir phosphate) 30 mg Tamiflu 30mg capsules | 10 capsule [PoM] £7.71 DT = £7.71
  Oseltamivir (as Oseltamivir phosphate) 45 mg Tamiflu 45mg capsules | 10 capsule [PoM] £15.41 DT = £15.41
  Oseltamivir (as Oseltamivir phosphate) 75 mg Tamiflu 75mg capsules | 10 capsule [PoM] £15.41 DT = £15.41

Zanamivir

16-Jul-2024

- ● **DRUG ACTION** Reduces replication of influenza A and B viruses by inhibiting viral neuraminidase.

- ● **INDICATIONS AND DOSE**

Post-exposure prophylaxis of influenza
- ▸ BY INHALATION OF POWDER
- ▸ Child 5-17 years: 10 mg once daily for 10 days
- ▸ Adult: 10 mg once daily for 10 days

Prevention of influenza during an epidemic
- ▸ BY INHALATION OF POWDER
- ▸ Child 5-17 years: 10 mg once daily for up to 28 days
- ▸ Adult: 10 mg once daily for up to 28 days

Treatment of influenza
- ▸ BY INHALATION OF POWDER
- ▸ Child 5-17 years: 10 mg twice daily for 5 days
- ▸ Adult: 10 mg twice daily for 5 days

Treatment of influenza [complicated and potentially life-threatening, resistant to other treatments, and/or other treatments are unsuitable] | Treatment of influenza [uncomplicated, resistant to other treatments, and inhaled formulation unsuitable]
▶ BY INTRAVENOUS INFUSION
▶ **Child 6 months–5 years:** 14 mg/kg twice daily for 5 to 10 days
▶ **Child 6–17 years:** 12 mg/kg twice daily (max. per dose 600 mg) for 5 to 10 days
▶ **Adult:** 600 mg twice daily for 5 to 10 days

● UNLICENSED USE Public Health England advises intravenous zanamivir may be used for the treatment of uncomplicated influenza, but it is not licensed for this indication.

● CAUTIONS
▶ When used by inhalation Asthma · chronic pulmonary disease · uncontrolled chronic illness

CAUTIONS, FURTHER INFORMATION
▶ Asthma and chronic pulmonary disease
▶ When used by inhalation Risk of bronchospasm—short-acting bronchodilator should be available. Avoid in severe asthma unless close monitoring possible and appropriate facilities available to treat bronchospasm.

● INTERACTIONS → Appendix 1: zanamivir

● SIDE-EFFECTS

GENERAL SIDE-EFFECTS
▶ **Common or very common** Skin reactions
▶ **Uncommon** Oropharyngeal oedema
▶ **Rare or very rare** Face oedema · severe cutaneous adverse reactions (SCARs)
▶ **Frequency not known** Behaviour abnormal · delirium · hallucination · level of consciousness decreased · seizure

SPECIFIC SIDE-EFFECTS
▶ **Common or very common**
▶ With intravenous use Diarrhoea · hepatocellular injury
▶ **Uncommon**
▶ When used by inhalation Bronchospasm · dehydration · dyspnoea · presyncope · throat tightness
▶ **Frequency not known**
▶ When used by inhalation Psychiatric disorder

SIDE-EFFECTS, FURTHER INFORMATION Neurological and psychiatric disorders occur more commonly in children and adolescents.

● PREGNANCY Manufacturer advises avoid unless potential benefit outweighs risk (e.g. during a pandemic)—limited information available; *animal* studies do not indicate toxicity.

● BREAST FEEDING Manufacturer advises use only if potential benefit outweighs risk (e.g. during a pandemic)—limited information available; present in low levels in milk in *animal* studies.

● RENAL IMPAIRMENT
Dose adjustments
▶ With intravenous use Manufacturer advises reduce dose if creatinine clearance less than 80 mL/minute—consult product literature for details. See p. 21.

● DIRECTIONS FOR ADMINISTRATION
▶ When used by inhalation Manufacturer advises other inhaled drugs should be administered before zanamivir.
▶ With intravenous use Manufacturer advises for *intermittent intravenous infusion*, give undiluted or dilute to a concentration of not less than 200 micrograms/mL with Sodium Chloride 0.9%; give over 30 minutes.

● NATIONAL FUNDING/ACCESS DECISIONS
For full details see funding body website
NICE decisions
▶ Oseltamivir, zanamivir, and amantadine for prophylaxis of influenza (September 2008) NICE TA158 Recommended with restrictions
▶ Oseltamivir, zanamivir, and amantadine for treatment of influenza (February 2009) NICE TA168 Recommended with restrictions

Scottish Medicines Consortium (SMC) decisions
▶ Zanamivir (*Dectova*®) for the treatment of complicated and potentially life-threatening influenza A or B virus infection in patients (aged 6 months and older) when the patient's influenza virus is known or suspected to be resistant to anti-influenza medicinal products other than zanamivir, and/or other anti-viral medicinal products for treatment of influenza, including inhaled zanamivir, are not suitable for the individual patient (December 2019) SMC No. SMC2204 Recommended

All Wales Medicines Strategy Group (AWMSG) decisions
▶ Zanamivir (*Dectova*®) for the treatment of complicated and potentially life-threatening influenza A or B virus infection in patients (aged 6 months and older) when the patient's influenza virus is known or suspected to be resistant to anti-influenza medicinal products other than zanamivir, and/or other anti-viral medicinal products for treatment of influenza, including inhaled zanamivir, are not suitable for the individual patient (October 2019) AWMSG No. 4130 Recommended

NHS restrictions
▶ When used by inhalation *Relenza*® is not prescribable in NHS primary care except for the treatment and prophylaxis of influenza as indicated in the NICE guidance; endorse prescription 'SLS'.

● MEDICINAL FORMS There can be variation in the licensing of different medicines containing the same drug.
Solution for infusion
ELECTROLYTES: May contain Sodium
▶ Dectova (GlaxoSmithKline UK Ltd) ▼
Zanamivir 10 mg per 1 ml Dectova 200mg/20ml solution for infusion vials | 1 vial PoM £27.83 (Hospital only)
Inhalation powder
▶ Relenza (GlaxoSmithKline UK Ltd)
Zanamivir 5 mg Relenza 5mg inhalation powder blisters with Diskhaler | 20 blister PoM £16.36 DT = £16.36

6.7 Respiratory syncytial virus

Respiratory syncytial virus

Management in children

Ribavirin p. 722 is licensed for administration by inhalation for the treatment of severe bronchiolitis caused by the respiratory syncytial virus (RSV) in infants, especially when they have other serious diseases. However, there is no evidence that ribavirin produces clinically relevant benefit in RSV bronchiolitis.

Palivizumab p. 762 is a monoclonal antibody licensed for preventing serious lower respiratory-tract disease caused by respiratory syncytial virus in children at high risk of the disease; it should be prescribed under specialist supervision and on the basis of the likelihood of hospitalisation.

Palivizumab is recommended for:

- children under 9 months of age with chronic lung disease (defined as requiring oxygen for at least 28 days from birth) and who were born preterm;
- children under 6 months of age with haemodynamically significant, acyanotic congenital heart disease who were born preterm.

Palivizumab should be considered for:

- children under 2 years of age with severe combined immunodeficiency syndrome;
- children under 1 year of age who require long-term ventilation;
- children 1–2 years of age who require long-term ventilation and have an additional co-morbidity (including cardiac disease or pulmonary hypertension).

For details of the preterm age groups included in the recommendations, see *Immunisation against Infectious Disease* (2006), available at www.gov.uk/dh.

DRUGS FOR RESPIRATORY DISEASES >
MONOCLONAL ANTIBODIES

Palivizumab

01-May-2024

- **DRUG ACTION** Palivizumab is a humanised monoclonal antibody that binds to fusion protein A on the surface of respiratory syncytial virus (RSV), which inhibits the virus from entering the host cell, thereby preventing RSV infection.

- **INDICATIONS AND DOSE**

Prevention of serious lower respiratory-tract disease caused by respiratory syncytial virus in children at high risk of the disease [under 6 months of age (at the start of the RSV season) and born at 35 weeks corrected gestational age or less, or under 2 years of age who have received treatment for bronchopulmonary dysplasia in the last 6 months, or with haemodynamically significant congenital heart disease] (under expert supervision)
  - ► BY INTRAMUSCULAR INJECTION
  - ► Child 1–23 months: 15 mg/kg once a month, to be administered during season of RSV risk

Prevention of serious lower respiratory-tract disease caused by respiratory syncytial virus in children at high risk of the disease and undergoing cardiac bypass surgery [under 6 months of age (at the start of the RSV season) and born at 35 weeks corrected gestational age or less, or under 2 years of age who have received treatment for bronchopulmonary dysplasia in the last 6 months, or with haemodynamically significant congenital heart disease] (under expert supervision)
  - ► BY INTRAMUSCULAR INJECTION
  - ► Child 1–23 months: Initially 15 mg/kg, to be administered as soon as stable after surgery, then 15 mg/kg once a month, to be administered during season of RSV risk

- **CAUTIONS** Moderate to severe acute infection · moderate to severe febrile illness · serum-palivizumab concentration may be reduced after cardiac surgery · thrombocytopenia

- **SIDE-EFFECTS**
  - ► **Common or very common** Apnoea
  - ► **Uncommon** Seizure · thrombocytopenia · urticaria
  - ► **Frequency not known** Hypersensitivity

- **ALLERGY AND CROSS-SENSITIVITY** PHE advises avoid if previous anaphylactic reaction to another humanised monoclonal antibody.

- **DIRECTIONS FOR ADMINISTRATION** For *intramuscular injection*, administration into the anterolateral aspect of the thigh is preferred. EvGr Injection volume over 1 mL should be divided between more than one site. Ⓜ

- **PRESCRIBING AND DISPENSING INFORMATION** Palivizumab is a biological medicine. Biological medicines must be prescribed and dispensed by brand name, see *Biological medicines* and *Biosimilar medicines*, under Guidance on prescribing p. 1; record the brand name and batch number after each administration.

- **HANDLING AND STORAGE** Store in a refrigerator (2–8°C) and protect from light.

- **MEDICINAL FORMS** There can be variation in the licensing of different medicines containing the same drug.
  Solution for injection
  - ► Synagis (AstraZeneca UK Ltd)
    Palivizumab 100 mg per 1 ml Synagis 100mg/1ml solution for injection vials | 1 vial PoM £563.64
    Synagis 50mg/0.5ml solution for injection vials | 1 vial PoM £306.34 (Hospital only)

Chapter 6
Endocrine system

CONTENTS

1   Antidiuretic hormone disorders

Posterior pituitary hormones and antagonists

14-Sep-2020

Posterior pituitary hormones

Diabetes insipidus

Vasopressin p. 766 (antidiuretic hormone, ADH) is used in the treatment of *pituitary* ('cranial') *diabetes insipidus* as is its analogue desmopressin p. 764. Dosage is tailored to produce a slight diuresis every 24 hours to avoid water intoxication. Treatment may be required for a limited period only in diabetes insipidus following trauma or pituitary surgery.

Desmopressin is more potent and has a longer duration of action than vasopressin; unlike vasopressin it has no vasoconstrictor effect. It is given by mouth or intranasally for maintenance therapy, and by injection in the postoperative period or in unconscious patients. Desmopressin is also used in the differential diagnosis of diabetes insipidus. Following a dose intramuscularly or intranasally, restoration of the ability to concentrate urine after water deprivation confirms a diagnosis of cranial diabetes insipidus. Failure to respond occurs in nephrogenic diabetes insipidus.

In *nephrogenic* and *partial pituitary diabetes insipidus* benefit may be gained from the paradoxical antidiuretic effect of thiazides.

Carbamazepine p. 355 is sometimes useful in partial pituitary diabetes insipidus [unlicensed]; it may act by sensitising the renal tubules to the action of remaining endogenous vasopressin. The MHRA/CHM have released important safety information on the use of antiepileptic drugs and the risk of suicidal thoughts and behaviour. For further information, see Epilepsy p. 349.

Other uses

Desmopressin is also used to boost factor VIII concentration in mild to moderate haemophilia and in von Willebrand's disease; it is also used to test fibrinolytic response. Desmopressin may also have a role in nocturnal enuresis.

Vasopressin infusion is used to control variceal bleeding in portal hypertension, prior to more definitive treatment and with variable results. Terlipressin acetate, a derivative of vasopressin with reportedly less pressor and antidiuretic activity, is used similarly.

Oxytocin p. 950, another posterior pituitary hormone, is indicated in obstetrics.

Antidiuretic hormone antagonists

Demeclocycline hydrochloride p. 655 can be used in the treatment of hyponatraemia resulting from inappropriate secretion of antidiuretic hormone, if fluid restriction alone does not restore sodium concentration or is not tolerable. Demeclocycline hydrochloride is thought to act by directly blocking the renal tubular effect of antidiuretic hormone.

Tolvaptan p. 767 is a vasopressin V_2-receptor antagonist licensed for the treatment of hyponatraemia secondary to syndrome of inappropriate antidiuretic hormone secretion; treatment duration with tolvaptan is determined by the underlying disease and its treatment.

Rapid correction of hyponatraemia during tolvaptan therapy can cause osmotic demyelination, leading to serious neurological events; close monitoring of serum sodium concentration and fluid balance is essential.

1.1   Diabetes insipidus

Other drugs used for Diabetes insipidus Chlortalidone, p. 264

PITUITARY AND HYPOTHALAMIC HORMONES AND ANALOGUES >VASOPRESSIN AND ANALOGUES

Desmopressin

01-Sep-2023

● **DRUG ACTION** Desmopressin is an analogue of vasopressin.

● **INDICATIONS AND DOSE**

Diabetes insipidus, treatment

▸ BY MOUTH

▸ **Child 1–23 months:** Initially 10 micrograms 2–3 times a day, adjusted according to response; usual dose 30–150 micrograms daily

▸ **Child 2-11 years:** Initially 50 micrograms 2–3 times a day, adjusted according to response; usual dose 100–800 micrograms daily

▸ **Child 12-17 years:** Initially 100 micrograms 2–3 times a day, adjusted according to response; usual dose 0.2–1.2 mg daily

▸ **Adult:** Initially 100 micrograms 3 times a day; maintenance 100–200 micrograms 3 times a day; usual dose 0.2–1.2 mg daily

▸ BY SUBLINGUAL ADMINISTRATION

▸ **Child 2-17 years:** Initially 60 micrograms 3 times a day, adjusted according to response; usual dose 40–240 micrograms 3 times a day

▸ **Adult 18-65 years:** Initially 60 micrograms 3 times a day, adjusted according to response; usual dose 40–240 micrograms 3 times a day

▸ BY INTRANASAL ADMINISTRATION

▸ **Child 1-23 months:** Initially 2.5–5 micrograms 1–2 times a day, adjusted according to response

▸ **Child 2-11 years:** Initially 5–20 micrograms 1–2 times a day, adjusted according to response

▸ **Child 12-17 years:** Initially 10–20 micrograms 1–2 times a day, adjusted according to response

▸ **Adult:** 10–40 micrograms daily in 1–2 divided doses

▸ BY SUBCUTANEOUS INJECTION, OR BY INTRAVENOUS INJECTION, OR BY INTRAMUSCULAR INJECTION

▸ **Adult:** 1–4 micrograms daily

Primary nocturnal enuresis

▸ BY MOUTH USING TABLETS

▸ **Child 5-17 years:** 200 micrograms once daily, increased if necessary to 400 micrograms once daily, dose to be taken at bedtime, limit fluid intake from 1 hour before to 8 hours after administration, dose to be increased only if lower dose not effective, reassess after 3 months by withdrawing treatment for at least 1 week

▸ **Adult 18-65 years:** 200 micrograms once daily, increased if necessary to 400 micrograms once daily, dose to be taken at bedtime, limit fluid intake from 1 hour before to 8 hours after administration, dose to be increased only if lower dose not effective, reassess after 3 months by withdrawing treatment for at least 1 week

▸ BY MOUTH USING ORAL SOLUTION

▸ **Child 5-17 years:** 180 micrograms once daily, increased if necessary to 360 micrograms once daily, dose to be taken at bedtime, limit fluid intake from 1 hour before to 8 hours after administration, dose to be increased only if lower dose not effective, reassess after 3 months by withdrawing treatment for at least 1 week

▸ **Adult:** 180 micrograms once daily, increased if necessary to 360 micrograms once daily, dose to be taken at bedtime, limit fluid intake from 1 hour before to 8 hours after administration, dose to be increased only if lower dose not effective, reassess after 3 months by withdrawing treatment for at least 1 week

▸ BY SUBLINGUAL ADMINISTRATION

▸ **Child 5-17 years:** 120 micrograms once daily, increased if necessary to 240 micrograms once daily, dose to be taken at bedtime, limit fluid intake from 1 hour before to 8 hours after administration, dose to be increased only if lower dose not effective, reassess after 3 months by withdrawing treatment for at least 1 week

▸ **Adult 18-65 years:** 120 micrograms once daily, increased if necessary to 240 micrograms once daily, dose to be taken at bedtime, limit fluid intake from 1 hour before to 8 hours after administration, dose to be increased only if lower dose not effective, reassess after 3 months by withdrawing treatment for at least 1 week

Polyuria or polydipsia after hypophysectomy

▸ BY MOUTH USING TABLETS

▸ **Adult:** Dose to be adjusted according to urine osmolality

▸ BY SUBLINGUAL ADMINISTRATION

▸ **Adult 18-65 years:** Dose to be adjusted according to urine osmolality

Idiopathic nocturnal polyuria in females

▸ BY SUBLINGUAL ADMINISTRATION

▸ **Adult:** 25 micrograms daily, to be taken 1 hour before bedtime

Idiopathic nocturnal polyuria in males

▸ BY SUBLINGUAL ADMINISTRATION

▸ **Adult:** 50 micrograms daily, to be taken 1 hour before bedtime

Diabetes insipidus, diagnosis (water deprivation test)

▸ BY INTRANASAL ADMINISTRATION

▸ **Adult:** 20 micrograms, limit fluid intake to 500 mL from 1 hour before to 8 hours after administration

▸ BY INTRAMUSCULAR INJECTION, OR BY SUBCUTANEOUS INJECTION

▸ **Adult:** 2 micrograms for 1 dose, limit fluid intake to 500 mL from 1 hour before to 8 hours after administration

Nocturia associated with multiple sclerosis (when other treatments have failed)

▸ BY INTRANASAL ADMINISTRATION

▸ **Adult 18-65 years:** 10–20 micrograms once daily, to be taken at bedtime, dose not to be repeated within 24 hours, limit fluid intake from 1 hour before to 8 hours after administration

Renal function testing

▸ BY INTRANASAL ADMINISTRATION

▸ **Adult:** 40 micrograms, empty bladder at time of administration and limit fluid intake to 500 mL from 1 hour before until 8 hours after administration to avoid fluid overload

▸ BY SUBCUTANEOUS INJECTION, OR BY INTRAMUSCULAR INJECTION

▸ **Adult:** 2 micrograms, empty bladder at time of administration and restrict fluid intake to 500 mL from 1 hour before until 8 hours after administration to avoid fluid overload

Mild to moderate haemophilia and von Willebrand's disease

▸ BY INTRANASAL ADMINISTRATION

▸ **Adult:** 300 micrograms every 12 hours if required, one 150 microgram spray into each nostril, 30 minutes before surgery or when bleeding, dose may alternatively be repeated at intervals of at least 3 days, if self-administered

▸ BY INTRAVENOUS INFUSION, OR BY SUBCUTANEOUS INJECTION

▸ **Adult:** 300 nanograms/kg for 1 dose, to be administered immediately before surgery or after trauma; may be repeated at intervals of 12 hours

Fibrinolytic response testing

► BY INTRANASAL ADMINISTRATION

► Adult: 300 micrograms, blood to be sampled after 1 hour for fibrinolytic activity, one 150 microgram spray to be administered into each nostril

► BY INTRAVENOUS INFUSION, OR BY SUBCUTANEOUS INJECTION

► Adult: 300 nanograms/kg for 1 dose, blood to be sampled after 20 minutes for fibrinolytic activity

Lumbar-puncture-associated headache

► BY INTRAMUSCULAR INJECTION, OR BY SUBCUTANEOUS INJECTION

► Adult: (consult product literature)

DOSE EQUIVALENCE AND CONVERSION

► *Tablets, intranasal spray,* and *solution for injection* contain desmopressin acetate; doses are expressed as desmopressin acetate.

► *Sublingual tablets, oral lyophilisate,* and *oral solution* contain desmopressin acetate; doses are expressed as desmopressin. For example, 1 mL of *Demovo*® oral solution contains 400 micrograms of desmopressin acetate equivalent to 360 micrograms of desmopressin.

● UNLICENSED USE Desmopressin is used in the doses provided in BNF Publications for the treatment of diabetes insipidus, but these may differ from those licensed.

► In children Consult product literature for individual preparations. Oral use of *DDAVP*® intravenous injection is not licensed.

● CONTRA-INDICATIONS Cardiac insufficiency · conditions treated with diuretics · history of hyponatraemia · polydipsia in alcohol dependence · psychogenic polydipsia · syndrome of inappropriate ADH secretion · von Willebrand's Disease Type IIB (may result in pseudothrombocytopenia)

● CAUTIONS Avoid fluid overload · cardiovascular disease (not indicated for nocturia associated with multiple sclerosis) · conditions which might be aggravated by water retention · cystic fibrosis · elderly · epilepsy · hypertension (not indicated for nocturia associated with multiple sclerosis) · nocturia—limit fluid intake to minimum from 1 hour before dose until 8 hours afterwards · nocturnal enuresis—limit fluid intake to minimum from 1 hour before dose until 8 hours afterwards

CAUTIONS, FURTHER INFORMATION EvGr Elderly patients are at increased risk of hyponatraemia and renal impairment—measure baseline serum sodium concentration, then monitor regularly during treatment; discontinue treatment if levels fall below the normal range. Review treatment if no therapeutic benefit after 3 months. ⟨M⟩

● INTERACTIONS → Appendix 1: desmopressin

● SIDE-EFFECTS

GENERAL SIDE-EFFECTS

► **Common or very common** Headache · hyponatraemia (rare in children) · nausea

► **Rare or very rare** Allergic dermatitis · emotional disorder

► **Frequency not known** Aggression (in children) · fluid retention

SPECIFIC SIDE-EFFECTS

► **Common or very common**

► With intranasal use Asthenia · conjunctivitis

► With oral use Abdominal pain

► With sublingual use Diarrhoea (in adults) · dizziness (in adults) · dry mouth (in adults)

► **Uncommon**

► With intranasal use Epistaxis · gastrointestinal discomfort · nasal congestion · rhinitis · vomiting

► With sublingual use Constipation (in adults) · fatigue (in adults) · gastrointestinal discomfort (frequency not known in children) · peripheral oedema (in adults)

► **Rare or very rare**

► With intranasal use Brain oedema

► **Frequency not known**

► With intramuscular use Abdominal pain

► With intravenous use Abdominal pain · vasodilation

► With oral use Brain oedema (in children and young adults)

► With subcutaneous use Abdominal pain

SIDE-EFFECTS, FURTHER INFORMATION Treatment with desmopressin without restricting fluid intake may lead to fluid retention and/or hyponatraemia.

● PREGNANCY Small oxytocic effect in third trimester; increased risk of pre-eclampsia.

● BREAST FEEDING Amount too small to be harmful.

● RENAL IMPAIRMENT EvGr Caution with *injection, nasal spray,* and *tablets* (antidiuretic effect may be reduced). Avoid *oral lyophilisate, oral solution,* and *sublingual tablets* in moderate or severe impairment. ⟨M⟩

● MONITORING REQUIREMENTS In *nocturia*, periodic blood pressure and weight checks are needed to monitor for fluid overload.

● DIRECTIONS FOR ADMINISTRATION Desmopressin oral lyophilisates are for sublingual administration. Expert sources advise *DDAVP*® and *Desmotabs*® tablets may be crushed. Expert sources advise *DDAVP*® injection may be administered orally. EvGr For *intravenous infusion* (*DDAVP*®, *Octim*®), give intermittently in Sodium Chloride 0.9%; dilute with 50 mL and give over 20 minutes. ⟨M⟩

● PATIENT AND CARER ADVICE

Hyponatraemic convulsions Patients being treated for primary nocturnal enuresis should be warned to avoid fluid overload (including during swimming) and to stop taking desmopressin during an episode of vomiting or diarrhoea (until fluid balance normal).

Medicines for Children leaflet: Desmopressin for bedwetting www.medicinesforchildren.org.uk/medicines/desmopressin-for-bedwetting/

● NATIONAL FUNDING/ACCESS DECISIONS

For full details see funding body website

Scottish Medicines Consortium (SMC) decisions

► **Desmopressin oral lyophilisate (*Noqdirna*®) for symptomatic treatment of nocturia due to idiopathic nocturnal polyuria in adults (August 2017)** SMC No. 1218/17 Recommended with restrictions

All Wales Medicines Strategy Group (AWMSG) decisions

► **Desmopressin acetate (*Noqdirna*®) for treatment of nocturia due to idiopathic nocturnal polyuria in adults (October 2017)** AWMSG No. 3282 Recommended with restrictions

● MEDICINAL FORMS There can be variation in the licensing of different medicines containing the same drug. Forms available from special-order manufacturers include: oral capsule, oral suspension, oral solution, nasal drops, spray

Oral tablet

► **Desmopressin (Non-proprietary)**

Desmopressin acetate 100 microgram Desmopressin 100microgram tablets | 90 tablet PoM £76.62 DT = £51.34

Desmopressin acetate 200 microgram Desmopressin 200microgram tablets | 30 tablet PoM £32.00 DT = £19.91

► **DDAVP** (Ferring Pharmaceuticals Ltd)

Desmopressin acetate 100 microgram DDAVP 0.1mg tablets | 90 tablet PoM £44.12 DT = £51.34

Desmopressin acetate 200 microgram DDAVP 0.2mg tablets | 90 tablet PoM £88.23

► **Desmotabs** (Ferring Pharmaceuticals Ltd)

Desmopressin acetate 200 microgram Desmotabs 0.2mg tablets | 30 tablet PoM £29.43 DT = £19.91

Solution for injection

▸ **DDAVP** (Ferring Pharmaceuticals Ltd)
Desmopressin acetate 4 microgram per 1 ml DDAVP 4micrograms/1ml solution for injection ampoules | 10 ampoule [PoM] £13.16 DT = £13.16
▸ **Octim** (Ferring Pharmaceuticals Ltd)
Desmopressin acetate 15 microgram per 1 ml Octim 15micrograms/1ml solution for injection ampoules | 10 ampoule [PoM] £192.20 DT = £192.20

Spray

▸ **Desmopressin (Non-proprietary)**
Desmopressin acetate 2.5 microgram per 1 dose Minirin 2.5micrograms/dose nasal spray | 50 dose [PoM] [▣]
Desmopressin acetate 10 microgram per 1 dose Desmopressin 10micrograms/dose nasal spray | 60 dose [PoM] £35.76 DT = £31.36
Desmopressin acetate 150 microgram per 1 dose Desmopressin 150micrograms/dose nasal spray | 25 dose [PoM] [▣]

Oral solution

▸ **Demovo** (Alturix Ltd)
Desmopressin (as Desmopressin acetate) 360 microgram per 1 ml Demovo 360micrograms/ml oral solution | 15 ml [PoM] £19.95 DT = £19.95 [SF]

Sublingual tablet

CAUTIONARY AND ADVISORY LABELS 26
EXCIPIENTS: May contain Aspartame
▸ **Desmopressin (Non-proprietary)**
Desmopressin acetate 60 microgram Desmopressin 60microgram sublingual tablets sugar free | 100 tablet [PoM] £27.79–£55.78 DT = £27.79 [SF]
Desmopressin acetate 120 microgram Desmopressin 120microgram sublingual tablets sugar free | 30 tablet [PoM] £16.69–£30.34 DT = £16.69 [SF] | 100 tablet [PoM] £80.85 [SF]
Desmopressin acetate 240 microgram Desmopressin 240microgram sublingual tablets sugar free | 30 tablet [PoM] £33.37–£60.68 DT = £33.37 [SF] | 100 tablet [PoM] £111.14–£297.56 [SF]

Oral lyophilisate

CAUTIONARY AND ADVISORY LABELS 26
▸ **Desmopressin (Non-proprietary)**
Desmopressin (as Desmopressin acetate)
120 microgram Desmopressin 120microgram oral lyophilisates sugar free | 30 tablet [PoM] £30.34–£54.62 DT = £30.34 [SF]
Desmopressin (as Desmopressin acetate)
240 microgram Desmopressin 240microgram oral lyophilisates sugar free | 30 tablet [PoM] £60.68–£109.22 DT = £60.68 [SF]
▸ **DDAVP Melt** (Ferring Pharmaceuticals Ltd)
Desmopressin (as Desmopressin acetate) 60 microgram DDAVP Melt 60microgram oral lyophilisates | 100 tablet [PoM] £50.53 DT = £50.53 [SF]
Desmopressin (as Desmopressin acetate) 120 microgram DDAVP Melt 120microgram oral lyophilisates | 100 tablet [PoM] £101.07 DT = £101.07 [SF]
Desmopressin (as Desmopressin acetate) 240 microgram DDAVP Melt 240microgram oral lyophilisates | 100 tablet [PoM] £202.14 [SF]
▸ **DesmoMelt** (Ferring Pharmaceuticals Ltd)
Desmopressin (as Desmopressin acetate)
120 microgram DesmoMelt 120microgram oral lyophilisates | 30 tablet [PoM] £30.34 DT = £30.34 [SF]
Desmopressin (as Desmopressin acetate)
240 microgram DesmoMelt 240microgram oral lyophilisates | 30 tablet [PoM] £60.68 DT = £60.68 [SF]
▸ **Noqdirna** (Ferring Pharmaceuticals Ltd)
Desmopressin (as Desmopressin acetate) 25 microgram Noqdirna 25microgram oral lyophilisates | 30 tablet [PoM] £15.16 DT = £15.16 [SF]
Desmopressin (as Desmopressin acetate)
50 microgram Noqdirna 50microgram oral lyophilisates | 30 tablet [PoM] £15.16 DT = £15.16 [SF]

Vasopressin

17-Sep-2024

(ADH; Antidiuretic hormone)

● **DRUG ACTION** Vasopressin is an endogenous hormone with a direct antidiuretic effect on the kidney; it is given in the synthetic form of argipressin.

● **INDICATIONS AND DOSE**

Pituitary diabetes insipidus
▸ BY INTRAMUSCULAR INJECTION, OR BY SUBCUTANEOUS INJECTION
▸ Adult: 5–20 units every 4 hours, dose expressed as argipressin

Initial control of oesophageal variceal bleeding
▸ BY INTRAVENOUS INFUSION
▸ Adult: 20 units, dose to be administered over 15 minutes, dose expressed as argipressin

DOSE EQUIVALENCE AND CONVERSION
▸ Argipressin 1 unit is equivalent to vasopressin 1 unit.

● **CONTRA-INDICATIONS** Chronic nephritis (until reasonable blood nitrogen concentrations attained) · vascular disease (especially disease of coronary arteries) unless extreme caution

● **CAUTIONS** Asthma · avoid fluid overload · conditions which might be aggravated by water retention · epilepsy · heart failure · hypertension · migraine

● **INTERACTIONS** → Appendix 1: vasopressin

● **SIDE-EFFECTS** Abdominal pain · angina pectoris · bronchospasm · cardiac arrest · chest pain · diarrhoea · flatulence · fluid imbalance · gangrene · headache · hyperhidrosis · hypertension · musculoskeletal chest pain · nausea · pallor · peripheral ischaemia · tremor · urticaria · vertigo · vomiting

● **PREGNANCY** Oxytocic effect in third trimester.

● **BREAST FEEDING** Not known to be harmful.

● **DIRECTIONS FOR ADMINISTRATION** For *intravenous infusion* (argipressin), manufacturer advises give intermittently in Glucose 5%; suggested concentration 20 units/100 mL given over 15 minutes.

● **MEDICINAL FORMS** There can be variation in the licensing of different medicines containing the same drug. Forms available from special-order manufacturers include: solution for injection

Solution for injection

▸ **Vasopressin (Non-proprietary)**
Argipressin 20 unit per 1 ml Argipressin 20units/1ml solution for injection ampoules | 10 ampoule [PoM] £750.00–£754.86 (Hospital only)

1.2 Syndrome of inappropriate antidiuretic hormone secretion

Other drugs used for Syndrome of inappropriate antidiuretic hormone secretion Demeclocycline hydrochloride, p. 655

DIURETICS › SELECTIVE VASOPRESSIN V$_2$-RECEPTOR ANTAGONISTS

Tolvaptan

20-Apr-2022

- **DRUG ACTION** Tolvaptan is a vasopressin V$_2$-receptor antagonist.

- **INDICATIONS AND DOSE**

JINARC®

Autosomal dominant polycystic kidney disease in adults with CKD stage 1 to 4 at initiation of treatment with evidence of rapidly progressing disease (initiated by a specialist)
- ▸ BY MOUTH
- ▸ Adult: Initially 60 mg daily in 2 divided doses for at least a week, 45 mg in the morning before breakfast, and then 15 mg taken 8 hours later; increased to 90 mg daily in 2 divided doses for at least a week, 60 mg in the morning before breakfast, and then 30 mg taken 8 hours later, then increased if tolerated to 120 mg daily in 2 divided doses, 90 mg in the morning before breakfast, and then 30 mg taken 8 hours later, dose titration should be performed cautiously; patients may down-titrate to lower doses based on tolerability

DOSE ADJUSTMENTS DUE TO INTERACTIONS
- ▸ For *Jinarc*®, manufacturer advises reduce dose with concurrent use of potent CYP3A4 inhibitors—if daily dose 90 mg or 120 mg, reduce to 30 mg once daily (can be further reduced to 15 mg once daily if not tolerated); if daily dose 60 mg, reduce to 15 mg once daily. Manufacturer also advises reduce dose with concurrent use of moderate CYP3A4 inhibitors or ciprofloxacin—if daily dose 120 mg, reduce to 60 mg daily (45 mg in morning and 15 mg taken 8 hours later); if daily dose 90 mg, reduce to 45 mg daily (30 mg in morning and 15 mg taken 8 hours later); if daily dose 60 mg, reduce to 30 mg daily (15 mg in morning and 15 mg taken 8 hours later).

SAMSCA®

Hyponatraemia secondary to syndrome of inappropriate antidiuretic hormone secretion (initiated in hospital or under specialist supervision)
- ▸ BY MOUTH
- ▸ Adult: Initially 15 mg once daily, increased if necessary up to 60 mg once daily, a reduced starting dose of 7.5 mg once daily should be considered for patients at risk of overly rapid correction of serum-sodium concentration

- **CONTRA-INDICATIONS** Anuria · hypernatraemia · hypovolaemic hyponatraemia · impaired perception of thirst · volume depletion

- **CAUTIONS**

GENERAL CAUTIONS Abnormal liver function tests and/or signs or symptoms of liver injury (do not initiate if the criteria for permanent discontinuation are met—consult product literature) · diabetes mellitus · patients at risk of dehydration (ensure adequate fluid intake) · urinary outflow obstruction (increased risk of acute retention)

SPECIFIC CAUTIONS
- ▸ When used for Autosomal dominant polycystic kidney disease Serum-sodium abnormalities (correct before treatment initiation)
- ▸ When used for Hyponatraemia secondary to syndrome of inappropriate antidiuretic hormone secretion Patients at risk of demyelination syndromes (e.g hypoxia, alcoholism and malnutrition)

- **INTERACTIONS** → Appendix 1: tolvaptan

- **SIDE-EFFECTS**
- ▸ **Common or very common** Appetite decreased · asthenia · constipation · dehydration · diarrhoea · dizziness · dry mouth · dyspnoea · gastrointestinal discomfort · gastrooesophageal reflux disease · gout · headache · hepatic disorders · hyperglycaemia · hypernatraemia · hyperuricaemia · insomnia · muscle spasms · palpitations · polydipsia · skin reactions · thirst · urinary disorders · weight decreased
- ▸ **Frequency not known** Acute hepatic failure (cases requiring liver transplantation reported)

SIDE-EFFECTS, FURTHER INFORMATION Interrupt treatment and perform liver-function tests promptly if symptoms of hepatic impairment occur (anorexia, nausea, vomiting, fatigue, abdominal pain, jaundice, dark urine, pruritus)—consult product literature.

- **PREGNANCY** Avoid—toxicity in *animal* studies.

- **BREAST FEEDING** Avoid—present in milk in *animal* studies.

- **HEPATIC IMPAIRMENT** Manufacturer advises caution in severe impairment; avoid if abnormal liver-function tests and/or signs or symptoms of liver injury meet the requirements for permanent discontinuation—consult product literature.

- **RENAL IMPAIRMENT** No information available in severe impairment. EvGr For *Jinarc*®, discontinue if progression to CKD stage 5. Ⓜ

- **MONITORING REQUIREMENTS**
- ▸ Manufacturer advises monitor volume, fluid and electrolyte status (risk of dehydration); monitor electrolytes at least every 3 months during long-term therapy.
- ▸ When used for Autosomal dominant polycystic kidney disease Manufacturer advises monitor liver function tests and for symptoms of liver injury. Liver enzymes and bilirubin must be measured and reviewed before treatment initiation, monthly for 18 months, and every 3 months thereafter; interrupt treatment if abnormalities occur—consult product literature for further information including the criteria for permanent discontinuation. Manufacturer advises evaluate uric acid concentration before treatment initiation and as clinically indicated during treatment; monitor urine osmolality periodically.
- ▸ When used for Hyponatraemia secondary to syndrome of inappropriate antidiuretic hormone secretion Manufacturer advises monitor liver function tests and for symptoms of liver injury; interrupt treatment if abnormalities occur. Manufacturer advises monitor serum-sodium concentration no later than 6 hours after treatment initiation, then monitor serum-sodium and volume status at least every 6 hours during the first 1–2 days of treatment and until dose stabilised. If serum-sodium correction exceeds 6 mmol/litre during the first 6 hours or 8 mmol/litre in the first 6–12 hours, frequency of monitoring should be increased; interrupt or discontinue treatment if serum-sodium increases by 12 mmol/litre or greater in 24 hours or 18 mmol/litre or greater in 48 hours.

- **PRESCRIBING AND DISPENSING INFORMATION** The manufacturer of *Jinarc*® has provided training materials for healthcare professionals to use prior to prescribing tolvaptan in order to minimise the risk of irreversible hepatotoxicity and to highlight the importance of pregnancy prevention.

- **PATIENT AND CARER ADVICE** For *Jinarc*®, morning dose to be taken 30 minutes before food, second dose can be taken with or without food.
Risk minimisation materials For *Jinarc*®, a patient brochure and alert card should be provided.

- **NATIONAL FUNDING/ACCESS DECISIONS**
  For full details see funding body website
  NICE decisions
  ▶ Tolvaptan for treating autosomal dominant polycystic kidney disease (October 2015) NICE TA358 Recommended with restrictions

- **MEDICINAL FORMS** There can be variation in the licensing of different medicines containing the same drug.
  Oral tablet
  CAUTIONARY AND ADVISORY LABELS 27
  ▶ Jinarc (Otsuka Pharmaceuticals (U.K.) Ltd) ▼
    Tolvaptan 15 mg Jinarc 15mg tablets | 7 tablet PoM £302.05 (Hospital only)
    Tolvaptan 30 mg Jinarc 30mg tablets | 7 tablet PoM £302.05 (Hospital only)
    Tolvaptan 45 mg Jinarc 45mg tablets | 7 tablet PoM 🅢
    Tolvaptan 60 mg Jinarc 60mg tablets | 7 tablet PoM 🅢
    Tolvaptan 90 mg Jinarc 90mg tablets | 7 tablet PoM 🅢
  ▶ Samsca (Otsuka Pharmaceuticals (U.K.) Ltd)
    Tolvaptan 15 mg Samsca 15mg tablets | 10 tablet PoM £746.80
    Tolvaptan 30 mg Samsca 30mg tablets | 10 tablet PoM £746.80

2 Bone metabolism disorders

Osteoporosis

03-Feb-2021

Description of condition

Osteoporosis is a progressive bone disease characterised by low bone mass measured by bone mineral density (BMD), and microarchitectural deterioration of bone tissue. This leads to an increased risk of fragility fractures (fractures resulting from low-level trauma). Osteoporosis is considered severe if there have been one or more fragility fractures.

Osteoporosis occurs most commonly in postmenopausal women, men over 50 years, and in patients taking long-term oral corticosteroids (glucocorticoids). Other risk factors for osteoporosis include increasing age, vitamin D deficiency and low calcium intake, lack of physical activity, low body mass index (BMI), cigarette smoking, excess alcohol intake, parental history of hip fractures, a previous fracture at a site characteristic of osteoporotic fractures, and early menopause. Some diseases are also known to be associated with osteoporosis such as rheumatoid arthritis and diabetes. Certain medications may also increase the risk of fracture in some patients, through mechanisms such as induction of liver enzymes which interfere with vitamin D metabolism.

Aims of treatment

A combination of lifestyle changes and drug treatment aims to prevent fragility fractures in patients with osteoporosis.

Lifestyle changes

EvGr Patients should be encouraged to increase their level of physical activity, stop smoking, maintain a normal BMI level (between 20–25 kg/m^2), and reduce their alcohol intake to improve their bone health and reduce the risk of fragility fractures. Ⓐ For guidance on stopping smoking, see Smoking cessation p. 565.

EvGr Patients at risk of osteoporosis should also ensure an adequate intake of calcium and vitamin D. Calcium should preferably be obtained through increasing dietary intake; supplements may be used if necessary. A daily dietary supplement of vitamin D may be considered for those at increased risk of deficiency.

Elderly patients, especially those who are housebound or live in residential or nursing homes, are at high risk of vitamin D deficiency and may benefit from calcium and vitamin D treatment. Ⓐ Elderly patients also have an increased risk of falls (see Prescribing in the elderly p. 31).

Drug treatment

EvGr Choice of treatment is generally determined by the spectrum of anti-fracture effects across skeletal sites, patient preference and suitability. Ⓐ

Some recommendations on the management of osteoporosis from the National Osteoporosis Guideline Group (NOGG)—Clinical guideline for the prevention and treatment of osteoporosis (July 2019), and Scottish Intercollegiate Guidelines Network (SIGN)—Management of osteoporosis and the prevention of fragility fractures (SIGN 142, January 2021) differ. Recommendations in BNF publications are based on the NOGG guideline, and differences with SIGN (2021) have been highlighted.

Postmenopausal osteoporosis

EvGr The oral bisphosphonates alendronic acid p. 770 and risedronate sodium p. 773 are considered as first-line options for most patients with postmenopausal osteoporosis due to their broad spectrum of anti-fracture efficacy. Alendronic acid and risedronate sodium have been shown to reduce occurrence of vertebral, non-vertebral and hip fractures. SIGN (2021) also recommend that ibandronic acid p. 771 may be considered as an alternative oral bisphosphonate. Parenteral bisphosphonates or denosumab p. 777 are alternative options for women who are intolerant of oral bisphosphonates or in whom they are unsuitable, with raloxifene hydrochloride p. 868 or strontium ranelate p. 775 as additional alternative options.

Hormone replacement therapy (HRT) may also be considered as an additional alternative option, but its use is generally restricted to younger postmenopausal women with menopausal symptoms who are at high risk of fractures. This is due to the risk of adverse effects such as cardiovascular disease and cancer in older postmenopausal women and women on long-term HRT therapy. SIGN (2021) also recommend tibolone p. 874 as an option in younger postmenopausal women, particularly those with menopausal symptoms.

Teriparatide p. 776 is reserved for postmenopausal women with severe osteoporosis at very high risk of fractures, particularly vertebral fractures. SIGN (2021) also recommend romosozumab p. 779 as an option for postmenopausal women with severe osteoporosis who have previously experienced a fragility fracture and are at imminent risk of another (within 24 months). In postmenopausal women with at least one severe or two moderate low-trauma vertebral fractures, teriparatide or romosozumab are recommended over oral bisphosphonates. Ⓐ

Glucocorticoid-induced osteoporosis

Glucocorticoid treatment is strongly associated with bone loss and increased risk of fractures. The greatest rate of bone loss occurs early after initiation of glucocorticoids and increases with the dose and duration of therapy. EvGr Bone-protection treatment should be started at the onset of glucocorticoid treatment in patients who are at high risk of a fracture.

Women aged ≥70 years, OR with a previous fragility fracture, OR who are taking large doses of glucocorticoids (prednisolone ≥7.5 mg daily or equivalent) should be considered for bone-protection treatment. Men aged ≥70 years with a previous fragility fracture, OR who are taking large doses of glucocorticoids, should also be considered for treatment. For some premenopausal women and younger men (particularly those with a previous history of fracture or who are receiving large doses of glucocorticoids), bone-protection treatment may be appropriate. SIGN (2021) recommends that bone-protection treatment should be considered in all men and women taking large doses of glucocorticoids (prednisolone ≥7.5 mg daily or equivalent) for 3 months or longer.

The oral bisphosphonates alendronic acid or risedronate sodium are first-line treatment options. Zoledronic acid

p. 774, denosumab or teriparatide are alternative options in patients intolerant of oral bisphosphonates or in whom they are unsuitable.

If glucocorticoid treatment is stopped, the need to continue bone-protection treatment should be reviewed. However, bone-protection treatment should be continued with long-term glucocorticoid treatment. Complex cases of glucocorticoid-induced osteoporosis should be referred to a specialist. (A)

Osteoporosis in men

[EvGr] The oral bisphosphonates alendronic acid or risedronate sodium are recommended as first-line treatments for osteoporosis in men. Zoledronic acid or denosumab are alternatives in men who are intolerant of oral bisphosphonates or in whom they are unsuitable; teriparatide or strontium ranelate are additional alternative options. (A)

Men having androgen deprivation therapy for prostate cancer have an increased fracture risk. [EvGr] Fracture risk assessment should be considered when starting this therapy. A bisphosphonate can be offered to men with confirmed osteoporosis; denosumab may be considered as an alternative if bisphosphonates are unsuitable or not tolerated. (A)

Bisphosphonates: treatment duration

[EvGr] Some patients may benefit from a bisphosphonate-free period as their therapeutic effects last for some time after cessation of treatment, although there is limited evidence to support this.

Bisphosphonate treatment should be reviewed after 5 years of treatment with alendronic acid, risedronate sodium or ibandronic acid, and after 3 years of treatment with zoledronic acid. Based on fracture-risk assessment, continuation beyond this period can generally be recommended for patients who are over 75 years of age, have a history of previous hip or vertebral fracture, have had one or more fragility fractures during treatment, or who are taking long-term glucocorticoid treatment. Due to limited evidence, recommendations on duration are based on limited extension studies in postmenopausal women. There is no evidence for treatment beyond 10 years; management of these patients should be on a case-by-case basis with specialist input as appropriate. (A)

Useful Resources

Clinical guideline for the prevention and treatment of osteoporosis. The National Osteoporosis Guideline Group (NOGG). 2017 (updated July 2019).
www.sheffield.ac.uk/NOGG/downloads.html

Management of osteoporosis and the prevention of fragility fractures. Scottish Intercollegiate Guidelines Network. Clinical guideline 142. June 2020 (updated January 2021).
www.sign.ac.uk/our-guidelines/management-of-osteoporosis-and-the-prevention-of-fragility-fractures

---

Other drugs used for Bone metabolism disorders
Calcitriol, p. 1241

Bisphosphonates 

- **DRUG ACTION** Bisphosphonates are adsorbed onto hydroxyapatite crystals in bone, slowing both their rate of growth and dissolution, and therefore reducing the rate of bone turnover.

> **IMPORTANT SAFETY INFORMATION**
>
> **MHRA/CHM ADVICE: BISPHOSPHONATES: ATYPICAL FEMORAL FRACTURES (JUNE 2011)**
>
> Atypical femoral fractures have been reported rarely with bisphosphonate treatment, mainly in patients receiving long-term treatment for osteoporosis.
>
> The need to continue bisphosphonate treatment for osteoporosis should be re-evaluated periodically based on an assessment of the benefits and risks of treatment for individual patients, particularly after 5 or more years of use.
>
> Patients should be advised to report any thigh, hip, or groin pain during treatment with a bisphosphonate.
>
> Discontinuation of bisphosphonate treatment in patients suspected to have an atypical femoral fracture should be considered after an assessment of the benefits and risks of continued treatment.
>
> **MHRA/CHM ADVICE: BISPHOSPHONATES: OSTEONECROSIS OF THE JAW (NOVEMBER 2009) AND INTRAVENOUS BISPHOSPHONATES: OSTEONECROSIS OF THE JAW—FURTHER MEASURES TO MINIMISE RISK (JULY 2015)**
>
> The risk of osteonecrosis of the jaw is substantially greater for patients receiving intravenous bisphosphonates in the treatment of cancer than for patients receiving oral bisphosphonates for osteoporosis or Paget's disease.
>
> Risk factors for developing osteonecrosis of the jaw that should be considered are: potency of bisphosphonate (highest for zoledronate), route of administration, cumulative dose, duration and type of malignant disease, concomitant treatment, smoking, comorbid conditions, and history of dental disease.
>
> All patients with cancer and patients with poor dental status should have a dental check-up (and any necessary remedial work should be performed) before bisphosphonate treatment, or as soon as possible after starting treatment. Patients should also maintain good oral hygiene, receive routine dental check-ups, and report any oral symptoms such as dental mobility, pain, or swelling, non-healing sores or discharge to a doctor and dentist during treatment.
>
> Before prescribing an intravenous bisphosphonate, patients should be given a patient reminder card and informed of the risk of osteonecrosis of the jaw. Advise patients to tell their doctor if they have any problems with their mouth or teeth before starting treatment, and if the patient wears dentures, they should make sure their dentures fit properly. Patients should tell their doctor and dentist that they are receiving an intravenous bisphosphonate if they need dental treatment or dental surgery.
>
> Guidance for dentists in primary care is included in *Oral Health Management of Patients at Risk of Medication-related Osteonecrosis of the Jaw: Dental Clinical Guidance*, Scottish Dental Clinical Effectiveness Programme, March 2017 (available at www.sdcep.org.uk/published-guidance/medication-related-osteonecrosis-of-the-jaw/).
>
> **MHRA/CHM ADVICE: BISPHOSPHONATES: OSTEONECROSIS OF THE EXTERNAL AUDITORY CANAL (DECEMBER 2015)**
>
> Benign idiopathic osteonecrosis of the external auditory canal has been reported very rarely with bisphosphonate treatment, mainly in patients receiving long-term therapy (2 years or longer).

The possibility of osteonecrosis of the external auditory canal should be considered in patients receiving bisphosphonates who present with ear symptoms, including chronic ear infections, or suspected cholesteatoma.

Risk factors for developing osteonecrosis of the external auditory canal include: steroid use, chemotherapy, infection, an ear operation, or cotton-bud use.

Patients should be advised to report any ear pain, discharge from the ear, or an ear infection during treatment with a bisphosphonate.

- **CAUTIONS**
- **Elderly with oral use** Screening Tool of Older Persons' potentially inappropriate Prescriptions (STOPP) criteria to aid medication reviews (see Prescribing in the elderly p. 31 for information): potentially inappropriate in patients with a current or recent history of upper gastro-intestinal disease or bleeding (risk of relapse/exacerbation of oesophagitis, oesophageal ulcer, or oesophageal stricture).
- **SIDE-EFFECTS**
- **Common or very common** Alopecia · anaemia · appetite decreased · arthralgia · asthenia · chills · constipation · diarrhoea · dizziness · dysphagia · electrolyte imbalance · eye inflammation · fever · gastritis · gastrointestinal discomfort · headache · influenza like illness · malaise · myalgia · nausea · oesophageal ulcer (discontinue) · oesophagitis (discontinue) · pain · peripheral oedema · renal impairment · skin reactions · taste altered · vomiting
- **Uncommon** Anaphylactic reaction · angioedema · bronchospasm · oesophageal stenosis (discontinue) · osteonecrosis
- **Rare or very rare** Atypical femur fracture · Stevens-Johnson syndrome
- **PATIENT AND CARER ADVICE**
  Atypical femoral fractures Patients should be advised to report any thigh, hip, or groin pain during treatment with a bisphosphonate.
  Osteonecrosis of the jaw During bisphosphonate treatment patients should maintain good oral hygiene, receive routine dental check-ups, and report any oral symptoms.
  Osteonecrosis of the external auditory canal Patients should be advised to report any ear pain, discharge from ear or an ear infection during treatment with a bisphosphonate.

▶ 769

Alendronic acid

16-Nov-2022

(Alendronate)

- **INDICATIONS AND DOSE**

Treatment of postmenopausal osteoporosis
- BY MOUTH
- Adult (female): 10 mg once daily, alternatively 70 mg once weekly.

Treatment of osteoporosis in men
- BY MOUTH
- Adult (male): 10 mg once daily.

Prevention and treatment of corticosteroid-induced osteoporosis in postmenopausal women not receiving hormone replacement therapy
- BY MOUTH
- Adult (female): 10 mg once daily.

- **CONTRA-INDICATIONS** Abnormalities of oesophagus · hypocalcaemia · other factors which delay emptying (e.g. stricture or achalasia)
- **CAUTIONS** Active gastro-intestinal bleeding · atypical femoral fractures · duodenitis · dysphagia · exclude other causes of osteoporosis · gastritis · history (within 1 year) of ulcers · surgery of the upper gastro-intestinal tract ·

symptomatic oesophageal disease · ulcers · upper gastro-intestinal disorders

- **INTERACTIONS** → Appendix 1: bisphosphonates
- **SIDE-EFFECTS**
- **Common or very common** Gastrointestinal disorders · joint swelling · vertigo
- **Uncommon** Haemorrhage
- **Rare or very rare** Femoral stress fracture · oropharyngeal ulceration · photosensitivity reaction · severe cutaneous adverse reactions (SCARs)

  SIDE-EFFECTS, FURTHER INFORMATION Severe oesophageal reactions (oesophagitis, oesophageal ulcers, oesophageal stricture and oesophageal erosions) have been reported; patients should be advised to stop taking the tablets and to seek medical attention if they develop symptoms of oesophageal irritation such as dysphagia, new or worsening heartburn, pain on swallowing or retrosternal pain.
- **PREGNANCY** Avoid.
- **BREAST FEEDING** Manufacturer advises avoid—no information available.
- **RENAL IMPAIRMENT** EvGr Avoid if creatinine clearance less than 35 mL/minute. Ⓜ See p. 21.
- **MONITORING REQUIREMENTS** Correct disturbances of calcium and mineral metabolism (e.g. vitamin-D deficiency, hypocalcaemia) before starting treatment. Monitor serum-calcium concentration during treatment.
- **DIRECTIONS FOR ADMINISTRATION** Manufacturer advises tablets should be swallowed whole and oral solution should be swallowed as a single 100 mL dose. Doses should be taken with plenty of water while sitting or standing, on an empty stomach at least 30 minutes before breakfast (or another oral medicine); patient should stand or sit upright for at least 30 minutes after administration.
- **PATIENT AND CARER ADVICE** Patients or their carers should be given advice on how to administer alendronic acid tablets and oral solution.
  Oesophageal reactions Patients (or their carers) should be advised to stop taking alendronic acid and to seek medical attention if they develop symptoms of oesophageal irritation such as dysphagia, new or worsening heartburn, pain on swallowing or retrosternal pain.
- **NATIONAL FUNDING/ACCESS DECISIONS**
  For full details see funding body website
  NICE decisions
- **Bisphosphonates for treating osteoporosis (updated July 2019)** NICE TA464 Recommended with restrictions
  Scottish Medicines Consortium (SMC) decisions
- **Alendronic acid (*Binosto*®) for the treatment of postmenopausal osteoporosis (April 2016)** SMC No. 1137/16 Recommended with restrictions

- **MEDICINAL FORMS** There can be variation in the licensing of different medicines containing the same drug. Forms available from special-order manufacturers include: oral solution

Oral tablet
- **Alendronic acid (Non-proprietary)**
  Alendronic acid (as Alendronate sodium) 10 mg Alendronic acid 10mg tablets | 28 tablet PoM £7.50 DT = £7.50
  Alendronic acid (as Alendronate sodium) 70 mg Alendronic acid 70mg tablets | 4 tablet PoM £1.78 DT = £0.94
- **Fosamax Once Weekly** (Organon Pharma (UK) Ltd)
  Alendronic acid (as Alendronate sodium) 70 mg Fosamax Once Weekly 70mg tablets | 4 tablet PoM £22.80 DT = £0.94

Oral solution
- **Alendronic acid (Non-proprietary)**
  Alendronic acid 700 microgram per 1 ml Alendronic acid 70mg/100ml oral solution unit dose sugar free | 4 unit dose PoM £29.80 DT = £26.07 SF

Effervescent tablet

- **Binosto** (Internis Pharmaceuticals Ltd)
  Alendronic acid (as Alendronate sodium) 70 mg Binosto 70mg effervescent tablets | 4 tablet [PoM] £11.60 DT = £11.60 [SF]

Alendronic acid with colecalciferol

12-Nov-2020

The properties listed below are those particular to the combination only. For the properties of the components please consider, alendronic acid p. 770, colecalciferol p. 1242.

- **INDICATIONS AND DOSE**

Treatment of postmenopausal osteoporosis in women at risk of vitamin D deficiency

- BY MOUTH
  - Adult (female): 1 tablet once weekly.

- **INTERACTIONS** → Appendix 1: bisphosphonates · vitamin D substances
- **DIRECTIONS FOR ADMINISTRATION** Manufacturer advises tablets should be swallowed whole with plenty of water while sitting or standing; to be taken on an empty stomach at least 30 minutes before breakfast (or another oral medicine); patient should stand or sit upright for at least 30 minutes after taking tablet.
- **PATIENT AND CARER ADVICE** Patients or carers should be given advice on how to administer alendronic acid with colecalciferol tablets.
- **MEDICINAL FORMS** There can be variation in the licensing of different medicines containing the same drug.

Oral tablet

- **Fosavance** (Organon Pharma (UK) Ltd)
  Colecalciferol 70 microgram, Alendronic acid (as Alendronate sodium) 70 mg Fosavance tablets | 4 tablet [PoM] £22.80 DT = £22.80

F 769

Ibandronic acid

27-Oct-2021

- **INDICATIONS AND DOSE**

Reduction of bone damage in bone metastases in breast cancer

- INITIALLY BY MOUTH
  - Adult: 50 mg daily, alternatively (by intravenous infusion) 6 mg every 3–4 weeks

Hypercalcaemia of malignancy

- BY INTRAVENOUS INFUSION
  - Adult: 2–4 mg as a single infusion, dose to be adjusted according to serum calcium concentration

Treatment of postmenopausal osteoporosis

- INITIALLY BY MOUTH
  - Adult (female): 150 mg once a month, alternatively (by intravenous injection) 3 mg every 3 months, to be administered over 15–30 seconds.

- **CONTRA-INDICATIONS**
  GENERAL CONTRA-INDICATIONS Hypocalcaemia
  SPECIFIC CONTRA-INDICATIONS
  - With oral use Abnormalities of the oesophagus · other factors which delay emptying (e.g. stricture or achalasia)
- **CAUTIONS**
  GENERAL CAUTIONS Atypical femoral fractures
  SPECIFIC CAUTIONS
  - With intravenous use Cardiac disease (avoid fluid overload)
  - With oral use Upper gastro-intestinal disorders
- **INTERACTIONS** → Appendix 1: bisphosphonates
- **SIDE-EFFECTS**
  GENERAL SIDE-EFFECTS
  - **Common or very common** Acute phase reaction
  - **Uncommon** Asthma exacerbated
  - **Rare or very rare** Face oedema

  SPECIFIC SIDE-EFFECTS
  - **Common or very common**
    - With intravenous use Bundle branch block · cataract · increased risk of infection · joint disorder · oral disorders · osteoarthritis · parathyroid disorder · thirst
    - With oral use Gastrointestinal disorders · muscle cramps · musculoskeletal stiffness
  - **Uncommon**
    - With intravenous use Acrochordon · affective disorder · altered smell sensation · anxiety · blood disorder · cardiovascular disorder · cerebrovascular disorder · cholelithiasis · cystitis · deafness · hyperaesthesia · hypothermia · injury · memory loss · migraine · muscle tone increased · myocardial ischaemia · palpitations · pelvic pain · pulmonary oedema · radiculopathy · renal cyst · sleep disorder · stridor · thrombophlebitis · urinary retention · weight decreased
  - **Rare or very rare**
    - With intravenous use Anaphylactic shock
  - **Frequency not known**
    - With oral use Oesophagitis erosive (discontinue)
- **PREGNANCY** Avoid.
- **BREAST FEEDING** Avoid—present in milk in *animal* studies.
- **RENAL IMPAIRMENT** [EvGr] When used for postmenopausal osteoporosis, avoid if creatinine clearance less than 30 mL/minute. (M)
  Dose adjustments See p. 21.
  - With intravenous use [EvGr] When used for bone metastases, if creatinine clearance 30–49 mL/minute reduce dose to 4 mg; if creatinine clearance less than 30 mL/minute reduce dose to 2 mg. Dilute requisite dose in 500 mL infusion fluid and give over 1 hour. (M)
  - With oral use [EvGr] When used for bone metastases, if creatinine clearance 30–49 mL/minute reduce dose to 50 mg on alternative days; if creatinine clearance less than 30 mL/minute reduce dose to 50 mg once weekly. (M)
- **MONITORING REQUIREMENTS** Monitor renal function and serum calcium, phosphate and magnesium.
- **DIRECTIONS FOR ADMINISTRATION** Manufacturers advise tablets should be swallowed whole with plenty of water while sitting or standing; to be taken on an empty stomach at least 30 minutes (for most ibandronic acid tablets, 50 mg) or 1 hour (for *Bonviva*® tablets, 150 mg) before first food or drink (other than water) of the day, or another oral medicine; patient should stand or sit upright for at least 1 hour after taking tablet.
  For *intravenous infusion* (*Bondronat*®), manufacturer advises give intermittently in Glucose 5% or Sodium chloride 0.9%; for hypercalcaemia of malignancy, dilute requisite dose in 500 mL infusion fluid and give over 2 hours. For the reduction of bone damage in bone metastases, dilute requisite dose in 100 mL infusion fluid and give over at least 15 minutes.
- **PATIENT AND CARER ADVICE** Patients or carers should be given advice on how to administer ibandronic acid tablets.
  Oesophageal reactions Patients and carers should be advised to stop tablets and seek medical attention for symptoms of oesophageal irritation such as dysphagia, pain on swallowing, retrosternal pain, or heartburn.
  Patient reminder card A patient reminder card should be provided to patients receiving intravenous ibandronic acid (risk of osteonecrosis of the jaw).

● **NATIONAL FUNDING/ACCESS DECISIONS**
For full details see funding body website
NICE decisions
▸ **Bisphosphonates for treating osteoporosis (updated July 2019)** NICE TA464 Recommended with restrictions

● **MEDICINAL FORMS** There can be variation in the licensing of different medicines containing the same drug.
Solution for injection
▸ **Ibandronic acid (Non-proprietary)**
Ibandronic acid (as Ibandronic sodium monohydrate) 1 mg per 1 ml Ibandronic acid 3mg/3ml solution for injection pre-filled syringes | 1 pre-filled disposable injection PoM £65.40 DT = £65.40 (Hospital only) | 1 pre-filled disposable injection PoM £65.40 DT = £65.40
▸ **Bonviva** (Atnahs Pharma UK Ltd)
Ibandronic acid (as Ibandronic sodium monohydrate) 1 mg per 1 ml Bonviva 3mg/3ml solution for injection pre-filled syringes | 1 pre-filled disposable injection PoM £68.64 DT = £65.40
Solution for infusion
▸ **Ibandronic acid (Non-proprietary)**
Ibandronic acid (as Ibandronic sodium monohydrate) 1 mg per 1 ml Ibandronic acid 6mg/6ml concentrate for solution for infusion vials | 1 vial PoM £130.42 (Hospital only)
▸ **Bondronat** (Atnahs Pharma UK Ltd)
Ibandronic acid (as Ibandronic sodium monohydrate) 1 mg per 1 ml Bondronat 6mg/6ml concentrate for solution for infusion vials | 1 vial PoM £183.69 (Hospital only)
Oral tablet
▸ **Ibandronic acid (Non-proprietary)**
**Ibandronic acid (as Ibandronic sodium monohydrate)
50 mg** Ibandronic acid 50mg tablets | 28 tablet PoM £186.69 DT = £24.35
**Ibandronic acid (as Ibandronic sodium monohydrate)
150 mg** Ibandronic acid 150mg tablets | 1 tablet PoM £18.40 DT = £1.28 | 3 tablet PoM £3.84–£55.21
▸ **Bondronat** (Atnahs Pharma UK Ltd)
**Ibandronic acid (as Ibandronic sodium monohydrate)
50 mg** Bondronat 50mg tablets | 28 tablet PoM £183.69 DT = £24.35
▸ **Bonviva** (Atnahs Pharma UK Ltd)
**Ibandronic acid (as Ibandronic sodium monohydrate)
150 mg** Bonviva 150mg tablets | 1 tablet PoM £18.40 DT = £1.28

F 769

Pamidronate disodium

21-Jul-2021

(Formerly called aminohydroxypropylidenediphosphonate disodium (APD))

● **INDICATIONS AND DOSE**
Hypercalcaemia of malignancy
▸ BY INTRAVENOUS INFUSION
▸ Adult: 15–60 mg, to be given (via cannula in a relatively large vein) as a single infusion or in divided doses over 2–4 days, dose adjusted according to serum calcium concentration; maximum 90 mg per course
Osteolytic lesions and bone pain in bone metastases associated with breast cancer or multiple myeloma
▸ BY INTRAVENOUS INFUSION
▸ Adult: 90 mg every 4 weeks, to be administered via cannula in a relatively large vein, dose may alternatively be administered every 3 weeks, to coincide with chemotherapy in breast cancer
Paget's disease of bone
▸ BY INTRAVENOUS INFUSION
▸ Adult: 30 mg every week for a 6 week course (total dose 180 mg), alternatively initially 30 mg once weekly for 1 week, then increased to 60 mg every 2 weeks (max. per dose 60 mg) for a 6 week course (total dose 210 mg), to be administered via cannula in a relatively large vein, course may be repeated every 6 months; maximum 360 mg per course

● **CAUTIONS** Atypical femoral fractures · cardiac disease (especially in elderly) · ensure adequate hydration · previous thyroid surgery (risk of hypocalcaemia)
● **INTERACTIONS** → Appendix 1: bisphosphonates
● **SIDE-EFFECTS**
▸ **Common or very common** Decreased leucocytes · drowsiness · flushing · hypertension · insomnia · paraesthesia · tetany · thrombocytopenia
▸ **Uncommon** Agitation · dyspnoea · hypotension · muscle cramps · seizure
▸ **Rare or very rare** Acute respiratory distress syndrome (ARDS) · confusion · glomerulonephritis · haematuria · heart failure · interstitial lung disease · nephritis tubulointerstitial · nephrotic syndrome · oedema · pulmonary oedema · reactivation of infections · renal disorder exacerbated · renal tubular disorder · visual hallucinations · xanthopsia
▸ **Frequency not known** Atrial fibrillation

SIDE-EFFECTS, FURTHER INFORMATION Oral supplements are advised to minimise potential risk of hypocalcaemia for those with mainly lytic bone metastases or multiple myeloma at risk of calcium or vitamin D deficiency (e.g. through malabsorption or lack of exposure to sunlight) and in those with Paget's disease.

● **PREGNANCY** Avoid—toxicity in *animal* studies.
● **BREAST FEEDING** Avoid.
● **HEPATIC IMPAIRMENT** Manufacturer advises caution in severe hepatic impairment (no information available).
● **RENAL IMPAIRMENT**
Dose adjustments EvGr Max. infusion rate 20 mg/hour. Avoid if creatinine clearance less than 30 mL/minute, except in life-threatening hypercalcaemia if benefit outweighs risk. Ⓜ See p. 21.
EvGr If renal function deteriorates in patients with bone metastases, withhold dose until serum creatinine returns to within 10% of baseline value. Ⓜ
● **MONITORING REQUIREMENTS**
▸ Monitor serum electrolytes, calcium and phosphate—possibility of convulsions due to electrolyte changes.
▸ Assess renal function before each dose.
● **DIRECTIONS FOR ADMINISTRATION** For *slow intravenous infusion* (*Pamidronate disodium*, Hospira, Medac, Wockhardt), manufacturer advises give intermittently in Glucose 5% or Sodium chloride 0.9%; give at a rate not exceeding 1 mg/minute; not to be given with infusion fluids containing calcium. For *Pamidronate disodium* (Medac, Hospira, Wockhardt), manufacturer advises dilute with infusion fluid to a concentration of not more than 90 mg in 250 mL.
● **PATIENT AND CARER ADVICE** A patient reminder card should be provided (risk of osteonecrosis of the jaw).
Driving and skilled tasks Patients should be warned against performing skilled tasks (e.g. cycling, driving or operating machinery) immediately after treatment (somnolence or dizziness can occur).

● **MEDICINAL FORMS** There can be variation in the licensing of different medicines containing the same drug.
Solution for infusion
▸ **Pamidronate disodium (Non-proprietary)**
Pamidronate disodium 3 mg per 1 ml Pamidronate disodium 30mg/10ml solution for infusion vials | 1 vial PoM £59.66 (Hospital only)
Pamidronate disodium 9 mg per 1 ml Pamidronate disodium 90mg/10ml solution for infusion vials | 1 vial PoM £170.45 (Hospital only)

Risedronate sodium

21-Jul-2021

● **INDICATIONS AND DOSE**

Paget's disease of bone
▸ BY MOUTH
▸ Adult: 30 mg daily for 2 months, course may be repeated if necessary after at least 2 months

Treatment of postmenopausal osteoporosis to reduce risk of vertebral or hip fractures
▸ BY MOUTH
▸ Adult (female): 5 mg daily, alternatively 35 mg once weekly.

Prevention of osteoporosis (including corticosteroid-induced osteoporosis) in postmenopausal women
▸ BY MOUTH
▸ Adult (female): 5 mg daily.

Treatment of osteoporosis in men at high risk of fractures
▸ BY MOUTH
▸ Adult (male): 35 mg once weekly.

● **CONTRA-INDICATIONS** Hypocalcaemia

● **CAUTIONS** Atypical femoral fractures · oesophageal abnormalities · other factors which delay transit or emptying (e.g. stricture or achalasia) · upper gastro-intestinal disorders

● **INTERACTIONS** → Appendix 1: bisphosphonates

● **SIDE-EFFECTS**
▸ **Uncommon** Gastrointestinal disorders
▸ **Rare or very rare** Glossitis
▸ **Frequency not known** Amblyopia · apnoea · chest pain · corneal lesion · dry eye · hypersensitivity · hypersensitivity vasculitis · increased risk of infection · leg cramps · liver disorder · muscle weakness · neoplasms · nocturia · tinnitus · toxic epidermal necrolysis · weight decreased

● **PREGNANCY** Avoid.

● **BREAST FEEDING** Avoid.

● **RENAL IMPAIRMENT** [EvGr] Avoid if creatinine clearance less than 30 mL/minute. ⟨M⟩ See p. 21.

● **MONITORING REQUIREMENTS**
▸ Correct hypocalcaemia before starting.
▸ Correct other disturbances of bone and mineral metabolism (e.g. vitamin-D deficiency) at onset of treatment.

● **DIRECTIONS FOR ADMINISTRATION** Manufacturer advises swallow tablets whole with full glass of water; on rising, take on an empty stomach at least 30 minutes before first food or drink of the day **or**, if taking at any other time of the day, avoid food and drink for at least 2 hours before or after risedronate (particularly avoid calcium-containing products e.g. milk; also avoid iron and mineral supplements and antacids); stand or sit upright for at least 30 minutes; do not take tablets at bedtime or before rising.

● **PATIENT AND CARER ADVICE** Patients or carers should be given advice on how to administer risedronate sodium tablets.
Oesophageal reactions Patients should be advised to stop taking the tablets and seek medical attention if they develop symptoms of oesophageal irritation such as dysphagia, pain on swallowing, retrosternal pain, or heartburn.

● **NATIONAL FUNDING/ACCESS DECISIONS**
For full details see funding body website
NICE decisions
▸ **Bisphosphonates for treating osteoporosis (updated July 2019)** NICE TA464 Recommended with restrictions

● **MEDICINAL FORMS** There can be variation in the licensing of different medicines containing the same drug. Forms available from special-order manufacturers include: oral suspension, oral solution
Oral tablet
▸ **Risedronate sodium (Non-proprietary)**
  Risedronate sodium 5 mg Risedronate sodium 5mg tablets | 28 tablet [PoM] £26.21 DT = £25.88
  Risedronate sodium 30 mg Risedronate sodium 30mg tablets | 28 tablet [PoM] £143.83 DT = £143.83
  Risedronate sodium 35 mg Risedronate sodium 35mg tablets | 4 tablet [PoM] £19.12 DT = £1.12
▸ **Actonel** (Teva UK Ltd)
  Risedronate sodium 35 mg Actonel 35mg tablets | 4 tablet [PoM] 🅧 DT = £1.12

Risedronate with calcium carbonate and colecalciferol

09-Nov-2020

The properties listed below are those particular to the combination only. For the properties of the components please consider, risedronate sodium above, calcium carbonate p. 1188, colecalciferol p. 1242.

● **INDICATIONS AND DOSE**

Treatment of postmenopausal osteoporosis to reduce risk of vertebral or hip fractures
▸ BY MOUTH
▸ Adult: 1 tablet once weekly on day 1 of the weekly cycle, followed by 1 sachet daily on days 2–6 of the weekly cycle

● **INTERACTIONS** → Appendix 1: bisphosphonates · calcium salts · vitamin D substances

● **DIRECTIONS FOR ADMINISTRATION** Manufacturer advises tablets should be swallowed whole with plenty of water while sitting or standing; to be taken on an empty stomach at least 30 minutes before breakfast (or another oral medicine); patient should stand or sit upright for at least 30 minutes after taking tablet. Manufacturer advises granules should be stirred into a glass of water and after dissolution complete taken immediately.

● **PRESCRIBING AND DISPENSING INFORMATION** *Actonel Combi* ® effervescent granules contain calcium carbonate 2.5 g (calcium 1 g or Ca^{2+} 25 mmol) and colecalciferol 22 micrograms (880 units)/sachet.

● **PATIENT AND CARER ADVICE** Patients or carers should be given advice on how to administer risedronate with calcium carbonate and colecalciferol tablets and granules.

● **MEDICINAL FORMS** No licensed medicines listed.

Sodium clodronate

05-Aug-2021

● **INDICATIONS AND DOSE**

Osteolytic lesions, hypercalcaemia and bone pain associated with skeletal metastases in patients with breast cancer or multiple myeloma
▸ BY MOUTH
▸ Adult: 1.6 g daily in 1–2 divided doses, then increased if necessary up to 3.2 g daily in 2 divided doses

LORON 520 ®

Osteolytic lesions, hypercalcaemia and bone pain associated with skeletal metastases in patients with breast cancer or multiple myeloma
▸ BY MOUTH
▸ Adult: Initially 2 tablets daily in 1–2 divided doses, increased if necessary up to 4 tablets daily

● **CONTRA-INDICATIONS** Acute severe gastro-intestinal inflammatory conditions

- **CAUTIONS** Atypical femoral fractures · maintain adequate fluid intake during treatment · upper gastro-intestinal disorders

- **INTERACTIONS** → Appendix 1: bisphosphonates

- **SIDE-EFFECTS** Proteinuria · respiratory disorder

- **PREGNANCY** Avoid.

- **BREAST FEEDING** Manufacturer advises avoid—no information available.

- **RENAL IMPAIRMENT** Manufacturer advises avoid if creatinine clearance less than 10 mL/minute.
  Dose adjustments See p. 21.
     Manufacturer advises reduce dose to 1200 mg daily if creatinine clearance 30–50 mL/minute (consult product literature).
     Manufacturer advises use half normal dose if creatinine clearance 10–30 mL/minute.

- **MONITORING REQUIREMENTS** Monitor renal function, serum calcium and serum phosphate before and during treatment.

- **DIRECTIONS FOR ADMINISTRATION** Manufacturer advises avoid food or fluids (other than plain water) for 2 hours before and 1 hour after treatment, particularly calcium-containing products e.g. milk; also avoid iron and mineral supplements and antacids; maintain adequate fluid intake.

- **PATIENT AND CARER ADVICE** Patients or carers should be given advice on how to administer sodium clodronate capsules and tablets.

- **MEDICINAL FORMS** There can be variation in the licensing of different medicines containing the same drug.
  Oral tablet
  CAUTIONARY AND ADVISORY LABELS 10
  ▶ **Clasteon** (Kent Pharma (UK) Ltd)
     Sodium clodronate 800 mg Clasteon 800mg tablets | 60 tablet [PoM] £146.43 DT = £146.43
  ▶ **Loron** (Esteve Pharmaceuticals Ltd)
     Sodium clodronate 520 mg Loron 520mg tablets | 60 tablet [PoM] £114.44 DT = £114.44
  Oral capsule
  ▶ **Clasteon** (Kent Pharma (UK) Ltd)
     Sodium clodronate 400 mg Clasteon 400mg capsules | 30 capsule [PoM] £34.96 | 120 capsule [PoM] £139.83 DT = £139.83

⟨F⟩ 769

Zoledronic acid

05-Aug-2024

- **INDICATIONS AND DOSE**

Prevention of skeletal related events in advanced malignancies involving bone (specialist use only)
▶ BY INTRAVENOUS INFUSION
▶ Adult: 4 mg every 3–4 weeks, calcium 500 mg daily and vitamin D 400 units daily should also be taken

Tumour-induced hypercalcaemia (specialist use only)
▶ BY INTRAVENOUS INFUSION
▶ Adult: 4 mg for 1 dose

Paget's disease of bone (specialist use only)
▶ BY INTRAVENOUS INFUSION
▶ Adult: 5 mg for 1 dose, at least 500 mg elemental calcium twice daily (with vitamin D) for at least 10 days is recommended following infusion

Osteoporosis (including corticosteroid-induced osteoporosis) in men and postmenopausal women
▶ BY INTRAVENOUS INFUSION
▶ Adult: 5 mg once yearly as a single dose, in patients with a recent low-trauma hip fracture, the dose should be given at least 2 weeks after hip fracture repair; before first infusion give 50 000–125 000 units of vitamin D

Fracture prevention in osteopenia [hip or femoral neck]
▶ BY INTRAVENOUS INFUSION
▶ Elderly (female): 5 mg once every 18 months as a single dose.

- **UNLICENSED USE** [EvGr] Zoledronic acid is used for fracture prevention in women with osteopenia, ⟨Ⓐ⟩ but is not licensed for this indication.

- **CONTRA-INDICATIONS**
▶ When used for Paget's disease of bone or Osteoporosis (including corticosteroid-induced osteoporosis) in men and postmenopausal women or Fracture prevention in osteopenia [hip or femoral neck] Hypocalcaemia

- **CAUTIONS** Atypical femoral fractures · cardiac disease (avoid fluid overload) · concomitant medicines that affect renal function

- **INTERACTIONS** → Appendix 1: bisphosphonates

- **SIDE-EFFECTS**
▶ **Common or very common** Flushing
▶ **Uncommon** Anaphylactic shock · anxiety · arrhythmias · bronchoconstriction · chest pain · circulatory collapse · cough · drowsiness · dry mouth · dyspnoea · haematuria · hyperhidrosis · hypertension · hypotension · leucopenia · muscle spasms · proteinuria · sensation abnormal · sleep disorder · stomatitis · syncope · thrombocytopenia · tremor · vision blurred · weight increased
▶ **Rare or very rare** Confusion · Fanconi syndrome acquired · interstitial lung disease · pancytopenia
▶ **Frequency not known** Acute phase reaction

  SIDE-EFFECTS, FURTHER INFORMATION Renal impairment and renal failure have been reported; ensure patient is hydrated before each dose and assess renal function.

- **CONCEPTION AND CONTRACEPTION** Contra-indicated in women of child-bearing potential.

- **PREGNANCY** Avoid—toxicity in *animal* studies.

- **BREAST FEEDING** Avoid—no information available.

- **HEPATIC IMPAIRMENT** Manufacturer advises caution in severe hepatic impairment (limited information available).

- **RENAL IMPAIRMENT** [EvGr] Avoid in tumour-induced hypercalcaemia if serum creatinine above 400 micromol/litre. Avoid in advanced malignancies involving bone if creatinine clearance less than 30 mL/minute (or if serum creatinine greater than 265 micromol/litre). Avoid in Paget's disease, treatment of postmenopausal osteoporosis and osteoporosis in men if creatinine clearance less than 35 mL/minute. ⟨Ⓜ⟩
  Dose adjustments [EvGr] In advanced malignancies involving bone, if creatinine clearance 50–60 mL/minute reduce dose to 3.5 mg every 3–4 weeks; if creatinine clearance 40–50 mL/minute reduce dose to 3.3 mg every 3–4 weeks; if creatinine clearance 30–40 mL/minute reduce dose to 3 mg every 3–4 weeks; if renal function deteriorates in patients with bone metastases, withhold dose until serum creatinine returns to within 10% of baseline value. ⟨Ⓜ⟩ See p. 21.

- **MONITORING REQUIREMENTS**
▶ Correct disturbances of calcium metabolism (e.g. vitamin D deficiency, hypocalcaemia) before starting. Monitor serum electrolytes, calcium, phosphate and magnesium.
▶ Monitor renal function in patients at risk, such as those with pre-existing renal impairment, those of advanced age, those taking concomitant nephrotoxic drugs or diuretics, or those who are dehydrated.

- **DIRECTIONS FOR ADMINISTRATION**
▶ When used for Prevention of skeletal related events in advanced malignancies involving bone or Tumour-induced hypercalcaemia For *intravenous infusion*, infuse over at least 15 minutes; administer as a single intravenous solution in a separate infusion line. If using 4 *mg/5 mL concentrate for solution for infusion* or preparing a reduced dose of

4 mg/100 mL solution for infusion for patients with renal impairment, dilute requisite dose according to product literature.

▸ When used for Paget's disease of bone or Osteoporosis (including corticosteroid-induced osteoporosis) in men and postmenopausal women For *intravenous infusion*, give via a vented infusion line over at least 15 minutes.

● PATIENT AND CARER ADVICE A patient reminder card should be provided (risk of osteonecrosis of the jaw).

● NATIONAL FUNDING/ACCESS DECISIONS
For full details see funding body website
NICE decisions
▸ Bisphosphonates for treating osteoporosis (updated July 2019) NICE TA464 Recommended with restrictions
Scottish Medicines Consortium (SMC) decisions
▸ Zoledronic acid (*Zometa*®) for patients with breast cancer and multiple myeloma (May 2003) SMC No. 29/02 Recommended with restrictions
▸ Zoledronic acid (*Aclasta*®) for Paget's disease of bone (October 2006) SMC No. 317/06 Recommended
▸ Zoledronic acid (*Aclasta*®) for the treatment of osteoporosis in postmenopausal women at increased risk of fractures (March 2008) SMC No. 447/08 Recommended with restrictions

● MEDICINAL FORMS There can be variation in the licensing of different medicines containing the same drug.
Infusion
▸ Zoledronic acid (Non-proprietary)
Zoledronic acid (as Zoledronic acid monohydrate) 40 microgram per 1 ml Zoledronic acid 4mg/100ml infusion bags | 1 bag [PoM] £174.14 (Hospital only)
Zoledronic acid (as Zoledronic acid monohydrate) 50 microgram per 1 ml Zoledronic acid 5mg/100ml infusion bags | 1 bag [PoM] £266.72 (Hospital only)
Solution for infusion
▸ Zoledronic acid (Non-proprietary)
Zoledronic acid (as Zoledronic acid monohydrate) 40 microgram per 1 ml Zoledronic acid 4mg/100ml solution for infusion vials | 1 vial [PoM] £172.85-£174.14 (Hospital only)
Zoledronic acid (as Zoledronic acid monohydrate) 50 microgram per 1 ml Zoledronic acid 5mg/100ml solution for infusion vials | 1 vial [PoM] £234.00-£266.72 (Hospital only)
Zoledronic acid (as Zoledronic acid monohydrate)
800 microgram per 1 ml Zoledronic acid 4mg/5ml concentrate for solution for infusion vials | 1 vial [PoM] £2.73-£222.29 (Hospital only) | 1 vial [PoM] £174.14
▸ Zometa (Phoenix Labs Ltd)
Zoledronic acid (as Zoledronic acid monohydrate) 40 microgram per 1 ml Zometa 4mg/100ml solution for infusion bottles | 1 bottle [PoM] £174.14
Zoledronic acid (as Zoledronic acid monohydrate)
800 microgram per 1 ml Zometa 4mg/5ml solution for infusion vials | 1 vial [PoM] £174.14 (Hospital only)

CALCIUM REGULATING DRUGS › BONE RESORPTION INHIBITORS

Calcitonin (salmon)
01-Jun-2021

(Salcatonin)

● INDICATIONS AND DOSE
Hypercalcaemia of malignancy
▸ BY SUBCUTANEOUS INJECTION, OR BY INTRAMUSCULAR INJECTION
▸ Adult: 100 units every 6–8 hours (max. per dose 400 units every 6–8 hours), adjusted according to response
▸ BY INTRAVENOUS INFUSION
▸ Adult: Up to 10 units/kg, in severe or emergency cases, to be administered by slow intravenous infusion over at least 6 hours

Paget's disease of bone
▸ BY SUBCUTANEOUS INJECTION, OR BY INTRAMUSCULAR INJECTION
▸ Adult: 100 units daily, adjusted according to response for maximum 3 months (6 months in exceptional circumstances), a minimum dosage regimen of 50 units three times a week has been shown to achieve clinical and biochemical improvement
Prevention of acute bone loss due to sudden immobility
▸ BY SUBCUTANEOUS INJECTION, OR BY INTRAMUSCULAR INJECTION
▸ Adult: Initially 100 units daily in 1–2 divided doses, then reduced to 50 units daily at the start of mobilisation, usual duration of treatment is 2 weeks; maximum 4 weeks

● CONTRA-INDICATIONS Hypocalcaemia

● CAUTIONS History of allergy (skin test advised) · risk of malignancy—avoid prolonged use (use lowest effective dose for shortest possible time)

● INTERACTIONS → Appendix 1: calcitonins

● SIDE-EFFECTS
▸ **Common or very common** Abdominal pain · arthralgia · diarrhoea · dizziness · fatigue · flushing · headache · musculoskeletal pain · nausea · secondary malignancy (long term use) · taste altered · vomiting
▸ **Uncommon** Hypersensitivity · hypertension · influenza like illness · oedema · polyuria · skin reactions · visual impairment
▸ **Rare or very rare** Bronchospasm · throat swelling · tongue swelling
▸ **Frequency not known** Hypocalcaemia · tremor

● PREGNANCY Avoid unless potential benefit outweighs risk (toxicity in *animal* studies).

● BREAST FEEDING Avoid; inhibits lactation in *animals*.

● RENAL IMPAIRMENT [EvGr] Use with caution in end-stage renal disease (reduced renal metabolism; limited information available). ⟨M⟩

● DIRECTIONS FOR ADMINISTRATION For *intravenous infusion*, manufacturer advises give intermittently in Sodium Chloride 0.9%. Diluted solution given without delay. Dilute in 500 mL give over at least 6 hours; glass or hard plastic containers should not be used.

● MEDICINAL FORMS There can be variation in the licensing of different medicines containing the same drug.
Solution for injection
▸ Calcitonin (salmon) (Non-proprietary)
Calcitonin (salmon) 100 unit per 1 ml Calcitonin (salmon) 100units/1ml solution for injection ampoules | 5 ampoule [PoM] £246.00-£246.02

Strontium ranelate
09-Oct-2020

● DRUG ACTION Strontium ranelate stimulates bone formation and reduces bone resorption.

● INDICATIONS AND DOSE
Severe osteoporosis in men and postmenopausal women at increased risk of fractures [when other treatments are contra-indicated or not tolerated] (initiated by a specialist)
▸ BY MOUTH
▸ Adult: 2 g once daily, dose to be taken in water and at bedtime

● CONTRA-INDICATIONS Cerebrovascular disease · current or previous venous thromboembolic event · ischaemic heart disease · peripheral arterial disease · temporary or permanent immobilisation · uncontrolled hypertension

- **CAUTIONS** Risk factors for cardiovascular disease—assess before and every 6–12 months during treatment · Risk factors for venous thromboembolism (discontinue in patients who become immobile)

  CAUTIONS, FURTHER INFORMATION
  ▸ **Risk of cardiovascular events** Manufacturer advises treatment should be stopped if ischaemic heart disease, peripheral arterial disease, or cerebrovascular disease develops, or if hypertension is uncontrolled.

- **INTERACTIONS** → Appendix 1: strontium

- **SIDE-EFFECTS**
  ▸ **Common or very common** Angioedema · arthralgia · bronchial hyperreactivity · consciousness impaired · constipation · diarrhoea · dizziness · embolism and thrombosis · gastrointestinal discomfort · gastrointestinal disorders · headache · hepatitis · hypercholesterolaemia · insomnia · memory loss · muscle complaints · myocardial infarction · nausea · pain · paraesthesia · peripheral oedema · skin reactions · vertigo · vomiting
  ▸ **Uncommon** Alopecia · confusion · dry mouth · fever · lymphadenopathy · malaise · oral disorders · seizure
  ▸ **Rare or very rare** Bone marrow failure · eosinophilia · severe cutaneous adverse reactions (SCARs)

- **PREGNANCY** Manufacturer advises avoid—toxicity in *animal* studies.

- **BREAST FEEDING** Manufacturer advises avoid—data suggest present in human milk.

- **RENAL IMPAIRMENT** Manufacturer advises avoid if creatinine clearance less than 30 mL/minute. See p. 21.

- **EFFECT ON LABORATORY TESTS** Manufacturer advises may interfere with colorimetric assay of calcium in blood and urine—consult product literature.

- **DIRECTIONS FOR ADMINISTRATION** Granules should be stirred into at least 30mL of water, and taken immediately at bedtime on an empty stomach; avoid food for at least 2 hours before treatment, particularly calcium-containing products e.g. milk.

- **PATIENT AND CARER ADVICE** Patients or carers should be given advice on how to administer strontium ranelate granules.
  Severe allergic reactions Patients should be advised to stop taking strontium ranelate and consult their doctor immediately if skin rash develops.

- **MEDICINAL FORMS** No licensed medicines listed.

CALCIUM REGULATING DRUGS > PARATHYROID HORMONES AND ANALOGUES

Abaloparatide
03-Sep-2024

- **DRUG ACTION** Abaloparatide is a parathyroid hormone analogue that activates osteoblasts, thereby stimulating bone formation.

- **INDICATIONS AND DOSE**

  Osteoporosis in postmenopausal women at increased risk of fractures
  ▸ BY SUBCUTANEOUS INJECTION
  ▸ Adult (female): 80 micrograms once daily for maximum duration of treatment 18 months.

- **CONTRA-INDICATIONS** Bone metastases · pre-existing hypercalcaemia · previous radiation therapy to the skeleton · risk factors for osteosarcoma · skeletal malignancies · unexplained raised alkaline phosphatase

- **CAUTIONS** Cardiac disease (monitor for worsening disease—discontinue if severe cardiovascular symptoms occur)

- **SIDE-EFFECTS**
  ▸ **Common or very common** Arrhythmias · arthralgia · asthenia · constipation · diarrhoea · dizziness · gastrointestinal discomfort · headache · hypercalcaemia · hypercalciuria · hypertension · hyperuricaemia · insomnia · malaise · muscle spasms · nausea · nephrolithiasis · pain · palpitations · skin reactions · vomiting
  ▸ **Uncommon** Postural hypotension

- **PREGNANCY** [EvGr] Avoid (no information available). ⟨M⟩

- **BREAST FEEDING** [EvGr] Avoid (no information available). ⟨M⟩

- **RENAL IMPAIRMENT** [EvGr] Avoid in severe impairment (increased risk of exposure). ⟨M⟩

- **MONITORING REQUIREMENTS** [EvGr] Assess blood pressure, cardiac status, and ECG prior to initiation. ⟨M⟩

- **DIRECTIONS FOR ADMINISTRATION** For *subcutaneous injection*, inject into the lower abdomen (except for the 5 cm around the navel); rotate injection site and avoid skin that is tender, bruised, red, scaly, scarred, or hardened. Patients may self-administer *Eladynos*® after appropriate training in subcutaneous injection technique.

- **HANDLING AND STORAGE** Store in a refrigerator (2–8°C)—consult product literature for further information regarding storage outside the refrigerator.

- **PATIENT AND CARER ADVICE**
  Self administration Patients or their carers should be given training in subcutaneous injection technique.
  Missed doses If a dose is more than 12 hours late, the missed dose should not be administered and the next dose should be administered at the normal time.
  Driving and skilled tasks Patients and carers should be counselled on the effects on driving and performance of skilled tasks—increased risk of dizziness.

- **NATIONAL FUNDING/ACCESS DECISIONS**
  For full details see funding body website
  NICE decisions
  ▸ **Abaloparatide for treating osteoporosis after menopause (August 2024)** NICE TA991 Recommended with restrictions

- **MEDICINAL FORMS** There can be variation in the licensing of different medicines containing the same drug.
  Solution for injection
  ▸ Eladynos (Theramex HQ UK Ltd) ▼
  Abaloparatide 2 mg per 1 ml Eladynos 80micrograms/40microlitres solution for injection 1.5ml pre-filled pens | 1 pre-filled disposable injection [PoM] £294.54 (Hospital only)

Teriparatide
01-Jun-2021

- **INDICATIONS AND DOSE**

  Treatment of osteoporosis in postmenopausal women and in men at increased risk of fractures | Treatment of corticosteroid-induced osteoporosis
  ▸ BY SUBCUTANEOUS INJECTION
  ▸ Adult: 20 micrograms daily for maximum duration of treatment 24 months (course not to be repeated)

- **CONTRA-INDICATIONS** Bone metastases · hyperparathyroidism · metabolic bone diseases · Paget's disease · pre-existing hypercalcaemia · previous radiation therapy to the skeleton · skeletal malignancies · unexplained raised alkaline phosphatase

- **SIDE-EFFECTS**
  ▸ **Common or very common** Anaemia · asthenia · chest pain · depression · dizziness · dyspnoea · gastrointestinal disorders · headache · hypercholesterolaemia · hyperhidrosis · hypotension · muscle complaints · nausea · pain · palpitations · sciatica · syncope · vertigo · vomiting

▶ **Uncommon** Arthralgia · emphysema · hypercalcaemia · hyperuricaemia · nephrolithiasis · tachycardia · urinary disorders · weight increased

▶ **Rare or very rare** Oedema · renal impairment · urticaria generalised

● PREGNANCY Avoid.

● BREAST FEEDING Avoid.

● RENAL IMPAIRMENT EvGr Caution in moderate impairment; avoid if severe. ◆M◆

● PRESCRIBING AND DISPENSING INFORMATION Teriparatide is a biological medicine. Biological medicines must be prescribed and dispensed by brand name, see *Biological medicines* and *Biosimilar medicines*, under Guidance on prescribing p. 1.

● NATIONAL FUNDING/ACCESS DECISIONS
For full details see funding body website

NICE decisions

▶ **Raloxifene and teriparatide for the secondary prevention of osteoporotic fragility fractures in postmenopausal women** (updated February 2018) NICE TA161 Recommended with restrictions

● MEDICINAL FORMS There can be variation in the licensing of different medicines containing the same drug.

Solution for injection

▶ Teriparatide (Non-proprietary)
Teriparatide 250 microgram per 1 ml Teriparatide 20micrograms/80microlitres dose solution for injection 2.4ml pre-filled disposable devices | 1 pre-filled disposable injection PoM £200.00 DT = £271.88 (Hospital only) | 1 pre-filled disposable injection PoM £231.10 DT = £271.88 | 3 pre-filled disposable injection PoM £600.00 (Hospital only)

▶ Forsteo (Eli Lilly and Company Ltd)
Teriparatide 250 microgram per 1 ml Forsteo 20micrograms/80microlitres dose solution for injection 2.4ml pre-filled pens | 1 pre-filled disposable injection PoM £271.88 DT = £271.88

▶ Movymia (Genus Pharmaceuticals Holdings Ltd) ▼
Teriparatide 250 microgram per 1 ml Movymia 20micrograms/80microlitres dose solution for injection 2.4ml cartridge with pen | 1 cartridge PoM £235.00
Movymia 20micrograms/80microlitres dose solution for injection 2.4ml cartridge | 1 cartridge PoM £235.00

▶ Sondelbay (Accord-UK Ltd) ▼
Teriparatide 250 microgram per 1 ml Sondelbay 20micrograms/80microlitres dose solution for injection 2.4ml pre-filled pens | 1 pre-filled disposable injection PoM £271.87 DT = £271.88 | 3 pre-filled disposable injection PoM £815.61

▶ Terrosa (Gedeon Richter (UK) Ltd) ▼
Teriparatide 250 microgram per 1 ml Terrosa 20micrograms/80microlitres dose solution for injection 2.4ml cartridge with pen | 1 cartridge PoM £239.25
Terrosa 20micrograms/80microlitres dose solution for injection 2.4ml cartridge | 1 cartridge PoM £239.25 | 3 cartridge PoM £717.75

DRUGS AFFECTING BONE STRUCTURE AND MINERALISATION ⟩ MONOCLONAL ANTIBODIES

Denosumab
25-May-2022

● DRUG ACTION Denosumab is a human monoclonal antibody that inhibits osteoclast formation, function, and survival, thereby decreasing bone resorption.

● INDICATIONS AND DOSE

PROLIA ®

Osteoporosis in postmenopausal women and in men at increased risk of fractures | Bone loss associated with hormone ablation in men with prostate cancer at increased risk of fractures | Bone loss associated with long-term systemic glucocorticoid therapy in patients at increased risk of fracture

▶ BY SUBCUTANEOUS INJECTION

▶ Adult: 60 mg every 6 months, supplement with calcium and Vitamin D, to be administered into the thigh, abdomen or upper arm

XGEVA ®

Prevention of skeletal related events in patients with bone metastases

▶ BY SUBCUTANEOUS INJECTION

▶ Adult: 120 mg every 4 weeks, supplementation of at least calcium 500 mg and Vitamin D 400 units daily should also be taken unless hypercalcaemia is present, to be administered into the thigh, abdomen or upper arm

Giant cell tumour of bone that is unresectable or where surgical resection is likely to result in severe morbidity

▶ BY SUBCUTANEOUS INJECTION

▶ Adult: 120 mg every 4 weeks, give additional dose on days 8 and 15 of the first month of treatment only, supplementation of at least calcium 500 mg and Vitamin D 400 units daily should also be taken unless hypercalcaemia is present, to be administered into the thigh, abdomen or upper arm

---

IMPORTANT SAFETY INFORMATION

MHRA/CHM ADVICE: DENOSUMAB: ATYPICAL FEMORAL FRACTURES (FEBRUARY 2013)
Atypical femoral fractures have been reported rarely in patients receiving denosumab for the long-term treatment (2.5 or more years) of postmenopausal osteoporosis.
Patients should be advised to report any new or unusual thigh, hip, or groin pain during treatment with denosumab.
Discontinuation of denosumab in patients suspected to have an atypical femoral fracture should be considered after an assessment of the benefits and risks of continued treatment.

MHRA/CHM ADVICE: DENOSUMAB: MINIMISING THE RISK OF OSTEONECROSIS OF THE JAW; MONITORING FOR HYPOCALCAEMIA—UPDATED RECOMMENDATIONS (SEPTEMBER 2014) AND DENOSUMAB: OSTEONECROSIS OF THE JAW—FURTHER MEASURES TO MINIMISE RISK (JULY 2015)
Denosumab is associated with a risk of osteonecrosis of the jaw (ONJ) and with a risk of hypocalcaemia.
Osteonecrosis of the jaw Osteonecrosis of the jaw is a well-known and common side-effect in patients receiving denosumab 120 mg for cancer. Risk factors include smoking, old age, poor oral hygiene, invasive dental procedures (including tooth extractions, dental implants, oral surgery), comorbidity (including dental disease, anaemia, coagulopathy, infection), advanced cancer, previous treatment with bisphosphonates, and concomitant treatments (including chemotherapy, anti-angiogenic biologics, corticosteroids, and radiotherapy

to head and neck). The following precautions are now recommended to reduce the risk of ONJ:

Denosumab 120 mg (cancer indication)

- A dental examination and appropriate preventative dentistry before starting treatment are now recommended for all patients
- Do not start denosumab in patients with a dental or jaw condition requiring surgery, or in patients who have unhealed lesions from dental or oral surgery

Denosumab 60 mg (osteoporosis indication)

- Check for ONJ risk factors before starting treatment. A dental examination and appropriate preventative dentistry are now recommended for patients with risk factors

All patients should be given a patient reminder card and informed of the risk of ONJ. Advise patients to tell their doctor if they have any problems with their mouth or teeth before starting treatment, if they wear dentures they should make sure their dentures fit properly before starting treatment, to maintain good oral hygiene, receive routine dental check-ups during treatment, and immediately report any oral symptoms such as dental mobility, pain, swelling, non-healing sores or discharge to a doctor and dentist. Patients should tell their doctor and dentist that they are receiving denosumab if they need dental treatment or dental surgery.

Hypocalcaemia Denosumab is associated with a risk of hypocalcaemia. This risk increases with the degree of renal impairment. Hypocalcaemia usually occurs in the first weeks of denosumab treatment, but it can also occur later in treatment.

Plasma-calcium concentration monitoring is recommended for denosumab 120 mg (cancer indication):

- before the first dose
- within two weeks after the initial dose
- if suspected symptoms of hypocalcaemia occur
- consider monitoring more frequently in patients with risk factors for hypocalcaemia (e.g. severe renal impairment, creatinine clearance less than 30 mL/minute)

Plasma-calcium concentration monitoring is recommended for denosumab 60 mg (osteoporosis indication):

- before each dose
- within two weeks after the initial dose in patients with risk factors for hypocalcaemia (e.g. severe renal impairment, creatinine clearance less than 30 mL/minute)
- if suspected symptoms of hypocalcaemia occur

All patients should be advised to report symptoms of hypocalcaemia to their doctor (e.g. muscle spasms, twitches, cramps, numbness or tingling in the fingers, toes, or around the mouth).

MHRA/CHM ADVICE: DENOSUMAB: REPORTS OF OSTEONECROSIS OF THE EXTERNAL AUDITORY CANAL (JUNE 2017)

Osteonecrosis of the external auditory canal has been reported with denosumab and this should be considered in patients who present with ear symptoms including chronic ear infections or in those with suspected cholesteatoma. Possible risk factors include steroid use and chemotherapy, with or without local risk factors such as infection or trauma. The MHRA recommends advising patients to report any ear pain, discharge from the ear, or an ear infection during denosumab treatment.

MHRA/CHM ADVICE: DENOSUMAB (*XGEVA* ®) FOR GIANT CELL TUMOUR OF BONE: RISK OF CLINICALLY SIGNIFICANT HYPERCALCAEMIA FOLLOWING DISCONTINUATION (JUNE 2018)

Cases of clinically significant hypercalcaemia (rebound hypercalcaemia) have been reported up to 9 months after discontinuation of denosumab treatment for giant cell tumour of bone. The MHRA recommends that prescribers should monitor patients for signs and symptoms of hypercalcaemia after discontinuation, consider periodic assessment of serum calcium, re-evaluate the patient's calcium and vitamin D supplementation requirements, and advise patients to report symptoms of hypercalcaemia.

Denosumab is not recommended in patients with growing skeletons.

MHRA/CHM ADVICE: DENOSUMAB (*XGEVA* ®) FOR ADVANCED MALIGNANCIES INVOLVING BONE: STUDY DATA SHOW NEW PRIMARY MALIGNANCIES REPORTED MORE FREQUENTLY COMPARED TO ZOLEDRONIC ACID (ZOLEDRONATE) (JUNE 2018)

A pooled analysis has shown an increased rate of new primary malignancies in patients given *Xgeva* ® (1-year cumulative incidence 1.1%) compared with those given zoledronic acid (0.6%), when used for the prevention of skeletal-related events with advanced malignancies involving bone. No treatment-related pattern in individual cancers or cancer groupings were apparent.

MHRA/CHM ADVICE: DENOSUMAB 60 MG (*PROLIA* ®): INCREASED RISK OF MULTIPLE VERTEBRAL FRACTURES AFTER STOPPING OR DELAYING ONGOING TREATMENT (AUGUST 2020)

Cases of multiple vertebral fractures have been reported in patients within 18 months of discontinuation or interruption of ongoing denosumab 60 mg treatment for osteoporosis. The MHRA advises healthcare professionals not to discontinue denosumab without a specialist review, and to evaluate patients' individual risk and benefit factors before initiating treatment, particularly in those at increased risk of vertebral fractures (such as patients with previous vertebral fracture). Healthcare professionals should re-evaluate the need for continued treatment periodically based on expected benefits and potential risks of treatment on an individual basis, particularly after 5 or more years of use.

MHRA/CHM ADVICE: DENOSUMAB 60 MG (*PROLIA* ®): SHOULD NOT BE USED IN PATIENTS UNDER 18 YEARS DUE TO THE RISK OF SERIOUS HYPERCALCAEMIA (MAY 2022)

Cases of serious and life-threatening hypercalcaemia requiring hospitalisation and leading to acute kidney injury have been reported in children and adolescents aged under 18 years who were given denosumab 60 mg in clinical trials and during off-label use. Hypercalcaemia occurred during treatment or in the weeks to months after the last dose.

Healthcare professionals are reminded that:
- *Prolia* ® is only licensed for the treatment of osteoporosis and other bone loss conditions in patients aged 18 years and older;
- patients younger than 18 years currently receiving *Prolia* ® in clinical trials or off-label should be counselled alongside their carers to seek advice from healthcare professionals.

- **CONTRA-INDICATIONS** Hypocalcaemia

  XGEVA ® Unhealed lesions from dental or oral surgery

- **CAUTIONS** Risk factors for osteonecrosis of the external auditory canal · risk factors for osteonecrosis of the jaw— consider temporary interruption of denosumab if occurs during treatment

  PROLIA ®
  ‣ When used for Osteoporosis in postmenopausal women Rebound increase in bone turnover on discontinuation (increased risk of fracture)

  CAUTIONS, FURTHER INFORMATION
  ‣ Rebound increase in bone turnover on discontinuation
  ‣ When used for Osteoporosis in postmenopausal women EvGr Following discontinuation, transition to an alternative antiresorptive therapy should be considered to prevent rebound increase in bone turnover, bone loss and increased fracture risk. Ⓐ

- **INTERACTIONS** → Appendix 1: denosumab
- **SIDE-EFFECTS**
  - ▶ **Common or very common** Abdominal discomfort · alopecia · constipation · diarrhoea · dyspnoea · hyperhidrosis · hypocalcaemia (including fatal cases) · hypophosphataemia · increased risk of infection · osteonecrosis · pain · sciatica · second primary malignancy · skin reactions
  - ▶ **Uncommon** Atypical femur fracture · cellulitis (seek prompt medical attention) · hypercalcaemia (on discontinuation)
  - ▶ **Rare or very rare** Hypersensitivity · hypersensitivity vasculitis
  - ▶ **Frequency not known** Facial swelling
- **CONCEPTION AND CONTRACEPTION** Ensure effective contraception in women of child-bearing potential, during treatment and for at least 5 months after stopping treatment.
- **PREGNANCY** Manufacturer advises avoid—toxicity in *animal* studies; risk of toxicity increases with each trimester.
- **BREAST FEEDING** Manufacturer advises avoid.
- **RENAL IMPAIRMENT** Increased risk of hypocalcaemia if creatinine clearance less than 30 mL/minute, see p. 21.
- **MONITORING REQUIREMENTS** Correct hypocalcaemia and vitamin D deficiency before starting. Monitor plasma-calcium concentration during therapy.
- **PATIENT AND CARER ADVICE**
  Atypical femoral fractures Patients should be advised to report any new or unusual thigh, hip, or groin pain during treatment with denosumab.
  Osteonecrosis of the jaw All patients should be informed to maintain good oral hygiene, receive routine dental check-ups, and immediately report any oral symptoms such as dental mobility, pain, or swelling to a doctor and dentist.
  Hypocalcaemia All patients should be advised to report symptoms of hypocalcaemia to their doctor (e.g. muscle spasms, twitches, cramps, numbness or tingling in the fingers, toes, or around the mouth).
  Patient reminder card A patient reminder card should be provided (risk of osteonecrosis of the jaw).

  PROLIA® **Missed doses**
  ▶ When used for Osteoporosis in postmenopausal women [EvGr] Treatment should be given within 1 month of scheduled date. Ⓐ
- **NATIONAL FUNDING/ACCESS DECISIONS**
  For full details see funding body website

  NICE decisions
  - ▶ **Denosumab for the prevention of osteoporotic fractures in postmenopausal women (October 2010)** NICE TA204 Recommended with restrictions
  - ▶ **Denosumab for the prevention of skeletal-related events in adults with bone metastases from solid tumours (October 2012)** NICE TA265 Recommended with restrictions

  Scottish Medicines Consortium (SMC) decisions
  - ▶ **Denosumab (*Prolia*®) for osteoporosis in postmenopausal women at increased risk of fractures (December 2010)** SMC No. 651/10 Recommended with restrictions

---

- **MEDICINAL FORMS** There can be variation in the licensing of different medicines containing the same drug.

  Solution for injection
  CAUTIONARY AND ADVISORY LABELS 10
  EXCIPIENTS: May contain Sorbitol
  - ▶ Prolia (Amgen Ltd)
    Denosumab 60 mg per 1 ml Prolia 60mg/1ml solution for injection pre-filled syringes | 1 pre-filled disposable injection [PoM] £183.00 DT = £183.00
  - ▶ Xgeva (Amgen Ltd)
    Denosumab 70 mg per 1 ml Xgeva 120mg/1.7ml solution for injection vials | 1 vial [PoM] £309.86 DT = £309.86

Romosozumab
27-May-2022

- **DRUG ACTION** Romosozumab is a humanised monoclonal antibody that inhibits sclerostin, thereby increasing bone formation and decreasing bone resorption.
- **INDICATIONS AND DOSE**
  Severe osteoporosis in postmenopausal women at increased risk of fractures (specialist use only)
  - ▶ BY SUBCUTANEOUS INJECTION
  - ▶ Adult: 210 mg once a month for 12 months, supplement with calcium and vitamin D, to be administered as two consecutive 105 mg injections at different injection sites into the thigh, abdomen or upper arm
- **CONTRA-INDICATIONS** History of myocardial infarction or stroke—discontinue if occurs during treatment · hypocalcaemia
- **CAUTIONS** Risk factors for cardiovascular disease · risk factors for osteonecrosis of the jaw—consider temporary interruption of romosozumab if occurs during treatment
- **SIDE-EFFECTS**
  - ▶ **Common or very common** Arthralgia · headache · hypersensitivity · increased risk of infection · muscle spasms · neck pain · skin reactions
  - ▶ **Uncommon** Cataract · hypocalcaemia · myocardial infarction · stroke
  - ▶ **Rare or very rare** Angioedema
  - ▶ **Frequency not known** Atypical femur fracture · cardiovascular event · osteonecrosis of jaw
- **RENAL IMPAIRMENT** Manufacturer advises monitor serum calcium concentration in patients with severe renal impairment, or in those receiving dialysis—increased risk of hypocalcaemia.
- **MONITORING REQUIREMENTS** Manufacturer advises to correct hypocalcaemia before therapy is initiated. Monitor for signs and symptoms of hypocalcaemia during therapy.
- **PRESCRIBING AND DISPENSING INFORMATION**
  Romosozumab is a biological medicine. Biological medicines must be prescribed and dispensed by brand name, see *Biological medicines* and *Biosimilar medicines*, under Guidance on prescribing p. 1.
  The manufacturer of *Evenity*® has provided a *Prescriber Guide*.
- **HANDLING AND STORAGE** Manufacturer advises store in a refrigerator (2-8°C) and protect from light—consult product literature for further information regarding storage outside the refrigerator.
- **PATIENT AND CARER ADVICE**
  Atypical femoral fractures Manufacturer advises patients should be advised to report any new or unusual thigh, hip, or groin pain during treatment.
  Osteonecrosis of the jaw Manufacturer advises patients should be informed to maintain good oral hygiene, receive routine dental check-ups, and immediately report any oral symptoms such as dental mobility, pain, or swelling.
  Hypocalcaemia Manufacturer advises patients should be advised to report symptoms of hypocalcaemia.
  Patients should receive a package leaflet and patient alert card.
- **NATIONAL FUNDING/ACCESS DECISIONS**
  For full details see funding body website

  NICE decisions
  - ▶ **Romosozumab for treating severe osteoporosis (May 2022)** NICE TA791 Recommended with restrictions

  Scottish Medicines Consortium (SMC) decisions
  - ▶ **Romosozumab (*Evenity*®) for the treatment of severe osteoporosis in postmenopausal women at high risk of fracture (November 2020)** SMC No. SMC2280 Recommended with restrictions

6 Endocrine system

- MEDICINAL FORMS There can be variation in the licensing of different medicines containing the same drug.

Solution for injection
EXCIPIENTS: May contain Polysorbates
- ▸ **Evenity** (UCB Pharma Ltd)
  Romosozumab 90 mg per 1 ml Evenity 105mg/1.17ml solution for injection pre-filled pens | 2 pre-filled disposable injection [PoM] £427.75

---

3 Corticosteroid responsive conditions

CORTICOSTEROIDS

Corticosteroids, general use
22-Mar-2022

Overview

Dosages of corticosteroids vary widely in different diseases and in different patients. If the use of a corticosteroid can save or prolong life, as in exfoliative dermatitis, pemphigus, acute leukaemia or acute transplant rejection, high doses may need to be given, because the complications of therapy are likely to be less serious than the effects of the disease itself.

When long-term corticosteroid therapy is used in some chronic diseases, the adverse effects of treatment may become greater than the disabilities caused by the disease. To minimise side-effects the maintenance dose should be kept as low as possible.

When potentially less harmful measures are ineffective, corticosteroids are used topically for the treatment of inflammatory conditions of the skin. Corticosteroids should be avoided or used only under specialist supervision in psoriasis.

Corticosteroids are used both topically (by rectum) and systemically (by mouth or intravenously) in the management of ulcerative colitis and Crohn's disease. They are also included in locally applied creams for haemorrhoids.

Use can be made of the mineralocorticoid activity of fludrocortisone acetate p. 787 to treat postural hypotension in autonomic neuropathy.

High-dose corticosteroids should be avoided for the management of septic shock. However, there is evidence that administration of lower doses of hydrocortisone p. 787 and fludrocortisone acetate is of benefit in adrenal insufficiency resulting from septic shock.

Dexamethasone p. 786 and betamethasone p. 785 have little if any mineralocorticoid action and their long duration of action makes them particularly suitable for suppressing corticotropin secretion in congenital adrenal hyperplasia where the dose should be tailored to clinical response and by measurement of adrenal androgens and 17-hydroxyprogesterone. In common with all glucocorticoids their suppressive action on the hypothalamic- pituitary-adrenal axis is greatest and most prolonged when they are given at night. In most individuals a single dose of dexamethasone at night, is sufficient to inhibit corticotropin secretion for 24 hours. This is the basis of the 'overnight dexamethasone suppression test' for diagnosing Cushing's syndrome.

Betamethasone and dexamethasone are also appropriate for conditions where water retention would be a disadvantage.

A corticosteroid may be used in the management of raised intracranial pressure or cerebral oedema that occurs as a result of malignancy (see Prescribing in palliative care p. 26). However, a corticosteroid should not be used for the management of head injury or stroke because it is unlikely to be of benefit and may even be harmful.

Corticosteroids are no longer recommended for the routine emergency treatment of anaphylaxis. For guidance on the management of anaphylaxis, see Antihistamines, allergen immunotherapy and allergic emergencies p. 316.

[EvGr] Corticosteroids are preferably used by inhalation in the management of asthma and chronic obstructive pulmonary disease (COPD). Systemic therapy along with bronchodilators is required for treatment of acute asthma attacks, in some very severe cases of chronic asthma, and exacerbations of COPD. Ⓐ

Corticosteroids may also be useful in conditions such as autoimmune hepatitis, rheumatoid arthritis and sarcoidosis; they may also lead to remissions of acquired haemolytic anaemia, and some cases of the nephrotic syndrome (particularly in children) and thrombocytopenic purpura.

Corticosteroids can improve the prognosis of serious conditions such as systemic lupus erythematosus, temporal arteritis, and polyarteritis nodosa; the effects of the disease process may be suppressed and symptoms relieved, but the underlying condition is not cured, although it may ultimately remit. It is usual to begin therapy in these conditions at fairly high dose, and then to reduce the dose to the lowest commensurate with disease control.

For other references to the use of corticosteroids see: Prescribing in palliative care, immunosuppression, rheumatic diseases, eye, otitis externa, allergic rhinitis, and aphthous ulcers.

Side-effects

MHRA/CHM advice: Corticosteroids: rare risk of central serous chorioretinopathy with local as well as systemic administration (August 2017)
Central serous chorioretinopathy is a retinal disorder that has been linked to the systemic use of corticosteroids. Recently, it has also been reported after local administration of corticosteroids via inhaled and intranasal, epidural, intra-articular, topical dermal, and periocular routes. The MHRA recommends that patients should be advised to report any blurred vision or other visual disturbances with corticosteroid treatment given by any route; consider referral to an ophthalmologist for evaluation of possible causes if a patient presents with vision problems.

Overdosage or prolonged use can exaggerate some of the normal physiological actions of corticosteroids leading to mineralocorticoid and glucocorticoid side-effects.

Mineralocorticoid side effects

- hypertension
- sodium retention
- water retention
- potassium loss
- calcium loss

Mineralocorticoid side effects are most marked with fludrocortisone, but are significant with hydrocortisone, corticotropin, and tetracosactide. Mineralocorticoid actions are negligible with the high potency glucocorticoids, betamethasone and dexamethasone, and occur only slightly with methylprednisolone, prednisolone, and triamcinolone.

Glucocorticoid side effects

- diabetes
- osteoporosis, which is a danger, particularly in the elderly, as it can result in osteoporotic fractures for example of the hip or vertebrae
- in addition high doses are associated with avascular necrosis of the femoral head
- muscle wasting (proximal myopathy) can also occur
- corticosteroid therapy is also weakly linked with peptic ulceration and perforation
- psychiatric reactions may also occur

Managing side-effects
Side-effects can be minimised by using the lowest effective dose for the minimum period possible. The suppressive

action of a corticosteroid on cortisol secretion is least when it is given as a single dose in the morning. In an attempt to reduce pituitary-adrenal suppression further, the total dose for two days can sometimes be taken as a single dose on alternate days; alternate-day administration has not been very successful in the management of asthma. Pituitary-adrenal suppression can also be reduced by means of intermittent therapy with short courses. In some conditions it may be possible to reduce the dose of corticosteroid by adding a small dose of an immunosuppressive drug.

For information on the cessation of oral corticosteroid treatment, see *Treatment cessation*, for systemic corticosteroids (e.g. prednisolone p. 791).

Whenever possible *local treatment* with creams, intra-articular injections, inhalations, eye-drops, or enemas should be used in preference to *systemic treatment*.

Inhaled corticosteroids have considerably fewer systemic effects than oral corticosteroids, but adverse effects including adrenal suppression have been reported. Use of other corticosteroid therapy (including topical) or concurrent use of drugs which inhibit corticosteroid metabolism should be taken into account when assessing systemic risk.

For guidance on the management of adrenal insufficiency and adrenal crisis (acute adrenal insufficiency), see Adrenal insufficiency below.

Adrenal insufficiency   22-Mar-2022

Description of condition

Adrenal insufficiency occurs as a result of inadequate production of steroid hormones in the adrenal cortex of the adrenal glands. Glucocorticoids (e.g. cortisol) and mineralocorticoids (e.g. aldosterone) are the two main groups of steroid hormones produced by the adrenal cortex; their production is primarily regulated by the hypothalamic-pituitary-adrenal (HPA) axis and renin-angiotensin system, respectively. These hormones affect a number of body systems such as those involved in metabolic activity, water and electrolyte balance, and the body's response to stress. Symptoms of adrenal insufficiency can be mild, non-specific, and may include fatigue, gastrointestinal upset, anorexia, weight loss, musculoskeletal symptoms, salt cravings, and dizziness or syncope due to hypotension.

Adrenal insufficiency is classified as either primary, secondary, or tertiary, and results from disorders that affect the adrenal cortex (e.g. Addison's disease, congenital adrenal hyperplasia), the anterior pituitary gland (e.g. pituitary tumour or subarachnoid haemorrhage), or the hypothalamus (e.g. HPA axis suppression), respectively.

Some drugs can also cause adrenal insufficiency, with the systemic use of glucocorticoids being the most common cause due to suppression of the HPA axis. If glucocorticoids are stopped or decreased too quickly after prolonged use, endogenous glucocorticoid production may not be sufficient to meet the body's needs. Some patients on glucocorticoid therapy (oral, inhaled, topical, intranasal, and intra-articular) are at particular risk of adrenal insufficiency. For further information on those at risk, see The Society for Endocrinology Steroid Emergency Card Working Group and Specialist Pharmacy Services guidance: **Exogenous steroids, adrenal insufficiency and adrenal crisis-who is at risk and how should they be managed safely** (see *Useful resources*).

Adrenal insufficiency can lead to adrenal crisis (acute adrenal insufficiency) if not identified and treated. Adrenal crisis can also occur in patients at risk of adrenal insufficiency when glucocorticoid levels are insufficient, such as when exogenous glucocorticoids have been omitted, delayed, or given at inadequate doses. This may occur particularly during times of increased need (e.g. surgery,

infection, or trauma) as patients are unable to mount a stress response by increasing endogenous glucocorticoid production. Life-threatening symptoms such as severe dehydration, hypotension, hypovolaemic shock, altered consciousness, seizures, stroke, or cardiac arrest may develop; if left untreated, adrenal crisis may lead to death or permanent disability.

NHS Improvement Patient Safety Alert: Steroid Emergency Card to support early recognition and treatment of adrenal crisis in adults (August 2020)

A patient-held **Steroid Emergency Card** has been developed for patients with adrenal insufficiency and steroid dependence who are at risk of adrenal crisis. It aims to support healthcare staff with the early recognition of patients at risk of adrenal crisis and the emergency treatment of adrenal crisis. All eligible patients should be issued a Steroid Emergency Card. Providers that treat patients with acute physical illness or trauma, or who may require emergency treatment, elective surgery, or other invasive procedures, should establish processes to check for risk of adrenal crisis and confirm if the patient has a Steroid Emergency Card. For further information, see NHS Improvement Patient Safety Alert: **Steroid Emergency Card to support early recognition and treatment of adrenal crisis in adults** (available at: www.england.nhs.uk/publication/national-patient-safety-alert-steroid-emergency-card-to-support-early-recognition-and-treatment-of-adrenal-crisis-in-adults/).

The Steroid Treatment Card is unaffected by the introduction of the Steroid Emergency Card. For further information on the Steroid Emergency Card and Steroid Treatment Card, see *Patient and carer advice* in drug monographs.

Aims of treatment

Treatment aims to reduce symptoms, reduce the risk of complications such as adrenal crisis, and to improve overall quality of life.

Management of adrenal insufficiency

Recommendations on the management of adrenal insufficiency are from the *Royal College of Physicians Patient Safety Committee and Society for Endocrinology Clinical Committee—Guidance for the prevention and emergency management of adult patients with adrenal insufficiency (July 2020).*

If adrenal crisis (acute adrenal insufficiency) is suspected, prompt treatment should be given without delay. For further information, see *Adrenal Crisis*.

Adrenal insufficiency is treated by physiological glucocorticoid replacement with mainly hydrocortisone p. 787 (most similar to cortisol), prednisolone, or rarely dexamethasone. Patients with primary adrenal insufficiency usually also require mineralocorticoid replacement with fludrocortisone acetate p. 787 due to aldosterone deficiency.

Some patients, usually those with secondary or tertiary adrenal insufficiency, including treatment with exogenous steroids or other drugs (such as some antifungals and antiretroviral medication), may have a suboptimal cortisol response but do not require maintenance glucocorticoid replacement.

Glucocorticoid replacement during stress

All patients with adrenal insufficiency and patients considered to be at risk of adrenal insufficiency should be educated on the importance of 'stress' glucocorticoid doses (increased doses) for the prevention of adrenal crisis during times of stress (e.g. surgical or invasive procedures), in order to maintain cortisol levels as close to the physiological concentration as possible. Patients with adrenal insufficiency who do not usually require maintenance glucocorticoids should still be advised of the likely need for glucocorticoid replacement during times of stress.

In patients with adrenal insufficiency and intercurrent illness, 'sick day rules' should be followed. For patients who are unwell with moderate intercurrent illness (e.g. fever or infection requiring antibacterials), the patient's daily glucocorticoid dose should generally be doubled. Patients with adrenal insufficiency on long-acting hydrocortisone preparations should switch to short-acting, more rapidly absorbed preparations during an intercurrent illness. For severe intercurrent illness (e.g. persistent vomiting from gastrointestinal viral illnesses), intramuscular or intravenous hydrocortisone should be given. Patients with adrenal insufficiency are at higher risk of glucocorticoid deficiency if they are vomiting or have diarrhoea. Patients with established adrenal insufficiency, and their family/carers, should be provided with a hydrocortisone emergency injection kit, be trained in the administration of intramuscular hydrocortisone, and advised to go to hospital if vomiting or diarrhoeal illness persist.

For further information on the management of patients who are undergoing surgery or an invasive procedure, or those with intercurrent illness, see the Royal College of Physicians Patient Safety Committee and Society for Endocrinology Clinical Committee: **Guidance for the prevention and emergency management of adult patients with adrenal insufficiency** (see *Useful resources*).

For information on glucocorticoid cover during stress and sick day rules for patients on exogenous steroids who are at an increased risk of adrenal insufficiency, see the Society for Endocrinology Steroid Emergency Card Working Group and Specialist Pharmacy Services guidance: **Exogenous steroids, adrenal insufficiency and adrenal crisis-who is at risk and how should they be managed safely** (see *Useful resources*).

Management of adrenal crisis

Recommendations on the management of adrenal crisis are from the *Royal College of Physicians Patient Safety Committee and Society for Endocrinology Clinical Committee—Guidance for the prevention and emergency management of adult patients with adrenal insufficiency (July 2020)*.

Adrenal crisis (acute adrenal insufficiency) is a medical emergency. All patients who are considered to be at risk of, or suspected of having adrenal crisis should be treated immediately, especially pregnant women; investigations can be initiated once the patient is clinically stable. There is no adverse consequence of initiating a life-saving bolus dose of hydrocortisone treatment.

Treatment involves prompt glucocorticoid replacement with hydrocortisone p. 787, and rehydration using a crystalloid fluid (e.g. sodium chloride 0.9%). For patients usually on fludrocortisone, high-dose hydrocortisone has sufficient mineralocorticoid effect to cover this.

Particular care is required in patients with diabetes insipidus and adrenal insufficiency related to hypothalamic-pituitary disease who are treated with desmopressin, as they are at risk of uncontrolled diabetes insipidus if doses of desmopressin are omitted, or hyponatraemia if excess fluid is given.

All patients should be referred to an endocrinologist for advice on ongoing treatment and education around 'sick day rules' prior to hospital discharge.

Useful Resources

Guidance for the prevention and emergency management of adult patients with adrenal insufficiency. Royal College of Physicians Patient Safety Committee and Society for Endocrinology Clinical Committee. July 2020.
www.rcpjournals.org/content/clinmedicine/20/4/371

Exogenous steroids, adrenal insufficiency and adrenal crisis-who is at risk and how should they be managed safely. Society for Endocrinology Steroid Emergency Card Working Group and Specialist Pharmacy Services. March 2021.
www.endocrinology.org/adrenal-crisis

Glucocorticoid therapy

Glucocorticoid and mineralocorticoid activity

In comparing the relative potencies of corticosteroids in terms of their anti-inflammatory (glucocorticoid) effects it should be borne in mind that high glucocorticoid activity in itself is of no advantage unless it is accompanied by relatively low mineralocorticoid activity (see Disadvantages of Corticosteroids). The mineralocorticoid activity of fludrocortisone acetate p. 787 is so high that its anti-inflammatory activity is of no clinical relevance.

Equivalent anti-inflammatory doses of corticosteroids
This table takes no account of mineralocorticoid effects, nor does it take account of variations in duration of action
Prednisolone 5 mg
≡ Betamethasone 750 micrograms
≡ Deflazacort 6 mg
≡ Dexamethasone 750 micrograms
≡ Hydrocortisone 20 mg
≡ Methylprednisolone 4 mg
≡ Prednisone 5 mg
≡ Triamcinolone 4 mg

The relatively high mineralocorticoid activity of hydrocortisone p. 787, and the resulting fluid retention, makes it unsuitable for disease suppression on a long-term basis. However, hydrocortisone can be used for adrenal replacement therapy. Hydrocortisone is used on a short-term basis by intravenous injection for the emergency management of some conditions. The relatively moderate anti-inflammatory potency of hydrocortisone also makes it a useful topical corticosteroid for the management of inflammatory skin conditions because side-effects (both topical and systemic) are less marked.

Prednisolone p. 791 and prednisone have predominantly glucocorticoid activity. Prednisolone is the corticosteroid most commonly used by mouth for long-term disease suppression.

Betamethasone p. 785 and dexamethasone p. 786 have very high glucocorticoid activity in conjunction with insignificant mineralocorticoid activity. This makes them particularly suitable for high-dose therapy in conditions where fluid retention would be a disadvantage.

Betamethasone and dexamethasone also have a long duration of action and this, coupled with their lack of mineralocorticoid action makes them particularly suitable for conditions which require suppression of corticotropin (corticotrophin) secretion (e.g. congenital adrenal hyperplasia).

Some esters of betamethasone and of beclometasone dipropionate (beclomethasone) exert a considerably more marked topical effect (e.g. on the skin or the lungs) than when given by mouth; use is made of this to obtain topical effects whilst minimising systemic side-effects (e.g. for skin applications and asthma inhalations).

Deflazacort p. 785 has a high glucocorticoid activity; it is derived from prednisolone.

Corticosteroids (systemic) 

● **CONTRA-INDICATIONS** Avoid injections containing benzyl alcohol in neonates · avoid live virus vaccines in those receiving immunosuppressive doses (serum antibody response diminished) · systemic infection (unless specific therapy given)

CONTRA-INDICATIONS, FURTHER INFORMATION For further information on contra-indications associated with intra-articular, intradermal and intralesional preparations, consult product literature.

● **CAUTIONS** Congestive heart failure · diabetes mellitus (including a family history of) · diverticular disease (increased risk of diverticular perforation) · diverticulitis · epilepsy · glaucoma (including a family history of or susceptibility to) · history of steroid myopathy · history of tuberculosis or X-ray changes (frequent monitoring required) · hypertension · hypothyroidism · infection (particularly untreated) · long-term use · myasthenia gravis · ocular herpes simplex (risk of corneal perforation) · osteoporosis (in children) · osteoporosis (postmenopausal women and the elderly at risk) · peptic ulcer · psychiatric reactions · recent intestinal anastomoses · recent myocardial infarction (rupture reported) · severe affective disorders (particularly if history of steroid-induced psychosis) · thromboembolic disorders · ulcerative colitis

CAUTIONS, FURTHER INFORMATION For further information on cautions associated with intra-articular, intradermal, and intralesional preparations, consult product literature.

▶ **Elderly** Screening Tool of Older Persons' potentially inappropriate Prescriptions (STOPP) criteria to aid medication reviews (see Prescribing in the elderly p. 31 for information). Potentially inappropriate:
- if used instead of inhaled corticosteroids for maintenance therapy in moderate to severe COPD (unnecessary exposure to long-term side-effects)
- as long-term (longer than 3 months) monotherapy for rheumatoid arthritis (risk of side-effects)
- for treatment of osteoarthritis other than for periodic intra-articular injections for monoarticular pain (risk of side-effects)
- with concurrent NSAIDs without proton pump inhibitor prophylaxis (increased risk of peptic ulcer disease)

● **SIDE-EFFECTS**

▶ **Common or very common** Anxiety · appetite increased · behaviour abnormal · cataract subcapsular · cognitive impairment · Cushing's syndrome · electrolyte imbalance · fluid retention · gastrointestinal discomfort · headache · healing impaired · hirsutism · hypertension · increased risk of infection · menstrual cycle irregularities · mood altered · nausea · osteoporosis · peptic ulcer · psychotic disorder · skin reactions · sleep disorder · weight increased

▶ **Uncommon** Adrenal suppression · alkalosis hypokalaemic · bone fractures · diabetic control impaired · glaucoma · haemorrhage · heart failure · hyperhidrosis · leucocytosis · myopathy · osteonecrosis · pancreatitis · papilloedema · seizure · thromboembolism · tuberculosis reactivation · vertigo · vision blurred

▶ **Rare or very rare** Tendon rupture

▶ **Frequency not known** Chorioretinopathy · eye disorders · growth retardation (very common in children) · intracranial pressure increased with papilloedema (usually after withdrawal)

SIDE-EFFECTS, FURTHER INFORMATION **Adrenal suppression** During prolonged therapy with corticosteroids, particularly with systemic use, adrenal atrophy develops and can persist for years after stopping. Abrupt withdrawal after a prolonged period can lead to acute adrenal insufficiency, hypotension, or death. To compensate for a diminished adrenocortical response caused by prolonged corticosteroid treatment, any significant intercurrent illness, trauma, or surgical procedure requires a temporary increase in corticosteroid dose, or if already stopped, a temporary reintroduction of corticosteroid treatment. For vamorolone, there is no evidence on the effects of increasing the dose, and temporary supplementation with hydrocortisone is advised.

Infections Prolonged courses of corticosteroids increase susceptibility to infections and severity of infections; clinical presentation of infections may also be atypical. Serious infections e.g. septicaemia and tuberculosis may reach an advanced stage before being recognised, and amoebiasis or strongyloidiasis may be activated or exacerbated (exclude before initiating a corticosteroid in those at risk or with suggestive symptoms). Fungal or viral ocular infections may also be exacerbated.

Chickenpox Unless they have had chickenpox, patients receiving oral or parenteral corticosteroids for purposes other than replacement should be regarded as being at risk of severe chickenpox. Manifestations of fulminant illness include pneumonia, hepatitis and disseminated intravascular coagulation; rash is not necessarily a prominent feature. Passive immunisation with varicella–zoster immunoglobulin is needed for exposed non–immune patients receiving systemic corticosteroids or for those who have used them within the previous 3 months. Confirmed chickenpox warrants specialist care and urgent treatment. Corticosteroids should not be stopped and dosage may need to be increased.

Measles Patients taking corticosteroids should be advised to take particular care to avoid exposure to measles and to seek immediate medical advice if exposure occurs. Prophylaxis with intramuscular normal immunoglobulin may be needed.

Psychiatric reactions Systemic corticosteroids, particularly in high doses, are linked to psychiatric reactions including euphoria, insomnia, irritability, mood lability, suicidal thoughts, psychotic reactions, and behavioural disturbances. These reactions frequently subside on reducing the dose or discontinuing the corticosteroid but they may also require specific management. Patients should be advised to seek medical advice if psychiatric symptoms (especially depression and suicidal thoughts) occur and they should also be alert to the rare possibility of such reactions during withdrawal of corticosteroid treatment. Systemic corticosteroids should be prescribed with care in those predisposed to psychiatric reactions, including those who have previously suffered corticosteroid–induced psychosis, or who have a personal or family history of psychiatric disorders.

● **PREGNANCY** The benefit of treatment with corticosteroids during pregnancy outweighs the risk. Corticosteroid cover is required during labour. Following a review of the data on the safety of systemic corticosteroids used in pregnancy and breast-feeding the CSM (May 1998) concluded that corticosteroids vary in their ability to cross the placenta but there is no convincing evidence that systemic corticosteroids increase the incidence of congenital abnormalities such as cleft palate or lip. When administration is prolonged or repeated during pregnancy, systemic corticosteroids increase the risk of intra-uterine growth restriction; there is no evidence of intra-uterine growth restriction following short-term treatment (e.g. prophylactic treatment for neonatal respiratory distress syndrome). Any adrenal suppression in the neonate following prenatal exposure usually resolves spontaneously after birth and is rarely clinically important. **Monitoring** Pregnant women with pre-eclampsia or fluid retention should be monitored closely when given systemic corticosteroids.

● **BREAST FEEDING** The benefit of treatment with corticosteroids during breast-feeding outweighs the risk.

● **HEPATIC IMPAIRMENT** In general, manufacturers advise caution (risk of increased exposure).

● **RENAL IMPAIRMENT** In general, manufacturers advise caution.

● **MONITORING REQUIREMENTS**

▶ EvGr The following baseline measurements should be taken before starting treatment and at regular intervals during the course of long-term treatment: Ⓐ
  • blood pressure
  • body weight
  • BMI
  • height (children and adolescents)
  • HbA$_{1c}$
  • triglycerides
  • potassium
  • eye examination (for glaucoma and cataract)
▶ EvGr In addition monitor the following during treatment, depending on clinical judgement: Ⓐ
  • osteoporosis risk
  • falls risk assessment
  • adrenal suppression

● **EFFECT ON LABORATORY TESTS** May suppress skin test reactions.

● **TREATMENT CESSATION**

▶ In adults Abrupt withdrawal after a prolonged period can lead to acute adrenal insufficiency, hypotension or death. Withdrawal can also be associated with fever, myalgia, arthralgia, rhinitis, conjunctivitis, painful itchy skin nodules and weight loss. The magnitude and speed of dose reduction in corticosteroid withdrawal should be determined on a case-by–case basis, taking into consideration the underlying condition that is being treated, and individual patient factors such as the likelihood of relapse and the duration of corticosteroid treatment. *Gradual* withdrawal of systemic corticosteroids should be considered in those whose disease is unlikely to relapse and have:
  • received more than 40 mg prednisolone (or equivalent) daily for more than 1 week;
  • been given repeat doses in the evening;
  • received more than 3 weeks' treatment;
  • recently received repeated courses (particularly if taken for longer than 3 weeks);
  • taken a short course within 1 year of stopping long-term therapy;
  • other possible causes of adrenal suppression.

Systemic corticosteroids may be stopped abruptly in those whose disease is unlikely to relapse *and* who have received treatment for 3 weeks or less *and* who are not included in the patient groups described above.

During corticosteroid withdrawal the dose may be reduced rapidly down to physiological doses (equivalent to prednisolone 7.5 mg daily) and then reduced more slowly. Assessment of the disease may be needed during withdrawal to ensure that relapse does not occur.

▶ In children The magnitude and speed of dose reduction in corticosteroid withdrawal should be determined on a case-by–case basis, taking into consideration the underlying condition that is being treated, and individual patient factors such as the likelihood of relapse and the duration of corticosteroid treatment. *Gradual* withdrawal of systemic corticosteroids should be considered in those whose disease is unlikely to relapse and have:
  • received more than 40 mg prednisolone (or equivalent) daily for more than 1 week *or* 2 mg/kg daily for 1 week *or* 1 mg/kg daily for 1 month;
  • been given repeat doses in the evening;
  • received more than 3 weeks' treatment;
  • recently received repeated courses (particularly if taken for longer than 3 weeks);
  • taken a short course within 1 year of stopping long-term therapy;
  • other possible causes of adrenal suppression.

Systemic corticosteroids may be stopped abruptly in those whose disease is unlikely to relapse *and* who have received treatment for 3 weeks or less *and* who are not included in the patient groups described above.

During corticosteroid withdrawal the dose may be reduced rapidly down to physiological doses (equivalent to prednisolone 2–2.5 mg/m^2 daily) and then reduced more slowly. Assessment of the disease may be needed during withdrawal to ensure that relapse does not occur.

● **PATIENT AND CARER ADVICE**

Advice for patients A patient information leaflet should be supplied to every patient when a systemic corticosteroid is prescribed. Patients should especially be advised of potential side-effects including adrenal suppression, immunosuppression, and psychiatric reactions (for further details, see *Side-effects, further information*).

Steroid Treatment Card Steroid Treatment Cards should be issued where appropriate to support communication of the risks associated with treatment and to record details of the prescriber, drug, dosage, and duration of treatment. Steroid treatment cards are available for purchase from the NHS Print online ordering portal cmswebshop.corp.xerox.com/NHS/Login.aspx.

GP practices can obtain supplies through Primary Care Support England. NHS Trusts can order supplies via the online ordering portal.

In **Scotland,** steroid treatment cards can be obtained from APS Group Scotland by emailing stockorders.dppas@apsgroup.co.uk or by fax on 0131 629 9967.

Steroid Emergency Card

▸ In adults Steroid Emergency Cards should be issued to patients with adrenal insufficiency and steroid dependence for whom missed doses, illness, or surgery puts them at risk of adrenal crisis. The Royal College of Physicians and the Society for Endocrinology advise that the following patients are considered at risk of adrenal insufficiency and should be given a Steroid Emergency Card:

- those with primary adrenal insufficiency;
- those with adrenal insufficiency due to hypopituitarism requiring corticosteroid replacement;
- those taking corticosteroids at doses equivalent to, or exceeding, prednisolone 5 mg daily for 4 weeks or longer across all routes of administration (oral, topical, inhaled, intranasal, or intra-articular);
- those taking corticosteroids at doses equivalent to, or exceeding, prednisolone 40 mg daily for longer than 1 week, or repeated short oral courses;
- those taking a course of oral corticosteroids within 1 year of stopping long-term therapy.

The card includes a management summary for the emergency treatment of adrenal crisis and can be issued by any healthcare professional managing such patients.

Steroid Emergency Cards are available online at www.endocrinology.org/adrenal-crisis or are available for purchase from the NHS Print online ordering portal cmswebshop.corp.xerox.com/NHS/Login.aspx or Primary Care Support England (PCSE) online.

In **Northern Ireland** see: niformulary.hscni.net/wpfd_file/hscb-steroid-emergency-card/.

In **Scotland** see: www.healthcareimprovementscotland.scot/publications/steroid-emergency-card-to-support-early-recognition-and-treatment-of-adrenal-crisis-in-adults/.

In **Wales** see: www.weds-wales.co.uk/steroid-therapy/.

Adrenal Insufficiency Card

▸ In children The British Society for Paediatric Endocrinology and Diabetes (BSPED) has developed an Adrenal Insufficiency Card which should be issued to children with adrenal insufficiency and steroid dependence. The card includes a management summary for the emergency treatment of adrenal crisis and sick day dosing, and can be issued by any healthcare professional managing such patients. The BSPED Adrenal Insufficiency Card is available at: www.bsped.org.uk/adrenal-insufficiency. In **Wales** see: www.weds-wales.co.uk/steroid-therapy/.

▣ 783

Betamethasone
08-Oct-2024

- **DRUG ACTION** Betamethasone has very high glucocorticoid activity and insignificant mineralocorticoid activity.

- **INDICATIONS AND DOSE**

Suppression of inflammatory and allergic disorders | Congenital adrenal hyperplasia

▸ BY MOUTH

▸ Adult: Usual dose 0.5–5 mg once daily

▸ BY INTRAMUSCULAR INJECTION, OR BY SLOW INTRAVENOUS INJECTION, OR BY INTRAVENOUS INFUSION

▸ Adult: 4–20 mg, dose may be repeated up to 4 times in 24 hours

- **INTERACTIONS** → Appendix 1: corticosteroids

- **SIDE-EFFECTS** Hiccups · malaise · myocardial rupture (following recent myocardial infarction) · oedema · Stevens-Johnson syndrome

- **PREGNANCY** Readily crosses the placenta. Transient effect on fetal movements and heart rate.

- **DIRECTIONS FOR ADMINISTRATION** For *intravenous infusion* (as sodium phosphate) (*Betnesol*®), give continuously or intermittently *or via* drip tubing *in* Glucose 5% *or* Sodium chloride 0.9%.

- **MEDICINAL FORMS** There can be variation in the licensing of different medicines containing the same drug.

Soluble tablet

CAUTIONARY AND ADVISORY LABELS 10, 13, 21 (not for use as mouthwash for oral ulceration)

▸ Betamethasone (Non-proprietary)

Betamethasone (as Betamethasone sodium phosphate) 500 microgram Betamethasone 500microgram soluble tablets sugar free | 30 tablet PoM £7.00 SF | 100 tablet PoM £58.15 DT = £15.28 SF

Solution for injection

CAUTIONARY AND ADVISORY LABELS 10

▸ Betamethasone (Non-proprietary)

Betamethasone (as Betamethasone sodium phosphate) 4 mg per 1 ml Betamethasone 4mg/1ml solution for injection ampoules | 5 ampoule PoM £112.36-£126.54

▣ 783

Deflazacort
20-Jul-2023

- **DRUG ACTION** Deflazacort is derived from prednisolone; it has predominantly glucocorticoid activity.

- **INDICATIONS AND DOSE**

Suppression of inflammatory and allergic disorders

▸ BY MOUTH

▸ Adult: Maintenance 3–18 mg daily

Suppression of inflammatory and allergic disorders (acute disorders)

▸ BY MOUTH

▸ Adult: Initially up to 120 mg daily

Inflammatory and allergic disorders

▸ BY MOUTH

▸ Child 1 month–11 years: 0.25–1.5 mg/kg once daily or on alternate days; increased if necessary up to 2.4 mg/kg daily (max. per dose 120 mg), in emergency situations

▸ Child 12–17 years: 3–18 mg once daily or on alternate days; increased if necessary up to 2.4 mg/kg daily (max. per dose 120 mg), in emergency situations

- **INTERACTIONS** → Appendix 1: corticosteroids

- **SIDE-EFFECTS**

▸ **Uncommon** Carbohydrate intolerance · depressed mood · oedema

▸ **Frequency not known** Confusion · delusions · epilepsy exacerbated · hallucination · hypertrophic cardiomyopathy (in preterm infants) · idiopathic intracranial hypertension · memory loss · peptic ulcer perforation · schizophrenia exacerbated · severe cutaneous adverse reactions (SCARs) · suicidal thoughts · telangiectasia · tendinitis · tumour lysis syndrome

- **HEPATIC IMPAIRMENT**

Dose adjustments Manufacturer advises adjust to the minimum effective dose.

- **MEDICINAL FORMS** There can be variation in the licensing of different medicines containing the same drug. Forms available from special-order manufacturers include: oral tablet

Oral tablet

CAUTIONARY AND ADVISORY LABELS 5, 10

▸ Calcort (Neon Healthcare Ltd)

Deflazacort 6 mg Calcort 6mg tablets | 60 tablet PoM £15.82 DT = £15.82

📌 783

Dexamethasone

24-Jul-2024

- **DRUG ACTION** Dexamethasone has very high glucocorticoid activity and insignificant mineralocorticoid activity.

- **INDICATIONS AND DOSE**

Suppression of inflammatory and allergic disorders
▸ BY MOUTH
▸ Adult: 0.5–10 mg daily

Mild croup
▸ BY MOUTH
▸ Child: 150 micrograms/kg for 1 dose

Severe croup (or mild croup that might cause complications)
▸ INITIALLY BY MOUTH
▸ Child: Initially 150 micrograms/kg for 1 dose, to be given before transfer to hospital, then (by mouth or by intravenous injection) 150 micrograms/kg for 1 dose, then (by mouth or by intravenous injection) 150 micrograms/kg for 1 dose, to be given 12 hours after previous dose if required

Congenital adrenal hyperplasia (under expert supervision)
▸ BY MOUTH
▸ Adult: Consult specialist for advice on dosing
▸ BY INTRAMUSCULAR INJECTION, OR BY SLOW INTRAVENOUS INJECTION, OR BY INTRAVENOUS INFUSION
▸ Adult: Consult specialist for advice on dosing

Overnight dexamethasone suppression test
▸ BY MOUTH
▸ Adult: 1 mg for 1 dose, to be given at night

Adjunctive treatment of suspected bacterial meningitis
▸ BY INTRAVENOUS INJECTION
▸ Adult: 10 mg every 6 hours, to be started before or up to 12 hours after the first dose of antibacterial—seek specialist advice if more than 12 hours have elapsed after starting antibacterials, continued for 4 days in patients with meningitis caused by *Streptococcus pneumoniae* (pneumococcus) or *Haemophilus influenzae* type b—discontinue treatment if another cause is suspected or confirmed

Symptom control of anorexia in palliative care
▸ Adult: 2–4 mg daily

Dysphagia due to obstruction by tumour in palliative care
▸ Adult: 8 mg daily

Dyspnoea due to bronchospasm or partial obstruction in palliative care
▸ Adult: 4–8 mg daily

Adjunct in the treatment of nausea and vomiting in palliative care
▸ BY MOUTH
▸ Adult: 8–16 mg daily

Headaches due to raised intracranial pressure in palliative care
▸ Adult: 16 mg daily for 4–5 days, then reduced to 4–6 mg daily, reduce dose if possible. To be given before 6pm to reduce the risk of insomnia

Pain due to nerve compression in palliative care
▸ Adult: 8 mg daily

Cerebral oedema associated with brain tumours
▸ BY MOUTH
▸ Adult: 0.5–10 mg daily
▸ INITIALLY BY INTRAVENOUS INJECTION
▸ Adult: Initially 8.3 mg for 1 dose, then (by intramuscular injection) 3.3 mg every 6 hours until symptoms subside, subsequently, dose may be reduced

after 2–4 days and then gradually discontinued over 5–7 days

Life-threatening cerebral oedema
▸ BY INTRAVENOUS INJECTION
▸ Adult: Initially 41.5 mg for 1 dose, then 6.6 mg every 2 hours for 3 days, then 3.3 mg every 2 hours for 1 day, then 3.3 mg every 4 hours for 4 days, dose then reduced in steps of 3.3 mg per day, continue dose reduction to discontinue over the following 7–10 days or change to oral dexamethasone maintenance if required

COVID-19 requiring supplemental oxygen
▸ BY MOUTH, OR BY INTRAVENOUS INJECTION
▸ Adult: 6 mg once daily for 10 days, or until the day of discharge if this is sooner

Reduction of peri- and neonatal morbidity and mortality [in established preterm labour, planned preterm birth, or preterm prelabour rupture of membranes]
▸ BY INTRAMUSCULAR INJECTION
▸ Adult: 4.95 mg every 12 hours for 48 hours, to be given within 7 days prior to birth, treatment course may be repeated once as clinically indicated at least 7 days after completion of the first course, alternatively 9.9 mg every 24 hours for 48 hours, to be given within 7 days prior to birth, treatment course may be repeated once as clinically indicated at least 7 days after completion of the first course

DOSE EQUIVALENCE AND CONVERSION
▸ Doses expressed as dexamethasone base.
▸ Dexamethasone base 3.3 mg is equivalent to dexamethasone phosphate 4 mg.
▸ Dexamethasone base 3.3 mg is equivalent to dexamethasone sodium phosphate 4.3 mg.

- **UNLICENSED USE** EvGr Dexamethasone is used for the treatment of suspected bacterial meningitis, Ⓐ but is not licensed for this indication.
▸ With intramuscular use EvGr Dexamethasone is used to reduce peri- and neonatal morbidity and mortality in women with established preterm labour, planned preterm birth, or preterm prelabour rupture of membranes, Ⓐ but is not licensed for this indication.

- **INTERACTIONS** → Appendix 1: corticosteroids

- **SIDE-EFFECTS**
▸ With oral use Hiccups · hyperglycaemia · hypotension · malaise · myocardial rupture (following recent myocardial infarction) · protein catabolism · telangiectasia
▸ With parenteral use Hypotension · perineal irritation (may occur following the intravenous injection of large doses of the phosphate ester) · telangiectasia

- **PREGNANCY** Dexamethasone readily crosses the placenta.

- **DIRECTIONS FOR ADMINISTRATION**
▸ With oral use in children For administration *by mouth* tablets may be dispersed in water or injection solution given by mouth.
▸ With intravenous use in children For *intravenous infusion* dilute with Glucose 5% or Sodium Chloride 0.9%; give over 15–20 minutes.
▸ With intravenous use in adults For *intravenous infusion* (*Dexamethasone*, Hospira) give continuously *or* intermittently *or via* drip tubing *in* Glucose 5% *or* Sodium Chloride 0.9%.

- **PRESCRIBING AND DISPENSING INFORMATION** Dexamethasone 3.8 mg/mL Injection has replaced dexamethasone 4 mg/mL Injection.

Palliative care For further information on the use of dexamethasone in palliative care, see www.medicinescomplete.com/#/content/palliative/systemic-corticosteroids.

6

Endocrine system

- **PATIENT AND CARER ADVICE**
  Medicines for Children leaflet: Dexamethasone for croup
  www.medicinesforchildren.org.uk/medicines/dexamethasone-
  for-croup/

- **MEDICINAL FORMS** There can be variation in the licensing of
  different medicines containing the same drug. Forms available
  from special-order manufacturers include: oral capsule, oral
  suspension, oral solution
  Oral tablet
  CAUTIONARY AND ADVISORY LABELS 10, 21
  - ▸ Dexamethasone (Non-proprietary)
    Dexamethasone 500 microgram Dexamethasone 500microgram
    tablets | 28 tablet [PoM] £54.08 DT = £1.97 | 30 tablet [PoM] £2.11–
    £77.78
    Dexamethasone 1 mg Dexamethasone 1mg tablets |
    30 tablet [PoM] £3.54–£5.66 DT = £3.54
    Dexamethasone 2 mg Dexamethasone 2mg tablets |
    28 tablet [PoM] £1.88–£24.00 | 50 tablet [PoM] £42.85 DT = £3.35 |
    100 tablet [PoM] £6.74–£8.49
    Dexamethasone 4 mg Dexamethasone 4mg tablets |
    30 tablet [PoM] £42.79–£61.48 | 50 tablet [PoM] £120.00 DT = £71.32
    | 100 tablet [PoM] £142.64–£204.94
  Soluble tablet
  CAUTIONARY AND ADVISORY LABELS 10, 13, 21
  ELECTROLYTES: May contain Sodium
  - ▸ Dexamethasone (Non-proprietary)
    **Dexamethasone (as Dexamethasone sodium phosphate)
    2 mg** Dexamethasone 2mg soluble tablets sugar free |
    50 tablet [PoM] £29.99–£41.70 DT = £41.70 [SF]
    **Dexamethasone (as Dexamethasone sodium phosphate)
    4 mg** Dexamethasone 4mg soluble tablets sugar free |
    50 tablet [PoM] £60.00 DT = £60.00 [SF]
    **Dexamethasone (as Dexamethasone sodium phosphate)
    8 mg** Dexamethasone 8mg soluble tablets sugar free |
    50 tablet [PoM] £120.00 DT = £120.00 [SF]
    **Dexamethasone (as Dexamethasone sodium phosphate)
    10 mg** Dexamethasone 10mg soluble tablets sugar free |
    10 tablet [PoM] £10.00–£16.00 DT = £10.00 [SF]
    **Dexamethasone (as Dexamethasone sodium phosphate)
    20 mg** Dexamethasone 20mg soluble tablets sugar free |
    10 tablet [PoM] £20.00–£32.00 DT = £20.00 [SF]
  Solution for injection
  CAUTIONARY AND ADVISORY LABELS 10
  EXCIPIENTS: May contain Disodium edetate, propylene glycol
  - ▸ Dexamethasone (Non-proprietary)
    **Dexamethasone (as Dexamethasone sodium phosphate) 3.3 mg
    per 1 ml** Dexamethasone (base) 6.6mg/2ml solution for injection
    ampoules | 10 ampoule [PoM] £24.59–£28.00
    Dexamethasone (base) 6.6mg/2ml solution for injection vials |
    5 vial [PoM] £24.00 DT = £24.00
    Dexamethasone (base) 3.3mg/1ml solution for injection ampoules |
    10 ampoule [PoM] £24.00 DT = £6.65 | 10 ampoule [PoM] £28.79 DT =
    £6.65 (Hospital only)
    **Dexamethasone (as Dexamethasone sodium phosphate) 3.8 mg
    per 1 ml** Dexamethasone (base) 3.8mg/1ml solution for injection vials
    | 10 vial [PoM] £19.99 DT = £19.99
  Oral solution
  CAUTIONARY AND ADVISORY LABELS 10, 21
  - ▸ Dexamethasone (Non-proprietary)
    **Dexamethasone (as Dexamethasone sodium phosphate)
    400 microgram per 1 ml** Dexamethasone 2mg/5ml oral solution
    sugar free | 150 ml [PoM] £42.30 DT = £42.30 [SF]
    **Dexamethasone (as Dexamethasone sodium phosphate) 2 mg per
    1 ml** Dexamethasone 10mg/5ml oral solution sugar free |
    50 ml [PoM] £28.00 [SF] | 150 ml [PoM] £156.79 DT = £156.79 [SF]
    **Dexamethasone (as Dexamethasone sodium phosphate) 4 mg
    per 1 ml** Dexamethasone 20mg/5ml oral solution sugar free |
    50 ml [PoM] £42.00 DT = £42.00 [SF]
  - ▸ Dexsol (Rosemont Pharmaceuticals Ltd)
    **Dexamethasone (as Dexamethasone sodium phosphate)
    400 microgram per 1 ml** Dexsol 2mg/5ml oral solution |
    75 ml [PoM] £21.15 [SF] | 150 ml [PoM] £42.30 DT = £42.30 [SF]

[⚑ 783]

Fludrocortisone acetate   20-Jul-2023

- **DRUG ACTION** Fludrocortisone has very high
  mineralocorticoid activity and insignificant glucocorticoid
  activity.

- **INDICATIONS AND DOSE**
  Neuropathic postural hypotension
  - ▸ BY MOUTH
  - ▸ Adult: 100–400 micrograms daily
  **Mineralocorticoid replacement in adrenocortical
  insufficiency**
  - ▸ BY MOUTH
  - ▸ Adult: 50–300 micrograms once daily
  **Adrenocortical insufficiency resulting from septic shock
  (in combination with hydrocortisone)**
  - ▸ BY MOUTH
  - ▸ Adult: 50 micrograms daily

- **UNLICENSED USE** Not licensed for use in neuropathic
  postural hypotension.

- **INTERACTIONS** → Appendix 1: corticosteroids

- **SIDE-EFFECTS** Conjunctivitis · fatigue · idiopathic
  intracranial hypertension · insomnia · muscle weakness ·
  thrombophlebitis

- **HEPATIC IMPAIRMENT**
  Monitoring Monitor patient closely in hepatic impairment.

- **MEDICINAL FORMS** There can be variation in the licensing of
  different medicines containing the same drug. Forms available
  from special-order manufacturers include: oral capsule, oral
  suspension
  Oral tablet
  CAUTIONARY AND ADVISORY LABELS 10
  - ▸ Fludrocortisone acetate (Non-proprietary)
    Fludrocortisone acetate 50 microgram Fludrocortisone
    50microgram tablets | 30 tablet [PoM] £13.60–£24.48
    Fludrocortisone acetate 100 microgram Fludrocortisone
    100microgram tablets | 30 tablet [PoM] £17.10 DT = £4.56 |
    100 tablet [PoM] £12.00–£17.73

[⚑ 783]

Hydrocortisone   08-Oct-2024

- **DRUG ACTION** Hydrocortisone has equal glucocorticoid
  and mineralocorticoid activity.

- **INDICATIONS AND DOSE**
  Thyrotoxic crisis [thyroid storm]
  - ▸ BY INTRAVENOUS INJECTION
  - ▸ Adult: 100 mg every 6 hours, to be administered as
    sodium succinate
  Adrenocortical insufficiency resulting from septic shock
  - ▸ BY INTRAVENOUS INJECTION
  - ▸ Adult: 50 mg every 6 hours, to be given in combination
    with fludrocortisone
  **Acute hypersensitivity reactions such as angioedema of
  the upper respiratory tract and anaphylaxis [adjunct to
  adrenaline]**
  - ▸ BY INTRAVENOUS INJECTION
  - ▸ Adult: 100–300 mg, to be administered as sodium
    succinate
  **Corticosteroid replacement [patients who have taken
  more than 10 mg prednisolone per day or equivalent
  within 3 months of minor surgery under general
  anaesthesia]**
  - ▸ BY INTRAVENOUS INJECTION, OR BY INTRAVENOUS INFUSION
  - ▸ Adult: Initially 25–50 mg for 1 dose, to be administered
    at induction of surgery, the patient's usual oral
    corticosteroid dose is recommenced after surgery

continued →

Corticosteroid replacement [patients who have taken more than 10 mg prednisolone per day or equivalent within 3 months of moderate or major surgery]

▶ INITIALLY BY INTRAVENOUS INJECTION, OR BY INTRAVENOUS INFUSION

▶ Adult: Initially 25–50 mg for 1 dose, to be administered at induction of surgery (following usual oral corticosteroid dose on the morning of surgery), followed by (by intravenous injection) 25–50 mg 3 times a day for 24 hours after moderate surgery and for 48–72 hours after major surgery

Adrenocortical insufficiency in Addison's disease or following adrenalectomy

▶ BY MOUTH USING IMMEDIATE-RELEASE MEDICINES

▶ Adult: 20–30 mg daily in 2 divided doses, a larger dose to be given in the morning and a smaller dose in the evening, mimicking the normal diurnal rhythm of cortisol secretion, the optimum daily dose is determined on the basis of clinical response

Adrenal crisis [in patients with adrenal insufficiency who are steroid-dependent]

▶ INITIALLY BY INTRAMUSCULAR INJECTION, OR BY INTRAVENOUS INJECTION

▶ Child 16–17 years: Initially 100 mg for 1 dose, then (by continuous intravenous infusion) 200 mg/24 hours, dilute in Glucose 5%, alternatively (by intramuscular injection or by intravenous injection) 50 mg every 6 hours, dose increased to 100 mg every 6 hours in patients who are severely obese

▶ Adult: Initially 100 mg for 1 dose, then (by continuous intravenous infusion) 200 mg/24 hours, dilute in Glucose 5%, alternatively (by intramuscular injection or by intravenous injection) 50 mg every 6 hours, dose increased to 100 mg every 6 hours in patients who are severely obese

Adrenal crisis in the community [in patients with adrenal insufficiency who are steroid-dependent]

▶ BY INTRAMUSCULAR INJECTION, OR BY INTRAVENOUS INJECTION

▶ Child 1–11 months: 25 mg for 1 dose, patients should be admitted to hospital after the first dose, steroid treatment must not be stopped

▶ Child 1–5 years: 50 mg for 1 dose, patients should be admitted to hospital after the first dose, steroid treatment must not be stopped

▶ Child 6–15 years: 100 mg for 1 dose, patients should be admitted to hospital after the first dose, steroid treatment must not be stopped

Adrenal crisis in hospital when illness is severe [in patients with adrenal insufficiency who are steroid-dependent]

▶ INITIALLY BY INTRAMUSCULAR INJECTION, OR BY INTRAVENOUS INJECTION

▶ Child 1–11 months: Initially 25 mg for 1 dose, alternatively (by intravenous injection or by intravenous infusion) initially 2 mg/kg for 1 dose, then (by intravenous injection or by intravenous infusion) 2 mg/kg every 4–6 hours

▶ Child 1–5 years: Initially 50 mg for 1 dose, alternatively (by intravenous injection or by intravenous infusion) initially 2 mg/kg for 1 dose (max. per dose 100 mg), then (by intravenous injection or by intravenous infusion) 2 mg/kg every 4–6 hours (max. per dose 100 mg)

▶ Child 6–15 years: Initially 100 mg for 1 dose, alternatively (by intravenous injection or by intravenous infusion) initially 2 mg/kg for 1 dose (max. per dose 100 mg), then (by intravenous injection or by intravenous infusion) 2 mg/kg every 4–6 hours (max. per dose 100 mg)

Adrenal crisis in hospital when stable and improving [in patients with adrenal insufficiency who are steroid-dependent]

▶ BY INTRAVENOUS INJECTION, OR BY INTRAVENOUS INFUSION

▶ Child 1 month–15 years: 1 mg/kg every 4–6 hours (max. per dose 50 mg)

Adrenal crisis in hospital when stable and tolerating drinks and diet [in patients with adrenal insufficiency who are steroid-dependent]

▶ BY MOUTH

▶ Child 1 month–15 years: 7.5 mg/m^2 4 times a day, restart fludrocortisone if indicated

Severe inflammatory bowel disease

▶ BY SLOW INTRAVENOUS INJECTION, OR BY INTRAVENOUS INFUSION

▶ Adult: 100–500 mg 3–4 times a day or when required

Replacement in adrenocortical insufficiency

▶ BY MOUTH USING MODIFIED-RELEASE TABLETS

▶ Adult: 20–30 mg once daily, dose to be taken in the morning, to be adjusted according to response

▶ BY MOUTH USING IMMEDIATE-RELEASE MEDICINES

▶ Adult: 20–30 mg daily in 2 divided doses, a larger dose to be given in the morning and a smaller dose in the evening, to be adjusted according to response

Congenital adrenal hyperplasia

▶ BY MOUTH USING MODIFIED-RELEASE CAPSULES

▶ Adult: 15–25 mg daily in 2 divided doses, take morning dose 1 hour before food and the evening dose at least 2 hours after last meal, at initiation, give two-thirds to three-quarters of the dose in the evening, and the remainder in the morning; adjust dose thereafter based on response. A lower dose may be sufficient in patients with remaining endogenous cortisol production

Acute hypersensitivity reactions | Angioedema

▶ BY INTRAMUSCULAR INJECTION, OR BY INTRAVENOUS INJECTION

▶ Child 1–5 months: Initially 25 mg 3 times a day, dose to be adjusted according to response

▶ Child 6 months–5 years: Initially 50 mg 3 times a day, dose to be adjusted according to response

▶ Child 6–11 years: Initially 100 mg 3 times a day, dose to be adjusted according to response

▶ Child 12–17 years: Initially 200 mg 3 times a day, dose to be adjusted according to response

Severe acute asthma | Life-threatening acute asthma

▶ BY INTRAVENOUS INJECTION

▶ Child 1 month–1 year: 4 mg/kg every 6 hours (max. per dose 100 mg) until conversion to oral prednisolone is possible, dose given, preferably, as sodium succinate, alternatively 25 mg every 6 hours until conversion to oral prednisolone is possible, dose given, preferably, as sodium succinate

▶ Child 2–4 years: 4 mg/kg every 6 hours (max. per dose 100 mg) until conversion to oral prednisolone is possible, dose given, preferably, as sodium succinate, alternatively 50 mg every 6 hours until conversion to oral prednisolone is possible, dose given, preferably, as sodium succinate

▶ Child 5–11 years: 4 mg/kg every 6 hours (max. per dose 100 mg) until conversion to oral prednisolone is possible, dose given, preferably, as sodium succinate, alternatively 100 mg every 6 hours until conversion to oral prednisolone is possible, dose given, preferably, as sodium succinate

▶ Child 12–17 years: 4 mg/kg every 6 hours (max. per dose 100 mg) until conversion to oral prednisolone is possible, dose given, preferably, as sodium succinate, alternatively 100 mg every 6 hours until conversion to oral prednisolone is possible, dose given, preferably, as sodium succinate

▸ Adult: 100 mg every 6 hours until conversion to oral prednisolone is possible, dose given, preferably, as sodium succinate

COVID-19 requiring supplemental oxygen [when dexamethasone cannot be used or is unavailable]
▸ BY INTRAVENOUS INJECTION, OR BY INTRAVENOUS INFUSION
▸ Adult: 50 mg every 8 hours for 10 days, or until the day of discharge if this is sooner; may be continued for up to 28 days in patients with septic shock

DOSE EQUIVALENCE AND CONVERSION
▸ With oral use
▸ For *Replacement in adrenocortical insufficiency*, when switching from immediate-release tablets to *Plenadren*® modified-release tablets use same total daily dose. Bioavailability of *Plenadren*® lower than immediate-release tablets—monitor clinical response.

IMPORTANT SAFETY INFORMATION

MHRA/CHM ADVICE: HYDROCORTISONE MUCO-ADHESIVE BUCCAL TABLETS: SHOULD NOT BE USED OFF-LABEL FOR ADRENAL INSUFFICIENCY IN CHILDREN DUE TO SERIOUS RISKS (DECEMBER 2018)

The MHRA has received reports of off-label use of hydrocortisone muco-adhesive buccal tablets for adrenal insufficiency in children. Healthcare professionals are advised that:
● hydrocortisone muco-adhesive buccal tablets are indicated only for local use in the mouth for aphthous ulceration and should not be used to treat adrenal insufficiency;
● substitution of licensed oral hydrocortisone formulations with muco-adhesive buccal tablets can result in insufficient cortisol absorption and, in stress situations, life-threatening adrenal crisis;
● only hydrocortisone products licensed for adrenal replacement therapy should be used.

MHRA/CHM ADVICE: *ALKINDI*® (HYDROCORTISONE GRANULES): RISK OF ACUTE ADRENAL INSUFFICIENCY IN CHILDREN WHEN SWITCHING FROM HYDROCORTISONE TABLET FORMULATIONS TO GRANULES (FEBRUARY 2021)

▸ In children
Adrenal crisis has been reported in an infant who was switched from hydrocortisone soluble tablets to hydrocortisone granules (*Alkindi*®). Acute adrenal insufficiency could also occur when switching from crushed hydrocortisone tablets to granules due to a potential risk of inaccurate dosing. Healthcare professionals should advise parents or carers of children switching from hydrocortisone tablets to *Alkindi*® to carefully observe the child for symptoms of adrenal insufficiency during the first week. They should be counselled on what to do if symptoms of adrenal insufficiency develop, including the need to seek immediate medical advice and administer extra doses of *Alkindi*® if appropriate. A long-term increase in the daily dose of *Alkindi*® should be considered if additional doses are required during the first week after switching.

● INTERACTIONS → Appendix 1: corticosteroids

● SIDE-EFFECTS
▸ With oral use Dyslipidaemia · fatigue · hypotension · malaise · myocardial rupture (following recent myocardial infarction) · oedema
▸ With parenteral use Hiccups · Kaposi's sarcoma · lipomatosis · malaise · myocardial rupture (following recent myocardial infarction)

● DIRECTIONS FOR ADMINISTRATION
▸ With intravenous use in children EvGr For *intravenous administration*, dilute with Glucose 5% or Sodium Chloride 0.9%. M For *intermittent infusion* give over 20–30 minutes.

▸ With oral use in children EvGr For *Alkindi*®, capsules should be opened and granules either administered directly into the mouth and then followed immediately with a drink, or sprinkled onto a spoonful of soft food (such as yoghurt) and given immediately. Granules should not be chewed or added to liquid before administration due to the bitter taste, and they should not be given via an enteral tube as it may cause blockage. M
▸ With intravenous use in adults EvGr For *intravenous infusion* (*SoluCortef*®), give continuously *or* intermittently *or* via drip tubing *in* Glucose 5% *or* Sodium chloride 0.9%. M

● PRESCRIBING AND DISPENSING INFORMATION
▸ When used for Asthma For choice of therapy, see Asthma, acute p. 274 and Asthma, chronic p. 271.
▸ With oral use in children The RCPCH and NPPG recommend that, when a liquid special of hydrocortisone is required, the following strength is used: 5 mg/5 mL.

● NATIONAL FUNDING/ACCESS DECISIONS
For full details see funding body website

Scottish Medicines Consortium (SMC) decisions
▸ **Hydrocortisone (*Plenadren*®) for the treatment of adrenal insufficiency in adults (December 2016)** SMC No. 848/12 Not recommended
▸ **Hydrocortisone (*Alkindi*®) for the replacement therapy of adrenal insufficiency in infants, children and adolescents (aged from birth to less than 18 years old) (October 2018)** SMC No. SMC2088 Recommended with restrictions
▸ **Hydrocortisone modified-release (*Efmody*®) for the treatment of congenital adrenal hyperplasia (CAH) in adolescents aged 12 years and over and adults (March 2022)** SMC No. SMC2414 Not recommended

All Wales Medicines Strategy Group (AWMSG) decisions
▸ **Hydrocortisone MR (*Efmody*®) for the treatment of congenital adrenal hyperplasia (CAH) in adolescents aged 12 years and over and adults (October 2022)** AWMSG No. 3017 Recommended with restrictions

● LESS SUITABLE FOR PRESCRIBING
▸ With intravenous use Hydrocortisone as the sodium phosphate is less suitable for prescribing as paraesthesia and pain (particularly in the perineal region) may follow intravenous injection.

● EXCEPTIONS TO LEGAL CATEGORY
▸ With intramuscular use or intravenous use Prescription only medicine restriction does not apply where administration is for saving life in emergency.

● MEDICINAL FORMS There can be variation in the licensing of different medicines containing the same drug. Forms available from special-order manufacturers include: oral capsule, oral suspension, oral solution

Oral tablet
CAUTIONARY AND ADVISORY LABELS 10, 21
▸ Hydrocortisone (Non-proprietary)
Hydrocortisone 2.5 mg Hydrocortisone 2.5mg tablets | 30 tablet PoM £33.68–£35.44 DT = £35.44
Hydrocortisone 5 mg Hydrocortisone 5mg tablets | 30 tablet PoM £43.00 DT = £26.41
Hydrocortisone 10 mg Hydrocortisone 10mg tablets | 30 tablet PoM £19.99 DT = £1.91
Hydrocortisone 15 mg Hydrocortisone 15mg tablets | 30 tablet PoM £33.51–£44.78 DT = £33.51
Hydrocortisone 20 mg Hydrocortisone 20mg tablets | 30 tablet PoM £4.60 DT = £3.86
▸ Hydventia (GlucoRx Ltd)
Hydrocortisone 10 mg Hydventia 10mg tablets | 30 tablet PoM £10.47 DT = £1.91
Hydrocortisone 20 mg Hydventia 20mg tablets | 30 tablet PoM £20.94 DT = £3.86

Modified-release tablet
CAUTIONARY AND ADVISORY LABELS 10, 22, 25
▸ Plenadren (Takeda UK Ltd)
Hydrocortisone 5 mg Plenadren 5mg modified-release tablets | 50 tablet PoM £242.50 DT = £242.50

Hydrocortisone 20 mg Plenadren 20mg modified-release tablets | 50 tablet [PoM] £400.00 DT = £400.00

Soluble tablet

CAUTIONARY AND ADVISORY LABELS 10, 13, 21

ELECTROLYTES: May contain Sodium

▸ **Hydrocortisone (Non-proprietary)**

Hydrocortisone (as Hydrocortisone sodium phosphate)

10 mg Hydrocortisone 10mg soluble tablets sugar free | 30 tablet [PoM] £37.50–£60.00 DT = £37.50 [SF]

Powder for solution for injection

▸ **Hydrocortisone (Non-proprietary)**

Hydrocortisone (as Hydrocortisone sodium succinate)

100 mg Hydrocortisone sodium succinate 100mg powder for solution for injection vials | 10 vial [PoM] £9.17–£18.00 DT = £9.17

▸ **Solu-Cortef** (Pfizer Ltd)

Hydrocortisone (as Hydrocortisone sodium succinate)

100 mg Solu-Cortef 100mg powder for solution for injection vials | 10 vial [PoM] £9.17 DT = £9.17

Powder and solvent for solution for injection

CAUTIONARY AND ADVISORY LABELS 10

▸ **Hydrocortisone (Non-proprietary)**

Hydrocortisone (as Hydrocortisone sodium succinate)

100 mg Hydrocortisone sodium succinate 100mg powder and solvent for solution for injection vials | 1 vial [PoM] £1.16 DT = £1.16

▸ **Solu-Cortef** (Pfizer Ltd)

Hydrocortisone (as Hydrocortisone sodium succinate)

100 mg Solu-Cortef 100mg powder and solvent for solution for injection vials | 1 vial [PoM] £1.16 DT = £1.16

Solution for injection

CAUTIONARY AND ADVISORY LABELS 10

▸ **Hydrocortisone (Non-proprietary)**

Hydrocortisone (as Hydrocortisone sodium phosphate) 100 mg per 1 ml Hydrocortisone sodium phosphate 100mg/1ml solution for injection ampoules | 5 ampoule [PoM] £10.60 DT = £10.60

Modified-release capsule

CAUTIONARY AND ADVISORY LABELS 10, 23, 25

▸ **Efmody** (Neurocrine UK Ltd)

Hydrocortisone 5 mg Efmody 5mg modified-release capsules | 50 capsule [PoM] £135.00 DT = £135.00

Hydrocortisone 10 mg Efmody 10mg modified-release capsules | 50 capsule [PoM] £275.00 DT = £275.00

Oral solution

▸ **Hydrocortisone (Non-proprietary)**

Hydrocortisone sodium phosphate 1 mg per 1 ml Hydrocortisone 5mg/5ml oral solution sugar free | 100 ml [PoM] £135.00–£242.70 DT = £135.00 [SF]

Hydrocortisone sodium phosphate 2 mg per 1 ml Hydrocortisone 10mg/5ml oral solution sugar free | 100 ml [PoM] £270.00–£486.00 DT = £270.00 [SF]

Oral granules

CAUTIONARY AND ADVISORY LABELS 10

▸ **Alkindi** (Neurocrine UK Ltd)

Hydrocortisone 500 microgram Alkindi 0.5mg granules in capsules for opening | 50 capsule [PoM] £33.75 DT = £33.75

Hydrocortisone 1 mg Alkindi 1mg granules in capsules for opening | 50 capsule [PoM] £67.50 DT = £67.50

Hydrocortisone 2 mg Alkindi 2mg granules in capsules for opening | 50 capsule [PoM] £135.00 DT = £135.00

Hydrocortisone 5 mg Alkindi 5mg granules in capsules for opening | 50 capsule [PoM] £337.50 DT = £337.50

⏷ 783

Methylprednisolone

20-Jul-2023

● **DRUG ACTION** Methylprednisolone exerts predominantly glucocorticoid effects with minimal mineralcorticoid effects.

● **INDICATIONS AND DOSE**

Suppression of inflammatory and allergic disorders | Cerebral oedema associated with malignancy

▸ BY MOUTH

▸ Adult: Initially 2–40 mg daily

▸ BY INTRAMUSCULAR INJECTION, OR BY SLOW INTRAVENOUS INJECTION, OR BY INTRAVENOUS INFUSION

▸ Adult: Initially 10–500 mg

Treatment of graft rejection reactions

▸ BY INTRAVENOUS INFUSION

▸ Adult: Up to 1 g daily for up to 3 days

Treatment of relapse in multiple sclerosis

▸ BY MOUTH

▸ Adult: 500 mg once daily for 5 days

Treatment of relapse in multiple sclerosis (when oral steroids have failed or have not been tolerated, or in those who require hospital admission)

▸ BY INTRAVENOUS INFUSION

▸ Adult: 1 g once daily for 3–5 days

DEPO-MEDRONE ®

Suppression of inflammatory and allergic disorders

▸ BY DEEP INTRAMUSCULAR INJECTION

▸ Adult: 40–120 mg, then 40–120 mg after 2–3 weeks if required, to be injected into the gluteal muscle

● **UNLICENSED USE** [EvGr] Not licensed for use by mouth for the treatment of multiple sclerosis relapse. Not licensed for use by intravenous infusion for the treatment of multiple sclerosis relapse for durations longer than 3 days. [A] Methylprednisolone doses in the BNF may differ from those in product literature.

IMPORTANT SAFETY INFORMATION

MHRA/CHM ADVICE: METHYLPREDNISOLONE INJECTABLE MEDICINE CONTAINING LACTOSE (*SOLU-MEDRONE* ® 40 MG): DO NOT USE IN PATIENTS WITH COWS' MILK ALLERGY (OCTOBER 2017)

▸ With intramuscular use or intravenous use

An EU-wide review has concluded that *Solu-Medrone* ® 40 mg may contain trace amounts of milk proteins and should not be used in patients with a known or suspected allergy to cows' milk. Serious allergic reactions, including bronchospasm and anaphylaxis, have been reported in patients allergic to cows' milk proteins. If a patient's symptoms worsen or new allergic symptoms occur, administration should be stopped and the patient treated accordingly.

MHRA/CHM ADVICE: *SOLU-MEDRONE* ® 40 MG (METHYLPREDNISOLONE AS SODIUM SUCCINATE): CHANGE FROM LACTOSE-CONTAINING TO A LACTOSE-FREE FORMULATION—RISK OF SERIOUS ALLERGIC REACTIONS IF FORMULATIONS ARE CONFUSED (NOVEMBER 2020)

▸ With intramuscular use or intravenous use

Solu-Medrone ® 40 mg powder and solvent for solution for injection has been reformulated to a lactose-free preparation in which the lactose is replaced with sucrose. There is a risk of serious allergic reactions if the new lactose-free preparation is confused with the lactose-containing preparation. Healthcare professionals should take extra care to ensure that patients who have been treated with the lactose-free preparation do not inadvertently receive the lactose-containing preparation. They should also be aware of the transition to the lactose-free preparation in their respective practices, and the precautionary measures taken by the manufacturer to differentiate between the packaging and labelling of the old (lactose-containing) and new (lactose-free) formulations to help avoid potential medication errors. Prescribers are advised to ensure patients who are allergic to cow's milk proteins and require the new lactose-free formulation are prescribed *Solu-Medrone* ® injection 40 mg lactose free or methylprednisolone injection 40 mg lactose free.

● **CAUTIONS**

▸ With intravenous use Rapid intravenous administration of large doses associated with cardiovascular collapse

▸ With systemic use Systemic sclerosis (increased incidence of scleroderma renal crisis)

● **INTERACTIONS** → Appendix 1: corticosteroids

- **SIDE-EFFECTS**
▶ **Common or very common**
▶ With oral use Depressed mood
▶ **Frequency not known**
▶ With oral use Confusion · delusions · diarrhoea · dizziness · dyslipidaemia · fatigue · hallucination · hiccups · hypotension · insomnia · Kaposi's sarcoma · lipomatosis · malaise · myocardial rupture (following recent myocardial infarction) · oedema · schizophrenia · suicidal ideation · telangiectasia · withdrawal syndrome
▶ With parenteral use Confusion · delusions · depressed mood · diarrhoea · dizziness · dyslipidaemia · fatigue · hallucination · hiccups · hypotension · Kaposi's sarcoma · lipomatosis · malaise · oedema · schizophrenia · suicidal thoughts · telangiectasia · vomiting · withdrawal syndrome

- **MONITORING REQUIREMENTS** Manufacturer advises monitor blood pressure and renal function (s-creatinine) routinely in patients with systemic sclerosis—increased incidence of scleroderma renal crisis.

- **DIRECTIONS FOR ADMINISTRATION** For *intravenous infusion* (as sodium succinate) (*Solu-Medrone*®), give continuously *or* intermittently *or via* drip tubing in Glucose 5% *or* Sodium chloride 0.9%. Reconstitute initially with water for injections; doses up to 250 mg should be given over at least 5 minutes, high doses over at least 30 minutes.

- **PRESCRIBING AND DISPENSING INFORMATION**
▶ With intramuscular use or intravenous use For warnings about the different formulations of *Solu-Medrone*® 40 mg, see *Important safety information.*

- **MEDICINAL FORMS** There can be variation in the licensing of different medicines containing the same drug. Forms available from special-order manufacturers include: oral suspension

Oral tablet
CAUTIONARY AND ADVISORY LABELS 10, 21
▶ **Medrone** (Pfizer Ltd)
Methylprednisolone 2 mg Medrone 2mg tablets | 30 tablet [PoM] £3.88 DT = £3.88
Methylprednisolone 4 mg Medrone 4mg tablets | 30 tablet [PoM] £6.19 DT = £6.19
Methylprednisolone 16 mg Medrone 16mg tablets | 30 tablet [PoM] £17.17 DT = £17.17
Methylprednisolone 100 mg Medrone 100mg tablets | 20 tablet [PoM] £48.32 DT = £48.32

Powder and solvent for solution for injection
CAUTIONARY AND ADVISORY LABELS 10
▶ **Methylprednisolone (Non-proprietary)**
Methylprednisolone (as Methylprednisolone sodium succinate) 40 mg Methylprednisolone sodium succinate 40mg powder and solvent for solution for injection vials | 1 vial [PoM] £1.58 DT = £1.58
Methylprednisolone (as Methylprednisolone sodium succinate) 125 mg Methylprednisolone sodium succinate 125mg powder and solvent for solution for injection vials | 1 vial [PoM] £4.75 DT = £4.75
Methylprednisolone (as Methylprednisolone sodium succinate) 500 mg Methylprednisolone sodium succinate 500mg powder and solvent for solution for injection vials | 1 vial [PoM] £9.60 DT = £9.60
Methylprednisolone (as Methylprednisolone sodium succinate) 1 gram Methylprednisolone sodium succinate 1g powder and solvent for solution for injection vials | 1 vial [PoM] £17.30 DT = £17.30
▶ **Solu-Medrone** (Pfizer Ltd)
Methylprednisolone (as Methylprednisolone sodium succinate) 40 mg Solu-Medrone 40mg powder and solvent for solution for injection vials | 1 vial [PoM] £1.58 DT = £1.58
Methylprednisolone (as Methylprednisolone sodium succinate) 125 mg Solu-Medrone 125mg powder and solvent for solution for injection vials | 1 vial [PoM] £4.75 DT = £4.75
Methylprednisolone (as Methylprednisolone sodium succinate) 500 mg Solu-Medrone 500mg powder and solvent for solution for injection vials | 1 vial [PoM] £9.60 DT = £9.60
Methylprednisolone (as Methylprednisolone sodium succinate) 1 gram Solu-Medrone 1g powder and solvent for solution for injection vials | 1 vial [PoM] £17.30 DT = £17.30

Suspension for injection
CAUTIONARY AND ADVISORY LABELS 10
▶ **Depo-Medrone** (Pfizer Ltd)
Methylprednisolone acetate 40 mg per 1 ml Depo-Medrone 40mg/1ml suspension for injection vials | 1 vial [PoM] £3.44 DT = £3.44 | 10 vial [PoM] £34.04
Depo-Medrone 80mg/2ml suspension for injection vials | 1 vial [PoM] £6.18 DT = £6.18 | 10 vial [PoM] £61.39
Depo-Medrone 120mg/3ml suspension for injection vials | 1 vial [PoM] £8.96 DT = £8.96 | 10 vial [PoM] £88.81

F 783

Prednisolone

24-Jun-2024

- **DRUG ACTION** Prednisolone exerts predominantly glucocorticoid effects with minimal mineralocorticoid effects.

- **INDICATIONS AND DOSE**

Acute exacerbation of chronic obstructive pulmonary disease (if increased breathlessness interferes with daily activities)
▶ BY MOUTH
▶ Adult: 30 mg once daily for 5 days

Severe croup (before transfer to hospital) | Mild croup that might cause complications (before transfer to hospital)
▶ BY MOUTH
▶ Child: 1–2 mg/kg

Mild to moderate acute asthma (when oral corticosteroid taken for more than a few days) | Severe or life-threatening acute asthma (when oral corticosteroid taken for more than a few days)
▶ BY MOUTH
▶ Child 1 month-11 years: 2 mg/kg once daily (max. per dose 60 mg) for up to 3 days, longer if necessary

Mild to moderate acute asthma | Severe or life-threatening acute asthma
▶ BY MOUTH
▶ Child 1 month-11 years: 1–2 mg/kg once daily (max. per dose 40 mg) for up to 3 days, longer if necessary
▶ Child 12-17 years: 40–50 mg once daily for at least 5 days
▶ Adult: 40–50 mg once daily for at least 5 days

Suppression of inflammatory and allergic disorders
▶ BY MOUTH
▶ Adult: Initially 10–20 mg once daily, dose preferably taken in the morning after breakfast, dose can often be reduced within a few days but may need to be continued for several weeks or months; maintenance 2.5–15 mg per day, higher doses may be needed; cushingoid side-effects increasingly likely with doses above 7.5 mg per day

Suppression of inflammatory and allergic disorders (initial dose in severe disease)
▶ BY MOUTH
▶ Adult: Initially up to 60 mg once daily, dose preferably taken in the morning after breakfast, dose can often be reduced within a few days but may need to be continued for several weeks or months

Idiopathic thrombocytopenic purpura
▶ BY MOUTH
▶ Adult: 1 mg/kg daily, gradually reduce dose over several weeks

Ulcerative colitis | Crohn's disease
▶ BY MOUTH
▶ Adult: Initially 20–40 mg once daily until remission occurs, followed by reducing doses, doses preferably taken in the morning after breakfast, doses up to 60 mg per day may be used in some cases   continued →

Neuritic pain or weakness heralding rapid onset of permanent nerve damage (during reversal reactions multibacillary leprosy)
▶ BY MOUTH
▶ Adult: Initially 40–60 mg daily, dose to be instituted at once

Generalised myasthenia gravis (when given on alternate days)
▶ BY MOUTH
▶ Adult: Initially 10 mg once daily on alternate days, dose then increased in steps of 10 mg once daily on alternate days to 1–1.5 mg/kg once daily on alternate days (max. per dose 100 mg)

Generalised myasthenia gravis in ventilated patients (when given on alternate days)
▶ BY MOUTH
▶ Adult: Initially 1.5 mg/kg once daily on alternate days (max. per dose 100 mg)

Generalised myasthenia gravis (when giving daily)
▶ BY MOUTH
▶ Adult: Initially 5 mg daily, increased in steps of 5 mg daily. maintenance 60–80 mg daily, alternatively maintenance 0.75–1 mg/kg daily, ventilated patients may be started on 1.5 mg/kg (max. 100 mg) on alternate days

Ocular myasthenia
▶ BY MOUTH
▶ Adult: Usual dose 10–40 mg once daily on alternate days, reduce to minimum effective dose

Reduction in rate of joint destruction in moderate to severe rheumatoid arthritis of less than 2 years' duration
▶ BY MOUTH
▶ Adult: 7.5 mg daily

Polymyalgia rheumatica
▶ BY MOUTH
▶ Adult: 10–15 mg daily until remission of disease activity; maintenance 7.5–10 mg daily, reduce gradually to maintenance dose. Many patients require treatment for at least 2 years and in some patients it may be necessary to continue long term low-dose corticosteroid treatment

Giant cell (temporal) arteritis
▶ BY MOUTH
▶ Adult: 40–60 mg daily until remission of disease activity, the higher dose being used if visual symptoms occur; maintenance 7.5–10 mg daily, reduce gradually to maintenance dose. Many patients require treatment for at least 2 years and in some patients it may be necessary to continue long term low-dose corticosteroid treatment

Polyarteritis nodosa | Polymyositis | Systemic lupus erythematosus
▶ BY MOUTH
▶ Adult: Initially 60 mg daily, to be reduced gradually; maintenance 10–15 mg daily

Symptom control of anorexia in palliative care
▶ BY MOUTH
▶ Adult: 15–30 mg daily

Pneumocystis pneumonia in moderate to severe infections associated with HIV infection
▶ BY MOUTH
▶ Adult: 50–80 mg daily for 5 days, the dose is then reduced to complete 21 days of treatment, corticosteroid treatment should ideally be started at the same time as the anti-pneumocystis therapy and certainly no later than 24–72 hours afterwards. The corticosteroid should be withdrawn before anti-pneumocystis treatment is complete

Short-term prophylaxis of episodic cluster headache as monotherapy or in combination with verapamil during verapamil titration
▶ BY MOUTH
▶ Adult: 60–100 mg once daily for 2–5 days, dose then reduced in steps of 10 mg every 2–3 days until prednisolone is discontinued

Proctitis
▶ BY RECTUM USING RECTAL FOAM
▶ Adult: 1 metered application 1–2 times a day for 2 weeks, continued for further 2 weeks if good response, to be inserted into the rectum, 1 metered application contains 20 mg prednisolone
▶ BY RECTUM USING SUPPOSITORIES
▶ Adult: 5 mg twice daily, to be inserted into the rectum morning and night, after a bowel movement

Distal ulcerative colitis
▶ BY RECTUM USING RECTAL FOAM
▶ Adult: 1 metered application 1–2 times a day for 2 weeks, continued for further 2 weeks if good response, to be inserted into the rectum, 1 metered application contains 20 mg prednisolone

Rectal complications of Crohn's disease
▶ BY RECTUM USING SUPPOSITORIES
▶ Adult: 5 mg twice daily, to be inserted into the rectum morning and night, after a bowel movement

Rectal and rectosigmoidal ulcerative colitis | Rectal and rectosigmoidal Crohn's disease
▶ BY RECTUM USING ENEMA
▶ Adult: 20 mg once daily for 2–4 weeks, continued if response good, to be used at bedtime

COVID-19 requiring supplemental oxygen [when dexamethasone cannot be used or is unavailable]
▶ BY MOUTH
▶ Adult: 40 mg once daily for 10 days, or until the day of discharge if this is sooner

---

IMPORTANT SAFETY INFORMATION

SAFE PRACTICE
▶ With systemic use
Prednisolone has been confused with propranolol; care must be taken to ensure the correct drug is prescribed and dispensed.

● CONTRA-INDICATIONS
▶ With rectal use Abdominal or local infection · bowel perforation · extensive fistulas · intestinal obstruction · recent intestinal anastomoses

● CAUTIONS
▶ With rectal use Systemic absorption may occur with rectal preparations
▶ With systemic use Duchenne's muscular dystrophy (possible transient rhabdomyolysis and myoglobinuria following strenuous physical activity) · systemic sclerosis (increased incidence of scleroderma renal crisis with a daily dose of 15 mg or more)

● INTERACTIONS → Appendix 1: corticosteroids

● SIDE-EFFECTS
▶ With oral use Diarrhoea · dizziness · dyslipidaemia · fatigue · insomnia · lipomatosis · malaise · protein catabolism · scleroderma renal crisis · telangiectasia

SIDE-EFFECTS, FURTHER INFORMATION Since systemic absorption can follow rectal use, also consider the side-effects of systemic corticosteroids.

● PREGNANCY As it crosses the placenta 88% of prednisolone is inactivated.
Monitoring ▶ With systemic use Pregnant women with fluid retention should be monitored closely.

- **BREAST FEEDING** Prednisolone appears in small amounts in breast milk but maternal doses of up to 40 mg daily are unlikely to cause systemic effects in the infant.
  Monitoring ▸ With systemic use Infant should be monitored for adrenal suppression if mother is taking a dose higher than 40 mg.
- **MONITORING REQUIREMENTS**
▸ With systemic use Manufacturer advises monitor blood pressure and renal function (s-creatinine) routinely in patients with systemic sclerosis—increased incidence of scleroderma renal crisis.
▸ With oral use in children [EvGr] Monitor blood pressure and urinary glucose weekly. (A)
- **PRESCRIBING AND DISPENSING INFORMATION**
▸ When used for Asthma For choice of therapy, see Asthma, acute p. 274 and Asthma, chronic p. 271.

  Palliative care For further information on the use of prednisolone in palliative care, see www.medicinescomplete. com/#/content/palliative/systemic-corticosteroids.
- **PATIENT AND CARER ADVICE**
  Medicines for Children leaflet: Prednisolone for asthma
  www.medicinesforchildren.org.uk/medicines/prednisolone-for-asthma/

- **MEDICINAL FORMS** There can be variation in the licensing of different medicines containing the same drug. Forms available from special-order manufacturers include: oral suspension, oral solution, enema

Oral tablet
CAUTIONARY AND ADVISORY LABELS 10, 21
▸ Prednisolone (Non-proprietary)
  Prednisolone 500 microgram Prednisolone 500microgram tablets | 28 tablet [PoM] £4.75–£8.08 DT = £4.75
  Prednisolone 1 mg Prednisolone 1mg tablets | 28 tablet [PoM] £1.31 DT = £0.66 | 28 tablet [PoM] £0.20 DT = £0.66 (Hospital only)
  Prednisolone 2 mg Prednisolone 2mg tablets | 28 tablet [PoM] £5.00–£8.50 DT = £5.00
  Prednisolone 2.5 mg Prednisolone 2.5mg tablets | 28 tablet [PoM] £6.00 DT = £3.94
  Prednisolone 3 mg Prednisolone 3mg tablets | 28 tablet [PoM] £5.50–£9.36 DT = £5.50
  Prednisolone 4 mg Prednisolone 4mg tablets | 28 tablet [PoM] £5.75–£11.85
  Prednisolone 5 mg Prednisolone 5mg tablets | 28 tablet [PoM] £9.86 DT = £0.74 | 28 tablet [PoM] £0.28 DT = £0.74 (Hospital only)
  Prednisolone 10 mg Prednisolone 10mg tablets | 28 tablet [PoM] £14.60 DT = £9.70
  Prednisolone 20 mg Prednisolone 20mg tablets | 28 tablet [PoM] £29.40 DT = £19.46
  Prednisolone 25 mg Prednisolone 25mg tablets | 56 tablet [PoM] £50.00 DT = £50.00
  Prednisolone 30 mg Prednisolone 30mg tablets | 28 tablet [PoM] £29.12–£47.00 DT = £29.12

Gastro-resistant tablet
CAUTIONARY AND ADVISORY LABELS 5, 10, 25
▸ Prednisolone (Non-proprietary)
  Prednisolone 1 mg Prednisolone 1mg gastro-resistant tablets | 100 tablet [PoM] £32.49–£51.70 DT = £32.49
  Prednisolone 2.5 mg Prednisolone 2.5mg gastro-resistant tablets | 28 tablet [PoM] £3.90 DT = £1.06 | 30 tablet [PoM] £1.14–£1.30
  Prednisolone 5 mg Prednisolone 5mg gastro-resistant tablets | 28 tablet [PoM] £6.50 DT = £1.17 | 30 tablet [PoM] £1.25–£4.12
▸ Dilacort (Crescent Pharma Ltd)
  Prednisolone 2.5 mg Dilacort 2.5mg gastro-resistant tablets | 28 tablet [PoM] £1.14 DT = £1.06
  Prednisolone 5 mg Dilacort 5mg gastro-resistant tablets | 28 tablet [PoM] £1.41 DT = £1.17

Soluble tablet
CAUTIONARY AND ADVISORY LABELS 10, 13, 21
▸ Prednisolone (Non-proprietary)
  Prednisolone (as Prednisolone sodium phosphate)
  5 mg Prednisolone 5mg soluble tablets sugar free | 30 tablet [PoM] £71.13 DT = £53.48 [SF]

Suppository
▸ Prednisolone (Non-proprietary)
  Prednisolone (as Prednisolone sodium phosphate)
  5 mg Prednisolone sodium phosphate 5mg suppositories | 10 suppository [PoM] £263.78 DT = £250.57

Rectal foam
▸ Prednisolone (Non-proprietary)
  Prednisolone (as Prednisolone sodium metasulfobenzoate)
  20 mg per 1 application Prednisolone 20mg/application foam enema | 14 dose [PoM] £237.00–£334.44 DT = £439.11

Oral solution
CAUTIONARY AND ADVISORY LABELS 10
▸ Prednisolone (Non-proprietary)
  Prednisolone 1 mg per 1 ml Prednisolone 5mg/5ml oral solution unit dose | 10 unit dose [PoM] £11.41 DT = £16.45
  Prednisolone 10 mg per 1 ml Prednisolone 10mg/ml oral solution sugar free | 30 ml [PoM] £55.50–£100.00 DT = £55.50 [SF]

Enema
▸ Prednisolone (Non-proprietary)
  Prednisolone sodium phosphate 200 microgram per 1 ml Prednisolone 20mg/100ml rectal solution | 7 enema [PoM] £29.95 DT = £29.95

▸ **783**

Triamcinolone acetonide
20-Jul-2023

- **DRUG ACTION** Triamcinolone exerts predominantly glucocorticoid effects with minimal mineralcorticoid effect.

- **INDICATIONS AND DOSE**
Suppression of inflammatory and allergic disorders
▸ BY DEEP INTRAMUSCULAR INJECTION
▸ Adult: 40 mg (max. per dose 100 mg), repeated if necessary, dose given for depot effect, to be administered into gluteal muscle; repeated at intervals according to patient's response

- **CAUTIONS** High dosage (may cause proximal myopathy), avoid in chronic therapy
- **INTERACTIONS** → Appendix 1: corticosteroids
- **SIDE-EFFECTS**
▸ **Uncommon** Dizziness · fatigue · flushing · hyperglycaemia · hypotension · insomnia

- **MEDICINAL FORMS** There can be variation in the licensing of different medicines containing the same drug.
Suspension for injection
CAUTIONARY AND ADVISORY LABELS 10
EXCIPIENTS: May contain Benzyl alcohol
▸ Triamcinolone acetonide (Non-proprietary)
  Triamcinolone acetonide 10 mg per 1 ml Triamcinolone acetonide 10mg/1ml suspension for injection ampoules | 1 ampoule [PoM] [℞]
  Triamcinolone acetonide 40 mg per 1 ml Triamcinolone acetonide 40mg/1ml suspension for injection vials | 1 vial [PoM] [℞]
▸ Kenalog (Bristol-Myers Squibb Pharmaceuticals Ltd)
  Triamcinolone acetonide 40 mg per 1 ml Kenalog Intra-articular / Intramuscular 40mg/1ml suspension for injection vials | 5 vial [PoM] £7.45 DT = £7.45

3.1 Cushing's syndrome and disease

Cushing's syndrome
07-Apr-2021

Management
Cushing's syndrome results from chronic exposure to excess cortisol; exogenous corticosteroid use is the most common cause. Endogenous causes include adrenocorticotrophic hormone (ACTH)-secreting pituitary tumours (Cushing's disease), cortisol-secreting adrenal tumours, and rarely,

ectopic ACTH-secreting tumours. Most types of endogenous Cushing's syndrome are treated surgically.

Metyrapone p. 795 is licensed for the management of Cushing's syndrome.

Ketoconazole below is licensed for the treatment of endogenous Cushing's syndrome.

> **Other drugs used for Cushing's syndrome and disease**
> Pasireotide, p. 1082

ENZYME INHIBITORS

Ketoconazole
30-May-2023

- **DRUG ACTION** An imidazole derivative which acts as a potent inhibitor of cortisol and aldosterone synthesis by inhibiting the activity of 17α-hydroxylase, 11-hydroxylation steps and at higher doses the cholesterol side-chain cleavage enzyme. It also inhibits the activity of adrenal C17-20 lyase enzymes resulting in androgen synthesis inhibition, and may have a direct effect on corticotropic tumour cells in patients with Cushing's disease.

- **INDICATIONS AND DOSE**

Endogenous Cushing's syndrome (specialist use only)
> BY MOUTH
> Adult: Initially 400–600 mg daily in 2–3 divided doses, increased to 800–1200 mg daily; maintenance 400–800 mg daily in 2–3 divided doses, for dose titrations in patients with established dose, adjustments in adrenal insufficiency, or concomitant corticosteroid replacement therapy, consult product literature; maximum 1200 mg per day

DOSE ADJUSTMENTS DUE TO INTERACTIONS
> EvGr Max. dose 200 mg daily with concurrent use of cobicistat-boosted regimens. Ⓜ

IMPORTANT SAFETY INFORMATION

CHMP ADVICE: KETOCONAZOLE (JULY 2013)
The CHMP has recommended that the marketing authorisation for oral ketoconazole to treat fungal infections should be suspended. The CHMP concluded that the risk of hepatotoxicity associated with oral ketoconazole is greater than the benefit in treating fungal infections. Doctors should review patients who are being treated with oral ketoconazole for fungal infections, with a view to stopping treatment or choosing an alternative treatment. Patients with a prescription of oral ketoconazole for fungal infections should be referred back to their doctors.

Oral ketoconazole for Cushing's syndrome and topical products containing ketoconazole are not affected by this advice.

- **CONTRA-INDICATIONS** Acquired QTc prolongation · Acute porphyrias p. 1202 · avoid concomitant use of hepatotoxic drugs · congenital QTc prolongation

- **CAUTIONS** Pre-treatment liver enzymes should not exceed 2 times the normal upper limit · risk of adrenal insufficiency

- **INTERACTIONS** → Appendix 1: antifungals, azoles

- **SIDE-EFFECTS**
> **Common or very common** Adrenal insufficiency · diarrhoea · gastrointestinal discomfort · nausea · skin reactions · vomiting
> **Uncommon** Allergic conditions · alopecia · angioedema · asthenia · dizziness · drowsiness · headache · thrombocytopenia
> **Rare or very rare** Fever · hepatic disorders · taste altered

> **Frequency not known** Alcohol intolerance · appetite abnormal · arthralgia · azoospermia · dry mouth · epistaxis · flatulence · fontanelle bulging · gynaecomastia · hot flush · insomnia · intracranial pressure increased · malaise · menstrual disorder · myalgia · nervousness · papilloedema · paraesthesia · peripheral oedema · photophobia · photosensitivity reaction · tongue discolouration

SIDE-EFFECTS, FURTHER INFORMATION Potentially life-threatening hepatotoxicity reported rarely with oral use. Manufacturer advises reduce dose if hepatic enzymes increased to less than 3 times the upper limit of normal—consult product literature; discontinue permanently if hepatic enzymes at least 3 times the upper limit of normal.

- **CONCEPTION AND CONTRACEPTION** Effective contraception must be used in women of child-bearing potential.

- **PREGNANCY** Manufacturer advises avoid—teratogenic in *animal* studies.

- **BREAST FEEDING** Manufacturer advises avoid—present in breast milk.

- **HEPATIC IMPAIRMENT** Manufacturer advises avoid.

- **MONITORING REQUIREMENTS**
> Monitor ECG before and one week after initiation, and then as clinically indicated thereafter.
> Adrenal insufficiency Monitor adrenal function within one week of initiation, then regularly thereafter. When cortisol levels are normalised or close to target and effective dose established, monitor every 3–6 months as there is a risk of autoimmune disease development or exacerbation after normalisation of cortisol levels. If symptoms suggestive of adrenal insufficiency such as fatigue, anorexia, nausea, vomiting, hypotension, hyponatraemia, hyperkalaemia, and/or hypoglycaemia occur, measure cortisol levels and discontinue treatment temporarily (can be resumed thereafter at lower dose) or reduce dose and if necessary, initiate corticosteroid substitution.
> Hepatotoxicity Monitor liver function before initiation of treatment, then weekly for 1 month after initiation, then monthly for 6 months—more frequently if dose adjusted or abnormal liver function detected.

- **PATIENT AND CARER ADVICE** Patients or their carers should be told how to recognise signs of liver disorder, and advised to discontinue treatment and seek prompt medical attention if symptoms such as anorexia, nausea, vomiting, fatigue, jaundice, abdominal pain, or dark urine develop. Patients or their carers should also be told how to recognise signs of adrenal insufficiency.
Driving and skilled tasks Dizziness and somnolence may affect the performance of skilled tasks (e.g. driving).

- **MEDICINAL FORMS** There can be variation in the licensing of different medicines containing the same drug. Forms available from special-order manufacturers include: oral suspension

Oral tablet
CAUTIONARY AND ADVISORY LABELS 2, 5, 21
> **Ketoconazole (non-proprietary)** ▼
> **Ketoconazole 200 mg** Ketoconazole 200mg tablets | 60 tablet PoM £515.00 DT = £515.00

Metyrapone
14-Dec-2020

- **DRUG ACTION** Metyrapone is a competitive inhibitor of 11β-hydroxylation in the adrenal cortex; the resulting inhibition of cortisol (and to a lesser extent aldosterone) production leads to an increase in ACTH production which, in turn, leads to increased synthesis and release of cortisol precursors. Metyrapone may be used as a test of anterior pituitary function.

- **INDICATIONS AND DOSE**

Differential diagnosis of ACTH-dependent Cushing's syndrome (specialist supervision in hospital)
  - ▶ BY MOUTH
  - ▶ Adult: 750 mg every 4 hours for 6 doses

Management of Cushing's syndrome (specialist supervision in hospital)
  - ▶ BY MOUTH
  - ▶ Adult: Usual dose 0.25–6 g daily, dose to be tailored to cortisol production, dose is either low, and tailored to cortisol production, or high, in which case corticosteroid replacement therapy is also needed

Resistant oedema due to increased aldosterone secretion in cirrhosis, nephrotic syndrome, and congestive heart failure (with glucocorticoid replacement therapy) (specialist supervision in hospital)
  - ▶ BY MOUTH
  - ▶ Adult: 3 g daily in divided doses

- **CONTRA-INDICATIONS** Adrenocortical insufficiency

- **CAUTIONS** Avoid in Acute porphyrias p. 1202 · gross hypopituitarism (risk of precipitating acute adrenal failure) · hypertension on long-term administration · hypothyroidism (delayed response)

- **INTERACTIONS** → Appendix 1: metyrapone

- **SIDE-EFFECTS**
  - ▶ **Common or very common** Dizziness · headache · hypotension · nausea · sedation · vomiting
  - ▶ **Rare or very rare** Abdominal pain · adrenal insufficiency · allergic dermatitis · hirsutism
  - ▶ **Frequency not known** Alopecia · bone marrow failure · hypertension

- **PREGNANCY** Avoid (may impair biosynthesis of fetal-placental steroids).

- **BREAST FEEDING** Avoid—no information available.

- **HEPATIC IMPAIRMENT** Manufacturer advises caution (risk of delayed response).

- **PATIENT AND CARER ADVICE**
Driving and skilled tasks Drowsiness may affect the performance of skilled tasks (e.g. driving).

- **MEDICINAL FORMS** There can be variation in the licensing of different medicines containing the same drug.
Oral capsule
CAUTIONARY AND ADVISORY LABELS 21
  - ▶ Metyrapone (Non-proprietary)
    Metyrapone 250 mg Metyrapone 250mg capsules | 100 capsule [PoM] £438.57 DT = £438.57

Osilodrostat
30-Jun-2021

- **DRUG ACTION** Osilodrostat is a potent inhibitor of 11β-hydroxylase, the enzyme that catalyses the last step of cortisol synthesis in the adrenal gland, thereby lowering cortisol levels.

- **INDICATIONS AND DOSE**

Endogenous Cushing's syndrome (under expert supervision)
  - ▶ BY MOUTH
  - ▶ Adult: 2 mg twice daily, increased, if tolerated, in steps of 1–2 mg initially, no more frequently than once every 1–2 weeks, adjusted according to response; usual maintenance 2–7 mg twice daily (max. per dose 30 mg twice daily), for dose reduction or treatment interruption due to low cortisol levels or QT-interval prolongation—consult product literature
  - ▶ Adult (patients of Asian origin): 1 mg twice daily, increased, if tolerated, in steps of 1–2 mg initially, no more frequently than once every 1–2 weeks, adjusted according to response; usual maintenance 2–7 mg twice daily (max. per dose 30 mg twice daily), for dose reduction or treatment interruption due to low cortisol levels or QT-interval prolongation—consult product literature.

- **CAUTIONS** Patients of Asian origin (increased bioavailability) · risk factors for QT-interval prolongation

- **INTERACTIONS** → Appendix 1: osilodrostat

- **SIDE-EFFECTS**
  - ▶ **Common or very common** Abdominal pain · adrenal hypofunction · appetite decreased · diarrhoea · dizziness · fatigue · headache · hirsutism · hypokalaemia · hypotension · malaise · nausea · oedema · QT interval prolongation · skin reactions · syncope · tachycardia · vomiting

- **CONCEPTION AND CONTRACEPTION** [EvGr] Females of childbearing potential should use effective contraception during treatment and for at least 1 week after last treatment. ⟨M⟩

- **PREGNANCY** [EvGr] Avoid—toxicity in *animal* studies. ⟨M⟩

- **BREAST FEEDING** [EvGr] Discontinue breast-feeding during treatment and for at least 1 week after last treatment—no information available. ⟨M⟩

- **HEPATIC IMPAIRMENT** [EvGr] Caution (limited information available)—consider more frequent monitoring of adrenal function during dose titration. ⟨M⟩
Dose adjustments [EvGr] In moderate impairment, a starting dose of 1 mg twice daily is recommended. In severe impairment, a starting dose of 1 mg once daily in the evening, increased initially to 1 mg twice daily, is recommended. ⟨M⟩

- **MONITORING REQUIREMENTS**
  - ▶ [EvGr] Measure cortisol levels every 1–2 weeks until adequate response maintained, and as clinically indicated thereafter, with additional monitoring during periods of increased cortisol demand. Dose reduction or treatment interruption may be required—consult product literature.
  - ▶ Obtain ECG prior to treatment, within the first week, and as clinically indicated thereafter; monitor more frequently if risk factors for QT-interval prolongation are present. If the QTc interval exceeds 480 milliseconds prior to or during treatment, cardiology consultation is recommended. Dose reduction or treatment interruption may be required—consult product literature.
  - ▶ Monitor electrolyte concentrations periodically during treatment. ⟨M⟩

- **PATIENT AND CARER ADVICE** Patients and carers should be counselled on the signs and symptoms of hypocortisolism.

Driving and skilled tasks Patients and carers should be cautioned on the effects on driving and performance of skilled tasks—increased risk of dizziness and fatigue.

● MEDICINAL FORMS There can be variation in the licensing of different medicines containing the same drug.

Oral tablet

▶ Isturisa (Recordati Rare Diseases UK Ltd) ▼

Osilodrostat (as Osilodrostat phosphate) **1 mg** Isturisa 1mg tablets | 60 tablet [PoM] £1,603.00 (Hospital only)

Osilodrostat (as Osilodrostat phosphate) **5 mg** Isturisa 5mg tablets | 60 tablet [PoM] £6,414.00 (Hospital only)

Osilodrostat (as Osilodrostat phosphate) **10 mg** Isturisa 10mg tablets | 60 tablet [PoM] £6,735.00 (Hospital only)

4 Diabetes mellitus and hypoglycaemia

4.1 Diabetes mellitus

Diabetes

10-Aug-2022

Description of condition

Diabetes mellitus is a group of metabolic disorders in which persistent hyperglycaemia is caused by deficient insulin secretion or by resistance to the action of insulin. This leads to the abnormalities of carbohydrate, fat and protein metabolism that are characteristic of diabetes mellitus.

Type 1 diabetes p. 797 and Type 2 diabetes p. 800 are the two most common classifications of diabetes. Other common types of diabetes are gestational diabetes (develops during pregnancy and resolves after delivery, see Diabetes, pregnancy and breast-feeding p. 805) and secondary diabetes (may be caused by pancreatic damage, hepatic cirrhosis, or endocrine disease). Treatment with endocrine, antiviral, or antipsychotic drugs may also cause secondary diabetes.

Driving

Drivers with diabetes may be required to notify the Driver and Vehicle Licensing Agency (DVLA) of their condition depending on their treatment, the type of licence they hold, and whether they have diabetic complications (including episodes of hypoglycaemia). All drivers who are treated with insulin must inform the DVLA, with some exceptions for temporary treatment. Detailed guidance on notification requirements, eligibility to drive, and precautions required, is available from the DVLA at www.gov.uk/guidance/diabetes-mellitus-assessing-fitness-to-drive.

Advice from the DVLA

The DVLA recommends (2022) that drivers with diabetes need to be particularly careful to avoid hypoglycaemia and should be informed of the warning signs and actions to take. Drivers treated with insulin should always carry a capillary blood-glucose meter and test strips when driving, even if they use a continuous glucose monitoring (CGM) system. Drivers using a CGM system who experience hypoglycemia symptoms or have a CGM reading of 4 mmol/litre or below, should confirm their blood-glucose concentration with a capillary blood-glucose reading. Blood-glucose concentration should be checked no more than 2 hours before driving and every 2 hours while driving. More frequent self-monitoring may be required if, for any reason, there is a greater risk of hypoglycaemia, such as after physical activity or altered meal routine.

Blood-glucose concentration should be at least 5 mmol/litre while driving. If blood-glucose is 5 mmol/litre or below, a snack should be taken. Drivers treated with insulin should ensure that a supply of fast-acting carbohydrate is always available in the vehicle. If blood-glucose is less than 4 mmol/litre, or warning signs of hypoglycaemia develop, the driver should not drive. If already driving, the driver should stop the vehicle in a safe place as soon as possible, and turn off the engine, remove the keys from the ignition, and move from the driver's seat; drivers should wait until 45 minutes after their blood-glucose has returned to normal (at least 5 mmol/litre), before continuing their journey.

Notification to the DVLA and monitoring of blood-glucose concentrations may also be necessary for some drivers taking oral antidiabetic drugs, particularly those which carry a risk of hypoglycaemia (e.g. sulfonylureas and meglitinides).

Drivers must not drive if hypoglycaemia awareness has been lost and the DVLA must be notified; driving may resume if a medical report confirms that awareness has been regained.

Note: additional criteria apply for drivers of large goods or passenger carrying vehicles—consult DVLA guidance.

Alcohol

Alcohol can make the signs of hypoglycaemia less clear, and can cause delayed hypoglycaemia; specialist sources recommend that patients with diabetes should drink alcohol only in moderation, and when accompanied by food.

Oral glucose tolerance tests

The oral glucose tolerance test is used mainly for diagnosis of impaired glucose tolerance; it is **not** recommended or necessary for routine diagnostic use when severe symptoms of hyperglycaemia are present. In patients who have less severe symptoms and a blood-glucose concentration that does not establish or exclude diabetes (e.g. impaired fasting glycaemia), an oral glucose tolerance test may be required. It is also used to establish the presence of gestational diabetes.

An oral glucose tolerance test involves measuring the blood-glucose concentration after fasting, and then 2 hours after drinking a standard anhydrous glucose drink. Anhydrous glucose may alternatively be given as the appropriate amount of *Polycal*® or as *Rapilose*® OGTT oral solution.

HbA1c measurement

Glycated haemoglobin (HbA1c) forms when red blood cells are exposed to glucose in the plasma. The HbA1c test reflects average plasma glucose over the previous 2 to 3 months and provides a good indicator of glycaemic control. Unlike the oral glucose tolerance test, an HbA1c test can be performed at any time of the day and does not require any special preparation such as fasting.

HbA1c values are expressed in *mmol of glycated haemoglobin per mol of haemoglobin (mmol/mol)*, a standardised unit specific for HbA1c created by the International Federation of Clinical Chemistry and Laboratory Medicine (IFCC). HbA1c values were previously aligned to the assay used in the Diabetes Control and Complications Trial (DCCT) and expressed as a percentage.

Equivalent values	
IFCC-HbA1c (mmol/mol)	DCCT-HbA1c (%)
42	6.0
48	6.5
53	7.0
59	7.5
64	8.0
69	8.5
75	9.0

Diagnosis

The HbA1c test is used for monitoring glycaemic control in both Type 1 diabetes p. 797 and Type 2 diabetes p. 800 and is now also used for diagnosis of type 2 diabetes. EvGr HbA1c should not be used for diagnosis in those with suspected type 1 diabetes, in children, during pregnancy, or in women who are up to two months postpartum. It should also not be used for patients who have:

- had symptoms of diabetes for less than 2 months;
- a high diabetes risk and are acutely ill;
- treatment with medication that may cause hyperglycaemia;
- acute pancreatic damage;
- end-stage chronic kidney disease;
- HIV infection.

HbA1c used for diagnosis of diabetes should be interpreted with caution in patients with abnormal haemoglobin, anaemia, altered red cell lifespan, or who have had a recent blood transfusion. A

Monitoring

EvGr HbA1c is also a reliable predictor of microvascular and macrovascular complications and mortality. Lower HbA1c is associated with a lower risk of long term vascular complications and patients should be supported to aim for an individualised HbA1c target (see Type 1 diabetes below and Type 2 diabetes p. 800).

HbA1c should usually be measured in patients with type 1 diabetes every 3 to 6 months, and more frequently if blood-glucose control is thought to be changing rapidly. Patients with type 2 diabetes should be monitored every 3 to 6 months until HbA1c and medication are stable when monitoring can be reduced to every 6 months. A

HbA1c monitoring is invalid for patients with disturbed erythrocyte turnover or for patients with a lack of, or abnormal haemoglobin. In these cases, quality-controlled plasma glucose profiles, total glycated haemoglobin estimation (if there is abnormal haemoglobin), or fructosamine estimation can be used.

Laboratory measurement of fructosamine concentration measures the glycated fraction of all plasma proteins over the previous 14 to 21 days but is a less accurate measure of glycaemic control than HbA1c.

Type 1 diabetes

17-Apr-2024

Description of condition

Type 1 diabetes describes an absolute insulin deficiency in which there is little or no endogenous insulin secretory capacity due to destruction of insulin-producing beta-cells in the pancreatic islets of Langerhans. This form of the disease has an auto-immune basis in most cases, and it can occur at any age, but most commonly before adulthood.

Loss of insulin secretion results in hyperglycaemia and other metabolic abnormalities. If poorly managed, the resulting tissue damage has both short-term and long-term adverse effects on health; this can result in retinopathy, nephropathy, neuropathy, premature cardiovascular disease, and peripheral arterial disease.

Typical features in adult patients presenting with type 1 diabetes are hyperglycaemia (random blood-glucose concentration above 11 mmol/litre), ketosis, rapid weight loss, a body mass index below 25 kg/m^2, age younger than 50 years, and a personal/family history of autoimmune disease (though not all features may be present).

Aims of treatment

Treatment is aimed at using insulin regimens to achieve as optimal a level of blood-glucose control as is feasible, while avoiding or reducing the frequency of hypoglycaemic episodes, in order to minimise the risk of long-term microvascular and macrovascular complications.

Disability from complications can often be prevented by early detection and active management of the disease (see

Diabetic complications p. 802). EvGr The target for glycaemic control should be individualised for each patient, considering factors such as daily activities, aspirations, likelihood of complications, adherence to treatment, comorbidities, occupation, and history of hypoglycaemia.

Aim for a target glycated haemoglobin (HbA1c) level of 48 mmol/mol (6.5%) or lower in patients with type 1 diabetes. A For further information on HbA1c, including monitoring frequency, see Diabetes p. 796.

EvGr Continuous glucose monitoring (CGM) should be offered to support patients to self-manage their diabetes. Patients using CGM will still need to take capillary blood-glucose measurements, but can do this less often. Patients unwilling to or unable to use CGM should be offered capillary blood-glucose monitoring and be advised to measure their blood-glucose concentration at least four times a day, including before each meal and before bed. Patients should aim for:

- a fasting blood-glucose concentration of 5–7 mmol/litre on waking;
- a blood-glucose concentration of 4–7 mmol/litre before meals at other times of the day;
- a blood-glucose concentration of 5–9 mmol/litre at least 90 minutes after eating; A
- a blood-glucose concentration of at least 5 mmol/litre when driving, as recommended by the Driver and Vehicle Licensing Agency (DVLA).

For further guidance on blood-glucose management, see NICE guideline: **Type 1 diabetes in adults: diagnosis and management** (see *Useful resources*).

Management

EvGr Type 1 diabetes requires insulin replacement, supported by active management of other cardiovascular risk factors, such as hypertension and high circulating lipids (see Diabetic complications p. 802). A Insulin replacement therapy aims to recreate normal fluctuations in circulating insulin concentrations while supporting a flexible lifestyle with minimal restrictions. Flexible insulin therapy usually involves self-injecting multiple daily doses of insulin, with doses adjusted according to planned exercise, intended food intake and other factors, including current blood-glucose, which the patient needs to test on a regular basis.

EvGr In patients who have a BMI of 25 kg/m^2 or above (23 kg/m^2 or above for patients of South Asian or related ethnicity) who wish to improve their blood-glucose control while minimising their effective insulin dose, consider metformin hydrochloride p. 807 [unlicensed indication] as an addition to insulin therapy. A EvGr The dose of standard-release metformin should be increased gradually to minimise the risk of gastro-intestinal side-effects. E EvGr Modified-release metformin should be offered if the patient experiences gastro-intestinal side-effects with standard treatment.

Dietary control is important in both type 1 and type 2 diabetes and patients should receive advice from a dietitian. Dietary advice should include information on weight control, cardiovascular risk, hyperglycaemic effects of different foods and appropriate changes in insulin doses according to food intake. Healthy eating can reduce cardiovascular risk and dietary modifications may be recommended to account for various associated features of diabetes such as excess weight and obesity, low body-weight, disordered eating, hypertension, and renal failure. Patients with type 1 diabetes should be offered carbohydrate-counting training as part of a structured education programme. A

Insulin therapy in type 1 diabetes

EvGr All patients with type 1 diabetes require insulin therapy (**see also Insulin p. 799**). Treatment should be initiated and managed by clinicians with relevant expertise; there are several different types of regimens. A

Multiple daily injection basal-bolus insulin regimens
One or more separate daily injections of intermediate-acting insulin or long-acting insulin analogue as the basal insulin; alongside multiple bolus injections of short-acting insulin before meals. This regimen offers flexibility to tailor insulin therapy with the carbohydrate load of each meal.

Mixed (biphasic) regimen
One, two, or three insulin injections per day of short-acting insulin mixed with intermediate-acting insulin. The insulin preparations may be mixed by the patient at the time of injection, or a premixed product can be used.

Continuous subcutaneous insulin infusion (insulin pump)
A regular or continuous amount of insulin (usually in the form of a rapid-acting insulin analogue or soluble insulin), delivered by a programmable pump and insulin storage reservoir via a subcutaneous needle or cannula.

Recommended insulin regimens
[EvGr] Patients with type 1 diabetes should be offered multiple daily injection basal-bolus insulin regimens as the **first-line choice**. Twice-daily insulin detemir p. 839 should be offered as the long-acting basal insulin therapy, unless the patient is already meeting their agreed treatment goals on another insulin regimen. Once-daily insulin glargine (100 units/ml) p. 839 may be prescribed if insulin detemir is not tolerated, or if a twice-daily regimen is not acceptable to the patient. Insulin degludec p. 838 may also be offered as an alternative once-daily regimen if there is particular concern about nocturnal hypoglycaemia. A once-daily ultra-long acting insulin (such as insulin degludec, or insulin glargine 300 units/ml) may be offered as an alternative for patients who need help with injection administration from a carer or healthcare professional.

Other basal insulin regimens should be considered only if the recommended regimens do not deliver agreed treatment goals. Non-basal-bolus insulin regimens (e.g. twice-daily mixed [biphasic], basal-only, or bolus-only regimens) are **not** recommended for adults with *newly diagnosed* type 1 diabetes.

A rapid-acting insulin analogue is recommended as the mealtime insulin replacement, rather than soluble human insulin or animal insulin (rarely used). The rapid-acting insulin analogue should be injected before meals—routine use after meals should be discouraged. Patients who have a strong preference for an alternative mealtime insulin should be offered their preferred insulin.

Alternatively, if a multiple daily injection basal–bolus regimen is not possible, a twice-daily mixed insulin regimen should be considered if it is preferred.

In patients who are using a twice-daily *human* mixed insulin regimen and have hypoglycaemia that affects their quality of life, a trial of a twice-daily analogue mixed insulin regimen should be considered.

Continuous subcutaneous insulin infusion (insulin pump) therapy, should only be offered to patients who suffer disabling hypoglycaemia while attempting to achieve their target HbA1c level, or, who have high HbA1c levels (69 mmol/mol [8.5%] or above) with multiple daily injection therapy (including, if appropriate, the use of long-acting insulin analogues) despite a high level of care. Insulin pump therapy should be initiated by a specialist team. ⟨A⟩

Insulin requirements
[EvGr] The dosage of insulin must be determined individually for each patient and should be adjusted as necessary according to the results of regular monitoring of blood-glucose concentrations. ⟨A⟩

Persistent poor glucose control, leading to erratic insulin requirements or episodes of hypoglycaemia, may be due to many factors, including adherence, injection technique, injection site problems, blood-glucose monitoring skills, lifestyle issues (including diet, exercise and alcohol intake), psychological issues, and organic causes such as renal disease, thyroid disorders, coeliac disease, Addison's disease or gastroparesis. These factors should be considered before changes are made to a previously optimised regimen.

Infection, stress, accidental or surgical trauma can all increase the required insulin dose. Insulin requirements may be decreased (and therefore susceptibility to hypoglycaemia increased) by physical activity, intercurrent illness, reduced food intake, impaired renal function, and in certain endocrine disorders.

Risks of hypoglycaemia with insulin
[EvGr] Hypoglycaemia is an inevitable adverse effect of insulin treatment, and patients should be advised of the warning signs and actions to take (for guidance on management, see Hypoglycaemia p. 845).

Impaired awareness of hypoglycaemia can occur when the ability to recognise usual symptoms is lost, or when the symptoms are blunted or no longer present. Patients' awareness of hypoglycaemia should be assessed annually using the Gold score or the Clarke score. ⟨A⟩

An increase in the frequency of hypoglycaemic episodes may reduce the warning symptoms experienced by the patient. Impaired awareness of symptoms below 3 mmol/litre is associated with a significantly increased risk of severe hypoglycaemia. Beta-blockers can also blunt hypoglycaemic awareness, by reducing warning signs such as tremor.

Loss of warning of hypoglycaemia among insulin-treated patients can be a serious hazard, especially for drivers and those in dangerous occupations. Advice should be given in line with the Driver and Vehicle Licensing Agency (DVLA) guidance (see *Driving* under Diabetes p. 796).

[EvGr] To restore the warning signs, episodes of hypoglycaemia must be minimised. Insulin regimens, doses and blood-glucose targets should be reviewed and continuous subcutaneous insulin infusion therapy and real-time continuous blood-glucose monitoring should be considered. Patients should receive structured education to ensure they are following the principles of a flexible insulin regimen correctly, with additional education regarding avoiding and treating hypoglycaemia for those who continue to have impaired awareness. Relaxation of individualised blood-glucose targets should be avoided as a strategy to improve impaired hypoglycaemia awareness. If recurrent severe episodes of hypoglycaemia continue despite appropriate interventions, the patient should be referred to a specialist centre. ⟨A⟩

There is conflicting evidence regarding reports that some patients may experience loss of awareness of hypoglycaemia after transfer from animal to human insulin; clinical studies do not confirm that human insulin decreases hypoglycaemia awareness.

Manufacturers advise any switch between brands or formulation of insulin (including switching from animal to human insulin) should be done under strict supervision; a change in dose may be required.

Hypodermic equipment

[EvGr] Patients should be advised on the safe disposal of lancets, single-use syringes, and needles, and should be provided with suitable disposal containers. Arrangements should be made for the suitable disposal of these containers. ⟨A⟩

Lancets, needles, syringes, and accessories are listed under Hypodermic Equipment in Part IXA of the Drug Tariff (Part III of the Northern Ireland Drug Tariff, Part 3 of the Scottish Drug Tariff). The Drug Tariffs can be access online at:

• National Health Service Drug Tariff for England and Wales:
www.nhsbsa.nhs.uk/pharmacies-gp-practices-and-appliance-contractors/drug-tariff

• Health and Personal Social Services for Northern Ireland Drug Tariff:
hscbusiness.hscni.net/services/2034.htm

- Scottish Drug Tariff:
publichealthscotland.scot/services/scottish-drug-tariff/
introduction-and-contents/

Useful Resources

Type 1 diabetes in adults: diagnosis and management.
National Institute for Health and Care Excellence. NICE
guideline NG17. August 2015, updated June 2022.
www.nice.org.uk/guidance/ng17

Insulin

16-Sep-2021

Overview

For recommended insulin regimens see Type 1 diabetes
p. 797 and Type 2 diabetes p. 800.

Insulin is a polypeptide hormone secreted by pancreatic
beta-cells. Insulin increases glucose uptake by adipose tissue
and muscles, and suppresses hepatic glucose release. The
role of insulin is to lower blood-glucose concentrations in
order to prevent hyperglycaemia and its associated
microvascular, macrovascular and metabolic complications.

The natural profile of insulin secretion in the body consists
of basal insulin (a low and steady secretion of background
insulin that controls the glucose continuously released from
the liver) and meal-time bolus insulin (secreted in response
to glucose absorbed from food and drink).

Sources of insulin

Three types of insulin are available in the UK: human
insulin, human insulin analogues, and animal insulin.
Animal insulins are extracted and purified from animal
sources (bovine or porcine insulin). Although widely used in
the past, animal insulins are no longer initiated in people
with diabetes but may still be used by some adult patients
who cannot, or do not wish to, change to human insulins.

Human insulins are produced by recombinant DNA
technology and have the same amino acid sequence as
endogenous human insulin. Human insulin analogues are
produced in the same way as human insulins, but the insulin
is modified to produce a desired kinetic characteristic, such
as an extended duration of action or faster absorption and
onset of action.

Immunological resistance to insulin is uncommon and
true insulin allergy is rare. Human insulin and insulin
analogues are less immunogenic than animal insulins.

Administration of insulin

Insulin is inactivated by gastro-intestinal enzymes and must
therefore be given by injection; the subcutaneous route is
ideal in most circumstances. Insulin should be injected into a
body area with plenty of subcutaneous fat—usually the
abdomen (fastest absorption rate) or outer thighs/buttocks
(slower absorption compared with the abdomen or inner
thighs).

Absorption from a limb site can vary considerably (by as
much as 20–40%) day-to-day, particularly in children. Local
tissue reactions, changes in insulin sensitivity, injection site,
blood flow, depth of injection, and the amount of insulin
injected can all affect the rate of absorption. Increased blood
flow around the injection site due to exercise can also
increase insulin absorption.

[EvGr] Lipohypertrophy can occur due to repeatedly
injecting into the same small area, and can cause erratic
absorption of insulin, and contribute to poor glycaemic
control. Patients should be advised not to use affected areas
for further injection until the skin has recovered.
Lipohypertrophy can be minimised by using different
injection sites in rotation. Injection sites should be checked
for signs of infection, swelling, bruising, and
lipohypertrophy before administration. Ⓐ

Insulin preparations

Insulin preparations can be broadly categorised into three
groups based on their time-action profiles: short-acting
insulins (including soluble insulin and rapid-acting insulins),
intermediate-acting insulins and long-acting insulins. The
duration of action of each particular type of insulin varies
considerably from one patient to another, and needs to be
assessed individually.

Short-acting insulins

Short-acting insulins have a short duration and a relatively
rapid onset of action, to replicate the insulin normally
produced by the body in response to glucose absorbed from a
meal. These are available as soluble Insulin below (human
and, bovine or porcine—both rarely used), and the rapid-
acting insulin analogues (insulin aspart p. 835, insulin
glulisine p. 836 and insulin lispro p. 836).

Soluble insulin

Soluble insulin is usually given subcutaneously but some
preparations can be given intravenously and
intramuscularly. For maintenance regimens, it is usual to
inject the insulin 15 to 30 minutes before meals, depending
on the insulin preparation used.

When injected subcutaneously, soluble insulin has a rapid
onset of action (30 to 60 minutes), a peak action between 1
and 4 hours, and a duration of action of up to 9 hours.

When injected intravenously, soluble insulin has a short
half-life of only a few minutes and its onset of action is
instantaneous.

Soluble insulin administered intravenously is the most
appropriate form of insulin for use in diabetic emergencies
e.g. diabetic ketoacidosis and peri-operatively.

Rapid-acting insulin

Insulin aspart, insulin glulisine, and insulin lispro have a
faster onset of action (within 15 minutes) and shorter
duration of action (approximately 2–5 hours) than soluble
insulin, and are usually given by subcutaneous injection.

[EvGr] For maintenance regimens, these insulins should
ideally be injected immediately before meals. Rapid-acting
insulin, administered before meals, has an advantage over
short-acting soluble insulin in terms of improved glucose
control, reduction of HbA1c, and reduction in the incidence
of severe hypoglycaemia, including nocturnal
hypoglycaemia.

The routine use of *post-meal* injections of rapid-acting
insulin should be avoided—when given during or after meals,
they are associated with poorer glucose control, an increased
risk of high postprandial-glucose concentration, and
subsequent hypoglycaemia. Ⓐ

Intermediate-acting insulin

Intermediate-acting insulins (isophane insulin p. 837) have
an intermediate duration of action, designed to mimic the
effect of endogenous basal insulin. When given by
subcutaneous injection, they have an onset of action of
approximately 1–2 hours, a maximal effect at 3–12 hours,
and a duration of action of 11–24 hours.

Isophane insulin is a suspension of insulin with
protamine; it may be given as one or more daily injections
alongside separate meal-time short-acting insulin
injections, or mixed with a short-acting (soluble or rapid-
acting) insulin in the same syringe—for recommended
insulin regimens see Type 1 diabetes p. 797 and Type 2
diabetes p. 800. Isophane insulin may be mixed with a short-
acting insulin by the patient, or a pre-mixed biphasic insulin
can be supplied (biphasic isophane insulin p. 837, biphasic
insulin aspart p. 838 and biphasic insulin lispro p. 838).

Biphasic insulins (biphasic isophane insulin, biphasic
insulin aspart, biphasic insulin lispro) are pre-mixed insulin
preparations containing various combinations of short-
acting insulin (soluble insulin or rapid-acting analogue
insulin) and an intermediate-acting insulin.

The percentage of short-acting insulin varies from 15% to 50%. These preparations should be administered by subcutaneous injection immediately before a meal.

Long-acting insulin

Like intermediate-acting insulins, the long-acting insulins (protamine zinc insulin, insulin zinc suspension, insulin detemir p. 839, insulin glargine p. 839, insulin degludec p. 838) mimic endogenous basal insulin secretion, but their duration of action may last up to 36 hours. They achieve a steady-state level after 2–4 days to produce a constant level of insulin.

Insulin glargine and insulin degludec are given once daily and insulin detemir is given once or twice daily according to individual requirements. The older long-acting insulins, (insulin zinc suspension and protamine zinc insulin) are now rarely prescribed.

Type 2 diabetes

15-Jan-2024

Description of condition

Type 2 diabetes is a chronic metabolic condition characterised by insulin resistance and insufficient pancreatic insulin production, resulting in high blood-glucose levels (hyperglycaemia).

It is commonly associated with obesity, physical inactivity, raised blood pressure, dyslipidaemia, and a tendency to develop thrombosis; therefore it increases cardiovascular risk. It is associated with long-term microvascular and macrovascular complications, together with reduced quality of life and life expectancy.

Aims of treatment

Treatment is aimed at minimising the risk of long-term microvascular and macrovascular complications by effective blood-glucose control and maintenance of glycated haemoglobin (HbA1c) at or below the target value set for each individual patient.

Management

[EvGr] Lifestyle modifications (such as weight loss, eating a healthy diet, smoking cessation, and regular exercise) can help reduce hyperglycaemia and cardiovascular risk, and should be encouraged where appropriate. Nutritional advice should be provided by a healthcare professional with specific expertise and competencies in nutrition. For further guidance on reducing cardiovascular risk, see Cardiovascular disease risk assessment and prevention p. 219.

The choice of drug treatment for patients with type 2 diabetes should be based on the patient's preference and clinical circumstances (such as weight, comorbidities and concomitant medication), and the effectiveness, safety, tolerability, and monitoring requirements of the treatment. When reviewing or considering changing treatment, consider ways to optimise the patient's current treatment regimen (e.g. managing side-effects, supporting adherence, and reinforcing lifestyle advice), and discuss stopping treatment that has had no impact on glycaemic control or weight, unless there is an additional clinical benefit (such as cardiovascular or renal protection) from continued treatment. [A]

For guidance on the management of diabetes in pregnancy and breastfeeding, see Diabetes, pregnancy and breast-feeding p. 805.

For guidance on the management of complications associated with diabetes, see Diabetic complications p. 802.

Targets and monitoring

[EvGr] Lifestyle interventions, and antidiabetic drugs should be offered to support patients to control blood-glucose and to reach and maintain their HbA1c target.

A target HbA1c level of 48 mmol/mol (6.5%) is generally recommended when type 2 diabetes is managed by diet and lifestyle alone, or when combined with a single antidiabetic drug not associated with hypoglycaemia (such as metformin hydrochloride p. 807). Patients prescribed a single drug associated with hypoglycaemia (such as a sulfonylurea) should usually aim for an HbA1c level of 53 mmol/mol (7.0%). Targets may differ and should be individualised and agreed with each patient.

If HbA1c levels are poorly controlled despite treatment with a single drug and rise to 58 mmol/mol (7.5%) or higher, drug treatment should be intensified, alongside reinforcement of advice regarding diet, lifestyle, and adherence to drug treatment.

When two or more antidiabetic drugs are prescribed, a target HbA1c level of 53 mmol/mol (7.0%) is recommended for patients in which it is appropriate. [A]

Note: [EvGr] Consider relaxing the target HbA1c level on a case-by-case basis, with particular consideration for patients who are older or frail, those unlikely to achieve longer-term risk-reduction benefits, or where tight blood-glucose control is not appropriate or poses a high risk of the consequences of hypoglycaemia.

If patients reach a lower HbA1c level than their target and are not experiencing hypoglycaemia, encourage them to maintain it. Be aware of other possible reasons for a low HbA1c level, for example deteriorating renal function or sudden weight loss. [A]

For further guidance on HbA1c, including monitoring frequency, see Diabetes p. 796; and for guidance on self-monitoring of capillary blood-glucose, and continuous glucose monitoring, see NICE guideline: **Type 2 diabetes in adults: management** (see *Useful resources*).

Antidiabetic drugs

There are several classes of non-insulin antidiabetic drugs available for the treatment of type 2 diabetes. For recommended treatment regimens and the place in therapy of each drug, see *Drug treatment, antidiabetic drugs*.

Metformin hydrochloride has an anti-hyperglycaemic effect, lowering both basal and postprandial blood-glucose concentrations. It is not associated with weight gain, and does not stimulate insulin secretion and therefore, when given alone, does not cause hypoglycaemia.

Sulfonylureas, such as gliclazide p. 831, glimepiride p. 831, glipizide p. 832, and tolbutamide p. 832, may cause hypoglycaemia; it is more likely with long-acting sulfonylureas such as glimepiride, which have been associated with severe, prolonged and sometimes fatal cases of hypoglycaemia. Sulfonylureas are also associated with modest weight gain, probably due to increased plasma-insulin concentrations.

Acarbose p. 806 has a poorer anti-hyperglycaemic effect than many other antidiabetic drugs.

Meglitinides, such as repaglinide p. 822, have a rapid onset of action and short duration of activity. These drugs can be used flexibly around mealtimes and adjusted to fit around individual eating habits which may be beneficial for some patients, but generally are a less preferred option than the sulfonylureas.

The thiazolidinedione, pioglitazone p. 832, is associated with weight gain and several long-term risks, and its ongoing benefit to the patient should be reviewed regularly and treatment stopped if response is insufficient.

Dipeptidylpeptidase-4 (DPP-4) inhibitors, such as alogliptin p. 809, linagliptin p. 809, sitagliptin p. 811, saxagliptin p. 810, and vildagliptin p. 812, do not appear to be associated with weight gain and have less incidence of hypoglycaemia than the sulfonylureas.

Sodium-glucose co-transporter 2 (SGLT2) inhibitors, such as canagliflozin p. 824, dapagliflozin p. 826, empagliflozin p. 827, and ertugliflozin p. 829, in addition to lowering blood-glucose, may promote weight loss and improve cardiovascular outcomes in certain patients. There is greater uncertainty around the cardiovascular benefits associated with ertugliflozin than there is for canagliflozin, dapagliflozin, and empagliflozin. SGLT2 inhibitors are associated with a risk of diabetic ketoacidosis. For information on the use of SGLT2 inhibitors in patients with type 2 diabetes and chronic kidney disease, see *Diabetic nephropathy* in Diabetic complications p. 802.

Glucagon-like peptide-1 (GLP-1) receptor agonists, such as dulaglutide p. 813, exenatide p. 814, liraglutide p. 816, lixisenatide p. 818, and semaglutide p. 819, should be reserved for combination therapy when other treatment options have failed. GLP-1 receptor agonists promote weight loss, and for some patients may improve cardiovascular outcomes.

Dual glucose-dependent insulinotropic polypeptide (GIP) and GLP-1 receptor agonists, such as tirzepatide p. 822, promote weight loss and can be used as an alternative to GLP-1 receptor agonists in combination with other drugs when other treatments have failed.

Drug treatment, antidiabetic drugs

[EvGr] Consider rescue therapy with insulin or a sulfonylurea for patients who become symptomatically hyperglycaemic at any stage of treatment. Treatment should be reviewed when blood-glucose control has been achieved. ⟨A⟩

Initial treatment

[EvGr] Standard-release metformin hydrochloride is recommended as the first choice for initial drug treatment for all patients, due to its positive effect on weight loss, reduced risk of hypoglycaemic events, and the additional long-term cardiovascular benefits associated with its use.

The dose of standard-release metformin should be increased gradually to minimise the risk of gastro-intestinal side-effects. Modified-release metformin should be offered if the patient experiences gastro-intestinal side-effects with standard treatment.

In addition to metformin, patients with chronic heart failure or established atherosclerotic cardiovascular disease should also be offered a sodium glucose co-transporter 2 (SGLT2) inhibitor with proven cardiovascular benefit as initial drug treatment. An SGLT2 inhibitor should also be considered for patients who are at high risk of developing cardiovascular disease. Metformin should be initiated first, with the SGLT2 inhibitor started as soon as tolerability to metformin is confirmed. ⟨A⟩

If metformin is contra-indicated or not tolerated, see *Non-metformin regimens* below.

Further treatment options

[EvGr] At any stage after starting initial treatment, an SGLT2 inhibitor with proven cardiovascular benefit should be offered to patients who develop chronic heart failure or established atherosclerotic cardiovascular disease, and should be considered in patients who become at high risk of developing cardiovascular disease.

If monotherapy with metformin hydrochloride p. 807 (alongside modification to diet) does not control HbA1c to below the agreed threshold, consider metformin hydrochloride in combination with either a dipeptidylpeptidase-4 (DPP-4) inhibitor, or pioglitazone p. 832, or a sulfonylurea. A sodium glucose co-transporter 2 (SGLT2) inhibitor may be considered in combination with metformin, when sulfonylureas are contra-indicated or not tolerated, or if the patient is at significant risk of hypoglycaemia or its consequences.

If dual therapy is unsuccessful, consider a triple therapy regimen by adding in either a DPP-4 inhibitor, or pioglitazone, or a sulfonylurea. An SGLT2 inhibitor may be considered in the following triple therapy regimens:

- Metformin hydrochloride and a sulfonylurea, and either canagliflozin p. 824, dapagliflozin p. 826, or empagliflozin p. 827; **or**
- Metformin hydrochloride and pioglitazone, and either canagliflozin or empagliflozin; **or**
- Metformin hydrochloride and a DPP-4 inhibitor and ertugliflozin p. 829 (only if a sulfonylurea or pioglitazone is not appropriate).

Alternatively, if dual therapy is unsuccessful, it may be appropriate to start **insulin**-based treatment—see *Drug treatment, insulin.* ⟨A⟩

[EvGr] Elderly patients or those with renal impairment are at particular risk of hypoglycaemia; if a sulfonylurea is indicated, a shorter-acting sulfonylurea, such as gliclazide p. 831 or tolbutamide p. 832 should be prescribed. ⟨E⟩

Glucagon-like peptide-1 receptor agonists or dual glucose-dependent insulinotropic polypeptide and glucagon-like peptide-1 receptor agonists

[EvGr] If triple therapy with metformin hydrochloride and two other oral drugs is tried and is ineffective, or is unsuitable, a GLP-1 receptor agonist or tirzepatide p. 822 may be considered as part of a triple therapy regimen as an alternative to one of the other drugs.

These drugs should only be considered for patients who have a BMI of 35 kg/m^2 or above (adjusted for ethnicity) and specific psychological or medical problems associated with obesity; *or* for those who have a BMI less than 35 kg/m^2 and for whom insulin therapy would have significant occupational implications, or if the weight loss associated with these drugs would benefit other significant obesity-related comorbidities.

GLP-1 receptor agonist therapies with proven cardiovascular benefit (such as liraglutide) should be considered in patients with established cardiovascular disease.

After 6 months, the GLP-1 receptor agonist should be reviewed and only continued if there has been a beneficial metabolic response (a reduction of at least 11 mmol/mol [1.0%] in HbA1c and a weight loss of at least 3% of initial body-weight).

Insulin should only be prescribed in combination with a GLP-1 receptor agonist under specialist care advice and with ongoing support from a consultant-led multidisciplinary team. ⟨A⟩

Non-metformin regimens

[EvGr] If metformin is contra-indicated or not tolerated, a sodium glucose co-transporter 2 (SGLT2) inhibitor with proven cardiovascular benefit should be offered as first-line treatment for patients who have chronic heart failure or established atherosclerotic cardiovascular disease. An SGLT2 inhibitor should also be considered for patients who are at high risk of developing cardiovascular disease.

For all other patients, consider a dipeptidylpeptidase-4 (DPP-4) inhibitor, or pioglitazone, or a sulfonylurea as first-line drug treatment if metformin is contra-indicated or not tolerated. An SGLT2 inhibitor may be considered as an alternative option to a DPP-4 inhibitor, if neither a sulfonylurea or pioglitazone are appropriate.

Repaglinide p. 822 is also an effective alternative option for single therapy, but it has a limited role in treatment because, should an intensification of treatment be required, it is not licensed to be used in any combination other than with metformin hydrochloride; it would therefore require a complete change of treatment in those patients who have started it due to intolerance or contra-indication to metformin. ⟨A⟩

Further treatment options

[EvGr] At any stage after starting initial treatment, an SGLT2 inhibitor with proven cardiovascular benefit should be offered to patients who develop chronic heart failure or established atherosclerotic cardiovascular disease, and should be considered in patients who become at high risk of developing cardiovascular disease.

If initial monotherapy does not control HbA1c to below the patient's agreed threshold, consider adding either a dipeptidylpeptidase-4 (DPP-4) inhibitor, pioglitazone, or a sulfonylurea.

If dual therapy does not provide adequate glucose control, insulin-based treatment should be considered—see *Drug treatment, insulin*. Ⓐ

Drug treatment, insulin

EvGr When indicated for intensification of treatment, insulin (see also, Insulin p. 799) should be started with a structured support programme covering insulin dose titration, injection technique, self-monitoring, and knowledge of dietary effects and glucose control. Metformin hydrochloride should be continued unless it is contra-indicated or not tolerated. Other antidiabetic drugs should be reviewed and stopped if necessary.

Recommended insulin regimens include:

- human isophane insulin p. 837 injected once or twice daily, according to requirements;
- a human isophane insulin in combination with a short-acting insulin, administered either separately or as a pre-mixed (biphasic) human insulin preparation (this may be particularly appropriate if HbA1c is 75 mmol/mol (9.0%) or higher);
- Insulin detemir p. 839 or insulin glargine p. 839 as an alternative to human isophane insulin. This can be preferable if a *once daily* injection would be beneficial (for example if assistance is required to inject insulin), or if recurrent symptomatic hypoglycaemic episodes are problematic, or if the patient would otherwise need twice-daily human isophane insulin injections in combination with oral glucose-lowering drugs. Also consider switching to insulin detemir or insulin glargine from human isophane insulin if significant hypoglycaemia is problematic, or in patients who cannot use the device needed to inject human isophane insulin;
- biphasic preparations (pre-mixed) that include a short-acting human *analogue* insulin (rather than short-acting human *soluble insulin*) can be preferable for patients who prefer injecting insulin immediately before a meal, or if hypoglycaemia is a problem, or if blood-glucose concentrations rise markedly after meals.

When starting insulin therapy, bedtime basal insulin should be initiated and the dose titrated against morning (fasting) glucose. Patients who are prescribed a basal insulin regimen (human isophane insulin p. 837, insulin detemir p. 839 or insulin glargine p. 839) should be monitored for the need for short-acting insulin before meals (or a biphasic insulin preparation).

Patients who are prescribed a biphasic insulin should be monitored for the need for a further injection of short-acting insulin before meals or for a change to a basal-bolus regimen with human isophane insulin or insulin detemir or insulin glargine if blood-glucose control remains inadequate. Ⓐ

Useful Resources

Type 2 diabetes in adults: management. National Institute for Health and Care Excellence. NICE guideline 28. June 2022.
www.nice.org.uk/guidance/ng28

Pharmacological management of glycaemic control in people with type 2 diabetes. Scottish Intercollegiate Guidelines Network. Clinical guideline 154. November 2017.
www.sign.ac.uk/our-guidelines/pharmacological-management-of-glycaemic-control-in-people-with-type-2-diabetes/

Diabetic complications

18-Dec-2023

See also

Diabetes p. 796
  Type 1 diabetes p. 797
  Type 2 diabetes p. 800
  Diabetic foot infections, antibacterial therapy p. 581. For guidance on other diabetic foot problems, see NICE guideline **Diabetic foot problems** (available at: www.nice.org.uk/guidance/ng19).

Diabetes and cardiovascular disease

Diabetes is a strong risk factor for cardiovascular disease. EvGr Other risk factors for cardiovascular disease that should also be addressed are: smoking, hypertension, obesity, and dyslipidaemia. Ⓐ Cardiovascular risk in patients with diabetes can be further reduced by the use of an ACE inhibitor (or an angiotensin-II receptor antagonist) and lipid-regulating drugs. For full guidance on the assessment and prevention of cardiovascular disease, see Cardiovascular disease risk assessment and prevention p. 219.

Diabetic nephropathy

EvGr In diabetic patients with nephropathy, blood pressure should be reduced to the lowest achievable level to slow the rate of decline of glomerular filtration rate and reduce proteinuria. Provided there are no contra-indications, all diabetic patients who have confirmed nephropathy with an albumin:creatinine ratio (ACR) of 3 mg/mmol or more should be treated with an ACE inhibitor or an angiotensin-II receptor antagonist, even if the blood pressure is normal. In patients with chronic kidney disease (CKD) and proteinuria, ACE inhibitors or angiotensin-II receptor antagonists should be given as monotherapy to reduce the rate of progression of CKD. For patients with type 2 diabetes and CKD who are already on an ACE inhibitor or angiotensin-II receptor antagonist, add on therapy with a sodium glucose co-transporter 2 (SGLT2) inhibitor should be offered if the ACR is over 30 mg/mmol; for patients with an ACR of 3–30 mg/mmol, add on therapy should be considered. For patients with type 2 diabetes and stage 3 or 4 CKD with albuminuria who are on optimised treatment with an ACE inhibitor or angiotensin-II receptor antagonist, and an SGLT2 inhibitor (unless these are unsuitable), add on therapy with finerenone p. 948 is recommended. Ⓐ

ACE inhibitors can potentiate the hypoglycaemic effect of insulin and oral antidiabetic drugs; this effect is more likely during the first weeks of combined treatment and in patients with renal impairment.

See also treatment of hypertension in diabetes in Hypertension p. 166.

Diabetic neuropathy

Optimal diabetic control is beneficial for the management of painful neuropathy. EvGr However, *acute* painful diabetic neuropathy can occur in patients with type 1 diabetes who have a rapid improvement in blood-glucose control. This is usually self-limiting and simple analgesics (such as paracetamol p. 507) along with other measures (such as bed cradles) are recommended as first line treatments. If the response is inadequate, other treatment options for painful diabetic neuropathy should be considered. Simple analgesia may be continued until the effects of additional treatments have been established.

Monotherapy with antidepressant drugs, including tricyclics (such as amitriptyline hydrochloride p. 431 and imipramine hydrochloride p. 435 [unlicensed use]), duloxetine p. 426, and venlafaxine p. 427 [unlicensed use] should be considered in patients for the treatment of painful diabetic peripheral neuropathy. Antiepileptic drugs, such as pregabalin p. 374 and gabapentin p. 362, can also be considered. Opioid analgesics in combination with gabapentin can be considered if pain is not controlled with monotherapy. Ⓐ

In *autonomic neuropathy*, diabetic diarrhoea can often be managed by tetracycline p. 659 [unlicensed use], or codeine phosphate p. 517 as the best alternative; other antidiarrhoeal preparations can also be tried. Erythromycin p. 624 (especially when given intravenously) may be beneficial for gastroparesis [unlicensed use]. EvGr Patients with suspected gastroparesis should be considered for referral to specialist services if the differential diagnosis is in doubt or the patient has persistent or severe vomiting. Ⓐ

In *neuropathic postural hypotension*, increased salt intake and the use of the mineralcorticoid fludrocortisone acetate p. 787 [unlicensed use] may help by increasing plasma volume, but uncomfortable oedema is a common side-effect. Fludrocortisone can also be combined with flurbiprofen p. 1301 and ephedrine hydrochloride p. 311 [both unlicensed]. Midodrine [unlicensed], an alpha agonist, may also be useful in postural hypotension.

Gustatory sweating can be treated with an antimuscarinic such as propantheline bromide p. 97; side-effects are common. See also, the management of hyperhidrosis (Hyperhidrosis p. 1435).

In some patients with *neuropathic oedema*, ephedrine hydrochloride [unlicensed use] offers effective relief.

See also the management of Erectile dysfunction p. 938.

Visual impairment

EvGr Optimal diabetic and blood pressure control should be maintained to prevent onset and progression of diabetic eye disease, Ⓐ see Hypertension p. 166, Type 1 diabetes p. 797, and Type 2 diabetes p. 800 for target thresholds.

Diabetic hyperglycaemic emergencies

13-May-2024

Description of condition

Diabetic ketoacidosis (DKA) and the hyperosmolar hyperglycaemic state ((HHS), previously referred to as hyperosmolar non-ketotic (HONK) coma) are medical emergencies with significant morbidity and mortality. HHS has a higher mortality than DKA.

The major precipitating factor for both DKA and HHS is infection. Other precipitating factors for DKA include discontinuation of or inadequate insulin therapy, acute illness such as myocardial infarction and pancreatitis, new onset of diabetes, or stress (e.g. trauma, surgery); and for HHS, these include inadequate insulin or oral antidiabetic therapy, acute illness in a patient with known diabetes, or stress.

DKA develops rapidly (within hours), and mainly occurs in individuals with type 1 diabetes, with around a third of cases occurring in those with type 2 diabetes. Unlike DKA, HHS can take days to develop and consequently the dehydration and metabolic disturbances are more severe at presentation. HHS typically occurs in individuals aged over 45 years, but can also occur in younger adults and adolescents, often as the initial presentation of type 2 diabetes.

DKA is characterised by **hyperglycaemia** (blood glucose above 11 mmol/L or known diabetes mellitus), **ketonaemia** (capillary or blood ketone above 3 mmol/L or significant ketonuria of 2+ or more), and **acidosis** (bicarbonate less than 15 mmol/L and/or venous pH less than 7.3). Common signs and symptoms of DKA include dehydration due to polydipsia and polyuria, weight loss, excessive tiredness, nausea, vomiting, abdominal pain, Kussmaul respiration (rapid and deep respiration) with acetone breath, and reduced consciousness.

Characteristic features of HHS are **marked hypovolaemia**, **marked hyperglycaemia** (blood glucose of 30 mmol/L or

above without significant hyperketonaemia or acidosis), and **hyperosmolality** (osmolality of 320 mOsm/kg or above); however, a mixed picture of DKA and HHS occurs relatively frequently. Common signs and symptoms of HHS include dehydration due to polyuria and polydipsia, weakness, weight loss, tachycardia, dry mucous membranes, poor skin turgor, hypotension, acute cognitive impairment, and in severe cases, shock.

Aims of treatment

The treatment of DKA aims to restore circulatory volume, correct electrolyte imbalance and hyperglycaemia, clear ketones and suppress ketogenesis, identify and treat any precipitating causes, and prevent complications.

The treatment of HHS aims to correct fluid and electrolyte losses, hyperosmolality and hyperglycaemia, identify and treat any underlying or precipitating causes, and prevent complications.

Diabetic ketoacidosis

Individuals with suspected DKA should be diagnosed promptly and managed intensively—the diabetes specialist team should be involved as soon as possible after admission to hospital (ideally within 24 hours). Those who are elderly, pregnant, aged 18–25 years, have heart or renal failure, or other serious comorbidities, require specialist input.

The initial drug management of DKA involves intravenous fluid replacement, followed by intravenous insulin; patients who normally take long-acting insulin should continue their usual dose(s) throughout treatment. Potassium replacement and glucose administration may also be required to prevent subsequent hypokalaemia and hypoglycaemia, depending on potassium levels and blood glucose concentrations, respectively.

For further information on the management of DKA, see JBDS guideline: **The Management of Diabetic Ketoacidosis in Adults** (see *Useful resources*); this guideline can also be used for individuals aged 16–18 years being managed by an adult diabetes team. If these individuals are being managed by a paediatric diabetes team, the BSPED guideline: **Guideline for the Management of Children and Young People under the age of 18 years with Diabetic Ketoacidosis**, and NICE guideline: **Diabetes (type 1 and type 2) in children and young people** (see *Useful resources*) should be followed.

Hyperosmolar hyperglycaemic state

Individuals with suspected HHS should be diagnosed promptly and managed intensively—the diabetes specialist team should be involved as soon as possible after admission to hospital. All patients should be reviewed promptly by a senior clinician familiar with the treatment of HHS.

The initial drug management of HHS involves intravenous fluid replacement, followed by intravenous insulin. For patients with significant ketonaemia or ketonuria, insulin can be started earlier. Potassium should be replaced or omitted as required.

For further information on the management of HHS, see JBDS guideline: **The Management of the Hyperosmolar Hyperglycaemic State (HHS) in Adults with Diabetes** (see *Useful resources*); this guideline can also be used for individuals aged 16–18 years being managed by an adult diabetes team. If these individuals are being managed by a paediatric diabetes team, the ACDC and BSPED guideline: **Practical Management of Hyperglycaemic Hyperosmolar State (HHS) in children** (see *Useful resources*) should be followed.

Useful Resources

Recommendations reflect The Management of Diabetic Ketoacidosis in Adults Guideline. Joint British Diabetes Societies for Inpatient Care Group. March 2023.

abcd.care/joint-british-diabetes-societies-jbds-inpatient-care-group

The Management of the Hyperosmolar Hyperglycaemic State (HHS) in Adults with diabetes Guideline. Joint British Diabetes Societies for Inpatient Care Group. February 2022. abcd.care/joint-british-diabetes-societies-jbds-inpatient-care-group

BSPED Guideline for the Management of Children and Young People under the age of 18 years with Diabetic Ketoacidosis. British Society for Paediatric Endocrinology and Diabetes. November 2021.
www.bsped.org.uk/clinical-resources/guidelines/#diabetes

Diabetes (type 1 and type 2) in children and young people: diagnosis and management. National Institute for Health and Care Excellence. NICE guideline 18. August 2015 (updated May 2023).
www.nice.org.uk/guidance/ng18

Practical Management of Hyperglycaemic Hyperosmolar State (HHS) in children. Association of Children's Diabetes Clinicians, British Society for Paediatric Endocrinology and Diabetes, and Children and Young People's National Diabetes Network. Clinical guideline. April 2021
www.a-c-d-c.org/endorsed-guidelines/

Diabetes, surgery and medical illness

16-Sep-2021

Management of diabetes during surgery

Peri-operative management of blood-glucose concentrations depends on factors including the required duration of fasting, timing of surgery (morning or afternoon), usual treatment regimen (insulin, antidiabetic drugs or diet), prior glycaemic control, other co-morbidities, and the likelihood that the patient will be capable of self-managing their diabetes in the immediate post-operative period. EvGr All patients should have emergency treatment for hypoglycaemia written on their drug chart on admission. Ⓔ

Note: The following recommendations provide general guidance for the management of diabetes during surgery. **Local protocols and guidelines should be followed where they exist**.

Use of insulin during surgery

Elective surgery—minor procedures in patients with good glycaemic control

EvGr Patients usually treated with insulin who have good glycaemic control (HbA1c less than 69 mmol/mol or 8.5 %) and are undergoing *minor procedures*, can be managed during the operative period by adjustment of their usual insulin regimen, which should be adjusted depending on the type of insulin usually prescribed, following detailed local protocols (which should also include intravenous fluid management, monitoring and control of electrolytes and avoidance of hyperchloraemic metabolic acidosis). On the day before the surgery, the patient's usual insulin should be given as normal, other than once daily long-acting insulin analogues, which should be given at a dose reduced by 20 %. Ⓔ

Elective surgery—major procedures or poor glycaemic control

EvGr Patients usually treated with insulin, who are either undergoing *major procedures* (surgery requiring a long fasting period of more than one missed meal) or whose diabetes is poorly controlled, will usually require a variable rate intravenous insulin infusion (continued until the patient is eating/drinking and stabilised on their previous glucose-lowering medication).

The aim is to achieve and maintain glucose concentration within the usual target range (6–10 mmol/litre; but up to 12 mmol/litre is acceptable) by infusing a constant rate of glucose-containing fluid as a substrate, while also infusing insulin at a variable rate. Detailed local protocols should be consulted. In general, the following steps should be followed:

- on the *day before surgery*, once daily long-acting insulin analogues should be given at 80 % of the usual dose; otherwise the patient's usual insulin should be given as normal;
- on the *day of surgery and throughout the intra-operative period*, once daily long-acting insulin analogues should be continued at 80 % of the usual dose; all other insulin should be stopped until the patient is eating and drinking again after surgery;
- on the *day of surgery*, start an intravenous substrate infusion of potassium chloride with glucose and sodium chloride p. 1180 (based on serum electrolytes which must be measured frequently), and infuse at a rate appropriate to the patient's fluid requirements. To prevent hypoglycaemia, this infusion must **not** be stopped while the insulin infusion is running;
- a variable rate intravenous insulin infusion of soluble human insulin p. 835 in sodium chloride 0.9 % p. 1180 (made either according to locally agreed protocols or using prefilled syringes) should be given via a syringe pump at an initial infusion rate determined by bedside capillary blood-glucose measurement. Hourly blood-glucose measurement should be taken to ensure that the intravenous insulin infusion rate is correct for at least the first 12 hours; the insulin infusion rate should be adjusted according to local protocol to maintain blood-glucose concentrations within the usual target range (6–10 mmol/litre; up to 12 mmol/litre is acceptable);
- intravenous glucose 20 % p. 1182 should be given if blood-glucose drops below 6 mmol/litre, and blood-glucose checked every hour, to prevent a drop below 4 mmol/litre. If blood-glucose drops below 4 mmol/litre, intravenous glucose 20 % should be adjusted and blood-glucose checked every 15 minutes, until blood-glucose is above 6 mmol/litre (testing can then revert to hourly). If blood-glucose rises above 12 mmol/litre, check ketones and consider other signs of diabetic ketoacidosis.

Conversion back to a subcutaneous insulin should not begin until the patient can eat and drink without nausea or vomiting. Once the patient's previous insulin regimen is re-started, the usual insulin dose may require adjustment, as insulin requirements can change due to post-operative stress, infection or altered food intake.

Previous subcutaneous basal-bolus regimens, should be restarted when the first postoperative meal-time insulin dose is due (e.g. with breakfast or lunch); doses may need adjustment due to postoperative stress, infection or altered food intake. The variable rate intravenous insulin infusion and intravenous fluids should be continued until 30–60 minutes **after** the first meal-time short-acting insulin dose. If the patient was previously on a **long-acting insulin analogue**, this should have been continued throughout the operative period at 80 % of the normal dose, and should now just continue at that same dose until the patient leaves hospital; only the short-acting insulin needs to be restarted as above.

Previous subcutaneous twice-daily mixed insulin regimens, should be restarted before breakfast or an evening meal (not at any other time). The variable rate intravenous insulin infusion should be maintained for 30–60 minutes after the first subcutaneous insulin dose has been given.

Patients who were **previously managed with a continuous subcutaneous insulin infusion** should be referred to a specialist team. The subcutaneous infusion should be restarted at the normal basal rate, not at bedtime, and the insulin infusion continued until the next meal bolus has been given.

Patients **not previously prescribed insulin**, who are to start a subcutaneous insulin regimen post-surgery, should have an insulin dose calculated with advice from a specialist diabetes team, considering the patient's sensitivity to insulin, degree of glycaemic control, weight, age, and the average hourly insulin dose used in the peri-operative period. ⟨E⟩

Emergency surgery

⟨EvGr⟩ Patients with diabetes (type 1 and 2) requiring emergency surgery, should always have their blood-glucose, blood or urinary ketone concentration, serum electrolytes and serum bicarbonate checked before surgery. If ketones are high or bicarbonate is low, blood gases should also be checked. If ketoacidosis is present, recommendations for diabetes ketoacidosis should be followed immediately, and surgery delayed if possible. If there is no acidosis, intravenous fluids and an insulin infusion should be started and managed as for *major elective surgery* (above). ⟨E⟩

Use of antidiabetic drugs during surgery

⟨EvGr⟩ Manipulation of antidiabetic drug may **not** be appropriate for all surgery or for all patients; particularly when fasting time is more than one missed meal, in patients with poor glycaemic control, and when there is risk of renal injury. In these cases, a *variable rate intravenous insulin infusion* p. 835 should be used as for *major elective surgery* (above), and usual antidiabetic medication adjusted in the peri-operative period. Insulin is almost always required in medical and surgical emergencies.

When insulin is required and given during surgery, acarbose p. 806, meglitinides, sulfonylureas, pioglitazone p. 832, dipeptidyl peptidase-4 inhibitors (gliptins) and sodium glucose co-transporter 2 inhibitors should be stopped once the insulin infusion is commenced and not restarted until the patient is eating and drinking normally. Glucagon-like peptide-1 receptor agonists can be continued as normal during the insulin infusion.

If elective *minor surgical procedures* only require a short-fasting period (just one missed meal), it may be possible to adjust antidiabetic drugs to avoid a switch to a variable rate intravenous insulin infusion; normal drug treatment can continue.

In suitable cases, acarbose, nateglinide and repaglinide p. 822 can be continued with just the dose omitted on the morning of surgery if fasting (the morning dose may be given if the patient is not fasting and surgery is in the afternoon).

Pioglitazone, **dipeptidylpeptidase-4 inhibitors (gliptins)** and **glucagon-like peptide-1 receptor agonists** can be taken as normal during the whole peri-operative period.

Sodium glucose co-transporter 2 inhibitors should be omitted on the day of surgery and not restarted until the patient is stable; their use during periods of dehydration and acute illness is associated with an increased risk of developing diabetic ketoacidosis.

Sulfonylureas are associated with hypoglycaemia in the fasted state and therefore should always be omitted on the day of surgery until the patient is eating and drinking again. Capillary blood-glucose should be checked hourly. If hyperglycaemia occurs, an appropriate dose of subcutaneous rapid-acting insulin may be given. A second dose may be given 2 hours later, and a variable rate intravenous insulin infusion considered if hyperglycaemia persists.

Metformin hydrochloride p. 807 is renally excreted; renal impairment may lead to accumulation and lactic acidosis during surgery. If only one meal will be missed during surgery, and the patient has an eGFR greater than 60 mL/minute/1.73m^2 and a low risk of acute kidney injury (and the procedure does not involve administration of contrast media), it may be possible to continue metformin hydrochloride throughout the peri-operative period—just the lunchtime dose should be omitted if the usual dose is prescribed three times a day.

If the patient will miss more than one meal or there is significant risk of the patient developing acute kidney injury,

metformin hydrochloride should be stopped when the pre-operative fast begins. A variable rate intravenous insulin infusion should be started if the metformin hydrochloride dose is more than once daily. Otherwise insulin should only be started if blood-glucose concentration is greater than 12 mmol/litre on two consecutive occasions. Metformin should not be recommenced until the patient is eating and drinking again, and normal renal function has been assured.

There is no need to stop metformin hydrochloride after contrast medium in patients missing only one meal or who have an eGFR greater than 60 mL/minute/1.73m^2. If contrast medium is to be used, and eGFR is less than 60 mL/minute/1.73m^2, metformin should be omitted on the day of the procedure and for the following 48 hours. ⟨E⟩

Use of antidiabetic drugs during medical illness

Manufacturers of some antidiabetic drugs recommend that they may need to be replaced temporarily with insulin during intercurrent illness when the drug is unlikely to control hyperglycaemia (such as myocardial infarction, coma, severe infection, trauma and other medical emergencies). Consult individual product literature.

Sodium glucose co-transporter 2 inhibitors are associated with increased risk of developing diabetic ketoacidosis during periods of dehydration, stress, surgery, trauma, acute medical illness or any other catabolic state, and should be used with caution during these times. The MHRA has advised (2016) that these drugs should be temporarily stopped in patients who are hospitalised for acute serious illness until the patient is medically stable.

Diabetes, pregnancy and breast-feeding

04-Apr-2022

Description of condition

Diabetes in pregnancy is associated with increased risks to the woman (such as pre-eclampsia and rapidly worsening retinopathy), and to the developing fetus, compared with pregnancy in non-diabetic women. Effective blood-glucose control before conception and throughout pregnancy reduces (but does not eliminate) the risk of adverse outcomes such as miscarriage, congenital malformation, stillbirth, and neonatal death.

Management of pre-existing diabetes

⟨EvGr⟩ Women with pre-existing diabetes who are planning on becoming pregnant should aim to keep their HbA1c concentration below 48 mmol/mol (6.5%) if possible without causing problematic hypoglycaemia. Any reduction towards this target is likely to reduce the risk of congenital malformations in the newborn.

Women with pre-existing diabetes who are planning to become pregnant should be advised to take folic acid at the dose for women who are at high-risk of conceiving a child with a neural tube defect, see folic acid p. 1161. ⟨A⟩

Overview

Oral antidiabetic drugs

⟨EvGr⟩ All oral antidiabetic drugs, except metformin hydrochloride p. 807, should be discontinued before pregnancy (or as soon as an unplanned pregnancy is identified) and substituted with insulin therapy. Women with diabetes may be treated with metformin hydrochloride p. 807 as an adjunct or alternative to insulin in the preconception period and during pregnancy when the likely benefits from improved blood-glucose control outweigh the potential for harm. Metformin hydrochloride p. 807 can be continued immediately after birth and during breast-feeding for those with pre-existing Type 2 diabetes p. 800. All other antidiabetic drugs should be avoided while breast-feeding. ⟨A⟩

Insulin

Limited evidence suggests that the rapid-acting insulin analogues (insulin aspart p. 835 and insulin lispro p. 836) can be associated with fewer episodes of hypoglycaemia, a reduction in postprandial glucose excursions and an improvement in overall glycaemic control compared with regular human insulin.

[EvGr] Isophane insulin p. 837 is the first-choice for long-acting insulin during pregnancy, however in women who have good blood-glucose control before pregnancy with the long-acting insulin analogues (insulin detemir p. 839 or insulin glargine p. 839), it may be appropriate to continue using them throughout pregnancy.

Continuous subcutaneous insulin infusion p. 835 (insulin pump therapy) may be appropriate for pregnant women who have difficulty achieving glycaemic control with multiple daily injections of insulin p. 835 without significant disabling hypoglycaemia.

All women treated with insulin p. 835 during pregnancy should be aware of the risks of hypoglycaemia, particularly in the first trimester, and should be advised to always carry a fast-acting form of glucose, such as dextrose tablets or a glucose-containing drink. Pregnant women with Type 1 diabetes p. 797 should also be prescribed glucagon p. 845 for use if needed.

Women with pre-existing diabetes treated with insulin p. 835 during pregnancy are at increased risk of hypoglycaemia in the postnatal period and should reduce their insulin immediately after birth. Blood-glucose levels should be monitored carefully to establish the appropriate dose. Ⓐ

Medication for diabetic complications

[EvGr] Angiotensin-converting enzyme inhibitors and angiotensin II receptor antagonists should be discontinued and replaced with an alternative antihypertensive suitable for use in pregnancy before conception or as soon as pregnancy is confirmed (see *Hypertension in pregnancy* under Hypertension p. 166). Statins should not be prescribed during pregnancy and should be discontinued before a planned pregnancy. Ⓐ

Gestational diabetes

[EvGr] Women with gestational diabetes who have a fasting plasma glucose below 7 mmol/litre at diagnosis, should first attempt a change in diet and exercise alone in order to reduce blood-glucose. If blood-glucose targets are not met within 1 to 2 weeks, metformin hydrochloride p. 807 may be prescribed. Insulin p. 835 may be prescribed if metformin is contra-indicated or not acceptable, and may also be added to treatment if metformin is not effective alone.

Women who have a fasting plasma glucose above 7 mmol/litre at diagnosis should be treated with insulin p. 835 immediately, with or without metformin hydrochloride p. 807, in addition to a change in diet and exercise.

Women who have a fasting plasma glucose between 6 and 6.9 mmol/litre alongside complications such as macrosomia or hydramnios should be considered for immediate insulin p. 835 treatment, with or without metformin hydrochloride p. 807.

Women with gestational diabetes should discontinue hypoglycaemic treatment immediately after giving birth. Ⓐ

Useful Resources

Diabetes in pregnancy: management from preconception to the postnatal period. National Institute for Health and Care Excellence. NICE guideline NG3. February 2015 (updated December 2020).
www.nice.org.uk/guidance/ng3

BLOOD GLUCOSE LOWERING DRUGS 〉 ALPHA GLUCOSIDASE INHIBITORS

Acarbose

14-Mar-2025

- **DRUG ACTION** Acarbose, an inhibitor of intestinal alpha glucosidases, delays the digestion and absorption of starch and sucrose; it has a small but significant effect in lowering blood glucose.

- **INDICATIONS AND DOSE**

Diabetes mellitus inadequately controlled by diet or by diet with oral antidiabetic drugs
▸ BY MOUTH
▸ Adult: Initially 50 mg 1–2 times a day, then increased to 50 mg 3 times a day for 6–8 weeks, then increased if necessary to 100 mg 3 times a day; increased if necessary to 200 mg 3 times a day

- **CONTRA-INDICATIONS** Disorders of digestion or absorption · hernia (condition may deteriorate) · inflammatory bowel disease · predisposition to intestinal obstruction

- **CAUTIONS** May enhance hypoglycaemic effects of insulin and sulfonylureas (hypoglycaemic episodes may be treated with oral glucose but not with sucrose)

- **INTERACTIONS** → Appendix 1: acarbose

- **SIDE-EFFECTS**
▸ **Common or very common** Diarrhoea (may need to reduce dose) · gastrointestinal discomfort · gastrointestinal disorders
▸ **Uncommon** Nausea · vomiting
▸ **Rare or very rare** Hepatic disorders · oedema
▸ **Frequency not known** Acute generalised exanthematous pustulosis (AGEP) · thrombocytopenia

SIDE-EFFECTS, FURTHER INFORMATION Antacids containing magnesium and aluminium salts unlikely to be beneficial for treating side effects.

- **PREGNANCY** Avoid.

- **BREAST FEEDING** Avoid.

- **HEPATIC IMPAIRMENT** Manufacturer advises avoid in severe impairment.

- **RENAL IMPAIRMENT** [EvGr] Avoid if creatinine clearance less than 25 mL/minute. Ⓜ See p. 21.

- **MONITORING REQUIREMENTS** Monitor liver function.

- **DIRECTIONS FOR ADMINISTRATION** Manufacturer advises tablets should be chewed with first mouthful of food or swallowed whole with a little liquid immediately before food.

- **PATIENT AND CARER ADVICE** Antacids unlikely to be beneficial for treating side-effects. To counteract possible hypoglycaemia, patients receiving insulin or a sulfonylurea as well as acarbose need to carry glucose (not sucrose—acarbose interferes with sucrose absorption). Patients should be given advice on how to administer acarbose tablets.

- **MEDICINAL FORMS** There can be variation in the licensing of different medicines containing the same drug.
Oral tablet
▸ Acarbose (Non-proprietary)
Acarbose **50 mg** Acarbose 50mg tablets | 90 tablet [PoM] £31.29 DT = £30.16
Acarbose **100 mg** Acarbose 100mg tablets | 90 tablet [PoM] £45.06 DT = £41.43

BLOOD GLUCOSE LOWERING DRUGS ›
BIGUANIDES

Metformin hydrochloride
07-May-2024

- **DRUG ACTION** Metformin exerts its effect mainly by decreasing gluconeogenesis and by increasing peripheral utilisation of glucose; since it acts only in the presence of endogenous insulin it is effective only if there are some residual functioning pancreatic islet cells.

- **INDICATIONS AND DOSE**

Type 2 diabetes mellitus [monotherapy or in combination with other antidiabetic drugs (including insulin)]
▶ BY MOUTH USING IMMEDIATE-RELEASE MEDICINES
▶ Child 10-17 years (specialist use only): Initially 500 mg once daily; increased if necessary to 2 g daily in 2–3 divided doses, dose to be adjusted according to response at intervals of at least 1 week
▶ Adult: Initially 500 mg once daily for at least 1 week, dose to be taken with breakfast, then 500 mg twice daily for at least 1 week, dose to be taken with breakfast and evening meal, then 500 mg 3 times a day, dose to be taken with breakfast, lunch and evening meal, dose can be increased if necessary up to maximum 2 g per day
▶ BY MOUTH USING MODIFIED-RELEASE MEDICINES
▶ Adult: Initially 500 mg once daily, dose to be taken with evening meal, then increased if necessary up to 2 g once daily, dose to be taken with evening meal, dose increased gradually, every 10–15 days; 2 g total daily dose may alternatively be given as 1 g twice daily with meals only if control not achieved with once daily dose regimen. If control still not achieved then change to standard release tablets

Type 2 diabetes mellitus [reduction in risk or delay of onset]
▶ BY MOUTH USING MODIFIED-RELEASE MEDICINES
▶ Adult 18-74 years: Initially 500 mg once daily, dose to be taken with evening meal, then increased if necessary up to 2 g once daily, dose to be taken with evening meal, dose increased gradually, every 10–15 days. For further information on risk factors—consult product literature

Type 1 diabetes mellitus [in combination with insulin in individuals with a BMI of 25 kg/m^2 or more (23 kg/m^2 or more for individuals from South Asian and related family backgrounds)]
▶ BY MOUTH USING IMMEDIATE-RELEASE MEDICINES
▶ Adult: Initially 500 mg once daily for at least 1 week, dose to be taken with breakfast, then 500 mg twice daily for at least 1 week, dose to be taken with breakfast and evening meal, then 500 mg 3 times a day, dose to be taken with breakfast, lunch and evening meal, dose can be increased if necessary up to maximum 2 g per day
▶ BY MOUTH USING MODIFIED-RELEASE MEDICINES
▶ Adult: Initially 500 mg once daily, dose to be taken with evening meal, then increased if necessary up to 2 g daily in 1–2 divided doses, dose to be taken with meal (s), dose increased gradually, every 10–15 days

Polycystic ovary syndrome
▶ BY MOUTH USING IMMEDIATE-RELEASE MEDICINES
▶ Adult (initiated by a specialist): Initially 500 mg once daily for 1 week, dose to be taken with breakfast, then 500 mg twice daily for 1 week, dose to be taken with breakfast and evening meal, then 1.5–1.7 g daily in 2–3 divided doses, dose to be taken with meals

- **UNLICENSED USE** EvGr Metformin is used in the doses provided in BNF publications for the treatment of type 2 diabetes mellitus, ‹E› but these may differ from those

licensed. EvGr Metformin is used for the treatment of polycystic ovary syndrome, ‹E› but is not licensed for this indication. EvGr Metformin may be used for the treatment of type 1 diabetes mellitus, ‹E› but is not licensed for this indication.

> **IMPORTANT SAFETY INFORMATION**
>
> **MHRA/CHM ADVICE: METFORMIN IN PREGNANCY: STUDY SHOWS NO SAFETY CONCERNS (MARCH 2022)**
> European and CHM reviews of data from a large cohort study of Finnish population registries did not identify any safety issues with the use of metformin during pregnancy. Product literature for single-ingredient metformin preparations was subsequently updated to permit its use as an adjunct or alternative to insulin during pregnancy and the periconception period, if clinically indicated.
>
> **MHRA/CHM ADVICE: METFORMIN AND REDUCED VITAMIN B$_{12}$ LEVELS: NEW ADVICE FOR MONITORING PATIENTS AT RISK (JUNE 2022)**
> A European review, with input from the MHRA, has found vitamin B$_{12}$ deficiency to be a common side-effect in patients treated with metformin, especially in those receiving a higher dose or longer treatment duration and in those with risk factors for vitamin B$_{12}$ deficiency.
>
> Healthcare professionals are advised to check serum-vitamin B$_{12}$ levels if deficiency is suspected and consider periodic monitoring in patients with risk factors for deficiency. Vitamin B$_{12}$ deficiency should be treated according to current guidelines and treatment with metformin continued for as long as it is tolerated. Patients and their carers should be counselled on the signs and symptoms of vitamin B$_{12}$ deficiency and advised to seek medical advice if these occur. Patients should continue taking metformin unless they are advised to stop.

- **CONTRA-INDICATIONS** Acute metabolic acidosis (including lactic acidosis and diabetic ketoacidosis)

- **CAUTIONS**
  GENERAL CAUTIONS Risk factors for lactic acidosis
  SPECIFIC CAUTIONS
  ▶ When used for Type 1 diabetes mellitus in adults Recurrent lactic acidosis

  CAUTIONS, FURTHER INFORMATION
  ▶ Risk factors for lactic acidosis Manufacturer advises caution in chronic stable heart failure (monitor cardiac function), and concomitant use of drugs that can acutely impair renal function; interrupt treatment if dehydration occurs, and avoid in conditions that can acutely worsen renal function, or cause tissue hypoxia.
  ▶ Elderly Screening Tool of Older Persons' potentially inappropriate Prescriptions (STOPP) criteria to aid medication reviews (see Prescribing in the elderly p. 31 for information): potentially inappropriate if eGFR less than 30 mL/minute/1.73 m^2 (contra-indicated in severe renal impairment; risk of lactic acidosis).

- **INTERACTIONS** → Appendix 1: metformin

- **SIDE-EFFECTS**
  ▶ **Common or very common** Abdominal pain · appetite decreased · diarrhoea · gastrointestinal disorder · nausea · taste altered · vitamin B12 deficiency · vomiting
  ▶ **Rare or very rare** Hepatitis · lactic acidosis (discontinue) · skin reactions

  SIDE-EFFECTS, FURTHER INFORMATION Gastrointestinal side-effects are most frequent during treatment initiation and usually resolve spontaneously. A slow increase in dose may improve tolerability.

- **PREGNANCY** EvGr Can be used in pregnancy for both pre-existing and gestational diabetes. Women with gestational

6
Endocrine system

diabetes should discontinue treatment after giving birth.
ⒶSee also *Important safety information.*

● **BREAST FEEDING** EvGr May be used during breast-feeding in women with pre-existing diabetes. Ⓐ

● **HEPATIC IMPAIRMENT** Withdraw if tissue hypoxia likely.

● **RENAL IMPAIRMENT** See p. 21.
▸ In adults Manufacturer advises avoid if eGFR is less than 30 mL/minute/1.73 m².
▸ In children Manufacturer advises avoid if estimated glomerular filtration rate is less than 30 mL/minute/1.73 m².

Dose adjustments
▸ In children Manufacturer advises consider dose reduction in moderate impairment.
▸ In adults Manufacturer advises reduce dose in moderate impairment—consult product literature.

● **MONITORING REQUIREMENTS** Determine renal function before treatment and at least annually (at least twice a year in patients with additional risk factors for renal impairment, or if deterioration suspected).

● **PRESCRIBING AND DISPENSING INFORMATION**
▸ When used for Type 2 diabetes mellitus in adults The maximum dose for metformin immediate-release medicines in the BNF differs from product licence and is based on clinical experience. Patients taking up to 2 g daily of the standard-release metformin may start with the same daily dose of metformin modified release; not suitable if dose of standard-release tablets more than 2 g daily.

● **PATIENT AND CARER ADVICE** Manufacturer advises that patients and their carers should be informed of the risk of lactic acidosis and told to seek immediate medical attention if symptoms such as dyspnoea, muscle cramps, abdominal pain, hypothermia, or asthenia occur.
Medicines for Children leaflet: Metformin for diabetes
www.medicinesforchildren.org.uk/medicines/metformin-for-diabetes/

● **NATIONAL FUNDING/ACCESS DECISIONS**

GLUCOPHAGE ® SR For full details see funding body website

Scottish Medicines Consortium (SMC) decisions
▸ Metformin hydrochloride (*Glucophage SR*®) for type 2 diabetes mellitus (October 2009) SMC No. 148/04
Recommended with restrictions

● **MEDICINAL FORMS** There can be variation in the licensing of different medicines containing the same drug. Forms available from special-order manufacturers include: oral capsule, oral suspension, oral solution

Oral tablet
CAUTIONARY AND ADVISORY LABELS 21
▸ **Metformin hydrochloride (Non-proprietary)**
Metformin hydrochloride 500 mg Metformin 500mg tablets | 28 tablet PoM £1.42 DT = £0.60 | 84 tablet PoM £1.80–£2.88 | 500 tablet PoM £10.71–£14.11 | 1000 tablet PoM £9.75–£32.96
Metformin hydrochloride 850 mg Metformin 850mg tablets | 56 tablet PoM £3.20 DT = £0.94 | 200 tablet PoM £2.69 | 300 tablet PoM £4.10–£10.00
Metformin hydrochloride 1 gram Metformin 1g tablets | 28 tablet PoM £51.42 DT = £35.20
▸ **Axpinet** (GlucoRx Ltd)
Metformin hydrochloride 500 mg Axpinet 500mg tablets | 28 tablet PoM £0.50 DT = £0.60
Metformin hydrochloride 850 mg Axpinet 850mg tablets | 56 tablet PoM £0.95 DT = £0.94
▸ **Glucophage** (Merck Serono Ltd)
Metformin hydrochloride 500 mg Glucophage 500mg tablets | 84 tablet PoM £2.88
Metformin hydrochloride 850 mg Glucophage 850mg tablets | 56 tablet PoM £3.20 DT = £0.94

Modified-release tablet
CAUTIONARY AND ADVISORY LABELS 21, 25
▸ **Metformin hydrochloride (Non-proprietary)**
Metformin hydrochloride 500 mg Metformin 500mg modified-release tablets | 28 tablet PoM £0.90–£2.61 | 56 tablet PoM £5.22 DT = £2.52
Metformin hydrochloride 750 mg Metformin 750mg modified-release tablets | 28 tablet PoM £3.20–£4.31 | 56 tablet PoM £6.80 DT = £6.40
Metformin hydrochloride 1 gram Metformin 1g modified-release tablets | 28 tablet PoM £1.14–£4.53 | 56 tablet PoM £9.06 DT = £3.18
▸ **Diagemet XL** (Genus Pharmaceuticals Ltd)
Metformin hydrochloride 500 mg Diagemet XL 500mg tablets | 28 tablet PoM £1.49
▸ **Glucophage SR** (Merck Serono Ltd)
Metformin hydrochloride 500 mg Glucophage SR 500mg tablets | 28 tablet PoM £1.99 | 56 tablet PoM £4.00 DT = £2.52
Metformin hydrochloride 750 mg Glucophage SR 750mg tablets | 28 tablet PoM £3.20 | 56 tablet PoM £6.40 DT = £6.40
Metformin hydrochloride 850 mg Glucophage SR 850mg tablets | 30 tablet PoM £3.20 DT = £3.20
Metformin hydrochloride 1 gram Glucophage SR 1000mg tablets | 28 tablet PoM £3.20 | 56 tablet PoM £6.40 DT = £3.18
▸ **Glucorex SR** (GlucoRx Ltd)
Metformin hydrochloride 500 mg Glucorex SR 500mg tablets | 28 tablet PoM £0.95
▸ **Jesacrin** (Key Pharmaceuticals Ltd)
Metformin hydrochloride 500 mg Jesacrin 500mg modified-release tablets | 28 tablet PoM £0.90 | 56 tablet PoM £1.75 DT = £2.52
Metformin hydrochloride 750 mg Jesacrin 750mg modified-release tablets | 28 tablet PoM £3.20 | 56 tablet PoM £6.40 DT = £6.40
Metformin hydrochloride 1 gram Jesacrin 1000mg modified-release tablets | 28 tablet PoM £4.26 | 56 tablet PoM £8.52 DT = £3.18
▸ **Meijumet** (Medreich Plc)
Metformin hydrochloride 500 mg Meijumet 500mg modified-release tablets | 28 tablet PoM £1.50 | 56 tablet PoM £3.00 DT = £2.52
Metformin hydrochloride 750 mg Meijumet 750mg modified-release tablets | 28 tablet PoM £3.20 | 56 tablet PoM £6.40 DT = £6.40
Metformin hydrochloride 1 gram Meijumet 1000mg modified-release tablets | 28 tablet PoM £3.20 | 56 tablet PoM £6.40 DT = £3.18
▸ **Metabet SR** (Morningside Healthcare Ltd)
Metformin hydrochloride 500 mg Metabet SR 500mg tablets | 28 tablet PoM £1.99 | 56 tablet PoM £4.00 DT = £2.52
Metformin hydrochloride 1 gram Metabet SR 1000mg tablets | 28 tablet PoM £3.20 | 56 tablet PoM £6.40 DT = £3.18
▸ **Rudimet** (Rudipharm Ltd)
Metformin hydrochloride 500 mg Rudimet 500mg prolonged-release tablets | 56 tablet PoM Ⓧ DT = £2.52
Metformin hydrochloride 750 mg Rudimet 750mg prolonged-release tablets | 56 tablet PoM Ⓧ DT = £6.40
Metformin hydrochloride 1 gram Rudimet 1000mg prolonged-release tablets | 56 tablet PoM Ⓧ DT = £3.18
▸ **Sukkarto SR** (Morningside Healthcare Ltd)
Metformin hydrochloride 500 mg Sukkarto SR 500mg tablets | 28 tablet PoM £1.73 | 56 tablet PoM £3.46 DT = £2.52
Metformin hydrochloride 750 mg Sukkarto SR 750mg tablets | 56 tablet PoM £2.87 DT = £6.40
Metformin hydrochloride 1 gram Sukkarto SR 1000mg tablets | 28 tablet PoM £2.77 | 56 tablet PoM £5.24 DT = £3.18
▸ **Yaltormin SR** (Wockhardt UK Ltd)
Metformin hydrochloride 500 mg Yaltormin SR 500mg tablets | 28 tablet PoM £1.20 | 56 tablet PoM £2.39 DT = £2.52
Metformin hydrochloride 750 mg Yaltormin SR 750mg tablets | 28 tablet PoM £1.44 | 56 tablet PoM £2.88 DT = £6.40
Metformin hydrochloride 1 gram Yaltormin SR 1000mg tablets | 28 tablet PoM £1.92 | 56 tablet PoM £3.83 DT = £3.18

Oral solution
CAUTIONARY AND ADVISORY LABELS 21
▸ **Metformin hydrochloride (Non-proprietary)**
Metformin hydrochloride 100 mg per 1 ml Metformin 500mg/5ml oral solution sugar free | 100 ml PoM £13.56–£30.00 SF | 150 ml PoM £31.34 DT = £12.91 SF | 300 ml PoM £45.10 SF
Metformin hydrochloride 170 mg per 1 ml Metformin 850mg/5ml oral solution sugar free | 150 ml PoM £68.00 DT = £68.00 SF
Metformin hydrochloride 200 mg per 1 ml Metformin 1g/5ml oral solution sugar free | 150 ml PoM £76.00–£144.02 DT = £144.02 SF

Powder for oral solution
CAUTIONARY AND ADVISORY LABELS 13
- ▸ **Metformin hydrochloride (Non-proprietary)**
  Metformin hydrochloride 500 mg Metformin 500mg oral powder sachets sugar free | 30 sachet [PoM] £6.30-£11.34 DT = £6.30 [SF]
  Metformin hydrochloride 1 gram Metformin 1g oral powder sachets sugar free | 30 sachet [PoM] £12.60 [SF]

Combinations available: *Alogliptin with metformin,* below · *Canagliflozin with metformin,* p. 825 · *Dapagliflozin with metformin,* p. 827 · *Empagliflozin with metformin,* p. 829 · *Linagliptin with metformin,* p. 810 · *Pioglitazone with metformin,* p. 833 · *Saxagliptin with metformin,* p. 811 · *Sitagliptin with metformin,* p. 812 · *Vildagliptin with metformin,* p. 812

BLOOD GLUCOSE LOWERING DRUGS ›
DIPEPTIDYLPEPTIDASE-4 INHIBITORS (GLIPTINS)

Alogliptin
04-Jul-2022

- ● **DRUG ACTION** Inhibits dipeptidylpeptidase-4 to increase insulin secretion and lower glucagon secretion.

● **INDICATIONS AND DOSE**

Type 2 diabetes mellitus in combination with other antidiabetic drugs (including insulin) if existing treatment fails to achieve adequate glycaemic control
- ▸ BY MOUTH
- ▸ Adult: 25 mg once daily, for further information on use with other antidiabetic drugs—consult product literature

DOSE ADJUSTMENTS DUE TO INTERACTIONS
- ▸ Dose of concomitant sulfonylurea or insulin may need to be reduced.
- ▸ Caution with use in combination with both metformin and pioglitazone—risk of hypoglycaemia (dose of metformin or pioglitazone may need to be reduced).

- ● **CAUTIONS** History of pancreatitis · not recommended in moderate to severe heart failure (limited experience)
- ● **INTERACTIONS** → Appendix 1: dipeptidylpeptidase-4 inhibitors
- ● **SIDE-EFFECTS**
- ▸ **Common or very common** Abdominal pain · gastrooesophageal reflux disease · headache · increased risk of infection · skin reactions
- ▸ **Frequency not known** Angioedema · bullous pemphigoid (discontinue) · hepatic function abnormal · pancreatitis acute · Stevens-Johnson syndrome

SIDE-EFFECTS, FURTHER INFORMATION Discontinue if symptoms of acute pancreatitis occur such as persistent, severe abdominal pain.
- ● **ALLERGY AND CROSS-SENSITIVITY** [EvGr] Contra-indicated if history of serious hypersensitivity to dipeptidylpeptidase-4 inhibitors. [M]
- ● **PREGNANCY** Manufacturer advises avoid—no information available.
- ● **BREAST FEEDING** Avoid—present in milk in *animal* studies.
- ● **HEPATIC IMPAIRMENT** Manufacturer advises avoid in severe impairment—no information available.
- ● **RENAL IMPAIRMENT**
  Dose adjustments [EvGr] Reduce dose to 12.5 mg once daily if creatinine clearance 30–50 mL/minute.
  Reduce dose to 6.25 mg once daily if creatinine clearance less than 30 mL/minute. [M]
  See p. 21.
- ● **MONITORING REQUIREMENTS** Determine renal function before treatment and periodically thereafter.

- ● **MEDICINAL FORMS** There can be variation in the licensing of different medicines containing the same drug.
  Oral tablet
- ▸ **Alogliptin (Non-proprietary)**
  Alogliptin (as Alogliptin benzoate) 6.25 mg Alogliptin 6.25mg tablets | 28 tablet [PoM] £26.60 DT = £26.60
  Alogliptin (as Alogliptin benzoate) 12.5 mg Alogliptin 12.5mg tablets | 28 tablet [PoM] £26.60 DT = £26.60
  Alogliptin (as Alogliptin benzoate) 25 mg Alogliptin 25mg tablets | 28 tablet [PoM] £26.60 DT = £26.60
- ▸ **Vipidia** (Takeda UK Ltd)
  Alogliptin (as Alogliptin benzoate) 6.25 mg Vipidia 6.25mg tablets | 28 tablet [PoM] £26.60 DT = £26.60
  Alogliptin (as Alogliptin benzoate) 12.5 mg Vipidia 12.5mg tablets | 28 tablet [PoM] £26.60 DT = £26.60
  Alogliptin (as Alogliptin benzoate) 25 mg Vipidia 25mg tablets | 28 tablet [PoM] £26.60 DT = £26.60

Alogliptin with metformin
03-Feb-2020

The properties listed below are those particular to the combination only. For the properties of the components please consider, alogliptin above, metformin hydrochloride p. 807.

● **INDICATIONS AND DOSE**

Type 2 diabetes mellitus not controlled by metformin alone or by metformin in combination with either pioglitazone or insulin
- ▸ BY MOUTH
- ▸ Adult: 1 tablet twice daily, based on patient's current metformin dose

- ● **INTERACTIONS** → Appendix 1: dipeptidylpeptidase-4 inhibitors · metformin

- ● **MEDICINAL FORMS** There can be variation in the licensing of different medicines containing the same drug.
  Oral tablet
  CAUTIONARY AND ADVISORY LABELS 21
- ▸ **Alogliptin with metformin (Non-proprietary)**
  Alogliptin (as Alogliptin benzoate) 12.5 mg, Metformin hydrochloride 1 gram Alogliptin 12.5mg / Metformin 1g tablets | 56 tablet [PoM] £26.60 DT = £26.60
- ▸ **Vipdomet** (Takeda UK Ltd)
  Alogliptin (as Alogliptin benzoate) 12.5 mg, Metformin hydrochloride 1 gram Vipdomet 12.5mg/1000mg tablets | 56 tablet [PoM] £26.60 DT = £26.60

Linagliptin
27-Apr-2022

- ● **DRUG ACTION** Inhibits dipeptidylpeptidase-4 to increase insulin secretion and lower glucagon secretion.

● **INDICATIONS AND DOSE**

Type 2 diabetes mellitus as monotherapy (if metformin inappropriate), or in combination with other antidiabetic drugs (including insulin) if existing treatment fails to achieve adequate glycaemic control
- ▸ BY MOUTH
- ▸ Adult: 5 mg once daily, for further information on use with other antidiabetic drugs—consult product literature

DOSE ADJUSTMENTS DUE TO INTERACTIONS
- ▸ Dose of concomitant sulfonylurea or insulin may need to be reduced.

- ● **CAUTIONS** History of pancreatitis
- ● **INTERACTIONS** → Appendix 1: dipeptidylpeptidase-4 inhibitors
- ● **SIDE-EFFECTS**
- ▸ **Uncommon** Cough · nasopharyngitis
- ▸ **Rare or very rare** Angioedema · bullous pemphigoid (discontinue) · skin reactions

▸ **Frequency not known** Pancreatitis

SIDE-EFFECTS, FURTHER INFORMATION Discontinue if symptoms of acute pancreatitis occur such as persistent, severe abdominal pain.

● PREGNANCY Avoid—no information available.

● BREAST FEEDING Avoid—present in milk in *animal* studies.

● NATIONAL FUNDING/ACCESS DECISIONS
For full details see funding body website

Scottish Medicines Consortium (SMC) decisions

▸ Linagliptin (*Trajenta*®) for the treatment of type 2 diabetes mellitus to improve glycaemic control in adults (January 2012) SMC No. 746/11 Recommended with restrictions

▸ Linagliptin (*Trajenta*®) for the treatment of type 2 diabetes mellitus to improve glycaemic control in adults in combination with insulin with or without metformin, when this regimen alone, with diet and exercise, does not provide adequate glycaemic control (May 2015) SMC No. 850/13 Recommended

● MEDICINAL FORMS There can be variation in the licensing of different medicines containing the same drug.

Oral tablet

▸ Trajenta (Boehringer Ingelheim Ltd)
Linagliptin 5 mg Trajenta 5mg tablets | 28 tablet [PoM] £33.26 DT = £33.26

Combinations available: *Empagliflozin with linagliptin,* p. 829

Linagliptin with metformin
20-Nov-2020

The properties listed below are those particular to the combination only. For the properties of the components please consider, linagliptin p. 809, metformin hydrochloride p. 807.

● INDICATIONS AND DOSE

Type 2 diabetes mellitus not controlled by metformin alone or by metformin in combination with either a sulfonylurea or insulin

▸ BY MOUTH

▸ Adult: 1 tablet twice daily, based on patient's current metformin dose

● INTERACTIONS → Appendix 1: dipeptidylpeptidase-4 inhibitors · metformin

● NATIONAL FUNDING/ACCESS DECISIONS
For full details see funding body website

Scottish Medicines Consortium (SMC) decisions

▸ Linagliptin with metformin (*Jentadueto*®) for the treatment of adult patients with type 2 diabetes mellitus in combination with insulin (i.e. triple combination therapy) as an adjunct to diet and exercise to improve glycaemic control when insulin and metformin alone do not provide adequate glycaemic control (June 2015) SMC No. 1057/15 Recommended with restrictions

● MEDICINAL FORMS There can be variation in the licensing of different medicines containing the same drug.

Oral tablet
CAUTIONARY AND ADVISORY LABELS 21

▸ Jentadueto (Boehringer Ingelheim Ltd)
Linagliptin 2.5 mg, Metformin hydrochloride 850 mg Jentadueto 2.5mg/850mg tablets | 56 tablet [PoM] £33.26 DT = £33.26
Linagliptin 2.5 mg, Metformin hydrochloride 1000 mg Jentadueto 2.5mg/1000mg tablets | 56 tablet [PoM] £33.26 DT = £33.26

Saxagliptin
24-May-2022

● DRUG ACTION Inhibits dipeptidylpeptidase-4 to increase insulin secretion and lower glucagon secretion.

● INDICATIONS AND DOSE

Type 2 diabetes mellitus as monotherapy (if metformin inappropriate), or in combination with other antidiabetic drugs (including insulin) if existing treatment fails to achieve adequate glycaemic control

▸ BY MOUTH

▸ Adult: 5 mg once daily, for further information on use with other antidiabetic drugs—consult product literature

DOSE ADJUSTMENTS DUE TO INTERACTIONS

▸ Dose of concomitant sulfonylurea or insulin may need to be reduced.

● CAUTIONS History of pancreatitis · moderate to severe heart failure (limited experience)

● INTERACTIONS → Appendix 1: dipeptidylpeptidase-4 inhibitors

● SIDE-EFFECTS

▸ **Common or very common** Abdominal pain · dizziness · fatigue · headache · increased risk of infection · skin reactions · vomiting

▸ **Uncommon** Pancreatitis

▸ **Rare or very rare** Angioedema

▸ **Frequency not known** Bullous pemphigoid (discontinue) · constipation · nausea

SIDE-EFFECTS, FURTHER INFORMATION Discontinue if symptoms of acute pancreatitis occur such as persistent, severe abdominal pain.

● ALLERGY AND CROSS-SENSITIVITY [EvGr] Contra-indicated if patient has a history of serious hypersensitivity to dipeptidylpeptidase-4 inhibitors. ⟨M⟩

● PREGNANCY Avoid unless essential—toxicity in *animal* studies.

● BREAST FEEDING Avoid—present in milk in *animal* studies.

● HEPATIC IMPAIRMENT Manufacturer advises caution in moderate impairment; avoid in severe impairment (risk of increased exposure).

● RENAL IMPAIRMENT [EvGr] Caution if eGFR less than 45 mL/minute/1.73 m². Avoid in end-stage renal disease requiring haemodialysis. ⟨M⟩
Dose adjustments [EvGr] Reduce dose to 2.5 mg once daily if eGFR less than 45 mL/minute/1.73 m²; ⟨M⟩ see p. 21.

● MONITORING REQUIREMENTS Determine renal function before treatment and periodically thereafter.

● NATIONAL FUNDING/ACCESS DECISIONS
For full details see funding body website

Scottish Medicines Consortium (SMC) decisions

▸ Saxagliptin (*Onglyza*®) in adults with type 2 diabetes mellitus to improve glycaemic control as triple oral therapy in combination with metformin plus a sulfonylurea when this regimen alone, with diet and exercise, does not provide adequate glycaemic control (December 2013) SMC No. 918/13 Recommended with restrictions

● MEDICINAL FORMS There can be variation in the licensing of different medicines containing the same drug.

Oral tablet

▸ Onglyza (AstraZeneca UK Ltd)
Saxagliptin (as Saxagliptin hydrochloride) 2.5 mg Onglyza 2.5mg tablets | 28 tablet [PoM] £31.60 DT = £31.60
Saxagliptin (as Saxagliptin hydrochloride) 5 mg Onglyza 5mg tablets | 28 tablet [PoM] £31.60 DT = £31.60

Saxagliptin with dapagliflozin   25-Aug-2020

The properties listed below are those particular to the combination only. For the properties of the components please consider, saxagliptin p. 810, dapagliflozin p. 826.

- **INDICATIONS AND DOSE**

  Type 2 diabetes mellitus not controlled by metformin and/or a sulfonylurea with either saxagliptin or dapagliflozin
  - ▸ BY MOUTH
  - ▸ Adult 18–74 years: 5/10 mg once daily
  - ▸ Adult 75 years and over: Initiation not recommended

  DOSE ADJUSTMENTS DUE TO INTERACTIONS
  - ▸ Dose of concomitant sulfonylurea may need to be reduced.

  DOSE EQUIVALENCE AND CONVERSION
  - ▸ Dose expressed as *x*/*y* mg saxagliptin/dapagliflozin.

- **INTERACTIONS** → Appendix 1: dipeptidylpeptidase-4 inhibitors · sodium glucose co-transporter 2 inhibitors

- **HEPATIC IMPAIRMENT** Manufacturer advises caution in moderate impairment; avoid in severe impairment.

- **RENAL IMPAIRMENT**
  Dose adjustments Manufacturer advises avoid if eGFR less than 60 mL/minute/1.73 m^2 (ineffective).

- **PATIENT AND CARER ADVICE**
  Missed doses Manufacturer advises if a dose is more than 12 hours late, the missed dose should not be taken and the next dose should be taken at the normal time.

- **NATIONAL FUNDING/ACCESS DECISIONS**
  For full details see funding body website

  Scottish Medicines Consortium (SMC) decisions
  - ▸ Saxagliptin/dapagliflozin (*Qtern*®) in adults with type 2 diabetes mellitus: to improve glycaemic control when metformin and/or sulfonylurea and one of the monocomponents of *Qtern*® do not provide adequate glycaemic control; when already being treated with the free combination of dapagliflozin and saxagliptin (July 2017) SMC No. 1255/17 Recommended with restrictions

- **MEDICINAL FORMS** There can be variation in the licensing of different medicines containing the same drug.
  Oral tablet
  - ▸ Qtern (AstraZeneca UK Ltd)
    Saxagliptin (as Saxagliptin hydrochloride) 5 mg, Dapagliflozin (as Dapagliflozin propanediol monohydrate) 10 mg Qtern 5mg/10mg tablets | 28 tablet [PoM] £49.56 DT = £49.56

Saxagliptin with metformin   25-Aug-2020

The properties listed below are those particular to the combination only. For the properties of the components please consider, saxagliptin p. 810, metformin hydrochloride p. 807.

- **INDICATIONS AND DOSE**

  Type 2 diabetes mellitus not controlled by metformin alone or by metformin in combination with either a sulfonylurea or insulin
  - ▸ BY MOUTH
  - ▸ Adult: 1 tablet twice daily, based on patient's current metformin dose

- **INTERACTIONS** → Appendix 1: dipeptidylpeptidase-4 inhibitors · metformin

- **NATIONAL FUNDING/ACCESS DECISIONS**
  For full details see funding body website

  Scottish Medicines Consortium (SMC) decisions
  - ▸ Saxagliptin with metformin (*Komboglyze*®) as an adjunct to diet and exercise to improve glycaemic control in adults with type 2 diabetes mellitus inadequately controlled on their maximally tolerated dose of metformin alone or those already being treated with the combination of saxagliptin and metformin as separate tablets (June 2013) SMC No. 870/13 Recommended with restrictions

- **MEDICINAL FORMS** No licensed medicines listed.

Sitagliptin   04-May-2022

- **DRUG ACTION** Inhibits dipeptidylpeptidase-4 to increase insulin secretion and lower glucagon secretion.

- **INDICATIONS AND DOSE**

  Type 2 diabetes mellitus as monotherapy (if metformin inappropriate), or in combination with other antidiabetic drugs (including insulin) if existing treatment fails to achieve adequate glycaemic control
  - ▸ BY MOUTH
  - ▸ Adult: 100 mg once daily, for further information on use with other antidiabetic drugs—consult product literature

  DOSE ADJUSTMENTS DUE TO INTERACTIONS
  - ▸ Dose of concomitant sulfonylurea or insulin may need to be reduced.

- **CAUTIONS** History of pancreatitis

- **INTERACTIONS** → Appendix 1: dipeptidylpeptidase-4 inhibitors

- **SIDE-EFFECTS**
  - ▸ **Common or very common** Headache
  - ▸ **Uncommon** Constipation · dizziness · skin reactions
  - ▸ **Frequency not known** Angioedema · back pain · bullous pemphigoid (discontinue) · cutaneous vasculitis · interstitial lung disease · joint disorders · myalgia · pancreatitis acute · renal impairment · Stevens-Johnson syndrome · vomiting

  SIDE-EFFECTS, FURTHER INFORMATION Discontinue if symptoms of acute pancreatitis occur such as persistent, severe abdominal pain.

- **PREGNANCY** Avoid—toxicity in *animal* studies.

- **BREAST FEEDING** Avoid—present in milk in *animal* studies.

- **RENAL IMPAIRMENT**
  Dose adjustments [EvGr] Reduce dose to 50 mg once daily if eGFR 30–45 mL/minute/1.73 m^2.
  Reduce dose to 25 mg once daily if eGFR less than 30 mL/minute/1.73 m^2. ⟨M⟩
  See p. 21.

- **MONITORING REQUIREMENTS** [EvGr] Determine renal function before treatment and periodically thereafter. ⟨M⟩

- **NATIONAL FUNDING/ACCESS DECISIONS**
  For full details see funding body website

  Scottish Medicines Consortium (SMC) decisions
  - ▸ Sitagliptin (*Januvia*®) as monotherapy for type 2 diabetes mellitus (July 2010) SMC No. 607/10 Recommended with restrictions
  - ▸ Sitagliptin (*Januvia*®) for the treatment of type 2 diabetes mellitus to improve glycaemic control in adults as add-on to insulin (with or without metformin) when diet and exercise plus stable dose of insulin do not provide adequate glycaemic control (September 2015) SMC No. 1083/15 Recommended

- **MEDICINAL FORMS** There can be variation in the licensing of different medicines containing the same drug.
  Oral tablet
  - ▸ Sitagliptin (Non-proprietary)
    Sitagliptin 25 mg Sitagliptin 25mg tablets | 28 tablet [PoM] £39.84 DT = £0.97
    Sitagliptin 50 mg Sitagliptin 50mg tablets | 28 tablet [PoM] £39.84 DT = £0.99
    Sitagliptin 100 mg Sitagliptin 100mg tablets | 28 tablet [PoM] £39.84 DT = £1.38

▸ **Januvia** (Merck Sharp & Dohme (UK) Ltd)
Sitagliptin 25 mg Januvia 25mg tablets | 28 tablet [PoM] £33.26 DT = £0.97
Sitagliptin 50 mg Januvia 50mg tablets | 28 tablet [PoM] £33.26 DT = £0.99
Sitagliptin 100 mg Januvia 100mg tablets | 28 tablet [PoM] £33.26 DT = £1.38

Sitagliptin with metformin

18-Nov-2020

The properties listed below are those particular to the combination only. For the properties of the components please consider, sitagliptin p. 811, metformin hydrochloride p. 807.

● **INDICATIONS AND DOSE**

Type 2 diabetes mellitus not controlled by metformin alone or by metformin in combination with either a sulfonylurea or pioglitazone or insulin
▸ BY MOUTH
▸ Adult: 1 tablet twice daily

● INTERACTIONS → Appendix 1: dipeptidylpeptidase-4 inhibitors · metformin

● NATIONAL FUNDING/ACCESS DECISIONS
For full details see funding body website
Scottish Medicines Consortium (SMC) decisions
▸ Sitagliptin/metformin (*Janumet*®) for type 2 diabetes (May 2010) SMC No. 492/08 Recommended with restrictions
▸ Sitagliptin/metformin (*Janumet*®) in combination with a sulfonylurea (i.e. triple combination therapy) as an adjunct to diet and exercise in patients inadequately controlled on their maximal tolerated dose of metformin and a sulfonylurea (August 2010) SMC No. 627/10 Recommended

● MEDICINAL FORMS There can be variation in the licensing of different medicines containing the same drug.
Oral tablet
CAUTIONARY AND ADVISORY LABELS 21
▸ **Sitagliptin with metformin (Non-proprietary)**
Sitagliptin 50 mg, Metformin hydrochloride 1 gram Metformin 1g / Sitagliptin 50mg tablets | 56 tablet [PoM] £33.26 DT = £8.19
▸ **Janumet** (Merck Sharp & Dohme (UK) Ltd)
Sitagliptin 50 mg, Metformin hydrochloride 1 gram Janumet 50mg/1000mg tablets | 56 tablet [PoM] £33.26 DT = £8.19

Vildagliptin

27-Apr-2022

● **DRUG ACTION** Inhibits dipeptidylpeptidase-4 to increase insulin secretion and lower glucagon secretion.

● **INDICATIONS AND DOSE**

Type 2 diabetes mellitus as monotherapy (if metformin inappropriate), or in combination with other antidiabetic drugs (including insulin) if existing treatment fails to achieve adequate glycaemic control
▸ BY MOUTH
▸ Adult: 50 mg twice daily, reduce dose to 50 mg once daily in the morning when used in dual combination with a sulfonylurea. For further information on use with other antidiabetic drugs—consult product literature

DOSE ADJUSTMENTS DUE TO INTERACTIONS
▸ Dose of concomitant sulfonylurea or insulin may need to be reduced.

● CAUTIONS History of pancreatitis · manufacturer advises avoid in severe heart failure—no information available
● INTERACTIONS → Appendix 1: dipeptidylpeptidase-4 inhibitors
● SIDE-EFFECTS
▸ **Common or very common** Dizziness

▸ **Uncommon** Arthralgia · constipation · headache · hypoglycaemia · peripheral oedema
▸ **Rare or very rare** Increased risk of infection
▸ **Frequency not known** Bullous pemphigoid (discontinue) · hepatitis · myalgia · pancreatitis · skin reactions
SIDE-EFFECTS, FURTHER INFORMATION **Pancreatitis** Discontinue if symptoms of acute pancreatitis occur, such as persistent severe abdominal pain.
  Liver toxicity Rare reports of liver dysfunction; discontinue if jaundice or other signs of liver dysfunction occur.

● PREGNANCY Avoid—toxicity in *animal* studies.
● BREAST FEEDING Avoid—present in milk in *animal* studies.
● HEPATIC IMPAIRMENT Manufacturer advises avoid.
● RENAL IMPAIRMENT
Dose adjustments [EvGr] Reduce dose to 50 mg once daily if creatinine clearance less than 50 mL/minute. ⋈ See p. 21.
● MONITORING REQUIREMENTS Monitor liver function before treatment and every 3 months for first year and periodically thereafter.
● PATIENT AND CARER ADVICE
Liver toxicity Patients should be advised to seek prompt medical attention if symptoms such as nausea, vomiting, abdominal pain, fatigue, and dark urine develop.
● NATIONAL FUNDING/ACCESS DECISIONS
For full details see funding body website
Scottish Medicines Consortium (SMC) decisions
▸ Vildagliptin (*Galvus*®) for the treatment of type 2 diabetes mellitus [as dual oral therapy in combination with metformin] (April 2008) SMC No. 435/07 Recommended with restrictions
▸ Vildagliptin (*Galvus*®) for the treatment of type 2 diabetes mellitus [as dual oral therapy in combination with a sulphonylurea] (October 2009) SMC No. 571/09 Recommended
▸ Vildagliptin (*Galvus*®) as monotherapy for the treatment of type 2 diabetes mellitus, in patients inadequately controlled by diet and exercise alone and for whom metformin is inappropriate due to contra-indications or intolerance (January 2013) SMC No. 826/12 Recommended with restrictions
▸ Vildagliptin (*Galvus*®) for the treatment of type 2 diabetes mellitus in adults as triple oral therapy in combination with a sulphonylurea and metformin when diet and exercise plus dual therapy with these medicinal products do not provide adequate glycaemic control (December 2013) SMC No. 875/13 Recommended with restrictions

● MEDICINAL FORMS There can be variation in the licensing of different medicines containing the same drug.
Oral tablet
▸ **Vildagliptin (Non-proprietary)**
Vildagliptin 50 mg Vildagliptin 50mg tablets | 56 tablet [PoM] £24.21 DT = £11.11
▸ **Galvus** (Novartis Pharmaceuticals UK Ltd)
Vildagliptin 50 mg Galvus 50mg tablets | 56 tablet [PoM] £33.35 DT = £11.11

Vildagliptin with metformin

16-Nov-2020

The properties listed below are those particular to the combination only. For the properties of the components please consider, vildagliptin above, metformin hydrochloride p. 807.

● **INDICATIONS AND DOSE**

Type 2 diabetes mellitus not controlled by metformin alone or by metformin in combination with either a sulfonylurea or insulin
▸ BY MOUTH
▸ Adult: 1 tablet twice daily, based on patient's current metformin dose

- **INTERACTIONS** → Appendix 1: dipeptidylpeptidase-4 inhibitors · metformin

- **NATIONAL FUNDING/ACCESS DECISIONS**
  For full details see funding body website
  Scottish Medicines Consortium (SMC) decisions
  ▸ Vildagliptin with metformin (*Eucreas*®) for the treatment of type 2 diabetes (July 2008) SMC No. 477/08 Recommended with restrictions

- **MEDICINAL FORMS** There can be variation in the licensing of different medicines containing the same drug.
  Oral tablet
  CAUTIONARY AND ADVISORY LABELS 21
  ▸ Vildagliptin with metformin (Non-proprietary)
     Vildagliptin 50 mg, Metformin hydrochloride 850 mg Vildagliptin 50mg / Metformin 850mg tablets | 60 tablet PoM £35.68 DT = £35.68
     Vildagliptin 50 mg, Metformin hydrochloride 1 gram Vildagliptin 50mg / Metformin 1g tablets | 60 tablet PoM £38.47 DT = £35.68
  ▸ Eucreas (Novartis Pharmaceuticals UK Ltd)
     Vildagliptin 50 mg, Metformin hydrochloride 850 mg Eucreas 50mg/850mg tablets | 60 tablet PoM £35.68 DT = £35.68
     Vildagliptin 50 mg, Metformin hydrochloride 1 gram Eucreas 50mg/1000mg tablets | 60 tablet PoM £35.68 DT = £35.68

BLOOD GLUCOSE LOWERING DRUGS ›
GLUCAGON-LIKE PEPTIDE-1 RECEPTOR AGONISTS

Dulaglutide
04-Feb-2025

- **DRUG ACTION** Dulaglutide is a long-acting glucagon-like peptide 1 (GLP-1) receptor agonist that augments glucose-dependent insulin secretion, and slows gastric emptying.

- **INDICATIONS AND DOSE**

  Type 2 diabetes mellitus as monotherapy (if metformin inappropriate)
  ▸ BY SUBCUTANEOUS INJECTION
  ▸ Adult: 0.75 mg once weekly

  Type 2 diabetes mellitus in combination with other antidiabetic drugs (including insulin) if existing treatment fails to achieve adequate glycaemic control
  ▸ BY SUBCUTANEOUS INJECTION
  ▸ Adult: 1.5 mg once weekly; increased if necessary to 3 mg once weekly after at least 4 weeks, then increased if necessary to 4.5 mg once weekly after another 4 weeks, a starting dose of 0.75 mg once weekly may be considered for potentially vulnerable patients; maximum 4.5 mg per week

  DOSE ADJUSTMENTS DUE TO INTERACTIONS
  ▸ Dose of concomitant insulin or drugs that stimulate insulin secretion may need to be reduced.

IMPORTANT SAFETY INFORMATION

MHRA/CHM ADVICE: GLP-1 RECEPTOR AGONISTS: REPORTS OF DIABETIC KETOACIDOSIS WHEN CONCOMITANT INSULIN WAS RAPIDLY REDUCED OR DISCONTINUED (JUNE 2019)
Serious and life-threatening cases of diabetic ketoacidosis have been reported in patients with type 2 diabetes mellitus on a combination of a glucagon-like peptide-1 (GLP-1) receptor agonist and insulin, particularly after discontinuation or rapid dose reduction of concomitant insulin. Healthcare professionals are advised that any dose reduction of insulin should be done in a stepwise manner with careful blood glucose self-monitoring, particularly when GLP-1 receptor agonist therapy is initiated. Patients should be informed of the risk factors for and signs and symptoms of diabetic ketoacidosis, and advised to seek immediate medical attention if these develop.

MHRA/CHM ADVICE: GLP-1 RECEPTOR AGONISTS: REMINDER OF THE POTENTIAL SIDE EFFECTS AND TO BE AWARE OF THE POTENTIAL FOR MISUSE (OCTOBER 2024)
The MHRA reminds healthcare professionals to ensure that patients are aware of potential side-effects associated with glucagon-like peptide-1 (GLP-1) receptor agonists following anecdotal evidence and Yellow Card reports suggesting misuse of these medicines for weight management outside of their licence. The only GLP-1 receptor agonists licensed for weight management are liraglutide p. 816 (*Saxenda*®), semaglutide p. 819 (*Wegovy*®), and tirzepatide p. 822 (*Mounjaro*®), which is also a glucose-dependent insulinotropic polypeptide (GIP) receptor agonist. The benefits and risks of these medicines for weight loss in individuals who are not obese, or who are not overweight with weight-related co-morbidities, have not been studied.

Healthcare professionals should inform patients and carers upon initial prescription and at any dose increase about the common risk of gastro-intestinal side-effects (including nausea, vomiting, diarrhoea, and constipation) associated with GLP-1 receptor agonists; these are usually non-serious but can persist for several days and may lead to serious complications such as severe dehydration and kidney damage, resulting in hospitalisation. For this reason, patients should be advised to stay well hydrated by drinking plenty of fluids throughout treatment. They should also be informed of other serious but less common side-effects, including acute gallstone disease, pancreatitis, and serious allergic reactions.

Patients and carers should be advised to ensure that prescriptions are only obtained from registered healthcare professionals and that private prescriptions are dispensed from authorised sources to avoid the risk of receiving falsified pens. Patients and carers should consult the patient information leaflet for instructions on the use of GLP-1 receptor agonists, and be advised to only administer the prescribed dose.

MHRA/CHM ADVICE: GLP-1 AND DUAL GIP/GLP-1 RECEPTOR AGONISTS: POTENTIAL RISK OF PULMONARY ASPIRATION DURING GENERAL ANAESTHESIA OR DEEP SEDATION (JANUARY 2025)
An EU review has concluded that glucagon-like peptide-1 (GLP-1) and dual glucose-dependent insulinotropic polypeptide (GIP)/GLP-1 receptor agonists are associated with a potential risk of pulmonary aspiration in patients undergoing surgery or procedures requiring general anaesthesia or deep sedation. These medicines are known to slow gastric emptying, thereby increasing the risk of residual gastric contents despite preoperative fasting, which could lead to pulmonary aspiration and other severe complications, such as aspiration pneumonia.

The MHRA advises healthcare professionals to identify the increased risk of aspiration as early as possible, ideally at the pre-assessment clinic before surgery, in patients using GLP-1 or dual GIP/GLP-1 receptor agonists. Anaesthetists should complete an individualised preoperative risk assessment and consider the following:
- patients with underlying diabetic gastroparesis, as well as other co-morbidities such as obesity or gastroesophageal reflux disease, and symptoms of delayed gastric emptying (such as nausea, vomiting and abdominal pain) may have a higher risk of aspiration;
- directly asking patients or their carers about their use of GLP-1 or dual GIP/GLP-1 receptor agonists, as private prescriptions may not be included in the patient's medical notes or drug history, and patients who may have purchased these medications for use in

aesthetic weight loss may not readily disclose this information (see also advice issued in October 2024, above).

There is limited evidence to support any recommendations on a time frame to withhold GLP-1 or dual GIP/GLP-1 receptor agonists prior to anaesthesia, new fasting guidelines, or an appropriate medical procedure to confirm an empty stomach. Anaesthetists should manage aspiration risk in line with usual anaesthetic practice and retain flexibility to provide individualised assessment.

Healthcare professionals should counsel patients or their carers to continue taking their prescribed medicines and not stop treatment without first discussing with their doctor. They should also be advised regarding the risk of aspiration and that there may be a need to modify pre-procedure instruction and anaesthetic technique.

● CONTRA-INDICATIONS Severe gastro-intestinal disease—no information available

● CAUTIONS General anaesthesia or deep sedation (risk of pulmonary aspiration due to delayed gastric emptying)

● INTERACTIONS → Appendix 1: glucagon-like peptide-1 receptor agonists

● SIDE-EFFECTS
▸ **Common or very common** Appetite decreased · atrioventricular block · burping · constipation · diarrhoea · fatigue · gastrointestinal discomfort · gastrointestinal disorders · hypoglycaemia · nausea · sinus tachycardia · vomiting
▸ **Uncommon** Dehydration · gallbladder disorders
▸ **Rare or very rare** Angioedema · pancreatitis acute

SIDE-EFFECTS, FURTHER INFORMATION Discontinue if symptoms of acute pancreatitis occur, such as persistent, severe abdominal pain. If pancreatitis confirmed, do not restart treatment.

● PREGNANCY Manufacturer advises avoid—toxicity in *animal* studies.

● BREAST FEEDING Manufacturer advises avoid— no information available.

● RENAL IMPAIRMENT [EvGr] Avoid if eGFR less than 15 mL/minute/1.73 m² (limited information available), [M] see p. 21.

● PRESCRIBING AND DISPENSING INFORMATION Dulaglutide is a biological medicine. Biological medicines must be prescribed and dispensed by brand name, see *Biological medicines* and *Biosimilar medicines*, under Guidance on prescribing p. 1; record the brand name and batch number after each administration.

For choice of therapy, see Type 2 diabetes p. 800.

● HANDLING AND STORAGE **Refrigerated storage** is usually necessary (2 °C – 8 °C). Once in use, may be stored unrefrigerated for up to 14 days at a temperature not above 30 °C.

● PATIENT AND CARER ADVICE Patients or carers should be given advice on how to administer dulaglutide injection.
Acute pancreatitis Patients should be told how to recognise signs and symptoms of acute pancreatitis and advised to seek medical attention if symptoms such as persistent, severe abdominal pain develop.
Dehydration Patients should be informed of the potential risk of dehydration in relation to gastro-intestinal side-effects and advised to take precautions to avoid fluid depletion.
Missed doses If a dose is missed, it should be administered as soon as possible only if there are at least 3 days until the next scheduled dose; if less than 3 days remain before the next scheduled dose, the missed dose should not be taken and the next dose should be taken at the normal time.

● NATIONAL FUNDING/ACCESS DECISIONS
For full details see funding body website
Scottish Medicines Consortium (SMC) decisions
▸ Dulaglutide (*Trulicity*®) for use in adults with type 2 diabetes mellitus to improve glycaemic control as add-on therapy in combination with other glucose-lowering medicinal products including insulin, when these, together with diet and exercise, do not provide adequate glycaemic control (January 2016) SMC No. 1110/15 Recommended with restrictions

● MEDICINAL FORMS There can be variation in the licensing of different medicines containing the same drug.
Solution for injection
EXCIPIENTS: May contain Polysorbates
▸ **Trulicity** (Eli Lilly and Company Ltd)
Dulaglutide 1.5 mg per 1 ml Trulicity 0.75mg/0.5ml solution for injection pre-filled pens | 4 pre-filled disposable injection [PoM] £73.25 DT = £73.25
Dulaglutide 3 mg per 1 ml Trulicity 1.5mg/0.5ml solution for injection pre-filled pens | 4 pre-filled disposable injection [PoM] £73.25 DT = £73.25
Dulaglutide 6 mg per 1 ml Trulicity 3mg/0.5ml solution for injection pre-filled pens | 4 pre-filled disposable injection [PoM] £73.25 DT = £73.25
Dulaglutide 9 mg per 1 ml Trulicity 4.5mg/0.5ml solution for injection pre-filled pens | 4 pre-filled disposable injection [PoM] £73.25 DT = £73.25

Exenatide
04-Feb-2025

● DRUG ACTION Binds to, and activates, the GLP-1 (glucagon-like peptide-1) receptor to increase insulin secretion, suppresses glucagon secretion, and slows gastric emptying.

● INDICATIONS AND DOSE

Type 2 diabetes mellitus in combination with other antidiabetic drugs (including insulin) if existing treatment fails to achieve adequate glycaemic control
▸ BY SUBCUTANEOUS INJECTION USING IMMEDIATE-RELEASE MEDICINES
▸ **Adult:** Initially 5 micrograms twice daily for at least 1 month, then increased if necessary up to 10 micrograms twice daily, dose to be taken within 1 hour before 2 main meals (at least 6 hours apart)
▸ BY SUBCUTANEOUS INJECTION USING MODIFIED-RELEASE MEDICINES
▸ **Adult:** 2 mg once weekly

DOSE ADJUSTMENTS DUE TO INTERACTIONS
▸ Dose of concomitant sulfonylurea may need to be reduced.

PHARMACOKINETICS
▸ Effect of *modified-release* exenatide injection (*Bydureon*®) may persist for 10 weeks after discontinuation.

IMPORTANT SAFETY INFORMATION
MHRA/CHM ADVICE: GLP-1 RECEPTOR AGONISTS: REPORTS OF DIABETIC KETOACIDOSIS WHEN CONCOMITANT INSULIN WAS RAPIDLY REDUCED OR DISCONTINUED (JUNE 2019)
Serious and life-threatening cases of diabetic ketoacidosis have been reported in patients with type 2 diabetes mellitus on a combination of a glucagon-like peptide-1 (GLP-1) receptor agonist and insulin, particularly after discontinuation or rapid dose reduction of concomitant insulin. Healthcare professionals are advised that any dose reduction of insulin should be done in a stepwise manner with careful blood glucose self-monitoring, particularly when GLP-1 receptor agonist therapy is initiated. Patients should be informed of the risk factors for and signs and symptoms of diabetic ketoacidosis, and advised to seek immediate medical attention if these develop.

The MHRA reminds healthcare professionals to ensure that patients are aware of potential side-effects associated with glucagon-like peptide-1 (GLP-1) receptor agonists following anecdotal evidence and Yellow Card reports suggesting misuse of these medicines for weight management outside of their licence. The only GLP-1 receptor agonists licensed for weight management are liraglutide p. 816 (*Saxenda*®), semaglutide p. 819 (*Wegovy*®), and tirzepatide p. 822 (*Mounjaro*®), which is also a glucose-dependent insulinotropic polypeptide (GIP) receptor agonist. The benefits and risks of these medicines for weight loss in individuals who are not obese, or who are not overweight with weight-related co-morbidities, have not been studied.

Healthcare professionals should inform patients and carers upon initial prescription and at any dose increase about the common risk of gastro-intestinal side-effects (including nausea, vomiting, diarrhoea, and constipation) associated with GLP-1 receptor agonists; these are usually non-serious but can persist for several days and may lead to serious complications such as severe dehydration and kidney damage, resulting in hospitalisation. For this reason, patients should be advised to stay well hydrated by drinking plenty of fluids throughout treatment. They should also be informed of other serious but less common side-effects, including acute gallstone disease, pancreatitis, and serious allergic reactions.

Patients and carers should be advised to ensure that prescriptions are only obtained from registered healthcare professionals and that private prescriptions are dispensed from authorised sources to avoid the risk of receiving falsified pens. Patients and carers should consult the patient information leaflet for instructions on the use of GLP-1 receptor agonists, and be advised to only administer the prescribed dose.

An EU review has concluded that glucagon-like peptide-1 (GLP-1) and dual glucose-dependent insulinotropic polypeptide (GIP)/GLP-1 receptor agonists are associated with a potential risk of pulmonary aspiration in patients undergoing surgery or procedures requiring general anaesthesia or deep sedation. These medicines are known to slow gastric emptying, thereby increasing the risk of residual gastric contents despite preoperative fasting, which could lead to pulmonary aspiration and other severe complications, such as aspiration pneumonia.

The MHRA advises healthcare professionals to identify the increased risk of aspiration as early as possible, ideally at the pre-assessment clinic before surgery, in patients using GLP-1 or dual GIP/GLP-1 receptor agonists. Anaesthetists should complete an individualised preoperative risk assessment and consider the following:

- patients with underlying diabetic gastroparesis, as well as other co-morbidities such as obesity or gastroesophageal reflux disease, and symptoms of delayed gastric emptying (such as nausea, vomiting and abdominal pain) may have a higher risk of aspiration;
- directly asking patients or their carers about their use of GLP-1 or dual GIP/GLP-1 receptor agonists, as private prescriptions may not be included in the patient's medical notes or drug history, and patients who may have purchased these medications for use in aesthetic weight loss may not readily disclose this information (see also advice issued in October 2024, above).

There is limited evidence to support any recommendations on a time frame to withhold GLP-1 or dual GIP/GLP-1 receptor agonists prior to anaesthesia, new fasting guidelines, or an appropriate medical procedure to confirm an empty stomach. Anaesthetists should manage aspiration risk in line with usual anaesthetic practice and retain flexibility to provide individualised assessment.

Healthcare professionals should counsel patients or their carers to continue taking their prescribed medicines and not stop treatment without first discussing with their doctor. They should also be advised regarding the risk of aspiration and that there may be a need to modify pre-procedure instruction and anaesthetic technique.

- **CONTRA-INDICATIONS** Ketoacidosis · severe gastro-intestinal disease
- **CAUTIONS** Elderly · general anaesthesia or deep sedation (risk of pulmonary aspiration due to delayed gastric emptying) · may cause weight loss greater than 1.5 kg weekly · pancreatitis
- **INTERACTIONS** → Appendix 1: glucagon-like peptide-1 receptor agonists
- **SIDE-EFFECTS**
  - ▶ **Common or very common** Appetite decreased · asthenia · constipation · diarrhoea · dizziness · gastrointestinal discomfort · gastrointestinal disorders · headache · nausea · skin reactions · vomiting
  - ▶ **Uncommon** Alopecia · burping · drowsiness · gallbladder disorders · hyperhidrosis · hypoglycaemia · pancreatitis acute · renal impairment · taste altered
  - ▶ **Frequency not known** Angioedema · pancreatitis haemorrhagic

  SIDE-EFFECTS, FURTHER INFORMATION Discontinue if symptoms of acute pancreatitis occur, such as persistent, severe abdominal pain. If pancreatitis confirmed, do not restart treatment.
- **CONCEPTION AND CONTRACEPTION** Women of child-bearing age should use effective contraception during treatment with modified-release exenatide and for 12 weeks after discontinuation.
- **PREGNANCY** Avoid—toxicity in *animal* studies.
- **BREAST FEEDING** Avoid—no information available.
- **RENAL IMPAIRMENT** EvGr For *immediate-release* injection, use with caution if creatinine clearance 30–50 mL/minute; avoid if creatinine clearance less than 30 mL/minute. For *modified-release* injection, avoid if eGFR less than 30 mL/minute/1.73 m². ⟨M⟩ See p. 21.
- **PRESCRIBING AND DISPENSING INFORMATION** For choice of therapy, see Type 2 diabetes p. 800.
- **PATIENT AND CARER ADVICE** Patients or their carers should be given advice on how to administer exenatide injection. Patients changing from immediate-release to modified-release exenatide formulation may experience initial transient increase in blood glucose. For *immediate-release injections*, some oral medications should be taken at least 1 hour before or 4 hours after exenatide injection—consult product literature for details. Patients or their carers should be told how to recognise signs and symptoms of pancreatitis and advised to seek prompt medical attention if symptoms such as abdominal pain, nausea, and vomiting develop.

  Patients should be given a user manual.

  Missed doses If a dose of the *immediate-release injection* is missed, treatment should be continued with the next scheduled dose—do not administer **after** a meal.

If a dose of the *modified-release injection* is missed, it should be administered as soon as practical, provided the next regularly scheduled dose is due in 3 days or more; thereafter, patients can resume their usual once weekly dosing schedule.

● **NATIONAL FUNDING/ACCESS DECISIONS**
For full details see funding body website
Scottish Medicines Consortium (SMC) decisions
▸ Exenatide (*Byetta*®) for the treatment of type 2 diabetes mellitus (July 2007) SMC No. 376/07 Recommended with restrictions
▸ Exenatide (*Byetta*®) for the treatment of type 2 diabetes mellitus in combination with metformin and a thiazolidinedione (March 2011) SMC No. 684/11 Recommended with restrictions
▸ Exenatide (*Bydureon*®) for the treatment of type 2 diabetes mellitus (January 2012) SMC No. 748/11 Recommended with restrictions
▸ Exenatide (*Byetta*®) as adjunctive therapy to basal insulin with or without metformin and/or pioglitazone in adults with type 2 diabetes who have not achieved adequate glycaemic control with these agents (June 2012) SMC No. 785/12 Recommended

● **MEDICINAL FORMS** There can be variation in the licensing of different medicines containing the same drug.
Prolonged-release suspension for injection
CAUTIONARY AND ADVISORY LABELS 10
EXCIPIENTS: May contain Sucrose
▸ Bydureon (AstraZeneca UK Ltd)
Exenatide 2.353 mg per 1 ml Bydureon BCise 2mg/0.85ml prolonged-release suspension for injection pre-filled pens | 4 pre-filled disposable injection [PoM] £73.36 DT = £73.36

Liraglutide

04-Feb-2025

● **DRUG ACTION** Liraglutide binds to, and activates, the GLP-1 (glucagon-like peptide-1) receptor to increase insulin secretion, suppresses glucagon secretion, and slows gastric emptying.

● **INDICATIONS AND DOSE**
DOSE ADJUSTMENTS DUE TO INTERACTIONS
▸ Dose of concomitant insulin or sulfonylurea may need to be reduced.

SAXENDA ®
Adjunct in weight management [in conjunction with dietary measures and increased physical activity in individuals with a body mass index (BMI) of 30 kg/m^2 or more, or in individuals with a BMI of 27 kg/m^2 or more in the presence of at least one weight-related co-morbidity]
▸ BY SUBCUTANEOUS INJECTION
▸ Adult: Initially 0.6 mg once daily, then increased in steps of 0.6 mg, dose to be increased at intervals of at least 1 week up to a maintenance dose of 3 mg once daily or the maximum tolerated dose has been reached. Consider discontinuation if escalation to the next dose is not tolerated for 2 consecutive weeks. Discontinue if at least 5% of initial body-weight has not been lost after 12 weeks at maximum dose; maximum 3 mg per day

VICTOZA ®
Type 2 diabetes mellitus as monotherapy (if metformin inappropriate), or in combination with other antidiabetic drugs, (including insulin) if existing treatment fails to achieve adequate glycaemic control
▸ BY SUBCUTANEOUS INJECTION
▸ Adult: Initially 0.6 mg once daily for at least 1 week, then increased to 1.2 mg once daily for at least 1 week, then increased if necessary to 1.8 mg once daily

IMPORTANT SAFETY INFORMATION
MHRA/CHM ADVICE: GLP-1 RECEPTOR AGONISTS: REPORTS OF DIABETIC KETOACIDOSIS WHEN CONCOMITANT INSULIN WAS RAPIDLY REDUCED OR DISCONTINUED (JUNE 2019)
▸ When used for Type 2 diabetes mellitus
Serious and life-threatening cases of diabetic ketoacidosis have been reported in patients with type 2 diabetes mellitus on a combination of a glucagon-like peptide-1 (GLP-1) receptor agonist and insulin, particularly after discontinuation or rapid dose reduction of concomitant insulin. Healthcare professionals are advised that any dose reduction of insulin should be done in a stepwise manner with careful blood glucose self-monitoring, particularly when GLP-1 receptor agonist therapy is initiated. Patients should be informed of the risk factors for and signs and symptoms of diabetic ketoacidosis, and advised to seek immediate medical attention if these develop.

MHRA/CHM ADVICE: *SAXENDA* ® (LIRAGLUTIDE): VIGILANCE REQUIRED DUE TO POTENTIALLY HARMFUL FALSIFIED PRODUCTS (NOVEMBER 2023)
Falsified *Saxenda*® preparations, some containing insulin, have been found in the UK. Healthcare professionals are advised to remind patients to always obtain prescription medicines from qualified healthcare providers, and not to use preparations they suspect are falsified as this may lead to serious harm. Healthcare professionals should remain vigilant for symptoms associated with hypoglycaemia in patients who may have obtained a falsified preparation containing insulin; patients should be advised to seek immediate medical attention if such symptoms occur. Suspected falsified preparations should be quarantined and reported to the Yellow Card scheme.

MHRA/CHM ADVICE: GLP-1 RECEPTOR AGONISTS: REMINDER OF THE POTENTIAL SIDE EFFECTS AND TO BE AWARE OF THE POTENTIAL FOR MISUSE (OCTOBER 2024)
The MHRA reminds healthcare professionals to ensure that patients are aware of potential side-effects associated with glucagon-like peptide-1 (GLP-1) receptor agonists following anecdotal evidence and Yellow Card reports suggesting misuse of these medicines for weight management outside of their licence. The only GLP-1 receptor agonists licensed for weight management are liraglutide above (*Saxenda*®), semaglutide p. 819 (*Wegovy*®), and tirzepatide p. 822 (*Mounjaro*®), which is also a glucose-dependent insulinotropic polypeptide (GIP) receptor agonist. The benefits and risks of these medicines for weight loss in individuals who are not obese, or who are not overweight with weight-related co-morbidities, have not been studied.

Healthcare professionals should inform patients and carers upon initial prescription and at any dose increase about the common risk of gastro-intestinal side-effects (including nausea, vomiting, diarrhoea, and constipation) associated with GLP-1 receptor agonists; these are usually non-serious but can persist for several days and may lead to serious complications such as severe dehydration and kidney damage, resulting in hospitalisation. For this reason, patients should be advised to stay well hydrated by drinking plenty of fluids throughout treatment. They should also be informed of other serious but less common side-effects, including acute gallstone disease, pancreatitis, and serious allergic reactions. Healthcare professionals are advised that hypoglycaemia can occur in non-diabetic patients using liraglutide for weight management and therefore to ensure patients and carers know the signs and symptoms to be aware of, and to seek immediate medical attention if these occur.

Patients and carers should be advised to ensure that prescriptions are only obtained from registered healthcare professionals and that private prescriptions are dispensed from authorised sources to avoid the risk of receiving falsified pens (see also advice issued in November 2023, above). Patients and carers should consult the patient information leaflet for instructions on the use of GLP-1 receptor agonists, and be advised to only administer the prescribed dose.

MHRA/CHM ADVICE: GLP-1 AND DUAL GIP/GLP-1 RECEPTOR AGONISTS: POTENTIAL RISK OF PULMONARY ASPIRATION DURING GENERAL ANAESTHESIA OR DEEP SEDATION (JANUARY 2025)
An EU review has concluded that glucagon-like peptide-1 (GLP-1) and dual glucose-dependent insulinotropic polypeptide (GIP)/GLP-1 receptor agonists are associated with a potential risk of pulmonary aspiration in patients undergoing surgery or procedures requiring general anaesthesia or deep sedation. These medicines are known to slow gastric emptying, thereby increasing the risk of residual gastric contents despite preoperative fasting, which could lead to pulmonary aspiration and other severe complications, such as aspiration pneumonia.

The MHRA advises healthcare professionals to identify the increased risk of aspiration as early as possible, ideally at the pre-assessment clinic before surgery, in patients using GLP-1 or dual GIP/GLP-1 receptor agonists. Anaesthetists should complete an individualised preoperative risk assessment and consider the following:
- patients with underlying diabetic gastroparesis, as well as other co-morbidities such as obesity or gastroesophageal reflux disease, and symptoms of delayed gastric emptying (such as nausea, vomiting and abdominal pain) may have a higher risk of aspiration;
- directly asking patients or their carers about their use of GLP-1 or dual GIP/GLP-1 receptor agonists, as private prescriptions may not be included in the patient's medical notes or drug history, and patients who may have purchased these medications for use in aesthetic weight loss may not readily disclose this information (see also advice issued in October 2024, above).

There is limited evidence to support any recommendations on a time frame to withhold GLP-1 or dual GIP/GLP-1 receptor agonists prior to anaesthesia, new fasting guidelines, or an appropriate medical procedure to confirm an empty stomach. Anaesthetists should manage aspiration risk in line with usual anaesthetic practice and retain flexibility to provide individualised assessment.

Healthcare professionals should counsel patients or their carers to continue taking their prescribed medicines and not stop treatment without first discussing with their doctor. They should also be advised regarding the risk of aspiration and that there may be a need to modify pre-procedure instruction and anaesthetic technique.

- **CONTRA-INDICATIONS** Diabetic gastroparesis · inflammatory bowel disease

SAXENDA® Concomitant use with other products for weight management · elderly 75 years or over (limited information) · obesity secondary to endocrinological or eating disorders

VICTOZA® Diabetic ketoacidosis

- **CAUTIONS** General anaesthesia or deep sedation (risk of pulmonary aspiration due to delayed gastric emptying) · severe congestive heart failure (no information available) · thyroid disease

- **INTERACTIONS** → Appendix 1: glucagon-like peptide-1 receptor agonists

- **SIDE-EFFECTS**
- ▸ **Common or very common** Appetite decreased (in patients with type 2 diabetes) · asthenia · burping · constipation · diarrhoea · dizziness · dry mouth · gallbladder disorders · gastrointestinal discomfort · gastrointestinal disorders · headache · hypoglycaemia · increased risk of infection · insomnia · nausea · skin reactions · taste altered · toothache · vomiting
- ▸ **Uncommon** Dehydration · malaise · pancreatitis · renal impairment · tachycardia
- ▸ **Frequency not known** Angioedema · cutaneous amyloidosis · thyroid disorder

   SIDE-EFFECTS, FURTHER INFORMATION Discontinue if symptoms of acute pancreatitis occur, such as persistent, severe abdominal pain. If pancreatitis confirmed, do not restart treatment.

- **PREGNANCY** Manufacturer advises avoid—toxicity in *animal* studies (recommendation also supported by tertiary sources).

- **BREAST FEEDING** Manufacturer advises avoid—no information available; *animal* studies suggest that transfer into milk is low, but excretion into human milk not known (a tertiary source confirms lack of information in human lactation, but also states that risk to infants appears to be negligible. [EvGr] Blood glucose monitoring of the infant should be considered) ◈D◈.

- **HEPATIC IMPAIRMENT**

   SAXENDA® Manufacturer advises use with caution in mild to moderate impairment; avoid in severe impairment (risk of decreased exposure).

   VICTOZA® Manufacturer advises avoid in severe impairment (risk of decreased exposure).

- **RENAL IMPAIRMENT**

   SAXENDA® Manufacturer advises avoid if creatinine clearance less than 30 mL/minute. See p. 21.

   VICTOZA® Manufacturer advises avoid in end-stage renal disease.

- **PRESCRIBING AND DISPENSING INFORMATION** Liraglutide is a biological medicine. Biological medicines must be prescribed and dispensed by brand name, see *Biological medicines* and *Biosimilar medicines*, under Guidance on prescribing p. 1; record the brand name and batch number after each administration.

   VICTOZA® For choice of therapy, see Type 2 diabetes p. 800.

- **HANDLING AND STORAGE** Manufacturer advises store in a refrigerator (2–8°C)—after first use can also be stored below 30°C and used within 1 month; keep cap on pen to protect from light.

- **PATIENT AND CARER ADVICE** Patients and their carers should be given advice on how to administer liraglutide injection. Patients and their carers should be told how to recognise signs and symptoms of acute pancreatitis and advised to seek immediate medical attention if symptoms develop. Patients and their carers should be informed of the potential risk of dehydration in relation to gastro-intestinal side-effects and advised to take precautions to avoid fluid depletion; they should also be informed of the

6 Endocrine system

symptoms of cholelithiasis and cholecystitis, and of increased heart rate.

SAXENDA ®

Missed doses Manufacturer advises if a dose is more than 12 hours late, the missed dose should not be taken and the next dose should be taken at the normal time.

Driving and skilled tasks Patients and carers should be cautioned on the effects of driving and performance of skilled tasks—increased risk of dizziness, particularly during first 3 months of treatment.

- **NATIONAL FUNDING/ACCESS DECISIONS**
For full details see funding body website

NICE decisions
▸ Liraglutide for managing overweight and obesity (December 2020) NICE TA664 Recommended with restrictions

Scottish Medicines Consortium (SMC) decisions
▸ Liraglutide (*Saxenda* ®) as an adjunct to a reduced-calorie diet and increased physical activity for weight management in adult patients with an initial Body Mass Index (BMI) of 30 kg/m² or more (obese), or 27 kg/m² to less than 30 kg/m² (overweight) in the presence of at least one weight-related co-morbidity (May 2022) SMC No. SMC2455 Recommended with restrictions

- **MEDICINAL FORMS** There can be variation in the licensing of different medicines containing the same drug.

Solution for injection
EXCIPIENTS: May contain Propylene glycol
▸ Saxenda (Novo Nordisk Ltd)
Liraglutide 6 mg per 1 ml Saxenda 6mg/ml solution for injection 3ml pre-filled pens | 5 pre-filled disposable injection [PoM] £196.20

Combinations available: *Insulin degludec with liraglutide,* p. 839

Lixisenatide

04-Feb-2025

- **DRUG ACTION** Binds to, and activates, the GLP-1 (glucagon-like peptide-1) receptor to increase insulin secretion, suppresses glucagon secretion, and slows gastric emptying.

- **INDICATIONS AND DOSE**

Type 2 diabetes mellitus in combination with other antidiabetic drugs (including insulin) if existing treatment fails to achieve adequate glycaemic control
▸ BY SUBCUTANEOUS INJECTION
▸ Adult: Initially 10 micrograms once daily for 14 days, then increased to 20 micrograms once daily, dose to be taken within 1 hour before a meal

DOSE ADJUSTMENTS DUE TO INTERACTIONS
▸ Dose of concomitant sulfonylurea or insulin may need to be reduced.

IMPORTANT SAFETY INFORMATION
MHRA/CHM ADVICE: GLP-1 RECEPTOR AGONISTS: REPORTS OF DIABETIC KETOACIDOSIS WHEN CONCOMITANT INSULIN WAS RAPIDLY REDUCED OR DISCONTINUED (JUNE 2019)
Serious and life-threatening cases of diabetic ketoacidosis have been reported in patients with type 2 diabetes mellitus on a combination of insulin and the glucagon-like peptide-1 (GLP-1) receptor agonist exenatide, liraglutide, or dulaglutide, particularly after discontinuation or rapid dose reduction of concomitant insulin. The MHRA has not currently received any UK reports of diabetic ketoacidosis with the GLP-1 receptor agonists lixisenatide and semaglutide but this risk cannot be excluded. Healthcare professionals are advised that any dose reduction of insulin should be done in a stepwise manner with careful blood glucose self-monitoring, particularly when GLP-1 receptor agonist therapy is initiated. Patients should be informed of the

risk factors for and signs and symptoms of diabetic ketoacidosis, and advised to seek immediate medical attention if these develop.

MHRA/CHM ADVICE: GLP-1 RECEPTOR AGONISTS: REMINDER OF THE POTENTIAL SIDE EFFECTS AND TO BE AWARE OF THE POTENTIAL FOR MISUSE (OCTOBER 2024)
The MHRA reminds healthcare professionals to ensure that patients are aware of potential side-effects associated with glucagon-like peptide-1 (GLP-1) receptor agonists following anecdotal evidence and Yellow Card reports suggesting misuse of these medicines for weight management outside of their licence. The only GLP-1 receptor agonists licensed for weight management are liraglutide p. 816 (*Saxenda* ®), semaglutide p. 819 (*Wegovy* ®), and tirzepatide p. 822 (*Mounjaro* ®), which is also a glucose-dependent insulinotropic polypeptide (GIP) receptor agonist. The benefits and risks of these medicines for weight loss in individuals who are not obese, or who are not overweight with weight-related co-morbidities, have not been studied.

Healthcare professionals should inform patients and carers upon initial prescription and at any dose increase about the common risk of gastro-intestinal side-effects (including nausea, vomiting, diarrhoea, and constipation) associated with GLP-1 receptor agonists; these are usually non-serious but can persist for several days and may lead to serious complications such as severe dehydration and kidney damage, resulting in hospitalisation. For this reason, patients should be advised to stay well hydrated by drinking plenty of fluids throughout treatment. They should also be informed of other serious but less common side-effects, including acute gallstone disease, pancreatitis, and serious allergic reactions.

Patients and carers should be advised to ensure that prescriptions are only obtained from registered healthcare professionals and that private prescriptions are dispensed from authorised sources to avoid the risk of receiving falsified pens. Patients and carers should consult the patient information leaflet for instructions on the use of GLP-1 receptor agonists, and be advised to only administer the prescribed dose.

MHRA/CHM ADVICE: GLP-1 AND DUAL GIP/GLP-1 RECEPTOR AGONISTS: POTENTIAL RISK OF PULMONARY ASPIRATION DURING GENERAL ANAESTHESIA OR DEEP SEDATION (JANUARY 2025)
An EU review has concluded that glucagon-like peptide-1 (GLP-1) and dual glucose-dependent insulinotropic polypeptide (GIP)/GLP-1 receptor agonists are associated with a potential risk of pulmonary aspiration in patients undergoing surgery or procedures requiring general anaesthesia or deep sedation. These medicines are known to slow gastric emptying, thereby increasing the risk of residual gastric contents despite preoperative fasting, which could lead to pulmonary aspiration and other severe complications, such as aspiration pneumonia.

The MHRA advises healthcare professionals to identify the increased risk of aspiration as early as possible, ideally at the pre-assessment clinic before surgery, in patients using GLP-1 or dual GIP/GLP-1 receptor agonists. Anaesthetists should complete an individualised preoperative risk assessment and consider the following:
- patients with underlying diabetic gastroparesis, as well as other co-morbidities such as obesity or gastroesophageal reflux disease, and symptoms of delayed gastric emptying (such as nausea, vomiting and abdominal pain) may have a higher risk of aspiration;
- directly asking patients or their carers about their use of GLP-1 or dual GIP/GLP-1 receptor agonists, as

private prescriptions may not be included in the patient's medical notes or drug history, and patients who may have purchased these medications for use in aesthetic weight loss may not readily disclose this information (see also advice issued in October 2024, above).

There is limited evidence to support any recommendations on a time frame to withhold GLP-1 or dual GIP/GLP-1 receptor agonists prior to anaesthesia, new fasting guidelines, or an appropriate medical procedure to confirm an empty stomach. Anaesthetists should manage aspiration risk in line with usual anaesthetic practice and retain flexibility to provide individualised assessment.

Healthcare professionals should counsel patients or their carers to continue taking their prescribed medicines and not stop treatment without first discussing with their doctor. They should also be advised regarding the risk of aspiration and that there may be a need to modify pre-procedure instruction and anaesthetic technique.

● **CONTRA-INDICATIONS** Ketoacidosis · severe gastro-intestinal disease

● **CAUTIONS** General anaesthesia or deep sedation (risk of pulmonary aspiration due to delayed gastric emptying) · history of pancreatitis

● **INTERACTIONS** → Appendix 1: glucagon-like peptide-1 receptor agonists

● **SIDE-EFFECTS**
▸ **Common or very common** Back pain · cystitis · diarrhoea · dizziness · drowsiness · dyspepsia · headache · increased risk of infection · nausea · vomiting
▸ **Uncommon** Gallbladder disorders · urticaria
▸ **Rare or very rare** Impaired gastric emptying
▸ **Frequency not known** Arrhythmia · pancreatitis acute

SIDE-EFFECTS, FURTHER INFORMATION Discontinue if symptoms of acute pancreatitis occur, such as persistent, severe abdominal pain. If pancreatitis confirmed, do not restart treatment.

● **CONCEPTION AND CONTRACEPTION** Women of child-bearing age should use effective contraception.

● **PREGNANCY** Avoid—toxicity in *animal* studies.

● **BREAST FEEDING** Avoid—no information available.

● **RENAL IMPAIRMENT** [EvGr] Avoid if creatinine clearance less than 30 mL/minute (no information available). Ⓜ See p. 21.

● **PRESCRIBING AND DISPENSING INFORMATION** For choice of therapy, see Type 2 diabetes p. 800.

● **PATIENT AND CARER ADVICE** Patients or their carers should be given advice on how to administer lixisenatide injection. Some oral medications should be taken at least 1 hour before or 4 hours after lixisenatide injection—consult product literature for details.
Acute pancreatitis Patients and their carers should be told how to recognise signs and symptoms of acute pancreatitis and advised to seek prompt medical attention if symptoms such as persistent, severe abdominal pain develop.
Dehydration Patients and their carers should be informed of the potential risk of dehydration in relation to gastro-intestinal side-effects and advised to take precautions to avoid fluid depletion.
Missed doses If a dose is missed, inject within 1 hour before the next meal—do not administer **after** a meal.

● **NATIONAL FUNDING/ACCESS DECISIONS**
For full details see funding body website
Scottish Medicines Consortium (SMC) decisions
▸ Lixisenatide (*Lyxumia* ®) for the treatment of adults with type 2 diabetes mellitus to achieve glycaemic control in combination with oral glucose-lowering medicinal products

and/or basal insulin when these, together with diet and exercise, do not provide adequate glycaemic control (September 2013) SMC No. 903/13 Recommended with restrictions

● **MEDICINAL FORMS** No licensed medicines listed.

Combinations available: *Insulin glargine with lixisenatide,* p. 840

Semaglutide
04-Feb-2025

● **DRUG ACTION** Semaglutide binds to, and activates, the GLP-1 (glucagon-like peptide-1) receptor to increase insulin secretion, suppress glucagon secretion, and slow gastric emptying.

● **INDICATIONS AND DOSE**
DOSE ADJUSTMENTS DUE TO INTERACTIONS
▸ Dose of concomitant insulin or sulfonylurea may need to be reduced.

OZEMPIC ®

Type 2 diabetes mellitus as monotherapy (if metformin inappropriate), or in combination with other antidiabetic drugs (including insulin) if existing treatment fails to achieve adequate glycaemic control
▸ BY SUBCUTANEOUS INJECTION
▸ Adult: Initially 0.25 mg once weekly for 4 weeks, then increased to 0.5 mg once weekly for at least 4 weeks, then increased if necessary to 1 mg once weekly for at least 4 weeks, then increased if necessary to 2 mg once weekly

DOSE EQUIVALENCE AND CONVERSION
▸ For *Ozempic* ®: Subcutaneous semaglutide 0.5 mg once weekly is comparable to oral semaglutide 14 mg once daily. Due to the high pharmacokinetic variability of oral semaglutide, the effect of switching between oral and subcutaneous semaglutide cannot easily be predicted.

RYBELSUS ®

Type 2 diabetes mellitus as monotherapy (if metformin inappropriate), or in combination with other antidiabetic drugs (including insulin) if existing treatment fails to achieve adequate glycaemic control
▸ BY MOUTH
▸ Adult: Initially 3 mg once daily for 1 month, then increased to 7 mg once daily for at least 1 month, then increased if necessary to 14 mg once daily, one 14 mg tablet should be used to achieve a 14 mg dose; use of two 7 mg tablets to achieve a 14 mg dose has not been studied and is therefore not recommended

DOSE EQUIVALENCE AND CONVERSION
▸ For *Rybelsus* ®: Oral semaglutide 14 mg once daily is comparable to subcutaneous semaglutide 0.5 mg once weekly. Due to the high pharmacokinetic variability of oral semaglutide, the effect of switching between oral and subcutaneous semaglutide cannot easily be predicted.

continued →

WEGOVY ®

Weight management [in conjunction with dietary measures and increased physical activity in individuals with a BMI of 30 kg/m^2 or more, or in individuals with a BMI of 27 kg/m^2 or more in the presence of at least one weight-related co-morbidity] | Cardiovascular risk reduction [in conjunction with dietary measures and increased physical activity in individuals with established cardiovascular disease and a BMI of 27 kg/m^2 or more]

▸ BY SUBCUTANEOUS INJECTION

▸ Adult: 0.25 mg once weekly for at least 4 weeks, then increased if tolerated to 0.5 mg once weekly for at least 4 weeks, then increased if tolerated to 1 mg once weekly for at least 4 weeks, then increased if tolerated to 1.7 mg once weekly for at least 4 weeks, then maintenance 2.4 mg once weekly

IMPORTANT SAFETY INFORMATION

MHRA/CHM ADVICE: GLP-1 RECEPTOR AGONISTS: REPORTS OF DIABETIC KETOACIDOSIS WHEN CONCOMITANT INSULIN WAS RAPIDLY REDUCED OR DISCONTINUED (JUNE 2019)

Serious and life-threatening cases of diabetic ketoacidosis have been reported in patients with type 2 diabetes mellitus on a combination of insulin and the glucagon-like peptide-1 (GLP-1) receptor agonist exenatide, liraglutide, or dulaglutide, particularly after discontinuation or rapid dose reduction of concomitant insulin. The MHRA has not currently received any UK reports of diabetic ketoacidosis with the GLP-1 receptor agonists lixisenatide and semaglutide but this risk cannot be excluded. Healthcare professionals are advised that any dose reduction of insulin should be done in a stepwise manner with careful blood glucose self-monitoring, particularly when GLP-1 receptor agonist therapy is initiated. Patients should be informed of the risk factors for and signs and symptoms of diabetic ketoacidosis, and advised to seek immediate medical attention if these develop.

MHRA/CHM ADVICE: *OZEMPIC*® (SEMAGLUTIDE): VIGILANCE REQUIRED DUE TO POTENTIALLY HARMFUL FALSIFIED PRODUCTS (NOVEMBER 2023)

Falsified *Ozempic*® preparations, some containing insulin, have been found in the UK. Healthcare professionals are advised to remind patients to always obtain prescription medicines from qualified healthcare providers, and not to use preparations they suspect are falsified as this may lead to serious harm. Healthcare professionals should remain vigilant for symptoms associated with hypoglycaemia in patients who may have obtained a falsified preparation containing insulin; patients should be advised to seek immediate medical attention if such symptoms occur. Suspected falsified preparations should be quarantined and reported to the Yellow Card scheme.

MHRA/CHM ADVICE: GLP-1 RECEPTOR AGONISTS: REMINDER OF THE POTENTIAL SIDE EFFECTS AND TO BE AWARE OF THE POTENTIAL FOR MISUSE (OCTOBER 2024)

The MHRA reminds healthcare professionals to ensure that patients are aware of potential side-effects associated with glucagon-like peptide-1 (GLP-1) receptor agonists following anecdotal evidence and Yellow Card reports suggesting misuse of these medicines for weight management outside of their licence. The only GLP-1 receptor agonists licensed for weight management are liraglutide p. 816 (*Saxenda*®), semaglutide p. 819 (*Wegovy*®), and tirzepatide p. 822 (*Mounjaro*®), which is also a glucose-dependent insulinotropic polypeptide (GIP) receptor agonist. The benefits and risks of these medicines for weight loss in individuals who are not obese, or who are not overweight with weight-related co-morbidities, have not been studied.

Healthcare professionals should inform patients and carers upon initial prescription and at any dose increase about the common risk of gastro-intestinal side-effects (including nausea, vomiting, diarrhoea, and constipation) associated with GLP-1 receptor agonists; these are usually non-serious but can persist for several days and may lead to serious complications such as severe dehydration and kidney damage, resulting in hospitalisation. For this reason, patients should be advised to stay well hydrated by drinking plenty of fluids throughout treatment. They should also be informed of other serious but less common side-effects, including acute gallstone disease, pancreatitis, and serious allergic reactions. Healthcare professionals are advised that hypoglycaemia can occur in non-diabetic patients using semaglutide for weight management and therefore to ensure patients and carers know the signs and symptoms to be aware of, and to seek immediate medical attention if these occur.

Patients and carers should be advised to ensure that prescriptions are only obtained from registered healthcare professionals and that private prescriptions are dispensed from authorised sources to avoid the risk of receiving falsified pens (see also advice issued in November 2023, above). Patients and carers should consult the patient information leaflet for instructions on the use of GLP-1 receptor agonists, and be advised to only administer the prescribed dose.

MHRA/CHM ADVICE: GLP-1 AND DUAL GIP/GLP-1 RECEPTOR AGONISTS: POTENTIAL RISK OF PULMONARY ASPIRATION DURING GENERAL ANAESTHESIA OR DEEP SEDATION (JANUARY 2025)

An EU review has concluded that glucagon-like peptide-1 (GLP-1) and dual glucose-dependent insulinotropic polypeptide (GIP)/GLP-1 receptor agonists are associated with a potential risk of pulmonary aspiration in patients undergoing surgery or procedures requiring general anaesthesia or deep sedation. These medicines are known to slow gastric emptying, thereby increasing the risk of residual gastric contents despite preoperative fasting, which could lead to pulmonary aspiration and other severe complications, such as aspiration pneumonia.

The MHRA advises healthcare professionals to identify the increased risk of aspiration as early as possible, ideally at the pre-assessment clinic before surgery, in patients using GLP-1 or dual GIP/GLP-1 receptor agonists. Anaesthetists should complete an individualised preoperative risk assessment and consider the following:

● patients with underlying diabetic gastroparesis, as well as other co-morbidities such as obesity or gastroesophageal reflux disease, and symptoms of delayed gastric emptying (such as nausea, vomiting and abdominal pain) may have a higher risk of aspiration;

● directly asking patients or their carers about their use of GLP-1 or dual GIP/GLP-1 receptor agonists, as private prescriptions may not be included in the patient's medical notes or drug history, and patients who may have purchased these medications for use in aesthetic weight loss may not readily disclose this information (see also advice issued in October 2024, above).

There is limited evidence to support any recommendations on a time frame to withhold GLP-1 or dual GIP/GLP-1 receptor agonists prior to anaesthesia, new fasting guidelines, or an appropriate medical procedure to confirm an empty stomach. Anaesthetists should manage aspiration risk in line with usual anaesthetic practice and retain flexibility to provide individualised assessment.

Healthcare professionals should counsel patients or their carers to continue taking their prescribed medicines and not stop treatment without first discussing with their doctor. They should also be advised regarding the risk of aspiration and that there may be a need to modify pre-procedure instruction and anaesthetic technique.

● **CONTRA-INDICATIONS**
▶ When used for Type 2 diabetes mellitus Diabetic ketoacidosis

● **CAUTIONS** Diabetic retinopathy (in patients treated with insulin) · general anaesthesia or deep sedation (risk of pulmonary aspiration due to delayed gastric emptying) · history of pancreatitis · severe congestive heart failure (no information available)

● **INTERACTIONS** → Appendix 1: glucagon-like peptide-1 receptor agonists

● **SIDE-EFFECTS**
GENERAL SIDE-EFFECTS
▶ **Common or very common** Appetite decreased (in patients with type 2 diabetes) · burping · cholelithiasis · constipation · diarrhoea · fatigue · gastrointestinal discomfort · gastrointestinal disorders · nausea · vomiting · weight decreased (in patients with type 2 diabetes)
▶ **Uncommon** Pancreatitis acute · taste altered

SPECIFIC SIDE-EFFECTS
▶ **Common or very common**
▶ With subcutaneous use Alopecia · diabetic retinopathy (in patients with type 2 diabetes) · dizziness · headache · hypoglycaemia
▶ **Rare or very rare**
▶ With subcutaneous use Angioedema

SIDE-EFFECTS, FURTHER INFORMATION Discontinue if symptoms of acute pancreatitis occur, such as persistent, severe abdominal pain. If pancreatitis confirmed, do not restart treatment.

● **CONCEPTION AND CONTRACEPTION** Manufacturer advises women of childbearing potential should use effective contraception during and for at least two months after stopping treatment.

● **PREGNANCY** Manufacturer advises avoid—toxicity in *animal* studies.

● **BREAST FEEDING** Manufacturer advises avoid—present in milk in *animal* studies.

● **HEPATIC IMPAIRMENT** Manufacturer advises caution (limited information in severe impairment).

● **RENAL IMPAIRMENT** Manufacturer advises avoid in end-stage renal disease.

● **DIRECTIONS FOR ADMINISTRATION** For *subcutaneous injection*, inject into the abdomen, thigh, or upper arm.

For administration by *mouth*, tablets should be swallowed whole with a sip of water (up to half a glass, equivalent to 120 mL) on an empty stomach; wait at least 30 minutes before eating, drinking, or taking other oral medicines—intake with food or large volumes of water decreases absorption of semaglutide.

● **PRESCRIBING AND DISPENSING INFORMATION** Semaglutide is a biological medicine. Biological medicines must be prescribed and dispensed by brand name, see *Biological medicines* and *Biosimilar medicines*, under Guidance on prescribing p. 1; manufacturer advises to record the brand name and batch number after each administration.
▶ When used for Type 2 diabetes mellitus For choice of therapy, see Type 2 diabetes p. 800.

WEGOVY ® EvGr If patient is unable to lose at least 5% of their initial body-weight after 6 months on treatment, consider whether to continue treatment. ◆M◆

● **HANDLING AND STORAGE**
▶ With subcutaneous use Store injection pens in a refrigerator (2–8°C)—after first use can also be stored at room temperature (below 30°C) for up to 6 weeks; keep cap on pen to protect from light.

● **PATIENT AND CARER ADVICE** Patients and their carers should be given advice on how to administer semaglutide tablets and injection.
Acute pancreatitis Patients and their carers should be told how to recognise signs and symptoms of acute pancreatitis and advised to seek immediate medical attention if symptoms develop.
Dehydration Patients and their carers should be informed of the potential risk of dehydration in relation to gastro-intestinal side-effects and advised to take precautions to avoid fluid depletion.
Missed doses
▶ With subcutaneous use If a dose is more than 5 days late, the missed dose should not be administered and the next dose should be administered at the normal time. If more doses of *Wegovy* ® are missed, consider re-starting at a reduced dose.
▶ With oral use If a dose is missed, the missed dose should not be taken and the next dose should be taken at the normal time.
Driving and skilled tasks Patients and carers should be counselled on the effects on driving and performance of skilled tasks—increased risk of dizziness, particularly during the dose escalation period.

● **NATIONAL FUNDING/ACCESS DECISIONS**
For full details see funding body website
NICE decisions
▶ **Semaglutide for managing overweight and obesity (September 2023)** NICE TA875 Recommended with restrictions
Scottish Medicines Consortium (SMC) decisions
▶ **Semaglutide (*Ozempic* ®) for the treatment of adults with insufficiently controlled type 2 diabetes mellitus as an adjunct to diet and exercise (January 2019)** SMC No. SMC2092 Recommended with restrictions
▶ **Semaglutide (*Rybelsus* ®) for the treatment of adults with insufficiently controlled type 2 diabetes to improve glycaemic control as an adjunct to diet and exercise: as monotherapy when metformin is considered inappropriate due to intolerance or contra-indications; or in combination with other medicinal products for the treatment of diabetes (September 2020)** SMC No. SMC2287 Recommended with restrictions
▶ **Semaglutide (*Wegovy* ®) as an adjunct to a reduced-calorie diet and increased physical activity for weight management, including weight loss and weight maintenance, in adults with an initial BMI of 30 kg/m^2 or more (obese), or 27 kg/m^2 to less than 30 kg/m^2 (overweight) in the presence of at least one weight-related co-morbidity (October 2023)** SMC No. SMC2497 Recommended with restrictions
All Wales Medicines Strategy Group (AWMSG) decisions
▶ **Semaglutide (*Ozempic* ®) for the treatment of insufficiently controlled type 2 diabetes mellitus in adults as an add-on therapy to oral antidiabetic medicines or basal insulin (November 2018)** AWMSG No. 1842 Recommended with restrictions

● **MEDICINAL FORMS** There can be variation in the licensing of different medicines containing the same drug.
Solution for injection
EXCIPIENTS: May contain Propylene glycol
▶ **Ozempic** (Novo Nordisk Ltd)
Semaglutide 1.34 mg per 1 ml Ozempic 0.25mg/0.19ml solution for injection 1.5ml pre-filled pens | 1 pre-filled disposable injection PoM £73.25 DT = £73.25
Ozempic 0.5mg/0.37ml solution for injection 1.5ml pre-filled pens | 1 pre-filled disposable injection PoM £73.25 DT = £73.25

6

Endocrine system

Ozempic 1mg/0.74ml solution for injection 3ml pre-filled pens | 1 pre-filled disposable injection [PoM] £73.25 DT = £73.25

▸ **Wegovy FlexTouch** (Novo Nordisk Ltd) ▼
Semaglutide 676 microgram per 1 ml Wegovy FlexTouch 0.25mg/0.37ml solution for injection 1.5ml pre-filled pens | 1 pre-filled disposable injection [PoM] £73.25
Semaglutide 1.34 mg per 1 ml Wegovy FlexTouch 1mg/0.75ml solution for injection 3ml pre-filled pens | 1 pre-filled disposable injection [PoM] £73.25
Wegovy FlexTouch 0.5mg/0.37ml solution for injection 1.5ml pre-filled pens | 1 pre-filled disposable injection [PoM] £73.25 DT = £73.25
Semaglutide 2.27 mg per 1 ml Wegovy FlexTouch 1.7mg/0.75ml solution for injection 3ml pre-filled pens | 1 pre-filled disposable injection [PoM] £124.53
Semaglutide 3.2 mg per 1 ml Wegovy FlexTouch 2.4mg/0.75ml solution for injection 3ml pre-filled pens | 1 pre-filled disposable injection [PoM] £175.80

Oral tablet
CAUTIONARY AND ADVISORY LABELS 25

▸ **Rybelsus** (Novo Nordisk Ltd)
Semaglutide 3 mg Rybelsus 3mg tablets | 30 tablet [PoM] £78.48 DT = £78.48
Semaglutide 7 mg Rybelsus 7mg tablets | 30 tablet [PoM] £78.48 DT = £78.48
Semaglutide 14 mg Rybelsus 14mg tablets | 30 tablet [PoM] £78.48 DT = £78.48

BLOOD GLUCOSE LOWERING DRUGS ›
MEGLITINIDES

Repaglinide

04-Jun-2021

● **DRUG ACTION** Repaglinide stimulates insulin secretion.

● **INDICATIONS AND DOSE**

Type 2 diabetes mellitus (as monotherapy or in combination with metformin when metformin alone inadequate)

▸ BY MOUTH

▸ Adult: Initially 500 micrograms (max. per dose 4 mg), adjusted according to response, dose to be taken within 30 minutes before main meals and adjusted at intervals of 1–2 weeks; maximum 16 mg per day

Type 2 diabetes mellitus (as monotherapy or in combination with metformin when metformin alone inadequate), if transferring from another oral antidiabetic drug

▸ BY MOUTH

▸ Adult: Initially 1 mg (max. per dose 4 mg), adjusted according to response, dose to be taken within 30 minutes before main meals and adjusted at intervals of 1–2 weeks; maximum 16 mg per day

● **CONTRA-INDICATIONS** Ketoacidosis

● **CAUTIONS** Debilitated patients · elderly (no information available) · malnourished patients

CAUTIONS, FURTHER INFORMATION Manufacturer advises patients exposed to stress (including fever, trauma, infection or surgery) may require treatment interruption and temporary replacement with insulin to maintain glycaemic control.

● **INTERACTIONS** → Appendix 1: meglitinides

● **SIDE-EFFECTS**

▸ **Common or very common** Abdominal pain · diarrhoea · hypoglycaemia

▸ **Rare or very rare** Cardiovascular disease · constipation · hepatic function abnormal · vasculitis · vision disorders · vomiting

▸ **Frequency not known** Acute coronary syndrome · hypoglycaemic coma · nausea · skin reactions

● **PREGNANCY** Avoid.

● **BREAST FEEDING** Avoid—present in milk in *animal* studies.

● **HEPATIC IMPAIRMENT** Manufacturer advises avoid in severe impairment (risk of increased exposure).

● **RENAL IMPAIRMENT** [EvGr] Use with caution. ⟨M⟩

● **PATIENT AND CARER ADVICE**
Driving and skilled tasks Drivers need to be particularly careful to avoid hypoglycaemia and should be warned of the problems.

● **MEDICINAL FORMS** There can be variation in the licensing of different medicines containing the same drug.
Oral tablet

▸ **Repaglinide (Non-proprietary)**
Repaglinide 500 microgram Repaglinide 500microgram tablets | 30 tablet [PoM] £1.08-£3.53 | 90 tablet [PoM] £10.00 DT = £3.25
Repaglinide 1 mg Repaglinide 1mg tablets | 30 tablet [PoM] £2.98-£3.53 | 90 tablet [PoM] £8.95-£10.50 DT = £8.95
Repaglinide 2 mg Repaglinide 2mg tablets | 90 tablet [PoM] £10.62 DT = £10.62

BLOOD GLUCOSE LOWERING DRUGS › OTHER

Tirzepatide

04-Feb-2025

● **DRUG ACTION** Tirzepatide is a long-acting GIP (glucose-dependent insulinotropic polypeptide) receptor and GLP-1 (glucagon-like peptide-1) receptor agonist that increases insulin sensitivity and secretion, suppresses glucagon secretion, and slows gastric emptying.

● **INDICATIONS AND DOSE**

Type 2 diabetes mellitus as monotherapy [if metformin inappropriate] | Type 2 diabetes mellitus in combination with other antidiabetic drugs (including insulin) [if existing treatment fails to achieve adequate glycaemic control]

▸ BY SUBCUTANEOUS INJECTION

▸ Adult: Initially 2.5 mg once weekly for 4 weeks, then increased to 5 mg once weekly for at least 4 weeks, then increased if necessary up to 15 mg once weekly, dose to be increased in steps of 2.5 mg at intervals of at least 4 weeks

Weight management [in conjunction with dietary measures and increased physical activity in individuals with a BMI of 30 kg/m^2 or more, or in individuals with a BMI of 27 kg/m^2 or more in the presence of at least one weight-related co-morbidity]

▸ BY SUBCUTANEOUS INJECTION

▸ Adult: Initially 2.5 mg once weekly for 4 weeks, then increased to 5 mg once weekly for at least 4 weeks, then increased if necessary up to 15 mg once weekly, dose to be increased in steps of 2.5 mg at intervals of at least 4 weeks. Assess benefit of continuing treatment if at least 5% of initial body-weight has not been lost after 6 months at highest tolerated dose

DOSE ADJUSTMENTS DUE TO INTERACTIONS

▸ Dose of concomitant insulin or sulfonylurea may need to be reduced.

IMPORTANT SAFETY INFORMATION

MHRA/CHM ADVICE: GLP-1 RECEPTOR AGONISTS: REPORTS OF DIABETIC KETOACIDOSIS WHEN CONCOMITANT INSULIN WAS RAPIDLY REDUCED OR DISCONTINUED (JUNE 2019)

Serious and life-threatening cases of diabetic ketoacidosis have been reported in patients with type 2 diabetes mellitus on a combination of insulin and the glucagon-like peptide-1 (GLP-1) receptor agonist exenatide, liraglutide, or dulaglutide, particularly after discontinuation or rapid dose reduction of concomitant insulin. The MHRA has not currently received any UK reports of diabetic ketoacidosis with the GLP-1 receptor agonists lixisenatide and semaglutide but this risk cannot be excluded. Similarly, this risk cannot be excluded for the GIP (glucose-dependent insulinotropic polypeptide) receptor and GLP-1 receptor agonist tirzepatide. Healthcare professionals are advised that any dose reduction of insulin should be done in a stepwise manner with careful blood glucose self-monitoring, particularly when GLP-1 receptor agonist therapy is initiated. Patients should be informed of the risk factors for and signs and symptoms of diabetic ketoacidosis, and advised to seek immediate medical attention if these develop.

MHRA/CHM ADVICE: GLP-1 RECEPTOR AGONISTS: REMINDER OF THE POTENTIAL SIDE EFFECTS AND TO BE AWARE OF THE POTENTIAL FOR MISUSE (OCTOBER 2024)

The MHRA reminds healthcare professionals to ensure that patients are aware of potential side-effects associated with glucagon-like peptide-1 (GLP-1) receptor agonists following anecdotal evidence and Yellow Card reports suggesting misuse of these medicines for weight management outside of their licence. The only GLP-1 receptor agonists licensed for weight management are liraglutide p. 816 (*Saxenda*®), semaglutide p. 819 (*Wegovy*®), and tirzepatide p. 822 (*Mounjaro*®), which is also a glucose-dependent insulinotropic polypeptide (GIP) receptor agonist. The benefits and risks of these medicines for weight loss in individuals who are not obese, or who are not overweight with weight-related co-morbidities, have not been studied.

Healthcare professionals should inform patients and carers upon initial prescription and at any dose increase about the common risk of gastro-intestinal side-effects (including nausea, vomiting, diarrhoea, and constipation) associated with GLP-1 receptor agonists; these are usually non-serious but can persist for several days and may lead to serious complications such as severe dehydration and kidney damage, resulting in hospitalisation. For this reason, patients should be advised to stay well hydrated by drinking plenty of fluids throughout treatment. They should also be informed of other serious but less common side-effects, including acute gallstone disease, pancreatitis, and serious allergic reactions.

Patients and carers should be advised to ensure that prescriptions are only obtained from registered healthcare professionals and that private prescriptions are dispensed from authorised sources to avoid the risk of receiving falsified pens. Patients and carers should consult the patient information leaflet for instructions on the use of GLP-1 receptor agonists, and be advised to only administer the prescribed dose.

MHRA/CHM ADVICE: GLP-1 AND DUAL GIP/GLP-1 RECEPTOR AGONISTS: POTENTIAL RISK OF PULMONARY ASPIRATION DURING GENERAL ANAESTHESIA OR DEEP SEDATION (JANUARY 2025)

An EU review has concluded that glucagon-like peptide-1 (GLP-1) and dual glucose-dependent insulinotropic polypeptide (GIP)/GLP-1 receptor agonists are associated with a potential risk of pulmonary aspiration in patients undergoing surgery or procedures requiring general anaesthesia or deep sedation. These medicines are known to slow gastric emptying, thereby increasing the risk of residual gastric contents despite preoperative fasting, which could lead to pulmonary aspiration and other severe complications, such as aspiration pneumonia.

The MHRA advises healthcare professionals to identify the increased risk of aspiration as early as possible, ideally at the pre-assessment clinic before surgery, in patients using GLP-1 or dual GIP/GLP-1 receptor agonists. Anaesthetists should complete an individualised preoperative risk assessment and consider the following:

- patients with underlying diabetic gastroparesis, as well as other co-morbidities such as obesity or gastroesophageal reflux disease, and symptoms of delayed gastric emptying (such as nausea, vomiting

and abdominal pain) may have a higher risk of aspiration;
- directly asking patients or their carers about their use of GLP-1 or dual GIP/GLP-1 receptor agonists, as private prescriptions may not be included in the patient's medical notes or drug history, and patients who may have purchased these medications for use in aesthetic weight loss may not readily disclose this information (see also advice issued in October 2024, above).

There is limited evidence to support any recommendations on a time frame to withhold GLP-1 or dual GIP/GLP-1 receptor agonists prior to anaesthesia, new fasting guidelines, or an appropriate medical procedure to confirm an empty stomach. Anaesthetists should manage aspiration risk in line with usual anaesthetic practice and retain flexibility to provide individualised assessment.

Healthcare professionals should counsel patients or their carers to continue taking their prescribed medicines and not stop treatment without first discussing with their doctor. They should also be advised regarding the risk of aspiration and that there may be a need to modify pre-procedure instruction and anaesthetic technique.

● **CAUTIONS** Delayed gastric emptying · diabetic retinopathy · general anaesthesia or deep sedation (risk of pulmonary aspiration due to delayed gastric emptying) · history of pancreatitis · severe gastro-intestinal disease

CAUTIONS, FURTHER INFORMATION
▸ Delayed gastric emptying [EvGr] Tirzepatide delays gastric emptying, particularly following the first dose. This has the potential to slow the rate of absorption of concomitant oral medicines. The risk of a delayed effect should be considered for oral medicines where a rapid onset of action is important. Monitor patients on oral medicines with a narrow therapeutic index, especially at the start of tirzepatide treatment and after dose increases. ◈ See also *Conception and Contraception*, below.

● **INTERACTIONS** → Appendix 1: glucagon-like peptide-1 receptor agonists

● **SIDE-EFFECTS**
▸ **Common or very common** Alopecia · appetite decreased (in patients with type 2 diabetes) · asthenia · burping · constipation · diarrhoea · dizziness · gastrointestinal discomfort · gastrointestinal disorders · hypersensitivity · hypotension · lethargy · malaise · nausea · vomiting
▸ **Uncommon** Gallbladder disorders · pancreatitis acute · taste altered · weight decreased (in patients with type 2 diabetes)
▸ **Rare or very rare** Angioedema
▸ **Frequency not known** Hypoglycaemia

SIDE-EFFECTS, FURTHER INFORMATION Discontinue if symptoms of acute pancreatitis occur, such as persistent, severe abdominal pain. If pancreatitis confirmed, do not restart treatment.

● **ALLERGY AND CROSS-SENSITIVITY** [EvGr] *Mounjaro Kwikpen*® contains benzyl alcohol which may cause allergic reactions. ◈

● **CONCEPTION AND CONTRACEPTION** [EvGr] Tirzepatide delays gastric emptying which may affect absorption of concomitant oral medicines. Since reduced efficacy of oral contraceptives cannot be excluded, it is advised that female patients who are overweight or obese and using an oral contraceptive should add a barrier method of contraception or switch to a non-oral contraceptive method for the first 4 weeks of treatment, and for 4 weeks after *each* dose increase. Discontinue treatment at least one month before planned pregnancy. ◈

● **PREGNANCY** [EvGr] Avoid—toxicity in *animal* studies. ◈

6

- **BREAST FEEDING** Specialist sources indicate use with caution—no information available. Large molecular weight suggests limited excretion into milk and drug molecule likely to be partially destroyed in the infant's gastro-intestinal tract.
- **HEPATIC IMPAIRMENT** [EvGr] Use *Mounjaro Kwikpen*® with caution (potential risk of metabolic acidosis due to accumulation of benzyl alcohol excipient over time). ⓜ
- **RENAL IMPAIRMENT** [EvGr] Use *Mounjaro Kwikpen*® with caution (potential risk of metabolic acidosis due to accumulation of benzyl alcohol excipient over time). ⓜ
- **HANDLING AND STORAGE** *Mounjaro Kwikpen*® should be stored in a refrigerator (2–8°C); may be stored at 30°C or below for up to 30 days.
- **PATIENT AND CARER ADVICE** Patients or their carers should be given advice on how to administer tirzepatide injection. Acute pancreatitis Patients and their carers should be told how to recognise signs and symptoms of acute pancreatitis and advised to seek immediate medical attention if symptoms develop.
  Dehydration Patients and their carers should be informed of the potential risk of dehydration in relation to gastro-intestinal side-effects and advised to take precautions to avoid fluid depletion.
  A patient leaflet and user manual should be provided.
  Missed doses If a dose is more than 4 days late, the missed dose should be omitted and the next dose administered at the normal time.
- **NATIONAL FUNDING/ACCESS DECISIONS**
  For full details see funding body website
  NICE decisions
  ▸ **Tirzepatide for treating type 2 diabetes (October 2023)** NICE TA924 Recommended with restrictions
  ▸ **Tirzepatide for managing overweight and obesity (December 2024)** NICE TA1026 Recommended with restrictions
  Scottish Medicines Consortium (SMC) decisions
  ▸ **Tirzepatide (*Mounjaro*®) for the treatment of adults with insufficiently controlled type 2 diabetes mellitus as an adjunct to diet and exercise: as monotherapy when metformin is considered inappropriate due to intolerance or contra-indications; or in addition to other medicinal products for the treatment of diabetes (April 2024)** SMC No. SMC2633 Recommended with restrictions
  ▸ **Tirzepatide (*Mounjaro*®) for weight management, including weight loss and weight maintenance, as an adjunct to a reduced-calorie diet and increased physical activity in adults with an initial BMI of 30 kg/m² or more, or 27 kg/m² to less than 30 kg/m² in the presence of at least one weight-related co-morbid condition (June 2024)** SMC No. SMC2653 Recommended with restrictions
- **MEDICINAL FORMS** There can be variation in the licensing of different medicines containing the same drug.
  Solution for injection
  CAUTIONARY AND ADVISORY LABELS 10
  EXCIPIENTS: May contain Benzyl alcohol
  ▸ **Mounjaro KwikPen** (Eli Lilly and Company Ltd) ▼
  Tirzepatide 4.167 mg per 1 ml Mounjaro KwikPen 2.5mg/0.6ml solution for injection 2.4ml pre-filled pens | 1 pre-filled disposable injection [PoM] £92.00 DT = £92.00
  Tirzepatide 8.333 mg per 1 ml Mounjaro KwikPen 5mg/0.6ml solution for injection 2.4ml pre-filled pens | 1 pre-filled disposable injection [PoM] £92.00 DT = £92.00
  Tirzepatide 12.5 mg per 1 ml Mounjaro KwikPen 7.5mg/0.6ml solution for injection 2.4ml pre-filled pens | 1 pre-filled disposable injection [PoM] £107.00 DT = £107.00
  Tirzepatide 16.667 mg per 1 ml Mounjaro KwikPen 10mg/0.6ml solution for injection 2.4ml pre-filled pens | 1 pre-filled disposable injection [PoM] £107.00 DT = £107.00
  Tirzepatide 20.833 mg per 1 ml Mounjaro KwikPen 12.5mg/0.6ml solution for injection 2.4ml pre-filled pens | 1 pre-filled disposable injection [PoM] £122.00 DT = £122.00

Tirzepatide 25 mg per 1 ml Mounjaro KwikPen 15mg/0.6ml solution for injection 2.4ml pre-filled pens | 1 pre-filled disposable injection [PoM] £122.00 DT = £122.00

BLOOD GLUCOSE LOWERING DRUGS ❯ SODIUM GLUCOSE CO-TRANSPORTER 2 INHIBITORS

Canagliflozin

01-Feb-2024

- **DRUG ACTION** Reversibly inhibits sodium-glucose co-transporter 2 (SGLT2) in the renal proximal convoluted tubule to reduce glucose reabsorption and increase urinary glucose excretion.

- **INDICATIONS AND DOSE**

Type 2 diabetes mellitus as monotherapy (if metformin inappropriate) | Type 2 diabetes mellitus in combination with insulin or other antidiabetic drugs (if existing treatment fails to achieve adequate glycaemic control)
▸ BY MOUTH
▸ Adult: 100 mg once daily; increased if tolerated to 300 mg once daily if required, dose to be taken preferably before breakfast

DOSE ADJUSTMENTS DUE TO INTERACTIONS
▸ Manufacturer advises increase dose if tolerated to 300 mg once daily with concurrent use of rifampicin.
▸ Dose of concomitant insulin or drugs that stimulate insulin secretion may need to be reduced.

IMPORTANT SAFETY INFORMATION

MHRA/CHM ADVICE (UPDATED APRIL 2016): RISK OF DIABETIC KETOACIDOSIS WITH SODIUM-GLUCOSE CO-TRANSPORTER 2 (SGLT2) INHIBITORS (CANAGLIFLOZIN, DAPAGLIFLOZIN OR EMPAGLIFLOZIN)
A review by the European Medicines Agency has concluded that serious, life-threatening, and fatal cases of diabetic ketoacidosis (DKA) have been reported rarely in patients taking an SGLT2 inhibitor. In several cases, the presentation of DKA was atypical with patients having only moderately elevated blood glucose levels, and some of them occurred during off-label use.
To minimise the risk of such effects when treating patients with a SGLT2 inhibitor, the European Medicines Agency has issued the following advice:
- inform patients of the signs and symptoms of DKA, (including rapid weight loss, nausea or vomiting, abdominal pain, fast and deep breathing, sleepiness, a sweet smell to the breath, a sweet or metallic taste in the mouth, or a different odour to urine or sweat), and advise them to seek immediate medical advice if they develop any of these
- test for raised ketones in patients with signs and symptoms of DKA, even if plasma glucose levels are near-normal
- use canagliflozin with caution in patients with risk factors for DKA, (including a low beta cell reserve, conditions leading to restricted food intake or severe dehydration, sudden reduction in insulin, increased insulin requirements due to acute illness, surgery or alcohol abuse), and discuss these risk factors with patients
- discontinue treatment if DKA is suspected or diagnosed
- do not restart treatment with any SGLT2 inhibitor in patients who experienced DKA during use, unless another cause for DKA was identified and resolved
- interrupt SGLT2 inhibitor treatment in patients who are hospitalised for major surgery or acute serious illnesses; treatment may be restarted once the patient's condition has stabilised

MHRA/CHM ADVICE: SGLT2 INHIBITORS: MONITOR KETONES IN BLOOD DURING TREATMENT INTERRUPTION FOR SURGICAL PROCEDURES OR ACUTE SERIOUS MEDICAL ILLNESS (MARCH 2020)

New recommendations have been issued following a European review of peri-operative diabetic ketoacidosis in patients taking SGLT2 inhibitors. Healthcare professionals are advised to monitor ketone levels during SGLT2 inhibitor treatment interruption in patients who have been hospitalised for major surgery or acute serious illness—measurement of blood ketone levels is preferred to urine. Treatment may be restarted once ketone levels are normal and the patient's condition has stabilised.

MHRA/CHM ADVICE (UPDATED MARCH 2017): INCREASED RISK OF LOWER-LIMB AMPUTATION (MAINLY TOES)

Canagliflozin may increase the risk of lower-limb amputation (mainly toes) in patients with type 2 diabetes. Preventive foot care is important for all patients with diabetes. The MHRA has issued the following advice while clinical trials are ongoing:
- consider stopping canagliflozin if a patient develops a significant lower limb complication (e.g. skin ulcer, osteomyelitis, or gangrene)
- carefully monitor patients who have risk factors for amputation (e.g. previous amputations, existing peripheral vascular disease, or neuropathy)
- monitor all patients for signs and symptoms of water or salt loss; ensure patients stay sufficiently hydrated to prevent volume depletion in line with the manufacturer's recommendations
- advise patients to stay well hydrated, carry out routine preventive foot care, and seek medical advice promptly if they develop skin ulceration, discolouration, or new pain or tenderness
- start treatment for foot problems (e.g. ulceration, infection, or new pain or tenderness) as early as possible
- continue to follow standard treatment guidelines for routine preventive foot care for people with diabetes.

MHRA/CHM ADVICE: SGLT2 INHIBITORS: REPORTS OF FOURNIER'S GANGRENE (NECROTISING FASCIITIS OF THE GENITALIA OR PERINEUM) (FEBRUARY 2019)

Fournier's gangrene, a rare but serious and potentially life-threatening infection, has been associated with the use of sodium-glucose co-transporter 2 (SGLT2) inhibitors. If Fournier's gangrene is suspected, stop the SGLT2 inhibitor and urgently start treatment (including antibiotics and surgical debridement).

Patients should be advised to seek urgent medical attention if they experience severe pain, tenderness, erythema, or swelling in the genital or perineal area, accompanied by fever or malaise—urogenital infection or perineal abscess may precede necrotising fasciitis.

- **CONTRA-INDICATIONS** Diabetic ketoacidosis · type 1 diabetes mellitus (increased risk of diabetic ketoacidosis)
- **CAUTIONS** Elderly (risk of volume depletion) · elevated haematocrit · hypotension · risk of volume depletion
  CAUTIONS, FURTHER INFORMATION
- Volume depletion Correct hypovolaemia before starting treatment.
- **INTERACTIONS** → Appendix 1: sodium glucose co-transporter 2 inhibitors
- **SIDE-EFFECTS**
- **Common or very common** Balanoposthitis · constipation · dyslipidaemia · hypoglycaemia (in combination with insulin or sulfonylurea) · increased risk of infection · nausea · thirst · urinary disorders · urosepsis

- **Uncommon** Dehydration · dizziness postural · hypotension · lower limb amputations · renal failure · skin reactions · syncope
- **Rare or very rare** Anaphylactic reaction · angioedema · diabetic ketoacidosis (discontinue immediately)
- **Frequency not known** Fournier's gangrene (discontinue and initiate treatment promptly)
  SIDE-EFFECTS, FURTHER INFORMATION Consider interrupting treatment if volume depletion occurs.
- **PREGNANCY** Avoid—toxicity in *animal* studies.
- **BREAST FEEDING** Avoid—present in milk in *animal* studies.
- **HEPATIC IMPAIRMENT** Manufacturer advises avoid in severe impairment—no information available.
- **RENAL IMPAIRMENT** [EvGr] Caution if eGFR less than $60 \, mL/minute/1.73 \, m^2$. Avoid initiation when baseline eGFR less than $30 \, mL/minute/1.73 \, m^2$. [M]
  Dose adjustments [EvGr] Limit dose to 100 mg once daily when eGFR less than $60 \, mL/minute/1.73 \, m^2$; consider addition of other hypoglycaemic agents if further glycaemic control needed. If eGFR falls to less than $30 \, mL/minute/1.73 \, m^2$ during treatment, continue with 100 mg once daily. [M] See p. 21.
- **MONITORING REQUIREMENTS** [EvGr] Determine renal function before treatment and at least annually thereafter, and before initiation of concomitant drugs that reduce renal function and periodically thereafter. [M]
- **PATIENT AND CARER ADVICE** Patients should be advised to report symptoms of volume depletion including postural hypotension and dizziness. Patients should be informed of the signs and symptoms of diabetic ketoacidosis, see MHRA advice.
- **NATIONAL FUNDING/ACCESS DECISIONS** For full details see funding body website
  NICE decisions
- **Canagliflozin, dapagliflozin and empagliflozin as monotherapies for treating type 2 diabetes (May 2016)** NICE TA390 Recommended with restrictions
- **Canagliflozin in combination therapy for treating type 2 diabetes (June 2014)** NICE TA315 Recommended with restrictions

- **MEDICINAL FORMS** There can be variation in the licensing of different medicines containing the same drug.
  Oral tablet
- **Invokana** (A. Menarini Farmaceutica Internazionale SRL)
  Canagliflozin (as Canagliflozin hemihydrate) 100 mg Invokana 100mg tablets | 30 tablet [PoM] £39.20 DT = £39.20
  Canagliflozin (as Canagliflozin hemihydrate) 300 mg Invokana 300mg tablets | 30 tablet [PoM] £39.20 DT = £39.20

Canagliflozin with metformin　　23-Jul-2021

The properties listed below are those particular to the combination only. For the properties of the components please consider, canagliflozin p. 824, metformin hydrochloride p. 807.

- **INDICATIONS AND DOSE**

Type 2 diabetes mellitus not controlled by metformin alone or by metformin in combination with insulin or other antidiabetic drugs
- BY MOUTH
- Adult: 1 tablet twice daily, dose based on patient's current metformin dose, daily dose of metformin should not exceed 2 g

DOSE ADJUSTMENTS DUE TO INTERACTIONS
- Dose of concomitant insulin or drugs that stimulate insulin secretion may need to be reduced.

- **INTERACTIONS** → Appendix 1: metformin · sodium glucose co-transporter 2 inhibitors

- **RENAL IMPAIRMENT** [EvGr] Avoid if eGFR less than 60 mL/minute/1.73 m^2 (consult product literature). (M) See p. 21.
- **NATIONAL FUNDING/ACCESS DECISIONS** For full details see funding body website
  Scottish Medicines Consortium (SMC) decisions
  ▶ Canagliflozin plus metformin (*Vokanamet*®) in adults aged 18 years and older with type 2 diabetes mellitus as an adjunct to diet and exercise to improve glycaemic control (January 2015) SMC No. 1019/14 Recommended with restrictions
- **MEDICINAL FORMS** There can be variation in the licensing of different medicines containing the same drug.
  Oral tablet
  CAUTIONARY AND ADVISORY LABELS 21
  ▶ **Vokanamet** (A. Menarini Farmaceutica Internazionale SRL)
    Canagliflozin (as Canagliflozin hemihydrate) 50 mg, Metformin hydrochloride 850 mg Vokanamet 50mg/850mg tablets | 60 tablet [PoM] £39.20 DT = £39.20
    Canagliflozin (as Canagliflozin hemihydrate) 50 mg, Metformin hydrochloride 1 gram Vokanamet 50mg/1000mg tablets | 60 tablet [PoM] £39.20 DT = £39.20

Dapagliflozin

25-Apr-2025

- **DRUG ACTION** Reversibly inhibits sodium-glucose co-transporter 2 (SGLT2) in the renal proximal convoluted tubule to reduce glucose reabsorption and increase urinary glucose excretion.

- **INDICATIONS AND DOSE**

Type 2 diabetes mellitus [as monotherapy if metformin inappropriate] | Type 2 diabetes mellitus [in combination with insulin or other antidiabetic drugs] | Symptomatic chronic heart failure | Chronic kidney disease
  ▶ BY MOUTH
  ▶ Adult: 10 mg once daily

DOSE ADJUSTMENTS DUE TO INTERACTIONS
  ▶ Dose of concomitant insulin or drugs that stimulate insulin secretion may need to be reduced (risk of hypoglycaemia)—consult product literature.

IMPORTANT SAFETY INFORMATION
MHRA/CHM ADVICE (UPDATED APRIL 2016): RISK OF DIABETIC KETOACIDOSIS WITH SODIUM-GLUCOSE CO-TRANSPORTER 2 (SGLT2) INHIBITORS (CANAGLIFLOZIN, DAPAGLIFLOZIN OR EMPAGLIFLOZIN)
A review by the European Medicines Agency has concluded that serious, life-threatening, and fatal cases of diabetic ketoacidosis (DKA) have been reported rarely in patients taking an SGLT2 inhibitor. In several cases, the presentation of DKA was atypical with patients having only moderately elevated blood glucose levels, and some of them occurred during off-label use.

To minimise the risk of such effects when treating patients with a SGLT2 inhibitor, the European Medicines Agency has issued the following advice:
- inform patients of the signs and symptoms of DKA, (including rapid weight loss, nausea or vomiting, abdominal pain, fast and deep breathing, sleepiness, a sweet smell to the breath, a sweet or metallic taste in the mouth, or a different odour to urine or sweat), and advise them to seek immediate medical advice if they develop any of these
- test for raised ketones in patients with signs and symptoms of DKA, even if plasma glucose levels are near-normal
- use dapagliflozin with caution in patients with risk factors for DKA, (including a low beta cell reserve, conditions leading to restricted food intake or severe dehydration, sudden reduction in insulin, increased insulin requirements due to acute illness, surgery or

alcohol abuse), and discuss these risk factors with patients
- discontinue treatment if DKA is suspected or diagnosed
- do not restart treatment with any SGLT2 inhibitor in patients who experienced DKA during use, unless another cause for DKA was identified and resolved
- interrupt SGLT2 inhibitor treatment in patients who are hospitalised for major surgery or acute serious illnesses; treatment may be restarted once the patient's condition has stabilised

MHRA/CHM ADVICE: SGLT2 INHIBITORS: MONITOR KETONES IN BLOOD DURING TREATMENT INTERRUPTION FOR SURGICAL PROCEDURES OR ACUTE SERIOUS MEDICAL ILLNESS (MARCH 2020)
New recommendations have been issued following a European review of peri-operative diabetic ketoacidosis in patients taking SGLT2 inhibitors. Healthcare professionals are advised to monitor ketone levels during SGLT2 inhibitor treatment interruption in patients who have been hospitalised for major surgery or acute serious illness—measurement of blood ketone levels is preferred to urine. Treatment may be restarted once ketone levels are normal and the patient's condition has stabilised.

MHRA/CHM ADVICE: SGLT2 INHIBITORS: REPORTS OF FOURNIER'S GANGRENE (NECROTISING FASCIITIS OF THE GENITALIA OR PERINEUM) (FEBRUARY 2019)
Fournier's gangrene, a rare but serious and potentially life-threatening infection, has been associated with the use of sodium-glucose co-transporter 2 (SGLT2) inhibitors. If Fournier's gangrene is suspected, stop the SGLT2 inhibitor and urgently start treatment (including antibiotics and surgical debridement).

Patients should be advised to seek urgent medical attention if they experience severe pain, tenderness, erythema, or swelling in the genital or perineal area, accompanied by fever or malaise—urogenital infection or perineal abscess may precede necrotising fasciitis.

MHRA/CHM ADVICE: *FORXIGA* ® (DAPAGLIFLOZIN) 5 MG SHOULD NO LONGER BE USED FOR THE TREATMENT OF TYPE 1 DIABETES MELLITUS (NOVEMBER 2021)
Dapagliflozin 5 mg is no longer authorised for the treatment of patients with type 1 diabetes mellitus (T1DM) and should no longer be used in this population. Discontinuation of dapagliflozin in patients with T1DM must be made by or in consultation with a physician specialised in diabetes care as soon as clinically practical. After stopping dapagliflozin, frequent blood glucose monitoring is recommended, and the insulin dose should be increased carefully to minimise the risk of hypoglycaemia.

- **CONTRA-INDICATIONS** Diabetic ketoacidosis · type 1 diabetes mellitus (increased risk of diabetic ketoacidosis)
- **CAUTIONS** Elderly · hypotension · risk of volume depletion
  CAUTIONS, FURTHER INFORMATION
  ▶ Volume depletion Correct hypovolaemia before starting treatment.
- **INTERACTIONS** → Appendix 1: sodium glucose co-transporter 2 inhibitors
- **SIDE-EFFECTS**
  ▶ **Common or very common** Back pain · balanoposthitis · cystitis · dizziness · dyslipidaemia · hypoglycaemia (in combination with insulin or sulfonylurea) · increased risk of infection · prostatitis · skin reactions · urinary disorders · vulvovaginal disorders
  ▶ **Uncommon** Constipation · dry mouth · fluid imbalance · genital pruritus · hypotension · thirst · weight decreased
  ▶ **Rare or very rare** Angioedema · diabetic ketoacidosis (discontinue immediately) · Fournier's gangrene

(discontinue and initiate treatment promptly) · nephritis tubulointerstitial

SIDE-EFFECTS, FURTHER INFORMATION **Volume depletion** Interrupt treatment if volume depletion occurs.

Urinary tract infections Urinary glucose excretion may be associated with an increased risk of urinary tract infection. Consider temporarily interrupting treatment with dapagliflozin when treating pyelonephritis or urosepsis.

Renal function changes Creatinine levels may increase during initial treatment. These increases in creatinine are generally transient with continued treatment or reversible after stopping treatment.

● **PREGNANCY** Avoid—toxicity in *animal* studies.

● **BREAST FEEDING** Avoid—present in milk in *animal* studies.

● **HEPATIC IMPAIRMENT** [EvGr] Caution in severe impairment (risk of increased exposure; limited information available). ⟨M⟩
Dose adjustments [EvGr] Initially 5 mg daily in severe impairment, increased if tolerated to 10 mg daily. ⟨M⟩

● **RENAL IMPAIRMENT** See p. 21. [EvGr] Avoid initiation if eGFR less than 15 mL/minute/1.73 m^2. ⟨M⟩
▸ When used for Type 2 diabetes mellitus [EvGr] Consider additional antidiabetic drugs with dapagliflozin if eGFR less than 45 mL/minute/1.73 m^2 (reduced efficacy). ⟨M⟩

● **PATIENT AND CARER ADVICE** Patients should be informed of the signs and symptoms of diabetic ketoacidosis, see MHRA advice.

● **NATIONAL FUNDING/ACCESS DECISIONS**
For full details see funding body website
NICE decisions
▸ **Dapagliflozin in combination therapy for treating type 2 diabetes (updated November 2016)** NICE TA288 Recommended with restrictions
▸ **Canagliflozin, dapagliflozin and empagliflozin as monotherapies for treating type 2 diabetes (May 2016)** NICE TA390 Recommended with restrictions
▸ **Dapagliflozin in triple therapy for treating type 2 diabetes (November 2016)** NICE TA418 Recommended with restrictions
▸ **Dapagliflozin for treating chronic heart failure with reduced ejection fraction (February 2021)** NICE TA679 Recommended with restrictions
▸ **Dapagliflozin for treating chronic heart failure with preserved or mildly reduced ejection fraction (June 2023)** NICE TA902 Recommended
▸ **Dapagliflozin for treating chronic kidney disease (March 2022)** NICE TA775 Recommended with restrictions
Scottish Medicines Consortium (SMC) decisions
▸ **Dapagliflozin (*Forxiga*®) in adults for the treatment of symptomatic chronic heart failure with reduced ejection fraction (April 2021)** SMC No. SMC2322 Recommended
▸ **Dapagliflozin (*Forxiga*®) in adults for the treatment of symptomatic chronic heart failure with left ventricular ejection fraction of less than 40% (August 2023)** SMC No. SMC2577 Recommended
▸ **Dapagliflozin (*Forxiga*®) in adults for the treatment of chronic kidney disease (May 2022)** SMC No. SMC2428 Recommended with restrictions
▸ **Dapagliflozin (*Forxiga*®) in adults for the treatment of chronic kidney disease [in an extended patient population] (April 2025)** SMC No. SMC2763 Recommended with restrictions

● **MEDICINAL FORMS** There can be variation in the licensing of different medicines containing the same drug.
Oral tablet
▸ Forxiga (AstraZeneca UK Ltd)
Dapagliflozin (as Dapagliflozin propanediol monohydrate) 5 mg Forxiga 5mg tablets | 28 tablet [PoM] £36.59 DT = £36.59

Dapagliflozin (as Dapagliflozin propanediol monohydrate) 10 mg Forxiga 10mg tablets | 28 tablet [PoM] £36.59 DT = £36.59

Combinations available: *Saxagliptin with dapagliflozin*, p. 811

Dapagliflozin with metformin   04-Nov-2020

The properties listed below are those particular to the combination only. For the properties of the components please consider, dapagliflozin p. 826, metformin hydrochloride p. 807.

● **INDICATIONS AND DOSE**
Type 2 diabetes mellitus [not controlled by metformin alone, or by metformin in combination with other antidiabetic drugs (including insulin)]
▸ BY MOUTH
▸ Adult: 1 tablet twice daily, based on patient's current metformin dose

● **INTERACTIONS** → Appendix 1: metformin · sodium glucose co-transporter 2 inhibitors

● **HEPATIC IMPAIRMENT** Manufacturer advises avoid (increased risk of lactic acidosis).

● **NATIONAL FUNDING/ACCESS DECISIONS**
For full details see funding body website
Scottish Medicines Consortium (SMC) decisions
▸ **Dapagliflozin with metformin (*Xigduo*®) for use in adults with type 2 diabetes mellitus as an adjunct to diet and exercise to improve glycaemic control: in patients inadequately controlled on their maximally tolerated dose of metformin alone; in combination with other glucose-lowering medicinal products, including insulin, in patients inadequately controlled with metformin and these medicinal products; in patients already being treated with the combination of dapagliflozin and metformin as separate tablets (August 2014)** SMC No. 983/14 Recommended with restrictions

● **MEDICINAL FORMS** There can be variation in the licensing of different medicines containing the same drug.
Oral tablet
CAUTIONARY AND ADVISORY LABELS 21
▸ Xigduo (AstraZeneca UK Ltd)
Dapagliflozin (as Dapagliflozin propanediol monohydrate) 5 mg, Metformin hydrochloride 850 mg Xigduo 5mg/850mg tablets | 56 tablet [PoM] £36.59 DT = £36.59
Dapagliflozin (as Dapagliflozin propanediol monohydrate) 5 mg, Metformin hydrochloride 1 gram Xigduo 5mg/1000mg tablets | 56 tablet [PoM] £36.59 DT = £36.59

Empagliflozin   01-Aug-2024

● **DRUG ACTION** Reversibly inhibits sodium-glucose co-transporter 2 (SGLT2) in the renal proximal convoluted tubule to reduce glucose reabsorption and increase urinary glucose excretion.

● **INDICATIONS AND DOSE**
Type 2 diabetes mellitus [as monotherapy if metformin inappropriate] | Type 2 diabetes mellitus [in combination with insulin or other antidiabetic drugs]
▸ BY MOUTH
▸ Adult: 10 mg once daily, increased to 25 mg once daily, dose increased if necessary and if tolerated
Symptomatic chronic heart failure | Chronic kidney disease
▸ BY MOUTH
▸ Adult: 10 mg once daily   continued →

DOSE ADJUSTMENTS DUE TO INTERACTIONS
▸ Dose of concomitant insulin or drugs that stimulate insulin secretion may need to be reduced.

IMPORTANT SAFETY INFORMATION
MHRA/CHM ADVICE (UPDATED APRIL 2016): RISK OF DIABETIC KETOACIDOSIS WITH SODIUM-GLUCOSE CO-TRANSPORTER 2 (SGLT2) INHIBITORS (CANAGLIFLOZIN, DAPAGLIFLOZIN OR EMPAGLIFLOZIN)
A review by the European Medicines Agency has concluded that serious, life-threatening, and fatal cases of diabetic ketoacidosis (DKA) have been reported rarely in patients taking an SGLT2 inhibitor. In several cases, the presentation of DKA was atypical with patients having only moderately elevated blood glucose levels, and some of them occurred during off-label use.

To minimise the risk of such effects when treating patients with a SGLT2 inhibitor, the European Medicines Agency has issued the following advice:
- inform patients of the signs and symptoms of DKA, (including rapid weight loss, nausea or vomiting, abdominal pain, fast and deep breathing, sleepiness, a sweet smell to the breath, a sweet or metallic taste in the mouth, or a different odour to urine or sweat), and advise them to seek immediate medical advice if they develop any of these
- test for raised ketones in patients with signs and symptoms of DKA, even if plasma glucose levels are near-normal
- use empagliflozin with caution in patients with risk factors for DKA, (including a low beta cell reserve, conditions leading to restricted food intake or severe dehydration, sudden reduction in insulin, increased insulin requirements due to acute illness, surgery or alcohol abuse), and discuss these risk factors with patients
- discontinue treatment if DKA is suspected or diagnosed
- do not restart treatment with any SGLT2 inhibitor in patients who experienced DKA during use, unless another cause for DKA was identified and resolved
- interrupt SGLT2 inhibitor treatment in patients who are hospitalised for major surgery or acute serious illnesses; treatment may be restarted once the patient's condition has stabilised

MHRA/CHM ADVICE: SGLT2 INHIBITORS: MONITOR KETONES IN BLOOD DURING TREATMENT INTERRUPTION FOR SURGICAL PROCEDURES OR ACUTE SERIOUS MEDICAL ILLNESS (MARCH 2020)
New recommendations have been issued following a European review of peri-operative diabetic ketoacidosis in patients taking SGLT2 inhibitors. Healthcare professionals are advised to monitor ketone levels during SGLT2 inhibitor treatment interruption in patients who have been hospitalised for major surgery or acute serious illness—measurement of blood ketone levels is preferred to urine. Treatment may be restarted once ketone levels are normal and the patient's condition has stabilised.

MHRA/CHM ADVICE: SGLT2 INHIBITORS: REPORTS OF FOURNIER'S GANGRENE (NECROTISING FASCIITIS OF THE GENITALIA OR PERINEUM) (FEBRUARY 2019)
Fournier's gangrene, a rare but serious and potentially life-threatening infection, has been associated with the use of sodium-glucose co-transporter 2 (SGLT2) inhibitors. If Fournier's gangrene is suspected, stop the SGLT2 inhibitor and urgently start treatment (including antibiotics and surgical debridement).

Patients should be advised to seek urgent medical attention if they experience severe pain, tenderness, erythema, or swelling in the genital or perineal area, accompanied by fever or malaise—urogenital infection or perineal abscess may precede necrotising fasciitis.

- **CONTRA-INDICATIONS** Diabetic ketoacidosis · type 1 diabetes mellitus (increased risk of diabetic ketoacidosis)
- **CAUTIONS** Complicated urinary tract infections—consider temporarily interrupting treatment · elderly · hypotension · risk of volume depletion
  CAUTIONS, FURTHER INFORMATION
  ▸ Volume depletion EvGr Correct hypovolaemia before starting treatment. Consider interrupting treatment if volume depletion occurs. Ⓜ
  ▸ Elderly EvGr Increased risk of volume depletion in patients aged 75 years and older. Ⓜ
- **INTERACTIONS** → Appendix 1: sodium glucose co-transporter 2 inhibitors
- **SIDE-EFFECTS**
  ▸ **Common or very common** Balanoposthitis · constipation · hypoglycaemia (in combination with insulin or sulfonylurea) · hypovolaemia (more common in elderly) · increased risk of infection · skin reactions · thirst · urinary disorders · urosepsis
  ▸ **Uncommon** Angioedema · ketoacidosis (discontinue immediately)
  ▸ **Rare or very rare** Fournier's gangrene (discontinue and initiate treatment promptly) · nephritis tubulointerstitial
- **PREGNANCY** Manufacturer advises avoid—toxicity in *animal* studies.
- **BREAST FEEDING** Manufacturer advises avoid—present in milk in *animal* studies.
- **HEPATIC IMPAIRMENT** EvGr Avoid in severe impairment (risk of increased exposure; limited information available). Ⓜ
- **RENAL IMPAIRMENT** EvGr Avoid initiation if eGFR less than 20 mL/minute/1.73 m². Ⓜ
  Dose adjustments
  ▸ When used for Type 2 diabetes mellitus EvGr Limit dose to 10 mg once daily if eGFR less than 60 mL/minute/1.73 m². Consider addition of other hypoglycemic agents if eGFR less than 45 mL/minute/1.73 m² (reduced efficacy). Ⓜ See p. 21.
- **MONITORING REQUIREMENTS** Determine renal function before treatment and before initiation of concomitant drugs that may reduce renal function, then at least annually thereafter.
- **PATIENT AND CARER ADVICE** Patients should be informed of the signs and symptoms of diabetic ketoacidosis, see MHRA advice.
- **NATIONAL FUNDING/ACCESS DECISIONS**
  For full details see funding body website
  NICE decisions
  ▸ Canagliflozin, dapagliflozin and empagliflozin as monotherapies for treating type 2 diabetes (May 2016) NICE TA390 Recommended with restrictions
  ▸ Empagliflozin in combination therapy for treating type 2 diabetes (March 2015) NICE TA336 Recommended with restrictions
  ▸ Empagliflozin for treating chronic heart failure with reduced ejection fraction (March 2022) NICE TA773 Recommended with restrictions
  ▸ Empagliflozin for treating chronic heart failure with preserved or mildly reduced ejection fraction (November 2023) NICE TA929 Recommended
  ▸ Empagliflozin for treating chronic kidney disease (December 2023) NICE TA942 Recommended with restrictions
  Scottish Medicines Consortium (SMC) decisions
  ▸ Empagliflozin (*Jardiance*®) in adults for the treatment of symptomatic chronic heart failure with reduced ejection fraction (October 2021) SMC No. SMC2396 Recommended

▶ Empagliflozin (*Jardiance®*) in adults for the treatment of symptomatic chronic heart failure with preserved ejection fraction (left ventricular ejection fraction of more than 40%) (May 2023) SMC No. SMC2523 Recommended
▶ Empagliflozin (*Jardiance®*) in adults for the treatment of chronic kidney disease (July 2024) SMC No. SMC2642 Recommended with restrictions

● MEDICINAL FORMS　There can be variation in the licensing of different medicines containing the same drug.

Oral tablet

▶ Jardiance (Boehringer Ingelheim Ltd)
Empagliflozin 10 mg　Jardiance 10mg tablets | 28 tablet [PoM] £36.59 DT = £36.59
Empagliflozin 25 mg　Jardiance 25mg tablets | 28 tablet [PoM] £36.59 DT = £36.59

Empagliflozin with linagliptin　04-Nov-2020

The properties listed below are those particular to the combination only. For the properties of the components please consider, empagliflozin p. 827, linagliptin p. 809.

● INDICATIONS AND DOSE

Type 2 diabetes mellitus [not controlled by metformin and/or a sulfonylurea with either empagliflozin or linagliptin]

▶ BY MOUTH
▶ Adult 18-74 years:　10/5 mg once daily, increased to 25/5 mg once daily if necessary and if tolerated
▶ Adult 75 years and over:　Initiation not recommended

DOSE ADJUSTMENTS DUE TO INTERACTIONS
▶ Dose of concomitant insulin or drugs that stimulate insulin secretion may need to be reduced.

DOSE EQUIVALENCE AND CONVERSION
▶ Dose expressed as *x/y* mg of empagliflozin/linagliptin.

● INTERACTIONS → Appendix 1: dipeptidylpeptidase-4 inhibitors · sodium glucose co-transporter 2 inhibitors

● PATIENT AND CARER ADVICE
Missed doses　Manufacturer advises if a dose is more than 12 hours late, the missed dose should not be taken and the next dose should be taken at the normal time.

● NATIONAL FUNDING/ACCESS DECISIONS
For full details see funding body website

Scottish Medicines Consortium (SMC) decisions
▶ Empagliflozin with linagliptin (*Glyxambi®*) is indicated in adults aged 18 years and older with type 2 diabetes mellitus: to improve glycaemic control when metformin and/or sulphonylurea (SU) and one of the monocomponents of *Glyxambi®* do not provide adequate glycaemic control; or when already being treated with the free combination of empagliflozin and linagliptin (August 2019) SMC No. SMC1236/17 Recommended with restrictions

● MEDICINAL FORMS　There can be variation in the licensing of different medicines containing the same drug.

Oral tablet

▶ Glyxambi (Boehringer Ingelheim Ltd)
Linagliptin 5 mg, Empagliflozin 10 mg　Glyxambi 10mg/5mg tablets | 28 tablet [PoM] £55.88 DT = £55.88
Linagliptin 5 mg, Empagliflozin 25 mg　Glyxambi 25mg/5mg tablets | 28 tablet [PoM] £55.88 DT = £55.88

Empagliflozin with metformin　09-Nov-2020

The properties listed below are those particular to the combination only. For the properties of the components please consider, empagliflozin p. 827, metformin hydrochloride p. 807.

● INDICATIONS AND DOSE

Type 2 diabetes mellitus not controlled by metformin alone or by metformin in combination with other antidiabetic drugs or insulin

▶ BY MOUTH
▶ Adult 18-84 years:　5/850–5/1000 mg twice daily, based on patient's current metformin dose, increased if necessary to 12.5/850–12.5/1000 mg twice daily
▶ Adult 85 years and over:　Initiation not recommended

DOSE ADJUSTMENTS DUE TO INTERACTIONS
▶ Dose of concomitant insulin or drugs that stimulate insulin secretion may need to be reduced.

DOSE EQUIVALENCE AND CONVERSION
▶ The proportions are expressed in the form "x"/"y" where "x" and "y" are the strengths in milligrams of empagliflozin and metformin respectively.

● INTERACTIONS → Appendix 1: metformin · sodium glucose co-transporter 2 inhibitors

● NATIONAL FUNDING/ACCESS DECISIONS
For full details see funding body website

Scottish Medicines Consortium (SMC) decisions
▶ Empagliflozin with metformin (*Synjardy®*) in adults with type 2 diabetes mellitus as an adjunct to diet and exercise to improve glycaemic control: in patients inadequately controlled on their maximally tolerated dose of metformin alone; in patients inadequately controlled with metformin in combination with other glucose-lowering medicinal products, including insulin; in patients already being treated with the combination of empagliflozin and metformin as separate tablets (October 2015) SMC No. 1092/15 Recommended with restrictions

● MEDICINAL FORMS　There can be variation in the licensing of different medicines containing the same drug.

Oral tablet

CAUTIONARY AND ADVISORY LABELS　21

▶ Synjardy (Boehringer Ingelheim Ltd)
Empagliflozin 12.5 mg, Metformin hydrochloride 850 mg　Synjardy 12.5mg/850mg tablets | 56 tablet [PoM] £36.59 DT = £36.59
Empagliflozin 5 mg, Metformin hydrochloride 850 mg　Synjardy 5mg/850mg tablets | 56 tablet [PoM] £36.59 DT = £36.59
Empagliflozin 12.5 mg, Metformin hydrochloride 1 gram　Synjardy 12.5mg/1000mg tablets | 56 tablet [PoM] £36.59 DT = £36.59
Empagliflozin 5 mg, Metformin hydrochloride 1 gram　Synjardy 5mg/1000mg tablets | 56 tablet [PoM] £36.59 DT = £36.59

Ertugliflozin　01-Feb-2024

● DRUG ACTION　Reversibly inhibits sodium-glucose co-transporter 2 (SGLT2) in the renal proximal convoluted tubule to reduce glucose reabsorption and increase urinary glucose excretion.

● INDICATIONS AND DOSE

Type 2 diabetes mellitus as monotherapy (if metformin inappropriate) | Type 2 diabetes mellitus in combination with insulin or other antidiabetic drugs (if existing treatment fails to achieve adequate glycaemic control)

▶ BY MOUTH
▶ Adult:　5 mg once daily; increased to 15 mg once daily if necessary and if tolerated, dose to be taken in the morning

continued →

DOSE ADJUSTMENTS DUE TO INTERACTIONS
▸ Manufacturer advises dose of concomitant insulin or drugs that stimulate insulin secretion may need to be reduced.

IMPORTANT SAFETY INFORMATION

MHRA/CHM ADVICE (UPDATED APRIL 2016): RISK OF DIABETIC KETOACIDOSIS WITH SODIUM-GLUCOSE CO-TRANSPORTER 2 (SGLT2) INHIBITORS

A review by the European Medicines Agency has concluded that serious, life-threatening, and fatal cases of diabetic ketoacidosis (DKA) have been reported rarely in patients taking an SGLT2 inhibitor. In several cases, the presentation of DKA was atypical with patients having only moderately elevated blood glucose levels, and some of them occurred during off-label use.

To minimise the risk of such effects when treating patients with a SGLT2 inhibitor, the European Medicines Agency has issued the following advice:

• inform patients of the signs and symptoms of DKA, (including rapid weight loss, nausea or vomiting, abdominal pain, fast and deep breathing, sleepiness, a sweet smell to the breath, a sweet or metallic taste in the mouth, or a different odour to urine or sweat), and advise them to seek immediate medical advice if they develop any of these

• test for raised ketones in patients with signs and symptoms of DKA, even if plasma glucose levels are near-normal

• use ertugliflozin with caution in patients with risk factors for DKA, (including a low beta cell reserve, conditions leading to restricted food intake or severe dehydration, sudden reduction in insulin, increased insulin requirements due to acute illness, surgery or alcohol abuse), and discuss these risk factors with patients

• discontinue treatment if DKA is suspected or diagnosed

• do not restart treatment with any SGLT2 inhibitor in patients who experienced DKA during use, unless another cause for DKA was identified and resolved

• interrupt SGLT2 inhibitor treatment in patients who are hospitalised for major surgery or acute serious illnesses; treatment may be restarted once the patient's condition has stabilised

MHRA/CHM ADVICE: SGLT2 INHIBITORS: MONITOR KETONES IN BLOOD DURING TREATMENT INTERRUPTION FOR SURGICAL PROCEDURES OR ACUTE SERIOUS MEDICAL ILLNESS (MARCH 2020)

New recommendations have been issued following a European review of peri-operative diabetic ketoacidosis in patients taking SGLT2 inhibitors. Healthcare professionals are advised to monitor ketone levels during SGLT2 inhibitor treatment interruption in patients who have been hospitalised for major surgery or acute serious illness—measurement of blood ketone levels is preferred to urine. Treatment may be restarted once ketone levels are normal and the patient's condition has stabilised.

MHRA/CHM ADVICE: SGLT2 INHIBITORS: REPORTS OF FOURNIER'S GANGRENE (NECROTISING FASCIITIS OF THE GENITALIA OR PERINEUM) (FEBRUARY 2019)

Fournier's gangrene, a rare but serious and potentially life-threatening infection, has been associated with the use of sodium-glucose co-transporter 2 (SGLT2) inhibitors. If Fournier's gangrene is suspected, stop the SGLT2 inhibitor and urgently start treatment (including antibiotics and surgical debridement).

Patients should be advised to seek urgent medical attention if they experience severe pain, tenderness, erythema, or swelling in the genital or perineal area, accompanied by fever or malaise—urogenital infection or perineal abscess may precede necrotising fasciitis.

● **CONTRA-INDICATIONS** Diabetic ketoacidosis · type 1 diabetes mellitus (increased risk of diabetic ketoacidosis)

● **CAUTIONS** Dehydration · elderly (risk of volume depletion) · history of hypotension

CAUTIONS, FURTHER INFORMATION
▸ Volume depletion Manufacturer advises correct hypovolaemia before starting treatment—consider interrupting treatment if volume depletion occurs.

● **INTERACTIONS** → Appendix 1: sodium glucose co-transporter 2 inhibitors

● **SIDE-EFFECTS**
▸ **Common or very common** Hypoglycaemia · hypovolaemia · increased risk of infection · polydipsia · thirst · urinary disorders · vulvovaginal pruritus
▸ **Rare or very rare** Diabetic ketoacidosis (discontinue immediately)
▸ **Frequency not known** Fournier's gangrene (discontinue and initiate treatment promptly) · lower limb amputations · phimosis

SIDE-EFFECTS, FURTHER INFORMATION Consider interrupting treatment if volume depletion occurs.

● **PREGNANCY** Manufacturer advises avoid—toxicity in *animal* studies.

● **BREAST FEEDING** Manufacturer advises avoid—present in milk in *animal* studies.

● **HEPATIC IMPAIRMENT** Manufacturer advises avoid in severe impairment (no information available).

● **RENAL IMPAIRMENT** EvGr Avoid initiation if eGFR less than 60 mL/minute/1.73 m^2. Frequent monitoring of renal function required if eGFR less than 60 mL/minute/1.73 m^2. Avoid if eGFR is persistently less than 45 mL/minute/1.73 m^2. ⓜ See p. 21.

● **MONITORING REQUIREMENTS**
▸ Manufacturer advises to determine renal function before treatment and periodically thereafter.
▸ Manufacturer advises monitor volume status and electrolytes during treatment in patients at risk of volume depletion.

● **PATIENT AND CARER ADVICE** Manufacturer advises that patients should be informed of the signs and symptoms of diabetic ketoacidosis, see MHRA advice.

● **NATIONAL FUNDING/ACCESS DECISIONS** For full details see funding body website

NICE decisions
▸ **Ertugliflozin as monotherapy or with metformin for treating type 2 diabetes (March 2019)** NICE TA572 Recommended with restrictions
▸ **Ertugliflozin with metformin and a dipeptidyl peptidase-4 inhibitor for treating type 2 diabetes (June 2019)** NICE TA583 Recommended with restrictions

Scottish Medicines Consortium (SMC) decisions
▸ **Ertugliflozin (*Steglatro*®) in adults with type 2 diabetes mellitus as an adjunct to diet and exercise to improve glycaemic control: as monotherapy in patients for whom the use of metformin is considered inappropriate due to intolerance or contra-indications; in addition to other medicinal products for the treatment of diabetes (January 2019)** SMC No. SMC2102 Recommended with restrictions

● **MEDICINAL FORMS** There can be variation in the licensing of different medicines containing the same drug.

Oral tablet
▸ **Steglatro** (Merck Sharp & Dohme (UK) Ltd) ▼
 Ertugliflozin (as Ertugliflozin L-pyroglutamic acid) 5 mg Steglatro 5mg tablets | 28 tablet PoM £29.40 DT = £29.40
 Ertugliflozin (as Ertugliflozin L-pyroglutamic acid) 15 mg Steglatro 15mg tablets | 28 tablet PoM £29.40 DT = £29.40

BLOOD GLUCOSE LOWERING DRUGS >
SULFONYLUREAS

Sulfonylureas 

- **DRUG ACTION** The sulfonylureas act mainly by augmenting insulin secretion and consequently are effective only when some residual pancreatic beta-cell activity is present; during long-term administration they also have an extrapancreatic action.

- **CONTRA-INDICATIONS** Presence of ketoacidosis

- **CAUTIONS** Can encourage weight gain · elderly · G6PD deficiency

CAUTIONS, FURTHER INFORMATION
▸ Elderly Screening Tool of Older Persons' potentially inappropriate Prescriptions (STOPP) criteria to aid medication reviews (see Prescribing in the elderly p. 31 for information): potentially inappropriate if prescribed a **long-acting** sulfonylurea (e.g. glibenclamide, chlorpropamide, glimepiride) in type 2 diabetes mellitus (risk of prolonged hypoglycaemia).

- **SIDE-EFFECTS**
▸ **Common or very common** Abdominal pain · diarrhoea · hypoglycaemia · nausea
▸ **Uncommon** Hepatic disorders · vomiting
▸ **Rare or very rare** Agranulocytosis · erythropenia · granulocytopenia · haemolytic anaemia · leucopenia · pancytopenia · thrombocytopenia
▸ **Frequency not known** Allergic dermatitis (usually in the first 6–8 weeks of therapy) · constipation · photosensitivity reaction · skin reactions · visual impairment

- **HEPATIC IMPAIRMENT** In general, manufacturers advise avoid in severe impairment (increased risk of hypoglycaemia).

- **RENAL IMPAIRMENT** Sulfonylureas should be used with care in those with mild to moderate renal impairment, because of the hazard of hypoglycaemia. Care is required to use the lowest dose that adequately controls blood glucose. Avoid where possible in severe renal impairment.

- **PATIENT AND CARER ADVICE** The risk of hypoglycaemia associated with sulfonylureas should be discussed with the patient, especially when concomitant glucose-lowering drugs are prescribed.
Driving and skilled tasks Drivers need to be particularly careful to avoid hypoglycaemia and should be warned of the problems.

▶ **above**

Gliclazide
17-Mar-2025

- **INDICATIONS AND DOSE**
Type 2 diabetes mellitus
▸ BY MOUTH USING IMMEDIATE-RELEASE MEDICINES
▸ Adult: Initially 40–80 mg once daily, dose to be taken with breakfast, increased if necessary up to 160 mg 1–2 times a day, dose to be adjusted according to response
▸ BY MOUTH USING MODIFIED-RELEASE MEDICINES
▸ Adult: Initially 30 mg once daily, dose to be taken with breakfast, increased if necessary up to 120 mg once daily, dose to be taken with breakfast, dose to be adjusted according to response every 4 weeks (after 2 weeks if no decrease in blood glucose)

DOSE EQUIVALENCE AND CONVERSION
▸ Gliclazide modified release 30 mg may be considered to be approximately equivalent in therapeutic effect to standard formulation gliclazide 80 mg.

- **CONTRA-INDICATIONS** Avoid where possible in Acute porphyrias p. 1202

- **INTERACTIONS** → Appendix 1: sulfonylureas
- **SIDE-EFFECTS** Anaemia · angioedema · dyspepsia · gastrointestinal disorder · hypersensitivity vasculitis · hyponatraemia · severe cutaneous adverse reactions (SCARs)

- **PREGNANCY** The use of sulfonylureas in pregnancy should generally be avoided because of the risk of neonatal hypoglycaemia.

- **BREAST FEEDING** Avoid—theoretical possibility of hypoglycaemia in the infant.

- **RENAL IMPAIRMENT** If necessary, gliclazide which is principally metabolised in the liver, can be used in renal impairment but careful monitoring of blood-glucose concentration is essential.

- **MEDICINAL FORMS** There can be variation in the licensing of different medicines containing the same drug. Forms available from special-order manufacturers include: oral suspension
Oral tablet
CAUTIONARY AND ADVISORY LABELS 21
▸ **Gliclazide (Non-proprietary)**
Gliclazide 40 mg Gliclazide 40mg tablets | 28 tablet PoM £3.36 DT = £0.89
Gliclazide 80 mg Gliclazide 80mg tablets | 28 tablet PoM £3.50 DT = £0.78 | 60 tablet PoM £0.81-£1.85
Gliclazide 160 mg Gliclazide 160mg tablets | 28 tablet PoM £3.27 DT = £3.27
▸ **Glydex** (Medreich Plc)
Gliclazide 160 mg Glydex 160mg tablets | 28 tablet PoM £3.27 DT = £3.27
▸ **Zicron** (Bristol Laboratories Ltd)
Gliclazide 40 mg Zicron 40mg tablets | 28 tablet PoM £3.36 DT = £0.89
Modified-release tablet
CAUTIONARY AND ADVISORY LABELS 21, 25
▸ **Gliclazide (Non-proprietary)**
Gliclazide 30 mg Gliclazide 30mg modified-release tablets | 28 tablet PoM £1.66-£5.21 DT = £1.64 | 56 tablet PoM £3.33-£5.90
Gliclazide 60 mg Gliclazide 60mg modified-release tablets | 28 tablet PoM £15.60 DT = £15.60 | 56 tablet PoM £31.20
▸ **Diamicron MR** (Servier Laboratories Ltd)
Gliclazide 30 mg Diamicron 30mg MR tablets | 28 tablet PoM £2.81 DT = £1.64 | 56 tablet PoM £5.62
▸ **Edicil MR** (Teva UK Ltd)
Gliclazide 30 mg Edicil MR 30mg tablets | 28 tablet PoM £1.99 DT = £1.64 | 56 tablet PoM £5.24
▸ **Lamzarin** (Key Pharmaceuticals Ltd)
Gliclazide 30 mg Lamzarin 30mg modified-release tablets | 28 tablet PoM £2.81 DT = £1.64 | 56 tablet PoM £5.62
Gliclazide 60 mg Lamzarin 60mg modified-release tablets | 28 tablet PoM £4.77 DT = £15.60
▸ **Xywin** (Ipca Laboratories UK Ltd)
Gliclazide 30 mg Xywin 30mg modified-release tablets | 28 tablet PoM £4.34 DT = £1.64 | 56 tablet PoM £4.92
▸ **Ziclaseg** (Lupin Healthcare (UK) Ltd)
Gliclazide 30 mg Ziclaseg 30mg modified-release tablets | 28 tablet PoM £2.38 DT = £1.64 | 56 tablet PoM £4.77
▸ **Zicron PR** (Bristol Laboratories Ltd)
Gliclazide 30 mg Zicron PR 30mg tablets | 28 tablet PoM £2.81 DT = £1.64 | 56 tablet PoM £3.90

▶ **above**

Glimepiride
27-Feb-2020

- **INDICATIONS AND DOSE**
Type 2 diabetes mellitus
▸ BY MOUTH
▸ Adult: Initially 1 mg daily, adjusted according to response, then increased in steps of 1 mg every 1–2 weeks, increased to 4 mg daily, dose to be taken shortly before or with first main meal, the daily dose may be increased further, in exceptional circumstances; maximum 6 mg per day

● **CAUTIONS**
▸ Porphyria Sulfonylureas should be avoided where possible in Acute porphyrias p. 1202 but glimepiride is thought to be safe.

● **INTERACTIONS** → Appendix 1: sulfonylureas

● **SIDE-EFFECTS**
▸ **Rare or very rare** Gastrointestinal discomfort · hypersensitivity vasculitis
▸ **Frequency not known** Drug cross-reactivity

● **PREGNANCY** The use of sulfonylureas in pregnancy should generally be avoided because of the risk of neonatal hypoglycaemia.

● **BREAST FEEDING** Avoid—theoretical possibility of hypoglycaemia in the infant.

● **MONITORING REQUIREMENTS** Manufacturer recommends regular hepatic and haematological monitoring but limited evidence of clinical value.

● **MEDICINAL FORMS** There can be variation in the licensing of different medicines containing the same drug. Forms available from special-order manufacturers include: oral suspension, oral solution
Oral tablet
▸ Glimepiride (Non-proprietary)
  Glimepiride 1 mg Glimepiride 1mg tablets | 30 tablet PoM £4.33 DT = £1.20
  Glimepiride 2 mg Glimepiride 2mg tablets | 30 tablet PoM £7.13 DT = £1.24
  Glimepiride 3 mg Glimepiride 3mg tablets | 30 tablet PoM £10.75 DT = £1.27
  Glimepiride 4 mg Glimepiride 4mg tablets | 30 tablet PoM £14.24 DT = £1.58

⟨ 831

Glipizide

27-Feb-2020

● **INDICATIONS AND DOSE**

Type 2 diabetes mellitus
▸ BY MOUTH
▸ Adult: Initially 2.5–5 mg daily, adjusted according to response, dose to be taken shortly before breakfast or lunch, doses up to 15 mg may be given as a single dose, higher doses to be given in divided doses; maximum 20 mg per day

● **CAUTIONS**
▸ Porphyria Sulfonylureas should be avoided where possible in Acute porphyrias p. 1202 but glipizide is thought to be safe.

● **INTERACTIONS** → Appendix 1: sulfonylureas

● **SIDE-EFFECTS**
▸ **Common or very common** Abdominal pain upper
▸ **Uncommon** Dizziness · drowsiness · tremor · vision disorders
▸ **Frequency not known** Confusion · headache · hyponatraemia · malaise

● **PREGNANCY** The use of sulfonylureas in pregnancy should generally be avoided because of the risk of neonatal hypoglycaemia.

● **BREAST FEEDING** Avoid—theoretical possibility of hypoglycaemia in the infant.

● **HEPATIC IMPAIRMENT** Manufacturer advises caution in mild to moderate impairment.
Dose adjustments Manufacturer advises consider initial dose of 2.5 mg daily and conservative maintenance dosing in mild to moderate impairment.

● **MEDICINAL FORMS** There can be variation in the licensing of different medicines containing the same drug.
Oral tablet
▸ Minodiab (Pfizer Ltd)
  Glipizide 5 mg Minodiab 5mg tablets | 28 tablet PoM £1.26 DT = £1.26

⟨ 831

Tolbutamide

● **INDICATIONS AND DOSE**

Type 2 diabetes mellitus
▸ BY MOUTH
▸ Adult: 0.5–1.5 g daily in divided doses, dose to be taken with or immediately after meals, alternatively 0.5–1.5 g once daily, dose to be taken with or immediately after breakfast; maximum 2 g per day

● **CONTRA-INDICATIONS** Avoid where possible in Acute porphyrias p. 1202

● **INTERACTIONS** → Appendix 1: sulfonylureas

● **SIDE-EFFECTS**
▸ **Rare or very rare** Aplastic anaemia · blood disorder
▸ **Frequency not known** Alcohol intolerance · appetite abnormal · erythema multiforme (usually in the first 6–8 weeks of therapy) · exfoliative dermatitis (usually in the first 6–8 weeks of therapy) · fever (usually in the first 6–8 weeks of therapy) · headache · hypersensitivity (usually in the first 6–8 weeks of therapy) · paraesthesia · tinnitus · weight increased

● **PREGNANCY** The use of sulfonylureas in pregnancy should generally be avoided because of the risk of neonatal hypoglycaemia.

● **BREAST FEEDING** The use of sulfonylureas in breast-feeding should be avoided because there is a theoretical possibility of hypoglycaemia in the infant.

● **RENAL IMPAIRMENT** If necessary, the short-acting drug tolbutamide can be used in renal impairment but careful monitoring of blood-glucose concentration is essential.

● **MEDICINAL FORMS** There can be variation in the licensing of different medicines containing the same drug. Forms available from special-order manufacturers include: oral suspension
Oral tablet
▸ Tolbutamide (Non-proprietary)
  Tolbutamide 500 mg Tolbutamide 500mg tablets | 28 tablet PoM £120.00 DT = £84.00

BLOOD GLUCOSE LOWERING DRUGS ⟩
THIAZOLIDINEDIONES

Pioglitazone

15-Apr-2024

● **DRUG ACTION** The thiazolidinedione, pioglitazone, reduces peripheral insulin resistance, leading to a reduction of blood-glucose concentration.

● **INDICATIONS AND DOSE**

Type 2 diabetes mellitus as monotherapy (if metformin inappropriate), or in combination with other antidiabetic drugs (including insulin) if existing treatment fails to achieve adequate glycaemic control
▸ BY MOUTH
▸ Adult: Initially 15–30 mg once daily, adjusted according to response to 45 mg once daily, review treatment after 3–6 months and regularly thereafter. In elderly patients, initiate with lowest possible dose and increase gradually

DOSE ADJUSTMENTS DUE TO INTERACTIONS
▶ Dose of concomitant sulfonylurea or insulin may need to be reduced.

IMPORTANT SAFETY INFORMATION

MHRA/CHM ADVICE: PIOGLITAZONE CARDIOVASCULAR SAFETY (DECEMBER 2007 AND JANUARY 2011)

Incidence of heart failure is increased when pioglitazone is combined with insulin especially in patients with predisposing factors e.g. previous myocardial infarction. Patients who take pioglitazone should be closely monitored for signs of heart failure; treatment should be discontinued if any deterioration in cardiac status occurs.

Pioglitazone should not be used in patients with heart failure or a history of heart failure.

PIOGLITAZONE: RISK OF BLADDER CANCER (JULY 2011)

The European Medicines Agency has advised that there is a small increased risk of bladder cancer associated with pioglitazone use. However, in patients who respond adequately to treatment, the benefits of pioglitazone continue to outweigh the risks.

Pioglitazone should not be used in patients with active bladder cancer or a past history of bladder cancer, or in those who have uninvestigated macroscopic haematuria. Pioglitazone should be used with caution in elderly patients as the risk of bladder cancer increases with age.

Before initiating treatment with pioglitazone, patients should be assessed for risk factors of bladder cancer (including age, smoking status, exposure to certain occupational or chemotherapy agents, or previous radiation therapy to the pelvic region) and any macroscopic haematuria should be investigated. The safety and efficacy of pioglitazone should be reviewed after 3–6 months and pioglitazone should be stopped in patients who do not respond adequately to treatment.

Patients already receiving treatment with pioglitazone should be assessed for risk factors of bladder cancer and treatment should be reviewed after 3–6 months, as above.

Patients should be advised to report promptly any haematuria, dysuria, or urinary urgency during treatment.

● **CONTRA-INDICATIONS** Diabetic ketoacidosis · history of heart failure · previous or active bladder cancer · uninvestigated macroscopic haematuria

● **CAUTIONS** Concomitant use with insulin (risk of heart failure) · elderly (increased risk of heart failure, fractures, and bladder cancer) · increased risk of bone fractures, particularly in women · risk factors for bladder cancer · risk factors for heart failure

CAUTIONS, FURTHER INFORMATION

▶ Elderly For thiazolidinediones, Screening Tool of Older Persons' potentially inappropriate Prescriptions (STOPP) criteria to aid medication reviews (see Prescribing in the elderly p. 31 for information): potentially inappropriate in patients with heart failure (contra-indicated; risk of exacerbation).

● **INTERACTIONS** → Appendix 1: pioglitazone

● **SIDE-EFFECTS**
▶ **Common or very common** Bone fracture · increased risk of infection · numbness · visual impairment · weight increased
▶ **Uncommon** Bladder cancer · insomnia
▶ **Frequency not known** Macular oedema

  SIDE-EFFECTS, FURTHER INFORMATION Rare reports of liver dysfunction; discontinue if jaundice occurs.

● **PREGNANCY** Avoid—toxicity in *animal* studies.

● **BREAST FEEDING** Avoid—present in milk in *animal* studies.

● **HEPATIC IMPAIRMENT** Manufacturer advises avoid.

● **MONITORING REQUIREMENTS** Monitor liver function before treatment and periodically thereafter.

● **PATIENT AND CARER ADVICE**
Liver toxicity Patients should be advised to seek immediate medical attention if symptoms such as nausea, vomiting, abdominal pain, fatigue and dark urine develop.

● **NATIONAL FUNDING/ACCESS DECISIONS**
For full details see funding body website

Scottish Medicines Consortium (SMC) decisions
▶ Pioglitazone (*Actos*®) in combination with metformin and a sulfonylurea for type 2 diabetes mellitus (March 2007)
SMC No. 354/07 Recommended with restrictions

● **MEDICINAL FORMS** There can be variation in the licensing of different medicines containing the same drug. Forms available from special-order manufacturers include: oral suspension

Oral tablet
▶ Pioglitazone (Non-proprietary)
   Pioglitazone (as Pioglitazone hydrochloride) 15 mg Pioglitazone 15mg tablets | 28 tablet [PoM] £25.83 DT = £0.99
   Pioglitazone (as Pioglitazone hydrochloride) 30 mg Pioglitazone 30mg tablets | 28 tablet [PoM] £35.89 DT = £1.31
   Pioglitazone (as Pioglitazone hydrochloride) 45 mg Pioglitazone 45mg tablets | 28 tablet [PoM] £39.55 DT = £2.04

Pioglitazone with metformin   03-Feb-2020

The properties listed below are those particular to the combination only. For the properties of the components please consider, pioglitazone p. 832, metformin hydrochloride p. 807.

● **INDICATIONS AND DOSE**

Type 2 diabetes not controlled by metformin alone
▶ BY MOUTH
▶ Adult: 1 tablet twice daily, titration with the individual components (pioglitazone and metformin) desirable before initiation

● **INTERACTIONS** → Appendix 1: metformin · pioglitazone

● **MEDICINAL FORMS** There can be variation in the licensing of different medicines containing the same drug.
Oral tablet
CAUTIONARY AND ADVISORY LABELS 21
▶ Pioglitazone with metformin (Non-proprietary)
   Pioglitazone (as Pioglitazone hydrochloride) 15 mg, Metformin hydrochloride 850 mg Pioglitazone 15mg / Metformin 850mg tablets | 56 tablet [PoM] £42.61 DT = £42.61
▶ Competact (Neon Healthcare Ltd)
   Pioglitazone (as Pioglitazone hydrochloride) 15 mg, Metformin hydrochloride 850 mg Competact 15mg/850mg tablets | 56 tablet [PoM] £35.89 DT = £42.61

INSULINS

Insulins 

IMPORTANT SAFETY INFORMATION

NHS IMPROVEMENT PATIENT SAFETY ALERT: RISK OF SEVERE HARM AND DEATH DUE TO WITHDRAWING INSULIN FROM PEN DEVICES (NOVEMBER 2016)

Insulin should not be extracted from insulin pen devices.

The strength of insulin in pen devices can vary by multiples of 100 units/mL. Insulin syringes have graduations only suitable for calculating doses of standard 100 units/mL. If insulin extracted from a pen or cartridge is of a higher strength, and that is not considered in determining the volume required, it can lead to a significant and potentially fatal overdose.

NHS NEVER EVENT: OVERDOSE OF INSULIN DUE TO ABBREVIATIONS OR INCORRECT DEVICE (JANUARY 2018)

The words 'unit' or 'international units' should **not** be abbreviated.

Specific insulin administration devices should always be used to measure insulin i.e. insulin syringes and pens.

Insulin should **not** be withdrawn from an insulin pen or pen refill and then administered using a syringe and needle.

HEALTH SERVICES SAFETY INVESTIGATIONS BODY (HSSIB) PATIENT SAFETY INVESTIGATIONS: ADMINISTERING HIGH-STRENGTH INSULIN FROM A PEN DEVICE IN HOSPITAL (JULY 2022)

A review of an accidental overdose of high-strength insulin, leading to hypoglycaemia, identified that high-strength insulin was extracted from an insulin pen device using an insulin syringe. To reduce the risk of similar incidents occurring, the HSSIB has issued advice: www.hssib.org.uk/patient-safety-investigations/administering-high-strength-insulin-from-a-pen-device-in-hospital/.

MHRA/CHM ADVICE: INSULINS (ALL TYPES): RISK OF CUTANEOUS AMYLOIDOSIS AT INJECTION SITE (SEPTEMBER 2020)

A European review concluded that injection of insulin (all types) can lead to deposits of amyloid protein under the skin (cutaneous amyloidosis) at the injection site. Insulin-derived cutaneous amyloidosis interferes with insulin absorption, and administration of insulin at an affected site may affect glycaemic control. The MHRA advises healthcare professionals should consider cutaneous amyloidosis as a differential diagnosis to lipodystrophy when patients present with subcutaneous lumps at an insulin injection site. Patients should be reminded to rotate injection sites within the same body region to reduce or prevent the risk of cutaneous amyloidosis and other skin reactions. Patients should also be advised that injecting into an affected 'lumpy' area may reduce the effectiveness of insulin. Those currently injecting into a 'lumpy' area should contact their doctor before changing injection site due to the risk of hypoglycaemia; blood glucose should be closely monitored after changing injection site, and dose adjustment of insulin or other antidiabetic medication may be required.

● **SIDE-EFFECTS**
▸ **Common or very common** Oedema
▸ **Uncommon** Lipodystrophy
▸ **Frequency not known** Cutaneous amyloidosis

Overdose Overdose causes hypoglycaemia.

● **PREGNANCY**
Dose adjustments During pregnancy, insulin requirements may alter and doses should be assessed frequently by an experienced diabetes physician.

The dose of insulin generally needs to be increased in the second and third trimesters of pregnancy.

● **BREAST FEEDING**
Dose adjustments During breast-feeding, insulin requirements may alter and doses should be assessed frequently by an experienced diabetes physician.

● **HEPATIC IMPAIRMENT** Insulin requirements may be decreased.

● **RENAL IMPAIRMENT** The compensatory response to hypoglycaemia is impaired in renal impairment.
Dose adjustments [EvGr] Insulin requirements may decrease in patients with renal impairment and therefore dose reduction may be necessary. ⟨M⟩

● **MONITORING REQUIREMENTS**
▸ Many patients now monitor their own blood-glucose concentrations; all carers and children need to be trained to do this.

▸ Since blood-glucose concentration varies substantially throughout the day, 'normoglycaemia' cannot always be achieved throughout a 24-hour period without causing damaging hypoglycaemia.
▸ It is therefore best to recommend that patients should maintain a blood-glucose concentration of between 4 and 9 mmol/litre for most of the time (4–7 mmol/litre before meals and less than 9 mmol/litre after meals).
▸ While accepting that on occasions, for brief periods, the blood-glucose concentration will be above these values; strenuous efforts should be made to prevent it from falling below 4 mmol/litre. Patients using multiple injection regimens should understand how to adjust their insulin dose according to their carbohydrate intake. With fixed-dose insulin regimens, the carbohydrate intake needs to be regulated, and should be distributed throughout the day to match the insulin regimen. The intake of energy and of simple and complex carbohydrates should be adequate to allow normal growth and development but obesity must be avoided.

● **DIRECTIONS FOR ADMINISTRATION** Insulin is generally given by *subcutaneous injection*; the injection site should be rotated to prevent lipodystrophy and cutaneous amyloidosis. Injection devices ('pens'), which hold the insulin in a cartridge and meter the required dose, are convenient to use. Insulin syringes (for use with needles) are required for insulins not available in cartridge form, but are less popular with children and carers.

● **PRESCRIBING AND DISPENSING INFORMATION** Insulins must be prescribed and dispensed by brand name.

Show container to patient or carer and confirm the expected version is dispensed.
Units The word 'unit' should **not** be abbreviated.

● **PATIENT AND CARER ADVICE**
Hypoglycaemia Hypoglycaemia is a potential problem with insulin therapy. All patients must be carefully instructed on how to avoid it; this involves appropriate adjustment of insulin type, dose and frequency together with suitable timing and quantity of meals and snacks.
Insulin Passport Insulin Passports and patient information booklets should be offered to patients receiving insulin. The Insulin Passport provides a record of the patient's current insulin preparations and contains a section for emergency information. The patient information booklet provides advice on the safe use of insulin. They are available for purchase from:

3M Security Print and Systems Limited
Gorse Street, Chadderton
Oldham
OL9 9QH
Tel: 0845 610 1112

GP practices can obtain supplies through their Local Area Team stores.

NHS Trusts can order supplies from cmswebshop.corp.xerox.com/NHS/Login.aspx. Further information is available at www.england.nhs.uk/improvement-hub/wp-content/uploads/sites/44/2017/11/Safe-use-of-insulin-and-you-patient-info-booklet.pdf.

Driving and skilled tasks Drivers need to be particularly careful to avoid hypoglycaemia and should be warned of the problems.

INSULINS › RAPID-ACTING

Insulin
26-Feb-2025

(Neutral Insulin; Soluble Insulin)

- **DRUG ACTION** Soluble insulin is a natural or recombinant insulin with a short duration of action.

- **INDICATIONS AND DOSE**

Diabetes mellitus
▶ BY SUBCUTANEOUS INJECTION, OR BY INTRAMUSCULAR INJECTION, OR BY INTRAVENOUS INJECTION, OR BY INTRAVENOUS INFUSION
▶ Adult: According to requirements

Diabetic ketoacidosis | Diabetes during surgery
▶ BY INTRAVENOUS INFUSION
▶ Adult: (consult local protocol)

- **INTERACTIONS** → Appendix 1: insulin
- **SIDE-EFFECTS**
▶ **Uncommon** Skin reactions
▶ **Rare or very rare** Refraction disorder

- **DIRECTIONS FOR ADMINISTRATION** Short-acting injectable insulins can be given by continuous subcutaneous infusion using a portable infusion pump. This device delivers a continuous basal insulin infusion and patient-activated bolus doses at meal times. This technique can be useful for patients who suffer recurrent hypoglycaemia or marked morning rise in blood-glucose concentration despite optimised multiple-injection regimens. Patients on subcutaneous insulin infusion must be highly motivated, able to monitor their blood-glucose concentration, and have expert training, advice and supervision from an experienced healthcare team. Some insulin preparations are not recommended for use in subcutaneous insulin infusion pumps—may precipitate in catheter or needle—consult product literature.

  For *intravenous infusion* give continuously in Sodium chloride 0.9%. Adsorbed to some extent by plastic infusion set; ensure insulin is not injected into 'dead space' of injection port of the infusion bag.

- **PRESCRIBING AND DISPENSING INFORMATION** A sterile solution of insulin (i.e. bovine or porcine) or of human insulin; pH 6.6–8.0.

- **NATIONAL FUNDING/ACCESS DECISIONS**
For full details see funding body website
NICE decisions
▶ **Continuous subcutaneous insulin infusion for the treatment of diabetes mellitus (type 1) (July 2008)** NICE TA151
Recommended
▶ **Hybrid closed loop systems for managing blood glucose levels in type 1 diabetes (December 2023)** NICE TA943
Recommended with restrictions

- **MEDICINAL FORMS** There can be variation in the licensing of different medicines containing the same drug. Forms available from special-order manufacturers include: solution for injection, solution for infusion

Solution for injection
▶ **Insulin (Non-proprietary)**
Insulin human 500 unit per 1 ml Humulin R 500units/ml solution for injection 20ml vials | 1 vial [PoM] 💷
Humulin R KwikPen 500units/ml solution for injection 3ml pre-filled pens | 2 pre-filled disposable injection [PoM] 💷
▶ **Actrapid** (Novo Nordisk Ltd)
Insulin human (as Insulin soluble human) 100 unit per 1 ml Actrapid 100units/ml solution for injection 10ml vials | 1 vial [PoM] £7.48 DT = £15.68
▶ **Humulin S** (Eli Lilly and Company Ltd)
Insulin human (as Insulin soluble human) 100 unit per 1 ml Humulin S 100units/ml solution for injection 10ml vials | 1 vial [PoM] £15.68 DT = £15.68

Humulin S 100units/ml solution for injection 3ml cartridges | 5 cartridge [PoM] £19.08 DT = £19.08
▶ **Hypurin Porcine Neutral** (Wockhardt UK Ltd)
Insulin porcine (as Insulin soluble porcine) 100 unit per 1 ml Hypurin Porcine Neutral 100units/ml solution for injection 10ml vials | 1 vial [PoM] £39.39 DT = £39.39
Hypurin Porcine Neutral 100units/ml solution for injection 3ml cartridges | 5 cartridge [PoM] £59.08 DT = £59.08

Combinations available: *Biphasic insulin aspart,* p. 838 · *Biphasic insulin lispro,* p. 838 · *Biphasic isophane insulin,* p. 837 · *Insulin degludec,* p. 838 · *Insulin degludec with liraglutide,* p. 839 · *Insulin detemir,* p. 839 · *Insulin glargine,* p. 839 · *Insulin glargine with lixisenatide,* p. 840 · *Isophane insulin,* p. 837

Insulin aspart
26-Feb-2025

- **DRUG ACTION** Insulin aspart is a recombinant human insulin analogue with a rapid onset and short duration of action.

- **INDICATIONS AND DOSE**
FIASP ®
Diabetes mellitus
▶ BY SUBCUTANEOUS INJECTION
▶ Child 1–17 years: Administer immediately before meals or when necessary shortly after meals, according to requirements
▶ Adult: Administer immediately before meals or when necessary shortly after meals, according to requirements
▶ BY SUBCUTANEOUS INFUSION, OR BY INTRAVENOUS INFUSION
▶ Child 1–17 years: According to requirements
▶ Adult: According to requirements

NOVORAPID ®
Diabetes mellitus
▶ BY SUBCUTANEOUS INJECTION
▶ Child: Administer immediately before meals or when necessary shortly after meals, according to requirements
▶ Adult: Administer immediately before meals or when necessary shortly after meals, according to requirements
▶ BY SUBCUTANEOUS INFUSION, OR BY INTRAVENOUS INFUSION
▶ Child: According to requirements
▶ Adult: According to requirements

PHARMACOKINETICS
▶ *Fiasp ®* and *NovoRapid ®* are **not** interchangeable due to differences in bioavailability; *Fiasp ®* has a quicker onset of action and shorter duration.

- **UNLICENSED USE** Not licensed for use in children under 1 year.

- **INTERACTIONS** → Appendix 1: insulin
- **SIDE-EFFECTS**
▶ **Common or very common** Skin reactions
▶ **Uncommon** Refraction disorder

- **PREGNANCY** Not known to be harmful—may be used during pregnancy.

- **BREAST FEEDING** Not known to be harmful—may be used during lactation.

- **DIRECTIONS FOR ADMINISTRATION** Short-acting injectable insulins can be given by continuous subcutaneous infusion using a portable infusion pump. This device delivers a continuous basal insulin infusion and patient-activated bolus doses at meal times. This technique can be useful for patients who suffer recurrent hypoglycaemia or marked morning rise in blood-glucose concentration despite optimised multiple-injection regimens. Patients on subcutaneous insulin infusion must be highly motivated, able to monitor their blood-glucose concentration, and have expert training, advice and supervision from an experienced healthcare team.

Manufacturer advises for *intravenous infusion* of *Fiasp®*, give continuously in Glucose 5% or Sodium Chloride 0.9%; dilute to 0.5-1 unit/mL with infusion fluid.

Manufacturer advises for *intravenous infusion* of *NovoRapid®*, give continuously in Glucose 5% or Sodium Chloride 0.9%; dilute to 0.05-1 unit/mL with infusion fluid; adsorbed to some extent by plastics of infusion set.

- **PRESCRIBING AND DISPENSING INFORMATION** Insulin aspart is a biological medicine. Biological medicines must be prescribed and dispensed by brand name, see *Biological medicines* and *Biosimilar medicines*, under Guidance on prescribing p. 1. Dose adjustments and close metabolic monitoring is recommended if switching between insulin aspart preparations.

- **NATIONAL FUNDING/ACCESS DECISIONS**
For full details see funding body website
NICE decisions
▶ Continuous subcutaneous insulin infusion for the treatment of diabetes mellitus (type 1) (July 2008) NICE TA151 Recommended
Scottish Medicines Consortium (SMC) decisions
▶ Insulin aspart (*Fiasp®*) for the treatment of diabetes mellitus in adults (April 2017) SMC No. 1227/17 Recommended

- **MEDICINAL FORMS** There can be variation in the licensing of different medicines containing the same drug.
Solution for injection
▶ Fiasp (Novo Nordisk Ltd)
Insulin aspart 100 unit per 1 ml Fiasp 100units/ml solution for injection 10ml vials | 1 vial PoM £14.08 DT = £14.08
▶ Fiasp FlexTouch (Novo Nordisk Ltd)
Insulin aspart 100 unit per 1 ml Fiasp FlexTouch 100units/ml solution for injection 3ml pre-filled pens | 5 pre-filled disposable injection PoM £30.60 DT = £30.60
▶ Fiasp Penfill (Novo Nordisk Ltd)
Insulin aspart 100 unit per 1 ml Fiasp Penfill 100units/ml solution for injection 3ml cartridges | 5 cartridge PoM £28.31 DT = £28.31
▶ NovoRapid (Novo Nordisk Ltd)
Insulin aspart 100 unit per 1 ml NovoRapid 100units/ml solution for injection 10ml vials | 1 vial PoM £14.08 DT = £14.08
▶ NovoRapid FlexPen (Novo Nordisk Ltd)
Insulin aspart 100 unit per 1 ml NovoRapid FlexPen 100units/ml solution for injection 3ml pre-filled pens | 5 pre-filled disposable injection PoM £30.60 DT = £30.60
▶ NovoRapid FlexTouch (Novo Nordisk Ltd)
Insulin aspart 100 unit per 1 ml NovoRapid FlexTouch 100units/ml solution for injection 3ml pre-filled pens | 5 pre-filled disposable injection PoM £32.13 DT = £30.60
▶ NovoRapid Penfill (Novo Nordisk Ltd)
Insulin aspart 100 unit per 1 ml NovoRapid Penfill 100units/ml solution for injection 3ml cartridges | 5 cartridge PoM £28.31 DT = £28.31
▶ NovoRapid PumpCart (Novo Nordisk Ltd)
Insulin aspart 100 unit per 1 ml NovoRapid PumpCart 100units/ml solution for injection 1.6ml cartridges | 5 cartridge PoM £15.10 DT = £15.10

F 833

Insulin glulisine

26-Feb-2025

- **DRUG ACTION** Insulin glulisine is a recombinant human insulin analogue with a rapid onset and short duration of action.

- **INDICATIONS AND DOSE**
Diabetes mellitus
▶ BY SUBCUTANEOUS INJECTION
▶ Child: Administer immediately before meals or when necessary shortly after meals, according to requirements

▶ Adult: Administer immediately before meals or when necessary shortly after meals, according to requirements
▶ BY SUBCUTANEOUS INFUSION, OR BY INTRAVENOUS INFUSION
▶ Child: According to requirements
▶ Adult: According to requirements

- **UNLICENSED USE** Not licensed for children under 6 years.

- **INTERACTIONS** → Appendix 1: insulin

- **DIRECTIONS FOR ADMINISTRATION** Short-acting injectable insulins can be given by continuous subcutaneous infusion using a portable infusion pump. This device delivers a continuous basal insulin infusion and patient-activated bolus doses at meal times. This technique can be useful for patients who suffer recurrent hypoglycaemia or marked morning rise in blood-glucose concentration despite optimised multiple-injection regimens. Patients on subcutaneous insulin infusion must be highly motivated, able to monitor their blood-glucose concentration, and have expert training, advice and supervision from an experienced healthcare team.
▶ With intravenous use in adults For *intravenous infusion* (*Apidra®*), give continuously in Sodium chloride 0.9%; dilute to 1 unit/mL with infusion fluid; use a co-extruded polyolefin/polyamide plastic infusion bag with a dedicated infusion line.

- **NATIONAL FUNDING/ACCESS DECISIONS**
For full details see funding body website
NICE decisions
▶ Continuous subcutaneous insulin infusion for the treatment of diabetes mellitus (type 1) (July 2008) NICE TA151 Recommended
Scottish Medicines Consortium (SMC) decisions
▶ Insulin glulisine (*Apidra®*) for adolescents and children with diabetes mellitus (November 2008) SMC No. 512/08 Recommended with restrictions

- **MEDICINAL FORMS** There can be variation in the licensing of different medicines containing the same drug.
Solution for injection
▶ Apidra (Sanofi)
Insulin glulisine 100 unit per 1 ml Apidra 100units/ml solution for injection 10ml vials | 1 vial PoM £16.00 DT = £16.00
Apidra 100units/ml solution for injection 3ml cartridges | 5 cartridge PoM £28.30 DT = £28.30
▶ Apidra SoloStar (Sanofi)
Insulin glulisine 100 unit per 1 ml Apidra 100units/ml solution for injection 3ml pre-filled SoloStar pens | 5 pre-filled disposable injection PoM £28.30 DT = £28.30

F 833

Insulin lispro

26-Feb-2025

- **DRUG ACTION** Insulin lispro is a recombinant human insulin analogue with a rapid onset and short duration of action.

- **INDICATIONS AND DOSE**
Diabetes mellitus
▶ BY SUBCUTANEOUS INJECTION
▶ Child 2-17 years: Administer shortly before meals or when necessary shortly after meals, according to requirements
▶ Adult: Administer shortly before meals or when necessary shortly after meals, according to requirements
▶ BY SUBCUTANEOUS INFUSION, OR BY INTRAVENOUS INFUSION, OR BY INTRAVENOUS INJECTION
▶ Child 2-17 years: According to requirements
▶ Adult: According to requirements

- **INTERACTIONS** → Appendix 1: insulin

- **PREGNANCY** Not known to be harmful—may be used during pregnancy.
- **BREAST FEEDING** Not known to be harmful—may be used during lactation.
- **DIRECTIONS FOR ADMINISTRATION** Short-acting injectable insulins can be given by continuous subcutaneous infusion using a portable infusion pump. This device delivers a continuous basal insulin infusion and patient-activated bolus doses at meal times. This technique can be useful for patients who suffer recurrent hypoglycaemia or marked morning rise in blood-glucose concentration despite optimised multiple-injection regimens (see also NICE guidance, below). Patients on subcutaneous insulin infusion must be highly motivated, able to monitor their blood-glucose concentration, and have expert training, advice and supervision from an experienced healthcare team.
  - With intravenous use in adults For *intravenous infusion* give continuously in Glucose 5% or Sodium chloride 0.9%. Adsorbed to some extent by plastics of infusion set.
  - With intravenous use in children For *intravenous infusion*, dilute to a concentration of 0.1–1 unit/mL with Glucose 5% or Sodium Chloride 0.9% and mix thoroughly; insulin may be adsorbed by plastics, flush giving set with 5 mL of infusion fluid containing insulin.
- **PRESCRIBING AND DISPENSING INFORMATION** Insulin lispro is a biological medicine. Biological medicines must be prescribed and dispensed by brand name, see *Biological medicines* and *Biosimilar medicines*, under Guidance on prescribing p. 1.
- **NATIONAL FUNDING/ACCESS DECISIONS** For full details see funding body website
  NICE decisions
  - Continuous subcutaneous insulin infusion for the treatment of diabetes mellitus (type 1) (July 2008) NICE TA151 Recommended

- **MEDICINAL FORMS** There can be variation in the licensing of different medicines containing the same drug.
  Solution for injection
  - Admelog (Sanofi)
    Insulin lispro 100 unit per 1 ml Admelog 100units/ml solution for injection 10ml vials | 1 vial [PoM] £14.12 DT = £16.61
    Admelog 100units/ml solution for injection 3ml cartridges | 5 cartridge [PoM] £21.23 DT = £28.31
    Admelog 100units/ml solution for injection 3ml pre-filled pens | 5 pre-filled disposable injection [PoM] £22.10 DT = £29.46
  - Humalog (Insulin lispro) (Eli Lilly and Company Ltd)
    Insulin lispro 100 unit per 1 ml Humalog 100units/ml solution for injection 10ml vials | 1 vial [PoM] £16.61 DT = £16.61
    Humalog 100units/ml solution for injection 3ml cartridges | 5 cartridge [PoM] £28.31 DT = £28.31
  - Humalog Junior KwikPen (Eli Lilly and Company Ltd)
    Insulin lispro 100 unit per 1 ml Humalog Junior KwikPen 100units/ml solution for injection 3ml pre-filled pens | 5 pre-filled disposable injection [PoM] £29.46 DT = £29.46
  - Humalog KwikPen (Eli Lilly and Company Ltd)
    Insulin lispro 100 unit per 1 ml Humalog KwikPen 100units/ml solution for injection 3ml pre-filled pens | 5 pre-filled disposable injection [PoM] £29.46 DT = £29.46
    Insulin lispro 200 unit per 1 ml Humalog KwikPen 200units/ml solution for injection 3ml pre-filled pens | 5 pre-filled disposable injection [PoM] £58.92 DT = £58.92
  - Lyumjev (Eli Lilly and Company Ltd) ▼
    Insulin lispro 100 unit per 1 ml Lyumjev 100units/ml solution for injection 3ml cartridges | 5 cartridge [PoM] £28.31 DT = £28.31
    Lyumjev 100units/ml solution for injection 10ml vials | 1 vial [PoM] £16.61 DT = £16.61
  - Lyumjev Junior KwikPen (Eli Lilly and Company Ltd) ▼
    Insulin lispro 100 unit per 1 ml Lyumjev Junior KwikPen 100units/ml solution for injection 3ml pre-filled pens | 5 pre-filled disposable injection [PoM] £29.46 DT = £29.46

- Lyumjev KwikPen (Eli Lilly and Company Ltd) ▼
  Insulin lispro 100 unit per 1 ml Lyumjev KwikPen 100units/ml solution for injection 3ml pre-filled pens | 5 pre-filled disposable injection [PoM] £29.46 DT = £29.46
  Insulin lispro 200 unit per 1 ml Lyumjev KwikPen 200units/ml solution for injection 3ml pre-filled pens | 5 pre-filled disposable injection [PoM] £58.92 DT = £58.92

INSULINS > INTERMEDIATE-ACTING

⬛ 6
Endocrine system

F 833

Biphasic isophane insulin
26-Feb-2025

- **DRUG ACTION** Biphasic isophane insulin is a mixture of natural or recombinant insulins with a short onset and intermediate duration of action.

- **INDICATIONS AND DOSE**
  Diabetes mellitus
  - BY SUBCUTANEOUS INJECTION
  - Child: Dose according to requirements
  - Adult: Dose according to requirements

- **INTERACTIONS** → Appendix 1: insulin
- **SIDE-EFFECTS**
  - **Rare or very rare** Angioedema
  - **Frequency not known** Hypokalaemia · weight increased

- **PRESCRIBING AND DISPENSING INFORMATION** A sterile buffered suspension of either porcine or human insulin complexed with protamine sulfate (or another suitable protamine) in a solution of insulin of the same species.
  Check product container—the proportions of the two components should be checked carefully (the order in which the proportions are stated may not be the same in other countries).

- **MEDICINAL FORMS** There can be variation in the licensing of different medicines containing the same drug.
  Suspension for injection
  - Humulin M3 (Eli Lilly and Company Ltd)
    Insulin human (as Insulin soluble human) 30 unit per 1 ml, Insulin human (as Insulin isophane human) 70 unit per 1 ml Humulin M3 100units/ml suspension for injection 3ml cartridges | 5 cartridge [PoM] £19.08 DT = £19.08
    Humulin M3 100units/ml suspension for injection 10ml vials | 1 vial [PoM] £15.68 DT = £15.68
  - Humulin M3 KwikPen (Eli Lilly and Company Ltd)
    Insulin human (as Insulin soluble human) 30 unit per 1 ml, Insulin human (as Insulin isophane human) 70 unit per 1 ml Humulin M3 KwikPen 100units/ml suspension for injection 3ml pre-filled pens | 5 pre-filled disposable injection [PoM] £21.70 DT = £21.70
  - Hypurin Porcine 30/70 Mix (Wockhardt UK Ltd)
    Insulin porcine (as Insulin soluble porcine) 30 unit per 1 ml, Insulin porcine (as Insulin isophane porcine) 70 unit per 1 ml Hypurin Porcine 30/70 Mix 100units/ml suspension for injection 3ml cartridges | 5 cartridge [PoM] £59.08 DT = £59.08
    Hypurin Porcine 30/70 Mix 100units/ml suspension for injection 10ml vials | 1 vial [PoM] £39.39 DT = £39.39

F 833

Isophane insulin
26-Feb-2025

(Isophane Protamine Insulin; NPH Insulin)

- **DRUG ACTION** Isophane insulin is a natural or recombinant insulin with an intermediate duration of action.

- **INDICATIONS AND DOSE**
  Diabetes mellitus
  - BY SUBCUTANEOUS INJECTION
  - Child: According to requirements
  - Adult: According to requirements

- **INTERACTIONS** → Appendix 1: insulin
- **PREGNANCY** Recommended where longer-acting insulins are needed.

6

Endocrine system

- **PRESCRIBING AND DISPENSING INFORMATION** A sterile suspension of bovine or porcine insulin or of human insulin in the form of a complex obtained by the addition of protamine sulfate or another suitable protamine.

- **MEDICINAL FORMS** There can be variation in the licensing of different medicines containing the same drug.

Suspension for injection

▸ **Humulin I** (Eli Lilly and Company Ltd)
Insulin human (as Insulin isophane human) 100 unit per 1 ml Humulin I 100units/ml suspension for injection 10ml vials | 1 vial [PoM] £15.68 DT = £15.68
Humulin I 100units/ml suspension for injection 3ml cartridges | 5 cartridge [PoM] £19.08 DT = £19.08

▸ **Humulin I KwikPen** (Eli Lilly and Company Ltd)
Insulin human (as Insulin isophane human) 100 unit per 1 ml Humulin I KwikPen 100units/ml suspension for injection 3ml pre-filled pens | 5 pre-filled disposable injection [PoM] £21.70 DT = £21.70

▸ **Hypurin Porcine Isophane** (Wockhardt UK Ltd)
Insulin porcine (as Insulin isophane porcine) 100 unit per 1 ml Hypurin Porcine Isophane 100units/ml suspension for injection 10ml vials | 1 vial [PoM] £39.39 DT = £39.39
Hypurin Porcine Isophane 100units/ml suspension for injection 3ml cartridges | 5 cartridge [PoM] £59.08 DT = £59.08

▸ **Insulatard** (Novo Nordisk Ltd)
Insulin human (as Insulin isophane human) 100 unit per 1 ml Insulatard 100units/ml suspension for injection 10ml vials | 1 vial [PoM] £7.48 DT = £15.68

▸ **Insulatard Penfill** (Novo Nordisk Ltd)
Insulin human (as Insulin isophane human) 100 unit per 1 ml Insulatard Penfill 100units/ml suspension for injection 3ml cartridges | 5 cartridge [PoM] £22.90 DT = £19.08

INSULINS > INTERMEDIATE-ACTING COMBINED WITH RAPID-ACTING

⚑ 833

Biphasic insulin aspart

26-Feb-2025

- **DRUG ACTION** Biphasic insulin aspart is a mixture of recombinant human insulin analogues with a rapid onset and intermediate duration of action.

- **INDICATIONS AND DOSE**

Diabetes mellitus
▸ BY SUBCUTANEOUS INJECTION
▸ Child: Administer up to 10 minutes before or soon after a meal, according to requirements
▸ Adult: Administer up to 10 minutes before or soon after a meal, according to requirements

- **INTERACTIONS** → Appendix 1: insulin

- **SIDE-EFFECTS**
▸ **Uncommon** Skin reactions

- **PRESCRIBING AND DISPENSING INFORMATION** Check product container—the proportions of the two components should be checked carefully (the order in which the proportions are stated may not be the same in other countries).

- **MEDICINAL FORMS** There can be variation in the licensing of different medicines containing the same drug.

Suspension for injection

▸ **NovoMix 30 FlexPen** (Novo Nordisk Ltd)
Insulin aspart 30 unit per 1 ml, Insulin aspart (as Insulin aspart protamine) 70 unit per 1 ml NovoMix 30 FlexPen 100units/ml suspension for injection 3ml pre-filled pens | 5 pre-filled disposable injection [PoM] £29.89 DT = £29.89

▸ **NovoMix 30 Penfill** (Novo Nordisk Ltd)
Insulin aspart 30 unit per 1 ml, Insulin aspart (as Insulin aspart protamine) 70 unit per 1 ml NovoMix 30 Penfill 100units/ml suspension for injection 3ml cartridges | 5 cartridge [PoM] £28.79 DT = £28.79

⚑ 833

Biphasic insulin lispro

26-Feb-2025

- **DRUG ACTION** Biphasic insulin lispro is a mixture of recombinant human insulin analogues with a rapid onset and intermediate duration of action.

- **INDICATIONS AND DOSE**

Diabetes mellitus
▸ BY SUBCUTANEOUS INJECTION
▸ Child: Administer up to 15 minutes before or soon after a meal, according to requirements
▸ Adult: Administer up to 15 minutes before or soon after a meal, according to requirements

- **CAUTIONS** Children under 12 years (use only if benefit likely compared to soluble insulin)

- **INTERACTIONS** → Appendix 1: insulin

- **PRESCRIBING AND DISPENSING INFORMATION** Check product container—the proportions of the two components should be checked carefully (the order in which the proportions are stated may not be the same in other countries).

- **MEDICINAL FORMS** There can be variation in the licensing of different medicines containing the same drug.

Suspension for injection

▸ **Humalog Mix25** (Eli Lilly and Company Ltd)
Insulin lispro 25 unit per 1 ml, Insulin lispro (as Insulin lispro protamine) 75 unit per 1 ml Humalog Mix25 100units/ml suspension for injection 10ml vials | 1 vial [PoM] £16.61 DT = £16.61
Humalog Mix25 100units/ml suspension for injection 3ml cartridges | 5 cartridge [PoM] £29.46 DT = £29.46

▸ **Humalog Mix25 KwikPen** (Eli Lilly and Company Ltd)
Insulin lispro 25 unit per 1 ml, Insulin lispro (as Insulin lispro protamine) 75 unit per 1 ml Humalog Mix25 KwikPen 100units/ml suspension for injection 3ml pre-filled pens | 5 pre-filled disposable injection [PoM] £30.98 DT = £30.98

▸ **Humalog Mix50** (Eli Lilly and Company Ltd)
Insulin lispro 50 unit per 1 ml, Insulin lispro (as Insulin lispro protamine) 50 unit per 1 ml Humalog Mix50 100units/ml suspension for injection 3ml cartridges | 5 cartridge [PoM] £29.46 DT = £29.46

▸ **Humalog Mix50 KwikPen** (Eli Lilly and Company Ltd)
Insulin lispro 50 unit per 1 ml, Insulin lispro (as Insulin lispro protamine) 50 unit per 1 ml Humalog Mix50 KwikPen 100units/ml suspension for injection 3ml pre-filled pens | 5 pre-filled disposable injection [PoM] £30.98 DT = £30.98

INSULINS > LONG-ACTING

⚑ 833

Insulin degludec

26-Feb-2025

- **DRUG ACTION** Insulin degludec is a recombinant human insulin analogue with a long duration of action.

- **INDICATIONS AND DOSE**

Diabetes mellitus
▸ BY SUBCUTANEOUS INJECTION
▸ Child 1-17 years: Dose to be given according to requirements
▸ Adult: Dose to be given according to requirements

IMPORTANT SAFETY INFORMATION

NATIONAL PATIENT SAFETY ALERT: POTENTIAL FOR INAPPROPRIATE DOSING OF INSULIN WHEN SWITCHING *TRESIBA*® (INSULIN DEGLUDEC) PRODUCTS (DECEMBER 2023)

In response to a shortage of *Tresiba*® FlexTouch® 100 units/mL pre-filled pens, some patients may have been switched to *Tresiba*® FlexTouch® 200 units/mL pre-filled pens. However, there have been reports of patients being incorrectly advised to reduce the number of units of insulin, resulting in one patient requiring hospitalisation for diabetic ketoacidosis.

Healthcare professionals are reminded that *Tresiba®* FlexTouch® pen delivery devices show the number of **units** that will be injected rather than the volume of solution, therefore no dose conversion is necessary when switching patients from one strength to another. Patients who have been switched to a different *Tresiba®* FlexTouch® pen must be made aware of this.

When prescribing *Tresiba®* 100 units/mL Penfill® **cartridges**, patients should also be given a compatible Novo Nordisk insulin delivery system and appropriate needles.

All patients initiated on a new device should be counselled on the change and given training on use, including signposting to training videos, and the potential need for closer monitoring of blood glucose concentration.

- **INTERACTIONS** → Appendix 1: insulin

- **SIDE-EFFECTS**
▸ **Rare or very rare** Urticaria

- **PREGNANCY** Evidence of the safety of long-acting insulin analogues in pregnancy is limited, therefore isophane insulin is recommended where longer-acting insulins are needed; insulin detemir may also be considered.

- **PRESCRIBING AND DISPENSING INFORMATION** Insulin degludec (*Tresiba®*) is available in strengths of 100 units/mL (allows 1-unit dose adjustment) and 200 units/mL (allows 2-unit dose adjustment)—ensure correct strength prescribed.

- **NATIONAL FUNDING/ACCESS DECISIONS** For full details see funding body website
All Wales Medicines Strategy Group (AWMSG) decisions
▸ **Insulin degludec (*Tresiba®*) for the treatment of diabetes mellitus in adults, adolescents and children from the age of 1 year (October 2022)** AWMSG No. 5196 Recommended

- **MEDICINAL FORMS** There can be variation in the licensing of different medicines containing the same drug.
Solution for injection
▸ Tresiba FlexTouch (Novo Nordisk Ltd)
Insulin degludec 100 unit per 1 ml Tresiba FlexTouch 100units/ml solution for injection 3ml pre-filled pens | 5 pre-filled disposable injection [PoM] £46.60 DT = £46.60
Insulin degludec 200 unit per 1 ml Tresiba FlexTouch 200units/ml solution for injection 3ml pre-filled pens | 3 pre-filled disposable injection [PoM] £55.92 DT = £55.92
▸ Tresiba Penfill (Novo Nordisk Ltd)
Insulin degludec 100 unit per 1 ml Tresiba Penfill 100units/ml solution for injection 3ml cartridges | 5 cartridge [PoM] £46.60 DT = £46.60

Insulin degludec with liraglutide

22-Oct-2020

The properties listed below are those particular to the combination only. For the properties of the components please consider, insulin degludec p. 838, liraglutide p. 816.

- **INDICATIONS AND DOSE**
As add-on to oral antidiabetics in type 2 diabetes mellitus not controlled by oral antidiabetics alone
▸ BY SUBCUTANEOUS INJECTION
▸ Adult: Initially 10 dose-steps once daily, adjusted according to response; maximum 50 dose-steps per day
When transferring from basal insulin in type 2 diabetes mellitus not controlled by oral antidiabetics in combination with basal insulin
▸ BY SUBCUTANEOUS INJECTION
▸ Adult: Initially 16 dose-steps once daily, adjusted according to response; maximum 50 dose-steps per day

- **INTERACTIONS** → Appendix 1: glucagon-like peptide-1 receptor agonists · insulin

- **PATIENT AND CARER ADVICE** Counselling advised on administration. Show container to patient and confirm that patient is expecting the version dispensed.

- **NATIONAL FUNDING/ACCESS DECISIONS** For full details see funding body website
Scottish Medicines Consortium (SMC) decisions
▸ **Insulin degludec/liraglutide (*Xultophy®*) for treatment of adults with type 2 diabetes mellitus to improve glycaemic control in combination with oral glucose-lowering medicinal products when these alone or combined with a GLP-1 receptor agonist or with basal insulin do not provide adequate glycaemic control (October 2015)** SMC No. 1088/15 Recommended with restrictions

- **MEDICINAL FORMS** There can be variation in the licensing of different medicines containing the same drug.
Solution for injection
▸ Xultophy (Novo Nordisk Ltd)
Liraglutide 3.6 mg per 1 ml, Insulin degludec 100 unit per 1 ml Xultophy 100units/ml / 3.6mg/ml solution for injection 3ml pre-filled pens | 3 pre-filled disposable injection [PoM] £95.53 DT = £95.53

⚑ 833

Insulin detemir

26-Feb-2025

- **DRUG ACTION** Insulin detemir is a recombinant human insulin analogue with a long duration of action.

- **INDICATIONS AND DOSE**
Diabetes mellitus
▸ BY SUBCUTANEOUS INJECTION
▸ Child 1-17 years: According to requirements
▸ Adult: According to requirements

- **INTERACTIONS** → Appendix 1: insulin

- **SIDE-EFFECTS**
▸ **Uncommon** Refraction disorder

- **PREGNANCY** Evidence of the safety of long-acting insulin analogues in pregnancy is limited, therefore isophane insulin p. 837 is recommended where longer-acting insulins are needed; insulin detemir may also be considered where longer-acting insulins are needed.

- **NATIONAL FUNDING/ACCESS DECISIONS** For full details see funding body website
Scottish Medicines Consortium (SMC) decisions
▸ **Insulin detemir (*Levemir®*) for the treatment of diabetes mellitus (March 2016)** SMC No. 1126/16 Recommended with restrictions

- **MEDICINAL FORMS** There can be variation in the licensing of different medicines containing the same drug.
Solution for injection
▸ Levemir FlexPen (Novo Nordisk Ltd)
Insulin detemir 100 unit per 1 ml Levemir FlexPen 100units/ml solution for injection 3ml pre-filled pens | 5 pre-filled disposable injection [PoM] £42.00 DT = £42.00
▸ Levemir Penfill (Novo Nordisk Ltd)
Insulin detemir 100 unit per 1 ml Levemir Penfill 100units/ml solution for injection 3ml cartridges | 5 cartridge [PoM] £42.00 DT = £42.00

⚑ 833

Insulin glargine

26-Feb-2025

- **DRUG ACTION** Insulin glargine is a recombinant human insulin analogue with a long duration of action.

- **INDICATIONS AND DOSE**
Diabetes mellitus
▸ BY SUBCUTANEOUS INJECTION
▸ Child 2-17 years: According to requirements   continued →

‣ Adult: According to requirements

TOUJEO ®

Diabetes mellitus
‣ BY SUBCUTANEOUS INJECTION
‣ Adult: According to requirements

● **INTERACTIONS** → Appendix 1: insulin

● **SIDE-EFFECTS**
▸ **Rare or very rare** Myalgia · taste altered
▸ **Frequency not known** Sodium retention

● **PREGNANCY** Evidence of the safety of long-acting insulin analogues in pregnancy is limited, therefore isophane insulin is recommended where longer-acting insulins are needed; insulin detemir may also be considered.

● **PRESCRIBING AND DISPENSING INFORMATION** Insulin glargine is a biological medicine. Biological medicines must be prescribed and dispensed by brand name, see *Biological medicines* and *Biosimilar medicines*, under Guidance on prescribing p. 1. Dose adjustments and close metabolic monitoring is recommended if switching between insulin glargine preparations.

● **NATIONAL FUNDING/ACCESS DECISIONS**
For full details see funding body website

Scottish Medicines Consortium (SMC) decisions
‣ Insulin glargine (*Lantus*®) for the treatment of diabetes mellitus in adults, adolescents and children aged 2 years and above (April 2013) SMC No. 860/13 Recommended with restrictions
‣ Insulin glargine (*Toujeo*®) for the treatment of type 1 or type 2 diabetes mellitus in adults aged 18 years and above (September 2015) SMC No. 1078/15 Recommended with restrictions

● **MEDICINAL FORMS** There can be variation in the licensing of different medicines containing the same drug.

Solution for injection
▸ **Abasaglar** (Eli Lilly and Company Ltd)
Insulin glargine 100 unit per 1 ml Abasaglar 100units/ml solution for injection 3ml cartridges | 5 cartridge [PoM] £35.28 DT = £34.75
▸ **Abasaglar KwikPen** (Eli Lilly and Company Ltd)
Insulin glargine 100 unit per 1 ml Abasaglar KwikPen 100units/ml solution for injection 3ml pre-filled pens | 5 pre-filled disposable injection [PoM] £35.28 DT = £34.75
▸ **Lantus** (Sanofi)
Insulin glargine 100 unit per 1 ml Lantus 100units/ml solution for injection 3ml cartridges | 5 cartridge [PoM] £34.75 DT = £34.75
Lantus 100units/ml solution for injection 3ml pre-filled SoloStar pens | 5 pre-filled disposable injection [PoM] £34.75 DT = £34.75
Lantus 100units/ml solution for injection 10ml vials | 1 vial [PoM] £25.69 DT = £25.69
▸ **Semglee** (Biosimilar Collaborations Ireland Ltd)
Insulin glargine 100 unit per 1 ml Semglee 100units/ml solution for injection 3ml pre-filled pens | 5 pre-filled disposable injection [PoM] £29.99 DT = £34.75
▸ **Toujeo** (Sanofi)
Insulin glargine 300 unit per 1 ml Toujeo 300units/ml solution for injection 1.5ml pre-filled SoloStar pens | 3 pre-filled disposable injection [PoM] £32.14 DT = £32.14 | 5 pre-filled disposable injection [PoM] £53.57
▸ **Toujeo DoubleStar** (Sanofi)
Insulin glargine 300 unit per 1 ml Toujeo 300units/ml solution for injection 3ml pre-filled DoubleStar pens | 3 pre-filled disposable injection [PoM] £64.27 DT = £64.27

Insulin glargine with lixisenatide

09-Nov-2020

The properties listed below are those particular to the combination only. For the properties of the components please consider, insulin glargine p. 839, lixisenatide p. 818.

● **INDICATIONS AND DOSE**
Type 2 diabetes mellitus [in combination with metformin]
▸ BY SUBCUTANEOUS INJECTION
▸ Adult: (consult product literature)

● **INTERACTIONS** → Appendix 1: glucagon-like peptide-1 receptor agonists · insulin

● **PRESCRIBING AND DISPENSING INFORMATION** *Suliqua*® is available in two pen strengths, providing different dosing options. To avoid medication errors, the prescriber must ensure that the correct strength and number of dose steps is prescribed. The manufacturer of *Suliqua*® has provided a healthcare professional guide and letter which includes important information on dosing.

● **PATIENT AND CARER ADVICE** Manufacturer advises check pen label before each administration to avoid medication error.
A patient guide should be provided.

● **NATIONAL FUNDING/ACCESS DECISIONS**
For full details see funding body website

Scottish Medicines Consortium (SMC) decisions
▸ Insulin glargine with lixisenatide (*Suliqua*®) in combination with metformin for the treatment of adults with type II diabetes mellitus (T2DM), to improve glycaemic control when this has not been provided by metformin alone or metformin combined with another oral glucose-lowering medicinal product or with basal insulin (April 2020) SMC No. SMC2235 Recommended with restrictions

● **MEDICINAL FORMS** No licensed medicines listed.

4.1a Diabetes, diagnosis and monitoring

Diabetes mellitus, diagnostic and monitoring devices

24-May-2022

Urinalysis: urinary glucose

Reagent strips are available for measuring for glucose in the urine. Tests for ketones by patients are rarely required unless they become unwell—see Blood Monitoring.

Microalbuminuria can be detected with *Micral-Test II*® but this should be followed by confirmation in the laboratory, since false positive results are common.

Blood glucose monitoring

In the UK blood-glucose concentration is expressed in mmol/litre and Diabetes UK advises that these units should be used for self-monitoring of blood-glucose. In other European countries units of mg/100 mL (or mg/dL) are commonly used.

It is advisable to check that the meter is pre-set in the correct units.

Capillary blood-glucose monitoring using a meter gives a direct measure of the glucose concentration at the time of the test and can detect hypoglycaemia as well as hyperglycaemia. Patients should be properly trained in the use of blood-glucose monitoring systems and to take appropriate action on the results obtained. Inadequate understanding of the normal fluctuations in blood-glucose can lead to confusion and inappropriate action.

Continuous glucose monitoring may be appropriate in certain patients with diabetes. A continuous glucose monitor is a device that measures interstitial fluid glucose levels and sends the readings to a display device or smartphone.

For further information on self-monitoring of capillary blood-glucose, and continuous glucose monitoring, see NICE guidelines: **Type 1 diabetes in adults: diagnosis and management** (available at: www.nice.org.uk/guidance/ng17) and **Type 2 diabetes in adults: management** (available at: www.nice.org.uk/guidance/ng28).

Patients using multiple injection regimens should understand how to adjust their insulin dose according to their carbohydrate intake. With fixed-dose insulin regimens, the carbohydrate intake needs to be regulated, and should be distributed throughout the day to match the insulin regimen.

If the patient is unwell and diabetic ketoacidosis is suspected, blood **ketones** should be measured according to local guidelines. Patients and their carers should be trained in the use of blood ketone monitoring systems and to take appropriate action on the results obtained, including when to seek medical attention.

> **Other drugs used for Diabetes, diagnosis and monitoring**
> Glucose, p. 1182

Meters and test strips

Meter (all NHS)	Type of monitoring	Compatible test strips	Test strip net price	Sensitivity range (mmol/litre)	Manufacturer
Accu-Chek® Active	Blood glucose	Active®	50 strip= £0.00	0.6– 33.3 mmol/litre	Roche Diabetes Care Ltd
Accu-Chek® Aviva	Blood glucose	Aviva®	50 strip= £12.99	0.6– 33.3 mmol/litre	Roche Diabetes Care Ltd
Accu-Chek® Aviva Expert	Blood glucose	Aviva®	50 strip= £12.99	0.6– 33.3 mmol/litre	Roche Diabetes Care Ltd
Accu-Chek® Mobile	Blood glucose	Mobile®	50 device= £10.24	0.3– 33.3 mmol/litre	Roche Diabetes Care Ltd
Accu-Chek® Aviva Nano	Blood glucose	Aviva®	50 strip= £12.99	0.6– 33.3 mmol/litre	Roche Diabetes Care Ltd
BGStar® Free of charge from diabetes healthcare professionals	Blood glucose	BGStar®	50 strip= £0.00	1.1– 33.3 mmol/litre	Sanofi
Breeze 2®	Blood glucose	Breeze 2®	50 strip= £15.00	0.6– 33.3 mmol/litre	Bayer Plc
CareSens N® Free of charge from diabetes healthcare professionals	Blood glucose	CareSens N®	50 strip= £12.75	1.1– 33.3 mmol/litre	Spirit Healthcare Ltd
Contour®	Blood glucose	Contour®	50 strip= £10.15	0.6– 33.3 mmol/litre	Ascensia Diabetes Care UK Ltd
Contour® XT	Blood glucose	Contour® Next	50 strip= £16.21	0.6– 33.3 mmol/litre	Ascensia Diabetes Care UK Ltd
Element®	Blood glucose	Element®	50 strip= £9.89	0.55– 33.3 mmol/litre	Neon Diagnostics Ltd
FreeStyle® Meter no longer available	Blood glucose	FreeStyle®	50 strip= £16.40	1.1– 27.8 mmol/litre	Abbott Laboratories Ltd
FreeStyle Freedom® Meter no longer available	Blood glucose	FreeStyle®	50 strip= £16.40	1.1– 27.8 mmol/litre	Abbott Laboratories Ltd
FreeStyle Freedom Lite®	Blood glucose	FreeStyle Lite®	50 strip= £16.41	1.1– 27.8 mmol/litre	Abbott Laboratories Ltd
FreeStyle InsuLinx®	Blood glucose	FreeStyle Lite®	50 strip= £16.41	1.1– 27.8 mmol/litre	Abbott Laboratories Ltd
FreeStyle Lite®	Blood glucose	FreeStyle Lite®	50 strip= £16.41	1.1– 27.8 mmol/litre	Abbott Laboratories Ltd
FreeStyle Mini® Meter no longer available	Blood glucose	FreeStyle®	50 strip= £16.40	1.1– 27.8 mmol/litre	Abbott Laboratories Ltd
FreeStyle Optium®	Blood glucose	FreeStyle Optium®	50 strip= £16.30	1.1– 27.8 mmol/litre	Abbott Laboratories Ltd
FreeStyle Optium®	Blood ketones	FreeStyle Optium® β-ketone	10 strip= £21.94	0– 8.0 mmol/litre	Abbott Laboratories Ltd
FreeStyle Optium Neo®	Blood glucose	FreeStyle Optium®	50 strip= £16.30	1.1– 27.8 mmol/litre	Abbott Laboratories Ltd
FreeStyle Optium Neo®	Blood ketones	FreeStyle Optium® β-ketone	10 strip= £21.94	0– 8.0 mmol/litre	Abbott Laboratories Ltd

Meter (all NHS)	Type of monitoring	Compatible test strips	Test strip net price	Sensitivity range (mmol/litre)	Manufacturer
GlucoDock® module For use with iPhone®, iPod touch®, and iPad®	Blood glucose	GlucoDock®	50 strip= £14.90	1.1– 33.3 mmol/litre	Medisana Healthcare (UK) Ltd
GlucoLab®	Blood glucose	GlucoLab®	50 strip= £9.89	0.55– 33.3 mmol/litre	Neon Diagnostics Ltd
GlucoRx® Free of charge from diabetes healthcare professionals	Blood glucose	GlucoRx®	50 strip= £5.45	1.1– 33.3 mmol/litre	GlucoRx Ltd
GlucoRx Nexus® Free of charge from diabetes healthcare professionals	Blood glucose	GlucoRx Nexus®	50 strip= £8.95	1.1– 33.3 mmol/litre	GlucoRx Ltd
Glucotrend® Meter no longer available	Blood glucose	Active®	50 strip= £0.00	0.6– 33.3 mmol/litre	Roche Diabetes Care Ltd
iBGStar®	Blood glucose	BGStar®	50 strip= £0.00	1.1– 33.3 mmol/litre	Sanofi
Mendor Discreet®	Blood glucose	Mendor Discreet®	50 strip= £14.75	1.1– 33.3 mmol/litre	SpringMed Solutions Ltd
Microdot®+ Free of charge from diabetes healthcare professionals	Blood glucose	Microdot®+	50 strip= £9.49	1.1– 29.2 mmol/litre	Cambridge Sensors Ltd
MyGlucoHealth®	Blood glucose	MyGlucoHealth®	50 strip= £15.50	0.6– 33.3 mmol/litre	Entra Health Systems Ltd
One Touch® VerioPro Free of charge from diabetes healthcare professionals	Blood glucose	One Touch® Verio	50 strip= £15.12	1.1– 33.3 mmol/litre	LifeScan
SD CodeFree®	Blood glucose	SD CodeFree®	50 strip= £7.40	0.6– 33.3 mmol/litre	Home Health (UK) Ltd
Sensocard Plus® Meter no longer available	Blood glucose	Sensocard®	50 strip= £16.30	1.1– 33.3 mmol/litre	BBI Healthcare Ltd
TRUEyou mini®	Blood glucose	TRUEyou®	50 strip= £0.00	1.1– 33.3 mmol/litre	Trividia Health UK Ltd
WaveSense JAZZ® Free of charge from diabetes healthcare professionals	Blood glucose	WaveSense JAZZ®	50 strip= £8.74	1.1– 33.3 mmol/litre	AgaMatrix Europe Ltd

Blood glucose testing strips

● **BLOOD GLUCOSE TESTING STRIPS**

4SURE testing strips (Nipro Diagnostics (UK) Ltd)
50 strip · NHS indicative price = £7.99 · Drug Tariff (Part IXr)

Accu-Chek Inform II testing strips (Roche Diagnostics Ltd)
50 strip · No NHS indicative price available · Drug Tariff (Part IXr)

Advocate Redi-Code+ testing strips (Diabetes Care Technology Ltd)
50 strip · NHS indicative price = £9.95 · Drug Tariff (Part IXr)

AgaMatrix Agile testing strips (AgaMatrix Europe Ltd)
50 strip · NHS indicative price = £5.99 · Drug Tariff (Part IXr)

AutoSense testing strips (Advance Diagnostic Products (NI) Ltd)
25 strip · NHS indicative price = £4.50 · Drug Tariff (Part IXr)

Aviva testing strips (Roche Diabetes Care Ltd)
50 strip · NHS indicative price = £12.99 · Drug Tariff (Part IXr)

Betachek C50 cassette (National Diagnostic Products)
50 device · NHS indicative price = £9.95 · Drug Tariff (Part IXr)100 device · NHS indicative price = £19.90 · Drug Tariff (Part IXr)

Betachek G5 testing strips (National Diagnostic Products)
50 strip · NHS indicative price = £5.50 · Drug Tariff (Part IXr)

Betachek Visual testing strips (National Diagnostic Products)
50 strip · NHS indicative price = £5.50 · Drug Tariff (Part IXr)

Breeze 2 testing discs (Bayer Plc)
50 strip · NHS indicative price = £15.00 · Drug Tariff (Part IXr)

CareSens N testing strips (Spirit Healthcare Ltd)
50 strip · NHS indicative price = £12.75 · Drug Tariff (Part IXr)

CareSens PRO testing strips (Spirit Healthcare Ltd)
50 strip · NHS indicative price = £9.95 · Drug Tariff (Part IXr)

CareSens S testing strips (Spirit Healthcare Ltd)
50 strip · NHS indicative price = £5.45 · Drug Tariff (Part IXr)

Contour Next testing strips (Ascensia Diabetes Care UK Ltd)
50 strip · NHS indicative price = £16.21 · Drug Tariff (Part IXr)

Contour Plus testing strips (Ascensia Diabetes Care UK Ltd)
50 strip · NHS indicative price = £5.95 · Drug Tariff (Part IXr)

Contour testing strips (Ascensia Diabetes Care UK Ltd)
50 strip · NHS indicative price = £10.15 · Drug Tariff (Part IXr)

Dario Lite testing strips (LabStyle Innovations Ltd)
50 strip · NHS indicative price = £9.95 · Drug Tariff (Part IXr)

Dario testing strips (LabStyle Innovations Ltd)
50 strip · NHS indicative price = £14.95 · Drug Tariff (Part IXr)

Element testing strips (Neon Diagnostics Ltd)
50 strip · NHS indicative price = £9.89 · Drug Tariff (Part IXr)

Finetest Lite testing strips (Neon Diagnostics Ltd)
50 strip · NHS indicative price = £5.15 · Drug Tariff (Part IXr)

Fora Advanced pro GD40 testing strips (Miller Medical Supplies Ltd)
50 strip · NHS indicative price = £7.95 · Drug Tariff (Part IXr)

FreeStyle Lite testing strips (Abbott Laboratories Ltd)
50 strip · NHS indicative price = £16.41 · Drug Tariff (Part IXr)

FreeStyle Optium H testing strips (Abbott Laboratories Ltd)
100 strip · No NHS indicative price available · Drug Tariff (Part IXr)

FreeStyle Optium Neo H testing strips (Abbott Laboratories Ltd)
100 strip · No NHS indicative price available · Drug Tariff (Part IXr)

FreeStyle Optium testing strips (Abbott Laboratories Ltd)
50 strip · NHS indicative price = £16.30 · Drug Tariff (Part IXr)

FreeStyle Precision Pro testing strips (Abbott Laboratories Ltd)
100 strip · No NHS indicative price available · Drug Tariff (Part IXr)

FreeStyle testing strips (Abbott Laboratories Ltd)
50 strip · NHS indicative price = £16.40 · Drug Tariff (Part IXr)

GluNEO testing strips (Neon Diagnostics Ltd)
50 strip · NHS indicative price = £9.89 · Drug Tariff (Part IXr)

GlucoDock testing strips (Medisana Healthcare (UK) Ltd)
50 strip · NHS indicative price = £14.90 · Drug Tariff (Part IXr)

GlucoLab testing strips (Neon Diagnostics Ltd)
50 strip · NHS indicative price = £9.89 · Drug Tariff (Part IXr)

GlucoMen areo Sensor testing strips (A. Menarini Diagnostics Ltd)
50 strip · NHS indicative price = £7.25 · Drug Tariff (Part IXr)

GlucoRx GO Professional testing strips (GlucoRx Ltd)
50 strip · NHS indicative price = £9.95 · Drug Tariff (Part IXr)

GlucoRx GO testing strips (GlucoRx Ltd)
50 strip · NHS indicative price = £9.95 · Drug Tariff (Part IXr)

GlucoRx HCT Glucose testing strips (GlucoRx Ltd)
50 strip · NHS indicative price = £8.95 · Drug Tariff (Part IXr)

GlucoRx Nexus testing strips (GlucoRx Ltd)
50 strip · NHS indicative price = £8.95 · Drug Tariff (Part IXr)

GlucoRx Q testing strips (GlucoRx Ltd)
50 strip · NHS indicative price = £5.45 · Drug Tariff (Part IXr)

GlucoRx Vivid testing strips (GlucoRx Ltd)
50 strip · NHS indicative price = £5.45 · Drug Tariff (Part IXr)

GlucoRx X6 Glucose testing strips (GlucoRx Ltd)
50 strip · NHS indicative price = £15.95 · Drug Tariff (Part IXr)

GlucoZen.auto testing strips (GlucoZen Ltd)
50 strip · NHS indicative price = £7.64 · Drug Tariff (Part IXr)100 strip · NHS indicative price = £10.85 · Drug Tariff (Part IXr)

Glucofix Tech Sensor testing strips (A. Menarini Diagnostics Ltd)
50 strip · NHS indicative price = £5.95 · Drug Tariff (Part IXr)

Glucoflex-R testing strips (National Diagnostic Products)
50 strip · NHS indicative price = £5.50 · Drug Tariff (Part IXr)

Guide testing strips (Roche Diabetes Care Ltd)
50 strip · NHS indicative price = £16.21 · Drug Tariff (Part IXr)

Instant testing strips (Roche Diabetes Care Ltd)
50 strip · NHS indicative price = £5.95 · Drug Tariff (Part IXr)

Kinetik Wellbeing AG-607 testing strips (Kinetik Medical Devices Ltd)
50 strip · NHS indicative price = £8.49 · Drug Tariff (Part IXr)100 strip · NHS indicative price = £13.98 · Drug Tariff (Part IXr)

Kinetik Wellbeing BG-710/BG-710b testing strips (Kinetik Medical Devices Ltd)
50 strip · NHS indicative price = £7.50 · Drug Tariff (Part IXr)100 strip · NHS indicative price = £13.00 · Drug Tariff (Part IXr)

MODZ testing strips (Modz Oy)
50 strip · NHS indicative price = £14.00 · Drug Tariff (Part IXr)

MediTouch 2 testing strips (Medisana Healthcare (UK) Ltd)
50 strip · NHS indicative price = £12.49 · Drug Tariff (Part IXr)

MediTouch testing strips (Medisana Healthcare (UK) Ltd)
50 strip · NHS indicative price = £14.90 · Drug Tariff (Part IXr)

Mendor Discreet testing strips (SpringMed Solutions Ltd)
50 strip · NHS indicative price = £14.75 · Drug Tariff (Part IXr)

Microdot+ testing strips (Cambridge Sensors Ltd)
50 strip · NHS indicative price = £9.49 · Drug Tariff (Part IXr)

Mobile cassette (Roche Diabetes Care Ltd)
50 device · NHS indicative price = £10.24 · Drug Tariff (Part IXr)

MySugarWatch testing strips (MySugarWatch Ltd)
50 strip · NHS indicative price = £14.86 · Drug Tariff (Part IXr)

Myglucohealth testing strips (Entra Health Systems Ltd)
50 strip · NHS indicative price = £15.50 · Drug Tariff (Part IXr)

Mylife Aveo testing strips (Ypsomed Ltd)
50 strip · NHS indicative price = £6.95 · Drug Tariff (Part IXr)

Mylife Pura testing strips (Ypsomed Ltd)
50 strip · NHS indicative price = £9.50 · Drug Tariff (Part IXr)

Mylife Unio testing strips (Ypsomed Ltd)
50 strip · NHS indicative price = £9.50 · Drug Tariff (Part IXr)

OKmeter Core testing strips (Syringa UK Ltd)
50 strip · NHS indicative price = £9.90 · Drug Tariff (Part IXr)

Oh'Care Lite testing strips (Neon Diagnostics Ltd)
50 strip · NHS indicative price = £8.88 · Drug Tariff (Part IXr)

On Call Extra testing strips (Connect2Pharma Ltd)
50 strip · NHS indicative price = £5.20 · Drug Tariff (Part IXr)

On Call Sure testing strips (Connect2Pharma Ltd)
50 strip · NHS indicative price = £8.50 · Drug Tariff (Part IXr)

On-Call Advanced testing strips (Point Of Care Testing Ltd)
50 strip · NHS indicative price = £13.65 · Drug Tariff (Part IXr)

OneTouch Select Plus testing strips (LifeScan)
50 strip · NHS indicative price = £9.99 · Drug Tariff (Part IXr)

OneTouch Verio testing strips (LifeScan)
50 strip · NHS indicative price = £15.12 · Drug Tariff (Part IXr)

Performa testing strips (Roche Diabetes Care Ltd)
50 strip · NHS indicative price = £5.99 · Drug Tariff (Part IXr)

SD CodeFree testing strips (Home Health (UK) Ltd)
50 strip · NHS indicative price = £7.40 · Drug Tariff (Part IXr)

SURESIGN Resure testing strips (Ciga Healthcare Ltd)
50 strip · NHS indicative price = £8.49 · Drug Tariff (Part IXr)

Sensocard testing strips (BBI Healthcare Ltd)
50 strip · NHS indicative price = £16.30 · Drug Tariff (Part IXr)

StatStrip testing strips (Nova Biomedical)
50 strip · No NHS indicative price available · Drug Tariff (Part IXr)

TEE2 testing strips (Spirit Healthcare Ltd)
50 strip · NHS indicative price = £7.75 · Drug Tariff (Part IXr)

True Metrix testing strips (Trividia Health UK Ltd)
50 strip · NHS indicative price = £5.95 · Drug Tariff (Part IXr)100 strip · NHS indicative price = £11.00 · Drug Tariff (Part IXr)

VivaChek Ino testing strips (JR Biomedical Ltd)
50 strip · NHS indicative price = £8.99 · Drug Tariff (Part IXr)

WaveSense JAZZ Duo testing strips (AgaMatrix Europe Ltd)
50 strip · NHS indicative price = £8.74 · Drug Tariff (Part IXr)

WaveSense JAZZ testing strips (AgaMatrix Europe Ltd)
50 strip · NHS indicative price = £8.74 · Drug Tariff (Part IXr)

Xceed Precision Pro testing strips (Abbott Laboratories Ltd)
10 strip · No NHS indicative price available50 strip · No NHS indicative price available · Drug Tariff (Part IXr)100 strip · No NHS indicative price available · Drug Tariff (Part IXr)

palmdoc iCare Advanced Solo testing strips (Palmdoc Ltd)
50 strip · NHS indicative price = £13.50 · Drug Tariff (Part IXr)

palmdoc iCare Advanced testing strips (Palmdoc Ltd)
50 strip · NHS indicative price = £9.70 · Drug Tariff (Part IXr)

palmdoc testing strips (Palmdoc Ltd)
50 strip · NHS indicative price = £5.90 · Drug Tariff (Part IXr)

Blood ketones testing strips

● **BLOOD KETONES TESTING STRIPS**

4SURE beta-ketone testing strips (Nipro Diagnostics (UK) Ltd) |
10 strip · NHS indicative price = £9.92 · Drug Tariff (Part IXr)

Fora Advanced pro GD40 Ketone testing strips (Miller Medical Supplies Ltd) | 10 strip · NHS indicative price = £8.95 · Drug Tariff (Part IXr)

FreeStyle Optium H beta-ketone testing strips (Abbott Laboratories Ltd) | 10 strip · No NHS indicative price available · Drug Tariff (Part IXr)

FreeStyle Optium beta-ketone testing strips (Abbott Laboratories Ltd) | 10 strip · NHS indicative price = £21.94 · Drug Tariff (Part IXr)

FreeStyle Precision Pro beta-ketone testing strips (Abbott Laboratories Ltd) | 50 strip · No NHS indicative price available

GlucoMen areo Ketone Sensor testing strips (A. Menarini Diagnostics Ltd) | 10 strip · NHS indicative price = £9.95 · Drug Tariff (Part IXr)

GlucoRx HCT Ketone testing strips (GlucoRx Ltd) | 10 strip · NHS indicative price = £9.95 · Drug Tariff (Part IXr)

GlucoRx X6 Ketone testing strips (GlucoRx Ltd) | 10 strip · NHS indicative price = £15.95 · Drug Tariff (Part IXr)

Glucofix Tech beta-ketone Sensor testing strips (A. Menarini Diagnostics Ltd) | 10 strip · NHS indicative price = £9.95 · Drug Tariff (Part IXr)

KetoSens testing strips (Spirit Healthcare Ltd) | 10 strip • NHS indicative price = £9.95 • Drug Tariff (Part IXr)

MySugarWatch beta-ketone testing strips (MySugarWatch Ltd) | 10 strip • NHS indicative price = £8.95 • Drug Tariff (Part IXr)

StatStrip beta-ketone testing strips (Nova Biomedical) | 50 strip • No NHS indicative price available

Xceed Precision Pro beta-ketone testing strips (Abbott Laboratories Ltd) | 10 strip • No NHS indicative price available • Drug Tariff (Part IXr) | 50 strip • No NHS indicative price available | 100 strip • No NHS indicative price available

Glucose interstitial fluid detection sensors

● **GLUCOSE INTERSTITIAL FLUID DETECTION SENSORS**

A8 TouchCare Nano Sensor (Medtrum Ltd)
2 kit • No NHS indicative price available • Drug Tariff (Part IXa)

A8 TouchCare Nano Transmitter (Medtrum Ltd)
1 device • No NHS indicative price available • Drug Tariff (Part IXa)

CareSens Air Sensor (Spirit Healthcare Ltd)
1 kit • NHS indicative price = £31.87 • Drug Tariff (Part IXa)

Dexcom G6 Receiver (Dexcom International Ltd)
1 device • No NHS indicative price available • Drug Tariff (Part IXa)

Dexcom G6 Sensor (Dexcom International Ltd)
1 kit • No NHS indicative price available • Drug Tariff (Part IXa)3 kit • No NHS indicative price available • Drug Tariff (Part IXa)

Dexcom G6 Transmitter (Dexcom International Ltd)
1 device • No NHS indicative price available • Drug Tariff (Part IXa)

Dexcom G7 Receiver (Dexcom International Ltd)
1 device • No NHS indicative price available • Drug Tariff (Part IXa)

Dexcom G7 Sensor (Dexcom International Ltd)
1 kit • No NHS indicative price available • Drug Tariff (Part IXa)3 kit • No NHS indicative price available • Drug Tariff (Part IXa)

Dexcom One Sensor (Dexcom International Ltd)
1 kit • NHS indicative price = £23.00 • Drug Tariff (Part IXa)3 kit • NHS indicative price = £69.00 • Drug Tariff (Part IXa)

Dexcom One Transmitter (Dexcom International Ltd)
1 device • NHS indicative price = £18.00 • Drug Tariff (Part IXa)

Dexcom One+ Sensor (Dexcom International Ltd)
1 kit • NHS indicative price = £24.97 • Drug Tariff (Part IXa)

FreeStyle Libre 2 Plus Sensor (Abbott Laboratories Ltd)
1 kit • NHS indicative price = £37.50 • Drug Tariff (Part IXa)

FreeStyle Libre 2 Sensor (Abbott Laboratories Ltd)
1 kit • NHS indicative price = £35.00 • Drug Tariff (Part IXa)

FreeStyle Libre 3 Plus Sensor (Abbott Laboratories Ltd)
1 kit • NHS indicative price = £45.00 • Drug Tariff (Part IXa)

FreeStyle Libre 3 Sensor (Abbott Laboratories Ltd)
1 kit • NHS indicative price = £42.00 • Drug Tariff (Part IXa)

GlucoRx AiDEX Sensor (GlucoRx Ltd)
1 kit • NHS indicative price = £29.76 • Drug Tariff (Part IXa)

GlucoRx AiDEX Transmitter (GlucoRx Ltd)
1 device • NHS indicative price = £19.95 • Drug Tariff (Part IXa)

Guardian 4 Link Transmitter Replacement (Medtronic Ltd)
1 device • No NHS indicative price available • Drug Tariff (Part IXa)

Guardian 4 Sensor (Medtronic Ltd)
1 device • No NHS indicative price available • Drug Tariff (Part IXa)
5 device • No NHS indicative price available10 device • No NHS indicative price available15 device • No NHS indicative price available

Hypodermic insulin injection pens

● **HYPODERMIC INSULIN INJECTION PENS**
AUTOPEN ® 24
Autopen® 24 (for use with Sanofi- Aventis 3-mL insulin cartridges), allowing 1-unit dosage adjustment, max. 21 units (single-unit version) or 2-unit dosage adjustment, max. 42 units (2- unit version).

AUTOPEN ® CLASSIC
Autopen® Classic (for use with Lilly and Wockhardt 3-mL insulin cartridges), allowing 1-unit dosage adjustment, max. 21 units (single-unit version) or 2-unit dosage adjustment, max. 42 units (2-unit version).

Autopen Classic hypodermic insulin injection pen reusable for 3ml cartridge 1 unit dial up / range 1-21 units (Owen Mumford Ltd)
1 device • NHS indicative price = £18.20 • Drug Tariff (Part IXa)

Autopen Classic hypodermic insulin injection pen reusable for 3ml cartridge 2 unit dial up / range 2-42 units (Owen Mumford Ltd)
1 device • NHS indicative price = £18.20 • Drug Tariff (Part IXa)

HUMAPEN ® LUXURA HD
For use with *Humulin*® and *Humalog*® 3-mL cartridges; allowing 0.5-unit dosage adjustment, max. 30 units.

NOVOPEN ECHO ® PLUS
For use with *Penfill*® 3-mL insulin cartridges; allowing 0.5-unit dosage adjustment, max. 30 units.

NovoPen Echo Plus hypodermic insulin injection pen reusable for 3ml cartridge 0.5 unit dial up / range 0.5-30 units (Novo Nordisk Ltd)
1 device • NHS indicative price = £26.86 • Drug Tariff (Part IXa)

NovoPen Echo Plus hypodermic insulin injection pen reusable for 3ml cartridge 0.5 unit dial up / range 0.5-30 units (Novo Nordisk Ltd)
1 device • NHS indicative price = £26.86 • Drug Tariff (Part IXa)

NOVOPEN ® 6
For use with *Penfill*® 3-mL insulin cartridges; allowing 1-unit dosage adjustment, max. 60 units.

NovoPen 6 hypodermic insulin injection pen reusable for 3ml cartridge 1 unit dial up / range 1-60 units (Novo Nordisk Ltd)
1 device • NHS indicative price = £26.86 • Drug Tariff (Part IXa)

NovoPen 6 hypodermic insulin injection pen reusable for 3ml cartridge 1 unit dial up / range 1-60 units (Novo Nordisk Ltd)
1 device • NHS indicative price = £26.86 • Drug Tariff (Part IXa)

Needle free insulin delivery systems

● **NEEDLE FREE INSULIN DELIVERY SYSTEMS**
INSUJET ®
For use with any 10-mL vial or 3-mL cartridge of insulin, allowing 1-unit dosage adjustment, max 40 units. Available as *starter set* (*InsuJet*® device, nozzle cap, nozzle and piston, 1 × 10-mL adaptor, 1 × 3-mL adaptor, 1 cartridge cap removal key), *nozzle pack* (15 nozzles), *cartridge adaptor pack* (15 adaptors), or *vial adaptor pack* (15 adaptors).

InsuJet starter set (Reliance Medical Ltd)
1 pack • NHS indicative price = £90.00 • Drug Tariff (Part IXa)

Urine glucose testing strips

● **URINE GLUCOSE TESTING STRIPS**

Diastix testing strips (Ascensia Diabetes Care UK Ltd)
50 strip • NHS indicative price = £2.96 • Drug Tariff (Part IXr)

Medi-Test Glucose testing strips (BHR Pharmaceuticals Ltd)
50 strip • NHS indicative price = £2.36 • Drug Tariff (Part IXr)

Urine ketone testing strips

● **URINE KETONES TESTING STRIPS**

GlucoRx KetoRx Sticks 2GK testing strips (GlucoRx Ltd)
50 strip • NHS indicative price = £2.25 • Drug Tariff (Part IXr)

Ketostix testing strips (Ascensia Diabetes Care UK Ltd)
50 strip • NHS indicative price = £3.13 • Drug Tariff (Part IXr)

Urine protein testing strips

● **URINE PROTEIN TESTING STRIPS**

Albustix testing strips (Siemens Medical Solutions Diagnostics Ltd)
50 strip • NHS indicative price = £4.42 • Drug Tariff (Part IXr)

Medi-Test Protein 2 testing strips (BHR Pharmaceuticals Ltd)
50 strip • NHS indicative price = £3.31 • Drug Tariff (Part IXr)

4.2 Hypoglycaemia

Hypoglycaemia

17-Jun-2021

Description of condition

Hypoglycaemia is a lower than normal blood-glucose concentration. It results from an imbalance between glucose supply, glucose utilisation, and existing insulin concentration. It can be defined as 'mild' if the episode is self-treated and 'severe' if assistance is required. For the purposes of hospital inpatients diagnosed with diabetes, anyone with a blood-glucose concentration less than 4 mmol/litre should be treated.

Hypoglycaemia is the most common side-effect of insulin and sulfonylureas in the treatment of all types of diabetes mellitus and presents a major barrier to satisfactory long-term glycaemic control. Metformin hydrochloride p. 807, pioglitazone p. 832, the dipeptidylpeptidase-4 inhibitors (gliptins), sodium-glucose co-transporter-2 inhibitors, and glucagon-like peptide-1 receptor agonists, prescribed without insulin or sulfonylurea therapy, are unlikely to result in hypoglycaemia. Hypoglycaemia should be excluded in any person with diabetes who is acutely unwell, drowsy, unconscious, unable to co-operate, or presenting with aggressive behaviour or seizures.

Treatment of hypoglycaemia

For a quick reference resource with doses for the treatment of hypoglycaemia, see *Hypoglycaemia* in Medical emergencies in the community p. 2028.

[EvGr] Adults with symptoms of hypoglycaemia who have a blood-glucose concentration greater than 4 mmol/litre, should be treated with a small carbohydrate snack such as a slice of bread or a normal meal, if due.

Any patient with a blood-glucose concentration less than 4 mmol/litre, with or without symptoms, and who is **conscious and able to swallow**, should be treated with a fast-acting carbohydrate by mouth. Fast-acting carbohydrates include *Lift*® glucose liquid (previously *Glucojuice*®), glucose tablets, glucose 40% gels (e.g. *Glucogel*®, *Dextrogel*®, or *Rapilose*®), pure fruit juice, and sugar (sucrose) dissolved in an appropriate volume of water. Oral glucose formulations p. 1182 are preferred as absorption occurs more quickly. Orange juice should not be given to patients following a low-potassium diet due to chronic kidney disease, and sugar dissolved in water is not effective for patients taking acarbose which prevents the breakdown of sucrose to glucose. [E][EvGr] Chocolates and biscuits should be avoided if possible, as they have a lower sugar content and their high fat content may delay stomach emptying. [A]

[EvGr] If necessary, repeat treatment after 15 minutes, up to a maximum of 3 treatments in total. Once blood-glucose concentration is above 4 mmol/litre and the patient has recovered, a snack providing a long-acting carbohydrate should be given to prevent blood glucose from falling again (e.g. two biscuits, one slice of bread, 200–300 mL of milk (not soya or other forms of 'alternative' milk, e.g. almond or coconut), or a normal carbohydrate-containing meal if due). Insulin should not be omitted if due, but the dose regimen may need review.

Hypoglycaemia which does not respond (blood-glucose concentration remains below 4 mmol/litre after 30–45 minutes or after 3 treatment cycles), should be treated with intramuscular glucagon below or glucose 10% intravenous infusion. In alcoholic patients, thiamine supplementation should be given with, or following, the administration of intravenous glucose to minimise the risk of Wernicke's encephalopathy. [E]

Glucagon is a polypeptide hormone produced by the alpha cells of the islets of Langerhans, which increases blood-glucose concentration by mobilising glycogen stored in the liver. The manufacturer advises that it is ineffective in patients whose liver glycogen is depleted, therefore should not be used in anyone who has fasted for a prolonged period or has adrenal insufficiency, chronic hypoglycaemia, or alcohol-induced hypoglycaemia. [EvGr] Glucagon may also be less effective in patients taking a sulfonylurea; in these cases, intravenous glucose will be required. [E]

[EvGr] In an emergency, if the patient has a decreased level of consciousness caused by hypoglycaemia, intramuscular glucagon can be given by a family member or friend who has been shown how to use it. [A][EvGr] If glucagon is not effective after 10 minutes, glucose 10% intravenous infusion should be given. [E]

Hypoglycaemia which causes **unconsciousness** is an emergency. [EvGr] Patients who are unconscious, having seizures, or who are very aggressive, should have any intravenous insulin stopped, and be treated initially with glucagon. If glucagon is unsuitable, or there is no response after 10 minutes, glucose 10% intravenous infusion, or alternatively glucose 20% intravenous infusion should be given. [E] Glucose 50% intravenous infusion is not recommended as it is hypertonic, thus increases the risk of extravasation injury, and is viscous, making administration difficult.

[EvGr] A long-acting carbohydrate should be given as soon as possible once the patient has recovered and their blood-glucose concentration is above 4 mmol/litre (e.g. two biscuits, one slice of bread, 200–300 mL of milk (not soya or other forms of 'alternative' milk, e.g. almond or coconut), or a normal carbohydrate-containing meal if due). Patients who have received glucagon require a larger portion of long-acting carbohydrate to replenish glycogen stores (e.g. four biscuits, two slices of bread, 400–600 mL of milk (not soya or other forms of 'alternative' milk, e.g. almond or coconut), or a normal carbohydrate containing meal if due). Glucose 10% intravenous infusion should be given to patients who are nil by mouth.

If an insulin injection is due, it should **not** be omitted; however, a review of the usual insulin regimen may be required. Patients who self-manage their insulin pump may need to adjust their pump infusion rate. If the patient was on intravenous insulin, continue to check blood-glucose concentration every 15 minutes until above 3.5 mmol/litre, then re-start intravenous insulin after review of the dose regimen. Concurrent glucose 10% intravenous infusion should be considered. [E]

Hypoglycaemia caused by a sulfonylurea or long-acting insulin, may persist for up to 24–36 hours following the last dose, especially if there is concurrent renal impairment.

[EvGr] Blood-glucose monitoring should be continued for at least 24–48 hours. [E]

GLYCOGENOLYTIC HORMONES

Glucagon

17-Jun-2022

● INDICATIONS AND DOSE

Diabetic hypoglycaemia

▶ BY SUBCUTANEOUS INJECTION, OR BY INTRAMUSCULAR INJECTION

▶ Child 1 month-8 years (body-weight up to 25 kg): 500 micrograms, if no response within 10 minutes intravenous glucose must be given

▶ Child 9-17 years (body-weight 25 kg and above): 1 mg, if no response within 10 minutes intravenous glucose must be given

▶ Adult: 1 mg, if no response within 10 minutes intravenous glucose must be given   continued →

Severe hypotension, heart failure or cardiogenic shock due to acute overdosage of beta-blockers
▸ INITIALLY BY INTRAVENOUS INJECTION
▸ Child: 50–150 micrograms/kg (max. per dose 10 mg), administered over 1–2 minutes, followed by (by intravenous infusion) 50 micrograms/kg/hour, titrated according to response
▸ Adult: 5–10 mg, administered over 1–2 minutes, followed by (by intravenous infusion) 50–150 micrograms/kg/hour, titrated according to response

Diagnostic aid
▸ BY INTRAVENOUS INJECTION, OR BY INTRAMUSCULAR INJECTION
▸ Adult: (consult product literature)

DOSE EQUIVALENCE AND CONVERSION
▸ 1 unit of glucagon = 1 mg of glucagon.

OGLUO ®

Diabetic hypoglycaemia
▸ BY SUBCUTANEOUS INJECTION
▸ Child 2–5 years (body-weight up to 25 kg): 500 micrograms, if no response within 15 minutes an additional dose may be administered whilst waiting for emergency assistance
▸ Child 2–5 years (body-weight 25 kg and above): 1 mg, if no response within 15 minutes an additional dose may be administered whilst waiting for emergency assistance
▸ Child 6-17 years: 1 mg, if no response within 15 minutes an additional dose may be administered whilst waiting for emergency assistance
▸ Adult: 1 mg, if no response within 15 minutes an additional dose may be administered whilst waiting for emergency assistance

● UNLICENSED USE TOXBASE advises glucagon is used for the treatment of severe hypotension, heart failure or cardiogenic shock due to acute overdosage of beta-blockers, but it is not licensed for this indication.

● CONTRA-INDICATIONS Phaeochromocytoma

● CAUTIONS Glucagonoma · ineffective in chronic hypoglycaemia, starvation, and adrenal insufficiency · insulinoma

● INTERACTIONS → Appendix 1: glucagon

● SIDE-EFFECTS
▸ **Common or very common** Nausea
▸ **Uncommon** Vomiting
▸ **Rare or very rare** Abdominal pain · hypertension · hypotension · tachycardia

● DIRECTIONS FOR ADMINISTRATION For *intravenous infusion*, TOXBASE advises reconstituted solution may be used undiluted or diluted in Glucose 5%. Incompatibility For *intravenous infusion*, expert sources advise do not add to infusion fluids containing calcium—precipitation may occur.
OGLUO ® *Ogluo* ® is administered by subcutaneous injection into the lower abdomen, outer thigh or outer upper arm.

● PATIENT AND CARER ADVICE
Medicines for Children leaflet: Glucagon for hypoglycaemia www.medicinesforchildren.org.uk/medicines/glucagon-for-hypoglycaemia/

● EXCEPTIONS TO LEGAL CATEGORY Prescription-only medicine restriction does not apply where administration is for saving life in emergency.

● MEDICINAL FORMS There can be variation in the licensing of different medicines containing the same drug.
Solution for injection
▸ **Ogluo** (Tetris Pharma Ltd)
Glucagon 5 mg per 1 ml Ogluo 500micrograms/0.1ml solution for injection pre-filled pens | 1 pre-filled disposable injection PoM £73.00 DT = £73.00
Ogluo 1mg/0.2ml solution for injection pre-filled pens | 1 pre-filled disposable injection PoM £73.00 DT = £73.00
Powder and solvent for solution for injection
▸ **GlucaGen Hypokit** (Novo Nordisk Ltd)
Glucagon hydrochloride 1 mg GlucaGen Hypokit 1mg powder and solvent for solution for injection | 1 vial PoM £11.52 DT = £11.52

4.2a Chronic hypoglycaemia

GLYCOGENOLYTIC HORMONES

Diazoxide
17-May-2021

● **INDICATIONS AND DOSE**
Chronic intractable hypoglycaemia
▸ BY MOUTH
▸ Adult: Initially 5 mg/kg daily in 2–3 divided doses, adjusted according to response; maintenance 3–8 mg/kg daily in 2–3 divided doses

● CAUTIONS Aortic coarctation · aortic stenosis · arteriovenous shunt · heart failure · hyperuricaemia · impaired cardiac circulation · impaired cerebral circulation

● INTERACTIONS → Appendix 1: diazoxide

● SIDE-EFFECTS Abdominal pain · albuminuria · appetite decreased (long term use) · arrhythmia · azotaemia · cardiomegaly · cataract · constipation · diabetic hyperosmolar coma · diarrhoea · dizziness · dyspnoea · eosinophilia · extrapyramidal symptoms · fever · fluid retention · galactorrhoea · haemorrhage · headache · heart failure · hirsutism · hyperglycaemia · hyperuricaemia (long term use) · hypogammaglobulinaemia · hypotension · ileus · ketoacidosis · leucopenia · libido decreased · musculoskeletal pain · nausea · nephritic syndrome · oculogyric crisis · pancreatitis · parkinsonism · pulmonary hypertension · skin reactions · sodium retention · taste altered · thrombocytopenia · tinnitus · vision disorders · voice alteration (long term use) · vomiting

● PREGNANCY Use only if essential; alopecia and hypertrichosis reported in neonates with prolonged use; may inhibit uterine activity during labour.

● BREAST FEEDING Manufacturer advises avoid—no information available.

● RENAL IMPAIRMENT
Dose adjustments EvGr Dose reduction may be required. Ⓜ

● MONITORING REQUIREMENTS
▸ Monitor blood pressure.
▸ Monitor white cell and platelet count during prolonged use.

● MEDICINAL FORMS There can be variation in the licensing of different medicines containing the same drug. Forms available from special-order manufacturers include: oral capsule, oral suspension, oral solution
Oral tablet
▸ **Eudemine** (RPH Pharmaceuticals AB)
Diazoxide 50 mg Eudemine 50mg tablets | 100 tablet PoM £108.61 DT = £108.61
Oral capsule
▸ **Diazoxide (Non-proprietary)**
Diazoxide 25 mg Proglycem 25 capsules | 100 capsule PoM Ⓢ

5   Dopamine responsive conditions

DOPAMINERGIC DRUGS > DOPAMINE RECEPTOR AGONISTS

Dopamine-receptor agonists

Overview

Bromocriptine p. 482 is used for the treatment of galactorrhoea, and for the treatment of prolactinomas (when it reduces both plasma prolactin concentration and tumour size). Bromocriptine also inhibits the release of growth hormone and is sometimes used in the treatment of acromegaly, but somatostatin analogues (such as octreotide p. 1081) are more effective.

Cabergoline p. 484 has similar side-effects to bromocriptine, however patients intolerant of bromocriptine may be able to tolerate cabergoline (and *vice versa*).

Quinagolide below has actions and uses similar to those of ergot-derived dopamine agonists, but its side-effects differ slightly.

Suppression of lactation

Although bromocriptine and cabergoline are licensed to suppress lactation, they are **not** recommended for routine suppression (or for the relief of symptoms of postpartum pain and engorgement) that can be adequately treated with simple analgesics and breast support. If a dopamine-receptor agonist is required, cabergoline is preferred. Quinagolide is not licensed for the suppression of lactation.

Quinagolide

05-Jan-2024

- **DRUG ACTION** Quinagolide is a non-ergot dopamine D_2 agonist.

- **INDICATIONS AND DOSE**

Hyperprolactinaemia
▸ BY MOUTH
▸ Adult: Initially 25 micrograms once daily for 3 days, dose to be taken at bedtime, increased in steps of 25 micrograms every 3 days; usual dose 75–150 micrograms daily, for doses higher than 300 micrograms daily increase in steps of 75–150 micrograms at intervals of not less than 4 weeks

- **UNLICENSED USE** Not licensed for the suppression of lactation.

> **IMPORTANT SAFETY INFORMATION**
> IMPULSE CONTROL DISORDERS
> Treatment with dopamine-receptor agonists is associated with impulse control disorders, including pathological gambling, binge eating, and hypersexuality. Patients and their carers should be informed about the risk of impulse control disorders.

- **CAUTIONS** Acute porphyrias p. 1202 · history of psychotic illness · history of serious mental disorders

CAUTIONS, FURTHER INFORMATION
▸ Hyperprolactinemic patients In hyperprolactinaemic patients, the source of the hyperprolactinaemia should be established (i.e. exclude pituitary tumour before treatment).

- **INTERACTIONS** → Appendix 1: dopamine receptor agonists

- **SIDE-EFFECTS**
▸ **Common or very common** Abdominal pain · appetite decreased · constipation · diarrhoea · dizziness · fatigue · flushing · headache · hypotension · insomnia · nasal congestion · nausea · oedema · syncope · vomiting
▸ **Rare or very rare** Acute psychosis · drowsiness

- **CONCEPTION AND CONTRACEPTION** Advise non-hormonal contraception if pregnancy not desired.

- **PREGNANCY** Discontinue when pregnancy confirmed unless medical reason for continuing (specialist advice needed).

- **BREAST FEEDING** Suppresses lactation.

- **HEPATIC IMPAIRMENT** Manufacturer advises avoid (no information available).

- **RENAL IMPAIRMENT** EvGr Avoid (no information available). ⟨M⟩

- **MONITORING REQUIREMENTS** Monitor blood pressure for a few days after starting treatment and following dosage increase.

- **PATIENT AND CARER ADVICE**
Driving and skilled tasks
Sudden onset of sleep Excessive daytime sleepiness and sudden onset of sleep can occur with dopamine-receptor agonists.

Patients starting treatment with these drugs should be warned of the risk and of the need to exercise caution when driving or operating machinery. Those who have experienced excessive sedation or sudden onset of sleep should refrain from driving or operating machines until these effects have stopped occurring.

Management of excessive daytime sleepiness should focus on the identification of an underlying cause, such as depression or concomitant medication. Patients should be counselled on improving sleep behaviour.
Hypotensive reactions Hypotensive reactions can be disturbing in some patients during the first few days of treatment with dopamine-receptor agonists, particular care should be exercised when driving or operating machinery.

- **MEDICINAL FORMS** There can be variation in the licensing of different medicines containing the same drug.
Oral tablet
CAUTIONARY AND ADVISORY LABELS 10, 21
▸ **Quinagolide (Non-proprietary)**
Quinagolide (as Quinagolide hydrochloride)
25 microgram Quinagolide 25microgram tablets | 3 tablet PoM ⟨S⟩
Quinagolide (as Quinagolide hydrochloride)
50 microgram Quinagolide 50microgram tablets | 3 tablet PoM ⟨S⟩
Quinagolide (as Quinagolide hydrochloride)
75 microgram Quinagolide 75microgram tablets | 30 tablet PoM £156.90 DT = £156.90
▸ **Norprolac** (Ferring Pharmaceuticals Ltd)
Quinagolide (as Quinagolide hydrochloride)
25 microgram Norprolac 25microgram tablets | 3 tablet PoM ⟨S⟩
Quinagolide (as Quinagolide hydrochloride)
50 microgram Norprolac 50microgram tablets | 3 tablet PoM ⟨S⟩
Form unstated
▸ **Quinagolide (Non-proprietary)**
Quinagolide 50microgram tablets and Quinagolide 25microgram tablets | 6 tablet PoM £60.00 DT = £30.00

6 Gonadotrophin responsive conditions

Gonadotrophins

Gonadotrophin-affecting drugs

Danazol is licensed for the treatment of *endometriosis* and for the relief of severe pain and tenderness in *benign fibrocystic breast disease* where other measures have proved unsatisfactory. It may also be effective in the long-term management of *hereditary angioedema* [unlicensed indication].

Cetrorelix below and ganirelix below are luteinising hormone releasing hormone antagonists, which inhibit the release of gonadotrophins (luteinising hormone and follicle stimulating hormone). They are used in the treatment of infertility by assisted reproductive techniques.

Gonadorelin analogues

Gonadorelin analogues are used in the treatment of endometriosis, precocious puberty, infertility, male hypersexuality with severe sexual deviation, anaemia due to uterine fibroids (together with iron supplementation), breast cancer, prostate cancer and before intra-uterine surgery. Use of leuprorelin acetate and triptorelin for 3 to 4 months before surgery reduces the uterine volume, fibroid size and associated bleeding.

Breast pain (mastalgia)

Once any serious underlying cause for breast pain has been ruled out, most women will respond to reassurance and reduction in dietary fat; withdrawal of an oral contraceptive or of hormone replacement therapy may help to resolve the pain.

Mild, non-cyclical breast pain is treated with simple analgesics; moderate to severe pain, cyclical pain or symptoms that persist for longer than 6 months may require specific drug treatment.

Danazol is licensed for the relief of severe pain and tenderness in benign fibrocystic breast disease which has not responded to other treatment.

Tamoxifen p. 1085 may be a useful adjunct in the treatment of mastalgia [unlicensed indication] especially when symptoms can definitely be related to cyclic oestrogen production; it may be given on the days of the cycle when symptoms are predicted.

Treatment for breast pain should be reviewed after 6 months and continued if necessary. Symptoms recur in about 50% of women within 2 years of withdrawal of therapy but may be less severe.

PITUITARY AND HYPOTHALAMIC HORMONES AND ANALOGUES > ANTI-GONADOTROPHIN-RELEASING HORMONES

Cetrorelix

22-Apr-2021

● **INDICATIONS AND DOSE**

Adjunct in the treatment of female infertility (initiated under specialist supervision)

▸ BY SUBCUTANEOUS INJECTION

▸ Adult (female): 250 micrograms once daily, dose to be administered in the morning, starting on day 5 or 6 of ovarian stimulation with gonadotrophins (or each evening starting on day 5 of ovarian stimulation), continue throughout administration of gonadotrophin including day of ovulation induction (or evening before ovulation induction), dose to be injected into the lower abdominal wall.

● **SIDE-EFFECTS**

▸ **Common or very common** Ovarian hyperstimulation syndrome

▸ **Uncommon** Headache · hypersensitivity · nausea

● **PREGNANCY** Avoid in confirmed pregnancy.

● **BREAST FEEDING** Avoid.

● **HEPATIC IMPAIRMENT** Manufacturer advises use with caution—no information available.

● **RENAL IMPAIRMENT** [EvGr] Use with caution in mild to moderate impairment; avoid in severe impairment (no information available). ⟨M⟩

● **MEDICINAL FORMS** There can be variation in the licensing of different medicines containing the same drug.

Powder and solvent for solution for injection

▸ **Cetrotide** (Merck Serono Ltd)
Cetrorelix (as Cetrorelix acetate) 250 microgram Cetrotide 250microgram powder and solvent for solution for injection vials | 1 vial [PoM] £27.13 DT = £27.13

Ganirelix

22-Apr-2021

● **INDICATIONS AND DOSE**

Adjunct in the treatment of female infertility (initiated under specialist supervision)

▸ BY SUBCUTANEOUS INJECTION

▸ Adult: 250 micrograms once daily, dose to be administered in the morning (or each afternoon) starting on day 5 or day 6 of ovarian stimulation with gonadotrophins, continue throughout administration of gonadotrophins including day of ovulation induction (if administering in afternoon, give last dose in afternoon before ovulation induction), dose to be injected preferably into the upper leg (rotate injection sites to prevent lipoatrophy)

● **SIDE-EFFECTS**

▸ **Common or very common** Skin reactions

▸ **Uncommon** Headache · malaise · nausea

▸ **Rare or very rare** Dyspnoea · facial swelling · hypersensitivity

▸ **Frequency not known** Abdominal distension · ovarian hyperstimulation syndrome · pelvic pain

● **PREGNANCY** Avoid in confirmed pregnancy—toxicity in *animal* studies.

● **BREAST FEEDING** Avoid—no information available.

● **HEPATIC IMPAIRMENT** Manufacturer advises avoid in moderate to severe impairment (no information available).

● **RENAL IMPAIRMENT** [EvGr] Avoid in moderate to severe renal impairment (no information available). ⟨M⟩

● **MEDICINAL FORMS** There can be variation in the licensing of different medicines containing the same drug.

Solution for injection

▸ **Ganirelix** (Non-proprietary)
Ganirelix 500 microgram per 1 ml Ganirelix 250micrograms/0.5ml solution for injection pre-filled syringes | 1 pre-filled disposable injection [PoM] £27.13 (Hospital only)

▸ **Fyremadel** (Ferring Pharmaceuticals Ltd)
Ganirelix 500 microgram per 1 ml Fyremadel 250micrograms/0.5ml solution for injection pre-filled syringes | 1 pre-filled disposable injection [PoM] £19.35 (Hospital only) | 5 pre-filled disposable injection [PoM] £96.75 (Hospital only)

▸ **Ovamex** (Theramex HQ UK Ltd)
Ganirelix 500 microgram per 1 ml Ovamex 250micrograms/0.5ml solution for injection pre-filled syringes | 1 pre-filled disposable injection [PoM] £19.35 (Hospital only)

Linzagolix
26-Nov-2024

- **DRUG ACTION** Linzagolix is a non-peptide gonadotrophin-releasing hormone (GnRH) receptor antagonist that competitively binds to GnRH receptors in the pituitary gland, thereby reducing production of oestrogen and progesterone.

- **INDICATIONS AND DOSE**

  Moderate to severe uterine fibroids [in combination with add-back hormone replacement therapy] (under expert supervision)
  - BY MOUTH
  - Adult 18–56 years: 100–200 mg once daily, to be taken in combination with *estradiol* 1 mg and *norethisterone* 500 micrograms once daily, dose to be started preferably in the first week of the menstrual cycle

  Moderate to severe uterine fibroids [without add-back hormone replacement therapy] (under expert supervision)
  - BY MOUTH
  - Adult 18–56 years: 100 mg once daily, dose to be started preferably in the first week of the menstrual cycle, alternatively 200 mg once daily for maximum duration of 6 months, to be given for reduction of uterine and fibroid volume, dose to be started preferably in the first week of the menstrual cycle

- **CONTRA-INDICATIONS** Genital bleeding of unknown cause · osteoporosis

- **CAUTIONS** Cardiovascular disease · history of depression and/or suicidal ideation (discontinue if severe depression recurs) · risk factors for osteoporosis (dual X-ray absorptiometry (DXA) scan recommended before starting) · risk factors for QT-interval prolongation

- **INTERACTIONS** → Appendix 1: linzagolix

- **SIDE-EFFECTS**
  - **Common or very common** Anxiety · arthralgia · asthenia · constipation · depression · haemorrhage · headache · hot flush · libido decreased · menstrual cycle irregularities · mood altered · nausea · pelvic pain · sweat changes · vomiting · vulvovaginal dryness
  - **Uncommon** Abdominal pain upper · hypertension

- **CONCEPTION AND CONTRACEPTION** [EvGr] Linzagolix therapy does **not** provide contraception, however it may change menstrual bleeding patterns (e.g. reduction in blood loss often resulting in amenorrhoea) and reduce the ability to recognise the occurrence of a pregnancy. Hormonal contraception must be stopped prior to beginning treatment and pregnancy excluded. Females of childbearing potential should use effective non-hormonal contraception during treatment. ◈

- **PREGNANCY** [EvGr] Avoid (embryotoxic in *animal* studies). ◈

- **BREAST FEEDING** [EvGr] Avoid (present in milk in *animal* studies). ◈

- **HEPATIC IMPAIRMENT** [EvGr] Caution in patients with a history of abnormal hepatic function (no information available); avoid in severe impairment (risk of increased exposure). ◈

- **RENAL IMPAIRMENT** [EvGr] Caution in mild impairment (risk of increased exposure); avoid in moderate to severe impairment. ◈

- **MONITORING REQUIREMENTS** [EvGr] A dual X-ray absorptiometry (DXA) scan is recommended after 1 year of treatment. Thereafter, bone mineral density (BMD) should be assessed according to individual risk and previous BMD assessment in patients taking linzagolix in combination with add-back hormone replacement therapy, and annually in those taking linzagolix without add-back hormone replacement therapy. ◈

- **PATIENT AND CARER ADVICE** Patients should be advised to seek medical attention if any signs or symptoms of liver injury occur.

- **NATIONAL FUNDING/ACCESS DECISIONS** For full details see funding body website
  NICE decisions
  - Linzagolix for treating moderate to severe symptoms of uterine fibroids (August 2024) NICE TA996 Recommended with restrictions
  Scottish Medicines Consortium (SMC) decisions
  - Linzagolix (*Yselty*®) for the treatment of moderate to severe symptoms of uterine fibroids in adult women of reproductive age (November 2024) SMC No. SMC2631 Recommended with restrictions

- **MEDICINAL FORMS** There can be variation in the licensing of different medicines containing the same drug.
  Oral tablet
  - **Yselty** (Theramex HQ UK Ltd) ▼
    Linzagolix (as Linzagolix choline) 100 mg Yselty 100mg tablets | 28 tablet [PoM] £80.00
    Linzagolix (as Linzagolix choline) 200 mg Yselty 200mg tablets | 28 tablet [PoM] £80.00

Relugolix with estradiol and norethisterone acetate
25-Apr-2025

The properties listed below are those particular to the combination only. For the properties of the components please consider, estradiol p. 870, norethisterone p. 878.

- **DRUG ACTION** Relugolix is a non-peptide gonadotrophin-releasing hormone (GnRH) receptor antagonist that prevents follicular growth and development, thereby reducing production of oestrogen and progesterone. Relugolix is combined with the oestrogen estradiol to reduce symptoms related to lowered levels of oestrogen, and the progestogen norethisterone to counteract estradiol-induced endometrial hyperplasia.

- **INDICATIONS AND DOSE**

  Moderate to severe uterine fibroids (under expert supervision) | Endometriosis (under expert supervision)
  - BY MOUTH
  - Adult: 1 tablet once daily, dose to be taken at around the same time each day, starting within 5 days of the onset of menstrual bleeding, consider discontinuing treatment when patient enters menopause

- **CONTRA-INDICATIONS** Osteoporosis

- **CAUTIONS** History of depression (discontinue if severe depression recurs) · risk factors for osteoporosis (dual X-ray absorptiometry (DXA) scan recommended before starting)

- **INTERACTIONS** → Appendix 1: estradiol · norethisterone · relugolix

- **SIDE-EFFECTS**
  - **Common or very common** Alopecia · breast cyst · dyspepsia · hot flush · irritability · libido decreased · menstrual cycle irregularities · sweat changes · uterine haemorrhage
  - **Uncommon** Uterine myoma expulsion
  - **Frequency not known** Arterial thromboembolism · bone loss · uterine leiomyoma prolapse

- **CONCEPTION AND CONTRACEPTION** [EvGr] *Ryeqo*® inhibits ovulation and provides adequate contraception when used for at least 1 month at the recommended dose. Effective non-hormonal contraception is recommended for the first month after initiation of treatment and for 7 days following 2 or more consecutive missed doses. Patients should not take other hormonal contraceptives while being treated with *Ryeqo*®. Ovulation returns rapidly after discontinuing *Ryeqo*®. An alternative method of

contraception should start immediately after discontinuing treatment. ⓜ
- PREGNANCY [EvGr] Avoid—relugolix showed embryotoxicity in *animal* studies. ⓜ
- BREAST FEEDING [EvGr] Avoid during treatment and for 2 weeks following last treatment—relugolix present in milk in *animal* studies. ⓜ
- MONITORING REQUIREMENTS [EvGr] A dual X-ray absorptiometry (DXA) scan is recommended after 1 year of treatment. ⓜ
- PATIENT AND CARER ADVICE Advise patients to contact their doctor if they experience mood changes and depressive symptoms during treatment.
- NATIONAL FUNDING/ACCESS DECISIONS For full details see funding body website

NICE decisions
▸ Relugolix–estradiol–norethisterone acetate for treating moderate to severe symptoms of uterine fibroids (October 2022) NICE TA832 Recommended
▸ Relugolix–estradiol–norethisterone for treating symptoms of endometriosis (April 2025) NICE TA1057 Recommended

Scottish Medicines Consortium (SMC) decisions
▸ Relugolix with estradiol and norethisterone acetate tablets (*Ryeqo*®) for the treatment of moderate to severe symptoms of uterine fibroids in adult women of reproductive age (June 2022) SMC No. SMC2442 Recommended with restrictions
▸ Relugolix with estradiol and norethisterone acetate tablets (*Ryeqo*®) in adult women of reproductive age for symptomatic treatment of endometriosis in women with a history of previous medical or surgical treatment for their endometriosis (January 2025) SMC No. SMC2666 Recommended

- MEDICINAL FORMS There can be variation in the licensing of different medicines containing the same drug.
  Oral tablet
  ▸ Ryeqo (Gedeon Richter (UK) Ltd) ▼
    Norethisterone acetate 500 microgram, Estradiol (as Estradiol hemihydrate) 1 mg, Relugolix 40 mg Ryeqo 40mg/1mg/0.5mg tablets | 28 tablet [PoM] £72.00 | 84 tablet [PoM] £216.00

PITUITARY AND HYPOTHALAMIC HORMONES AND ANALOGUES ❭ GONADOTROPHIN-RELEASING HORMONES

Buserelin

04-Sep-2020

- DRUG ACTION Administration of gonadorelin analogues produces an initial phase of stimulation; continued administration is followed by down-regulation of gonadotrophin-releasing hormone receptors, thereby reducing the release of gonadotrophins (follicle stimulating hormone and luteinising hormone) which in turn leads to inhibition of androgen and oestrogen production.

- INDICATIONS AND DOSE
Endometriosis
▸ BY INTRANASAL ADMINISTRATION
▸ Adult: 300 micrograms 3 times a day maximum duration of treatment 6 months (do not repeat), to be started on days 1 or 2 of menstruation; administer one 150 microgram spray into each nostril

Pituitary desensitisation before induction of ovulation by gonadotrophins for in vitro fertilisation (under expert supervision)
▸ BY SUBCUTANEOUS INJECTION
▸ Adult: 200–500 micrograms once daily, increased if necessary up to 500 micrograms twice daily, starting in early follicular phase (day 1) or, after exclusion of pregnancy, in midluteal phase (day 21) and continued

until down-regulation achieved (usually 1–3 weeks) then maintained during gonadotrophin administration (stopping gonadotrophin and buserelin on administration of chorionic gonadotrophin at appropriate stage of follicular development)
▸ BY INTRANASAL ADMINISTRATION
▸ Adult: 150–300 micrograms 4 times a day, (150 micrograms equivalent to one spray), to be administered during waking hours. Start in early follicular phase (day 1) or, after exclusion of pregnancy, in the midluteal phase (day 21) and continued until down-regulation achieved (usually about 2–3 weeks) then maintained during gonadotrophin administration (stopping gonadotrophin and buserelin on administration of chorionic gonadotrophin at appropriate stage of follicular development)

Advanced prostate cancer
▸ INITIALLY BY SUBCUTANEOUS INJECTION
▸ Adult: 500 micrograms every 8 hours for 7 days, then (by intranasal administration) 200 micrograms 6 times a day, (a single 100 microgram spray to be administered into each nostril)

- CONTRA-INDICATIONS
▸ When used for Endometriosis Undiagnosed vaginal bleeding · use longer than 6 months (do not repeat)
▸ When used for Pituitary desensitisation Undiagnosed vaginal bleeding

- CAUTIONS Depression · diabetes · hypertension · patients with metabolic bone disease (decrease in bone mineral density can occur) · polycystic ovarian disease

- SIDE-EFFECTS
GENERAL SIDE-EFFECTS
▸ **Common or very common** Depression · mood altered
▸ **Rare or very rare** Auditory disorder · hypotension · leucopenia · pituitary tumour benign · thrombocytopenia · tinnitus
▸ **Frequency not known** Alopecia · anxiety · appetite change · breast abnormalities · broken nails · concentration impaired · constipation · diarrhoea · dizziness · drowsiness · dry eye · dysuria · embolism and thrombosis · fatigue · feeling of pressure behind the eyes · follicle recruitment increased · galactorrhoea · gastrointestinal discomfort · gynaecomastia · hair changes · headache · hot flush · hydronephrosis · hyperhidrosis · increased risk of fracture · lymphostasis · memory loss · menopausal symptoms · menstrual cycle irregularities · muscle weakness in legs · musculoskeletal discomfort · nausea · oedema · osteoporosis · ovarian and fallopian tube disorders · pain · painful sexual intercourse · palpitations · paraesthesia · QT interval prolongation · sexual dysfunction · shock · skin reactions · sleep disorder · testicular atrophy · thirst · tumour activation temporary · uterine leiomyoma degeneration · vision disorders · vomiting · vulvovaginal disorders · weight changes

SPECIFIC SIDE-EFFECTS
▸ With intranasal use Altered smell sensation · epistaxis · hoarseness · nasal irritation · taste altered

SIDE-EFFECTS, FURTHER INFORMATION During the initial stage (1–2 weeks) increased production of testosterone may be associated with progression of prostate cancer. In susceptible patients this tumour 'flare' may cause spinal cord compression, ureteric obstruction or increased bone pain.

- CONCEPTION AND CONTRACEPTION Non-hormonal, barrier methods of contraception should be used during entire treatment period. Pregnancy should be excluded before treatment, the first injection should be given during menstruation or shortly afterwards or use barrier contraception for 1 month beforehand.

- **PREGNANCY** Avoid.
- **BREAST FEEDING** Avoid.
- **DIRECTIONS FOR ADMINISTRATION**
▶ With intranasal use Manufacturer advises avoid use of nasal decongestants before and for at least 30 minutes after treatment.
▶ With subcutaneous use Rotate injection site to prevent atrophy and nodule formation.
- **PATIENT AND CARER ADVICE** Patients or carers should be given advice on how to administer buserelin nasal spray.

- **MEDICINAL FORMS** There can be variation in the licensing of different medicines containing the same drug.

  Solution for injection
  ▶ Buserelin (Non-proprietary)
  Buserelin (as Buserelin acetate) 1 mg per 1 ml Buserelin 5.5mg/5.5ml solution for injection vials | 2 vial [PoM] £43.00 DT = £34.37
  ▶ Suprefact (Neon Healthcare Ltd)
  Buserelin (as Buserelin acetate) 1 mg per 1 ml Suprefact 5.5mg/5.5ml solution for injection vials | 2 vial [PoM] £34.37 DT = £34.37

Goserelin

16-Jul-2024

- **DRUG ACTION** Administration of gonadorelin analogues produces an initial phase of stimulation; continued administration is followed by down-regulation of gonadotrophin-releasing hormone receptors, thereby reducing the release of gonadotrophins (follicle stimulating hormone and luteinising hormone) which in turn leads to inhibition of androgen and oestrogen production.

- **INDICATIONS AND DOSE**

  ZOLADEX LA ®

  Locally advanced prostate cancer as an alternative to surgical castration | Adjuvant treatment to radiotherapy or radical prostatectomy in patients with high-risk localised or locally advanced prostate cancer | Neoadjuvant treatment prior to radiotherapy in patients with high-risk localised or locally advanced prostate cancer | Metastatic prostate cancer
  ▶ BY SUBCUTANEOUS INJECTION
  ▶ Adult: 10.8 mg every 12 weeks, to be administered into the anterior abdominal wall

  ZOLADEX ®

  Locally advanced prostate cancer as an alternative to surgical castration | Adjuvant treatment to radiotherapy or radical prostatectomy in patients with high-risk localised or locally advanced prostate cancer | Neoadjuvant treatment prior to radiotherapy in patients with high-risk localised or locally advanced prostate cancer | Metastatic prostate cancer | Advanced breast cancer | Oestrogen-receptor-positive early breast cancer
  ▶ BY SUBCUTANEOUS INJECTION
  ▶ Adult: 3.6 mg every 28 days, to be administered into the anterior abdominal wall

  Endometriosis
  ▶ BY SUBCUTANEOUS INJECTION
  ▶ Adult: 3.6 mg every 28 days maximum duration of treatment 6 months (do not repeat), to be administered into the anterior abdominal wall

  Endometrial thinning before intra-uterine surgery
  ▶ BY SUBCUTANEOUS INJECTION
  ▶ Adult: 3.6 mg, dose may be repeated after 28 days if uterus is large or to allow flexible surgical timing, to be administered into the anterior abdominal wall

  Before surgery in women who have anaemia due to uterine fibroids
  ▶ BY SUBCUTANEOUS INJECTION
  ▶ Adult: 3.6 mg every 28 days maximum duration of treatment 3 months, to be given with supplementary iron, to be administered into the anterior abdominal wall

  Pituitary desensitisation before induction of ovulation by gonadotrophins for in vitro fertilisation (after exclusion of pregnancy) (under expert supervision)
  ▶ BY SUBCUTANEOUS INJECTION
  ▶ Adult: 3.6 mg, dose given to achieve pituitary down-regulation (usually 1–3 weeks) then gonadotrophin is administered (stopping gonadotrophin on administration of chorionic gonadotrophin at appropriate stage of follicular development), to be administered into the anterior abdominal wall

- **CONTRA-INDICATIONS** Undiagnosed vaginal bleeding · use longer than 6 months in endometriosis (do not repeat)
- **CAUTIONS** Depression · diabetes · hypertension · patients with metabolic bone disease (decrease in bone mineral density can occur) · polycystic ovarian disease · risk of spinal cord compression in men · risk of ureteric obstruction in men
- **SIDE-EFFECTS**
▶ **Common or very common** Alopecia · arthralgia · bone pain · breast abnormalities · depression · glucose tolerance impaired · gynaecomastia · headache · heart failure · hot flush · hyperhidrosis · mood altered · myocardial infarction · neoplasm complications · paraesthesia · sexual dysfunction · skin reactions · spinal cord compression · vulvovaginal disorders · weight increased
▶ **Uncommon** Hypercalcaemia (in women) · ureteral obstruction
▶ **Rare or very rare** Ovarian and fallopian tube disorders · pituitary haemorrhage · pituitary tumour · psychotic disorder
▶ **Frequency not known** Abdominal cramps · body hair change · constipation · diarrhoea · fatigue · hepatic function abnormal · interstitial pneumonia · muscle complaints · nausea · nervousness · peripheral oedema (when used for gynaecological conditions) · premature menopause · pulmonary embolism · QT interval prolongation · sleep disorder · uterine leiomyoma degeneration · voice alteration · vomiting · vulvovaginal infection · withdrawal bleed

  SIDE-EFFECTS, FURTHER INFORMATION Tumour flare can occur when androgen deprivation therapy is initiated.

- **CONCEPTION AND CONTRACEPTION** Non-hormonal, barrier methods of contraception should be used during entire treatment period. Pregnancy should be excluded before treatment, the first injection should be given during menstruation or shortly afterwards or use barrier contraception for 1 month beforehand.
- **PREGNANCY** Avoid.
- **BREAST FEEDING** Avoid.
- **MONITORING REQUIREMENTS** Men at risk of tumour 'flare' should be monitored closely during the first month of therapy for prostate cancer.
- **DIRECTIONS FOR ADMINISTRATION** Rotate injection site to prevent atrophy and nodule formation.

- **MEDICINAL FORMS** There can be variation in the licensing of different medicines containing the same drug.

  Prolonged-release subcutaneous implant
  ▶ Zoladex (AstraZeneca UK Ltd)
  Goserelin (as Goserelin acetate) 3.6 mg Zoladex 3.6mg implant SafeSystem pre-filled syringes | 1 pre-filled disposable injection [PoM] £70.00 DT = £70.00

› **Zoladex LA** (AstraZeneca UK Ltd)
Goserelin (as Goserelin acetate) **10.8 mg** Zoladex LA 10.8mg
implant SafeSystem pre-filled syringes | 1 pre-filled disposable
injection [PoM] £235.00 DT = £235.00

Leuprorelin acetate

14-Jan-2025

● **DRUG ACTION** Administration of gonadorelin analogues
produces an initial phase of stimulation; continued
administration is followed by down-regulation of
gonadotrophin-releasing hormone receptors, thereby
reducing the release of gonadotrophins (follicle
stimulating hormone and luteinising hormone) which in
turn leads to inhibition of androgen and oestrogen
production.

● **INDICATIONS AND DOSE**

PROSTAP 3 DCS ®

Prostate cancer (specialist use only)
▶ BY SUBCUTANEOUS INJECTION
▶ Adult: 11.25 mg every 3 months

Endometriosis (specialist use only)
▶ BY INTRAMUSCULAR INJECTION
▶ Adult: 11.25 mg every 3 months for maximum duration
  of 6 months (not to be repeated), to be started during
  first 5 days of menstrual cycle

**Pre- and perimenopausal breast cancer (specialist use
only)**
▶ BY SUBCUTANEOUS INJECTION
▶ Adult: 11.25 mg every 3 months, for further
  information on use with adjuvant treatments, consult
  product literature

PROSTAP SR DCS ®

Prostate cancer (specialist use only)
▶ BY SUBCUTANEOUS INJECTION, OR BY INTRAMUSCULAR
  INJECTION
▶ Adult: 3.75 mg every month

Endometriosis (specialist use only)
▶ BY SUBCUTANEOUS INJECTION, OR BY INTRAMUSCULAR
  INJECTION
▶ Adult: 3.75 mg every month for maximum duration of
  6 months (not to be repeated), to be started during first
  5 days of menstrual cycle

**Endometrial thinning before intra-uterine surgery
(specialist use only)**
▶ BY SUBCUTANEOUS INJECTION, OR BY INTRAMUSCULAR
  INJECTION
▶ Adult: 3.75 mg for 1 dose, dose to be given as a single
  dose between day 3 and 5 of menstrual cycle,
  5–6 weeks before surgery

**Reduction of size of uterine fibroids and of associated
bleeding before surgery (specialist use only)**
▶ BY SUBCUTANEOUS INJECTION, OR BY INTRAMUSCULAR
  INJECTION
▶ Adult: 3.75 mg every month usually for 3–4 months
  (maximum 6 months)

Preservation of ovarian function (specialist use only)
▶ BY SUBCUTANEOUS INJECTION, OR BY INTRAMUSCULAR
  INJECTION
▶ Adult: Initially 3.75 mg as a single dose 2 weeks before
  starting chemotherapy, followed by 3.75 mg every
  month for the duration of chemotherapy treatment

**Pre- and perimenopausal breast cancer (specialist use
only)**
▶ BY SUBCUTANEOUS INJECTION
▶ Adult: 3.75 mg every month, for further information on
  use with adjuvant treatments, consult product
  literature

STALADEX ® 11.25MG

Prostate cancer (specialist use only)
▶ BY SUBCUTANEOUS INJECTION
▶ Adult: 11.25 mg every 3 months

● **CONTRA-INDICATIONS**
PROSTAP 3 DCS ® Undiagnosed vaginal bleeding
PROSTAP SR DCS ® Undiagnosed vaginal bleeding

● **CAUTIONS** Diabetes · family history of osteoporosis ·
patients with metabolic bone disease (decrease in bone
mineral density can occur) · risk of spinal cord
compression in men with prostate cancer · risk of ureteric
obstruction in men with prostate cancer

● **SIDE-EFFECTS**
▶ **Common or very common** Appetite decreased · arthralgia ·
  bone pain · breast abnormalities · depression · dizziness ·
  fatigue · gynaecomastia · headache · hepatic disorders · hot
  flush · hyperhidrosis · insomnia · mood altered · muscle
  weakness · nausea · paraesthesia · peripheral oedema ·
  sexual dysfunction · testicular atrophy · vulvovaginal
  dryness · weight change
▶ **Uncommon** Alopecia · diarrhoea · fever · myalgia ·
  palpitations · visual impairment · vomiting
▶ **Rare or very rare** Haemorrhage
▶ **Frequency not known** Anaemia · dyslipidaemia · glucose
  tolerance impaired · hypertension · hypotension ·
  idiopathic intracranial hypertension · insulin resistance ·
  interstitial lung disease · leucopenia · metabolic syndrome
  · osteoporosis · paralysis · pulmonary embolism · QT
  interval prolongation · seizure · severe cutaneous adverse
  reactions (SCARs) · skin reactions · spinal fracture ·
  thrombocytopenia · urinary tract obstruction ·
  vulvovaginal infection

SIDE-EFFECTS, FURTHER INFORMATION In prostate cancer,
during the initial stage (1–2 weeks) increased production
of testosterone may be associated with progression of
prostate cancer. In susceptible patients this tumour 'flare'
may cause spinal cord compression, ureteric obstruction or
increased bone pain.

● **CONCEPTION AND CONTRACEPTION** Non-hormonal, barrier
methods of contraception should be used during entire
treatment period. Pregnancy should be excluded before
treatment, the first injection should be given during
menstruation or shortly afterwards or use barrier
contraception for 1 month beforehand.

● **PREGNANCY** Avoid—teratogenic in *animal* studies.

● **BREAST FEEDING** Avoid.

● **MONITORING REQUIREMENTS**
▶ Monitor liver function.
▶ Monitor prostate-specific antigen serum levels.

● **DIRECTIONS FOR ADMINISTRATION** Rotate injection site to
prevent atrophy and nodule formation.
STALADEX ® 11.25MG To be administered under the skin of
the abdomen.

● **PATIENT AND CARER ADVICE** Patients and carers should be
counselled on the signs and symptoms of idiopathic
intracranial hypertension (such as severe or recurrent
headache, vision disturbances and tinnitus)—consider
discontinuing treatment if these occur. Patients and carers
should be informed of the increased risk of depression
during treatment.

PROSTAP 3 DCS ® Patients and carers should be counselled
on the signs and symptoms of severe cutaneous adverse
reactions (SCARs) when starting treatment—treatment
should be immediately discontinued if these occur.

PROSTAP SR DCS ® Patients and carers should be
counselled on the signs and symptoms of severe cutaneous
adverse reactions (SCARs) when starting treatment—

treatment should be immediately discontinued if these occur.

- **NATIONAL FUNDING/ACCESS DECISIONS**
  For full details see funding body website
  Scottish Medicines Consortium (SMC) decisions
  - Leuprorelin acetate (*Prostap*® DCS) as adjuvant treatment in combination with tamoxifen or an aromatase inhibitor, of endocrine responsive early stage breast cancer in pre- and perimenopausal women at higher risk of disease recurrence (February 2021) SMC No. SMC2319 Recommended
  - Leuprorelin acetate (*Prostap*® DCS) as treatment in pre- and perimenopausal women with advanced breast cancer suitable for hormonal manipulation (February 2021) SMC No. SMC2320 Recommended

- **MEDICINAL FORMS** There can be variation in the licensing of different medicines containing the same drug.
  Prolonged-release subcutaneous implant
  - **Staladex** (Aspire Pharma Ltd)
    Leuprorelin acetate 11.25 mg Staladex 11.25mg implant pre-filled syringes | 1 pre-filled disposable injection [PoM] £206.00 DT = £206.00

  Powder and solvent for prolonged-release suspension for inj
  EXCIPIENTS: May contain Polysorbates
  - **Prostap 3 DCS** (Takeda UK Ltd)
    Leuprorelin acetate 11.25 mg Prostap 3 DCS 11.25mg powder and solvent for prolonged-release suspension for injection pre-filled syringes | 1 pre-filled disposable injection [PoM] £225.72 DT = £225.72
  - **Prostap SR DCS** (Takeda UK Ltd)
    Leuprorelin acetate 3.75 mg Prostap SR DCS 3.75mg powder and solvent for prolonged-release suspension for injection pre-filled syringes | 1 pre-filled disposable injection [PoM] £75.24 DT = £75.24

Nafarelin
04-Aug-2020

- **DRUG ACTION** Administration of gonadorelin analogues produces an initial phase of stimulation; continued administration is followed by down-regulation of gonadotrophin-releasing hormone receptors, thereby reducing the release of gonadotrophins (follicle stimulating hormone and luteinising hormone) which in turn leads to inhibition of androgen and oestrogen production.

- **INDICATIONS AND DOSE**
  Endometriosis
  - BY INTRANASAL ADMINISTRATION
  - Adult (female): 200 micrograms twice daily for maximum 6 months (do not repeat), one spray in one nostril in the morning, and one spray in the other nostril in the evening (starting on days 2–4 of menstruation).

  Pituitary desensitisation before induction of ovulation by gonadotrophins for in vitro fertilisation (under expert supervision)
  - BY INTRANASAL ADMINISTRATION
  - Adult: 400 micrograms twice daily, one spray in each nostril, to be started in early follicular phase (day 2) or, after exclusion of pregnancy, in midluteal phase (day 21) and continued until down regulation achieved (usually within 4 weeks) then maintained (usually for 8–12 days) during gonadotrophin administration (stopping gonadotrophin and nafarelin on administration of chorionic gonadotrophin at follicular maturity), discontinue if down-regulation not achieved within 12 weeks

- **CONTRA-INDICATIONS** Undiagnosed vaginal bleeding · use longer than 6 months in the treatment of endometriosis (do not repeat)

- **CAUTIONS** Patients with metabolic bone disease (decrease in bone mineral density can occur)

- **SIDE-EFFECTS**
  - **Common or very common** Artificial menopause · breast abnormalities · chest pain · depression · dyspnoea · emotional lability · headaches · hirsutism · hot flush · hypersensitivity · hypertension · hypotension · insomnia · myalgia · oedema · oestrogen deficiency · paraesthesia · rhinitis · seborrhoea · sexual dysfunction · skin reactions · uterine haemorrhage · vulvovaginal dryness · weight changes
  - **Uncommon** Alopecia · arthralgia · ovarian cyst (may require discontinuation)
  - **Frequency not known** Ovarian hyperstimulation syndrome · palpitations · vision blurred

- **CONCEPTION AND CONTRACEPTION** Non-hormonal, barrier methods of contraception should be used during entire treatment period. Pregnancy should be excluded before treatment, the first dose should be given during menstruation or shortly afterwards or use barrier contraception for 1 month beforehand.

- **PREGNANCY** Avoid.

- **BREAST FEEDING** Avoid.

- **DIRECTIONS FOR ADMINISTRATION** Manufacturer advises avoid use of nasal decongestants before and for at least 30 minutes after treatment; repeat dose if sneezing occurs during or immediately after administration.

- **PATIENT AND CARER ADVICE** Patients or carers should be given advice on how to administer nafarelin nasal spray.

- **MEDICINAL FORMS** There can be variation in the licensing of different medicines containing the same drug.
  Spray
  CAUTIONARY AND ADVISORY LABELS 10
  - **Synarel** (Pfizer Ltd)
    Nafarelin (as Nafarelin acetate) 200 microgram per 1 dose Synarel 200micrograms/dose nasal spray | 60 dose [PoM] £52.43 DT = £52.43

Triptorelin
23-Jan-2025

- **DRUG ACTION** Administration of gonadorelin analogues produces an initial phase of stimulation; continued administration is followed by down-regulation of gonadotrophin-releasing hormone receptors, thereby reducing the release of gonadotrophins (follicle stimulating hormone and luteinising hormone) which in turn leads to inhibition of androgen and oestrogen production.

- **INDICATIONS AND DOSE**
  DECAPEPTYL® SR 11.25MG
  Advanced prostate cancer (specialist use only)
  - BY INTRAMUSCULAR INJECTION
  - Adult: 11.25 mg every 3 months
  Endometriosis
  - BY INTRAMUSCULAR INJECTION
  - Adult: 11.25 mg every 3 months for maximum 6 months (not to be repeated), to be started during first 5 days of menstrual cycle

  DECAPEPTYL® SR 22.5MG
  Advanced prostate cancer (specialist use only)
  - BY INTRAMUSCULAR INJECTION
  - Adult: 22.5 mg every 6 months

  DECAPEPTYL® SR 3MG
  Advanced prostate cancer (specialist use only)
  - BY INTRAMUSCULAR INJECTION
  - Adult: 3 mg every 4 weeks　　　　　　continued →

Endocrine system

6

Endometriosis
▶ BY INTRAMUSCULAR INJECTION
▶ Adult: 3 mg every 4 weeks maximum duration of 6 months (not to be repeated), to be started during first 5 days of menstrual cycle

Reduction in size of uterine fibroids
▶ BY INTRAMUSCULAR INJECTION
▶ Adult: 3 mg every 4 weeks for at least 3 months, maximum duration of treatment 6 months (not to be repeated), to be started during first 5 days of menstrual cycle

Premenopausal breast cancer [as combination therapy] (specialist use only)
▶ BY INTRAMUSCULAR INJECTION
▶ Adult: 3 mg every 4 weeks for up to 5 years, initiated 6–8 weeks before starting aromatase inhibitor—for further information, consult product literature

GONAPEPTYL DEPOT ®

Advanced prostate cancer
▶ BY SUBCUTANEOUS INJECTION, OR BY DEEP INTRAMUSCULAR INJECTION
▶ Adult: 3.75 mg every 4 weeks

Endometriosis | Reduction in size of uterine fibroids
▶ BY SUBCUTANEOUS INJECTION, OR BY DEEP INTRAMUSCULAR INJECTION
▶ Adult: 3.75 mg every 4 weeks maximum duration of 6 months (not to be repeated), to be started during first 5 days of menstrual cycle

SALVACYL ®

Male hypersexuality with severe sexual deviation
▶ BY INTRAMUSCULAR INJECTION
▶ Adult: 11.25 mg every 12 weeks

● **CONTRA-INDICATIONS** In endometriosis do not use for longer than 6 months (do not repeat) · undiagnosed vaginal bleeding

SALVACYL ® Severe osteoporosis

● **CAUTIONS**

GENERAL CAUTIONS History of depression · patients with metabolic bone disease (decrease in bone mineral density can occur)

SPECIFIC CAUTIONS
▶ When used for Breast cancer Risk factors for osteoporosis
▶ When used for Male hypersexuality with severe sexual deviation Risk factors for osteoporosis
▶ When used for Prostate cancer Risk factors for osteoporosis · risk of spinal cord compression in men · risk of ureteric obstruction in men

SALVACYL ® Increased risk of sensitivity to restored testosterone if treatment interrupted—consider administration of an anti-androgen before stopping treatment · transient increase in serum testosterone occurs on initiation—consider administration of an anti-androgen

● **SIDE-EFFECTS**

GENERAL SIDE-EFFECTS
▶ **Common or very common** Anxiety · asthenia · depression · diabetes mellitus · dizziness · dry mouth · embolism · gastrointestinal discomfort · gynaecomastia · haemorrhage · headache · hot flush · hyperhidrosis · hypersensitivity · hypertension · joint disorders · menstrual cycle irregularities · mood altered · muscle complaints · nausea · oedema · ovarian and fallopian tube disorders · pain · painful sexual intercourse · pelvic pain · sexual dysfunction · skin reactions · sleep disorders · weight changes
▶ **Uncommon** Alopecia · appetite abnormal · asthma exacerbated · chills · confusion · constipation · diarrhoea · drowsiness · dyspnoea · flatulence · gout · muscle weakness

· taste altered · testicular disorders · tinnitus · vertigo · vision disorders · vomiting
▶ **Rare or very rare** Abnormal sensation in eye · chest pain · difficulty standing · fever · hypotension · influenza like illness · musculoskeletal stiffness · nasopharyngitis · orthopnoea · osteoarthritis · QT interval prolongation
▶ **Frequency not known** Angioedema · malaise

SPECIFIC SIDE-EFFECTS
▶ **Common or very common**
▶ With intramuscular use Bone disorders · bone fracture · breast abnormalities · glucose tolerance impaired · hyperglycaemia · musculoskeletal disorder · seborrhoea · sensation abnormal · urinary disorders · vulvovaginal disorders
▶ With subcutaneous use Dysuria · vulvovaginal dryness
▶ **Uncommon**
▶ With intramuscular use Broken nails · central nervous system haemorrhage · cerebral ischaemia · concentration impaired · cystocele · dry eye · fluid retention · hirsutism · hyperlipidaemia · memory impairment · myocardial ischaemia · oral ulceration · palpitations · syncope · thrombocytosis · tremor
▶ With subcutaneous use Paraesthesia
▶ **Frequency not known**
▶ With subcutaneous use Bone disorder · breast pain · memory loss

SIDE-EFFECTS, FURTHER INFORMATION During the initial stage increased production of testosterone may be associated with progression of prostate cancer. In susceptible patients this tumour 'flare' may cause spinal cord compression, ureteric obstruction or increased pain.

● **CONCEPTION AND CONTRACEPTION** Non-hormonal, barrier methods of contraception should be used during entire treatment period. Pregnancy should be excluded before treatment, the first injection should be given during menstruation or shortly afterwards or use barrier contraception for 1 month beforehand.

● **PREGNANCY** Avoid.

● **BREAST FEEDING** Avoid.

● **MONITORING REQUIREMENTS**
▶ When used for Prostate cancer Men at risk of tumour 'flare' should be monitored closely during the first month of therapy.

● **DIRECTIONS FOR ADMINISTRATION** Rotate injection site to prevent atrophy and nodule formation.

● **PRESCRIBING AND DISPENSING INFORMATION**
DECAPEPTYL ® SR 11.25MG Each vial includes an overage to allow accurate administration of an 11.25 mg dose.
DECAPEPTYL ® SR 22.5MG Each vial includes an overage to allow accurate administration of a 22.5 mg dose.
DECAPEPTYL ® SR 3MG Each vial includes an overage to allow accurate administration of 3 mg dose.

● **NATIONAL FUNDING/ACCESS DECISIONS**
For full details see funding body website

Scottish Medicines Consortium (SMC) decisions
▶ Triptorelin (*Decapeptyl* ® *SR* 3 mg) as adjuvant treatment, in combination with tamoxifen or an aromatase inhibitor, of endocrine responsive early stage breast cancer in women at high risk of recurrence who are confirmed as premenopausal after completion of chemotherapy (October 2019) SMC No. SMC2186 Recommended

All Wales Medicines Strategy Group (AWMSG) decisions
▶ Triptorelin (*Decapeptyl* ® *SR*) as adjuvant treatment to radiotherapy in patients with high-risk localised or locally advanced prostate cancer and as neoadjuvant treatment prior to radiotherapy in patients with high-risk localised or locally advanced prostate cancer (March 2017) AWMSG No. 1658 Recommended

- **MEDICINAL FORMS** There can be variation in the licensing of different medicines containing the same drug.

  Powder and solvent for prolonged-release suspension for inj

  ▸ **Decapeptyl SR** (Ipsen Ltd)
    Triptorelin (as Triptorelin acetate) 3 mg Decapeptyl SR 3mg powder and solvent for suspension for injection vials | 1 vial [PoM] £69.00 DT = £69.00
    Triptorelin 11.25 mg Decapeptyl SR 11.25mg powder and solvent for suspension for injection vials | 1 vial [PoM] £207.00 DT = £207.00
    Triptorelin (as Triptorelin embonate) 22.5 mg Decapeptyl SR 22.5mg powder and solvent for suspension for injection vials | 1 vial [PoM] £414.00 DT = £414.00
  ▸ **Gonapeptyl Depot** (Ferring Pharmaceuticals Ltd)
    Triptorelin (as Triptorelin acetate) 3.75 mg Gonapeptyl Depot 3.75mg powder and solvent for suspension for injection pre-filled syringes | 1 pre-filled disposable injection [PoM] £81.69 DT = £81.69
  ▸ **Salvacyl** (Ipsen Ltd)
    Triptorelin 11.25 mg Salvacyl 11.25mg powder and solvent for prolonged-release suspension for injection vials | 1 vial [PoM] £248.00 DT = £207.00

7   Hypothalamic and anterior pituitary hormone related disorders

Hypothalamic and anterior pituitary hormones

17-Jun-2022

Anterior pituitary hormones

Corticotrophins

Tetracosactide below (tetracosactrin), an analogue of corticotropin (ACTH), is used to test adrenocortical function; failure of the plasma cortisol concentration to rise after administration of tetracosactide indicates adrenal insufficiency. For guidance on the management of adrenal insufficiency, see Adrenal insufficiency p. 781.

Both corticotropin and tetracosactide were formerly used as alternatives to corticosteroids in conditions such as Crohn's disease; their value was limited by the variable and unpredictable therapeutic response and by the waning of their effect with time.

Gonadotrophins

Follicle-stimulating hormone (FSH) and luteinising hormone (LH) together, or follicle-stimulating hormone alone (as in follitropin), are used in the treatment of infertility in women with proven hypopituitarism or who have not responded to clomifene citrate p. 881, or in superovulation treatment for assisted conception (such as *in vitro* fertilisation).

The gonadotrophins are also occasionally used in the treatment of hypogonadotrophic hypogonadism and associated oligospermia. There is no justification for their use in primary gonadal failure.

Growth hormone

Growth hormone is used to treat deficiency of the hormone in children and in adults. In children it is used in Prader-Willi syndrome, Turner syndrome, chronic renal insufficiency, short children considered small for gestational age at birth, and short stature homeobox-containing gene (SHOX) deficiency.

Growth hormone of human origin (HGH; somatotrophin) has been replaced by recombinant growth hormone of human sequence; somatropin p. 861 is licensed for use in adults and children, and somatrogon (a long-acting form) is licensed for growth hormone deficiency in children.

Mecasermin, a human insulin-like growth factor-I (rhIGF-I), is licensed to treat growth failure in children with severe primary insulin-like growth factor-I deficiency.

Hypothalamic hormones

Gonadorelin p. 856 when injected intravenously in normal subjects leads to a rapid rise in plasma concentrations of both luteinising hormone (LH) and follicle-stimulating hormone (FSH). It has not proved to be very helpful, however, in distinguishing hypothalamic from pituitary lesions. **Gonadorelin analogues** are indicated in endometriosis and infertility and in breast and prostate cancer.

7.1   Adrenocortical function testing

PITUITARY AND HYPOTHALAMIC HORMONES AND ANALOGUES ⟩ CORTICOTROPHINS

Tetracosactide

30-Sep-2022

(Tetracosactrin)

- **INDICATIONS AND DOSE**

  Diagnosis of adrenocortical insufficiency (diagnostic 30-minute test)
  ▸ BY INTRAVENOUS INJECTION, OR BY INTRAMUSCULAR INJECTION
  ▸ Adult: 250 micrograms for 1 dose

  Diagnosis of adrenocortical insufficiency (diagnostic 5-hour test)
  ▸ BY INTRAMUSCULAR INJECTION USING DEPOT INJECTION
  ▸ Adult: 1 mg for 1 dose

  Alternative to corticosteroids in conditions such as Crohn's disease or rheumatoid arthritis (formerly used but value was limited by the variable and unpredictable therapeutic response and by the waning of effect with time)
  ▸ BY INTRAMUSCULAR INJECTION USING DEPOT INJECTION
  ▸ Adult: Initially 1 mg daily, alternatively initially 1 mg every 12 hours, (in acute cases), then reduced to 1 mg every 2–3 days, followed by 1 mg once weekly, alternatively 500 micrograms every 2–3 days

- **CONTRA-INDICATIONS** Acute psychosis · adrenogenital syndrome · allergic disorders · asthma · Cushing's syndrome · infectious diseases · peptic ulcer · primary adrenocortical insufficiency · refractory heart failure

- **CAUTIONS** Active infectious diseases (should not be used unless adequate disease-specific therapy is being given) · active systemic diseases (should not be used unless adequate disease-specific therapy is being given) · diabetes mellitus · diverticulitis · history of asthma · history of atopic allergy · history of eczema · history of hayfever · history of hypersensitivity · hypertension · latent amoebiasis (may become activated) · latent tuberculosis (may become activated) · myasthenia gravis · ocular herpes simplex · osteoporosis · predisposition to thromboembolism · pscyhological disturbances may be triggered · recent intestinal anastomosis · reduced immune response (should not be used unless adequate disease-specific therapy is being given) · ulcerative colitis

  CAUTIONS, FURTHER INFORMATION
  ▸ Risk of anaphylaxis Should only be administered under medical supervision—consult product literature.
  ▸ Hypertension Patients already receiving medication for moderate to severe hypertension must have their dosage adjusted if treatment started.
  ▸ Diabetes mellitus Patients already receiving medication for diabetes mellitus must have their dosage adjusted if treatment started.

- **SIDE-EFFECTS** Abdominal distension · abscess · adrenocortical unresponsiveness · angioedema · appetite increased · bone fractures · congestive heart failure · Cushing's syndrome · diabetes mellitus exacerbated · dizziness · dyspnoea · electrolyte imbalance · exophthalmos · fluid retention · flushing · gastrointestinal disorders · glaucoma · growth retardation · haemorrhage · headache · healing impaired · hirsutism · hyperglycaemia · hyperhidrosis · hypersensitivity (may be more severe in patients susceptible to allergies, especially asthma) · hypertension · idiopathic intracranial hypertension exacerbated · increased risk of infection · leucocytosis · malaise · menstruation irregular · muscle weakness · myopathy · nausea · osteonecrosis · osteoporosis · pancreatitis · papilloedema · pituitary unresponsiveness · posterior subcapsular cataract · protein catabolism · psychiatric disorder · seizure · skin reactions · tendon rupture · thromboembolism · vasculitis necrotising · vertigo · vomiting · weight increased

- **ALLERGY AND CROSS-SENSITIVITY** [EvGr] Contra-indicated in patients with history of hypersensitivity to tetracosactide/corticotrophins or excipients. [M]

- **PREGNANCY** Avoid (but may be used diagnostically if essential).

- **BREAST FEEDING** Avoid (but may be used diagnostically if essential).

- **HEPATIC IMPAIRMENT** For *depot injection*, manufacturer advises caution in cirrhosis (may enhance effect of tetracosactide therapy).

- **RENAL IMPAIRMENT** [EvGr] Use with caution in renal failure. [M]

- **EFFECT ON LABORATORY TESTS** May suppress skin test reactions.

  Post administration total plasma cortisol levels during 30-minute test for diagnosis of adrenocotical insufficiency might be misleading due to altered cortisol binding globulin levels in some special clinical situations including, patients on oral contraceptives, post-operative patients, critical illness, severe liver disease and nephrotic syndrome.

- **MEDICINAL FORMS** There can be variation in the licensing of different medicines containing the same drug.

  Solution for injection
  - Synacthen (Atnahs Pharma UK Ltd)
    Tetracosactide acetate 250 microgram per 1 ml Synacthen 250micrograms/1ml solution for injection ampoules | 1 ampoule [PoM] £38.00 DT = £38.00

  Suspension for injection
  EXCIPIENTS: May contain Benzyl alcohol
  - Synacthen Depot (Atnahs Pharma UK Ltd)
    Tetracosactide acetate 1 mg per 1 ml Synacthen Depot 1mg/1ml suspension for injection ampoules | 1 ampoule [PoM] £346.28 DT = £346.28

7.2 Assessment of pituitary function

PITUITARY AND HYPOTHALAMIC HORMONES AND ANALOGUES > GONADOTROPHIN-RELEASING HORMONES

Gonadorelin

16-Jul-2024

(Gonadotrophin-releasing hormone; GnRH; LH–RH)

- **INDICATIONS AND DOSE**
  Assessment of pituitary function
  - BY SUBCUTANEOUS INJECTION, OR BY INTRAVENOUS INJECTION
  - Adult: 100 micrograms for 1 dose

- **CAUTIONS** Pituitary adenoma

- **SIDE-EFFECTS**
  - **Uncommon** Pain · skin reactions · swelling
  - **Rare or very rare** Abdominal discomfort · bronchospasm · dizziness · eye erythema · flushing · headache · nausea · tachycardia
  - **Frequency not known** Menorrhagia · sepsis · thrombophlebitis

- **PREGNANCY** Avoid.

- **BREAST FEEDING** Avoid.

- **MEDICINAL FORMS** There can be variation in the licensing of different medicines containing the same drug.
  Powder for solution for injection
  - Gonadorelin (Non-proprietary)
    Gonadorelin (as Gonadorelin hydrochloride)
    100 microgram Gonadorelin 100microgram powder for solution for injection vials | 1 vial [PoM] £75.00 (Hospital only)

7.3 Gonadotrophin replacement therapy

GONADOTROPHINS

Choriogonadotropin alfa

22-May-2020

(Human chorionic gonadotropin)

- **INDICATIONS AND DOSE**
  Treatment of infertility in women with proven hypopituitarism or who have not responded to clomifene | Superovulation treatment for assisted conception (such as in vitro fertilisation)
  - BY SUBCUTANEOUS INJECTION
  - Adult (female): Adjusted according to response.

- **CONTRA-INDICATIONS** Active thromboembolic disorders · ectopic pregnancy in previous 3 months · hypothalamus malignancy · mammary malignancy · ovarian enlargement or cyst (unless caused by polycystic ovarian disease) · ovarian malignancy · pituitary malignancy · undiagnosed vaginal bleeding · uterine malignancy

- **CAUTIONS** Acute porphyrias p. 1202

- **SIDE-EFFECTS**
  - **Common or very common** Abdominal pain · fatigue · headache · nausea · ovarian hyperstimulation syndrome · vomiting
  - **Uncommon** Breast pain · depression · diarrhoea · irritability · restlessness
  - **Rare or very rare** Rash · shock · thromboembolism

● **MEDICINAL FORMS** There can be variation in the licensing of different medicines containing the same drug.

Solution for injection

▸ Ovitrelle (Merck Serono Ltd)

Choriogonadotropin alfa 500 microgram per 1 ml Ovitrelle 250micrograms/0.5ml solution for injection pre-filled syringes | 1 pre-filled disposable injection [PoM] £37.66 DT = £37.66 [CD4–2]

Follitropin alfa

06-Oct-2020

(Recombinant human follicle stimulating hormone)

● **INDICATIONS AND DOSE**

Infertility in women with proven hypopituitarism or who have not responded to clomifene | Superovulation treatment for assisted conception (such as in vitro fertilisation)

▸ BY SUBCUTANEOUS INJECTION

▸ Adult (female): Adjusted according to response.

Hypogonadotrophic hypogonadism

▸ BY SUBCUTANEOUS INJECTION

▸ Adult (male): (consult product literature).

● **CONTRA-INDICATIONS** Ovarian cysts (not caused by polycystic ovarian syndrome) · ovarian enlargement (not caused by polycystic ovarian syndrome) · tumours of breast · tumours of hypothalamus · tumours of ovaries · tumours of pituitary · tumours of prostate · tumours of testes · tumours of uterus · vaginal bleeding of unknown cause

● **CAUTIONS** Acute porphyrias p. 1202 · history of tubal disease

● **SIDE-EFFECTS**

▸ **Common or very common** Acne · diarrhoea · gastrointestinal discomfort · gynaecomastia · headache · nausea · ovarian and fallopian tube disorders · varicocele · vomiting · weight increased

▸ **Rare or very rare** Asthma exacerbated · thromboembolism

● **PREGNANCY** Avoid.

● **BREAST FEEDING** Avoid.

● **PRESCRIBING AND DISPENSING INFORMATION** Follitropin alfa is a biological medicine. Biological medicines must be prescribed and dispensed by brand name, see *Biological medicines* and *Biosimilar medicines*, under Guidance on prescribing p. 1.

● **PATIENT AND CARER ADVICE**

Conception and contraception Patients planning to conceive should be warned that there is a risk of multiple pregnancy.

● **MEDICINAL FORMS** There can be variation in the licensing of different medicines containing the same drug.

Solution for injection

▸ Bemfola (Gedeon Richter (UK) Ltd)

Follitropin alfa 600 unit per 1 ml Bemfola 75units/0.125ml solution for injection pre-filled pens | 1 pre-filled disposable injection [PoM] £25.85 DT = £25.85
Bemfola 225units/0.375ml solution for injection pre-filled pens | 1 pre-filled disposable injection [PoM] £77.55 DT = £77.55
Bemfola 450units/0.75ml solution for injection pre-filled pens | 1 pre-filled disposable injection [PoM] £155.10
Bemfola 300units/0.5ml solution for injection pre-filled pens | 1 pre-filled disposable injection [PoM] £103.40
Bemfola 150units/0.25ml solution for injection pre-filled pens | 1 pre-filled disposable injection [PoM] £51.70 DT = £51.70

▸ Gonal-f (Merck Serono Ltd)

Follitropin alfa 625 unit per 1 ml Gonal-f 450units/0.72ml solution for injection pre-filled pens | 1 pre-filled disposable injection [PoM] £169.20 DT = £169.20
Gonal-f 900units/1.44ml solution for injection pre-filled pens | 1 pre-filled disposable injection [PoM] £338.40 DT = £338.40
Gonal-f 300units/0.48ml solution for injection pre-filled pens | 1 pre-filled disposable injection [PoM] £112.80 DT = £112.80

▸ Ovaleap (Theramex HQ UK Ltd)

Follitropin alfa 600 unit per 1 ml Ovaleap 450units/0.75ml solution for injection cartridges | 1 cartridge [PoM] £141.00 (Hospital only)
Ovaleap 900units/1.5ml solution for injection cartridges | 1 cartridge [PoM] £282.00 (Hospital only)
Ovaleap 300units/0.5ml solution for injection cartridges | 1 cartridge [PoM] £94.00 (Hospital only)

Powder and solvent for solution for injection

▸ Gonal-f (Merck Serono Ltd)

Follitropin alfa 75 unit Gonal-f 75unit powder and solvent for solution for injection vials | 1 vial [PoM] £25.22 DT = £25.22

Follitropin alfa with lutropin alfa

07-Jun-2022

The properties listed below are those particular to the combination only. For the properties of the components please consider, follitropin alfa above, lutropin alfa p. 858.

● **INDICATIONS AND DOSE**

Infertility in women with proven hypopituitarism or who have not responded to clomifene | Superovulation treatment for assisted conception (such as in vitro fertilisation)

▸ BY SUBCUTANEOUS INJECTION

▸ Adult (female): Adjusted according to response.

● **MEDICINAL FORMS** There can be variation in the licensing of different medicines containing the same drug.

Solution for injection

▸ Pergoveris (Merck Serono Ltd)

Lutropin alfa 312.5 unit per 1 ml, Follitropin alfa 625 unit per 1 ml Pergoveris 450units/225units/0.72ml solution for injection pre-filled pens | 1 pre-filled disposable injection [PoM] £217.04
Pergoveris 900units/450units/1.44ml solution for injection pre-filled pens | 1 pre-filled disposable injection [PoM] £434.09 (Hospital only)
Pergoveris 300units/150units/0.48ml solution for injection pre-filled pens | 1 pre-filled disposable injection [PoM] £144.70 (Hospital only)

Powder and solvent for solution for injection

ELECTROLYTES: May contain Sodium

▸ Pergoveris (Merck Serono Ltd)

Lutropin alfa 75 unit, Follitropin alfa 150 unit Pergoveris 150unit/75unit powder and solvent for solution for injection vials | 1 vial [PoM] £72.35

Follitropin delta

01-Aug-2024

● **DRUG ACTION** Follitropin delta is a recombinant human follicle stimulating hormone, which causes development of multiple mature follicles.

● **INDICATIONS AND DOSE**

Superovulation treatment for assisted conception (such as in vitro fertilisation) (initiated under specialist supervision)

▸ BY SUBCUTANEOUS INJECTION

▸ Adult (female): Initial dosing based on serum anti-Müllerian hormone concentration and body-weight—consult product literature.

● **CONTRA-INDICATIONS** Ovarian cysts (not caused by polycystic ovarian syndrome) · ovarian enlargement (not caused by polycystic ovarian syndrome) · tumours of breast · tumours of hypothalamus · tumours of ovaries · tumours of pituitary · tumours of uterus · vaginal bleeding of unknown cause

● **CAUTIONS** Acute porphyrias p. 1202 · history of tubal disease (increased risk of ectopic pregnancy)

● **SIDE-EFFECTS**

▸ **Common or very common** Fatigue · headache · nausea · ovarian hyperstimulation syndrome · pelvic disorders · uterine pain

Endocrine system · 6

▶ **Uncommon** Abdominal discomfort · breast abnormalities · constipation · diarrhoea · dizziness · drowsiness · mood swings · vaginal haemorrhage · vomiting

SIDE-EFFECTS, FURTHER INFORMATION If ovarian hyperstimulation syndrome occurs, the patient should be advised to withhold hCG and avoid intercourse or use barrier contraceptive methods for at least 4 days.

● **PREGNANCY** Manufacturer advises avoid—not indicated during pregnancy.

● **BREAST FEEDING** Manufacturer advises avoid—not indicated during breastfeeding.

● **MONITORING REQUIREMENTS** Manufacturer advises regular monitoring of ovarian response with ultrasound alone, or in combination with serum estradiol levels. Frequent monitoring of follicular development is required to reduce the risk of ovarian hyperstimulation syndrome during treatment, and for at least 2 weeks after triggering of final follicular maturation—consult product literature.

● **DIRECTIONS FOR ADMINISTRATION** Manufacturer recommends the cartridge should be used with the *Rekovelle*® injection pen. The first injection should be performed under direct medical supervision; self-administration should only be performed by patients who are well motivated, adequately trained and have access to expert advice.

● **PRESCRIBING AND DISPENSING INFORMATION** Follitropin delta is a biological medicine. Biological medicines must be prescribed and dispensed by brand name, see *Biological medicines* and *Biosimilar medicines*, under Guidance on prescribing p. 1.

● **HANDLING AND STORAGE** Manufacturer advises store in a refrigerator (2–8 °C)—consult product literature for further information regarding storage conditions outside refrigerator.

● **PATIENT AND CARER ADVICE**
Conception and contraception Manufacturer advises that patients planning to conceive should be warned that there is a risk of multiple pregnancy.

● **NATIONAL FUNDING/ACCESS DECISIONS**
For full details see funding body website
Scottish Medicines Consortium (SMC) decisions
▶ Follitropin delta (*Rekovelle*®) for controlled ovarian stimulation for the development of multiple follicles in women undergoing assisted reproductive technologies such as an in vitro fertilisation or intracytoplasmic sperm injection cycle (July 2024) SMC No. SMC2670 Recommended with restrictions

● **MEDICINAL FORMS** There can be variation in the licensing of different medicines containing the same drug.
Solution for injection
▶ Rekovelle (Ferring Pharmaceuticals Ltd)
Follitropin delta 33.33 microgram per 1 ml Rekovelle 36micrograms/1.08ml solution for injection pre-filled pens | 1 pre-filled disposable injection [PoM] £354.94
Rekovelle 72micrograms/2.16 ml solution for injection pre-filled pens | 1 pre-filled disposable injection [PoM] £709.89
Rekovelle 12micrograms/0.36ml solution for injection pre-filled pens | 1 pre-filled disposable injection [PoM] £118.31

Lutropin alfa

22-May-2020

(Recombinant human luteinising hormone)

● **INDICATIONS AND DOSE**
Treatment of infertility in women with proven hypopituitarism or who have not responded to clomifene (in conjunction with follicle-stimulating hormone) | Superovulation treatment for assisted conception (such as in vitro fertilisation) (in conjunction with follicle-stimulating hormone)
▶ BY SUBCUTANEOUS INJECTION
▶ Adult (female): Adjusted according to response.

● **CONTRA-INDICATIONS** Mammary carcinoma · ovarian carcinoma · ovarian enlargement or cyst (unless caused by polycystic ovarian disease) · tumours of hypothalamus · tumours of pituitary · undiagnosed vaginal bleeding · uterine carcinoma

● **CAUTIONS** Acute porphyrias p. 1202

● **SIDE-EFFECTS**
▶ **Common or very common** Breast pain · diarrhoea · gastrointestinal discomfort · headache · nausea · ovarian and fallopian tube disorders · pelvic pain · vomiting
▶ **Rare or very rare** Thromboembolism

● **MEDICINAL FORMS** There can be variation in the licensing of different medicines containing the same drug.
Powder and solvent for solution for injection
▶ Luveris (Merck Serono Ltd)
Lutropin alfa 75 unit Luveris 75unit powder and solvent for solution for injection vials | 1 vial [PoM] £31.38

Menotrophin

06-Oct-2020

● **INDICATIONS AND DOSE**
Infertility in women with proven hypopituitarism or who have not responded to clomifene | Superovulation treatment for assisted conception (such as in vitro fertilisation)
▶ BY SUBCUTANEOUS INJECTION, OR BY DEEP INTRAMUSCULAR INJECTION
▶ Adult (female): Adjusted according to response.
Hypogonadotrophic hypogonadism
▶ BY DEEP INTRAMUSCULAR INJECTION, OR BY SUBCUTANEOUS INJECTION
▶ Adult (male): (consult product literature).

● **CONTRA-INDICATIONS** Ovarian cysts (not caused by polycystic ovarian syndrome) · ovarian enlargement (not caused by polycystic ovarian syndrome) · tumours of breast · tumours of hypothalamus · tumours of ovaries · tumours of pituitary · tumours of prostate · tumours of testes · tumours of uterus · vaginal bleeding of unknown cause

● **CAUTIONS** Acute porphyrias p. 1202 · history of tubal disease

● **SIDE-EFFECTS**
▶ **Common or very common** Gastrointestinal discomfort · headache · nausea · ovarian and fallopian tube disorders · pelvic pain · uterine pain
▶ **Uncommon** Breast abnormalities · diarrhoea · dizziness · fatigue · hot flush · vomiting
▶ **Rare or very rare** Skin reactions
▶ **Frequency not known** Arthralgia · pain · thromboembolism · vision disorder

● **PREGNANCY** Avoid.

● **BREAST FEEDING** Avoid.

● **PRESCRIBING AND DISPENSING INFORMATION** Menotrophin is purified extract of human post-menopausal urine containing follicle-stimulating hormone (FSH) and luteinising hormone (LH) in a ratio of 1:1

- **PATIENT AND CARER ADVICE**
  Conception and contraception Patients planning to conceive should be warned that there is a risk of multiple pregnancy.

- **MEDICINAL FORMS** There can be variation in the licensing of different medicines containing the same drug.
  Powder and solvent for solution for injection
  ▸ Menopur (Ferring Pharmaceuticals Ltd)
    Menotrophin 75 unit Menopur 75unit powder and solvent for solution for injection vials | 10 vial [PoM] £180.18 DT = £180.18
    Menotrophin 150 unit Menopur 150unit powder and solvent for solution for injection vials | 10 vial [PoM] £360.36 DT = £360.36
    Menotrophin 600 unit Menopur 600unit powder and solvent for solution for injection vials | 1 vial [PoM] £144.14 DT = £144.14
    Menotrophin 1200 unit Menopur 1,200unit powder and solvent for solution for injection vials | 1 vial [PoM] £288.29 DT = £288.29
  ▸ Meriofert (IBSA Pharma Ltd)
    Menotrophin 75 unit Meriofert 75unit powder and solvent for solution for injection vials | 10 vial [PoM] £279.00 DT = £180.18
    Menotrophin 150 unit Meriofert 150unit powder and solvent for solution for injection vials | 10 vial [PoM] £558.00 DT = £360.36
  ▸ Meriofert PFS (IBSA Pharma Ltd)
    Menotrophin 900 unit Meriofert PFS 900unit powder and solvent for solution for injection pre-filled syringes | 1 pre-filled disposable injection [PoM] £334.80 (Hospital only)

Urofollitropin

02-Sep-2020

- **INDICATIONS AND DOSE**
  Infertility in women with proven hypopituitarism or who have not responded to clomifene | Superovulation treatment for assisted conception (such as in vitro fertilisation)
  ▸ BY SUBCUTANEOUS INJECTION, OR BY DEEP INTRAMUSCULAR INJECTION
  ▸ Adult (female): Adjusted according to response.

- **CONTRA-INDICATIONS** Ovarian cysts (not caused by polycystic ovarian syndrome) · tumours of breast · tumours of hypothalamus · tumours of ovaries · tumours of pituitary · tumours of uterus · vaginal bleeding of unknown cause

- **CAUTIONS** Acute porphyrias p. 1202

- **SIDE-EFFECTS**
  ▸ **Common or very common** Breast tenderness · constipation · diarrhoea · gastrointestinal discomfort · headache · hot flush · increased risk of infection · muscle spasms · nausea · ovarian hyperstimulation syndrome · pain · pelvic pain · rash · vaginal discharge · vaginal haemorrhage · vomiting

- **PREGNANCY** Avoid.

- **BREAST FEEDING** Avoid.

- **PRESCRIBING AND DISPENSING INFORMATION**
  Urofollitropin is purified extract of human post-menopausal urine containing follicle-stimulating hormone (FSH).

- **PATIENT AND CARER ADVICE**
  Conception and contraception Patients planning to conceive should be warned that there is a risk of multiple pregnancy.

- **MEDICINAL FORMS** There can be variation in the licensing of different medicines containing the same drug.
  Powder and solvent for solution for injection
  ▸ Fostimon (IBSA Pharma Ltd)
    Follicle stimulating hormone human (as Urofollitropin) 75 unit Fostimon 75unit powder and solvent for solution for injection vials | 10 vial [PoM] £279.00 DT = £279.00
    Follicle stimulating hormone human (as Urofollitropin) 150 unit Fostimon 150unit powder and solvent for solution for injection vials | 10 vial [PoM] £558.00 DT = £558.00

7.4   Growth hormone disorders

PITUITARY AND HYPOTHALAMIC HORMONES AND ANALOGUES ⟩ GROWTH HORMONE RECEPTOR ANTAGONISTS

Pegvisomant

08-Apr-2021

- **DRUG ACTION** Pegvisomant is a genetically modified analogue of human growth hormone and is a highly selective growth hormone receptor antagonist.

- **INDICATIONS AND DOSE**
  Treatment of acromegaly in patients with inadequate response to surgery, radiation, or both, and to treatment with somatostatin analogues (initiated by a specialist)
  ▸ BY SUBCUTANEOUS INJECTION
  ▸ Adult: Initially 80 mg for 1 dose, followed by 10 mg daily, then increased in steps of 5 mg daily, adjusted according to response; maximum 30 mg per day

- **CAUTIONS** Abnormal liver function tests and/or signs or symptoms of liver injury (further investigations may be required before treatment initiation—consult product literature) · diabetes mellitus (adjustment of antidiabetic therapy may be necessary)

- **SIDE-EFFECTS**
  ▸ **Common or very common** Arthralgia · arthritis · asthenia · constipation · diarrhoea · dizziness · drowsiness · dyslipidaemia · dyspnoea · eye pain · fever · gastrointestinal discomfort · gastrointestinal disorders · haemorrhage · headaches · hyperglycaemia · hypertension · hypoglycaemia · influenza like illness · lipohypertrophy · myalgia · nausea · numbness · oedema · skin reactions · sleep disorders · sweat changes · tremor · vomiting · weight increased
  ▸ **Uncommon** Apathy · confusion · dry mouth · eye strain · feeling abnormal · healing impaired · hunger · leucocytosis · leucopenia · libido increased · memory loss · Meniere's disease · oral disorders · panic attack · polyuria · proteinuria · renal impairment · taste altered · thrombocytopenia
  ▸ **Frequency not known** Anger · angioedema · hepatic function abnormal · laryngospasm

  SIDE-EFFECTS, FURTHER INFORMATION **Injection-site reactions** Rotate injection sites to avoid lipohypertrophy.
  Abnormal hepatic function Manufacturer advises interrupt treatment if liver function tests at least 5 times the upper limit of normal *or* transaminase levels at least 3 times the upper limit of normal **and** blood bilirubin increased—consult product literature. Discontinue if liver injury is confirmed.

- **CONCEPTION AND CONTRACEPTION** Possible increase in female fertility.

- **PREGNANCY** Avoid.

- **BREAST FEEDING** Avoid.

- **HEPATIC IMPAIRMENT** Manufacturer advises caution (no information available); temporary or permanent withdrawal may be needed—consult product literature.

- **MONITORING REQUIREMENTS**
  ▸ Manufacturer advises assess liver function tests before treatment initiation and monitor liver function tests during treatment—consult product literature.
  ▸ Manufacturer advises monitor serum IGF-I concentrations.

- **NATIONAL FUNDING/ACCESS DECISIONS**
  For full details see funding body website
  Scottish Medicines Consortium (SMC) decisions
  ▸ Pegvisomant (*Somavert*®) for the treatment of adult patients with acromegaly who have had an inadequate response to

surgery and/or radiation therapy and in whom an appropriate medical treatment with somatostatin analogues did not normalize insulin-like growth factor type 1 (IGF-1) concentrations or was not tolerated (November 2017) SMC No. 158/05 Recommended

All Wales Medicines Strategy Group (AWMSG) decisions
▶ Pegvisomant (*Somavert®*) for the treatment of adult patients with acromegaly who have had an inadequate response to surgery and/or radiation therapy and in whom an appropriate medical treatment with somatostatin analogues did not normalise insulin-like growth factor-1 (IGF-1) concentrations or was not tolerated (November 2017) AWMSG No. 3545 Recommended

● **MEDICINAL FORMS** There can be variation in the licensing of different medicines containing the same drug.

Powder and solvent for solution for injection
▶ Somavert (Pfizer Ltd)
Pegvisomant 10 mg Somavert 10mg powder and solvent for solution for injection vials | 30 vial [PoM] £1,500.00 (Hospital only)
Pegvisomant 15 mg Somavert 15mg powder and solvent for solution for injection vials | 30 vial [PoM] £2,250.00 (Hospital only)
Pegvisomant 20 mg Somavert 20mg powder and solvent for solution for injection vials | 1 vial [PoM] £100.00 (Hospital only) | 30 vial [PoM] £3,000.00 (Hospital only)
Pegvisomant 25 mg Somavert 25mg powder and solvent for solution for injection vials | 30 vial [PoM] £3,750.00 (Hospital only)
Pegvisomant 30 mg Somavert 30mg powder and solvent for solution for injection vials | 30 vial [PoM] £4,500.00 (Hospital only)

PITUITARY AND HYPOTHALAMIC HORMONES AND ANALOGUES > HUMAN GROWTH HORMONES

Somapacitan

26-Nov-2024

(Recombinant human growth hormone, long-acting)

● **INDICATIONS AND DOSE**

Deficiency of growth hormone in treatment-naïve patients (under expert supervision)
▶ BY SUBCUTANEOUS INJECTION
▶ Adult 18–59 years: Initially 1.5 mg once weekly, then maintenance dose to be increased in steps of 0.5–1.5 mg every 2–4 weeks, adjusted according to response, up to 8 mg once weekly, for advice on dose adjustments and treatment evaluation or discontinuation—consult product literature
▶ Adult 60 years and over: Initially 1 mg once weekly, then maintenance dose to be increased in steps of 0.5–1.5 mg every 2–4 weeks, adjusted according to response, up to 8 mg once weekly, for advice on dose adjustments and treatment evaluation or discontinuation—consult product literature

Deficiency of growth hormone in treatment-naïve females on oral oestrogen therapy (under expert supervision)
▶ BY SUBCUTANEOUS INJECTION
▶ Adult: Initially 2 mg once weekly, then maintenance dose to be increased in steps of 0.5–1.5 mg every 2–4 weeks, adjusted according to response, up to 8 mg once weekly, for advice on dose adjustments and treatment evaluation or discontinuation—consult product literature

Deficiency of growth hormone in patients switching from another growth hormone therapy (under expert supervision)
▶ BY SUBCUTANEOUS INJECTION
▶ Adult 18-59 years: Initially 2 mg once weekly, then maintenance dose to be increased in steps of 0.5–1.5 mg every 2–4 weeks, adjusted according to response, up to 8 mg once weekly, for advice on dose adjustments and treatment evaluation or discontinuation—consult product literature
▶ Adult 60 years and over: Initially 1.5 mg once weekly, then maintenance dose to be increased in steps of 0.5–1.5 mg every 2–4 weeks, adjusted according to response, up to 8 mg once weekly, for advice on dose adjustments and treatment evaluation or discontinuation—consult product literature

Deficiency of growth hormone in females on oral oestrogen therapy switching from another growth hormone therapy (under expert supervision)
▶ BY SUBCUTANEOUS INJECTION
▶ Adult: Initially 4 mg once weekly, then maintenance dose to be increased in steps of 0.5–1.5 mg every 2–4 weeks, adjusted according to response, up to 8 mg once weekly, for advice on dose adjustments and treatment evaluation or discontinuation—consult product literature

DOSE EQUIVALENCE AND CONVERSION
▶ For patients switching from another growth hormone therapy, the initial dose of somapacitan should be administered at least 8 hours after the last dose of daily growth hormone or 1 week after the last dose of weekly growth hormone.

● **CONTRA-INDICATIONS** Complications in acute critical illness (consult product literature) · evidence of tumour activity (complete antitumour therapy and ensure intracranial lesions are inactive before starting)

● **CAUTIONS** Diabetes mellitus (adjustment of antidiabetic therapy may be necessary) · glucose intolerance or risk factors for diabetes (additional monitoring may be necessary) · history of malignant disease or benign tumour · hypoadrenalism (initiation or adjustment of glucocorticoid replacement therapy may be necessary) · hypothyroidism (periodic thyroid function tests recommended) · resolved intracranial hypertension (monitor closely)

● **INTERACTIONS** → Appendix 1: somapacitan

● **SIDE-EFFECTS**
▶ **Common or very common** Adrenal insufficiency · asthenia · headache · hyperglycaemia · hypothyroidism · joint disorders · muscle complaints · paraesthesia · peripheral oedema · skin reactions
▶ **Uncommon** Carpal tunnel syndrome · lipohypertrophy

● **PREGNANCY** [EvGr] Avoid (toxicity in *animal* studies). Ⓜ

● **BREAST FEEDING** [EvGr] Avoid (present in milk in *animal* studies). Ⓜ

● **MONITORING REQUIREMENTS** Monitor serum insulin-like growth factor-1 concentrations during treatment—consult product literature.

● **DIRECTIONS FOR ADMINISTRATION** Inject into the abdomen, thighs, buttocks, or upper arms; rotate injection site weekly to prevent lipoatrophy. *Sogroya®* may be self-administered or administered by a carer after appropriate training in subcutaneous injection technique.

● **PRESCRIBING AND DISPENSING INFORMATION** Somapacitan is a biological medicine. Biological medicines must be prescribed and dispensed by brand name, see *Biological medicines* and *Biosimilar medicines*, under Guidance on prescribing p. 1; record the brand name and batch number after each administration.

● **HANDLING AND STORAGE** Store in a refrigerator (2–8°C) and protect from light—consult product literature for further information regarding storage outside the refrigerator.

● **PATIENT AND CARER ADVICE**
Self-administration Patients and their carers should be given training in subcutaneous injection technique, if appropriate.

Missed doses If a dose is more than 3 days late, the missed dose should not be administered and the next dose should be administered on the usual scheduled day.

If two or more doses are missed, the next dose should be administered on the usual scheduled day.

● **NATIONAL FUNDING/ACCESS DECISIONS**
For full details see funding body website
Scottish Medicines Consortium (SMC) decisions
▶ Somapacitan (*Sogroya*®) for the replacement of endogenous growth hormone in children aged 3 years and above, and adolescents with growth failure due to growth hormone deficiency, and in adults with growth hormone deficiency (November 2024) SMC No. SMC2629 Recommended with restrictions

● **MEDICINAL FORMS** There can be variation in the licensing of different medicines containing the same drug.
Solution for injection
▶ Sogroya (Novo Nordisk Ltd) ▼
Somapacitan 6.7 mg per 1 ml Sogroya 10mg/1.5ml solution for injection pre-filled pens | 1 pre-filled disposable injection [PoM] £285.45
Somapacitan 10 mg per 1 ml Sogroya 15mg/1.5ml solution for injection pre-filled pens | 1 pre-filled disposable injection [PoM] £428.18

Somatropin
29-Sep-2023
(Recombinant Human Growth Hormone)

● **INDICATIONS AND DOSE**
Gonadal dysgenesis (Turner syndrome)
▶ BY SUBCUTANEOUS INJECTION
▶ Adult: 1.4 mg/m^2 daily, alternatively 45–50 micrograms/kg daily
Deficiency of growth hormone
▶ BY SUBCUTANEOUS INJECTION
▶ Adult: Initially 150–300 micrograms daily, then increased if necessary up to 1 mg daily, dose to be increased gradually, use minimum effective dose (requirements may decrease with age)
DOSE EQUIVALENCE AND CONVERSION
▶ Dose formerly expressed in units; somatropin 1 mg ≡ 3 units.

● **CONTRA-INDICATIONS** Evidence of tumour activity (complete antitumour therapy and ensure intracranial lesions inactive before starting)
● **CAUTIONS** Diabetes mellitus (adjustment of antidiabetic therapy may be necessary) · disorders of the epiphysis of the hip (monitor for limping) · history of malignant disease · hypoadrenalism (initiation or adjustment of glucocorticoid replacement therapy may be necessary) · initiation of treatment close to puberty not recommended in child born small for corrected gestational age · papilloedema · resolved intracranial hypertension (monitor closely) · risk of hypothyroidism—manufacturers recommend periodic thyroid function tests · Silver-Russell syndrome
● **INTERACTIONS** → Appendix 1: somatropin
● **SIDE-EFFECTS**
▶ **Common or very common** Carpal tunnel syndrome · fluid retention · headache · joint disorders · lipoatrophy · myalgia · oedema · paraesthesia
▶ **Uncommon** Gynaecomastia · idiopathic intracranial hypertension
▶ **Rare or very rare** Hyperglycaemia · hyperinsulinism · hypothyroidism · osteonecrosis of femur · pancreatitis · slipped capital femoral epiphysis
▶ **Frequency not known** Leukaemia · musculoskeletal stiffness

● **SIDE-EFFECTS, FURTHER INFORMATION** Funduscopy for papilloedema recommended if severe or recurrent headache, visual problems, nausea and vomiting occur—if papilloedema confirmed consider benign intracranial hypertension (rare cases reported).
● **PREGNANCY** Discontinue if pregnancy occurs—no information available.
● **BREAST FEEDING** No information available. Absorption from milk unlikely.
● **DIRECTIONS FOR ADMINISTRATION** Rotate subcutaneous injection sites to prevent lipoatrophy.
● **PRESCRIBING AND DISPENSING INFORMATION** Somatropin is a biological medicine. Biological medicines must be prescribed and dispensed by brand name, see *Biological medicines* and *Biosimilar medicines*, under Guidance on prescribing p. 1.
GENOTROPIN® PREPARATIONS Cartridges are for use with *Genotropin*® Pen device (non-NHS but available free of charge from clinics).
NORDITROPIN® PREPARATIONS Cartridges are for use with appropriate *NordiPen*® device (non-NHS but available free of charge from clinics).
Multidose disposable prefilled pens for use with *NovoFine*® or *NovoTwist*® needles.
NUTROPINAQ® For use with *NutropinAq*® Pen device (non-NHS but available free of charge from clinics).
OMNITROPE® For use with *Omnitrope Pen* 5® and *Omnitrope Pen* 10® devices (non-NHS but available free of charge from clinics).
SAIZEN® POWDER AND SOLVENT FOR SOLUTION FOR INJECTION For use with *one. click*® autoinjector device or *cool.click*® needle-free autoinjector device or *easypod*® autoinjector device (non-NHS but available free of charge from clinics).
SAIZEN® SOLUTION FOR INJECTION For use with *cool.click*® needle-free autoinjector device or *easypod*® autoinjector device (non-NHS but available free of charge from clinics).
ZOMACTON® 4 mg vial for use with *ZomaJet 2*® *Vision* needle-free device (non-NHS but available free of charge from clinics) or with needles and syringes.
10 mg vial for use with *ZomaJet Vision X*® needle-free device (non-NHS but available free of charge from clinics) or with needles and syringes.

● **NATIONAL FUNDING/ACCESS DECISIONS**
For full details see funding body website
NICE decisions
▶ Somatropin for adults with growth hormone deficiency (August 2003) NICE TA64 Recommended with restrictions

● **MEDICINAL FORMS** There can be variation in the licensing of different medicines containing the same drug.
Solution for injection
EXCIPIENTS: May contain Benzyl alcohol
▶ Norditropin FlexPro (Novo Nordisk Ltd)
Somatropin (epr) 3.3 mg per 1 ml Norditropin FlexPro 5mg/1.5ml solution for injection pre-filled pens | 1 pre-filled disposable injection [PoM] £106.35 [CD4-2]
Somatropin (epr) 6.7 mg per 1 ml Norditropin FlexPro 10mg/1.5ml solution for injection pre-filled pens | 1 pre-filled disposable injection [PoM] £212.70 DT = £212.70 [CD4-2]
Somatropin (epr) 10 mg per 1 ml Norditropin FlexPro 15mg/1.5ml solution for injection pre-filled pens | 1 pre-filled disposable injection [PoM] £319.05 DT = £319.05 [CD4-2]
▶ Omnitrope SurePal (Sandoz Ltd)
Somatropin (rbe) 3.333 mg per 1 ml Omnitrope SurePal 5 5mg/1.5ml solution for injection cartridges | 5 cartridge [PoM] £368.74 DT = £368.74 [CD4-2]
Somatropin (rbe) 6.667 mg per 1 ml Omnitrope SurePal 10 10mg/1.5ml solution for injection cartridges | 5 cartridge [PoM] £737.49 DT = £737.49 [CD4-2]

Somatropin (rbe) 10 mg per 1 ml Omnitrope SurePal 15 15mg/1.5ml solution for injection cartridges | 5 cartridge [PoM] £1,106.22 DT = £1,106.22 [CD4–2]

▶ **Saizen** (Merck Serono Ltd)
Somatropin (rmc) 5.825 mg per 1 ml Saizen 6mg/1.03ml solution for injection cartridges | 1 cartridge [PoM] £139.08 DT = £139.08 [CD4–2]
Somatropin (rmc) 8 mg per 1 ml Saizen 12mg/1.5ml solution for injection cartridges | 1 cartridge [PoM] £278.16 DT = £278.16 [CD4–2] Saizen 20mg/2.5ml solution for injection cartridges | 1 cartridge [PoM] £463.60 DT = £463.60 [CD4–2]

Powder and solvent for solution for injection
EXCIPIENTS: May contain Benzyl alcohol

▶ **Genotropin** (Pfizer Ltd)
Somatropin (rbe) 5.3 mg Genotropin 5.3mg powder and solvent for solution for injection cartridges | 1 cartridge [PoM] £92.15 DT = £92.15 [CD4–2]
Somatropin (rbe) 12 mg Genotropin 12mg powder and solvent for solution for injection cartridges | 1 cartridge [PoM] £208.65 DT = £208.65 [CD4–2]

▶ **Genotropin GoQuick** (Pfizer Ltd)
Somatropin (rbe) 5.3 mg Genotropin GoQuick 5.3mg powder and solvent for solution for injection pre-filled pens | 1 pre-filled disposable injection [PoM] £92.15 DT = £92.15 [CD4–2]
Somatropin (rbe) 12 mg Genotropin GoQuick 12mg powder and solvent for solution for injection pre-filled pens | 1 pre-filled disposable injection [PoM] £208.65 DT = £208.65 [CD4–2]

▶ **Genotropin MiniQuick** (Pfizer Ltd)
Somatropin (rbe) 200 microgram Genotropin MiniQuick 200microgram powder and solvent for solution for injection pre-filled disposable devices | 7 pre-filled disposable injection [PoM] £24.35 DT = £24.35 [CD4–2]
Somatropin (rbe) 400 microgram Genotropin MiniQuick 400microgram powder and solvent for solution for injection pre-filled disposable devices | 7 pre-filled disposable injection [PoM] £48.68 DT = £48.68 [CD4–2]
Somatropin (rbe) 600 microgram Genotropin MiniQuick 600microgram powder and solvent for solution for injection pre-filled disposable devices | 7 pre-filled disposable injection [PoM] £73.03 DT = £73.03 [CD4–2]
Somatropin (rbe) 800 microgram Genotropin MiniQuick 800microgram powder and solvent for solution for injection pre-filled disposable devices | 7 pre-filled disposable injection [PoM] £97.37 DT = £97.37 [CD4–2]
Somatropin (rbe) 1 mg Genotropin MiniQuick 1mg powder and solvent for solution for injection pre-filled disposable devices | 7 pre-filled disposable injection [PoM] £121.71 DT = £121.71 [CD4–2]
Somatropin (rbe) 1.2 mg Genotropin MiniQuick 1.2mg powder and solvent for solution for injection pre-filled disposable devices | 7 pre-filled disposable injection [PoM] £146.06 DT = £146.06 [CD4–2]
Somatropin (rbe) 1.4 mg Genotropin MiniQuick 1.4mg powder and solvent for solution for injection pre-filled disposable devices | 7 pre-filled disposable injection [PoM] £170.39 DT = £170.39 [CD4–2]
Somatropin (rbe) 1.6 mg Genotropin MiniQuick 1.6mg powder and solvent for solution for injection pre-filled disposable devices | 7 pre-filled disposable injection [PoM] £194.74 DT = £194.74 [CD4–2]
Somatropin (rbe) 1.8 mg Genotropin MiniQuick 1.8mg powder and solvent for solution for injection pre-filled disposable devices | 7 pre-filled disposable injection [PoM] £219.08 DT = £219.08 [CD4–2]
Somatropin (rbe) 2 mg Genotropin MiniQuick 2mg powder and solvent for solution for injection pre-filled disposable devices | 7 pre-filled disposable injection [PoM] £243.42 DT = £243.42 [CD4–2]

▶ **Zomacton** (Ferring Pharmaceuticals Ltd)
Somatropin (rbe) 4 mg Zomacton 4mg powder and solvent for solution for injection vials | 1 vial [PoM] £68.28 DT = £68.28 [CD4–2]

8   Sex hormone responsive conditions

Sex hormones

14-Nov-2023

Oestrogens and HRT

Oestrogens are necessary for the development of female secondary sexual characteristics; they also stimulate myometrial hypertrophy with endometrial hyperplasia.

In terms of oestrogenic activity *natural oestrogens* (estradiol p. 870 (oestradiol), estrone (oestrone), and estriol p. 960 (oestriol)) have a more appropriate profile for hormone replacement therapy (HRT) than *synthetic oestrogens* (ethinylestradiol p. 874 (ethinyloestradiol) and mestranol). Tibolone p. 874 has oestrogenic, progestogenic and weak androgenic activity.

Oestrogen therapy is given cyclically or continuously for a number of gynaecological conditions. If long-term therapy is required in women with a uterus, a progestogen should normally be added to reduce the risk of cystic hyperplasia of the endometrium (or of endometriotic foci in women who have had a hysterectomy) and possible transformation to cancer.

Oestrogens are no longer used to suppress lactation because of their association with thromboembolism.

Hormone replacement therapy

Hormone replacement therapy (HRT) with small doses of an oestrogen (together with a progestogen in women with a uterus) is appropriate for alleviating menopausal symptoms such as vaginal atrophy or vasomotor instability. Oestrogen given systemically in the perimenopausal and postmenopausal period or tibolone given in the postmenopausal period also diminish postmenopausal osteoporosis but other drugs are preferred; for further information, see Osteoporosis p. 768. Menopausal atrophic vaginitis may respond to a short course of a topical vaginal oestrogen preparation used for a few weeks and repeated if necessary.

Systemic therapy with an oestrogen or drugs with oestrogenic properties alleviates the symptoms of oestrogen deficiency such as vasomotor symptoms. Tibolone combines oestrogenic and progestogenic activity with weak androgenic activity; it is given continuously, without cyclical progestogen.

HRT may be used in women with early natural or surgical menopause (before age 45 years), since they are at high risk of osteoporosis. For early menopause, HRT can be given until the approximate age of natural menopause (i.e. until age 50 years). Alternatives to HRT should be considered if osteoporosis is the main concern.

Clonidine hydrochloride p. 172 may be used to reduce vasomotor symptoms in women who cannot take an oestrogen, but clonidine hydrochloride may cause unacceptable side-effects.

HRT increases the risk of venous thromboembolism, stroke, endometrial cancer (reduced by a progestogen), breast cancer, and ovarian cancer; there is an increased risk of coronary heart disease in women who start combined HRT more than 10 years after menopause. For details of these risks see HRT Risk table.

The Medicines and Healthcare products Regulatory Agency (MHRA) advises that HRT should only be prescribed to relieve post-menopausal symptoms that are adversely affecting quality of life and treatment should be reviewed regularly to ensure the minimum effective dose is used for the shortest duration. For osteoporosis, consider alternative treatments. HRT does not prevent coronary heart disease or protect against a decline in cognitive function and it should not be prescribed for these purposes. Experience of treating women over 65 years with HRT is limited.

For the treatment of menopausal symptoms the benefits of short-term HRT outweigh the risks in the majority of women, especially in those aged under 60 years.

For the treatment of menopausal symptoms in women with breast cancer, see Breast cancer p. 1072.

Risk of breast cancer

All types of *systemic* (oral or transdermal) HRT treatment increase the risk of breast cancer after 1 year of use. This risk is higher for combined oestrogen-progestogen HRT (particularly for continuous HRT preparations where both

6

Endocrine system

oestrogen and progestogen are taken throughout each month) than for oestrogen-only HRT, but is irrespective of the type of oestrogen or progestogen. Longer duration of HRT use (but not the age at which HRT is started) further increases risk.

Although the risk of breast cancer is lower after stopping HRT than it is during current use, the excess risk persists for more than 10 years after stopping compared with women who have never used HRT. Vaginal preparations containing low doses of oestrogen to treat local symptoms are not thought to be associated with an effect on breast cancer risk.

The MHRA advises discussing the updated information on the risk of breast cancer with women who use or are considering starting HRT, at their next routine appointment. The MHRA advises encouraging current and past HRT users to be vigilant for signs of breast cancer and to attend routine breast screening. If a decision is made to stop treatment, in the absence of contra-indications, the MHRA recommends this should be done gradually to minimise recurrence of menopausal symptoms. For more information, see estradiol p. 870, conjugated oestrogens (equine) p. 869 and the MHRA Drug Safety Update: www.gov.uk/drug-safety-update/hormone-replacement-therapy-hrt-further-information-on-the-known-increased-risk-of-breast-cancer-with-hrt-and-its-persistence-after-stopping.

Radiological detection of breast cancer can be made more difficult as mammographic density can increase with HRT use especially oestrogen-progestogen combined treatment, but this is not thought to be the case with tibolone p. 874.

Tibolone p. 874 has also been associated with an increased risk of breast cancer during treatment, although the extent of risk and its persistence after stopping is currently inconclusive.

Risk of endometrial cancer

The increased risk of endometrial cancer depends on the dose and duration of oestrogen-only HRT. In women with a uterus, the addition of a progestogen cyclically (for at least 10 days per 28-day cycle) reduces the additional risk of endometrial cancer; this additional risk is eliminated if a progestogen is given continuously. However, this should be weighed against the increased risk of breast cancer.

The risk of endometrial cancer in women who have not used HRT increases with body mass index (BMI); the increased risk of endometrial cancer in users of oestrogen-only HRT or tibolone is more apparent in women who are not overweight.

Evidence suggests an increased risk of endometrial cancer with tibolone. After 2.7 years of use (in women of average age 68 years), 1 extra case of endometrial hyperplasia and 4 extra cases of endometrial cancer were diagnosed compared with placebo users.

Risk of ovarian cancer

Long-term use of combined HRT or oestrogen-only HRT is associated with a small increased risk of ovarian cancer; this excess risk disappears within a few years of stopping.

Risk of venous thromboembolism

Women using combined or oestrogen-only HRT are at an increased risk of deep vein thrombosis and of pulmonary embolism especially in the first year of use. In women who have predisposing factors (such as a personal or family history of deep vein thrombosis or pulmonary embolism, severe varicose veins, obesity, trauma, or prolonged bed-rest) it is prudent to review the need for HRT, as in some cases the risks of HRT may exceed the benefits. Travel involving prolonged immobility further increases the risk of deep vein thrombosis.

Although the level of risk of thromboembolism associated with non-oral routes of administration of HRT has not been established, it may be lower for the transdermal route compared to the oral route; studies have found the risk

associated with transdermal HRT to be no greater than the baseline population risk of thromboembolism.

Limited data does not suggest an increased risk of thromboembolism with tibolone compared with combined HRT or women not taking HRT.

Risk of stroke

Risk of stroke increases with age, therefore older women have a greater absolute risk of stroke. Combined HRT or oestrogen-only HRT slightly increases the risk of stroke.

Tibolone increases the risk of stroke about 2.2 times from the first year of treatment; risk of stroke is age-dependent and therefore the absolute risk of stroke with tibolone increases with age.

Risk of coronary heart disease

HRT does not prevent coronary heart disease and should not be prescribed for this purpose. There is an increased risk of coronary heart disease in women who start combined HRT more than 10 years after menopause. Although very little information is available on the risk of coronary heart disease in younger women who start HRT close to the menopause, studies suggest a lower relative risk compared with older women.

There is insufficient data to draw a conclusion on the risk of coronary heart disease with tibolone.

Choice

The choice of HRT for an individual depends on an overall balance of indication, risk, and convenience. A woman with a uterus normally requires oestrogen with cyclical progestogen for the last 12 to 14 days of the cycle or a preparation which involves continuous administration of an oestrogen and a progestogen (or one which provides both oestrogenic and progestogenic activity in a single preparation). Continuous combined preparations or tibolone p. 874 are **not suitable** for use in the perimenopause or within 12 months of the last menstrual period; women who use such preparations may bleed irregularly in the early stages of treatment—if bleeding continues endometrial abnormality should be ruled out and consideration given to changing to cyclical HRT.

An oestrogen alone is suitable for continuous use in women without a uterus. However, in endometriosis, endometrial foci may remain despite hysterectomy and the addition of a progestogen should be considered in these circumstances.

An oestrogen may be given by mouth or by transdermal administration, which avoids first-pass metabolism.

Considerations in the elderly

The use of oestrogens in elderly patients is potentially inappropriate (STOPP criteria) if prescribed in patients with a history of breast cancer or venous thromboembolism (increased risk of recurrence). Oral oestrogens may be inappropriate if prescribed without concurrent progestogen in those with an intact uterus (risk of endometrial cancer).

For further information, see *STOPP/START criteria* in Prescribing in the elderly p. 31.

Surgery

Major surgery under general anaesthesia, including orthopaedic and vascular leg surgery, is a predisposing factor for venous thromboembolism and it may be prudent to stop HRT 4–6 weeks before surgery; it should be restarted only after full mobilisation. If HRT is continued or if discontinuation is not possible (e.g. in non-elective surgery), prophylaxis with unfractionated or low molecular weight heparin and graduated compression hosiery is advised.

Reasons to stop HRT

Hormone replacement therapy should be stopped (pending investigation and treatment), if any of the following occur:

- sudden severe chest pain (even if not radiating to left arm);
- sudden breathlessness (or cough with blood-stained sputum);

- unexplained swelling or severe pain in calf of one leg;
- severe stomach pain;
- serious neurological effects including unusual severe, prolonged headache especially if first time or getting progressively worse or sudden partial or complete loss of vision or sudden disturbance of hearing or other perceptual disorders or dysphasia or bad fainting attack or collapse or first unexplained epileptic seizure or weakness, motor disturbances, very marked numbness suddenly affecting one side or one part of body;
- hepatitis, jaundice, liver enlargement;

- blood pressure above systolic 160 mmHg or diastolic 95 mmHg;
- prolonged immobility after surgery or leg injury;
- detection of a risk factor which contra-indicates treatment.

Ethinylestradiol

Ethinylestradiol p. 874 (ethinyloestradiol) is licensed for short-term treatment of symptoms of oestrogen deficiency, for osteoporosis prophylaxis if other drugs cannot be used and for the treatment of female hypogonadism and menstrual disorders.

Table 1: Summary of HRT risks and benefits* during current use and current use plus post-treatment from age of menopause up to age 69 years, per 1000 women with 5 years or 10 years use of HRT

	Risks over 5 years use (with no use or 5 years current HRT use)		Total risks up to age 69 (after no use or after 5 years HRT use[†])		Risks over 10 years (with no use or 10 years current HRT use)		Total risks up to age 69 (after no use or after 10 years HRT use[†])	
	Cases per 1000 women with no HRT use	Extra cases per 1000 women using HRT	Cases per 1000 women with no HRT use	Extra cases per 1000 women using HRT	Cases per 1000 women with no HRT use	Extra cases per 1000 women using HRT	Cases per 1000 women with no HRT use	Extra cases per 1000 women using HRT
Risks associated with combined estrogen-progestogen HRT								
Breast cancer	13	+8	63	+17	27	+20	63	+34
Sequential HRT	13	+7	63	+14	27	+17	63	+29
Continuous combined HRT	13	+10	63	+20	27	+25	63	+40
Endometrial cancer	2	-	10	-	4	-	10	-
Ovarian cancer	2	+ <1	10	+ <1	4	+1	10	+1
Venous thromboembolism (VTE)[§]	5	+7	26	+7	8	+13	26	+13
Stroke	4	+1	26	+1	8	+2	26	+2
Coronary heart disease (CHD)	14	-	88	-	28	-	88	-
Fracture of femur	1.5	-	12	-	1	-	12	-
Risks associated with estrogen-only HRT								
Breast cancer	13	+3	63	+5	27	+7	63	+11
Endometrial cancer	2	+4	10	+4	4	+32	10	+32
Ovarian cancer	2	+ <1	10	+ <1	4	+1	10	+1
Venous thromboembolism (VTE)[§]	5	+2	26	+2	10	+3	26	+3
Stroke	4	+1	26	+1	8	+2	26	+2
Coronary heart disease (CHD)	14	-	88	-	28	-	88	-
Fracture of femur	0.5	-	12	-	1	-	12	-

*Menopausal symptom relief is not included in this table, but is a key benefit of HRT and will play a major part in the decision to prescribe HRT.

[†]Best estimates based on relative risks of HRT use from age 50 (see DSU table 2 for relative risks). For breast cancer this includes cases diagnosed during current HRT use and diagnosed after HRT use until age 69 years; for other risks, this assumes no residual effects after stopping HRT use.

[§]Latest evidence suggests that transdermal HRT products have a lower risk of VTE than oral preparations.

Table 2: Detailed summary of relative and absolute risks and benefits during current use from age of menopause and up to age 69, per 1000 women with 5 years or 10 years use of HRT

	Duration of HRT use (years)	Total cases per 1000 women with no HRT use* (RR= 1)	Total cases (range) per 1000 women using HRT†	Extra cases per 1000 women using HRT	Risk ratio (RR) (95% CI)‡
Risks associated with combined estrogen–progestogen HRT					
Cancer risks					
Breast cancer					
Overall combined HRT					
Current use from age 50	5	13	21	+8	1.62
	10	27	47	+20	1.74
Total risk from age 50 to 69 (HRT use + past use)	5	63	80	+17	1.27
	10	63	97	+34	1.54
Sequential HRT					
Current use from age 50	5	13	20	+7	1.54
	10	27	44	+17	1.63
Total risk from age 50 to 69 (HRT use + past use)	5	63	77	+14	1.22
	10	63	92	+29	1.46
Continuous combined HRT					
Current use from age 50	5	13	23	+10	1.77
	10	27	52	+25	1.93
Total risk to from age 50 to 69 (HRT use + past use)	5	63	83	+20	1.32
	10	63	103	+40	1.63
Endometrial Cancer					
age 50–59	5	2	2 (2–3)	NS	1·0 (0·8–1·2)[4]
	10	4	4 (4–5)	NS	1·1 (0·9–1·2)
age 60–69	5	3	3 (2–4)	NS	1·0 (0·8–1·2)[4]
	10	6	7 (5–7)	NS	1·1 (0·9–1·2)
Ovarian Cancer					
age 50–59	5	2	2 (2–3)	+ <1	1.1 (1.0–1.3)
	10	4	5 (4–6)	+1	1·3 (1·1–1·5)
age 60–69	5	3	3 (3–4)	+ <1	1.1 (1.0–1.3)
	10	6	8 (7–9)	+2	1·3 (1·1–1·5)
Cardiovascular risks					
Venous thromboembolism (VTE)§					
age 50–59	5	5	12 (10–15)	+7	2·3 (1·8–3·0)
age 60–69	5	8	18 (15–24)	+10	
Stroke					
age 50–59	5	4	5 (5–6)	+1	1.3 (1.1–1.4)
age 60–69	5	9	12 (10–13)	+3	
Coronary heart disease (CHD)					
age 50–59	5	9	12 (7–19)	NS	1·3 (0·8–2·1)
age 60–69	5	18	18 (13–25)	NS	1·0 (0·7–1·4)
age 70–79	5	29	44 (29–61)	+15	1·5 (1·0–2·1)
Benefits?					
Fracture of femur					
age 50–59	5	1.5	1 (0.8–1.5)	NS	0·7 (0·5–1.0)
age 60-69	5	5.5	4 (3-5.5)	NS	

	Duration of HRT use (years)	Total cases per 1000 women with no HRT use* (RR= 1)	Total cases (range) per 1000 women using HRT†	Extra cases per 1000 women using HRT	Risk ratio (RR) (95% CI)‡
Risks associated with estrogen-only HRT use					
Cancer risks					
Breast cancer					
Current use from age 50	5	13	16	+3	1.2
	10	27	34	+7	1.33
Total risk from age 50 to age 69 (HRT use + past use)	5	63	68	+5	1.08
	10	63	74	+11	1.17
Endometrial cancer					
age 50–59	5	2	6 (5–7)	+4	3.0 (2.5–3.6)
	10	4	36 (25–52)	+32	9.0 (6.3–12.9)
age 60–69	5	3	9 (8–11)	+6	3.0 (2.5–3.6)
	10	6	54 (38–77)	+48	9.0 (6.3–12.9)
Ovarian cancer					
age 50–59	5	2	2	+ <1	1.1 (1.0–1.3)
	10	4	5 (5–6)	+1	1·3 (1·2–1·5)
age 60–69	5	3	3	+ <1	1.1 (1.0–1.3)
	10	6	8 (7–9)	+2	1·3 (1·2–1·5)
Cardiovascular risks					
Venous thromboembolism (VTE)					
age 50–59	5	5	7 (5–9)	+2	1.3 (1.0–1.7)
age 60–69	5	8	10 (8–14)	+2	
Stroke					
age 50–59	5	4	5 (5–6)	+1	1.3 (1.0–1.4)
age 60–69	5	9	12 (10–13)	+3	
Coronary heart disease (CHD)					
age 50–59	5	14	8 (6–15)	NS	0·6 (0·4–1·1)
age 60–69	5	31	28 (22–37)	NS	0·9 (0·7–1·2)
age 70–79	5	44	48 (35–66)	NS	1·1 (0·8–1·5)
Benefits♭					
Fracture of femur					
age 50–59	5	0.5	0.3 (0.2–0.5)	0	0·6 (0·4–0·9)
age 60-69	5	5.5	3 (2-5)	−2	

* Background incidence from: Hospital Admissions in England (HES) for stroke and VTE; placebo arms of Women's Health Initiative (WHI) trial for coronary heart disease (CHD) and fracture; the International Agency Research on Cancer (IARC) for ovarian cancer and endometrial cancer; and from Office for National Statistics (ONS) for England for 2015, calculated for never-users in the Collaborative Group on Hormonal Factors in Breast Cancer meta-analysis for breast cancer.

† Best estimate and range based on relative risk and 95% confidence intervals (CI).

‡ Risk ratios and 95% CI from: meta-analysis of prospective observational studies for breast cancer (95% CI not available); meta-analyses of RCTs and observational studies for endometrial cancer, ovarian cancer and VTE; meta-analyses of randomised controlled trials (RCTs) for stroke; and from WHI trial for CHD and fracture risk.

§ Latest evidence suggests that transdermal HRT products have a lower risk of VTE than oral preparations.

♭ Menopausal symptom relief is not included in this table but is a key benefit of HRT and will play a major part in the decision to prescribe HRT.

NS=non-significant difference.

Ethinylestradiol is occasionally used under **specialist supervision** for the management of *hereditary haemorrhagic telangiectasia* (but evidence of benefit is limited). It is also used licensed for the palliative treatment of prostate cancer.

Raloxifene

Raloxifene hydrochloride p. 868 is licensed for the treatment and prevention of *postmenopausal osteoporosis*; unlike hormone replacement therapy, raloxifene hydrochloride does not reduce menopausal vasomotor symptoms.

Progestogens and progesterone receptor modulators

There are two main groups of progestogen, progesterone and its analogues (dydrogesterone and medroxyprogesterone acetate p. 936) and testosterone analogues (norethisterone p. 878 and norgestrel). The newer progestogens (desogestrel p. 930, norgestimate, and gestodene) are all derivatives of norgestrel; levonorgestrel p. 932 is the active isomer of norgestrel and has twice its potency. Progesterone p. 880 and its analogues are less androgenic than the testosterone derivatives and neither progesterone nor dydrogesterone causes virilisation.

Where endometriosis requires drug treatment, it may respond to a progestogen, e.g. norethisterone, administered on a continuous basis. Danazol and gonadorelin analogues are also licensed for endometriosis.

Although oral progestogens have been used widely for menorrhagia (see Heavy menstrual bleeding p. 868) they are relatively ineffective compared with tranexamic acid p. 127 or, particularly where dysmenorrhoea is also a factor, mefenamic acid p. 1308; the levonorgestrel-releasing intra-uterine device may be particularly useful for women also requiring contraception. Oral progestogens have also been used for severe dysmenorrhoea, but where contraception is also required in younger women the best choice is a combined oral contraceptive.

Progestogens have also been advocated for the alleviation of premenstrual symptoms, but no convincing physiological basis for such treatment has been shown.

For guidance on the use of progestogens in preventing miscarriage, and preterm labour, see Obstetrics p. 949.

Hormone replacement therapy

In women with a uterus a progestogen needs to be added to long-term oestrogen therapy for hormone replacement, to prevent cystic hyperplasia of the endometrium and possible transformation to cancer; it can be added on a cyclical or a continuous basis. Combined packs incorporating suitable progestogen tablets are available.

Oral contraception

Desogestrel, gestodene, levonorgestrel, norethisterone, and norgestimate are used in combined oral contraceptives and in progestogen-only contraceptives.

Cancer

Progestogens also have a role in neoplastic disease.

Progesterone receptor modulators

Ulipristal acetate p. 929 is a progesterone receptor modulator with a partial progesterone antagonist effect. Intermittent ulipristal acetate can be used to treat moderate to severe symptoms of uterine fibroids in premenopausal women where surgery and uterine artery embolisation are unsuitable, or have failed. Ulipristal acetate is also used as a emergency hormonal contraceptive.

Endometriosis

27-Jun-2024

Description of condition

Endometriosis is the growth of endometrial-like tissue outside the uterus. Endometriosis is a condition affecting women mainly of reproductive age and, although its exact cause is unknown, it is an oestrogen-dependent condition and is associated with menstruation. Endometriosis is typically associated with symptoms such as pelvic pain, painful periods and subfertility. Women with endometriosis report pain, which can be frequent, chronic and severe, as well as tiredness, more sick days, and a significant physical, sexual, psychological and social impact. Endometriosis is an important cause of subfertility and this can also have a significant effect on quality of life.

Women may also have endometriosis without symptoms, so it is difficult to know how common the disease is in the population. It is also unclear whether endometriosis is always progressive or can remain stable or improve with time.

Aims of treatment

The aim of treatment is to reduce the severity of symptoms, improve the quality of life, and to improve fertility if this is affected.

Drug treatment

Management options for endometriosis include drug treatment and surgery. Most drug treatments for endometriosis work by suppressing ovarian function and are contraceptive. Surgical treatment aims to remove or destroy endometriotic lesions. The choice of treatment depends on the woman's preferences and priorities in terms of pain management and fertility.

[EvGr] A short trial (such as 3 months) of paracetamol or an NSAID alone or in combination should be considered for first-line management of endometriosis-related pain. If pain relief is inadequate, consider other forms of pain management and referral for further assessment.

Hormonal treatment (with a combined oral contraceptive or a progestogen) should be offered to women with suspected, confirmed or recurrent endometriosis. The patient should be informed that hormonal treatment for endometriosis can reduce pain and has no permanent negative effect on subsequent fertility. If initial hormonal treatment for endometriosis is not effective, not tolerated or is contra-indicated, the woman should be referred to a gynaecologist or specialist endometriosis service for possible further treatment, which could include other hormonal treatments or surgery. ⟨A⟩ For use of drugs to treat neuropathic pain, see Neuropathic pain.

[EvGr] If fertility is a priority, the management of endometriosis-related subfertility should have multidisciplinary involvement with input from a fertility specialist. Women with endometriosis who are trying to conceive should not be offered hormonal treatment alone, or in combination with surgery, because it does not improve spontaneous pregnancy rates. ⟨A⟩ For further information on the management of endometriosis when fertility is a priority, see NICE guideline: **Endometriosis: diagnosis and management** (see *Useful resources*).

Surgery

[EvGr] Women with suspected or confirmed endometriosis should be asked about their symptoms, preferences and priorities with respect to pain and fertility, to guide surgical decision-making. For deep endometriosis involving the bowel, bladder or ureter, gonadotropin-releasing hormones given for 3 months before surgery should be considered. Excision rather than ablation should be considered to treat endometriomas, taking into account the woman's desire for fertility and her ovarian reserve. After laparoscopic excision or ablation of endometriosis, consider hormonal treatment (with, for example, a combined hormonal contraceptive), to prolong the benefits of surgery and manage symptoms.

A hysterectomy may be indicated if, for example, the woman has adenomyosis or heavy menstrual bleeding that has not responded to other treatments. Ⓐ

Useful Resources

Endometriosis: diagnosis and management. National Institute for Health and Care Excellence guideline NG73. February 2017 (updated April 2024).
www.nice.org.uk/guidance/ng73

Patient decision aid: Hormone treatment for endometriosis symptoms—what are my options? National Institute for Health and Care Excellence. September 2017.
www.nice.org.uk/guidance/ng73/resources/patient-decision-aid-information-4595573199

Heavy menstrual bleeding

11-Jun-2021

Description of condition

Heavy menstrual bleeding, also known as menorrhagia, is excessive menstrual blood loss of 80 mL or more, and/or for a duration of more than 7 days, which results in the need to change menstrual products every 1–2 hours. Heavy menstrual bleeding occurs regularly, every 24–35 days.

Drug treatment

EvGr The choice of treatment should be guided by the presence or absence of fibroids (including size, number and location), polyps, endometrial pathology or adenomyosis, other symptoms (such as pressure or pain), co-morbidities, and patient preference.

In females with heavy menstrual bleeding and unidentified pathology, fibroids less than 3 cm in diameter causing no distortion of the uterine cavity, or suspected or diagnosed adenomyosis, a levonorgestrel-releasing intra-uterine system p. 932 is the first-line treatment option. Patients should be advised that irregular menstrual bleeding can occur particularly during the first months of use and that the full benefit of treatment may take at least 6 months.

If a levonorgestrel-releasing intra-uterine system p. 932 is unsuitable, either tranexamic acid p. 127, an NSAID, a combined hormonal contraceptive, or a cyclical oral progestogen should be considered. Progestogen-only contraceptives may suppress menstruation and be beneficial to females with heavy menstrual bleeding. A non-hormonal treatment is recommended in patients actively trying to conceive.

If drug treatment is unsuccessful or declined by the patient, or if symptoms are severe, referral to a specialist for alternative drug treatment or surgery should be considered.

In females with fibroids of 3 cm or more in diameter, referral to a specialist should be considered. Treatment options include tranexamic acid, an NSAID, a levonorgestrel-releasing intra-uterine system p. 932, a combined hormonal contraceptive, a cyclical oral progestogen, ulipristal acetate p. 929, uterine artery embolisation, or surgery. Treatment choice depends on the size, number and location of the fibroids, and severity of symptoms. If drug treatment is required while investigations and definitive treatment is being organised, either tranexamic acid, or an NSAID, or both, can be given. Intermittent ulipristal acetate can be offered to treat moderate to severe symptoms of uterine fibroids in premenopausal women where surgery and uterine artery embolisation are unsuitable, or have failed.

The effectiveness of drug treatment for heavy menstrual bleeding may be limited in females with fibroids that are substantially greater than 3 cm in diameter. Treatment with a gonadotrophin-releasing hormone analogue before

hysterectomy and myomectomy should be considered if uterine fibroids are causing an enlarged or distorted uterus. Ⓐ

Useful Resources

Heavy menstrual bleeding: assessment and management. National Institute for Health and Care Excellence. NICE guideline 88. March 2018 (updated May 2021).
www.nice.org.uk/guidance/ng88

8.1 Female sex hormone responsive conditions

> **Other drugs used for Female sex hormone responsive conditions** Clonidine hydrochloride, p. 172

CALCIUM REGULATING DRUGS > BONE RESORPTION INHIBITORS

Raloxifene hydrochloride

01-Jun-2021

● INDICATIONS AND DOSE

Treatment and prevention of postmenopausal osteoporosis
▶ BY MOUTH
▶ Adult: 60 mg once daily

Breast cancer [chemoprevention in postmenopausal women at moderate to high risk] (initiated under specialist supervision)
▶ BY MOUTH
▶ Adult: 60 mg once daily for 5 years

● **UNLICENSED USE** Not licensed for chemoprevention of breast cancer in the UK. Licensed for this indication in USA.

● **CONTRA-INDICATIONS** Cholestasis · endometrial cancer · history of venous thromboembolism · undiagnosed uterine bleeding

● **CAUTIONS** Avoid in Acute porphyrias p. 1202 · breast cancer (manufacturer advises avoid during treatment for breast cancer) · history of oestrogen-induced hypertriglyceridaemia (monitor serum triglycerides) · risk factors for stroke · risk factors for venous thromboembolism (discontinue if prolonged immobilisation)

● **INTERACTIONS** → Appendix 1: raloxifene

● **SIDE-EFFECTS**
▶ **Common or very common** Influenza · leg cramps · peripheral oedema · vasodilation
▶ **Uncommon** Embolism and thrombosis
▶ **Rare or very rare** Breast abnormalities · gastrointestinal discomfort · gastrointestinal disorder · headaches · nausea · rash · thrombocytopenia · vomiting

● **HEPATIC IMPAIRMENT** Manufacturer advises avoid (risk of increased exposure).

● **RENAL IMPAIRMENT** EvGr Caution in mild to moderate impairment. Avoid in severe impairment. Ⓜ

● **NATIONAL FUNDING/ACCESS DECISIONS**
For full details see funding body website
NICE decisions
▶ **Raloxifene for the primary prevention of osteoporotic fragility fractures in postmenopausal women (updated February 2018)** NICE TA160 Not recommended
▶ **Raloxifene and teriparatide for the secondary prevention of osteoporotic fragility fractures in postmenopausal women (updated February 2018)** NICE TA161 Recommended with restrictions

- **MEDICINAL FORMS** There can be variation in the licensing of different medicines containing the same drug.
  ### Oral tablet
  ▸ **Raloxifene hydrochloride (Non-proprietary)**
  Raloxifene hydrochloride 60 mg Raloxifene 60mg tablets | 28 tablet PoM £17.06 DT = £5.34

NEUROKININ-3 RECEPTOR ANTAGONISTS

Fezolinetant
25-Apr-2025

- **DRUG ACTION** Fezolinetant is a non-hormonal neurokinin 3-receptor antagonist that modulates neuronal activity in the hypothalamic thermoregulatory centre.

- **INDICATIONS AND DOSE**

  Moderate to severe vasomotor symptoms associated with menopause
  ▸ BY MOUTH
  ▸ Adult 18–65 years: 45 mg once daily

> **IMPORTANT SAFETY INFORMATION**
> MHRA/CHM ADVICE: FEZOLINETANT (*VEOZA*®): RISK OF LIVER INJURY; NEW RECOMMENDATIONS TO MINIMISE RISK (APRIL 2025)
> An EU-wide review of safety data found serious drug-induced liver injury associated with fezolinetant. Serum alanine aminotransferase (ALT) and/or aspartate aminotransferase (AST) levels exceeding 10 times the upper limit of normal (ULN) with concurrent elevations in bilirubin and/or alkaline phosphatase (ALP) have been reported, including signs and symptoms suggestive of liver injury in some cases. These were generally reversible on stopping fezolinetant.
>   Healthcare professionals are advised that liver-function tests (LFTs) must be performed before treatment initiation, then monthly for the first 3 months and periodically thereafter, as clinically indicated, during treatment. LFTs must also be performed when signs or symptoms suggestive of liver injury occur. Monitoring should continue until LFTs normalise.
>   Treatment with fezolinetant:
> - should be avoided in patients with known, or at higher risk of, liver disease;
> - must not be started if ALT or AST, or total bilirubin is 2 times the ULN or more.
> Treatment must be discontinued if serum transaminases are:
> - exceeding 5 times the ULN;
> - 3 times ULN or more **and** either total bilirubin exceeds 2 times the ULN, or symptoms of liver injury develop.
> Patients or their carers should be advised to seek immediate medical attention if signs or symptoms of liver injury occur.

- **INTERACTIONS** → Appendix 1: fezolinetant

- **SIDE-EFFECTS**
  ▸ **Common or very common** Abdominal pain · diarrhoea · insomnia
  ▸ **Frequency not known** Drug-induced liver injury · endometrial adenocarcinoma

- **CONCEPTION AND CONTRACEPTION** EvGr Perimenopausal females of childbearing potential should use effective non-hormonal contraception during treatment. Ⓜ

- **PREGNANCY** EvGr Avoid (toxicity in *animal* studies). Ⓜ

- **BREAST FEEDING** EvGr Avoid (present in milk in *animal* studies). Ⓜ

- **HEPATIC IMPAIRMENT** EvGr Avoid in moderate to severe impairment (risk of increased exposure). Ⓜ See also *Important safety information.*

- **RENAL IMPAIRMENT** EvGr Avoid if eGFR less than 30 mL/minute/1.73 m^2 (limited information available). Ⓜ See p. 21.

- **PATIENT AND CARER ADVICE**
  Missed doses If a dose is more than 12 hours late, the missed dose should not be taken and the next dose should be taken at the normal time.

- **MEDICINAL FORMS** There can be variation in the licensing of different medicines containing the same drug.
  ### Oral tablet
  ▸ **Veoza** (Astellas Pharma Ltd) ▼
  Fezolinetant 45 mg Veoza 45mg tablets | 28 tablet PoM £44.80 DT = £44.80

OESTROGENS

Conjugated oestrogens (equine)
07-Jun-2023

- **INDICATIONS AND DOSE**

  PREMARIN® TABLETS
  Menopausal symptoms
  ▸ BY MOUTH
  ▸ Adult: 0.3–1.25 mg daily continuously; with cyclical progestogen for 12–14 days of each cycle in women with a uterus

  Postmenopausal osteoporosis prophylaxis
  ▸ BY MOUTH
  ▸ Adult: 0.625–1.25 mg daily continuously; with cyclical progestogen for 12–14 days of each cycle in women with a uterus

> **IMPORTANT SAFETY INFORMATION**
> MHRA/CHM ADVICE: HORMONE REPLACEMENT THERAPY (HRT): FURTHER INFORMATION ON THE KNOWN INCREASED RISK OF BREAST CANCER WITH HRT AND ITS PERSISTENCE AFTER STOPPING (SEPTEMBER 2019)
> Data from a meta-analysis of more than 100 000 women with breast cancer have confirmed that the risk of breast cancer is increased with the use of all forms of systemic HRT, except vaginal oestrogens, for longer than 1 year. Findings have shown that the risk increases further with longer duration of use, is higher for combined oestrogen-progestogen HRT than with oestrogen-only HRT, and persists for more than 10 years after stopping HRT. Healthcare professionals are advised to only prescribe HRT for the relief of postmenopausal symptoms that adversely affect quality of life, and to regularly review patients to ensure that it is used for the shortest time and at the lowest dose. Patients currently and previously on HRT should be informed of the risk and to be vigilant for signs of breast cancer; they should also be encouraged to attend breast screening appointments.

- **CONTRA-INDICATIONS** Active arterial thromboembolic disease (e.g. angina or myocardial infarction) · history of breast cancer · history of venous thromboembolism · liver disease (where liver function tests have failed to return to normal) · oestrogen-dependent cancer · recent arterial thromboembolic disease (e.g. angina or myocardial infarction) · thrombophilic disorder · undiagnosed vaginal bleeding · untreated endometrial hyperplasia

- **CAUTIONS** Acute porphyrias p. 1202 · diabetes (increased risk of heart disease) · factors predisposing to thromboembolism · history of breast nodules (closely monitor breast status—risk of breast cancer) · history of endometrial hyperplasia · history of fibrocystic disease (closely monitor breast status—risk of breast cancer) · hypophyseal tumours · increased risk of gall-bladder

6
Endocrine system

disease reported · migraine · migraine-like headaches · presence of antiphospholipid antibodies (increased risk of thrombotic events) · risk factors for oestrogen-dependent tumours (e.g. breast cancer in first-degree relative) · risk of breast cancer · symptoms of endometriosis may be exacerbated · uterine fibroids may increase in size

CAUTIONS, FURTHER INFORMATION
▶ **Risk of breast cancer** HRT use is associated with an increased risk of breast cancer—see *Important safety information*.

Radiological detection of breast cancer can be made more difficult as mammographic density can increase with HRT use.
▶ **Risk of endometrial cancer** The increased risk of endometrial cancer depends on the dose and duration of oestrogen-only HRT.

In women with a uterus, the addition of a progestogen cyclically (for at least 10 days per 28-day cycle) reduces the additional risk of endometrial cancer; this additional risk is eliminated if a progestogen is given continuously. However, this should be weighed against the increased risk of breast cancer.
▶ **Risk of ovarian cancer** Long-term use of combined HRT or oestrogen-only HRT is associated with a small increased risk of ovarian cancer. This excess risk disappears within a few years of stopping.
▶ **Risk of venous thromboembolism** Women using combined or oestrogen-only HRT are at an increased risk of deep vein thrombosis and of pulmonary embolism especially in the first year of use.

In *women who have predisposing factors* (such as a personal or family history of deep vein thrombosis or pulmonary embolism, severe varicose veins, obesity, trauma, or prolonged bed-rest) it is prudent to review the need for HRT, as in some cases the risks of HRT may exceed the benefits.

Travel involving prolonged immobility further increases the risk of deep vein thrombosis.
▶ **Risk of stroke** Risk of stroke increases with age, therefore older women have a greater absolute risk of stroke. Combined HRT or oestrogen-only HRT increases the risk of stroke.
▶ **Risk of coronary heart disease** HRT does not prevent coronary heart disease and should not be prescribed for this purpose. There is an increased risk of coronary heart disease in women who start combined HRT more than 10 years after menopause. Although very little information is available on the risk of coronary heart disease in younger women who start HRT close to the menopause, studies suggest a lower relative risk compared with older women.

● INTERACTIONS → Appendix 1: hormone replacement therapy

● SIDE-EFFECTS
▶ **Common or very common** Alopecia · arthralgia · breast abnormalities · depression · leg cramps · menstrual cycle irregularities · vaginal discharge · weight changes
▶ **Uncommon** Anxiety · cervical abnormalities · contact lens intolerance · dizziness · embolism and thrombosis · gallbladder disorder · gastrointestinal discomfort · headaches · hirsutism · libido disorder · mood altered · nausea · oedema · skin reactions · vulvovaginal candidiasis
▶ **Rare or very rare** Angioedema · asthma exacerbated · cerebrovascular insufficiency · chorea exacerbated · colitis ischaemic · epilepsy exacerbated · galactorrhoea · glucose tolerance impaired · hypocalcaemia · jaundice cholestatic · myocardial infarction · neoplasms · pancreatitis · pelvic pain · vomiting
▶ **Frequency not known** Endometrial hyperplasia · erythema nodosum

SIDE-EFFECTS, FURTHER INFORMATION Cyclical HRT (where a progestogen is taken for 12–14 days of each

28-day oestrogen treatment cycle) usually results in regular withdrawal bleeding towards the end of the progestogen. Continuous combined HRT commonly produces irregular breakthrough bleeding in the first 4–6 months of treatment. Bleeding beyond 6 months or after a spell of amenorrhoea requires further investigation to exclude serious gynaecological pathology.

● CONCEPTION AND CONTRACEPTION HRT does **not** provide contraception and a woman is considered potentially fertile for 2 years after her last menstrual period if she is under 50 years, and for 1 year if she is over 50 years. A woman who is under 50 years and free of all risk factors for venous and arterial disease can use a low-oestrogen combined oral contraceptive pill to provide both relief of menopausal symptoms and contraception; it is recommended that the oral contraceptive be stopped at 50 years of age since there are more suitable alternatives. If any potentially fertile woman needs HRT, non-hormonal contraceptive measures (such as condoms) are necessary. Measurement of follicle-stimulating hormone can help to determine fertility, but high measurements alone (particularly in women aged under 50 years) do not necessarily preclude the possibility of becoming pregnant.

● PREGNANCY Manufacturer advises avoid—not indicated during pregnancy.

● BREAST FEEDING Avoid until weaning or for 6 months after birth (adverse effects on lactation).

● HEPATIC IMPAIRMENT Manufacturer advises caution; avoid in acute or active disease.

● PATIENT AND CARER ADVICE
Information sheet The MHRA has provided a patient information sheet to aid healthcare professionals when counselling women on the risk of breast cancer with HRT use.

● MEDICINAL FORMS There can be variation in the licensing of different medicines containing the same drug.
Oral tablet
▶ **Premarin** (Pfizer Ltd)
Conjugated oestrogens 300 microgram Premarin 0.3mg tablets | 84 tablet [PoM] £14.94 DT = £24.02
Conjugated oestrogens 625 microgram Premarin 0.625mg tablets | 84 tablet [PoM] £17.50 DT = £26.87
Conjugated oestrogens 1.25 mg Premarin 1.25mg tablets | 84 tablet [PoM] £33.89 DT = £52.56

Combinations available: *Conjugated oestrogens with medroxyprogesterone*, p. 875

Estradiol
07-Jun-2023

● INDICATIONS AND DOSE
BEDOL ®

Menopausal symptoms | Osteoporosis prophylaxis
▶ BY MOUTH
▶ Adult: 2 mg daily, started on day 1–5 of menstruation (or at any time if cycles have ceased or are infrequent), to be taken with cyclical progestogen for 12–14 days of each cycle in women with a uterus

ELLESTE SOLO ® MX

Menopausal symptoms
▶ BY TRANSDERMAL APPLICATION
▶ Adult: Apply 1 patch twice weekly continuously, started within 5 days of onset of menstruation (or at any time if cycles have ceased or are infrequent), to be used with cyclical progestogen for 12–14 days of each cycle in women with a uterus, initiate therapy with MX 40 patch, subsequently adjust according to response

Osteoporosis prophylaxis
▶ BY TRANSDERMAL APPLICATION
▶ Adult: Apply 1 patch twice weekly continuously, started within 5 days of onset of menstruation (or at any time if cycles have ceased or are infrequent), to be used with cyclical progestogen for 12–14 days of each cycle in women with a uterus, initiate therapy with *MX* 80 patch, subsequently adjust according to response

ELLESTE-SOLO ® 1-MG
Menopausal symptoms
▶ BY MOUTH
▶ Adult: 1 mg daily, starting on day 1 of menstruation (or at any time if cycles have ceased or are infrequent), to be taken with cyclical progestogen for 12–14 days of each cycle in women with a uterus

ELLESTE-SOLO ® 2-MG
Menopausal symptoms not controlled with lower strength | Osteoporosis prophylaxis
▶ BY MOUTH
▶ Adult: 2 mg daily, started on day 1 of menstruation (or at any time if cycles have ceased or are infrequent), to be given with cyclical progestogen for 12–14 days of each cycle in women with a uterus

ESTRADERM MX ®
Menopausal symptoms
▶ BY TRANSDERMAL APPLICATION
▶ Adult: Apply 1 patch twice weekly continuously, started within 5 days of onset of menstruation (or at any time if cycles have ceased or are infrequent), to be used with cyclical progestogen for at least 12 days of each cycle in women with a uterus, initiate therapy with *MX* 25 patch for first 3 months; subsequently adjust according to response

Osteoporosis prophylaxis
▶ BY TRANSDERMAL APPLICATION
▶ Adult: Apply 1 patch twice weekly continuously, started within 5 days of onset of menstruation (or at any time if cycles have ceased or are infrequent), to be used with cyclical progestogen for at least 12 days of each cycle in women with a uterus, initiate therapy with *MX* 50 patch; subsequently adjust according to response

ESTRADOT ®
Menopausal symptoms
▶ BY TRANSDERMAL APPLICATION
▶ Adult: Apply 1 patch twice weekly continuously, to be used with cyclical progestogen for 12–14 days of each cycle in women with a uterus, initiate therapy with *Estradot* 25 patch for 3 months; subsequently adjust according to response

Osteoporosis prophylaxis
▶ BY TRANSDERMAL APPLICATION
▶ Adult: Apply 1 patch twice weekly continuously, to be used with cyclical progestogen for 12–14 days of each cycle in women with a uterus, initiate therapy with *Estradot* 50 patch; subsequently adjust according to response

EVOREL ®
Menopausal symptoms | Osteoporosis prophylaxis
▶ BY TRANSDERMAL APPLICATION
▶ Adult: Apply 1 patch twice weekly continuously, started within 5 days of onset of menstruation (or at any time if cycles have ceased or are infrequent), to be used with cyclical progestogen for 12–14 days of each cycle in women with a uterus, therapy should be initiated with *Evorel* 50 patch; subsequently adjust according to response; dose may be reduced to *Evorel* 25 patch after first month if necessary for menopausal symptoms **only**

FEMSEVEN ®
Menopausal symptoms | Osteoporosis prophylaxis
▶ BY TRANSDERMAL APPLICATION
▶ Adult: Apply 1 patch once weekly continuously, to be used with cyclical progestogen for 12–14 days of each cycle in women with a uterus, initiate therapy with *FemSeven* 50 patch for the first few months, subsequently adjust according to response

LENZETTO ®
Menopausal symptoms
▶ BY TRANSDERMAL APPLICATION
▶ Adult: Apply 1 spray once daily, increased if necessary to 2 sprays once daily after at least 4 weeks of continuous treatment, to be used with cyclical progestogen for 12–14 days of each cycle in women with a uterus, max. dose 3 sprays daily

OESTROGEL ®
Menopausal symptoms
▶ TO THE SKIN
▶ Adult: Apply 1.5 mg once daily continuously, increased if necessary up to 3 mg after 1 month continuously, to be applied over a large area, to be used with cyclical progestogen for at least 12 days of each cycle in women with a uterus. If switching from cyclical HRT, start at end of regimen; otherwise start at any time

Osteoporosis prophylaxis
▶ TO THE SKIN
▶ Adult: Apply 1.5 mg once daily continuously, to be applied over a large area, to be used with cyclical progestogen for at least 12 days of each cycle in women with a uterus. If switching from cyclical HRT, start at end of regimen; otherwise start at any time

DOSE EQUIVALENCE AND CONVERSION
▶ For *Oestrogel* ®: 2 measures is equivalent to estradiol 1.5 mg.

PROGYNOVA ®
Menopausal symptoms
▶ BY MOUTH
▶ Adult: 1–2 mg daily continuously, to be started on day 1 of menstruation (or at any time if cycles have ceased or are infrequent), to be taken with cyclical progestogen for 12–14 days of each cycle in women with a uterus

Osteoporosis prophylaxis
▶ BY MOUTH
▶ Adult: 2 mg daily continuously, to be taken with cyclical progestogen for 12–14 days of each cycle in women with a uterus

PROGYNOVA ® TS
Menopausal symptoms | Osteoporosis prophylaxis
▶ BY TRANSDERMAL APPLICATION
▶ Adult: Apply 1 patch once weekly continuously, alternatively apply 1 patch once weekly for 3 weeks, followed by a 7-day patch-free interval (cyclical), to be used with cyclical progestogen for 12–14 days of each cycle in women with a uterus, initiate therapy with *TS* 50 patch, subsequently adjust according to response, women receiving *TS* 100 patches for menopausal symptoms may continue with this strength for osteoporosis prophylaxis

SANDRENA ®
Menopausal symptoms
▶ TO THE SKIN
▶ Adult: Apply 1 mg once daily, to be applied over area 1–2 times size of hand; with cyclical progestogen for 12–14 days of each cycle in women with

continued →

a uterus, dose may be adjusted after 2–3 cycles to lowest effective dose; usual dose 0.5–1.5 mg daily

ZUMENON ®

Menopausal symptoms
▸ BY MOUTH
▸ Adult: Initially 1 mg daily, to be started on day 1 of menstruation (or any time if cycles have ceased or are infrequent), increased if necessary to 2 mg daily, to be taken with a cyclical progestogen for 12–14 days of each cycle in women with a uterus

Osteoporosis prophylaxis
▸ BY MOUTH
▸ Adult: 2 mg daily, to be taken with a cyclical progestogen for 12–14 days of each cycle in women with a uterus

IMPORTANT SAFETY INFORMATION

MHRA/CHM ADVICE: HORMONE REPLACEMENT THERAPY (HRT): FURTHER INFORMATION ON THE KNOWN INCREASED RISK OF BREAST CANCER WITH HRT AND ITS PERSISTENCE AFTER STOPPING (SEPTEMBER 2019)

Data from a meta-analysis of more than 100 000 women with breast cancer have confirmed that the risk of breast cancer is increased with the use of all forms of systemic HRT, except vaginal oestrogens, for longer than 1 year. Findings have shown that the risk increases further with longer duration of use, is higher for combined oestrogen-progestogen HRT than with oestrogen-only HRT, and persists for more than 10 years after stopping HRT. Healthcare professionals are advised to only prescribe HRT for the relief of postmenopausal symptoms that adversely affect quality of life, and to regularly review patients to ensure that it is used for the shortest time and at the lowest dose. Patients currently and previously on HRT should be informed of the risk and to be vigilant for signs of breast cancer; they should also be encouraged to attend breast screening appointments.

● CONTRA-INDICATIONS Active arterial thromboembolic disease (e.g. angina or myocardial infarction) · history of breast cancer · history of venous thromboembolism · oestrogen-dependent cancer · recent arterial thromboembolic disease (e.g. angina or myocardial infarction) · thrombophilic disorder · undiagnosed vaginal bleeding · untreated endometrial hyperplasia

● CAUTIONS Acute porphyrias p. 1202 · diabetes (increased risk of heart disease) · factors predisposing to thromboembolism · history of breast nodules—closely monitor breast status (risk of breast cancer) · history of endometrial hyperplasia · history of fibrocystic disease—closely monitor breast status (risk of breast cancer) · hypophyseal tumours · increased risk of gall-bladder disease · migraine (or migraine-like headaches) · presence of antiphospholipid antibodies (increased risk of thrombotic events) · prolonged exposure to unopposed oestrogens may increase risk of developing endometrial cancer · risk factors for oestrogen-dependent tumours (e.g. breast cancer in first-degree relative) · symptoms of endometriosis may be exacerbated · uterine fibroids may increase in size

CAUTIONS, FURTHER INFORMATION
▸ Risk of endometrial cancer The increased risk of endometrial cancer depends on the dose and duration of oestrogen-only HRT.

In women with a uterus using *systemic* preparations, the addition of a progestogen cyclically (for at least 10 days per 28-day cycle) reduces the additional risk of endometrial cancer; this additional risk is eliminated if a progestogen is given continuously. However, this should be weighed against the increased risk of breast cancer.

▸ Risk of ovarian cancer Long-term use of combined HRT or oestrogen-only HRT is associated with a small increased risk of ovarian cancer. This excess risk disappears within a few years of stopping.
▸ Risk of venous thromboembolism Women using combined or oestrogen-only HRT are at an increased risk of deep vein thrombosis and of pulmonary embolism especially in the first year of use.

In *women who have predisposing factors* (such as a personal or family history of deep vein thrombosis or pulmonary embolism, severe varicose veins, obesity, trauma, or prolonged bed-rest) it is prudent to review the need for HRT, as in some cases the risks of HRT may exceed the benefits.

Travel involving prolonged immobility further increases the risk of deep vein thrombosis.

Although the level of risk of thromboembolism associated with non-oral routes of administration of HRT has not been established, it may be lower for the transdermal route compared to the oral route; studies have found the risk associated with transdermal HRT to be no greater than the baseline population risk of thromboembolism.
▸ Risk of stroke Risk of stroke increases with age, therefore older women have a greater absolute risk of stroke. Combined HRT or oestrogen-only HRT increases the risk of stroke.
▸ Risk of coronary heart disease HRT does not prevent coronary heart disease and should not be prescribed for this purpose. There is an increased risk of coronary heart disease in women who start combined HRT more than 10 years after menopause. Although very little information is available on the risk of coronary heart disease in younger women who start HRT close to the menopause, studies suggest a lower relative risk compared with older women.
▸ Risk of breast cancer with systemic use HRT use is associated with an increased risk of breast cancer—see *Important safety information*. Radiological detection of breast cancer can be made more difficult as mammographic density can increase with HRT use.

● INTERACTIONS → Appendix 1: hormone replacement therapy

● SIDE-EFFECTS

GENERAL SIDE-EFFECTS
▸ **Common or very common** Headaches · nausea · skin reactions
▸ **Uncommon** Hypertension

SPECIFIC SIDE-EFFECTS
▸ **Common or very common**
▸ With oral use Asthenia · gastrointestinal discomfort · gastrointestinal disorders · haemorrhage · menstrual cycle irregularities · muscle complaints · pelvic pain · weight changes
▸ With transdermal use Abdominal pain · breast abnormalities · menstrual cycle irregularities · uterine disorders · vaginal discharge · weight changes
▸ **Uncommon**
▸ With oral use Anxiety · back pain · breast abnormalities · cervical abnormalities · cystitis-like symptom · depression · dizziness · embolism and thrombosis · erythema nodosum · gallbladder disorder · oedema · palpitations · peripheral vascular disease · tumour growth · visual impairment · vulvovaginal candidiasis
▸ With transdermal use Asthenia · breast neoplasm benign · depression · flatulence · increased risk of infection · leiomyoma · mood swings · vertigo · vomiting
▸ **Rare or very rare**
▸ With oral use Angioedema · cerebrovascular insufficiency · chorea · contact lens intolerance · haemolytic anaemia · hepatic disorders · hirsutism · malaise · myocardial

infarction · sexual dysfunction · steepening of corneal curvature · vaginal discharge · vomiting

▸ With transdermal use Epilepsy exacerbated · galactorrhoea · glucose tolerance impaired · libido disorder

▸ **Frequency not known**

▸ With oral use Carbohydrate metabolism change · epilepsy exacerbated · hypertriglyceridaemia · increased risk of coronary artery disease · neoplasms · pancreatitis · systemic lupus erythematosus (SLE)

SIDE-EFFECTS, FURTHER INFORMATION Cyclical HRT (where a progestogen is taken for 12–14 days of each 28-day oestrogen treatment cycle) usually results in regular withdrawal bleeding towards the end of the progestogen. Continuous combined HRT commonly produces irregular breakthrough bleeding in the first 4–6 months of treatment. Bleeding beyond 6 months or after a spell of amenorrhoea requires further investigation to exclude serious gynaecological pathology.

● CONCEPTION AND CONTRACEPTION HRT does **not** provide contraception and a woman is considered potentially fertile for 2 years after her last menstrual period if she is under 50 years, and for 1 year if she is over 50 years. A woman who is under 50 years and free of all risk factors for venous and arterial disease can use a low-oestrogen combined oral contraceptive pill to provide both relief of menopausal symptoms and contraception; it is recommended that the oral contraceptive be stopped at 50 years of age since there are more suitable alternatives. If any potentially fertile woman needs HRT, non-hormonal contraceptive measures (such as condoms) are necessary. Measurement of follicle-stimulating hormone can help to determine fertility, but high measurements alone (particularly in women aged under 50 years) do not necessarily preclude the possibility of becoming pregnant.

● PREGNANCY Not known to be harmful.

● BREAST FEEDING Avoid; adverse effects on lactation.

● HEPATIC IMPAIRMENT Manufacturer advises caution; avoid in acute or active disease.

● MONITORING REQUIREMENTS

▸ History of breast nodules or fibrocystic disease—closely monitor breast status (risk of breast cancer).

▸ The endometrial safety of long-term or repeated use of topical vaginal oestrogens is uncertain; treatment should be reviewed at least annually, with special consideration given to any symptoms of endometrial hyperplasia or carcinoma.

● DIRECTIONS FOR ADMINISTRATION

▸ With transdermal use Manufacturer advises patch should be removed after 3–4 days (or once a week in case of 7-day patch) and replaced with fresh patch on slightly different site; recommended sites: clean, dry, unbroken areas of skin on trunk below waistline; not to be applied on or near breasts or under waistband. If patch falls off in bath allow skin to cool before applying new patch.

● PATIENT AND CARER ADVICE

▸ With transdermal use Patient counselling is advised for estradiol patches and spray (administration).

▸ With topical use Patient counselling is advised for estradiol gels (administration).
Information sheet

▸ With oral use or topical use or transdermal use The MHRA has provided a patient information sheet to aid healthcare professionals when counselling women on the risk of breast cancer with HRT use.

LENZETTO ® ▸ With transdermal use Apply to dry, healthy skin of the inner forearm or alternatively the inner thigh and allow to dry for 2 minutes before covering with clothing. Avoid skin contact with another person (particularly children) or pets and avoid washing the area for at least 1 hour after application. If a sunscreen is needed, apply at least 1 hour before Lenzetto ®.

OESTROGEL ® ▸ With topical use Apply gel to clean, dry, intact skin such as arms, shoulders or inner thighs and allow to dry for 5 minutes before covering with clothing. Not to be applied on or near breasts or on vulval region. Avoid skin contact with another person (particularly male) and avoid other skin products or washing the area for at least 1 hour after application.

SANDRENA ® ▸ With topical use Apply gel to intact areas of skin such as lower trunk or thighs, using right and left sides on alternate days. Wash hands after application. Not to be applied on the breasts or face and avoid contact with eyes. Allow area of application to dry for 5 minutes and do not wash area for at least 1 hour.

● MEDICINAL FORMS There can be variation in the licensing of different medicines containing the same drug.

Oral tablet

▸ **Elleste Solo** (Exeltis UK Ltd)
Estradiol 1 mg Elleste Solo 1mg tablets | 84 tablet [PoM] £5.06 DT = £5.06
Estradiol 2 mg Elleste Solo 2mg tablets | 84 tablet [PoM] £5.06 DT = £5.06

▸ **Progynova** (Bayer Plc)
Estradiol valerate 1 mg Progynova 1mg tablets | 84 tablet [PoM] £7.30 DT = £7.30
Estradiol valerate 2 mg Progynova 2mg tablets | 84 tablet [PoM] £7.30 DT = £7.30

▸ **Zumenon** (Viatris UK Healthcare Ltd)
Estradiol 1 mg Zumenon 1mg tablets | 84 tablet [PoM] £6.89 DT = £5.06
Estradiol 2 mg Zumenon 2mg tablets | 84 tablet [PoM] £6.89 DT = £5.06

Spray

CAUTIONARY AND ADVISORY LABELS 15
EXCIPIENTS: May contain Ethanol

▸ **Lenzetto** (Gedeon Richter (UK) Ltd)
Estradiol (as Estradiol hemihydrate) 1.53 mg per 1 dose Lenzetto 1.53mg/dose transdermal spray | 56 dose [PoM] £6.90 DT = £6.90 | 168 dose [PoM] £20.70 DT = £20.70

Transdermal gel

EXCIPIENTS: May contain Propylene glycol

▸ **Oestrogel** (Besins Healthcare (UK) Ltd)
Estradiol 600 microgram per 1 gram Oestrogel Pump-Pack 0.06% gel | 80 gram [PoM] £9.15 DT = £9.15

▸ **Sandrena** (Orion Pharma (UK) Ltd)
Estradiol (as Estradiol hemihydrate) 500 microgram Sandrena 500microgram gel sachets | 28 sachet [PoM] £5.08 DT = £5.08
Estradiol (as Estradiol hemihydrate) 1 mg Sandrena 1mg gel sachets | 28 sachet [PoM] £5.85 DT = £5.85 | 91 sachet [PoM] £17.57

Transdermal patch

▸ **Estraderm MX** (Norgine Pharmaceuticals Ltd)
Estradiol 25 microgram per 24 hour Estraderm MX 25 patches | 8 patch [PoM] £5.50 DT = £4.07 | 24 patch [PoM] £16.46 DT = £16.46
Estradiol 50 microgram per 24 hour Estraderm MX 50 patches | 8 patch [PoM] £5.51 DT = £4.62 | 24 patch [PoM] £16.46 DT = £13.87
Estradiol 75 microgram per 24 hour Estraderm MX 75 patches | 8 patch [PoM] £6.42 DT = £4.90 | 24 patch [PoM] £19.27 DT = £19.27
Estradiol 100 microgram per 24 hour Estraderm MX 100 patches | 8 patch [PoM] £6.66 DT = £5.09 | 24 patch [PoM] £19.99 DT = £19.99

▸ **Estradot** (Sandoz Ltd)
Estradiol 25 microgram per 24 hour Estradot 25micrograms/24hours patches | 8 patch [PoM] £7.38 DT = £4.07
Estradiol 37.5 microgram per 24 hour Estradot 37.5micrograms/24hours patches | 8 patch [PoM] £7.39 DT = £7.39
Estradiol 50 microgram per 24 hour Estradot 50micrograms/24hours patches | 8 patch [PoM] £7.41 DT = £4.62
Estradiol 75 microgram per 24 hour Estradot 75micrograms/24hours patches | 8 patch [PoM] £8.62 DT = £4.90
Estradiol 100 microgram per 24 hour Estradot 100micrograms/24hours patches | 8 patch [PoM] £8.95 DT = £5.09

▸ **Evorel** (Theramex HQ UK Ltd)
Estradiol 25 microgram per 24 hour Evorel 25 patches | 8 patch [PoM] £4.07 DT = £4.07
Estradiol 50 microgram per 24 hour Evorel 50 patches | 4 patch [PoM] [£] DT = £6.04 | 8 patch [PoM] £4.62 DT = £4.62 | 24 patch [PoM] £13.87 DT = £13.87
Estradiol 75 microgram per 24 hour Evorel 75 patches | 8 patch [PoM] £4.90 DT = £4.90

Estradiol 100 microgram per 24 hour Evorel 100 patches | 8 patch [PoM] £5.09 DT = £5.09

▸ **FemSeven** (Theramex HQ UK Ltd)
Estradiol 50 microgram per 24 hour FemSeven 50 patches | 4 patch [PoM] £6.04 DT = £6.04
Estradiol 75 microgram per 24 hour FemSeven 75 patches | 4 patch [PoM] £6.98
Estradiol 100 microgram per 24 hour FemSeven 100 patches | 4 patch [PoM] £7.28 DT = £7.28

▸ **Progynova TS** (Bayer Plc)
Estradiol 50 microgram per 24 hour Progynova TS 50micrograms/24hours transdermal patches | 12 patch [PoM] £18.90 DT = £18.02
Estradiol 100 microgram per 24 hour Progynova TS 100micrograms/24hours transdermal patches | 12 patch [PoM] £20.70 DT = £20.70

Combinations available: *Estradiol with dydrogesterone*, p. 875 · *Estradiol with levonorgestrel*, p. 876 · *Estradiol with medroxyprogesterone*, p. 876 · *Estradiol with norethisterone*, p. 876 · *Estradiol with progesterone*, p. 877

Ethinylestradiol

22-May-2020

(Ethinyloestradiol)

● **INDICATIONS AND DOSE**

Short-term treatment of symptoms of oestrogen deficiency | Osteoporosis prophylaxis if other drugs cannot be used
▸ BY MOUTH
▸ Adult (female): 10–50 micrograms daily for 21 days, repeated after 7-day tablet-free period, to be given with progestogen for 12–14 days per cycle in women with intact uterus.

Female hypogonadism
▸ BY MOUTH
▸ Adult (female): 10–50 micrograms daily usually on cyclical basis, initial oestrogen therapy should be followed by combined oestrogen and progestogen therapy.

Menstrual disorders
▸ BY MOUTH
▸ Adult (female): 20–50 micrograms daily from day 5 to 25 of each cycle, to be given with progestogen, added either throughout the cycle or from day 15 to 25.

Palliative treatment of prostate cancer
▸ BY MOUTH
▸ Adult (male): 0.15–1.5 mg daily.

● **CONTRA-INDICATIONS** Active or recent arterial thromboembolic disease (e.g. angina or myocardial infarction) · Acute porphyrias p. 1202 · history of breast cancer · history of venous thromboembolism · liver disease (where liver function tests have failed to return to normal) · oestrogen-dependent cancer · thrombophilic disorder · undiagnosed vaginal bleeding · untreated endometrial hyperplasia

CONTRA-INDICATIONS, FURTHER INFORMATION
▸ Combined hormonal contraception For more information on contra-indications for ethinylestradiol in *contraception* see combined hormonal contraceptive preparations containing ethinylestradiol.
▸ Hormone replacement therapy For more information on contra-indications for hormone replacement therapy see Sex hormones p. 862

● **CAUTIONS** Cardiovascular disease (risk of fluid retention) · diabetes (increased risk of heart disease) · history of breast nodules or fibrocystic disease—closely monitor breast status (risk of breast cancer) · history of endometrial hyperplasia · history of hypertriglyceridaemia (increased risk of pancreatitis) · hypophyseal tumours · increased risk of gall-bladder disease · migraine (migraine-like

headaches) · presence of antiphospholipid antibodies (increased risk of thrombotic events) · prolonged exposure to unopposed oestrogens may increase risk of developing endometrial cancer · risk factors for oestrogen-dependent tumours (e.g. breast cancer in first-degree relative) · risk factors for venous thromboembolism · symptoms of endometriosis may be exacerbated · uterine fibroids may increase in size

CAUTIONS, FURTHER INFORMATION
▸ Combined hormonal contraception For more information on cautions for ethinylestradiol in *contraception* see combined hormonal contraceptive preparations containing ethinylestradiol.
▸ Hormone replacement therapy For more information on cautions for hormone replacement therapy see Sex hormones p. 862

● **INTERACTIONS** → Appendix 1: hormone replacement therapy

● **SIDE-EFFECTS** Breast abnormalities · cervical mucus increased · cholelithiasis · contact lens intolerance · depression · electrolyte imbalance · embolism and thrombosis · erythema nodosum · feminisation · fluid retention · headaches · hypertension · jaundice cholestatic · metrorrhagia · mood altered · myocardial infarction · nausea · neoplasms · skin reactions · stroke · uterine disorders · vomiting · weight change

SIDE-EFFECTS, FURTHER INFORMATION Cyclical HRT (where a progestogen is taken for 12–14 days of each 28-day oestrogen treatment cycle) usually results in regular withdrawal bleeding towards the end of the progestogen. Continuous combined HRT commonly produces irregular breakthrough bleeding in the first 4–6 months of treatment. Bleeding beyond 6 months or after a spell of amenorrhoea requires further investigation to exclude serious gynaecological pathology.

● **PREGNANCY** Not known to be harmful.

● **BREAST FEEDING** Avoid until weaning or for 6 months after birth (adverse effects on lactation).

● **HEPATIC IMPAIRMENT** Manufacturer advises caution; avoid in acute or active disease.

● **MEDICINAL FORMS** Forms available from special-order manufacturers include: oral tablet, oral capsule, oral suspension

Tibolone

25-Mar-2024

● **INDICATIONS AND DOSE**

Short-term treatment of symptoms of oestrogen deficiency (including women being treated with gonadotrophin releasing hormone analogues) | Osteoporosis prophylaxis in women at high risk of fractures when other prophylaxis contra-indicated or not tolerated
▸ BY MOUTH
▸ Adult: 2.5 mg daily

● **CONTRA-INDICATIONS** Acute porphyrias p. 1202 · history of arterial thromboembolic disease (e.g. angina, myocardial infarction, stroke, or TIA) · history of breast cancer · oestrogen-dependent cancer · thrombophilic disorder · undiagnosed vaginal bleeding · untreated endometrial hyperplasia · venous thromboembolism

● **CAUTIONS** Diabetes (increased risk of heart disease) · epilepsy · factors predisposing to thromboembolism · history of breast nodules—closely monitor breast status (risk of breast cancer) · history of endometrial hyperplasia · history of fibrocystic disease—closely monitor breast status (risk of breast cancer) · hypertriglyceridaemia · hypophyseal tumours · migraine (or migraine-like headaches) · presence of antiphospholipid antibodies (increased risk of thrombotic events) · prolonged exposure to unopposed oestrogens may increase risk of developing endometrial cancer · risk factors for oestrogen-dependent tumours (e.g. breast cancer in first-degree relative) · risk of stroke

● **SIDE-EFFECTS**
▸ **Common or very common** Breast abnormalities · cervical dysplasia · endometrial thickening · gastrointestinal discomfort · genital abnormalities · hair growth abnormal · increased risk of infection · pelvic pain · postmenopausal haemorrhage · vaginal discharge · vaginal haemorrhage · weight increased
▸ **Uncommon** Oedema · skin reactions
▸ **Frequency not known** Arthralgia · dementia · depression · dizziness · erythema nodosum · gallbladder disorder · headaches · increased risk of ischaemic stroke · myalgia · neoplasms · vision disorders

  SIDE-EFFECTS, FURTHER INFORMATION **Vaginal bleeding** Investigate for endometrial cancer if bleeding continues beyond 6 months or after stopping treatment.

  Reasons to withdraw treatment Withdraw treatment if signs of thromboembolic disease, abnormal liver function tests, or signs of cholestatic jaundice.

● **PREGNANCY** Avoid; toxicity in *animal* studies.

● **BREAST FEEDING** Avoid.

● **HEPATIC IMPAIRMENT** [EvGr] Avoid in acute or history of liver disease, where liver function tests have failed to return to normal. Caution in liver disorders e.g. liver adenoma. Ⓜ

● **RENAL IMPAIRMENT** [EvGr] Caution (risk of fluid retention). Ⓜ

● **PRESCRIBING AND DISPENSING INFORMATION** Unsuitable for use in the premenopause (unless being treated with gonadotrophin-releasing hormone analogue) and as (or with) an oral contraceptive.

  Also unsuitable for use within 12 months of last menstrual period (may cause irregular bleeding).

  If transferring from cyclical HRT, start at end of regimen; if transferring from continuous-combined HRT, start at any time.

● **MEDICINAL FORMS** There can be variation in the licensing of different medicines containing the same drug.
  Oral tablet
  ▸ **Tibolone (Non-proprietary)**
    Tibolone 2.5 mg Tibolone 2.5mg tablets | 28 tablet [PoM] £10.36 DT = £2.95 | 84 tablet [PoM] £9.69–£31.08
  ▸ **Livial** (Organon Pharma (UK) Ltd)
    Tibolone 2.5 mg Livial 2.5mg tablets | 28 tablet [PoM] £10.36 DT = £2.95 | 84 tablet [PoM] £31.08

OESTROGENS COMBINED WITH PROGESTOGENS

Conjugated oestrogens with medroxyprogesterone

The properties listed below are those particular to the combination only. For the properties of the components please consider, conjugated oestrogens (equine) p. 869, medroxyprogesterone acetate p. 936.

● **INDICATIONS AND DOSE**

PREMIQUE ® LOW DOSE TABLETS

Menopausal symptoms in women with a uterus
  ▸ BY MOUTH
  ▸ Adult: 1 tablet daily continuously

● **INTERACTIONS** → Appendix 1: hormone replacement therapy · medroxyprogesterone

● **MEDICINAL FORMS** There can be variation in the licensing of different medicines containing the same drug.
  Modified-release tablet
  ▸ **Premique** (Pfizer Ltd)
    Conjugated oestrogens 300 microgram, Medroxyprogesterone acetate 1.5 mg Premique Low Dose 0.3mg/1.5mg modified-release tablets | 84 tablet [PoM] £21.01 DT = £34.13

Estradiol with dydrogesterone   18-Jun-2021

The properties listed below are those particular to the combination only. For the properties of the components please consider, estradiol p. 870.

● **INDICATIONS AND DOSE**

FEMOSTON ® 1 MG/10 MG

Menopausal symptoms in women with a uterus
  ▸ BY MOUTH
  ▸ Adult: 1 tablet daily for 14 days, white tablet to be taken and started within 5 days of onset of menstruation (or any time if cycles have ceased or are infrequent), then 1 tablet daily for 14 days, grey tablet to be taken, subsequent courses repeated without interval, *Femoston* ® 1 *mg*/10 *mg* given initially and *Femoston* ® 2 *mg*/10 *mg* substituted if symptoms not controlled

Osteoporosis prophylaxis in women with a uterus
  ▸ BY MOUTH
  ▸ Adult: 1 tablet daily for 14 days, white tablet to be taken and started within 5 days of onset of menstruation (or any time if cycles have ceased or are infrequent), then 1 tablet daily for 14 days, grey tablet to be taken, subsequent courses repeated without interval

FEMOSTON ® 2 MG/10 MG

Menopausal symptoms in women with a uterus
  ▸ BY MOUTH
  ▸ Adult: 1 tablet daily for 14 days, red tablet to be taken and started within 5 days of onset of menstruation (or any time if cycles have ceased or are infrequent), then 1 tablet daily for 14 days, yellow tablet to be taken, subsequent courses repeated without interval, *Femoston* ® 1 *mg*/10 *mg* given initially and *Femoston* ® 2 *mg*/10 *mg* substituted if symptoms not controlled

Osteoporosis prophylaxis in women with a uterus
  ▸ BY MOUTH
  ▸ Adult: 1 tablet daily for 14 days, red tablet to be taken and started within 5 days of onset of menstruation (or any time if cycles have ceased or are infrequent), then 1 tablet daily for 14 days, yellow tablet to be taken, subsequent courses repeated without interval

FEMOSTON ®-CONTI 0.5 MG/2.5MG

Menopausal symptoms in women with a uterus whose last menstrual period occurred over 12 months previously
  ▸ BY MOUTH
  ▸ Adult: 1 tablet daily continuously, if changing from cyclical HRT begin treatment the day after finishing oestrogen plus progestogen phase

FEMOSTON ®-CONTI 1 MG/5MG

Menopausal symptoms in women with a uterus whose last menstrual period occurred over 12 months previously | Osteoporosis prophylaxis in women with a uterus whose last menstrual period occurred over 12 months previously
  ▸ BY MOUTH
  ▸ Adult: 1 tablet daily continuously, if changing from cyclical HRT begin treatment the day after finishing oestrogen plus progestogen phase

- **INTERACTIONS** → Appendix 1: estradiol · hormone replacement therapy
- **SIDE-EFFECTS**
  - **Common or very common** Asthenia · breast abnormalities · cervical abnormalities · depression · dizziness · flatulence · gastrointestinal discomfort · headaches · malaise · menstrual cycle irregularities · nausea · nervousness · pain · pelvic pain · peripheral oedema · postmenopausal haemorrhage · skin reactions · vomiting · vulvovaginal candidiasis · weight changes
  - **Uncommon** Cystitis-like symptom · embolism and thrombosis · gallbladder disorder · hepatic function abnormal · hypertension · libido disorder · peripheral vascular disease · tumour growth · varicose veins
  - **Rare or very rare** Angioedema · myocardial infarction
  - **Frequency not known** Chorea · contact lens intolerance · dementia · epilepsy exacerbated · erythema nodosum · haemolytic anaemia · hypertriglyceridaemia · leg cramps · neoplasms · pancreatitis · steepening of corneal curvature · systemic lupus erythematosus (SLE) · urinary incontinence
- **HEPATIC IMPAIRMENT** Manufacturer advises caution; avoid in acute or active disease.
- **RENAL IMPAIRMENT** EvGr Use with caution. Ⓜ

- **MEDICINAL FORMS** There can be variation in the licensing of different medicines containing the same drug.
  Oral tablet
  - **Femoston-conti** (Exeltis UK Ltd)
  Estradiol 500 microgram, Dydrogesterone 2.5 mg Femoston-conti 0.5mg/2.5mg tablets | 84 tablet PoM £24.43 DT = £24.43
  Estradiol 1 mg, Dydrogesterone 5 mg Femoston-conti 1mg/5mg tablets | 84 tablet PoM £24.43 DT = £24.43
  Form unstated
  - **Femoston 1/10** (Exeltis UK Ltd)
  Femoston 1/10mg tablets | 84 tablet PoM £16.16
  - **Femoston 2/10** (Exeltis UK Ltd)
  Femoston 2/10mg tablets | 84 tablet PoM £16.16

Estradiol with levonorgestrel

The properties listed below are those particular to the combination only. For the properties of the components please consider, estradiol p. 870, levonorgestrel p. 932.

- **INDICATIONS AND DOSE**
  FEMSEVEN CONTI ®
  Menopausal symptoms in women with a uterus whose last menstrual period occurred over 12 months previously
  - BY TRANSDERMAL APPLICATION
  - Adult: Apply 1 patch once weekly continuously

- **INTERACTIONS** → Appendix 1: estradiol · hormone replacement therapy · levonorgestrel

- **PATIENT AND CARER ADVICE** Patient counselling is advised for estradiol with levonorgestrel patches (application).

- **MEDICINAL FORMS** There can be variation in the licensing of different medicines containing the same drug.
  Transdermal patch
  - **FemSeven Conti** (Theramex HQ UK Ltd)
  Levonorgestrel 7 microgram per 24 hour, Estradiol 50 microgram per 24 hour FemSeven Conti patches | 4 patch PoM £15.48 DT = £15.48

Estradiol with medroxyprogesterone

05-Oct-2021

The properties listed below are those particular to the combination only. For the properties of the components please consider, estradiol p. 870, medroxyprogesterone acetate p. 936.

- **INDICATIONS AND DOSE**
  INDIVINA ® TABLETS
  Menopausal symptoms in women with a uterus whose last menstrual period occurred over 3 years previously | Osteoporosis prophylaxis in women with a uterus whose last menstrual period occurred over 3 years previously
  - BY MOUTH
  - Adult: Initially 1/2.5 mg daily taken continuously, adjust according to response, to be started at end of scheduled bleed if changing from cyclical HRT

- **INTERACTIONS** → Appendix 1: estradiol · hormone replacement therapy · medroxyprogesterone

- **MEDICINAL FORMS** There can be variation in the licensing of different medicines containing the same drug.
  Oral tablet
  - **Indivina** (Orion Pharma (UK) Ltd)
  Estradiol valerate 1 mg, Medroxyprogesterone acetate 2.5 mg Indivina 1mg/2.5mg tablets | 84 tablet PoM £20.58 DT = £20.58
  Estradiol valerate 2 mg, Medroxyprogesterone acetate 5 mg Indivina 2mg/5mg tablets | 84 tablet PoM £20.58 DT = £20.58
  Estradiol valerate 1 mg, Medroxyprogesterone acetate 5 mg Indivina 1mg/5mg tablets | 84 tablet PoM £20.58 DT = £20.58

Estradiol with norethisterone

11-Dec-2020

The properties listed below are those particular to the combination only. For the properties of the components please consider, estradiol p. 870, norethisterone p. 878.

- **INDICATIONS AND DOSE**
  CLINORETTE ®
  Menopausal symptoms in women with a uterus
  - BY MOUTH
  - Adult: 1 tablet daily for 16 days, white tablet to be taken, starting on day 5 of menstruation (or at any time if cycles have ceased or are infrequent), then 1 tablet daily for 12 days, pink tablet to be taken, subsequent courses repeated without interval

  ELLESTE-DUET ® 1-MG
  Menopausal symptoms
  - BY MOUTH
  - Adult: 1 tablet daily for 16 days, white tablet to be taken and started on day 1 of menstruation (or at any time if cycles have ceased or are infrequent), then 1 tablet daily for 12 days, green tablet to be taken, subsequent courses are repeated without interval

  ELLESTE-DUET ® 2-MG
  Menopausal symptoms | Osteoporosis prophylaxis
  - BY MOUTH
  - Adult: 1 tablet daily for 16 days, orange tablet to be taken, to be started on day 1 of menstruation (or at any time if cycles have ceased or are infrequent), then 1 tablet daily for 12 days, grey tablet to be taken, subsequent courses are repeated without interval

ELLESTE-DUET ® CONTI

Menopausal symptoms in women whose last menstrual period occurred over 12 months previously | Osteoporosis prophylaxis

▶ BY MOUTH

▶ Adult: 1 tablet daily continuously, to be started at end of scheduled bleed if changing from cyclical HRT

EVOREL ® CONTI

Menopausal symptoms in women whose last menstrual period occurred over 18 months previously | Osteoporosis prophylaxis

▶ BY TRANSDERMAL APPLICATION

▶ Adult: Apply 1 patch twice weekly continuously, to be started at end of scheduled bleed if changing from cyclical HRT

EVOREL ® SEQUI

Menopausal symptoms | Osteoporosis prophylaxis

▶ BY TRANSDERMAL APPLICATION

▶ Adult: Apply 1 patch twice weekly for 2 weeks, *Evorel®* 50 patch to be applied and started within 5 days of onset of menstruation (or at any time if cycles have ceased or are infrequent), then apply 1 patch twice weekly for the following 2 weeks, *Evorel®* Conti patch to be applied, subsequent courses are repeated without interval.

KLIOFEM ®

Menopausal symptoms in women with a uterus whose last menstrual period occurred over 12 months previously | Osteoporosis prophylaxis in women with a uterus

▶ BY MOUTH

▶ Adult: 1 tablet daily continuously, to be started at end of scheduled bleed if changing from cyclical HRT

KLIOVANCE ®

Menopausal symptoms in women with a uterus whose last menstrual period occurred over 12 months previously | Osteoporosis prophylaxis in women with a uterus

▶ BY MOUTH

▶ Adult: 1 tablet daily continuously, to be started at end of scheduled bleed if changing from cyclical HRT

NOVOFEM ®

Menopausal symptoms in women whose last menstrual period occurred over 6 months previously | Osteoporosis prophylaxis

▶ BY MOUTH

▶ Adult: 1 tablet daily for 16 days, red tablet to be taken, then 1 tablet daily for 12 days, white tablet to be taken, subsequent courses are repeated without interval; start treatment with red tablet at any time or if changing from cyclical HRT, start treatment the day after finishing previous regimen

TRISEQUENS ®

Menopausal symptoms in women whose last menstrual period occurred over 6 months previously | Osteoporosis prophylaxis

▶ BY MOUTH

▶ Adult: 1 tablet daily for 12 days, blue tablet to be taken, followed by 1 tablet daily for 10 days, white tablet to be taken, then 1 tablet daily for 6 days, red tablet to be taken, subsequent courses are repeated without interval; start treatment with blue tablet at any time or if changing from cyclical HRT, start treatment the day after finishing previous regimen

● INTERACTIONS → Appendix 1: estradiol · hormone replacement therapy · norethisterone

● **PATIENT AND CARER ADVICE**

EVOREL ® SEQUI Patients and carers should be advised on the application of *Evorel®* Sequi patches.

● **MEDICINAL FORMS** There can be variation in the licensing of different medicines containing the same drug.

Oral tablet

▶ **Elleste Duet** (Exeltis UK Ltd)
  Norethisterone acetate 1 mg, Estradiol 2 mg Elleste Duet Conti tablets | 84 tablet [PoM] £17.02 DT = £17.02

▶ **Kliofem** (Novo Nordisk Ltd)
  Norethisterone acetate 1 mg, Estradiol 2 mg Kliofem tablets | 84 tablet [PoM] £11.43 DT = £17.02

▶ **Kliovance** (Novo Nordisk Ltd)
  Norethisterone acetate 500 microgram, Estradiol 1 mg Kliovance tablets | 84 tablet [PoM] £13.20 DT = £13.20

Form unstated

▶ **Elleste Duet** (Exeltis UK Ltd)
  Elleste Duet 1mg tablets | 84 tablet [PoM] £9.20
  Elleste Duet 2mg tablets | 84 tablet [PoM] £9.20

▶ **Evorel Sequi** (Theramex HQ UK Ltd)
  Evorel Sequi patches | 8 patch [PoM] £13.20

▶ **Novofem** (Novo Nordisk Ltd)
  Novofem tablets | 84 tablet [PoM] £11.43

▶ **Trisequens** (Novo Nordisk Ltd)
  Trisequens tablets | 84 tablet [PoM] £11.10

Transdermal patch

▶ **Evorel Conti** (Theramex HQ UK Ltd)
  Estradiol 50 microgram per 24 hour, Norethisterone acetate 170 microgram per 24 hour Evorel Conti patches | 8 patch [PoM] £15.47 | 24 patch [PoM] £44.28 DT = £44.28

Estradiol with progesterone   04-Oct-2022

The properties listed below are those particular to the combination only. For the properties of the components please consider, estradiol p. 870, progesterone p. 880.

● **INDICATIONS AND DOSE**

BIJUVE ®

Menopausal symptoms in women with a uterus whose last menstrual period occurred over 12 months previously

▶ BY MOUTH

▶ Adult: 1 capsule daily continuously, dose to be taken in the evening with food, if changing from continuous sequential or cyclical HRT, start treatment the day after finishing the 28-day cycle. Treatment may start immediately after surgical menopause or if changing from another continuous combined HRT

● INTERACTIONS → Appendix 1: estradiol · hormone replacement therapy

● **SIDE-EFFECTS**

▶ **Common or very common** Alopecia · breast abnormalities · dizziness · fatigue · gastrointestinal discomfort · haemorrhage · headaches · nausea · pain · pelvic pain · skin reactions · uterine disorders · vulvovaginal disorders · weight changes

▶ **Uncommon** Altered smell sensation · anaemia · anxiety · arthralgia · cervical abnormalities · chills · concentration impaired · constipation · depression · diarrhoea · drowsiness · dry mouth · flatulence · fluid retention · hirsutism · hot flush · hyperlipidaemia · hyperphagia · hypertension · hyperuricaemia · increased risk of infection · leiomyoma · libido increased · memory impairment · metrorrhagia · mood altered · muscle spasms · neoplasms · oral discomfort · pancreatitis acute · paraesthesia · postmenopausal haemorrhage · sleep disorders · taste altered · telangiectasia · thrombophlebitis · vertigo · visual impairment · vomiting

● **NATIONAL FUNDING/ACCESS DECISIONS**
For full details see funding body website

Scottish Medicines Consortium (SMC) decisions

▶ Estradiol / micronised progesterone (*Bijuve®*) as continuous combined hormone replacement therapy (HRT) for estrogen deficiency symptoms in postmenopausal women with intact

6   Endocrine system

uterus and with at least 12 months since last menses (September 2022) SMC No. SMC2502 Recommended

- **MEDICINAL FORMS** There can be variation in the licensing of different medicines containing the same drug.
  Oral capsule
  ▸ **Bijuve** (Theramex HQ UK Ltd)
    Estradiol 1 mg, Progesterone 100 mg Bijuve 1mg/100mg capsules | 28 capsule [PoM] £8.14 DT = £8.14

PROGESTOGENS

Dienogest   17-Feb-2020

- **DRUG ACTION** Dienogest is a nortestosterone derivative that has a progestogenic effect in the uterus, reducing the production of estradiol and thereby suppressing endometriotic lesions.

- **INDICATIONS AND DOSE**
  Endometriosis
  ▸ BY MOUTH
  ▸ Females of childbearing potential: 2 mg once daily, can be started on any day of cycle, dose should be taken continuously at the same time each day

- **CONTRA-INDICATIONS** Arterial disease (past or present) · cardiovascular disease (past or present) · diabetes with vascular involvement · liver tumours (past or present) · sex hormone-dependent malignancies (confirmed or suspected) · undiagnosed vaginal bleeding · venous thromboembolism (active)

- **CAUTIONS** Diabetes (progestogens can decrease glucose tolerance—monitor patient closely) · history of depression · history of ectopic pregnancy · history of gestational diabetes · patients at risk of osteoporosis · patients at risk of venous thromboembolism

  CAUTIONS, FURTHER INFORMATION
  ▸ Immobilisation Manufacturer advises to discontinue treatment during prolonged immobilisation. For elective surgery, treatment should be discontinued at least 4 weeks before surgery; treatment may be restarted 2 weeks after complete remobilisation.

- **INTERACTIONS** → Appendix 1: dienogest

- **SIDE-EFFECTS**
  ▸ **Common or very common** Alopecia · anxiety · asthenic conditions · breast abnormalities · depression · gastrointestinal discomfort · gastrointestinal disorders · haemorrhage · headaches · hot flush · libido loss · mood altered · nausea · ovarian cyst · pain · skin reactions · sleep disorder · vomiting · vulvovaginal disorders · weight changes
  ▸ **Uncommon** Anaemia · appetite increased · autonomic dysfunction · broken nails · circulatory system disorder · concentration impaired · constipation · dandruff · diarrhoea · dry eye · dyspnoea · genital discharge · hair changes · hyperhidrosis · hypotension · increased risk of infection · limb discomfort · muscle spasms · oedema · palpitations · pelvic pain · photosensitivity reaction · tinnitus
  ▸ **Frequency not known** Glucose tolerance impaired · insulin resistance · menstrual cycle irregularities

- **CONCEPTION AND CONTRACEPTION** Manufacturer advises that, if contraception is required, females of childbearing potential should use non-hormonal contraception during treatment. The menstrual cycle usually returns to normal within 2 months after stopping treatment.

- **BREAST FEEDING** Manufacturer advises avoid—present in milk in *animal* studies.

- **HEPATIC IMPAIRMENT** Manufacturer advises avoid in severe impairment (no information available).

- **PATIENT AND CARER ADVICE** Manufacturer advises patients with a history of chloasma gravidarum to avoid sunlight or UV radiation exposure during treatment.
  Missed doses Manufacturer advises if one or more tablets are missed, or if vomiting and/or diarrhoea occurs within 3–4 hours of taking a tablet, another tablet should be taken as soon as possible and the next dose taken at the normal time.

- **MEDICINAL FORMS** There can be variation in the licensing of different medicines containing the same drug.
  Oral tablet
  ▸ **Dienogest (Non-proprietary)**
    Dienogest 2 mg Dienogest 2mg tablets | 28 tablet [PoM] £20.50-£26.00 DT = £20.50 | 84 tablet [PoM] £61.50
  ▸ **Dimetrum** (Besins Healthcare (UK) Ltd)
    Dienogest 2 mg Dimetrum 2mg tablets | 28 tablet [PoM] £16.40 DT = £20.50
  ▸ **Sawis** (Gedeon Richter (UK) Ltd)
    Dienogest 2 mg Sawis 2mg tablets | 28 tablet [PoM] £20.50 DT = £20.50

Norethisterone   19-Dec-2023

- **INDICATIONS AND DOSE**
  Endometriosis
  ▸ BY MOUTH
  ▸ Adult: 10–15 mg daily for 4–6 months or longer, to be started on day 5 of cycle; increased to 20–25 mg daily if required, dose only increased if spotting occurs and reduced once bleeding has stopped

  Dysfunctional uterine bleeding (to arrest bleeding) | Menorrhagia (to arrest bleeding)
  ▸ BY MOUTH
  ▸ Adult: 5 mg 3 times a day for 10 days

  Dysfunctional uterine bleeding (to prevent bleeding) | Menorrhagia (to prevent bleeding)
  ▸ BY MOUTH
  ▸ Adult: 5 mg twice daily, to be taken from day 19 to day 26 of cycle

  Dysmenorrhoea
  ▸ BY MOUTH
  ▸ Adult: 5 mg 3 times a day for 3–4 cycles, to be taken from day 5–24 of cycle

  Premenstrual syndrome (but not recommended)
  ▸ BY MOUTH
  ▸ Adult: 5 mg 2–3 times a day for several cycles, to be taken from day 19–26 of cycle

  Postponement of menstruation
  ▸ BY MOUTH
  ▸ Females of childbearing potential: 5 mg 3 times a day, to be started 3 days before expected onset (menstruation occurs 2–3 days after stopping)

  Breast cancer
  ▸ BY MOUTH
  ▸ Adult: 40 mg daily, increased if necessary to 60 mg daily

  Short-term contraception
  ▸ BY DEEP INTRAMUSCULAR INJECTION
  ▸ Females of childbearing potential: 200 mg, to be administered within first 5 days of cycle or immediately after parturition (duration 8 weeks). To be injected into the gluteal muscle, then 200 mg after 8 weeks if required

  Contraception
  ▸ BY MOUTH
  ▸ Females of childbearing potential: 350 micrograms daily, dose to be taken at same time each day, starting on day 1 of cycle then continuously, if administration delayed for 3 hours or more it should be regarded as a 'missed pill'

- **CONTRA-INDICATIONS**

  GENERAL CONTRA-INDICATIONS Acute porphyrias p. 1202 · current breast cancer (unless progestogens are being used in the management of this condition) · history during pregnancy of idiopathic jaundice (non-contraceptive indications) · history during pregnancy of pemphigoid gestationis (non-contraceptive indications) · history during pregnancy of severe pruritus (non-contraceptive indications)

  SPECIFIC CONTRA-INDICATIONS
  ▸ With oral use History of thromboembolism (non-contraceptive indications) · undiagnosed vaginal bleeding (non-contraceptive indications)

- **CAUTIONS**

  GENERAL CAUTIONS Cardiac dysfunction · conditions that may worsen with fluid retention · diabetes (progestogens can decrease glucose tolerance—monitor patient closely) · history of breast cancer—seek specialist advice before use · hypertension · liver tumours—seek specialist advice before use · migraine · multiple risk factors for cardiovascular disease—seek specialist advice before intramuscular use · positive antiphospholipid antibodies · rheumatoid arthritis · risk factors for venous thromboembolism · systemic lupus erythematosus

  SPECIFIC CAUTIONS
  ▸ With intramuscular use Cervical cancer
  ▸ When used for Contraception History of stroke (including transient ischaemic attack)—seek specialist advice before intramuscular use · ischaemic heart disease—seek specialist advice before intramuscular use · undiagnosed vaginal bleeding—seek specialist advice before intramuscular use
  ▸ With oral use for Contraception Malabsorption syndromes

- **INTERACTIONS** → Appendix 1: norethisterone

- **SIDE-EFFECTS**

  GENERAL SIDE-EFFECTS
  ▸ **Common or very common** Menstrual cycle irregularities
  ▸ **Uncommon** Breast tenderness
  ▸ **Frequency not known** Hepatic cancer · thromboembolism

  SPECIFIC SIDE-EFFECTS
  ▸ **Common or very common**
  ▸ With intramuscular use Dizziness · haemorrhage · headache · hypersensitivity · nausea · skin reactions · weight increased
  ▸ **Uncommon**
  ▸ With intramuscular use Abdominal distension · depressed mood
  ▸ **Frequency not known**
  ▸ With oral use Appetite change · depression · fatigue · gastrointestinal disorder · headaches · hypertension · libido disorder · nervousness · rash · weight change

  SIDE-EFFECTS, FURTHER INFORMATION **Breast cancer risk with contraceptive use** The benefits of using progestogen-only contraceptives (POCs), such as norethisterone, should be weighed against the possible risks for each individual woman.

  There is a possible small increase in the risk of breast cancer in women using, or who have recently used, progestogen-only contraception. Causal association is not clearly established, and absolute risk remains very small, and is like that of current or recent use of combined hormonal contraception.

  The most important risk factor for breast cancer appears to be the age the contraceptive is stopped rather than the duration of use; the risk gradually disappears during the 10 years after stopping.

- **PREGNANCY**
  ▸ With oral use Masculinisation of female fetuses and other defects reported with non-contraceptive use.

- **BREAST FEEDING** Progestogen-only contraceptives do not affect lactation. Higher doses (used in malignant conditions) may suppress lactation and alter milk composition—use lowest effective dose.
  ▸ With intramuscular use Withhold breast-feeding for neonates with severe or persistent jaundice requiring medical treatment.

- **HEPATIC IMPAIRMENT** Manufacturers advise caution; avoid in severe or active disease.
  ▸ When used for Breast cancer Manufacturer advises avoid.

- **RENAL IMPAIRMENT**
  ▸ With oral use EvGr Use with caution. M

- **PATIENT AND CARER ADVICE**
  ▸ Diarrhoea and vomiting with oral contraceptives Vomiting and persistent, severe diarrhoea can interfere with the absorption of oral progestogen-only contraceptives. If vomiting occurs within 2 hours of taking an oral progestogen-only contraceptive, another pill should be taken as soon as possible. If a replacement pill is not taken within 3 hours of the normal time for taking the progestogen-only pill, or in cases of persistent vomiting or very severe diarrhoea, additional precautions should be used during illness and for 2 days after recovery.
  ▸ Starting routine for oral contraceptives One tablet daily, on a continuous basis, starting on day 1 of cycle and taken at the same time each day (if delayed by longer than 3 hours contraceptive protection may be lost). Additional contraceptive precautions are not required if norethisterone is started up to and including day 5 of the menstrual cycle; if started after this time, additional contraceptive precautions are required for 2 days.
  ▸ Changing from a combined oral contraceptive Start on the day following completion of the combined oral contraceptive course without a break (or in the case of *everyday* (ED) tablets, omitting the inactive tablets).
  ▸ After childbirth (not breast-feeding) Oral progestogen-only contraceptives can be started before 21 days postpartum without the need for additional contraceptive precautions. If started 21 days or more postpartum, additional contraceptive precautions are required for 2 days.
  ▸ Contraceptives by injection Full counselling backed by *patient information leaflet* required before administration—likelihood of menstrual disturbance and the potential for a delay in return to full fertility. Delayed return of fertility and irregular cycles may occur after discontinuation of treatment but there is no evidence of permanent infertility.

  Missed doses

  Missed oral contraceptive pill The following advice is recommended: 'If you forget a pill, take it as soon as you remember and carry on with the next pill at the right time (this may mean taking 2 pills at the same time). If the pill was more than 3 hours overdue you are not protected. Continue normal pill-taking but you must also use another method, such as the condom, for the next 2 days'.

  The Faculty of Sexual and Reproductive Healthcare recommends emergency contraception if one or more progestogen-only contraceptive tablets are missed or taken more than 3 hours late and unprotected intercourse has occurred before 2 further tablets have been correctly taken.

- **MEDICINAL FORMS** There can be variation in the licensing of different medicines containing the same drug. Forms available from special-order manufacturers include: oral suspension

  Solution for injection
  ▸ Noristerat (Bayer Plc)
    Norethisterone enantate 200 mg per 1 ml Noristerat 200mg/1ml solution for injection ampoules | 1 ampoule PoM £4.05 DT = £4.05

  Oral tablet
  ▸ Norethisterone (Non-proprietary)
    Norethisterone 5 mg Norethisterone 5mg tablets | 30 tablet PoM £11.00 DT = £7.05

▶ **Noriday** (Pfizer Ltd)
Norethisterone 350 microgram Noriday 350microgram tablets |
84 tablet [PoM] £2.10 DT = £2.10
▶ **Primolut N** (Bayer Plc)
Norethisterone 5 mg Primolut N 5mg tablets | 30 tablet [PoM]
£2.26 DT = £7.05
▶ **Utovlan** (Pfizer Ltd)
Norethisterone 5 mg Utovlan 5mg tablets | 30 tablet [PoM] £1.40
DT = £7.05 | 90 tablet [PoM] £4.21

Combinations available: *Estradiol with norethisterone,* p. 876

Progesterone

30-Nov-2023

● **INDICATIONS AND DOSE**

CRINONE ® VAGINAL GEL

**Supplementation of luteal phase in infertility (under
expert supervision)**
▶ BY VAGINA
▶ Adult: 1 applicatorful daily, start either after
documented ovulation or on day 18–21 of cycle

**Adjunct in in-vitro fertilisation [when mainly tubal,
idiopathic, or endometriosis related infertility is
associated with normal ovulatory cycles] (under expert
supervision)**
▶ BY VAGINA
▶ Adult: 1 applicatorful daily, dose to be inserted
preferably in the morning, start from the day of embryo
transfer and continue for a total of 30 days once
pregnancy is confirmed

CYCLOGEST ® PESSARIES

Premenstrual syndrome | Post-natal depression
▶ BY VAGINA, OR BY RECTUM
▶ Adult: 200–800 mg daily, doses above 200 mg to be
given in 2 divided doses, for premenstrual syndrome
start on day 12–14 and continue until onset of
menstruation (but not recommended); rectally if
barrier methods of contraception are used, in patients
who have recently given birth or in those who suffer
from vaginal infection or recurrent cystitis

**Supplementation of luteal phase during assisted
reproductive technology (ART) treatment (under expert
supervision)**
▶ BY VAGINA
▶ Adult: 400 mg twice daily, start at oocyte retrieval, and
continue for 38 days once pregnancy is confirmed

**Threatened miscarriage [with vaginal bleeding and
previous miscarriage] (initiated by a specialist)**
▶ BY VAGINA
▶ Adult: 400 mg twice daily from when intra-uterine
pregnancy is confirmed until week 16 of pregnancy if
fetal heartbeat confirmed, offer a repeat scan within
2 weeks if fetal heartbeat is not seen on an initial scan

LUBION ®

**Supplementation of luteal phase during assisted
reproductive technology (ART) treatment in women for
whom vaginal preparations are inappropriate**
▶ BY SUBCUTANEOUS INJECTION, OR BY INTRAMUSCULAR
INJECTION
▶ Adult: 25 mg once daily from day of oocyte retrieval up
to week 12 of pregnancy

LUTIGEST ®

**Supplementation of luteal phase during assisted
reproductive technology (ART) treatment (under expert
supervision)**
▶ BY VAGINA
▶ Adult: 100 mg 3 times a day, start the day after oocyte
retrieval, and continue for 30 days once pregnancy is
confirmed

UTROGESTAN ® CAPSULES

Progestogenic opposition of oestrogen HRT
▶ BY MOUTH
▶ Adult: 200 mg once daily on days 15–26 of each 28-day
oestrogen HRT cycle, alternatively 100 mg once daily
on days 1–25 of each 28-day oestrogen HRT cycle

UTROGESTAN ® VAGINAL CAPSULES

**Supplementation of luteal phase during assisted
reproductive technology (ART) cycles**
▶ BY VAGINA
▶ Adult: 200 mg 3 times a day from day of embryo
transfer until at least week 7 of pregnancy up to week
12 of pregnancy

**Threatened miscarriage [with vaginal bleeding and
previous miscarriage] (initiated by a specialist)**
▶ BY VAGINA
▶ Adult: 400 mg twice daily from when intra-uterine
pregnancy is confirmed until week 16 of pregnancy if
fetal heartbeat confirmed, offer a repeat scan within
2 weeks if fetal heartbeat is not seen on an initial scan

**Prevention of preterm birth [with cervical length ≤25 mm
and/or history of spontaneous preterm birth or loss]**
▶ BY VAGINA
▶ Adult: 200 mg once daily to be given at bedtime, from
between week 16 and 24 of pregnancy until at least
week 34 of pregnancy as clinically indicated

● **UNLICENSED USE** [EvGr] *Cyclogest*® pessaries and
Utrogestan® vaginal capsules are used in the prevention of
threatened miscarriage, Ⓐbut are not licensed for this
indication.

UTROGESTAN® **VAGINAL CAPSULES** [EvGr] Progesterone is
used for the prevention of preterm birth from week 16 of
pregnancy, Ⓐbut this may differ from that licensed.

● **CONTRA-INDICATIONS** Acute porphyrias p. 1202 · breast
cancer · genital cancer · history during pregnancy of
idiopathic jaundice · history during pregnancy of
pemphigoid gestationis · history during pregnancy of
severe pruritus · history of thromboembolism · missed
miscarriage · thrombophlebitis · undiagnosed vaginal
bleeding

● **CAUTIONS** Conditions that may worsen with fluid
retention · diabetes (progestogens can decrease glucose
tolerance—monitor patient closely) · history of depression
· migraine · risk factors for thromboembolism

● **SIDE-EFFECTS**
▶ **Common or very common**
▶ With oral use Headache · menstrual cycle irregularities
▶ With vaginal use Breast pain · drowsiness · gastrointestinal
discomfort
▶ **Uncommon**
▶ With oral use Breast pain · constipation · diarrhoea ·
dizziness · drowsiness · jaundice cholestatic · skin reactions
· vomiting
▶ **Rare or very rare**
▶ With oral use Depression · nausea
▶ **Frequency not known**
▶ With intramuscular use Alopecia · breast changes · cervical
abnormalities · depression · drowsiness · fever · hirsutism ·
insomnia · jaundice cholestatic · menstrual cycle
irregularities · nausea · oedema · protein catabolism · skin
reactions · weight increased
▶ With rectal use Diarrhoea · flatulence
▶ With vaginal use Leakage of the pessary base · menstrual
cycle irregularities · vulvovaginal pain

● **ALLERGY AND CROSS-SENSITIVITY** For *Utrogestan*® *oral and
vaginal capsules*, manufacturer advises contra-indicated in
patients with hypersensitivity to soy or peanut products—
contains soya lecithin.

● **PREGNANCY** Not known to be harmful.

- **BREAST FEEDING** Avoid—present in milk.
- **HEPATIC IMPAIRMENT** Manufacturer advises caution; avoid in severe impairment. For *Utrogestan®* *oral capsules*, manufacturer advises avoid in acute or active liver disease. For *Crinone® vaginal gel*, manufacturer advises caution in severe impairment.
- **RENAL IMPAIRMENT** EvGr Caution (risk of fluid retention; no information available). ⟨M⟩
- **DIRECTIONS FOR ADMINISTRATION**
- With oral use Manufacturer advises capsules should be taken at bedtime on an empty stomach.
- **PRESCRIBING AND DISPENSING INFORMATION** *Cyclogest®* pessaries and *Utrogestan®* oral and vaginal capsules contain micronised progesterone.
- **PATIENT AND CARER ADVICE**
- With oral use Patient counselling is advised for progesterone capsules (administration).
- **NATIONAL FUNDING/ACCESS DECISIONS** For full details see funding body website
  Scottish Medicines Consortium (SMC) decisions
- Progesterone (*Lutigest®*) for luteal support as part of an assisted reproductive technology (ART) treatment program for infertile women (October 2016) SMC No. 1185/16 Recommended
- Micronised progesterone (*Utrogestan Vaginal®*) in women for supplementation of the luteal phase during Assisted Reproductive Technology (ART) cycles (May 2017) SMC No. 935/13 Recommended
- Progesterone (*Lubion®*) is indicated in adults for luteal support as part of an Assisted Reproductive Technology (ART) treatment program in infertile women who are unable to use or tolerate vaginal preparations (July 2018) SMC No. SMC2017 Recommended
- Micronised progesterone (*Utrogestan®*) for adjunctive use with oestrogen in post-menopausal women with an intact uterus, as hormone replacement therapy (HRT) (December 2022) SMC No. SMC2529 Recommended
- **LESS SUITABLE FOR PRESCRIBING**
- With vaginal use Progesterone pessaries are less suitable for prescribing.

- **MEDICINAL FORMS** There can be variation in the licensing of different medicines containing the same drug.

  Pessary
  - Cyclogest (L.D. Collins & Co. Ltd)
    Progesterone 200 mg Cyclogest 200mg pessaries | 15 pessary PoM £8.95 DT = £8.95
    Progesterone 400 mg Cyclogest 400mg pessaries | 15 pessary PoM £12.96 DT = £12.96
  - Lutigest (Ferring Pharmaceuticals Ltd)
    Progesterone 100 mg Lutigest 100mg vaginal tablets | 21 pessary PoM £19.50 DT = £19.50

  Vaginal capsule
  - Utrogestan (Besins Healthcare (UK) Ltd)
    Progesterone 200 mg Utrogestan 200mg vaginal capsules with applicators | 21 capsule PoM £21.00 DT = £21.00

  Solution for injection
  - Lubion (IBSA Pharma Ltd)
    Progesterone 22.48 mg per 1 ml Lubion 25mg/1.112ml solution for injection vials | 7 vial PoM £56.00 DT = £56.00

  Vaginal gel
  - Crinone (Merck Serono Ltd)
    Progesterone 80 mg per 1 gram Crinone 8% progesterone vaginal gel | 15 unit dose PoM £30.83 DT = £30.83

  Oral capsule
  - Utrogestan (Besins Healthcare (UK) Ltd)
    Progesterone 100 mg Utrogestan 100mg capsules | 30 capsule PoM £6.60 DT = £4.16

  Combinations available: *Estradiol with progesterone,* p. 877

8.1a Anti-oestrogens

OVULATION STIMULANTS

Clomifene citrate
(Clomiphene citrate)   23-Nov-2020

- **DRUG ACTION** Anti-oestrogen which induces gonadotrophin release by occupying oestrogen receptors in the hypothalamus, thereby interfering with feedback mechanisms; chorionic gonadotrophin is sometimes used as an adjunct.

- **INDICATIONS AND DOSE**

  Female infertility due to ovulatory dysfunction
  - BY MOUTH
  - Adult (female): 50 mg once daily for 5 days, to be started at any time if no recent uterine bleeding or on or around the fifth day of cycle if progestogen-induced bleeding is planned or if spontaneous uterine bleeding occurs, then 100 mg once daily if required for 5 days, this second course to be given at least 30 days after the first course, only in the absence of ovulation; most patients who are going to respond will do so to first course, 3 courses should constitute adequate therapeutic trial; long-term cyclical therapy not recommended (beyond a total of 6 cycles).

  IMPORTANT SAFETY INFORMATION
  Manufacturer advises clomifene should not normally be used for longer than 6 cycles (possible increased risk of ovarian cancer).

- **CONTRA-INDICATIONS** Abnormal uterine bleeding of undetermined cause · hormone-dependent tumours · ovarian cysts
- **CAUTIONS** Ectopic pregnancy · incidence of multiple births increased · ovarian hyperstimulation syndrome · polycystic ovary syndrome (cysts may enlarge during treatment, also risk of exaggerated response to usual doses) · uterine fibroids
- **SIDE-EFFECTS** Abdominal distension · alopecia · angioedema · anxiety · breast tenderness · cataract · cerebral thrombosis · depression · disorientation · dizziness · fatigue · headache · hot flush · hypertriglyceridaemia · insomnia · jaundice cholestatic · menstrual cycle irregularities · mood altered · nausea · neoplasms · nervous system disorders · optic neuritis · ovarian and fallopian tube disorders · palpitations · pancreatitis · paraesthesia · psychosis · seizure · skin reactions · speech disorder · stroke · syncope · tachycardia · uterine disorders · vertigo · vision disorders · visual impairment (discontinue and initiate ophthalmological examination) · vomiting
- **CONCEPTION AND CONTRACEPTION** Exclude pregnancy before treatment.
- **PREGNANCY** Possible effects on fetal development.
- **BREAST FEEDING** May inhibit lactation.
- **HEPATIC IMPAIRMENT** Manufacturer advises avoid in liver disease or history of liver dysfunction.
- **PATIENT AND CARER ADVICE**
  Conception and contraception Patients planning to conceive should be warned that there is a risk of multiple pregnancy (*rarely* more than twins).

- **MEDICINAL FORMS** There can be variation in the licensing of different medicines containing the same drug.

Oral tablet

▶ Clomifene citrate (Non-proprietary)

Clomifene citrate 50 mg Clomifene 50mg tablets | 30 tablet [PoM] £18.00 DT = £10.15

▶ Clomid (Sanofi)

Clomifene citrate 50 mg Clomid 50mg tablets | 5 tablet [PoM] £1.69 | 30 tablet [PoM] £10.15 DT = £10.15

8.2 Male sex hormone responsive conditions

Androgens, anti-androgens and anabolic steroids

14-Aug-2020

Androgens

Androgens cause masculinisation; they may be used as replacement therapy in castrated adults and in those who are hypogonadal due to either pituitary or testicular disease. In the normal male they inhibit pituitary gonadotrophin secretion and depress spermatogenesis. Androgens also have an anabolic action which led to the development of anabolic steroids.

Androgens are useless as a treatment of impotence and impaired spermatogenesis unless there is associated hypogonadism; they should not be given until the hypogonadism has been properly investigated. Treatment should be under expert supervision.

When given to patients with hypopituitarism they can lead to normal sexual development and potency but not to fertility. If fertility is desired, the usual treatment is with gonadotrophins or pulsatile gonadotrophin-releasing hormone which will stimulate spermatogenesis as well as androgen production.

Intramuscular depot preparations of **testosterone esters** are preferred for replacement therapy. Testosterone enantate, propionate or undecanoate, or alternatively *Sustanon*®, which consists of a mixture of testosterone esters and has a longer duration of action, may be used.

Anti-androgens

Cyproterone acetate

Cyproterone acetate p. 885 is an anti-androgen used in the treatment of severe hypersexuality and sexual deviation in the male. It inhibits spermatogenesis and produces reversible infertility (but is not a male contraceptive); abnormal sperm forms are produced. Fully informed consent is recommended and an initial spermatogram. As hepatic tumours have been produced in *animal* studies, careful consideration should be given to the risk/benefit ratio before treatment. Cyproterone acetate is also licensed for use alone in patients with metastatic prostate cancer refractory to gonadorelin analogue therapy, and has been used as an adjunct in prostatic cancer and in the treatment of acne and hirsutism in women.

The MHRA/CHM have released important safety information on the use of cyproterone acetate and risk of meningioma. For further information, see *Important safety information* for cyproterone acetate.

Dutasteride and finasteride

Dutasteride p. 907 and finasteride p. 907 are alternatives to alpha-blockers particularly in men with a significantly enlarged prostate. Finasteride is also licensed for use with doxazosin p. 903 in the management of benign prostatic hyperplasia.

A low strength of finasteride is licensed for treating male-pattern baldness in men.

Anabolic steroids

Anabolic steroids have some androgenic activity but they cause less virilisation than androgens in women. They are used in the treatment of some *aplastic anaemias*. Anabolic steroids have been given for osteoporosis in women but they are no longer advocated for this purpose.

The protein-building properties of anabolic steroids have not proved beneficial in the clinical setting. Their use as body builders or tonics is unjustified; some athletes abuse them.

ANDROGENS

Androgens 

- **CONTRA-INDICATIONS** Breast cancer in males · history of liver tumours · hypercalcaemia · prostate cancer
- **CAUTIONS** Cardiac impairment · diabetes mellitus · elderly · epilepsy · hypertension · ischaemic heart disease · migraine · risk factors for venous thromboembolism · skeletal metastases—risk of hypercalcaemia or hypercalciuria (if this occurs, treat appropriately and restart treatment once normal serum calcium concentration restored) · sleep apnoea · stop treatment or reduce dose if severe polycythaemia occurs · thrombophilia—increased risk of thrombosis · tumours—risk of hypercalcaemia or hypercalciuria (if this occurs, treat appropriately and restart treatment once normal serum calcium concentration restored)

CAUTIONS, FURTHER INFORMATION

▶ Elderly Screening Tool of Older Persons' potentially inappropriate Prescriptions (STOPP) criteria to aid medication reviews (see Prescribing in the elderly p. 31 for information): potentially inappropriate in the absence of primary or secondary hypogonadism (risk of androgen toxicity; no proven benefit outside of the hypogonadism indication).

- **SIDE-EFFECTS**

▶ **Common or very common** Hot flush · hypertension · polycythaemia · prostate abnormalities · skin reactions · weight increased

▶ **Uncommon** Alopecia · asthenia · behaviour abnormal · depression · dizziness · dyspnoea · dysuria · gynaecomastia · headache · hyperhidrosis · insomnia · nausea · sexual dysfunction

▶ **Rare or very rare** Pulmonary oil microembolism

▶ **Frequency not known** Anxiety · epiphyses premature fusion · fluid retention · jaundice · oedema · oligozoospermia · paraesthesia · precocious puberty · prostate cancer · seborrhoea · sleep apnoea · urinary tract obstruction

SIDE-EFFECTS, FURTHER INFORMATION Stop treatment or reduce dose if severe polycythaemia occurs.

- **PREGNANCY** Avoid—causes masculinisation of female fetus.
- **BREAST FEEDING** Avoid.
- **HEPATIC IMPAIRMENT** In general, manufacturers advise caution (increased risk of fluid retention and heart failure).
- **RENAL IMPAIRMENT** In general, manufacturers advise caution (increased risk of fluid retention and heart failure).
- **MONITORING REQUIREMENTS**

▶ Monitor haematocrit and haemoglobulin before treatment, every three months for the first year, and yearly thereafter.

▶ Monitor prostate and PSA in men over 45 years.

- **PATIENT AND CARER ADVICE**

Androgenic effects in women Women should be advised to report any signs of virilisation e.g. deepening of the voice or hirsutism.

Testosterone

▶ 882

28-Mar-2023

● **INDICATIONS AND DOSE**

Low sexual desire in postmenopausal women (administered on expert advice)

▶ BY TRANSDERMAL APPLICATION

▶ Adult: Apply 50 mg every week, the contents of a 5-g sachet or 5-g tube (containing 50 mg/5 g of testosterone) to be divided for daily dosing and applied to non-hair areas, such as the abdomen or upper thighs, over the period of 1 week

TESTAVAN ®

Hypogonadism due to androgen deficiency in men

▶ BY TRANSDERMAL APPLICATION

▶ Adult: Apply 23 mg once daily; increased in steps of 23 mg, adjusted according to response; maximum 69 mg per day

DOSE EQUIVALENCE AND CONVERSION

▶ For *Testavan* ®: one pump actuation delivers 1.15 g of gel containing 23 mg of testosterone.

TESTIM ®

Hypogonadism due to testosterone deficiency in men

▶ BY TRANSDERMAL APPLICATION

▶ Adult: Apply 50 mg once daily, subsequent application adjusted according to response; maximum 100 mg per day

DOSE EQUIVALENCE AND CONVERSION

▶ For *Testim* ®: one tube of 5 g contains 50 mg testosterone.

TESTOGEL ® 16.2MG/G

Hypogonadism due to androgen deficiency in men

▶ BY TRANSDERMAL APPLICATION

▶ Adult: Apply 40.5 mg once daily; increased in steps of 20.25 mg, adjusted according to response; maximum 81 mg per day

DOSE EQUIVALENCE AND CONVERSION

▶ For *Testogel* ® 16.2 mg/g: one pump actuation delivers 1.25 g of gel containing 20.25 mg of testosterone.

TESTOGEL ® 40.5MG/2.5G

Hypogonadism due to androgen deficiency in men

▶ BY TRANSDERMAL APPLICATION

▶ Adult: Apply 40.5 mg once daily; adjusted in steps of 20.25 mg, dose to be adjusted according to response; maximum 81 mg per day

DOSE EQUIVALENCE AND CONVERSION

▶ For *Testogel* ® 40.5 mg/2.5 g: one sachet of 2.5 g contains 40.5 mg of testosterone.

TESTOGEL ® 50MG/5G

Hypogonadism due to androgen deficiency in men

▶ BY TRANSDERMAL APPLICATION

▶ Adult: Apply 50 mg once daily; increased in steps of 25 mg, adjusted according to response; maximum 100 mg per day

DOSE EQUIVALENCE AND CONVERSION

▶ For *Testogel* ® 50 mg/5 g: one sachet of 5 g contains 50 mg of testosterone.

TOSTRAN ®

Hypogonadism due to testosterone deficiency in men

▶ BY TRANSDERMAL APPLICATION

▶ Adult: Apply 60 mg once daily, subsequent application adjusted according to response; maximum 80 mg per day

DOSE EQUIVALENCE AND CONVERSION

▶ For *Tostran* ®: 1 g of gel contains 20 mg testosterone.

● **UNLICENSED USE** [EvGr] Testosterone is used for the treatment of low sexual desire in postmenopausal women, [E] but is not licensed for this indication.

> **IMPORTANT SAFETY INFORMATION**
>
> MHRA/CHM ADVICE: TOPICAL TESTOSTERONE (*TESTOGEL* ®): RISK OF HARM TO CHILDREN FOLLOWING ACCIDENTAL EXPOSURE (JANUARY 2023)
>
> The CHM has reviewed reports of topical testosterone being repeatedly accidentally transferred to children, resulting in genital enlargement and premature puberty due to increased blood-testosterone levels. Repeated accidental exposure in adult females may also result in facial and/or body hair growth, deepening of voice, and menstrual cycle changes.
>
> Healthcare professionals are advised to counsel patients or their carers on:
> * the risks and possible side-effects of accidental transfer of topical testosterone to others;
> * methods to reduce these risks, such as washing hands with soap and water after application, covering the application site with clean clothing once the gel has dried, and washing the application site with soap and water (after the recommended time period) before physical contact with others;
> * being alert for signs of accidental exposure, and to seek medical advice if this is suspected.

● **INTERACTIONS** → Appendix 1: testosterone

● **SIDE-EFFECTS**

▶ **Common or very common** Hypertriglyceridaemia

▶ **Frequency not known** Anaemia · deep vein thrombosis · electrolyte imbalance · frontal balding (in women) · hair growth unwanted (in women) · hypertrichosis · malaise · muscle cramps · musculoskeletal pain · testicular disorder · vasodilation · voice lowered (in women)

SIDE-EFFECTS, FURTHER INFORMATION **When used for low sexual desire in post-menopausal women** The long-term effects of testosterone in this patient group are largely unknown, but side-effects can include growth of unwanted hair, frontal balding and deepening of the voice.

● **DIRECTIONS FOR ADMINISTRATION** [EvGr] Avoid skin contact with gel application sites to prevent accidental testosterone transfer to other people, especially pregnant women and children ⟨M⟩—consult product literature. See also *Important safety information*.

TESTAVAN ® Manufacturer advises apply one pump actuation of gel evenly onto clean, dry, intact skin over upper arm and shoulder using the applicator, without getting any gel on the hands—repeat on opposite upper arm and shoulder if two pump actuations are required, and repeat again on initial upper arm and shoulder if three pump actuations are required. Allow to dry completely before dressing and cover application site with clothing. Wash hands with soap and water immediately if gel was touched during application; avoid shower or bath for at least 2 hours.

TESTIM ® Manufacturer advises squeeze entire content of tube on to one palm and apply as a thin layer on clean, dry, healthy skin of shoulder or upper arm, preferably in the morning after washing or bathing (if 2 tubes required use 1 per shoulder or upper arm); rub in and allow to dry before putting on clothing to cover site; wash hands with soap after application; avoid washing application site for at least 6 hours.

TESTOGEL ® 16.2MG/G Apply thin layer of gel on clean, dry, healthy skin over right and left upper arms and shoulders. Not to be applied on genital area as high alcohol content may cause local irritation. Allow to dry for 3–5 minutes before dressing. Wash hands with soap and water after applying gel, and cover the site with clothing once gel dried; avoid shower or bath for at least 2 hours.

TESTOGEL ® 40.5MG/2.5G Apply thin layer of gel on clean, dry, healthy skin over right and left upper arms and shoulders immediately after sachet is opened. Not to be applied on genital area as high alcohol content may cause local irritation. Allow to dry for 3–5 minutes before dressing. Wash hands with soap and water after applying gel, and cover the site with clothing once gel dried; avoid shower or bath for at least 1 hour.

TESTOGEL ® 50MG/5G Manufacturer advises apply thin layer of gel on clean, dry, healthy skin such as shoulders, arms or abdomen, immediately after sachet is opened. Not to be applied on genital area as high alcohol content may cause local irritation. Allow to dry for 3–5 minutes before dressing. Wash hands with soap and water after applying gel, avoid shower or bath for at least 6 hours.

TOSTRAN ® Manufacturer advises apply gel on clean, dry, intact skin of abdomen or both inner thighs, preferably in the morning. Gently rub in with a finger until dry before dressing. Wash hands with soap and water after applying gel; avoid washing application site for at least 2 hours. Not to be applied on genital area.

- **PATIENT AND CARER ADVICE** Patient or carer should be given advice on how to administer testosterone gel.

- **NATIONAL FUNDING/ACCESS DECISIONS** For full details see funding body website

Scottish Medicines Consortium (SMC) decisions
- Testosterone (*Testavan* ®) as replacement therapy for adult male hypogonadism, when testosterone deficiency has been confirmed by clinical features and biochemical tests (April 2019) SMC No. SMC2152 Recommended with restrictions

- **MEDICINAL FORMS** There can be variation in the licensing of different medicines containing the same drug.

Transdermal gel
CAUTIONARY AND ADVISORY LABELS 15
EXCIPIENTS: May contain Butylated hydroxytoluene, propylene glycol
- Testavan (The Simple Pharma Company UK Ltd)
   Testosterone 20 mg per 1 gram Testavan 20mg/g transdermal gel | 85.5 gram [PoM] £25.22 DT = £25.22 [CD4-2] | 256.5 gram [PoM] £75.66 [CD4-2]
   Testavan 20mg/g transdermal gel refill | 85.5 gram [PoM] £25.22 [CD4-2]
- Testogel (Besins Healthcare (UK) Ltd)
   Testosterone 40.5 mg Testogel 40.5mg/2.5g transdermal gel sachets | 30 sachet [PoM] £39.94 DT = £39.94 [CD4-2]
   Testosterone 16.2 mg per 1 gram Testogel 16.2mg/g gel | 88 gram [PoM] £39.94 DT = £39.94 [CD4-2]
- Tostran (Advanz Pharma Germany GmbH)
   Testosterone 20 mg per 1 gram Tostran 2% gel | 60 gram [PoM] £28.63 DT = £28.63 [CD4-2]

Testosterone decanoate, isocaproate, phenylpropionate and propionate

14-Jul-2020

The properties listed below are those particular to the combination only. For the properties of the components please consider, testosterone propionate below.

- **INDICATIONS AND DOSE**

Androgen deficiency
- BY DEEP INTRAMUSCULAR INJECTION
- Adult: 1 mL every 3 weeks, adjusted according to response

DOSE EQUIVALENCE AND CONVERSION
- Each 1 mL dose of *Sustanon* ® 250 solution for injection contains 100 mg testosterone decanoate, 60 mg testosterone isocaproate, 60 mg testosterone phenylpropionate and 30 mg testosterone propionate.

- **INTERACTIONS** → Appendix 1: testosterone

- **MEDICINAL FORMS** There can be variation in the licensing of different medicines containing the same drug.
Solution for injection
EXCIPIENTS: May contain Arachis (peanut) oil, benzyl alcohol
- Sustanon (Aspen Pharma Trading Ltd)
   Testosterone propionate 30 mg per 1 ml, Testosterone isocaproate 60 mg per 1 ml, Testosterone phenylpropionate 60 mg per 1 ml, Testosterone decanoate 100 mg per 1 ml Sustanon 250mg/1ml solution for injection ampoules | 1 ampoule [PoM] £2.45 [CD4-2]

⟜ 882

Testosterone enantate

13-May-2020

- **INDICATIONS AND DOSE**

Hypogonadism
- BY SLOW INTRAMUSCULAR INJECTION
- Adult: Initially 250 mg every 2–3 weeks; maintenance 250 mg every 3–6 weeks

Breast cancer
- BY SLOW INTRAMUSCULAR INJECTION
- Adult: 250 mg every 2–3 weeks

- **UNLICENSED USE** Not licensed for use in breast cancer.

- **INTERACTIONS** → Appendix 1: testosterone

- **SIDE-EFFECTS** Bone formation increased · circulatory system disorder · gastrointestinal disorder · gastrointestinal haemorrhage · hepatomegaly · hypercalcaemia · neoplasms · spermatogenesis abnormal

- **MEDICINAL FORMS** There can be variation in the licensing of different medicines containing the same drug.
Solution for injection
- Testosterone enantate (Non-proprietary)
   Testosterone enantate 250 mg per 1 ml Testosterone enantate 250mg/1ml solution for injection ampoules | 3 ampoule [PoM] £101.33 DT = £101.33 [CD4-2]

⟜ 882

Testosterone propionate

13-May-2020

- **INDICATIONS AND DOSE**

Androgen deficiency
- BY INTRAMUSCULAR INJECTION
- Adult: 50 mg 2–3 times a week

Delayed puberty in males
- BY INTRAMUSCULAR INJECTION
- Adult: 50 mg once weekly

Breast cancer in women
- BY INTRAMUSCULAR INJECTION
- Adult: 100 mg 2–3 times a week

- **INTERACTIONS** → Appendix 1: testosterone

- **MEDICINAL FORMS** Forms available from special-order manufacturers include: solution for injection

⟜ 882

Testosterone undecanoate

13-May-2020

- **INDICATIONS AND DOSE**

Androgen deficiency
- BY MOUTH
- Adult: 120–160 mg daily for 2–3 weeks; maintenance 40–120 mg daily

Hypogonadism
- BY DEEP INTRAMUSCULAR INJECTION
- Adult (male): 1 g every 10–14 weeks, to be given over 2 minutes, if necessary, second dose may be given after 6 weeks to achieve rapid steady state plasma testosterone levels and then every 10–14 weeks.

● **INTERACTIONS** → Appendix 1: testosterone
● **SIDE-EFFECTS**
   GENERAL SIDE-EFFECTS
► **Uncommon** Diarrhoea · mood altered
   SPECIFIC SIDE-EFFECTS
► **Uncommon**
► With intramuscular use Appetite increased · arthralgia · breast abnormalities · cardiovascular disorder · cough · dysphonia · hypercholesterolaemia · increased risk of infection · migraine · muscle complaints · muscle disorder · musculoskeletal stiffness · night sweats · pain in extremity · snoring · testicular disorders · tremor · urinary disorders · urinary tract disorder
► **Frequency not known**
► With intramuscular use Hair growth increased · spermatogenesis reduced
► With oral use Azoospermia · fluid imbalance · gastrointestinal discomfort · hepatic function abnormal · lipid metabolism change · myalgia

● **MEDICINAL FORMS** There can be variation in the licensing of different medicines containing the same drug.
   Solution for injection
► **Testosterone undecanoate (Non-proprietary)**
   Testosterone undecanoate 250 mg per 1 ml Testosterone undecanoate 1g/4ml solution for injection vials | 1 vial PoM £87.11 DT = £87.11 CD4-2
► **Nebido** (Grunenthal Ltd)
   Testosterone undecanoate 250 mg per 1 ml Nebido 1000mg/4ml solution for injection vials | 1 vial PoM £87.11 DT = £87.11 CD4-2
► **Roxadin** (Galvany Pharma Ltd)
   Testosterone undecanoate 250 mg per 1 ml Roxadin 1000mg/4ml solution for injection vials | 1 vial PoM £65.33 DT = £87.11 CD4-2

8.2a Male sex hormone antagonism

ANTI-ANDROGENS

Cyproterone acetate   01-Dec-2020

● **INDICATIONS AND DOSE**
Hyper-sexuality in males | Sexual deviation in males
► BY MOUTH
► Adult: 50 mg twice daily, to be taken after food
Prevention of tumour flare with initial gonadorelin analogue therapy
► BY MOUTH
► Adult (male): 200 mg daily in 2–3 divided doses for 5–7 days before initiation of gonadorelin analogue, followed by 200 mg daily in 2–3 divided doses for 3–4 weeks after initiation of gonadorelin analogue; maximum 300 mg per day.
Long-term palliative therapy where gonadorelin analogues or orchidectomy contra-indicated, not tolerated, or where oral therapy preferred
► BY MOUTH
► Adult (male): 200–300 mg daily in 2–3 divided doses.

Hot flushes with gonadorelin analogue therapy or after orchidectomy
► BY MOUTH
► Adult (male): Initially 50 mg daily, then adjusted according to response to 50–150 mg daily in 1–3 divided doses.

IMPORTANT SAFETY INFORMATION
MHRA/CHM ADVICE: CYPROTERONE ACETATE: NEW ADVICE TO MINIMISE RISK OF MENINGIOMA (JUNE 2020)
Cyproterone acetate has been associated with an overall rare, but cumulative dose-dependent, increased risk of meningioma (single and multiple), mainly at doses of 25 mg/day and higher. Healthcare professionals are advised to monitor patients for meningiomas, and to permanently discontinue treatment if diagnosed. Use of cyproterone acetate, including co-cyprindiol, for all indications is contra-indicated in those with meningioma or a history of meningioma. Treatment with high doses of cyproterone acetate for any indication, except prostate cancer, should be restricted to when alternative treatments or interventions are unavailable or considered inappropriate.

● **CONTRA-INDICATIONS**
   GENERAL CONTRA-INDICATIONS Dubin-Johnson syndrome · existing or history of thromboembolic disorders · malignant diseases (except for carcinoma of the prostate) · meningioma or history of meningioma · previous or existing liver tumours (not due to metastases from carcinoma of the prostate) · Rotor syndrome · wasting diseases (except for inoperable carcinoma of the prostate)
   SPECIFIC CONTRA-INDICATIONS
► When used for Hypersexuality Severe depression · severe diabetes (with vascular changes) · sickle-cell anaemia
● **CAUTIONS** Diabetes mellitus · in prostate cancer, severe depression · in prostate cancer, sickle-cell anaemia · ineffective for male hypersexuality in chronic alcoholism (relevance to prostate cancer not known)
● **INTERACTIONS** → Appendix 1: anti-androgens
● **SIDE-EFFECTS**
► **Common or very common** Depressed mood · dyspnoea · fatigue · gynaecomastia · hepatic disorders · hot flush · hyperhidrosis · nipple pain · restlessness · weight change
► **Uncommon** Skin reactions
► **Rare or very rare** Galactorrhoea · meningioma (increased risk with increasing cumulative dose) · neoplasms
► **Frequency not known** Adrenocortical suppression · anaemia · azoospermia · hair changes · hypotrichosis · osteoporosis · sebaceous gland underactivity (may clear acne) · thromboembolism

   SIDE-EFFECTS, FURTHER INFORMATION Direct hepatic toxicity including jaundice, hepatitis and hepatic failure have been reported (fatalities reported, usually after several months, at dosages of 100 mg and above). If hepatotoxicity is confirmed, cyproterone should normally be withdrawn unless the hepatotoxicity can be explained by another cause such as metastatic disease (in which case cyproterone should be continued only if the perceived benefit exceeds the risk).

● **HEPATIC IMPAIRMENT** Manufacturer advises avoid (unless used for prostate cancer).
● **MONITORING REQUIREMENTS**
► Monitor blood counts initially and throughout treatment.
► Monitor adrenocortical function regularly.
► Monitor hepatic function regularly—liver function tests should be performed before and regularly during treatment and whenever symptoms suggestive of hepatotoxicity occur.

6
Endocrine system

- **PATIENT AND CARER ADVICE**
  Driving and skilled tasks Fatigue and lassitude may impair performance of skilled tasks (e.g. driving).

- **MEDICINAL FORMS** There can be variation in the licensing of different medicines containing the same drug. Forms available from special-order manufacturers include: oral tablet, oral capsule, oral suspension, oral solution
  Oral tablet
  CAUTIONARY AND ADVISORY LABELS 21
  ▸ **Cyproterone acetate (Non-proprietary)**
    Cyproterone acetate 50 mg Cyproterone 50mg tablets | 56 tablet [PoM] £101.71 DT = £101.71
    Cyproterone acetate 100 mg Cyproterone 100mg tablets | 84 tablet [PoM] £250.00 DT = £132.57
  ▸ **Androcur** (Advanz Pharma)
    Cyproterone acetate 50 mg Androcur 50mg tablets | 60 tablet [PoM] £31.34
  ▸ **Cyprostat** (Advanz Pharma)
    Cyproterone acetate 50 mg Cyprostat 50mg tablets | 160 tablet [PoM] £82.86

9 Thyroid disorders

PITUITARY AND HYPOTHALAMIC HORMONES AND ANALOGUES › THYROID STIMULATING HORMONES

Thyrotropin alfa

02-Dec-2020

(Recombinant human thyroid stimulating hormone; rhTSH)

- **DRUG ACTION** Thyrotropin alfa is a recombinant form of thyrotrophin (thyroid stimulating hormone).

- **INDICATIONS AND DOSE**
  Detection of thyroid remnants and thyroid cancer in post-thyroidectomy patients, together with serum thyroglobulin testing (with or without radioiodine imaging) | To increase radio-iodine uptake for the ablation of thyroid remnant tissue in suitable post-thyroidectomy patients
  ▸ BY INTRAMUSCULAR INJECTION
  ▸ Adult: 900 micrograms every 24 hours for 2 doses, dose to be administered into the gluteal muscle, consult product literature for further information on indications and dose

- **CAUTIONS** Presence of thyroglobulin autoantibodies may give false negative results

- **SIDE-EFFECTS**
  ▸ **Common or very common** Asthenia · dizziness · headache · nausea · vomiting
  ▸ **Uncommon** Chills · diarrhoea · feeling hot · fever · flushing · hypersensitivity · influenza · influenza like illness · pain · paraesthesia · pulmonary reaction · skin reactions · taste altered
  ▸ **Rare or very rare** Atrial fibrillation · hyperthyroidism
  ▸ **Frequency not known** Arthralgia · dyspnoea · goitre · hyperhidrosis · myalgia · neoplasm complications · palpitations · residual metastases enlarged · stroke · tremor

- **ALLERGY AND CROSS-SENSITIVITY** [EvGr] Contra-indicated if previous hypersensitivity to bovine or human thyrotrophin. ⓜ

- **PREGNANCY** Avoid.

- **BREAST FEEDING** Avoid.

- **MEDICINAL FORMS** There can be variation in the licensing of different medicines containing the same drug.
  Powder for solution for injection
  ▸ **Thyrogen** (Sanofi)
    Thyrotropin alfa 900 microgram Thyrogen 900microgram powder for solution for injection vials | 2 vial [PoM] £583.04

9.1 Hyperthyroidism

Hyperthyroidism

09-Dec-2019

Description of condition

Hyperthyroidism results from the excessive production and secretion of thyroid hormones leading to thyrotoxicosis (an excess of circulating thyroid hormones). Signs and symptoms of hyperthyroidism include a goitre, hyperactivity, disturbed sleep, fatigue, palpitations, anxiety, heat intolerance, increased appetite with unintentional weight loss, and diarrhoea. Complications include Graves' orbitopathy, thyroid storm (thyrotoxic crisis), pregnancy complications, reduced bone mineral density, heart failure, and atrial fibrillation. Risk factors include smoking, a family history of thyroid disease, co-existent autoimmune conditions, and low iodine intake.

Primary hyperthyroidism refers to when the condition arises from the thyroid gland rather than due to a pituitary or hypothalamic disorder. It is mainly caused by Graves' disease (an autoimmune disorder mediated by antibodies that stimulate the thyroid-stimulating hormone (TSH) receptor). Other causes include toxic nodular goitre (autonomously functioning thyroid nodules that secrete excess thyroid hormone), or drug-induced thyrotoxicosis.

Primary hyperthyroidism is more common in females than males and can be classified as either overt or subclinical; both of which may or may not be symptomatic. Overt hyperthyroidism is characterised by TSH levels below the reference range and free thyroxine (FT4) and/or free tri-iodothyronine (FT3) levels above the reference range. In subclinical hyperthyroidism, TSH is suppressed but FT4 and FT3 are within the reference range.

Thyrotoxicosis can also occur without hyperthyroidism; this is usually transient, and can occur due to excess intake of levothyroxine or over-the-counter supplements containing thyroid hormone, or thyroiditis.

Aims of treatment

Treatment aims to alleviate symptoms, align thyroid function tests within or close to the reference range, and to reduce the risk of long-term complications.

Non-drug treatment

[EvGr] Radioactive iodine or surgery (such as total thyroidectomy or hemithyroidectomy) may be considered by specialists in the management of Graves' disease or toxic nodular goitre. Whilst awaiting these treatments, antithyroid drugs should be offered to control hyperthyroidism, see *Graves' disease* and *Toxic nodular goitre* in *Primary hyperthyroidism*. Ⓐ

Primary Hyperthyroidism

[EvGr] Patients with symptoms of thyroid storm should be treated as a medical emergency. Refer patients urgently to an endocrinologist if a pituitary or hypothalamic disorder is suspected, and refer or discuss with an endocrinologist all patients with new-onset hyperthyroidism (base urgency on clinical judgement). If malignancy is suspected, refer patients using a suspected cancer pathway.

Explain to patients, and their family or carers if appropriate, that:

- Some patients may feel well even when their thyroid function tests are outside the reference range;
- Even when they have no symptoms, treatment may be advised to reduce the risk of long-term complications;
- Symptoms may lag behind treatment changes for several weeks to months.

Consider antithyroid drugs alongside supportive treatment (for example, beta-blockers) for patients with hyperthyroidism awaiting specialist assessment and further treatment. Carbimazole below is the recommended choice of antithyroid drug, with propylthiouracil p. 888 considered for those in whom carbimazole is unsuitable. For further information, see *Graves' disease* and *Toxic nodular goitre*.

Before starting antithyroid drugs, check full blood count and liver function tests. Ⓐ

The MHRA/CHM have released important safety information regarding the use of carbimazole below and the risk of acute pancreatitis. For further information, see *Important safety information* for carbimazole below.

For guidance on follow up and monitoring of hyperthyroidism, see NICE guideline: **Thyroid disease** (see *Useful resources*).

Graves' disease

EvGr Under specialist care, radioactive iodine is recommended as first-line definitive treatment unless it is unsuitable or remission is likely to be achieved with antithyroid drugs. For patients in whom an antithyroid drug is likely to achieve remission (such as in mild and uncomplicated cases), a choice of either carbimazole below or radioactive iodine should be offered. Carbimazole below should be offered as first-line definitive treatment if radioactive iodine and surgery are unsuitable treatment options.

Offer carbimazole below as a 12–18 month course using either a block and replace regimen (combination of fixed high-dose carbimazole with levothyroxine sodium p. 890), or a titration regimen (dose based on thyroid function tests), and review the need for further treatment. If patients have persistent or relapsed hyperthyroidism despite antithyroid drug treatment, consider radioactive iodine or surgery.

Consider propylthiouracil for patients who experience side-effects to carbimazole below, are pregnant or are trying to conceive within the following 6 months, or have a history of pancreatitis.

If agranulocytosis develops during antithyroid treatment, stop and do not restart treatment. Ⓐ

Toxic nodular goitre

EvGr Under specialist care, radioactive iodine is recommended as first-line definitive treatment for patients with hyperthyroidism secondary to multiple nodules; offer total thyroidectomy or life-long antithyroid drugs if radioactive iodine is unsuitable. For patients with hyperthyroidism secondary to a single nodule, offer radioactive iodine or surgery (hemithyroidectomy) as first-line definitive treatment; if these options are unsuitable, offer life-long antithyroid drugs. Consider treatment with a titration regimen of carbimazole below when offering life-long antithyroid drugs.

Consider propylthiouracil for patients who experience side-effects to carbimazole, are pregnant or are trying to conceive within the following 6 months, or have a history of pancreatitis.

If agranulocytosis develops during antithyroid treatment, stop and do not restart treatment. Ⓐ

Subclinical hyperthyroidism

EvGr For patients who have 2 TSH readings lower than 0.1 mIU/litre at least 3 months apart and evidence of thyroid disease or symptoms of thyrotoxicosis, consider seeking specialist advice.

Consider measuring TSH every 6 months for patients with untreated subclinical hyperthyroidism. For further information on monitoring in subclinical hyperthyroidism, see NICE guideline: **Thyroid disease** (see *Useful resources*). Ⓐ

Thyrotoxicosis without hyperthyroidism

EvGr Transient thyrotoxicosis without hyperthyroidism usually only needs supportive treatment (for example, beta-blockers). Ⓐ

Hyperthyroidism in pregnancy

EvGr Females with hyperthyroidism who are planning a pregnancy should be referred to an endocrinologist and advised to use effective contraception until specialist advice has been sought; advise patients to seek immediate medical advice if pregnancy is suspected or confirmed. All pregnant females should be referred urgently to a specialist. If there is uncertainty whether current antithyroid drug treatment should be continued or changed, or if the patient has adrenergic symptoms (such as tremor or tachycardia), seek urgent advice from an endocrinologist whilst awaiting specialist assessment. Pregnant females with severe signs and symptoms of hyperthyroidism (such as thyroid storm) should be admitted to hospital. Females who have recently received radioactive iodine should be advised to avoid becoming pregnant for at least 6 months after treatment. Ⓐ

The MHRA/CHM have released important safety information regarding the use of carbimazole below, with strengthened advice on contraception due to an increased risk of congenital malformations. For further information, see *Conception and contraception*, *Pregnancy*, and *Important safety information* for carbimazole below.

Useful Resources

Thyroid disease: assessment and management. National Institute for Health and Care Excellence. NICE guideline 145. November 2019, updated February 2020. www.nice.org.uk/guidance/ng145

Other drugs used for Hyperthyroidism Metoprolol tartrate, p. 182 · Nadolol, p. 177 · Propranolol hydrochloride, p. 178

ANTITHYROID DRUGS ❯ SULFUR-CONTAINING IMIDAZOLES

Carbimazole   02-Sep-2020

● INDICATIONS AND DOSE

Hyperthyroidism
- ▸ BY MOUTH
- ▸ Adult: 15–40 mg daily continue until the patient becomes euthyroid, usually after 4 to 8 weeks, higher doses should be prescribed under specialist supervision only, then reduced to 5–15 mg daily, reduce dose gradually, therapy usually given for 12 to 18 months

Hyperthyroidism (blocking-replacement regimen) in combination with levothyroxine
- ▸ BY MOUTH
- ▸ Adult: 40–60 mg daily, therapy usually given for 18 months

DOSE EQUIVALENCE AND CONVERSION
- ▸ When substituting, carbimazole 1 mg is considered equivalent to propylthiouracil 10 mg but the dose may need adjusting according to response.

IMPORTANT SAFETY INFORMATION
NEUTROPENIA AND AGRANULOCYTOSIS
Manufacturer advises of the importance of recognising bone marrow suppression induced by carbimazole and the need to stop treatment promptly.

- Patient should be asked to report symptoms and signs suggestive of infection, especially sore throat.
- A white blood cell count should be performed if there is any clinical evidence of infection.
- Carbimazole should be stopped promptly if there is clinical or laboratory evidence of neutropenia.

MHRA/CHM ADVICE: CARBIMAZOLE: INCREASED RISK OF CONGENITAL MALFORMATIONS; STRENGTHENED ADVICE ON CONTRACEPTION (FEBRUARY 2019)

Carbimazole is associated with an increased risk of congenital malformations when used during pregnancy, especially in the first trimester and at high doses (daily dose of 15 mg or more).

Women of childbearing potential should use effective contraception during treatment with carbimazole. It should only be considered in pregnancy after a thorough benefit-risk assessment, and at the lowest effective dose without additional administration of thyroid hormones—close maternal, fetal, and neonatal monitoring is recommended.

MHRA/CHM ADVICE: CARBIMAZOLE: RISK OF ACUTE PANCREATITIS (FEBRUARY 2019)

Cases of acute pancreatitis have been reported during treatment with carbimazole. It should be stopped immediately and permanently if acute pancreatitis occurs.

Carbimazole should not be used in patients with a history of acute pancreatitis associated with previous treatment—re-exposure may result in life-threatening acute pancreatitis with a decreased time to onset.

- **CONTRA-INDICATIONS** Severe blood disorders
- **INTERACTIONS** → Appendix 1: carbimazole
- **SIDE-EFFECTS**
▸ **Rare or very rare** Bone marrow disorders · haemolytic anaemia · severe cutaneous adverse reactions (SCARs) · thrombocytopenia
▸ **Frequency not known** Agranulocytosis · alopecia · angioedema · dyspepsia · eosinophilia · fever · gastrointestinal disorder · generalised lymphadenopathy · haemorrhage · headache · hepatic disorders · insulin autoimmune syndrome · leucopenia · malaise · myopathy · nausea · nerve disorders · neutropenia · pancreatitis acute (discontinue permanently) · salivary gland enlargement · skin reactions · taste loss
- **CONCEPTION AND CONTRACEPTION** The MHRA advises that females of childbearing potential should use effective contraception during treatment.
- **PREGNANCY** The MHRA advises consider use only after a thorough benefit-risk assessment. See *Important Safety Information* for further information.
- **BREAST FEEDING** Present in breast milk but this does not preclude breast-feeding as long as neonatal development is closely monitored and the lowest effective dose is used. Amount in milk may be sufficient to affect neonatal thyroid function therefore lowest effective dose should be used.
- **HEPATIC IMPAIRMENT** Manufacturer advises use with caution in mild to moderate insufficiency—half-life may be prolonged; avoid in severe insufficiency.
- **PATIENT AND CARER ADVICE** Warn patient or carers to tell doctor **immediately** if sore throat, mouth ulcers, bruising, fever, malaise, or non-specific illness develops.

- **MEDICINAL FORMS** There can be variation in the licensing of different medicines containing the same drug. Forms available from special-order manufacturers include: oral capsule, oral suspension, oral solution

Oral tablet
▸ **Carbimazole (Non-proprietary)**
Carbimazole 5 mg Carbimazole 5mg tablets | 100 tablet [PoM] £87.20 DT = £3.81

Carbimazole 10 mg Carbimazole 10mg tablets | 100 tablet [PoM] £93.74 DT = £91.28
Carbimazole 15 mg Carbimazole 15mg tablets | 100 tablet [PoM] £360.88 DT = £355.90
Carbimazole 20 mg Carbimazole 20mg tablets | 100 tablet [PoM] £208.17 DT = £2.22

ANTITHYROID DRUGS › THIOURACILS

Propylthiouracil

18-Aug-2021

- **INDICATIONS AND DOSE**
Hyperthyroidism
▸ BY MOUTH
▸ Adult: Initially 200–400 mg daily in divided doses until the patient becomes euthyroid, then reduced to 50–150 mg daily in divided doses, initial dose should be gradually reduced to the maintenance dose

DOSE EQUIVALENCE AND CONVERSION
▸ When substituting, carbimazole 1 mg is considered equivalent to propylthiouracil 10 mg but the dose may need adjusting according to response.

- **INTERACTIONS** → Appendix 1: propylthiouracil
- **SIDE-EFFECTS**
▸ **Rare or very rare** Agranulocytosis · bone marrow disorders · glomerulonephritis acute · hearing impairment · leucopenia · thrombocytopenia · vomiting
▸ **Frequency not known** Alopecia · arthralgia · arthritis · encephalopathy · fever · gastrointestinal disorder · haemorrhage · headache · hepatic disorders · hypoprothrombinaemia · interstitial pneumonitis · lupus-like syndrome · lymphadenopathy · myopathy · nausea · nephritis · skin reactions · taste altered · vasculitis

SIDE-EFFECTS, FURTHER INFORMATION Severe hepatic reactions have been reported, including fatal cases and cases requiring liver transplant—discontinue if significant liver-enzyme abnormalities develop.

- **PREGNANCY** Propylthiouracil can be given but the blocking-replacement regimen is **not** suitable. Propylthiouracil crosses the placenta and in high doses may cause fetal goitre and hypothyroidism—the lowest dose that will control the hyperthyroid state should be used (requirements in Graves' disease tend to fall during pregnancy).
- **BREAST FEEDING** Present in breast milk but this does not preclude breast-feeding as long as neonatal development is closely monitored and the lowest effective dose is used. Amount in milk probably too small to affect infant; high doses may affect neonatal thyroid function.
Monitoring Monitor infant's thyroid status.
- **HEPATIC IMPAIRMENT** Manufacturer advises caution (risk of increased half life).
Dose adjustments Manufacturer advises consider dose reduction.
- **RENAL IMPAIRMENT**
Dose adjustments See p. 21.
[EvGr] Use three-quarters normal dose if eGFR 10–50 mL/minute/1.73 m^2.
Use half normal dose if eGFR less than 10 mL/minute/1.73 m^2. ⟨M⟩
- **MONITORING REQUIREMENTS** Monitor for hepatotoxicity.
- **PATIENT AND CARER ADVICE** Patients should be told how to recognise signs of liver disorder and advised to seek prompt medical attention if symptoms such as anorexia, nausea, vomiting, fatigue, abdominal pain, jaundice, dark urine, or pruritus develop.

- **MEDICINAL FORMS** There can be variation in the licensing of different medicines containing the same drug. Forms available from special-order manufacturers include: oral suspension, oral solution

Oral tablet

▶ **Propylthiouracil** (Non-proprietary)

Propylthiouracil 25 mg Propylthiouracil 25mg tablets |
28 tablet [PoM] £27.65–£44.00 DT = £27.65
Propylthiouracil 50 mg Propylthiouracil 50mg tablets |
56 tablet [PoM] £58.19 DT = £4.52 | 100 tablet [PoM] £8.00–£59.20
Propylthiouracil 100 mg Propylthiouracil 100mg tablets |
56 tablet [PoM] £46.71 DT = £46.71

VITAMINS AND TRACE ELEMENTS

Iodide with iodine

(Lugol's Solution; Aqueous Iodine Oral Solution)

- **INDICATIONS AND DOSE**

Thyrotoxicosis (pre-operative)

▶ BY MOUTH USING ORAL SOLUTION
▶ Adult: 0.1–0.3 mL 3 times a day

DOSE EQUIVALENCE AND CONVERSION

▶ Doses based on the use of an aqueous oral solution containing iodine 50 mg/mL and potassium iodide 100 mg/mL.

- **CAUTIONS** Not for long-term treatment
- **SIDE-EFFECTS** Conjunctivitis · depression (long term use) · erectile dysfunction (long term use) · excessive tearing · headache · hypersensitivity · increased risk of infection · influenza like illness · insomnia (long term use) · rash · salivary gland pain
- **PREGNANCY** Neonatal goitre and hypothyroidism.
- **BREAST FEEDING** Stop breast-feeding. Danger of neonatal hypothyroidism or goitre. Appears to be concentrated in milk.
- **DIRECTIONS FOR ADMINISTRATION** For oral solution, dilute well with milk or water.

- **MEDICINAL FORMS** There can be variation in the licensing of different medicines containing the same drug. Forms available from special-order manufacturers include: oral solution

Oral solution

CAUTIONARY AND ADVISORY LABELS 27

9.2 Hypothyroidism

Hypothyroidism

18-Jun-2024

Description of condition

Hypothyroidism results from the underproduction and secretion of thyroid hormones. Signs and symptoms of hypothyroidism include fatigue, weight gain, constipation, menstrual irregularities, depression, dry skin, intolerance to the cold, and reduced body and scalp hair. Complications include dyslipidaemia, coronary heart disease, heart failure, impaired fertility, pregnancy complications, impaired concentration and/or memory, and rarely myxoedema coma (which is a life-threatening medical emergency).

Primary hypothyroidism refers to when the condition arises from the thyroid gland and may be caused by iodine deficiency, autoimmune disease (such as Hashimoto's thyroiditis), radiotherapy, surgery or drugs, rather than due to a pituitary or hypothalamic disorder (secondary hypothyroidism).

Primary hypothyroidism is more common in females than males and can be classified as either overt or subclinical; both of which may or may not be symptomatic. Overt hypothyroidism is characterised by thyroid stimulating hormone (TSH) levels above the reference range and free thyroxine (FT4) levels below the reference range. In subclinical hypothyroidism, TSH levels are above the reference range but FT4 and free tri-iodothyronine (FT3) levels are within the reference range. In pregnancy, it is defined as overt based on elevated TSH levels (using trimester-specific reference ranges) regardless of FT4 levels.

Aims of treatment

The aims of treatment are to alleviate symptoms, align thyroid function tests within or close to the reference range, and to reduce the risk of long-term complications.

Management of primary hypothyroidism

[EvGr] Explain to patients, and their family or carers if appropriate, that:

- Some patients may feel well even when their thyroid function tests are outside the reference range;
- Even when they have no symptoms, treatment may be advised to reduce the risk of long-term complications;
- Symptoms may lag behind treatment changes for several weeks to months. ⟨A⟩

Overt hypothyroidism

[EvGr] Offer levothyroxine sodium p. 890 as first-line treatment and aim to maintain thyroid-stimulating hormone (TSH) levels within the reference range. If symptoms persist, even after achieving normal TSH levels, consider adjusting the dose to achieve optimal well-being whilst avoiding doses that cause TSH suppression or thyrotoxicosis.

For patients whose TSH level was very high before starting treatment or who have had a prolonged period of untreated disease, the TSH level can take up to 6 months to return to the reference range.

Consider measuring TSH levels every 3 months until a stable level has been achieved, then yearly thereafter. Monitoring free thyroxine (FT4) should also be considered in those who continue to be symptomatic.

Due to the uncertainty around the long-term adverse effects and the insufficient evidence of benefit over levothyroxine monotherapy, the use of natural thyroid extract is not recommended. Liothyronine (either alone or in combination with levothyroxine) is not routinely recommended for the same reasons. NHS England have produced guidance on the prescribing of liothyronine, for further information see: www.england.nhs.uk/long-read/liothyronine-advice-for-prescribers/. ⟨A⟩

Subclinical hypothyroidism

[EvGr] When considering whether to start treatment for subclinical hypothyroidism, take into account features suggesting underlying thyroid disease.

For patients who have a TSH level of 10 mIU/L or higher on 2 separate occasions 3 months apart, consider levothyroxine sodium p. 890. If symptoms persist, even after achieving normal TSH levels, consider adjusting the dose to achieve optimal well-being whilst avoiding doses that cause TSH suppression or thyrotoxicosis.

For patients whose TSH level was very high before starting treatment or who have had a prolonged period of untreated disease, the TSH level can take up to 6 months to return to the reference range.

For patients in whom treatment is started, consider measuring TSH levels every 3 months until a stable level has been achieved, then yearly thereafter. Monitoring free thyroxine (FT4) should also be considered in those who continue to be symptomatic.

For symptomatic patients aged under 65 years with a TSH level above the reference range, but lower than 10 mIU/L on 2 separate occasions 3 months apart, consider a 6-month trial of levothyroxine sodium p. 890. If symptoms do not improve after starting levothyroxine, re-measure TSH and if the level remains elevated, adjust the dose. If symptoms persist when serum TSH is within the reference range, consider stopping levothyroxine and follow the recommendations on *Monitoring untreated subclinical hypothyroidism and monitoring after stopping treatment* in the NICE guideline: **Thyroid disease** (see *Useful resources*). Ⓐ

Management of secondary hypothyroidism

EvGr If secondary hypothyroidism is suspected, refer the patient urgently to an endocrinologist to assess the underlying cause. Ⓐ

Hypothyroidism in pregnancy

EvGr Refer all females with hypothyroidism who are planning a pregnancy or are pregnant, to an endocrinologist. For those planning a pregnancy and whose thyroid function tests (TFTs) are not within range, advise delaying conception until stabilised on levothyroxine sodium treatment below. If there is any uncertainty about treatment initiation or dosing, discuss this with an endocrinologist whilst awaiting review.

TFTs may produce misleading results in pregnancy and trimester-related reference ranges should be used. If pregnancy is confirmed, urgently measure TFTs; discuss the initiation, or changes to levothyroxine sodium treatment below and TFT monitoring with an endocrinologist whilst awaiting review, to reduce the risk of obstetric and neonatal complications. Ⓐ

Useful Resources

Thyroid disease: assessment and management. National Institute for Health and Care Excellence. NICE guideline 145. November 2019, updated February 2020
www.nice.org.uk/guidance/ng145

THYROID HORMONES

▌Levothyroxine sodium

08-Jun-2021

(Thyroxine sodium)

● INDICATIONS AND DOSE

Primary hypothyroidism
▸ BY MOUTH
▸ Adult: Initially 1.6 micrograms/kg once daily, adjusted according to response, round dose to the nearest 25 micrograms, dose to be taken preferably 30–60 minutes before breakfast, caffeine-containing liquids (e.g. coffee, tea), or other medication
▸ Elderly: Initially 25–50 micrograms once daily; adjusted in steps of 25 micrograms every 4 weeks, adjusted according to response; maintenance 50–200 micrograms once daily, dose to be taken preferably 30–60 minutes before breakfast, caffeine-containing liquids (e.g. coffee, tea), or other medication

Primary hypothyroidism in patients with cardiac disease
▸ BY MOUTH
▸ Adult: Initially 25–50 micrograms once daily; adjusted in steps of 25 micrograms every 4 weeks, adjusted according to response; maintenance 50–200 micrograms once daily, dose to be taken preferably 30–60 minutes before breakfast, caffeine-containing liquids (e.g. coffee, tea), or other medication

Hyperthyroidism (blocking-replacement regimen) in combination with carbimazole
▸ BY MOUTH
▸ Adult: 50–150 micrograms daily therapy usually given for 18 months

● UNLICENSED USE EvGr Levothyroxine is used in the doses provided in the BNF for the treatment of primary

hypothyroidism, Ⓐ but these may differ from those licensed.

> **IMPORTANT SAFETY INFORMATION**
>
> **MHRA/CHM ADVICE: LEVOTHYROXINE: NEW PRESCRIBING ADVICE FOR PATIENTS WHO EXPERIENCE SYMPTOMS ON SWITCHING BETWEEN DIFFERENT LEVOTHYROXINE PRODUCTS (MAY 2021)**
> A small proportion of patients treated with levothyroxine report symptoms, often consistent with thyroid dysfunction, when switching between different tablet formulations of levothyroxine. Healthcare professionals are advised that if a patient reports symptoms after changing to a different tablet of levothyroxine, a thyroid function test should be considered; if a patient is persistently symptomatic, whether they are biochemically euthyroid or have evidence of abnormal thyroid function, consistently prescribing a specific levothyroxine tablet known to be well tolerated by the patient should be considered. If symptoms or poor control of thyroid function persist despite adhering to a specific tablet, consider prescribing levothyroxine in an oral solution formulation.

● CONTRA-INDICATIONS Thyrotoxicosis

● CAUTIONS Cardiovascular disorders · diabetes insipidus · diabetes mellitus (dose of antidiabetic drugs including insulin may need to be increased) · elderly · hypertension · long-standing hypothyroidism · myocardial infarction · myocardial insufficiency · panhypopituitarism (initiate corticosteroid therapy before starting levothyroxine) · predisposition to adrenal insufficiency (initiate corticosteroid therapy before starting levothyroxine)

CAUTIONS, FURTHER INFORMATION
▸ Cardiovascular disorders Baseline ECG is valuable because changes induced by hypothyroidism can be confused with ischaemia.

● INTERACTIONS → Appendix 1: thyroid hormones

● SIDE-EFFECTS Angina pectoris · anxiety · arrhythmias · arthralgia · diarrhoea · dyspnoea · fever · flushing · headache · hyperhidrosis · insomnia · malaise · menstruation irregular · muscle spasms · muscle weakness · oedema · palpitations · skin reactions · thyrotoxic crisis · tremor · vomiting · weight decreased

SIDE-EFFECTS, FURTHER INFORMATION **Initial dosage in patients with cardiovascular disorders** If metabolism increases too rapidly (causing diarrhoea, nervousness, rapid pulse, insomnia, tremors and sometimes anginal pain where there is latent myocardial ischaemia), reduce dose or withhold for 1–2 days and start again at a lower dose.

● PREGNANCY Levothyroxine may cross the placenta. Excessive or insufficient maternal thyroid hormones can be detrimental to fetus.
Dose adjustments Levothyroxine requirement may increase during pregnancy.
Monitoring Assess maternal thyroid function before conception (if possible), at diagnosis of pregnancy, at antenatal booking, during both the second and third trimesters, and after delivery (more frequent monitoring required on initiation or adjustment of levothyroxine).

● BREAST FEEDING Amount too small to affect tests for neonatal hypothyroidism.

● MONITORING REQUIREMENTS
▸ When used for Primary hypothyroidism EvGr Consider measuring thyroid stimulating hormone (TSH) level every three months until stabilised (two similar measurements within the reference range, 3 months apart), then yearly thereafter. Consider measuring free thyroxine (FT4) if symptoms of hypothyroidism persist after starting levothyroxine. Ⓐ

- **MEDICINAL FORMS** There can be variation in the licensing of different medicines containing the same drug. Forms available from special-order manufacturers include: oral capsule, oral suspension, oral solution

Oral tablet

▸ **Levothyroxine sodium (Non-proprietary)**
Levothyroxine sodium anhydrous 12.5 microgram Levothyroxine sodium 12.5microgram tablets | 28 tablet [PoM] £21.00 DT = £12.34
Levothyroxine sodium anhydrous 25 microgram Levothyroxine sodium 25microgram tablets | 28 tablet [PoM] £3.05 DT = £0.73 | 500 tablet [PoM] £41.61–£54.46
Levothyroxine sodium 25microgram tablets lactose free | 100 tablet [PoM] [S]
Levothyroxine sodium anhydrous 50 microgram Levothyroxine sodium 50microgram tablets lactose free | 100 tablet [PoM] [S]
Levothyroxine sodium 50microgram tablets | 28 tablet [PoM] £1.28 DT = £0.60 | 1000 tablet [PoM] £21.43–£47.85
Levothyroxine sodium anhydrous 75 microgram Levothyroxine sodium 75microgram tablets | 28 tablet [PoM] £3.60 DT = £2.68
Levothyroxine sodium anhydrous 100 microgram Levothyroxine sodium 100microgram tablets lactose free | 100 tablet [PoM] [S]
Levothyroxine sodium 100microgram tablets | 28 tablet [PoM] £1.24 DT = £0.61 | 1000 tablet [PoM] £21.79–£43.57

▸ **Eltroxin** (Advanz Pharma)
Levothyroxine sodium anhydrous 25 microgram Eltroxin 25microgram tablets | 28 tablet [PoM] £2.54 DT = £0.73
Levothyroxine sodium anhydrous 50 microgram Eltroxin 50microgram tablets | 28 tablet [PoM] £1.77 DT = £0.60
Levothyroxine sodium anhydrous 100 microgram Eltroxin 100microgram tablets | 28 tablet [PoM] £1.78 DT = £0.61

▸ **Vencamil** (Aristo Pharma Ltd)
Levothyroxine sodium anhydrous 25 microgram Vencamil 25microgram tablets | 28 tablet [PoM] £2.53 DT = £0.73
Levothyroxine sodium anhydrous 50 microgram Vencamil 50microgram tablets | 28 tablet [PoM] £1.76 DT = £0.60
Levothyroxine sodium anhydrous 75 microgram Vencamil 75microgram tablets | 28 tablet [PoM] £2.53 DT = £2.68
Levothyroxine sodium anhydrous 100 microgram Vencamil 100microgram tablets | 28 tablet [PoM] £1.77 DT = £0.61

Oral capsule

▸ **Levothyroxine sodium (Non-proprietary)**
Levothyroxine sodium anhydrous 25 microgram Tirosint 25microgram capsules | 28 capsule [PoM] [S] DT = £70.08
Levothyroxine sodium anhydrous 50 microgram Tirosint 50microgram capsules | 28 capsule [PoM] [S] DT = £39.93
Levothyroxine sodium anhydrous 100 microgram Tirosint 100microgram capsules | 28 capsule [PoM] [S]

Oral solution

▸ **Levothyroxine sodium (Non-proprietary)**
Levothyroxine sodium anhydrous 5 microgram per 1 ml Levothyroxine sodium 25micrograms/5ml oral solution sugar free | 100 ml [PoM] £95.00 DT = £58.34 [SF]
Levothyroxine sodium anhydrous 10 microgram per 1 ml Levothyroxine sodium 50micrograms/5ml oral solution sugar free | 100 ml [PoM] £91.27 DT = £51.94 [SF]
Levothyroxine sodium anhydrous 15 microgram per 1 ml Levothyroxine sodium 75micrograms/5ml oral solution sugar free | 100 ml [PoM] £163.50 DT = £163.50 [SF]
Levothyroxine sodium anhydrous 20 microgram per 1 ml Levothyroxine sodium 100micrograms/5ml oral solution sugar free | 100 ml [PoM] £165.00 DT = £103.02 [SF]
Levothyroxine sodium anhydrous 25 microgram per 1 ml Levothyroxine sodium 125micrograms/5ml oral solution sugar free | 100 ml [PoM] £185.00-£296.00 DT = £185.00 [SF]

Liothyronine sodium

08-Jul-2019

(L-Tri-iodothyronine sodium)

- **INDICATIONS AND DOSE**

Hypothyroidism

▸ BY MOUTH
▸ Adult: Initially 10–20 micrograms daily; increased to 60 micrograms daily in 2–3 divided doses, dose should be increased gradually, smaller initial doses given for the elderly

Hypothyroid coma

▸ BY SLOW INTRAVENOUS INJECTION
▸ Adult: 5–20 micrograms every 12 hours, increased to 5–20 micrograms every 4 hours if required, alternatively initially 50 micrograms for 1 dose, then 25 micrograms every 8 hours, reduced to 25 micrograms twice daily

DOSE EQUIVALENCE AND CONVERSION

▸ 20–25 micrograms of liothyronine sodium is equivalent to approximately 100 micrograms of levothyroxine sodium.
▸ Brands without a UK licence may not be bioequivalent and dose adjustment may be necessary.

- **CONTRA-INDICATIONS** Thyrotoxicosis

- **CAUTIONS** Cardiovascular disorders · diabetes insipidus · diabetes mellitus (dose of antidiabetic drugs including insulin may need to be increased) · elderly · hypertension · long-standing hypothyroidism · myocardial infarction · myocardial insufficiency · panhypopituitarism (initiate corticosteroid therapy before starting liothyronine) · predisposition to adrenal insufficiency (initiate corticosteroid therapy before starting liothyronine)

CAUTIONS, FURTHER INFORMATION

▸ Cardiovascular disorders Baseline ECG is valuable because changes induced by hypothyroidism can be confused with ischaemia.

- **INTERACTIONS** → Appendix 1: thyroid hormones

- **SIDE-EFFECTS**

GENERAL SIDE-EFFECTS Angina pectoris · anxiety · arrhythmias · diarrhoea · fever · flushing · headache · hyperhidrosis · insomnia · muscle cramps · muscle weakness · palpitations · tremor · vomiting · weight decreased

SPECIFIC SIDE-EFFECTS

▸ With intravenous use Menstruation irregular
▸ With oral use Heat intolerance

SIDE-EFFECTS, FURTHER INFORMATION **Initial dosage in patients with cardiovascular disorders** If metabolism increases too rapidly (causing diarrhoea, nervousness, rapid pulse, insomnia, tremors and sometimes anginal pain where there is latent myocardial ischaemia), reduce dose or withhold for 1–2 days and start again at a lower dose.

- **PREGNANCY** Does not cross the placenta in significant amounts. Excessive or insufficient maternal thyroid hormones can be detrimental to fetus.
Dose adjustments Liothyronine requirement may increase during pregnancy.
Monitoring Assess maternal thyroid function before conception (if possible), at diagnosis of pregnancy, at antenatal booking, during both the second and third trimesters, and after delivery (more frequent monitoring required on initiation or adjustment of liothyronine).

- **BREAST FEEDING** Amount too small to affect tests for neonatal hypothyroidism.

- **PRESCRIBING AND DISPENSING INFORMATION**
Switching to a different brand Patients switched to a different brand should be monitored (particularly if pregnant or if heart disease present) as brands without a UK licence may not be bioequivalent. Pregnant women or those with heart disease should undergo an early review of thyroid status, and other patients should have thyroid function assessed if experiencing a significant change in symptoms. If liothyronine is continued long-term, thyroid function tests should be repeated 1–2 months after any change in brand.

- **MEDICINAL FORMS** There can be variation in the licensing of different medicines containing the same drug. Forms available from special-order manufacturers include: oral tablet, oral capsule, oral suspension, oral solution, solution for injection

Oral tablet

▸ **Liothyronine sodium (Non-proprietary)**

Liothyronine sodium 5 microgram Liothyronine 5microgram tablets | 28 tablet [PoM] £123.38 DT = £83.37

Liothyronine sodium 10 microgram Liothyronine 10microgram tablets | 28 tablet [PoM] £289.64 DT = £152.44

Liothyronine sodium 20 microgram Liothyronine 20microgram tablets | 28 tablet [PoM] £147.14 DT = £62.20

Liothyronine sodium 25 microgram Cytomel 25microgram tablets | 100 tablet [PoM] ⓢ

Powder for solution for injection

▸ **Liothyronine sodium (Non-proprietary)**

Liothyronine sodium 20 microgram Liothyronine 20microgram powder for solution for injection vials | 5 vial [PoM] £1,567.50

Oral capsule

▸ **Liothyronine sodium (Non-proprietary)**

Liothyronine sodium 5 microgram Liothyronine 5microgram capsules | 28 capsule [PoM] £55.00 DT = £55.00

Liothyronine sodium 10 microgram Liothyronine 10microgram capsules | 28 capsule [PoM] £65.00 DT = £65.00

Liothyronine sodium 20 microgram Liothyronine 20microgram capsules | 28 capsule [PoM] £55.00 DT = £55.00

Oral solution

▸ **Enolio** (Eclosix Ltd)

Liothyronine sodium 10 microgram per 1 ml Enolio 10micrograms/ml oral solution | 50 ml [PoM] £42.20

Chapter 7
Genito-urinary system

CONTENTS

1 Bladder and urinary disorders

Lower urinary tract symptoms in males

21-Oct-2024

Description of condition

Lower urinary tract symptoms (LUTS) in males include voiding symptoms (weak or intermittent urinary stream, straining, hesitancy, terminal dribbling, and incomplete emptying), storage symptoms (urinary frequency, urgency, urgency incontinence, and nocturia), and post-micturition symptoms (predominantly post-micturition dribbling, and sensation of incomplete emptying). Causes include bladder outflow obstruction (BOO), often secondary to benign prostatic hyperplasia (BPH), bladder dysfunction, structural and functional abnormalities of the urinary tract, and non-urological conditions.

Age is an important risk factor for LUTS, with prevalence rising with increasing age; bothersome LUTS can occur in up to 30% of males aged over 65 years.

Management

For guidance on the management of acute urinary retention, and catheterisation in chronic urinary retention, see Urinary retention p. 902.

For guidance on urinary incontinence in neurological disease, see NICE guideline CG148: **Urinary incontinence in neurological disease: assessment and management**, available at: www.nice.org.uk/guidance/cg148.

[EvGr] Validated symptom score questionnaires, bladder diaries, and frequency volume charts are used to assess patients' baseline lower urinary tract symptoms, and to monitor treatment outcomes.

Conservative measures such as pelvic floor exercises, bladder training, and lifestyle changes are usually tried first for the management of non-neurogenic LUTS.

Where conservative management options are unsuccessful or unsuitable, first-line treatment for males with moderate to severe LUTS is usually an alpha-adrenoceptor blocker, due to their efficacy, rapid onset of action, and low rate and severity of side-effects.

An antimuscarinic may be added for males who continue to experience storage symptoms despite the use of an alpha-adrenoceptor blocker alone, or may be used alone in males with predominantly storage symptoms. A beta-3 adrenoceptor agonist such as mirabegron p. 901 or vibegron p. 901 can be used instead where use of an antimuscarinic is ineffective or unsuitable.

For moderate to severe LUTS in males with an enlarged prostate (>30 g) and/or raised prostate specific antigen level (>1.4 ng/mL) who are considered to be at high risk of disease progression, a 5α-reductase inhibitor (5ARI) is the treatment option of choice; this may be used in combination with an alpha-adrenoceptor blocker depending on symptom severity. If combination treatment is given, consider stopping the alpha-adrenoceptor blocker after 6 months in those with moderate symptoms. ⓐ

[EvGr] Under specialist advice or in accordance with local policy, the phosphodiesterase type-5 inhibitor tadalafil p. 941 may be considered instead of an alpha-adrenoceptor blocker for males with both erectile dysfunction and moderate to severe LUTS. It may also be considered in males with moderate-severe LUTS without erectile dysfunction when alpha-adrenoceptor blockers are ineffective or not tolerated. ⓔ

[EvGr] In males with nocturnal polyuria, the use of an afternoon loop diuretic may be of benefit. Desmopressin p. 764 may also be considered if other medical causes have been excluded and other treatments have been ineffective. ⓐ

For further guidance on the management of LUTS, including assessment, specialist referral, and surgical options, see NICE guideline CG97: **Lower urinary tract symptoms in men: management** (see *Useful resources*).

7

Genito-urinary system

Drug treatment considerations

Alpha-adrenoceptor blockers (such as alfuzosin hydrochloride p. 902, doxazosin p. 903, tamsulosin hydrochloride p. 905, or terazosin p. 906)

Alpha-adrenoceptor blockers are effective for both voiding and storage symptoms, however they do not alter the progression of BPH. The onset of effect is rapid, with a benefit in symptoms seen within hours to days, although it can take a few weeks for the full effect to develop. They have similar efficacy at appropriate doses, but their side-effect profiles differ. Vasodilatory effects are more pronounced with doxazosin and terazosin than with alfuzosin and tamsulosin and patients, particularly the elderly, should be warned about the risk of postural hypotension. The occurrence of floppy iris syndrome (which is an issue for those requiring cataract surgery) is a risk with all alpha-adrenoceptor blockers but is much greater with tamsulosin in comparison to the other drugs. Alpha-adrenoceptor blockers do not affect libido, or erectile function, but can cause abnormal ejaculation, with ejaculatory disturbance occurring much more commonly with tamsulosin.

Antimuscarinics (such as darifenacin p. 897, fesoterodine fumarate p. 897, oxybutynin hydrochloride p. 898, propiverine hydrochloride p. 899, solifenacin succinate p. 899, tolterodine tartrate p. 900, or trospium chloride p. 900)

The full benefit of antimuscarinics on storage symptoms may take up to 4 weeks to be seen. Evidence for the long-term use of antimuscarinics for LUTS in males is lacking. Their use may be associated with urinary retention, so should be avoided in patients with a high post-void residual volume (>150 mL). Patients should be advised to discontinue medication if worsening voiding LUTS or urinary stream is noted after initiation of therapy.

Where an antimuscarinic is effective but cannot be tolerated, changing the formulation or switching to an alternative antimuscarinic may be of benefit; due to its long half-life, an interval of approximately one week should be allowed after stopping treatment with solifenacin before commencing another antimuscarinic.

Elderly and frail males are more susceptible to the side-effects of antimuscarinics; given these drugs are associated with an increased risk of falls, cognitive decline, confusion, and agitation, they should be used with caution and alternative treatment options (e.g. beta-3 adrenoceptor agonists) considered in high-risk patients (such as those with dementia or chronic cognitive impairment). As other commonly prescribed medications may also have antimuscarinic properties, the patient's overall antimuscarinic burden should be assessed using a validated tool such as the Anticholinergic Cognitive Burden Scale when prescribing or reviewing treatment.

5α-reductase inhibitors (such as dutasteride p. 907, or finasteride p. 907)

Unlike alpha-adrenoceptor blockers, in patients with BPH, 5ARIs reduce prostate size, the risk of acute urinary retention, and the need for BPH surgery. Finasteride and dutasteride have similar efficacy; symptom reduction depends on initial prostate size, but the onset of effect is slow, and it may take at least 6 months for a clinical benefit to be seen. The risks of sexual side-effects of these drugs, including reduced libido, erectile dysfunction and ejaculation disturbance should be discussed with patients before commencing treatment as part of shared-decision making.

Deprescribing

Deprescribing of drugs for LUTS should be considered if there is no improvement in symptoms, side-effects outweigh the benefits, use is inappropriate/unsuitable, or because of patient preference.

Where treatment with an antimuscarinic is being discontinued, it can generally be stopped outright without the need for weaning. However, gradual weaning, e.g. reducing the daily dose by 25–50% every 1 to 4 weeks according to response, may be considered if troublesome withdrawal symptoms occur. Withdrawal symptoms that may be experienced range from mild (such as anxiety, irritability, insomnia, sweating, or nausea) to severe (such as tachycardia, orthostatic hypotension, severe anxiety, or severe insomnia).

Useful Resources

Lower urinary tract symptoms in men: management. National Institute for Health and Care Excellence. Clinical guideline 97. May 2010, updated June 2015. www.nice.org.uk/guidance/cg97

1.1 Urinary frequency, enuresis, and incontinence

Urinary incontinence and pelvic organ prolapse in women

16-Jun-2019

Description of condition

Urinary incontinence is the involuntary leakage of urine and can range in severity and nature. It can impact the person, as well as their families and carers, and can be detrimental to an individual's physical, psychological, and social well-being. Urinary incontinence can be the result of functional abnormalities in the lower urinary tract, or due to other illnesses. It can be sub-classified into four main types: stress, urgency, mixed, and overflow incontinence.

Stress incontinence is the involuntary leakage on effort or exertion, or on sneezing or coughing, and is associated with the loss of pelvic floor support and/or damage to the urethral sphincter.

Urgency incontinence is involuntary leakage which is accompanied, or immediately preceded by a sudden compelling desire to pass urine that is difficult to delay. It is often part of a larger symptom complex known as overactive bladder syndrome. This syndrome is defined as urinary urgency, which may or may not be accompanied by urgency incontinence, but is usually associated with increased frequency and nocturia. The symptoms are thought to be caused by involuntary contractions of the detrusor muscle.

Mixed urinary incontinence is involuntary leakage associated with both urgency and stress, however, one type tends to be predominant.

Overflow incontinence is a complication of chronic urinary retention and occurs when a person cannot empty their bladder completely and it becomes over distended. This may result in continuous, or frequent loss of small quantities of urine. For further information, see Urinary retention p. 902.

Other types include continuous urinary incontinence, where there is constant leakage of urine which may be due to the severity of the persons' condition or may be due to an underlying cause, such as a fistula. Incontinence may also be situational, for example during sexual intercourse or when a person is giggling.

The main risk factor for developing any type of incontinence is older age; this is due to the physiological changes that occur with natural aging. Some other risk factors for *stress* incontinence include pregnancy, vaginal delivery, obesity, constipation, family history, smoking, lack of supporting tissue (such as in prolapse or hysterectomy) and use of some drugs such as ACE inhibitors (can cause cough) and alpha-adrenergic blockers (relax the bladder outlet and urethra).

Some conditions can increase detrusor muscle overactivity and therefore worsen *urgency* incontinence. These include conditions that affect the lower urinary tract such as; Urinary-tract infections p. 681, urinary obstruction, or oestrogen deficiency, those affecting the nervous system such as; stroke, dementia, and Parkinson's disease, and systemic conditions such as; diabetes mellitus or hypercalcaemia. Side-effects of some drugs may also increase detrusor muscle overactivity or indirectly contribute to urgency incontinence; these include cholinesterase inhibitors, drugs that cause constipation, and those with anticholinergic effects. Diuretics, alcohol, and caffeine all increase urine production and can cause polyuria, frequency, urgency, and nocturia.

Aims of treatment

Manage urinary incontinence and the symptoms of overactive bladder syndrome.

Non-drug treatment

[EvGr] Women with urinary incontinence should modify their fluid intake, and if their BMI is 30 kg/m^2 or greater, be advised to lose weight. For those with an overactive bladder, a reduction in caffeine intake should be trialled.

Absorbent products, hand-held urinals and toileting aids should not be used to treat urinary incontinence, unless the person has severe cognitive or mobility impairment that may prevent further treatment. They may be used in some women as a coping strategy whilst awaiting treatment, as an adjunct to ongoing therapy, or as long-term management after all treatment options have been considered; their use should be reviewed at least annually. Intravaginal and intraurethral devices should only be used when required to prevent leakage at specific times, for example during exercise.

Surgical management may be an option for some women and will depend on a number of factors. Discussion around the details of the procedures and subsequent shared decision making should be carried out. ⟨A⟩

Urgency incontinence

[EvGr] Women should be offered bladder training for at least 6 weeks as first-line treatment. If frequency is a problem and satisfactory benefit from bladder training is not achieved, drug treatment for an overactive bladder should be added. ⟨A⟩

Stress incontinence

[EvGr] Women should trial supervised pelvic floor muscle training for at least 3 months, which should include at least 8 contractions performed 3 times per day. ⟨A⟩

Mixed incontinence

[EvGr] Women should trial both bladder training for at least 6 weeks and supervised pelvic floor muscle training for at least 3 months, which should include at least 8 contractions performed 3 times per day. If frequency is a problem and satisfactory benefit from bladder training is not achieved, drug treatment for an overactive bladder should be added. ⟨A⟩

Drug treatment

[EvGr] When considering drug treatment in women with incontinence exclude any possible causes, including drugs or conditions that may exacerbate incontinence or overactive bladder.

A urine dipstick test should be performed in all women presenting with incontinence to test for active infection or haematuria, and analysed along with the patients symptoms. For further information, see Urinary-tract infections p. 681. Women should be referred to a specialist if there is:

- persistent bladder or urethral pain;
- pelvic mass that is clinically benign;
- associated faecal incontinence;
- suspected neurological disease, or urogenital fistulae;
- history of previous incontinence surgery, pelvic cancer surgery or pelvic radiation therapy;
- recurrent or persistant UTI for those aged over 60; ⟨A⟩ see Urinary-tract infections p. 681
- [EvGr] palpable bladder after voiding, or symptoms of voiding difficulty.

Urgent referral should occur in women aged 45 years or older if there is unexplained visible haematuria without UTI, or visible haematuria persisting or recurring despite successful treatment of UTI. Urgent referral is also required in women aged 60 years or older with unexplained non-visible haematuria and either dysuria or raised white cell count. ⟨A⟩

Urgency incontinence

[EvGr] An anticholinergic drug should be considered for women who have trialled bladder training, where frequency is a problem and symptoms persist. Consider the total anticholinergic load, coexisting conditions, such as cognitive impairment or poor bladder emptying, and the risk of side-effects when offering anticholinergic medicine. When prescribing an anticholinergic in those with dementia, see Dementia p. 343. Immediate release oxybutynin hydrochloride p. 898, immediate release tolterodine tartrate p. 900, or darifenacin p. 897 can be used first-line. Immediate release oxybutynin should not be used in frail, older women at risk of sudden deterioration in their physical or mental health. The lowest dose should be used and titrated upwards if necessary. *Transdermal* oxybutynin hydrochloride p. 898 may be used in those unable to tolerate oral treatment. Mirabegron p. 901 may be used if treatment with an anticholinergic is contra-indicated, ineffective, or not tolerated, for further information, see *National funding/access decisions* in mirabegron.

Treatment should be reviewed after 4 weeks, or sooner if required. If treatment is effective review the woman again at 12 weeks, then annually thereafter, or every 6 months if the woman is over 75 years of age. If treatment has not been effective or is not tolerated an alternative anticholinergic drug can be used, the current dose adjusted or, mirabegron trialled; review again after 4 weeks. Alternative anticholinergics include, an untried first-line drug, or one of the following; fesoterodine fumarate p. 897, propiverine hydrochloride p. 899, solifenacin succinate p. 899, trospium chloride p. 900, or an *extended release* formulation of either oxybutynin hydrochloride or tolterodine tartrate. Women who have tried taking medicine for overactive bladder, but treatment has failed, should be referred to secondary care, where treatment with botulinum toxin type A p. 469 or surgical methods may be considered.

Flavoxate hydrochloride p. 897, propantheline bromide p. 97, or imipramine hydrochloride p. 435 should not be used as treatment options.

In women who have troublesome nocturia, desmopressin p. 764 may also be used. *Intravaginal* oestrogen therapy can be used in those women who are post-menopausal and have vaginal atrophy. Treatment with an intravaginal oestrogen should be reviewed at least annually to re-assess the need for continued treatment and monitor for symptoms of endometrial hyperplasia or carcinoma. ⟨A⟩

Stress incontinence

[EvGr] Duloxetine p. 426 is **not** recommended as first-line treatment for women with stress incontinence. It may be used second-line where conservative treatment including pelvic floor training has failed, and only if surgery is not appropriate or the woman prefers pharmacological treatment, but should not be offered routinely. ⟨A⟩

Mixed incontinence

Women with mixed urinary incontinence should be treated according to the predominant type, refer to *Urgency incontinence* or *Stress incontinence* for drug treatment options.

Pelvic organ prolapse

Pelvic organ prolapse is the symptomatic descent of part of the wall of the vagina or uterus. Symptoms can include a vaginal bulge or sensation of something coming down, urinary, bowel and sexual symptoms, and pelvic and back pain. These can all affect a woman's quality of life.

EvGr Women who present to primary care with symptoms, or an incidental finding of vaginal prolapse should be examined to rule out pelvic mass or other pathology, and a full history taken. Treatment preferences should be discussed and referral made where necessary. Women in secondary care should be considered for referral to a clinician with expertise in prolapse if experiencing incidental symptoms, or on incidental finding of vaginal prolapse. A validated pelvic floor symptom questionnaire may aid assessment and decision making.

Women should be given advice on minimising heavy lifting, preventing or treating constipation, and if their BMI is 30 kg/m^2 or greater, encouraged to lose weight. A programme of supervised pelvic floor muscle training for at least 16 weeks may also be tried for some women.

A vaginal oestrogen may be used for women with prolapse and signs of vaginal atrophy, an oestrogen-releasing ring may be more appropriate for those women who have cognitive or physical impairments.

A vaginal pessary may be used alone, or in conjunction with pelvic floor muscle training for those with symptomatic pelvic organ prolapse. Surgical management may be required in women whose symptoms have not improved with non-surgical methods, or who have declined non-surgical treatment. Ⓐ

Nocturnal enuresis in children

23-May-2017

Description of condition

Nocturnal enuresis is the involuntary discharge of urine during sleep, which is common in young children. Children are generally expected to be dry by a developmental age of 5 years, and historically it has been common practice to consider children for treatment only when they reach 7 years; however, symptoms may still persist in a small proportion by the age of 10 years.

Treatment

Children under 5 years

EvGr For children under 5 years, treatment is usually unnecessary as the condition is likely to resolve spontaneously. Reassurance and advice can be useful for some families. Ⓐ

Non Drug Treatment

EvGr Initially, advice should be given on fluid intake, diet, toileting behaviour, and use of reward systems. For children who do not respond to this advice (more than 1–2 wet beds per week), an enuresis alarm should be the recommended treatment for motivated, well-supported children. Alarms in children under 7 years should be considered depending on the child's maturity, motivation and understanding of the alarm. Alarms have a lower relapse rate than drug treatment when discontinued.

Treatment using an alarm should be reviewed after 4 weeks and continued until a minimum of 2 weeks' uninterrupted dry nights have been achieved. If complete dryness is not achieved after 3 months but the condition is still improving and the child remains motivated to use the alarm, it is recommended to continue the treatment. Combined treatment with desmopressin p. 764, or the use of desmopressin alone, is recommended if the initial alarm treatment is unsuccessful or it is no longer appropriate or desirable. Ⓐ

Drug Treatment

EvGr Treatment with oral or sublingual desmopressin is recommended for children over 5 years of age when alarm use is inappropriate or undesirable, or when rapid or short-term results are the priority (for example, to cover periods away from home). Desmopressin alone can also be used if there has been a partial response to a combination of desmopressin and an alarm following initial treatment with an alarm alone. Treatment should be assessed after 4 weeks and continued for 3 months if there are signs of response. Repeated courses of desmopressin can be used in responsive children who experience repeated recurrences of bedwetting, but should be withdrawn **gradually** at regular intervals (for 1 week every 3 months) for full reassessment.

Under specialist supervision, nocturnal enuresis associated with daytime symptoms (overactive bladder) can be managed with desmopressin alone or in combination with an antimuscarinic drug (such as oxybutynin hydrochloride p. 898 or tolterodine tartrate p. 900 [unlicensed indication]). Treatment should be continued for 3 months; the course can be repeated if necessary.

The tricyclic antidepressant imipramine hydrochloride p. 435 can be considered for children who have not responded to all other treatments and have undergone specialist assessment, however relapse is common after withdrawal and children and their carers should be aware of the dangers of overdose. Initial treatment should continue for 3 months; further courses can be considered following a medical review every 3 months. Tricyclic antidepressants should be withdrawn gradually. Ⓐ

Useful Resources

Bedwetting in under 19s. National Institute for Health and Care Excellence. Clinical guideline CG111. October 2010. www.nice.org.uk/guidance/cg111

ANTIMUSCARINICS

Antimuscarinics (systemic)   

- **CONTRA-INDICATIONS** Angle-closure glaucoma · gastro-intestinal obstruction · intestinal atony · myasthenia gravis (but some antimuscarinics may be used to decrease muscarinic side-effects of anticholinesterases) · paralytic ileus · pyloric stenosis · severe ulcerative colitis · significant bladder outflow obstruction · toxic megacolon · urinary retention

- **CAUTIONS** Acute myocardial infarction (in adults) · arrhythmias (may be worsened) · autonomic neuropathy · cardiac insufficiency (due to association with tachycardia) · cardiac surgery (due to association with tachycardia) · children (increased risk of side-effects) · conditions characterised by tachycardia · congestive heart failure (may be worsened) · coronary artery disease (may be worsened) · diarrhoea · elderly (especially if frail) · gastro-oesophageal reflux disease · hiatus hernia with reflux oesophagitis · hypertension · hyperthyroidism (due to association with tachycardia) · individuals susceptible to angle-closure glaucoma · prostatic hyperplasia · pyrexia · ulcerative colitis

CAUTIONS, FURTHER INFORMATION
▶ Elderly Screening Tool of Older Persons' potentially inappropriate Prescriptions (STOPP) criteria to aid medication reviews (see Prescribing in the elderly p. 31 for information). Potentially inappropriate:
  - if treating extrapyramidal side-effects of antipsychotic medications (risk of antimuscarinic toxicity)
  - with delirium or dementia (risk of exacerbation of cognitive impairment), angle-closure glaucoma (contra-

indicated; risk of acute exacerbation of glaucoma), or chronic prostatism (risk of urinary retention)
- if two or more antimuscarinic drugs prescribed concomitantly (risk of increased antimuscarinic toxicity)

- **SIDE-EFFECTS**
  - **Common or very common** Constipation · dizziness · drowsiness · dry mouth · dyspepsia · flushing · headache · nausea · palpitations · skin reactions · tachycardia · urinary disorders · vision disorders · vomiting
  - **Rare or very rare** Angioedema · confusion (more common in elderly)

- **PATIENT AND CARER ADVICE**
  Driving and skilled tasks Antimuscarinics can affect the performance of skilled tasks (e.g. driving).

ANTIMUSCARINICS › URINARY

Darifenacin

13-May-2020

- **INDICATIONS AND DOSE**

Urinary frequency | Urinary urgency | Incontinence
- ► BY MOUTH
- ► Adult: Initially 7.5 mg once daily, increased if necessary to 15 mg after 2 weeks

- **INTERACTIONS** → Appendix 1: darifenacin

- **SIDE-EFFECTS**
  - **Common or very common** Abdominal pain · dry eye · nasal dryness
  - **Uncommon** Asthenia · bladder pain · cough · diarrhoea · dyspnoea · erectile dysfunction · flatulence · hyperhidrosis · hypertension · increased risk of infection · injury · insomnia · oedema · oral ulceration · taste altered · thinking abnormal · urinary tract disorder

- **PREGNANCY** Manufacturer advises avoid—toxicity in *animal* studies.

- **BREAST FEEDING** Present in milk in *animal* studies—manufacturer advises caution.

- **HEPATIC IMPAIRMENT** Manufacturer advises caution in moderate impairment; avoid in severe impairment (risk of increased exposure).
  Dose adjustments Manufacturer advises maximum 7.5 mg daily in moderate impairment.

- **PRESCRIBING AND DISPENSING INFORMATION** The need for continuing therapy for urinary incontinence should be reviewed every 4–6 weeks until symptoms stabilise, and then every 6–12 months.

- **MEDICINAL FORMS** There can be variation in the licensing of different medicines containing the same drug.
  Modified-release tablet
  CAUTIONARY AND ADVISORY LABELS 3, 25
  - ► Darifenacin (Non-proprietary)
    Darifenacin (as Darifenacin hydrobromide) 7.5 mg Darifenacin 7.5mg modified-release tablets | 28 tablet [PoM] £36.00 DT = £25.48
    Darifenacin (as Darifenacin hydrobromide) 15 mg Darifenacin 15mg modified-release tablets | 28 tablet [PoM] £36.00 DT = £25.48
  - ► Emselex (pharmaand GmbH)
    Darifenacin (as Darifenacin hydrobromide) 7.5 mg Emselex 7.5mg modified-release tablets | 28 tablet [PoM] £25.48 DT = £25.48
    Darifenacin (as Darifenacin hydrobromide) 15 mg Emselex 15mg modified-release tablets | 28 tablet [PoM] £25.48 DT = £25.48

Fesoterodine fumarate

03-Aug-2021

- **INDICATIONS AND DOSE**

Urinary frequency | Urinary urgency | Urge incontinence
- ► BY MOUTH
- ► Adult: 4 mg once daily, increased if necessary up to 8 mg once daily

DOSE ADJUSTMENTS DUE TO INTERACTIONS
- ► Manufacturer advises max. 4 mg daily with concurrent use of potent inhibitors of CYP3A4; avoid concurrent use in patients who also have hepatic or renal impairment.
- ► For dose adjustments with concurrent use of moderate inhibitors of CYP3A4 in patients with hepatic or renal impairment, consult product literature.

- **INTERACTIONS** → Appendix 1: fesoterodine

- **SIDE-EFFECTS**
  - **Common or very common** Diarrhoea · dry eye · gastrointestinal discomfort · insomnia · throat complaints
  - **Uncommon** Cough · fatigue · gastrointestinal disorders · nasal dryness · taste altered · urinary tract infection · vertigo

- **PREGNANCY** Manufacturer advises avoid—toxicity in *animal* studies.

- **BREAST FEEDING** Manufacturer advises avoid—no information available.

- **HEPATIC IMPAIRMENT** Manufacturer advises caution in mild to moderate impairment; avoid in severe impairment (no information available).
  Dose adjustments Manufacturer advises increase dose cautiously in mild impairment; maximum 4 mg daily in moderate impairment.

- **RENAL IMPAIRMENT** [EvGr] Use with caution. ⟨M⟩
  Dose adjustments [EvGr] Increase dose cautiously if eGFR 30–80 mL/minute/1.73 m^2; max. 4 mg daily if eGFR less than 30 mL/minute/1.73 m^2. ⟨M⟩ See p. 21.

- **PRESCRIBING AND DISPENSING INFORMATION** The need for continuing therapy for urinary incontinence should be reviewed every 4–6 weeks until symptoms stabilise, and then every 6–12 months.

- **NATIONAL FUNDING/ACCESS DECISIONS**
  For full details see funding body website

  Scottish Medicines Consortium (SMC) decisions
  - ► **Fesoterodine fumarate (*Toviaz*®) for treatment of the symptoms of increased urinary frequency (and/or urgency incontinence) that may occur in patients with overactive bladder (OAB) syndrome (July 2008)** SMC No. 480/08 Recommended with restrictions

- **MEDICINAL FORMS** There can be variation in the licensing of different medicines containing the same drug.
  Modified-release tablet
  CAUTIONARY AND ADVISORY LABELS 3, 25
  - ► Fesoterodine fumarate (Non-proprietary)
    Fesoterodine fumarate 4 mg Fesoterodine 4mg modified-release tablets | 28 tablet [PoM] £25.78 DT = £2.74
    Fesoterodine fumarate 8 mg Fesoterodine 8mg modified-release tablets | 28 tablet [PoM] £25.78 DT = £2.82
  - ► Teraleve (Dr Reddy's Laboratories (UK) Ltd)
    Fesoterodine fumarate 4 mg Teraleve 4mg modified-release tablets | 28 tablet [PoM] £16.76 DT = £2.74
    Fesoterodine fumarate 8 mg Teraleve 8mg modified-release tablets | 28 tablet [PoM] £16.76 DT = £2.82
  - ► Toviaz (Pfizer Ltd)
    Fesoterodine fumarate 4 mg Toviaz 4mg modified-release tablets | 28 tablet [PoM] £25.78 DT = £2.74
    Fesoterodine fumarate 8 mg Toviaz 8mg modified-release tablets | 28 tablet [PoM] £25.78 DT = £2.82

Flavoxate hydrochloride

13-May-2020

- **INDICATIONS AND DOSE**

Urinary frequency | Urinary incontinence | Dysuria | Urinary urgency | Bladder spasm due to catheterisation, cytoscopy, or surgery
- ► BY MOUTH
- ► Adult: 200 mg 3 times a day

F 896

7

Genito-urinary system

- **CONTRA-INDICATIONS** Gastro-intestinal haemorrhage
- **INTERACTIONS** → Appendix 1: flavoxate
- **SIDE-EFFECTS** Diarrhoea · dysphagia · eosinophilia · fatigue · hyperpyrexia · hypersensitivity · leucopenia · nervousness · vertigo
- **PREGNANCY** Manufacturer advises avoid unless no safer alternative.
- **BREAST FEEDING** Manufacturer advises caution—no information available.
- **PRESCRIBING AND DISPENSING INFORMATION** The need for continuing therapy for urinary incontinence should be reviewed every 4–6 weeks until symptoms stabilise, and then every 6–12 months.

- **MEDICINAL FORMS** There can be variation in the licensing of different medicines containing the same drug. Forms available from special-order manufacturers include: oral suspension, oral solution

Oral tablet

CAUTIONARY AND ADVISORY LABELS 3

▸ Urispas (Recordati Pharmaceuticals Ltd)
  Flavoxate hydrochloride 200 mg Urispas 200 tablets | 90 tablet [PoM] £11.67 DT = £11.67

▶ 896

Oxybutynin hydrochloride

16-Oct-2024

- **INDICATIONS AND DOSE**

Urinary frequency | Urinary urgency | Urinary incontinence | Neurogenic bladder instability

▸ BY MOUTH USING IMMEDIATE-RELEASE MEDICINES

▸ Child 5-11 years: Initially 2.5–3 mg twice daily, increased to 5 mg 2–3 times a day

▸ Child 12-17 years: Initially 5 mg 2–3 times a day, increased if necessary up to 5 mg 4 times a day

▸ Adult: Initially 5 mg 2–3 times a day, increased if necessary up to 5 mg 4 times a day

▸ Elderly: Initially 2.5–3 mg twice daily, increased if tolerated to 5 mg twice daily, adjusted according to response

▸ BY MOUTH USING MODIFIED-RELEASE TABLETS

▸ Child 5-17 years: Initially 5 mg once daily, adjusted in steps of 5 mg every week, adjusted according to response; maximum 15 mg per day

▸ Adult: Initially 5 mg once daily, increased in steps of 5 mg every week, adjusted according to response; maximum 20 mg per day

Neurogenic detrusor overactivity (under expert supervision)

▸ BY INTRAVESICAL INSTILLATION

▸ Adult: Initially 5 mg twice daily, higher starting doses may be necessary—consult product literature, increased if necessary up to 10 mg 4 times a day, dose to be adjusted according to response

▸ Elderly: Initially 5 mg twice daily, higher starting doses may be necessary—consult product literature, increased if necessary up to 10 mg 3 times a day, dose to be adjusted according to response

Urinary frequency | Urinary urgency | Urinary incontinence

▸ BY TRANSDERMAL APPLICATION USING PATCHES

▸ Adult: Apply 1 patch twice weekly, patch is to be applied to clean, dry unbroken skin on abdomen, hip or buttock. Patch should be removed every 3–4 days and site replacement patch on a different area. The same area should be avoided for 7 days

Nocturnal enuresis associated with overactive bladder

▸ BY MOUTH USING IMMEDIATE-RELEASE MEDICINES

▸ Child 5-17 years: 2.5–3 mg twice daily, increased to 5 mg 2–3 times a day, last dose to be taken before bedtime

▸ BY MOUTH USING MODIFIED-RELEASE TABLETS

▸ Child 5-17 years: Initially 5 mg once daily, adjusted in steps of 5 mg every week, adjusted according to response; maximum 15 mg per day

- **CAUTIONS** Acute porphyrias p. 1202
- **INTERACTIONS** → Appendix 1: oxybutynin
- **SIDE-EFFECTS**

GENERAL SIDE-EFFECTS

▸ **Common or very common** Diarrhoea

SPECIFIC SIDE-EFFECTS

▸ **Common or very common**
▸ With oral use Dry eye
▸ With transdermal use Gastrointestinal discomfort · increased risk of infection
▸ **Uncommon**
▸ With oral use Abdominal discomfort · appetite decreased · dysphagia
▸ With transdermal use Back pain · hot flush · injury
▸ **Frequency not known**
▸ With intravesical use Abnormal sensation in eye · agoraphobia · akathisia · anticholinergic syndrome · apathy · chest discomfort · cognitive disorder · concentration impaired · consciousness impaired · dry eye · fatigue · feeling cold · gastrointestinal discomfort · haematuria · hallucination · hyperprolactinaemia · hypotension · increased risk of infection · insomnia · proteinuria · seizure · supraventricular tachycardia · sweat changes · taste altered · thirst · vertigo
▸ With oral use Anxiety · arrhythmia · cognitive disorder · depressive symptom · drug dependence · gastrointestinal disorders · glaucoma · hallucination · heat stroke · hypohidrosis · mydriasis · nightmare · paranoia · photosensitivity reaction · seizure · urinary tract infection

SIDE-EFFECTS, FURTHER INFORMATION Since systemic absorption can follow transdermal use, also consider the side-effects of systemic antimuscarinics.

- **PREGNANCY** Manufacturers advise avoid unless essential—toxicity in *animal* studies.
- **BREAST FEEDING** Specialist sources indicate probably compatible (limited information available). High plasma-protein binding suggests limited excretion into milk and poor oral bioavailability suggests limited absorption by the infant; monitor breast-fed infants for adverse reactions.
- **HEPATIC IMPAIRMENT** Manufacturer advises caution.
- **RENAL IMPAIRMENT** Manufacturer advises caution.
- **DIRECTIONS FOR ADMINISTRATION**
▸ With transdermal use Manufacturer advises apply patches to clean, dry, unbroken skin on abdomen, hip or buttock; remove after every 3–4 days and site replacement patch on a different area (avoid using same area for 7 days).
- **PRESCRIBING AND DISPENSING INFORMATION**
▸ In adults The need for continuing therapy for urinary incontinence should be reviewed every 4–6 weeks until symptoms stabilise, and then every 6–12 months.
▸ In children The need for therapy for urinary indications should be reviewed soon after it has been commenced and then at regular intervals; a response usually occurs within 6 months but may take longer.
- **PATIENT AND CARER ADVICE** Patients or carers should be trained on administration of *intravesical* solution.
  Patients or carers should be given advice on how to apply *transdermal* patches.
Medicines for Children leaflet: Oxybutynin for daytime urinary symptoms www.medicinesforchildren.org.uk/medicines/oxybutynin-for-daytime-urinary-symptoms/

- **NATIONAL FUNDING/ACCESS DECISIONS**
  For full details see funding body website
  Scottish Medicines Consortium (SMC) decisions
  ▶ Oxybutynin (*Kentera*®) for treatment of urge incontinence and/or increased urinary frequency and urgency (August 2005) SMC No. 190/05 Recommended with restrictions

- **MEDICINAL FORMS** There can be variation in the licensing of different medicines containing the same drug. Forms available from special-order manufacturers include: oral suspension, oral solution

Oral tablet
CAUTIONARY AND ADVISORY LABELS 3
  ▶ Oxybutynin hydrochloride (Non-proprietary)
    Oxybutynin hydrochloride 2.5 mg Oxybutynin 2.5mg tablets | 56 tablet PoM £6.58 DT = £1.00 | 84 tablet PoM £1.39–£7.00
    Oxybutynin hydrochloride 5 mg Oxybutynin 5mg tablets | 56 tablet PoM £5.53 DT = £1.26 | 84 tablet PoM £1.80–£6.50
  ▶ Ditropan (Neon Healthcare Ltd)
    Oxybutynin hydrochloride 2.5 mg Ditropan 2.5mg tablets | 84 tablet PoM £1.60
    Oxybutynin hydrochloride 5 mg Ditropan 5mg tablets | 84 tablet PoM £2.90

Modified-release tablet
CAUTIONARY AND ADVISORY LABELS 3, 25
  ▶ Oxybutynin hydrochloride (Non-proprietary)
    Oxybutynin hydrochloride 5 mg Oxybutynin 5mg modified-release tablets | 28 tablet PoM £13.77–£28.16 DT = £28.16
    Oxybutynin hydrochloride 10 mg Oxybutynin 10mg modified-release tablets | 28 tablet PoM £27.54–£53.36 DT = £53.36

Oral solution
CAUTIONARY AND ADVISORY LABELS 3
  ▶ Oxybutynin hydrochloride (Non-proprietary)
    Oxybutynin hydrochloride 500 microgram per 1 ml Oxybutynin 2.5mg/5ml oral solution sugar free | 150 ml PoM £256.73 DT = £226.74 SF
    Oxybutynin hydrochloride 1 mg per 1 ml Oxybutynin 5mg/5ml oral solution sugar free | 150 ml PoM £266.99 DT = £255.97 SF

Transdermal patch
CAUTIONARY AND ADVISORY LABELS 3
  ▶ Kentera (Accord-UK Ltd)
    Oxybutynin 3.9 mg per 24 hour Kentera 3.9mg/24hours patches | 8 patch PoM £27.20 DT = £27.20

Intravesical solution
CAUTIONARY AND ADVISORY LABELS 3
  ▶ Velariq (Medice UK Ltd)
    Oxybutynin hydrochloride 1 mg per 1 ml Velariq 10mg/10ml intravesical solution pre-filled syringes | 12 pre-filled disposable injection PoM £204.00 | 96 pre-filled disposable injection PoM £1,632.00

◤ 896

Propiverine hydrochloride

15-Jul-2021

- **INDICATIONS AND DOSE**

Urinary frequency, urgency and incontinence associated with overactive bladder
  ▶ BY MOUTH USING IMMEDIATE-RELEASE MEDICINES
  ▶ Adult: 15 mg 1–2 times a day, increased if necessary up to 15 mg 3 times a day
  ▶ BY MOUTH USING MODIFIED-RELEASE CAPSULES
  ▶ Adult: 30 mg once daily

Urinary frequency, urgency and incontinence associated with neurogenic bladder instability
  ▶ BY MOUTH USING IMMEDIATE-RELEASE MEDICINES
  ▶ Adult: 15 mg 3 times a day

- **INTERACTIONS** → Appendix 1: propiverine
- **SIDE-EFFECTS**
  ▶ **Common or very common** Abdominal pain · fatigue
  ▶ **Uncommon** Taste altered · tremor
  ▶ **Rare or very rare** Restlessness
  ▶ **Frequency not known** Hallucination
- **PREGNANCY** Manufacturer advises avoid (restriction of skeletal development in *animals*).

- **BREAST FEEDING** Manufacturer advises avoid—present in milk in *animal* studies.
- **HEPATIC IMPAIRMENT** Manufacturer advises caution in mild impairment; avoid in moderate to severe impairment (no information available).
- **RENAL IMPAIRMENT** EvGr Use with caution. ◈M◈
  Dose adjustments EvGr Max. daily dose 30 mg if creatinine clearance less than 30 mL/minute. ◈M◈ See p. 21.
- **PRESCRIBING AND DISPENSING INFORMATION** The need for continuing therapy for urinary incontinence should be reviewed every 4–6 weeks until symptoms stabilise, and then every 6–12 months.

- **MEDICINAL FORMS** There can be variation in the licensing of different medicines containing the same drug.

Oral tablet
CAUTIONARY AND ADVISORY LABELS 3
  ▶ Propiverine hydrochloride (Non-proprietary)
    Propiverine hydrochloride 15 mg Propiverine 15mg tablets | 56 tablet PoM £18.00–£69.16 DT = £58.83
  ▶ Detrunorm (Consilient Health Ltd)
    Propiverine hydrochloride 15 mg Detrunorm 15mg tablets | 56 tablet PoM £18.00 DT = £58.83

Modified-release capsule
CAUTIONARY AND ADVISORY LABELS 3, 25
  ▶ Detrunorm XL (Consilient Health Ltd)
    Propiverine hydrochloride 30 mg Detrunorm XL 30mg capsules | 28 capsule PoM £24.45 DT = £24.45
    Propiverine hydrochloride 45 mg Detrunorm XL 45mg capsules | 28 capsule PoM £27.90 DT = £27.90

◤ 896

Solifenacin succinate

23-Jul-2020

- **INDICATIONS AND DOSE**

Urinary frequency | Urinary urgency | Urinary incontinence
  ▶ BY MOUTH
  ▶ Adult: 5 mg once daily, increased if necessary to 10 mg once daily

DOSE ADJUSTMENTS DUE TO INTERACTIONS
  ▶ Manufacturer advises maximum 5 mg once daily with concurrent use of potent inhibitors of CYP3A4; avoid concurrent use in patients who also have moderate hepatic impairment or severe renal impairment.

- **CAUTIONS** Susceptibility to QT-interval prolongation
- **INTERACTIONS** → Appendix 1: solifenacin
- **SIDE-EFFECTS**
  ▶ **Common or very common** Gastrointestinal discomfort
  ▶ **Uncommon** Cystitis · dry eye · dry throat · fatigue · gastrointestinal disorders · nasal dryness · peripheral oedema · taste altered · urinary tract infection
  ▶ **Rare or very rare** Hallucination
  ▶ **Frequency not known** Anaphylactic reaction · appetite decreased · arrhythmias · delirium · dysphonia · glaucoma · hyperkalaemia · liver disorder · muscle weakness · QT interval prolongation · renal impairment
- **PREGNANCY** Manufacturer advises caution—no information available.
- **BREAST FEEDING** Manufacturer advises avoid—present in milk in *animal* studies.
- **HEPATIC IMPAIRMENT** Manufacturer advises caution in moderate impairment (risk of increased half-life); avoid in severe impairment (no information available).
  Dose adjustments Manufacturer advises maximum 5 mg once daily in moderate impairment.
- **RENAL IMPAIRMENT** Manufacturer advises caution in severe impairment.
  Dose adjustments See p. 21.
  Manufacturer advises maximum 5 mg once daily if creatinine clearance 30 mL/minute or less.

- **DIRECTIONS FOR ADMINISTRATION** Manufacturer advises for *oral suspension*, doses should be followed by a glass of water—ingestion with food or other drinks may lead to the release of solifenacin in the mouth, causing a bitter taste and numbness in the mouth.

- **PRESCRIBING AND DISPENSING INFORMATION** The need for continuing therapy for urinary incontinence should be reviewed every 4–6 weeks until symptoms stabilise, and then every 6–12 months.

- **MEDICINAL FORMS** There can be variation in the licensing of different medicines containing the same drug. Forms available from special-order manufacturers include: oral suspension, oral solution

Oral tablet

CAUTIONARY AND ADVISORY LABELS 3

▸ **Solifenacin succinate (Non-proprietary)**
Solifenacin succinate 5 mg Solifenacin 5mg tablets |
30 tablet [PoM] £33.14 DT = £1.18 | 250 tablet [PoM] £276.20
Solifenacin succinate 10 mg Solifenacin 10mg tablets |
30 tablet [PoM] £43.09 DT = £1.41 | 250 tablet [PoM] £359.10

▸ **Vesicare** (Astellas Pharma Ltd)
Solifenacin succinate 5 mg Vesicare 5mg tablets | 30 tablet [PoM]
£27.62 DT = £1.18
Solifenacin succinate 10 mg Vesicare 10mg tablets |
30 tablet [PoM] £35.91 DT = £1.41

Oral solution

CAUTIONARY AND ADVISORY LABELS 3

▸ **Solifenacin succinate (Non-proprietary)**
Solifenacin succinate 1 mg per 1 ml Solifenacin 5mg/5ml oral
solution sugar free | 150 ml [PoM] £182.53 DT = £182.53 [SF]

Oral suspension

CAUTIONARY AND ADVISORY LABELS 3
EXCIPIENTS: May contain Ethanol, hydroxybenzoates (parabens), propylene glycol

▸ **Vesicare** (Astellas Pharma Ltd)
Solifenacin succinate 1 mg per 1 ml Vesicare 1mg/ml oral
suspension | 150 ml [PoM] £27.62 DT = £27.62 [SF]

⚑ 896

Tolterodine tartrate

25-Feb-2022

- **INDICATIONS AND DOSE**

Urinary frequency | Urinary urgency | Urinary incontinence
▸ BY MOUTH USING IMMEDIATE-RELEASE MEDICINES
▸ Adult: 2 mg twice daily, reduced if not tolerated to 1 mg twice daily
▸ BY MOUTH USING MODIFIED-RELEASE CAPSULES
▸ Adult: 4 mg once daily

- **CAUTIONS** History of QT-interval prolongation

- **INTERACTIONS** → Appendix 1: tolterodine

- **SIDE-EFFECTS**
▸ **Common or very common** Abdominal pain · bronchitis · chest pain · diarrhoea · dry eye · fatigue · gastrointestinal disorders · paraesthesia · peripheral oedema · vertigo · weight increased
▸ **Uncommon** Arrhythmia · heart failure · memory loss · nervousness
▸ **Frequency not known** Hallucination

- **PREGNANCY** Manufacturer advises avoid—toxicity in *animal* studies.

- **BREAST FEEDING** Manufacturer advises avoid—no information available.

- **HEPATIC IMPAIRMENT** Manufacturer advises caution (risk of increased exposure).
Dose adjustments For *immediate-release medicines*, manufacturer advises dose reduction to 1 mg twice daily. For *modified-release capsules*, manufacturer advises dose reduction to 2 mg once daily.

- **RENAL IMPAIRMENT** Manufacturer advises caution (risk of increased exposure).

Dose adjustments See p. 21.
For *immediate-release medicines*, manufacturer advises dose reduction to 1 mg twice daily if eGFR less than or equal to 30 mL/minute/1.73 m^2.
For *modified-release capsules*, manufacturer advises dose reduction to 2 mg once daily if eGFR less than or equal to 30 mL/minute/1.73 m^2.

- **PRESCRIBING AND DISPENSING INFORMATION** The need for continuing therapy for urinary incontinence should be reviewed every 4–6 weeks until symptoms stabilise, and then every 6–12 months.

- **MEDICINAL FORMS** There can be variation in the licensing of different medicines containing the same drug. Forms available from special-order manufacturers include: oral suspension, oral solution, oral powder

Oral tablet

CAUTIONARY AND ADVISORY LABELS 3

▸ **Tolterodine tartrate (Non-proprietary)**
Tolterodine tartrate 1 mg Tolterodine 1mg tablets | 56 tablet [PoM]
£29.03 DT = £1.64
Tolterodine tartrate 2 mg Tolterodine 2mg tablets | 56 tablet [PoM]
£30.56 DT = £2.19

▸ **Detrusitol** (Viatris UK Healthcare Ltd)
Tolterodine tartrate 1 mg Detrusitol 1mg tablets | 56 tablet [PoM]
£29.03 DT = £1.64
Tolterodine tartrate 2 mg Detrusitol 2mg tablets | 56 tablet [PoM]
£30.56 DT = £2.19

Modified-release capsule

CAUTIONARY AND ADVISORY LABELS 3, 25

▸ **Blerone XL** (Zentiva Pharma UK Ltd)
Tolterodine tartrate 4 mg Blerone XL 4mg capsules |
28 capsule [PoM] £6.90 DT = £12.89

▸ **Detrusitol XL** (Viatris UK Healthcare Ltd)
Tolterodine tartrate 4 mg Detrusitol XL 4mg capsules |
28 capsule [PoM] £25.78 DT = £12.89 | 30 capsule [PoM] £25.78

▸ **Mariosea XL** (Teva UK Ltd)
Tolterodine tartrate 2 mg Mariosea XL 2mg capsules |
28 capsule [PoM] £11.59 DT = £11.60
Tolterodine tartrate 4 mg Mariosea XL 4mg capsules |
28 capsule [PoM] £12.79 DT = £12.89

▸ **Neditol XL** (Aspire Pharma Ltd)
Tolterodine tartrate 2 mg Neditol XL 2mg capsules |
28 capsule [PoM] £11.60 DT = £11.60
Tolterodine tartrate 4 mg Neditol XL 4mg capsules |
28 capsule [PoM] £12.89 DT = £12.89

▸ **Preblacon XL** (Accord-UK Ltd)
Tolterodine tartrate 4 mg Preblacon XL 4mg capsules |
28 capsule [PoM] £25.78 DT = £12.89

▸ **Tolterma XL** (Macleods Pharma UK Ltd)
Tolterodine tartrate 2 mg Tolterma XL 2mg capsules |
28 capsule [PoM] £12.74 DT = £11.60
Tolterodine tartrate 4 mg Tolterma XL 4mg capsules |
28 capsule [PoM] £24.89 DT = £12.89

▸ **Tolthen XL** (Northumbria Pharma Ltd)
Tolterodine tartrate 2 mg Tolthen XL 2mg capsules |
28 capsule [PoM] £6.99 DT = £11.60
Tolterodine tartrate 4 mg Tolthen XL 4mg capsules |
28 capsule [PoM] £6.99 DT = £12.89

⚑ 896

Trospium chloride

11-Dec-2018

- **INDICATIONS AND DOSE**

Urinary frequency | Urinary urgency | Urge incontinence
▸ BY MOUTH USING IMMEDIATE-RELEASE MEDICINES
▸ Adult: 20 mg twice daily, to be taken before food
▸ BY MOUTH USING MODIFIED-RELEASE MEDICINES
▸ Adult: 60 mg once daily

- **INTERACTIONS** → Appendix 1: trospium

- **SIDE-EFFECTS**
▸ **Common or very common** Abdominal pain
▸ **Uncommon** Chest pain · diarrhoea · flatulence
▸ **Rare or very rare** Arthralgia · asthenia · dyspnoea · myalgia

▸ **Frequency not known** Agitation · anaphylactic reaction · hallucination · severe cutaneous adverse reactions (SCARs)
● **PREGNANCY** Manufacturer advises caution.
● **BREAST FEEDING** Manufacturer advises caution.
● **HEPATIC IMPAIRMENT** Manufacturer advises caution in mild to moderate impairment; avoid in severe impairment (no information available).
● **RENAL IMPAIRMENT** Use with caution. Avoid *Regurin*® XL.
  Dose adjustments Reduce dose to 20 mg once daily or 20 mg on alternate days if eGFR 10–30 mL/minute/1.73m^2.
● **PRESCRIBING AND DISPENSING INFORMATION** The need for continuing therapy for urinary incontinence should be reviewed every 4–6 weeks until symptoms stabilise, and then every 6–12 months.

● **MEDICINAL FORMS** There can be variation in the licensing of different medicines containing the same drug. Forms available from special-order manufacturers include: oral solution
Oral tablet
CAUTIONARY AND ADVISORY LABELS 23
  ▸ Trospium chloride (Non-proprietary)
    Trospium chloride 20 mg Trospium chloride 20mg tablets | 60 tablet PoM £11.49–£19.99 DT = £10.27
  ▸ Regurin (Viatris UK Healthcare Ltd)
    Trospium chloride 20 mg Regurin 20mg tablets | 60 tablet PoM £26.00 DT = £10.27
Modified-release capsule
CAUTIONARY AND ADVISORY LABELS 23, 25
  ▸ Regurin XL (Viatris UK Healthcare Ltd)
    Trospium chloride 60 mg Regurin XL 60mg capsules | 28 capsule PoM £23.05 DT = £23.05

BETA₃-ADRENOCEPTOR AGONISTS

Mirabegron
05-Aug-2021

● **INDICATIONS AND DOSE**
Urinary frequency, urgency, and urge incontinence
  ▸ BY MOUTH
  ▸ Adult: 50 mg once daily
  DOSE ADJUSTMENTS DUE TO INTERACTIONS
  ▸ Manufacturer advises reduce dose to 25 mg once daily in patients with mild hepatic impairment with concurrent use of potent inhibitors of CYP3A4; avoid in moderate impairment.
  ▸ Manufacturer advises reduce dose to 25 mg once daily if eGFR 30–89 mL/minute/1.73 m^2 with concurrent use of potent inhibitors of CYP3A4; avoid if eGFR less than 30 mL/minute/1.73 m^2.

● **CONTRA-INDICATIONS** Severe uncontrolled hypertension (systolic blood pressure ≥180 mmHg or diastolic blood pressure ≥110 mmHg)
● **CAUTIONS** History of QT-interval prolongation · stage 2 hypertension
● **INTERACTIONS** → Appendix 1: mirabegron
● **SIDE-EFFECTS**
  ▸ **Common or very common** Arrhythmias · constipation · diarrhoea · dizziness · headache · increased risk of infection · nausea
  ▸ **Uncommon** Cystitis · dyspepsia · gastritis · joint swelling · palpitations · skin reactions · vulvovaginal pruritus
  ▸ **Rare or very rare** Angioedema · eyelid oedema · hypersensitivity vasculitis · hypertensive crisis · lip swelling · urinary retention
  ▸ **Frequency not known** Insomnia
● **CONCEPTION AND CONTRACEPTION** Contraception advised in women of child-bearing potential.
● **PREGNANCY** Avoid—toxicity in *animal* studies.
● **BREAST FEEDING** Avoid—present in milk in *animal* studies.

● **HEPATIC IMPAIRMENT** Manufacturer advises caution in moderate impairment (risk of increased exposure); avoid in severe impairment (no information available).
  Dose adjustments Manufacturer advises dose reduction to 25 mg once daily in moderate impairment.
● **RENAL IMPAIRMENT** EvGr Avoid if eGFR less than 15 mL/minute/1.73 m^2 (no information available). Ⓜ
  Dose adjustments EvGr Reduce dose to 25 mg once daily if eGFR 15–29 mL/minute/1.73 m^2. Ⓜ See p. 21.
● **MONITORING REQUIREMENTS** Blood pressure should be monitored before starting treatment and regularly during treatment, especially in patients with pre-existing hypertension.
● **NATIONAL FUNDING/ACCESS DECISIONS**
  For full details see funding body website
  NICE decisions
  ▸ **Mirabegron for treating symptoms of overactive bladder (June 2013)** NICE TA290 Recommended with restrictions

● **MEDICINAL FORMS** There can be variation in the licensing of different medicines containing the same drug.
Modified-release tablet
CAUTIONARY AND ADVISORY LABELS 25
  ▸ Mirabegron (Non-proprietary)
    Mirabegron 25 mg Mirabegron 25mg modified-release tablets | 30 tablet PoM £29.00 DT = £29.00
    Mirabegron 50 mg Mirabegron 50mg modified-release tablets | 30 tablet PoM £29.00 DT = £29.00

Vibegron
30-Dec-2024

● **DRUG ACTION** Vibegron, a selective beta₃-adrenoceptor agonist, relaxes the detrusor muscle during filling, thereby increasing bladder capacity.

● **INDICATIONS AND DOSE**
Symptomatic treatment of overactive bladder syndrome
  ▸ BY MOUTH
  ▸ Adult: 75 mg once daily

● **SIDE-EFFECTS**
  ▸ **Common or very common** Constipation · diarrhoea · headache · nausea · urinary tract infection
  ▸ **Uncommon** Hot flush · skin reactions · urinary disorders
● **PREGNANCY** EvGr Avoid (toxicity in *animal* studies). Ⓜ
● **BREAST FEEDING** EvGr Avoid (present in milk in *animal* studies). Ⓜ
● **HEPATIC IMPAIRMENT** EvGr Avoid in severe impairment (no information available). Ⓜ
● **RENAL IMPAIRMENT** EvGr Avoid if creatinine clearance less than 15 mL/minute (no information available). Ⓜ
● **DIRECTIONS FOR ADMINISTRATION** EvGr Tablets may be swallowed whole with a glass of water. Alternatively, tablets may also be crushed, mixed with a tablespoon (approx. 15 mL) of soft food (e.g. apple sauce), and taken immediately with a glass of water. Ⓜ
● **NATIONAL FUNDING/ACCESS DECISIONS**
  For full details see funding body website
  NICE decisions
  ▸ **Vibegron for treating symptoms of overactive bladder syndrome (September 2024)** NICE TA999 Recommended with restrictions
  Scottish Medicines Consortium (SMC) decisions
  ▸ **Vibegron (*Obgemsa*®) for the symptomatic treatment of adult patients with overactive bladder syndrome (December 2024)** SMC No. SMC2696 Recommended

7

Genito-urinary system

- **MEDICINAL FORMS** There can be variation in the licensing of different medicines containing the same drug.

Oral tablet

▶ Obgemsa (Pierre Fabre Ltd) ▼
Vibegron 75 mg Obgemsa 75mg tablets | 30 tablet [PoM] £26.68 DT = £26.68

1.2 Urinary retention

Urinary retention

14-Oct-2024

Description of condition

Urinary retention is the inability to voluntarily urinate. It may be secondary to urethral blockage, benign prostatic hyperplasia, drug treatment (such as use of antimuscarinic drugs, sympathomimetics, tricyclic antidepressants), conditions that reduce detrusor contractions or interfere with relaxation of the urethra, neurogenic causes, or it may occur postpartum or postoperatively.

Acute urinary retention is a medical emergency characterised by the abrupt development of the inability to pass urine, pain, and a palpable or percussible bladder.

Chronic urinary retention is the gradual (over months or years) development of the inability to empty the bladder completely, characterised by a residual volume greater than one litre or associated with the presence of a distended or palpable bladder.

Treatment

Treatment of urinary retention depends on the underlying condition. Catheterisation is used to relieve acute painful urinary retention or when no cause can be found. Surgical procedures or dilatation are often used to correct mechanical outflow obstructions.

Acute urinary retention

[EvGr] Acute retention is painful and requires immediate treatment by catheterisation. Before the catheter is removed an alpha-adrenoceptor blocker (such as alfuzosin hydrochloride below, doxazosin p. 903, tamsulosin hydrochloride p. 905, prazosin p. 904, indoramin p. 903 or terazosin p. 906) should be given for at least two days to manage acute urinary retention ⒶⒶ.

Chronic urinary retention

[EvGr] In patients with chronic urinary retention, intermittent bladder catheterisation should be offered before an indwelling catheter. Catheters may be used as a long-term solution where persistent urinary retention is causing incontinence, infection, or renal dysfunction and a surgical solution is not feasible. Ⓐ Their use is associated with an increased risk of adverse events including recurrent urinary infections, trauma to the urethra, pain, and stone formation.

The parasympathomimetic bethanechol chloride p. 906 increases detrusor muscle contraction. It is licensed for acute postoperative, postpartum and neurogenic urinary retention but its use has largely been superseded by catheterisation.

Other drugs used for urinary retention include neostigmine p. 1286, and pyridostigmine bromide p. 1286.

For further guidance on the non-catheterisation management of urinary retention and other lower urinary tract symptoms in males, see Lower urinary tract symptoms in males p. 893.

Useful Resources

Lower urinary tract symptoms in men. National Institute for Health and Care Excellence. Clinical guideline CG97. May 2010 (updated June 2015).
www.nice.org.uk/guidance/cg97

> **Other drugs used for Urinary retention** Tadalafil, p. 941

ALPHA-ADRENOCEPTOR BLOCKERS

Alfuzosin hydrochloride

15-Apr-2024

- **INDICATIONS AND DOSE**

Benign prostatic hyperplasia

▶ BY MOUTH USING IMMEDIATE-RELEASE MEDICINES
▶ Adult: 2.5 mg 3 times a day; maximum 10 mg per day
▶ Elderly: Initially 2.5 mg twice daily, adjusted according to response; maximum 10 mg per day
▶ BY MOUTH USING MODIFIED-RELEASE MEDICINES
▶ Adult: 10 mg once daily

Acute urinary retention associated with benign prostatic hyperplasia

▶ BY MOUTH USING MODIFIED-RELEASE TABLETS
▶ Elderly: 10 mg once daily for 2–3 days during catheterisation and for one day after removal; max. 4 days

- **CONTRA-INDICATIONS** Avoid if history of micturition syncope · avoid if history of postural hypotension
- **CAUTIONS** Acute heart failure · cerebrovascular disease · concomitant antihypertensives (reduced dosage and specialist supervision may be required) · discontinue if angina worsens · elderly · history of QT-interval prolongation · patients undergoing cataract surgery (risk of intra-operative floppy iris syndrome)

CAUTIONS, FURTHER INFORMATION
▶ Elderly For alpha$_1$-selective adrenoceptor blockers, Screening Tool of Older Persons' potentially inappropriate Prescriptions (STOPP) criteria to aid medication reviews (see Prescribing in the elderly p. 31 for information). Potentially inappropriate:
  - in those with symptomatic postural hypotension or micturition syncope (risk of precipitating recurrent syncope)
  - in those with persistent postural hypotension i.e. recurrent drop in systolic blood pressure ≥ 20 mmHg (risk of syncope and falls).

- **INTERACTIONS** → Appendix 1: alpha blockers
- **SIDE-EFFECTS**
▶ **Common or very common** Asthenia · diarrhoea · dizziness · dry mouth · headache · malaise · nausea · postural hypotension · vertigo · vomiting
▶ **Uncommon** Abdominal pain · arrhythmias · chest pain · drowsiness · flushing · oedema · palpitations · rhinitis · skin reactions · syncope · visual impairment
▶ **Rare or very rare** Angina pectoris · angioedema
▶ **Frequency not known** Cerebral ischaemia · floppy iris syndrome · hepatic disorders · neutropenia · priapism · thrombocytopenia

SIDE-EFFECTS, FURTHER INFORMATION First dose may cause collapse due to hypotensive effect (therefore should be taken on retiring to bed). Patient should be warned to lie down if symptoms such as dizziness, fatigue or sweating develop, and to remain lying down until they abate completely.

- **HEPATIC IMPAIRMENT** For *immediate-release* preparations manufacturer advises caution in mild to moderate hepatic failure; avoid in severe hepatic failure (risk of increased half-life). For *modified-release* preparations manufacturer advises avoid in hepatic failure.
Dose adjustments For *immediate-release* preparations manufacturer advises initial dose of 2.5 mg once daily, increased to 2.5 mg twice daily according to response in mild to moderate hepatic failure.
- **RENAL IMPAIRMENT** [EvGr] Avoid use of *modified-release* preparations if creatinine clearance less than 30 mL/minute as limited experience. Ⓜ See p. 21.

Dose adjustments [EvGr] For *immediate-release* preparations, initial dose 2.5 mg twice daily and adjust according to response. [M]

- **PATIENT AND CARER ADVICE** Patient should be counselled on the first dose effect.
  Driving and skilled tasks May affect performance of skilled tasks e.g. driving.

- **MEDICINAL FORMS** There can be variation in the licensing of different medicines containing the same drug. Forms available from special-order manufacturers include: oral solution

Oral tablet
- **Alfuzosin hydrochloride (Non-proprietary)**
  Alfuzosin hydrochloride 2.5 mg Alfuzosin 2.5mg tablets | 60 tablet [PoM] £21.20 DT = £1.27

Modified-release tablet
CAUTIONARY AND ADVISORY LABELS 21, 25
- **Besavar XL** (Zentiva Pharma UK Ltd)
  Alfuzosin hydrochloride 10 mg Besavar XL 10mg tablets | 30 tablet [PoM] £7.50 DT = £12.51
- **Fuzatal XL** (Teva UK Ltd)
  Alfuzosin hydrochloride 10 mg Fuzatal XL 10mg tablets | 30 tablet [PoM] £12.76 DT = £12.51
- **Vasran XL** (Sun Pharma UK Ltd)
  Alfuzosin hydrochloride 10 mg Vasran XL 10mg tablets | 30 tablet [PoM] £11.48 DT = £12.51
- **Xatral XL** (Sanofi)
  Alfuzosin hydrochloride 10 mg Xatral XL 10mg tablets | 30 tablet [PoM] £12.51 DT = £12.51
- **Zochek** (Milpharm Ltd)
  Alfuzosin hydrochloride 10 mg Zochek 10mg modified-release tablets | 30 tablet [PoM] £12.51 DT = £12.51

Doxazosin
19-Jan-2024

- **INDICATIONS AND DOSE**

Hypertension
- BY MOUTH USING IMMEDIATE-RELEASE MEDICINES
- Adult: Initially 1 mg once daily for 1–2 weeks, then increased to 2 mg once daily, then increased if necessary to 4 mg once daily, usual dose up to 4 mg once daily; increased if necessary up to 16 mg once daily
- BY MOUTH USING MODIFIED-RELEASE MEDICINES
- Adult: Initially 4 mg once daily, then increased if necessary to 8 mg once daily, dose can be adjusted after 4 weeks

Benign prostatic hyperplasia
- BY MOUTH USING IMMEDIATE-RELEASE MEDICINES
- Adult: Initially 1 mg once daily, usual maintenance 2–4 mg once daily, dose may be doubled at intervals of 1–2 weeks according to response; increased if necessary up to 8 mg once daily
- BY MOUTH USING MODIFIED-RELEASE MEDICINES
- Adult: Initially 4 mg once daily, then increased if necessary to 8 mg once daily, dose can be adjusted after 4 weeks

- **CONTRA-INDICATIONS** History of micturition syncope (in patients with benign prostatic hypertrophy) · history of postural hypotension · monotherapy in patients with overflow bladder or anuria

- **CAUTIONS** Care with initial dose (postural hypotension) · cataract surgery (risk of intra-operative floppy iris syndrome) · elderly · heart failure · pulmonary oedema due to aortic or mitral stenosis

- **INTERACTIONS** → Appendix 1: alpha blockers

- **SIDE-EFFECTS**
- **Common or very common** Arrhythmias · asthenia · chest pain · cough · cystitis · dizziness · drowsiness · dry mouth · dyspnoea · gastrointestinal discomfort · headache · hypotension · increased risk of infection · influenza like illness · muscle complaints · nausea · oedema · pain · palpitations · skin reactions · urinary disorders · vertigo
- **Uncommon** Angina pectoris · anxiety · appetite abnormal · arthralgia · constipation · depression · diarrhoea · gastrointestinal disorders · gout · haemorrhage · insomnia · myocardial infarction · sensation abnormal · sexual dysfunction · stroke · syncope · tinnitus · tremor · vomiting · weight increased
- **Rare or very rare** Alopecia · bronchospasm · flushing · gynaecomastia · hepatic disorders · leucopenia · malaise · muscle weakness · thrombocytopenia · vision blurred
- **Frequency not known** Floppy iris syndrome

- **PREGNANCY** No evidence of teratogenicity; manufacturers advise use only when potential benefit outweighs risk.

- **BREAST FEEDING** Accumulates in milk in *animal* studies—manufacturer advises avoid.

- **HEPATIC IMPAIRMENT** Manufacturer advises caution in mild to moderate impairment (limited information available); avoid in severe impairment (no information available).

- **PATIENT AND CARER ADVICE** Patient counselling is advised for doxazosin tablets (initial dose).
  Driving and skilled tasks May affect performance of skilled tasks e.g. driving.

- **MEDICINAL FORMS** There can be variation in the licensing of different medicines containing the same drug. Forms available from special-order manufacturers include: oral capsule, oral suspension, oral solution

Oral tablet
- **Doxazosin (Non-proprietary)**
  Doxazosin (as Doxazosin mesilate) 1 mg Doxazosin 1mg tablets | 28 tablet [PoM] £10.56 DT = £0.70
  Doxazosin (as Doxazosin mesilate) 2 mg Doxazosin 2mg tablets | 28 tablet [PoM] £14.08 DT = £0.69
  Doxazosin (as Doxazosin mesilate) 4 mg Doxazosin 4mg tablets | 28 tablet [PoM] £14.08 DT = £0.77
  Doxazosin (as Doxazosin mesilate) 8 mg Doxazosin 8mg tablets | 28 tablet [PoM] £20.49 DT = £20.49
- **Cardura** (Viatris UK Healthcare Ltd)
  Doxazosin (as Doxazosin mesilate) 1 mg Cardura 1mg tablets | 28 tablet [PoM] £10.56 DT = £0.70
  Doxazosin (as Doxazosin mesilate) 2 mg Cardura 2mg tablets | 28 tablet [PoM] £14.08 DT = £0.69
- **Doxadura** (Dexcel-Pharma Ltd)
  Doxazosin (as Doxazosin mesilate) 4 mg Doxadura 4mg tablets | 28 tablet [PoM] £1.11 DT = £0.77

Modified-release tablet
CAUTIONARY AND ADVISORY LABELS 25
- **Cardura XL** (Viatris UK Healthcare Ltd)
  Doxazosin (as Doxazosin mesilate) 4 mg Cardura XL 4mg tablets | 28 tablet [PoM] £5.00 DT = £5.00
  Doxazosin (as Doxazosin mesilate) 8 mg Cardura XL 8mg tablets | 28 tablet [PoM] £9.98 DT = £9.98
- **Doxadura XL** (Dexcel-Pharma Ltd)
  Doxazosin (as Doxazosin mesilate) 4 mg Doxadura XL 4mg tablets | 28 tablet [PoM] £4.75 DT = £5.00
- **Larbex XL** (Teva UK Ltd)
  Doxazosin (as Doxazosin mesilate) 4 mg Larbex XL 4mg tablets | 28 tablet [PoM] £6.08 DT = £5.00
- **Raporsin XL** (Accord-UK Ltd)
  Doxazosin (as Doxazosin mesilate) 4 mg Raporsin XL 4mg tablets | 28 tablet [PoM] £5.70 DT = £5.00

Indoramin
15-Apr-2024

- **INDICATIONS AND DOSE**

Hypertension
- BY MOUTH
- Adult: Initially 25 mg twice daily, increased in steps of 25–50 mg every 2 weeks, maximum daily dose should be given in divided doses; maximum 200 mg per day

continued →

Benign prostatic hyperplasia
▶ BY MOUTH
▸ Adult: 20 mg twice daily, increased in steps of 20 mg every 2 weeks if required, increased if necessary up to 100 mg daily in divided doses
▸ Elderly: 20 mg daily may be adequate, dose to be taken at night

DOSE ADJUSTMENTS DUE TO INTERACTIONS
▸ Caution with concomitant antihypertensives in benign prostatic hyperplasia—reduced dosage and specialist supervision may be required.

● CONTRA-INDICATIONS Established heart failure · history micturition syncope (when used for benign prostatic hyperplasia) · history of postural hypotension (when used for benign prostatic hyperplasia)

● CAUTIONS Cataract surgery (risk of intra-operative floppy iris syndrome) · control incipient heart failure before initiating indoramin · elderly · epilepsy (convulsions in *animal* studies) · history of depression · Parkinson's disease (extrapyramidal disorders reported)

CAUTIONS, FURTHER INFORMATION
▸ Elderly For alpha$_1$-selective adrenoceptor blockers, Screening Tool of Older Persons' potentially inappropriate Prescriptions (STOPP) criteria to aid medication reviews (see Prescribing in the elderly p. 31 for information). Potentially inappropriate:
  ● in those with symptomatic postural hypotension or micturition syncope (risk of precipitating recurrent syncope)
  ● in those with persistent postural hypotension i.e. recurrent drop in systolic blood pressure $\geq$ 20 mmHg (risk of syncope and falls).

● INTERACTIONS → Appendix 1: alpha blockers

● SIDE-EFFECTS
▸ **Rare or very rare** Parkinson's disease exacerbated
▸ **Frequency not known** Depression · dizziness · drowsiness · dry mouth · ejaculation failure · fatigue · headache · nasal congestion · weight increased

● PREGNANCY No evidence of teratogenicity; manufacturers advise use only when potential benefit outweighs risk.

● BREAST FEEDING No information available.

● HEPATIC IMPAIRMENT Manufacturer advises caution.

● RENAL IMPAIRMENT [EvGr] Use with caution. ⓜ

● PATIENT AND CARER ADVICE
Driving and skilled tasks Drowsiness may affect performance of skilled tasks (e.g. driving); effects of alcohol may be enhanced.

● MEDICINAL FORMS There can be variation in the licensing of different medicines containing the same drug.
Oral tablet
CAUTIONARY AND ADVISORY LABELS 2
▸ Indoramin (Non-proprietary)
  Indoramin (as Indoramin hydrochloride) 20 mg Indoramin 20mg tablets | 56 tablet [PoM] £10.65 | 60 tablet [PoM] £74.99 DT = £42.36

Prazosin

15-Apr-2024

● **INDICATIONS AND DOSE**
Hypertension
▶ BY MOUTH
▸ Adult: Initially 500 micrograms 2–3 times a day for 3–7 days, the initial dose should be taken on retiring to bed at night to avoid collapse, increased to 1 mg 2–3 times a day for a further 3–7 days, then increased if necessary up to 20 mg daily in divided doses

Congestive heart failure (rarely used)
▶ BY MOUTH
▸ Adult: 500 micrograms 2–4 times a day, initial dose to be taken at bedtime, then increased to 4 mg daily in divided doses; maintenance 4–20 mg daily in divided doses

Raynaud's syndrome (but efficacy not established)
▶ BY MOUTH
▸ Adult: Initially 500 micrograms twice daily, initial dose to be taken at bedtime, dose may be increased after 3–7 days, then increased if necessary to 1–2 mg twice daily

Benign prostatic hyperplasia
▶ BY MOUTH
▸ Adult: Initially 500 micrograms twice daily for 3–7 days, subsequent doses should be adjusted according to response, maintenance 2 mg twice daily, initiate with lowest possible dose in elderly patients

DOSE ADJUSTMENTS DUE TO INTERACTIONS
▸ Caution with concomitant antihypertensives in benign prostatic hyperplasia—reduced dosage and specialist supervision may be required.

● CONTRA-INDICATIONS History of micturition syncope (in patients with benign prostatic hyperplasia) · history of postural hypotension · not recommended for congestive heart failure due to mechanical obstruction (e.g. aortic stenosis)

● CAUTIONS Cataract surgery (risk of intra-operative floppy iris syndrome) · elderly · first dose hypotension

CAUTIONS, FURTHER INFORMATION
▸ Elderly For alpha$_1$-selective adrenoceptor blockers, Screening Tool of Older Persons' potentially inappropriate Prescriptions (STOPP) criteria to aid medication reviews (see Prescribing in the elderly p. 31 for information). Potentially inappropriate:
  ● in those with symptomatic postural hypotension or micturition syncope (risk of precipitating recurrent syncope)
  ● in those with persistent postural hypotension i.e. recurrent drop in systolic blood pressure $\geq$ 20 mmHg (risk of syncope and falls).

● INTERACTIONS → Appendix 1: alpha blockers

● SIDE-EFFECTS
▸ **Common or very common** Asthenia · constipation · depression · diarrhoea · dizziness · drowsiness · dry mouth · dyspnoea · headache · nasal congestion · nausea · nervousness · oedema · palpitations · postural hypotension · sexual dysfunction · skin reactions · syncope · urinary disorders · vertigo · vision blurred · vomiting
▸ **Uncommon** Angina pectoris · arrhythmias · arthralgia · epistaxis · eye pain · eye redness · gastrointestinal discomfort · hyperhidrosis · paraesthesia · sleep disorders · tinnitus
▸ **Rare or very rare** Alopecia · fever · flushing · gynaecomastia · hallucination · hepatic function abnormal · pain · pancreatitis · vasculitis

● PREGNANCY No evidence of teratogenicity; manufacturers advise use only when potential benefit outweighs risk.

● BREAST FEEDING Present in milk, amount probably too small to be harmful; manufacturer advises use with caution.

● HEPATIC IMPAIRMENT Manufacturer advises caution (no information available).
Dose adjustments Manufacturer advises initial dose reduction to 500 micrograms daily; increased with caution.

● RENAL IMPAIRMENT
Dose adjustments Manufacturer advises initial dose reduction to 500 micrograms daily in moderate to severe impairment; increase with caution.

● **PATIENT AND CARER ADVICE**
First dose effect First dose may cause collapse due to hypotensive effect (therefore should be taken on retiring to bed). Patients should be warned to lie down if symptoms such as dizziness, fatigue or sweating develop, and to remain lying down until they abate completely.
Driving and skilled tasks May affect performance of skilled tasks e.g. driving.

● **MEDICINAL FORMS** There can be variation in the licensing of different medicines containing the same drug. Forms available from special-order manufacturers include: oral tablet, oral suspension, oral solution
Oral tablet
▸ Prazosin (Non-proprietary)
Prazosin (as Prazosin hydrochloride) 2 mg Minipress 2mg tablets | 100 tablet [PoM] [⬛] DT = £129.46
Prazosin (as Prazosin hydrochloride) 5 mg Minipress 5mg tablets | 100 tablet [PoM] [⬛] DT = £63.40
▸ Hypovase (Pfizer Ltd)
Prazosin (as Prazosin hydrochloride) 500 microgram Hypovase 500microgram tablets | 60 tablet [PoM] £2.69 DT = £2.69

Tamsulosin hydrochloride
14-Jan-2025

● **INDICATIONS AND DOSE**

Benign prostatic hyperplasia
▸ BY MOUTH USING MODIFIED-RELEASE MEDICINES
▸ Adult: 400 micrograms once daily

● **CONTRA-INDICATIONS** History of micturition syncope · history of postural hypotension

● **CAUTIONS** Care with initial dose (postural hypotension) · cataract surgery (risk of intra-operative floppy iris syndrome) · concomitant antihypertensives (reduced dosage and specialist supervision may be required) · elderly

CAUTIONS, FURTHER INFORMATION
▸ Elderly For alpha$_1$-selective adrenoceptor blockers, Screening Tool of Older Persons' potentially inappropriate Prescriptions (STOPP) criteria to aid medication reviews (see Prescribing in the elderly p. 31 for information). Potentially inappropriate:
● in those with symptomatic postural hypotension or micturition syncope (risk of precipitating recurrent syncope)
● in those with persistent postural hypotension i.e. recurrent drop in systolic blood pressure ≥ 20 mmHg (risk of syncope and falls).

● **INTERACTIONS** → Appendix 1: alpha blockers

● **SIDE-EFFECTS**
▸ **Common or very common** Dizziness · sexual dysfunction
▸ **Uncommon** Asthenia · constipation · diarrhoea · headache · nausea · palpitations · postural hypotension · rhinitis · skin reactions · vomiting
▸ **Rare or very rare** Angioedema · Stevens-Johnson syndrome · syncope
▸ **Frequency not known** Dry mouth · epistaxis · vision disorders

● **HEPATIC IMPAIRMENT** Manufacturer advises avoid in severe impairment.

● **RENAL IMPAIRMENT** [EvGr] Use with caution if creatinine clearance less than 10 mL/minute. ⓜ See p. 21.

● **PATIENT AND CARER ADVICE**
Driving and skilled tasks May affect performance of skilled tasks e.g. driving.

● **MEDICINAL FORMS** There can be variation in the licensing of different medicines containing the same drug.
Modified-release tablet
CAUTIONARY AND ADVISORY LABELS 25
▸ Cositam XL (Consilient Health Ltd)
Tamsulosin hydrochloride 400 microgram Cositam XL 400microgram tablets | 30 tablet [PoM] £8.89 DT = £10.47
▸ Faramsil (Sandoz Ltd)
Tamsulosin hydrochloride 400 microgram Faramsil 400microgram modified-release tablets | 30 tablet [PoM] £8.89 DT = £10.47
▸ Flomaxtra XL (Astellas Pharma Ltd)
Tamsulosin hydrochloride 400 microgram Flomaxtra XL 400microgram tablets | 30 tablet [PoM] £10.47 DT = £10.47
Modified-release capsule
CAUTIONARY AND ADVISORY LABELS 25
▸ Tamsulosin hydrochloride (Non-proprietary)
Tamsulosin hydrochloride 400 microgram Tamsulosin 400microgram modified-release capsules | 30 capsule [PoM] £1.88-£3.80 DT = £1.28 | 200 capsule [PoM] £16.00-£67.60
▸ Contiflo XL (Sun Pharma UK Ltd)
Tamsulosin hydrochloride 400 microgram Contiflo XL 400microgram capsules | 30 capsule [PoM] £7.44 DT = £1.28
▸ Pamsvax XL (Accord-UK Ltd)
Tamsulosin hydrochloride 400 microgram Pamsvax XL 400microgram capsules | 30 capsule [PoM] £1.28 DT = £1.28
▸ Tabphyn MR (Genus Pharmaceuticals Ltd)
Tamsulosin hydrochloride 400 microgram Tabphyn MR 400microgram capsules | 30 capsule [PoM] £4.45 DT = £1.28
▸ Tamfrex XL (Milpharm Ltd)
Tamsulosin hydrochloride 400 microgram Tamfrex XL 400microgram capsules | 30 capsule [PoM] £28.51 DT = £1.28
▸ Tamsumac (Macleods Pharma UK Ltd)
Tamsulosin hydrochloride 400 microgram Tamsumac 0.4mg modified-release capsules | 30 capsule [PoM] £3.87 DT = £1.28
▸ Tamurex (Somex Pharma)
Tamsulosin hydrochloride 400 microgram Tamurex 400microgram modified-release capsules | 30 capsule [PoM] £3.87 DT = £1.28

Tamsulosin with dutasteride
03-Nov-2020

The properties listed below are those particular to the combination only. For the properties of the components please consider, tamsulosin hydrochloride above, dutasteride p. 907.

● **INDICATIONS AND DOSE**

Benign prostatic hyperplasia
▸ BY MOUTH
▸ Adult (male): 1 capsule daily.

● **INTERACTIONS** → Appendix 1: alpha blockers · dutasteride
● **PATIENT AND CARER ADVICE**
Driving and skilled tasks May affect performance of skilled tasks e.g. driving.

● **MEDICINAL FORMS** There can be variation in the licensing of different medicines containing the same drug.
Oral capsule
CAUTIONARY AND ADVISORY LABELS 25
▸ Tamsulosin with dutasteride (Non-proprietary)
Tamsulosin hydrochloride 400 microgram, Dutasteride 500 microgram Tamsulosin 400microgram / Dutasteride 500microgram capsules | 30 capsule [PoM] £19.80 DT = £5.94
▸ Combodart (Recordati Pharmaceuticals Ltd)
Tamsulosin hydrochloride 400 microgram, Dutasteride 500 microgram Combodart 0.5mg/0.4mg capsules | 30 capsule [PoM] £19.80 DT = £5.94
▸ Dutrozen (Zentiva Pharma UK Ltd)
Tamsulosin hydrochloride 400 microgram, Dutasteride 500 microgram Dutrozen 0.5mg/0.4mg capsules | 30 capsule [PoM] £18.81 DT = £5.94

Genito-urinary system

7

Tamsulosin with solifenacin
06-Jul-2021

The properties listed below are those particular to the combination only. For the properties of the components please consider, tamsulosin hydrochloride p. 905, solifenacin succinate p. 899.

- **INDICATIONS AND DOSE**

  Moderate to severe urinary frequency, urgency, and obstructive symptoms associated with benign prostatic hyperplasia when monotherapy ineffective
  - BY MOUTH
  - Adult (male): 1 tablet daily.

  DOSE ADJUSTMENTS DUE TO INTERACTIONS
  - Manufacturer advises max. 1 *Vesomni*® tablet daily with concurrent use of potent inhibitors of CYP3A4; avoid concurrent use in patients who also have moderate hepatic impairment, severe renal impairment, are poor metabolisers of CYP2D6, or in patients also taking a potent inhibitor of CYP2D6.

- **INTERACTIONS** → Appendix 1: alpha blockers · solifenacin

- **HEPATIC IMPAIRMENT** Manufacturer advises caution in moderate impairment; avoid in severe impairment (no information available).
  Dose adjustments Manufacturer advises max. 1 *Vesomni*® tablet daily in moderate impairment.

- **RENAL IMPAIRMENT** [EvGr] Caution in severe impairment. (M)
  Dose adjustments [EvGr] Max. 1 *Vesomni*® tablet daily if creatinine clearance 30 mL/minute or less. (M) See p. 21.

- **MEDICINAL FORMS** There can be variation in the licensing of different medicines containing the same drug.
  Modified-release tablet
  CAUTIONARY AND ADVISORY LABELS 3, 25
  - **Tamsulosin with solifenacin (Non-proprietary)**
    Tamsulosin hydrochloride 400 microgram, Solifenacin succinate 6 mg Solifenacin 6mg / Tamsulosin 400microgram modified-release tablets | 30 tablet [PoM] £29.00 DT = £27.62
  - **Vecit** (Celix Pharma Ltd)
    Tamsulosin hydrochloride 400 microgram, Solifenacin succinate 6 mg Vecit 6mg/0.4mg modified-release tablets | 30 tablet [PoM] £23.48 DT = £27.62
  - **Vesomni** (Astellas Pharma Ltd)
    Tamsulosin hydrochloride 400 microgram, Solifenacin succinate 6 mg Vesomni 6mg/0.4mg modified-release tablets | 30 tablet [PoM] £27.62 DT = £27.62

Terazosin
15-Apr-2024

- **INDICATIONS AND DOSE**

  Mild to moderate hypertension
  - BY MOUTH
  - Adult: 1 mg daily for 7 days, then increased if necessary to 2 mg daily, dose should be taken at bedtime; maintenance 2–10 mg once daily, doses above 20 mg rarely improve efficacy

  Benign prostatic hyperplasia
  - BY MOUTH
  - Adult: Initially 1 mg daily, dose should be taken at bedtime, if necessary dose may be doubled at intervals of 1–2 weeks according to response; maintenance 5–10 mg daily; maximum 10 mg per day

- **CONTRA-INDICATIONS** History of micturition syncope (in benign prostatic hyperplasia) · history of postural hypotension (in benign prostatic hyperplasia)

- **CAUTIONS** Cataract surgery (risk of intra-operative floppy iris syndrome) · elderly · first dose

CAUTIONS, FURTHER INFORMATION
- First dose First dose may cause collapse due to hypotension within 30–90 minutes, therefore should be taken on retiring to bed; may also occur with rapid dose increase.
- Elderly For alpha₁-selective adrenoceptor blockers, Screening Tool of Older Persons' potentially inappropriate Prescriptions (STOPP) criteria to aid medication reviews (see Prescribing in the elderly p. 31 for information). Potentially inappropriate:
  - in those with symptomatic postural hypotension or micturition syncope (risk of precipitating recurrent syncope)
  - in those with persistent postural hypotension i.e. recurrent drop in systolic blood pressure ≥ 20 mmHg (risk of syncope and falls).

- **INTERACTIONS** → Appendix 1: alpha blockers

- **SIDE-EFFECTS** Angioedema · anxiety · arrhythmias · arthritis · asthenia · chest pain · conjunctivitis · constipation · cough · depression · diarrhoea · dizziness · drowsiness · dry mouth · dyspnoea · epistaxis · fever · flatulence · gastrointestinal discomfort · gout · headache · hyperhidrosis · increased risk of infection · insomnia · joint disorders · myalgia · nasal congestion · nausea · oedema · pain · palpitations · paraesthesia · postural hypotension · sexual dysfunction · skin reactions · syncope · thrombocytopenia · tinnitus · urinary disorders · vasodilation · vertigo · vision disorders · vomiting · weight increased

- **PREGNANCY** No evidence of teratogenicity; manufacturers advise use only when potential benefit outweighs risk.

- **BREAST FEEDING** No information available.

- **PATIENT AND CARER ADVICE** Patient counselling is advised for terazosin tablets (initial dose).
  First dose effect First dose may cause collapse due to hypotensive effect (therefore should be taken on retiring to bed). Patient should be warned to lie down if symptoms such as dizziness, fatigue or sweating develop, and to remain lying down until they abate completely.
  Driving and skilled tasks May affect performance of skilled tasks e.g. driving.

- **MEDICINAL FORMS** There can be variation in the licensing of different medicines containing the same drug.
  Oral tablet
  - **Terazosin (Non-proprietary)**
    Terazosin (as Terazosin hydrochloride) 2 mg Terazosin 2mg tablets | 28 tablet [PoM] £2.80 DT = £2.25
    Terazosin (as Terazosin hydrochloride) 5 mg Terazosin 5mg tablets | 28 tablet [PoM] £6.56 DT = £4.69
    Terazosin (as Terazosin hydrochloride) 10 mg Terazosin 10mg tablets | 28 tablet [PoM] £8.11 DT = £7.64
  - **Hytrin** (Advanz Pharma)
    Terazosin (as Terazosin hydrochloride) 1 mg Hytrin 1mg tablets | 7 tablet [PoM] [S]
    Terazosin (as Terazosin hydrochloride) 2 mg Hytrin 2mg tablets | 28 tablet [PoM] £2.20 DT = £2.25
    Terazosin (as Terazosin hydrochloride) 5 mg Hytrin 5mg tablets | 28 tablet [PoM] £4.13 DT = £4.69
    Terazosin (as Terazosin hydrochloride) 10 mg Hytrin 10mg tablets | 28 tablet [PoM] £7.87 DT = £7.64

CHOLINE ESTERS

Bethanechol chloride
09-Dec-2020

- **INDICATIONS AND DOSE**

  Urinary retention
  - BY MOUTH
  - Adult: 10–25 mg 3–4 times a day, to be taken 30 minutes before food

- **CONTRA-INDICATIONS** Bradycardia · conditions where increased motility of the gastro-intestinal tract could be harmful · conditions where increased motility of the urinary tract could be harmful · epilepsy · heart block · hyperthyroidism · hypotension · intestinal obstruction · obstructive airways disease · parkinsonism · peptic ulcer · recent myocardial infarction · urinary obstruction

- **CAUTIONS** Autonomic neuropathy (use lower initial dose)
- **SIDE-EFFECTS** Abdominal pain · hyperhidrosis · nausea · vomiting
- **PREGNANCY** Manufacturer advises avoid—no information available.
- **BREAST FEEDING** Manufacturer advises avoid; gastrointestinal disturbances in infant reported.
- **LESS SUITABLE FOR PRESCRIBING** Less suitable for prescribing.

- **MEDICINAL FORMS** There can be variation in the licensing of different medicines containing the same drug. Forms available from special-order manufacturers include: oral suspension, oral solution

Oral tablet

CAUTIONARY AND ADVISORY LABELS 22

▸ Myotonine (Glenwood GmbH)
  Bethanechol chloride 10 mg Myotonine 10mg tablets | 100 tablet [PoM] £18.51 DT = £18.51
  Bethanechol chloride 25 mg Myotonine 25mg tablets | 100 tablet [PoM] £27.26 DT = £27.26

5α-REDUCTASE INHIBITORS

Dutasteride
02-Sep-2020

- **DRUG ACTION** A specific inhibitor of the enzyme 5α-reductase, which metabolises testosterone into the more potent androgen, dihydrotestosterone.

- **INDICATIONS AND DOSE**

Benign prostatic hyperplasia
▸ BY MOUTH
▸ Adult: 500 micrograms daily, review treatment at 3–6 months and then every 6–12 months (may require several months treatment before benefit is obtained)

- **INTERACTIONS** → Appendix 1: dutasteride

- **SIDE-EFFECTS**
▸ **Common or very common** Breast disorder · sexual dysfunction
▸ **Uncommon** Alopecia · hypertrichosis
▸ **Frequency not known** Angioedema · depressed mood · hypersensitivity · localised oedema · skin reactions · testicular disorders

- **CONCEPTION AND CONTRACEPTION** Dutasteride is excreted in semen and use of a condom is recommended if sexual partner is pregnant or likely to become pregnant.

- **HEPATIC IMPAIRMENT** Manufacturer advises caution in mild to moderate impairment; avoid in severe impairment (no information available).

- **MONITORING REQUIREMENTS** Manufacturer advises that patients should be regularly evaluated for prostate cancer.

- **EFFECT ON LABORATORY TESTS** May decrease serum concentration of prostate cancer markers such as prostate-specific antigen; reference values may need adjustment.

- **HANDLING AND STORAGE** Women of childbearing potential should avoid handling leaking capsules of dutasteride.

- **PATIENT AND CARER ADVICE** Cases of male breast cancer have been reported. Patients or their carers should be told to promptly report to their doctor any changes in breast tissue such as lumps, pain, or nipple discharge.

- **MEDICINAL FORMS** There can be variation in the licensing of different medicines containing the same drug. Forms available from special-order manufacturers include: oral solution

Oral capsule

CAUTIONARY AND ADVISORY LABELS 25

▸ Dutasteride (Non-proprietary)
  Dutasteride 500 microgram Dutasteride 500microgram capsules | 30 capsule [PoM] £13.90 DT = £2.07
▸ Avodart (Recordati Pharmaceuticals Ltd)
  Dutasteride 500 microgram Avodart 500microgram capsules | 30 capsule [PoM] £14.60 DT = £2.07

Combinations available: *Tamsulosin with dutasteride,* p. 905

Finasteride
03-May-2024

- **DRUG ACTION** A specific inhibitor of the enzyme 5α-reductase, which metabolises testosterone into the more potent androgen, dihydrotestosterone.

- **INDICATIONS AND DOSE**

Benign prostatic hyperplasia
▸ BY MOUTH
▸ Adult: 5 mg once daily, review treatment at 3–6 months and then every 6–12 months (may require several months treatment before benefit is obtained)

Androgenetic alopecia in men
▸ BY MOUTH
▸ Adult: 1 mg once daily, continuous use for 3–6 months is required before benefit is seen, and effects are reversed 6–12 months after treatment is discontinued

IMPORTANT SAFETY INFORMATION

MHRA/CHM ADVICE: RARE REPORTS OF DEPRESSION AND SUICIDAL THOUGHTS (MAY 2017)

The MHRA has received reports of depression and, in rare cases, suicidal thoughts in men taking finasteride (*Propecia*®) for male pattern hair loss; depression is also associated with *Proscar*® for benign prostatic hyperplasia.

MHRA/CHM ADVICE: FINASTERIDE: REMINDER OF THE RISK OF PSYCHIATRIC SIDE EFFECTS AND OF SEXUAL SIDE EFFECTS (WHICH MAY PERSIST AFTER DISCONTINUATION OF TREATMENT) (APRIL 2024)

Following a safety review of the available evidence, a patient alert card highlighting the risk of psychiatric and sexual side-effects associated with finasteride is being introduced to increase awareness. Healthcare professionals are reminded that finasteride has been associated with depression, suicidal thoughts, and sexual dysfunction (including decreased libido and erectile dysfunction, with some cases reported to persist after treatment discontinuation). Healthcare professionals are advised to ask patients if they have a history of depression or suicidal ideation before prescribing finasteride, and to monitor for these side-effects after starting treatment.

Patients and caregivers should be counselled to seek medical advice if the patient develops depression, suicidal thoughts, or sexual dysfunction. Those taking *Propecia*® should stop treatment immediately if depression or suicidal thoughts occur.

- **CAUTIONS** Obstructive uropathy

- **SIDE-EFFECTS**
▸ **Common or very common** Sexual dysfunction
▸ **Uncommon** Breast abnormalities · depression · skin reactions
▸ **Frequency not known** Angioedema · infertility male · palpitations · suicidal behaviours · testicular pain

- **CONCEPTION AND CONTRACEPTION** Finasteride is excreted in semen and use of a condom is recommended if sexual partner is pregnant or likely to become pregnant.
- **EFFECT ON LABORATORY TESTS** Decreases serum concentration of prostate cancer markers such as prostate-specific antigen; reference values may need adjustment.
- **HANDLING AND STORAGE** Women of childbearing potential should avoid handling crushed or broken tablets of finasteride.
- **PATIENT AND CARER ADVICE** Cases of male breast cancer have been reported. Patients or their carers should be told to promptly report to their doctor any changes in breast tissue such as lumps, pain, or nipple discharge.
- **NATIONAL FUNDING/ACCESS DECISIONS**
  NHS restrictions Finasteride is not prescribable in NHS primary care for the treatment of androgenetic alopecia in men.

- **MEDICINAL FORMS** There can be variation in the licensing of different medicines containing the same drug. Forms available from special-order manufacturers include: oral suspension, oral powder

  Oral tablet
  CAUTIONARY AND ADVISORY LABELS 25
  ▸ **Finasteride (Non-proprietary)**
  Finasteride 1 mg Finasteride 1mg tablets | 28 tablet [PoM] £3.00–£33.68 | 30 tablet [PoM] £8.00 | 84 tablet [PoM] £40.50–£88.40 | 90 tablet [PoM] £19.00
  Finasteride 5 mg Finasteride 5mg tablets | 28 tablet [PoM] £14.95 DT = £1.06
  ▸ **Propecia** (Organon Pharma (UK) Ltd)
  Finasteride 1 mg Propecia 1mg tablets | 28 tablet [PoM] £33.68 | 84 tablet [PoM] £88.40
  ▸ **Proscar** (Organon Pharma (UK) Ltd)
  Finasteride 5 mg Proscar 5mg tablets | 30 tablet [PoM] £14.94

1.3 Urolithiasis

Renal and ureteric stones

03-Apr-2019

Description of condition

Renal and ureteric stones are crystalline calculi that may form anywhere in the upper urinary tract. They are often asymptomatic but may cause pain when they move or obstruct the flow of urine. Most stones are composed of calcium salts (calcium oxalate, calcium phosphate or both). The rest are composed of struvite, uric acid, cystine and other substances. Patients are susceptible to stone formation when there is a decrease in urine volume and/or an excess of stone forming substances in the urine.

The following are risk factors that have been associated with stone formation: dehydration, change in urine pH, males aged between 40–60 years, positive family history, obesity, urinary anatomical abnormalities, and excessive dietary intake of oxalate, urate, sodium, and animal protein. Certain diseases which alter urinary volume, pH, and concentrations of certain ions (such as calcium, phosphate, oxalate, sodium, and uric acid) may also increase the risk of stone formation. Certain drugs such as calcium or vitamin D supplements, protease inhibitors, or diuretics may also increase the risk of stone formation.

Symptoms of acute renal or ureteric stones can include an abrupt onset of severe unilateral abdominal pain radiating to the groin (known as renal colic) that may be accompanied with nausea, vomiting, haematuria, increased urinary frequency, dysuria and fever (if concomitant urinary infection is present).

Stones can pass spontaneously and will depend on a number of factors, including the size of the stone (stones greater than 6 mm have a very low chance of spontaneous passage), the location (distal ureteral stones are more likely to pass than proximal ureteral stones), and the degree of obstruction.

Aims of treatment

[EvGr] The aim of treatment is to improve the detection, clearance and prevention of renal and ureteric stones thereby reducing pain and improving quality of life. [A]

Non-drug treatment

[EvGr] Consider watchful waiting for asymptomatic renal stones if they are less than 5mm in diameter. If they are larger; the risk and benefit of this option should be discussed with the patient.

Options for surgical stone removal should be discussed by the specialist hospital team depending on severity of obstruction, patient factors, size and site of stone. Options include shockwave lithotripsy, percutaneous nephrolithotomy and ureteroscopy.

Consider stone analysis and measure serum calcium in patients with recurring renal or ureteric stones.

Along with maintaining a healthy lifestyle, advise patients to drink 2.5–3 litres of water a day with the addition of fresh lemon juice and to avoid carbonated drinks. Maintain a normal daily calcium intake of 700–1,200mg and salt intake of no more than 6g a day. For patients with recurrent calcium stones avoid excessive intake of oxalate-rich products, such as rhubarb, spinach, cocoa, tea, nuts, soy products, strawberries, and wheat bran. For patients with recurrent uric acid stones, avoid excessive dietary intake of urate rich products, such as liver, kidney, calf thymus, poultry skin, and certain fish (herring with skin, sardines and anchovies). [A]

Pain Management

[EvGr] Offer NSAIDs as first line treatment for the management of pain associated with suspected renal colic or renal and ureteric stones. If NSAIDs are contra-indicated or not sufficiently controlling the pain, consider intravenous paracetamol. Subsequently, opioids can be used if both paracetamol and NSAIDs are contra-indicated or not sufficiently controlling the pain. Do not offer antispasmodics to patients with suspected renal colic. [A]

Medical Expulsive Therapy

[EvGr] Consider alpha-adrenoceptor blockers for patients with distal ureteric stones less than 10mm in diameter. Alpha-adrenoceptor blockers may also be considered as adjunctive therapy for patients having shockwave lithotripsy for ureteric stones less than 10mm. [A]

Prevention of recurrence of stones

[EvGr] Alongside lifestyle advice, consider potassium citrate [unlicensed] in patients with recurrent stones composed of at least 50% calcium oxalate. Thiazides [unlicensed] may be given if patients also have hypercalciuria after restricting their sodium intake to no more than 6g a day. [A]

1.4 Urological pain

Urological pain

03-Apr-2019

Treatment

Lidocaine hydrochloride gel is a useful topical application in *urethral pain* or to relieve the discomfort of catheterisation.

For information on the management of pain in renal and ureteric stones, see Renal and ureteric stones above.

Alkalinisation of urine

Alkalinisation of urine can be undertaken with potassium citrate. The alkalinising action may relieve the discomfort of *cystitis* caused by lower urinary tract infections. Sodium bicarbonate p. 1178 is used as a urinary alkalinising agent in some metabolic and renal disorders.

ALKALISING DRUGS > URINARY

Citric acid with potassium citrate

25-Apr-2022

● **INDICATIONS AND DOSE**

Relief of discomfort in mild urinary-tract infections | Alkalinisation of urine
▸ BY MOUTH USING ORAL SOLUTION
▸ Adult: 10 mL 3 times a day, to be diluted well with water

● **CONTRA-INDICATIONS** Addison's disease · dehydration · hyperkalaemia · ventricular arrhythmia

● **CAUTIONS** Cardiac disease · elderly

● **INTERACTIONS** → Appendix 1: potassium citrate

● **SIDE-EFFECTS** Hyperkalaemia · nausea · vomiting

● **RENAL IMPAIRMENT** [EvGr] Consider avoiding (risk of hyperkalaemia). ⟨M⟩

● **PRESCRIBING AND DISPENSING INFORMATION** When prepared extemporaneously, the BP states Potassium Citrate Mixture BP consists of potassium citrate 30%, citric acid monohydrate 5% in a suitable vehicle with a lemon flavour. Extemporaneous preparations should be recently prepared according to the following formula: potassium citrate 3 g, citric acid monohydrate 500 mg, syrup 2.5 mL, quillaia tincture 0.1 mL, lemon spirit 0.05 mL, double-strength chloroform water 3 mL, water to 10 mL. Contains about 28 mmol K^+/10 mL.

● **EXCEPTIONS TO LEGAL CATEGORY** Proprietary brands of potassium citrate are on sale to the public for the relief of discomfort in mild urinary-tract infections.

● **MEDICINAL FORMS** There can be variation in the licensing of different medicines containing the same drug.
Oral solution
CAUTIONARY AND ADVISORY LABELS 27
▸ Citric acid with potassium citrate (Non-proprietary)
Citric acid monohydrate 50 mg per 1 ml, Potassium citrate 300 mg per 1 ml Potassium citrate mixture | 200 ml [P] £2.45 DT = £3.54
Effervescent tablet
▸ Effercitrate (Cambridge Healthcare Supplies Ltd)
Citric acid 250 mg, Potassium citrate 1.5 gram Effercitrate tablets | 12 tablet [GSL] £6.29 DT = £6.29 [SF]

Sodium citrate

18-Nov-2021

● **INDICATIONS AND DOSE**

Bladder washouts
▸ Adult: (consult product literature)

Relief of discomfort in mild urinary-tract infections
▸ BY MOUTH
▸ Adult: (consult product literature)

Constipation (dose approved for use by community practitioner nurse prescribers)
▸ BY RECTUM
▸ Child 3-17 years: 5 mL for 1 dose
▸ Adult: 5 mL for 1 dose

MICOLETTE ®
Constipation
▸ BY RECTUM
▸ Child 3-17 years: 5–10 mL for 1 dose
▸ Adult: 5–10 mL for 1 dose

MICRALAX ®
Constipation
▸ BY RECTUM
▸ Child 3-17 years: 5 mL for 1 dose
▸ Adult: 5 mL for 1 dose

RELAXIT ®
Constipation
▸ BY RECTUM
▸ Child 1 month-2 years: 5 mL for 1 dose, insert only half the nozzle length
▸ Child 3-17 years: 5 mL for 1 dose
▸ Adult: 5 mL for 1 dose

● **CONTRA-INDICATIONS**
▸ With oral use Conditions where excess sodium or glucose should be avoided (e.g. cardiac disease, hypertension, patients on a sodium-restricted diet or diabetes)
▸ With rectal use Acute gastro-intestinal conditions

● **CAUTIONS**
▸ With oral use Elderly
▸ With rectal use Debilitated patients (in adults) · sodium and water retention in susceptible individuals

● **INTERACTIONS** → Appendix 1: sodium citrate

● **SIDE-EFFECTS** Polyuria

● **PREGNANCY**
▸ With oral use Use with caution.

● **RENAL IMPAIRMENT**
▸ With oral use [EvGr] Caution (contains sodium). ⟨M⟩

● **PRESCRIBING AND DISPENSING INFORMATION** Sodium citrate 300 mmol/litre (88.2 mg/mL) oral solution is licensed for use before general anaesthesia for caesarean section (available from Viridian).

● **EXCEPTIONS TO LEGAL CATEGORY** Proprietary brands of sodium citrate are on sale to the public for the relief of discomfort in mild urinary-tract infections.

● **MEDICINAL FORMS** There can be variation in the licensing of different medicines containing the same drug. Forms available from special-order manufacturers include: oral solution
Oral solution
▸ Sodium citrate (Non-proprietary)
Sodium citrate 88.23 mg per 1 ml Sodium citrate 0.3M oral solution | 30 ml [PoM] £4.70 DT = £4.70
Granules for oral solution
▸ Sodium citrate (Non-proprietary)
Sodium citrate 4 gram Cystitis Relief 4g granules for oral solution sachets | 6 sachet [GSL] £3.16 DT = £3.16
▸ Brands may include CanesOasis, Cystocalm
Powder for oral solution
▸ Sodium citrate (Non-proprietary)
Sodium citrate 4 gram Numark cystitis treatment 4g oral powder sachets | 6 sachet [GSL] £1.85 DT = £1.85
Irrigation solution
▸ Sodium citrate (Non-proprietary)
Sodium citrate 3% irrigation solution 1litre bags | 1 bag [⊠]
Enema
▸ Micralax Micro-enema (RPH Pharmaceuticals AB)
Sodium citrate 90 mg per 1 ml Micralax Micro-enema 5ml | 12 enema [P] £8.49
▸ Relaxit (Supra Enterprises Ltd)
Sodium citrate 90 mg per 1 ml Relaxit Micro-enema 5ml | 12 enema £5.21

Genito-urinary system

7

HEPARINOIDS

Pentosan polysulfate sodium
05-Oct-2021

● **INDICATIONS AND DOSE**

Bladder pain syndrome

▶ BY MOUTH

▶ Adult: 100 mg 3 times a day, review treatment after 6 months and discontinue if no response

IMPORTANT SAFETY INFORMATION

MHRA/CHM ADVICE (UPDATED SEPTEMBER 2019): *ELMIRON*®
(PENTOSAN POLYSULFATE SODIUM): RARE RISK OF PIGMENTARY
MACULOPATHY

Cases of pigmentary maculopathy have been reported
rarely with pentosan polysulfate sodium, especially after
long-term use at high doses. Healthcare professionals
are advised that patients should have regular ophthalmic
examinations during treatment, and to consider
stopping treatment if pigmentary maculopathy develops.
Patients should be advised to seek immediate medical
attention if visual changes occur.

● **CONTRA-INDICATIONS** Active bleeding

● **CAUTIONS** Patients at increased risk of bleeding

● **INTERACTIONS** → Appendix 1: pentosan

● **SIDE-EFFECTS**

▶ **Common or very common** Alopecia · asthenia · back pain ·
diarrhoea · dizziness · gastrointestinal discomfort ·
haemorrhage · headache · increased risk of infection ·
nausea · pelvic pain · peripheral oedema

▶ **Uncommon** Amblyopia · anaemia · appetite decreased ·
arthralgia · constipation · depression · dyspnoea ·
emotional lability · eye disorders · flatulence ·
hyperhidrosis · hyperkinesia · insomnia · leucopenia ·
melanocytic naevus size increased · myalgia · oral
ulceration · paraesthesia · photosensitivity reaction · skin
reactions · thrombocytopenia · tinnitus · vomiting · weight
changes

▶ **Frequency not known** Coagulation disorder · hepatic
function abnormal

● **PREGNANCY** Manufacturer advises avoid—no information
available.

● **BREAST FEEDING** Manufacturer advises avoid—no
information available.

● **HEPATIC IMPAIRMENT** Manufacturer advises caution—
evidence of hepatic involvement in elimination.

● **RENAL IMPAIRMENT** Manufacturer advises caution—
evidence of renal involvement in elimination.

● **MONITORING REQUIREMENTS** Manufacturer advises
careful monitoring in patients with history of heparin or
pentosan polysulfate sodium induced thrombocytopenia.

● **NATIONAL FUNDING/ACCESS DECISIONS**
For full details see funding body website

NICE decisions

▶ Pentosan polysulfate sodium for treating bladder pain
syndrome (November 2019) NICE TA610 Recommended with
restrictions

Scottish Medicines Consortium (SMC) decisions

▶ Pentosan polysulfate sodium (*Elmiron*®) for the treatment of
adults with bladder pain syndrome characterised by either
glomerulations or Hunner's lesions with moderate to severe
pain, urgency and frequency of micturition (November 2019)
SMC No. SMC2194 Recommended

● **MEDICINAL FORMS** There can be variation in the licensing of
different medicines containing the same drug.

Oral capsule

CAUTIONARY AND ADVISORY LABELS 23

▶ Pentosan polysulfate sodium (Non-proprietary)
Pentosan polysulfate sodium 50 mg Fibrase 50mg capsules |
50 capsule PoM Ⓢ

▶ Elmiron (Consilient Health Ltd)
Pentosan polysulfate sodium 100 mg Elmiron 100mg capsules |
90 capsule PoM £450.00 DT = £450.00

TERPENES

Anethol with borneol, camphene, cineole, fenchone and pinene

● **INDICATIONS AND DOSE**

Urolithiasis for the expulsion of calculi

▶ BY MOUTH

▶ Adult: 1–2 capsules 3–4 times a day, to be taken before
food

● **LESS SUITABLE FOR PRESCRIBING** Preparation is less
suitable for prescribing.

● **MEDICINAL FORMS** No licensed medicines listed.

2 Bladder instillations and urological surgery

Bladder instillations and urological surgery
19-Jul-2020

Bladder infection

Chlorhexidine solution p. 911 given as bladder irrigation is
licensed for the management of common infections of the
bladder in patients with an indwelling urinary catheter.
Chlorhexidine has broad spectrum activity against many
Gram-positive and Gram-negative bacteria but it is
ineffective against most *Pseudomonas spp*. Solutions
containing chlorhexidine 1 in 5000 (0.02%) are used but they
may irritate the mucosa and cause burning on micturition (in
which case they should be discontinued). Sterile sodium
chloride solution 0.9% p. 1180 (physiological saline) is
licensed for use as a routine mechanical irrigant to flush out
debris, small blood clots, or tissue in catheters.

Continuous bladder irrigation with amphotericin B p. 689
(*Fungizone*®) 50 micrograms/mL is licensed to treat some
fungal infections (e.g. candiduria).

Bladder cancer

Bladder installations of doxorubicin hydrochloride p. 1038
and mitomycin p. 1054 are licensed for the management of
superficial bladder tumours. Such instillations reduce
systemic side-effects; adverse effects on the bladder (e.g.
micturition disorders and reduction in bladder capacity) may
occur. Instillation of epirubicin hydrochloride p. 1039 is also
licensed for the treatment and prophylaxis of certain forms
of superficial bladder cancer.

Instillation of BCG (Bacillus Calmette-Guérin p. 1089), a
live attenuated strain derived from *Mycobacterium bovis*, is
licensed for the treatment of primary or recurrent bladder
carcinoma *in-situ* and for the prevention of recurrence
following transurethral resection.

Urological surgery

Glycine irrigation solution 1.5% p. 911 is licensed for use in
transurethral surgical procedures such as prostatic resection;

EvGr sterile sodium chloride solution 0.9% (physiological saline) is used for irrigation in percutaneous renal surgery (e.g. nephrolithotomy, ureteroscopy). ◇A

> **Other drugs used for Bladder instillations and urological surgery** Sodium citrate, p. 909

ANTISEPTICS AND DISINFECTANTS

| Chlorhexidine
                                            23-Feb-2022

● **INDICATIONS AND DOSE**
Bladder irrigation and catheter patency solutions
▶ BY INTRAVESICAL INSTILLATION
▶ Adult: (consult product literature)

● **MEDICINAL FORMS** There can be variation in the licensing of different medicines containing the same drug. Forms available from special-order manufacturers include: irrigation solution
Cutaneous or intravesical irrigation solution
▶ Chlorhexidine (Non-proprietary)
   Chlorhexidine acetate 200 microgram per 1 ml Chlorhexidine acetate 0.02% irrigation solution 1litre bottles | 1 bottle P Ⓢ
   Chlorhexidine acetate 500 microgram per 1 ml Chlorhexidine acetate 0.05% irrigation solution 1litre bottles | 1 bottle P Ⓢ

| Chlorhexidine with lidocaine

The properties listed below are those particular to the combination only. For the properties of the components please consider, chlorhexidine above, lidocaine hydrochloride p. 1547.

● **INDICATIONS AND DOSE**
Urethral sounding and catheterisation
▶ BY URETHRAL APPLICATION
▶ Adult: 6–11 mL
Cystoscopy
▶ BY URETHRAL APPLICATION
▶ Adult: 11 mL, then 6–11 mL if required
Surface anaesthesia (dose approved for use by community practitioner nurse prescribers) (on doctor's advice only)
▶ BY URETHRAL APPLICATION
▶ Adult: 6–11 mL

● **INTERACTIONS** → Appendix 1: antiarrhythmics

● **MEDICINAL FORMS** There can be variation in the licensing of different medicines containing the same drug.
Gel
EXCIPIENTS: May contain Hydroxybenzoates (parabens)
▶ Instillagel (CliniMed Ltd)
   Chlorhexidine gluconate 500 microgram per 1 ml, Lidocaine hydrochloride 20 mg per 1 ml Instillagel gel | 60 ml P £10.50 DT = £10.50 | 110 ml P £11.00 DT = £11.00

IRRIGATING SOLUTIONS

| Glycine
                                            23-Nov-2020

● **INDICATIONS AND DOSE**
Bladder irrigation during urological surgery | Irrigation for transurethral resection of the prostate gland and bladder tumours
▶ Adult: (consult product literature)

● **CAUTIONS**
▶ Urological surgery There is a high risk of fluid absorption from the irrigant used in endoscopic surgery within the urinary tract.

● **SIDE-EFFECTS** Cardiovascular disorder · electrolyte depletion · fluid overload · pulmonary disorder · seizure · vision blurred

● **MEDICINAL FORMS** There can be variation in the licensing of different medicines containing the same drug.
Irrigation solution
▶ Glycine (Non-proprietary)
   Glycine 1.5% irrigation solution 3litre Easyflow bags | 1 bag Ⓢ
   Glycine 1.5% irrigation solution 1litre Flowfusor bottles | 1 bottle Ⓢ
   Glycine 1.5% irrigation solution 1litre Easyflow bags | 1 bag Ⓢ
   Glycine 1.5% irrigation solution 2litre Flowfusor bottles | 1 bottle Ⓢ

| Catheter maintenance solutions

● **CATHETER MAINTENANCE SOLUTIONS**
Curion CuriFlush Solutio G citric acid 3.23% catheter maintenance solution (Mediq Healthcare UK Ltd)
50 ml · NHS indicative price = £3.49 · Drug Tariff (Part IXa)100 ml · NHS indicative price = £3.49 · Drug Tariff (Part IXa)

Curion CuriFlush Solutio R citric acid 6% catheter maintenance solution (Mediq Healthcare UK Ltd)
50 ml · NHS indicative price = £3.49 · Drug Tariff (Part IXa)100 ml · NHS indicative price = £3.49 · Drug Tariff (Part IXa)

OptiFlo G citric acid 3.23% catheter maintenance solution (Bard Ltd)
50 ml · NHS indicative price = £3.99 · Drug Tariff (Part IXa)100 ml · NHS indicative price = £3.99 · Drug Tariff (Part IXa)

OptiFlo R citric acid 6% catheter maintenance solution (Bard Ltd)
50 ml · NHS indicative price = £3.99 · Drug Tariff (Part IXa)100 ml · NHS indicative price = £3.99 · Drug Tariff (Part IXa)

Uro-Tainer PHMB polihexanide 0.02% catheter maintenance solution (B.Braun Medical Ltd)
100 ml · NHS indicative price = £3.86 · Drug Tariff (Part IXa)

Uro-Tainer Twin Solutio R citric acid 6% catheter maintenance solution (B.Braun Medical Ltd)
60 ml · NHS indicative price = £5.45 · Drug Tariff (Part IXa)

Uro-Tainer Twin Suby G citric acid 3.23% catheter maintenance solution (B.Braun Medical Ltd)
60 ml · NHS indicative price = £5.45 · Drug Tariff (Part IXa)

UroFlush G citric acid 3.23% catheter maintenance solution (TriOn Pharma Ltd)
50 ml · NHS indicative price = £3.15 · Drug Tariff (Part IXa)100 ml · NHS indicative price = £3.15 · Drug Tariff (Part IXa)

UroFlush R citric acid 6% catheter maintenance solution (TriOn Pharma Ltd)
100 ml · NHS indicative price = £3.15 · Drug Tariff (Part IXa)

Curion CuriFlush sodium chloride 0.9% catheter maintenance solution (Mediq Healthcare UK Ltd) **Sodium chloride 9 mg per 1 ml**
50 ml · NHS indicative price = £3.49 · Drug Tariff (Part IXa)100 ml · NHS indicative price = £3.49 · Drug Tariff (Part IXa)

OptiFlo S saline 0.9% catheter maintenance solution (Bard Ltd)
Sodium chloride 9 mg per 1 ml 50 ml · NHS indicative price = £3.76 · Drug Tariff (Part IXa)100 ml · NHS indicative price = £3.76 · Drug Tariff (Part IXa)

Uro-Tainer M sodium chloride 0.9% catheter maintenance solution (B.Braun Medical Ltd) **Sodium chloride 9 mg per 1 ml** 50 ml · No NHS indicative price available · Drug Tariff (Part IXa)100 ml · No NHS indicative price available · Drug Tariff (Part IXa)

Uro-Tainer sodium chloride 0.9% catheter maintenance solution (B.Braun Medical Ltd) **Sodium chloride 9 mg per 1 ml** 50 ml · NHS indicative price = £3.82 · Drug Tariff (Part IXa)100 ml · NHS indicative price = £3.82 · Drug Tariff (Part IXa)

UroFlush Saline 0.9% catheter maintenance solution (TriOn Pharma Ltd) **Sodium chloride 9 mg per 1 ml** 50 ml · NHS indicative price = £3.15 · Drug Tariff (Part IXa)100 ml · NHS indicative price = £3.15 · Drug Tariff (Part IXa)

3 Contraception

Contraceptives, hormonal

21-Feb-2025

Overview

Hormonal contraception includes combined hormonal contraception (containing an oestrogen and a progestogen) and progestogen-only contraception.

[EvGr] When prescribing contraception, information should be given on all available methods taking into consideration medical eligibility. This should include contraceptive effectiveness (including factors that alter efficacy), non-contraceptive benefits, health risks, and side-effects to allow an informed decision to be made on the most suitable choice. [A]

In adolescents, hormonal contraception is used after menarche. When prescribing contraception for females aged under 16 years, it is considered good practice for health professionals to follow the criteria commonly known as the Fraser Guidelines, available at: www.fsrh.org/standards-and-guidance/documents/cec-ceu-guidance-young-people-mar-2010/.

For information on contraceptive use in specific populations such as young people, females aged over 40 years, overweight or obese individuals, individuals with eating disorders, those with cardiac disease or inflammatory bowel disease, and after pregnancy, see FSRH guidance available at: www.fsrh.org/standards-and-guidance/fsrh-guidelines-and-statements/contraception-for-specific-populations/.

For the UK Medical Eligibility Criteria for Contraceptive Use, which includes information on risk categorisation for patients with pre-existing medical conditions, see FSRH guidance available at: www.fsrh.org/standards-and-guidance/uk-medical-eligibility-criteria-for-contraceptive-use-ukmec/.

Contraception in patients taking medication with teratogenic potential: FSRH (February 2018) and MHRA (March 2019) guidance

Females of childbearing potential should be advised to use highly effective contraception if they or their male partners are taking known teratogenic drugs or drugs with potential teratogenic effects. Highly effective contraception should be used both during treatment and for the recommended duration after discontinuation to avoid unintended pregnancy. Pregnancy testing should be performed before treatment initiation to exclude pregnancy and repeat testing may be required.

Methods of contraception considered to be 'highly effective' include male and female sterilisation, and the long-acting reversible contraceptives (LARC)—copper intra-uterine device (Cu-IUD), levonorgestrel intra-uterine device (LNG-IUD) and progestogen-only implant (IMP). Females using the IMP must not take any interacting drugs that could reduce contraceptive effectiveness; for further information see Contraceptives, interactions p. 917.

For further guidance, see the FSRH CEU statement (www.fsrh.org/standards-and-guidance/documents/fsrh-ceu-statement-contraception-for-women-using-known/), MHRA drug safety update (www.gov.uk/drug-safety-update/medicines-with-teratogenic-potential-what-is-effective-contraception-and-how-often-is-pregnancy-testing-needed), and the UK teratogenic information service (www.uktis.org).

Combined hormonal contraceptives

Combined hormonal contraceptives (CHC) are available as tablets (COC), transdermal patches (CTP), and vaginal rings (CVR). They are highly user-dependant methods where the failure rate if used perfectly (i.e. correctly and consistently) is less than 1%. Certain factors such as the person's weight, malabsorption (COC only), and drug interactions may contribute to contraceptive failure. Prescriptions of up to 12 months' supply for CHC initiation or continuation may be appropriate to avoid unwanted discontinuation and increased risk of pregnancy.

For information on advice to give to patients on the management of incorrect CHC use, see FSRH clinical guidance: **Incorrect use of Combined Hormonal Contraception** (see *Useful resources*).

[EvGr] It is recommended that combined hormonal contraceptives are not continued beyond 50 years of age as safer alternatives exist. [A]

CHC use may be associated with some health benefits such as:

- Reduced risk of ovarian, endometrial and colorectal cancer;
- Predictable bleeding patterns;
- Reduced dysmenorrhoea and menorrhagia;
- Management of symptoms of polycystic ovary syndrome (PCOS), endometriosis and premenstrual syndrome;
- Improvement of acne;
- Reduced menopausal symptoms;
- Maintaining bone mineral density in peri-menopausal females under the age of 50 years.

However, the use of CHC is also associated with health risks. For information on these risks, and further information on the benefits, see FSRH clinical guideline: **Combined Hormonal Contraception** (see *Useful resources*).

[EvGr] As CHC use is associated with a reduction in ovarian cancer risk, NICE recommends that following a discussion on the benefits and risks, a COC [unlicensed use] can be considered as preventive treatment for at-risk females (those with genetic or familial risk factors), where use for reduction of ovarian cancer risk outweighs the increased risk of developing breast cancer, and after taking into account the timing of any risk-reducing surgery. [A] For further information, see NICE guideline: **Ovarian cancer: identifying and managing familial and genetic risk**, available at: www.nice.org.uk/guidance/ng241.

Preparation choice

COCs containing a fixed amount of an oestrogen and a progestogen in each active tablet are termed 'monophasic'; those with varying amounts of the two hormones are termed 'multiphasic'.

COCs usually contain ethinylestradiol as the oestrogen component; mestranol, estetrol and estradiol are also used. The ethinylestradiol content of COCs range from 20–40 micrograms. [EvGr] A monophasic preparation containing 30 micrograms or less of ethinylestradiol in combination with levonorgestrel or norethisterone (to minimise cardiovascular risk), is generally used as the first line option. However, choice should be made taking into account the patients medical history, personal preference, previous contraceptive experience, and any age related considerations.

Due to potential reduced efficacy, non-oral CHC should be considered if there are concerns over absorption. In females who weigh 90 kg or more, consider non-topical options or use additional precautions with CTP. [A]

Combined Oral Contraceptives Monophasic 21-day preparations

Oestrogen content	Progestogen content	Brand
Ethinylestradiol 20 micrograms	Desogestrel 150 micrograms	Bimizza®
Ethinylestradiol 20 micrograms	Desogestrel 150 micrograms	Gedarel® 20/150
Ethinylestradiol 20 micrograms	Desogestrel 150 micrograms	Mercilon®
Ethinylestradiol 20 micrograms	Gestodene 75 micrograms	Akizza® 20/75
Ethinylestradiol 20 micrograms	Gestodene 75 micrograms	Femodette®
Ethinylestradiol 20 micrograms	Gestodene 75 micrograms	Millinette® 20/75
Ethinylestradiol 20 micrograms	Gestodene 75 micrograms	Sunya® 20/75
Ethinylestradiol 30 micrograms	Desogestrel 150 micrograms	Cimizt®
Ethinylestradiol 30 micrograms	Desogestrel 150 micrograms	Gedarel® 30/150
Ethinylestradiol 30 micrograms	Desogestrel 150 micrograms	Marvelon®
Ethinylestradiol 30 micrograms	Drospirenone 3 mg	Dretine®
Ethinylestradiol 30 micrograms	Drospirenone 3 mg	Lucette®
Ethinylestradiol 30 micrograms	Drospirenone 3 mg	Yacella®
Ethinylestradiol 30 micrograms	Drospirenone 3 mg	Yasmin®
Ethinylestradiol 30 micrograms	Drospirenone 3 mg	Yiznell®
Ethinylestradiol 30 micrograms	Gestodene 75 micrograms	Akizza® 30/75
Ethinylestradiol 30 micrograms	Gestodene 75 micrograms	Femodene®
Ethinylestradiol 30 micrograms	Gestodene 75 micrograms	Katya® 30/75
Ethinylestradiol 30 micrograms	Gestodene 75 micrograms	Millinette® 30/75
Ethinylestradiol 30 micrograms	Levonorgestrel 150 micrograms	Ambelina®
Ethinylestradiol 30 micrograms	Levonorgestrel 150 micrograms	Elevin®
Ethinylestradiol 30 micrograms	Levonorgestrel 150 micrograms	Levest®
Ethinylestradiol 30 micrograms	Levonorgestrel 150 micrograms	Maexeni®
Ethinylestradiol 30 micrograms	Levonorgestrel 150 micrograms	Microgynon® 30
Ethinylestradiol 30 micrograms	Levonorgestrel 150 micrograms	Ovranette®
Ethinylestradiol 30 micrograms	Levonorgestrel 150 micrograms	Rigevidon®
Ethinylestradiol 35 micrograms	Norethisterone 500 micrograms	Brevinor®
Ethinylestradiol 35 micrograms	Norethisterone 1 mg	Norimin®
Ethinylestradiol 35 micrograms	Norgestimate 250 micrograms	Cilique®
Ethinylestradiol 35 micrograms	Norgestimate 250 micrograms	Lizinna®
Mestranol 50 micrograms	Norethisterone 1 mg	Norinyl-1®

Combined Oral Contraceptives Monophasic 28-day preparations

Oestrogen content	Progestogen content	Brand
Estetrol 14.2 mg	Drospirenone 3 mg	Drovelis®
Estradiol (as hemihydrate) 1.5 mg	Nomegestrol acetate 2.5 mg	Zoely®
Ethinylestradiol 20 micrograms	Drospirenone 3 mg	Eloine®
Ethinylestradiol 30 micrograms	Gestodene 75 micrograms	Femodene® ED
Ethinylestradiol 30 micrograms	Levonorgestrel 150 micrograms	Microgynon® 30 ED

Combined Oral Contraceptives Multiphasic 21-day preparations

Oestrogen content	Progestogen content	Brand
Ethinylestradiol 30 micrograms	Levonorgestrel 50 micrograms	
Ethinylestradiol 40 micrograms	Levonorgestrel 75 micrograms	Logynon®
Ethinylestradiol 30 micrograms	Levonorgestrel 125 micrograms	
Ethinylestradiol 30 micrograms	Levonorgestrel 50 micrograms	
Ethinylestradiol 40 micrograms	Levonorgestrel 75 micrograms	TriRegol®
Ethinylestradiol 30 micrograms	Levonorgestrel 125 micrograms	
Ethinylestradiol 35 micrograms	Norethisterone 500 micrograms	
Ethinylestradiol 35 micrograms	Norethisterone 1 mg	Synphase®
Ethinylestradiol 35 micrograms	Norethisterone 500 micrograms	

Combined Oral Contraceptives Multiphasic 28-day preparations

Oestrogen content	Progestogen content	Brand
Estradiol valerate 3 mg		
Estradiol valerate 2 mg	Dienogest 2 mg	
Estradiol valerate 2 mg	Dienogest 3 mg	Qlaira®
Estradiol valerate 1 mg		
Ethinylestradiol 30 micrograms	Levonorgestrel 50 micrograms	
Ethinylestradiol 40 micrograms	Levonorgestrel 75 micrograms	Logynon® ED
Ethinylestradiol 30 micrograms	Levonorgestrel 125 micrograms	

Regimen choice

[EvGr] Information should be given to females on both the traditional 21 day CHC regimen with a monthly withdrawal bleed during the 7 day hormone free interval (HFI), and 'tailored' CHC regimens [unlicensed use]. Tailored CHC regimens can only be used with monophasic CHC containing ethinylestradiol [unlicensed use]; they offer the choice of either a shortened, or less frequent, or no hormone free interval based on the person's preference.

The following tailored regimens may be used [unlicensed use]:

- Shortened HFI: 21 days of continuous use followed by a 4 day HFI;
- Extended use (tricycling): 9 weeks of continuous use followed by a 4 or 7 day HFI;
- Flexible extended use: continuous use for 21 days or more followed by a 4 day HFI when breakthrough bleeding occurs;
- Continuous use: continuous CHC use with no HFI. [A]

Withdrawal bleeds do not represent physiological menstruation and there is no difference in efficacy or safety of using the traditional 21 day regimen, which mimics the natural menstrual cycle, over using extended or continuous regimens. Use of the traditional regimen may be associated with disadvantages such as heavy or painful withdrawal bleeds, headaches, mood changes, and increased risk of incorrect use with subsequent unplanned pregnancy. [EvGr] Withdrawal bleeds during traditional CHC use has been reported in females who are pregnant and should therefore not be relied on as reassurance of a person's pregnancy status. [A]

Follow up

[EvGr] A review of continued medical eligibility, satisfaction and adherence, drug interactions, and consideration of alternative contraception should be undertaken annually. Body mass index and blood pressure should also be checked annually. [A]

Surgery

[EvGr] CHC use should be discontinued at least 4 weeks prior to major elective surgery, any surgery to the legs or pelvis, or surgery that involves prolonged immobilisation of a lower limb. An alternative method of contraception should be used to prevent unintentional pregnancy, and CHC may be recommenced 2 weeks after full remobilisation. When discontinuation is not possible, e.g. after trauma or if a patient admitted for an elective procedure is still on CHC, thromboprophylaxis should be considered. [M]

When to seek further advice

[EvGr] All females should be advised to seek advice from a healthcare professional if they experience any troublesome side-effects, have a significant health event, start any new medication, would like to discontinue CHC, or to discuss alternative methods at any time. For further information, see FSRH guidance: **Combined Hormonal Contraception** (see *Useful resources*). [A]

Progestogen-only contraceptives

Progestogen-only contraceptive options are available in oral, injectable, subdermal, and intra-uterine form. Some forms are highly user-dependent (e.g. oral tablet), whilst others rely on timely re-administration (e.g. depot injection); the failure rate if used perfectly (i.e. correctly and consistently) is less than 1%. The primary mechanism of action differs between contraceptive options, however progestogenic effects leading to contraceptive action include changes to the cervical mucus affecting sperm penetration, endometrial changes affecting implantation, effects on tubal motility, and ovulation suppression.

Oral progestogen-only contraceptives

Oral progestogen-only preparations contain either levonorgestrel p. 932, norethisterone p. 878, desogestrel p. 930, or drospirenone p. 931. [EvGr] Desogestrel and drospirenone suppress ovulation more consistently and may improve symptoms of dysmenorrhoea, however there is insufficient evidence to compare the contraceptive effectiveness of oral progestogen-only contraceptives with each other. Incorrect use, vomiting or severe diarrhoea, and drug interactions may contribute to contraceptive failure. Prescriptions of up to 12 months' supply at initial and subsequent visits may be appropriate. Follow-up in the form of an annual review is recommended, with the advice to return at any time if any problems arise. [A]

For further information on progestogen-only pills, see FSRH guidance: **Progestogen-only Pills** (see *Useful resources*).

Parenteral progestogen-only contraceptives

Parenteral long-acting progestogens include the injections medroxyprogesterone acetate p. 936 and norethisterone enantate, and the implant etonogestrel p. 935. These are long-acting reversible contraceptive options that work primarily by suppressing ovulation along with other progestogenic effects. [EvGr] As they often lead to amenorrhoea or reduced bleeding, they may benefit those with menstrual problems (such as heavy bleeding or dysmenorrhoea). [A]

Injections

The failure rate for injectable progestogen-only contraception during the first year is approximately only 0.2% with perfect use (used consistently and correctly), the failure rate with typical use (includes incorrect/inconsistent use) is approximately 6%. The typical failure rates are higher compared to other long-acting methods and may be due to the relative frequency of repeat injections.

[EvGr] Depot medroxyprogesterone acetate is administered every 13 weeks. Its use is associated with a small loss of bone mineral density, which largely recovers after discontinuation. However, due to the concerns and uncertainties around bone-loss the following is advised regarding its use:

- Females aged under 18 years may use depot medroxyprogesterone acetate after all options have been discussed and are considered unsuitable or unacceptable.
- In all females, although there is no definitive upper duration limit, use should be reviewed every 2 years and continuation benefits and risks discussed.
- Females aged 50 years and over should switch to another contraceptive method; if they do not wish to discontinue

use, continuation may be considered following a discussion of the benefits and risks.
- In females with significant risk factors for osteoporosis, other methods of contraception should be considered.

Patients should be informed that there can be a delayed return of fertility of up to 1 year after discontinuation of depot medroxyprogesterone acetate. However, patients who discontinue use and do not wish to conceive, should be advised to start an alternative contraceptive method before or at the time of their next scheduled injection. ⟨A⟩

Norethisterone enantate is less commonly used in the UK. [EvGr] It is used for short-term contraception (duration of 8 weeks) for females whose partners undergo a vasectomy until the vasectomy is effective, and after rubella immunisation. ⟨A⟩

For further information on progestogen-only injections including dosing interval of repeat injections and management of side-effects, see FSRH guidance: **Progestogen-only Injectable Contraception** (see *Useful resources*).

Implant
[EvGr] The etonogestrel implant p. 935 is inserted subdermally and provides highly effective contraception for up to 3 years. The contraceptive failure rate for both perfect and typical use is approximately 0.05% in the first year of use. Routine follow-up during implant use, removal or replacement is not generally required, however patients should be advised to see their healthcare professional if the implant cannot be felt or problematic bleeding occurs. ⟨A⟩

For further information on progestogen-only implant, see FSRH guidance: **Progestogen-only Implant** (see *Useful resources*).

Intra-uterine progestogen-only devices
Intra-uterine devices (IUDs) containing levonorgestrel p. 932 are long-acting reversible contraceptive options that have a duration of use that ranges from 3–10 years depending on the device used, and the age of the female at insertion. A foreign-body effect may be a contributing factor to the contraceptive action, in addition to progestogenic effects. Ovulation is not suppressed in the majority of females (over 75%) who use an IUD. An IUD releasing 20mcg/24hour of levonorgestrel may also have health benefits such as improving pain associated with dysmenorrhoea, endometriosis or adenomyosis.

FSRH CEU have issued recommendations on the management of pain and anxiety associated with insertion of intra-uterine contraception, available at: www.fsrh.org/Public/Documents/fsrh-statement-pain-associated-with-insertion-of-intrauterine.aspx.

[EvGr] Patients should be advised to seek medical advice if they develop symptoms of pelvic infection, pain, abnormal bleeding, non-palpable threads or they can feel the stem of the IUD. ⟨A⟩

For further information on progestogen-only IUDs, see FSRH guidance: **Intra-uterine Contraception** (see *Useful resources*).

Surgery
In accordance with the UK Medical Eligibility Criteria for Contraceptive Use, progestogen-only pills, injections, implants, and intra-uterine devices are suitable for use as contraceptives in females undergoing surgery. For further information, see FSRH guidance: **UK Medical Eligibility Criteria for Contraceptive Use** (available at: www.fsrh.org/standards-and-guidance/uk-medical-eligibility-criteria-for-contraceptive-use-ukmec/).

Useful Resources

Combined Hormonal Contraception. The Faculty of Sexual & Reproductive Healthcare. Clinical guideline. January 2019, updated October 2023.

www.fsrh.org/standards-and-guidance/documents/combined-hormonal-contraception/

Recommended actions after incorrect use of combined hormonal contraception (e.g. late or missed pills, ring and patch). The Faculty of Sexual & Reproductive Healthcare Clinical Effectiveness Unit. Guidance. March 2020.
www.fsrh.org/Public/Documents/fsrh-ceu-guidance-recommended-actions-after-incorrect-use.aspx

Progestogen-only Pills. The Faculty of Sexual & Reproductive Healthcare. Clinical guidance. August 2022, updated July 2023.
www.fsrh.org/Public/Documents/ceu-guideline-progestogen-only-pills.aspx

Progestogen-only Injectable Contraception. The Faculty of Sexual & Reproductive Healthcare. Clinical guidance. December 2014, updated July 2023.
www.fsrh.org/standards-and-guidance/documents/cec-ceu-guidance-injectables-dec-2014/

Progestogen-only Implant. The Faculty of Sexual & Reproductive Healthcare. Clinical guidance. February 2021, updated July 2023.
www.fsrh.org/standards-and-guidance/documents/cec-ceu-guidance-implants-feb-2014/

Intra-uterine Contraception. The Faculty of Sexual & Reproductive Healthcare. Clinical guidance. March 2023, updated July 2023.
www.fsrh.org/standards-and-guidance/documents/ceuguidanceintrauterinecontraception/

Contraceptives, non-hormonal

01-Dec-2024

Contraception in patients taking medication with teratogenic potential: FSRH (February 2018) and MHRA (March 2019) guidance

Females of childbearing potential should be advised to use highly effective contraception if they or their male partners are taking known teratogenic drugs or drugs with potential teratogenic effects. Highly effective contraception should be used both during treatment and for the recommended duration after discontinuation to avoid unintended pregnancy. Pregnancy testing should be performed before treatment initiation to exclude pregnancy and repeat testing may be required.

Methods of contraception considered to be 'highly effective' include male and female sterilisation, and the long-acting reversible contraceptives (LARC)—copper intra-uterine device (Cu-IUD), levonorgestrel intra-uterine device (LNG-IUD) and progestogen-only implant (IMP). Females using the IMP must not take any interacting drugs that could reduce contraceptive effectiveness; for further information, see Contraceptives, interactions p. 917.

For further guidance, see the FSRH Clinical Effectiveness Unit (CEU) statement (www.fsrh.org/standards-and-guidance/documents/fsrh-ceu-statement-contraception-for-women-using-known/), MHRA drug safety update (www.gov.uk/drug-safety-update/medicines-with-teratogenic-potential-what-is-effective-contraception-and-how-often-is-pregnancy-testing-needed), and the UK teratogenic information service (www.uktis.org).

Barrier methods

Barrier methods include condoms (male and female), diaphragms and cervical caps. Male condoms are less effective than some other contraception methods but are effective when used consistently and correctly, and provide significant protection against some sexually transmitted infections (STIs). Female condoms are also available; they are pre-lubricated with a non-spermicidal lubricant.

There is no evidence that condoms lubricated with spermicide provide additional protection against pregnancy or STIs. [EvGr] Diaphragms and caps must be used in conjunction with a **spermicide** and should not be removed until at least 6 hours after the last episode of intercourse. [A]

Spermicidal contraceptives

Spermicidal contraceptives are useful additional safeguards but do **not** give adequate protection if used alone. They have two components: a spermicide and a vehicle for its delivery (e.g. vaginal gel). [EvGr] They are suitable for use with barrier methods, such as diaphragms or caps; however, spermicidal contraceptives are not recommended for use with condoms, as there is no evidence of any additional protection compared with non-spermicidal lubricants.

Spermicidal contraceptives are not suitable for use in those with or at high risk of sexually transmitted infections (including HIV); [A] high frequency use of the spermicide nonoxinol '9' p. 938 has been associated with genital lesions, which may increase the risk of acquiring these infections.

Contraceptive devices

Intra-uterine devices

[EvGr] The intra-uterine device (IUD) is a suitable contraceptive for women of all ages irrespective of parity; [A] however they may be unsuitable in women with certain conditions such as those with pelvic inflammatory disease or unexplained vaginal bleeding. The UK Medical Eligibility Criteria for Contraceptive Use (published by FSRH) provides guidance on safe use of contraceptive methods including restrictions for intra-uterine devices; full guidance is available at: www.fsrh.org/standards-and-guidance/uk-medical-eligibility-criteria-for-contraceptive-use-ukmec/.

[EvGr] Copper intra-uterine devices (Cu-IUDs) are effective immediately after insertion and can be used for contraception for 5 or 10 years depending on the device. [A] Framed Cu-IUDs in the UK have a copper surface area of $300\ mm^2$ or more, with either banded copper arms, a copper stem only, or copper arms with a silver-containing stem. A frameless, copper-bearing intra-uterine device (*GyneFix*®) is also available.

[EvGr] Fertility declines with age and therefore a Cu-IUD with a copper surface area of $300\ mm^2$ or more, which is fitted in a woman aged 40 years and over, can remain in the uterus and be used for contraception until menopause. [A] For further information on Cu-IUDs, see FSRH guidance: **Intra-uterine Contraception** (see *Useful resources*).

[EvGr] Cu-IUDs are also highly effective emergency contraception that can be retained to provide ongoing contraception. [A] For further information, see Emergency contraception below.

For guidance on the management of pain and anxiety associated with insertion of intra-uterine contraception, see FSRH Clinical Effectiveness Unit (CEU) statement: **Pain associated with insertion of intra-uterine contraception**, available at: www.fsrh.org/Public/Documents/fsrh-statement-pain-associated-with-insertion-of-intrauterine.aspx.

Caution with oil-based lubricants

Products such as petroleum jelly (*Vaseline*®), baby oil and oil-based vaginal and rectal preparations are likely to damage condoms, contraceptive diaphragms and caps made from latex rubber, and may render them less effective as a barrier method of contraception and as a protection from sexually transmitted infections (including HIV).

Useful resources

Barrier Methods for Contraception and STI Prevention. The Faculty of Sexual & Reproductive Healthcare. Clinical guidance. August 2012, updated October 2015.

www.fsrh.org/standards-and-guidance/documents/ceuguidancebarriermethodscontraceptionsdi/

Intra-uterine Contraception. The Faculty of Sexual & Reproductive Healthcare. Clinical guidance. March 2023, updated July 2023.

www.fsrh.org/standards-and-guidance/fsrh-guidelines-and-statements/method-specific/intrauterine-contraception/

Emergency contraception

01-Dec-2024

Overview

[EvGr] Emergency contraception is intended for occasional use, to reduce the risk of pregnancy after unprotected sexual intercourse (UPSI). It does not replace effective regular contraception.

Females of childbearing potential who do not wish to conceive should be offered emergency contraception after UPSI that has taken place on any day of a natural menstrual cycle. Emergency contraception should also be offered after UPSI from day 21 after childbirth (unless the criteria for lactational amenorrhoea are met), and from day 5 after abortion, miscarriage, ectopic pregnancy or uterine evacuation for gestational trophoblastic disease.

Emergency contraception should also be offered to females whose regular contraception has been compromised or has been used incorrectly. [A]

Emergency contraceptive methods

Copper intra-uterine devices

[EvGr] Insertion of a copper intra-uterine device (see intra-uterine contraceptive devices (copper) p. 928) is the most effective form of emergency contraception and should be offered (if appropriate) to all females who have had UPSI and do not wish to conceive. A copper intra-uterine contraceptive device can be inserted up to 120 hours (5 days) after the first UPSI in a natural menstrual cycle, or up to 5 days after the earliest estimated date of ovulation (i.e. within the minimum period before implantation), whichever is later. [A] For information on the use of copper intra-uterine devices as emergency contraception in women using hormonal contraception, see FSRH guideline: **Emergency Contraception** (see *Useful resources*).

[EvGr] Antibacterial cover may be considered for copper intra-uterine contraceptive device insertion if there is a significant risk of sexually transmitted infection that could be associated with ascending pelvic infection.

A copper intra-uterine device is not known to be affected by body mass index (BMI), body-weight, or by other drugs. [A]

For further guidance on the use of copper intra-uterine devices as emergency contraception, see FSRH guideline: **Emergency Contraception** (see *Useful resources*).

For guidance on the management of pain and anxiety associated with insertion of intra-uterine contraception, see FSRH Clinical Effectiveness Unit (CEU) statement: **Pain associated with insertion of intra-uterine contraception**, available at: www.fsrh.org/Public/Documents/fsrh-statement-pain-associated-with-insertion-of-intrauterine.aspx.

Due to the current shortage of banded copper intra-uterine devices, which is thought to be due to a shortfall in global copper supply, the FSRH CEU have issued guidance to support clinical practice during this time, available at: www.fsrh.org/standards-and-guidance/documents/fsrh-statement-copper-intrauterine-device-shortage/.

Hormonal methods

[EvGr] Oral emergency hormonal contraceptives (includes levonorgestrel p. 932 and ulipristal acetate p. 929) should be offered as soon as possible if a copper intra-uterine device is not appropriate or is not acceptable to the patient and there has been UPSI within the last 5 days; either drug should be taken as soon as possible to increase efficacy. Oral emergency contraception administered after ovulation is ineffective.

Levonorgestrel is effective if taken within 72 hours (3 days) of UPSI and may also be used between 72 and 96 hours after UPSI [unlicensed use], but efficacy decreases with time. Ulipristal acetate is effective if taken within 120 hours (5 days) of UPSI. Ulipristal acetate has been demonstrated to be more effective than levonorgestrel for emergency contraception.

There is the possibility that a higher body-weight or BMI could reduce the effectiveness of oral emergency contraception, particularly levonorgestrel. If the patient's BMI is greater than 26 kg/m^2 or their body-weight is greater than 70 kg, it is recommended that either ulipristal acetate or a double dose of levonorgestrel [unlicensed indication] is given (see *Emergency contraception* under levonorgestrel). It is unknown which is more effective.

Ulipristal acetate should be considered as the first-line oral emergency contraceptive for females who have had UPSI within the last 96–120 hours (even if they have also had additional instances of UPSI within the last 96 hours). It should also be considered first line for females who have had UPSI within the last 5 days if it is likely to have taken place during the 5 days before the estimated day of ovulation.

Levonorgestrel may be considered for oral emergency contraception in females on a regular combined hormonal contraceptive who have missed contraception within the first week of restarting their contraceptive. ⟨A⟩ See FSRH guideline: **Emergency Contraception** (see *Useful resources*) for further information.

[EvGr] Ulipristal acetate and levonorgestrel can be used as oral emergency contraception more than once in the same cycle. ⟨A⟩ Note that the manufacturer of levonorgestrel advises that there may be an increased risk of side-effects (such as menstrual irregularities) with repeated administration of levonorgestrel as emergency contraception more than once in the same cycle.

For further information on the use of oral hormonal methods as emergency contraception, see FSRH guideline: **Emergency Contraception** (see *Useful resources*).

Emergency hormonal contraception interactions
See Contraceptives, interactions below.

Starting hormonal contraception after emergency hormonal contraception

The copper intra-uterine device immediately provides effective ongoing contraception, whereas oral emergency hormonal contraception methods do **not**.

[EvGr] After taking levonorgestrel, females should start suitable hormonal contraception immediately. They must use condoms reliably or abstain from intercourse until contraception becomes effective.

Females should wait 5 days after taking ulipristal acetate before starting suitable hormonal contraception; they must use condoms reliably or abstain from intercourse during the 5 day waiting period and also until their contraceptive method is effective. However, hormonal contraception can be started immediately in females who are on a regular combined hormonal contraceptive who have missed contraception within the first week of restarting after a scheduled hormone-free interval, and have taken ulipristal acetate as emergency contraception; they must use condoms reliably or abstain from intercourse for 7 days until contraception becomes effective. ⟨A⟩ For further information on delaying versus immediately restarting combined hormonal contraception after taking ulipristal acetate, see FSRH CEU statement: **Response to recent publication** (available at: www.fsrh.org/standards-and-guidance/documents/fsrh-ceu-statement-response-to-recent-publication-regarding/).

Useful Resources

Emergency Contraception. The Faculty of Sexual and Reproductive Healthcare. FSRH guideline. March 2017, updated July 2023.
www.fsrh.org/Public/Documents/ceu-clinical-guidance-emergency-contraception-march-2017.aspx

Contraceptives, interactions   01-Dec-2024

Overview

Contraceptive providers should take a drug history (including any herbal products) and check for drug interactions prior to provision of hormonal contraception. The effectiveness of *combined* oral contraceptives, *progestogen-only* oral contraceptives, contraceptive patches, vaginal rings, subdermal implants, and emergency hormonal contraception can be considerably reduced by interaction with drugs that induce hepatic enzyme activity (e.g. carbamazepine p. 355, eslicarbazepine acetate p. 359, efavirenz p. 741, nevirapine p. 742, oxcarbazepine p. 370, phenytoin p. 372, phenobarbital p. 388, primidone p. 389, rifabutin p. 673, rifampicin p. 674, ritonavir p. 756, St John's wort, and topiramate p. 384), requiring additional or alternative methods of contraception to be used (see below). A condom together with a long-acting method (such as an injectable contraceptive) may be more suitable for patients with HIV infection or at risk of HIV infection; advice on the possibility of interaction with antiretroviral drugs should be sought from HIV specialists. Note that the MHRA recommends that concurrent use of St John's wort with any form of hormonal contraception should be avoided; for further guidance, see MHRA drug safety update: **St John's wort: interaction with hormonal contraceptives, including implants** (available at: www.gov.uk/drug-safety-update/st-john-s-wort-interaction-with-hormonal-contraceptives-including-implants).

For further information on other drug interactions with hormonal contraceptives, see the *Interactions* section of the relevant drug monograph.

Hormonal contraception with concurrent use of enzyme-inducing and teratogenic drugs

In females taking a teratogenic or potentially teratogenic drug that is an enzyme inducer, or if an enzyme-inducing drug is also being taken with a teratogen or potential teratogen, the preferred method of contraception is a copper intra-uterine device (IUD) or a progestogen-only IUD (levonorgestrel p. 932). If a progestogen-only injectable contraceptive (such as medroxyprogesterone acetate p. 936) is used, this should be in combination with reliable use of condoms. Use of combined hormonal contraception, progestogen-only pills, and the etonogestrel implant is not recommended; for further guidance, see FSRH Clinical Effectiveness Unit (CEU) statement (www.fsrh.org/standards-and-guidance/documents/fsrh-ceu-statement-contraception-for-women-using-known/), MHRA drug safety update (www.gov.uk/drug-safety-update/medicines-with-teratogenic-potential-what-is-effective-contraception-and-how-often-is-pregnancy-testing-needed), and the UK teratogenic information service (www.uktis.org).

Combined hormonal contraceptive interactions

Interactions with enzyme-inducing drugs
Females using combined hormonal contraceptive patches, vaginal rings, or oral tablets who require enzyme-inducing drugs should always be advised to change to a reliable contraceptive method that is unaffected by enzyme-inducers, such as a copper IUD, a progestogen-only IUD (levonorgestrel), or a progestogen-only injectable contraceptive (such as medroxyprogesterone acetate). This

should be continued for the duration of treatment and for 4 weeks after stopping.

If a change in contraceptive method is undesirable or inappropriate, the following options should be discussed:

Short-term use (2 months or less) of an enzyme-inducing drug (except rifampicin or rifabutin)
Continuing the combined hormonal contraceptive method may be considered if used in combination with consistent and careful use of condoms for the duration of treatment and for 4 weeks after stopping the enzyme-inducing drug.

Continued use (over 2 months) of an enzyme-inducing drug (except rifampicin or rifabutin)
In exceptional circumstances, the use of a monophasic combined oral contraceptive containing ethinylestradiol p. 874 at a higher daily dose [unlicensed use] may be considered and used either continuously or 'tricycled' (i.e. taking three packets of monophasic tablets without a break followed by a shortened tablet-free interval of 4 days [unlicensed use]); continue for the duration of treatment with the interacting drug and for 4 weeks after stopping. However, contraceptive effectiveness is not guaranteed. For further guidance, see FSRH guidance: **Drug Interactions with Hormonal Contraception** (see *Useful resources*).

If breakthrough bleeding occurs (and all other causes are ruled out) additional precautions should be used, or contraception should be changed to a method unaffected by the interacting drugs.

Use of contraceptive patches and vaginal rings (including concurrent use of two patches or two vaginal rings) is not recommended for females taking enzyme-inducing drugs over a long period.

Females taking rifampicin or rifabutin
An alternative method of contraception that is unaffected by enzyme-inducers is **always** recommended because they are such potent enzyme-inducing drugs; the alternative method of contraception should be continued for 4 weeks after stopping the enzyme-inducing drug.

Interactions with HIV-protease inhibitors
Note that despite ritonavir being an enzyme inducer, the FSRH suggests that concurrent use of HIV-protease inhibitors boosted with ritonavir are not expected to affect the efficacy of the combined hormonal contraceptives, but some caution is required if they are given with combined hormonal contraceptives because the increased risk of side-effects might impact adherence.

For HIV-protease inhibitors boosted with cobicistat, FSRH recommends caution or an alternative effective method of contraception.

Interactions with lamotrigine
It is possible that lamotrigine p. 366 could reduce the efficacy of combined hormonal contraceptives, therefore the additional reliable use of condoms is recommended. However, combined hormonal contraceptives can decrease lamotrigine concentrations, which might result in reduced efficacy (e.g. seizure control). If combined hormonal contraceptive use is unavoidable, consider increasing the lamotrigine dose and monitoring lamotrigine concentrations. A continuous combined hormonal contraceptive regimen (with no hormone-free interval) could be used to avoid cyclical changes in lamotrigine concentrations [unlicensed use].

Oral progestogen-only contraceptives interactions

Interactions with enzyme-inducing drugs
The efficacy of oral progestogen-only preparations is reduced by enzyme-inducing drugs and an alternative contraceptive method, unaffected by the interacting drug, such as a copper IUD, a progestogen-only IUD (levonorgestrel), or a progestogen-only injectable contraceptive (such as medroxyprogesterone acetate) is

recommended during treatment with an interacting drug and for at least 4 weeks afterwards.

For short-term use of an enzyme-inducing drug (less than 2 months), continuing the progestogen-only oral method may be appropriate if used in combination with consistent and careful use of condoms for the duration of treatment and for 4 weeks after stopping the enzyme-inducing drug.

Note that despite ritonavir being an enzyme inducer, the FSRH suggests that concurrent use of HIV-protease inhibitors boosted with ritonavir are not expected to affect the efficacy of the oral progestogen-only contraceptives but might increase their concentrations. They therefore state that no extra precautions are needed in those taking HIV-protease inhibitors boosted with ritonavir.

Interactions with lamotrigine
It is possible that lamotrigine could reduce the efficacy of progestogen-only oral contraceptives, therefore the additional reliable use of condoms is recommended. Desogestrel p. 930 might increase lamotrigine concentrations, but evidence for other oral progestogen-only contraceptives is lacking. Patients should be advised to be vigilant for signs of lamotrigine toxicity if starting progestogen-only contraceptives and consideration given to monitoring lamotrigine concentrations on stopping the contraceptive.

Parenteral (including *subdermal*) progestogen-only contraceptives interactions

Interactions with enzyme-inducing drugs
The effectiveness of intramuscular norethisterone injection p. 878 and intramuscular and subcutaneous medroxyprogesterone acetate injections p. 936 is not affected by enzyme-inducing drugs and they may be continued as normal during courses of these drugs. FSRH guidance on drug interactions between HIV antiretroviral therapy and contraception (see *Useful resources*) suggests that for patients with a high BMI or those taking efavirenz and rifampicin, the use of intra-uterine contraception, or additional use of condoms, or shortening the dosing interval of medroxyprogesterone acetate injection might be considered.

Effectiveness of the etonogestrel-releasing subdermal implant p. 935 may be reduced by enzyme-inducing drugs and an alternative contraceptive method, unaffected by the interacting drug, such as a copper IUD, a progestogen-only IUD (levonorgestrel p. 932), or a progestogen-only injectable contraceptive (such as medroxyprogesterone acetate), is recommended during treatment with the interacting drug and for at least 4 weeks after stopping. For a short course of an enzyme-inducing drug, if a change in contraceptive method is undesirable or inappropriate, continued contraception with the implant may be appropriate if used in combination with consistent and careful use of condoms for the duration of treatment and for 4 weeks after stopping the enzyme-inducing drug. Note that despite ritonavir being an enzyme inducer, the FSRH suggests that concurrent use of HIV-protease inhibitors boosted with ritonavir are not expected to affect the efficacy of the etonogestrel implant but might increase etonogestrel concentrations. They therefore state that no extra precautions are needed in those taking HIV-protease inhibitors boosted with ritonavir.

Interactions with lamotrigine
It is possible that lamotrigine could reduce the efficacy of the progestogen-only subdermal implant, therefore the additional reliable use of condoms is recommended. Contraceptive effectiveness of progestogen-only injectable contraceptives is not expected to be affected by lamotrigine, however progestogen-only contraceptives might increase lamotrigine concentrations. Patients should be advised to be vigilant for signs of lamotrigine toxicity if starting progestogen-only contraceptives and consideration given to

monitoring lamotrigine concentrations on stopping the contraceptive.

Emergency hormonal contraception interactions

The effectiveness of levonorgestrel and ulipristal acetate p. 929 could be reduced in females taking enzyme-inducing drugs (and for at least 4 weeks after stopping). ⬚EvGr A copper IUD can be offered instead. If the copper IUD is declined or unsuitable, the dose of levonorgestrel should be increased (See *Dose adjustments due to interactions* under levonorgestrel). ⬘Ⓐ If levonorgestrel is also unsuitable, a standard dose of ulipristal acetate may be considered. Females should be advised that the effectiveness of emergency hormonal contraception when enzyme-inducing drugs are being taken is unknown. Note that despite ritonavir being an enzyme inducer, the FSRH suggests that concurrent use of HIV-protease inhibitors boosted with ritonavir do not affect the efficacy of levonorgestrel emergency hormonal contraception but might increase levonorgestrel concentrations. They therefore do not extend the advice for enzyme inducers to HIV-protease inhibitors boosted with ritonavir.

The effectiveness of ulipristal acetate for emergency contraception in females using drugs that increase gastric pH is unknown. A copper IUD or levonorgestrel can be offered instead. If these are unsuitable, ulipristal acetate can be offered, but it is possible that effectiveness could be reduced.

⬚EvGr Hormonal contraception should not be newly initiated in a patient until 5 days after administration of ulipristal acetate as emergency hormonal contraception— the contraceptive effect of ulipristal acetate will be reduced. Consistent and careful use of condoms is recommended. Females on a regular combined oral contraceptive may in certain circumstances be able to restart regular contraception immediately after administration of ulipristal acetate as emergency hormonal contraception. ⬘Ⓐ For further information, see *Starting hormonal contraception after emergency hormonal contraception* under *Emergency contraceptive methods* in Emergency contraception p. 916.

When a progestogen (including levonorgestrel for emergency contraception) is given 7 days before, or 5 days after administration of ulipristal acetate as emergency hormonal contraception, the contraceptive effect of ulipristal acetate may be reduced.

Antibacterials that do not induce liver enzymes

Due to anecdotal reports of contraceptive failures, there had been concerns that some antibacterials that do not induce liver enzymes (e.g. ampicillin p. 637, doxycycline p. 655) reduce the efficacy of *combined* oral contraceptives by impairing the bacterial flora responsible for recycling ethinylestradiol p. 874 from the large bowel. However, there is a lack of evidence to support this interaction. It is recommended by the FSRH that no additional contraceptive precautions are required when hormonal contraceptives, including emergency hormonal contraceptives, are used with antibacterials that do not induce liver enzymes, unless diarrhoea or vomiting occur when using oral contraceptives. These recommendations should be discussed with the female, who should also be advised that guidance in patient information leaflets may differ.

Useful Resources

Drug Interactions with Hormonal Contraception. The Faculty of Sexual and Reproductive Healthcare Clinical Effectiveness Unit. Clinical guidance. May 2022.
www.fsrh.org/Public/Documents/ceu-clinical-guidance-drug-interactions-with-hormonal.aspx

Emergency Contraception. The Faculty of Sexual and Reproductive Healthcare. FSRH guideline. March 2017, updated December 2020.

www.fsrh.org/Public/Documents/ceu-clinical-guidance-emergency-contraception-march-2017.aspx

Drug Interactions Between HIV Antiretroviral Therapy (ART) and Contraception. The Faculty of Sexual and Reproductive Healthcare Clinical Effectiveness Unit. Clinical guidance. February 2023.
www.fsrh.org/Public/Documents/fsrh-ceu-guidance-drug-interactions-between-hiv-art-and-contraception.aspx

3.1 Contraception, combined

OESTROGENS COMBINED WITH PROGESTOGENS

Combined hormonal contraceptives

- **CONTRA-INDICATIONS** Acute porphyrias p. 1202 · atrial fibrillation · benign hepatocellular adenoma · Budd-Chiari syndrome · cardiomyopathy with impaired cardiac function · complicated congenital heart disease · complicated valvular heart disease · current breast cancer · hepatocellular carcinoma · hypertension (blood pressure systolic 160 mmHg or diastolic 100 mmHg or higher) · hypertensive retinopathy · ischaemic heart disease · known thrombogenic mutations (e.g. factor V Leiden, prothrombin mutation, protein S, protein C and antithrombin deficiencies) · less than 3 weeks postpartum in non-breastfeeding women with other risk factors for venous thromboembolism · less than 6 weeks postpartum in breastfeeding women · major surgery with prolonged immobilisation · migraine with aura · peripheral vascular disease with intermittent claudication · positive antiphospholipid antibodies · previous or current venous thrombosis · smoking in patients aged 35 years and over (15 or more cigarettes daily) · stroke · systemic lupus erythematosus with antiphospholipid antibodies · transient ischaemic attack

- **CAUTIONS**

  GENERAL CAUTIONS Carrier of breast cancer gene mutations e.g. BRCA1, BRCA2—seek specialist advice before use · cervical intraepithelial neoplasia or cancer · cholestasis during pregnancy · cholestasis with previous use of combined hormonal contraception—seek specialist advice before use · focal nodular hyperplasia · gallbladder disease—if medically treated or current, seek specialist advice before use · history of breast cancer—seek specialist advice before use · history of negative mood changes induced by hormonal contraceptive (a product containing an alternative progestogen may be tried) · inflammatory bowel disease · organ transplantation—when complicated, seek specialist advice before use · personal or family history of hypertriglyceridaemia (increased risk of pancreatitis) · prolactinoma—seek specialist advice before use · risk factors for cardiovascular disease · risk factors for venous thromboembolism · sickle-cell disease · undiagnosed mass or breast symptoms during combined hormonal contraception treatment—if symptoms exist prior to initiation, seek specialist advice before use · undiagnosed vaginal bleeding · viral hepatitis during combined hormonal contraception treatment—if condition exists prior to initiation, seek specialist advice before use

  SPECIFIC CAUTIONS

  ► With oral use Bariatric surgery with body mass index 30 kg/m² to 34 kg/m² (possible reduction in contraceptive efficacy)—if body mass index ≥ 35 kg/m², seek specialist advice before use · severe diarrhoea (possible reduction in

Genito-urinary system

contraceptive efficacy) · vomiting (possible reduction in contraceptive efficacy)

CAUTIONS, FURTHER INFORMATION

▶ Risk of venous thromboembolism There is an increased risk of venous thromboembolic disease in users of combined hormonal contraceptives particularly during the first year and possibly after restarting combined hormonal contraceptives following a break of four weeks or more. This risk is smaller than that associated with pregnancy and the postpartum period. In all cases the risk of venous thromboembolism increases with age and in the presence of other risk factors, such as obesity. The risk also varies depending on the type of progestogen and oestrogen dose.

▶ Risk factors for venous thromboembolism Use with **caution** if any of following factors present. If multiple risk factors are present, clinical judgement must be applied to decide whether the risk of using the combined hormonal contraceptive outweighs the benefit; referral to a specialist contraceptive provider may be required (for risk factors where treatment with combined hormonal contraceptives should be avoided, see *Contra-indications*).

- *Age* 40 years and older—if 50 years and older, seek specialist advice before use;
- 6 weeks to 6 months *postpartum in breastfeeding women*;
- 3 to 6 weeks *postpartum in non-breastfeeding women* in the absence of additional risk factors for venous thromboembolism—if 3 to 6 weeks postpartum with risk factors, or if less than 3 weeks postpartum without risk factors, seek specialist advice before use;
- *Smoking* if age under 35 years, or if 35 years and older and have stopped smoking at least 1 year ago—if 35 years and older smoking less than 15 cigarettes a day or stopped smoking less than 1 year ago, seek specialist advice before use;
- *Obesity* with body mass index 30 kg/m^2 to 34 kg/m^2—if body mass index $\geq$ 35 kg/m^2, seek specialist advice before use;
- *History of hypertension during pregnancy* in currently normotensive women;
- *Family history of venous thromboembolism* in a first-degree relative aged 45 years and older—if first-degree relative is under 45 years, seek specialist advice before use;
- *Major surgery* without prolonged immobilisation;
- *Long-term immobility* (e.g. wheelchair use, debilitating illness)—seek specialist advice before use;
- *Superficial venous thrombosis*;
- *Uncomplicated valvular heart disease*;
- *Uncomplicated congenital heart disease*;
- *Cardiomyopathy* with normal cardiac function;
- *Long QT syndrome*;
- *Systemic lupus erythematosus* with no antiphospholipid antibodies;
- *High altitudes*: women travelling above 4500 m or 14500 feet for more than 1 week should consider alternative contraceptive methods (risk of thrombosis).

Combined Hormonal Contraception and Risk of Venous Thromboembolism

Progestogen in Combined Hormonal Contraceptive	Estimated incidence per 10 000 women per year of use
Non-pregnant, not using combined hormonal contraception	2
Levonorgestrel[1]	5–7
Norgestimate[1]	5–7
Norethisterone[1]	5–7
Etonogestrel[1]	6–12
Norelgestromin[1]	6–12
Gestodene[1]	9–12
Desogestrel[1]	9–12
Drospirenone[1]	9–12
Dienogest[2]	Not known—insufficient data
Nomegestrol[2]	Not known—insufficient data

[1] Combined with ethinylestradiol [2] Combined with estradiol

▶ Risk of cardiovascular disease Combined hormonal contraceptives also slightly increase the risk of *cardiovascular disease* such as myocardial infarction and ischaemic stroke; risk appears to be greater with higher oestrogen doses.

▶ Risk factors for cardiovascular disease Use with **caution** if any one of following factors present. If multiple risk factors are present, clinical judgement must be applied to decide whether the risk of using the combined hormonal contraceptive outweighs the benefit; referral to a specialist contraceptive provider may be required (for risk factors where treatment with combined hormonal contraceptives should be avoided, see *Contra-indications*).

- *Age* 40 years and older—if 50 years and older, seek specialist advice before use;
- *Smoking* if age under 35 years, or if 35 years and older and have stopped smoking at least 1 year ago—if 35 years and older smoking less than 15 cigarettes a day, or stopped smoking less than 1 year ago, seek specialist advice before use;
- *Hypertension* if adequately controlled or if blood pressure systolic 140–159 *mmHg* or *diastolic* 90–99 *mmHg*, seek specialist advice before use;
- *History of hypertension during pregnancy* in currently normotensive women;
- *Dyslipidaemias*;
- *Non-migrainous headache (mild or severe)* during combined hormonal contraceptive use;
- *Migraine without aura* prior to initiation of combined hormonal contraceptives—if *migraine without aura* occurs during combined hormonal contraceptive use or when history of *migraine with aura* is 5 or more years ago, seek specialist advice;
- *Idiopathic intracranial hypertension*;
- *Uncomplicated valvular heart disease*;
- *Uncomplicated congenital heart disease*;
- *Cardiomyopathy* with normal cardiac function;
- *Long QT syndrome*;
- *Diabetes mellitus*—if vascular disease present, seek specialist advice before use;
- *Rheumatoid arthritis*;
- *Systemic lupus erythematosus* without antiphospholipid antibodies.

● SIDE-EFFECTS

▶ **Common or very common** Abdominal pain · breast abnormalities · diarrhoea · fluid retention · headaches · metrorrhagia · mood altered · nausea · sexual dysfunction ·

skin reactions · vaginal discharge · vomiting · weight increased
▸ **Uncommon** Alopecia
▸ **Rare or very rare** Embolism and thrombosis

SIDE-EFFECTS, FURTHER INFORMATION **Breast cancer** There is a small increase in the risk of having breast cancer diagnosed in women taking the combined oral contraceptive pill; this relative risk may be due to an earlier diagnosis. In users of combined oral contraceptive pills the cancers are more likely to be localised to the breast. The most important factor for diagnosing breast cancer appears to be the age at which the contraceptive is stopped rather than the duration of use; any increase in the rate of diagnosis diminishes gradually during the 10 years after stopping and disappears by 10 years.

Cervical cancer Use of combined oral contraceptives for 5 years or longer is associated with a small increased risk of cervical cancer; the risk diminishes after stopping and disappears by about 10 years. The possible small increase in the risk of breast cancer and cervical cancer should be weighed against the protective effect against cancers of the ovary and endometrium.

● **PREGNANCY** Not known to be harmful.

● **BREAST FEEDING** FSRH advises usually suitable for use from 6 weeks postpartum (benefits generally outweigh risks); safe for use 6 months or more postpartum.

● **HEPATIC IMPAIRMENT** In general, manufacturer advises caution; avoid in acute disease, severe chronic disease, or liver tumour.

● **DIRECTIONS FOR ADMINISTRATION**
▸ With oral use Each tablet should be taken at approximately same time each day; if delayed, contraceptive protection may be lost. FSRH advises if reasonably certain woman is not pregnant, first course can be started on any day of cycle—if starting on day 6 of cycle or later, additional precautions (barrier methods) necessary during first 7 days; for estradiol-containing preparations, additional precautions (barrier methods) necessary for 7 days (9 days for *Qlaira* ®) if started after day 1 of cycle.
Changing to combined preparation containing different progestogen
▸ With oral use FSRH advises if previous contraceptive used correctly, or pregnancy can reasonably be excluded, start the first active tablet of new brand immediately. Consult product literature for requirements of specific preparations.
Changing from progestogen-only tablet
▸ With oral use FSRH advises if previous contraceptive used correctly, or pregnancy can reasonably be excluded, start new brand immediately, additional precautions (barrier methods) necessary for first 7 days (9 days for *Qlaira* ®).
Secondary amenorrhoea (exclude pregnancy)
▸ With oral use FSRH advises start any day, additional precautions (barrier methods) necessary during first 7 days (9 days for *Qlaira* ®).
After childbirth (not breast-feeding)
▸ With oral use FSRH advises start 3 weeks after childbirth except on specialist advice in the absence of additional risk factors for thromboembolism, or 6 weeks after childbirth in the presence of additional risk factors for thromboembolism (increased risk of thrombosis if started earlier); additional precautions (barrier methods) necessary for first 7 days (9 days for *Qlaira* ®).
After abortion, miscarriage, ectopic pregnancy or gestational trophoblastic disease
▸ With oral use FSRH advises additional contraceptive precautions (barrier methods) required for 7 days if started after day 5 following treatment; for estradiol-containing preparations, additional contraceptive precautions (barrier methods) required for 7 days (9 days for *Qlaira* ®) if started after day 1 following treatment.

● **PATIENT AND CARER ADVICE**
Travel Women taking oral contraceptives or using the patch or vaginal ring are at an increased risk of deep vein thrombosis during travel involving long periods of immobility (over 3 hours). The risk may be reduced by appropriate exercise during the journey and possibly by wearing graduated compression hosiery.
Diarrhoea and vomiting
▸ With oral use Vomiting and severe diarrhoea can interfere with the absorption of combined oral contraceptives. The FSRH advises following the instructions for missed pills if vomiting occurs within 3 hours of taking a combined oral contraceptive or severe diarrhoea occurs for more than 24 hours. Use of non-oral contraception should be considered if diarrhoea or vomiting persist.
Missed doses
▸ With oral use The critical time for loss of contraceptive protection is when a pill is omitted at the *beginning* or *end* of a cycle (which lengthens the pill-free interval). If a woman forgets to take a pill, it should be taken as soon as she remembers, and the next one taken at the normal time (even if this means taking 2 pills together). A missed pill is one that is 24 or more hours late. If a woman misses only one pill, she should take an active pill as soon as she remembers and then resume normal pill-taking. No additional precautions are necessary. If a woman misses 2 or more pills (especially from the first 7 in a packet), she may not be protected. She should take an active pill as soon as she remembers and then resume normal pill-taking. In addition, she must either abstain from sex or use an additional method of contraception such as a condom for the next 7 days. If these 7 days run beyond the end of the packet, the next packet should be started at once, omitting the pill-free interval (or, in the case of *everyday* (ED) pills, omitting the 7 inactive tablets). Emergency contraception is recommended if 2 or more combined oral contraceptive tablets are missed from the first 7 tablets in a packet and unprotected intercourse has occurred since finishing the last packet.

▸ 919

Dienogest with estradiol valerate

17-Feb-2021

● **INDICATIONS AND DOSE**

Contraception with 28-day combined preparations | Menstrual symptoms with 28-day combined preparations
▸ BY MOUTH
▸ Females of childbearing potential: 1 active tablet daily for 26 days, followed by 1 inactive tablet daily for 2 days, to be started on day 1 of cycle with first active tablet (withdrawal bleeding may occur during the 2-day interval of inactive tablets); subsequent courses repeated without interval

● **INTERACTIONS** → Appendix 1: combined hormonal contraceptives

● **SIDE-EFFECTS**
▸ **Common or very common** Gastrointestinal discomfort · increased risk of infection · menstrual cycle irregularities
▸ **Uncommon** Appetite increased · cervical abnormalities · crying · depression · dizziness · fatigue · haemorrhage · hot flush · hyperhidrosis · hypertension · muscle spasms · neoplasms · oedema · ovarian and fallopian tube disorders · painful sexual intercourse · pelvic disorders · sleep disorders · uterine cramps · vulvovaginal disorders · weight decreased
▸ **Rare or very rare** Aggression · anxiety · asthma · chest pain · cholecystitis chronic · concentration impaired · constipation · contact lens intolerance · dry eye · dry mouth · dyspnoea · eye swelling · fever · galactorrhoea ·

gastrooesophageal reflux disease · genital discharge · hair changes · hypertriglyceridaemia · hypotension · lymphadenopathy · malaise · myocardial infarction · pain · palpitations · paraesthesia · seborrhoea · sensation of pressure · urinary tract pain · vascular disorders · vertigo

● **DIRECTIONS FOR ADMINISTRATION**
Changing to *Qlaira*® Start the first active *Qlaira*® tablet on the day after taking the last active tablet of the previous brand.

● **PATIENT AND CARER ADVICE**
Diarrhoea and vomiting In cases of persistent vomiting or severe diarrhoea lasting more than 12 hours in women taking *Qlaira*®, refer to product literature.
Missed doses A missed pill for a patient taking *Qlaira*® is one that is 12 hours or more late; for information on how to manage missed pills in women taking *Qlaira*®, refer to product literature.

● **MEDICINAL FORMS** There can be variation in the licensing of different medicines containing the same drug.
Form unstated
▸ Qlaira (Bayer Plc)
Qlaira tablets | 84 tablet [PoM] £25.18

Drospirenone with estetrol
19-Dec-2023 ⚑ 919

● **INDICATIONS AND DOSE**
Contraception
▸ BY MOUTH
▸ Females of childbearing potential: 1 active tablet once daily for 24 days, followed by 1 inactive tablet once daily for 4 days, to be started on day 1 of cycle with first active tablet (withdrawal bleeding may occur during the 4-day interval of inactive tablets) —if starting on day 2 to 5 of cycle, additional precautions (barrier methods) necessary during first 7 days; subsequent courses repeated without interval, see Contraceptives, hormonal p. 912 for recommendations from the FSRH on 'tailored' regimens in which there is a shortened, less frequent, or no interval where *inactive* tablets are taken.

● **INTERACTIONS** → Appendix 1: combined hormonal contraceptives · drospirenone

● **SIDE-EFFECTS**
▸ **Common or very common** Anger · haemorrhage · menstrual cycle irregularities · weight change
▸ **Uncommon** Anxiety · appetite disorder · chest pain · crying · depression · dizziness · drowsiness · dry mouth · fatigue · feeling abnormal · gastrointestinal discomfort · hot flush · increased risk of infection · insomnia · oedema · pain · painful sexual intercourse · paraesthesia · sweat changes · uterine disorders · vulvovaginal disorders
▸ **Rare or very rare** Bladder spasm · breast fibroadenoma · constipation · dry eye · facial swelling · gastrointestinal disorders · hirsutism · hyperkalaemia · hypertension · hyperthermia · hypotension · joint swelling · lactation disorder · limb discomfort · lip swelling · malaise · memory loss · muscle spasms · ovarian cyst · pelvic pain · performance status decreased · seborrhoea · urine odour abnormal · varicose veins · vertigo · vision disorders

● **MEDICINAL FORMS** There can be variation in the licensing of different medicines containing the same drug.
Oral tablet
▸ Drovelis (Gedeon Richter (UK) Ltd) ▼
Drospirenone 3 mg, Estetrol (as Estetrol monohydrate) **14.2 mg** Drovelis 3mg/14.2mg tablets | 28 tablet [PoM] £8.60 DT = £8.60

Estradiol with nomegestrol
13-Sep-2020 ⚑ 919

● **INDICATIONS AND DOSE**
Contraception
▸ BY MOUTH
▸ Females of childbearing potential: 1 active tablet daily for 24 days, followed by 1 inactive tablet daily for 4 days, to be started on day 1 of cycle with first active tablet (withdrawal bleeding occurs when inactive tablets being taken); subsequent courses repeated without interval

● **INTERACTIONS** → Appendix 1: combined hormonal contraceptives · estradiol

● **SIDE-EFFECTS**
▸ **Common or very common** Depression · menstrual cycle irregularities · pelvic pain
▸ **Uncommon** Abdominal distension · appetite abnormal · galactorrhoea · hot flush · hyperhidrosis · oedema · painful sexual intercourse · seborrhoea · sensation of pressure · uterine cramps · vulvovaginal disorders
▸ **Rare or very rare** Cerebrovascular insufficiency · concentration impaired · contact lens intolerance · dry eye · dry mouth · gallbladder disorders · hypertrichosis
▸ **Frequency not known** Meningioma

● **PREGNANCY** Toxicity in *animal* studies.

● **DIRECTIONS FOR ADMINISTRATION** *Zoely*® (every day (ED) combined (monophasic) preparation), 1 *active* tablet daily for 24 days, followed by 1 *inactive* tablet daily for 4 days, starting on day 1 of cycle with first *active* tablet; subsequent courses repeated without interval (withdrawal bleeding occurs when *inactive* tablets being taken). Changing to *Zoely*® Start the first active *Zoely*® tablet on the day after taking the last active tablet of the previous brand or, at the latest, the day after the tablet-free or inactive tablet interval of the previous brand.

● **PATIENT AND CARER ADVICE**
Diarrhoea and vomiting In cases of persistent vomiting or severe diarrhoea lasting more than 12 hours in women taking *Zoely*®, refer to product literature.
Missed doses A missed pill for a patient taking *Zoely*® is one that is 12 hours or more late; for information on how to manage missed pills in women taking *Zoely*®, refer to product literature.

● **MEDICINAL FORMS** There can be variation in the licensing of different medicines containing the same drug.
Oral tablet
▸ Zoely (Theramex HQ UK Ltd)
Estradiol (as Estradiol hemihydrate) 1.5 mg, Nomegestrol acetate **2.5 mg** Zoely 2.5mg/1.5mg tablets | 84 tablet [PoM] £19.80 DT = £19.80

Ethinylestradiol with desogestrel
14-Mar-2021 ⚑ 919

● **INDICATIONS AND DOSE**
Menstrual symptoms with 21-day combined preparations
▸ BY MOUTH
▸ Females of childbearing potential: 1 tablet once daily for 21 days; subsequent courses repeated after 7-day interval, withdrawal bleeding occurs during the 7-day interval, if reasonably certain woman is not pregnant, first course can be started on any day of cycle—if starting on day 6 of cycle or later, additional precautions (barrier methods) necessary during first 7 days, tablets should be taken at approximately the same time each day

Contraception with 21-day combined preparations
▶ BY MOUTH
▶ Females of childbearing potential: 1 tablet once daily for 21 days; subsequent courses repeated after hormone-free interval, withdrawal bleeding occurs during the hormone-free interval, if reasonably certain woman is not pregnant, first course can be started on any day of cycle—if starting on day 6 of cycle or later, additional precautions (barrier methods) necessary during first 7 days, tablets should be taken at approximately the same time each day, see Contraceptives, hormonal p. 912 for recommendations from the FSRH on 'traditional' and 'tailored' regimens in which there is a shortened, less frequent, or no hormone-free interval.

● INTERACTIONS → Appendix 1: combined hormonal contraceptives · desogestrel · ethinylestradiol

● SIDE-EFFECTS
▶ **Common or very common** Depressed mood
▶ **Rare or very rare** Contact lens intolerance · erythema nodosum · weight decreased
▶ **Frequency not known** Angioedema aggravated

● MEDICINAL FORMS There can be variation in the licensing of different medicines containing the same drug.

Oral tablet
▶ Bimizza (Morningside Healthcare Ltd)
  Ethinylestradiol 20 microgram, Desogestrel 150 microgram Bimizza 150microgram/20microgram tablets | 63 tablet [PoM] £5.04 DT = £5.98
▶ Cimizt (Morningside Healthcare Ltd)
  Ethinylestradiol 30 microgram, Desogestrel 150 microgram Cimizt 30microgram/150microgram tablets | 63 tablet [PoM] £3.80 DT = £4.93
▶ Gedarel (Gedeon Richter (UK) Ltd)
  Ethinylestradiol 20 microgram, Desogestrel 150 microgram Gedarel 20microgram/150microgram tablets | 63 tablet [PoM] £5.98 DT = £5.98
  Ethinylestradiol 30 microgram, Desogestrel 150 microgram Gedarel 30microgram/150microgram tablets | 63 tablet [PoM] £4.93 DT = £4.93
▶ Marvelon (Organon Pharma (UK) Ltd)
  Ethinylestradiol 30 microgram, Desogestrel 150 microgram Marvelon tablets | 63 tablet [PoM] £7.10 DT = £4.93
▶ Mercilon (Organon Pharma (UK) Ltd)
  Ethinylestradiol 20 microgram, Desogestrel 150 microgram Mercilon 150microgram/20microgram tablets | 63 tablet [PoM] £8.44 DT = £5.98

F 919

Ethinylestradiol with drospirenone

19-Dec-2023

● INDICATIONS AND DOSE

Menstrual symptoms with 21-day combined preparations
▶ BY MOUTH
▶ Females of childbearing potential: 1 tablet once daily for 21 days; subsequent courses repeated after 7-day interval, withdrawal bleeding occurs during the 7-day interval

Contraception with 21-day combined preparations
▶ BY MOUTH
▶ Females of childbearing potential: 1 tablet once daily for 21 days; subsequent courses repeated after hormone-free interval, withdrawal bleeding occurs during the hormone-free interval, see Contraceptives, hormonal p. 912 for recommendations from the FSRH on 'traditional' and 'tailored' regimens in which there is a shortened, less frequent, or no hormone-free interval.

Menstrual symptoms with 28-day combined preparations
▶ BY MOUTH
▶ Females of childbearing potential: 1 active tablet once daily for 24 days, followed by 1 inactive tablet once

daily for 4 days, to be started on day 1 of cycle with first active tablet (withdrawal bleeding may occur during the 4-day interval of inactive tablets); subsequent courses repeated without interval

Contraception with 28-day combined preparations
▶ BY MOUTH
▶ Females of childbearing potential: 1 active tablet once daily for 24 days, followed by 1 inactive tablet once daily for 4 days, to be started on day 1 of cycle with first active tablet (withdrawal bleeding may occur during the 4-day interval of inactive tablets); subsequent courses repeated without interval, see Contraceptives, hormonal p. 912 for recommendations from the FSRH on 'tailored' regimens in which there is a shortened, less frequent, or no interval where *inactive* tablets are taken.

● INTERACTIONS → Appendix 1: combined hormonal contraceptives · drospirenone · ethinylestradiol

● SIDE-EFFECTS
▶ **Common or very common** Depressed mood · increased risk of infection · menstrual disorder
▶ **Uncommon** Hypertension · hypotension · weight decreased
▶ **Rare or very rare** Asthma · erythema nodosum · hearing impairment

● PATIENT AND CARER ADVICE
  Pill-free interval Withdrawal bleeding can occur during the 7-day tablet-free interval.

● MEDICINAL FORMS There can be variation in the licensing of different medicines containing the same drug.

Oral tablet
▶ Dretine (Theramex HQ UK Ltd)
  Ethinylestradiol 30 microgram, Drospirenone 3 mg Dretine 0.03mg/3mg tablets | 63 tablet [PoM] £8.34 DT = £14.70
▶ ELOINE (Bayer Plc)
  Ethinylestradiol 20 microgram, Drospirenone 3 mg Eloine 0.02mg/3mg tablets | 84 tablet [PoM] £14.70 DT = £14.70
▶ Ellanite (Kent Pharma (UK) Ltd)
  Ethinylestradiol 30 microgram, Drospirenone 3 mg Ellanite 0.03mg/3mg tablets | 63 tablet [PoM] £14.20 DT = £14.70
▶ Lucette (Gedeon Richter (UK) Ltd)
  Ethinylestradiol 30 microgram, Drospirenone 3 mg Lucette 0.03mg/3mg tablets | 63 tablet [PoM] £11.00 DT = £14.70
▶ Yacella (Morningside Healthcare Ltd)
  Ethinylestradiol 30 microgram, Drospirenone 3 mg Yacella 0.03mg/3mg tablets | 63 tablet [PoM] £8.30 DT = £14.70
▶ Yasmin (Bayer Plc)
  Ethinylestradiol 30 microgram, Drospirenone 3 mg Yasmin tablets | 63 tablet [PoM] £14.70 DT = £14.70

F 919

Ethinylestradiol with etonogestrel

14-Mar-2021

● INDICATIONS AND DOSE

Menstrual symptoms
▶ BY VAGINA
▶ Females of childbearing potential: 1 unit, insert the ring into the vagina on day 1 of cycle and leave in for 3 weeks; remove ring on day 22; subsequent courses repeated after 7-day ring free interval (during which withdrawal bleeding occurs)

Contraception
▶ BY VAGINA
▶ Females of childbearing potential: 1 unit, insert the ring into the vagina on day 1 of cycle and leave in for 3 weeks; remove ring on day 22; subsequent courses repeated after 7-day ring free interval (during which withdrawal bleeding occurs), see Contraceptives, hormonal p. 912 for recommendations from the FSRH on 'tailored' regimens in which there is a shortened, less frequent, or no ring-free interval.

- **INTERACTIONS** → Appendix 1: combined hormonal contraceptives · ethinylestradiol · etonogestrel
- **SIDE-EFFECTS**
  ▶ **Common or very common** Depression · device complications · genital pruritus · increased risk of infection · menstrual cycle irregularities · pelvic disorders
  ▶ **Uncommon** Abdominal distension · appetite increased · cervical abnormalities · constipation · cystitis · dizziness · fatigue · hot flush · malaise · muscle spasms · oedema · pain · painful sexual intercourse · sensation abnormal · urinary disorders · uterine cramps · visual impairment · vulvovaginal disorders
  ▶ **Rare or very rare** Galactorrhoea
  ▶ **Frequency not known** Angioedema aggravated · penis disorder
- **DIRECTIONS FOR ADMINISTRATION**
  Changing from combined hormonal contraception to vaginal ring Manufacturer advises insert ring at the latest on the day after the usual tablet-free, patch-free, or inactive-tablet interval. If previous contraceptive used correctly, or pregnancy can reasonably be excluded, can switch to ring on any day of cycle.
  Changing from progestogen-only method to vaginal ring From an implant or intra-uterine progestogen-only device, manufacturer advises insert ring on the day implant or intra-uterine progestogen-only device removed; from an injection, insert ring when next injection due; from oral preparation, first ring may be inserted on any day after stopping pill. For all methods additional precautions (barrier methods) should be used concurrently for first 7 days.
- **PATIENT AND CARER ADVICE** Patients or carers should be given advice on how to administer vaginal ring.
  Counselling The presence of the ring should be checked regularly.
  Missed doses
  Expulsion, delayed insertion or removal, or broken vaginal ring If the vaginal ring is expelled for *less than* 3 *hours*, rinse the ring with cool water and reinsert immediately; no additional contraception is needed.
    If the ring remains outside the vagina for *more than* 3 *hours* or if the user does not know when the ring was expelled, contraceptive protection may be reduced:
  - If ring expelled during week 1 or 2 of cycle, rinse ring with cool water and reinsert; use additional precautions (barrier methods) for next 7 days;
  - If ring expelled during week 3 of cycle, either insert a new ring to start a new cycle *or* allow a withdrawal bleed and insert a new ring no later than 7 days after ring was expelled; latter option only available if ring was used continuously for at least 7 days before expulsion.
  If insertion of a new ring at the start of a new cycle is delayed, contraceptive protection is lost. A new ring should be inserted as soon as possible; additional precautions (barrier methods) should be used for the first 7 days of the new cycle. If intercourse occurred during the extended ring-free interval, pregnancy should be considered.
    No additional contraception is required if removal of the ring is delayed by up to 1 week (4 weeks of continuous use). The 7-day ring-free interval should be observed and subsequently a new ring should be inserted. Contraceptive protection may be reduced with continuous use of the ring for more than 4 weeks—pregnancy should be ruled out before inserting a new ring.
    If the ring breaks during use, remove it and insert a new ring immediately; additional precautions (barrier methods) should be used for the first 7 days of the new cycle.

- **MEDICINAL FORMS** There can be variation in the licensing of different medicines containing the same drug.
  Vaginal delivery system
  ▶ **NuvaRing** (Organon Pharma (UK) Ltd)
    Ethinylestradiol 2.7 mg, Etonogestrel 11.7 mg NuvaRing 0.12mg/0.015mg per day vaginal delivery system | 3 system [PoM] £29.70 DT = £29.70
  ▶ **SyreniRing** (Crescent Pharma Ltd)
    Ethinylestradiol 2.7 mg, Etonogestrel 11.7 mg SyreniRing 0.12mg/0.015mg per day vaginal delivery system | 3 system [PoM] £23.76 DT = £29.70

☛ 919

Ethinylestradiol with gestodene
14-Mar-2021

- **INDICATIONS AND DOSE**

Menstrual symptoms with 21-day combined preparations
▶ BY MOUTH
▶ Females of childbearing potential: 1 tablet once daily for 21 days; subsequent courses repeated after 7-day interval, withdrawal bleeding occurs during the 7-day interval, if reasonably certain woman is not pregnant, first course can be started on any day of cycle—if starting on day 6 of cycle or later, additional precautions (barrier methods) necessary during first 7 days, tablets should be taken at approximately the same time each day

Contraception with 21-day combined preparations
▶ BY MOUTH
▶ Females of childbearing potential: 1 tablet once daily for 21 days; subsequent courses repeated after hormone-free interval, withdrawal bleeding occurs during the hormone-free interval, if reasonably certain woman is not pregnant, first course can be started on any day of cycle—if starting on day 6 of cycle or later, additional precautions (barrier methods) necessary during first 7 days, tablets should be taken at approximately the same time each day, see Contraceptives, hormonal p. 912 for recommendations from the FSRH on 'traditional' and 'tailored' regimens in which there is a shortened, less frequent, or no hormone-free interval.

Menstrual symptoms with 28-day combined preparations
▶ BY MOUTH
▶ Females of childbearing potential: 1 active tablet once daily for 21 days, followed by 1 inactive tablet daily for 7 days; subsequent courses repeated without interval, withdrawal bleeding occurs during the 7-day interval of *inactive* tablets being taken, if reasonably certain woman is not pregnant, first course can be started on any day of cycle—if starting on day 6 of cycle or later, additional precautions (barrier methods) necessary during first 7 days, tablets should be taken at approximately the same time each day

Contraception with 28-day combined preparations
▶ BY MOUTH
▶ Females of childbearing potential: 1 active tablet once daily for 21 days, followed by 1 inactive tablet daily for 7 days; subsequent courses repeated without interval, withdrawal bleeding occurs during the interval of *inactive* tablets being taken, if reasonably certain woman is not pregnant, first course can be started on any day of cycle—if starting on day 6 of cycle or later, additional precautions (barrier methods) necessary during first 7 days, tablets should be taken at approximately the same time each day, see Contraceptives, hormonal p. 912 for recommendations from the FSRH on 'tailored' regimens in which *inactive* tablets are taken for a shortened, less frequent, or absent interval.

- **INTERACTIONS** → Appendix 1: combined hormonal contraceptives · ethinylestradiol

- **SIDE-EFFECTS**
- **Common or very common** Depression · dizziness · increased risk of infection · menstrual cycle irregularities · nervousness
- **Uncommon** Appetite abnormal · hirsutism · hypertension · hypertriglyceridaemia
- **Rare or very rare** Angioedema · chorea exacerbated · ear disorders · erythema nodosum · eye irritation · gallbladder disorders · gastrointestinal disorders · haemolytic uraemic syndrome · hepatic disorders · hypersensitivity · inflammatory bowel disease · neoplasms · optic neuritis · pancreatitis · systemic lupus erythematosus exacerbated · varicose veins exacerbated · weight decreased

- **MEDICINAL FORMS** There can be variation in the licensing of different medicines containing the same drug.

Oral tablet

- **Ethinylestradiol with gestodene (Non-proprietary)**
  **Ethinylestradiol 30 microgram, Gestodene
  50 microgram** Ethinylestradiol 30microgram / Gestodene 50microgram tablets | 18 tablet [PoM] ⓢ
  **Ethinylestradiol 40 microgram, Gestodene
  70 microgram** Ethinylestradiol 40microgram / Gestodene 70microgram tablets | 15 tablet [PoM] ⓢ
  **Ethinylestradiol 30 microgram, Gestodene
  100 microgram** Ethinylestradiol 30microgram / Gestodene 100microgram tablets | 30 tablet [PoM] ⓢ
- **Akizza** (Morningside Healthcare Ltd)
  Ethinylestradiol 30 microgram, Gestodene 75 microgram Akizza 75microgram/30microgram tablets | 63 tablet [PoM] £8.85 DT = £6.73
  Ethinylestradiol 20 microgram, Gestodene 75 microgram Akizza 75microgram/20microgram tablets | 63 tablet [PoM] £6.73 DT = £8.85
- **Femodene** (Bayer Plc)
  **Ethinylestradiol 30 microgram, Gestodene
  75 microgram** Femodene tablets | 63 tablet [PoM] £6.73 DT = £6.73
- **Femodette** (Bayer Plc)
  **Ethinylestradiol 20 microgram, Gestodene
  75 microgram** Femodette tablets | 63 tablet [PoM] £8.85 DT = £8.85
- **Katya** (Kent Pharma (UK) Ltd)
  Ethinylestradiol 30 microgram, Gestodene 75 microgram Katya 30/75 tablets | 63 tablet [PoM] £5.03 DT = £6.73
- **Millinette** (Gedeon Richter (UK) Ltd)
  **Ethinylestradiol 30 microgram, Gestodene
  75 microgram** Millinette 30microgram/75microgram tablets | 63 tablet [PoM] £4.85 DT = £6.73
  **Ethinylestradiol 20 microgram, Gestodene
  75 microgram** Millinette 20microgram/75microgram tablets | 63 tablet [PoM] £6.37 DT = £8.85
- **Sunya** (Kent Pharma (UK) Ltd)
  Ethinylestradiol 20 microgram, Gestodene 75 microgram Sunya 20/75 tablets | 63 tablet [PoM] £6.62 DT = £8.85

▶ 919

Ethinylestradiol with levonorgestrel

14-Mar-2021

- **INDICATIONS AND DOSE**

Menstrual symptoms with 21-day combined preparations
- BY MOUTH
- Females of childbearing potential: 1 tablet once daily for 21 days; subsequent courses repeated after 7-day interval, withdrawal bleeding occurs during the 7-day interval, if reasonably certain woman is not pregnant, first course can be started on any day of cycle—if starting on day 6 of cycle or later, additional precautions (barrier methods) necessary during first 7 days, tablets should be taken at approximately the same time each day

Contraception with 21-day combined preparations
- BY MOUTH
- Females of childbearing potential: 1 tablet once daily for 21 days; subsequent courses repeated after hormone-free interval, withdrawal bleeding occurs during the hormone-free interval, if reasonably certain woman is not pregnant, first course can be started on any day of cycle—if starting on day 6 of cycle or later, additional precautions (barrier methods) necessary during first 7 days, tablets should be taken at approximately the same time each day, see Contraceptives, hormonal p. 912 for recommendations from the FSRH on 'traditional' and 'tailored' regimens in which there is a shortened, less frequent, or no hormone-free interval.

Menstrual symptoms with 28-day combined preparations
- BY MOUTH
- Females of childbearing potential: 1 active tablet once daily for 21 days, followed by 1 inactive tablet once daily for 7 days, withdrawal bleeding occurs during the 7-day interval of *inactive* tablets being taken, if reasonably certain woman is not pregnant, first course can be started on any day of cycle—if starting on day 6 of cycle or later, additional precautions (barrier methods) necessary during first 7 days, tablets should be taken at approximately the same time each day. Subsequent courses repeated without interval

Contraception with 28-day combined preparations
- BY MOUTH
- Females of childbearing potential: 1 active tablet once daily for 21 days, followed by 1 inactive tablet once daily for 7 days, withdrawal bleeding occurs during the interval of *inactive* tablets being taken, if reasonably certain woman is not pregnant, first course can be started on any day of cycle—if starting on day 6 of cycle or later, additional precautions (barrier methods) necessary during first 7 days, tablets should be taken at approximately the same time each day. Subsequent courses repeated without interval, see Contraceptives, hormonal p. 912 for recommendations from the FSRH on 'tailored' regimens in which there is a shortened, less frequent, or no interval where *inactive* tablets are taken.

- **INTERACTIONS** → Appendix 1: combined hormonal contraceptives · ethinylestradiol · levonorgestrel

- **SIDE-EFFECTS**
- **Common or very common** Depressed mood
- **Rare or very rare** Contact lens intolerance · erythema nodosum · weight decreased
- **Frequency not known** Angioedema aggravated · chorea exacerbated · hepatic function abnormal · hypertriglyceridaemia · inflammatory bowel disease · menstrual cycle irregularities

- **MEDICINAL FORMS** There can be variation in the licensing of different medicines containing the same drug.

Oral tablet

- **Ethinylestradiol with levonorgestrel (Non-proprietary)**
  **Ethinylestradiol 30 microgram, Levonorgestrel
  50 microgram** Ethinylestradiol 30microgram / Levonorgestrel 50microgram tablets | 6 tablet [PoM] ⓢ
  **Ethinylestradiol 40 microgram, Levonorgestrel
  75 microgram** Ethinylestradiol 40microgram / Levonorgestrel 75microgram tablets | 5 tablet [PoM] ⓢ
  **Ethinylestradiol 30 microgram, Levonorgestrel
  125 microgram** Ethinylestradiol 30microgram / Levonorgestrel 125microgram tablets | 10 tablet [PoM] ⓢ
- **Ambelina** (Crescent Pharma Ltd)
  **Ethinylestradiol 30 microgram, Levonorgestrel
  150 microgram** Ambelina 150microgram/30microgram tablets | 63 tablet [PoM] £2.60 DT = £2.82
- **Elevin** (Genesis Pharmaceuticals Ltd)
  **Ethinylestradiol 30 microgram, Levonorgestrel
  150 microgram** Elevin 150microgram/30microgram tablets | 63 tablet [PoM] £29.25 DT = £2.82

▶ **Levest** (Morningside Healthcare Ltd)
**Ethinylestradiol 30 microgram, Levonorgestrel
150 microgram** Levest 150/30 tablets | 63 tablet [PoM] £1.80 DT = £2.82

▶ **Maexeni** (Lupin Healthcare (UK) Ltd)
**Ethinylestradiol 30 microgram, Levonorgestrel
150 microgram** Maexeni 150microgram/30microgram tablets | 63 tablet [PoM] £1.88 DT = £2.82

▶ **Microgynon 30** (Bayer Plc)
**Ethinylestradiol 30 microgram, Levonorgestrel
150 microgram** Microgynon 30 tablets | 63 tablet [PoM] £2.82 DT = £2.82

▶ **Ovranette** (Pfizer Ltd)
**Ethinylestradiol 30 microgram, Levonorgestrel
150 microgram** Ovranette 150microgram/30microgram tablets | 63 tablet [PoM] £2.20 DT = £2.82

▶ **Rigevidon** (Gedeon Richter (UK) Ltd)
**Ethinylestradiol 30 microgram, Levonorgestrel
150 microgram** Rigevidon tablets | 63 tablet [PoM] £1.89 DT = £2.82

⚑ 919

Ethinylestradiol with norelgestromin

14-Mar-2021

● **INDICATIONS AND DOSE**

Menstrual symptoms
▶ BY TRANSDERMAL APPLICATION
▶ Females of childbearing potential: Apply 1 patch once weekly for 3 weeks, apply first patch on day 1 of cycle, change patch on days 8 and 15; remove third patch on day 22 and apply new patch after 7-day patch-free interval to start subsequent contraceptive cycle, subsequent courses repeated after a 7-day patch free interval (during which withdrawal bleeding occurs)

Contraception
▶ BY TRANSDERMAL APPLICATION
▶ Females of childbearing potential: Apply 1 patch once weekly for 3 weeks, apply first patch on day 1 of cycle, change patch on days 8 and 15; remove third patch on day 22 and apply new patch after a patch-free interval to start subsequent contraceptive cycle, subsequent courses repeated after a patch-free interval (during which withdrawal bleeding occurs), see Contraceptives, hormonal p. 912 for recommendations from the FSRH on 'traditional' and 'tailored' regimens in which there is a shortened, less frequent, or no patch-free interval.

● **CAUTIONS** Body-weight 90 kg and above (possible reduction in contraceptive efficacy)

● **INTERACTIONS** → Appendix 1: combined hormonal contraceptives · ethinylestradiol

● **SIDE-EFFECTS**
▶ **Common or very common** Abdominal distension · anxiety · dizziness · fatigue · increased risk of infection · malaise · menstrual cycle irregularities · muscle spasms · uterine cramps · vaginal haemorrhage
▶ **Uncommon** Appetite increased · dyslipidaemia · hypertension · insomnia · lactation disorders · oedema · photosensitivity reaction · vulvovaginal dryness
▶ **Rare or very rare** Gallbladder disorders · genital discharge · neoplasms · stroke · swelling
▶ **Frequency not known** Anger · angioedema · cervical dysplasia · colitis · contact lens intolerance · erythema nodosum · hepatic disorders · hyperglycaemia · intracranial haemorrhage · myocardial infarction · pulmonary artery thrombosis · taste altered

● **DIRECTIONS FOR ADMINISTRATION** Manufacturer advises adhesives or bandages should not be used to hold patch in place. If no longer sticky do not reapply but use a new patch.
Changing to a transdermal combined hormonal contraceptive
Changing from combined oral contraception
Manufacturer advises apply patch on the first day of

withdrawal bleeding; if no withdrawal bleeding within 5 days of taking last *active* tablet, rule out pregnancy before applying first patch. Unless patch is applied on first day of withdrawal bleeding, additional precautions (barrier methods) should be used concurrently for first 7 days.
Changing from progestogen-only method
Manufacturer advises
● from an implant, apply first patch on the day implant removed
● from an injection, apply first patch when next injection due
● from oral progestogen, first patch may be applied on any day after stopping pill
For all methods additional precautions (barrier methods) should be used concurrently for first 7 days.
After childbirth (not breast-feeding) Manufacturer advises start 4 weeks after birth; if started later than 4 weeks after birth additional precautions (barrier methods) should be used for first 7 days.
After abortion or miscarriage Manufacturer advises before 20 weeks' gestation start immediately; no additional contraception required if started immediately. After 20 weeks' gestation start on day 21 after abortion or on the first day of first spontaneous menstruation; additional precautions (barrier methods) should be used for first 7 days after applying the patch.

● **PATIENT AND CARER ADVICE** Patients and carers should be given advice on how to administer patches.
Travel Women using patches are at an increased risk of deep vein thrombosis during travel involving long periods of immobility (over 3 hours). The risk may be reduced by appropriate exercise during the journey and possibly by wearing graduated compression hosiery.
Missed doses
Delayed application or detached patch If a patch is partly detached for less than 24 hours, reapply to the same site or replace with a new patch immediately; no additional contraception is needed and the next patch should be applied on the usual 'change day'. If a patch remains detached for more than 24 hours or if the user is not aware when the patch became detached, then stop the current contraceptive cycle and start a new cycle by applying a new patch, giving a new 'Day 1'; an additional non-hormonal contraceptive must be used concurrently for the first 7 days of the new cycle.
If application of a new patch at the start of a new cycle is delayed, contraceptive protection is lost. A new patch should be applied as soon as remembered giving a new 'Day 1'; additional non-hormonal methods of contraception should be used for the first 7 days of the new cycle. If application of a patch in the middle of the cycle is delayed (i.e. the patch is not changed on day 8 or day 15):
● for up to 48 hours, apply a new patch immediately; next patch 'change day' remains the same and no additional contraception is required;
● for more than 48 hours, contraceptive protection may have been lost. Stop the current cycle and start a new 4-week cycle immediately by applying a new patch giving a new 'Day 1'; additional non-hormonal contraception should be used for the first 7 days of the new cycle.
If the patch is not removed at the end of the cycle (day 22), remove it as soon as possible and start the next cycle on the usual 'change day', the day after day 28; no additional contraception is required.

● **NATIONAL FUNDING/ACCESS DECISIONS**
For full details see funding body website

Scottish Medicines Consortium (SMC) decisions
▶ **Ethinylestradiol with norelgestromin (***Evra***®) for use as female contraception** (September 2003) SMC No. 48/03
Recommended with restrictions

- **MEDICINAL FORMS** There can be variation in the licensing of different medicines containing the same drug.
  ### Transdermal patch
  - ▸ Evra (Gedeon Richter (UK) Ltd)
    Ethinylestradiol 33.9 microgram per 24 hour, Norelgestromin 203 microgram per 24 hour Evra transdermal patches | 9 patch [PoM] £19.51 DT = £19.51

☞ 919

Ethinylestradiol with norethisterone
14-Mar-2021

- **INDICATIONS AND DOSE**

Menstrual symptoms with 21-day combined preparations
- ▸ BY MOUTH
- ▸ Females of childbearing potential: 1 tablet once daily for 21 days; subsequent courses repeated after 7-day interval, withdrawal bleeding occurs during the 7-day interval, if reasonably certain woman is not pregnant, first course can be started on any day of cycle—if starting on day 6 of cycle or later, additional precautions (barrier methods) necessary during first 7 days, tablets should be taken at approximately the same time each day

Contraception with 21-day combined preparations
- ▸ BY MOUTH
- ▸ Females of childbearing potential: 1 tablet once daily for 21 days; subsequent courses repeated after hormone-free interval, withdrawal bleeding occurs during the hormone-free interval, if reasonably certain woman is not pregnant, first course can be started on any day of cycle—if starting on day 6 of cycle or later, additional precautions (barrier methods) necessary during first 7 days, tablets should be taken at approximately the same time each day, see Contraceptives, hormonal p. 912 for recommendations from the FSRH on 'traditional' and 'tailored' regimens in which there is a shortened, less frequent, or no hormone-free interval.

- **INTERACTIONS** → Appendix 1: combined hormonal contraceptives · ethinylestradiol · norethisterone

- **SIDE-EFFECTS** Angioedema aggravated

- **MEDICINAL FORMS** There can be variation in the licensing of different medicines containing the same drug.
  ### Oral tablet
  - ▸ Ethinylestradiol with norethisterone (Non-proprietary)
    Ethinylestradiol 35 microgram, Norethisterone 500 microgram Ethinylestradiol 35microgram / Norethisterone 500microgram tablets | 5 tablet [PoM] [⊠]
    Ethinylestradiol 35 microgram, Norethisterone 750 microgram Ethinylestradiol 35microgram / Norethisterone 750microgram tablets | 21 tablet [PoM] [⊠]
    Ethinylestradiol 35 microgram, Norethisterone 1 mg Ethinylestradiol 35microgram / Norethisterone 1mg tablets | 9 tablet [PoM] [⊠]
  - ▸ Brevinor (Pfizer Ltd)
    Ethinylestradiol 35 microgram, Norethisterone 500 microgram Brevinor 500microgram/35microgram tablets | 63 tablet [PoM] £1.99 DT = £1.99
  - ▸ Norimin (Pfizer Ltd)
    Ethinylestradiol 35 microgram, Norethisterone 1 mg Norimin 1mg/35microgram tablets | 63 tablet [PoM] £2.28 DT = £2.28

☞ 919

Ethinylestradiol with norgestimate
15-Mar-2021

- **INDICATIONS AND DOSE**

Menstrual symptoms with 21-day combined preparations
- ▸ BY MOUTH
- ▸ Females of childbearing potential: 1 tablet once daily for 21 days; subsequent courses repeated after 7-day interval, withdrawal bleeding occurs during the 7-day interval, if reasonably certain woman is not pregnant, first course can be started on any day of cycle—if starting on day 6 of cycle or later, additional precautions (barrier methods) necessary during first 7 days, tablets should be taken at approximately the same time each day

Contraception with 21-day combined preparations
- ▸ BY MOUTH
- ▸ Females of childbearing potential: 1 tablet once daily for 21 days; subsequent courses repeated after hormone-free interval, withdrawal bleeding occurs during the hormone-free interval, if reasonably certain woman is not pregnant, first course can be started on any day of cycle—if starting on day 6 of cycle or later, additional precautions (barrier methods) necessary during first 7 days, tablets should be taken at approximately the same time each day, see Contraceptives, hormonal p. 912 for recommendations from the FSRH on 'traditional' and 'tailored' regimens in which there is a shortened, less frequent, or no hormone-free interval.

- **INTERACTIONS** → Appendix 1: combined hormonal contraceptives · ethinylestradiol

- **SIDE-EFFECTS**
- ▸ **Common or very common** Anxiety · asthenic conditions · chest pain · constipation · depression · dizziness · gastrointestinal discomfort · gastrointestinal disorders · genital discharge · hypersensitivity · increased risk of infection · insomnia · menstrual cycle irregularities · muscle complaints · oedema · pain
- ▸ **Uncommon** Appetite abnormal · cervical dysplasia · dry eye · dyspnoea · hirsutism · hot flush · hypertension · ovarian cyst · palpitations · paraesthesia · syncope · visual impairment · vulvovaginal dryness · weight changes
- ▸ **Rare or very rare** Hepatic disorders · pancreatitis · photosensitivity reaction · sweat changes · tachycardia · vertigo
- ▸ **Frequency not known** Angioedema · contact lens intolerance · dyslipidaemia · erythema nodosum · neoplasms · seizure · suppressed lactation

- **MEDICINAL FORMS** There can be variation in the licensing of different medicines containing the same drug.
  ### Oral tablet
  - ▸ Cilique (Gedeon Richter (UK) Ltd)
    Ethinylestradiol 35 microgram, Norgestimate 250 microgram Cilique 250microgram/35microgram tablets | 63 tablet [PoM] £4.65 DT = £4.65
  - ▸ Lizinna (Morningside Healthcare Ltd)
    Ethinylestradiol 35 microgram, Norgestimate 250 microgram Lizinna 250microgram/35microgram tablets | 63 tablet [PoM] £4.64 DT = £4.65

☞ 919

Norethisterone with mestranol

- **INDICATIONS AND DOSE**

Contraception | Menstrual symptoms
- ▸ BY MOUTH
- ▸ Females of childbearing potential: 1 tablet once daily for 21 days; subsequent courses repeated after 7-day interval, withdrawal bleeding can occur during the 7-day interval, if reasonably certain woman is not pregnant, first course can be started on any day of cycle—if starting on day 6 of cycle or later, additional precautions (barrier methods) necessary during first 7 days, tablets should be taken at the same time each day

- **INTERACTIONS** → Appendix 1: combined hormonal contraceptives · norethisterone

- **MEDICINAL FORMS** No licensed medicines listed.

7   Genito-urinary system

3.2 Contraception, devices

Other drugs used for Contraception, devices
Levonorgestrel, p. 932

CONTRACEPTIVE DEVICES

Intra-uterine contraceptive devices (copper)

06-Mar-2024

● **INDICATIONS AND DOSE**
Contraception
▶ BY INTRA-UTERINE ADMINISTRATION
▶ Females of childbearing potential: (consult product literature)

IMPORTANT SAFETY INFORMATION
MHRA/CHM ADVICE (JUNE 2015) INTRA-UTERINE CONTRACEPTION: UTERINE PERFORATION—UPDATED INFORMATION ON RISK FACTORS
Uterine perforation most often occurs during insertion, but might not be detected until sometime later. The risk of uterine perforation is increased when the device is inserted up to 36 weeks postpartum or in patients who are breastfeeding. Before inserting an intra-uterine contraceptive device, inform patients that perforation occurs in approximately 1 in every 1000 insertions and signs and symptoms include:
● severe pelvic pain after insertion (worse than period cramps);
● pain or increased bleeding after insertion which continues for more than a few weeks;
● sudden changes in periods;
● pain during intercourse;
● unable to feel the threads.
Patients should be informed on how to check their threads and to arrange a check-up if threads cannot be felt, especially if they also have significant pain. Partial perforation may occur even if the threads can be seen; consider this if there is severe pain following insertion and perform an ultrasound.

● **CONTRA-INDICATIONS** Active trophoblastic disease (until return to normal of urine and plasma-gonadotrophin concentration) · genital malignancy · medical diathermy · pelvic inflammatory disease · post-abortion sepsis · postpartum sepsis · recent sexually transmitted infection (if not fully investigated and treated) · severe anaemia · unexplained uterine bleeding · Wilson's disease

● **CAUTIONS** Anaemia · anatomical abnormalities—seek specialist advice · anticoagulant therapy · cardiac disease—seek specialist advice · endometriosis · epilepsy (risk of seizure at time of insertion) · immunosuppression (risk of infection)—seek specialist advice · menorrhagia (progestogen intra-uterine device might be preferable) · postpartum—seek specialist advice · risk of sexually transmitted infections · severe primary dysmenorrhoea · young age

CAUTIONS, FURTHER INFORMATION EvGr If removal is after day 7 of the menstrual cycle, intercourse should be avoided or another method of contraception used for at least 7 days before removal of intra-uterine device. Ⓜ
▶ Sexually transmitted infections and pelvic inflammatory disease The main excess risk of pelvic infection occurs in the first 3 weeks after insertion and is believed to be related to existing carriage of a sexually transmitted infection.
  The FSRH advises pre-insertion screening (for chlamydia and, depending on sexual history and local prevalence of

disease, *Neisseria gonorrhoeae*) be performed in women at risk of sexually transmitted infections. If results are unavailable at the time of fitting an intra-uterine device for emergency contraception, consider appropriate prophylactic antibacterial cover.

● **SIDE-EFFECTS** Abdominal pain lower · anaemia · back pain · device complications · menstrual cycle irregularities · pelvic inflammatory disease · uterine injuries

● **ALLERGY AND CROSS-SENSITIVITY** EvGr Contra-indicated if patient has a copper allergy. Ⓜ

● **PREGNANCY** If an intra-uterine device fails and the woman wishes to continue to full-term the device should be removed in the first trimester if possible. Remove device; if pregnancy occurs, increased likelihood that it may be ectopic.

● **BREAST FEEDING** Not known to be harmful.

● **MONITORING REQUIREMENTS** Gynaecological examination before insertion, 6–8 weeks after insertion, then annually.

● **DIRECTIONS FOR ADMINISTRATION** The healthcare professional inserting (or removing) the device should be fully trained in the technique and should provide full counselling backed, where available, by the patient information leaflet.

● **PRESCRIBING AND DISPENSING INFORMATION**
ANCORA ® 375 CU For uterine length over 6.5 cm; replacement every 5 years.
COPPER T380 A ® For uterine length 6.5–9 cm; replacement every 10 years.
EUROGINE T 380 ® AG '*Mini*' size for minimum uterine length 5 cm; '*Normal*' size for uterine length 6.5–9 cm; replacement every 5 years.
EUROGINE T 380 ® CU '*Mini*' size for minimum uterine length 5 cm; '*Normal*' size for uterine length 6.5–9 cm; replacement every 5 years.
FLEXI-T ® 300 For uterine length over 5 cm; replacement every 5 years.
FLEXI-T ®+ 380 For uterine length over 6 cm; replacement every 5 years.
GYNEFIX ® Suitable for all uterine sizes; replacement every 5 years.
IUB BALLERINE MIDI ® For uterine length over 6 cm; replacement every 5 years.
LOAD ® 375 For uterine length over 7 cm; replacement every 5 years.
MINI TT380 ® SLIMLINE For minimum uterine length 5 cm; replacement every 5 years.
MULTI-SAFE ® 375 For uterine length 6–9 cm; replacement every 5 years.
MULTILOAD ® CU375 For uterine length 6–9 cm; replacement every 5 years.
NEO-SAFE ® T380 For uterine length 6.5–9 cm; replacement every 5 years.
NOVA-T ® 380 For uterine length 6.5–9 cm; replacement every 5 years.
T-SAFE ® 380A QL For uterine length 6.5–9 cm; replacement every 10 years.
TT380 ® SLIMLINE For uterine length 6.5–9 cm; replacement every 10 years.
UT380 SHORT ® For uterine length 5–7 cm; replacement every 5 years.
UT380 STANDARD ® For uterine length 6.5–9 cm; replacement every 5 years.

- **MEDICINAL FORMS** There can be variation in the licensing of different medicines containing the same drug.

  Products without form

  ▶ **Intra-uterine contraceptive devices** (R.F. Medical Supplies Ltd, Farla Medical Ltd, Durbin Plc, Williams Medical Supplies Ltd, Bayer Plc)
  Copper T380 A intra-uterine contraceptive device | 1 device £8.95
  Steriload intra-uterine contraceptive device | 1 device £9.65
  Load 375 intra-uterine contraceptive device | 1 device £8.52
  T-Safe 380A QL intra-uterine contraceptive device | 1 device £11.38
  UT380 Standard intra-uterine contraceptive device | 1 device £11.22
  Nova-T 380 intra-uterine contraceptive device | 1 device £15.20
  Flexi-T+ 380 intra-uterine contraceptive device | 1 device £10.06
  Eurogine T 380 Cu intra-uterine contraceptive device normal | 1 device £10.95
  Mini TT380 Slimline intra-uterine contraceptive device | 1 device £12.46
  Eurogine T 380 Ag intra-uterine contraceptive device mini | 1 device £12.50
  Eurogine T 380 Ag intra-uterine contraceptive device normal | 1 device £12.50
  Flexi-T 300 intra-uterine contraceptive device | 1 device £9.47
  Eurogine T 380 Cu intra-uterine contraceptive device mini | 1 device £10.95
  Multi-Safe 375 intra-uterine contraceptive device | 1 device £8.96
  Optima TCu 380A intra-uterine contraceptive device | 1 device £9.65
  GyneFix intra-uterine contraceptive device | 1 device £27.11
  TT380 Slimline intra-uterine contraceptive device | 1 device £12.46
  Ancora 375 Cu intra-uterine contraceptive device | 1 device £7.95
  Neo-Safe T380 intra-uterine contraceptive device | 1 device £13.40
  UT380 Short intra-uterine contraceptive device | 1 device £11.22

Silicone contraceptive pessaries

- **SILICONE CONTRACEPTIVE PESSARIES**

  FemCap 22mm (Durbin Plc)
  | 1 device · NHS indicative price = £15.29 · Drug Tariff (Part IXa)

  FemCap 26mm (Durbin Plc)
  | 1 device · NHS indicative price = £15.29 · Drug Tariff (Part IXa)

  FemCap 30mm (Durbin Plc)
  | 1 device · NHS indicative price = £15.29 · Drug Tariff (Part IXa)

3.3 Contraception, emergency

> **Other drugs used for Contraception, emergency** Intra-uterine contraceptive devices (copper), p. 928 · Levonorgestrel, p. 932

PROGESTERONE RECEPTOR MODULATORS

Uliprital acetate   13-Apr-2021

- **DRUG ACTION** Ulipristal acetate is a synthetic, selective progesterone receptor modulator with a partial progesterone antagonist effect.

- **INDICATIONS AND DOSE**

  Emergency contraception
  ▶ BY MOUTH
  ▶ Females of childbearing potential: 30 mg for 1 dose, to be taken as soon as possible after coitus, but no later than after 120 hours

  Uterine fibroids (under expert supervision)
  ▶ BY MOUTH
  ▶ Adult: 5 mg once daily for up to 3 months, to be started during the first week of menstruation, treatment course may be repeated if necessary; re-treatment should start no sooner than during the first week of the second menstruation following completion of the previous course; maximum 4 courses

> **IMPORTANT SAFETY INFORMATION**
>
> **MHRA/CHM ADVICE: ULIPRISTAL ACETATE 5 MG (*ESMYA*®): FURTHER RESTRICTIONS DUE TO RISK OF SERIOUS LIVER INJURY (FEBRUARY 2021)**
>
> Rare but serious cases of liver injury and hepatic failure requiring liver transplantation have been reported worldwide in women treated with *Esmya*® for symptoms of uterine fibroids. Its licence was temporarily suspended in March 2020 to allow a further review of these risks. Although the temporary suspension has been lifted, further restrictions have been introduced.
>
> Healthcare professionals are advised that *Esmya*® should only be used for intermittent treatment of moderate to severe uterine fibroid symptoms before menopause and when surgical procedures (including uterine fibroid embolisation) are not suitable or have failed. If considered to be appropriate therapy, the risks and benefits of *Esmya*® should be discussed with patients before prescribing so that they can make an informed decision about treatment options. Liver function should be monitored before, during, and after treatment courses (see *Monitoring requirements*); *Esmya*® should not be used in those with an underlying liver disorder. Patients should be advised to stop therapy and seek immediate medical advice if any signs of liver damage develop.
>
> There are currently no concerns with the use of the emergency contraceptive *ellaOne*®—see *Indications and dose*.

- **CONTRA-INDICATIONS**

  GENERAL CONTRA-INDICATIONS Breast cancer · cervical cancer · ovarian cancer · severe asthma controlled by oral glucocorticoids · undiagnosed vaginal bleeding · uterine cancer

  SPECIFIC CONTRA-INDICATIONS
  ▶ When used for Uterine fibroids   Vaginal bleeding not caused by uterine fibroids

- **INTERACTIONS** → Appendix 1: ulipristal

- **SIDE-EFFECTS**
  ▶ **Common or very common** Asthenia · breast abnormalities · dizziness · endometrial thickening · gastrointestinal discomfort · headaches · hot flush · menstrual cycle irregularities · mood altered · myalgia · nausea · ovarian and fallopian tube disorders · pain · pelvic pain · skin reactions · vertigo · vomiting · weight increased
  ▶ **Uncommon** Alopecia · anxiety · appetite disorder · chills · concentration impaired · constipation · diarrhoea · drowsiness · dry mouth · fever · flatulence · genital abnormalities · hyperhidrosis · increased risk of infection · insomnia · libido disorder · malaise · oedema · urinary incontinence · vision disorders · vulvovaginal disorders
  ▶ **Rare or very rare** Abnormal sensation in eye · disorientation · dry throat · epistaxis · eye erythema · painful sexual intercourse · syncope · taste altered · thirst · tremor
  ▶ **Frequency not known** Angioedema · hepatic disorders

- **CONCEPTION AND CONTRACEPTION**
  ▶ When used for Uterine fibroids EvGr Non-hormonal contraceptive methods should be used during treatment and for 12 days after stopping, if required. ◈

- **PREGNANCY**
  ▶ When used for Emergency contraception EvGr Limited information available—if pregnancy occurs, report to the *ellaOne*® pregnancy registry. ◈
  ▶ When used for Uterine fibroids EvGr Avoid—limited information available. ◈

● **BREAST FEEDING**
▸ When used for Emergency contraception EvGr Avoid for 1 week after administration—present in milk. Ⓜ
▸ When used for Uterine fibroids EvGr Avoid—present in milk but no further information available. Ⓜ

● **HEPATIC IMPAIRMENT**
▸ When used for Emergency contraception EvGr Avoid in severe impairment—no information available. Ⓜ
▸ When used for Uterine fibroids EvGr Avoid—risk of increased exposure. Ⓜ

● **RENAL IMPAIRMENT**
▸ When used for Uterine fibroids EvGr Avoid in severe impairment unless patient is closely monitored—no information available. Ⓜ

● **MONITORING REQUIREMENTS**
▸ When used for Uterine fibroids EvGr Perform liver function tests before treatment initiation—do not initiate if serum transaminases exceed 2 times the upper limit of normal. During the first 2 treatment courses, monitor liver function monthly; for further treatment courses, perform liver function tests once before each new treatment course and when clinically indicated. At the end of each treatment course, perform liver function tests after 2-4 weeks. Discontinue treatment if serum transaminases exceed 3 times the upper limit of normal and closely monitor patient. Periodically monitor the endometrium following repeated intermittent treatment. Ⓜ

● **PATIENT AND CARER ADVICE**
▸ When used for Emergency contraception When prescribing or supplying hormonal emergency contraception, women should be told:
  ● if vomiting occurs within 3 hours of taking a dose, a replacement dose should be taken;
  ● that their next period may be early or late;
  ● to seek medical attention promptly if any lower abdominal pain occurs because this could signify an ectopic pregnancy.
The Faculty of Sexual and Reproductive Healthcare also advises women should be told:
  ● that a barrier method of contraception needs to be used—see Emergency contraception p. 916 for further information;
  ● that a pregnancy test should be performed if the next menstrual period is delayed by more than 7 days, is lighter than usual, or is associated with abdominal pain that is not typical of the woman's usual dysmenorrhoea;
  ● that a pregnancy test should be performed if hormonal contraception is started soon after use of emergency contraception even if they have bleeding; bleeding associated with the contraceptive method may not represent menstruation.
▸ When used for Uterine fibroids Prescribers should explain to patients the requirement for treatment-free intervals—see also *Important safety information*.
Patient card
▸ When used for Uterine fibroids A patient card should be provided.
Missed doses
  ▸ When used for Uterine fibroids If a dose is more than 12 hours late, the missed dose should not be taken and the next dose should be taken at the normal time.
Driving and skilled tasks
  ▸ When used for Emergency contraception Patients and carers should be counselled on the effects on driving and performance of skilled tasks—increased risk of dizziness.

● **MEDICINAL FORMS** There can be variation in the licensing of different medicines containing the same drug.
Oral tablet
▸ Ulipristal acetate (Non-proprietary)
  Ulipristal acetate 30 mg Ulipristal 30mg tablets | 1 tablet Ⓟ
  £11.50–£19.60 DT = £14.05

▸ Ellaone (Omega Pharma Ltd)
  Ulipristal acetate 30 mg EllaOne 30mg tablets | 1 tablet Ⓟ £14.05
  DT = £14.05

3.4 Contraception, oral progestogen-only

Other drugs used for **Contraception, oral progestogen-only** Norethisterone, p. 878

PROGESTOGENS

Desogestrel

02-May-2024

● **INDICATIONS AND DOSE**
Contraception
▸ BY MOUTH
▸ Females of childbearing potential: 75 micrograms daily, dose to be taken at same time each day, starting on day 1 of cycle then continuously, if administration delayed for 12 hours or more it should be regarded as a 'missed pill'

● **CONTRA-INDICATIONS** Acute porphyrias p. 1202 · current breast cancer

● **CAUTIONS** Cardiac dysfunction · diabetes (progestogens can decrease glucose tolerance—monitor patient closely) · history of breast cancer—seek specialist advice before use · history of stroke (including transient ischaemic attack) · history of venous thromboembolism · ischaemic heart disease · liver tumours—seek specialist advice before use · malabsorption states · migraine with aura · multiple risk factors for cardiovascular disease · positive antiphospholipid antibodies · rheumatoid arthritis · systemic lupus erythematosus · undiagnosed vaginal bleeding

● **INTERACTIONS** → Appendix 1: desogestrel

● **SIDE-EFFECTS**
▸ **Common or very common** Breast abnormalities · depressed mood · headache · libido decreased · menstrual cycle irregularities · mood altered · nausea · skin reactions · weight increased
▸ **Uncommon** Alopecia · contact lens intolerance · fatigue · ovarian cyst · vomiting · vulvovaginal infection
▸ **Rare or very rare** Erythema nodosum
▸ **Frequency not known** Angioedema · arterial thromboembolism · neoplasms

SIDE-EFFECTS, FURTHER INFORMATION The benefits of using progestogen-only contraceptives (POCs), such as desogestrel, should be weighed against the possible risks for each individual woman.

There is a possible small increase in the risk of breast cancer in women using, or who have recently used, progestogen-only contraception. Causal association is not clearly established, and absolute risk remains very small, and is like that of current or recent use of combined hormonal contraception.

The most important risk factor for breast cancer appears to be the age the contraceptive is stopped rather than the duration of use; the risk gradually disappears during the 10 years after stopping.

● **ALLERGY AND CROSS-SENSITIVITY** EvGr *Feanolla* ®, *Lovima* ® and *Moonia* ® tablets contra-indicated in patients with hypersensitivity or allergy to peanuts or soya. Ⓜ

● **PREGNANCY** Not known to be harmful.

● **BREAST FEEDING** EvGr Suitable for use, however, a small amount of its active metabolite etonogestrel is present in milk Ⓜ (recommendation also supported by primary literature). [EvGr] A decrease in milk production has been reported infrequently. ⟨M⟩

- **HEPATIC IMPAIRMENT** Manufacturer advises caution; avoid in severe or active disease.

- **PATIENT AND CARER ADVICE**
Surgery All progestogen-only contraceptives are suitable for use as an alternative to combined hormonal contraceptives before major elective surgery, before all surgery to the legs, or before surgery which involves prolonged immobilisation of a lower limb.
Starting routine One tablet daily, on a continuous basis, starting on day 1 of cycle and taken at the same time each day (if delayed by longer than 12 hours contraceptive protection may be lost). Additional contraceptive precautions are not required if desogestrel is started up to and including day 5 of the menstrual cycle; if started after this time, additional contraceptive precautions are required for 2 days.
Changing from a combined oral contraceptive Start on the day following completion of the combined oral contraceptive course without a break (or in the case of *everyday* (ED) tablets, omitting the inactive tablets).
After childbirth (not breast-feeding) Oral progestogen-only contraceptives can be started before 21 days postpartum without the need for additional contraceptive precautions. If started 21 days or more postpartum, additional contraceptive precautions are required for 2 days.
Diarrhoea and vomiting Vomiting and persistent, severe diarrhoea can interfere with the absorption of oral progestogen-only contraceptives. If vomiting occurs within 2 hours of taking desogestrel, another pill should be taken as soon as possible. If a replacement pill is not taken within 12 hours of the normal time for taking desogestrel, or in cases of persistent vomiting or very severe diarrhoea, additional precautions should be used during illness and for 2 days after recovery.
Missed doses The following advice is recommended: 'If you forget a pill, take it as soon as you remember and carry on with the next pill at the right time (this may mean taking 2 pills at the same time). If the pill was more than 12 hours overdue you are not protected. Continue normal pill-taking but you must also use another method, such as the condom, for the next 2 days'.
   The Faculty of Sexual and Reproductive Healthcare recommends emergency contraception if one or more tablets are missed or taken more than 12 hours late and unprotected intercourse has occurred before 2 further tablets have been correctly taken.

- **NATIONAL FUNDING/ACCESS DECISIONS**
For full details see funding body website
Scottish Medicines Consortium (SMC) decisions
▶ Desogestrel (*Cerazette*®) for use as contraception (September 2003) SMC No. 36/03 Recommended with restrictions

- **EXCEPTIONS TO LEGAL CATEGORY** *Hana*® 75 microgram tablets and *Lovima*® 75 microgram tablets can be sold to the public for use as oral contraception in females of childbearing potential, following a clinical assessment.

- **MEDICINAL FORMS** There can be variation in the licensing of different medicines containing the same drug.

Oral tablet
▶ **Desogestrel (Non-proprietary)**
Desogestrel 75 microgram Desogestrel 75microgram tablets |
84 tablet [PoM] £9.55 DT = £2.09
▶ **Cerazette** (Organon Pharma (UK) Ltd)
Desogestrel 75 microgram Cerazette 75microgram tablets |
84 tablet [PoM] £9.55 DT = £2.09
▶ **Cerelle** (Gedeon Richter (UK) Ltd)
Desogestrel 75 microgram Cerelle 75microgram tablets |
84 tablet [PoM] £4.30 DT = £2.09
▶ **Desorex** (Somex Pharma)
Desogestrel 75 microgram Desorex 75microgram tablets |
84 tablet [PoM] £2.45 DT = £2.09

▶ **Zelleta** (Morningside Healthcare Ltd)
Desogestrel 75 microgram Zelleta 75microgram tablets |
84 tablet [PoM] £3.51 DT = £2.09

Drospirenone
19-Dec-2023

- **INDICATIONS AND DOSE**
Contraception
▶ BY MOUTH
▶ Females of childbearing potential: 1 active tablet once daily for 24 days, followed by 1 inactive tablet once daily for 4 days, to be started on day 1 of cycle with first active tablet (withdrawal bleeding may occur during the 4-day interval of inactive tablets); subsequent courses repeated without interval, if administration delayed for 24 hours or more it should be regarded as a 'missed pill'

- **CONTRA-INDICATIONS** Acute porphyrias p. 1202 · current breast cancer
- **CAUTIONS** Diabetes (progestogens can decrease glucose tolerance—monitor patient closely) · history of breast cancer—seek specialist advice before use · history of stroke (including transient ischaemic attack) · history of venous thromboembolism · hyperkalaemia · hypoaldosteronism— consider assessing urea and electrolytes, and blood pressure · ischaemic heart disease · liver tumours—seek specialist advice before use · multiple risk factors for cardiovascular disease · undiagnosed vaginal bleeding
- **INTERACTIONS** → Appendix 1: drospirenone
- **SIDE-EFFECTS**
▶ **Common or very common** Abdominal pain · breast abnormalities · headache · libido disorder · menstrual cycle irregularities · mood altered · nausea · skin reactions · vaginal haemorrhage · weight changes
▶ **Uncommon** Alopecia · anaemia · anxiety · appetite disorder · constipation · depression · diarrhoea · dizziness · fatigue · hot flush · hyperhidrosis · hyperkalaemia · hypertension · ovarian cyst · pelvic pain · peripheral oedema · seborrhoea · uterine leiomyoma · vomiting · vulvovaginal disorders · vulvovaginal infection
▶ **Rare or very rare** Cervical dysplasia · contact lens intolerance · galactorrhoea · polyuria
- **PREGNANCY** [EvGr] Not known to be harmful. ⟨M⟩
- **BREAST FEEDING** [EvGr] Progestogen-only contraceptives do not affect lactation. ⟨M⟩
- **HEPATIC IMPAIRMENT** [EvGr] Avoid in severe disease. ⟨M⟩
- **RENAL IMPAIRMENT** [EvGr] Avoid in severe renal insufficiency or acute renal failure (potential risk of hyperkalaemia). ⟨M⟩ The FSRH advises caution in mild to moderate impairment, or significant risk factors for chronic kidney disease particularly if aged over 50 years— consider assessing urea and electrolytes, and blood pressure.

- **PATIENT AND CARER ADVICE**
Surgery All progestogen-only contraceptives are suitable for use as an alternative to combined hormonal contraceptives before major elective surgery, before all surgery to the legs, or before surgery which involves prolonged immobilisation of a lower limb.
Starting routine One tablet daily, on a continuous basis, starting on day 1 of cycle and taken at the same time each day (if delayed by longer than 24 hours contraceptive protection may be lost). If started at any other time, additional contraceptive precautions are required for 7 days.
Changing from a combined oral contraceptive Start on the day following completion of the combined oral contraceptive course without a break (or in the case of *everyday* (ED) tablets, omitting the inactive tablets).

After childbirth (not breast-feeding) Oral progestogen-only contraceptives can be started before 21 days postpartum without the need for additional contraceptive precautions. If started 21 days or more postpartum, additional contraceptive precautions are required for 7 days.
Diarrhoea and vomiting Vomiting and persistent, severe diarrhoea can interfere with the absorption of oral progestogen-only contraceptives. If vomiting occurs within 3–4 hours of taking drospirenone, another pill should be taken as soon as possible. If a replacement pill is not taken within 24 hours of the normal time for taking drospirenone, or in cases of persistent vomiting or very severe diarrhoea, additional precautions should be used during illness and for 7 days after recovery.
Missed doses The following advice is recommended: 'If you forget any active pill, take it as soon as you remember and carry on with the next pill at the right time (this may mean taking 2 pills at the same time). If the active pill was more than 24 hours overdue you are not protected. Continue normal pill-taking but you must also use another method, such as the condom, for the next 7 days. If these 7 days run into or beyond the end of the packet, the next packet should be started at once, omitting the 4 inactive pills'.

The FSRH recommends emergency contraception if:
- any active tablets are missed or taken more than 24 hours late and unprotected intercourse has occurred before 7 further tablets have been correctly taken *or*
- active tablets are missed or taken more than 24 hours late on days 1–7 and unprotected intercourse has occurred during the preceding 4-day interval of inactive tablets or during week 1.

- **MEDICINAL FORMS** There can be variation in the licensing of different medicines containing the same drug.
Oral tablet
  - **Slynd** (Exeltis UK Ltd)
    Drospirenone 4 mg Slynd 4mg tablets | 84 tablet PoM £14.70 DT = £14.70

Levonorgestrel

02-Aug-2024

- **INDICATIONS AND DOSE**
Emergency contraception
- BY MOUTH
- Females of childbearing potential: 1.5 mg for 1 dose, taken as soon as possible after coitus, preferably within 12 hours and no later than after 72 hours (may also be used between 72–96 hours after coitus but efficacy decreases with time), alternatively 3 mg for 1 dose, taken as soon as possible after coitus, preferably within 12 hours and no later than after 72 hours (may also be used between 72–96 hours after coitus but efficacy decreases with time). Higher dose should be considered for patients with body-weight over 70 kg or BMI over 26 kg/m^2

Contraception
- BY MOUTH
- Females of childbearing potential: 30 micrograms daily starting on day 1 of the cycle then continuously, dose is to be taken at the same time each day, if administration delayed for 3 hours or more it should be regarded as a "missed pill"

BENILEXA ® ONE HANDED 20MICROGRAMS/24HOURS INTRA-UTERINE DELIVERY SYSTEM

Contraception | Menorrhagia
- BY INTRA-UTERINE ADMINISTRATION
- Females of childbearing potential: Insert within 5 days of onset of menstruation, post-abortion or miscarriage, or at any time if replacement within licensed duration of use or if reasonably certain female is not pregnant and there is no risk of conception; postpartum insertions should be performed ≤48 hours after delivery, or delayed until ≥4 weeks and, either inserted within 5 days of onset of menstruation, or at any time if criteria for lactational amenorrhoea method are met. If the above criteria are not met, additional contraceptive precautions, e.g. barrier methods, should be used for at least 7 days before replacement or following insertion. Effective for 8 years when used for contraception if age <45, or until age 55 if age ≥45 at time of insertion; effective for 3 years when used for menorrhagia

Prevention of endometrial hyperplasia during oestrogen replacement therapy
- BY INTRA-UTERINE ADMINISTRATION
- Females of childbearing potential: Insert during last days of menstruation or withdrawal bleeding or at any time if amenorrhoeic; effective for 5 years

JAYDESS ® 13.5MG INTRA-UTERINE DEVICE

Contraception
- BY INTRA-UTERINE ADMINISTRATION
- Females of childbearing potential: Insert within 5 days of onset of menstruation, post-abortion or miscarriage, or at any time if replacement within licensed duration of use or if reasonably certain female is not pregnant and there is no risk of conception; postpartum insertions should be performed ≤48 hours after delivery, or delayed until ≥4 weeks and, either inserted within 5 days of onset of menstruation, or at any time if criteria for lactational amenorrhoea method are met. If the above criteria are not met, additional contraceptive precautions, e.g. barrier methods, should be used for at least 7 days before replacement or following insertion. Effective for 3 years

KYLEENA ® 19.5MG INTRA-UTERINE DEVICE

Contraception
- BY INTRA-UTERINE ADMINISTRATION
- Females of childbearing potential: Insert within 5 days of onset of menstruation, post-abortion or miscarriage, or at any time if replacement within licensed duration of use or if reasonably certain female is not pregnant and there is no risk of conception; postpartum insertions should be performed ≤48 hours after delivery, or delayed until ≥4 weeks and, either inserted within 5 days of onset of menstruation, or at any time if criteria for lactational amenorrhoea method are met. If the above criteria are not met, additional contraceptive precautions, e.g. barrier methods, should be used for at least 7 days before replacement or following insertion. Effective for 5 years

LEVOSERT ® 20MICROGRAMS/24HOURS INTRA-UTERINE DEVICE

Contraception | Menorrhagia
- BY INTRA-UTERINE ADMINISTRATION
- Females of childbearing potential: Insert within 5 days of onset of menstruation, post-abortion or miscarriage, or at any time if replacement within licensed duration of use or if reasonably certain female is not pregnant and there is no risk of conception; postpartum insertions should be performed ≤48 hours after delivery, or delayed until ≥4 weeks and, either inserted within 5 days of onset of menstruation, or at any time if criteria for lactational amenorrhoea method are met. If the above criteria are not met, additional contraceptive precautions, e.g. barrier methods, should be used for at least 7 days before replacement or following insertion. Effective for 8 years when used for contraception if age <45, or until age 55 if age ≥45 at time of insertion; effective for 3 years when used for menorrhagia

Prevention of endometrial hyperplasia during oestrogen replacement therapy

▸ BY INTRA-UTERINE ADMINISTRATION

▸ Females of childbearing potential: Insert during last days of menstruation or withdrawal bleeding or at any time if amenorrhoeic; effective for 5 years

MIRENA ® 20MICROGRAMS/24HOURS INTRA-UTERINE DEVICE

Contraception | Menorrhagia

▸ BY INTRA-UTERINE ADMINISTRATION

▸ Females of childbearing potential: Insert within 5 days of onset of menstruation, post-abortion or miscarriage, or at any time if replacement within licensed duration of use or if reasonably certain female is not pregnant and there is no risk of conception; postpartum insertions should be performed ≤48 hours after delivery, or delayed until ≥4 weeks and, either inserted within 5 days of onset of menstruation, or at any time if criteria for lactational amenorrhoea method are met. If the above criteria are not met, additional contraceptive precautions, e.g. barrier methods, should be used for at least 7 days before replacement or following insertion. Effective for 8 years when used for contraception if age <45, or until age 55 if age ≥45 at time of insertion; effective for 5 years when used for menorrhagia

Prevention of endometrial hyperplasia during oestrogen replacement therapy

▸ BY INTRA-UTERINE ADMINISTRATION

▸ Females of childbearing potential: Insert during last days of menstruation or withdrawal bleeding or at any time if amenorrhoeic; effective for 5 years

DOSE ADJUSTMENTS DUE TO INTERACTIONS

▸ When used orally as an emergency contraceptive, the effectiveness of levonorgestrel could be reduced in women taking enzyme-inducing drugs (and for up to 4 weeks after stopping); a copper intra-uterine device should preferably be used instead. If the copper intra-uterine device is undesirable or inappropriate, the dose of levonorgestrel should be increased to a total of 3 mg taken as a single dose; pregnancy should be excluded following use, and medical advice sought if pregnancy occurs.

● **UNLICENSED USE**

▸ With intra-uterine use The FSRH advises levonorgestrel is used as detailed below, although these situations are considered unlicensed:
  - Insertion at any time if reasonably certain the woman is not pregnant or at risk of pregnancy;
  - Additional precautions (e.g. barrier methods) for at least 7 days before replacement even if immediate replacement is intended;
  - Insertion immediately following termination of pregnancy if successful expulsion is confirmed;
  - Postpartum insertions within 48 hours or 4 weeks after delivery;
  - Duration of use for 52 mg levonorgestrel intra-uterine devices for contraception and prevention of endometrial hyperplasia during oestrogen replacement therapy.

▸ With oral use The FSRH advises levonorgestrel is used as detailed below, although these situations are considered unlicensed:
  - Higher dose option for emergency contraception in patients with body-weight over 70 kg or BMI over 26 kg/m^2;
  - Use for emergency contraception between 72–96 hours after coitus.

▸ With intra-uterine use or oral use in children Consult product literature for licensing status of individual preparations.

BENILEXA ® ONE HANDED 20MICROGRAMS/24HOURS INTRA-UTERINE DELIVERY SYSTEM The FSRH advises *Benilexa* ® is used for the prevention of endometrial hyperplasia, although this is considered unlicensed.

LEVOSERT ® 20MICROGRAMS/24HOURS INTRA-UTERINE DEVICE The FSRH advises *Levosert* ® is used for the prevention of endometrial hyperplasia, although this is considered unlicensed.

> **IMPORTANT SAFETY INFORMATION**
>
> **MHRA/CHM ADVICE (JUNE 2015) INTRA-UTERINE CONTRACEPTION: UTERINE PERFORATION—UPDATED INFORMATION ON RISK FACTORS**
>
> Uterine perforation most often occurs during insertion, but might not be detected until sometime later. The risk of uterine perforation is increased when the device is inserted up to 36 weeks postpartum or in patients who are breastfeeding. Before inserting an intra-uterine contraceptive device, inform patients that perforation occurs in approximately 1 in every 1000 insertions and signs and symptoms include:
> - severe pelvic pain after insertion (worse than period cramps);
> - pain or increased bleeding after insertion which continues for more than a few weeks;
> - sudden changes in periods;
> - pain during intercourse;
> - unable to feel the threads.
>
> Patients should be informed on how to check their threads and to arrange a check-up if threads cannot be felt, especially if they also have significant pain. Partial perforation may occur even if the threads can be seen; consider this if there is severe pain following insertion and perform an ultrasound.

● **CONTRA-INDICATIONS**

GENERAL CONTRA-INDICATIONS Current breast cancer (use with caution for emergency contraception)

SPECIFIC CONTRA-INDICATIONS

▸ With intra-uterine use Active trophoblastic disease (until return to normal of urine- and plasma-gonadotrophin concentration) · acute malignancies affecting the blood (use with caution in remission) · not suitable for emergency contraception · pelvic inflammatory disease · post-abortion sepsis · postpartum sepsis · recent sexually transmitted infection (if not fully investigated and treated) · unexplained uterine bleeding · uterine or cervical malignancy

▸ With oral use Acute porphyrias p. 1202

● **CAUTIONS**

GENERAL CAUTIONS Cardiac disease—seek specialist advice for intra-uterine insertion · diabetes · history of breast cancer—seek specialist advice before use · history of stroke (including transient ischaemic attack) · history of venous thromboembolism · ischaemic heart disease · migraine · multiple risk factors for cardiovascular disease · positive antiphospholipid antibodies · rheumatoid arthritis · systemic lupus erythematosus

SPECIFIC CAUTIONS

▸ With intra-uterine use Anatomical abnormalities—seek specialist advice before use · cervical intraepithelial neoplasia · epilepsy (risk of seizure at time of insertion) · immunosuppression (risk of infection)—seek specialist advice before use · postpartum—seek specialist advice before use · risk of sexually transmitted infections · young age

▸ With oral use Malabsorption states

▸ With oral use for Contraception Undiagnosed vaginal bleeding

CAUTIONS, FURTHER INFORMATION
▶ With intra-uterine use [EvGr] If removal is after day 7 of the menstrual cycle, intercourse should be avoided or another method of contraception used for at least 7 days before removal of intra-uterine device. ⟨M⟩
▶ Sexually transmitted infections and pelvic inflammatory disease
▶ With intra-uterine use The main excess risk of pelvic infection occurs in the first 3 weeks after insertion and is believed to be related to existing carriage of a sexually transmitted infection. The FSRH advises pre-insertion screening (for chlamydia and, depending on sexual history and local prevalence of disease, *Neisseria gonorrhoeae*) be performed in women at risk of sexually transmitted infections.

MIRENA ® 20MICROGRAMS/24HOURS INTRA-UTERINE DEVICE Advanced uterine atrophy

● INTERACTIONS → Appendix 1: levonorgestrel

● SIDE-EFFECTS
GENERAL SIDE-EFFECTS
▶ **Common or very common** Dizziness · gastrointestinal discomfort · haemorrhage · headaches · menstrual cycle irregularities · nausea · skin reactions
SPECIFIC SIDE-EFFECTS
▶ **Common or very common**
▶ With intra-uterine use Back pain · breast abnormalities · depression · device expulsion · hirsutism · increased risk of infection · libido decreased · nervousness · ovarian cyst · pelvic disorders · vulvovaginal disorders · weight increased
▶ With oral use Breast tenderness · diarrhoea · fatigue · vomiting
▶ **Uncommon**
▶ With intra-uterine use Alopecia · endometritis · oedema · uterine rupture
▶ **Rare or very rare**
▶ With oral use Face oedema · pelvic pain
▶ **Frequency not known**
▶ With intra-uterine use Breast cancer
▶ With oral use Arterial thromboembolism · cerebrovascular insufficiency · depressed mood · diabetes mellitus · neoplasms · sexual dysfunction · weight changes

SIDE-EFFECTS, FURTHER INFORMATION **Breast cancer risk with contraceptive use** The benefits of using progestogen-only contraceptives (POCs), such as levonorgestrel, should be weighed against the possible risks for each individual woman.

There is a possible small increase in the risk of breast cancer in women using, or who have recently used, progestogen-only contraception. Causal association is not clearly established, and absolute risk remains very small, and is like that of current or recent use of combined hormonal contraception.

The most important risk factor for breast cancer appears to be the age the contraceptive is stopped rather than the duration of use; the risk gradually disappears during the 10 years after stopping.

With intra-uterine use Patients should be informed about the device that has been inserted and when it should be removed or replaced (including referring them to a patient information leaflet and other sources of information).

Patients may experience irregular, prolonged or infrequent menstrual bleeding in the 3–6 months following insertion; bleeding pattern improves with time but persists in some patients.

Progestogenic side-effects resolve with time (after the first few months).

● PREGNANCY
▶ With oral use Not known to be harmful.
▶ With intra-uterine use If an intra-uterine device fails and the woman wishes to continue to full-term, the device should

be removed in the first trimester if possible. Avoid—if pregnancy occurs remove intra-uterine device.

● BREAST FEEDING Progestogen-only contraceptives do not affect lactation.

● HEPATIC IMPAIRMENT
▶ With intra-uterine use or oral use for Contraception Manufacturer advises avoid in liver tumour.
▶ With oral use for Contraception or Emergency contraception Manufacturer advises avoid in severe impairment.
▶ With intra-uterine use Manufacturer advises avoid in acute hepatic disease or in severe impairment (no information available)—consult product literature.

● MONITORING REQUIREMENTS
▶ With intra-uterine use Gynaecological examination before insertion, 4–6 weeks after insertion, then annually.

● DIRECTIONS FOR ADMINISTRATION
▶ With intra-uterine use The doctor or nurse inserting (or removing) the device should be fully trained in the technique and should provide full counselling reinforced by the patient information leaflet.

● PRESCRIBING AND DISPENSING INFORMATION
▶ With intra-uterine use Levonorgestrel-releasing intra-uterine devices vary in licensed indication, duration of use and insertion technique—the MHRA recommends to prescribe and dispense by brand name to avoid inadvertent switching.

● PATIENT AND CARER ADVICE
Diarrhoea and vomiting with use as an oral contraceptive Vomiting and persistent, severe diarrhoea can interfere with the absorption of oral progestogen-only contraceptives. If vomiting occurs within 2 hours of taking an oral progestogen-only contraceptive, another pill should be taken as soon as possible. If a replacement pill is not taken within 3 hours of the normal time for taking the progestogen-only pill, or in cases of persistent vomiting or very severe diarrhoea, additional precautions should be used during illness and for 2 days after recovery.
Starting routine
▶ With oral use for Contraception One tablet daily, on a continuous basis, starting on day 1 of cycle and taken at the same time each day (if delayed by longer than 3 hours contraceptive protection may be lost). Additional contraceptive precautions are not required if levonorgestrel is started up to and including day 5 of the menstrual cycle; if started after this time, additional contraceptive precautions are required for 2 days.
Changing from a combined oral contraceptive Start on the day following completion of the combined oral contraceptive course without a break (or in the case of *everyday* (ED) tablets, omitting the inactive tablets).
After childbirth (not breast-feeding) Oral progestogen-only contraceptives can be started before 21 days postpartum without the need for additional contraceptive precautions. If started 21 days or more postpartum, additional contraceptive precautions are required for 2 days.
▶ With oral use for Emergency contraception When prescribing or supplying hormonal emergency contraception, manufacturer advises women should be told:
● if vomiting occurs within 3 hours, a replacement dose should be taken;
● that their next period may be early or late;
● to seek medical attention promptly if any lower abdominal pain occurs because this could signify an ectopic pregnancy.
The Faculty of Sexual and Reproductive Healthcare also advises women should be told:
● that a barrier method of contraception needs to be used—see Emergency contraception p. 916 for further information;
● that a pregnancy test should be performed if the next menstrual period is delayed by more than 7 days, is

lighter than usual, or is associated with abdominal pain that is not typical of the woman's usual dysmenorrhoea;

- that a pregnancy test should be performed if hormonal contraception is started soon after use of emergency contraception even if they have bleeding; bleeding associated with the contraceptive method may not represent menstruation.

▸ With intra-uterine use   Counsel women on the signs, symptoms and risks of perforation and ectopic pregnancy. **Missed doses**   When used as an oral contraceptive, the following advice is recommended 'If you forget a pill, take it as soon as you remember and carry on with the next pill at the right time (this may mean taking 2 pills at the same time). If the pill was more than 3 hours overdue you are not protected. Continue normal pill-taking but you must also use another method, such as the condom, for the next 2 days'.

The Faculty of Sexual and Reproductive Healthcare recommends emergency contraception if one or more progestogen-only contraceptive tablets are missed or taken more than 3 hours late and unprotected intercourse has occurred before 2 further tablets have been correctly taken.

- **NATIONAL FUNDING/ACCESS DECISIONS**
For full details see funding body website
Scottish Medicines Consortium (SMC) decisions
▸ **Levonorgestrel (*Kyleena*®) for contraception for up to 5 years (February 2018)** SMC No. 1299/18 Recommended
All Wales Medicines Strategy Group (AWMSG) decisions
▸ **Levonorgestrel (*Kyleena*®) for contraception for up to 5 years (September 2018)** AWMSG No. 3582 Recommended

- **EXCEPTIONS TO LEGAL CATEGORY**   *Levonelle*® *One Step* can be sold to women over 16 years; when supplying emergency contraception to the public, pharmacists should refer to guidance issued by the Royal Pharmaceutical Society.

- **MEDICINAL FORMS**   There can be variation in the licensing of different medicines containing the same drug.

Oral tablet
▸ **Levonorgestrel (Non-proprietary)**
Levonorgestrel 1.5 mg   Levonorgestrel 1.5mg tablets | 1 tablet [PoM] £2.74–£3.74 DT = £2.74
▸ **Emerres** (Morningside Healthcare Ltd)
Levonorgestrel 1.5 mg   Emerres 1.5mg tablets | 1 tablet [PoM] £3.65 DT = £2.74
▸ **Levonelle** (Bayer Plc)
Levonorgestrel 1.5 mg   Levonelle 1500microgram tablets | 1 tablet [PoM] £5.20 DT = £2.74
▸ **Melkine** (Crescent Pharma Ltd)
Levonorgestrel 1.5 mg   Melkine 1.5mg tablets | 1 tablet [PoM] £4.16 DT = £2.74
▸ **Norgeston** (Bayer Plc)
Levonorgestrel 30 microgram   Norgeston 30microgram tablets | 35 tablet [PoM] £0.92 DT = £0.92
▸ **Upostelle** (Gedeon Richter (UK) Ltd)
Levonorgestrel 1.5 mg   Upostelle 1500microgram tablets | 1 tablet [PoM] £3.75 DT = £2.74

Intra-uterine device
▸ **Benilexa One Handed** (Gedeon Richter (UK) Ltd)
Levonorgestrel 20 microgram per 24 hour   Benilexa One Handed 20micrograms/24hours intra-uterine delivery system | 1 device [PoM] £71.00 DT = £88.00
▸ **Jaydess** (Bayer Plc) ▼
Levonorgestrel 13.5 mg   Jaydess 13.5mg intra-uterine device | 1 device [PoM] £69.22 DT = £69.22
▸ **Kyleena** (Bayer Plc)
Levonorgestrel 19.5 mg   Kyleena 19.5mg intra-uterine device | 1 device [PoM] £76.00 DT = £76.00
▸ **Levosert** (Gedeon Richter (UK) Ltd)
Levonorgestrel 20 microgram per 24 hour   Levosert 20micrograms/24hours intra-uterine device | 1 device [PoM] £66.00 DT = £88.00

▸ **Mirena** (Bayer Plc)
Levonorgestrel 20 microgram per 24 hour   Mirena 20micrograms/24hours intra-uterine device | 1 device [PoM] £88.00 DT = £88.00

3.5 Contraception, parenteral progestogen-only

> **Other drugs used for Contraception, parenteral progestogen-only** Norethisterone, p. 878

PROGESTOGENS

Etonogestrel
11-Mar-2021

- **INDICATIONS AND DOSE**

Contraception [no hormonal contraceptive use in previous month]
▸ BY SUBDERMAL IMPLANTATION
▸ Females of childbearing potential: 1 implant, which can be left in place for up to 3 years, when inserted during the first 5 days of cycle, no additional contraceptive precautions are needed, when inserted at any other time, additional precautions (e.g. barrier methods) advised for next 7 days

Contraception [postpartum]
▸ BY SUBDERMAL IMPLANTATION
▸ Females of childbearing potential: 1 implant, which can be left in place for up to 3 years, when inserted within 20 days after delivery (or up to 6 months postpartum if fully breast-feeding and amenorrhoeic), no additional contraceptive precautions are needed, when inserted at any other time, additional precautions (e.g. barrier methods) advised for next 7 days

Contraception [following abortion or miscarriage]
▸ BY SUBDERMAL IMPLANTATION
▸ Females of childbearing potential: 1 implant, which can be left in place for up to 3 years, when inserted within 5 days after abortion or miscarriage, no additional contraceptive precautions are needed, when inserted at any other time, additional precautions (e.g. barrier methods) advised for next 7 days

Contraception [changing from other hormonal contraceptive]
▸ BY SUBDERMAL IMPLANTATION
▸ Females of childbearing potential: 1 implant, which can be left in place for up to 3 years, consult product literature for advice on when to insert and additional contraceptive precautions

- **UNLICENSED USE**   The FSRH advises that the etonogestrel implant is used as detailed below, although these situations are considered unlicensed:
  - females outside the age range of 18–40 years;
  - postpartum insertions within 20 days after delivery (or up to 6 months postpartum if fully breast-feeding and amenorrhoeic);
  - insertion within 5 days after abortion or miscarriage in the second trimester.

> **IMPORTANT SAFETY INFORMATION**
>
> MHRA/CHM ADVICE (UPDATED FEBRUARY 2020): *NEXPLANON*® (ETONOGESTREL) CONTRACEPTIVE IMPLANTS: NEW INSERTION SITE TO REDUCE RARE RISK OF NEUROVASCULAR INJURY AND IMPLANT MIGRATION
>
> There have been reports of neurovascular injury and migration of *Nexplanon*® implants from the insertion site to the vasculature, including the pulmonary artery in rare cases. Correct subdermal insertion by an

7
Genito-urinary system

appropriately trained and accredited healthcare professional is recommended to reduce the risk of these events. Healthcare professionals are advised to review the updated guidance from the manufacturer and the statement from the Faculty of Sexual and Reproductive Healthcare (FSRH) on how to correctly insert the implant. Patients should be advised on how to locate the implant, informed to check this occasionally and report any concerns. An implant that cannot be palpated at its insertion site should be located and removed as soon as possible; if unable to locate implant within the arm, the MHRA recommends using chest imaging. Implants inserted at a previous site that can be palpated should not pose a risk and should only be replaced if there are issues with its location or if a routine replacement is due.

- **CONTRA-INDICATIONS** Acute porphyrias p. 1202 · current breast cancer

- **CAUTIONS** Cardiac dysfunction · cervical cancer · diabetes (progestogens can decrease glucose tolerance—monitor patient closely) · history of breast cancer—seek specialist advice before use · history of stroke (including transient ischaemic attack) · history of venous thromboembolism · ischaemic heart disease · liver tumours—seek specialist advice before use · migraine · multiple risk factors for cardiovascular disease · positive antiphospholipid antibodies · rheumatoid arthritis · systemic lupus erythematosus · undiagnosed vaginal bleeding—seek specialist advice before use

- **INTERACTIONS** → Appendix 1: etonogestrel

- **SIDE-EFFECTS**
- ▸ **Common or very common** Abdominal pain · alopecia · anxiety · appetite increased · breast abnormalities · depressed mood · dizziness · emotional lability · fatigue · flatulence · headaches · hot flush · increased risk of infection · influenza like illness · libido decreased · menstrual cycle irregularities · nausea · ovarian cyst · pain · skin reactions · weight changes
- ▸ **Uncommon** Arthralgia · constipation · diarrhoea · drowsiness · dysuria · fever · galactorrhoea · genital abnormalities · hypertrichosis · insomnia · myalgia · oedema · vomiting · vulvovaginal discomfort
- ▸ **Frequency not known** Abscess · angioedema · embolism and thrombosis · haemorrhage · insulin resistance · neoplasms · paraesthesia · seborrhoea

SIDE-EFFECTS, FURTHER INFORMATION The benefits of using progestogen-only contraceptives (POCs), such as etonogestrel, should be weighed against the possible risks for each individual woman.

There is a possible small increase in the risk of breast cancer in women using, or who have recently used, progestogen-only contraception. Causal association is not clearly established, and absolute risk remains very small, and is like that of current or recent use of combined hormonal contraception.

The most important risk factor for breast cancer appears to be the age the contraceptive is stopped rather than the duration of use; the risk gradually disappears during the 10 years after stopping.

- **PREGNANCY** Not known to be harmful, remove implant if pregnancy occurs.

- **BREAST FEEDING** Progestogen-only contraceptives do not affect lactation.

- **DIRECTIONS FOR ADMINISTRATION** The doctor or nurse administering (or removing) the system should be fully trained in the technique and should provide full counselling reinforced by the patient information leaflet.

- **PATIENT AND CARER ADVICE** Full counselling backed by patient information leaflet required before administration.

- **MEDICINAL FORMS** There can be variation in the licensing of different medicines containing the same drug.

Prolonged-release subcutaneous implant
- ▸ **Nexplanon** (Organon Pharma (UK) Ltd)
  Etonogestrel 68 mg Nexplanon 68mg implant | 1 device [PoM]
  £83.43 DT = £83.43

Medroxyprogesterone acetate
05-Dec-2024

- **INDICATIONS AND DOSE**

Dysfunctional uterine bleeding
- ▸ BY MOUTH
- ▸ Adult: 2.5–10 mg daily for 5–10 days, repeated for 2 cycles, begin treatment on day 16–21 of cycle

Secondary amenorrhoea
- ▸ BY MOUTH
- ▸ Adult: 2.5–10 mg daily for 5–10 days, repeated for 3 cycles, begin treatment on day 16–21 of cycle

Mild to moderate endometriosis
- ▸ BY MOUTH
- ▸ Adult: 10 mg 3 times a day for 90 consecutive days, begin treatment on day 1 of cycle

Progestogenic opposition of oestrogen HRT
- ▸ BY MOUTH
- ▸ Adult: 10 mg daily for the last 14 days of each 28-day oestrogen HRT cycle

Endometrial cancer | Renal cell cancer
- ▸ BY MOUTH
- ▸ Adult: 200–600 mg daily

Breast cancer
- ▸ BY MOUTH
- ▸ Adult: 0.4–1.5 g daily

Contraception
- ▸ BY DEEP INTRAMUSCULAR INJECTION
- ▸ Females of childbearing potential: 150 mg, to be administered within the first 5 days of cycle or within first 5 days after parturition (delay until 6 weeks after parturition if breast-feeding)
- ▸ BY SUBCUTANEOUS INJECTION
- ▸ Females of childbearing potential: 104 mg, to be administered within first 5 days of cycle or within 5 days postpartum (delay until 6 weeks postpartum if breast-feeding), injected into anterior thigh or abdomen, dose only suitable if no hormonal contraceptive use in previous month

Long-term contraception
- ▸ BY DEEP INTRAMUSCULAR INJECTION
- ▸ Females of childbearing potential: 150 mg every 12 weeks, first dose to be administered within the first 5 days of cycle or within first 5 days after parturition (delay until 6 weeks after parturition if breast-feeding)
- ▸ BY SUBCUTANEOUS INJECTION
- ▸ Females of childbearing potential: 104 mg every 13 weeks, first dose to be administered within first 5 days of cycle or within 5 days postpartum (delay until 6 weeks postpartum if breast-feeding), injected into anterior thigh or abdomen, dose only suitable if no hormonal contraceptive use in previous month

Contraception (when patient changing from other hormonal contraceptive)
- ▸ BY SUBCUTANEOUS INJECTION
- ▸ Females of childbearing potential: (consult product literature)

Hot flushes caused by long-term androgen suppression in men with prostate cancer
- ▸ BY MOUTH
- ▸ Adult: 20 mg once daily initially for 10 weeks, evaluate effect at the end of the treatment period

- **UNLICENSED USE** [EvGr] Medroxyprogesterone acetate is used for the treatment of hot flushes caused by long-term androgen suppression in men, (A) but it is not licensed for this indication.

> **IMPORTANT SAFETY INFORMATION**
>
> **MHRA/CHM ADVICE: MEDROXYPROGESTERONE ACETATE: RISK OF MENINGIOMA AND MEASURES TO MINIMISE THIS RISK (OCTOBER 2024)**
>
> A French epidemiological study has identified a small increased risk of developing meningioma with high-dose medroxyprogesterone acetate (all parenteral preparations and oral preparations containing 100 mg or more), mainly after prolonged use of several years. When used for contraception, high-dose medroxyprogesterone acetate is contra-indicated in patients with meningioma or a history of meningioma—if meningioma is diagnosed, it must be stopped. When used for cancer, if meningioma is diagnosed during treatment, continuation of high-dose medroxyprogesterone acetate should be reconsidered on an individual basis, taking into account the benefits and risks.
>
> This advice does not apply to lower doses (less than 100 mg) or combination preparations.

- **CONTRA-INDICATIONS**

  GENERAL CONTRA-INDICATIONS Acute porphyrias p. 1202 · current breast cancer (unless progestogens are being used in the management of this condition)

  SPECIFIC CONTRA-INDICATIONS
  - With oral use History of thromboembolism · undiagnosed vaginal bleeding
  - When used for Contraception Current or history of meningioma

- **CAUTIONS**

  GENERAL CAUTIONS Cardiac dysfunction · conditions that may worsen with fluid retention · diabetes (progestogens can decrease glucose tolerance—monitor patient closely) · history of breast cancer—seek specialist advice before use · hypertension · liver tumours—seek specialist advice before use · migraine · positive antiphospholipid antibodies · rheumatoid arthritis · risk factors for thromboembolism · systemic lupus erythematosus

  SPECIFIC CAUTIONS
  - With intramuscular use or subcutaneous use Cervical cancer · history of stroke (including transient ischaemic attack)—seek specialist advice before use · history of venous thromboembolism · ischaemic heart disease—seek specialist advice before use · multiple risk factors for cardiovascular disease—seek specialist advice before use · undiagnosed vaginal bleeding—seek specialist advice before use
  - With oral use History of depression

- **INTERACTIONS** → Appendix 1: medroxyprogesterone

- **SIDE-EFFECTS**

  GENERAL SIDE-EFFECTS
  - **Common or very common** Alopecia · breast abnormalities · depression · dizziness · fluid retention · insomnia · menstrual cycle irregularities · nausea · sexual dysfunction · skin reactions · weight changes
  - **Uncommon** Drowsiness · embolism and thrombosis · fever · galactorrhoea · hirsutism · muscle spasms · tachycardia
  - **Frequency not known** Meningioma (with high doses, particularly in long term use)

  SPECIFIC SIDE-EFFECTS
  - **Common or very common**
  - With oral use Appetite increased · cervical abnormalities · constipation · fatigue · headache · hyperhidrosis · hypersensitivity · nervousness · oedema · tremor · vomiting

- With parenteral use Anxiety · asthenia · gastrointestinal discomfort · headaches · mood altered · pain · vulvovaginal infection
- **Uncommon**
- With oral use Congestive heart failure · corticoid-like effects · diabetes mellitus exacerbated · diarrhoea · dry mouth · euphoric mood · hypercalcaemia
- With parenteral use Appetite abnormal · arthralgia · hot flush · hypertension · ovarian cyst · painful sexual intercourse · uterine haemorrhage · varicose veins · vertigo · vulvovaginal disorders
- **Rare or very rare**
- With oral use Cerebral infarction · jaundice · malaise · myocardial infarction
- With parenteral use Breast cancer · lipodystrophy
- **Frequency not known**
- With oral use Adrenergic-like effects · cataract diabetic · concentration impaired · confusion · glycosuria · palpitations · visual impairment (discontinue if papilloedema or retinal vascular lesions)
- With parenteral use Hepatic disorders · osteoporosis · osteoporotic fractures · seizure

  SIDE-EFFECTS, FURTHER INFORMATION **With oral use** In general, side effects may be more common with high doses such as those used in malignant disease.

  With parenteral use Reduction in bone mineral density is greater with increasing duration of use. The loss is mostly recovered on discontinuation.

  Breast cancer risk with contraceptive use The benefits of using progestogen-only contraceptives (POCs), such as medroxyprogesterone acetate, should be weighed against the possible risks for each individual woman.

  There is a possible small increase in the risk of breast cancer in women using, or who have recently used, progestogen-only contraception. Causal association is not clearly established, and absolute risk remains very small, and is like that of current or recent use of combined hormonal contraception.

  The most important risk factor for breast cancer appears to be the age the contraceptive is stopped rather than the duration of use; the risk gradually disappears during the 10 years after stopping.

- **CONCEPTION AND CONTRACEPTION**
- With intramuscular use If interval between dose is greater than 12 weeks and 5 days (in long-term contraception), rule out pregnancy before next injection and advise patient to use additional contraceptive measures (e.g. barrier) for 14 days after the injection.
- With subcutaneous use If interval between dose is greater than 13 weeks and 7 days (in long-term contraception), rule out pregnancy before next injection.

- **PREGNANCY**
- With oral use Avoid—genital malformations and cardiac defects reported.
- With intramuscular use or subcutaneous use Not known to be harmful.

- **BREAST FEEDING** Present in milk—no adverse effects reported. Progestogen-only contraceptives do not affect lactation.
- With intramuscular use or subcutaneous use The manufacturers advise that in women who are breast-feeding, the first dose should be delayed until 6 weeks after birth; however, evidence suggests no harmful effect to infant if given earlier. The benefits of using medroxyprogesterone acetate in breast-feeding women outweigh any risks.

- **HEPATIC IMPAIRMENT**
- With oral use Manufacturer advises caution; avoid in acute or active disease.
- With intramuscular use or subcutaneous use Manufacturer advises caution; avoid in severe or active disease.

- **RENAL IMPAIRMENT**
  - With oral use [EvGr] Use with caution. [M]
- **PATIENT AND CARER ADVICE**
  - With intramuscular use or subcutaneous use Full counselling backed by *patient information leaflet* required before administration—likelihood of menstrual disturbance and the potential for a delay in return to full fertility. Delayed return of fertility and irregular cycles may occur after discontinuation of treatment but there is no evidence of permanent infertility.

- **MEDICINAL FORMS** There can be variation in the licensing of different medicines containing the same drug. Forms available from special-order manufacturers include: oral suspension, oral solution

Oral tablet
- Medroxyprogesterone acetate (Non-proprietary)
  Medroxyprogesterone acetate 2.5 mg Medroxyprogesterone 2.5mg tablets | 30 tablet [PoM] £1.84 DT = £1.84
  Medroxyprogesterone acetate 5 mg Medroxyprogesterone 5mg tablets | 10 tablet [PoM] £1.23 DT = £1.23 | 100 tablet [PoM] £12.32
  Medroxyprogesterone acetate 10 mg Medroxyprogesterone 10mg tablets | 10 tablet [PoM] £2.47 DT = £2.47 | 90 tablet [PoM] £22.16 DT = £22.16 | 100 tablet [PoM] £24.73 DT = £24.73
  Medroxyprogesterone acetate 100 mg Medroxyprogesterone 100mg tablets | 60 tablet [PoM] £29.98 | 100 tablet [PoM] £49.94 DT = £49.94
  Medroxyprogesterone acetate 200 mg Medroxyprogesterone 200mg tablets | 30 tablet [PoM] £29.65 DT = £29.65
  Medroxyprogesterone acetate 400 mg Medroxyprogesterone 400mg tablets | 30 tablet [PoM] £58.67 DT = £58.67
- Provera (Pfizer Ltd)
  Medroxyprogesterone acetate 2.5 mg Provera 2.5mg tablets | 30 tablet [PoM] £1.84 DT = £1.84
  Medroxyprogesterone acetate 5 mg Provera 5mg tablets | 10 tablet [PoM] £1.23 DT = £1.23 | 100 tablet [PoM] £12.32
  Medroxyprogesterone acetate 10 mg Provera 10mg tablets | 10 tablet [PoM] £2.47 DT = £2.47 | 90 tablet [PoM] £22.16 DT = £22.16 | 100 tablet [PoM] £24.73 DT = £24.73
  Medroxyprogesterone acetate 100 mg Provera 100mg tablets | 60 tablet [PoM] £29.98 | 100 tablet [PoM] £49.94 DT = £49.94
  Medroxyprogesterone acetate 200 mg Provera 200mg tablets | 30 tablet [PoM] £29.65 DT = £29.65
  Medroxyprogesterone acetate 400 mg Provera 400mg tablets | 30 tablet [PoM] £58.67 DT = £58.67

Suspension for injection
- Depo-Provera (Pfizer Ltd)
  Medroxyprogesterone acetate 150 mg per 1 ml Depo-Provera 150mg/1ml suspension for injection pre-filled syringes | 1 pre-filled disposable injection [PoM] £6.01 DT = £6.01
- Sayana Press (Pfizer Ltd)
  Medroxyprogesterone acetate 160 mg per 1 ml Sayana Press 104mg/0.65 ml suspension for injection pre-filled disposable devices | 1 pre-filled disposable injection [PoM] £6.90 DT = £6.90

3.6 Contraception, spermicidal

SPERMICIDALS

Nonoxinol

- **INDICATIONS AND DOSE**

Spermicidal contraceptive in conjunction with barrier methods of contraception such as diaphragms or caps
- BY VAGINA
- Females of childbearing potential: (consult product literature)

- **SIDE-EFFECTS** Genital erosion · increased risk of HIV infection · pain · paraesthesia · skin reactions · vaginal redness

SIDE-EFFECTS, FURTHER INFORMATION High frequency use of the spermicide nonoxinol-9 has been associated with genital lesions, which may increase the risk of acquiring sexually transmitted infections.

- **CONCEPTION AND CONTRACEPTION** No evidence of harm to diaphragms.
- **PREGNANCY** Toxicity in *animal* studies.
- **BREAST FEEDING** Present in milk in *animal* studies.

- **MEDICINAL FORMS** No licensed medicines listed.

4 Erectile and ejaculatory conditions
4.1 Erectile dysfunction

Erectile dysfunction

06-Mar-2017

Description of condition

Erectile dysfunction (impotence) is the persistent inability to attain and maintain an erection that is sufficient to permit satisfactory sexual performance. It can have physical or psychological causes. Erectile dysfunction can also be a side-effect of drugs such as antihypertensives, antidepressants, antipsychotics, cytotoxic drugs and recreational drugs (including alcohol).

Risk factors for erectile dysfunction include sedentary lifestyle, obesity, smoking, hypercholesterolaemia and metabolic syndrome. Erectile dysfunction increases the risk of cardiovascular disease. All men with unexplained erectile dysfunction should be evaluated for the presence of cardiovascular risk factors and any identified risk should be addressed.

Drug treatment

[EvGr] The recommended approach for the management of erectile dysfunction is a combination of drug treatment and lifestyle changes (including regular exercise, reduction in body mass index, Smoking cessation p. 565, and reduced alcohol consumption).

An oral phosphodiesterase type-5 inhibitor is the first-line drug treatment for erectile dysfunction, regardless of the cause. [A] These drugs act by increasing the blood flow to the penis. They do not initiate an erection—sexual stimulation is required.

The choice of oral phosphodiesterase type-5 inhibitor depends on the frequency of intercourse and response to treatment. [EvGr] Avanafil p. 939, sildenafil p. 940 and vardenafil p. 942 are short-acting drugs and are suitable for occasional use as required. Tadalafil p. 941 is a longer-acting drug. It can be used as required, but can also be used as a regular lower daily dose to allow for spontaneous (rather than scheduled) sexual activity or in those who have frequent sexual activity. A patient with erectile dysfunction should receive six doses of an individual phosphodiesterase type-5 inhibitor at the maximum dose (with sexual stimulation) before being classified as a non-responder. Patients who fail to respond to the maximum dose of at least two different phosphodiesterase type-5 inhibitors should be referred to a specialist.

Intracavernosal, intraurethral or topical application of alprostadil p. 943 (prostaglandin E_1) is recommended as second-line therapy under careful medical supervision. Intracavernosal or intraurethral preparations can also be used to aid diagnosis. [A]

Priapism associated with alprostadil

Manufacturers advise that patients should seek medical help if a prolonged erection lasting four hours or more occurs; application of an ice pack to the upper-inner thigh (alternating between the left and right thighs every two minutes for up to ten minutes) may result in reflex opening of the venous valves.

If priapism has lasted more than six hours, treatment should not be delayed; manufacturer advises management as follows:

- Initial therapy by penile aspiration: using aseptic technique, 20–50mL of blood should be aspirated using a 19–21 gauge butterfly needle inserted into the *corpus cavernosum*; if necessary the procedure may be repeated on the opposite side;
- Lavage: if initial aspiration is unsuccessful, a second 19–21 gauge butterfly needle can be inserted into the opposite *corpus cavernosum*; sterile physiological saline can be injected through the first needle and drained through the second;
- If aspiration and lavage of are unsuccessful, intracavernosal injection of a sympathomimetic with action on alpha-adrenergic receptors can be given, with continuous monitoring of blood pressure and pulse— see phenylephrine hydrochloride p. 946 [unlicensed indication], adrenaline/epinephrine p. 945 [unlicensed indication], and metaraminol p. 945 [unlicensed indication]. Extreme **caution** is required in patients with coronary heart disease, hypertension, cerebral ischaemia and in patients taking a monoamine-oxidase inhibitor (facilities for managing hypertensive crisis should be available when administered to patients taking MAOIs);
- If necessary the sympathomimetic injections can be followed by further aspiration of blood through the same butterfly needle;
- If administration of a sympathomimetic drug is unsuccessful, urgent referral for surgical management is required.

Prescribing on the NHS

Some drug treatments for erectile dysfunction may only be prescribed on the NHS under certain circumstances; for details see the criteria listed in part XVIIIB of the Drug Tariff (Part XIb of the Northern Ireland Drug Tariff, Part 12 of the Scottish Drug Tariff). The Drug Tariffs can be accessed online at: National Health Service Drug Tariff for England and Wales: www.nhsbsa.nhs.uk/pharmacies-gp-practices-and-appliance-contractors/drug-tariff.

Health and Personal Social Services for Northern Ireland Drug Tariff: www.hscbusiness.hscni.net/services/2034.htm.

Scottish Drug Tariff: www.isdscotland.org/Health-Topics/Prescribing-and-Medicines/Scottish-Drug-Tariff/.

Related drugs

Other drugs used for Erectile dysfunction: aviptadil with phentolamine mesilate p. 946.

PHOSPHODIESTERASE TYPE-5 INHIBITORS

Avanafil
15-Apr-2024

- **INDICATIONS AND DOSE**

Erectile dysfunction
- BY MOUTH
- Adult: Initially 100 mg, to be taken approximately 15–30 minutes before sexual activity, then adjusted according to response to 50–200 mg (max. per dose 200 mg), to be taken as a single dose as needed; maximum 1 dose per day

Erectile dysfunction in patients on alpha-blocker therapy
- BY MOUTH
- Adult: Initially 50 mg, to be taken approximately 15–30 minutes before sexual activity, then adjusted according to response to 50–200 mg (max. per dose 200 mg), to be taken as a single dose as needed; maximum 1 dose per day

DOSE ADJUSTMENTS DUE TO INTERACTIONS
- Manufacturer advises max. 100 mg once every 48 hours with concurrent use of moderate inhibitors of CYP3A4.

- **CONTRA-INDICATIONS** Avoid if systolic blood pressure below 90 mmHg (no information available) · blood pressure >170/100 mmHg · hereditary degenerative retinal disorders · history of non-arteritic anterior ischaemic optic neuropathy · life-threatening arrhythmia in previous 6 months · mild to severe heart failure · patients in whom vasodilation or sexual activity are inadvisable · recent history of myocardial infarction · recent history of stroke · recent unstable angina

- **CAUTIONS** Active peptic ulceration · anatomical deformation of the penis (e.g. angulation, cavernosal fibrosis, Peyronie's disease) · bleeding disorders · cardiovascular disease · left ventricular outflow obstruction · predisposition to priapism (e.g. in sickle-cell disease, multiple myeloma, or leukaemia)

  CAUTIONS, FURTHER INFORMATION
- Elderly For phosphodiesterase type-5 inhibitors, Screening Tool of Older Persons' potentially inappropriate Prescriptions (STOPP) criteria to aid medication reviews (see Prescribing in the elderly p. 31 for information): potentially inappropriate in severe heart failure characterised by hypotension i.e. systolic blood pressure less than 90 mmHg, or concurrent nitrate therapy for angina (risk of cardiovascular collapse).

- **INTERACTIONS** → Appendix 1: phosphodiesterase type-5 inhibitors

- **SIDE-EFFECTS**
- **Common or very common** Headaches · nasal complaints · vasodilation
- **Uncommon** Asthenia · dizziness · drowsiness · dyspnoea exertional · gastrointestinal discomfort · muscle complaints · nausea · pain · palpitations · respiratory disorders · vision blurred · vomiting
- **Rare or very rare** Akathisia · angina pectoris · chest pain · diarrhoea · dry mouth · emotional disorder · gastritis · genital pruritus · gout · haematuria · hypertension · increased risk of infection · influenza like illness · insomnia · penis disorder · peripheral oedema · rash · seasonal allergy · sexual dysfunction · tachycardia · urinary frequency increased · weight increased

- **HEPATIC IMPAIRMENT** Manufacturer advises avoid in severe impairment.
  Dose adjustments Manufacturer advises use lowest effective initial dose in mild to moderate impairment and adjust according to tolerance.

- **RENAL IMPAIRMENT** [EvGr] Avoid if creatinine clearance less than 30 mL/minute. ⟨M⟩ See p. 21.

- **PATIENT AND CARER ADVICE** Onset of effect may be delayed if taken with food.

- **NATIONAL FUNDING/ACCESS DECISIONS**
  For full details see funding body website
  Scottish Medicines Consortium (SMC) decisions
- Avanafil (*Spedra*®) for the treatment of erectile dysfunction (ED) in adult men (September 2015) SMC No. 980/14 Not recommended
  All Wales Medicines Strategy Group (AWMSG) decisions
- Avanafil (*Spedra*®) for the treatment of erectile dysfunction in adult men (July 2015) AWMSG No. 1261 Recommended
  NHS restrictions *Spedra*® is not prescribable in NHS primary care for the treatment of erectile dysfunction except in men who meet the criteria listed in part XVIIIB of the Drug Tariff. The prescription must be endorsed 'SLS'. For more information see *Prices in the BNF*, under How to use the BNF.

- **MEDICINAL FORMS** There can be variation in the licensing of different medicines containing the same drug.
  Oral tablet
- Spedra (A. Menarini Farmaceutica Internazionale SRL)
  Avanafil 50 mg Spedra 50mg tablets | 4 tablet [PoM] £10.94 DT = £10.94 | 8 tablet [PoM] £19.70 DT = £19.70

Avanafil 100 mg Spedra 100mg tablets | 4 tablet [PoM] £14.08 DT = £14.08 | 8 tablet [PoM] £26.26 DT = £26.26

Avanafil 200 mg Spedra 200mg tablets | 4 tablet [PoM] £21.90 DT = £21.90 | 8 tablet [PoM] £39.40 DT = £39.40

Sildenafil

15-Apr-2024

● **INDICATIONS AND DOSE**

Pulmonary arterial hypertension (initiated under specialist supervision)

▸ BY MOUTH

▸ Adult: 20 mg 3 times a day

▸ BY INTRAVENOUS INJECTION

▸ Adult: 10 mg 3 times a day, use intravenous route when the oral route is not appropriate

Erectile dysfunction

▸ BY MOUTH

▸ Adult: Initially 50 mg, to be taken approximately 1 hour before sexual activity, adjusted according to response to 25–100 mg (max. per dose 100 mg) as required, to be taken as a single dose; maximum 1 dose per day

Digital ulcers [associated with systemic sclerosis]

▸ BY MOUTH

▸ Adult: 25 mg 3 times a day, increased to 50 mg 3 times a day

DOSE ADJUSTMENTS DUE TO INTERACTIONS

▸ When used for Erectile dysfunction Manufacturer advises a starting dose of 25 mg with concurrent use of moderate and potent inhibitors of CYP3A4. Manufacturer advises if concurrent use of ritonavir is unavoidable, the max. dose should not exceed 25 mg within 48 hours.

▸ With oral use for Pulmonary arterial hypertension Manufacturer advises reduce dose to 20 mg twice daily with concurrent use of moderate inhibitors of CYP3A4. Manufacturer advises reduce dose to 20 mg once daily with concurrent use of some potent inhibitors of CYP3A4 (avoid with ketoconazole, itraconazole and ritonavir).

▸ With intravenous use for Pulmonary arterial hypertension Manufacturer advises reduce dose to 10 mg twice daily with concurrent use of moderate inhibitors of CYP3A4. Manufacturer advises reduce dose to 10 mg once daily with concurrent use of some potent inhibitors of CYP3A4 (avoid with ketoconazole, itraconazole and ritonavir).

● **UNLICENSED USE** [EvGr] Sildenafil is used for the treatment of digital ulcer, [E] but is not licensed for this indication.

● **CONTRA-INDICATIONS**

GENERAL CONTRA-INDICATIONS Hereditary degenerative retinal disorders · history of non-arteritic anterior ischaemic optic neuropathy · recent history of myocardial infarction · recent history of stroke

SPECIFIC CONTRA-INDICATIONS

▸ When used for Erectile dysfunction Avoid if systolic blood pressure below 90 mmHg (no information available) · patients in whom vasodilation or sexual activity are inadvisable · recent unstable angina

▸ When used for Pulmonary arterial hypertension Sickle-cell anaemia

● **CAUTIONS**

GENERAL CAUTIONS Active peptic ulceration · anatomical deformation of the penis (e.g. angulation, cavernosal fibrosis, Peyronie's disease) · autonomic dysfunction · bleeding disorders · cardiovascular disease · left ventricular outflow obstruction · predisposition to priapism (e.g. in sickle-cell disease, multiple myeloma, or leukaemia)

SPECIFIC CAUTIONS

▸ When used for Pulmonary arterial hypertension Hypotension (avoid if systolic blood pressure below 90 mmHg) · intravascular volume depletion · pulmonary veno-occlusive disease

CAUTIONS, FURTHER INFORMATION

▸ Elderly For phosphodiesterase type-5 inhibitors, Screening Tool of Older Persons' potentially inappropriate Prescriptions (STOPP) criteria to aid medication reviews (see Prescribing in the elderly p. 31 for information): potentially inappropriate in severe heart failure characterised by hypotension i.e. systolic blood pressure less than 90 mmHg, or concurrent nitrate therapy for angina (risk of cardiovascular collapse).

● **INTERACTIONS** → Appendix 1: phosphodiesterase type-5 inhibitors

● **SIDE-EFFECTS**

▸ **Common or very common** Alopecia · anaemia · anxiety · cough · diarrhoea · dizziness · fluid retention · gastrointestinal discomfort · gastrointestinal disorders · headaches · increased risk of infection · insomnia · nasal complaints · nausea · night sweats · pain · skin reactions · tremor · vasodilation · vision disorders

▸ **Uncommon** Arrhythmias · chest pain · drowsiness · dry eye · dry mouth · eye discomfort · eye disorders · eye inflammation · fatigue · feeling hot · gynaecomastia · haemorrhage · hypertension · hypotension · myalgia · numbness · palpitations · sinus congestion · tinnitus · vertigo · vomiting

▸ **Rare or very rare** Acute coronary syndrome · arteriosclerotic retinopathy · cerebrovascular insufficiency · glaucoma · haematospermia · hearing impairment · irritability · optic neuropathy (discontinue if sudden visual impairment occurs) · oral hypoaesthesia · priapism · retinal occlusion · scleral discolouration · seizure · severe cutaneous adverse reactions (SCARs) · sudden cardiac death · syncope · throat tightness

● **PREGNANCY** Use only if potential benefit outweighs risk—no evidence of harm in *animal* studies.

● **BREAST FEEDING** Manufacturer advises avoid—no information available.

● **HEPATIC IMPAIRMENT** Manufacturer advises caution in mild to moderate impairment; avoid in severe impairment (no information available).

Dose adjustments

▸ With intravenous use for Pulmonary arterial hypertension Manufacturer advises if usual dose not tolerated, consider dose reduction to 10 mg twice daily in mild to moderate impairment.

▸ With oral use for Pulmonary arterial hypertension Manufacturer advises if usual dose not tolerated, consider dose reduction to 20 mg twice daily in mild to moderate impairment.

▸ When used for Erectile dysfunction Manufacturer advises consider initial dose reduction to 25 mg in mild to moderate impairment; adjust according to response.

● **RENAL IMPAIRMENT**

Dose adjustments

▸ When used for Erectile dysfunction [EvGr] Consider initial dose of 25 mg if creatinine clearance less than 30 mL/minute. [M] See p. 21.

▸ With oral use for Pulmonary arterial hypertension [EvGr] If usual dose not tolerated, consider dose reduction to 20 mg twice daily. [M]

▸ With intravenous use for Pulmonary arterial hypertension [EvGr] If usual dose not tolerated, consider dose reduction to 10 mg twice daily. [M]

● **TREATMENT CESSATION**

▸ When used for Pulmonary arterial hypertension Consider gradual withdrawal.

● **PATIENT AND CARER ADVICE**

▸ When used for Erectile dysfunction Onset of effect may be delayed if taken with food.

- **NATIONAL FUNDING/ACCESS DECISIONS**
For full details see funding body website
Scottish Medicines Consortium (SMC) decisions
- Sildenafil tablets (*Revatio*®) for the treatment of pulmonary arterial hypertension (February 2010) SMC No. 596/10 Recommended with restrictions
- Sildenafil injection (*Revatio*®) for the treatment of pulmonary arterial hypertension (PAH) in patients who are unable to take sildenafil orally (March 2011) SMC No. 688/11 Recommended with restrictions
NHS restrictions *Viagra*® is not prescribable in NHS primary care for treatment of erectile dysfunction except in men who meet the criteria listed in part XVIIIB of the Drug Tariff (Part XIb of the Northern Ireland Drug Tariff, Part 12 of the Scottish Drug Tariff). The prescription must be endorsed 'SLS'. For more information see *Prices in the BNF*, under How to use the BNF.

- **MEDICINAL FORMS** There can be variation in the licensing of different medicines containing the same drug. Forms available from special-order manufacturers include: oral suspension, oral solution

Oral tablet
- **Sildenafil (Non-proprietary)**
Sildenafil (as Sildenafil citrate) 20 mg Sildenafil 20mg tablets | 90 tablet PoM £446.33 DT = £446.33
Sildenafil (as Sildenafil citrate) 25 mg Sildenafil 25mg tablets | 4 tablet PoM £14.10 DT = £0.62 | 8 tablet PoM £1.19–£28.21
Sildenafil (as Sildenafil citrate) 50 mg Sildenafil 50mg tablets | 4 tablet PoM £18.08 DT = £0.60 | 8 tablet PoM £0.80–£42.54
Sildenafil (as Sildenafil citrate) 100 mg Sildenafil 100mg tablets | 4 tablet PoM £23.50 DT = £0.67 | 8 tablet PoM £1.34–£46.99
- **Granpidam** (Accord-UK Ltd)
Sildenafil (as Sildenafil citrate) 20 mg Granpidam 20mg tablets | 90 tablet PoM £424.01 DT = £446.33
- **Revatio** (Viatris UK Healthcare Ltd)
Sildenafil (as Sildenafil citrate) 20 mg Revatio 20mg tablets | 90 tablet PoM £446.33 DT = £446.33
- **Viagra** (Viatris UK Healthcare Ltd)
Sildenafil (as Sildenafil citrate) 25 mg Viagra 25mg tablets | 4 tablet PoM £16.59 DT = £0.62 | 8 tablet PoM £33.19
Sildenafil (as Sildenafil citrate) 50 mg Viagra 50mg tablets | 4 tablet PoM £21.27 DT = £0.60 | 8 tablet PoM £42.54
Sildenafil (as Sildenafil citrate) 100 mg Viagra 100mg tablets | 4 tablet PoM £23.50 DT = £0.67 | 8 tablet PoM £46.99

Solution for injection
- **Revatio** (Viatris UK Healthcare Ltd)
Sildenafil (as Sildenafil citrate) 800 microgram per 1 ml Revatio 10mg/12.5ml solution for injection vials | 1 vial PoM £45.28 (Hospital only)

Oral suspension
- **Sildenafil (Non-proprietary)**
Sildenafil (as Sildenafil citrate) 10 mg per 1 ml Sildenafil 10mg/ml oral suspension sugar free | 122 ml PoM £186.75 DT = £186.75 SF
- **Revatio** (Viatris UK Healthcare Ltd)
Sildenafil (as Sildenafil citrate) 10 mg per 1 ml Revatio 10mg/ml oral suspension | 90 ml PoM £186.75 DT = £186.75 SF

Tadalafil

15-Apr-2024

- **INDICATIONS AND DOSE**
Pulmonary arterial hypertension (initiated under specialist supervision)
- BY MOUTH
- Adult: 40 mg once daily

Erectile dysfunction
- BY MOUTH
- Adult: Initially 10 mg (max. per dose 20 mg), to be taken at least 30 minutes before sexual activity, subsequent doses adjusted according to response, the effect of intermittent dosing may persist for longer than 24 hours, continuous daily use not recommended; maximum 1 dose per day

Erectile dysfunction; for patients who anticipate sexual activity at least twice a week
- BY MOUTH
- Adult: 5 mg once daily, reduced to 2.5 mg once daily, adjusted according to response

Benign prostatic hyperplasia
- BY MOUTH
- Adult: 5 mg once daily

- **CONTRA-INDICATIONS**
GENERAL CONTRA-INDICATIONS Acute myocardial infarction in past 90 days · history of non-arteritic anterior ischaemic optic neuropathy · hypotension (avoid if systolic blood pressure below 90 mmHg)
SPECIFIC CONTRA-INDICATIONS
- When used for Benign prostatic hyperplasia or Erectile dysfunction Mild to severe heart failure · patients in whom vasodilation or sexual activity are inadvisable · recent stroke · uncontrolled arrhythmias · uncontrolled hypertension · unstable angina

- **CAUTIONS**
- When used for Benign prostatic hyperplasia or Erectile dysfunction Anatomical deformation of the penis (e.g. angulation, cavernosal fibrosis, Peyronie's disease) · cardiovascular disease · left ventricular outflow obstruction · predisposition to priapism (e.g. in sickle-cell disease, multiple myeloma, or leukaemia)
- When used for Pulmonary arterial hypertension Anatomical deformation of the penis · aortic and mitral valve disease · congestive cardiomyopathy · coronary artery disease · hereditary degenerative retinal disorders · left ventricular dysfunction · life-threatening arrhythmias · pericardial constriction · predisposition to priapism · pulmonary veno-occlusive disease · uncontrolled hypertension
CAUTIONS, FURTHER INFORMATION
- Elderly For phosphodiesterase type-5 inhibitors, Screening Tool of Older Persons' potentially inappropriate Prescriptions (STOPP) criteria to aid medication reviews (see Prescribing in the elderly p. 31 for information): potentially inappropriate in severe heart failure characterised by hypotension i.e. systolic blood pressure less than 90 mmHg, or concurrent nitrate therapy for angina (risk of cardiovascular collapse).

- **INTERACTIONS** → Appendix 1: phosphodiesterase type-5 inhibitors

- **SIDE-EFFECTS**
- **Common or very common** Flushing · gastrointestinal discomfort · headaches · myalgia · nasal congestion · pain
- **Uncommon** Arrhythmias · chest pain · dizziness · dyspnoea · eye pain · fatigue · gastrooesophageal reflux disease · haemorrhage · hypertension · hypotension · nausea · oedema · palpitations · skin reactions · tinnitus · vision disorders · vomiting
- **Rare or very rare** Acute coronary syndrome · angioedema · cerebrovascular insufficiency · eye erythema · eye swelling · haematospermia · hyperhidrosis · memory loss · optic neuropathy (discontinue if sudden visual impairment occurs) · priapism · retinal occlusion · seizure · Stevens-Johnson syndrome · sudden cardiac death · sudden hearing loss (discontinue drug and seek medical advice) · syncope

- **PREGNANCY** Manufacturer advises avoid.

- **BREAST FEEDING** Manufacturer advises avoid—present in milk in *animal* studies.

- **HEPATIC IMPAIRMENT**
- When used for Pulmonary arterial hypertension Manufacturer advises caution in mild to moderate impairment (limited information available); avoid in severe impairment (no information available).
- When used for Benign prostatic hyperplasia or Erectile dysfunction Manufacturer advises caution for regular once-daily

dosing (no information available), and in severe impairment for intermittent use (limited information available).

Dose adjustments
▸ When used for Pulmonary arterial hypertension Manufacturer advises consider initial dose reduction to 20 mg once daily in mild to moderate impairment.
▸ When used for Erectile dysfunction Manufacturer advises dose of 10 mg for intermittent use (no information available for higher doses).

● RENAL IMPAIRMENT
▸ When used for Pulmonary arterial hypertension [EvGr] Avoid in severe impairment. ◈
▸ When used for Erectile dysfunction or Benign prostatic hyperplasia [EvGr] Avoid regular once-daily dosing in severe impairment. ◈

Dose adjustments
▸ When used for Pulmonary arterial hypertension [EvGr] Initial dose of 20 mg once daily in mild-to-moderate impairment; dose may be increased to 40 mg once daily if tolerated. ◈
▸ When used for Erectile dysfunction [EvGr] Maximum dose of 10 mg for intermittent use in severe impairment. ◈

● NATIONAL FUNDING/ACCESS DECISIONS
For full details see funding body website

Scottish Medicines Consortium (SMC) decisions
▸ Tadalafil (*Adcirca* ®) for the treatment of pulmonary arterial hypertension (PAH) classified as WHO functional class II and III, to improve exercise capacity (July 2012) SMC No. 710/11 Recommended with restrictions
NHS restrictions   *Cialis* ® is not prescribable in NHS primary care for the treatment of erectile dysfunction except in men who meet the criteria listed in part XVIIIB of the Drug Tariff (Part XIb of the Northern Ireland Drug Tariff, Part 12 of the Scottish Drug Tariff). The prescription must be endorsed 'SLS'. For more information see *Prices in the BNF*, under How to use the BNF.

● MEDICINAL FORMS There can be variation in the licensing of different medicines containing the same drug.

Oral tablet
▸ Tadalafil (Non-proprietary)
   Tadalafil 2.5 mg Tadalafil 2.5mg tablets | 28 tablet [PoM] £54.99 DT = £20.06
   Tadalafil 5 mg Tadalafil 5mg tablets | 28 tablet [PoM] £54.99 DT = £3.68
   Tadalafil 10 mg Tadalafil 10mg tablets | 4 tablet [PoM] £0.20 DT = £0.90 (Hospital only) | 4 tablet [PoM] £28.88 DT = £0.90
   Tadalafil 20 mg Tadalafil 20mg tablets | 4 tablet [PoM] £54.99 DT = £0.99 | 4 tablet [PoM] £0.29 DT = £0.99 (Hospital only) | 8 tablet [PoM] £1.98–£109.98 | 56 tablet [PoM] £390.00
▸ Adcirca (Eli Lilly and Company Ltd)
   Tadalafil 20 mg Adcirca 20mg tablets | 56 tablet [PoM] £491.22
▸ Cialis (Eli Lilly and Company Ltd)
   Tadalafil 2.5 mg Cialis 2.5mg tablets | 28 tablet [PoM] £54.99 DT = £20.06
   Tadalafil 5 mg Cialis 5mg tablets | 28 tablet [PoM] £54.99 DT = £3.68
   Tadalafil 10 mg Cialis 10mg tablets | 4 tablet [PoM] £28.88 DT = £0.90
   Tadalafil 20 mg Cialis 20mg tablets | 4 tablet [PoM] £28.88 DT = £0.99 | 8 tablet [PoM] £57.76
▸ Talmanco (Viatris UK Healthcare Ltd)
   Tadalafil 20 mg Talmanco 20mg tablets | 56 tablet [PoM] £417.54

Vardenafil

15-Apr-2024

● INDICATIONS AND DOSE
Erectile dysfunction
▸ BY MOUTH USING TABLETS
▸ Adult: Initially 10 mg (max. per dose 20 mg), to be taken approximately 25–60 minutes before sexual activity, subsequent doses adjusted according to

response, onset of effect may be delayed if taken with high-fat meal; maximum 1 dose per day
▸ BY MOUTH USING ORODISPERSIBLE TABLET
▸ Adult: 10 mg, to be taken approximately 25–60 minutes before sexual activity; maximum 10 mg per day

Erectile dysfunction (patients on alpha-blocker therapy)
▸ BY MOUTH USING TABLETS
▸ Adult: Initially 5 mg (max. per dose 20 mg), to be taken approximately 25–60 minutes before sexual activity, subsequent doses adjusted according to response, onset of effect may be delayed if taken with high-fat meal; maximum 1 dose per day

● DOSE EQUIVALENCE AND CONVERSION
▸ *Orodispersible* tablets and *film-coated* tablets are **not** bioequivalent.

● CONTRA-INDICATIONS Avoid if systolic blood pressure below 90 mmHg · hereditary degenerative retinal disorders · myocardial infarction · patients in whom vasodilation or sexual activity are inadvisable · previous history of non-arteritic anterior ischaemic optic neuropathy · recent stroke · unstable angina

● CAUTIONS Active peptic ulceration · anatomical deformation of the penis (e.g. angulation, cavernosal fibrosis, Peyronie's disease) · bleeding disorders · cardiovascular disease · elderly · left ventricular outflow obstruction · predisposition to priapism (e.g. in sickle-cell disease, multiple myeloma, or leukaemia) · susceptibility to prolongation of QT interval

CAUTIONS, FURTHER INFORMATION
▸ Elderly For phosphodiesterase type-5 inhibitors, Screening Tool of Older Persons' potentially inappropriate Prescriptions (STOPP) criteria to aid medication reviews (see Prescribing in the elderly p. 31 for information): potentially inappropriate in severe heart failure characterised by hypotension i.e. systolic blood pressure less than 90 mmHg, or concurrent nitrate therapy for angina (risk of cardiovascular collapse).

● INTERACTIONS → Appendix 1: phosphodiesterase type-5 inhibitors

● SIDE-EFFECTS
▸ **Common or very common** Dizziness · flushing · gastrointestinal discomfort · headache · nasal congestion
▸ **Uncommon** Allergic oedema · angioedema · arrhythmias · back pain · diarrhoea · drowsiness · dry mouth · dyspnoea · eye discomfort · eye disorders · gastrointestinal disorders · malaise · muscle complaints · muscle tone increased · nausea · palpitations · sensation abnormal · sinus congestion · skin reactions · sleep disorder · tinnitus · vertigo · vision disorders · vomiting
▸ **Rare or very rare** Angina pectoris · anxiety · chest pain · conjunctivitis · haemorrhage · hypertension · hypotension · memory loss · myocardial infarction · photosensitivity reaction · priapism · seizure · syncope
▸ **Frequency not known** Haematospermia · optic neuropathy (discontinue if sudden visual impairment occurs) · QT interval prolongation · sudden hearing loss

● HEPATIC IMPAIRMENT For *film-coated tablets*, manufacturer advises caution in mild to moderate impairment; avoid in severe impairment. For *orodispersible tablets*, manufacturer advises caution in mild impairment; avoid in moderate to severe impairment.
Dose adjustments For *film-coated tablets*, manufacturer advises initial dose reduction to 5 mg in mild to moderate impairment, increase according to response; max. 10 mg in moderate impairment.

   For *orodispersible tablets*, manufacturer advises initial dose reduction to 5 mg using *film-coated tablets* in mild impairment, increase according to response.

- **RENAL IMPAIRMENT**
  Dose adjustments [EvGr] Consider initial dose of 5 mg if creatinine clearance less than 30 mL/minute; *orodispersible tablets* not suitable for initial doses. ⟨M⟩ See p. 21.
- **PRESCRIBING AND DISPENSING INFORMATION**
  Orodispersible tablets not suitable for initiation of therapy in patients taking alpha-blockers.
- **NATIONAL FUNDING/ACCESS DECISIONS**
  For full details see funding body website
  Scottish Medicines Consortium (SMC) decisions
- Vardenafil orodispersible tablet (*Levitra*®) for the treatment of erectile dysfunction (October 2011) SMC No. 727/11
  Recommended with restrictions
  NHS restrictions   *Levitra*® is not prescribable in NHS primary care for the treatment of erectile dysfunction except in men who meet the criteria listed in part XVIIIB of the Drug Tariff (Part XIb of the Northern Ireland Drug Tariff, Part 12 of the Scottish Drug Tariff). The prescription must be endorsed 'SLS'. For more information see *Prices in the BNF*, under How to use the BNF.

- **MEDICINAL FORMS**   There can be variation in the licensing of different medicines containing the same drug.
  Oral tablet
  - Vardenafil (Non-proprietary)
    Vardenafil (as Vardenafil hydrochloride trihydrate)
    5 mg   Vardenafil 5mg tablets | 4 tablet [PoM] £7.90 DT = £7.49 | 8 tablet [PoM] £11.36
    Vardenafil (as Vardenafil hydrochloride trihydrate)
    10 mg   Vardenafil 10mg tablets | 4 tablet [PoM] £13.30 DT = £8.95
    Vardenafil (as Vardenafil hydrochloride trihydrate)
    20 mg   Vardenafil 20mg tablets | 4 tablet [PoM] £40.00 DT = £9.49 | 8 tablet [PoM] £8.83–£42.52

PROSTAGLANDINS AND ANALOGUES

Alprostadil
20-Jul-2020

- **INDICATIONS AND DOSE**

Erectile dysfunction (initiated under specialist supervision)
- BY URETHRAL APPLICATION
- Adult: Initially 250 micrograms, adjusted according to response; usual dose 0.125–1 mg; maximum 2 doses per day; maximum 7 doses per week

Aid to diagnosis of erectile dysfunction
- BY URETHRAL APPLICATION
- Adult: 500 micrograms for 1 dose

Erectile dysfunction
- TO THE SKIN
- Adult: Apply 300 micrograms, to the tip of the penis, 5–30 minutes before sexual activity; max 1 dose in 24 hours not more than 2–3 times per week

CAVERJECT®
Erectile dysfunction
- BY INTRACAVERNOSAL INJECTION
- Adult: Initially 2.5 micrograms for 1 dose (first dose), followed by 5 micrograms for 1 dose (second dose), to be given if some response to first dose, alternatively 7.5 micrograms for 1 dose (second dose), to be given if no response to first dose, then increased in steps of 5–10 micrograms, to obtain a dose suitable for producing erection lasting not more than 1 hour; if no response to dose then next higher dose can be given within 1 hour, if there is a response the next dose should not be given for at least 24 hours; usual dose 5–20 micrograms (max. per dose 60 micrograms), maximum frequency of injection not more than 3 times per week with at least 24 hour interval between injections

Erectile dysfunction associated with neurological dysfunction
- BY INTRACAVERNOSAL INJECTION
- Adult: Initially 1.25 micrograms for 1 dose (first dose), then 2.5 micrograms for 1 dose (second dose), then 5 micrograms for 1 dose (third dose), increased in steps of 5–10 micrograms, to obtain a dose suitable for producing erection lasting not more than 1 hour; if no response to dose then next higher dose can be given within 1 hour, if there is a response the next dose should not be given for at least 24 hours; usual dose 5–20 micrograms (max. per dose 60 micrograms), maximum frequency of injection not more than 3 times per week with at least 24 hour interval between injections

Aid to diagnosis
- BY INTRACAVERNOSAL INJECTION
- Adult: 10–20 micrograms for 1 dose (consult product literature)

Aid to diagnosis where evidence of neurological dysfunction
- BY INTRACAVERNOSAL INJECTION
- Adult: Initially 5 micrograms (max. per dose 10 micrograms) for 1 dose, (consult product literature)

CAVERJECT® DUAL CHAMBER
Erectile dysfunction
- BY INTRACAVERNOSAL INJECTION
- Adult: Initially 2.5 micrograms for 1 dose (first dose), followed by 5 micrograms for 1 dose (second dose), to be given if some response to first dose, alternatively 7.5 micrograms for 1 dose (second dose), to be given if no response to first dose, then increased in steps of 5–10 micrograms, to obtain a dose suitable for producing erection lasting not more than 1 hour; if no response to dose then next higher dose can be given within 1 hour, if there is a response the next dose should not be given for at least 24 hours; usual dose 5–20 micrograms (max. per dose 60 micrograms), maximum frequency of injection not more than 3 times per week with at least 24 hour interval between injections

Erectile dysfunction associated with neurological dysfunction
- BY INTRACAVERNOSAL INJECTION
- Adult: Initially 1.25 micrograms for 1 dose (first dose), then 2.5 micrograms for 1 dose (second dose), then 5 micrograms for 1 dose (third dose), increased in steps of 5–10 micrograms, to obtain a dose suitable for producing erection lasting not more than 1 hour; if no response to dose then next higher dose can be given within 1 hour, if there is a response the next dose should not be given for at least 24 hours; usual dose 5–20 micrograms (max. per dose 60 micrograms), maximum frequency of injection not more than 3 times per week with at least 24 hour interval between injections

Aid to diagnosis
- BY INTRACAVERNOSAL INJECTION
- Adult: 10–20 micrograms for 1 dose (consult product literature)

Aid to diagnosis where evidence of neurological dysfunction
- BY INTRACAVERNOSAL INJECTION
- Adult: Initially 5 micrograms (max. per dose 10 micrograms) for 1 dose, (consult product literature)

continued →

VIRIDAL ® DUO

Neurogenic erectile dysfunction

▶ BY INTRACAVERNOSAL INJECTION

▶ **Adult:** Initially 1.25 micrograms, increased in steps of 2.5–5 micrograms, to obtain dose suitable for producing erection not lasting more than 1 hour; usual dose 10–20 micrograms (max. per dose 40 micrograms), maximum frequency of injection not more than 3 times per week with at least 24 hour interval between injections; reduce dose if erection lasts longer than 2 hours

Erectile dysfunction

▶ BY INTRACAVERNOSAL INJECTION

▶ **Adult:** Initially 2.5 micrograms, increased in steps of 2.5–5 micrograms, to obtain dose suitable for producing erection not lasting more than 1 hour; usual dose 10–20 micrograms (max. per dose 40 micrograms), maximum frequency of injection not more than 3 times per week with at least 24 hour interval between injections; reduce dose if erection lasts longer than 2 hours

● **CONTRA-INDICATIONS**

GENERAL CONTRA-INDICATIONS Not for use in patients with penile implants or when sexual activity medically inadvisable (e.g. orthostatic hypotension, myocardial infarction, and syncope) · not for use with other agents for erectile dysfunction · predisposition to prolonged erection (as in thrombocythaemia, polycythaemia, sickle cell anaemia, multiple myeloma or leukaemia) · urethral application contra-indicated in balanitis · urethral application contra-indicated in severe curvature · urethral application contra-indicated in severe hypospadia · urethral application contra-indicated in urethral stricture · urethral application contra-indicated in urethritis

SPECIFIC CONTRA-INDICATIONS

▶ With topical use Balanitis · severe curvature · severe hypospadia · urethral stricture · urethritis

● **CAUTIONS** Anatomical deformations of penis (painful erection more likely)—follow up regularly to detect signs of penile fibrosis (consider discontinuation if angulation, cavernosal fibrosis or Peyronie's disease develop) · priapism (patients should be instructed to report any erection lasting 4 hours or longer) · risk factors for cardiovascular disorders · risk factors for cerebrovascular disorders

● **INTERACTIONS** → Appendix 1: alprostadil

● **SIDE-EFFECTS**

GENERAL SIDE-EFFECTS

▶ **Common or very common** Balanoposthitis · hypotension · penile disorders · sexual dysfunction

SPECIFIC SIDE-EFFECTS

▶ **Common or very common**

▶ With intracavernosal use Haemorrhage · muscle spasms · skin reactions

▶ With topical use Genital abnormalities · rash · urinary tract pain

▶ With urethral use Dizziness · haemorrhage · headache · muscle spasms · urethral burning

▶ **Uncommon**

▶ With intracavernosal use Asthenia · dry mouth · extrasystole · hyperhidrosis · increased risk of infection · inflammation · mydriasis · nausea · oedema · pelvic pain · peripheral vascular disease · presyncope · scrotal disorders · sensation abnormal · spermatocele · testicular disorders · urinary disorders · vascular disorders · vasodilation

▶ With topical use Dizziness · hyperaesthesia · pain in extremity · scrotal pain · syncope · urinary tract disorders

▶ With urethral use Hyperhidrosis · increased risk of infection · leg pain · nausea · pelvic pain · perineal pain · peripheral vascular disease · scrotal disorders · sensation abnormal ·

skin reactions · spermatocele · syncope · testicular disorders · urinary disorders · vascular disorders · vasodilation

▶ **Frequency not known**

▶ With intracavernosal use Myocardial ischaemia · stroke

● **CONCEPTION AND CONTRACEPTION**

▶ With urethral use If partner is pregnant, barrier contraception should be used. No evidence of harm to latex condoms and diaphragms.

▶ With topical use Condoms should be used to avoid exposure to women of child-bearing age, pregnant or lactating women. No evidence of harm to latex condoms.

● **DIRECTIONS FOR ADMINISTRATION**

▶ With intracavernosal use Manufacturer advises the first dose of the intracavernosal injection must be given by medically trained personnel; self-administration may only be undertaken after proper training.

▶ With urethral use Manufacturer advises during initiation of treatment the urethral application should be used under medical supervision; self-administration may only be undertaken after proper training.

● **PATIENT AND CARER ADVICE** Patients should be instructed to report any erection lasting 4 hours or longer.

▶ With topical use Counsel patients that condoms should be used to avoid local reactions and exposure of alprostadil to women of childbearing age, pregnant, or lactating women.

● **NATIONAL FUNDING/ACCESS DECISIONS**

NHS restrictions Caverject®, Viridal® Duo, Vitaros® and MUSE® are not prescribable in NHS primary care for the treatment of erectile dysfunction except in men who meet the criteria listed in part XVIIIB of the Drug Tariff (Part XIb of the Northern Ireland Drug Tariff, Part 12 of the Scottish Drug Tariff). The prescription must be endorsed 'SLS'. For more information see Prices in the BNF, under How to use BNF publications.

● **MEDICINAL FORMS** There can be variation in the licensing of different medicines containing the same drug.

Cutaneous cream

▶ Vitaros (The Simple Pharma Company UK Ltd)
Alprostadil 3 mg per 1 gram Vitaros 3mg/g cream | 4 applicator [PoM] £40.00 DT = £40.00

Stick

▶ Muse (Viatris UK Healthcare Ltd)
Alprostadil 500 microgram Muse 500microgram urethral sticks | 1 applicator [PoM] £11.30 DT = £11.30 | 6 applicator [PoM] £67.79
Alprostadil 1 mg Muse 1000microgram urethral sticks | 1 applicator [PoM] £11.56 DT = £11.56 | 6 applicator [PoM] £65.67

Powder and solvent for solution for injection

▶ Alprostadil (Non-proprietary)
Alprostadil 10 microgram Alprostadil 10microgram powder and solvent for solution for injection vials | 1 vial [PoM] £9.24 DT = £9.24
Alprostadil 20 microgram Alprostadil 20microgram powder and solvent for solution for injection vials | 1 vial [PoM] £11.94 DT = £11.94

▶ Caverject (Pfizer Ltd)
Alprostadil 10 microgram Caverject 10microgram powder and solvent for solution for injection vials | 1 vial [PoM] £9.24 DT = £9.24
Caverject Dual Chamber 10microgram powder and solvent for injection | 2 pre-filled disposable injection [PoM] £14.70 DT = £14.70
Alprostadil 20 microgram Caverject Dual Chamber 20microgram powder and solvent for solution for injection | 2 pre-filled disposable injection [PoM] £19.00 DT = £19.00
Caverject 20microgram powder and solvent for solution for injection vials | 1 vial [PoM] £11.94 DT = £11.94

▶ Viridal (Advanz Pharma)
Alprostadil 10 microgram Viridal Duo Starter Pack 10microgram powder and solvent for solution for injection cartridges with device | 2 cartridge [PoM] £35.55 DT = £35.55
Alprostadil 20 microgram Viridal Duo Starter Pack 20microgram powder and solvent for solution for injection cartridges with device | 2 cartridge [PoM] £35.55 DT = £35.55

Alprostadil 40 microgram Viridal Duo Starter Pack 40microgram powder and solvent for solution for injection cartridges with device | 2 cartridge [PoM] £35.55 DT = £35.55

SYMPATHOMIMETICS > VASOCONSTRICTOR

Adrenaline/epinephrine
10-Apr-2025

- **DRUG ACTION** Acts on both alpha and beta receptors and increases both heart rate and contractility (beta$_1$ effects); it can cause peripheral vasodilation (a beta$_2$ effect) or vasoconstriction (an alpha effect).

- **INDICATIONS AND DOSE**

  Priapism associated with alprostadil, if aspiration and lavage of corpora are unsuccessful (alternative to phenylephrine or metaraminol)
  - BY INTRACAVERNOSAL INJECTION
  - Adult: 10–20 micrograms every 5–10 minutes, using a 20 microgram/mL solution, **Important:** if suitable strength of adrenaline not available may be specially prepared by diluting 0.1 mL of the adrenaline 1 in 1000 (1 mg/mL) injection to 5 mL with sodium chloride 0.9%, continuously monitor blood pressure and pulse; maximum 100 micrograms per course

- **UNLICENSED USE**
  - When used for Priapism The use of adrenaline is an unlicensed indication.

- **CAUTIONS** Arteriosclerosis · arrhythmias · cerebrovascular disease · cor pulmonale · diabetes mellitus · elderly · hypercalcaemia · hyperreflexia · hypertension · hyperthyroidism · hypokalaemia · ischaemic heart disease · obstructive cardiomyopathy · occlusive vascular disease · organic brain damage · phaeochromocytoma · prostate disorders · psychoneurosis · severe angina · susceptibility to angle-closure glaucoma

  CAUTIONS, FURTHER INFORMATION Cautions listed are only for non-life-threatening situations.

- **INTERACTIONS** → Appendix 1: sympathomimetics, vasoconstrictor

- **SIDE-EFFECTS**
  - **Rare or very rare** Cardiomyopathy
  - **Frequency not known** Angina pectoris · angle closure glaucoma · anxiety · appetite decreased · arrhythmias · asthenia · CNS haemorrhage · confusion · dizziness · dry mouth · dyspnoea · headache · hepatic necrosis · hyperglycaemia · hyperhidrosis · hypersalivation · hypertension (increased risk of cerebral haemorrhage) · hypokalaemia · injection site necrosis · insomnia · intestinal necrosis · metabolic acidosis · mydriasis · myocardial infarction · nausea · pallor · palpitations · peripheral coldness · psychosis · pulmonary oedema (on excessive dosage or extreme sensitivity) · renal necrosis · soft tissue necrosis · tremor · urinary disorders · vomiting

- **RENAL IMPAIRMENT** Manufacturers advise use with caution in severe impairment.

- **MONITORING REQUIREMENTS** Monitor blood pressure and ECG.

- **MEDICINAL FORMS** There can be variation in the licensing of different medicines containing the same drug. Forms available from special-order manufacturers include: solution for injection

Solution for injection
EXCIPIENTS: May contain Sulfites
- Adrenaline/epinephrine (Non-proprietary)
  Adrenaline 1 mg per 1 ml Adrenaline (base) 10mg/10ml (1 in 1,000) solution for injection ampoules | 10 ampoule [PoM] £162.98-£281.10 DT = £162.98
  Adrenaline (base) for anaphylaxis 1mg/1ml (1 in 1,000) solution for injection pre-filled syringes | 1 pre-filled disposable injection [PoM] £15.77 DT = £15.77

Adrenaline (base) 1mg/1ml (1 in 1,000) solution for injection pre-filled syringes | 1 pre-filled disposable injection [PoM] £12.98-£15.77 DT = £15.77
Adrenaline (as Adrenaline acid tartrate) 1 mg per 1 ml Adrenaline (base) 5mg/5ml (1 in 1,000) solution for injection ampoules | 10 ampoule [PoM] £199.90 DT = £166.15
Adrenaline (base) 500micrograms/0.5ml (1 in 1,000) solution for injection ampoules | 10 ampoule [PoM] £333.46-£533.52 DT = £333.46
Adrenaline (base) 1mg/1ml (1 in 1,000) solution for injection ampoules | 10 ampoule [PoM] £11.81 DT = £11.81 (Hospital only) | 10 ampoule [PoM] £6.00-£11.81 DT = £11.81

Metaraminol
28-Apr-2020

- **INDICATIONS AND DOSE**

  Priapism (alternative to intracavernosal injections of phenylephrine and adrenaline)
  - BY INTRACAVERNOSAL INJECTION
  - Adult: 1 mg every 15 minutes

- **UNLICENSED USE** Use for priapism is an unlicensed indication.

- **CAUTIONS** Associated with fatal hypertensive crises · cirrhosis · coronary vascular thrombosis · diabetes mellitus · elderly · extravasation at injection site may cause necrosis · following myocardial infarction · hypercapnia · hypertension · hyperthyroidism · hypoxia · mesenteric vascular thrombosis · peripheral vascular thrombosis · Prinzmetal's variant angina · uncorrected hypovolaemia

- **INTERACTIONS** → Appendix 1: sympathomimetics, vasoconstrictor

- **SIDE-EFFECTS**
  - **Common or very common** Headache · hypertension
  - **Rare or very rare** Skin exfoliation · soft tissue necrosis
  - **Frequency not known** Abscess · arrhythmias · nausea · palpitations · peripheral ischaemia

- **MONITORING REQUIREMENTS** Monitor blood pressure and rate of flow frequently.

- **DIRECTIONS FOR ADMINISTRATION** For *intracavernosal injection*, dilute 1 mg (0.1 mL of 10 mg/mL) metaraminol injection to 50 mL with Sodium Chloride injection 0.9% and give carefully by slow injection into the corpora in 5 mL injections.

- **MEDICINAL FORMS** There can be variation in the licensing of different medicines containing the same drug. Forms available from special-order manufacturers include: solution for injection

Solution for injection
- Metaraminol (Non-proprietary)
  Metaraminol (as Metaraminol tartrate) 500 microgram per 1 ml Metaraminol 2.5mg/5ml solution for injection ampoules | 10 ampoule [PoM] £52.90 (Hospital only)
  Metaraminol 5mg/10ml solution for injection ampoules | 10 ampoule [PoM] £107.40 (Hospital only)
  Metaraminol 2.5mg/5ml solution for injection pre-filled syringes | 10 pre-filled disposable injection [PoM] £95.00 (Hospital only)
  Metaraminol 5mg/10ml solution for injection vials | 10 vial [PoM] £55.00 (Hospital only)
  Metaraminol (as Metaraminol tartrate) 10 mg per 1 ml Metaraminol 10mg/1ml solution for injection vials | 10 vial [PoM] £20.50 (Hospital only)
  Metaraminol 10mg/1ml solution for injection ampoules | 5 ampoule [PoM] £25.00 | 10 ampoule [PoM] £70.60 | 10 ampoule [PoM] £21.50 (Hospital only)

Phenylephrine hydrochloride

- **INDICATIONS AND DOSE**

Priapism associated with alprostadil, if aspiration and lavage of the corpora are unsuccessful (alternative to adrenaline or metaraminol)
▶ BY INTRACAVERNOSAL INJECTION
▶ Adult: 100–200 micrograms every 5–10 minutes, dose to be administered using a 200 micrograms/mL solution; maximum 1 mg per course

- **UNLICENSED USE** Use of phenylephrine hydrochloride injection in priapism is an unlicensed indication.
- **CONTRA-INDICATIONS** Hypertension
- **INTERACTIONS** → Appendix 1: sympathomimetics, vasoconstrictor
- **SIDE-EFFECTS** Angle closure glaucoma · anxiety · appetite decreased · arrhythmias · asthenia · confusion · dyspnoea · headache · hypertension · hypoxia · insomnia · nausea · palpitations · peripheral ischaemia · psychosis · tremor · urinary retention · vomiting
- **DIRECTIONS FOR ADMINISTRATION** For *intracavernosal injection*, if suitable strength of phenylephrine injection is not available, it may be specially prepared by diluting 0.1 mL of the phenylephrine 1% (10 mg/mL) injection to 5 mL with Sodium Chloride 0.9%.

- **MEDICINAL FORMS** There can be variation in the licensing of different medicines containing the same drug. Forms available from special-order manufacturers include: solution for injection

Solution for injection
▶ Phenylephrine hydrochloride (Non-proprietary)
Phenylephrine (as Phenylephrine hydrochloride) 50 microgram per 1 ml Phenylephrine 500micrograms/10ml solution for injection pre-filled syringes | 10 pre-filled disposable injection PoM £150.00 (Hospital only)
Phenylephrine hydrochloride 100 microgram per 1 ml Phenylephrine 1mg/10ml solution for injection ampoules | 10 ampoule PoM £47.59 (Hospital only)
Phenylephrine 2mg/20ml solution for injection vials | 10 vial PoM £110.00 (Hospital only)
Phenylephrine hydrochloride 10 mg per 1 ml Phenylephrine 10mg/1ml solution for injection ampoules | 10 ampoule PoM £99.00–£99.12 (Hospital only)
Phenylephrine 10mg/1ml concentrate for solution for injection ampoules | 10 ampoule PoM £102.09 (Hospital only)

VASODILATORS ⟩ PERIPHERAL VASODILATORS

Aviptadil with phentolamine mesilate

16-Oct-2020

- **DRUG ACTION** Phentolamine is a short-acting alpha-adrenoceptor antagonist that acts directly on vascular smooth muscle, resulting in vasodilatation; aviptadil is a vasoactive intestinal polypeptide that acts as a smooth muscle relaxant.

- **INDICATIONS AND DOSE**

Erectile dysfunction
▶ BY INTRACAVERNOSAL INJECTION
▶ Adult: 25/2000 micrograms, frequency of injection should not exceed once daily or three times weekly, duration of erection should not exceed 1 hour

DOSE EQUIVALENCE AND CONVERSION
▶ Dose expressed as *x/y* micrograms of aviptadil/phentolamine.

- **CONTRA-INDICATIONS** Anatomical deformation of the penis (e.g. angulation, cavernosal fibrosis, Peyronie's disease) · not for use with other agents for erectile dysfunction · patients for whom sexual activity is inadvisable · penile implants · predisposition to priapism (e.g. in sickle cell anaemia or trait, multiple myeloma, or leukaemia)

- **CAUTIONS** Concomitant treatment with anticoagulants (potential increased risk of bleeding) · history of psychiatric disorder or addiction (potential for abuse) · severe cardiovascular disease · severe cerebrovascular disease

- **SIDE-EFFECTS**
▶ **Common or very common** Bruising · flushing
▶ **Uncommon** Dizziness · haematoma · headache · palpitations · tachycardia
▶ **Rare or very rare** Angina pectoris · myocardial infarction · penile fibrosis (following multiple injections) · penile nodules · sexual dysfunction

- **MONITORING REQUIREMENTS** Manufacturer advises monitor regularly (e.g. every 3 months), particularly in the initial stages of self-injection therapy; careful examination of the penis is recommended to detect signs of penile fibrosis or Peyronie's disease—discontinue treatment in patients who develop penile angulation, cavernosal fibrosis, or Peyronie's disease.

- **DIRECTIONS FOR ADMINISTRATION** Manufacturer advises that the initial injections of *Invicorp*® must be administered by medically trained personnel; self-administration may only be undertaken after proper training.

- **HANDLING AND STORAGE** Manufacturer advises store in a refrigerator (2–8°C).

- **PATIENT AND CARER ADVICE** Manufacturer advises that patients should be instructed to report any erection lasting 4 hours or longer.

- **NATIONAL FUNDING/ACCESS DECISIONS**
For full details see funding body website
Scottish Medicines Consortium (SMC) decisions
▶ Aviptadil/phentolamine mesilate (*Invicorp*®) for the **symptomatic treatment of erectile dysfunction in adult males due to neurogenic, vasculogenic, psychogenic, or mixed aetiology (December 2017)** SMC No. 1284/17 Recommended with restrictions
All Wales Medicines Strategy Group (AWMSG) decisions
▶ Aviptadil/phentolamine mesilate (*Invicorp*®) for the **symptomatic treatment of erectile dysfunction in adult males due to neurogenic, vasculogenic, psychogenic, or mixed aetiology (July 2017)** AWMSG No. 3435 Recommended with restrictions

- **MEDICINAL FORMS** There can be variation in the licensing of different medicines containing the same drug.
Solution for injection
▶ Invicorp (Evolan Pharma AB)
Aviptadil 71.43 microgram per 1 ml, Phentolamine mesilate 5.71 mg per 1 ml Invicorp 25micrograms/2mg/0.35ml solution for injection ampoules | 5 ampoule PoM £61.23 DT = £47.50

4.2 Premature ejaculation

Premature ejaculation

01-Aug-2017

Description of condition

Premature ejaculation is a common male sexual disorder characterised by brief ejaculatory latency, loss of control, and psychological distress.

Treatment

EvGr Non-drug treatment (including psychosexual counselling, education, and behavioural treatments) are recommended in patients for whom premature ejaculation causes few (if any) problems or in patients who prefer not to take drug treatment. These techniques can also be used in addition to a drug treatment.

For patients with life-long premature ejaculation, drug treatment is the recommended approach. ⟨A⟩ Dapoxetine below, a short-acting selective serotonin re-uptake inhibitor, is licensed to be used when required for this condition (not continuous daily use).

[EvGr] Other selective serotonin re-uptake inhibitors (citalopram p. 422, fluoxetine p. 424, fluvoxamine maleate p. 424, escitalopram p. 423, paroxetine p. 425, sertraline p. 425 [unlicensed indications]) and the tricyclic antidepressant clomipramine [unlicensed indication] have been widely used as regular, daily treatment. Caution is suggested in prescribing selective serotonin re-uptake inhibitors for young adolescents with premature ejaculation, and to men who also have a depressive disorder, particularly when associated with suicidal ideation. Ejaculation delay may start a few days after the start of treatment, but it is more evident after 1 to 2 weeks, since receptor desensitisation requires time to occur.

If premature ejaculation is secondary to Erectile dysfunction p. 938, the erectile dysfunction should be treated first. ⟨A⟩

Topical anaesthetic preparations for the management of premature ejaculation are available without prescription.

SELECTIVE SEROTONIN RE-UPTAKE INHIBITORS

Dapoxetine
19-Jul-2021

- **DRUG ACTION** Dapoxetine is a short-acting selective serotonin re-uptake inhibitor.

- **INDICATIONS AND DOSE**

  Premature ejaculation in men who meet all the following criteria: poor control over ejaculation, a history of premature ejaculation over the past 6 months, marked distress or interpersonal difficulty as a consequence of premature ejaculation, and an intravaginal ejaculatory latency time of less than two minutes
  - BY MOUTH
  - Adult: Initially 30 mg, to be taken approximately 1–3 hours before sexual activity, subsequent doses adjusted according to response; review treatment after 4 weeks (or 6 doses) and at least every 6 months thereafter, not recommended for adults 65 years and over; maximum 1 dose per day; maximum 60 mg per day

  DOSE ADJUSTMENTS DUE TO INTERACTIONS
  - Manufacturer advises max. dose 30 mg with concurrent use of moderate inhibitors of CYP3A4 except in patients verified to be extensive CYP2D6 metabolisers where manufacturer recommends max. dose 60 mg.
  - Manufacturer advises avoid with concurrent use of potent inhibitors of CYP3A4 except in patients verified to be extensive CYP2D6 metabolisers where manufacturer recommends max. dose 30 mg.

- **CONTRA-INDICATIONS** History of bipolar disorder · history of mania · history of severe depression · history of syncope · postural hypotension · significant cardiac disease · uncontrolled epilepsy

- **CAUTIONS** Bleeding disorders · epilepsy (discontinue if convulsions develop) · susceptibility to angle-closure glaucoma

- **INTERACTIONS** → Appendix 1: SSRIs

- **SIDE-EFFECTS**
- **Common or very common** Anxiety · asthenia · concentration impaired · constipation · diarrhoea · dizziness · drowsiness · dry mouth · gastrointestinal discomfort · gastrointestinal disorders · headache · hypotension · mood altered · nausea · paraesthesia · sexual dysfunction · sinus congestion · sleep disorders · sweat changes · syncope · tinnitus · tremor · vasodilation · vision blurred · vomiting · yawning
- **Uncommon** Akathisia · arrhythmias · behaviour abnormal · confusion · depression · eye pain · feeling abnormal · feeling hot · hypertension · level of consciousness decreased · mydriasis · pruritus · taste altered · thinking abnormal · vertigo
- **Rare or very rare** Sudden onset of sleep
- **Frequency not known** Increased risk of fracture
  SIDE-EFFECTS, FURTHER INFORMATION Discontinue if psychiatric disorder develops.
- **HEPATIC IMPAIRMENT** Manufacturer advises avoid in moderate to severe impairment.
- **RENAL IMPAIRMENT** [EvGr] Use with caution if creatinine clearance 30–80 mL/minute; avoid if creatinine clearance less than 30 mL/minute (limited information available). Ⓜ See p. 21.
- **PRE-TREATMENT SCREENING** Test for postural hypotension before starting treatment.
- **TREATMENT CESSATION** The dose should preferably be reduced gradually over about 4 weeks, or longer if withdrawal symptoms emerge (6 months in patients who have been on long-term maintenance treatment).
- **PATIENT AND CARER ADVICE**
  Postural hypotension and syncope Patients should be advised to maintain hydration and to sit or lie down until prodromal symptoms such as nausea, dizziness, and sweating abate.

- **MEDICINAL FORMS** There can be variation in the licensing of different medicines containing the same drug.
  Oral tablet
  CAUTIONARY AND ADVISORY LABELS 2, 25
  - **Dapoxetine (Non-proprietary)**
    Dapoxetine 30 mg Dapoxetine 30mg tablets | 3 tablet [PoM] £14.71-£23.00 DT = £14.71 | 6 tablet [PoM] £26.48-£42.00 DT = £26.48
    Dapoxetine 60 mg Dapoxetine 60mg tablets | 3 tablet [PoM] £19.12-£28.60 DT = £19.12 | 6 tablet [PoM] £34.42-£45.60 DT = £34.42
  - **Priligy** (A. Menarini Farmaceutica Internazionale SRL)
    Dapoxetine 30 mg Priligy 30mg tablets | 3 tablet [PoM] £14.71 DT = £14.71 | 6 tablet [PoM] £26.48 DT = £26.48
    Dapoxetine 60 mg Priligy 60mg tablets | 3 tablet [PoM] £19.12 DT = £19.12 | 6 tablet [PoM] £34.42 DT = £34.42

5   Gynaecological conditions
5.1   Polycystic ovary syndrome

Polycystic ovary syndrome
20-Sep-2021

Description of condition

Polycystic ovary syndrome (PCOS) is one of the most common endocrine disorders affecting females of childbearing potential. Clinical features may include ovulation disorders, polycystic ovarian morphology, and hyperandrogenism (with the clinical manifestations of acne, hirsutism and oligomenorrhoea). Complications of PCOS include cardiovascular disease, obstructive sleep apnoea, psychological disorders (such as anxiety and depression), infertility, endometrial cancer, pregnancy complications (such as gestational diabetes and pre-eclampsia), and metabolic disorders (such as insulin resistance and type 2 diabetes).

Aims of treatment

Treatment aims to manage the clinical features of PCOS and prevent the development of complications.

Non-drug treatment

[EvGr] Lifestyle modifications are recommended first line in the management of PCOS; healthy eating, regular physical exercise and maintaining a healthy weight should be encouraged. For females who are overweight or obese, weight loss advice should be offered or referral to a dietician considered, as weight loss may achieve menstrual regularity and reduce insulin resistance, hyperandrogenism, and the risk of type 2 diabetes and cardiovascular disease. For further information on weight management, see Obesity p. 104. Cardiovascular disease risk factors should be assessed (noting that conventional cardiovascular risk calculators have not been validated in females with PCOS) and managed appropriately; specialist referral is required if dyslipidaemia requires treatment. (A) For further information, see Cardiovascular disease risk assessment and prevention p. 219.

Drug treatment

[EvGr] Combined oral contraceptives [unlicensed] are commonly used in PCOS for the treatment of acne, hirsutism, and menstrual irregularity in females who are not planning a pregnancy. Alternative treatment options for menstrual irregularities include a cyclical progestogen [unlicensed] or a levonorgestrel intra-uterine system [unlicensed]. (A) For the management of acne in females with PCOS, see Acne p. 1438.

[EvGr] Treatment with insulin-sensitising drugs, such as metformin, should only be initiated by a specialist. Metformin hydrochloride p. 807 can be considered for females with PCOS who have impaired glucose tolerance or are already undergoing lifestyle modifications with no improvement in impaired glucose tolerance [unlicensed indication]. Metformin hydrochloride may improve short-term insulin sensitivity and reduce androgen concentrations, but there is limited supporting evidence on the long-term benefits.

For the management of infertility, consider referral for fertility treatment.

In females with PCOS who are pregnant or are considering a pregnancy, consider referral for gestational diabetes screening, and whether any changes to drug treatment(s) are required. (A)

6   Kidney disorders

> **Other drugs used for Kidney disorders** Dapagliflozin, p. 826 · Empagliflozin, p. 827 · Tolvaptan, p. 767

DIURETICS > POTASSIUM-SPARING DIURETICS > MINERALOCORTICOID RECEPTOR ANTAGONISTS

| Finerenone
04-Apr-2023

- **DRUG ACTION** Finerenone is a non-steroidal mineralocorticoid receptor antagonist that inhibits receptor-mediated sodium reabsorption and decreases receptor overactivation, thereby reducing the inflammation and fibrosis that lead to kidney damage.

- **INDICATIONS AND DOSE**

Chronic kidney disease (stage 3 and 4 with albuminuria) associated with type 2 diabetes [if serum-potassium ≤5 mmol/L and eGFR ≥60 mL/min/1.73 m^2]
- ▸ BY MOUTH
- ▸ Adult: 20 mg once daily, for dose adjustments and interruption according to serum-potassium levels—consult product literature

Chronic kidney disease (stage 3 and 4 with albuminuria) associated with type 2 diabetes [if serum-potassium ≤5 mmol/L and eGFR 25 to 59 mL/min/1.73 m^2]
- ▸ BY MOUTH
- ▸ Adult: Initially 10 mg once daily; increased if necessary up to 20 mg once daily, dose to be adjusted according to serum-potassium levels and eGFR, for dose adjustments, interruption, and discontinuation according to serum-potassium levels and eGFR— consult product literature

- **CONTRA-INDICATIONS** Addison's disease · hyperkalaemia

 CONTRA-INDICATIONS, FURTHER INFORMATION
- ▸ Hyperkalaemia [EvGr] Do not initiate treatment if serum-potassium > 5 mmol/L.
 Withhold if serum-potassium increases to > 5.5 mmol/L during treatment. (M)

- **INTERACTIONS** → Appendix 1: mineralocorticoid receptor antagonists

- **SIDE-EFFECTS**
- ▸ **Common or very common** Electrolyte imbalance · hypotension · pruritus

- **PREGNANCY** [EvGr] Avoid unless potential benefit outweighs risk—reproductive toxicity in *animal* studies. (M)

- **BREAST FEEDING** [EvGr] Avoid unless potential benefit outweighs risk— *animal* studies have reported excretion into milk with adverse reactions in the exposed offspring. (M)

- **HEPATIC IMPAIRMENT** [EvGr] Avoid in severe impairment (no information available). Consider additional serum-potassium monitoring in moderate impairment. (M)

- **RENAL IMPAIRMENT** [EvGr] Avoid initiation if eGFR less than 25 mL/minute/1.73 m^2 (limited information available). Discontinue if eGFR falls persistently below 15 mL/minute/1.73 m^2 (end-stage renal disease) during treatment (limited information available). (M) See p. 21.

- **MONITORING REQUIREMENTS**
- ▸ [EvGr] Measure serum-potassium and eGFR at baseline; if serum-potassium > 4.8 to 5 mmol/L at initiation, additional monitoring of serum-potassium required during first 4 weeks of treatment.
- ▸ Remeasure serum-potassium and eGFR 4 weeks after initiation or when restarting treatment or increasing dose; thereafter remeasure serum-potassium periodically and as clinically indicated—consult product literature. (M)

- **DIRECTIONS FOR ADMINISTRATION** [EvGr] *Kerendia*® tablets may be crushed and mixed with water or soft foods, such as apple sauce, immediately before administration. (M)

- **NATIONAL FUNDING/ACCESS DECISIONS**
 For full details see funding body website
 NICE decisions
- ▸ Finerenone for treating chronic kidney disease in type 2 diabetes (March 2023) NICE TA877 Recommended with restrictions
 Scottish Medicines Consortium (SMC) decisions
- ▸ Finerenone (*Kerendia*®) for the treatment of chronic kidney disease (stage 3 and 4 with albuminuria) associated with type 2 diabetes in adults (November 2022) SMC No. SMC2486 Recommended

- **MEDICINAL FORMS** There can be variation in the licensing of different medicines containing the same drug.
 Oral tablet
- ▸ Kerendia (Bayer Plc) ▼
 Finerenone 10 mg Kerendia 10mg tablets | 28 tablet [PoM] £36.68 DT = £36.68
 Finerenone 20 mg Kerendia 20mg tablets | 28 tablet [PoM] £36.68 DT = £36.68

7 Obstetrics

Obstetrics

06-Dec-2023

Induction of abortion

[EvGr] Pre-treatment with mifepristone p. 954 can facilitate the process of medical abortion. [A] It sensitises the uterus to subsequent administration of a prostaglandin and, therefore, abortion occurs in a shorter time and with a lower dose of prostaglandin.

[EvGr] The prostaglandin misoprostol p. 955 is given by mouth, buccally, sublingually, or vaginally, to induce medical abortion following sequential use with mifepristone; it is also used for cervical priming before surgical abortion.
[A]

Gemeprost p. 955, a prostaglandin administered vaginally as pessaries, is licensed for the medical induction of abortion in the second trimester of pregnancy; it is also licensed to soften and dilate the cervix before surgical abortion in early pregnancy.

Miscarriage

[EvGr] Vaginal micronised progesterone p. 880 [unlicensed use] is used for the prevention of miscarriage and should be offered following vaginal bleeding in females with an intra-uterine pregnancy confirmed by a scan, if they have previously had a miscarriage. If a fetal heartbeat is confirmed, continue progesterone until 16 completed weeks of pregnancy. [A]

In pregnant females with antiphospholipid antibody syndrome who have suffered recurrent miscarriage, administration of low-dose aspirin p. 142 and a prophylactic dose of a low molecular weight heparin may decrease the risk of fetal loss (use under specialist supervision only).

[EvGr] For the medical management of missed miscarriage, mifepristone [unlicensed use] followed by misoprostol [unlicensed use] may be offered, unless the gestational sac has already been passed. Misoprostol [unlicensed use] may be used for the medical management of incomplete miscarriage. [A] For further guidance on the management of miscarriage, see NICE guideline: **Ectopic pregnancy and miscarriage: diagnosis and initial management** (see *Useful resources*).

Ectopic pregnancy

[EvGr] Systemic methotrexate [unlicensed use] is used for the management of ectopic pregnancy. [A]

Preterm labour

Antibacterials for the prevention of intra-uterine infection in preterm prelabour rupture of membranes (P PROM)
For guidance on the use of antibacterials to prevent intra-uterine infection in females with P PROM, see Antibacterials, use for prophylaxis p. 574.

Progesterone
[EvGr] Prophylactic progesterone may be offered as an alternative to cervical cerclage in pregnant females with either a history of spontaneous preterm birth (up to 34 +0 weeks of pregnancy) or loss (from 16+0 weeks of pregnancy onwards), and a short cervix, to reduce the risk of preterm birth. In females with only one of these risk factors, the use of prophylactic progesterone should be considered. Treatment with progesterone should be initiated between 16 +0 and 24+0 weeks of pregnancy, and continued until at least 34 weeks. [A] For further guidance on the use of progesterone, see NICE guideline: **Preterm labour and birth** (see *Useful resources*).

Myometrial relaxants
Tocolytic drugs postpone preterm labour and they are used with the aim of reducing harm to the child. The greatest benefit is gained by using the delay to administer corticosteroid therapy or to implement other measures which improve perinatal health (including transfer to a unit with neonatal intensive care facility).

[EvGr] Females between 24+0 and 33+6 weeks of gestation who have intact membranes and are in suspected or diagnosed preterm labour can be given nifedipine p. 189 [unlicensed use] for tocolysis. An oxytocin receptor antagonist (such as atosiban p. 953) is an alternative if nifedipine is contra-indicated or unsuitable.

The beta$_2$ agonists salbutamol and terbutaline sulfate are no longer recommended for inhibiting uncomplicated preterm labour. [A] Use of high-dose short acting beta$_2$ agonists in obstetric indications has been associated with serious, sometimes fatal cardiovascular events in the mother and fetus, particularly when used for a prolonged period of time.

Corticosteroids
[EvGr] Depending on the stage of pregnancy, individual circumstances, and the balance of risks and benefits, corticosteroids such as dexamethasone p. 786 [unlicensed use] may be offered to females who are in suspected or established preterm labour, or who are having a planned preterm birth, or who have preterm prelabour rupture of membranes (P-PROM). [A] For further guidance on the use of corticosteroids, see Royal College of Obstetricians and Gynaecologists guideline: **Antenatal corticosteroids to reduce neonatal morbidity and mortality** (available at: www.rcog.org.uk/guidance/browse-all-guidance/green-top-guidelines/antenatal-corticosteroids-to-reduce-neonatal-morbidity-and-mortality-green-top-guideline-no-74) and NICE guideline: **Preterm labour and birth** (see *Useful resources*).

Magnesium
[EvGr] Magnesium sulfate p. 1193 [unlicensed use], for neuroprotection of the baby, may be offered to females who are in established preterm labour or who are having a planned preterm birth within 24 hours (depending on the stage of pregnancy and individual circumstances). [A] For further guidance on the use of magnesium, see NICE guideline: **Preterm labour and birth** (see *Useful resources*).

Induction of labour

[EvGr] If a pharmacological method of induction is considered suitable, offer dinoprostone p. 951 or misoprostol for females with a Bishop score of 6 or less.

For females with a Bishop score of more than 6, oxytocin p. 950 may be offered in conjunction with amniotomy. [A] Uterine activity must be monitored carefully and hyperstimulation avoided. Large doses of oxytocin may result in excessive fluid retention.

[EvGr] Mifepristone [unlicensed use], followed by either misoprostol [unlicensed use] or dinoprostone [unlicensed use] can be given for the induction of labour following intra-uterine fetal death in females with no uterine scarring. [A]

Prevention and treatment of haemorrhage

[EvGr] Active management of the third stage of labour reduces the risk of postpartum haemorrhage. Females having a vaginal delivery who have chosen to have an active third stage, should be informed that prophylactic ergometrine with oxytocin p. 952 may be more effective than oxytocin alone in reducing the risk of postpartum haemorrhage, but that it is more likely to cause nausea and vomiting. Ergometrine with oxytocin is advised if there are risk factors which could increase the risk of postpartum haemorrhage. Females receiving ergometrine with oxytocin should be offered an antiemetic, such as cyclizine p. 492. Carbetocin p. 952 is the recommended uterotonic for the prevention of postpartum haemorrhage following caesarean birth. The selected uterotonic should be given immediately after the birth of the baby and before the cord is clamped and cut.

Uterotonic drugs are used to treat postpartum haemorrhage caused by uterine atony; treatment options include oxytocin, ergometrine maleate p. 952, or a combination of ergometrine with oxytocin. Carbetocin [unlicensed use], carboprost p. 953, and misoprostol [unlicensed use] are alternative options. Tranexamic acid p. 127 [unlicensed use] should be given in addition to uterotonic drugs to manage postpartum haemorrhage. Ⓐ

For further guidance on the management of postpartum haemorrhage, see NICE guideline: **Intrapartum care** (see *Useful resources*).

Useful resources

Abortion care. National Institute for Health and Care Excellence. NICE guideline 140. September 2019.
www.nice.org.uk/guidance/ng140

Intrapartum care. National Institute for Health and Care Excellence. NICE guideline 235. September 2023.
www.nice.org.uk/guidance/ng235

Inducing labour. National Institute for Health and Care Excellence. NICE guideline 207. November 2021.
www.nice.org.uk/guidance/ng207

Preterm labour and birth. National Institute for Health and Care Excellence. NICE guideline 25. November 2015 (updated June 2022).
www.nice.org.uk/guidance/ng25

Ectopic pregnancy and miscarriage: diagnosis and initial management. National Institute for Health and Care Excellence. NICE guideline 126. April 2019 (updated August 2023).
www.nice.org.uk/guidance/ng126

7.1 Induction of labour

> **Other drugs used for Induction of labour** Misoprostol, p. 955

OXYTOCIN AND ANALOGUES

Oxytocin

24-Sep-2024

● **INDICATIONS AND DOSE**

Induction of labour for medical reasons | Stimulation of labour in hypotonic uterine inertia
▶ BY INTRAVENOUS INFUSION
▶ Adult: Initially 0.001–0.004 unit/minute, not to be started for at least 6 hours after administration of vaginal prostaglandin, dose increased at intervals of at least 30 minutes until a maximum of 3–4 contractions occur every 10 minutes (0.01 units/minute is often adequate) up to max. 0.02 units/minute, if regular contractions not established after a total 5 units, stop induction attempt (may be repeated next day starting again at 0.001–0.004 units/minute)

Caesarean section
▶ BY SLOW INTRAVENOUS INJECTION
▶ Adult: 5 units immediately after delivery

Active management of the third stage of labour
▶ BY SLOW INTRAVENOUS INJECTION
▶ Adult: 5 units for 1 dose, to be administered immediately after delivery and before the cord is clamped and cut. Dose to be given only if oxytocin was used for induction of labour
▶ BY INTRAMUSCULAR INJECTION
▶ Adult: 10 units for 1 dose, to be administered immediately after delivery and before the cord is clamped and cut

Treatment of postpartum haemorrhage
▶ BY SLOW INTRAVENOUS INJECTION
▶ Adult: 5 units, repeated if necessary

Treatment of severe cases of postpartum haemorrhage (following intravenous injection)
▶ BY INTRAVENOUS INFUSION
▶ Adult: 40 units, given in 500 mL infusion fluid given at a rate sufficient to control uterine atony

Incomplete, inevitable, or missed miscarriage
▶ INITIALLY BY SLOW INTRAVENOUS INJECTION
▶ Adult: 5 units, followed by (by intravenous infusion) 0.02–0.04 unit/minute if required, the rate of infusion can be faster if necessary

● **UNLICENSED USE** Oxytocin doses in the BNF may differ from those in the product literature. Administration by intramuscular injection is an unlicensed use.

> **IMPORTANT SAFETY INFORMATION**
> Prolonged intravenous administration at high doses with large volume of fluid (which is possible in inevitable or missed miscarriage or postpartum haemorrhage) may cause water intoxication with hyponatraemia. To avoid: manufacturer advises use electrolyte-containing diluent (i.e. not glucose), increase oxytocin concentration to reduce fluid, restrict fluid intake by mouth; monitor fluid and electrolytes.
>
> NATIONAL PATIENT SAFETY ALERT: RISK OF OXYTOCIN OVERDOSE DURING LABOUR AND CHILDBIRTH (SEPTEMBER 2024)
> Following a comprehensive review of patient safety incident data, a number of oxytocin-related incidents have been reported including accounts of postpartum oxytocin regimens being accidentally administered during labour or in theatre before caesarean section. One incident reported oxytocin infusion and IV fluids being confused during labour causing the baby's heart rate to slow down, and requiring delivery by an emergency caesarean section due to a placental abruption; the baby was born in poor condition and needed close monitoring in the neonatal intensive care unit.
>
> To mitigate the risks associated with preparing oxytocin infusions in advance, the NHS England National Patient Safety Team are instructing all relevant maternity care providers to review and update local clinical procedures to ensure:
> ● Oxytocin infusions for any indication are **not** pre-prepared at ward level in any clinical area (including delivery suites and theatres).
> ● Post-partum haemorrhage (PPH) kits or trolleys are immediately available in all clinical areas where it may be required.
> ● Roles and responsibilities of staff groups in the labour setting, including theatres, are clearly defined in terms of prescribing, preparation, administration, and disposal of oxytocin infusions (including intrapartum oxytocin infusions, postpartum oxytocin infusions, and unused or pre-prepared oxytocin infusions).
> ● Where a female is identified to be at high risk of PPH:
>   ● the PPH kit/trolley should be brought into the labour/delivery room/theatre during the second stage of labour;
>   ● the postpartum oxytocin infusion should be prepared at the time of birth and not before;
>   ● a second midwife should be available to support the administration of the postpartum oxytocin infusion.

● **CONTRA-INDICATIONS** Any condition where spontaneous labour and/or vaginal delivery inadvisable (e.g. presence of a uterine scar resulting from major surgery including classical caesarean section) · avoid intravenous injection during labour · avoid prolonged administration in oxytocin-resistant uterine inertia · avoid rapid intravenous

injection (may transiently reduce blood pressure) · fetal
distress (discontinue immediately if this occurs) ·
hypertonic uterine contractions (discontinue immediately
if this occurs) · severe cardiovascular disease · severe pre-
eclamptic toxaemia

- **CAUTIONS**
  GENERAL CAUTIONS Avoid large infusion volumes and
  restrict fluid intake by mouth (risk of hyponatraemia and
  water-intoxication) · cardiovascular disease
  SPECIFIC CAUTIONS
  ▸ When used for Induction of labour for medical reasons or
    Stimulation of labour in hypotonic uterine inertia History of
    lower-uterine segment caesarean section · mild
    pregnancy-induced cardiac disease · mild pregnancy-
    induced hypertension · moderate pregnancy-induced
    cardiac disease · moderate pregnancy-induced
    hypertension · presence of borderline cephalopelvic
    disproportion (avoid if significant) · risk factors for
    disseminated intravascular coagulation · secondary uterine
    inertia · women over 35 years

- **INTERACTIONS** → Appendix 1: oxytocin

- **SIDE-EFFECTS**
  ▸ **Common or very common** Arrhythmias · headache · nausea ·
    vomiting
  ▸ **Rare or very rare** Dyspnoea · hypotension · rash
  ▸ **Frequency not known** Angioedema · disseminated
    intravascular coagulation · electrolyte imbalance · flushing
    · haemorrhage · myocardial ischaemia · pulmonary oedema
    · QT interval prolongation · uterine rupture · water
    intoxication

  SIDE-EFFECTS, FURTHER INFORMATION Avoid rapid
  intravenous injection (may transiently reduce blood
  pressure).
     Uterine hyperstimulation -usually with excessive
  doses—may cause fetal distress, asphyxia, and death, or
  may lead to hypertonicity, tetanic contractions, soft-tissue
  damage or uterine rupture.

  Overdose Placental abruption and amniotic fluid embolism
  reported on overdose.

- **MONITORING REQUIREMENTS**
  ▸ Careful monitoring of fetal heart rate and uterine motility
    essential for dose titration.
  ▸ Monitor for disseminated intravascular coagulation after
    parturition.

- **DIRECTIONS FOR ADMINISTRATION** For *intravenous infusion*
  (*Syntocinon*®), manufacturer advises give continuously in
  Glucose 5% *or* Sodium chloride 0.9%. Preferably given *via* a
  variable-speed infusion pump in a concentration
  appropriate to the pump; if given by drip infusion for
  induction or *enhancement of labour*, dilute 5 units in 500 mL
  infusion fluid or for higher doses, 10 units in 500 mL. [EvGr]
  For *treatment of postpartum uterine haemorrhage* dilute
  40 units in 500 mL infusion fluid. Ⓐ If high doses given
  for prolonged period (e.g. for inevitable or missed abortion
  or for postpartum haemorrhage), manufacturer advises use
  low volume of an electrolyte-containing infusion fluid (not
  Glucose 5%) given at higher concentration than for
  induction or enhancement of labour; close attention to
  patient's fluid and electrolyte status essential.
  ▸ When used for Active management of the third stage of labour
    [EvGr] Give over 3–5 minutes if administered via *slow
    intravenous injection.* Ⓐ

- **MEDICINAL FORMS** There can be variation in the licensing of
  different medicines containing the same drug. Forms available
  from special-order manufacturers include: infusion, solution
  for infusion
  Solution for injection
  ▸ **Oxytocin (Non-proprietary)**
    Oxytocin 5 unit per 1 ml Oxytocin 5units/1ml solution for injection
    ampoules | 5 ampoule [PoM] £4.00 (Hospital only) |
    10 ampoule [PoM] £8.03
    Oxytocin 10 unit per 1 ml Oxytocin 10units/1ml solution for infusion
    ampoules | 5 ampoule [PoM] £25.00 | 10 ampoule [PoM] £50.00
    Oxytocin 10units/1ml concentrate for solution for infusion ampoules |
    5 ampoule [PoM] £9.10 (Hospital only) | 10 ampoule [PoM] £9.90 |
    10 ampoule [PoM] £9.90 (Hospital only)
  ▸ **Syntocinon** (Exeltis UK Ltd)
    Oxytocin 5 unit per 1 ml Syntocinon 5units/1ml solution for injection
    ampoules | 5 ampoule [PoM] £4.01 (Hospital only)
    Oxytocin 10 unit per 1 ml Syntocinon 10units/1ml solution for
    injection ampoules | 5 ampoule [PoM] £4.53 (Hospital only)

PROSTAGLANDINS AND ANALOGUES

Dinoprostone
24-Jun-2021

- **INDICATIONS AND DOSE**
  PROPESS®
  Cervical ripening and induction of labour at term
  ▸ BY VAGINA
  ▸ Adult: 1 pessary, insert pessary (in retrieval device)
    high into posterior fornix and remove when cervical
    ripening adequate; if oxytocin necessary, remove
    30 minutes before oxytocin infusion; remove if cervical
    ripening inadequate after 24 hours (dose not to be
    repeated)

  PROSTIN E2® VAGINAL GEL
  Induction of labour
  ▸ BY VAGINA
  ▸ Adult: 1 mg, inserted high into the posterior fornix
    (avoid administration into the cervical canal), followed
    by 1–2 mg after 6 hours if required; maximum 3 mg per
    course

  Induction of labour (unfavourable primigravida)
  ▸ BY VAGINA
  ▸ Adult: 2 mg, inserted high into the posterior fornix
    (avoid administration into the cervical canal), followed
    by 1–2 mg if required, after 6 hours; maximum 4 mg
    per course

  PROSTIN E2® VAGINAL TABLETS
  Induction of labour
  ▸ BY VAGINA
  ▸ Adult: 3 mg, inserted high into the posterior fornix,
    followed by 3 mg after 6–8 hours, to be given if labour
    not established; maximum 6 mg per course

  DOSE EQUIVALENCE AND CONVERSION
  ▸ *Prostin E2 Vaginal tablets* and *Vaginal Gel* are not
    bioequivalent.

- **CONTRA-INDICATIONS** Active cardiac disease · active
  pulmonary disease · avoid extra-amniotic route in
  cervicitis or vaginitis · fetal distress · fetal malpresentation
  · grand multiparas · history of caesarean section · history of
  difficult or traumatic delivery · history of major uterine
  surgery · major cephalopelvic disproportion · multiple
  pregnancy · placenta praevia or unexplained vaginal
  bleeding during pregnancy · ruptured membranes ·
  untreated pelvic infection

- **CAUTIONS** Effect of oxytocin enhanced · history of asthma
  · history of epilepsy · history of glaucoma and raised intra-
  ocular pressure · hypertension · risk factors for
  disseminated intravascular coagulation · uterine rupture ·
  uterine scarring

- **SIDE-EFFECTS**
  - ► **Uncommon** Amniotic cavity infection · febrile disorders · headache · hyperbilirubinaemia neonatal · hypotension · pruritus · uterine atony · vaginal burning
  - ► **Frequency not known** Abdominal pain · diarrhoea · disseminated intravascular coagulation · genital oedema · nausea · uterine rupture · vomiting
- **HEPATIC IMPAIRMENT** Manufacturer advises avoid.
- **RENAL IMPAIRMENT** EvGr Avoid. ◇Ⓜ
- **MONITORING REQUIREMENTS**
  - ► Monitor for disseminated intravascular coagulation after parturition.
  - ► Monitor uterine activity and fetal status (particular care if history of uterine hypertony)
  - ► Care needed in monitoring uterine activity when used in sequence following oxytocin.
- **PRESCRIBING AND DISPENSING INFORMATION** **Important:** Do not confuse dose of *Prostin E2* ® **vaginal gel** with that of *Prostin E2* ® **vaginal tablets**—not bioequivalent.

- **MEDICINAL FORMS** There can be variation in the licensing of different medicines containing the same drug.
  Pessary
  - ► Prostin E2 (Pfizer Ltd)
    Dinoprostone 3 mg Prostin E2 3mg vaginal tablets | 8 pessary PoM £106.23 (Hospital only)
  Vaginal gel
  - ► Prostin E2 (Pfizer Ltd)
    Dinoprostone 400 microgram per 1 ml Prostin E2 1mg vaginal gel | 2.5 ml PoM £13.28 (Hospital only)
    Dinoprostone 800 microgram per 1 ml Prostin E2 2mg vaginal gel | 2.5 ml PoM £13.28 (Hospital only)

7.2 Postpartum haemorrhage

Other drugs used for Postpartum haemorrhage Factor VIIa (recombinant), p. 129 · Misoprostol, p. 955 · Oxytocin, p. 950 · Tranexamic acid, p. 127

ERGOT ALKALOIDS

Ergometrine maleate

05-Jan-2024

- **INDICATIONS AND DOSE**
  Postpartum haemorrhage caused by uterine atony
  - ► BY INTRAMUSCULAR INJECTION
  - ► Adult: 200–500 micrograms for 1 dose, intramuscular injection is the preferred route of administration
  - ► BY SLOW INTRAVENOUS INJECTION
  - ► Adult: 250–500 micrograms for 1 dose

- **CONTRA-INDICATIONS** Eclampsia · first stage of labour · induction of labour · second stage of labour · sepsis · severe cardiac disease · severe hypertension · vascular disease
- **CAUTIONS** Acute porphyrias p. 1202 · cardiac disease · hypertension · multiple pregnancy
- **INTERACTIONS** → Appendix 1: ergometrine
- **SIDE-EFFECTS** Abdominal pain · arrhythmias · chest pain · coronary vasospasm · dizziness · dyspnoea · headache · hypertension · myocardial infarction · nausea · palpitations · pulmonary oedema · rash · tinnitus · vasoconstriction · vomiting
- **HEPATIC IMPAIRMENT** Manufacturer advises caution in mild to moderate impairment; avoid in severe impairment.
- **RENAL IMPAIRMENT** Manufacturer advises caution in mild or moderate impairment. Manufacturer advises avoid in severe impairment.

- **MEDICINAL FORMS** There can be variation in the licensing of different medicines containing the same drug.
  Solution for injection
  - ► Ergometrine maleate (Non-proprietary)
    Ergometrine maleate 500 microgram per 1 ml Ergometrine 500micrograms/1ml solution for injection ampoules | 10 ampoule PoM £26.00

Ergometrine with oxytocin

05-Jan-2024

The properties listed below are those particular to the combination only. For the properties of the components please consider, ergometrine maleate above, oxytocin p. 950.

- **INDICATIONS AND DOSE**
  Postpartum haemorrhage caused by uterine atony
  - ► BY INTRAMUSCULAR INJECTION
  - ► Adult: 1 mL for 1 dose
  Active management of the third stage of labour
  - ► BY INTRAMUSCULAR INJECTION
  - ► Adult: 1 mL for 1 dose, to be administered immediately after delivery and before the cord is clamped and cut
  Bleeding due to incomplete miscarriage or abortion
  - ► BY INTRAMUSCULAR INJECTION
  - ► Adult: Adjusted according to response to, the patient's condition and blood loss

- **INTERACTIONS** → Appendix 1: ergometrine · oxytocin

- **MEDICINAL FORMS** There can be variation in the licensing of different medicines containing the same drug.
  Solution for injection
  - ► Syntometrine (Alliance Pharmaceuticals Ltd)
    Ergometrine maleate 500 microgram per 1 ml, Oxytocin 5 unit per 1 ml Syntometrine 500micrograms/1ml solution for injection ampoules | 5 ampoule PoM £7.87

OXYTOCIN AND ANALOGUES

Carbetocin

05-Jan-2024

- **INDICATIONS AND DOSE**
  Prevention of postpartum haemorrhage after caesarean section
  - ► BY SLOW INTRAVENOUS INJECTION
  - ► Adult: 100 micrograms for 1 dose, to be administered as soon as possible after delivery, preferably before removal of placenta
  Prevention of postpartum haemorrhage after vaginal delivery
  - ► BY SLOW INTRAVENOUS INJECTION, OR BY INTRAMUSCULAR INJECTION
  - ► Adult: 100 micrograms for 1 dose, to be administered as soon as possible after delivery, preferably before removal of placenta

- **CONTRA-INDICATIONS** Epilepsy
- **CAUTIONS** Asthma · cardiovascular disease (avoid if severe) · hyponatraemia · migraine
- **SIDE-EFFECTS**
  - ► **Common or very common** Abdominal pain · chest pain · chills · dizziness · dyspnoea · feeling hot · flushing · headache · hypotension · nausea · pain · pruritus · taste metallic · tremor · vomiting
  - ► **Uncommon** Arrhythmias · fever · muscle weakness
  - ► **Rare or very rare** Urinary retention
  - ► **Frequency not known** Hyperhidrosis
- **HEPATIC IMPAIRMENT** Manufacturer advises avoid in hepatic disease.
- **RENAL IMPAIRMENT** Manufacturer advises avoid.

- **DIRECTIONS FOR ADMINISTRATION** For *slow intravenous injection*, give over 1 minute.
- **NATIONAL FUNDING/ACCESS DECISIONS**
  For full details see funding body website
  Scottish Medicines Consortium (SMC) decisions
  ► Carbetocin (*Pabal*®) for the prevention of uterine atony following delivery of the infant by Caesarean section under epidural or spinal anaesthesia (January 2018) SMC No. 309/06 Not recommended

- **MEDICINAL FORMS** There can be variation in the licensing of different medicines containing the same drug.
  Solution for injection
  ► Carbetocin (Non-proprietary)
    Carbetocin 100 microgram per 1 ml Carbetocin 100micrograms/1ml solution for injection pre-filled syringes | 5 pre-filled disposable injection PoM £88.20 (Hospital only)
  ► Pabal (Ferring Pharmaceuticals Ltd)
    Carbetocin 100 microgram per 1 ml Pabal 100micrograms/1ml solution for injection vials | 5 vial PoM £88.20 (Hospital only)

PROSTAGLANDINS AND ANALOGUES

Carboprost

08-Nov-2021

- **INDICATIONS AND DOSE**
  Postpartum haemorrhage due to uterine atony in patients unresponsive to ergometrine and oxytocin
  ► BY DEEP INTRAMUSCULAR INJECTION
  ► Adult: 250 micrograms, repeated if necessary, to be given at intervals of not less than 15 minutes. Total dose should not exceed 2 mg (8 doses)

- **CONTRA-INDICATIONS** Cardiac disease · pulmonary disease · untreated pelvic infection
- **CAUTIONS** Excessive dosage may cause uterine rupture · history of anaemia · history of asthma · history of cardiovascular disease · history of diabetes · history of epilepsy · history of glaucoma · history of hypertension · history of hypotension · history of jaundice · history of pulmonary disease · history of raised intra-ocular pressure · uterine scars
- **SIDE-EFFECTS**
  ► **Common or very common** Chills · cough · diarrhoea · headache · nausea · uterine disorders · vasodilation · vomiting
  ► **Uncommon** Abdominal pain upper · asthma · back pain · breast tenderness · chest discomfort · dizziness · drowsiness · dry mouth · dyspnoea · eye pain · haemorrhage · hiccups · hyperhidrosis · hypertension · increased risk of infection · movement disorders · muscle complaints · paraesthesia · pelvic pain · respiratory disorders · septic shock · sleep disorder · syncope · tachycardia · taste altered · tinnitus · uterine injuries · vertigo · vision blurred
  ► **Frequency not known** Anxiety · asthenia · blepharospasm · choking sensation · palpitations · rash · thirst · throat complaints · thyrotoxic crisis
- **HEPATIC IMPAIRMENT** Manufacturer advises avoid in active hepatic disease.
- **RENAL IMPAIRMENT** Manufacturer advises avoid.

- **MEDICINAL FORMS** There can be variation in the licensing of different medicines containing the same drug.
  Solution for injection
  ► Hemabate (Pfizer Ltd)
    Carboprost (as Carboprost trometamol) 250 microgram per 1 ml Hemabate 250micrograms/1ml solution for injection ampoules | 10 ampoule PoM £182.01 (Hospital only)

7.3 Preterm labour

Other drugs used for Preterm labour Nifedipine, p. 189 · Salbutamol, p. 287 · Terbutaline sulfate, p. 290

OXYTOCIN RECEPTOR ANTAGONISTS

Atosiban

24-May-2021

- **INDICATIONS AND DOSE**
  Uncomplicated premature labour between 24 and 33 weeks of gestation
  ► INITIALLY BY INTRAVENOUS INJECTION
  ► Adult: Initially 6.75 mg over 1 minute, then (by intravenous infusion) 18 mg/hour for 3 hours, then (by intravenous infusion) reduced to 6 mg/hour for up to 45 hours. Maximum duration of treatment is 48 hours

- **CONTRA-INDICATIONS** Abnormal fetal heart rate · abruptio placenta · antepartum haemorrhage (requiring immediate delivery) · eclampsia · intra-uterine fetal death · intra-uterine infection · placenta praevia · premature rupture of membranes after 30 weeks' gestation · severe pre-eclampsia
- **CAUTIONS** Intra-uterine growth restriction
- **SIDE-EFFECTS**
  ► **Common or very common** Dizziness · headache · hot flush · hyperglycaemia · hypotension · nausea · tachycardia · vomiting
  ► **Uncommon** Fever · insomnia · skin reactions
  ► **Rare or very rare** Uterine atony · uterine haemorrhage
  ► **Frequency not known** Dyspnoea · pulmonary oedema
- **HEPATIC IMPAIRMENT** Manufacturer advises caution—no information available.
- **MONITORING REQUIREMENTS** Monitor blood loss after delivery.
- **DIRECTIONS FOR ADMINISTRATION** For *intravenous infusion* (*Tractocile*® concentrate for intravenous infusion), manufacturer advises give continuously *in* Glucose 5% *or* Sodium chloride 0.9%. Withdraw 10 mL infusion fluid from 100-mL bag and replace with 10 mL atosiban concentrate (7.5 mg/mL) to produce a final concentration of 750 micrograms/mL.

- **MEDICINAL FORMS** There can be variation in the licensing of different medicines containing the same drug.
  Solution for injection
  ► Tractocile (Ferring Pharmaceuticals Ltd)
    Atosiban (as Atosiban acetate) 7.5 mg per 1 ml Tractocile 6.75mg/0.9ml solution for injection vials | 1 vial PoM £18.41 (Hospital only)
  Solution for infusion
  ► Atosiban (Non-proprietary)
    Atosiban (as Atosiban acetate) 7.5 mg per 1 ml Atosiban 37.5mg/5ml concentrate for solution for infusion vials | 1 vial PoM £51.99–£52.82 (Hospital only)
    Atosiban 6.75mg/0.9ml solution for injection ampoules | 1 ampoule PoM £17.99 (Hospital only)
  ► Tractocile (Ferring Pharmaceuticals Ltd)
    Atosiban (as Atosiban acetate) 7.5 mg per 1 ml Tractocile 37.5mg/5ml solution for infusion vials | 1 vial PoM £52.82 (Hospital only)

7.4 Termination of pregnancy

PROGESTERONE RECEPTOR MODULATORS

Mifepristone

30-Aug-2023

- **DRUG ACTION** Mifepristone, an antiprogestogenic steroid, sensitises the myometrium to prostaglandin-induced contractions and ripens the cervix.

- **INDICATIONS AND DOSE**

Cervical ripening before mechanical cervical dilatation for termination of pregnancy of up to 84 days gestation (under close medical supervision)
▸ BY MOUTH
▸ Adult: 200 mg for 1 dose, to be taken 36-48 hours before procedure

Induction of labour in intra-uterine fetal death in women without uterine scarring (under close medical supervision)
▸ BY MOUTH
▸ Adult: 200 mg for 1 dose, dose followed by dinoprostone *or* misoprostol, given in accordance with national protocols

Medical termination of intra-uterine pregnancy of up to 49 days gestation (under close medical supervision)
▸ BY MOUTH
▸ Adult: 600 mg for 1 dose, dose followed 36–48 hours later (unless abortion already complete) by gemeprost 1 mg by vagina *or* misoprostol 400 micrograms by mouth, alternatively 200 mg for 1 dose, dose followed 36–48 hours later (unless abortion already complete) by gemeprost 1 mg by vagina; observe for at least 3 hours (or until bleeding or pain at acceptable level); follow-up visit within 2 weeks to verify complete expulsion and to assess vaginal bleeding

Medical termination of intra-uterine pregnancy of 50–63 days gestation (under close medical supervision)
▸ BY MOUTH
▸ Adult: 600 mg for 1 dose, alternatively 200 mg for 1 dose, dose followed 36–48 hours later (unless abortion already complete) by gemeprost 1 mg by vagina; observe for at least 3 hours (or until bleeding or pain at acceptable level); follow-up visit within 2 weeks to verify complete expulsion and to assess vaginal bleeding

Termination of pregnancy of 13–24 weeks gestation (in combination with a prostaglandin) (under close medical supervision)
▸ BY MOUTH
▸ Adult: 600 mg for 1 dose, alternatively 200 mg for 1 dose, dose followed 36–48 hours later by gemeprost 1 mg by vagina every 3 hours up to max. 5 mg *or* misoprostol; if abortion does not occur, 24 hours after start of treatment repeat course of gemeprost 1 mg by vagina up to max. 5 mg; follow-up visit after appropriate interval to assess vaginal bleeding recommended

Missed miscarriage
▸ BY MOUTH
▸ Adult: 200 mg for 1 dose, dose followed 48 hours later (unless expulsion of gestational sac already complete) by misoprostol 800 micrograms by vagina, by mouth, or by sublingual administration

- **UNLICENSED USE** EvGr Mifepristone is used in the doses provided in the BNF for the induction of labour in intra-uterine fetal death in women without uterine scarring Ⓐ, but these may differ from those licensed. EvGr

Mifepristone is used as a treatment for missed miscarriage Ⓐ, but is not licensed for this indication.

- **CONTRA-INDICATIONS** Acute porphyrias p. 1202 · chronic adrenal failure · suspected ectopic pregnancy (use other specific means of termination) · uncontrolled severe asthma

- **CAUTIONS** Adrenal suppression (may require corticosteroid) · anticoagulant therapy · asthma (avoid if severe and uncontrolled) · existing cardiovascular disease · haemorrhagic disorders · history of endocarditis · prosthetic heart valve · risk factors for cardiovascular disease

- **INTERACTIONS** → Appendix 1: mifepristone

- **SIDE-EFFECTS**
▸ **Common or very common** Abdominal cramps · diarrhoea · infection · nausea · pelvic inflammatory disease · uterine disorders · vaginal haemorrhage (sometimes severe) · vomiting
▸ **Uncommon** Hypotension
▸ **Rare or very rare** Angioedema · chills · dizziness · erythema nodosum · fever · headache · hot flush · malaise · skin reactions · toxic epidermal necrolysis · toxic shock syndrome · uterine rupture

- **HEPATIC IMPAIRMENT** Manufacturer advises avoid in hepatic failure (no information available).

- **RENAL IMPAIRMENT** EvGr Avoid in renal failure (no information available). Ⓜ

- **MONITORING REQUIREMENTS** Careful monitoring of blood pressure and pulse essential for 3 hours after administration of gemeprost pessary (risk of profound hypotension).

- **PRESCRIBING AND DISPENSING INFORMATION** Supplied to NHS hospitals and premises approved under Abortion Act 1967.

Mifepristone 200 mg oral tablet is also available in *Medabon*® *Combipack* with misoprostol 200 micrograms vaginal tablets.

- **PATIENT AND CARER ADVICE**
▸ When used for Missed miscarriage Patients should be advised to contact their healthcare professional if bleeding has not started 48 hours after completing treatment with mifepristone followed by misoprostol.

Patient information leaflet to be provided.

- **MEDICINAL FORMS** There can be variation in the licensing of different medicines containing the same drug.
Oral tablet
CAUTIONARY AND ADVISORY LABELS 10
▸ **Mifepristone (Non-proprietary)**
Mifepristone 200 mg Mifepristone 200mg tablets | 1 tablet PoM £10.14 | 30 tablet PoM £252.00 (Hospital only)

Mifepristone and misoprostol

15-Sep-2022

The properties listed below are those particular to the combination only. For the properties of the components please consider, misoprostol p. 955, mifepristone above.

- **INDICATIONS AND DOSE**

Medical termination of intra-uterine pregnancy of up to 63 days gestation (under close medical supervision)
▸ BY MOUTH, OR BY VAGINA
▸ Adult: (consult product literature)

- **INTERACTIONS** → Appendix 1: mifepristone · misoprostol

- **SIDE-EFFECTS**
▸ **Common or very common** Diarrhoea · gastrointestinal discomfort · haemorrhage · nausea · uterine disorders · vomiting
▸ **Uncommon** Infection · skin reactions

▸ **Rare or very rare** Chills · dizziness · erythema nodosum · fever · headache · hot flush · hypotension · malaise · severe cutaneous adverse reactions (SCARs) · uterine rupture

▸ **Frequency not known** Cardiac arrest · cardiovascular event · coronary vasospasm · myocardial infarction · pelvic inflammatory disease · toxic shock syndrome

● PRESCRIBING AND DISPENSING INFORMATION *Medabon®* *Combipack* contains mifepristone 200 mg oral tablet and misoprostol 200 micrograms vaginal tablets.

● PATIENT AND CARER ADVICE Patient information leaflet to be provided.

● MEDICINAL FORMS There can be variation in the licensing of different medicines containing the same drug.

Form unstated

▸ Medabon Combipack (Sun Pharma UK Ltd)
Medabon Combipack tablets | 1 pack [PoM] £17.00 (Hospital only)

PROSTAGLANDINS AND ANALOGUES

Gemeprost

28-May-2021

● **INDICATIONS AND DOSE**

Cervical ripening prior to first trimester surgical abortion

▸ BY VAGINA

▸ Adult: 1 mg, dose to be inserted into posterior fornix 3 hours before surgery

Second trimester abortion

▸ BY VAGINA

▸ Adult: 1 mg every 3 hours for maximum 5 administrations, to be inserted into posterior fornix, second course may begin 24 hours after start of treatment (if treatment fails, pregnancy should be terminated by another method)

Second trimester intra-uterine death

▸ BY VAGINA

▸ Adult: 1 mg every 3 hours for maximum 5 administrations only, to be inserted into posterior fornix

Medical termination of intra-uterine pregnancy of up to 49 days gestation following mifepristone | Medical termination of intra-uterine pregnancy of 50–63 days gestation following mifepristone

▸ BY VAGINA

▸ Adult: 1 mg

Termination of pregnancy of 13–24 weeks gestation (in combination with a prostaglandin) following mifepristone

▸ BY VAGINA

▸ Adult: 1 mg every 3 hours, if abortion does not occur, 24 hours after start of treatment repeat course of gemeprost 1 mg by vagina up to max. 5 mg; follow-up visit after appropriate interval to assess vaginal bleeding recommended, careful monitoring of blood pressure and pulse essential for 3 hours after administration of gemeprost pessary (risk of profound hypotension); maximum 5 mg per course

● CONTRA-INDICATIONS Placenta praevia · unexplained vaginal bleeding · uterine scarring

● CAUTIONS Cardiovascular insufficiency · cervicitis · obstructive airways disease · raised intra-ocular pressure · vaginitis

● SIDE-EFFECTS Back pain · chest pain · chills · coronary vasospasm · diarrhoea · dizziness · dyspnoea · fever · flushing · headache · hypotension · muscle weakness · myocardial infarction · nausea · palpitations · uterine pain · uterine rupture · vaginal haemorrhage · vomiting

● RENAL IMPAIRMENT Manufacturer advises avoid.

● MONITORING REQUIREMENTS

▸ If used in combination with mifepristone, carefully monitor blood pressure and pulse for 3 hours.

▸ When used for second trimester intra-uterine death, monitor for coagulopathy during treatment.

● MEDICINAL FORMS No licensed medicines listed.

Misoprostol

10-Jan-2025

● DRUG ACTION Misoprostol is a synthetic prostaglandin analogue that acts as a potent uterine stimulant.

● **INDICATIONS AND DOSE**

Termination of pregnancy following mifepristone (gestation up to 49 days)

▸ BY MOUTH

▸ Adult: 400 micrograms for 1 dose, dose to be given 24–48 hours after mifepristone

Termination of pregnancy following mifepristone (gestation 50 to 63 days)

▸ INITIALLY BY VAGINA, OR BY BUCCAL ADMINISTRATION, OR BY SUBLINGUAL ADMINISTRATION

▸ Adult: 800 micrograms for 1 dose, dose to be given 24–48 hours after mifepristone, if abortion has not occurred 4 hours after first misoprostol dose a further dose may be given, (by mouth or by vagina) 400 micrograms for 1 dose

Termination of pregnancy following mifepristone (gestation of 9 to 13 weeks)

▸ INITIALLY BY VAGINA

▸ Adult: 800 micrograms for 1 dose, dose to be given 36–48 hours after mifepristone, followed by (by vagina or by mouth) 400 micrograms every 3 hours if required for a maximum of 4 doses

Termination of pregnancy following mifepristone (gestation of 13 to 24 weeks)

▸ INITIALLY BY VAGINA

▸ Adult: 800 micrograms for 1 dose, dose to be given 36–48 hours after mifepristone, followed by (by vagina or by mouth) 400 micrograms every 3 hours if required for a maximum of 4 doses, if abortion has not occurred 3 hours after the last dose of misoprostol, a further dose of mifepristone may be given, and misoprostol may be recommended 12 hours later

Missed miscarriage [if expulsion of gestational sac incomplete following mifepristone]

▸ BY VAGINA, OR BY MOUTH, OR BY SUBLINGUAL ADMINISTRATION

▸ Adult: 800 micrograms for 1 dose, dose to be given 48 hours after mifepristone

Incomplete miscarriage

▸ BY VAGINA, OR BY MOUTH, OR BY SUBLINGUAL ADMINISTRATION

▸ Adult: 600 micrograms for 1 dose, alternatively 800 micrograms for 1 dose

Treatment of postpartum haemorrhage

▸ BY SUBLINGUAL ADMINISTRATION, OR BY RECTUM

▸ Adult: 800 micrograms for 1 dose

ANGUSTA ®

Induction of labour (specialist supervision in hospital)

▸ BY MOUTH

▸ Adult: 25 micrograms every 2 hours, alternatively 50 micrograms every 4 hours, to be given in accordance with local protocols; maximum 200 micrograms per day

● UNLICENSED USE Misoprostol is used in the doses provided in the BNF for termination of pregnancy, but these may differ from those licensed.

[EvGr] Misoprostol is used as a treatment for missed or incomplete miscarriage, (A) but is not licensed for these indications.

[EvGr] Misoprostol is used for the treatment of postpartum haemorrhage, (A) but is not licensed for this indication.

- **CONTRA-INDICATIONS**

ANGUSTA ® Active labour · fetal malpresentation · placenta praevia · suspicion or evidence of fetal compromise · unexplained vaginal bleeding after 24 weeks gestation · uterine abnormality · uterine scar

- **CAUTIONS**
- When used for Termination of pregnancy Established cardiovascular disease · risk factors for cardiovascular disease (e.g. over 35 years of age with chronic smoking, hyperlipidaemia, or diabetes)

ANGUSTA ® Before 37 weeks' gestation (limited information available) · chorioamnionitis · modified Bishop score greater than 6 (limited information available)

- **INTERACTIONS** → Appendix 1: misoprostol
- **SIDE-EFFECTS**
- **Common or very common** Chills · constipation · diarrhoea · dizziness · fever · flatulence · gastrointestinal discomfort · haemorrhage · headache · muscle cramps · nausea · post abortion infection · skin reactions · uterine cramps · vomiting
- **Uncommon** Menstrual cycle irregularities · postmenopausal haemorrhage
- **Rare or very rare** Angioedema · erythema nodosum · malaise · toxic epidermal necrolysis · uterine rupture
- **Frequency not known** Back pain · cardiac arrest · cardiovascular event · coronary vasospasm · hypotension · myocardial infarction
- **BREAST FEEDING** Manufacturer advises avoid—present in milk, and may cause diarrhoea in nursing infants. [EvGr] Tertiary sources state present in milk but amount probably too small to be harmful; to further reduce risk following termination of pregnancy, consider interrupting breastfeeding for 5 hours after a dose. (D)

ANGUSTA ® [EvGr] Avoid for 4 hours after administration of the last dose. (M)

- **HEPATIC IMPAIRMENT**

ANGUSTA ® [EvGr] Caution in impairment—risk of increased exposure. (M)
Dose adjustments [EvGr] Consider dose reduction and/or prolonged dosing interval in impairment. (M)

- **RENAL IMPAIRMENT**

ANGUSTA ® [EvGr] Caution in impairment—risk of increased exposure; avoid if eGFR less than 15 ml/min/1.73 m². (M) See p. 21.
Dose adjustments [EvGr] Consider dose reduction and/or prolonged dosing interval in impairment. (M)

- **PRESCRIBING AND DISPENSING INFORMATION** Misoprostol 200 micrograms vaginal tablets are not available as a single-ingredient preparation but are in *Medabon* ® *Combipack* with mifepristone 200 mg oral tablet.

- **PATIENT AND CARER ADVICE**
- When used for Missed miscarriage or Incomplete miscarriage Patients should be advised to contact their healthcare professional if bleeding has not started 48 hours after treatment.
Driving and skilled tasks Patients should be cautioned on the effects on driving and performance of skilled tasks— increased risk of dizziness.

- **MEDICINAL FORMS** There can be variation in the licensing of different medicines containing the same drug.
Oral tablet
- **Angusta** (Norgine Pharmaceuticals Ltd)
Misoprostol 25 microgram Angusta 25microgram tablets | 8 tablet [PoM] £83.14 (Hospital only)
Vaginal tablet
- **Misoprostol (Non-proprietary)**
Misoprostol 200 microgram Misoprostol 200microgram vaginal tablets | 4 tablet [PoM] [S] (Hospital only)

Combinations available: *Mifepristone and misoprostol,* p. 954

8 Vaginal and vulval conditions

Vaginal and vulval conditions
07-Jul-2023

Vaginal and vulval changes

Topical oestrogen for vaginal atrophy
Topical oestrogens are available as estradiol pessaries and vaginal rings p. 959, and as estriol pessaries, cream and gel p. 960. [EvGr] They are used to treat the symptoms of vaginal atrophy related to oestrogen deficiency in postmenopausal women. (A) Systemic effects of oestrogen are minimised by using the lowest effective dose to control symptoms; [EvGr] the dose may be increased on the advice of a healthcare professional with expertise in menopause if there is inadequate symptom control. Treatment is continued for as long as needed to relieve symptoms and reviewed initially at 3 months, then at least annually.

Vaginal oestrogens can also be considered in women with pelvic organ prolapse who have signs of vaginal atrophy. (A) For further information, see Urinary incontinence and pelvic organ prolapse in women p. 894.

Non-hormonal preparations for vaginal atrophy
Several non-hormonal vaginal moisturisers are available and some are prescribable on the NHS (consult Drug Tariff). [EvGr] Menopausal women with vaginal dryness can use vaginal moisturisers and lubricants alone or in addition to vaginal oestrogen. (A)

Vaginal and vulval infections

Vulvovaginal candidiasis
Vulvovaginal candidiasis (genital thrush) is symptomatic inflammation of the vagina and/or vulva caused by a superficial fungal infection; most cases are caused by *Candida albicans.*

[EvGr] Acute vulvovaginal candidiasis is treated with either an oral azole drug (such as fluconazole p. 690 or itraconazole p. 692), or with an intravaginal imidazole pessary or cream (e.g. clotrimazole p. 958 or econazole nitrate p. 958) inserted high into the vagina. (A) [EvGr] Treatment may be supplemented with a topical antifungal cream for vulvitis and to treat other superficial sites of infection. (M) Local irritation may occur on application of intravaginal imidazole drug preparations and may be mistaken for treatment failure.

Intravaginal imidazole drugs are effective against candida in short courses of 1 to 14 days according to the preparation used. [EvGr] Treatment can be repeated if the initial course fails to control symptoms or if symptoms recur after 7 days. (M)

Vulvovaginal candidiasis in pregnancy
[EvGr] Symptomatic vulvovaginal candidiasis is common during pregnancy and can be treated with intravaginal application of an imidazole (such as clotrimazole). Pregnant women need a longer duration of treatment, usually about 7 days, to clear the infection. (A) There is limited systemic

absorption of imidazoles from the vagina. EvGr Treatment with an oral azole drug should be avoided during pregnancy. Ⓐ

Recurrent vulvovaginal candidiasis

Recurrence of vulvovaginal candidiasis is particularly likely if there are predisposing factors, such as recent (up to 3 months before) antibacterial therapy, poorly controlled diabetes mellitus, pregnancy, immunosuppression, HRT use, or possibly oral contraceptive use.

EvGr Treatment of recurrent vulvovaginal candidiasis involves initial treatment with oral fluconazole (induction regimen) to ensure clinical remission, followed immediately by a maintenance regimen for 6 months. When oral fluconazole treatment is unsuitable, an intravaginal imidazole can be given. Ⓐ

Other infections

Systemic drugs are required in the treatment of infections such as gonorrhoea and syphilis. Oral or intravaginal antibacterial drugs may be required for the treatment of bacterial vaginosis. For further information, see Genital system infections, antibacterial therapy p. 584.

EvGr Trichomonal infections commonly involve the lower urinary tract as well as the genital system and need systemic treatment with metronidazole p. 628.

The antiviral drugs aciclovir p. 729, famciclovir p. 730, and valaciclovir p. 731 can be used in the treatment of genital infection due to herpes simplex virus; they have a beneficial effect on virus shedding, and reducing the severity and duration of episodes. Ⓐ For further information, see Herpesvirus infections p. 727.

For information on the human papillomavirus vaccine, see Human papillomavirus vaccine p. 1483.

8.1   Vaginal and vulval infections

8.1a   Vaginal and vulval bacterial infections

ANTIBACTERIALS › LINCOSAMIDES

❙ Clindamycin

22-Mar-2024

- **INDICATIONS AND DOSE**

DALACIN ® CREAM

Bacterial vaginosis
- ▸ BY VAGINA
- ▸ Adult: 1 applicatorful once daily for 3–7 nights, dose to be administered at night

DOSE EQUIVALENCE AND CONVERSION
- ▸ For *Dalacin* ® 2% cream: 1 applicatorful delivers a 5 g dose of clindamycin 2%.

- **INTERACTIONS** → Appendix 1: clindamycin

- **SIDE-EFFECTS**
- ▸ **Common or very common** Diarrhoea (discontinue) · skin reactions
- ▸ **Frequency not known** Constipation · dizziness · gastrointestinal discomfort · headache · increased risk of infection · nausea · vertigo · vomiting · vulvovaginal irritation

   SIDE-EFFECTS, FURTHER INFORMATION Clindamycin 2% cream is poorly absorbed into the blood—low risk of systemic effects.

- **CONCEPTION AND CONTRACEPTION** Damages latex condoms and diaphragms.

- **PRESCRIBING AND DISPENSING INFORMATION** For choice of antibacterial therapy, see Genital system infections, antibacterial therapy p. 584.

- **MEDICINAL FORMS** There can be variation in the licensing of different medicines containing the same drug.
Vaginal cream
EXCIPIENTS: May contain Benzyl alcohol, cetostearyl alcohol (including cetyl and stearyl alcohol), polysorbates, propylene glycol
- ▸ **Dalacin** (Pfizer Ltd)
  Clindamycin (as Clindamycin phosphate) 20 mg per 1 gram   Dalacin 2% cream | 40 gram PoM £10.86 DT = £10.86

ANTISEPTICS AND DISINFECTANTS

❙ Dequalinium chloride

20-Aug-2020

- **DRUG ACTION** Dequalinium chloride is a bactericidal anti-infective which causes bacterial cell death by increasing cell permeability and reducing enzyme activity.

- **INDICATIONS AND DOSE**

Bacterial vaginosis
- ▸ BY VAGINA
- ▸ Adult 18–55 years: 10 mg once daily for 6 days, inserted at night

- **CONTRA-INDICATIONS** Vaginal ulceration

- **SIDE-EFFECTS**
- ▸ **Common or very common** Increased risk of infection · vulvovaginal disorders
- ▸ **Uncommon** Haemorrhage · headache · nausea
- ▸ **Frequency not known** Cystitis · fever

- **CONCEPTION AND CONTRACEPTION** Does not affect efficacy of latex condoms; however, manufacturer advises avoid use of non-latex condoms and intravaginal devices—no information available.

- **PREGNANCY** Manufacturer advises avoid unless essential—limited information available.

- **NATIONAL FUNDING/ACCESS DECISIONS**
For full details see funding body website
Scottish Medicines Consortium (SMC) decisions
- ▸ Dequalinium chloride (*Fluomizin* ®) for treatment of bacterial vaginosis (November 2016) SMC No. 1194/16 Recommended with restrictions
All Wales Medicines Strategy Group (AWMSG) decisions
- ▸ Dequalinium chloride (*Fluomizin* ®) for treatment of bacterial vaginosis after initial treatment is ineffective or not tolerated as an alternative option to clindamycin vaginal cream (November 2016) AWMSG No. 2775 Recommended with restrictions

- **MEDICINAL FORMS** There can be variation in the licensing of different medicines containing the same drug.
Vaginal tablet
- ▸ **Fluomizin** (Gedeon Richter (UK) Ltd)
  Dequalinium chloride 10 mg   Fluomizin 10mg vaginal tablets | 6 tablet PoM £6.95 DT = £6.95

CARBOXYLIC ACIDS

❙ Lactic acid

24-Nov-2020

- **INDICATIONS AND DOSE**

BALANCE ACTIV RX ® GEL

Prevention of bacterial vaginosis
- ▸ BY VAGINA
- ▸ Adult: 5 mL 1–2 times a week, insert the content of 1 tube (5 mL)

RELACTAGEL ® GEL

Prevention of bacterial vaginosis
- ▸ BY VAGINA
- ▸ Adult: 5 mL daily for 2–3 nights after menstruation, insert the contents of one tube

continued →

Genito-urinary system · 7

Treatment of bacterial vaginosis
▸ BY VAGINA
▸ Adult: 5 mL daily for 7 nights, insert the contents of one tube

● **ALLERGY AND CROSS-SENSITIVITY** [EvGr] Contra-indicated in shellfish allergy. Ⓜ

● **CONCEPTION AND CONTRACEPTION**
RELACTAGEL ® GEL Not recommended if trying to conceive.

● **MEDICINAL FORMS** There can be variation in the licensing of different medicines containing the same drug.
Products without form
EXCIPIENTS: May contain Propylene glycol
▸ **Balance Activ** (BBI Healthcare Ltd)
Balance Activ BV vaginal pH correction gel | 7 device £5.25
▸ **Relactagel** (Arok Healthcare)
Relactagel vaginal pH correction gel | 7 device £5.25

8.1b Vaginal and vulval fungal infections

Other drugs used for Vaginal and vulval fungal infections
Fluconazole, p. 690 · Itraconazole, p. 692

ANTIFUNGALS > IMIDAZOLE ANTIFUNGALS

Clotrimazole
10-Nov-2021

● **INDICATIONS AND DOSE**

Superficial sites of infection in vaginal and vulval candidiasis (dose for 1% or 2% cream)
▸ BY VAGINA USING CREAM
▸ Adult: Apply 2–3 times a day, to be applied to anogenital area

Vaginal candidiasis (dose for 10% intravaginal cream)
▸ BY VAGINA USING VAGINAL CREAM
▸ Adult: 5 g for 1 dose, one applicatorful to be inserted into the vagina at night, dose can be repeated once if necessary

Vaginal candidiasis
▸ BY VAGINA USING PESSARIES
▸ Adult: 200 mg once daily for 3 nights, course can be repeated once if necessary, alternatively 100 mg once daily for 6 nights, course can be repeated once if necessary, alternatively 500 mg once daily for 1 night, dose can be repeated once if necessary

Recurrent vulvovaginal candidiasis
▸ BY VAGINA USING PESSARIES
▸ Adult: 500 mg every week for 6 months, dose to be administered following topical imidazole for 10–14 days

● **INTERACTIONS** → Appendix 1: antifungals, azoles

● **SIDE-EFFECTS** Abdominal pain · discomfort · genital peeling · oedema · paraesthesia · pelvic pain · skin reactions · vaginal haemorrhage

● **CONCEPTION AND CONTRACEPTION** Cream and pessaries may damage latex condoms and diaphragms.

● **PREGNANCY**
Dose adjustments Pregnant women need a longer duration of treatment, usually about 7 days, to clear the infection. Oral antifungal treatment should be avoided during pregnancy.

● **EXCEPTIONS TO LEGAL CATEGORY** Brands for sale to the public include *Canesten* ® Internal Cream.

● **MEDICINAL FORMS** There can be variation in the licensing of different medicines containing the same drug.
Pessary
EXCIPIENTS: May contain Benzyl alcohol, cetostearyl alcohol (including cetyl and stearyl alcohol), polysorbates
▸ **Canesten (clotrimazole)** (Bayer Plc)
Clotrimazole 100 mg Canesten 100mg pessaries | 6 pessary P £3.85 DT = £3.85
Clotrimazole 200 mg Canesten 200mg pessaries | 3 pessary P £3.41 DT = £3.41
Clotrimazole 500 mg Canesten 500mg pessaries | 1 pessary PoM £2.00 DT = £6.88
Cutaneous cream
EXCIPIENTS: May contain Benzyl alcohol, cetostearyl alcohol (including cetyl and stearyl alcohol), polysorbates
▸ **Clotrimazole (Non-proprietary)**
Clotrimazole 10 mg per 1 gram Clotrimazole 1% cream | 20 gram P £2.33 DT = £1.43 | 50 gram P £6.00 DT = £3.58
▸ **Canesten (clotrimazole)** (Bayer Plc)
Clotrimazole 10 mg per 1 gram Canesten 1% cream | 20 gram P £2.89 DT = £1.43 | 50 gram P £4.71 DT = £3.58
Canesten Antifungal cream | 20 gram P £2.22 DT = £1.43
Clotrimazole 20 mg per 1 gram Canesten Thrush External 2% cream | 20 gram P £6.41 DT = £5.71
Vaginal cream
EXCIPIENTS: May contain Benzyl alcohol, cetostearyl alcohol (including cetyl and stearyl alcohol), polysorbates
▸ **Canesten (clotrimazole)** (Bayer Plc)
Clotrimazole 100 mg per 1 gram Canesten 10% vaginal cream | 5 gram PoM £4.50 DT = £7.48

Econazole nitrate
30-Nov-2023

● **INDICATIONS AND DOSE**

GYNO-PEVARYL ® ONCE

Vaginal and vulval candidiasis
▸ BY VAGINA
▸ Adult: 1 pessary for 1 dose, pessary to be inserted at night, dose to be repeated once if necessary

GYNO-PEVARYL ® CREAM

Vaginal and vulval candidiasis
▸ INITIALLY BY VAGINA USING VAGINAL CREAM
▸ Adult: 1 applicatorful daily for at least 14 days, dose to be inserted vaginally at night and (to the skin) apply daily for at least 14 days, to be applied to vulva at night, course can be repeated once if necessary

GYNO-PEVARYL ® PESSARY

Vaginal and vulval candidiasis
▸ BY VAGINA
▸ Adult: 1 pessary daily for 3 days, pessary to be inserted at night, course can be repeated once if necessary

● **SIDE-EFFECTS**
▸ **Common or very common** Skin reactions
▸ **Uncommon** Vaginal burning
▸ **Frequency not known** Angioedema

● **CONCEPTION AND CONTRACEPTION** Cream and pessaries damage latex condoms and diaphragms.

● **PREGNANCY** Pregnant women need a longer duration of treatment, usually about 7 days, to clear the infection.

● **MEDICINAL FORMS** There can be variation in the licensing of different medicines containing the same drug.
Pessary
▸ **Gyno-Pevaryl** (Karo Healthcare UK Ltd)
Econazole nitrate 150 mg Gyno-Pevaryl 150mg vaginal pessaries | 3 pessary PoM £4.17 DT = £4.17
Vaginal cream
EXCIPIENTS: May contain Butylated hydroxyanisole
▸ **Gyno-Pevaryl** (Karo Healthcare UK Ltd)
Econazole nitrate 10 mg per 1 gram Gyno-Pevaryl 1% cream | 30 gram PoM £3.78 DT = £3.78

Ketoconazole

30-May-2023

● **INDICATIONS AND DOSE**

Vaginal and vulva candidiasis
▸ BY VAGINA USING CREAM
▸ Adult: Apply 1–2 times a day, to be applied to the anogenital area

● **CONTRA-INDICATIONS** Acute porphyrias p. 1202
● **INTERACTIONS** → Appendix 1: antifungals, azoles
● **SIDE-EFFECTS**
▸ **Common or very common** Skin reactions
▸ **Uncommon** Alopecia · angioedema
▸ **Rare or very rare** Taste altered
● **CONCEPTION AND CONTRACEPTION** Effect on latex condoms and diaphragms not yet known.

● **MEDICINAL FORMS** There can be variation in the licensing of different medicines containing the same drug.

Cutaneous cream
EXCIPIENTS: May contain Cetostearyl alcohol (including cetyl and stearyl alcohol), polysorbates, propylene glycol
▸ **Nizoral** (Thornton & Ross Ltd)
Ketoconazole 20 mg per 1 gram Nizoral 2% cream | 30 gram [PoM] £4.24 DT = £4.24

8.2 Vaginal atrophy

OESTROGENS

Estradiol

07-Jun-2023

● **INDICATIONS AND DOSE**

Vaginal atrophy in postmenopausal women | Prophylaxis of recurrent urinary-tract infection in postmenopausal women
▸ BY VAGINA USING PESSARIES
▸ Adult: 10 micrograms daily for 2 weeks, then reduced to 10 micrograms twice weekly

ESTRING ®

Postmenopausal urogenital conditions (not suitable for vasomotor symptoms or osteoporosis prophylaxis)
▸ BY VAGINA
▸ Adult: To be inserted into upper third of vagina and worn continuously; replace after 3 months; max. duration of continuous treatment 2 years

Prophylaxis of recurrent urinary-tract infection in postmenopausal women
▸ BY VAGINA
▸ Adult: To be inserted into upper third of vagina and worn continuously; replace after 3 months

● **UNLICENSED USE** [EvGr] Estradiol pessaries or vaginal tablets, and *Estring*® are used for the prophylaxis of recurrent urinary-tract infection in postmenopausal women, ⟨Ε⟩ but are not licensed for this indication.

● **CONTRA-INDICATIONS** Active arterial thromboembolic disease (e.g. angina or myocardial infarction) · history of breast cancer · history of venous thromboembolism · oestrogen-dependent cancer · recent arterial thromboembolic disease (e.g. angina or myocardial infarction) · thrombophilic disorder · undiagnosed vaginal bleeding · untreated endometrial hyperplasia

● **CAUTIONS** Acute porphyrias p. 1202 · diabetes (increased risk of heart disease) · factors predisposing to thromboembolism · history of breast nodules—closely monitor breast status (risk of breast cancer) · history of endometrial hyperplasia · history of fibrocystic disease—closely monitor breast status (risk of breast cancer) · hypophyseal tumours · increased risk of gall-bladder disease · migraine (or migraine-like headaches) · presence of antiphospholipid antibodies (increased risk of thrombotic events) · prolonged exposure to unopposed oestrogens may increase risk of developing endometrial cancer · review treatment at least annually to assess need for continued treatment · risk factors for oestrogen-dependent tumours (e.g. breast cancer in first-degree relative) · symptoms of endometriosis may be exacerbated · uterine fibroids may increase in size

CAUTIONS, FURTHER INFORMATION
▸ **Risk of endometrial cancer** The increased risk of endometrial cancer depends on the dose and duration of oestrogen-only HRT.
▸ **Risk of ovarian cancer** Long-term use of combined HRT or oestrogen-only HRT is associated with a small increased risk of ovarian cancer. This excess risk disappears within a few years of stopping.
▸ **Risk of venous thromboembolism** Women using combined or oestrogen-only HRT are at an increased risk of deep vein thrombosis and of pulmonary embolism especially in the first year of use.

In *women who have predisposing factors* (such as a personal or family history of deep vein thrombosis or pulmonary embolism, severe varicose veins, obesity, trauma, or prolonged bed-rest) it is prudent to review the need for HRT, as in some cases the risks of HRT may exceed the benefits.

Travel involving prolonged immobility further increases the risk of deep vein thrombosis.

Although the level of risk of thromboembolism associated with non-oral routes of administration of HRT has not been established, it may be lower for the transdermal route compared to the oral route; studies have found the risk associated with transdermal HRT to be no greater than the baseline population risk of thromboembolism.
▸ **Risk of stroke** Risk of stroke increases with age, therefore older women have a greater absolute risk of stroke. Combined HRT or oestrogen-only HRT increases the risk of stroke.
▸ **Risk of coronary heart disease** HRT does not prevent coronary heart disease and should not be prescribed for this purpose. There is an increased risk of coronary heart disease in women who start combined HRT more than 10 years after menopause. Although very little information is available on the risk of coronary heart disease in younger women who start HRT close to the menopause, studies suggest a lower relative risk compared with older women.

● **INTERACTIONS** → Appendix 1: hormone replacement therapy
● **SIDE-EFFECTS**
GENERAL SIDE-EFFECTS
▸ **Common or very common** Abdominal pain · headaches · nausea · skin reactions · vaginal haemorrhage · vulvovaginal disorders
▸ **Uncommon** Hypertension · vulvovaginal fungal infection · weight increased
▸ **Rare or very rare** Diarrhoea · embolism and thrombosis · endometrial hyperplasia · fluid retention · genital pruritus · increased risk of ischaemic stroke · insomnia · neoplasm malignant · neoplasms · vaginismus

● **CONCEPTION AND CONTRACEPTION** For estradiol pessaries or vaginal tablets, no evidence of damage to latex condoms and diaphragms.
● **PREGNANCY** Not known to be harmful.
● **BREAST FEEDING** Avoid; adverse effects on lactation.
● **HEPATIC IMPAIRMENT** Manufacturer advises caution; avoid in acute or active disease.

7
Genito-urinary system

- **MONITORING REQUIREMENTS**
- ▶ History of breast nodules or fibrocystic disease—closely monitor breast status (risk of breast cancer).
- ▶ The endometrial safety of long-term or repeated use of topical vaginal oestrogens is uncertain; treatment should be reviewed at least annually, with special consideration given to any symptoms of endometrial hyperplasia or carcinoma.

- **MEDICINAL FORMS** There can be variation in the licensing of different medicines containing the same drug.

  Pessary
  - ▶ Estradiol (Non-proprietary)
    Estradiol 10 microgram Estradiol 10microgram pessaries | 24 pessary PoM £15.00 DT = £10.82
  - ▶ Vagifem (Novo Nordisk Ltd)
    Estradiol 10 microgram Vagifem 10microgram vaginal tablets | 24 pessary PoM £16.72 DT = £10.82
  - ▶ Vagirux (Gedeon Richter (UK) Ltd)
    Estradiol 10 microgram Vagirux 10microgram vaginal tablets | 24 pessary PoM £11.34 DT = £10.82

  Vaginal delivery system
  CAUTIONARY AND ADVISORY LABELS 10
  - ▶ Estring (Pfizer Ltd)
    Estradiol (as Estradiol hemihydrate) 7.5 microgram per 24 hour Estring 7.5micrograms/24hours vaginal delivery system | 1 device PoM £31.42 DT = £31.42

Estriol

07-Jun-2023

- **INDICATIONS AND DOSE**

Vaginal atrophy in postmenopausal women
- ▶ INITIALLY BY VAGINA USING VAGINAL CREAM, OR BY VAGINA USING VAGINAL GEL
- ▶ Adult: Apply 1 applicatorful daily for 3–4 weeks, then (by vagina) reduced to 1 applicatorful twice weekly, to be applied at bedtime, treatment should be evaluated after 12 weeks

Vaginal atrophy in postmenopausal women
- ▶ INITIALLY BY VAGINA USING PESSARIES
- ▶ Adult: 1 pessary daily for 3 weeks, then (by vagina) 1 pessary twice weekly, to be inserted at bedtime

Prophylaxis of recurrent urinary-tract infection in postmenopausal women
- ▶ BY VAGINA USING VAGINAL CREAM
- ▶ Adult: Apply 1 applicatorful daily for 3–4 weeks, then reduced to 1 applicatorful twice weekly, to be applied at bedtime

OVESTIN ®

Vaginal surgery for prolapse when there is epithelial atrophy in postmenopausal women (before surgery)
- ▶ BY VAGINA
- ▶ Adult: Apply 1 applicatorful daily for 2 weeks before surgery, resume 2 weeks after surgery

DOSE EQUIVALENCE AND CONVERSION
- ▶ For *Ovestin*® cream, 1 applicatorful contains 500 micrograms estriol; for *Blissel*® gel, 1 applicatorful contains 50 micrograms estriol; for *Imvaggis*® pessary, 1 pessary contains 30 micrograms estriol.

- **UNLICENSED USE** EvGr Estriol vaginal cream is used for the prophylaxis of recurrent urinary-tract infection in postmenopausal women, ⓔ but is not licensed for this indication.

- **CONTRA-INDICATIONS** Active arterial thromboembolic disease (e.g. angina or myocardial infarction) · history of breast cancer · history of venous thromboembolism · oestrogen-dependent cancer · recent arterial thromboembolic disease (e.g. angina or myocardial infarction) · thrombophilic disorder · undiagnosed vaginal bleeding · untreated endometrial hyperplasia

- **CAUTIONS** Acute porphyrias p. 1202 · diabetes (increased risk of heart disease) · factors predisposing to thromboembolism · history of breast nodules—closely monitor breast status (risk of breast cancer) · history of endometrial hyperplasia · history of fibrocystic disease— closely monitor breast status (risk of breast cancer) · hypophyseal tumours · increased risk of gall-bladder disease · migraine (or migraine-like headaches) · presence of antiphospholipid antibodies (increased risk of thrombotic events) · prolonged exposure to unopposed oestrogens may increase risk of developing endometrial cancer · review treatment at least annually to assess need for continued treatment · risk factors for oestrogen-dependent tumours (e.g. breast cancer in first-degree relative) · symptoms of endometriosis may be exacerbated · uterine fibroids may increase in size

  CAUTIONS, FURTHER INFORMATION
  - ▶ Risk of endometrial cancer The increased risk of endometrial cancer depends on the dose and duration of oestrogen-only HRT.
  - ▶ Risk of ovarian cancer Long-term use of combined HRT or oestrogen-only HRT is associated with a small increased risk of ovarian cancer. This excess risk disappears within a few years of stopping.
  - ▶ Risk of venous thromboembolism Women using combined or oestrogen-only HRT are at an increased risk of deep vein thrombosis and of pulmonary embolism especially in the first year of use.

    In *women who have predisposing factors* (such as a personal or family history of deep vein thrombosis or pulmonary embolism, severe varicose veins, obesity, trauma, or prolonged bed-rest) it is prudent to review the need for HRT, as in some cases the risks of HRT may exceed the benefits.

    Travel involving prolonged immobility further increases the risk of deep vein thrombosis.

    Although the level of risk of thromboembolism associated with non-oral routes of administration of HRT has not been established, it may be lower for the transdermal route compared to the oral route; studies have found the risk associated with transdermal HRT to be no greater than the baseline population risk of thromboembolism.
  - ▶ Risk of stroke Risk of stroke increases with age, therefore older women have a greater absolute risk of stroke. Combined HRT or oestrogen-only HRT increases the risk of stroke.
  - ▶ Risk of coronary heart disease HRT does not prevent coronary heart disease and should not be prescribed for this purpose. There is an increased risk of coronary heart disease in women who start combined HRT more than 10 years after menopause. Although very little information is available on the risk of coronary heart disease in younger women who start HRT close to the menopause, studies suggest a lower relative risk compared with older women.

- **INTERACTIONS** → Appendix 1: hormone replacement therapy

- **SIDE-EFFECTS**
- ▶ **Common or very common** Dysuria · genital abnormalities · skin reactions · vulvovaginal disorders
- ▶ **Uncommon** Anorectal discomfort · candida infection · headache · pelvic pain
- ▶ **Frequency not known** Breast abnormalities · cervical mucus increased · dementia · erythema nodosum · gallbladder disorder · increased risk of coronary artery disease · increased risk of ischaemic stroke · increased risk of venous thromboembolism · nausea · neoplasms · vaginal haemorrhage · vomiting

- **CONCEPTION AND CONTRACEPTION** *Imvaggis*® pessary may damage latex condoms (decreases tensile strength).

OVESTIN® Effect on latex condoms and diaphragms not yet known.

- **PREGNANCY** Not known to be harmful.
- **BREAST FEEDING** Avoid; adverse effects on lactation.
- **HEPATIC IMPAIRMENT** Manufacturer advises caution; avoid in acute or active disease.
- **RENAL IMPAIRMENT** EvGr Use with caution. ⟨M⟩
- **MONITORING REQUIREMENTS**
  ▸ Closely monitor breast status if history of breast nodules or fibrocystic disease (risk of breast cancer).
  ▸ The endometrial safety of long-term or repeated use of topical vaginal oestrogens is uncertain; treatment should be reviewed at least annually, with special consideration given to any symptoms of endometrial hyperplasia or carcinoma.

- **MEDICINAL FORMS** There can be variation in the licensing of different medicines containing the same drug.

  Pessary
  EXCIPIENTS: May contain Butylated hydroxytoluene
  ▸ **Estriol (Non-proprietary)**
  Estriol 500 microgram Estriol 500microgram pessaries | 15 pessary PoM £5.45
  ▸ **Imvaggis** (Besins Healthcare (UK) Ltd)
  Estriol 30 microgram Imvaggis 0.03mg pessaries | 24 pessary PoM £13.38 DT = £13.38

  Vaginal gel
  EXCIPIENTS: May contain Hydroxybenzoates (parabens)
  ▸ **Blissel** (Consilient Health Ltd)
  Estriol 50 microgram per 1 gram Blissel 50micrograms/g vaginal gel with applicator | 30 gram PoM £18.90 DT = £18.90

  Vaginal cream
  EXCIPIENTS: May contain Arachis (peanut) oil, cetostearyl alcohol (including cetyl and stearyl alcohol), polysorbates
  ▸ **Estriol (Non-proprietary)**
  Estriol 100 microgram per 1 gram Estriol 0.01% vaginal cream | 80 gram PoM ⊠
  Estriol 1 mg per 1 gram Estriol 1mg/g vaginal cream with applicator | 15 gram PoM £5.45 DT = £5.45

Prasterone

25-Mar-2024

- **DRUG ACTION** Prasterone is biochemically and biologically identical to endogenous dehydroepiandrosterone (DHEA), and is converted to oestrogens and androgens.

- **INDICATIONS AND DOSE**

  Vulvar and vaginal atrophy [in postmenopausal women with moderate to severe symptoms]
  ▸ BY VAGINA USING PESSARIES
  ▸ Adult: 6.5 mg once daily, at bedtime. Treatment should be reassessed at least every 6 months

- **CONTRA-INDICATIONS** Active or recent arterial thromboembolic disease (e.g. angina or myocardial infarction) · Acute porphyrias p. 1202 · history of breast cancer · oestrogen-dependent cancer · thrombophilic disorder · undiagnosed vaginal bleeding · untreated endometrial hyperplasia · venous thromboembolism

- **CAUTIONS** Assess need for continued treatment at least every 6 months · cholelithiasis · diabetes mellitus · factors predisposing to thromboembolism · history of endometrial hyperplasia · hypertriglyceridaemia · migraine (or migraine-like headaches) · prolonged exposure to unopposed oestrogens may increase risk of developing endometrial cancer · risk factors for oestrogen-dependent tumours (e.g. breast cancer in first-degree relative) · symptoms of endometriosis may be exacerbated · uterine fibroids may increase in size

  CAUTIONS, FURTHER INFORMATION
  ▸ **Risk of endometrial cancer** The increased risk of endometrial cancer depends on the dose and duration of oestrogen-only HRT.

Bleeding or spotting occurring during treatment should be investigated.

For oestrogen products for vaginal application, where systemic exposure to oestrogen remains within the normal postmenopausal range, it is not recommended to add a progestogen.

▸ **Risk of ovarian cancer** Long-term use of combined HRT or oestrogen-only HRT is associated with a small increased risk of ovarian cancer. This excess risk disappears within a few years of stopping.

▸ **Risk of venous thromboembolism** Women using combined or oestrogen-only HRT are at an increased risk of deep vein thrombosis and of pulmonary embolism especially in the first year of use.

In *women who have predisposing factors* (such as a personal or family history of deep vein thrombosis or pulmonary embolism, severe varicose veins, obesity, trauma, major surgery or prolonged bed-rest) it is prudent to review the need for HRT, as in some cases the risks of HRT may exceed the benefits.

Travel involving prolonged immobility further increases the risk of deep vein thrombosis.

Although the level of risk of thromboembolism associated with non-oral routes of administration of HRT has not been established, it may be lower for the transdermal route compared to the oral route; studies have found the risk associated with transdermal HRT to be no greater than the baseline population risk of thromboembolism.

▸ **Risk of stroke** Risk of stroke increases with age, therefore older women have a greater absolute risk of stroke. Combined HRT or oestrogen-only HRT slightly increases the risk of stroke.

▸ **Other conditions** The product literature advises caution in other conditions including hypertension, asthma, epilepsy, otosclerosis, and systemic lupus erythematosus. Evidence for caution in these conditions is unsatisfactory and many women with these conditions may stand to benefit from HRT.

- **SIDE-EFFECTS**
  ▸ **Common or very common** Cervical abnormalities · weight change
  ▸ **Uncommon** Breast neoplasm benign · uterine polyp

- **CONCEPTION AND CONTRACEPTION** Manufacturer advises avoid use with condoms, diaphragms or cervical caps made of latex—may damage rubber.

- **PREGNANCY** Manufacturer advises avoid—no information available.

- **BREAST FEEDING** Manufacturer advises avoid—no information available.

- **HEPATIC IMPAIRMENT** EvGr Avoid in acute or history of liver disease, where liver function tests have failed to return to normal. Caution in liver disorders e.g. liver adenoma. ⟨M⟩

- **PATIENT AND CARER ADVICE**
  Missed doses Manufacturer advises if a dose is more than 16 hours late, the missed dose should not be taken and the next dose should be taken at the normal time.

- **MEDICINAL FORMS** There can be variation in the licensing of different medicines containing the same drug.

  Pessary
  ▸ **Intrarosa** (Theramex HQ UK Ltd)
  Prasterone 6.5 mg Intrarosa 6.5mg pessaries | 28 pessary PoM £15.94 DT = £15.94 CD4-2

SELECTIVE OESTROGEN RECEPTOR MODULATORS

Ospemifene

31-Aug-2020

- **DRUG ACTION** Ospemifene is a selective oestrogen receptor modulator that has an oestrogen-like effect in the vagina, increasing the cellular maturation and mucification of the vaginal epithelium.

- **INDICATIONS AND DOSE**

Moderate to severe symptomatic vulvar and vaginal atrophy [in post-menopausal women who are not candidates for local vaginal oestrogen therapy]
  - BY MOUTH
  - Adult: 60 mg once daily

- **CONTRA-INDICATIONS** Breast cancer (suspected or actively treated) · endometrial hyperplasia · history of venous thromboembolism · sex-hormone dependent malignancy (suspected or active) · unexplained vaginal bleeding

- **CAUTIONS** Risk factors for stroke · risk factors for venous thromboembolism (discontinue if prolonged immobilisation)

- **INTERACTIONS** → Appendix 1: ospemifene

- **SIDE-EFFECTS**
  - **Common or very common** Genital discharge · hot flush · increased risk of infection · muscle spasms · skin reactions · vaginal discharge · vaginal haemorrhage
  - **Uncommon** Endometrial thickening · hypersensitivity · tongue swelling

- **PREGNANCY** Manufacturer advises avoid—toxicity in *animal* studies.

- **HEPATIC IMPAIRMENT** Manufacturer advises avoid in severe impairment—no information available.

- **PATIENT AND CARER ADVICE** Manufacturer advises patients and their carers should be advised to seek immediate medical attention if they experience symptoms of thromboembolism (such as sudden chest pain, dyspnoea or swelling of a leg).

- **NATIONAL FUNDING/ACCESS DECISIONS**
  For full details see funding body website

  Scottish Medicines Consortium (SMC) decisions
  - Ospemifene (*Senshio*®) for the treatment of moderate to severe symptomatic vulvar and vaginal atrophy in post-menopausal women who are not candidates for local vaginal oestrogen therapy (September 2019) SMC No. SMC2170 Recommended

- **MEDICINAL FORMS** There can be variation in the licensing of different medicines containing the same drug.
  Oral tablet
  CAUTIONARY AND ADVISORY LABELS 21
  - **Senshio** (Shionogi BV)
    Ospemifene 60 mg Senshio 60mg tablets | 28 tablet PoM £39.50
    DT = £39.50

Chapter 8
Immune system and malignant disease

CONTENTS

Immune system

1   Immune system disorders and transplantation

Immune response
16-May-2022

Inflammatory bowel disease

Azathioprine p. 965, ciclosporin p. 966, mercaptopurine p. 1047, and methotrexate p. 1048 have a role in the treatment of inflammatory bowel disease.

Folic acid p. 1161 should be given to reduce the possibility of methotrexate toxicity [unlicensed indication]. Folic acid is usually given weekly on a different day to the methotrexate; alternative regimens may be used in some settings.

Immunosuppressant therapy

Immunosuppressants are used to suppress rejection in organ transplant recipients and to treat a variety of chronic inflammatory and autoimmune diseases. Solid organ transplant patients are maintained on drug regimens, which may include antiproliferative drugs (azathioprine or mycophenolate mofetil p. 977), calcineurin inhibitors (ciclosporin or tacrolimus p. 969), corticosteroids, or sirolimus p. 968. Choice is dependent on the type of organ, time after transplantation, and clinical condition of the patient. Specialist management is required and other immunomodulators may be used to initiate treatment or to treat rejection.

Impaired immune responsiveness

Modification of tissue reactions caused by corticosteroids and other immunosuppressants may result in the rapid *spread of infection*. Corticosteroids may suppress clinical signs of infection and allow diseases such as septicaemia or tuberculosis to reach an advanced stage before being recognised— **important**: normal immunoglobulin administration should be considered as soon as possible after measles exposure, and an antiviral [unlicensed] or varicella-zoster immunoglobulin may be required for individuals exposed to varicella (chickenpox) or herpes zoster (shingles); for further information, see Herpesvirus infections p. 727 and Immunoglobulins p. 1462. Wherever possible, immunisation or additional booster doses for individuals with immunosuppression should be carried out either before immunosuppression occurs or deferred until an improvement in immunity has been seen. Specialist advice should be sought on the use of live vaccines for those being treated with immunosuppressive drugs.

Antiproliferative immunosuppressants

Azathioprine is widely used for transplant recipients and it is also used to treat a number of auto-immune conditions, usually when corticosteroid therapy alone provides inadequate control. It is metabolised to mercaptopurine, and doses should be reduced when allopurinol p. 1280 is given concurrently.

Mycophenolate mofetil is metabolised to mycophenolic acid which has a more selective mode of action than azathioprine.

There is evidence that compared with similar regimens incorporating azathioprine, mycophenolate mofetil reduces the risk of acute rejection episodes; the risk of opportunistic infections (particularly due to tissue-invasive cytomegalovirus) and the occurrence of blood disorders such as leucopenia may be higher.

Cyclophosphamide p. 1032 is less commonly prescribed as an immunosuppressant.

Corticosteroids and other immunosuppressants

Prednisolone p. 791 is widely used in oncology. It has a marked antitumour effect in acute lymphoblastic leukaemia, Hodgkin's disease, and the non-Hodgkin lymphomas. It has a role in the palliation of symptomatic end-stage malignant disease when it may enhance appetite and produce a sense of well-being.

The corticosteroids are also powerful immunosuppressants. They are used to prevent organ transplant rejection, and in high dose to treat rejection episodes.

Ciclosporin a calcineurin inhibitor, is a potent immunosuppressant which is virtually non-myelotoxic but markedly nephrotoxic. It has an important role in organ and tissue transplantation, for prevention of graft rejection following bone marrow, kidney, liver, pancreas, heart, lung, and heart-lung transplantation, and for prophylaxis and treatment of graft-versus-host disease.

Tacrolimus is also a calcineurin inhibitor. Although not chemically related to ciclosporin it has a similar mode of action and side-effects, but the incidence of neurotoxicity appears to be greater; cardiomyopathy has also been reported. Disturbance of glucose metabolism also appears to be significant.

Sirolimus is a non-calcineurin inhibiting immunosuppressant licensed for renal transplantation.

Basiliximab p. 975 is used for prophylaxis of acute rejection in allogeneic renal transplantation. It is given with ciclosporin and corticosteroid immunosuppression regimens; its use should be confined to specialist centres.

Belatacept p. 978 is a fusion protein and co-stimulation blocker that prevents T-cell activation; it is licensed for prophylaxis of graft rejection in adults undergoing renal transplantation who are seropositive for the Epstein-Barr virus. It is used with interleukin-2 receptor antagonist induction, in combination with corticosteroids and a mycophenolic acid.

Antithymocyte immunoglobulin (rabbit) below is licensed for the prophylaxis of organ rejection in renal and heart allograft recipients and for the treatment of corticosteroid-resistant allograft rejection in renal transplantation. Tolerability is increased by pretreatment with an intravenous corticosteroid and antihistamine; an antipyretic drug such as paracetamol may also be beneficial.

> **Other drugs used for Immune system disorders and transplantation** Anakinra, p. 1256 · Budesonide, p. 47 · Chloroquine, p. 710 · Eculizumab, p. 1152 · Everolimus, p. 1109 · Hydroxychloroquine sulfate, p. 1253 · Rituximab, p. 1019 · Tocilizumab, p. 1258

IMMUNE SERA AND IMMUNOGLOBULINS >
IMMUNOGLOBULINS

Antithymocyte immunoglobulin (rabbit)

17-Jul-2020

● **INDICATIONS AND DOSE**

Prophylaxis of organ rejection in heart allograft recipients
▶ BY INTRAVENOUS INFUSION
▸ Adult: 1–2.5 mg/kg daily for 3–5 days, to be given over at least 6 hours

Prophylaxis of organ rejection in renal allograft recipients
▶ BY INTRAVENOUS INFUSION
▸ Adult: 1–1.5 mg/kg daily for 3–9 days, to be given over at least 6 hours

Treatment of corticosteroid-resistant allograft rejection in renal transplantation
▶ BY INTRAVENOUS INFUSION
▸ Adult: 1.5 mg/kg daily for 7–14 days, to be given over at least 6 hours

DOSES AT EXTREMES OF BODY-WEIGHT
▸ To avoid excessive dosage in obese patients, calculate dose on the basis of ideal body weight.

● **CONTRA-INDICATIONS** Infection

● **INTERACTIONS** → Appendix 1: immunoglobulins

● **SIDE-EFFECTS**
▸ **Common or very common** Chills · diarrhoea · dysphagia · dyspnoea · fever · hypotension · infection · lymphopenia · myalgia · nausea · neoplasm malignant · neoplasms · neutropenia · reactivation of infection · secondary malignancy · sepsis · skin reactions · thrombocytopenia · vomiting
▸ **Uncommon** Cytokine release syndrome · hepatic disorders · hypersensitivity · infusion related reaction

SIDE-EFFECTS, FURTHER INFORMATION Tolerability is increased by pretreatment with an intravenous corticosteroid and antihistamine; an antipyretic drug such as paracetamol may also be beneficial.

● **PREGNANCY** Manufacturer advises use only if potential benefit outweighs risk—no information available.

● **BREAST FEEDING** Manufacturer advises avoid—no information available.

● **MONITORING REQUIREMENTS** Monitor blood count.

● **DIRECTIONS FOR ADMINISTRATION** For *continuous intravenous infusion* (*Thymoglobuline®*), manufacturer advises give in Glucose 5% or Sodium Chloride 0.9%; reconstitute each vial with 5 mL Water for Injections to produce a solution of 5 mg/mL; gently rotate to dissolve. Dilute requisite dose with infusion fluid to a total volume of 50–500 mL (usually 50 mL/vial); begin infusion immediately after dilution; give through an in-line filter (pore size 0.22 micron); not to be given with unfractionated heparin and hydrocortisone in glucose infusion—precipitation reported.

● **NATIONAL FUNDING/ACCESS DECISIONS**
For full details see funding body website
NICE decisions
▶ **Immunosuppressive therapy for kidney transplant in adults (October 2017)** NICE TA481 Not recommended

● **MEDICINAL FORMS** There can be variation in the licensing of different medicines containing the same drug.
Solution for infusion
▶ **Antithymocyte immunoglobulin (rabbit) (Non-proprietary)**
Antithymocyte immunoglobulin (rabbit) 20 mg per 1 ml Grafalon 100mg/5ml concentrate for solution for infusion vials | 1 vial PoM ℥ (Hospital only)

Powder and solvent for solution for infusion
▶ **Thymoglobulin** (Sanofi)
Antithymocyte immunoglobulin (rabbit) 25 mg Thymoglobuline 25mg powder and solvent for solution for infusion vials | 1 vial PoM £158.77 (Hospital only)

IMMUNOSTIMULANTS > PROTEIN KINASE
INHIBITORS

Leniolisib

29-Apr-2025

● **DRUG ACTION** Leniolisib is an inhibitor of the delta isoform of phosphoinositide-3 kinase (PI3Kδ) that restores normal development and proliferation of B- and T-lymphocytes, thereby normalising the hyperactive PI3Kδ pathway.

● **INDICATIONS AND DOSE**

Activated phosphoinositide 3-kinase delta (PI3Kδ) syndrome (APDS)
▶ BY MOUTH
▸ Adult (body-weight 45 kg and above): 70 mg twice daily, dose to be given approx. 12 hours apart

● **INTERACTIONS** → Appendix 1: leniolisib

● **SIDE-EFFECTS**
▸ **Common or very common** Alopecia · arrhythmias · diarrhoea · fatigue · fever · headache · pain · sinusitis · skin reactions

● **CONCEPTION AND CONTRACEPTION** EvGr Females of childbearing potential should use effective contraception during treatment and for at least 1 week after last treatment. Ⓜ

● **PREGNANCY** EvGr Avoid (embryotoxic in *animal* studies). Ⓜ

● **BREAST FEEDING** EvGr Avoid during treatment and for 1 week after last treatment (present in milk in *animal* studies). Ⓜ

● **HEPATIC IMPAIRMENT** EvGr Avoid in moderate to severe impairment (no information available but leniolisib is extensively metabolised in the liver). Ⓜ

● **PATIENT AND CARER ADVICE**
Missed doses If a dose is more than 6 hours late, the missed dose should not be taken and the next dose should be taken at the normal time.

- **NATIONAL FUNDING/ACCESS DECISIONS**
For full details see funding body website
NICE decisions
- Leniolisib for treating activated phosphoinositide 3-kinase delta syndrome in people 12 years and over (April 2025) NICE HST33 Recommended

- **MEDICINAL FORMS** There can be variation in the licensing of different medicines containing the same drug.
   Oral tablet
   - Joenja (Pharming Technologies B.V.) ▼
     Leniolisib (as Leniolisib phosphate) 70 mg Joenja 70mg tablets | 60 tablet [PoM] £29,000.00 (Hospital only)

IMMUNOSUPPRESSANTS > ANTIMETABOLITES

Azathioprine
18-Nov-2021

- **DRUG ACTION** Azathioprine is metabolised to mercaptopurine.

INDICATIONS AND DOSE

Severe acute Crohn's disease | Maintenance of remission of Crohn's disease | Maintenance of remission of acute ulcerative colitis
- BY MOUTH
- Adult: 2–2.5 mg/kg daily, some patients may respond to lower doses

Rheumatoid arthritis that has not responded to other disease-modifying drugs | Severe systemic lupus erythematosus and other connective tissue disorders | Polymyositis in cases of corticosteroid resistance
- BY MOUTH
- Adult: Initially up to 2.5 mg/kg daily in divided doses, adjusted according to response, rarely more than 3 mg/kg daily; maintenance 1–3 mg/kg daily, consider withdrawal if no improvement within 3 months

Autoimmune conditions
- BY MOUTH, OR BY INTRAVENOUS INJECTION, OR BY INTRAVENOUS INFUSION
- Adult: 1–3 mg/kg daily, adjusted according to response, consider withdrawal if no improvement within 3 months, oral administration preferable, if not possible then can be given by intravenous injection (intravenous solution very irritant) *or* by intravenous infusion

Suppression of transplant rejection
- BY MOUTH, OR BY INTRAVENOUS INJECTION, OR BY INTRAVENOUS INFUSION
- Adult: 1–2.5 mg/kg daily, adjusted according to response, oral administration preferable, if not possible then can be given by intravenous injection (intravenous solution very irritant) *or* by intravenous infusion

Severe refractory eczema, normal or high TPMT activity
- BY MOUTH
- Adult: 1–3 mg/kg daily

Severe refractory eczema, intermediate TPMT activity
- BY MOUTH
- Adult: 0.5–1.5 mg/kg daily

Generalised myasthenia gravis
- BY MOUTH, OR BY INTRAVENOUS INJECTION, OR BY INTRAVENOUS INFUSION
- Adult: Initially 0.5–1 mg/kg daily, then increased to 2–2.5 mg/kg daily, dose is increased over 3–4 weeks, azathioprine is usually started at the same time as the corticosteroid and allows a lower maintenance dose of the corticosteroid to be used, oral administration preferable, if not possible then can be given by intravenous injection (intravenous solution very irritant) *or* by intravenous infusion

DOSE ADJUSTMENTS DUE TO INTERACTIONS
- Manufacturer advises reduce dose to one-quarter of the usual dose with concurrent use of allopurinol.

- **UNLICENSED USE** Azathioprine doses given in BNF for suppression of transplant rejection and autoimmune conditions may differ from those in product literature. Use for severe refractory eczema is unlicensed.

- **CONTRA-INDICATIONS**
- When used for Severe refractory eczema Absent thiopurine methyltransferase (TPMT) activity · very low thiopurine methyltransferase (TPMT) activity

- **CAUTIONS** Reduce dose in elderly · reduced thiopurine methyltransferase activity

- **INTERACTIONS** → Appendix 1: azathioprine

- **SIDE-EFFECTS**

GENERAL SIDE-EFFECTS
- **Common or very common** Bone marrow depression (dose-related) · increased risk of infection · leucopenia · pancreatitis · thrombocytopenia
- **Uncommon** Anaemia · hepatic disorders · hypersensitivity
- **Rare or very rare** Agranulocytosis · alopecia · bone marrow disorders · diarrhoea · gastrointestinal disorders · neoplasms · photosensitivity reaction · pneumonitis · severe cutaneous adverse reactions (SCARs)
- **Frequency not known** Nodular regenerative hyperplasia · sinusoidal obstruction syndrome

SPECIFIC SIDE-EFFECTS
- With oral use Nausea

SIDE-EFFECTS, FURTHER INFORMATION Side-effects may require drug withdrawal.
   Hypersensitivity reactions Hypersensitivity reactions (including malaise, dizziness, vomiting, diarrhoea, fever, rigors, myalgia, arthralgia, rash, hypotension and renal dysfunction) call for immediate withdrawal.
   Neutropenia and thrombocytopenia Neutropenia is dose-dependent. Management of neutropenia and thrombocytopenia requires careful monitoring and dose adjustment.
   Nausea Nausea is common early in the course of treatment and usually resolves after a few weeks without an alteration in dose. Moderate nausea can be managed by using divided daily doses, taking doses after food, prescribing concurrent antiemetics or temporarily reducing the dose.

- **ALLERGY AND CROSS-SENSITIVITY** [EvGr] Contra-indicated in hypersensitivity to mercaptopurine. ⟨M⟩

- **PREGNANCY** Transplant patients immunosuppressed with azathioprine should not discontinue it on becoming pregnant. However, there have been reports of premature birth and low birth-weight following exposure to azathioprine, particularly in combination with corticosteroids. Spontaneous abortion has been reported following maternal or paternal exposure. Azathioprine is teratogenic in *animal* studies. The use of azathioprine during pregnancy needs to be supervised in specialist units. Treatment should not generally be initiated during pregnancy.

- **BREAST FEEDING** Present in milk in low concentration. No evidence of harm in small studies—use if potential benefit outweighs risk.

- **HEPATIC IMPAIRMENT** Manufacturer advises caution (impaired metabolism)—monitor liver function and complete blood count more frequently in those with severe impairment.
   Dose adjustments Manufacturer advises use doses at lower end of the dose range in hepatic failure; reduce dose if hepatic or haematological toxicity occur.

- **RENAL IMPAIRMENT** [EvGr] Caution (may result in slower elimination)—monitor complete blood count more frequently in those with severe impairment. ⟨M⟩
Dose adjustments [EvGr] Consider reducing starting dose (limited information available). ⟨M⟩

- **PRE-TREATMENT SCREENING**
Thiopurine methyltransferase The enzyme thiopurine methyltransferase (TPMT) metabolises thiopurine drugs (azathioprine, mercaptopurine, tioguanine); the risk of myelosuppression is increased in patients with reduced activity of the enzyme, particularly for the few individuals in whom TPMT activity is undetectable. Manufacturer advises consider measuring TPMT activity before starting azathioprine, mercaptopurine, or tioguanine therapy. Seek specialist advice for those with reduced or absent TPMT activity.

- **MONITORING REQUIREMENTS**
▸ Monitor for toxicity throughout treatment.
▸ Monitor full blood count weekly (more frequently with higher doses or if severe renal impairment) for first 4 weeks (manufacturer advises weekly monitoring for 8 weeks but evidence of practical value unsatisfactory), thereafter reduce frequency of monitoring to at least every 3 months.
▸ Blood tests and monitoring for signs of myelosuppression are essential in long-term treatment.

- **DIRECTIONS FOR ADMINISTRATION** For *intravenous injection*, manufacturer advises give over at least 1 minute (followed by 50 mL sodium chloride intravenous infusion). For *intravenous infusion* (*Imuran*®), manufacturer advises reconstitute 50 mg with 5–15 mL Water for Injections; dilute requisite dose to a volume of 20–200 mL with infusion fluid. Expert sources advise give in Glucose 5% *or* Sodium Chloride 0.9%. Intravenous injection is alkaline and very irritant. Manufacturer advises intravenous route should therefore be used **only** if oral route not feasible.

- **PATIENT AND CARER ADVICE** Patients and their carers should be warned to report immediately any signs or symptoms of bone marrow suppression e.g. inexplicable bruising or bleeding, infection.

- **MEDICINAL FORMS** There can be variation in the licensing of different medicines containing the same drug. Forms available from special-order manufacturers include: oral capsule, oral suspension, oral solution

Oral tablet
CAUTIONARY AND ADVISORY LABELS 21
▸ **Azathioprine (Non-proprietary)**
  Azathioprine 25 mg Azathioprine 25mg tablets | 28 tablet [PoM] £2.67 DT = £1.01 | 100 tablet [PoM] £3.61–£9.52
  Azathioprine 50 mg Azathioprine 50mg tablets | 56 tablet [PoM] £5.50 DT = £1.44 | 100 tablet [PoM] £2.57–£12.77
  Azathioprine 75 mg Azathioprine 75mg tablets | 100 tablet [PoM] £32.97
  Azathioprine 100 mg Azathioprine 100mg tablets | 100 tablet [PoM] £43.96
▸ **Imuran** (Aspen Pharma Trading Ltd)
  Azathioprine 25 mg Imuran 25mg tablets | 100 tablet [PoM] £10.99

Oral suspension
▸ **Jayempi** (Nova Laboratories Ltd)
  Azathioprine 10 mg per 1 ml Jayempi 10mg/ml oral suspension | 200 ml [PoM] £250.00 DT = £250.00 [SF]

IMMUNOSUPPRESSANTS > CALCINEURIN INHIBITORS AND RELATED DRUGS

Ciclosporin

(Cyclosporin)

28-Jan-2025

- **DRUG ACTION** Ciclosporin inhibits production and release of lymphokines, thereby suppressing cell-mediated immune response.

- **INDICATIONS AND DOSE**

Severe acute ulcerative colitis refractory to corticosteroid treatment
▸ BY CONTINUOUS INTRAVENOUS INFUSION
▸ Adult: 2 mg/kg, to be given over 24 hours, dose adjusted according to blood-ciclosporin concentration and response

Severe active rheumatoid arthritis (administered on expert advice)
▸ BY MOUTH
▸ Adult: Initially 1.5 mg/kg twice daily, increased if necessary up to 2.5 mg/kg twice daily after 6 weeks, dose increases should be made gradually, for maintenance treatment, titrate dose individually to the lowest effective dose according to tolerability, treatment may be required for up to 12 weeks

Severe active rheumatoid arthritis [in combination with low-dose methotrexate, when methotrexate monotherapy has been ineffective] (administered on expert advice)
▸ BY MOUTH
▸ Adult: Initially 1.25 mg/kg twice daily, increased if necessary up to 2.5 mg/kg twice daily after 6 weeks, dose increases should be made gradually, for maintenance treatment, titrate dose individually to the lowest effective dose according to tolerability, treatment may be required for up to 12 weeks

Short-term treatment of severe atopic dermatitis where conventional therapy ineffective or inappropriate (administered on expert advice)
▸ BY MOUTH
▸ Adult: Initially 1.25 mg/kg twice daily (max. per dose 2.5 mg/kg twice daily) usual maximum duration of 8 weeks but may be used for longer under specialist supervision, if good initial response not achieved within 2 weeks, increase dose rapidly up to maximum

Short-term treatment of very severe atopic dermatitis where conventional therapy ineffective or inappropriate (administered on expert advice)
▸ BY MOUTH
▸ Adult: 2.5 mg/kg twice daily usual maximum duration of 8 weeks but may be used for longer under specialist supervision

Severe psoriasis where conventional therapy ineffective or inappropriate (administered on expert advice)
▸ BY MOUTH
▸ Adult: Initially 1.25 mg/kg twice daily (max. per dose 2.5 mg/kg twice daily), increased gradually to maximum if no improvement within 1 month, initial dose of 2.5 mg/kg twice daily justified if condition requires rapid improvement; discontinue if inadequate response after 3 months at the optimum dose; max. duration of treatment usually 1 year unless other treatments cannot be used

Organ transplantation (used alone)
▸ BY MOUTH
▸ Adult: 10–15 mg/kg, to be administered 4–12 hours before transplantation, followed by 10–15 mg/kg daily for 1–2 weeks postoperatively, then maintenance 2–6 mg/kg daily, reduce dose gradually to

maintenance. Dose should be adjusted according to blood-ciclosporin concentration and renal function; dose is lower if given concomitantly with other immunosuppressant therapy (e.g. corticosteroids); if necessary one-third corresponding oral dose can be given by intravenous infusion over 2–6 hours

Bone-marrow transplantation | Prevention and treatment of graft-versus-host disease

▸ INITIALLY BY INTRAVENOUS INFUSION

▸ Adult: 3–5 mg/kg daily, to be administered over 2–6 hours from day before transplantation to 2 weeks postoperatively, alternatively (by mouth) initially 12.5–15 mg/kg daily, then (by mouth) 12.5 mg/kg daily for 3-6 months and then tailed off (may take up to a year after transplantation)

Nephrotic syndrome

▸ BY MOUTH

▸ Adult: 5 mg/kg daily in 2 divided doses, for maintenance reduce to lowest effective dose according to proteinuria and serum creatinine measurements; discontinue after 3 months if no improvement in glomerulonephritis or glomerulosclerosis (after 6 months in membranous glomerulonephritis)

DOSE ADJUSTMENTS DUE TO INTERACTIONS

▸ With oral use Manufacturer advises increase dose by 50% or switch to intravenous administration with concurrent use of octreotide.

● UNLICENSED USE Not licensed for use in severe acute ulcerative colitis refractory to corticosteroid treatment.

IMPORTANT SAFETY INFORMATION

MHRA/CHM ADVICE: CICLOSPORIN MUST BE PRESCRIBED AND DISPENSED BY BRAND NAME (DECEMBER 2009)

Patients should be stabilised on a particular brand of oral ciclosporin because switching between formulations without close monitoring may lead to clinically important changes in blood-ciclosporin concentration.

● CONTRA-INDICATIONS Malignancy (in non-transplant indications) · uncontrolled hypertension (in non-transplant indications) · uncontrolled infections (in non-transplant indications)

● CAUTIONS Elderly—monitor renal function · hyperuricaemia · in atopic dermatitis, active herpes simplex infections—allow infection to clear before starting (if they occur during treatment withdraw if severe) · in atopic dermatitis, *Staphylococcus aureus* skin infections—not absolute contra-indication providing controlled (but avoid erythromycin unless no other alternative) · in psoriasis treat, patients with malignant or pre-malignant conditions of skin only after appropriate treatment (and if no other option) · in uveitis, Behcet's syndrome (monitor neurological status) · lymphoproliferative disorders (discontinue treatment) · malignancy

CAUTIONS, FURTHER INFORMATION

▸ Malignancy In psoriasis, exclude malignancies (including those of skin and cervix) before starting (biopsy any lesions not typical of psoriasis) and treat patients with malignant or pre-malignant conditions of skin only after appropriate treatment (and if no other option); discontinue if lymphoproliferative disorder develops.

● INTERACTIONS → Appendix 1: ciclosporin

● SIDE-EFFECTS

SPECIFIC SIDE-EFFECTS

▸ **Common or very common** Appetite decreased · diarrhoea · electrolyte imbalance · eye inflammation · fatigue · fever · flushing · gastrointestinal discomfort · gingival hyperplasia · hair changes · headaches · hepatic disorders · hyperglycaemia · hyperlipidaemia · hypertension · hyperuricaemia · leucopenia · muscle complaints · nausea ·

paraesthesia · peptic ulcer · renal impairment (renal structural changes on long-term administration) · seizure · skin reactions · tremor · vomiting

▸ **Uncommon** Anaemia · encephalopathy · oedema · thrombocytopenia · weight increased

▸ **Rare or very rare** Gynaecomastia · haemolytic anaemia · idiopathic intracranial hypertension · menstrual disorder · multifocal motor neuropathy · muscle weakness · myopathy · pancreatitis

▸ **Frequency not known** Pain in extremity · thrombotic microangiopathy

● PREGNANCY Crosses placenta; manufacturer advises avoid unless potential benefit outweighs risk—toxicity in *animal* studies.

● BREAST FEEDING Manufacturer advises avoid—present in milk.

● HEPATIC IMPAIRMENT Manufacturer advises caution in severe impairment (risk of increased exposure).
Dose adjustments Manufacturer advises consider dose reduction in severe impairment to maintain blood-ciclosporin concentration in target range—monitor until concentration stable.

● RENAL IMPAIRMENT In non-transplant indications, manufacturer advises establishing baseline renal function before initiation of treatment; if baseline function is impaired in non-transplant indications, except nephrotic syndrome—avoid.
Dose adjustments See p. 21. In nephrotic syndrome, manufacturer advises initial dose should not exceed 2.5 mg/kg daily in patients with baseline renal impairment. *During treatment* for non-transplant indications, manufacturer recommends if eGFR decreases by more than 25% below baseline on more than one measurement, reduce dose by 25–50%. If the eGFR decrease from baseline exceeds 35%, further dose reduction should be considered (even if within normal range); discontinue if reduction not successful within 1 month.

● MONITORING REQUIREMENTS

▸ Monitor whole blood ciclosporin concentration (trough level dependent on indication—consult local treatment protocol for details).

▸ Dermatological and physical examination, including blood pressure and renal function measurements required at least twice before starting treatment for psoriasis or atopic dermatitis. Monitor liver function. Monitor serum potassium, especially in renal dysfunction (risk of hyperkalaemia). Monitor serum magnesium. Measure blood lipids before treatment and after the first month of treatment. In psoriasis and atopic dermatitis monitor serum creatinine every 2 weeks for first 3 months then every month. Investigate lymphadenopathy that persists despite improvement in atopic dermatitis. Monitor kidney function—dose dependent increase in serum creatinine and urea during first few weeks may necessitate dose reduction in transplant patients (exclude rejection if kidney transplant) or discontinuation in non-transplant patients. Monitor blood pressure—discontinue if hypertension develops that cannot be controlled by antihypertensives. In long-term management of nephrotic syndrome, perform renal biopsies at yearly intervals. In rheumatoid arthritis measure serum creatinine at least twice before treatment. During treatment, monitor serum creatinine every 2 weeks for first 3 months, then every month for a further 3 months, then every 4–8 weeks depending on the stability of the disease, concomitant medication, and concomitant diseases (or more frequently if dose increased or concomitant NSAIDs introduced or increased). Monitor hepatic function if concomitant NSAIDs given.

Immune system and malignant disease

Immune system and malignant disease 8

DIRECTIONS FOR ADMINISTRATION
▶ With oral use Manufacturer advises mix solution with orange or apple juice, or other soft drink (to improve taste) immediately before taking (and rinse with more to ensure total dose). Do not mix with grapefruit juice. Total daily dose should be taken in 2 divided doses.
▶ With intravenous use For *intravenous infusion* (*Sandimmun*®), manufacturer advises give intermittently *or* continuously *in* Glucose 5% *or* Sodium Chloride 0.9%; dilute to a concentration of 50 mg in 20–100 mL; give intermittent infusion over 2–6 hours; not to be used with PVC equipment. Observe patient for signs of anaphylaxis for at least 30 minutes after starting infusion and at frequent intervals thereafter.

PRESCRIBING AND DISPENSING INFORMATION
Brand name prescribing Prescribing and dispensing of ciclosporin should be by brand name to avoid inadvertent switching. If it is necessary to switch a patient to a different brand of ciclosporin, the patient should be monitored closely for changes in blood-ciclosporin concentration, serum creatinine, blood pressure, and transplant function (for transplant indications). *Sandimmun*® capsules and oral solution are available direct from Novartis for patients who cannot be transferred to a different oral preparation.

PATIENT AND CARER ADVICE Patients and carers should be counselled on the administration of different formulations of ciclosporin. Manufacturer advises avoid excessive exposure to UV light, including sunlight. In psoriasis and atopic dermatitis, avoid use of UVB or PUVA.

MEDICINAL FORMS There can be variation in the licensing of different medicines containing the same drug.

Oral capsule
CAUTIONARY AND ADVISORY LABELS 11
EXCIPIENTS: May contain Ethanol, ethyl lactate, propylene glycol
▶ **Ciclosporin** (Non-proprietary)
Ciclosporin 25 mg Ciclosporin 25mg capsules | 30 capsule [PoM] [₤] DT = £18.37
Ciclosporin 50 mg Ciclosporin 50mg capsules | 30 capsule [PoM] [₤] DT = £35.97
Ciclosporin 100 mg Ciclosporin 100mg capsules | 30 capsule [PoM] [₤] DT = £68.28
▶ **Capimune** (Viatris UK Healthcare Ltd)
Ciclosporin 25 mg Capimune 25mg capsules | 30 capsule [PoM] £13.05 DT = £18.37
Ciclosporin 50 mg Capimune 50mg capsules | 30 capsule [PoM] £25.50 DT = £35.97
Ciclosporin 100 mg Capimune 100mg capsules | 30 capsule [PoM] £48.50 DT = £68.28
▶ **Capsorin** (Morningside Healthcare Ltd)
Ciclosporin 25 mg Capsorin 25mg capsules | 30 capsule [PoM] £11.14 DT = £18.37
Ciclosporin 50 mg Capsorin 50mg capsules | 30 capsule [PoM] £21.80 DT = £35.97
Ciclosporin 100 mg Capsorin 100mg capsules | 30 capsule [PoM] £41.59 DT = £68.28
▶ **Deximune** (Dexcel-Pharma Ltd)
Ciclosporin 25 mg Deximune 25mg capsules | 30 capsule [PoM] £13.06 DT = £18.37
Ciclosporin 50 mg Deximune 50mg capsules | 30 capsule [PoM] £25.60 DT = £35.97
Ciclosporin 100 mg Deximune 100mg capsules | 30 capsule [PoM] £48.90 DT = £68.28
▶ **Neoral** (Novartis Pharmaceuticals UK Ltd)
Ciclosporin 10 mg Neoral 10mg capsules | 60 capsule [PoM] £18.25 DT = £18.25
Ciclosporin 25 mg Neoral 25mg capsules | 30 capsule [PoM] £18.37 DT = £18.37
Ciclosporin 50 mg Neoral 50mg capsules | 30 capsule [PoM] £35.97 DT = £35.97
Ciclosporin 100 mg Neoral 100mg capsules | 30 capsule [PoM] £68.28 DT = £68.28
▶ **Sandimmun** (Novartis Pharmaceuticals UK Ltd)
Ciclosporin 25 mg Sandimmun 25mg capsules | 30 capsule [PoM] £29.58 DT = £18.37
Ciclosporin 50 mg Sandimmun 50mg capsules | 30 capsule [PoM] £57.92 DT = £35.97
Ciclosporin 100 mg Sandimmun 100mg capsules | 30 capsule [PoM] £109.93 DT = £68.28
▶ **Vanquoral** (Teva UK Ltd)
Ciclosporin 10 mg Vanquoral 10mg capsules | 60 capsule [PoM] £12.75 DT = £18.25
Ciclosporin 25 mg Vanquoral 25mg capsules | 30 capsule [PoM] £13.05 DT = £18.37
Ciclosporin 50 mg Vanquoral 50mg capsules | 30 capsule [PoM] £25.59 DT = £35.97
Ciclosporin 100 mg Vanquoral 100mg capsules | 30 capsule [PoM] £48.89 DT = £68.28

Solution for infusion
CAUTIONARY AND ADVISORY LABELS 11
EXCIPIENTS: May contain Alcohol, polyoxyl castor oils
▶ **Sandimmun** (Novartis Pharmaceuticals UK Ltd)
Ciclosporin 50 mg per 1 ml Sandimmun 250mg/5ml concentrate for solution for infusion ampoules | 10 ampoule [PoM] £110.05
Sandimmun 50mg/1ml concentrate for solution for infusion ampoules | 10 ampoule [PoM] £23.23 DT = £23.23

Oral solution
CAUTIONARY AND ADVISORY LABELS 11
EXCIPIENTS: May contain Alcohol, propylene glycol
▶ **Neoral** (Novartis Pharmaceuticals UK Ltd)
Ciclosporin 100 mg per 1 ml Neoral 100mg/ml oral solution | 50 ml [PoM] £102.30 DT = £164.72 [SF]

Sirolimus
19-Mar-2025

DRUG ACTION Sirolimus is a non-calcineurin inhibiting immunosuppressant.

INDICATIONS AND DOSE
Prophylaxis of organ rejection in kidney allograft recipients
▶ BY MOUTH
▶ Adult: Initially 6 mg for 1 dose, to be given after surgery once wound has healed, then 2 mg once daily; to be given in combination with ciclosporin and corticosteroid for 2–3 months (sirolimus doses should be given 4 hours after ciclosporin), ciclosporin should then be withdrawn over 4–8 weeks (if not possible, sirolimus should be discontinued and an alternate immunosuppressive regimen used), dose to be adjusted according to whole blood-sirolimus trough concentration

DOSE EQUIVALENCE AND CONVERSION
▶ For *tablets*, the 500 microgram strength tablet is not bioequivalent to the 1 mg and 2 mg strength tablets. Multiples of 500 microgram tablets should **not** be used as a substitute for other tablet strengths.

CAUTIONS Hyperlipidaemia · increased susceptibility to infection (especially urinary-tract infection) · increased susceptibility to lymphoma and other malignancies, particularly of the skin (limit exposure to UV light)

INTERACTIONS → Appendix 1: sirolimus

SIDE-EFFECTS
▶ **Common or very common** Abdominal pain · anaemia · arthralgia · ascites · constipation · diabetes mellitus · diarrhoea · dyslipidaemia · electrolyte imbalance · embolism and thrombosis · fever · haemolytic uraemic syndrome · haemorrhage · headache · healing impaired · hyperglycaemia · hypertension · increased risk of infection · interstitial lung disease · leucopenia · lymphatic vessel disorders · menstrual cycle irregularities · nausea · neoplasms · neutropenia · oedema · osteonecrosis · ovarian cyst · pain · pancreatitis · pericardial effusion · pleural effusion · proteinuria · sepsis · skin reactions · stomatitis · tachycardia · thrombocytopenia
▶ **Uncommon** Clostridioides difficile colitis · focal segmental glomerulosclerosis · hepatic failure · nephrotic syndrome ·

pancytopenia · post transplant lymphoproliferative disorder

- ► **Frequency not known** Posterior reversible encephalopathy syndrome (PRES)
- ● **CONCEPTION AND CONTRACEPTION** [EvGr] Ensure effective contraception during and for 12 weeks after treatment. ⟨M⟩
- ● **PREGNANCY** [EvGr] Avoid unless essential (toxicity in *animal* studies). ⟨M⟩
- ● **BREAST FEEDING** [EvGr] Discontinue breast-feeding (no information available). ⟨M⟩ Specialist sources also note a lack of data and that safer alternatives are preferable, especially with regards to premature infants, or in the neonatal period. However, the large molecular weight and high plasma-protein binding mean excretion into milk is unlikely, and poor oral bioavailability would suggest limited absorption by an infant, and so it may be compatible in some circumstances.
- ● **HEPATIC IMPAIRMENT** [EvGr] Caution (risk of increased exposure) ⟨M⟩.
  Dose adjustments [EvGr] Maintenance dose reduction of approx. 50% in severe impairment—monitor whole blood-sirolimus trough concentration every 5–7 days until 3 consecutive measurements have shown stable blood-sirolimus concentration. ⟨M⟩
- ● **MONITORING REQUIREMENTS**
- ► Monitor whole blood-sirolimus trough concentration (Afro-Caribbean patients may require higher doses).
- ► Manufacturer advises pre-dose ('trough') whole blood-sirolimus concentration (using **chromatographic** assay) when used with ciclosporin should be 4–12 micrograms/litre (local treatment protocols may differ); after withdrawal of ciclosporin pre-dose whole blood-sirolimus concentration should be 12–20 micrograms/litre (local treatment protocols may differ).
- ► Close monitoring of whole blood-sirolimus concentration required if concomitant treatment with potent inducers or inhibitors of metabolism and after discontinuing them, or if ciclosporin dose reduced significantly or stopped.
- ► When changing between oral solution and tablets, measurement of whole blood 'trough' sirolimus concentration after 1–2 weeks is recommended.
- ► Therapeutic drug monitoring assays Sirolimus whole-blood concentration is measured using either high performance liquid chromatography (HPLC) or immunoassay. Switching between different immunoassays or between an immunoassay and HPLC can lead to clinically significant differences in results and therefore incorrect dose adjustments. Adjustment to the target therapeutic dose range should be made with knowledge of the assay used and corresponding reference range.
- ► Monitor kidney function when given with ciclosporin; monitor lipids; monitor urine proteins.
- ● **DIRECTIONS FOR ADMINISTRATION** [EvGr] Food may affect absorption (take at the same time with respect to food). Sirolimus oral solution should be mixed with at least 60 mL water or orange juice in a glass or plastic container immediately before taking; refill container with at least 120 mL of water or orange juice and drink immediately (to ensure total dose). Do not mix with any other liquids. ⟨M⟩
- ● **HANDLING AND STORAGE** Protect from light. Oral solution and topical gel: store in a refrigerator (2-8°C).
- ● **PATIENT AND CARER ADVICE** Advise patients to avoid excessive exposure to UV light including sunlight.
- ● **NATIONAL FUNDING/ACCESS DECISIONS** For full details see funding body website
  NICE decisions
- ► **Immunosuppressive therapy for kidney transplant in adults (October 2017)** NICE TA481 Not recommended

Scottish Medicines Consortium (SMC) decisions
- ► Sirolimus (*Hyftor*®) for the treatment of adult and paediatric patients aged 6 and above with facial angiofibroma associated with tuberous sclerosis complex (January 2025) SMC No. SMC2710 Recommended

- ● **MEDICINAL FORMS** There can be variation in the licensing of different medicines containing the same drug.
  Oral tablet
- ► **Sirolimus (Non-proprietary)**
  Sirolimus 500 microgram Sirolimus 500microgram tablets | 30 tablet [PoM] £69.00 DT = £69.00
  Sirolimus 1 mg Sirolimus 1mg tablets | 30 tablet [PoM] £86.49 DT = £86.49
  Sirolimus 2 mg Sirolimus 2mg tablets | 30 tablet [PoM] £172.98 DT = £172.98
- ► **Rapamune** (Pfizer Ltd)
  Sirolimus 500 microgram Rapamune 0.5mg tablets | 30 tablet [PoM] £69.00 DT = £69.00
  Sirolimus 1 mg Rapamune 1mg tablets | 30 tablet [PoM] £86.49 DT = £86.49
  Sirolimus 2 mg Rapamune 2mg tablets | 30 tablet [PoM] £172.98 DT = £172.98
  Oral solution
  EXCIPIENTS: May contain Ethanol
- ► **Rapamune** (Pfizer Ltd)
  Sirolimus 1 mg per 1 ml Rapamune 1mg/ml oral solution | 60 ml [PoM] £162.41 DT = £162.41 [SF]

Tacrolimus

27-Sep-2024

- ● **DRUG ACTION** Tacrolimus is a calcineurin inhibitor.

- ● **INDICATIONS AND DOSE**
  ADOPORT®
  Prophylaxis of graft rejection following liver transplantation, starting 12 hours after transplantation
- ► BY MOUTH
- ► Adult: Initially 100–200 micrograms/kg daily in 2 divided doses, then maintenance, dose to be adjusted according to response and whole blood-tacrolimus trough concentrations—doses are usually reduced in the post-transplant period

  Prophylaxis of graft rejection following kidney transplantation, starting within 24 hours of transplantation
- ► BY MOUTH
- ► Adult: Initially 200–300 micrograms/kg daily in 2 divided doses, then maintenance, dose to be adjusted according to response and whole blood-tacrolimus trough concentrations—doses are usually reduced in the post-transplant period

  Prophylaxis of graft rejection following heart transplantation following antibody induction, starting within 5 days of transplantation
- ► BY MOUTH
- ► Adult: Initially 75 micrograms/kg daily in 2 divided doses, then maintenance, dose to be adjusted according to response and whole blood-tacrolimus trough concentrations—doses are usually reduced in the post-transplant period

  Prophylaxis of graft rejection following heart transplantation without antibody induction, starting within 12 hours of transplantation
- ► BY MOUTH
- ► Adult: Initially 75 micrograms/kg daily in 2 divided doses, then maintenance, dose to be adjusted according to response and whole blood-tacrolimus trough concentrations—doses are usually reduced in the post-transplant period continued →

continued →

8

Immune system and malignant disease

Allograft rejection resistant to conventional immunosuppressive therapy
▶ BY MOUTH
▶ Adult: Seek specialist advice

ADVAGRAF ®

Prophylaxis of graft rejection following liver transplantation, starting 12–18 hours after transplantation
▶ BY MOUTH
▶ Adult: Initially 100–200 micrograms/kg once daily, dose to be taken in the morning, then maintenance, dose to be adjusted according to response and whole blood-tacrolimus trough concentrations—doses are usually reduced in the post-transplant period, dose to be taken in the morning

Prophylaxis of graft rejection following kidney transplantation, starting within 24 hours of transplantation
▶ BY MOUTH
▶ Adult: Initially 200–300 micrograms/kg once daily, dose to be taken in the morning, then maintenance, dose to be adjusted according to response and whole blood-tacrolimus trough concentrations—doses are usually reduced in the post-transplant period, dose to be taken in the morning

Allograft rejection resistant to conventional immunosuppressive therapy
▶ BY MOUTH
▶ Adult: Seek specialist advice

DAILIPORT ®

Prophylaxis of graft rejection following liver transplantation, starting 12–18 hours after transplantation
▶ BY MOUTH
▶ Adult: Initially 100–200 micrograms/kg once daily, dose to be taken in the morning, then maintenance, dose to be adjusted according to response and whole blood-tacrolimus trough concentrations—doses are usually reduced in the post-transplant period, dose to be taken in the morning

Prophylaxis of graft rejection following kidney transplantation, starting within 24 hours of transplantation
▶ BY MOUTH
▶ Adult: Initially 200–300 micrograms/kg once daily, dose to be taken in the morning, then maintenance, dose to be adjusted according to response and whole blood-tacrolimus trough concentrations—doses are usually reduced in the post-transplant period, dose to be taken in the morning

Allograft rejection resistant to conventional immunosuppressive therapy
▶ BY MOUTH
▶ Adult: Seek specialist advice

ENVARSUS ® MODIFIED-RELEASE TABLETS

Prophylaxis of graft rejection following liver transplantation, starting within 24 hours of transplantation
▶ BY MOUTH
▶ Adult: Initially 110–130 micrograms/kg once daily, dose to be taken in the morning, then maintenance, dose to be adjusted according to response and whole blood-tacrolimus trough concentrations—doses are usually reduced in the post-transplant period, dose to be taken in the morning

Prophylaxis of graft rejection following kidney transplantation, starting within 24 hours of transplantation
▶ BY MOUTH
▶ Adult: Initially 170 micrograms/kg once daily, dose to be taken in the morning, then maintenance, dose to be adjusted according to response and whole blood-tacrolimus trough concentrations—doses are usually reduced in the post-transplant period, dose to be taken in the morning

Rejection therapy
▶ BY MOUTH
▶ Adult: Seek specialist advice

MODIGRAF ®

Prophylaxis of graft rejection following liver transplantation, starting 12 hours after transplantation
▶ BY MOUTH
▶ Adult: Initially 100–200 micrograms/kg daily in 2 divided doses, then maintenance, dose to be adjusted according to response and whole blood-tacrolimus trough concentrations—doses are usually reduced in the post-transplant period

Prophylaxis of graft rejection following kidney transplantation, starting within 24 hours of transplantation
▶ BY MOUTH
▶ Adult: Initially 200–300 micrograms/kg daily in 2 divided doses, then maintenance, dose to be adjusted according to response and whole blood-tacrolimus trough concentrations—doses are usually reduced in the post-transplant period

Prophylaxis of graft rejection following heart transplantation following antibody induction, starting within 5 days of transplantation
▶ BY MOUTH
▶ Adult: Initially 75 micrograms/kg daily in 2 divided doses, then maintenance, dose to be adjusted according to response and whole blood-tacrolimus trough concentrations—doses are usually reduced in the post-transplant period

Prophylaxis of graft rejection following heart transplantation without antibody induction, starting within 12 hours of transplantation
▶ BY MOUTH
▶ Adult: Initially 75 micrograms/kg daily in 2 divided doses, then maintenance, dose to be adjusted according to response and whole blood-tacrolimus trough concentrations—doses are usually reduced in the post-transplant period

Rejection therapy
▶ BY MOUTH
▶ Adult: Seek specialist advice

PROGRAF ® CAPSULES

Prophylaxis of graft rejection following liver transplantation, starting 12 hours after transplantation
▶ BY MOUTH
▶ Adult: Initially 100–200 micrograms/kg daily in 2 divided doses, then maintenance, dose to be adjusted according to response and whole blood-tacrolimus trough concentrations—doses are usually reduced in the post-transplant period

Prophylaxis of graft rejection following kidney transplantation, starting within 24 hours of transplantation
▶ BY MOUTH
▶ Adult: Initially 200–300 micrograms/kg daily in 2 divided doses, then maintenance, dose to be adjusted according to response and whole blood-tacrolimus

trough concentrations—doses are usually reduced in the post-transplant period

Prophylaxis of graft rejection following heart transplantation following antibody induction, starting within 5 days of transplantation
▶ BY MOUTH
▶ Adult: Initially 75 micrograms/kg daily in 2 divided doses, then maintenance, dose to be adjusted according to response and whole blood-tacrolimus trough concentrations—doses are usually reduced in the post-transplant period

Prophylaxis of graft rejection following heart transplantation without antibody induction, starting within 12 hours of transplantation
▶ BY MOUTH
▶ Adult: Initially 75 micrograms/kg daily in 2 divided doses, then maintenance, dose to be adjusted according to response and whole blood-tacrolimus trough concentrations—doses are usually reduced in the post-transplant period

Allograft rejection resistant to conventional immunosuppressive therapy
▶ BY MOUTH
▶ Adult: Seek specialist advice

PROGRAF ® INFUSION

Prophylaxis of graft rejection following liver transplantation, starting 12 hours after transplantation when oral route not appropriate
▶ BY INTRAVENOUS INFUSION
▶ Adult: Initially 10–50 micrograms/kg daily for up to 7 days (then transfer to oral therapy), dose to be administered over 24 hours

Prophylaxis of graft rejection following kidney transplantation, starting within 24 hours of transplantation when oral route not appropriate
▶ BY INTRAVENOUS INFUSION
▶ Adult: Initially 50–100 micrograms/kg daily for up to 7 days (then transfer to oral therapy), dose to be administered over 24 hours

Prophylaxis of graft rejection following heart transplantation following antibody induction, starting within 5 days of transplantation
▶ BY INTRAVENOUS INFUSION
▶ Adult: Initially 10–20 micrograms/kg daily for up to 7 days (then transfer to oral therapy), dose to be administered over 24 hours

Prophylaxis of graft rejection following heart transplantation without antibody induction, starting within 12 hours of transplantation
▶ BY INTRAVENOUS INFUSION
▶ Adult: Initially 10–20 micrograms/kg daily for up to 7 days (then transfer to oral therapy), dose to be administered over 24 hours

Allograft rejection resistant to conventional immunosuppressive therapy
▶ BY CONTINUOUS INTRAVENOUS INFUSION
▶ Adult: Seek specialist advice (consult local protocol)

DOSE EQUIVALENCE AND CONVERSION
▶ For *Prograf*®: intravenous and oral doses are **not** interchangeable due to differences in bioavailability.

Follow correct dosing recommendations for the dosage form when switching formulations.

> **IMPORTANT SAFETY INFORMATION**
> **MHRA/CHM ADVICE: ORAL TACROLIMUS PRODUCTS: PRESCRIBE AND DISPENSE BY BRAND NAME ONLY, TO MINIMISE THE RISK OF INADVERTENT SWITCHING BETWEEN PRODUCTS, WHICH HAS BEEN ASSOCIATED WITH REPORTS OF TOXICITY AND GRAFT REJECTION (JUNE 2012; NOVEMBER 2017)**
> ▶ With oral use
> Inadvertent switching between oral tacrolimus products has been associated with reports of toxicity and graft rejection. To ensure maintenance of therapeutic response when a patient is stabilised on a particular brand, oral tacrolimus products should be prescribed and dispensed by brand name only.
> - *Adoport*® and *Prograf*® are immediate-release capsules that are taken twice daily, once in the morning and once in the evening;
> - *Modigraf*® granules are used to prepare an immediate-release oral suspension which is taken twice daily, once in the morning and once in the evening;
> - *Advagraf*® and *Dailiport*® are prolonged-release capsules that are taken once daily in the morning. Switching between tacrolimus brands requires careful supervision and therapeutic monitoring by an appropriate specialist.
> Important: *Envarsus*® is not interchangeable with other oral tacrolimus containing products; the MHRA has advised (June 2012) that oral tacrolimus products should be prescribed and dispensed by brand only.

● CAUTIONS Increased risk of infections · increased susceptibility to lymphoproliferative disorders · malignancies · neurotoxicity · risk factors for cardiomyopathies · risk factors for QT-interval prolongation · UV light (avoid excessive exposure to sunlight and sunlamps)

● INTERACTIONS → Appendix 1: tacrolimus

● SIDE-EFFECTS

GENERAL SIDE-EFFECTS
▶ **Common or very common** Alopecia · anaemia · anxiety · appetite decreased · arrhythmias · ascites · asthenic conditions · bile duct disorders · confusion · consciousness impaired · constipation · coronary artery disease · cough · depression · diabetes mellitus · diarrhoea · dizziness · dysgraphia · dyslipidaemia · dyspnoea · electrolyte imbalance · embolism and thrombosis · eye disorder · febrile disorders · fluid imbalance · gastrointestinal discomfort · gastrointestinal disorders · gastrointestinal inflammatory disorders · haemorrhage · hallucination · headache · hepatic disorders · hyperglycaemia · hyperhidrosis · hypertension · hyperuricaemia · hypotension · increased risk of infection · interstitial lung disease · ischaemia · joint disorders · leucocytosis · leucopenia · metabolic acidosis · mood altered · muscle spasms · nasal complaints · nausea · nephropathy · nerve disorders · nervous system disorder · oedema · oral disorders · pain · peripheral vascular disease · primary transplant dysfunction · psychiatric disorder · renal impairment · renal tubular necrosis · respiratory disorders · seizure · sensation abnormal · skin reactions · sleep disorders · temperature sensation altered · thrombocytopenia · tinnitus · tremor · urinary tract disorder · urine abnormal · vision disorders · vomiting · weight changes
▶ **Uncommon** Asthma · cardiac arrest · cardiomyopathy · cataract · central nervous system haemorrhage · chest discomfort · coagulation disorders · coma · dysmenorrhoea · encephalopathy · feeling abnormal · haemolytic anaemia · hearing impairment · heart failure · hypoglycaemia · hypoproteinaemia · influenza like illness · memory loss ·

multi organ failure · neutropenia · palpitations · pancreatitis · pancytopenia · paralysis · paresis · photosensitivity reaction · psychotic disorder · shock · speech disorder · stroke · ventricular hypertrophy
▶ **Rare or very rare** Fall · hirsutism · mobility decreased · muscle tone increased · muscle weakness · pancreatic pseudocyst · pericardial effusion · QT interval prolongation · severe cutaneous adverse reactions (SCARs) · sinusoidal obstruction syndrome · thirst · ulcer
▶ **Frequency not known** Agranulocytosis · neoplasm malignant · neoplasms · polyomavirus-associated nephropathy · progressive multifocal leukoencephalopathy (PML) · pure red cell aplasia

SPECIFIC SIDE-EFFECTS
▶ With intravenous use Anaphylactoid reaction (due to excipient)

SIDE-EFFECTS, FURTHER INFORMATION Cardiomyopathy has been reported to occur primarily in children with tacrolimus blood trough concentrations much higher than the recommended maximum levels. Patients should be monitored by echocardiography for hypertrophic changes—consider dose reduction or discontinuation if these occur.

● ALLERGY AND CROSS-SENSITIVITY EvGr Contra-indicated if history of hypersensitivity to macrolides. M
▶ With oral use EvGr For *Advagraf*®, *Dailiport*® and *Prograf*® capsules, use only if benefit outweighs potential risk in patients with hypersensitivity to peanuts or soya (printing ink on the capsules contains soya lecithin). M

● CONCEPTION AND CONTRACEPTION Exclude pregnancy before treatment.

● PREGNANCY Specialist sources indicate avoid unless benefit outweighs potential risk—crosses the placenta and risk of premature delivery, intra-uterine growth restriction, hyperkalaemia and renal toxicity. Maternal risk of hyperglycaemia, hypertension, pre-eclampsia and renal impairment.

● BREAST FEEDING Specialist sources indicate present in milk (following systemic administration) but amount probably too small to be harmful—monitor exclusively breastfed infants, including blood concentrations, if there are concerns regarding toxicity.

● HEPATIC IMPAIRMENT Manufacturer advises caution in severe impairment.
Dose adjustments Manufacturer advises consider dose reduction in severe impairment.

● MONITORING REQUIREMENTS
▶ EvGr After initial dosing, and for maintenance treatment, tacrolimus doses should be adjusted according to response and whole blood-tacrolimus trough concentrations (especially during episodes of diarrhoea). Patients of black African or African–Caribbean family origin may require higher doses. Consult local treatment protocols for further details of therapeutic drug monitoring.
▶ Monitor blood pressure, ECG (for hypertrophic changes— risk of cardiomyopathy), fasting blood-glucose concentration, haematological and coagulation parameters, plasma protein, electrolytes, neurological (including visual) status, hepatic and renal function. Monitor for posterior reversible encephalopathy syndrome (PRES). M

● DIRECTIONS FOR ADMINISTRATION For *intravenous infusion* (*Prograf*®); manufacturer advises give continuously in Glucose 5% *or* Sodium Chloride 0.9%. Dilute concentrate in infusion fluid to a final concentration of 4–100 micrograms/mL; give over 24 hours. Tacrolimus is incompatible with PVC.

● PATIENT AND CARER ADVICE Advise patients to avoid excessive exposure to UV light including sunlight and to report symptoms of eye disorders for prompt evaluation by an ophthalmologist.
Driving and skilled tasks May affect performance of skilled tasks (e.g. driving).

● NATIONAL FUNDING/ACCESS DECISIONS
For full details see funding body website
NICE decisions
▶ **Immunosuppressive therapy for kidney transplant in adults [for immediate-release tacrolimus] (October 2017)** NICE TA481 Recommended with restrictions
▶ **Immunosuppressive therapy for kidney transplant in adults [for prolonged-release tacrolimus] (October 2017)** NICE TA481 Not recommended

Scottish Medicines Consortium (SMC) decisions
▶ Tacrolimus granules for suspension (*Modigraf*®) for prophylaxis of transplant rejection in adult and paediatric, kidney, liver or heart allograft recipients or for treatment of allograft rejection resistant to treatment with other immunosuppressive medicinal products in adult and paediatric patients (December 2010) SMC No. 657/10 Recommended with restrictions
▶ Tacrolimus (*Envarsus*®) for prophylaxis of transplant rejection in adult kidney or liver allograft recipients and treatment of allograft rejection resistant to treatment with other immunosuppressive medicinal products in adult patients (April 2015) SMC No. 1041/15 Recommended

● MEDICINAL FORMS There can be variation in the licensing of different medicines containing the same drug.
Modified-release tablet
CAUTIONARY AND ADVISORY LABELS 23, 25
EXCIPIENTS: May contain Butylated hydroxytoluene
▶ **Envarsus** (Chiesi Ltd)
Tacrolimus (as Tacrolimus monohydrate)
750 microgram Envarsus 750microgram modified-release tablets | 30 tablet PoM £44.33 DT = £44.33
Tacrolimus (as Tacrolimus monohydrate) 1 mg Envarsus 1mg modified-release tablets | 30 tablet PoM £59.10 DT = £59.10
Tacrolimus (as Tacrolimus monohydrate) 4 mg Envarsus 4mg modified-release tablets | 30 tablet PoM £236.40 DT = £236.40

Modified-release capsule
CAUTIONARY AND ADVISORY LABELS 23, 25
EXCIPIENTS: May contain Gelatin, lecithin, propylene glycol, tartrazine
▶ **Advagraf** (Astellas Pharma Ltd)
Tacrolimus (as Tacrolimus monohydrate)
500 microgram Advagraf 0.5mg modified-release capsules | 50 capsule PoM £35.79 DT = £35.79
Tacrolimus (as Tacrolimus monohydrate) 1 mg Advagraf 1mg modified-release capsules | 50 capsule PoM £71.59 DT = £71.59 | 100 capsule PoM £143.17 DT = £143.17
Tacrolimus (as Tacrolimus monohydrate) 3 mg Advagraf 3mg modified-release capsules | 50 capsule PoM £214.76 DT = £214.76
Tacrolimus (as Tacrolimus monohydrate) 5 mg Advagraf 5mg modified-release capsules | 50 capsule PoM £266.92 DT = £266.92
▶ **Dailiport** (Sandoz Ltd)
Tacrolimus (as Tacrolimus monohydrate)
500 microgram Dailiport 0.5mg modified-release capsules | 50 capsule PoM £28.63 DT = £35.79
Tacrolimus (as Tacrolimus monohydrate) 1 mg Dailiport 1mg modified-release capsules | 50 capsule PoM £57.27 DT = £71.59 | 100 capsule PoM £114.54 DT = £143.17
Tacrolimus (as Tacrolimus monohydrate) 2 mg Dailiport 2mg modified-release capsules | 50 capsule PoM £110.40 (Hospital only)
Tacrolimus (as Tacrolimus monohydrate) 3 mg Dailiport 3mg modified-release capsules | 50 capsule PoM £171.81 DT = £214.76
Tacrolimus (as Tacrolimus monohydrate) 5 mg Dailiport 5mg modified-release capsules | 50 capsule PoM £213.54 DT = £266.92

Oral capsule
CAUTIONARY AND ADVISORY LABELS 23
EXCIPIENTS: May contain Gelatin, lecithin, propylene glycol
▶ **Adoport** (Sandoz Ltd)
Tacrolimus 500 microgram Adoport 0.5mg capsules | 50 capsule PoM £42.92 DT = £61.88
Tacrolimus 1 mg Adoport 1mg capsules | 50 capsule PoM £55.69 DT = £80.28 | 100 capsule PoM £111.36

Tacrolimus 5 mg Adoport 5mg capsules | 50 capsule [PoM] £205.74 DT = £296.58

▸ **Prograf** (Astellas Pharma Ltd)
Tacrolimus 500 microgram Prograf 500microgram capsules | 50 capsule [PoM] £61.88 DT = £61.88
Tacrolimus 1 mg Prograf 1mg capsules | 50 capsule [PoM] £80.28 DT = £80.28 | 100 capsule [PoM] £160.54
Tacrolimus 5 mg Prograf 5mg capsules | 50 capsule [PoM] £296.58 DT = £296.58

Solution for infusion
EXCIPIENTS: May contain Polyoxyl castor oils

▸ **Prograf** (Astellas Pharma Ltd)
Tacrolimus 5 mg per 1 ml Prograf 5mg/1ml solution for infusion ampoules | 10 ampoule [PoM] £584.51

Granules for oral suspension
CAUTIONARY AND ADVISORY LABELS 13, 23

▸ **Modigraf** (Astellas Pharma Ltd)
Tacrolimus (as Tacrolimus monohydrate)
200 microgram Modigraf 0.2mg granules for oral suspension sachets | 50 sachet [PoM] £71.30 DT = £71.30 [SF]
Tacrolimus (as Tacrolimus monohydrate) 1 mg Modigraf 1mg granules for oral suspension sachets | 50 sachet [PoM] £356.65 DT = £356.65 [SF]

Voclosporin
10-Nov-2023

- **DRUG ACTION** Voclosporin is a calcineurin inhibitor that inhibits production and release of lymphokines, thereby suppressing cell-mediated immune response.

- **INDICATIONS AND DOSE**

Lupus nephritis (under expert supervision)
▸ BY MOUTH
▸ Adult 18-75 years: 23.7 mg twice daily, dose adjusted according to renal function—consult product literature, evaluate treatment continuation after at least 24 weeks

DOSE ADJUSTMENTS DUE TO INTERACTIONS
▸ [EvGr] Reduce dose to 15.8 mg in the morning and 7.9 mg in the evening with concurrent use of moderate CYP3A4 inhibitors. ◈

- **CAUTIONS** Hypertension · increased risk of infections · increased risk of malignancy · increased risk of neurotoxicity · QT-interval prolongation

- **INTERACTIONS** → Appendix 1: voclosporin

- **SIDE-EFFECTS**
▸ **Common or very common** Alopecia · anaemia · appetite decreased · cough · diarrhoea · gastrointestinal discomfort · gingival haemorrhage · hair changes · headache · hyperkalaemia · hypertension · increased risk of infection · nausea · oral disorders · renal impairment · seizure · tremor

- **ALLERGY AND CROSS-SENSITIVITY** [EvGr] Contra-indicated in patients with hypersensitivity to peanuts or soya (may contain trace amounts of soya lecithin). ◈

- **PREGNANCY** [EvGr] Avoid (toxicity in *animal* studies). ◈

- **BREAST FEEDING** Specialist sources indicate large molecular weight suggests limited excretion into milk. Consider an alternative drug, especially if breast-feeding a pre- or full-term neonate (no information available).

- **HEPATIC IMPAIRMENT** [EvGr] Avoid in severe impairment (no information available). ◈
Dose adjustments [EvGr] Reduce starting dose to 15.8 mg twice daily in mild to moderate impairment. ◈

- **RENAL IMPAIRMENT** [EvGr] Use with caution if eGFR less than 45 mL/minute/1.73 m^2 and only if potential benefit outweighs risk. ◈
Dose adjustments [EvGr] Reduce starting dose to 15.8 mg twice daily if eGFR less than 30 mL/minute/1.73 m^2. ◈
See p. 21.

- **MONITORING REQUIREMENTS**
▸ [EvGr] Obtain eGFR at baseline before treatment initiation and assess every 2 weeks for the first month, then every 4 weeks thereafter, during treatment. For dose adjustment if eGFR falls below 60 mL/minute/1.73 m^2—consult product literature.
▸ Monitor serum-potassium concentrations periodically during treatment.
▸ Monitor blood pressure every 2 weeks for the first month, then as clinically indicated thereafter, during treatment—consult product literature.
▸ Monitor neurological status including seizures, tremors, or signs and symptoms suggestive of posterior reversible encephalopathy syndrome (PRES)—consider dose reduction or treatment discontinuation if these occur. ◈

- **PATIENT AND CARER ADVICE** Patients should be advised to avoid excessive exposure to UV light, including sunlight. **Missed doses** If a dose is more than 4 hours late, the missed dose should not be taken and the next dose should be taken at the normal time.

- **NATIONAL FUNDING/ACCESS DECISIONS**
For full details see funding body website
NICE decisions
▸ **Voclosporin with mycophenolate mofetil for treating lupus nephritis (May 2023)** NICE TA882 Recommended
Scottish Medicines Consortium (SMC) decisions
▸ **Voclosporin (*Lupkynis*®) in combination with mycophenolate mofetil for the treatment of adult patients with active class III, IV or V (including mixed class III/V and IV/V) lupus nephritis (October 2023)** SMC No. SMC2570 Recommended

- **MEDICINAL FORMS** There can be variation in the licensing of different medicines containing the same drug.
Oral capsule
EXCIPIENTS: May contain Ethanol, sorbitol, vitamin e
▸ **Lupkynis** (Otsuka Pharmaceuticals (U.K.) Ltd) ▼
Voclosporin 7.9 mg Lupkynis 7.9mg capsules | 180 capsule [PoM] £1,000.00 (Hospital only)

IMMUNOSUPPRESSANTS ❯ COMPLEMENT INHIBITORS

Avacopan
28-Mar-2024

- **DRUG ACTION** Avacopan is a complement 5a receptor (C5aR1) antagonist that inhibits C5a-mediated neutrophil activation, thereby reducing the pro-inflammatory effects of the C5a protein on blood vessels.

- **INDICATIONS AND DOSE**

Granulomatosis with polyangiitis (under expert supervision) | Microscopic polyangiitis (under expert supervision)
▸ BY MOUTH
▸ Adult: 30 mg twice daily, dose to be taken with food, for dose interruption or treatment discontinuation due to side-effects—consult product literature

- **CONTRA-INDICATIONS** Absolute neutrophil count less than 1.5 × 10^9/litre (do not initiate) · lymphocyte count less than 0.5 × 10^9/litre (do not initiate) · signs of liver disease—consult product literature · white blood cell count less than 3.5 × 10^9/litre (do not initiate)

- **CAUTIONS** Immunisation · serious infections
CAUTIONS, FURTHER INFORMATION
▸ Immunisation [EvGr] Administer vaccinations preferably before starting treatment or during quiescent phase of the disease—safety of immunisation with live viral vaccines unknown. ◈
▸ Infection [EvGr] Use with caution in patients with a history of

Immune system and malignant disease

hepatitis B or C, HIV infection, or tuberculosis—no information available.

Pneumocystis jirovecii pneumonia prophylaxis is recommended—consult local protocol. ⓜ

● **INTERACTIONS** → Appendix 1: avacopan

● **SIDE-EFFECTS**
▶ **Common or very common** Abdominal pain upper · diarrhoea · headache · hepatic disorders · increased risk of infection · leucopenia · nausea · neutropenia · vomiting
▶ **Uncommon** Angioedema
▶ **Frequency not known** Cardiac disorder · vanishing bile duct syndrome

● **PREGNANCY** [EvGr] Avoid—toxicity in animal studies. ⓜ

● **BREAST FEEDING** [EvGr] Avoid—limited information available. ⓜ

● **HEPATIC IMPAIRMENT** [EvGr] Avoid in severe impairment (no information available). ⓜ

● **MONITORING REQUIREMENTS**
▶ [EvGr] Obtain white blood cell count at baseline and monitor during treatment as clinically indicated—consult product literature.
▶ Obtain hepatic transaminases and total bilirubin at baseline and monitor during treatment as clinically indicated—consult product literature. ⓜ

● **PATIENT AND CARER ADVICE** Patients should be advised to immediately report any evidence of bone marrow failure such as infection, unexpected bruising, or bleeding. Patients should be advised to seek immediate medical attention if any symptoms of angioedema develop.
Missed doses If a dose is more than 9 hours late, the missed dose should not be taken and the next dose should be taken at the normal time.

● **NATIONAL FUNDING/ACCESS DECISIONS**
For full details see funding body website
NICE decisions
▶ Avacopan for treating severe active granulomatosis with polyangiitis or microscopic polyangiitis (September 2022) NICE TA825 Recommended
Scottish Medicines Consortium (SMC) decisions
▶ Avacopan (*Tavneos*®) in combination with a rituximab or cyclophosphamide regimen for the treatment of adult patients with severe, active granulomatosis with polyangiitis or microscopic polyangiitis (November 2023) SMC No. SMC2578 Recommended

● **MEDICINAL FORMS** There can be variation in the licensing of different medicines containing the same drug.
Oral capsule
CAUTIONARY AND ADVISORY LABELS 21, 25
EXCIPIENTS: May contain Polyoxyl castor oils
▶ Tavneos (Vifor Fresenius Medical Care Renal Pharma UK Ltd) ▼
Avacopan 10 mg Tavneos 10mg capsules | 180 capsule [PoM]
£5,547.95 (Hospital only)

IMMUNOSUPPRESSANTS › INTERLEUKIN INHIBITORS

Satralizumab
11-Mar-2024

● **DRUG ACTION** Satralizumab is a recombinant humanised monoclonal antibody that inhibits interleukin-6 signalling.

● **INDICATIONS AND DOSE**
Neuromyelitis optica spectrum disorder (initiated under specialist supervision)
▶ BY SUBCUTANEOUS INJECTION
▶ Adult: Initially 120 mg every 2 weeks for the first 3 doses, followed by maintenance 120 mg every 4 weeks

● **CAUTIONS** Active infection (delay treatment until infection is controlled) · immunisation
CAUTIONS, FURTHER INFORMATION
▶ Immunisation [EvGr] Patients should receive all recommended vaccinations before starting treatment—immunisation during treatment has not been studied. Live or live attenuated vaccines should be avoided during treatment—safety is unknown. ⓜ

● **INTERACTIONS** → Appendix 1: monoclonal antibodies

● **SIDE-EFFECTS**
▶ **Common or very common** Allergic rhinitis · arthralgia · bradycardia · gastritis · headaches · hyperlipidaemia · hypertension · hypofibrinogenaemia · injection related reaction · insomnia · musculoskeletal stiffness · peripheral oedema · skin reactions · weight increased

SIDE-EFFECTS, FURTHER INFORMATION If increased liver transaminase, low platelet count, or low neutrophil count occurs treatment should be interrupted or discontinued—consult product literature.

● **PREGNANCY** [EvGr] Avoid (limited information available). ⓜ

● **BREAST FEEDING** Specialist sources indicate use with caution, especially if breast-feeding a newborn or premature infant (limited information available). Risk of transfer to infant may be minimised by resuming treatment at least 2 weeks postpartum.

● **MONITORING REQUIREMENTS**
▶ [EvGr] Monitor liver transaminases every 4 weeks for the first 3 months of treatment, then every 3 months for 1 year, and as clinically indicated thereafter ⓜ—consult product literature for further information.
▶ [EvGr] Monitor neutrophil count 4 to 8 weeks after starting treatment and as clinically indicated thereafter ⓜ—consult product literature for further information.

● **DIRECTIONS FOR ADMINISTRATION** Inject into the thigh or abdomen (except for the 5 cm around the navel); rotate injection site and avoid moles, scars, or skin that is tender, bruised, red, hardened, or broken.
Patients may self-administer *Enspryng*® after appropriate training in subcutaneous injection technique.

● **PRESCRIBING AND DISPENSING INFORMATION**
Satralizumab is a biological medicine. Biological medicines must be prescribed and dispensed by brand name, see *Biological medicines* and *Biosimilar medicines*, under Guidance on prescribing p. 1; record the brand name and batch number after each administration.

● **HANDLING AND STORAGE** Store in a refrigerator (2–8°C) and protect from light and moisture—consult product literature for further information regarding storage outside refrigerator.

● **PATIENT AND CARER ADVICE** Patients and their carers should be instructed to seek early medical attention if signs and symptoms of infection develop during treatment.
Self-administration Patients and their carers should be given training in subcutaneous injection technique if appropriate.
A patient card should be provided.
Missed doses For information on delayed or missed doses—consult product literature.

● **MEDICINAL FORMS** There can be variation in the licensing of different medicines containing the same drug.
Solution for injection
▶ Enspryng (Roche Products Ltd) ▼
Satralizumab 120 mg per 1 ml Enspryng 120mg/1ml solution for injection pre-filled syringes | 1 pre-filled disposable injection [PoM]
£7,030.00 (Hospital only)

IMMUNOSUPPRESSANTS › MONOCLONAL ANTIBODIES

Canakinumab   17-May-2021

● **DRUG ACTION** Canakinumab is a recombinant human monoclonal antibody that selectively inhibits interleukin-1 beta receptor binding.

● **INDICATIONS AND DOSE**

Gouty arthritis [in patients whose condition has not responded adequately to treatment with NSAIDs or colchicine, or in those with contra-indications or intolerances to them, and in whom repeated courses of corticosteroids are inappropriate]
▸ BY SUBCUTANEOUS INJECTION
▸ Adult: 150 mg for 1 dose, in patients who respond, dose may be repeated after at least 12 weeks if symptoms recur, to be administered to the upper thigh, abdomen, upper arm or buttocks

Cryopyrin-associated periodic syndromes (specialist use only)
▸ BY SUBCUTANEOUS INJECTION
▸ Adult (body-weight 41 kg and above): 150 mg every 8 weeks, to be administered to the upper thigh, abdomen, upper arm or buttocks, additional doses may be considered if clinical response not achieved within 7 days—consult product literature

Tumour necrosis factor receptor associated periodic syndrome (specialist use only) | Hyperimmunoglobulin D syndrome (specialist use only) | Familial Mediterranean fever (specialist use only)
▸ BY SUBCUTANEOUS INJECTION
▸ Adult (body-weight 41 kg and above): 150 mg every 4 weeks, to be administered to the upper thigh, abdomen, upper arm or buttocks, a second dose may be considered if clinical response not achieved within 7 days—consult product literature

Still's disease (specialist use only)
▸ BY SUBCUTANEOUS INJECTION
▸ Adult: 4 mg/kg every 4 weeks (max. per dose 300 mg), to be administered to the upper thigh, abdomen, upper arm or buttocks

● **CONTRA-INDICATIONS** Active severe infection · leucopenia · neutropenia

● **CAUTIONS** History of recurrent infection · latent and active tuberculosis · predisposition to infection

CAUTIONS, FURTHER INFORMATION
▸ Vaccinations [EvGr] Patients should receive all recommended vaccinations (including pneumococcal and inactivated influenza vaccine) before starting treatment; avoid live vaccines unless potential benefit outweighs risk—consult product literature for further information. ◈

● **INTERACTIONS** → Appendix 1: monoclonal antibodies

● **SIDE-EFFECTS**
▸ **Common or very common** Abdominal pain upper · arthralgia · asthenia · dizziness · increased risk of infection · leucopenia · neutropenia · pain · proteinuria · vertigo
▸ **Uncommon** Gastrooesophageal reflux disease

● **CONCEPTION AND CONTRACEPTION** Effective contraception required during treatment and for up to 3 months after last dose.

● **PREGNANCY** Manufacturer advises avoid unless potential benefit outweighs risk.

● **BREAST FEEDING** Consider if benefit outweighs risk—not known if present in human milk.

● **PRE-TREATMENT SCREENING** Patients should be evaluated for latent and active tuberculosis before starting treatment.

● **MONITORING REQUIREMENTS**
▸ Manufacturer advises monitor full blood count including neutrophil count before starting treatment, 1–2 months after starting treatment, and periodically thereafter.
▸ Manufacturer advises monitor for signs and symptoms of infection (including tuberculosis) during and after treatment.

● **HANDLING AND STORAGE** Manufacturer advises store in a refrigerator (2–8 °C).

● **PATIENT AND CARER ADVICE** Manufacturer advises patients and carers should be instructed to seek medical advice if signs or symptoms suggestive of tuberculosis (including persistent cough, weight loss and subfebrile temperature) occur.
Driving and skilled tasks Manufacturer advises patients and carers should be counselled on the effects on driving and performance of skilled tasks—increased risk of dizziness and drowsiness.

● **MEDICINAL FORMS** There can be variation in the licensing of different medicines containing the same drug.
Solution for injection
▸ Ilaris (Novartis Pharmaceuticals UK Ltd)
Canakinumab 150 mg per 1 ml Ilaris 150mg/1ml solution for injection vials | 1 vial [PoM] £9,927.80

IMMUNOSUPPRESSANTS › MONOCLONAL ANTIBODIES › ANTI-LYMPHOCYTE

Basiliximab   23-Mar-2021

● **DRUG ACTION** Basiliximab is a monoclonal antibody that acts as an interleukin-2 receptor antagonist and prevents T-lymphocyte proliferation.

● **INDICATIONS AND DOSE**

Prophylaxis of acute rejection in allogeneic renal transplantation used in combination with ciclosporin and corticosteroid-containing immunosuppression regimens (specialist use only)
▸ BY INTRAVENOUS INJECTION, OR BY INTRAVENOUS INFUSION
▸ Adult: Initially 20 mg, administered within 2 hours before transplant surgery, followed by 20 mg after 4 days, dose to be administered after surgery, withhold second dose if severe hypersensitivity or graft loss occurs

● **CAUTIONS** Off-label use in cardiac transplantation—increased risk of serious cardiac side-effects

● **INTERACTIONS** → Appendix 1: monoclonal antibodies

● **SIDE-EFFECTS** Anaemia · capillary leak syndrome · constipation · cytokine release syndrome · diarrhoea · dyspnoea · electrolyte imbalance · headache · heart failure · hypercholesterolaemia · hypersensitivity · hypertension · hypotension · increased risk of infection · myocardial infarction · nausea · pain · peripheral oedema · post procedural wound complication · pulmonary oedema · respiratory disorders · skin reactions · sneezing · tachycardia · weight increased

● **CONCEPTION AND CONTRACEPTION** Adequate contraception must be used during treatment and for 16 weeks after last dose.

● **PREGNANCY** Manufacturer advises avoid—no information available.

● **BREAST FEEDING** Manufacturer advises avoid—no information available.

● **DIRECTIONS FOR ADMINISTRATION** For *intravenous infusion* (*Simulect®*), manufacturer advises give intermittently in Glucose 5% or Sodium Chloride 0.9%; reconstitute 10 mg with 2.5 mL Water for Injections then dilute to at least 25 mL with infusion fluid; reconstitute 20 mg with 5 mL

Water for Injections then dilute to at least 50 mL with infusion fluid; give over 20-30 minutes.

- **NATIONAL FUNDING/ACCESS DECISIONS**
For full details see funding body website
NICE decisions
▶ Immunosuppressive therapy for kidney transplant in adults (October 2017) NICE TA481 Recommended

- **MEDICINAL FORMS** There can be variation in the licensing of different medicines containing the same drug.
Powder and solvent for solution for injection
- ▶ Simulect (Novartis Pharmaceuticals UK Ltd)
Basiliximab 10 mg Simulect 10mg powder and solvent for solution for injection vials | 1 vial [PoM] £758.69 (Hospital only)

Belimumab

28-Nov-2022

- **INDICATIONS AND DOSE**

Systemic lupus erythematosus (under expert supervision)
- ▶ BY INTRAVENOUS INFUSION
- ▶ Adult: 10 mg/kg every 2 weeks for 3 doses, then 10 mg/kg every 4 weeks, review treatment if no response within 6 months
- ▶ BY SUBCUTANEOUS INJECTION
- ▶ Adult: 200 mg once weekly, review treatment if no response within 6 months

Lupus nephritis (under expert supervision)
- ▶ BY INTRAVENOUS INFUSION
- ▶ Adult: 10 mg/kg every 2 weeks for 3 doses, then 10 mg/kg every 4 weeks
- ▶ BY SUBCUTANEOUS INJECTION
- ▶ Adult: 400 mg once weekly for 4 doses, then 200 mg once weekly

IMPORTANT SAFETY INFORMATION

MHRA/CHM ADVICE: BELIMUMAB (*BENLYSTA*®): INCREASED RISK OF SERIOUS PSYCHIATRIC EVENTS SEEN IN CLINICAL TRIALS (APRIL 2019)

Clinical trials show an increased risk of depression, suicidal ideation or behaviour, or self-injury in patients with systemic lupus erythematosus on belimumab. Healthcare professionals should assess patients for these risks before starting treatment, monitor for new or worsening signs of these risks during treatment, and advise patients to seek immediate medical attention if new or worsening symptoms occur.

- **CAUTIONS** Do not initiate until active infections controlled · history or development of malignancy · predisposition to infection

- **INTERACTIONS** → Appendix 1: monoclonal antibodies

- **SIDE-EFFECTS**
- ▶ **Common or very common** Depression · diarrhoea · fever · hypersensitivity · increased risk of infection · infusion related reaction · leucopenia · migraine · nausea · pain in extremity · skin reactions
- ▶ **Uncommon** Angioedema · suicidal behaviours
- ▶ **Frequency not known** Progressive multifocal leukoencephalopathy (PML) · psychiatric disorder · self-injurious behaviour · severe cutaneous adverse reactions (SCARs)

SIDE-EFFECTS, FURTHER INFORMATION Hypersensitivity reactions and infusion reactions can occur, and can be severe or life-threatening. Hypersensitivity reactions are possible several days after administration. Before infusion, premedication with an antihistamine, with or without an antipyretic may be considered.

- **CONCEPTION AND CONTRACEPTION** Manufacturer advises adequate contraception during treatment and for at least 4 months after last dose.

- **PREGNANCY** Avoid unless essential.

- **BREAST FEEDING** Avoid—present in milk in *animal* studies.

- **RENAL IMPAIRMENT** [EvGr] Caution in severe impairment (limited information available). [M]

- **MONITORING REQUIREMENTS** Delay in the onset of acute hypersensitivity reactions has been observed; patients should remain under clinical supervision for several hours following at least the first 2 infusions.

- **DIRECTIONS FOR ADMINISTRATION** [EvGr] For *intravenous infusion*, give intermittently in Sodium Chloride 0.9%; reconstitute with Water for Injections (120 mg in 1.5 mL, 400 mg in 4.8 mL) to produce a solution containing 80 mg/mL; gently swirl vial for 60 seconds, then allow to stand; swirl vial (without shaking) for 60 seconds every 5 minutes until dissolved; dilute requisite dose with infusion fluid to a final volume of 250 mL and give over 1 hour.

  For *subcutaneous injection*, allow the pre-filled device to reach room temperature prior to administration. Inject into the thigh or abdomen (except for the 5 cm around the navel); rotate injection site and avoid injecting into areas of the skin that are tender, bruised, red, or hard. If 2 injections are administered at the same site, they should be injected at least 5 cm apart. [M]

  Patients may self-administer *Benlysta*® pre-filled device after appropriate training in subcutaneous injection technique.

- **PRESCRIBING AND DISPENSING INFORMATION** Belimumab is a biological medicine. Biological medicines must be prescribed and dispensed by brand name, see *Biological medicines* and *Biosimilar medicines*, under Guidance on prescribing p. 1; record the brand name and batch number after each administration.
Switching between formulations [EvGr] For advice about switching from intravenous to subcutaneous administration—consult product literature. [M]

- **HANDLING AND STORAGE** Store in a refrigerator (2–8°C) and protect from light.
  A single *Benlysta*® pre-filled device may be stored at room temperature (below 25°C) for max. 12 hours, then discarded.

- **PATIENT AND CARER ADVICE** Patients and their carers should be advised to seek immediate medical attention if signs or symptoms of infection or hypersensitivity reaction occur.
Self-administration Patients and their carers should be given training in subcutaneous injection technique if appropriate.

- **NATIONAL FUNDING/ACCESS DECISIONS**
For full details see funding body website
NICE decisions
▶ Belimumab for treating active autoantibody-positive systemic lupus erythematosus (December 2021) NICE TA752 Recommended with restrictions

Scottish Medicines Consortium (SMC) decisions
▶ Belimumab solution for injection (*Benlysta*®) as add-on therapy in adult patients with active, autoantibody-positive systemic lupus erythematosus (SLE) with a high degree of disease activity (e.g. positive anti-dsDNA and low complement) despite standard therapy (November 2022) SMC No. SMC2530 Recommended with restrictions
▶ Belimumab powder for concentrate for solution for infusion (*Benlysta*®) as add-on therapy in patients aged 5 years and older with active, autoantibody-positive systemic lupus erythematosus (SLE) with a high degree of disease activity (e.g., positive anti-dsDNA and low complement) despite standard therapy (November 2022) SMC No. SMC2477 Recommended with restrictions

- **MEDICINAL FORMS** There can be variation in the licensing of different medicines containing the same drug.

Solution for injection
EXCIPIENTS: May contain Polysorbates

▸ Benlysta (GlaxoSmithKline UK Ltd) ▼

Belimumab 200 mg per 1 ml Benlysta 200mg/1ml solution for injection pre-filled pens | 4 pre-filled disposable injection [PoM] £891.00 (Hospital only)

Powder for solution for infusion
EXCIPIENTS: May contain Polysorbates

▸ Benlysta (GlaxoSmithKline UK Ltd) ▼

Belimumab 120 mg Benlysta 120mg powder for concentrate for solution for infusion vials | 1 vial [PoM] £121.50 (Hospital only)
Belimumab 400 mg Benlysta 400mg powder for concentrate for solution for infusion vials | 1 vial [PoM] £405.00 (Hospital only)

IMMUNOSUPPRESSANTS > PURINE SYNTHESIS INHIBITORS

Mycophenolate mofetil
05-Oct-2021

- **INDICATIONS AND DOSE**

Prophylaxis of acute rejection in renal transplantation (in combination with a corticosteroid and ciclosporin) (under expert supervision)

▸ BY MOUTH

▸ Adult: 1 g twice daily, to be started within 72 hours of transplantation

▸ BY INTRAVENOUS INFUSION

▸ Adult: 1 g twice daily for maximum 14 days, then transfer to oral therapy, to be started within 24 hours of transplantation

Prophylaxis of acute rejection in cardiac transplantation (in combination with ciclosporin and corticosteroids) (under expert supervision)

▸ BY MOUTH

▸ Adult: 1.5 g twice daily, to be started within 5 days of transplantation

Prophylaxis of acute rejection in hepatic transplantation (in combination with ciclosporin and corticosteroids) (under expert supervision)

▸ INITIALLY BY INTRAVENOUS INFUSION

▸ Adult: 1 g twice daily for 4 days, up to a maximum of 14 days, to be started within 24 hours of transplantation, then (by mouth) 1.5 g twice daily, the dose route should be changed as soon as is tolerated

CEPTAVA ®

Renal transplantation (specialist use only)

▸ BY MOUTH

▸ Adult: 720 mg twice daily, to be started within 72 hours of transplantation

DOSE EQUIVALENCE AND CONVERSION

▸ For *Ceptava* ®: mycophenolic acid 720 mg is approximately equivalent to mycophenolate mofetil 1 g but avoid unnecessary switching because of pharmacokinetic differences.

MYFORTIC ®

Renal transplantation (specialist use only)

▸ BY MOUTH

▸ Adult: 720 mg twice daily, to be started within 72 hours of transplantation

DOSE EQUIVALENCE AND CONVERSION

▸ For *Myfortic* ®: mycophenolic acid 720 mg is approximately equivalent to mycophenolate mofetil 1 g

but avoid unnecessary switching because of pharmacokinetic differences.

IMPORTANT SAFETY INFORMATION

MHRA/CHM ADVICE: MYCOPHENOLATE MOFETIL, MYCOPHENOLIC ACID: UPDATED CONTRACEPTION ADVICE FOR MALE PATIENTS (FEBRUARY 2018)

Available clinical evidence does not indicate an increased risk of malformations or miscarriage in pregnancies where the father was taking mycophenolate medicines, however mycophenolate mofetil and mycophenolic acid are genotoxic and a risk cannot be fully excluded; for further information, see *Conception and contraception* and *Patient and carer advice.*

- **CAUTIONS** Active serious gastro-intestinal disease (risk of haemorrhage, ulceration and perforation) · delayed graft function · elderly (increased risk of infection, gastro-intestinal haemorrhage and pulmonary oedema) · increased susceptibility to skin cancer (avoid exposure to strong sunlight) · risk of hypogammaglobulinaemia or bronchiectasis when used in combination with other immunosuppressants

CAUTIONS, FURTHER INFORMATION

▸ Hypogammaglobulinaemia or bronchiectasis Measure serum immunoglobulin levels if recurrent infections develop, and consider bronchiectasis or pulmonary fibrosis if persistent respiratory symptoms such as cough and dyspnoea develop.

- **INTERACTIONS** → Appendix 1: mycophenolate
- **SIDE-EFFECTS**

GENERAL SIDE-EFFECTS

▸ **Common or very common** Acidosis · alopecia · anaemia · appetite decreased · arthralgia · asthenia · bone marrow disorders · chills · constipation · cough · depression · diarrhoea · drowsiness · dyslipidaemia · dyspnoea · electrolyte imbalance · fever · gastrointestinal discomfort · gastrointestinal disorders · gastrointestinal haemorrhage · headache · hyperglycaemia · hypertension · hypotension · increased risk of infection · insomnia · leucocytosis · leucopenia · malaise · nausea · neoplasms · oedema · oral disorders · pain · pancreatitis · paraesthesia · renal impairment · respiratory disorders · seizure · sepsis · skin reactions · tachycardia · thinking abnormal · thrombocytopenia · tremor · vomiting · weight decreased

▸ **Uncommon** Agranulocytosis

▸ **Frequency not known** Endocarditis · hypogammaglobulinaemia · interstitial lung disease · malignancy · meningitis · neutropenia · polyomavirus-associated nephropathy · progressive multifocal leukoencephalopathy (PML) · pulmonary fibrosis · pure red cell aplasia

SPECIFIC SIDE-EFFECTS

▸ **Common or very common**

▸ With intravenous use Hepatitis · muscle tone increased

▸ With oral use Anxiety · burping · confusion · dizziness · gout · hepatic disorders · hyperbilirubinaemia · hyperuricaemia · neuromuscular dysfunction · taste altered · vasodilation

SIDE-EFFECTS, FURTHER INFORMATION Cases of pure red cell aplasia have been reported with mycophenolate mofetil; dose reduction or discontinuation should be considered under specialist supervision.

- **CONCEPTION AND CONTRACEPTION**

Pregnancy prevention The MHRA advises to exclude pregnancy in females of child-bearing potential before treatment—2 pregnancy tests 8–10 days apart are recommended. Women should use at least 1 method of effective contraception before and during treatment, and for 6 weeks after discontinuation—2 methods of effective contraception are preferred. Male patients or their female partner should use effective contraception during treatment and for 90 days after discontinuation.

- **PREGNANCY** Avoid unless no suitable alternative—congenital malformations and spontaneous abortions reported.
- **BREAST FEEDING** Manufacturer advises avoid—present in milk in *animal* studies.
- **RENAL IMPAIRMENT** No data available in cardiac or hepatic transplant patients with renal impairment.
- **MONITORING REQUIREMENTS** Monitor full blood count every week for 4 weeks then twice a month for 2 months then every month in the first year (consider interrupting treatment if neutropenia develops).
- **DIRECTIONS FOR ADMINISTRATION** For *intravenous infusion* (*CellCept*®), manufacturer advises give intermittently in Glucose 5%; reconstitute each 500–mg vial with 14 mL Glucose 5% and dilute the contents of 2 vials in 140 mL infusion fluid; give over 2 hours.
- **PATIENT AND CARER ADVICE**
Pregnancy prevention advice The MHRA advises that prescribers should ensure that female patients understand the need to comply with the pregnancy prevention advice, and they should be informed to seek immediate medical attention if there is a possibility of pregnancy; male patients planning to conceive children should be informed of the implications of both immunosuppression and the effect of the prescribed medications on the pregnancy. Bone marrow suppression Patients should be warned to report immediately any signs or symptoms of bone marrow suppression e.g. infection or inexplicable bruising or bleeding.
- **NATIONAL FUNDING/ACCESS DECISIONS**
For full details see funding body website
NICE decisions
- Immunosuppressive therapy for kidney transplant in adults [mycophenolate mofetil, when used as part of an immunosuppressive regimen, as an initial option] (October 2017) NICE TA481 Recommended
- Immunosuppressive therapy for kidney transplant in adults [mycophenolate sodium (*Ceptava*®, *Myfortic*®) as an initial treatment] (October 2017) NICE TA481 Not recommended

---

- **MEDICINAL FORMS** There can be variation in the licensing of different medicines containing the same drug. Forms available from special-order manufacturers include: oral suspension

Oral tablet
- Mycophenolate mofetil (Non-proprietary)
Mycophenolate mofetil 500 mg Mycophenolate mofetil 500mg tablets | 50 tablet PoM £74.03 DT = £5.81
- CellCept (Roche Products Ltd)
Mycophenolate mofetil 500 mg CellCept 500mg tablets | 50 tablet PoM £82.26 DT = £5.81
- Myfenax (Teva UK Ltd)
Mycophenolate mofetil 500 mg Myfenax 500mg tablets | 50 tablet PoM £78.15 DT = £5.81

Gastro-resistant tablet
CAUTIONARY AND ADVISORY LABELS 25
- Mycophenolate mofetil (Non-proprietary)
Mycophenolic acid (as Mycophenolate sodium) 180 mg Mycophenolic acid 180mg gastro-resistant tablets | 120 tablet PoM £96.72 DT = £96.72
Mycophenolic acid (as Mycophenolate sodium) 360 mg Mycophenolic acid 360mg gastro-resistant tablets | 120 tablet PoM £193.43 DT = £193.43
- Ceptava (Sandoz Ltd)
Mycophenolic acid (as Mycophenolate sodium) 180 mg Ceptava 180mg gastro-resistant tablets | 120 tablet PoM £77.38 DT = £96.72
Mycophenolic acid (as Mycophenolate sodium) 360 mg Ceptava 360mg gastro-resistant tablets | 120 tablet PoM £154.75 DT = £193.43
- Myfortic (Novartis Pharmaceuticals UK Ltd)
Mycophenolic acid (as Mycophenolate sodium) 180 mg Myfortic 180mg gastro-resistant tablets | 120 tablet PoM £96.72 DT = £96.72

Mycophenolic acid (as Mycophenolate sodium) 360 mg Myfortic 360mg gastro-resistant tablets | 120 tablet PoM £193.43 DT = £193.43

Oral suspension
EXCIPIENTS: May contain Aspartame
- Mycophenolate mofetil (Non-proprietary)
Mycophenolate mofetil 200 mg per 1 ml Mycophenolate mofetil 1g/5ml oral suspension sugar free | 175 ml PoM £115.16–£180.00 SF
- CellCept (Roche Products Ltd)
Mycophenolate mofetil 200 mg per 1 ml CellCept 1g/5ml oral suspension | 160 ml PoM £115.16 DT = £115.16 SF

Oral capsule
- Mycophenolate mofetil (Non-proprietary)
Mycophenolate mofetil 250 mg Mycophenolate mofetil 250mg capsules | 100 capsule PoM £82.26 DT = £82.26
- CellCept (Roche Products Ltd)
Mycophenolate mofetil 250 mg CellCept 250mg capsules | 100 capsule PoM £82.26 DT = £82.26
- Myfenax (Teva UK Ltd)
Mycophenolate mofetil 250 mg Myfenax 250mg capsules | 100 capsule PoM £78.15 DT = £82.26

Powder for solution for infusion
- CellCept (Roche Products Ltd)
Mycophenolate mofetil (as Mycophenolate mofetil hydrochloride) 500 mg CellCept 500mg powder for solution for infusion vials | 4 vial PoM £36.49 (Hospital only)

IMMUNOSUPPRESSANTS › T-CELL ACTIVATION INHIBITORS

Belatacept

01-Sep-2020

- **INDICATIONS AND DOSE**

Prophylaxis of graft rejection in adults undergoing renal transplantation who are seropositive for the Epstein-Barr virus
- BY INTRAVENOUS INFUSION
- Adult: (consult product literature)

- **CAUTIONS** Increased risk of acute graft rejection—with tapering of corticosteroid, particularly in patients with high immunologic risk · increased risk of infection · latent and active tuberculosis · risk factors for post-transplant lymphoproliferative disorder
- **INTERACTIONS** → Appendix 1: belatacept
- **SIDE-EFFECTS**
- **Common or very common** Acidosis · alopecia · anaemia · angina pectoris · arrhythmias · arterial fibrosis · cataract · chest pain · constipation · cough · Cushing's syndrome · decreased leucocytes · diabetes mellitus · diarrhoea · dizziness · dyslipidaemia · dyspnoea · ear pain · electrolyte imbalance · embolism and thrombosis · eye erythema · fatigue · fever · fluid imbalance · gastrointestinal discomfort · gastrointestinal disorders · haemorrhage · headaches · healing impaired · heart failure · hepatic disorders · hypercapnia · hyperglycaemia · hypertension · hypoproteinaemia · hypotension · increased risk of infection · intervertebral disc disorder · joint disorders · lethargy · leucocytosis · lymphocele · malaise · muscle complaints · muscle weakness · nausea · neoplasms · nerve disorders · neutropenia · oral disorders · oropharyngeal complaints · osteoarthritis · pain · paraesthesia · peripheral oedema · polyomavirus infections · pulmonary oedema · red blood cell abnormalities · renal disorders · renal tubular necrosis · respiratory disorders · scrotal disorders · sepsis · shock · skin reactions · stroke · sweat changes · syncope · thrombocytopenia · tinnitus · transplant rejection · tremor · urinary disorders · urine abnormalities · vascular disorders · ventricular hypertrophy · vertigo · vesicoureteric reflux · vision disorders · vomiting · weight changes
- **Uncommon** Acute coronary syndrome · adrenal insufficiency · agranulocytosis · alkalosis · anxiety · aortic valve disease · appetite decreased · arterial stenosis ·

atrioventricular block · attention deficit/hyperactivity disorder · bone disorders · bone fracture · breast mass · broken nails · cervical dysplasia · cholelithiasis · cognitive disorder · demyelination · depression · diabetic foot · diabetic ketoacidosis · disease recurrence · dysphonia · encephalopathy · endocarditis · eye inflammation · facial paralysis · facial swelling · feeling hot · fibrosis · flushing · haemolysis · hair changes · hearing impairment · hemiparesis · hypercoagulation · hypogammaglobulinaemia · infertility · inflammation · infusion related reaction · intermittent claudication · intracranial pressure increased · lymphangitis · memory loss · mood altered · nephritis · nephrosclerosis · pancreatitis · penile ulceration · pneumonitis · post procedural haematoma · procedural complications · progressive multifocal leukoencephalopathy (PML) · pulmonary hypertension · renal tubular atrophy · restless legs · seasonal allergy · seizure · sexual dysfunction · sleep apnoea · sleep disorders · taste altered · tendon rupture · testicular pain · ulcer · vitamin D deficiency · vulvovaginal disorders · wound dehiscence

SIDE-EFFECTS, FURTHER INFORMATION Side effects are reported when used in combination with basiliximab, mycophenolate mofetil and corticosteroids.

● **CONCEPTION AND CONTRACEPTION** Adequate contraception must be used during treatment and for up to 8 weeks after last dose.

● **PREGNANCY** Use only if essential.

● **BREAST FEEDING** Avoid—no information available.

● **PRE-TREATMENT SCREENING** Patients should be evaluated for latent and active tuberculosis before starting treatment.

● **MONITORING REQUIREMENTS** Patients should be monitored for signs and symptoms of tuberculosis during and after treatment.

● **PATIENT AND CARER ADVICE** Patients should be advised to avoid excessive exposure to UV light including sunlight.

● **NATIONAL FUNDING/ACCESS DECISIONS**
For full details see funding body website
NICE decisions
▸ Immunosuppressive therapy for kidney transplant in adults (October 2017) NICE TA481 Not recommended

● **MEDICINAL FORMS** There can be variation in the licensing of different medicines containing the same drug.
Powder for solution for infusion
▸ Nulojix (Bristol-Myers Squibb Pharmaceuticals Ltd)
Belatacept 250 mg Nulojix 250mg powder for concentrate for solution for infusion vials | 1 vial [PoM] £354.52 (Hospital only) | 2 vial [PoM] £709.04 (Hospital only)

RHO KINASE INHIBITORS

Belumosudil   05-Mar-2024

● **INDICATIONS AND DOSE**
Chronic graft-versus-host disease (under expert supervision)
▸ BY MOUTH
▸ Adult: 200 mg once daily
DOSE ADJUSTMENTS DUE TO INTERACTIONS
▸ [EvGr] Increase dose to 200 mg twice daily with concurrent use of potent CYP3A4 inducers or proton pump inhibitors. ◈

● **INTERACTIONS** → Appendix 1: belumosudil

● **SIDE-EFFECTS**
▸ **Common or very common** Anaemia · appetite decreased · arthralgia · asthenia · constipation · cough · diarrhoea · dizziness · dyspnoea · fever · gastrointestinal discomfort · headache · hyperglycaemia · hypertension · increased risk

of infection · leucopenia · malaise · muscle spasms · nausea · neutropenia · oedema · pain · peripheral neuropathy · pruritus · swelling · vomiting · weight decreased
▸ **Frequency not known** Microangiopathic haemolytic anaemia · multi organ failure

● **CONCEPTION AND CONTRACEPTION** [EvGr] Females of childbearing potential and male patients, if their female partner is of childbearing potential, should use highly effective contraception during treatment and for at least 1 week after the last treatment. ◈

● **PREGNANCY** [EvGr] Avoid—toxicity in *animal* studies. ◈

● **BREAST FEEDING** [EvGr] Avoid during treatment and for at least 1 week after the last treatment—no information available. ◈

● **HEPATIC IMPAIRMENT** [EvGr] Caution in severe impairment (no information available); increased exposure in mild or moderate impairment—no dose adjustment required. ◈

● **MONITORING REQUIREMENTS**
▸ [EvGr] A complete blood count should be performed before starting treatment.
▸ Monitor liver function tests before starting treatment and at least monthly during treatment. Treatment should be withheld or permanently discontinued in patients who develop hepatotoxicity—consult product literature. ◈

● **PATIENT AND CARER ADVICE**
Vomiting If vomiting occurs after taking tablets, no additional dose should be taken on that day and the next dose should be taken at the usual time.
Missed doses If a dose is more than 12 hours late, the missed dose should not be taken and the next dose should be taken at the normal time.
Driving and skilled tasks Patients and carers should be cautioned on the effects on driving and performance of skilled tasks—increased risk of fatigue and dizziness.

● **NATIONAL FUNDING/ACCESS DECISIONS**
For full details see funding body website
NICE decisions
▸ **Belumosudil for treating chronic graft-versus-host disease after 2 or more systemic treatments in people 12 years and over (February 2024) NICE TA949 Recommended**

● **MEDICINAL FORMS** There can be variation in the licensing of different medicines containing the same drug.
Oral tablet
CAUTIONARY AND ADVISORY LABELS 21
▸ Rezurock (Sanofi) ▼
Belumosudil (as Belumosudil mesilate) 200 mg Rezurock 200mg tablets | 30 tablet [PoM] £6,708.00

1.1   Multiple sclerosis

Multiple sclerosis   18-Nov-2022

Description of condition

Multiple sclerosis is a chronic, immune-mediated, demyelinating inflammatory condition of the central nervous system, which affects the brain, optic nerves and spinal cord, and leads to progressive severe disability.

Relapsing-remitting multiple sclerosis is the most common pattern of the disease. It is characterised by periods of exacerbation of symptoms (relapses) followed by unpredictable periods of stability (remission). The severity and frequency of relapses varies greatly between patients. Disease activity is defined as *Active* if at least two clinically significant relapses occur within the last 2 years. *Highly active* disease is characterised by an unchanged/increased relapse rate or by ongoing severe relapses compared with the previous year, despite disease-modifying drug treatment. *Rapidly-evolving severe* relapsing-remitting multiple sclerosis is defined by two or more disabling relapses in 1 year, and one or more gadolinium-enhancing lesions on brain magnetic resonance imaging (MRI) or a significant increase in T2 lesion load compared with a previous MRI. The clinical pattern of relapsing-remitting multiple sclerosis often develops into *secondary-progressive* multiple sclerosis, with progressive disability unrelated to relapses.

Primary-progressive multiple sclerosis follows a gradual course, with the development of symptoms that worsen over time, without relapses and remissions.

Progressive-relapsing multiple sclerosis follows a course of steadily worsening neurological function from onset, in addition to acute relapses.

Aims of treatment

There is no cure for multiple sclerosis. The overall aims of treatment are to modify the course of the disease and manage symptoms, in order to improve quality of life. Treatment is aimed at reducing the frequency and duration of relapses and at preventing or slowing disability.

Drug treatment

Shared decision-making between the patient and their clinicians is particularly important in the treatment of multiple sclerosis, due to the unpredictability of the condition and the lack of evidence of long-term benefit of treatments. A discussion about treatment options, risks and benefits of treatment, the patient's disability status, and disease severity and activity should take place to ensure that treatment choices are right for the patient and their circumstances. [EvGr] Treatment should be initiated as early as possible, under the supervision of a specialist. Ⓐ

Low levels of vitamin D are believed to be a risk factor for developing multiple sclerosis. Patients with multiple sclerosis are usually given regular vitamin D after assessment of their serum levels of vitamin D, but there is insufficient evidence to support its use as a treatment for multiple sclerosis. [EvGr] Patients should not be offered vitamin D solely for the purpose of treating multiple sclerosis. Ⓐ

Relapsing-remitting multiple sclerosis

[EvGr] Under specialist care, disease-modifying drugs such as anti-lymphocyte monoclonal antibodies, antimetabolites, immunomodulators, immunostimulants, and interferons may be used for the treatment of relapsing-remitting multiple sclerosis. Ⓐ

Secondary progressive multiple sclerosis

Under specialist care, disease-modifying drugs such as immunomodulators and interferons may be used for the treatment of secondary progressive multiple sclerosis.

Primary progressive multiple sclerosis

Under specialist care, disease-modifying drugs such as anti-lymphocyte monoclonal antibodies may be used for the treatment of primary progressive multiple sclerosis.

Progressive-relapsing multiple sclerosis

There are no specific treatment options for this type of multiple sclerosis. None of the currently licensed disease-modifying drugs are recommended in non-relapsing progressive disease.

Management of symptoms

Other than episodes of neurological dysfunction, chronic symptoms and complications (such as fatigue, spasticity, visual, cognitive and memory problems, bladder disorders, pain, emotional lability, depression, and anxiety) produce much of the disability in multiple sclerosis. [EvGr] Smoking increases the progression of disability in multiple sclerosis, therefore Smoking cessation p. 565 should be encouraged. Ⓐ

Relapses

Patients with suspected relapses should be referred to a specialist for diagnosis and treatment. [EvGr] Corticosteroids are recommended for reducing inflammation and accelerating recovery in acute relapses of relapsing-remitting multiple sclerosis. Oral methylprednisolone p. 790 is recommended as the first-line option. Intravenous methylprednisolone should be considered as an alternative if oral methylprednisolone has failed or is not tolerated, or if hospitalisation is required. Ⓐ

Fatigue and impaired mobility

[EvGr] Personalised support should be offered to help patients with multiple sclerosis and fatigue. Regular exercise may have beneficial effects on mobility and fatigue, and should be encouraged. Cognitive behavioural techniques and mindfulness for fatigue, stress management, and well-being should also be considered in combination with exercise. For patients who wish to try drug treatment for fatigue (on specialist initiation), amantadine hydrochloride p. 480 [unlicensed use], a selective serotonin re-uptake inhibitor [unlicensed use], or modafinil p. 559 [unlicensed use] may be used to treat fatigue related to multiple sclerosis. Vitamin B_{12} injections are **not** recommended as a treatment for fatigue in patients with multiple sclerosis. Ⓐ Fampridine p. 981 is licensed for the improvement of walking in patients with multiple sclerosis who have a walking disability, but NICE do not consider it to be a cost-effective treatment and do not recommend its use.

Spasticity

Many factors may aggravate spasticity in multiple sclerosis, including infection, bladder and bowel dysfunction, poor posture or positioning, pressure ulcers, and pain. [EvGr] These causes should be managed appropriately. The first-line option for managing spasticity in multiple sclerosis is baclofen p. 1289. If baclofen is ineffective or not tolerated, gabapentin p. 362 [unlicensed use] may be considered as a second-line option.). Both drugs may be used cautiously in combination if the individual drugs are ineffective or if side-effects prevent an increase in the dose of either drug. A 4-week trial of cannabis extract p. 1288 can be offered as adjunctive treatment for moderate to severe spasticity in multiple sclerosis if other pharmacological treatments are not effective. Treatment with cannabis extract should be initiated and supervised by a specialist. For further information, see NICE clinical guideline: **Cannabis-based medicinal products** (see *Useful resources*). Ⓐ

Oscillopsia

[EvGr] Gabapentin [unlicensed use] is recommended as first-line treatment for oscillopsia; memantine hydrochloride p. 349 [unlicensed use] may be considered as a second-line option. Ⓐ

Emotional lability

[EvGr] Amitriptyline hydrochloride p. 431 [unlicensed use] may be used to treat emotional lability in patients with multiple sclerosis. Ⓐ

Useful Resources

Clinical Commissioning Policy: disease modifying therapies for patients with multiple sclerosis. NHS England. May 2014. www.england.nhs.uk/specialised-commissioning-document-library/routinely-commissioned-policies/

Multiple sclerosis in adults: management. National Institute for Health and Care Excellence. NICE guideline 220. June 2022. www.nice.org.uk/guidance/ng220

Cannabis-based medicinal products. National Institute for Health and Care Excellence. Clinical guideline 144. November 2019 (updated March 2021). www.nice.org.uk/guidance/ng144

Other drugs used for Multiple sclerosis Cladribine, p. 1043

CHOLINERGIC RECEPTOR STIMULATING DRUGS

Fampridine

19-Aug-2021

- ● **INDICATIONS AND DOSE**

Improvement of walking disability in multiple sclerosis (specialist use only)
- ▶ BY MOUTH
- ▶ Adult: 10 mg every 12 hours, discontinue treatment if no improvement within 2 weeks

- ● **CONTRA-INDICATIONS** History of seizures (discontinue treatment if seizures occur)
- ● **CAUTIONS** Atrioventricular conduction disorders · predisposition to seizures · sinoatrial conduction disorders · symptomatic cardiac rhythm disorders
- ● **INTERACTIONS** → Appendix 1: fampridine
- ● **SIDE-EFFECTS**
- ▶ **Common or very common** Anxiety · asthenia · balance impaired · constipation · dizziness · dyspepsia · dyspnoea · headache · insomnia · laryngeal pain · nausea · pain · palpitations · paraesthesia · tremor · urinary tract infection · vomiting
- ▶ **Uncommon** Seizure · skin reactions · tachycardia
- ● **PREGNANCY** Avoid—toxicity in *animal* studies.
- ● **BREAST FEEDING** Avoid—no information available.
- ● **RENAL IMPAIRMENT** EvGr Caution in mild impairment; avoid if creatinine clearance less than 50 mL/minute, Ⓜ see p. 21.
- ● **PRESCRIBING AND DISPENSING INFORMATION** Dispense in original container (pack contains a desiccant) and discard any tablets remaining 7 days after opening.
- ● **NATIONAL FUNDING/ACCESS DECISIONS**
For full details see funding body website

Scottish Medicines Consortium (SMC) decisions
- ▶ Fampridine (*Fampyra*®) for the improvement of walking in adult patients with multiple sclerosis (MS) with walking disability (EDSS [expanded disability status scale] 4 to 7) (April 2020) SMC No. SMC2253 Recommended

All Wales Medicines Strategy Group (AWMSG) decisions
- ▶ Fampridine (*Fampyra*®) for improvement of walking in adult patients with multiple sclerosis with walking disability (Expanded Disability Status Scale 4 to 7) (December 2019) AWMSG No. 3942 Recommended

- ● **MEDICINAL FORMS** There can be variation in the licensing of different medicines containing the same drug. Forms available from special-order manufacturers include: oral capsule

Modified-release tablet
CAUTIONARY AND ADVISORY LABELS 23, 25
- ▶ Fampyra (Merz Pharma UK Ltd)
Fampridine 10 mg Fampyra 10mg modified-release tablets | 56 tablet PoM £362.00 (Hospital only)

IMMUNOSTIMULANTS › INTERFERONS

Interferon beta

21-Mar-2025

- ● **INDICATIONS AND DOSE**

AVONEX® INJECTION

For relapsing, remitting multiple sclerosis | For a single demyelinating event with an active inflammatory process (if severe enough to require intravenous corticosteroid and patient at high risk of developing multiple sclerosis)
- ▶ BY INTRAMUSCULAR INJECTION
- ▶ Adult: (consult product literature)

BETAFERON® INJECTION

For relapsing, remitting multiple sclerosis | For secondary progressive multiple sclerosis with active disease | For a single demyelinating event with an active inflammatory process (if severe enough to require intravenous corticosteroid and patient at high risk of developing multiple sclerosis)
- ▶ BY SUBCUTANEOUS INJECTION
- ▶ Adult: (consult product literature)

EXTAVIA®

For relapsing, remitting multiple sclerosis | For secondary progressive multiple sclerosis with active disease | For a single demyelinating event with an active inflammatory process (if severe enough to require intravenous corticosteroid and patient at high risk of developing multiple sclerosis)
- ▶ BY SUBCUTANEOUS INJECTION
- ▶ Adult: (consult product literature)

REBIF® CARTRIDGE

For relapsing, remitting multiple sclerosis | For a single demyelinating event with an active inflammatory process (if at high risk of developing multiple sclerosis)
- ▶ BY SUBCUTANEOUS INJECTION
- ▶ Adult: (consult product literature)

REBIF® PRE-FILLED PEN AND SYRINGE

For relapsing, remitting multiple sclerosis | For a single demyelinating event with an active inflammatory process (if at high risk of developing multiple sclerosis)
- ▶ BY SUBCUTANEOUS INJECTION
- ▶ Adult: (consult product literature)

- ● **CONTRA-INDICATIONS** Severe depressive illness
CONTRA-INDICATIONS, FURTHER INFORMATION Consult product literature for further information on contra-indications.
- ● **CAUTIONS** History of cardiac disorders · history of depressive disorders (avoid in severe depression or in those with suicidal ideation) · history of seizures · history of severe myelosupression
CAUTIONS, FURTHER INFORMATION Consult product literature for further information on cautions.
- ● **INTERACTIONS** → Appendix 1: interferons
- ● **SIDE-EFFECTS**
GENERAL SIDE-EFFECTS
- ▶ **Common or very common** Alopecia · appetite decreased · arthralgia · asthenia · chills · confusion · depression · diarrhoea · fever · headaches · hypothyroidism · influenza like illness (decreasing over time) · insomnia · malaise · menstrual cycle irregularities · nausea · pain · skin reactions · vasodilation · vomiting · weight changes
- ▶ **Uncommon** Emotional lability · glomerulosclerosis · hepatic disorders · nephrotic syndrome · seizure · thrombocytopenia
- ▶ **Rare or very rare** Cardiomyopathy · dyspnoea · haemolytic uraemic syndrome · hyperthyroidism · thrombotic microangiopathy
- ▶ **Frequency not known** Anxiety · chest pain · dizziness · injection site necrosis · muscle weakness · palpitations · pulmonary arterial hypertension
SPECIFIC SIDE-EFFECTS
- ▶ **Common or very common**
- ▶ With intramuscular use Muscle complaints · musculoskeletal stiffness · neuromuscular dysfunction · rhinorrhoea · sensation abnormal · sweat changes
- ▶ With subcutaneous use Anaemia · tachycardia
- ▶ **Uncommon**
- ▶ With subcutaneous use Suicide attempt

8

Immune system and malignant disease

▶ **Rare or very rare**

▶ With subcutaneous use Bronchospasm · pancreatitis · thyroid disorder

▶ **Frequency not known**

▶ With intramuscular use Angioedema · arrhythmias · arthritis · congestive heart failure · hypersensitivity · neurological effects · pancytopenia · psychosis · suicide · syncope · systemic lupus erythematosus (SLE)

▶ With subcutaneous use Abdominal pain · abscess · capillary leak syndrome · conjunctivitis · constipation · cough aggravated · ear pain · erectile dysfunction · eye disorder · hyperhidrosis · hypertension · increased risk of infection · lupus-like syndrome · lymphadenopathy · muscle tone increased · myalgia · paraesthesia · peripheral oedema · urinary disorders · visual impairment

● **PREGNANCY** Manufacturer advises use if clinically needed—possible toxicity in *animal* studies, but limited human data do not suggest an increased risk.

● **BREAST FEEDING** Manufacturer advises suitable for use during breast feeding—amount in milk probably too small to be harmful (recommendation also supported by specialist sources).

● **HEPATIC IMPAIRMENT** Manufacturer advises caution; avoid in decompensated liver disease.

● **RENAL IMPAIRMENT** Manufacturer advises caution in severe impairment.

● **MONITORING REQUIREMENTS**

▶ Liver Function Manufacturer advises monitor liver function at baseline, then 1 month, 3 months and 6 months after initiation of therapy. Consider dose reduction if alanine aminotransferase (ALT) exceeds 5 times the upper limit of normal (consult product literature).

▶ Thrombotic Microangiopathy Manufacturer advises patients should be monitored for clinical features of thrombotic microangiopathy (TMA), including thrombocytopenia, new onset hypertension, fever, central nervous system symptoms (e.g. confusion and paresis), and impaired renal function. Any signs of TMA should be investigated fully and, if diagnosed, interferon beta should be stopped immediately and treatment for TMA promptly initiated (consult product literature for details).

▶ Nephrotic Syndrome Manufacturer advises patients should also be monitored for signs and symptoms of nephrotic syndrome, including oedema, proteinuria, and impaired renal function—monitor renal function periodically. If nephrotic syndrome develops, treat promptly and consider stopping interferon beta treatment.

▶ Thyroid Function Manufacturer advises baseline thyroid function tests and repeat if signs or symptoms of thyroid dysfunction occur.

● **PRESCRIBING AND DISPENSING INFORMATION** Interferon beta is a biological medicine. Biological medicines must be prescribed and dispensed by brand name, see *Biological medicines* and *Biosimilar medicines*, under Guidance on prescribing p. 1; manufacturer advises to record the brand name and batch number after each administration.

● **NATIONAL FUNDING/ACCESS DECISIONS**
For full details see funding body website
NICE decisions

▶ Beta interferons [*Avonex*®, *Extavia*®, *Rebif*®] and glatiramer acetate for treating multiple sclerosis (June 2018) NICE TA527 Recommended with restrictions

▶ Beta interferons [*Betaferon*®] and glatiramer acetate for treating multiple sclerosis (June 2018) NICE TA527 Not recommended
NHS restrictions
NHS England Clinical Commissioning Policy NHS England (May 2014) has provided guidance on the use of interferon beta p. 981 for the treatment of multiple sclerosis in England. An NHS England Clinical Commissioning Policy outlines the funding arrangements and the criteria for initiating and discontinuing this treatment option, see www.england.nhs.uk/commissioning/spec-services/npc-crg/group-d/neurology/.

● **MEDICINAL FORMS** There can be variation in the licensing of different medicines containing the same drug.
Solution for injection
EXCIPIENTS: May contain Benzyl alcohol

▶ **Avonex** (Biogen Idec Ltd)
Interferon beta-1a 12 mega unit per 1 ml Avonex 30micrograms/0.5ml (6million units) solution for injection pre-filled syringes | 4 pre-filled disposable injection PoM £654.00 | 12 pre-filled disposable injection PoM £1,962.00
Avonex 30micrograms/0.5ml (6million units) solution for injection pre-filled pens | 4 pre-filled disposable injection PoM £654.00 | 12 pre-filled disposable injection PoM £1,962.00

▶ **Rebif** (Merck Serono Ltd)
Interferon beta-1a 12 mega unit per 1 ml Rebif 22micrograms/0.5ml (6million units) solution for injection pre-filled syringes | 12 pre-filled disposable injection PoM £613.52
Rebif 22micrograms/0.5ml (6million units) solution for injection 1.5ml cartridges | 4 cartridge PoM £613.52
Rebif 8.8micrograms/0.2ml (2.4million units) solution for injection pre-filled syringes | 6 pre-filled disposable injection PoM ⓈⒽ
Rebif 22micrograms/0.5ml (6million units) solution for injection pre-filled pens | 12 pre-filled disposable injection PoM £613.52
Interferon beta-1a 24 mega unit per 1 ml Rebif 44micrograms/0.5ml (12million units) solution for injection pre-filled syringes | 12 pre-filled disposable injection PoM £813.21
Rebif 44micrograms/0.5ml (12million units) solution for injection pre-filled pens | 12 pre-filled disposable injection PoM £813.21
Rebif 44micrograms/0.5ml (12million units) solution for injection 1.5ml cartridges | 4 cartridge PoM £813.21
Interferon beta-1a 48 mega unit per 1 ml Rebif 8.8micrograms/0.1ml (2.4million units) with 22micrograms/0.25ml (6million units) solution for injection 1.5ml cartridges initiation pack | 2 cartridge PoM £406.61
Powder and solvent for solution for injection

▶ **Betaferon** (Bayer Plc)
Interferon beta-1b 300 microgram Betaferon 300microgram powder and solvent for solution for injection vials | 15 vial PoM £596.63 DT = £596.63 (Hospital only)

Peginterferon beta-1a
25-May-2021

● **DRUG ACTION** Peginterferon beta-1a is a polyethylene glycol-conjugated ('pegylated') derivative of interferon beta; pegylation increases the persistence of interferon in the blood.

● **INDICATIONS AND DOSE**
Treatment of relapsing, remitting multiple sclerosis

▶ BY SUBCUTANEOUS INJECTION

▶ Adult: (consult product literature)

● **CONTRA-INDICATIONS** Severe depression · suicidal ideation

● **CAUTIONS** History of cardiac disorders · history of depressive disorders (avoid in severe depression or in those with suicidal ideation) · history of seizures · history of severe myelosupression

CAUTIONS, FURTHER INFORMATION Consult product literature for further information about cautions.

● **SIDE-EFFECTS**

▶ **Common or very common** Arthralgia · asthenia · chills · depression · fever · headache · hyperthermia · influenza like illness · myalgia · nausea · pain · skin reactions · vomiting

▶ **Uncommon** Seizure · thrombocytopenia

▶ **Rare or very rare** Glomerulosclerosis · haemolytic uraemic syndrome · injection site necrosis · nephrotic syndrome · thrombotic microangiopathy

▶ **Frequency not known** Pulmonary arterial hypertension

● **CONCEPTION AND CONTRACEPTION** Effective contraception required during treatment—consult product literature.

- **PREGNANCY** Do not initiate during pregnancy. Avoid unless potential benefit outweighs risk.
- **BREAST FEEDING** Avoid—no information available.
- **HEPATIC IMPAIRMENT** Manufacturer advises caution in severe hepatic impairment.
- **RENAL IMPAIRMENT** [EvGr] Use with caution in severe renal impairment. ⟨M⟩
- **MONITORING REQUIREMENTS**
- ▸ Monitor for signs of hepatic injury—hepatic failure has been reported rarely.
- ▸ Thrombotic microangiopathy Patients should be monitored for clinical features of thrombotic microangiopathy (TMA), including thrombocytopenia, new onset hypertension, fever, central nervous system symptoms (e.g. confusion and paresis), and impaired renal function. Any signs of TMA should be investigated fully and, if diagnosed, interferon beta should be stopped immediately and treatment for TMA promptly initiated (consult product literature for details).
- ▸ Nephrotic syndrome Patients should also be monitored for signs and symptoms of nephrotic syndrome, including oedema, proteinuria, and impaired renal function— monitor renal function periodically. If nephrotic syndrome develops, treat promptly and consider stopping interferon beta treatment.
- **NATIONAL FUNDING/ACCESS DECISIONS** For full details see funding body website

NICE decisions
- ▸ **Peginterferon beta-1a for treating relapsing-remitting multiple sclerosis (February 2020)** NICE TA624 Recommended

- **MEDICINAL FORMS** There can be variation in the licensing of different medicines containing the same drug.

Solution for injection
- ▸ Plegridy (Biogen Idec Ltd)
  Interferon beta-1a (as Peginterferon beta-1a) 126 microgram per 1 ml Plegridy 63micrograms/0.5ml solution for injection pre-filled pens | 1 pre-filled disposable injection [PoM] [◪]
  Interferon beta-1a (as Peginterferon beta-1a) 188 microgram per 1 ml Plegridy 94micrograms/0.5ml solution for injection pre-filled pens | 1 pre-filled disposable injection [PoM] [◪]
  Interferon beta-1a (as Peginterferon beta-1a) 250 microgram per 1 ml Plegridy 125micrograms/0.5ml solution for injection pre-filled syringes | 2 pre-filled disposable injection [PoM] £654.00 (Hospital only)
  Plegridy 125micrograms/0.5ml solution for injection pre-filled pens | 2 pre-filled disposable injection [PoM] £654.00 (Hospital only)

IMMUNOSTIMULANTS ⟩ OTHER

▌Glatiramer acetate
29-Nov-2024

- **DRUG ACTION** Glatiramer is an immunomodulating drug comprising synthetic polypeptides.

● INDICATIONS AND DOSE

Multiple sclerosis [relapsing-remitting] (initiated under specialist supervision)
- ▸ BY SUBCUTANEOUS INJECTION
- ▸ Adult: 20 mg once daily, alternatively 40 mg 3 times a week, doses to be separated by an interval of at least 48 hours

IMPORTANT SAFETY INFORMATION

MHRA/CHM ADVICE: GLATIRAMER ACETATE: ANAPHYLACTIC REACTIONS MAY OCCUR MONTHS TO YEARS AFTER TREATMENT INITIATION (OCTOBER 2024)
An EU- and UK-wide review has concluded that glatiramer acetate is associated with anaphylactic reactions that may occur shortly following administration. These reactions can occur months or years after treatment initiation, and cases with a fatal outcome have been reported. Glatiramer acetate can also cause post-injection reactions, the signs and symptoms of which may delay identification of anaphylactic reactions. Healthcare professionals are advised to inform patients and their carers of the signs and symptoms of anaphylactic reactions, and to seek immediate emergency medical attention if these develop. If an anaphylactic reaction occurs, treatment must be discontinued.

- **CAUTIONS** Cardiac disorders
- **SIDE-EFFECTS**
- ▸ **Common or very common** Anxiety · appetite decreased · arrhythmias · asthenia · chest pain · chills · constipation · cough · depression · dyspepsia · dysphagia · dyspnoea (may occur within minutes of injection) · ear disorder · eye disorders · fever · gastrointestinal disorders · headaches · hyperhidrosis · hypersensitivity · increased risk of infection · joint disorders · local reaction · lymphadenopathy · nausea · neoplasms · neuromuscular dysfunction · oedema · oral disorders · pain · palpitations · rhinitis seasonal · skin reactions · speech disorder · syncope · taste altered · tremor · urinary disorders · vasodilation · vision disorders · vomiting · weight increased
- ▸ **Uncommon** Abnormal dreams · abscess · alcohol intolerance · anaphylactic reaction (may occur months to years after initiation) · angioedema · apnoea · arthritis · breast engorgement · burping · cataract · choking sensation · cholelithiasis · cognitive disorder · confusion · cyst · dry eye · dysgraphia · dyslexia · erythema nodosum · goitre · gout · haemorrhage · hallucination · hangover · hepatic disorders · hostility · hyperlipidaemia · hyperthyroidism · hypothermia · immediate post-injection reaction · inflammation · injection site necrosis · leucocytosis · leucopenia · mood altered · movement disorders · mucous membrane disorder · muscle atrophy · nephrolithiasis · nerve disorders · paralysis · pelvic prolapse · personality disorder · post vaccination syndrome · prostatic disorder · respiratory disorders · seizure · sexual dysfunction · skin nodule · splenomegaly · stupor · suicide attempt · testicular disorder · thrombocytopenia · urinary tract disorder · urine abnormal · varicose veins · vulvovaginal disorder
- **PREGNANCY** Manufacturer advises avoid—no information available.
- **BREAST FEEDING** Manufacturer advises caution—no information available.
- **RENAL IMPAIRMENT** [EvGr] Use with caution (no information available). ⟨M⟩
- **NATIONAL FUNDING/ACCESS DECISIONS** For full details see funding body website

NICE decisions
- ▸ **Beta interferons and glatiramer acetate for treating multiple sclerosis (June 2018)** NICE TA527 Recommended with restrictions

Scottish Medicines Consortium (SMC) decisions
- ▸ **Glatiramer acetate 40 mg/mL (*Copaxone*®) for the treatment of relapsing forms of multiple sclerosis (MS) (December 2015)** SMC No. 1108/15 Recommended

NHS restrictions
NHS England Clinical Commissioning Policy NHS England (May 2014) has provided guidance on the use of glatiramer acetate for the treatment of multiple sclerosis in England. An NHS England Clinical Commissioning Policy outlines the funding arrangements and the criteria for initiating and discontinuing this treatment option, see www.england. nhs.uk/commissioning/spec-services/npc-crg/group-d/ neurology/.

8

Immune system and malignant disease

Immune system and malignant disease

8

- **MEDICINAL FORMS** There can be variation in the licensing of different medicines containing the same drug.

Solution for injection

▸ Brabio (Viatris UK Healthcare Ltd)

Glatiramer acetate 20 mg per 1 ml Brabio 20mg/1ml solution for injection pre-filled syringes | 28 pre-filled disposable injection [PoM] £462.56 DT = £513.95

Glatiramer acetate 40 mg per 1 ml Brabio 40mg/1ml solution for injection pre-filled syringes | 12 pre-filled disposable injection [PoM] £462.56 DT = £513.95

▸ Copaxone (Teva UK Ltd)

Glatiramer acetate 20 mg per 1 ml Copaxone 20mg/1ml solution for injection pre-filled syringes | 28 pre-filled disposable injection [PoM] £513.95 DT = £513.95

Glatiramer acetate 40 mg per 1 ml Copaxone 40mg/1ml solution for injection pre-filled syringes | 12 pre-filled disposable injection [PoM] £513.95 DT = £513.95

IMMUNOSUPPRESSANTS ›
IMMUNOMODULATING DRUGS

| Dimethyl fumarate

29-Mar-2022

- **DRUG ACTION** Dimethyl fumarate is converted into active monomethyl fumarate which is thought to work by activating the nuclear factor (erythroid-derived 2)-like 2 (Nrf2) pathway, resulting in immunomodulatory and anti-inflammatory effects.

- **INDICATIONS AND DOSE**

SKILARENCE®

Plaque psoriasis [moderate-to-severe] (under expert supervision)

▸ BY MOUTH

▸ Adult: Initially 30 mg once daily for 1 week, dose to be taken in the evening, then increased in steps of 30 mg every week for 3 weeks, then increased in steps of 120 mg every week for 5 weeks, for further information on the dose titration and administration schedule, advice on establishing a maintenance dose, and for dose adjustments due to side-effects, consult product literature; maximum 720 mg per day

TECFIDERA®

Multiple sclerosis [relapsing-remitting] (initiated by a specialist)

▸ BY MOUTH

▸ Adult: Initially 120 mg twice daily for 7 days, then increased to 240 mg twice daily, for dose adjustments due to side effects—consult product literature

IMPORTANT SAFETY INFORMATION

MHRA/CHM ADVICE: DIMETHYL FUMARATE (*TECFIDERA*®): UPDATED ADVICE ON THE RISK OF PROGRESSIVE MULTIFOCAL LEUKOENCEPHALOPATHY (PML) ASSOCIATED WITH MILD LYMPHOPENIA (JANUARY 2021)

A European review of safety data identified 11 cases of PML with lymphopenia associated with *Tecfidera*® treatment, including 3 cases in patients with mild lymphopenia (lymphocyte count between 0.8×10^9/litre and the lower limit of normal); previously, PML had only been confirmed in the setting of moderate to severe lymphopenia.

Healthcare professionals are advised that *Tecfidera*® is contra-indicated in patients with suspected or confirmed PML and should not be initiated in those with severe lymphopenia (lymphocyte count below 0.5×10^9/litre); patients with low lymphocyte counts should be investigated for underlying causes before initiating treatment. During treatment, all patients should have a lymphocyte count at least every 3 months. Treatment should be re-evaluated in those with sustained moderate reductions of absolute lymphocyte counts (between 0.5 and 0.8×10^9/litre) for longer than 6 months. *Tecfidera*® should be stopped in those with severe lymphopenia persisting for more than 6 months, and permanently discontinued if a patient develops PML.

Patients should be advised to be vigilant for any new or worsening neurological or psychiatric symptoms, and to seek urgent medical attention if these occur. They should also inform their family or carer about the risks and when to seek medical attention, as they may notice symptoms of which the patient is unaware. Symptoms of PML can resemble those of a multiple sclerosis relapse.

- **CONTRA-INDICATIONS**

SKILARENCE® Do not initiate if leucocyte count below 3×10^9/litre · do not initiate if lymphocyte count below 1×10^9/litre · do not initiate if pathological haematological abnormalities identified · severe gastro-intestinal disorders

TECFIDERA® See *Important safety information.*

- **CAUTIONS** Reduced lymphocyte count

SKILARENCE® Significant infection (consider avoiding initiation until infection resolved and suspending treatment if infection develops)

TECFIDERA® Serious infection (do not initiate until infection resolved; consider suspending treatment if infection develops) · severe active gastro-intestinal disease

- **INTERACTIONS** → Appendix 1: dimethyl fumarate

- **SIDE-EFFECTS**

▸ **Common or very common** Appetite decreased · asthenia · constipation · decreased leucocytes · diarrhoea · eosinophilia · feeling hot · gastrointestinal discomfort · gastrointestinal disorders · headache · increased risk of infection · leucocytosis · nausea · paraesthesia · skin reactions · urine abnormalities · vasodilation · vomiting

▸ **Uncommon** Dizziness · thrombocytopenia

▸ **Rare or very rare** Acute lymphocytic leukaemia · pancytopenia

▸ **Frequency not known** Angioedema · drug-induced liver injury · dyspnoea · hypotension · hypoxia · JC virus infection · progressive multifocal leukoencephalopathy (PML) · renal failure · rhinorrhoea

SIDE-EFFECTS, FURTHER INFORMATION Severe prolonged lymphopenia reported, and patients are exposed to a potential risk of PML. Treatment should be stopped immediately if PML is suspected.

- **PREGNANCY**

SKILARENCE® Manufacturer advises avoid—toxicity in *animal* studies.

TECFIDERA® Manufacturer advises avoid unless essential and potential benefit outweighs risk—toxicity in *animal* studies.

- **BREAST FEEDING** Specialist sources indicate present in milk but amount probably too small to be harmful. Monitor breastfed infants for flushing, vomiting, diarrhoea, adequate weight gain, and developmental milestones, especially younger, exclusively breastfed infants.

- **HEPATIC IMPAIRMENT**

SKILARENCE® Manufacturer advises avoid in severe impairment (no information available).

TECFIDERA® Manufacturer advises caution in severe impairment (no information available).

- **RENAL IMPAIRMENT**

SKILARENCE® Manufacturer advises avoid in severe impairment—no information available.

TECFIDERA® Manufacturer advises caution in severe impairment—no information available.

- **MONITORING REQUIREMENTS**
▶ Manufacturer advises monitor full blood count before treatment initiation then every 3 months thereafter—consult product information for further information.
▶ Manufacturer advises monitor patient closely for features of progressive multifocal leukoencephalopathy (PML) (e.g. signs and symptoms of neurological dysfunction) and other opportunistic infections.
▶ Manufacturer advises monitor renal and hepatic function before treatment initiation and during treatment—consult product literature for further information.
▶ Manufacturer of *Tecfidera*® advises perform a baseline MRI as a reference and repeat as required during treatment.

- **PRESCRIBING AND DISPENSING INFORMATION**
SKILARENCE® The manufacturer of *Skilarence*® has provided a *Healthcare Professional Guideline*, which includes important safety information on the risk of serious infections.

- **PATIENT AND CARER ADVICE** Manufacturer advises patients and their carers should be informed of the possibility of experiencing symptoms of flushing; they should also be advised to report symptoms of infection to their doctor. The MHRA recommends that patients and their carers should be counselled on the risk of progressive multifocal leukoencephalopathy and advised to seek immediate medical attention if symptoms develop.

- **NATIONAL FUNDING/ACCESS DECISIONS**
SKILARENCE® For full details see funding body website
NICE decisions
▶ **Dimethyl fumarate for treating moderate-to-severe plaque psoriasis (September 2017)** NICE TA475 Recommended with restrictions

Scottish Medicines Consortium (SMC) decisions
▶ **Dimethyl fumarate (*Skilarence*®) for the treatment of moderate to severe plaque psoriasis in adults in need of systemic medicinal therapy (April 2018)** SMC No. 1313/18 Recommended with restrictions

TECFIDERA® For full details see funding body website
NICE decisions
▶ **Dimethyl fumarate (*Tecfidera*®) for treating relapsing-remitting multiple sclerosis (August 2014)** NICE TA320 Recommended with restrictions

Scottish Medicines Consortium (SMC) decisions
▶ **Dimethyl fumarate (*Tecfidera*®) for the treatment of adult patients with relapsing remitting multiple sclerosis (April 2014)** SMC No. 886/13 Recommended

- **MEDICINAL FORMS** There can be variation in the licensing of different medicines containing the same drug.

Gastro-resistant capsule
CAUTIONARY AND ADVISORY LABELS 21, 25
　▶ Tecfidera (Biogen Idec Ltd)
　Dimethyl fumarate 120 mg Tecfidera 120mg gastro-resistant capsules | 14 capsule [PoM] £343.00 (Hospital only)
　Dimethyl fumarate 240 mg Tecfidera 240mg gastro-resistant capsules | 56 capsule [PoM] £1,373.00 (Hospital only)

Gastro-resistant tablet
CAUTIONARY AND ADVISORY LABELS 21, 25
　▶ Skilarence (Almirall Ltd)
　Dimethyl fumarate 30 mg Skilarence 30mg gastro-resistant tablets | 42 tablet [PoM] £89.04 DT = £89.04
　Dimethyl fumarate 120 mg Skilarence 120mg gastro-resistant tablets | 90 tablet [PoM] £190.80 DT = £190.80 | 180 tablet [PoM] £381.60 DT = £381.60

Diroximel fumarate
07-Jul-2022

- **DRUG ACTION** Diroximel fumarate is converted into active monomethyl fumarate which is thought to work by activating the nuclear factor (erythroid-derived 2)-like 2 (Nrf2) pathway, resulting in immunomodulatory and anti-inflammatory effects.

- **INDICATIONS AND DOSE**
Multiple sclerosis (initiated under specialist supervision)
▶ BY MOUTH
▶ Adult: Initially 231 mg twice daily for 7 days, then maintenance 462 mg twice daily, for dose adjustments due to side effects—consult product literature

- **CONTRA-INDICATIONS** Progressive multifocal leukoencephalopathy (suspected or confirmed) · severe lymphopenia (lymphocyte count below 0.5×10^9/litre)—consult product literature

- **CAUTIONS** Reduced lymphocyte count—consult product literature · risk factors for progressive multifocal leukoencephalopathy · serious infection (do not initiate until infection resolved; consider suspending treatment if infection develops) · severe active gastrointestinal disease (no information available)
CAUTIONS, FURTHER INFORMATION
▶ Progressive Multifocal Leukoencephalopathy [EvGr] There is an increased risk of opportunistic infection and progressive multifocal leukoencephalopathy (PML) caused by JC virus associated with dimethyl fumarate and other fumarates. Prolonged moderate to severe lymphopenia increases the risk of PML, although risk cannot be excluded in patients with mild lymphopenia. Other factors that may increase the risk include treatment duration, profound decreases in CD4+ and CD8+ T cell count, and previous immunosuppressant or immunomodulatory treatment. ◈

- **INTERACTIONS** → Appendix 1: diroximel fumarate
- **SIDE-EFFECTS**
▶ **Common or very common** Alopecia · decreased leucocytes · diarrhoea · feeling hot · gastrointestinal discomfort · gastrointestinal disorders · increased risk of infection · nausea · paraesthesia · skin reactions · urine abnormalities · vasodilation · vomiting
▶ **Uncommon** Thrombocytopenia
▶ **Frequency not known** Angioedema · drug-induced liver injury · dyspnoea · hypotension · hypoxia · progressive multifocal leukoencephalopathy (PML) · rhinorrhoea

- **PREGNANCY** [EvGr] Avoid unless potential benefit outweighs risk—toxicity in animal studies. ◈

- **BREAST FEEDING** Specialist sources indicate present in milk but amount probably too small to be harmful. Monitor breastfed infants for flushing, vomiting, diarrhoea, adequate weight gain, and developmental milestones, especially younger, exclusively breastfed infants.

- **HEPATIC IMPAIRMENT** [EvGr] Caution in severe impairment (no information available). ◈

- **RENAL IMPAIRMENT** [EvGr] Caution in moderate or severe impairment (no information available). ◈

- **MONITORING REQUIREMENTS**
▶ [EvGr] Monitor full blood count, including lymphocytes, before treatment initiation then every 3 months thereafter—consult product literature.
▶ Monitor patient closely for features of progressive multifocal leukoencephalopathy (e.g. signs and symptoms of neurological dysfunction) and other opportunistic infections.
▶ Monitor renal and hepatic function before treatment initiation and during treatment—consult product literature.
▶ Perform baseline MRI and repeat as required during treatment. ◈

Immune system and malignant disease

8

Immune system and malignant disease

8

● PATIENT AND CARER ADVICE Patients and their carers should be informed of the possibility of experiencing symptoms of flushing; they should also be advised to report symptoms of infection to their doctor. Patients and their carers should be counselled on the risk of progressive multifocal leukoencephalopathy and advised to seek immediate medical attention if symptoms develop. **Missed doses** If a dose is more than 8 hours late, the missed dose should not be taken and the next dose should be taken at the normal time.

● NATIONAL FUNDING/ACCESS DECISIONS
For full details see funding body website
NICE decisions
▸ Diroximel fumarate for treating relapsing-remitting multiple sclerosis (June 2022) NICE TA794 Recommended with restrictions

Scottish Medicines Consortium (SMC) decisions
▸ Diroximel fumarate (*Vumerity*®) for the treatment of adult patients with relapsing-remitting multiple sclerosis (RRMS) (February 2022) SMC No. SMC2444 Recommended

● MEDICINAL FORMS There can be variation in the licensing of different medicines containing the same drug.
Gastro-resistant capsule
CAUTIONARY AND ADVISORY LABELS 25
▸ **Vumerity** (Biogen Idec Ltd)
   Diroximel fumarate 231 mg Vumerity 231mg gastro-resistant capsules | 120 capsule [PoM] £1,471.07 (Hospital only)

Fingolimod

18-Jan-2023

● DRUG ACTION Fingolimod is a sphingosine-1-phosphate receptor modulator, which prevents movement of lymphocytes out of lymph nodes, thereby limiting inflammation in the central nervous system.

● **INDICATIONS AND DOSE**
Multiple sclerosis (initiated by a specialist)
▸ BY MOUTH
▸ Adult: 500 micrograms once daily

IMPORTANT SAFETY INFORMATION
MHRA/CHM ADVICE: FINGOLIMOD—NOT RECOMMENDED FOR PATIENTS AT KNOWN RISK OF CARDIOVASCULAR EVENTS. ADVICE FOR EXTENDED MONITORING FOR THOSE WITH SIGNIFICANT BRADYCARDIA OR HEART BLOCK AFTER THE FIRST DOSE AND FOLLOWING TREATMENT INTERRUPTION (JANUARY 2013)
Fingolimod is known to cause transient bradycardias and heart block after the first dose—see *Cautions*, *Contra-indications*, and *Monitoring* for further information.

MHRA/CHM ADVICE: FINGOLIMOD: NEW CONTRA-INDICATIONS IN RELATION TO CARDIAC RISK (DECEMBER 2017)
Fingolimod can cause persistent bradycardia, which can increase the risk of serious cardiac arrhythmias. New contra-indications have been introduced for patients with pre-existing cardiac disorders—see *Contra-indications* for further information.

MHRA/CHM ADVICE: MULTIPLE SCLEROSIS THERAPIES: SIGNAL OF REBOUND EFFECT AFTER STOPPING OR SWITCHING THERAPY (APRIL 2017)
A signal of rebound syndrome in multiple sclerosis patients whose treatment with fingolimod was stopped or switched to other treatments has been reported in two recently published articles. The MHRA advise to be vigilant for such events and report any suspected adverse effects relating to fingolimod, or other treatments for multiple sclerosis, via the Yellow Card Scheme, while this report is under investigation.

MHRA/CHM ADVICE: FINGOLIMOD: UPDATED ADVICE ABOUT RISK OF CANCERS AND SERIOUS INFECTIONS (DECEMBER 2017)
Fingolimod has an immunosuppressive effect and can increase the risk of skin cancers and lymphoma.

Following a recent EU review, the MHRA has recommended the following strengthened warnings:
● re-assess the benefit-risk balance of fingolimod therapy in individual patients, particularly those with additional risk factors for malignancy—either closely monitor for skin cancers or consider discontinuation on a case-by-case basis
● examine all patients for skin lesions before they start fingolimod and then re-examine at least every 6 to 12 months
● advise patients to protect themselves against UV radiation exposure and seek urgent medical advice if they notice any skin lesions
● refer patients with suspicious lesions to a dermatologist
Fingolimod has also been associated with risk of fatal fungal infections and reports of progressive multifocal leukoencephalopathy (PML)—see *Monitoring* and *Side effects* for further information.

MHRA/CHM ADVICE: FINGOLIMOD (*GILENYA*®): INCREASED RISK OF CONGENITAL MALFORMATIONS; NEW CONTRA-INDICATION DURING PREGNANCY AND IN WOMEN OF CHILDBEARING POTENTIAL NOT USING EFFECTIVE CONTRACEPTION (SEPTEMBER 2019)
An increased risk of major congenital malformations, including cardiac, renal, and musculoskeletal defects, has been associated with the use of fingolimod in pregnancy. Females of childbearing potential must use effective contraception during, and for 2 months after stopping, treatment. Healthcare professionals are advised that fingolimod is contra-indicated in pregnancy and that female patients should be informed of the risk of congenital malformations and given a pregnancy-specific patient reminder card. Pregnancy should be excluded before starting treatment, and pregnancy testing repeated at suitable intervals during treatment. Fingolimod should be stopped 2 months before planning a pregnancy. If a female taking fingolimod becomes pregnant, treatment should be stopped immediately, and the patient referred to an obstetrician for close monitoring. Exposed pregnancies should be enrolled on the pregnancy registry.

MHRA/CHM ADVICE: FINGOLIMOD (*GILENYA*®): UPDATED ADVICE ABOUT THE RISKS OF SERIOUS LIVER INJURY AND HERPES MENINGOENCEPHALITIS (JANUARY 2021)
A European review of safety data identified 7 cases of clinically significant liver injury that developed between 10 days and 5 years of starting fingolimod, including 3 reports of acute hepatic failure requiring liver transplantation. The guidance for monitoring liver function and criteria for discontinuation have been strengthened to minimise the risks of liver injury.
   Liver function tests including serum bilirubin should be performed before starting and during treatment at months 1, 3, 6, 9, and 12, then periodically thereafter until 2 months after discontinuation.
   In the absence of clinical symptoms, if liver transaminases (AST or ALT) exceed:
● 3 times the upper limit of normal (ULN) but less than 5 times the ULN without increase in serum bilirubin, liver function tests should be monitored more frequently;
● 5 times the ULN or at least 3 times the ULN with any increase in serum bilirubin, fingolimod should be discontinued; treatment may be restarted when serum levels have returned to normal, after careful benefit-risk assessment of the underlying cause.
In the presence of clinical symptoms suggestive of hepatic dysfunction, liver function tests should be checked promptly and fingolimod discontinued if significant liver injury is confirmed; further treatment may be restarted after recovery, only if an alternative cause of hepatic dysfunction is established.

The review also considered reported cases of herpes zoster/herpes simplex infections with visceral or CNS dissemination (e.g. herpes meningoencephalitis), some of which were fatal. Healthcare professionals are reminded to continue to be vigilant for infections with fingolimod.

Patients should be advised to seek urgent medical attention if they develop any signs or symptoms of liver injury or brain infection (during fingolimod treatment and for 8 weeks after the last dose in the case of the latter).

● **CONTRA-INDICATIONS** Active malignancies · baseline QTc interval 500 milliseconds or greater · cerebrovascular disease (including transient ischaemic attack) in the previous 6 months · decompensated heart failure (requiring inpatient treatment) in the previous 6 months · heart failure in the previous 6 months (New York Heart Association class III/IV) · increased risk for opportunistic infections (including immunosuppression) · myocardial infarction in the previous 6 months · second-degree Mobitz type II atrioventricular block or third-degree AV block, or sick-sinus syndrome, if the patient does not have a pacemaker · severe active infection · severe cardiac arrhythmias requiring treatment with class Ia or class III anti-arrhythmic drugs · unstable angina in the previous 6 months

● **CAUTIONS** Check varicella zoster virus status—consult product literature for further information · chronic obstructive pulmonary disease · elderly (limited information available) · history of myocardial infarction · history of symptomatic bradycardia or recurrent syncope · patients receiving anti-arrhythmic or heart-rate lowering drugs, including beta-blockers and heart rate-lowering calcium-channel blockers (seek advice from cardiologist regarding switching to alternative drugs, or appropriate monitoring if unable to switch) · pulmonary fibrosis · severe respiratory disease · severe sleep apnoea · significant QT prolongation (QTc greater than 470 milliseconds in women, or QTc greater than 450 milliseconds in men); if QTc 500 milliseconds or greater—see *Contra-indications* · susceptibility to QT-interval prolongation (including electrolyte disturbances) · uncontrolled hypertension

CAUTIONS, FURTHER INFORMATION

▸ **Washout period** A washout period is recommended when switching treatment from some disease modifying therapies—consult product literature for further information.

▸ **Bradycardia and cardiac rhythm disturbance** Fingolimod may cause transient bradycardia, atrioventricular conduction delays and heart block after the first dose. Fingolimod is not recommended in patients with the cardiovascular risks listed above unless the anticipated benefits outweigh the potential risks, and advice from a cardiologist (including monitoring advice) is sought before initiation.

● **INTERACTIONS** → Appendix 1: fingolimod

● **SIDE-EFFECTS**

▸ **Common or very common** Alopecia · arthralgia · asthenia · atrioventricular block · back pain · bradycardia · cough · decreased leucocytes · depression · diarrhoea · dizziness · dyspnoea · headaches · hypertension · increased risk of infection · myalgia · neoplasms · skin reactions · vision blurred · weight decreased

▸ **Uncommon** Macular oedema · nausea · seizures · thrombocytopenia

▸ **Rare or very rare** Posterior reversible encephalopathy syndrome (PRES)

▸ **Frequency not known** Autoimmune haemolytic anaemia · haemophagocytic lymphohistiocytosis · hepatic disorders ·

peripheral oedema · progressive multifocal leukoencephalopathy (PML)

SIDE-EFFECTS, FURTHER INFORMATION **Basal-cell carcinoma** Patients should be advised to seek medical advice if they have any signs of basal-cell carcinoma including skin nodules, patches or open sores that do not heal within weeks.

Progressive multifocal leukoencephalopathy (PML) and other opportunistic infections Patients should be advised to seek medical attention if they have any signs of PML or any other infections. Suspension of treatment should be considered if a patient develops a severe infection, taking into consideration the risk-benefit.

● **CONCEPTION AND CONTRACEPTION** Manufacturer advises females of childbearing potential should use effective contraception during treatment and for 2 months after last treatment—see *Important safety information* for further information.

● **PREGNANCY** Manufacturer advises avoid—teratogenic.

● **BREAST FEEDING** Avoid.

● **HEPATIC IMPAIRMENT** Manufacturer advises caution when initiating treatment in mild to moderate impairment; avoid in severe impairment.

● **MONITORING REQUIREMENTS**

▸ **All** patients receiving fingolimod should be monitored at treatment initiation, (first dose monitoring—before, during and after dose), and after treatment interruption (see note below); monitoring should include:

▸ **Pre-treatment**
 ● an ECG and blood pressure measurement before starting

▸ **During the first 6 hours of treatment**
 ● continuous ECG monitoring for 6 hours
 ● blood pressure and heart rate measurement every hour

▸ **After 6 hours of treatment**
 ● a further ECG and blood pressure measurement

▸ If heart rate at the end of the 6 hour period is at its lowest since fingolimod was first administered, monitoring should be extended by at least 2 hours and until heart rate increases.

▸ If post-dose bradyarrhythmia-related symptoms occur, appropriate clinical management should be initiated and monitoring should be continued until the symptoms have resolved. If pharmacological intervention is required during the first-dose monitoring, overnight monitoring should follow, and the first-dose monitoring should then be repeated after the second dose.

▸ If after 6 hours, the heart rate is less than 45 beats per minute, or the ECG shows new onset second degree or higher grade AV block, or a QTc interval of 500 milliseconds or greater, monitoring should be extended (at least overnight, until side-effect resolution).

▸ The occurrence at any time of third degree AV block requires extended monitoring (at least overnight, until side-effect resolution).

▸ In case of T-wave inversion, ensure there are no associated signs or symptoms of myocardial ischaemia—if suspected seek advice from a cardiologist.

▸ **Note**

▸ First dose monitoring as above **should be repeated** in all patients whose treatment is interrupted for:
 ● 1 day or more during the first 2 weeks of treatment
 ● more than 7 days during weeks 3 and 4 of treatment
 ● more than 2 weeks after one month of treatment

▸ If the treatment interruption is of shorter duration than the above, treatment should be continued with the next dose as planned.

▸ Manufacturer advises eye examination recommended 3–4 months after initiation of treatment (and before initiation of treatment in patients with diabetes or history of uveitis).

▶ Manufacturer advises skin examination for skin lesions before starting treatment and then every 6 to 12 months thereafter or as clinically indicated.

▶ The MHRA advises to monitor liver function—see *Important Safety Information*.

▶ Monitor full blood count before treatment, at 3 months, then at least yearly thereafter and if signs of infection (interrupt treatment if lymphocyte count reduced)— consult product literature.

▶ Monitor for signs and symptoms of haemophagocytic syndrome (including pyrexia, asthenia, hepato-splenomegaly and adenopathy—may be associated with hepatic failure and respiratory distress; also progressive cytopenia, elevated serum-ferritin concentrations, hypertriglyceridaemia, hypofibrinogenaemia, coagulopathy, hepatic cytolysis, hyponatraemia)—initiate treatment immediately.

▶ Manufacturer advises to monitor routine MRI for lesions suggestive of progressive multifocal leukoencephalopathy (PML), particularly in patients considered at increased risk; monitor for signs and symptoms of new neurological dysfunction.

● **PRESCRIBING AND DISPENSING INFORMATION** The manufacturer of *Gilenya*® has provided a *Prescriber's checklist*.

● **PATIENT AND CARER ADVICE**
Patient reminder card Patients should be given a patient reminder card.
Female patients of childbearing potential should also be given a pregnancy-specific patient reminder card.

● **NATIONAL FUNDING/ACCESS DECISIONS**
For full details see funding body website
NICE decisions
▶ Fingolimod for the treatment of highly active relapsing-remitting multiple sclerosis (April 2012) NICE TA254 Recommended with restrictions

Scottish Medicines Consortium (SMC) decisions
▶ Fingolimod (*Gilenya*®) as a single disease modifying therapy in highly active relapsing remitting multiple sclerosis [in patients with high disease activity despite treatment with a beta-interferon with an unchanged or increased relapse rate or ongoing severe relapses as compared to the previous year] (September 2012) SMC No. 763/12 Recommended with restrictions
▶ Fingolimod (*Gilenya*®) as a single disease modifying therapy in highly active relapsing remitting multiple sclerosis [for patients with rapidly evolving severe relapsing remitting multiple sclerosis] (October 2014) SMC No. 992/14 Recommended with restrictions
▶ Fingolimod (*Gilenya*®) as a single disease modifying therapy in highly active relapsing remitting multiple sclerosis for patients with high disease activity despite treatment with at least one disease modifying therapy (April 2015) SMC No. 1038/15 Recommended

All Wales Medicines Strategy Group (AWMSG) decisions
▶ Fingolimod (*Gilenya*®) as a single disease modifying therapy in highly active relapsing remitting multiple sclerosis in adults with rapidly evolving severe relapsing remitting multiple sclerosis (January 2017) AWMSG No. 3135 Recommended
NHS restrictions
NHS England Clinical Commissioning Policy NHS England (May 2014) has provided guidance on the use of fingolimod for the treatment of multiple sclerosis in England. An NHS England Clinical Commissioning Policy outlines the funding arrangements and the criteria for initiating and discontinuing this treatment option, see www.england.nhs. uk/commissioning/spec-services/npc-crg/group-d/neurology/.

● **MEDICINAL FORMS** There can be variation in the licensing of different medicines containing the same drug.
Oral capsule
▶ **Fingolimod (non-proprietary)** ▼
Fingolimod (as Fingolimod hydrochloride)
500 microgram Fingolimod 500microgram capsules |
7 capsule PoM £312.00–£367.50 | 7 capsule PoM £312.38–£330.75 (Hospital only) | 28 capsule PoM £1,470.00 DT = £1,470.00 (Hospital only) | 28 capsule PoM £1,250.00–£1,470.00 DT = £1,470.00
▶ **Gilenya** (Novartis Pharmaceuticals UK Ltd)
Fingolimod (as Fingolimod hydrochloride)
250 microgram Gilenya 0.25mg capsules | 28 capsule PoM £1,470.00
Fingolimod (as Fingolimod hydrochloride)
500 microgram Gilenya 0.5mg capsules | 7 capsule PoM £367.50 | 28 capsule PoM £1,470.00 DT = £1,470.00

Ozanimod

10-Feb-2023

● **DRUG ACTION** Ozanimod is a sphingosine-1-phosphate receptor modulator, which prevents movement of lymphocytes out of lymph nodes, thereby limiting inflammation in the central nervous system and intestine.

● **INDICATIONS AND DOSE**

Multiple sclerosis (initiated by a specialist) | Ulcerative colitis (initiated by a specialist)
▶ BY MOUTH
▶ Adult: Initially 0.23 mg once daily on days 1–4, then increased to 0.46 mg once daily on days 5–7, then increased to 0.92 mg once daily from day 8 onwards, the same dose escalation regimen is recommended when treatment is interrupted for 1 day or more during the first 14 days of treatment, for more than 7 consecutive days between days 15–28, or for more than 14 consecutive days after day 28. For interruptions of shorter duration, treatment may be continued with the next planned dose

● **CONTRA-INDICATIONS** Active malignancy · decompensated heart failure (requiring inpatient treatment) in the previous 6 months · heart failure (New York Heart Association class III or IV) in the previous 6 months · immunodeficiency · myocardial infarction in the previous 6 months · phototherapy with UV-B radiation or PUVA-photochemotherapy (increased risk of cutaneous neoplasm) · posterior reversible encephalopathy syndrome (suspected or confirmed) · progressive multifocal leukoencephalopathy · second-degree Mobitz type II atrioventricular (AV) block, third-degree AV block, or sick sinus syndrome, if the patient does not have a pacemaker · severe active infection · stroke (including transient ischaemic attack) in the previous 6 months · unstable angina in the previous 6 months

● **CAUTIONS** Administration of vaccinations · cerebrovascular disease · chronic obstructive pulmonary disease · diabetes mellitus (increased risk of macular oedema) · elderly (limited information available) · heart failure · immunosuppression or other risk factors for infection · myocardial infarction · patients receiving QT-prolonging or heart rate-lowering drugs, including beta-blockers and heart rate-lowering calcium-channel blockers · pulmonary fibrosis · recurrent syncope · retinal disease (increased risk of macular oedema) · risk of discontinuation effects, including disease rebound · second-degree Mobitz type I atrioventricular block · severe respiratory disease · severe untreated sleep apnoea · significant QT prolongation (QTc greater than 500 milliseconds) · sinus bradycardia (heart rate below 55 beats per minute) · uncontrolled hypertension · uveitis (increased risk of macular oedema)

CAUTIONS, FURTHER INFORMATION

▸ Bradycardia and cardiac rhythm disturbance [EvGr] Ozanimod may cause transient bradycardia, atrioventricular conduction delays and heart block after the first dose. It is not recommended in patients with a history of cardiac arrest, cerebrovascular disease, symptomatic bradycardia or recurrent syncope, uncontrolled hypertension, severe untreated sleep apnoea, or significant QT prolongation or other risk factors for QT prolongation unless the anticipated benefits outweigh the potential risks, and advice from a cardiologist (including monitoring advice) is sought before initiation. ◈M◈

▸ Vaccinations [EvGr] Vaccination may be less effective during and for up to 3 months after treatment. Live attenuated vaccines should be avoided during and for 3 months after treatment; if they are required they should be given at least 1 month prior to initiation. Immunisation against varicella zoster is recommended prior to treatment in those without documented immunity. ◈M◈

● INTERACTIONS → Appendix 1: ozanimod

● SIDE-EFFECTS

▸ **Common or very common** Bradycardia · headache · hypertension · increased risk of infection · lymphopenia · peripheral oedema · postural hypotension

▸ **Rare or very rare** Progressive multifocal leukoencephalopathy (PML)

▸ **Frequency not known** Non-melanoma skin cancer

● CONCEPTION AND CONTRACEPTION [EvGr] Exclude pregnancy before treatment; females of childbearing potential should use effective contraception during treatment and for 3 months after last dose. ◈M◈

● PREGNANCY [EvGr] Avoid—toxicity in *animal* studies. ◈M◈

● BREAST FEEDING [EvGr] Avoid—present in milk in *animal* studies. ◈M◈

● HEPATIC IMPAIRMENT [EvGr] Avoid in severe impairment (no information available). ◈M◈

● MONITORING REQUIREMENTS

▸ [EvGr] Patients with certain pre-existing cardiac conditions should be monitored for bradycardia for 6 hours after the first dose. An ECG should be obtained before dosing and after 6 hours ◈M◈—consult product literature for further information.

▸ [EvGr] Monitor blood pressure regularly during treatment.

▸ Monitor hepatic transaminases and bilirubin before initiation of treatment and then at months 1, 3, 6, 9 and 12 and periodically thereafter (interrupt treatment if significant liver injury occurs: liver transaminases above 5 times the upper limit of normal).

▸ Monitor full blood count before initiation and periodically during treatment (interrupt treatment if lymphocyte count reduced) ◈M◈—consult product literature.

▸ [EvGr] Eye examination recommended in patients with diabetes or history of uveitis or retinal disease before initiation and periodically during treatment (interrupt treatment if macular oedema occurs). ◈M◈

● PRESCRIBING AND DISPENSING INFORMATION The manufacturer of *Zeposia*® has provided a *Prescriber's Checklist*.

● PATIENT AND CARER ADVICE Patients should be advised to avoid exposure to sunlight without protection. Patients should be advised to promptly report symptoms of infection during and for up to 3 months after stopping treatment.
Patient reminder card Patients should be given a *Patient/Caregiver Guide*.
　Female patients of childbearing potential should be given a *Pregnancy Reminder Card*.

● NATIONAL FUNDING/ACCESS DECISIONS
For full details see funding body website
NICE decisions

▸ **Ozanimod for treating relapsing-remitting multiple sclerosis (June 2021)** NICE TA706 Not recommended

▸ **Ozanimod for treating moderately to severely active ulcerative colitis (October 2022)** NICE TA828 Recommended with restrictions

Scottish Medicines Consortium (SMC) decisions

▸ **Ozanimod (*Zeposia*®) for the treatment of adult patients with relapsing remitting multiple sclerosis (February 2021)** SMC No. SMC2309 Recommended with restrictions

▸ **Ozanimod (*Zeposia*®) for the treatment of adult patients with moderately to severely active ulcerative colitis who have had an inadequate response, lost response, or were intolerant to either conventional therapy or a biologic agent (October 2022)** SMC No. SMC2478 Recommended

● MEDICINAL FORMS There can be variation in the licensing of different medicines containing the same drug.

Oral capsule
EXCIPIENTS: May contain Gelatin

▸ Zeposia (Bristol-Myers Squibb Pharmaceuticals Ltd) ▼
　Ozanimod (as Ozanimod hydrochloride) 230 microgram Zeposia 0.23mg capsules | 4 capsule [PoM] ⚹
　Ozanimod (as Ozanimod hydrochloride) 460 microgram Zeposia 0.46mg capsules | 3 capsule [PoM] ⚹
　Ozanimod (as Ozanimod hydrochloride) 920 microgram Zeposia 0.92mg capsules | 28 capsule [PoM] £1,373.00

Ponesimod

01-Mar-2022

● DRUG ACTION Ponesimod is a sphingosine-1-phosphate receptor modulator, which prevents movement of lymphocytes out of lymph nodes, thereby limiting inflammation in the central nervous system.

● INDICATIONS AND DOSE

Multiple sclerosis (initiated under specialist supervision)

▸ BY MOUTH

▸ Adult: Initially 2 mg once daily on days 1–2, then increased to 3 mg once daily on days 3–4, then increased to 4 mg once daily on days 5–6, then increased in steps of 1 mg once daily from days 7–11, then increased to 10 mg once daily on days 12–14; maintenance 20 mg once daily from day 15 onwards, for re-initiation after treatment interruption—consult product literature

● CONTRA-INDICATIONS Active chronic infections · active malignancies · decompensated heart failure (requiring inpatient treatment) in the previous 6 months · heart failure (New York Heart Association class III or IV) in the previous 6 months · immunodeficiency · macular oedema · myocardial infarction in the previous 6 months · phototherapy with UV-B radiation or PUVA-photochemotherapy (increased risk of cutaneous neoplasm) · second-degree Mobitz type II AV block, third-degree AV block, or sick sinus syndrome, unless pacemaker fitted · severe active infections · stroke (including transient ischaemic attack) in the previous 6 months · unstable angina in the previous 6 months

● CAUTIONS Administration of vaccinations · cerebrovascular disease (including transient ischaemic attack or stroke more than 6 months ago) · chronic obstructive pulmonary disease · decompensated heart failure (more than 6 months ago) · diabetes mellitus (increased risk of macular oedema) · elderly (no information available) · history of cardiac arrest · history of second-degree Mobitz type II AV block, third-degree AV block, sick sinus syndrome, or sino-atrial heart block · history of significant liver disease · history of uveitis (increased risk of macular oedema) · immunosuppression or other risk factors for infection · patients receiving QT-prolonging or heart rate-lowering drugs, including beta-blockers and heart rate-lowering calcium-channel blockers · pulmonary fibrosis · recurrent syncope · risk of discontinuation effects, including disease rebound · severe respiratory disease · significant QT prolongation (QTc greater than 500 milliseconds) or other risk factors for QT prolongation · sinus bradycardia (heart rate below 55 beats per minute) · uncontrolled hypertension · unstable ischaemic heart disease

● CAUTIONS, FURTHER INFORMATION
▶ Bradycardia and cardiac rhythm disturbance [EvGr] Ponesimod may cause transient bradycardia, AV conduction delays, and heart block after the first dose. It is not recommended in patients with the cardiovascular risks listed above unless the anticipated benefits outweigh the potential risks, and advice from a cardiologist (including monitoring advice) is sought before initiation. ◆M◆
▶ Vaccinations [EvGr] Vaccination may be less effective during treatment. Live attenuated vaccines should be avoided during treatment; if they are required treatment should be stopped 1 week before and restarted 4 weeks after vaccination. Immunisation against varicella zoster is recommended prior to treatment in those without documented immunity. ◆M◆

● INTERACTIONS → Appendix 1: ponesimod

● SIDE-EFFECTS
▶ **Common or very common** Anxiety · chest discomfort · cough · depression · dizziness · drowsiness · dyspepsia · dyspnoea · fatigue · fever · hypercholesterolaemia · hypertension · increased risk of infection · insomnia · joint disorders · ligament sprain · lymphopenia · macular oedema · migraine · numbness · pain · peripheral oedema · vertigo
▶ **Uncommon** Bradycardia · dry mouth · hyperkalaemia
▶ **Frequency not known** Atrioventricular block · neoplasms · seizure

● CONCEPTION AND CONTRACEPTION [EvGr] Exclude pregnancy before treatment; females of childbearing potential should use effective contraception during treatment and for 1 week after last dose. ◆M◆

● PREGNANCY [EvGr] Avoid—toxicity in *animal* studies. ◆M◆

● BREAST FEEDING [EvGr] Avoid—present in milk in *animal* studies. ◆M◆

● HEPATIC IMPAIRMENT [EvGr] Avoid in moderate to severe impairment (increased exposure). ◆M◆

● MONITORING REQUIREMENTS
▶ [EvGr] An ECG should be obtained before initiation of treatment. Patients with certain pre-existing cardiac conditions should be monitored for bradycardia for at least 4 hours after the first dose ◆M◆—consult product literature for further information.
▶ [EvGr] Monitor blood pressure regularly during treatment.
▶ Monitor full blood count before initiation and periodically during treatment ◆M◆—consult product literature for further information.
▶ [EvGr] Monitor hepatic transaminases and bilirubin before initiation of treatment and then as clinically indicated (discontinue treatment if significant liver injury occurs).
▶ Eye examination recommended in all patients before initiation of treatment and then as clinically indicated (interrupt treatment if macular oedema occurs); patients with diabetes or history of uveitis to have eye examination periodically during treatment. ◆M◆

● PRESCRIBING AND DISPENSING INFORMATION The manufacturer of *Ponvory*® has provided a *Prescriber's Checklist*.

● PATIENT AND CARER ADVICE Patients should be advised to avoid exposure to sunlight without protection. Patients should be advised to promptly report symptoms of infection during and for up to 1 week after last dose. Patient reminder card Patients should be given a *Patient/Caregiver Guide*.

Female patients of childbearing potential should be given a *Pregnancy Reminder Card*.

● NATIONAL FUNDING/ACCESS DECISIONS
For full details see funding body website
NICE decisions
▶ Ponesimod for treating relapsing-remitting multiple sclerosis (February 2022) NICE TA767 Recommended
Scottish Medicines Consortium (SMC) decisions
▶ Ponesimod (*Ponvory*®) for the treatment of adult patients with relapsing forms of multiple sclerosis (RMS) with active disease defined by clinical or imaging features (November 2021) SMC No. SMC2384 Recommended with restrictions

● MEDICINAL FORMS There can be variation in the licensing of different medicines containing the same drug.
Oral tablet
▶ Ponvory (Janssen-Cilag Ltd) ▼
Ponesimod 2 mg Ponvory 2mg tablets | 2 tablet [PoM] [📋] (Hospital only)
Ponesimod 3 mg Ponvory 3mg tablets | 2 tablet [PoM] [📋] (Hospital only)
Ponesimod 4 mg Ponvory 4mg tablets | 2 tablet [PoM] [📋] (Hospital only)
Ponesimod 5 mg Ponvory 5mg tablets | 1 tablet [PoM] [📋] (Hospital only)
Ponesimod 6 mg Ponvory 6mg tablets | 1 tablet [PoM] [📋] (Hospital only)
Ponesimod 7 mg Ponvory 7mg tablets | 1 tablet [PoM] [📋] (Hospital only)
Ponesimod 8 mg Ponvory 8mg tablets | 1 tablet [PoM] [📋] (Hospital only)
Ponesimod 9 mg Ponvory 9mg tablets | 1 tablet [PoM] [📋] (Hospital only)
Ponesimod 10 mg Ponvory 10mg tablets | 3 tablet [PoM] [📋] (Hospital only)
Ponesimod 20 mg Ponvory 20mg tablets | 28 tablet [PoM] £1,073.97 (Hospital only)

Siponimod

03-Dec-2020

● DRUG ACTION Siponimod is a sphingosine-1-phosphate receptor modulator, which prevents movement of lymphocytes out of lymph nodes, thereby limiting inflammation in the central nervous system.

● INDICATIONS AND DOSE
Multiple sclerosis [secondary progressive, with active disease] (initiated by a specialist)
▶ BY MOUTH
▶ Adult: Initially 0.25 mg once daily on days 1 and 2, followed by 0.5 mg once daily on day 3, followed by 0.75 mg once daily on day 4, followed by 1.25 mg once daily on day 5, dose to be taken in the morning for the first 5 days; maintenance 2 mg once daily from day 6 onwards, in patients with a CYP2C9*1*3 or CYP2C9*2*3 genotype a reduced maintenance dose of 1 mg once daily is used from day 6 onwards. For dose adjustments based on lymphocyte count—consult product literature

● CONTRA-INDICATIONS Active malignancies · cryptococcal meningitis · decompensated heart failure (requiring inpatient treatment) in the previous 6 months · heart failure in the previous 6 months (New York Heart Association class III or IV) · immunodeficiency syndrome · macular oedema · myocardial infarction in the previous 6 months · patients homozygous for CYP2C9*3*3 genotype (poor metabolisers) · phototherapy with UV-B radiation or PUVA-photochemotherapy (increased risk of cutaneous neoplasms) · progressive multifocal leukoencephalopathy ·

second-degree Mobitz type II atrioventricular block or third-degree AV block, or sick-sinus syndrome, if the patient does not have a pacemaker · severe active infection · stroke (including transient ischaemic attack) in the previous 6 months · unstable angina pectoris in the previous 6 months

- CAUTIONS Administration of vaccinations (may be less effective during siponimod treatment—consult product literature for further information) · diabetes mellitus (increased risk of macular oedema) · elderly (limited information available) · exposure to sunlight (increased risk of cutaneous neoplasms) · first- or second-degree Mobitz type I atrioventricular block · heart failure (New York Heart Association class I and II) · myocardial infarction · patients receiving QT-prolonging or heart rate-lowering drugs, including beta-blockers and heart rate-lowering calcium-channel blockers (seek advice from cardiologist regarding switching to alternative drugs or appropriate monitoring) · recurrent syncope · retinal disease (increased risk of macular oedema) · risk of discontinuation effects, including disease rebound · severe sleep apnoea · significant QT prolongation (QTc greater than 500 milliseconds) · sinus bradycardia (heart rate below 55 beats per minute) · uncontrolled hypertension · uveitis (increased risk of macular oedema)

CAUTIONS, FURTHER INFORMATION

▸ **Bradycardia and cardiac rhythm disturbance** Siponimod may cause transient bradycardia, atrioventricular conduction delays and heart block after the first dose. Siponimod is not recommended in patients with a history of symptomatic bradycardia or recurrent syncope, uncontrolled hypertension, severe untreated sleep apnoea, or significant QT prolongation unless the anticipated benefits outweigh the potential risks, and advice from a cardiologist (including monitoring advice) is sought before initiation.

- INTERACTIONS → Appendix 1: siponimod

- SIDE-EFFECTS

▸ **Common or very common** Arrhythmias · asthenia · atrioventricular block · diarrhoea · dizziness · headache · hypertension · increased risk of infection · lymphopenia · macular oedema · nausea · neoplasms · pain in extremity · peripheral oedema · seizure · tremor

▸ **Frequency not known** Meningitis cryptococcal · vision disorders

- ALLERGY AND CROSS-SENSITIVITY Manufacturer advises contra-indicated in patients with hypersensitivity to peanut or soya products.

- CONCEPTION AND CONTRACEPTION Manufacturer advises exclude pregnancy before treatment; females of childbearing potential should use effective contraception during treatment and for 10 days after last dose.

- PREGNANCY Manufacturer advises avoid—toxicity in *animal* studies.

- BREAST FEEDING Manufacturer advises avoid—present in milk in *animal* studies.

- HEPATIC IMPAIRMENT Manufacturer advises caution when initiating treatment in mild to moderate impairment; avoid in severe impairment.

- PRE-TREATMENT SCREENING Manufacturer advises CYP2C9 genotyping before treatment initiation—consult product literature. Manufacturer advises check varicella zoster virus status in patients with unconfirmed or incomplete vaccination history. A full course of vaccination against varicella zoster is required 1 month before initiating treatment in antibody-negative patients.

- MONITORING REQUIREMENTS

▸ Manufacturer advises regular monitoring of heart rate, particularly during treatment initiation, and of blood pressure.

▸ Manufacturer advises patients with certain pre-existing cardiac conditions should be monitored for bradycardia for 6 hours after the first dose. An ECG should be obtained before dosing and after 6 hours—consult product literature for further information.

▸ Manufacturer advises monitor full blood count before initiation and periodically during treatment (reduce dosage or interrupt treatment if lymphocyte count reduced)—consult product literature.

▸ Manufacturer advises monitor hepatic transaminases and bilirubin before initiation of treatment and then as clinically indicated (interrupt treatment if significant liver injury occurs).

▸ Manufacturer advises eye examination recommended 3–4 months after initiation of treatment (and before initiation of treatment in patients with diabetes or history of uveitis or retinal disease).

- PRESCRIBING AND DISPENSING INFORMATION The manufacturer of *Mayzent*® has provided a *Physician Education Pack*.

- PATIENT AND CARER ADVICE Manufacturer advises patients to avoid exposure to sunlight without protection. Manufacturer advises patients should promptly report symptoms of infection.
Missed doses Manufacturer advises if a dose is missed during treatment initiation (days 1–6), the initial titration regimen should be restarted. If a maintenance dose is missed (after day 6), the missed dose should not be taken, and the next dose should be taken at the normal time. If 4 or more consecutive doses are missed, the initial titration regimen should be used to restart treatment.
Driving and skilled tasks Manufacturer advises patients should be counselled on the effects on driving and performance of skilled tasks—increased risk of dizziness during treatment initiation.

- NATIONAL FUNDING/ACCESS DECISIONS
For full details see funding body website
NICE decisions

▸ **Siponimod for treating secondary progressive multiple sclerosis (November 2020)** NICE TA656 Recommended

Scottish Medicines Consortium (SMC) decisions

▸ **Siponimod (*Mayzent*®) for the treatment of adult patients with secondary progressive multiple sclerosis (SPMS) with active disease evidenced by relapses or imaging features of inflammatory activity (October 2020)** SMC No. SMC2265 Recommended

- MEDICINAL FORMS There can be variation in the licensing of different medicines containing the same drug.
Oral tablet
EXCIPIENTS: May contain Lecithin
▸ **Mayzent** (Novartis Pharmaceuticals UK Ltd) ▼
Siponimod (as Siponimod fumaric acid) 250 microgram Mayzent 0.25mg tablets | 12 tablet [PoM] £293.52 (Hospital only) | 120 tablet [PoM] £1,761.12 (Hospital only)
Siponimod (as Siponimod fumaric acid) 1 mg Mayzent 1mg tablets | 28 tablet [PoM] £1,643.72 (Hospital only)
Siponimod (as Siponimod fumaric acid) 2 mg Mayzent 2mg tablets | 28 tablet [PoM] £1,643.72 (Hospital only)

IMMUNOSUPPRESSANTS ❭ MONOCLONAL ANTIBODIES ❭ ANTI-LYMPHOCYTE

Anti-lymphocyte monoclonal antibodies 

- DRUG ACTION The anti-lymphocyte monoclonal antibodies cause lysis of B lymphocytes.

IMPORTANT SAFETY INFORMATION
All anti-lymphocyte monoclonal antibodies should be given under the supervision of an experienced specialist,

in an environment where full resuscitation facilities are immediately available.

- **SIDE-EFFECTS**
▶ **Common or very common** Anaemia · anaphylactic reaction · arthralgia · conjunctivitis · cough · hypersensitivity (discontinue permanently) · increased risk of infection · infusion related reaction · neutropenia · pain in extremity
▶ **Uncommon** Haemolytic anaemia

SIDE-EFFECTS, FURTHER INFORMATION **Infusion-related side-effects** In rare cases infusion reactions may be fatal. Infusion-related side-effects occur predominantly during the first infusion. Patients should receive premedication before administration of anti-lymphocyte monoclonal antibodies to reduce these effects—consult product literature for details of individual regimens. The infusion may have to be stopped temporarily and the infusion-related effects treated—consult product literature for appropriate management.

Cytokine release syndrome Fatalities following severe cytokine release syndrome (characterised by severe dyspnoea) and associated with features of tumour lysis syndrome have occurred after infusions of anti-lymphocyte monoclonal antibodies. Patients with a high tumour burden as well as those with pulmonary insufficiency or infiltration are at increased risk and should be monitored very closely (and a slower rate of infusion considered).

Progressive Multifocal Leukoencephalopathy (PML) If suspected, treatment should be suspended until PML has been excluded. If a patient develops an opportunistic infection or PML, anti-lymphocyte monoclonal antibodies should be permanently discontinued.

- **PRE-TREATMENT SCREENING** All patients should be screened for hepatitis B before treatment.
- **MONITORING REQUIREMENTS** Patients should also be monitored for cytopenias—consult product literature for specific recommendations.

▶ 991

Alemtuzumab

28-May-2024

- **INDICATIONS AND DOSE**

Treatment of adults with relapsing-remitting multiple sclerosis with active disease defined by clinical or imaging features
▶ BY INTRAVENOUS INFUSION
▶ Adult: (consult product literature)

- **UNLICENSED USE** Although no longer licensed for oncological and transplant indications, alemtuzumab is also available through a patient access programme for these indications.

IMPORTANT SAFETY INFORMATION
MHRA/CHM ADVICE (UPDATED FEBRUARY 2020): *LEMTRADA*® **(ALEMTUZUMAB): UPDATED RESTRICTIONS AND STRENGTHENED MONITORING REQUIREMENTS FOLLOWING REVIEW OF SERIOUS CARDIOVASCULAR AND IMMUNE-MEDIATED REACTIONS**
Following a review of alemtuzumab by the European Medicines Agency, a revised indication, additional contra-indications (see *Contra-indications*), and strengthened monitoring requirements before, during, and after treatment have been recommended. Healthcare professionals are advised that alemtuzumab should only be used for the treatment of patients with relapsing-remitting multiple sclerosis (RRMS) that is highly active despite a full and adequate course of treatment with at least one disease-modifying agent, or in patients with rapidly evolving severe RRMS.

Healthcare professionals should monitor patients before, during, and after treatment for cardiovascular reactions and non-immune thrombocytopenia (see *Monitoring requirements*). Patients should be informed of serious cardiovascular symptoms that can occur within a few days of treatment, signs of autoimmune disorders that can occur 48 months or more after treatment, and symptoms of hepatic injury; immediate medical attention should be sought by patients if they experience any of these symptoms.

- **CONTRA-INDICATIONS** Angina (past history) · autoimmune diseases (excluding multiple sclerosis) · cervicocephalic arterial dissection (past history) · clotting abnormalities (including patients on anticoagulant therapy) · human immunodeficiency virus · hypertension (uncontrolled) · myocardial infarction (past history) · severe active infection (until complete resolution) · stroke (past history)

- **CAUTIONS** Hepatitis B carriers · hepatitis C carriers · not recommended for inactive disease · not recommended for stable disease · patients should receive oral prophylaxis for herpes infection starting on the first day of treatment and continuing for at least a month following each treatment course · pretreatment before administration is required (consult product literature)

CAUTIONS, FURTHER INFORMATION For full details of cautions, consult product literature.
▶ **Autoimmune mediated conditions** The risk of autoimmune mediated conditions may increase during treatment, including immune thrombocytopenic purpura, thyroid disorders, nephropathies, cytopenias, autoimmune hepatitis, and acquired haemophilia A. Manufacturer advises monitoring for autoimmune mediated conditions throughout the course of treatment (consult product literature).

- **INTERACTIONS** → Appendix 1: monoclonal antibodies

- **SIDE-EFFECTS**
▶ **Common or very common** Abdominal pain · alopecia · anxiety · asthenia · asthma · cytokine release syndrome · decreased leucocytes · depression · diarrhoea · endocrine ophthalmopathy · goitre · haemorrhage · hiccups · hyperthyroidism · hypothyroidism · influenza like illness · leucocytosis · lymphadenopathy · malaise · meningitis · menstrual cycle irregularities · multiple sclerosis exacerbated · muscle complaints · muscle weakness · neoplasms · nephropathy · oropharyngeal pain · pain · peripheral oedema · sensation abnormal · skin reactions · stomatitis · sweat changes · thrombocytopenia · thyroiditis · tremor · urine abnormalities · vertigo · vision disorders · vomiting
▶ **Uncommon** Acquired haemophilia · appetite decreased · cervical dysplasia · constipation · dry mouth · dysphagia · ear pain · facial swelling · gallbladder disorders · gastrointestinal disorders · Goodpasture's syndrome · limb discomfort · musculoskeletal stiffness · nephrolithiasis · pancytopenia · pneumonitis · tension headache · throat irritation · weight changes
▶ **Rare or very rare** Haemophagocytic lymphohistiocytosis
▶ **Frequency not known** Artery dissection · cerebrovascular insufficiency · hepatitis autoimmune (including fatal cases) · liver injury · myocardial infarction · myocardial ischaemia · reactivation of infections · thyroid disorder autoimmune

- **CONCEPTION AND CONTRACEPTION** Women of childbearing potential should use effective contraception during and for 4 months after treatment.

- **PREGNANCY** Manufacturer advises avoid unless potential benefit outweighs risk—toxicity in *animal* studies. Autoimmune thyroid disease during treatment may affect fetus (consult product literature).

- **BREAST FEEDING** Manufacturer advises avoid during and for 4 months after each treatment course unless potential benefit outweighs risk.

- **PRE-TREATMENT SCREENING** Screening patients at high risk of hepatitis B or C is recommended before treatment. All patients should be evaluated for active or latent tuberculosis before starting treatment.
- **MONITORING REQUIREMENTS**
  ▸ The MHRA advises to check liver, thyroid, and kidney function, urinalysis with microscopy, blood counts, and vital signs (including blood pressure, heart rate, and ECG) before infusions.
  ▸ The MHRA advises monitor blood pressure and heart rate continuously or at least once every hour during infusions—discontinue infusion if severe adverse reactions occur.
  ▸ The MHRA advises monitor patients for infusion-related reactions for at least 2 hours after infusions; patients should be informed of the risk of delayed infusion-related reactions and to seek immediate medical attention if these occur.
  ▸ The MHRA advises monitor platelet counts after treatment—consult product literature.
  ▸ For further information on monitoring, see *Important safety information*.
  ▸ HPV screening should be carried out annually in female patients.
- **PRESCRIBING AND DISPENSING INFORMATION** All patients should receive oral prophylaxis for herpes infection starting on the first day of treatment and continuing for at least a month following each treatment course.
- **PATIENT AND CARER ADVICE** Patients should be provided with a patient alert card and patient guide.
- **NATIONAL FUNDING/ACCESS DECISIONS** For full details see funding body website
  NICE decisions
  ▸ **Alemtuzumab for treating highly active relapsing-remitting multiple sclerosis (updated May 2024)** NICE TA312 Recommended

- **MEDICINAL FORMS** There can be variation in the licensing of different medicines containing the same drug.
  Solution for infusion
  ▸ **Lemtrada** (Sanofi) ▼
  Alemtuzumab 10 mg per 1 ml Lemtrada 12mg/1.2ml concentrate for solution for infusion vials | 1 vial PoM £7,045.00 (Hospital only)

⯀ 991

Natalizumab
28-May-2024

- **INDICATIONS AND DOSE**
  Highly active relapsing-remitting multiple sclerosis despite treatment with at least one disease-modifying drug, or those patients with rapidly-evolving severe relapsing-remitting multiple sclerosis (initiated under specialist supervision)
  ▸ BY INTRAVENOUS INFUSION
  ▸ Adult 18-65 years: 300 mg every 4 weeks, consider discontinuing treatment if no response after 6 months

- **CONTRA-INDICATIONS** Active infection · active malignancies (except cutaneous basal cell carcinoma) · immunosuppression · progressive multifocal leukoencephalopathy

- **CAUTIONS**
  ▸ Progressive Multifocal Leukoencephalopathy Natalizumab is associated with an increased risk of opportunistic infection and progressive multifocal leukoencephalopathy (PML) caused by JC virus. The risk of developing PML increases with the presence of anti-JCV antibodies, previous use of immunosuppressant therapy, and treatment duration (especially beyond 2 years of treatment). Patients with all three risk factors should only be treated with natalizumab if the benefits of treatment outweigh the risks. Manufacturer advises treatment should be suspended until

PML has been excluded. Manufacturer also advises if a patient develops an opportunistic infection or PML, natalizumab should be permanently discontinued.
　For information on cautions consult product literature.

- **INTERACTIONS** → Appendix 1: monoclonal antibodies
- **SIDE-EFFECTS**
  ▸ **Common or very common** Fatigue · fever · headache
  ▸ **Uncommon** Progressive multifocal leukoencephalopathy (PML)
  ▸ **Frequency not known** Acute retinal necrosis · basophil count increased · eosinophilia · hyperbilirubinaemia · JC virus granule cell neuronopathy · liver injury · meningitis herpes · nucleated red cells

  SIDE-EFFECTS, FURTHER INFORMATION **Liver injury** Discontinue treatment if significant liver injury occurs.
  　Infusion-related reactions Infusion-related reactions including dizziness, nausea, urticaria, chills, vomiting and flushing have been reported either during infusion or within 1 hour after completion of infusion.

- **PREGNANCY** Avoid unless essential—toxicity in *animal* studies.
- **BREAST FEEDING** Present in milk in *animal* studies—avoid.
- **PRE-TREATMENT SCREENING**
  Progressive Multifocal Leukoencephalopathy A magnetic resonance image (MRI) scan is recommended before starting treatment with natalizumab.
  　Testing for serum anti-JCV antibodies before starting treatment or in those with unknown antibody status already receiving natalizumab is recommended and should be repeated every 6 months (consult product literature for full details).

- **MONITORING REQUIREMENTS**
  ▸ Monitor liver function.
  ▸ Progressive Multifocal Leukoencephalopathy A magnetic resonance image (MRI) scan is recommended annually. Patients should be monitored for new or worsening neurological symptoms, and for cognitive and psychiatric signs of PML.
  All patients should continue to be monitored for signs and symptoms that may be suggestive of PML for approximately 6 months following discontinuation of treatment.
  ▸ Hypersensitivity reactions Patients should be observed for hypersensitivity reactions, including anaphylaxis, during the infusion and for 1 hour after completion of the infusion.

- **DIRECTIONS FOR ADMINISTRATION** For *intravenous infusion* (*Tysabri* ®), manufacturer advises give intermittently in Sodium Chloride 0.9%; dilute 300 mg in 100 mL infusion fluid; gently invert to mix, do not shake. Use within 8 hours of dilution and give over 1 hour.

- **PATIENT AND CARER ADVICE**
  Hypersensitivity reactions Patients should be told the importance of uninterrupted dosing, particularly in the early months of treatment (intermittent therapy may increase risk of sensitisation).
  Progressive Multifocal Leukoencephalopathy Patients should be informed about the risks of PML before starting treatment with natalizumab and again after 2 years; they should be given an alert card which includes information about the symptoms of PML.
  Liver toxicity Advise patients to seek immediate medical attention if symptoms such as jaundice or dark urine develop.
  Alert card A patient alert card should be provided.

- **NATIONAL FUNDING/ACCESS DECISIONS**
  For full details see funding body website
  NICE decisions
  ▸ **Natalizumab for the treatment of adults with highly active relapsing-remitting multiple sclerosis (updated May 2024)** NICE TA127 Recommended with restrictions

Immune system and malignant disease

Scottish Medicines Consortium (SMC) decisions
▶ Natalizumab (*Tysabri*®) for use as single disease modifying therapy in highly active relapsing remitting multiple sclerosis (RRMS) (September 2007) SMC No. 329/06 Recommended with restrictions
NHS restrictions
NHS England Clinical Commissioning Policy NHS England (May 2014) has provided guidance on the use of natalizumab for the treatment of multiple sclerosis in England. An NHS England Clinical Commissioning Policy outlines the funding arrangements and the criteria for initiating and discontinuing this treatment option, see www.england.nhs.uk/commissioning/spec-services/npc-crg/group-d/neurology/.

● MEDICINAL FORMS There can be variation in the licensing of different medicines containing the same drug.
Solution for infusion
ELECTROLYTES: May contain Sodium
  ▶ Tyruko (Sandoz Ltd) ▼
    Natalizumab 20 mg per 1 ml Tyruko 300mg/15ml concentrate for solution for infusion vials | 1 vial [PoM] £1,017.00 (Hospital only)
  ▶ Tysabri (Biogen Idec Ltd)
    Natalizumab 20 mg per 1 ml Tysabri 300mg/15ml concentrate for solution for infusion vials | 1 vial [PoM] £1,130.00 (Hospital only)

⊩ 991

Ocrelizumab

11-Nov-2020

● **INDICATIONS AND DOSE**

Multiple sclerosis (specialist use only)
▶ BY INTRAVENOUS INFUSION
▶ Adult: Initially 300 mg, then 300 mg after 2 weeks; maintenance 600 mg every 6 months, the first maintenance dose should be given 6 months after the first initial dose; a minimum interval of 5 months should be maintained between each maintenance dose, for dose interruption, adjustment of infusion rate or discontinuation of treatment due to infusion-related reactions or side-effects—consult product literature

● CONTRA-INDICATIONS Active infection · active malignancies · severely immunocompromised patients
● CAUTIONS Complete required vaccinations at least 6 weeks before treatment initiation · hepatitis B reactivation
● INTERACTIONS → Appendix 1: monoclonal antibodies
● SIDE-EFFECTS
▶ **Common or very common** Catarrh
▶ **Frequency not known** Malignancy
● CONCEPTION AND CONTRACEPTION Manufacturer advises women of childbearing potential should use contraception during treatment and for 12 months after the last dose.
● PREGNANCY Manufacturer advises avoid unless potential benefit outweighs risk—limited information available; monitor infants for B-cell depletion.
● BREAST FEEDING Manufacturer advises avoid—present in milk in *animal* studies.
● MONITORING REQUIREMENTS
▶ Manufacturer advises monitor for signs and symptoms of progressive multifocal leukoencephalopathy (PML) (including any new onset or worsening of neurological symptoms)—if PML is suspected, interrupt treatment; discontinue treatment permanently if PML is confirmed.
▶ Manufacturer advises monitor for infusion-related reactions during the infusion and observe patients for 1 hour after completion of the infusion—if severe pulmonary symptoms occur, permanently discontinue treatment.
● PRESCRIBING AND DISPENSING INFORMATION Manufacturer advises to record the batch number after each administration.

● HANDLING AND STORAGE Manufacturer advises store in a refrigerator (2–8°C)—consult product literature for further information regarding storage conditions after preparation of the infusion.
● PATIENT AND CARER ADVICE Manufacturer advises patients and carers should be advised that infusion-related reactions can occur within 24 hours of infusion.
● NATIONAL FUNDING/ACCESS DECISIONS
For full details see funding body website
NICE decisions
▶ Ocrelizumab for treating relapsing–remitting multiple sclerosis (July 2018) NICE TA533 Recommended with restrictions
▶ Ocrelizumab for treating primary progressive multiple sclerosis (June 2019) NICE TA585 Recommended with restrictions
Scottish Medicines Consortium (SMC) decisions
▶ Ocrelizumab (*Ocrevus*®) for the treatment of adult patients with relapsing forms of multiple sclerosis (RMS) with active disease defined by clinical or imaging features (December 2018) SMC No. SMC2121 Recommended with restrictions
▶ Ocrelizumab (*Ocrevus*®) for treatment of adult patients with early primary progressive multiple sclerosis (PPMS) in terms of disease duration and level of disability, and with imaging features characteristic of inflammatory activity (January 2020) SMC No. SMC2223 Recommended

● MEDICINAL FORMS There can be variation in the licensing of different medicines containing the same drug.
Solution for infusion
  ▶ Ocrevus (Roche Products Ltd)
    Ocrelizumab 30 mg per 1 ml Ocrevus 300mg/10ml concentrate for solution for infusion vials | 1 vial [PoM] £4,790.00 (Hospital only)

Ofatumumab

20-May-2022

● DRUG ACTION The anti-lymphocyte monoclonal antibodies cause lysis of B lymphocytes.

● **INDICATIONS AND DOSE**

Multiple sclerosis (initiated by a specialist)
▶ BY SUBCUTANEOUS INJECTION
▶ Adult: Initially 20 mg once weekly for 3 doses (weeks 0, 1 and 2), then maintenance 20 mg once a month, starting on week 4 (2 weeks after the third dose)

● CONTRA-INDICATIONS Active hepatitis B infection · active malignancies · severe active infection · severely immunocompromised patients
● CAUTIONS Active infection · hepatitis B carriers (seek expert advice before starting) · history of progressive multifocal leukoencephalopathy
CAUTIONS, FURTHER INFORMATION
▶ Immunisation [EvGr] Patients should receive all recommended vaccinations before starting treatment; live vaccines should be given at least 4 weeks before, and inactivated vaccines ideally at least 2 weeks before, starting ofatumumab. Ⓜ
● INTERACTIONS → Appendix 1: monoclonal antibodies
● SIDE-EFFECTS
▶ **Common or very common** Cystitis · increased risk of infection · injection related reaction
▶ **Frequency not known** Hepatitis B reactivation · JC virus infection · progressive multifocal leukoencephalopathy (PML)

SIDE-EFFECTS, FURTHER INFORMATION If progressive multifocal leukoencephalopathy (PML) is suspected, treatment should be suspended until PML has been excluded. If a patient develops an opportunistic infection or PML, ofantumumab should be permanently discontinued.

- **CONCEPTION AND CONTRACEPTION** [EvGr] Females of childbearing potential should use effective contraception during treatment and for 6 months after the last dose. ⟨M⟩

- **PREGNANCY** [EvGr] Avoid unless potential benefit outweighs risk—no information available; if exposed during pregnancy, monitor infant for B-cell depletion. ⟨M⟩

- **BREAST FEEDING** [EvGr] Avoid during first few days after birth—possible risk from transfer of antibodies to infant. After this time, use during breast-feeding only if clinically needed. If ofatumumab is used throughout the third trimester, breast-feeding can start immediately after birth. ⟨M⟩

- **PRE-TREATMENT SCREENING** [EvGr] All patients should be screened for hepatitis B before treatment. ⟨M⟩

- **MONITORING REQUIREMENTS** [EvGr] Monitor for signs or symptoms of progressive multifocal leukoencephalopathy (withhold treatment if suspected). ⟨M⟩

- **DIRECTIONS FOR ADMINISTRATION** [EvGr] Usual sites for subcutaneous injection are the abdomen, thigh or upper outer arm. ⟨M⟩ After an initial dose administered under medical guidance, patients may self-administer *Kesimpta*® if they have been given the appropriate training in subcutaneous injection technique.

- **PRESCRIBING AND DISPENSING INFORMATION** Ofatumumab is a biological medicine. Biological medicines must be prescribed and dispensed by brand name, see *Biological medicines* and *Biosimilar medicines*, under Guidance on prescribing p. 1.

- **HANDLING AND STORAGE** Store in a refrigerator (2–8°C) and protect from light.

- **PATIENT AND CARER ADVICE**
  Self-administration [EvGr] Patients and their carers should be given training in subcutaneous injection technique if appropriate. ⟨M⟩

- **NATIONAL FUNDING/ACCESS DECISIONS**
  For full details see funding body website
  NICE decisions
  ▸ **Ofatumumab for treating relapsing multiple sclerosis (May 2021) NICE TA699 Recommended**

  Scottish Medicines Consortium (SMC) decisions
  ▸ **Ofatumumab (*Kesimpta*®) for the treatment of adult patients with relapsing forms of multiple sclerosis with active disease defined by clinical or imaging features (July 2021) SMC No. SMC2357 Recommended with restrictions**

- **MEDICINAL FORMS** There can be variation in the licensing of different medicines containing the same drug.
  Solution for injection
  EXCIPIENTS: May contain Disodium edetate, polysorbates
  ▸ **Kesimpta Sensoready** (Novartis Pharmaceuticals UK Ltd) ▼
  Ofatumumab 50 mg per 1 ml Kesimpta Sensoready 20mg/0.4ml solution for injection pre-filled pens | 1 pre-filled disposable injection [PoM] £1,492.50

[F 991]

Ublituximab
08-Apr-2025

- **INDICATIONS AND DOSE**
  Multiple sclerosis (under expert supervision)
  ▸ BY INTRAVENOUS INFUSION
  ▸ Adult: Initially 150 mg for 1 dose, then 450 mg after 2 weeks; maintenance 450 mg every 6 months, the first maintenance dose should be given 6 months after the first initial dose; a minimum interval of 5 months should be kept between each maintenance dose, for dose interruption, adjustment of infusion rate or discontinuation of treatment due to infusion-related reactions or side-effects—consult product literature

- **CONTRA-INDICATIONS** Active malignancies · severe active infection · severely immunocompromised patients

- **CAUTIONS** Hepatitis B carriers (seek expert advice before starting) · immunisation
  CAUTIONS, FURTHER INFORMATION
  ▸ Immunisation [EvGr] Patients should receive all recommended vaccinations before starting treatment; live vaccines should be given at least 4 weeks before, and inactivated vaccines ideally at least 2 weeks before, starting ublituximab. ⟨M⟩

- **INTERACTIONS** → Appendix 1: monoclonal antibodies

- **CONCEPTION AND CONTRACEPTION** [EvGr] Females of childbearing potential should use effective contraception during treatment and for at least 4 months after last treatment. ⟨M⟩

- **PREGNANCY** [EvGr] Avoid unless potential benefit outweighs risk (toxicity in *animal* studies); if exposed during pregnancy, monitor infant for B-lymphocyte depletion. ⟨M⟩

- **BREAST FEEDING** Specialist sources indicate use with caution, especially if breast-feeding a neonate or preterm infant (no information available). Large molecular weight suggests limited excretion into milk and drug molecule likely to be partially destroyed in the infant's gastro-intestinal tract; waiting for at least 2 weeks postpartum to resume treatment may minimise transfer to infant.

- **MONITORING REQUIREMENTS**
  ▸ [EvGr] Monitor for new onset or worsening neurological signs and symptoms of progressive multifocal leukoencephalopathy (PML)—interrupt treatment if PML is suspected; discontinue treatment if PML is confirmed.
  ▸ Monitor for infusion-related reactions during infusions, and for at least 1 hour after completion of the first 2 infusions. ⟨M⟩

- **DIRECTIONS FOR ADMINISTRATION** For *intravenous infusion*, dilute with Sodium Chloride 0.9% to give a final concentration of 0.6 mg/mL for the first infusion and 1.8 mg/mL for subsequent infusions. For duration of infusion—consult product literature.

- **PRESCRIBING AND DISPENSING INFORMATION** Ublituximab is a biological medicine. Biological medicines must be prescribed and dispensed by brand name, see *Biological medicines* and *Biosimilar medicines*, under Guidance on prescribing p. 1; record the brand name and batch number after each administration.

- **HANDLING AND STORAGE** Store in a refrigerator (2–8°C) and protect from light—consult product literature for further information regarding storage conditions after preparation of the infusion.

- **PATIENT AND CARER ADVICE** Patients and carers should be advised that infusion-related reactions can occur within 24 hours of infusion.

- **NATIONAL FUNDING/ACCESS DECISIONS**
  For full details see funding body website
  NICE decisions
  ▸ **Ublituximab for treating relapsing multiple sclerosis (December 2024) NICE TA1025 Recommended with restrictions**

  Scottish Medicines Consortium (SMC) decisions
  ▸ **Ublituximab (*Briumvi*®) for the treatment of adult patients with relapsing forms of multiple sclerosis with active disease defined by clinical or imaging features (January 2025) SMC No. SMC2731 Recommended with restrictions**

- **MEDICINAL FORMS** There can be variation in the licensing of different medicines containing the same drug.
  Solution for infusion
  EXCIPIENTS: May contain Polysorbates
  ▸ **Briumvi** (Neuraxpharm UK Ltd) ▼
  Ublituximab 25 mg per 1 ml Briumvi 150mg/6ml concentrate for solution for infusion vials | 1 vial [PoM] £2,947.00 (Hospital only)

Immune system and malignant disease

8

IMMUNOSUPPRESSANTS > PYRIMIDINE SYNTHESIS INHIBITORS

Teriflunomide

23-Jun-2022

- **DRUG ACTION** Teriflunomide is a metabolite of leflunomide which has immunomodulating and anti-inflammatory properties.

- **INDICATIONS AND DOSE**

Multiple sclerosis (initiated by a specialist)
- BY MOUTH
- Adult: 14 mg once daily

- **CONTRA-INDICATIONS** Anaemia · leucopenia · neutropenia · serious infection · severe hypoproteinaemia · severe immunodeficiency · significantly impaired bone-marrow function · thrombocytopenia

- **CAUTIONS** Adult over 65 years (limited information available) · anaemia · dyspnoea—assess for interstitial lung disease and consider suspending treatment · hypoproteinaemia (avoid if severe) · impaired bone-marrow function (avoid if severe) · latent tuberculosis · leucopenia · persistent cough—assess for interstitial lung disease and consider suspending treatment · severe infection—delay or suspend treatment until resolved · significant alcohol consumption · signs or symptoms of serious skin reactions (including ulcerative stomatitis, Stevens-Johnson syndrome, and toxic epidermal necrolysis)—discontinue treatment · switching between other immunomodulating drugs · thrombocytopenia

- **INTERACTIONS** → Appendix 1: teriflunomide

- **SIDE-EFFECTS**
- **Common or very common** Abdominal pain upper · alopecia · anaemia · anxiety · arthralgia · cystitis · diarrhoea · headache · hypersensitivity · hypertension · increased risk of infection · menorrhagia · myalgia · nausea · nerve disorders · neutropenia · oral disorders · pain · palpitations · sensation abnormal · skin reactions · urinary frequency increased · vomiting · weight decreased
- **Uncommon** Colitis · dyslipidaemia · interstitial lung disease · nail disorder · pancreatitis · sepsis · severe cutaneous adverse reactions (SCARs) · thrombocytopenia
- **Rare or very rare** Hepatic disorders
- **Frequency not known** Pulmonary hypertension

SIDE-EFFECTS, FURTHER INFORMATION **Hepatic injury** Discontinue treatment if signs or symptoms of hepatic injury, or if liver enzymes exceed 3 times the upper limit of reference range.

Important: accelerated elimination procedure recommended following discontinuation due to serious adverse effects (consult product literature).

- **CONCEPTION AND CONTRACEPTION** Effective contraception essential for women of child-bearing potential during treatment and for up to 2 years after treatment. In patients undergoing treatment with teriflunomide that are planning to conceive, the accelerated elimination procedure should be used prior to conception. Use of non-oral contraception is recommended during the accelerated elimination procedure—consult product literature.

- **PREGNANCY** Avoid—toxicity in animal studies.

- **BREAST FEEDING** Present in milk in *animal* studies—manufacturer advises avoid.

- **HEPATIC IMPAIRMENT** EvGr Avoid in severe impairment. M Monitoring EvGr In patients with pre-existing liver disease, monitor liver function every 2 weeks for the first 6 months during treatment, then every 8 weeks thereafter for at least 2 years. Increase to weekly monitoring if alanine aminotransferase (ALT) is 2–3 times the upper limit of normal; discontinue treatment if signs or symptoms of

hepatic injury occur, or if liver enzymes exceed 3 times the upper limit of normal. M

- **MONITORING REQUIREMENTS**
- EvGr Monitor full blood count (including differential white cell count and platelet count) before treatment and as clinically indicated during treatment.
- Monitor blood pressure before treatment and periodically thereafter.
- Monitor liver function before treatment and every 4 weeks for the first 6 months during treatment, then as clinically indicated. M Additional monitoring required in pre-existing liver disease or if alanine aminotransferase (ALT) increases during treatment, see *Hepatic impairment*.

- **TREATMENT CESSATION**
Accelerated elimination procedures To aid drug elimination in case of serious adverse effect or before conception, stop treatment and give *either* colestyramine p. 229 *or* charcoal, activated p. 1561. After the accelerated elimination procedure a plasma concentration of less than 20 micrograms/litre (measured on 2 occasions at least 14 days apart) and a waiting period of one and a half months are necessary before conception.

- **PRESCRIBING AND DISPENSING INFORMATION** The manufacturer of *Aubagio*® has provided a guide for healthcare professionals.

- **PATIENT AND CARER ADVICE** Patients and their carers should be advised to report symptoms of infections to a doctor.
Patients or their carers should be given a patient card.

- **NATIONAL FUNDING/ACCESS DECISIONS**
For full details see funding body website

NICE decisions
- **Teriflunomide for treating relapsing-remitting multiple sclerosis (January 2014)** NICE TA303 Recommended with restrictions

Scottish Medicines Consortium (SMC) decisions
- **Teriflunomide (*Aubagio*®) for adults with relapsing-remitting multiple sclerosis (March 2014)** SMC No. 940/14 Recommended with restrictions

- **MEDICINAL FORMS** There can be variation in the licensing of different medicines containing the same drug.
Oral tablet
- **Teriflunomide (Non-proprietary)**
  Teriflunomide 14 mg Teriflunomide 14mg tablets | 28 tablet [PoM] £870.00–£1,037.84 (Hospital only) | 28 tablet [PoM] £705.00–£934.05
- **Aubagio** (Sanofi)
  Teriflunomide 7 mg Aubagio 7mg tablets | 28 tablet [PoM] £1,037.84 (Hospital only)
  Teriflunomide 14 mg Aubagio 14mg tablets | 28 tablet [PoM] £1,037.84 (Hospital only)

Malignant disease

1   Antibody responsive malignancy

ANTINEOPLASTIC DRUGS › MONOCLONAL ANTIBODIES

Amivantamab [Specialist drug]
03-Jan-2023

● **INDICATIONS AND DOSE**

Non-small cell lung cancer
▸ BY INTRAVENOUS INFUSION
▸ Adult: Specialist drug – access specialist resources for dosing information

IMPORTANT SAFETY INFORMATION
Resuscitation facilities should be available during administration.

● **SIDE-EFFECTS**
▸ **Common or very common** Appetite decreased · asthenia · constipation · diarrhoea · dizziness · dry eye · electrolyte imbalance · eye discomfort · eye disorders · eye inflammation · facial swelling · gastrointestinal discomfort · hypoalbuminaemia · increased risk of infection · infusion related reaction · interstitial lung disease · mucositis · myalgia · nail disorders · nausea · oedema · onycholysis · oral disorders · perineal rash · peripheral swelling · skin reactions · vertigo · vision disorders · vomiting
▸ **Uncommon** Toxic epidermal necrolysis
▸ **Frequency not known** Back pain · dyspnoea · fever · muscle weakness · pleural effusion · pulmonary embolism

● **CONCEPTION AND CONTRACEPTION** [EvGr] Females of childbearing potential should use effective contraception during treatment and for at least 3 months after last treatment. ⓜ

● **PATIENT AND CARER ADVICE** Patients should be advised to limit sun exposure during treatment and for 2 months after last treatment; protective clothing and use of sunscreen are advisable. Patients should be advised to discontinue contact lens use until worsening eye symptoms are evaluated.
Driving and skilled tasks Patients and carers should be counselled on the effects on driving and performance of skilled tasks—increased risk of dizziness and visual impairment.

● **NATIONAL FUNDING/ACCESS DECISIONS**
For full details see funding body website
NICE decisions
▸ Amivantamab for treating EGFR exon 20 insertion mutation-positive advanced non-small-cell lung cancer after platinum-based chemotherapy (December 2022) NICE TA850 Not recommended

● **MEDICINAL FORMS** There can be variation in the licensing of different medicines containing the same drug.
Solution for infusion
EXCIPIENTS: May contain Edetic acid (edta), polysorbates
▸ Rybrevant (Janssen-Cilag Ltd) ▼
Amivantamab 50 mg per 1 ml Rybrevant 350mg/7ml concentrate for solution for infusion vials | 1 vial [PoM] £1,079.00 (Hospital only)

Atezolizumab [Specialist drug]
04-Oct-2022

● **INDICATIONS AND DOSE**

Urothelial carcinoma | Non-small cell lung cancer | Small cell lung cancer | Breast cancer | Hepatocellular carcinoma
▸ BY INTRAVENOUS INFUSION
▸ Adult: Specialist drug – access specialist resources for dosing information

IMPORTANT SAFETY INFORMATION
MHRA/CHM ADVICE: ATEZOLIZUMAB (*TECENTRIQ*®) AND OTHER IMMUNE-STIMULATORY ANTI-CANCER DRUGS: RISK OF SEVERE CUTANEOUS ADVERSE REACTIONS (SCARS) (JUNE 2021)
Severe cutaneous adverse reactions (SCARs), including cases of Stevens-Johnson syndrome (SJS) and toxic epidermal necrolysis (TEN), have been reported in patients treated with immunostimulant antineoplastic drugs, such as atezolizumab. Healthcare professionals are advised to monitor patients for suspected severe skin reactions and exclude other causes. Patients should be advised to seek urgent medical attention if severe skin reactions occur. If a SCAR is suspected, atezolizumab therapy should be withheld and the patient referred to a specialist for diagnosis and treatment. Atezolizumab should be permanently discontinued for any grade confirmed SJS or TEN, and for any grade 4 SCAR. Caution is recommended when considering the use of atezolizumab in patients with a history of severe or life-threatening SCAR associated with other immunostimulant antineoplastic drugs.

● **INTERACTIONS** → Appendix 1: monoclonal antibodies
● **SIDE-EFFECTS**
▸ **Common or very common** Abdominal pain · appetite decreased · arthralgia · ascites · asthenia · cardiac inflammation · chills · cough · cystitis · cytokine release syndrome · diarrhoea · dry mouth · dysphagia · dyspnoea · electrolyte imbalance · euthyroid sick syndrome · eye disorders · fever · gastrointestinal disorders · goitre · haemorrhage · headache · hepatic disorders · hypercreatininaemia · hyperglycaemia · hypersensitivity · hyperthyroidism · hypotension · hypothyroidism · hypoxia · immune-mediated lung disease · increased risk of infection · influenza like illness · infusion related reaction · interstitial lung disease · myalgia · myxoedema · myxoedema coma · nasal complaints · nausea · oesophageal varices · oral disorders · oropharyngeal complaints · pain · pericardial disorders · radiation pneumonitis · renal abscess · respiratory disorders · skin reactions · skin ulcer · throat irritation · thrombocytopenia · thyroid disorder · thyroiditis · ulcerative colitis · vomiting
▸ **Uncommon** Adrenal hypofunction · connective tissue disorders · cutaneous vasculitis · diabetes mellitus · diabetic ketoacidosis · encephalitis autoimmune · ketoacidosis · meningitis · muscle abscess · myopathy · nephritis · nerve disorders · pancreatitis · paraneoplastic glomerulonephritis · photophobia · severe cutaneous adverse reactions (SCARs)
▸ **Rare or very rare** Facial paresis · hypophysitis · neuromuscular dysfunction · temperature regulation disorder · uveitis

SIDE-EFFECTS, FURTHER INFORMATION **Immune-related reactions** Manufacturer advises most immune-related adverse reactions are reversible and managed by temporarily stopping treatment and administration of a corticosteroid.
  Infusion-related reactions Manufacturer advises permanently discontinue treatment in patients with severe infusion reactions.

- **CONCEPTION AND CONTRACEPTION** Manufacturer advises effective contraception in women of childbearing potential, during treatment and for 5 months after stopping treatment.
- **PATIENT AND CARER ADVICE** An alert card should be provided.
  Driving and skilled tasks Manufacturer advises patients should be counselled on the effects on driving and performance of skilled tasks—increased risk of drowsiness.
- **NATIONAL FUNDING/ACCESS DECISIONS**
  For full details see funding body website
  NICE decisions
  ▸ Atezolizumab for treating locally advanced or metastatic urothelial carcinoma after platinum-containing chemotherapy (June 2018) NICE TA525 Recommended with restrictions
  ▸ Atezolizumab for untreated PD-L1-positive advanced urothelial cancer when cisplatin is unsuitable (October 2021) NICE TA739 Recommended
  ▸ Atezolizumab for treating locally advanced or metastatic non-small-cell lung cancer after chemotherapy (May 2018) NICE TA520 Recommended with restrictions
  ▸ Atezolizumab in combination for treating metastatic non-squamous non-small-cell lung cancer (June 2019) NICE TA584 Recommended with restrictions
  ▸ Atezolizumab monotherapy for untreated advanced non-small-cell lung cancer (June 2021) NICE TA705 Recommended
  ▸ Atezolizumab for adjuvant treatment of resected non-small-cell lung cancer (September 2022) NICE TA823 Recommended
  ▸ Atezolizumab with carboplatin and etoposide for untreated extensive-stage small-cell lung cancer (July 2020) NICE TA638 Recommended with restrictions
  ▸ Atezolizumab with nab-paclitaxel for untreated PD-L1-positive, locally advanced or metastatic, triple-negative breast cancer (July 2020) NICE TA639 Recommended
  ▸ Atezolizumab with bevacizumab for treating advanced or unresectable hepatocellular carcinoma (December 2020) NICE TA666 Recommended with restrictions
  Scottish Medicines Consortium (SMC) decisions
  ▸ Atezolizumab (*Tecentriq*®) for the treatment of adult patients with locally advanced or metastatic non-small cell lung cancer (NSCLC) after prior chemotherapy. Patients with EGFR activating mutations or ALK-positive tumour mutations should also have received targeted therapy before receiving *Tecentriq*® (July 2018) SMC No. 1336/18 Recommended with restrictions
  ▸ Atezolizumab (*Tecentriq*®), in combination with bevacizumab, paclitaxel and carboplatin, is indicated for the first-line treatment of adult patients with metastatic non-squamous non-small cell lung cancer (NSCLC) (November 2019) SMC No. SMC2208 Not recommended
  ▸ Atezolizumab (*Tecentriq*®) as monotherapy for the first-line treatment of adult patients with metastatic non-small cell lung cancer (NSCLC) whose tumours have a PD-L1 expression on 50% or more tumour cells (TC) or 10% or more tumour-infiltrating immune cells (IC) and who do not have epidermal growth factor receptor (EGFR) mutant or anaplastic lymphoma kinase (ALK)-positive NSCLC (November 2021) SMC No. SMC2379 Recommended
  ▸ Atezolizumab (*Tecentriq*®) monotherapy as adjuvant treatment following complete resection for adult patients with Stage II to IIIA non-small cell lung cancer (NSCLC) whose tumours have PD-L1 expression on 50% or more tumour cells (TC) and whose disease has not progressed following platinum-based adjuvant chemotherapy (August 2022) SMC No. SMC2492 Recommended
  ▸ Atezolizumab (*Tecentriq*®) in combination with carboplatin and etoposide, is indicated for the first-line treatment of adult patients with extensive-stage small cell lung cancer (November 2020) SMC No. SMC2279 Recommended
  ▸ Atezolizumab (*Tecentriq*®) as monotherapy for the treatment of adult patients with locally advanced or metastatic urothelial carcinoma: after prior platinum-containing chemotherapy, or who are considered cisplatin ineligible (November 2018) SMC No. SMC2103 Not recommended
  ▸ Atezolizumab (*Tecentriq*®) in combination with nab-paclitaxel for the treatment of adult patients with unresectable locally advanced or metastatic triple-negative breast cancer whose tumours have PD-L1 expression at a level of 1% or more and who have not received prior chemotherapy for metastatic disease (November 2020) SMC No. SMC2267 Recommended
  ▸ Atezolizumab (*Tecentriq*®) in combination with bevacizumab for the treatment of adult patients with advanced or unresectable hepatocellular carcinoma who have not received prior systemic therapy (July 2021) SMC No. SMC2349 Recommended

- **MEDICINAL FORMS** There can be variation in the licensing of different medicines containing the same drug.
  Solution for infusion
  EXCIPIENTS: May contain Polysorbates, sucrose
  ▸ **Tecentriq** (Roche Products Ltd)
    Atezolizumab 60 mg per 1 ml Tecentriq 840mg/14ml concentrate for solution for infusion vials | 1 vial PoM £2,665.38 (Hospital only)
    Tecentriq 1200mg/20ml concentrate for solution for infusion vials | 1 vial PoM £3,807.69 (Hospital only)

Avelumab [Specialist drug]

27-May-2022

- **INDICATIONS AND DOSE**

Merkel cell carcinoma | Renal cell carcinoma | Urothelial carcinoma

▸ BY INTRAVENOUS INFUSION
▸ Adult: Specialist drug – access specialist resources for dosing information

---

IMPORTANT SAFETY INFORMATION

MHRA/CHM ADVICE: ATEZOLIZUMAB (*TECENTRIQ*®) AND OTHER IMMUNE-STIMULATORY ANTI-CANCER DRUGS: RISK OF SEVERE CUTANEOUS ADVERSE REACTIONS (SCARS) (JUNE 2021)

Severe cutaneous adverse reactions (SCARs), including cases of Stevens-Johnson syndrome (SJS) and toxic epidermal necrolysis (TEN), have been reported in patients treated with immunostimulant antineoplastic drugs, such as avelumab. Healthcare professionals are advised to monitor patients for suspected severe skin reactions and exclude other causes. Patients should be advised to seek urgent medical attention if severe skin reactions occur. If a SCAR is suspected, avelumab therapy should be withheld and the patient referred to a specialist for diagnosis and treatment. Avelumab should be permanently discontinued for any grade confirmed SJS or TEN, and for any grade 4 SCAR. Caution is recommended when considering the use of avelumab in patients with a history of severe or life-threatening SCAR associated with other immunostimulant antineoplastic drugs.

- **INTERACTIONS** → Appendix 1: monoclonal antibodies
- **SIDE-EFFECTS**
  ▸ **Common or very common** Anaemia · appetite decreased · arthralgia · asthenia · back pain · chills · constipation · cough · diarrhoea · dizziness · dry mouth · dyspnoea · fever · gastrointestinal discomfort · headache · hypertension · hyperthyroidism · hyponatraemia · hypothyroidism · influenza like illness · infusion related reaction · interstitial lung disease · lymphopenia · myalgia · nausea · nerve disorders · peripheral oedema · skin reactions · thrombocytopenia · vomiting · weight decreased
  ▸ **Uncommon** Adrenal hypofunction · arthritis · eosinophilia · flushing · gastrointestinal disorders · hepatic disorders · hyperglycaemia · hypersensitivity · hypotension · myositis · nephritis · neuromuscular dysfunction · renal failure · thyroiditis

‣ **Rare or very rare** Cardiac inflammation · diabetes mellitus · hypopituitarism · pancreatitis · systemic inflammatory response syndrome · uveitis

‣ **Frequency not known** Endocrine disorders

SIDE-EFFECTS, FURTHER INFORMATION **Infusion-related reactions** Manufacturer advises permanently discontinue treatment in patients with grade 3 or 4 infusion-related reactions.

   Immune-related reactions Most immune-related adverse reactions are reversible and managed by temporarily stopping treatment and administration of a corticosteroid.

● CONCEPTION AND CONTRACEPTION Manufacturer advises women of child-bearing potential should use effective contraception during treatment and for at least 1 month after stopping treatment.

● PATIENT AND CARER ADVICE Patients should be provided with an alert card. A patient information brochure highlighting important safety information to minimise the risk of immune-related side-effects is also available. **Driving and skilled tasks** Patients and carers should be counselled on the effects on driving and performance of skilled tasks—increased risk of fatigue.

● NATIONAL FUNDING/ACCESS DECISIONS
For full details see funding body website
NICE decisions
‣ **Avelumab for treating metastatic Merkel cell carcinoma (updated April 2021)** NICE TA517 Recommended with restrictions
‣ **Avelumab for untreated metastatic Merkel cell carcinoma (April 2021)** NICE TA691 Recommended with restrictions
‣ **Avelumab with axitinib for untreated advanced renal cell carcinoma (September 2020)** NICE TA645 Recommended
‣ **Avelumab for maintenance treatment of locally advanced or metastatic urothelial cancer after platinum-based chemotherapy (May 2022)** NICE TA788 Recommended with restrictions
Scottish Medicines Consortium (SMC) decisions
‣ **Avelumab (*Bavencio*®) as monotherapy for the treatment of adult patients with metastatic Merkel cell carcinoma (May 2018)** SMC No. 1315/18 Recommended
‣ **Avelumab (*Bavencio*®) in combination with axitinib for the first-line treatment of adult patients with advanced renal cell carcinoma (October 2020)** SMC No. SMC2248 Recommended
‣ **Avelumab (*Bavencio*®) as monotherapy for the first-line maintenance treatment of adult patients with locally advanced or metastatic urothelial carcinoma who are progression-free following platinum-based chemotherapy (August 2021)** SMC No. SMC2359 Recommended

● MEDICINAL FORMS There can be variation in the licensing of different medicines containing the same drug.
Solution for infusion
  ‣ Bavencio (Merck Serono Ltd)
    Avelumab 20 mg per 1 ml Bavencio 200mg/10ml concentrate for solution for infusion vials | 1 vial [PoM] £768.00

Bevacizumab [Specialist drug]
20-Mar-2025

● **INDICATIONS AND DOSE**
Colorectal cancer | Breast cancer | Renal cell carcinoma | Non-small cell lung cancer | Epithelial ovarian cancer | Fallopian tube cancer | Peritoneal cancer | Cervical carcinoma
  ‣ BY INTRAVENOUS INFUSION
  ‣ Adult: Specialist drug – access specialist resources for dosing information

DOSE EQUIVALENCE AND CONVERSION
‣ Bevacizumab for intravenous infusion and bevacizumab gamma for intravitreal injection are **not** interchangeable.

IMPORTANT SAFETY INFORMATION
MHRA/CHM ADVICE: BEVACIZUMAB AND SUNITINIB: RISK OF OSTEONECROSIS OF THE JAW (JANUARY 2011)
Treatment with bevacizumab or sunitinib may be a risk factor for the development of osteonecrosis of the jaw.
   Patients treated with bevacizumab or sunitinib, who have previously received bisphosphonates, or are treated concurrently with bisphosphonates, may be particularly at risk.
   Dental examination and appropriate preventive dentistry should be considered before treatment with bevacizumab or sunitinib.
   If possible, invasive dental procedures should be avoided in patients treated with bevacizumab or sunitinib who have previously received, or who are currently receiving, intravenous bisphosphonates.

MHRA/CHM ADVICE: SYSTEMICALLY ADMINISTERED VEGF PATHWAY INHIBITORS: RISK OF ANEURYSM AND ARTERY DISSECTION (JULY 2020)
A European review of worldwide data concluded that systemically administered VEGF pathway inhibitors may lead to aneurysm and artery dissection in patients with or without hypertension. Some fatal cases have been reported, mainly in relation to aortic aneurysm rupture and aortic dissection. The MHRA advises healthcare professionals to carefully consider the risk of aneurysm and artery dissection in patients with risk factors before initiating treatment with bevacizumab; any modifiable risk factors (such as smoking and hypertension) should be reduced as much as possible. Blood pressure should be monitored regularly, and product literature should be consulted if hypertension occurs during treatment.

● INTERACTIONS → Appendix 1: monoclonal antibodies

● SIDE-EFFECTS
‣ **Common or very common** Abscess · anaemia · appetite decreased · arthralgia · asthenia · congestive heart failure · constipation · cough · decreased leucocytes · dehydration · diarrhoea · drowsiness · dysarthria · dysphonia · dyspnoea · electrolyte imbalance · embolism and thrombosis · eye disorders · fever · fistula · gastrointestinal discomfort · gastrointestinal disorders · haemorrhage · headache · healing impaired · hypersensitivity · hypertension · hypoxia · increased risk of infection · infusion related reaction · mucositis · muscle weakness · myalgia · nausea · neutropenia · ovarian failure · pain · pelvic pain · peripheral neuropathy · proteinuria · rectovaginal fistula · sepsis · skin reactions · stomatitis · stroke · supraventricular tachycardia · syncope · taste altered · thrombocytopenia · vomiting · weight decreased
‣ **Rare or very rare** Encephalopathy · necrotising fasciitis (discontinue and initiate treatment promptly)
‣ **Frequency not known** Aneurysm · artery dissection · chest pain · chills · flushing · gallbladder perforation · hyperglycaemia · hypotension · nasal septum perforation · osteonecrosis of jaw · pulmonary hypertension · renal thrombotic microangiopathy

● CONCEPTION AND CONTRACEPTION Effective contraception required during and for at least 6 months after treatment in females.

● NATIONAL FUNDING/ACCESS DECISIONS
For full details see funding body website
NICE decisions
‣ **Bevacizumab and cetuximab for the treatment of metastatic colorectal cancer (January 2007)** NICE TA118 Not recommended

▶ Bevacizumab in combination with oxaliplatin and either fluorouracil plus folinic acid or capecitabine for the treatment of metastatic colorectal cancer (December 2010) NICE TA212 Not recommended

▶ Cetuximab, bevacizumab and panitumumab for the treatment of metastatic colorectal cancer after first-line chemotherapy (January 2012) NICE TA242 Not recommended

▶ Bevacizumab (first-line), sorafenib (first and second-line), sunitinib (second-line) and temsirolimus (first-line) for the treatment of advanced and/or metastatic renal cell carcinoma (August 2009) NICE TA178 Not recommended

▶ Bevacizumab in combination with a taxane for the first-line treatment of metastatic breast cancer (February 2011) NICE TA214 Not recommended

▶ Bevacizumab in combination with capecitabine for the first-line treatment of metastatic breast cancer (August 2012) NICE TA263 Not recommended

▶ Bevacizumab in combination with paclitaxel and carboplatin for the first-line treatment of advanced ovarian cancer (May 2013) NICE TA284 Not recommended

▶ Bevacizumab in combination with gemcitabine and carboplatin for the treatment of the first recurrence of platinum-sensitive advanced ovarian cancer (May 2013) NICE TA285 Not recommended

▶ Atezolizumab with bevacizumab for treating advanced or unresectable hepatocellular carcinoma (December 2020) NICE TA666 Recommended with restrictions

▶ Olaparib with bevacizumab for maintenance treatment of advanced high-grade epithelial ovarian, fallopian tube or primary peritoneal cancer (January 2024) NICE TA946 Recommended

Scottish Medicines Consortium (SMC) decisions

▶ Bevacizumab (*Avastin*®) in combination with capecitabine for first-line treatment of metastatic breast cancer (May 2012) SMC No. 778/12 Not recommended

▶ Bevacizumab (*Avastin*®) in combination with paclitaxel, topotecan, or pegylated liposomal doxorubicin for the treatment of platinum-resistant recurrent ovarian, fallopian tube, or primary peritoneal cancer (September 2015) SMC No. 1063/15 Recommended with restrictions

▶ Bevacizumab (*Avastin*®) in combination with carboplatin and paclitaxel, for the front-line treatment of advanced (International Federation of Gynaecology and Obstetrics (FIGO) stages IIIB, IIIC and IV) epithelial ovarian, fallopian tube, or primary peritoneal cancer (November 2015) SMC No. 806/12 Recommended with restrictions

All Wales Medicines Strategy Group (AWMSG) decisions

▶ Bevacizumab (*Avastin*®) in combination with paclitaxel and cisplatin, for the treatment of adult patients with persistent, recurrent, or metastatic carcinoma of the cervix (June 2022) AWMSG No. 5044 Recommended with restrictions

▶ Bevacizumab (*Avastin*®) in combination with paclitaxel and topotecan in patients who cannot receive platinum therapy, for the treatment of adult patients with persistent, recurrent, or metastatic carcinoma of the cervix (June 2022) AWMSG No. 5044 Not recommended

● **MEDICINAL FORMS** There can be variation in the licensing of different medicines containing the same drug. Forms available from special-order manufacturers include: solution for injection

Solution for infusion

▶ Abevmy (Biosimilar Collaborations Ireland Ltd) ▼
Bevacizumab 25 mg per 1 ml Abevmy 400mg/16ml concentrate for solution for infusion vials | 1 vial PoM £810.00 (Hospital only)
Abevmy 100mg/4ml concentrate for solution for infusion vials | 1 vial PoM £202.50 (Hospital only)

▶ Alymsys (Zentiva Pharma UK Ltd) ▼
Bevacizumab 25 mg per 1 ml Alymsys 400mg/16ml concentrate for solution for infusion vials | 1 vial PoM £810.10 (Hospital only)
Alymsys 100mg/4ml concentrate for solution for infusion vials | 1 vial PoM £205.55 (Hospital only)

▶ Avastin (Roche Products Ltd)
Bevacizumab 25 mg per 1 ml Avastin 400mg/16ml solution for infusion vials | 1 vial PoM £924.40 (Hospital only)
Avastin 100mg/4ml solution for infusion vials | 1 vial PoM £242.66 (Hospital only)

▶ Aybintio (Organon Pharma (UK) Ltd) ▼
Bevacizumab 25 mg per 1 ml Aybintio 100mg/4ml solution for infusion vials | 1 vial PoM £218.39 (Hospital only)
Aybintio 400mg/16ml solution for infusion vials | 1 vial PoM £831.96 (Hospital only)

▶ Oyavas (Thornton & Ross Ltd) ▼
Bevacizumab 25 mg per 1 ml Oyavas 400mg/16ml concentrate for solution for infusion vials | 1 vial PoM £877.80 (Hospital only)
Oyavas 100mg/4ml concentrate for solution for infusion vials | 1 vial PoM £230.00 (Hospital only)

▶ Vegzelma (Celltrion Healthcare UK Ltd) ▼
Bevacizumab 25 mg per 1 ml Vegzelma 400mg/16ml concentrate for solution for infusion vials | 1 vial PoM £810.00 (Hospital only)
Vegzelma 100mg/4ml concentrate for solution for infusion vials | 1 vial PoM £205.00 (Hospital only)

▶ Versavo (Dr Reddy's Laboratories (UK) Ltd) ▼
Bevacizumab 25 mg per 1 ml Versavo 400mg/16ml concentrate for solution for infusion vials | 1 vial PoM £924.40 (Hospital only)
Versavo 100mg/4ml concentrate for solution for infusion vials | 1 vial PoM £242.66 (Hospital only)

▶ Zirabev (Pfizer Ltd)
Bevacizumab 25 mg per 1 ml Zirabev 400mg/16ml solution for infusion vials | 1 vial PoM £902.70 (Hospital only)
Zirabev 100mg/4ml solution for infusion vials | 1 vial PoM £225.67 (Hospital only)

Blinatumomab [Specialist drug]

01-Apr-2025

● **INDICATIONS AND DOSE**

Acute lymphoblastic leukaemia

▶ BY CONTINUOUS INTRAVENOUS INFUSION

▶ Adult: Specialist drug – access specialist resources for dosing information

● **INTERACTIONS** → Appendix 1: monoclonal antibodies

● **SIDE-EFFECTS**

▶ **Common or very common** Abdominal pain · anaemia · arrhythmias · ataxia · chest discomfort · chills · cognitive disorder · confusion · constipation · cough · cranial nerve disorder · cytokine release syndrome · decreased leucocytes · diarrhoea · dizziness · drowsiness · dyspnoea · encephalopathy · facial swelling · fever · flushing · headache · hyperbilirubinaemia · hypersensitivity · hypertension · hypogammaglobulinaemia · hypoglobulinaemia · hypotension · increased risk of infection · infusion related reaction · insomnia · leucocytosis · memory loss · nausea · neutropenia · oedema · pain · respiratory disorders · seizure · sensation abnormal · sepsis · skin reactions · speech impairment · thrombocytopenia · tremor · tumour lysis syndrome · vomiting · weight increased

▶ **Uncommon** Capillary leak syndrome · cytokine storm · haemophagocytic lymphohistiocytosis · lymphadenopathy · pancreatitis

▶ **Frequency not known** Consciousness impaired · psychiatric disorder · viral infection reactivation

SIDE-EFFECTS, FURTHER INFORMATION **Cytokine release syndrome, infusion-reactions, and tumour lysis syndrome** Life-threatening (including fatal) cases of cytokine release syndrome and tumour lysis syndrome have been reported in patients taking blinatumomab; temporary interruption or discontinuation might be required.

Neurological events There is potentially a higher risk of neurological events in patients with clinically relevant CNS pathology.

Pancreatitis Life-threatening or fatal cases of pancreatitis have been reported; temporary interruption or discontinuation might be required.

- **CONCEPTION AND CONTRACEPTION** Manufacturer advises effective contraception during treatment and for at least 48 hours after treatment in women of child-bearing potential.

- **PATIENT AND CARER ADVICE** A patient alert card should be provided. Educational materials should be provided to patients and carers to ensure blinatumomab is used in a safe and effective way, and to prevent the risk of medication errors and neurological events—consult product information.
  Driving and skilled tasks Manufacturer advises patients and carers should be counselled about the effects on driving and performance of skilled tasks—increased risk of confusion, disorientation, co-ordination and balance disorders, seizures and disturbances in consciousness.

- **NATIONAL FUNDING/ACCESS DECISIONS**
  For full details see funding body website
  NICE decisions
  - Blinatumomab for previously treated Philadelphia-chromosome-negative acute lymphoblastic leukaemia (June 2017) NICE TA450 Recommended
  - Blinatumomab for treating acute lymphoblastic leukaemia in remission with minimal residual disease activity (July 2019) NICE TA589 Recommended with restrictions
  - Blinatumomab with chemotherapy for consolidation treatment of Philadelphia-chromosome-negative CD19-positive minimal residual disease-negative B-cell precursor acute lymphoblastic leukaemia (March 2025) NICE TA1049 Recommended with restrictions

  Scottish Medicines Consortium (SMC) decisions
  - Blinatumomab (*Blincyto*®) as monotherapy for the treatment of adults with Philadelphia chromosome-negative CD19 positive B-precursor acute lymphoblastic leukaemia in first or second complete remission with minimal residual disease greater than or equal to 0.1% (March 2020) SMC No. SMC2234 Recommended with restrictions

- **MEDICINAL FORMS** There can be variation in the licensing of different medicines containing the same drug.
  Powder for solution for infusion
  EXCIPIENTS: May contain Polysorbates
  - Blincyto (Amgen Ltd) ▼
    Blinatumomab 38.5 microgram Blincyto 38.5micrograms powder for concentrate and solution for solution for infusion vials | 1 vial [PoM] £2,017.00 (Hospital only)

Brentuximab vedotin [Specialist drug]

03-Feb-2021

- **INDICATIONS AND DOSE**
  Hodgkin lymphoma | Systemic anaplastic large cell lymphoma | Cutaneous T-cell lymphoma
  - BY INTRAVENOUS INFUSION
  - Adult: Specialist drug – access specialist resources for dosing information

- **INTERACTIONS** → Appendix 1: monoclonal antibodies

- **SIDE-EFFECTS**
  - **Common or very common** Abdominal pain · alopecia · anaemia · arthralgia · back pain · chills · constipation · cough · diarrhoea · dizziness · dyspnoea · fatigue · fever · hyperglycaemia · increased risk of infection · infusion related reaction · myalgia · nausea · nerve disorders · neutropenia · skin reactions · thrombocytopenia · vomiting · weight decreased
  - **Uncommon** Anaphylactic reaction · cytomegalovirus infection reactivation · pancreatitis acute (sometimes fatal, discontinue) · sepsis · severe cutaneous adverse reactions (SCARs) · tumour lysis syndrome
  - **Frequency not known** Acute respiratory distress syndrome (ARDS) · disease recurrence · gastrointestinal disorders ·

gastrointestinal haemorrhage · interstitial lung disease · progressive multifocal leukoencephalopathy (PML)

- **CONCEPTION AND CONTRACEPTION** Effective contraception required during treatment and for 6 months after treatment in men and women.

- **NATIONAL FUNDING/ACCESS DECISIONS**
  For full details see funding body website
  NICE decisions
  - Brentuximab vedotin for treating relapsed or refractory systemic anaplastic large cell lymphoma (October 2017) NICE TA478 Recommended with restrictions
  - Brentuximab vedotin in combination for untreated systemic anaplastic large cell lymphoma (August 2020) NICE TA641 Recommended
  - Brentuximab vedotin for treating CD30-positive Hodgkin lymphoma (June 2018) NICE TA524 Recommended with restrictions
  - Brentuximab vedotin for treating CD30-positive cutaneous T-cell lymphoma (April 2019) NICE TA577 Recommended with restrictions

  Scottish Medicines Consortium (SMC) decisions
  - Brentuximab vedotin (*Adcetris*®) for the treatment of adult patients with CD30-positive cutaneous T-cell lymphoma (CTCL) after at least one prior systemic therapy (January 2020) SMC No. SMC2229 Recommended with restrictions
  - Brentuximab vedotin (*Adcetris*®) in combination with cyclophosphamide, doxorubicin and prednisone for adult patients with previously untreated systemic anaplastic large cell lymphoma (sALCL) (January 2021) SMC No. SMC2310 Recommended

- **MEDICINAL FORMS** There can be variation in the licensing of different medicines containing the same drug.
  Powder for solution for infusion
  EXCIPIENTS: May contain Polysorbates
  ELECTROLYTES: May contain Sodium
  - Adcetris (Takeda UK Ltd)
    Brentuximab vedotin 50 mg Adcetris 50mg powder for concentrate for solution for infusion vials | 1 vial [PoM] £2,500.00 (Hospital only)

Cemiplimab [Specialist drug]

05-Mar-2025

- **INDICATIONS AND DOSE**
  Cutaneous squamous cell carcinoma | Basal cell carcinoma | Non-small cell lung cancer | Cervical cancer
  - BY INTRAVENOUS INFUSION
  - Adult: Specialist drug – access specialist resources for dosing information

---

IMPORTANT SAFETY INFORMATION

MHRA/CHM ADVICE: ATEZOLIZUMAB (*TECENTRIQ*®) AND OTHER IMMUNE-STIMULATORY ANTI-CANCER DRUGS: RISK OF SEVERE CUTANEOUS ADVERSE REACTIONS (SCARS) (JUNE 2021)
Severe cutaneous adverse reactions (SCARs), including cases of Stevens-Johnson syndrome (SJS) and toxic epidermal necrolysis (TEN), have been reported in patients treated with immunostimulant antineoplastic drugs, such as cemiplimab. Healthcare professionals are advised to monitor patients for suspected severe skin reactions and exclude other causes. Patients should be advised to seek urgent medical attention if severe skin reactions occur. If a SCAR is suspected, cemiplimab therapy should be withheld and the patient referred to a specialist for diagnosis and treatment. Cemiplimab should be permanently discontinued for any grade confirmed SJS or TEN, and for any grade 4 SCAR. Caution is recommended when considering the use of cemiplimab in patients with a history of severe or life-threatening SCAR associated with other immunostimulant antineoplastic drugs.

- INTERACTIONS → Appendix 1: monoclonal antibodies
- SIDE-EFFECTS
  ▶ **Common or very common** Anaemia · appetite decreased · arthralgia · asthenia · constipation · cough · cystitis · diarrhoea · dyspnoea · erythema nodosum · facial swelling · fever · gastrointestinal discomfort · gastrointestinal disorders · headache · hepatic disorders · hyperbilirubinaemia · hyperpyrexia · hypertension · hyperthermia · hyperthyroidism · hypothyroidism · immune-mediated lung disease · increased risk of infection · inflammation · infusion related reaction · interstitial lung disease · malaise · musculoskeletal discomfort · myalgia · nausea · nephritis · nephrotoxicity · nerve disorders · oedema · pain · paraesthesia · pulmonary fibrosis · renal impairment · skin reactions · stomatitis · urosepsis · vomiting
  ▶ **Uncommon** Adrenal insufficiency · arthritis · cardiac inflammation · connective tissue disorders · hypophysitis · lymphocytic hypophysitis · muscle weakness · myositis · thrombocytopenia · thyroiditis
  ▶ **Rare or very rare** Diabetic ketoacidosis · eye inflammation · meningitis · myasthenia gravis · paraneoplastic encephalomyelitis · type 1 diabetes mellitus
  ▶ **Frequency not known** Haemophagocytic lymphohistiocytosis · severe cutaneous adverse reactions (SCARs) · solid organ transplant rejection
- CONCEPTION AND CONTRACEPTION Manufacturer advises females of childbearing potential should use effective contraception during treatment and for at least 4 months after the last dose.
- PATIENT AND CARER ADVICE
  Risk of immune-related side-effects A patient alert card and patient guide should be provided.
- NATIONAL FUNDING/ACCESS DECISIONS
  For full details see funding body website
  NICE decisions
  ▶ **Cemiplimab for treating advanced cutaneous squamous cell carcinoma (June 2022)** NICE TA802 Recommended with restrictions
  Scottish Medicines Consortium (SMC) decisions
  ▶ **Cemiplimab (*Libtayo*®) as monotherapy for the treatment of adult patients with metastatic or locally advanced cutaneous squamous cell carcinoma (CSCC) who are not candidates for curative surgery or curative radiation (December 2023)** SMC No. SMC2584 Recommended
  ▶ **Cemiplimab (*Libtayo*®) as monotherapy for the treatment of adult patients with recurrent or metastatic cervical cancer and disease progression on or after platinum-based chemotherapy (February 2025)** SMC No. SMC2719 Recommended

- MEDICINAL FORMS There can be variation in the licensing of different medicines containing the same drug.
  Solution for infusion
  EXCIPIENTS: May contain L-proline, polysorbates, sucrose
  ▶ **Libtayo** (Regeneron UK Ltd) ▼
  Cemiplimab 50 mg per 1 ml Libtayo 350mg/7ml concentrate for solution for infusion vials | 1 vial [PoM] £4,650.00 (Hospital only)

Cetuximab [Specialist drug]   20-May-2021

- **INDICATIONS AND DOSE**
  Colorectal cancer | Squamous cell cancer of the head and neck
  ▶ BY INTRAVENOUS INFUSION
  ▶ Adult: Specialist drug – access specialist resources for dosing information

---

IMPORTANT SAFETY INFORMATION
Patients must receive an antihistamine and a corticosteroid at least one hour before infusion. Resuscitation facilities should be available during administration.

MHRA/CHM ADVICE: EPIDERMAL GROWTH FACTOR RECEPTOR (EGFR) INHIBITORS: SERIOUS CASES OF KERATITIS AND ULCERATIVE KERATITIS (MAY 2012)
Keratitis and ulcerative keratitis have been reported following treatment with epidermal growth factor receptor (EGFR) inhibitors for cancer (cetuximab, erlotinib, gefitinib and panitumumab). In rare cases, this has resulted in corneal perforation and blindness. Patients undergoing treatment with EGFR inhibitors who present with acute or worsening signs and symptoms suggestive of keratitis should be referred promptly to an ophthalmology specialist. Treatment should be interrupted or discontinued if ulcerative keratitis is diagnosed.

- CONTRA-INDICATIONS *RAS* mutated colorectal tumours (or if *RAS* tumour status unknown)
- INTERACTIONS → Appendix 1: monoclonal antibodies
- SIDE-EFFECTS
  ▶ **Common or very common** Appetite decreased · cytokine release syndrome · dehydration · diarrhoea · electrolyte imbalance · eye inflammation · fatigue · headache · hypersensitivity · infusion related reaction · mucositis · nausea · skin eruption · vomiting
  ▶ **Uncommon** Embolism and thrombosis · interstitial lung disease (discontinue)
  ▶ **Rare or very rare** Severe cutaneous adverse reactions (SCARs)
  ▶ **Frequency not known** Meningitis aseptic · superinfection of skin lesions
  SIDE-EFFECTS, FURTHER INFORMATION Infusion-related reactions may be delayed; consult product literature for details.
- CONCEPTION AND CONTRACEPTION Contraceptive advice required.
- NATIONAL FUNDING/ACCESS DECISIONS
  For full details see funding body website
  NICE decisions
  ▶ **Cetuximab for the treatment of locally advanced squamous cell cancer of the head and neck (June 2008)** NICE TA145 Recommended
  ▶ **Cetuximab for treating recurrent or metastatic squamous cell cancer of the head and neck (August 2017)** NICE TA473 Recommended
  ▶ **Cetuximab, bevacizumab and panitumumab for the treatment of metastatic colorectal cancer after first-line chemotherapy (January 2012)** NICE TA242 Not recommended
  ▶ **Cetuximab and panitumumab for previously untreated metastatic colorectal cancer (updated September 2017)** NICE TA439 Recommended with restrictions
  ▶ **Encorafenib plus cetuximab for previously treated BRAF V600E mutation-positive metastatic colorectal cancer (January 2021)** NICE TA668 Recommended

- **MEDICINAL FORMS** There can be variation in the licensing of different medicines containing the same drug.

Solution for infusion

▶ **Erbitux** (Merck Serono Ltd)

Cetuximab 5 mg per 1 ml Erbitux 100mg/20ml solution for infusion vials | 1 vial [PoM] £178.10 (Hospital only)
Erbitux 500mg/100ml solution for infusion vials | 1 vial [PoM] £890.50 (Hospital only)

Daratumumab
03-Apr-2024

- **DRUG ACTION** Daratumumab is a monoclonal antibody that binds to CD38, a cell-surface protein, resulting in tumour cell death by immune-mediated actions and apoptosis.

- **INDICATIONS AND DOSE**

Multiple myeloma (specialist use only)

▶ BY INTRAVENOUS INFUSION, OR BY SUBCUTANEOUS INJECTION
▶ Adult: Specialist indication – access specialist resources for dosing information

Light-chain (AL) amyloidosis (under expert supervision)

▶ BY SUBCUTANEOUS INJECTION
▶ Adult: (consult product literature or local protocols)

IMPORTANT SAFETY INFORMATION

MHRA/CHM ADVICE: DARATUMUMAB (*DARZALEX*®): RISK OF REACTIVATION OF HEPATITIS B VIRUS (AUGUST 2019)
An EU cumulative review of worldwide data has identified reports of hepatitis B virus (HBV) reactivation in patients treated with daratumumab, including several fatal cases. Healthcare professionals are advised to screen all patients for hepatitis B before starting treatment; patients with unknown serology already being treated with daratumumab should also be screened. Those with positive serology should be monitored for signs of HBV reactivation during, and for at least 6 months after, treatment; immediate medical attention should be sought if signs and symptoms of HBV reactivation develop. Daratumumab should be stopped in patients with HBV reactivation and appropriate treatment initiated, based on expert advice. Experts should be consulted before resuming daratumumab in patients with adequately controlled viral reactivation.

- **CAUTIONS** History of obstructive pulmonary disorder (consider additional post-medication—consult product literature) · patients may need pre-medication to minimise adverse reactions · risk of herpes zoster reactivation (consider antiviral prophylaxis)

CAUTIONS, FURTHER INFORMATION

▶ Infusion-related reactions Serious infusion-related reactions can occur following either intravenous or subcutaneous injection, and daratumumab should only be administered by appropriately trained staff where resuscitation facilities are available; manufacturer advises pre-medication with a corticosteroid, an antihistamine and an anti-pyretic and post-medication with oral corticosteroids—consult product literature. Manufacturer advises patients should be closely monitored for signs of infusion-related reactions during and after administration; in the event of a hypersensitivity reaction, treatment should be stopped immediately and appropriate management initiated.

- **INTERACTIONS** → Appendix 1: monoclonal antibodies

- **SIDE-EFFECTS**

▶ **Common or very common** Anaemia · appetite decreased · arthralgia · asthenia · atrial fibrillation · chills · constipation · cough · decreased leucocytes · dehydration · diarrhoea · dizziness · dyspnoea · fever · headache · hyperglycaemia · hypertension · hypocalcaemia · hypogammaglobulinaemia · increased risk of infection · infusion related reaction · insomnia · muscle spasms · nausea · neutropenia · pain · pancreatitis · paraesthesia · peripheral neuropathy · peripheral oedema · pulmonary oedema · sepsis · skin reactions · syncope · thrombocytopenia · vomiting

▶ **Uncommon** Hepatitis B reactivation

▶ **Rare or very rare** Anaphylactic reaction

SIDE-EFFECTS, FURTHER INFORMATION Manufacturer advises treatment should be immediately interrupted if an infusion-related reaction of any grade or severity occurs—consult product literature for specific management recommendations.

- **CONCEPTION AND CONTRACEPTION** Manufacturer advises effective contraception in women of childbearing potential during treatment and for 3 months after stopping treatment. See also *Pregnancy and reproductive function* in Cytotoxic drugs p. 1027.

- **PREGNANCY** [EvGr] Avoid—no information available. ⓜ See also *Pregnancy and reproductive function* in Cytotoxic drugs p. 1027.

- **BREAST FEEDING** Manufacturer advises avoid—no information available.

- **EFFECT ON LABORATORY TESTS** Possible positive indirect Coombs test (may affect antibody screening).

- **HANDLING AND STORAGE** Manufacturer advises store in a refrigerator at 2–8°C; consult product literature for storage advice following dilution.

- **NATIONAL FUNDING/ACCESS DECISIONS**
For full details see funding body website

NICE decisions

▶ **Daratumumab in combination for untreated multiple myeloma when a stem cell transplant is suitable (February 2022)** NICE TA763 Recommended

▶ **Daratumumab monotherapy for treating relapsed and refractory multiple myeloma (April 2022)** NICE TA783 Recommended with restrictions

▶ **Daratumumab with bortezomib and dexamethasone for previously treated multiple myeloma (June 2023)** NICE TA897 Recommended with restrictions

▶ **Daratumumab with lenalidomide and dexamethasone for untreated multiple myeloma when a stem cell transplant is unsuitable (October 2023)** NICE TA917 Recommended

▶ **Daratumumab in combination for treating newly diagnosed systemic amyloid light-chain amyloidosis (March 2024)** NICE TA959 Recommended with restrictions

Scottish Medicines Consortium (SMC) decisions

▶ **Daratumumab (*Darzalex*®) as monotherapy, for the treatment of adult patients with relapsed and refractory multiple myeloma, whose prior therapy included a proteasome inhibitor and an immunomodulatory agent and have demonstrated disease progression on the last therapy (October 2017)** SMC No. 1205/17 Recommended with restrictions

▶ **Daratumumab (*Darzalex*®) in combination with lenalidomide and dexamethasone, or bortezomib and dexamethasone, for the treatment of adult patients with multiple myeloma who have received at least one prior therapy (July 2019)** SMC No. SMC2180 Recommended with restrictions

▶ **Daratumumab subcutaneous injection (*Darzalex*®) in combination with lenalidomide and dexamethasone, or bortezomib and dexamethasone, for the treatment of adult patients with multiple myeloma who have received at least one prior therapy (October 2020)** SMC No. SMC2301 Recommended with restrictions

▶ **Daratumumab subcutaneous injection (*Darzalex*®) as monotherapy, for the treatment of adult patients with relapsed and refractory multiple myeloma, whose prior therapy included a proteasome inhibitor and an immunomodulatory agent and have demonstrated disease

progression on the last therapy (October 2020)
SMC No. SMC2304 Recommended with restrictions
▶ Daratumumab (*Darzalex*®) in combination with bortezomib, thalidomide and dexamethasone for the treatment of adult patients with newly diagnosed multiple myeloma who are eligible for autologous stem cell transplant (January 2021) SMC No. SMC2302 Recommended
▶ Daratumumab subcutaneous injection (*Darzalex*®) in combination with bortezomib, thalidomide and dexamethasone for the treatment of adult patients with newly diagnosed multiple myeloma who are eligible for autologous stem cell transplant (January 2021) SMC No. SMC2326 Recommended
▶ Daratumumab (*Darzalex*®) in combination with bortezomib, melphalan and prednisone for the treatment of adult patients with newly diagnosed multiple myeloma who are ineligible for autologous stem cell transplant (May 2022) SMC No. SMC2416 Not recommended
▶ Daratumumab (*Darzalex*®) in combination with lenalidomide and dexamethasone for the treatment of adult patients with newly diagnosed multiple myeloma who are ineligible for autologous stem cell transplant (September 2023) SMC No. SMC2536 Recommended
▶ Daratumumab subcutaneous injection (*Darzalex*®) in combination with cyclophosphamide, bortezomib and dexamethasone for the treatment of adult patients with newly diagnosed systemic light chain amyloidosis (August 2022) SMC No. SMC2447 Recommended

● **MEDICINAL FORMS** There can be variation in the licensing of different medicines containing the same drug.
Solution for injection
EXCIPIENTS: May contain Polysorbates, sorbitol
▶ **Darzalex** (Janssen-Cilag Ltd)
Daratumumab 120 mg per 1 ml Darzalex 1800mg/15ml solution for injection vials | 1 vial PoM £4,320.00 (Hospital only)
Solution for infusion
EXCIPIENTS: May contain Polysorbates
ELECTROLYTES: May contain Sodium
▶ **Darzalex** (Janssen-Cilag Ltd)
Daratumumab 20 mg per 1 ml Darzalex 400mg/20ml concentrate for solution for infusion vials | 1 vial PoM £1,440.00 (Hospital only)
Darzalex 100mg/5ml concentrate for solution for infusion vials | 1 vial PoM £360.00 (Hospital only)

Dinutuximab beta [Specialist drug]

04-Nov-2020

● **INDICATIONS AND DOSE**

Neuroblastoma
▶ BY INTRAVENOUS INFUSION
▶ Adult: Specialist drug – access specialist resources for dosing information

IMPORTANT SAFETY INFORMATION
Resuscitation facilities should be available during administration.

● **CONTRA-INDICATIONS** Acute grade 3 or 4, or extensive chronic graft-versus-host disease
● **INTERACTIONS** → Appendix 1: monoclonal antibodies
● **SIDE-EFFECTS**
▶ **Common or very common** Anaemia · anxiety · appetite decreased · arthralgia · ascites · capillary leak syndrome · chest pain · chills · constipation · cough · cytokine release syndrome · decreased leucocytes · device related infection · diarrhoea · dizziness · dyspnoea · electrolyte imbalance · eye disorders · eye inflammation · fever · fluid imbalance · gastrointestinal discomfort · gastrointestinal disorders · haematuria · headache · heart failure · hyperhidrosis · hypersensitivity · hypertension · hypertriglyceridaemia ·

hypoalbuminaemia · hypotension · hypoxia · increased risk of infection · left ventricular dysfunction · muscle spasms · nausea · neutropenia · oedema · oral disorders · pain · paraesthesia · pericardial effusion · peripheral neuropathy · photosensitivity reaction · pulmonary oedema · renal impairment · respiratory disorders · seizure · sepsis · skin reactions · tachycardia · thrombocytopenia · tremor · urinary retention · urine abnormalities · vision disorders · vomiting · weight changes
▶ **Uncommon** Disseminated intravascular coagulation · eosinophilia · hepatocellular injury · hypovolaemic shock · intracranial pressure increased · peripheral vascular disease · posterior reversible encephalopathy syndrome (PRES)
▶ **Frequency not known** Erythropenia
● **CONCEPTION AND CONTRACEPTION** Manufacturer advises women of childbearing potential should use contraception during and for 6 months after stopping treatment.
● **PATIENT AND CARER ADVICE**
Driving and skilled tasks Manufacturer advises patients should not use or drive machines during treatment.
● **NATIONAL FUNDING/ACCESS DECISIONS**
For full details see funding body website
NICE decisions
▶ Dinutuximab beta for treating neuroblastoma (August 2018) NICE TA538 Recommended with restrictions
Scottish Medicines Consortium (SMC) decisions
▶ Dinutuximab beta (*Qarziba*®) for the treatment of high-risk neuroblastoma in patients aged 12 months and above, who have previously received induction chemotherapy and achieved at least a partial response, followed by myeloablative therapy and stem cell transplantation, as well as patients with history of relapsed or refractory neuroblastoma, with or without residual disease (November 2018) SMC No. SMC2105 Recommended

● **MEDICINAL FORMS** There can be variation in the licensing of different medicines containing the same drug.
Solution for infusion
▶ **Qarziba** (Recordati UK Ltd) ▼
Dinutuximab beta 4.5 mg per 1 ml Qarziba 20mg/4.5ml concentrate for solution for infusion vials | 1 vial PoM £7,610.00 (Hospital only)

Dostarlimab [Specialist drug]

03-May-2024

● **INDICATIONS AND DOSE**
Endometrial cancer
▶ BY INTRAVENOUS INFUSION
▶ Adult: Specialist drug – access specialist resources for dosing information

● **INTERACTIONS** → Appendix 1: monoclonal antibodies
● **SIDE-EFFECTS**
▶ **Common or very common** Adrenal insufficiency · anaemia · arthralgia · autoimmune haemolytic anaemia · chills · diarrhoea · enterocolitis haemorrhagic · fever · gastrointestinal disorders · hyperthyroidism · hypertransaminasaemia · hypothyroidism · infusion related reaction · interstitial lung disease · myalgia · nausea · pancreatitis · skin reactions · vomiting
▶ **Uncommon** Diabetic ketoacidosis · eye inflammation · hepatic disorders · hypophysitis · nephritis · thyroiditis · type 1 diabetes mellitus
▶ **Frequency not known** Hypersensitivity

SIDE-EFFECTS, FURTHER INFORMATION **Immune-related reactions** Manufacturer advises most immune-related adverse reactions are reversible and managed by temporarily stopping treatment and administration of a corticosteroid.

Infusion-related reactions Manufacturer advises permanently discontinue treatment in patients with severe infusion reactions.

● **CONCEPTION AND CONTRACEPTION** EvGr Females of childbearing potential should use effective contraception during treatment and for 4 months after last treatment. ◈M◈

● **PATIENT AND CARER ADVICE** A patient card should be provided.

● **NATIONAL FUNDING/ACCESS DECISIONS**
For full details see funding body website
NICE decisions
▸ Dostarlimab for previously treated advanced or recurrent endometrial cancer with high microsatellite instability or mismatch repair deficiency (March 2022) NICE TA779 Recommended
▸ Dostarlimab with platinum-based chemotherapy for treating advanced or recurrent endometrial cancer with high microsatellite instability or mismatch repair deficiency (April 2024) NICE TA963 Recommended

Scottish Medicines Consortium (SMC) decisions
▸ Dostarlimab (*Jemperli*®) as monotherapy for the treatment of adult patients with recurrent or advanced mismatch repair deficient or microsatellite instability-high endometrial cancer that has progressed on or following prior treatment with a platinum-containing regimen (March 2022) SMC No. SMC2404 Recommended
▸ Dostarlimab (*Jemperli*®) in combination with platinum-containing chemotherapy for the treatment of adult patients with mismatch repair deficient or microsatellite instability-high primary advanced or recurrent endometrial cancer and who are candidates for systemic therapy (April 2024) SMC No. SMC2635 Recommended

● **MEDICINAL FORMS** There can be variation in the licensing of different medicines containing the same drug.
Solution for infusion
EXCIPIENTS: May contain Polysorbates
▸ Jemperli (GlaxoSmithKline UK Ltd) ▼
Dostarlimab 50 mg per 1 ml Jemperli 500mg/10ml concentrate for solution for infusion vials | 1 vial PoM £5,887.33 (Hospital only)

Durvalumab [Specialist drug]

27-Feb-2025

● **INDICATIONS AND DOSE**
Non-small cell lung cancer | Small cell lung cancer | Biliary tract cancer
▸ BY INTRAVENOUS INFUSION
▸ Adult: Specialist drug – access specialist resources for dosing information

IMPORTANT SAFETY INFORMATION
MHRA/CHM ADVICE: ATEZOLIZUMAB (*TECENTRIQ*®) AND OTHER IMMUNE-STIMULATORY ANTI-CANCER DRUGS: RISK OF SEVERE CUTANEOUS ADVERSE REACTIONS (SCARS) (JUNE 2021)
Severe cutaneous adverse reactions (SCARs), including cases of Stevens-Johnson syndrome (SJS) and toxic epidermal necrolysis (TEN), have been reported in patients treated with immunostimulant antineoplastic drugs, such as durvalumab. Healthcare professionals are advised to monitor patients for suspected severe skin reactions and exclude other causes. Patients should be advised to seek urgent medical attention if severe skin reactions occur. If a SCAR is suspected, durvalumab therapy should be withheld and the patient referred to a specialist for diagnosis and treatment. Durvalumab should be permanently discontinued for any grade confirmed SJS or TEN, and for any grade 4 SCAR. Caution is recommended when considering the use of durvalumab in patients with a history of severe or life-threatening SCAR associated with other immunostimulant antineoplastic drugs.

● **SIDE-EFFECTS**
▸ **Common or very common** Arthralgia · cough · diarrhoea · dysphonia · dysuria · fever · flank pain · gastrointestinal discomfort · hyperthyroidism · hypothyroidism · increased risk of infection · infusion related reaction · interstitial lung disease · myalgia · night sweats · peripheral oedema · peripheral swelling · skin reactions
▸ **Uncommon** Adrenal insufficiency · gastrointestinal disorders · glomerulonephritis · hepatic disorders · immune-mediated pancreatitis · myopathy · nephritis · pancreatitis · thyroiditis
▸ **Rare or very rare** Cystitis · diabetes insipidus · hypophysitis · hypopituitarism · immune thrombocytopenic purpura · immune-mediated arthritis · meningitis · meningitis non-infective · myasthenia gravis · myocarditis · polymyalgia rheumatica · type 1 diabetes mellitus · uveitis
▸ **Frequency not known** Encephalitis non-infective · Guillain-Barre syndrome · transverse myelitis

SIDE-EFFECTS, FURTHER INFORMATION **Immune-related reactions** Manufacturer advises that most immune-related adverse reactions resolved with appropriate management, including initiation of immunosuppressive treatment and treatment modifications.

Infusion-related reactions Manufacturer advises to permanently discontinue treatment in patients with severe infusion reactions.

● **CONCEPTION AND CONTRACEPTION** Manufacturer advises effective contraception in women of childbearing potential during treatment and for at least 3 months after stopping treatment.

● **NATIONAL FUNDING/ACCESS DECISIONS**
For full details see funding body website
NICE decisions
▸ Durvalumab for maintenance treatment of unresectable non-small-cell lung cancer after platinum-based chemoradiation (June 2022) NICE TA798 Recommended with restrictions
▸ Durvalumab with chemotherapy before surgery (neoadjuvant) then alone after surgery (adjuvant) for treating resectable non-small-cell lung cancer (January 2025) NICE TA1030 Recommended
▸ Durvalumab with etoposide and either carboplatin or cisplatin for untreated extensive-stage small-cell lung cancer (February 2025) NICE TA1041 Recommended with restrictions
▸ Durvalumab with gemcitabine and cisplatin for treating unresectable or advanced biliary tract cancer (January 2024) NICE TA944 Recommended

Scottish Medicines Consortium (SMC) decisions
▸ Durvalumab (*Imfinzi*®) for locally advanced, unresectable non-small cell lung cancer after platinum-based chemoradiation in adults (June 2019) SMC No. SMC2156 Recommended
▸ Durvalumab (*Imfinzi*®) in combination with platinum-based chemotherapy as neoadjuvant treatment, followed by durvalumab as monotherapy after surgery, is indicated for the treatment of adults with resectable (tumours 4 cm or more and/or node-positive) non-small cell lung cancer and no known EGFR mutations or ALK rearrangements (December 2024) SMC No. SMC2677 Not recommended
▸ Durvalumab (*Imfinzi*®) in combination with etoposide and either carboplatin or cisplatin is indicated for the first-line treatment of adults with extensive-stage small cell lung cancer (February 2025) SMC No. SMC2734 Recommended
▸ Durvalumab (*Imfinzi*®) in combination with gemcitabine and cisplatin for the first-line treatment of adults with locally advanced, unresectable, or metastatic biliary tract cancer (November 2023) SMC No. SMC2582 Recommended

● **MEDICINAL FORMS** There can be variation in the licensing of different medicines containing the same drug.
Solution for infusion
EXCIPIENTS: May contain Polysorbates
▸ **Imfinzi** (AstraZeneca UK Ltd)
   Durvalumab 50 mg per 1 ml Imfinzi 120mg/2.4ml concentrate for solution for infusion vials | 1 vial [PoM] £592.00 (Hospital only)
   Imfinzi 500mg/10ml concentrate for solution for infusion vials | 1 vial [PoM] £2,466.00 (Hospital only)

Elotuzumab [Specialist drug]

12-Apr-2019

● **INDICATIONS AND DOSE**
Multiple myeloma
▸ BY INTRAVENOUS INFUSION
▸ Adult: Specialist drug – access specialist resources for dosing information

● **INTERACTIONS** → Appendix 1: monoclonal antibodies

● **SIDE-EFFECTS**
▸ **Common or very common** Chest pain · cough · decreased leucocytes · deep vein thrombosis · diarrhoea · fatigue · fever · headache · hypersensitivity · increased risk of infection · infusion related reaction · mood altered · night sweats · numbness · oropharyngeal pain · weight decreased
▸ **Frequency not known** Second primary malignancy

   SIDE-EFFECTS, FURTHER INFORMATION Side-effects reported when used in combination with lenalidomide and dexamethasone, bortezomib and dexamethasone, or pomalidomide and dexamethasone.
   Infusion-related reactions Manufacturer advises for mild-to-moderate infusion reactions interrupt treatment or reduce infusion rate; permanently discontinue therapy in severe infusion reactions.

● **CONCEPTION AND CONTRACEPTION** Manufacturer advises effective contraception in men and women of childbearing potential; male patients should continue effective contraceptive measures for 180 days after stopping treatment if their partner is pregnant or of childbearing potential.

● **MEDICINAL FORMS** There can be variation in the licensing of different medicines containing the same drug.
Powder for solution for infusion
EXCIPIENTS: May contain Polysorbates, sucrose
▸ **Empliciti** (Bristol-Myers Squibb Pharmaceuticals Ltd)
   Elotuzumab 300 mg Empliciti 300mg powder for concentrate for solution for infusion vials | 1 vial [PoM] £1,085.00 (Hospital only)
   Elotuzumab 400 mg Empliciti 400mg powder for concentrate for solution for infusion vials | 1 vial [PoM] £1,446.00 (Hospital only)

Elranatamab [Specialist drug]

30-Dec-2024

● **INDICATIONS AND DOSE**
Multiple myeloma
▸ BY SUBCUTANEOUS INJECTION
▸ Adult: Specialist drug – access specialist resources for dosing information

   IMPORTANT SAFETY INFORMATION
   Resuscitation facilities should be available during administration.

● **CONTRA-INDICATIONS** Active infection

● **INTERACTIONS** → Appendix 1: monoclonal antibodies

● **SIDE-EFFECTS**
▸ **Common or very common** Anaemia · appetite decreased · arthralgia · cytokine release syndrome · decreased leucocytes · device complications · diarrhoea · dyspnoea · electrolyte imbalance · fatigue · fever · headache ·

hypogammaglobulinaemia · immune effector cell-associated neurotoxicity syndrome · increased risk of infection · nausea · nerve disorders · neuralgia · neutropenia · sensation abnormal · sepsis · skin reactions · thrombocytopenia
▸ **Frequency not known** Progressive multifocal leukoencephalopathy (PML)

● **CONCEPTION AND CONTRACEPTION** [EvGr] Females of childbearing potential should use effective contraception during treatment and for 6 months after last treatment. Ⓜ

● **PATIENT AND CARER ADVICE** Patients should be counselled to seek urgent medical attention if signs or symptoms of cytokine release syndrome or neurotoxicity occur.
   A patient alert card should be provided.
Driving and skilled tasks Patients should be cautioned on the effects on driving and performance of skilled tasks—consult product literature.

● **NATIONAL FUNDING/ACCESS DECISIONS**
   For full details see funding body website
NICE decisions
▸ **Elranatamab for treating relapsed and refractory multiple myeloma after 3 or more treatments (December 2024)**
NICE TA1023 Recommended

Scottish Medicines Consortium (SMC) decisions
▸ **Elranatamab (*Elrexfio*®) as monotherapy for the treatment of adult patients with relapsed and refractory multiple myeloma, who have received at least three prior therapies, including an immunomodulatory agent, a proteasome inhibitor, and an anti-CD38 antibody and have demonstrated disease progression on the last therapy (September 2024)**
SMC No. SMC2669 Recommended

● **MEDICINAL FORMS** There can be variation in the licensing of different medicines containing the same drug.
Solution for injection
EXCIPIENTS: May contain Disodium edetate, polysorbates
▸ **Elrexfio** (Pfizer Ltd) ▼
   Elranatamab 40 mg per 1 ml Elrexfio 44mg/1.1ml solution for injection vials | 1 vial [PoM] £2,456.00 (Hospital only)
   Elrexfio 76mg/1.9ml solution for injection vials | 1 vial [PoM] £4,242.50 (Hospital only)

Enfortumab vedotin [Specialist drug]

29-Jul-2022

● **INDICATIONS AND DOSE**
Urothelial carcinoma
▸ BY INTRAVENOUS INFUSION
▸ Adult: Specialist drug – access specialist resources for dosing information

● **INTERACTIONS** → Appendix 1: enfortumab vedotin

● **SIDE-EFFECTS**
▸ **Common or very common** Alopecia · anaemia · appetite decreased · conjunctivitis · diarrhoea · dry eye · fatigue · gait abnormal · hyperglycaemia · infusion related reaction · interstitial lung disease · muscle weakness · nausea · nerve disorders · sensation abnormal · sepsis · skin reactions · stomatitis · taste altered · vomiting · weight decreased
▸ **Uncommon** Motor dysfunction · muscle atrophy · neuralgia · neurotoxicity · peroneal nerve palsy
▸ **Frequency not known** Diabetic ketoacidosis · neutropenia · severe cutaneous adverse reactions (SCARs)

   SIDE-EFFECTS, FURTHER INFORMATION Hyperglycaemia and diabetic ketoacidosis, including fatal events, have been reported in those with and without pre-existing diabetes mellitus; manufacturer advises treatment should be withheld if blood glucose is more than 13.9 mmol/L.

● **CONCEPTION AND CONTRACEPTION** [EvGr] Females of childbearing potential should have a pregnancy test within 7 days before starting treatment and use effective contraception during and for at least 12 months after last treatment. Male patients should avoid fathering a child during and for up to 9 months after last treatment. Ⓜ

● **PATIENT AND CARER ADVICE** Patients and their carers should be advised to seek immediate medical attention if signs or symptoms of severe skin reactions occur.
Patient card A patient card should be provided.

● **MEDICINAL FORMS** There can be variation in the licensing of different medicines containing the same drug.

Powder for solution for infusion
EXCIPIENTS: May contain Polysorbates

▸ **Padcev** (Astellas Pharma Ltd) ▼
Enfortumab vedotin 20 mg Padcev 20mg powder for concentrate for solution for infusion vials | 1 vial PoM £578.00 (Hospital only)
Enfortumab vedotin 30 mg Padcev 30mg powder for concentrate for solution for infusion vials | 1 vial PoM £867.00 (Hospital only)

Epcoritamab [Specialist drug]
25-Jun-2024

● **INDICATIONS AND DOSE**
Diffuse large B-cell lymphoma
▸ BY SUBCUTANEOUS INJECTION
▸ Adult: Specialist drug – access specialist resources for dosing information

● **CONTRA-INDICATIONS** Concomitant use of live or live attenuated vaccines (no information available) · infection (active)

● **SIDE-EFFECTS**
▸ **Common or very common** Anaemia · asthenia · cytokine release syndrome · diarrhoea · electrolyte imbalance · fever · gastrointestinal discomfort · headache · immune effector cell-associated neurotoxicity syndrome (may be delayed) · increased risk of infection · lethargy · nausea · neutropenia · oedema · peripheral swelling · skin reactions · thrombocytopenia · tumour flare · tumour lysis syndrome · vomiting
▸ **Frequency not known** Progressive multifocal leukoencephalopathy (PML) · sepsis

● **CONCEPTION AND CONTRACEPTION** EvGr Females of childbearing potential should use effective contraception during treatment and for at least 4 months after last treatment. Ⓜ

● **PATIENT AND CARER ADVICE** Patients and carers should be counselled on the signs and symptoms of cytokine release syndrome and immune effector cell-associated neurotoxicity syndrome, and advised to seek immediate medical attention if these occur.
Patient card A patient card should be provided.
Driving and skilled tasks Patients and carers should be counselled on the effects on driving and performance of skilled tasks—increased risk of neurological side-effects.

● **NATIONAL FUNDING/ACCESS DECISIONS**
For full details see funding body website
NICE decisions
▸ **Epcoritamab for treating relapsed or refractory diffuse large B-cell lymphoma after 2 or more systemic treatments (March 2024) NICE TA954 Recommended with restrictions**
Scottish Medicines Consortium (SMC) decisions
▸ **Epcoritamab (Tepkinly®) as monotherapy for the treatment of adult patients with relapsed or refractory diffuse large B-cell lymphoma after two or more lines of systemic therapy (June 2024) SMC No. SMC2632 Recommended**

● **MEDICINAL FORMS** There can be variation in the licensing of different medicines containing the same drug.

Solution for injection
EXCIPIENTS: May contain Polysorbates, sorbitol

▸ **Tepkinly** (AbbVie Ltd) ▼
Epcoritamab 5 mg per 1 ml Tepkinly 4mg/0.8 ml concentrate for solution for injection vials | 1 vial PoM £547.33 (Hospital only)
Epcoritamab 60 mg per 1 ml Tepkinly 48mg/0.8ml solution for injection vials | 1 vial PoM £6,568.00 (Hospital only)

Gemtuzumab ozogamicin [Specialist drug]
06-Nov-2020

● **INDICATIONS AND DOSE**
Acute myeloid leukaemia
▸ BY INTRAVENOUS INFUSION
▸ Adult: Specialist drug – access specialist resources for dosing information

> **IMPORTANT SAFETY INFORMATION**
> Resuscitation facilities should be available during administration.

● **INTERACTIONS** → Appendix 1: gemtuzumab ozogamicin

● **SIDE-EFFECTS**
▸ **Common or very common** Anaemia · appetite decreased · arrhythmias · ascites · asthenia · bone marrow disorders · bronchospasm · central nervous system haemorrhage · chills · constipation · decreased leucocytes · diarrhoea · dyspnoea · facial swelling · fever · gastrointestinal discomfort · gastrointestinal disorders · haemorrhage · headache · hepatic disorders · hyperbilirubinaemia · hyperglycaemia · hypersensitivity · hypertension · hyperthermia · hypotension · increased risk of infection · infusion related reaction (including fatal cases) · lethargy · malaise · mucositis · multi organ failure · nausea · neutropenia · oedema · oral disorders · oropharyngeal complaints · periorbital oedema · sepsis · sinusoidal obstruction syndrome · skin reactions · thrombocytopenia · tumour lysis syndrome (including fatal cases) · vomiting
▸ **Frequency not known** Interstitial pneumonia

SIDE-EFFECTS, FURTHER INFORMATION Infusion-related reactions (including fatal cases) can occur during the first 24 hours after administration. Manufacturer advises interrupt treatment immediately and treat as clinically indicated; permanent discontinuation should be strongly considered in patients who develop signs and symptoms of anaphylaxis.

● **CONCEPTION AND CONTRACEPTION** Manufacturer advises women of childbearing potential should use 2 methods of effective contraception during treatment and for at least 7 months after the last dose; male patients should use 2 methods of effective contraception during treatment and for at least 4 months after the last dose if their partner is of childbearing potential.

● **PATIENT AND CARER ADVICE**
Driving and skilled tasks Manufacturer advises patients and carers should be counselled on the effects on driving and performance of skilled tasks—increased risk of fatigue and headache.

● **NATIONAL FUNDING/ACCESS DECISIONS**
For full details see funding body website
NICE decisions
▸ **Gemtuzumab ozogamicin for untreated acute myeloid leukaemia (November 2018) NICE TA545 Recommended with restrictions**
Scottish Medicines Consortium (SMC) decisions
▸ **Gemtuzumab ozogamicin (Mylotarg®) as combination therapy with daunorubicin and cytarabine for the treatment of**

patients age 15 years and above with previously untreated, *de novo* CD33-positive acute myeloid leukaemia, except acute promyelocytic leukaemia (October 2018) SMC No. SMC2089 Recommended with restrictions

- **MEDICINAL FORMS** There can be variation in the licensing of different medicines containing the same drug.
  Powder for solution for infusion
  ▶ Mylotarg (Pfizer Ltd)
    Gemtuzumab ozogamicin 5 mg Mylotarg 5mg powder for concentrate for solution for infusion vials | 1 vial PoM £6,300.00 (Hospital only)

Glofitamab [Specialist drug]

25-Jun-2024

- **INDICATIONS AND DOSE**
  Diffuse large B-cell lymphoma
  ▶ BY INTRAVENOUS INFUSION
  ▶ Adult: Specialist drug – access specialist resources for dosing information

- **CONTRA-INDICATIONS** Active infection
- **INTERACTIONS** → Appendix 1: glofitamab
- **SIDE-EFFECTS**
  ▶ **Common or very common** Anaemia · biliary tract infection bacterial · confusion · constipation · cytokine release syndrome · diarrhoea · drowsiness · electrolyte imbalance · fever · haemorrhage · headache · increased risk of infection · lymphopenia · nausea · neutropenia · sepsis · skin reactions · thrombocytopenia · tremor · tumour flare · tumour lysis syndrome · vascular device infection · vomiting
  ▶ **Frequency not known** Pleural effusion

- **CONCEPTION AND CONTRACEPTION** EvGr Females of childbearing potential should use effective contraception during treatment and for at least 2 months after last treatment. ⓜ

- **PATIENT AND CARER ADVICE** Patients and carers should be advised to seek immediate medical attention if signs or symptoms of cytokine release syndrome or infection occur. Patient card A patient card should be provided.
  Driving and skilled tasks Patients and carers should be counselled on the effects on driving and performance of skilled tasks—increased risk of cytokine release syndrome, drowsiness, headache, and tremor.

- **NATIONAL FUNDING/ACCESS DECISIONS**
  For full details see funding body website
  NICE decisions
  ▶ Glofitamab for treating relapsed or refractory diffuse large B-cell lymphoma after 2 or more systemic treatments (October 2023) NICE TA927 Recommended
  Scottish Medicines Consortium (SMC) decisions
  ▶ Glofitamab (*Columvi*®) as monotherapy for the treatment of adult patients with relapsed or refractory diffuse large B-cell lymphoma, after two or more lines of systemic therapy (June 2024) SMC No. SMC2614 Recommended

- **MEDICINAL FORMS** There can be variation in the licensing of different medicines containing the same drug.
  Solution for infusion
  EXCIPIENTS: May contain Polysorbates, sucrose
  ▶ Columvi (Roche Products Ltd) ▼
    Glofitamab 1 mg per 1 ml Columvi 10mg/10ml concentrate for solution for infusion vials | 1 vial PoM £2,748.00 (Hospital only)
    Columvi 2.5mg/2.5ml concentrate for solution for infusion vials | 1 vial PoM £687.00 (Hospital only)

Inotuzumab ozogamicin [Specialist drug]

09-Nov-2020

- **INDICATIONS AND DOSE**
  Acute lymphoblastic leukaemia
  ▶ BY INTRAVENOUS INFUSION
  ▶ Adult: Specialist drug – access specialist resources for dosing information

IMPORTANT SAFETY INFORMATION
Resuscitation facilities should be available during administration.

- **CONTRA-INDICATIONS** Prior confirmed severe or ongoing sinusoidal obstruction syndrome
- **INTERACTIONS** → Appendix 1: monoclonal antibodies
- **SIDE-EFFECTS**
  ▶ **Common or very common** Anaemia · appetite decreased · ascites · bone marrow disorders · central nervous system haemorrhage · chills · constipation · decreased leucocytes · diarrhoea · fatigue · fever · gastrointestinal discomfort · haemorrhage · headache · hyperbilirubinaemia · hypersensitivity · hyperuricaemia · increased risk of infection · infusion related reaction · nausea · neutropenia · QT interval prolongation · sepsis · sinusoidal obstruction syndrome · stomatitis · thrombocytopenia · tumour lysis syndrome · vomiting
  ▶ **Frequency not known** Hepatotoxicity

  SIDE-EFFECTS, FURTHER INFORMATION Manufacturer advises interrupt treatment if an infusion related reaction occurs; depending on the severity, discontinuation of the infusion or administration of corticosteroids and antihistamines should be considered; permanently discontinue treatment in severe or life-threatening infusion reactions.

- **CONCEPTION AND CONTRACEPTION** Manufacturer advises effective contraception in women of childbearing potential during treatment and for at least 8 months after the last dose; male patients should use effective contraception during treatment and for at least 5 months after the last dose if their partner is of childbearing potential.

- **PATIENT AND CARER ADVICE**
  Driving and skilled tasks Manufacturer advises patients and carers should be counselled on the effects on driving and performance of skilled tasks—increased risk of fatigue.

- **NATIONAL FUNDING/ACCESS DECISIONS**
  For full details see funding body website
  NICE decisions
  ▶ Inotuzumab ozogamicin for treating relapsed or refractory B-cell acute lymphoblastic leukaemia (September 2018) NICE TA541 Recommended with restrictions
  Scottish Medicines Consortium (SMC) decisions
  ▶ Inotuzumab ozogamicin (*Besponsa*®) as monotherapy for the treatment of adults with relapsed or refractory CD22-positive B cell precursor acute lymphoblastic leukaemia (ALL). Adult patients with Philadelphia chromosome positive relapsed or refractory B cell precursor ALL should have failed treatment with at least 1 tyrosine kinase inhibitor (June 2018) SMC No. 1328/18 Recommended with restrictions

- **MEDICINAL FORMS** There can be variation in the licensing of different medicines containing the same drug.
  Powder for solution for infusion
  ELECTROLYTES: May contain Sodium
  ▶ Besponsa (Pfizer Ltd) ▼
    Inotuzumab ozogamicin 1 mg Besponsa 1mg powder for concentrate for solution for infusion vials | 1 vial PoM £8,048.00 (Hospital only)

Ipilimumab [Specialist drug]

13-Sep-2022

● INDICATIONS AND DOSE

Melanoma | Renal cell carcinoma | Non-small cell lung cancer | Malignant pleural mesothelioma | Colorectal cancer

▶ BY INTRAVENOUS INFUSION

▸ Adult: Specialist drug – access specialist resources for dosing information

---

IMPORTANT SAFETY INFORMATION

MHRA/CHM ADVICE: IPILIMUMAB (*YERVOY*®): REPORTS OF CYTOMEGALOVIRUS (CMV) GASTROINTESTINAL INFECTION OR REACTIVATION (JANUARY 2019)

There have been post-marketing cases of gastrointestinal CMV infection or reactivation in ipilimumab-treated patients reported to have corticosteroid-refractory immune-related colitis, including fatal cases.

Patients should be advised to contact their healthcare professional immediately at the onset of symptoms of colitis. Possible causes, including infections, should be investigated; a stool infection work-up should be performed and patients screened for CMV. For patients with corticosteroid-refractory immune-related colitis, use of an additional immunosuppressive agent should only be considered if other causes are excluded using viral PCR on biopsy, and eliminating other viral, bacterial, and parasitic causes.

MHRA/CHM ADVICE: ATEZOLIZUMAB (*TECENTRIQ*®) AND OTHER IMMUNE-STIMULATORY ANTI-CANCER DRUGS: RISK OF SEVERE CUTANEOUS ADVERSE REACTIONS (SCARS) (JUNE 2021)

Severe cutaneous adverse reactions (SCARs), including cases of Stevens-Johnson syndrome (SJS) and toxic epidermal necrolysis (TEN), have been reported in patients treated with immunostimulant antineoplastic drugs, such as ipilimumab. Healthcare professionals are advised to monitor patients for suspected severe skin reactions and exclude other causes. Patients should be advised to seek urgent medical attention if severe skin reactions occur. If a SCAR is suspected, ipilimumab therapy should be withheld and the patient referred to a specialist for diagnosis and treatment. Ipilimumab should be permanently discontinued for any grade confirmed SJS or TEN, and for any grade 4 SCAR. Caution is recommended when considering the use of ipilimumab in patients with a history of severe or life-threatening SCAR associated with other immunostimulant antineoplastic drugs.

● INTERACTIONS → Appendix 1: monoclonal antibodies

● SIDE-EFFECTS

▶ **Common or very common** Alopecia · anaemia · appetite decreased · arthralgia · asthenia · cancer pain · chills · confusion · constipation · cough · dehydration · diarrhoea · dizziness · dyspnoea · electrolyte imbalance · eye discomfort · fever · gastrointestinal discomfort · gastrointestinal disorders · haemorrhage · headache · hepatic disorders · hypophysitis · hypopituitarism · hypotension · hypothyroidism · influenza like illness · lethargy · lymphopenia · mucositis · muscle complaints · musculoskeletal discomfort · nausea · nerve disorders · night sweats · oedema · pain · skin reactions · vasodilation · vision disorders · vomiting · weight decreased

▶ **Uncommon** Adrenal hypofunction · alkalosis · allergic rhinitis · amenorrhoea · arrhythmias · arthritis · brain oedema · depression · dysarthria · eosinophilia · eye inflammation · glomerulonephritis · haemolytic anaemia · hair colour changes · hypersensitivity · hyperthyroidism · hypogonadism · increased risk of infection · infusion related reaction · libido decreased · meningitis aseptic ·

movement disorders · multi organ failure · muscle weakness · myopathy · nephritis autoimmune · neutropenia · pancreatitis · paraneoplastic syndrome · peripheral ischaemia · pneumonitis · polymyalgia rheumatica · psychiatric disorder · pulmonary oedema · renal failure · renal tubular acidosis · respiratory disorders · sepsis · severe cutaneous adverse reactions (SCARs) · stomatitis · syncope · systemic inflammatory response syndrome · thrombocytopenia · tremor · tumour lysis syndrome · vascular disorders · vasculitis

▶ **Rare or very rare** Myasthenia gravis · proteinuria · serous retinal detachment · thyroiditis

▶ **Frequency not known** Cytomegalovirus infection reactivation · haemophagocytic lymphohistiocytosis · solid organ transplant rejection

SIDE-EFFECTS, FURTHER INFORMATION A corticosteroid can be used after starting ipilimumab, to treat immune-related reactions.

● CONCEPTION AND CONTRACEPTION Use effective contraception.

● PATIENT AND CARER ADVICE A patient information guide and alert card should be provided.

Driving and skilled tasks Patients and carers should be counselled on the effects on driving and performance of skilled tasks—increased risk of fatigue.

● NATIONAL FUNDING/ACCESS DECISIONS

For full details see funding body website

NICE decisions

▶ **Ipilimumab for previously treated advanced (unresectable or metastatic) melanoma (December 2012)** NICE TA268 Recommended with restrictions

▶ **Ipilimumab for previously untreated advanced (unresectable or metastatic) melanoma (July 2014)** NICE TA319 Recommended with restrictions

▶ **Nivolumab in combination with ipilimumab for treating advanced melanoma (July 2016)** NICE TA400 Recommended with restrictions

▶ **Nivolumab with ipilimumab for previously treated metastatic colorectal cancer with high microsatellite instability or mismatch repair deficiency (July 2021)** NICE TA716 Recommended

▶ **Nivolumab with ipilimumab and chemotherapy for untreated metastatic non-small-cell lung cancer (September 2021)** NICE TA724 Not recommended

▶ **Nivolumab with ipilimumab for untreated advanced renal cell carcinoma (March 2022)** NICE TA780 Recommended

▶ **Nivolumab with ipilimumab for untreated unresectable malignant pleural mesothelioma (August 2022)** NICE TA818 Recommended with restrictions

Scottish Medicines Consortium (SMC) decisions

▶ **Ipilimumab (*Yervoy*®) for the treatment of advanced (unresectable or metastatic) melanoma in adults who have received prior therapy (April 2013)** SMC No. 779/12 Recommended

▶ **Ipilimumab (*Yervoy*®) for the treatment of advanced (unresectable or metastatic) melanoma in adults (first-line use) (November 2014)** SMC No. 997/14 Recommended

---

● MEDICINAL FORMS There can be variation in the licensing of different medicines containing the same drug.

Solution for infusion

ELECTROLYTES: May contain Sodium

▸ Yervoy (Bristol-Myers Squibb Pharmaceuticals Ltd)
Ipilimumab 5 mg per 1 ml Yervoy 50mg/10ml concentrate for solution for infusion vials | 1 vial [PoM] £3,750.00 (Hospital only)
Yervoy 200mg/40ml concentrate for solution for infusion vials | 1 vial [PoM] £15,000.00 (Hospital only)

Isatuximab [Specialist drug]
10-Feb-2022

- **INDICATIONS AND DOSE**

Multiple myeloma
▸ BY INTRAVENOUS INFUSION
▸ Adult: Specialist drug – access specialist resources for dosing information

IMPORTANT SAFETY INFORMATION
Resuscitation facilities should be available during administration.

- **SIDE-EFFECTS**
▸ **Common or very common** Appetite decreased · atrial fibrillation · diarrhoea · dyspnoea · fatigue · increased risk of infection · infusion related reaction · nausea · neoplasms · neutropenia · vomiting · weight decreased
▸ **Uncommon** Anaphylactic reaction

- **CONCEPTION AND CONTRACEPTION** Manufacturer advises effective contraception in female patients of childbearing potential during treatment and for 5 months after last treatment.

- **PATIENT AND CARER ADVICE** A patient alert card should be provided.

- **NATIONAL FUNDING/ACCESS DECISIONS**
For full details see funding body website
NICE decisions
▸ Isatuximab with pomalidomide and dexamethasone for treating relapsed and refractory multiple myeloma (November 2020) NICE TA658 Recommended with restrictions
Scottish Medicines Consortium (SMC) decisions
▸ Isatuximab (*Sarclisa*®) in combination with pomalidomide and dexamethasone for the treatment of adult patients with relapsed and refractory multiple myeloma who have received at least two prior therapies, including lenalidomide and a proteasome inhibitor, and have demonstrated disease progression on the last therapy (April 2021) SMC No. SMC2303 Recommended with restrictions

- **MEDICINAL FORMS** There can be variation in the licensing of different medicines containing the same drug.
Solution for infusion
EXCIPIENTS: May contain Polysorbates, sucrose
▸ Sarclisa (Sanofi)
Isatuximab 20 mg per 1 ml Sarclisa 500mg/25ml concentrate for solution for infusion vials | 1 vial [PoM] £2,534.69 (Hospital only)
Sarclisa 100mg/5ml concentrate for solution for infusion vials | 1 vial [PoM] £506.94 (Hospital only)

Loncastuximab tesirine [Specialist drug]
05-Mar-2024

- **INDICATIONS AND DOSE**

Diffuse large B-cell lymphoma | High-grade B-cell lymphoma
▸ BY INTRAVENOUS INFUSION
▸ Adult: Specialist drug – access specialist resources for dosing information

- **INTERACTIONS** → Appendix 1: monoclonal antibodies

- **SIDE-EFFECTS**
▸ **Common or very common** Anaemia · appetite decreased · ascites · asthenia · constipation · diarrhoea · dyspnoea · facial swelling · fluid imbalance · gastrointestinal discomfort · increased risk of infection · inflammation · lethargy · myalgia · nausea · neutropenia · oedema · pain · pericardial effusion · photosensitivity reaction · pleural effusion · skin reactions · thrombocytopenia · vomiting
▸ **Uncommon** Limb discomfort · musculoskeletal discomfort · pericarditis

▸ **Frequency not known** Bone marrow depression · effusion · telangiectasia

- **CONCEPTION AND CONTRACEPTION** [EvGr] Females of childbearing potential should use effective contraception during treatment and for at least 10 months after last treatment; male patients should use effective contraception during treatment and for at least 7 months after last treatment if their partner is of childbearing potential. ⟨M⟩

- **PATIENT AND CARER ADVICE** Patients should be advised to minimise or avoid exposure to sunlight, and protect skin by wearing sun-protective clothing and/or using sunscreen.
Patient card A patient card should be provided.
Driving and skilled tasks Patients and carers should be counselled on the effects on driving and performance of skilled tasks—increased risk of fatigue.

- **NATIONAL FUNDING/ACCESS DECISIONS**
For full details see funding body website
NICE decisions
▸ Loncastuximab tesirine for treating relapsed or refractory diffuse large B-cell lymphoma and high-grade B-cell lymphoma after 2 or more systemic treatments (January 2024) NICE TA947 Recommended with restrictions
Scottish Medicines Consortium (SMC) decisions
▸ Loncastuximab tesirine (*Zynlonta*®) as monotherapy for the treatment of adult patients with relapsed or refractory diffuse large B-cell lymphoma and high-grade B-cell lymphoma, after two or more lines of systemic therapy (February 2024) SMC No. SMC2609 Recommended with restrictions

- **MEDICINAL FORMS** There can be variation in the licensing of different medicines containing the same drug.
Powder for solution for infusion
EXCIPIENTS: May contain Polysorbates
▸ Zynlonta (Swedish Orphan Biovitrum Ltd) ▼
Loncastuximab tesirine 10 mg Zynlonta 10mg powder for concentrate for solution for infusion vials | 1 vial [PoM] £15,200.00 (Hospital only)

Mogamulizumab [Specialist drug]
04-Jan-2022

- **INDICATIONS AND DOSE**

Mycosis fungoides | Sézary syndrome
▸ BY INTRAVENOUS INFUSION
▸ Adult: Specialist drug – access specialist resources for dosing information

IMPORTANT SAFETY INFORMATION
Resuscitation facilities should be available during administration.

HEPATITIS B INFECTION
Manufacturer advises patients should be tested for hepatitis B infection before treatment initiation; expert advice on measures against hepatitis B reactivation should be sought for patients with positive hepatitis B serology.

- **INTERACTIONS** → Appendix 1: monoclonal antibodies

- **SIDE-EFFECTS**
▸ **Common or very common** Anaemia · constipation · diarrhoea · fatigue · fever · headache · hypothyroidism · increased risk of infection · infusion related reaction · leucopenia · nausea · neutropenia · peripheral oedema · sepsis · skin reactions · stomatitis · thrombocytopenia · vomiting
▸ **Uncommon** Hepatic disorders · tumour lysis syndrome
▸ **Frequency not known** Cardiomyopathy · myocardial infarction · polymyositis · severe cutaneous adverse reactions (SCARs) · viral infection reactivation

● **CONCEPTION AND CONTRACEPTION** Manufacturer advises effective contraception in male and female patients of childbearing potential during treatment and for at least 6 months after last treatment.

● **PATIENT AND CARER ADVICE**
Driving and skilled tasks Manufacturer advises patients and carers should be counselled on the effects on driving and performance of skilled tasks—increased risk of fatigue.

● **NATIONAL FUNDING/ACCESS DECISIONS**
For full details see funding body website

NICE decisions
▸ Mogamulizumab for previously treated mycosis fungoides and Sézary syndrome [in adults with mycosis fungoides] (December 2021) NICE TA754 Recommended with restrictions
▸ Mogamulizumab for previously treated mycosis fungoides and Sézary syndrome [in adults with Sézary syndrome] (December 2021) NICE TA754 Recommended

Scottish Medicines Consortium (SMC) decisions
▸ Mogamulizumab (*Poteligeo*®) for the treatment of adult patients with mycosis fungoides or Sézary syndrome who have received at least one prior systemic therapy (June 2021) SMC No. SMC2336 Recommended with restrictions

● **MEDICINAL FORMS** There can be variation in the licensing of different medicines containing the same drug.
Solution for infusion
EXCIPIENTS: May contain Polysorbates
▸ Poteligeo (Kyowa Kirin Ltd)
Mogamulizumab 4 mg per 1 ml Poteligeo 20mg/5ml concentrate for solution for infusion vials | 1 vial [PoM] £1,329.00 (Hospital only)

Mosunetuzumab [Specialist drug] 18-Sep-2023

● **INDICATIONS AND DOSE**
Follicular lymphoma
▸ BY INTRAVENOUS INFUSION
▸ Adult: Specialist drug – access specialist resources for dosing information

● **CONTRA-INDICATIONS** Active infection

● **INTERACTIONS** → Appendix 1: monoclonal antibodies

● **SIDE-EFFECTS**
▸ **Common or very common** Anaemia · chills · cytokine release syndrome · diarrhoea · electrolyte imbalance · fever · headache · increased risk of infection · neutropenia · skin reactions · thrombocytopenia · tumour flare
▸ **Uncommon** Haemophagocytic lymphohistiocytosis · tumour lysis syndrome
▸ **Frequency not known** Sepsis

● **CONCEPTION AND CONTRACEPTION** [EvGr] Females of childbearing potential should use effective contraception during treatment and for at least 3 months after last treatment. ⓜ

● **PATIENT AND CARER ADVICE** A patient alert card should be provided.

● **NATIONAL FUNDING/ACCESS DECISIONS**
For full details see funding body website

NICE decisions
▸ **Mosunetuzumab for treating relapsed or refractory follicular lymphoma (May 2023)** NICE TA892 Not recommended
Scottish Medicines Consortium (SMC) decisions
▸ **Mosunetuzumab (*Lunsumio*®) as monotherapy for the treatment of adult patients with relapsed or refractory follicular lymphoma who have received at least two prior systemic therapies (September 2023)** SMC No. SMC2542 Not recommended

● **MEDICINAL FORMS** There can be variation in the licensing of different medicines containing the same drug.
Solution for infusion
EXCIPIENTS: May contain Polysorbates
▸ Lunsumio (Roche Products Ltd) ▼
Mosunetuzumab 1 mg per 1 ml Lunsumio 1mg/1ml concentrate for solution for infusion vials | 1 vial [PoM] £220.00 (Hospital only)
Lunsumio 30mg/30ml concentrate for solution for infusion vials | 1 vial [PoM] £6,600.00 (Hospital only)

Nivolumab [Specialist drug] 03-May-2024

● **INDICATIONS AND DOSE**
Melanoma | Renal cell carcinoma | Non-small cell lung cancer | Malignant pleural mesothelioma | Urothelial carcinoma | Squamous cell cancer of the head and neck | Classical Hodgkin lymphoma | Gastrointestinal cancer
▸ BY INTRAVENOUS INFUSION
▸ Adult: Specialist drug – access specialist resources for dosing information

---

IMPORTANT SAFETY INFORMATION
MHRA/CHM ADVICE: NIVOLUMAB (*OPDIVO*®): REPORTS OF ORGAN TRANSPLANT REJECTION (JULY 2017)
A European review of worldwide data concluded that nivolumab may increase the risk of rejection in organ transplant recipients. The MHRA recommends considering the benefit of treatment with nivolumab versus the risk of possible organ transplant rejection for each patient.

MHRA/CHM ADVICE: NIVOLUMAB (*OPDIVO*®): REPORTS OF CYTOMEGALOVIRUS (CMV) GASTROINTESTINAL INFECTION OR REACTIVATION (OCTOBER 2019)
A European review of worldwide data identified cases suggestive of gastrointestinal CMV infection or reactivation in nivolumab-treated patients, including fatal cases.

Patients should be advised to contact their healthcare professional immediately at the onset of symptoms of colitis. Possible causes, including infections, should be investigated; a stool infection work-up should be performed and patients screened for CMV. For patients with corticosteroid-refractory immune-related colitis, use of an additional immunosuppressive agent should only be considered if other causes are excluded using viral PCR on biopsy, and eliminating other viral, bacterial, and parasitic causes.

MHRA/CHM ADVICE: ATEZOLIZUMAB (*TECENTRIQ*®) AND OTHER IMMUNE-STIMULATORY ANTI-CANCER DRUGS: RISK OF SEVERE CUTANEOUS ADVERSE REACTIONS (SCARS) (JUNE 2021)
Severe cutaneous adverse reactions (SCARs), including cases of Stevens-Johnson syndrome (SJS) and toxic epidermal necrolysis (TEN), have been reported in patients treated with immunostimulant antineoplastic drugs, such as nivolumab. Healthcare professionals are advised to monitor patients for suspected severe skin reactions and exclude other causes. Patients should be advised to seek urgent medical attention if severe skin reactions occur. If a SCAR is suspected, nivolumab therapy should be withheld and the patient referred to a specialist for diagnosis and treatment. Nivolumab should be permanently discontinued for any grade confirmed SJS or TEN, and for any grade 4 SCAR. Caution is recommended when considering the use of nivolumab in patients with a history of severe or life-threatening SCAR associated with other immunostimulant antineoplastic drugs.

● **INTERACTIONS** → Appendix 1: monoclonal antibodies

Immune system and malignant disease

- SIDE-EFFECTS
▶ **Common or very common** Abdominal pain · alopecia · anaemia · appetite decreased · arrhythmias · arthralgia · arthritis · chest pain · constipation · cough · cytokine release syndrome · decreased leucocytes · dehydration · diarrhoea · dizziness · dry eye · dry mouth · dyspnoea · electrolyte imbalance · fatigue · fever · gastrointestinal disorders · haemolytic anaemia · headache · hyperglycaemia · hypersensitivity · hypertension · hyperthyroidism · hypoalbuminaemia · hypoglycaemia · hypothyroidism · increased risk of infection · inflammation · infusion related reaction · interstitial lung disease · muscle complaints · musculoskeletal discomfort · nausea · nerve disorders · neutropenia · oedema · pain · renal impairment · respiratory disorders · skin reactions · stomatitis · thrombocytopenia · thyroiditis · vision blurred · vomiting · weight decreased
▶ **Uncommon** Adrenal hypofunction · cardiac inflammation · connective tissue disorders · diabetes mellitus · eosinophilia · eye inflammation · hepatic disorders · hypophysitis · hypopituitarism · metabolic acidosis · pancreatitis · paresis · pericardial disorders · sarcoidosis
▶ **Rare or very rare** Cystitis · demyelination · diabetic ketoacidosis · histiocytic necrotising lymphadenitis · hypoparathyroidism · meningitis aseptic · myopathy · nephritis · neuromuscular dysfunction · severe cutaneous adverse reactions (SCARs) · vasculitis
▶ **Frequency not known** Cytomegalovirus infection reactivation · haemophagocytic lymphohistiocytosis · solid organ transplant rejection · thyroid disorder · tumour lysis syndrome

SIDE-EFFECTS, FURTHER INFORMATION **Immune-related reactions** Manufacturer advises that most immune-related adverse reactions improved or resolved with appropriate management, including initiation of corticosteroids and treatment modifications.

Infusion-related reactions Manufacturer advises that patients with mild or moderate infusion reactions can continue treatment with close monitoring and use of pre-medication according to local guidelines; discontinue treatment if severe infusion reactions occur.

- CONCEPTION AND CONTRACEPTION [EvGr] Ensure effective contraception during and for at least 5 months after treatment in females of childbearing potential. Ⓜ

- PATIENT AND CARER ADVICE Patients should be provided with a patient alert card with each prescription.
Driving and skilled tasks Patients and carers should be counselled on the effects on driving and performance of skilled tasks—increased risk of fatigue.

- NATIONAL FUNDING/ACCESS DECISIONS
For full details see funding body website

NICE decisions
▶ Nivolumab for treating advanced (unresectable or metastatic) melanoma (February 2016) NICE TA384 Recommended
▶ Nivolumab in combination with ipilimumab for treating advanced melanoma (July 2016) NICE TA400 Recommended with restrictions
▶ Nivolumab for adjuvant treatment of completely resected melanoma with lymph node involvement or metastatic disease (March 2021) NICE TA684 Recommended
▶ Nivolumab for previously treated advanced renal cell carcinoma (updated November 2017) NICE TA417 Recommended
▶ Nivolumab with ipilimumab for untreated advanced renal cell carcinoma (March 2022) NICE TA780 Recommended
▶ Cabozantinib with nivolumab for untreated advanced renal cell carcinoma (April 2024) NICE TA964 Recommended with restrictions
▶ Nivolumab for treating relapsed or refractory classical Hodgkin lymphoma (updated November 2017) NICE TA462 Recommended with restrictions

▶ Nivolumab for advanced squamous non-small-cell lung cancer after chemotherapy (October 2020) NICE TA655 Recommended with restrictions
▶ Nivolumab for advanced non-squamous non-small-cell lung cancer after chemotherapy (July 2021) NICE TA713 Recommended with restrictions
▶ Nivolumab with ipilimumab and chemotherapy for untreated metastatic non-small-cell lung cancer (September 2021) NICE TA724 Not recommended
▶ Nivolumab with chemotherapy for neoadjuvant treatment of resectable non-small-cell lung cancer (March 2023) NICE TA876 Recommended
▶ Nivolumab for treating locally advanced unresectable or metastatic urothelial cancer after platinum-containing chemotherapy (July 2018) NICE TA530 Not recommended
▶ Nivolumab for adjuvant treatment of invasive urothelial cancer at high risk of recurrence (August 2022) NICE TA817 Recommended with restrictions
▶ Nivolumab for previously treated unresectable advanced or recurrent oesophageal cancer (June 2021) NICE TA707 Recommended
▶ Nivolumab for adjuvant treatment of resected oesophageal or gastro-oesophageal junction cancer (November 2021) NICE TA746 Recommended
▶ Nivolumab with platinum- and fluoropyrimidine-based chemotherapy for untreated HER2-negative advanced gastric, gastro-oesophageal junction or oesophageal adenocarcinoma (January 2023) NICE TA857 Recommended
▶ Nivolumab with fluoropyrimidine- and platinum-based chemotherapy for untreated unresectable advanced, recurrent, or metastatic oesophageal squamous cell carcinoma (February 2023) NICE TA865 Recommended with restrictions
▶ Nivolumab with ipilimumab for previously treated metastatic colorectal cancer with high microsatellite instability or mismatch repair deficiency (July 2021) NICE TA716 Recommended
▶ Nivolumab for treating recurrent or metastatic squamous cell carcinoma of the head and neck after platinum-based chemotherapy (October 2021) NICE TA736 Recommended with restrictions
▶ Nivolumab with ipilimumab for untreated unresectable malignant pleural mesothelioma (August 2022) NICE TA818 Recommended with restrictions

Scottish Medicines Consortium (SMC) decisions
▶ Nivolumab (Opdivo®) for the treatment of locally advanced or metastatic squamous non-small cell lung cancer (NSCLC) after prior chemotherapy in adults (July 2016) SMC No. 1144/16 Recommended
▶ Nivolumab (Opdivo®) for the treatment of locally advanced or metastatic non-squamous non-small cell lung cancer (NSCLC) after prior chemotherapy in adults (October 2016) SMC No. 1180/16 Recommended with restrictions
▶ Nivolumab (Opdivo®) in combination with ipilimumab and 2 cycles of platinum-based doublet chemotherapy for the first-line treatment of metastatic non-small cell lung cancer in adults whose tumours have no sensitising epidermal growth factor receptor mutations or anaplastic lymphoma kinase translocations (January 2022) SMC No. SMC2397 Not recommended
▶ Nivolumab (Opdivo®) in combination with platinum-based chemotherapy for the neoadjuvant treatment of resectable non-small cell lung cancer in adults (tumours 4 cm and above, or node positive) (December 2023) SMC No. SMC2619 Recommended
▶ Nivolumab (Opdivo®) for use as monotherapy for the treatment of advanced (unresectable or metastatic) melanoma in adults (August 2016) SMC No. 1120/16 Recommended with restrictions
▶ Nivolumab (Opdivo®) in combination with ipilimumab for the treatment of advanced (unresectable or metastatic)

melanoma in adults (November 2016) SMC No. 1187/16 Recommended with restrictions

▸ Nivolumab (*Opdivo*®) as monotherapy for the adjuvant treatment of adults with melanoma with involvement of lymph nodes or metastatic disease who have undergone complete resection (December 2018) SMC No. SMC2112 Recommended

▸ Nivolumab (*Opdivo*®) as monotherapy for the treatment of advanced renal cell carcinoma after prior therapy in adults (June 2017) SMC No. 1188/16 Recommended

▸ Nivolumab (*Opdivo*®) in combination with ipilimumab for the first-line treatment of adult patients with intermediate/poor-risk advanced renal cell carcinoma (June 2019) SMC No. SMC2153 Recommended

▸ Nivolumab (*Opdivo*®) for the treatment of adult patients with relapsed or refractory classical Hodgkin lymphoma (cHL) after autologous stem cell transplant (ASCT) and treatment with brentuximab vedotin (July 2017) SMC No. 1240/17 Recommended

▸ Nivolumab (*Opdivo*®) as monotherapy for the treatment of squamous cell cancer of the head and neck (SCCHN) in adults progressing on or after platinum-based therapy (September 2017) SMC No. 1261/17 Recommended with restrictions

▸ Nivolumab (*Opdivo*®) as monotherapy for the treatment of locally advanced unresectable or metastatic urothelial carcinoma in adults after failure of prior platinum-containing therapy (January 2018) SMC No. 1285/18 Not recommended

▸ Nivolumab (*Opdivo*®) as monotherapy for the adjuvant treatment of adults with muscle invasive urothelial carcinoma (MIUC) with tumour cell PD-L1 expression at a level of 1% or more, who are at high risk of recurrence after undergoing radical resection of MIUC (February 2023) SMC No. SMC2503 Recommended

▸ Nivolumab (*Opdivo*®) as monotherapy for the treatment of adult patients with unresectable advanced, recurrent or metastatic oesophageal squamous cell carcinoma after prior fluoropyrimidine and platinum-based combination chemotherapy (August 2021) SMC No. SMC2362 Recommended

▸ Nivolumab (*Opdivo*®) in combination with fluoropyrimidine- and platinum-based combination chemotherapy for the first-line treatment of adult patients with unresectable advanced, recurrent or metastatic oesophageal squamous cell carcinoma with tumour cell PD-L1 expression at a level of 1% or more (June 2023) SMC No. SMC2519 Recommended

▸ Nivolumab (*Opdivo*®) as monotherapy for the adjuvant treatment of adult patients with completely resected oesophageal or gastro-oesophageal junction cancer who have residual pathologic disease following prior neoadjuvant chemoradiotherapy (May 2022) SMC No. SMC2429 Recommended

▸ Nivolumab (*Opdivo*®) in combination with fluoropyrimidine and platinum-based combination chemotherapy for the first-line treatment of adults with HER2-negative advanced or metastatic gastric, gastro-oesophageal junction or oesophageal adenocarcinoma whose tumours express PD-L1 with a combined positive score of 5 or more (September 2022) SMC No. SMC2458 Recommended

▸ Nivolumab (*Opdivo*®) in combination with ipilimumab for the treatment of adults with mismatch repair deficient or microsatellite instability-high metastatic colorectal cancer who have been previously treated with fluoropyrimidine-based combination chemotherapy (December 2021) SMC No. SMC2394 Recommended

▸ Nivolumab (*Opdivo*®) in combination with ipilimumab for the first-line treatment of adult patients with unresectable malignant pleural mesothelioma (MPM) (February 2022) SMC No. SMC2385 Recommended

● **MEDICINAL FORMS** There can be variation in the licensing of different medicines containing the same drug.

Solution for infusion

EXCIPIENTS: May contain Polysorbates

ELECTROLYTES: May contain Sodium

▸ Opdivo (Bristol-Myers Squibb Pharmaceuticals Ltd)

Nivolumab 10 mg per 1 ml Opdivo 40mg/4ml concentrate for solution for infusion vials | 1 vial [PoM] £439.00 (Hospital only)
Opdivo 120mg/12ml concentrate for solution for infusion vials | 1 vial [PoM] £1,317.00 (Hospital only)
Opdivo 100mg/10ml concentrate for solution for infusion vials | 1 vial [PoM] £1,097.00 (Hospital only)
Opdivo 240mg/24ml concentrate for solution for infusion vials | 1 vial [PoM] £2,633.00 (Hospital only)

Nivolumab with relatlimab
[Specialist drug]   01-Aug-2024

The properties listed below are those particular to the combination only. For the properties of the components please consider, nivolumab p. 1011.

● **INDICATIONS AND DOSE**

Melanoma

▸ BY INTRAVENOUS INFUSION

▸ Adult: Specialist drug – access specialist resources for dosing information

● **INTERACTIONS** → Appendix 1: monoclonal antibodies

● **SIDE-EFFECTS**

▸ **Common or very common** Abdominal pain · adrenal hypofunction · alopecia · anaemia · appetite decreased · arthralgia · arthritis · chills · confusion · constipation · cough · decreased leucocytes · dehydration · diabetes mellitus · diarrhoea · dizziness · dry eye · dry mouth · dysphagia · dyspnoea · electrolyte imbalance · eosinophilia · eye disorders · eye inflammation · fatigue · fever · gastrointestinal disorders · headache · hepatitis · hyperthyroidism · hyperuricaemia · hypoalbuminaemia · hypoglycaemia · hypophysitis · hypothyroidism · increased risk of infection · influenza like illness · infusion related reaction · interstitial lung disease · muscle spasms · muscle weakness · myocarditis · nasal congestion · nausea · nerve disorders · neutropenia · oedema · pain · pancreatitis · photosensitivity reaction · proteinuria · renal impairment · skin reactions · stomatitis · taste altered · thrombocytopenia · thyroiditis · visual impairment · vomiting · weight decreased

▸ **Uncommon** Asthma · azoospermia · cholangitis · connective tissue disorders · haemolytic anaemia · hypogonadism · hypopituitarism · myopathy · nephritis · pericardial effusion · systemic lupus erythematosus (SLE)

▸ **Frequency not known** Endocrine disorders · haemophagocytic lymphohistiocytosis · hypersensitivity · lung infiltration

● **PATIENT AND CARER ADVICE** A patient card should be provided.

● **NATIONAL FUNDING/ACCESS DECISIONS**

For full details see funding body website

NICE decisions

▸ Nivolumab–relatlimab for untreated unresectable or metastatic melanoma in people 12 years and over (February 2024) NICE TA950 Recommended with restrictions

Scottish Medicines Consortium (SMC) decisions

▸ Nivolumab with relatlimab (*Opdualag*®) for first-line treatment of advanced (unresectable or metastatic) melanoma in adults and adolescents 12 years of age and over (July 2024) SMC No. SMC2645 Recommended

- **MEDICINAL FORMS** There can be variation in the licensing of different medicines containing the same drug.
Solution for infusion
EXCIPIENTS: May contain Polysorbates
▸ **Opdualag** (Bristol-Myers Squibb Pharmaceuticals Ltd) ▼
Relatlimab 4 mg per 1 ml, Nivolumab 12 mg per 1 ml Opdualag 240mg/20ml / 80mg/20ml concentrate for solution for infusion vials | 1 vial PoM £6,134.75 (Hospital only)

Obinutuzumab [Specialist drug]

11-Nov-2020

- **INDICATIONS AND DOSE**

Chronic lymphocytic leukaemia | Follicular lymphoma
▸ BY INTRAVENOUS INFUSION
▸ Adult: Specialist drug – access specialist resources for dosing information

IMPORTANT SAFETY INFORMATION

All anti-lymphocyte monoclonal antibodies should be given under the supervision of an experienced specialist, in an environment where full resuscitation facilities are immediately available.

HEPATITIS B INFECTION AND REACTIVATION
Hepatitis B infection and reactivation (including fatal cases) have been reported in patients taking **obinutuzumab**. Manufacturer advises patients with positive hepatitis B serology should be referred to a liver specialist for monitoring and initiation of antiviral therapy before treatment initiation; treatment should not be initiated in patients with evidence of current hepatitis B infection until the infection has been adequately treated. Manufacturer also advises patients should be closely monitored for clinical and laboratory signs of active hepatitis B infection (consult product literature).

- **CONTRA-INDICATIONS** For obinutuzumab contra-indications, consult product literature.
- **INTERACTIONS** → Appendix 1: monoclonal antibodies
- **SIDE-EFFECTS**
▸ **Common or very common** Alopecia · anaemia · arrhythmias · arthralgia · asthenia · chest pain · constipation · cough · depression · diarrhoea · dyspepsia · eye erythema · fever · gastrointestinal disorders · heart failure · hypertension · hyperuricaemia · increased risk of infection · infusion related reaction · leucopenia · lymph node pain · nasal complaints · neutropenia · night sweats · pain · skin reactions · squamous cell carcinoma · thrombocytopenia · tumour lysis syndrome · urinary disorders · weight increased
▸ **Frequency not known** Acute coronary syndrome · angina pectoris · chills · dizziness · dyspnoea · flushing · headache · hypersensitivity · hypotension · nausea · progressive multifocal leukoencephalopathy (PML) · reactivation of infections · vomiting

SIDE-EFFECTS, FURTHER INFORMATION **Cytokine release syndrome** Fatalities following severe cytokine release syndrome (characterised by severe dyspnoea) and associated with features of tumour lysis syndrome have occurred after infusions of anti-lymphocyte monoclonal antibodies. Patients with a high tumour burden as well as those with pulmonary insufficiency or infiltration are at increased risk and should be monitored very closely (and a slower rate of infusion considered).

Infusion-related side-effects In rare cases infusion reactions can be fatal. Infusion-related side-effects occur predominantly during the first infusion. Patients should receive premedication before administration of anti-lymphocyte monoclonal antibodies to reduce these effects.

The infusion might need to be stopped temporarily and the infusion-related effects treated.

Progressive Multifocal Leukoencephalopathy (PML) If suspected, treatment should be suspended until PML has been excluded. If a patient develops an opportunistic infection or PML, obinutuzumab should be permanently discontinued.

- **CONCEPTION AND CONTRACEPTION** Use effective contraception during and for 18 months after treatment.
- **NATIONAL FUNDING/ACCESS DECISIONS**
For full details see funding body website
NICE decisions
▸ Obinutuzumab in combination with chlorambucil for untreated chronic lymphocytic leukaemia (June 2015) NICE TA343 Recommended with restrictions
▸ Obinutuzumab for untreated advanced follicular lymphoma (March 2018) NICE TA513 Recommended with restrictions
▸ Obinutuzumab with bendamustine for treating follicular lymphoma after rituximab (May 2020) NICE TA629 Recommended
Scottish Medicines Consortium (SMC) decisions
▸ Obinutuzumab (*Gazyvaro*®) in combination with bendamustine followed by obinutuzumab maintenance is indicated for the treatment of patients with follicular lymphoma who did not respond or who progressed during or up to six months after treatment with rituximab or a rituximab-containing regimen (March 2017) SMC No. 1219/17 Recommended
▸ Obinutuzumab (*Gazyvaro*®) in combination with chemotherapy, followed by maintenance therapy in patients achieving a response, for the treatment of patients with previously untreated advanced follicular lymphoma (FL) (September 2018) SMC No. SMC2015 Not recommended

- **MEDICINAL FORMS** There can be variation in the licensing of different medicines containing the same drug.
Solution for infusion
▸ **Gazyvaro** (Roche Products Ltd)
Obinutuzumab 25 mg per 1 ml Gazyvaro 1000mg/40ml concentrate for solution for infusion vials | 1 vial PoM £3,312.00 (Hospital only)

Panitumumab [Specialist drug]

21-Jul-2020

- **INDICATIONS AND DOSE**

Colorectal cancer
▸ BY INTRAVENOUS INFUSION
▸ Adult: Specialist drug – access specialist resources for dosing information

IMPORTANT SAFETY INFORMATION
MHRA/CHM ADVICE: SEVERE SKIN REACTIONS
Severe skin reactions have been reported very commonly in patients treated with panitumumab. Patients receiving panitumumab who have severe skin reactions or develop worsening skin reactions should be monitored for the development of inflammatory or infectious sequelae (including cellulitis, sepsis, and necrotising fasciitis). Appropriate treatment should be promptly initiated and panitumumab withheld or discontinued.

MHRA/CHM ADVICE: EPIDERMAL GROWTH FACTOR RECEPTOR (EGFR) INHIBITORS: SERIOUS CASES OF KERATITIS AND ULCERATIVE KERATITIS (MAY 2012)
Keratitis and ulcerative keratitis have been reported following treatment with epidermal growth factor receptor (EGFR) inhibitors for cancer (cetuximab, erlotinib, gefitinib and panitumumab). In rare cases, this has resulted in corneal perforation and blindness. Patients undergoing treatment with EGFR inhibitors who present with acute or worsening signs and

symptoms suggestive of keratitis should be referred promptly to an ophthalmology specialist. Treatment should be interrupted or discontinued if ulcerative keratitis is diagnosed.

● **CONTRA-INDICATIONS** Interstitial pulmonary disease · the combination of panitumumab with oxaliplatin-containing chemotherapy is contra-indicated in patients with mutant *RAS* metastatic colorectal cancer or for whom *RAS* status is unknown

● **INTERACTIONS** → Appendix 1: monoclonal antibodies

● **SIDE-EFFECTS**

▶ **Common or very common** Alopecia · anaemia · anxiety · appetite decreased · asthenia · chest pain · chills · constipation · cough · dehydration · diarrhoea · dizziness · dry eye · dry mouth · dyspnoea · electrolyte imbalance · embolism and thrombosis · eye discomfort · eye disorders · eye inflammation · fever · flushing · gastrointestinal discomfort · gastrooesophageal reflux disease · haemorrhage · hair changes · headache · hyperglycaemia · hyperhidrosis · hypersensitivity (may be delayed) · hypertension · hypotension · increased risk of infection · insomnia · leucopenia · mucositis · nail disorders · nausea · oral disorders · pain · peripheral oedema · skin reactions · skin ulcer · tachycardia · vomiting · weight decreased

▶ **Uncommon** Angioedema · bronchospasm · cyanosis · infusion related reaction · nasal dryness · onycholysis · severe cutaneous adverse reactions (SCARs)

▶ **Rare or very rare** Anaphylactic reaction

▶ **Frequency not known** Interstitial lung disease

● **CONCEPTION AND CONTRACEPTION** Manufacturer advises effective contraception during and for 6 months after treatment.

● **NATIONAL FUNDING/ACCESS DECISIONS** For full details see funding body website

NICE decisions

▶ **Cetuximab, bevacizumab and panitumumab for the treatment of metastatic colorectal cancer after first-line chemotherapy (January 2012)** NICE TA242 Not recommended

▶ **Cetuximab and panitumumab for previously untreated metastatic colorectal cancer (updated September 2017)** NICE TA439 Recommended with restrictions

● **MEDICINAL FORMS** There can be variation in the licensing of different medicines containing the same drug.

Solution for infusion
ELECTROLYTES: May contain Sodium
▶ Vectibix (Amgen Ltd)
Panitumumab 20 mg per 1 ml Vectibix 400mg/20ml concentrate for solution for infusion vials | 1 vial [PoM] £1,517.16 (Hospital only)
Vectibix 100mg/5ml concentrate for solution for infusion vials | 1 vial [PoM] £379.29 (Hospital only)

Pembrolizumab [Specialist drug]   27-Feb-2025

● **INDICATIONS AND DOSE**

Melanoma | Non-small cell lung cancer | Urothelial carcinoma | Classical Hodgkin lymphoma | Head and neck squamous cell carcinoma | Renal cell carcinoma | Colorectal cancer | Oesophageal carcinoma | Breast cancer | Endometrial carcinoma | Cervical cancer | Gastric cancer | Small intestine cancer | Biliary cancer

▶ BY INTRAVENOUS INFUSION

▶ **Adult:** Specialist drug – access specialist resources for dosing information

IMPORTANT SAFETY INFORMATION

● **INTERACTIONS** → Appendix 1: monoclonal antibodies

● **SIDE-EFFECTS**

▶ **Common or very common** Alopecia · anaemia · appetite decreased · arrhythmias · arthritis · asthenia · chills · connective tissue disorders · constipation · cough · cytokine release syndrome · decreased leucocytes · diarrhoea · dizziness · dry eye · dry mouth · dyspnoea · electrolyte imbalance · enterocolitis haemorrhagic · eye inflammation · eyelid hypopigmentation · fever · fluid imbalance · gastrointestinal discomfort · gastrointestinal disorders · genital abnormalities · headache · hepatic disorders · hypersensitivity · hypertension · hyperthyroidism · hypothyroidism · immune-mediated lung disease · increased risk of infection · influenza like illness · infusion related reaction · insomnia · interstitial lung disease · joint disorders · lethargy · lip swelling · musculoskeletal discomfort · myalgia · myopathy · myxoedema · nausea · nerve disorders · neutropenia · oedema · pain · severe cutaneous adverse reactions (SCARs) · skin reactions · taste altered · thrombocytopenia · torticollis · vomiting

▶ **Uncommon** Adrenal hypofunction · cardiac inflammation · diabetic ketoacidosis · eosinophilia · epilepsy · glomerulonephritis · hair colour changes · hypophysitis · hypopituitarism · immune-mediated pancreatitis · lymphocytic hypophysitis · nephritis · nephrotic syndrome · neuromuscular dysfunction · pancreatitis · pericardial effusion · renal impairment · sarcoidosis · tendon disorders · thyroid disorder · thyroiditis · type 1 diabetes mellitus

▶ **Rare or very rare** Aortitis · cholangitis sclerosing · cystitis · encephalitis non-infective · erythema nodosum · haemolytic anaemia · haemophagocytic lymphohistiocytosis · hypoparathyroidism · meningitis · meningitis non-infective · pure red cell aplasia · transverse myelitis · vasculitis

▶ **Frequency not known** Solid organ transplant rejection

SIDE-EFFECTS, FURTHER INFORMATION **Immune-related reactions** Most immune-related adverse reactions are reversible and managed by temporarily stopping treatment and administration of a corticosteroid.

  Infusion-related reactions Manufacturer advises to permanently discontinue treatment in patients with severe infusion reactions.

● **CONCEPTION AND CONTRACEPTION** Manufacturer recommends effective contraception during treatment and for at least 4 months after treatment in women of childbearing potential.

● **PATIENT AND CARER ADVICE** Patients should be provided with an alert card and advised to keep it with them at all times. A patient information brochure highlighting important safety information to minimise the risk of immune-related side-effects is also available.
Driving and skilled tasks Patients should be counselled on the effects on driving and performance of skilled tasks—increased risk of dizziness and fatigue.

● **NATIONAL FUNDING/ACCESS DECISIONS**
For full details see funding body website
NICE decisions
▸ Pembrolizumab for treating advanced melanoma after disease progression with ipilimumab (updated September 2017) NICE TA357 Recommended with restrictions
▸ Pembrolizumab for advanced melanoma not previously treated with ipilimumab (updated September 2017) NICE TA366 Recommended with restrictions
▸ Pembrolizumab for adjuvant treatment of completely resected stage 3 melanoma (February 2022) NICE TA766 Recommended
▸ Pembrolizumab for adjuvant treatment of resected stage 2B or 2C melanoma (October 2022) NICE TA837 Recommended
▸ Pembrolizumab for treating PD-L1-positive non-small-cell lung cancer after chemotherapy (updated September 2017) NICE TA428 Recommended with restrictions
▸ Pembrolizumab for untreated PD-L1-positive metastatic non-small-cell lung cancer (July 2018) NICE TA531 Recommended with restrictions
▸ Pembrolizumab with pemetrexed and platinum chemotherapy for untreated, metastatic, non-squamous non-small-cell lung cancer (March 2021) NICE TA683 Recommended with restrictions
▸ Pembrolizumab with carboplatin and paclitaxel for untreated metastatic squamous non-small-cell lung cancer (February 2022) NICE TA770 Recommended with restrictions
▸ Pembrolizumab with chemotherapy before surgery (neoadjuvant) then alone after surgery (adjuvant) for treating resectable non-small-cell lung cancer (November 2024) NICE TA1017 Recommended
▸ Pembrolizumab for adjuvant treatment of resected non-small-cell lung cancer (February 2025) NICE TA1037 Recommended
▸ Pembrolizumab for treating locally advanced or metastatic urothelial carcinoma after platinum-containing chemotherapy (April 2021) NICE TA692 Not recommended
▸ Pembrolizumab for treating relapsed or refractory classical Hodgkin lymphoma after stem cell transplant or at least 2 previous therapies (February 2022) NICE TA772 Recommended with restrictions
▸ Pembrolizumab for treating relapsed or refractory classical Hodgkin lymphoma (updated May 2024) NICE TA540 Not recommended
▸ Pembrolizumab for treating relapsed or refractory classical Hodgkin lymphoma in people 3 years and over (May 2024) NICE TA967 Recommended with restrictions
▸ Pembrolizumab with axitinib for untreated advanced renal cell carcinoma (September 2020) NICE TA650 Not recommended
▸ Pembrolizumab for adjuvant treatment of renal cell carcinoma (October 2022) NICE TA830 Recommended
▸ Lenvatinib with pembrolizumab for untreated advanced renal cell carcinoma (January 2023) NICE TA858 Recommended with restrictions
▸ Pembrolizumab for untreated metastatic or unresectable recurrent head and neck squamous cell carcinoma (November 2020) NICE TA661 Recommended with restrictions
▸ Pembrolizumab for untreated metastatic colorectal cancer with high microsatellite instability or mismatch repair deficiency (June 2021) NICE TA709 Recommended with restrictions
▸ Pembrolizumab for previously treated endometrial, biliary, colorectal, gastric or small intestine cancer with high microsatellite instability or mismatch repair deficiency

(September 2023) NICE TA914 Recommended with restrictions
▸ Pembrolizumab with trastuzumab and chemotherapy for untreated locally advanced unresectable or metastatic HER2-positive gastric or gastro-oesophageal junction adenocarcinoma (June 2024) NICE TA983 Not recommended
▸ Pembrolizumab with platinum- and fluoropyrimidine-based chemotherapy for untreated advanced oesophageal and gastro-oesophageal junction cancer (updated August 2024) NICE TA737 Recommended
▸ Pembrolizumab with platinum- and fluoropyrimidine-based chemotherapy for untreated advanced HER2-negative gastric or gastro-oesophageal junction adenocarcinoma (August 2024) NICE TA997 Recommended
▸ Pembrolizumab plus chemotherapy for untreated, triple-negative, locally recurrent unresectable or metastatic breast cancer (June 2022) NICE TA801 Recommended with restrictions
▸ Pembrolizumab for neoadjuvant and adjuvant treatment of triple-negative early or locally advanced breast cancer (December 2022) NICE TA851 Recommended
▸ Pembrolizumab plus chemotherapy with or without bevacizumab for persistent, recurrent or metastatic cervical cancer (December 2023) NICE TA939 Recommended with restrictions
▸ Pembrolizumab with lenvatinib for previously treated advanced or recurrent endometrial cancer (June 2023) NICE TA904 Recommended

Scottish Medicines Consortium (SMC) decisions
▸ Pembrolizumab (*Keytruda*®) as monotherapy for the treatment of advanced (unresectable or metastatic) melanoma in adults previously untreated with ipilimumab (November 2015) SMC No. 1086/15 Recommended
▸ Pembrolizumab (*Keytruda*®) as monotherapy for the treatment of advanced (unresectable or metastatic) melanoma in adults previously treated with ipilimumab (December 2016) SMC No. 1087/15 Not recommended
▸ Pembrolizumab (*Keytruda*®) as monotherapy for the adjuvant treatment of adults with stage III melanoma and lymph node involvement who have undergone complete resection (May 2019) SMC No. SMC2144 Recommended
▸ Pembrolizumab (*Keytruda*®) as monotherapy for the adjuvant treatment of adults and adolescents aged 12 years and older with stage 2B or 2C melanoma and who have undergone complete resection (April 2023) SMC No. SMC2526 Recommended
▸ Pembrolizumab (*Keytruda*®) for the treatment of locally advanced or metastatic non-small cell lung carcinoma (NSCLC) in adults whose tumours express programmed death ligand 1 (PD-L1) and who have received at least one prior chemotherapy regimen (January 2017) SMC No. 1204/17 Recommended with restrictions
▸ Pembrolizumab (*Keytruda*®) as monotherapy for the first-line treatment of metastatic non-small cell lung carcinoma in adults whose tumours express programmed death ligand 1 with a 50% or more tumour proportion score with no epidermal growth factor receptor or anaplastic lymphoma kinase (ALK)-positive tumour mutations (July 2017) SMC No. 1239/17 Recommended with restrictions
▸ Pembrolizumab (*Keytruda*®) in combination with carboplatin and either paclitaxel or nab-paclitaxel, for the first-line treatment of metastatic squamous non-small cell lung cancer in adults (September 2019) SMC No. SMC2187 Recommended with restrictions
▸ Pembrolizumab (*Keytruda*®) in combination with pemetrexed and platinum chemotherapy for the first-line treatment of metastatic non-squamous non-small cell lung carcinoma in adults whose tumours have no epidermal growth factor receptor or anaplastic lymphoma kinase (ALK)-positive mutations (October 2019) SMC No. SMC2207 Recommended with restrictions

► Pembrolizumab (*Keytruda*®) as monotherapy for the adjuvant treatment of adults with non-small cell lung carcinoma who are at high risk of recurrence following complete resection and platinum-based chemotherapy (October 2024) SMC No. SMC2689 Recommended with restrictions

► Pembrolizumab (*Keytruda*®) in combination with platinum-containing chemotherapy as neoadjuvant treatment, and then continued as monotherapy as adjuvant treatment, for the treatment of resectable non-small cell lung carcinoma at high risk of recurrence in adults (November 2024) SMC No. SMC2688 Not recommended

► Pembrolizumab (*Keytruda*®) as monotherapy for the treatment of locally advanced or metastatic urothelial carcinoma in adults who have received prior platinum-containing chemotherapy (February 2018) SMC No. 1291/18 Recommended with restrictions

► Pembrolizumab (*Keytruda*®) as monotherapy for the treatment of locally advanced or metastatic urothelial carcinoma in adults who are not eligible for cisplatin-containing chemotherapy (first line) (September 2018) SMC No. 1339/18 Not recommended

► Pembrolizumab (*Keytruda*®) as monotherapy for the treatment of adult patients with relapsed or refractory classical Hodgkin lymphoma who have failed autologous stem cell transplant and brentuximab vedotin, or who are transplant-ineligible and have failed brentuximab vedotin (March 2018) SMC No. 1296/18 Recommended with restrictions

► Pembrolizumab (*Keytruda*®) as monotherapy for the treatment of adult and paediatric patients aged 3 years and older with relapsed or refractory classical Hodgkin lymphoma who have failed autologous stem cell transplant (ASCT), or following at least two prior therapies when ASCT is not a treatment option (November 2021) SMC No. SMC2380 Recommended with restrictions

► Pembrolizumab (*Keytruda*®) in combination with axitinib for the first-line treatment of advanced renal cell carcinoma (RCC) in adults (September 2020) SMC No. SMC2247 Recommended with restrictions

► Pembrolizumab (*Keytruda*®) as monotherapy for the adjuvant treatment of adults with renal cell carcinoma at increased risk of recurrence following nephrectomy, or following nephrectomy and resection of metastatic lesions (October 2022) SMC No. SMC2479 Recommended

► Pembrolizumab (*Keytruda*®) as monotherapy or in combination with platinum and 5-fluorouracil chemotherapy, for the first-line treatment of metastatic or unresectable recurrent head and neck squamous cell carcinoma in adults whose tumours express programmed death ligand 1 with a combined positive score of 1 or more (September 2020) SMC No. SMC2257 Recommended with restrictions

► Pembrolizumab (*Keytruda*®) as monotherapy for the first-line treatment of metastatic microsatellite instability-high or mismatch repair deficient colorectal cancer in adults (September 2021) SMC No. SMC2375 Recommended with restrictions

► Pembrolizumab (*Keytruda*®) as monotherapy for the treatment of microsatellite instability-high or mismatch repair deficient tumours in adults with previously treated: unresectable or metastatic colorectal cancer; advanced or recurrent endometrial carcinoma with disease progression; unresectable or metastatic gastric, small intestine, or biliary cancer with disease progression (January 2024) SMC No. SMC2589 Recommended

► Pembrolizumab (*Keytruda*®) in combination with platinum and fluoropyrimidine based chemotherapy, for the first-line treatment of patients with locally advanced unresectable or metastatic carcinoma of the oesophagus in adults whose tumours express PD-L1 with a combined positive score of 10 or more (May 2022) SMC No. SMC2420 Recommended with restrictions

► Pembrolizumab (*Keytruda*®) in combination with fluoropyrimidine and platinum-containing chemotherapy, for the first-line treatment of locally advanced unresectable or metastatic HER2-negative gastric or gastro-oesophageal junction adenocarcinoma in adults whose tumours express PD-L1 with a combined positive score of 1 or more (July 2024) SMC No. SMC2660 Recommended

► Pembrolizumab (*Keytruda*®) in combination with trastuzumab, fluoropyrimidine and platinum-containing chemotherapy for the first-line treatment of locally advanced unresectable or metastatic HER2-positive gastric or gastro-oesophageal junction adenocarcinoma in adults whose tumours express PD-L1 with a combined positive score of 1 or more (July 2024) SMC No. SMC2644 Not recommended

► Pembrolizumab (*Keytruda*®) in combination with chemotherapy, for the treatment of locally recurrent unresectable or metastatic triple-negative breast cancer in adults whose tumours express PD-L1 with a combined positive score of 10 or more and who have not received prior chemotherapy for metastatic disease (October 2022) SMC No. SMC2460 Recommended with restrictions

► Pembrolizumab (*Keytruda*®) in combination with chemotherapy as neoadjuvant treatment, and then continued as monotherapy as adjuvant treatment after surgery, for the treatment of adults with locally advanced, or early stage triple-negative breast cancer at high risk of recurrence (June 2023) SMC No. SMC2538 Recommended

► Pembrolizumab (*Keytruda*®) in combination with lenvatinib, for the treatment of advanced or recurrent endometrial carcinoma in adults who have disease progression on or following prior treatment with a platinum-containing therapy in any setting and who are not candidates for curative surgery or radiation (October 2022) SMC No. SMC2474 Recommended with restrictions

► Pembrolizumab (*Keytruda*®) in combination with chemotherapy, with or without bevacizumab, for the treatment of persistent, recurrent, or metastatic cervical cancer in adults whose tumours express programmed death ligand 1 with a combined positive score of 1 or more (February 2023) SMC No. SMC2501 Recommended with restrictions

● MEDICINAL FORMS There can be variation in the licensing of different medicines containing the same drug.

Solution for infusion
EXCIPIENTS: May contain Polysorbates
► Keytruda (Merck Sharp & Dohme (UK) Ltd)
  Pembrolizumab 25 mg per 1 ml Keytruda 100mg/4ml concentrate for solution for infusion vials | 1 vial [PoM] £2,630.00 (Hospital only)

Pertuzumab [Specialist drug]

17-May-2021

● **INDICATIONS AND DOSE**
Breast cancer
► BY INTRAVENOUS INFUSION
► Adult: Specialist drug – access specialist resources for dosing information

---

IMPORTANT SAFETY INFORMATION
Resuscitation facilities should be available during administration.

● INTERACTIONS → Appendix 1: monoclonal antibodies
● SIDE-EFFECTS
► **Common or very common** Alopecia · anaemia · appetite decreased · arthralgia · asthenia · chills · constipation · cough · diarrhoea · dizziness · dyspnoea · epistaxis · excessive tearing · fever · gastrointestinal discomfort · headache · hot flush · hypersensitivity · increased risk of infection · infusion related reaction · insomnia · left ventricular dysfunction · leucopenia · mucositis · myalgia · nail disorder · nausea · neutropenia · oedema · pain ·

paraesthesia · peripheral neuropathy · skin reactions · stomatitis · taste altered · vomiting

▶ **Uncommon** Heart failure · interstitial lung disease · pleural effusion

▶ **Rare or very rare** Cytokine release syndrome · tumour lysis syndrome

▶ **Frequency not known** Hypomagnesaemia · neutropenic sepsis · weight decreased

SIDE-EFFECTS, FURTHER INFORMATION Side-effects mostly described for pertuzumab in combination with other antineoplastic drugs.

Heart failure Withhold treatment if signs and symptoms suggestive of congestive heart failure occur; discontinue treatment if symptomatic heart failure confirmed.

● CONCEPTION AND CONTRACEPTION Ensure effective contraception during and for six months after treatment in women of childbearing potential.

● NATIONAL FUNDING/ACCESS DECISIONS
For full details see funding body website
NICE decisions

▶ Pertuzumab for the neoadjuvant treatment of HER2-positive breast cancer (December 2016) NICE TA424 Recommended with restrictions

▶ Pertuzumab with trastuzumab and docetaxel for treating HER2-positive breast cancer (March 2018) NICE TA509 Recommended with restrictions

▶ Pertuzumab for adjuvant treatment of HER2-positive early stage breast cancer (March 2019) NICE TA569 Recommended with restrictions

Scottish Medicines Consortium (SMC) decisions

▶ Pertuzumab (*Perjeta*®) for use in combination with trastuzumab and chemotherapy for the neoadjuvant treatment of adult patients with human epidermal growth factor receptor 2 (HER2)-positive, locally advanced, inflammatory, or early stage breast cancer at high risk of recurrence (December 2018) SMC No. SMC2119 Recommended

▶ Pertuzumab (*Perjeta*®) for use in combination with trastuzumab and docetaxel in adult patients with HER2-positive metastatic or locally recurrent unresectable breast cancer, who have not received previous anti-HER2 therapy or chemotherapy for their metastatic disease (January 2019) SMC No. SMC2120 Recommended

▶ Pertuzumab (*Perjeta*®) for use in combination with trastuzumab and chemotherapy for the adjuvant treatment of adult patients with human epidermal growth factor receptor 2 (HER2)-positive early breast cancer (eBC) at high risk of recurrence (September 2020) SMC No. SMC2284 Recommended with restrictions

● MEDICINAL FORMS There can be variation in the licensing of different medicines containing the same drug.
Solution for infusion
▶ Perjeta (Roche Products Ltd)
Pertuzumab 30 mg per 1 ml Perjeta 420mg/14ml concentrate for solution for infusion vials | 1 vial [PoM] £2,395.00 (Hospital only)

Pertuzumab with trastuzumab [Specialist drug]

06-Aug-2021

The properties listed below are those particular to the combination only. For the properties of the components please consider, pertuzumab p. 1017, trastuzumab p. 1023.

● INDICATIONS AND DOSE
Breast cancer
▶ BY SUBCUTANEOUS INJECTION
▶ Adult: Specialist drug – access specialist resources for dosing information

● INTERACTIONS → Appendix 1: monoclonal antibodies

● CONCEPTION AND CONTRACEPTION [EvGr] Ensure effective contraception during and for 7 months after treatment in females of childbearing potential. (M)

● PATIENT AND CARER ADVICE
Driving and skilled tasks [EvGr] Patients and carers should be counselled on the effects on driving and other skilled tasks—increased risk of injection-related reactions and dizziness. (M)

● NATIONAL FUNDING/ACCESS DECISIONS
For full details see funding body website
Scottish Medicines Consortium (SMC) decisions
▶ Pertuzumab/trastuzumab (*Phesgo*®) used in combination with chemotherapy for the treatment of adults with HER2-positive early stage breast cancer or in combination with docetaxel for the treatment of adults with HER2-positive metastatic or locally recurrent unresectable breast cancer (July 2021) SMC No. SMC2364 Recommended with restrictions

● MEDICINAL FORMS There can be variation in the licensing of different medicines containing the same drug.
Solution for injection
EXCIPIENTS: May contain Polysorbates, sucrose
▶ Phesgo (Roche Products Ltd) ▼
Pertuzumab 60 mg per 1 ml, Trastuzumab 60 mg per 1 ml Phesgo 600mg/600mg/10ml solution for injection vials | 1 vial [PoM] £3,617.00 (Hospital only)
Trastuzumab 40 mg per 1 ml, Pertuzumab 80 mg per 1 ml Phesgo 1200mg/600mg/15ml solution for injection vials | 1 vial [PoM] £6,012.00 (Hospital only)

Polatuzumab vedotin [Specialist drug]

25-Jul-2023

● INDICATIONS AND DOSE
Diffuse large B-cell lymphoma
▶ BY INTRAVENOUS INFUSION
▶ Adult: Specialist drug – access specialist resources for dosing information

● CONTRA-INDICATIONS Active severe infection

● INTERACTIONS → Appendix 1: monoclonal antibodies

● SIDE-EFFECTS
▶ **Common or very common** Anaemia · appetite decreased · arthralgia · asthenia · bone marrow disorders · chills · constipation · cough · decreased leucocytes · diarrhoea · dizziness · electrolyte imbalance · fever · gait abnormal · gastrointestinal discomfort · hypoalbuminaemia · increased risk of infection · infusion related reaction · nausea · neutropenia · peripheral neuropathy · pneumonitis · pruritus · sensation abnormal · sepsis · thrombocytopenia · vision blurred · vomiting · weight decreased

▶ **Frequency not known** Gastrointestinal toxicity · hepatic disorders · progressive multifocal leukoencephalopathy (PML) · reactivation of infection

SIDE-EFFECTS, FURTHER INFORMATION Infusion-related reactions, including severe cases and delayed reactions up to 24 hours, have been reported. Pre-medication might be required to minimise reactions; interrupt and manage as appropriate; discontinue if severe infusion reaction.

● CONCEPTION AND CONTRACEPTION Manufacturer advises females of childbearing potential should confirm pregnancy status before treatment and use effective contraception during treatment and for 9 months after last treatment; male patients should use effective contraception during treatment and for 6 months after last treatment if their partner is pregnant or of childbearing potential.

● PATIENT AND CARER ADVICE
Driving and skilled tasks Manufacturer advises patients and carers should be counselled on the effects on driving and

other skilled tasks—increased risk of infusion-related reactions, peripheral neuropathy, fatigue, and dizziness.

● **NATIONAL FUNDING/ACCESS DECISIONS**
For full details see funding body website
NICE decisions
▸ **Polatuzumab vedotin with rituximab and bendamustine for treating relapsed or refractory diffuse large B-cell lymphoma (September 2020)** NICE TA649 Recommended
▸ **Polatuzumab vedotin in combination for untreated diffuse large B-cell lymphoma (March 2023)** NICE TA874 Recommended with restrictions
Scottish Medicines Consortium (SMC) decisions
▸ **Polatuzumab vedotin (*Polivy*®) in combination with rituximab, cyclophosphamide, doxorubicin, and prednisone for the treatment of adult patients with previously untreated diffuse large B-cell lymphoma (DLBCL) (June 2023)** SMC No. SMC2525 Recommended with restrictions
▸ **Polatuzumab vedotin (*Polivy*®) in combination with bendamustine and rituximab for the treatment of adult patients with relapsed/refractory diffuse large B-cell lymphoma who are not candidates for haematopoietic stem cell transplant (July 2023)** SMC No. SMC2524 Recommended

● **MEDICINAL FORMS** There can be variation in the licensing of different medicines containing the same drug.
Powder for solution for infusion
EXCIPIENTS: May contain Polysorbates, sucrose
▸ **Polivy** (Roche Products Ltd) ▼
Polatuzumab vedotin 30 mg Polivy 30mg powder for concentrate for solution for infusion vials | 1 vial [PoM] £2,370.00 (Hospital only)
Polatuzumab vedotin 140 mg Polivy 140mg powder for concentrate for solution for infusion vials | 1 vial [PoM] £11,060.00 (Hospital only)

Ramucirumab [Specialist drug]
20-Aug-2020

● **INDICATIONS AND DOSE**
Gastric cancer | Colorectal cancer | Non-small cell lung cancer | Hepatocellular carcinoma
▸ BY INTRAVENOUS INFUSION
▸ Adult: Specialist drug – access specialist resources for dosing information

IMPORTANT SAFETY INFORMATION
MHRA/CHM ADVICE: SYSTEMICALLY ADMINISTERED VEGF PATHWAY INHIBITORS: RISK OF ANEURYSM AND ARTERY DISSECTION (JULY 2020)
A European review of worldwide data concluded that systemically administered VEGF pathway inhibitors may lead to aneurysm and artery dissection in patients with or without hypertension. Some fatal cases have been reported, mainly in relation to aortic aneurysm rupture and aortic dissection. The MHRA advises healthcare professionals to carefully consider the risk of aneurysm and artery dissection in patients with risk factors before initiating treatment with ramucirumab; any modifiable risk factors (such as smoking and hypertension) should be reduced as much as possible. Blood pressure should be monitored regularly, and product literature should be consulted if hypertension occurs during treatment.

● **INTERACTIONS** → Appendix 1: monoclonal antibodies
● **SIDE-EFFECTS**
▸ **Common or very common** Arterial thromboembolism · diarrhoea · electrolyte imbalance · encephalopathy · epistaxis · gastrointestinal discomfort · gastrointestinal disorders · headache · hepatic coma · hepatic pain · hypertension · hypoalbuminaemia · infusion related reaction · nephrotic syndrome · neutropenia · peripheral oedema · proteinuria · rash · thrombocytopenia

▸ **Frequency not known** Aneurysm · artery dissection · cardiac arrest · cerebrovascular insufficiency · haemangioma · myocardial infarction · thrombotic microangiopathy

SIDE-EFFECTS, FURTHER INFORMATION Infusion-related hypersensitivity reactions have been reported with ramucirumab, particularly during or following the first or second infusion—if the patient experiences a grade 1 or 2 infusion-related reaction, the manufacturer advises to reduce rate of infusion and give premedication for all subsequent infusions; permanently discontinue treatment in grade 3 or 4 infusion-related reactions.

● **CONCEPTION AND CONTRACEPTION** Manufacturer advises effective contraception during treatment and for up to 3 months after treatment in women of childbearing potential.

● **NATIONAL FUNDING/ACCESS DECISIONS**
For full details see funding body website
NICE decisions
▸ **Ramucirumab for treating advanced gastric cancer or gastro-oesophageal junction adenocarcinoma previously treated with chemotherapy (January 2016)** NICE TA378 Not recommended
▸ **Ramucirumab for previously treated locally advanced or metastatic non-small-cell lung cancer (August 2016)** NICE TA403 Not recommended

● **MEDICINAL FORMS** There can be variation in the licensing of different medicines containing the same drug.
Solution for infusion
ELECTROLYTES: May contain Sodium
▸ **Cyramza** (Eli Lilly and Company Ltd)
Ramucirumab 10 mg per 1 ml Cyramza 100mg/10ml concentrate for solution for infusion vials | 1 vial [PoM] £500.00 (Hospital only)
Cyramza 500mg/50ml concentrate for solution for infusion vials | 1 vial [PoM] £2,500.00 (Hospital only)

⟦☞ 991⟧

Rituximab
11-Nov-2022

● **INDICATIONS AND DOSE**
Rheumatoid arthritis (under expert supervision)
▸ BY INTRAVENOUS INFUSION
▸ Adult: 1 g, then 1 g after 2 weeks, consult product literature for information on retreatment
Granulomatosis with polyangiitis and microscopic polyangiitis (under expert supervision)
▸ BY INTRAVENOUS INFUSION
▸ Adult: (consult product literature)
Non-Hodgkin's lymphoma (specialist use only) | Chronic lymphocytic leukaemia (specialist use only)
▸ BY INTRAVENOUS INFUSION
▸ Adult: Specialist indication – access specialist resources for dosing information
Non-Hodgkin's lymphoma (specialist use only)
▸ BY SUBCUTANEOUS INJECTION
▸ Adult: Specialist indication – access specialist resources for dosing information
Pemphigus vulgaris (under expert supervision)
▸ BY INTRAVENOUS INFUSION
▸ Adult: 1 g, then 1 g after 2 weeks; maintenance 0.5 g, at months 12 and 18, and then every 6 months thereafter if needed, consult product literature for the treatment of relapse

● **CONTRA-INDICATIONS**
GENERAL CONTRA-INDICATIONS Severe infection
SPECIFIC CONTRA-INDICATIONS
▸ When used for Rheumatoid arthritis or Granulomatosis with polyangiitis and microscopic polyangiitis or Pemphigus vulgaris Severe heart failure · severe, uncontrolled heart disease

CONTRA-INDICATIONS, FURTHER INFORMATION For full details on contra-indications, consult product literature.

● **CAUTIONS**

GENERAL CAUTIONS History of cardiovascular disease (exacerbation of angina, arrhythmia, and heart failure have been reported) · patients receiving cardiotoxic chemotherapy (exacerbation of angina, arrhythmia, and heart failure have been reported) · pre-medication recommended to minimise adverse reactions (consult product literature) · predisposition to infection · transient hypotension occurs frequently during infusion (anti-hypertensives may need to be withheld for 12 hours before infusion)

SPECIFIC CAUTIONS

▸ When used for Granulomatosis with polyangiitis and microscopic polyangiitis or Pemphigus vulgaris *Pneumocystis jirovecii* pneumonia—consult product literature for prophylaxis requirements

CAUTIONS, FURTHER INFORMATION For full details on cautions, consult product literature or local treatment protocol.

▸ Hepatitis B infection and reactivation Hepatitis B infection and reactivation (including fatal cases) have been reported in patients taking **rituximab**. Manufacturer advises patients with positive hepatitis B serology should be referred to a liver specialist for monitoring and initiation of antiviral therapy before treatment initiation; treatment should not be initiated in patients with evidence of current hepatitis B infection until the infection has been adequately treated. Manufacturer also advises patients should be closely monitored for clinical and laboratory signs of active hepatitis B infection (consult product literature).

● **INTERACTIONS** → Appendix 1: monoclonal antibodies

● **SIDE-EFFECTS**

▸ **Common or very common** Alopecia · angioedema · anxiety · appetite decreased · arrhythmias · asthenia · bone marrow disorders · bursitis · cancer pain · cardiac disorder · chest pain · chills · constipation · depression · diarrhoea · dizziness · dysphagia · dyspnoea · ear pain · electrolyte imbalance · fever · gastrointestinal discomfort · gastrointestinal disorders · headaches · hepatitis B · hypercholesterolaemia · hyperglycaemia · hypertension · hypotension · insomnia · lacrimation disorder · leucopenia · malaise · multi organ failure · muscle complaints · muscle tone increased · myocardial infarction · nausea · nerve disorders · oedema · oral disorders · osteoarthritis · pain · respiratory disorders · sensation abnormal · sepsis · skin reactions · sweat changes · throat irritation · thrombocytopenia · tinnitus · vasodilation · vomiting · weight decreased

▸ **Uncommon** Asthma · coagulation disorder · heart failure · hypoxia · ischaemic heart disease · lymphadenopathy · taste altered

▸ **Rare or very rare** Cytokine release syndrome · facial paralysis · hepatitis B reactivation · interstitial lung disease · progressive multifocal leukoencephalopathy (PML) · renal failure · Stevens-Johnson syndrome (discontinue) · toxic epidermal necrolysis · tumour lysis syndrome · vasculitis · vision disorders

▸ **Frequency not known** Epistaxis · hearing loss · hypogammaglobulinaemia · infective thrombosis · influenza like illness · irritability · muscle weakness · nasal congestion · posterior reversible encephalopathy syndrome (PRES) · psychiatric disorder · seizure · skin papilloma · tremor

SIDE-EFFECTS, FURTHER INFORMATION Associated with infections, sometimes severe, including tuberculosis, septicaemia, and hepatitis B reactivation.

Progressive multifocal leukoencephalopathy has been reported in association with rituximab; patients should be monitored for cognitive, neurological, or psychiatric signs

and symptoms. If progressive multifocal leukoencephalopathy is suspected, suspend treatment until it has been excluded.

● **CONCEPTION AND CONTRACEPTION** Effective contraception in females of childbearing potential required during and for 12 months after treatment.

● **PREGNANCY** Avoid unless potential benefit to mother outweighs risk of B-lymphocyte depletion in fetus.

● **BREAST FEEDING** Avoid breast-feeding during and for 12 months after treatment.

● **MONITORING REQUIREMENTS** For full details on monitoring requirements consult product literature.

● **DIRECTIONS FOR ADMINISTRATION** For *intravenous infusion*, give intermittently in Glucose 5% or Sodium Chloride 0.9%; dilute to 1–4 mg/mL and gently invert bag to avoid foaming; for further information, consult product literature.

● **PRESCRIBING AND DISPENSING INFORMATION** Rituximab is a biological medicine. Biological medicines must be prescribed and dispensed by brand name, see *Biological medicines* and *Biosimilar medicines*, under Guidance on prescribing p. 1.

● **PATIENT AND CARER ADVICE**

Alert card

▸ When used for Rheumatoid arthritis or Granulomatosis with polyangiitis and microscopic polyangiitis or Pemphigus vulgaris Patients should be provided with a patient alert card with each infusion.

● **NATIONAL FUNDING/ACCESS DECISIONS**

For full details see funding body website

NICE decisions

▸ **Rituximab in combination with glucocorticoids for treating anti-neutrophil cytoplasmic antibody-associated vasculitis (March 2014)** NICE TA308 Recommended with restrictions

▸ **Adalimumab, etanercept, infliximab, rituximab, and abatacept for the treatment of rheumatoid arthritis after the failure of a TNF inhibitor (August 2010)** NICE TA195 Recommended with restrictions

▸ **Rituximab for the first-line treatment of stage III-IV follicular lymphoma (January 2012)** NICE TA243 Recommended

▸ **Rituximab for the treatment of relapsed or refractory stage III or IV follicular non-Hodgkin's lymphoma (February 2008)** NICE TA137 Recommended with restrictions

▸ **Rituximab for the treatment of relapsed or refractory chronic lymphocytic leukaemia (July 2010)** NICE TA193 Recommended with restrictions

▸ **Rituximab for the first-line maintenance treatment of follicular non-Hodgkin's lymphoma (June 2011)** NICE TA226 Recommended

▸ **Rituximab for the first-line treatment of chronic lymphocytic leukaemia (July 2009)** NICE TA174 Recommended

▸ **Idelalisib for treating chronic lymphocytic leukaemia [in combination with rituximab] (October 2015)** NICE TA359 Recommended

▸ **Venetoclax with rituximab for previously treated chronic lymphocytic leukaemia (February 2019)** NICE TA561 Recommended with restrictions

Scottish Medicines Consortium (SMC) decisions

▸ Rituximab (*MabThera*®) for use in combination with glucocorticoids for the induction of remission in adult patients with severe, active granulomatosis with polyangiitis (Wegener's) and microscopic polyangiitis (September 2013) SMC No. 894/13 Recommended with restrictions

▸ Rituximab (*MabThera*®) subcutaneous injection for the treatment of non-Hodgkin's lymphoma in adults (July 2014) SMC No. 975/14 Recommended with restrictions

All Wales Medicines Strategy Group (AWMSG) decisions

▸ Rituximab (*MabThera*®) for the treatment of patients with moderate to severe pemphigus vulgaris (October 2022) AWMSG No. 3192 Recommended

● **MEDICINAL FORMS** There can be variation in the licensing of different medicines containing the same drug.

Solution for injection

▸ **MabThera** (Roche Products Ltd)

Rituximab 119.66 mg per 1 ml MabThera 1400mg/11.7ml solution for injection vials | 1 vial [PoM] £1,344.65 (Hospital only)

Solution for infusion

EXCIPIENTS: May contain Polysorbates
ELECTROLYTES: May contain Sodium

▸ **MabThera** (Roche Products Ltd)

Rituximab 10 mg per 1 ml MabThera 100mg/10ml concentrate for solution for infusion vials | 2 vial [PoM] £349.25 (Hospital only)
MabThera 500mg/50ml concentrate for solution for infusion vials | 1 vial [PoM] £873.15 (Hospital only)

▸ **Rixathon** (Sandoz Ltd)

Rituximab 10 mg per 1 ml Rixathon 100mg/10ml concentrate for solution for infusion vials | 3 vial [PoM] £471.50 (Hospital only)
Rixathon 500mg/50ml concentrate for solution for infusion vials | 2 vial [PoM] £1,571.67 (Hospital only)

▸ **Ruxience** (Pfizer Ltd) ▼

Rituximab 10 mg per 1 ml Ruxience 100mg/10ml concentrate for solution for infusion vials | 1 vial [PoM] £157.17 (Hospital only)
Ruxience 500mg/50ml concentrate for solution for infusion vials | 1 vial [PoM] £785.84 (Hospital only)

▸ **Truxima** (Celltrion Healthcare UK Ltd)

Rituximab 10 mg per 1 ml Truxima 100mg/10ml concentrate for solution for infusion vials | 2 vial [PoM] £314.33 (Hospital only)
Truxima 500mg/50ml concentrate for solution for infusion vials | 1 vial [PoM] £785.84 (Hospital only)

Sacituzumab govitecan [Specialist drug]

13-Sep-2022

● **INDICATIONS AND DOSE**

Breast cancer

▸ BY INTRAVENOUS INFUSION

▸ Adult: Specialist drug – access specialist resources for dosing information

---

IMPORTANT SAFETY INFORMATION
Resuscitation facilities should be available during administration.

● **INTERACTIONS** → Appendix 1: sacituzumab govitecan

● **SIDE-EFFECTS**

▸ **Common or very common** Allergic rhinitis · alopecia · anaemia · appetite decreased · arthralgia · asthma · back pain · chest discomfort · choking · constipation · cough · decreased leucocytes · dehydration · diarrhoea · dizziness · dyspnoea · electrolyte imbalance · epistaxis · eye inflammation · eye pruritus · facial swelling · fatigue · fever · flushing · gastrointestinal discomfort · headache · hyperglycaemia · hypersensitivity · hypotension · increased risk of infection · insomnia · nausea · neutropenia · oedema · oral disorders · respiratory disorders · scrotal oedema · seasonal allergy · skin reactions · swelling · taste altered · throat tightness · vomiting · weight decreased

● **ALLERGY AND CROSS-SENSITIVITY** [EvGr] Contra-indicated in patients with hypersensitivity to previous irinotecan therapy. ⟨M⟩

● **CONCEPTION AND CONTRACEPTION** [EvGr] Females of childbearing potential should use effective contraception during treatment and for 6 months after last treatment; male patients should use effective contraception during treatment and for 3 months after last treatment if their partner is of childbearing potential. Female fertility may be impaired—impairment of fertility has been observed in *animal* studies. ⟨M⟩

● **PATIENT AND CARER ADVICE** Patients and their carers should be advised to seek immediate medical attention if they have black stools, rectal bleeding, dehydration or are unable to tolerate oral fluids.

Driving and skilled tasks Patients and carers should be counselled on the effects on driving and performance of skilled tasks—increased risk of dizziness.

● **NATIONAL FUNDING/ACCESS DECISIONS**
For full details see funding body website

NICE decisions

▸ Sacituzumab govitecan for treating unresectable triple-negative advanced breast cancer after 2 or more therapies (August 2022) NICE TA819 Recommended

Scottish Medicines Consortium (SMC) decisions

▸ Sacituzumab govitecan (*Trodelvy*®) for the treatment of adult patients with unresectable locally advanced or metastatic triple-negative breast cancer (mTNBC) who have received two or more prior lines of systemic therapies, at least one of them given for unresectable locally advanced or metastatic disease (March 2022) SMC No. SMC2446 Recommended

● **MEDICINAL FORMS** There can be variation in the licensing of different medicines containing the same drug.

Powder for solution for infusion

EXCIPIENTS: May contain Polysorbates

▸ **Trodelvy** (Gilead Sciences Ltd) ▼

Sacituzumab govitecan 180 mg Trodelvy 180mg powder for concentrate for solution for infusion vials | 1 vial [PoM] £793.00 (Hospital only)

Siltuximab

30-Jul-2020

● **DRUG ACTION** Siltuximab is a monoclonal antibody that inhibits interleukin-6 receptor binding.

● **INDICATIONS AND DOSE**

Treatment of multicentric Castleman's disease (MCD) in patients who are human immunodeficiency virus (HIV) negative and human herpesvirus-8 (HHV-8) negative

▸ BY INTRAVENOUS INFUSION

▸ Adult: 11 mg/kg every 3 weeks

● **CAUTIONS** Patients at increased risk of gastrointestinal perforation—promptly investigate those presenting with symptoms suggestive of gastrointestinal perforation · severe infection—withhold treatment until resolved · treat infection prior to treatment

CAUTIONS, FURTHER INFORMATION

▸ Hypersensitivity reactions Infusion-related side-effects are reported commonly with siltuximab; resuscitation facilities should be available during treatment.
Consult product literature for further information about siltuximab cautions.

● **INTERACTIONS** → Appendix 1: monoclonal antibodies

● **SIDE-EFFECTS**

▸ **Common or very common** Abdominal pain · arthralgia · constipation · diarrhoea · dizziness · dyslipidaemia · gastrooesophageal reflux disease · headache · hypersensitivity · hypertension · hyperuricaemia · increased risk of infection · infusion related reaction · localised oedema · nausea · neutropenia · oral ulceration · oropharyngeal pain · pain in extremity · renal impairment · skin reactions · thrombocytopenia · vomiting · weight increased

SIDE-EFFECTS, FURTHER INFORMATION Siltuximab therapy should be discontinued permanently in the event of a severe infusion-related reaction, anaphylaxis, a severe allergic reaction, or the occurrence of cytokine-release syndrome. Mild to moderate infusion-related reactions may improve by temporarily reducing the rate or stopping the infusion. When restarting treatment, a reduced infusion rate and the administration of antihistamines, paracetamol, and corticosteroids may be considered. Consider discontinuation of siltuximab if more than 2 doses are delayed due to treatment-related toxicities during the first 48 weeks—for full details consult product literature.

- **CONCEPTION AND CONTRACEPTION** Women of childbearing potential should use effective contraception during and for 3 months after treatment.
- **PREGNANCY** Manufacturer advises avoid unless potential benefit outweighs risk.
- **BREAST FEEDING** Manufacturer advises avoid—no information available.
- **HEPATIC IMPAIRMENT** Manufacturer advises caution (no information).
- **MONITORING REQUIREMENTS**
  - Monitor neutrophil and platelet count, and haemoglobin levels prior to each dose of siltuximab treatment for the first 12 months and thereafter prior to every third dosing cycle. Consider delaying treatment if required neutrophil, platelet, and haemoglobin levels not achieved—consult product literature for details.
  - Monitor for infection during treatment.
- **DIRECTIONS FOR ADMINISTRATION** For *intravenous infusion* (*Sylvant ®*), manufacturer advises give intermittently *in* Glucose 5%. Allow vials to reach room temperature over approximately 30 minutes, then reconstitute each 100 mg vial with 5.2 mL of Water for Injections, and each 400 mg vial with 20 mL of Water for Injections, to produce a 20 mg/mL solution. Gently swirl without shaking to dissolve. Further dilute to 250 mL with Glucose 5% and gently mix. Use within 6 hours of dilution and give over 60 minutes using an administration set lined with polyvinyl chloride or polyurethane, through a low-protein binding in-line 0.2 micron filter.

- **MEDICINAL FORMS** There can be variation in the licensing of different medicines containing the same drug.
  Powder for solution for infusion
  - Sylvant (Recordati UK Ltd) ▼
    Siltuximab 100 mg Sylvant 100mg powder for concentrate for solution for infusion vials | 1 vial [PoM] £502.15 (Hospital only)
    Siltuximab 400 mg Sylvant 400mg powder for concentrate for solution for infusion vials | 1 vial [PoM] £2,009.81 (Hospital only)

Tafasitamab [Specialist drug]
24-May-2023

- **INDICATIONS AND DOSE**

Diffuse large B-cell lymphoma
  - BY INTRAVENOUS INFUSION
  - Adult: Specialist drug – access specialist resources for dosing information

- **INTERACTIONS** → Appendix 1: monoclonal antibodies

- **SIDE-EFFECTS**
  - **Common or very common** Abdominal pain · alopecia · anaemia · appetite decreased · arthralgia · asthenia · basal cell carcinoma · constipation · COPD exacerbated · cough · decreased leucocytes · diarrhoea · dyspnoea · electrolyte imbalance · fever · headache · hyperbilirubinaemia · hyperhidrosis · hypogammaglobulinaemia · increased risk of infection · infusion related reaction · malaise · mucositis · muscle spasms · nasal congestion · nausea · neutropenia · pain · paraesthesia · peripheral oedema · sepsis · skin reactions · taste altered · thrombocytopenia · vomiting · weight decreased
  - **Frequency not known** Bone marrow depression · tumour lysis syndrome

- **CONCEPTION AND CONTRACEPTION** [EvGr] Females of childbearing potential should use effective contraception during treatment and for at least 3 months after last treatment. [M]

- **PATIENT AND CARER ADVICE**
  Driving and skilled tasks Patients and carers should be counselled on the effects on driving and performance of skilled tasks—increased risk of fatigue.

- **NATIONAL FUNDING/ACCESS DECISIONS**
  For full details see funding body website
  NICE decisions
  - Tafasitamab with lenalidomide for treating relapsed or refractory diffuse large B-cell lymphoma (May 2023) NICE TA883 Not recommended

  Scottish Medicines Consortium (SMC) decisions
  - Tafasitamab (*Minjuvi®*) in combination with lenalidomide, followed by tafasitamab monotherapy, for the treatment of adult patients with relapsed or refractory diffuse large B-cell lymphoma who are not eligible for autologous stem cell transplant (May 2023) SMC No. SMC2522 Not recommended

- **MEDICINAL FORMS** There can be variation in the licensing of different medicines containing the same drug.
  Powder for solution for infusion
  EXCIPIENTS: May contain Polysorbates
  - Minjuvi (Incyte Biosciences UK Ltd) ▼
    Tafasitamab 200 mg Minjuvi 200mg powder for concentrate for solution for infusion vials | 1 vial [PoM] £705.00 (Hospital only)

Talquetamab [Specialist drug]
13-Nov-2023

- **INDICATIONS AND DOSE**

Multiple myeloma
  - BY SUBCUTANEOUS INJECTION
  - Adult: Specialist drug – access specialist resources for dosing information

- **CONTRA-INDICATIONS** Active serious infection

- **SIDE-EFFECTS**
  - **Common or very common** Abdominal pain · alopecia · anaemia · anxiety · aphasia · appetite decreased · bradyphrenia · chills · confusion · constipation · cough · cytokine release syndrome · decreased leucocytes · delirium · diarrhoea · dizziness · drowsiness · dry eye · dry mouth · dysgraphia · dysphagia · dysphonia · dyspnoea · electrolyte imbalance · encephalopathy · fatigue · fever · fluid imbalance · gait abnormal · haemorrhage · hallucination · headache · hypogammaglobulinaemia · immune effector cell-associated neurotoxicity syndrome · increased risk of infection · inflammation · joint swelling · memory impairment · motor dysfunction · muscle spasms · muscle weakness · nail disorder · nausea · nerve disorders · neutropenia · oedema · oral disorders · pain · periorbital oedema · respiratory disorders · sensation abnormal · sepsis · skin reactions · sleep disorder · subdural haematoma · taste altered · thrombocytopenia · tremor · vomiting · weight decreased

- **CONCEPTION AND CONTRACEPTION** [EvGr] Females of childbearing potential should use effective contraception during treatment and for at least 3 months after last treatment. [M]

- **PATIENT AND CARER ADVICE** Patients and their carers should be advised to seek medical attention if signs or symptoms of cytokine release syndrome, oral or neurologic toxicity, or infection occur.
  Patient card A patient card should be provided.
  Driving and skilled tasks Patients and their carers should be counselled on the effects on driving and performance of skilled tasks—increased risk of depressed level of consciousness and neurologic toxicity (consult product literature).

- **MEDICINAL FORMS** There can be variation in the licensing of different medicines containing the same drug.
  Solution for injection
  EXCIPIENTS: May contain Disodium edetate, polysorbates, sucrose
  ▸ **Talvey** (Janssen-Cilag Ltd) ▼
    Talquetamab 2 mg per 1 ml Talvey 3mg/1.5ml solution for injection vials | 1 vial [PoM] £326.41 (Hospital only)
    Talquetamab 40 mg per 1 ml Talvey 40mg/1ml solution for injection vials | 1 vial [PoM] £4,352.00 (Hospital only)

Tarlatamab [Specialist drug]
18-Mar-2025

- **INDICATIONS AND DOSE**
  Small cell lung cancer
  ▸ BY INTRAVENOUS INFUSION
  ▸ Adult: Specialist drug – access specialist resources for dosing information

- **INTERACTIONS** → Appendix 1: tarlatamab

- **SIDE-EFFECTS**
  ▸ **Common or very common** Anaemia · appetite decreased · asthenia · confusion · constipation · cytokine release syndrome · delirium · dyspnoea · encephalopathy · fever · hyponatraemia · immune effector cell-associated neurotoxicity syndrome (may occur up to several weeks after administration) · nausea · neurotoxicity · neutropenia · taste altered · tremor
  ▸ **Uncommon** Ataxia · seizure
  ▸ **Frequency not known** Hypersensitivity

- **CONCEPTION AND CONTRACEPTION** [EvGr] Females of childbearing potential should use effective contraception during treatment and for at least 28 days after last treatment. ⟨M⟩

- **PATIENT AND CARER ADVICE** Patients and carers should be counselled on the signs and symptoms of cytokine release syndrome and immune effector cell-associated neurotoxicity syndrome, and advised to seek immediate medical attention if these occur.
  A patient alert card should be provided.
  Driving and skilled tasks Patients and carers should be counselled on the effects on driving and performance of skilled tasks—increased risk of neurological side-effects.

- **MEDICINAL FORMS** There can be variation in the licensing of different medicines containing the same drug.
  Powder and solution for solution for infusion
  EXCIPIENTS: May contain Polysorbates
  ▸ **Imdylltra** (Amgen Ltd) ▼
    Tarlatamab 1 mg Imdylltra 1mg powder for concentrate and solution for solution for infusion vials | 1 vial [PoM] £955.00 (Hospital only)
    Tarlatamab 10 mg Imdylltra 10mg powder for concentrate and solution for solution for infusion vials | 1 vial [PoM] £9,550.00 (Hospital only)

Teclistamab [Specialist drug]
26-Nov-2024

- **INDICATIONS AND DOSE**
  Multiple myeloma
  ▸ BY SUBCUTANEOUS INJECTION
  ▸ Adult: Specialist drug – access specialist resources for dosing information

- **CONTRA-INDICATIONS** Active infection (do not initiate until resolved)

- **INTERACTIONS** → Appendix 1: monoclonal antibodies

- **SIDE-EFFECTS**
  ▸ **Common or very common** Acute respiratory failure · anaemia · appetite decreased · arthralgia · asthenia · cancer pain · confusion · constipation · cough · cytokine release syndrome · decreased leucocytes · diarrhoea · drowsiness · dyspnoea · ear pain · electrolyte imbalance ·

encephalopathy · fever · fluid overload · haemorrhage · headache · hyperamylasaemia · hypertension · hypoalbuminaemia · hypofibrinogenaemia · hypogammaglobulinaemia · hypoglobulinaemia · hypoxia · immune effector cell-associated neurotoxicity syndrome · increased risk of infection · iron deficiency · level of consciousness decreased · malaise · memory impairment · myalgia · nausea · nerve disorders · neutropenia · oedema · oral disorders · oropharyngeal pain · pain · peripheral swelling · sensation abnormal · sepsis · subdural haematoma · thrombocytopenia · vomiting
  ▸ **Frequency not known** Acute kidney injury · progressive multifocal leukoencephalopathy (PML) · viral infection reactivation

- **CONCEPTION AND CONTRACEPTION** [EvGr] Females of childbearing potential and male patients with a partner of childbearing potential should use effective contraception during treatment and for 3 months after last treatment. ⟨M⟩

- **PATIENT AND CARER ADVICE** Patients and carers should be advised to seek immediate medical attention if signs or symptoms of cytokine release syndrome or neurologic toxicity occur.
  Patient card A patient card should be provided.
  Driving and skilled tasks Patients and carers should be counselled on the effects on driving and performance of skilled tasks—increased risk of depressed level of consciousness (consult product literature).

- **NATIONAL FUNDING/ACCESS DECISIONS**
  For full details see funding body website
  NICE decisions
  ▸ **Teclistamab for treating relapsed and refractory multiple myeloma after 3 or more treatments (November 2024)**
  NICE TA1015 Recommended
  Scottish Medicines Consortium (SMC) decisions
  ▸ **Teclistamab (*Tecvayli®*) as monotherapy for the treatment of adult patients with relapsed and refractory multiple myeloma, who have received at least three prior therapies, including an immunomodulatory agent, a proteasome inhibitor, and an anti-CD38 antibody and have demonstrated disease progression on the last therapy (September 2024)**
  SMC No. SMC2668 Recommended

- **MEDICINAL FORMS** There can be variation in the licensing of different medicines containing the same drug.
  Solution for injection
  EXCIPIENTS: May contain Disodium edetate, polysorbates
  ▸ **Tecvayli** (Janssen-Cilag Ltd) ▼
    Teclistamab 10 mg per 1 ml Tecvayli 30mg/3ml solution for injection vials | 1 vial [PoM] £775.14 (Hospital only)
    Teclistamab 90 mg per 1 ml Tecvayli 153mg/1.7ml solution for injection vials | 1 vial [PoM] £3,952.78 (Hospital only)

Trastuzumab [Specialist drug]
20-Apr-2021

- **INDICATIONS AND DOSE**
  Breast cancer
  ▸ BY INTRAVENOUS INFUSION, OR BY SUBCUTANEOUS INJECTION
  ▸ Adult: Specialist drug – access specialist resources for dosing information
  Gastric cancer
  ▸ BY INTRAVENOUS INFUSION
  ▸ Adult: Specialist drug – access specialist resources for dosing information

IMPORTANT SAFETY INFORMATION
Resuscitation facilities should be available during administration.
  When prescribing, dispensing, or administering, check that this is the correct preparation—trastuzumab is **not**

interchangeable with trastuzumab emtansine or trastuzumab deruxtecan.

- **CONTRA-INDICATIONS** Severe dyspnoea at rest
- **INTERACTIONS** → Appendix 1: monoclonal antibodies
- **SIDE-EFFECTS**
- **Common or very common** Alopecia · anaemia · angioedema · anxiety · appetite decreased · arrhythmias · arthralgia · arthritis · asthenia · asthma · breast abnormalities · cardiomyopathy · chest pain · chills · constipation · cough · cystitis · depression · diarrhoea · dizziness · drowsiness · dry eye · dry mouth · dyspnoea · excessive tearing · eye inflammation · fever · gastrointestinal discomfort · haemorrhage · haemorrhoids · headache · heart failure · hepatic disorders · hyperhidrosis · hypersensitivity · hypotension · increased risk of infection · influenza like illness · infusion related reaction (may be delayed) · insomnia · leucopenia · malaise · mucositis · muscle complaints · muscle tone increased · nail disorders · nausea · neutropenia · neutropenic sepsis · oedema · oral disorders · pain · palpitations · paraesthesia · peripheral neuropathy · renal disorder · respiratory disorders · rhinorrhoea · skin reactions · taste altered · thrombocytopenia · tremor · vasodilation · vomiting · weight decreased
- **Uncommon** Deafness · interstitial lung disease · pericardial effusion
- **Frequency not known** Cardiac disorder · cardiogenic shock · glomerulonephritis · haematotoxicity · hyperkalaemia · hypertension · hypoprothrombinaemia · hypoxia · left ventricular dysfunction · post procedural infection · pulmonary fibrosis · pulmonary oedema · renal failure · tumour lysis syndrome

SIDE-EFFECTS, FURTHER INFORMATION **Heart failure** Consider discontinuing treatment in cases of left ventricular dysfunction.

Interstitial lung disease and pneumonitis Interstitial lung disease and pneumonitis, including fatal events, have been reported; if confirmed treatment should be discontinued.

- **CONCEPTION AND CONTRACEPTION** Manufacturer advises effective contraception in women of childbearing potential during and for 7 months after treatment.
- **NATIONAL FUNDING/ACCESS DECISIONS** For full details see funding body website

NICE decisions
- **Guidance on the use of trastuzumab for the treatment of advanced breast cancer (March 2002)** NICE TA34 Recommended with restrictions
- **Lapatinib or trastuzumab in combination with an aromatase inhibitor for the first-line treatment of metastatic hormone-receptor-positive breast cancer that overexpresses HER2 (June 2012)** NICE TA257 Not recommended
- **Pertuzumab with trastuzumab and docetaxel for treating HER2-positive breast cancer (March 2018)** NICE TA509 Recommended with restrictions
- **Trastuzumab for the treatment of HER2-positive metastatic gastric cancer (November 2010)** NICE TA208 Recommended with restrictions

Scottish Medicines Consortium (SMC) decisions
- **Trastuzumab (*Herceptin*®) for the treatment of adult patients with HER2 positive metastatic breast cancer and early breast cancer (January 2014)** SMC No. 928/13 Recommended with restrictions
- **Trastuzumab (*Herceptin*®) in combination with capecitabine or fluorouracil and cisplatin for the treatment of patients with HER2 positive metastatic adenocarcinoma of the stomach or gastro-oesophageal junction who have not received prior anti-cancer treatment for their metastatic disease (October 2015)** SMC No. 623/10 Recommended with restrictions

- **MEDICINAL FORMS** There can be variation in the licensing of different medicines containing the same drug.

Solution for injection
- **Herceptin** (Roche Products Ltd)
  Trastuzumab 120 mg per 1 ml Herceptin 600mg/5ml solution for injection vials | 1 vial PoM £1,222.20 (Hospital only)

Powder for solution for infusion
- **Herceptin** (Roche Products Ltd)
  Trastuzumab 150 mg Herceptin 150mg powder for concentrate for solution for infusion vials | 1 vial PoM £407.40 (Hospital only)
- **Herzuma** (Celltrion Healthcare UK Ltd) ▼
  Trastuzumab 150 mg Herzuma 150mg powder for concentrate for solution for infusion vials | 1 vial PoM £366.66 (Hospital only)
  Trastuzumab 420 mg Herzuma 420mg powder for concentrate for solution for infusion vials | 1 vial PoM £1,026.65 (Hospital only)
- **Ogivri** (Biosimilar Collaborations Ireland Ltd)
  Trastuzumab 150 mg Ogivri 150mg powder for concentrate for solution for infusion vials | 1 vial PoM £366.00 (Hospital only)
  Trastuzumab 420 mg Ogivri 420mg powder for concentrate for solution for infusion vials | 1 vial PoM £1,026.00 (Hospital only)
- **Ontruzant** (Organon Pharma (UK) Ltd)
  Trastuzumab 150 mg Ontruzant 150mg powder for concentrate for solution for infusion vials | 1 vial PoM £366.66 (Hospital only)
- **Trazimera** (Pfizer Ltd)
  Trastuzumab 150 mg Trazimera 150mg powder for concentrate for solution for infusion vials | 1 vial PoM £366.66 (Hospital only)
  Trastuzumab 420 mg Trazimera 420mg powder for concentrate for solution for infusion vials | 1 vial PoM £1,026.65 (Hospital only)
- **Zercepac** (Accord-UK Ltd) ▼
  Trastuzumab 60 mg Zercepac 60mg powder for concentrate for solution for infusion vials | 1 vial PoM £146.66 (Hospital only)
  Trastuzumab 150 mg Zercepac 150mg powder for concentrate for solution for infusion vials | 1 vial PoM £366.65 (Hospital only)
  Trastuzumab 420 mg Zercepac 420mg powder for concentrate for solution for infusion vials | 1 vial PoM £1,026.62 (Hospital only)

Trastuzumab deruxtecan [Specialist drug]

19-Dec-2024

- **INDICATIONS AND DOSE**

Breast cancer
- BY INTRAVENOUS INFUSION
- Adult: Specialist drug – access specialist resources for dosing information

IMPORTANT SAFETY INFORMATION
When prescribing, dispensing, or administering, check that this is the correct preparation—trastuzumab deruxtecan is **not** interchangeable with trastuzumab or trastuzumab emtansine.

- **INTERACTIONS** → Appendix 1: monoclonal antibodies
- **SIDE-EFFECTS**
- **Common or very common** Alopecia · anaemia · appetite decreased · asthenia · constipation · cough · decreased leucocytes · diarrhoea · dizziness · dry eye · dyspnoea · epistaxis · flushing · gastrointestinal discomfort · headaches · heart failure · hypersensitivity · hypokalaemia · increased risk of infection · influenza like illness · infusion related reaction · interstitial lung disease · lymphangitis · nausea · neutropenia · oral disorders · respiratory disorders · skin reactions · thrombocytopenia · vomiting

SIDE-EFFECTS, FURTHER INFORMATION **Heart failure** Delay or discontinue treatment in cases of left ventricular dysfunction; discontinue treatment if symptomatic heart failure occurs.

Interstitial lung disease and pneumonitis Interstitial lung disease and pneumonitis, including fatal events, have been reported; if confirmed treatment should be discontinued.

- **CONCEPTION AND CONTRACEPTION** EvGr Females of childbearing potential should use effective contraception during treatment and for at least 7 months after last treatment; male patients should use effective contraception during treatment and for at least 4 months after last treatment if their partner is of childbearing potential. ⓜ

- **PATIENT AND CARER ADVICE** Patients and carers should be advised to seek immediate medical attention if signs or symptoms of interstitial lung disease or pneumonitis occur.

  Patient Card A patient card should be provided.

- **NATIONAL FUNDING/ACCESS DECISIONS**
  For full details see funding body website

  NICE decisions
  ▶ Trastuzumab deruxtecan for treating HER2-positive unresectable or metastatic breast cancer after 2 or more anti-HER2 therapies (May 2021) NICE TA704 Recommended
  ▶ Trastuzumab deruxtecan for treating HER2-positive unresectable or metastatic breast cancer after 1 or more anti-HER2 treatments (February 2023) NICE TA862 Recommended
  ▶ Trastuzumab deruxtecan for treating HER2-low metastatic or unresectable breast cancer after chemotherapy (July 2024) NICE TA992 Not recommended

  Scottish Medicines Consortium (SMC) decisions
  ▶ Trastuzumab deruxtecan (*Enhertu*®) as monotherapy for the treatment of adult patients with unresectable or metastatic HER2-positive breast cancer who have received two or more prior anti-HER2-based regimens (January 2022) SMC No. SMC2388 Recommended
  ▶ Trastuzumab deruxtecan (*Enhertu*®) as monotherapy for the treatment of adult patients with unresectable or metastatic HER2-positive breast cancer who have received one or more prior anti-HER2-based regimens (April 2023) SMC No. SMC2545 Recommended with restrictions
  ▶ Trastuzumab deruxtecan (*Enhertu*®) as monotherapy for the treatment of adult patients with unresectable or metastatic HER2-low breast cancer who have received prior chemotherapy in the metastatic setting or developed disease recurrence during or within 6 months of completing adjuvant chemotherapy (December 2023) SMC No. SMC2608 Recommended

- **MEDICINAL FORMS** There can be variation in the licensing of different medicines containing the same drug.

  Powder for solution for infusion
  EXCIPIENTS: May contain Polysorbates
  ▶ Enhertu (Daiichi Sankyo UK Ltd) ▼
  Trastuzumab deruxtecan 100 mg Enhertu 100mg powder for concentrate for solution for infusion vials | 1 vial PoM £1,455.00 (Hospital only)

Trastuzumab emtansine [Specialist drug]

17-May-2021

- **INDICATIONS AND DOSE**

  Breast cancer
  ▶ BY INTRAVENOUS INFUSION
  ▶ Adult: Specialist drug – access specialist resources for dosing information

  IMPORTANT SAFETY INFORMATION
  Resuscitation facilities should be available during administration.
      When prescribing, dispensing, or administering, check that this is the correct preparation—trastuzumab emtansine is **not** interchangeable with trastuzumab or trastuzumab deruxtecan.

- **INTERACTIONS** → Appendix 1: monoclonal antibodies

- **SIDE-EFFECTS**
  ▶ **Common or very common** Alopecia · anaemia · arthralgia · asthenia · chills · conjunctivitis · constipation · cough · diarrhoea · dizziness · dry eye · dry mouth · dyspnoea · excessive tearing · fever · gastrointestinal discomfort · haemorrhage · headache · hypersensitivity · hypertension · hypokalaemia · infusion related reaction · insomnia · left ventricular dysfunction · leucopenia · memory loss · musculoskeletal pain · myalgia · nail disorder · nausea · neutropenia · peripheral neuropathy · peripheral oedema · skin reactions · stomatitis · taste altered · thrombocytopenia · urinary tract infection · vision blurred · vomiting
  ▶ **Uncommon** Hepatic disorders · nodular regenerative hyperplasia · pneumonitis

  SIDE-EFFECTS, FURTHER INFORMATION **Heart failure** Delay or discontinue treatment in cases of left ventricular dysfunction; discontinue treatment if symptomatic heart failure occurs.
      Interstitial lung disease and pneumonitis Interstitial lung disease and pneumonitis, including fatal events, have been reported; if confirmed treatment should be discontinued.
      Peripheral neuropathy Temporarily discontinue treatment if peripheral neuropathy occurs; if restarting, consider dose adjustment.

- **CONCEPTION AND CONTRACEPTION** Manufacturer advises effective contraception must be used during and for 7 months after stopping treatment in women and men.

- **NATIONAL FUNDING/ACCESS DECISIONS**
  For full details see funding body website

  NICE decisions
  ▶ Trastuzumab emtansine for treating HER2-positive advanced breast cancer after trastuzumab and a taxane (updated November 2017) NICE TA458 Recommended with restrictions
  ▶ Trastuzumab emtansine for adjuvant treatment of HER2-positive early breast cancer (June 2020) NICE TA632 Recommended

  Scottish Medicines Consortium (SMC) decisions
  ▶ Trastuzumab emtansine (*Kadcyla*®) for HER2-positive, unresectable locally advanced or metastatic breast cancer after trastuzumab and a taxane (April 2017) SMC No. 990/14 Recommended
  ▶ Trastuzumab emtansine (*Kadcyla*®) as a single agent, for the adjuvant treatment of adult patients with HER2-positive early breast cancer who have residual invasive disease, in the breast and/or lymph nodes, after neoadjuvant taxane-based and HER2-targeted therapy (November 2020) SMC No. SMC2298 Recommended

- **MEDICINAL FORMS** There can be variation in the licensing of different medicines containing the same drug.

  Powder for solution for infusion
  ▶ Kadcyla (Roche Products Ltd)
  Trastuzumab emtansine 100 mg Kadcyla 100mg powder for concentrate for solution for infusion vials | 1 vial PoM £1,641.01
  Trastuzumab emtansine 160 mg Kadcyla 160mg powder for concentrate for solution for infusion vials | 1 vial PoM £2,625.62

Tremelimumab [Specialist drug]

25-Oct-2023

- **INDICATIONS AND DOSE**

  Hepatocellular carcinoma
  ▶ BY INTRAVENOUS INFUSION
  ▶ Adult: Specialist drug – access specialist resources for dosing information

- **SIDE-EFFECTS**
  ▶ **Common or very common** Adrenal insufficiency · cough · diarrhoea · dysuria · fever · flank pain · gastrointestinal discomfort · gastrointestinal disorders · hepatic disorders ·

8

Immune system and malignant disease

hyperthyroidism · hypothyroidism · immune-mediated lung disease · increased risk of infection · infusion related reaction · interstitial lung disease · myalgia · night sweats · pancreatitis · peripheral oedema · peripheral swelling · skin reactions · thyroiditis
▶ **Uncommon** Cardiac inflammation · dysphonia · hypophysitis · hypopituitarism · immune thrombocytopenic purpura · immune-mediated arthritis · meningitis · myasthenia gravis · myopathy · nephritis · type 1 diabetes mellitus
▶ **Rare or very rare** Cystitis · diabetes insipidus · Guillain-Barre syndrome · uveitis
▶ **Frequency not known** Transverse myelitis

● CONCEPTION AND CONTRACEPTION [EvGr] Females of childbearing potential should use effective contraception during treatment and for at least 3 months after last treatment. Ⓜ

● PATIENT AND CARER ADVICE A patient card should be provided.

● MEDICINAL FORMS There can be variation in the licensing of different medicines containing the same drug.

Solution for infusion
EXCIPIENTS: May contain Disodium edetate, polysorbates
▶ Imjudo (AstraZeneca UK Ltd) ▼
Tremelimumab 20 mg per 1 ml Imjudo 300mg/15ml concentrate for solution for infusion vials | 1 vial [PoM] £20,610.00 (Hospital only)

Zolbetuximab [Specialist drug]

01-Apr-2025

● **INDICATIONS AND DOSE**

Gastric cancer
▶ BY INTRAVENOUS INFUSION
▶ Adult: Specialist drug – access specialist resources for dosing information

● SIDE-EFFECTS
▶ **Common or very common** Abdominal pain upper · appetite decreased · hypersalivation · hypersensitivity · hypoalbuminaemia · infusion related reaction · malaise · nausea · peripheral oedema · vomiting · weight decreased

● NATIONAL FUNDING/ACCESS DECISIONS
For full details see funding body website

NICE decisions
▶ Zolbetuximab with chemotherapy for untreated claudin-18.2-positive HER2-negative unresectable advanced gastric or gastro-oesophageal junction adenocarcinoma (March 2025) NICE TA1046 Not recommended

● MEDICINAL FORMS There can be variation in the licensing of different medicines containing the same drug.
Powder for solution for infusion
EXCIPIENTS: May contain Polysorbates, sucrose
▶ Vyloy (Astellas Pharma Ltd) ▼
Zolbetuximab 100 mg Vyloy 100mg powder for concentrate for solution for infusion vials | 1 vial [PoM] £410.00 (Hospital only)

2 Carcinoid syndrome

ENZYME INHIBITORS

Telotristat ethyl

23-Oct-2020

● DRUG ACTION Telotristat ethyl and its active metabolite inhibit L-tryptophan hydroxylases TPH-1 and TPH-2 which reduces the production of serotonin, thereby alleviating symptoms associated with carcinoid syndrome.

● **INDICATIONS AND DOSE**

Carcinoid syndrome diarrhoea (specialist use only)
▶ BY MOUTH
▶ Adult: 250 mg 3 times a day, review treatment if no response after 12 weeks

● INTERACTIONS → Appendix 1: telotristat ethyl

● SIDE-EFFECTS
▶ **Common or very common** Appetite decreased · depression · fatigue · fever · gastrointestinal discomfort · gastrointestinal disorders · headache · nausea · peripheral oedema

● PREGNANCY Manufacturer advises avoid—toxicity in *animal* studies.

● BREAST FEEDING Manufacturer advises avoid—no information available.

● HEPATIC IMPAIRMENT Manufacturer advises caution in mild to moderate impairment; avoid in severe impairment (no information available).
Dose adjustments Manufacturer advises consider dose reduction to 250 mg twice daily in mild impairment and to 250 mg once daily in moderate impairment, according to tolerability.

● RENAL IMPAIRMENT Manufacturer advises caution in mild-to-moderate impairment; avoid in severe impairment—no information available.

● MONITORING REQUIREMENTS Manufacturer advises monitor liver function at initiation and during treatment as clinically indicated—discontinue if liver injury suspected.

● PATIENT AND CARER ADVICE Manufacturer advises inform patients to report any symptoms of depression or decreased interest.

● NATIONAL FUNDING/ACCESS DECISIONS
For full details see funding body website

Scottish Medicines Consortium (SMC) decisions
▶ Telotristat ethyl (*Xermelo*®) for the treatment of carcinoid syndrome diarrhoea in combination with somatostatin analogue (SSA) therapy in adults inadequately controlled by SSA therapy (June 2018) SMC No. 1327/18 Recommended with restrictions

All Wales Medicines Strategy Group (AWMSG) decisions
▶ Telotristat ethyl (*Xermelo*®) for the treatment of carcinoid syndrome diarrhoea in combination with somatostatin analogue (SSA) therapy in adults inadequately controlled by SSA therapy (July 2018) AWMSG No. 2037 Recommended with restrictions

● MEDICINAL FORMS There can be variation in the licensing of different medicines containing the same drug.
Oral tablet
CAUTIONARY AND ADVISORY LABELS 3, 21
▶ Xermelo (SERB)
Telotristat ethyl (as Telotristat etiprate) 250 mg Xermelo 250mg tablets | 90 tablet [PoM] £1,120.00

3   Cytotoxic responsive malignancy

Cytotoxic drugs

07-Sep-2023

Overview

The chemotherapy of cancer is complex and should be confined to specialists in oncology. Cytotoxic drugs have both anti-cancer activity and the potential to damage normal tissue; most cytotoxic drugs are teratogenic. Chemotherapy may be given with a curative intent or it may aim to prolong life or to palliate symptoms. In an increasing number of cases chemotherapy may be combined with radiotherapy or surgery or both as either neoadjuvant treatment (initial chemotherapy aimed at shrinking the primary tumour, thereby rendering local therapy less destructive or more effective) or as adjuvant treatment (which follows definitive treatment of the primary disease, when the risk of subclinical metastatic disease is known to be high). All cytotoxic drugs cause side-effects and a balance has to be struck between likely benefit and acceptable toxicity.

Combinations of cytotoxic drugs, as continuous or pulsed cycles of treatment, are frequently more toxic than single drugs but have the advantage in certain tumours of enhanced response, reduced development of drug resistance and increased survival. However for some tumours, single-agent chemotherapy remains the treatment of choice.

Cytotoxic drugs fall into a number of classes, each with characteristic antitumour activity, sites of action, and toxicity. A knowledge of sites of metabolism and excretion is important because impaired drug handling as a result of disease is not uncommon and may result in enhanced toxicity.

Cytotoxic drug handling guidelines

- Trained personnel should reconstitute cytotoxics
- Reconstitution should be carried out in designated pharmacy areas
- Protective clothing (including gloves, gowns, and masks) should be worn
- The eyes should be protected and means of first aid should be specified
- Pregnant staff should avoid exposure to cytotoxic drugs (all females of child-bearing age should be informed of the reproductive hazard)
- Use local procedures for dealing with spillages and safe disposal of waste material, including syringes, containers, and absorbent material
- Staff exposure to cytotoxic drugs should be monitored

Intrathecal chemotherapy

A Health Service Circular (HSC 2008/001) provides guidance on the introduction of safe practice in NHS Trusts where intrathecal chemotherapy is administered; written local guidance covering all aspects of national guidance should be available. Support for training programmes is also available. Copies, and further information may be obtained from the Department of Health and Social Care website (www.gov.uk/government/organisations/department-of-health-and-social-care).

Safe systems for cytotoxic medicines

NHS cancer networks have been established across the UK to bring together all stakeholders in all sectors of care, to work collaboratively to plan and deliver high quality cancer services for a given population. NHS cancer networks have websites containing information on local chemotherapy services and treatment.

Safe system requirements:
- cytotoxic drugs for the treatment of cancer should be given as part of a wider pathway of care coordinated by a multidisciplinary team
- cytotoxic drugs should be prescribed, dispensed, and administered only in the context of a written protocol or treatment plan
- injectable cytotoxic drugs should only be dispensed if they are prepared for administration
- oral cytotoxic medicines should be dispensed with clear directions for use

Cytotoxic drugs: important safety information

Risk of incorrect dosing of oral anti-cancer medicines

The National Patient Safety Agency has advised (January 2008) that the prescribing and use of oral cytotoxic medicines should be carried out to the same standard as parenteral cytotoxic therapy.

- non-specialists who prescribe or administer on-going oral cytotoxic medication should have access to written protocols and treatment plans, including guidance on the monitoring and treatment of toxicity;
- staff dispensing oral cytotoxic medicines should confirm that the prescribed dose is appropriate for the patient. Patients should have written information that includes details of the intended oral anti-cancer regimen, the treatment plan, and arrangements for monitoring, taken from the original protocol from the initiating hospital. Staff dispensing oral cytotoxic medicines should also have access to this information, and to advice from an experienced cancer pharmacist in the initiating hospital.

Cytotoxic drug doses

Doses of cytotoxic drugs are determined using a variety of different methods including body-surface area or body-weight. Alternatively, doses may be fixed. Doses may be further adjusted following consideration of a patient's neutrophil count, renal and hepatic function, and history of previous adverse effects to the cytotoxic drug. Doses may also differ depending on whether a drug is used alone or in combination.

Because of the complexity of dosage regimens in the treatment of malignant disease, dose statements have been omitted from some of the drug entries in this chapter. However, even where dose statements have been provided, detailed specialist literature, individual hospital chemotherapy protocols, or local cancer networks should be consulted before prescribing, dispensing, or administering cytotoxic drugs.

Prescriptions should **not** be repeated except on the instructions of a specialist.

Cytotoxic drug side-effects

Side-effects common to most cytotoxic drugs are discussed below whilst side-effects characteristic of a particular drug or class of drugs (e.g. neurotoxicity with vinca alkaloids) are mentioned in the appropriate sections. Manufacturers' product literature, hospital-trust protocols, and cancer-network protocols should be consulted for full details of side-effects associated with individual drugs and specific chemotherapy regimes.

Many side-effects of cytotoxic drugs often do not occur at the time of administration, but days or weeks later. It is therefore important that patients and healthcare professionals can identify symptoms that cause concern and can contact an expert for advice. Toxicities should be accurately recorded using a recognised scoring system such as the Common Toxicity Criteria for Adverse Events (CTCAE) developed by the National Cancer Institute.

Extravasation of intravenous drugs

A number of cytotoxic drugs will cause severe local tissue necrosis if leakage into the extravascular compartment occurs. To reduce the risk of extravasation injury it is recommended that cytotoxic drugs are administered by appropriately trained staff. See information on the prevention and management of extravasation injury.

Oral mucositis

A sore mouth is a common complication of cancer chemotherapy; it is most often associated with fluorouracil p. 1046, methotrexate p. 1048, and the anthracyclines. It is best to prevent the complication. Good oral hygiene (rinsing the mouth frequently and effective brushing of the teeth with a soft brush 2–3 times daily) is probably beneficial. For fluorouracil p. 1046, sucking ice chips during short infusions of the drug is also helpful.

Once a sore mouth has developed, treatment is much less effective. Saline mouthwashes should be used but there is no good evidence to support the use of antiseptic or anti-inflammatory mouthwashes. In general, mucositis is self-limiting but with poor oral hygiene it can be a focus for blood-borne infection.

Tumour lysis syndrome

Tumour lysis syndrome occurs secondary to spontaneous or treatment-related rapid destruction of malignant cells. Patients at risk of tumour lysis syndrome include those with non-Hodgkin's lymphoma (especially if high grade and bulky disease), Burkitt's lymphoma, acute lymphoblastic leukaemia and acute myeloid leukaemia (particularly if high white blood cell counts or bulky disease), and occasionally those with solid tumours. Pre-existing hyperuricaemia, dehydration, and renal impairment are also predisposing factors. Features include hyperkalaemia, hyperuricaemia (see below), and hyperphosphataemia with hypocalcaemia; renal damage and arrhythmias can follow. Early identification of patients at risk, and initiation of prophylaxis or therapy for tumour lysis syndrome, is essential.

Hyperuricaemia

Hyperuricaemia, which may be present in high-grade lymphoma and leukaemia, can be markedly worsened by chemotherapy and is associated with acute renal failure. Allopurinol p. 1280 should be started 24 hours before treating such tumours and patients should be adequately hydrated. The dose of mercaptopurine p. 1047 or azathioprine p. 965 should be reduced if allopurinol needs to be given concomitantly. Febuxostat p. 1280 may also be used and should be started 2 days before cytotoxic therapy is initiated.

Rasburicase p. 1072, a recombinant urate oxidase, is licensed for hyperuricaemia in patients with haematological malignancy. It rapidly reduces plasma-uric acid concentration and may be of particular value in preventing complications following treatment of leukaemias or bulky lymphomas.

Bone-marrow suppression

All cytotoxic drugs except vincristine sulfate p. 1061 and bleomycin p. 1054 cause bone-marrow suppression. This commonly occurs 7 to 10 days after administration, but is delayed for certain drugs, such as carmustine p. 1031, lomustine p. 1034, and melphalan p. 1035. Peripheral blood counts must be checked before each treatment, and doses should be reduced or therapy delayed if bone-marrow has not recovered.

Cytotoxic drugs may be contra-indicated in patients with acute infection; any infection should be treated before, or when starting, cytotoxic drugs.

Fever in a neutropenic patient (neutrophil count less than 1.06×10^9/litre) requires immediate broad-spectrum antibacterial therapy. Appropriate bacteriological investigations should be conducted as soon as possible. Patients taking cytotoxic drugs who have signs or symptoms of infection should be advised to seek prompt medical attention. All patients should initially be investigated and

treated under the supervision of the appropriate oncology or haematology specialist.

In selected patients, the duration and the severity of neutropenia can be reduced by the use of recombinant human granulocyte-colony stimulating factors.

Symptomatic anaemia is usually treated with red blood cell transfusions. For guidance on the use of erythropoietins in patients with cancer, see MHRA/CHM advice and NICE guidance.

Alopecia

Reversible hair loss is a common complication, although it varies in degree between drugs and individual patients. No pharmacological methods of preventing this are available.

Thromboembolism

Venous thromboembolism can be a complication of cancer itself, but chemotherapy increases the risk.

Cytotoxic drugs: effect on pregnancy and reproductive function

Most cytotoxic drugs are teratogenic and should not be administered during pregnancy, especially during the first trimester. Considerable caution is necessary if a pregnant woman presents with cancer requiring chemotherapy, and specialist advice should always be sought.

Exclude pregnancy before treatment with cytotoxic drugs. Contraceptive advice should be given before cytotoxic therapy begins- women of childbearing age should use effective contraception during and after treatment.

Regimens that do not contain an alkylating drug or procarbazine may have less effect on fertility, but those with an alkylating drug or procarbazine carry the risk of causing permanent male sterility (there is no effect on potency). Pretreatment counselling and consideration of sperm storage may be appropriate. Women are less severely affected, though the span of reproductive life may be shortened by the onset of a premature menopause. No increase in fetal abnormalities or abortion rate has been recorded in patients who remain fertile after cytotoxic chemotherapy.

Cytotoxic drugs: nausea and vomiting

Nausea and vomiting cause considerable distress to many patients who receive chemotherapy and to a lesser extent abdominal radiotherapy, and may lead to refusal of further treatment; prophylaxis of nausea and vomiting is therefore extremely important. Symptoms may be acute (occurring within 24 hours of treatment), delayed (first occurring more than 24 hours after treatment), or anticipatory (occurring prior to subsequent doses). Delayed and anticipatory symptoms are more difficult to control than acute symptoms and require different management.

Patients vary in their susceptibility to drug-induced nausea and vomiting; those affected more often include women, patients under 50 years of age, anxious patients, and those who experience motion sickness. Susceptibility also increases with repeated exposure to the cytotoxic drug.

Drugs may be divided according to their emetogenic potential and some examples are given below, but the symptoms vary according to the dose, to other drugs administered and to the individual's susceptibility to emetogenic stimuli.

Mildly emetogenic treatment—fluorouracil, etoposide p. 1057, methotrexate p. 1048 (less than $100 \, \text{mg/m}^2$, low dose in children), the vinca alkaloids, and abdominal radiotherapy.

Moderately emetogenic treatment—the taxanes, doxorubicin hydrochloride p. 1038, intermediate and low doses of cyclophosphamide p. 1032, mitoxantrone p. 1040, and high doses of methotrexate ($0.1–1.2 \, \text{g/m}^2$).

Highly emetogenic treatment— cisplatin p. 1056, dacarbazine p. 1033, and high doses of cyclophosphamide.

Prevention of acute symptoms
For patients at *low risk of emesis*, pretreatment with dexamethasone p. 786 or lorazepam p. 393 may be used.

For patients at *high risk of emesis*, a $5HT_3$-receptor antagonist, usually given by mouth in combination with dexamethasone and the neurokinin receptor antagonist aprepitant p. 495 is effective.

Prevention of delayed symptoms
For delayed symptoms associated with moderately emetogenic chemotherapy, a combination of dexamethasone and $5HT_3$-receptor antagonist is effective; for highly emetogenic chemotherapy, a combination of dexamethasone and aprepitant is effective. Rolapitant and metoclopramide hydrochloride p. 494 are also licensed for delayed chemotherapy-induced nausea and vomiting.

Prevention of anticipatory symptoms
Good symptom control is the best way to prevent anticipatory symptoms. Lorazepam can be helpful for its amnesic, sedative, and anxiolytic effects.

For information on the treatment of nausea and vomiting, see Nausea and labyrinth disorders p. 491.

Treatment of cytotoxic-induced side-effects
Anthracycline side-effects
Anthracycline-induced cardiotoxicity
The anthracycline cytotoxic drugs are associated with dose-related, cumulative, and potentially life-threatening cardiotoxic side-effects.

Anthracycline extravasation
Local guidelines for the management of extravasation should be followed or specialist advice sought.

See further information on the prevention and management of extravasation injury.

Chemotherapy-induced mucositis and myelosuppression
Folinic acid p. 1071 (given as calcium folinate) is used to counteract the folate-antagonist action of methotrexate p. 1048 and thus speed recovery from methotrexate-induced mucositis or myelosuppression ('folinic acid rescue').

Folinic acid is also used in the management of methotrexate overdose, together with other measures to maintain fluid and electrolyte balance, and to manage possible renal failure.

Folinic acid does not counteract the antibacterial activity of folate antagonists such as trimethoprim p. 665.

When folinic acid and fluorouracil p. 1046 are used together in metastatic colorectal cancer the response-rate improves compared to that with fluorouracil alone.

The calcium salt of levofolinic acid p. 1071, a single isomer of folinic acid, is also used for rescue therapy following methotrexate administration, for cases of methotrexate overdose, and for use with fluorouracil for colorectal cancer. The dose of calcium levofolinate is generally half that of calcium folinate.

The disodium salts of folinic acid and levofolinic acid are also used for rescue therapy following methotrexate therapy, and for use with fluorouracil for colorectal cancer.

Urothelial toxicity
Haemorrhagic cystitis is a common manifestation of urothelial toxicity which occurs with the oxazaphosphorines, cyclophosphamide p. 1032 and ifosfamide p. 1034; it is caused by the metabolite acrolein. Mesna p. 1070 reacts specifically with this metabolite in the urinary tract, preventing toxicity. Mesna is used routinely (preferably by mouth) in patients receiving ifosfamide, and in patients receiving cyclophosphamide by the intravenous route at a high dose (e.g. more than 2 g) or in those who experienced urothelial toxicity when given cyclophosphamide previously.

Anthracyclines and other cytotoxic antibiotics
Drugs in this group are widely used. Many cytotoxic antibiotics act as radiomimetics and simultaneous use of radiotherapy should be **avoided** because it may markedly increased toxicity. Daunorubicin p. 1037, doxorubicin hydrochloride p. 1038, epirubicin hydrochloride p. 1039 and idarubicin hydrochloride p. 1040 are anthracycline antibiotics. Mitoxantrone p. 1040 is an anthracycline derivative.

Doxorubicin hydrochloride is available as both *conventional* and *liposomal* formulations. The different formulations vary in their licensed indications, pharmacokinetics, dosage and administration, and are not interchangeable. *Conventional* doxorubicin hydrochloride is used to treat the acute leukaemias, Hodgkin's and non-Hodgkin's lymphomas, paediatric malignancies, and some solid tumours including breast cancer.

Epirubicin hydrochloride is structurally related to doxorubicin hydrochloride and can be used to treat breast cancer.

Idarubicin hydrochloride has general properties similar to those of doxorubicin hydrochloride; it is mostly used in the treatment of haematological malignancies.

Daunorubicin also has general properties similar to those of doxorubicin hydrochloride.

Mitoxantrone is structurally related to doxorubicin hydrochloride.

Pixantrone p. 1041 is licensed as monotherapy for the treatment of refractory or multiply relapsed aggressive non-Hodgkin B-cell lymphomas, although the benefits of using it as a fifth-line or greater chemotherapy in refractory patients has not been established.

Bleomycin p. 1054 is given intravenously or intramuscularly to treat metastatic germ cell cancer and, in some regimens, non-Hodgkin's lymphoma.

Dactinomycin is principally used to treat paediatric cancers. Its side-effects are similar to those of doxorubicin, except that cardiac toxicity is not a problem.

Mitomycin p. 1054 can be given intravenously to treat gastro-intestinal, breast, non-small cell lung, and metastatic pancreatic cancers; and by bladder instillation for superficial bladder tumours. It causes delayed bone marrow toxicity.

Vinca alkaloids
The vinca alkaloids, vinblastine sulfate p. 1061, vincristine sulfate p. 1061, and vindesine sulfate p. 1062, are used to treat a variety of cancers including leukaemias, lymphomas, and some solid tumours. Vinorelbine p. 1062 is a semi-synthetic vinca alkaloid. See also, role of vinorelbine in the treatment of breast cancer.

Antimetabolites
Antimetabolites are incorporated into new nuclear material or combine irreversibly with cellular enzymes, preventing normal cellular division.

Alkylating drugs
Extensive experience is available with these drugs, which are among the most widely used in cancer chemotherapy. They act by damaging DNA, thus interfering with cell replication.

Cyclophosphamide is used mainly in combination with other agents for treating a wide range of malignancies, including some leukaemias, lymphomas, and solid tumours. It is given by mouth or intravenously; it is inactive until metabolised by the liver.

Ifosfamide is related to cyclophosphamide and is given intravenously.

Melphalan p. 1035 is licensed for the treatment of multiple myeloma, polycythaemia vera, childhood neuroblastoma, advanced ovarian adenocarcinoma, and advanced breast cancer. However, in practice, melphalan is rarely used for ovarian adenocarcinoma; it is no longer used for advanced breast cancer. Melphalan is also licensed for regional arterial perfusion in localised malignant melanoma of the extremities and localised soft-tissue sarcoma of the extremities.

Lomustine p. 1034 is a lipid-soluble nitrosourea and the drug is given at intervals of 4 to 6 weeks.

Carmustine p. 1031 has similar activity to lomustine; it is given to patients with multiple myeloma, non-Hodgkin's lymphomas, Hodgkin's disease, and brain tumours. Carmustine implants are licensed for intralesional use in adults for the treatment of recurrent glioblastoma multiforme as an adjunct to surgery. Carmustine implants are also licensed for high-grade malignant glioma as adjunctive treatment to surgery and radiotherapy.

Estramustine phosphate p. 1034 is a combination of an oestrogen and chlormethine used predominantly in prostate cancer. It is given by mouth and has both an antimitotic effect and (by reducing testosterone concentration) a hormonal effect.

Mitobronitol is occasionally used to treat chronic myeloid leukaemia; it is available on a named-patient basis from specialist importing companies.

ANTINEOPLASTIC DRUGS > ALKYLATING AGENTS

Bendamustine hydrochloride
[Specialist drug]

02-Aug-2021

● **INDICATIONS AND DOSE**

Chronic lymphocytic leukaemia | Non-Hodgkin's lymphoma | Multiple myeloma

▸ BY INTRAVENOUS INFUSION

▸ Adult: Specialist drug – access specialist resources for dosing information

IMPORTANT SAFETY INFORMATION

MHRA/CHM ADVICE: BENDAMUSTINE (*LEVACT*®): INCREASED MORTALITY OBSERVED IN RECENT CLINICAL STUDIES IN OFF-LABEL USE; MONITOR FOR OPPORTUNISTIC INFECTIONS, HEPATITIS B REACTIVATION (JULY 2017)

Recent clinical trials have shown increased mortality when bendamustine was used in combination treatments outside its approved indications. In addition, a recent European review of post-marketing data has suggested that the risk of opportunistic infections for all patients receiving bendamustine treatment may be greater than previously recognised.

The MHRA recommends monitoring patients for opportunistic infections as well as cardiac, neurological, and respiratory adverse events; known carriers of hepatitis B virus (HBV) should be monitored for signs and symptoms of active HBV infection. Patients should be advised to report promptly new signs of infection; consider discontinuing bendamustine if there are signs of opportunistic infections.

MHRA/CHM ADVICE: BENDAMUSTINE (*LEVACT*®): INCREASED RISK OF NON-MELANOMA SKIN CANCER AND PROGRESSIVE MULTIFOCAL ENCEPHALOPATHY (PML) (MARCH 2021)

Evidence from clinical trials and a European review of safety data found an increased risk of non-melanoma skin cancers (basal and squamous cell carcinoma) in patients treated with bendamustine-containing regimens. Healthcare professionals are advised to perform periodic skin examinations in these patients, particularly those with risk factors for skin cancer.

The review also identified very rare cases of PML in patients treated with bendamustine, usually in combination with rituximab or obinutuzumab. Healthcare professionals should consider PML in the differential diagnosis for these patients with new or worsening neurological, cognitive, or behavioural signs or symptoms. If PML is suspected, appropriate diagnostic evaluation should be undertaken and treatment suspended until PML is excluded.

● **CONTRA-INDICATIONS** Jaundice · low leucocyte count · low platelet count · major surgery less than 30 days before start of treatment · severe bone marrow suppression

● **INTERACTIONS** → Appendix 1: alkylating agents

● **SIDE-EFFECTS**

▸ **Common or very common** Alopecia · amenorrhoea · anaemia · angina pectoris · appetite decreased · arrhythmias · cardiac disorder · chills · constipation · decreased leucocytes · dehydration · diarrhoea · dizziness · fatigue · fever · haemorrhage · headache · hepatitis B reactivation · hypersensitivity · hypertension · hypokalaemia · hypotension · increased risk of infection · insomnia · mucositis · nausea · neutropenia · pain · palpitations · pulmonary disorder · skin reactions · stomatitis · thrombocytopenia · tumour lysis syndrome · vomiting

▸ **Uncommon** Bone marrow disorders · heart failure · myocardial infarction · neoplasms · pericardial effusion

▸ **Rare or very rare** Anticholinergic syndrome · aphonia · ataxia · circulatory collapse · drowsiness · haemolysis · hyperhidrosis · infertility · multi organ failure · nervous system disorder · paraesthesia · peripheral neuropathy · pulmonary fibrosis · sepsis · taste altered

▸ **Frequency not known** Extravasation necrosis · hepatic failure · necrosis · progressive multifocal leukoencephalopathy (PML) · renal failure · severe cutaneous adverse reactions (SCARs)

SIDE-EFFECTS, FURTHER INFORMATION **Secondary malignancy** Use of bendamustine is associated with an increased incidence of acute leukaemias.

Infections Serious and fatal infections are reported, including opportunistic infections such as Pneumocystis jirovecii pneumonia (PJP), varicella zoster virus (VZV) and cytomegalovirus (CMV)—manufacturer advises monitoring for respiratory signs and symptoms throughout treatment; patients should be advised to report new signs of infection, including fever or respiratory symptoms, promptly. Reactivation of hepatitis B is reported in patients who are chronic carriers of the virus—manufacturer advises monitoring for signs and symptoms of active hepatitis B during treatment and for several months after stopping treatment.

● **CONCEPTION AND CONTRACEPTION** Effective contraception is required during treatment in men or women, and for 6 months after treatment in men.

● **NATIONAL FUNDING/ACCESS DECISIONS**
For full details see funding body website

NICE decisions

▸ **Bendamustine for the first-line treatment of chronic lymphocytic leukaemia (February 2011)** NICE TA216 Recommended

▸ **Obinutuzumab with bendamustine for treating follicular lymphoma refractory to rituximab (August 2017)** NICE TA472 Recommended with restrictions

Scottish Medicines Consortium (SMC) decisions

▸ **Bendamustine hydrochloride (*Levact*®) for chronic lymphocytic leukaemia (CLL) (April 2011)** SMC No. 694/11 Recommended

● **MEDICINAL FORMS** There can be variation in the licensing of different medicines containing the same drug.

Powder for solution for infusion

▸ **Bendamustine hydrochloride (Non-proprietary)**
Bendamustine hydrochloride 25 mg Bendamustine 25mg powder for concentrate for solution for infusion vials | 5 vial [PoM] £329.90–£347.26 (Hospital only)

Bendamustine hydrochloride 100 mg Bendamustine 100mg powder for concentrate for solution for infusion vials | 1 vial [PoM]

£1,300.00–£1,379.04 (Hospital only) | 5 vial PoM £1,310.09 (Hospital only)

Busulfan [Specialist drug]

08-Jul-2020

(Busulphan)

- **INDICATIONS AND DOSE**

Chronic myeloid leukaemia
- ▸ BY MOUTH
- ▸ Adult: Specialist drug – access specialist resources for dosing information

Conditioning treatment before haematopoietic progenitor cell transplantation
- ▸ BY MOUTH, OR BY INTRAVENOUS INFUSION
- ▸ Adult: Specialist drug – access specialist resources for dosing information

> **IMPORTANT SAFETY INFORMATION**
> RISKS OF INCORRECT DOSING OF ORAL ANTI-CANCER MEDICINES
> See Cytotoxic drugs p. 1027.

- **CONTRA-INDICATIONS** Acute porphyrias p. 1202
- **INTERACTIONS** → Appendix 1: alkylating agents
- **SIDE-EFFECTS**

GENERAL SIDE-EFFECTS
- ▸ **Common or very common** Alopecia · diarrhoea · hepatic disorders · interstitial lung disease · nausea · sinusoidal obstruction syndrome · skin reactions · thrombocytopenia · vomiting
- ▸ **Uncommon** Seizure
- ▸ **Rare or very rare** Cataract · eye disorders

SPECIFIC SIDE-EFFECTS
- ▸ **Common or very common**
- ▸ With intravenous use Anaemia · anxiety · appetite decreased · arrhythmias · arthralgia · ascites · asthenia · asthma · cardiomegaly · chest pain · chills · confusion · constipation · cough · depression · dizziness · dyspnoea · dysuria · electrolyte imbalance · embolism and thrombosis · fever · gastrointestinal discomfort · gastrointestinal disorders · haemorrhage · headache · hiccups · hyperglycaemia · hypersensitivity · hypertension · hypoalbuminaemia · hypotension · increased risk of infection · insomnia · mucositis · myalgia · nervous system disorder · neutropenia · oedema · pain · pancytopenia · pericardial effusion · pericarditis · reactivation of infections · renal disorder · renal impairment · respiratory disorders · stomatitis · vasodilation · weight increased
- ▸ With oral use Amenorrhoea (may be reversible) · azoospermia · bone marrow disorders · cardiac tamponade · delayed puberty · hyperbilirubinaemia · infertility male · leucopenia · leukaemia · menopausal symptoms · oral disorders · ovarian and fallopian tube disorders · testicular atrophy
- ▸ **Uncommon**
- ▸ With intravenous use Capillary leak syndrome · delirium · encephalopathy · hallucination · hypoxia · intracranial haemorrhage
- ▸ **Rare or very rare**
- ▸ With oral use Dry mouth · erythema nodosum · gynaecomastia · myasthenia gravis · radiation injury · Sjögren's syndrome
- ▸ **Frequency not known**
- ▸ With intravenous use Hypogonadism · ovarian failure · premature menopause · sepsis

SIDE-EFFECTS, FURTHER INFORMATION **Lung toxicity**
Discontinue if lung toxicity develops.

Secondary malignancy Use of busulfan is associated with an increased incidence of secondary malignancy.

- **CONCEPTION AND CONTRACEPTION** Manufacturers advise effective contraception during and for 6 months after treatment in men or women.

- **MEDICINAL FORMS** There can be variation in the licensing of different medicines containing the same drug. Forms available from special-order manufacturers include: oral capsule, oral suspension, oral solution

Oral tablet
- ▸ Busulfan (Non-proprietary)
  Busulfan 2 mg Busulfan 2mg tablets | 25 tablet PoM £14.43

Solution for infusion
- ▸ Busulfan (Non-proprietary)
  Busulfan 6 mg per 1 ml Busulfan 60mg/10ml concentrate for solution for infusion vials | 8 vial PoM £1,529.50–£2,816.40 (Hospital only)

Carmustine [Specialist drug]

13-Jul-2020

- **INDICATIONS AND DOSE**

Brain tumours | Multiple myeloma | Non-Hodgkin's lymphomas | Hodgkin's disease
- ▸ BY INTRAVENOUS INFUSION
- ▸ Adult: Specialist drug – access specialist resources for dosing information

Glioblastoma multiforme | Malignant glioma
- ▸ BY INTRALESIONAL IMPLANTATION
- ▸ Adult: Specialist drug – access specialist resources for dosing information

- **CONTRA-INDICATIONS** Acute porphyrias p. 1202
- **INTERACTIONS** → Appendix 1: alkylating agents
- **SIDE-EFFECTS**

GENERAL SIDE-EFFECTS
- ▸ **Common or very common** Alopecia · anaemia · ataxia · constipation · diarrhoea · dizziness · headache · nausea · seizures · vomiting

SPECIFIC SIDE-EFFECTS
- ▸ **Common or very common**
- ▸ When used by implant Abdominal pain · abscess · anxiety · asthenia · chest pain · coma · confusion · conjunctival oedema · depression · diabetes mellitus · drowsiness · dysphagia · electrolyte imbalance · embolism and thrombosis · eye pain · faecal incontinence · fever · gait abnormal · haemorrhage · hallucination · healing impaired · hydrocephalus · hyperglycaemia · hypersensitivity · hypertension · hypotension · increased risk of infection · injury · insomnia · intracranial pressure increased · leucocytosis · memory loss · meningitis · oedema · pain · paralysis · paranoia · peripheral neuropathy · personality disorder · rash · sensation abnormal · sepsis · speech impairment · stupor · thinking abnormal · thrombocytopenia · tremor · urinary incontinence · vision disorders
- ▸ With intravenous use Acute leukaemia · appetite decreased · bone marrow depression · encephalopathy (with high doses) · hepatotoxicity · interstitial lung disease · myelodysplastic syndrome (following long term use) · ocular toxicity · pulmonary fibrosis · respiratory disorders · retinal haemorrhage · stomatitis
- ▸ **Uncommon**
- ▸ When used by implant Cerebral infarction · intracranial haemorrhage
- ▸ **Rare or very rare**
- ▸ With intravenous use Gynaecomastia · nephrotoxicity (cumulative) · peripheral vascular disease (with high doses)
- ▸ **Frequency not known**
- ▸ With intravenous use Infertility · myalgia

SIDE-EFFECTS, FURTHER INFORMATION **Pulmonary toxicity** Lung infiltration, pulmonary fibrosis, pneumonitis, and interstitial lung disease have been reported with intravenous use, some of which have been fatal. These appear to be dose-related, cumulative, and may be delayed.

Hepatotoxicity Hepatotoxicity has been reported to occur with high intravenous doses, and may be delayed up to 60 days after administration; usually reversible.

● **CONCEPTION AND CONTRACEPTION** Manufacturer advises effective contraception during treatment in men or women.

● **NATIONAL FUNDING/ACCESS DECISIONS**
For full details see funding body website
NICE decisions
▶ **Carmustine implants and temozolomide for the treatment of newly diagnosed high-grade glioma (June 2007)** NICE TA121 Recommended with restrictions

● **MEDICINAL FORMS** There can be variation in the licensing of different medicines containing the same drug.
Prolonged-release intralesional implant
  ▸ **Gliadel** (Clinigen Healthcare Ltd)
    Carmustine 7.7 mg Gliadel 7.7mg implant | 8 device PoM £5,203.00 (Hospital only)

Chlorambucil [Specialist drug]
13-Jul-2020

● **INDICATIONS AND DOSE**

Lymphomas and chronic leukaemias
▶ BY MOUTH
▸ Adult: Specialist drug – access specialist resources for dosing information

---

IMPORTANT SAFETY INFORMATION
RISKS OF INCORRECT DOSING OF ORAL ANTI-CANCER MEDICINES
See Cytotoxic drugs p. 1027.

● **INTERACTIONS** → Appendix 1: alkylating agents

● **SIDE-EFFECTS**
▶ **Common or very common** Anaemia · bone marrow disorders · diarrhoea · gastrointestinal disorder · leucopenia · nausea · neoplasms · neutropenia · oral ulceration · seizures · thrombocytopenia · vomiting
▶ **Uncommon** Skin reactions
▶ **Rare or very rare** Cystitis · fever · hepatic disorders · interstitial pneumonia · movement disorders · muscle twitching · peripheral neuropathy · pulmonary fibrosis · severe cutaneous adverse reactions (SCARs) · tremor
▶ **Frequency not known** Amenorrhoea · azoospermia

SIDE-EFFECTS, FURTHER INFORMATION **Secondary malignancy** Use of chlorambucil is associated with an increased incidence of acute leukaemia, particularly with prolonged use.

Skin reactions Manufacturer advises assessing continued use if rash occurs—has been reported to progress to Stevens-Johnson syndrome and toxic epidermal necrolysis.

● **CONCEPTION AND CONTRACEPTION** Contraceptive advice required.

● **NATIONAL FUNDING/ACCESS DECISIONS**
For full details see funding body website
NICE decisions
▶ **Obinutuzumab in combination with chlorambucil for untreated chronic lymphocytic leukaemia (June 2015)** NICE TA343 Recommended with restrictions
▶ **Ofatumumab in combination with chlorambucil or bendamustine for untreated chronic lymphocytic leukaemia (June 2015)** NICE TA344 Recommended with restrictions

● **MEDICINAL FORMS** There can be variation in the licensing of different medicines containing the same drug.
Oral tablet
  ▸ **Chlorambucil (Non-proprietary)**
    Chlorambucil 2 mg Chlorambucil 2mg tablets | 25 tablet PoM £11.15

Chlormethine [Specialist drug]
10-Sep-2021

● **INDICATIONS AND DOSE**

Mycosis fungoides-type cutaneous T-cell lymphoma
▶ TO THE SKIN
▸ Adult: Specialist drug – access specialist resources for dosing information

● **INTERACTIONS** → Appendix 1: chlormethine
● **SIDE-EFFECTS**
▶ **Common or very common** Hypersensitivity · skin infection · skin reactions · skin ulcer

● **CONCEPTION AND CONTRACEPTION** Manufacturer advises contraception in women of child-bearing potential during treatment.

● **PATIENT AND CARER ADVICE** Patients and carers should be advised to wash hands after each application and should wear nitrile gloves for each application. If non-affected areas are exposed, these areas should be washed. Occlusive dressings should not be applied over the treated area.

● **NATIONAL FUNDING/ACCESS DECISIONS**
For full details see funding body website
NICE decisions
▶ **Chlormethine gel for treating mycosis fungoides-type cutaneous T-cell lymphoma (August 2021)** NICE TA720 Recommended with restrictions
Scottish Medicines Consortium (SMC) decisions
▶ **Chlormethine hydrochloride (*Ledaga*®) for the topical treatment of mycosis fungoides-type cutaneous T-cell lymphoma (MF-type CTCL) in adult patients (May 2021)** SMC No. SMC2318 Recommended

● **MEDICINAL FORMS** There can be variation in the licensing of different medicines containing the same drug.
Cutaneous gel
EXCIPIENTS: May contain Butylated hydroxytoluene, propylene glycol
  ▸ **Ledaga** (Recordati Rare Diseases UK Ltd)
    Chlormethine hydrochloride 160 microgram per 1 gram Ledaga 160micrograms/g gel | 60 gram PoM £1,000.00

Cyclophosphamide
04-Aug-2023

● **INDICATIONS AND DOSE**

Rheumatoid arthritis with severe systemic manifestations (under expert supervision)
▶ BY MOUTH
▸ Adult: 1–1.5 mg/kg daily

Severe systemic rheumatoid arthritis (under expert supervision) | Other connective tissue diseases (especially with active vasculitis) (under expert supervision)
▶ BY INTRAVENOUS INJECTION
▸ Adult: 0.5–1 g every 2 weeks, then reduced to 0.5–1 g every month, frequency adjusted according to clinical response and haematological monitoring. To be given with prophylactic mesna

Malignant disease (specialist use only)
▶ BY MOUTH, OR BY INTRAVENOUS INFUSION
▸ Adult: Specialist indication – access specialist resources for dosing information

- **UNLICENSED USE** Not licensed for rheumatoid arthritis with severe systemic manifestations.

> **IMPORTANT SAFETY INFORMATION**
> RISKS OF INCORRECT DOSING OF ORAL ANTI-CANCER MEDICINES
> See Cytotoxic drugs p. 1027.

- **CAUTIONS** Avoid in Acute porphyrias p. 1202 · diabetes mellitus · haemorrhagic cystitis · previous or concurrent mediastinal irradiation—risk of cardiotoxicity

- **INTERACTIONS** → Appendix 1: alkylating agents

- **SIDE-EFFECTS**
  GENERAL SIDE-EFFECTS
  ▸ **Common or very common** Agranulocytosis · alopecia · anaemia · asthenia · bone marrow disorders · cystitis · decreased leucocytes · fever · haemolytic uraemic syndrome · haemorrhage · hepatic disorders · immunosuppression · increased risk of infection · mucosal abnormalities · neutropenia · progressive multifocal leukoencephalopathy (PML) · reactivation of infections · sperm abnormalities · thrombocytopenia
  ▸ **Uncommon** Appetite decreased · embolism and thrombosis · flushing · hypersensitivity · ovarian and fallopian tube disorders · sepsis
  ▸ **Rare or very rare** Bladder disorders · chest pain · confusion · constipation · diarrhoea · disseminated intravascular coagulation · dizziness · eye inflammation · fluid imbalance · headache · hyponatraemia · menstrual cycle irregularities · nail discolouration · nausea · neoplasms · oral disorders · pancreatitis acute · renal failure · rhabdomyolysis · secondary neoplasm · seizure · severe cutaneous adverse reactions (SCARs) · SIADH · skin reactions · visual impairment · vomiting
  ▸ **Frequency not known** Abdominal pain · altered smell sensation · arrhythmias · arthralgia · ascites · cardiac inflammation · cardiogenic shock · cardiomyopathy · cough · deafness · dyspnoea · encephalopathy · excessive tearing · facial swelling · gastrointestinal disorders · heart failure · hyperhidrosis · hypoxia · infertility · influenza like illness · interstitial lung disease · multi organ failure · muscle complaints · myelopathy · myocardial infarction · nasal complaints · nephrogenic diabetes insipidus · nephrotoxicity · nerve disorders · neuralgia · neurotoxicity · oedema · oropharyngeal pain · palpitations · pericardial effusion · peripheral ischaemia · pulmonary fibrosis · pulmonary hypertension · pulmonary oedema · QT interval prolongation · radiation injuries · renal tubular disorder · renal tubular necrosis · respiratory disorders · scleroderma · sensation abnormal · sinusoidal obstruction syndrome · taste altered · testicular atrophy · tinnitus · tremor · tumour lysis syndrome · vasculitis

  SPECIFIC SIDE-EFFECTS
  ▸ With intravenous use Infusion site necrosis · injection site necrosis

  SIDE-EFFECTS, FURTHER INFORMATION **Haemorrhagic cystitis** A urinary metabolite of cyclophosphamide, acrolein, can cause haemorrhagic cystitis; this is a rare but serious complication that may be prevented by increasing fluid intake for 24–48 hours after intravenous injection. Mesna can also help prevent cystitis when high-dose therapy (e.g. more than 2 g intravenously) is used or when the patient is considered to be at high risk of cystitis (e.g. because of pelvic irradiation).
      Secondary malignancy As with all cytotoxic therapy, treatment with cyclophosphamide is associated with an increased incidence of secondary malignancies.

- **CONCEPTION AND CONTRACEPTION** EvGr Females of childbearing potential should use effective contraception during treatment and for at least 12 months after last treatment; male patients should use effective contraception during treatment and for at least 6 months

after last treatment if their partner is of childbearing potential. M See also *Pregnancy and reproductive function* in Cytotoxic drugs p. 1027.

- **PREGNANCY** Avoid. See also *Pregnancy and reproductive function* in Cytotoxic drugs p. 1027.

- **BREAST FEEDING** Discontinue breast-feeding during and for 36 hours after stopping treatment.

- **HEPATIC IMPAIRMENT** Manufacturer advises caution (risk of decreased cyclophosphamide activation and increased risk of veno-occlusive liver disease).
  Dose adjustments Manufacturer advises consider dose adjustment in severe impairment—consult product literature.

- **RENAL IMPAIRMENT**
  Dose adjustments EvGr Consider dose reduction (consult product literature). M

- **DIRECTIONS FOR ADMINISTRATION** For *intravenous infusion* (cyclophosphamide injection; *Baxter*), manufacturer advises give via drip tubing in Glucose 5% or Sodium Chloride 0.9%; reconstitute 500 mg with 25 mL Sodium Chloride 0.9%; reconstitute 1 g with 50 mL Sodium Chloride 0.9%.

- **MEDICINAL FORMS** There can be variation in the licensing of different medicines containing the same drug. Forms available from special-order manufacturers include: oral tablet, oral suspension, oral solution, solution for injection, solution for infusion

  Oral tablet
  CAUTIONARY AND ADVISORY LABELS 25, 27
  ▸ Cyclophosphamide (Non-proprietary)
    Cyclophosphamide (as Cyclophosphamide monohydrate)
    50 mg Cyclophosphamide 50mg tablets | 100 tablet [PoM] £153.00
    DT = £153.00
  ▸ Cytoxan (Imported (United States))
    Cyclophosphamide 25 mg Cytoxan 25mg tablets |
    100 tablet [PoM] [Ⓢ]

  Powder for solution for injection
  ▸ Cyclophosphamide (Non-proprietary)
    Cyclophosphamide (as Cyclophosphamide monohydrate)
    500 mg Cyclophosphamide 500mg powder for solution for injection vials | 1 vial [PoM] £8.21-£10.63 (Hospital only)
    Cyclophosphamide (as Cyclophosphamide monohydrate)
    1 gram Cyclophosphamide 1g powder for solution for injection vials | 1 vial [PoM] £15.22-£19.70 (Hospital only)
    Cyclophosphamide (as Cyclophosphamide monohydrate)
    2 gram Cyclophosphamide 2g powder for solution for injection vials | 1 vial [PoM] £28.22 (Hospital only)

Dacarbazine [Specialist drug]   24-Jun-2021

- **INDICATIONS AND DOSE**

Melanoma | Soft-tissue sarcomas | Hodgkin's disease
  ▸ BY INTRAVENOUS INFUSION, OR BY INTRAVENOUS INJECTION
  ▸ Adult: Specialist drug – access specialist resources for dosing information

- **INTERACTIONS** → Appendix 1: alkylating agents

- **SIDE-EFFECTS**
  ▸ **Common or very common** Anaemia · appetite decreased · leucopenia · nausea · thrombocytopenia · vomiting
  ▸ **Uncommon** Alopecia · infection · influenza like illness · photosensitivity reaction · skin reactions
  ▸ **Rare or very rare** Agranulocytosis · confusion · diarrhoea · flushing · headache · hepatic disorders · lethargy · pancytopenia · paraesthesia · renal impairment · seizure · visual impairment

- **CONCEPTION AND CONTRACEPTION** Ensure effective contraception during and for at least 6 months after treatment in men or women.

- **MEDICINAL FORMS** There can be variation in the licensing of different medicines containing the same drug.
  Powder for solution for infusion
  ▸ Dacarbazine (Non-proprietary)
    Dacarbazine (as Dacarbazine citrate) 500 mg Dacarbazine 500mg powder for solution for infusion vials | 1 vial [PoM] £37.50
    Dacarbazine (as Dacarbazine citrate) 1 gram Dacarbazine 1g powder for solution for infusion vials | 1 vial [PoM] £70.00
  Powder for solution for injection
  ▸ Dacarbazine (Non-proprietary)
    Dacarbazine (as Dacarbazine citrate) 100 mg Dacarbazine 100mg powder for solution for injection vials | 10 vial [PoM] £90.00
    Dacarbazine (as Dacarbazine citrate) 200 mg Dacarbazine 200mg powder for solution for injection vials | 10 vial [PoM] £160.00

Estramustine phosphate [Specialist drug]

10-May-2021

- **INDICATIONS AND DOSE**
Prostate cancer
▸ BY MOUTH
▸ Adult: Specialist drug – access specialist resources for dosing information

IMPORTANT SAFETY INFORMATION
RISKS OF INCORRECT DOSING OF ORAL ANTI-CANCER MEDICINES
See Cytotoxic drugs p. 1027.

- **CONTRA-INDICATIONS** Peptic ulceration · severe cardiovascular disease · thromboembolic disorders
- **INTERACTIONS** → Appendix 1: alkylating agents
- **SIDE-EFFECTS**
▸ **Common or very common** Anaemia · congestive heart failure · diarrhoea · embolism · fluid retention · gynaecomastia · headache · hepatic function abnormal · lethargy · leucopenia · myocardial infarction · nausea · thrombocytopenia · vomiting
▸ **Frequency not known** Allergic dermatitis · angioedema · confusion · depression · erectile dysfunction · hypertension · muscle weakness · myocardial ischaemia
- **CONCEPTION AND CONTRACEPTION** Men should use effective contraceptive methods during treatment.
- **PATIENT AND CARER ADVICE** Patients should be given advice on how to administer estramustine capsules.

- **MEDICINAL FORMS** No licensed medicines listed.

Ifosfamide [Specialist drug]

30-Jan-2022

- **INDICATIONS AND DOSE**
Malignant disease
▸ BY INTRAVENOUS INFUSION
▸ Adult: Specialist drug – access specialist resources for dosing information

- **CONTRA-INDICATIONS** Acute infection · Acute porphyrias p. 1202 · cystitis · urinary-tract obstruction · urothelial damage
- **INTERACTIONS** → Appendix 1: alkylating agents
- **SIDE-EFFECTS**
▸ **Common or very common** Alopecia · appetite decreased · bone marrow disorders · haemorrhage · hepatic disorders · infection · leucopenia · nausea · reactivation of infection · renal impairment · thrombocytopenia · vomiting
▸ **Uncommon** Cardiotoxicity · diarrhoea · hypotension · oral disorders
▸ **Rare or very rare** Skin reactions
▸ **Frequency not known** Abdominal pain · agranulocytosis · amenorrhoea · anaemia · angina pectoris · angioedema ·

arrhythmias · arthralgia · asterixis · behaviour abnormal · blood disorders · bone disorders · cancer progression · capillary leak syndrome · cardiac arrest · cardiomyopathy · chills · conjunctivitis · constipation · cough · deafness · delirium · delusions · disseminated intravascular coagulation · dysarthria · dyspnoea · electrolyte imbalance · embolism and thrombosis · encephalopathy · eye irritation · fatigue · fever · flushing · gait abnormal · gastrointestinal disorders · growth retardation · haemolytic anaemia · heart failure · hyperglycaemia · hyperhidrosis · hyperphosphaturia · hypertension · hypoxia · immunosuppression · infertility · interstitial lung disease · malaise · mania · memory loss · metabolic acidosis · movement disorders · mucosal ulceration · multi organ failure · muscle complaints · myocardial infarction · nail disorder · neoplasms · nephritis tubulointerstitial · nephrogenic diabetes insipidus · neurotoxicity · oedema · ovarian and fallopian tube disorders · pain · pancreatitis · panic attack · peripheral neuropathy · polydipsia · premature menopause · psychiatric disorders · pulmonary fibrosis · pulmonary hypertension · pulmonary oedema · radiation recall reaction · respiratory disorders · rhabdomyolysis · secondary malignancy · sensation abnormal · sepsis · severe cutaneous adverse reactions (SCARs) · SIADH · sinusoidal obstruction syndrome · sperm abnormalities · status epilepticus · tinnitus · tumour lysis syndrome · urinary disorders · vasculitis · vertigo · visual impairment

SIDE-EFFECTS, FURTHER INFORMATION Urothelial toxicity Mesna is routinely given with ifosfamide to reduce urothelial toxicity.
  Secondary malignancy Use of ifosfamide is associated with an increased incidence of acute leukaemia.
- **CONCEPTION AND CONTRACEPTION** Manufacturer advises adequate contraception during and for at least 6 months after treatment in men or women.

- **MEDICINAL FORMS** There can be variation in the licensing of different medicines containing the same drug.
Powder for solution for injection
▸ Ifosfamide (Non-proprietary)
  Ifosfamide 1 gram Ifosfamide 1g powder for concentrate for solution for injection vials | 1 vial [PoM] £151.49
  Ifosfamide 2 gram Ifosfamide 2g powder for concentrate for solution for injection vials | 1 vial [PoM] £298.41

Lomustine [Specialist drug]

10-May-2021

- **INDICATIONS AND DOSE**
Hodgkin's disease | Malignant melanoma | Certain solid tumours
▸ BY MOUTH
▸ Adult: Specialist drug – access specialist resources for dosing information

IMPORTANT SAFETY INFORMATION
RISKS OF INCORRECT DOSING OF ORAL ANTI-CANCER MEDICINES
See Cytotoxic drugs p. 1027.

- **CONTRA-INDICATIONS** Coeliac disease
- **INTERACTIONS** → Appendix 1: alkylating agents
- **SIDE-EFFECTS**
▸ **Common or very common** Leucopenia
▸ **Frequency not known** Alopecia · anaemia · apathy · appetite decreased · azotaemia · bone marrow failure (delayed) · confusion · coordination abnormal · diarrhoea · hepatic disorders · interstitial pneumonia · lethargy · lung infiltration · nausea · neoplasms · neurological effects · pulmonary fibrosis · renal disorders · renal impairment · speech impairment · stomatitis · thrombocytopenia · vision loss (irreversible) · vomiting

SIDE-EFFECTS, FURTHER INFORMATION Prolonged use of lomustine is associated with an increased incidence of acute leukaemias.

- **CONCEPTION AND CONTRACEPTION** Manufacturer advises effective contraception during and for at least 6 months after treatment in men or women.

- **MEDICINAL FORMS** There can be variation in the licensing of different medicines containing the same drug. Forms available from special-order manufacturers include: oral capsule
  Oral capsule
  ▸ Lomustine (Non-proprietary)
    Lomustine 10 mg CeeNU 10mg capsules | 20 capsule [PoM] ⒮
    Lomustine 40 mg Lomustine 40mg capsules | 20 capsule [PoM]
    £780.82 (Hospital only)
    Lomustine 100 mg CeeNU 100mg capsules | 20 capsule [PoM] ⒮

Melphalan [Specialist drug]
21-Mar-2023

- **INDICATIONS AND DOSE**
Multiple myeloma
▸ BY MOUTH, OR BY INTRAVENOUS INJECTION, OR BY INTRAVENOUS INFUSION
▸ Adult: Specialist drug – access specialist resources for dosing information
Polycythaemia vera
▸ BY MOUTH
▸ Adult: Specialist drug – access specialist resources for dosing information
Localised malignant melanoma of the extremities | Localised soft-tissue sarcoma of the extremities
▸ BY REGIONAL ARTERIAL PERFUSION
▸ Adult: Specialist drug – access specialist resources for dosing information

> **IMPORTANT SAFETY INFORMATION**
> RISKS OF INCORRECT DOSING OF ORAL ANTI-CANCER MEDICINES
> See Cytotoxic drugs p. 1027.

- **INTERACTIONS** → Appendix 1: alkylating agents
- **SIDE-EFFECTS**
  GENERAL SIDE-EFFECTS
▸ **Common or very common** Alopecia · anaemia · bone marrow depression (delayed) · diarrhoea · nausea · stomatitis · thrombocytopenia · vomiting
▸ **Rare or very rare** Haemolytic anaemia · hepatic disorders · interstitial pneumonitis · pulmonary fibrosis · skin reactions
  SPECIFIC SIDE-EFFECTS
▸ **Common or very common**
▸ With oral use Leucopenia
▸ With parenteral use Feeling hot · myalgia · myopathy · paraesthesia
▸ **Rare or very rare**
▸ With parenteral use Peripheral vascular disease
  SIDE-EFFECTS, FURTHER INFORMATION Use of melphalan is associated with an increased incidence of acute leukaemias.

- **CONCEPTION AND CONTRACEPTION** Manufacturer advises adequate contraception during treatment in men or women.

- **MEDICINAL FORMS** There can be variation in the licensing of different medicines containing the same drug.
  Oral tablet
  ▸ Melphalan (Non-proprietary)
    Melphalan 2 mg Melphalan 2mg tablets | 25 tablet [PoM] £16.48

Powder and solvent for solution for injection
▸ Melphalan (Non-proprietary)
  Melphalan (as Melphalan hydrochloride) 50 mg Melphalan 50mg powder and solvent for solution for injection vials | 1 vial [PoM] £26.64–£105.00 (Hospital only)
▸ Phelinun (Adienne Pharma & Biotech)
  Melphalan (as Melphalan hydrochloride) 50 mg Phelinun 50mg powder and solvent for concentrate for solution for infusion vials | 1 vial [PoM] £129.81 (Hospital only)

Streptozocin [Specialist drug]
09-Oct-2018

- **INDICATIONS AND DOSE**
Neuroendocrine tumours of pancreatic origin
▸ BY INTRAVENOUS INFUSION
▸ Adult: Specialist drug – access specialist resources for dosing information

- **INTERACTIONS** → Appendix 1: streptozocin
- **SIDE-EFFECTS**
▸ **Common or very common** Acute kidney injury · diarrhoea · nausea · nephrotoxicity · renal tubular injury · urinary disorder · urine abnormalities · vomiting
▸ **Frequency not known** Confusion · depression · extravasation necrosis · fever · glucose tolerance impaired · hepatotoxicity · hypoalbuminaemia · lethargy · nephrogenic diabetes insipidus

- **CONCEPTION AND CONTRACEPTION** Manufacturer advises women of childbearing potential should use effective contraception during treatment and for 30 days after last treatment; male patients should use effective contraception during treatment and for 90 days after last treatment if their partner is of childbearing potential.

- **MEDICINAL FORMS** There can be variation in the licensing of different medicines containing the same drug.
  Powder for solution for infusion
  ▸ Zanosar (Esteve Pharmaceuticals Ltd)
    Streptozocin 1 gram Zanosar 1g powder for concentrate for solution for infusion vials | 1 vial [PoM] £570.00 (Hospital only)

Temozolomide [Specialist drug]
10-May-2021

- **INDICATIONS AND DOSE**
Glioblastoma multiforme | Malignant glioma
▸ BY MOUTH
▸ Adult: Specialist drug – access specialist resources for dosing information

> **IMPORTANT SAFETY INFORMATION**
> RISKS OF INCORRECT DOSING OF ORAL ANTI-CANCER MEDICINES
> See Cytotoxic drugs p. 1027.

- **INTERACTIONS** → Appendix 1: alkylating agents
- **SIDE-EFFECTS**
▸ **Common or very common** Alopecia · anaemia · anxiety · appetite decreased · arthralgia · asthenia · cognitive impairment · concentration impaired · confusion · constipation · cough · Cushing's syndrome · decreased leucocytes · depression · diarrhoea · dizziness · drowsiness · dysphagia · dyspnoea · ear pain · embolism and thrombosis · eye pain · fever · gastrointestinal discomfort · haemorrhage · headache · hearing impairment · hemiparesis · hyperglycaemia · hypersensitivity · hypertension · increased risk of infection · influenza like illness · insomnia · level of consciousness decreased · malaise · memory loss · movement disorders · muscle weakness · myalgia · myopathy · nausea · nerve disorders · neutropenia · oedema · oral disorders · pain · peripheral swelling · radiation injuries · seizures · sensation abnormal · skin reactions · speech impairment · taste altered ·

Immune system and malignant disease

thrombocytopenia · tinnitus · tremor · urinary disorders · vertigo · vision disorders · vomiting · weight changes
▶ **Uncommon** Altered smell sensation · angioedema · aplastic anaemia (sometimes fatal) · behaviour disorder · breast pain · chills · condition aggravated · diabetes insipidus · dry eye · dry mouth · emotional lability · erectile dysfunction · gait abnormal · gastrointestinal disorders · hallucination · hemiplegia · hepatic disorders · hepatic failure (sometimes fatal) · hepatitis B reactivation (sometimes fatal) · hyperacusia · hyperbilirubinaemia · hyperhidrosis · hypokalaemia · interstitial lung disease · intracranial haemorrhage · meningoencephalitis herpetic (sometimes fatal) · menstrual cycle irregularities · nasal congestion · neoplasms · nervous system disorder · palpitations · pancytopenia (sometimes prolonged) · photosensitivity reaction · pulmonary fibrosis · reactivation of infections · respiratory failure (sometimes fatal) · secondary malignancy · sepsis (sometimes fatal) · severe cutaneous adverse reactions (SCARs) · thirst · tongue discolouration · vasodilation

● **CONCEPTION AND CONTRACEPTION** Manufacturer advises adequate contraception during treatment. Men should avoid fathering a child during and for at least 6 months after treatment.

● **NATIONAL FUNDING/ACCESS DECISIONS**
For full details see funding body website
NICE decisions
▶ **Temozolomide for the treatment of recurrent malignant glioma (brain cancer) (April 2001)** NICE TA23 Recommended with restrictions
▶ **Carmustine implants and temozolomide for the treatment of newly diagnosed high-grade glioma (June 2007)** NICE TA121 Recommended with restrictions

● **MEDICINAL FORMS** There can be variation in the licensing of different medicines containing the same drug. Forms available from special-order manufacturers include: oral suspension
Oral capsule
CAUTIONARY AND ADVISORY LABELS 23, 25
▶ **Temozolomide (Non-proprietary)**
Temozolomide 5 mg Temozolomide 5mg capsules | 5 capsule PoM £10.06–£16.00 (Hospital only)
Temozolomide 20 mg Temozolomide 20mg capsules | 5 capsule PoM £40.23–£65.00 (Hospital only)
Temozolomide 100 mg Temozolomide 100mg capsules | 5 capsule PoM £201.18–£325.00 (Hospital only)
Temozolomide 140 mg Temozolomide 140mg capsules | 5 capsule PoM £296.47–£465.00 (Hospital only)
Temozolomide 180 mg Temozolomide 180mg capsules | 5 capsule PoM £381.18–£586.00 (Hospital only)
Temozolomide 250 mg Temozolomide 250mg capsules | 5 capsule PoM £529.42–£814.00 (Hospital only)
▶ **Temodal** (Merck Sharp & Dohme (UK) Ltd)
Temozolomide 5 mg Temodal 5mg capsules | 5 capsule PoM £10.59 (Hospital only)
Temozolomide 20 mg Temodal 20mg capsules | 5 capsule PoM £42.35 (Hospital only)
Temozolomide 100 mg Temodal 100mg capsules | 5 capsule PoM £211.77 (Hospital only)
Temozolomide 140 mg Temodal 140mg capsules | 5 capsule PoM £296.48 (Hospital only)
Temozolomide 180 mg Temodal 180mg capsules | 5 capsule PoM £381.19 (Hospital only)
Temozolomide 250 mg Temodal 250mg capsules | 5 capsule PoM £529.43 (Hospital only)

Thiotepa [Specialist drug]

16-Nov-2020

● **INDICATIONS AND DOSE**
Conditioning treatment before haematopoietic stem cell transplantation in the treatment of haematological disease or solid tumours
▶ BY INTRAVENOUS INFUSION
▶ Adult: Specialist drug – access specialist resources for dosing information

● **CONTRA-INDICATIONS** Acute porphyrias p. 1202
● **INTERACTIONS** → Appendix 1: alkylating agents
● **SIDE-EFFECTS**
▶ **Common or very common** Alopecia · amenorrhoea · anaemia · anxiety · appetite decreased · arrhythmias · arthralgia · asthenia · azoospermia · cataract · chills · cognitive disorder · confusion · conjunctivitis · constipation · cough · cystitis · delirium · diarrhoea · dizziness · dysuria · embolism · encephalopathy · extrapyramidal symptoms · fever · gastrointestinal discomfort · gastrointestinal disorders · generalised oedema · graft versus host disease · haemorrhage · headache · hearing impairment · heart failure · hepatic disorders · hyperglycaemia · hypersensitivity · hypertension · hypopituitarism · increased risk of infection · infertility · interstitial lung disease · intracranial aneurysm · intracranial haemorrhage · leucopenia · lymphoedema · menopausal symptoms · mucositis · multi organ failure · myalgia · nausea · neutropenia · ototoxicity · pain · pancytopenia · paraesthesia · psychiatric disorder · pulmonary oedema · renal impairment · secondary malignancy · seizure · sepsis · sinusoidal obstruction syndrome · skin reactions · stomatitis · thrombocytopenia · toxic shock syndrome · vision blurred · vomiting · weight increased
▶ **Uncommon** Cardiomyopathy · hallucination · hypoxia · myocarditis
▶ **Frequency not known** Severe cutaneous adverse reactions (SCARs)

● **CONCEPTION AND CONTRACEPTION** Contraceptive advice required.

● **NATIONAL FUNDING/ACCESS DECISIONS**
For full details see funding body website
Scottish Medicines Consortium (SMC) decisions
▶ **Thiotepa (***Tepadina***®) in combination with other chemotherapy as conditioning treatment in adults or children with haematological diseases, or solid tumours prior to haematopoietic stem cell transplantation (July 2012)** SMC No. 790/12 Not recommended

● **MEDICINAL FORMS** There can be variation in the licensing of different medicines containing the same drug.
Powder for solution for infusion
▶ **Thiotepa (Non-proprietary)**
Thiotepa 15 mg Thiotepa 15mg powder for concentrate for solution for infusion vials | 1 vial PoM £123.00–£250.00 (Hospital only)
Thiotepa 100 mg Thiotepa 100mg powder for concentrate for solution for infusion vials | 1 vial PoM £736.00–£850.00 (Hospital only)
▶ **Tepadina** (Adienne Pharma & Biotech)
Thiotepa 15 mg Tepadina 15mg powder for concentrate for solution for infusion vials | 1 vial PoM £123.00 (Hospital only)
Thiotepa 100 mg Tepadina 100mg powder for concentrate for solution for infusion vials | 1 vial PoM £736.00 (Hospital only)

Treosulfan [Specialist drug]
05-Jul-2023

● **INDICATIONS AND DOSE**

Ovarian cancer
▶ BY MOUTH, OR BY INTRAVENOUS INJECTION, OR BY INTRAVENOUS INFUSION, OR BY INTRAPERITONEAL INSTILLATION
▶ Adult: Specialist drug – access specialist resources for dosing information

TRECONDI ®

Conditioning treatment before allogeneic haematopoietic stem cell transplantation in patients with malignant and non-malignant disease
▶ BY INTRAVENOUS INFUSION
▶ Adult: Specialist drug – access specialist resources for dosing information

---

IMPORTANT SAFETY INFORMATION
RISKS OF INCORRECT DOSING OF ORAL ANTI-CANCER MEDICINES
See Cytotoxic drugs p. 1027.

● **CONTRA-INDICATIONS**

GENERAL CONTRA-INDICATIONS Acute porphyrias p. 1202 · concomitant use of live vaccines

SPECIFIC CONTRA-INDICATIONS
▶ When used for Conditioning treatment before allogeneic haematopoietic stem cell transplantation Active uncontrolled infection · Fanconi anaemia and other DNA repair disorders · severe concomitant cardiac, lung, liver and renal impairment

● **INTERACTIONS** → Appendix 1: alkylating agents

● **SIDE-EFFECTS**

GENERAL SIDE-EFFECTS
▶ **Common or very common** Alopecia · anaemia · bone marrow disorders · leucopenia · nausea · sepsis · skin reactions · thrombocytopenia · vomiting
▶ **Uncommon** Neoplasms · treatment related secondary malignancy
▶ **Rare or very rare** Addison's disease · cardiomyopathy · hypoglycaemia · influenza like illness · paraesthesia · pneumonia · pulmonary fibrosis · scleroderma

SPECIFIC SIDE-EFFECTS
▶ **Common or very common**
▶ With intravenous use Appetite decreased · arrhythmia · arthralgia · asthenia · chills · constipation · diarrhoea · dizziness · dysphagia · dyspnoea · febrile neutropenia · fever · flushing · gastrointestinal discomfort · gastrointestinal disorders · haemorrhage · headache · hypersensitivity · hypertension · insomnia · lethargy · myalgia · oedema · oral disorders · pain · renal impairment · weight changes
▶ **Uncommon**
▶ With intravenous use Confusion · cough · dry mouth · hepatic disorders · hiccups · hyperglycaemia · hyperhidrosis · hypotension · interstitial lung disease · laryngeal pain · oesophageal pain · peripheral neuropathy · respiratory disorders · sinusoidal obstruction syndrome
▶ With oral use Stomatitis
▶ **Rare or very rare**
▶ With intravenous use Inflammation localised
▶ With oral use Alveolitis · cystitis haemorrhagic
▶ **Frequency not known**
▶ With intravenous use Acidosis · agitation · amenorrhoea · cardiac arrest · cystitis · dry eye · dysphonia · dysuria · electrolyte imbalance · embolism · encephalopathy · extrapyramidal symptoms · feeling cold · glucose tolerance impaired · heart failure · hypoxia · intracranial haemorrhage · muscle weakness · myocardial infarction · oropharyngeal pain · ovarian suppression · pericardial effusion · skin ulcer · syncope

SIDE-EFFECTS, FURTHER INFORMATION Prolonged use of treosulfan is associated with an increased incidence of acute non-lymphocytic leukaemia.

● **CONCEPTION AND CONTRACEPTION** Manufacturer advises females of childbearing potential and male patients with partners of childbearing potential should use effective contraception during and for 6 months after treatment.

● **PATIENT AND CARER ADVICE**
Driving and skilled tasks Patients and carers should be counselled on the effects on driving and performance of skilled tasks—increased risk of nausea, vomiting or dizziness.

● **NATIONAL FUNDING/ACCESS DECISIONS**
For full details see funding body website
NICE decisions
▶ Treosulfan with fludarabine for malignant disease before allogeneic stem cell transplant (August 2020) NICE TA640 Recommended

Scottish Medicines Consortium (SMC) decisions
▶ Treosulfan (*Trecondi*®) in combination with fludarabine as part of conditioning treatment prior to allogeneic haematopoietic stem cell transplantation in adult patients with malignant and non-malignant diseases, and in paediatric patients older than one month with malignant diseases (June 2023) SMC No. SMC2527 Recommended with restrictions

● **MEDICINAL FORMS** There can be variation in the licensing of different medicines containing the same drug.
Powder for solution for injection
▶ **Treosulfan (Non-proprietary)**
Treosulfan 5 gram Treosulfan 5g powder for solution for injection vials | 1 vial PoM £486.50 | 5 vial PoM £2,434.00
▶ **Trecondi** (medac UK)
Treosulfan 1 gram Trecondi 1g powder for solution for infusion | 5 vial PoM £494.40 (Hospital only)
Treosulfan 5 gram Trecondi 5g powder for solution for infusion | 5 vial PoM £2,434.25 (Hospital only)

ANTINEOPLASTIC DRUGS > ANTHRACYCLINES AND RELATED DRUGS

Daunorubicin [Specialist drug]
19-Dec-2021

● **INDICATIONS AND DOSE**

Acute myelogenous leukaemia | Acute lymphocytic leukaemia
▶ BY INTRAVENOUS INFUSION
▶ Adult: Specialist drug – access specialist resources for dosing information

AIDS-related Kaposi's sarcoma (liposomal formulation only)
▶ BY INTRAVENOUS INFUSION
▶ Adult: Specialist drug – access specialist resources for dosing information

DOSE EQUIVALENCE AND CONVERSION
▶ Daunorubicin is available as *conventional* and *liposomal* formulations; these formulations are **not** interchangeable.

IMPORTANT SAFETY INFORMATION
MHRA/CHM ADVICE: LIPOSOMAL AND LIPID-COMPLEX FORMULATIONS: NAME CHANGE TO REDUCE MEDICATION ERRORS (JULY 2020)
Serious harm and fatal overdoses have occurred following confusion between liposomal, pegylated-liposomal, lipid-complex, and conventional formulations of the same drug substance. Medicines with these formulations will explicitly include 'liposomal', 'pegylated-liposomal', or 'lipid-complex' within their

---

Immune system and malignant disease

name to reduce the risk of potentially fatal medication errors.

The MHRA reminds healthcare professionals that liposomal, pegylated-liposomal, lipid-complex, and conventional formulations containing the same drug substance are **not** interchangeable. Healthcare professionals are advised to make a clear distinction between formulations when prescribing, dispensing, administering, and communicating about daunorubicin. The product name and dose should be verified before administration and the maximum dose should not be exceeded.

- **CONTRA-INDICATIONS** Myocardial insufficiency · previous treatment with maximum cumulative doses of daunorubicin or other anthracycline · recent myocardial infarction · severe arrhythmia

- **INTERACTIONS** → Appendix 1: anthracyclines

- **SIDE-EFFECTS** Abdominal pain · alopecia · amenorrhoea · anaemia · arrhythmias · ascites · atrioventricular block · azoospermia · bone marrow disorders · cardiac inflammation · cardiomyopathy · chills · congestive heart failure · cyanosis · death · dehydration · diarrhoea · dyspnoea · extravasation necrosis · fever · flushing · gastrointestinal disorders · haemorrhage · hepatomegaly · hyperpyrexia · hyperuricaemia · hypoxia · infection · ischaemic heart disease · leucopenia · mucositis · myocardial infarction · nail discolouration · nausea · nephropathy · neutropenia · oedema · pain · paraesthesia · pleural effusion · posterior reversible encephalopathy syndrome (PRES) · radiation injuries · shock · skin reactions · stomatitis · thrombocytopenia · thrombophlebitis · urine discolouration · venous sclerosis · vomiting

SIDE-EFFECTS, FURTHER INFORMATION Cardiotoxicity is cumulative and may be irreversible, however responds to treatment if detected early.

- **CONCEPTION AND CONTRACEPTION** Contraceptive advice required.

- **MEDICINAL FORMS** There can be variation in the licensing of different medicines containing the same drug.
Powder for solution for infusion
▸ Daunorubicin (Non-proprietary)
Daunorubicin (as Daunorubicin hydrochloride)
20 mg Daunorubicin 20mg powder for solution for infusion vials | 10 vial PoM £715.00 (Hospital only)

Daunorubicin with cytarabine
[Specialist drug]

06-Feb-2025

The properties listed below are those particular to the combination only. For the properties of the components please consider, daunorubicin p. 1037, cytarabine p. 1045.

- **INDICATIONS AND DOSE**
Acute myeloid leukaemia
▸ BY INTRAVENOUS INFUSION
▸ Adult: Specialist drug – access specialist resources for dosing information
DOSE EQUIVALENCE AND CONVERSION
▸ Daunorubicin with cytarabine is available as a *liposomal* formulation; it is **not** interchangeable with other daunorubicin- or cytarabine-containing preparations.

IMPORTANT SAFETY INFORMATION
MHRA/CHM ADVICE: LIPOSOMAL AND LIPID-COMPLEX FORMULATIONS: NAME CHANGE TO REDUCE MEDICATION ERRORS (JULY 2020)
Serious harm and fatal overdoses have occurred following confusion between liposomal, pegylated-

liposomal, lipid-complex, and conventional formulations of the same drug substance. Medicines with these formulations will explicitly include 'liposomal', 'pegylated-liposomal', or 'lipid-complex' within their name to reduce the risk of potentially fatal medication errors.

The MHRA reminds healthcare professionals that liposomal, pegylated-liposomal, lipid-complex, and conventional formulations containing the same drug substance are **not** interchangeable. Healthcare professionals are advised to make a clear distinction between formulations when prescribing, dispensing, administering, and communicating about daunorubicin with cytarabine. The product name and dose should be verified before administration and the maximum dose should not be exceeded.

- **INTERACTIONS** → Appendix 1: anthracyclines · cytarabine
- **NATIONAL FUNDING/ACCESS DECISIONS**
For full details see funding body website
NICE decisions
▸ Liposomal cytarabine–daunorubicin for untreated acute myeloid leukaemia (December 2018) NICE TA552
Recommended with restrictions
Scottish Medicines Consortium (SMC) decisions
▸ Liposomal daunorubicin and cytarabine (*Vyxeos*®) for the treatment of adults with newly diagnosed, therapy-related acute myeloid leukaemia (t-AML) or AML with myelodysplasia-related changes (March 2019) SMC No. SMC2130
Recommended

- **MEDICINAL FORMS** There can be variation in the licensing of different medicines containing the same drug.
Powder for solution for infusion
▸ Vyxeos (Jazz Pharmaceuticals UK Ltd)
Daunorubicin (liposomal) 44 mg, Cytarabine (liposomal) 100 mg Vyxeos liposomal 44mg/100mg powder for concentrate for solution for infusion vials | 1 vial PoM £4,581.00 (Hospital only)

Doxorubicin hydrochloride
[Specialist drug]

05-Oct-2021

- **INDICATIONS AND DOSE**
Acute leukaemias | Hodgkin's lymphoma | Non-Hodgkin's lymphoma | Solid tumours [including breast cancer] | Soft-tissue sarcoma
▸ BY INTRAVENOUS INJECTION
▸ Adult: Specialist drug – access specialist resources for dosing information
Bladder cancer
▸ BY INTRAVESICAL INSTILLATION
▸ Adult: Specialist drug – access specialist resources for dosing information
DOSE EQUIVALENCE AND CONVERSION
▸ Doxorubicin is available as *conventional* and *pegylated liposomal* formulations; these formulations are **not** interchangeable.

CAELYX ®

AIDS-related Kaposi's sarcoma | Ovarian cancer | Multiple myeloma | Breast cancer
▸ BY INTRAVENOUS INFUSION
▸ Adult: Specialist drug – access specialist resources for dosing information

DOSE EQUIVALENCE AND CONVERSION
- *Caelyx*® is a *pegylated liposomal* formulation; it is **not** interchangeable with other formulations of doxorubicin.

IMPORTANT SAFETY INFORMATION
MHRA/CHM ADVICE: LIPOSOMAL AND LIPID-COMPLEX FORMULATIONS: NAME CHANGE TO REDUCE MEDICATION ERRORS (JULY 2020)
Serious harm and fatal overdoses have occurred following confusion between liposomal, pegylated-liposomal, lipid-complex, and conventional formulations of the same drug substance. Medicines with these formulations will explicitly include 'liposomal', 'pegylated-liposomal', or 'lipid-complex' within their name to reduce the risk of potentially fatal medication errors.

The MHRA reminds healthcare professionals that liposomal, pegylated-liposomal, lipid-complex, and conventional formulations containing the same drug substance are **not** interchangeable. Healthcare professionals are advised to make a clear distinction between formulations when prescribing, dispensing, administering, and communicating about doxorubicin. The product name and dose should be verified before administration and the maximum dose should not be exceeded.

- **CONTRA-INDICATIONS** Consult product literature
- **INTERACTIONS** → Appendix 1: anthracyclines
- **SIDE-EFFECTS**
- **Common or very common** Alopecia · anaemia · anxiety · appetite decreased · arrhythmias · arthralgia · asthenia · bone marrow depression · breast pain · cachexia · cardiovascular disorder · chest discomfort · chills · constipation · cough · decreased leucocytes · dehydration · depression · diarrhoea · dizziness · drowsiness · dry mouth · dysphagia · dyspnoea · dysuria · electrolyte imbalance · epistaxis · eye inflammation · fever · gastrointestinal discomfort · gastrointestinal disorders · headache · hyperhidrosis · hypersensitivity · hypertension · hyperthermia · hypotension · increased risk of infection · influenza like illness · infusion related reaction · insomnia · malaise · mucosal abnormalities · muscle complaints · muscle tone increased · muscle weakness · nail disorder · nausea · nerve disorders · neutropenia · oedema · oral disorders · pain · scrotal erythema · sensation abnormal · sepsis · skin reactions · skin ulcer · syncope · taste altered · thrombocytopenia · vasodilation · vision blurred · vomiting · weight decreased
- **Uncommon** Confusion · embolism and thrombosis
- **Rare or very rare** Secondary oral neoplasms · severe cutaneous adverse reactions (SCARs)
- **Frequency not known** Asthma · congestive heart failure · secondary malignancy · throat tightness

SIDE-EFFECTS, FURTHER INFORMATION Extravasation can cause tissue necrosis.

Cardiomyopathy Higher cumulative doses are associated with cardiomyopathy and it is usual to limit total cumulative doses to 450 mg/m^2.

Liposomal formulations Liposomal formulations of doxorubicin may reduce the incidence of cardiotoxicity and lower the potential for local necrosis, but infusion reactions, sometimes severe, may occur. Hand-foot syndrome (painful, macular reddening skin eruptions) occurs commonly with liposomal doxorubicin and may be dose limiting. It can occur after 2–3 treatment cycles and may be prevented by cooling hands and feet and avoiding socks, gloves, or tight-fitting footwear. It may also occur with non-liposomal formulations.

Elevated bilirubin concentrations Doxorubicin is largely excreted in the bile and an elevated bilirubin concentration is an indication for reducing the dose.

- **CONCEPTION AND CONTRACEPTION** Manufacturer advises effective contraception during and for at least 6 months after treatment in men or women.

- **NATIONAL FUNDING/ACCESS DECISIONS**
For full details see funding body website
NICE decisions
- **Topotecan, pegylated liposomal doxorubicin hydrochloride, paclitaxel, trabectedin and gemcitabine for treating recurrent ovarian cancer (April 2016)** NICE TA389 Recommended
- **Olaratumab in combination with doxorubicin for treating advanced soft tissue sarcoma (August 2017)** NICE TA465 Recommended with restrictions

- **MEDICINAL FORMS** There can be variation in the licensing of different medicines containing the same drug. Forms available from special-order manufacturers include: solution for injection, solution for infusion

Solution for injection
- **Doxorubicin hydrochloride (Non-proprietary)**
Doxorubicin hydrochloride 2 mg per 1 ml Doxorubicin 50mg/25ml solution for injection Cytosafe vials | 1 vial [PoM] £103.00 (Hospital only)
Doxorubicin 50mg/25ml solution for infusion vials | 1 vial [PoM] £103.00 (Hospital only)
Doxorubicin 10mg/5ml solution for injection Cytosafe vials | 1 vial [PoM] £20.60 (Hospital only)
Doxorubicin 10mg/5ml concentrate for solution for infusion vials | 1 vial [PoM] £19.57-£20.60 (Hospital only)
Doxorubicin 10mg/5ml solution for infusion vials | 1 vial [PoM] £20.60 (Hospital only)
Doxorubicin 50mg/25ml concentrate for solution for infusion vials | 1 vial [PoM] £96.00-£97.85 (Hospital only)

Solution for infusion
- **Doxorubicin hydrochloride (Non-proprietary)**
Doxorubicin hydrochloride 2 mg per 1 ml Doxorubicin 200mg/100ml solution for infusion vials | 1 vial [PoM] £412.00 (Hospital only)
Doxorubicin 20mg/10ml concentrate for solution for infusion vials | 1 vial [PoM] £22.00 (Hospital only)
Doxorubicin 100mg/50ml concentrate for solution for infusion vials | 1 vial [PoM] £235.00 (Hospital only)
Doxorubicin 200mg/100ml solution for injection Cytosafe vials | 1 vial [PoM] £412.00 (Hospital only)
Doxorubicin 200mg/100ml concentrate for solution for infusion vials | 1 vial [PoM] £389.00-£391.40 (Hospital only)
Doxorubicin hydrochloride (as Doxorubicin hydrochloride pegylated liposomal) 2 mg per 1 ml Doxorubicin pegylated liposomal 50mg/25ml concentrate for solution for infusion vials | 1 vial [PoM] £712.00-£712.49 (Hospital only) | 1 vial [PoM] £712.48
Doxorubicin pegylated liposomal 20mg/10ml concentrate for solution for infusion vials | 1 vial [PoM] £360.00-£360.23 (Hospital only) | 1 vial [PoM] £360.22

Epirubicin hydrochloride [Specialist drug]

21-May-2021

- **INDICATIONS AND DOSE**
Breast cancer | Gastric cancer | Small cell lung cancer | Ovarian cancer | Colorectal cancer | Lymphoma | Leukaemia | Multiple myeloma
- BY INTRAVENOUS INJECTION, OR BY INTRAVENOUS INFUSION
- Adult: Specialist drug – access specialist resources for dosing information

Bladder cancer
- BY INTRAVESICAL INSTILLATION
- Adult: Specialist drug – access specialist resources for dosing information

- **CONTRA-INDICATIONS** Bladder inflammation or contraction (when used as a bladder instillation) · catheterisation difficulties (when used as a bladder instillation) · haematuria (when used as a bladder instillation) · invasive tumours penetrating the bladder (when used as a bladder instillation) · myocardiopathy · previous treatment with maximum cumulative doses of epirubicin or other anthracycline · recent myocardial infarction · severe arrhythmia · severe myocardial insufficiency · unstable angina · urinary tract infections (when used as a bladder instillation)

- **INTERACTIONS** → Appendix 1: anthracyclines
- **SIDE-EFFECTS**
- **Common or very common**
- With intravesical use Chemical cystitis
- With parenteral use Alopecia · amenorrhoea · anaemia · appetite decreased · arrhythmias · cardiac conduction disorders · chills · congestive heart failure · dehydration · diarrhoea · eye inflammation · fever · gastrointestinal discomfort · gastrointestinal disorders · haemorrhage · increased risk of infection · leucopenia · malaise · mucositis · nail discolouration · nausea · neutropenia · oral disorders · skin reactions · thrombocytopenia · urine discolouration · vasodilation · vomiting
- **Uncommon**
- With parenteral use Asthenia · embolism and thrombosis · sepsis
- **Rare or very rare**
- With parenteral use Hyperuricaemia
- **Frequency not known**
- With parenteral use Bone marrow depression · cardiomyopathy · cardiotoxicity · photosensitivity reaction · radiation injuries · shock

SIDE-EFFECTS, FURTHER INFORMATION Manufacturer advises extreme caution with cumulative doses exceeding 900 mg/m^2—risk of congestive heart failure increased.

- **CONCEPTION AND CONTRACEPTION** [EvGr] Females of childbearing potential should use effective contraception during treatment and for at least 6.5 months after last dose; male patients should use effective contraception during treatment and for at least 3.5 months after last dose. Ⓜ

- **MEDICINAL FORMS** There can be variation in the licensing of different medicines containing the same drug. Forms available from special-order manufacturers include: solution for injection, solution for infusion

Solution for injection
- **Epirubicin hydrochloride (Non-proprietary)**
  Epirubicin hydrochloride 2 mg per 1 ml Epirubicin 50mg/25ml solution for injection vials | 1 vial [PoM] £86.89-£106.19 (Hospital only)
  Epirubicin 10mg/5ml solution for injection vials | 1 vial [PoM] £17.38-£21.24 (Hospital only)
- **Pharmorubicin** (Pfizer Ltd)
  Epirubicin hydrochloride 2 mg per 1 ml Pharmorubicin 50mg/25ml solution for injection Cytosafe vials | 1 vial [PoM] £106.19 (Hospital only)
  Pharmorubicin 10mg/5ml solution for injection Cytosafe vials | 1 vial [PoM] £21.24 (Hospital only)

Solution for infusion
- **Epirubicin hydrochloride (Non-proprietary)**
  Epirubicin hydrochloride 2 mg per 1 ml Epirubicin 100mg/50ml solution for infusion vials | 1 vial [PoM] £201.76 (Hospital only)
  Epirubicin 200mg/100ml solution for infusion vials | 1 vial [PoM] £347.55-£366.85 (Hospital only)

Idarubicin hydrochloride [Specialist drug]

25-Jun-2020

- **INDICATIONS AND DOSE**

Acute non-lymphocytic leukaemias | Breast cancer
- BY MOUTH
- Adult: Specialist drug – access specialist resources for dosing information

Acute leukaemias | Breast cancer
- BY INTRAVENOUS INJECTION
- Adult: Specialist drug – access specialist resources for dosing information

IMPORTANT SAFETY INFORMATION
RISKS OF INCORRECT DOSING OF ORAL ANTI-CANCER MEDICINES
See Cytotoxic drugs p. 1027.

- **CONTRA-INDICATIONS** Previous treatment with maximum cumulative dose of idarubicin or other anthracycline · recent myocardial infarction · severe arrhythmias · severe myocardial insufficiency
- **INTERACTIONS** → Appendix 1: anthracyclines
- **SIDE-EFFECTS**
GENERAL SIDE-EFFECTS
- **Common or very common** Alopecia · anaemia · appetite decreased · arrhythmias · cardiomyopathy · chills · congestive heart failure · diarrhoea · embolism and thrombosis · fever · haemorrhage · headache · increased risk of infection · leucopenia · nausea · neutropenia · skin reactions · stomatitis · thrombocytopenia · urine discolouration · vomiting
- **Uncommon** Dehydration · gastrointestinal disorders · hyperuricaemia · leukaemia secondary · myocardial infarction · nail discolouration · sepsis · shock · soft tissue necrosis
- **Rare or very rare** Cardiac conduction disorders · cardiac inflammation · flushing · intracranial haemorrhage
- **Frequency not known** Bone marrow disorders · tumour lysis syndrome
SPECIFIC SIDE-EFFECTS
- **Common or very common**
- With intravenous use Abdominal pain · mucosal abnormalities · paraesthesia · radiation injuries
- With oral use Gastrointestinal discomfort · mucositis · radiation skin sensitivity
- **CONCEPTION AND CONTRACEPTION** [EvGr] Females of childbearing potential should use effective contraception during treatment and for at least 6 and a half months after last treatment; male patients should use effective contraception during treatment and for at least 3 and a half months after last treatment. Ⓜ

- **MEDICINAL FORMS** There can be variation in the licensing of different medicines containing the same drug.
Oral capsule
CAUTIONARY AND ADVISORY LABELS 25
- Zavedos (Pfizer Ltd)
  Idarubicin hydrochloride 5 mg Zavedos 5mg capsules | 1 capsule [PoM] £41.47
  Idarubicin hydrochloride 10 mg Zavedos 10mg capsules | 1 capsule [PoM] £69.12

Mitoxantrone [Specialist drug]

25-Jun-2020

(Mitozantrone)

- **INDICATIONS AND DOSE**

Breast cancer | Non-Hodgkin's lymphoma | Acute myeloid leukaemia | Chronic myeloid leukaemia | Prostate cancer
- BY INTRAVENOUS INFUSION
- Adult: Specialist drug – access specialist resources for dosing information

- **INTERACTIONS** → Appendix 1: anthracyclines
- **SIDE-EFFECTS**
- **Uncommon** Urine discolouration
- **Frequency not known** Abdominal pain · acute leukaemia · alopecia · amenorrhoea · anxiety · appetite decreased · arrhythmia · asthenia · bone marrow depression ·

confusion · constipation · diarrhoea · drowsiness · dyspnoea · fever · gastrointestinal haemorrhage · heart failure · mucositis · nail discolouration · nail dystrophy · nausea · neurological effects · paraesthesia · scleral discolouration · skin discolouration · stomatitis · thrombocytopenia · vomiting

● **SIDE-EFFECTS, FURTHER INFORMATION** Cardiac toxicity, including irreversible and fatal congestive heart failure, may occur either during treatment with mitoxantrone or months to years after discontinuation; the risk increases with cumulative dose.

● **CONCEPTION AND CONTRACEPTION** Manufacturer advises effective contraception during and for at least 6 months after treatment in men or women.

● **MEDICINAL FORMS** There can be variation in the licensing of different medicines containing the same drug.

Solution for infusion
▶ Onkotrone (Baxter Healthcare Ltd)
Mitoxantrone (as Mitoxantrone hydrochloride) 2 mg per 1 ml Onkotrone 20mg/10ml solution for infusion vials | 1 vial [PoM] £121.85 (Hospital only)
Onkotrone 25mg/12.5ml solution for infusion vials | 1 vial [PoM] £152.33

Pixantrone [Specialist drug]   21-May-2021

● **INDICATIONS AND DOSE**

Non-Hodgkin B-cell lymphomas
▶ BY INTRAVENOUS INFUSION
▶ Adult: Specialist drug – access specialist resources for dosing information

● **CONTRA-INDICATIONS** Active severe infection · risk factors for severe infection

● **INTERACTIONS** → Appendix 1: anthracyclines

● **SIDE-EFFECTS**
▶ **Common or very common** Alopecia · anaemia · appetite decreased · arrhythmias · asthenia · blood disorder · bundle branch block · cancer progression · cardiac disorder (during or following treatment) · chest pain · congestive heart failure · constipation · cough · decreased leucocytes · diarrhoea · drowsiness · dry mouth · dyspnoea · electrolyte imbalance · eye inflammation · fever · gastrointestinal discomfort · haemorrhage · headache · hypotension · increased risk of infection · left ventricular dysfunction · mucositis · nail disorder · nausea · neutropenia · oedema · oral disorders · pain · paraesthesia · proteinuria · secondary malignancy · skin reactions · taste altered · thrombocytopenia · urine discolouration · vascular disorders · vomiting
▶ **Uncommon** Anxiety · arthralgia · arthritis · bone marrow failure · chills · dizziness · dry eye · eosinophilia · hyperbilirubinaemia · hyperuricaemia · local reaction · meningitis · muscle weakness · musculoskeletal stiffness · night sweats · oesophagitis · oliguria · pleural effusion · pneumonitis · rhinorrhoea · septic shock · skin ulcer · sleep disorders · spontaneous penile erection · vertigo · weight decreased

● **CONCEPTION AND CONTRACEPTION** Ensure effective contraception during and for at least 6 months after treatment in men or women.

● **PATIENT AND CARER ADVICE** Photosensitivity is a theoretical risk and patients should be advised to follow sun protection strategies.

● **NATIONAL FUNDING/ACCESS DECISIONS**
For full details see funding body website
NICE decisions
▶ Pixantrone monotherapy for treating multiply relapsed or refractory aggressive non-Hodgkin's B-cell lymphoma (February 2014) NICE TA306 Recommended with restrictions

● **MEDICINAL FORMS** No licensed medicines listed.

ANTINEOPLASTIC DRUGS > ANTIMETABOLITES

Azacitidine [Specialist drug]   25-Jul-2023

● **INDICATIONS AND DOSE**

Myelodysplastic syndromes | Chronic myelomonocytic leukaemia
▶ BY SUBCUTANEOUS INJECTION
▶ Adult: Specialist drug – access specialist resources for dosing information

Acute myeloid leukaemia
▶ BY MOUTH, OR BY SUBCUTANEOUS INJECTION
▶ Adult: Specialist drug – access specialist resources for dosing information

DOSE EQUIVALENCE AND CONVERSION
▶ Oral and injectable azacitidine preparations are not interchangeable.

● **CONTRA-INDICATIONS**
▶ With subcutaneous use Advanced malignant hepatic tumour

● **INTERACTIONS** → Appendix 1: azacitidine

● **SIDE-EFFECTS**
GENERAL SIDE-EFFECTS
▶ **Common or very common** Anxiety · appetite decreased · arthralgia · asthenia · constipation · diarrhoea · gastrointestinal discomfort · increased risk of infection · leucopenia · nausea · neutropenia · pain · thrombocytopenia · vomiting · weight decreased

SPECIFIC SIDE-EFFECTS
▶ **Common or very common**
▶ With oral use Cystitis
▶ With subcutaneous use Alopecia · anaemia · bone marrow disorders · chest pain · chills · confusion · dehydration · dizziness · drowsiness · dyspnoea · fever · haemorrhage · headache · hypertension · hypokalaemia · hypotension · induration · inflammation · insomnia · intracranial haemorrhage · laryngeal pain · malaise · muscle complaints · pleural effusion · renal failure · sepsis · skin reactions · stomatitis · syncope
▶ **Uncommon**
▶ With subcutaneous use Hepatic coma · hepatic failure · pyoderma gangrenosum · renal tubular acidosis
▶ **Rare or very rare**
▶ With subcutaneous use Injection site necrosis · interstitial lung disease · tumour lysis syndrome

● **CONCEPTION AND CONTRACEPTION** [EvGr] Females of childbearing potential should use effective contraception during treatment and for 6 months after treatment; male patients should use effective contraception during treatment and for 3 months after treatment. Ⓜ

● **PATIENT AND CARER ADVICE** Patients should be advised to promptly report any febrile episodes or signs and symptoms of bleeding.
Driving and skilled tasks Patients and carers should be cautioned on the effects on driving and performance of skilled tasks—increased risk of fatigue.

● **NATIONAL FUNDING/ACCESS DECISIONS**
For full details see funding body website
NICE decisions
▶ Azacitidine for the treatment of myelodysplastic syndromes, chronic myelomonocytic leukaemia and acute myeloid leukaemia (March 2011) NICE TA218 Recommended with restrictions
▶ Azacitidine for treating acute myeloid leukaemia with more than 30% bone marrow blasts (July 2016) NICE TA399 Not recommended

Immune system and malignant disease

▶ Oral azacitidine for maintenance treatment of acute myeloid leukaemia after induction therapy (October 2022) NICE TA827 Recommended

Scottish Medicines Consortium (SMC) decisions
▶ Azacitidine (*Onureg*®) as maintenance therapy in adults with acute myeloid leukaemia who have achieved complete remission or complete remission with incomplete blood count recovery following induction therapy with or without consolidation treatment and who are not candidates for, including those who choose not to proceed to, hematopoietic stem cell transplantation (July 2023) SMC No. SMC2533 Recommended

● **MEDICINAL FORMS** There can be variation in the licensing of different medicines containing the same drug.
Powder for suspension for injection
▶ **Azacitidine (Non-proprietary)**
Azacitidine 100 mg Azacitidine 100mg powder for suspension for injection vials | 1 vial [PoM] £220.00-£321.00 (Hospital only)
Azacitidine 150 mg Azacitidine 150mg powder for suspension for injection vials | 1 vial [PoM] £433.35-£481.50 (Hospital only)
▶ **Vidaza** (Bristol-Myers Squibb Pharmaceuticals Ltd)
Azacitidine 100 mg Vidaza 100mg powder for suspension for injection vials | 1 vial [PoM] £321.00 (Hospital only)
Oral tablet
CAUTIONARY AND ADVISORY LABELS 25
▶ **Onureg** (Bristol-Myers Squibb Pharmaceuticals Ltd)
Azacitidine 200 mg Onureg 200mg tablets | 7 tablet [PoM] £5,867.00 (Hospital only)
Azacitidine 300 mg Onureg 300mg tablets | 7 tablet [PoM] £5,867.00 (Hospital only)

Capecitabine [Specialist drug]

27-Jul-2021

● **INDICATIONS AND DOSE**

Colorectal cancer | Gastric cancer | Breast cancer
▶ BY MOUTH
▶ Adult: Specialist drug – access specialist resources for dosing information

IMPORTANT SAFETY INFORMATION
RISKS OF INCORRECT DOSING OF ORAL ANTI-CANCER MEDICINES
See Cytotoxic drugs p. 1027.

MHRA/CHM ADVICE: 5-FLUOROURACIL (INTRAVENOUS), CAPECITABINE, TEGAFUR: DPD TESTING RECOMMENDED BEFORE INITIATION TO IDENTIFY PATIENTS AT INCREASED RISK OF SEVERE AND FATAL TOXICITY (OCTOBER 2020)
Patients with partial or complete dihydropyrimidine dehydrogenase (DPD) deficiency are at increased risk of severe and fatal toxicity during treatment with fluoropyrimidines. Healthcare professionals are advised to test all patients for DPD deficiency before initiating treatment and confirm their, including family, history of complete or partial DPD deficiency. Capecitabine is contra-indicated in patients with known complete DPD deficiency; in those with partial DPD deficiency, a reduced starting dose is recommended. Patients should be monitored for toxicity, particularly during the first cycle of treatment or after a dose increase; severe toxicity can occur even in those with negative test results for DPD deficiency. Healthcare professionals should also counsel patients on the benefits and risks of their treatment and ensure they are provided with the patient information leaflet.

● **CONTRA-INDICATIONS** Complete dihydropyrimidine dehydrogenase deficiency (increased risk of severe, life-threatening, or fatal toxicity)—consult product literature

● **INTERACTIONS** → Appendix 1: capecitabine

● **SIDE-EFFECTS**
▶ **Common or very common** Alopecia · anaemia · appetite abnormal · asthenia · chest pain · constipation · cough ·

dehydration · depression · diarrhoea · dizziness · dry mouth · dyspnoea · embolism and thrombosis · eye disorders · eye inflammation · eye irritation · fever · gastrointestinal discomfort · gastrointestinal disorders · haemorrhage · headache · hyperbilirubinaemia · increased risk of infection · insomnia · joint disorders · lethargy · malaise · nail disorder · nausea · neutropenia · oedema · pain · rhinorrhoea · sensation abnormal · skin reactions · stomatitis · taste altered · vomiting · weight decreased
▶ **Uncommon** Acute coronary syndrome · aphasia · arrhythmias · ascites · asthma · chills · confusion · diabetes mellitus · dysphagia · ear pain · facial swelling · haemolytic anaemia · hepatic disorders · hot flush · hydronephrosis · hypertension · hypertriglyceridaemia · hypokalaemia · hypotension · influenza like illness · ischaemic heart disease · leucopenia · libido decreased · lipoma · malnutrition · memory loss · movement disorders · muscle weakness · musculoskeletal stiffness · palpitations · pancytopenia · panic attack · peripheral coldness · peripheral neuropathy · photosensitivity reaction · pneumothorax · radiation recall reaction · sepsis · skin ulcer · syncope · thrombocytopenia · urinary disorders · vertigo · vision disorders
▶ **Rare or very rare** Cutaneous lupus erythematosus · encephalopathy · QT interval prolongation · severe cutaneous adverse reactions (SCARs) · vasospasm
▶ **Frequency not known** Cardiomyopathy · heart failure · sudden death

SIDE-EFFECTS, FURTHER INFORMATION Interrupt treatment if grade 2 or 3 hand and foot syndrome (palmar-plantar erythrodysaesthesia syndrome) occurs; review ongoing dosing as needed.

● **CONCEPTION AND CONTRACEPTION** Contraceptive advice required.

● **NATIONAL FUNDING/ACCESS DECISIONS**
For full details see funding body website
NICE decisions
▶ Bevacizumab in combination with capecitabine for the first-line treatment of metastatic breast cancer (August 2012) NICE TA263 Not recommended
▶ Bevacizumab in combination with oxaliplatin and either fluorouracil plus folinic acid or capecitabine for the treatment of metastatic colorectal cancer (December 2010) NICE TA212 Not recommended
▶ Capecitabine for the treatment of advanced gastric cancer (July 2010) NICE TA191 Recommended
▶ Capecitabine and tegafur with uracil for metastatic colorectal cancer (May 2003) NICE TA61 Recommended
▶ Capecitabine and oxaliplatin in the adjuvant treatment of stage III (Dukes' C) colon cancer (April 2006) NICE TA100 Recommended

● **MEDICINAL FORMS** There can be variation in the licensing of different medicines containing the same drug.
Oral tablet
CAUTIONARY AND ADVISORY LABELS 21
▶ **Capecitabine (Non-proprietary)**
Capecitabine 150 mg Capecitabine 150mg tablets | 60 tablet [PoM] £30.00 DT = £30.00 | 60 tablet [PoM] £38.02 DT = £30.00 (Hospital only)
Capecitabine 300 mg Capecitabine 300mg tablets | 60 tablet [PoM] £76.04 (Hospital only)
Capecitabine 500 mg Capecitabine 500mg tablets | 120 tablet [PoM] £225.72 DT = £225.72 | 120 tablet [PoM] £240.00 DT = £225.72 (Hospital only)

Cladribine

21-May-2025

- **DRUG ACTION** Cladribine is a nucleoside analogue that is cytotoxic particularly to lymphocytes and monocytes, inhibiting both DNA synthesis and repair. Its effect on B- and T-lymphocytes is thought to interrupt the cascade of immune events central to multiple sclerosis.

● INDICATIONS AND DOSE

Hairy cell leukaemia (specialist use only)
- ▶ BY SUBCUTANEOUS INJECTION, OR BY INTRAVENOUS INFUSION
- ▸ Adult: Specialist indication – access specialist resources for dosing information

B-cell chronic lymphocytic leukaemia (specialist use only)
- ▶ BY INTRAVENOUS INFUSION
- ▸ Adult: Specialist indication – access specialist resources for dosing information

Multiple sclerosis (under expert supervision)
- ▶ BY MOUTH
- ▸ Adult: (consult product literature or local protocols)

IMPORTANT SAFETY INFORMATION

MHRA/CHM ADVICE: CLADRIBINE FOR LEUKAEMIA: REPORTS OF PROGRESSIVE MULTIFOCAL ENCEPHALOPATHY (PML); STOP TREATMENT IF PML SUSPECTED (DECEMBER 2017)
- ▶ With intravenous use or subcutaneous use

The MHRA is aware of 3 confirmed cases of progressive multifocal encephalopathy (PML) that developed 6 months to several years after cladribine treatment for haematological conditions. An association between cladribine and prolonged lymphopenia has been reported. PML should be considered in the differential diagnosis for patients with new or worsening neurological signs or symptoms. Patients should be monitored for signs and symptoms of new neurological dysfunction, and advised to seek urgent medical attention if they experience symptoms—stop treatment immediately if PML is suspected and ensure specialist investigation is received.

MHRA/CHM ADVICE: CLADRIBINE (*MAVENCLAD*®): NEW ADVICE TO MINIMISE RISK OF SERIOUS LIVER INJURY (MARCH 2022)
- ▶ With oral use

A small number of cases of clinically significant liver injury have been reported during cladribine treatment for multiple sclerosis. Time to onset varied but most cases occurred within 8 weeks of starting the first treatment course. Some patients had underlying hepatic disorders or a history of drug-related hepatic injury; a causal mechanism had not been identified. Healthcare professionals are advised to:
- ● check the patient's history for liver disorders;
- ● monitor liver function tests (including total bilirubin) before each treatment course in years 1 and 2, and during treatment if clinically indicated;
- ● urgently check liver function tests (including bilirubin) in patients with signs or symptoms of liver injury;
- ● discontinue or interrupt treatment in patients with hepatic dysfunction or unexplained increases in liver enzymes.

Patients and carers should be informed of the risk of serious liver injury and advised to seek immediate medical attention if signs of liver problems develop.

● CONTRA-INDICATIONS
- ▶ With oral use Active chronic hepatitis · active chronic tuberculosis · active malignancy · HIV infection · immunocompromised patients

● CAUTIONS

GENERAL CAUTIONS Acute infection · use irradiated blood only (haematology consultation advised)

SPECIFIC CAUTIONS
- ▶ With intravenous use or subcutaneous use High tumour burden—consult product literature · symptomatic or severe bone marrow depression
- ▶ With oral use No prior exposure to varicella zoster virus · prior malignancy (consider if potential benefit outweighs risk)

CAUTIONS, FURTHER INFORMATION
- ▶ Immunosuppressive effect of cladribine
- ▶ With intravenous use or subcutaneous use Cladribine has potent and prolonged myelosuppressive and immunosuppressive effects. Patients treated with cladribine are more prone to serious bacterial, opportunistic fungal, and viral infections, and prophylactic therapy should be considered in those at risk. Acute infections should be treated before initiating cladribine. To prevent potentially fatal transfusion-related graft-versus-host reaction, only irradiated blood products should be administered. Prescribers should consult specialist literature when using highly immunosuppressive drugs.
- ▶ Varicella zoster virus
- ▶ With oral use Manufacturer advises vaccination prior to initiation of therapy in patients who have no history of exposure to varicella zoster virus; delay treatment for 4–6 weeks after vaccination.

● INTERACTIONS → Appendix 1: cladribine

● SIDE-EFFECTS

GENERAL SIDE-EFFECTS
- ▶ **Common or very common** Increased risk of infection

SPECIFIC SIDE-EFFECTS
- ▶ **Common or very common**
- ▶ With intravenous use Anaemia · anxiety · appetite decreased · arrhythmias · arthritis · asthenia · chest pain · chills · confusion · conjunctivitis · constipation · cough · diarrhoea · dizziness · dyspnoea · febrile neutropenia · fever · flatulence · gastrointestinal discomfort · haemolytic anaemia · headache · hyperhidrosis · hypersensitivity · insomnia · interstitial lung disease · joint disorders · malaise · muscle weakness · myalgia · myocardial ischaemia · nausea · neoplasms · oedema · pain · pulmonary fibrosis · renal impairment · respiratory disorders · secondary malignancy · septic shock · skin reactions · thrombocytopenia · vomiting
- ▶ With oral use Alopecia · lymphopenia · rash
- ▶ With subcutaneous use Anaemia · anxiety · appetite decreased · arrhythmias · arthralgia · arthritis · asthenia · bone marrow disorders · chills · constipation · cough · diarrhoea · dizziness · dyspnoea · fever · gastrointestinal disorders · gastrointestinal pain · haemorrhage · headache · hyperhidrosis · hypotension · immunosuppression · insomnia · lymphopenia · malaise · mucositis · myalgia · myocardial ischaemia · nausea · neutropenia · oedema · pain · respiratory disorders · secondary malignancy · sepsis · skin reactions · thrombocytopenia · vomiting
- ▶ **Uncommon**
- ▶ With intravenous use Bone marrow disorders · hypereosinophilia · level of consciousness decreased · nerve disorders · neurotoxicity (with high doses) · paralysis · paraparesis · Stevens-Johnson syndrome · tumour lysis syndrome
- ▶ With oral use Liver injury
- ▶ With subcutaneous use Ataxia · cachexia · confusion · drowsiness · eye inflammation · haemolytic anaemia · paraesthesia · polyneuropathy
- ▶ **Rare or very rare**
- ▶ With intravenous use Heart failure
- ▶ With subcutaneous use Amyloidosis · cholecystitis · depression · dysphagia · epilepsy · graft versus host disease · heart failure · hepatic failure · hypereosinophilia · pulmonary embolism · renal failure · severe cutaneous

Immune system and malignant disease

adverse reactions (SCARs) · speech disorder · tumour lysis syndrome
▶ **Frequency not known**
▶ With oral use Malignancy
● CONCEPTION AND CONTRACEPTION Manufacturer advises effective contraception during treatment and for at least 6 months after the last dose in men and women of childbearing potential.
▶ With oral use Manufacturer advises exclude pregnancy before each treatment course; if using a hormonal contraceptive, a barrier method should also be used for at least 4 weeks after the last dose of each course.
● PREGNANCY Manufacturer advises avoid—teratogenic in *animal* studies. See also *Pregnancy and reproductive function* in Cytotoxic drugs p. 1027.
● BREAST FEEDING
▶ With intravenous use or subcutaneous use Manufacturer advises avoid during treatment and for 6 months after the last dose—no information available.
▶ With oral use Manufacturer advises avoid during treatment and for 1 week after the last dose—no information available.
● HEPATIC IMPAIRMENT
▶ With intravenous use Manufacturer advises caution (limited information available).
▶ With subcutaneous use Manufacturer advises caution in mild impairment; avoid in moderate to severe impairment (no information available).
▶ With oral use Manufacturer advises avoid in moderate to severe impairment (no information available).
● RENAL IMPAIRMENT
▶ With subcutaneous use Manufacturer advises caution in mild impairment; avoid in moderate-to-severe impairment.
▶ With oral use Manufacturer advises avoid in moderate-to-severe impairment—no information available.
▶ With intravenous use Manufacturer advises caution—limited information available.
● PRE-TREATMENT SCREENING
▶ With oral use Manufacturer advises exclude HIV infection, active or latent tuberculosis and active or latent hepatitis before starting each treatment course—delay treatment until infection adequately treated.
● MONITORING REQUIREMENTS
▶ EvGr Monitor for malignancy—follow routine cancer screening guidelines.
▶ Monitor for progressive multifocal leukoencephalopathy—perform a baseline MRI.
▶ Monitor for haemolysis in patients who are or who become Coombs' positive.
▶ Haematological monitoring required—consult product literature. Ⓜ
▶ With intravenous use or subcutaneous use EvGr Renal and hepatic function should be monitored periodically as clinically indicated. Ⓜ
▶ With oral use EvGr Hepatic function should be monitored Ⓜ—see *Important safety information*.
● DIRECTIONS FOR ADMINISTRATION *Litak* ® for subcutaneous use only—no dilution required; manufacturer advises patients may self-administer, after appropriate training.
    Leustat ® for infusion use only.
● PRESCRIBING AND DISPENSING INFORMATION
▶ With oral use The manufacturer of *Mavenclad* ® has provided a *Prescriber Guide*.
● HANDLING AND STORAGE
    LEUSTAT ® Manufacturer advises store in a refrigerator (2–8°C).
    LITAK ® Manufacturer advises store in a refrigerator (2–8°C).

● PATIENT AND CARER ADVICE
▶ With oral use A patient guide should be provided.
Driving and skilled tasks
▶ With intravenous use or subcutaneous use Patients and carers should be counselled on the effects on driving and performance of skilled tasks—increased risk of dizziness and drowsiness.
● NATIONAL FUNDING/ACCESS DECISIONS
For full details see funding body website
NICE decisions
▶ **Cladribine for treating relapsing-remitting multiple sclerosis (updated May 2024)** NICE TA616 Recommended with restrictions
▶ **Cladribine for treating active relapsing forms of multiple sclerosis (April 2025)** NICE TA1053 Recommended with restrictions
Scottish Medicines Consortium (SMC) decisions
▶ **Cladribine (*Mavenclad* ®) for the treatment of adult patients with highly active relapsing multiple sclerosis (MS) as defined by clinical or imaging features (February 2018)** SMC No. 1300/18 Recommended with restrictions

● MEDICINAL FORMS There can be variation in the licensing of different medicines containing the same drug.
Solution for injection
▶ Litak (Lipomed GmbH)
    Cladribine 2 mg per 1 ml Litak 10mg/5ml solution for injection vials | 1 vial PoM £165.00 (Hospital only)
Solution for infusion
ELECTROLYTES: May contain Sodium
▶ Leustat (Atnahs Pharma UK Ltd)
    Cladribine 1 mg per 1 ml Leustat 10mg/10ml solution for infusion vials | 1 vial PoM £159.70
Oral tablet
▶ Mavenclad (Merck Serono Ltd)
    Cladribine 10 mg Mavenclad 10mg tablets | 1 tablet PoM £2,047.24 | 4 tablet PoM £8,188.97 | 6 tablet PoM £12,283.46

Clofarabine [Specialist drug]

13-Dec-2021

● **INDICATIONS AND DOSE**
Acute lymphoblastic leukaemia
▶ BY INTRAVENOUS INFUSION
▶ Adult 18-20 years: Specialist drug – access specialist resources for dosing information

● INTERACTIONS → Appendix 1: clofarabine
● SIDE-EFFECTS
▶ **Common or very common** Alopecia · anxiety · appetite decreased · arthralgia · capillary leak syndrome · chills · cough · dehydration · diarrhoea · dizziness · drowsiness · dyspnoea · fatigue · feeling abnormal · feeling hot · fever · flushing · gastrointestinal discomfort · haemorrhage · headache · hearing impairment · hepatic disorders · hyperbilirubinaemia · hyperhidrosis · hypersensitivity · hypotension · increased risk of infection · irritability · mucositis · multi organ failure · myalgia · nausea · neutropenia · oedema · oral disorders · pain · paraesthesia · pericardial effusion · peripheral neuropathy · psychiatric disorder · renal impairment · respiratory disorders · sepsis · sinusoidal obstruction syndrome · skin reactions · systemic inflammatory response syndrome · tachycardia · tremor · tumour lysis syndrome · vomiting · weight decreased
▶ **Frequency not known** Clostridioides difficile colitis · gastrointestinal disorders · hyponatraemia · pancreatitis · severe cutaneous adverse reactions (SCARs)
● CONCEPTION AND CONTRACEPTION Contraceptive advice required.

- **MEDICINAL FORMS** There can be variation in the licensing of different medicines containing the same drug.

Solution for infusion

ELECTROLYTES: May contain Sodium

▸ **Clofarabine (Non-proprietary)**

Clofarabine 1 mg per 1 ml Clofarabine 20mg/20ml concentrate for solution for infusion vials | 1 vial [PoM] £1,300.00 (Hospital only)

Cytarabine [Specialist drug]

05-Oct-2021

- **INDICATIONS AND DOSE**

Acute myeloid leukaemia

▸ BY INTRAVENOUS INFUSION, OR BY INTRAVENOUS INJECTION, OR BY SUBCUTANEOUS INJECTION

▸ Adult: Specialist drug – access specialist resources for dosing information

Lymphomatous meningitis

▸ BY INTRATHECAL INJECTION

▸ Adult: Specialist drug – access specialist resources for dosing information

---

IMPORTANT SAFETY INFORMATION

Not all cytarabine preparations can be given by intrathecal injection—consult product literature.

- **INTERACTIONS** → Appendix 1: cytarabine
- **SIDE-EFFECTS**
▸ **Common or very common** Alopecia · anaemia · appetite decreased · consciousness impaired · diarrhoea · dysarthria · dysphagia · eye disorders · eye inflammation · eye stinging · fever · gastrointestinal discomfort · gastrointestinal disorders · haemorrhagic conjunctivitis (consider prophylactic corticosteroid eye drops) · hyperuricaemia · leucopenia · nausea · oral disorders · renal impairment · skin reactions · thrombocytopenia · urinary retention · vasculitis · vision disorders · vomiting
▸ **Uncommon** Arthralgia · dyspnoea · headache · increased risk of infection · myalgia · nerve disorders · pain · paralysis · pericarditis · sepsis · skin ulcer · throat pain
▸ **Rare or very rare** Arrhythmias
▸ **Frequency not known** Acute respiratory distress syndrome (ARDS) · amenorrhoea · ataxia · azoospermia · bone marrow disorders · cardiomyopathy · cerebellar dysfunction · chest pain · coma · confusion · cytarabine syndrome · dizziness · drowsiness · haemorrhage · hand and foot syndrome (palmar-plantar erythrodysaesthesia syndrome) · hepatic disorders · hyperbilirubinaemia · neurotoxicity · neurotoxicity rash · neutropenia · pancreatitis · personality change · pulmonary oedema · reticulocytopenia · rhabdomyolysis · seizure · tremor
- **CONCEPTION AND CONTRACEPTION** Contraceptive advice required.

- **MEDICINAL FORMS** There can be variation in the licensing of different medicines containing the same drug. Forms available from special-order manufacturers include: solution for injection

Solution for injection

▸ **Cytarabine (Non-proprietary)**

Cytarabine 20 mg per 1 ml Cytarabine 100mg/5ml solution for injection vials | 5 vial [PoM] £20.48–£30.00 (Hospital only)

Cytarabine 100 mg per 1 ml Cytarabine 500mg/5ml solution for injection vials | 5 vial [PoM] £89.78 (Hospital only)

Cytarabine 100mg/1ml solution for injection vials | 5 vial [PoM] £26.93 (Hospital only)

Cytarabine 2g/20ml solution for injection vials | 1 vial [PoM] £73.63–£79.00 (Hospital only)

Cytarabine 1g/10ml solution for injection vials | 1 vial [PoM] £37.05–£40.00 (Hospital only)

Combinations available: *Daunorubicin with cytarabine [Specialist drug]*, p. 1038

Decitabine [Specialist drug]

13-Aug-2021

- **INDICATIONS AND DOSE**

Acute myeloid leukaemia

▸ BY INTRAVENOUS INFUSION

▸ Adult: Specialist drug – access specialist resources for dosing information

- **INTERACTIONS** → Appendix 1: decitabine
- **SIDE-EFFECTS**
▸ **Common or very common** Anaemia · diarrhoea · epistaxis · fever · headache · hypersensitivity · increased risk of infection · leucopenia · nausea · neutropenia · sepsis · stomatitis · thrombocytopenia · vomiting
▸ **Uncommon** Acute febrile neutrophilic dermatosis · pancytopenia
▸ **Frequency not known** Gastrointestinal disorders · interstitial lung disease
- **CONCEPTION AND CONTRACEPTION** [EvGr] Females of childbearing potential should use effective contraception during treatment and for 6 months after stopping treatment; male patients should use effective contraception and avoid fathering a child during treatment and for 3 months after stopping treatment. ⟨M⟩
- **MEDICINAL FORMS** There can be variation in the licensing of different medicines containing the same drug.

Powder for solution for infusion

ELECTROLYTES: May contain Potassium, sodium

▸ **Dacogen** (Janssen-Cilag Ltd)

Decitabine 50 mg Dacogen 50mg powder for concentrate for solution for infusion vials | 1 vial [PoM] £970.86

Decitabine with cedazuridine [Specialist drug]

06-Feb-2024

The properties listed below are those particular to the combination only. For the properties of the components please consider, decitabine above.

- **INDICATIONS AND DOSE**

Acute myeloid leukaemia

▸ BY MOUTH

▸ Adult: Specialist drug – access specialist resources for dosing information

---

IMPORTANT SAFETY INFORMATION

RISKS OF INCORRECT DOSING OF ORAL ANTI-CANCER MEDICINES

See Cytotoxic drugs p. 1027.

- **INTERACTIONS** → Appendix 1: cedazuridine · decitabine
- **SIDE-EFFECTS**
▸ **Common or very common** Anaemia · chills · cystitis · diarrhoea · dysuria · epistaxis · erythema · fever · gastrointestinal disorders · headache · hyperglycaemia · increased risk of infection · leucopenia · nasal congestion · nausea · neutropenia · oral disorders · oropharyngeal complaints · polyserositis · sepsis · thrombocytopenia · vomiting
▸ **Frequency not known** Bone marrow depression
- **MEDICINAL FORMS** There can be variation in the licensing of different medicines containing the same drug.

Oral tablet

CAUTIONARY AND ADVISORY LABELS 25

▸ **Inaqovi** (Otsuka Pharmaceuticals (U.K.) Ltd) ▼

Decitabine 35 mg, Cedazuridine 100 mg Inaqovi 35mg/100mg tablets | 5 tablet [PoM] £3,595.00 (Hospital only)

Fludarabine phosphate [Specialist drug]

13-Aug-2021

● **INDICATIONS AND DOSE**

Chronic lymphocytic leukaemia

▶ BY MOUTH, OR BY INTRAVENOUS INJECTION, OR BY INTRAVENOUS INFUSION
▶ Adult: Specialist drug – access specialist resources for dosing information

IMPORTANT SAFETY INFORMATION

RISKS OF INCORRECT DOSING OF ORAL ANTI-CANCER MEDICINES
See Cytotoxic drugs p. 1027.

● **CONTRA-INDICATIONS** Haemolytic anaemia
● **INTERACTIONS** → Appendix 1: fludarabine
● **SIDE-EFFECTS**

GENERAL SIDE-EFFECTS

▶ **Common or very common** Anaemia · appetite decreased · asthenia · bone marrow depression (may be cumulative) · chills · cough · diarrhoea · fever · increased risk of infection · malaise · mucositis · nausea · neoplasms · nerve disorders · neutropenia · oedema · stomatitis · thrombocytopenia · vision disorders · vomiting
▶ **Uncommon** Autoimmune disorder · confusion · dyspnoea · haemorrhage · pneumonitis · pulmonary fibrosis · pulmonary toxicity · tumour lysis syndrome
▶ **Rare or very rare** Agitation · arrhythmia · coma · heart failure · seizure · severe cutaneous adverse reactions (SCARs)

SPECIFIC SIDE-EFFECTS

▶ **Common or very common**
▶ With oral use Progressive multifocal leukoencephalopathy (PML) · skin reactions · viral infection reactivation
▶ With parenteral use Rash
▶ **Uncommon**
▶ With oral use Acquired haemophilia · crystalluria · electrolyte imbalance · haemolytic anaemia · hyperuricaemia · metabolic acidosis · renal failure
▶ **Frequency not known**
▶ With oral use Posterior reversible encephalopathy syndrome (PRES)
▶ With parenteral use Encephalopathy · intracranial haemorrhage

● **CONCEPTION AND CONTRACEPTION** Manufacturer advises effective contraception during and for at least 6 months after treatment in men or women.

● **NATIONAL FUNDING/ACCESS DECISIONS**
For full details see funding body website

NICE decisions

▶ Fludarabine monotherapy for the first-line treatment of chronic lymphocytic leukaemia (February 2007) NICE TA119 Not recommended
▶ Fludarabine for B-cell chronic lymphocytic leukaemia (September 2001) NICE TA29 Recommended

Scottish Medicines Consortium (SMC) decisions

▶ Fludarabine phosphate (*Fludara*®) for B-cell chronic lymphocytic leukaemia (November 2006) SMC No. 176/05 Recommended with restrictions

● **MEDICINAL FORMS** There can be variation in the licensing of different medicines containing the same drug.

Solution for injection

▶ Fludarabine phosphate (Non-proprietary)
Fludarabine phosphate 25 mg per 1 ml Fludarabine phosphate 50mg/2ml concentrate for solution for injection vials | 1 vial [PoM] £155.00–£156.00 (Hospital only)

Oral tablet

▶ Fludara (Sanofi)
Fludarabine phosphate 10 mg Fludara 10mg tablets | 20 tablet [PoM] £403.31 (Hospital only)

Powder for solution for injection

▶ Fludara (Sanofi)
Fludarabine phosphate 50 mg Fludara 50mg powder for solution for injection vials | 5 vial [PoM] £735.34 (Hospital only)

Fluorouracil [Specialist drug]

19-Jan-2021

● **INDICATIONS AND DOSE**

Solid tumours [including gastro-intestinal tract cancers and breast cancer] | Colorectal cancer

▶ BY INTRAVENOUS INJECTION, OR BY INTRAVENOUS INFUSION, OR BY INTRA-ARTERIAL INFUSION
▶ Adult: Specialist drug – access specialist resources for dosing information

IMPORTANT SAFETY INFORMATION

MHRA/CHM ADVICE: 5-FLUOROURACIL (INTRAVENOUS), CAPECITABINE, TEGAFUR: DPD TESTING RECOMMENDED BEFORE INITIATION TO IDENTIFY PATIENTS AT INCREASED RISK OF SEVERE AND FATAL TOXICITY (OCTOBER 2020)

▶ With intravenous use
Patients with partial or complete dihydropyrimidine dehydrogenase (DPD) deficiency are at increased risk of severe and fatal toxicity during treatment with fluoropyrimidines. Healthcare professionals are advised to test all patients for DPD deficiency before initiating treatment and confirm their, including family, history of complete or partial DPD deficiency. Fluorouracil is contra-indicated in patients with known complete DPD deficiency; in those with partial DPD deficiency, a reduced starting dose is recommended. Patients should be monitored for toxicity, particularly during the first cycle of treatment or after a dose increase; severe toxicity can occur even in those with negative test results for DPD deficiency. Therapeutic drug monitoring may improve clinical outcomes in patients receiving continuous fluorouracil infusions. Healthcare professionals should also counsel patients on the benefits and risks of their treatment and ensure they are provided with the patient information leaflet.

● **CONTRA-INDICATIONS** Bone marrow depression (after treatment with radiotherapy or other antineoplastic agents) · complete or near complete absence of dihydropyrimidine dehydrogenase activity (increased risk of severe, life-threatening, or fatal toxicity)—consult product literature · serious infections

● **INTERACTIONS** → Appendix 1: fluorouracil

● **SIDE-EFFECTS**

▶ **Common or very common** Agranulocytosis · alopecia · anaemia · anal inflammation · appetite decreased · asthenia · bone marrow disorders · bronchospasm · diarrhoea · gastrointestinal disorders · haemorrhage · hand and foot syndrome (long term use) · healing impaired · immunosuppression · increased risk of infection · ischaemic heart disease · leucopenia · malaise · mucositis · nausea · neutropenia · skin reactions · stomatitis · thrombocytopenia · vomiting
▶ **Uncommon** Arrhythmias · cardiac inflammation · cardiogenic shock · cardiomyopathy congestive · dehydration · dizziness · drowsiness · euphoric mood · eye disorders · eye inflammation · headache · heart failure · hepatic disorders · hypotension · movement disorders · myocardial infarction · nail discolouration · nail disorders · nerve disorders · ovulation disorder · parkinsonism · photosensitivity reaction · sepsis · spermatogenesis disorder · vision disorders

▶ **Rare or very rare** Biliary sclerosis · cardiac arrest · cerebral ischaemia · cholecystitis · coma · confusion · embolism and thrombosis · encephalopathy · fever · muscle weakness · peripheral vascular disease · renal failure · seizure · speech impairment · sudden cardiac death

▶ **Frequency not known** Vein discolouration

● **CONCEPTION AND CONTRACEPTION** Contraceptive advice required.

● **MEDICINAL FORMS** There can be variation in the licensing of different medicines containing the same drug. Forms available from special-order manufacturers include: solution for injection

Solution for injection

CAUTIONARY AND ADVISORY LABELS　11

▶ Fluorouracil (Non-proprietary)
  Fluorouracil (as Fluorouracil sodium) 25 mg per 1 ml Fluorouracil 500mg/20ml solution for injection vials | 10 vial [PoM] £64.00 (Hospital only)
  Fluorouracil (as Fluorouracil sodium) 50 mg per 1 ml Fluorouracil 1g/20ml solution for injection vials | 1 vial [PoM] £12.16 (Hospital only) | 1 vial [PoM] £12.80
  Fluorouracil 500mg/10ml solution for injection vials | 1 vial [PoM] £6.08-£6.40 (Hospital only)

Solution for infusion

CAUTIONARY AND ADVISORY LABELS　11

▶ Fluorouracil (Non-proprietary)
  Fluorouracil (as Fluorouracil sodium) 25 mg per 1 ml Fluorouracil 2.5g/100ml solution for infusion vials | 1 vial [PoM] £32.00 (Hospital only)
  Fluorouracil (as Fluorouracil sodium) 50 mg per 1 ml Fluorouracil 5g/100ml solution for infusion vials | 1 vial [PoM] £60.80-£64.00 (Hospital only)
  Fluorouracil 2.5g/50ml solution for infusion vials | 1 vial [PoM] £30.40-£32.00 (Hospital only)

Gemcitabine [Specialist drug]

09-May-2021

● **INDICATIONS AND DOSE**

Non-small cell lung cancer | Pancreatic cancer | Bladder cancer | Ovarian cancer | Breast cancer
▶ BY INTRAVENOUS INFUSION
▶ Adult: Specialist drug – access specialist resources for dosing information

● **INTERACTIONS** → Appendix 1: gemcitabine

● **SIDE-EFFECTS**
▶ **Common or very common** Alopecia · anaemia · appetite decreased · asthenia · back pain · bone marrow depression · chills · constipation · cough · diarrhoea · drowsiness · dyspnoea · fever · haematuria · headache · hyperhidrosis · influenza like illness · insomnia · leucopenia · myalgia · nausea · neutropenia · oedema · oral disorders · proteinuria · rhinitis · skin reactions · thrombocytopenia · vomiting
▶ **Uncommon** Interstitial pneumonitis · respiratory disorders
▶ **Rare or very rare** Capillary leak syndrome · hypotension · myocardial infarction · posterior reversible encephalopathy syndrome (PRES) · severe cutaneous adverse reactions (SCARs) · skin ulcer · thrombocytosis
▶ **Frequency not known** Arrhythmias · colitis ischaemic · gangrene · haemolytic uraemic syndrome · heart failure · hepatic disorders · pulmonary oedema · radiation injuries · renal failure · stroke · vasculitis

SIDE-EFFECTS, FURTHER INFORMATION Gemcitabine should be discontinued if signs of microangiopathic haemolytic anaemia occur.

● **CONCEPTION AND CONTRACEPTION** Manufacturer advises effective contraception during treatment. Men must avoid fathering a child during and for 6 months after treatment.

● **NATIONAL FUNDING/ACCESS DECISIONS**
For full details see funding body website

NICE decisions
▶ Gemcitabine for the treatment of pancreatic cancer (May 2001) NICE TA25 Recommended
▶ Gemcitabine for the treatment of metastatic breast cancer (January 2007) NICE TA116 Recommended with restrictions
▶ Bevacizumab in combination with gemcitabine and carboplatin for treating the first recurrence of platinum-sensitive advanced ovarian cancer (May 2013) NICE TA285 Not recommended
▶ Topotecan, pegylated liposomal doxorubicin hydrochloride, paclitaxel, trabectedin and gemcitabine for treating recurrent ovarian cancer (April 2016) NICE TA389 Not recommended
▶ Paclitaxel as albumin-bound nanoparticles with gemcitabine for untreated metastatic pancreatic cancer (September 2017) NICE TA476 Recommended with restrictions

● **MEDICINAL FORMS** There can be variation in the licensing of different medicines containing the same drug.

Solution for infusion

▶ Gemcitabine (Non-proprietary)
  Gemcitabine (as Gemcitabine hydrochloride) 38 mg per 1 ml Gemcitabine 200mg/5.3ml concentrate for solution for infusion vials | 1 vial [PoM] £32.00 (Hospital only)
  Gemcitabine 1g/26.3ml concentrate for solution for infusion vials | 1 vial [PoM] £162.00-£209.26 (Hospital only)
  Gemcitabine 2g/52.6ml concentrate for solution for infusion vials | 1 vial [PoM] £324.00-£418.55 (Hospital only)
  Gemcitabine 200mg/5.26ml concentrate for solution for infusion vials | 1 vial [PoM] £33.69-£41.89 (Hospital only)
  Gemcitabine (as Gemcitabine hydrochloride) 100 mg per 1 ml Gemcitabine 2g/20ml concentrate for solution for infusion vials | 1 vial [PoM] £324.00 (Hospital only)
  Gemcitabine 1g/10ml concentrate for solution for infusion vials | 1 vial [PoM] £162.00 (Hospital only)
  Gemcitabine 200mg/2ml concentrate for solution for infusion vials | 1 vial [PoM] £32.00 (Hospital only)

Powder for solution for infusion

▶ Gemcitabine (Non-proprietary)
  Gemcitabine (as Gemcitabine hydrochloride) 200 mg Gemcitabine 200mg powder for solution for infusion vials | 1 vial [PoM] £14.00
  Gemcitabine (as Gemcitabine hydrochloride) 1 gram Gemcitabine 1g powder for solution for infusion vials | 1 vial [PoM] £162.76 (Hospital only) | 1 vial [PoM] £25.00

Mercaptopurine

09-May-2021

(6-Mercaptopurine)

● **INDICATIONS AND DOSE**

Severe acute Crohn's disease (under expert supervision) | Maintenance of remission of Crohn's disease (under expert supervision) | Maintenance of remission of ulcerative colitis (under expert supervision)
▶ BY MOUTH
▶ Adult: 1–1.5 mg/kg daily, some patients may respond to lower doses

Acute leukaemias (specialist use only) | Chronic myeloid leukaemia (specialist use only)
▶ BY MOUTH
▶ Adult: Specialist indication – access specialist resources for dosing information

DOSE ADJUSTMENTS DUE TO INTERACTIONS
▶ Manufacturer advises reduce dose to one-quarter of the usual dose with concurrent use of allopurinol.

DOSE EQUIVALENCE AND CONVERSION
▶ Mercaptopurine tablets and *Xaluprine*® oral suspension are **not** bioequivalent.

8

Immune system and malignant disease

- **UNLICENSED USE** Not licensed for use in ulcerative colitis and Crohn's disease.

> **IMPORTANT SAFETY INFORMATION**
>
> **SAFE PRACTICE**
> Mercaptopurine has been confused with mercaptamine; care must be taken to ensure the correct drug is prescribed and dispensed.
>
> **RISKS OF INCORRECT DOSING OF ORAL ANTI-CANCER MEDICINES**
> See Cytotoxic drugs p. 1027.

- **CONTRA-INDICATIONS**
  ▸ When used for Non-cancer indications Absent thiopurine methyltransferase activity
- **CAUTIONS** Reduced thiopurine methyltransferase activity
  CAUTIONS, FURTHER INFORMATION
  ▸ Thiopurine methyltransferase The enzyme thiopurine methyltransferase (TPMT) metabolises thiopurine drugs (azathioprine, mercaptopurine, tioguanine); the risk of myelosuppression is increased in patients with reduced activity of the enzyme, particularly for the few individuals in whom TPMT activity is undetectable. Those with reduced TPMT activity may be treated under specialist supervision.
- **INTERACTIONS** → Appendix 1: mercaptopurine
- **SIDE-EFFECTS**
  ▸ **Common or very common** Anaemia · appetite decreased · bone marrow depression · diarrhoea · hepatic disorders · hepatotoxicity (more common at high doses) · leucopenia · nausea · oral disorders · pancreatitis · thrombocytopenia · vomiting
  ▸ **Uncommon** Arthralgia · fever · increased risk of infection · neutropenia · rash
  ▸ **Rare or very rare** Alopecia · face oedema · intestinal ulcer · neoplasms · oligozoospermia
  ▸ **Frequency not known** Photosensitivity reaction
- **CONCEPTION AND CONTRACEPTION** Contraceptive advice required, see *Pregnancy and reproductive function* in Cytotoxic drugs p. 1027.
- **PREGNANCY** Avoid (teratogenic). See also *Pregnancy and reproductive function* in Cytotoxic drugs p. 1027.
- **BREAST FEEDING** Discontinue breast-feeding.
- **HEPATIC IMPAIRMENT** Manufacturer advises caution (risk of increased exposure).
  Dose adjustments Manufacturer advises consider dose reduction.
- **RENAL IMPAIRMENT** [EvGr] Use with caution. ⓜ
  Dose adjustments [EvGr] Consider dose reduction. ⓜ
- **PRE-TREATMENT SCREENING** Manufacturer advises consider measuring thiopurine methyltransferase (TPMT) activity before starting mercaptopurine therapy.
- **MONITORING REQUIREMENTS** Monitor liver function.
- **PRESCRIBING AND DISPENSING INFORMATION** Flavours of oral liquid formulations may include raspberry.

- **MEDICINAL FORMS** There can be variation in the licensing of different medicines containing the same drug. Forms available from special-order manufacturers include: oral tablet, oral capsule, oral suspension
  Oral tablet
  ▸ Mercaptopurine (Non-proprietary)
    Mercaptopurine 10 mg Mercaptopurine 10mg tablets | 100 tablet [PoM] Ⓧ DT = £123.30
    Mercaptopurine 50 mg Mercaptopurine 50mg tablets | 25 tablet [PoM] £9.42 DT = £9.64
  ▸ Hanixol (Fontus Health Ltd)
    Mercaptopurine 50 mg Hanixol 50mg tablets | 25 tablet [PoM] £34.39 DT = £9.64

Oral suspension
EXCIPIENTS: May contain Aspartame
▸ Xaluprine (Nova Laboratories Ltd)
  Mercaptopurine 20 mg per 1 ml Xaluprine 20mg/ml oral suspension | 100 ml [PoM] £170.00 DT = £170.00

▌Methotrexate

15-Apr-2025

- **DRUG ACTION** Methotrexate inhibits the enzyme dihydrofolate reductase, essential for the synthesis of purines and pyrimidines.

- **INDICATIONS AND DOSE**

  Mild to moderate Crohn's disease refractory or intolerant to thiopurines (under expert supervision)
  ▸ BY SUBCUTANEOUS INJECTION
  ▸ Adult: Initially 25 mg once weekly until remission induced; maintenance 15 mg once weekly

  Severe Crohn's disease (under expert supervision)
  ▸ BY INTRAMUSCULAR INJECTION
  ▸ Adult: Initially 25 mg once weekly until remission induced; maintenance 15 mg once weekly

  Maintenance of remission of severe Crohn's disease (under expert supervision)
  ▸ BY MOUTH
  ▸ Adult: 10–25 mg once weekly

  Moderate to severe active rheumatoid arthritis (under expert supervision)
  ▸ BY MOUTH
  ▸ Adult: 7.5 mg once weekly, adjusted according to response; maximum 20 mg per week

  Severe active rheumatoid arthritis (under expert supervision)
  ▸ BY INTRAMUSCULAR INJECTION, OR BY SUBCUTANEOUS INJECTION
  ▸ Adult: Initially 7.5 mg once weekly, then increased in steps of 2.5 mg once weekly, adjusted according to response; maximum 25 mg per week

  Neoplastic diseases (specialist use only)
  ▸ BY MOUTH, OR BY INTRAVENOUS INJECTION, OR BY INTRAVENOUS INFUSION, OR BY INTRA-ARTERIAL INFUSION, OR BY INTRAMUSCULAR INJECTION, OR BY INTRATHECAL INJECTION
  ▸ Adult: Specialist indication – access specialist resources for dosing information

  Severe psoriasis unresponsive to conventional therapy (under expert supervision)
  ▸ BY MOUTH, OR BY INTRAMUSCULAR INJECTION, OR BY INTRAVENOUS INJECTION, OR BY SUBCUTANEOUS INJECTION
  ▸ Adult: Initially 2.5–10 mg once weekly, then increased in steps of 2.5–5 mg, adjusted according to response, dose to be adjusted at intervals of at least 1 week; usual dose 7.5–15 mg once weekly, stop treatment if inadequate response after 3 months at the optimum dose; maximum 30 mg per week

- **UNLICENSED USE** Not licensed for use in severe Crohn's disease.

> **IMPORTANT SAFETY INFORMATION**
>
> **NHS NEVER EVENT: OVERDOSE OF METHOTREXATE FOR NON-CANCER TREATMENT (JANUARY 2018)**
> Patients given methotrexate, by any route, for non-cancer treatment should not be given more than their intended weekly dose.
>
> **WEEKLY DOSING**
> Note that the dose is a **weekly** dose. To avoid error with low-dose methotrexate, it is recommended that:
> - the patient or their carer is carefully advised of the **dose** and **frequency** and the reason for taking

methotrexate and any other prescribed medication (e.g. folic acid);

- only one strength of methotrexate tablet (usually 2.5 mg) is prescribed and dispensed;
- the prescription and the dispensing label clearly show the dose and frequency of methotrexate administration;
- the patient or their carer is warned to report immediately the onset of any feature of blood disorders (e.g. sore throat, bruising, and mouth ulcers), liver toxicity (e.g. nausea, vomiting, abdominal discomfort, and dark urine), and respiratory effects (e.g. shortness of breath).

MHRA/CHM ADVICE: METHOTREXATE ONCE-WEEKLY FOR AUTOIMMUNE DISEASES: NEW MEASURES TO REDUCE RISK OF FATAL OVERDOSE DUE TO INADVERTENT DAILY INSTEAD OF WEEKLY DOSING (SEPTEMBER 2020)

▶ With oral use

Methotrexate should be taken **once a week** in autoimmune conditions and, less commonly, in some cancer therapy regimens. A European review highlighted continued reports of inadvertent overdose due to more frequent dosing (including daily administration), which has resulted in some fatalities. Subsequently, new measures have been implemented by the MHRA. Prescribers are advised to:

- ensure patients can understand and comply with once-weekly dosing before prescribing methotrexate, decide with the patient which day of the week they will take their dose, and note this down in full on the prescription;
- consider the patient's overall polypharmacy burden when deciding which formulation to prescribe, especially in those with a high pill burden;
- inform patients and carers of the potentially fatal risk of accidental overdose if methotrexate is taken more frequently than once a week, and reaffirm that it should not be taken daily;
- advise patients and carers to seek immediate medical attention if overdose is suspected.

The MHRA further advises dispensers to remind patients of the once-weekly dosing and the risks of potentially fatal overdose if they take more than directed. Where possible, the day of the week for dosing should be written in full in the space provided on the outer packaging. Patients should be encouraged to write the day of the week for dosing in their patient alert card and carry it with them.

MHRA/CHM ADVICE: METHOTREXATE: ADVISE PATIENTS TO TAKE PRECAUTIONS IN THE SUN TO AVOID PHOTOSENSITIVITY REACTIONS (AUGUST 2023)

Photosensitivity reactions, including phototoxicity, are known side-effects of methotrexate that may occur with low- and high-dose treatment. These reactions are distinct from radiation recall reactions, and can appear as severe sunburn (e.g. rashes with papules or blistering, and sometimes swelling); rarely, photosensitivity reactions have contributed to deaths from secondary infections.

Healthcare professionals are reminded to inform patients and their carers of the risk and signs of photosensitivity reactions during methotrexate treatment, and advise them to:

- avoid exposure to UV light (including intense sunlight, especially between 11 a.m. and 3 p.m., sunlamps, and sunbeds);
- use a sunscreen with a high sun protection factor (SPF) and wear protective clothing during sun exposure;
- speak to a healthcare professional if they have concerns about a skin reaction.

● **CONTRA-INDICATIONS** Active infection · ascites · immunodeficiency syndromes · significant pleural effusion

● **CAUTIONS** Dehydration (increased risk of toxicity) · diarrhoea · extreme caution in blood disorders (avoid if severe) · peptic ulceration (avoid in active disease) · photosensitivity · risk of accumulation in pleural effusion or ascites—drain before treatment · ulcerative colitis · ulcerative stomatitis

CAUTIONS, FURTHER INFORMATION

▶ Blood count Bone marrow suppression can occur abruptly; factors likely to increase toxicity include advanced age, renal impairment, and concomitant use with another anti-folate drug (e.g. trimethoprim). Manufacturer advises a clinically significant drop in white cell count or platelet count calls for immediate withdrawal of methotrexate and introduction of supportive therapy.

▶ Gastro-intestinal toxicity Manufacturer advises withdraw treatment if stomatitis or diarrhoea develops—may be first sign of gastro-intestinal toxicity.

▶ Photosensitivity Psoriasis lesions may be aggravated by UV radiation—skin ulceration has been reported.
  Radiation recall reaction has been reported in both radiation- and sun-damaged skin.

▶ Liver toxicity Liver cirrhosis reported. Manufacturer advises treatment should not be started or should be discontinued if any abnormality of liver function or liver biopsy is present or develops during therapy. Abnormalities can return to normal within 2 weeks after which treatment may be recommended if judged appropriate. Persistent increases in liver transaminases may necessitate dose reduction or discontinuation.

▶ Pulmonary toxicity Pulmonary toxicity may be a special problem in rheumatoid arthritis. Manufacturer advises patients to seek medical attention if dyspnoea, cough or fever develops; monitor for symptoms at each visit—discontinue if pneumonitis suspected.

● **INTERACTIONS** → Appendix 1: methotrexate

● **SIDE-EFFECTS**

GENERAL SIDE-EFFECTS

▶ **Uncommon** Seizure

SPECIFIC SIDE-EFFECTS

▶ **Common or very common**

▶ With systemic use Anaemia · appetite decreased · diarrhoea · drowsiness · fatigue · gastrointestinal discomfort · headache · increased risk of infection · interstitial lung disease · leucopenia · nausea · oral disorders · respiratory disorders · skin reactions · throat ulcer · thrombocytopenia · vomiting

▶ **Uncommon**

▶ With parenteral use Drug toxicity · local reaction

▶ With systemic use Agranulocytosis · alopecia · arthralgia · bone marrow disorders · chills · confusion · cystitis · depression · diabetes mellitus · dysuria · fever · gastrointestinal disorders · haemorrhage · healing impaired · hepatic disorders · myalgia · neoplasms · nephropathy · osteoporosis · photosensitivity reaction · pulmonary fibrosis · rheumatoid arthritis aggravated · severe cutaneous adverse reactions (SCARs) · vasculitis · vertigo · vulvovaginal disorders

▶ **Rare or very rare**

▶ With oral use Asthma · brain oedema · cognitive impairment · paresis · psychosis · speech impairment

▶ With parenteral use Apnoea · asthma-like conditions

▶ With systemic use Azotaemia · conjunctivitis · cough · dyspnoea · embolism and thrombosis · eosinophilia · gynaecomastia · hypotension · immune deficiency · infertility · insomnia · lymphadenopathy · meningism · meningitis aseptic · menstrual cycle irregularities · mood altered · muscle weakness · nail discolouration · neutropenia · pain · pancreatitis · pericardial disorders · pericarditis · proteinuria · radiation injuries · reactivation of infection · renal impairment · retinopathy · sensation abnormal · sepsis · sexual dysfunction · sperm abnormalities · stress fracture · taste altered · telangiectasia · tinnitus · vision disorders

▸ **Frequency not known**
▸ With intrathecal use Arachnoiditis · cerebrospinal fluid pressure increased · Guillain-Barre syndrome · leukoencephalopathy · paresis · pulmonary oedema
▸ With oral use Chest pain · death · electrolyte imbalance · encephalopathy · neurotoxicity · pulmonary oedema
▸ With parenteral use Aphasia · cognitive disorder · hemiparesis · injection site necrosis · leukoencephalopathy · metabolic change · necrosis · sudden death
▸ With systemic use Defective oogenesis · dizziness · mucositis · oedema · progressive multifocal leukoencephalopathy (PML) · skin ulcer

SIDE-EFFECTS, FURTHER INFORMATION Give folic acid to reduce side-effects. Folic acid decreases mucosal and gastrointestinal side-effects of methotrexate and may prevent hepatotoxicity; there is no evidence of a reduction in haematological side-effects.

Withdraw treatment if ulcerative stomatitis develops—may be first sign of gastro-intestinal toxicity.

Treatment with folinic acid (as calcium folinate) may be required in acute toxicity.

● CONCEPTION AND CONTRACEPTION Manufacturer advises effective contraception during and for at least 6 months after treatment in men and women.

● PREGNANCY Avoid (teratogenic; fertility may be reduced during therapy but this may be reversible).

● BREAST FEEDING Discontinue breast-feeding—present in milk.

● HEPATIC IMPAIRMENT When used for malignancy, avoid in severe hepatic impairment—consult local treatment protocol for details. Avoid with hepatic impairment in non-malignant conditions—dose-related toxicity.

● RENAL IMPAIRMENT Risk of nephrotoxicity at high doses. EvGr Use with caution; avoid in severe impairment. Ⓜ
Dose adjustments EvGr Reduce dose (consult product literature). Ⓜ

● PRE-TREATMENT SCREENING Exclude pregnancy before treatment.
Patients should have full blood count and renal and liver function tests before starting treatment.

● MONITORING REQUIREMENTS
▸ In view of reports of blood dyscrasias (including fatalities) and liver cirrhosis with low-dose methotrexate patients should:
 • have full blood count and renal and liver function tests repeated every 1–2 weeks until therapy stabilised, thereafter patients should be monitored every 2–3 months.
 • be advised to report all symptoms and signs suggestive of infection, especially sore throat
▸ Local protocols for frequency of monitoring may vary.
▸ Treatment with folinic acid (as calcium folinate) may be required in acute toxicity.

● PRESCRIBING AND DISPENSING INFORMATION Folinic acid following methotrexate administration helps to prevent methotrexate-induced mucositis and myelosuppression.
The licensed routes of administration for parenteral preparations vary—further information can be found in the product literature for the individual preparations.
Risk minimisation materials documents are available for healthcare professionals.

● PATIENT AND CARER ADVICE Patients and their carers should be warned to report immediately the onset of any feature of blood disorders (e.g. sore throat, bruising, and mouth ulcers), liver toxicity (e.g. nausea, vomiting, abdominal discomfort and dark urine), and respiratory

effects (e.g. shortness of breath). Patients and their carers should be advised to avoid exposure to UV light (including intense sunlight, sunlamps, and sunbeds)—see *Important safety information*.
Patients should be advised to avoid self-medication with over-the-counter aspirin or ibuprofen.
Patients should be counselled on the dose, treatment booklet, and the use of NSAIDs.
▸ With oral use A patient alert card should be provided to patients on once-weekly dosing—see also *Important safety information*.
Methotrexate treatment booklets Methotrexate treatment booklets should be issued where appropriate.
In **England**, **Wales**, and **Northern Ireland**, they are available for purchase from:

3M Security Print and Systems Limited
Gorse Street, Chadderton
Oldham
OL9 9QH
Tel: 0845 610 1112

GP practices can obtain supplies through their Local Area Team stores.
NHS Hospitals can order supplies from cmswebshop.corp.xerox.com/NHS/Login.aspx.
In **Scotland**, treatment booklets can be obtained by emailing stockorders.dppas@theapsgroup.com or by fax on 0131 629 9967.
These booklets include advice for adults taking oral methotrexate for inflammatory conditions, and a section for recording results of blood tests and dosage information.

● MEDICINAL FORMS There can be variation in the licensing of different medicines containing the same drug. Forms available from special-order manufacturers include: oral suspension, oral solution, solution for injection

Oral tablet
CAUTIONARY AND ADVISORY LABELS 10, 11
▸ **Methotrexate (Non-proprietary)**
 Methotrexate 2.5 mg Methotrexate 2.5mg tablets | 24 tablet PoM £1.70–£3.27 | 28 tablet PoM ⚠ DT = £1.57 | 100 tablet PoM £5.61–£14.01
 Methotrexate 10 mg Methotrexate 10mg tablets | 100 tablet PoM £55.74 DT = £38.85

Solution for injection
▸ **Methotrexate (Non-proprietary)**
 Methotrexate (as Methotrexate sodium) 2.5 mg per 1 ml Methotrexate 5mg/2ml solution for injection vials | 5 vial PoM £36.00 (Hospital only)
 Methotrexate (as Methotrexate sodium) 25 mg per 1 ml Methotrexate 1g/40ml solution for injection vials | 1 vial PoM £1,452.55 (Hospital only)
 Methotrexate 500mg/20ml solution for injection vials | 1 vial PoM £48.00 (Hospital only)
 Methotrexate 50mg/2ml solution for injection vials | 1 vial PoM £72.63 (Hospital only) | 5 vial PoM £35.00 (Hospital only)
 Methotrexate (as Methotrexate sodium) 100 mg per 1 ml Methotrexate 1g/10ml solution for injection vials | 1 vial PoM £80.75–£85.00 (Hospital only)
▸ **Methofill** (Accord-UK Ltd)
 Methotrexate 50 mg per 1 ml Methofill 12.5mg/0.25ml solution for injection pre-filled injector | 1 pre-filled disposable injection PoM £14.34 = £14.35
 Methofill 30mg/0.6ml solution for injection pre-filled syringes | 1 pre-filled disposable injection PoM £14.55 DT = £14.55
 Methofill 22.5mg/0.45ml solution for injection pre-filled injector | 1 pre-filled disposable injection PoM £16.10 DT = £16.11
 Methofill 30mg/0.6ml solution for injection pre-filled injector | 1 pre-filled disposable injection PoM £16.55 DT = £16.56
 Methofill 27.5mg/0.55ml solution for injection pre-filled injector | 1 pre-filled disposable injection PoM £16.49 DT = £16.50
 Methofill 7.5mg/0.15ml solution for injection pre-filled injector | 1 pre-filled disposable injection PoM £12.86 DT = £12.87
 Methofill 20mg/0.4ml solution for injection pre-filled injector | 1 pre-filled disposable injection PoM £15.55 DT = £15.56

Methofill 10mg/0.2ml solution for injection pre-filled injector | 1 pre-filled disposable injection [PoM] £13.25 DT = £13.26

Methofill 15mg/0.3ml solution for injection pre-filled injector | 1 pre-filled disposable injection [PoM] £14.40 DT = £14.41

Methofill 17.5mg/0.35ml solution for injection pre-filled injector | 1 pre-filled disposable injection [PoM] £15.24 DT = £15.25

Methofill 25mg/0.5ml solution for injection pre-filled injector | 1 pre-filled disposable injection [PoM] £16.12 DT = £16.13

Methotrexate (as Methotrexate sodium) 50 mg per 1 ml Methofill 15mg/0.3ml solution for injection pre-filled syringes | 1 pre-filled disposable injection [PoM] £12.40 DT = £12.40

Methofill 25mg/0.5ml solution for injection pre-filled syringes | 1 pre-filled disposable injection [PoM] £14.24 DT = £14.24

Methofill 10mg/0.2ml solution for injection pre-filled syringes | 1 pre-filled disposable injection [PoM] £11.25 DT = £11.25

Methofill 7.5mg/0.15ml solution for injection pre-filled syringes | 1 pre-filled disposable injection [PoM] £10.86 DT = £10.86

Methofill 17.5mg/0.35ml solution for injection pre-filled syringes | 1 pre-filled disposable injection [PoM] £13.24 DT = £13.24

Methofill 27.5mg/0.55ml solution for injection pre-filled syringes | 1 pre-filled disposable injection [PoM] £14.49 DT = £14.49

Methofill 22.5mg/0.45ml solution for injection pre-filled syringes | 1 pre-filled disposable injection [PoM] £14.10 DT = £14.10

Methofill 12.5mg/0.25ml solution for injection pre-filled syringes | 1 pre-filled disposable injection [PoM] £12.34 DT = £12.34

Methofill 20mg/0.4ml solution for injection pre-filled syringes | 1 pre-filled disposable injection [PoM] £13.55 DT = £13.55

▸ **Metoject PEN** (medac UK)

Methotrexate 50 mg per 1 ml Metoject PEN 27.5mg/0.55ml solution for injection pre-filled pens | 1 pre-filled disposable injection [PoM] £16.50 DT = £16.50

Metoject PEN 17.5mg/0.35ml solution for injection pre-filled pens | 1 pre-filled disposable injection [PoM] £15.25 DT = £15.25

Metoject PEN 30mg/0.6ml solution for injection pre-filled pens | 1 pre-filled disposable injection [PoM] £16.56 DT = £16.56

Metoject PEN 12.5mg/0.25ml solution for injection pre-filled pens | 1 pre-filled disposable injection [PoM] £14.35 DT = £14.35

Metoject PEN 10mg/0.2ml solution for injection pre-filled pens | 1 pre-filled disposable injection [PoM] £13.26 DT = £13.26

Metoject PEN 15mg/0.3ml solution for injection pre-filled pens | 1 pre-filled disposable injection [PoM] £14.41 DT = £14.41

Metoject PEN 22.5mg/0.45ml solution for injection pre-filled pens | 1 pre-filled disposable injection [PoM] £16.11 DT = £16.11

Metoject PEN 7.5mg/0.15ml solution for injection pre-filled pens | 1 pre-filled disposable injection [PoM] £12.87 DT = £12.87

Metoject PEN 25mg/0.5ml solution for injection pre-filled pens | 1 pre-filled disposable injection [PoM] £16.13 DT = £16.13

Metoject PEN 20mg/0.4ml solution for injection pre-filled pens | 1 pre-filled disposable injection [PoM] £15.56 DT = £15.56

▸ **Nordimet** (Nordic Pharma Ltd)

Methotrexate 25 mg per 1 ml Nordimet 15mg/0.6ml solution for injection pre-filled pens | 1 pre-filled disposable injection [PoM] £14.92 DT = £14.92

Nordimet 20mg/0.8ml solution for injection pre-filled pens | 1 pre-filled disposable injection [PoM] £16.06 DT = £16.06

Nordimet 22.5mg/0.9ml solution for injection pre-filled pens | 1 pre-filled disposable injection [PoM] £16.61 DT = £16.61

Nordimet 12.5mg/0.5ml solution for injection pre-filled pens | 1 pre-filled disposable injection [PoM] £14.85 DT = £14.85

Nordimet 10mg/0.4ml solution for injection pre-filled pens | 1 pre-filled disposable injection [PoM] £13.77 DT = £13.77

Nordimet 17.5mg/0.7ml solution for injection pre-filled pens | 1 pre-filled disposable injection [PoM] £15.75 DT = £15.75

Nordimet 25mg/1ml solution for injection pre-filled pens | 1 pre-filled disposable injection [PoM] £16.64 DT = £16.64

Nordimet 7.5mg/0.3ml solution for injection pre-filled pens | 1 pre-filled disposable injection [PoM] £13.37 DT = £13.37

▸ **Zlatal** (Nordic Pharma Ltd)

Methotrexate (as Methotrexate sodium) 25 mg per 1 ml Zlatal 17.5mg/0.7ml solution for injection pre-filled syringes | 1 pre-filled disposable injection [PoM] £15.75 DT = £15.75

Zlatal 10mg/0.4ml solution for injection pre-filled syringes | 1 pre-filled disposable injection [PoM] £13.77 DT = £13.77

Zlatal 25mg/1ml solution for injection pre-filled syringes | 1 pre-filled disposable injection [PoM] £16.64 DT = £16.64

Zlatal 20mg/0.8ml solution for injection pre-filled syringes | 1 pre-filled disposable injection [PoM] £16.06 DT = £16.06

Zlatal 12.5mg/0.5ml solution for injection pre-filled syringes | 1 pre-filled disposable injection [PoM] £14.85 DT = £14.85

Zlatal 7.5mg/0.3ml solution for injection pre-filled syringes | 1 pre-filled disposable injection [PoM] £13.37 DT = £13.37

Zlatal 22.5mg/0.9ml solution for injection pre-filled syringes | 1 pre-filled disposable injection [PoM] £16.61 DT = £16.61

Zlatal 15mg/0.6ml solution for injection pre-filled syringes | 1 pre-filled disposable injection [PoM] £14.92 DT = £14.92

Oral suspension
CAUTIONARY AND ADVISORY LABELS 10, 11

Solution for infusion
▸ **Methotrexate (Non-proprietary)**

Methotrexate (as Methotrexate sodium) 100 mg per 1 ml Methotrexate 5g/50ml solution for infusion vials | 1 vial [PoM] £380.00–£400.00 (Hospital only)

Oral solution
CAUTIONARY AND ADVISORY LABELS 10, 11

▸ **Methotrexate (Non-proprietary)**

Methotrexate (as Methotrexate sodium) 2 mg per 1 ml Methotrexate 2mg/ml oral solution sugar free | 35 ml [PoM] £95.00–£152.00 DT = £95.00 [SF] | 65 ml [PoM] £125.00 DT = £125.00 [SF]

▸ **Jylamvo** (Esteve Pharmaceuticals Ltd)

Methotrexate (as Methotrexate sodium) 2 mg per 1 ml Jylamvo 2mg/ml oral solution | 60 ml [PoM] £112.50 [SF]

Nelarabine [Specialist drug]
10-Nov-2020

● **INDICATIONS AND DOSE**

T-cell acute lymphoblastic leukaemia | T-cell lymphoblastic lymphoma

▸ BY INTRAVENOUS INFUSION

▸ Adult: Specialist drug – access specialist resources for dosing information

● **INTERACTIONS** → Appendix 1: nelarabine

● **SIDE-EFFECTS**

▸ **Common or very common** Abdominal pain · anaemia · appetite decreased · arthralgia · asthenia · confusion · constipation · cough · diarrhoea · dizziness · drowsiness · dyspnoea · electrolyte imbalance · fever · gait abnormal · headache · hyperbilirubinaemia · hypotension · increased risk of infection · leucopenia · memory loss · movement disorders · muscle weakness · myalgia · nausea · neutropenia · oedema · pain · peripheral neuropathy · respiratory disorders · seizures · sensation abnormal · sepsis · stomatitis · taste altered · thrombocytopenia · tremor · tumour lysis syndrome · vision blurred · vomiting

▸ **Rare or very rare** Rhabdomyolysis

▸ **Frequency not known** Progressive multifocal leukoencephalopathy (PML)

SIDE-EFFECTS, FURTHER INFORMATION If signs or symptoms of neurotoxicity occur, treatment should be discontinued immediately.

● **CONCEPTION AND CONTRACEPTION** Manufacturer advises effective contraception during and for at least 3 months after treatment in men and women.

● **PATIENT AND CARER ADVICE**

Driving and skilled tasks Drowsiness may affect performance of skilled tasks (e.g. cycling or driving).

● **NATIONAL FUNDING/ACCESS DECISIONS**

For full details see funding body website

Scottish Medicines Consortium (SMC) decisions

▸ Nelarabine (*Atriance*®) for the treatment of patients with T-cell acute lymphoblastic leukaemia (T-ALL) and T-cell lymphoblastic lymphoma (T-LBL) (April 2008) SMC No. 454/08 Recommended with restrictions

● **MEDICINAL FORMS** There can be variation in the licensing of different medicines containing the same drug.

Solution for infusion
ELECTROLYTES: May contain Sodium

▸ **Atriance** (Sandoz Ltd) ▼

Nelarabine 5 mg per 1 ml Atriance 250mg/50ml solution for infusion vials | 1 vial [PoM] £222.00 (Hospital only)

Pemetrexed [Specialist drug]

13-Aug-2021

● **INDICATIONS AND DOSE**

Malignant pleural mesothelioma | Non-small cell lung cancer
▶ BY INTRAVENOUS INFUSION
▸ Adult: Specialist drug – access specialist resources for dosing information

● **INTERACTIONS** → Appendix 1: pemetrexed

● **SIDE-EFFECTS**
▶ **Common or very common** Appetite decreased · fatigue · mucositis · nausea · neuropathy sensory · oedema · pain · renal disorder · skin reactions · stomatitis · vomiting

● **CONCEPTION AND CONTRACEPTION** [EvGr] Females of childbearing potential must use effective contraception during treatment and for 6 months after last treatment; male patients should use effective contraception and avoid fathering a child during treatment and for 3 months after treatment. [M]

● **NATIONAL FUNDING/ACCESS DECISIONS**
For full details see funding body website
NICE decisions
▸ **Pemetrexed for the treatment of non-small cell lung cancer (August 2007)** NICE TA124 Not recommended
▸ **Pemetrexed for the first-line treatment of non-small cell lung cancer (September 2009)** NICE TA181 Recommended with restrictions
▸ **Pemetrexed maintenance treatment for non-squamous non-small cell lung cancer after pemetrexed and cisplatin (August 2016)** NICE TA402 Recommended with restrictions
▸ **Pemetrexed for the maintenance treatment of non-small-cell lung cancer (updated August 2017)** NICE TA190 Recommended
▸ **Pemetrexed for the treatment of malignant pleural mesothelioma (January 2008)** NICE TA135 Recommended with restrictions
Scottish Medicines Consortium (SMC) decisions
▸ **Pemetrexed (*Alimta*®) as monotherapy for the second line treatment of patients with locally advanced or metastatic non-small cell lung cancer other than predominantly squamous cell histology (September 2008)** SMC No. 342/07 Recommended with restrictions
▸ **Pemetrexed (*Alimta*®) for the first line treatment of patients with locally advanced or metastatic non-small cell lung cancer (February 2010)** SMC No. 531/09 Recommended with restrictions
▸ **Pemetrexed (*Alimta*®) as monotherapy for the maintenance treatment of locally advanced or metastatic non-small cell lung cancer other than predominantly squamous cell histology in patients whose disease has not progressed immediately following platinum-based chemotherapy (December 2014)** SMC No. 770/12 Recommended

● **MEDICINAL FORMS** There can be variation in the licensing of different medicines containing the same drug.
Solution for infusion
▸ Pemetrexed (Non-proprietary)
    Pemetrexed 25 mg per 1 ml Pemetrexed 1g/40ml concentrate for solution for infusion vials | 1 vial [PoM] £1,280.00–£1,600.00 (Hospital only)
    Pemetrexed 100mg/4ml concentrate for solution for infusion vials | 1 vial [PoM] £128.00–£160.00 (Hospital only)
    Pemetrexed 500mg/20ml concentrate for solution for infusion vials | 1 vial [PoM] £640.00–£800.00 (Hospital only)
    Pemetrexed 850mg/34ml concentrate for solution for infusion vials | 1 vial [PoM] £1,360.00 (Hospital only)
Powder for solution for infusion
ELECTROLYTES: May contain Sodium
▸ Pemetrexed (Non-proprietary)
    Pemetrexed 100 mg Pemetrexed 100mg powder for concentrate for solution for infusion vials | 1 vial [PoM] £125.00 (Hospital only)
    Pemetrexed 500 mg Pemetrexed 500mg powder for concentrate for solution for infusion vials | 1 vial [PoM] £450.00 (Hospital only)

▸ Alimta (Eli Lilly and Company Ltd)
    Pemetrexed 100 mg Alimta 100mg powder for concentrate for solution for infusion vials | 1 vial [PoM] £160.00 (Hospital only)
    Pemetrexed 500 mg Alimta 500mg powder for concentrate for solution for infusion vials | 1 vial [PoM] £800.00 (Hospital only)

Tegafur with gimeracil and oteracil [Specialist drug]

27-Jul-2021

● **INDICATIONS AND DOSE**

Gastric cancer
▶ BY MOUTH
▸ Adult: Specialist drug – access specialist resources for dosing information

IMPORTANT SAFETY INFORMATION
RISKS OF INCORRECT DOSING OF ORAL ANTI-CANCER MEDICINES
See Cytotoxic drugs p. 1027.

MHRA/CHM ADVICE: 5-FLUOROURACIL (INTRAVENOUS), CAPECITABINE, TEGAFUR: DPD TESTING RECOMMENDED BEFORE INITIATION TO IDENTIFY PATIENTS AT INCREASED RISK OF SEVERE AND FATAL TOXICITY (OCTOBER 2020)
Patients with partial or complete dihydropyrimidine dehydrogenase (DPD) deficiency are at increased risk of severe and fatal toxicity during treatment with fluoropyrimidines. Healthcare professionals are advised to test all patients for DPD deficiency before initiating treatment and confirm their, including family, history of complete or partial DPD deficiency. Tegafur with gimeracil and oteracil is contra-indicated in patients with known complete DPD deficiency; in those with partial DPD deficiency, a reduced starting dose is recommended. Patients should be monitored for toxicity, particularly during the first cycle of treatment or after a dose increase; severe toxicity can occur even in those with negative test results for DPD deficiency. Healthcare professionals should also counsel patients on the benefits and risks of their treatment and ensure they are provided with the patient information leaflet.

● **CONTRA-INDICATIONS** Complete dihydropyrimidine dehydrogenase deficiency (increased risk of severe, life-threatening, or fatal toxicity)—consult product literature

● **INTERACTIONS** → Appendix 1: tegafur

● **SIDE-EFFECTS**
▶ **Common or very common** Anaemia · appetite abnormal · asthenia · constipation · cough · decreased leucocytes · dehydration · diarrhoea · dizziness · dry mouth · dysphagia · dyspnoea · electrolyte imbalance · embolism and thrombosis · eye disorders · eye inflammation · gastrointestinal discomfort · gastrointestinal disorders · haemorrhage · headache · hearing impairment · hiccups · hyperbilirubinaemia · hypertension · hypoproteinaemia · hypotension · insomnia · nausea · nerve disorders · neutropenia · oral disorders · taste altered · thrombocytopenia · vision disorders · vomiting
▶ **Uncommon** Aerophagia · allergic rhinitis · alopecia · angina pectoris · anxiety · aphasia · arrhythmias · ascites · breast abnormalities · burping · cerebrovascular insufficiency · chills · coagulation disorders · confusion · depression · drowsiness · dysphonia · ear discomfort · encephalopathy · eosinophilia · fever · gout · hallucination · heart failure · hemiparesis · hyperaemia · hyperglobulinaemia · hyperglycaemia · hyperlipidaemia · hypertrichosis · hypovolaemic shock · increased leucocytes · increased risk of infection · joint disorders · limb discomfort · loss of consciousness · memory loss · movement disorders · mucositis · muscle complaints · muscle weakness · myocardial infarction · nail disorders · nasal complaints · neoplasm complications · nephrotoxicity · oedema · oesophageal spasm · pain · palpitations · pancytopenia ·

pericardial effusion · personality disorder · renal
impairment · seizure · sensation abnormal · sepsis · sexual
dysfunction · skin reactions · smell altered · sweat changes ·
syncope · throat complaints · thrombocytosis · tremor ·
urinary frequency increased · vasodilation · vertigo · weight
changes

▶ **Rare or very rare** Acute hepatic failure · chest discomfort ·
feeling cold · interstitial lung disease · local swelling ·
malaise · multi organ failure · pancreatitis acute ·
performance status decreased · photosensitivity reaction ·
rhabdomyolysis · severe cutaneous adverse reactions
(SCARs)

● **CONCEPTION AND CONTRACEPTION** Manufacturer advises
effective contraception during and for up to 6 months after
treatment.

● **NATIONAL FUNDING/ACCESS DECISIONS**
For full details see funding body website
Scottish Medicines Consortium (SMC) decisions
▶ **Tegafur with gimeracil and oteracil (*Teysuno*®) for the
treatment of advanced gastric cancer when given in
combination with cisplatin (September 2012) SMC No. 802/12
Recommended with restrictions**

● **MEDICINAL FORMS** No licensed medicines listed.

Tioguanine [Specialist drug]   10-May-2021

(Thioguanine)

● **INDICATIONS AND DOSE**

Acute leukaemia | Chronic myeloid leukaemia
▶ BY MOUTH
▶ Adult: Specialist drug – access specialist resources for
dosing information

> **IMPORTANT SAFETY INFORMATION**
> RISKS OF INCORRECT DOSING OF ORAL ANTI-CANCER MEDICINES
> See Cytotoxic drugs p. 1027.

● **INTERACTIONS** → Appendix 1: tioguanine

● **SIDE-EFFECTS**
▶ **Common or very common** Bone marrow failure ·
gastrointestinal disorders · hepatic disorders ·
hyperbilirubinaemia · hyperuricaemia · hyperuricosuria ·
nodular regenerative hyperplasia · oesophageal varices ·
sinusoidal obstruction syndrome · splenomegaly ·
stomatitis · thrombocytopenia · uric acid nephropathy ·
weight increased
▶ **Frequency not known** Photosensitivity reaction
SIDE-EFFECTS, FURTHER INFORMATION Manufacturer
advises tioguanine is not recommended for maintenance
or long-term continuous therapy because of the high risk
of hepatic toxicity. If hepatic toxicity develops,
discontinue treatment.

● **CONCEPTION AND CONTRACEPTION** Ensure effective
contraception during treatment in men or women.

● **MEDICINAL FORMS** There can be variation in the licensing of
different medicines containing the same drug. Forms available
from special-order manufacturers include: oral capsule
Oral tablet
▶ Tioguanine (Non-proprietary)
Tioguanine 40 mg Tioguanine 40mg tablets | 25 tablet [PoM]
£76.35 DT = £76.35

Trifluridine with tipiracil [Specialist drug]
01-Oct-2024

● **INDICATIONS AND DOSE**

Gastric cancer | Colorectal cancer
▶ BY MOUTH
▶ Adult: Specialist drug – access specialist resources for
dosing information

> **IMPORTANT SAFETY INFORMATION**
> RISKS OF INCORRECT DOSING OF ORAL ANTI-CANCER MEDICINES
> See Cytotoxic drugs p. 1027.

● **SIDE-EFFECTS**
▶ **Common or very common** Alopecia · anaemia · appetite
decreased · asthenia · constipation · decreased leucocytes ·
diarrhoea · dyspnoea · fever · gastrointestinal discomfort ·
hyperbilirubinaemia · hypoalbuminaemia · increased risk
of infection · malaise · mucositis · nausea · neutropenia ·
oedema · oral disorders · peripheral neuropathy · skin
reactions · taste altered · thrombocytopenia · urine
abnormalities · vomiting · weight decreased
▶ **Uncommon** Angina pectoris · anxiety · arrhythmia · ascites ·
bile duct disorders · cancer pain · cataract · conjunctivitis ·
cough · cystitis · dehydration · dizziness · dry eye ·
dysphonia · ear discomfort · electrolyte imbalance ·
embolism · erythropenia · feeling of body temperature
change · flushing · gastrointestinal disorders · gout ·
haemorrhage · headache · hepatotoxicity · hyperglycaemia
· hyperhidrosis · hypertension · hypotension · increased
leucocytes · insomnia · joint disorders · lethargy ·
menstrual disorder · muscle complaints · muscle weakness
· nail disorder · neurotoxicity · neutropenic sepsis ·
oropharyngeal pain · pain · palpitations · pancreatitis acute
· pancytopenia · photosensitivity reaction · pleural effusion
· pulmonary embolism (including fatal cases) · QT interval
prolongation · renal failure · rhinorrhoea · sensation
abnormal · septic shock (including fatal cases) · syncope ·
urinary disorder · vertigo · vision disorders
▶ **Frequency not known** Interstitial lung disease

● **CONCEPTION AND CONTRACEPTION** Manufacturer advises
effective contraception in women of child-bearing
potential and in men with a partner of child-bearing
potential, during treatment and for 6 months after
stopping treatment. Manufacturer also advises use of an
additional barrier method in women using hormonal
contraceptives—effect of trifluridine with tipiracil on
hormonal contraception unknown.

● **NATIONAL FUNDING/ACCESS DECISIONS**
For full details see funding body website
NICE decisions
▶ **Trifluridine with tipiracil for previously treated metastatic
colorectal cancer (August 2016) NICE TA405 Recommended
with restrictions**
▶ **Trifluridine with tipiracil with bevacizumab for treating
metastatic colorectal cancer after 2 systemic treatments
(September 2024) NICE TA1008 Recommended**
▶ **Trifluridine with tipiracil for treating metastatic gastric cancer
or gastro-oesophageal junction adenocarcinoma after 2 or
more treatments (December 2022) NICE TA852 Recommended**
Scottish Medicines Consortium (SMC) decisions
▶ **Trifluridine with tipiracil (*Lonsurf*®) for the treatment of adult
patients with metastatic colorectal cancer who have been
previously treated with, or are not considered candidates for,
available therapies including fluoropyrimidine-, oxaliplatin-
and irinotecan-based chemotherapies, anti-vascular
endothelial growth factor agents, and anti-epidermal growth
factor receptor agents (February 2017) SMC No. 1221/17
Recommended**

▶ Trifluridine with tipiracil (*Lonsurf*®) in combination with bevacizumab for the treatment of adult patients with metastatic colorectal cancer who have received two prior anti-cancer treatment regimens including fluoropyrimidine-, oxaliplatin- and irinotecan-based chemotherapies, anti-vascular endothelial growth factor agents, and/or anti-epidermal growth factor receptor agents (August 2024) SMC No. SMC2654 Recommended

▶ Trifluridine with tipiracil (*Lonsurf*®) as monotherapy for the treatment of adult patients with metastatic gastric cancer including adenocarcinoma of the gastroesophageal junction, who have been previously treated with at least two prior systemic treatment regimens for advanced disease (June 2021) SMC No. SMC2329 Recommended with restrictions

● **MEDICINAL FORMS** There can be variation in the licensing of different medicines containing the same drug.
Oral tablet
CAUTIONARY AND ADVISORY LABELS 21
▶ Lonsurf (Servier Laboratories Ltd)
Tipiracil (as Tipiracil hydrochloride) 6.14 mg, Trifluridine 15 mg Lonsurf 15mg/6.14mg tablets | 20 tablet [PoM] £500.00 (Hospital only) | 60 tablet [PoM] £1,500.00 (Hospital only)
Tipiracil (as Tipiracil hydrochloride) 8.19 mg, Trifluridine 20 mg Lonsurf 20mg/8.19mg tablets | 20 tablet [PoM] £666.67 (Hospital only) | 60 tablet [PoM] £2,000.00 (Hospital only)

ANTINEOPLASTIC DRUGS > CYTOTOXIC ANTIBIOTICS AND RELATED SUBSTANCES

Bleomycin [Specialist drug]

19-Sep-2023

● **INDICATIONS AND DOSE**
Squamous cell carcinoma of the head and neck, cervix and external genitalia | Testicular cancer | Non-Hodgkin's lymphoma | Hodgkin's lymphoma
▶ BY INTRAMUSCULAR INJECTION, OR BY INTRAVENOUS INJECTION, OR BY INTRAVENOUS INFUSION, OR BY INTRA-ARTERIAL INJECTION, OR BY INTRA-ARTERIAL INFUSION, OR BY SUBCUTANEOUS INJECTION
▶ Adult: Specialist drug – access specialist resources for dosing information

● **CONTRA-INDICATIONS** Ataxia telangiectasia · pulmonary infection · significantly reduced lung function
● **INTERACTIONS** → Appendix 1: bleomycin
● **SIDE-EFFECTS**
▶ **Common or very common** Alopecia · appetite decreased · chills · dyspnoea · embolism and thrombosis · fever (after administration) · fingertip swelling · fingertip tenderness · headache · hypersensitivity · idiosyncratic drug reaction · induration · interstitial lung disease · malaise · mucositis · nausea · oedema · pulmonary fibrosis · respiratory disorders · skin reactions · stomatitis · vomiting · weight decreased
▶ **Uncommon** Angular cheilitis · arthralgia · bone marrow disorders · cancer pain · confusion · diarrhoea · dizziness · haemorrhage · hypotension · leucopenia · myalgia · nail discolouration · nail disorder · neutropenia · oliguria · thrombocytopenia · urinary disorders · vein wall hypertrophy
▶ **Rare or very rare** Cerebrovascular insufficiency · chest pain · haemolytic uraemic syndrome · hepatic impairment · myocardial infarction · pericarditis · peripheral vascular disease · scleroderma · thrombotic microangiopathy · tumour lysis syndrome
▶ **Frequency not known** Anaemia · sepsis

SIDE-EFFECTS, FURTHER INFORMATION Pulmonary reactions, including interstitial pneumonitis, pulmonary fibrosis, and pulmonary toxicity have been reported. Pulmonary toxicity occurs more frequently in those over 70 years, and in those who have received total doses greater than 400 units. If pulmonary changes occur, discontinue treatment and investigate.

● **CONCEPTION AND CONTRACEPTION** [EvGr] Ensure effective contraception during and for 6 months after treatment in male and female patients. ⓜ

● **MEDICINAL FORMS** There can be variation in the licensing of different medicines containing the same drug.
Powder for solution for injection
▶ Bleomycin (Non-proprietary)
Bleomycin (as Bleomycin sulfate) 15000 unit Bleomycin 15,000unit powder for solution for injection vials | 1 vial [PoM] £19.06 (Hospital only)

Mitomycin [Specialist drug]

28-Jul-2020

● **INDICATIONS AND DOSE**
Bladder tumours
▶ BY INTRAVESICAL INSTILLATION
▶ Adult: Specialist drug – access specialist resources for dosing information
Gastric cancer | Breast cancer | Non-small cell lung cancer | Pancreatic cancer
▶ BY INTRAVENOUS INJECTION
▶ Adult: Specialist drug – access specialist resources for dosing information

> **IMPORTANT SAFETY INFORMATION**
> MHRA/CHM ADVICE: *MITOMYCIN-C KYOWA*® 40 MG RESTRICTED TO INTRAVESICAL ADMINISTRATION ONLY FOR TREATMENT OF SUPERFICIAL BLADDER CANCER (SEPTEMBER 2019)
> Sub-visible particles, at levels above specification limits, have been observed after reconstitution of *Mitomycin-C Kyowa*® 40 mg; healthcare professionals are advised that its use has been restricted to the treatment of superficial bladder cancer via the intravesical route only.

● **INTERACTIONS** → Appendix 1: mitomycin
● **SIDE-EFFECTS**
GENERAL SIDE-EFFECTS
▶ **Common or very common** Bone marrow disorders · cough · cystitis · haemorrhage · leucopenia · malaise · nausea · skin reactions · thrombocytopenia · vomiting
▶ **Uncommon** Alopecia · appetite decreased · diarrhoea · fever
▶ **Rare or very rare** Hepatic disorders · increased risk of infection · renal disorder · sepsis
▶ **Frequency not known** Anaemia · asthenia · chills · constipation · eosinophilia · erythropenia · flushing · hypertension · lethargy · neutropenia · oedema · respiratory disorders · weight decreased

SPECIFIC SIDE-EFFECTS
▶ **Common or very common**
▶ With intravenous use Dyspnoea · extravasation necrosis · glomerulonephropathy · interstitial pneumonia · nephropathy · renal impairment
▶ With intravesical use Hypersensitivity · urinary disorders · urinary tract discomfort
▶ **Uncommon**
▶ With intravenous use Mucositis · oral disorders
▶ **Rare or very rare**
▶ With intravenous use Haemolytic anaemia · heart failure · pulmonary hypertension · sinusoidal obstruction syndrome
▶ With intravesical use Acute kidney injury · bladder disorders · interstitial lung disease · urinary tract stenosis
▶ **Frequency not known**
▶ With intravenous use Abdominal discomfort · cholecystitis · injection site necrosis · neoplasms · shock · urine abnormalities · vascular pain
▶ With intravesical use Pain · penile necrosis · proteinuria · pulmonary fibrosis · pulmonary oedema · ulcer

SIDE-EFFECTS, FURTHER INFORMATION Mitomycin is usually administered at 6-weekly intervals because it causes delayed bone-marrow toxicity. Prolonged use may result in a cumulative effect.

- CONCEPTION AND CONTRACEPTION Contraceptive advice required.

- MEDICINAL FORMS There can be variation in the licensing of different medicines containing the same drug.

Powder and solvent for intravesical solution

ELECTROLYTES: May contain Sodium

▸ Mitomycin (Non-proprietary)

Mitomycin 40 mg Mitomycin 40mg powder and solvent for intravesical solution vials | 1 vial PoM £135.00 (Hospital only)

Powder for solution for injection

▸ Mitomycin (Non-proprietary)

Mitomycin 5 mg Mitomycin 5mg powder for solution for injection vials | 1 vial PoM (Hospital only)

Mitomycin 10 mg Mitomycin 10mg powder for solution for injection vials | 1 vial PoM £20.30

Mitomycin 40 mg Mitomycin 40mg powder for solution for injection vials | 1 vial PoM £75.89 (Hospital only)

▸ Mitocin (Vygoris Ltd)

Mitomycin 20 mg Mitocin 20mg powder for solution for injection vials | 1 vial PoM £39.00 (Hospital only)

Pentostatin [Specialist drug]

02-Aug-2021

- INDICATIONS AND DOSE

Hairy cell leukaemia

▸ BY INTRAVENOUS INJECTION, OR BY INTRAVENOUS INFUSION

▸ Adult: Specialist drug – access specialist resources for dosing information

- INTERACTIONS → Appendix 1: pentostatin

- SIDE-EFFECTS

▸ **Common or very common** Agranulocytosis · alopecia · amenorrhoea · anaemia · angina pectoris · anxiety · appetite decreased · arrhythmias · arthritis · asthenia · asthma · atrioventricular block · blood disorder · bone disorder · bone marrow disorders · breast mass · cardiac arrest · chest pain · chills · confusion · constipation · cough · deafness · death · depersonalisation · depression · diarrhoea · dizziness · drowsiness · dry eye · dry mouth · dysarthria · dysphagia · dyspnoea · ear pain · electrolyte imbalance · embolism and thrombosis · emotional lability · eosinophilia · eye disorders · eye inflammation · eye pain · febrile neutropenia · fever · fluid imbalance · flushing · gastrointestinal discomfort · gastrointestinal disorders · gout · graft versus host disease · haemorrhage · hallucination · hangover · headaches · heart failure · hostility · hyperbilirubinaemia · hyperglycaemia · hyperhidrosis · hypersensitivity · hypertension · hypotension · increased risk of infection · influenza like illness · jaundice · joint disorders · leucopenia · lymphadenopathy · malaise · memory loss · meningism · movement disorders · muscle complaints · nausea · neoplasms · nephrolithiasis · nephropathy · nerve disorders · neurotoxicity (withhold or discontinue) · oedema · oral disorders · pain · paralysis · pericardial effusion · photosensitivity reaction · pulmonary oedema · rash (withhold if severe) · renal impairment · respiratory disorders · retinopathy · seborrhoea · seizures · sensation abnormal · sepsis · sexual dysfunction · skin reactions · sleep disorders · splenomegaly · syncope · taste altered · thinking abnormal · thrombocytopenia · tinnitus · tremor · urinary disorders · urogenital disorder · vasculitis · vertigo · vision disorders · vomiting · weight changes

▸ **Uncommon** Angioedema · capillary leak syndrome · cardiomyopathy · Clostridioides difficile colitis · cystitis · haemolytic anaemia · mucositis · multi organ failure · myocardial infarction · pure red cell aplasia · transplant failure · tumour lysis syndrome

▸ **Rare or very rare** Alveolar fibrosis · dementia · interstitial lung disease · pericarditis · shock · Stevens-Johnson syndrome · systemic inflammatory response syndrome

SIDE-EFFECTS, FURTHER INFORMATION Pentostatin can cause myelosuppression, immunosuppression, and a number of other side-effects that may be severe. Treatment should be withheld in patients who develop a severe rash, and withheld or discontinued in patients showing signs of neurotoxicity.

- CONCEPTION AND CONTRACEPTION EvGr Females of childbearing potential should use effective contraception; male patients should avoid fathering a child during treatment and for 6 months after treatment. ⟨M⟩

- MEDICINAL FORMS There can be variation in the licensing of different medicines containing the same drug.

Powder for solution for injection

▸ Nipent (Pfizer Ltd)

Pentostatin 10 mg Nipent 10mg powder for solution for injection vials | 1 vial PoM £734.21 (Hospital only)

ANTINEOPLASTIC DRUGS › PLANT ALKALOIDS

Trabectedin [Specialist drug]

04-Aug-2021

- INDICATIONS AND DOSE

Soft-tissue sarcoma | Ovarian cancer

▸ BY INTRAVENOUS INFUSION

▸ Adult: Specialist drug – access specialist resources for dosing information

- CONTRA-INDICATIONS Elevated creatine phosphokinase (consult product literature)

- INTERACTIONS → Appendix 1: trabectedin

- SIDE-EFFECTS

▸ **Common or very common** Alopecia · anaemia · appetite decreased · arthralgia · asthenia · back pain · constipation · cough · dehydration · diarrhoea · dizziness · dyspnoea · fever · flushing · gastrointestinal discomfort · headache · hyperbilirubinaemia · hypersensitivity · hypokalaemia · hypotension · infection · insomnia · leucopenia · mucositis · myalgia · nausea · neutropenia · oedema · paraesthesia · peripheral neuropathy · skin reactions · stomatitis · taste altered · thrombocytopenia · vomiting · weight decreased

▸ **Uncommon** Capillary leak syndrome · rhabdomyolysis (discontinue) · septic shock

▸ **Rare or very rare** Hepatic failure

▸ **Frequency not known** Extravasation necrosis

SIDE-EFFECTS, FURTHER INFORMATION A corticosteroid, such as dexamethasone by intravenous infusion, must be given 30 minutes before therapy for its antiemetic and hepatoprotective effects.

- CONCEPTION AND CONTRACEPTION Effective contraception recommended during and for at least 3 months after treatment in women and during and for at least 5 months after treatment in men.

- NATIONAL FUNDING/ACCESS DECISIONS

For full details see funding body website

NICE decisions

▸ **Trabectedin for the treatment of advanced soft tissue sarcoma (updated February 2021)** NICE TA185 Recommended

▸ **Topotecan, pegylated liposomal doxorubicin hydrochloride, paclitaxel, trabectedin and gemcitabine for treating recurrent ovarian cancer (April 2016)** NICE TA389 Not recommended

Scottish Medicines Consortium (SMC) decisions

▸ **Trabectedin (*Yondelis*®) for the treatment of adult patients with advanced soft tissue sarcoma, after failure of anthracyclines and ifosfamide, or who are unsuited to receive these agents (November 2020)** SMC No. SMC2283 Recommended

- **MEDICINAL FORMS** There can be variation in the licensing of different medicines containing the same drug.

Powder for solution for infusion

▸ **Trabectedin (Non-proprietary)**
Trabectedin 250 microgram Trabectedin 250 microgram powder for concentrate for solution for infusion vials | 1 vial PoM £326.70 (Hospital only)
Trabectedin 1 mg Trabectedin 1mg powder for concentrate for solution for infusion vials | 1 vial PoM £1,229.40 (Hospital only)

▸ **Yondelis** (Immedica Pharma AB)
Trabectedin 250 microgram Yondelis 0.25mg powder for concentrate for solution for infusion vials | 1 vial PoM £363.00 (Hospital only)
Trabectedin 1 mg Yondelis 1mg powder for concentrate for solution for infusion vials | 1 vial PoM £1,366.00 (Hospital only)

ANTINEOPLASTIC DRUGS > PLATINUM COMPOUNDS

Carboplatin [Specialist drug]

16-Aug-2021

● **INDICATIONS AND DOSE**

Ovarian cancer | Small cell lung cancer | Testicular germ cell tumours
▸ BY INTRAVENOUS INFUSION
▸ Adult: Specialist drug – access specialist resources for dosing information

● **INTERACTIONS** → Appendix 1: platinum compounds

● **SIDE-EFFECTS**
▸ **Common or very common** Alopecia · anaemia · asthenia · cardiovascular disorder · constipation · diarrhoea · gastrointestinal discomfort · haemorrhage · hypersensitivity · increased risk of infection · interstitial lung disease · leucopenia · mucosal abnormalities · musculoskeletal disorder · nausea · neutropenia · ototoxicity · peripheral neuropathy · reflexes decreased · respiratory disorders · sensation abnormal · skin reactions · taste altered · thrombocytopenia · urogenital disorder · vision disorders · vomiting
▸ **Rare or very rare** Angioedema
▸ **Frequency not known** Appetite decreased · bone marrow failure · chills · dehydration · embolism · encephalopathy · extravasation necrosis · fever · haemolytic uraemic syndrome · heart failure · hypertension · hyponatraemia · hypotension · injection site necrosis · malaise · pancreatitis · pulmonary fibrosis · stomatitis · stroke · treatment related secondary malignancy · tumour lysis syndrome

● **CONCEPTION AND CONTRACEPTION** Contraceptive advice required.

● **NATIONAL FUNDING/ACCESS DECISIONS**
For full details see funding body website

NICE decisions
▸ **Bevacizumab in combination with paclitaxel and carboplatin for the first-line treatment of advanced ovarian cancer (May 2013)** NICE TA284 Not recommended
▸ **Bevacizumab in combination with gemcitabine and carboplatin for treating the first recurrence of platinum-sensitive advanced ovarian cancer (May 2013)** NICE TA285 Not recommended

● **MEDICINAL FORMS** There can be variation in the licensing of different medicines containing the same drug.

Solution for infusion
▸ **Carboplatin (Non-proprietary)**
Carboplatin 10 mg per 1 ml Carboplatin 50mg/5ml concentrate for solution for infusion vials | 1 vial PoM £20.20–£28.33 (Hospital only)
Carboplatin 150mg/15ml concentrate for solution for infusion vials | 1 vial PoM £56.92–£73.17 (Hospital only)
Carboplatin 600mg/60ml concentrate for solution for infusion vials | 1 vial PoM £232.64–£334.29 (Hospital only)
Carboplatin 600mg/60ml solution for infusion vials | 1 vial PoM £260.00 (Hospital only)

Carboplatin 450mg/45ml concentrate for solution for infusion vials | 1 vial PoM £168.85–£217.13 (Hospital only)
Carboplatin 450mg/45ml solution for infusion vials | 1 vial PoM £197.48 (Hospital only)
Carboplatin 150mg/15ml solution for infusion vials | 1 vial PoM £65.83 (Hospital only)
Carboplatin 50mg/5ml solution for infusion vials | 1 vial PoM £22.86 (Hospital only)

Cisplatin [Specialist drug]

07-Feb-2022

● **INDICATIONS AND DOSE**

Testicular cancer | Ovarian cancer | Lung cancer | Bladder cancer | Squamous cell carcinoma of the head and neck | Cervical carcinoma
▸ BY INTRAVENOUS INFUSION
▸ Adult: Specialist drug – access specialist resources for dosing information

● **INTERACTIONS** → Appendix 1: platinum compounds

● **SIDE-EFFECTS**
▸ **Common or very common** Anaemia · arrhythmias · bone marrow failure · electrolyte imbalance · extravasation necrosis · fever · leucopenia · nephrotoxicity (dose-related and potentially cumulative) · sepsis · thrombocytopenia
▸ **Uncommon** Anaphylactoid reaction · ototoxicity (dose-related and potentially cumulative) · spermatogenesis abnormal
▸ **Rare or very rare** Acute leukaemia · cardiac arrest · encephalopathy · myocardial infarction · nerve disorders · seizure · stomatitis
▸ **Frequency not known** Alopecia · appetite decreased · asthenia · autonomic dysfunction · cardiac disorder · cerebrovascular insufficiency · deafness · dehydration · diarrhoea · haemolytic anaemia · hiccups · hyperuricaemia · infection · Lhermitte's sign · malaise · muscle spasms · myelopathy · nausea · papilloedema · pulmonary embolism · rash · Raynaud's phenomenon · renal impairment · renal tubular disorder · retinal discolouration · SIADH · taste loss · tetany · thrombotic microangiopathy · tinnitus · vision disorders · vomiting

● **CONCEPTION AND CONTRACEPTION** Manufacturer advises effective contraception during and for at least 6 months after treatment in men or women.

● **MEDICINAL FORMS** There can be variation in the licensing of different medicines containing the same drug.

Solution for infusion
▸ **Cisplatin (Non-proprietary)**
Cisplatin 1 mg per 1 ml Cisplatin 50mg/50ml concentrate for solution for infusion vials | 1 vial PoM £26.70–£28.11 (Hospital only)
Cisplatin 100mg/100ml solution for infusion vials | 1 vial PoM £50.22 (Hospital only)
Cisplatin 50mg/50ml solution for infusion vials | 1 vial PoM £25.37 (Hospital only)
Cisplatin 10mg/10ml concentrate for solution for infusion vials | 1 vial PoM £5.36 (Hospital only)
Cisplatin 100mg/100ml concentrate for solution for infusion vials | 1 vial PoM £52.86–£55.64 (Hospital only)

Oxaliplatin [Specialist drug]

26-Aug-2021

● **INDICATIONS AND DOSE**

Colorectal cancer
▸ BY INTRAVENOUS INFUSION
▸ Adult: Specialist drug – access specialist resources for dosing information

● **CONTRA-INDICATIONS** Peripheral neuropathy with functional impairment

● **INTERACTIONS** → Appendix 1: platinum compounds

SIDE-EFFECTS

▶ **Common or very common** Alopecia · anaemia · appetite decreased · arthralgia · asthenia · chills · conjunctivitis · constipation · cough · decreased leucocytes · dehydration · depression · diarrhoea · dizziness · dyspnoea · electrolyte imbalance · embolism and thrombosis · fever · flushing · gastrointestinal discomfort · gastrointestinal disorders · haemorrhage · headache · hiccups · hyperglycaemia · hyperhidrosis · hypersensitivity · hypertension · increased risk of infection · insomnia · meningism · mucositis · nail disorder · nausea · necrosis · nerve disorders · neutropenia · neutropenic sepsis · pain · peripheral neuropathy (dose-limiting) · sensation abnormal · skin reactions · stomatitis · taste altered · thrombocytopenia · urinary disorders · vision disorders · vomiting · weight changes

▶ **Uncommon** Metabolic acidosis · nervousness · ototoxicity

▶ **Rare or very rare** Acute kidney injury · acute tubular necrosis · Clostridioides difficile colitis · deafness · disseminated intravascular coagulation · dysarthria · haemolytic anaemia · hepatic disorders · immuno-allergic thrombocytopenia · interstitial lung disease · nephritis acute interstitial · nodular regenerative hyperplasia · pancreatitis · posterior reversible encephalopathy syndrome (PRES) (with oxaliplatin combination chemotherapy) · pulmonary fibrosis · sinusoidal obstruction syndrome · vision loss (reversible on discontinuation)

▶ **Frequency not known** Autoimmune pancytopenia · chest discomfort · dysphagia · extravasation necrosis · gait abnormal · hypersensitivity vasculitis · movement disorders · muscle complaints · muscle contractions involuntary · QT interval prolongation · respiratory disorders · rhabdomyolysis · throat complaints

SIDE-EFFECTS, FURTHER INFORMATION Neurotoxicity is dose limiting.

Respiratory symptoms If unexplained respiratory symptoms occur, oxaliplatin should be discontinued until investigations exclude interstitial lung disease and pulmonary fibrosis.

● **CONCEPTION AND CONTRACEPTION** Effective contraception required during and for 4 months after treatment in women and 6 months after treatment in men.

● **NATIONAL FUNDING/ACCESS DECISIONS** For full details see funding body website

NICE decisions

▶ **Capecitabine and oxaliplatin in the adjuvant treatment of stage III (Dukes' C) colon cancer (April 2006)** NICE TA100 Recommended

▶ **Irinotecan, oxaliplatin, and raltitrexed for advanced colorectal cancer (August 2005)** NICE TA93 Recommended with restrictions

● **MEDICINAL FORMS** There can be variation in the licensing of different medicines containing the same drug.

Solution for infusion

▶ Oxaliplatin (Non-proprietary)

Oxaliplatin 5 mg per 1 ml Oxaliplatin 50mg/10ml concentrate for solution for infusion vials | 1 vial [PoM] £147.82–£213.80 (Hospital only)
Oxaliplatin 100mg/20ml concentrate for solution for infusion vials | 1 vial [PoM] £289.50–£428.15 (Hospital only)
Oxaliplatin 200mg/40ml concentrate for solution for infusion vials | 1 vial [PoM] £591.26–£856.25 (Hospital only)

ANTINEOPLASTIC DRUGS › PODOPHYLLOTOXIN DERIVATIVES

Etoposide [Specialist drug]   21-Jun-2021

● **INDICATIONS AND DOSE**

Testicular cancer | Small cell lung cancer | Hodgkin's lymphoma | Non-Hodgkin's lymphoma | Acute myeloid leukaemia | Ovarian cancer

▶ BY MOUTH, OR BY INTRAVENOUS INFUSION

▶ Adult: Specialist drug – access specialist resources for dosing information

Gestational trophoblastic neoplasia

▶ BY INTRAVENOUS INFUSION

▶ Adult: Specialist drug – access specialist resources for dosing information

---

IMPORTANT SAFETY INFORMATION

RISKS OF INCORRECT DOSING OF ORAL ANTI-CANCER MEDICINES
See Cytotoxic drugs p. 1027.

● **INTERACTIONS** → Appendix 1: etoposide

● **SIDE-EFFECTS**

GENERAL SIDE-EFFECTS

▶ **Common or very common** Abdominal pain · acute leukaemia · alopecia · anaemia · appetite decreased · arrhythmia · asthenia · bone marrow depression · constipation · diarrhoea · dizziness · hepatotoxicity · hypertension · leucopenia · malaise · mucositis · myocardial infarction · nausea · neutropenia · skin reactions · thrombocytopenia · vomiting

▶ **Uncommon** Nerve disorders

▶ **Rare or very rare** Dysphagia · interstitial pneumonitis · neurotoxicity · pulmonary fibrosis · radiation recall reaction · seizure · severe cutaneous adverse reactions (SCARs) · taste altered · vision loss

SPECIFIC SIDE-EFFECTS

▶ **Common or very common**

▶ With intravenous use Anaphylactic reaction · hypotension · infection

▶ With oral use Oesophagitis · stomatitis · transient systolic hypotension

▶ **Uncommon**

▶ With intravenous use Haemorrhage

▶ **Rare or very rare**

▶ With intravenous use Fever

▶ With oral use Drowsiness

▶ **Frequency not known**

▶ With intravenous use Angioedema · bronchospasm · extravasation necrosis · infertility · tumour lysis syndrome

● **CONCEPTION AND CONTRACEPTION** Contraceptive advice required.

● **MEDICINAL FORMS** There can be variation in the licensing of different medicines containing the same drug.

Solution for infusion

▶ Etoposide (Non-proprietary)

Etoposide 20 mg per 1 ml Etoposide 100mg/5ml concentrate for solution for infusion vials | 1 vial [PoM] £11.50–£21.25 (Hospital only)
Etoposide 500mg/25ml concentrate for solution for infusion vials | 1 vial [PoM] £60.70–£102.69 (Hospital only)

Oral capsule

CAUTIONARY AND ADVISORY LABELS 23

▶ Etoposide (Non-proprietary)

Etoposide 50 mg Etoposide 50mg capsules | 20 capsule [PoM] £194.65 DT = £194.65

Etoposide 100 mg Etoposide 100mg capsules | 10 capsule [PoM] £170.11 DT = £170.11

Powder for solution for injection

▶ Etopophos (Neon Healthcare Ltd)

Etoposide (as Etoposide phosphate) 100 mg Etopophos 100mg powder for solution for injection vials | 10 vial [PoM] £261.68

Immune system and malignant disease

ANTINEOPLASTIC DRUGS > TAXANES

Cabazitaxel [Specialist drug]
02-Nov-2021

- **INDICATIONS AND DOSE**

Prostate cancer
▸ BY INTRAVENOUS INFUSION
▸ Adult: Specialist drug – access specialist resources for dosing information

- **CONTRA-INDICATIONS** Acute porphyrias p. 1202
- **INTERACTIONS** → Appendix 1: taxanes
- **SIDE-EFFECTS**
▸ **Common or very common** Acute kidney injury · alopecia · anaemia · anxiety · appetite decreased · arrhythmias · arthralgia · asthenia · chest pain · chills · confusion · conjunctivitis · constipation · cough · cystitis · deep vein thrombosis · dehydration · diarrhoea · dizziness · dry mouth · dyspnoea · excessive tearing · fever · gastrointestinal discomfort · gastrointestinal disorders · haemorrhage · headache · hydronephrosis · hyperglycaemia · hypersensitivity · hypertension · hypokalaemia · hypotension · increased risk of infection · lethargy · leucopenia · malaise · mucositis · muscle complaints · nausea · nerve disorders · neutropenia · oedema · oropharyngeal pain · pain · pelvic pain · renal colic · renal failure (fatal cases of renal failure reported) · sensation abnormal · sepsis · skin reactions · taste altered · thrombocytopenia · tinnitus · ureteral obstruction · urinary disorders · vasodilation · vertigo · vomiting · weight decreased
▸ **Frequency not known** Interstitial lung disease

SIDE-EFFECTS, FURTHER INFORMATION Manufacturer advises pretreatment with a corticosteroid, antihistamine and histamine H2-receptor antagonist to reduce the risk and severity of hypersensitivity reactions.

- **CONCEPTION AND CONTRACEPTION** Ensure effective contraception during treatment (women) and for up to 6 months after treatment (men).

- **NATIONAL FUNDING/ACCESS DECISIONS**
For full details see funding body website

NICE decisions
▸ Cabazitaxel for hormone-relapsed metastatic prostate cancer treated with docetaxel (updated August 2016) NICE TA391 Recommended with restrictions

Scottish Medicines Consortium (SMC) decisions
▸ Cabazitaxel (*Jevtana*®) in combination with prednisone or prednisolone is indicated for the treatment of adult patients with hormone refractory metastatic prostate cancer previously treated with a docetaxel-containing regimen (December 2016) SMC No. 735/11 Recommended with restrictions

- **MEDICINAL FORMS** There can be variation in the licensing of different medicines containing the same drug.
Solution for infusion
EXCIPIENTS: May contain Ethanol
▸ **Cabazitaxel (Non-proprietary)**
Cabazitaxel (as Cabazitaxel monohydrate) 10 mg per 1 ml Cabazitaxel 45mg/4.5ml concentrate for solution for infusion vials | 1 vial [PoM] £2,772.00–£3,141.60 (Hospital only)
Cabazitaxel 50mg/5ml concentrate for solution for infusion vials | 1 vial [PoM] £3,080.00 (Hospital only)
Cabazitaxel 60mg/6ml concentrate for solution for infusion vials | 1 vial [PoM] £3,141.60–£3,696.00 (Hospital only)
Cabazitaxel 20 mg per 1 ml Cabazitaxel 60mg/3ml concentrate for solution for infusion vials | 1 vial [PoM] £3,326.40–£3,696.00 (Hospital only)
Cabazitaxel 40 mg per 1 ml Cabazitaxel 60mg/1.5ml concentrate and solvent for solution for infusion vials | 1 vial [PoM] £3,696.00–£3,697.00 (Hospital only)

Docetaxel [Specialist drug]
06-Jul-2020

- **INDICATIONS AND DOSE**

Breast cancer | Non-small cell lung cancer | Prostate cancer | Gastric adenocarcinoma | Squamous cell carcinoma of the head and neck
▸ BY INTRAVENOUS INFUSION
▸ Adult: Specialist drug – access specialist resources for dosing information

- **CONTRA-INDICATIONS** Acute porphyrias p. 1202
- **INTERACTIONS** → Appendix 1: taxanes
- **SIDE-EFFECTS**
▸ **Common or very common** Abdominal pain · alopecia · anaemia · appetite decreased · arrhythmia · arthralgia · asthenia · constipation · diarrhoea · dyspnoea · fluid imbalance · haemorrhage · hypersensitivity · hypertension · hypotension · increased risk of infection · myalgia · nail disorders · nausea · neutropenia · pain · peripheral neuropathy · sepsis · skin reactions · stomatitis · taste altered · thrombocytopenia · vomiting
▸ **Uncommon** Gastrointestinal disorders · heart failure
▸ **Frequency not known** Ascites · bone marrow depression · chest tightness · chills · cutaneous lupus erythematosus · disseminated intravascular coagulation · eye disorders · eye inflammation · fever · hearing impairment · hepatitis · hyponatraemia · interstitial lung disease · loss of consciousness · multi organ failure · myocardial infarction · nail discolouration · neurotoxicity · ototoxicity · pericardial effusion · peripheral lymphoedema · peripheral oedema · pulmonary fibrosis · pulmonary oedema · radiation injuries · renal impairment · respiratory disorders · sclerodermal-like changes · seizure · sensation abnormal · severe cutaneous adverse reactions (SCARs) · vasodilation · venous thromboembolism · vision disorders · weight increased

SIDE-EFFECTS, FURTHER INFORMATION Pretreatment with dexamethasone by mouth is recommended for reducing fluid retention and hypersensitivity reactions.

- **CONCEPTION AND CONTRACEPTION** Manufacturer advises effective contraception for men and women during treatment, and for at least 6 months after stopping treatment in men.

- **NATIONAL FUNDING/ACCESS DECISIONS**
For full details see funding body website

NICE decisions
▸ Docetaxel for the treatment of hormone-refractory metastatic prostate cancer (June 2006) NICE TA101 Recommended
▸ Pertuzumab with trastuzumab and docetaxel for treating HER2-positive breast cancer (March 2018) NICE TA509 Recommended with restrictions

- **MEDICINAL FORMS** There can be variation in the licensing of different medicines containing the same drug.
Solution for infusion
EXCIPIENTS: May contain Ethanol
▸ **Docetaxel (Non-proprietary)**
Docetaxel 10 mg per 1 ml Docetaxel 80mg/8ml concentrate for solution for infusion vials | 1 vial [PoM] £534.75 (Hospital only)
Docetaxel 160mg/16ml concentrate for solution for infusion vials | 1 vial [PoM] £1,069.50 (Hospital only)
Docetaxel 20mg/2ml concentrate for solution for infusion vials | 1 vial [PoM] £162.75 (Hospital only)
Docetaxel 20 mg per 1 ml Docetaxel 80mg/4ml concentrate for solution for infusion vials | 1 vial [PoM] £479.06–£504.27 (Hospital only)
Docetaxel 160mg/8ml concentrate for solution for infusion vials | 1 vial [PoM] £950.00–£958.11 (Hospital only)
Docetaxel 20mg/1ml concentrate for solution for infusion vials | 1 vial [PoM] £145.80–£160.00 (Hospital only)

Paclitaxel [Specialist drug]

15-Feb-2022

● **INDICATIONS AND DOSE**

Ovarian cancer [conventional paclitaxel only] | Non-small cell lung cancer [conventional paclitaxel only] | AIDS-related Kaposi's sarcoma [conventional paclitaxel only] | Breast cancer [conventional paclitaxel and albumin-bound paclitaxel] | Pancreatic adenocarcinoma [albumin-bound paclitaxel only]

▸ BY INTRAVENOUS INFUSION

▸ Adult: Specialist drug – access specialist resources for dosing information

DOSE EQUIVALENCE AND CONVERSION

▸ Paclitaxel is available as *conventional* and *albumin-bound* formulations; these formulations are **not** interchangeable.

IMPORTANT SAFETY INFORMATION

MHRA/CHM ADVICE: PACLITAXEL FORMULATIONS (CONVENTIONAL AND NAB-PACLITAXEL): CAUTION REQUIRED DUE TO POTENTIAL FOR MEDICATION ERROR (JANUARY 2022)

The MHRA reminds healthcare professionals that albumin-bound paclitaxel formulations (nab-paclitaxel; brand names *Abraxane®*, *Pazenir®*) differ from conventional paclitaxel formulations and are **not** interchangeable. Healthcare professionals are advised to make a clear distinction between formulations when prescribing, dispensing, administering, and communicating about paclitaxel. The use of brand names is advised for albumin-bound paclitaxel formulations to prevent medication errors. The product name and dose should be verified before administration and product literature followed for preparation and administration.

● **CONTRA-INDICATIONS** Acute porphyrias p. 1202

● **INTERACTIONS** → Appendix 1: taxanes

● **SIDE-EFFECTS**

▸ **Common or very common** Alopecia · anaemia · anxiety · appetite decreased · arrhythmias · arthralgia · asthenia · bone marrow disorders · chest discomfort · chills · constipation · cough · decreased leucocytes · depression · diarrhoea · dizziness · drowsiness · dry eye · dyspnoea · electrolyte imbalance · excessive tearing · extravasation necrosis · eye inflammation · fever · fluid imbalance · gastrointestinal discomfort · gastrointestinal disorders · haemorrhage · headache · hyperpyrexia · hypertension · increased risk of infection · influenza like illness · insomnia · interstitial pneumonitis · laryngeal pain · lymphoedema · malaise · movement disorders · mucositis · muscle complaints · nail discolouration · nail disorders · nasal complaints · nausea · nerve disorders · neutropenia · oedema · oral disorders · pain · performance status decreased · sensation abnormal · skin reactions · taste altered · thrombocytopenia · vasodilation · vertigo · vision disorders · vomiting · weight changes

▸ **Uncommon** Allergic rhinitis · breast pain · catheter related infection · dry mouth · dysphagia · ear pain · embolism and thrombosis · eye discomfort · facial swelling · gait abnormal · hepatomegaly · hoarseness · hyperglycaemia · hypoalbuminaemia · hypoglycaemia · hypotension · limb discomfort · muscle weakness · neoplasm complications · peripheral coldness · photosensitivity reaction · polydipsia · reflexes abnormal · respiratory disorders · sepsis · sweat changes · swelling · syncope · tinnitus · tremor · urinary disorders

▸ **Rare or very rare** Atrioventricular block · cardiac arrest · congestive heart failure · left ventricular dysfunction · radiation injuries · severe cutaneous adverse reactions (SCARs)

SIDE-EFFECTS, FURTHER INFORMATION Manufacturer advises routine premedication with a corticosteroid, an antihistamine and a histamine H2-receptor antagonist is recommended to prevent severe hypersensitivity reactions; hypersensitivity reactions may occur rarely despite premedication.

● **CONCEPTION AND CONTRACEPTION** Ensure effective contraception during and for at least 6 months after treatment in men or women.

● **NATIONAL FUNDING/ACCESS DECISIONS**
For full details see funding body website

NICE decisions

▸ **Guidance on the use of paclitaxel in the treatment of ovarian cancer (updated May 2005)** NICE TA55 Recommended

▸ **Bevacizumab in combination with paclitaxel and carboplatin for the first-line treatment of advanced ovarian cancer (May 2013)** NICE TA284 Not recommended

▸ **Topotecan, pegylated liposomal doxorubicin hydrochloride, paclitaxel, trabectedin and gemcitabine for treating recurrent ovarian cancer (April 2016)** NICE TA389 Recommended

▸ **Paclitaxel as albumin-bound nanoparticles with gemcitabine for untreated metastatic pancreatic cancer (September 2017)** NICE TA476 Recommended with restrictions

Scottish Medicines Consortium (SMC) decisions

▸ **Paclitaxel albumin (*Abraxane®*) for the treatment of metastatic breast cancer (April 2010)** SMC No. 556/09 Recommended with restrictions

▸ **Paclitaxel albumin (*Abraxane®*) in combination with gemcitabine for the first-line treatment of adult patients with metastatic adenocarcinoma of the pancreas (February 2015)** SMC No. 968/14 Recommended

---

● **MEDICINAL FORMS** There can be variation in the licensing of different medicines containing the same drug.

Solution for infusion

EXCIPIENTS: May contain Polyoxyl castor oils

▸ **Paclitaxel (Non-proprietary)**

Paclitaxel 6 mg per 1 ml Paclitaxel 150mg/25ml concentrate for solution for infusion vials | 1 vial PoM £300.52–£704.37 (Hospital only)

Paclitaxel 30mg/5ml concentrate for solution for infusion vials | 1 vial PoM £66.85–£156.68 (Hospital only)

Paclitaxel 100mg/16.7ml concentrate for solution for infusion vials | 1 vial PoM £200.35–£469.59 (Hospital only)

Paclitaxel 300mg/50ml concentrate for solution for infusion vials | 1 vial PoM £601.03–£1,408.74 (Hospital only)

ANTINEOPLASTIC DRUGS > TOPOISOMERASE I INHIBITORS

Irinotecan hydrochloride [Specialist drug]

26-Aug-2020

● **INDICATIONS AND DOSE**

Colorectal cancer

▸ BY INTRAVENOUS INFUSION

▸ Adult: Specialist drug – access specialist resources for dosing information

Adenocarcinoma of the pancreas

▸ BY INTRAVENOUS INFUSION USING LIPID FORMULATION

▸ Adult: Specialist drug – access specialist resources for dosing information

continued →

DOSE EQUIVALENCE AND CONVERSION
▶ Irinotecan is available as *conventional* and *liposomal* formulations; these formulations are **not** interchangeable.

IMPORTANT SAFETY INFORMATION
MHRA/CHM ADVICE: *ONIVYDE*® (IRINOTECAN, LIPOSOMAL FORMULATIONS): REPORTS OF SERIOUS AND FATAL THROMBOEMBOLIC EVENTS (MARCH 2019)
Onivyde® has been associated with reports of serious thromboembolic events, such as pulmonary embolism, venous thrombosis, and arterial thromboembolism. Healthcare professionals are advised to obtain a thorough medical history to identify patients with multiple risk factors. Patients should be advised to seek medical advice immediately if signs or symptoms of thromboembolism occur, such as sudden pain and swelling in a leg or an arm, sudden onset of coughing, chest pain or difficulty breathing.

MHRA/CHM ADVICE: LIPOSOMAL AND LIPID-COMPLEX FORMULATIONS: NAME CHANGE TO REDUCE MEDICATION ERRORS (JULY 2020)
Serious harm and fatal overdoses have occurred following confusion between liposomal, pegylated-liposomal, lipid-complex, and conventional formulations of the same drug substance. Medicines with these formulations will explicitly include 'liposomal', 'pegylated-liposomal', or 'lipid-complex' within their name to reduce the risk of potentially fatal medication errors.

The MHRA reminds healthcare professionals that liposomal, pegylated-liposomal, lipid-complex, and conventional formulations containing the same drug substance are **not** interchangeable. Healthcare professionals are advised to make a clear distinction between formulations when prescribing, dispensing, administering, and communicating about irinotecan. The product name and dose should be verified before administration and the maximum dose should not be exceeded.

● **CONTRA-INDICATIONS** Bowel obstruction · chronic inflammatory bowel disease

● **INTERACTIONS** → Appendix 1: irinotecan

● **SIDE-EFFECTS**
▶ **Common or very common** Alopecia · anaemia (dose-limiting) · appetite decreased · asthenia · cholinergic syndrome · constipation · decreased leucocytes · diarrhoea (delayed diarrhoea requires prompt treatment) · dizziness · dysphonia · dyspnoea · electrolyte imbalance · embolism and thrombosis · febrile neutropenia (dose-limiting) · fever · fluid imbalance · gastrointestinal discomfort · gastrointestinal disorders · hypoalbuminaemia · hypoglycaemia · hypotension · increased risk of infection · infusion related reaction · insomnia · mucositis · nausea · neutropenia (dose-limiting) · oedema · renal impairment · sepsis · stomatitis · taste altered · thrombocytopenia (dose-limiting) · vomiting · weight decreased
▶ **Uncommon** Hypersensitivity · hypoxia · nail discolouration · skin reactions
▶ **Frequency not known** Circulatory collapse · Clostridioides difficile colitis · gastrointestinal haemorrhage · hiccups · hypertension · interstitial lung disease · muscle cramps · paraesthesia · pseudomembranous enterocolitis · speech disorder · ulcerative colitis

● **CONCEPTION AND CONTRACEPTION** For *conventional* formulations, manufacturer advises effective contraception during treatment and for up to 1 month after treatment in women of child-bearing potential, and up to 3 months after treatment in men. For *liposomal* formulations, manufacturer advises effective

contraception during treatment and for up to 1 month after treatment in women of child-bearing potential, and up to 4 months after treatment in men.

● **PATIENT AND CARER ADVICE**
Driving and skilled tasks Manufacturer advises patients and carers should be counselled on the effects on driving and performance of skilled tasks—increased risk of dizziness and visual disturbances within 24 hours of administration.

● **NATIONAL FUNDING/ACCESS DECISIONS**
For full details see funding body website
NICE decisions
▶ **Pegylated liposomal irinotecan for treating pancreatic cancer after gemcitabine (April 2017)** NICE TA440 Not recommended
Scottish Medicines Consortium (SMC) decisions
▶ **Liposomal irinotecan (*Onivyde*®) for treatment of metastatic adenocarcinoma of the pancreas, in combination with fluorouracil (5-FU) and leucovorin (folinic acid), in adult patients who have progressed following gemcitabine based therapy (March 2017)** SMC No. 1217/17 Not recommended

● **MEDICINAL FORMS** There can be variation in the licensing of different medicines containing the same drug.
Solution for infusion
EXCIPIENTS: May contain Sorbitol
▶ **Irinotecan hydrochloride (Non-proprietary)**
Irinotecan hydrochloride trihydrate 20 mg per 1 ml Irinotecan 500mg/25ml concentrate for solution for infusion vials | 1 vial [PoM] £600.00–£867.29 (Hospital only)
Irinotecan 40mg/2ml concentrate for solution for infusion vials | 1 vial [PoM] £49.03–£54.06 (Hospital only)
Irinotecan 300mg/15ml concentrate for solution for infusion vials | 1 vial [PoM] £370.50–£455.87 (Hospital only)
Irinotecan 100mg/5ml concentrate for solution for infusion vials | 1 vial [PoM] £120.25–£151.97 (Hospital only)
▶ **Campto** (Pfizer Ltd)
Irinotecan hydrochloride trihydrate 20 mg per 1 ml Campto 100mg/5ml concentrate for solution for infusion vials | 1 vial [PoM] £130.00 (Hospital only)
Campto 40mg/2ml concentrate for solution for infusion vials | 1 vial [PoM] £53.00 (Hospital only)
Campto 300mg/15ml concentrate for solution for infusion vials | 1 vial [PoM] £390.00 (Hospital only)
Dispersion for infusion
ELECTROLYTES: May contain Sodium
▶ **Onivyde** (Servier Laboratories Ltd)
Irinotecan (as Irinotecan sucrosofate salt pegylated liposomal) 4.3 mg per 1 ml Onivyde pegylated liposomal 43mg/10ml concentrate for dispersion for infusion vials | 1 vial [PoM] £615.35 (Hospital only)

Topotecan [Specialist drug]

17-Sep-2021

● **INDICATIONS AND DOSE**
Ovarian cancer | Cervical carcinoma
▶ BY INTRAVENOUS INFUSION
▶ Adult: Specialist drug – access specialist resources for dosing information
Small-cell lung cancer
▶ BY INTRAVENOUS INFUSION, OR BY MOUTH
▶ Adult: Specialist drug – access specialist resources for dosing information

IMPORTANT SAFETY INFORMATION
RISKS OF INCORRECT DOSING OF ORAL ANTI-CANCER MEDICINES
See Cytotoxic drugs p. 1027.

● **INTERACTIONS** → Appendix 1: topotecan

● **SIDE-EFFECTS**
▶ **Common or very common** Alopecia · anaemia · appetite decreased · asthenia · colitis neutropenic · constipation · diarrhoea · fever · gastrointestinal discomfort · hyperbilirubinaemia · hypersensitivity · infection · leucopenia · malaise · mucositis · nausea · neutropenia ·

pancytopenia · sepsis · skin reactions · thrombocytopenia · vomiting
▶ **Rare or very rare** Angioedema · interstitial lung disease
▶ **Frequency not known** Bone marrow depression (dose-limiting) · haemorrhage

● **CONCEPTION AND CONTRACEPTION** Contraceptive advice required.

● **NATIONAL FUNDING/ACCESS DECISIONS**
For full details see funding body website
NICE decisions
▶ Topotecan for the treatment of recurrent and stage IVB cervical cancer (October 2009) NICE TA183 Recommended
▶ Topotecan for the treatment of relapsed small-cell lung cancer (November 2009) NICE TA184 Recommended
▶ Topotecan, pegylated liposomal doxorubicin hydrochloride, paclitaxel, trabectedin and gemcitabine for treating recurrent ovarian cancer (April 2016) NICE TA389 Not recommended
Scottish Medicines Consortium (SMC) decisions
▶ Topotecan (*Hycamtin*®) in combination with cisplatin for patients with carcinoma of the cervix recurrent after radiotherapy and for patients with stage IVB disease (December 2007) SMC No. 421/07 Recommended with restrictions

● **MEDICINAL FORMS** There can be variation in the licensing of different medicines containing the same drug.
Solution for infusion
▶ Topotecan (Non-proprietary)
Topotecan (as Topotecan hydrochloride) 1 mg per 1 ml　Topotecan 4mg/4ml concentrate for solution for infusion vials | 1 vial PoM £290.00 | 5 vial PoM £1,453.10 (Hospital only)
Topotecan 1mg/1ml concentrate for solution for infusion vials | 1 vial PoM £97.00
Oral capsule
CAUTIONARY AND ADVISORY LABELS 25
▶ Hycamtin (Sandoz Ltd)
Topotecan (as Topotecan hydrochloride)
250 microgram　Hycamtin 0.25mg capsules | 10 capsule PoM £75.00 (Hospital only)
Topotecan (as Topotecan hydrochloride) 1 mg　Hycamtin 1mg capsules | 10 capsule PoM £360.00 (Hospital only)

ANTINEOPLASTIC DRUGS > VINCA ALKALOIDS

Vinblastine sulfate [Specialist drug]

02-Jul-2020

● **INDICATIONS AND DOSE**
Variety of cancers including leukaemias, lymphomas, and some solid tumours (e.g. breast and lung cancer)
▶ BY INTRAVENOUS INJECTION
▶ Adult: Specialist drug – access specialist resources for dosing information

---

IMPORTANT SAFETY INFORMATION
Vinblastine is for **intravenous administration only**. Inadvertent intrathecal administration can cause severe neurotoxicity, which is usually fatal.
　The National Patient Safety Agency has advised (August 2008) that adult and teenage patients treated in an adult or adolescent unit should receive their vinca alkaloid dose in a 50 mL minibag. Teenagers and children treated in a child unit may receive their vinca alkaloid dose in a syringe.

● **CONTRA-INDICATIONS** Intrathecal injection **contra-indicated**.
● **INTERACTIONS** → Appendix 1: vinca alkaloids
● **SIDE-EFFECTS**
▶ **Rare or very rare** Hearing impairment · nerve disorders · vestibular damage

▶ **Frequency not known** Abdominal pain · alopecia (reversible) · anaemia · appetite decreased · asthenia · balance impaired · cancer pain · constipation · depression · diarrhoea · dizziness · dyspnoea · haemorrhage · headache · hypertension · ileus · increased risk of infection · leucopenia (dose-limiting) · malaise · myalgia · myocardial infarction · nausea · nystagmus · oral blistering · pain · Raynaud's phenomenon · reflexes absent · respiratory disorders · seizure · sensation abnormal · SIADH · skin reactions · stroke · thrombocytopenia · vertigo · vomiting

● **CONCEPTION AND CONTRACEPTION** Contraceptive advice required.

● **MEDICINAL FORMS** There can be variation in the licensing of different medicines containing the same drug.
Solution for injection
▶ Vinblastine sulfate (Non-proprietary)
Vinblastine sulfate 1 mg per 1 ml　Vinblastine 10mg/10ml solution for injection vials | 5 vial PoM £85.00 (Hospital only)

Vincristine sulfate [Specialist drug]　03-Jul-2020

● **INDICATIONS AND DOSE**
Leukaemias | Lymphomas | Solid tumours [including breast cancer and lung cancer]
▶ BY INTRAVENOUS INJECTION, OR BY INTRAVENOUS INFUSION
▶ Adult: Specialist drug – access specialist resources for dosing information

---

IMPORTANT SAFETY INFORMATION
Vincristine injections are for **intravenous administration only**. Inadvertent intrathecal administration can cause severe neurotoxicity, which is usually fatal.
　The National Patient Safety Agency has advised (August 2008) that adult and teenage patients treated in an adult or adolescent unit should receive their vinca alkaloid dose in a 50 mL minibag. Teenagers and children treated in a child unit may receive their vinca alkaloid dose in a syringe.

● **CONTRA-INDICATIONS** Intrathecal injection **contra-indicated**.
● **INTERACTIONS** → Appendix 1: vinca alkaloids
● **SIDE-EFFECTS**
▶ **Rare or very rare** Hypersensitivity · rash · SIADH
▶ **Frequency not known** Abdominal cramps · adrenal disorder · alopecia · anaemia · appetite decreased · azotaemia · bladder atony · bronchospasm · connective tissue disorders · constipation · coronary artery disease · dehydration · diarrhoea · dizziness · dyspnoea · eighth cranial nerve damage · eye disorders · fever · gait abnormalities · gastrointestinal disorders · haemolytic anaemia · headache · hearing impairment · hypertension · hyponatraemia · hypotension · infection · leucopenia · movement disorders · muscle atrophy · myalgia · myocardial infarction · nausea · neuromuscular effects (dose-limiting) · neutropenia · oedema · oral ulceration · pain · paralysis · paresis · reflexes absent · renal disorder · secondary malignancy · sensation abnormal · sepsis · throat pain · thrombocytopenia · urinary disorders · vertigo · vestibular damage · vision loss · vomiting · weight decreased

SIDE-EFFECTS, FURTHER INFORMATION **Bronchospasm** Severe bronchospasm following administration is more common when used in combination with mitomycin-C.
　Neurotoxicity Sensory and motor neuropathies are common and are cumulative. Manufacturer advises monitoring patients for symptoms of neuropathy, such as hypoesthesia, hyperesthesia, paresthesia, hyporeflexia, areflexia, neuralgia, jaw pain, decreased vibratory sense, cranial neuropathy, ileus, burning sensation, arthralgia,

myalgia, muscle spasm, or weakness, both before and during treatment—requires dose reduction, treatment interruption or treatment discontinuation, depending on severity.

Motor weakness can also occur and dose reduction or discontinuation of therapy may be appropriate if motor weakness increases. Recovery from neurotoxic effects is usually slow but complete.

● CONCEPTION AND CONTRACEPTION Contraceptive advice required.

● MEDICINAL FORMS There can be variation in the licensing of different medicines containing the same drug.
Solution for injection
  ▸ Vincristine sulfate (Non-proprietary)
    Vincristine sulfate 1 mg per 1 ml Vincristine 1mg/1ml solution for injection vials | 1 vial [PoM] £13.47 (Hospital only) | 5 vial [PoM] £67.35 (Hospital only)
    Vincristine 2mg/2ml solution for injection vials | 1 vial [PoM] £26.66 (Hospital only) | 5 vial [PoM] £133.30 (Hospital only)

Vindesine sulfate [Specialist drug]
03-Jul-2020

● INDICATIONS AND DOSE
Variety of cancers including leukaemias, lymphomas, and some solid tumours (e.g. breast and lung cancer)
  ▸ BY INTRAVENOUS INJECTION
  ▸ Adult: Specialist drug – access specialist resources for dosing information

IMPORTANT SAFETY INFORMATION
Vindesine injections are for **intravenous administration only**. Inadvertent intrathecal administration can cause severe neurotoxicity, which is usually fatal.

The National Patient Safety Agency has advised (August 2008) that adult and teenage patients treated in an adult or adolescent unit should receive their vinca alkaloid dose in a 50 mL minibag. Teenagers and children treated in a child unit may receive their vinca alkaloid dose in a syringe.

● CONTRA-INDICATIONS Intrathecal injection **contra-indicated**.

● INTERACTIONS → Appendix 1: vinca alkaloids

● SIDE-EFFECTS
  ▸ **Common or very common** Alopecia
  ▸ **Frequency not known** Anaemia · appetite decreased · asthenia · balance impaired · cellulitis · chills · constipation · depression · diarrhoea · dizziness · dysphagia · fever · gastrointestinal discomfort · gastrointestinal disorders · granulocytopenia (dose-limiting) · headache · hearing impairment · malaise · nausea · nerve disorders · nystagmus · oral disorders · pain · peroneal nerve palsy · rash maculopapular · reflexes absent · seizure · sensation abnormal · thrombocytopenia · thrombocytosis · vertigo · vestibular damage · vision loss · vomiting

SIDE-EFFECTS, FURTHER INFORMATION Neurotoxicity, usually as peripheral or autonomic neuropathy; it occurs less often with vindesine than with vincristine. Patients with neurotoxicity commonly have peripheral paraesthesia, loss of deep tendon reflexes; and ototoxicity has been reported. There have been instances in which neurotoxicity has made it necessary to reduce the dosage or temporarily discontinue use of vindesine.

● CONCEPTION AND CONTRACEPTION Contraceptive advice required.

● MEDICINAL FORMS There can be variation in the licensing of different medicines containing the same drug.
Powder for solution for injection
  ▸ Eldisine (Genus Pharmaceuticals Ltd)
    Vindesine sulfate 5 mg Eldisine 5mg powder for solution for injection vials | 1 vial [PoM] £78.30 (Hospital only)

Vinorelbine [Specialist drug]
04-Jul-2020

● INDICATIONS AND DOSE
Breast cancer | Non-small cell lung cancer
  ▸ BY MOUTH, OR BY INTRAVENOUS INJECTION, OR BY INTRAVENOUS INFUSION
  ▸ Adult: Specialist drug – access specialist resources for dosing information

IMPORTANT SAFETY INFORMATION
Vinorelbine injections are for **intravenous administration only**. Inadvertent intrathecal administration can cause severe neurotoxicity, which is usually fatal.

The National Patient Safety Agency has advised (August 2008) that adult and teenage patients treated in an adult or adolescent unit should receive their vinca alkaloid dose in a 50 mL minibag. Teenagers and children treated in a child unit may receive their vinca alkaloid dose in a syringe.

RISKS OF INCORRECT DOSING OF ORAL ANTI-CANCER MEDICINES See Cytotoxic drugs p. 1027.

● CONTRA-INDICATIONS
GENERAL CONTRA-INDICATIONS Concurrent radiotherapy if treating the liver
SPECIFIC CONTRA-INDICATIONS
  ▸ With oral use Long-term oxygen therapy · previous significant surgical resection of small bowel · previous significant surgical resection of stomach
CONTRA-INDICATIONS, FURTHER INFORMATION Intrathecal injection **contra-indicated**.

● INTERACTIONS → Appendix 1: vinca alkaloids

● SIDE-EFFECTS
GENERAL SIDE-EFFECTS
  ▸ **Common or very common** Alopecia · anaemia · appetite decreased · arthralgia · bone marrow depression (dose-limiting) · constipation · diarrhoea · dyspnoea · fever · hypertension · hypotension · increased risk of infection · leucopenia · myalgia · nausea · neutropenia (dose-limiting) · pain · reflexes absent · stomatitis · thrombocytopenia · vomiting
  ▸ **Uncommon** Bronchospasm · flushing · peripheral coldness · sepsis
  ▸ **Rare or very rare** Circulatory collapse · hyponatraemia · interstitial lung disease · myocardial infarction · pancreatitis
  ▸ **Frequency not known** SIADH
SPECIFIC SIDE-EFFECTS
  ▸ **Common or very common**
  ▸ With intravenous use Asthenia · cancer pain · chest pain · muscle weakness in legs · nervous system disorder · vein discolouration
  ▸ With oral use Abdominal pain · chills · cough · dizziness · dysphagia · dysuria · fatigue · gastrointestinal disorders · headache · insomnia · liver disorder · neuromuscular disorders · sensory disorder · skin eruption · taste altered · urogenital disorder · vision disorder · weight changes
  ▸ **Uncommon**
  ▸ With intravenous use Paraesthesia
  ▸ With oral use Ataxia

▶ **Rare or very rare**
▶ With intravenous use Arrhythmias · ischaemic heart disease · necrosis · palpitations · paralytic ileus · skin reactions
▶ **Frequency not known**
▶ With intravenous use Febrile neutropenia
▶ With oral use Gastrointestinal haemorrhage · hypersensitivity

SIDE-EFFECTS, FURTHER INFORMATION **Bronchospasm** Severe bronchospasm following administration of the vinca alkaloids is more common when used in combination with mitomycin-C.
   Neurotoxicity Neurotoxicity reported in clinical trials, most commonly as constipation, paresthesia, hypersthesia, and hyporeflexia.

● CONCEPTION AND CONTRACEPTION Manufacturer advises effective contraception during and for 3 months after treatment; men must avoid fathering a child during and for at least 3 months after treatment.

● MEDICINAL FORMS There can be variation in the licensing of different medicines containing the same drug.
Solution for infusion
▶ Vinorelbine (Non-proprietary)
   Vinorelbine (as Vinorelbine tartrate) 10 mg per 1 ml Vinorelbine 50mg/5ml concentrate for solution for infusion vials | 1 vial [PoM] £139.00 (Hospital only) | 10 vial [PoM] £1,539.80 (Hospital only)
   Vinorelbine 10mg/1ml concentrate for solution for infusion vials | 1 vial [PoM] £29.00 (Hospital only) | 10 vial [PoM] £329.50 (Hospital only)
▶ Navelbine (Pierre Fabre Ltd)
   Vinorelbine (as Vinorelbine tartrate) 10 mg per 1 ml Navelbine 10mg/1ml concentrate for solution for infusion vials | 10 vial [PoM] £297.45 (Hospital only)
   Navelbine 50mg/5ml concentrate for solution for infusion vials | 10 vial [PoM] £1,399.79 (Hospital only)
Oral capsule
CAUTIONARY AND ADVISORY LABELS 21, 25
▶ Vinorelbine (Non-proprietary)
   Vinorelbine (as Vinorelbine tartrate) 20 mg Vinorelbine 20mg capsules | 1 capsule [PoM] £41.68-£43.98 (Hospital only)
   Vinorelbine (as Vinorelbine tartrate) 30 mg Vinorelbine 30mg capsules | 1 capsule [PoM] £62.68-£65.98 (Hospital only)
   Vinorelbine (as Vinorelbine tartrate) 80 mg Vinorelbine 80mg capsules | 1 capsule [PoM] £167.12-£175.92 (Hospital only)
▶ Navelbine (Pierre Fabre Ltd)
   Vinorelbine (as Vinorelbine tartrate) 20 mg Navelbine 20mg capsules | 1 capsule [PoM] £43.98 (Hospital only)
   Vinorelbine (as Vinorelbine tartrate) 30 mg Navelbine 30mg capsules | 1 capsule [PoM] £65.98 (Hospital only)
   Vinorelbine (as Vinorelbine tartrate) 80 mg Navelbine 80mg capsules | 1 capsule [PoM] £175.92 (Hospital only)

ANTINEOPLASTIC DRUGS ＞ OTHER

Amsacrine [Specialist drug]
15-Nov-2018

● **INDICATIONS AND DOSE**
Acute leukaemia
▶ BY INTRAVENOUS INFUSION
▶ Adult: Specialist drug – access specialist resources for dosing information

● INTERACTIONS → Appendix 1: amsacrine
● SIDE-EFFECTS
▶ **Common or very common** Abdominal pain · alopecia · arrhythmias · bone marrow disorders · cardiotoxicity · congestive heart failure · diarrhoea · dyspnoea · emotional lability · fever · generalised tonic-clonic seizure · haemorrhage · hepatic disorders · hypokalaemia · hypotension · infection · nausea · necrosis · skin reactions · stomatitis · thrombocytopenia · vomiting
▶ **Rare or very rare** Anaemia · cardiomyopathy · confusion · dizziness · granulocytopenia · headache · lethargy · leucopenia · numbness · peripheral neuropathy ·

proteinuria · renal impairment · visual impairment · weight changes
▶ **Frequency not known** Cardiac arrest · hyperuricaemia
● CONCEPTION AND CONTRACEPTION Manufacturer advises effective contraception during and for 3 months after treatment in women of child-bearing potential, and during and for 6 months after treatment in men.

● MEDICINAL FORMS No licensed medicines listed.

Arsenic trioxide [Specialist drug]
10-Nov-2021

● **INDICATIONS AND DOSE**
Acute promyelocytic leukaemia
▶ BY INTRAVENOUS INFUSION
▶ Adult: Specialist drug – access specialist resources for dosing information

● INTERACTIONS → Appendix 1: arsenic trioxide
● SIDE-EFFECTS
▶ **Common or very common** Abdominal pain · alveolar haemorrhage · anaemia · arrhythmias · arthralgia · chest pain · chills · diarrhoea · differentiation syndrome · dizziness · dyspnoea · electrolyte imbalance · fatigue · fever · headache · hyperbilirubinaemia · hyperglycaemia · hypotension · hypoxia · increased leucocytes · increased risk of infection · ketoacidosis · myalgia · nausea · neutropenia · oedema · pain · pancytopenia · paraesthesia · pericardial effusion · QT interval prolongation · renal failure · respiratory disorders · seizure · skin reactions · thrombocytopenia · vasculitis · vision blurred · vomiting · weight increased
▶ **Frequency not known** Confusion · decreased leucocytes · encephalopathy · fluid imbalance · heart failure · hepatotoxicity · peripheral neuropathy · pneumonitis · sepsis

SIDE-EFFECTS, FURTHER INFORMATION Signs and symptoms of differentiation syndrome (leucocyte activation syndrome) include unexplained fever, dyspnoea, weight gain, pulmonary infiltrates, pleural or pericardial effusions, with or without leucocytosis—treat with high dose corticosteroids, consult product literature.

● CONCEPTION AND CONTRACEPTION Manufacturer advises effective contraception during treatment in men and women.

● **NATIONAL FUNDING/ACCESS DECISIONS**
For full details see funding body website
NICE decisions
▶ Arsenic trioxide for treating acute promyelocytic leukaemia (June 2018) NICE TA526 Recommended
Scottish Medicines Consortium (SMC) decisions
▶ Arsenic trioxide (*Trisenox*®) for newly diagnosed, low-to-intermediate risk acute promyelocytic leukaemia (July 2019) SMC No. SMC2181 Recommended

● MEDICINAL FORMS There can be variation in the licensing of different medicines containing the same drug.
Solution for infusion
▶ Arsenic trioxide (Non-proprietary)
   Arsenic trioxide 1 mg per 1 ml Arsenic 10mg/10ml concentrate for solution for infusion vials | 10 vial [PoM] £2,700.00 (Hospital only)
   Arsenic 20mg/20ml concentrate for solution for infusion vials | 5 vial [PoM] £945.00 (Hospital only)
   Arsenic 10mg/10ml concentrate for solution for infusion ampoules | 10 ampoule [PoM] £2,920.00 (Hospital only)
▶ Trisenox (Teva UK Ltd)
   Arsenic trioxide 2 mg per 1 ml Trisenox 12mg/6ml concentrate for solution for infusion vials | 10 vial [PoM] £2,480.00 (Hospital only)

Asparaginase [Specialist drug]

03-Nov-2020

- **INDICATIONS AND DOSE**

Acute lymphoblastic leukaemia
- ▸ BY INTRAVENOUS INFUSION
- ▸ Adult: Specialist drug – access specialist resources for dosing information

---

IMPORTANT SAFETY INFORMATION
Resuscitation facilities should be available during administration.

- **CONTRA-INDICATIONS** History of pancreatitis related to asparaginase therapy · history of serious haemorrhage related to asparaginase therapy · history of serious thrombosis related to asparaginase therapy · pancreatitis · pre-existing known coagulopathy
- **INTERACTIONS** → Appendix 1: asparaginase
- **SIDE-EFFECTS**
- ▸ **Common or very common** Agitation · anaemia · angioedema · appetite decreased · arthralgia · bronchospasm · coagulation disorders · confusion · depression · diarrhoea · dizziness · drowsiness · dyspnoea · embolism and thrombosis · fatigue · flushing · gastrointestinal discomfort · haemorrhage · hallucination · hyperglycaemia · hypersensitivity · hypoalbuminaemia · hypoglycaemia · hypotension · increased risk of infection · leucopenia · nausea · neurological effects · oedema · pain · pancreatitis acute · skin reactions · thrombocytopenia · vomiting · weight decreased
- ▸ **Uncommon** Headache · hyperammonaemia · hyperuricaemia
- ▸ **Rare or very rare** Coma · consciousness impaired · diabetic ketoacidosis · hepatic disorders · hyperparathyroidism · hypoparathyroidism · ischaemic stroke · necrotising pancreatitis · pancreatic pseudocyst · pancreatitis (sometimes fatal) · posterior reversible encephalopathy syndrome (PRES) · secondary hypothyroidism · seizure · tremor

SIDE-EFFECTS, FURTHER INFORMATION There have been rare reports of cholestasis, icterus, hepatic cell necrosis and hepatic failure with fatal outcome; manufacturer advises interrupt treatment if these symptoms develop.

- **CONCEPTION AND CONTRACEPTION** Manufacturer advises effective contraception in men and women of child-bearing potential during treatment and for at least 3 months after last dose; asparaginase may reduce effectiveness of oral contraceptives—additional precautions (e.g. barrier method) are required.
- **PATIENT AND CARER ADVICE**
Driving and skilled tasks Manufacturer advises asparaginase has moderate influence on driving and performance of skilled tasks—increased risk of dizziness and somnolence.
- **NATIONAL FUNDING/ACCESS DECISIONS**
For full details see funding body website
Scottish Medicines Consortium (SMC) decisions
- ▸ Asparaginase (*Spectrila*®) as a component of antineoplastic combination therapy for the treatment of acute lymphoblastic leukaemia in paediatric patients from birth to 18 years and adult patients (April 2018) SMC No. 1319/18 Recommended

---

- **MEDICINAL FORMS** There can be variation in the licensing of different medicines containing the same drug.
Powder for solution for infusion
- ▸ Spectrila (medac UK)
Asparaginase 10000 unit Spectrila 10,000unit powder for concentrate for solution for infusion vials | 1 vial PoM £450.00 (Hospital only)

Crisantaspase [Specialist drug]

07-Aug-2020

- **INDICATIONS AND DOSE**

Acute lymphoblastic leukaemia
- ▸ BY INTRAVENOUS INFUSION, OR BY INTRAMUSCULAR INJECTION
- ▸ Adult: Specialist drug – access specialist resources for dosing information

---

IMPORTANT SAFETY INFORMATION
Resuscitation facilities should be available during administration.

- **CONTRA-INDICATIONS** History of pancreatitis related to asparaginase therapy
- **INTERACTIONS** → Appendix 1: crisantaspase
- **SIDE-EFFECTS**
- ▸ **Common or very common** Chills · coagulation disorders · confusion · diarrhoea · dizziness · drowsiness · dyspnoea · face oedema · fever · headache · hepatic disorders · hypersensitivity · limb swelling · lip swelling · neurotoxicity · pain · pallor · pancreatitis · seizures · skin reactions · thrombosis
- ▸ **Uncommon** Diabetic ketoacidosis · hyperglycaemia · hyperlipidaemia · hypoxia · increased risk of infection · respiratory disorders
- ▸ **Rare or very rare** Arthritis reactive · coma · dysphagia · dysphasia · encephalopathy · haemorrhage · level of consciousness decreased · myalgia · myocardial infarction · necrotising pancreatitis · neutropenia · paresis · sepsis · thrombocytopenia
- ▸ **Frequency not known** Abdominal pain · flushing · hyperammonaemia · hypertension · hypotension · nausea · pseudocyst · vomiting
- **CONCEPTION AND CONTRACEPTION** Contraceptive advice required.
- **MEDICINAL FORMS** There can be variation in the licensing of different medicines containing the same drug.
Powder for solution for injection
- ▸ Erwinase (Porton Biopharma Ltd)
Crisantaspase 10000 unit Erwinase 10,000unit powder for solution for injection vials | 5 vial PoM £3,822.50 (Hospital only)

Eribulin [Specialist drug]

25-Aug-2021

- **INDICATIONS AND DOSE**

Breast cancer
- ▸ BY INTRAVENOUS INJECTION
- ▸ Adult: Specialist drug – access specialist resources for dosing information

- **CONTRA-INDICATIONS** Congenital long QT syndrome
- **INTERACTIONS** → Appendix 1: eribulin
- **SIDE-EFFECTS**
- ▸ **Common or very common** Alopecia · anaemia · appetite decreased · arthralgia · asthenia · chest pain · chills · conjunctivitis · constipation · cough · decreased leucocytes · dehydration · depression · diarrhoea · dizziness · dry mouth · dyspnoea · dysuria · electrolyte imbalance · embolism and thrombosis · excessive tearing · fever · gastrointestinal discomfort · gastrooesophageal reflux disease · haemorrhage · headache · hot flush · hyperbilirubinaemia · hyperglycaemia · increased risk of infection · influenza like illness · insomnia · lethargy · mucositis · muscle complaints · muscle weakness · nail disorder · nausea · nerve disorders · neurotoxicity · neutropenia · oral disorders · oropharyngeal pain · pain · peripheral oedema · rhinorrhoea · sensation abnormal · skin reactions · sweat changes · tachycardia · taste altered ·

thrombocytopenia · tinnitus · vertigo · vomiting · weight decreased

▸ **Uncommon** Angioedema · hepatotoxicity · interstitial lung disease · pancreatitis · proteinuria · renal failure · sepsis
▸ **Rare or very rare** Disseminated intravascular coagulation
▸ **Frequency not known** QT interval prolongation · severe cutaneous adverse reactions (SCARs)

● CONCEPTION AND CONTRACEPTION Ensure effective contraception during and for up to 3 months after treatment in men or women.

● NATIONAL FUNDING/ACCESS DECISIONS
For full details see funding body website
NICE decisions
▸ **Eribulin for treating locally advanced or metastatic breast cancer after 2 or more chemotherapy regimens (December 2016)** NICE TA423 Recommended with restrictions
▸ **Eribulin for treating locally advanced or metastatic breast cancer after 1 chemotherapy regimen (March 2018)** NICE TA515 Not recommended
Scottish Medicines Consortium (SMC) decisions
▸ **Eribulin (*Halaven*®) for the treatment of adult patients with locally advanced or metastatic breast cancer who have progressed after at least one chemotherapeutic regimen for advanced disease (March 2016)** SMC No. 1065/15 Recommended with restrictions

● MEDICINAL FORMS There can be variation in the licensing of different medicines containing the same drug.
Solution for injection
EXCIPIENTS: May contain Ethanol
▸ Eribulin (Non-proprietary)
Eribulin (as Eribulin mesilate) 440 microgram per 1 ml Eribulin 880micrograms/2ml solution for injection vials | 1 vial [PoM] £324.90-£361.00 (Hospital only)
▸ Halaven (Eisai Ltd)
Eribulin (as Eribulin mesilate) 440 microgram per 1 ml Halaven 0.88mg/2ml solution for injection vials | 1 vial [PoM] £361.00 (Hospital only)

Hydroxycarbamide
04-Sep-2020

(Hydroxyurea)

● INDICATIONS AND DOSE

Polycythaemia vera (specialist use only) | Essential thrombocythaemia (specialist use only) | Chronic myeloid leukaemia (specialist use only)
▸ BY MOUTH
▸ Adult: Specialist indication – access specialist resources for dosing information

HYDREA ®

Chronic myeloid leukaemia (specialist use only) | Cancer of the cervix (specialist use only)
▸ BY MOUTH
▸ Adult: Specialist indication – access specialist resources for dosing information

SIKLOS ®

Sickle-cell disease [prevention of recurrent vaso-occlusive crises] (initiated by a specialist)
▸ BY MOUTH
▸ Adult: Initially 15 mg/kg daily, increased in steps of 2.5–5 mg/kg daily, dose to be increased every 12 weeks according to response; usual dose 15–30 mg/kg daily; maximum 35 mg/kg per day

XROMI ®

Sickle-cell disease [prevention of vaso-occlusive complications] (under expert supervision)
▸ BY MOUTH
▸ Adult: Initially 15 mg/kg daily, increased in steps of 5 mg/kg daily, dose to be increased every 8 weeks according to response; usual maintenance 20–25 mg/kg daily; maximum 35 mg/kg per day

---

> **IMPORTANT SAFETY INFORMATION**
> RISKS OF INCORRECT DOSING OF ORAL ANTI-CANCER MEDICINES
> See Cytotoxic drugs p. 1027.

● CAUTIONS Leg ulcers (review treatment if cutaneous vasculitic ulcerations develop)

● INTERACTIONS → Appendix 1: hydroxycarbamide

● SIDE-EFFECTS
▸ **Common or very common** Alopecia · anaemia · appetite decreased · asthenia · bone marrow disorders · chills · constipation · cutaneous vasculitis · dermatomyositis · diarrhoea · disorientation · dizziness · drowsiness · dyspnoea · dysuria · fever · gastrointestinal discomfort · haemorrhage · hallucination · headache · hepatic disorders · leucopenia · lung infiltration · malaise · mucositis · nail discolouration · nail disorder · nausea · neoplasms · neutropenia · oral disorders · pancreatitis · peripheral neuropathy · pulmonary fibrosis · pulmonary oedema · red blood cell abnormalities · seizure · skin reactions · skin ulcers · sperm abnormalities · thrombocytopenia · vomiting
▸ **Rare or very rare** Cutaneous lupus erythematosus · gangrene · systemic lupus erythematosus (SLE)
▸ **Frequency not known** Amenorrhoea · gastrointestinal disorders · hypomagnesaemia · Parvovirus B19 infection · vitamin D deficiency · weight increased

● CONCEPTION AND CONTRACEPTION Manufacturer advises effective contraception before and during treatment. See also *Pregnancy and reproductive function* in Cytotoxic drugs p. 1027.

● PREGNANCY Avoid (teratogenic in *animal* studies). See also *Pregnancy and reproductive function* in Cytotoxic drugs p. 1027.

● BREAST FEEDING Discontinue breast-feeding.

● HEPATIC IMPAIRMENT Manufacturer advises caution in mild to moderate impairment; avoid in severe impairment (unless used for malignant conditions).

● RENAL IMPAIRMENT In sickle-cell disease, avoid if eGFR less than 30 mL/minute/1.73 m^2. Use with caution in malignant disease.
Dose adjustments In sickle-cell disease, reduce initial dose by 50% if eGFR less than 60 mL/minute/1.73 m^2.

● MONITORING REQUIREMENTS
▸ Monitor renal and hepatic function before and during treatment.
▸ Monitor full blood count before treatment, and repeatedly throughout use; in sickle-cell disease monitor every 2 weeks for the first 2 months and then every 2 to 3 months thereafter (or every 2 weeks if on maximum dose).
▸ Patients receiving long-term therapy for malignant disease should be monitored for secondary malignancies.

● PATIENT AND CARER ADVICE Patients receiving long-term therapy with hydroxycarbamide should be advised to protect skin from sun exposure.

● NATIONAL FUNDING/ACCESS DECISIONS
For full details see funding body website
Scottish Medicines Consortium (SMC) decisions
▸ **Hydroxycarbamide oral solution (*Xromi*®) for the prevention of vaso-occlusive complications of sickle-cell disease in patients over 2 years of age (August 2020)** SMC No. SMC2271 Recommended with restrictions
All Wales Medicines Strategy Group (AWMSG) decisions
▸ **Hydroxycarbamide oral solution (*Xromi*®) for the prevention of vaso-occlusive complications of sickle-cell disease in patients over 2 years of age (August 2020)** AWMSG No. 4264 Recommended with restrictions

- **MEDICINAL FORMS** There can be variation in the licensing of different medicines containing the same drug. Forms available from special-order manufacturers include: oral capsule, oral suspension, oral solution

Oral tablet
- ▸ Siklos (Masters Pharmaceuticals Ltd)
  Hydroxycarbamide 100 mg Siklos 100mg tablets | 60 tablet [PoM] £100.00 DT = £100.00
  Hydroxycarbamide 1 gram Siklos 1000mg tablets | 30 tablet [PoM] £500.00 DT = £500.00

Oral solution
CAUTIONARY AND ADVISORY LABELS 27
EXCIPIENTS: May contain Hydroxybenzoates (parabens)
- ▸ Xromi (Nova Laboratories Ltd)
  Hydroxycarbamide 100 mg per 1 ml Xromi 100mg/ml oral solution | 150 ml [PoM] £250.00 DT = £250.00 [SF]

Oral capsule
- ▸ Hydroxycarbamide (Non-proprietary)
  Hydroxycarbamide 500 mg Hydroxycarbamide 500mg capsules | 100 capsule [PoM] £86.00 DT = £16.14
- ▸ Droxia (Imported (United States))
  Hydroxycarbamide 300 mg Droxia 300mg capsules | 60 capsule [PoM] [⊠]
- ▸ Hydrea (Neon Healthcare Ltd)
  Hydroxycarbamide 500 mg Hydrea 500mg capsules | 100 capsule [PoM] £10.47 DT = £16.14

Mitotane [Specialist drug]

09-Sep-2021

- **INDICATIONS AND DOSE**

Adrenocortical carcinoma
- ▸ BY MOUTH
- ▸ Adult: Specialist drug – access specialist resources for dosing information

---
IMPORTANT SAFETY INFORMATION
RISKS OF INCORRECT DOSING OF ORAL ANTI-CANCER MEDICINES
See Cytotoxic drugs p. 1027.

- **CONTRA-INDICATIONS** Acute porphyrias p. 1202
- **INTERACTIONS** → Appendix 1: mitotane
- **SIDE-EFFECTS**
- ▸ **Common or very common** Adrenal insufficiency · anaemia · appetite decreased · asthenia · cognitive impairment · confusion · diarrhoea · dizziness · drowsiness · dyslipidaemia · gastrointestinal discomfort · gynaecomastia · headache · hepatic disorders · leucopenia · movement disorders · mucositis · muscle weakness · nausea · paraesthesia · polyneuropathy · rash · thrombocytopenia · vertigo · vomiting
- ▸ **Frequency not known** Encephalopathy · eye disorders · flushing · fungal infection · generalised pain · growth retardation · haemorrhage · hyperpyrexia · hypersalivation · hypertension · hypothyroidism · hypouricaemia · lens opacity · neuro-psychological retardation · ovarian cyst · postural hypotension · proteinuria · taste altered · thyroid disorder · vision disorders
- **CONCEPTION AND CONTRACEPTION** Contraceptive advice required.
- **PATIENT AND CARER ADVICE** Patients should be warned to contact doctor immediately if injury, infection, or illness occurs (because of risk of acute adrenal insufficiency— treatment may need to be temporarily discontinued and exogenous steroids administered).
  Patient card A patient card should be provided.
  Driving and skilled tasks Central nervous system toxicity may affect performance of skilled tasks (e.g. driving).

- **MEDICINAL FORMS** There can be variation in the licensing of different medicines containing the same drug.

Oral tablet
CAUTIONARY AND ADVISORY LABELS 2, 10, 21
- ▸ Lysodren (Esteve RD UK & Ireland Ltd)
  Mitotane 500 mg Lysodren 500mg tablets | 100 tablet [PoM] £590.97 DT = £590.97

Panobinostat [Specialist drug]

28-Jul-2020

- **INDICATIONS AND DOSE**

Multiple myeloma
- ▸ BY MOUTH
- ▸ Adult: Specialist drug – access specialist resources for dosing information

---
IMPORTANT SAFETY INFORMATION
RISKS OF INCORRECT DOSING OF ORAL ANTI-CANCER MEDICINES
See Cytotoxic drugs p. 1027.

- **INTERACTIONS** → Appendix 1: panobinostat
- **SIDE-EFFECTS**
- ▸ **Common or very common** Anaemia · appetite decreased · arrhythmias · asthenia · cheilitis · chills · Clostridioides difficile colitis · cough · decreased leucocytes · diarrhoea · dizziness · dry mouth · dyspnoea · electrolyte imbalance · fever · fluid imbalance · gastrointestinal discomfort · gastrointestinal disorders · haemorrhage · headache · hepatic disorders · hyperbilirubinaemia · hyperglycaemia · hypertension · hyperuricaemia · hypoalbuminaemia · hypotension · hypothyroidism · increased risk of infection · insomnia · intracranial haemorrhage · joint swelling · malaise · nausea · neutropenia · palpitations · pancytopenia · peripheral oedema · QT interval prolongation · renal failure · respiratory disorders · sepsis · skin reactions · syncope · taste altered · thrombocytopenia · tremor · urinary incontinence · vomiting · weight decreased
- ▸ **Uncommon** Haemorrhagic shock · myocardial infarction

  SIDE-EFFECTS, FURTHER INFORMATION Side-effects are reported when used in combination with bortezomib and dexamethasone.

  Gastro-intestinal disorders Manufacturer advises that patients are treated with anti-diarrhoeals, or any additional treatment, in accordance with local treatment guidelines at the first sign of abdominal cramping or onset of diarrhoea.
- **CONCEPTION AND CONTRACEPTION** Manufacturer advises exclude pregnancy before starting treatment in women of child-bearing potential, and ensure highly effective contraception used during treatment and for 3 months after last dose. Women using hormonal contraceptives should also use a barrier method of contraception. Highly effective contraception also required for men and their female partners during treatment and for 6 months after last dose.
- **PATIENT AND CARER ADVICE** Manufacturer advises that patients and their carers should be told to seek medical advice if severe gastro-intestinal toxicity occurs.
  Missed doses Manufacturer advises if a dose is missed, it can be taken up to 12 hours after the specified dose time.
  Driving and skilled tasks Dizziness may affect performance of skilled tasks (e.g. driving).
- **NATIONAL FUNDING/ACCESS DECISIONS**
  For full details see funding body website

  NICE decisions
- ▸ **Panobinostat for treating multiple myeloma after at least 2 previous treatments (January 2016)** NICE TA380
  Recommended with restrictions

- **MEDICINAL FORMS** There can be variation in the licensing of different medicines containing the same drug.
  Oral capsule
  CAUTIONARY AND ADVISORY LABELS 25
  ▸ Farydak (pharmaand GmbH)
    Panobinostat (as Panobinostat lactate anhydrous)
    10 mg Farydak 10mg capsules | 6 capsule [PoM] £3,492.00
    Panobinostat (as Panobinostat lactate anhydrous) **15 mg** Farydak
    15mg capsules | 6 capsule [PoM] £3,492.00
    Panobinostat (as Panobinostat lactate anhydrous)
    20 mg Farydak 20mg capsules | 6 capsule [PoM] £4,656.00

Pegaspargase [Specialist drug]　　　25-Aug-2020

- **INDICATIONS AND DOSE**

Acute lymphoblastic leukaemia
▸ BY INTRAMUSCULAR INJECTION, OR BY INTRAVENOUS INFUSION
▸ Adult: Specialist drug – access specialist resources for dosing information

> **IMPORTANT SAFETY INFORMATION**
> Resuscitation facilities should be available during administration.

- **CONTRA-INDICATIONS** History of pancreatitis · history of serious haemorrhagic event with previous L-asparaginase therapy · history of serious thrombosis with previous L-asparaginase therapy

- **INTERACTIONS** → Appendix 1: pegaspargase

- **SIDE-EFFECTS**
▸ **Common or very common** Abdominal pain · anaemia · appetite decreased · ascites · coagulation disorders · diarrhoea · dyslipidaemia · embolism and thrombosis · febrile neutropenia · hepatic disorders · hyperglycaemia · hypersensitivity · hypoalbuminaemia · hypokalaemia · hypoxia · increased risk of infection · nausea · pain in extremity · pancreatitis (discontinue if suspected and do not restart if confirmed) · peripheral neuropathy · seizure · sepsis · skin reactions · stomatitis · syncope · vomiting · weight decreased
▸ **Rare or very rare** Encephalopathy · haemorrhage · necrotising pancreatitis
▸ **Frequency not known** Acute kidney injury · bone marrow disorders · confusion · diabetic ketoacidosis · drowsiness · fever · hyperammonaemia (monitor if symptoms present) · hyperglycaemic hyperosmolar nonketotic syndrome · hypoglycaemia · pancreatic pseudocyst · stroke · toxic epidermal necrolysis · tremor
  SIDE-EFFECTS, FURTHER INFORMATION There have been rare reports of cholestasis, icterus, hepatic cell necrosis and hepatic failure with fatal outcome in patients receiving pegaspargase.

- **CONCEPTION AND CONTRACEPTION** Manufacturer advises effective contraception in men and women of child-bearing potential during treatment and for at least 6 months after discontinuing treatment; pegaspargase may reduce effectiveness of oral contraceptives—additional precautions (e.g. barrier method) are required.

- **PATIENT AND CARER ADVICE**
  Pancreatitis Manufacturer advises patients and carers should be told how to recognise signs and symptoms of pancreatitis and advised to seek medical attention if symptoms such as persistent, severe abdominal pain develop.
  Driving and skilled tasks Manufacturer advises patients and carers should be counselled on the effects on driving and performance of skilled tasks—increased risk of confusion and somnolence.

- **NATIONAL FUNDING/ACCESS DECISIONS**
  For full details see funding body website
  NICE decisions
  ▸ Pegaspargase for treating acute lymphoblastic leukaemia (September 2016) NICE TA408 Recommended
  Scottish Medicines Consortium (SMC) decisions
  ▸ Pegaspargase (*Oncaspar*®) as a component of antineoplastic combination therapy in acute lymphoblastic leukaemia (ALL) in paediatric patients from birth to 18 years, and adult patients (November 2016) SMC No. 1197/16 Recommended

- **MEDICINAL FORMS** There can be variation in the licensing of different medicines containing the same drug.
  Powder for solution for injection
  ▸ Oncaspar (Servier Laboratories Ltd)
    Pegaspargase 3750 unit Oncaspar 3,750unit powder for solution for injection vials | 1 vial [PoM] £1,296.19 (Hospital only)

Procarbazine [Specialist drug]　　　16-Nov-2021

- **INDICATIONS AND DOSE**

Hodgkin's lymphoma
▸ BY MOUTH
▸ Adult: Specialist drug – access specialist resources for dosing information

> **IMPORTANT SAFETY INFORMATION**
> RISKS OF INCORRECT DOSING OF ORAL ANTI-CANCER MEDICINES
> See Cytotoxic drugs p. 1027.

- **CONTRA-INDICATIONS** Pre-existing severe leucopenia · pre-existing severe thrombocytopenia

- **INTERACTIONS** → Appendix 1: procarbazine

- **SIDE-EFFECTS**
▸ **Common or very common** Appetite decreased
▸ **Frequency not known** Azoospermia · hepatic disorders · infection · lethargy · leucopenia · nausea · neutropenia · ovarian failure · pneumonitis · skin reactions · thrombocytopenia · vomiting

- **CONCEPTION AND CONTRACEPTION** Contraceptive advice required.

- **MEDICINAL FORMS** There can be variation in the licensing of different medicines containing the same drug.
  Oral capsule
  CAUTIONARY AND ADVISORY LABELS 4
  ▸ Procarbazine (Non-proprietary)
    Procarbazine (as Procarbazine hydrochloride)
    50 mg Procarbazine 50mg capsules | 50 capsule [PoM] £503.61-£555.23 DT = £528.79

Raltitrexed [Specialist drug]　　　10-Aug-2021

- **INDICATIONS AND DOSE**

Colorectal cancer
▸ BY INTRAVENOUS INFUSION
▸ Adult: Specialist drug – access specialist resources for dosing information

- **INTERACTIONS** → Appendix 1: raltitrexed

- **SIDE-EFFECTS**
▸ **Common or very common** Alopecia · anaemia · appetite decreased · arthralgia · asthenia · cellulitis · conjunctivitis · constipation · dehydration · diarrhoea · fever · gastrointestinal discomfort · headache · hyperbilirubinaemia · hyperhidrosis · influenza like illness · leucopenia · malaise · mucositis · muscle cramps · muscle tone increased · nausea · neutropenia · oral disorders · pain · peripheral oedema · sepsis · skin reactions · taste altered · thrombocytopenia · vomiting · weight decreased

▸ **Frequency not known** Gastrointestinal haemorrhage

● **CONCEPTION AND CONTRACEPTION** Ensure effective contraception during and for at least 6 months after treatment in men or women.

● **MEDICINAL FORMS** There can be variation in the licensing of different medicines containing the same drug.

Powder for solution for infusion
▸ Tomudex (Pfizer Ltd)
Raltitrexed 2 mg Tomudex 2mg powder for solution for infusion vials | 1 vial [PoM] £148.75 (Hospital only)

IMMUNOSTIMULANTS › INTERFERONS

Ropeginterferon alfa-2b [Specialist drug]

25-Jul-2023

● **INDICATIONS AND DOSE**

Polycythaemia vera
▸ BY SUBCUTANEOUS INJECTION
▸ Adult: Specialist drug – access specialist resources for dosing information

● **CONTRA-INDICATIONS** History or presence of autoimmune disease · immunosuppressed transplant patients · severe cardiovascular disease · severe psychiatric disorders (or history of), particularly severe depression, suicidal ideation or attempts · uncontrolled diabetes · uncontrolled thyroid disease

● **INTERACTIONS** → Appendix 1: interferons

● **SIDE-EFFECTS**
▸ **Common or very common** Alopecia · anaemia · anxiety · appetite decreased · arthralgia · arthritis · asthenia · atrial fibrillation · chills · constipation · depression · diarrhoea · dizziness · drowsiness · dry eye · dry mouth · dyspnoea · fever · gastrointestinal discomfort · hepatic disorders · hyperhidrosis · hyperthyroidism · hypertriglyceridaemia · hypothyroidism · increased risk of infection · influenza like illness · leucopenia · mood altered · muscle complaints · nausea · neutropenia · pain · pancytopenia · sensation abnormal · Sjögren's syndrome · skin reactions · sleep disorders · thrombocytopenia · thyroiditis
▸ **Uncommon** Abdominal wall disorder · aortic valve incompetence · atrioventricular block · cardiovascular disorder · cognitive impairment · coronary thrombosis · cough · deafness · erectile dysfunction · eye discomfort · flushing · gastrointestinal disorders · haematospermia · haemorrhage · hallucination · headaches · hypertension · muscle weakness · nail dystrophy · nerve disorders · odynophagia · photosensitivity reaction · pneumonitis · Raynaud's phenomenon · sarcoidosis · sensitivity to weather change · throat irritation · tinnitus · tremor · urinary disorders · vertigo · vision disorders · weight decreased

● **CONCEPTION AND CONTRACEPTION** [EvGr] Females of childbearing potential should use effective contraception during treatment. ⟨M⟩

● **PATIENT AND CARER ADVICE**
Driving and skilled tasks Patients and carers should be counselled on the effects on driving and performance of skilled tasks—increased risk of dizziness and somnolence.

● **NATIONAL FUNDING/ACCESS DECISIONS**
For full details see funding body website
Scottish Medicines Consortium (SMC) decisions
▸ **Ropeginterferon alfa-2b (***Besremi*®**) as monotherapy in adults for the treatment of polycythaemia vera without symptomatic splenomegaly (July 2023)** SMC No. SMC2563 Not recommended

● **MEDICINAL FORMS** There can be variation in the licensing of different medicines containing the same drug.
Solution for injection
EXCIPIENTS: May contain Benzyl alcohol, polysorbates
▸ Besremi (AOP Orphan Ltd) ▼
Interferon alfa-2b (as Ropeginterferon alfa-2b) 500 microgram per 1 ml Besremi 250micrograms/0.5ml solution for injection pre-filled pens | 1 pre-filled disposable injection [PoM] £1,782.14

RETINOID AND RELATED DRUGS

Bexarotene [Specialist drug]

28-Jun-2023

● **INDICATIONS AND DOSE**

Cutaneous T-cell lymphoma
▸ BY MOUTH
▸ Adult: Specialist drug – access specialist resources for dosing information

IMPORTANT SAFETY INFORMATION
RISKS OF INCORRECT DOSING OF ORAL ANTI-CANCER MEDICINES
See Cytotoxic drugs p. 1027.

MHRA/CHM ADVICE: ORAL RETINOID MEDICINES: REVISED AND SIMPLIFIED PREGNANCY PREVENTION EDUCATIONAL MATERIALS FOR HEALTHCARE PROFESSIONALS AND WOMEN (JUNE 2019)
Materials to support the Pregnancy Prevention Programme in women and girls of childbearing potential taking oral acitretin, alitretinoin, or isotretinoin have been updated. Oral tretinoin and bexarotene do not have a Pregnancy Prevention Programme in light of their oncology indication and specialist care setting. However, healthcare professionals are advised that these medicines are extremely teratogenic and product information should be consulted for contraceptive and pregnancy testing requirements when used in females of childbearing potential.

Neuropsychiatric reactions have been reported in patients taking oral retinoids. Healthcare professionals are advised to monitor patients for signs of depression or suicidal ideation and refer for appropriate treatment, if necessary; particular care is needed in those with a history of depression. Patients should be advised to speak to their doctor if they experience any changes in mood or behaviour, and encouraged to ask family and friends to look out for any change in mood.

● **CONTRA-INDICATIONS** Acute porphyrias p. 1202 · history of pancreatitis · hypervitaminosis A · uncontrolled hyperlipidaemia · uncontrolled hypothyroidism

● **INTERACTIONS** → Appendix 1: retinoids

● **SIDE-EFFECTS**
▸ **Common or very common** Alopecia · anaemia · appetite decreased · arthralgia · asthenia · chills · constipation · deafness · diarrhoea · dizziness · dry eye · dry mouth · dyslipidaemia · eye disorders · gastrointestinal discomfort · gastrointestinal disorders · headaches · hyperhidrosis · hypersensitivity · hypoproteinaemia · hypothyroidism · increased risk of infection · insomnia · leucopenia · lymphadenopathy · muscle complaints · nausea · oedema · oral disorders · pain · pseudolymphoma · sensation abnormal · skin nodule · skin reactions · skin ulcer · thyroid disorder · vomiting · weight changes
▸ **Uncommon** Albuminuria · anxiety · arrhythmias · ataxia · blood disorder · cataract · coagulation disorder · depression · ear disorder · eosinophilia · eye inflammation · fever · gout · haemorrhage · hair disorder · hepatic failure · hyperbilirubinaemia · hypertension · hyperthyroidism · increased leucocytes · mucous membrane disorder · muscle weakness · nail disorder · neoplasms · nerve disorders · pancreatitis · renal impairment · serous drainage ·

Immune system and malignant disease

thrombocytopenia · thrombocytosis · varicose veins · vasodilation · vertigo · vision disorders

▶ **Frequency not known** Burping · chest pain · confusion · cough aggravated · dehydration · drowsiness · dysphagia · dyspnoea · emotional lability · hypercalcaemia · hyperuricaemia · libido decreased · muscle tone increased · pelvic pain · peripheral vascular disease · red blood cell abnormality · taste altered · thirst · tinnitus · white blood cell abnormalities

● **ALLERGY AND CROSS-SENSITIVITY** [EvGr] Caution— hypersensitivity to retinoids. ◈

● **CONCEPTION AND CONTRACEPTION** [EvGr] Ensure effective contraception during and for at least 1 month after treatment in male and female patients. ◈

● **PATIENT AND CARER ADVICE**
Risk of neuropsychiatric reactions The MHRA advises patients and carers to seek medical attention if changes in mood or behaviour occur.

● **NATIONAL FUNDING/ACCESS DECISIONS**
For full details see funding body website
Scottish Medicines Consortium (SMC) decisions
▶ Bexarotene (*Targretin*®) for skin manifestations of advanced stage cutaneous T-cell lymphoma (November 2002) SMC No. 14/02 Recommended with restrictions

● **MEDICINAL FORMS** There can be variation in the licensing of different medicines containing the same drug.
Oral capsule
▶ Bexarotene (Non-proprietary)
Bexarotene 75 mg Bexarotene 75mg capsules | 100 capsule [PoM] £843.75 (Hospital only) | 100 capsule [PoM] £703.00
▶ Targretin (Eisai Ltd)
Bexarotene 75 mg Targretin 75mg capsules | 100 capsule [PoM] £937.50 (Hospital only)

Tretinoin [Specialist drug]

06-Nov-2023

(Retinoic acid; Vitamin A acid)

● **INDICATIONS AND DOSE**
Acute promyelocytic leukaemia
▶ BY MOUTH
▶ Adult: Specialist drug – access specialist resources for dosing information

IMPORTANT SAFETY INFORMATION
MHRA/CHM ADVICE: ORAL RETINOID MEDICINES: REVISED AND SIMPLIFIED PREGNANCY PREVENTION EDUCATIONAL MATERIALS FOR HEALTHCARE PROFESSIONALS AND WOMEN (JUNE 2019)
Materials to support the Pregnancy Prevention Programme in women and girls of childbearing potential taking oral acitretin, alitretinoin, or isotretinoin have been updated. Oral tretinoin and bexarotene do not have a Pregnancy Prevention Programme in light of their oncology indication and specialist care setting. However, healthcare professionals are advised that these medicines are extremely teratogenic and product information should be consulted for contraceptive and pregnancy testing requirements when used in females of childbearing potential.

Neuropsychiatric reactions have been reported in patients taking oral retinoids. Healthcare professionals are advised to monitor patients for signs of depression or suicidal ideation and refer for appropriate treatment, if necessary; particular care is needed in those with a history of depression. Patients should be advised to speak to their doctor if they experience any changes in mood or behaviour, and encouraged to ask family and friends to look out for any change in mood.

● **INTERACTIONS** → Appendix 1: retinoids

● **SIDE-EFFECTS**
▶ **Common or very common** Abdominal pain · alopecia · anxiety · appetite decreased · arrhythmia · asthma · bone pain · cheilitis · chest pain · chills · confusion · conjunctival disorder · constipation · depression · diarrhoea · dizziness · dry mouth · flushing · headache · hearing impairment · hyperhidrosis · insomnia · intracranial pressure increased · malaise · nasal dryness · nausea · pancreatitis · paraesthesia · respiratory disorders · skin reactions · visual impairment · vomiting
▶ **Frequency not known** Embolism and thrombosis · erythema nodosum · genital ulceration · hypercalcaemia · increased leucocytes · mood altered · myocardial infarction · myositis · necrotising fasciitis · stroke · thrombocytosis · vasculitis

SIDE-EFFECTS, FURTHER INFORMATION **Retinoic acid syndrome** Fever, dyspnoea, acute respiratory distress, pulmonary infiltrates, pleural effusion, hyperleucocytosis, hypotension, oedema, weight gain, hepatic, renal and multi-organ failure requires immediate treatment— consult product literature.

● **ALLERGY AND CROSS-SENSITIVITY** [EvGr] Contra-indicated in patients with hypersensitivity to peanuts or soya (capsule filling contains soya-bean oil). ◈

● **CONCEPTION AND CONTRACEPTION** [EvGr] Ensure effective contraception during and for at least 1 month after treatment. ◈

● **PATIENT AND CARER ADVICE**
Risk of neuropsychiatric reactions The MHRA advises patients and carers to seek medical attention if changes in mood or behaviour occur.

● **MEDICINAL FORMS** There can be variation in the licensing of different medicines containing the same drug.
Oral capsule
CAUTIONARY AND ADVISORY LABELS 21, 25
▶ Tretinoin (Non-proprietary)
Tretinoin 10 mg Tretinoin 10mg capsules | 100 capsule [PoM] £350.00 DT = £350.00

3.1 Cytotoxic drug-induced side effects

ANTIDOTES AND CHELATORS ⟩ IRON CHELATORS

Dexrazoxane

13-Sep-2021

● **DRUG ACTION** Dexrazoxane is an iron chelator.

● **INDICATIONS AND DOSE**
CARDIOXANE ®
Prevention of chronic cumulative cardiotoxicity caused by doxorubicin or epirubicin treatment in advanced or metastatic breast cancer patients who have received a prior cumulative dose of 300 mg/m² of doxorubicin or a prior cumulative dose of 540 mg/m² of epirubicin when further anthracycline treatment is required
▶ BY INTRAVENOUS INFUSION
▶ Adult: Administer 10 times the doxorubicin-equivalent dose or 10 times the epirubicin-equivalent dose, dose to be given 30 minutes before anthracycline administration

SAVENE ®
Anthracycline extravasation
▶ BY INTRAVENOUS INFUSION
▶ Adult: Initially 1 g/m² daily (max. per dose 2 g) for 2 days, then 500 mg/m² for 1 day, first dose to be given as soon as possible and within 6 hours after injury

● **CAUTIONS** Myelosuppression (effects may be additive to those of chemotherapy)

CARDIOXANE ® Heart failure—no information available · myocardial infarction in previous 12 months—no information available · symptomatic valvular heart disease—no information available · uncontrolled angina—no information available

- **INTERACTIONS** → Appendix 1: iron chelators
- **SIDE-EFFECTS**
- ▶ **Common or very common** Alopecia · anaemia · appetite decreased · asthenia · constipation · cough · diarrhoea · dizziness · drowsiness · dry mouth · dyspnoea · embolism and thrombosis · fever · gastrointestinal discomfort · headache · increased risk of infection · leucopenia · myalgia · nail disorder · nausea · neutropenia · peripheral neuropathy · peripheral oedema · post procedural infection · sensation abnormal · skin reactions · stomatitis · syncope · tachycardia · thrombocytopenia · tremor · vaginal haemorrhage · vomiting · weight decreased · wound complications
- ▶ **Uncommon** Acute myeloid leukaemia · lymphoedema · sepsis · thirst · vertigo
- ▶ **Frequency not known** Anaphylactic reaction
- **CONCEPTION AND CONTRACEPTION** Ensure effective contraception during and for at least 3 months after treatment in men and women.
- **PREGNANCY** Avoid unless essential (toxicity in *animal* studies).
- **BREAST FEEDING** Discontinue breast-feeding.
- **HEPATIC IMPAIRMENT**

CARDIOXANE ® Manufacturer advises caution (no information available).
Dose adjustments Manufacturer advises if anthracycline dose is reduced, reduce the *Cardioxane* ® dose by a similar ratio.

SAVENE ® Manufacturer advises avoid (no information available).

- **RENAL IMPAIRMENT**
Dose adjustments EvGr Reduce dose by 50% if creatinine clearance less than 40 mL/minute. M See p. 21.
- **MONITORING REQUIREMENTS**
- ▶ Monitor full blood count.
- ▶ Monitor for cardiac toxicity.
- ▶ Monitor liver function.
- **DIRECTIONS FOR ADMINISTRATION**

CARDIOXANE ® For *intravenous infusion*, give intermittently *in* Compound Sodium Lactate; reconstitute each vial with 25 mL Water for Injections and dilute each vial with 25–100 mL infusion fluid; give requisite dose over 15 minutes.

SAVENE ® For *intravenous infusion*, give intermittently *in* diluent; reconstitute each 500-mg vial with 25 mL of diluent; dilute requisite dose further in remaining diluent and give over 1–2 hours into a large vein in an area other than the one affected. Local coolants such as ice packs should be removed at least 15 minutes before administration.

- **MEDICINAL FORMS** There can be variation in the licensing of different medicines containing the same drug.
Powder for solution for infusion
- ▶ Cardioxane (CNX Therapeutics Ltd)
Dexrazoxane 500 mg Cardioxane 500mg powder for solution for infusion vials | 1 vial PoM £156.57
Powder and solvent for solution for infusion
ELECTROLYTES: May contain Potassium, sodium
- ▶ Savene (CNX Therapeutics Ltd)
Dexrazoxane 500 mg Savene 500mg powder for concentrate and solvent for solution for infusion vials | 10 vial PoM £6,750.00 (Hospital only)

ANTIDOTES AND CHELATORS ＞OTHER

Glucarpidase

16-Nov-2023

- **DRUG ACTION** Glucarpidase is a recombinant bacterial enzyme that converts methotrexate to its inactive metabolites.

- **INDICATIONS AND DOSE**
Reduction of toxic plasma-methotrexate concentration
- ▶ BY INTRAVENOUS INJECTION
- ▶ Adult: 50 units/kg for 1 dose, dose to be given without delay; the optimal administration timeframe for patients with delayed methotrexate elimination is within 48–60 hours from the start of high-dose methotrexate infusion, folinic acid rescue should continue to be given at least 2 hours after glucarpidase administration—see also *Interactions*

- **INTERACTIONS** → Appendix 1: glucarpidase
- **SIDE-EFFECTS**
- ▶ **Uncommon** Feeling hot · flushing · headache · sensation abnormal
- ▶ **Rare or very rare** Abdominal pain upper · crystalluria · diarrhoea · drowsiness · fever · hypersensitivity · hypotension · nausea · pleural effusion · skin reactions · tachycardia · throat tightness · tremor · vomiting
- **PREGNANCY** Specialist sources indicate probably compatible (no information available).
- **BREAST FEEDING** Specialist sources indicate probably compatible (no information available).
- **EFFECT ON LABORATORY TESTS** May interfere with measurement of methotrexate concentration by immunoassay if carried out within 48 hours of administration—consult product literature.
- **DIRECTIONS FOR ADMINISTRATION** For *intravenous injection*, reconstitute each vial with 1 mL Sodium Chloride 0.9% and give over 5 minutes.
- **PRESCRIBING AND DISPENSING INFORMATION** Glucarpidase is a biological medicine. Biological medicines must be prescribed and dispensed by brand name, see *Biological medicines* and *Biosimilar medicines*, under Guidance on prescribing p. 1; record the brand name and batch number after each administration.
- **HANDLING AND STORAGE** Store in a refrigerator (2–8°C)—consult product literature for storage conditions after reconstitution.

- **MEDICINAL FORMS** There can be variation in the licensing of different medicines containing the same drug.
Powder for solution for injection
- ▶ Voraxaze (Protherics Medicines Development Ltd) ▼
Glucarpidase 1000 unit Voraxaze 1,000unit powder for solution for injection vials | 1 vial PoM £25,385.00 (Hospital only)

DETOXIFYING DRUGS ＞UROPROTECTIVE DRUGS

Mesna

16-Dec-2020

- **INDICATIONS AND DOSE**
Cytotoxic induced urothelial toxicity
- ▶ BY MOUTH, OR BY INTRAVENOUS INJECTION
- ▶ Adult: Dose to be calculated according to oxazaphosphorine (cyclophosphamide or ifosfamide) treatment (consult product literature)

- **SIDE-EFFECTS**
- ▶ **Common or very common** Appetite decreased · arthralgia · asthenia · chest pain · chills · concentration impaired · conjunctivitis · constipation · cough · dehydration · diarrhoea · dizziness · drowsiness · dry mouth · dyspnoea · dysuria · fever · flatulence · flushing · gastrointestinal

discomfort · haemorrhage · headache · hyperhidrosis · influenza like illness · laryngeal discomfort · lymphadenopathy · malaise · mucosal irritation · myalgia · nasal congestion · nausea · oral irritation · pain · palpitations · respiratory disorders · sensation abnormal · skin reactions · sleep disorders · syncope · vision disorders · vomiting

▸ **Frequency not known** Acute kidney injury · angioedema · drug reaction with eosinophilia and systemic symptoms (DRESS) · hypotension · hypoxia · oedema · tachycardia · ulcer

● **ALLERGY AND CROSS-SENSITIVITY** EvGr Caution if history of hypersensitivity to thiol-containing compounds. ⟨M⟩

● **PREGNANCY** Not known to be harmful. See also *Pregnancy and reproductive function* in Cytotoxic drugs p. 1027.

● **EFFECT ON LABORATORY TESTS** False positive urinary ketones. False positive or false negative urinary erythrocytes.

● **DIRECTIONS FOR ADMINISTRATION** Manufacturer advises for administration *by mouth*, injection solution may be given in a flavoured drink such as orange juice or cola which may be stored in a refrigerator for up to 24 hours in a sealed container.

● **MEDICINAL FORMS** There can be variation in the licensing of different medicines containing the same drug. Forms available from special-order manufacturers include: oral solution

Solution for injection
▸ **Mesna (Non-proprietary)**
Mesna 100 mg per 1 ml Mesna 1g/10ml solution for injection ampoules | 15 ampoule PoM £527.10 (Hospital only)
Mesna 400mg/4ml solution for injection ampoules | 15 ampoule PoM £240.30 (Hospital only)

Oral tablet
▸ **Mesna (Non-proprietary)**
Mesna 400 mg Mesna 400mg tablets | 10 tablet PoM £160.04–£160.40
Mesna 600 mg Mesna 600mg tablets | 10 tablet PoM £227.70

VITAMINS AND TRACE ELEMENTS › FOLATES

Folinic acid
17-Feb-2021

● **INDICATIONS AND DOSE**
Prevention of methotrexate-induced adverse effects
▸ BY INTRAMUSCULAR INJECTION, OR BY INTRAVENOUS INJECTION, OR BY INTRAVENOUS INFUSION
▸ Adult: 15 mg every 6 hours for 24 hours, to be started usually 12–24 hours after start of methotrexate infusion, dose may be continued by mouth, consult local treatment protocol for further information

Suspected methotrexate overdosage
▸ BY INTRAVENOUS INJECTION, OR BY INTRAVENOUS INFUSION
▸ Adult: Initial dose equal to or exceeding dose of methotrexate, to be given at a maximum rate of 160 mg/minute, consult poisons information centres for advice on continuing management

Adjunct to fluorouracil in colorectal cancer
▸ BY SLOW INTRAVENOUS INJECTION
▸ Adult: (consult product literature)

SODIOFOLIN ®
As an antidote to methotrexate
▸ BY INTRAVENOUS INFUSION, OR BY INTRAVENOUS INJECTION
▸ Adult: (consult product literature)

Adjunct to fluorouracil in colorectal cancer
▸ BY INTRAVENOUS INJECTION, OR BY INTRAVENOUS INFUSION
▸ Adult: (consult product literature)

● **CONTRA-INDICATIONS** Intrathecal injection

● **CAUTIONS** Avoid simultaneous administration of methotrexate · **not** indicated for pernicious anaemia or

other megaloblastic anaemias caused by vitamin B_{12} deficiency

● **INTERACTIONS** → Appendix 1: folates

● **SIDE-EFFECTS**
GENERAL SIDE-EFFECTS
▸ **Uncommon** Fever
▸ **Rare or very rare** Agitation (with high doses) · depression (with high doses) · epilepsy exacerbated · gastrointestinal disorder · insomnia (with high doses)

SPECIFIC SIDE-EFFECTS
▸ **Common or very common**
▸ With intravenous use Bone marrow failure · dehydration · diarrhoea · mucositis · nausea · oral disorders · skin reactions · vomiting
▸ **Rare or very rare**
▸ With intramuscular use Urticaria
▸ With intravenous use Sensitisation
▸ **Frequency not known**
▸ With intravenous use Hyperammonaemia

● **PREGNANCY** Not known to be harmful; benefit outweighs risk.

● **BREAST FEEDING** Presence in milk unknown but benefit outweighs risk.

● **NATIONAL FUNDING/ACCESS DECISIONS**
For full details see funding body website
NICE decisions
▸ **Bevacizumab in combination with oxaliplatin and either fluorouracil plus folinic acid or capecitabine for the treatment of metastatic colorectal cancer (December 2010)** NICE TA212 Not recommended

● **MEDICINAL FORMS** There can be variation in the licensing of different medicines containing the same drug. Forms available from special-order manufacturers include: oral suspension, oral solution
Oral tablet
▸ **Folinic acid (Non-proprietary)**
Folinic acid (as Calcium folinate) 15 mg Calcium folinate 15mg tablets | 10 tablet PoM £66.80 DT = £37.85
▸ **Refolinon** (Pfizer Ltd)
Folinic acid (as Calcium folinate) 15 mg Refolinon 15mg tablets | 30 tablet PoM £85.74 DT = £85.74

Solution for injection
▸ **Folinic acid (Non-proprietary)**
Folinic acid (as Calcium folinate) 10 mg per 1 ml Calcium folinate 200mg/20ml solution for injection vials | 10 vial PoM ⬧ (Hospital only)
Calcium folinate 300mg/30ml solution for injection vials | 1 vial PoM £100.00 (Hospital only)
Calcium folinate 350mg/35ml solution for injection vials | 1 vial PoM £166.79 (Hospital only) | 10 vial PoM £1,667.90 (Hospital only)
Calcium folinate 100mg/10ml solution for injection vials | 1 vial PoM £37.50–£54.31 (Hospital only) | 10 vial PoM £543.10 (Hospital only)
Calcium folinate 50mg/5ml solution for injection vials | 1 vial PoM £20.00 (Hospital only) | 1 vial PoM £30.56 | 10 vial PoM £305.60
▸ **Sodiofolin** (medac UK)
Folinic acid (as Disodium folinate) 50 mg per 1 ml Sodiofolin 400mg/8ml solution for injection vials | 1 vial PoM £126.25 (Hospital only)
Sodiofolin 100mg/2ml solution for injection vials | 1 vial PoM £35.09 (Hospital only)

Levofolinic acid
17-Feb-2021

● **DRUG ACTION** Levofolinic acid is an isomer of folinic acid.

● **INDICATIONS AND DOSE**
Prevention of methotrexate-induced adverse effects
▸ BY INTRAMUSCULAR INJECTION, OR BY INTRAVENOUS INJECTION, OR BY INTRAVENOUS INFUSION
▸ Adult: Usual dose 7.5 mg every 6 hours for 10 doses, usually started 12–24 hours after beginning of methotrexate infusion

continued →

8   Immune system and malignant disease

Suspected methotrexate overdosage
► BY INTRAVENOUS INFUSION, OR BY INTRAVENOUS INJECTION
► Adult: Initial dose at least 50% of the dose of methotrexate, intravenous infusion to be administered at a maximum rate of 160 mg/minute, consult poisons information centres for advice on continuing management

Adjunct to fluorouracil in colorectal cancer
► BY SLOW INTRAVENOUS INJECTION
► Adult: (consult product literature)

● **CONTRA-INDICATIONS** Intrathecal injection
● **CAUTIONS** Avoid simultaneous administration of methotrexate · **not** indicated for pernicious anaemia or other megaloblastic anaemias caused by vitamin B_{12} deficiency
● **INTERACTIONS** → Appendix 1: folates
● **SIDE-EFFECTS**
► **Common or very common** Dehydration · diarrhoea · mucosal toxicity · nausea · vomiting
► **Uncommon** Fever
► **Rare or very rare** Agitation (with high doses) · depression (with high doses) · epilepsy exacerbated · gastrointestinal disorder · insomnia (with high doses) · urticaria
● **PREGNANCY** Not known to be harmful; benefit outweighs risk.
● **BREAST FEEDING** Presence in milk unknown but benefit outweighs risk.

● **MEDICINAL FORMS** There can be variation in the licensing of different medicines containing the same drug.
Solution for injection
► Levofolinic acid (Non-proprietary)
Levofolinic acid (as Disodium levofolinate) 50 mg per 1 ml Levofolinic acid 50mg/1ml solution for injection vials | 1 vial PoM £24.70 (Hospital only)
Levofolinic acid 200mg/4ml solution for injection vials | 1 vial PoM £80.40 (Hospital only)
► Isovorin (Pfizer Ltd)
Levofolinic acid (as Calcium levofolinate) 10 mg per 1 ml Isovorin 175mg/17.5ml solution for injection vials | 1 vial PoM £81.33 (Hospital only)

3.1a Hyperuricaemia associated with cytotoxic drugs

> **Other drugs used for Hyperuricaemia associated with cytotoxic drugs** Allopurinol, p. 1280 · Febuxostat, p. 1280

DETOXIFYING DRUGS › URATE OXIDASES

Rasburicase
21-Nov-2020

● **INDICATIONS AND DOSE**
Prophylaxis and treatment of acute hyperuricaemia, before and during initiation of chemotherapy, in patients with haematological malignancy and high tumour burden at risk of rapid lysis
► BY INTRAVENOUS INFUSION
► Adult: 200 micrograms/kg once daily for up to 7 days according to plasma-uric acid concentration

● **CONTRA-INDICATIONS** G6PD deficiency
● **CAUTIONS** Atopic allergies
● **SIDE-EFFECTS**
► **Common or very common** Diarrhoea · fever · headache · nausea · skin reactions · vomiting

► **Uncommon** Bronchospasm · haemolysis · haemolytic anaemia · hypersensitivity · hypotension · methaemoglobinaemia · seizure
► **Rare or very rare** Rhinitis
► **Frequency not known** Muscle contractions involuntary
● **PREGNANCY** Manufacturer advises avoid—no information available.
● **BREAST FEEDING** Manufacturer advises avoid—no information available.
● **MONITORING REQUIREMENTS** Monitor closely for hypersensitivity.
● **EFFECT ON LABORATORY TESTS** May interfere with test for uric acid—consult product literature.
● **DIRECTIONS FOR ADMINISTRATION** For *intravenous infusion* (*Fasturtec®*), manufacturer advises give intermittently in Sodium Chloride 0.9%; reconstitute with solvent provided; gently swirl vial without shaking to dissolve; dilute requisite dose to 50 mL with infusion fluid and give over 30 minutes.

● **MEDICINAL FORMS** There can be variation in the licensing of different medicines containing the same drug.
Powder and solvent for solution for infusion
► Fasturtec (Sanofi)
Rasburicase 1.5 mg Fasturtec 1.5mg powder and solvent for solution for infusion vials | 3 vial PoM £208.39 (Hospital only)
Rasburicase 7.5 mg Fasturtec 7.5mg powder and solvent for solution for infusion vials | 1 vial PoM £347.32 (Hospital only)

4 Hormone responsive malignancy

Breast cancer
14-Nov-2023

Description of condition

Breast cancer is the most common form of malignancy in women, especially in those aged over 50 years. Established risk factors include age, early onset of menstruation, late menopause, older age at first completed pregnancy, and a family history of breast cancer. The use of oral contraceptives or hormone replacement therapy (HRT) is also associated with an increased risk of breast cancer.

Breast cancer in men is rare. Although risk factors are not fully understood, it may be associated with abnormalities of sex hormone metabolism, including those caused by liver disease or testicular trauma, genetic predisposition, and environmental risk factors such as industrial exposure to chronic heat.

Additional risk factors include obesity and alcohol consumption.

Physical activity and breast-feeding protect against breast cancer.

Non-invasive breast cancer, also known as ductal carcinoma *in situ*, is when the cancer remains localised in the ducts. However, in most cases, the cancer is invasive at the time of diagnosis, which means that malignant cells are liable to spread beyond the immediate area of the tumour. Invasive breast cancer, where malignant cells spread beyond the ducts, can be defined as early breast cancer (stage I/II), locally advanced disease (stage III) and advanced disease (stage IV).

Aims of treatment

Reducing mortality, increasing progression-free and disease-free survival and improving quality of life are the main aims of treatment, and are dependent on the stage of the disease.

Surgery and radiotherapy aim to remove the tumour mass, whilst adjuvant drug therapy (drug treatment following surgery) aims to reduce the risk of disease recurrence and the risk of developing invasive disease. Neoadjuvant drug therapy (drug treatment before surgery) aims to reduce the size of the tumour to allow breast-conserving surgery to be possible and to reduce axillary lymph node involvement. Advanced breast cancer is not curable, and treatment aims to prolong survival, relieve symptoms and improve quality of life.

Overview

The management of patients with breast cancer involves surgery, radiotherapy, drug therapy, or a combination of these. The course of the disease and the therapeutic approach vary depending on the characteristics of the cancer. Factors such as patient age, menopausal status, tumour size and grade, involvement of axillary lymph nodes or skin, and the presence of hormone receptors within the tumour, may inform the extent and aggressiveness of the disease. [EvGr] The risks and benefits of each therapy should be discussed with the patient before being started. ⓐ

Early and locally advanced breast cancer

For operable breast cancer, treatment involves surgery to the breast (breast-conserving surgery or mastectomy) and to the axillary lymph nodes, with or without radiotherapy to reduce local recurrence rates. This is often followed by adjuvant drug therapy to eradicate the micro-metastases that cause relapses. [EvGr] In women with invasive breast cancer, radiotherapy is recommended after breast-conserving surgery with clear margins (no cancer cells are found at the edges of the removed tissue), as it reduces local recurrence rates. However, the use of radiotherapy may be omitted if risk of local recurrence is very low and the woman is willing to take adjuvant endocrine therapy for a minimum of 5 years. Radiotherapy is also recommended after mastectomy in patients with node-positive invasive breast cancer or involved resection margins (cancer cells are found at the edges of the removed tissue). It should also be considered in patients with node-negative T3 or T4 invasive breast cancer. ⓐ

Adjuvant drug therapy

Adjuvant drug therapy may include the use of chemotherapy, endocrine therapy, biological therapy, or bisphosphonate therapy. [EvGr] The decision to use adjuvant drug therapy should be based on the risks and benefits of treatment, disease prognosis and predictive factors such as oestrogen receptor (ER), progesterone receptor (PR), and human epidermal growth receptor 2 (HER2) status of the primary tumour.

In women with invasive breast cancer in only one breast who have not received treatment, including the use of neoadjuvant chemotherapy, NICE clinical guideline 101 recommends the use of the PREDICT tool to estimate prognosis and the absolute benefits of adjuvant therapy (www.predict.nhs.uk). ⓐ

Chemotherapy

[EvGr] Adjuvant anthracycline–taxane combination chemotherapy is recommended in patients with invasive breast cancer who are at sufficient risk of disease recurrence to require chemotherapy. ⓐ The choice of chemotherapy regimen is usually guided by local policy, Cancer Alliances, and the National Cancer Drugs Fund list.

Biological therapy

[EvGr] Trastuzumab p. 1023 should be offered to patients with tumour size T1c and above HER2-positive invasive breast cancer, in combination with surgery, chemotherapy, or radiotherapy. It should also be considered in patients with a smaller tumour size (T1a or T1b) depending on their co-morbidities, prognosis, and possible toxicity with concomitant chemotherapy. Cardiac function should be regularly assessed in patients receiving trastuzumab p. 1023, and particular caution should be taken in patients with

underlying cardiac disease (consult product literature for further details). ⓐ

Endocrine therapy

[EvGr] Tamoxifen p. 1085 should be used as initial adjuvant endocrine therapy in men and premenopausal women with oestrogen-receptor-positive invasive breast cancer. In addition, ovarian function suppression with a gonadotropin-releasing hormone (GnRH) should be considered in premenopausal women, taking into account the risk of temporary menopause. ⓐ Ovarian function suppression aims to stop the production of circulating oestrogen, which can stimulate breast cancer progression. It may be most beneficial in women who are at sufficient risk of disease recurrence to have been offered chemotherapy.

[EvGr] In postmenopausal women with oestrogen-receptor positive invasive breast cancer who are at medium or high-risk of disease recurrence, an aromatase inhibitor should be given as first-line therapy. Alternatively, tamoxifen should be given if an aromatase inhibitor is not tolerated or is contra-indicated, or if the risk of disease recurrence is low. ⓐ

Extended endocrine therapy

[EvGr] Extended endocrine therapy (total duration longer than 5 years) with an aromatase inhibitor [unlicensed indication] should be offered to postmenopausal women with oestrogen-receptor-positive invasive breast cancer at medium or high-risk of disease recurrence who have been taking tamoxifen for 2 to 5 years. Extended therapy should also be considered in postmenopausal women at low risk of disease recurrence.

Extended tamoxifen therapy for longer than 5 years can also be considered in both premenopausal and postmenopausal women with oestrogen-receptor-positive invasive breast cancer. ⓐ

Endocrine therapy for ductal carcinoma in situ

[EvGr] Following breast-conserving surgery, endocrine therapy should be offered to women with oestrogen-positive ductal carcinoma *in situ*, if radiotherapy is recommended but not given. If radiotherapy is **not** recommended, the use of endocrine therapy should also be considered. ⓐ

Bisphosphonate therapy

Zoledronic acid p. 774 and sodium clodronate p. 773 have been shown to improve disease-free survival and overall survival in postmenopausal women with node-positive invasive breast cancer. However, there is insufficient evidence to recommend their use in premenopausal women. [EvGr] Intravenous zoledronic acid [unlicensed indication] or oral sodium clodronate [unlicensed indication] should be offered to postmenopausal women with lymph-node-positive invasive breast cancer. Treatment should be considered in those with lymph-node-negative invasive breast cancer who are at high-risk of recurrence.

Bisphosphonate therapy is also recommended in women at high-risk of osteoporosis due to the use of aromatase inhibitors in postmenopausal women, or in women with treatment-induced premature menopause. For further information, see Guidance for the management of breast cancer treatment-induced bone loss: a consensus position statement from a UK expert group, 2008. ⓐ

Neoadjuvant drug therapy

Neoadjuvant drug therapy may involve the use of chemotherapy or endocrine therapy.

Chemotherapy

[EvGr] Neoadjuvant chemotherapy should be offered to reduce tumour size in patients with oestrogen-receptor-negative invasive breast cancer. In patients with oestrogen-receptor-positive invasive breast cancer, chemotherapy should be considered. In patients with HER2-positive invasive breast cancer, neoadjuvant chemotherapy should be offered in combination with trastuzumab p. 1023 and pertuzumab p. 1017.

8
Immune system and malignant disease

A chemotherapy regimen containing both a platinum [unlicensed indication] and an anthracycline should be considered in patients with triple-negative invasive breast cancer (oestrogen-receptor-negative, progesterone-receptor negative and HER2-negative). Ⓐ

Endocrine therapy

EvGr If chemotherapy is not indicated, neoadjuvant endocrine therapy should be considered as an alternative in postmenopausal women with oestrogen-receptor-positive invasive breast cancer. Ⓐ Chemotherapy and endocrine therapy are equally effective in postmenopausal women in terms of breast-conservation and shrinking of the tumour. Although chemotherapy is more effective than endocrine therapy at shrinking the tumour in premenopausal women, some tumours may respond to endocrine treatment.

Advanced breast cancer

Treatment of advanced breast cancer depends on the patient's treatment history, disease severity, and oestrogen receptor and HER2 status.

Endocrine therapy

EvGr For the majority of patients with oestrogen-receptor-positive advanced breast cancer, endocrine therapy is recommended as first-line treatment. Aromatase inhibitors should be offered to postmenopausal women with no previous history of endocrine treatment, or to those previously treated with tamoxifen p. 1085.

Tamoxifen in combination with ovarian function suppression should be offered as first-line treatment to pre- and perimenopausal women with oestrogen-receptor-positive advanced breast cancer not previously treated with tamoxifen.

Ovarian function suppression should be offered to pre- and perimenopausal women who have had disease progression despite treatment with tamoxifen.

Tamoxifen should be offered as first-line treatment to men with oestrogen-receptor-positive advanced breast cancer. Ⓐ

Chemotherapy

EvGr Chemotherapy should be offered as first-line treatment in patients with oestrogen-receptor-positive advanced breast cancer that is imminently life-threatening or requires early relief of symptoms because of significant visceral organ involvement. Once chemotherapy treatment is completed, endocrine therapy should be offered. Ⓐ The choice of chemotherapy regimen is usually guided by local policy, Cancer Alliances, and the National Cancer Drugs Fund list.

Biological therapy

EvGr Trastuzumab is recommended for the treatment of HER2-positive advanced breast cancer. It is used in combination with paclitaxel p. 1059 in those who have not received chemotherapy for metastatic breast cancer, and as monotherapy for patients who have received at least two chemotherapy regimens for metastatic breast cancer (see trastuzumab *National funding/access decisions*). Ⓐ

Bisphosphonate therapy

EvGr The use of bisphosphonates should be considered in patients with metastatic breast cancer to reduce pain and prevent skeletal complications of bone metastases. Ⓐ

Familial breast cancer

EvGr Chemoprevention should be offered to all women who have been identified as being at high-risk of developing breast cancer. Chemoprevention should also be considered in women at moderate-risk. Other strategies to reduce breast cancer risk should also be considered, for example bilateral mastectomy or bilateral oophorectomy. Women who were at high-risk of breast cancer and have undergone a bilateral mastectomy should not receive chemoprevention. Ⓐ

Treatment options for chemoprevention

EvGr Chemoprevention should only be continued for 5 years.

Tamoxifen is recommended for premenopausal women who do not have a history of, or increased risk of thromboembolic disease or endometrial cancer.

Anastrozole p. 1086 is recommended in postmenopausal women who do not have severe osteoporosis, see Osteoporosis p. 768. In women who have severe osteoporosis, or who do not wish to take anastrozole, treatment with tamoxifen can be given, provided there is no history, or increased risk of thromboembolic disease or endometrial cancer. Alternatively, raloxifene hydrochloride p. 868 is an option [unlicensed indication] in postmenopausal women with a uterus who do not wish to take tamoxifen, unless there is a history or increased risk of thromboembolic disease. Ⓐ

Treatment of menopausal symptoms

EvGr Some treatments used in the management of breast cancer, such as tamoxifen or ovarian function suppression may lead to menopausal symptoms or early menopause, and women should be counselled about these side-effects prior to starting any of these treatments.

Women diagnosed with breast cancer should discontinue their hormone replacement therapy (HRT) because of possible tumour stimulation and interference with adjuvant endocrine therapy. HRT should not be offered routinely to women with menopausal symptoms if they have a history of breast cancer; however, in exceptional circumstances, HRT can be offered to women with severe menopausal symptoms once the associated risks have been discussed.

Selective serotonin re-uptake inhibitor (SSRIs) antidepressants may be offered to relieve menopausal symptoms such as hot flushes in women with breast cancer who are not taking tamoxifen. Ⓐ Clonidine hydrochloride p. 172, venlafaxine p. 427 [unlicensed indication] and gabapentin p. 362 [unlicensed indication] are sometimes used for the treatment of hot flushes in women with breast cancer after discussion with the patient and information given about side effects. The MHRA/CHM have released important safety information on the use of antiepileptic drugs and the risk of suicidal thoughts and behaviour. For further information, see Epilepsy p. 349.

Useful Resources

Early and locally advanced breast cancer: diagnosis and management. National Institute for Health and Care Excellence. Clinical guideline 101. July 2018.
www.nice.org.uk/guidance/ng101

Advanced breast cancer: diagnosis and treatment. National Institute for Health and Care Excellence. Clinical guideline 81. August 2017.
www.nice.org.uk/guidance/cg81

Familial breast cancer: classification, care and managing breast cancer and related risks in people with a family history of breast cancer. National Institute for Health and Care Excellence. Clinical guideline 164. June 2013 (updated November 2023).
www.nice.org.uk/guidance/cg164

Guidance for the management of breast cancer treatment-induced bone loss: a consensus position statement from a UK expert group, 2008.
theros.org.uk/clinical-publications-and-resources/

Patient decision aids: Taking a medicine to reduce the chance of developing breast cancer: postmenopausal women at moderately increased risk; Taking a medicine to reduce the chance of developing breast cancer: postmenopausal women at high risk. National Institute for Health and Care Excellence. March 2017.
www.nice.org.uk/about/what-we-do/our-programmes/nice-guidance/nice-guidelines/shared-decision-making

Prostate cancer

26-Nov-2021

Description of condition

Prostate cancer is the most common form of cancer affecting men. It can also affect transgender women, as the prostate is usually conserved after gender-confirming surgery. The main risk factors are age (most cases being diagnosed in men over 70 years of age), ethnicity (more common in black African-Caribbean men), obesity, and a familial component. Prostate cancer is usually slow-growing and asymptomatic at diagnosis, however, the presenting symptoms of advanced disease are usually urinary outflow obstruction, or, pelvic or back pain due to bone metastases. Treatment decisions are guided by baseline prostate specific antigen (PSA) levels, tumour grade (Gleason score), the stage of the tumour, the patient's life expectancy (based on age and comorbid conditions), treatment morbidity, and patient preference.

Aims of treatment

Reducing mortality, increasing progression-free and disease-free survival and improving quality of life are the main aims of treatment, and are dependent on the stage of disease.

Watchful waiting or active surveillance aim to monitor for disease progression, while radical treatments such as prostatectomy and radiotherapy aim to eliminate the malignancy. Hormone therapy and chemotherapy aim to slow the progression of prostate cancer and to control symptoms. In metastatic disease, treatment is aimed at prolonging survival and relieving symptoms.

Overview

[EvGr] Treatment options for patients with prostate cancer include watchful waiting, active surveillance, prostatectomy, radiotherapy (such as external beam), brachytherapy, hormone therapy, and chemotherapy. The benefits and risks of each option should be discussed with patients. Ⓐ

Watchful waiting is a strategy for 'controlling' rather than 'curing' prostate cancer and is aimed at patients in whom curative treatment is unsuitable or declined. It involves monitoring for disease progression and is often suitable in patients not likely to suffer significant morbidity from their prostate cancer. Active surveillance, a 'curative' strategy, is aimed at patients who do not wish to have immediate treatment. It involves the deferred use of radical treatment until disease progression occurs or until the patient requests treatment. For information on monitoring in watchful waiting or the protocol for active surveillance, see NICE clinical guideline **Prostate cancer** (see *Useful resources*).

[EvGr] At any stage of care, when moving from active surveillance to radical treatment, patient preferences, comorbidities and life expectancy should be taken into account. Ⓐ

Hormone therapy includes anti-androgen therapy—to block the effects of androgens, androgen deprivation therapy such as a luteinising hormone-releasing hormone (LHRH) agonist, or a gonadorelin antagonist—to reduce androgen levels, and bilateral orchidectomy—to remove the endogenous supply of androgens.

In patients with localised prostate cancer, the choice of treatment is guided by whether the disease is considered low, intermediate, or high risk according to the Gleason score, the serum PSA level, and the tumour clinical stage. High risk localised prostate cancer is also included in the definition of locally advanced prostate cancer. For further information on risk stratification, see NICE clinical guideline **Prostate cancer** (see *Useful resources*).

Localised or locally advanced prostate cancer

[EvGr] In patients with **low-risk localised prostate cancer**, offer a choice between active surveillance, radical prostatectomy or radiotherapy.

Radical treatment should be offered to patients with localised prostate cancer undergoing active surveillance who show evidence of disease progression.

In patients with **intermediate-risk localised prostate cancer**, radical treatments (prostatectomy or radiotherapy) should be offered, and for those who decline them, active surveillance can be considered.

In patients with **high-risk localised prostate cancer** (when there is a realistic prospect of long-term disease control), and in those with **locally advanced disease**, radical prostatectomy or radiotherapy should be offered.

In patients with **intermediate-risk** and **high-risk localised prostate cancer** who have chosen radical radiotherapy, this should be offered in combination with androgen deprivation therapy. Androgen deprivation therapy should be given for 6 months before, during or after radiotherapy; in patients with **high-risk localised prostate cancer**, consider continuing therapy for up to 3 years. Brachytherapy in combination with radiotherapy can also be considered in these patients.

In patients with newly diagnosed **non-metastatic prostate cancer** discuss the option of chemotherapy with docetaxel p. 1058 [unlicensed indication] if they are starting long term androgen deprivation therapy, have no significant co-morbidities and have high-risk disease.

In patients with **hormone-relapsed non-metastatic prostate cancer** who are at high risk of developing metastatic disease, darolutamide p. 1078 or apalutamide p. 1077, with androgen deprivation therapy is recommended as a treatment option. Ⓐ If a patient's prostate cancer metastasised while on treatment with darolutamide or apalutamide, it would be expected to be resistant to treatment with enzalutamide or abiraterone for metastatic disease because of the similar way these drugs work.

[EvGr] Pelvic radiotherapy should be considered in those with **locally advanced prostate cancer** who have a higher than 15% risk of pelvic lymph node involvement and are to receive neoadjuvant hormonal therapy and radical radiotherapy. Ⓐ

Metastatic prostate cancer

[EvGr] Patients with newly diagnosed **metastatic prostate cancer** who do not have significant comorbidities, should be offered chemotherapy with docetaxel.

Bilateral orchidectomy should be offered to all patients with **metastatic prostate cancer** as an alternative to continuous LHRH agonist treatment. Anti-androgen monotherapy with bicalutamide p. 1077 [unlicensed indication] can be offered to those who are willing to accept the adverse impact on overall survival and gynaecomastia, in the hope of retaining sexual function. However, if satisfactory sexual function is not maintained, stop bicalutamide and start androgen deprivation therapy.

Abiraterone acetate p. 1076 (in combination with prednisone or prednisolone p. 791) and enzalutamide p. 1078 are both recommended as options for the treatment of **hormone-relapsed metastatic prostate cancer** in patients who have no or mild symptoms after androgen deprivation therapy has failed, and before chemotherapy is indicated.

In patients with **hormone-relapsed metastatic prostate cancer**, chemotherapy with docetaxel can be used. It is recommended that treatment with docetaxel is stopped after 10 cycles, or if severe adverse events occur, or if there is evidence of disease progression.

Abiraterone acetate (in combination with prednisone or prednisolone) and enzalutamide are also recommended in **hormone-relapsed metastatic prostate cancer** if disease has progressed during or after treatment with a docetaxel-containing chemotherapy regimen.

In patients with **hormone-relapsed metastatic prostate cancer**, a corticosteroid such as dexamethasone p. 786 can be offered as third line therapy after androgen deprivation therapy and anti-androgen therapy.

In patients with **hormone-relapsed metastatic prostate cancer**, zoledronic acid p. 774 can be considered to prevent or reduce skeletal-related events.

Bisphosphonates can be considered for pain relief in **hormone-relapsed metastatic prostate cancer** when other treatments have failed to give satisfactory pain relief. Ⓐ

Management of side-effects of treatment

[EvGr] Patients should be informed about the side-effects of treatment; particularly urinary and sexual dysfunction, loss of fertility, radiation-induced enteropathy, osteoporosis, gynaecomastia, fatigue, and hot flushes. Ⓐ

Tumour flare due to an initial surge in testosterone concentrations has been reported in the initial stages of treatment with LHRH agonists; the manufacturers advise that the use of prophylactic anti-androgen therapy (such as cyproterone acetate p. 885) should be considered.

[EvGr] Medroxyprogesterone acetate p. 936 [unlicensed indication] can be used, initially for up to 10 weeks, to manage troublesome hot flushes caused by long-term androgen suppression; cyproterone acetate can be considered as an alternative if medroxyprogesterone acetate is not effective or not tolerated. Ⓐ

The MHRA/CHM have issued important safety information on the use of cyproterone acetate and risk of meningioma. For further information, see *Important safety information* for cyproterone acetate.

[EvGr] Patients who experience loss of sexual function should have access to specialist erectile dysfunction services and be considered for treatment with a phosphodiesterase type-5 inhibitor.

Patients who are on androgen deprivation therapy should be offered a supervised exercise program (at least twice a week for 12 weeks) to reduce fatigue and improve quality of life.

A bisphosphonate should be offered to patients who have osteoporosis and who are having androgen deprivation therapy; denosumab p. 777 is an alternative if bisphosphonates are not appropriate.

Although there is limited evidence, intermittent therapy may be considered for patients who are having long-term androgen deprivation therapy to reduce side-effects.

Gynaecomastia can occur with long-term (longer than 6 months) bicalutamide p. 1077 treatment. Prophylactic radiotherapy (within the first month of treatment) should be offered; or if radiotherapy is unsuccessful, weekly tamoxifen p. 1085 [unlicensed indication] can be considered. Ⓐ

Useful Resources

Prostate cancer: diagnosis and management. National Institute for Health and Care Excellence. NICE guideline 131. May 2019.
www.nice.org.uk/guidance/ng131

> **Other drugs used for Hormone responsive malignancy**
> Buserelin, p. 850 · Ethinylestradiol, p. 874 · Goserelin, p. 851 · Leuprorelin acetate, p. 852 · Norethisterone, p. 878 · Triptorelin, p. 853

ANTINEOPLASTIC DRUGS > ANTI-ANDROGENS

Abiraterone acetate

10-Sep-2021

● **INDICATIONS AND DOSE**

Metastatic castration-resistant prostate cancer in patients whose disease has progressed during or after treatment with a docetaxel-containing chemotherapy regimen (in combination with prednisone or prednisolone) | Metastatic castration-resistant prostate cancer in patients who are asymptomatic or mildly symptomatic after failure of androgen deprivation therapy in whom chemotherapy is not yet clinically indicated (in combination with prednisone or prednisolone) | High risk metastatic hormone-sensitive prostate cancer in newly diagnosed patients (in combination with androgen deprivation therapy, and prednisone or prednisolone)

▸ BY MOUTH
▸ Adult: 1 g once daily, for dose of concurrent prednisone or prednisolone—consult product literature

● **CAUTIONS** Diabetes (increased risk of hyperglycaemia— monitor blood sugar frequently) · history of cardiovascular disease

CAUTIONS, FURTHER INFORMATION
▸ Cardiovascular disease Manufacturer advises correct hypertension and hypokalaemia before treatment (if significant risk of congestive heart failure, such as history of cardiac failure, uncontrolled hypertension or cardiac events, consult product literature for management and increased monitoring).

● **INTERACTIONS** → Appendix 1: anti-androgens

● **SIDE-EFFECTS**
▸ **Common or very common** Angina pectoris · arrhythmias · bone fracture · diarrhoea · dyspepsia · haematuria · heart failure · hepatic disorders · hypertension · hypertriglyceridaemia · hypokalaemia · left ventricular dysfunction · osteoporosis · peripheral oedema · rash · sepsis · urinary tract infection
▸ **Uncommon** Adrenal insufficiency · myopathy
▸ **Rare or very rare** Alveolitis allergic
▸ **Frequency not known** Fluid retention · myocardial infarction · QT interval prolongation

● **CONCEPTION AND CONTRACEPTION** Men should use condoms if their partner is pregnant, and use condoms in combination with another effective contraceptive method if their partner is of child-bearing potential—toxicity in *animal* studies.

● **HEPATIC IMPAIRMENT** Manufacturer advises use with caution in moderate impairment and only if benefit clearly outweighs risk; avoid in severe impairment.

● **RENAL IMPAIRMENT** [EvGr] Caution in severe impairment (no information available). Ⓜ

● **MONITORING REQUIREMENTS**
▸ Monitor blood pressure, serum potassium concentration, and fluid balance before treatment, and at least monthly during treatment—consult product literature for management of hypertension, hypokalaemia and oedema.
▸ Monitor liver function before treatment, then every 2 weeks for the first 3 months of treatment, then monthly thereafter—interrupt treatment if serum alanine aminotransferase or aspartate aminotransferase greater than 5 times the upper limit (consult product literature for details of restarting treatment at a lower dose) and discontinue permanently if 20 times the upper limit.

● **NATIONAL FUNDING/ACCESS DECISIONS**
For full details see funding body website
NICE decisions
▸ **Abiraterone for castration-resistant metastatic prostate cancer previously treated with a docetaxel-containing regimen (updated July 2016)** NICE TA259 Recommended with restrictions
▸ **Abiraterone for treating metastatic hormone-relapsed prostate cancer before chemotherapy is indicated (updated July 2016)** NICE TA387 Recommended with restrictions
▸ **Abiraterone for treating newly diagnosed high-risk hormone-sensitive metastatic prostate cancer (August 2021)** NICE TA721 Not recommended

Scottish Medicines Consortium (SMC) decisions
▸ **Abiraterone acetate (*Zytiga*®) with prednisone or prednisolone for the treatment of metastatic castration-resistant prostate cancer (mCRPC) in adult men whose disease has progressed on or after a docetaxel-based chemotherapy regimen (August 2012)** SMC No. 764/12 Recommended with restrictions
▸ **Abiraterone acetate (*Zytiga*®) is indicated with prednisone or prednisolone for the treatment of metastatic castration-resistant prostate cancer (mCRPC) in adult men who are asymptomatic or mildly symptomatic after failure of androgen deprivation therapy in whom chemotherapy is not yet clinically indicated (October 2015)** SMC No. 873/13 Recommended
▸ **Abiraterone acetate (*Zytiga*®) with prednisone or prednisolone for the treatment of adult men with newly diagnosed high-risk metastatic hormone-sensitive prostate cancer (mHSPC) in combination with androgen deprivation therapy (ADT) (January 2020)** SMC No. SMC2215 Recommended

● **MEDICINAL FORMS** There can be variation in the licensing of different medicines containing the same drug.
Oral tablet
CAUTIONARY AND ADVISORY LABELS 23
  ▸ **Abiraterone acetate (Non-proprietary)**
    Abiraterone acetate 250 mg Abiraterone 250mg tablets | 120 tablet PoM £2,735.00 (Hospital only)
    Abiraterone acetate 500 mg Abiraterone 500mg tablets | 56 tablet PoM £1,914.50-£2,735.00 (Hospital only) | 56 tablet PoM £460.00-£3,281.99
  ▸ **Zytiga** (Janssen-Cilag Ltd)
    Abiraterone acetate 500 mg Zytiga 500mg tablets | 56 tablet PoM £2,735.00

Apalutamide
         25-Jul-2023

● **DRUG ACTION** Apalutamide is an androgen receptor inhibitor that decreases tumour cell proliferation and increases apoptosis.

● **INDICATIONS AND DOSE**
Prostate cancer (specialist use only)
▸ BY MOUTH
▸ Adult: 240 mg once daily, for dose adjustments due to side-effects—consult product literature

● **CONTRA-INDICATIONS** History or risk of seizures
● **CAUTIONS** History or risk of QT-interval prolongation · recent cardiovascular disease
● **INTERACTIONS** → Appendix 1: anti-androgens
● **SIDE-EFFECTS**
▸ **Common or very common** Acute coronary syndrome · alopecia · appetite decreased · arteriosclerosis · arthralgia · autoimmune thyroiditis · bone fractures · cardiovascular insufficiency · cerebrovascular insufficiency · conjunctivitis · costal cartilage fracture · diarrhoea · dyslipidaemia · fall · fatigue · genital rash · hemiparesis · hot flush · hypertension · hypothyroidism · ischaemic heart disease ·

muscle spasms · oral disorders · rash pustular · sacrum fracture · skin reactions · taste altered · weight decreased
▸ **Uncommon** Seizure (discontinue permanently) · tongue biting
▸ **Frequency not known** QT interval prolongation · severe cutaneous adverse reactions (SCARs)
● **CONCEPTION AND CONTRACEPTION** Manufacturer advises men should use condoms in combination with another highly effective contraceptive method during treatment and for 3 months after stopping treatment if their partner is of childbearing potential.
● **HEPATIC IMPAIRMENT** Manufacturer advises avoid in severe impairment (no information available).
● **RENAL IMPAIRMENT** Manufacturer advises caution in severe impairment (no information available).
● **NATIONAL FUNDING/ACCESS DECISIONS**
For full details see funding body website
NICE decisions
▸ **Apalutamide with androgen deprivation therapy for treating high-risk hormone-relapsed non-metastatic prostate cancer (October 2021)** NICE TA740 Recommended
▸ **Apalutamide with androgen deprivation therapy for treating hormone-sensitive metastatic prostate cancer (October 2021)** NICE TA741 Recommended with restrictions

Scottish Medicines Consortium (SMC) decisions
▸ **Apalutamide (*Erleada*®) for the treatment of adults with metastatic hormone-sensitive prostate cancer in combination with androgen deprivation therapy (September 2022)** SMC No. SMC2472 Recommended
▸ **Apalutamide (*Erleada*®) for the treatment of adults with non-metastatic castration-resistant prostate cancer who are at high risk of developing metastatic disease (July 2023)** SMC No. SMC2579 Recommended

● **MEDICINAL FORMS** There can be variation in the licensing of different medicines containing the same drug.
Oral tablet
  ▸ **Erleada** (Janssen-Cilag Ltd) ▼
    Apalutamide 60 mg Erleada 60mg tablets | 112 tablet PoM £2,735.00 (Hospital only)
    Apalutamide 240 mg Erleada 240mg tablets | 28 tablet PoM £2,735.00 (Hospital only)

Bicalutamide
         01-Sep-2020

● **INDICATIONS AND DOSE**
Locally advanced prostate cancer at high risk of disease progression either alone or as adjuvant treatment to prostatectomy or radiotherapy | Locally advanced, non-metastatic prostate cancer when surgical castration or other medical intervention inappropriate
▸ BY MOUTH
▸ Adult: 150 mg once daily

Advanced prostate cancer, in combination with gonadorelin analogue or surgical castration
▸ BY MOUTH
▸ Adult: 50 mg once daily, to be started at the same time as surgical castration or at least 3 days before gonadorelin therapy

Prostate cancer (metastatic) with the aim of retaining sexual function.
▸ BY MOUTH
▸ Adult: 150 mg once daily

● **UNLICENSED USE** EvGr Bicalutamide is used in prostate cancer (metastatic) with the aim of retaining sexual function, Ⓐ but it is not licensed for this indication.
● **CAUTIONS** Risk of photosensitivity—avoid excessive exposure to UV light and sunlight
● **INTERACTIONS** → Appendix 1: anti-androgens

Immune system and malignant disease

- **SIDE-EFFECTS**
▶ **Common or very common** Alopecia · anaemia · appetite decreased · asthenia · breast tenderness · chest pain · constipation · depression · dizziness · drowsiness · flatulence · gastrointestinal discomfort · gynaecomastia · haematuria · hair changes · hepatic disorders · hot flush · hypertransaminasaemia · nausea · oedema · sexual dysfunction · skin reactions · weight increased
▶ **Uncommon** Angioedema · interstitial lung disease
▶ **Rare or very rare** Photosensitivity reaction
▶ **Frequency not known** QT interval prolongation

- **HEPATIC IMPAIRMENT** Manufacturer advises caution in moderate to severe impairment (increased risk of accumulation).

- **MONITORING REQUIREMENTS** Consider periodic liver function tests.

- **PATIENT AND CARER ADVICE**
Risk of photosensitivity Patients should be advised to consider the use of sunscreen.

- **MEDICINAL FORMS** There can be variation in the licensing of different medicines containing the same drug. Forms available from special-order manufacturers include: oral suspension

Oral tablet
▶ **Bicalutamide (Non-proprietary)**
Bicalutamide 50 mg Bicalutamide 50mg tablets | 28 tablet [PoM] £119.79 DT = £1.67
Bicalutamide 150 mg Bicalutamide 150mg tablets | 28 tablet [PoM] £240.00 DT = £2.38
▶ **Casodex** (AstraZeneca UK Ltd)
Bicalutamide 50 mg Casodex 50mg tablets | 28 tablet [PoM] £119.79 DT = £1.67
Bicalutamide 150 mg Casodex 150mg tablets | 28 tablet [PoM] £240.00 DT = £2.38

Darolutamide

09-Nov-2023

- **DRUG ACTION** Darolutamide is an androgen receptor inhibitor that decreases tumour cell proliferation.

- **INDICATIONS AND DOSE**
Prostate cancer (specialist use only)
▶ BY MOUTH
▶ Adult: 600 mg twice daily, for dose adjustments or interruption due to side-effects—consult product literature

- **CAUTIONS** History or risk of QT-interval prolongation · recent cardiovascular disease

- **INTERACTIONS** → Appendix 1: anti-androgens

- **SIDE-EFFECTS**
▶ **Common or very common** Acute coronary syndrome · asthenia · atherosclerosis coronary artery · bone fracture · cardiogenic shock · heart failure · ischaemic heart disease · lethargy · malaise · pain · rash
▶ **Frequency not known** Neutropenia

- **CONCEPTION AND CONTRACEPTION** Manufacturer advises men use condoms during and for 1 week after stopping treatment if their partner is pregnant, and highly effective contraception if their partner is of childbearing potential.

- **HEPATIC IMPAIRMENT** Manufacturer advises caution in moderate and severe impairment.
Dose adjustments Manufacturer advises reduce initial dose in moderate or severe impairment to 300 mg twice daily.

- **RENAL IMPAIRMENT** Manufacturer advises caution in severe impairment.
Dose adjustments Manufacturer advises reduce initial dose in severe impairment to 300 mg twice daily.

- **NATIONAL FUNDING/ACCESS DECISIONS**
For full details see funding body website
NICE decisions
▶ **Darolutamide with androgen deprivation therapy for treating hormone-relapsed non-metastatic prostate cancer (November 2020)** NICE TA660 Recommended
▶ **Darolutamide with androgen deprivation therapy and docetaxel for treating hormone-sensitive metastatic prostate cancer (June 2023)** NICE TA903 Recommended
Scottish Medicines Consortium (SMC) decisions
▶ **Darolutamide (*Nubeqa*®) for the treatment of adult men with non-metastatic castration-resistant prostate cancer who are at high risk of developing metastatic disease (November 2020)** SMC No. SMC2297 Recommended
▶ **Darolutamide (*Nubeqa*®) for the treatment of adults with metastatic hormone-sensitive prostate cancer in combination with docetaxel (October 2023)** SMC No. SMC2604 Recommended

- **MEDICINAL FORMS** There can be variation in the licensing of different medicines containing the same drug.
Oral tablet
CAUTIONARY AND ADVISORY LABELS 21
▶ **Nubeqa** (Bayer Plc)
Darolutamide 300 mg Nubeqa 300mg tablets | 112 tablet [PoM] £4,040.00 (Hospital only)

Enzalutamide

01-Mar-2022

- **INDICATIONS AND DOSE**
Prostate cancer (specialist use only)
▶ BY MOUTH
▶ Adult: 160 mg once daily, for dose adjustments due to side-effects—consult product literature

DOSE ADJUSTMENTS DUE TO INTERACTIONS
▶ Manufacturer advises if concurrent use of potent inhibitors of CYP2C8 is unavoidable, reduce dose to 80 mg daily.

- **CAUTIONS** History or risk of QT-interval prolongation · history or risk of seizure · recent cardiovascular disease

- **INTERACTIONS** → Appendix 1: anti-androgens

- **SIDE-EFFECTS**
▶ **Common or very common** Acute coronary syndrome · anxiety · asthenia · atherosclerosis coronary artery · bone fracture · concentration impaired · fall · gynaecomastia · headache · hot flush · hypertension · ischaemic heart disease · memory loss · restless legs · skin reactions · taste altered
▶ **Uncommon** Cognitive disorder · leucopenia · neutropenia · seizures · visual hallucinations
▶ **Frequency not known** Back pain · diarrhoea · face oedema · muscle complaints · muscle weakness · nausea · oral disorders · posterior reversible encephalopathy syndrome (PRES) · QT interval prolongation · second primary malignancy · severe cutaneous adverse reactions (SCARs) · throat oedema · thrombocytopenia · vomiting

- **CONCEPTION AND CONTRACEPTION** [EvGr] Men should use condoms during treatment and for 3 months after stopping treatment if their partner is pregnant, and use condoms in combination with another effective contraceptive method if their partner is of child-bearing potential—toxicity in *animal* studies. Ⓜ

- **RENAL IMPAIRMENT** [EvGr] Caution in severe impairment and end-stage renal disease—no information available. Ⓜ

- **HANDLING AND STORAGE** Women of childbearing potential should avoid handling enzalutamide tablets.

• **PATIENT AND CARER ADVICE**
Missed doses Manufacturer advises if a dose is not taken at the usual time, the missed dose should be taken as close as possible to the usual time; if a dose is missed entirely for the day, the missed dose should be taken the following day at the usual dose.
Driving and skilled tasks Manufacturer advises patients and carers should be counselled on the effects on driving and performance of skilled tasks—risk of psychiatric or neurological events, including seizures.

• **NATIONAL FUNDING/ACCESS DECISIONS**
For full details see funding body website
NICE decisions
▸ **Enzalutamide for metastatic hormone-relapsed prostate cancer previously treated with a docetaxel-containing regimen (July 2014)** NICE TA316 Recommended with restrictions
▸ **Enzalutamide for treating metastatic hormone-relapsed prostate cancer before chemotherapy is indicated (January 2016)** NICE TA377 Recommended with restrictions
▸ **Enzalutamide for hormone-relapsed non-metastatic prostate cancer (May 2019)** NICE TA580 Not recommended
▸ **Enzalutamide for treating hormone-sensitive metastatic prostate cancer (July 2021)** NICE TA712 Recommended
Scottish Medicines Consortium (SMC) decisions
▸ **Enzalutamide (*Xtandi*®) for the treatment of adult men with high-risk non-metastatic castration-resistant prostate cancer (October 2019)** SMC No. SMC2195 Not recommended
▸ **Enzalutamide (*Xtandi*®) for the treatment of adult men with metastatic hormone-sensitive prostate cancer in combination with androgen deprivation therapy (February 2022)** SMC No. SMC2400 Recommended

• **MEDICINAL FORMS** There can be variation in the licensing of different medicines containing the same drug.
Oral tablet
CAUTIONARY AND ADVISORY LABELS 25
  ▸ Xtandi (Astellas Pharma Ltd)
  Enzalutamide 40 mg Xtandi 40mg tablets | 112 tablet [PoM]
  £2,734.67 DT = £2,734.67

Flutamide

04-Jun-2020

• **INDICATIONS AND DOSE**
Advanced prostate cancer | Metastatic prostate cancer refractory to gonadorelin analogue therapy (monotherapy)
▸ BY MOUTH
▸ Adult: 250 mg 3 times a day

• **CONTRA-INDICATIONS** Do not initiate if serum transaminases greater than 2–3 times the upper limit of normal

• **CAUTIONS** Avoid excessive alcohol consumption · avoid in Acute porphyrias p. 1202 · cardiac disease (oedema reported) · diabetes (decreased tolerance to glucose)

• **INTERACTIONS** → Appendix 1: anti-androgens

• **SIDE-EFFECTS**
▸ **Common or very common** Appetite abnormal · asthenia · breast abnormalities · diarrhoea · drowsiness · galactorrhoea · gynaecomastia · hepatic function abnormal (sometimes fatal) · hepatitis (sometimes fatal) · insomnia · nausea · vomiting
▸ **Rare or very rare** Alopecia · anxiety · breast neoplasm · cardiovascular disorder · chest pain · constipation · cough · depression · dizziness · dyspnoea · gastrointestinal discomfort · gastrointestinal disorders · hair growth abnormal · headache · herpes zoster · hot flush · hypertension · interstitial pneumonitis · libido decreased · lupus-like syndrome · lymphoedema · malaise · muscle

cramps · oedema · photosensitivity reaction · skin reactions · thirst · vision blurred
▸ **Frequency not known** QT interval prolongation

• **HEPATIC IMPAIRMENT** Manufacturer advises caution.

• **RENAL IMPAIRMENT** Manufacturer advises caution.

• **MONITORING REQUIREMENTS**
▸ Manufacturer advises monitor liver function before starting treatment, monthly for the first 4 months, and thereafter as clinically indicated.
▸ Manufacturer advises monitor bone mineral density before starting treatment, after 1 year of treatment, and thereafter as clinically indicated.
▸ Manufacturer advises monitor for respiratory symptoms during the first few weeks of treatment (interstitial pneumonitis reported).

• **PATIENT AND CARER ADVICE** Manufacturer advises patients and their carers should be told to discontinue treatment and seek immediate medical attention if signs or symptoms of hepatic toxicity occur.

• **MEDICINAL FORMS** There can be variation in the licensing of different medicines containing the same drug.
Oral tablet
  ▸ Flutamide (Non-proprietary)
  Flutamide 250 mg Flutamide 250mg tablets | 84 tablet [PoM]
  £200.00 DT = £167.88

OESTROGENS

Diethylstilbestrol

21-May-2020

(Stilboestrol)

• **INDICATIONS AND DOSE**
Breast cancer in postmenopausal women
▸ BY MOUTH
▸ Adult: 10–20 mg daily
Prostate cancer
▸ BY MOUTH
▸ Adult: 1–3 mg daily

• **CAUTIONS** Cardiovascular disease

• **SIDE-EFFECTS** Bone pain (in breast cancer) · breast abnormalities · cervical mucus increased · cholelithiasis · contact lens intolerance · depression · erectile dysfunction · erythema nodosum · feminisation · fluid retention · gynaecomastia · headaches · hypercalcaemia (in breast cancer) · hypertension · increased risk of thrombosis · jaundice cholestatic · mood altered · nausea · neoplasms · skin reactions · sodium retention · testicular atrophy · uterine disorders · vomiting · weight changes · withdrawal bleed

• **PREGNANCY** In first trimester, high doses associated with vaginal carcinoma, urogenital abnormalities, and reduced fertility in female offspring. Increased risk of hypospadias in male offspring.

• **HEPATIC IMPAIRMENT** Manufacturer advises caution in mild to moderate impairment; avoid in severe or active impairment.

• **MEDICINAL FORMS** There can be variation in the licensing of different medicines containing the same drug.
Oral tablet
  ▸ Diethylstilbestrol (Non-proprietary)
  Diethylstilbestrol 1 mg Diethylstilbestrol 1mg tablets | 28 tablet [PoM] £209.95 DT = £209.95

PITUITARY AND HYPOTHALAMIC HORMONES AND ANALOGUES > ANTI-GONADOTROPHIN-RELEASING HORMONES

Degarelix

18-Dec-2023

- **INDICATIONS AND DOSE**

Advanced hormone-dependent prostate cancer
▶ BY SUBCUTANEOUS INJECTION
▶ Adult: Initially 240 mg, to be administered as 2 injections of 120 mg, then 80 mg every 28 days, dose to be administered into the abdominal region

- **CAUTIONS** Diabetes · susceptibility to QT-interval prolongation

- **SIDE-EFFECTS**
▶ **Common or very common** Anaemia · chills · diarrhoea · dizziness · fatigue · fever · gynaecomastia · headache · hot flush · influenza like illness · insomnia · musculoskeletal discomfort · musculoskeletal pain · nausea · sexual dysfunction · skin reactions · sweat changes · testicular disorders · weight changes
▶ **Uncommon** Alopecia · appetite decreased · arrhythmias · bone disorders · breast pain · cognitive impairment · constipation · depression · diabetes mellitus · dry mouth · dyspnoea · gastrointestinal discomfort · genital discomfort · hyperglycaemia · hypertension · hypotension · joint disorders · malaise · muscle spasms · muscle weakness · numbness · palpitations · pelvic pain · peripheral oedema · QT interval prolongation · renal impairment · urinary disorders · vision blurred · vomiting
▶ **Rare or very rare** Febrile neutropenia · heart failure · injection site necrosis · myocardial infarction · rhabdomyolysis

- **HEPATIC IMPAIRMENT** Manufacturer advises caution (limited information available)—monitor liver function.

- **RENAL IMPAIRMENT** Manufacturer advises caution in severe impairment—no information available.

- **MONITORING REQUIREMENTS** Monitor bone density.

- **NATIONAL FUNDING/ACCESS DECISIONS**
For full details see funding body website
NICE decisions
▶ Degarelix for treating advanced hormone-dependent prostate cancer (August 2016) NICE TA404 Recommended with restrictions
Scottish Medicines Consortium (SMC) decisions
▶ Degarelix (*Firmagon*®) for treatment of high-risk localised and locally advanced hormone-dependent prostate cancer in combination with radiotherapy or as neo-adjuvant treatment prior to radiotherapy in patients with high-risk localised or locally advanced hormone-dependent prostate cancer (December 2023) SMC No. SMC2625 Recommended

- **MEDICINAL FORMS** There can be variation in the licensing of different medicines containing the same drug.
Powder and solvent for solution for injection
▶ Degarelix (Non-proprietary)
Degarelix (as Degarelix acetate) 80 mg Degarelix 80mg powder and solvent for solution for injection vials | 1 vial PoM £80.11 DT = £89.01
Degarelix (as Degarelix acetate) 120 mg Degarelix 120mg powder and solvent for solution for injection vials | 2 vial PoM £158.51 DT = £176.12
▶ Firmagon (Ferring Pharmaceuticals Ltd)
Degarelix (as Degarelix acetate) 80 mg Firmagon 80mg powder and solvent for solution for injection vials | 1 vial PoM £89.01 DT = £89.01
Degarelix (as Degarelix acetate) 120 mg Firmagon 120mg powder and solvent for solution for injection vials | 2 vial PoM £176.12 DT = £176.12

Relugolix

21-Oct-2024

- **DRUG ACTION** Relugolix is a non-peptide gonadotrophin-releasing hormone (GnRH) receptor antagonist that reduces the release of luteinising hormone and follicle-stimulating hormone, thereby reducing production of testosterone.

- **INDICATIONS AND DOSE**

Prostate cancer (under expert supervision)
▶ BY MOUTH
▶ Adult: Loading dose 360 mg for 1 dose, then maintenance 120 mg once daily

- **CAUTIONS** History or risk of QT-interval prolongation · risk factors for cardiovascular disease · risk factors for osteoporosis

- **INTERACTIONS** → Appendix 1: relugolix

- **SIDE-EFFECTS**
▶ **Common or very common** Anaemia · arthralgia · arthritis · asthenia · colitis · constipation · depression · diarrhoea · dizziness · gynaecomastia · headache · hot flush · hyperhidrosis · hypertension · insomnia · libido decreased · musculoskeletal discomfort · myalgia · nausea · pain · rash · weight increased
▶ **Uncommon** Bone disorders
▶ **Rare or very rare** Myocardial infarction
▶ **Frequency not known** QT interval prolongation

- **CONCEPTION AND CONTRACEPTION** EvGr Male patients should use effective contraception during treatment and for 2 weeks after last treatment if their partner is of childbearing potential. Male fertility may be impaired (reduced testes weight has been observed in *animal* studies). M

- **RENAL IMPAIRMENT** EvGr Use with caution in severe impairment (risk of increased exposure). M

- **PRESCRIBING AND DISPENSING INFORMATION** Dispense in original container (contains desiccant).

- **PATIENT AND CARER ADVICE**
Missed doses If a dose is more than 12 hours late, the missed dose should not be taken and the next dose should be taken at the normal time.
  If treatment is interrupted for more than 7 days, the loading dose should be used to restart treatment.
Driving and skilled tasks Patients and carers should be counselled on the effects on driving and performance of skilled tasks—increased risk of dizziness and fatigue.

- **NATIONAL FUNDING/ACCESS DECISIONS**
For full details see funding body website
NICE decisions
▶ Relugolix for treating hormone-sensitive prostate cancer (August 2024) NICE TA995 Recommended
Scottish Medicines Consortium (SMC) decisions
▶ Relugolix (*Orgovyx*®) for the treatment of adult patients with advanced hormone-sensitive prostate cancer, high-risk localised and locally advanced hormone-dependent prostate cancer in combination with radiotherapy, or as neo-adjuvant treatment prior to radiotherapy in patients with high-risk localised or locally advanced hormone-dependent prostate cancer (October 2024) SMC No. SMC2678 Recommended

- **MEDICINAL FORMS** There can be variation in the licensing of different medicines containing the same drug.
Oral tablet
▶ Orgovyx (Accord-UK Ltd) ▼
Relugolix 120 mg Orgovyx 120mg tablets | 30 tablet PoM £87.45

PITUITARY AND HYPOTHALAMIC HORMONES AND ANALOGUES > SOMATOSTATIN ANALOGUES

Somatostatin analogues 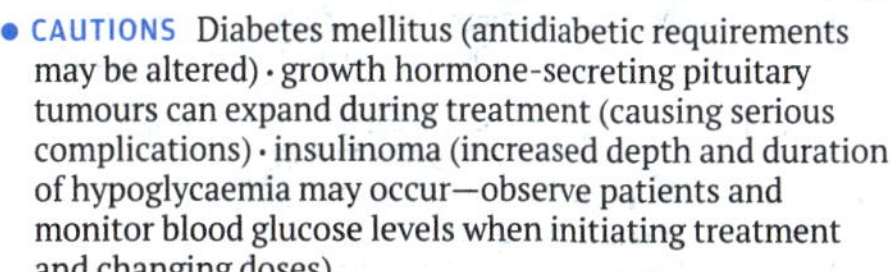

- **CAUTIONS** Diabetes mellitus (antidiabetic requirements may be altered) · growth hormone-secreting pituitary tumours can expand during treatment (causing serious complications) · insulinoma (increased depth and duration of hypoglycaemia may occur—observe patients and monitor blood glucose levels when initiating treatment and changing doses)

- **SIDE-EFFECTS**
  - ▸ **Common or very common** Alopecia · appetite decreased · asthenia · cholecystitis · cholelithiasis (following long term use) · cholestasis · constipation · diabetes mellitus · diarrhoea · dizziness · gastrointestinal discomfort · gastrointestinal disorders · glucose tolerance impaired (following long term use) · headache · hyperglycaemia (long term use) · hypoglycaemia · myalgia · nausea · pruritus · sinus bradycardia · vomiting

- **MONITORING REQUIREMENTS**
  - ▸ Monitor for signs of tumour expansion (e.g. visual field defects).
  - ▸ Ultrasound examination of the gallbladder is recommended before treatment and at intervals of 6–12 months during treatment.

- **DIRECTIONS FOR ADMINISTRATION** Injection sites should be rotated.

⌐ above

Lanreotide

07-Apr-2021

- **INDICATIONS AND DOSE**

SOMATULINE AUTOGEL ®

Acromegaly (if somatostatin analogue not given previously)
- ▸ BY DEEP SUBCUTANEOUS INJECTION
- ▸ Adult: Initially 60 mg every 28 days, adjusted according to response, (consult product literature), for patients treated previously with somatostatin analogue, consult product literature for initial dose, dose to be given in the gluteal region

Neuroendocrine (particularly carcinoid) tumours
- ▸ BY DEEP SUBCUTANEOUS INJECTION
- ▸ Adult: Initially 60–120 mg every 28 days, adjusted according to response, dose to be given in the gluteal region

Unresectable locally advanced or metastatic gastroenteropancreatic neuroendocrine tumours of midgut, pancreatic or unknown origin where hindgut sites of origin have been excluded
- ▸ BY DEEP SUBCUTANEOUS INJECTION
- ▸ Adult: 120 mg every 28 days

- **CAUTIONS** Cardiac disorders (including bradycardia)

- **INTERACTIONS** → Appendix 1: lanreotide

- **SIDE-EFFECTS**
  - ▸ **Common or very common** Biliary dilatation · lethargy · musculoskeletal pain · weight decreased
  - ▸ **Uncommon** Hot flush · insomnia
  - ▸ **Frequency not known** Pancreatitis

- **PREGNANCY** Manufacturer advises use only if potential benefit outweighs risk.

- **BREAST FEEDING** Manufacturer advises caution—no information available.

- **MONITORING REQUIREMENTS** Monitor for hypothyroidism when clinically indicated.

- **NATIONAL FUNDING/ACCESS DECISIONS**
  For full details see funding body website
  All Wales Medicines Strategy Group (AWMSG) decisions
  - ▸ Lanreotide (*Somatuline® Autogel®*) for treatment of grade 1 and a subset of grade 2 (Ki67 index up to 10 %) gastroenteropancreatic neuroendocrine tumours (GEP-NETs) of midgut, pancreatic or unknown origin where hindgut sites of origin have been excluded, in adult patients with unresectable locally advanced or metastatic disease (September 2018) AWMSG No. 1988 Recommended

- **MEDICINAL FORMS** There can be variation in the licensing of different medicines containing the same drug.
  Solution for injection
  - ▸ Lanreotide (Non-proprietary)
    Lanreotide (as Lanreotide acetate) 120 mg per 1 ml Lanreotide 60mg/0.5ml solution for injection pre-filled syringes | 1 pre-filled disposable injection [PoM] £551.00 DT = £551.00
    Lanreotide (as Lanreotide acetate) 180 mg per 1 ml Lanreotide 90mg/0.5ml solution for injection pre-filled syringes | 1 pre-filled disposable injection [PoM] £736.00 DT = £736.00
    Lanreotide (as Lanreotide acetate) 240 mg per 1 ml Lanreotide 120mg/0.5ml solution for injection pre-filled syringes | 1 pre-filled disposable injection [PoM] £749.60–£937.00 DT = £937.00

⌐ above

Octreotide

14-Sep-2020

- **INDICATIONS AND DOSE**

Symptoms associated with carcinoid tumours with features of carcinoid syndrome, VIPomas, glucagonomas
- ▸ BY SUBCUTANEOUS INJECTION
- ▸ Adult: Initially 50 micrograms 1–2 times a day, adjusted according to response; increased to 200 micrograms 3 times a day, higher doses may be required exceptionally; maintenance doses are variable; in carcinoid tumours, discontinue after 1 week if no effect, if rapid response required, initial dose may be given by intravenous injection (with ECG monitoring and after dilution)

Acromegaly, short-term treatment before pituitary surgery or long-term treatment in those inadequately controlled by other treatment or until radiotherapy becomes fully effective
- ▸ BY SUBCUTANEOUS INJECTION
- ▸ Adult: 100–200 micrograms 3 times a day, discontinue if no improvement within 3 months

Prevention of complications following pancreatic surgery
- ▸ BY SUBCUTANEOUS INJECTION
- ▸ Adult: (consult product literature)

Test dose before use of depot preparation
- ▸ BY SUBCUTANEOUS INJECTION
- ▸ Adult: Test dose 50–100 micrograms for 1 dose, test dose should be given if subcutanous octreotide not previously given

Acromegaly | Neuroendocrine (particularly carcinoid) tumour adequately controlled by subcutaneous octreotide
- ▸ BY DEEP INTRAMUSCULAR INJECTION USING DEPOT INJECTION
- ▸ Adult: Initially 20 mg every 4 weeks for 3 months then adjusted according to response, increased if necessary up to 30 mg every 4 weeks, to be administered into the gluteal muscle, for *acromegaly*, start depot 1 day after the last dose of subcutaneous octreotide, for *neuroendocrine tumours*, continue subcutaneous octreotide for 2 weeks after first dose of depot octreotide

Advanced neuroendocrine tumours of the midgut, or tumours of unknown primary origin where non-midgut sites of origin have been excluded
- ▸ BY DEEP INTRAMUSCULAR INJECTION USING DEPOT INJECTION
- ▸ Adult: 30 mg every 4 weeks   continued →

Immune system and malignant disease

Reduce intestinal secretions in palliative care | Reduce vomiting due to bowel obstruction in palliative care
▶ BY CONTINUOUS SUBCUTANEOUS INFUSION
▸ Adult: 0.25–0.5 mg/24 hours (max. per dose 0.75 mg/24 hours), occasionally doses higher than the maximum are sometimes required

● INTERACTIONS → Appendix 1: octreotide

● SIDE-EFFECTS
▶ **Common or very common** Arrhythmias · biliary sludge · dyspnoea · hyperbilirubinaemia · hypothyroidism · skin reactions · thyroid disorder
▶ **Uncommon** Dehydration
▶ **Frequency not known** Hepatic disorders · pancreatitis acute (after administration) · thrombocytopenia

SIDE-EFFECTS, FURTHER INFORMATION Administering non-depot injections of octreotide between meals and at bedtime may reduce gastrointestinal side-effects.

● CONCEPTION AND CONTRACEPTION Effective contraception required during treatment.

● PREGNANCY Possible effect on fetal growth; manufacturer advises use only if potential benefit outweighs risk.

● BREAST FEEDING Manufacturer advises avoid—present in milk in *animal* studies.

● HEPATIC IMPAIRMENT Manufacturer advises caution (risk of increased half-life in cirrhosis).
Dose adjustments Manufacturer advises consider dose reduction—consult product literature.

● MONITORING REQUIREMENTS
▶ Monitor thyroid function on long-term therapy.
▶ Monitor liver function.
▸ With intravenous use ECG monitoring required with intravenous administration.

● TREATMENT CESSATION Avoid abrupt withdrawal of short-acting subcutaneous octreotide (associated with biliary colic and pancreatitis).

● DIRECTIONS FOR ADMINISTRATION For *intravenous injection or intravenous infusion*, manufacturer advises dilute requisite dose to a ratio of at least 1:1 and up to a maximum of 1:9 by volume with Sodium Chloride 0.9%.

● PRESCRIBING AND DISPENSING INFORMATION
Palliative care For further information on the use of octreotide in palliative care, see www.medicinescomplete.com/#/content/palliative/octreotide.

● NATIONAL FUNDING/ACCESS DECISIONS
For full details see funding body website
All Wales Medicines Strategy Group (AWMSG) decisions
▸ Octreotide (*Sandostatin® LAR®*) for the treatment of patients with advanced neuroendocrine tumours of the midgut or of unknown primary origin where non-midgut sites of origin have been excluded (September 2018) AWMSG No. 3732 Recommended

● MEDICINAL FORMS There can be variation in the licensing of different medicines containing the same drug.
Solution for injection
▸ Octreotide (Non-proprietary)
Octreotide (as Octreotide acetate) 50 microgram per 1 ml Octreotide 50micrograms/1ml solution for injection pre-filled syringes | 5 pre-filled disposable injection PoM £35.00–£58.00 DT = £35.00
Octreotide 50micrograms/1ml solution for injection ampoules | 5 ampoule PoM £12.64–£18.60 DT = £14.87
Octreotide (as Octreotide acetate) 100 microgram per 1 ml Octreotide 100micrograms/1ml solution for injection ampoules | 5 ampoule PoM £27.75–£32.65 DT = £27.97
Octreotide 100micrograms/1ml solution for injection pre-filled syringes | 5 pre-filled disposable injection PoM £98.00 DT = £55.00
Octreotide 100micrograms/1ml solution for injection vials | 1 vial PoM £31.85 (Hospital only) | 5 vial PoM £32.65 DT = £32.65

Octreotide (as Octreotide acetate) 200 microgram per 1 ml Octreotide 1mg/5ml solution for injection vials | 1 vial PoM £65.00 DT = £65.00
Octreotide (as Octreotide acetate) 500 microgram per 1 ml Octreotide 500micrograms/1ml solution for injection vials | 5 vial PoM £158.25 DT = £158.25
Octreotide 500micrograms/1ml solution for injection pre-filled syringes | 5 pre-filled disposable injection PoM £250.00–£440.00 DT = £250.00
Octreotide 500micrograms/1ml solution for injection ampoules | 5 ampoule PoM £115.15–£169.35 DT = £135.47
▸ Sandostatin (Novartis Pharmaceuticals UK Ltd)
Octreotide (as Octreotide acetate) 50 microgram per 1 ml Sandostatin 50micrograms/1ml solution for injection ampoules | 5 ampoule PoM £14.87 DT = £14.87
Octreotide (as Octreotide acetate) 100 microgram per 1 ml Sandostatin 100micrograms/1ml solution for injection ampoules | 5 ampoule PoM £27.97 DT = £27.97
Octreotide (as Octreotide acetate) 500 microgram per 1 ml Sandostatin 500micrograms/1ml solution for injection ampoules | 5 ampoule PoM £135.47 DT = £135.47
Powder and solvent for suspension for injection
▸ Olatuton (Teva UK Ltd)
Octreotide (as Octreotide acetate) 10 mg Olatuton 10mg powder and solvent for prolonged-release suspension for injection vials | 1 vial PoM £494.74 DT = £549.71
Octreotide (as Octreotide acetate) 20 mg Olatuton 20mg powder and solvent for prolonged-release suspension for injection vials | 1 vial PoM £719.40 DT = £799.33
Octreotide (as Octreotide acetate) 30 mg Olatuton 30mg powder and solvent for prolonged-release suspension for injection vials | 1 vial PoM £898.57 DT = £998.41
▸ Sandostatin LAR (Novartis Pharmaceuticals UK Ltd)
Octreotide (as Octreotide acetate) 10 mg Sandostatin LAR 10mg powder and solvent for suspension for injection vials | 1 vial PoM £549.71 DT = £549.71
Octreotide (as Octreotide acetate) 20 mg Sandostatin LAR 20mg powder and solvent for suspension for injection vials | 1 vial PoM £799.33 DT = £799.33
Octreotide (as Octreotide acetate) 30 mg Sandostatin LAR 30mg powder and solvent for suspension for injection vials | 1 vial PoM £998.41 DT = £998.41

⚐ 1081

Pasireotide

22-Jan-2019

● INDICATIONS AND DOSE
Cushing's disease [when surgery has failed or is inappropriate]
▶ BY SUBCUTANEOUS INJECTION
▸ Adult: Initially 600 micrograms twice daily for 2 months, then increased if necessary to 900 micrograms twice daily, consider discontinuation if no response after 2 months of treatment, for dose adjustment due to side-effects—consult product literature
▶ BY DEEP INTRAMUSCULAR INJECTION
▸ Adult: Initially 10 mg every 4 weeks, increased if necessary up to 40 mg every 4 weeks, dose may be titrated every 2–4 months based on response and tolerability, consider discontinuation if no clinical benefit observed, for dose adjustment due to side-effects—consult product literature

Acromegaly [when surgery has failed or is inappropriate, and control with another somatostatin analogue is inadequate]
▶ BY DEEP INTRAMUSCULAR INJECTION
▸ Adult: Initially 40 mg every 4 weeks, increased if necessary up to 60 mg every 4 weeks, dose may be increased if levels of growth hormone and/or insulin-like growth factor-1 are not fully controlled after 3 months of initial dosing, for dose adjustment due to side-effects—consult product literature

- **CAUTIONS** Cardiac disorders (including bradycardia) · susceptibility to QT-interval prolongation (including electrolyte disturbances)
- **INTERACTIONS** → Appendix 1: pasireotide
- **SIDE-EFFECTS**
▶ **Common or very common** Adrenal insufficiency · arthralgia · hypotension · QT interval prolongation
▶ **Uncommon** Anaemia
- **PREGNANCY** Manufacturer advises avoid—toxicity in *animal* studies.
- **BREAST FEEDING** Manufacturer advises avoid—present in milk in *animal* studies.
- **HEPATIC IMPAIRMENT** Manufacturer advises caution in moderate impairment (risk of increased exposure); avoid in severe impairment.
  Dose adjustments
  ▶ With subcutaneous use for Cushing's disease Manufacturer advises reduce initial dose to 300 micrograms twice daily (max. dose 600 micrograms twice daily) in moderate impairment.
  ▶ With intramuscular use for Cushing's disease Manufacturer advises max. dose 20 mg every four weeks in moderate impairment.
  ▶ When used for Acromegaly Manufacturer advises reduce initial dose to 20 mg every four weeks (max. dose 40 mg every four weeks) in moderate impairment.
- **RENAL IMPAIRMENT** Manufacturer advises caution in severe impairment—increased plasma-pasireotide exposure.
- **MONITORING REQUIREMENTS**
▶ Manufacturer advises consider monitoring pituitary function before treatment initiation and periodically thereafter.
▶ With subcutaneous use Manufacturer advises monitor liver function before treatment initiation, after 1, 2, 4, 8, and 12 weeks of treatment, and thereafter as clinically indicated. Manufacturer advises assess glycaemic status before treatment initiation, weekly for the first 2–3 months of treatment, over the first 2–4 weeks after any dose increase, periodically thereafter, and 3 months after treatment is complete—if glycaemic control is poor, diabetes management and monitoring should be intensified before and during treatment. Manufacturer advises monitor ECG and electrolytes before treatment initiation, after one week of treatment, and periodically thereafter.
▶ With intramuscular use Manufacturer advises monitor liver function before treatment initiation, after the first 2–3 weeks of treatment, then monthly for 3 months, and thereafter as clinically indicated. Manufacturer advises assess glycaemic status before treatment initiation, weekly for the first 3 months of treatment, over the first 4–6 weeks after any dose increase, periodically thereafter, and 3 months after treatment is complete—if glycaemic control is poor, diabetes management and monitoring should be intensified before and during treatment. Manufacturer advises monitor ECG and electrolytes before treatment initiation, after 3 weeks of treatment, and periodically thereafter.
- **PRESCRIBING AND DISPENSING INFORMATION**
  Switching between formulations
  ▶ When used for Cushing's disease There are no clinical data available on switching between formulations; if a switch is required, manufacturer advises to maintain an interval of at least 28 days between the last intramuscular injection and the first subcutaneous injection—for further information, consult product literature.
- **PATIENT AND CARER ADVICE** Manufacturer advises patients and their carers should be informed of the signs and symptoms of hypocortisolism (including weakness, fatigue, anorexia, nausea, vomiting, hypotension, hyperkalaemia, hyponatraemia, hypoglycaemia).
  Driving and skilled tasks Manufacturer advises patients and carers should be counselled on the effects on driving and performance of skilled tasks—increased risk of fatigue and dizziness.

- **MEDICINAL FORMS** There can be variation in the licensing of different medicines containing the same drug.
  Solution for injection
  ▶ Signifor (Recordati Rare Diseases UK Ltd)
  Pasireotide (as Pasireotide diaspartate) 300 microgram per 1 ml Signifor 0.3mg/1ml solution for injection ampoules | 60 ampoule [PoM] £2,800.00
  Pasireotide (as Pasireotide diaspartate) 600 microgram per 1 ml Signifor 0.6mg/1ml solution for injection ampoules | 60 ampoule [PoM] £3,240.00
  Pasireotide (as Pasireotide diaspartate) 900 microgram per 1 ml Signifor 0.9mg/1ml solution for injection ampoules | 60 ampoule [PoM] £3,240.00
  Powder and solvent for suspension for injection
  ▶ Signifor (Recordati Rare Diseases UK Ltd)
  Pasireotide (as Pasireotide pamoate) 10 mg Signifor 10mg powder and solvent for suspension for injection vials | 1 vial [PoM] £2,300.00
  Pasireotide (as Pasireotide pamoate) 20 mg Signifor 20mg powder and solvent for suspension for injection vials | 1 vial [PoM] £2,300.00
  Pasireotide (as Pasireotide pamoate) 30 mg Signifor 30mg powder and solvent for suspension for injection vials | 1 vial [PoM] £2,300.00
  Pasireotide (as Pasireotide pamoate) 40 mg Signifor 40mg powder and solvent for suspension for injection vials | 1 vial [PoM] £2,300.00
  Pasireotide (as Pasireotide pamoate) 60 mg Signifor 60mg powder and solvent for suspension for injection vials | 1 vial [PoM] £2,300.00

PROGESTOGENS

Megestrol acetate
31-Jan-2020

- **INDICATIONS AND DOSE**
  Treatment of breast cancer
  ▶ BY MOUTH
  ▶ Adult: 160 mg once daily

- **CONTRA-INDICATIONS** Acute porphyrias p. 1202
- **CAUTIONS** Elderly · history of thrombophlebitis
- **SIDE-EFFECTS**
▶ **Common or very common** Adrenal insufficiency · alopecia · appetite increased · asthenia · carpal tunnel syndrome · constipation · Cushing's syndrome · diabetes mellitus · diarrhoea · dyspnoea · embolism and thrombosis · erectile dysfunction · flatulence · glucose tolerance impaired · heart failure · hot flush · hypercalcaemia · hyperglycaemia · hypertension · lethargy · menorrhagia · mood altered · nausea · oedema · pain · skin reactions · tumour flare · urinary frequency increased · vomiting · weight increased
- **PREGNANCY** Avoid. Reversible feminisation of male fetuses reported in *animal* studies. Risk of hypospadias in male fetuses and masculinisation of female fetuses.
- **BREAST FEEDING** Discontinue breast-feeding.
- **HEPATIC IMPAIRMENT** Manufacturer advises caution in severe impairment.

- **MEDICINAL FORMS** There can be variation in the licensing of different medicines containing the same drug. Forms available from special-order manufacturers include: oral tablet, oral capsule, oral suspension
  Oral tablet
  ▶ Megestrol acetate (Non-proprietary)
  Megestrol acetate 40 mg Megestrol 40mg tablets | 100 tablet [E] DT = £184.53
  Megestrol acetate 160 mg Megestrol 160mg tablets | 1 tablet [PoM] [E]

▸ **Megace** (Alliance Pharmaceuticals Ltd)
Megestrol acetate 160 mg Megace 160mg tablets | 30 tablet [PoM]
£19.52 DT = £19.52
Oral suspension
▸ **Megestrol acetate (Non-proprietary)**
Megestrol acetate 40 mg per 1 ml Megestrol 200mg/5ml oral
suspension | 240 ml [PoM] [⚠]

4.1 Hormone responsive breast cancer

ANTINEOPLASTIC DRUGS › ANTI-OESTROGENS

Elacestrant
27-Feb-2025

● **DRUG ACTION** Elacestrant is a selective oestrogen
receptor-α (ERα) antagonist that decreases tumour cell
proliferation.

● **INDICATIONS AND DOSE**

**Oestrogen-receptor-positive breast cancer (initiated by a
specialist)**
▸ BY MOUTH
▸ Adult: 345 mg once daily, for dose adjustments or
interruption due to side-effects—consult product
literature

DOSE ADJUSTMENTS DUE TO INTERACTIONS
▸ [EvGr] Reduce dose to 86 mg once daily if concurrent use
of potent CYP3A4 inhibitors is unavoidable.
▸ Reduce dose to 172 mg once daily if concurrent use of
moderate CYP3A4 inhibitors, ciprofloxacin,
ciclosporin, or fluvoxamine is unavoidable. [M]

● **INTERACTIONS** → Appendix 1: elacestrant
● **SIDE-EFFECTS**
▸ **Common or very common** Anaemia · appetite decreased ·
arthralgia · asthenia · constipation · cough · diarrhoea ·
dizziness · dyspnoea · gastrointestinal discomfort ·
headache · hot flush · insomnia · nausea · pain · rash ·
stomatitis · syncope · urinary tract infection · vomiting
▸ **Uncommon** Acute hepatic failure · embolism and
thrombosis

● **CONCEPTION AND CONTRACEPTION** [EvGr] Females of
childbearing potential should use effective contraception
during treatment and for 1 week after last treatment.
Fertility may be impaired in males and females of
reproductive potential—impairment of fertility has been
observed in *animal* studies. [M]
● **PREGNANCY** [EvGr] Avoid (toxicity in *animal* studies). [M]
● **BREAST FEEDING** [EvGr] Avoid during treatment and for
1 week after last treatment (no information available). [M]
● **HEPATIC IMPAIRMENT** [EvGr] Caution in mild to moderate
impairment (risk of increased exposure); avoid in severe
impairment (no information available). [M]
Dose adjustments [EvGr] Reduce dose to 258 mg once daily
in moderate impairment. [M]
● **PATIENT AND CARER ADVICE**
Vomiting If vomiting occurs after taking tablets, no
additional dose should be taken on that day and the next
dose should be taken at the usual time.
Missed doses If a dose is more than 6 hours late, the
missed dose should not be taken and the next dose should
be taken at the normal time.
Driving and skilled tasks Patients and carers should be
cautioned on the effects on driving and performance of
skilled tasks—increased risk of fatigue, asthenia, and
insomnia.

● **NATIONAL FUNDING/ACCESS DECISIONS**
For full details see funding body website
NICE decisions
▸ **Elacestrant for treating oestrogen receptor-positive
HER2-negative advanced breast cancer with an ESR1 mutation
after endocrine treatment (February 2025)** NICE TA1036
Recommended with restrictions

● **MEDICINAL FORMS** There can be variation in the licensing of
different medicines containing the same drug.
Oral tablet
CAUTIONARY AND ADVISORY LABELS 21
▸ **Korserdu** (Menarini Stemline UK Ltd) ▼
Elacestrant (as Elacestrant dihydrochloride) 86 mg Korserdu
86mg tablets | 28 tablet [PoM] £2,447.00 (Hospital only)
Elacestrant (as Elacestrant dihydrochloride) 345 mg Korserdu
345mg tablets | 28 tablet [PoM] £7,340.00 (Hospital only)

Fulvestrant
10-Aug-2021

● **INDICATIONS AND DOSE**

Oestrogen-receptor-positive breast cancer
▸ BY DEEP INTRAMUSCULAR INJECTION
▸ Adult: 500 mg every 2 weeks for the first 3 doses, then
500 mg every month, to be administered into the
buttock

● **SIDE-EFFECTS**
▸ **Common or very common** Appetite decreased · arthralgia ·
asthenia · diarrhoea · headache · hot flush · hypersensitivity
· increased risk of infection · nausea · pain · rash · vaginal
haemorrhage · venous thromboembolism · vomiting
▸ **Uncommon** Hepatic disorders · vaginal discharge
▸ **Frequency not known** Myalgia
● **PREGNANCY** Manufacturer advises avoid—increased
incidence of fetal abnormalities and death in *animal*
studies.
● **BREAST FEEDING** Manufacturer advises avoid—present in
milk in *animal* studies.
● **HEPATIC IMPAIRMENT** Manufacturer advises caution in
mild to moderate impairment—risk of increased exposure;
avoid in severe impairment—no information available.
● **RENAL IMPAIRMENT** Manufacturer advises caution if
creatinine clearance less than 30 mL/minute—no
information available. See p. 21.
● **DIRECTIONS FOR ADMINISTRATION** Manufacturer advises
500 mg dose should be administered as one 250-mg
injection (slowly over 1–2 minutes) into each buttock.
● **NATIONAL FUNDING/ACCESS DECISIONS**
For full details see funding body website
NICE decisions
▸ **Fulvestrant for untreated locally advanced or metastatic
oestrogen-receptor positive breast cancer (January 2018)**
NICE TA503 Not recommended

● **MEDICINAL FORMS** There can be variation in the licensing of
different medicines containing the same drug.
Solution for injection
▸ **Fulvestrant (Non-proprietary)**
Fulvestrant 50 mg per 1 ml Fulvestrant 250mg/5ml solution for
injection pre-filled syringes | 2 pre-filled disposable injection [PoM]
£522.41 DT = £522.41 (Hospital only) | 2 pre-filled disposable
injection [PoM] £520.00 DT = £522.41
▸ **Faslodex** (AstraZeneca UK Ltd)
Fulvestrant 50 mg per 1 ml Faslodex 250mg/5ml solution for
injection pre-filled syringes | 2 pre-filled disposable injection [PoM]
£522.41 DT = £522.41

Tamoxifen

28-Jul-2020

- **DRUG ACTION** An anti-oestrogen which induces gonadotrophin release by occupying oestrogen receptors in the hypothalamus, thereby interfering with feedback mechanisms; chorionic gonadotrophin is sometimes used as an adjunct in the treatment of female infertility.

- ## INDICATIONS AND DOSE

Pre- and perimenopausal women with oestrogen-receptor-positive breast cancer not previously treated with tamoxifen
- ▸ BY MOUTH
- ▸ Adult: 20 mg daily

Anovulatory infertility
- ▸ BY MOUTH
- ▸ Adult: Initially 20 mg daily on days 2, 3, 4 and 5 of cycle, if necessary the daily dose may be increased to 40 mg then 80 mg for subsequent courses; if cycles irregular, start initial course on any day, with subsequent course starting 45 days later or on day 2 of cycle if menstruation occurs

Gynaecomastia [prevention in men undergoing long-term bicalutamide treatment, if radiotherapy unsuccessful]
- ▸ BY MOUTH
- ▸ Adult: 20 mg once weekly

Breast cancer [chemoprevention in women at moderate-to-high risk]
- ▸ BY MOUTH
- ▸ Adult: 20 mg daily for 5 years

- **UNLICENSED USE** Tamoxifen may be used as detailed below, although considered outside the scope of its licence:
  - ● EvGr the prevention of gynaecomastia in men Ⓐ.

- **CONTRA-INDICATIONS** Treatment of infertility contra-indicated if personal or family history of idiopathic venous thromboembolism or genetic predisposition to thromboembolism

- **CAUTIONS** Acute porphyrias p. 1202

- **INTERACTIONS** → Appendix 1: tamoxifen

- **SIDE-EFFECTS**
- ▸ **Common or very common** Alopecia · anaemia · cataract · cerebral ischaemia · constipation · diarrhoea · dizziness · embolism and thrombosis · fatigue · fluid retention · headache · hepatic disorders · hot flush · hypersensitivity · hypertriglyceridaemia · muscle complaints · nausea · neoplasms · retinopathy · sensation abnormal · skin reactions · taste altered · uterine disorders · vaginal haemorrhage · vomiting · vulvovaginal disorders
- ▸ **Uncommon** Hypercalcaemia · interstitial pneumonitis · leucopenia · pancreatitis · thrombocytopenia · vision disorders
- ▸ **Rare or very rare** Agranulocytosis · angioedema · corneal changes · cutaneous lupus erythematosus · cutaneous vasculitis · cystic ovarian swelling · nerve disorders · neutropenia · radiation recall reaction · Stevens-Johnson syndrome · tumour flare
- ▸ **Frequency not known** Amenorrhoea

  SIDE-EFFECTS, FURTHER INFORMATION **Endometrial changes** Increased endometrial changes, including hyperplasia, polyps, cancer, and uterine sarcoma reported; prompt investigation required if abnormal vaginal bleeding including menstrual irregularities, vaginal discharge, and pelvic pain or pressure in those receiving (or who have received) tamoxifen.

  Risk of thromboembolism Tamoxifen can increase the risk of thromboembolism particularly during and immediately after major surgery or periods of immobility (consider interrupting treatment and initiating anticoagulant measures).

- **CONCEPTION AND CONTRACEPTION** Unless being used in the treatment of female infertility, effective contraception must be used during treatment and for 2 months after stopping. Patients being treated for infertility should be warned that there is a risk of multiple pregnancy (*rarely* more than twins).

- **PREGNANCY** Avoid—possible effects on fetal development.

- **BREAST FEEDING** Suppresses lactation. Avoid unless potential benefit outweighs risk.

- **PRESCRIBING AND DISPENSING INFORMATION** Patient decision aids Taking tamoxifen to reduce the chance of developing breast cancer: premenopausal women at moderately increased risk; Taking tamoxifen to reduce the chance of developing breast cancer: premenopausal women at high risk. National Institute for Health and Care Excellence. March 2017.
  www.nice.org.uk/about/what-we-do/our-programmes/nice-guidance/nice-guidelines/shared-decision-making

- **PATIENT AND CARER ADVICE** Endometrial changes Patients should be informed of the risk of endometrial cancer and told to report relevant symptoms promptly.
  Thromboembolism Patients should be made aware of the symptoms of thromboembolism and advised to report sudden breathlessness and any pain in the calf of one leg.

- **MEDICINAL FORMS** There can be variation in the licensing of different medicines containing the same drug. Forms available from special-order manufacturers include: oral suspension, oral solution

  Oral tablet
- ▸ **Tamoxifen (Non-proprietary)**
  Tamoxifen (as Tamoxifen citrate) 10 mg Tamoxifen 10mg tablets | 30 tablet PoM £49.45 DT = £7.19
  Tamoxifen (as Tamoxifen citrate) 20 mg Tamoxifen 20mg tablets | 30 tablet PoM £13.00 DT = £2.12
  Tamoxifen (as Tamoxifen citrate) 40 mg Tamoxifen 40mg tablets | 30 tablet PoM £98.93 DT = £98.93

  Oral solution
- ▸ **Tamoxifen (Non-proprietary)**
  Tamoxifen (as Tamoxifen citrate) 2 mg per 1 ml Tamoxifen 10mg/5ml oral solution sugar free | 150 ml PoM £116.42 DT = £116.42 SF

Toremifene

25-Aug-2020

- ## INDICATIONS AND DOSE

Hormone-dependent metastatic breast cancer in postmenopausal women
- ▸ BY MOUTH
- ▸ Adult: 60 mg daily

- **CONTRA-INDICATIONS** Bradycardia · electrolyte disturbances (particularly uncorrected hypokalaemia) · endometrial hyperplasia · heart failure with reduced left-ventricular ejection fraction · history of arrhythmias · QT prolongation

- **CAUTIONS** Avoid in Acute porphyrias p. 1202 · history of severe thromboembolic disease

- **INTERACTIONS** → Appendix 1: toremifene

- **SIDE-EFFECTS**
- ▸ **Common or very common** Dizziness · fatigue · hot flush · hyperhidrosis · nausea · oedema · skin reactions · vaginal discharge · vomiting
- ▸ **Uncommon** Appetite decreased · constipation · depression · dyspnoea · headache · insomnia · thromboembolism · uterine disorders · weight increased
- ▸ **Rare or very rare** Alopecia · corneal opacity · endometrial cancer · hepatic disorders · uterine haemorrhage · vertigo
- ▸ **Frequency not known** Anaemia · leucopenia · thrombocytopenia

SIDE-EFFECTS, FURTHER INFORMATION Increased endometrial changes, including hyperplasia, polyps and cancer reported.

- **PREGNANCY** Avoid.
- **BREAST FEEDING** Avoid.
- **HEPATIC IMPAIRMENT** Manufacturer advises caution; avoid in severe hepatic failure (risk of decreased elimination).

- **MEDICINAL FORMS** There can be variation in the licensing of different medicines containing the same drug.
  Oral tablet
  ▸ Fareston (Orion Pharma (UK) Ltd)
    Toremifene (as Toremifene citrate) 60 mg Fareston 60mg tablets | 30 tablet [PoM] £29.08 DT = £29.08

HORMONE ANTAGONISTS AND RELATED AGENTS ⟩ AROMATASE INHIBITORS

Anastrozole

02-Jul-2024

- **INDICATIONS AND DOSE**

Adjuvant treatment of oestrogen-receptor-positive early invasive breast cancer in postmenopausal women | Adjuvant treatment of oestrogen-receptor-positive early invasive breast cancer in postmenopausal women following 2–3 years of tamoxifen therapy | Oestrogen-receptor-positive advanced breast cancer in postmenopausal women
  ▸ BY MOUTH
  ▸ Adult: 1 mg once daily

Breast cancer [chemoprevention in postmenopausal women at moderate to high risk] (initiated by a specialist)
  ▸ BY MOUTH
  ▸ Adult: 1 mg once daily for 5 years

- **CONTRA-INDICATIONS** Not for premenopausal women
- **CAUTIONS** Susceptibility to osteoporosis
- **SIDE-EFFECTS**
▸ **Common or very common** Alopecia · appetite decreased · arthritis · asthenia · bone pain · carpal tunnel syndrome · depression · diarrhoea · drowsiness · headache · hot flush · hypercholesterolaemia · hypersensitivity · joint disorders · myalgia · nausea · osteoporosis · sensation abnormal · skin reactions · taste altered · vaginal haemorrhage · vomiting · vulvovaginal dryness
▸ **Uncommon** Hepatitis · hypercalcaemia · trigger finger
▸ **Rare or very rare** Angioedema · Stevens-Johnson syndrome · vasculitis
- **PREGNANCY** Avoid.
- **BREAST FEEDING** Avoid.
- **HEPATIC IMPAIRMENT** Manufacturer advises use with caution in moderate-to-severe impairment.
- **RENAL IMPAIRMENT** [EvGr] Caution if eGFR less than 30 mL/minute/1.73 m^2 (limited information available). Ⓜ See p. 21.
- **PRE-TREATMENT SCREENING** Laboratory test for menopause if doubt.
- **MONITORING REQUIREMENTS**
▸ Osteoporosis Assess bone mineral density before treatment and at regular intervals.
- **PATIENT AND CARER ADVICE**
  Driving and skilled tasks Asthenia and drowsiness may affect ability to drive or operate machinery.
- **NATIONAL FUNDING/ACCESS DECISIONS**
  For full details see funding body website
  Scottish Medicines Consortium (SMC) decisions
▸ Anastrozole (*Arimidex*®) for the adjuvant treatment of postmenopausal women with oestrogen receptor-positive

early invasive breast cancer (September 2005) SMC No. 198/05 Recommended with restrictions
▸ Anastrozole (*Arimidex*®) for early breast cancer in hormone receptor-positive postmenopausal women who have received 2 to 3 years of adjuvant tamoxifen (November 2006) SMC No. 322/06 Recommended with restrictions

- **MEDICINAL FORMS** There can be variation in the licensing of different medicines containing the same drug.
  Oral tablet
  ▸ Anastrozole (Non-proprietary)
    Anastrozole 1 mg Anastrozole 1mg tablets | 28 tablet [PoM] £68.56 DT = £1.37
  ▸ Arimidex (AstraZeneca UK Ltd)
    Anastrozole 1 mg Arimidex 1mg tablets | 28 tablet [PoM] £68.56 DT = £1.37

Exemestane

11-Jun-2021

- **INDICATIONS AND DOSE**

Adjuvant treatment of oestrogen-receptor-positive early breast cancer in postmenopausal women following 2–3 years of tamoxifen therapy | Advanced breast cancer in postmenopausal women in whom anti-oestrogen therapy has failed
  ▸ BY MOUTH
  ▸ Adult: 25 mg daily

- **CONTRA-INDICATIONS** Not indicated for premenopausal women
- **INTERACTIONS** → Appendix 1: exemestane
- **SIDE-EFFECTS**
▸ **Common or very common** Alopecia · appetite decreased · arthralgia · asthenia · bone fracture · carpal tunnel syndrome · constipation · depression · diarrhoea · dizziness · gastrointestinal discomfort · headache · hot flush · hyperhidrosis · insomnia · leucopenia · nausea · osteoporosis · pain · paraesthesia · peripheral oedema · skin reactions · thrombocytopenia · vomiting
▸ **Rare or very rare** Acute generalised exanthematous pustulosis (AGEP) · drowsiness · hepatic disorders
- **PREGNANCY** Avoid.
- **BREAST FEEDING** Avoid.
- **HEPATIC IMPAIRMENT** Manufacturer advises caution.
- **RENAL IMPAIRMENT** Manufacturer advises caution.

- **MEDICINAL FORMS** There can be variation in the licensing of different medicines containing the same drug.
  Oral tablet
  CAUTIONARY AND ADVISORY LABELS 21
  ▸ Exemestane (Non-proprietary)
    Exemestane 25 mg Exemestane 25mg tablets | 30 tablet [PoM] £88.80 DT = £5.40
  ▸ Aromasin (Pfizer Ltd)
    Exemestane 25 mg Aromasin 25mg tablets | 30 tablet [PoM] £88.80 DT = £5.40

Letrozole

- **INDICATIONS AND DOSE**

First-line treatment in postmenopausal women with hormone-dependent advanced breast cancer | Adjuvant treatment of oestrogen-receptor-positive invasive early breast cancer in postmenopausal women | Advanced breast cancer in postmenopausal women (naturally or artificially induced menopause) in whom other anti-oestrogen therapy has failed | Extended adjuvant treatment of hormone-dependent invasive breast cancer in postmenopausal women who have received standard adjuvant tamoxifen therapy for 5 years | Neo-adjuvant treatment in postmenopausal women with localised hormone-receptor-positive, human epidermal growth factor-2 negative breast cancer where chemotherapy is not suitable and surgery not yet indicated

- ▸ BY MOUTH
- ▸ Adult: 2.5 mg daily

- **CONTRA-INDICATIONS** Not indicated for premenopausal women

- **CAUTIONS** Susceptibility to osteoporosis

- **SIDE-EFFECTS**
- ▸ **Common or very common** Alopecia · appetite abnormal · arthralgia · asthenia · bone fracture · bone pain · constipation · depression · diarrhoea · dizziness · gastrointestinal discomfort · headache · hot flush · hypercholesterolaemia · hyperhidrosis · hypertension · malaise · myalgia · nausea · oedema · osteoporosis · skin reactions · vaginal haemorrhage · vomiting · weight changes
- ▸ **Uncommon** Anxiety · arthritis · breast pain · cancer pain · carpal tunnel syndrome · cataract · cerebrovascular insufficiency · cough · drowsiness · dry mouth · dysaesthesia · dyspnoea · embolism and thrombosis · eye irritation · fever · insomnia · irritability · ischaemic heart disease · leucopenia · memory loss · mucosal dryness · myocardial infarction · palpitations · stomatitis · tachycardia · taste altered · thirst · urinary frequency increased · urinary tract infection · vision blurred · vulvovaginal disorders
- ▸ **Frequency not known** Angioedema · hepatitis · toxic epidermal necrolysis · trigger finger

- **CONCEPTION AND CONTRACEPTION** Manufacturer advises effective contraception required until postmenopausal status fully established (return of ovarian function reported in postmenopausal women).

- **PREGNANCY** Avoid (isolated cases of birth defects reported).

- **BREAST FEEDING** Manufacturer advises avoid.

- **HEPATIC IMPAIRMENT** Manufacturer advises caution in severe impairment (increased exposure and half-life).

- **RENAL IMPAIRMENT** EvGr Use with caution if creatinine clearance less than 10 mL/minute (limited information available), Ⓜ see p. 21.

- **MONITORING REQUIREMENTS**
- ▸ Osteoporosis Assess bone mineral density before treatment and at regular intervals.

- **MEDICINAL FORMS** There can be variation in the licensing of different medicines containing the same drug.

Oral tablet
- ▸ Letrozole (Non-proprietary)
Letrozole 2.5 mg Letrozole 2.5mg tablets | 14 tablet PoM £2.58–£90.92 | 28 tablet PoM £90.92 DT = £1.48
- ▸ Femara (Novartis Pharmaceuticals UK Ltd)
Letrozole 2.5 mg Femara 2.5mg tablets | 30 tablet PoM £90.92

---

5   Immunotherapy responsive malignancy

ANTINEOPLASTIC DRUGS

Talimogene laherparepvec
[Specialist drug]

- **INDICATIONS AND DOSE**

Melanoma
- ▸ BY INTRALESIONAL INJECTION
- ▸ Adult: Specialist drug – access specialist resources for dosing information

- **CONTRA-INDICATIONS** Severely immunocompromised patients

CONTRA-INDICATIONS, FURTHER INFORMATION
Manufacturer advises avoid in patients who are severely immunocompromised, for example, those with severe congenital or acquired cellular and/or humoral immune deficiency—may be at increased risk of disseminated herpetic infection.

- **SIDE-EFFECTS**
- ▸ **Common or very common** Anaemia · anxiety · arthralgia · chills · confusion · constipation · cough · deep vein thrombosis · dehydration · depression · diarrhoea · dizziness · dyspnoea · ear pain · fatigue · fever · flushing · gastrointestinal discomfort · headache · hypertension · immune-mediated events · increased risk of infection · influenza like illness · insomnia · malaise · myalgia · nausea · neoplasm complications · oropharyngeal pain · pain · peripheral oedema · procedural pain · secretion discharge · skin reactions · tachycardia · vomiting · weight decreased · wound complications
- ▸ **Uncommon** Glomerulonephritis · injection site plasmacytoma · obstructive airway disorder · pneumonitis · post procedural infection · vasculitis

SIDE-EFFECTS, FURTHER INFORMATION Necrosis or ulceration of tumour tissue may occur, and impaired healing at the injection site has been reported. Manufacturer advises careful wound care and infection precautions; if persistent infection or delayed healing develops, the risks and benefits of continuing treatment should be considered.

- **CONCEPTION AND CONTRACEPTION** Manufacturer advises use of latex condoms.

- **PATIENT AND CARER ADVICE** Manufacturer advises that patients and carers should be informed about the risks of treatment, advised to avoid touching or scratching injection sites, and to keep these sites covered with occlusive dressings. Close contacts should avoid direct contact with injected lesions or body fluids of treated patients during treatment and for up to 30 days after last treatment—if exposed, clean the affected area and seek medical attention if symptoms of herpetic infection develop; close contacts who are immunocompromised or pregnant should not be exposed to potentially contaminated materials. For further information, see the *Information for Patients and Close Contacts* provided by the manufacturer.

Provide patient alert card—record batch number for each administration of *Imlygic*®.

Driving and skilled tasks Manufacturer advises that patients and their carers should be counselled on the effects on driving and performance of skilled tasks—risk of dizziness and confusion.

- **NATIONAL FUNDING/ACCESS DECISIONS**
For full details see funding body website
NICE decisions
▸ Talimogene laherparepvec for treating unresectable metastatic melanoma (September 2016) NICE TA410 Recommended

- **MEDICINAL FORMS** There can be variation in the licensing of different medicines containing the same drug.
Solution for injection
EXCIPIENTS: May contain Sorbitol
ELECTROLYTES: May contain Sodium
▸ Imlygic (Amgen Ltd)
Talimogene laherparepvec 1 million plaque forming units per 1 ml Imlygic 1million plaque forming units/1ml solution for injection vials | 1 vial PoM £1,670.00 (Hospital only)
Talimogene laherparepvec 100 million plaque forming units per 1 ml Imlygic 100million plaque forming units/1ml solution for injection vials | 1 vial PoM £1,670.00 (Hospital only)

IMMUNOSTIMULANTS > INTERFERONS

Interferon gamma-1b

25-May-2021

(Immune interferon)

- **INDICATIONS AND DOSE**

To reduce the frequency of serious infection in chronic granulomatous disease
▸ BY SUBCUTANEOUS INJECTION
▸ Adult: 50 micrograms/m^2 3 times a week

To reduce the frequency of serious infection in severe malignant osteopetrosis
▸ BY SUBCUTANEOUS INJECTION
▸ Adult: 50 micrograms/m^2 3 times a week

- **CONTRA-INDICATIONS** Simultaneous administration of foreign proteins including immunological products (such as vaccines)—risk of exaggerated immune response
- **CAUTIONS** Arrhythmias · cardiac disease · congestive heart failure · ischaemia · seizure disorders (including seizures associated with fever)
- **SIDE-EFFECTS**
▸ **Common or very common** Abdominal pain · arthralgia · back pain · chills · depression · diarrhoea · fatigue · fever · headache · nausea · rash · vomiting
▸ **Frequency not known** Atrioventricular block · chest discomfort · confusion · connective tissue disorders · embolism and thrombosis · gait abnormal · gastrointestinal haemorrhage · hallucination · heart failure · hepatic failure · hypertriglyceridaemia · hypoglycaemia · hyponatraemia · hypotension · influenza like illness · interstitial lung disease · myocardial infarction · neutropenia · pancreatitis · parkinsonism · proteinuria · renal failure · respiratory disorders · seizure · syncope · systemic lupus erythematosus (SLE) · tachycardia · thrombocytopenia · transient ischaemic attack
- **CONCEPTION AND CONTRACEPTION** Effective contraception required during treatment—consult product literature.
- **PREGNANCY** Manufacturers recommend avoid unless potential benefit outweighs risk (toxicity in *animal* studies).
- **BREAST FEEDING** Manufacturers advise avoid—no information available.
- **HEPATIC IMPAIRMENT** Manufacturer advises caution in severe impairment (increased risk of accumulation).
- **RENAL IMPAIRMENT** Manufacturer advises caution in severe impairment—risk of accumulation.
- **MONITORING REQUIREMENTS** Monitor before and during treatment: haematological tests (including full blood count, differential white cell count, and platelet count),

blood chemistry tests (including renal and liver function tests) and urinalysis.

- **MEDICINAL FORMS** There can be variation in the licensing of different medicines containing the same drug.
Solution for injection
▸ Immukin (Clinigen Healthcare Ltd)
Interferon gamma-1b (recombinant human) 200 microgram per 1 ml Immukin 100micrograms/0.5ml solution for injection vials | 6 vial PoM £930.00

IMMUNOSTIMULANTS > INTERLEUKINS

Aldesleukin [Specialist drug]

24-Jul-2020

- **INDICATIONS AND DOSE**

Renal cell carcinoma
▸ BY SUBCUTANEOUS INJECTION, OR BY CONTINUOUS INTRAVENOUS INFUSION
▸ Adult: Specialist drug – access specialist resources for dosing information

- **UNLICENSED USE** Aldesleukin is not licensed for use in patients in whom all three of the following prognostic factors are present: performance status of Eastern Co-operative Oncology Group of 1 or greater, more than one organ with metastatic disease sites, and a period of less than 24 months between initial diagnosis of primary tumour and date of evaluation of treatment.
- **CONTRA-INDICATIONS** Consult product literature
- **INTERACTIONS** → Appendix 1: aldesleukin
- **SIDE-EFFECTS**
▸ **Common or very common** Acidosis · alopecia · anaemia · anxiety · appetite decreased · arrhythmias · arthralgia · ascites · asthenia · cardiovascular disorders · chest pain · chills · coagulation disorders · confusion · conjunctivitis · constipation · cough · cyanosis · dehydration · depression · diarrhoea · dizziness · drowsiness · dyspepsia · dysphagia · dyspnoea · electrolyte imbalance · eosinophilia · fever · gastrointestinal disorders · haemorrhage · hallucination · headache · heart failure · hepatic disorders · hyperbilirubinaemia · hyperglycaemia · hyperhidrosis · hypertension · hyperthyroidism · hypotension · hypothermia · hypothyroidism · hypoxia · increased risk of infection · insomnia · irritability · ischaemic heart disease · leucopenia · malaise · mucositis · myalgia · nasal congestion · nausea · nerve disorders · oedema · oral disorders · pain · palpitations · paraesthesia · pulmonary oedema · renal impairment · respiratory disorders · sepsis · skin reactions · speech disorder · syncope · taste loss · thrombocytopenia · vomiting · weight changes
▸ **Uncommon** Angioedema · cardiac arrest · cardiac inflammation · cardiomyopathy · coma · embolism and thrombosis · hypoglycaemia · muscle weakness · myopathy · neutropenia · pancreatitis · paralysis · pericardial disorders · seizure
▸ **Rare or very rare** Agranulocytosis · aplastic anaemia · cholecystitis · Crohn's disease aggravated · diabetes mellitus · haemolytic anaemia · injection site necrosis · Stevens-Johnson syndrome · ventricular dysfunction
▸ **Frequency not known** Capillary leak syndrome (less common and less severe with subcutaneous injection) · central nervous system vasculitis · immune complex RPGN · inflammatory arthritis · intracranial haemorrhage · leukoencephalopathy · myocardial infarction · oculo-bulbar myasthenia gravis · psychiatric disorder · stroke · thyroiditis
- **CONCEPTION AND CONTRACEPTION** Ensure effective contraception during treatment in men and women.

- **MEDICINAL FORMS** There can be variation in the licensing of different medicines containing the same drug.
Powder for solution for injection
  - Proleukin (Clinigen Healthcare Ltd)
    Aldesleukin 18 mega unit Proleukin 18million unit powder for solution for injection vials | 1 vial [PoM] £636.00

IMMUNOSTIMULANTS > OTHER

Bacillus Calmette-Guérin [Specialist drug]
01-Aug-2024

- **INDICATIONS AND DOSE**
Bladder carcinoma
  - BY INTRAVESICAL INSTILLATION
  - Adult: Specialist drug – access specialist resources for dosing information

- **CONTRA-INDICATIONS** Fever of unknown origin · gross haematuria · HIV infection · impaired immune response · tuberculosis (active) · urinary-tract infection

- **SIDE-EFFECTS**
  - **Common or very common** Anaemia · arthritis · chills · cystitis · diarrhoea · fatigue · fever · gastrointestinal discomfort · haematuria · increased risk of infection · influenza like illness · joint disorders · malaise · myalgia · nausea · pneumonitis · urinary disorders · vomiting
  - **Uncommon** Bladder constriction · hepatitis · pancytopenia · pyuria · skin reactions · thrombocytopenia · ureteral obstruction
  - **Rare or very rare** Acute kidney injury · alopecia · appetite decreased · balanoposthitis · chest pain · confusion · conjunctivitis · cough · dizziness · drowsiness · dyspnoea · gastrointestinal disorders · granuloma · headache · hyperhidrosis · hypotension · lymphadenopathy · muscle tone increased · pain · peripheral oedema · prostatitis · sensation abnormal · vascular fistula · vertigo · vulvovaginal discomfort · weight decreased
  - **Frequency not known** Haemophagocytic lymphohistiocytosis · sperm abnormalities

- **PATIENT AND CARER ADVICE** Patients should be advised to refrain from intercourse or to use a condom during and for 1 week after each treatment to prevent potential sexual transmission of Bacillus Calmette-Guérin (BCG). Patients and carers should be counselled on the actions to be taken if symptoms of a late flare-up of latent BCG infection occur.

- **MEDICINAL FORMS** There can be variation in the licensing of different medicines containing the same drug.
Powder and solvent for intravesical suspension
EXCIPIENTS: May contain Polysorbates
  - BCG-medac (medac UK)
    RIVM strain Bacillus of Calmette-Guerin 850 million colony forming units per 1 ml BCG-medac 200million-1,500million colony forming units powder and solvent for intravesical suspension vials with conical adaptor | 1 vial [PoM] £150.00 (Hospital only)
Powder for reconstitution for instillation
  - OncoTICE (Merck Sharp & Dohme (UK) Ltd)
    TICE strain Bacillus of Calmette-Guerin 12.5 mg OncoTICE 12.5mg powder for reconstitution for instillation vials | 1 vial [PoM] £96.51 (Hospital only)

Mifamurtide [Specialist drug]
20-Sep-2024

- **INDICATIONS AND DOSE**
Osteosarcoma
  - BY INTRAVENOUS INFUSION
  - Adult 18-30 years: Specialist drug – access specialist resources for dosing information

- **INTERACTIONS** → Appendix 1: mifamurtide

- **SIDE-EFFECTS**
  - **Common or very common** Alopecia · anaemia · anxiety · appetite decreased · arthralgia · asthenia · cancer pain · chest discomfort · chills · confusion · constipation · cough · cyanosis · dehydration · depression · diarrhoea · dizziness · drowsiness · dysmenorrhoea · dyspnoea · feeling cold · fever · flushing · gastrointestinal discomfort · haemorrhage · headache · hearing loss · hepatic pain · hyperhidrosis · hypertension · hypokalaemia · hypotension · hypothermia · increased risk of infection · insomnia · laryngeal pain · leucopenia · malaise · mucositis · muscle complaints · musculoskeletal stiffness · nasal congestion · nausea · neutropenia · oedema · pain · pallor · palpitations · respiratory disorders · sensation abnormal · sepsis · skin reactions · tachycardia · thrombocytopenia · tinnitus · tremor · urinary disorders · vertigo · vision blurred · vomiting · weight decreased
  - **Frequency not known** Pericardial effusion

- **CONCEPTION AND CONTRACEPTION** [EvGr] Females of childbearing potential should use effective contraception. ⟨M⟩

- **PATIENT AND CARER ADVICE**
Driving and skilled tasks Patients and carers should be counselled on the effects on driving and performance of skilled tasks—increased risk of dizziness, vertigo, fatigue, and blurred vision.

- **NATIONAL FUNDING/ACCESS DECISIONS**
For full details see funding body website
NICE decisions
  - Mifamurtide for the treatment of osteosarcoma (October 2011) NICE TA235 Recommended

- **MEDICINAL FORMS** There can be variation in the licensing of different medicines containing the same drug.
Powder for dispersion for infusion
  - Mifamurtide (Non-proprietary)
    Mifamurtide 4 mg Mifamurtide 4mg powder for concentrate for dispersion for infusion vials | 1 vial [PoM] £2,375.00 (Hospital only)
  - Mepact (Takeda UK Ltd)
    Mifamurtide 4 mg Mepact 4mg powder for concentrate for dispersion for infusion vials | 1 vial [PoM] £2,375.00 (Hospital only)

IMMUNOSUPPRESSANTS > THALIDOMIDE AND RELATED ANALOGUES

Lenalidomide [Specialist drug]
28-Feb-2023

- **INDICATIONS AND DOSE**
Multiple myeloma | Myelodysplastic syndromes | Mantle cell lymphoma | Follicular lymphoma
  - BY MOUTH
  - Adult: Specialist drug – access specialist resources for dosing information

IMPORTANT SAFETY INFORMATION
PREGNANCY PREVENTION PROGRAMME
Important: teratogenic risk. Lenalidomide is structurally related to thalidomide and there is a risk of teratogenesis.

Patients, prescribers, and pharmacists must comply with the manufacturer's Pregnancy Prevention Programme. Every prescription must be accompanied by a completed Prescription Authorisation Form.

For females of childbearing potential, each prescription for lenalidomide should be limited to a maximum supply of 4 weeks' treatment. Pregnancy testing should ideally be carried out on the same day as prescription issuing and dispensing.

MHRA/CHM ADVICE: IMMUNOMODULATORY DRUGS AND PREGNANCY PREVENTION: TEMPORARY ADVICE FOR MANAGEMENT DURING CORONAVIRUS (COVID-19) (MAY 2020)
The MHRA has issued temporary guidance for female patients on lenalidomide during the coronavirus (COVID-19) pandemic to support adherence to the Pregnancy Prevention Programme (see *Conception and contraception*), particularly for those who are shielding due to other health conditions, and should be followed until further notice.

MHRA/CHM ADVICE: RISK OF THROMBOSIS AND THROMBOEMBOLISM (DECEMBER 2014)
The MHRA advises that patients treated with lenalidomide for the management of multiple myeloma should be closely monitored for evidence of arterial and venous thromboembolic events, and risk factors for thromboembolism (such as smoking, hypertension, hyperlipidaemia) should be minimised. Healthcare professionals should consider appropriate thrombotic prophylactic medication during treatment with lenalidomide after assessment of the risks and benefits.

● INTERACTIONS → Appendix 1: lenalidomide
● SIDE-EFFECTS
▶ **Common or very common** Anaemia · appetite decreased · arthralgia · asthenia · atrial fibrillation · chills · constipation · cough · decreased leucocytes · dehydration · diarrhoea · dizziness · dry mouth · dyspnoea · electrolyte imbalance · embolism and thrombosis · fall · fever · gastrointestinal discomfort · haemorrhage · headache · heart failure · hyperglycaemia · hypertension · hyperthyroidism · hypotension · hypothyroidism · increased risk of infection · influenza like illness · insomnia · interstitial lung disease · iron overload · lethargy · mood altered · muscle complaints · muscle weakness · myocardial infarction · nausea · neoplasms · nerve disorders · neutropenia · night sweats · pain · pancytopenia · paraesthesia · peripheral oedema · renal failure · respiratory disorder · rhinorrhoea · sepsis · skin reactions · taste altered · thrombocytopenia · toothache · tumour flare · vertigo · vomiting · weight decreased
▶ **Uncommon** Angioedema
▶ **Rare or very rare** Hypersensitivity · severe cutaneous adverse reactions (SCARs) · tumour lysis syndrome
▶ **Frequency not known** Acquired haemophilia · gastrointestinal disorders · hepatic disorders · hypersensitivity vasculitis · pancreatitis · progressive multifocal leukoencephalopathy (PML) · reactivation of infections · solid organ transplant rejection

SIDE-EFFECTS, FURTHER INFORMATION Patients aged 75 years and over—increased risk of serious side-effects.

Hepatic disorders Hepatic failure, including fatal cases, have been reported. Abnormal liver function tests are generally reversible upon dosing interruption; once returned to baseline, consider restarting treatment at a reduced dose.

Neutropenia and thrombocytopenia Reduce dose or interrupt treatment if neutropenia or thrombocytopenia develop.

Rash If grade 2 or 3 rash occurs, treatment should be discontinued and only restarted following appropriate clinical evaluation. Discontinue permanently if grade 4, exfoliative, or bullous rash, or if drug reaction with eosinophilia and systemic symptoms (DRESS), Stevens-Johnson syndrome, or toxic epidermal necrolysis is suspected.

Thromboembolism If thromboembolic event occurs, discontinue lenalidomide and treat with standard anticoagulation therapy; consider restarting with continued anticoagulation therapy once thromboembolic event resolved.

● CONCEPTION AND CONTRACEPTION [EvGr] Pregnancy must be excluded in female patients of childbearing potential before starting treatment with lenalidomide. A medically supervised pregnancy test should be performed on, or within 3 days prior to, initiation and repeated every 4 weeks thereafter (including 4 weeks after the last dose), except in the case of confirmed tubal sterilisation. Females of childbearing potential must use effective contraception for at least 4 weeks before, during, and for at least 4 weeks after stopping treatment (including during dose interruptions), unless the patient is committed to absolute and continuous abstinence confirmed on a monthly basis; oral combined hormonal contraceptives and copper-releasing intra-uterine devices are not recommended. As lenalidomide is present in semen, male patients, even after successful vasectomy, must use condoms during treatment (including during dose interruptions) and for at least 1 week after stopping, if their partner is pregnant or is of childbearing potential and not using effective contraception. Ⓜ

● PATIENT AND CARER ADVICE
Thromboembolism Patients and their carers should be made aware of the symptoms of thromboembolism and advised to report sudden breathlessness, chest pain, or swelling of a limb.
Neutropenia and thrombocytopenia Patients and their carers should be made aware of the symptoms of neutropenia and advised to seek medical advice if symptoms suggestive of neutropenia (such as fever, sore throat) or of thrombocytopenia (such as bleeding) develop.

Patients should be given a patient card and information leaflet about the Pregnancy Prevention Programme.
Conception and contraception Patient counselling is advised for lenalidomide capsules (pregnancy and contraception).

● NATIONAL FUNDING/ACCESS DECISIONS
For full details see funding body website
NICE decisions
▶ **Lenalidomide for treating myelodysplastic syndromes associated with an isolated deletion 5q cytogenetic abnormality (updated June 2019)** NICE TA322 Recommended with restrictions
▶ **Lenalidomide for the treatment of multiple myeloma in people who have received at least 2 prior therapies (updated June 2019)** NICE TA171 Recommended with restrictions
▶ **Lenalidomide plus dexamethasone for multiple myeloma after 1 treatment with bortezomib (June 2019)** NICE TA586 Recommended with restrictions
▶ **Lenalidomide plus dexamethasone for previously untreated multiple myeloma (June 2019)** NICE TA587 Recommended with restrictions
▶ **Lenalidomide with rituximab for previously treated follicular lymphoma (April 2020)** NICE TA627 Recommended
▶ **Lenalidomide maintenance treatment after an autologous stem cell transplant for newly diagnosed multiple myeloma (March 2021)** NICE TA680 Recommended with restrictions

Scottish Medicines Consortium (SMC) decisions
▶ **Lenalidomide (*Revlimid*®) for third line treatment of multiple myeloma (May 2010)** SMC No. 441/08 Recommended with restrictions
▶ **Lenalidomide (*Revlimid*®) in combination with dexamethasone, for the treatment of multiple myeloma in adult patients who have received at least one prior therapy (April 2014)** SMC No. 441/08 Recommended with restrictions
▶ **Lenalidomide (*Revlimid*®) for the treatment of adult patients with previously untreated multiple myeloma who are not eligible for transplant (December 2015)** SMC No. 1096/15 Recommended with restrictions
▶ **Lenalidomide (*Revlimid*®) as monotherapy for the maintenance treatment of adult patients with newly diagnosed multiple myeloma who have undergone autologous

stem cell transplantation (October 2020) SMC No. SMC2289 Recommended

▶ Lenalidomide (*Revlimid*®) in combination with rituximab (anti-CD20 antibody) for the treatment of adult patients with previously treated follicular lymphoma (Grade 1 to 3a) (October 2020) SMC No. SMC2281 Recommended

● **MEDICINAL FORMS** There can be variation in the licensing of different medicines containing the same drug.

Oral capsule
CAUTIONARY AND ADVISORY LABELS 25

▶ **Lenalidomide** (Non-proprietary)

Lenalidomide 2.5 mg Lenalidomide 2.5mg capsules | 7 capsule [PoM] £1,027.80 (Hospital only) | 21 capsule [PoM] £3,426.00 | 21 capsule [PoM] £2,912.10–£3,426.00 (Hospital only)
Lenalidomide 5 mg Lenalidomide 5mg capsules | 21 capsule [PoM] £3,570.00 | 21 capsule [PoM] £3,034.50–£3,570.00 (Hospital only)
Lenalidomide 7.5 mg Lenalidomide 7.5mg capsules | 21 capsule [PoM] £3,675.00 | 21 capsule [PoM] £3,123.75–£3,675.00 (Hospital only)
Lenalidomide 10 mg Lenalidomide 10mg capsules | 21 capsule [PoM] £3,780.00 DT = £3,780.00 (Hospital only) | 21 capsule [PoM] £3,780.00 DT = £3,780.00
Lenalidomide 15 mg Lenalidomide 15mg capsules | 21 capsule [PoM] £3,969.00 DT = £3,969.00 | 21 capsule [PoM] £3,969.00 DT = £3,969.00 (Hospital only)
Lenalidomide 20 mg Lenalidomide 20mg capsules | 21 capsule [PoM] £4,168.50 | 21 capsule [PoM] £3,543.23–£4,168.50 (Hospital only)
Lenalidomide 25 mg Lenalidomide 25mg capsules | 21 capsule [PoM] £4,368.00 | 21 capsule [PoM] £3,712.80–£4,368.00 (Hospital only)

▶ **Revlimid** (Bristol-Myers Squibb Pharmaceuticals Ltd) ▼

Lenalidomide 2.5 mg Revlimid 2.5mg capsules | 7 capsule [PoM] £1,142.00 | 21 capsule [PoM] £3,426.00
Lenalidomide 5 mg Revlimid 5mg capsules | 7 capsule [PoM] £1,190.00 | 21 capsule [PoM] £3,570.00
Lenalidomide 7.5 mg Revlimid 7.5mg capsules | 21 capsule [PoM] £3,675.00
Lenalidomide 10 mg Revlimid 10mg capsules | 21 capsule [PoM] £3,780.00 DT = £3,780.00
Lenalidomide 15 mg Revlimid 15mg capsules | 21 capsule [PoM] £3,969.00 DT = £3,969.00
Lenalidomide 20 mg Revlimid 20mg capsules | 21 capsule [PoM] £4,168.50
Lenalidomide 25 mg Revlimid 25mg capsules | 21 capsule [PoM] £4,368.00

Pomalidomide [Specialist drug]   25-May-2021

● **INDICATIONS AND DOSE**

Multiple myeloma
▶ BY MOUTH
▶ Adult: Specialist drug – access specialist resources for dosing information

---

IMPORTANT SAFETY INFORMATION

MHRA/CHM ADVICE: RISK OF HEPATITIS B REACTIVATION (MAY 2016)
An EU wide review has concluded that pomalidomide can cause hepatitis B reactivation; the MHRA recommends to establish hepatitis B virus status in all patients before initiation of treatment. Patients with a history of hepatitis B infection should be closely monitored for signs and symptoms of active infection throughout treatment; expert advice should be sought for patients who test positive for active infection.

PREGNANCY PREVENTION PROGRAMME
Important: teratogenic risk.
Patients, prescribers, and pharmacists must comply with the manufacturer's Pregnancy Prevention Programme. Every prescription must be accompanied by a completed Prescription Authorisation Form.

For females of childbearing potential, each prescription for pomalidomide should be limited to a maximum supply of 4 weeks' treatment. Pregnancy testing should ideally be carried out on the same day as prescription issuing and dispensing.

MHRA/CHM ADVICE: IMMUNOMODULATORY DRUGS AND PREGNANCY PREVENTION: TEMPORARY ADVICE FOR MANAGEMENT DURING CORONAVIRUS (COVID-19) (MAY 2020)
The MHRA has issued temporary guidance for female patients on pomalidomide during the coronavirus (COVID-19) pandemic to support adherence to the Pregnancy Prevention Programme (see *Conception and contraception*), particularly for those who are shielding due to other health conditions, and should be followed until further notice.

THROMBOEMBOLISM
[EvGr] Risk factors for thromboembolism (such as smoking, hypertension, hyperlipidaemia) should be minimised. Thromboprophylaxis should be considered, particularly in patients with additional risk factors. ⟨M⟩

● **INTERACTIONS** → Appendix 1: pomalidomide

● **SIDE-EFFECTS**
▶ **Common or very common** Anaemia · angioedema · appetite decreased · atrial fibrillation · cataract · Clostridioides difficile colitis · confusion · constipation · cough · decreased leucocytes · depression · diarrhoea · dizziness · dry mouth · dyspnoea · electrolyte imbalance · embolism and thrombosis · fall · fatigue · fever · gastrointestinal discomfort · haemorrhage · heart failure · hyperglycaemia · hypertension · hyperuricaemia · hypotension · increased risk of infection · insomnia · interstitial lung disease · intracranial haemorrhage · level of consciousness decreased · muscle spasms · muscle weakness · myocardial infarction · nausea · neoplasms · neutropenia · oedema · pain · pancytopenia · paraesthesia · pelvic pain · peripheral neuropathy · renal impairment · sepsis · skin reactions · stomatitis · syncope · taste altered · thrombocytopenia · tremor · urinary retention · vertigo · vomiting · weight decreased
▶ **Uncommon** Hepatitis · hyperbilirubinaemia · stroke · tumour lysis syndrome
▶ **Frequency not known** Hepatitis B reactivation · severe cutaneous adverse reactions (SCARs)

● **CONCEPTION AND CONTRACEPTION** [EvGr] Pregnancy must be excluded in female patients of childbearing potential before starting treatment with pomalidomide. A medically supervised pregnancy test should be performed on, or within 3 days prior to, initiation and repeated every 4 weeks thereafter (including 4 weeks after the last dose), except in the case of confirmed tubal sterilisation. Females of childbearing potential must use effective contraception for at least 4 weeks before, during, and for at least 4 weeks after stopping treatment (including during dose interruptions), unless the patient is committed to absolute and continuous abstinence confirmed on a monthly basis; oral combined hormonal contraceptives and copper-releasing intra-uterine devices are not recommended. As pomalidomide is present in semen, male patients, even after successful vasectomy, must use condoms during treatment (including during dose interruptions) and for at least 1 week after stopping, if their partner is pregnant or is of childbearing potential and not using effective contraception. ⟨M⟩

● **PATIENT AND CARER ADVICE** Patients and their carers should be made aware of the symptoms of thromboembolism and advised to report sudden breathlessness, chest pain, or swelling of a limb.

Patients and their carers should be made aware of the symptoms of neutropenia and advised to seek medical advice if symptoms suggestive of neutropenia (such as

Immune system and malignant disease

fever, sore throat) or of thrombocytopenia (such as bleeding) develop.

Patients should be given a patient card and information leaflet about the Pregnancy Prevention Programme.

Conception and contraception Patient counselling is advised for pomalidomide capsules (pregnancy and contraception).

● **NATIONAL FUNDING/ACCESS DECISIONS**

For full details see funding body website

NICE decisions

▸ **Pomalidomide for multiple myeloma previously treated with lenalidomide and bortezomib (January 2017)** NICE TA427 Recommended with restrictions

● **MEDICINAL FORMS** There can be variation in the licensing of different medicines containing the same drug.

Oral capsule

CAUTIONARY AND ADVISORY LABELS 3, 25

EXCIPIENTS: May contain Propylene glycol

▸ **Pomalidomide (non-proprietary)** ▼

Pomalidomide 1 mg Pomalidomide 1mg capsules |
21 capsule PoM £7,995.60–£8,884.00 (Hospital only)
Pomalidomide 2 mg Pomalidomide 2mg capsules |
21 capsule PoM £7,995.60–£8,884.00 (Hospital only)
Pomalidomide 3 mg Pomalidomide 3mg capsules |
21 capsule PoM £7,995.60–£8,884.00 (Hospital only)
Pomalidomide 4 mg Pomalidomide 4mg capsules |
21 capsule PoM £7,995.60–£8,884.00 (Hospital only)

▸ **Imnovid** (Bristol-Myers Squibb Pharmaceuticals Ltd) ▼

Pomalidomide 1 mg Imnovid 1mg capsules | 21 capsule PoM
£8,884.00 (Hospital only)
Pomalidomide 2 mg Imnovid 2mg capsules | 21 capsule PoM
£8,884.00 (Hospital only)
Pomalidomide 3 mg Imnovid 3mg capsules | 21 capsule PoM
£8,884.00
Pomalidomide 4 mg Imnovid 4mg capsules | 21 capsule PoM
£8,884.00

Thalidomide [Specialist drug]

24-May-2021

● **INDICATIONS AND DOSE**

Multiple myeloma

▸ BY MOUTH

▸ Adult: Specialist drug – access specialist resources for dosing information

IMPORTANT SAFETY INFORMATION

PREGNANCY PREVENTION PROGRAMME

Important: teratogenic risk.

Patients, prescribers, and pharmacists must comply with the manufacturer's Pregnancy Prevention Programme. Every prescription must be accompanied by a completed Prescription Authorisation Form.

For females of childbearing potential, each prescription for thalidomide should be limited to a maximum supply of 4 weeks' treatment. Pregnancy testing should ideally be carried out on the same day as prescription issuing and dispensing.

MHRA/CHM ADVICE: IMMUNOMODULATORY DRUGS AND PREGNANCY PREVENTION: TEMPORARY ADVICE FOR MANAGEMENT DURING CORONAVIRUS (COVID-19) (MAY 2020)

The MHRA has issued temporary guidance for female patients on thalidomide during the coronavirus (COVID-19) pandemic to support adherence to the Pregnancy Prevention Programme (see *Conception and contraception*), particularly for those who are shielding due to other health conditions, and should be followed until further notice.

MHRA/CHM ADVICE: RISK OF ARTERIAL AND VENOUS THROMBOEMBOLISM (DECEMBER 2014)

Patients treated with thalidomide have an increased risk of arterial thromboembolism, including myocardial

infarction and cerebrovascular events, in addition to the established risk of venous thromboembolism. The MHRA advises to minimise risk factors for thromboembolism (such as smoking, hypertension, hyperlipidaemia). Healthcare professionals should consider venous and arterial thrombotic risk and administer antithrombotic prophylaxis for at least the first 5 months of treatment.

● **INTERACTIONS** → Appendix 1: thalidomide

● **SIDE-EFFECTS**

▸ **Common or very common** Anaemia · arrhythmias · asthenia · bronchopneumopathy · confusion · constipation · decreased leucocytes · depression · dizziness · drowsiness · dry mouth · dyspnoea · embolism and thrombosis · fever · heart failure · increased risk of infection · interstitial lung disease · malaise · movement disorders · neutropenia · peripheral neuropathy · peripheral oedema · sensation abnormal · skin reactions · thrombocytopenia · tremor · vomiting

▸ **Frequency not known** Atrioventricular block · gastrointestinal disorders · gastrointestinal haemorrhage · hearing impairment · hypothyroidism · liver disorder · menstrual cycle irregularities · myocardial infarction · neoplasms · pancreatitis · pancytopenia · posterior reversible encephalopathy syndrome (PRES) · pulmonary hypertension · reactivation of infections · renal failure · seizure · severe cutaneous adverse reactions (SCARs) · sexual dysfunction · tumour lysis syndrome

SIDE-EFFECTS, FURTHER INFORMATION Patients aged 76 years and over—increased risk of serious side-effects.

Neutropenia and thrombocytopenia Reduce dose or interrupt treatment if neutropenia or thrombocytopenia develop.

Peripheral neuropathy If symptoms suggestive of peripheral neuropathy develop (such as paraesthesia, abnormal coordination, or weakness) dose reduction, dose interruption, or treatment discontinuation might be necessary.

Rash If rash occurs, treatment should be discontinued and only restarted following appropriate clinical evaluation.

● **CONCEPTION AND CONTRACEPTION** EvGr Pregnancy must be excluded in female patients of childbearing potential before starting treatment with thalidomide. A medically supervised pregnancy test should be performed on, or within 3 days prior to, initiation and repeated every 4 weeks thereafter (including 4 weeks after the last dose), except in the case of confirmed tubal sterilisation. Females of childbearing potential must use effective contraception for at least 4 weeks before, during, and for at least 4 weeks after stopping treatment (including during dose interruptions), unless the patient is committed to absolute and continuous abstinence confirmed on a monthly basis; oral combined hormonal contraceptives and copper-releasing intra-uterine devices are not recommended. As thalidomide is present in semen, male patients, even after successful vasectomy, must use condoms during treatment (including during dose interruptions) and for at least 1 week after stopping, if their partner is pregnant or is of childbearing potential and not using effective contraception. Ⓜ

● **PATIENT AND CARER ADVICE** Patients and their carers should be made aware of the symptoms of thromboembolism and advised to report sudden breathlessness, chest pain, or swelling of a limb.

Patients and their carers should be made aware of the symptoms of neutropenia and advised to seek medical advice if symptoms suggestive of neutropenia (such as fever, sore throat) or of thrombocytopenia (such as bleeding) develop.

Patients and their carers should be advised to seek medical advice if symptoms of peripheral neuropathy such as paraesthesia, abnormal coordination, or weakness develop.

Patients should be given a patient card and information leaflet about the Pregnancy Prevention Programme. **Conception and contraception** Patient counselling advised for thalidomide capsules (pregnancy and contraception).

- **NATIONAL FUNDING/ACCESS DECISIONS**
For full details see funding body website
NICE decisions
► **Bortezomib and thalidomide for the first-line treatment of multiple myeloma (July 2011)** NICE TA228 Recommended

- **MEDICINAL FORMS** There can be variation in the licensing of different medicines containing the same drug. Forms available from special-order manufacturers include: oral tablet, oral suspension, oral solution
Oral tablet
  ► **Talidex** (Special Order)
  Thalidomide 25 mg Talidex 25mg tablets | 30 tablet 🄴
Oral capsule
  CAUTIONARY AND ADVISORY LABELS 2
  ► **Thalidomide (Non-proprietary)**
  Thalidomide 50 mg Thalidomide 50mg capsules | 28 capsule [PoM] £253.70-£298.48 DT = £298.48 (Hospital only)
  Thalidomide BMS 50mg capsules | 28 capsule [PoM] £298.48 DT = £298.48

6 **Photodynamic therapy responsive malignancy**

PHOTOSENSITISERS

Temoporfin [Specialist drug]
03-Sep-2020

- **INDICATIONS AND DOSE**
Squamous cell carcinoma of the head and neck
  ► BY SLOW INTRAVENOUS INJECTION
  ► Adult: Specialist drug – access specialist resources for dosing information

- **CONTRA-INDICATIONS** Acute porphyrias p. 1202 · concomitant photosensitising treatment · diseases exacerbated by light · elective surgery · ophthalmic slit-lamp examination for 30 days after administration

- **SIDE-EFFECTS**
► **Common or very common** Anaemia · constipation · dizziness · dysphagia · fever · haemorrhage · headache · local infection · nausea · oedema · oral disorders · pain · paraesthesia · photosensitivity reaction (sunscreens ineffective) · skin reactions · stomatitis necrotising · sunburn · vomiting
► **Frequency not known** Fistula · obstructive airway disorder · sepsis · vascular rupture

- **CONCEPTION AND CONTRACEPTION** Manufacturer advises avoid pregnancy for at least 3 months after treatment.

- **PATIENT AND CARER ADVICE**
Photosensitivity Avoid exposure of skin and eyes to direct sunlight or bright indoor light for at least 15 days after administration.

Avoid prolonged exposure of injection site arm to direct sunlight for 6 months after administration.

If extravasation occurs protect area from light for at least 3 months.

- **MEDICINAL FORMS** There can be variation in the licensing of different medicines containing the same drug.
Solution for injection
  ► **Foscan** (Biolitec Pharma Ltd)
  Temoporfin 1 mg per 1 ml Foscan 3mg/3ml solution for injection vials | 1 vial [PoM] £1,800.00 (Hospital only)

Foscan 6mg/6ml solution for injection vials | 1 vial [PoM] £3,400.00 (Hospital only)

7 **Targeted therapy responsive malignancy**

ANTINEOPLASTIC DRUGS > PROTEASOME INHIBITORS

Bortezomib [Specialist drug]
03-Nov-2020

- **INDICATIONS AND DOSE**
Multiple myeloma | Mantle cell lymphoma
  ► BY INTRAVENOUS INJECTION, OR BY SUBCUTANEOUS INJECTION
  ► Adult: Specialist drug – access specialist resources for dosing information

IMPORTANT SAFETY INFORMATION
Bortezomib injection is for **intravenous or subcutaneous administration** only. Inadvertent intrathecal administration with fatal outcome has been reported.

- **CONTRA-INDICATIONS** Acute diffuse infiltrative pulmonary disease · pericardial disease
- **INTERACTIONS** → Appendix 1: bortezomib
- **SIDE-EFFECTS**
► **Common or very common** Anaemia · anxiety · appetite abnormal · arrhythmias · asthenia · chills · constipation · cough · decreased leucocytes · diabetes mellitus · diarrhoea · dizziness · dysphagia · dyspnoea · electrolyte imbalance · encephalopathy · enzyme abnormality · eye inflammation · fever · fluid imbalance · gastrointestinal discomfort · gastrointestinal disorders · haemorrhage · hair disorder · headaches · hearing impairment · heart failure · hepatic disorders · hiccups · hyperbilirubinaemia · hypersensitivity · hypertension · hypotension · increased risk of infection · ischaemic heart disease · lethargy · loss of consciousness · malaise · mood altered · muscle complaints · muscle weakness · nausea · nerve disorders · neuromuscular dysfunction · neutropenia · oedema · oral disorders · oropharyngeal complaints · pain · renal impairment · sensation abnormal · sepsis · skin reactions · sleep disorder · syncope · taste altered · thrombocytopenia · tinnitus · ventricular dysfunction · vertigo · vision disorders · vomiting · weight changes
► **Uncommon** Altered smell sensation · angioedema · arthritis · azotaemia · cardiac arrest · cardiomyopathy · cardiovascular disorder · cerebrovascular insufficiency · chest discomfort · circulation impaired · circulatory collapse · Clostridioides difficile colitis · coagulation disorders · concentration impaired · confusion · Cushing's syndrome · dry eye · dysphonia · ear discomfort · embolism and thrombosis · eye discomfort · eye disorders · failure to thrive · gait abnormal · gas exchange abnormal · genital pain · haemolytic anaemia · hallucination · hyperthyroidism · increased leucocytes · injury · irritable bowel syndrome · joint disorders · lymphadenopathy · memory loss · movement disorders · mucous membrane disorder · myopathy · neurotoxicity · palpitations · pancreatitis · pancytopenia · pericardial disorders · pericarditis · pneumonitis · posterior reversible encephalopathy syndrome (PRES) (discontinue) · proteinuria · psychiatric disorders · psychotic disorder · pulmonary hypertension · pulmonary oedema · reflexes abnormal · respiratory disorders · rhinorrhoea · seizure · sensation of pressure · severe cutaneous adverse reactions (SCARs) · sexual dysfunction · shock · SIADH · skin mass · skin ulcers · speech disorder · sweat changes · temperature

Immune system and malignant disease

sensation altered · thirst change · tremor · tumour lysis syndrome · urinary disorders · urinary tract disorder · vascular disorders · vasculitis · vasodilation
▸ **Rare or very rare** Acidosis · acute coronary syndrome · alcohol intolerance · amyloidosis · apnoea · ascites · atrioventricular block · bladder irritation · blood disorders · bone disorder · bone fracture · brain oedema · breast disorder · cardiac valve disorder · cholelithiasis · CNS haemorrhage · cognitive disorder · coma · coronary artery insufficiency · delirium · drooling · ear disorder · erythromelalgia · fistula · gout · healing impaired · hypothyroidism · inflammation · interstitial lung disease (sometimes fatal) · lymphoedema · macrophage activation · mass · meningitis · metabolic disorder · multi organ failure · nail disorder · neoplasm malignant · neoplasms · nervous system disorder · paralysis · paresis · pelvic pain · perforation · photosensitivity reaction · platelet abnormalities · procedural complications · prostatitis · pulmonary fibrosis · radiation injury · seborrhoea · sudden death · suicidal ideation · testicular disorders · throat complaints · ulcer · vaginal ulceration · venous insufficiency · vitamin deficiencies
▸ **Frequency not known** Herpes zoster reactivation · JC virus infection · progressive multifocal leukoencephalopathy (PML) (discontinue)
● **CONCEPTION AND CONTRACEPTION** Manufacturer advises effective contraception during and for 3 months after treatment in men or women.
● **NATIONAL FUNDING/ACCESS DECISIONS** For full details see funding body website

NICE decisions
▸ **Bortezomib for previously untreated mantle cell lymphoma (December 2015)** NICE TA370 Recommended
▸ **Bortezomib for induction therapy in multiple myeloma before high-dose chemotherapy and autologous stem cell transplantation (April 2014)** NICE TA311 Recommended
▸ **Bortezomib and thalidomide for the first-line treatment of multiple myeloma (July 2011)** NICE TA228 Recommended with restrictions
▸ **Bortezomib monotherapy for relapsed multiple myeloma (October 2007)** NICE TA129 Recommended with restrictions

Scottish Medicines Consortium (SMC) decisions
▸ **Bortezomib (*Velcade*®) in combination with dexamethasone, or with dexamethasone and thalidomide, for the induction treatment of adult patients with previously untreated multiple myeloma who are eligible for high-dose chemotherapy with haematopoietic stem cell transplantation (January 2014)** SMC No. 927/13 Recommended with restrictions

● **MEDICINAL FORMS** There can be variation in the licensing of different medicines containing the same drug. Forms available from special-order manufacturers include: solution for injection

Solution for injection
▸ Bortezomib (Non-proprietary)
  Bortezomib 2.5 mg per 1 ml Bortezomib 3.5mg/1.4ml solution for injection vials | 1 vial [PoM] £495.55 (Hospital only)
  Bortezomib 7mg/2.8ml solution for injection vials | 1 vial [PoM] £991.10 (Hospital only)

Powder for solution for injection
▸ Bortezomib (Non-proprietary)
  Bortezomib 1 mg Bortezomib 1mg powder for solution for injection vials | 1 vial [PoM] £217.82 (Hospital only)
  Bortezomib 2.5 mg Bortezomib 2.5mg powder for solution for injection vials | 1 vial [PoM] £544.56 (Hospital only)
  Bortezomib 3.5 mg Bortezomib 3.5mg powder for solution for injection vials | 1 vial [PoM] £495.55–£910.91 (Hospital only)
▸ Velcade (Janssen-Cilag Ltd)
  Bortezomib 3.5 mg Velcade 3.5mg powder for solution for injection vials | 1 vial [PoM] £762.38 (Hospital only)

Carfilzomib [Specialist drug]
07-Oct-2022

● **INDICATIONS AND DOSE**
Multiple myeloma
▸ BY INTRAVENOUS INFUSION
▸ Adult: Specialist drug – access specialist resources for dosing information

IMPORTANT SAFETY INFORMATION
MHRA/CHM ADVICE: CARFILZOMIB (*KYPROLIS*®): REMINDER OF RISK OF POTENTIALLY FATAL CARDIAC EVENTS (AUGUST 2019)
Cases of cardiac arrest, cardiac failure, and myocardial infarction, including fatalities, have been reported in patients with or without pre-existing cardiac disorders receiving carfilzomib. Healthcare professionals are advised to monitor patients for signs and symptoms of cardiac disorders before and during carfilzomib treatment. Carfilzomib should be discontinued if severe or life-threatening cardiac events occur; restarting treatment may be considered at a lower dose once the condition is controlled and the patient is stable.

MHRA/CHM ADVICE: CARFILZOMIB (*KYPROLIS*®): RISK OF REACTIVATION OF HEPATITIS B VIRUS (NOVEMBER 2019)
An EU review of worldwide data has identified reports of hepatitis B virus (HBV) reactivation in patients treated with carfilzomib. Healthcare professionals are advised to screen all patients for HBV before initiating treatment; those with unknown serology already being treated with carfilzomib should also be screened. Patients with positive serology should be considered for antiviral prophylaxis, and be monitored for signs of HBV reactivation during and after treatment; immediate medical attention should be sought if signs and symptoms of HBV reactivation develop. Experts should be consulted for advice about HBV treatment and the continuation, interruption, or resumption of carfilzomib in patients with HBV reactivation.

● **INTERACTIONS** → Appendix 1: carfilzomib
● **SIDE-EFFECTS**
▸ **Common or very common** Anaemia · anxiety · appetite decreased · arrhythmias · arthralgia · asthenia · cataract · chest pain · chills · confusion · constipation · cough · decreased leucocytes · dehydration · diarrhoea · dizziness · dysphonia · dyspnoea · electrolyte imbalance · embolism and thrombosis · fever · flushing · gastrointestinal discomfort · haemorrhage · headache · heart failure · hyperbilirubinaemia · hyperglycaemia · hyperhidrosis · hypertension · hyperuricaemia · hypoalbuminaemia · hypotension · increased risk of infection · influenza like illness · infusion related reaction · insomnia · malaise · muscle complaints · muscle weakness · myocardial infarction · nausea · neutropenia · oropharyngeal pain · pain · palpitations · peripheral neuropathy · peripheral oedema · pulmonary hypertension · pulmonary oedema · renal impairment · respiratory disorders · sensation abnormal · sepsis · skin reactions · thrombocytopenia · tinnitus · toothache · vision blurred · vomiting
▸ **Uncommon** Cardiac arrest · cardiomyopathy · Clostridioides difficile colitis · gastrointestinal perforation · haemolytic uraemic syndrome · hepatic disorders · hepatitis B reactivation · interstitial lung disease · intracranial haemorrhage · multi organ failure · myocardial ischaemia · pericardial effusion · pericarditis · stroke · tumour lysis syndrome
▸ **Rare or very rare** Angioedema · posterior reversible encephalopathy syndrome (PRES) · thrombotic microangiopathy
▸ **Frequency not known** Progressive multifocal leukoencephalopathy (PML) · QT interval prolongation

SIDE-EFFECTS, FURTHER INFORMATION **Progressive multifocal leukoencephalopathy (PML)** Interrupt treatment if suspected and discontinue if confirmed.

Thrombotic microangiopathy Thrombotic microangiopathy, including thrombotic thrombocytopenic purpura and haemolytic uraemic syndrome, including fatal events, have been reported; interrupt treatment if suspected.

Tumour lysis syndrome Tumour lysis syndrome, including fatal cases, have been reported; interrupt treatment if suspected.

● CONCEPTION AND CONTRACEPTION Manufacturer recommends effective contraception during and for 1 month after treatment in women of childbearing potential; hormonal contraceptives associated with a risk of thrombosis should be avoided. Male patients should use effective contraception during and for 3 months after treatment if their partner is pregnant or of childbearing potential.

● PATIENT AND CARER ADVICE Manufacturer advises that patients and carers are warned to report signs and symptoms of thromboembolism (such as dyspnoea, chest pain, arm or leg swelling or pain).

Driving and skilled tasks Patients and their carers should be counselled on the effects on driving and skilled tasks—increased risk of dizziness, hypotension and blurred vision.

● NATIONAL FUNDING/ACCESS DECISIONS
For full details see funding body website

NICE decisions

▸ **Carfilzomib for previously treated multiple myeloma (November 2020)** NICE TA657 Recommended with restrictions

▸ **Carfilzomib with dexamethasone and lenalidomide for previously treated multiple myeloma (April 2021)** NICE TA695 Recommended with restrictions

Scottish Medicines Consortium (SMC) decisions

▸ Carfilzomib (*Kyprolis*®) in combination with dexamethasone alone for the treatment of adult patients with multiple myeloma who have received at least one prior therapy (August 2017) SMC No. 1242/17 Recommended

▸ Carfilzomib (*Kyprolis*®) in combination with lenalidomide and dexamethasone for the treatment of adult patients with multiple myeloma who have received at least one prior therapy (October 2020) SMC No. SMC2290 Recommended with restrictions

● MEDICINAL FORMS There can be variation in the licensing of different medicines containing the same drug.

Powder for solution for infusion
EXCIPIENTS: May contain Sulfobutylether beta cyclodextrin sodium
ELECTROLYTES: May contain Sodium

▸ Kyprolis (Amgen Ltd)
Carfilzomib 10 mg Kyprolis 10mg powder for solution for infusion vials | 1 vial PoM £176.00 (Hospital only)
Carfilzomib 30 mg Kyprolis 30mg powder for solution for infusion vials | 1 vial PoM £528.00 (Hospital only)
Carfilzomib 60 mg Kyprolis 60mg powder for solution for infusion vials | 1 vial PoM £1,056.00 (Hospital only)

Ixazomib [Specialist drug]
28-Feb-2023

● **INDICATIONS AND DOSE**

Multiple myeloma
▸ BY MOUTH
▸ Adult: Specialist drug – access specialist resources for dosing information

IMPORTANT SAFETY INFORMATION
RISKS OF INCORRECT DOSING OF ORAL ANTI-CANCER MEDICINES
See Cytotoxic drugs p. 1027.

● INTERACTIONS → Appendix 1: ixazomib

● SIDE-EFFECTS

▸ **Common or very common** Back pain · constipation · diarrhoea · herpes zoster reactivation · increased risk of infection · nausea · neutropenia · peripheral neuropathy (monitor for symptoms) · peripheral oedema · skin reactions · thrombocytopenia · vomiting

▸ **Rare or very rare** Posterior reversible encephalopathy syndrome (PRES) (discontinue) · Stevens-Johnson syndrome · thrombotic microangiopathy · transverse myelitis · tumour lysis syndrome

▸ **Frequency not known** Appetite decreased · conjunctivitis · dizziness · dry eye · fatigue · hepatic disorders · hypokalaemia

● CONCEPTION AND CONTRACEPTION Manufacturer advises effective contraception in women of child-bearing potential and in men with a partner of child-bearing potential, during treatment and for at least 90 days after stopping treatment; additional barrier method recommended in women using hormonal contraceptives.

● PATIENT AND CARER ADVICE
Missed doses Manufacturer advises if less than 72 hours remain before the next scheduled dose, the missed dose should not be taken and the next dose should be taken at the normal time.

● NATIONAL FUNDING/ACCESS DECISIONS
For full details see funding body website

NICE decisions

▸ **Ixazomib with lenalidomide and dexamethasone for treating relapsed or refractory multiple myeloma (February 2023)** NICE TA870 Recommended with restrictions

● MEDICINAL FORMS There can be variation in the licensing of different medicines containing the same drug.

Oral capsule
CAUTIONARY AND ADVISORY LABELS 23, 25
▸ Ninlaro (Takeda UK Ltd)
Ixazomib (as Ixazomib citrate) 2.3 mg Ninlaro 2.3mg capsules | 3 capsule PoM £6,336.00 (Hospital only)
Ixazomib (as Ixazomib citrate) 3 mg Ninlaro 3mg capsules | 3 capsule PoM £6,336.00 (Hospital only)
Ixazomib (as Ixazomib citrate) 4 mg Ninlaro 4mg capsules | 3 capsule PoM £6,336.00 (Hospital only)

ANTINEOPLASTIC DRUGS › PROTEIN KINASE INHIBITORS

Abemaciclib [Specialist drug]
19-Dec-2022

● **INDICATIONS AND DOSE**

Breast cancer
▸ BY MOUTH
▸ Adult: Specialist drug – access specialist resources for dosing information

IMPORTANT SAFETY INFORMATION
RISKS OF INCORRECT DOSING OF ORAL ANTI-CANCER MEDICINES
See Cytotoxic drugs p. 1027.

MHRA/CHM ADVICE: CDK4/6 INHIBITORS (ABEMACICLIB, PALBOCICLIB, RIBOCICLIB): REPORTS OF INTERSTITIAL LUNG DISEASE AND PNEUMONITIS, INCLUDING SEVERE CASES (JUNE 2021)

Interstitial lung disease and pneumonitis, in some cases severe or fatal, have been reported in patients being treated with CDK4/6 inhibitors, such as abemaciclib. Healthcare professionals are advised to ask patients taking abemaciclib about pulmonary symptoms indicative of interstitial lung disease and pneumonitis, such as cough or dyspnoea. Patients should be advised to seek advice right away if these symptoms occur. Healthcare professionals should ensure patients have a copy of the Patient Information Leaflet (PIL) for abemaciclib.

● INTERACTIONS → Appendix 1: abemaciclib

● SIDE-EFFECTS
► **Common or very common** Alopecia · anaemia · appetite decreased · decreased leucocytes · diarrhoea · dizziness · dyspepsia · embolism and thrombosis · excessive tearing · fatigue · fever · headache · increased risk of infection · interstitial lung disease · muscle weakness · nail disorder · nausea · neutropenia · obliterative bronchiolitis · pulmonary fibrosis · skin reactions · stomatitis · taste altered · thrombocytopenia · vomiting
► **Frequency not known** Neutropenic sepsis

● **CONCEPTION AND CONTRACEPTION** Manufacturer advises highly effective contraception in women of childbearing potential during treatment and for at least 3 weeks after completing treatment.

● **PATIENT AND CARER ADVICE** Patients should be instructed to start an antidiarrhoeal such as loperamide, increase oral fluids, and seek medical advice at the first sign of loose stools. Patients should also be instructed to seek medical advice if fever occurs.
Driving and skilled tasks Patients should be cautioned on the effects on driving and performance of skilled tasks—increased risk of fatigue and dizziness.

● **NATIONAL FUNDING/ACCESS DECISIONS**
For full details see funding body website
NICE decisions
► **Abemaciclib with an aromatase inhibitor for previously untreated, hormone receptor-positive, HER2-negative, locally advanced or metastatic breast cancer (February 2019)** NICE TA563 Recommended with restrictions
► **Abemaciclib with fulvestrant for treating hormone receptor-positive, HER2-negative advanced breast cancer after endocrine therapy (September 2021)** NICE TA725 Recommended with restrictions
► **Abemaciclib with endocrine therapy for adjuvant treatment of hormone receptor-positive, HER2-negative, node-positive early breast cancer at high risk of recurrence (July 2022)** NICE TA810 Recommended
Scottish Medicines Consortium (SMC) decisions
► Abemaciclib (*Verzenios*®) for the treatment of women with hormone receptor (HR) positive, human epidermal growth factor receptor 2 (HER2) negative locally advanced or metastatic breast cancer in combination with an aromatase inhibitor as initial endocrine-based therapy, or in women who have received prior endocrine therapy (May 2019) SMC No. SMC2135 Recommended
► Abemaciclib (*Verzenios*®) for the treatment of women with hormone receptor (HR) positive, human epidermal growth factor receptor 2 (HER2) negative locally advanced or metastatic breast cancer in combination with fulvestrant as initial endocrine-based therapy or in women who have received prior endocrine therapy (May 2019) SMC No. SMC2179 Recommended with restrictions
► Abemaciclib (*Verzenios*®) in combination with endocrine therapy for the adjuvant treatment of adult patients with hormone receptor (HR)-positive, human epidermal growth factor receptor 2 (HER2)-negative, node-positive early breast cancer at high risk of recurrence (December 2022) SMC No. SMC2494 Recommended

● **MEDICINAL FORMS** There can be variation in the licensing of different medicines containing the same drug.
Oral tablet
CAUTIONARY AND ADVISORY LABELS 3, 25
► **Verzenios** (Eli Lilly and Company Ltd)
Abemaciclib 50 mg Verzenios 50mg tablets | 28 tablet [PoM] £1,475.00 (Hospital only) | 56 tablet [PoM] £2,950.00 (Hospital only)
Abemaciclib 100 mg Verzenios 100mg tablets | 28 tablet [PoM] £1,475.00 (Hospital only) | 56 tablet [PoM] £2,950.00 (Hospital only)
Abemaciclib 150 mg Verzenios 150mg tablets | 28 tablet [PoM] £1,475.00 (Hospital only) | 56 tablet [PoM] £2,950.00 (Hospital only)

Acalabrutinib [Specialist drug]

25-Jun-2021

● **INDICATIONS AND DOSE**
Chronic lymphocytic leukaemia
► BY MOUTH
► Adult: Specialist drug – access specialist resources for dosing information

IMPORTANT SAFETY INFORMATION
RISKS OF INCORRECT DOSING OF ORAL ANTI-CANCER MEDICINES
See Cytotoxic drugs p. 1027.

● INTERACTIONS → Appendix 1: acalabrutinib

● SIDE-EFFECTS
► **Common or very common** Abdominal pain · anaemia · arrhythmias · arthralgia · asthenia · constipation · diarrhoea · dizziness · haemorrhage · headache · increased risk of infection · intracranial haemorrhage · musculoskeletal pain · nausea · neutropenia · second primary malignancy · skin reactions · thrombocytopenia · vomiting
► **Uncommon** Hepatitis B reactivation · lymphocytosis · tumour lysis syndrome
► **Frequency not known** Cough · leucopenia · progressive multifocal leukoencephalopathy (PML) · sepsis

● **CONCEPTION AND CONTRACEPTION** [EvGr] Females of childbearing potential should use effective contraception during treatment. [M]

● **PATIENT AND CARER ADVICE** [EvGr] Patients should be advised to protect skin from exposure to sun (risk of skin cancer). [M]
Missed doses [EvGr] If a dose is more than 3 hours late, the missed dose should not be taken and the next dose should be taken at the normal time. [M]
Driving and skilled tasks [EvGr] Patients and carers should be counselled on the effects on driving and performance of skilled tasks—increased risk of dizziness and fatigue. [M]

● **NATIONAL FUNDING/ACCESS DECISIONS**
For full details see funding body website
NICE decisions
► **Acalabrutinib for treating chronic lymphocytic leukaemia [in adults with untreated chronic lymphocytic leukaemia] (April 2021)** NICE TA689 Recommended with restrictions
► **Acalabrutinib for treating chronic lymphocytic leukaemia [in adults with previously treated chronic lymphocytic leukaemia] (April 2021)** NICE TA689 Recommended
Scottish Medicines Consortium (SMC) decisions
► Acalabrutinib (*Calquence*®) as monotherapy or in combination with obinutuzumab for the treatment of adult patients with previously untreated chronic lymphocytic leukaemia (CLL) [and in whom chemo-immunotherapy is unsuitable] (April 2021) SMC No. SMC2346 Recommended with restrictions

► Acalabrutinib (*Calquence*®) as monotherapy for the treatment of adult patients with chronic lymphocytic leukaemia (CLL) who have received at least one prior therapy (April 2021) SMC No. SMC2348 Recommended with restrictions

► Acalabrutinib (*Calquence*®) as monotherapy or in combination with obinutuzumab for the treatment of adult patients with previously untreated chronic lymphocytic leukaemia (CLL) [and who are ineligible for fludarabine, cyclophosphamide and rituximab therapy] (June 2021) SMC No. SMC2347 Recommended with restrictions

● **MEDICINAL FORMS** There can be variation in the licensing of different medicines containing the same drug.

Oral tablet

► Calquence (AstraZeneca UK Ltd) ▼

Acalabrutinib (as Acalabrutinib maleate) **100 mg** Calquence 100mg tablets | 60 tablet PoM £5,059.00 (Hospital only)

Afatinib [Specialist drug]

30-Sep-2021

● **INDICATIONS AND DOSE**

Non-small cell lung cancer

► BY MOUTH

► Adult: Specialist drug – access specialist resources for dosing information

IMPORTANT SAFETY INFORMATION
RISKS OF INCORRECT DOSING OF ORAL ANTI-CANCER MEDICINES
See Cytotoxic drugs p. 1027.

● **INTERACTIONS** → Appendix 1: afatinib

● **SIDE-EFFECTS**

► **Common or very common** Appetite decreased · cystitis · dehydration · diarrhoea · dry eye · dyspepsia · epistaxis · eye inflammation · fever · hypokalaemia · muscle spasms · nausea · oral disorders · paronychia · renal impairment · rhinorrhoea · skin reactions · taste altered · vomiting · weight decreased

► **Uncommon** Interstitial lung disease · pancreatitis

► **Rare or very rare** Severe cutaneous adverse reactions (SCARs)

SIDE-EFFECTS, FURTHER INFORMATION Interstitial lung disease, including fatal events, has been reported; if new or worsening respiratory symptoms (including dyspnoea, cough, and fever) occur, withhold treatment and discontinue if confirmed.

● **CONCEPTION AND CONTRACEPTION** Ensure effective contraception during and for at least one month after treatment in women of childbearing potential.

● **PATIENT AND CARER ADVICE** Patient counselling advised (administration).

Patients should be advised to protect skin from exposure to sun—wear protective clothing and/or sunscreen.
Driving and skilled tasks Ocular adverse reactions may affect performance of skilled tasks e.g. driving.

● **NATIONAL FUNDING/ACCESS DECISIONS**
For full details see funding body website

NICE decisions

► Afatinib for treating epidermal growth factor receptor mutation-positive locally advanced or metastatic non-small-cell lung cancer (April 2014) NICE TA310 Recommended with restrictions

● **MEDICINAL FORMS** There can be variation in the licensing of different medicines containing the same drug.

Oral tablet
CAUTIONARY AND ADVISORY LABELS 25

► Giotrif (Boehringer Ingelheim Ltd)

Afatinib (as Afatinib dimaleate) **20 mg** Giotrif 20mg tablets | 28 tablet PoM £2,023.28 (Hospital only)

Afatinib (as Afatinib dimaleate) **30 mg** Giotrif 30mg tablets | 28 tablet PoM £2,023.28 (Hospital only)
Afatinib (as Afatinib dimaleate) **40 mg** Giotrif 40mg tablets | 28 tablet PoM £2,023.28 (Hospital only)

Alectinib [Specialist drug]

25-Apr-2025

● **INDICATIONS AND DOSE**

Non-small cell lung cancer

► BY MOUTH

► Adult: Specialist drug – access specialist resources for dosing information

IMPORTANT SAFETY INFORMATION
RISKS OF INCORRECT DOSING OF ORAL ANTI-CANCER MEDICINES
See Cytotoxic drugs p. 1027.

● **INTERACTIONS** → Appendix 1: alectinib

● **SIDE-EFFECTS**

► **Common or very common** Acute kidney injury · anaemia · arrhythmias · arthralgia · constipation · diarrhoea · eye disorders · eye inflammation · hyperbilirubinaemia · interstitial lung disease · musculoskeletal pain · myalgia · nausea · oedema · oral disorders · photosensitivity reaction · skin reactions · taste altered · vision disorders · vomiting · weight increased

► **Uncommon** Drug-induced liver injury · haemolytic anaemia

● **CONCEPTION AND CONTRACEPTION** Manufacturer advises women of child-bearing potential should use effective contraception during and for at least 3 months after stopping treatment.

● **PATIENT AND CARER ADVICE**
Photosensitivity Manufacturer advises patients should use a broad spectrum sunscreen and lip balm and be advised to avoid prolonged sun exposure during treatment, and for 7 days after discontinuation.
Myalgia Manufacturer advises patients should advised to report any unexplained muscle pain, tenderness or weakness.
Vomiting Manufacturer advises if vomiting occurs after taking tablets, no additional dose should be taken on that day and the next dose should be taken at the usual time.
Missed doses Manufacturer advises if a dose is more than 6 hours late, the missed dose should not be taken and the next dose should be taken at the normal time.
Driving and skilled tasks Manufacturer advises patients and carers should be counselled on the effects on driving and performance of skilled tasks—increased risk of symptomatic bradycardia and vision disorders.

● **NATIONAL FUNDING/ACCESS DECISIONS**
For full details see funding body website

NICE decisions

► Alectinib (*Alecensa*®) for untreated ALK-positive advanced non-small cell lung cancer (August 2018) NICE TA536 Recommended

► Alectinib for adjuvant treatment of ALK-positive non-small cell lung cancer (November 2024) NICE TA1014 Recommended

Scottish Medicines Consortium (SMC) decisions

► Alectinib hydrochloride (*Alecensa*®) as monotherapy for the first-line treatment of adult patients with anaplastic lymphoma kinase (ALK)-positive advanced non-small cell lung cancer (NSCLC) (August 2018) SMC No. SMC2012 Recommended

► Alectinib hydrochloride (*Alecensa*®) as monotherapy as adjuvant treatment for adult patients with Stage IB (tumours 4cm or greater) to IIIA anaplastic lymphoma kinase (ALK)-positive non-small cell lung cancer (NSCLC) following complete tumour resection (April 2025) SMC No. SMC2749 Recommended

Immune system and malignant disease

- **MEDICINAL FORMS** There can be variation in the licensing of different medicines containing the same drug.

Oral capsule

CAUTIONARY AND ADVISORY LABELS 11, 21
ELECTROLYTES: May contain Sodium

▸ **Alecensa** (Roche Products Ltd)
  Alectinib (as Alectinib hydrochloride) 150 mg Alecensa 150mg capsules | 224 capsule [PoM] £5,032.00

Alpelisib [Specialist drug]

19-Dec-2022

- **INDICATIONS AND DOSE**

Breast cancer

▸ BY MOUTH
▸ Adult: Specialist drug – access specialist resources for dosing information

---

IMPORTANT SAFETY INFORMATION

RISKS OF INCORRECT DOSING OF ORAL ANTI-CANCER MEDICINES
See Cytotoxic drugs p. 1027.

- **CONTRA-INDICATIONS** History of severe cutaneous reactions · osteonecrosis of the jaw
- **INTERACTIONS** → Appendix 1: alpelisib
- **SIDE-EFFECTS**
▸ **Common or very common** Acute kidney injury · alopecia · anaemia · angioedema · appetite decreased · asthenia · dehydration · diarrhoea · dry eye · dry mouth · electrolyte imbalance · eyelid oedema · fever · gastrointestinal discomfort · headache · hypersensitivity · hypertension · increased risk of infection · insomnia · interstitial lung disease · lymphoedema · mucosal abnormalities · muscle complaints · nausea · oedema · oral disorders · osteonecrosis of jaw · skin reactions · taste altered · urosepsis · vision blurred · vomiting · vulvovaginal dryness · weight decreased
▸ **Uncommon** Diabetic ketoacidosis · ketoacidosis · pancreatitis · severe cutaneous adverse reactions (SCARs)
▸ **Frequency not known** Dyspnoea · gastrointestinal disorders · hyperglycaemia · hyperglycaemic hyperosmolar nonketotic syndrome · pleural effusion
- **CONCEPTION AND CONTRACEPTION** Manufacturer advises male patients should use effective contraception during treatment and for one week after last dose if their partner is pregnant or of childbearing potential. The effect on human fertility is not known—impairment of fertility has been observed in *animal* studies.
- **PATIENT AND CARER ADVICE**
Vomiting Manufacturer advises if vomiting occurs after taking tablets, no additional dose should be taken on that day and the next dose should be taken at the usual time.
Missed doses Manufacturer advises if dose is more than 9 hours late, the missed dose should not be taken and the next dose should be taken at the usual time.
Driving and skilled tasks Manufacturer advises patients and carers should be cautioned on the effects on driving and performance of skilled tasks—increased risk of fatigue or blurred vision.
- **NATIONAL FUNDING/ACCESS DECISIONS**
For full details see funding body website
NICE decisions
▸ Alpelisib with fulvestrant for treating hormone receptor-positive, HER2-negative, PIK3CA-mutated advanced breast cancer (August 2022) NICE TA816 Recommended with restrictions
Scottish Medicines Consortium (SMC) decisions
▸ Alpelisib (*Piqray®*) in combination with fulvestrant for the treatment of postmenopausal women, and men, with hormone receptor (HR)-positive, human epidermal growth factor receptor 2 (HER2)-negative, locally advanced or metastatic

breast cancer with a PIK3CA mutation after disease progression following endocrine-based therapy (December 2022) SMC No. SMC2481 Not recommended

---

- **MEDICINAL FORMS** There can be variation in the licensing of different medicines containing the same drug.

Oral tablet

CAUTIONARY AND ADVISORY LABELS 25, 21

▸ **Piqray** (Novartis Pharmaceuticals UK Ltd) ▼
  Alpelisib 50 mg Piqray 50mg tablets | 28 tablet [PoM] [Ṡ] (Hospital only)
  Alpelisib 150 mg Piqray 150mg tablets | 56 tablet [PoM] £4,082.14 (Hospital only)
  Alpelisib 200 mg Piqray 200mg tablets | 28 tablet [PoM] £4,082.14 (Hospital only)

Asciminib [Specialist drug]

16-Nov-2022

- **INDICATIONS AND DOSE**

Chronic myeloid leukaemia

▸ BY MOUTH
▸ Adult: Specialist drug – access specialist resources for dosing information

---

IMPORTANT SAFETY INFORMATION

RISKS OF INCORRECT DOSING OF ORAL ANTI-CANCER MEDICINES
See Cytotoxic drugs p. 1027.

MHRA/CHM ADVICE: RISK OF HEPATITIS B VIRUS REACTIVATION
WITH BCR-ABL TYROSINE KINASE INHIBITORS (MAY 2016)
An EU wide review has concluded that BCR-ABL tyrosine kinase inhibitors can cause hepatitis B reactivation; the MHRA recommends establishing hepatitis B virus status in all patients before initiation of treatment.

The MHRA advises that patients who are carriers of hepatitis B virus should be closely monitored for signs and symptoms of active infection throughout treatment with BCR-ABL tyrosine kinase inhibitors, and for several months after stopping treatment; expert advice should be sought for patients who test positive for hepatitis B virus and in those with active infection.

- **INTERACTIONS** → Appendix 1: asciminib
- **SIDE-EFFECTS**
▸ **Common or very common** Anaemia · appetite decreased · arthralgia · asthenia · cough · diarrhoea · dizziness · dry eye · dyslipidaemia · dyspnoea · fever · gastrointestinal discomfort · headache · hyperbilirubinaemia · hyperlipasaemia · hypertension · increased risk of infection · musculoskeletal discomfort · myalgia · nausea · neutropenia · oedema · pain · palpitations · pancreatitis · pleural effusion · skin reactions · thrombocytopenia · vision blurred · vomiting
▸ **Uncommon** QT interval prolongation
- **CONCEPTION AND CONTRACEPTION** [EvGr] Females of childbearing potential should use effective contraception during and for at least 3 days after last treatment. ◈
- **PATIENT AND CARER ADVICE** Patients or carers should be given advice on how to administer *Scemblix®* tablets.
Missed doses If a once-daily dose is more than 12 hours late, or a twice-daily dose is more than 6 hours late, the missed dose should not be taken and the next dose should be taken at the normal time.
- **NATIONAL FUNDING/ACCESS DECISIONS**
For full details see funding body website
NICE decisions
▸ Asciminib for treating chronic myeloid leukaemia after 2 or more tyrosine kinase inhibitors (August 2022) NICE TA813 Recommended

Scottish Medicines Consortium (SMC) decisions

▶ Asciminib (*Scemblix®*) for the treatment of adult patients with Philadelphia chromosome-positive chronic myeloid leukaemia in chronic phase, previously treated with two or more tyrosine kinase inhibitors, and without a known T315I mutation (November 2022) SMC No. SMC2482 Recommended

● MEDICINAL FORMS There can be variation in the licensing of different medicines containing the same drug.

Oral tablet

CAUTIONARY AND ADVISORY LABELS 23, 25

▶ Scemblix (Novartis Pharmaceuticals UK Ltd) ▼
  Asciminib (as Asciminib hydrochloride) 20 mg Scemblix 20mg tablets | 60 tablet PoM £4,050.37 (Hospital only)
  Asciminib (as Asciminib hydrochloride) 40 mg Scemblix 40mg tablets | 60 tablet PoM £4,050.37 (Hospital only)

Avapritinib [Specialist drug]
02-Dec-2024

● **INDICATIONS AND DOSE**

Gastro-intestinal stromal tumours | Advanced systemic mastocytosis

▶ BY MOUTH

▶ Adult: Specialist drug – access specialist resources for dosing information

---

IMPORTANT SAFETY INFORMATION

RISKS OF INCORRECT DOSING OF ORAL ANTI-CANCER MEDICINES
See Cytotoxic drugs p. 1027.

● INTERACTIONS → Appendix 1: avapritinib

● SIDE-EFFECTS

▶ **Common or very common** Abdominal pain · acute kidney injury · alopecia · anaemia · anxiety · appetite decreased · arthralgia · ascites · asthenia · CNS haemorrhage · cognitive impairment · concentration impaired · confusion · constipation · cough · dementia · depression · diarrhoea · dizziness · drowsiness · dry mouth · dysphagia · dyspnoea · electrolyte imbalance · excessive tearing · eye inflammation · facial swelling · feeling cold · fever · fluid imbalance · gastrointestinal disorders · haemorrhage · hair colour changes · headache · hyperbilirubinaemia · hypertension · hypoalbuminaemia · insomnia · leucopenia · malaise · memory impairment · movement disorders · muscle complaints · nasal congestion · nausea · neutropenia · oedema · oral disorders · pain · peripheral neuropathy · peripheral swelling · photosensitivity reaction · psychiatric disorder · QT interval prolongation · respiratory disorders · sensation abnormal · skin reactions · speech impairment · taste altered · thrombocytopenia · tremor · vertigo · vision disorders · vomiting · weight changes

▶ **Uncommon** Encephalopathy · pericardial effusion · tumour haemorrhage

▶ **Frequency not known** Libido decreased · premature menopause

● **CONCEPTION AND CONTRACEPTION** EvGr Females of childbearing potential should use effective contraception during treatment and for six weeks after last treatment. Male patients should use effective contraception during treatment and for two weeks after last treatment, if their partner is of childbearing potential. Ⓜ

● **PATIENT AND CARER ADVICE**

Vomiting EvGr If vomiting occurs after taking tablets, no additional dose should be taken on that day and the next dose should be taken at the usual time. Ⓜ
Photosensitivity EvGr Avoid or minimise exposure to direct sunlight; patients should be advised to use a high protection sunscreen and wear protective clothing. Ⓜ

Missed doses EvGr If a dose is more than 16 hours late, the missed dose should not be taken and the next dose should be taken at the usual time. Ⓜ
Driving and skilled tasks EvGr Patients and carers should be cautioned on the effects on driving and performance of skilled tasks—increased risk of cognitive effects. Ⓜ

● NATIONAL FUNDING/ACCESS DECISIONS
For full details see funding body website

NICE decisions

▶ Avapritinib for treating advanced systemic mastocytosis (November 2024) NICE TA1012 Recommended

---

● MEDICINAL FORMS There can be variation in the licensing of different medicines containing the same drug.

Oral tablet

CAUTIONARY AND ADVISORY LABELS 23, 25

▶ Ayvakyt (Blueprint Medicines (UK) Ltd) ▼
  Avapritinib 25 mg Ayvakyt 25mg tablets | 30 tablet PoM £26,667.00 (Hospital only)
  Avapritinib 50 mg Ayvakyt 50mg tablets | 30 tablet PoM £26,667.00 (Hospital only)
  Avapritinib 100 mg Ayvakyt 100mg tablets | 30 tablet PoM £26,667.00 (Hospital only)
  Avapritinib 200 mg Ayvakyt 200mg tablets | 30 tablet PoM £26,667.00 (Hospital only)
  Avapritinib 300 mg Ayvakyt 300mg tablets | 30 tablet PoM £26,667.00 (Hospital only)

Axitinib [Specialist drug]
15-Oct-2020

● **INDICATIONS AND DOSE**

Renal cell carcinoma

▶ BY MOUTH

▶ Adult: Specialist drug – access specialist resources for dosing information

---

IMPORTANT SAFETY INFORMATION

MHRA/CHM ADVICE: SYSTEMICALLY ADMINISTERED VEGF PATHWAY INHIBITORS: RISK OF ANEURYSM AND ARTERY DISSECTION (JULY 2020)
A European review of worldwide data concluded that systemically administered VEGF pathway inhibitors may lead to aneurysm and artery dissection in patients with or without hypertension. Some fatal cases have been reported, mainly in relation to aortic aneurysm rupture and aortic dissection. The MHRA advises healthcare professionals to carefully consider the risk of aneurysm and artery dissection in patients with risk factors before initiating treatment with axitinib; any modifiable risk factors (such as smoking and hypertension) should be reduced as much as possible. Blood pressure should be monitored regularly, and product literature should be consulted if hypertension occurs during treatment.

RISKS OF INCORRECT DOSING OF ORAL ANTI-CANCER MEDICINES
See Cytotoxic drugs p. 1027.

● CONTRA-INDICATIONS Recent active gastro-intestinal bleeding · untreated brain metastases

● INTERACTIONS → Appendix 1: axitinib

● SIDE-EFFECTS

▶ **Common or very common** Alopecia · anaemia · appetite decreased · arthralgia · asthenia · Budd-Chiari syndrome · cerebrovascular insufficiency · CNS haemorrhage · constipation · cough · dehydration · diarrhoea · dizziness · dysphonia · dyspnoea · electrolyte imbalance · embolism and thrombosis · fistula · gallbladder disorders · gastrointestinal anastomotic leak · gastrointestinal discomfort · gastrointestinal disorders · haemorrhage · headache · heart failure · hyperbilirubinaemia · hypertension · hyperthyroidism · hypothyroidism · increased risk of infection · left ventricular dysfunction ·

8

Immune system and malignant disease

mucositis · myalgia · myocardial infarction · nausea · oesophagobronchial fistula · oral disorders · oropharyngeal pain · pain in extremity · polycythaemia · proteinuria · renal impairment · scrotal haematocoele · skin reactions · splenic haematoma · splinter haemorrhages · taste altered · thrombocytopenia · tinnitus · uterine bleeding abnormal · vomiting · weight decreased
► **Uncommon** Encephalopathy · leucopenia · neutropenia
► **Frequency not known** Aneurysm · artery dissection
● **CONCEPTION AND CONTRACEPTION** Effective contraception required during and for up to 1 week after treatment.
● **NATIONAL FUNDING/ACCESS DECISIONS**
For full details see funding body website
NICE decisions
► Axitinib for treating advanced renal cell carcinoma after failure of prior systemic treatment (February 2015) NICE TA333 Recommended with restrictions
► Avelumab with axitinib for untreated advanced renal cell carcinoma (September 2020) NICE TA645 Recommended
► Pembrolizumab with axitinib for untreated advanced renal cell carcinoma (September 2020) NICE TA650 Not recommended

---

● **MEDICINAL FORMS** There can be variation in the licensing of different medicines containing the same drug.
Oral tablet
CAUTIONARY AND ADVISORY LABELS 25
► **Inlyta** (Pfizer Ltd)
Axitinib 1 mg Inlyta 1mg tablets | 56 tablet [PoM] £703.40 (Hospital only)
Axitinib 3 mg Inlyta 3mg tablets | 56 tablet [PoM] £2,110.20 (Hospital only)
Axitinib 5 mg Inlyta 5mg tablets | 56 tablet [PoM] £3,517.00 (Hospital only)
Axitinib 7 mg Inlyta 7mg tablets | 56 tablet [PoM] £4,923.80 (Hospital only)

Binimetinib [Specialist drug]   05-Mar-2019

● **INDICATIONS AND DOSE**
Melanoma
► BY MOUTH
► Adult: Specialist drug – access specialist resources for dosing information

IMPORTANT SAFETY INFORMATION
RISKS OF INCORRECT DOSING OF ORAL ANTI-CANCER MEDICINES
See Cytotoxic drugs p. 1027.

● **CONTRA-INDICATIONS** History of retinal vein occlusion
● **SIDE-EFFECTS**
► **Common or very common** Alopecia · anaemia · angioedema · arthralgia · constipation · diarrhoea · dizziness · embolism and thrombosis · eye disorders · eye inflammation · fatigue · fever · fluid retention · gastrointestinal discomfort · gastrointestinal disorders · haemorrhage · headache · heart failure · hypersensitivity · hypersensitivity vasculitis · hypertension · intracranial haemorrhage · left ventricular dysfunction · lip squamous cell carcinoma · muscle complaints · muscle weakness · myopathy · nausea · neoplasms · nerve disorders · oedema · pain · panniculitis · photosensitivity reaction · renal failure · skin reactions · taste altered · ulcerative colitis · vision disorders · vomiting
► **Uncommon** Facial paralysis · facial paresis · pancreatitis
► **Frequency not known** Interstitial lung disease · retinal occlusion (discontinue permanently) · retinopathy
● **CONCEPTION AND CONTRACEPTION** Manufacturer advises women of child-bearing potential should use effective contraception during and for at least one month after stopping treatment.

● **PATIENT AND CARER ADVICE**
Missed doses Manufacturer advises if a dose is more than 6 hours late, the missed dose should not be taken and the next dose should be taken at the normal time.
Driving and skilled tasks Manufacturer advises patients and carers should be counselled on the effects on driving and performance of skilled tasks—increased risk of visual disturbances.
● **NATIONAL FUNDING/ACCESS DECISIONS**
For full details see funding body website
NICE decisions
► **Encorafenib with binimetinib for unresectable or metastatic BRAF V600 mutation-positive melanoma (February 2019)** NICE TA562 Recommended with restrictions

---

● **MEDICINAL FORMS** There can be variation in the licensing of different medicines containing the same drug.
Oral tablet
CAUTIONARY AND ADVISORY LABELS 25
► **Mektovi** (Pierre Fabre Ltd)
Binimetinib 15 mg Mektovi 15mg tablets | 84 tablet [PoM] £2,240.00 (Hospital only)
Binimetinib 45 mg Mektovi 45mg tablets | 28 tablet [PoM] £2,240.00

Bosutinib [Specialist drug]   05-Dec-2019

● **INDICATIONS AND DOSE**
Chronic myeloid leukaemia
► BY MOUTH
► Adult: Specialist drug – access specialist resources for dosing information

IMPORTANT SAFETY INFORMATION
RISKS OF INCORRECT DOSING OF ORAL ANTI-CANCER MEDICINES
See Cytotoxic drugs p. 1027.

MHRA/CHM ADVICE (MAY 2016): RISK OF HEPATITIS B VIRUS REACTIVATION WITH BCR-ABL TYROSINE KINASE INHIBITORS
An EU wide review has concluded that bosutinib can cause hepatitis B reactivation; the MHRA recommends establishing hepatitis B virus status in all patients before initiation of treatment. Patients who are carriers of hepatitis B virus should be closely monitored for signs and symptoms of active infection throughout treatment and for several months after stopping treatment; expert advice should be sought for patients who test positive for hepatitis B virus and in those with active infection.

● **INTERACTIONS** → Appendix 1: bosutinib
● **SIDE-EFFECTS**
► **Common or very common** Anaemia · appetite decreased · arthralgia · asthenia · chest discomfort · cough · dehydration · diarrhoea · dizziness · dyspnoea · electrolyte imbalance · fever · gastritis · gastrointestinal discomfort · haemorrhage · headache · hepatic disorders · hyperbilirubinaemia · hyperlipasaemia · hypertension · increased risk of infection · leucopenia · long QT syndrome · malaise · myalgia · nausea · neutropenia · oedema · pain · pericardial effusion · QT interval prolongation · renal impairment · respiratory disorders · skin reactions · taste altered · thrombocytopenia · tinnitus · vomiting
► **Uncommon** Pancreatitis · pericarditis · pulmonary hypertension · pulmonary oedema · tumour lysis syndrome
► **Frequency not known** Hepatitis B reactivation · interstitial lung disease · severe cutaneous adverse reactions (SCARs)
● **CONCEPTION AND CONTRACEPTION** Effective contraception required during treatment in women.

● **NATIONAL FUNDING/ACCESS DECISIONS**
For full details see funding body website
NICE decisions
▸ **Bosutinib for previously treated chronic myeloid leukaemia (August 2016)** NICE TA401 Recommended with restrictions

● **MEDICINAL FORMS** There can be variation in the licensing of different medicines containing the same drug.
Oral tablet
CAUTIONARY AND ADVISORY LABELS 21
▸ **Bosutinib (Non-proprietary)**
Bosutinib 100 mg Bosutinib 100mg tablets | 28 tablet [PoM]
£773.25–£859.17 (Hospital only) | 28 tablet [PoM] £773.26
Bosutinib 400 mg Bosutinib 400mg tablets | 28 tablet [PoM]
£3,093.00–£3,436.67 (Hospital only) | 28 tablet [PoM] £3,093.00
Bosutinib 500 mg Bosutinib 500mg tablets | 28 tablet [PoM]
£3,093.00–£3,436.67 (Hospital only) | 28 tablet [PoM] £3,093.00
▸ **Bosulif** (Pfizer Ltd)
Bosutinib 100 mg Bosulif 100mg tablets | 28 tablet [PoM] £859.17
(Hospital only)
Bosutinib 400 mg Bosulif 400mg tablets | 28 tablet [PoM]
£3,436.67 (Hospital only)
Bosutinib 500 mg Bosulif 500mg tablets | 28 tablet [PoM]
£3,436.67 (Hospital only)

Brigatinib [Specialist drug]
12-Feb-2021

● **INDICATIONS AND DOSE**
Non-small cell lung cancer
▸ BY MOUTH
▸ Adult: Specialist drug – access specialist resources for dosing information

IMPORTANT SAFETY INFORMATION
RISKS OF INCORRECT DOSING OF ORAL ANTI-CANCER MEDICINES
See Cytotoxic drugs p. 1027.

● **INTERACTIONS** → Appendix 1: brigatinib
● **SIDE-EFFECTS**
▸ **Common or very common** Anaemia · angioedema · appetite decreased · arrhythmias · arthralgia · asthenia · cataract · chest discomfort · constipation · cough · diarrhoea · dizziness · dry mouth · dyspnoea · electrolyte imbalance · eye disorders · eye inflammation · fever · flatulence · gastrointestinal discomfort · genital pruritus · glaucoma · headaches · hyperbilirubinaemia · hypercholesterolaemia · hyperglycaemia · hyperinsulinaemia · hypertension · increased risk of infection · insomnia · interstitial lung disease · memory impairment · muscle complaints · musculoskeletal discomfort · nausea · nerve disorders · neurotoxicity · oedema · oral disorders · pain · palpitations · peripheral swelling · photosensitivity · QT interval prolongation · sensation abnormal · skin reactions · taste altered · vision disorders · vomiting · vulvovaginal pruritus · weight decreased
▸ **Uncommon** Pancreatitis
▸ **Frequency not known** Hypoxia · respiratory disorders

● **CONCEPTION AND CONTRACEPTION** Manufacturer advises effective non-hormonal contraception in females of childbearing potential during and for at least 4 months after treatment. Male patients with partners of childbearing potential should use effective contraception during and for at least 3 months after treatment.

● **PATIENT AND CARER ADVICE** Manufacturer advises patients and carers should be told to report symptoms of visual disturbance, or unexplained muscle pain, tenderness, or weakness.
Driving and skilled tasks Manufacturer advises patients and carers should be counselled on the effects on driving and performance of skilled tasks—increased risk of visual disturbance, dizziness, or fatigue.

● **NATIONAL FUNDING/ACCESS DECISIONS**
For full details see funding body website
NICE decisions
▸ **Brigatinib for treating ALK-positive advanced non-small-cell lung cancer after crizotinib (March 2019)** NICE TA571 Recommended with restrictions
▸ **Brigatinib for ALK-positive advanced non-small-cell lung cancer that has not been previously treated with an ALK inhibitor (January 2021)** NICE TA670 Recommended
Scottish Medicines Consortium (SMC) decisions
▸ **Brigatinib (*Alunbrig*®) as monotherapy for the treatment of adult patients with anaplastic lymphoma kinase positive (ALK+) advanced non-small cell lung cancer (NSCLC) previously treated with crizotinib (June 2019)** SMC No. SMC2147 Recommended
▸ **Brigatinib (*Alunbrig*®) as monotherapy for the treatment of adult patients with anaplastic lymphoma kinase (ALK)-positive advanced non-small cell lung cancer (NSCLC) previously not treated with an ALK inhibitor (January 2021)** SMC No. SMC2314 Recommended

● **MEDICINAL FORMS** There can be variation in the licensing of different medicines containing the same drug.
Oral tablet
CAUTIONARY AND ADVISORY LABELS 25
▸ **Alunbrig** (Takeda UK Ltd)
Brigatinib 30 mg Alunbrig 30mg tablets | 28 tablet [PoM] £1,225.00
Brigatinib 90 mg Alunbrig 90mg tablets | 28 tablet [PoM] £3,675.00
Brigatinib 180 mg Alunbrig 180mg tablets | 28 tablet [PoM] £4,900.00
Form unstated
CAUTIONARY AND ADVISORY LABELS 25
▸ **Alunbrig** (Takeda UK Ltd)
Alunbrig 90mg/180mg tablets treatment initiation pack | 28 tablet [PoM] £4,900.00

Cabozantinib [Specialist drug]
01-Apr-2025

● **INDICATIONS AND DOSE**
Medullary thyroid carcinoma
▸ BY MOUTH USING CAPSULES
▸ Adult: Specialist drug – access specialist resources for dosing information
Renal cell carcinoma | Hepatocellular carcinoma | Differentiated thyroid carcinoma
▸ BY MOUTH USING TABLETS
▸ Adult: Specialist drug – access specialist resources for dosing information
DOSE EQUIVALENCE AND CONVERSION
▸ Cabozantinib tablets and capsules are **not** bioequivalent.

IMPORTANT SAFETY INFORMATION
Cabozantinib formulations are not bioequivalent and should **not** be used interchangeably.

MHRA/CHM ADVICE: SYSTEMICALLY ADMINISTERED VEGF PATHWAY INHIBITORS: RISK OF ANEURYSM AND ARTERY DISSECTION (JULY 2020)
A European review of worldwide data concluded that systemically administered VEGF pathway inhibitors may lead to aneurysm and artery dissection in patients with or without hypertension. Some fatal cases have been reported, mainly in relation to aortic aneurysm rupture and aortic dissection. The MHRA advises healthcare professionals to carefully consider the risk of aneurysm and artery dissection in patients with risk factors before initiating treatment with cabozantinib; any modifiable risk factors (such as smoking and hypertension) should

be reduced as much as possible. Monitor blood pressure regularly—consult product literature if hypertension occurs during treatment.

RISKS OF INCORRECT DOSING OF ORAL ANTI-CANCER MEDICINES See Cytotoxic drugs p. 1027.

- **CONTRA-INDICATIONS** Reversible posterior leukoencephalopathy syndrome
- **INTERACTIONS** → Appendix 1: cabozantinib
- **SIDE-EFFECTS**
- ▶ **Common or very common** Abscess · alopecia · anaemia · anxiety · appetite decreased · arrhythmias · arthralgia · asthenia · chills · cholelithiasis · confusion · constipation · cough · dehydration · depression · diarrhoea · dizziness · dry mouth · dysphagia · dysphonia · dyspnoea · dysuria · ear pain · electrolyte imbalance · embolism and thrombosis · encephalopathy · fistula · gastrointestinal discomfort · gastrointestinal disorders · haemorrhage · hair changes · headache · healing impaired · hyperbilirubinaemia · hyperglycaemia · hypertension · hypoalbuminaemia · hypoglycaemia · hypotension · hypothyroidism · increased risk of infection · lymphopenia · mucositis · muscle spasms · nausea · nerve disorders · neutropenia · oedema · oral disorders · oropharyngeal pain · osteonecrosis of jaw (discontinue) · pain · pallor · pancreatitis · paraesthesia · peripheral coldness · proteinuria · respiratory disorders · skin reactions · stroke · taste altered · thrombocytopenia · tinnitus · tracheo-oesophageal fistula · tremor · vision blurred · vomiting · weight decreased
- ▶ **Uncommon** Abnormal dreams · amenorrhoea · angina pectoris · ataxia · cataract · concentration impaired · conjunctivitis · cyst · delirium · eosinophilia · hearing impairment · hepatic disorders · loss of consciousness · myocardial infarction · pneumonitis · renal impairment · rhabdomyolysis · seizure · skin ulcer · speech disorder · telangiectasia · throat oedema · thrombocytosis · wound complications
- ▶ **Frequency not known** Aneurysm · artery dissection · cutaneous vasculitis · QT interval prolongation

SIDE-EFFECTS, FURTHER INFORMATION Discontinue if nephrotic syndrome occurs.

Hand and foot syndrome (palmar-plantar erythrodysaesthesia syndrome) Consider treatment interruption if severe and restart at a lower dose when resolved to grade 1.

Haemorrhage Severe, sometimes fatal, haemorrhage has been reported—discontinue.

Perforations and fistulas Discontinue if fistulas, such as gastrointestinal fistula, tracheal fistula, and tracheo-oesophageal fistula, or gastrointestinal perforation occurs.

Thromboembolic events Discontinue if symptoms develop, including myocardial infarction or other significant thromboembolic complications.

Wound Complications Discontinue if wound healing complications requiring medical intervention occur.

- **CONCEPTION AND CONTRACEPTION** Patients and their sexual partners must use effective contraception (in addition to barrier method) during treatment and for at least 4 months after the last dose.
- **PATIENT AND CARER ADVICE** Food should not be consumed for at least 2 hours before and at least 1 hour after each dose.

Missed doses If a dose is more than 12 hours late, the missed dose should not be taken and the next dose should be taken at the normal time.

Driving and skilled tasks Patients and carers should be cautioned on the effects on driving and performance of skilled tasks— increased risk of dizziness and weakness.

- **NATIONAL FUNDING/ACCESS DECISIONS** For full details see funding body website

NICE decisions
- ▶ **Cabozantinib for previously treated advanced renal cell carcinoma (August 2017)** NICE TA463 Recommended
- ▶ **Cabozantinib for untreated advanced renal cell carcinoma (October 2018)** NICE TA542 Recommended with restrictions
- ▶ **Cabozantinib with nivolumab for untreated advanced renal cell carcinoma (April 2024)** NICE TA964 Recommended with restrictions
- ▶ **Cabozantinib for treating medullary thyroid cancer (March 2018)** NICE TA516 Recommended with restrictions
- ▶ **Cabozantinib for previously treated advanced differentiated thyroid cancer unsuitable for or refractory to radioactive iodine (November 2023)** NICE TA928 Not recommended
- ▶ **Cabozantinib for previously treated advanced hepatocellular carcinoma (December 2022)** NICE TA849 Recommended with restrictions

Scottish Medicines Consortium (SMC) decisions
- ▶ Cabozantinib (*Cabometyx*®) for the treatment of advanced renal cell carcinoma (RCC) in adults following prior vascular endothelial growth factor (VEGF)-targeted therapy (June 2017) SMC No. 1234/17 Recommended
- ▶ Cabozantinib (*Cabometyx*®) for treatment of advanced renal cell carcinoma (RCC) in treatment-naïve adults with intermediate or poor risk per IMDC criteria (February 2019) SMC No. SMC2136 Not recommended
- ▶ Cabozantinib (*Cabometyx*®) in combination with nivolumab for the first-line treatment of advanced renal cell carcinoma in adults (October 2021) SMC No. SMC2386 Recommended
- ▶ Cabozantinib (*Cabometyx*®) as monotherapy for the treatment of adult patients with locally advanced or metastatic differentiated thyroid carcinoma, refractory or not eligible to radioactive iodine who have progressed during or after prior systemic therapy (February 2024) SMC No. SMC2590 Not recommended
- ▶ Cabozantinib (Cabozantinib Ipsen) as monotherapy for the treatment of hepatocellular carcinoma in adults who have previously been treated with sorafenib (March 2025) SMC No. SMC2754 Recommended

- **MEDICINAL FORMS** There can be variation in the licensing of different medicines containing the same drug.

Oral tablet
CAUTIONARY AND ADVISORY LABELS 23, 25
- ▶ **Cabozantinib (Non-proprietary)**
  Cabozantinib (as Cabozantinib s-malate) **20 mg** Cabozantinib 20mg tablets | 30 tablet [PoM] £5,143.00 (Hospital only)
  Cabozantinib (as Cabozantinib s-malate) **40 mg** Cabozantinib 40mg tablets | 30 tablet [PoM] £5,143.00 (Hospital only)
  Cabozantinib (as Cabozantinib s-malate) **60 mg** Cabozantinib 60mg tablets | 30 tablet [PoM] £5,143.00 (Hospital only)
- ▶ **Cabometyx** (Ipsen Ltd)
  Cabozantinib (as Cabozantinib s-malate) **20 mg** Cabometyx 20mg tablets | 30 tablet [PoM] £5,143.00 (Hospital only)
  Cabozantinib (as Cabozantinib s-malate) **40 mg** Cabometyx 40mg tablets | 30 tablet [PoM] £5,143.00 (Hospital only)
  Cabozantinib (as Cabozantinib s-malate) **60 mg** Cabometyx 60mg tablets | 30 tablet [PoM] £5,143.00 (Hospital only)

Form unstated
CAUTIONARY AND ADVISORY LABELS 23, 25
- ▶ **Cometriq** (Ipsen Ltd)
  Cometriq 20mg capsules and Cometriq 80mg capsules | 56 capsule [PoM] £4,800.00 | 112 capsule [PoM] £4,800.00

Oral capsule
CAUTIONARY AND ADVISORY LABELS 23, 25
EXCIPIENTS: May contain Gelatin
- ▶ **Cometriq** (Ipsen Ltd)
  Cabozantinib (as Cabozantinib s-malate) **20 mg** Cometriq 20mg capsules | 84 capsule [PoM] £4,800.00
  Cabozantinib (as Cabozantinib s-malate) **80 mg** Cometriq 80mg capsules | 7 capsule [PoM] [▨]

Capivasertib [Specialist drug]

10-Oct-2024

● INDICATIONS AND DOSE

Breast cancer

▶ BY MOUTH

▶ Adult: Specialist drug – access specialist resources for dosing information

---

IMPORTANT SAFETY INFORMATION

RISKS OF INCORRECT DOSING OF ORAL ANTI-CANCER MEDICINES
See Cytotoxic drugs p. 1027.

● INTERACTIONS → Appendix 1: capivasertib

● SIDE-EFFECTS

▶ **Common or very common** Anaemia · appetite decreased · asthenia · cystitis · diabetes mellitus · diabetic ketoacidosis · diabetic metabolic decompensation · diarrhoea · drug reaction with eosinophilia and systemic symptoms (DRESS) · dyspepsia · frequent bowel movements · hyperglycaemia · hypersensitivity · malaise · mucositis · nausea · oral disorders · pyuria · skin reactions · taste altered · urinary tract infection · vomiting

● CONCEPTION AND CONTRACEPTION [EvGr] Females of childbearing potential should use effective contraception during treatment and for at least 4 weeks after last treatment; male patients should use effective contraception during treatment and for 16 weeks after last treatment if their partner is of childbearing potential. ⟨M⟩

● PATIENT AND CARER ADVICE
Vomiting If vomiting occurs after taking tablets, no additional dose should be taken on that day and the next dose should be taken at the usual time.
Missed doses If a dose is more than 4 hours late, the missed dose should not be taken and the next dose should be taken at the normal time.
Driving and skilled tasks Patients and carers should be cautioned on the effects on driving and performance of skilled tasks—increased risk of fatigue.

● MEDICINAL FORMS There can be variation in the licensing of different medicines containing the same drug.

Oral tablet

CAUTIONARY AND ADVISORY LABELS 25

▶ Truqap (AstraZeneca UK Ltd) ▼
Capivasertib 160 mg Truqap 160mg tablets | 64 tablet [PoM]
£5,850.00 (Hospital only)
Capivasertib 200 mg Truqap 200mg tablets | 64 tablet [PoM]
£5,850.00 (Hospital only)

Ceritinib [Specialist drug]

10-Jun-2021

● INDICATIONS AND DOSE

Non-small cell lung cancer

▶ BY MOUTH

▶ Adult: Specialist drug – access specialist resources for dosing information

---

IMPORTANT SAFETY INFORMATION

RISKS OF INCORRECT DOSING OF ORAL ANTI-CANCER MEDICINES
See Cytotoxic drugs p. 1027.

● CONTRA-INDICATIONS Congenital long QT syndrome

● INTERACTIONS → Appendix 1: ceritinib

● SIDE-EFFECTS

▶ **Common or very common** Anaemia · appetite decreased · arrhythmias · asthenia · azotaemia · constipation · diarrhoea · dysphagia · gastrointestinal discomfort · gastrooesophageal reflux disease · hepatic disorders · hyperbilirubinaemia · hyperglycaemia · hypophosphataemia · interstitial lung disease · nausea ·

oesophageal disorder · pericardial effusion · pericarditis · QT interval prolongation · renal impairment · skin reactions · vision disorders · vitreous floater · vomiting · weight decreased

▶ **Uncommon** Pancreatitis

SIDE-EFFECTS, FURTHER INFORMATION **Gastro-intestinal effects** Consider interrupting treatment, and reduce dose as appropriate.
　Interstitial lung disease Interstitial lung disease and pneumonitis, including fatal events, have been reported; permanently discontinue treatment if diagnosed.

● CONCEPTION AND CONTRACEPTION Manufacturer recommends effective contraception in women of childbearing potential during treatment and for up to 3 months after discontinuation of treatment.

● PATIENT AND CARER ADVICE Patients and carers should be counselled on the administration of tablets.
Missed doses Manufacturer advises if a patient vomits during a course of treatment or if a dose is more than 12 hours late, the replacement or missed dose should not be taken and the next dose should be taken at the normal time.
Driving and skilled tasks Manufacturer advises patients and their carers should be counselled on the effects on driving and skilled tasks—increased risk of fatigue and vision disorders.

● NATIONAL FUNDING/ACCESS DECISIONS
For full details see funding body website

NICE decisions

▶ Ceritinib for previously treated anaplastic lymphoma kinase-positive non-small cell lung cancer (June 2016) NICE TA395 Recommended with restrictions

▶ Ceritinib for untreated ALK-positive non-small cell lung cancer (January 2018) NICE TA500 Recommended with restrictions

Scottish Medicines Consortium (SMC) decisions

▶ Ceritinib (*Zykadia*®) for treatment of adult patients with anaplastic lymphoma kinase (ALK)-positive advanced non-small cell lung cancer (NSCLC) previously treated with crizotinib (December 2015) SMC No. 1097/15 Recommended

---

● MEDICINAL FORMS There can be variation in the licensing of different medicines containing the same drug.

Oral tablet

CAUTIONARY AND ADVISORY LABELS 21, 25

▶ Zykadia (Novartis Pharmaceuticals UK Ltd)
Ceritinib 150 mg Zykadia 150mg tablets | 84 tablet [PoM] £2,757.13 (Hospital only)

Cobimetinib [Specialist drug]

30-Apr-2019

● INDICATIONS AND DOSE

Melanoma

▶ BY MOUTH

▶ Adult: Specialist drug – access specialist resources for dosing information

---

IMPORTANT SAFETY INFORMATION

RISKS OF INCORRECT DOSING OF ORAL ANTI-CANCER MEDICINES
See Cytotoxic drugs p. 1027.

● INTERACTIONS → Appendix 1: cobimetinib

● SIDE-EFFECTS

▶ **Common or very common** Anaemia · basal cell carcinoma · chills · dehydration · diarrhoea · electrolyte imbalance · fever · haemorrhage · hyperglycaemia · hypertension · nausea · photosensitivity · pneumonitis · retinal detachment · retinopathy · skin reactions · sunburn · vision disorders · vomiting

▶ **Uncommon** Rhabdomyolysis

▶ **Frequency not known** Intracranial haemorrhage

- **CONCEPTION AND CONTRACEPTION** Manufacturer advises use of two effective contraceptive methods during treatment and for at least 3 months after stopping treatment.
- **PATIENT AND CARER ADVICE**
Vomiting Manufacturer advises if vomiting occurs after taking tablets, no additional dose should be taken on that day and the next dose should be taken at the usual time.
Missed doses Manufacturer advises if a dose is more than 12 hours late, the missed dose should not be taken and the next dose should be taken at the normal time.
Driving and skilled tasks Manufacturer advises patients should be counselled on the effects on driving and performance of skilled tasks—increased risk of visual disturbances.
- **NATIONAL FUNDING/ACCESS DECISIONS**
For full details see funding body website
NICE decisions
▶ Cobimetinib in combination with vemurafenib for treating unresectable or metastatic BRAF V600 mutation-positive melanoma (October 2016) NICE TA414 Not recommended

- **MEDICINAL FORMS** There can be variation in the licensing of different medicines containing the same drug.
Oral tablet
▶ Cotellic (Roche Products Ltd)
Cobimetinib (as Cobimetinib hemifumarate) **20 mg** Cotellic 20mg tablets | 63 tablet PoM £4,275.67

Crizotinib [Specialist drug]

07-Jan-2025

- **INDICATIONS AND DOSE**
Non-small cell lung cancer
▶ BY MOUTH
▶ Adult: Specialist drug – access specialist resources for dosing information

---

IMPORTANT SAFETY INFORMATION
RISKS OF INCORRECT DOSING OF ORAL ANTI-CANCER MEDICINES
See Cytotoxic drugs p. 1027.

MHRA/CHM ADVICE (NOVEMBER 2015): RISK OF CARDIAC FAILURE
Severe, sometimes fatal cases of cardiac failure have been reported in adult patients treated with crizotinib. The MHRA has issued the following advice:
- monitor all patients for signs and symptoms of heart failure (including dyspnoea, oedema, or rapid weight gain from fluid retention)
- consider reducing the dose, or interrupting or stopping treatment if symptoms of heart failure occur

---

- **INTERACTIONS** → Appendix 1: crizotinib
- **SIDE-EFFECTS**
▶ **Common or very common** Acute respiratory distress syndrome (ARDS) · anaemia · appetite decreased · arrhythmias · constipation · diarrhoea · dizziness · fatigue · gait abnormal · gastrointestinal discomfort · gastrointestinal disorders · gonadal hypofunction · heart failure · hepatic disorders · hypophosphataemia · interstitial lung disease · leucopenia · local swelling · movement disorders · muscle atrophy · muscle tone decreased · muscle weakness · nausea · nerve disorders · neuralgia · neurotoxicity · neutropenia · oedema · periorbital oedema · peroneal nerve palsy · pulmonary oedema · QT interval prolongation · renal abscess · renal disorders · sensation abnormal · skin reactions · syncope · taste altered · vision disorders · vitreous floater · vomiting
▶ **Uncommon** Gastrointestinal perforation (including fatal cases, discontinue) · hepatic failure (including fatal cases) · photosensitivity reaction · renal impairment

SIDE-EFFECTS, FURTHER INFORMATION **Heart failure** Consider reducing the dose, or interrupting or stopping treatment, if symptoms of heart failure occur.
Interstitial lung disease Interstitial lung disease and pneumonitis, including fatal events, have been reported; withdraw treatment if suspected, and permanently discontinue treatment if diagnosed.
- **CONCEPTION AND CONTRACEPTION** EvGr Ensure effective contraception during and for at least 90 days after treatment. Ⓜ
- **PATIENT AND CARER ADVICE**
Gastrointestinal perforation Patients and carers should be counselled on the signs and symptoms of gastrointestinal perforation and advised to seek immediate medical attention if symptoms develop.
Vision disorders Patients and carers should be counselled on the signs and symptoms of vision disorders and advised to seek immediate medical attention if symptoms develop— risk of severe visual loss.
Photosensitivity Patients and carers should be advised to minimise exposure to sunlight, and protect skin by wearing sun-protective clothing and/or using sunscreen.
Patient Information Booklet A patient information booklet, including a patient alert card, should be provided.
Missed doses If a dose is more than 6 hours late, the missed dose should not be taken and the next dose should be taken at the normal time.
Driving and skilled tasks Patients and carers should be cautioned on the effects on driving and performance of skilled tasks—increased risk of symptomatic bradycardia (including syncope, dizziness, and hypotension), vision disorder and fatigue.
- **NATIONAL FUNDING/ACCESS DECISIONS**
For full details see funding body website
NICE decisions
▶ Crizotinib for untreated anaplastic lymphoma kinase-positive advanced non-small-cell lung cancer (September 2016) NICE TA406 Recommended with restrictions
▶ Crizotinib for previously treated anaplastic lymphoma kinase-positive advanced non-small-cell lung cancer (December 2016) NICE TA422 Recommended with restrictions
▶ Crizotinib for treating ROS1-positive advanced non-small-cell lung cancer (December 2024) NICE TA1021 Recommended with restrictions
Scottish Medicines Consortium (SMC) decisions
▶ Crizotinib (Xalkori®) for treatment of adults with ROS1-positive advanced non-small cell lung cancer (June 2018) SMC No. 1329/18 Recommended

- **MEDICINAL FORMS** There can be variation in the licensing of different medicines containing the same drug.
Oral capsule
CAUTIONARY AND ADVISORY LABELS 11, 25
▶ Xalkori (Pfizer Ltd)
Crizotinib **200 mg** Xalkori 200mg capsules | 60 capsule PoM £4,689.00 (Hospital only)
Crizotinib **250 mg** Xalkori 250mg capsules | 60 capsule PoM £4,689.00 (Hospital only)

Dabrafenib [Specialist drug]

18-Sep-2024

- **INDICATIONS AND DOSE**
Melanoma | Non-small cell lung cancer
▶ BY MOUTH USING CAPSULES
▶ Adult: Specialist drug – access specialist resources for dosing information

---

IMPORTANT SAFETY INFORMATION
RISKS OF INCORRECT DOSING OF ORAL ANTI-CANCER MEDICINES
See Cytotoxic drugs p. 1027.

- **CONTRA-INDICATIONS** BRAF wild-type melanoma · BRAF wild-type non-small cell lung cancer
- **INTERACTIONS** → Appendix 1: dabrafenib
- **SIDE-EFFECTS**
  - **Common or very common** Alopecia · appetite decreased · arthralgia · asthenia · chills · constipation · cough · diarrhoea · dizziness · electrolyte imbalance · fever · headache · hyperglycaemia · hypotension · increased risk of infection · influenza like illness · leucopenia · muscle complaints · musculoskeletal stiffness · nausea · neoplasms · neutropenia · pain in extremity · photosensitivity reaction · skin reactions · sweat changes · thrombocytopenia · vomiting
  - **Uncommon** Eye inflammation · nephritis · pancreatitis · panniculitis · renal impairment · sarcoidosis
  - **Rare or very rare** Haemophagocytic lymphohistiocytosis
  - **Frequency not known** Malignancy · myocarditis · severe cutaneous adverse reactions (SCARs)
- **CONCEPTION AND CONTRACEPTION** [EvGr] Females of childbearing potential should use effective non-hormonal contraception during treatment and for 2 weeks after last treatment. [M]
- **PATIENT AND CARER ADVICE** Patients and carers should be informed to immediately report new skin lesions—risk of cutaneous squamous cell carcinoma and new primary melanoma. Patients and carers should be counselled on the administration of dabrafenib.

  If vomiting occurs after taking dabrafenib, no additional dose should be taken and the next dose should be taken at the normal time.

  Missed doses If a dose is more than 6 hours late, the missed dose should not be taken and the next dose should be taken at the normal time.

  Driving and skilled tasks Patients and carers should be counselled on the effects on driving and performance of skilled tasks—increased risk of fatigue, dizziness, and visual disturbances.

- **NATIONAL FUNDING/ACCESS DECISIONS**
  For full details see funding body website
  NICE decisions
  - **Dabrafenib for treating unresectable or metastatic BRAF V600 mutation-positive melanoma (October 2014)** NICE TA321 Recommended with restrictions
  - **Trametinib in combination with dabrafenib for treating unresectable or metastatic melanoma (June 2016)** NICE TA396 Recommended with restrictions
  - **Dabrafenib with trametinib for adjuvant treatment of resected BRAF V600 mutation-positive melanoma (October 2018)** NICE TA544 Recommended with restrictions
  - **Dabrafenib plus trametinib for treating BRAF V600 mutation-positive advanced non-small-cell lung cancer (June 2023)** NICE TA898 Recommended with restrictions

  Scottish Medicines Consortium (SMC) decisions
  - **Dabrafenib (*Tafinlar*®) for the monotherapy of adult patients with unresectable or metastatic melanoma with a BRAF V600 mutation (March 2015)** SMC No. 1023/15 Recommended with restrictions
  - **Dabrafenib (*Tafinlar*®) in combination with trametinib for the adjuvant treatment of adult patients with Stage III melanoma with a BRAF V600 mutation, following complete resection (February 2019)** SMC No. SMC2131 Recommended

- **MEDICINAL FORMS** There can be variation in the licensing of different medicines containing the same drug.
  Oral capsule
  CAUTIONARY AND ADVISORY LABELS 23, 25
  - Tafinlar (Novartis Pharmaceuticals UK Ltd)
    Dabrafenib (as Dabrafenib mesilate) 50 mg Tafinlar 50mg capsules | 28 capsule [PoM] £933.33 (Hospital only)
    Dabrafenib (as Dabrafenib mesilate) 75 mg Tafinlar 75mg capsules | 28 capsule [PoM] £1,400.00 (Hospital only)

Dacomitinib [Specialist drug]

22-Mar-2023

- **INDICATIONS AND DOSE**

  Non-small cell lung cancer
  - BY MOUTH
  - Adult: Specialist drug – access specialist resources for dosing information

> **IMPORTANT SAFETY INFORMATION**
> RISKS OF INCORRECT DOSING OF ORAL ANTI-CANCER MEDICINES
> See Cytotoxic drugs p. 1027.

- **INTERACTIONS** → Appendix 1: dacomitinib
- **SIDE-EFFECTS**
  - **Common or very common** Alopecia · appetite decreased · asthenia · dehydration · diarrhoea · dry eye · dry mouth · eye inflammation · hypertrichosis · hypokalaemia · increased risk of infection · interstitial lung disease (discontinue permanently) · mucositis · nail discolouration · nail disorders · nausea · oral disorders · oropharyngeal pain · pneumonitis (discontinue permanently) · skin reactions · taste altered · vomiting · weight decreased
- **CONCEPTION AND CONTRACEPTION** Manufacturer advises females of childbearing potential should use effective contraception during treatment and for at least 17 days after stopping treatment.
- **PATIENT AND CARER ADVICE**
  Photosensitivity Manufacturer advises patients should wear protective clothing and apply sunscreen before sun exposure.
  Driving and skilled tasks Manufacturer advises patients and carers should be cautioned on the effects on driving and performance of skilled tasks—increased risk of fatigue and ocular side-effects.
- **NATIONAL FUNDING/ACCESS DECISIONS**
  For full details see funding body website
  NICE decisions
  - **Dacomitinib for untreated EGFR mutation-positive non-small cell lung cancer (August 2019)** NICE TA595 Recommended

  Scottish Medicines Consortium (SMC) decisions
  - **Dacomitinib (*Vizimpro*®) as monotherapy for the first-line treatment of adult patients with locally advanced or metastatic non-small cell lung cancer (NSCLC) with epidermal growth factor receptor (EGFR)-activating mutations (September 2019)** SMC No. SMC2184 Recommended

- **MEDICINAL FORMS** There can be variation in the licensing of different medicines containing the same drug.
  Oral tablet
  - Vizimpro (Pfizer Ltd)
    Dacomitinib (as Dacomitinib monohydrate) 15 mg Vizimpro 15mg tablets | 30 tablet [PoM] £2,703.00 (Hospital only)
    Dacomitinib (as Dacomitinib monohydrate) 30 mg Vizimpro 30mg tablets | 30 tablet [PoM] £2,703.00 (Hospital only)
    Dacomitinib (as Dacomitinib monohydrate) 45 mg Vizimpro 45mg tablets | 30 tablet [PoM] £2,703.00 (Hospital only)

Dasatinib [Specialist drug]

15-Jul-2022

- **INDICATIONS AND DOSE**

  Chronic myeloid leukaemia | Acute lymphoblastic leukaemia
  - BY MOUTH
  - Adult: Specialist drug – access specialist resources for dosing information

  DOSE EQUIVALENCE AND CONVERSION
  - *Sprycel*® film-coated tablets and *Sprycel*® powder for oral suspension are **not** bioequivalent.   continued →

Immune system and malignant disease

UXIL ®

Acute lymphoblastic leukaemia
‣ BY MOUTH
‣ Adult: Specialist drug – access specialist resources for dosing information

DOSE EQUIVALENCE AND CONVERSION
‣ *Uxil*® film-coated tablets and other dasatinib preparations are **not** bioequivalent.

IMPORTANT SAFETY INFORMATION
Sprycel® formulations are **not** bioequivalent and should not be used interchangeably.
Uxil® film-coated tablets and other dasatinib preparations are **not** bioequivalent and should not be used interchangeably.

RISKS OF INCORRECT DOSING OF ORAL ANTI-CANCER MEDICINES
See Cytotoxic drugs p. 1027.

MHRA/CHM ADVICE (MAY 2016): RISK OF HEPATITIS B VIRUS REACTIVATION WITH BCR-ABL TYROSINE KINASE INHIBITORS
An EU wide review has concluded that dasatinib can cause hepatitis B reactivation; the MHRA recommends establishing hepatitis B virus status in all patients before initiation of treatment. Patients who are carriers of hepatitis B virus should be closely monitored for signs and symptoms of active infection throughout treatment and for several months after stopping treatment; expert advice should be sought for patients who test positive for hepatitis B virus and in those with active infection.

● INTERACTIONS → Appendix 1: dasatinib
● SIDE-EFFECTS
‣ **Common or very common** Alopecia · anaemia · appetite abnormal · arrhythmias · arthralgia · asthenia · bone marrow depression · cardiac disorder · cardiomyopathy · chest pain · chills · constipation · cough · depression · diarrhoea · dizziness · drowsiness · dry eye · dyspnoea · eye inflammation · facial swelling · fever · fluid imbalance · flushing · gastrointestinal discomfort · gastrointestinal disorders · genital abnormalities · haemorrhage · headache · heart failure · hypertension · hyperuricaemia · increased risk of infection · insomnia · interstitial lung disease · milia · mucositis · muscle complaints · muscle weakness · musculoskeletal stiffness · myocardial dysfunction · nausea · nerve disorders · neutropenia · oedema · oral disorders · pain · palpitations · pericardial effusion · perinephric effusion · peripheral swelling · pulmonary hypertension · pulmonary oedema · respiratory disorders · sepsis · skin reactions · sweat changes · taste altered · thrombocytopenia · tinnitus · vision disorders · vomiting · weight changes
‣ **Uncommon** Acute coronary syndrome · anxiety · arthritis · ascites · asthma · cardiac inflammation · cardiomegaly · cerebrovascular insufficiency · cholecystitis · CNS haemorrhage · confusion · dysphagia · embolism and thrombosis · emotional lability · excessive tearing · gynaecomastia · hair disorder · hearing loss · hepatic disorders · hypercholesterolaemia · hypoalbuminaemia · hypotension · hypothyroidism · ischaemic heart disease · libido decreased · lymphadenopathy · lymphopenia · malaise · memory loss · menstrual disorder · movement disorders · myopathy · nail disorder · osteonecrosis · pancreatitis · panniculitis · penile disorders · photosensitivity reaction · proteinuria · QT interval prolongation · renal impairment · scrotal oedema · skin ulcer · syncope · tendinitis · testicular swelling · tremor · tumour lysis syndrome · urinary frequency increased · vertigo · vulvovaginal swelling
‣ **Rare or very rare** Cardiac arrest · dementia · diabetes mellitus · epiphyses delayed fusion · facial paralysis · gait abnormal · growth retardation · hypersensitivity vasculitis · hyperthyroidism · pure red cell aplasia · seizure · thyroiditis

‣ **Frequency not known** Electrolyte imbalance · hepatitis B reactivation · nephrotic syndrome · Stevens-Johnson syndrome · thrombotic microangiopathy
● CONCEPTION AND CONTRACEPTION Effective contraception required during treatment.
● NATIONAL FUNDING/ACCESS DECISIONS
For full details see funding body website
NICE decisions
‣ Dasatinib, nilotinib and imatinib for untreated chronic myeloid leukaemia (CML) (December 2016) NICE TA426 Recommended with restrictions
‣ Dasatinib, nilotinib and high-dose imatinib for treating imatinib-resistant or intolerant chronic myeloid leukaemia (CML) (December 2016) NICE TA425 Recommended with restrictions
Scottish Medicines Consortium (SMC) decisions
‣ Dasatinib (*Sprycel*®) tablets for the treatment of adult patients with chronic, accelerated or blast phase chronic myelogenous leukaemia (CML) with resistance or intolerance to prior therapy including imatinib mesilate (September 2016) SMC No. 370/07 Recommended
‣ Dasatinib (*Sprycel*®) tablets for the treatment of adult patients with newly diagnosed Philadelphia chromosome positive (Ph+) chronic myelogenous leukaemia (CML) in the chronic phase (September 2016) SMC No. 1170/16 Recommended

● MEDICINAL FORMS There can be variation in the licensing of different medicines containing the same drug.
Oral tablet
CAUTIONARY AND ADVISORY LABELS 5, 25
‣ Dasatinib (Non-proprietary)
  Dasatinib (as Dasatinib monohydrate) 20 mg Dasatinib 20mg tablets | 60 tablet PoM £626.24–£1,127.23 DT = £1,252.48 (Hospital only) | 60 tablet PoM £650.00 DT = £1,252.48
  Dasatinib (as Dasatinib monohydrate) 50 mg Dasatinib 50mg tablets | 60 tablet PoM £1,200.00 DT = £2,504.96 | 60 tablet PoM £1,252.48–£2,254.46 DT = £2,504.96 (Hospital only)
  Dasatinib (as Dasatinib monohydrate) 80 mg Dasatinib 80mg tablets | 30 tablet PoM £1,252.48–£2,254.46 DT = £2,504.96 (Hospital only) | 30 tablet PoM £1,200.00 DT = £2,504.96
  Dasatinib (as Dasatinib monohydrate) 100 mg Dasatinib 100mg tablets | 30 tablet PoM £1,252.48–£2,254.46 DT = £2,504.96 (Hospital only) | 30 tablet PoM £1,200.00 DT = £2,504.96
  Dasatinib (as Dasatinib monohydrate) 140 mg Dasatinib 140mg tablets | 30 tablet PoM £2,129.22–£2,254.46 DT = £2,504.96 (Hospital only) | 30 tablet PoM £1,200.00 DT = £2,504.96
‣ Sprycel (Bristol-Myers Squibb Pharmaceuticals Ltd)
  Dasatinib (as Dasatinib monohydrate) 20 mg Sprycel 20mg tablets | 60 tablet PoM £1,252.48 DT = £1,252.48
  Dasatinib (as Dasatinib monohydrate) 50 mg Sprycel 50mg tablets | 60 tablet PoM £2,504.96 DT = £2,504.96
  Dasatinib (as Dasatinib monohydrate) 80 mg Sprycel 80mg tablets | 30 tablet PoM £2,504.96 DT = £2,504.96
  Dasatinib (as Dasatinib monohydrate) 100 mg Sprycel 100mg tablets | 30 tablet PoM £2,504.96 DT = £2,504.96
  Dasatinib (as Dasatinib monohydrate) 140 mg Sprycel 140mg tablets | 30 tablet PoM £2,504.96 DT = £2,504.96
Oral suspension
CAUTIONARY AND ADVISORY LABELS 5
EXCIPIENTS: May contain Benzyl alcohol, sucrose
‣ Sprycel (Imported (Germany))
  Dasatinib (as Dasatinib monohydrate) 10 mg per 1 ml Sprycel 10mg/ml oral suspension | 90 ml PoM Ⓔ

Encorafenib [Specialist drug]
28-May-2021

● **INDICATIONS AND DOSE**

Melanoma | Colorectal cancer
▶ BY MOUTH
▶ Adult: Specialist drug – access specialist resources for dosing information

> **IMPORTANT SAFETY INFORMATION**
> RISKS OF INCORRECT DOSING OF ORAL ANTI-CANCER MEDICINES
> See Cytotoxic drugs p. 1027.

● **CONTRA-INDICATIONS** BRAF wild-type colorectal cancer · BRAF wild-type malignant melanoma

● **INTERACTIONS** → Appendix 1: encorafenib

● **SIDE-EFFECTS**
▶ **Common or very common** Alopecia · anaphylactic reaction · angioedema · appetite decreased · arrhythmias · arthralgia · arthritis · constipation · facial paralysis · facial paresis · fatigue · fever · headache · hypersensitivity · hypersensitivity vasculitis · insomnia · muscle complaints · muscle weakness · nausea · neoplasms · nerve disorders · pain · photosensitivity reaction · renal impairment · skin reactions · taste altered · vomiting
▶ **Uncommon** Eye inflammation · pancreatitis
▶ **Frequency not known** Haemorrhage · QT interval prolongation · visual impairment

● **CONCEPTION AND CONTRACEPTION** Manufacturer advises women of child-bearing potential should use effective contraception during and for at least one month after stopping treatment; additional barrier method recommended in women using hormonal contraceptives.

● **PATIENT AND CARER ADVICE** Manufacturer advises patients should be informed to immediately report new skin lesions—risk of cutaneous squamous cell carcinoma and new primary melanoma.
Missed doses Manufacturer advises if a dose is more than 12 hours late, the missed dose should not be taken and the next dose should be taken at the normal time.
Driving and skilled tasks Manufacturer advises patients and carers should be counselled on the effects on driving and performance of skilled tasks—increased risk of visual disturbances.

● **NATIONAL FUNDING/ACCESS DECISIONS**
For full details see funding body website
NICE decisions
▶ Encorafenib with binimetinib for unresectable or metastatic BRAF V600 mutation-positive melanoma (February 2019) NICE TA562 Recommended with restrictions
▶ Encorafenib plus cetuximab for previously treated BRAF V600E mutation-positive metastatic colorectal cancer (January 2021) NICE TA668 Recommended

Scottish Medicines Consortium (SMC) decisions
▶ Encorafenib (*Braftovi*®) in combination with binimetinib for the treatment of adult patients with unresectable or metastatic melanoma with a BRAF V600 mutation (February 2020) SMC No. SMC2238 Recommended
▶ Encorafenib (*Braftovi*®) in combination with cetuximab, for the treatment of adult patients with metastatic colorectal cancer with a BRAF V600E mutation, who have received prior systemic therapy (May 2021) SMC No. SMC2312 Recommended

● **MEDICINAL FORMS** There can be variation in the licensing of different medicines containing the same drug.
Oral capsule
CAUTIONARY AND ADVISORY LABELS 25
▶ Braftovi (Pierre Fabre Ltd)
Encorafenib 50 mg Braftovi 50mg capsules | 28 capsule [PoM]
£622.22 (Hospital only)
Encorafenib 75 mg Braftovi 75mg capsules | 42 capsule [PoM]
£1,400.00 (Hospital only)

Entrectinib [Specialist drug]
22-Mar-2023

● **INDICATIONS AND DOSE**

Solid tumours | Non-small cell lung cancer
▶ BY MOUTH
▶ Adult: Specialist drug – access specialist resources for dosing information

> **IMPORTANT SAFETY INFORMATION**
> RISKS OF INCORRECT DOSING OF ORAL ANTI-CANCER MEDICINES
> See Cytotoxic drugs p. 1027.

● **CONTRA-INDICATIONS** Congenital long QT syndrome
● **INTERACTIONS** → Appendix 1: entrectinib
● **SIDE-EFFECTS**
▶ **Common or very common** Abdominal pain · anaemia · anxiety · appetite decreased · arthralgia · asthenia · bone fractures · cognitive disorder · concentration impaired · confusion · constipation · cough · delirium · depression · diarrhoea · dizziness · drowsiness · dysphagia · dyspnoea · fever · fluid imbalance · gait abnormal · hallucinations · headache · heart failure · hyperuricaemia · hypotension · increased risk of infection · memory impairment · mood altered · movement disorders · muscle weakness · myalgia · nausea · neutropenia · oedema · pain · peripheral neuropathy · peripheral swelling · photosensitivity reaction · pleural effusion · psychiatric disorders · pulmonary oedema · QT interval prolongation · sensation abnormal · skin reactions · sleep disorders · syncope · taste altered · urinary disorders · vertigo · vision disorders · vomiting · weight increased
▶ **Uncommon** Tumour lysis syndrome

● **CONCEPTION AND CONTRACEPTION** Manufacturer advises females of childbearing potential should use effective contraception during treatment and for 5 weeks after last treatment; male patients should use effective contraception during treatment and for 3 months after last treatment if their partner is of childbearing potential. Additional barrier method recommended in females using hormonal contraceptives.

● **PATIENT AND CARER ADVICE**
Missed doses Manufacturer advises if a dose is more than 12 hours late, the missed dose should not be taken and the next dose should be taken at the normal time. If vomiting occurs immediately after a dose is taken, patients may repeat the dose.
Driving and skilled tasks Manufacturer advises patients and carers should be counselled on the effects on driving and performance of skilled tasks—increased risk of cognitive disorders, syncope, blurred vision, or dizziness.

● **NATIONAL FUNDING/ACCESS DECISIONS**
For full details see funding body website
NICE decisions
▶ Entrectinib for treating ROS1-positive advanced non-small-cell lung cancer (August 2020) NICE TA643 Recommended
▶ Entrectinib for treating NTRK fusion-positive solid tumours (August 2020) NICE TA644 Recommended

Scottish Medicines Consortium (SMC) decisions
▶ Entrectinib (*Rozlytrek*®) for the treatment of adult patients with ROS1-positive, advanced non-small cell lung cancer (NSCLC) not previously treated with ROS-1 inhibitors (January 2021) SMC No. SMC2294 Recommended
▶ Entrectinib (*Rozlytrek*®) for the treatment of adult and paediatric patients 12 years of age and older, with solid tumours that have a neurotrophic tyrosine receptor kinase (NTRK) gene fusion (March 2021) SMC No. SMC2295 Recommended

- **MEDICINAL FORMS** There can be variation in the licensing of different medicines containing the same drug.
Oral capsule
CAUTIONARY AND ADVISORY LABELS 25
  ▸ Rozlytrek (Roche Products Ltd) ▼
    Entrectinib 100 mg Rozlytrek 100mg capsules | 30 capsule [PoM] £860.00 (Hospital only)
    Entrectinib 200 mg Rozlytrek 200mg capsules | 90 capsule [PoM] £5,160.00 (Hospital only)

Erdafitinib [Specialist drug]
21-Jan-2025

- **INDICATIONS AND DOSE**
Urothelial carcinoma
  ▸ BY MOUTH
  ▸ Adult: Specialist drug – access specialist resources for dosing information

> **IMPORTANT SAFETY INFORMATION**
> RISKS OF INCORRECT DOSING OF ORAL ANTI-CANCER MEDICINES
> See Cytotoxic drugs p. 1027.

- **INTERACTIONS** → Appendix 1: erdafitinib
- **SIDE-EFFECTS**
  ▸ **Common or very common** Alopecia · anaemia · appetite decreased · asthenia · constipation · diarrhoea · dry eye · dry mouth · electrolyte imbalance · epistaxis · eye disorders · eye inflammation · gastrointestinal discomfort · hepatic disorders · hyperbilirubinaemia · hyperparathyroidism · nail discolouration · nail disorders · nasal dryness · nausea · oral disorders · paronychia · renal impairment · retinopathy · skin reactions · taste altered · vision disorders · vomiting · weight decreased
  ▸ **Uncommon** Mucosal dryness · vascular calcification
  ▸ **Frequency not known** Gastrointestinal disorder
- **CONCEPTION AND CONTRACEPTION** [EvGr] Females of childbearing potential should use highly effective contraception during treatment and for 1 month after last treatment; an additional barrier method of contraception or an alternative non-hormonal method of contraception (e.g. intra-uterine device), should be used in females using hormonal contraceptives. Male patients should use effective contraception during treatment and for 1 month after last treatment. ⓜ
- **PATIENT AND CARER ADVICE** Patients and carers should be counselled on preventative treatment and care for dry eye symptoms, nail disorders, and skin disorders. Patients and carers should be counselled to seek medical attention if signs and symptoms of dry mouth or stomatitis worsen.
  Photosensitivity Patients should be advised to wear protective clothing and apply sunscreen before sun exposure, due to the potential risk of photosensitivity reactions.
  Vomiting If vomiting occurs after taking erdafitinib, no additional dose should be taken on that day and the next dose should be taken at the usual time.
  Driving and skilled tasks Patients and carers should be counselled on the effects on driving and performance of skilled tasks—increased risk of eye disorders such as central serous retinopathy or keratitis.

- **MEDICINAL FORMS** There can be variation in the licensing of different medicines containing the same drug.
Oral tablet
CAUTIONARY AND ADVISORY LABELS 25
  ▸ Balversa (Janssen-Cilag Ltd) ▼
    Erdafitinib 3 mg Balversa 3mg tablets | 56 tablet [PoM] £12,750.00 (Hospital only) | 84 tablet [PoM] £12,750.00 (Hospital only)
    Erdafitinib 4 mg Balversa 4mg tablets | 28 tablet [PoM] £12,750.00 (Hospital only) | 56 tablet [PoM] £12,750.00 (Hospital only)
    Erdafitinib 5 mg Balversa 5mg tablets | 28 tablet [PoM] £12,750.00 (Hospital only)

Erlotinib [Specialist drug]
18-May-2021

- **INDICATIONS AND DOSE**
Non-small cell lung cancer | Pancreatic cancer
  ▸ BY MOUTH
  ▸ Adult: Specialist drug – access specialist resources for dosing information

> **IMPORTANT SAFETY INFORMATION**
> MHRA/CHM ADVICE: EPIDERMAL GROWTH FACTOR RECEPTOR (EGFR) INHIBITORS: SERIOUS CASES OF KERATITIS AND ULCERATIVE KERATITIS (MAY 2012)
> Keratitis and ulcerative keratitis have been reported following treatment with epidermal growth factor receptor (EGFR) inhibitors for cancer (cetuximab, erlotinib, gefitinib and panitumumab). In rare cases, this has resulted in corneal perforation and blindness. Patients undergoing treatment with EGFR inhibitors who present with acute or worsening signs and symptoms suggestive of keratitis should be referred promptly to an ophthalmology specialist. Treatment should be interrupted or discontinued if ulcerative keratitis is diagnosed.
>
> RISKS OF INCORRECT DOSING OF ORAL ANTI-CANCER MEDICINES
> See Cytotoxic drugs p. 1027.

- **INTERACTIONS** → Appendix 1: erlotinib
- **SIDE-EFFECTS**
  ▸ **Common or very common** Alopecia · diarrhoea · eye inflammation · haemorrhage · increased risk of infection · renal failure · skin reactions
  ▸ **Uncommon** Brittle nails · eye disorders · gastrointestinal disorders · hair changes · interstitial lung disease · nephritis · proteinuria
  ▸ **Rare or very rare** Hepatic failure · severe cutaneous adverse reactions (SCARs)
  ▸ **Frequency not known** Appetite decreased · chills · cough · depression · dyspnoea · fatigue · fever · gastrointestinal discomfort · headache · nausea · neuropathy sensory · stomatitis · vomiting · weight decreased
- **CONCEPTION AND CONTRACEPTION** Effective contraception required during and for at least 2 weeks after treatment.
- **NATIONAL FUNDING/ACCESS DECISIONS**
  For full details see funding body website
  NICE decisions
  ▸ **Erlotinib monotherapy for maintenance treatment of non-small-cell lung cancer (June 2011)** NICE TA227 Not recommended
  ▸ **Erlotinib for the first-line treatment of locally advanced or metastatic EGFR-TK mutation-positive non-small-cell lung cancer (June 2012)** NICE TA258 Recommended with restrictions
  ▸ **Erlotinib and gefitinib for treating non-small-cell lung cancer that has progressed after prior chemotherapy [in patients with tumours that are EGFR-TK mutation-negative] (December 2015)** NICE TA374 Not recommended
  ▸ **Erlotinib and gefitinib for treating non-small-cell lung cancer that has progressed after prior chemotherapy [in patients with tumours of unknown EGFR-TK mutation status] (December 2015)** NICE TA374 Recommended with restrictions

- **MEDICINAL FORMS** There can be variation in the licensing of different medicines containing the same drug.
Oral tablet
CAUTIONARY AND ADVISORY LABELS 23
  ▸ Erlotinib (Non-proprietary)
    Erlotinib (as Erlotinib hydrochloride) 25 mg Erlotinib 25mg tablets | 30 tablet [PoM] £200.00 | 30 tablet [PoM] £88.40–£139.00 (Hospital only)

Erlotinib (as Erlotinib hydrochloride) 100 mg Erlotinib 100mg tablets | 30 tablet [PoM] £704.00-£800.00 | 30 tablet [PoM] £378.33-£704.00 (Hospital only)

Erlotinib (as Erlotinib hydrochloride) 150 mg Erlotinib 150mg tablets | 30 tablet [PoM] £900.00 | 30 tablet [PoM] £163.15-£815.00 (Hospital only)

▸ **Tarceva** (Neon Healthcare Ltd)
Erlotinib (as Erlotinib hydrochloride) 25 mg Tarceva 25mg tablets | 30 tablet [PoM] £378.33

Erlotinib (as Erlotinib hydrochloride) 100 mg Tarceva 100mg tablets | 30 tablet [PoM] £1,324.14

Erlotinib (as Erlotinib hydrochloride) 150 mg Tarceva 150mg tablets | 30 tablet [PoM] £1,631.53

Everolimus

19-Dec-2022

● **DRUG ACTION** Everolimus is a protein kinase inhibitor.

● **INDICATIONS AND DOSE**

Neuroendocrine tumours of pancreatic origin (specialist use only) | Neuroendocrine tumours of gastro-intestinal origin (specialist use only)
▸ BY MOUTH
▸ Adult: Specialist indication – access specialist resources for dosing information

AFINITOR ®

Neuroendocrine tumours of pancreatic origin (specialist use only) | Neuroendocrine tumours of lung origin (specialist use only) | Neuroendocrine tumours of gastro-intestinal origin (specialist use only) | Renal cell carcinoma (specialist use only) | Breast cancer (specialist use only)
▸ BY MOUTH
▸ Adult: Specialist indication – access specialist resources for dosing information

CERTICAN ®

Liver transplantation (under expert supervision)
▸ BY MOUTH
▸ Adult: Initially 1 mg twice daily, to be started approximately 4 weeks after transplantation; maintenance, dose adjusted according to response and whole blood everolimus concentration; dose adjustments can be made every 4–5 days

Renal transplantation (under expert supervision) | Heart transplantation (under expert supervision)
▸ BY MOUTH
▸ Adult: Initially 750 micrograms twice daily, to be started as soon as possible after transplantation; maintenance, dose adjusted according to response and whole blood everolimus concentration; dose adjustments can be made every 4–5 days

VOTUBIA ® **DISPERSIBLE TABLETS**

Subependymal giant cell astrocytoma associated with tuberous sclerosis complex (initiated by a specialist)
▸ BY MOUTH USING DISPERSIBLE TABLETS
▸ Adult: (consult product literature)

Adjunctive treatment of refractory partial-onset seizures, with or without secondary generalisation, associated with tuberous sclerosis complex (initiated by a specialist)
▸ BY MOUTH USING DISPERSIBLE TABLETS
▸ Adult: (consult product literature)

VOTUBIA ® **TABLETS**

Subependymal giant cell astrocytoma associated with tuberous sclerosis complex (initiated by a specialist)
▸ BY MOUTH USING TABLETS
▸ Adult: (consult product literature)

Renal angiomyolipoma associated with tuberous sclerosis complex (initiated by a specialist)
▸ BY MOUTH USING TABLETS
▸ Adult: (consult product literature)

> **IMPORTANT SAFETY INFORMATION**
>
> RISKS OF INCORRECT DOSING OF ORAL ANTI-CANCER MEDICINES
> See Cytotoxic drugs p. 1027.
>
> MHRA/CHM ADVICE: ANTIEPILEPTICS: RISK OF SUICIDAL THOUGHTS AND BEHAVIOUR (AUGUST 2008)
> See Epilepsy p. 349.
>
> MHRA/CHM ADVICE: ANTIEPILEPTIC DRUGS: UPDATED ADVICE ON SWITCHING BETWEEN DIFFERENT MANUFACTURERS' PRODUCTS (NOVEMBER 2017)
> See Epilepsy p. 349 and see also *Prescribing and dispensing information*.
>
> MHRA/CHM ADVICE: ANTIEPILEPTIC DRUGS IN PREGNANCY: UPDATED ADVICE FOLLOWING COMPREHENSIVE SAFETY REVIEW (JANUARY 2021)
> See Epilepsy p. 349.

● **CAUTIONS** History of bleeding disorders · peri-surgical period (impaired wound healing)

● **INTERACTIONS** → Appendix 1: everolimus

● **SIDE-EFFECTS**
▸ **Common or very common** Alopecia · anaemia · appetite decreased · arthralgia · asthenia · cough · decreased leucocytes · dehydration · diabetes mellitus · diarrhoea · dry mouth · dyslipidaemia · dysphagia · dyspnoea · electrolyte imbalance · eye inflammation · fever · gastrointestinal discomfort · haemorrhage · headache · hyperglycaemia · hypertension · increased risk of infection · insomnia · interstitial lung disease · menstrual cycle irregularities · mucositis · nail disorders · nausea · neutropenia · oral disorders · peripheral oedema · proteinuria · renal impairment · respiratory disorders · skin reactions · taste altered · thrombocytopenia · vomiting · weight decreased
▸ **Uncommon** Congestive heart failure · embolism and thrombosis · flushing · healing impaired · hepatitis B · musculoskeletal chest pain · pancytopenia · rhabdomyolysis · sepsis · urinary frequency increased
▸ **Rare or very rare** Pure red cell aplasia
▸ **Frequency not known** Hepatitis B reactivation · suicidal behaviours

SIDE-EFFECTS, FURTHER INFORMATION Reduce dose or discontinue if severe side-effects occur—consult product literature.

● **CONCEPTION AND CONTRACEPTION** Effective contraception must be used during and for up to 8 weeks after treatment. See also *Pregnancy and reproductive function* in Cytotoxic drugs p. 1027.

● **PREGNANCY** Manufacturer advises avoid (toxicity in *animal* studies). See also *Pregnancy and reproductive function* in Cytotoxic drugs p. 1027. See also *Pregnancy* in Epilepsy p. 349.

● **BREAST FEEDING** Manufacturer advises avoid.

● **HEPATIC IMPAIRMENT** Consult product literature.

● **MONITORING REQUIREMENTS**
▸ For *Votubia* ® preparations: manufacturer advises everolimus blood concentration monitoring is required—consult product literature.
▸ For *Certican* ®: manufacturer advises pre-dose ('trough') whole blood everolimus concentration should be 3–8 nanograms/mL; monitoring should be performed every 4–5 days (using **chromatographic** assay) after initiation or dose adjustment until 2 consecutive stable concentrations; monitor patients with hepatic impairment taking concomitant strong CYP3A4 inducers and

inhibitors when switching formulation, and/or if concomitant ciclosporin dose is reduced.

▶ Manufacturer advises monitor blood-glucose concentration, complete blood count, serum-triglycerides and serum-cholesterol before treatment and periodically thereafter.

▶ Manufacturer advises monitor renal function before treatment and periodically thereafter.

▶ Manufacturer advises monitor for signs and symptoms of infection before and during treatment.

● DIRECTIONS FOR ADMINISTRATION

VOTUBIA ® DISPERSIBLE TABLETS Manufacturer advises tablets must be dispersed in water before administration— consult product literature for details.

VOTUBIA ® TABLETS Manufacturer advises tablets may be dispersed in approximately 30 mL of water by gently stirring, immediately before drinking. After solution has been swallowed, any residue must be re-dispersed in the same volume of water and swallowed.

● PRESCRIBING AND DISPENSING INFORMATION *Votubia*® is available as both *tablets* and *dispersible tablets*. These formulations vary in their licensed indications and are not interchangeable—consult product literature for information on switching between formulations.

● PATIENT AND CARER ADVICE

Pneumonitis Non-infectious pneumonitis reported. Manufacturer advises patients and their carers should be informed to seek urgent medical advice if new or worsening respiratory symptoms occur.

Infections Manufacturer advises patients and their carers should be informed of the risk of infection.

● NATIONAL FUNDING/ACCESS DECISIONS

For full details see funding body website

NICE decisions

▶ **Everolimus with exemestane for treating advanced breast cancer after endocrine therapy (December 2016)** NICE TA421 Recommended with restrictions

▶ **Everolimus for advanced renal cell carcinoma after previous treatment (February 2017)** NICE TA432 Recommended with restrictions

▶ **Everolimus and sunitinib for treating unresectable or metastatic neuroendocrine tumours in people with progressive disease (June 2017)** NICE TA449 Recommended with restrictions

Scottish Medicines Consortium (SMC) decisions

▶ Everolimus dispersible tablets (*Votubia*®) for the adjunctive treatment of patients aged 2 years and older whose refractory partial-onset seizures, with or without secondary generalisation, are associated with tuberous sclerosis complex (June 2018) SMC No. 1331/18 Recommended

All Wales Medicines Strategy Group (AWMSG) decisions

▶ Everolimus dispersible tablets (*Votubia*®) for the adjunctive treatment of patients aged 2 years and older whose refractory partial-onset seizures, with or without secondary generalisation, are associated with tuberous sclerosis complex (TSC) (September 2021) AWMSG No. 2142 Recommended

▶ Everolimus tablets and dispersible tablets (*Votubia*®) for the treatment of adult and paediatric patients with subependymal giant cell astrocytoma (SEGA) associated with tuberous sclerosis complex (TSC) who require therapeutic intervention but are not amenable to surgery (December 2022) AWMSG No. 1156 Recommended

▶ Everolimus tablets (*Votubia*®) for the treatment of adult patients with renal angiomyolipoma associated with tuberous sclerosis complex (TSC) who are at risk of complications (based on factors such as tumour size or presence of aneurysm, or presence of multiple or bilateral tumours) but who do not require immediate surgery (December 2022) AWMSG No. 1156 Recommended

AFINITOR ® For full details see funding body website

NICE decisions

▶ **Lenvatinib with everolimus for previously treated advanced renal cell carcinoma (January 2018)** NICE TA498 Recommended with restrictions

CERTICAN ® For full details see funding body website

NICE decisions

▶ **Everolimus for preventing organ rejection in liver transplantation (July 2015)** NICE TA348 Not recommended

▶ **Immunosuppressive therapy for kidney transplant in adults (October 2017)** NICE TA481 Not recommended

● MEDICINAL FORMS There can be variation in the licensing of different medicines containing the same drug.

Dispersible tablet

CAUTIONARY AND ADVISORY LABELS 13

▶ Votubia (Novartis Pharmaceuticals UK Ltd)

Everolimus 2 mg Votubia 2mg dispersible tablets | 30 tablet PoM £960.00 SF

Everolimus 3 mg Votubia 3mg dispersible tablets | 30 tablet PoM £1,440.00 SF

Everolimus 5 mg Votubia 5mg dispersible tablets | 30 tablet PoM £2,250.00 SF

Oral tablet

CAUTIONARY AND ADVISORY LABELS 25

▶ Everolimus (Non-proprietary)

Everolimus 2.5 mg Everolimus 2.5mg tablets | 30 tablet PoM £1,020.00-£1,200.00 | 30 tablet PoM £1,080.00-£1,200.00 (Hospital only)

Everolimus 5 mg Everolimus 5mg tablets | 30 tablet PoM £2,250.00 | 30 tablet PoM £1,912.50-£2,250.00 (Hospital only)

Everolimus 10 mg Everolimus 10mg tablets | 30 tablet PoM £2,272.05-£2,673.00 | 30 tablet PoM £2,405.70-£2,673.00 (Hospital only)

▶ Afinitor (Novartis Pharmaceuticals UK Ltd)

Everolimus 2.5 mg Afinitor 2.5mg tablets | 30 tablet PoM £1,200.00

Everolimus 5 mg Afinitor 5mg tablets | 30 tablet PoM £2,250.00

Everolimus 10 mg Afinitor 10mg tablets | 30 tablet PoM £2,673.00

▶ Certican (Novartis Pharmaceuticals UK Ltd)

Everolimus 250 microgram Certican 0.25mg tablets | 60 tablet PoM £148.50

Everolimus 750 microgram Certican 0.75mg tablets | 60 tablet PoM £445.50

▶ Votubia (Novartis Pharmaceuticals UK Ltd)

Everolimus 2.5 mg Votubia 2.5mg tablets | 30 tablet PoM £1,200.00

Everolimus 5 mg Votubia 5mg tablets | 30 tablet PoM £2,250.00

Everolimus 10 mg Votubia 10mg tablets | 30 tablet PoM £2,970.00

Fedratinib [Specialist drug]

26-Nov-2024

● INDICATIONS AND DOSE

Disease-related splenomegaly or symptoms [in patients with primary myelofibrosis, post-polycythaemia vera myelofibrosis, or post-essential thrombocythaemia myelofibrosis]

▶ BY MOUTH

▶ Adult: Specialist drug – access specialist resources for dosing information

> **IMPORTANT SAFETY INFORMATION**
> RISKS OF INCORRECT DOSING OF ORAL ANTI-CANCER MEDICINES
> See Cytotoxic drugs p. 1027.

● CONTRA-INDICATIONS Absolute neutrophil count less than 1×10^9 cells/litre (do not initiate) · platelet count less than 50×10^9/litre (do not initiate) · thiamine deficiency

● INTERACTIONS → Appendix 1: fedratinib

● SIDE-EFFECTS

▶ Common or very common Anaemia · asthenia · constipation · diarrhoea · dizziness · dyspepsia · dysuria · haemorrhage · headache · hypertension · muscle spasms · nausea ·

neutropenia · pain · thrombocytopenia · urinary tract infection · vomiting · weight increased · Wernicke's encephalopathy
► **Frequency not known** Hepatic failure · pancreatitis
SIDE-EFFECTS, FURTHER INFORMATION Nausea is very common, often occurring within 2 days of starting treatment. Nausea can be managed by prescribing concurrent antiemetics (consult product literature), and/or taking doses with a high fat meal.
● **CONCEPTION AND CONTRACEPTION** [EvGr] Females of childbearing potential should use effective contraception during treatment and for at least 1 month after last treatment. ⟨M⟩
● **PATIENT AND CARER ADVICE**
Driving and skilled tasks Patients and carers should be counselled on the effects on driving and performance of skilled tasks—increased risk of dizziness.
● **NATIONAL FUNDING/ACCESS DECISIONS**
For full details see funding body website
NICE decisions
► Fedratinib for treating disease-related splenomegaly or symptoms in myelofibrosis (November 2024) NICE TA1018 Recommended with restrictions
Scottish Medicines Consortium (SMC) decisions
► Fedratinib (*Inrebic*®) for the treatment of disease-related splenomegaly or symptoms in adult patients with primary myelofibrosis, post-polycythaemia vera myelofibrosis or post-essential thrombocythaemia myelofibrosis who are Janus-associated kinase inhibitor-naive or who have been treated with ruxolitinib (April 2022) SMC No. SMC2462 Recommended

● **MEDICINAL FORMS** There can be variation in the licensing of different medicines containing the same drug.
Oral capsule
CAUTIONARY AND ADVISORY LABELS 25
► **Inrebic** (Bristol-Myers Squibb Pharmaceuticals Ltd) ▼
Fedratinib (as Fedratinib dihydrochloride monohydrate)
100 mg Inrebic 100mg capsules | 120 capsule [PoM] £6,119.68 (Hospital only)

Fruquintinib [Specialist drug]
12-Mar-2025

● **INDICATIONS AND DOSE**
Colorectal cancer
► BY MOUTH
► Adult: Specialist drug – access specialist resources for dosing information

---

IMPORTANT SAFETY INFORMATION
MHRA/CHM ADVICE: SYSTEMICALLY ADMINISTERED VEGF PATHWAY INHIBITORS: RISK OF ANEURYSM AND ARTERY DISSECTION (JULY 2020)
A European review of worldwide data concluded that systemically administered VEGF pathway inhibitors may lead to aneurysm and artery dissection in patients with or without hypertension. Some fatal cases have been reported, mainly in relation to aortic aneurysm rupture and aortic dissection. The MHRA advises healthcare professionals to carefully consider the risk of aneurysm and artery dissection in patients with risk factors before initiating treatment; any modifiable risk factors (such as smoking and hypertension) should be reduced as much as possible. Blood pressure should be monitored regularly, and product literature should be consulted if hypertension occurs during treatment.

RISKS OF INCORRECT DOSING OF ORAL ANTI-CANCER MEDICINES
See Cytotoxic drugs p. 1027.

● **CONTRA-INDICATIONS** Thromboembolic events

CONTRA-INDICATIONS, FURTHER INFORMATION
[EvGr] Avoid starting treatment in patients with a history of deep vein thrombosis or pulmonary embolism in the last 6 months, or a history of stroke or transient ischaemic attack in the last 12 months. Immediately discontinue treatment if arterial thrombosis is suspected. ⟨M⟩
● **INTERACTIONS** → Appendix 1: fruquintinib
● **SIDE-EFFECTS**
► **Common or very common** Anastomotic haemorrhage · aphonia · appetite decreased · arthralgia · asthenia · diarrhoea · dysphonia · gastrointestinal disorders · haemorrhage · hepatic disorders · hyperamylasaemia · hyperbilirubinaemia · hyperlipasaemia · hypertension · hypokalaemia · hypothyroidism · increased risk of infection · leucopenia · mucositis · muscle spasms · musculoskeletal discomfort · neutropenia · oral disorders · oropharyngeal complaints · pain · skin reactions · throat complaints · thrombocytopenia · urine abnormalities · weight decreased
► **Uncommon** Pancreatitis · posterior reversible encephalopathy syndrome (PRES)
► **Frequency not known** Healing impaired
● **CONCEPTION AND CONTRACEPTION** [EvGr] Females of childbearing potential and male patients with female partners of childbearing potential should use effective contraception during treatment and for at least 2 weeks after last treatment. ⟨M⟩
● **PATIENT AND CARER ADVICE**
Vomiting If vomiting occurs after taking a dose, no additional dose should be taken on that day and the next dose should be taken at the usual time.
Missed doses If a dose is more than 12 hours late, the missed dose should not be taken and the next dose should be taken at the normal time.
Driving and skilled tasks Patients and carers should be cautioned on the effects on driving and performance of skilled tasks—increased risk of fatigue.

● **MEDICINAL FORMS** There can be variation in the licensing of different medicines containing the same drug.
Oral capsule
CAUTIONARY AND ADVISORY LABELS 25
EXCIPIENTS: May contain Tartrazine
► **Fruzaqla** (Takeda UK Ltd) ▼
Fruquintinib 1 mg Fruzaqla 1mg capsules | 21 capsule [PoM] £790.00 (Hospital only)
Fruquintinib 5 mg Fruzaqla 5mg capsules | 21 capsule [PoM] £3,950.00 (Hospital only)

Gefitinib [Specialist drug]
19-Jul-2021

● **INDICATIONS AND DOSE**
Non-small cell lung cancer
► BY MOUTH
► Adult: Specialist drug – access specialist resources for dosing information

---

IMPORTANT SAFETY INFORMATION
MHRA/CHM ADVICE: EPIDERMAL GROWTH FACTOR RECEPTOR (EGFR) INHIBITORS: SERIOUS CASES OF KERATITIS AND ULCERATIVE KERATITIS (MAY 2012)
Keratitis and ulcerative keratitis have been reported following treatment with epidermal growth factor receptor (EGFR) inhibitors for cancer (cetuximab, erlotinib, gefitinib and panitumumab). In rare cases, this has resulted in corneal perforation and blindness. Patients undergoing treatment with EGFR inhibitors who present with acute or worsening signs and symptoms suggestive of keratitis should be referred promptly to an ophthalmology specialist. Treatment

should be interrupted or discontinued if ulcerative keratitis is diagnosed.

RISKS OF INCORRECT DOSING OF ORAL ANTI-CANCER MEDICINES
See Cytotoxic drugs p. 1027.

● INTERACTIONS → Appendix 1: gefitinib
● SIDE-EFFECTS
▸ **Common or very common** Alopecia · angioedema · appetite decreased · asthenia · cystitis · dehydration · diarrhoea · dry eye · dry mouth · eye inflammation · fever · haemorrhage · hypersensitivity · interstitial lung disease (discontinue) · nail disorder · nausea · proteinuria · rash pustular · skin reactions · stomatitis · vomiting
▸ **Uncommon** Corneal erosion · gastrointestinal perforation · hepatic disorders · pancreatitis
▸ **Rare or very rare** Cutaneous vasculitis · severe cutaneous adverse reactions (SCARs)
● CONCEPTION AND CONTRACEPTION Contraceptive advice required.
● NATIONAL FUNDING/ACCESS DECISIONS
For full details see funding body website
NICE decisions
▸ Gefitinib for the first-line treatment of locally advanced or metastatic non-small-cell lung cancer (July 2010) NICE TA192 Recommended with restrictions
▸ Erlotinib and gefitinib for treating non-small-cell lung cancer that has progressed after prior chemotherapy (December 2015) NICE TA374 Not recommended
Scottish Medicines Consortium (SMC) decisions
▸ Gefitinib (*Iressa*®) for the treatment of adult patients with locally advanced or metastatic non-small cell lung cancer with activating mutations of epidermal growth factor receptor tyrosine kinase (December 2015) SMC No. 615/10 Recommended with restrictions

● MEDICINAL FORMS There can be variation in the licensing of different medicines containing the same drug.
Oral tablet
▸ Gefitinib (Non-proprietary)
Gefitinib 250 mg Gefitinib 250mg tablets | 30 tablet PoM £2,166.10–£2,167.71
▸ Iressa (AstraZeneca UK Ltd)
Gefitinib 250 mg Iressa 250mg tablets | 30 tablet PoM £2,167.71

Gilteritinib [Specialist drug]

22-Mar-2023

● INDICATIONS AND DOSE
Acute myeloid leukaemia
▸ BY MOUTH
▸ Adult: Specialist drug – access specialist resources for dosing information

IMPORTANT SAFETY INFORMATION
RISKS OF INCORRECT DOSING OF ORAL ANTI-CANCER MEDICINES
See Cytotoxic drugs p. 1027.

● INTERACTIONS → Appendix 1: gilteritinib
● SIDE-EFFECTS
▸ **Common or very common** Acute kidney injury · anaphylactic reaction · arthralgia · asthenia · constipation · cough · diarrhoea · differentiation syndrome · dizziness · dyspnoea · heart failure · hypotension · malaise · myalgia · nausea · pain · pericardial effusion · pericarditis · peripheral oedema · QT interval prolongation
▸ **Uncommon** Posterior reversible encephalopathy syndrome (PRES)
▸ **Frequency not known** Pancreatitis
● CONCEPTION AND CONTRACEPTION Manufacturer advises perform pregnancy test in females of childbearing potential within 7 days prior to treatment initiation;

effective contraception should be used during treatment and for at least 6 months after last treatment—additional barrier method recommended in those using hormonal contraceptives. Male patients should use effective contraception during treatment and for at least 4 months after last treatment if their partner is of childbearing potential.

● PATIENT AND CARER ADVICE
Vomiting Manufacturer advises if vomiting occurs after taking tablets, no additional dose should be taken on that day and the next dose should be taken at the usual time.
A patient alert card should be provided.
Missed doses Manufacturer advises if a dose is missed or not taken at the usual time, the missed dose should be taken as soon as possible on the same day. The next dose should be taken at the usual time.
Driving and skilled tasks Manufacturer advises patients and their carers should be counselled on the effects on driving and performance of skilled tasks—increased risk of dizziness.

● NATIONAL FUNDING/ACCESS DECISIONS
For full details see funding body website
NICE decisions
▸ Gilteritinib for treating relapsed or refractory acute myeloid leukaemia (August 2020) NICE TA642 Recommended
Scottish Medicines Consortium (SMC) decisions
▸ Gilteritinib (*Xospata*®) as monotherapy for the treatment of adult patients who have relapsed or refractory acute myeloid leukaemia with a FLT3 mutation (September 2020) SMC No. SMC2252 Recommended

● MEDICINAL FORMS There can be variation in the licensing of different medicines containing the same drug.
Oral tablet
CAUTIONARY AND ADVISORY LABELS 25
▸ Xospata (Astellas Pharma Ltd)
Gilteritinib (as Gilteritinib fumarate) 40 mg Xospata 40mg tablets | 84 tablet PoM £14,188.00 (Hospital only)

Ibrutinib [Specialist drug]

18-Sep-2023

● INDICATIONS AND DOSE
Mantle cell lymphoma | Chronic lymphocytic leukaemia | Waldenström's macroglobulinaemia
▸ BY MOUTH
▸ Adult: Specialist drug – access specialist resources for dosing information

IMPORTANT SAFETY INFORMATION
RISKS OF INCORRECT DOSING OF ORAL ANTI-CANCER MEDICINES
See Cytotoxic drugs p. 1027.

MHRA/CHM ADVICE: IBRUTINIB (*IMBRUVICA*®): REPORTS OF VENTRICULAR TACHYARRHYTHMIA; RISK OF HEPATITIS B REACTIVATION AND OF OPPORTUNISTIC INFECTIONS (AUGUST 2017)
Cases of ventricular tachyarrhythmia have been reported with the use of ibrutinib. The MHRA advises that ibrutinib should be temporarily discontinued in patients who develop symptoms suggestive of ventricular arrhythmia and to assess benefit-risk before restarting therapy.
Hepatitis B virus status should be established before initiating therapy—for patients with positive hepatitis B serology, consultation with a liver disease expert is recommended before the start of treatment; monitor and manage patients according to local protocols to minimise the risk of hepatitis B virus reactivation. Prophylaxis should be considered for those at an increased risk of opportunistic infections.

MHRA/CHM ADVICE: *IMBRUVICA*® (IBRUTINIB): NEW RISK MINIMISATION MEASURES, INCLUDING DOSE MODIFICATION RECOMMENDATIONS, DUE TO THE INCREASED RISK FOR SERIOUS CARDIAC EVENTS (NOVEMBER 2022)

An assessment of available clinical trial data found that ibrutinib therapy increased the risk of fatal and serious cardiac arrhythmias and cardiac failure. Patients with advanced age, Eastern Cooperative Oncology Group (ECOG) performance status ≥ 2, or cardiac co-morbidities may be at greater risk of such events, including sudden fatal cardiac events.

Healthcare professionals are advised to:
- evaluate a patient's cardiac history and function before starting therapy—benefit-risk should be assessed in those with risk factors for cardiac events and alternative treatment may be considered;
- carefully monitor patients during therapy for signs of cardiac function deterioration—further evaluation should be considered where there are cardiovascular concerns;
- discontinue therapy in patients with grade 3 or 4 cardiac failure, or grade 4 cardiac arrhythmias;
- withhold therapy in patients with any new-onset or worsening grade 2 cardiac failure or grade 3 cardiac arrhythmias—treatment may be resumed, if appropriate, at a lower dose once symptoms have resolved to grade 1 or baseline.

- **INTERACTIONS** → Appendix 1: ibrutinib

- **SIDE-EFFECTS**
  - **Common or very common** Arrhythmias · arthralgia · broken nails · constipation · diarrhoea · dizziness · dyspepsia · fever · haemorrhage · headache · heart failure · hypertension · hyperuricaemia · increased leucocytes · increased risk of infection · interstitial lung disease · muscle spasms · musculoskeletal pain · nausea · neoplasms · neutropenia · peripheral neuropathy · peripheral oedema · sepsis · skin reactions · stomatitis · thrombocytopenia · vision blurred · vomiting
  - **Uncommon** Angioedema · cardiac arrest · cerebrovascular insufficiency · CNS haemorrhage · hepatic disorders · hepatitis B reactivation · panniculitis · tumour lysis syndrome
  - **Rare or very rare** Leukostasis syndrome (withhold treatment) · Stevens-Johnson syndrome
  - **Frequency not known** Anaemia · asthenia · haemophagocytic lymphohistiocytosis · progressive multifocal leukoencephalopathy (PML) · splenic rupture (on discontinuation)

- **CONCEPTION AND CONTRACEPTION** Highly effective contraception (must include a non-hormonal method) required during and for 3 months after stopping treatment.

- **NATIONAL FUNDING/ACCESS DECISIONS**
  For full details see funding body website

  NICE decisions
  - Ibrutinib for previously treated chronic lymphocytic leukaemia and untreated chronic lymphocytic leukaemia with 17p deletion or TP53 mutation (January 2017) NICE TA429 Recommended with restrictions
  - Ibrutinib with venetoclax for untreated chronic lymphocytic leukaemia (May 2023) NICE TA891 Recommended
  - Ibrutinib for treating relapsed or refractory mantle cell lymphoma (January 2018) NICE TA502 Recommended with restrictions
  - Ibrutinib for treating Waldenstrom's macroglobulinaemia (June 2022) NICE TA795 Not recommended

  Scottish Medicines Consortium (SMC) decisions
  - Ibrutinib (*Imbruvica*®) for the treatment of adult patients with chronic lymphocytic leukaemia who have received at least one prior therapy (April 2017) SMC No. 1151/16 Recommended with restrictions
  - Ibrutinib (*Imbruvica*®) in combination with venetoclax for the treatment of adult patients with previously untreated chronic lymphocytic leukaemia (September 2023) SMC No. SMC2543 Recommended
  - Ibrutinib (*Imbruvica*®) in combination with rituximab for the treatment of adult patients with Waldenström's macroglobulinaemia (October 2020) SMC No. SMC2259 Recommended with restrictions
  - Ibrutinib (*Imbruvica*®) as a single agent for the treatment of adult patients with Waldenström's macroglobulinaemia who have received at least one prior therapy, or in first line treatment for patients unsuitable for chemo-immunotherapy (December 2021) SMC No. SMC2387 Recommended with restrictions

- **MEDICINAL FORMS** There can be variation in the licensing of different medicines containing the same drug.

  Oral tablet
  CAUTIONARY AND ADVISORY LABELS 25
  - **Imbruvica** (Janssen-Cilag Ltd)
    Ibrutinib 140 mg Imbruvica 140mg tablets | 28 tablet PoM £1,430.80 (Hospital only)
    Ibrutinib 280 mg Imbruvica 280mg tablets | 28 tablet PoM £2,861.60 (Hospital only)
    Ibrutinib 420 mg Imbruvica 420mg tablets | 28 tablet PoM £4,292.40 (Hospital only)
    Ibrutinib 560 mg Imbruvica 560mg tablets | 28 tablet PoM £5,723.20 (Hospital only)

Idelalisib [Specialist drug]

16-Oct-2020

- **INDICATIONS AND DOSE**

  Chronic lymphocytic leukaemia | Follicular lymphoma
  - BY MOUTH
  - Adult: Specialist drug – access specialist resources for dosing information

IMPORTANT SAFETY INFORMATION

RISKS OF INCORRECT DOSING OF ORAL ANTI-CANCER MEDICINES
See Cytotoxic drugs p. 1027.

MHRA/CHM ADVICE: IDELALISIB (ZYDELIG®): UPDATED INDICATIONS AND ADVICE ON MINIMISING THE RISK OF INFECTION (SEPTEMBER 2016)
In light of a recent safety review the indications for idelalisib have been updated. Manufacturer recommendations regarding monitoring for infection and prophylaxis of *Pneumocystis jirovecii* pneumonia have also been updated. Patients should be advised on the risk of serious or fatal infections during treatment, and idelalisib should not be initiated in patients with any evidence of infection.

- **INTERACTIONS** → Appendix 1: idelalisib

- **SIDE-EFFECTS**
  - **Common or very common** Colitis · diarrhoea · fever · infection · interstitial lung disease · neutropenia · rash
  - **Rare or very rare** Severe cutaneous adverse reactions (SCARs)

  SIDE-EFFECTS, FURTHER INFORMATION Pneumonitis and organising pneumonia, including fatal events, have been reported. Treatment should be interrupted if suspected and discontinued if pneumonitis or organising pneumonia confirmed.

- **CONCEPTION AND CONTRACEPTION** Highly effective contraception (in addition to barrier method) required during and for one month after treatment.

- **NATIONAL FUNDING/ACCESS DECISIONS**
For full details see funding body website
NICE decisions
▶ **Idelalisib for treating chronic lymphocytic leukaemia (October 2015)** NICE TA359 Recommended
▶ **Idelalisib for treating refractory follicular lymphoma (October 2019)** NICE TA604 Not recommended
Scottish Medicines Consortium (SMC) decisions
▶ **Idelalisib (*Zydelig*®) in combination with rituximab for the treatment of adult patients with chronic lymphocytic leukaemia (CLL): who have received at least one prior therapy, or as first line treatment in the presence of 17p deletion or TP53 mutation in patients unsuitable for chemo-immunotherapy (March 2015)** SMC No. 1026/15 Recommended with restrictions
▶ **Idelalisib (*Zydelig*®) as monotherapy for the treatment of adult patients with follicular lymphoma (FL) that is refractory to two prior lines of treatment (May 2015)** SMC No. 1039/15 Recommended with restrictions

- **MEDICINAL FORMS** There can be variation in the licensing of different medicines containing the same drug.
Oral tablet
CAUTIONARY AND ADVISORY LABELS 25
▶ **Zydelig** (Gilead Sciences Ltd)
Idelalisib 100 mg Zydelig 100mg tablets | 60 tablet [PoM] £3,114.75 (Hospital only)
Idelalisib 150 mg Zydelig 150mg tablets | 60 tablet [PoM] £3,114.75 (Hospital only)

Imatinib [Specialist drug]

25-Aug-2021

- **INDICATIONS AND DOSE**
Chronic myeloid leukaemia | Acute lymphoblastic leukaemia | Gastro-intestinal stromal tumours | Myelodysplastic/myeloproliferative diseases | Dermatofibrosarcoma protuberans | Hypereosinophilic syndrome | Chronic eosinophilic leukaemia
▶ BY MOUTH
▶ **Adult:** Specialist drug – access specialist resources for dosing information

IMPORTANT SAFETY INFORMATION
RISKS OF INCORRECT DOSING OF ORAL ANTI-CANCER MEDICINES
See Cytotoxic drugs p. 1027.

MHRA/CHM ADVICE (MAY 2016): RISK OF HEPATITIS B VIRUS REACTIVATION WITH BCR-ABL TYROSINE KINASE INHIBITORS
An EU wide review has concluded that imatinib can cause hepatitis B reactivation; the MHRA recommends establishing hepatitis B virus status in all patients before initiation of treatment. Patients who are carriers of hepatitis B virus should be closely monitored for signs and symptoms of active infection throughout treatment and for several months after stopping treatment; expert advice should be sought for patients who test positive for hepatitis B virus and in those with active infection.

- **INTERACTIONS** → Appendix 1: imatinib
- **SIDE-EFFECTS**
▶ **Common or very common** Alopecia · anaemia · appetite abnormal · asthenia · bone marrow disorders · chills · constipation · cough · diarrhoea · dizziness · dry eye · dry mouth · dyspnoea · excessive tearing · eye inflammation · fever · fluid imbalance · flushing · gastrointestinal discomfort · gastrointestinal disorders · haemorrhage · headaches · insomnia · joint disorders · muscle complaints · nausea · neutropenia · oedema · pain · photosensitivity reaction · sensation abnormal · skin reactions · sweat changes · taste altered · thrombocytopenia · vision blurred · vomiting · weight changes

▶ **Uncommon** Anxiety · arrhythmias · ascites · breast abnormalities · broken nails · burping · chest pain · CNS haemorrhage · congestive heart failure · depression · drowsiness · dysphagia · electrolyte imbalance · eosinophilia · eye discomfort · gout · gynaecomastia · hearing loss · hepatic disorders · hyperbilirubinaemia · hyperglycaemia · hypertension · hyperuricaemia · hypotension · increased risk of infection · laryngeal pain · lymphadenopathy · lymphopenia · malaise · memory loss · menstrual cycle irregularities · nerve disorders · oral disorders · palpitations · pancreatitis · peripheral coldness · pulmonary oedema · Raynaud's phenomenon · renal impairment · renal pain · respiratory disorders · restless legs · scrotal oedema · sepsis · sexual dysfunction · syncope · thrombocytosis · tinnitus · tremor · urinary frequency increased · vertigo
▶ **Rare or very rare** Angina pectoris · angioedema · arthritis · cardiac arrest · cataract · confusion · glaucoma · haemolytic anaemia · haemorrhagic ovarian cyst · hepatic failure (including fatal cases) · hypersensitivity vasculitis · inflammatory bowel disease · intracranial pressure increased · muscle weakness · myocardial infarction · myopathy · nail discolouration · pericardial disorders · pulmonary fibrosis · pulmonary hypertension · seizure · severe cutaneous adverse reactions (SCARs) · thrombotic microangiopathy · tumour lysis syndrome
▶ **Frequency not known** Embolism and thrombosis · hepatitis B reactivation · interstitial lung disease · neoplasm complications · osteonecrosis · pericarditis

- **CONCEPTION AND CONTRACEPTION** [EvGr] Females of childbearing potential should use effective contraception during treatment and for at least 15 days after last treatment. ⟨M⟩
- **PATIENT AND CARER ADVICE** Patients or carers should be given advice on how to administer imatinib tablets.
- **NATIONAL FUNDING/ACCESS DECISIONS**
For full details see funding body website
NICE decisions
▶ **Imatinib for the adjuvant treatment of gastro-intestinal stromal tumours (November 2014)** NICE TA326 Recommended
▶ **Imatinib for chronic myeloid leukaemia (updated January 2016)** NICE TA70 Recommended
▶ **Imatinib for the treatment of unresectable and/or metastatic gastro-intestinal stromal tumours (updated November 2010)** NICE TA86 Recommended with restrictions
▶ **Imatinib for the treatment of unresectable and/or metastatic gastro-intestinal stromal tumours (November 2010)** NICE TA209 Not recommended
▶ **Dasatinib, nilotinib and imatinib for untreated chronic myeloid leukaemia (CML) (December 2016)** NICE TA426 Recommended
▶ **Dasatinib, nilotinib and high-dose imatinib for treating imatinib-resistant or intolerant chronic myeloid leukaemia (CML) (December 2016)** NICE TA425 Not recommended
Scottish Medicines Consortium (SMC) decisions
▶ **Imatinib (*Glivec*®) for chronic myeloid leukaemia (January 2003)** SMC No. 26/02 Recommended with restrictions
▶ **Imatinib (*Glivec*®) for the adjuvant treatment of gastrointestinal stromal tumours (September 2010)** SMC No. 584/09 Recommended with restrictions

- **MEDICINAL FORMS** There can be variation in the licensing of different medicines containing the same drug.
Oral tablet
CAUTIONARY AND ADVISORY LABELS 21, 27
▶ **Imatinib (Non-proprietary)**
Imatinib (as Imatinib mesilate) 100 mg Imatinib 100mg tablets | 60 tablet [PoM] £104.49–£333.41 (Hospital only) | 60 tablet [PoM] £152.25–£924.65
Imatinib (as Imatinib mesilate) 400 mg Imatinib 400mg tablets | 30 tablet [PoM] £254.49–£1,849.34 | 30 tablet [PoM] £208.98–£664.58 (Hospital only)

Imatinib (as Imatinib mesilate) 600 mg Imatinib 600mg tablets | 30 tablet [PoM] ⚠ (Hospital only)

▸ **Glivec** (Novartis Pharmaceuticals UK Ltd)
Imatinib (as Imatinib mesilate) 100 mg Glivec 100mg tablets | 60 tablet [PoM] £973.32
Imatinib (as Imatinib mesilate) 400 mg Glivec 400mg tablets | 30 tablet [PoM] £1,946.67

Lapatinib [Specialist drug]
13-Feb-2023

● **INDICATIONS AND DOSE**

Breast cancer
▸ BY MOUTH
▸ Adult: Specialist drug – access specialist resources for dosing information

IMPORTANT SAFETY INFORMATION
RISKS OF INCORRECT DOSING OF ORAL ANTI-CANCER MEDICINES
See Cytotoxic drugs p. 1027.

● INTERACTIONS → Appendix 1: lapatinib

● SIDE-EFFECTS
▸ **Common or very common** Alopecia · appetite decreased · arthralgia · asthenia · constipation · cough · dehydration · diarrhoea (treat promptly; withhold if severe) · dyspnoea · epistaxis · gastrointestinal discomfort · headache · hepatotoxicity (discontinue permanently if severe) · hot flush · hyperbilirubinaemia · insomnia · mucositis · nail disorder · nausea · pain · paronychia · skin reactions · stomatitis · vomiting
▸ **Uncommon** Interstitial lung disease
▸ **Frequency not known** Severe cutaneous adverse reactions (SCARs)

● CONCEPTION AND CONTRACEPTION Contraceptive advice required.

● PATIENT AND CARER ADVICE Counselling advised (administration). Patients should be advised to report any unexpected changes in bowel habit.

● NATIONAL FUNDING/ACCESS DECISIONS
For full details see funding body website
NICE decisions
▸ **Lapatinib or trastuzumab in combination with an aromatase inhibitor for the first-line treatment of metastatic hormone-receptor-positive breast cancer that overexpresses HER2 (June 2012)** NICE TA257 Not recommended

● MEDICINAL FORMS There can be variation in the licensing of different medicines containing the same drug.
Oral tablet
▸ Tyverb (Novartis Pharmaceuticals UK Ltd)
Lapatinib (as Lapatinib ditosylate monohydrate) 250 mg Tyverb 250mg tablets | 84 tablet [PoM] £965.16 | 105 tablet [PoM] £1,206.45

Larotrectinib [Specialist drug]
03-Jun-2020

● **INDICATIONS AND DOSE**

Solid tumours
▸ BY MOUTH
▸ Adult: Specialist drug – access specialist resources for dosing information

IMPORTANT SAFETY INFORMATION
RISKS OF INCORRECT DOSING OF ORAL ANTI-CANCER MEDICINES
See Cytotoxic drugs p. 1027.

● INTERACTIONS → Appendix 1: larotrectinib

● SIDE-EFFECTS
▸ **Common or very common** Anaemia · constipation · dizziness · fatigue · gait abnormal · leucopenia · muscle weakness · myalgia · nausea · neutropenia · paraesthesia · taste altered · vomiting · weight increased
SIDE-EFFECTS, FURTHER INFORMATION Increases in ALT and AST have been reported in patients receiving larotrectinib; withhold treatment or permanently discontinue depending on severity. The majority of ALT and AST increases occurred in the first 3 months of treatment.

● CONCEPTION AND CONTRACEPTION Manufacturer advises effective contraception in females of childbearing potential and in men with a partner of childbearing potential, during treatment and for 1 month after last treatment; additional barrier method recommended in women using hormonal contraceptives.

● PATIENT AND CARER ADVICE
Driving and skilled tasks Manufacturer advises patients and carers should be counselled on the effects on driving and performance of skilled tasks—increased risk of dizziness and fatigue.

● NATIONAL FUNDING/ACCESS DECISIONS
For full details see funding body website
NICE decisions
▸ **Larotrectinib for treating NTRK fusion-positive solid tumours (May 2020)** NICE TA630 Recommended with restrictions

● MEDICINAL FORMS There can be variation in the licensing of different medicines containing the same drug.
Oral solution
EXCIPIENTS: May contain Hydroxybenzoates (parabens), potassium sorbate, propylene glycol, sorbitol, sucrose
▸ Vitrakvi (Bayer Plc) ▼
Larotrectinib (as Larotrectinib sulfate) 20 mg per 1 ml Vitrakvi 20mg/ml oral solution sugar free | 100 ml [PoM] £5,000.00 (Hospital only) [SF]
Oral capsule
CAUTIONARY AND ADVISORY LABELS 25
EXCIPIENTS: May contain Gelatin, propylene glycol
▸ Vitrakvi (Bayer Plc) ▼
Larotrectinib (as Larotrectinib sulfate) 25 mg Vitrakvi 25mg capsules | 56 capsule [PoM] £3,500.00 (Hospital only)
Larotrectinib (as Larotrectinib sulfate) 100 mg Vitrakvi 100mg capsules | 56 capsule [PoM] £14,000.00 (Hospital only)

Lenvatinib [Specialist drug]
28-Jun-2023

● **INDICATIONS AND DOSE**

KISPLYX ®

Renal cell carcinoma
▸ BY MOUTH
▸ Adult: Specialist drug – access specialist resources for dosing information

LENVIMA ®

Differentiated thyroid carcinoma | Hepatocellular carcinoma | Endometrial carcinoma
▸ BY MOUTH
▸ Adult: Specialist drug – access specialist resources for dosing information

IMPORTANT SAFETY INFORMATION
MHRA/CHM ADVICE: SYSTEMICALLY ADMINISTERED VEGF PATHWAY INHIBITORS: RISK OF ANEURYSM AND ARTERY DISSECTION (JULY 2020)
A European review of worldwide data concluded that systemically administered VEGF pathway inhibitors may lead to aneurysm and artery dissection in patients with or without hypertension. Some fatal cases have been reported, mainly in relation to aortic aneurysm rupture and aortic dissection. The MHRA advises healthcare

professionals to carefully consider the risk of aneurysm and artery dissection in patients with risk factors before initiating treatment with lenvatinib; any modifiable risk factors (such as smoking and hypertension) should be reduced as much as possible. Blood pressure should be monitored regularly, and product literature should be consulted if hypertension occurs during treatment.

RISKS OF INCORRECT DOSING OF ORAL ANTI-CANCER MEDICINES See Cytotoxic drugs p. 1027.

- **CONTRA-INDICATIONS** Fistulae
- **INTERACTIONS** → Appendix 1: lenvatinib
- **SIDE-EFFECTS**
▶ **Common or very common** Alopecia · appetite decreased · arthralgia · asthenia · cerebrovascular insufficiency · cholecystitis · constipation · decreased leucocytes · dehydration · diarrhoea · dizziness · dry mouth · dysphonia · electrolyte imbalance · embolism and thrombosis · encephalopathy · gastrointestinal discomfort · gastrointestinal disorders · haemorrhage · headache · heart failure · hepatic coma · hepatic disorders · hyperbilirubinaemia · hypercholesterolaemia · hypertension · hypoalbuminaemia · hypotension · hypothyroidism · increased risk of infection · insomnia · malaise · mucositis · myalgia · myocardial infarction · nausea · neutropenia · oral disorders · oropharyngeal complaints · pain · peripheral oedema · proteinuria · QT interval prolongation · renal impairment · renal tubular necrosis · skin reactions · taste altered · thrombocytopenia · vomiting · weight decreased
▶ **Uncommon** Adrenal insufficiency · healing impaired · nephrotic syndrome · osteonecrosis of jaw · pancreatitis · paresis · pneumothorax · splenic infarction
▶ **Frequency not known** Aneurysm · anxiety · artery dissection · cardiac disorder · cardiogenic shock · fistula · intracranial haemorrhage · neoplasm complications

SIDE-EFFECTS, FURTHER INFORMATION Manufacturer advises gastrointestinal toxicity should be actively managed — dehydration and/or hypovolaemia caused by gastrointestinal toxicity are identified as primary risk factors for renal impairment or failure.

- **CONCEPTION AND CONTRACEPTION** Manufacturer advises women of child-bearing potential should use highly effective contraception during treatment and for 1 month after the last dose, an additional barrier method of contraception should be used in women using oral hormonal contraceptives.
- **PATIENT AND CARER ADVICE**
Missed doses Manufacturer advises if a dose is more than 12 hours late, the missed dose should not be taken and the next dose should be taken at the normal time.
Driving and skilled tasks Manufacturer advises patients and carers should be counselled on the effects on driving and performance of skilled tasks—increased risk of fatigue and dizziness.
- **NATIONAL FUNDING/ACCESS DECISIONS**
For full details see funding body website
NICE decisions
▶ **Lenvatinib and sorafenib for treating differentiated thyroid cancer after radioactive iodine (August 2018)** NICE TA535 Recommended with restrictions
▶ **Lenvatinib for untreated advanced hepatocellular carcinoma (December 2018)** NICE TA551 Recommended with restrictions
▶ **Lenvatinib with everolimus for previously treated advanced renal cell carcinoma (January 2018)** NICE TA498 Recommended with restrictions
▶ **Lenvatinib with pembrolizumab for untreated advanced renal cell carcinoma (January 2023)** NICE TA858 Recommended with restrictions

▶ **Pembrolizumab with lenvatinib for previously treated advanced or recurrent endometrial cancer (June 2023)** NICE TA904 Recommended
Scottish Medicines Consortium (SMC) decisions
▶ **Lenvatinib (*Lenvima*®) for the treatment of adult patients with progressive, locally advanced or metastatic, differentiated (papillary/follicular/Hürthle cell) thyroid carcinoma (DTC), refractory to radioactive iodine (RAI) (October 2016)** SMC No. 1179/16 Recommended
▶ **Lenvatinib (*Lenvima*®) as monotherapy for the treatment of adult patients with advanced or unresectable hepatocellular carcinoma (HCC) who have received no prior systemic therapy (April 2019)** SMC No. SMC2138 Recommended
▶ **Lenvatinib (*Kisplyx*®) in combination with everolimus for the treatment of adult patients with advanced renal cell carcinoma (RCC) following one prior vascular endothelial growth factor (VEGF)-targeted therapy (November 2019)** SMC No. SMC2199 Recommended
▶ **Lenvatinib (*Kisplyx*®) in combination with pembrolizumab for the first-line treatment of adult patients with advanced renal cell carcinoma (June 2022)** SMC No. SMC2476 Recommended with restrictions

- **MEDICINAL FORMS** There can be variation in the licensing of different medicines containing the same drug.
Oral capsule
CAUTIONARY AND ADVISORY LABELS 25
▶ **Kisplyx** (Eisai Ltd)
Lenvatinib (as Lenvatinib mesilate) 4 mg Kisplyx 4mg capsules | 30 capsule [PoM] £1,437.00 (Hospital only)
Lenvatinib (as Lenvatinib mesilate) 10 mg Kisplyx 10mg capsules | 30 capsule [PoM] £1,437.00 (Hospital only)
▶ **Lenvima** (Eisai Ltd)
Lenvatinib (as Lenvatinib mesilate) 4 mg Lenvima 4mg capsules | 30 capsule [PoM] £1,437.00 (Hospital only)
Lenvatinib (as Lenvatinib mesilate) 10 mg Lenvima 10mg capsules | 30 capsule [PoM] £1,437.00 (Hospital only)

Lorlatinib [Specialist drug]

25-Jul-2023

- **INDICATIONS AND DOSE**
Non-small cell lung cancer
▶ BY MOUTH
▶ Adult: Specialist drug – access specialist resources for dosing information

IMPORTANT SAFETY INFORMATION
RISKS OF INCORRECT DOSING OF ORAL ANTI-CANCER MEDICINES See Cytotoxic drugs p. 1027.

- **INTERACTIONS** → Appendix 1: lorlatinib
- **SIDE-EFFECTS**
▶ **Common or very common** Anaemia · anxiety · arthralgia · asthenia · behaviour abnormal · cognitive disorder · concentration impaired · confusion · constipation · delirium · dementia · depression · diarrhoea · dyslipidaemia · gait abnormal · hallucinations · headache · inflammation · interstitial lung disease · learning disability · memory loss · mental impairment (thought disturbance) · mood altered · muscle weakness · myalgia · nausea · nerve disorders · neurotoxicity · oedema · pain · peroneal nerve palsy · sensation abnormal · skin reactions · speech impairment · vision disorders · vitreous floater · weight increased
▶ **Frequency not known** Atrioventricular block

SIDE-EFFECTS, FURTHER INFORMATION If worsening respiratory symptoms indicative of interstitial lung disease or pneumonitis (including dyspnoea, cough, and fever)— withhold or permanently discontinue treatment based on severity.

- **CONCEPTION AND CONTRACEPTION** Manufacturer advises females of childbearing potential should use effective non-hormonal contraception during treatment and for 35 days after last treatment; male patients should use effective contraception during treatment and for 14 weeks after last treatment if their partner is pregnant or of childbearing potential.

- **PATIENT AND CARER ADVICE**
Missed doses Manufacturer advises if a dose is more than 20 hours late, the missed dose should not be taken and the next dose should be taken at the normal time.
Driving and skilled tasks Manufacturer advises patients and carers should be counselled on the effects on driving and performance of skilled tasks—increased risk of CNS effects.

- **NATIONAL FUNDING/ACCESS DECISIONS**
For full details see funding body website
NICE decisions
▸ Lorlatinib for previously treated ALK-positive advanced non-small-cell lung cancer (May 2020) NICE TA628 Recommended
▸ Lorlatinib for untreated ALK-positive advanced non-small-cell lung cancer (July 2023) NICE TA909 Not recommended
Scottish Medicines Consortium (SMC) decisions
▸ Lorlatinib (*Lorviqua*®) as monotherapy for the treatment of adult patients with anaplastic lymphoma kinase (ALK)-positive advanced non-small cell lung cancer whose disease has progressed after alectinib or ceritinib as the first ALK tyrosine kinase inhibitor (TKI) therapy or crizotinib and at least one other ALK TKI (March 2020) SMC No. SMC2239 Recommended
▸ Lorlatinib (*Lorviqua*®) as monotherapy for the treatment of adult patients with anaplastic lymphoma kinase (ALK)-positive advanced non-small cell lung cancer previously not treated with an ALK inhibitor (March 2022) SMC No. SMC2415 Recommended

- **MEDICINAL FORMS** There can be variation in the licensing of different medicines containing the same drug.
Oral tablet
CAUTIONARY AND ADVISORY LABELS 25
▸ Lorviqua (Pfizer Ltd) ▼
Lorlatinib 25 mg Lorviqua 25mg tablets | 90 tablet [PoM] £5,283.00 (Hospital only)
Lorlatinib 100 mg Lorviqua 100mg tablets | 30 tablet [PoM] £5,283.00 (Hospital only)

Midostaurin [Specialist drug]
01-Oct-2021

- **INDICATIONS AND DOSE**
Acute myeloid leukaemia | Systemic mastocytosis | Mast cell leukaemia
▸ BY MOUTH
▸ Adult: Specialist drug – access specialist resources for dosing information

IMPORTANT SAFETY INFORMATION
RISKS OF INCORRECT DOSING OF ORAL ANTI-CANCER MEDICINES
See Cytotoxic drugs p. 1027.

- **INTERACTIONS** → Appendix 1: midostaurin
- **SIDE-EFFECTS**
▸ **Common or very common** Asthenia · bruising · chills · concentration impaired · constipation · cough · cystitis · diarrhoea · dizziness · dyspepsia · dyspnoea · fall · febrile neutropenia · fever · haemorrhage · headache · hyperglycaemia · hypersensitivity · hypotension · increased risk of infection · interstitial lung disease · nausea · oedema · oropharyngeal pain · pleural effusion · QT interval prolongation · sepsis · tremor · vertigo · vomiting · weight increased
▸ **Frequency not known** Cardiac disorder · congestive heart failure

- **CONCEPTION AND CONTRACEPTION** Manufacturer advises perform pregnancy test in women of childbearing potential within 7 days prior to treatment initiation; effective contraception must be used during treatment and for at least 4 months after stopping treatment—additional barrier method recommended in women using hormonal contraceptives.

- **NATIONAL FUNDING/ACCESS DECISIONS**
For full details see funding body website
NICE decisions
▸ Midostaurin for untreated acute myeloid leukaemia (June 2018) NICE TA523 Recommended with restrictions
▸ Midostaurin for treating advanced systemic mastocytosis (September 2021) NICE TA728 Recommended
Scottish Medicines Consortium (SMC) decisions
▸ Midostaurin (*Rydapt*®) for treatment of adult patients with newly diagnosed acute myeloid leukaemia who are FLT3 mutation positive in combination with standard daunorubicin and cytarabine induction and high dose cytarabine consolidation chemotherapy, and for patients in complete response followed by midostaurin single agent maintenance therapy (June 2018) SMC No. 1330/18 Recommended

- **MEDICINAL FORMS** There can be variation in the licensing of different medicines containing the same drug.
Oral capsule
CAUTIONARY AND ADVISORY LABELS 21, 25
EXCIPIENTS: May contain Alcohol
▸ Rydapt (Novartis Pharmaceuticals UK Ltd)
Midostaurin 25 mg Rydapt 25mg capsules | 56 capsule [PoM] £5,609.94

Mobocertinib [Specialist drug]
18-Jan-2023

- **INDICATIONS AND DOSE**
Non-small cell lung cancer
▸ BY MOUTH
▸ Adult: Specialist drug – access specialist resources for dosing information

IMPORTANT SAFETY INFORMATION
RISKS OF INCORRECT DOSING OF ORAL ANTI-CANCER MEDICINES
See Cytotoxic drugs p. 1027.

- **INTERACTIONS** → Appendix 1: mobocertinib
- **SIDE-EFFECTS**
▸ **Common or very common** Alopecia · anaemia · appetite decreased · asthenia · cardiomyopathy · conjunctival haemorrhage · cough · dehydration · diarrhoea · dry eye · dyspnoea · electrolyte imbalance · eye discomfort · eye disorders · eye inflammation · heart failure · hypertension · increased risk of infection · insomnia · interstitial lung disease (discontinue permanently) · mucositis · nail disorders · nausea · odynophagia · onycholysis · oral disorders · pneumonitis (discontinue permanently) · QT interval prolongation · renal impairment · respiratory failure · rhinorrhoea · skin reactions · ventricular arrhythmia · vision blurred · vomiting · weight decreased
▸ **Uncommon** Torsade de pointes (discontinue permanently)
SIDE-EFFECTS, FURTHER INFORMATION Diarrhoea might be severe (or life-threatening) and associated with dehydration. Diarrhoea should be managed appropriately by anti-diarrhoeal treatment, interruption, or discontinuation of treatment, and dose modifications. An anti-diarrhoeal should be initiated at first onset of loose stools or increased frequency of bowel movements.

- **CONCEPTION AND CONTRACEPTION** [EvGr] Females of childbearing potential should use effective non-hormonal contraception during and for 1 month after last treatment; male patients should use effective contraception during and for 1 week after last treatment if their partner is of childbearing potential. (M)

● **PATIENT AND CARER ADVICE** Patients should be advised to have anti-diarrhoeals readily available.
Vomiting If vomiting occurs after taking capsules, no additional dose should be taken on that day and the next dose should be taken at the usual time.
Missed doses If a dose is more than 6 hours late, the missed dose should not be taken and the next dose should be taken at the normal time.
Driving and skilled tasks Patients and carers should be counselled on the effects on driving and performance of skilled tasks—increased risk of fatigue and visual disturbances.

● **NATIONAL FUNDING/ACCESS DECISIONS**
For full details see funding body website
NICE decisions
▸ Mobocertinib for treating EGFR exon 20 insertion mutation-positive advanced non-small-cell lung cancer after platinum-based chemotherapy (January 2023) NICE TA855 Recommended

Scottish Medicines Consortium (SMC) decisions
▸ Mobocertinib (*Exkivity*®) as monotherapy for the treatment of adult patients with epidermal growth factor receptor (EGFR) exon 20 insertion mutation-positive locally advanced or metastatic non-small cell lung cancer (NSCLC), who have received prior platinum-based chemotherapy (January 2023) SMC No. SMC2516 Recommended

● **MEDICINAL FORMS** No licensed medicines listed.

Momelotinib [Specialist drug]
25-Jun-2024

● **INDICATIONS AND DOSE**
Disease-related splenomegaly or symptoms [in patients with moderate to severe anaemia who have primary myelofibrosis, post-polycythaemia vera myelofibrosis, or post-essential thrombocythaemia myelofibrosis]
▸ BY MOUTH
▸ Adult: Specialist drug – access specialist resources for dosing information

IMPORTANT SAFETY INFORMATION
RISKS OF INCORRECT DOSING OF ORAL ANTI-CANCER MEDICINES
See Cytotoxic drugs p. 1027.

● **CONTRA-INDICATIONS** Active infection (do not initiate)

● **INTERACTIONS** → Appendix 1: momelotinib

● **SIDE-EFFECTS**
▸ **Common or very common** Abdominal pain · arthralgia · asthenia · bruising · constipation · cough · cystitis · diarrhoea · dizziness · fever · flushing · haematoma · headache · hypotension · increased risk of infection · nausea · nerve disorders · neutropenia · pain · paraesthesia · sepsis · syncope · thrombocytopenia · vertigo · vision blurred · vomiting
▸ **Frequency not known** Drug-induced liver injury

● **CONCEPTION AND CONTRACEPTION** [EvGr] Females of childbearing potential should use effective contraception during treatment and for at least 1 week after last treatment; additional barrier method recommended in females using hormonal contraceptives. (M)

● **PATIENT AND CARER ADVICE**
Driving and skilled tasks Patients and carers should be counselled on the effects on driving and performance of skilled tasks—increased risk of dizziness and blurred vision.

● **NATIONAL FUNDING/ACCESS DECISIONS**
For full details see funding body website
NICE decisions
▸ Momelotinib for treating myelofibrosis-related splenomegaly or symptoms (March 2024) NICE TA957 Recommended with restrictions

Scottish Medicines Consortium (SMC) decisions
▸ Momelotinib (*Omjjara*®) for the treatment of disease-related splenomegaly or symptoms in adult patients with moderate to severe anaemia who have primary myelofibrosis, post-polycythaemia vera myelofibrosis or post-essential thrombocythaemia myelofibrosis and who are Janus-associated kinase inhibitor-naïve or have been treated with ruxolitinib (June 2024) SMC No. SMC2636 Recommended

● **MEDICINAL FORMS** There can be variation in the licensing of different medicines containing the same drug.
Oral tablet
▸ **Omjjara** (GlaxoSmithKline UK Ltd) ▼
**Momelotinib (as Momelotinib dihydrochloride monohydrate)
100 mg** Omjjara 100mg tablets | 30 tablet [PoM] £5,650.00 (Hospital only)
**Momelotinib (as Momelotinib dihydrochloride monohydrate)
150 mg** Omjjara 150mg tablets | 30 tablet [PoM] £5,650.00 (Hospital only)
**Momelotinib (as Momelotinib dihydrochloride monohydrate)
200 mg** Omjjara 200mg tablets | 30 tablet [PoM] £5,650.00 (Hospital only)

Neratinib [Specialist drug]
22-Mar-2023

● **INDICATIONS AND DOSE**
Breast cancer
▸ BY MOUTH
▸ Adult: Specialist drug – access specialist resources for dosing information

IMPORTANT SAFETY INFORMATION
RISKS OF INCORRECT DOSING OF ORAL ANTI-CANCER MEDICINES
See Cytotoxic drugs p. 1027.

● **INTERACTIONS** → Appendix 1: neratinib

● **SIDE-EFFECTS**
▸ **Common or very common** Appetite decreased · dehydration · diarrhoea · dry mouth · epistaxis · fatigue · gastrointestinal discomfort · increased risk of infection · mucositis · muscle spasms · nail discolouration · nail disorders · nausea · oral disorders · skin reactions · vomiting · weight decreased
▸ **Uncommon** Renal failure
▸ **Frequency not known** Hepatotoxicity

SIDE-EFFECTS, FURTHER INFORMATION Diarrhoea
Diarrhoea can be severe and associated with dehydration; it is more likely to occur during initiation and can be recurrent. Diarrhoea should be managed appropriately by anti-diarrhoeal treatment, interruption or discontinuation of treatment, dose modifications, and dietary changes. An anti-diarrhoeal should be initiated with the first dose, and maintained during the first 1 to 2 months of treatment, aiming for 1 to 2 bowel motions per day.
Hepatotoxicity If hepatotoxicity occurs, manufacturer advises treatment should be withheld or permanently discontinued, based on severity.

● **CONCEPTION AND CONTRACEPTION** Manufacturer advises females of childbearing potential should use highly effective contraception during treatment and for 1 month after last treatment; an additional barrier method of contraception should be used in females using hormonal contraceptives. Male patients should use effective contraception during treatment and for 3 months after last treatment if their partner is of childbearing potential.

● **PATIENT AND CARER ADVICE** A patient alert card, patient treatment journal, and patient guide should be provided.
Missed doses Manufacturer advises if a dose is missed, the missed dose should not be taken and the next dose should be taken at the normal time.
Driving and skilled tasks Manufacturer advises patients and carers should be counselled on the effects on driving and performance of skilled tasks—increased risk of fatigue, dizziness, dehydration, and syncope.

● **NATIONAL FUNDING/ACCESS DECISIONS**
For full details see funding body website
NICE decisions
▸ **Neratinib for extended adjuvant treatment of hormone receptor-positive, HER2-positive early stage breast cancer after adjuvant trastuzumab (November 2019)** NICE TA612 Recommended with restrictions
Scottish Medicines Consortium (SMC) decisions
▸ **Neratinib (*Nerlynx*®) for extended adjuvant treatment of adult patients with early-stage hormone receptor positive HER2-overexpressed/amplified breast cancer and who completed adjuvant trastuzumab-based therapy less than one year ago (August 2020)** SMC No. SMC2251 Recommended

● **MEDICINAL FORMS** There can be variation in the licensing of different medicines containing the same drug.
Oral tablet
CAUTIONARY AND ADVISORY LABELS 21, 25
▸ Nerlynx (Pierre Fabre Ltd)
Neratinib (as Neratinib maleate) 40 mg Nerlynx 40mg tablets | 180 tablet [PoM] £4,500.00 (Hospital only)

Nilotinib [Specialist drug]

22-Feb-2021

● **INDICATIONS AND DOSE**
Chronic myeloid leukaemia
▸ BY MOUTH
▸ Adult: Specialist drug – access specialist resources for dosing information

---

IMPORTANT SAFETY INFORMATION
RISKS OF INCORRECT DOSING OF ORAL ANTI-CANCER MEDICINES
See Cytotoxic drugs p. 1027.

MHRA/CHM ADVICE (MAY 2016): RISK OF HEPATITIS B VIRUS REACTIVATION WITH TYROSINE KINASE INHIBITORS
An EU wide review has concluded that nilotinib can cause hepatitis B virus reactivation; the MHRA recommends establishing hepatitis B virus status in all patients before initiation of treatment. Patients who are carriers of hepatitis B virus should be closely monitored for signs and symptoms of active infection throughout treatment and for several months after stopping treatment; expert advice should be sought for patients who test positive for hepatitis B virus and in those with active infection.

● **INTERACTIONS** → Appendix 1: nilotinib

● **SIDE-EFFECTS**
▸ **Common or very common** Alopecia · anaemia · anxiety · appetite abnormal · arrhythmias · asthenia · cardiac conduction disorders · chest discomfort · chills · constipation · cough · decreased leucocytes · depression · diabetes mellitus · diarrhoea · dizziness · dry eye · dyslipidaemia · dyspnoea · ear pain · electrolyte imbalance · erectile dysfunction · eye discomfort · eye disorders · eye inflammation · fever · flushing · gastrointestinal discomfort · gastrointestinal disorders · gout · haemorrhage · headaches · hepatic disorders · hyperaemia · hyperbilirubinaemia · hyperglycaemia · hypertension · hyperuricaemia · hypothyroidism · increased risk of infection · influenza like illness · insomnia · ischaemic

heart disease · joint disorders · leucocytosis · malaise · menorrhagia · muscle complaints · muscle weakness · nausea · neutropenia · oedema · oral disorders · oropharyngeal pain · pain · palpitations · pancreatitis · peripheral vascular disease · QT interval prolongation · sensation abnormal · skin reactions · sweat changes · thrombocytopenia · thrombocytosis · tinnitus · urinary disorders · vertigo · vision disorders · vomiting · weight changes
▸ **Uncommon** Arthritis · atherosclerosis · breast abnormalities · cerebrovascular insufficiency · concentration impaired · confusion · dry mouth · dysphonia · eosinophilia · erythema nodosum · facial paralysis · facial swelling · fluid imbalance · gynaecomastia · hearing impairment · heart failure · hyperthyroidism · hypoglycaemia · hypotension · interstitial lung disease · intracranial haemorrhage · lethargy · loss of consciousness · memory loss · musculoskeletal stiffness · myocardial dysfunction · myocardial infarction · neoplasms · nerve disorders · oesophageal pain · pancytopenia · pericardial effusion · pericarditis · photosensitivity reaction · pulmonary hypertension · pulmonary oedema · renal failure · respiratory disorders · restless legs · sepsis · skin ulcer · syncope · taste altered · temperature sensation altered · throat complaints · thrombosis · tremor · urine discolouration
▸ **Rare or very rare** Brain oedema · chorioretinopathy · cyanosis · haemorrhagic shock · hepatitis B reactivation · hyperparathyroidism · sebaceous hyperplasia · sudden death · thyroiditis · tumour lysis syndrome

● **CONCEPTION AND CONTRACEPTION** Manufacturer advises highly effective contraception in women of childbearing potential during treatment and for up to two weeks after stopping treatment.

● **PATIENT AND CARER ADVICE** Manufacturer advises patients and carers should seek immediate medical attention if signs or symptoms of cardiovascular events occur.
All patients should be provided with the *Important Information About How to Take Your Medication* leaflet provided by the manufacturer.

● **NATIONAL FUNDING/ACCESS DECISIONS**
For full details see funding body website
NICE decisions
▸ **Dasatinib, nilotinib and imatinib for untreated chronic myeloid leukaemia (CML) (December 2016)** NICE TA426 Recommended with restrictions
▸ **Dasatinib, nilotinib and high-dose imatinib for treating imatinib-resistant or intolerant chronic myeloid leukaemia (CML) (December 2016)** NICE TA425 Recommended with restrictions

---

● **MEDICINAL FORMS** There can be variation in the licensing of different medicines containing the same drug.
Oral capsule
CAUTIONARY AND ADVISORY LABELS 25, 27
▸ Tasigna (Novartis Pharmaceuticals UK Ltd)
Nilotinib (as Nilotinib hydrochloride monohydrate)
50 mg Tasigna 50mg capsules | 120 capsule [PoM] £2,432.85 DT = £2,432.85
Nilotinib (as Nilotinib hydrochloride monohydrate)
150 mg Tasigna 150mg capsules | 112 capsule [PoM] £2,432.85 DT = £2,432.85
Nilotinib (as Nilotinib hydrochloride monohydrate)
200 mg Tasigna 200mg capsules | 112 capsule [PoM] £2,432.85 DT = £2,432.85

Nintedanib

04-Apr-2023

- **DRUG ACTION** Nintedanib is a tyrosine protein kinase inhibitor.

- **INDICATIONS AND DOSE**

OFEV®

Idiopathic pulmonary fibrosis (initiated by a specialist) | Chronic fibrosing interstitial lung disease with a progressive phenotype (initiated by a specialist) | Systemic sclerosis-associated interstitial lung disease (initiated by a specialist)
▶ BY MOUTH
▸ Adult: 150 mg twice daily, reduced if not tolerated to 100 mg twice daily, for dose adjustments due to side-effects, consult product literature

VARGATEF®

Non-small cell lung cancer (specialist use only)
▶ BY MOUTH
▸ Adult: Specialist indication – access specialist resources for dosing information

---

IMPORTANT SAFETY INFORMATION

MHRA/CHM ADVICE: SYSTEMICALLY ADMINISTERED VEGF PATHWAY INHIBITORS: RISK OF ANEURYSM AND ARTERY DISSECTION (JULY 2020)

A European review of worldwide data concluded that systemically administered VEGF pathway inhibitors may lead to aneurysm and artery dissection in patients with or without hypertension. Some fatal cases have been reported, mainly in relation to aortic aneurysm rupture and aortic dissection. The MHRA advises healthcare professionals to carefully consider the risk of aneurysm and artery dissection in patients with risk factors before initiating treatment with nintedanib; any modifiable risk factors (such as smoking and hypertension) should be reduced as much as possible. Patients should be monitored and treated for hypertension as required.

RISKS OF INCORRECT DOSING OF ORAL ANTI-CANCER MEDICINES
See Cytotoxic drugs p. 1027.

- **CONTRA-INDICATIONS**
OFEV® Severe pulmonary hypertension

- **CAUTIONS** History or risk factors for QT prolongation · hypertension · impaired wound healing · increased risk of bleeding · patients at high risk of cardiovascular disease · previous abdominal surgery · recent history of hollow organ perforation · risk factors for aneurysm or artery dissection · theoretical increased risk of gastrointestinal perforation · theoretical increased risk of venous thromboembolism

OFEV® Mild to moderate pulmonary hypertension

- **INTERACTIONS** → Appendix 1: nintedanib

- **SIDE-EFFECTS**
▶ **Common or very common** Abdominal pain · abscess · alopecia · appetite decreased · dehydration · diarrhoea · drug-induced liver injury · electrolyte imbalance · haemorrhage · headache · hyperbilirubinaemia · hypertension · mucositis · nausea · neutropenia · peripheral neuropathy · sepsis · skin reactions · stomatitis · thrombocytopenia · venous thromboembolism · vomiting · weight decreased
▶ **Uncommon** Gastrointestinal disorders · myocardial infarction · pancreatitis · renal impairment
▶ **Frequency not known** Aneurysm · artery dissection

- **ALLERGY AND CROSS-SENSITIVITY** EvGr Contra-indicated in patients with peanut or soya hypersensitivity. Ⓜ

- **CONCEPTION AND CONTRACEPTION** Manufacturer advises exclude pregnancy before treatment and ensure effective contraception (in addition to barrier method) during treatment and for at least 3 months after last dose.

- **PREGNANCY** Manufacturer advises avoid—toxicity in *animal* studies. See also *Pregnancy and reproductive function* in Cytotoxic drugs p. 1027.

- **BREAST FEEDING** Manufacturer advises avoid—present in milk in *animal* studies.

- **HEPATIC IMPAIRMENT** Manufacturer advises caution in mild impairment (risk of increased exposure); avoid in moderate to severe impairment (limited information available).

OFEV® **Dose adjustments** Manufacturer advises dose reduction to 100 mg twice daily in mild impairment.

- **RENAL IMPAIRMENT** EvGr Caution in severe impairment (no information available). Ⓜ

- **MONITORING REQUIREMENTS**
▶ The MHRA advises to monitor blood pressure regularly.
▶ For *Vargatef®*, manufacturer advises monitor full blood count before each treatment cycle and regularly thereafter; monitor hepatic function before each treatment cycle during combination therapy and monthly during monotherapy; monitor renal function during treatment; monitor for thromboembolic events; monitor prothrombin time, INR and for bleeding if used concomitantly with anticoagulants; monitor for cerebral bleeding in patients with stable brain metastases.
▶ For *Ofev®* manufacturer advises monitor hepatic function before treatment initiation and during the first month of treatment, then at regular intervals during the subsequent 2 months and as clinically indicated thereafter; monitor renal function during treatment.

- **PRESCRIBING AND DISPENSING INFORMATION**
VARGATEF® Not to be taken on the same day as docetaxel therapy.

- **NATIONAL FUNDING/ACCESS DECISIONS**
For full details see funding body website
NICE decisions
▶ Nintedanib for previously treated locally advanced, metastatic, or locally recurrent non-small-cell lung cancer (July 2015) NICE TA347 Recommended with restrictions
▶ Nintedanib for treating idiopathic pulmonary fibrosis (January 2016) NICE TA379 Recommended with restrictions
▶ Nintedanib for treating idiopathic pulmonary fibrosis when forced vital capacity is above 80% predicted (February 2023) NICE TA864 Recommended with restrictions
▶ Nintedanib for treating progressive fibrosing interstitial lung diseases (November 2021) NICE TA747 Recommended
Scottish Medicines Consortium (SMC) decisions
▶ Nintedanib (*Ofev®*) in adults for the treatment of idiopathic pulmonary fibrosis [in patients with a predicted forced vital capacity less than or equal to 80%] (October 2015) SMC No. 1076/15 Recommended with restrictions
▶ Nintedanib (*Ofev®*) in adults for the treatment of idiopathic pulmonary fibrosis [in patients with a predicted forced vital capacity of more than 80%] (March 2023) SMC No. SMC2513 Recommended with restrictions
▶ Nintedanib (*Ofev®*) for the treatment of other chronic fibrosing interstitial lung diseases with a progressive phenotype in adults (June 2021) SMC No. SMC2331 Recommended

---

- **MEDICINAL FORMS** There can be variation in the licensing of different medicines containing the same drug.
Oral capsule
CAUTIONARY AND ADVISORY LABELS 21, 25
EXCIPIENTS: May contain Lecithin
▸ Ofev (Boehringer Ingelheim Ltd)
  Nintedanib (as Nintedanib esilate) 100 mg Ofev 100mg capsules | 60 capsule PoM £2,151.10 (Hospital only)
  Nintedanib (as Nintedanib esilate) 150 mg Ofev 150mg capsules | 60 capsule PoM £2,151.10 (Hospital only)

▶ Vargatef (Boehringer Ingelheim Ltd)
Nintedanib (as Nintedanib esilate) 100 mg Vargatef 100mg
capsules | 120 capsule [PoM] £2,151.10 (Hospital only)
Nintedanib (as Nintedanib esilate) 150 mg Vargatef 150mg
capsules | 60 capsule [PoM] £2,151.10 (Hospital only)

Osimertinib [Specialist drug]   05-Mar-2025

● **INDICATIONS AND DOSE**

Non-small cell lung cancer

▶ BY MOUTH

▶ Adult: Specialist drug – access specialist resources for
dosing information

IMPORTANT SAFETY INFORMATION

RISKS OF INCORRECT DOSING OF ORAL ANTI-CANCER MEDICINES
See Cytotoxic drugs p. 1027.

● **CONTRA-INDICATIONS** Congenital long QT syndrome

● **INTERACTIONS** → Appendix 1: osimertinib

● **SIDE-EFFECTS**

▶ **Common or very common** Diarrhoea · eyelid pruritus ·
increased risk of infection · interstitial lung disease · nail
discolouration · nail disorders · skin reactions · stomatitis

▶ **Uncommon** Cutaneous vasculitis · eye disorders · eye
inflammation · QT interval prolongation

▶ **Rare or very rare** Stevens-Johnson syndrome

▶ **Frequency not known** Decreased leucocytes · neutropenia ·
thrombocytopenia

● **CONCEPTION AND CONTRACEPTION** Manufacturer advises
use of effective, non-hormonal, contraception during and
for 2 months after treatment in women, and 4 months
after treatment in men.

● **PATIENT AND CARER ADVICE**

Missed doses Manufacturer advises if a dose is more than
12 hours late, the missed dose should not be taken and the
next dose should be taken at the normal time.

● **NATIONAL FUNDING/ACCESS DECISIONS**
For full details see funding body website

NICE decisions

▶ **Osimertinib for treating EGFR T790M mutation-positive
advanced non-small-cell lung cancer (October 2020)**
NICE TA653 Recommended with restrictions

▶ **Osimertinib for untreated EGFR mutation-positive non-small-
cell lung cancer (October 2020)** NICE TA654 Recommended

▶ **Osimertinib for adjuvant treatment of EGFR mutation-positive
non-small-cell lung cancer after complete tumour resection
(February 2025)** NICE TA1043 Recommended with
restrictions

Scottish Medicines Consortium (SMC) decisions

▶ **Osimertinib (*Tagrisso*®) for the treatment of adult patients
with locally advanced or metastatic epidermal growth factor
receptor (EGFR) T790M mutation-positive non-small-cell lung
cancer (NSCLC) (February 2017)** SMC No. 1214/17
Recommended with restrictions

▶ **Osimertinib (*Tagrisso*®) for adjuvant treatment after
complete tumour resection in adult patients with stage IB-IIIA
non-small cell lung cancer (NSCLC) whose tumours have
epidermal growth factor receptor (EGFR) exon 19 deletions or
exon 21 (L858R) substitution mutations (November 2021)**
SMC No. SMC2383 Recommended with restrictions

▶ **Osimertinib (*Tagrisso*®) as monotherapy for the first-line
treatment of adult patients with locally advanced or
metastatic non-small cell lung cancer (NSCLC) with activating
epidermal growth factor receptor (EGFR) mutations (January
2022)** SMC No. SMC2382 Recommended

● **MEDICINAL FORMS** There can be variation in the licensing of
different medicines containing the same drug.

Oral tablet

▶ Tagrisso (AstraZeneca UK Ltd)
Osimertinib (as Osimertinib mesylate) 40 mg Tagrisso 40mg
tablets | 30 tablet [PoM] £5,770.00
Osimertinib (as Osimertinib mesylate) 80 mg Tagrisso 80mg
tablets | 30 tablet [PoM] £5,770.00 (Hospital only)

Palbociclib [Specialist drug]   15-Nov-2022

● **INDICATIONS AND DOSE**

Breast cancer

▶ BY MOUTH

▶ Adult: Specialist drug – access specialist resources for
dosing information

IMPORTANT SAFETY INFORMATION

RISKS OF INCORRECT DOSING OF ORAL ANTI-CANCER MEDICINES
See Cytotoxic drugs p. 1027.

MHRA/CHM ADVICE: CDK4/6 INHIBITORS (ABEMACICLIB,
PALBOCICLIB, RIBOCICLIB): REPORTS OF INTERSTITIAL LUNG
DISEASE AND PNEUMONITIS, INCLUDING SEVERE CASES (JUNE
2021)
Interstitial lung disease and pneumonitis, in some cases
severe or fatal, have been reported in patients being
treated with CDK4/6 inhibitors, such as palbociclib.
Healthcare professionals are advised to ask patients
taking palbociclib about pulmonary symptoms indicative
of interstitial lung disease and pneumonitis, such as
cough or dyspnoea. Patients should be advised to seek
advice right away if these symptoms occur. Healthcare
professionals should ensure patients have a copy of the
Patient Information Leaflet (PIL) for palbociclib.

● **INTERACTIONS** → Appendix 1: palbociclib

● **SIDE-EFFECTS**

▶ **Common or very common** Alopecia · anaemia · appetite
decreased · asthenia · diarrhoea · dry eye · epistaxis ·
excessive tearing · fever · infection · interstitial lung
disease · leucopenia · mucositis · nausea · neutropenia · oral
disorders · oropharyngeal complaints · skin reactions ·
taste altered · thrombocytopenia · vision blurred · vomiting

SIDE-EFFECTS, FURTHER INFORMATION Side-effects are
reported when used in combination with letrozole or
fulvestrant.

● **CONCEPTION AND CONTRACEPTION** Manufacturer advises
effective contraception in women of childbearing potential
during treatment and for at least 3 weeks after completing
treatment. Male patients should use effective
contraception during treatment and for at least 14 weeks
after completing treatment if their partner is of
childbearing potential.

● **PATIENT AND CARER ADVICE**

Missed doses Manufacturer advises to take palbociclib at
the same time each day; if a dose is missed, the missed
dose should not be taken and the next dose should be
taken at the usual time.

● **NATIONAL FUNDING/ACCESS DECISIONS**
For full details see funding body website

NICE decisions

▶ **Palbociclib with an aromatase inhibitor for previously
untreated, hormone receptor-positive, HER2-negative, locally
advanced or metastatic breast cancer (December 2017)**
NICE TA495 Recommended with restrictions

▶ **Palbociclib with fulvestrant for treating hormone receptor-
positive, HER2-negative advanced breast cancer after
endocrine therapy (October 2022)** NICE TA836 Recommended
with restrictions

Scottish Medicines Consortium (SMC) decisions

▶ Palbociclib (*Ibrance*®) for the treatment of hormone receptor (HR)-positive, human epidermal growth factor receptor 2 (HER2)-negative locally advanced or metastatic breast cancer: in combination with an aromatase inhibitor; or in combination with fulvestrant in women who have received prior endocrine therapy (December 2017) SMC No. 1276/17 Recommended with restrictions

▶ Palbociclib (*Ibrance*®) for the treatment of hormone receptor (HR)-positive, human epidermal growth factor receptor 2 (HER2)-negative locally advanced or metastatic breast cancer -in combination with fulvestrant in women who have received prior endocrine therapy (July 2019) SMC No. SMC2149 Recommended

● **MEDICINAL FORMS** There can be variation in the licensing of different medicines containing the same drug.

Oral tablet

CAUTIONARY AND ADVISORY LABELS 25

▶ Ibrance (Pfizer Ltd)
Palbociclib 75 mg Ibrance 75mg tablets | 21 tablet [PoM] £2,950.00 (Hospital only) | 63 tablet [PoM] £8,850.00 (Hospital only)
Palbociclib 100 mg Ibrance 100mg tablets | 21 tablet [PoM] £2,950.00 (Hospital only) | 63 tablet [PoM] £8,850.00 (Hospital only)
Palbociclib 125 mg Ibrance 125mg tablets | 21 tablet [PoM] £2,950.00 (Hospital only) | 63 tablet [PoM] £8,850.00 (Hospital only)

Pazopanib [Specialist drug]

07-Jul-2021

● **INDICATIONS AND DOSE**

Renal cell carcinoma | Soft-tissue sarcoma

▶ BY MOUTH

▶ Adult: Specialist drug – access specialist resources for dosing information

IMPORTANT SAFETY INFORMATION

MHRA/CHM ADVICE: SYSTEMICALLY ADMINISTERED VEGF PATHWAY INHIBITORS: RISK OF ANEURYSM AND ARTERY DISSECTION (JULY 2020)

A European review of worldwide data concluded that systemically administered VEGF pathway inhibitors may lead to aneurysm and artery dissection in patients with or without hypertension. Some fatal cases have been reported, mainly in relation to aortic aneurysm rupture and aortic dissection. The MHRA advises healthcare professionals to carefully consider the risk of aneurysm and artery dissection in patients with risk factors before initiating treatment with pazopanib; any modifiable risk factors (such as smoking and hypertension) should be reduced as much as possible. Blood pressure should be monitored regularly, and product literature should be consulted if hypertension occurs during treatment.

RISKS OF INCORRECT DOSING OF ORAL ANTI-CANCER MEDICINES
See Cytotoxic drugs p. 1027.

● **INTERACTIONS** → Appendix 1: pazopanib

● **SIDE-EFFECTS**

▶ **Common or very common** Alopecia · appetite decreased · arthralgia · asthenia · bradycardia · cancer pain · cardiac disorder · chest pain · chills · cough · dehydration · diarrhoea · dizziness · drowsiness · dry mouth · dysphonia · dyspnoea · electrolyte imbalance · gastrointestinal discomfort · gastrointestinal disorders · haemorrhage · hair colour changes · headache · hepatic disorders · hiccups · hyperbilirubinaemia · hyperhidrosis · hypertension · hypoalbuminaemia · hypothyroidism · increased risk of infection · insomnia · left ventricular dysfunction · leucopenia · mucosal abnormalities · muscle complaints · musculoskeletal pain · nail disorder · nausea · neutropenia · oedema · oral disorders · peripheral neuropathy · pneumothorax · proteinuria · sensation abnormal · skin reactions · taste altered · thrombocytopenia · vasodilation ·

venous thromboembolism · vision blurred · vomiting · weight decreased

▶ **Uncommon** Cerebrovascular insufficiency · eye disorders · haemolytic uraemic syndrome · menstrual cycle irregularities · myocardial infarction · myocardial ischaemia · oropharyngeal pain · pancreatitis · photosensitivity reaction · polycythaemia · QT interval prolongation · rhinorrhoea · skin ulcer · thrombotic microangiopathy (discontinue permanently)

▶ **Rare or very rare** Interstitial lung disease · posterior reversible encephalopathy syndrome (PRES) (discontinue permanently)

▶ **Frequency not known** Aneurysm · artery dissection

● **CONCEPTION AND CONTRACEPTION** Effective contraception advised during treatment.

● **NATIONAL FUNDING/ACCESS DECISIONS**
For full details see funding body website

NICE decisions

▶ **Pazopanib for the first-line treatment of advanced renal cell carcinoma (updated August 2013)** NICE TA215 Recommended with restrictions

Scottish Medicines Consortium (SMC) decisions

▶ **Pazopanib (*Votrient*®) for the first-line treatment of advanced renal cell carcinoma (RCC) and for patients who have received prior cytokine therapy for advanced disease (March 2011)** SMC No. 676/11 Recommended with restrictions

▶ **Pazopanib (*Votrient*®) for the treatment of adult patients with selective subtypes of advanced soft tissue sarcoma (STS) who have received prior chemotherapy for metastatic disease or who have progressed within 12 months after (neo)adjuvant therapy (December 2012)** SMC No. 820/12 Not recommended

● **MEDICINAL FORMS** There can be variation in the licensing of different medicines containing the same drug.

Oral tablet

CAUTIONARY AND ADVISORY LABELS 23, 25

▶ Votrient (Novartis Pharmaceuticals UK Ltd)
Pazopanib (as Pazopanib hydrochloride) 200 mg Votrient 200mg tablets | 30 tablet [PoM] £560.50
Pazopanib (as Pazopanib hydrochloride) 400 mg Votrient 400mg tablets | 30 tablet [PoM] £1,121.00

Pemigatinib [Specialist drug]

01-Mar-2022

● **INDICATIONS AND DOSE**

Cholangiocarcinoma

▶ BY MOUTH

▶ Adult: Specialist drug – access specialist resources for dosing information

IMPORTANT SAFETY INFORMATION

RISKS OF INCORRECT DOSING OF ORAL ANTI-CANCER MEDICINES
See Cytotoxic drugs p. 1027.

● **INTERACTIONS** → Appendix 1: pemigatinib

● **SIDE-EFFECTS**

▶ **Common or very common** Alopecia · arthralgia · constipation · diarrhoea · dry eye · dry mouth · electrolyte imbalance · eye disorders · fatigue · hair growth abnormal · increased risk of infection · nail discolouration · nail disorders · nausea · punctate keratitis · skin reactions · stomatitis · taste altered · vision blurred

▶ **Frequency not known** Soft tissue calcification

● **CONCEPTION AND CONTRACEPTION** [EvGr] Females of childbearing potential and male patients with a partner of childbearing potential should use effective contraception during and for 1 week after stopping treatment; additional barrier method recommended in women using hormonal contraceptives. Ⓜ

● **PATIENT AND CARER ADVICE**

Missed doses If a dose is more than 4 hours late or vomiting occurs after taking a dose, no additional dose should be taken and the next dose should be taken at the normal scheduled time.

Driving and skilled tasks Patients and carers should be counselled on the effects on driving and performance of skilled tasks—increased risk of fatigue and visual disturbances.

● **NATIONAL FUNDING/ACCESS DECISIONS**

For full details see funding body website

NICE decisions

▸ Pemigatinib for treating relapsed or refractory advanced cholangiocarcinoma with FGFR2 fusion or rearrangement (August 2021) NICE TA722 Recommended

Scottish Medicines Consortium (SMC) decisions

▸ Pemigatinib (*Pemazyre®*) as monotherapy for the treatment of adults with locally advanced or metastatic cholangiocarcinoma with a fibroblast growth factor receptor 2 gene fusion or rearrangement that have progressed after at least one prior line of systemic therapy (February 2022) SMC No. SMC2399 Recommended

● **MEDICINAL FORMS** There can be variation in the licensing of different medicines containing the same drug.

Oral tablet

CAUTIONARY AND ADVISORY LABELS 25

▸ **Pemazyre** (Incyte Biosciences UK Ltd) ▼

Pemigatinib 4.5 mg Pemazyre 4.5mg tablets | 14 tablet [PoM] £7,159.00 (Hospital only)

Pemigatinib 9 mg Pemazyre 9mg tablets | 14 tablet [PoM] £7,159.00 (Hospital only)

Pemigatinib 13.5 mg Pemazyre 13.5mg tablets | 14 tablet [PoM] £7,159.00 (Hospital only)

Ponatinib [Specialist drug]

19-Jul-2021

● **INDICATIONS AND DOSE**

Chronic myeloid leukaemia | Acute lymphoblastic leukaemia

▸ BY MOUTH

▸ Adult: Specialist drug – access specialist resources for dosing information

---

IMPORTANT SAFETY INFORMATION

MHRA/CHM ADVICE: RISK OF HEPATITIS B VIRUS REACTIVATION WITH BCR-ABL TYROSINE KINASE INHIBITORS (MAY 2016)

An EU wide review has concluded that ponatinib can cause hepatitis B reactivation; the MHRA recommends establishing hepatitis B virus status in all patients before initiation of treatment. Patients who are carriers of hepatitis B virus should be closely monitored for signs and symptoms of active infection throughout treatment and for several months after stopping treatment; expert advice should be sought for patients who test positive for hepatitis B virus and in those with active infection.

MHRA/CHM ADVICE (UPDATED APRIL 2017): PONATINIB: RISK OF VASCULAR OCCLUSIVE EVENTS—UPDATED ADVICE ON POSSIBLE DOSE REDUCTION

The benefits and risks of ponatinib were reviewed by the European Medicines Agency's Committee on Medicinal Products for Human Use in 2014, which recommended that strengthened warnings should be added to the product information aimed at minimising the risk of blood clots and blockages in the arteries. Additional long-term follow-up data are now available that support new advice on dose modification to reduce this risk. The MHRA advises that although the recommended starting dose of ponatinib remains unchanged, prescribers should consider reducing the dose for patients with chronic phase chronic myeloid leukaemia (CP-CML) who have achieved a major cytogenetic response while on treatment. The following factors should be taken into account in the individual patient assessment:

● cardiovascular risk;

● side-effects of ponatinib therapy (including cardiovascular and other dose-related toxicity);

● time to cytogenetic response;

● BCR-ABL transcript levels.

The MHRA recommends close monitoring of response, if dose reduction is undertaken.

MHRA/CHM ADVICE: PONATINIB (*ICLUSIG®*): REPORTS OF POSTERIOR REVERSIBLE ENCEPHALOPATHY SYNDROME (OCTOBER 2018)

Post-marketing cases of posterior reversible encephalopathy syndrome (PRES) have been reported in patients receiving ponatinib.

Treatment should be interrupted if PRES is confirmed and resumed only once the event is resolved and if the benefit of continued treatment outweighs the risk.

Patients should be advised to contact their healthcare professional immediately if they develop sudden-onset severe headache, confusion, seizures, or vision changes.

MHRA/CHM ADVICE: SYSTEMICALLY ADMINISTERED VEGF PATHWAY INHIBITORS: RISK OF ANEURYSM AND ARTERY DISSECTION (JULY 2020)

A European review of worldwide data concluded that systemically administered VEGF pathway inhibitors may lead to aneurysm and artery dissection in patients with or without hypertension. Some fatal cases have been reported, mainly in relation to aortic aneurysm rupture and aortic dissection. The MHRA advises healthcare professionals to carefully consider the risk of aneurysm and artery dissection in patients with risk factors before initiating treatment with ponatinib; any modifiable risk factors (such as smoking and hypertension) should be reduced as much as possible. Blood pressure should be monitored regularly, and product literature should be consulted if hypertension occurs during treatment.

RISKS OF INCORRECT DOSING OF ORAL ANTI-CANCER MEDICINES See Cytotoxic drugs p. 1027.

● **INTERACTIONS** → Appendix 1: ponatinib

● **SIDE-EFFECTS**

▸ **Common or very common** Acute coronary syndrome · alopecia · anaemia · appetite decreased · arrhythmias · arthralgia · asthenia · cerebrovascular insufficiency · chills · constipation · cough · diarrhoea · dizziness · dry eye · dry mouth · dysphonia · dyspnoea · electrolyte imbalance · embolism and thrombosis · erectile dysfunction · eye inflammation · fever · fluid imbalance · gastrointestinal discomfort · gastrooesophageal reflux disease · haemorrhage · headaches · heart failure · hyperglycaemia · hypertension · hypertriglyceridaemia · hyperuricaemia · hypothyroidism · increased risk of infection · influenza like illness · insomnia · ischaemic heart disease · lethargy · mass · muscle complaints · nausea · neutropenia · oedema · pain · pancreatitis · pancytopenia · pericardial effusion · peripheral neuropathy · peripheral vascular disease · pleural effusion · pulmonary hypertension · sensation abnormal · sepsis · skin reactions · stomatitis · sweat changes · vasodilation · vision disorders · vomiting · weight decreased

▸ **Uncommon** Cardiac discomfort · cardiomyopathy ischaemic · coronary vasospasm · hepatic disorders · hepatic failure (including fatal cases) · intracranial haemorrhage · left ventricular dysfunction · posterior reversible encephalopathy syndrome (PRES) · renal artery stenosis · splenic infarction · tumour lysis syndrome

▸ **Rare or very rare** Panniculitis

▸ **Frequency not known** Acute kidney injury · aneurysm · artery dissection · thrombocytopenia

SIDE-EFFECTS, FURTHER INFORMATION **Heart failure** If signs and symptoms of heart failure develop, withhold treatment; consider stopping treatment if severe heart failure develops.

Thromboembolism Withhold treatment immediately if arterial occlusion or thromboembolism suspected.

● CONCEPTION AND CONTRACEPTION Ensure effective contraception during treatment in men and women; effectiveness of hormonal contraception unknown—alternative or additional methods of contraception should be used.

● NATIONAL FUNDING/ACCESS DECISIONS
For full details see funding body website
NICE decisions
► **Ponatinib for treating chronic myeloid leukaemia and acute lymphoblastic leukaemia (June 2017)** NICE TA451 Recommended

● MEDICINAL FORMS There can be variation in the licensing of different medicines containing the same drug.
Oral tablet
CAUTIONARY AND ADVISORY LABELS 3, 25
► Ponatinib (Non-proprietary)
Ponatinib (as Ponatinib hydrochloride) 15 mg Ponatinib 15mg tablets | 30 tablet [PoM] £2,525.00
Ponatinib (as Ponatinib hydrochloride) 30 mg Ponatinib 30mg tablets | 30 tablet [PoM] £5,050.00
Ponatinib (as Ponatinib hydrochloride) 45 mg Ponatinib 45mg tablets | 30 tablet [PoM] £5,050.00

Pralsetinib [Specialist drug]

21-Mar-2023

● **INDICATIONS AND DOSE**
Non-small cell lung cancer
► BY MOUTH
► Adult: Specialist drug – access specialist resources for dosing information

IMPORTANT SAFETY INFORMATION
RISKS OF INCORRECT DOSING OF ORAL ANTI-CANCER MEDICINES
See Cytotoxic drugs p. 1027.

● CONTRA-INDICATIONS Uncontrolled hypertension
● INTERACTIONS → Appendix 1: pralsetinib
● SIDE-EFFECTS
► **Common or very common** Anaemia · aplastic anaemia · arthralgia · asthenia · constipation · cough · decreased leucocytes · diarrhoea · dry mouth · dyspnoea · electrolyte imbalance · eye inflammation · facial swelling · fever · gastrointestinal discomfort · haemorrhage · headaches · hyperbilirubinaemia · hypertension · hypoalbuminaemia · increased risk of infection · inflammation · interstitial lung disease · long QT syndrome · musculoskeletal stiffness · myalgia · nausea · neutropenia · oedema · oral disorders · pain · QT interval prolongation · skin reactions · taste altered · thrombocytopenia · vomiting
► **Frequency not known** Sepsis

● CONCEPTION AND CONTRACEPTION [EvGr] Females of childbearing potential should use highly effective non-hormonal contraception during treatment and for at least 2 weeks after last treatment; male patients should use effective contraception during treatment and for at least 1 week after last treatment if their partner is of childbearing potential. (M) The effect on human fertility is not known—impairment of fertility has been observed in *animal* studies.

● PATIENT AND CARER ADVICE Patients should be advised to report new or worsening respiratory symptoms immediately.

Vomiting If vomiting occurs after taking capsules, no additional dose should be taken on that day and the next dose should be taken at the usual time.
Driving and skilled tasks Patients and their carers should be counselled on the effects on driving and performance of skilled tasks—increased risk of fatigue.

● NATIONAL FUNDING/ACCESS DECISIONS
For full details see funding body website
NICE decisions
► **Pralsetinib for treating RET fusion-positive advanced non-small-cell lung cancer (August 2022)** NICE TA812 Not recommended

Scottish Medicines Consortium (SMC) decisions
► **Pralsetinib (*Gavreto*®) as monotherapy for the treatment of adult patients with rearranged during transfection (RET) fusion-positive advanced non-small cell lung cancer (NSCLC) not previously treated with a RET inhibitor (March 2023)** SMC No. SMC2496 Recommended

● MEDICINAL FORMS No licensed medicines listed.

Quizartinib [Specialist drug]

26-Nov-2024

● **INDICATIONS AND DOSE**
Acute myeloid leukaemia
► BY MOUTH
► Adult: Specialist drug – access specialist resources for dosing information

IMPORTANT SAFETY INFORMATION
RISKS OF INCORRECT DOSING OF ORAL ANTI-CANCER MEDICINES
See Cytotoxic drugs p. 1027.

● CONTRA-INDICATIONS Congenital long QT syndrome · QTc interval more than 450 milliseconds derived using Fridericia's formula (do not initiate)
● INTERACTIONS → Appendix 1: quizartinib
● SIDE-EFFECTS
► **Common or very common** Anaemia · appetite decreased · device related bacteraemia · diarrhoea · facial swelling · fluid overload · gastrointestinal discomfort · haemorrhage · headaches · increased risk of infection · nausea · neutropenia · oedema · pancytopenia · peripheral swelling · QT interval prolongation · thrombocytopenia · vomiting
► **Uncommon** Cardiac arrest · ventricular fibrillation

● CONCEPTION AND CONTRACEPTION [EvGr] Females of childbearing potential should use effective contraception during treatment and for at least 7 months after last treatment; male patients should use effective contraception during treatment and for at least 4 months after last treatment if their partner is of childbearing potential. (M)

● PATIENT AND CARER ADVICE
Patient card A patient card should be provided.

● NATIONAL FUNDING/ACCESS DECISIONS
For full details see funding body website
NICE decisions
► **Quizartinib for induction, consolidation and maintenance treatment of newly diagnosed FLT3-ITD-positive acute myeloid leukaemia (October 2024)** NICE TA1013 Recommended
Scottish Medicines Consortium (SMC) decisions
► **Quizartinib (*Vanflyta*®) in combination with standard cytarabine and anthracycline induction and standard cytarabine consolidation chemotherapy, followed by quizartinib single-agent maintenance therapy for adult patients with newly diagnosed acute myeloid leukaemia that is FLT3-ITD positive (November 2024)** SMC No. SMC2699 Recommended

- **MEDICINAL FORMS** There can be variation in the licensing of different medicines containing the same drug.

Oral tablet

- ▶ **Vanflyta** (Daiichi Sankyo UK Ltd) ▼
  Quizartinib (as Quizartinib dihydrochloride) 17.7 mg Vanflyta 17.7mg tablets | 28 tablet [PoM] £6,451.00
  Quizartinib (as Quizartinib dihydrochloride) 26.5 mg Vanflyta 26.5mg tablets | 56 tablet [PoM] £12,902.00

Regorafenib [Specialist drug]   10-Nov-2023

- **INDICATIONS AND DOSE**

Colorectal cancer | Gastrointestinal stromal tumours | Hepatocellular carcinoma

- ▶ BY MOUTH
- ▶ Adult: Specialist drug – access specialist resources for dosing information

> **IMPORTANT SAFETY INFORMATION**
>
> MHRA/CHM ADVICE: SYSTEMICALLY ADMINISTERED VEGF PATHWAY INHIBITORS: RISK OF ANEURYSM AND ARTERY DISSECTION (JULY 2020)
>
> A European review of worldwide data concluded that systemically administered VEGF pathway inhibitors may lead to aneurysm and artery dissection in patients with or without hypertension. Some fatal cases have been reported, mainly in relation to aortic aneurysm rupture and aortic dissection. The MHRA advises healthcare professionals to carefully consider the risk of aneurysm and artery dissection in patients with risk factors before initiating treatment with regorafenib; any modifiable risk factors (such as smoking and hypertension) should be reduced as much as possible. Blood pressure should be monitored regularly, and product literature should be consulted if hypertension occurs during treatment.
>
> RISKS OF INCORRECT DOSING OF ORAL ANTI-CANCER MEDICINES
> See Cytotoxic drugs p. 1027.

- **INTERACTIONS** → Appendix 1: regorafenib

- **SIDE-EFFECTS**
- ▶ **Common or very common** Alopecia · anaemia · appetite decreased · asthenia · diarrhoea · dry mouth · dysphonia · electrolyte imbalance · fever · gastrooesophageal reflux disease · haemorrhage · headache · hyperbilirubinaemia · hypertension · hyperuricaemia · hypothyroidism · increased risk of infection · leucopenia · mucositis · musculoskeletal stiffness · nausea · pain · proteinuria · skin reactions · stomatitis · taste altered · thrombocytopenia · tremor · vomiting · weight decreased
- ▶ **Uncommon** Gastrointestinal fistula (discontinue) · gastrointestinal perforation (including fatal cases, discontinue) · hepatic disorders · myocardial infarction (withhold treatment) · myocardial ischaemia (withhold treatment) · nail disorder
- ▶ **Rare or very rare** Neoplasms · posterior reversible encephalopathy syndrome (PRES) (discontinue) · severe cutaneous adverse reactions (SCARs)
- ▶ **Frequency not known** Aneurysm · artery dissection

- **CONCEPTION AND CONTRACEPTION** Women of childbearing potential and men must use effective contraception during treatment and up to 8 weeks after last dose.

- **PATIENT AND CARER ADVICE** Counselling advised (administration).

- **NATIONAL FUNDING/ACCESS DECISIONS**
  For full details see funding body website

NICE decisions

- ▶ **Regorafenib for previously treated unresectable or metastatic gastrointestinal stromal tumours (November 2017)** NICE TA488 Recommended with restrictions

- ▶ **Regorafenib for previously treated advanced hepatocellular carcinoma (January 2019)** NICE TA555 Recommended with restrictions
- ▶ **Regorafenib for previously treated metastatic colorectal cancer (February 2023)** NICE TA866 Recommended

Scottish Medicines Consortium (SMC) decisions

- ▶ **Regorafenib** (*Stivarga*®) as a monotherapy for the treatment of adult patients with hepatocellular carcinoma (HCC) who have been previously treated with sorafenib (May 2018) SMC No. 1316/18 Recommended
- ▶ **Regorafenib** (*Stivarga*®) as monotherapy for the treatment of adult patients with metastatic colorectal cancer (CRC) who have been previously treated with, or are not considered candidates for, available therapies (October 2023) SMC No. SMC2562 Recommended

- **MEDICINAL FORMS** There can be variation in the licensing of different medicines containing the same drug.

Oral tablet

CAUTIONARY AND ADVISORY LABELS 21
ELECTROLYTES: May contain Sodium

- ▶ **Stivarga** (Bayer Plc)
  Regorafenib 40 mg Stivarga 40mg tablets | 84 tablet [PoM] £3,744.00 (Hospital only)

Ribociclib [Specialist drug]   19-Jul-2021

- **INDICATIONS AND DOSE**

Breast cancer

- ▶ BY MOUTH
- ▶ Adult: Specialist drug – access specialist resources for dosing information

> **IMPORTANT SAFETY INFORMATION**
>
> RISKS OF INCORRECT DOSING OF ORAL ANTI-CANCER MEDICINES
> See Cytotoxic drugs p. 1027.
>
> MHRA/CHM ADVICE: CDK4/6 INHIBITORS (ABEMACICLIB, PALBOCICLIB, RIBOCICLIB): REPORTS OF INTERSTITIAL LUNG DISEASE AND PNEUMONITIS, INCLUDING SEVERE CASES (JUNE 2021)
>
> Interstitial lung disease and pneumonitis, in some cases severe or fatal, have been reported in patients being treated with CDK4/6 inhibitors, such as ribociclib. Healthcare professionals are advised to ask patients taking ribociclib about pulmonary symptoms indicative of interstitial lung disease and pneumonitis, such as cough or dyspnoea. Patients should be advised to seek advice right away if these symptoms occur. Healthcare professionals should ensure patients have a copy of the Patient Information Leaflet (PIL) for ribociclib.

- **CONTRA-INDICATIONS** Pre-existing QTc prolongation · risk factors for QTc prolongation (including concomitant use of drugs known to prolong QTc interval)

- **INTERACTIONS** → Appendix 1: ribociclib

- **SIDE-EFFECTS**
- ▶ **Common or very common** Alopecia · anaemia · appetite decreased · asthenia · back pain · constipation · cough · decreased leucocytes · diarrhoea · dizziness · dry eye · dry mouth · dyspnoea · electrolyte imbalance · excessive tearing · fever · gastrointestinal discomfort · headache · hepatic disorders · increased risk of infection · nausea · neutropenia · oropharyngeal pain · peripheral oedema · QT interval prolongation · sepsis · skin reactions · stomatitis · syncope · taste altered · thrombocytopenia · vertigo · vomiting
- ▶ **Frequency not known** Interstitial lung disease · toxic epidermal necrolysis

- **ALLERGY AND CROSS-SENSITIVITY** Contra-indicated in patients with hypersensitivity to peanut or soya products.

- **CONCEPTION AND CONTRACEPTION** [EvGr] Females of childbearing potential should use effective contraception during treatment and for at least 21 days after last treatment. [M]

- **NATIONAL FUNDING/ACCESS DECISIONS**
For full details see funding body website
NICE decisions
  ▶ Ribociclib with an aromatase inhibitor for previously untreated, hormone receptor-positive, HER2-negative, locally advanced or metastatic breast cancer (December 2017) NICE TA496 Recommended
  ▶ Ribociclib with fulvestrant for treating hormone receptor-positive, HER2-negative advanced breast cancer after endocrine therapy (March 2021) NICE TA687 Recommended with restrictions

Scottish Medicines Consortium (SMC) decisions
  ▶ Ribociclib (*Kisqali*®) for use in combination with an aromatase inhibitor, for the treatment of postmenopausal women with hormone receptor (HR)-positive, human epidermal growth factor receptor 2 (HER2)-negative locally advanced or metastatic breast cancer as initial endocrine-based therapy (March 2018) SMC No. 1295/18 Recommended
  ▶ Ribociclib (*Kisqali*®) for the treatment of women with hormone receptor (HR)-positive, human epidermal growth factor receptor 2 (HER2)-negative locally advanced or metastatic breast cancer in combination with fulvestrant as initial endocrine-based therapy, or in women who have received prior endocrine therapy (November 2019) SMC No. SMC2198 Recommended with restrictions

- **MEDICINAL FORMS** There can be variation in the licensing of different medicines containing the same drug.
Oral tablet
CAUTIONARY AND ADVISORY LABELS 3, 25
  ▶ Kisqali (Novartis Pharmaceuticals UK Ltd)
  Ribociclib (as Ribociclib succinate) 200 mg Kisqali 200mg tablets | 21 tablet [PoM] £983.33 (Hospital only) | 42 tablet [PoM] £1,966.67 (Hospital only) | 63 tablet [PoM] £2,950.00 (Hospital only)

Ripretinib [Specialist drug]
01-Apr-2025

- **INDICATIONS AND DOSE**

Gastro-intestinal stromal tumour
  ▶ BY MOUTH
  ▶ Adult: Specialist drug – access specialist resources for dosing information

---

IMPORTANT SAFETY INFORMATION
RISKS OF INCORRECT DOSING OF ORAL ANTI-CANCER MEDICINES
See Cytotoxic drugs p. 1027.

- **CONTRA-INDICATIONS** Hypertension (do not initiate unless blood pressure adequately controlled)

- **INTERACTIONS** → Appendix 1: ripretinib

- **SIDE-EFFECTS**
  ▶ **Common or very common** Alopecia · arthralgia · constipation · cough · depression · diarrhoea · diastolic dysfunction · dyspnoea · fatigue · gastrointestinal discomfort · headache · heart failure · hypertension · hypophosphataemia · hypothyroidism · muscle complaints · muscle weakness · nausea · neoplasms · pain · peripheral neuropathy · peripheral oedema · skin reactions · stomatitis · tachycardia · vomiting · weight decreased
  ▶ **Frequency not known** Anaemia

  SIDE-EFFECTS, FURTHER INFORMATION Permanently discontinue treatment if grade 3 or 4 left ventricular systolic dysfunction occurs.
  If hypertension occurs, withhold treatment or permanently discontinue.

- **CONCEPTION AND CONTRACEPTION** [EvGr] Females of childbearing potential and male patients with female partners of childbearing potential should use effective contraception during treatment and for at least 1 week after last treatment (important: effects of ripretinib on oral contraceptives have not been studied; barrier contraception should also be used). [M]

- **PATIENT AND CARER ADVICE**
Phototoxicity Patients and carers should be advised to avoid or minimise exposure to direct sunlight or other sources of ultraviolet radiation due to the risk of phototoxicity; protective clothing and high SPF sunscreen should be used.
Driving and skilled tasks Patients and carers should be cautioned on the effects on driving and performance of skilled tasks—increased risk of fatigue.

- **NATIONAL FUNDING/ACCESS DECISIONS**
For full details see funding body website
NICE decisions
  ▶ Ripretinib for treating advanced gastrointestinal stromal tumour after 3 or more treatments (May 2023) NICE TA881 Not recommended

Scottish Medicines Consortium (SMC) decisions
  ▶ Ripretinib (*Qinlock*®) for the treatment of adult patients with advanced gastrointestinal stromal tumour who have received prior treatment with three or more kinase inhibitors, including imatinib (March 2025) SMC No. SMC2722 Not recommended

- **MEDICINAL FORMS** There can be variation in the licensing of different medicines containing the same drug.
Oral tablet
CAUTIONARY AND ADVISORY LABELS 3, 11, 25
  ▶ Qinlock (Deciphera Pharmaceuticals (Netherlands) B.V.) ▼
  Ripretinib 50 mg Qinlock 50mg tablets | 90 tablet [PoM] £18,400.00 (Hospital only)

Ruxolitinib [Specialist drug]
10-Nov-2023

- **INDICATIONS AND DOSE**

Disease-related splenomegaly or symptoms [in patients with primary myelofibrosis, post-polycythaemia vera myelofibrosis, or post-essential thrombocythaemia myelofibrosis] | Polycythaemia vera
  ▶ BY MOUTH
  ▶ Adult: Specialist drug – access specialist resources for dosing information

---

IMPORTANT SAFETY INFORMATION
RISKS OF INCORRECT DOSING OF ORAL ANTI-CANCER MEDICINES
See Cytotoxic drugs p. 1027.

- **INTERACTIONS** → Appendix 1: ruxolitinib

- **SIDE-EFFECTS**
  ▶ **Common or very common** Anaemia · bruising · constipation · dizziness · dyslipidaemia · flatulence · haemorrhage · headache · hypertension · increased risk of infection · intracranial haemorrhage · neutropenia · sepsis · thrombocytopenia · weight increased
  ▶ **Frequency not known** Progressive multifocal leukoencephalopathy (PML) (withhold treatment)

- **CONCEPTION AND CONTRACEPTION** [EvGr] Females of childbearing potential should use effective contraception during treatment. [M]

- **NATIONAL FUNDING/ACCESS DECISIONS**
For full details see funding body website
NICE decisions
  ▶ Ruxolitinib for treating disease-related splenomegaly or symptoms in adults with myelofibrosis (March 2016) NICE TA386 Recommended with restrictions

- Ruxolitinib for treating polycythaemia vera (October 2023) NICE TA921 Recommended

Scottish Medicines Consortium (SMC) decisions

- Ruxolitinib (*Jakavi*®) for the treatment of adult patients with polycythaemia vera (PV) who are resistant to or intolerant of hydroxyurea (HU) (December 2019) SMC No. SMC2213 Recommended

- **MEDICINAL FORMS** There can be variation in the licensing of different medicines containing the same drug.

Oral tablet

- Jakavi (Novartis Pharmaceuticals UK Ltd)
  Ruxolitinib (as Ruxolitinib phosphate) 5 mg   Jakavi 5mg tablets | 56 tablet PoM £1,428.00 DT = £1,428.00
  Ruxolitinib (as Ruxolitinib phosphate) 10 mg   Jakavi 10mg tablets | 56 tablet PoM £2,856.00 DT = £2,856.00
  Ruxolitinib (as Ruxolitinib phosphate) 15 mg   Jakavi 15mg tablets | 56 tablet PoM £2,856.00 DT = £2,856.00
  Ruxolitinib (as Ruxolitinib phosphate) 20 mg   Jakavi 20mg tablets | 56 tablet PoM £2,856.00 DT = £2,856.00

Selpercatinib [Specialist drug]
27-Feb-2025

- **INDICATIONS AND DOSE**

Non-small cell lung cancer | Thyroid cancer

- BY MOUTH
- Adult: Specialist drug – access specialist resources for dosing information

IMPORTANT SAFETY INFORMATION

RISKS OF INCORRECT DOSING OF ORAL ANTI-CANCER MEDICINES
See Cytotoxic drugs p. 1027.

- **CONTRA-INDICATIONS** Uncontrolled hypertension
- **INTERACTIONS** → Appendix 1: selpercatinib
- **SIDE-EFFECTS**
- **Common or very common** Abdominal pain · appetite decreased · arthralgia · constipation · diarrhoea · dizziness · dry mouth · fatigue · fever · haemorrhage · headache · hypersensitivity · hypertension · myalgia · nausea · oedema · QT interval prolongation · skin reactions · vomiting
- **Frequency not known** Intracranial haemorrhage · thrombocytopenia

- **CONCEPTION AND CONTRACEPTION** EvGr Females of childbearing potential and men with a partner of childbearing potential should use effective contraception during treatment and for one week after the last dose. Ⓜ The effect on human fertility is not known—impairment of fertility has been observed in *animal* studies.

- **PATIENT AND CARER ADVICE** EvGr If vomiting occurs after administration, no additional dose should be taken and the next dose should be taken at the normal time. Ⓜ
  Missed doses EvGr If a dose is missed, the missed dose should not be taken and the next dose should be taken at the normal time. Ⓜ
  Driving and skilled tasks EvGr Patients and their carers should be counselled on the effects on driving and skilled tasks—increased risk of fatigue and dizziness Ⓜ

- **NATIONAL FUNDING/ACCESS DECISIONS**
  For full details see funding body website

NICE decisions

- Selpercatinib for previously treated RET fusion-positive advanced non-small-cell lung cancer (January 2022) NICE TA760 Recommended
- Selpercatinib for untreated RET fusion-positive advanced non-small-cell lung cancer (July 2023) NICE TA911 Recommended with restrictions
- Selpercatinib for previously treated RET fusion-positive advanced non-small-cell lung cancer (February 2025) NICE TA1042 Recommended with restrictions

- Selpercatinib for advanced thyroid cancer with RET alterations after treatment with a targeted cancer drug in people 12 years and over (February 2025) NICE TA1038 Recommended with restrictions
- Selpercatinib for advanced thyroid cancer with RET alterations untreated with a targeted cancer drug in people 12 years and over (February 2025) NICE TA1039 Recommended with restrictions

Scottish Medicines Consortium (SMC) decisions

- Selpercatinib (*Retsevmo*®) as monotherapy for the treatment of adults and adolescents 12 years and older with advanced RET-mutant medullary thyroid cancer (MTC) who require systemic therapy following prior treatment with cabozantinib and/or vandetanib (September 2021) SMC No. SMC2370 Recommended
- Selpercatinib (*Retsevmo*®) as monotherapy for the treatment of adults with advanced RET fusion-positive thyroid cancer (TC) who require systemic therapy following prior treatment with sorafenib and/or lenvatinib (September 2021) SMC No. SMC2370 Recommended
- Selpercatinib (*Retsevmo*®) as monotherapy for the treatment of adults with advanced rearranged during transfection (RET) fusion-positive non-small cell lung cancer (NSCLC) who require systemic therapy following prior treatment with immunotherapy and/or platinum-based chemotherapy (November 2021) SMC No. SMC2371 Not recommended
- Selpercatinib (*Retsevmo*®) as monotherapy for the treatment of adults with advanced rearranged during transfection (RET) fusion-positive non-small cell lung cancer not previously treated with a RET inhibitor (November 2023) SMC No. SMC2573 Recommended with restrictions

- **MEDICINAL FORMS** There can be variation in the licensing of different medicines containing the same drug.

Oral capsule

CAUTIONARY AND ADVISORY LABELS 25
EXCIPIENTS: May contain Gelatin

- Retsevmo (Eli Lilly and Company Ltd) ▼
  Selpercatinib 40 mg   Retsevmo 40mg capsules | 56 capsule PoM £2,184.00 (Hospital only) | 168 capsule PoM £6,552.00 (Hospital only)
  Selpercatinib 80 mg   Retsevmo 80mg capsules | 56 capsule PoM £4,368.00 (Hospital only) | 112 capsule PoM £8,736.00 (Hospital only)

Sorafenib [Specialist drug]
13-Nov-2020

- **INDICATIONS AND DOSE**

Renal cell carcinoma | Differentiated thyroid carcinoma | Hepatocellular carcinoma

- BY MOUTH
- Adult: Specialist drug – access specialist resources for dosing information

IMPORTANT SAFETY INFORMATION

MHRA/CHM ADVICE: SYSTEMICALLY ADMINISTERED VEGF PATHWAY INHIBITORS: RISK OF ANEURYSM AND ARTERY DISSECTION (JULY 2020)

A European review of worldwide data concluded that systemically administered VEGF pathway inhibitors may lead to aneurysm and artery dissection in patients with or without hypertension. Some fatal cases have been reported, mainly in relation to aortic aneurysm rupture and aortic dissection. The MHRA advises healthcare professionals to carefully consider the risk of aneurysm and artery dissection in patients with risk factors before initiating treatment with sorafenib; any modifiable risk factors (such as smoking and hypertension) should be reduced as much as possible. Blood pressure should be

8

monitored regularly, and product literature should be consulted if hypertension occurs during treatment.

RISKS OF INCORRECT DOSING OF ORAL ANTI-CANCER MEDICINES
See Cytotoxic drugs p. 1027.

● **INTERACTIONS** → Appendix 1: sorafenib

● **SIDE-EFFECTS**

▶ **Common or very common** Alopecia · anaemia · appetite decreased · arthralgia · asthenia · congestive heart failure · constipation · decreased leucocytes · depression · diarrhoea · dry mouth · dysphagia · dysphonia · electrolyte imbalance · erectile dysfunction · fever · flushing · gastrointestinal discomfort · gastrointestinal disorders · haemorrhage · headache · hypertension · hypothyroidism · increased risk of infection · influenza like illness · intracranial haemorrhage · mucositis · muscle complaints · myocardial infarction · myocardial ischaemia · nausea · neoplasms · neutropenia · oral disorders · pain · peripheral neuropathy · proteinuria · renal failure · rhinorrhoea · skin reactions · taste altered · thrombocytopenia · tinnitus · vomiting · weight decreased

▶ **Uncommon** Acute respiratory distress syndrome (ARDS) · cholangitis · cholecystitis · dehydration · encephalopathy · gynaecomastia · hepatic disorders · hyperthyroidism · interstitial lung disease · pancreatitis · radiation injuries

▶ **Rare or very rare** Angioedema · hypersensitivity vasculitis · nephrotic syndrome · QT interval prolongation · rhabdomyolysis · severe cutaneous adverse reactions (SCARs)

▶ **Frequency not known** Aneurysm · artery dissection

● **CONCEPTION AND CONTRACEPTION** Contraceptive advice required.

● **NATIONAL FUNDING/ACCESS DECISIONS**
For full details see funding body website

NICE decisions

▶ Bevacizumab (first-line), sorafenib (first- and second-line), sunitinib (second-line) and temsirolimus (first-line) for the treatment of advanced and/or metastatic renal cell carcinoma (August 2009) NICE TA178 Not recommended

▶ Sorafenib for treating advanced hepatocellular carcinoma (September 2017) NICE TA474 Recommended with restrictions

▶ Lenvatinib and sorafenib for treating differentiated thyroid cancer after radioactive iodine (August 2018) NICE TA535 Recommended with restrictions

Scottish Medicines Consortium (SMC) decisions

▶ Sorafenib (*Nexavar*®) for the treatment of hepatocellular carcinoma (January 2016) SMC No. 482/08 Recommended with restrictions

● **MEDICINAL FORMS** There can be variation in the licensing of different medicines containing the same drug.

Oral tablet

CAUTIONARY AND ADVISORY LABELS 23

▶ Sorafenib (Non-proprietary)
Sorafenib (as Sorafenib tosylate) 200 mg Sorafenib 200mg tablets | 112 tablet PoM £2,567.00–£3,576.56 (Hospital only)

▶ Nexavar (Bayer Plc)
Sorafenib (as Sorafenib tosylate) 200 mg Nexavar 200mg tablets | 112 tablet PoM £3,576.56 (Hospital only)

Sunitinib [Specialist drug]

26-Nov-2020

● **INDICATIONS AND DOSE**

Gastro-intestinal stromal tumours | Renal cell carcinoma | Pancreatic neuroendocrine tumours

▶ BY MOUTH

▶ Adult: Specialist drug – access specialist resources for dosing information

---

IMPORTANT SAFETY INFORMATION

MHRA/CHM ADVICE: BEVACIZUMAB AND SUNITINIB: RISK OF OSTEONECROSIS OF THE JAW (JANUARY 2011)

Treatment with bevacizumab or sunitinib may be a risk factor for the development of osteonecrosis of the jaw.

Patients treated with bevacizumab or sunitinib, who have previously received bisphosphonates, or are treated concurrently with bisphosphonates, may be particularly at risk.

Dental examination and appropriate preventive dentistry should be considered before treatment with bevacizumab or sunitinib.

If possible, invasive dental procedures should be avoided in patients treated with bevacizumab or sunitinib who have previously received, or who are currently receiving, intravenous bisphosphonates.

MHRA/CHM ADVICE: SYSTEMICALLY ADMINISTERED VEGF PATHWAY INHIBITORS: RISK OF ANEURYSM AND ARTERY DISSECTION (JULY 2020)

A European review of worldwide data concluded that systemically administered VEGF pathway inhibitors may lead to aneurysm and artery dissection in patients with or without hypertension. Some fatal cases have been reported, mainly in relation to aortic aneurysm rupture and aortic dissection. The MHRA advises healthcare professionals to carefully consider the risk of aneurysm and artery dissection in patients with risk factors before initiating treatment with sunitinib; any modifiable risk factors (such as smoking and hypertension) should be reduced as much as possible. Blood pressure should be monitored regularly, and product literature should be consulted if hypertension occurs during treatment.

RISKS OF INCORRECT DOSING OF ORAL ANTI-CANCER MEDICINES
See Cytotoxic drugs p. 1027.

● **INTERACTIONS** → Appendix 1: sunitinib

● **SIDE-EFFECTS**

▶ **Common or very common** Abscess · alopecia · anaemia · appetite decreased · arthralgia · burping · chest pain · chills · constipation · cough · dehydration · depression · diarrhoea · dizziness · dry mouth · dysphagia · dyspnoea · embolism and thrombosis · excessive tearing · eye inflammation · fatigue · fever · gastrointestinal discomfort · gastrointestinal disorders · haemorrhage · hair colour changes · headache · hypertension · hypoglycaemia · hypothyroidism · increased risk of infection · influenza like illness · insomnia · leucopenia · mucositis · muscle complaints · muscle weakness · myocardial ischaemia · nail disorder · nasal complaints · nausea · neutropenia · oedema · oral disorders · oropharyngeal pain · pain · peripheral neuropathy · proteinuria · renal impairment · respiratory disorders · sensation abnormal · sepsis · skin reactions · taste altered · thrombocytopenia · urine discolouration · vasodilation · vomiting · weight decreased

▶ **Uncommon** Anal fistula (interrupt treatment) · cardiomyopathy · cerebrovascular insufficiency · cholecystitis · fistula (interrupt treatment) · healing impaired · heart failure · hepatic disorders · hypersensitivity · hyperthyroidism · intracranial haemorrhage · myocardial infarction · osteonecrosis of jaw · pancreatitis · pancytopenia · pericardial effusion · QT interval prolongation · tumour haemorrhage

▶ **Rare or very rare** Angioedema · myopathy · nephrotic syndrome · posterior reversible encephalopathy syndrome (PRES) · pyoderma gangrenosum · severe cutaneous adverse reactions (SCARs) · thrombotic microangiopathy · thyroiditis · torsade de pointes · tumour lysis syndrome

▶ **Frequency not known** Aneurysm · artery dissection

SIDE-EFFECTS, FURTHER INFORMATION Heart failure, including fatal cases, has been reported; consider reducing the dose, or interrupting or stopping treatment, if symptoms of heart failure occur.

● CONCEPTION AND CONTRACEPTION Effective contraception required during treatment.

● NATIONAL FUNDING/ACCESS DECISIONS
For full details see funding body website

NICE decisions

▶ Sunitinib for the first-line treatment of advanced and/or metastatic renal cell carcinoma (March 2009) NICE TA169 Recommended

▶ Sunitinib for the treatment of gastrointestinal stromal tumours (September 2009) NICE TA179 Recommended with restrictions

▶ Bevacizumab (first-line), sorafenib (first- and second-line), sunitinib (second-line) and temsirolimus (first-line) for the treatment of advanced and/or metastatic renal cell carcinoma (August 2009) NICE TA178 Not recommended

▶ Everolimus and sunitinib for treating unresectable or metastatic neuroendocrine tumours in people with progressive disease (June 2017) NICE TA449 Recommended

Scottish Medicines Consortium (SMC) decisions

▶ Sunitinib (*Sutent*®) for unresectable and/or metastatic malignant gastrointestinal stromal tumour (GIST) after failure of imatinib mesylate treatment due to resistance or intolerance (November 2009) SMC No. 275/06 Recommended

● MEDICINAL FORMS There can be variation in the licensing of different medicines containing the same drug.

Oral capsule

CAUTIONARY AND ADVISORY LABELS 14

▶ Sunitinib (Non-proprietary)
Sunitinib (as Sunitinib malate) 12.5 mg Sunitinib 12.5mg capsules | 28 capsule PoM £620.00–£784.70 (Hospital only) | 28 capsule PoM £706.23–£784.70
Sunitinib (as Sunitinib malate) 25 mg Sunitinib 25mg capsules | 28 capsule PoM £1,220.00–£1,569.40 (Hospital only) | 28 capsule PoM £1,412.46–£1,569.40
Sunitinib (as Sunitinib malate) 50 mg Sunitinib 50mg capsules | 28 capsule PoM £2,505.00–£3,138.80 (Hospital only) | 28 capsule PoM £3,138.80

▶ Sutent (Pfizer Ltd)
Sunitinib (as Sunitinib malate) 12.5 mg Sutent 12.5mg capsules | 28 capsule PoM £784.70 (Hospital only)
Sunitinib (as Sunitinib malate) 25 mg Sutent 25mg capsules | 28 capsule PoM £1,569.40 (Hospital only)
Sunitinib (as Sunitinib malate) 50 mg Sutent 50mg capsules | 28 capsule PoM £3,138.80 (Hospital only)

Temsirolimus [Specialist drug]
11-Jun-2021

● **INDICATIONS AND DOSE**

Renal cell carcinoma | Mantle cell lymphoma

▶ BY INTRAVENOUS INFUSION

▶ Adult: Specialist drug – access specialist resources for dosing information

● **INTERACTIONS** → Appendix 1: temsirolimus

● **SIDE-EFFECTS**

▶ **Common or very common** Abscess · anaemia · anxiety · appetite decreased · arthralgia · asthenia · chest pain · chills · conjunctivitis · constipation · cough · cystitis · decreased leucocytes · dehydration · depression · diabetes mellitus · diarrhoea · dizziness · drowsiness · dyslipidaemia · dysphagia · dyspnoea · electrolyte imbalance · embolism and thrombosis · fever · gastrointestinal discomfort ·

gastrointestinal disorders · genital oedema · haemorrhage · headache · hypersensitivity · hypertension · increased risk of infection · insomnia · interstitial lung disease · lacrimation disorder · mucositis · myalgia · nail disorder · nausea · neutropenia · oedema · oral disorders · pain · paraesthesia · pleural effusion · post procedural infection · renal failure · scrotal oedema · sepsis · skin reactions · taste altered · thrombocytopenia · vomiting

▶ **Uncommon** Healing impaired · intracranial haemorrhage · pericardial effusion

▶ **Frequency not known** Rhabdomyolysis

SIDE-EFFECTS, FURTHER INFORMATION Infusion related reactions have been associated with temsirolimus therapy. Withhold the infusion and treat infusion-related effects; if appropriate, the infusion can be restarted at a slower rate.

● CONCEPTION AND CONTRACEPTION Ensure effective contraception during treatment in men and women.

● NATIONAL FUNDING/ACCESS DECISIONS
For full details see funding body website

NICE decisions

▶ Bevacizumab (first-line), sorafenib (first- and second-line), sunitinib (second-line) and temsirolimus (first-line) for the treatment of advanced and/or metastatic renal cell carcinoma (August 2009) NICE TA178 Not recommended

● MEDICINAL FORMS There can be variation in the licensing of different medicines containing the same drug.

Solution for infusion

EXCIPIENTS: May contain Ethanol, propylene glycol

▶ Torisel (Pfizer Ltd)
Temsirolimus 25 mg per 1 ml Torisel 30mg/1.2ml concentrate for solution for infusion vials and diluent | 1 vial PoM £620.00 (Hospital only)

Tepotinib [Specialist drug]
18-Jan-2023

● **INDICATIONS AND DOSE**

Non-small cell lung cancer

▶ BY MOUTH

▶ Adult: Specialist drug – access specialist resources for dosing information

---

IMPORTANT SAFETY INFORMATION

RISKS OF INCORRECT DOSING OF ORAL ANTI-CANCER MEDICINES
See Cytotoxic drugs p. 1027.

● **INTERACTIONS** → Appendix 1: tepotinib

● **SIDE-EFFECTS**

▶ **Common or very common** Asthenia · constipation · diarrhoea · gastrointestinal discomfort · hepatic disorders · hypoalbuminaemia · interstitial lung disease · nausea · oedema · respiratory disorders · vomiting

▶ **Frequency not known** Dyspnoea · musculoskeletal pain · pneumonia · pulmonary embolism

SIDE-EFFECTS, FURTHER INFORMATION Interstitial lung disease and pneumonitis, including fatal events, have been reported; if suspected withhold treatment and if confirmed treatment should be discontinued.

● CONCEPTION AND CONTRACEPTION EvGr Females of childbearing potential and male patients with female partners of childbearing potential should use effective contraception during treatment and for at least 1 week after last treatment. Ⓜ

● **PATIENT AND CARER ADVICE**

Missed doses If a dose is more than 16 hours late, the missed dose should not be taken and the next dose should be taken at the normal time.

Driving and skilled tasks Patients and carers should be cautioned on the effects on driving and performance of skilled tasks—increased risk of fatigue or asthenia.

- **NATIONAL FUNDING/ACCESS DECISIONS**
For full details see funding body website
NICE decisions
▸ Tepotinib for treating advanced non-small-cell lung cancer with MET gene alterations (May 2022) NICE TA789 Recommended
Scottish Medicines Consortium (SMC) decisions
▸ Tepotinib (*Tepmetko*®) for the treatment of adult patients with advanced non-small cell lung cancer harbouring mesenchymal-epithelial transition factor gene (MET) exon 14 skipping alterations (January 2023) SMC No. SMC2535 Recommended

- **MEDICINAL FORMS** There can be variation in the licensing of different medicines containing the same drug.
Oral tablet
CAUTIONARY AND ADVISORY LABELS 21, 25
▸ Tepmetko (Merck Serono Ltd) ▼
Tepotinib (as Tepotinib hydrochloride) 225 mg Tepmetko 225mg tablets | 60 tablet [PoM] £7,200.00 (Hospital only)

Tivozanib [Specialist drug]

11-Nov-2020

- **INDICATIONS AND DOSE**
Renal cell carcinoma
▸ BY MOUTH
▸ Adult: Specialist drug – access specialist resources for dosing information

---

IMPORTANT SAFETY INFORMATION

MHRA/CHM ADVICE: SYSTEMICALLY ADMINISTERED VEGF PATHWAY INHIBITORS: RISK OF ANEURYSM AND ARTERY DISSECTION (JULY 2020)

A European review of worldwide data concluded that systemically administered VEGF pathway inhibitors may lead to aneurysm and artery dissection in patients with or without hypertension. Some fatal cases have been reported, mainly in relation to aortic aneurysm rupture and aortic dissection. The MHRA advises healthcare professionals to carefully consider the risk of aneurysm and artery dissection in patients with risk factors before initiating treatment with tivozanib; any modifiable risk factors (such as smoking and hypertension) should be reduced as much as possible. Blood pressure should be monitored regularly, and product literature should be consulted if hypertension occurs during treatment.

RISKS OF INCORRECT DOSING OF ORAL ANTI-CANCER MEDICINES
See Cytotoxic drugs p. 1027.

- **INTERACTIONS** → Appendix 1: tivozanib
- **SIDE-EFFECTS**
▸ **Common or very common** Alopecia · anaemia · angina pectoris · appetite decreased · arrhythmias · arthralgia · asthenia · cancer pain · cerebrovascular insufficiency · chest pain · chills · constipation · cough · diarrhoea · dizziness · dry mouth · dysphonia · dyspnoea · embolism and thrombosis · fever · gastrointestinal discomfort · gastrointestinal disorders · haemorrhage · headache · hypertension · hypothermia · hypothyroidism · increased risk of infection · insomnia · ischaemia · myalgia · myocardial infarction · nasal complaints · nausea · nerve disorders · oral disorders · oropharyngeal pain · pain · pancreatitis · peripheral oedema · proteinuria · sensation abnormal · skin reactions · swallowing difficulty · taste altered · tinnitus · vasodilation · vertigo · vision disorders · vomiting · weight decreased
▸ **Uncommon** Coronary artery insufficiency · ear congestion · excessive tearing · goitre · hyperhidrosis · hyperthyroidism · memory loss · mucositis · muscle weakness · pulmonary oedema · QT interval prolongation · thrombocytopenia · toxic nodular goitre

▸ **Rare or very rare** Posterior reversible encephalopathy syndrome (PRES)
▸ **Frequency not known** Aneurysm · artery dissection · heart failure

- **CONCEPTION AND CONTRACEPTION** Manufacturer advises effective contraception in men, women of childbearing potential, and their partners during treatment and for at least one month after the last dose; an additional barrier method of contraception should be used in women using hormonal contraceptives.

- **NATIONAL FUNDING/ACCESS DECISIONS**
For full details see funding body website
NICE decisions
▸ Tivozanib for treating advanced renal cell carcinoma (March 2018) NICE TA512 Recommended with restrictions
Scottish Medicines Consortium (SMC) decisions
▸ Tivozanib (*Fotivda*®) for the first-line treatment of adult patients with advanced renal cell carcinoma (RCC) and for adult patients who are vascular endothelial growth factor receptor and mammalian target of rapamycin pathway inhibitor-naive following disease progression after one prior treatment with cytokine therapy for advanced RCC (July 2018) SMC No. 1335/18 Recommended with restrictions

- **MEDICINAL FORMS** There can be variation in the licensing of different medicines containing the same drug.
Oral capsule
CAUTIONARY AND ADVISORY LABELS 25
▸ Fotivda (Recordati UK Ltd)
Tivozanib (as Tivozanib hydrochloride monohydrate) **890 microgram** Fotivda 890microgram capsules | 21 capsule [PoM] £2,052.00 (Hospital only)
Tivozanib (as Tivozanib hydrochloride monohydrate) **1.34 mg** Fotivda 1340microgram capsules | 21 capsule [PoM] £2,052.00 (Hospital only)

Trametinib [Specialist drug]

20-Jun-2024

- **INDICATIONS AND DOSE**
Melanoma | Non-small cell lung cancer
▸ BY MOUTH USING FILM-COATED TABLETS
▸ Adult: Specialist drug – access specialist resources for dosing information

---

IMPORTANT SAFETY INFORMATION

MHRA/CHM ADVICE (MARCH 2016): TRAMETINIB: RISK OF GASTROINTESTINAL PERFORATION AND COLITIS

A review by EU medicines regulators has concluded that trametinib can cause gastrointestinal perforation or colitis.

Trametinib should be used with caution in patients with risk factors for gastrointestinal perforation, such as gastrointestinal metastases, diverticulitis, or use of concomitant medicines that can cause gastrointestinal perforation. Prescribers should be vigilant for signs and symptoms of gastrointestinal perforation and should advise patients to seek urgent medical attention if they develop severe abdominal pain.

RISKS OF INCORRECT DOSING OF ORAL ANTI-CANCER MEDICINES
See Cytotoxic drugs p. 1027.

- **CONTRA-INDICATIONS** History of retinal vein occlusion
- **INTERACTIONS** → Appendix 1: trametinib
- **SIDE-EFFECTS**
▸ **Common or very common** Abdominal pain · alopecia · anaemia · asthenia · bradycardia · constipation · cough · dehydration · diarrhoea · dizziness · dry mouth · dyspnoea · eye inflammation · fever · haemorrhage · hypersensitivity · hypertension · hyponatraemia · hypotension · increased risk of infection · interstitial lung disease · intracranial

haemorrhage · left ventricular dysfunction · leucopenia · lymphoedema · mucositis · muscle spasms · musculoskeletal stiffness · nausea · nerve disorders · neutropenia · oedema · skin reactions · stomatitis · sweat changes · thrombocytopenia · vision disorders · vomiting
▸ **Uncommon** Chorioretinopathy · embolism and thrombosis · eye disorders · gastrointestinal disorders · heart failure · rhabdomyolysis · sarcoidosis
▸ **Rare or very rare** Haemophagocytic lymphohistiocytosis
▸ **Frequency not known** Atrioventricular block · myocarditis · severe cutaneous adverse reactions (SCARs)
● **CONCEPTION AND CONTRACEPTION** [EvGr] Females of childbearing potential should use effective contraception during treatment and for 16 weeks after last treatment. ⟨M⟩
● **PATIENT AND CARER ADVICE** Patients and their carers should be told to seek immediate medical attention if symptoms of pulmonary embolism or deep vein thrombosis occur; patients and their carers should also be advised to report new visual disturbances. Patients and carers should be counselled on the administration of trametinib.

If vomiting occurs after taking trametinib, no additional dose should be taken and the next dose should be taken at the normal time.
Missed doses If a dose is more than 12 hours late, the missed dose should not be taken and the next dose should be taken at the normal time.
Driving and skilled tasks Patients and carers should be counselled on the effects on driving and performance of skilled tasks—increased risk of fatigue, dizziness, and visual disturbances.

● **NATIONAL FUNDING/ACCESS DECISIONS**
For full details see funding body website
NICE decisions
▸ **Trametinib in combination with dabrafenib for treating unresectable or metastatic melanoma (June 2016)** NICE TA396 Recommended with restrictions
▸ **Dabrafenib with trametinib for adjuvant treatment of resected BRAF V600 mutation-positive melanoma (October 2018)** NICE TA544 Recommended with restrictions

Scottish Medicines Consortium (SMC) decisions
▸ **Trametinib (*Mekinist*®) in combination with dabrafenib for the treatment of adult patients with unresectable or metastatic melanoma with a BRAF V600 mutation [for first-line treatment] (September 2016)** SMC No. 1161/16 Recommended with restrictions
▸ **Trametinib (*Mekinist*®) in combination with dabrafenib for the treatment of adult patients with unresectable or metastatic melanoma with a BRAF V600 mutation [after first-line treatment] (March 2021)** SMC No. SMC2328 Recommended with restrictions

● **MEDICINAL FORMS** There can be variation in the licensing of different medicines containing the same drug.
Oral tablet
CAUTIONARY AND ADVISORY LABELS 23, 25
▸ **Mekinist** (Novartis Pharmaceuticals UK Ltd)
Trametinib (as Trametinib dimethyl sulfoxide)
500 microgram Mekinist 0.5mg tablets | 7 tablet [PoM] £280.00 (Hospital only) | 30 tablet [PoM] £1,200.00 (Hospital only)
Trametinib (as Trametinib dimethyl sulfoxide) 2 mg Mekinist 2mg tablets | 7 tablet [PoM] £1,120.00 (Hospital only) | 30 tablet [PoM] £4,800.00 (Hospital only)

Tucatinib [Specialist drug]   04-May-2022

● **INDICATIONS AND DOSE**
Breast cancer
▸ BY MOUTH
▸ **Adult:** Specialist drug – access specialist resources for dosing information

---

IMPORTANT SAFETY INFORMATION
RISKS OF INCORRECT DOSING OF ORAL ANTI-CANCER MEDICINES
See Cytotoxic drugs p. 1027.

● **INTERACTIONS** → Appendix 1: tucatinib
● **SIDE-EFFECTS**
▸ **Common or very common** Arthralgia · diarrhoea · epistaxis · hyperbilirubinaemia · nausea · oral disorders · oropharyngeal pain · rash pustular · skin reactions · vomiting · weight decreased

SIDE-EFFECTS, FURTHER INFORMATION Diarrhoea may be severe and associated with dehydration, hypotension, acute kidney injury and death. For management of diarrhoea, consult product literature.
● **CONCEPTION AND CONTRACEPTION** [EvGr] Females of childbearing potential and male patients with a partner of childbearing potential should use effective contraception during treatment and for at least 7 days after last treatment. ⟨M⟩
● **NATIONAL FUNDING/ACCESS DECISIONS**
For full details see funding body website
NICE decisions
▸ **Tucatinib with trastuzumab and capecitabine for treating HER2-positive advanced breast cancer after 2 or more anti-HER2 therapies (April 2022)** NICE TA786 Recommended
Scottish Medicines Consortium (SMC) decisions
▸ **Tucatinib (*Tukysa*®) in combination with trastuzumab and capecitabine for the treatment of adult patients with HER2-positive locally advanced or metastatic breast cancer who have received at least two prior anti-HER2 treatment regimens (January 2022)** SMC No. SMC2398 Recommended

---

● **MEDICINAL FORMS** There can be variation in the licensing of different medicines containing the same drug.
Oral tablet
ELECTROLYTES: May contain Potassium, sodium
▸ **Tukysa** (Pfizer Ltd) ▼
Tucatinib 50 mg Tukysa 50mg tablets | 88 tablet [PoM] £1,968.42 (Hospital only)
Tucatinib 150 mg Tukysa 150mg tablets | 84 tablet [PoM] £5,636.84 (Hospital only)

Vandetanib [Specialist drug]   10-Aug-2021

● **INDICATIONS AND DOSE**
Medullary thyroid cancer
▸ BY MOUTH
▸ **Adult:** Specialist drug – access specialist resources for dosing information

---

IMPORTANT SAFETY INFORMATION
MHRA/CHM ADVICE: SYSTEMICALLY ADMINISTERED VEGF PATHWAY INHIBITORS: RISK OF ANEURYSM AND ARTERY DISSECTION (JULY 2020)
A European review of worldwide data concluded that systemically administered VEGF pathway inhibitors may lead to aneurysm and artery dissection in patients with or without hypertension. Some fatal cases have been reported, mainly in relation to aortic aneurysm rupture and aortic dissection. The MHRA advises healthcare professionals to carefully consider the risk of aneurysm and artery dissection in patients with risk factors before

Immune system and malignant disease

initiating treatment with vandetanib; any modifiable risk factors (such as smoking and hypertension) should be reduced as much as possible. Blood pressure should be monitored regularly, and product literature should be consulted if hypertension occurs during treatment.

RISKS OF INCORRECT DOSING OF ORAL ANTI-CANCER MEDICINES See Cytotoxic drugs p. 1027.

- **CONTRA-INDICATIONS** Congenital long QT syndrome · QT interval greater than 480 milliseconds
- **INTERACTIONS** → Appendix 1: vandetanib
- **SIDE-EFFECTS**
‣ **Common or very common** Alopecia · anxiety · appetite decreased · asthenia · cerebral ischaemia · cholelithiasis · constipation · corneal deposits · cystitis · dehydration · depression · diarrhoea · dizziness · dry eye · dry mouth · dysphagia · electrolyte imbalance · eye disorders · eye inflammation · fever · gastrointestinal discomfort · gastrointestinal disorders · glaucoma · haemorrhage · headache · hyperglycaemia · hypertension · hypothyroidism · increased risk of infection · insomnia · interstitial lung disease · lethargy · loss of consciousness · movement disorders · nail disorder · nausea · nephrolithiasis · oedema · pain · photosensitivity reaction · proteinuria · QT interval prolongation · renal impairment · sensation abnormal · sepsis · skin reactions · stomatitis · taste altered · tremor · urinary disorders · vision disorders · vomiting · weight decreased
‣ **Uncommon** Arrhythmias · brain oedema · cardiac arrest · cardiac conduction disorder · cataract · healing impaired · heart failure · malnutrition · pancreatitis · posterior reversible encephalopathy syndrome (PRES) · respiratory failure · seizure · urine discolouration
‣ **Frequency not known** Aneurysm · artery dissection · intracranial haemorrhage · severe cutaneous adverse reactions (SCARs)
- **CONCEPTION AND CONTRACEPTION** Effective contraception required during and for at least 4 months after treatment.
- **PATIENT AND CARER ADVICE** Patients or carers should be given advice on how to administer vandetanib tablets.
Phototoxicity reactions Patients should be advised to wear protective clothing and/or sunscreen.
Alert card An alert card should be provided.
- **NATIONAL FUNDING/ACCESS DECISIONS**
For full details see funding body website

NICE decisions
‣ Vandetanib for treating medullary thyroid cancer (December 2018) NICE TA550 Not recommended

- **MEDICINAL FORMS** There can be variation in the licensing of different medicines containing the same drug.
Oral tablet
‣ Caprelsa (Sanofi)
Vandetanib 100 mg Caprelsa 100mg tablets | 30 tablet [PoM] £2,500.00
Vandetanib 300 mg Caprelsa 300mg tablets | 30 tablet [PoM] £5,000.00

Vemurafenib [Specialist drug]

10-Jun-2021

- **INDICATIONS AND DOSE**
Melanoma
▶ BY MOUTH
▶ Adult: Specialist drug – access specialist resources for dosing information

---

IMPORTANT SAFETY INFORMATION
DRUG RASH WITH EOSINOPHILIA AND SYSTEMIC SYMPTOMS (DRESS SYNDROME)
DRESS syndrome has been reported in patients taking vemurafenib. DRESS syndrome starts with rash, fever, swollen glands, and increased white cell count, and it can affect the liver, kidneys and lungs; DRESS can also be fatal.

Patients should be advised to stop taking vemurafenib and consult their doctor immediately if skin rash develops. Treatment with vemurafenib should not be restarted.

MHRA/CHM ADVICE (NOVEMBER 2015): RISK OF POTENTIATION OF RADIATION TOXICITY
Potentiation of radiation toxicity has been reported in patients treated with vemurafenib before, during, or after radiotherapy— use with caution.

RISKS OF INCORRECT DOSING OF ORAL ANTI-CANCER MEDICINES See Cytotoxic drugs p. 1027.

- **CONTRA-INDICATIONS** QT interval greater than 500 milliseconds (do not initiate) · wild-type BRAF malignant melanoma
- **INTERACTIONS** → Appendix 1: vemurafenib
- **SIDE-EFFECTS**
‣ **Common or very common** 7th nerve paralysis · alopecia · appetite decreased · arthralgia · arthritis · asthenia · connective tissue disorders · constipation · cough · diarrhoea · dizziness · eye inflammation · fever · folliculitis · headache · myalgia · nausea · neoplasms · pain · panniculitis · peripheral oedema · photosensitivity reaction · QT interval prolongation · radiation injuries · skin reactions · taste altered · vomiting · weight decreased
‣ **Uncommon** Liver injury · neutropenia · pancreatitis · peripheral neuropathy · retinal occlusion · severe cutaneous adverse reactions (SCARs) · vasculitis
‣ **Rare or very rare** Acute tubular necrosis · nephritis acute interstitial
‣ **Frequency not known** Acute kidney injury
- **CONCEPTION AND CONTRACEPTION** [EvGr] Women of childbearing potential should use effective contraception during treatment and for at least 6 months after treatment. Ⓜ
- **PATIENT AND CARER ADVICE** Counselling advised (administration).
Drug rash with eosinophilia and systemic symptoms (DRESS syndrome) Patients should be advised to stop taking vemurafenib and consult their doctor immediately if skin rash develops.
- **NATIONAL FUNDING/ACCESS DECISIONS**
For full details see funding body website

NICE decisions
‣ Vemurafenib for treating locally advanced or metastatic BRAF V600 mutation-positive malignant melanoma (updated January 2015) NICE TA269 Recommended with restrictions

Scottish Medicines Consortium (SMC) decisions
‣ Vemurafenib (*Zelboraf*®) as monotherapy for the treatment of adult patients with BRAF V600 mutation-positive unresectable or metastatic melanoma (December 2013) SMC No. 792/12 Recommended with restrictions

- **MEDICINAL FORMS** There can be variation in the licensing of different medicines containing the same drug.

Oral tablet

CAUTIONARY AND ADVISORY LABELS 25

▸ **Zelboraf** (Roche Products Ltd)
Vemurafenib 240 mg Zelboraf 240mg tablets | 56 tablet [PoM] £1,750.00 (Hospital only)

Zanubrutinib [Specialist drug]
30-Dec-2024

- **INDICATIONS AND DOSE**

Waldenström's macroglobulinaemia | Marginal zone lymphoma | Chronic lymphocytic leukaemia

▸ BY MOUTH

▸ Adult: Specialist drug – access specialist resources for dosing information

IMPORTANT SAFETY INFORMATION

RISKS OF INCORRECT DOSING OF ORAL ANTI-CANCER MEDICINES

See Cytotoxic drugs p. 1027.

- **INTERACTIONS** → Appendix 1: zanubrutinib

- **SIDE-EFFECTS**

▸ **Common or very common** Anaemia · arrhythmias · arthralgia · asthenia · constipation · cough · diarrhoea · dizziness · haemorrhage · hypertension · increased risk of infection · neutropenia · pain · peripheral oedema · skin reactions · thrombocytopenia

▸ **Uncommon** Hepatitis B reactivation · tumour lysis syndrome

▸ **Frequency not known** Haemothorax · intracranial haemorrhage · neoplasms · sepsis

- **CONCEPTION AND CONTRACEPTION** [EvGr] Females of childbearing potential should use highly effective contraception during and for up to one month after stopping treatment; additional barrier method required if using hormonal contraceptives. ⟨M⟩

- **PATIENT AND CARER ADVICE** Patients should be advised to use sun protection—risk of secondary skin cancers.
Driving and skilled tasks Patients and carers should be counselled on the effects on driving and performance of skilled tasks—increased risk of dizziness, fatigue and asthenia.

- **NATIONAL FUNDING/ACCESS DECISIONS**
For full details see funding body website

NICE decisions

▸ Zanubrutinib for treating Waldenstrom's macroglobulinaemia (October 2022) NICE TA833 Recommended with restrictions

▸ Zanubrutinib for treating chronic lymphocytic leukaemia (November 2023) NICE TA931 Recommended with restrictions

▸ Zanubrutinib for treating marginal zone lymphoma after anti-CD20-based treatment (September 2024) NICE TA1001 Recommended

Scottish Medicines Consortium (SMC) decisions

▸ Zanubrutinib (*Brukinsa*®) as monotherapy for the treatment of adult patients with Waldenström's macroglobulinaemia who have received at least one prior therapy, or in first-line treatment for patients unsuitable for chemo-immunotherapy (November 2022) SMC No. SMC2528 Recommended

▸ Zanubrutinib (*Brukinsa*®) as monotherapy for the treatment of adult patients with chronic lymphocytic leukaemia (October 2023) SMC No. SMC2600 Recommended with restrictions

▸ Zanubrutinib (*Brukinsa*®) as monotherapy for the treatment of adult patients with marginal zone lymphoma who have received at least one prior anti-CD20-based therapy (December 2024) SMC No. SMC2684 Recommended

- **MEDICINAL FORMS** There can be variation in the licensing of different medicines containing the same drug.

Oral capsule

CAUTIONARY AND ADVISORY LABELS 25

▸ **Brukinsa** (BeiGene UK Ltd) ▼
Zanubrutinib 80 mg Brukinsa 80mg capsules | 120 capsule [PoM] £4,928.65 (Hospital only)

ANTINEOPLASTIC DRUGS › OTHER

Belzutifan [Specialist drug]
21-Oct-2024

- **INDICATIONS AND DOSE**

Von Hippel-Lindau disease-associated tumours

▸ BY MOUTH

▸ Adult: Specialist drug – access specialist resources for dosing information

- **INTERACTIONS** → Appendix 1: belzutifan

- **SIDE-EFFECTS**

▸ **Common or very common** Anaemia · dizziness · dyspnoea · fatigue · hypoxia · nausea

- **CONCEPTION AND CONTRACEPTION** [EvGr] Females of childbearing potential and male patients, including their female partners of childbearing potential, should use highly effective contraception during treatment and for at least 1 week after last treatment; an additional barrier method of contraception should be used in female patients using hormonal contraceptives. ⟨M⟩

- **PATIENT AND CARER ADVICE** Patients should be counselled on smoking cessation—risk of hypoxia.
Alert card A patient alert card should be provided.
Driving and skilled tasks Patients and carers should be cautioned on the effects on driving and performance of skilled tasks—increased risk of dizziness and fatigue.

- **NATIONAL FUNDING/ACCESS DECISIONS**
For full details see funding body website

NICE decisions

▸ Belzutifan for treating tumours associated with von Hippel-Lindau disease (October 2024) NICE TA1011 Recommended

Scottish Medicines Consortium (SMC) decisions

▸ Belzutifan (*Welireg*®) for the treatment of adult patients with von Hippel-Lindau (VHL) disease who require therapy for VHL associated renal cell carcinoma, central nervous system hemangioblastomas, or pancreatic neuroendocrine tumours, and for whom localised procedures are unsuitable or undesirable (October 2023) SMC No. SMC2587 Recommended

- **MEDICINAL FORMS** There can be variation in the licensing of different medicines containing the same drug.

Oral tablet

▸ **Welireg** (Merck Sharp & Dohme (UK) Ltd) ▼
Belzutifan 40 mg Welireg 40mg tablets | 90 tablet [PoM] £11,936.70 (Hospital only)

Glasdegib [Specialist drug]
02-Mar-2022

- **INDICATIONS AND DOSE**

Acute myeloid leukaemia

▸ BY MOUTH

▸ Adult: Specialist drug – access specialist resources for dosing information

IMPORTANT SAFETY INFORMATION

RISKS OF INCORRECT DOSING OF ORAL ANTI-CANCER MEDICINES

See Cytotoxic drugs p. 1027.

- **INTERACTIONS** → Appendix 1: glasdegib

8
Immune system and malignant disease

- **SIDE-EFFECTS**
▶ **Common or very common** Alopecia · anaemia · appetite decreased · arrhythmias · arthralgia · CNS haemorrhage · constipation · diarrhoea · dyspnoea · eye contusion · fatigue · fever · gastrointestinal discomfort · haemorrhage · increased risk of infection · muscle complaints · muscle contractions involuntary · musculoskeletal pain · nausea · neutropenia · peripheral oedema · QT interval prolongation · sepsis · skin reactions · stomatitis · taste altered · thrombocytopenia · vomiting · weight decreased

- **CONCEPTION AND CONTRACEPTION** Manufacturer advises females of childbearing potential and male patients with a partner who is pregnant or of childbearing potential should use effective contraception (including condoms in males) during treatment and for at least 30 days after last dose. Fertility may be impaired in males and females—consult product literature.

- **PATIENT AND CARER ADVICE**
Vomiting Manufacturer advises if vomiting occurs after taking tablets, no additional dose should be taken on that day and the next dose should be taken at the usual time.
Missed doses Manufacturer advises if a dose is more than 10 hours late, the missed dose should not be taken and the next dose should be taken at the usual time.
Driving and skilled tasks Manufacturer advises patients and carers should be cautioned on the effects on driving and performance of skilled tasks—increased risk of fatigue, muscle cramps, pain, or nausea.

- **MEDICINAL FORMS** There can be variation in the licensing of different medicines containing the same drug.
Oral tablet
▶ **Daurismo** (Pfizer Ltd) ▼
Glasdegib (as Glasdegib maleate) 25 mg Daurismo 25mg tablets | 60 tablet PoM £10,517.00 (Hospital only)
Glasdegib (as Glasdegib maleate) 100 mg Daurismo 100mg tablets | 30 tablet PoM £10,517.00 (Hospital only)

Ivosidenib [Specialist drug]

18-Sep-2024

- **INDICATIONS AND DOSE**
Acute myeloid leukaemia | Cholangiocarcinoma
▶ BY MOUTH
▶ Adult: Specialist drug – access specialist resources for dosing information

IMPORTANT SAFETY INFORMATION
RISKS OF INCORRECT DOSING OF ORAL ANTI-CANCER MEDICINES
See Cytotoxic drugs p. 1027.

- **CONTRA-INDICATIONS** Congenital long QT syndrome · family history of sudden death or polymorphic ventricular arrhythmia · QT interval greater than 500 milliseconds
- **INTERACTIONS** → Appendix 1: ivosidenib
- **SIDE-EFFECTS**
▶ **Common or very common** Abdominal pain · anaemia · appetite decreased · ascites · diarrhoea · fall · fatigue · headache · hyperbilirubinaemia · hypersensitivity · jaundice cholestatic · nausea · peripheral neuropathy · QT interval prolongation · skin reactions · vomiting
▶ **Frequency not known** Differentiation syndrome
- **CONCEPTION AND CONTRACEPTION** EvGr Females of childbearing potential and male patients with a partner of childbearing potential should use effective contraception during treatment and for at least 1 month after last treatment; additional barrier method recommended in females using hormonal contraceptives. Ⓜ
- **PATIENT AND CARER ADVICE** Food should not be consumed for at least 2 hours before and at least 1 hour after each dose.

Vomiting If vomiting occurs after taking tablets, no additional dose should be taken on that day and the next dose should be taken at the usual time.
Alert card A patient alert card should be provided.
Missed doses If a dose is more than 12 hours late, the missed dose should not be taken and the next dose should be taken at the normal time.
Driving and skilled tasks Patients and carers should be counselled on the effects on driving and performance of skilled tasks—increased risk of fatigue and dizziness.

- **NATIONAL FUNDING/ACCESS DECISIONS**
For full details see funding body website
NICE decisions
▶ **Ivosidenib for treating advanced cholangiocarcinoma with an IDH1 R132 mutation after 1 or more systemic treatments (January 2024)** NICE TA948 Recommended
▶ **Ivosidenib with azacitidine for untreated acute myeloid leukaemia with an IDH1 R132 mutation (June 2024)** NICE TA979 Recommended

Scottish Medicines Consortium (SMC) decisions
▶ **Ivosidenib (*Tibsovo* ®) in combination with azacitidine for the treatment of adult patients with newly diagnosed acute myeloid leukaemia (AML) with an isocitrate dehydrogenase-1 (IDH1) R132 mutation who are not eligible to receive standard induction chemotherapy (March 2024)** SMC No. SMC2615 Recommended
▶ **Ivosidenib (*Tibsovo* ®) as monotherapy for the treatment of adult patients with locally advanced or metastatic cholangiocarcinoma with an isocitrate dehydrogenase-1 R132 mutation who were previously treated by at least one prior line of systemic therapy (September 2024)** SMC No. SMC2664 Recommended

- **MEDICINAL FORMS** There can be variation in the licensing of different medicines containing the same drug.
Oral tablet
▶ **Tibsovo** (Servier Laboratories Ltd) ▼
Ivosidenib 250 mg Tibsovo 250mg tablets | 60 tablet PoM £12,500.00 (Hospital only)

Niraparib [Specialist drug]

04-May-2022

- **INDICATIONS AND DOSE**
Ovarian cancer | Fallopian tube cancer | Peritoneal cancer
▶ BY MOUTH
▶ Adult: Specialist drug – access specialist resources for dosing information

IMPORTANT SAFETY INFORMATION
RISKS OF INCORRECT DOSING OF ORAL ANTI-CANCER MEDICINES
See Cytotoxic drugs p. 1027.

MHRA/CHM ADVICE: NIRAPARIB (*ZEJULA* ®): REPORTS OF SEVERE HYPERTENSION AND POSTERIOR REVERSIBLE ENCEPHALOPATHY SYNDROME (PRES), PARTICULARLY IN EARLY TREATMENT (OCTOBER 2020)
A European review of niraparib safety data identified worldwide reports of severe hypertension, including rare cases of hypertensive crisis, some with onset in the first month of treatment. Rare cases of PRES have also been reported, mostly associated with hypertension and within the first month of treatment.

Healthcare professionals are advised to control pre-existing hypertension before starting niraparib. Blood pressure should be monitored at least weekly for the first 2 months of treatment, then monthly for the first year, and periodically thereafter. Home blood pressure monitoring may be considered if appropriate; patients should be trained and advised to contact their doctor in case of an increase in blood pressure.

Hypertension during treatment should be managed with antihypertensives; treatment interruption or dose adjustment of niraparib may be required—consult product literature. Niraparib should be discontinued in case of hypertensive crisis or medically significant hypertension that cannot be adequately controlled with antihypertensive therapy. In cases of PRES, niraparib should also be discontinued and patients treated for specific symptoms (including hypertension).

● **INTERACTIONS** → Appendix 1: niraparib

● **SIDE-EFFECTS**
▸ **Common or very common** Anaemia · angioedema · anxiety · appetite decreased · arthralgia · asthenia · back pain · cognitive impairment · concentration impaired · conjunctivitis · constipation · cough · depression · diarrhoea · dizziness · dry mouth · dyspnoea · epistaxis · gastrointestinal discomfort · headache · hypersensitivity · hypertension · hypokalaemia · increased risk of infection · insomnia · leucopenia · memory impairment · mucositis · myalgia · nausea · neutropenia · palpitations · peripheral oedema · photosensitivity reaction · skin reactions · stomatitis · tachycardia · taste altered · thrombocytopenia · vomiting · weight decreased
▸ **Uncommon** Confusion · pancytopenia · pneumonitis
▸ **Rare or very rare** Posterior reversible encephalopathy syndrome (PRES)
▸ **Frequency not known** Acute myeloid leukaemia (discontinue permanently) · hot flush · myelodysplastic syndrome (discontinue permanently)

● **CONCEPTION AND CONTRACEPTION** Manufacturer advises effective contraception in women of childbearing potential during treatment and for 1 month after receiving the last dose.

● **PATIENT AND CARER ADVICE**
Driving and skilled tasks Manufacturer advises patients and their carers should be counselled on the effects on driving and skilled tasks—increased risk of dizziness and fatigue.

● **NATIONAL FUNDING/ACCESS DECISIONS**
For full details see funding body website
NICE decisions
▸ Niraparib for maintenance treatment of advanced ovarian, fallopian tube and peritoneal cancer after response to first-line platinum-based chemotherapy (February 2021) NICE TA673 Recommended
▸ Niraparib for maintenance treatment of relapsed, platinum-sensitive ovarian, fallopian tube and peritoneal cancer (April 2022) NICE TA784 Recommended with restrictions
Scottish Medicines Consortium (SMC) decisions
▸ Niraparib tosylate monohydrate (*Zejula*®) as monotherapy for the maintenance treatment of adult patients with platinum-sensitive relapsed high grade serous epithelial ovarian, fallopian tube, or primary peritoneal cancer who are in response (complete or partial) to platinum-based chemotherapy (August 2018) SMC No. 1341/18 Recommended with restrictions
▸ Niraparib (*Zejula*®) as monotherapy for the maintenance treatment of adult patients with advanced epithelial (FIGO Stages III and IV) high-grade ovarian, fallopian tube or primary peritoneal cancer who are in response (complete or partial) following completion of first-line platinum-based chemotherapy (May 2021) SMC No. SMC2338 Recommended

● **MEDICINAL FORMS** There can be variation in the licensing of different medicines containing the same drug.
Oral capsule
CAUTIONARY AND ADVISORY LABELS 25
▸ **Zejula** (GlaxoSmithKline UK Ltd)
Niraparib (as Niraparib tosylate monohydrate) 100 mg Zejula 100mg capsules | 56 capsule [PoM] £4,500.00 (Hospital only) | 84 capsule [PoM] £6,750.00 (Hospital only)

Olaparib [Specialist drug]

27-Feb-2025

● **INDICATIONS AND DOSE**
Breast cancer | Adenocarcinoma of the pancreas | Prostate cancer | Ovarian cancer | Fallopian tube cancer | Peritoneal cancer
▸ BY MOUTH
▸ Adult: Specialist drug – access specialist resources for dosing information

> **IMPORTANT SAFETY INFORMATION**
> RISKS OF INCORRECT DOSING OF ORAL ANTI-CANCER MEDICINES
> See Cytotoxic drugs p. 1027.

● **INTERACTIONS** → Appendix 1: olaparib

● **SIDE-EFFECTS**
▸ **Common or very common** Agranulocytosis · anaemia · appetite decreased · asthenia · cough · decreased leucocytes · diarrhoea · dizziness · dyspnoea · erythropenia · gastrointestinal discomfort · headache · nausea · neutropenia · neutropenic infection · neutropenic sepsis · oral disorders · skin reactions · taste altered · thrombocytopenia · vomiting
▸ **Uncommon** Angioedema
▸ **Rare or very rare** Erythema nodosum
▸ **Frequency not known** Haematotoxicity · neoplasms · pneumonitis

SIDE-EFFECTS, FURTHER INFORMATION **Haematological toxicity** Withhold treatment if severe haematological toxicity develops; further analysis recommended if toxicity still present 4 weeks after treatment withdrawal.

Pneumonitis If dyspnoea, cough and fever, or radiological abnormalities develop, withhold treatment and investigate; if pneumonitis confirmed, discontinue.

● **CONCEPTION AND CONTRACEPTION** Manufacturer advises females of childbearing potential should use 2 methods of effective contraception during treatment and for 1 month after last treatment; male patients should use effective contraception during treatment and for 3 months after last treatment if their partner is pregnant or of childbearing potential.

● **PATIENT AND CARER ADVICE**
Driving and skilled tasks Manufacturer advises patients should be counselled on the effects on driving and performance of skilled tasks—increased risk of malaise and dizziness.

● **NATIONAL FUNDING/ACCESS DECISIONS**
For full details see funding body website
NICE decisions
▸ Olaparib for maintenance treatment of relapsed, platinum-sensitive ovarian, fallopian tube or peritoneal cancer after 2 or more courses of platinum-based chemotherapy (July 2023) NICE TA908 Recommended with restrictions
▸ Olaparib with bevacizumab for maintenance treatment of advanced high-grade epithelial ovarian, fallopian tube or primary peritoneal cancer (January 2024) NICE TA946 Recommended
▸ Olaparib for maintenance treatment of BRCA mutation-positive advanced ovarian, fallopian tube or peritoneal cancer after response to first-line platinum-based chemotherapy (March 2024) NICE TA962 Recommended
▸ Olaparib for adjuvant treatment of BRCA mutation-positive HER2-negative high-risk early breast cancer after chemotherapy (May 2023) NICE TA886 Recommended
▸ Olaparib for treating BRCA mutation-positive HER2-negative advanced breast cancer after chemotherapy (February 2025) NICE TA1040 Recommended
▸ Olaparib for previously treated BRCA mutation-positive hormone-relapsed metastatic prostate cancer (May 2023) NICE TA887 Recommended

- Olaparib with abiraterone for untreated hormone-relapsed metastatic prostate cancer (February 2024) NICE TA951 Recommended

Scottish Medicines Consortium (SMC) decisions

- Olaparib (*Lynparza*®) tablets as monotherapy for the maintenance treatment of adult patients with newly diagnosed advanced (FIGO stages III and IV) BRCA1/2-mutated (germline and/or somatic) high-grade epithelial ovarian, fallopian tube or primary peritoneal cancer who are in response (complete or partial) following completion of first line platinum-based chemotherapy (December 2019) SMC No. SMC2209 Recommended
- Olaparib (*Lynparza*®) tablets as monotherapy for the maintenance treatment of adult patients with platinum-sensitive relapsed high-grade epithelial ovarian, fallopian tube, or primary peritoneal cancer who are in response (complete or partial) to platinum-based chemotherapy (August 2021) SMC No. SMC2367 Recommended with restrictions
- Olaparib (*Lynparza*®) tablets in combination with bevacizumab for the maintenance treatment of adults with advanced high-grade epithelial ovarian, fallopian tube or primary peritoneal cancer who are in response (complete or partial) following completion of first-line platinum-based chemotherapy in combination with bevacizumab, and whose cancer is associated with homologous recombination deficiency (December 2021) SMC No. SMC2368 Recommended
- Olaparib (*Lynparza*®) as monotherapy for the treatment of adult patients with metastatic castration-resistant prostate cancer and BRCA1/2-mutations (germline and/or somatic) who have progressed following prior therapy that included a new hormonal agent (October 2021) SMC No. SMC2366 Recommended
- Olaparib (*Lynparza*®) in combination with abiraterone and prednisone or prednisolone for the treatment of adult patients with metastatic castration-resistant prostate cancer in whom chemotherapy is not clinically indicated (March 2024) SMC No. SMC2617 Recommended
- Olaparib (*Lynparza*®) as monotherapy for the adjuvant treatment of adult patients with germline BRCA1/2-mutations who have HER2-negative, high-risk early breast cancer who have previously been treated with neoadjuvant or adjuvant chemotherapy (October 2023) SMC No. SMC2518 Recommended
- Olaparib (*Lynparza*®) as monotherapy for the treatment of adult patients with germline BRCA1/2-mutations, who have HER2-negative locally advanced or metastatic breast cancer and have previously been treated with an anthracycline and a taxane in the (neo)adjuvant or metastatic setting, unless not suitable. Patients with hormone receptor-positive breast cancer should also have progressed on or after prior endocrine therapy, unless not suitable (February 2025) SMC No. SMC2737 Recommended

- **MEDICINAL FORMS** There can be variation in the licensing of different medicines containing the same drug.

Oral tablet

CAUTIONARY AND ADVISORY LABELS 25

- Lynparza (AstraZeneca UK Ltd)

  Olaparib 100 mg Lynparza 100mg tablets | 56 tablet PoM £2,317.50 DT = £2,317.50

  Olaparib 150 mg Lynparza 150mg tablets | 56 tablet PoM £2,317.50 DT = £2,317.50

Rucaparib [Specialist drug]

25-Apr-2025

- **INDICATIONS AND DOSE**

Ovarian cancer | **Fallopian tube cancer** | **Peritoneal cancer**

- BY MOUTH
- Adult: Specialist drug – access specialist resources for dosing information

IMPORTANT SAFETY INFORMATION

RISKS OF INCORRECT DOSING OF ORAL ANTI-CANCER MEDICINES See Cytotoxic drugs p. 1027.

MHRA/CHM ADVICE: RUCAPARIB (*RUBRACA*®): WITHDRAWAL OF THIRD-LINE TREATMENT INDICATION (SEPTEMBER 2022)

A European review of the findings of the ARIEL4 study has recommended withdrawal of the third-line treatment indication of rucaparib for ovarian, fallopian tube, or peritoneal cancer, as a lower overall survival has been shown when compared with standard chemotherapy. Patients currently taking rucaparib for this indication should be informed of the latest data and offered alternative treatment options.

This advice does not affect its use as maintenance treatment of patients who are in complete or partial response to platinum-based chemotherapy.

- **INTERACTIONS** → Appendix 1: rucaparib
- **SIDE-EFFECTS**
- **Common or very common** Acute myeloid leukaemia (discontinue) · anaemia · appetite decreased · asthenia · decreased leucocytes · dehydration · diarrhoea · dizziness · dyspnoea · eye swelling · facial swelling · fever · gastrointestinal discomfort · hypercholesterolaemia · hypersensitivity · lethargy · myelodysplastic syndrome (discontinue) · nausea · neutropenia · photosensitivity reaction · skin reactions · taste altered · thrombocytopenia · vomiting
- **Frequency not known** Memory loss
- **CONCEPTION AND CONTRACEPTION** Manufacturer advises effective contraception in women of childbearing potential during treatment and for 6 months after receiving the last dose.
- **PATIENT AND CARER ADVICE**

Driving and skilled tasks Manufacturer advises patients and their carers should be counselled on the effects on driving and performance of skilled tasks—increased risk of dizziness and fatigue.

- **NATIONAL FUNDING/ACCESS DECISIONS** For full details see funding body website

NICE decisions

- Rucaparib for maintenance treatment of relapsed platinum-sensitive ovarian, fallopian tube or peritoneal cancer (September 2024) NICE TA1007 Recommended
- Rucaparib for maintenance treatment of advanced ovarian, fallopian tube and peritoneal cancer after response to first-line platinum-based chemotherapy (April 2025) NICE TA1055 Recommended with restrictions

Scottish Medicines Consortium (SMC) decisions

- Rucaparib (*Rubraca*®) as monotherapy for the maintenance treatment of adult patients with platinum-sensitive relapsed high-grade epithelial ovarian, fallopian tube, or primary peritoneal cancer who are in response (complete or partial) to platinum-based chemotherapy (March 2020) SMC No. SMC2224 Recommended with restrictions

- **MEDICINAL FORMS** There can be variation in the licensing of different medicines containing the same drug.

Oral tablet

- Rubraca (pharmaand GmbH)

  Rucaparib (as Rucaparib camsilate) 200 mg Rubraca 200mg tablets | 60 tablet PoM £3,562.00 (Hospital only)

Rucaparib (as Rucaparib camsilate) 250 mg Rubraca 250mg tablets | 60 tablet [PoM] £3,562.00 (Hospital only)
Rucaparib (as Rucaparib camsilate) 300 mg Rubraca 300mg tablets | 60 tablet [PoM] £3,562.00 (Hospital only)

Selinexor [Specialist drug]
21-Oct-2024

● INDICATIONS AND DOSE

Multiple myeloma
▸ BY MOUTH
▸ Adult: Specialist drug – access specialist resources for dosing information

---

IMPORTANT SAFETY INFORMATION
RISKS OF INCORRECT DOSING OF ORAL ANTI-CANCER MEDICINES
See Cytotoxic drugs p. 1027.

● SIDE-EFFECTS
▸ **Common or very common** Acute kidney injury · alopecia · anaemia · appetite decreased · asthenia · balance impaired · cataract · chills · cognitive disorder · concentration impaired · confusion · constipation · cough · decreased leucocytes · dehydration · delirium · diarrhoea · dizziness · dry mouth · dyspnoea · electrolyte imbalance · fall · fever · flatulence · gait abnormal · gastrointestinal discomfort · haemorrhage · hallucination · headache · hyperamylasaemia · hypercreatininaemia · hyperglycaemia · hyperlipasaemia · hyperuricaemia · hypotension · increased risk of infection · insomnia · malaise · memory impairment · muscle spasms · nausea · neutropenia · pain · peripheral neuropathy · sepsis · skin reactions · sweat changes · syncope · tachycardia · taste altered · thrombocytopenia · vertigo · vision disorders · vomiting · weight decreased
▸ **Uncommon** Encephalopathy · tumour lysis syndrome

● CONCEPTION AND CONTRACEPTION [EvGr] Effective contraception required during treatment and for at least 1 week after the last dose in male and female patients of reproductive potential. ⟨M⟩

● PATIENT AND CARER ADVICE
Driving and skilled tasks Patients and carers should be counselled on the effects on driving and performance of skilled tasks—increased risk of dizziness, fatigue, and confusion.

● NATIONAL FUNDING/ACCESS DECISIONS
For full details see funding body website
NICE decisions
▸ **Selinexor with dexamethasone for treating relapsed or refractory multiple myeloma after 4 or more treatments (May 2024)** NICE TA970 Recommended
▸ **Selinexor with bortezomib and dexamethasone for previously treated multiple myeloma (May 2024)** NICE TA974 Recommended with restrictions

Scottish Medicines Consortium (SMC) decisions
▸ **Selinexor (*Nexpovio*®) in combination with dexamethasone for the treatment of multiple myeloma in adult patients who have received at least four prior therapies and whose disease is refractory to at least two proteasome inhibitors, two immunomodulatory agents and an anti-CD38 monoclonal antibody, and who have demonstrated disease progression on the last therapy (October 2024)** SMC No. SMC2673 Recommended
▸ **Selinexor (*Nexpovio*®) in combination with bortezomib and dexamethasone for the treatment of adult patients with multiple myeloma who have received at least one prior therapy (October 2024)** SMC No. SMC2674 Recommended with restrictions

● MEDICINAL FORMS There can be variation in the licensing of different medicines containing the same drug.
Oral tablet
CAUTIONARY AND ADVISORY LABELS 25
▸ **Selinexor (Non-proprietary)**
   Selinexor 20 mg Xpovio 20mg tablets | 12 tablet [PoM] [▣] (Hospital only)
▸ **Nexpovio** (Menarini Stemline UK Ltd) ▼
   Selinexor 20 mg Nexpovio 20mg tablets | 8 tablet [PoM] £3,680.00 (Hospital only) | 12 tablet [PoM] £5,520.00 (Hospital only) | 16 tablet [PoM] £7,360.00 (Hospital only) | 20 tablet [PoM] £9,200.00 (Hospital only)

Sotorasib [Specialist drug]
31-Mar-2022

● INDICATIONS AND DOSE

Non-small cell lung cancer
▸ BY MOUTH
▸ Adult: Specialist drug – access specialist resources for dosing information

---

IMPORTANT SAFETY INFORMATION
RISKS OF INCORRECT DOSING OF ORAL ANTI-CANCER MEDICINES
See Cytotoxic drugs p. 1027.

● INTERACTIONS → Appendix 1: sotorasib

● SIDE-EFFECTS
▸ **Common or very common** Anaemia · appetite decreased · arthralgia · constipation · cough · diarrhoea · dyspnoea · electrolyte imbalance · fatigue · fever · gastrointestinal discomfort · headache · hepatic disorders · hypertension · increased risk of infection · myalgia · nausea · pain · peripheral oedema · rash · vomiting
▸ **Frequency not known** Interstitial lung disease

● PATIENT AND CARER ADVICE Patients and carers should be given advice on how to administer *Lumykras*® tablets.
Vomiting If vomiting occurs after taking tablets, no additional dose should be taken on that day and the next dose should be taken at the usual time.
Missed doses If a dose is more than 6 hours late, the missed dose should not be taken and the next dose should be taken at the normal time.

● NATIONAL FUNDING/ACCESS DECISIONS
For full details see funding body website
NICE decisions
▸ **Sotorasib for previously treated KRAS G12C mutation-positive advanced non-small-cell lung cancer (March 2022)** NICE TA781 Recommended

Scottish Medicines Consortium (SMC) decisions
▸ **Sotorasib (*Lumykras*®) as monotherapy for the treatment of adults with KRAS G12C-mutated, locally advanced or metastatic non-small cell lung cancer, who have progressed on, or are intolerant to, platinum-based chemotherapy and/or anti PD-1/PD-L1 immunotherapy (March 2022)** SMC No. SMC2443 Recommended

● MEDICINAL FORMS There can be variation in the licensing of different medicines containing the same drug.
Oral tablet
▸ **Lumykras** (Amgen Ltd) ▼
   Sotorasib 120 mg Lumykras 120mg tablets | 240 tablet [PoM] £6,907.35 (Hospital only)

Talazoparib [Specialist drug]

01-Apr-2025

● **INDICATIONS AND DOSE**

Breast cancer | Prostate cancer
▸ BY MOUTH
▸ Adult: Specialist drug – access specialist resources for dosing information

IMPORTANT SAFETY INFORMATION
RISKS OF INCORRECT DOSING OF ORAL ANTI-CANCER MEDICINES
See Cytotoxic drugs p. 1027.

● **INTERACTIONS** → Appendix 1: talazoparib

● **SIDE-EFFECTS**
▸ **Common or very common** Alopecia · anaemia · appetite decreased · asthenia · decreased leucocytes · diarrhoea · dizziness · gastrointestinal discomfort · headache · nausea · neutropenia · stomatitis · taste altered · thrombocytopenia · vomiting
▸ **Frequency not known** Bone marrow depression · neoplasms

● **CONCEPTION AND CONTRACEPTION** Manufacturer advises effective contraception in women of childbearing potential during treatment and for 7 months after receiving the last dose. Male patients should use effective contraception during and for at least 4 months after treatment if their partner is pregnant or of childbearing potential.

● **PATIENT AND CARER ADVICE**
Driving and skilled tasks Manufacturer advises patients and their carers should be counselled on the effects on driving and skilled tasks—increased risk of fatigue and dizziness.

● **NATIONAL FUNDING/ACCESS DECISIONS**
For full details see funding body website
NICE decisions
▸ Talazoparib for treating HER2-negative advanced breast cancer with germline BRCA mutations (February 2024) NICE TA952 Recommended

Scottish Medicines Consortium (SMC) decisions
▸ Talazoparib (*Talzenna*®) as monotherapy for the treatment of adult patients with germline BRCA1/2-mutations, who have HER2-negative locally advanced or metastatic breast cancer (March 2024) SMC No. SMC2607 Recommended
▸ Talazoparib (*Talzenna*®) in combination with enzalutamide for the treatment of adult patients with metastatic castration-resistant prostate cancer in whom chemotherapy is not clinically indicated (March 2025) SMC No. SMC2753 Recommended

● **MEDICINAL FORMS** There can be variation in the licensing of different medicines containing the same drug.
Oral capsule
CAUTIONARY AND ADVISORY LABELS 25
▸ Talzenna (Pfizer Ltd)
Talazoparib (as Talazoparib tosylate) 100 microgram Talzenna 0.1mg capsules | 30 capsule [PoM] £1,655.00 (Hospital only)
Talazoparib (as Talazoparib tosylate) 250 microgram Talzenna 0.25mg capsules | 30 capsule [PoM] £1,655.00 (Hospital only)
Talazoparib (as Talazoparib tosylate) 1 mg Talzenna 1mg capsules | 30 capsule [PoM] £4,965.00 (Hospital only)

Tebentafusp [Specialist drug]

25-Apr-2025

● **INDICATIONS AND DOSE**
Uveal melanoma
▸ BY INTRAVENOUS INFUSION
▸ Adult: Specialist drug – access specialist resources for dosing information

● **INTERACTIONS** → Appendix 1: tebentafusp

● **SIDE-EFFECTS**
▸ **Common or very common** Alopecia · anaemia · anxiety · appetite decreased · arrhythmias · arthralgia · asthenia · chills · constipation · cough · cytokine release syndrome · diarrhoea · dizziness · dyspnoea · electrolyte imbalance · eye inflammation · eyelash discolouration · facial swelling · fever · flushing · gastrointestinal discomfort · hair colour changes · headache · hepatic pain · hypertension · hypotension · hypoxia · inflammation · influenza like illness · insomnia · lip swelling · lymphopenia · muscle complaints · nasopharyngitis · nausea · night sweats · oedema · oropharyngeal pain · pain · paraesthesia · retinal discolouration · seborrhoea · skin reactions · solar dermatitis · taste altered · throat oedema · vomiting
▸ **Uncommon** Angina pectoris · tumour lysis syndrome
▸ **Frequency not known** QT interval prolongation

SIDE-EFFECTS, FURTHER INFORMATION Patients might need pre-medication to minimise the development of cytokine release syndrome; withhold or stop treatment depending on persistence and severity.

● **CONCEPTION AND CONTRACEPTION** [EvGr] Females of childbearing potential should use effective contraception during treatment and for at least 1 week after last treatment. Ⓜ

● **PATIENT AND CARER ADVICE** A patient guide should be provided.

● **NATIONAL FUNDING/ACCESS DECISIONS**
For full details see funding body website
NICE decisions
▸ Tebentafusp for treating advanced uveal melanoma (January 2025) NICE TA1027 Recommended

Scottish Medicines Consortium (SMC) decisions
▸ Tebentafusp (*Kimmtrak*®) as monotherapy for the treatment of human leukocyte antigen-A*02:01-positive adult patients with advanced (unresectable or metastatic) uveal melanoma (April 2025) SMC No. SMC2746 Not recommended

● **MEDICINAL FORMS** There can be variation in the licensing of different medicines containing the same drug.
Solution for infusion
EXCIPIENTS: May contain Polysorbates
▸ Kimmtrak (Immunocore Ltd) ▼
Tebentafusp 200 microgram per 1 ml Kimmtrak 100micrograms/0.5ml concentrate for solution for infusion vials | 1 vial [PoM] £10,114.00 (Hospital only)

Venetoclax [Specialist drug]

07-Jul-2022

● **INDICATIONS AND DOSE**

Chronic lymphocytic leukaemia | Acute myeloid leukaemia
▸ BY MOUTH
▸ Adult: Specialist drug – access specialist resources for dosing information

IMPORTANT SAFETY INFORMATION
RISKS OF INCORRECT DOSING OF ORAL ANTI-CANCER MEDICINES
See Cytotoxic drugs p. 1027.

MHRA/CHM ADVICE: VENETOCLAX (*VENCLYXTO*®): UPDATED RECOMMENDATIONS ON TUMOUR LYSIS SYNDROME (TLS) (DECEMBER 2021)
The MHRA reminds healthcare professionals about the risk of tumour lysis syndrome (TLS) associated with venetoclax, with fatal cases reported, some in patients with chronic lymphocytic leukaemia (CLL) receiving the lowest dose (a single dose of venetoclax 20 mg) used in the dose-titration phase and in patients with low-to-medium TLS risk. All patients prescribed venetoclax should have a TLS risk assessment. Healthcare professionals should adhere to guidance on appropriate prophylactic measures, routine laboratory tests, dose

titration, and drug interactions—consult product literature.

A patient alert card should be provided to each patient being treated for CLL. Patients should be advised about TLS including:
- the risk of developing TLS occurs in the first days or weeks of treatment with venetoclax, as the dose is increased;
- the importance of drinking plenty of water, having frequent blood tests, and taking medicines to prevent the build-up of uric acid;
- if they experience any symptoms of TLS listed in the patient information leaflet they should stop taking their tablets and contact a healthcare professional immediately.

- **INTERACTIONS** → Appendix 1: venetoclax
- **SIDE-EFFECTS**
- **Common or very common** Abdominal pain · anaemia · appetite decreased · arthralgia · asthenia · constipation · diarrhoea · dizziness · dyspnoea · electrolyte imbalance · gallbladder disorders · haemorrhage · headache · hyperuricaemia · hypotension · increased risk of infection · lymphopenia · nausea · neutropenia · sepsis (sometimes fatal) · stomatitis · syncope · thrombocytopenia · tumour lysis syndrome (sometimes fatal) · vomiting · weight decreased

- **CONCEPTION AND CONTRACEPTION** Manufacturer advises ensure effective, non-hormonal contraception during and for 30 days after treatment in women of child-bearing potential.

- **PATIENT AND CARER ADVICE**
Hydration Patients should be advised to drink 1.5–2 L of water daily, starting 2 days before and throughout the dose-titration phase; intravenous fluids should be administered for those who cannot maintain an adequate level of oral hydration with consideration of overall risk of tumour lysis syndrome.
Vomiting If vomiting occurs following dose administration, no additional doses should be taken on that day and the next dose should be taken at the normal time.
Chronic lymphocytic leukaemia (CLL) Patients should be provided with a patient alert card—see also *Important safety information*.
Missed doses If a dose is more than 8 hours late, the missed dose should not be taken and the next dose should be taken at the normal time.
Driving and skilled tasks Patients and carers should be counselled on the effects on driving and performance of skilled tasks—increased risk of dizziness and fatigue.

- **NATIONAL FUNDING/ACCESS DECISIONS**
For full details see funding body website
  NICE decisions
- **Venetoclax with rituximab for previously treated chronic lymphocytic leukaemia (February 2019)** NICE TA561 Recommended with restrictions
- **Venetoclax with obinutuzumab for untreated chronic lymphocytic leukaemia (December 2020)** NICE TA663 Recommended with restrictions
- **Venetoclax for treating chronic lymphocytic leukaemia (June 2022)** NICE TA796 Recommended
- **Venetoclax with azacitidine for untreated acute myeloid leukaemia when intensive chemotherapy is unsuitable (February 2022)** NICE TA765 Recommended
- **Venetoclax with low dose cytarabine for untreated acute myeloid leukaemia when intensive chemotherapy is unsuitable (April 2022)** NICE TA787 Recommended with restrictions
  Scottish Medicines Consortium (SMC) decisions
- **Venetoclax (*Venclyxto*®) as monotherapy for the treatment of chronic lymphocytic leukaemia in the presence of 17p deletion** or TP53 mutation in adult patients who are unsuitable for or have failed a B-cell receptor pathway inhibitor, or in the absence of 17p deletion or TP53 mutation in adult patients who have failed both chemoimmunotherapy and a B-cell receptor pathway inhibitor **(August 2017)** SMC No. 1249/17 Recommended
- **Venetoclax (*Venclyxto*®) in combination with rituximab for the treatment of adult patients with chronic lymphocytic leukaemia (CLL) who have received at least one prior therapy (August 2019)** SMC No. SMC2166 Recommended
- **Venetoclax (*Venclyxto*®) in combination with obinutuzumab for the treatment of adults with previously untreated chronic lymphocytic leukaemia [in the absence of 17p deletion or TP53 mutation in patients not fit to receive fludarabine, cyclophosphamide and rituximab chemo-immunotherapy, or in patients with the presence of 17p deletion or TP53 mutation] (December 2020)** SMC No. SMC2293 Recommended with restrictions
- **Venetoclax (*Venclyxto*®) in combination with obinutuzumab for the treatment of adults with previously untreated chronic lymphocytic leukaemia [in the absence of 17p deletion or TP53 mutation in patients who are fit to receive fludarabine, cyclophosphamide and rituximab chemo-immunotherapy] (May 2022)** SMC No. SMC2427 Recommended with restrictions
- **Venetoclax (*Venclyxto*®) in combination with a hypomethylating agent for the treatment of adult patients with newly diagnosed acute myeloid leukaemia who are ineligible for intensive chemotherapy (April 2022)** SMC No. SMC2412 Recommended

- **MEDICINAL FORMS** There can be variation in the licensing of different medicines containing the same drug.
  Oral tablet
  CAUTIONARY AND ADVISORY LABELS 21, 25
- **Venclyxto** (AbbVie Ltd)
  Venetoclax 10 mg Venclyxto 10mg tablets | 14 tablet PoM £59.87 (Hospital only)
  Venetoclax 50 mg Venclyxto 50mg tablets | 7 tablet PoM £149.67 (Hospital only)
  Venetoclax 100 mg Venclyxto 100mg tablets | 7 tablet PoM £299.34 (Hospital only) | 14 tablet PoM £598.68 (Hospital only) | 112 tablet PoM £4,789.47 (Hospital only)

Vismodegib [Specialist drug]

25-Jun-2021

- **INDICATIONS AND DOSE**
  Basal cell carcinoma
- ▸ BY MOUTH
- ▸ Adult: Specialist drug – access specialist resources for dosing information

---

IMPORTANT SAFETY INFORMATION
RISKS OF INCORRECT DOSING OF ORAL ANTI-CANCER MEDICINES
See Cytotoxic drugs p. 1027.

PREGNANCY PREVENTION PROGRAMME
Important: teratogenic risk—may cause severe birth defects and embryo-fetal death.

Prescribers and pharmacists must comply with prescribing and dispensing restrictions as specified in the manufacturer's Pregnancy Prevention Programme, and ensure that the patient fully acknowledges the programme's pregnancy prevention measures—consult product literature for further information.

- **INTERACTIONS** → Appendix 1: vismodegib
- **SIDE-EFFECTS**
- **Common or very common** Alopecia · amenorrhoea · appetite decreased · arthralgia · asthenia · constipation · dehydration · diarrhoea · gastrointestinal discomfort · hair

growth abnormal · muscle complaints · nausea · pain · skin reactions · taste altered · vomiting · weight decreased

▸ **Frequency not known** Epiphyses premature fusion

● **CONCEPTION AND CONTRACEPTION** For women of child-bearing potential, pregnancy must be excluded before initiation of treatment, and monthly during treatment. Women must use two contraceptive methods (including one highly effective method and one barrier method) during treatment and for 24 months after the final dose of vismodegib. Men must use a condom during treatment and for 2 months after the final dose.

● **PATIENT AND CARER ADVICE**
Conception and contraception Counselling on pregnancy and contraception advised. Patients must comply with the manufacturer's pregnancy prevention programme.

● **NATIONAL FUNDING/ACCESS DECISIONS**
For full details see funding body website
NICE decisions
▸ **Vismodegib for treating basal cell carcinoma (November 2017)** NICE TA489 Not recommended

● **MEDICINAL FORMS** There can be variation in the licensing of different medicines containing the same drug.
Oral capsule
CAUTIONARY AND ADVISORY LABELS 25
▸ **Erivedge** (Roche Products Ltd)
Vismodegib 150 mg Erivedge 150mg capsules | 28 capsule [PoM] £6,285.00 (Hospital only)

ANTINEOVASCULARISATION DRUGS ›

VASCULAR ENDOTHELIAL GROWTH FACTOR INHIBITORS

Aflibercept [Specialist drug]

12-Mar-2024

● **INDICATIONS AND DOSE**
Colorectal cancer
▸ BY INTRAVENOUS INFUSION
▸ Adult: Specialist drug – access specialist resources for dosing information

IMPORTANT SAFETY INFORMATION
MHRA/CHM ADVICE: SYSTEMICALLY ADMINISTERED VEGF PATHWAY INHIBITORS: RISK OF ANEURYSM AND ARTERY DISSECTION (JULY 2020)
A European review of worldwide data concluded that systemically administered VEGF pathway inhibitors may lead to aneurysm and artery dissection in patients with or without hypertension. Some fatal cases have been reported, mainly in relation to aortic aneurysm rupture and aortic dissection. The MHRA advises healthcare professionals to carefully consider the risk of aneurysm and artery dissection in patients with risk factors before initiating treatment with aflibercept; any modifiable risk

factors (such as smoking and hypertension) should be reduced as much as possible. Blood pressure should be monitored regularly, and product literature should be consulted if hypertension occurs during treatment.

● **CONTRA-INDICATIONS** Moderate or severe congestive heart failure · uncontrolled hypertension

● **INTERACTIONS** → Appendix 1: aflibercept

● **SIDE-EFFECTS**
▸ **Common or very common** Appetite decreased · asthenic conditions · dehydration · diarrhoea · dysphonia · dyspnoea · embolism and thrombosis · fistula (discontinue) · gastrointestinal discomfort · gastrointestinal disorders · haemorrhage · headache · hypersensitivity · hypertension · increased risk of infection · leucopenia · neutropenia · neutropenic sepsis · oral disorders · oropharyngeal pain · proteinuria · rhinorrhoea · skin reactions · thrombocytopenia · weight decreased
▸ **Uncommon** Gastrointestinal perforation (discontinue) · healing impaired · heart failure (discontinue) · nephrotic syndrome · osteonecrosis of jaw · posterior reversible encephalopathy syndrome (PRES) · thrombotic microangiopathy
▸ **Frequency not known** Alopecia · anaemia · anastomotic leak · aneurysm · angina pectoris · artery dissection · cerebrovascular insufficiency · constipation · hyperbilirubinaemia · myocardial infarction · nausea · vomiting · wound dehiscence

SIDE-EFFECTS, FURTHER INFORMATION Can impair wound healing—discontinue if wound healing complications requiring medical intervention occur. Haemorrhage, including fatal cases, have been reported.

● **CONCEPTION AND CONTRACEPTION** Exclude pregnancy before treatment. Effective contraception required during and for at least 6 months after treatment in men and women. Contraceptive advice should be given to men and women before therapy begins (and should cover the duration of contraception required after therapy has ended).

● **NATIONAL FUNDING/ACCESS DECISIONS**
For full details see funding body website
NICE decisions
▸ **Aflibercept in combination with irinotecan and fluorouracil-based therapy for treating metastatic colorectal cancer that has progressed following prior oxaliplatin-based chemotherapy (March 2014)** NICE TA307 Not recommended

● **MEDICINAL FORMS** There can be variation in the licensing of different medicines containing the same drug.
Solution for infusion
▸ **Zaltrap** (Sanofi)
Aflibercept 25 mg per 1 ml Zaltrap 100mg/4ml concentrate for solution for infusion vials | 1 vial [PoM] £295.65 (Hospital only)

Chapter 9
Blood and nutrition

CONTENTS

Blood and blood-forming organs

1   Anaemias

Anaemias

27-Nov-2024

Anaemia treatment considerations

Before initiating treatment for anaemia, it is essential to determine which type is present. Iron salts may be harmful if given to patients with anaemias other than those due to iron deficiency.

Sickle-cell anaemia

Sickle-cell disease is caused by a structural abnormality of haemoglobin resulting in deformed, less flexible red blood cells. Acute complications in the more severe forms include sickle-cell crisis, where infarction of the microvasculature and restricted blood supply to organs results in severe pain.

EvGr Sickle-cell crisis usually requires hospitalisation, fluid replacement, analgesia, and treatment of any concurrent infection. Patients who can be managed at home are often provided with a management plan from their secondary care team that should be followed, including when to seek medical advice. A Complications include anaemia, leg ulcers, renal failure, and increased susceptibility to infection. EvGr Pneumococcal vaccine, haemophilus influenzae type b vaccine, an annual influenza vaccine, and lifelong prophylactic penicillin reduce the risk of infection. Hepatitis B vaccine should also be given if the patient is not immune.

In most forms of sickle-cell disease, varying degrees of haemolytic anaemia are present which is accompanied by increased erythropoiesis; this may increase folate requirements and supplementation with folic acid is recommended. The optimum dose should be discussed with a specialist. A

Hydroxycarbamide p. 1065 can prevent acute chest syndrome, reduce the frequency of painful crises, and reduce transfusion requirements in sickle-cell disease. The beneficial effects of hydroxycarbamide may not become evident for several months.

G6PD deficiency

Glucose 6-phosphate dehydrogenase (G6PD) deficiency is common in individuals originating from Africa, Asia, the Mediterranean region, and the Middle East; it can also occur less frequently in all other individuals. G6PD deficiency is more common in males than it is in females.

Individuals with G6PD deficiency are susceptible to developing acute haemolytic anaemia when they take a number of common drugs or when they have an infection. They are also susceptible to developing acute haemolytic anaemia when they eat fava beans (broad beans); this is termed *favism*.

When prescribing drugs for patients with G6PD deficiency, the following three points should be kept in mind:

- G6PD deficiency is genetically heterogeneous; susceptibility to the haemolytic risk from drugs varies; thus, a drug found to be safe in some G6PD-deficient individuals may not be equally safe in others;
- manufacturers do not routinely test drugs for their effects in G6PD-deficient individuals;
- the risk and severity of haemolysis is almost always dose-related.

The lists below should be read with these points in mind. Ideally, information about G6PD deficiency should be available before prescribing drugs that are associated with a risk of haemolysis in G6PD-deficient patients, including those listed below. However, in the absence of this information, the possibility of haemolysis should be considered, especially if the patient belongs to a group in which G6PD deficiency is common.

Very few G6PD-deficient individuals with chronic non-spherocytic haemolytic anaemia have haemolysis even in the absence of an exogenous trigger. In these patients, exacerbation of haemolysis following oxidative stress, such as the administration of any of the drugs listed below, will occur.

Drugs with definite risk of haemolysis in most G6PD-deficient individuals

- Dapsone and other sulfones
- Fluoroquinolones (including ciprofloxacin, moxifloxacin, norfloxacin, and ofloxacin)
- Methylthioninium chloride
- Niridazole [not on UK market]
- Nitrofurantoin
- Pamaquin [not on UK market]
- Primaquine
- Quinolones
- Rasburicase
- Sulfonamides (including co-trimoxazole)

Drugs with possible risk of haemolysis in some G6PD-deficient individuals

- Aspirin
- Chloroquine
- Menadione, water-soluble derivatives (e.g. menadiol sodium phosphate)
- Quinine (may be acceptable in acute malaria)
- Sulfonylureas

Naphthalene in mothballs also causes haemolysis in individuals with G6PD deficiency.

Aplastic and renal anaemias

Intravenous horse antithymocyte globulin in combination with ciclosporin, may be used as immunosuppressive treatment for aplastic anaemia. The response rate for non-severe aplastic anaemia is higher with this combination than with ciclosporin alone. Prednisolone is used for the prevention of adverse effects associated with antithymocyte globulin treatment. Early reactions that may occur include fever, rash, fluid retention, rigors, acute respiratory distress syndrome, and anaphylaxis; serum sickness may occur

7–14 days later. Antithymocyte globulin should be given under specialist supervision with appropriate resuscitation facilities. Other treatment options for aplastic anaemia include ciclosporin alone or oxymetholone.

Pyridoxine hydrochloride p. 1237 is licensed for the treatment of idiopathic sideroblastic anaemia; the dose required is usually high.

Corticosteroids have an important place in the management of haematological disorders. For further information, see Corticosteroids, general use p. 780.

Erythropoietins

Epoetins (recombinant human erythropoietins) are used to treat anaemia associated with erythropoietin deficiency in chronic renal failure, to increase the yield of autologous blood in normal individuals and to shorten the period of symptomatic anaemia in patients receiving cytotoxic chemotherapy.

Epoetin beta p. 1145 is also licensed for the prevention of anaemia in preterm neonates of low birth-weight; a therapeutic response may take several weeks.

Darbepoetin alfa p. 1143 is a hyperglycosylated derivative of epoetin; it has a longer half-life and can be administered less frequently than epoetin.

Methoxy polyethylene glycol-epoetin beta p. 1147 is a continuous erythropoietin receptor activator that is licensed for the treatment of symptomatic anaemia associated with chronic kidney disease. It has a longer duration of action than epoetin.

For further guidance on the use of erythropoietins in patients with chronic kidney disease and anaemia, see NICE guideline: **Chronic kidney disease: assessment and management** (available at: www.nice.org.uk/guidance/ng203).

1.1 Hypoplastic, haemolytic, and renal anaemias

Other drugs used for Hypoplastic, haemolytic, and renal anaemias Eltrombopag, p. 1172

ANABOLIC STEROIDS

Oxymetholone

19-Oct-2023

- **INDICATIONS AND DOSE**

Aplastic anaemia
▶ BY MOUTH
▹ Adult: 1–5 mg/kg daily for 3 to 6 months

- **INTERACTIONS** → Appendix 1: oxymetholone

- **MEDICINAL FORMS** There can be variation in the licensing of different medicines containing the same drug. Forms available from special-order manufacturers include: oral suspension

Oral capsule
▶ Oxymetholone (Non-proprietary)
 Oxymetholone 50 mg Oxymetholone 50mg capsules |
 50 capsule [PoM] £475.00 [CD4-2]

EPOETINS

Epoetins 

IMPORTANT SAFETY INFORMATION

MHRA/CHM ADVICE: RECOMBINANT HUMAN ERYTHROPOIETINS: VERY RARE RISK OF SEVERE CUTANEOUS ADVERSE REACTIONS (UPDATED JANUARY 2018)

The MHRA is aware of very rare cases of severe cutaneous adverse reactions, including Stevens-Johnson syndrome and toxic epidermal necrolysis, in patients treated with erythropoietins; some cases were fatal. More severe cases were recorded with long-acting agents (darbepoetin alfa and methoxy polyethylene glycol-epoetin beta).

Patients and their carers should be advised of the signs and symptoms of severe skin reactions when starting treatment and instructed to stop treatment and seek immediate medical attention if they develop widespread rash and blistering; these rashes often follow fever or flu-like symptoms—discontinue treatment permanently if such reactions occur.

MHRA/CHM ADVICE (DECEMBER 2007) ERYTHROPOIETINS— HAEMOGLOBIN CONCENTRATION

Overcorrection of haemoglobin concentration in patients with chronic kidney disease may increase the risk of death and serious cardiovascular events, and in patients with cancer may increase the risk of thrombosis and related complications:

- patients should not be treated with erythropoietins for the licensed indications in chronic kidney disease or cancer in patients receiving chemotherapy *unless* symptoms of anaemia are present
- the haemoglobin concentration should be maintained within the range 10–12 g/100 mL
- haemoglobin concentrations higher than 12 g/100 mL should be avoided
- the aim of treatment is to relieve symptoms of anaemia, and in patients with chronic kidney disease to avoid the need for blood transfusion; the haemoglobin concentration should not be increased beyond that which provides adequate control of symptoms of anaemia (in some patients, this may be achieved at concentrations lower than the recommended range)

MHRA/CHM ADVICE (DECEMBER 2007 AND AUGUST 2008) ERYTHROPOIETINS—TUMOUR PROGRESSION AND SURVIVAL IN PATIENTS WITH CANCER

Clinical trial data show an unexplained excess mortality and increased risk of tumour progression in patients with anaemia associated with cancer who have been treated with erythropoietins. Many of these trials used erythropoietins outside of the licensed indications (i.e. overcorrected haemoglobin concentration or given to patients who have not received chemotherapy):

- erythropoietins licensed for the treatment of *symptomatic* anaemia associated with cancer, are licensed only for patients who are receiving chemotherapy
- the decision to use erythropoietins should be based on an assessment of the benefits and risks for individual patients; blood transfusion may be the preferred treatment for anaemia associated with cancer chemotherapy, particularly in those with a good cancer prognosis

● **CONTRA-INDICATIONS** Pure red cell aplasia following erythropoietin therapy · uncontrolled hypertension

● **CAUTIONS** Aluminium toxicity (can impair the response to erythropoietin) · concurrent infection (can impair the response to erythropoietin) · correct factors that contribute to the anaemia of chronic renal failure, such as iron or folate deficiency, before treatment · during dialysis (increase in unfractionated or low molecular weight heparin dose may be needed) · epilepsy · inadequately treated or poorly controlled blood pressure—interrupt treatment if blood pressure uncontrolled · ischaemic vascular disease · malignant disease · other inflammatory disease (can impair the response to erythropoietin) · risk factors for thromboembolism · risk of thrombosis may be increased when used for anaemia in adults receiving cancer chemotherapy · sickle-cell disease (lower target haemoglobin concentration may be appropriate) · sudden

stabbing migraine-like pain (warning of a hypertensive crisis) · thrombocytosis (monitor platelet count for first 8 weeks)

● **SIDE-EFFECTS**

▸ **Common or very common** Arthralgia · embolism and thrombosis · headache · hypertension (dose-dependent) · influenza like illness · skin reactions · stroke

▸ **Uncommon** Hypertensive crisis (in isolated patients with normal or low blood pressure) · respiratory tract congestion · seizure

▸ **Rare or very rare** Thrombocytosis

▸ **Frequency not known** Pure red cell aplasia (more common following subcutaneous administration in patients with chronic renal failure) · severe cutaneous adverse reactions (SCARs)

SIDE-EFFECTS, FURTHER INFORMATION **Hypertensive crisis** In isolated patients with normal or low blood pressure, hypertensive crisis with encephalopathy-like symptoms and generalised tonic-clonic seizures requiring immediate medical attention has occurred with epoetin.

Pure red cell aplasia There have been very rare reports of pure red cell aplasia in patients treated with erythropoietins. In patients who develop a lack of efficacy with erythropoietin therapy and with a diagnosis of pure red cell aplasia, treatment with erythropoietins must be discontinued and testing for erythropoietin antibodies considered. Patients who develop pure red cell aplasia should not be switched to another form of erythropoietin.

● **MONITORING REQUIREMENTS**

▸ Monitor closely blood pressure, reticulocyte counts, haemoglobin, and electrolytes—interrupt treatment if blood pressure uncontrolled.

▸ Other factors, such as iron or folate deficiency, that contribute to the anaemia of chronic renal failure should be corrected before treatment and monitored during therapy. Supplemental iron may improve the response in resistant patients.

⚑ 1142

Darbepoetin alfa
30-Apr-2019

● **INDICATIONS AND DOSE**

Symptomatic anaemia associated with chronic renal failure in patients on dialysis

▸ BY SUBCUTANEOUS INJECTION, OR BY INTRAVENOUS INJECTION

▸ Adult: Initially 450 nanograms/kg once weekly, dose to be adjusted according to response by approximately 25% at intervals of at least 4 weeks, maintenance dose to be given once weekly or once every 2 weeks, reduce dose by approximately 25% if rise in haemoglobin concentration exceeds 2 g/100 mL over 4 weeks or if haemoglobin concentration exceeds 12 g/100 mL; if haemoglobin concentration continues to rise, despite dose reduction, suspend treatment until haemoglobin concentration decreases and then restart at a dose approximately 25% lower than the previous dose, when changing route give same dose then adjust according to weekly or fortnightly haemoglobin measurements, adjust doses not more frequently than every 2 weeks during maintenance treatment

Symptomatic anaemia associated with chronic renal failure in patients not on dialysis

▸ BY SUBCUTANEOUS INJECTION

▸ Adult: Initially 450 nanograms/kg once weekly, alternatively initially 750 nanograms/kg every 2 weeks, dose to be adjusted according to response by approximately 25% at intervals of at least 4 weeks, maintenance dose can be given once weekly, every 2 weeks, or once a month, subcutaneous route preferred in patients not on haemodialysis, reduce dose by approximately 25% if rise in haemoglobin

continued →

9 Blood and nutrition

concentration exceeds 2 g/100 mL over 4 weeks or if haemoglobin concentration exceeds 12 g/100 mL; if haemoglobin concentration continues to rise, despite dose reduction, suspend treatment until haemoglobin concentration decreases and then restart at a dose approximately 25% lower than the previous dose, when changing route give same dose then adjust according to weekly or fortnightly haemoglobin measurements, adjust doses not more frequently than every 2 weeks during maintenance treatment

Symptomatic anaemia associated with chronic renal failure in patients not on dialysis

▶ BY INTRAVENOUS INJECTION

▶ Adult: Initially 450 nanograms/kg once weekly, dose to be adjusted according to response by approximately 25% at intervals of at least 4 weeks, maintenance dose given once weekly, subcutaneous route preferred in patients not on haemodialysis, reduce dose by approximately 25% if rise in haemoglobin concentration exceeds 2 g/100 mL over 4 weeks or if haemoglobin concentration exceeds 12 g/100 mL; if haemoglobin concentration continues to rise, despite dose reduction, suspend treatment until haemoglobin concentration decreases and then restart at a dose approximately 25% lower than the previous dose, when changing route give same dose then adjust according to weekly or fortnightly haemoglobin measurements, adjust doses not more frequently than every 2 weeks during maintenance treatment

Symptomatic anaemia in adults with non-myeloid malignancies receiving chemotherapy

▶ BY SUBCUTANEOUS INJECTION

▶ Adult: Initially 6.75 micrograms/kg every 3 weeks, alternatively initially 2.25 micrograms/kg once weekly, if response inadequate after 9 weeks further treatment may not be effective; if adequate response obtained then reduce dose by 25–50%, reduce dose by approximately 25–50% if rise in haemoglobin concentration exceeds 2 g/100 mL over 4 weeks or if haemoglobin concentration exceeds 12 g/100 mL; if haemoglobin concentration continues to rise, despite dose reduction, suspend treatment until haemoglobin concentration decreases and restart at a dose approximately 25% lower than the previous dose. Discontinue approximately 4 weeks after ending chemotherapy

● SIDE-EFFECTS

▶ Common or very common Hypersensitivity · oedema

● PREGNANCY No evidence of harm in *animal* studies—manufacturer advises caution.

● BREAST FEEDING Manufacturer advises avoid—no information available.

● HEPATIC IMPAIRMENT Manufacturer advises caution (no information available).

● NATIONAL FUNDING/ACCESS DECISIONS
For full details see funding body website

NICE decisions

▶ Erythropoiesis-stimulating agents (epoetin and darbepoetin) for treating anaemia in people with cancer having chemotherapy (November 2014) NICE TA323 Recommended with restrictions

● MEDICINAL FORMS There can be variation in the licensing of different medicines containing the same drug.

Solution for injection

▶ Aranesp (Amgen Ltd)
Darbepoetin alfa 25 microgram per 1 ml Aranesp 10micrograms/0.4ml solution for injection pre-filled syringes | 4 pre-filled disposable injection [PoM] £58.72 DT = £58.72

Darbepoetin alfa 40 microgram per 1 ml Aranesp 20micrograms/0.5ml solution for injection pre-filled syringes | 4 pre-filled disposable injection [PoM] £117.45 DT = £117.45
Darbepoetin alfa 100 microgram per 1 ml Aranesp 50micrograms/0.5ml solution for injection pre-filled syringes | 4 pre-filled disposable injection [PoM] £293.62 DT = £293.62
Aranesp 40micrograms/0.4ml solution for injection pre-filled syringes | 4 pre-filled disposable injection [PoM] £234.90 DT = £234.90
Aranesp 30micrograms/0.3ml solution for injection pre-filled syringes | 4 pre-filled disposable injection [PoM] £176.17 DT = £176.17
Darbepoetin alfa 200 microgram per 1 ml Aranesp 130micrograms/0.65ml solution for injection pre-filled syringes | 4 pre-filled disposable injection [PoM] £763.42 DT = £763.42
Aranesp 100micrograms/0.5ml solution for injection pre-filled syringes | 4 pre-filled disposable injection [PoM] £587.24 DT = £587.24
Aranesp 60micrograms/0.3ml solution for injection pre-filled syringes | 4 pre-filled disposable injection [PoM] £352.35 DT = £352.35
Aranesp 80micrograms/0.4ml solution for injection pre-filled syringes | 4 pre-filled disposable injection [PoM] £469.79 DT = £469.79
Darbepoetin alfa 500 microgram per 1 ml Aranesp 300micrograms/0.6ml solution for injection pre-filled syringes | 1 pre-filled disposable injection [PoM] £440.43 DT = £440.43
Aranesp 500micrograms/1ml solution for injection pre-filled syringes | 1 pre-filled disposable injection [PoM] £734.05 DT = £734.05
Aranesp 150micrograms/0.3ml solution for injection pre-filled syringes | 4 pre-filled disposable injection [PoM] £880.86 DT = £880.86

▶ Aranesp SureClick (Amgen Ltd)
Darbepoetin alfa 40 microgram per 1 ml Aranesp SureClick 20micrograms/0.5ml solution for injection pre-filled pens | 1 pre-filled disposable injection [PoM] £29.36 DT = £29.36
Darbepoetin alfa 100 microgram per 1 ml Aranesp SureClick 40micrograms/0.4ml solution for injection pre-filled pens | 1 pre-filled disposable injection [PoM] £58.72 DT = £58.72
Aranesp SureClick 80micrograms/0.4ml solution for injection pre-filled pens | 1 pre-filled disposable injection [PoM] £117.45 DT = £117.45
Darbepoetin alfa 200 microgram per 1 ml Aranesp SureClick 100micrograms/0.5ml solution for injection pre-filled pens | 1 pre-filled disposable injection [PoM] £146.81 DT = £146.81
Aranesp SureClick 60micrograms/0.3ml solution for injection pre-filled pens | 1 pre-filled disposable injection [PoM] £88.09 DT = £88.09
Darbepoetin alfa 500 microgram per 1 ml Aranesp SureClick 300micrograms/0.6ml solution for injection pre-filled pens | 1 pre-filled disposable injection [PoM] £440.43 DT = £440.43
Aranesp SureClick 150micrograms/0.3ml solution for injection pre-filled pens | 1 pre-filled disposable injection [PoM] £220.22 DT = £220.22
Aranesp SureClick 500micrograms/1ml solution for injection pre-filled pens | 1 pre-filled disposable injection [PoM] £734.05 DT = £734.05

F 1142

Epoetin alfa

11-Oct-2023

● INDICATIONS AND DOSE

EPREX ® PRE-FILLED SYRINGES

Symptomatic anaemia associated with chronic renal failure in patients on haemodialysis

▶ BY INTRAVENOUS INJECTION, OR BY SUBCUTANEOUS INJECTION

▶ Adult: Initially 50 units/kg 3 times a week, adjusted in steps of 25 units/kg 3 times a week, dose adjusted according to response at intervals of at least 4 weeks; maintenance 75–300 units/kg once weekly, intravenous route preferred, intravenous injection to be given over 1–5 minutes, subcutaneous injection, maximum 1 mL per injection site, maintenance dose can be given as a single dose or in divided doses, reduce dose by approximately 25% if rise in haemoglobin concentration exceeds 2 g/100 mL over 4 weeks or if haemoglobin concentration exceeds 12 g/100 mL; if haemoglobin concentration continues to rise, despite dose reduction, suspend treatment until haemoglobin concentration decreases and then restart at a dose approximately 25% lower than the previous dose

Symptomatic anaemia associated with chronic renal failure in adults on peritoneal dialysis

▸ BY INTRAVENOUS INJECTION, OR BY SUBCUTANEOUS INJECTION

▸ Adult: Initially 50 units/kg twice weekly; maintenance 25–50 units/kg twice weekly, intravenous route preferred, intravenous injection to be given over 1–5 minutes, subcutaneous injection, maximum 1 mL per injection site, reduce dose by approximately 25% if rise in haemoglobin concentration exceeds 2 g/100 mL over 4 weeks or if haemoglobin concentration exceeds 12 g/100 mL; if haemoglobin concentration continues to rise, despite dose reduction, suspend treatment until haemoglobin concentration decreases and then restart at a dose approximately 25% lower than the previous dose

Severe symptomatic anaemia of renal origin in adults with renal insufficiency not yet on dialysis

▸ BY INTRAVENOUS INJECTION, OR BY SUBCUTANEOUS INJECTION

▸ Adult: Initially 50 units/kg 3 times a week, increased in steps of 25 units/kg 3 times a week, adjusted according to response, dose to be increased at intervals of at least 4 weeks; maintenance 17–33 units/kg 3 times a week (max. per dose 200 units/kg 3 times a week), intravenous route preferred, intravenous injection to be given over 1–5 minutes, subcutaneous injection, maximum 1 mL per injection site, reduce dose by approximately 25% if rise in haemoglobin concentration exceeds 2 g/100 mL over 4 weeks or if haemoglobin concentration exceeds 12 g/100 mL; if haemoglobin concentration continues to rise, despite dose reduction, suspend treatment until haemoglobin concentration decreases and then restart at a dose approximately 25% lower than the previous dose

Symptomatic anaemia in adults receiving cancer chemotherapy

▸ BY SUBCUTANEOUS INJECTION

▸ Adult: Initially 150 units/kg 3 times a week, alternatively initially 450 units/kg once weekly, increased to 300 units/kg 3 times a week, increased if appropriate rise in haemoglobin (or reticulocyte count) not achieved after 4 weeks; discontinue if inadequate response after 4 weeks at higher dose, subcutaneous injection maximum 1 mL per injection site, reduce dose by approximately 25–50% if rise in haemoglobin concentration exceeds 2 g/100 mL over 4 weeks or if haemoglobin concentration exceeds 12 g/100 mL; if haemoglobin concentration continues to rise, despite dose reduction, suspend treatment until haemoglobin concentration decreases and then restart at a dose approximately 25% lower than the previous dose. Discontinue approximately 4 weeks after ending chemotherapy

To increase yield of autologous blood (to avoid homologous blood) in predonation programme in moderate anaemia either when large volume of blood required or when sufficient blood cannot be saved for elective major surgery

▸ BY INTRAVENOUS INJECTION

▸ Adult: 600 units/kg twice weekly for 3 weeks before surgery, consult product literature for details and advice on ensuring high iron stores, intravenous injection to be given over 1–5 minutes

Moderate anaemia (haemoglobin concentration 10–13 g/100 mL) before elective orthopaedic surgery in adults with expected moderate blood loss to reduce exposure to allogeneic blood transfusion or if autologous transfusion unavailable

▸ BY SUBCUTANEOUS INJECTION

▸ Adult: 600 units/kg once weekly for 3 weeks before surgery and on day of surgery, alternatively 300 units/kg daily for 15 days starting 10 days before surgery, consult product literature for details, subcutaneous injection maximum 1 mL per injection site

● CONTRA-INDICATIONS Surgical patients who cannot receive adequate antithrombotic prophylaxis

● CAUTIONS Risk of thrombosis may be increased when used for anaemia before orthopaedic surgery—avoid in cardiovascular disease including recent myocardial infarction or cerebrovascular accident

● SIDE-EFFECTS

▸ **Common or very common** Chills · cough · diarrhoea · fever · myalgia · nausea · pain · peripheral oedema · vomiting

▸ **Uncommon** Hyperkalaemia

● PREGNANCY No evidence of harm. Benefits probably outweigh risk of anaemia and of blood transfusion in pregnancy.

● BREAST FEEDING Unlikely to be present in milk. Minimal effect on infant.

● HEPATIC IMPAIRMENT Manufacturer advises caution in chronic hepatic failure.

● PRESCRIBING AND DISPENSING INFORMATION Epoetin alfa is a biological medicine. Biological medicines must be prescribed and dispensed by brand name, see *Biological medicines* and *Biosimilar medicines*, under Guidance on prescribing p. 1.

● NATIONAL FUNDING/ACCESS DECISIONS
For full details see funding body website

NICE decisions

▸ **Erythropoiesis-stimulating agents (epoetin and darbepoetin) for treating anaemia in people with cancer having chemotherapy (November 2014)** NICE TA323 Recommended with restrictions

● MEDICINAL FORMS There can be variation in the licensing of different medicines containing the same drug.

Solution for injection

▸ **Eprex** (Janssen-Cilag Ltd)
Epoetin alfa 4000 unit per 1 ml Eprex 2,000units/0.5ml solution for injection pre-filled syringes | 6 pre-filled disposable injection [PoM] £66.37 DT = £66.37
Epoetin alfa 10000 unit per 1 ml Eprex 6,000units/0.6ml solution for injection pre-filled syringes | 6 pre-filled disposable injection [PoM] £199.11 DT = £199.11
Eprex 4,000units/0.4ml solution for injection pre-filled syringes | 6 pre-filled disposable injection [PoM] £132.74 DT = £132.74
Eprex 5,000units/0.5ml solution for injection pre-filled syringes | 6 pre-filled disposable injection [PoM] £165.92 DT = £165.92
Eprex 3,000units/0.3ml solution for injection pre-filled syringes | 6 pre-filled disposable injection [PoM] £99.55 DT = £99.55
Eprex 10,000units/1ml solution for injection pre-filled syringes | 6 pre-filled disposable injection [PoM] £331.85 DT = £331.85
Eprex 8,000units/0.8ml solution for injection pre-filled syringes | 6 pre-filled disposable injection [PoM] £265.48 DT = £265.48
Epoetin alfa 40000 unit per 1 ml Eprex 20,000units/0.5ml solution for injection pre-filled syringes | 1 pre-filled disposable injection [PoM] £110.62 DT = £110.62
Eprex 30,000units/0.75ml solution for injection pre-filled syringes | 1 pre-filled disposable injection [PoM] £199.11 DT = £199.11
Eprex 40,000units/1ml solution for injection pre-filled syringes | 1 pre-filled disposable injection [PoM] £265.48 DT = £265.48

⌐ 1142

| Epoetin beta

06-Dec-2019

● INDICATIONS AND DOSE

Symptomatic anaemia associated with chronic renal failure

▸ BY SUBCUTANEOUS INJECTION

▸ Adult: Initially 20 units/kg 3 times a week for 4 weeks, increased in steps of 20 units/kg 3 times a week, according to response at intervals of 4 weeks, total weekly dose may be divided into daily doses;

continued →

maintenance dose, initially reduce dose by half then adjust according to response at intervals of 1–2 weeks, total weekly maintenance dose may be given as a single dose or in 3 or 7 divided doses. Subcutaneous route preferred in patients not on haemodialysis. Reduce dose by approximately 25% if rise in haemoglobin concentration exceeds 2 g/100 mL over 4 weeks or if haemoglobin concentration approaches or exceeds 12 g/100 mL; if haemoglobin concentration continues to rise, despite dose reduction, suspend treatment until haemoglobin concentration decreases and then restart at a dose approximately 25% lower than the previous dose; maximum 720 units/kg per week

▸ BY INTRAVENOUS INJECTION

▸ Adult: Initially 40 units/kg 3 times a week for 4 weeks, then increased to 80 units/kg 3 times a week, then increased in steps of 20 units/kg 3 times a week if required, at intervals of 4 weeks; maintenance dose, initially reduce dose by half then adjust according to response at intervals of 1–2 weeks. Intravenous injection to be administered over 2 minutes. Subcutaneous route preferred in patients not on haemodialysis. Reduce dose by approximately 25% if rise in haemoglobin concentration exceeds 2 g/100 mL over 4 weeks or if haemoglobin concentration approaches or exceeds 12 g/100 mL; if haemoglobin concentration continues to rise, despite dose reduction, suspend treatment until haemoglobin concentration decreases and then restart at a dose approximately 25% lower than the previous dose; maximum 720 units/kg per week

Symptomatic anaemia in adults with non-myeloid malignancies receiving chemotherapy

▸ BY SUBCUTANEOUS INJECTION

▸ Adult: Initially 450 units/kg once weekly for 4 weeks, dose to be given weekly as a single dose or in 3–7 divided doses, increase dose after 4 weeks (if a rise in haemoglobin of at least 1 g/100 mL not achieved), increased to 900 units/kg once weekly, dose to be given weekly as a single dose or in 3–7 divided doses, if adequate response obtained reduce dose by 25–50%, discontinue treatment if haemoglobin concentration does not increase by at least 1 g/100 mL after 8 weeks of therapy (response unlikely). Reduce dose by approximately 25–50% if rise in haemoglobin concentration exceeds 2 g/100 mL over 4 weeks or if haemoglobin concentration exceeds 12 g/100 mL; if haemoglobin concentration continues to rise, despite dose reduction, suspend treatment until haemoglobin concentration decreases and then restart at a dose approximately 25% lower than the previous dose. Discontinue approximately 4 weeks after ending chemotherapy; maximum 60 000 units per week

To increase yield of autologous blood (to avoid homologous blood) in predonation programme in moderate anaemia when blood-conserving procedures are insufficient or unavailable

▸ BY INTRAVENOUS INJECTION, OR BY SUBCUTANEOUS INJECTION

▸ Adult: (consult product literature)

● **PREGNANCY** No evidence of harm. Benefits probably outweigh risk of anaemia and of blood transfusion in pregnancy.

● **BREAST FEEDING** Unlikely to be present in milk. Minimal effect on infant.

● **HEPATIC IMPAIRMENT** Manufacturer advises caution in chronic hepatic failure.

● **NATIONAL FUNDING/ACCESS DECISIONS**
For full details see funding body website
NICE decisions
▸ **Erythropoiesis-stimulating agents (epoetin and darbepoetin) for treating anaemia in people with cancer having chemotherapy (November 2014)** NICE TA323 Recommended with restrictions

● **MEDICINAL FORMS** There can be variation in the licensing of different medicines containing the same drug.
Solution for injection
EXCIPIENTS: May contain Phenylalanine
▸ **NeoRecormon** (Roche Products Ltd)
  Epoetin beta 1667 unit per 1 ml NeoRecormon 500units/0.3ml solution for injection pre-filled syringes | 6 pre-filled disposable injection PoM £21.05 DT = £21.05
  Epoetin beta 6667 unit per 1 ml NeoRecormon 2,000units/0.3ml solution for injection pre-filled syringes | 6 pre-filled disposable injection PoM £84.17 DT = £84.17
  Epoetin beta 10000 unit per 1 ml NeoRecormon 3,000units/0.3ml solution for injection pre-filled syringes | 6 pre-filled disposable injection PoM £126.25 DT = £126.25
  Epoetin beta 13333 unit per 1 ml NeoRecormon 4,000units/0.3ml solution for injection pre-filled syringes | 6 pre-filled disposable injection PoM £168.34 DT = £168.34
  Epoetin beta 16667 unit per 1 ml NeoRecormon 10,000units/0.6ml solution for injection pre-filled syringes | 6 pre-filled disposable injection PoM £420.85 DT = £420.85
  NeoRecormon 5,000units/0.3ml solution for injection pre-filled syringes | 6 pre-filled disposable injection PoM £210.42 DT = £210.42
  Epoetin beta 20000 unit per 1 ml NeoRecormon 6,000units/0.3ml solution for injection pre-filled syringes | 6 pre-filled disposable injection PoM £252.50 DT = £252.50
  Epoetin beta 33333 unit per 1 ml NeoRecormon 20,000units/0.6ml solution for injection pre-filled syringes | 6 pre-filled disposable injection PoM £841.71 DT = £841.71
  Epoetin beta 50000 unit per 1 ml NeoRecormon 30,000units/0.6ml solution for injection pre-filled syringes | 4 pre-filled disposable injection PoM £841.71 DT = £841.71

⚑ 1142

Epoetin zeta
11-Oct-2023

● **INDICATIONS AND DOSE**

Symptomatic anaemia associated with chronic renal failure in patients on haemodialysis

▸ BY INTRAVENOUS INJECTION, OR BY SUBCUTANEOUS INJECTION

▸ Adult: Initially 50 units/kg 3 times a week, adjusted according to response, adjusted in steps of 25 units/kg 3 times a week, dose to be adjusted at intervals of at least 4 weeks; maintenance 25–100 units/kg 3 times a week, intravenous injection to be given over 1–5 minutes, if given by subcutaneous injection, a maximum of 1 mL can be given per injection site, avoid increasing haemoglobin concentration at a rate exceeding 2 g/100 mL over 4 weeks

Symptomatic anaemia associated with chronic renal failure in adults on peritoneal dialysis

▸ BY INTRAVENOUS INJECTION, OR BY SUBCUTANEOUS INJECTION

▸ Adult: Initially 50 units/kg twice weekly; maintenance 25–50 units/kg twice weekly, intravenous injection to be given over 1–5 minutes, if given by subcutaneous injection, a maximum of 1 mL can be given per injection site, avoid increasing haemoglobin concentration at a rate exceeding 2 g/100 mL over 4 weeks

Severe symptomatic anaemia of renal origin in adults with renal insufficiency not yet on dialysis

▸ BY INTRAVENOUS INJECTION, OR BY SUBCUTANEOUS INJECTION

▸ Adult: Initially 50 units/kg 3 times a week, adjusted according to response, adjusted in steps of 25 units/kg 3 times a week, dose to be increased at intervals of at least 4 weeks; maintenance 17–33 units/kg 3 times a week (max. per dose 200 units/kg 3 times a week), intravenous injection to be given over 1–5 minutes, if given by subcutaneous injection, a maximum of 1 mL can be given per injection site, avoid increasing haemoglobin concentration at a rate exceeding 2 g/100 mL over 4 weeks

Symptomatic anaemia in adults receiving cancer chemotherapy

▶ BY SUBCUTANEOUS INJECTION

▶ Adult: Initially 150 units/kg 3 times a week, alternatively initially 450 units/kg once weekly, increased to 300 units/kg 3 times a week, only increase dose if appropriate rise in haemoglobin (or reticulocyte count) not achieved after 4 weeks; discontinue if inadequate response after 4 weeks at higher dose, maximum 1 mL per injection site, reduce dose by approximately 25–50% if rise in haemoglobin concentration exceeds 2 g/100 mL over 4 weeks or if haemoglobin concentration exceeds 12 g/100 mL; if haemoglobin concentration continues to rise, despite dose reduction, suspend treatment until haemoglobin concentration decreases and then restart at a dose approximately 25% lower than the previous dose. Discontinue approximately 4 weeks after ending chemotherapy

To increase yield of autologous blood (to avoid homologous blood) in predonation programme in moderate anaemia either when large volume of blood required or when sufficient blood cannot be saved for elective major surgery

▶ BY INTRAVENOUS INJECTION

▶ Adult: 600 units/kg twice weekly for 3 weeks before surgery, intravenous injection to be given over 1–5 minutes, consult product literature for details and advice on ensuring high iron stores

Moderate anaemia (haemoglobin concentration 10–13 g/100 mL) before elective orthopaedic surgery in adults with expected moderate blood loss to reduce exposure to allogeneic blood transfusion or if autologous transfusion unavailable

▶ BY SUBCUTANEOUS INJECTION

▶ Adult: 600 units/kg every week for 3 weeks before surgery and on day of surgery, alternatively 300 units/kg daily for 15 days starting 10 days before surgery, maximum 1 mL per injection site, consult product literature for details

● **CONTRA-INDICATIONS** Surgical patients who cannot receive adequate antithrombotic prophylaxis

● **CAUTIONS** Risk of thrombosis may be increased when used for anaemia before orthopaedic surgery—avoid in cardiovascular disease including recent myocardial infarction or cerebrovascular accident

● **SIDE-EFFECTS**
▶ **Common or very common** Asthenia · dizziness
▶ **Uncommon** Intracranial haemorrhage
▶ **Rare or very rare** Angioedema
▶ **Frequency not known** Aneurysm · cerebrovascular insufficiency · hypertensive encephalopathy · myocardial infarction · myocardial ischaemia

● **PREGNANCY** No evidence of harm. Benefits probably outweigh risk of anaemia and of blood transfusion in pregnancy.

● **BREAST FEEDING** Unlikely to be present in milk. Minimal effect on infant.

● **HEPATIC IMPAIRMENT** Manufacturer advises caution in chronic hepatic failure.

● **PRESCRIBING AND DISPENSING INFORMATION** Epoetin zeta is a biological medicine. Biological medicines must be prescribed and dispensed by brand name, see *Biological medicines* and *Biosimilar medicines*, under Guidance on prescribing p. 1.

● **NATIONAL FUNDING/ACCESS DECISIONS**
For full details see funding body website
NICE decisions
▶ Erythropoiesis-stimulating agents (epoetin and darbepoetin) for treating anaemia in people with cancer having chemotherapy (November 2014) NICE TA323 Recommended with restrictions

● **MEDICINAL FORMS** There can be variation in the licensing of different medicines containing the same drug.
Solution for injection
EXCIPIENTS: May contain Phenylalanine

▶ **Retacrit** (Pfizer Ltd)
Epoetin zeta 3333 unit per 1 ml Retacrit 2,000units/0.6ml solution for injection pre-filled syringes | 6 pre-filled disposable injection PoM £57.70 DT = £57.70
Retacrit 3,000units/0.9ml solution for injection pre-filled syringes | 6 pre-filled disposable injection PoM £86.55 DT = £86.55
Retacrit 1,000units/0.3ml solution for injection pre-filled syringes | 6 pre-filled disposable injection PoM £28.85 DT = £28.85
Epoetin zeta 10000 unit per 1 ml Retacrit 6,000units/0.6ml solution for injection pre-filled syringes | 6 pre-filled disposable injection PoM £173.09 DT = £173.09
Retacrit 10,000units/1ml solution for injection pre-filled syringes | 6 pre-filled disposable injection PoM £288.48 DT = £288.48
Retacrit 8,000units/0.8ml solution for injection pre-filled syringes | 6 pre-filled disposable injection PoM £230.79 DT = £230.79
Retacrit 4,000units/0.4ml solution for injection pre-filled syringes | 6 pre-filled disposable injection PoM £115.40 DT = £115.40
Retacrit 5,000units/0.5ml solution for injection pre-filled syringes | 6 pre-filled disposable injection PoM £144.25 DT = £144.25
Epoetin zeta 40000 unit per 1 ml Retacrit 20,000units/0.5ml solution for injection pre-filled syringes | 1 pre-filled disposable injection PoM £96.16 DT = £96.16
Retacrit 40,000units/1ml solution for injection pre-filled syringes | 1 pre-filled disposable injection PoM £193.32 DT = £193.32
Retacrit 30,000units/0.75ml solution for injection pre-filled syringes | 1 pre-filled disposable injection PoM £144.25 DT = £144.25

Methoxy polyethylene glycol-epoetin beta

05-Oct-2021

● **INDICATIONS AND DOSE**

Symptomatic anaemia associated with chronic kidney disease in patients on dialysis and not currently treated with erythropoietins

▶ BY SUBCUTANEOUS INJECTION, OR BY INTRAVENOUS INJECTION

▶ Adult: Initially 600 nanograms/kg every 2 weeks, subcutaneous route preferred in patients not on haemodialysis, dose to be adjusted according to response at intervals of at least 1 month, maintenance dose of double the previous fortnightly dose may be given once a month if haemoglobin concentration is above 10 g/100 mL, reduce dose by approximately 25% if rate of rise in haemoglobin concentration exceeds 2 g/100 mL in 1 month or if haemoglobin concentration is increasing or approaching 12 g/100 mL; if haemoglobin concentration continues to rise, despite dose reduction, suspend treatment until haemoglobin concentration decreases and then restart at a dose approximately 25% lower than the previous dose, dose may be increased by approximately 25% if the rate of rise in haemoglobin concentration is less than 1 g/100 mL over 1 month; further increases of approximately 25% may be made at monthly intervals until the individual target haemoglobin concentration is obtained

Symptomatic anaemia associated with chronic kidney disease in patients not on dialysis and not currently treated with erythropoietins

▶ INITIALLY BY SUBCUTANEOUS INJECTION

▶ Adult: Initially 1.2 micrograms/kg every month, alternatively (by subcutaneous injection or by

continued →

9
Blood and nutrition

intravenous injection) initially 600 nanograms/kg every 2 weeks, subcutaneous route preferred in patients not on haemodialysis, dose to be adjusted according to response at intervals of at least 1 month, patients treated once every 2 weeks may be given a maintenance dose of double the previous fortnightly dose once a month if haemoglobin concentration is above 10 g/100 mL, reduce dose by approximately 25% if rate of rise in haemoglobin concentration exceeds 2 g/100 mL in 1 month or if haemoglobin concentration is increasing or approaching 12 g/100 mL; if haemoglobin concentration continues to rise, despite dose reduction, suspend treatment until haemoglobin concentration decreases and then restart at a dose approximately 25% lower than the previous dose, dose may be increased by approximately 25% if the rate of rise in haemoglobin concentration is less than 1 g/100 mL over 1 month; further increases of approximately 25% may be made at monthly intervals until the individual target haemoglobin concentration is obtained

Symptomatic anaemia associated with chronic kidney disease in patients currently treated with erythropoietins
▶ BY SUBCUTANEOUS INJECTION, OR BY INTRAVENOUS INJECTION
▶ Adult: (consult product literature)

IMPORTANT SAFETY INFORMATION

MHRA/CHM ADVICE: RECOMBINANT HUMAN ERYTHROPOIETINS: VERY RARE RISK OF SEVERE CUTANEOUS ADVERSE REACTIONS (UPDATED JANUARY 2018)

The MHRA is aware of very rare cases of severe cutaneous adverse reactions, including Stevens-Johnson syndrome and toxic epidermal necrolysis, in patients treated with erythropoietins; some cases were fatal. More severe cases were recorded with long-acting agents (darbepoetin alfa and methoxy polyethylene glycol-epoetin beta).

Patients and their carers should be advised of the signs and symptoms of severe skin reactions when starting treatment and instructed to stop treatment and seek immediate medical attention if they develop widespread rash and blistering; these rashes often follow fever or flu-like symptoms—discontinue treatment permanently if such reactions occur.

MHRA/CHM ADVICE (DECEMBER 2007) ERYTHROPOIETINS— HAEMOGLOBIN CONCENTRATION

Overcorrection of haemoglobin concentration in patients with chronic kidney disease may increase the risk of death and serious cardiovascular events, and in patients with cancer may increase the risk of thrombosis and related complications:
- patients should not be treated with erythropoietins for the licensed indications in chronic kidney disease or cancer in patients receiving chemotherapy *unless* symptoms of anaemia are present
- the haemoglobin concentration should be maintained within the range 10–12 g/100 mL
- haemoglobin concentrations higher than 12 g/100 mL should be avoided
- the aim of treatment is to relieve symptoms of anaemia, and in patients with chronic kidney disease to avoid the need for blood transfusion; the haemoglobin concentration should not be increased beyond that which provides adequate control of symptoms of anaemia (in some patients, this may be achieved at concentrations lower than the recommended range)

● CONTRA-INDICATIONS Pure red cell aplasia following erythropoietin therapy · uncontrolled hypertension

● CAUTIONS Bone marrow fibrosis (can impair the response to erythropoietin) · concurrent infection (can impair the response to erythropoietin) · haematological disease (can impair the response to erythropoietin) · haemolysis (can impair the response to erythropoietin) · inflammatory or traumatic episodes (can impair the response to erythropoietin) · malignant disease · occult blood loss (can impair the response to erythropoietin) · severe aluminium toxicity (can impair the response to erythropoietin)

● SIDE-EFFECTS
▶ **Common or very common** Hypertension (dose-dependent)
▶ **Uncommon** Embolism and thrombosis · headache
▶ **Rare or very rare** Hot flush · hypertensive encephalopathy · rash maculopapular
▶ **Frequency not known** Pure red cell aplasia (discontinue) · severe cutaneous adverse reactions (SCARs) · thrombocytopenia

● PREGNANCY No evidence of harm in *animal* studies— manufacturer advises caution.

● BREAST FEEDING Manufacturer advises use only if potential benefit outweighs risk—present in milk in *animal* studies.

● RENAL IMPAIRMENT Manufacturer advises caution with escalation of doses in chronic renal failure.

● MONITORING REQUIREMENTS
▶ Manufacturer advises monitor haemoglobin concentration every 2 weeks until stabilised and periodically thereafter— if patient fails to respond, check reticulocyte count, and search for causative factors such as deficiencies of iron, folic acid or vitamin B12, and correct if necessary. Monitor iron status before and during treatment.
▶ Manufacturer advises monitor blood pressure before and during treatment—if inadequately controlled, reduce dose or discontinue treatment.

● PRESCRIBING AND DISPENSING INFORMATION Methoxy polyethylene glycol-epoetin beta is a biological medicine. Biological medicines must be prescribed and dispensed by brand name, see *Biological medicines* and *Biosimilar medicines*, under Guidance on prescribing p. 1.

The manufacturer of *Mircera®* has provided a *Physician's Guide* which includes important safety information to minimise the risk of pure red cell aplasia.

● MEDICINAL FORMS There can be variation in the licensing of different medicines containing the same drug.

Solution for injection
▶ Mircera (Roche Products Ltd)
Methoxy polyethylene glycol-epoetin beta 100 microgram per 1 ml Mircera 30micrograms/0.3ml solution for injection pre-filled syringes | 1 pre-filled disposable injection PoM £44.05 DT = £44.05
Methoxy polyethylene glycol-epoetin beta 166.667 microgram per 1 ml Mircera 50micrograms/0.3ml solution for injection pre-filled syringes | 1 pre-filled disposable injection PoM £73.41 DT = £73.41
Methoxy polyethylene glycol-epoetin beta 250 microgram per 1 ml Mircera 75micrograms/0.3ml solution for injection pre-filled syringes | 1 pre-filled disposable injection PoM £110.11 DT = £110.11
Methoxy polyethylene glycol-epoetin beta 333.333 microgram per 1 ml Mircera 100micrograms/0.3ml solution for injection pre-filled syringes | 1 pre-filled disposable injection PoM £146.81 DT = £146.81
Methoxy polyethylene glycol-epoetin beta 400 microgram per 1 ml Mircera 120micrograms/0.3ml solution for injection pre-filled syringes | 1 pre-filled disposable injection PoM £176.18 DT = £176.18
Methoxy polyethylene glycol-epoetin beta 500 microgram per 1 ml Mircera 150micrograms/0.3ml solution for injection pre-filled syringes | 1 pre-filled disposable injection PoM £220.22 DT = £220.22
Methoxy polyethylene glycol-epoetin beta 600 microgram per 1 ml Mircera 360micrograms/0.6ml solution for injection pre-filled syringes | 1 pre-filled disposable injection PoM £528.56 DT = £528.56

Methoxy polyethylene glycol-epoetin beta 666.667 microgram per 1 ml Mircera 200micrograms/0.3ml solution for injection pre-filled syringes | 1 pre-filled disposable injection [PoM] £293.62 DT = £293.62

Methoxy polyethylene glycol-epoetin beta 833.333 microgram per 1 ml Mircera 250micrograms/0.3ml solution for injection pre-filled syringes | 1 pre-filled disposable injection [PoM] £367.03 DT = £367.03

HYPOXIA-INDUCIBLE FACTOR PROLYL HYDROXYLASE INHIBITORS

Roxadustat
14-Sep-2022

● **DRUG ACTION** Roxadustat is a hypoxia-inducible factor, prolyl hydroxylase inhibitor (HIF-PHI), which stimulates a coordinated erythropoietic response, thereby increasing haemoglobin production and improving iron bioavailability.

● **INDICATIONS AND DOSE**

Symptomatic anaemia associated with chronic kidney disease in patients not currently treated with an erythropoiesis-stimulating agent (initiated by a specialist)
▸ BY MOUTH
▸ Adult (body-weight up to 100 kg): Initially 70 mg 3 times a week, adjusted according to response; usual maintenance 20–400 mg 3 times a week, doses should not be taken on consecutive days, dose adjusted at intervals of 4 weeks to achieve haemoglobin concentration of 10 to 12 g/dL. For dose adjustments and maximum recommended dose—consult product literature, consider discontinuation of treatment if adequate increase in haemoglobin concentration not achieved in 24 weeks
▸ Adult (body-weight 100 kg and above): Initially 100 mg 3 times a week, adjusted according to response; usual maintenance 20–400 mg 3 times a week, doses should not be taken on consecutive days, dose adjusted at intervals of 4 weeks to achieve haemoglobin concentration of 10 to 12 g/dL. For dose adjustments and maximum recommended dose—consult product literature, consider discontinuation of treatment if adequate increase in haemoglobin concentration not achieved in 24 weeks

Symptomatic anaemia associated with chronic kidney disease in patients currently treated with an erythropoiesis-stimulating agent (initiated by a specialist)
▸ BY MOUTH
▸ Adult: (consult product literature)

● **CAUTIONS** Active infection · history of seizures, epilepsy and other medical conditions associated with a predisposition to seizures · risk factors for venous thromboembolism

● **INTERACTIONS** → Appendix 1: roxadustat

● **SIDE-EFFECTS**
▸ **Common or very common** Constipation · diarrhoea · embolism and thrombosis · headache · hyperkalaemia · hypertension · insomnia · nausea · peripheral oedema · seizure · sepsis · vomiting
▸ **Uncommon** Hyperbilirubinaemia
▸ **Frequency not known** Generalised exfoliative dermatitis · increased risk of infection · secondary hypothyroidism

● **CONCEPTION AND CONTRACEPTION** [EvGr] Females of childbearing potential should use highly effective contraception during treatment and for at least 1 week after last treatment. ⟨M⟩

● **PREGNANCY** [EvGr] Avoid—toxicity in *animal* studies. ⟨M⟩

● **BREAST FEEDING** [EvGr] Avoid—present in milk in *animal* studies. ⟨M⟩

● **HEPATIC IMPAIRMENT** [EvGr] Caution in moderate impairment; avoid in severe impairment (no information available). ⟨M⟩
Dose adjustments [EvGr] Use half the normal starting dose in moderate impairment. ⟨M⟩

● **PRE-TREATMENT SCREENING** [EvGr] Ensure adequate iron stores before treatment. ⟨M⟩

● **MONITORING REQUIREMENTS** [EvGr] Monitor haemoglobin concentration every 2 weeks until the desired haemoglobin concentration is achieved and stabilised, then every 4 weeks thereafter or as clinically indicated. ⟨M⟩

● **PATIENT AND CARER ADVICE** Patients and their carers should be advised to seek medical attention if symptoms of infection or venous thromboembolism develop during treatment.
Missed doses If a dose is missed, it should be administered as soon as possible only if there is more than 1 day until the next scheduled dose; if one day or less remains before the next scheduled dose, the missed dose should not be taken and the next dose should be taken on the next scheduled day.
Driving and skilled tasks Patients and carers should be cautioned on the effects on driving and performance of skilled tasks—increased risk of seizures.

● **NATIONAL FUNDING/ACCESS DECISIONS**
For full details see funding body website
NICE decisions
▸ **Roxadustat for treating symptomatic anaemia in chronic kidney disease (July 2022)** NICE TA807 Recommended with restrictions
Scottish Medicines Consortium (SMC) decisions
▸ **Roxadustat (*Evrenzo*®) for the treatment of adult patients with symptomatic anaemia associated with chronic kidney disease (August 2022)** SMC No. SMC2461 Recommended with restrictions

● **MEDICINAL FORMS** There can be variation in the licensing of different medicines containing the same drug.
Oral tablet
CAUTIONARY AND ADVISORY LABELS 25
EXCIPIENTS: May contain Lecithin
▸ **Evrehzo** (Astellas Pharma Ltd) ▼
Roxadustat 20 mg Evrenzo 20mg tablets | 12 tablet [PoM] £59.24 DT = £59.24
Roxadustat 50 mg Evrenzo 50mg tablets | 12 tablet [PoM] £148.11 DT = £148.11
Roxadustat 70 mg Evrenzo 70mg tablets | 12 tablet [PoM] £207.35 DT = £207.35
Roxadustat 100 mg Evrenzo 100mg tablets | 12 tablet [PoM] £296.21 DT = £296.21
Roxadustat 150 mg Evrenzo 150mg tablets | 12 tablet [PoM] £444.32

Vadadustat
28-Jan-2025

● **DRUG ACTION** Vadadustat is a hypoxia-inducible factor, prolyl hydroxylase inhibitor (HIF-PHI), which stimulates a coordinated erythropoietic response, thereby increasing iron mobilisation and haemoglobin production.

● **INDICATIONS AND DOSE**

Symptomatic anaemia associated with chronic kidney disease in patients on chronic maintenance dialysis (initiated by a specialist)
▸ BY MOUTH
▸ Adult: Initially 300 mg once daily, dose to be adjusted in increments of 150 mg, and increased no more frequently than every 4 weeks, to achieve or maintain a haemoglobin concentration of 10 to 12 g/dL. For

continued →

further information on dose titration and treatment interruption, or converting patients from an epoetin—consult product literature. Usual maintenance 150–600 mg once daily. Consider discontinuation of treatment if adequate increase in haemoglobin concentration not achieved in 24 weeks

- **CAUTIONS** Major adverse cardiovascular events · seizures (history of, or risk factors for) · thromboembolic events (history of, or risk factors for)
- **INTERACTIONS** → Appendix 1: vadadustat
- **SIDE-EFFECTS**
- ▶ **Common or very common** Constipation · cough · diarrhoea · embolism and thrombosis · headache · hypersensitivity · hypertension · hypotension · nausea · seizure · vomiting
- ▶ **Frequency not known** Cerebrovascular insufficiency · hepatocellular injury · myocardial infarction
- **PREGNANCY** EvGr Use only if potential benefit outweighs risk (limited information available). Ⓜ
- **BREAST FEEDING** EvGr Avoid (no information available). Ⓜ
- **HEPATIC IMPAIRMENT** EvGr Avoid in severe impairment (no information available). Ⓜ
- **MONITORING REQUIREMENTS**
- ▶ EvGr Monitor haemoglobin concentration every 2 weeks until the desired haemoglobin concentration is achieved and stabilised, then at least monthly thereafter.
- ▶ Monitor ALT, AST, and bilirubin before starting treatment, every month for the first 3 months after, and then as clinically indicated—discontinue treatment if ALT or AST persistently exceed 3 times the upper limit of normal, or are accompanied by bilirubin exceeding 2 times the upper limit of normal.
- ▶ Monitor iron stores before and during treatment.
- ▶ Monitor blood pressure before and during treatment as clinically indicated. Ⓜ
- **PATIENT AND CARER ADVICE** Patients and their carers should be advised to seek immediate medical attention if signs and symptoms of thromboembolism develop during treatment.
- **NATIONAL FUNDING/ACCESS DECISIONS** For full details see funding body website
  NICE decisions
- ▶ Vadadustat for treating symptomatic anaemia in adults having dialysis for chronic kidney disease (January 2025) NICE TA1035 Recommended

- **MEDICINAL FORMS** There can be variation in the licensing of different medicines containing the same drug.
  Oral tablet
  - ▶ Vafseo (Medice UK Ltd) ▼
    Vadadustat 150 mg Vafseo 150mg tablets | 28 tablet PoM £148.59 | 98 tablet PoM £520.08
    Vadadustat 300 mg Vafseo 300mg tablets | 28 tablet PoM £297.19 | 98 tablet PoM £1,040.16

1.1a Atypical haemolytic uraemic syndrome and paroxysmal nocturnal haemoglobinuria

IMMUNOSUPPRESSANTS > COMPLEMENT INHIBITORS

Crovalimab

14-Jan-2025

- **DRUG ACTION** Crovalimab is a recombinant monoclonal antibody that inhibits terminal complement activation at the C5 protein, thereby reducing haemolysis.

- **INDICATIONS AND DOSE**

Paroxysmal nocturnal haemoglobinuria (initiated under specialist supervision)
- ▶ INITIALLY BY INTRAVENOUS INFUSION
- ▶ Adult (body-weight 40–99 kg): Loading dose 1000 mg for 1 dose, to be given on day 1, then (by subcutaneous injection) 340 mg for 4 doses, to be given on days 2, 8, 15, and 22, followed by (by subcutaneous injection) maintenance 680 mg every 4 weeks, to be given from day 29 onwards
- ▶ Adult (body-weight 100 kg and above): Loading dose 1500 mg for 1 dose, to be given on day 1, then (by subcutaneous injection) 340 mg for 4 doses, to be given on days 2, 8, 15, and 22, followed by (by subcutaneous injection) maintenance 1020 mg every 4 weeks, to be given from day 29 onwards

DOSE EQUIVALENCE AND CONVERSION
- ▶ For patients switching from another complement inhibitor, the first loading dose of crovalimab should be administered at the time of the next scheduled complement inhibitor dose.

- **CONTRA-INDICATIONS** Patients unvaccinated against *Neisseria meningitidis* · unresolved infection caused by *Neisseria meningitidis*
- **CAUTIONS** Active systemic infections (monitor for signs and symptoms of worsening infection)
  CAUTIONS, FURTHER INFORMATION
- ▶ Vaccination against serious infection EvGr To reduce the risk of serious infection, it is advised that patients are vaccinated against *Neisseria meningitidis* (vaccines against serotypes A, C, Y, W135, and B, where available, are recommended), *Streptococcus pneumoniae*, and *Haemophilus influenzae* type b according to local guidelines, at least 2 weeks before starting treatment. If immediate treatment is needed, administer the required vaccines as soon as possible; treat with prophylactic antibiotics until 2 weeks after vaccination. Ⓜ
- **INTERACTIONS** → Appendix 1: crovalimab
- **SIDE-EFFECTS**
- ▶ **Common or very common** Abdominal pain · arthralgia · asthenia · diarrhoea · fever · headache · hypersensitivity · increased risk of infection · infusion related reaction · injection related reaction · rash · type III hypersensitivity reaction (complex-mediated) (when switching from another C5 inhibitor)
- ▶ **Uncommon** Sepsis

  SIDE-EFFECTS, FURTHER INFORMATION Monitor patients for symptoms of type III hypersensitivity reactions (such as arthralgia, rash, fever, fatigue, abdominal distress, headache and axonal neuropathy) for the first 30 days after switching between C5 inhibitors.

- **PREGNANCY** EvGr Use only if potential benefit outweighs risk (limited information available). Ⓜ Crovalimab is an immunoglobulin G (IgG) monoclonal antibody; human IgG antibodies are known to cross the placenta.

- **BREAST FEEDING** EvGr Avoid (limited information available). M

- **MONITORING REQUIREMENTS**
▶ EvGr Monitor for early signs of meningococcal infection caused by *Neisseria meningitidis*.
▶ Monitor for intravascular haemolysis (including serum-lactate dehydrogenase concentration) following treatment discontinuation; consider restarting appropriate treatment if haemolysis occurs. M

- **DIRECTIONS FOR ADMINISTRATION** For *intermittent intravenous infusion*, dilute requisite dose to a final concentration of 4–15 mg/mL with Sodium Chloride 0.9%; give over 60–90 minutes through a 0.2 micron in-line filter.

  For *subcutaneous injection*, administer into the abdomen (except for the 5 cm around the navel); rotate injection site and avoid moles, scars, and skin that is tender, bruised, red, hardened, or not intact.

  Piasky® may be self-administered or administered by a carer after appropriate training in subcutaneous injection technique.

- **PRESCRIBING AND DISPENSING INFORMATION** Crovalimab is a biological medicine. Biological medicines must be prescribed and dispensed by brand name, see *Biological medicines* and *Biosimilar medicines*, under Guidance on prescribing p. 1; record the brand name and batch number after each administration.

  The manufacturer of *Piasky*® has provided a *Healthcare Professional Guide*.

- **HANDLING AND STORAGE** Store in a refrigerator (2–8°C) and protect from light—consult product literature for further information regarding storage outside the refrigerator.

- **PATIENT AND CARER ADVICE** Patients and carers should be informed of the signs and symptoms of serious infections, especially meningococcal infection, and advised to seek immediate medical care if they occur.

  Self administration Patients or their carers should be given training in subcutaneous injection technique if appropriate.

  Patient card and guide A patient card and guide for patients and caregivers should be provided.

- **NATIONAL FUNDING/ACCESS DECISIONS**
  For full details see funding body website

  NICE decisions
▶ Crovalimab for treating paroxysmal nocturnal haemoglobinuria in people 12 years and over (November 2024) NICE TA1019 Recommended

  Scottish Medicines Consortium (SMC) decisions
▶ Crovalimab (*Piasky*®) as monotherapy for the treatment of adult and paediatric patients 12 years of age or older with a weight of 40 kg and above with paroxysmal nocturnal haemoglobinuria: in patients with haemolysis with clinical symptom(s) indicative of high disease activity; or who are clinically stable after having been treated with a complement component 5 inhibitor for at least the past 6 months (January 2025) SMC No. SMC2728 Recommended with restrictions

- **MEDICINAL FORMS** There can be variation in the licensing of different medicines containing the same drug.

  Solution for injection
  ▶ Piasky (Roche Products Ltd) ▼
    Crovalimab 170 mg per 1 ml Piasky 340mg/2ml solution for injection vials | 1 vial PoM £9,500.00 (Hospital only)

Danicopan
14-Jan-2025

- **DRUG ACTION** Danicopan is a complement inhibitor which binds to factor D and prevents activation of the complement alternative pathway, thereby inhibiting the complement cascade that leads to haemolysis.

- **INDICATIONS AND DOSE**

  Paroxysmal nocturnal haemoglobinuria (initiated by a specialist)
  ▶ BY MOUTH
  ▶ Adult: 150 mg 3 times a day, increased if necessary to 200 mg 3 times a day, dose may be increased after a minimum of 4 weeks, according to response

- **CONTRA-INDICATIONS** Patients unvaccinated against *Neisseria meningitidis* · unresolved *Neisseria meningitidis* infection

- **CAUTIONS** Active systemic infection · patients weighing less than 60 kg (risk of increased exposure)
  CAUTIONS, FURTHER INFORMATION
▶ Meningococcal infection EvGr Vaccinate against *Neisseria meningitidis* at least 2 weeks before treatment (vaccines against serotypes A, C, Y, W135, and B where available, are recommended); revaccinate according to current medical guidelines. Patients receiving danicopan less than 2 weeks after receiving meningococcal vaccine must be given prophylactic antibiotics until 2 weeks after vaccination. Other immunisations should also be up to date. M

- **INTERACTIONS** → Appendix 1: danicopan

- **SIDE-EFFECTS**
▶ **Common or very common** Fever · headache · hepatic function abnormal · hypertension · pain in extremity · vomiting

- **CONCEPTION AND CONTRACEPTION** EvGr The effect on human fertility is unknown (impairment of male and female fertility observed in *animal* studies). M

- **PREGNANCY** EvGr Avoid (limited information available). M

- **BREAST FEEDING** EvGr Avoid during and for 3 days after treatment (present in milk in *animal* studies). M

- **HEPATIC IMPAIRMENT** EvGr Avoid in severe impairment (no information available). M

- **RENAL IMPAIRMENT**
  Dose adjustments EvGr If eGFR less than 30 mL/minute/1.73 m^2, reduce dose to 100 mg 3 times a day; dose may be increased to 150 mg 3 times a day after a minimum of 4 weeks, according to response. Monitor for adverse reactions (risk of increased exposure). M
  See p. 21.

- **MONITORING REQUIREMENTS** EvGr Monitor for early signs and symptoms of meningococcal infection and sepsis. M

- **TREATMENT CESSATION** EvGr Treatment should be withdrawn gradually over 6 days to reduce the risk of alanine aminotransferase (ALT) elevations—consult product literature. M

- **PATIENT AND CARER ADVICE** Patients and carers should be informed of the signs and symptoms of serious infections, especially meningococcal infection, and advised to seek immediate medical care if they occur.

- **NATIONAL FUNDING/ACCESS DECISIONS**
  For full details see funding body website

  NICE decisions
▶ Danicopan with ravulizumab or eculizumab for treating paroxysmal nocturnal haemoglobinuria (October 2024) NICE TA1010 Recommended with restrictions

  Scottish Medicines Consortium (SMC) decisions
▶ Danicopan (*Voydeya*®) as an add-on to ravulizumab or eculizumab for the treatment of adult patients with paroxysmal nocturnal haemoglobinuria who have residual

9

Blood and nutrition

haemolytic anaemia (January 2025) SMC No. SMC2675 Recommended with restrictions

- **MEDICINAL FORMS** There can be variation in the licensing of different medicines containing the same drug.

Oral tablet
CAUTIONARY AND ADVISORY LABELS 21
▸ **Voydeya** (Alexion Pharma UK Ltd) ▼
Danicopan 50 mg Voydeya 50mg tablets | 90 tablet [PoM] [Ⓧ] (Hospital only)
Danicopan 100 mg Voydeya 100mg tablets | 180 tablet [PoM] £5,479.20 (Hospital only)

Form unstated
CAUTIONARY AND ADVISORY LABELS 21
▸ **Voydeya** (Alexion Pharma UK Ltd) ▼
Voydeya 50mg tablets and Voydeya 100mg tablets | 180 tablet [PoM] £4,109.40 (Hospital only)

Eculizumab

28-Mar-2024

- **DRUG ACTION** Eculizumab is a recombinant monoclonal antibody that inhibits terminal complement activation at the C5 protein and thereby reduces complement-mediated cell damage.

- **INDICATIONS AND DOSE**

Paroxysmal nocturnal haemoglobinuria (under expert supervision)
▸ BY INTRAVENOUS INFUSION
▸ Adult: Initially 600 mg once weekly for 4 weeks, then increased to 900 mg once weekly for 1 week, followed by maintenance 900 mg every 12–16 days

Atypical haemolytic uraemic syndrome (under expert supervision)
▸ BY INTRAVENOUS INFUSION
▸ Adult: Initially 900 mg once weekly for 4 weeks, then increased to 1.2 g once weekly for 1 week, followed by maintenance 1.2 g every 12–16 days

Myasthenia gravis (under expert supervision)
▸ BY INTRAVENOUS INFUSION
▸ Adult: Initially 900 mg once weekly for 4 weeks, then increased to 1.2 g once weekly for 1 week, followed by maintenance 1.2 g every 12–16 days, consider discontinuation if no response within 12 weeks after initial infusion

Neuromyelitis optica spectrum disorder (under expert supervision)
▸ BY INTRAVENOUS INFUSION
▸ Adult: Initially 900 mg once weekly for 4 weeks, then increased to 1.2 g once weekly for 1 week, followed by maintenance 1.2 g every 12–16 days

- **CONTRA-INDICATIONS** Patients unvaccinated against *Neisseria meningitidis* · unresolved *Neisseria meningitidis* infection

- **CAUTIONS** Active systemic infection
CAUTIONS, FURTHER INFORMATION
▸ Meningococcal infection Manufacturer advises vaccinate against *Neisseria meningitidis* at least 2 weeks before treatment (vaccines against serotypes A, C, Y, W135 and B where available, are recommended); revaccinate according to current medical guidelines. Patients receiving eculizumab less than 2 weeks after receiving meningococcal vaccine must be given prophylactic antibiotics until 2 weeks after vaccination. Advise patient to report promptly any signs of meningococcal infection. Other immunisations should also be up to date.

- **INTERACTIONS** → Appendix 1: monoclonal antibodies
- **SIDE-EFFECTS**
▸ **Common or very common** Alopecia · asthenia · cough · decreased leucocytes · diarrhoea · dizziness · fever · gastrointestinal discomfort · headache · hypertension ·

increased risk of infection · influenza like illness · joint disorders · muscle complaints · nausea · oropharyngeal pain · skin reactions · sleep disorders · taste altered · vomiting
▸ **Uncommon** Abscess · anxiety · appetite decreased · chest discomfort · chills · constipation · cystitis · depression · dysuria · haemorrhage · hepatosplenic abscess · hot flush · hyperhidrosis · hypersensitivity · hypotension · infusion related reaction · limb abscess · meningitis meningococcal · mood swings · nasal complaints · oedema · pain · palpitations · paraesthesia · renal abscess · sepsis · spontaneous penile erection · throat irritation · tinnitus · tremor · vascular disorders · vertigo · vision blurred
▸ **Rare or very rare** Abnormal clotting factor · conjunctival irritation · feeling hot · gastrooesophageal reflux disease · gingival discomfort · Grave's disease · jaundice · malignant melanoma · menstrual disorder · syncope · urogenital tract gonococcal infection

- **CONCEPTION AND CONTRACEPTION** Manufacturer advises effective contraception during and for 5 months after treatment.

- **PREGNANCY** Manufacturer advises use only if potential benefit outweighs risk—limited information available. Eculizumab is an immunoglobulin G (IgG) monoclonal antibody; human IgG antibodies are known to cross the placenta.

- **BREAST FEEDING** Manufacturer advises use with caution—limited information available; unlikely to be present in milk.

- **MONITORING REQUIREMENTS**
▸ Monitor for 1 hour after infusion.
▸ For *paroxysmal nocturnal haemoglobinuria*, monitor for intravascular haemolysis (including serum-lactate dehydrogenase concentration) during treatment and for at least 8 weeks after discontinuation.
▸ For *atypical haemolytic uraemic syndrome*, monitor for thrombotic microangiopathy (measure platelet count, serum-lactate dehydrogenase concentration, and serum creatinine) during treatment and for at least 12 weeks after discontinuation.

- **DIRECTIONS FOR ADMINISTRATION** For *intravenous infusion* (*Soliris*®), manufacturer advises give intermittently *in* Glucose 5% *or* Sodium Chloride 0.9%. Dilute requisite dose to a concentration of 5 mg/mL and mix gently; give over 25–45 minutes (infusion time may be increased to 2 hours if infusion-related reactions occur).

- **PRESCRIBING AND DISPENSING INFORMATION** Eculizumab is a biological medicine. Biological medicines must be prescribed and dispensed by brand name, see *Biological medicines* and *Biosimilar medicines*, under Guidance on prescribing p. 1.
Consult product literature for details of supplemental doses with concomitant plasmapheresis, plasma exchange, or plasma infusion.
The manufacturer of *Soliris*® has provided a *Physician's guide* and user manual for healthcare professionals.

- **HANDLING AND STORAGE** Store in a refrigerator (2-8°C) and protect from light—consult product literature for further information regarding storage outside refrigerator.

- **PATIENT AND CARER ADVICE** Patients or carers should be advised to report promptly any signs of meningococcal infection. Advice about prevention of gonorrhoea should also be given.
A patient information card and a patient safety card should be provided.

- **NATIONAL FUNDING/ACCESS DECISIONS**
For full details see funding body website
NICE decisions
▸ **Eculizumab for treating atypical haemolytic uraemic syndrome (January 2015)** NICE HST1 Recommended

- **MEDICINAL FORMS** There can be variation in the licensing of different medicines containing the same drug.

Solution for infusion

EXCIPIENTS: May contain Polysorbates

ELECTROLYTES: May contain Sodium

▸ **Bekemv** (Amgen Ltd) ▼

Eculizumab 10 mg per 1 ml Bekemv 300mg/30ml concentrate for solution for infusion vials | 1 vial [PoM] £3,150.00 (Hospital only)

▸ **Epysqli** (Samsung Bioepis NL B.V. Ltd) ▼

Eculizumab 10 mg per 1 ml Epysqli 300mg/30ml concentrate for solution for infusion vials | 1 vial [PoM] £3,150.00 (Hospital only)

▸ **Soliris** (Alexion Pharma UK Ltd)

Eculizumab 10 mg per 1 ml Soliris 300mg/30ml concentrate for solution for infusion vials | 1 vial [PoM] £3,150.00 (Hospital only)

Iptacopan
14-Jan-2025

- **DRUG ACTION** Iptacopan is a complement inhibitor which targets factor B and prevents the activation of C3 convertase, thereby inhibiting the complement cascade that leads to haemolysis.

- **INDICATIONS AND DOSE**

Paroxysmal nocturnal haemoglobinuria (under expert supervision)

▸ BY MOUTH

▸ Adult: 200 mg twice daily

DOSE EQUIVALENCE AND CONVERSION

▸ For patients switching from eculizumab, iptacopan should be initiated no later than 1 week after the last dose of eculizumab.

▸ For patients switching from ravulizumab, iptacopan should be initiated no later than 6 weeks after the last dose of ravulizumab.

- **CONTRA-INDICATIONS** Patients unvaccinated against *Neisseria meningitidis*, and *Streptococcus pneumoniae* · unresolved infection caused by encapsulated bacteria (including *Neisseria meningitidis*, *Streptococcus pneumoniae*, and *Haemophilus influenzae* type b)

CONTRA-INDICATIONS, FURTHER INFORMATION

▸ Vaccination against serious infection [EvGr] To reduce the risk of serious infection, it is advised that patients are vaccinated against *Neisseria meningitidis*, *Streptococcus pneumoniae*, and if appropriate, *Haemophilus influenzae* type b according to local guidelines, at least 2 weeks prior to starting treatment, unless the risk of delaying treatment outweighs the risk of developing an infection. If immediate treatment is needed, administer the required vaccines as soon as possible; treat with prophylactic antibiotics until 2 weeks after vaccination. Revaccinate according to local guidelines if necessary. ⟨M⟩

- **INTERACTIONS** → Appendix 1: iptacopan

- **SIDE-EFFECTS**

▸ **Common or very common** Arthralgia · diarrhoea · dizziness · gastrointestinal discomfort · headaches · increased risk of infection · nausea

▸ **Uncommon** Urticaria

- **PREGNANCY** [EvGr] Use only if potential benefit outweighs risk (limited information available). ⟨M⟩

- **BREAST FEEDING** [EvGr] Avoid (no information available). ⟨M⟩

- **HEPATIC IMPAIRMENT** [EvGr] Avoid in severe impairment. ⟨M⟩

- **MONITORING REQUIREMENTS**

▸ [EvGr] Monitor for early signs and symptoms of serious infection caused by encapsulated bacteria (including *Neisseria meningitidis*, *Streptococcus pneumoniae*, and *Haemophilus influenzae* type b).

▸ Monitor for signs and symptoms of haemolysis (including lactate dehydrogenase levels) during treatment and for at least 2 weeks after treatment discontinuation—consult product literature. ⟨M⟩

- **PRESCRIBING AND DISPENSING INFORMATION** The manufacturer of *Fabhalta*® has provided a *Healthcare Professionals Guide* and a *Vaccination Confirmation Form*.

- **PATIENT AND CARER ADVICE** Patients and carers should be informed of the signs and symptoms of serious infection and advised to seek immediate medical care if they occur. Patient card and guide A patient safety card and guide for patients and caregivers should be provided.

- **NATIONAL FUNDING/ACCESS DECISIONS**

For full details see funding body website

NICE decisions

▸ Iptacopan for treating paroxysmal nocturnal haemoglobinuria (September 2024) NICE TA1000 Recommended

Scottish Medicines Consortium (SMC) decisions

▸ Iptacopan (*Fabhalta*®) as monotherapy for the treatment of adult patients with paroxysmal nocturnal haemoglobinuria who have haemolytic anaemia (January 2025) SMC No. SMC2676 Recommended with restrictions

- **MEDICINAL FORMS** There can be variation in the licensing of different medicines containing the same drug.

Oral capsule

CAUTIONARY AND ADVISORY LABELS 8, 10

EXCIPIENTS: May contain Gelatin

▸ **Fabhalta** (Novartis Pharmaceuticals UK Ltd) ▼

Iptacopan (as Iptacopan hydrochloride monohydrate) 200 mg Fabhalta 200mg capsules | 56 capsule [PoM] £26,500.00 (Hospital only)

Pegcetacoplan
28-Mar-2024

- **DRUG ACTION** Pegcetacoplan is a pegylated peptide molecule, which binds to C3 and C3b complement proteins, thereby inhibiting the complement cascade that leads to haemolysis.

- **INDICATIONS AND DOSE**

Paroxysmal nocturnal haemoglobinuria (initiated by a specialist)

▸ BY SUBCUTANEOUS INFUSION

▸ Adult: 1080 mg twice weekly, administer on day 1 and day 4 of each treatment week, continue current dose of C5 inhibitor for the first 4 weeks of treatment, for dose adjustments due to lactate dehydrogenase levels—consult product literature

- **CONTRA-INDICATIONS** Patients unvaccinated against *Neisseria meningitidis*, *Streptococcus pneumoniae*, and *Haemophilus influenzae* · unresolved infection caused by encapsulated bacteria (including *Neisseria meningitidis*, *Streptococcus pneumoniae*, and *Haemophilus influenzae*)

CONTRA-INDICATIONS, FURTHER INFORMATION

▸ Vaccination against serious infection [EvGr] To reduce the risk of serious infection, it is advised that patients are vaccinated against *Neisseria meningitidis*, *Streptococcus pneumoniae*, and *Haemophilus influenzae* according to local guidelines, at least 2 weeks, but no longer than 2 years, prior to starting treatment, unless the risk of delaying treatment outweighs the risk of developing an infection. If immediate treatment is needed, administer the required vaccines as soon as possible; treat with prophylactic antibiotics until 2 weeks after vaccination. ⟨M⟩

- **SIDE-EFFECTS**

▸ **Common or very common** Asthenia · diarrhoea · dizziness · epistaxis · fever · gastrointestinal discomfort · headache · increased risk of infection · myalgia · nausea · pain · sepsis · skin reactions · thrombocytopenia

- **CONCEPTION AND CONTRACEPTION** [EvGr] Females of childbearing potential should use effective contraception during and for at least 8 weeks after treatment. ⓜ
- **PREGNANCY** [EvGr] Avoid—toxicity in *animal* studies. ⓜ
- **BREAST FEEDING** [EvGr] Avoid—no information available. ⓜ
- **MONITORING REQUIREMENTS**
  ▸ [EvGr] Monitor for early signs of infection caused by encapsulated bacteria (including *Neisseria meningitidis*, *Streptococcus pneumoniae*, and *Haemophilus influenzae*).
  ▸ Monitor for signs and symptoms of haemolysis including lactate dehydrogenase levels during treatment, and for at least 8 weeks after treatment discontinuation—consult product literature.
  ▸ Regularly monitor renal function (risk of polyethylene glycol (PEG) accumulation in kidneys). ⓜ
- **EFFECT ON LABORATORY TESTS** [EvGr] Pegcetacoplan may interfere with silica reagents in coagulation panels, resulting in artificially prolonged activated partial thromboplastin time (aPTT). ⓜ
- **TREATMENT CESSATION** Slow weaning and alternative therapy should be considered if treatment is to be discontinued due to the risk of serious intravascular haemolysis—consult product literature. Patients must be closely monitored for at least 8 weeks after treatment discontinuation.
- **DIRECTIONS FOR ADMINISTRATION** For *subcutaneous infusion*, administer into the abdomen, thighs, hips or upper arms over approximately 30 minutes if using two sites (ensuring sites are at least 7.5 cm apart), or approximately 60 minutes if using one site; rotate infusion sites. Patients may self-administer *Aspaveli*®, after appropriate training in subcutaneous infusion technique.
- **PRESCRIBING AND DISPENSING INFORMATION** The manufacturer of *Aspaveli*® has provided a *Guide for Healthcare Professionals*.
- **HANDLING AND STORAGE** Store in a refrigerator (2–8 °C) and protect from light.
- **PATIENT AND CARER ADVICE** If appropriate, patients and carers should be given training on how to administer pegcetacoplan subcutaneous infusion. Patients and carers should be informed of the signs and symptoms of serious infection and advised to seek immediate medical care if they occur.
  Patient card and guide A patient card and guide for patients and caregivers should be provided.
- **NATIONAL FUNDING/ACCESS DECISIONS**
  For full details see funding body website
  NICE decisions
  ▸ Pegcetacoplan for treating paroxysmal nocturnal haemoglobinuria (March 2022) NICE TA778 Recommended
  Scottish Medicines Consortium (SMC) decisions
  ▸ Pegcetacoplan (*Aspaveli*®) for the treatment of adult patients with paroxysmal nocturnal haemoglobinuria who are anaemic after treatment with a C5 inhibitor for at least 3 months (July 2022) SMC No. SMC2451 Recommended with restrictions

- **MEDICINAL FORMS** There can be variation in the licensing of different medicines containing the same drug.
  Solution for infusion
  EXCIPIENTS: May contain Sorbitol
  ▸ Aspaveli (Swedish Orphan Biovitrum Ltd) ▼
  Pegcetacoplan 54 mg per 1 ml Aspaveli 1080mg/20ml solution for infusion vials | 1 vial [PoM] £3,100.00 (Hospital only) | 8 vial [PoM] £24,800.00 (Hospital only)

Ravulizumab
28-Mar-2024

- **DRUG ACTION** Ravulizumab is a recombinant monoclonal antibody that inhibits terminal complement activation at the C5 protein, thereby reducing haemolysis and thrombotic microangiopathy.

- **INDICATIONS AND DOSE**
  Atypical haemolytic uraemic syndrome (under expert supervision) | Paroxysmal nocturnal haemoglobinuria (under expert supervision)
  ▸ BY INTRAVENOUS INFUSION
  ▸ Adult (body-weight 40–59 kg): Loading dose 2.4 g for 1 dose, then maintenance 3 g every 8 weeks, start maintenance dosing 2 weeks after the loading dose, a maintenance dose (except for the first maintenance dose) may be given up to 7 days before or after the scheduled date; the subsequent dose should be given according to the original schedule, for duration of infusion—consult product literature
  ▸ Adult (body-weight 60–99 kg): Loading dose 2.7 g for 1 dose, then maintenance 3.3 g every 8 weeks, start maintenance dosing 2 weeks after the loading dose, a maintenance dose (except for the first maintenance dose) may be given up to 7 days before or after the scheduled date; the subsequent dose should be given according to the original schedule, for duration of infusion—consult product literature
  ▸ Adult (body-weight 100 kg and above): Loading dose 3 g for 1 dose, then maintenance 3.6 g every 8 weeks, start maintenance dosing 2 weeks after the loading dose, a maintenance dose (except for the first maintenance dose) may be given up to 7 days before or after the scheduled date; the subsequent dose should be given according to the original schedule, for duration of infusion—consult product literature
  DOSE EQUIVALENCE AND CONVERSION
  ▸ For patients switching from eculizumab to ravulizumab, the initial loading dose of ravulizumab should be administered 2 weeks after the last eculizumab infusion.

- **CONTRA-INDICATIONS** Patients unvaccinated against *Neisseria meningitidis* · unresolved *Neisseria meningitidis* infection
- **CAUTIONS** Active systemic infection
  CAUTIONS, FURTHER INFORMATION
  ▸ Meningococcal infection [EvGr] Vaccinate against *Neisseria meningitidis* at least 2 weeks before treatment (vaccines against serotypes A, C, Y, W135 and B where available, are recommended); revaccinate according to current medical guidelines. Patients receiving ravulizumab less than 2 weeks after receiving meningococcal vaccine must be given prophylactic antibiotics until 2 weeks after vaccination. Other immunisations should also be up to date for all age groups. ⓜ
- **INTERACTIONS** → Appendix 1: ravulizumab
- **SIDE-EFFECTS**
  ▸ **Common or very common** Arthralgia · asthenia · back pain · diarrhoea · dizziness · fever · gastrointestinal discomfort · headache · increased risk of infection · influenza like illness · infusion related reaction · muscle complaints · nausea · skin reactions · vomiting
  ▸ **Uncommon** Chills · hypersensitivity · meningococcal sepsis
- **CONCEPTION AND CONTRACEPTION** Manufacturer advises effective contraception during and for up to 8 months after treatment.
- **PREGNANCY** Manufacturer advises use only if potential benefit outweighs risk—no information available. Ravulizumab is an immunoglobulin G (IgG) monoclonal

antibody; human IgG antibodies are known to cross the placenta.

- **BREAST FEEDING** Manufacturer advises avoid breast-feeding during and for up to 8 months after treatment—no information available.
- **MONITORING REQUIREMENTS**
- ▸ When used for Paroxysmal nocturnal haemoglobinuria EvGr Monitor for intravascular haemolysis (including serum-lactate dehydrogenase concentration) for at least 16 weeks after stopping treatment; consider restarting ravulizumab if haemolysis occurs. ⟨M⟩
- ▸ When used for Atypical haemolytic uraemic syndrome EvGr Monitor for thrombotic microangiopathy (measure platelet count, serum-lactate dehydrogenase concentration, and serum creatinine) after stopping treatment; consider restarting ravulizumab if thrombotic microangiopathy occurs. ⟨M⟩
- **DIRECTIONS FOR ADMINISTRATION** EvGr For *intravenous infusion* using *Ultomiris* ® 300 *mg/3 mL,* 1100 *mg/11 mL concentrate for infusion,* give intermittently in Sodium Chloride 0.9%. Dilute requisite dose with infusion fluid to a final concentration of 50 mg/mL and administer through an in-line filter (0.2 micron). For *intravenous infusion* using *Ultomiris* ® 300 *mg/30 mL concentrate for infusion,* give intermittently in Sodium Chloride 0.9%. Dilute requisite dose with infusion fluid to a final concentration of 5 mg/mL and administer through an in-line filter (0.2 micron). ⟨M⟩
- **PRESCRIBING AND DISPENSING INFORMATION** Ravulizumab is a biological medicine. Biological medicines must be prescribed and dispensed by brand name, see *Biological medicines* and *Biosimilar medicines,* under Guidance on prescribing p. 1; record the brand name and batch number after each administration.

  The manufacturer of *Ultomiris* ® has provided a *Physician's guide* for healthcare professionals.
- **HANDLING AND STORAGE** Store in a refrigerator (2-8°C) and protect from light—consult product literature for further information regarding storage outside refrigerator.
- **PATIENT AND CARER ADVICE** Patients or carers should be advised to report promptly any signs of meningococcal infection. Advice about prevention of gonorrhoea should also be given.

  A patient information card and a patient safety card should be provided.
- **NATIONAL FUNDING/ACCESS DECISIONS** For full details see funding body website
  NICE decisions
- ▸ Ravulizumab for treating paroxysmal nocturnal haemoglobinuria (May 2021) NICE TA698 Recommended
- ▸ Ravulizumab for treating atypical haemolytic uraemic syndrome (June 2021) NICE TA710 Recommended
  Scottish Medicines Consortium (SMC) decisions
- ▸ Ravulizumab (*Ultomiris* ®) for the treatment of adult patients with paroxysmal nocturnal haemoglobinuria (February 2021) SMC No. SMC2305 Recommended with restrictions
- ▸ Ravulizumab (*Ultomiris* ®) for the treatment of patients with a body weight of 10 kg or above with atypical haemolytic uremic syndrome who are complement inhibitor treatment-naive or have received eculizumab for at least 3 months and have evidence of response to eculizumab (May 2021) SMC No. SMC2330 Recommended with restrictions

- **MEDICINAL FORMS** There can be variation in the licensing of different medicines containing the same drug.
  Solution for infusion
  EXCIPIENTS: May contain Polysorbates
  ELECTROLYTES: May contain Sodium
  - ▸ **Ultomiris** (Alexion Pharma UK Ltd)
    Ravulizumab 100 mg per 1 ml Ultomiris 1,100mg/11ml concentrate for solution for infusion vials | 1 vial PoM £16,621.00

Ultomiris 300mg/3ml concentrate for solution for infusion vials | 1 vial PoM £4,533.00

1.2   Iron deficiency anaemia

Anaemia, iron deficiency   12-Feb-2025

Iron deficiency, treatment and prophylaxis

Iron deficiency anaemia is the reduction of red blood cell production due to low iron stores in the body.

Treatment with an iron preparation should be initiated for confirmed iron-deficiency anaemia. It is important to exclude any underlying causes of the anaemia (e.g. gastric erosion, gastro-intestinal cancer, coeliac disease, inflammatory bowel disease, or heavy menstrual bleeding), but iron treatment should not be delayed whilst awaiting investigations.

Prophylaxis with an iron preparation may be appropriate in malabsorption, menorrhagia, pregnancy, after subtotal or total gastrectomy, and in haemodialysis patients.

For further information on the management of iron-deficiency anaemia, including information on therapeutic trials of oral iron, see British Society of Gastroenterology guidance: **Guidelines for the Management of Iron Deficiency Anaemia in Adults** (available at: www.bsg.org. uk/clinical-resource/guidelines-iron-deficiency-anaemia-in-adults).

For information on the management of anaemia in peri-operative patients, see Centre for Perioperative Care guidance: **Guideline for the Management of Anaemia in the Perioperative Pathway** (available at: cpoc.org.uk/guidelines-resources-guidelines/anaemia-perioperative-pathway).

Oral iron

Iron salts should be given by mouth unless there are good reasons for using another route.

Ferrous salts show only marginal differences between one another in efficiency of absorption of iron. Haemoglobin regeneration rate is little affected by the type of salt used provided sufficient iron is given, and in most patients the speed of response is not critical. Choice of preparation is thus usually decided by the incidence of side-effects and cost.

EvGr An initial once-daily dose regimen of oral iron salts is recommended, as this may be just as effective as multiple daily dose regimens (such as two or three times a day dosing), with a lower incidence of side-effects and better compliance. Patients should be monitored in the first 4 weeks for a haemoglobin response to oral iron, and treatment continued for around 3 months after normalisation of haemoglobin concentration. ⟨A⟩ EvGr The dose of oral iron salts can be increased if the therapeutic response is slow and treatment is tolerated. ⟨E⟩ For guidance on iron dosing, see ferrous sulfate p. 1159, ferrous fumarate p. 1158, ferrous gluconate p. 1159, ferric maltol p. 1158, and sodium feredetate p. 1160.

Iron content of different iron salts

Iron salt/amount	Content of ferrous iron
ferrous fumarate 210 mg	69 mg
ferrous gluconate 300 mg	35 mg
ferrous sulfate, dried 200 mg	65 mg
sodium feredetate 190 mg/5 mL	27.5 mg/5 mL
ferric maltol 30 mg	30 mg

Compound preparations

Preparations containing iron and folic acid p. 1161 are used during pregnancy in women who are at high risk of developing iron and folic acid deficiency; they should be distinguished from those used for the prevention of neural tube defects in women planning a pregnancy.

It is important to note that the small doses of folic acid contained in these preparations are inadequate for the treatment of megaloblastic anaemias.

Some oral preparations contain ascorbic acid p. 1239 to aid absorption of the iron but the therapeutic advantage of such preparations is minimal and cost may be increased.

There is no justification for the inclusion of other ingredients, such as the **B group of vitamins** (except folic acid for pregnant women).

Modified-release preparations

Modified-release preparations of iron are licensed for once-daily dosage, but have no therapeutic advantage and should not be used. These preparations are formulated to release iron gradually; the low incidence of side-effects may reflect the small amounts of iron available for absorption as the iron is carried past the first part of the duodenum into an area of the gut where absorption may be poor.

Parenteral iron

Iron can be administered parenterally as iron dextran p. 1157, iron sucrose p. 1157, ferric carboxymaltose below, or ferric derisomaltose p. 1157. Parenteral iron is generally reserved for use when oral therapy is unsuccessful because the patient cannot tolerate oral iron, or does not take it reliably, or if there is continuing blood loss, or in malabsorption. Parenteral iron may also have a role in the management of chemotherapy-induced anaemia, when given with erythropoietins, in specific patient groups (see NICE guidance).

Many patients with chronic renal failure who are receiving haemodialysis (and some who are receiving peritoneal dialysis) also require iron by the intravenous route on a regular basis.

With the exception of patients with severe renal failure receiving haemodialysis, parenteral iron does not produce a faster haemoglobin response than oral iron provided that the oral iron preparation is taken reliably and is absorbed adequately. Depending on the preparation used, parenteral iron is given as a total dose or in divided doses. Further treatment should be guided by monitoring haemoglobin and serum iron concentrations.

MINERALS AND TRACE ELEMENTS > IRON, INJECTABLE

Iron (injectable)

IMPORTANT SAFETY INFORMATION

MHRA/CHM ADVICE: SERIOUS HYPERSENSITIVITY REACTIONS WITH INTRAVENOUS IRON (AUGUST 2013)

Serious hypersensitivity reactions, including life-threatening and fatal anaphylactic reactions, have been reported in patients receiving intravenous iron. These reactions can occur even when a previous administration has been tolerated (including a negative test dose). Test doses are no longer recommended and caution is needed with every dose of intravenous iron.

Intravenous iron products should only be administered when appropriately trained staff and resuscitation facilities are immediately available; patients should be closely monitored for signs of hypersensitivity during and for at least 30 minutes after every administration. In the event of a hypersensitivity reaction, treatment should be stopped immediately and appropriate management initiated.

The risk of hypersensitivity is increased in patients with known allergies, immune or inflammatory conditions, or those with a history of severe asthma, eczema, or other atopic allergy; in these patients,

intravenous iron should only be used if the benefits outweigh the risks.

Intravenous iron should be avoided in the first trimester of pregnancy and used in the second or third trimesters only if the benefit outweighs the potential risks for both mother and fetus.

- **CONTRA-INDICATIONS** Disturbances in utilisation of iron · iron overload
- **CAUTIONS** Allergic disorders · eczema · hepatic dysfunction · immune conditions · infection (discontinue if ongoing bacteraemia) · inflammatory conditions · oral iron should not be given until 5 days after the last injection · severe asthma
- **SIDE-EFFECTS**
- ▶ **Common or very common** Dizziness · flushing · headache · hypertension · hypophosphataemia · hypotension · nausea · skin reactions · taste altered
- ▶ **Uncommon** Arrhythmias · arthralgia · bronchospasm · chest pain · chills · constipation · diarrhoea · dyspnoea · fatigue · fever · gastrointestinal discomfort · hyperhidrosis · hypersensitivity · loss of consciousness · malaise · muscle complaints · pain · peripheral oedema · sensation abnormal · vision blurred · vomiting
- ▶ **Rare or very rare** Angioedema · anxiety · circulatory collapse · influenza like illness · pallor · palpitations · psychiatric disorder · seizure · syncope · tremor
- ▶ **Frequency not known** Kounis syndrome

SIDE-EFFECTS, FURTHER INFORMATION Anaphylactic reactions can occur with parenteral administration of iron complexes and facilities for cardiopulmonary resuscitation must be available.

Overdose For details on the management of poisoning, see Iron salts, under Emergency treatment of poisoning p. 1554.

- **PREGNANCY**
Monitoring in pregnancy EvGr Fetal monitoring is recommended during administration due to the risk of fetal bradycardia. ⟨M⟩

F above

Ferric carboxymaltose

28-Oct-2024

- **INDICATIONS AND DOSE**

Iron-deficiency anaemia

- ▶ BY SLOW INTRAVENOUS INJECTION, OR BY INTRAVENOUS INFUSION
- ▶ Adult: Dose calculated according to body-weight and iron deficit (consult product literature)

IMPORTANT SAFETY INFORMATION

MHRA/CHM ADVICE: FERRIC CARBOXYMALTOSE (*FERINJECT*®): RISK OF SYMPTOMATIC HYPOPHOSPHATAEMIA LEADING TO OSTEOMALACIA AND FRACTURES (NOVEMBER 2020)

A European review of worldwide data concluded that ferric carboxymaltose is associated with hypophosphataemia, resulting in hypophosphataemic osteomalacia and fractures, particularly in patients with existing risk factors and following prolonged exposure to high doses—some cases required clinical intervention, including surgery. The risk of persistent hypophosphatemia and osteomalacia may be higher with ferric carboxymaltose than with other intravenous iron formulations.

Healthcare professionals are advised to monitor serum phosphate levels in patients requiring multiple high-dose administrations, on long-term treatment, or with pre-existing risk factors for hypophosphataemia. Patients experiencing symptoms of hypophosphataemia (including new musculoskeletal symptoms or worsening tiredness) should seek medical advice—be aware that these symptoms may be confused with those of iron deficiency anaemia. If hypophosphataemia persists, ferric carboxymaltose treatment should be re-evaluated.

- **INTERACTIONS** → Appendix 1: iron
- **SIDE-EFFECTS**
  ▸ **Rare or very rare** Flatulence
  ▸ **Frequency not known** Face oedema
- **PREGNANCY** Avoid in first trimester; crosses the placenta in *animal* studies. May influence skeletal development.
- **HEPATIC IMPAIRMENT** Manufacturer advises caution— monitor iron status to avoid iron overload; avoid where iron overload increases risk of impairment (particularly porphyria cutanea tarda).
- **DIRECTIONS FOR ADMINISTRATION** For *intravenous infusion* (*Ferinject*®), give intermittently in Sodium Chloride 0.9%. Dilute 200–500 mg in up to 100 mL infusion fluid and give over at least 6 minutes; dilute 0.5–1 g in up to 250 mL infusion fluid and give over at least 15 minutes.
- **PRESCRIBING AND DISPENSING INFORMATION** A ferric carboxymaltose complex containing 5% (50 mg/mL) of iron.

- **MEDICINAL FORMS** There can be variation in the licensing of different medicines containing the same drug.
  Dispersion for injection
  ELECTROLYTES: May contain Sodium
  ▸ **Ferinject** (Vifor Pharma UK Ltd)
  Iron (as Ferric carboxymaltose) 50 mg per 1 ml Ferinject 1000mg/20ml dispersion for injection vials | 1 vial [PoM] £154.23 (Hospital only)
  Ferinject 500mg/10ml dispersion for injection vials | 5 vial [PoM] £477.50 (Hospital only)

F 1156

Ferric derisomaltose
03-Mar-2021

(Iron isomaltoside 1000)

- **INDICATIONS AND DOSE**
  Iron-deficiency anaemia
  ▸ BY INTRAVENOUS INJECTION
  ▸ Adult: (consult product literature)

- **INTERACTIONS** → Appendix 1: iron
- **SIDE-EFFECTS**
  ▸ **Uncommon** Fishbane reaction · infection
  ▸ **Rare or very rare** Dysphonia
- **PREGNANCY** [EvGr] Avoid in first trimester; use in second and third trimesters only if potential benefit outweighs risk—limited information available. [M]
- **HEPATIC IMPAIRMENT** Manufacturer advises caution in compensated hepatic disease—monitor iron status to avoid iron overload; avoid in decompensated hepatic disease, in hepatitis and where iron overload is a precipitating factor (particularly porphyria cutanea tarda).
- **NATIONAL FUNDING/ACCESS DECISIONS**
  For full details see funding body website
  Scottish Medicines Consortium (SMC) decisions
  ▸ Iron (III) isomaltoside 1000 5% (*Diafer*®) for iron deficiency in adults with chronic kidney disease (CKD) on dialysis, when oral iron preparations are ineffective or cannot be used (February 2017) SMC No. 1177/16 Recommended

- **MEDICINAL FORMS** There can be variation in the licensing of different medicines containing the same drug.
  Solution for injection
  ▸ **Ferric derisomaltose** (Non-proprietary)
  Iron (as Ferric derisomaltose) 100 mg per 1 ml Ferric derisomaltose 1g/10ml solution for injection vials | 2 vial [PoM] £339.00 (Hospital only)
  Ferric derisomaltose 500mg/5ml solution for injection vials | 5 vial [PoM] £423.75 (Hospital only)

Ferric derisomaltose 100mg/1ml solution for injection vials | 5 vial [PoM] £84.75 (Hospital only)
  ▸ **Diafer** (Pharmacosmos UK Ltd)
  Iron (as Ferric derisomaltose) 50 mg per 1 ml Diafer 100mg/2ml solution for injection ampoules | 25 ampoule [PoM] £423.75 (Hospital only)

F 1156

Iron dextran
28-Mar-2023

- **INDICATIONS AND DOSE**
  Iron-deficiency anaemia
  ▸ BY DEEP INTRAMUSCULAR INJECTION
  ▸ Adult: Intramuscular injection to be administered into the gluteal muscle, doses calculated according to body-weight and iron deficit (consult product literature)
  ▸ BY SLOW INTRAVENOUS INJECTION, OR BY INTRAVENOUS INFUSION
  ▸ Adult: Doses calculated according to body-weight and iron deficit (consult product literature)

> **IMPORTANT SAFETY INFORMATION**
> *CosmoFer*® should only be administered when appropriately trained staff and resuscitation facilities are immediately available; patients should be closely monitored during and for at least 30 minutes following each injection.

- **INTERACTIONS** → Appendix 1: iron
- **SIDE-EFFECTS**
  ▸ **Uncommon** Feeling hot
  ▸ **Rare or very rare** Deafness (transient) · haemolysis
  ▸ **Frequency not known** Injection site necrosis · rheumatoid arthritis aggravated
- **PREGNANCY** Avoid in first trimester.
- **HEPATIC IMPAIRMENT** Manufacturer advises avoid in decompensated cirrhosis and hepatitis.
- **RENAL IMPAIRMENT** [EvGr] Avoid in acute renal failure. [M]
- **DIRECTIONS FOR ADMINISTRATION** [EvGr] For *intravenous infusion* (*CosmoFer*®), give intermittently in Glucose 5% *or* Sodium Chloride 0.9%, dilute 100–200 mg in 100 mL infusion fluid; give 25 mg over 15 minutes initially, then give at a rate not exceeding 6.67 mg/minute; *total dose infusion* diluted in 500 mL infusion fluid and given over 4–6 hours (initial dose 25 mg over 15 minutes). [M]
- **PRESCRIBING AND DISPENSING INFORMATION** A complex of ferric hydroxide with dextran containing 5% (50 mg/mL) of iron.

- **MEDICINAL FORMS** There can be variation in the licensing of different medicines containing the same drug.
  Solution for injection
  ▸ **CosmoFer** (Pharmacosmos UK Ltd)
  Iron (as Iron dextran) 50 mg per 1 ml CosmoFer 500mg/10ml solution for injection ampoules | 2 ampoule [PoM] £79.70 DT = £79.70
  CosmoFer 100mg/2ml solution for injection ampoules | 5 ampoule [PoM] £39.85 DT = £39.85

F 1156

Iron sucrose
29-Nov-2019

- **INDICATIONS AND DOSE**
  Iron-deficiency anaemia
  ▸ BY SLOW INTRAVENOUS INJECTION, OR BY INTRAVENOUS INFUSION
  ▸ Adult: Doses calculated according to body-weight and iron deficit (consult product literature)

- **INTERACTIONS** → Appendix 1: iron
- **SIDE-EFFECTS**
  ▸ **Uncommon** Asthenia
  ▸ **Rare or very rare** Drowsiness · urine discolouration

- ▶ **Frequency not known** Cold sweat · confusion · level of consciousness decreased · thrombophlebitis
- • PREGNANCY Avoid in first trimester.
- • HEPATIC IMPAIRMENT Manufacturer advises caution—monitor iron status to avoid iron overload; avoid where iron overload is a precipitating factor (particularly porphyria cutanea tarda).
- • DIRECTIONS FOR ADMINISTRATION Manufacturer advises for *intermittent intravenous infusion* (*Venofer*®), dilute to a concentration of 1 mg/mL with Sodium Chloride 0.9%; give at a rate not exceeding 6.67 mg/minute (consult product literature). Manufacturer advises for *slow intravenous injection* (*Venofer*®), give undiluted at a rate of 1 mL/minute; do not exceed 10 mL (200 mg iron) per injection.
- • PRESCRIBING AND DISPENSING INFORMATION A complex of ferric hydroxide with sucrose containing 2% (20 mg/mL) of iron.

- • MEDICINAL FORMS There can be variation in the licensing of different medicines containing the same drug.

Solution for injection
- ▶ Venofer (Imported (United States), Vifor Pharma UK Ltd)
  Iron (as Iron sucrose) 20 mg per 1 ml Venofer 50mg/2.5ml solution for injection vials | 5 vial [PoM] ⓧ
  Venofer 100mg/5ml solution for injection vials | 5 vial [PoM] £51.20
  DT = £51.20

MINERALS AND TRACE ELEMENTS > IRON, ORAL

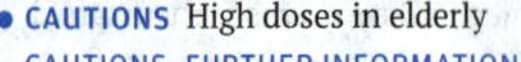

Iron (oral)

- • CAUTIONS High doses in elderly
  CAUTIONS, FURTHER INFORMATION
- ▶ Elderly Screening Tool of Older Persons' potentially inappropriate Prescriptions (STOPP) criteria to aid medication reviews (see Prescribing in the elderly p. 31 for information): potentially inappropriate at oral doses greater than 200 mg elemental iron daily (no evidence of enhanced iron absorption above these doses).

- • SIDE-EFFECTS
- ▶ **Common or very common** Constipation · diarrhoea · gastrointestinal discomfort · nausea
- ▶ **Uncommon** Vomiting
- ▶ **Frequency not known** Appetite decreased · gastrointestinal disorders

  SIDE-EFFECTS, FURTHER INFORMATION Iron can be constipating and occasionally lead to faecal impaction. Oral iron, particularly modified-release preparations, can exacerbate diarrhoea in patients with inflammatory bowel disease; care is also needed in patients with intestinal strictures and diverticular disease.

  Overdose For details on the management of poisoning, see Iron salts, under Emergency treatment of poisoning p. 1554.

- • MONITORING REQUIREMENTS
- ▶ [EvGr] Monitor haemoglobin concentration within the first 4 weeks of treatment, then regularly thereafter to assess response (e.g. every 4 weeks). Once haemoglobin is within the normal range, treatment should be continued for around a further 3 months to replenish the iron stores. After treatment, monitor blood count periodically (e.g. every 6 months) to detect recurrence. Ⓐ
- ▶ Therapeutic response [EvGr] For once daily dosing of most oral iron salts, the haemoglobin concentration should rise by at least 10 g/litre after 2 weeks of treatment, or 20 g/litre after 4 weeks of treatment. For alternate day dosing of most oral iron salts, the haemoglobin concentration should rise by at least 10 g/litre after 4 weeks of treatment. Ⓐ

- • PATIENT AND CARER ADVICE It is recommended to take iron on an empty stomach to allow for better absorption, although it can be taken after food to reduce gastro-intestinal side-effects if necessary. Certain food and drinks, such as milk or dairy products, unprocessed bran, tea, and coffee can reduce the absorption of oral iron. May discolour stools.

⯈ above

Ferric maltol
04-Apr-2023

- • INDICATIONS AND DOSE

Iron-deficiency anaemia [treatment and prophylaxis]
- ▶ BY MOUTH USING CAPSULES
- ▶ Adult: Initially 60 mg once daily, reduced if not tolerated to 60 mg once daily on alternate days, alternatively initially 30 mg twice daily, reduced if not tolerated to 30 mg once daily

DOSE EQUIVALENCE AND CONVERSION
- ▶ *Feraccru*® capsules contain ferric maltol 30 mg equivalent to 30 mg elemental iron.

- • UNLICENSED USE [EvGr] Ferric maltol is used in the doses provided in the BNF for the treatment and prophylaxis of iron-deficiency anaemia, Ⓔ but these may differ from those licensed.
- • CONTRA-INDICATIONS Exacerbation of inflammatory bowel disease · haemochromatosis · inflammatory bowel disease with haemoglobin less than 9.5 g/dL · iron overload syndromes · repeated blood transfusions
- • INTERACTIONS → Appendix 1: iron
- • SIDE-EFFECTS
- ▶ **Uncommon** Headache · joint stiffness · pain in extremity · skin reactions · small intestinal bacterial overgrowth · thirst
- • MONITORING REQUIREMENTS
- ▶ Therapeutic response [EvGr] Ferric maltol has a relatively low iron content and the rate of iron loading is slower than with other oral iron salts. For daily dosing, the haemoglobin concentration should rise by at least 10 g/litre after 6 weeks of treatment. Ⓐ
- • NATIONAL FUNDING/ACCESS DECISIONS
  For full details see funding body website

Scottish Medicines Consortium (SMC) decisions
- ▶ Ferric maltol (*Feraccru*®) for the treatment of iron deficiency in adults (January 2023) SMC No. SMC2500 Not recommended

All Wales Medicines Strategy Group (AWMSG) decisions
- ▶ Ferric maltol (*Feraccru*®) for the treatment of iron deficiency in adults (November 2022) AWMSG No. 5116 Recommended with restrictions

- • MEDICINAL FORMS There can be variation in the licensing of different medicines containing the same drug.

Oral capsule
CAUTIONARY AND ADVISORY LABELS 23
- ▶ Feraccru (Norgine Pharmaceuticals Ltd)
  Iron (as Ferric maltol) 30 mg Feraccru 30mg capsules |
  56 capsule [PoM] £47.60 DT = £47.60

⯈ above

Ferrous fumarate
27-Jan-2025

- • INDICATIONS AND DOSE

Iron-deficiency anaemia [treatment and prophylaxis]
- ▶ BY MOUTH USING TABLETS
- ▶ Adult: Initially 210 mg once daily, reduced if not tolerated to 210 mg once daily on alternate days, alternatively initially 322 mg once daily, reduced if not tolerated to 322 mg once daily on alternate days

▶ BY MOUTH USING CAPSULES
▶ Adult: 305 mg once daily, reduced if not tolerated to 305 mg once daily on alternate days
▶ BY MOUTH USING ORAL SOLUTION
▶ Adult: 5–10 mL once daily, reduced if not tolerated to 5–10 mL once daily on alternate days

DOSE EQUIVALENCE AND CONVERSION
▶ Tablets contain ferrous fumarate 210 mg (equivalent to 69 mg elemental iron) or ferrous fumarate 322 mg (equivalent to 106 mg elemental iron).
▶ Capsules contain ferrous fumarate 305 mg equivalent to 100 mg elemental iron.
▶ Oral solutions contain ferrous fumarate 28 mg/mL equivalent to 9 mg/mL elemental iron.

● UNLICENSED USE [EvGr] Ferrous fumarate is used in the doses provided in the BNF for the treatment and prophylaxis of iron-deficiency anaemia, Ⓐ but these may differ from those licensed.
● INTERACTIONS → Appendix 1: iron
● SIDE-EFFECTS Haemosiderosis

● MEDICINAL FORMS There can be variation in the licensing of different medicines containing the same drug.

Oral tablet
▶ Ferrous fumarate (Non-proprietary)
Ferrous fumarate 210 mg Ferrous fumarate 210mg tablets | 84 tablet Ⓟ £4.88 DT = £3.99
Ferrous fumarate 322 mg Ferrous fumarate 322mg tablets | 28 tablet Ⓟ £1.00 DT = £1.00

Oral solution
▶ Ferrous fumarate (Non-proprietary)
Ferrous fumarate 28 mg per 1 ml Ferrous fumarate 140mg/5ml oral solution | 200 ml Ⓟ £3.92 DT = £3.92
▶ Galfer (Thornton & Ross Ltd)
Ferrous fumarate 28 mg per 1 ml Galfer 140mg/5ml syrup | 300 ml Ⓟ £5.33 DT = £5.33 [SF]

Oral capsule
▶ Galfer (Thornton & Ross Ltd)
Ferrous fumarate 305 mg Galfer 305mg capsules | 100 capsule Ⓟ £5.00 DT = £5.00 | 250 capsule Ⓟ £12.50

Ferrous fumarate with folic acid

04-Apr-2023

The properties listed below are those particular to the combination only. For the properties of the components please consider, ferrous fumarate p. 1158, folic acid p. 1161.

● **INDICATIONS AND DOSE**
Iron-deficiency anaemia [treatment and prophylaxis]
▶ BY MOUTH USING TABLETS
▶ Adult: 1 tablet once daily

DOSE EQUIVALENCE AND CONVERSION
▶ Pregaday® tablets contain ferrous fumarate 322 mg (equivalent to 106 mg elemental iron) and folic acid 350 microgram.

● INTERACTIONS → Appendix 1: folates · iron

● MEDICINAL FORMS No licensed medicines listed.

▶ 1158

Ferrous gluconate

27-Jan-2025

● **INDICATIONS AND DOSE**
Iron-deficiency anaemia [treatment and prophylaxis]
▶ BY MOUTH USING TABLETS
▶ Adult: 600 mg once daily, reduced if not tolerated to 600 mg once daily on alternate days

DOSE EQUIVALENCE AND CONVERSION
▶ Tablets contain ferrous gluconate 300 mg equivalent to 35 mg elemental iron.

● UNLICENSED USE [EvGr] Ferrous gluconate is used in the doses provided in the BNF for the treatment and prophylaxis of iron-deficiency anaemia, Ⓐ but these may differ from those licensed.
● INTERACTIONS → Appendix 1: iron

● MEDICINAL FORMS There can be variation in the licensing of different medicines containing the same drug.

Oral tablet
▶ Ferrous gluconate (Non-proprietary)
Ferrous gluconate 300 mg Ferrous gluconate 300mg tablets | 28 tablet Ⓟ £6.00 DT = £1.19 | 1000 tablet Ⓟ £42.50–£119.64

▶ 1158

Ferrous sulfate

27-Jan-2025

● **INDICATIONS AND DOSE**
Iron-deficiency anaemia [treatment and prophylaxis]
▶ BY MOUTH USING TABLETS
▶ Adult: 200 mg once daily, reduced if not tolerated to 200 mg once daily on alternate days
▶ BY MOUTH USING MODIFIED-RELEASE TABLETS
▶ Adult: 325 mg once daily, reduced if not tolerated to 325 mg once daily on alternate days
▶ BY MOUTH USING ORAL DROPS
▶ Adult: 2–4 mL once daily, reduced if not tolerated to 2–4 mL once daily on alternate days

DOSE EQUIVALENCE AND CONVERSION
▶ Tablets contain ferrous sulfate 200 mg (equivalent to 65 mg elemental iron) or ferrous sulfate 325 mg (equivalent to 105 mg elemental iron).
▶ Oral drops contain ferrous sulfate 125 mg/mL equivalent to 25 mg/mL elemental iron.

● UNLICENSED USE [EvGr] Ferrous sulfate is used in the doses provided in the BNF for the treatment and prophylaxis of iron-deficiency anaemia, Ⓐ but these may differ from those licensed.
● INTERACTIONS → Appendix 1: iron
● SIDE-EFFECTS Tooth discolouration
● PRESCRIBING AND DISPENSING INFORMATION Modified-release preparations of iron are licensed for once-daily dosage, but have no therapeutic advantage and should not be used. These preparations are formulated to release iron gradually; the low incidence of side-effects may reflect the small amounts of iron available for absorption as the iron is carried past the first part of the duodenum into an area of the gut where absorption may be poor.
● LESS SUITABLE FOR PRESCRIBING Modified-release tablets such as Ferrograd® are less suitable for prescribing.

● MEDICINAL FORMS There can be variation in the licensing of different medicines containing the same drug.

Oral tablet
▶ Ferrous sulfate (Non-proprietary)
Ferrous sulfate dried 200 mg Ferrous sulfate 200mg tablets | 28 tablet Ⓟ £1.41 DT = £1.07 | 60 tablet Ⓟ £2.29–£3.05 | 100 tablet Ⓟ £3.81–£5.20 | 1000 tablet Ⓟ £38.21–£64.00

Modified-release tablet
CAUTIONARY AND ADVISORY LABELS 25
▶ Ferrograd (Teofarma S.r.l.)
Ferrous sulfate dried 325 mg Ferrograd 325mg modified-release tablets | 30 tablet Ⓟ £2.58 DT = £2.58

Oral drops
▶ Ironorm (Wallace Manufacturing Chemists Ltd)
Ferrous sulfate 125 mg per 1 ml Ironorm 125mg/ml oral drops | 15 ml Ⓟ £30.00 DT = £30.00 [SF]

Ferrous sulfate with ascorbic acid

24-May-2023

The properties listed below are those particular to the combination only. For the properties of the components please consider, ferrous sulfate p. 1159, ascorbic acid p. 1239.

● **INDICATIONS AND DOSE**

Iron-deficiency anaemia [treatment and prophylaxis]
► BY MOUTH USING MODIFIED-RELEASE TABLETS
► Adult: 1 tablet once daily, reduced if not tolerated to 1 tablet once daily on alternate days

DOSE EQUIVALENCE AND CONVERSION
► *Ferrograd C*® tablets contain ferrous sulfate 325 mg (equivalent to 105 mg elemental iron) and ascorbic acid 500 mg.

● UNLICENSED USE [EvGr] Ferrous sulfate with ascorbic acid is used in the doses provided in the BNF for the treatment and prophylaxis of iron-deficiency anaemia, Ⓐ but these may differ from those licensed.

● INTERACTIONS → Appendix 1: ascorbic acid · iron

● NATIONAL FUNDING/ACCESS DECISIONS
NHS restrictions *Ferrograd C*® is not prescribable in NHS primary care.

● LESS SUITABLE FOR PRESCRIBING Modified-release tablets such as *Ferrograd C*® are less suitable for prescribing.

● MEDICINAL FORMS There can be variation in the licensing of different medicines containing the same drug.
Modified-release tablet
CAUTIONARY AND ADVISORY LABELS 25
► Ferrograd C (Teofarma S.r.l.)
Ferrous sulfate dried 325 mg, Ascorbic acid (as Sodium ascorbate) 500 mg Ferrograd C modified-release tablets | 30 tablet Ⓟ £3.20

Ferrous sulfate with folic acid

27-Jan-2025

The properties listed below are those particular to the combination only. For the properties of the components please consider, ferrous sulfate p. 1159, folic acid p. 1161.

● **INDICATIONS AND DOSE**

Iron-deficiency anaemia [treatment and prophylaxis]
► BY MOUTH USING MODIFIED-RELEASE TABLETS
► Adult: 1 tablet once daily

DOSE EQUIVALENCE AND CONVERSION
► *Ferrograd Folic*® tablets contain ferrous sulfate 325 mg (equivalent to 105 mg elemental iron) and folic acid 350 microgram.

● INTERACTIONS → Appendix 1: folates · iron

● LESS SUITABLE FOR PRESCRIBING Modified-release tablets such as *Ferrograd Folic*® are less suitable for prescribing.

● MEDICINAL FORMS There can be variation in the licensing of different medicines containing the same drug.
Modified-release tablet
CAUTIONARY AND ADVISORY LABELS 25
► Ferrograd Folic (Teofarma S.r.l.)
Folic acid 350 microgram, Ferrous sulfate dried 325 mg Ferrograd Folic 325mg/350microgram modified-release tablets | 30 tablet Ⓟ £2.64 DT = £2.64

F 1158

Sodium feredetate

27-Jan-2025

(Sodium ironedetate)

● **INDICATIONS AND DOSE**

Iron-deficiency anaemia [treatment and prophylaxis]
► BY MOUTH USING ORAL SOLUTION
► Adult: 10–15 mL once daily, reduced if not tolerated to 10–15 mL once daily on alternate days

DOSE EQUIVALENCE AND CONVERSION
► *Feredet*® and *Sodifer*® oral solutions contain sodium feredetate 38 mg/mL equivalent to 5.5 mg/mL elemental iron.
► *Sytron*® oral solution contains sodium feredetate trihydrate 41.5 mg/mL equivalent to 5.5 mg/mL elemental iron.

● UNLICENSED USE [EvGr] Sodium feredetate is used in the doses provided in the BNF for the treatment and prophylaxis of iron-deficiency anaemia, Ⓐ but these may differ from those licensed.

● INTERACTIONS → Appendix 1: iron

● MEDICINAL FORMS There can be variation in the licensing of different medicines containing the same drug.
Oral solution
EXCIPIENTS: May contain Ethanol, hydroxybenzoates (parabens), sorbitol
► Sytron (Kyowa Kirin International UK NewCo Ltd)
Iron (as Sodium feredetate) 5.5 mg per 1 ml Sytron oral solution | 500 ml Ⓟ £14.95 DT = £14.95 [SF]

1.3 Megaloblastic anaemia

Anaemia, megaloblastic

12-Jul-2022

Overview

Most megaloblastic anaemias result from a lack of either vitamin B_{12} or folate, and it is essential to establish in every case which deficiency is present and the underlying cause. In emergencies, when delay might be dangerous, it is sometimes necessary to administer both substances after the bone marrow test while plasma assay results are awaited. Normally, however, appropriate treatment should not be instituted until the results of tests are available.

One cause of megaloblastic anaemia in the UK is *pernicious anaemia* in which lack of gastric intrinsic factor resulting from an autoimmune gastritis causes malabsorption of vitamin B_{12}.

Vitamin B_{12} is also needed in the treatment of megaloblastosis caused by *prolonged nitrous oxide anaesthesia*, which inactivates the vitamin, and in the rare syndrome of *congenital transcobalamin II deficiency*.

Vitamin B_{12} should be given prophylactically after *total gastrectomy* or *total ileal resection* (or after *partial gastrectomy* if a vitamin B_{12} absorption test shows vitamin B_{12} malabsorption).

Apart from dietary deficiency, all other causes of vitamin B_{12} deficiency are attributable to malabsorption. There is little place for the use of low-dose vitamin B_{12} orally and none for vitamin B_{12} intrinsic factor complexes given by mouth. Vitamin B_{12} in larger oral doses may be effective.

Hydroxocobalamin p. 1162 is retained in the body longer than cyanocobalamin p. 1162 and thus for maintenance therapy can be given at intervals of up to 3 months. Treatment is generally initiated with frequent administration of intramuscular injections to replenish the depleted body stores. Thereafter, maintenance treatment, which is usually for life, can be instituted. There is no evidence that doses larger than those recommended provide any additional benefit in vitamin B$_{12}$ neuropathy.

Folic acid below has few indications for long-term therapy since most causes of folate deficiency are self-limiting or will yield to a short course of treatment. It should not be used in undiagnosed megaloblastic anaemia unless vitamin B$_{12}$ is administered concurrently otherwise neuropathy may be precipitated.

In *folate-deficient megaloblastic anaemia* (e.g. because of poor nutrition, pregnancy, or antiepileptic drugs), daily folic acid supplementation for 4 months brings about haematological remission and replenishes body stores.

For prophylaxis in *chronic haemolytic states, malabsorption,* or *in renal dialysis,* folic acid is given daily or sometimes weekly, depending on the diet and the rate of haemolysis.

Folic acid is also used for the prevention of methotrexate-induced side-effects in severe Crohn's disease, rheumatic disease, and severe psoriasis.

Folinic acid p. 1071 is also effective in the treatment of folate deficient megaloblastic anaemia but it is generally used in association with cytotoxic drugs; it is given as calcium folinate.

There is **no** justification for prescribing multiple ingredient vitamin preparations containing vitamin B$_{12}$ or folic acid.

For the use of folic acid before and during pregnancy, see Neural tube defects (prevention in pregnancy) p. 1248.

VITAMINS AND TRACE ELEMENTS ＞ FOLATES

Folic acid
10-Nov-2021

- ● **INDICATIONS AND DOSE**

Folate-deficient megaloblastic anaemia
- ▶ BY MOUTH
- ▸ Child 1-11 months: Initially 500 micrograms/kg once daily (max. per dose 5 mg) for up to 4 months, doses up to 10 mg per day may be required in malabsorption states
- ▸ Child 1-17 years: 5 mg once daily for 4 months (until term in pregnant women), doses up to 15 mg per day may be required in malabsorption states
- ▸ Adult: 5 mg once daily for 4 months (until term in pregnant women), doses up to 15 mg per day may be required in malabsorption states

Prevention of neural tube defects [in those at a low risk of conceiving a child with a neural tube defect]
- ▶ BY MOUTH
- ▸ Females of childbearing potential: 400 micrograms once daily to be taken before conception and until week 12 of pregnancy

Prevention of neural tube defects [in those in the high-risk group who wish to become pregnant or who are at risk of becoming pregnant]
- ▶ BY MOUTH
- ▸ Females of childbearing potential: 5 mg once daily to be taken before conception and until week 12 of pregnancy

Prevention of neural tube defects [in those with sickle-cell disease]
- ▶ BY MOUTH
- ▸ Females of childbearing potential: 5 mg once daily, patient should continue taking their normal dose of folic acid 5 mg once daily (or increase the dose to 5 mg once daily) before conception and continue this throughout pregnancy

Prevention of methotrexate-induced side-effects in rheumatic disease
- ▶ BY MOUTH
- ▸ Adult: 5 mg once weekly, dose to be taken on a different day to methotrexate dose

Prevention of methotrexate side-effects in severe Crohn's disease | Prevention of methotrexate side-effects in severe psoriasis
- ▶ BY MOUTH
- ▸ Adult: 5 mg once weekly, dose to be taken on a different day to methotrexate dose

Prophylaxis in chronic haemolytic states
- ▶ BY MOUTH
- ▸ Adult: 5 mg every 1–7 days, frequency dependent on underlying disease

Prophylaxis of folate deficiency in dialysis
- ▶ BY MOUTH
- ▸ Child 1 month-11 years: 250 micrograms/kg once daily (max. per dose 10 mg)
- ▸ Child 12-17 years: 5–10 mg once daily
- ▸ Adult: 5 mg every 1–7 days

Prophylaxis of folate deficiency in patients receiving parenteral nutrition
- ▶ BY INTRAVENOUS INFUSION
- ▸ Adult: 15 mg 1–2 times a week, usually given by *intravenous infusion* in the parenteral nutrition solution

- ● **UNLICENSED USE** Not licensed for prevention of methotrexate-induced side-effects in severe Crohn's disease. Not licensed for prevention of methotrexate-induced side-effects in rheumatic disease. Not licensed for prevention of methotrexate-induced side-effects in severe psoriasis.

- ● **CAUTIONS** Should never be given alone for pernicious anaemia or other megaloblastic anaemias caused by vitamin B$_{12}$ deficiency (may precipitate subacute combined degeneration of the spinal cord)

- ● **INTERACTIONS** → Appendix 1: folates

- ● **SIDE-EFFECTS** Abdominal distension · appetite decreased · flatulence · nausea · vitamin B12 deficiency exacerbated

- ● **PATIENT AND CARER ADVICE**
Medicines for Children leaflet: Folic acid for megaloblastic anaemia caused by folate deficiency and haemolytic anaemia www.medicinesforchildren.org.uk/medicines/folic-acid-for-megaloblastic-anaemia-caused-by-folate-deficiency-and-haemolytic-anaemia/

- ● **EXCEPTIONS TO LEGAL CATEGORY**
- ▸ With oral use Can be sold to the public provided daily doses do not exceed 500 micrograms.

- ● **MEDICINAL FORMS** There can be variation in the licensing of different medicines containing the same drug. Forms available from special-order manufacturers include: oral capsule, oral suspension, oral solution, solution for injection

Oral tablet
- ▸ Folic acid (Non-proprietary)
Folic acid 400 microgram Folic acid 400microgram tablets | 90 tablet PoM Ⓢ DT = £1.78
Folic acid 5 mg Folic acid 5mg tablets | 28 tablet PoM £0.91 DT = £0.66

Oral solution
- ▸ Folic acid (Non-proprietary)
Folic acid 500 microgram per 1 ml Folic acid 2.5mg/5ml oral solution sugar free | 150 ml PoM £9.16 DT = £9.16 SF
Folic acid 1 mg per 1 ml Folic acid 5mg/5ml oral solution sugar free | 150 ml PoM £48.02-£75.00 DT = £92.25 SF
- ▸ Lexpec (Rosemont Pharmaceuticals Ltd)
Folic acid 500 microgram per 1 ml Lexpec Folic Acid 2.5mg/5ml oral solution | 150 ml PoM £9.16 DT = £9.16 SF

VITAMINS AND TRACE ELEMENTS > VITAMIN B GROUP

Cyanocobalamin

28-Mar-2024

● **INDICATIONS AND DOSE**

Prophylaxis of macrocytic anaemias associated with vitamin B$_{12}$ deficiency

▸ BY INTRAMUSCULAR INJECTION
▸ Adult: 0.25–1 mg once a month

Pernicious anaemia and other macrocytic anaemias without neurological involvement

▸ BY INTRAMUSCULAR INJECTION
▸ Adult: Initially 0.25–1 mg once daily on alternate days for 1 to 2 weeks, then 0.25 mg once weekly until blood count normal; maintenance 1 mg once a month

Pernicious anaemia and other macrocytic anaemias with neurological involvement

▸ BY INTRAMUSCULAR INJECTION
▸ Adult: 1 mg once daily on alternate days as long as improvement occurs; maintenance 1 mg once a month

Dietary vitamin B$_{12}$ deficiency

▸ BY MOUTH
▸ Adult: 50–150 micrograms once daily, dose to be taken between meals, dose may be increased as clinically indicated

Dietary vitamin B$_{12}$ deficiency during pregnancy or breast feeding

▸ BY MOUTH
▸ Adult: 1 mg once daily, dose to be taken between meals, dose may be increased as clinically indicated

OROBALIN ®

Dietary vitamin B$_{12}$ deficiency | Vitamin B$_{12}$ deficiency due to malabsorption

▸ BY MOUTH
▸ Adult: Initially 2 mg twice daily until remission, dose to be taken between meals, then maintenance 1 mg once daily, dose to be taken between meals

IMPORTANT SAFETY INFORMATION

MHRA/CHM ADVICE: VITAMIN B$_{12}$ (CYANOCOBALAMIN): ADVISE PATIENTS WITH KNOWN COBALT ALLERGY TO BE VIGILANT FOR SENSITIVITY REACTIONS (DECEMBER 2023)

Following a report via the Yellow Card Scheme, the MHRA conducted a review and found evidence in the literature of cobalt sensitivity-type reactions in patients being treated for vitamin B$_{12}$ deficiency; other similar reports have also been received. Such reactions typically present with cutaneous symptoms of chronic or subacute allergic contact dermatitis (an erythema multiforme-like eruption may infrequently be triggered); onset may be immediate or delayed up to 72 hours after vitamin B$_{12}$ administration. Vitamin B$_{12}$ (i.e. cyanocobalamin or hydroxocobalamin) contains cobalt and 1 to 3% of the general population is estimated to have cobalt allergy.

Healthcare professionals are recommended to assess the benefits and risks of continuing treatment in patients who develop cobalt sensitivity-type reactions and, if necessary to continue, advise such patients on appropriate symptom management. Patients with known cobalt allergy should be advised to speak to a healthcare professional if they are prescribed vitamin B$_{12}$ and be alert for symptoms of cobalt sensitivity-type reactions. All patients should be counselled to seek medical advice if they develop allergic skin reactions whilst on vitamin B$_{12}$ therapy; urgent medical attention must be sought if symptoms of a serious allergic reaction, such as extensive or blistering rash, wheeze, difficulty breathing, or feeling faint, occur.

● **PRESCRIBING AND DISPENSING INFORMATION** Currently available brands of the tablet may not be suitable for vegans.

The BP directs that when vitamin B$_{12}$ injection is prescribed or demanded hydroxocobalamin injection shall be dispensed or supplied.

● **NATIONAL FUNDING/ACCESS DECISIONS**

NHS restrictions *Cytamen* ® injection is not prescribable in NHS primary care.

● **LESS SUITABLE FOR PRESCRIBING** Cyanocobalamin injection is less suitable for prescribing.

● **MEDICINAL FORMS** There can be variation in the licensing of different medicines containing the same drug.

Oral tablet

▸ Cyanocobalamin (Non-proprietary)
  Cyanocobalamin 50 microgram Cyanocobalamin 50microgram tablets | 50 tablet [P] £30.00 DT = £2.60
  Cyanocobalamin 500 microgram Acyanocomin 500microgram tablets | 50 tablet £6.89
  Cyanocobalamin 1 mg Behepan 1mg tablets | 100 tablet [PoM] [Ⓔ]
▸ ActivB12 (MaN Pharma Ltd)
  Cyanocobalamin 100 microgram ActivB12 100microgram tablets | 28 tablet £1.95 | 50 tablet £3.22
▸ CyanocoB12 (TriOn Pharma Ltd)
  Cyanocobalamin 100 microgram CyanocoB12 100microgram tablets | 28 tablet £1.94 | 50 tablet £3.19
  Cyanocobalamin 500 microgram CyanocoB12 500microgram tablets | 50 tablet £6.89
▸ CyanocoMinn (Essential-Healthcare Ltd)
  Cyanocobalamin 100 microgram CyanocoMinn 100microgram tablets | 28 tablet £1.87 | 50 tablet £3.21
▸ Orobalin (Northumbria Pharma Ltd)
  Cyanocobalamin 1 mg Orobalin 1mg tablets | 30 tablet [PoM] £9.99 DT = £9.99
▸ SunVit-Pro (Cyanocobalamin) (SunVit-D3 Ltd)
  Cyanocobalamin 100 microgram SunVit-Pro Vitamin B12 100microgram tablets | 50 tablet £3.79

Hydroxocobalamin

29-Jan-2024

● **INDICATIONS AND DOSE**

Prophylaxis of macrocytic anaemias associated with vitamin B$_{12}$ deficiency

▸ BY INTRAMUSCULAR INJECTION
▸ Adult: 1 mg every 2–3 months

Pernicious anaemia and other macrocytic anaemias without neurological involvement

▸ BY INTRAMUSCULAR INJECTION
▸ Adult: Initially 1 mg 3 times a week for 2 weeks, then 1 mg every 2–3 months

Pernicious anaemia and other macrocytic anaemias with neurological involvement

▸ BY INTRAMUSCULAR INJECTION
▸ Adult: Initially 1 mg once daily on alternate days until no further improvement, then 1 mg every 2 months

Tobacco amblyopia

▸ BY INTRAMUSCULAR INJECTION
▸ Adult: Initially 1 mg daily for 2 weeks, then 1 mg twice weekly until no further improvement, then 1 mg every 1–3 months

Leber's optic atrophy

▸ BY INTRAMUSCULAR INJECTION
▸ Adult: Initially 1 mg daily for 2 weeks, then 1 mg twice weekly until no further improvement, then 1 mg every 1–3 months

CYANOKIT ®

Poisoning with cyanides

▸ BY INTRAVENOUS INFUSION
▸ Child (body-weight 5 kg and above): Initially 70 mg/kg (max. per dose 5 g), to be given over 15 minutes, then

70 mg/kg (max. per dose 5 g) if required, this second dose can be given over 15 minutes–2 hours depending on severity of poisoning and patient stability
▸ **Adult:** Initially 5 g, to be given over 15 minutes, then 5 g if required, this second dose can be given over 15 minutes–2 hours depending on severity of poisoning and patient stability

---

IMPORTANT SAFETY INFORMATION

MHRA/CHM ADVICE: VITAMIN B_{12} (HYDROXOCOBALAMIN): ADVISE PATIENTS WITH KNOWN COBALT ALLERGY TO BE VIGILANT FOR SENSITIVITY REACTIONS (DECEMBER 2023)

Following a report via the Yellow Card Scheme, the MHRA conducted a review and found evidence in the literature of cobalt sensitivity-type reactions in patients being treated for vitamin B_{12} deficiency; other similar reports have also been received. Such reactions typically present with cutaneous symptoms of chronic or subacute allergic contact dermatitis (an erythema multiforme-like eruption may infrequently be triggered); onset may be immediate or delayed up to 72 hours after vitamin B_{12} administration. Vitamin B_{12} (i.e. cyanocobalamin or hydroxocobalamin) contains cobalt and 1 to 3% of the general population is estimated to have cobalt allergy.

Healthcare professionals are recommended to assess the benefits and risks of continuing treatment in patients who develop cobalt sensitivity-type reactions and, if necessary to continue, advise such patients on appropriate symptom management. Patients with known cobalt allergy should be advised to speak to a healthcare professional if they are prescribed vitamin B_{12} and be alert for symptoms of cobalt sensitivity-type reactions. All patients should be counselled to seek medical advice if they develop allergic skin reactions whilst on vitamin B_{12} therapy; urgent medical attention must be sought if symptoms of a serious allergic reaction, such as extensive or blistering rash, wheeze, difficulty breathing, or feeling faint, occur.

Hydroxocobalamin preparations used for the treatment of known or suspected cyanide poisoning are excluded from these precautions because the potentially life-saving benefit of treatment in a medical emergency outweighs the risk of an allergic reaction.

● **CAUTIONS** Diagnosis of Vitamin B_{12} deficiency should be confirmed before giving hydroxocobalamin

● **SIDE-EFFECTS**

GENERAL SIDE-EFFECTS Diarrhoea · dizziness · headache · hot flush · nausea · skin reactions · urine discolouration

SPECIFIC SIDE-EFFECTS
▸ With intramuscular use Arrhythmia · chills · drug fever · hypokalaemia · malaise · pain · thrombocytosis · tremor · vomiting
▸ With intravenous use Angioedema · dysphagia · extrasystole · gastrointestinal discomfort · memory loss · mucosal discolouration red · peripheral oedema · pleural effusion · rash pustular · red discolouration of plasma · restlessness · swelling · throat complaints

● **BREAST FEEDING** Present in milk but not known to be harmful.

● **EFFECT ON LABORATORY TESTS**
▸ With intravenous use Deep red colour of hydroxocobalamin may interfere with laboratory tests.

● **DIRECTIONS FOR ADMINISTRATION** For *intravenous infusion* (*Cyanokit* ®), give intermittently in Sodium Chloride 0.9%, reconstitute 5 g vial with 200 mL Sodium Chloride 0.9%; gently invert vial for at least 1 minute to mix (do not shake).

● **PRESCRIBING AND DISPENSING INFORMATION**
▸ With intramuscular use The BP directs that when vitamin B_{12} injection is prescribed or demanded, hydroxocobalamin injection shall be dispensed or supplied.
Poisoning by cyanides
▸ With intravenous use *Cyanokit* ® is the only preparation of hydroxocobalamin that is suitable for use in victims of smoke inhalation who show signs of significant cyanide poisoning.

● **NATIONAL FUNDING/ACCESS DECISIONS**
NHS restrictions *Cobalin-H* ® is not prescribable in NHS primary care.
Neo-Cytamen ® is not prescribable in NHS primary care.

● **MEDICINAL FORMS** There can be variation in the licensing of different medicines containing the same drug.

Solution for injection
▸ **Hydroxocobalamin (Non-proprietary)**
Hydroxocobalamin 1 mg per 1 ml Hydroxocobalamin 1mg/1ml solution for injection ampoules | 5 ampoule [PoM] £19.70 DT = £11.16
Hydroxocobalamin 2.5 mg per 1 ml Hepavit 5mg/2ml solution for injection ampoules | 2 ampoule [PoM] 🅢 (Hospital only)
Hydroxocobalamin 5 mg per 1 ml Megamilbedoce 10mg/2ml solution for injection ampoules | 10 ampoule [PoM] 🅢
▸ **Cobalin** (Advanz Pharma)
Hydroxocobalamin 1 mg per 1 ml Cobalin-H 1mg/1ml solution for injection ampoules | 5 ampoule [PoM] £9.50 DT = £11.16
▸ **Neo-Cytamen** (RPH Pharmaceuticals AB)
Hydroxocobalamin 1 mg per 1 ml Neo-Cytamen 1000micrograms/1ml solution for injection ampoules | 5 ampoule [PoM] £12.49 DT = £11.16

Powder for solution for infusion
▸ **Cyanokit** (SERB)
Hydroxocobalamin 5 gram Cyanokit 5g powder for solution for infusion vials | 1 vial [PoM] £772.00 (Hospital only)

2　Iron overload

Iron overload

Overview

Severe tissue iron overload can occur in aplastic and other refractory anaemias, mainly as the result of repeated blood transfusions. It is a particular problem in refractory anaemias with hyperplastic bone marrow, especially *thalassaemia major*, where excessive iron absorption from the gut and inappropriate iron therapy can add to the tissue siderosis.

Iron overload associated with haemochromatosis can be treated with repeated venesection. Venesection may also be used for patients who have received multiple transfusions and whose bone marrow has recovered. Where venesection is contra-indicated, the long-term administration of the iron chelating compound desferrioxamine mesilate p. 1165 is useful. Desferrioxamine mesilate (up to 2 g per unit of blood) may also be given at the time of blood transfusion, provided that the desferrioxamine mesilate is **not** added to the blood and is **not** given through the same line as the blood (but the two may be given through the same cannula).

Iron excretion induced by desferrioxamine mesilate is enhanced by administration of ascorbic acid p. 1239 (vitamin C) daily by mouth; it should be given separately from food since it also enhances iron absorption. Ascorbic acid should not be given to patients with cardiac dysfunction; in patients with normal cardiac function ascorbic acid should be introduced 1 month after starting desferrioxamine mesilate.

Desferrioxamine mesilate infusion can be used to treat *aluminium overload* in dialysis patients; theoretically 100 mg of desferrioxamine binds with 4.1 mg of aluminium.

ANTIDOTES AND CHELATORS > IRON CHELATORS

Deferasirox
23-Nov-2020

- **DRUG ACTION** Deferasirox is an oral iron chelator.

● **INDICATIONS AND DOSE**

Transfusion-related chronic iron overload in patients with beta thalassaemia major who receive frequent blood transfusions (7 mL/kg/month or more of packed red blood cells) (specialist use only)
▸ BY MOUTH
▸ Adult: Initially 7–21 mg/kg once daily, dose adjusted according to serum-ferritin concentration and amount of transfused blood—consult product literature, then adjusted in steps of 3.5–7 mg/kg every 3–6 months, maintenance dose adjusted according to serum-ferritin concentration; maximum 28 mg/kg per day; Usual maximum 21 mg/kg

Transfusion-related chronic iron overload when desferrioxamine is contra-indicated or inadequate in patients with beta thalassaemia major who receive infrequent blood transfusions (less than 7 mL/kg/month of packed red blood cells) (specialist use only) | Transfusion-related chronic iron overload when desferrioxamine is contra-indicated or inadequate in patients with other anaemias (specialist use only)
▸ BY MOUTH
▸ Adult: Initially 7–21 mg/kg once daily, dose adjusted according to serum-ferritin concentration and amount of transfused blood—consult product literature, then adjusted in steps of 3.5–7 mg/kg every 3–6 months, maintenance dose adjusted according to serum-ferritin concentration; maximum 28 mg/kg per day; Usual maximum 21 mg/kg

Chronic iron overload when desferrioxamine is contra-indicated or inadequate in non-transfusion-dependent thalassaemia syndromes (specialist use only)
▸ BY MOUTH
▸ Adult: Initially 7 mg/kg once daily, then adjusted in steps of 3.5–7 mg/kg every 3–6 months, maintenance dose adjusted according to serum-ferritin concentration and liver-iron concentration (consult product literature); maximum 14 mg/kg per day

● **CAUTIONS** Elderly (increased risk of side-effects) · history of liver cirrhosis · not recommended in conditions which may reduce life expectancy (e.g. high-risk myelodysplastic syndromes) · platelet count less than 50×10^9/litre · risk of gastro-intestinal ulceration and haemorrhage · unexplained cytopenia—consider treatment interruption

● **INTERACTIONS** → Appendix 1: iron chelators

● **SIDE-EFFECTS**
▸ **Common or very common** Constipation · diarrhoea · gastrointestinal discomfort · headache · nausea · skin reactions · urine abnormalities · vomiting
▸ **Uncommon** Anxiety · cataract · cholelithiasis · dizziness · fatigue · fever · gastrointestinal disorders · gastrointestinal haemorrhage (including fatal cases) · hearing impairment · hepatic disorders · laryngeal pain · maculopathy · oedema · renal tubular disorders · sleep disorder
▸ **Rare or very rare** Optic neuritis · severe cutaneous adverse reactions (SCARs)
▸ **Frequency not known** Acute kidney injury · alopecia · anaemia aggravated · hyperammonaemic encephalopathy · hypersensitivity vasculitis · lens opacity · leucopenia · metabolic acidosis · nephritis tubulointerstitial · nephrolithiasis · neutropenia · pancreatitis acute · pancytopenia · renal tubular necrosis · thrombocytopenia

● **PREGNANCY** Manufacturer advises avoid unless essential— toxicity in *animal* studies.

● **BREAST FEEDING** Manufacturer advises avoid—present in milk in *animal* studies.

● **HEPATIC IMPAIRMENT** Manufacturer advises caution in moderate impairment; avoid in severe impairment.
Dose adjustments Manufacturer advises reduce initial dose considerably then gradually increase to max. 50% of normal dose in moderate impairment.

● **RENAL IMPAIRMENT** Manufacturer advises avoid if estimated creatinine clearance less than 60 mL/minute.
Dose adjustments See p. 21.
Manufacturer advises reduce dose if creatinine clearance less than 90 mL/minute and serum creatinine increased by more than 33% of baseline measurement on 2 consecutive occasions—consult product literature.

● **MONITORING REQUIREMENTS** Manufacturer advises monitoring of the following patient parameters: baseline serum creatinine twice and creatinine clearance once before initiation of treatment, weekly in the first month after treatment initiation or modification, then monthly thereafter; proteinuria before treatment initiation then monthly thereafter, and other markers of renal tubular function as needed; liver function before treatment initiation, every 2 weeks during the first month of treatment, then monthly thereafter; eye and ear examinations before treatment and annually during treatment; serum-ferritin concentration monthly.

● **DIRECTIONS FOR ADMINISTRATION** For *film-coated tablets*, manufacturer advises tablets may be crushed and sprinkled on to soft food (yoghurt or apple sauce), then administered immediately.

● **PATIENT AND CARER ADVICE** Patient or carers should be given advice on how to administer deferasirox tablets.

● **NATIONAL FUNDING/ACCESS DECISIONS**
For full details see funding body website
Scottish Medicines Consortium (SMC) decisions
▸ Deferasirox (*Exjade*®) for the treatment of chronic iron overload due to blood transfusions when deferoxamine therapy is contra-indicated or inadequate, in adult and paediatric patients aged 2 years and older with rare acquired or inherited anaemias (January 2017) SMC No. 347/07 Recommended with restrictions
▸ Deferasirox (*Exjade*®) for the treatment of chronic iron overload: due to frequent blood transfusions in patients with beta thalassaemia major aged 6 years and over; due to blood transfusions when deferoxamine therapy is contra-indicated or inadequate in other patient groups (June 2017) SMC No. 1246/17 Recommended with restrictions

● **MEDICINAL FORMS** There can be variation in the licensing of different medicines containing the same drug.
Oral tablet
CAUTIONARY AND ADVISORY LABELS 25
▸ **Deferasirox (Non-proprietary)**
Deferasirox 90 mg Deferasirox 90mg tablets | 30 tablet PoM £126.00 DT = £126.00 | 30 tablet PoM £105.00–£126.00 DT = £126.00 (Hospital only)
Deferasirox 180 mg Deferasirox 180mg tablets | 30 tablet PoM £252.00 DT = £252.00 | 30 tablet PoM £210.00–£252.00 DT = £252.00 (Hospital only)
Deferasirox 360 mg Deferasirox 360mg tablets | 30 tablet PoM £504.00 DT = £504.00 | 30 tablet PoM £424.00–£507.00 DT = £504.00 (Hospital only)
▸ **Exjade** (Novartis Pharmaceuticals UK Ltd) ▼
Deferasirox 90 mg Exjade 90mg tablets | 30 tablet PoM £126.00 DT = £126.00
Deferasirox 180 mg Exjade 180mg tablets | 30 tablet PoM £252.00 DT = £252.00
Deferasirox 360 mg Exjade 360mg tablets | 30 tablet PoM £504.00 DT = £504.00

Deferiprone
28-Jun-2021

- **DRUG ACTION** Deferiprone is an oral iron chelator.

- **INDICATIONS AND DOSE**

Treatment of iron overload in patients with thalassaemia major in whom desferrioxamine is contra-indicated or is inadequate
  - ▸ BY MOUTH
  - ▸ Adult: 25 mg/kg 3 times a day; maximum 100 mg/kg per day

- **CONTRA-INDICATIONS** History of agranulocytosis or recurrent neutropenia

- **INTERACTIONS** → Appendix 1: iron chelators

- **SIDE-EFFECTS**
  - ▸ **Common or very common** Abdominal pain (reducing dose and increasing gradually may improve tolerance) · agranulocytosis · appetite increased · arthralgia · diarrhoea (reducing dose and increasing gradually may improve tolerance) · fatigue · headache · nausea (reducing dose and increasing gradually may improve tolerance) · neutropenia · urine discolouration · vomiting (reducing dose and increasing gradually may improve tolerance)
  - ▸ **Frequency not known** Skin reactions · zinc deficiency

- **CONCEPTION AND CONTRACEPTION** Manufacturer advises avoid before intended conception—teratogenic and embryotoxic in *animal* studies. Contraception advised in females of child-bearing potential.

- **PREGNANCY** Manufacturer advises avoid during pregnancy—teratogenic and embryotoxic in *animal* studies.

- **BREAST FEEDING** Manufacturer advises avoid—no information available.

- **HEPATIC IMPAIRMENT** Manufacturer advises caution (no information available)—monitor hepatic function and consider interrupting treatment if persistent elevation in serum alanine aminotransferase. Manufacturer advises caution in patients with hepatitis C (ensure iron chelation is optimal)—monitor liver histology.

- **RENAL IMPAIRMENT** [EvGr] Caution in end-stage renal disease (no information available). ⟨M⟩

- **MONITORING REQUIREMENTS**
  - ▸ Monitor neutrophil count weekly and discontinue treatment if neutropenia develops.
  - ▸ Monitor plasma-zinc concentration.

- **PATIENT AND CARER ADVICE** Patients or their carers should be told how to recognise signs of neutropenia and advised to seek immediate medical attention if symptoms such as fever or sore throat develop.

- **MEDICINAL FORMS** There can be variation in the licensing of different medicines containing the same drug. Forms available from special-order manufacturers include: oral capsule, oral suspension, oral solution

Oral tablet
CAUTIONARY AND ADVISORY LABELS 14
  - ▸ **Deferiprone (Non-proprietary)**
    Deferiprone 500 mg Deferiprone 500mg tablets | 100 tablet [PoM] £78.00–£130.00 DT = £130.00
  - ▸ **Ferriprox** (Chiesi Ltd)
    Deferiprone 500 mg Ferriprox 500mg tablets | 100 tablet [PoM] £130.00 DT = £130.00
    Deferiprone 1 gram Ferriprox 1000mg tablets | 50 tablet [PoM] £130.00 DT = £130.00

Oral solution
CAUTIONARY AND ADVISORY LABELS 14
  - ▸ **Ferriprox** (Chiesi Ltd)
    Deferiprone 100 mg per 1 ml Ferriprox 100mg/ml oral solution | 500 ml [PoM] £152.39 DT = £152.39 [SF]

Desferrioxamine mesilate
09-Jun-2021

(Deferoxamine Mesilate)

- **INDICATIONS AND DOSE**

Iron poisoning
  - ▸ BY CONTINUOUS INTRAVENOUS INFUSION
  - ▸ Adult: Initially up to 15 mg/kg/hour, max. 80 mg/kg in 24 hours, dose to be reduced after 4–6 hours, in severe cases, higher doses may be given on advice from the National Poisons Information Service

Aluminium overload in dialysis patients
  - ▸ BY INTRAVENOUS INFUSION
  - ▸ Adult: (consult product literature or local protocols)

Chronic iron overload (low iron overload)
  - ▸ BY SUBCUTANEOUS INFUSION
  - ▸ Adult: The dose should reflect the degree of iron overload

Chronic iron overload (established overload)
  - ▸ BY SUBCUTANEOUS INFUSION
  - ▸ Adult: 20–50 mg/kg daily

- **CAUTIONS** Aluminium-related encephalopathy (may exacerbate neurological dysfunction)

- **INTERACTIONS** → Appendix 1: iron chelators

- **SIDE-EFFECTS**
  - ▸ **Common or very common** Arthralgia · bone disorder · fever · growth retardation · headache · muscle complaints · nausea · skin reactions
  - ▸ **Uncommon** Abdominal pain · asthma · deafness neurosensory · tinnitus · vomiting
  - ▸ **Rare or very rare** Angioedema · blood disorder · cataract · diarrhoea · dizziness · encephalopathy · eye disorders · hypersensitivity · hypotension (more common when given too rapidly by intravenous injection) · increased risk of infection · nerve disorders · nervous system disorder · paraesthesia · respiratory disorders · shock · tachycardia · thrombocytopenia · vision disorders
  - ▸ **Frequency not known** Acute kidney injury · hypocalcaemia · leucopenia · renal tubular disorder · seizure · urine discolouration

- **PREGNANCY** Teratogenic in *animal* studies. Manufacturer advises use only if potential benefit outweighs risk.

- **BREAST FEEDING** Manufacturer advises use only if potential benefit outweighs risk—no information available.

- **RENAL IMPAIRMENT** [EvGr] Use with caution. ⟨M⟩

- **MONITORING REQUIREMENTS** Eye and ear examinations before treatment and at 3-month intervals during treatment.

- **DIRECTIONS FOR ADMINISTRATION** For full details and warnings relating to administration, consult product literature.
  For *intravenous* or *subcutaneous* infusion (*Desferal*®), give continuously *or* intermittently in Glucose 5% or Sodium Chloride 0.9%. Reconstitute with Water for Injections to a concentration of 100 mg/mL; dilute with infusion fluid.

- **MEDICINAL FORMS** There can be variation in the licensing of different medicines containing the same drug.

Powder for solution for injection
  - ▸ **Desferrioxamine mesilate (Non-proprietary)**
    Desferrioxamine mesilate 500 mg Desferrioxamine 500mg powder for solution for injection vials | 10 vial [PoM] £51.29 DT = £46.63
    Desferrioxamine mesilate 2 gram Desferrioxamine 2g powder for solution for injection vials | 10 vial [PoM] £205.26
  - ▸ **Desferal** (Novartis Pharmaceuticals UK Ltd)
    Desferrioxamine mesilate 500 mg Desferal 500mg powder for solution for injection vials | 10 vial [PoM] £46.63 DT = £46.63

3 Neutropenia and stem cell mobilisation

3.1 Neutropenia

Neutropenia

05-Mar-2021

Management

Neutropenia is characterised by a low neutrophil count (absolute neutrophil count less than 1.5×10^9/litre). Neutropenia is a risk factor for the development of infection and sepsis, especially in patients receiving high-intensity chemotherapy regimens. Recombinant human granulocyte-colony stimulating factor (rhG-CSF) stimulates the production of neutrophils and may reduce the duration of chemotherapy-induced neutropenia and thereby reduce the incidence of associated febrile neutropenia; there is as yet no evidence that it improves overall survival. Granulocyte-colony stimulating factors include filgrastim below, lenograstim p. 1167, pegfilgrastim p. 1168 and lipegfilgrastim p. 1168.

Filgrastim (unglycosylated rhG-CSF) and lenograstim (glycosylated rhG-CSF) have similar effects; both have been used in a variety of clinical settings for the treatment of neutropenia. Pegfilgrastim and lipegfilgrastim are polyethylene glycol-conjugated ('pegylated') derivatives of filgrastim, which are longer-acting forms of filgrastim due to decreased renal clearance.

Granulocyte-colony stimulating factors should only be prescribed by those experienced in their use.

IMMUNOSTIMULANTS ❭ GRANULOCYTE-COLONY STIMULATING FACTORS

Granulocyte-colony stimulating factors

- **DRUG ACTION** Recombinant human granulocyte-colony stimulating factor (rhG-CSF) stimulates the production of neutrophils.

- **CAUTIONS** Malignant myeloid conditions · pre-malignant myeloid conditions · risk of splenomegaly and rupture— spleen size should be monitored · sickle-cell disease

  CAUTIONS, FURTHER INFORMATION
  - Acute respiratory distress syndrome There have been reports of pulmonary infiltrates leading to acute respiratory distress syndrome—patients with a recent history of pulmonary infiltrates or pneumonia may be at higher risk.

- **SIDE-EFFECTS**
  - **Common or very common** Arthralgia · cutaneous vasculitis · dyspnoea · haemoptysis · headache · hypersensitivity · leucocytosis · pain · spleen abnormalities · thrombocytopenia
  - **Uncommon** Acute febrile neutrophilic dermatosis · capillary leak syndrome · hypoxia · interstitial pneumonia · pulmonary fibrosis · pulmonary oedema · respiratory disorders · sickle cell anaemia with crisis

  SIDE-EFFECTS, FURTHER INFORMATION Treatment should be withdrawn in patients who develop signs of pulmonary infiltration.

- **PREGNANCY** Manufacturers advise avoid—toxicity in *animal* studies.

- **BREAST FEEDING** There is no evidence for the use of granulocyte-colony stimulating factors during breast-feeding and manufacturers advise avoiding their use.

- **MONITORING REQUIREMENTS**
  - Full blood counts including differential white cell and platelet counts should be monitored.
  - Spleen size should be monitored during treatment—risk of splenomegaly and rupture.

⚑ above

Filgrastim

24-Jul-2020

(Recombinant human granulocyte-colony stimulating factor; G-CSF)

- **INDICATIONS AND DOSE**

Reduction in duration of neutropenia and incidence of febrile neutropenia in cytotoxic chemotherapy for malignancy (except chronic myeloid leukaemia and myelodysplastic syndromes) (specialist use only)
  - ▶ BY SUBCUTANEOUS INJECTION, OR BY INTRAVENOUS INFUSION
  - ▶ Adult: 5 micrograms/kg daily until neutrophil count in normal range, usually for up to 14 days (up to 38 days in acute myeloid leukaemia), to be started at least 24 hours after cytotoxic chemotherapy. Preferably given by subcutaneous injection; if given by intravenous infusion, administer over 30 minutes

Reduction in duration of neutropenia (and associated sequelae) in myeloablative therapy followed by bone-marrow transplantation (specialist use only)
  - ▶ BY SUBCUTANEOUS INFUSION, OR BY INTRAVENOUS INFUSION
  - ▶ Adult: 10 micrograms/kg daily, to be started at least 24 hours following cytotoxic chemotherapy and within 24 hours of bone-marrow infusion, then adjusted according to neutrophil count— consult product literature, doses administered over 30 minutes or 24 hours via intravenous route and over 24 hours via subcutaneous route

Mobilisation of peripheral blood progenitor cells for autologous infusion, used alone (specialist use only)
  - ▶ BY SUBCUTANEOUS INFUSION, OR BY SUBCUTANEOUS INJECTION
  - ▶ Adult: 10 micrograms/kg daily for 5–7 days, to be administered over 24 hours if given by subcutaneous infusion

Mobilisation of peripheral blood progenitor cells for autologous infusion, used following adjunctive myelosuppressive chemotherapy—to improve yield (specialist use only)
  - ▶ BY SUBCUTANEOUS INJECTION
  - ▶ Adult: 5 micrograms/kg daily until neutrophil count in normal range, to be started the day after completing chemotherapy, for timing of leucopheresis, consult product literature

Mobilisation of peripheral blood progenitor cells in normal donors for allogeneic infusion (specialist use only)
  - ▶ BY SUBCUTANEOUS INJECTION
  - ▶ Adult 18-59 years: 10 micrograms/kg daily for 4–5 days, for timing of leucopheresis, consult product literature

Severe congenital neutropenia and history of severe or recurrent infections (distinguish carefully from other haematological disorders) (specialist use only)
  - ▶ BY SUBCUTANEOUS INJECTION
  - ▶ Adult: Initially 12 micrograms/kg daily, adjusted according to response, can be given in single or divided doses, consult product literature and local protocol

Severe cyclic neutropenia, or idiopathic neutropenia and history of severe or recurrent infections (distinguish carefully from other haematological disorders) (specialist use only)
▶ BY SUBCUTANEOUS INJECTION
▶ Adult: Initially 5 micrograms/kg daily, adjusted according to response, can be given in single or divided doses, consult product literature and local protocol

Persistent neutropenia in HIV infection (specialist use only)
▶ BY SUBCUTANEOUS INJECTION
▶ Adult: Initially 1 microgram/kg daily, subsequent doses increased as necessary until neutrophil count in normal range, then adjusted to maintain neutrophil count in normal range—consult product literature; maximum 4 micrograms/kg per day

● CONTRA-INDICATIONS Severe congenital neutropenia who develop leukaemia or have evidence of leukaemic evolution

● CAUTIONS Osteoporotic bone disease (monitor bone density if given for more than 6 months) · secondary acute myeloid leukaemia

● INTERACTIONS → Appendix 1: filgrastim

● SIDE-EFFECTS
▶ **Common or very common** Anaemia · diarrhoea · dysuria · haemorrhage · hepatomegaly · hyperuricaemia · hypotension · osteoporosis · rash
▶ **Uncommon** Fluid imbalance · graft versus host disease · interstitial lung disease · peripheral vascular disease · pseudogout · rheumatoid arthritis aggravated · urine abnormalities

● MONITORING REQUIREMENTS Regular morphological and cytogenetic bone-marrow examinations recommended in severe congenital neutropenia (possible risk of myelodysplastic syndromes or leukaemia).

● DIRECTIONS FOR ADMINISTRATION For *subcutaneous* or *intravenous infusion*, manufacturer advises give continuously *or* intermittently *in* Glucose 5%; for a filgrastim concentration of less than 1 500 000 units/mL (15 micrograms/mL) albumin solution (human albumin solution) is added to produce a final albumin concentration of 2 mg/mL; should not be diluted to a filgrastim concentration of less than 200 000 units/mL (2 micrograms/mL) and should not be diluted with sodium chloride solution.

● PRESCRIBING AND DISPENSING INFORMATION Filgrastim is a biological medicine. Biological medicines must be prescribed and dispensed by brand name, see *Biological medicines* and *Biosimilar medicines*, under Guidance on prescribing p. 1.
 1 million units of filgrastim solution for injection contains 10 micrograms filgrastim.

● MEDICINAL FORMS There can be variation in the licensing of different medicines containing the same drug.
Solution for injection
▶ Accofil (Accord-UK Ltd)
 Filgrastim 60 mega unit per 1 ml Accofil 30million units/0.5ml solution for injection pre-filled syringes | 5 pre-filled disposable injection PoM £284.20 DT = £250.75 (Hospital only) | 7 pre-filled disposable injection PoM £397.60 (Hospital only)
 Accofil 12million units/0.2ml solution for injection pre-filled syringes | 5 pre-filled disposable injection PoM £113.60 (Hospital only)
 Filgrastim 96 mega unit per 1 ml Accofil 48million units/0.5ml solution for injection pre-filled syringes | 5 pre-filled disposable injection PoM £455.70 DT = £399.50 (Hospital only) | 7 pre-filled disposable injection PoM £637.98 (Hospital only)
 Accofil 70million units/0.73ml solution for injection pre-filled syringes | 5 pre-filled disposable injection PoM £662.67 (Hospital only)
▶ Neupogen (Amgen Ltd)
 Filgrastim 30 mega unit per 1 ml Neupogen 30million units/1ml solution for injection vials | 5 vial PoM £263.52 DT = £263.52

▶ Neupogen Singleject (Amgen Ltd)
 Filgrastim 60 mega unit per 1 ml Neupogen Singleject 30million units/0.5ml solution for injection pre-filled syringes | 1 pre-filled disposable injection PoM £52.70
 Filgrastim 96 mega unit per 1 ml Neupogen Singleject 48million units/0.5ml solution for injection pre-filled syringes | 1 pre-filled disposable injection PoM £84.06
▶ Nivestim (Pfizer Ltd)
 Filgrastim 60 mega unit per 1 ml Nivestim 30million units/0.5ml solution for injection pre-filled syringes | 5 pre-filled disposable injection PoM £246.50 DT = £250.75
 Nivestim 12million units/0.2ml solution for injection pre-filled syringes | 5 pre-filled disposable injection PoM £153.00
 Filgrastim 96 mega unit per 1 ml Nivestim 48million units/0.5ml solution for injection pre-filled syringes | 5 pre-filled disposable injection PoM £395.25 DT = £399.50
▶ Zarzio (Sandoz Ltd)
 Filgrastim 60 mega unit per 1 ml Zarzio 30million units/0.5ml solution for injection pre-filled syringes | 5 pre-filled disposable injection PoM £250.75 DT = £250.75
 Filgrastim 96 mega unit per 1 ml Zarzio 48million units/0.5ml solution for injection pre-filled syringes | 5 pre-filled disposable injection PoM £399.50 DT = £399.50

 ⏴ 1166

Lenograstim
20-Jul-2020

(Recombinant human granulocyte-colony stimulating factor; rHuG-CSF)

● INDICATIONS AND DOSE
Reduction in the duration of neutropenia and associated complications following bone-marrow transplantation for non-myeloid malignancy (specialist use only) | Reduction in the duration of neutropenia and associated complications following peripheral stem cells transplantation for non-myeloid malignancy (specialist use only)
▶ BY INTRAVENOUS INFUSION, OR BY SUBCUTANEOUS INJECTION
▶ Adult: 150 micrograms/m^2 daily until neutrophil count stable in acceptable range (max. 28 days), to be started the day after transplantation. Intravenous infusion to be given over 30 minutes

Reduction in the duration of neutropenia and associated complications following treatment with cytotoxic chemotherapy associated with a significant incidence of febrile neutropenia (specialist use only)
▶ BY SUBCUTANEOUS INJECTION
▶ Adult: 150 micrograms/m^2 daily until neutrophil count stable in acceptable range (max. 28 days), to be started on the day after completion of chemotherapy

Mobilisation of peripheral blood progenitor cells for harvesting and subsequent infusion, used alone (specialist use only)
▶ BY SUBCUTANEOUS INJECTION
▶ Adult: 10 micrograms/kg daily for 4–6 days (5–6 days in healthy donors)

Mobilisation of peripheral blood progenitor cells, used following adjunctive myelosuppressive chemotherapy (to improve yield) (specialist use only)
▶ BY SUBCUTANEOUS INJECTION
▶ Adult: 150 micrograms/m^2 daily until neutrophil count stable in acceptable range, to be started 1–5 days after completion of chemotherapy, for timing of leucopheresis, consult product literature

● INTERACTIONS → Appendix 1: lenograstim

● SIDE-EFFECTS
▶ **Common or very common** Abdominal pain · asthenia
▶ **Rare or very rare** Erythema nodosum · pyoderma gangrenosum · toxic epidermal necrolysis

● DIRECTIONS FOR ADMINISTRATION For *intravenous infusion* (*Granocyte* ®), manufacturer advises give intermittently *in* Glucose 5% *or* Sodium Chloride 0.9%; initially reconstitute with 1 mL Water for Injection provided (do not shake vigorously) then dilute with up to 50 mL infusion fluid for each vial of *Granocyte*®-13 or up to 100 mL infusion fluid for *Granocyte*®-34; give over 30 minutes.

- **PRESCRIBING AND DISPENSING INFORMATION** *Granocyte*® solution for injection contains 105 micrograms of lenograstim per 13.4 mega unit vial and 263 micrograms lenograstim per 33.6 mega unit vial.

- **MEDICINAL FORMS** There can be variation in the licensing of different medicines containing the same drug.
  Powder and solvent for solution for injection
  EXCIPIENTS: May contain Phenylalanine
  ▸ Granocyte (Chugai Pharma UK Ltd)
   Lenograstim 13.4 mega unit Granocyte 13million unit powder and solvent for solution for injection pre-filled syringes | 1 pre-filled disposable injection PoM £40.11 DT = £40.11 | 5 pre-filled disposable injection PoM £200.55
   Lenograstim 33.6 mega unit Granocyte 34million unit powder and solvent for solution for injection pre-filled syringes | 1 pre-filled disposable injection PoM £62.54 DT = £62.54 | 5 pre-filled disposable injection PoM £312.69

▶ 1166

Lipegfilgrastim

10-Jun-2020

(Glycopegylated recombinant methionyl human granulocyte-colony stimulating factor)

- **INDICATIONS AND DOSE**

Reduction in duration of neutropenia and incidence of febrile neutropenia in cytotoxic chemotherapy for malignancy (except chronic myeloid leukaemia and myelodysplastic syndromes)
  ▸ BY SUBCUTANEOUS INJECTION
  ▸ Adult (specialist use only): 6 mg, for each chemotherapy cycle, given approximately 24 hours after chemotherapy, dose expressed as filgrastim

- **CAUTIONS** Myelosuppressive chemotherapy

- **INTERACTIONS** → Appendix 1: lipegfilgrastim

- **SIDE-EFFECTS**
  ▸ **Common or very common** Chest pain · hypokalaemia · skin eruption

- **MEDICINAL FORMS** There can be variation in the licensing of different medicines containing the same drug.
  Solution for injection
  ▸ Lonquex (Teva UK Ltd)
   Filgrastim (as Lipegfilgrastim) 10 mg per 1 ml Lonquex 6mg/0.6ml solution for injection pre-filled syringes | 1 pre-filled disposable injection PoM £652.06

▶ 1166

Pegfilgrastim

10-Jun-2020

(Pegylated recombinant methionyl human granulocyte-colony stimulating factor)

- **INDICATIONS AND DOSE**

Reduction in duration of neutropenia and incidence of febrile neutropenia in cytotoxic chemotherapy for malignancy (except chronic myeloid leukaemia and myelodysplastic syndromes) (specialist use only)
  ▸ BY SUBCUTANEOUS INJECTION
  ▸ Adult: 6 mg for each chemotherapy cycle, to be given at least 24 hours after chemotherapy, dose is expressed as filgrastim

- **CAUTIONS** Acute leukaemia · myelosuppressive chemotherapy

- **INTERACTIONS** → Appendix 1: pegfilgrastim

- **SIDE-EFFECTS**
  ▸ **Common or very common** Myalgia · nausea

- **Uncommon** Glomerulonephritis

- **MEDICINAL FORMS** There can be variation in the licensing of different medicines containing the same drug.
  Solution for injection
  ▸ Neulasta (Amgen Ltd)
   Filgrastim (as Pegfilgrastim) 10 mg per 1 ml Neulasta 6mg/0.6ml solution for injection pre-filled syringes | 1 pre-filled disposable injection PoM £686.38
  ▸ Pelgraz (Accord-UK Ltd)
   Filgrastim (as Pegfilgrastim) 10 mg per 1 ml Pelgraz 6mg/0.6ml solution for injection pre-filled injector | 1 pre-filled disposable injection PoM £686.37 (Hospital only)
   Pelgraz 6mg/0.6ml solution for injection pre-filled syringes | 1 pre-filled disposable injection PoM £686.37 (Hospital only)
  ▸ Pelmeg (Napp Pharmaceuticals Ltd)
   Filgrastim (as Pegfilgrastim) 10 mg per 1 ml Pelmeg 6mg/0.6ml solution for injection pre-filled syringes | 1 pre-filled disposable injection PoM £411.83 (Hospital only)

3.2 Stem cell mobilisation

IMMUNOSTIMULANTS ❭ CHEMOKINE RECEPTOR ANTAGONISTS

Plerixafor

22-Oct-2020

- **DRUG ACTION** Plerixafor is a chemokine receptor antagonist.

- **INDICATIONS AND DOSE**

Mobilise haematopoietic stem cells to peripheral blood for collection and subsequent autologous transplantation in patients with lymphoma or multiple myeloma (specialist use only)
  ▸ BY SUBCUTANEOUS INJECTION
  ▸ Adult (body-weight up to 84 kg): 240 micrograms/kg daily, alternatively 20 mg daily usually for 2–4 days (and up to 7 days), to be administered 6–11 hours before initiation of apheresis, dose to be given following 4 days treatment with a granulocyte-colony stimulating factor; maximum 40 mg per day
  ▸ Adult (body-weight 84 kg and above): 240 micrograms/kg daily usually for 2–4 days (and up to 7 days), to be administered 6–11 hours before initiation of apheresis, dose to be given following 4 days treatment with a granulocyte-colony stimulating factor; maximum 40 mg per day

- **SIDE-EFFECTS**
  ▸ **Common or very common** Arthralgia · constipation · diarrhoea · dizziness · dry mouth · erythema · fatigue · flatulence · gastrointestinal discomfort · headache · hyperhidrosis · malaise · musculoskeletal pain · nausea · oral hypoaesthesia · sleep disorders · vomiting
  ▸ **Frequency not known** Postural hypotension · splenomegaly · syncope

- **CONCEPTION AND CONTRACEPTION** Use effective contraception during treatment— teratogenic in *animal* studies.

- **PREGNANCY** Manufacturer advises avoid unless essential— teratogenic in *animal* studies.

- **BREAST FEEDING** Manufacturer advises avoid—no information available.

- **RENAL IMPAIRMENT** No information available if creatinine clearance less than 20 mL/minute.
  Dose adjustments Manufacturer advises reduce dose to 160 micrograms/kg (maximum 27 mg) daily if creatinine clearance 20–50 mL/minute. See p. 21.

- **MONITORING REQUIREMENTS** Monitor platelets and white blood cell count.

- **PATIENT AND CARER ADVICE**
Driving and skilled tasks Manufacturer advises patients and carers should be cautioned on the effects on driving and performance of skilled tasks—increased risk of dizziness, fatigue, or vasovagal reactions.

- **NATIONAL FUNDING/ACCESS DECISIONS**
For full details see funding body website
Scottish Medicines Consortium (SMC) decisions
▸ Plerixafor (*Mozobil*®) combined with G-CSF to enhance mobilisation of haematopoietic stem cells to the peripheral blood for collection & subsequent autologous transplantation in patients with lymphoma and multiple myeloma (January 2010) SMC No. 594/09 Recommended
All Wales Medicines Strategy Group (AWMSG) decisions
▸ Plerixafor (*Mozobil*®) in combination with G-CSF to enhance mobilisation of haematopoietic stem cells to the peripheral blood for collection and subsequent autologous transplantation in patients with lymphoma and multiple myeloma whose cells mobilise poorly (April 2010) AWMSG No. 249 Recommended with restrictions

- **MEDICINAL FORMS** There can be variation in the licensing of different medicines containing the same drug.
Solution for injection
▸ Plerixafor (Non-proprietary)
Plerixafor 20 mg per 1 ml Plerixafor 24mg/1.2ml solution for injection vials | 1 vial [PoM] £3,800.00–£4,882.77 (Hospital only)
▸ Mozobil (Sanofi)
Plerixafor 20 mg per 1 ml Mozobil 24mg/1.2ml solution for injection vials | 1 vial [PoM] £4,882.77

4   Platelet disorders
4.1 Essential thrombocythaemia

> **Other drugs used for Essential thrombocythaemia**
> Hydroxycarbamide, p. 1065

ANTITHROMBOTIC DRUGS › CYCLIC AMP PHOSPHODIESTERASE III INHIBITORS

Anagrelide [Specialist drug]   27-May-2022

- **INDICATIONS AND DOSE**
Essential thrombocythaemia [in patients at risk of thrombo-haemorrhagic events who have not responded adequately to other drugs or who cannot tolerate other drugs]
▸ BY MOUTH
▸ Adult: Specialist drug – access specialist resources for dosing information

> **IMPORTANT SAFETY INFORMATION**
> MHRA/CHM ADVICE: *XAGRID*® (ANAGRELIDE HYDROCHLORIDE): RISK OF THROMBOSIS, INCLUDING CEREBRAL INFARCTION, IF TREATMENT DISCONTINUED ABRUPTLY [ALSO APPLICABLE TO GENERIC FORMS] (APRIL 2022)
> There is an increased risk of potentially fatal thrombosis, including cerebral infarction, due to the rebound in platelet count when anagrelide treatment is discontinued abruptly. The platelet count will typically start to increase within 4 days after discontinuation and return to baseline levels within 1 to 2 weeks, but may rebound above these values.
> Healthcare professionals are advised to:
> - avoid abrupt treatment discontinuation;
> - monitor platelet counts frequently during dosage interruption or treatment withdrawal;

- counsel patients or their carers on how to recognise early signs and symptoms of thrombosis, including cerebral infarction, and to seek urgent medical advice if they occur.

- **INTERACTIONS** → Appendix 1: anagrelide
- **SIDE-EFFECTS**
▸ **Common or very common** Anaemia · arrhythmias · asthenia · diarrhoea · dizziness · fluid retention · gastrointestinal discomfort · gastrointestinal disorders · headaches · nausea · palpitations · skin reactions · vomiting
▸ **Uncommon** Alopecia · appetite decreased · arthralgia · chest pain · chills · confusion · congestive heart failure · constipation · depression · dry mouth · dyspnoea · erectile dysfunction · fever · haemorrhage · hypertension · insomnia · malaise · memory loss · myalgia · nervousness · oedema · pain · pancreatitis · pancytopenia · pneumonia · pulmonary hypertension · respiratory disorders · sensation abnormal · syncope · thrombocytopenia · weight changes
▸ **Rare or very rare** Angina pectoris · cardiomegaly · cardiomyopathy · coordination abnormal · drowsiness · dysarthria · influenza like illness · myocardial infarction · nocturia · pericardial effusion · postural hypotension · renal failure · tinnitus · vasodilation · vision disorders
▸ **Frequency not known** Hepatitis · interstitial lung disease · nephritis tubulointerstitial · thrombosis (on abrupt discontinuation)

- **CONCEPTION AND CONTRACEPTION** Effective contraception required during treatment.

- **PATIENT AND CARER ADVICE**
Driving and skilled tasks Dizziness may affect performance of skilled tasks (e.g. cycling, driving).

- **MEDICINAL FORMS** There can be variation in the licensing of different medicines containing the same drug.
Oral capsule
▸ Anagrelide (Non-proprietary)
Anagrelide (as Anagrelide hydrochloride)
500 microgram Anagrelide 500microgram capsules | 100 capsule [PoM] £404.57 DT = £404.57 | 100 capsule [PoM] [Σ] DT = £404.57 (Hospital only)
▸ Xagrid (Takeda UK Ltd)
Anagrelide (as Anagrelide hydrochloride) 500 microgram Xagrid 500microgram capsules | 100 capsule [PoM] £404.57 DT = £404.57

4.2 Thrombocytopenias

ANTIHAEMORRHAGICS › THROMBOPOIETIN RECEPTOR AGONISTS

Avatrombopag   03-Jan-2023

- **DRUG ACTION** Avatrombopag is a thrombopoietin receptor agonist that binds to and activates the thrombopoietin (TPO) receptor, thereby increasing platelet production.

- **INDICATIONS AND DOSE**
Thrombocytopenia [in patients with chronic liver disease undergoing invasive procedures and platelet count less than 40x10^9/litre] (under expert supervision)
▸ BY MOUTH
▸ Adult: 60 mg once daily for 5 days, treatment to be started 10 to 13 days before procedure; procedures to be carried out 5 to 8 days after the last dose of avatrombopag

Thrombocytopenia [in patients with chronic liver disease undergoing invasive procedures and platelet count between 40 to 50x10^9/litre] (under expert supervision)
▸ BY MOUTH
▸ Adult: 40 mg once daily for 5 days, treatment to be started 10 to 13 days before procedure;   continued →

procedures to be carried out 5 to 8 days after the last dose of avatrombopag

Chronic immune (idiopathic) thrombocytopenic purpura in patients refractory to other treatments (such as corticosteroids or immunoglobulins) (under expert supervision)

▸ BY MOUTH

▸ Adult: 20 mg once daily, dose to be adjusted to achieve a platelet count of 50×10^9/litre or more—consult product literature for dose adjustments, discontinue if inadequate response after 4 weeks treatment at maximum dose, or if platelet count more than 250×10^9/litre after 2 weeks of dosing at 20 mg once weekly; maximum 40 mg per day

DOSE ADJUSTMENTS DUE TO INTERACTIONS

▸ When used for Chronic immune (idiopathic) thrombocytopenic purpura [EvGr] Increase initial avatrombopag dose to 40 mg once daily in those already taking moderate CYP2C9 inducers. In those already taking avatrombopag, monitor platelet counts and adjust the avatrombopag dose as necessary when starting moderate CYP2C9 inducers. Decrease initial avatrombopag dose to 20 mg three times weekly in those already taking moderate CYP2C9 inhibitors. In those already taking avatrombopag, monitor platelet counts and adjust the avatrombopag dose as necessary when starting moderate CYP2C9 inhibitors. ⟨M⟩

● **CAUTIONS**

GENERAL CAUTIONS Known genetic polymorphisms— consult product literature · risk factors for thromboembolism

SPECIFIC CAUTIONS

▸ When used for Thrombocytopenia in patients with chronic liver disease undergoing invasive procedures Administration before laparotomy, thoracotomy, open-heart surgery, craniotomy, or excision of organs (no clinical experience)

● **INTERACTIONS** → Appendix 1: avatrombopag

● **SIDE-EFFECTS**

▸ **Common or very common** Fatigue

▸ **Uncommon** Anaemia · bone pain · fever · myalgia · portal vein thrombosis

● **PREGNANCY** [EvGr] Avoid—limited information available. ⟨M⟩

● **BREAST FEEDING** [EvGr] Avoid—present in milk in *animal* studies. ⟨M⟩

● **HEPATIC IMPAIRMENT** [EvGr] Caution in severe impairment (limited information available). ⟨M⟩

● **MONITORING REQUIREMENTS**

▸ [EvGr] Peripheral blood smear and complete blood counts are recommended before starting, and during, treatment. ⟨M⟩

▸ When used for Thrombocytopenia in patients with chronic liver disease undergoing invasive procedures [EvGr] Monitor platelet count before starting treatment and on the day of procedure. ⟨M⟩

▸ When used for Chronic immune (idiopathic) thrombocytopenic purpura [EvGr] Monitor platelet count at least once weekly until a stable platelet count of $50–150\times10^9$/litre achieved; monitor twice weekly during the first weeks of treatment in patients receiving once or twice weekly dosing, or after dose adjustments. After platelet count has stabilised, monitor platelet count at least monthly. After stopping treatment, monitor platelet counts weekly for at least 4 weeks (recurrence of thrombocytopenia likely). ⟨M⟩

● **NATIONAL FUNDING/ACCESS DECISIONS**

For full details see funding body website

NICE decisions

▸ Avatrombopag for treating thrombocytopenia in people with chronic liver disease needing a planned invasive procedure (June 2020) NICE TA626 Recommended

▸ Avatrombopag for treating primary chronic immune thrombocytopenia (December 2022) NICE TA853 Recommended

Scottish Medicines Consortium (SMC) decisions

▸ Avatrombopag (*Doptelet*®) for the treatment of severe thrombocytopenia in adult patients with chronic liver disease who are scheduled to undergo an invasive procedure (December 2020) SMC No. SMC2296 Recommended

▸ Avatrombopag (*Doptelet*®) for the treatment of primary chronic immune thrombocytopenia in adult patients who are refractory to other treatments (such as corticosteroids or immunoglobulins) (August 2021) SMC No. SMC2345 Recommended with restrictions

● **MEDICINAL FORMS** There can be variation in the licensing of different medicines containing the same drug.

Oral tablet

CAUTIONARY AND ADVISORY LABELS 21

▸ Doptelet (Swedish Orphan Biovitrum Ltd)
Avatrombopag (as Avatrombopag maleate) 20 mg Doptelet 20mg tablets | 10 tablet [PoM] £640.00 (Hospital only) | 15 tablet [PoM] £960.00 (Hospital only) | 30 tablet [PoM] £1,920.00 (Hospital only)

Lusutrombopag

27-Aug-2020

● **DRUG ACTION** Lusutrombopag is a thrombopoietin receptor agonist that binds to and activates the thrombopoietin (TPO) receptor, thereby increasing platelet production.

● **INDICATIONS AND DOSE**

Thrombocytopenia [in patients with chronic liver disease undergoing invasive procedures] (under expert supervision)

▸ BY MOUTH

▸ Adult: 3 mg once daily for 7 days, treatment to be started at least 8 days before procedure; in clinical trials procedures were carried out between 9 to 14 days after starting lusutrombopag

● **CAUTIONS** Administration before laparotomy, thoracotomy, open-heart surgery, craniotomy, or excision of organs (no clinical experience) · body-weight less than 45kg (limited information available) · history of splenectomy (no clinical experience) · risk factors for thromboembolism

CAUTIONS, FURTHER INFORMATION

▸ Body-weight less than 45kg Monitor platelet count approximately 5 days after the first dose and as necessary thereafter; stop treatment if the platelet count reaches 50×10^9/litre or more and has increased 20×10^9/litre from baseline.

● **SIDE-EFFECTS**

▸ **Common or very common** Headache · nausea · rash

▸ **Frequency not known** Embolism and thrombosis

● **PREGNANCY** Manufacturer advises avoid—no information available.

● **BREAST FEEDING** Manufacturer advises avoid—present in milk in *animal* studies.

● **HEPATIC IMPAIRMENT** Manufacturer advises caution in severe impairment (limited information available)— monitor platelet count approximately 5 days after the first dose and as necessary thereafter. Stop treatment if the platelet count reaches 50×10^9/litre or more and has increased 20×10^9/litre from baseline.

● **MONITORING REQUIREMENTS** Manufacturer advises monitor platelet count prior to procedure; more frequent monitoring may be required in some patients—see *Cautions* and *Hepatic Impairment* for further information.

● **NATIONAL FUNDING/ACCESS DECISIONS**
For full details see funding body website
NICE decisions
▸ Lusutrombopag for treating thrombocytopenia in people with chronic liver disease needing a planned invasive procedure (January 2020) NICE TA617 Recommended
Scottish Medicines Consortium (SMC) decisions
▸ Lusutrombopag (*Mulpleo*®) for the treatment of severe thrombocytopenia in adult patients with chronic liver disease undergoing invasive procedures (December 2019) SMC No. SMC2227 Recommended

● **MEDICINAL FORMS** There can be variation in the licensing of different medicines containing the same drug.
Oral tablet
▸ Mulpleo (Shionogi BV) ▼
Lusutrombopag 3 mg Mulpleo 3mg tablets | 7 tablet PoM £800.00

4.2a Acquired thrombotic thrombocytopenic purpura

ANTITHROMBOTIC DRUGS

▌Caplacizumab
12-Jan-2021

● **DRUG ACTION** Caplacizumab is a monoclonal antibody fragment (nanobody) that binds to von Willebrand factor, thereby inhibiting platelet adhesion.

● **INDICATIONS AND DOSE**
Acquired thrombotic thrombocytopenic purpura (specialist use only)
▸ INITIALLY BY INTRAVENOUS INJECTION
▸ Adult (body-weight 40 kg and above): Initially 10 mg for 1 dose, given before plasma exchange, followed by (by subcutaneous injection) 10 mg once daily given after each plasma exchange during, and for 30 days after finishing, daily plasma exchange therapy, treatment may be continued after this if there is evidence of unresolved immunological disease

● **CONTRA-INDICATIONS** Active bleeding (interrupt treatment)
● **CAUTIONS** Increased risk of bleeding
● **INTERACTIONS** → Appendix 1: caplacizumab
● **SIDE-EFFECTS**
▸ **Common or very common** Cerebral infarction · dyspnoea · fatigue · fever · haemorrhage · headache · menorrhagia · myalgia · subarachnoid haemorrhage · urticaria
● **PREGNANCY** Manufacturer advises avoid—no information available.
● **BREAST FEEDING** Manufacturer advises avoid—no information available.
● **HEPATIC IMPAIRMENT** Manufacturer advises caution in severe impairment (no information available).
● **DIRECTIONS FOR ADMINISTRATION** Manufacturer advises injection into the abdomen. Patients may self-administer *Cablivi*® after appropriate training in subcutaneous injection technique.
● **PRESCRIBING AND DISPENSING INFORMATION** Caplacizumab is a biological medicine. Biological medicines must be prescribed and dispensed by brand name, see *Biological medicines* and *Biosimilar medicines*, under Guidance on prescribing p. 1.
● **HANDLING AND STORAGE** Manufacturer advises store in a refrigerator (2-8°C) and protect from light—consult product literature for further information regarding storage outside refrigerator.

● **PATIENT AND CARER ADVICE**
Missed doses Manufacturer advises if a dose is more than 12 hours late, the missed dose should not be given and the next dose should be given at the normal time.
● **NATIONAL FUNDING/ACCESS DECISIONS**
For full details see funding body website
NICE decisions
▸ Caplacizumab with plasma exchange and immunosuppression for treating acute acquired thrombotic thrombocytopenic purpura (December 2020) NICE TA667 Recommended
Scottish Medicines Consortium (SMC) decisions
▸ Caplacizumab (*Cablivi*®) for the treatment of adults experiencing an episode of acquired thrombotic thrombocytopenic purpura (aTTP), in conjunction with plasma exchange and immunosuppression (September 2020) SMC No. SMC2266 Recommended

● **MEDICINAL FORMS** There can be variation in the licensing of different medicines containing the same drug.
Powder and solvent for solution for injection
EXCIPIENTS: May contain Polysorbates
▸ Cablivi (Sanofi)
Caplacizumab 10 mg Cablivi 10mg powder and solvent for solution for injection vials | 1 vial PoM £4,143.00 (Hospital only)

4.2b Immune thrombocytopenia

Immune thrombocytopenic purpura
12-Apr-2021

Overview

EvGr In adults with immune thrombocytopenic purpura, initial treatment is usually with a **corticosteroid**, such as prednisolone p. 791.

Intravenous normal immunoglobulin p. 1466, or intravenous anti-D (Rh₀) immunoglobulin [unlicensed use] may be appropriate in patients with immune thrombocytopenic purpura who are bleeding or at high-risk of bleeding, who require a surgical procedure, or who are unresponsive to corticosteroids. Immunoglobulin preparations may also be considered where a temporary rapid rise in platelets is needed, for example in pregnancy.

Treatment options for *persistent or chronic* immune thrombocytopenic purpura include thrombopoietin receptor agonists (avatrombopag p. 1169, eltrombopag p. 1172, and romiplostim p. 1174), rituximab [unlicensed use], or fostamatinib p. 1172. Ⓐ

Other therapies that have been tried in refractory immune thrombocytopenic purpura include: azathioprine, ciclosporin, cyclophosphamide, danazol, dapsone, mycophenolate mofetil, and vincristine sulfate.

EvGr Splenectomy can be considered as a treatment option only if drug therapy has failed; the patients age and co-morbidities should also be taken into account. Ⓐ

ANTIHAEMORRHAGICS › HAEMOSTATICS

Fostamatinib
15-Nov-2022

- **DRUG ACTION** Fostamatinib, through its metabolite R406, blocks the activity of the spleen tyrosine kinase (SYK) enzyme, thereby reducing immune-mediated destruction of platelets.

- **INDICATIONS AND DOSE**

Chronic immune thrombocytopenia in patients refractory to other treatments (under expert supervision)
- ▸ BY MOUTH
  - ▸ Adult: Initially 100 mg twice daily; increased if tolerated to 150 mg twice daily after 4 weeks, dose to be adjusted to achieve a platelet count of $50x10^9$/litre or more, discontinue if inadequate response after 12 weeks of treatment, for dose reduction, interruption or treatment discontinuation due to side-effects—consult product literature

- **INTERACTIONS** → Appendix 1: fostamatinib

- **SIDE-EFFECTS**
- ▸ **Common or very common** Chest pain · diarrhoea · dizziness · fatigue · frequent bowel movements · gastrointestinal discomfort · hypertension · increased risk of infection · influenza like illness · nausea · neutropenia · skin reactions · taste altered
- ▸ **Frequency not known** Hyperbilirubinaemia · hypoxia · nephrolithiasis · pain in extremity · syncope · toothache

- **CONCEPTION AND CONTRACEPTION** Manufacturer advises effective contraception during and for at least 1 month after stopping treatment in females of childbearing potential.

- **PREGNANCY** Manufacturer advises avoid—toxicity in *animal* studies.

- **BREAST FEEDING** Manufacturer advises avoid during and for at least 1 month after stopping treatment—metabolites present in milk in *animal* studies.

- **HEPATIC IMPAIRMENT** Manufacturer advises avoid in severe impairment; caution in mild to moderate impairment—monitor liver function monthly during treatment.
  Dose adjustments Manufacturer advises consider dose reduction, interruption or treatment discontinuation in mild to moderate impairment—consult product literature.

- **MONITORING REQUIREMENTS**
- ▸ Manufacturer advises monitor blood pressure every 2 weeks until stable, then monthly thereafter; antihypertensive therapy can be initiated or adjusted during treatment. If increased blood pressure persists, consider fostamatinib dose reduction, interruption or discontinuation—consult product literature.
- ▸ Manufacturer advises monitor full blood count, including neutrophils and platelet counts, monthly until a stable platelet count of at least $50x10^9$/litre is reached; monitor full blood counts regularly thereafter.
- ▸ Manufacturer advises monitor for any effects on bone remodelling or formation, especially in patients with osteoporosis, fractures or young adults where epiphyseal fusion has not yet occurred—limited information available.

- **NATIONAL FUNDING/ACCESS DECISIONS**
  For full details see funding body website
  NICE decisions
- ▸ **Fostamatinib for treating refractory chronic immune thrombocytopenia (October 2022)** NICE TA835 Recommended with restrictions

  Scottish Medicines Consortium (SMC) decisions
- ▸ **Fostamatinib (*Tavlesse*®) for the treatment of chronic immune thrombocytopenia in adult patients who are** refractory to other treatments (January 2021) SMC No. SMC2300 Recommended with restrictions

- **MEDICINAL FORMS** There can be variation in the licensing of different medicines containing the same drug.
  Oral tablet
- ▸ Tavlesse (Grifols UK Ltd) ▼
  Fostamatinib (as Fostamatinib disodium hexahydrate)
  100 mg Tavlesse 100mg tablets | 60 tablet [PoM] £3,090.00 (Hospital only)
  Fostamatinib (as Fostamatinib disodium hexahydrate)
  150 mg Tavlesse 150mg tablets | 60 tablet [PoM] £4,635.00 (Hospital only)

ANTIHAEMORRHAGICS › THROMBOPOIETIN RECEPTOR AGONISTS

Eltrombopag
29-Mar-2022

- **DRUG ACTION** Eltrombopag is a thrombopoietin receptor agonist that binds to and activates the thrombopoietin (TPO) receptor, thereby increasing platelet production.

- **INDICATIONS AND DOSE**

Chronic immune (idiopathic) thrombocytopenic purpura in patients of East or Southeast Asian origin refractory to other treatments (such as corticosteroids or immunoglobulins) (under expert supervision)
- ▸ BY MOUTH
  - ▸ Adult: Initially 25 mg once daily, dose to be adjusted to achieve a platelet count of $50x10^9$/litre or more—consult product literature for dose adjustments, discontinue if inadequate response after 4 weeks treatment at maximum dose; maximum 75 mg per day

Chronic immune (idiopathic) thrombocytopenic purpura in patients refractory to other treatments (such as corticosteroids or immunoglobulins) (under expert supervision)
- ▸ BY MOUTH
  - ▸ Adult: Initially 50 mg once daily, dose to be adjusted to achieve a platelet count of $50x10^9$/litre or more—consult product literature for dose adjustments, discontinue if inadequate response after 4 weeks treatment at maximum dose; maximum 75 mg per day

Treatment of thrombocytopenia associated with chronic hepatitis C infection, where the degree of thrombocytopenia is the main factor preventing the initiation or limiting the ability to maintain optimal interferon-based therapy (under expert supervision)
- ▸ BY MOUTH
  - ▸ Adult: Initially 25 mg once daily, dose to be adjusted to achieve a platelet count sufficient to initiate antiviral therapy then a platelet count of $50–75x10^9$/litre during antiviral therapy—consult product literature for dose adjustments, discontinue if inadequate response after 2 weeks treatment at maximum dose; maximum 100 mg per day

Acquired severe aplastic anaemia in patients of East or Southeast Asian origin either refractory to or heavily pretreated with prior immunosuppressive therapy and are unsuitable for haematopoietic stem cell transplantation (under expert supervision)
- ▸ BY MOUTH
  - ▸ Adult: Initially 25 mg once daily, dose to be adjusted to achieve a platelet count of $50x10^9$/litre or more—consult product literature for dose adjustments, discontinue if no haematological response after 16 weeks treatment; maximum 150 mg per day

Acquired severe aplastic anaemia in patients either refractory to or heavily pretreated with prior immunosuppressive therapy and are unsuitable for haematopoietic stem cell transplantation (under expert supervision)
- ▶ BY MOUTH
- ▶ Adult: Initially 50 mg once daily, dose to be adjusted to achieve a platelet count of $50x10^9$/litre or more—consult product literature for dose adjustments, discontinue if no haematological response after 16 weeks treatment; maximum 150 mg per day

DOSE EQUIVALENCE AND CONVERSION
- ▶ Powder for oral suspension may lead to higher eltrombopag exposure than oral tablet; platelet counts should be monitored weekly for 2 weeks when switching between preparations.

> **IMPORTANT SAFETY INFORMATION**
> MHRA/CHM ADVICE: ELTROMBOPAG (*REVOLADE*®): REPORTS OF INTERFERENCE WITH BILIRUBIN AND CREATININE TEST RESULTS (JULY 2018)
> See *Effect on laboratory tests*.

- ● CAUTIONS Patients of East or Southeast Asian origin · risk factors for thromboembolism
- ● INTERACTIONS → Appendix 1: eltrombopag
- ● SIDE-EFFECTS
- ▶ **Common or very common** Abnormal loss of weight · alopecia · anaemia · anxiety · appetite abnormal · arthralgia · asthenia · cataract · chest discomfort · chills · concentration impaired · constipation · cough · depression · diarrhoea · dizziness · drowsiness · dry eye · dry mouth · dysphagia · dyspnoea · ear pain · electrolyte imbalance · embolism and thrombosis · eosinophilia · eye disorders · eye pain · fever · gastrointestinal discomfort · gastrointestinal disorders · haemorrhage · headaches · hepatic disorders · hyperbilirubinaemia · hyperglycaemia · hypoglycaemia · increased leucocytes · increased risk of infection · influenza like illness · iron overload · lymphopenia · malaise · memory impairment · menorrhagia · mood altered · muscle complaints · nasal complaints · nausea · neutropenia · oedema · oral disorders · oropharyngeal complaints · pain · palpitations · renal impairment · renal thrombotic microangiopathy · sensation abnormal · skin reactions · sleep disorder · splenic infarction · sweat changes · syncope · taste altered · urine abnormalities · urine discolouration · vasodilation · vertigo · vision disorders · vomiting · weight decreased
- ▶ **Uncommon** Anisocytosis · arrhythmias · balance impaired · cardiovascular disorder · confusion · cyanosis · eye inflammation · feeling hot · feeling jittery · food poisoning · gout · haemolytic anaemia · hemiparesis · lens opacity · muscle weakness · myocardial infarction · nephritis lupus · nerve disorders · QT interval prolongation · rectosigmoid cancer · retinal pigment epitheliopathy · sinus disorder · sleep apnoea · speech disorder · sunburn · tremor · urinary disorders · wound inflammation
- ▶ **Frequency not known** Cerebral infarction · sepsis
- ● CONCEPTION AND CONTRACEPTION Ensure effective contraception during treatment.
- ● PREGNANCY Avoid—toxicity in *animal* studies.
- ● BREAST FEEDING Manufacturer advises avoid.
- ● HEPATIC IMPAIRMENT
- ▶ When used for Idiopathic thrombocytopenic purpura Manufacturer advises consider avoiding.
- ▶ When used for Severe aplastic anaemia Manufacturer advises caution.
- ▶ When used for Thrombocytopenia associated with chronic hepatitis C infection Manufacturer advises caution (increased risk of hepatic decompensation and thromboembolic events).

Dose adjustments
- ▶ When used for Idiopathic thrombocytopenic purpura Manufacturer advises initial dose reduction to 25 mg once daily and wait at least 3 weeks before upwards titration of dose.
- ▶ When used for Severe aplastic anaemia Manufacturer advises initial dose reduction to 25 mg once daily and wait at least 2 weeks before upwards titration of dose.
- ▶ When used for Thrombocytopenia associated with chronic hepatitis C infection Manufacturer advises initial dose reduction to 25 mg once daily in moderate to severe impairment and wait at least 2 weeks before upwards titration of dose.
- ● RENAL IMPAIRMENT EvGr Use with caution. Ⓜ
- ● PRE-TREATMENT SCREENING For *severe aplastic anaemia*, manufacturer advises do not initiate if patients have existing cytogenetic abnormalities of chromosome 7.
- ● MONITORING REQUIREMENTS
- ▶ Manufacturer advises monitor liver function before treatment, every two weeks when adjusting the dose, and monthly thereafter.
- ▶ Manufacturer advises regular ophthalmological examinations for cataract formation.
- ▶ Manufacturer advises peripheral blood smear prior to initiation to establish baseline level of cellular morphologic abnormalities; once stabilised, full blood count with white blood cell count differential should be performed monthly.
- ▶ For *idiopathic thrombocytopenic purpura*, manufacturer advises monitor full blood count including platelet count and peripheral blood smears every week during treatment until a stable platelet count is reached ($50x10^9$/litre or more for at least 4 weeks), then monthly thereafter; monitor platelet count weekly for 4 weeks following treatment discontinuation.
- ▶ For *severe aplastic anaemia*, manufacturer advises bone marrow examination with aspirations for cytogenetics prior to initiation, at 3 months of treatment and 6 months thereafter.
- ▶ For *thrombocytopenia associated with chronic hepatitis C infection*, manufacturer advises monitor platelet count every week before and during antiviral treatment until a stable platelet count is reached ($50–75x10^9$/litre), then monitor full blood count including platelet count and peripheral blood smears monthly thereafter.
- ● EFFECT ON LABORATORY TESTS Eltrombopag is highly coloured and can cause serum discolouration and interference with total bilirubin and creatinine testing. If laboratory results are inconsistent with clinical observations, manufacturer advises re-testing using another method to help determine the validity of the result.
- ● DIRECTIONS FOR ADMINISTRATION EvGr Each dose should be taken at least 2 hours before or 4 hours after any dairy products (or foods containing calcium), indigestion remedies, or medicines containing aluminium, calcium, iron, magnesium, zinc, or selenium to reduce possible interference with absorption. For *powder for oral suspension*, disperse dose in 20 mL of water and administer using an oral syringe. Discard suspension if not administered within 30 minutes of preparation. Ⓜ
- ● PATIENT AND CARER ADVICE Patients or carers should be given advice on how to administer eltrombopag tablets and powder for oral suspension.
- ● NATIONAL FUNDING/ACCESS DECISIONS
  For full details see funding body website
  NICE decisions
- ▶ **Eltrombopag for treating chronic immune (idiopathic) thrombocytopenic purpura (updated October 2018)** NICE TA293 Recommended with restrictions

Scottish Medicines Consortium (SMC) decisions
► Eltrombopag (*Revolade*®) for adult chronic immune (idiopathic) thrombocytopenic purpura (August 2010) SMC No. 625/10 Recommended with restrictions

● MEDICINAL FORMS There can be variation in the licensing of different medicines containing the same drug.
Oral tablet
► Eltrombopag (Non-proprietary)
Eltrombopag (as Eltrombopag olamine) 12.5 mg Promacta 12.5mg tablets | 30 tablet [PoM] Ⓢ (Hospital only)
► Revolade (Novartis Pharmaceuticals UK Ltd)
Eltrombopag (as Eltrombopag olamine) 25 mg Revolade 25mg tablets | 28 tablet [PoM] £770.00 DT = £770.00
Eltrombopag (as Eltrombopag olamine) 50 mg Revolade 50mg tablets | 28 tablet [PoM] £1,540.00 DT = £1,540.00
Eltrombopag (as Eltrombopag olamine) 75 mg Revolade 75mg tablets | 28 tablet [PoM] £2,310.00 DT = £2,310.00
Powder for oral suspension
CAUTIONARY AND ADVISORY LABELS 13
► Revolade (Novartis Pharmaceuticals UK Ltd)
Eltrombopag (as Eltrombopag olamine) 25 mg Revolade 25mg oral powder sachets | 30 sachet [PoM] £825.00 (Hospital only) [SF]

Romiplostim

22-Oct-2020

● DRUG ACTION Romiplostim is an Fc–peptide fusion protein that binds to and activates the thrombopoietin (TPO) receptor, thereby increasing platelet production.

● INDICATIONS AND DOSE
Chronic immune (idiopathic) thrombocytopenic purpura in patients refractory to other treatments (such as corticosteroids or immunoglobulins) (under expert supervision)
► BY SUBCUTANEOUS INJECTION
► Adult: Initially 1 microgram/kg once weekly, adjusted in steps of 1 microgram/kg once weekly (max. per dose 10 micrograms/kg once weekly) until a stable platelet count of $50x10^9$/litre or more is reached, consult product literature for further details of dose adjustments, discontinue treatment if inadequate response after 4 weeks at maximum dose

● CAUTIONS Risk factors for thromboembolism

● INTERACTIONS → Appendix 1: romiplostim

● SIDE-EFFECTS
► **Common or very common** Anaemia · angioedema · arthralgia · asthenia · bone marrow disorders · chills · constipation · diarrhoea · dizziness · embolism and thrombosis · fever · flushing · gastrointestinal discomfort · headaches · hypersensitivity · increased risk of infection · influenza like illness · muscle complaints · nausea · pain · palpitations · peripheral oedema · sensation abnormal · skin reactions · sleep disorders
► **Uncommon** Alopecia · appetite decreased · chest pain · clonus · cough · dehydration · depression · dry throat · dysphagia · dyspnoea · erythromelalgia · eye disorders · eye pruritus · feeling hot · feeling jittery · gastrooesophageal reflux disease · gout · haemorrhage · hair growth abnormal · hypotension · irritability · leucocytosis · malaise · muscle weakness · myocardial infarction · nasal complaints · neoplasms · oral disorders · papilloedema · peripheral ischaemia · peripheral neuropathy · photosensitivity reaction · pleuritic pain · portal vein thrombosis · skin nodule · splenomegaly · taste altered · thrombocytosis · tooth discolouration · vertigo · vision disorders · vomiting · weight changes

● PREGNANCY Manufacturer advises avoid—toxicity in *animal* studies.

● BREAST FEEDING Manufacturer advises avoid—no information available.

● HEPATIC IMPAIRMENT Manufacturer advises caution; consider avoiding in moderate to severe impairment (risk of thromboembolic complications).

● RENAL IMPAIRMENT Manufacturer advises caution—no information available.

● MONITORING REQUIREMENTS
► Manufacturer advises monitor full blood count and peripheral blood smears for morphological abnormalities before and during treatment.
► Manufacturer advises monitor platelet count weekly until platelet count reaches $50x10^9$/litre or more for at least 4 weeks without dose adjustment, then monthly thereafter.
► Manufacturer advises monitor platelet count following treatment discontinuation—risk of bleeding.

● PATIENT AND CARER ADVICE
Driving and skilled tasks Manufacturer advises that patients and their carers should be counselled on the effects on driving and the performance of skilled tasks—increased risk of dizziness.

● NATIONAL FUNDING/ACCESS DECISIONS
For full details see funding body website

NICE decisions
► Romiplostim for the treatment of chronic immune (idiopathic) thrombocytopenic purpura (updated October 2018) NICE TA221 Recommended with restrictions

Scottish Medicines Consortium (SMC) decisions
► Romiplostim (*Nplate*®) for adult chronic immune (idiopathic) thrombocytopenic purpura (October 2009) SMC No. 553/09 Recommended with restrictions

● MEDICINAL FORMS There can be variation in the licensing of different medicines containing the same drug.
Powder and solvent for solution for injection
► Nplate (Amgen Ltd)
Romiplostim 250 microgram Nplate 250microgram powder and solvent for solution for injection vials | 1 vial [PoM] £482.00 (Hospital only)
Powder for solution for injection
► Nplate (Amgen Ltd)
Romiplostim 125 microgram Nplate 125microgram powder for solution for injection vials | 1 vial [PoM] £241.00 (Hospital only)

Nutrition and metabolic disorders

1 Acid-base imbalance

1.1 Metabolic acidosis

ALKALISING DRUGS

Potassium citrate with potassium bicarbonate

13-Oct-2022

● INDICATIONS AND DOSE
Distal renal tubular acidosis
► BY MOUTH
► Adult: Initially 1 mEq/kg daily in 2 divided doses, adjusted in steps of 0.5 mEq/kg daily if required, to be adjusted until optimal response is achieved, use the lowest maximum daily dose; maximum 10 mEq/kg per day; maximum 336 mEq per day
DOSE EQUIVALENCE AND CONVERSION
► When switching from other alkalising therapy,

treatment should be initiated at the target dose used with the previous therapy, in mEq/kg per day, and adjusted as necessary.

- **CONTRA-INDICATIONS** Hyperkalaemia
- **CAUTIONS** Conditions predisposing to hyperkalaemia · gastrointestinal disorders

  CAUTIONS, FURTHER INFORMATION
- ▶ Gastrointestinal disorders EvGr Gastrointestinal disorders such as malabsorption, delayed gastric emptying, diarrhoea, nausea and vomiting could affect efficacy and safety. Monitor plasma bicarbonate levels regularly and adjust dose as clinically indicated. Ⓜ
- **SIDE-EFFECTS**
- ▶ **Common or very common** Diarrhoea · gastrointestinal discomfort · gastrointestinal disorder · nausea · vomiting
- **PREGNANCY** EvGr Use only if potential benefit outweighs risk—increased risk of developing hyperkalaemia. Ⓜ
- **BREAST FEEDING** EvGr Present in milk but not known to be harmful. Ⓜ
- **RENAL IMPAIRMENT** See p. 21. EvGr Avoid if eGFR is less than 45 mL/min/1.73m^2.

  Avoid if eGFR is between 45 and 59 mL/min/1.73m^2 and plasma potassium levels are elevated.

  Caution if eGFR is between 45 and 59 mL/min/1.73m^2— monitor renal function and plasma potassium levels prior to and after initiation of treatment or dose increase, then at least twice yearly thereafter. Ⓜ
- **DIRECTIONS FOR ADMINISTRATION** Granules should be swallowed whole with a large glass of water, preferably during meals. Alternatively, granules can be mixed (without crushing) with small amounts of soft food (e.g. yoghurt, fruit puree) and taken immediately without chewing. Do **not** mix granules with hot liquids, hot foods or alcohol. Granules should not be given via an enteral feeding tube as they may cause blockage.
- **PATIENT AND CARER ADVICE** Patients or carers should be given advice on how to administer *Sibnayal*® granules. **Missed doses** If vomiting occurs within 2 hours of taking a dose, a replacement dose should be taken.
- **NATIONAL FUNDING/ACCESS DECISIONS**
  For full details see funding body website

  Scottish Medicines Consortium (SMC) decisions
- ▶ **Potassium citrate and potassium hydrogen carbonate (*Sibnayal*®) for the treatment of distal renal tubular acidosis in adults, adolescents and children aged one year and older (August 2022) SMC No. SMC2409 Recommended**

- **MEDICINAL FORMS** There can be variation in the licensing of different medicines containing the same drug.

  Modified-release granules
  CAUTIONARY AND ADVISORY LABELS 25, 27
  ELECTROLYTES: May contain Potassium
  - ▶ Sibnayal (Advicenne S.A.)
    Potassium citrate 282 mg, Potassium bicarbonate 527 mg Sibnayal 8mEq prolonged-release granules sachets | 60 sachet PoM £120.00 (Hospital only) SF
    Potassium citrate 847 mg, Potassium bicarbonate 1.582 gram Sibnayal 24mEq prolonged-release granules sachets | 60 sachet PoM £360.00 (Hospital only) SF

2　Fluid and electrolyte imbalances

Fluids and electrolytes

15-Jan-2025

Electrolyte replacement therapy

The electrolyte concentrations (intravenous fluid) table and the electrolyte content (gastro-intestinal secretions) table

may be helpful in planning replacement electrolyte therapy; faeces, vomit, or aspiration should be saved and analysed where possible if abnormal losses are suspected.

Oral preparations for fluid and electrolyte imbalance

Sodium and potassium salts, may be given by mouth to prevent deficiencies or to treat established deficiencies of mild or moderate degree.

Oral potassium

Compensation for potassium loss is especially necessary:
- in those taking digoxin or anti-arrhythmic drugs, where potassium depletion may induce arrhythmias;
- in patients in whom secondary hyperaldosteronism occurs, e.g. renal artery stenosis, cirrhosis of the liver, the nephrotic syndrome, and severe heart failure;
- in patients with excessive losses of potassium in the faeces, e.g. chronic diarrhoea associated with intestinal malabsorption or laxative abuse.

Measures to compensate for potassium loss may also be required in the elderly since they frequently take inadequate amounts of potassium in the diet (but see **warning** on **renal insufficiency**). Measures may also be required during long-term administration of drugs known to induce potassium loss (e.g. corticosteroids). Potassium supplements are **seldom required** with the small doses of diuretics given to treat hypertension; **potassium-sparing diuretics** (rather than potassium supplements) are recommended for prevention of hypokalaemia due to diuretics such as furosemide p. 261 or the thiazides when these are given to eliminate oedema.

If potassium salts are used for the prevention of hypokalaemia, then doses of potassium chloride daily (in divided doses) by mouth are suitable in patients taking a normal diet. *Smaller doses* must be used if there is *renal insufficiency (common in the elderly)* to reduce the **risk** of **hyperkalaemia**.

Potassium salts cause nausea and vomiting and poor compliance is a major limitation to their effectiveness; when appropriate, potassium-sparing diuretics are preferable.

When there is *established potassium depletion* larger doses may be necessary, the quantity depending on the severity of any continuing potassium loss (monitoring of plasma-potassium concentration and specialist advice would be required). Potassium depletion is frequently associated with chloride depletion and with metabolic alkalosis, and these disorders require correction.

For guidance on the management of hyperkalaemia, see Hyperkalaemia p. 1198.

Oral sodium and water

Sodium chloride p. 1180 is indicated in states of sodium depletion and usually needs to be given intravenously. In chronic conditions associated with mild or moderate degrees of sodium depletion, e.g. in salt-losing bowel or renal disease, oral supplements of sodium chloride or sodium bicarbonate p. 1178, according to the acid-base status of the patient, may be sufficient.

Oral rehydration therapy (ORT)

As a worldwide problem *diarrhoea* is by far the most important indication for fluid and electrolyte replacement. Intestinal absorption of sodium and water is enhanced by glucose (and other carbohydrates). Replacement of fluid and electrolytes lost through diarrhoea can therefore be achieved by giving solutions containing sodium, potassium, and glucose or another carbohydrate such as rice starch.

Oral rehydration solutions should:
- enhance the absorption of water and electrolytes;
- replace the electrolyte deficit adequately and safely;
- contain an alkalinising agent to counter acidosis;
- be slightly hypo-osmolar (about 250 mmol/litre) to prevent the possible induction of osmotic diarrhoea;

- be simple to use in hospital and at home;
- be palatable and acceptable, especially to children;
- be readily available.

It is the policy of the World Health Organization (WHO) to promote a single oral rehydration solution but to use it flexibly (e.g. by giving extra water between drinks of oral rehydration solution to moderately dehydrated infants).

The WHO oral rehydration salts formulation contains sodium chloride 2.6 g, potassium chloride 1.5 g, sodium citrate 2.9 g, anhydrous glucose 13.5 g. It is dissolved in sufficient water to produce 1 litre (providing Na^+ 75 mmol, K^+ 20 mmol, Cl^- 65 mmol, citrate 10 mmol, glucose 75 mmol/litre). This formulation is recommended by the WHO and the United Nations Children's fund, but it is not commonly used in the UK.

Oral rehydration solutions used in the UK are lower in sodium (50–60 mmol/litre) than the WHO formulation since, in general, patients suffer less severe sodium loss.

Rehydration should be rapid over 3 to 4 hours (except in hypernatraemic dehydration in which case rehydration should occur more slowly over 12 hours). The patient should be reassessed after initial rehydration and if still dehydrated rapid fluid replacement should continue.

Once rehydration is complete further dehydration is prevented by encouraging the patient to drink normal volumes of an appropriate fluid and by replacing continuing losses with an oral rehydration solution; in infants, breast-feeding or formula feeds should be offered between oral rehydration drinks.

Oral bicarbonate

Sodium bicarbonate is given by mouth for *chronic acidotic states* such as uraemic acidosis or renal tubular acidosis. The dose for correction of metabolic acidosis is not predictable and the response must be assessed. For severe *metabolic acidosis*, sodium bicarbonate can be given intravenously.

Sodium bicarbonate may also be used to increase the pH of the urine; it is also used in dyspepsia.

Sodium supplements may increase blood pressure or cause fluid retention and pulmonary oedema in those at risk; hypokalaemia may be exacerbated.

Where *hyperchloraemic acidosis* is associated with potassium deficiency, as in some renal tubular and gastrointestinal disorders it may be appropriate to give oral **potassium bicarbonate**, although acute or severe deficiency should be managed by intravenous therapy.

Parenteral preparations for fluid and electrolyte imbalance

For guidance on intravenous fluids in the management of suspected sepsis, see Sepsis p. 579.

Electrolytes and water

Solutions of electrolytes are given intravenously, to meet normal fluid and electrolyte requirements or to replenish substantial deficits or continuing losses, when the patient is nauseated or vomiting and is unable to take adequate amounts by mouth. When intravenous administration is not possible, fluid (as sodium chloride 0.9% or glucose 5% p. 1182) can also be given by subcutaneous infusion (hypodermoclysis).

The nature and severity of the electrolyte imbalance must be assessed from the history and clinical and biochemical investigations. Sodium, potassium, chloride, magnesium, phosphate, and water depletion can occur singly and in combination with or without disturbances of acid-base balance.

Isotonic solutions may be infused safely into a peripheral vein. Solutions more concentrated than plasma, e.g. 20% glucose p. 1182, are best given through an indwelling catheter positioned in a large vein.

Intravenous sodium

Sodium chloride p. 1180 in isotonic solution provides the most important extracellular ions in near physiological concentrations and is indicated in *sodium depletion*, which can arise from such conditions as gastro-enteritis, diabetic ketoacidosis, ileus, and ascites. In a severe deficit of 4 to 8 litres, 2 to 3 litres of isotonic sodium chloride may be given over 2 to 3 hours; thereafter the infusion can usually be at a slower rate.

Chronic hyponatraemia arising from inappropriate secretion of antidiuretic hormone should ideally be corrected by fluid restriction. However, if sodium chloride is required for acute or chronic hyponatraemia, regardless of the cause, the deficit should be corrected slowly to avoid the risk of osmotic demyelination syndrome and the rise in plasma-sodium concentration should not exceed 10 mmol/litre in 24 hours. In severe hyponatraemia, sodium chloride 1.8% may be used cautiously.

Compound sodium lactate (Hartmann's solution) can be used instead of isotonic sodium chloride solution during or after surgery, or in the initial management of the injured or wounded; it may reduce the risk of hyperchloraemic acidosis.

Sodium chloride with glucose solutions p. 1181 are indicated when there is combined *water and sodium depletion*. A 1:1 mixture of isotonic sodium chloride and 5% glucose allows some of the water (free of sodium) to enter body cells which suffer most from dehydration while the sodium salt with a volume of water determined by the normal plasma Na^+ remains extracellular.

Combined sodium, potassium, chloride, and water depletion may occur, for example, with severe diarrhoea or persistent vomiting; replacement is carried out with sodium chloride intravenous infusion 0.9% and glucose intravenous infusion 5% with potassium as appropriate.

Intravenous glucose

Glucose solutions (5%) are used mainly to replace water deficit. Average water requirements in a healthy adult are 1.5 to 2.5 litres daily and this is needed to balance unavoidable losses of water through the skin and lungs and to provide sufficient for urinary excretion. Water depletion (dehydration) tends to occur when these losses are not matched by a comparable intake, as may occur in coma or dysphagia or in the elderly or apathetic who may not drink enough water on their own initiative.

Excessive loss of water without loss of electrolytes is uncommon, occurring in fevers, hyperthyroidism, and in uncommon water-losing renal states such as diabetes insipidus or hypercalcaemia. The volume of glucose solution needed to replace deficits varies with the severity of the disorder, but usually lies within the range of 2 to 6 litres.

Glucose solutions are also used to correct and prevent hypoglycaemia and to provide a source of energy in those too ill to be fed adequately by mouth; glucose solutions are a key component of parenteral nutrition.

Glucose solutions are given in regimens with calcium and insulin for the emergency management of Hyperkalaemia p. 1198. They are also given, after correction of hyperglycaemia, during treatment of diabetic ketoacidosis, when they must be accompanied by continuing insulin infusion.

Intravenous potassium

Potassium chloride with sodium chloride intravenous infusion p. 1180 is the initial treatment for the correction of *severe hypokalaemia* and when sufficient potassium cannot be taken by mouth.

Repeated measurement of plasma-potassium concentration is necessary to determine whether further infusions are required and to avoid the development of hyperkalaemia, which is especially likely in renal impairment.

Fluids and electrolytes

Electrolyte concentrations—intravenous fluids

Intravenous infusion	Millimoles per litre				
	Na$^+$	K$^+$	HCO$_3^-$	Cl$^-$	Ca^{2+}
Normal plasma values	142	4.5	26	103	2.5
Sodium Chloride 0.9%	150	-	-	150	-
Compound Sodium Lactate (Hartmann's)	131	5	29	111	2
Sodium Chloride 0.18% and Glucose 4% (Adults only)	30	-	-	30	-
Sodium Chloride 0.45% and Glucose 5% (Children only)	75	-	-	75	-
Potassium Chloride 0.15% and Glucose 5% (Children only)	-	20	-	20	-
Potassium Chloride 0.15% and Sodium Chloride 0.9% (Children only)	150	20	-	170	-
Potassium Chloride 0.3% and Glucose 5%	-	40	-	40	-
Potassium Chloride 0.3% and Sodium Chloride 0.9%	150	40	-	190	-
To correct metabolic acidosis					
Sodium Bicarbonate 1.26%	150	-	150	-	-
Sodium Bicarbonate 8.4% for cardiac arrest	1000	-	1000	-	-
Sodium Lactate (m/6)	167	-	167	-	-

Electrolyte content—gastro-intestinal secretions

Type of fluid	Millimoles per litre				
	H$^+$	Na$^+$	K$^+$	HCO$_3^-$	Cl$^-$
Gastric	40-60	20-80	5-20	-	100-150
Biliary	-	120-140	5-15	30-50	80-120
Pancreatic	-	120-140	5-15	70-110	40-80
Small bowel	-	120-140	5-15	20-40	90-130

Initial potassium replacement therapy should **not** involve glucose infusions, because glucose may cause a further decrease in the plasma-potassium concentration.

Bicarbonate and lactate
Sodium bicarbonate p. 1178 is used to control severe *metabolic acidosis* (pH <7.1) particularly that caused by loss of bicarbonate (as in renal tubular acidosis or from excessive gastro-intestinal losses). Mild metabolic acidosis associated with volume depletion should first be managed by appropriate fluid replacement because acidosis usually resolves as tissue and renal perfusion are restored. In more severe metabolic acidosis or when the acidosis remains unresponsive to correction of anoxia or hypovolaemia, sodium bicarbonate (1.26%) can be infused over 3–4 hours with plasma-pH and electrolyte monitoring. In severe shock, metabolic acidosis can develop without sodium or volume depletion; in these circumstances sodium bicarbonate is best given as a small volume of hypertonic solution, such as 50 mL of 8.4% solution intravenously.

Sodium lactate intravenous infusion is no longer used in metabolic acidosis because of the risk of producing lactic acidosis, particularly in seriously ill patients with poor tissue perfusion or impaired hepatic function.

For *chronic acidotic states*, sodium bicarbonate can be given by mouth.

Plasma and plasma substitutes
Plasma and plasma substitutes ('colloids') contain large molecules that do not readily leave the intravascular space where they exert osmotic pressure to maintain circulatory volume. Compared to fluids containing electrolytes such as sodium chloride and glucose ('crystalloids'), a smaller volume of colloid is required to produce the same expansion of blood volume, thereby shifting salt and water from the extravascular space. If resuscitation requires a volume of fluid that exceeds the maximum dose of the colloid then crystalloids can be given; packed red cells may also be required.

Albumin solution p. 1190, prepared from whole blood, contain soluble proteins and electrolytes but no clotting factors, blood group antibodies, or plasma cholinesterases; they may be given without regard to the recipient's blood group.

Albumin is usually used after the acute phase of illness, to correct a plasma-volume deficit; hypoalbuminaemia itself is not an appropriate indication. The use of albumin solution in acute plasma or blood loss may be wasteful; plasma substitutes are more appropriate. Concentrated albumin solution (20%) can be used under specialist supervision in patients with an intravascular fluid deficit and oedema because of interstitial fluid overload, to restore intravascular plasma volume with less exacerbation of the salt and water overload than isotonic solutions. Concentrated albumin solution may also be used to obtain a diuresis in hypoalbuminaemic patients (e.g. in hepatic cirrhosis).

Recent evidence does not support the previous view that the use of albumin increases mortality.

Plasma substitutes
Dextran, gelatin p. 1191, and the hydroxyethyl starch, tetrastarch, are macromolecular substances which are metabolised slowly. Dextran and gelatin may be used at the outset to expand and maintain blood volume in shock arising from conditions such as burns; they may also be used as an immediate short-term measure to treat haemorrhage until blood is available. Dextran and gelatin are rarely needed

when shock is due to sodium and water depletion because, in these circumstances, the shock responds to water and electrolyte repletion.

Hydroxyethyl starches should only be used for the treatment of hypovolaemia due to acute blood loss when crystalloids alone are not sufficient; they should be used at the lowest effective dose for the first 24 hours of fluid resuscitation.

Plasma substitutes should **not** be used to maintain plasma volume in conditions such as burns or peritonitis where there is loss of plasma protein, water, and electrolytes over periods of several days or weeks. In these situations, plasma or plasma protein fractions containing large amounts of albumin should be given.

Large volumes of *some* plasma substitutes can increase the risk of bleeding through depletion of coagulation factors.

BICARBONATE

Sodium bicarbonate

19-Apr-2022

● **INDICATIONS AND DOSE**

Alkalinisation of urine | Relief of discomfort in mild urinary-tract infections
▶ BY MOUTH
▶ Adult: 3 g every 2 hours until urinary pH exceeds 7, to be dissolved in water

Maintenance of alkaline urine
▶ BY MOUTH
▶ Adult: 5–10 g daily, to be dissolved in water

Chronic acidotic states such as uraemic acidosis or renal tubular acidosis
▶ BY MOUTH
▶ Adult: 4.8 g daily, (57 mmol each of Na^+ and HCO_3^-), higher doses may be required and should be adjusted according to response

Severe metabolic acidosis
▶ BY SLOW INTRAVENOUS INJECTION
▶ Adult: Administer an amount appropriate to the body base deficit, to be given using a strong solution (up to 8.4%)
▶ BY CONTINUOUS INTRAVENOUS INFUSION
▶ Adult: Administer an amount appropriate to the body base deficit, to be given using a weak solution (usually 1.26%)

NEPHROTRANS ®

Metabolic acidosis in patients with chronic renal impairment
▶ BY MOUTH
▶ Adult: 3–5 g daily in divided doses, adjusted according to response

● **CONTRA-INDICATIONS** Hypokalaemia · salt restricted diet
▶ With intravenous use for metabolic acidosis Conditions associated with sodium retention · history of urinary calculi
▶ With systemic use for metabolic acidosis Hypernatraemia · hypocalcaemia · hypochlorhydria · metabolic or respiratory alkalosis

● **CAUTIONS**
▶ With intravenous use Respiratory acidosis
▶ With oral use for metabolic acidosis Conditions associated with sodium retention
▶ With systemic use for metabolic acidosis Hypoventilation

● **INTERACTIONS** → Appendix 1: sodium bicarbonate

● **SIDE-EFFECTS**
▶ With intravenous use Skin exfoliation · soft tissue necrosis · ulcer
▶ With oral use Anxiety · appetite decreased · asthenia · dizziness · dyspnoea · flatulence · fluid retention ·

gastrointestinal discomfort · headache · hypertension · hypokalaemia · inflammation · metabolic alkalosis · mood altered · muscle complaints · nausea · nephrolithiasis (long term use) · pulmonary oedema · taste unpleasant · urinary frequency increased · vomiting

● **ALLERGY AND CROSS-SENSITIVITY**

NEPHROTRANS ® Contra-indicated in patients with hypersensitivity or allergy to peanuts or soya (contains soya lecithin and soya-bean oil).

● **PREGNANCY** EvGr Use with caution. ⟨M⟩

● **HEPATIC IMPAIRMENT**
▶ With oral use Manufacturer advises caution in cirrhosis.

● **RENAL IMPAIRMENT**
▶ With oral use EvGr Caution (risk of metabolic alkalosis, hypokalaemia and sodium retention). ⟨M⟩

● **MONITORING REQUIREMENTS** EvGr Monitor plasma-pH and electrolytes regularly during treatment. ⟨M⟩

● **DIRECTIONS FOR ADMINISTRATION**
▶ With intravenous use For *slow intravenous injection* use a small volume of hypertonic solution (such as 50 mL of 8.4%). For *continuous intravenous infusion* a weaker solution of 1.26% solution can be infused over 3–4 hours.
▶ With oral use Sodium bicarbonate may affect the stability or absorption of other drugs if administered at the same time. If possible, allow 1–2 hours before administering other drugs orally.

● **PRESCRIBING AND DISPENSING INFORMATION**
▶ With oral use *Sodium bicarbonate* 500*mg* capsules contain approximately 6 mmol each of Na^+ and HCO_3^-; *Sodium bicarbonate* 600*mg* capsules contain approximately 7 mmol each of Na^+ and HCO_3^-. Oral solutions of sodium bicarbonate are required occasionally; these are available from 'special-order' manufacturers or specialist importing companies; the strength of sodium bicarbonate should be stated on the prescription.
▶ With intravenous use Usual strength Sodium bicarbonate 1.26% (12.6 g, 150 mmol each of Na^+ and HCO_3^- /litre), various other strengths available.

● **PATIENT AND CARER ADVICE** Patients or carers should be given advice on the administration of sodium bicarbonate oral medicines.

● **MEDICINAL FORMS** There can be variation in the licensing of different medicines containing the same drug. Forms available from special-order manufacturers include: oral capsule, oral suspension, oral solution, solution for injection

Oral tablet
▶ Sodium bicarbonate (Non-proprietary)
Sodium bicarbonate 600 mg Sodium bicarbonate 600mg tablets | 100 tablet GSL ⟨£⟩

Gastro-resistant capsule
EXCIPIENTS: May contain Gelatin, polysorbates, propylene glycol, sorbitol
▶ Nephrotrans (Medice UK Ltd)
Sodium bicarbonate 500 mg Nephrotrans 500mg gastro-resistant capsules | 100 capsule PoM £18.75 DT = £18.75

Solution for injection
▶ Sodium bicarbonate (Non-proprietary)
Sodium bicarbonate 84 mg per 1 ml Sodium bicarbonate 8.4% (1mmol/ml) solution for infusion 100ml bottles | 10 bottle PoM £120.20 DT = £120.20 (Hospital only)
Sodium bicarbonate 8.4% (1mmol/ml) solution for injection 100ml bottles | 10 bottle PoM £120.20 DT = £120.20
Sodium bicarbonate 8.4% (1mmol/ml) solution for infusion 250ml bottles | 10 bottle PoM £120.20 DT = £120.20 (Hospital only)
Sodium bicarbonate 8.4% (1mmol/ml) solution for injection 10ml ampoules | 10 ampoule PoM £131.20–£196.64 DT = £176.22
Sodium bicarbonate 8.4% (1mmol/ml) solution for injection 250ml bottles | 10 bottle PoM £120.20 DT = £120.20

Oral capsule
▶ Sodium bicarbonate (Non-proprietary)
Sodium bicarbonate 500 mg Sodium bicarbonate 500mg capsules | 56 capsule PoM ⟨£⟩ DT = £2.89

Oral solution

▶ **Sodium bicarbonate (Non-proprietary)**
Sodium bicarbonate 84 mg per 1 ml S-Bicarb 420mg/5ml
(1mmol/ml) oral solution | 100 ml ⓢ
Sodium bicarbonate 420mg/5ml (1mmol/ml) oral solution sugar free
| 100 ml [PoM] £39.80 DT = £39.80 [SF]

▶ **Thamicarb** (Syri Ltd)
Sodium bicarbonate 84 mg per 1 ml Thamicarb 84mg/1ml oral
solution | 100 ml [PoM] £35.82 DT = £39.80 [SF] | 500 ml [PoM]
£179.28 DT = £199.20 [SF]

Infusion

▶ **Sodium bicarbonate (Non-proprietary)**
Sodium bicarbonate 12.6 mg per 1 ml Polyfusor sodium
bicarbonate 1.26% infusion 500ml bottles | 12 bottle [PoM] £376.56
Sodium bicarbonate 14 mg per 1 ml Polyfusor sodium bicarbonate
1.4% infusion 500ml bottles | 12 bottle [PoM] £376.56
Sodium bicarbonate 27.4 mg per 1 ml Polyfusor sodium
bicarbonate 2.74% infusion 500ml bottles | 12 bottle [PoM] £376.56
Sodium bicarbonate 42 mg per 1 ml Polyfusor sodium bicarbonate
4.2% infusion 500ml bottles | 12 bottle [PoM] £376.56
Sodium bicarbonate 84 mg per 1 ml Polyfusor sodium bicarbonate
8.4% infusion 200ml bottles | 12 bottle [PoM] £376.56

ELECTROLYTES AND MINERALS ⟩ POTASSIUM

Potassium chloride with calcium chloride dihydrate and sodium chloride

(Ringer's solution)

The properties listed below are those particular to the
combination only. For the properties of the components
please consider, potassium chloride p. 1201, sodium chloride
p. 1180.

● **INDICATIONS AND DOSE**

Electrolyte imbalance
▶ BY INTRAVENOUS INFUSION
▶ Adult: Dosed according to the deficit or daily
maintenance requirements (consult product literature)

● INTERACTIONS → Appendix 1: potassium chloride

● **PRESCRIBING AND DISPENSING INFORMATION** Ringer's
solution for injection provides the following ions (in
mmol/litre), Ca^{2+} 2.2, K^+ 4, Na^+ 147, Cl^- 156.

● MEDICINAL FORMS No licensed medicines listed.

Potassium chloride with calcium chloride, sodium chloride and sodium lactate

(Sodium Lactate Intravenous Infusion, Compound; Compound, Hartmann's Solution for Injection; Ringer-Lactate Solution for Injection)

The properties listed below are those particular to the
combination only. For the properties of the components
please consider, potassium chloride p. 1201, sodium chloride
p. 1180, calcium chloride p. 1188.

● **INDICATIONS AND DOSE**

**For prophylaxis, and replacement therapy, requiring the
use of sodium chloride and lactate, with minimal
amounts of calcium and potassium**
▶ BY INTRAVENOUS INFUSION
▶ Adult: (consult product literature)

● INTERACTIONS → Appendix 1: calcium salts · potassium
chloride

● **PRESCRIBING AND DISPENSING INFORMATION** Compound
sodium lactate intravenous infusion contains Na^+
131 mmol, K^+ 5 mmol, Ca^{2+} 2 mmol, HCO_3^- (as lactate)
29 mmol, Cl^- 111 mmol/litre.

● **MEDICINAL FORMS** There can be variation in the licensing of
different medicines containing the same drug.

Infusion

▶ **Potassium chloride with calcium chloride, sodium chloride and
sodium lactate (Non-proprietary)**
**Calcium chloride 270 microgram per 1 ml, Potassium chloride
400 microgram per 1 ml, Sodium lactate 3.17 mg per 1 ml,
Sodium chloride 6 mg per 1 ml** Sodium lactate compound
(Hartmann's Solution) infusion 1litre Cosinus bags | 10 bag [PoM]
£49.50
Sodium lactate compound (Hartmann's Solution) infusion 1litre bags |
10 bag [PoM] £21.00 (Hospital only)
Sodium lactate compound (Hartmann's Solution) infusion 1litre Viaflo
bags | 1 bag [PoM] ⓢ
Sodium lactate compound (Hartmann's Solution) infusion 1litre
Freeflex bags | 10 bag [PoM] £22.10
Ringer lactate (Hartmann's Solution) infusion 1litre Viaflo bags |
1 bag [PoM] £3.64 | 10 bag [PoM] £36.40

Potassium chloride with glucose

The properties listed below are those particular to the
combination only. For the properties of the components
please consider, potassium chloride p. 1201, glucose p. 1182.

● **INDICATIONS AND DOSE**

Electrolyte imbalance
▶ BY INTRAVENOUS INFUSION
▶ Adult: Dosed according to the deficit or daily
maintenance requirements

● INTERACTIONS → Appendix 1: potassium chloride

● **PRESCRIBING AND DISPENSING INFORMATION** Potassium
chloride 0.3% contains 40 mmol each of K^+ and Cl^-/litre or
0.15% contains 20 mmol each of K^+ and Cl^-/litre with 5% of
anhydrous glucose.

● **MEDICINAL FORMS** There can be variation in the licensing of
different medicines containing the same drug. Forms available
from special-order manufacturers include: infusion, solution
for infusion

Infusion

▶ **Potassium chloride with glucose (Non-proprietary)**
Presentations available from various suppliers include
**Potassium chloride 1.5 mg per 1 ml, Glucose anhydrous 50 mg
per 1 ml** Potassium chloride 0.15% (potassium 20mmol/1litre) /
Glucose 5% infusion | 1litre bags [PoM]
**Potassium chloride 1.5 mg per 1 ml, Glucose (as Glucose
monohydrate) 50 mg per 1 ml** Potassium chloride 0.15% (potassium
10mmol/500ml) / Glucose 5% infusion | 500ml bottles [PoM]
(Hospital only)
Potassium chloride 0.15% (potassium 20mmol/1litre) / Glucose 5%
infusion | 1litre bottles [PoM] (Hospital only)
**Potassium chloride 1.5 mg per 1 ml, Glucose anhydrous 100 mg
per 1 ml** Potassium chloride 0.15% (potassium 10mmol/500ml) /
Glucose 10% infusion | 500ml bags [PoM] (Hospital only)
**Potassium chloride 3 mg per 1 ml, Glucose anhydrous 50 mg per
1 ml** Potassium chloride 0.3% (potassium 20mmol/500ml) / Glucose
5% infusion | 500ml bags [PoM]
Potassium chloride 0.3% (potassium 40mmol/1litre) / Glucose 5%
infusion | 1litre bags [PoM]
**Potassium chloride 3 mg per 1 ml, Glucose (as Glucose
monohydrate) 50 mg per 1 ml** Potassium chloride 0.3% (potassium
20mmol/500ml) / Glucose 5% infusion | 500ml bottles [PoM]
(Hospital only)
Potassium chloride 0.3% (potassium 40mmol/1litre) / Glucose 5%
infusion | 1litre bottles [PoM] (Hospital only)

9

Blood and nutrition

Potassium chloride with glucose and sodium chloride

The properties listed below are those particular to the combination only. For the properties of the components please consider, potassium chloride p. 1201, glucose p. 1182, sodium chloride below.

● **INDICATIONS AND DOSE**

Electrolyte imbalance

▸ BY INTRAVENOUS INFUSION

▸ Adult: Dosed according to the deficit or daily maintenance requirements

● INTERACTIONS → Appendix 1: potassium chloride

● PRESCRIBING AND DISPENSING INFORMATION Concentration of potassium chloride to be specified by the prescriber (usually K^+ 10–40 mmol/litre).

● MEDICINAL FORMS There can be variation in the licensing of different medicines containing the same drug. Forms available from special-order manufacturers include: infusion, solution for infusion

Infusion

▸ Potassium chloride with glucose and sodium chloride (Non-proprietary)
  Presentations available from various suppliers include
  Potassium chloride 1.5 mg per 1 ml, Sodium chloride 1.8 mg per 1 ml, Glucose anhydrous 40 mg per 1 ml Potassium chloride 0.15% (potassium 20mmol/1litre) / Glucose 4% / Sodium chloride 0.18% infusion | 1litre bags PoM
  Potassium chloride 1.5 mg per 1 ml, Sodium chloride 1.8 mg per 1 ml, Glucose (as Glucose monohydrate) 40 mg per 1 ml Potassium chloride 0.15% (potassium 10mmol/500ml) / Glucose 4% / Sodium chloride 0.18% infusion | 500ml bottles PoM (Hospital only)
  Potassium chloride 0.15% (potassium 20mmol/1litre) / Glucose 4% / Sodium chloride 0.18% infusion | 1litre bottles PoM (Hospital only)
  Potassium chloride 1.5 mg per 1 ml, Sodium chloride 4.5 mg per 1 ml, Glucose anhydrous 50 mg per 1 ml Potassium chloride 0.15% (potassium 10mmol/500ml) / Glucose 5% / Sodium chloride 0.45% infusion | 500ml bags PoM
  Sodium chloride 1.8 mg per 1 ml, Potassium chloride 3 mg per 1 ml, Glucose anhydrous 40 mg per 1 ml Potassium chloride 0.3% (potassium 40mmol/1litre) / Glucose 4% / Sodium chloride 0.18% infusion | 1litre bags PoM
  Sodium chloride 1.8 mg per 1 ml, Potassium chloride 3 mg per 1 ml, Glucose (as Glucose monohydrate) 40 mg per 1 ml Potassium chloride 0.3% (potassium 20mmol/500ml) / Glucose 4% / Sodium chloride 0.18% infusion | 500ml bottles PoM (Hospital only)
  Potassium chloride 0.3% (potassium 40mmol/1litre) / Glucose 4% / Sodium chloride 0.18% infusion | 1litre bottles PoM (Hospital only)

Potassium chloride with potassium bicarbonate

30-Jul-2024

The properties listed below are those particular to the combination only. For the properties of the components please consider, potassium chloride p. 1201.

● **INDICATIONS AND DOSE**

Potassium depletion

▸ BY MOUTH

▸ Adult: Dosed according to the deficit or daily maintenance requirements (consult product literature)

● INTERACTIONS → Appendix 1: potassium chloride

● PRESCRIBING AND DISPENSING INFORMATION Each *Sando-K*® tablet contains potassium 470 mg (12 mmol of K^+) and chloride 285mg (8 mmol of Cl^-).

● MEDICINAL FORMS There can be variation in the licensing of different medicines containing the same drug.

Effervescent tablet

CAUTIONARY AND ADVISORY LABELS 13, 21

▸ **Aace K** (Essential-Healthcare Ltd)
  Potassium bicarbonate 400 mg, Potassium chloride 600 mg Aace K effervescent tablets | 100 tablet £7.97 SF

▸ **Sando-K** (Stirling Anglian Pharmaceuticals Ltd)
  Potassium bicarbonate 400 mg, Potassium chloride 600 mg Sando-K effervescent tablets | 100 tablet P £15.08 DT = £12.29

Potassium chloride with sodium chloride

The properties listed below are those particular to the combination only. For the properties of the components please consider, potassium chloride p. 1201, sodium chloride below.

● **INDICATIONS AND DOSE**

Electrolyte imbalance

▸ BY INTRAVENOUS INFUSION

▸ Adult: Depending on the deficit or the daily maintenance requirements (consult product literature)

● INTERACTIONS → Appendix 1: potassium chloride

● PRESCRIBING AND DISPENSING INFORMATION Potassium chloride 0.15% with sodium chloride 0.9% contains K^+ 20 mmol, Na^+ 150 mmol, and Cl^- 170 mmol/litre or potassium chloride 0.3% with sodium chloride 0.9% contains K^+ 40 mmol, Na^+ 150 mmol, and Cl^- 190 mmol/litre.

● MEDICINAL FORMS There can be variation in the licensing of different medicines containing the same drug. Forms available from special-order manufacturers include: infusion, solution for infusion

Infusion

▸ Potassium chloride with sodium chloride (Non-proprietary)
  Presentations available from various suppliers include
  Potassium chloride 1.5 mg per 1 ml, Sodium chloride 9 mg per 1 ml Potassium chloride 0.15% (potassium 10mmol/500ml) / Sodium chloride 0.9% infusion | 500ml bags PoM | 500ml bottles PoM (Hospital only)
  Potassium chloride 0.15% (potassium 20mmol/1litre) / Sodium chloride 0.9% infusion | 1litre bags PoM | 1litre bottles PoM (Hospital only)
  Potassium chloride 3 mg per 1 ml, Sodium chloride 9 mg per 1 ml Potassium chloride 0.3% (potassium 20mmol/500ml) / Sodium chloride 0.9% infusion | 500ml bags PoM | 500ml bottles PoM (Hospital only)
  Potassium chloride 0.3% (potassium 40mmol/1litre) / Sodium chloride 0.9% infusion | 1litre bags PoM | 1litre bottles PoM (Hospital only)

ELECTROLYTES AND MINERALS ❭ SODIUM CHLORIDE

Sodium chloride

21-Jun-2023

● **INDICATIONS AND DOSE**

Sodium deficiency

▸ BY MOUTH USING MODIFIED-RELEASE TABLETS

▸ Adult: Initially 4–8 tablets daily in divided doses, adjusted according to requirements; increased if necessary up to 20 tablets daily in divided doses, adjusted according to requirements, dose to be increased in severe depletion

▸ BY MOUTH USING ORAL SOLUTION

▸ Adult: Initially 40–80 mmol daily in divided doses, adjusted according to requirements

Chronic renal salt wasting
- BY MOUTH USING MODIFIED-RELEASE TABLETS
- Adult: Up to 20 tablets daily in divided doses, adjusted according to requirements

Fluid and electrolyte replacement
- BY INTRAVENOUS INFUSION
- Adult: The volume of sodium chloride solution needed to replace deficits may vary (consult product literature)

Diabetic ketoacidosis (when systolic blood pressure below 90 mmHg)
- BY INTRAVENOUS INFUSION
- Adult: Initially 500 mL, sodium chloride 0.9% to be given over 10–15 minutes, repeat dose if blood pressure remains below 90 mmHg. Seek specialist or senior medical advice and consult local protocol for guidance on further management

DOSE EQUIVALENCE AND CONVERSION
- With oral use
- Each *Slow Sodium*® modified-release tablet contains approx. 10 mmol each of Na$^+$ and Cl$^-$. Oral solution doses are expressed as mmol of sodium.

- **CAUTIONS**
- With intravenous use Avoid excessive administration · cardiac failure · dilutional hyponatraemia especially in the elderly · hypertension · peripheral oedema · pulmonary oedema · restrict intake in impaired renal function · toxaemia of pregnancy

- **SIDE-EFFECTS**
- With intravenous use Chills · fever · hypervolaemia · hyponatraemia · hyponatraemic encephalopathy · hypotension · local reaction · localised pain · paraesthesia · skin reactions · tremor · vascular irritation · venous thrombosis
- With oral use Abdominal cramps · acidosis hyperchloraemic · diarrhoea · generalised oedema · hyperhidrosis · hypertension · hypotension · irritability · muscle complaints · nausea · vomiting

- **MONITORING REQUIREMENTS**
- With intravenous use The jugular venous pressure should be assessed, the bases of the lungs should be examined for crepitations, and in elderly or seriously ill patients it is often helpful to monitor the right atrial (central) venous pressure.

- **DIRECTIONS FOR ADMINISTRATION** *Oral solution* may be diluted and thoroughly mixed into water before administration. *Slow Sodium*® modified-release tablets should be swallowed whole with water (approx. 70 mL per tablet in patients with normal kidney function).

- **PRESCRIBING AND DISPENSING INFORMATION** Sodium chloride 0.9% intravenous infusion contains Na$^+$ and Cl$^-$ each 150 mmol/litre. The term 'normal saline' should not be used to describe sodium chloride intravenous infusion 0.9%; the term 'physiological saline' is acceptable but it is preferable to give the composition (i.e. sodium chloride intravenous infusion 0.9%).

- **PATIENT AND CARER ADVICE** Patients or their carers should be advised on how to administer oral solutions and modified-release tablets.

- **PROFESSION SPECIFIC INFORMATION**
  Dental practitioners' formulary Compound Sodium Chloride Mouthwash may be prescribed—see sodium bicarbonate with sodium chloride p. 1378.

- **MEDICINAL FORMS** There can be variation in the licensing of different medicines containing the same drug. Forms available from special-order manufacturers include: oral solution, solution for injection, infusion, solution for infusion

Modified-release tablet
CAUTIONARY AND ADVISORY LABELS 25
- Slow Sodium (Stirling Anglian Pharmaceuticals Ltd)
  Sodium chloride 600 mg Slow Sodium 600mg tablets | 100 tablet [GSL] £13.17 DT = £10.91

Solution for injection
- Sodium chloride (Non-proprietary)
  Presentations available from various suppliers include
  Sodium chloride 9 mg per 1 ml Sodium chloride 0.9% solution for injection | 2ml, 5ml, 10ml, 20ml ampoules [PoM] | 50ml vials [PoM]
  Sodium chloride 300 mg per 1 ml Sodium chloride 30% solution for injection | 10ml ampoules [PoM]

Infusion
- Sodium chloride (Non-proprietary)
  Presentations available from various suppliers include
  Sodium chloride 1.8 mg per 1 ml Sodium chloride 0.18% infusion | 500ml bottles [PoM]
  Sodium chloride 4.5 mg per 1 ml Sodium chloride 0.45% infusion | 500ml bags [PoM]
  Sodium chloride 9 mg per 1 ml Sodium chloride 0.9% infusion | 50ml, 100ml, 250ml, 500ml, 1litre bags [PoM] | 50ml, 100ml, 250ml, 500ml, 1litre bottles [PoM] (Hospital only)
  Sodium chloride 18 mg per 1 ml Sodium chloride 1.8% infusion | 500ml bottles [PoM]
  Sodium chloride 27 mg per 1 ml Sodium chloride 2.7% infusion | 500ml bottles [PoM]
  Sodium chloride 50 mg per 1 ml Sodium chloride 5% infusion | 500ml bottles [PoM]

Oral solution
EXCIPIENTS: May contain Potassium sorbate
- Sodium chloride (Non-proprietary)
  Sodium chloride 58.5 mg per 1 ml Sodium chloride 292.5mg/5ml (1mmol/ml) oral solution | 100 ml [PoM] £33.16 DT = £33.16
  Sodium chloride 292 mg per 1 ml Sodium chloride 1.46g/5ml (5mmol/ml) oral solution | 100 ml [PoM] £22.00-£22.46 DT = £22.46
- Syrisal (Syri Ltd)
  Sodium chloride 58.5 mg per 1 ml Syrisal 292.5mg/5ml (1mmol/ml) oral solution | 100 ml [PoM] £30.20 DT = £33.16

Solution for infusion
- Sodium chloride (Non-proprietary)
  Presentations available from various suppliers include
  Sodium chloride 300 mg per 1 ml Sodium chloride 30% concentrate for solution for infusion | 10ml ampoules [PoM] (Hospital only) | 50ml, 100ml vials [PoM]

Combinations available: *Potassium chloride with calcium chloride dihydrate and sodium chloride*, p. 1179 · *Potassium chloride with calcium chloride, sodium chloride and sodium lactate*, p. 1179 · *Potassium chloride with glucose and sodium chloride*, p. 1180 · *Potassium chloride with sodium chloride*, p. 1180

| Sodium chloride with glucose

The properties listed below are those particular to the combination only. For the properties of the components please consider, sodium chloride p. 1180, glucose p. 1182.

- **INDICATIONS AND DOSE**

Combined water and sodium depletion
- BY INTRAVENOUS INFUSION
- Adult: (consult product literature)

- **MONITORING REQUIREMENTS** Maintenance fluid should accurately reflect daily requirements and close monitoring is required to avoid fluid and electrolyte imbalance.

- **MEDICINAL FORMS** There can be variation in the licensing of different medicines containing the same drug. Forms available from special-order manufacturers include: infusion, solution for infusion

Infusion

▸ Sodium chloride with glucose (Non-proprietary)
Presentations available from various suppliers include
Sodium chloride 1.8 mg per 1 ml, Glucose anhydrous 40 mg per 1 ml Sodium chloride 0.18% / Glucose 4% infusion | 500ml, 1litre bags [PoM]
Sodium chloride 1.8 mg per 1 ml, Glucose anhydrous 100 mg per 1 ml Sodium chloride 0.18% / Glucose 10% infusion | 500ml bags [PoM]
Sodium chloride 4.5 mg per 1 ml, Glucose anhydrous 25 mg per 1 ml Sodium chloride 0.45% / Glucose 2.5% infusion | 500ml bags [PoM]
Sodium chloride 4.5 mg per 1 ml, Glucose (as Glucose monohydrate) 25 mg per 1 ml Sodium chloride 0.45% / Glucose 2.5% infusion | 500ml bottles [PoM] (Hospital only)
Sodium chloride 4.5 mg per 1 ml, Glucose (as Glucose monohydrate) 50 mg per 1 ml Sodium chloride 0.45% / Glucose 5% infusion | 500ml bottles [PoM] (Hospital only)
Sodium chloride 9 mg per 1 ml, Glucose (as Glucose monohydrate) 50 mg per 1 ml Sodium chloride 0.9% / Glucose 5% infusion | 500ml bottles [PoM] (Hospital only)

NUTRIENTS ⟩ SUGARS

Glucose

22-Apr-2024

(Dextrose Monohydrate)

- **INDICATIONS AND DOSE**

Establish presence of gestational diabetes
▸ BY MOUTH
▸ Adult: Test dose 75 g, anhydrous glucose to be given to the fasting patient and blood-glucose concentrations measured at intervals, to be given with 200–300 mL fluid

Oral glucose tolerance test
▸ BY MOUTH
▸ Adult: Test dose 75 g, anhydrous glucose to be given to the fasting patient and blood-glucose concentrations measured at intervals, to be given with 200–300 mL fluid

Hypoglycaemia
▸ BY MOUTH
▸ Child up to 5 years: 5 g, repeated after 15 minutes if necessary, 5 g is available from 20 mL oral glucose liquid, 1.5 glucose tablets, or half a tube of glucose 40% oral gel. If oral glucose formulations are not available, the dose may be given using another fast-acting carbohydrate; 5 g is available from approximately 1 teaspoonful of sugar dissolved in an appropriate volume of water
▸ Child 5-11 years: 10 g, repeated after 15 minutes if necessary, 10 g is available from 40 mL oral glucose liquid, 3 glucose tablets, or 1 tube of glucose 40% oral gel. If oral glucose formulations are not available, the dose may be given using another fast-acting carbohydrate; 10 g is available from approximately 2 teaspoonfuls of sugar dissolved in an appropriate volume of water
▸ Child 12-17 years: 15 g, repeated after 15 minutes if necessary, 15 g is available from 60 mL oral glucose liquid, 4 glucose tablets, or 1.5 tubes of glucose 40% oral gel. If oral glucose formulations are not available, the dose may be given using another fast-acting carbohydrate; 15 g is available from approximately 3 teaspoonfuls of sugar dissolved in an appropriate volume of water
▸ Adult: 15–20 g, repeated after 15 minutes if necessary, 15–20 g is available from 60–80 mL oral glucose liquid, 4–5 glucose tablets, or 1.5–2 tubes of glucose 40% oral gel. If oral glucose formulations are not available, the dose may be given using another fast-acting carbohydrate; 15–20 g is available from approximately 3–4 teaspoonfuls of sugar dissolved in an appropriate volume of water, or 150–200 mL of pure fruit juice

▸ BY INTRAVENOUS INFUSION
▸ Child: 500 mg/kg, to be administered as Glucose 10% intravenous infusion into a large vein through a large-gauge needle; care is required since this concentration is irritant
▸ Adult: 15–20 g, to be administered over 15 minutes as Glucose 10% or 20% intravenous infusion into a large vein through a large-gauge needle; care is required since these concentrations are irritant

Hypoglycaemia [in conscious but uncooperative patients]
▸ BY BUCCAL ADMINISTRATION
▸ Child up to 5 years: 5 g, repeated after 15 minutes if necessary, to be given as half a tube of glucose 40% oral gel
▸ Child 5-11 years: 10 g, repeated after 15 minutes if necessary, to be given as 1 tube of glucose 40% oral gel
▸ Child 12-17 years: 15 g, repeated after 15 minutes if necessary, to be given as 1.5 tubes of glucose 40% oral gel
▸ Adult: 15–20 g, repeated after 15 minutes if necessary, to be given as 1.5–2 tubes of glucose 40% oral gel

Energy source
▸ BY INTRAVENOUS INFUSION
▸ Adult: 1–3 litres daily, solution concentration of 20–50% to be administered

Fluid and carbohydrate replacement
▸ BY INTRAVENOUS INFUSION
▸ Adult: The volume of glucose solution needed to replace deficits may vary (consult product literature)

Persistent cyanosis (in combination with propranolol) when blood glucose less than 3 mmol/litre (followed by morphine)
▸ BY INTRAVENOUS INFUSION
▸ Child: 200 mg/kg, to be administered as Glucose 10% intravenous infusion over 10 minutes

Diabetic ketoacidosis
▸ BY INTRAVENOUS INFUSION
▸ Adult: (consult local protocol)

DOSE EQUIVALENCE AND CONVERSION
▸ 75 g anhydrous glucose is equivalent to Glucose BP 82.5 g.
▸ For hypoglycaemia, examples of glucose preparations which can be used to give oral doses are based on the use of oral liquid containing glucose 250 mg/mL and tablets containing glucose 4 g per tablet. Buccal dosing is based on tubes of 40% oral gel containing glucose 10 g per tube.

- **CAUTIONS** Do not give alone except when there is no significant loss of electrolytes · prolonged administration of glucose solutions without electrolytes can lead to hyponatraemia and other electrolyte disturbances

- **SIDE-EFFECTS** Chills · electrolyte imbalance · fever · fluid imbalance · hypersensitivity · local reaction · localised pain · polyuria · rash · venous thrombosis

- **DIRECTIONS FOR ADMINISTRATION**
▸ With intravenous use [EvGr] Injections containing more than 10% glucose can be irritant and should generally be given into a central venous line except in emergencies. Ⓜ

- **PRESCRIBING AND DISPENSING INFORMATION** Glucose BP is the monohydrate but Glucose Intravenous Infusion BP is a sterile solution of anhydrous glucose or glucose monohydrate, potency being expressed in terms of anhydrous glucose.

- **EXCEPTIONS TO LEGAL CATEGORY**
  ‣ With intravenous use Prescription only medicine restriction does not apply to 50% solution where administration is for saving life in emergency.

- **MEDICINAL FORMS** There can be variation in the licensing of different medicines containing the same drug. Forms available from special-order manufacturers include: oral solution, solution for injection, solution for infusion

Solution for infusion
‣ **Glucose** (Non-proprietary)
  Glucose anhydrous 200 mg per 1 ml Glucose 20% solution for infusion 100ml vials | 1 vial [PoM] £9.00
  Glucose anhydrous 500 mg per 1 ml Glucose 50% solution for infusion 20ml ampoules | 10 ampoule [PoM] £18.94 DT = £18.94
  Glucose 50% solution for infusion 50ml vials | 25 vial [PoM] £85.00 DT = £85.00

Oral solution
‣ **Rapilose OGTT** (Penlan Healthcare Ltd)
  Glucose 250 mg per 1 ml Rapilose OGTT solution | 300 ml £3.98

Oral liquid
‣ **Glucojuice** (BBI Healthcare Ltd, Flavour Not Specified)
  Lift Fast Acting Glucose Shot liquid zesty lemon & lime | 60 ml £0.99
  Lift Fast Acting Glucose Shot liquid strawberry & lime | 60 ml £0.99
  Lift Fast Acting Glucose Shot liquid very berry | 60 ml £0.99
  Lift Fast Acting Glucose Shot liquid | 60 ml [⊠]
  Lift Fast Acting Glucose Shot liquid fruity tropical | 60 ml £0.99

Oral gel
‣ **AACE Gluco** (Essential-Healthcare Ltd)
  Glucose 400 mg per 1 gram AACE Gluco 40% gel | 75 gram £4.80 DT = £7.16
‣ **AddGluco** (TriOn Pharma Ltd)
  Glucose 400 mg per 1 gram AddGluco 40% gel | 75 gram £4.75 DT = £7.16
‣ **Dextrogel** (Neoceuticals Ltd)
  Glucose 400 mg per 1 gram Dextrogel 40% gel | 75 gram £5.38 DT = £7.16 | 80 gram £5.38
‣ **GlucoBoost** (Ennogen Healthcare International Ltd)
  Glucose 400 mg per 1 gram GlucoBoost 40% gel | 75 gram £7.16 DT = £7.16 | 80 gram £6.11
‣ **GlucoGel** (BBI Healthcare Ltd)
  Glucose 400 mg per 1 gram GlucoGel 40% gel original | 75 gram £7.16 DT = £7.16 | 80 gram £6.84
‣ **Rapilose** (Penlan Healthcare Ltd)
  Glucose 400 mg per 1 gram Rapilose 40% gel | 75 gram £5.49 DT = £7.16

Infusion
‣ **Glucose** (Non-proprietary)
  Presentations available from various suppliers include
  Glucose anhydrous 50 mg per 1 ml Glucose 5% infusion | 50ml, 100ml, 250ml, 500ml, 1litre bags [PoM] | 500ml, 1litre bottles [PoM]
  Glucose (as Glucose monohydrate) 50 mg per 1 ml Glucose 5% infusion | 50ml, 100ml, 250ml bottles [PoM] (Hospital only)
  Glucose anhydrous 100 mg per 1 ml Glucose 10% infusion | 500ml, 1litre bags [PoM]
  Glucose anhydrous 200 mg per 1 ml Glucose 20% infusion | 500ml bags [PoM]
  Glucose (as Glucose monohydrate) 300 mg per 1 ml Glucose 30% infusion | 500ml bottles [PoM] (Hospital only)
  Glucose anhydrous 400 mg per 1 ml Glucose 40% infusion | 500ml bags [PoM]
  Glucose anhydrous 500 mg per 1 ml Glucose 50% infusion | 500ml bags [PoM]
  Glucose anhydrous 700 mg per 1 ml Glucose 70% concentrate for solution for infusion | 500ml bags [PoM] (Hospital only)

Combinations available: *Potassium chloride with glucose*, p. 1179 · *Potassium chloride with glucose and sodium chloride*, p. 1180 · *Sodium chloride with glucose*, p. 1181

p. 1179 · p. 1180 · p. 1181

ORAL REHYDRATION SALTS

Disodium hydrogen citrate with glucose, potassium chloride and sodium chloride
09-May-2024

- **DRUG ACTION** Formulated as oral rehydration salts

- **INDICATIONS AND DOSE**

Fluid and electrolyte loss in diarrhoea
‣ BY MOUTH
‣ Child 1-11 months: 1–1½ times usual feed volume to be given
‣ Child 1-11 years: 200 mL, to be given after every loose motion
‣ Child 12-17 years: 200–400 mL, to be given after every loose motion, dose according to fluid loss
‣ Adult: 200–400 mL, to be given after every loose motion, dose according to fluid loss

- **DIRECTIONS FOR ADMINISTRATION** Manufacturer advises reconstitute 1 sachet with 200mL of water (freshly boiled and cooled for infants); 5 sachets reconstituted with 1 litre of water provide Na^+ 60 mmol, K^+ 20 mmol, Cl^- 60 mmol, citrate 10 mmol, and glucose 90 mmol.

- **PRESCRIBING AND DISPENSING INFORMATION** Flavours of oral powder formulations may include black currant, citrus, or natural.

- **PATIENT AND CARER ADVICE** After reconstitution any unused solution should be discarded no later than 1 hour after preparation unless stored in a refrigerator when it may be kept for up to 24 hours.
  Medicines for Children leaflet: Oral rehydration salts
  www.medicinesforchildren.org.uk/medicines/oral-rehydration-salts/

- **MEDICINAL FORMS** There can be variation in the licensing of different medicines containing the same drug.

Powder for oral solution
CAUTIONARY AND ADVISORY LABELS 13
‣ **Dioralyte** (Dendron Brands Ltd)
  Potassium chloride 300 mg, Sodium chloride 470 mg, Disodium hydrogen citrate 530 mg, Glucose 3.56 gram Dioralyte oral powder sachets blackcurrant | 20 sachet [P] £8.74
  Dioralyte oral powder sachets plain | 20 sachet [P] £8.74

Potassium chloride with rice powder, sodium chloride and sodium citrate
09-May-2024

- **DRUG ACTION** Formulated as oral rehydration salts

- **INDICATIONS AND DOSE**

Fluid and electrolyte loss in diarrhoea
‣ BY MOUTH
‣ Adult: 200–400 mL, to be given after every loose motion, dose according to fluid loss

- **DIRECTIONS FOR ADMINISTRATION** Manufacturer advises reconstitute 1 sachet with 200 mL of water (freshly boiled and cooled for infants); 5 sachets when reconstituted with 1 litre of water provide Na^+ 60 mmol, K^+ 20 mmol, Cl^- 50 mmol and citrate 10 mmol.

- **PRESCRIBING AND DISPENSING INFORMATION** Flavours of oral powder formulations may include apricot, black currant, or raspberry.

- **PATIENT AND CARER ADVICE** Patients and carers should be advised how to reconstitute *Dioralyte*® Relief oral powder. After reconstitution any unused solution should be discarded no later than 1 hour after preparation unless stored in a refrigerator when it may be kept for up to 24 hours.

- **MEDICINAL FORMS** There can be variation in the licensing of different medicines containing the same drug.
  Powder for oral solution
  CAUTIONARY AND ADVISORY LABELS 13
  EXCIPIENTS: May contain Aspartame
  ▸ Dioralyte Relief (Dendron Brands Ltd)
  Potassium chloride 300 mg, Sodium chloride 350 mg, Sodium citrate 580 mg, Rice powder pre-cooked 6 gram Dioralyte Relief oral powder sachets blackcurrant | 20 sachet Ⓟ £8.73 ⓈⒻ

2.1 Calcium imbalance

Calcium imbalance

22-Aug-2023

Calcium supplements

Calcium supplements are usually only required where dietary calcium intake is deficient. This dietary requirement varies with age and is relatively greater in childhood, pregnancy, and lactation, due to an increased demand, and in old age, due to impaired absorption. In osteoporosis, a calcium intake which is double the recommended amount reduces the rate of bone loss. If the actual dietary intake is less than the recommended amount, a supplement of as much as 40 mmol is appropriate.

In severe acute hypocalcaemia or hypocalcaemic tetany, an initial slow intravenous injection of calcium gluconate injection 10% p. 1189 should be given, with plasma-calcium and ECG monitoring (risk of arrhythmias if given too rapidly), and either repeated as required or, if only temporary improvement, followed by a continuous intravenous infusion to prevent recurrence. Calcium chloride injection p. 1188 is also available, but is more irritant; care should be taken to prevent extravasation. Oral supplements of calcium and vitamin D may also be required in persistent hypocalcaemia. Concurrent hypomagnesaemia should be corrected with magnesium sulfate p. 1193.

For guidance on the role of calcium gluconate 10% injection, or calcium chloride 10% injection [unlicensed use] in temporarily protecting the heart against the toxic effects of hyperkalaemia, see Hyperkalaemia p. 1198.

Severe hypercalcaemia

Severe hypercalcaemia calls for urgent treatment before detailed investigation of the cause. Dehydration should be corrected first with intravenous infusion of sodium chloride **0.9%** p. 1180. Drugs (such as thiazides and vitamin D compounds) which promote hypercalcaemia, should be discontinued and dietary calcium should be restricted.

If *severe hypercalcaemia persists* drugs which inhibit mobilisation of calcium from the skeleton may be required. The **bisphosphonates** are useful and pamidronate disodium p. 772 is probably the most effective.

Corticosteroids are widely given, but may only be useful where hypercalcaemia is due to sarcoidosis or vitamin D intoxication; they often take several days to achieve the desired effect.

Calcitonin (salmon) p. 775 can be used for the treatment of hypercalcaemia associated with malignancy; it is rarely effective where bisphosphonates have failed to reduce serum calcium adequately.

After treatment of severe hypercalcaemia the underlying cause must be established. *Further treatment* is governed by the same principles as for initial therapy. Salt and water depletion and drugs promoting hypercalcaemia should be avoided; oral administration of a bisphosphonate may be useful.

Hypercalciuria

Hypercalciuria should be investigated for an underlying cause, which should be treated. Where a cause is not identified (idiopathic hypercalciuria), the condition is managed by increasing fluid intake and giving bendroflumethiazide p. 193. Reducing dietary calcium intake may be beneficial but severe restriction of calcium intake has not proved beneficial and may even be harmful.

Hyperparathyroidism

07-Jul-2020

Hyperparathyroidism, primary

Primary hyperparathyroidism is a disorder of the parathyroid glands—most commonly caused by a non-cancerous tumour (adenoma) in one of the glands. The resulting excess secretion of parathyroid hormone leads to hypercalcaemia, hypophosphataemia and hypercalciuria. The main symptoms are a result of hypercalcaemia and include thirst, increased urine output, constipation, fatigue and memory impairment. Long term effects include cardiovascular disease, kidney stones, osteoporosis, and fractures.

Primary hyperparathyroidism is one of the leading causes of hypercalcaemia, and one of the most common endocrine disorders. It affects twice as many women than men and can develop at any age—with diagnosis most common in women aged 50 to 60 years.

Aims of treatment

Treatment is focused on cure through surgery; other treatment options aim to reduce long-term complications and improve quality of life.

Non-drug treatment

EvGr Information regarding the advantages and disadvantages of available treatments, ongoing monitoring, and advice on how to reduce the symptoms of primary hyperparathyroidism, should be given to all patients.

Parathyroidectomy surgery is the recommended first-line treatment of primary hyperparathyroidism, with unsuccessful surgery requiring multidisciplinary team review at a specialist centre.

For all patients with primary hyperparathyroidism, Cardiovascular disease risk assessment and prevention p. 219, and assessment of Osteoporosis p. 768 and fracture risk should be carried out. Ⓐ For further information on fracture risk assessment, see NICE clinical guideline: **Osteoporosis** (see *Useful resources*).

Women of childbearing age

EvGr For women with primary hyperparathyroidism who are considering pregnancy, parathyroid surgery should be offered; and for pregnant women the management and monitoring of primary hyperparathyroidism should be discussed with a multidisciplinary team at a specialist centre.

Women with primary hyperparathyroidism are at increased risk of hypertensive disease in pregnancy. Ⓐ For information on diagnosis and management, see *Hypertension in pregnancy* in Hypertension p. 166.

Drug treatment

EvGr Treatment with cinacalcet p. 1185 may be considered for patients with primary hyperparathyroidism if surgery has been unsuccessful [unlicensed indication], is unsuitable, or has been declined; and they have an elevated albumin-adjusted serum calcium level with or without symptoms of hypercalcaemia.

In secondary care, vitamin D levels should be measured and supplementation with vitamin D (see Vitamins p. 1235) offered for people with a probable diagnosis of primary hyperparathyroidism if needed.

To reduce fracture risk for people with primary hyperparathyroidism who have an increased fracture risk, a bisphosphonate can be considered. Do not offer bisphosphonates for chronic hypercalcaemia of primary hyperparathyroidism. Ⓐ

Useful Resources

Hyperparathyroidism (primary): diagnosis, assessment and initial management. National Institute of Health and Care Excellence. NICE guideline 132. May 2019.
www.nice.org.uk/guidance/ng132
   Osteoporosis: assessing the risk of fragility fracture. National Institute for Health and Care Excellence. Clinical guideline 146. February 2017.
www.nice.org.uk/guidance/cg146

2.1a Hypercalcaemia and hypercalciuria

CALCIUM REGULATING DRUGS › BONE RESORPTION INHIBITORS

▌Cinacalcet
25-Apr-2025

- **DRUG ACTION** Cinacalcet reduces parathyroid hormone which leads to a decrease in serum calcium concentrations.

- **INDICATIONS AND DOSE**

Secondary hyperparathyroidism [in patients with end-stage renal disease on dialysis] (under expert supervision)
  ▸ BY MOUTH
  ▸ Adult: Initially 30 mg once daily, increased if necessary up to 180 mg once daily, dose to be adjusted every 2–4 weeks according to response

Hypercalcaemia in parathyroid carcinoma | Primary hyperparathyroidism [in patients where parathyroidectomy is inappropriate]
  ▸ BY MOUTH
  ▸ Adult: Initially 30 mg twice daily, increased if necessary up to 90 mg 4 times a day, dose to be adjusted every 2–4 weeks according to response

- **CONTRA-INDICATIONS** Hypocalcaemia

- **CAUTIONS** Conditions that may worsen with a decrease in serum-calcium concentrations · switching from etelcalcetide

CAUTIONS, FURTHER INFORMATION
  ▸ Conditions that may worsen with a decrease in serum-calcium concentrations Manufacturer advises caution with use in patients with conditions that may worsen with a decrease in serum-calcium concentrations, including predisposition to QT-interval prolongation, history of seizures, and history of impaired cardiac function—serum-calcium concentration should be closely monitored.
  ▸ Switching from etelcalcetide Manufacturer advises that in patients who have discontinued etelcalcetide, do not initiate cinacalcet until at least three subsequent haemodialysis sessions are completed, and serum-calcium concentration is confirmed within normal range.

- **INTERACTIONS** → Appendix 1: cinacalcet

- **SIDE-EFFECTS**
  ▸ **Common or very common** Appetite decreased · asthenia · back pain · constipation · cough · diarrhoea · dizziness · dyspnoea · electrolyte imbalance · gastrointestinal discomfort · headache · hypersensitivity · hypotension · muscle complaints · nausea · paraesthesia · rash · seizure · upper respiratory tract infection · vomiting

  ▸ **Frequency not known** Heart failure aggravated · QT interval prolongation · ventricular arrhythmia

- **PREGNANCY** Manufacturer advises use only if potential benefit outweighs risk—no information available.

- **BREAST FEEDING** Manufacturer advises avoid—present in milk in *animal* studies.

- **HEPATIC IMPAIRMENT** Manufacturer advises caution in moderate to severe impairment.

- **MONITORING REQUIREMENTS**
  ▸ When used for Secondary hyperparathyroidism Manufacturer advises measure serum-calcium concentration before initiation of treatment and within 1 week after starting treatment or adjusting dose, then monthly thereafter. Measure parathyroid hormone concentration 1–4 weeks after starting treatment or adjusting dose, then every 1–3 months.
  ▸ When used for Primary hyperparathyroidism and parathyroid carcinoma Manufacturer advises measure serum-calcium concentration before initiation of treatment and within 1 week after starting treatment or adjusting dose, then every 2–3 months.

- **DIRECTIONS FOR ADMINISTRATION** Manufacturer advises capsules containing granules should be opened and the granules sprinkled on to a small amount of soft food (apple sauce or yogurt) or liquid, then administered immediately. Capsules should not be swallowed whole. For administration advice via nasogastric or gastrostomy tube—consult product literature.

- **PATIENT AND CARER ADVICE** Manufacturer advises patients and their carers should be counselled on the symptoms of hypocalcaemia and importance of serum-calcium monitoring.
Driving and skilled tasks Manufacturer advises patients and carers should be counselled on the effects on driving and performance of skilled tasks—increased risk of dizziness and seizures.

- **NATIONAL FUNDING/ACCESS DECISIONS**
For full details see funding body website
NICE decisions
  ▸ Cinacalcet for the treatment of secondary hyperparathyroidism in patients with end-stage renal disease on maintenance dialysis therapy [for routine treatment] (January 2007) NICE TA117 Not recommended
  ▸ Cinacalcet for the treatment of secondary hyperparathyroidism in patients with end-stage renal disease on maintenance dialysis therapy [in refractory secondary hyperparathyroidism] (January 2007) NICE TA117 Recommended with restrictions

- **MEDICINAL FORMS** There can be variation in the licensing of different medicines containing the same drug.
Oral tablet
CAUTIONARY AND ADVISORY LABELS 21
  ▸ Cinacalcet (Non-proprietary)
   Cinacalcet (as Cinacalcet hydrochloride) 30 mg Cinacalcet 30mg tablets | 28 tablet [PoM] £125.75 DT = £6.09
   Cinacalcet (as Cinacalcet hydrochloride) 60 mg Cinacalcet 60mg tablets | 28 tablet [PoM] £231.97 DT = £18.22
   Cinacalcet (as Cinacalcet hydrochloride) 90 mg Cinacalcet 90mg tablets | 28 tablet [PoM] £347.96 DT = £347.96

Etelcalcetide

26-Aug-2020

- **DRUG ACTION** Etelcalcetide reduces parathyroid hormone secretion, which leads to a decrease in serum calcium concentrations.

- **INDICATIONS AND DOSE**

Secondary hyperparathyroidism in patients with chronic kidney disease on haemodialysis
- ▶ BY INTRAVENOUS INJECTION
- ▶ Adult: Initially 5 mg 3 times a week, then increased in steps of 2.5–5 mg if required, dose to be increased at intervals of at least 4 weeks; usual maintenance 2.5–15 mg 3 times a week, max. dose 15 mg 3 times a week; consult product literature for information on missed doses, and for dose adjustment due to parathyroid hormone levels or serum-calcium concentrations

- **CAUTIONS** Conditions that may worsen with hypocalcaemia · hypocalcaemia (do not initiate if serum-calcium concentration is less than the lower limit of normal range) · switching from cinacalcet (do not initiate until 7 days after the last dose of cinacalcet)

CAUTIONS, FURTHER INFORMATION
- ▶ Conditions that may worsen with hypocalcaemia Manufacturer advises caution with use in patients with conditions that may worsen with hypocalcaemia, including predisposition to QT-interval prolongation, history of seizures, and history of congestive heart failure—serum-calcium concentration should be closely monitored.

- **INTERACTIONS** → Appendix 1: etelcalcetide

- **SIDE-EFFECTS**
- ▶ **Common or very common** Diarrhoea · electrolyte imbalance · headache · heart failure aggravated · hypotension · muscle complaints · nausea · QT interval prolongation · sensation abnormal · vomiting
- ▶ **Uncommon** Seizure
- ▶ **Frequency not known** Anaphylactic reaction

SIDE-EFFECTS, FURTHER INFORMATION Manufacturer advises if formation of anti-etelcalcetide antibodies with a clinically significant effect is suspected, contact manufacturer to discuss antibody testing.

- **PREGNANCY** Manufacturer advises avoid—limited information available.

- **BREAST FEEDING** Manufacturer advises avoid—present in milk in *animal* studies.

- **MONITORING REQUIREMENTS** Manufacturer advises monitor parathyroid hormone level 4 weeks after treatment initiation or dose adjustment and approximately every 1–3 months during maintenance treatment; monitor serum-calcium concentration before treatment initiation, within 1 week of initiation or dose adjustment, and then approximately every 4 weeks during maintenance treatment.

- **HANDLING AND STORAGE** Manufacturer advises store in a refrigerator (2–8°C)—consult product literature for further information regarding storage outside refrigerator.

- **PATIENT AND CARER ADVICE** Manufacturer advises patients and their carers should be told to seek medical advice if symptoms of hypocalcaemia occur.

- **NATIONAL FUNDING/ACCESS DECISIONS**
  For full details see funding body website
  NICE decisions
- ▶ Etelcalcetide for treating secondary hyperparathyroidism (June 2017) NICE TA448 Recommended with restrictions
  Scottish Medicines Consortium (SMC) decisions
- ▶ Etelcalcetide (*Parsabiv*®) for the treatment of secondary hyperparathyroidism (HPT) in adult patients with chronic

kidney disease (CKD) on haemodialysis therapy (September 2017) SMC No. 1262/17 Not recommended

- **MEDICINAL FORMS** There can be variation in the licensing of different medicines containing the same drug.

Solution for injection
- ▶ Parsabiv (Amgen Ltd)
  Etelcalcetide (as Etelcalcetide hydrochloride) 5 mg per 1 ml Parsabiv 2.5mg/0.5ml solution for injection vials | 6 vial [PoM] £136.87 (Hospital only)
  Parsabiv 10mg/2ml solution for injection vials | 6 vial [PoM] £327.84 (Hospital only)
  Parsabiv 5mg/1ml solution for injection vials | 6 vial [PoM] £163.92 (Hospital only)

2.1b Hypocalcaemia

CALCIUM REGULATING DRUGS › PARATHYROID HORMONES AND ANALOGUES

Palopegteriparatide

09-Dec-2024

- **DRUG ACTION** Palopegteriparatide is a prodrug of teriparatide, a shortened form of human parathyroid hormone.

- **INDICATIONS AND DOSE**

Chronic hypoparathyroidism (under expert supervision)
- ▶ BY SUBCUTANEOUS INJECTION
- ▶ Adult: Initially 18 micrograms once daily, dose should then be adjusted according to serum-calcium concentrations in steps of 3 micrograms every 7 days to a usual range of 6–60 micrograms daily. For advice on dose adjustments, treatment interruption or discontinuation, and calcium or vitamin D supplementation—consult product literature

- **CONTRA-INDICATIONS** Pseudohypoparathyroidism

- **CAUTIONS** Bone metastases (no information available) · concomitant use of cardiac glycosides (hypercalcaemia may predispose to digitalis toxicity)—monitor cardiac glycoside levels and check for signs and symptoms of digitalis toxicity · concomitant use of drugs that affect calcium levels · current or previous radiation therapy to skeleton (no information available) · increased risk factors for osteosarcoma including Paget's disease (no information available) · skeletal malignancy (no information available) · unexplained raised levels of bone-specific alkaline phosphatase (no information available)

- **SIDE-EFFECTS**
- ▶ **Common or very common** Arthralgia · asthenia · constipation · diarrhoea · dizziness · electrolyte imbalance · gastrointestinal discomfort · headache · muscle complaints · musculoskeletal pain · nausea · oropharyngeal pain · palpitations · paraesthesia · photosensitivity reaction · postural hypotension · postural orthostatic tachycardia syndrome · rash · syncope · thirst · vomiting
- ▶ **Uncommon** Chest discomfort · hypertension · urinary disorders

- **PREGNANCY** [EvGr] Avoid unless potential benefit outweighs risk (limited information available). [M]

- **BREAST FEEDING** [EvGr] Avoid unless potential benefit outweighs risk (no information available). No effects on the breast-fed infant are anticipated as not orally absorbed. [M]

- **HEPATIC IMPAIRMENT** [EvGr] Caution in severe impairment (no information available). [M]

- **RENAL IMPAIRMENT** [EvGr] Caution in moderate impairment (limited information available) and severe impairment (no information available). If eGFR less than 45 mL/minute, monitor serum-calcium concentrations more frequently when starting treatment (increased risk of hypercalcaemic reactions and transient eGFR decrease). ⟨M⟩

- **PRE-TREATMENT SCREENING** [EvGr] Confirm sufficient 25-hydroxyvitamin D stores (within normal range), and serum-calcium concentrations are stable (within or slightly below normal range) for at least 2 weeks before the first dose of treatment. ⟨M⟩
- **MONITORING REQUIREMENTS** [EvGr] Measure serum calcium 7 days after starting treatment and within 7 to 14 days after each dose adjustment during treatment; assess for signs and symptoms of hypo- and hypercalcaemia, and adjust active vitamin D and calcium supplement as necessary—consult product literature. ⟨M⟩
- **TREATMENT CESSATION** [EvGr] Abrupt interruption or discontinuation can result in hypocalcaemia—monitor for signs and symptoms if 3 or more consecutive doses are affected; consider measuring serum calcium and resume calcium supplement and active vitamin D treatment as required. ⟨M⟩
- **DIRECTIONS FOR ADMINISTRATION** For *subcutaneous injection*, remove prefilled pen from the refrigerator 20 minutes before administration. Inject into the abdomen or the front of the thigh; rotate injection site. Doses exceeding 30 micrograms daily should be given as 2 single doses administered consecutively at different sites. *Yorvipath*® may be self-administered or administered by a carer after appropriate training in subcutaneous injection technique.
- **HANDLING AND STORAGE** Store in a refrigerator (2-8°C) and protect from light; may be stored at room temperature (below 30°C) after opening and discarded within 14 days.
- **PATIENT AND CARER ADVICE**
  Self-administration Patients and their carers should be given training in subcutaneous injection technique, if appropriate.
  Missed doses If a dose is more than 12 hours late, the missed dose should not be administered and the next dose should be administered at the normal time.
  Driving and skilled tasks Patients and their carers should be cautioned on the effects on driving and performance of skilled tasks—increased risk of dizziness, orthostatic hypotension, syncope, or presyncope.

- **MEDICINAL FORMS** There can be variation in the licensing of different medicines containing the same drug.
  Solution for injection
  ▸ Yorvipath (Ascendis Pharma UK Ltd) ▼
  PTH(1-34) (as Palopegteriparatide) 300 microgram per 1 ml Yorvipath 294micrograms/0.98ml solution for injection pre-filled pens | 2 pre-filled disposable injection [PoM] £7,406.00 (Hospital only) Yorvipath 168micrograms/0.56ml solution for injection pre-filled pens | 2 pre-filled disposable injection [PoM] £7,406.00 (Hospital only) Yorvipath 420micrograms/1.4ml solution for injection pre-filled pens | 2 pre-filled disposable injection [PoM] £7,406.00 (Hospital only)

▌Parathyroid hormone
11-Jan-2023
(Human recombinant parathyroid hormone)

- **DRUG ACTION** Parathyroid hormone is produced by recombinant DNA technology; endogenous parathyroid hormone is involved in modulating serum calcium and phosphate levels, regulating renal calcium and phosphate excretion, activating vitamin D, and maintaining normal bone turnover.

- **INDICATIONS AND DOSE**
Chronic hypoparathyroidism (specialist use only)
  ▸ BY SUBCUTANEOUS INJECTION
  ▸ Adult: (consult product literature)

- **CONTRA-INDICATIONS** Bone metastases · current or previous radiation therapy to skeleton · increased risk factors for osteosarcoma (including Paget's disease or hereditary disorders) · pseudohypoparathyroidism · skeletal malignancy · unexplained raised levels of bone-specific alkaline phosphatase
- **CAUTIONS** Concomitant use of cardiac glycosides (hypercalcaemia may predispose to digitalis toxicity)— monitor cardiac glycoside levels and check for signs and symptoms of digitalis toxicity · concomitant use of drugs that affect calcium levels · young adults with open epiphyses—increased risk of osteosarcoma
- **INTERACTIONS** → Appendix 1: parathyroid hormone
- **SIDE-EFFECTS**
  ▸ **Common or very common** Abdominal pain upper · anxiety · arthralgia · asthenia · chest pain · cough · diarrhoea · drowsiness · electrolyte imbalance · headache · hypercalciuria · hypertension · insomnia · muscle complaints · nausea · pain · palpitations · sensation abnormal · tetany · thirst · urinary frequency increased · vomiting

  SIDE-EFFECTS, FURTHER INFORMATION Hypercalcaemia is more likely during initial dose titration; if severe hypercalcaemia develops, hydrate and consider suspending treatment (including calcium supplement and active vitamin D).
- **PREGNANCY** Manufacturer advises use only if potential benefit outweighs risk—no information available.
- **BREAST FEEDING** Manufacturer advises avoid—present in milk in *animal* studies.
- **HEPATIC IMPAIRMENT** Manufacturer advises caution in severe impairment (no information available).
- **RENAL IMPAIRMENT** Manufacturer advises caution in severe impairment—no information available.
- **PRE-TREATMENT SCREENING** Manufacturer advises confirm sufficient 25-hydroxyvitamin D stores and normal serum magnesium before treatment.
- **MONITORING REQUIREMENTS**
  ▸ Manufacturer advises monitor serum calcium and assess for signs and symptoms of hypocalcaemia and hypercalcaemia—adjust active vitamin D and calcium supplement as necessary; consult product literature.
  ▸ Manufacturer advises periodic monitoring of the response of serum calcium to treatment (response may decrease over time—if 25-hydroxyvitamin D is low, supplementation may restore serum calcium response).
- **TREATMENT CESSATION** Abrupt interruption or discontinuation can result in severe hypocalcaemia— manufacturer advises to monitor serum calcium and adjust calcium supplement and active vitamin D treatment.
- **PRESCRIBING AND DISPENSING INFORMATION** Manufacturer advises record the brand name and batch number after each administration.
- **HANDLING AND STORAGE** Manufacturer advises store in a refrigerator (2–8 °C); reconstituted solution may be stored for up to 14 days in a refrigerator, and up to 3 days outside of a refrigerator (below 25 °C), during the 14-day use period.
- **PATIENT AND CARER ADVICE** Patients may self-administer *Natpar*®, after appropriate training in subcutaneous injection technique.
  Missed doses Manufacturer advises missed doses should be administered as soon as possible, and additional treatment with calcium and/or active vitamin D must be taken, based on symptoms of hypocalcaemia.

- **MEDICINAL FORMS** There can be variation in the licensing of different medicines containing the same drug.

Powder and solvent for solution for injection
ELECTROLYTES: May contain Sodium
- ► **Natpar** (Takeda UK Ltd) ▼
  Parathyroid hormone 50 microgram Natpar 50micrograms/dose powder and solvent for solution for injection cartridges | 2 cartridge `PoM` £4,880.00 (Hospital only)
  Parathyroid hormone 75 microgram Natpar 75micrograms/dose powder and solvent for solution for injection cartridges | 2 cartridge `PoM` £4,880.00 (Hospital only)
  Parathyroid hormone 100 microgram Natpar 100micrograms/dose powder and solvent for solution for injection cartridges | 2 cartridge `PoM` £4,880.00 (Hospital only)

ELECTROLYTES AND MINERALS ⟩ CALCIUM

Calcium salts

- **CONTRA-INDICATIONS** Conditions associated with hypercalcaemia (e.g. some forms of malignant disease) · conditions associated with hypercalciuria (e.g. some forms of malignant disease)
- **CAUTIONS** History of nephrolithiasis · sarcoidosis
- **SIDE-EFFECTS**
- ► **Uncommon** Constipation · diarrhoea · hypercalcaemia · nausea
- **RENAL IMPAIRMENT** `EvGr` Use with caution. ◈

⚑ **above**

Calcium carbonate

17-Aug-2023

- **INDICATIONS AND DOSE**

Phosphate binding in renal failure and hyper-phosphataemia
- ► BY MOUTH
- ► Adult: (consult product literature)

Calcium deficiency
- ► BY MOUTH
- ► Adult: (consult product literature)

- **INTERACTIONS** → Appendix 1: calcium salts
- **SIDE-EFFECTS**
- ► **Uncommon** Hypercalciuria
- ► **Rare or very rare** Flatulence · gastrointestinal discomfort · milk-alkali syndrome · skin reactions
- **PRESCRIBING AND DISPENSING INFORMATION** *Adcal*® contains calcium carbonate 1.5 g (calcium 600 mg or Ca²⁺ 15 mmol); *Calcichew*® contains calcium carbonate 1.25 g (calcium 500 mg or Ca²⁺ 12.5 mmol); *Calcichew Forte*® contains calcium carbonate 2.5 g (calcium 1 g or Ca²⁺ 25 mmol); *Cacit*® contains calcium carbonate 1.25 g, providing calcium citrate when dispersed in water (calcium 500 mg or Ca²⁺ 12.5 mmol); consult product literature for details of other available products.
  Flavours of chewable tablet formulations may include orange or fruit flavour.

- **MEDICINAL FORMS** There can be variation in the licensing of different medicines containing the same drug. Forms available from special-order manufacturers include: oral tablet, oral capsule, oral suspension

Oral tablet
CAUTIONARY AND ADVISORY LABELS 25

Effervescent tablet
CAUTIONARY AND ADVISORY LABELS 13
- ► **Calcium carbonate (Non-proprietary)**
  Calcium carbonate 1.25 gram Calcium 500mg effervescent tablets sugar free | 76 tablet `P` £12.96 DT = £12.96 `SF`
- ► **A1-Cal** (TriOn Pharma Ltd)
  Calcium carbonate 625 mg A1-Cal 250mg effervescent tablets | 10 tablet £13.87 `SF`

Chewable tablet
CAUTIONARY AND ADVISORY LABELS 24
EXCIPIENTS: May contain Aspartame
- ► **Adcal** (Kyowa Kirin International UK NewCo Ltd)
  Calcium carbonate 1.5 gram Adcal 1500mg chewable tablets | 100 tablet `P` £8.70 DT = £8.70 `SF`
- ► **Calcichew** (Forum Health Products Ltd)
  Calcium carbonate 1.25 gram Calcichew 500mg chewable tablets | 100 tablet `P` £9.33 DT = £9.33 `SF`
  Calcium carbonate 2.5 gram Calcichew Forte chewable tablets | 60 tablet `P` £14.21 DT = £14.21 `SF`
- ► **Rennie** (Bayer Plc)
  Calcium carbonate 500 mg Rennie Orange 500mg chewable tablets | 24 tablet `GSL` £2.55 | 36 tablet `GSL` £3.19 | 72 tablet `GSL` £5.22
- ► **Setlers Antacid** (Thornton & Ross Ltd)
  Calcium carbonate 500 mg Setlers Antacid spearmint chewable tablets | 24 tablet `GSL` £2.04 | 36 tablet `GSL` £2.04 Setlers Antacid peppermint chewable tablets | 24 tablet `GSL` £2.04 | 36 tablet `GSL` £2.04

Calcium carbonate with calcium lactate gluconate

02-Mar-2023

The properties listed below are those particular to the combination only. For the properties of the components please consider, calcium carbonate above.

- **INDICATIONS AND DOSE**

Calcium deficiency
- ► BY MOUTH
- ► Adult: Dose according to requirements

- **INTERACTIONS** → Appendix 1: calcium salts
- **PRESCRIBING AND DISPENSING INFORMATION** Each *Calvive*® tablet contains 1 g calcium (Ca²⁺ 25 mmol); flavours of effervescent tablet formulations may include orange.

- **MEDICINAL FORMS** There can be variation in the licensing of different medicines containing the same drug.

Effervescent tablet
CAUTIONARY AND ADVISORY LABELS 13
EXCIPIENTS: May contain Aspartame
- ► **Calvive** (Haleon UK Trading Ltd)
  Calcium carbonate 1.75 gram, Calcium lactate gluconate 2.263 gram Calvive 1000 effervescent tablets | 30 tablet `P` £14.11 DT = £14.11 `SF`

⚑ **above**

Calcium chloride

10-Nov-2023

- **INDICATIONS AND DOSE**

Severe acute or symptomatic hypocalcaemia
- ► BY SLOW INTRAVENOUS INJECTION, OR BY INTRAVENOUS INFUSION
- ► Adult: Dose according to requirements

Acute severe hyperkalaemia (plasma-potassium concentration 6.5 mmol/litre or greater, or in the presence of ECG changes)
- ► BY SLOW INTRAVENOUS INJECTION
- ► Adult: 10 mL, calcium chloride 10% (providing approximately 6.8 mmol of calcium) should be administered as a single dose, repeat dose if no improvement in ECG within 5 to 10 minutes

- **UNLICENSED USE** EvGr Calcium chloride is used for the treatment of acute severe hyperkalaemia, ⒶA but is not licensed for this indication.

> **IMPORTANT SAFETY INFORMATION**
> MHRA/CHM ADVICE: CALCIUM CHLORIDE: POTENTIAL RISK OF UNDERDOSING WITH CALCIUM GLUCONATE IN SEVERE HYPERKALAEMIA (JUNE 2023)
> Healthcare professionals are advised that calcium chloride and calcium gluconate are not equivalent in terms of calcium dose—for further details, see *Important safety information* in calcium gluconate below.

- **CAUTIONS** Avoid in respiratory acidosis · avoid in respiratory failure
- **INTERACTIONS** → Appendix 1: calcium salts
- **SIDE-EFFECTS** Soft tissue calcification · taste unpleasant · vasodilation
- **DIRECTIONS FOR ADMINISTRATION** Care should be taken to avoid extravasation. Incompatible with bicarbonates, phosphates, or sulfates.

  For *slow intravenous injection*, may be given undiluted over 3 to 5 minutes.

- **PRESCRIBING AND DISPENSING INFORMATION** Non-proprietary *Calcium chloride dihydrate* 7.35% (calcium 20 mg or Ca^{2+} 500 micromol/mL); *Calcium chloride dihydrate* 10% (calcium 27.3 mg or Ca^{2+} 680 micromol/mL); *Calcium chloride dihydrate* 14.7% (calcium 40.1 mg or Ca^{2+} 1000 micromol/mL).

- **MEDICINAL FORMS** There can be variation in the licensing of different medicines containing the same drug. Forms available from special-order manufacturers include: solution for injection, solution for infusion

  Solution for injection
  - **Calcium chloride (Non-proprietary)**
    Calcium chloride dihydrate 100 mg per 1 ml Calcium chloride 10% solution for injection 10ml pre-filled syringes | 1 pre-filled disposable injection PoM £9.89–£12.43 DT = £12.08
    Calcium chloride dihydrate 147 mg per 1 ml Calcium chloride 14.7% solution for injection 5ml ampoules | 10 ampoule PoM £235.29
    Calcium chloride 14.7% solution for injection 10ml ampoules | 10 ampoule PoM £107.06–£159.95

F 1188

| Calcium gluconate

10-Nov-2023

- **INDICATIONS AND DOSE**

Severe acute or symptomatic hypocalcaemia
- INITIALLY BY SLOW INTRAVENOUS INJECTION
- Adult: Initially 10–20 mL, calcium gluconate injection 10% (providing approximately 2.25–4.5 mmol of calcium) should be administered, and either repeated as required or, if only temporary improvement, followed by a continuous intravenous infusion to prevent recurrence, alternatively (by continuous intravenous infusion), initially 50 mL/hour, adjusted according to response, infusion to be administered using 100 mL of calcium gluconate 10% diluted in 1 litre of glucose 5% or sodium chloride 0.9%

Acute severe hyperkalaemia [plasma-potassium concentration 6.5 mmol/litre or greater, or in the presence of ECG changes]
- BY SLOW INTRAVENOUS INJECTION
- Adult: 30 mL, calcium gluconate 10% (providing approximately 6.8 mmol of calcium) should be administered as a single dose, repeat dose if no improvement in ECG within 5 to 10 minutes

Calcium deficiency | Mild asymptomatic hypocalcaemia
- BY MOUTH
- Adult: Dose according to requirements

> **IMPORTANT SAFETY INFORMATION**
> MHRA/CHM ADVICE: CALCIUM GLUCONATE INJECTION IN SMALL-VOLUME GLASS CONTAINERS: NEW CONTRA-INDICATIONS DUE TO ALUMINIUM EXPOSURE RISK (AUGUST 2010)
> The MHRA has advised that repeated or prolonged administration of calcium gluconate injection packaged in 10 mL glass containers is contra-indicated in children under 18 years and in patients with renal impairment owing to the risk of aluminium accumulation; in these patients the use of calcium gluconate injection packaged in plastic containers is recommended.
>
> MHRA/CHM ADVICE: CALCIUM GLUCONATE: POTENTIAL RISK OF UNDERDOSING WITH CALCIUM GLUCONATE IN SEVERE HYPERKALAEMIA (JUNE 2023)
> An MHRA review of UK data in the context of severe hyperkalaemia and cardiac arrest has identified reports of incidents, including fatalities, associated with incorrect calcium gluconate dosing, a lack of potassium-lowering treatment, and lack of, or inappropriate, ECG monitoring.
> Healthcare professionals are advised that:
> - calcium gluconate and calcium chloride are not equivalent in terms of calcium dose;
> - there is a risk of inadvertent underdosing if calcium gluconate is given instead of calcium chloride—the salt should be verified before administration: 30 mL of calcium gluconate 10% provides 6.8 mmol of calcium (equivalent to 10 mL of calcium chloride 10%);
> - the dose of calcium gluconate must be administered by slow intravenous injection over 10 minutes;
> - repeat doses may be required 5–10 minutes after the initial dose as the effect of calcium is temporary, lasting 30–60 minutes.
> Healthcare professionals are also reminded that intravenous calcium salts should only be given in cases of documented severe hyperkalaemia and should not be routinely administered during cardiac arrest.

- **INTERACTIONS** → Appendix 1: calcium salts
- **SIDE-EFFECTS**
  GENERAL SIDE-EFFECTS Arrhythmias
  SPECIFIC SIDE-EFFECTS
  - With intravenous use Circulatory collapse · feeling hot · hyperhidrosis · hypotension · vasodilation · vomiting
  - With oral use Gastrointestinal disorder
- **MONITORING REQUIREMENTS**
  - With intravenous use for Severe acute or symptomatic hypocalcaemia EvGr Plasma-calcium and ECG monitoring required for administration by slow intravenous injection (risk of arrhythmias if given too rapidly). Ⓜ
- **DIRECTIONS FOR ADMINISTRATION** For *continuous intravenous infusion*, dilute 100 mL of calcium gluconate 10% in 1 litre of Glucose 5% or Sodium Chloride 0.9% and give at an initial rate of 50 mL/hour adjusted according to response. Incompatible with bicarbonates, phosphates, or sulfates. EvGr May be given undiluted (calcium gluconate 10%) by *slow intravenous injection* over 10 minutes. Ⓜ
- **PRESCRIBING AND DISPENSING INFORMATION** Calcium gluconate 1 g contains calcium 89 mg or Ca^{2+} 2.23 mmol.

- **MEDICINAL FORMS** There can be variation in the licensing of different medicines containing the same drug. Forms available from special-order manufacturers include: oral tablet, oral capsule, oral suspension, oral solution, solution for injection, solution for infusion

Solution for injection

- ▸ Calcium gluconate (Non-proprietary)
  Calcium gluconate 100 mg per 1 ml Calcium gluconate 10% solution for injection 10ml ampoules | 10 ampoule [PoM] £24.17-£28.21 | 20 ampoule [PoM] £30.00-£163.86 | 20 ampoule [PoM] £37.23 (Hospital only)

Effervescent tablet

CAUTIONARY AND ADVISORY LABELS 13
ELECTROLYTES: May contain Sodium

- ▸ Calcium gluconate (Non-proprietary)
  Calcium gluconate 1 gram Calcium gluconate 1g effervescent tablets | 28 tablet [GSL] £18.35-£23.60 DT = £18.35

↑ 1188

Calcium lactate

- **INDICATIONS AND DOSE**

Calcium deficiency

- ▸ BY MOUTH
- ▸ Adult: Dose according to requirements

- **INTERACTIONS** → Appendix 1: calcium salts

- **MEDICINAL FORMS** No licensed medicines listed.

↑ 1188

Calcium phosphate

- **INDICATIONS AND DOSE**

Indications listed in combination monographs (available in the UK only in combination with other drugs)

- ▸ BY MOUTH
- ▸ Adult: Doses listed in combination monographs

- **INTERACTIONS** → Appendix 1: calcium salts
- **SIDE-EFFECTS** Epigastric pain · gastrointestinal disorder · hypercalciuria

- **MEDICINAL FORMS** No licensed medicines listed.

2.2 Low blood volume

BLOOD AND RELATED PRODUCTS > PLASMA PRODUCTS

Albumin solution

09-Feb-2022

(Human Albumin Solution)

- **INDICATIONS AND DOSE**

Acute or sub-acute loss of plasma volume e.g. in burns, pancreatitis, trauma, and complications of surgery (with isotonic solutions) | Plasma exchange (with isotonic solutions) | Severe hypoalbuminaemia associated with low plasma volume and generalised oedema where salt and water restriction with plasma volume expansion are required (with concentrated solutions 20%) | Paracentesis of large volume ascites associated with portal hypertension (with concentrated solutions 20%)

- ▸ BY INTRAVENOUS INFUSION
- ▸ Adult: (consult product literature)

- **CAUTIONS** Correct dehydration when administering concentrated solution · history of cardiovascular disease · increased capillary permeability · risk of haemodilution (e.g. severe anaemia or haemorrhagic disorders) · risk of hypervolaemia (e.g. oesophageal varices or pulmonary oedema) · vaccination against hepatitis A and hepatitis B may be required

CAUTIONS, FURTHER INFORMATION

- ▸ Volume status Manufacturer advises adjust dose and rate of infusion to avoid fluid overload.

- **SIDE-EFFECTS**
- **Rare or very rare** Fever · flushing · nausea · shock · urticaria

- **MONITORING REQUIREMENTS** Plasma and plasma substitutes are often used in very ill patients whose condition is unstable. Therefore, close monitoring is required and fluid and electrolyte therapy should be adjusted according to the patient's condition at all times.

- **PRESCRIBING AND DISPENSING INFORMATION** A solution containing protein derived from plasma, serum, or normal placentas; at least 95% of the protein is albumin. The solution may be isotonic (containing 3.5–5% protein) or concentrated (containing 15–25% protein).

- **MEDICINAL FORMS** There can be variation in the licensing of different medicines containing the same drug.

Solution for infusion

- ▸ Albumin solution (Non-proprietary)
  Albumin solution human 200 mg per 1 ml Human Albumin Grifols 20% solution for infusion 50ml vials | 1 vial [PoM] £27.00 (Hospital only)
  Human Albumin Grifols 20% solution for infusion 100ml vials | 1 vial [PoM] £54.00 (Hospital only)
- ▸ Albunorm (Octapharma Ltd)
  Albumin solution human 50 mg per 1 ml Albunorm 5% solution for infusion 250ml bottles | 1 bottle [PoM] £33.75 (Hospital only)
  Albunorm 5% solution for infusion 100ml bottles | 1 bottle [PoM] £13.50 (Hospital only)
  Albunorm 5% solution for infusion 500ml bottles | 1 bottle [PoM] £67.50 (Hospital only)
  Albumin solution human 200 mg per 1 ml Albunorm 20% solution for infusion 100ml bottles | 1 bottle [PoM] £54.00 (Hospital only)
  Albunorm 20% solution for infusion 50ml bottles | 1 bottle [PoM] £27.00 (Hospital only)
- ▸ Alburex (CSL Behring UK Ltd)
  Albumin solution human 50 mg per 1 ml Alburex 5% solution for infusion 500ml vials | 1 vial [PoM] £67.50 (Hospital only)
  Albumin solution human 200 mg per 1 ml Alburex 20% solution for infusion 100ml vials | 1 vial [PoM] £54.00 (Hospital only)
- ▸ Biotest (Grifols UK Ltd)
  Albumin solution human 50 mg per 1 ml Human Albumin Biotest 5% solution for infusion 250ml vials | 1 vial [PoM] £33.75 (Hospital only)
  Albumin solution human 200 mg per 1 ml Human Albumin Biotest 20% solution for infusion 50ml vials | 1 vial [PoM] £27.00 (Hospital only)
  Human Albumin Biotest 20% solution for infusion 100ml vials | 1 vial [PoM] £54.00 (Hospital only)
- ▸ Grifols (Grifols UK Ltd)
  Albumin solution human 50 mg per 1 ml Human Albumin Grifols 5% solution for infusion 250ml bottles | 1 bottle [PoM] £33.75
  Human Albumin Grifols 5% solution for infusion 500ml bottles | 1 bottle [PoM] £67.50
- ▸ Octalbin (Octapharma Ltd)
  Albumin solution human 50 mg per 1 ml Octalbin 5% solution for infusion 250ml bottles | 1 bottle [PoM] £33.75 (Hospital only)
  Octalbin 5% solution for infusion 500ml bottles | 1 bottle [PoM] £67.50 (Hospital only)
  Albumin solution human 200 mg per 1 ml Octalbin 20% solution for infusion 100ml bottles | 1 bottle [PoM] £54.00 (Hospital only)
- ▸ Zenalb (Bio Products Laboratory Ltd)
  Albumin solution human 45 mg per 1 ml Zenalb 4.5% solution for infusion 250ml bottles | 1 bottle [PoM] £30.37
  Zenalb 4.5% solution for infusion 500ml bottles | 1 bottle [PoM] £60.75
  Albumin solution human 200 mg per 1 ml Zenalb 20% solution for infusion 100ml bottles | 1 bottle [PoM] £54.00
  Zenalb 20% solution for infusion 50ml bottles | 1 bottle [PoM] £27.00

PLASMA SUBSTITUTES

Gelatin

19-Apr-2021

- **INDICATIONS AND DOSE**

Low blood volume in hypovolaemic shock, burns and cardiopulmonary bypass
- ▶ BY INTRAVENOUS INFUSION
- ▶ Adult: Initially 500–1000 mL, use 3.5–4% solution

- **CAUTIONS** Cardiac disease · severe liver disease
- **SIDE-EFFECTS**
- ▶ **Rare or very rare** Chills · dyspnoea · fever · hyperhidrosis · hypersensitivity · hypertension · hypotension · hypoxia · tachycardia · tremor · urticaria · wheezing
- **PREGNANCY** Manufacturer of *Geloplasma*® advises avoid at the end of pregnancy.
- **HEPATIC IMPAIRMENT** Manufacturers advise avoid preparations that contain lactate (risk of impaired lactate metabolism).
- **RENAL IMPAIRMENT** EvGr Use with caution. ◈
- **MONITORING REQUIREMENTS**
- ▶ Urine output should be monitored. Care should be taken to avoid haematocrit concentration from falling below 25–30% and the patient should be monitored for hypersensitivity reactions.
- ▶ Plasma and plasma substitutes are often used in very ill patients whose condition is unstable. Therefore, close monitoring is required and fluid and electrolyte therapy should be adjusted according to the patient's condition at all times.
- **PRESCRIBING AND DISPENSING INFORMATION** The gelatin is partially degraded.

  Gelaspan® contains succinylated gelatin (modified fluid gelatin, average molecular weight 26 500) 40 g, Na^+ 151 mmol, K^+ 4 mmol, Mg^{2+} 1 mmol, Cl^- 103 mmol, Ca^{2+} 1 mmol, acetate 24 mmol/litre; *Gelofusine*® contains succinylated gelatin (modified fluid gelatin, average molecular weight 30 000) 40 g (4%), Na^+ 154 mmol, Cl^- 124 mmol/litre; *Geloplasma*® contains partially hydrolysed and succinylated gelatin (modified liquid gelatin) (as anhydrous gelatin) 30 g (3%), Na^+ 150 mmol, K^+ 5 mmol, Mg^{2+} 1.5mmol, Cl^- 100 mmol, lactate 30 mmol/litre; *Isoplex*® contains succinylated gelatin (modified fluid gelatin, average molecular weight 30 000) 40g (4%), Na^+ 145 mmol, K^+ 4 mmol, Mg^{2+} 0.9 mmol, Cl^- 105 mmol, lactate 25mmol/litre; *Volplex*® contains succinylated gelatin (modified fluid gelatin, average molecular weight 30 000) 40 g (4%), Na^+ 154 mmol, Cl^- 125 mmol/litre.

- **MEDICINAL FORMS** There can be variation in the licensing of different medicines containing the same drug.

  Infusion
  - ▶ **Gelaspan** (B.Braun Medical Ltd)
    Gelatin 40 mg per 1 ml Gelaspan 4% infusion 500ml Ecobags | 20 bag PoM £136.00 (Hospital only)
  - ▶ **Gelofusine** (B.Braun Medical Ltd)
    Gelatin 40 mg per 1 ml Gelofusine 4% infusion 1litre Ecobags | 10 bag PoM £87.90 (Hospital only)
    Gelofusine 4% infusion 500ml Ecobags | 20 bag PoM £94.00 (Hospital only)
  - ▶ **Geloplasma** (Fresenius Kabi Ltd)
    Gelatin 30 mg per 1 ml Geloplasma 3% infusion 500ml Freeflex bags | 20 bag PoM £85.50 (Hospital only)

2.3 Magnesium imbalance

Magnesium imbalance

08-Aug-2022

Overview

Magnesium is an essential constituent of many enzyme systems, particularly those involved in energy generation; the largest stores are in the skeleton.

Magnesium salts are not well absorbed from the gastro-intestinal tract, which explains the use of magnesium sulfate p. 1193 as an osmotic laxative.

EvGr Magnesium is excreted mainly by the kidneys and is therefore retained in renal failure, which can result in *hypermagnesaemia* (causing muscle weakness and arrhythmias). Calcium gluconate injection is used for the management of magnesium toxicity. ◈

Hypomagnesaemia

Since magnesium is secreted in large amounts in the gastro-intestinal fluid, excessive losses in diarrhoea, stoma or fistula can cause *hypomagnesaemia*; deficiency may also occur in alcoholism or as a result of treatment with certain drugs. Hypomagnesaemia often causes secondary hypocalcaemia, and also hypokalaemia.

Symptomatic hypomagnesaemia is usually associated with severe magnesium depletion. Magnesium can be given by intravenous infusion or by intramuscular injection of magnesium sulfate; the intramuscular injection is painful.

Patients with mild magnesium depletion are usually asymptomatic. Oral magnesium glycerophosphate p. 1192 is licensed for hypomagnesaemia. Oral magnesium aspartate below and magnesium citrate p. 1192 are licensed for the treatment and prevention of magnesium deficiency.

2.3a Hypomagnesaemia

ELECTROLYTES AND MINERALS > MAGNESIUM

Magnesium aspartate

24-Sep-2024

- **INDICATIONS AND DOSE**

  MAGNASPARTATE®

  Treatment and prevention of magnesium deficiency
  - ▶ BY MOUTH
  - ▶ Adult: 10–20 mmol once daily

  DOSE EQUIVALENCE AND CONVERSION
  - ▶ Each *Magnaspartate*® sachet contains magnesium aspartate equivalent to magnesium 243 mg *or* Mg^{2+} 10 mmol; dose expressed as Mg^{2+}.
  - ▶ Magnesium preparations may not be interchangeable due to differences in bioavailability, therefore caution should be exercised when switching preparations to ensure tolerability and to maintain therapeutic effect.

- **CONTRA-INDICATIONS** Disorders of cardiac conduction
- **INTERACTIONS** → Appendix 1: magnesium
- **SIDE-EFFECTS**
- ▶ **Uncommon** Diarrhoea · faeces soft
- ▶ **Rare or very rare** Fatigue · hypermagnesaemia
- ▶ **Frequency not known** Gastrointestinal irritation

  SIDE-EFFECTS, FURTHER INFORMATION Side-effects generally occur at higher doses; if side-effects (such as diarrhoea) occur, consider interrupting treatment and restarting at a reduced dose.

  Overdose Symptoms of hypermagnesaemia may include nausea, vomiting, flushing, thirst, hypotension, drowsiness, confusion, reflexes absent (due to neuromuscular blockade), respiratory depression, speech slurred, diplopia, muscle weakness, arrhythmias, coma, and cardiac arrest.

- RENAL IMPAIRMENT See p. 21. [EvGr] Avoid if eGFR less than 30 mL/minute/1.73 m². ⟨M⟩
- MONITORING REQUIREMENTS [EvGr] Monitor serum magnesium levels every 3–6 months. ⟨M⟩
- DIRECTIONS FOR ADMINISTRATION [EvGr] Dissolve contents of one *Magnaspartate*® sachet in 50–200 mL of water, tea, or orange juice and take immediately (or within 24 hours when dissolved in bottled water and stored below 25°C). *Magnaspartate*® may be dissolved in 200 mL of water and administered immediately (or within 24 hours when dissolved in bottled water and stored below 25°C) via a gastric, duodenal, or nasal feeding tube. ⟨M⟩
- PATIENT AND CARER ADVICE Patients and carers should be given advice on how to administer magnesium aspartate powder.

- MEDICINAL FORMS There can be variation in the licensing of different medicines containing the same drug.
Powder for oral solution
EXCIPIENTS: May contain Sucrose
▸ **Magnaspartate** (Kora Healthcare)
Magnesium (as Magnesium aspartate) 243 mg Magnaspartate 243mg (magnesium 10mmol) oral powder sachets | 10 sachet [PoM] £9.45 DT = £9.45 | 20 sachet [PoM] £18.89

Magnesium citrate
01-Aug-2022

- INDICATIONS AND DOSE
Treatment and prevention of magnesium deficiency
▸ BY MOUTH
▸ Adult: 4–8 mmol 3 times a day

DOSE EQUIVALENCE AND CONVERSION
▸ Each tablet contains magnesium citrate equivalent to magnesium 97.2 mg *or* Mg²⁺ 4 mmol; dose expressed as Mg²⁺.
▸ Magnesium preparations may not be interchangeable due to differences in bioavailability, therefore caution should be exercised when switching preparations to ensure tolerability and to maintain therapeutic effect.

- CAUTIONS Disorders of cardiac conduction
- INTERACTIONS → Appendix 1: magnesium
- SIDE-EFFECTS
▸ **Common or very common** Diarrhoea (with high doses) · faeces soft (with high doses)
▸ **Rare or very rare** Fatigue (long term use)
▸ **Frequency not known** Gastrointestinal irritation (with high doses)
- RENAL IMPAIRMENT [EvGr] Avoid in severe impairment. ⟨M⟩
- MONITORING REQUIREMENTS [EvGr] Monitor serum magnesium levels every 3–6 months. ⟨M⟩

- MEDICINAL FORMS There can be variation in the licensing of different medicines containing the same drug.
Oral tablet
▸ **Magnesium citrate (Non-proprietary)**
Magnesium (as Magnesium citrate) 97.2 mg Magnesium citrate (magnesium 97.2mg (4mmol)) tablets | 60 tablet [PoM] £24.00 DT = £24.00

Magnesium glycerophosphate
24-Sep-2024

- INDICATIONS AND DOSE
Prevent recurrence of magnesium deficit
▸ BY MOUTH
▸ Adult: 24 mmol daily in divided doses

DOSE EQUIVALENCE AND CONVERSION
▸ Magnesium glycerophosphate 1 g is approximately equivalent to magnesium 97.2 mg *or* Mg²⁺ 4 mmol; dose expressed as Mg²⁺.
▸ Magnesium preparations may not be interchangeable due to differences in bioavailability, therefore caution should be exercised when switching preparations to ensure tolerability and to maintain therapeutic effect.

NEOMAG® CHEWABLE TABLETS
Hypomagnesaemia
▸ BY MOUTH
▸ Adult: Initially 4–8 mmol 3 times a day, dose to be adjusted as necessary

DOSE EQUIVALENCE AND CONVERSION
▸ Each *Neomag*® chewable tablet contains magnesium glycerophosphate equivalent to magnesium 97.2 mg *or* Mg²⁺ 4 mmol; dose expressed as Mg²⁺.
▸ Magnesium preparations may not be interchangeable due to differences in bioavailability, therefore caution should be exercised when switching preparations to ensure tolerability and to maintain therapeutic effect.

- INTERACTIONS → Appendix 1: magnesium
- SIDE-EFFECTS Diarrhoea · hypermagnesaemia
Overdose Symptoms of hypermagnesaemia may include nausea, vomiting, flushing, thirst, hypotension, drowsiness, confusion, reflexes absent (due to neuromuscular blockade), respiratory depression, speech slurred, diplopia, muscle weakness, arrhythmias, coma, and cardiac arrest.
- RENAL IMPAIRMENT [EvGr] Caution (risk of hypermagnesaemia); avoid if creatinine clearance less than 30 mL/minute. ⟨M⟩ See p. 21.
- MONITORING REQUIREMENTS Manufacturer advises to monitor serum magnesium levels every 3–6 months.
- DIRECTIONS FOR ADMINISTRATION [EvGr] *Neomag*® chewable tablets may be broken into quarters and chewed or swallowed with water. ⟨M⟩
- NATIONAL FUNDING/ACCESS DECISIONS For full details see funding body website
Scottish Medicines Consortium (SMC) decisions
▸ Magnesium glycerophosphate (*Neomag*®) for use as an oral magnesium supplement for the treatment of patients with chronic magnesium loss, hypomagnesaemia, or drug-induced hypomagnesaemia (September 2017) SMC No. 1267/17 Recommended

- MEDICINAL FORMS There can be variation in the licensing of different medicines containing the same drug. Forms available from special-order manufacturers include: oral tablet, oral capsule, oral suspension, oral solution, oral powder
Oral tablet
▸ **Magnesium glycerophosphate (Non-proprietary)**
Magnesium (as Magnesium glycerophosphate) 97.2 mg Mag-4 (magnesium 97.2mg (4mmol)) tablets | 30 tablet £84.50
Oral capsule
▸ **Magnesium glycerophosphate (Non-proprietary)**
Magnesium (as Magnesium glycerophosphate) 48.6 mg Mag-4 (magnesium 48.6mg (2mmol)) capsules | 30 capsule £85.70
Magnesium (as Magnesium glycerophosphate) 97.2 mg Mag-4 (magnesium 97.2mg (4mmol)) capsules | 30 capsule £89.30
▸ **MagnEss Gly** (Essential-Healthcare Ltd)
Magnesium (as Magnesium glycerophosphate) 39.5 mg MagnEss Gly 39.5mg (1.6mmol) capsules | 50 capsule £28.17
Magnesium (as Magnesium glycerophosphate) 48.6 mg MagnEss Gly 48.6mg (2mmol) capsules | 50 capsule £35.87
Magnesium (as Magnesium glycerophosphate) 97.2 mg MagnEss Gly 97.2mg (4mmol) capsules | 50 capsule £37.87
▸ **MagnaPhos** (TriOn Pharma Ltd)
Magnesium (as Magnesium glycerophosphate) 39.5 mg MagnaPhos 39.5mg (1.6mmol) capsules | 50 capsule £28.32

Magnesium (as Magnesium glycerophosphate)
48.6 mg MagnaPhos 48.6mg (2mmol) capsules | 50 capsule £35.87
Magnesium (as Magnesium glycerophosphate)
97.2 mg MagnaPhos 97.2mg (4mmol) capsules | 50 capsule £37.75

Oral solution

▸ **LiquaMag GP** (Fontus Health Ltd)
Magnesium (as Magnesium glycerophosphate) 24.25 mg per
1 ml LiquaMag GP (magnesium 121.25mg/5ml (5mmol/5ml)) oral
solution | 200 ml £29.99 [SF]

▸ **MagnEss Gly** (Essential-Healthcare Ltd)
Magnesium (as Magnesium glycerophosphate) 19.44 mg per
1 ml MagnEss Gly 97.2mg/5ml (4mmol/5ml) oral solution | 200 ml
£29.97 [SF]
Magnesium (as Magnesium glycerophosphate) 24.25 mg per
1 ml MagnEss Gly 121.25mg/5ml (5mmol/5ml) oral solution | 200 ml
£31.97 [SF]

▸ **MagnaPhos** (TriOn Pharma Ltd)
Magnesium (as Magnesium glycerophosphate) 19.44 mg per
1 ml MagnaPhos 97.2mg/5ml (4mmol/5ml) oral solution | 200 ml
£25.57 DT = £10.91
Magnesium (as Magnesium glycerophosphate) 24.25 mg per
1 ml MagnaPhos 121.25mg/5ml (5mmol/5ml) oral solution | 200 ml
£37.87 DT = £37.87

Chewable tablet

EXCIPIENTS: May contain Aspartame

▸ **Magnesium glycerophosphate (Non-proprietary)**
Magnesium (as Magnesium glycerophosphate) 97.2 mg   Mag-4
(magnesium 97.2mg (4mmol)) chewable tablets | 30 tablet
£84.50 [SF]
Neomag (magnesium 97mg (4mmol)) chewable tablets |
50 tablet [PoM] £22.77 DT = £22.77 [SF]

▸ **MagnEss Gly** (Essential-Healthcare Ltd)
Magnesium (as Magnesium glycerophosphate) 97.2 mg   MagnEss
Gly 97.2mg (4mmol) chewable tablets | 50 tablet £15.44 DT =
£22.77 [SF]

▸ **MagnaPhate** (Arjun Products Ltd)
Magnesium (as Magnesium glycerophosphate)
97.2 mg MagnaPhate (magnesium 97.2mg (4mmol)) chewable tablets
| 50 tablet £22.64 DT = £22.77 [SF]

▸ **MagnaPhos** (TriOn Pharma Ltd)
Magnesium (as Magnesium glycerophosphate)
97.2 mg MagnaPhos 97.2mg (4mmol) chewable tablets | 50 tablet
£15.44 DT = £22.77 [SF]

Magnesium sulfate
12-Sep-2022

● INDICATIONS AND DOSE

**Severe acute asthma | Continuing respiratory
deterioration in anaphylaxis**
▸ BY INTRAVENOUS INFUSION
▸ Child 2-17 years: 40 mg/kg (max. per dose 2 g), to be
given over 20 minutes
▸ Adult: 1.2–2 g, to be given over 20 minutes

Prevention of seizures in pre-eclampsia
▸ INITIALLY BY INTRAVENOUS INJECTION
▸ Adult: Initially 4 g for 1 dose, to be given over
5–15 minutes, followed by (by continuous intravenous
infusion) 1 gram/hour for 24 hours, if seizure occurs,
give an additional dose of 2–4 g by intravenous
injection over 5–15 minutes

**Treatment of seizures and prevention of seizure
recurrence in eclampsia**
▸ INITIALLY BY INTRAVENOUS INJECTION
▸ Adult: Initially 4 g for 1 dose, to be given over
5–15 minutes, followed by (by continuous intravenous
infusion) 1 gram/hour for 24 hours after seizure or
delivery (whichever is later), if seizure recurs, give an
additional dose of 2–4 g by intravenous injection over
5–15 minutes

Hypomagnesaemia
▸ BY INTRAVENOUS INFUSION, OR BY INTRAMUSCULAR INJECTION
▸ Adult: Up to 40 g, given over a period of up to 5 days,
dose given depends on the amount required to replace
the deficit (allowing for urinary losses)

**Hypomagnesaemia maintenance (e.g. in intravenous
nutrition)**
▸ BY INTRAVENOUS INFUSION, OR BY INTRAMUSCULAR INJECTION
▸ Adult: 2.5–5 g daily, usual dose 3 g daily

Emergency treatment of serious arrhythmias
▸ BY INTRAVENOUS INJECTION
▸ Adult: 2 g, to be given over 10-15 minutes, dose may be
repeated once if necessary

Rapid bowel evacuation (acts in 2–4 hours)
▸ BY MOUTH
▸ Adult: 5–10 g, dose to be mixed in a glass of water,
taken preferably before breakfast

**Neuroprotection of neonate [in established preterm
labour or planned preterm birth within 24 hours]**
▸ INITIALLY BY INTRAVENOUS INJECTION
▸ Adult: Initially 4 g for 1 dose, to be given as a bolus
dose over 15 minutes, then (by continuous intravenous
infusion) 1 gram/hour until birth or for 24 hours,
whichever is sooner

DOSE EQUIVALENCE AND CONVERSION
▸ Magnesium sulfate heptahydrate 1 g equivalent to
Mg^{2+} approx. 4 mmol.

● **UNLICENSED USE** Magnesium sulfate may be used as
detailed below, although these situations are considered
unlicensed:
● severe acute asthma;
● continuing respiratory deterioration in anaphylaxis.
[EvGr] Magnesium sulfate is used for neuroprotection of
neonate in women with established preterm labour or
planned preterm birth within 24 hours, (A) but is not
licensed for this indication.

> **IMPORTANT SAFETY INFORMATION**
>
> MHRA/CHM ADVICE: MAGNESIUM SULFATE: RISK OF SKELETAL
> ADVERSE EFFECTS IN THE NEONATE FOLLOWING PROLONGED OR
> REPEATED USE IN PREGNANCY (MAY 2019)
> Maternal administration of magnesium sulfate for longer
> than 5–7 days in pregnancy has been associated with
> hypocalcaemia, hypermagnesaemia, and skeletal side-
> effects in neonates. Healthcare professionals are advised
> to consider monitoring neonates for abnormal calcium
> and magnesium levels, and skeletal side-effects if
> maternal treatment with magnesium sulfate during
> pregnancy is prolonged or repeated beyond current
> recommendations.

● **CONTRA-INDICATIONS**
▸ With oral use In rapid bowel evacuation—acute gastrointestinal conditions

● **CAUTIONS**
▸ With oral use In rapid bowel evacuation—elderly and
debilitated patients

● **INTERACTIONS** → Appendix 1: magnesium

● **SIDE-EFFECTS**
▸ **Rare or very rare**
▸ With oral use Paralytic ileus
▸ **Frequency not known**
▸ With intravenous use Bone demineralisation (reported in
neonates following prolonged or repeated use in
pregnancy) · electrolyte imbalance · osteopenia (reported
in neonates following prolonged or repeated use in
pregnancy)
▸ With oral use Diarrhoea · gastrointestinal discomfort ·
hypermagnesaemia

Overdose Symptoms of hypermagnesaemia may include
nausea, vomiting, flushing, thirst, hypotension,
drowsiness, confusion, reflexes absent (due to
neuromuscular blockade), respiratory depression, speech
slurred, diplopia, muscle weakness, arrhythmias, coma,
and cardiac arrest.

9
Blood and nutrition

- **PREGNANCY** For information on the risk of side-effects in neonates following prolonged or repeated maternal use of magnesium sulfate during pregnancy, see *Important Safety Information*.
- When used for Hypomagnesaemia or Arrhythmias or Prevention of seizures in pre-eclampsia or Treatment of seizures and prevention of seizure recurrence in eclampsia or Severe acute asthma or Continuing respiratory deterioration in anaphylaxis Not known to be harmful for short-term intravenous administration in eclampsia, but excessive doses in third trimester cause neonatal respiratory depression. Sufficient amount may cross the placenta in mothers treated with high doses e.g. in pre-eclampsia, causing hypotonia and respiratory depression in newborns.

- **HEPATIC IMPAIRMENT** Avoid in hepatic coma if risk of renal failure.

- **RENAL IMPAIRMENT**
- With intramuscular use or intravenous use [EvGr] Caution in mild to moderate impairment; avoid in severe impairment (increased risk of toxicity). [M]
- With oral use [EvGr] Avoid. [M]
  Dose adjustments
  - With intramuscular use or intravenous use [EvGr] Reduce dose (consult product literature). [M]

- **MONITORING REQUIREMENTS** Monitor blood pressure, respiratory rate, urinary output and for signs of overdosage (loss of patellar reflexes, weakness, nausea, sensation of warmth, flushing, drowsiness, double vision, and slurred speech).

- **DIRECTIONS FOR ADMINISTRATION**
- With intravenous use In severe hypomagnesaemia administer initially via controlled infusion device (preferably syringe pump). For *intravenous injection,* in arrhythmias, hypomagnesaemia, eclampsia, and pre-eclampsia, give continuously in Glucose 5% or Sodium Chloride 0.9%. Concentration of magnesium sulfate heptahydrate should not exceed 20% (200 mg/mL or 0.8 mmol/mL Mg^{2+}); dilute 1 part of magnesium sulfate injection 50% with at least 1.5 parts of Water for Injections. Max. rate 150 mg/minute (0.6 mmol/minute Mg^{2+}).

- **PRESCRIBING AND DISPENSING INFORMATION**
- With intramuscular use or intravenous use The BP directs that the label states the strength as the % w/v of magnesium sulfate heptahydrate and as the approximate concentration of magnesium ions (Mg^{2+}) in mmol/mL. Magnesium Sulfate Injection BP is a sterile solution of Magnesium Sulfate Heptahydrate.
- When used for Asthma For choice of therapy, see Asthma, acute p. 274 and Asthma, chronic p. 271.

- **EXCEPTIONS TO LEGAL CATEGORY**
- With oral use Magnesium sulfate is on sale to the public as Epsom Salts.

- **MEDICINAL FORMS** There can be variation in the licensing of different medicines containing the same drug. Forms available from special-order manufacturers include: oral capsule, solution for injection, infusion, solution for infusion

  Solution for injection
  - Magnesium sulfate (Non-proprietary)
    Magnesium sulfate heptahydrate 500 mg per 1 ml Magnesium sulfate 50% (magnesium 2mmol/ml) solution for injection 10ml ampoules | 10 ampoule [PoM] £21.71-£84.80 | 10 ampoule [PoM] £56.70 (Hospital only)
    Magnesium sulfate 50% (magnesium 2mmol/ml) solution for injection 20ml vials | 10 vial [PoM] £102.80
    Magnesium sulfate 50% (magnesium 2mmol/ml) solution for injection 5ml ampoules | 10 ampoule [PoM] £67.39-£75.10
    Magnesium sulfate 50% (magnesium 2mmol/ml) solution for injection 2ml ampoules | 10 ampoule [PoM] £17.35-£37.20

Solution for infusion
- Magnesium sulfate (Non-proprietary)
  Magnesium sulfate heptahydrate 100 mg per 1 ml Magnesium sulfate 10% (magnesium 0.4mmol/ml) solution for injection 10ml ampoules | 10 ampoule [PoM] £84.18-£97.23 DT = £54.00
  Magnesium sulfate 10% (magnesium 0.4mmol/ml) solution for infusion 10ml ampoules | 10 ampoule [PoM] £54.00 DT = £54.00
  Magnesium sulfate heptahydrate 200 mg per 1 ml Magnesium sulfate 20% (magnesium 0.8mmol/ml) solution for infusion 20ml ampoules | 5 ampoule [PoM] £99.00 (Hospital only)
  Magnesium sulfate 20% (magnesium 0.8mmol/ml) solution for infusion 10ml ampoules | 10 ampoule [PoM] £165.00 (Hospital only)
  Magnesium sulfate heptahydrate 500 mg per 1 ml Magnesium sulfate 50% (magnesium 2mmol/ml) solution for infusion 100ml vials | 10 vial [PoM] £141.40
  Magnesium sulfate 50% (magnesium 2mmol/ml) solution for infusion 50ml vials | 10 vial [PoM] £145.20

Powder
- Magnesium sulfate (Non-proprietary)
  Magnesium sulfate dried 1 mg per 1 mg Care Epsom Salts | 300 gram [GSL] £3.38

2.4 Phosphate imbalance

Phosphate imbalance
15-Dec-2021

Phosphate supplements

Oral phosphate supplements p. 1198 are licensed for the treatment of patients with vitamin D-resistant hypophosphataemic osteomalacia.

Phosphate deficiency may arise in patients with alcohol dependence. [EvGr] Phosphate depletion may also occur in patients with severe diabetic ketoacidosis, however phosphate replacement is not routinely recommended. [A]

Phosphate depletion in patients on total parenteral nutrition is common; for phosphate requirements in total parenteral nutrition regimens, see Intravenous nutrition p. 1227.

Phosphate-binding agents

[EvGr] For the management of hyperphosphataemia in patients with stage 4 or 5 chronic kidney disease (CKD), dietary management and dialysis (for patients who are having this) should be optimised prior to starting phosphate-binding agents. Both calcium-based and non-calcium-based preparations are used as phosphate-binding agents.

Calcium acetate p. 1195 should be offered as the first-line phosphate binder. If calcium acetate is not tolerated or is unsuitable (e.g. because of hypercalcaemia or low serum parathyroid hormone levels), sevelamer p. 1196 (a non-calcium-based phosphate binder) should be offered. For patients in whom sevelamer is unsuitable, consider calcium carbonate p. 1188 as an alternative if a calcium-based phosphate binder is needed, or sucroferric oxyhydroxide p. 1197 for patients who are on dialysis and do not need a calcium-based phosphate binder. Lanthanum p. 1195 (a non-calcium-based phosphate binder) should only be considered if other phosphate binders cannot be used.

For patients with stage 4 or 5 CKD who are on the maximum tolerated dose of a calcium-based phosphate binder but remain hyperphosphataemic, consider combining treatment with a non-calcium-based phosphate binder. [A]

For further guidance on the management of hyperphosphataemia in patients with CKD, see NICE guideline: **Chronic kidney disease: assessment and management** (available at: www.nice.org.uk/guidance/ng203).

2.4a Hyperphosphataemia

ELECTROLYTES AND MINERALS >
CALCIUM

▶ 1188

Calcium acetate
02-Dec-2021

- **INDICATIONS AND DOSE**

PHOSEX ® TABLETS

Hyperphosphataemia in patients with chronic renal failure on dialysis
▶ BY MOUTH
▸ Adult: Initially 1 tablet 3 times a day, to be taken with meals, dose to be adjusted according to serum-phosphate concentration, usual dose 4–6 tablets daily in divided doses, (1 or 2 tablets with each meal); maximum 12 tablets per day

RENACET ® TABLETS

Hyperphosphataemia in patients with chronic renal failure on dialysis
▶ BY MOUTH
▸ Adult: 475–950 mg, to be taken with breakfast and with a snack, 0.95–2.85 g, to be taken with a main meal and 0.95–1.9 g, to be taken with supper, dose to be adjusted according to serum-phosphate concentration; maximum 6.65 g per day

- **INTERACTIONS** → Appendix 1: calcium salts

- **SIDE-EFFECTS**
▸ **Uncommon** Vomiting

- **DIRECTIONS FOR ADMINISTRATION**

PHOSEX ® TABLETS Manufacturer advises *Phosex* ® tablets are taken with meals. Tablets can be broken to aid swallowing, but not chewed (bitter taste).

RENACET ® TABLETS Manufacturer advises that other drugs should be taken 1 to 2 hours before or after *Renacet* ® to reduce the possible interference with absorption of other drugs. *Renacet* ® tablets are taken with meals.

- **PRESCRIBING AND DISPENSING INFORMATION**

PHOSEX ® TABLETS *Phosex* ® tablets contain calcium acetate 1 g (equivalent to calcium 250 mg or Ca^{2+} 6.2 mmol).

RENACET ® TABLETS *Renacet* ® tablets contain calcium acetate 475 mg (equivalent to calcium 120.25 mg or Ca^{2+} 3 mmol).

- **PATIENT AND CARER ADVICE**

PHOSEX ® TABLETS Patients or carers should be given advice on how to administer *Phosex* ® tablets.

RENACET ® TABLETS Patients or carers should be given advice on how to administer *Renacet* ® tablets.

- **MEDICINAL FORMS** There can be variation in the licensing of different medicines containing the same drug.
Oral tablet
CAUTIONARY AND ADVISORY LABELS 25
▸ Phosex (Pharmacosmos UK Ltd)
Calcium acetate 1 gram Phosex 1g tablets | 180 tablet [PoM] £19.79 DT = £19.79
▸ Renacet (Stanningley Pharma Ltd)
Calcium acetate 475 mg Renacet 475mg tablets | 200 tablet [P] £14.95 DT = £14.95
Calcium acetate 950 mg Renacet 950mg tablets | 200 tablet [P] £19.75 DT = £19.75

Combinations available: *Calcium acetate with magnesium carbonate,* below

---

PHOSPHATE BINDERS

Calcium acetate with magnesium carbonate
04-Sep-2020

The properties listed below are those particular to the combination only. For the properties of the components please consider, calcium acetate above, magnesium carbonate p. 80.

- **INDICATIONS AND DOSE**

Hyperphosphataemia
▶ BY MOUTH
▸ Adult: Initially 1 tablet 3 times a day, adjusted according to serum-phosphate concentration, to be taken with food; usual dose 3–10 tablets daily; maximum 12 tablets per day

- **CONTRA-INDICATIONS** Hypercalcaemia · hypermagnesaemia · myasthenia gravis · third-degree AV block

- **INTERACTIONS** → Appendix 1: calcium salts · magnesium

- **DIRECTIONS FOR ADMINISTRATION** Manufacturer advises that other drugs should be taken at least 2 hours before or 3 hours after calcium acetate with magnesium carbonate to reduce possible interference with absorption of other drugs.

- **PATIENT AND CARER ADVICE** Patients or carers should be given advice on how to administer calcium acetate with magnesium carbonate tablets.

- **MEDICINAL FORMS** There can be variation in the licensing of different medicines containing the same drug.
Oral tablet
CAUTIONARY AND ADVISORY LABELS 25
▸ Rephoren (Vifor Fresenius Medical Care Renal Pharma UK Ltd)
Magnesium carbonate heavy 235 mg, Calcium acetate 435 mg Osvaren 435mg/235mg tablets | 180 tablet [PoM] £24.00 DT = £24.00

Lanthanum
09-Nov-2020

- **INDICATIONS AND DOSE**

Hyperphosphataemia in patients with chronic renal failure on haemodialysis or continuous ambulatory peritoneal dialysis (CAPD) | Hyperphosphataemia in patients with chronic kidney disease not on dialysis who have a serum-phosphate concentration of 1.78 mmol/litre or more that cannot be controlled by a low-phosphate diet
▶ BY MOUTH
▸ Adult: 1.5–3 g daily in divided doses, dose to be adjusted according to serum-phosphate concentration every 2–3 weeks, to be taken with or immediately after meals

- **CAUTIONS** Gastro-intestinal disorders

- **INTERACTIONS** → Appendix 1: lanthanum

- **SIDE-EFFECTS**
▸ **Common or very common** Constipation · diarrhoea · electrolyte imbalance · gastrointestinal discomfort · gastrointestinal disorders · headache · nausea · vomiting
▸ **Uncommon** Alopecia · appetite abnormal · arthralgia · asthenia · burping · chest pain · dizziness · dry mouth · eosinophilia · hyperglycaemia · hyperhidrosis · hyperparathyroidism · increased risk of infection · irritable bowel syndrome · malaise · myalgia · oral disorders · osteoporosis · pain · peripheral oedema · taste altered · thirst · vertigo · weight decreased

- **PREGNANCY** Manufacturer advises avoid—toxicity in *animal* studies.

- BREAST FEEDING Manufacturer advises caution—no information available.
- HEPATIC IMPAIRMENT Manufacturer advises caution (may be excreted in bile—possible risk of slower elimination and increased plasma concentrations in patients with reduced bile flow)—monitor liver function tests.
- DIRECTIONS FOR ADMINISTRATION Manufacturer advises tablets are to be chewed. Manufacturer advises each sachet of powder to be mixed with soft food and consumed within 15 minutes.
- PATIENT AND CARER ADVICE Patient and carers should be given advice on how to administer lanthanum tablets and powder.
- NATIONAL FUNDING/ACCESS DECISIONS
  For full details see funding body website
  Scottish Medicines Consortium (SMC) decisions
  ▸ Lanthanum carbonate chewable tablets (*Fosrenol®*) for the control of hyperphosphataemia in chronic renal failure patients (May 2007) SMC No. 286/06 Recommended with restrictions
  ▸ Lanthanum carbonate chewable tablets (*Fosrenol®*) for the control of hyperphosphataemia in adult patients with chronic renal failure not on dialysis with serum phosphate levels ≥1.78 mmol/L (October 2010) SMC No. 640/10 Not recommended
  ▸ Lanthanum carbonate oral powder (*Fosrenol®*) for the treatment of hyperphosphataemia in chronic renal failure patients (December 2012) SMC No. 821/12 Recommended with restrictions

- MEDICINAL FORMS There can be variation in the licensing of different medicines containing the same drug.
  Chewable tablet
  CAUTIONARY AND ADVISORY LABELS 21
  ▸ Lanthanum (Non-proprietary)
    Lanthanum (as Lanthanum carbonate) 500 mg Lanthanum carbonate 500mg chewable tablets | 90 tablet [PoM] £105.45–£198.50 DT = £124.06
    Lanthanum (as Lanthanum carbonate) 750 mg Lanthanum carbonate 750mg chewable tablets | 90 tablet [PoM] £155.21–£292.16 DT = £182.60
    Lanthanum (as Lanthanum carbonate) 1 gram Lanthanum carbonate 1g chewable tablets | 90 tablet [PoM] £164.55–£309.74 DT = £193.59
  ▸ Fosrenol (Takeda UK Ltd)
    Lanthanum (as Lanthanum carbonate) 500 mg Fosrenol 500mg chewable tablets | 90 tablet [PoM] £124.06 DT = £124.06
    Lanthanum (as Lanthanum carbonate) 750 mg Fosrenol 750mg chewable tablets | 90 tablet [PoM] £182.60 DT = £182.60
    Lanthanum (as Lanthanum carbonate) 1 gram Fosrenol 1000mg chewable tablets | 90 tablet [PoM] £193.59 DT = £193.59
  Oral powder
  CAUTIONARY AND ADVISORY LABELS 21
  ▸ Fosrenol (Takeda UK Ltd)
    Lanthanum (as Lanthanum carbonate) 750 mg Fosrenol 750mg oral powder sachets | 90 sachet [PoM] £182.60 DT = £182.60
    Lanthanum (as Lanthanum carbonate) 1 gram Fosrenol 1000mg oral powder sachets | 90 sachet [PoM] £193.59 DT = £193.59

Sevelamer

23-Apr-2024

- INDICATIONS AND DOSE
  RENAGEL®
  Hyperphosphataemia in patients on haemodialysis or peritoneal dialysis
  ▸ BY MOUTH
  ▸ Adult: Initially 2.4–4.8 g daily in 3 divided doses, dose to be given with meals and adjusted according to serum-phosphate concentration; usual dose 2.4–12 g daily in 3 divided doses

RENVELA® 2.4G ORAL POWDER SACHETS
Hyperphosphataemia in patients on haemodialysis or peritoneal dialysis | Hyperphosphataemia in patients with chronic kidney disease not on dialysis who have a serum-phosphate concentration of 1.78 mmol/litre or more
▸ BY MOUTH
▸ Adult: Initially 2.4–4.8 g daily in 3 divided doses, dose to be taken with meals and adjusted according to serum-phosphate concentration every 2–4 weeks—consult product literature; usual dose 6 g daily in 3 divided doses

RENVELA® 800MG TABLETS
Hyperphosphataemia in patients on haemodialysis or peritoneal dialysis | Hyperphosphataemia in patients with chronic kidney disease not on dialysis who have a serum-phosphate concentration of 1.78 mmol/litre or more
▸ BY MOUTH
▸ Adult: Initially 2.4–4.8 g daily in 3 divided doses, dose to be taken with meals and adjusted according to serum-phosphate concentration every 2–4 weeks; usual dose 6 g daily in 3 divided doses

- CONTRA-INDICATIONS Bowel obstruction
- CAUTIONS Gastro-intestinal disorders
- INTERACTIONS → Appendix 1: sevelamer
- SIDE-EFFECTS
  ▸ **Common or very common** Constipation · diarrhoea · gastrointestinal discomfort · gastrointestinal disorders · nausea · vomiting
  ▸ **Frequency not known** Skin reactions
- PREGNANCY Manufacturer advises use only if potential benefit outweighs risk.
- BREAST FEEDING
  RENAGEL® Manufacturer advises use only if potential benefit outweighs risk.
  RENVELA® 2.4G ORAL POWDER SACHETS Unlikely to be present in milk (however, manufacturer advises avoid).
  RENVELA® 800MG TABLETS Unlikely to be present in milk (however, manufacturer advises avoid).
- DIRECTIONS FOR ADMINISTRATION
  RENVELA® 2.4G ORAL POWDER SACHETS Manufacturer advises each sachet should be dispersed in 60 mL water, or mixed with a small amount of cool food (100 g), prior to administration and discarded if unused after 30 minutes.
- PATIENT AND CARER ADVICE
  RENVELA® 2.4G ORAL POWDER SACHETS Patients and carers should be advised on how to administer powder for oral suspension.
- NATIONAL FUNDING/ACCESS DECISIONS
  RENVELA® 2.4G ORAL POWDER SACHETS For full details see funding body website
  Scottish Medicines Consortium (SMC) decisions
  ▸ Sevelamer carbonate (*Renvela®*) for hyperphosphataemia in adult patients receiving haemodialysis (April 2011) SMC No. 641/10 Recommended with restrictions
  RENVELA® 800MG TABLETS For full details see funding body website
  Scottish Medicines Consortium (SMC) decisions
  ▸ Sevelamer carbonate (*Renvela®*) for hyperphosphataemia in adult patients receiving haemodialysis (April 2011) SMC No. 641/10 Recommended with restrictions

- **MEDICINAL FORMS** There can be variation in the licensing of different medicines containing the same drug.

Oral tablet

CAUTIONARY AND ADVISORY LABELS 25
EXCIPIENTS: May contain Propylene glycol

- ▸ **Renagel** (Sanofi)
  Sevelamer 800 mg Renagel 800mg tablets | 180 tablet [PoM]
  £167.04 DT = £28.45
- ▸ **Renvela** (Sanofi)
  Sevelamer 800 mg Renvela 800mg tablets | 180 tablet [PoM]
  £167.04 DT = £28.45

Powder for oral suspension

CAUTIONARY AND ADVISORY LABELS 13

- ▸ **Renvela** (Sanofi)
  Sevelamer carbonate 2.4 gram Renvela 2.4g oral powder sachets | 60 sachet [PoM] £167.04 DT = £167.04 [SF]

Sucroferric oxyhydroxide
07-Dec-2022

- **INDICATIONS AND DOSE**

Hyperphosphataemia in patients with chronic kidney disease on haemodialysis or peritoneal dialysis

- ▸ BY MOUTH
- ▸ **Adult:** Initially 1.5 g daily in 3 divided doses, dose to be taken with meals, then adjusted in steps of 500 mg every 2–4 weeks, dose adjusted according to serum-phosphate concentration; maintenance 1.5–2 g daily in divided doses; maximum 3 g per day

- **CONTRA-INDICATIONS** Haemochromatosis · iron accumulation disorders

- **CAUTIONS** Gastric disorders · hepatic disorders · major gastrointestinal surgery · peritonitis in the last 3 months

- **INTERACTIONS** → Appendix 1: iron

- **SIDE-EFFECTS**
- ▸ **Common or very common** Constipation · diarrhoea · gastrointestinal discomfort · gastrointestinal disorders · nausea · product taste abnormal · tooth discolouration · vomiting
- ▸ **Uncommon** Dysphagia · dyspnoea · electrolyte imbalance · fatigue · headache · skin reactions · tongue discolouration

  SIDE-EFFECTS, FURTHER INFORMATION Discoloured faeces may mask the visual signs of gastrointestinal bleeding.

- **PREGNANCY** Manufacturer advises use only if potential benefit outweighs risk—no information available.

- **BREAST FEEDING** Manufacturer advises avoid—no information available.

- **DIRECTIONS FOR ADMINISTRATION** Manufacturer advises *Velphoro*® tablets must be chewed or crushed, not swallowed whole.

- **PATIENT AND CARER ADVICE** Patients or carers should be counselled on administration of sucroferric oxyhydroxide tablets and advised that this medication can cause discoloured black stools.

- **MEDICINAL FORMS** There can be variation in the licensing of different medicines containing the same drug.

Chewable tablet

- ▸ **Velphoro** (Vifor Fresenius Medical Care Renal Pharma UK Ltd)
  Iron (as Sucroferric oxyhydroxide) 500 mg Velphoro 500mg chewable tablets | 90 tablet [PoM] £179.00 DT = £179.00

2.4b Hypophosphataemia

DRUGS AFFECTING BONE STRUCTURE AND MINERALISATION › MONOCLONAL ANTIBODIES

Burosumab
25-Apr-2025

- **DRUG ACTION** Burosumab is a human monoclonal antibody that inhibits the activity of fibroblast growth factor 23, thereby increasing renal tubular reabsorption of phosphate and increasing serum concentration of vitamin D.

- **INDICATIONS AND DOSE**

X-linked hypophosphataemia (initiated by a specialist)

- ▸ BY SUBCUTANEOUS INJECTION
- ▸ **Adult:** 1 mg/kg every 4 weeks (max. per dose 90 mg), dose may be administered 3 days either side of scheduled date if required, each dose should be rounded to the nearest 10 mg, dosing adjusted based on fasting serum-phosphate concentration—consult product literature

- **CONTRA-INDICATIONS** Concurrent use of oral phosphate or vitamin D analogues—discontinue 1 week before initiation of burosumab

- **SIDE-EFFECTS**
- ▸ **Common or very common** Back pain · constipation · dizziness · headaches · increased risk of infection · movement disorders · muscle spasms
- ▸ **Frequency not known** Hypersensitivity

- **PREGNANCY** Manufacturer advises avoid— toxicity in *animal* studies.

- **BREAST FEEDING** Manufacturer advises avoid—no information available.

- **RENAL IMPAIRMENT** Manufacturer advises avoid in severe impairment— no information available.

- **MONITORING REQUIREMENTS**
- ▸ [EvGr] Monitor fasting serum-phosphate concentration before treatment initiation, every 2 weeks for the first month, every 4 weeks for the following 2 months, 2 weeks after dose adjustment, and as appropriate thereafter— target the lower end of the normal reference range to decrease the risk of ectopic mineralisation. Periodic measurement of post-prandial serum-phosphate concentration is also advised.
- ▸ Monitor for signs and symptoms of nephrocalcinosis at treatment initiation, every 6 months for the first 12 months, and annually thereafter. Also monitor plasma alkaline phosphatase, calcium, parathyroid hormone, and creatinine every 6 months or as indicated, and urine calcium and phosphate every 3 months. Ⓜ

- **DIRECTIONS FOR ADMINISTRATION** [EvGr] Allow the vial to reach room temperature prior to administration. Inject into the upper arm, abdomen, buttock, or thigh. Maximum volume per injection site is 1.5 mL. If a volume over 1.5 mL is required on a given dosing day, the total volume should be split and given at 2 different injection sites. Ⓜ Patients or their carers may self-administer *Crysvita*® after appropriate training in subcutaneous injection technique.

- **PRESCRIBING AND DISPENSING INFORMATION** Burosumab is a biological medicine. Biological medicines must be prescribed and dispensed by brand name, see *Biological medicines* and *Biosimilar medicines*, under Guidance on prescribing p. 1; record the brand name and batch number after each administration.

- **HANDLING AND STORAGE** Store in a refrigerator (2-8°C) and protect from light.

- **PATIENT AND CARER ADVICE**
  Self-administration Patients or their carers should be given training in subcutaneous injection technique if appropriate.
  Driving and skilled tasks Patients and carers should be counselled on the effects on driving and performance of skilled tasks—increased risk of dizziness.

- **NATIONAL FUNDING/ACCESS DECISIONS**
  For full details see funding body website
  NICE decisions
  ▶ Burosumab for treating X-linked hypophosphataemia in adults (August 2024) NICE TA993 Recommended

- **MEDICINAL FORMS** There can be variation in the licensing of different medicines containing the same drug.
  Solution for injection
  EXCIPIENTS: May contain Polysorbates, sorbitol
  ▶ Crysvita (Kyowa Kirin Ltd)
    Burosumab 10 mg per 1 ml Crysvita 10mg/1ml solution for injection vials | 1 vial [PoM] £2,992.00 (Hospital only)
    Burosumab 20 mg per 1 ml Crysvita 20mg/1ml solution for injection vials | 1 vial [PoM] £5,984.00 (Hospital only)
    Burosumab 30 mg per 1 ml Crysvita 30mg/1ml solution for injection vials | 1 vial [PoM] £8,976.00 (Hospital only)

ELECTROLYTES AND MINERALS > PHOSPHATE

Phosphate

02-Mar-2023

- **INDICATIONS AND DOSE**
  Treatment of moderate to severe hypophosphataemia
  ▶ BY INTRAVENOUS INFUSION
  ▶ Adult: (consult product literature)
  Established hypophosphataemia (with monobasic potassium phosphate)
  ▶ BY INTRAVENOUS INFUSION
  ▶ Adult: 9 mmol every 12 hours, increased if necessary up to 0.5 mmol/kg (max. per dose 50 mmol), increased dose to be used in critically ill patients; dose to be infused over 6–12 hours, according to severity
  Vitamin D-resistant hypophosphataemic osteomalacia
  ▶ BY MOUTH USING EFFERVESCENT TABLETS
  ▶ Adult: 4–6 tablets daily, using *Phosphate Sandoz®*.

IMPORTANT SAFETY INFORMATION
  ▶ With intravenous use
  Some phosphate injection preparations also contain potassium. Expert sources advise for peripheral intravenous administration the *concentration* of potassium should not usually exceed 40 mmol/litre; the infusion solution should be **thoroughly mixed**. Local policies on avoiding inadvertent use of potassium concentrate should be followed. The potassium content of some phosphate preparations may also limit the *rate* at which they may be administered.

- **CAUTIONS**
  GENERAL CAUTIONS Cardiac disease · dehydration · diabetes mellitus · sodium and potassium concentrations of preparations
  SPECIFIC CAUTIONS
  ▶ With intravenous use Avoid extravasation · severe tissue necrosis

- **INTERACTIONS** → Appendix 1: phosphate

- **SIDE-EFFECTS**
  ▶ With intravenous use Electrolyte imbalance
  ▶ With oral use Abdominal distress · diarrhoea · nausea
  SIDE-EFFECTS, FURTHER INFORMATION Diarrhoea is a common side-effect and should prompt a reduction in dosage.

- **RENAL IMPAIRMENT**
  Dose adjustments Reduce dose.
  Monitoring Monitor closely in renal impairment.

- **MONITORING REQUIREMENTS** It is essential to monitor closely plasma concentrations of calcium, phosphate, potassium, and other electrolytes—excessive doses of phosphates may cause hypocalcaemia and metastatic calcification.

- **PRESCRIBING AND DISPENSING INFORMATION** *Phosphate Sandoz®* contains sodium dihydrogen phosphate anhydrous (anhydrous sodium acid phosphate) 1.936 g, sodium bicarbonate 350 mg, potassium bicarbonate 315 mg, equivalent to phosphorus 500 mg (phosphate 16.1 mmol), sodium 468.8 mg (Na^+ 20.4 mmol), potassium 123 mg (K^+ 3.1 mmol); *Polyfusor NA®* contains Na^+ 162 mmol/litre, K^+ 19 mmol/litre, PO_4^{3-} 100 mmol/litre; non-proprietary *potassium dihydrogen phosphate injection* (potassium acid phosphate) 13.6% may contain 1 mmol/mL phosphate, 1 mmol/mL potassium.

- **MEDICINAL FORMS** There can be variation in the licensing of different medicines containing the same drug. Forms available from special-order manufacturers include: infusion, solution for infusion
  Effervescent tablet
  CAUTIONARY AND ADVISORY LABELS 13
  ▶ Phosphate Sandoz (Stirling Anglian Pharmaceuticals Ltd)
    Sodium dihydrogen phosphate anhydrous 1.936 gram Phosphate Sandoz effervescent tablets | 100 tablet [GSL] £25.21 DT = £20.95
  Solution for infusion
  ▶ Phosphate (Non-proprietary)
    Potassium dihydrogen phosphate 136 mg per 1 ml Potassium dihydrogen phosphate 13.6% (potassium 10mmol/10ml) solution for infusion 10ml ampoules | 10 ampoule [PoM] £164.58 DT = £164.58
  Infusion
  ▶ Phosphate (Non-proprietary)
    Potassium dihydrogen phosphate 1.295 gram per 1 litre, Disodium hydrogen phosphate anhydrous 5.75 gram per 1 litre Polyfusor phosphates infusion 500ml bottles | 12 bottle [PoM] £223.32 (Hospital only)

2.5 Potassium imbalance

Hyperkalaemia

01-Jul-2024

Description of condition

Hyperkalaemia may be mild (serum-potassium concentration 5.5 – 5.9 mmol/litre), moderate (serum-potassium concentration 6.0 – 6.4 mmol/litre), or severe (serum-potassium concentration ≥ 6.5 mmol/litre). Patients most at risk of developing hyperkalaemia include those with chronic kidney disease (CKD), heart failure and diabetes. Some drugs can increase serum potassium concentration, these include ACE inhibitors, angiotensin-II receptor antagonists, mineralocorticoid receptor antagonists, potassium-sparing diuretics, NSAIDs, non-selective beta-adrenoceptor blockers, and trimethoprim.

Non-drug treatment

[EvGr] Non-dietary causes of hyperkalaemia such as constipation, acidosis, and poorly controlled diabetes should be managed accordingly. Patients with CKD and persistent hyperkalaemia should receive advice from a registered or specialist renal dietician on dietary strategies to reduce potassium intake after non-dietary measures have been addressed. [A]

Management of mild to moderate hyperkalaemia

[EvGr] Interventions to lower serum potassium should be initiated in patients with a serum potassium concentration ≥ 5.5 mmol/l. Most cases of mild or moderate hyperkalaemia detected in the community can be managed without the need for hospital admission, unless the patient is acutely unwell or has an acute kidney injury. For patients with moderate hyperkalaemia, their clinical condition, ECG and rate of potassium rise should be considered, and if necessary, treatment as for *severe hyperkalaemia* followed (see *Management of severe hyperkalaemia* below).

Drugs that exacerbate hyperkalaemia should be reviewed and managed as appropriate, taking into consideration both the risks and benefits of these drugs. Ⓐ For guidance on dose reduction or cessation of drugs contributing to hyperkalaemia, see the UK Kidney Association clinical practice guidelines **Management of Hyperkalaemia in Adults** (see *Useful resources*).

ᴱᵛᴳʳ For patients with CKD and a serum bicarbonate concentration < 22 mmol/litre, the use of sodium bicarbonate p. 1178 is recommended even in the absence of hyperkalaemia, as treatment of metabolic acidosis has additional benefits other than just lowering serum potassium.

A loop diuretic may be a useful adjunct for the treatment of chronic hyperkalaemia in patients who are non-oliguric and non-hypovolaemic.

On specialist initiation, a cation exchange compound such as patiromer calcium p. 1200 or sodium zirconium cyclosilicate p. 1201 may be used in certain patients with moderate hyperkalaemia who are otherwise unable to take an optimised dose of renin-angiotensin-aldosterone system (RAAS) inhibitors, or to take them at all, because of hyperkalaemia. Calcium polystyrene sulfonate below should no longer be routinely used, but it may be considered as a short-term option to treat chronic hyperkalaemia in non-hospitalised patients who do not meet the criteria for patiromer calcium or sodium zirconium cyclosilicate [unlicensed use]; however its effect is variable and unpredictable. Ⓐ

For further guidance on the management of mild to moderate hyperkalaemia, including cation exchange compounds, and monitoring of serum potassium concentrations, see the UK Kidney Association clinical practice guidelines **Management of Hyperkalaemia in Adults** (see *Useful resources*).

Management of severe hyperkalaemia

ᴱᵛᴳʳ Drugs exacerbating hyperkalaemia should be reviewed and withheld as appropriate.

Severe hyperkalaemia requires urgent hospital assessment as it can lead to life-threatening cardiac arrhythmias and cardiac arrest. Hyperkalaemia in the presence of ECG changes calls for urgent treatment with intravenous calcium chloride 10% p. 1188 [unlicensed use] or calcium gluconate 10% p. 1189, to temporarily protect against myocardial excitability. Calcium gluconate is the preferred calcium salt, except in a cardiac arrest/peri-arrest situation where calcium chloride is preferred.

An intravenous insulin-glucose infusion of 10 units soluble insulin [unlicensed use] and 25 g of intravenous glucose p. 1182 given over 5–30 minutes is recommended to move potassium into cells; this reduces serum-potassium concentration within 15 minutes (with the peak reduction occurring at 30–60 minutes). The patient's volume status and ease of administration should be considered when selecting the concentration of intravenous glucose solution (10%, 20%, or 50%) and the infusion rate. To reduce the risk of hypoglycaemia in patients with a pre-treatment blood glucose concentration < 7 mmol/litre, insulin-glucose treatment should be followed with an intravenous infusion of 10% glucose at a rate of 50 mL/hour for 5 hours (25 g); titrate the rate to maintain a blood glucose concentration of 4–7 mmol/litre. Adjunctive treatment with nebulised salbutamol p. 287 [unlicensed use] is also recommended as it has an additive effect on shifting potassium into the cells

when given with insulin and glucose. Consider repeating the insulin-glucose intravenous infusion if the serum-potassium concentration does not fall to < 6 mmol/litre within 2 hours after infusion or if rebound occurs. Seek specialist advice if the plasma-potassium concentration remains uncontrolled.

Sodium zirconium cyclosilicate or patiromer calcium are recommended in the emergency management of severe hyperkalaemia to remove potassium from the body. Calcium polystyrene sulfonate is no longer recommended for routine use in the management of acute hyperkalaemia, but may still have a role in certain circumstances such as intolerance of other cation exchange compounds. For some patients haemodialysis may be needed.

There is currently insufficient evidence to support the routine use of intravenous sodium bicarbonate for the acute treatment of hyperkalaemia, except in hyperkalaemic cardiac arrest. Ⓐ

For further guidance on the management of severe hyperkalaemia and strategies for preventing recurrence, and for guidance in hyperkalaemic cardiac arrest, see the UK Kidney Association clinical practice guidelines **Treatment of acute hyperkalaemia in adults** (see *Useful resources*).

Useful Resources

Clinical practice guidelines: treatment of acute hyperkalaemia in adults. UK Kidney Association. October 2023

ukkidney.org/health-professionals/guidelines/guidelines-commentaries

2.5a Hyperkalaemia

> **Other drugs used for Hyperkalaemia** Calcium chloride, p. 1188 · Calcium gluconate, p. 1189

ANTIDOTES AND CHELATORS ⟩ CATION EXCHANGE COMPOUNDS

▌Calcium polystyrene sulfonate   05-Oct-2021

● **INDICATIONS AND DOSE**

Hyperkalaemia associated with anuria or severe oliguria, and in dialysis patients

▸ BY MOUTH
▹ Adult: 15 g 3–4 times a day
▸ BY RECTUM
▹ Adult: 30 g, retained for 9 hours followed by irrigation to remove resin from colon

● **CONTRA-INDICATIONS** Hyperparathyroidism · metastatic carcinoma · multiple myeloma · obstructive bowel disease · sarcoidosis

● **INTERACTIONS** → Appendix 1: polystyrene sulfonate

● **SIDE-EFFECTS** Appetite decreased · constipation (discontinue—avoid magnesium-containing laxatives) · diarrhoea · electrolyte imbalance · epigastric discomfort · gastrointestinal disorders · gastrointestinal necrosis (in combination with sorbitol) · hypercalcaemia (in dialysed patients and occasionally in those with renal impairment) · increased risk of infection · nausea · vomiting

● **PREGNANCY** Manufacturers advise use only if potential benefit outweighs risk—no information available.

● **BREAST FEEDING** Manufacturers advise use only if potential benefit outweighs risk—no information available.

● **MONITORING REQUIREMENTS** Monitor for electrolyte disturbances (stop if plasma-potassium concentration below 5 mmol/litre).

● **DIRECTIONS FOR ADMINISTRATION**
▸ With rectal use Manufacturer advises mix each 30 g of resin with 150 mL of water or 10% glucose.

● **MEDICINAL FORMS** There can be variation in the licensing of different medicines containing the same drug. Forms available from special-order manufacturers include: enema
Powder for oral or rectal suspension
CAUTIONARY AND ADVISORY LABELS 13
▸ Calcium polystyrene sulfonate (Non-proprietary)
  Calcium polystyrene sulfonate 999 mg per 1 gram Calcium polystyrene sulfonate powder sugar free | 300 gram [PoM] £82.16 DT = £82.16 [SF]

Patiromer calcium
12-Apr-2023

● **DRUG ACTION** Patiromer is a non-absorbed cation-exchange polymer that acts as a potassium binder in the gastro-intestinal tract.

● **INDICATIONS AND DOSE**
Hyperkalaemia
▸ BY MOUTH
▸ Adult: Initially 8.4 g once daily; adjusted in steps of 8.4 g as required, dose adjustments should be made at intervals of at least one week; maximum 25.2 g per day
PHARMACOKINETICS
▸ Onset of action 4–7 hours.

● **CAUTIONS** Risk factors for hypercalcaemia (calcium partially released from counterion complex) · severe gastro-intestinal disorders (ischaemia, necrosis, and intestinal perforation reported with other potassium binders)

● **INTERACTIONS** → Appendix 1: patiromer

● **SIDE-EFFECTS**
▸ **Common or very common** Abdominal pain · constipation · diarrhoea · flatulence · hypomagnesaemia
▸ **Uncommon** Nausea · vomiting

● **PREGNANCY** Manufacturer advises avoid—no information available.

● **BREAST FEEDING** Manufacturer advises avoid—no information available (although no effects on the infant are anticipated).

● **MONITORING REQUIREMENTS** Manufacturer advises monitor for electrolyte disturbances, particularly plasma-potassium (as clinically indicated) and plasma-magnesium (continue to monitor for at least 1 month after initiation of treatment).

● **DIRECTIONS FOR ADMINISTRATION** Manufacturer advises *Veltassa* ® should be mixed with approx. 40 mL of water, then stirred and mixed with a further approx. 40 mL of water; the powder will not dissolve. More water may be added as needed. The mixture should be taken within 1 hour of preparation. Apple juice or cranberry juice may be used instead of water, other liquids should be avoided as they may contain high amounts of potassium.

● **HANDLING AND STORAGE** Store in a refrigerator (2–8°C) prior to dispensing; once dispensed, patient may store below 25°C for up to 6 months.

● **NATIONAL FUNDING/ACCESS DECISIONS**
For full details see funding body website
NICE decisions
▸ Patiromer for treating hyperkalaemia (February 2020)
NICE TA623 Recommended with restrictions
Scottish Medicines Consortium (SMC) decisions
▸ Patiromer sorbitex calcium (*Veltassa* ®) for the treatment of hyperkalaemia in adults [who have chronic kidney disease stage 3b to 5 and/or heart failure] (August 2021)
SMC No. SMC2381 Recommended with restrictions

▸ Patiromer sorbitex calcium (*Veltassa* ®) for the treatment of hyperkalaemia in adults [who have acute, life-threatening hyperkalaemia] (April 2023) SMC No. SMC2568 Recommended with restrictions

● **MEDICINAL FORMS** There can be variation in the licensing of different medicines containing the same drug.
Powder for oral suspension
CAUTIONARY AND ADVISORY LABELS 13
▸ Veltassa (Vifor Fresenius Medical Care Renal Pharma UK Ltd)
  Patiromer calcium (as Patiromer sorbitex calcium)
  8.4 gram Veltassa 8.4g oral powder sachets | 30 sachet [PoM] £172.50 DT = £172.50
  Patiromer calcium (as Patiromer sorbitex calcium)
  16.8 gram Veltassa 16.8g oral powder sachets | 30 sachet [PoM] £172.50 DT = £172.50

Sodium polystyrene sulfonate
05-Oct-2021

● **INDICATIONS AND DOSE**
Hyperkalaemia associated with anuria or severe oliguria, and in dialysis patients
▸ BY MOUTH
▸ Adult: 15 g 3–4 times a day
▸ BY RECTUM
▸ Adult: 30 g, retain for 9 hours followed by irrigation to remove resin from colon

● **CONTRA-INDICATIONS** Obstructive bowel disease

● **CAUTIONS** Congestive heart failure · hypertension · oedema

● **INTERACTIONS** → Appendix 1: polystyrene sulfonate

● **SIDE-EFFECTS** Appetite decreased · bezoar · constipation (discontinue—avoid magnesium-containing laxatives) · diarrhoea · electrolyte imbalance · epigastric discomfort · gastrointestinal disorders · increased risk of infection · nausea · necrosis (in combination with sorbitol) · vomiting

● **PREGNANCY** Manufacturers advise use only if potential benefit outweighs risk—no information available.

● **BREAST FEEDING** Manufacturers advise use only if potential benefit outweighs risk—no information available.

● **RENAL IMPAIRMENT** [EvGr] Use with caution. ◆M◆

● **MONITORING REQUIREMENTS** Monitor for electrolyte disturbances (stop if plasma-potassium concentration below 5 mmol/litre).

● **DIRECTIONS FOR ADMINISTRATION**
▸ With rectal use Manufacturer advises mix each 30 g of resin with 150 mL of water or 10% glucose.
▸ With oral use Manufacturer advises administer dose (powder) in a small amount of water or honey—do not give with fruit juice or squash, which have a high potassium content.

● **MEDICINAL FORMS** There can be variation in the licensing of different medicines containing the same drug. Forms available from special-order manufacturers include: oral suspension
Powder for oral or rectal suspension
CAUTIONARY AND ADVISORY LABELS 13
▸ Resonium A (Sanofi)
  Sodium polystyrene sulfonate 999.34 mg per 1 gram Resonium A powder | 454 gram [P] £81.11 DT = £81.11 [SF]

Sodium zirconium cyclosilicate
15-Nov-2022

- **DRUG ACTION** Sodium zirconium cyclosilicate is a non-absorbed cation-exchange compound that acts as a selective potassium binder in the gastro-intestinal tract.

- **INDICATIONS AND DOSE**

Hyperkalaemia
- ▸ BY MOUTH
  - ▸ Adult: Initially 10 g 3 times a day, for up to 72 hours, followed by maintenance 5 g once daily, adjusted according to serum-potassium concentrations. The usual maintenance dose range is 5 g once every other day to 10 g once daily

PHARMACOKINETICS
- ▸ Onset of action about 1 hour.

- **CAUTIONS** Abdominal X-ray (sodium zirconium cyclosilicate may be opaque to X-rays)

- **INTERACTIONS** → Appendix 1: sodium zirconium cyclosilicate

- **SIDE-EFFECTS**
- ▸ **Common or very common** Fluid imbalance · oedema · peripheral swelling
- ▸ **Frequency not known** Constipation · nausea

- **PREGNANCY** Manufacturer advises avoid—limited information; *animal* studies do not indicate toxicity.

- **MONITORING REQUIREMENTS** Manufacturer advises monitor serum potassium as clinically indicated.

- **DIRECTIONS FOR ADMINISTRATION** Manufacturer advises mix the contents of each 5- or 10-g sachet of powder with approx. 45 mL of water and stir well. The powder will not dissolve and the suspension should be taken while it is cloudy; if the powder settles it should be stirred again.

- **NATIONAL FUNDING/ACCESS DECISIONS**
For full details see funding body website
  NICE decisions
- ▸ Sodium zirconium cyclosilicate for treating hyperkalaemia (updated January 2022) NICE TA599 Recommended with restrictions

  Scottish Medicines Consortium (SMC) decisions
- ▸ Sodium zirconium cyclosilicate (*Lokelma*®) for the treatment of hyperkalaemia (HK) in adult patients [who have chronic kidney disease stage 3b to 5 and/or heart failure] (September 2020) SMC No. SMC2288 Recommended with restrictions
- ▸ Sodium zirconium cyclosilicate (*Lokelma*®) for the treatment of hyperkalaemia in adult patients [who have acute, life-threatening hyperkalaemia] (November 2022) SMC No. SMC2515 Recommended with restrictions

- **MEDICINAL FORMS** There can be variation in the licensing of different medicines containing the same drug.
  Powder for oral suspension
  CAUTIONARY AND ADVISORY LABELS 13
  - ▸ Lokelma (AstraZeneca UK Ltd)
    Sodium zirconium cyclosilicate 5 gram Lokelma 5g oral powder sachets | 30 sachet [PoM] £156.00 DT = £156.00
    Sodium zirconium cyclosilicate 10 gram Lokelma 10g oral powder sachets | 3 sachet [PoM] £31.20 DT = £31.20 | 30 sachet [PoM] £312.00 DT = £312.00

2.5b Hypokalaemia

ELECTROLYTES AND MINERALS ❭ POTASSIUM

Potassium bicarbonate with potassium acid tartrate
03-Aug-2020

- **INDICATIONS AND DOSE**

Hyperchloraemic acidosis associated with potassium deficiency (as in some renal tubular and gastro-intestinal disorders)
- ▸ BY MOUTH
- ▸ Adult: (consult product literature)

- **CONTRA-INDICATIONS** Hypochloraemia · plasma-potassium concentration above 5 mmol/litre

- **CAUTIONS** Cardiac disease · elderly

- **SIDE-EFFECTS** Diarrhoea · flatulence · gastrointestinal discomfort · nausea · vomiting

- **RENAL IMPAIRMENT** Avoid in severe impairment.
Monitoring Close monitoring required in renal impairment—high risk of hyperkalaemia.

- **DIRECTIONS FOR ADMINISTRATION** Manufacturer advises tablets to be dissolved in water before administration.

- **PRESCRIBING AND DISPENSING INFORMATION** These tablets do not contain chloride.

- **MEDICINAL FORMS** No licensed medicines listed.

Potassium chloride
29-Mar-2021

- **INDICATIONS AND DOSE**

Prevention of hypokalaemia (patients with normal diet)
- ▸ BY MOUTH
- ▸ Adult: 2–4 g daily in divided doses

Electrolyte imbalance
- ▸ BY INTRAVENOUS INFUSION
- ▸ Adult: Dose dependent on deficit or the daily maintenance requirements

> **IMPORTANT SAFETY INFORMATION**
> **SAFE PRACTICE**
> Potassium overdose can be fatal. Ready-mixed infusion solutions containing potassium should be used. Exceptionally, if potassium chloride concentrate is used for preparing an infusion, the infusion solution should be **thoroughly mixed**. Local policies on avoiding inadvertent use of potassium chloride concentrate should be followed.
>
> **NHS NEVER EVENT: MIS-SELECTION OF A STRONG POTASSIUM SOLUTION (JANUARY 2018)**
> Patients should not be inadvertently given a strong potassium solution (≥10% potassium w/v) intravenously, rather than the intended medication.

- **CONTRA-INDICATIONS** Plasma-potassium concentration above 5 mmol/litre

- **CAUTIONS**
- ▸ With intravenous use Seek specialist advice in very severe potassium depletion or difficult cases
- ▸ With oral use Cardiac disease · elderly · hiatus hernia (*with modified-release preparations*) · history of peptic ulcer (*with modified-release preparations*) · intestinal stricture (*with modified-release preparations*)

- **INTERACTIONS** → Appendix 1: potassium chloride

- **SIDE-EFFECTS**
  GENERAL SIDE-EFFECTS Hyperkalaemia
  SPECIFIC SIDE-EFFECTS
  ‣ With oral use Abdominal cramps · diarrhoea · gastrointestinal disorders · nausea · vomiting
- **RENAL IMPAIRMENT** Avoid in severe impairment.
  Dose adjustments Smaller doses must be used in the prevention of hypokalaemia, to reduce the risk of hyperkalaemia.
  Monitoring Close monitoring required in renal impairment—high risk of hyperkalaemia.
- **MONITORING REQUIREMENTS**
  ‣ Regular monitoring of plasma-potassium concentration is essential in those taking potassium supplements.
  ‣ With intravenous use ECG monitoring should be performed in difficult cases.
- **DIRECTIONS FOR ADMINISTRATION**
  ‣ With intravenous use Ready-mixed infusion solutions should be used where possible. EvGr If potassium chloride concentrate is used, it must be diluted and **thoroughly mixed** with Sodium Chloride 0.9% intravenous infusion, and given slowly. The maximum infusion rate is 20 mmol/hour. M For *peripheral intravenous infusion*, EvGr the concentration of potassium should not usually exceed 40 mmol/L. M Expert sources advise higher concentrations of potassium chloride may be given in very severe depletion, but require specialist advice.
- **PRESCRIBING AND DISPENSING INFORMATION** *Kay-Cee-L®* contains 1 mmol/mL each of K^+ and Cl^-.
  Potassium Tablets
  ‣ With oral use Do not confuse Effervescent Potassium Tablets BPC 1968 with effervescent potassium chloride tablets. Effervescent Potassium Tablets BPC 1968 do not contain chloride ions and their use should be restricted to hyperchloraemic states.
- **PATIENT AND CARER ADVICE** Patient or carers should be given advice on how to administer potassium chloride modified-release tablets.
  Salt substitutes A number of salt substitutes which contain significant amounts of potassium chloride are readily available as health food products (e.g. *LoSalt®* and *Ruthmol®*). These should not be used by patients with renal failure as potassium intoxication may result.
- **LESS SUITABLE FOR PRESCRIBING** Modified-release tablets are less suitable for prescribing. Modified-release preparations should be avoided unless effervescent tablets or liquid preparations inappropriate.

- **MEDICINAL FORMS** There can be variation in the licensing of different medicines containing the same drug. Forms available from special-order manufacturers include: modified-release tablet, oral solution, infusion, solution for infusion

Modified-release tablet
CAUTIONARY AND ADVISORY LABELS 25, 27
  ‣ Potassium chloride (Non-proprietary)
  Potassium chloride 600 mg Kaleorid LP 600mg tablets | 30 tablet PoM ⓧ
  Duro-K 600mg tablets | 100 tablet PoM ⓧ

Solution for infusion
  ‣ Potassium chloride (Non-proprietary)
  Potassium chloride 150 mg per 1 ml Potassium chloride 15% (potassium 20mmol/10ml) solution for infusion 10ml ampoules | 10 ampoule PoM £7.00 | 20 ampoule PoM £29.24 | 20 ampoule PoM £13.40 (Hospital only)
  Potassium chloride 15% (potassium 20mmol/10ml) concentrate for solution for infusion 10ml ampoules | 20 ampoule PoM £16.80
  Potassium chloride 200 mg per 1 ml Potassium chloride 20% (potassium 13.3mmol/5ml) solution for infusion 5ml ampoules | 10 ampoule PoM £14.00

Oral solution
CAUTIONARY AND ADVISORY LABELS 21
Infusion
  ‣ Potassium chloride (Non-proprietary)
  Potassium chloride 30 mg per 1 ml Potassium chloride 3% (potassium 40mmol/100ml) infusion 100ml bags | 1 bag PoM ⓧ (Hospital only)
  Potassium chloride 3% (potassium 20mmol/50ml) infusion 50ml bags | 1 bag PoM ⓧ (Hospital only)

3　Metabolic disorders

Metabolic disorders

29-Mar-2023

Use of medicines in metabolic disorders

Metabolic disorders should be managed under the guidance of a specialist. As many preparations are unlicensed and may be difficult to obtain, arrangements for continued prescribing and supply should be coordinated between the specialist centre, and local secondary and primary care.

Emergency management

For information on the emergency management of urea cycle disorders, consult the British Inherited Metabolic Disease Group (BIMDG) website at: www.bimdg.org.uk.

British Inherited Metabolic Disease Group (BIMDG) Metabolic Formulary

The BIMDG has developed a formulary to support healthcare professionals in the prescribing and monitoring of treatments for rare inherited metabolic disorders, see bimdg.org.uk/site/formularies.asp.

The formulary provides contact details of hospitals in the UK where access to specialist medications for metabolic disorders can be obtained in an emergency.

3.1　Acute porphyrias

Acute porphyrias

05-May-2022

Overview

The acute porphyrias (acute intermittent porphyria, variegate porphyria, hereditary coproporphyria, and 5-aminolaevulinic acid dehydratase deficiency porphyria) are hereditary disorders of haem biosynthesis; they have a prevalence of about 1 in 75 000 of the population.

Great care must be taken when prescribing for patients with acute porphyria, since certain drugs can induce acute porphyric crises. Since acute porphyrias are hereditary, relatives of affected individuals should be screened and advised about the potential danger of certain drugs.

EvGr Where there is no safe alternative, drug treatment for serious or life-threatening conditions should not be withheld from patients with acute porphyria. Where possible, the clinical situation should be discussed with a porphyria specialist for advice on how to proceed and monitor the patient. In the UK clinical advice can be obtained from the National Acute Porphyria Service or from the UK Porphyria Medicines Information Service (UKPMIS) (see *Useful resources*). E

Haem arginate p. 1204 is administered by short intravenous infusion as haem replacement in moderate, severe, or unremitting acute porphyria crises.

In the United Kingdom the National Acute Porphyria Service (NAPS) provides clinical support and treatment with haem arginate from two centres (Cardiff and Vale University

Health Board and King's College Hospital) (see *Useful resources*).

Drugs unsafe for use in acute porphyrias

[EvGr] The following list contains drugs that have been classified as 'unsafe' in porphyria because they have been shown to be porphyrinogenic in animals or in vitro, or have been associated with acute attacks in patients. Absence of a drug from the following lists does not necessarily imply that the drug is safe. For many drugs no information about porphyria is available. ⟨E⟩

An up-to-date list of drugs considered safe in acute porphyrias is available from the UKPMIS (see *Useful resources*).

Further information may be obtained from the European Porphyria Network (available at: porphyria.eu/) and UKPMIS (see *Useful resources*).

Quite modest changes in chemical structure can lead to changes in porphyrinogenicity but where possible general statements have been made about groups of drugs; these should be checked first.

Unsafe Drug Groups (check first)

- Anabolic steroids
- Antidepressants, MAOIs (contact UKPMIS for advice)
- Antidepressants, Tricyclic and related (contact UKPMIS for advice)
- Barbiturates (includes primidone and thiopental)
- Contraceptives, hormonal (for detailed advice contact UKPMIS or a porphyria specialist)
- Hormone replacement therapy (for detailed advice contact UKPMIS or a porphyria specialist)
- Imidazole antifungals (applies to oral and intravenous use; topical antifungals are thought to be safe due to low systemic exposure)
- Non-nucleoside reverse transcriptase inhibitors (contact UKPMIS for advice)
- Progestogens (for detailed advice contact UKPMIS or a porphyria specialist)
- Protease inhibitors (contact UKPMIS for advice)
- Sulfonamides (includes co-trimoxazole and sulfasalazine)
- Sulfonylureas (glipizide and glimepiride are thought to be safe)
- Taxanes (contact UKPMIS for advice)
- Triazole antifungals (applies to oral and intravenous use; topical antifungals are thought to be safe due to low systemic exposure)

Unsafe Drugs (check groups above first)

- Aceclofenac
- Alcohol
- Amiodarone
- Aprepitant
- Artemether with lumefantrine
- Bexarotene
- Bosentan
- Busulfan
- Carbamazepine
- Chloral hydrate (although evidence of hazard is uncertain, manufacturer advises avoid)
- Chloramphenicol
- Chloroform (small amounts in medicines probably safe)
- Clemastine
- Clindamycin
- Cocaine
- Danazol
- Dapsone
- Diltiazem
- Disopyramide
- Disulfiram
- Ergometrine
- Ergotamine
- Erythromycin
- Etamsylate
- Ethosuximide
- Etomidate
- Flutamide
- Fosaprepitant
- Fosphenytoin
- Griseofulvin
- Hydralazine
- Ifosfamide
- Indapamide
- Isometheptene mucate
- Isoniazid (safety uncertain, contact UKPMIS for advice)
- Ketamine
- Mefenamic acid (safety uncertain, contact UKPMIS for advice)
- Meprobamate
- Methyldopa
- Metolazone
- Metyrapone
- Mifepristone
- Minoxidil (safety uncertain, contact UKPMIS for advice)
- Mitotane
- Nalidixic acid
- Nitrazepam
- Nitrofurantoin
- Orphenadrine
- Oxcarbazepine
- Oxybutynin
- Pentazocine
- Pentoxifylline
- Pergolide
- Phenoxybenzamine
- Phenytoin
- Pivmecillinam
- Pizotifen
- Porfimer
- Raloxifene
- Rifabutin (safety uncertain, contact UKPMIS for advice)
- Rifampicin
- Riluzole
- Risperidone
- Spironolactone
- Sulfinpyrazone
- Tamoxifen
- Temoporfin
- Thiotepa
- Tiagabine
- Tibolone
- Topiramate
- Toremifene
- Trimethoprim
- Valproate
- Verapamil
- Xipamide

Useful Resources

Cardiff and Vale University Health Board National Acute Porphyria Service.
cavuhb.nhs.wales/our-services/laboratory-medicine/medical-biochemistry-and-immunology/porphyria-service-cardiff/national-acute-porphyria-service-naps/

King's College Hospital National Acute Porphyria Service.
www.kch.nhs.uk/service/a-z/porphyria

UK Porphyria Medicines Information Service. Drugs in porphyrias.
www.wmic.wales.nhs.uk/specialist-services/drugs-in-porphyria

BLOOD AND RELATED PRODUCTS > HAEM DERIVATIVES

Haem arginate
05-Oct-2021

(Human hemin)

- **INDICATIONS AND DOSE**

Acute porphyrias | Acute intermittent porphyria | Porphyria variegata | Hereditary coproporphyria
▸ BY INTRAVENOUS INFUSION
▸ Adult: Initially 3 mg/kg once daily for 4 days, if response inadequate, repeat 4-day course with close biochemical monitoring; maximum 250 mg per day

- **SIDE-EFFECTS**
▸ **Common or very common** Poor venous access
▸ **Rare or very rare** Fever
▸ **Frequency not known** Headache · injection site necrosis · skin discolouration · venous thrombosis

- **PREGNANCY** Manufacturer advises avoid unless essential.
- **BREAST FEEDING** Manufacturer advises avoid unless essential—no information available.
- **DIRECTIONS FOR ADMINISTRATION** For *intravenous infusion* (*Normosang* ®), manufacturer advises give intermittently in Sodium Chloride 0.9%; dilute requisite dose in 100 mL infusion fluid in glass bottle and give over at least 30 minutes through a filter *via* large antebrachial or central vein; administer within 1 hour after dilution.

- **MEDICINAL FORMS** There can be variation in the licensing of different medicines containing the same drug.
Solution for infusion
▸ **Normosang** (Recordati Rare Diseases UK Ltd)
Haem arginate 25 mg per 1 ml Normosang 250mg/10ml solution for infusion ampoules | 4 ampoule [PoM] £1,737.00 (Hospital only)

DRUGS FOR METABOLIC DISORDERS > SMALL INTERFERING RIBONUCLEIC ACID

Givosiran
13-May-2022

- **DRUG ACTION** Givosiran is a small interfering RNA, which reduces production of the enzyme ALAS1 involved in haem synthesis in the liver, thereby reducing accumulation of neurotoxic intermediates that cause acute porphyria attacks and symptoms.

- **INDICATIONS AND DOSE**

Acute hepatic porphyria (initiated under specialist supervision)
▸ BY SUBCUTANEOUS INJECTION
▸ Adult: 2.5 mg/kg once a month

- **INTERACTIONS** → Appendix 1: givosiran
- **SIDE-EFFECTS**
▸ **Common or very common** Fatigue · hypersensitivity · nausea · renal impairment · skin reactions

- **PREGNANCY** [EvGr] Use only if potential benefit outweighs risk—toxicity in *animal* studies. ◈
- **BREAST FEEDING** [EvGr] Avoid—present in milk in *animal* studies. ◈
- **RENAL IMPAIRMENT** [EvGr] Monitor renal function during treatment—progression of impairment reported. ◈
- **MONITORING REQUIREMENTS** [EvGr] Monitor liver function before treatment, every 4 weeks for the first 6 months of treatment, then as clinically indicated thereafter. For transaminase elevations consider discontinuing or interrupting treatment; restarting treatment at a reduced dose may be considered—consult product literature. ◈

- **DIRECTIONS FOR ADMINISTRATION** [EvGr] Maximum 1.5 mL per injection site; inject into the abdomen, thigh or upper arm and rotate injection site. Avoid injecting into scar tissue or skin that is reddened, inflamed or swollen. ◈
- **PRESCRIBING AND DISPENSING INFORMATION** [EvGr] The efficacy and safety data in acute hepatic porphyria (AHP) subtypes other than acute intermittent porphyria (hereditary coproporphyria, variegate porphyria and 5-aminolaevulinic acid dehydratase-deficient porphyria) are limited; this should be taken into consideration when assessing the individual benefit-risk in these rare AHP subtypes. ◈
- **NATIONAL FUNDING/ACCESS DECISIONS**
For full details see funding body website
NICE decisions
▸ **Givosiran for treating acute hepatic porphyria (November 2021)** NICE HST16 Recommended with restrictions

- **MEDICINAL FORMS** There can be variation in the licensing of different medicines containing the same drug.
Solution for injection
▸ **Givlaari** (Alnylam UK Ltd) ▼
Givosiran (as Givosiran sodium) 189 mg per 1 ml Givlaari 189mg/1ml solution for injection vials | 1 vial [PoM] £41,884.43 (Hospital only)

3.2 Alpha-mannosidosis

ENZYMES

Velmanase alfa
19-Dec-2023

- **DRUG ACTION** Velmanase alfa is an enzyme produced by recombinant DNA technology that provides replacement therapy for the treatment of alpha-mannosidosis, a lysosomal storage disorder caused by deficiency of alpha-mannosidase.

- **INDICATIONS AND DOSE**

Non-neurological manifestations of alpha-mannosidosis (under expert supervision)
▸ BY INTRAVENOUS INFUSION
▸ Adult: 1 mg/kg once weekly

- **CAUTIONS** Infusion-related reactions

CAUTIONS, FURTHER INFORMATION [EvGr] Infusion-related reactions can occur and velmanase alfa should only be administered when appropriately trained staff are available; pre-medication with an antihistamine and/or corticosteroid may prevent subsequent reactions in those who required symptomatic treatment. Patients should be closely monitored for signs of infusion-related reactions during and for at least 1 hour after administration, and managed appropriately—consult product literature. ◈

- **SIDE-EFFECTS**
▸ **Common or very common** Acute kidney injury · appetite increased · bradycardia · chills · confusion · cyanosis · diarrhoea · dizziness · epistaxis · eye erythema · eye irritation · eyelid oedema · fatigue · feeling hot · fever · gastrointestinal discomfort · headache · hyperhidrosis · hypersensitivity · insomnia · joint disorders · loss of consciousness · malaise · myalgia · nausea · pain · procedural headache · psychotic disorder · reflux gastritis · syncope · tremor · urticaria · vomiting · weight increased
▸ **Frequency not known** Hyperthermia · infusion related reaction

- **PREGNANCY** [EvGr] Avoid unless essential—limited information available. ◈
- **BREAST FEEDING** [EvGr] Suitable for use in breast-feeding—no information available but absorption by the infant is considered to be minimal. ◈

- **DIRECTIONS FOR ADMINISTRATION** EvGr For *intermittent intravenous infusion* (*Lamzede* ®), reconstitute each 10-mg vial with 5 mL Water for Injections to produce a 2 mg/mL solution; give requisite dose through a low-protein binding 0.22 micron in-line filter via an infusion pump, according to the recommended rate (max. 25 mL/hour) and duration (min. 50 minutes)—consult product literature. Patients tolerating their infusions well may be considered for home infusion—consult product literature. Ⓜ

- **PRESCRIBING AND DISPENSING INFORMATION** Velmanase alfa is a biological medicine. Biological medicines must be prescribed and dispensed by brand name, see *Biological medicines* and *Biosimilar medicines*, under Guidance on prescribing p. 1; record the brand name and batch number after each administration.

- **HANDLING AND STORAGE** Store in a refrigerator (2–8°C) and protect from light—consult product literature for storage conditions after reconstitution.

- **PATIENT AND CARER ADVICE** EvGr Patients or their carers should be given training in infusion technique, and be counselled on the signs and management of infusion-related reactions, if appropriate. Ⓜ

- **NATIONAL FUNDING/ACCESS DECISIONS**
  For full details see funding body website
  NICE decisions
  ▸ Velmanase alfa for treating alpha-mannosidosis (December 2023) NICE HST29 Recommended with restrictions

- **MEDICINAL FORMS** There can be variation in the licensing of different medicines containing the same drug.
  Powder for solution for infusion
  ▸ Lamzede (Chiesi Ltd) ▼
  Velmanase alfa 10 mg Lamzede 10mg powder for solution for infusion vials | 1 vial PoM £886.61 (Hospital only)

3.3 Amyloidosis

NEUROPROTECTIVE DRUGS

▌Eplontersen

25-Apr-2025

- **DRUG ACTION** Eplontersen is an antisense oligonucleotide inhibitor which inhibits transthyretin production.

- **INDICATIONS AND DOSE**
  Hereditary transthyretin amyloidosis (hATTR) [in patients with stage 1 or stage 2 polyneuropathy] (under expert supervision)
  ▸ BY SUBCUTANEOUS INJECTION
  ▸ Adult: 45 mg once a month, for information on vitamin A supplementation—consult product literature

- **SIDE-EFFECTS**
  ▸ **Common or very common** Cataract · proteinuria · vomiting

- **CONCEPTION AND CONTRACEPTION** EvGr Females of childbearing potential should use effective contraception during treatment; if conception is planned, eplontersen and vitamin A supplementation should be stopped and vitamin A levels monitored—consult product literature. Ⓜ

- **PREGNANCY** EvGr Avoid (limited information available— potential teratogenic risk due to unbalanced vitamin A levels, consult product literature). Ⓜ

- **BREAST FEEDING** EvGr Avoid (no information available). Ⓜ

- **HEPATIC IMPAIRMENT** EvGr Caution in moderate or severe impairment (no information available). Ⓜ

- **RENAL IMPAIRMENT** EvGr Use with caution if eGFR less than 45 mL/minute/1.73 m^2 (no information available). Ⓜ See p. 21.

- **PRE-TREATMENT SCREENING** EvGr Plasma vitamin A levels below the lower limit of normal should be corrected and any symptoms or signs of vitamin A deficiency should be evaluated before starting treatment. Ⓜ

- **DIRECTIONS FOR ADMINISTRATION** For *subcutaneous injection*, remove prefilled pen from the refrigerator at least 30 minutes before administration. Inject into the abdomen (except for the 5 cm around the navel), upper thigh, or back of upper arm (if not self-administered); rotate injection site and avoid skin that is scarred, red, bruised, tender, hard, or damaged. *Wainzua* ® may be self-administered or administered by a carer after appropriate training in subcutaneous injection technique.

- **HANDLING AND STORAGE** Store in a refrigerator (2–8°C) and protect from light—consult product literature about storage outside refrigerator.

- **PATIENT AND CARER ADVICE**
  Self-administration Patients and their carers should be given training in subcutaneous injection technique, if appropriate.
  User manual A user manual should be provided.

- **NATIONAL FUNDING/ACCESS DECISIONS**
  For full details see funding body website
  NICE decisions
  ▸ Eplontersen for treating hereditary transthyretin-related amyloidosis (November 2024) NICE TA1020 Recommended
  Scottish Medicines Consortium (SMC) decisions
  ▸ Eplontersen (*Wainzua* ®) for the treatment of hereditary transthyretin-mediated amyloidosis in adult patients with stage 1 and 2 polyneuropathy (April 2025) SMC No. SMC2755 Recommended

- **MEDICINAL FORMS** There can be variation in the licensing of different medicines containing the same drug.
  Solution for injection
  ▸ Wainzua (AstraZeneca UK Ltd) ▼
  Eplontersen (as Eplontersen sodium) 56 mg per 1 ml Wainzua 45mg/0.8ml solution for injection pre-filled pens | 1 pre-filled disposable injection PoM £31,954.12 (Hospital only)

▌Inotersen

27-Aug-2020

- **DRUG ACTION** Inotersen is an antisense oligonucleotide inhibitor which inhibits transthyretin production.

- **INDICATIONS AND DOSE**
  Stage 1 or stage 2 polyneuropathy in patients with hereditary transthyretin amyloidosis (hATTR) (initiated by a specialist)
  ▸ BY SUBCUTANEOUS INJECTION
  ▸ Adult: 284 mg once weekly, for dose adjustments due to side-effects and information on Vitamin A supplementation—consult product literature

- **CONTRA-INDICATIONS** Patients undergoing liver transplantation (no information available) · platelet count less than 100x10^9/litre before starting treatment · urine protein to creatinine ratio (UPCR) greater than or equal to 113 mg/mmol before starting treatment

- **CAUTIONS** Concomitant administration with nephrotoxic drugs · elderly · history of major bleeding

- **INTERACTIONS** → Appendix 1: inotersen

- **SIDE-EFFECTS**
  ▸ **Common or very common** Anaemia · appetite decreased · chills · eosinophilia · fever · glomerulonephritis · haematoma · headache · hypotension · influenza like illness · nausea · peripheral oedema · peripheral swelling · proteinuria · renal impairment · skin reactions · thrombocytopenia · vomiting
  ▸ **Frequency not known** Intracranial haemorrhage · solid organ transplant rejection · vitamin A deficiency

- **CONCEPTION AND CONTRACEPTION** Manufacturer advises women of childbearing potential should use effective contraception during treatment; if conception is planned, inotersen and vitamin A supplementation should be stopped and vitamin A levels monitored—consult product literature.

- **PREGNANCY** Manufacturer advises avoid unless essential (limited information available)—potential teratogenic risk due to unbalanced vitamin A levels, consult product literature.

- **BREAST FEEDING** Manufacturer advises avoid—present in milk in *animal* studies.

- **HEPATIC IMPAIRMENT** Manufacturer advises avoid in severe impairment (no information available).

- **RENAL IMPAIRMENT** Manufacturer advises avoid if eGFR less than 45 mL/minute/1.73 m^2. See p. 21.

- **PRE-TREATMENT SCREENING** Manufacturer advises plasma vitamin A levels below the lower limit of normal should be corrected and any ocular symptoms or signs of vitamin A deficiency should have resolved before starting treatment.

- **MONITORING REQUIREMENTS**
- ▶ Manufacturer advises monitor platelet count before starting treatment, every 2 weeks during treatment, and for 8 weeks after stopping treatment—consult product literature.
- ▶ Manufacturer advises monitor UPCR and eGFR before starting treatment, every 3 months or more frequently as clinically indicated during treatment, and for 8 weeks after stopping treatment—consult product literature.
- ▶ Manufacturer advises monitor hepatic enzymes before starting treatment, then 4 months after starting treatment, and annually thereafter or more frequently as clinically indicated.

- **DIRECTIONS FOR ADMINISTRATION** Manufacturer advises to take the syringe out of the refrigerator at least 30 minutes before administration. Patients may self-administer *Tegsedi*® after appropriate training in subcutaneous injection technique.

- **HANDLING AND STORAGE** Manufacturer advises store in a refrigerator (2–8°C) and protect from light—consult product literature for further information regarding storage outside refrigerator.

- **PATIENT AND CARER ADVICE** Manufacturer advises patients should immediately report any signs of unusual or prolonged bleeding, neck stiffness, or atypical severe headache.
  Self-administration Manufacturer advises patients and carers should be given training in subcutaneous injection technique.
  Missed doses If a dose is missed, the next dose should be administered as soon as possible, unless the next scheduled dose is within 2 days, in which case the missed dose should not be taken and the next dose should be taken at the normal time.

- **NATIONAL FUNDING/ACCESS DECISIONS**
  For full details see funding body website
  NICE decisions
- ▶ Inotersen for treating hereditary transthyretin amyloidosis **(May 2019)** NICE HST9 Recommended
  Scottish Medicines Consortium (SMC) decisions
- ▶ Inotersen (*Tegsedi*®) for the treatment of stage 1 or stage 2 polyneuropathy in adult patients with hereditary transthyretin amyloidosis (hATTR) **(August 2019)** SMC No. SMC2188 Recommended

- **MEDICINAL FORMS** There can be variation in the licensing of different medicines containing the same drug.
  Solution for injection
- ▶ **Tegsedi** (Swedish Orphan Biovitrum Ltd)
  Inotersen (as Inotersen sodium) 189.33 mg per 1 ml Tegsedi 284mg/1.5ml solution for injection pre-filled syringes | 4 pre-filled disposable injection PoM £23,700.00 (Hospital only)

Patisiran

31-Aug-2020

- **DRUG ACTION** Patisiran is a double-stranded small interfering RNA which reduces transthyretin production.

- **INDICATIONS AND DOSE**

  Stage 1 or stage 2 polyneuropathy in patients with hereditary transthyretin amyloidosis (hATTR) (initiated under specialist supervision)
  - ▶ BY INTRAVENOUS INFUSION
  - ▶ Adult: 300 micrograms/kg every 3 weeks (max. per dose 30 mg), dosage is based on actual body weight, for information on premedication, vitamin A supplementation, and missed doses—consult product literature

- **SIDE-EFFECTS**
- ▶ **Common or very common** Arthralgia · dyspepsia · dyspnoea · erythema · increased risk of infection · infusion related reaction · muscle spasms · peripheral oedema · vertigo
- ▶ **Frequency not known** Vitamin A deficiency

- **CONCEPTION AND CONTRACEPTION** Manufacturer advises women of childbearing potential should use effective contraception during treatment; if conception is planned, patisiran and vitamin A supplementation should be stopped and vitamin A levels monitored—consult product literature.

- **PREGNANCY** Manufacturer advises avoid unless essential (limited information available)—potential teratogenic risk due to unbalanced vitamin A levels, consult product literature.

- **BREAST FEEDING** Manufacturer advises avoid—present in milk in *animal* studies.

- **HEPATIC IMPAIRMENT** Manufacturer advises caution in moderate or severe impairment (no information available).

- **RENAL IMPAIRMENT** Manufacturer advises caution in severe impairment (no information available).

- **PRE-TREATMENT SCREENING** Manufacturer advises plasma vitamin A levels below the lower limit of normal should be corrected and any ocular symptoms or signs of vitamin A deficiency should be evaluated before starting treatment.

- **DIRECTIONS FOR ADMINISTRATION** Manufacturer advises for *intravenous infusion* (*Onpattro*®), filter through 0.45-micron syringe filter and dilute requisite dose with Sodium Chloride 0.9% to final volume of 200 mL; use a DEHP-free infusion set and give over about 80 minutes through an in-line filter (1.2 micron) at a rate of about 1 mL/minute for the first 15 minutes, then increase to about 3 mL/minute for the remainder of the infusion.

- **PRESCRIBING AND DISPENSING INFORMATION** Manufacturer advises patients should receive pre-medication (to reduce the risk of infusion-related reactions)—consult product literature.

- **HANDLING AND STORAGE** Manufacturer advises store in a refrigerator (2–8°C)—consult product literature for further information regarding storage outside refrigerator.

- **NATIONAL FUNDING/ACCESS DECISIONS**
  For full details see funding body website
  NICE decisions
- ▶ Patisiran for treating hereditary transthyretin amyloidosis **(August 2019)** NICE HST10 Recommended

Scottish Medicines Consortium (SMC) decisions
► Patisiran (*Onpattro*®) for the treatment of hereditary transthyretin-mediated amyloidosis (hATTR amyloidosis) in adult patients with stage 1 or stage 2 polyneuropathy (June 2019) SMC No. SMC2157 Recommended

● MEDICINAL FORMS There can be variation in the licensing of different medicines containing the same drug.
Solution for infusion
ELECTROLYTES: May contain Sodium
► Onpattro (Alnylam UK Ltd)
Patisiran (as Patisiran sodium) 2 mg per 1 ml Onpattro 10mg/5ml concentrate for solution for infusion vials | 1 vial PoM £7,676.47 (Hospital only)

Tafamidis
25-Jun-2024

● DRUG ACTION Tafamidis is a transthyretin stabiliser which inhibits amyloid formation, thereby delaying the development of nerve and cardiac muscle damage caused by transthyretin amyloidosis.

● INDICATIONS AND DOSE
Treatment of transthyretin amyloidosis in patients with stage 1 symptomatic polyneuropathy (ATTR-PN) [using 20 mg capsules] (initiated under specialist supervision)
► BY MOUTH
► Adult: 20 mg once daily

**Treatment of wild-type transthyretin amyloidosis in patients with cardiomyopathy (ATTR-CM) [using 61 mg capsules] (initiated under specialist supervision) |
Treatment of hereditary transthyretin amyloidosis in patients with cardiomyopathy (ATTR-CM) [using 61 mg capsules] (initiated under specialist supervision)**
► BY MOUTH
► Adult: 61 mg once daily

DOSE EQUIVALENCE AND CONVERSION
► Each 20 mg capsule contains tafamidis meglumine equivalent to 12.2 mg tafamidis.
► Each 61 mg capsule contains tafamidis equivalent to 80 mg tafamidis meglumine.
► Tafamidis and tafamidis meglumine are not interchangeable on a milligram-for-milligram basis.

● INTERACTIONS → Appendix 1: tafamidis

● SIDE-EFFECTS
► **Common or very common** Abdominal pain upper · diarrhoea · increased risk of infection
► **Frequency not known** Flatulence

● CONCEPTION AND CONTRACEPTION Exclude pregnancy before treatment and ensure effective contraception during and for one month after stopping treatment.

● PREGNANCY Avoid (toxicity in *animal* studies).

● BREAST FEEDING Avoid—present in milk in *animal* studies.

● HEPATIC IMPAIRMENT Manufacturer advises caution in severe impairment (no information available).

● PRESCRIBING AND DISPENSING INFORMATION Manufacturer advises tafamidis should be prescribed in addition to standard treatment, but before organ transplantation; it should be discontinued in patients who undergo organ transplantation.
The manufacturer of *Vyndaqel*® has provided a *Guide for Healthcare Professionals*.

● PATIENT AND CARER ADVICE
Missed doses Manufacturer advises if vomiting occurs after a dose is taken and the intact capsule is identified, another dose can be taken if possible; otherwise the next dose should be taken at the normal time.

● NATIONAL FUNDING/ACCESS DECISIONS
For full details see funding body website
NICE decisions
► Tafamidis for treating transthyretin amyloidosis with cardiomyopathy (June 2024) NICE TA984 Recommended
Scottish Medicines Consortium (SMC) decisions
► Tafamidis (*Vyndaqel*®) for the treatment of wild-type or hereditary transthyretin amyloidosis in adult patients with cardiomyopathy (November 2023) SMC No. SMC2585 Recommended

● MEDICINAL FORMS There can be variation in the licensing of different medicines containing the same drug.
Oral capsule
CAUTIONARY AND ADVISORY LABELS 25
EXCIPIENTS: May contain Sorbitol
► Vyndaqel (Pfizer Ltd) ▼
Tafamidis meglumine 20 mg Vyndaqel 20mg capsules | 30 capsule PoM £10,685.00 (Hospital only)
Tafamidis 61 mg Vyndaqel 61mg capsules | 30 capsule PoM £10,685.00 (Hospital only)

Vutrisiran
18-Sep-2023

● DRUG ACTION Vutrisiran is a double-stranded small interfering RNA which reduces transthyretin production.

● INDICATIONS AND DOSE
Hereditary transthyretin amyloidosis (hATTR) [stage 1 or stage 2 polyneuropathy] (initiated by a specialist)
► BY SUBCUTANEOUS INJECTION
► Adult: 25 mg every 3 months, for information on vitamin A supplementation and missed doses—consult product literature

● SIDE-EFFECTS
► **Common or very common** Arthralgia · dyspnoea · pain in extremity

● CONCEPTION AND CONTRACEPTION EvGr Females of childbearing potential should use effective contraception during treatment; if conception is planned, vutrisiran and vitamin A supplementation should be stopped and vitamin A levels monitored—consult product literature. Ⓜ

● PREGNANCY EvGr Avoid (limited information available—potential teratogenic risk due to unbalanced vitamin A levels, consult product literature). Ⓜ

● BREAST FEEDING EvGr Avoid (no information available). Ⓜ

● HEPATIC IMPAIRMENT EvGr Caution in moderate or severe impairment (no information available). Ⓜ

● RENAL IMPAIRMENT EvGr Caution in severe impairment (no information available). Ⓜ

● PRE-TREATMENT SCREENING EvGr Plasma vitamin A levels below the lower limit of normal should be corrected and any ocular symptoms or signs of vitamin A deficiency should be evaluated before starting treatment. Ⓜ

● DIRECTIONS FOR ADMINISTRATION Inject into the abdomen (except for around the navel), thigh, or upper arm; avoid skin that is scarred, red, inflamed, or swollen.

● NATIONAL FUNDING/ACCESS DECISIONS
For full details see funding body website
NICE decisions
► Vutrisiran for treating hereditary transthyretin-related amyloidosis (February 2023) NICE TA868 Recommended
Scottish Medicines Consortium (SMC) decisions
► Vutrisiran (*Amvuttra*®) for the treatment of hereditary transthyretin-mediated amyloidosis in adult patients with stage 1 or stage 2 polyneuropathy (September 2023) SMC No. SMC2596 Recommended

- **MEDICINAL FORMS** There can be variation in the licensing of different medicines containing the same drug.
  Solution for injection
  - **Amvuttra** (Alnylam UK Ltd) ▼
    Vutrisiran (as Vutrisiran sodium) 50 mg per 1 ml Amvuttra 25mg/0.5ml solution for injection pre-filled syringes | 1 pre-filled disposable injection [PoM] £95,862.36 (Hospital only)

3.4 Carnitine deficiency

AMINO ACIDS AND DERIVATIVES

Levocarnitine

29-Jun-2021

(Carnitine)

- **INDICATIONS AND DOSE**

Primary carnitine deficiency due to inborn errors of metabolism
  - BY MOUTH
  - Adult: Up to 200 mg/kg daily in 2–4 divided doses; maximum 3 g per day
  - BY SLOW INTRAVENOUS INJECTION
  - Adult: Up to 100 mg/kg daily in 2–4 divided doses, to be administered over 2–3 minutes

Secondary carnitine deficiency in haemodialysis patients
  - INITIALLY BY SLOW INTRAVENOUS INJECTION
  - Adult: 20 mg/kg, to be administered over 2–3 minutes, after each dialysis session, dosage adjusted according to plasma-carnitine concentration, then (by mouth) maintenance 1 g daily, administered if benefit is gained from first intravenous course

- **CAUTIONS** Diabetes mellitus
- **SIDE-EFFECTS**
  - **Rare or very rare** Abdominal cramps · diarrhoea · nausea · skin odour abnormal · vomiting

  SIDE-EFFECTS, FURTHER INFORMATION Side-effects may be dose-related—monitor tolerance during first week and after any dose increase.

- **PREGNANCY** Appropriate to use; no evidence of teratogenicity in *animal* studies.

- **RENAL IMPAIRMENT** Accumulation of metabolites may occur with chronic oral administration of high doses in severe impairment.

- **MONITORING REQUIREMENTS**
  - Monitoring of free and acyl carnitine in blood and urine recommended.

- **MEDICINAL FORMS** There can be variation in the licensing of different medicines containing the same drug. Forms available from special-order manufacturers include: oral capsule
  Oral solution
  - **Levocarnitine (Non-proprietary)**
    L-Carnitine 300 mg per 1 ml Levocarnitine 1.5g/5ml (30%) oral solution paediatric | 20 ml [PoM] [Ⓢ]
    Levocarnitine 1.5g/5ml (30%) oral solution paediatric sugar free | 20 ml [PoM] £46.99–£71.40 DT = £71.40 [SF] | 40 ml [PoM] £142.00 [SF] | 50 ml [PoM] £178.50 DT = £178.50 [SF] | 100 ml [PoM] £234.95 [SF]
  Oral capsule
  - **Levocarnitine (Non-proprietary)**
    L-Carnitine 250 mg Bio-Carnitine 250mg capsules | 125 capsule £17.04

3.5 Cystinosis

3.5a Nephropathic cystinosis

AMINO ACIDS AND DERIVATIVES

Mercaptamine

23-Nov-2023

(Cysteamine)

- **INDICATIONS AND DOSE**

Corneal cystine crystal deposits in patients with cystinosis (specialist use only)
  - TO THE EYE
  - Adult: Apply 1 drop 4 times a day, to be applied to both eyes (minimum 4 hours between doses); dose may be reduced according to response (minimum daily dose 1 drop in each eye)

CYSTAGON ®

Nephropathic cystinosis (specialist use only)
  - BY MOUTH
  - Adult (body-weight 50 kg and above): Initially one-sixth to one-quarter of the expected maintenance dose, increased gradually over 4–6 weeks to avoid intolerance, dose increased if there is adequate tolerance and the leucocyte-cystine concentration remains above 1 nanomol hemicystine/mg protein, maintenance 500 mg 4 times a day; maximum 1.95 g/m² per day

PROCYSBI ®

Nephropathic cystinosis (specialist use only)
  - BY MOUTH
  - Adult: Initially one-sixth to one-quarter of the expected maintenance dose, increased if there is adequate tolerance and the leucocyte-cystine concentration remains above 1 nanomol hemicystine/mg protein (measured using the mixed leucocyte assay), maintenance 650 mg/m² twice daily, administered every 12 hours; maximum 1.95 g/m² per day

---

IMPORTANT SAFETY INFORMATION

SAFE PRACTICE
Mercaptamine has been confused with mercaptopurine; care must be taken to ensure the correct drug is prescribed and dispensed.

- **CAUTIONS**
  - When used by eye Contact lens wearers
  - With oral use Dose of phosphate supplement may need to be adjusted if transferring from phosphocysteamine to mercaptamine

- **SIDE-EFFECTS**
  - **Common or very common**
  - When used by eye Dry eye · eye discomfort · eye disorders · vision blurred
  - With oral use Appetite decreased · asthenia · breath odour · diarrhoea · drowsiness · encephalopathy · fever · gastroenteritis · gastrointestinal discomfort · headache · nausea · skin reactions · vomiting
  - **Uncommon**
  - With oral use Compression fracture · gastrointestinal ulcer · hair colour changes · hallucination · joint hyperextension · leg pain · leucopenia · musculoskeletal disorders · nephrotic syndrome · nervousness · osteopenia · seizure
  - **Frequency not known**
  - With oral use Depression · intracranial pressure increased · papilloedema

- **ALLERGY AND CROSS-SENSITIVITY** [EvGr] Contra-indicated if history of hypersensitivity to penicillamine. ◈

- **PREGNANCY**
  ‣ With oral use Manufacturer advises avoid—teratogenic and toxic in *animal* studies.

- **BREAST FEEDING**
  ‣ With oral use Manufacturer advises avoid—no information available.

- **MONITORING REQUIREMENTS**
  ‣ With oral use Manufacturer advises leucocyte-cystine concentration, liver function, and haematological monitoring required—consult product literature. Manufacturer advises monitor for skin and bone abnormalities; dose reduction or treatment discontinuation may be required—consult product literature.

- **DIRECTIONS FOR ADMINISTRATION**
  PROCYSBI® Manufacturer advises capsules can be opened and contents sprinkled on food, water, acidic fruit juice or administered via an enteral feeding tube—consult product literature. Avoid dairy products and meals (rich in fats and protein) at least 1 hour before and after taking a dose.

- **PRESCRIBING AND DISPENSING INFORMATION**
  Mercaptamine has a very unpleasant taste and smell, which can affect compliance.

- **HANDLING AND STORAGE**
  ‣ When used by eye Manufacturer advises store in a refrigerator (2–8°C)—after opening store at room temperature up to 25°C for up to 7 days; protect from light.
  PROCYSBI® Manufacturer advises store in a refrigerator (2–8°C).

- **PATIENT AND CARER ADVICE**
  Driving and skilled tasks
  ‣ With oral use Manufacturer advises patients and carers should be counselled on the effects on driving and performance of skilled tasks—increased risk of drowsiness.
  ‣ When used by eye Manufacturer advises patients and carers should be counselled on the effects on driving and performance of skilled tasks—increased risk of blurred vision and visual disturbances.

  PROCYSBI® **Missed doses** Manufacturer advises if a dose is within 4 hours of the next dose, the missed dose should not be taken and the next dose should be taken at the normal time.

- **NATIONAL FUNDING/ACCESS DECISIONS**
  For full details see funding body website

  Scottish Medicines Consortium (SMC) decisions
  ‣ Mercaptamine (*Procysbi*®) for the treatment of proven nephropathic cystinosis (November 2023) SMC No. SMC2571
  Not recommended

  All Wales Medicines Strategy Group (AWMSG) decisions
  ‣ Mercaptamine bitartrate (*Procysbi*®) for the treatment of proven nephropathic cystinosis (May 2022) AWMSG No. 4804
  Recommended

- **MEDICINAL FORMS** There can be variation in the licensing of different medicines containing the same drug. Forms available from special-order manufacturers include: eye drops
  Gastro-resistant capsule
  CAUTIONARY AND ADVISORY LABELS 25
  ‣ Procysbi (Chiesi Ltd)
  Mercaptamine (as Mercaptamine bitartrate) 25 mg Procysbi 25mg gastro-resistant capsules | 60 capsule [PoM] £335.97 DT = £335.97
  Mercaptamine (as Mercaptamine bitartrate) 75 mg Procysbi 75mg gastro-resistant capsules | 250 capsule [PoM] £4,199.65 DT = £4,199.65

Eye drops
EXCIPIENTS: May contain Benzalkonium chloride, disodium edetate
‣ Mercaptamine (Non-proprietary)
Mercaptamine (as Mercaptamine hydrochloride) 4.4 mg per 1 ml Cystaran 0.44% eye drops | 15 ml [PoM] [Ⓢ] (Hospital only)
‣ Cystadrops (Recordati Rare Diseases UK Ltd)
Mercaptamine (as Mercaptamine hydrochloride) 3.8 mg per 1 ml Cystadrops 3.8mg/ml eye drops | 5 ml [PoM] £865.00 DT = £865.00

Oral capsule
CAUTIONARY AND ADVISORY LABELS 21
‣ Cystagon (Recordati Rare Diseases UK Ltd)
Mercaptamine (as Mercaptamine bitartrate) 50 mg Cystagon 50mg capsules | 100 capsule [PoM] £70.00 DT = £70.00
Mercaptamine (as Mercaptamine bitartrate) 150 mg Cystagon 150mg capsules | 100 capsule [PoM] £190.00 DT = £190.00

3.6 Fabry's disease

ENZYMES

Agalsidase alfa   21-Aug-2024

- **DRUG ACTION** Agalsidase alfa is a form of recombinant human alpha-galactosidase A used for long-term enzyme replacement therapy in Fabry's disease.

- **INDICATIONS AND DOSE**
  Fabry's disease (under expert supervision)
  ‣ BY INTRAVENOUS INFUSION
  ‣ Adult: 200 micrograms/kg every 2 weeks

- **INTERACTIONS** → Appendix 1: agalsidase alfa

- **SIDE-EFFECTS**
  ‣ **Common or very common** Arrhythmias · asthenia · chest discomfort · chills · cough · diarrhoea · dizziness · dyspnoea · excessive tearing · fever · flushing · gastrointestinal discomfort · headache · hoarseness · hypersomnia · hypertension · increased risk of infection · influenza like illness · joint disorders · malaise · musculoskeletal discomfort · myalgia · nausea · ototoxicity · pain · palpitations · peripheral oedema · peripheral swelling · rhinorrhoea · sensation abnormal · skin reactions · taste altered · temperature sensation altered · throat complaints · tremor · vomiting
  ‣ **Uncommon** Altered smell sensation · angioedema · hypersensitivity · sensation of pressure
  ‣ **Frequency not known** Heart failure · hyperhidrosis · hypotension · myocardial ischaemia

  SIDE-EFFECTS, FURTHER INFORMATION Infusion-related reactions; manage by interrupting the infusion, or minimise by pre-treatment with an antihistamine or corticosteroid — consult product literature.

- **PREGNANCY** Use with caution.

- **BREAST FEEDING** Use with caution—no information available.

- **DIRECTIONS FOR ADMINISTRATION** Administration for *intravenous infusion*, manufacturer advises give intermittently *in* Sodium Chloride 0.9%; dilute requisite dose with 100 mL infusion fluid and give over 40 minutes using an in-line filter.

- **MEDICINAL FORMS** There can be variation in the licensing of different medicines containing the same drug.
  Solution for infusion
  ‣ Replagal (Takeda UK Ltd)
  Agalsidase alfa 1 mg per 1 ml Replagal 3.5mg/3.5ml solution for infusion vials | 1 vial [PoM] £1,049.94 (Hospital only)

Agalsidase beta

21-Aug-2024

- **DRUG ACTION** Agalsidase beta is a form of recombinant human alpha-galactosidase A used for long-term enzyme replacement therapy in Fabry's disease.

- **INDICATIONS AND DOSE**

Fabry's disease (under expert supervision)
▸ BY INTRAVENOUS INFUSION
▸ Adult: 1 mg/kg every 2 weeks

- **INTERACTIONS** → Appendix 1: agalsidase beta
- **SIDE-EFFECTS**
▸ **Common or very common** Angioedema · arrhythmias · arthralgia · asthenia · chest discomfort · chills · cough · diarrhoea · dizziness · drowsiness · dyspnoea · eye disorders · fever · gastrointestinal discomfort · headache · hypertension · hyperthermia · hypotension · increased risk of infection · muscle complaints · musculoskeletal stiffness · nasal complaints · nausea · oedema · oral hypoaesthesia · pain · pallor · palpitations · respiratory disorders · sensation abnormal · skin reactions · syncope · temperature sensation altered · throat complaints · tinnitus · vasodilation · vertigo · vomiting
▸ **Uncommon** Dysphagia · ear discomfort · eye pruritus · influenza like illness · malaise · peripheral coldness · tremor
▸ **Frequency not known** Anaphylactoid reaction · hypersensitivity vasculitis · hypoxia

SIDE-EFFECTS, FURTHER INFORMATION Infusion-related reactions; manage by slowing the infusion rate, or minimise by pre-treatment with an antihistamine, antipyretic, or corticosteroid — consult product literature.

- **PREGNANCY** Use with caution.
- **BREAST FEEDING** Use with caution—no information available.
- **DIRECTIONS FOR ADMINISTRATION** For *intravenous infusion*, manufacturer advises give intermittently *in* Sodium Chloride 0.9%, reconstitute initially with Water for Injections (5 mg in 1.1 mL, 35 mg in 7.2 mL) to produce a solution containing 5 mg/mL. Dilute with Sodium Chloride 0.9% (for doses less than 35 mg dilute with at least 50 mL; doses 35–70 mg dilute with at least 100 mL; doses 70–100 mg dilute with at least 250 mL; doses greater than 100 mg dilute with 500 mL) and give through an in-line low protein-binding 0.2 micron filter at an initial rate of no more than 15 mg/hour; for subsequent infusions, infusion rate may be increased gradually once tolerance has been established.

- **MEDICINAL FORMS** There can be variation in the licensing of different medicines containing the same drug.

Powder for solution for infusion
▸ Fabrazyme (Sanofi)
Agalsidase beta 5 mg Fabrazyme 5mg powder for concentrate for solution for infusion vials | 1 vial PoM £315.08
Agalsidase beta 35 mg Fabrazyme 35mg powder for concentrate for solution for infusion vials | 1 vial PoM £2,196.59

Pegunigalsidase alfa

01-Aug-2024

- **DRUG ACTION** Pegunigalsidase alfa is a **pegylated** form of recombinant human alpha-galactosidase A used for long-term enzyme replacement therapy in Fabry's disease.

- **INDICATIONS AND DOSE**

Fabry's disease (under expert supervision)
▸ BY INTRAVENOUS INFUSION
▸ Adult: 1 mg/kg every 2 weeks

- **CAUTIONS** Infusion-related reactions

CAUTIONS, FURTHER INFORMATION
▸ Infusion-related reactions EvGr Infusion-related reactions can occur and pegunigalsidase alfa should only be administered when appropriately trained staff and resuscitation facilities are available; these reactions may be minimised by pre-medication with an antihistamine and corticosteroid. Patients should be closely monitored for signs of infusion-related reactions during and for 2 hours after administration, and managed appropriately—consult product literature. Ⓜ

- **SIDE-EFFECTS**
▸ **Common or very common** Anxiety · arrhythmias · arthralgia · asthenia · chest discomfort · chills · diarrhoea · dizziness · gastrointestinal discomfort · headache · hypersensitivity · infusion related reaction · malaise · musculoskeletal stiffness · myalgia · nausea · pain · paraesthesia · skin reactions · vertigo · vomiting
▸ **Uncommon** Bronchospasm · chronic kidney disease · dyspnoea · flushing · gastrointestinal disorders · glomerulonephritis membranoproliferative · hypertension · hypohidrosis · hypotension · influenza like illness · insomnia · lymphoedema · nasal complaints · nipple pain · oedema · peripheral neuropathy · proteinuria · restless legs · throat irritation · tremor · ventricular hypertrophy · weight increased

- **PREGNANCY** EvGr Use with caution (no information available). Ⓜ
- **BREAST FEEDING** Specialist sources indicate use with caution (no information available). Large molecular weight suggests limited excretion into milk and drug molecule likely to be partially destroyed in the infant's gastro-intestinal tract.

- **DIRECTIONS FOR ADMINISTRATION** EvGr For *intermittent intravenous infusion* (*Elfabrio*®), dilute requisite dose with Sodium Chloride 0.9% (for patients weighing up to 70 kg, dilute to at least 150 mL; for patients weighing 70–100 kg, dilute to at least 250 mL; for patients weighing more than 100 kg, dilute to at least 500 mL) and give over at least 3 hours initially using an in-line low-protein binding 0.2 micron filter—consult product literature. Patients who are stabilised may be considered for home infusion under the supervision of a healthcare professional—consult product literature. Ⓜ

- **PRESCRIBING AND DISPENSING INFORMATION** Pegunigalsidase alfa is a biological medicine. Biological medicines must be prescribed and dispensed by brand name, see *Biological medicines* and *Biosimilar medicines*, under Guidance on prescribing p. 1; record the brand name and batch number after each administration.

- **HANDLING AND STORAGE** Store in a refrigerator (2–8°C)—consult product literature for storage conditions after dilution.

- **PATIENT AND CARER ADVICE**
Driving and skilled tasks Patients and carers should be cautioned on the effects on driving and performance of skilled tasks—increased risk of dizziness or vertigo.

- **NATIONAL FUNDING/ACCESS DECISIONS**
For full details see funding body website

NICE decisions
▸ **Pegunigalsidase alfa for treating Fabry disease (October 2023)** NICE TA915 Recommended

Scottish Medicines Consortium (SMC) decisions
▸ **Pegunigalsidase alfa (*Elfabrio*®) as long-term enzyme replacement therapy in adult patients with confirmed diagnosis of Fabry disease (deficiency of alpha galactosidase) (July 2024)** SMC No. SMC2665 Recommended with restrictions

- **MEDICINAL FORMS** There can be variation in the licensing of different medicines containing the same drug.
Solution for infusion
ELECTROLYTES: May contain Sodium
  - ▸ **Elfabrio** (Chiesi Ltd) ▼
    Pegunigalsidase alfa 2 mg per 1 ml Elfabrio 5mg/2.5ml concentrate for solution for infusion vials | 1 vial [PoM] £313.80 (Hospital only)
    Elfabrio 20mg/10ml concentrate for solution for infusion vials | 1 vial [PoM] £1,255.19 (Hospital only)

ENZYME STABILISER

Migalastat
04-Oct-2023

- **DRUG ACTION** Migalastat is a pharmacological chaperone that binds to the active sites of certain mutant forms of alpha-galactosidase A, thereby stabilising these mutant forms in the endoplasmic reticulum, and facilitating normal trafficking to lysosomes.

- **INDICATIONS AND DOSE**
Fabry's disease (under expert supervision)
  - ▸ BY MOUTH
  - ▸ Adult: 123 mg once daily on alternate days, to be taken at the same time of day

IMPORTANT SAFETY INFORMATION
SAFE PRACTICE
Migalastat could be confused with miglustat; care must be taken to ensure the correct drug is prescribed and dispensed.

- **SIDE-EFFECTS**
- ▸ **Common or very common** Constipation · defaecation urgency · depression · diarrhoea · dizziness · dry mouth · dyspnoea · epistaxis · fatigue · gastrointestinal discomfort · headache · muscle complaints · nausea · pain · palpitations · proteinuria · sensation abnormal · skin reactions · torticollis · vertigo · weight increased
- **PREGNANCY** Manufacturer advises avoid—toxicity in *animal* studies.
- **BREAST FEEDING** Manufacturer advises avoid—present in milk in *animal* studies.
- **RENAL IMPAIRMENT** See p. 21. Manufacturer advises avoid if eGFR less than 30 mL/minute/1.73 m^2.
- **MONITORING REQUIREMENTS** Manufacturer advises monitor renal function, echocardiographic parameters and biochemical markers every 6 months.
- **DIRECTIONS FOR ADMINISTRATION** Food should not be consumed at least 2 hours before and 2 hours after taking *Galafold*® capsules (minimum 4 hours fast).
- **PATIENT AND CARER ADVICE** Patients or carers should be given advice on how to administer *Galafold*® capsules.
Missed doses If a dose is more than 12 hours late, the missed dose should not be taken and the next dose should be taken on the normal day and at the normal time (not to be taken on 2 consecutive days).
- **NATIONAL FUNDING/ACCESS DECISIONS**
For full details see funding body website
NICE decisions
- ▸ **Migalastat for treating Fabry disease (February 2017)** NICE HST4 Recommended with restrictions
Scottish Medicines Consortium (SMC) decisions
- ▸ **Migalastat (*Galafold*®) for long-term treatment of adults and adolescents aged 16 years and older with a confirmed diagnosis of Fabry disease (α-galactosidase A deficiency) and who have an amenable mutation (November 2016)** SMC No. 1196/16 Recommended with restrictions

- **MEDICINAL FORMS** There can be variation in the licensing of different medicines containing the same drug.
Oral capsule
CAUTIONARY AND ADVISORY LABELS 25
  - ▸ **Galafold** (Amicus Therapeutics UK Operations Ltd)
    Migalastat (as Migalastat hydrochloride) 123 mg Galafold 123mg capsules | 14 capsule [PoM] £16,153.85 (Hospital only)

3.7 Gaucher's disease

Other drugs used for Gaucher's disease Miglustat, p. 1217

ENZYME INHIBITORS ❯ GLUCOSYLCERAMIDE SYNTHASE INHIBITORS

Eliglustat
26-Aug-2020

- **DRUG ACTION** Eliglustat is an inhibitor of glucosylceramide synthase.

- **INDICATIONS AND DOSE**
Type 1 Gaucher disease (CYP2D6 poor metabolisers) (under expert supervision)
  - ▸ BY MOUTH
  - ▸ Adult: 84 mg once daily

Type 1 Gaucher disease (CYP2D6 intermediate or extensive metabolisers) (under expert supervision)
  - ▸ BY MOUTH
  - ▸ Adult: 84 mg twice daily

- **CONTRA-INDICATIONS** Cardiac disease (no information available) · concurrent use of Class IA and Class III antiarrhythmics · long QT syndrome (no information available)
- **INTERACTIONS** → Appendix 1: eliglustat
- **SIDE-EFFECTS**
- ▸ **Common or very common** Arthralgia · constipation · dry mouth · dry skin · dyspepsia · dysphagia · fatigue · gastrointestinal disorders · nausea · palpitations · taste altered · throat irritation
- **PREGNANCY** Manufacturer advises avoid—limited information available.
- **BREAST FEEDING** Manufacturer advises avoid—present in milk in *animal* studies.
- **PRE-TREATMENT SCREENING** Manufacturer advises CYP2D6 metaboliser status should be determined before initiation of treatment.
- **MONITORING REQUIREMENTS**
- ▸ For treatment-naive patients showing less than 20% spleen volume reduction after 9 months of treatment, manufacturer advises monitor for further improvement or consider an alternative treatment.
- ▸ For patients with stable disease who have switched from enzyme replacement therapy, manufacturer advises monitor for disease progression—consider reinstitution of enzyme replacement therapy or an alternative treatment if response sub-optimal.
- **PRESCRIBING AND DISPENSING INFORMATION** The manufacturer of *Cerdelga*® has provided a *Prescriber Guide*, which includes a prescriber checklist.
- **PATIENT AND CARER ADVICE** A patient alert card should be provided.
- **NATIONAL FUNDING/ACCESS DECISIONS**
For full details see funding body website
NICE decisions
- ▸ **Eliglustat for treating type 1 Gaucher disease (June 2017)** NICE HST5 Recommended

Scottish Medicines Consortium (SMC) decisions
► Eliglustat (*Cerdelga*®) for the long-term treatment of adult patients with Gaucher disease type 1 (GD1) who are CYP2D6 poor metabolisers, intermediate metabolisers or extensive metabolisers (December 2017) SMC No. 1277/17 Recommended

● MEDICINAL FORMS There can be variation in the licensing of different medicines containing the same drug.
Oral capsule
CAUTIONARY AND ADVISORY LABELS 10
► Cerdelga (Sanofi) ▼
Eliglustat (as Eliglustat tartrate) 84.4 mg Cerdelga 84mg capsules | 56 capsule [PoM] £19,164.96

ENZYMES

Imiglucerase

21-Jul-2020

● DRUG ACTION Imiglucerase is an enzyme produced by recombinant DNA technology that is administered as enzyme replacement therapy for non-neurological manifestations of type I or type III Gaucher's disease, a familial disorder affecting principally the liver, spleen, bone marrow, and lymph nodes.

● INDICATIONS AND DOSE

Non-neurological manifestations of type I Gaucher's disease (specialist use only) | Non-neurological manifestations of type III Gaucher's disease (specialist use only)
► BY INTRAVENOUS INFUSION
► Adult: Initially 60 units/kg every 2 weeks; maintenance, adjusted according to response, doses as low as 15 units/kg once every 2 weeks may improve haematological parameters and organomegaly

● SIDE-EFFECTS
► **Common or very common** Angioedema · cough · dyspnoea · hypersensitivity · skin reactions
► **Uncommon** Abdominal cramps · arthralgia · back pain · chest discomfort · chills · cyanosis · diarrhoea · dizziness · fatigue · fever · flushing · headache · hypotension · nausea · paraesthesia · tachycardia · vomiting

● PREGNANCY Manufacturer advises use with caution—limited information available.

● BREAST FEEDING No information available.

● MONITORING REQUIREMENTS
► Monitor for immunoglobulin G (IgG) antibodies to imiglucerase.
► When stabilised, monitor all parameters and response to treatment at intervals of 6–12 months.

● DIRECTIONS FOR ADMINISTRATION For *intravenous infusion* (*Cerezyme*®), manufacturer advises give intermittently in Sodium Chloride 0.9%; initially reconstitute with Water for Injections (400 units in 10.2 mL) to give 40 units/mL solution; dilute requisite dose with infusion fluid to a final volume of 100–200 mL and give initial dose at a rate not exceeding 0.5 units/kg/minute, subsequent doses to be given at a rate not exceeding 1 unit/kg/minute; administer within 3 hours after reconstitution.

● MEDICINAL FORMS There can be variation in the licensing of different medicines containing the same drug.
Powder for solution for infusion
ELECTROLYTES: May contain Sodium
► Cerezyme (Sanofi)
Imiglucerase 400 unit Cerezyme 400unit powder for concentrate for solution for infusion vials | 1 vial [PoM] £1,071.29 (Hospital only)

Velaglucerase alfa

29-Jul-2020

● DRUG ACTION Velaglucerase alfa is an enzyme produced by recombinant DNA technology that is administered as enzyme replacement therapy for the treatment of type I Gaucher's disease.

● INDICATIONS AND DOSE

Type I Gaucher's disease (specialist use only)
► BY INTRAVENOUS INFUSION
► Adult: Initially 60 units/kg every 2 weeks; adjusted according to response to 15–60 units/kg every 2 weeks

● SIDE-EFFECTS
► **Common or very common** Arthralgia · asthenia · chest discomfort · dizziness · dyspnoea · fever · flushing · gastrointestinal discomfort · headache · hypersensitivity · hypertension · hypotension · infusion related reaction · nausea · pain · skin reactions · tachycardia
SIDE-EFFECTS, FURTHER INFORMATION Infusion-related reactions are very common; manage by slowing the infusion rate, or interrupting the infusion, or minimise by pre-treatment with an antihistamine, antipyretic, or corticosteroid—consult product literature.

● PREGNANCY Manufacturer advises use with caution—limited information available.

● BREAST FEEDING Manufacturer advises use with caution—no information available.

● MONITORING REQUIREMENTS Monitor immunoglobulin G (IgG) antibody concentration in severe infusion-related reactions or if there is a lack or loss of effect with velaglucerase alfa.

● DIRECTIONS FOR ADMINISTRATION For *intravenous infusion* (*VPRIV*®), manufacturer advises give intermittently *in* Sodium Chloride 0.9%; reconstitute each 400-unit vial with 4.3 mL Water for Injections to produce a 100 units/mL solution; dilute requisite dose in 100 mL infusion fluid; give over 60 minutes through a 0.22 micron filter; start infusion within 24 hours of reconstitution.

● MEDICINAL FORMS There can be variation in the licensing of different medicines containing the same drug.
Powder for solution for infusion
ELECTROLYTES: May contain Sodium
► VPRIV (Takeda UK Ltd)
Velaglucerase alfa 400 unit VPRIV 400units powder for solution for infusion vials | 1 vial [PoM] £1,410.20 (Hospital only)

3.8 Homocystinuria

METHYL DONORS

Betaine

03-Nov-2020

● INDICATIONS AND DOSE

Adjunctive treatment of homocystinuria involving deficiencies or defects in cystathionine beta-synthase, 5,10-methylene-tetrahydrofolate reductase, or cobalamin cofactor metabolism (specialist use only)
► BY MOUTH
► Adult: 3 g twice daily (max. per dose 10 g), adjusted according to response; maximum 20 g per day

● SIDE-EFFECTS
► **Uncommon** Abdominal discomfort · agitation · alopecia · appetite decreased · brain oedema · diarrhoea · glossitis · irritability · nausea · skin reactions · urinary incontinence · vomiting

● PREGNANCY Manufacturer advises avoid unless essential—limited information available.

- **BREAST FEEDING** Manufacturer advises caution—no information available.
- **MONITORING REQUIREMENTS** Monitor plasma-methionine concentration before and during treatment—interrupt treatment if symptoms of cerebral oedema occur.
- **DIRECTIONS FOR ADMINISTRATION** Manufacturer advises powder should be mixed with water, juice, milk, formula, or food until completely dissolved and taken immediately; measuring spoons are provided to measure 1 g, 150 mg, and 100 mg of *Cystadane*® powder.
- **PRESCRIBING AND DISPENSING INFORMATION** Betaine should be used in conjunction with dietary restrictions and may be given with supplements of Vitamin B$_{12}$, pyridoxine, and folate under specialist advice.
- **NATIONAL FUNDING/ACCESS DECISIONS** For full details see funding body website

  Scottish Medicines Consortium (SMC) decisions
  ▸ Betaine anhydrous (*Cystadane*®) for the adjunctive treatment of homocystinuria involving deficiencies or defects in cystathionine beta-synthase (CBS), 5,10-methylene-tetrahydrofolate reductase (MTHFR) or cobalamin cofactor metabolism (cbl) (August 2010) SMC No. 407/07 Recommended with restrictions

- **MEDICINAL FORMS** There can be variation in the licensing of different medicines containing the same drug. Forms available from special-order manufacturers include: oral tablet, oral solution

  Oral powder
  ▸ Amversio (SERB)
     Betaine 1 gram per 1 gram Amversio oral powder | 180 gram [PoM] £305.00 DT = £347.00
  ▸ Cystadane (Recordati Rare Diseases UK Ltd)
     Betaine 1 gram per 1 gram Cystadane oral powder | 180 gram [PoM] £347.00 DT = £347.00

3.9 Hypophosphatasia

ENZYMES

| Asfotase alfa

21-Mar-2023

- **DRUG ACTION** Asfotase alfa is a human recombinant tissue-nonspecific alkaline phosphatase that promotes mineralisation of the skeleton.

- **INDICATIONS AND DOSE**

  Paediatric-onset hypophosphatasia (initiated by a specialist)
  ▸ BY SUBCUTANEOUS INJECTION
  ▸ Adult: 2 mg/kg 3 times a week, alternatively 1 mg/kg 6 times a week, dosing frequency depends on body-weight—consult product literature for further information

- **CAUTIONS** Hypersensitivity reactions

  CAUTIONS, FURTHER INFORMATION
  ▸ Hypersensitivity reactions Reactions, including signs and symptoms consistent with anaphylaxis, have occurred within minutes of administration and can occur in patients on treatment for more than one year; if these reactions occur, manufacturer advises immediate discontinuation of treatment and initiation of appropriate medical treatment. For information on re-administration, consult product literature.

- **SIDE-EFFECTS**
  ▸ **Common or very common** Bruising tendency · chills · cough · cutis laxa · fever · headache · hypersensitivity · hypocalcaemia · irritability · myalgia · nausea · nephrolithiasis · oral hypoaesthesia · pain · skin reactions · tachycardia · vasodilation · vomiting

SIDE-EFFECTS, FURTHER INFORMATION Injection-site reactions including hypertrophy, induration, skin discolouration, and cellulitis may occur, particularly in patients receiving treatment 6 times a week. Manufacturer advises rotation of injection sites to manage these reactions; interrupt treatment if severe reactions occur and administer appropriate medical therapy.

- **PREGNANCY** Manufacturer advises avoid—no information available.
- **BREAST FEEDING** Manufacturer advises avoid—no information available.
- **MONITORING REQUIREMENTS**
  ▸ Manufacturer advises monitor serum parathyroid hormone and calcium concentrations—supplements of calcium and oral vitamin D may be required.
  ▸ Manufacturer advises periodic ophthalmological examination and renal ultrasounds.
- **DIRECTIONS FOR ADMINISTRATION** Manufacturer advises max. 1 mL per injection site; administer multiple injections if more than 1 mL is required—consult product literature.
- **HANDLING AND STORAGE** Manufacturer advises store in a refrigerator (2–8 °C).
- **PATIENT AND CARER ADVICE**
  Injection guides The manufacturer has produced injection guides for patients and carers to support training given by health care professionals.
- **NATIONAL FUNDING/ACCESS DECISIONS** For full details see funding body website

  NICE decisions
  ▸ **Asfotase alfa for treating paediatric-onset hypophosphatasia (March 2023)** NICE HST23 Recommended with restrictions

- **MEDICINAL FORMS** There can be variation in the licensing of different medicines containing the same drug.

  Solution for injection
  ▸ Strensiq (Alexion Pharma UK Ltd) ▼
     Asfotase alfa 40 mg per 1 ml Strensiq 18mg/0.45ml solution for injection vials | 12 vial [PoM] £12,700.80 (Hospital only)
     Strensiq 28mg/0.7ml solution for injection vials | 12 vial [PoM] £19,756.80 (Hospital only)
     Strensiq 40mg/1ml solution for injection vials | 12 vial [PoM] £28,224.00 (Hospital only)
     Asfotase alfa 100 mg per 1 ml Strensiq 80mg/0.8ml solution for injection vials | 12 vial [PoM] £56,448.00 (Hospital only)

3.10 Leptin deficiency

DRUGS FOR METABOLIC DISORDERS › LEPTIN ANALOGUES

| Metreleptin

16-Mar-2021

- **DRUG ACTION** Metreleptin is a recombinant human leptin analogue which binds to, and activates the leptin receptor to increase fat breakdown in the blood, muscles and liver, thereby correcting some abnormalities in patients with lipodystrophy.

- **INDICATIONS AND DOSE**

  Leptin deficiency in lipodystrophy (specialist use only)
  ▸ BY SUBCUTANEOUS INJECTION
  ▸ Adult: (consult product literature)

- **CAUTIONS** Autoimmune disease · elderly (limited information available) · haematological abnormalities · severe infection
- **INTERACTIONS** → Appendix 1: metreleptin

- **SIDE-EFFECTS**
  ▶ **Common or very common** Alopecia · appetite abnormal · fatigue · gastrointestinal discomfort · headache · hypoglycaemia · menorrhagia · nausea · weight changes
  ▶ **Frequency not known** Arthralgia · cough · deep vein thrombosis · diabetes mellitus · diarrhoea · dyspnoea · increased risk of infection · insulin resistance · malaise · myalgia · pancreatitis · peripheral swelling · pleural effusion · skin reactions · tachycardia · vomiting

- **CONCEPTION AND CONTRACEPTION** [EvGr] May increase fertility due to restoration of luteinising hormone release. Females of childbearing potential should use additional, effective non-hormonal contraception during treatment. M

- **PREGNANCY** [EvGr] Avoid—toxicity in *animal* studies. M

- **BREAST FEEDING** Specialist sources indicate use with caution—no information available. Large molecular weight and short half-life suggest limited excretion into milk, but monitor breast-fed infants for adverse reactions such as hypoglycaemia, decreased weight and abdominal pain.

- **TREATMENT CESSATION** [EvGr] Treatment should be withdrawn gradually over 2 weeks in conjunction with a low fat diet, to reduce the risk of increased hypertriglyceridaemia and pancreatitis—monitor triglyceride levels and consider the initiation or adjustment of lipid-lowering therapies as needed. M

- **DIRECTIONS FOR ADMINISTRATION** [EvGr] Inject into the thigh, abdomen, or upper arm; rotate injection site—max. 1 mL per injection site. M Patients may self-administer *Myalepta*® after appropriate training in reconstitution and subcutaneous injection technique.

- **PRESCRIBING AND DISPENSING INFORMATION** The manufacturer of *Myalepta*® has provided a *Healthcare Professional Guide* and a *Specialist Prescriber Guide*.
  [EvGr] Prescribe the appropriate dose in milligrams and in millilitres—dosage should be based on actual body-weight. M

- **HANDLING AND STORAGE** Store in a refrigerator (2–8°C) and protect from light—consult product literature about storage after reconstitution.

- **PATIENT AND CARER ADVICE**
  Self-administration Patients and their carers should be given training on reconstitution and subcutaneous injection technique if appropriate—a review of technique is recommended every 6 months.
  Information for patients The manufacturer of *Myalepta*® has provided a *Patient Care Guide* and a *Patient Dose Information Card*.
  Missed doses If a dose is missed, it should be injected when remembered and the next dose should be injected at the normal time.
  Driving and skilled tasks Patients and their carers should be counselled on the effects on driving and performance of skilled tasks—increased risk of fatigue and dizziness.

- **NATIONAL FUNDING/ACCESS DECISIONS**
  For full details see funding body website
  NICE decisions
  ▶ Metreleptin for treating lipodystrophy [in patients aged 2 years and over with generalised lipodystrophy] (February 2021) NICE HST14 Recommended
  ▶ Metreleptin for treating lipodystrophy [in patients aged 12 years and over with partial lipodystrophy] (February 2021) NICE HST14 Recommended with restrictions

- **MEDICINAL FORMS** There can be variation in the licensing of different medicines containing the same drug.
  Powder for solution for injection
  CAUTIONARY AND ADVISORY LABELS 10
  EXCIPIENTS: May contain Polysorbates
  ▶ Myalepta (Chiesi Ltd) ▼
  Metreleptin 3 mg Myalepta 3mg powder for solution for injection vials | 30 vial [PoM] £17,512.50 (Hospital only)
  Metreleptin 5.8 mg Myalepta 5.8mg powder for solution for injection vials | 30 vial [PoM] £35,025.00 (Hospital only)
  Metreleptin 11.3 mg Myalepta 11.3mg powder for solution for injection vials | 30 vial [PoM] £70,050.00 (Hospital only)

3.11 Lysosomal acid lipase deficiency

ENZYMES

Sebelipase alfa

09-Jul-2024

- **DRUG ACTION** Sebelipase alfa is a recombinant human lysosomal acid lipase used as enzyme replacement therapy in lysosomal acid lipase deficiency (such as Wolman disease).

- **INDICATIONS AND DOSE**
  Lysosomal acid lipase deficiency (under expert supervision)
  ▶ BY INTRAVENOUS INFUSION
  ▶ Adult: 1 mg/kg every 2 weeks, then increased if necessary to 3 mg/kg every 2 weeks

- **CAUTIONS** Hypersensitivity reactions
  CAUTIONS, FURTHER INFORMATION
  ▶ Hypersensitivity reactions Hypersensitivity reactions, including anaphylaxis, have been reported, usually during or within 4 hours of an infusion; anaphylaxis has occurred during infusion as long as 1 year after treatment initiation. [EvGr] *Kanuma*® should only be administered by appropriately trained staff, and patients should be observed for 1 hour after the initial infusion or after any dose increase; manage hypersensitivity reactions by temporarily interrupting the infusion, reducing the rate of infusion and/or treatment with antihistamines, antipyretics, and/or corticosteroids. If a severe reaction occurs, stop infusion immediately and start appropriate medical treatment; caution is advised on re-administration. Pre-treatment with antipyretics and/or antihistamines may prevent subsequent reactions. M

- **SIDE-EFFECTS**
  ▶ **Common or very common** Chest discomfort · diarrhoea · dizziness · dyspnoea · fatigue · fever · gastrointestinal discomfort · hyperaemia · hypersensitivity · hypotension · skin reactions · tachycardia

- **ALLERGY AND CROSS-SENSITIVITY** [EvGr] *Kanuma*® is contra-indicated in patients with egg allergy (may contain traces of egg proteins). M

- **PREGNANCY** [EvGr] Avoid as a precaution (no information available). M

- **BREAST FEEDING** [EvGr] Avoid (no information available). M

- **DIRECTIONS FOR ADMINISTRATION** For *intravenous infusion* (*Kanuma*®), dilute requisite dose in Sodium Chloride 0.9% to a final concentration of 0.1–1.5 mg/mL and infuse over approximately 2 hours using a low protein-binding 0.2 micron in-line filter. For changes to duration of infusion—consult product literature.

- **PRESCRIBING AND DISPENSING INFORMATION** Sebelipase alfa is a biological medicine. Biological medicines must be prescribed and dispensed by brand name, see *Biological* *medicines* and *Biosimilar medicines*, under Guidance on prescribing p. 1; record the brand name and batch number after each administration.

The manufacturer of *Kanuma*® has provided a User Manual and a Guide for Healthcare Professionals.

● **HANDLING AND STORAGE** Store in a refrigerator (2–8°C) and protect from light—consult product literature for storage conditions after dilution.

● **PATIENT AND CARER ADVICE**
Driving and skilled tasks Patients and carers should be cautioned on the effects on driving and performance of skilled tasks—increased risk of dizziness.

● **MEDICINAL FORMS** There can be variation in the licensing of different medicines containing the same drug.
Solution for infusion
ELECTROLYTES: May contain Sodium
▸ **Kanuma** (Alexion Pharma UK Ltd) ▼
  Sebelipase alfa 2 mg per 1 ml Kanuma 20mg/10ml concentrate for solution for infusion vials | 1 vial [PoM] £6,286.00 (Hospital only)

3.12 Mucopolysaccharidosis

ENZYMES

| Elosulfase alfa   04-May-2022

● **DRUG ACTION** Elosulfase alfa is an enzyme produced by recombinant DNA technology that provides replacement therapy in conditions caused by N-acetylgalactosamine-6-sulfatase (GALNS) deficiency.

● **INDICATIONS AND DOSE**
Mucopolysaccharidosis IVA (specialist use only)
▸ BY INTRAVENOUS INFUSION
▸ Adult: 2 mg/kg once weekly

● **CAUTIONS** Elderly—no information available · infusion-related reactions

CAUTIONS, FURTHER INFORMATION
▸ Infusion-related reactions Infusion-related reactions can occur; manufacturer advises these may be minimised by pre-treatment with an antihistamine and antipyretic, given 30-60 minutes before treatment. If reaction is severe, stop infusion and start appropriate treatment. Caution and close monitoring is advised during re-administration following a severe reaction.

● **SIDE-EFFECTS**
▸ **Common or very common** Chills · diarrhoea · dizziness · dyspnoea · fever · gastrointestinal discomfort · headache · hypersensitivity · myalgia · nausea · oropharyngeal pain · vomiting
▸ **Frequency not known** Infusion related reaction

● **PREGNANCY** Manufacturer advises avoid unless essential—limited information available.

● **BREAST FEEDING** Manufacturer advises use only if potential benefit outweighs risk—present in milk in *animal* studies.

● **DIRECTIONS FOR ADMINISTRATION** For *intravenous infusion* (*Vimizim*®), manufacturer advises give intermittently *in* Sodium Chloride 0.9%; body-weight under 25 kg, dilute requisite dose to final volume of 100 mL infusion fluid and mix gently, give over 4 hours through in-line filter (0.2 micron) initially at a rate of 3 mL/hour, then increase to a rate of 6 mL/hour after 15 minutes, then increase gradually if tolerated every 15 minutes by 6 mL/hour to max. 36 mL/hour; body-weight 25 kg or over, dilute requisite dose to final volume of 250 mL and mix gently, give over 4 hours through in-line filter (0.2 micron) initially at a rate of 6 mL/hour, then increase to a rate of 12 mL/hour after 15 minutes, then increase gradually if

tolerated every 15 minutes by 12 mL/hour to max. 72 mL/hour.

● **HANDLING AND STORAGE** Manufacturer advises store in a refrigerator at 2–8°C. After dilution use immediately or, if necessary, store at 2-8°C for max. 24 hours, followed by up to 24 hours at 23–27°C.

● **PATIENT AND CARER ADVICE**
Driving and skilled tasks Manufacturer advises patients and carers should be counselled about the effects on driving and performance of skilled tasks—increased risk of dizziness.

● **NATIONAL FUNDING/ACCESS DECISIONS**
For full details see funding body website
NICE decisions
▸ **Elosulfase alfa for treating mucopolysaccharidosis type 4A (April 2022)** NICE HST19 Recommended

● **MEDICINAL FORMS** There can be variation in the licensing of different medicines containing the same drug.
Solution for infusion
EXCIPIENTS: May contain Polysorbates, sorbitol
ELECTROLYTES: May contain Sodium
▸ **Vimizim** (BioMarin (U.K.) Ltd) ▼
  Elosulfase alfa 1 mg per 1 ml Vimizim 5mg/5ml concentrate for solution for infusion vials | 1 vial [PoM] £750.00 (Hospital only)

| Galsulfase   21-Oct-2024

● **DRUG ACTION** Galsulfase is a recombinant form of human N-acetylgalactosamine-4-sulfatase.

● **INDICATIONS AND DOSE**
Mucopolysaccharidosis VI (specialist use only)
▸ BY INTRAVENOUS INFUSION
▸ Adult: 1 mg/kg once weekly

● **CAUTIONS** Acute febrile illness (consider delaying treatment) · acute respiratory illness (consider delaying treatment) · infusion-related reactions can occur · respiratory disease

● **SIDE-EFFECTS**
▸ **Common or very common** Abdominal pain · angioedema · apnoea · arthralgia · asthma · chest pain · chills · conjunctivitis · corneal opacity · cough · dyspnoea · ear pain · fever · headache · hearing impairment · hypertension · hypotension · increased risk of infection · malaise · nasal congestion · nausea · pain · reflexes absent · respiratory disorders · skin reactions · tremor · umbilical hernia · vomiting
▸ **Frequency not known** Arrhythmias · cyanosis · hypoxia · infusion related reaction · nerve disorders · pallor · paraesthesia · shock

SIDE-EFFECTS, FURTHER INFORMATION Infusion-related reactions often occur, they can be managed by slowing the infusion rate or interrupting the infusion, and can be minimised by pre-treatment with an antihistamine and an antipyretic. Recurrent infusion-related reactions may require pre-treatment with a corticosteroid — consult product literature for details.

● **PREGNANCY** Manufacturer advises avoid unless essential.

● **BREAST FEEDING** Manufacturer advises avoid—no information available.

● **DIRECTIONS FOR ADMINISTRATION** For *intravenous infusion* (*Naglazyme*®), manufacturer advises give intermittently *in* Sodium Chloride 0.9%; dilute requisite dose with infusion fluid to final volume of 250 mL and mix gently; infuse through a 0.2 micron in-line filter; give approx. 2.5% of the total volume over 1 hour, then infuse remaining volume over next 3 hours; if body-weight under 20 kg and at risk of fluid overload, dilute requisite dose in 100 mL infusion fluid and give over at least 4 hours.

- **NATIONAL FUNDING/ACCESS DECISIONS**
  For full details see funding body website
  All Wales Medicines Strategy Group (AWMSG) decisions
  ▶ Galsulfase (*Naglazyme*®) for long-term enzyme replacement therapy in patients with a confirmed diagnosis of mucopolysaccharidosis VI (October 2024) AWMSG No. 155 Recommended

- **MEDICINAL FORMS** There can be variation in the licensing of different medicines containing the same drug.
  Solution for infusion
  ▶ Naglazyme (BioMarin (U.K.) Ltd)
     Galsulfase 1 mg per 1 ml Naglazyme 5mg/5ml solution for infusion vials | 1 vial [PoM] £982.00 (Hospital only)

Idursulfase
16-Jul-2020

- **DRUG ACTION** Idursulfase is an enzyme produced by recombinant DNA technology licensed for long-term replacement therapy in mucopolysaccharidosis II (Hunter syndrome), a lysosomal storage disorder caused by deficiency of iduronate-2-sulfatase.

- **INDICATIONS AND DOSE**
  Mucopolysaccharidosis II (specialist use only)
  ▶ BY INTRAVENOUS INFUSION
  ▶ Adult: 500 micrograms/kg once weekly

- **CAUTIONS** Acute febrile respiratory illness (consider delaying treatment) · infusion-related reactions can occur · severe respiratory disease

- **SIDE-EFFECTS**
- **Common or very common** Arrhythmias · arthralgia · chest pain · cough · cyanosis · diarrhoea · dizziness · dyspnoea · fever · flushing · gastrointestinal discomfort · headache · hypertension · hypotension · hypoxia · infusion related reaction · nausea · oedema · respiratory disorders · skin reactions · tongue swelling · tremor · vomiting
- **Frequency not known** Hypersensitivity
  SIDE-EFFECTS, FURTHER INFORMATION Infusion-related reactions often occur, they can be managed by slowing the infusion rate or interrupting the infusion, and can be minimised by pre-treatment with an antihistamine and an antipyretic. Recurrent infusion-related reactions may require pre-treatment with a corticosteroid—consult product literature for details.

- **CONCEPTION AND CONTRACEPTION** Contra-indicated in women of child-bearing potential.

- **PREGNANCY** Manufacturer advises avoid.

- **BREAST FEEDING** Manufacturer advises avoid—present in milk in *animal* studies.

- **DIRECTIONS FOR ADMINISTRATION** For *intravenous infusion* (*Elaprase*®), manufacturer advises give intermittently *in* Sodium Chloride 0.9%; dilute requisite dose in 100 mL infusion fluid and mix gently (do not shake); give over 3 hours (gradually reduced to 1 hour if no infusion-related reactions).

- **MEDICINAL FORMS** There can be variation in the licensing of different medicines containing the same drug.
  Solution for infusion
  ▶ Elaprase (Takeda UK Ltd) ▼
     Idursulfase 2 mg per 1 ml Elaprase 6mg/3ml concentrate for solution for infusion vials | 1 vial [PoM] £1,985.00 (Hospital only)

Laronidase
09-Dec-2024

- **DRUG ACTION** Laronidase is an enzyme produced by recombinant DNA technology licensed for long-term replacement therapy in the treatment of non-neurological manifestations of mucopolysaccharidosis I, a lysosomal storage disorder caused by deficiency of alpha-L-iduronidase.

- **INDICATIONS AND DOSE**
  Non-neurological manifestations of mucopolysaccharidosis I (specialist use only)
  ▶ BY INTRAVENOUS INFUSION
  ▶ Adult: 100 units/kg once weekly

- **CAUTIONS** Infusion-related reactions can occur

- **INTERACTIONS** → Appendix 1: laronidase

- **SIDE-EFFECTS**
- **Common or very common** Abdominal pain · alopecia · anaphylactic reaction · angioedema · chills · cough · diarrhoea · dizziness · dyspnoea · fatigue · fever · flushing · headache · hypotension · influenza like illness · joint disorders · nausea · pain · pallor · paraesthesia · peripheral coldness · respiratory disorders · restlessness · skin reactions · sweat changes · tachycardia · temperature sensation altered · vomiting
- **Frequency not known** Cyanosis · hypoxia · oedema
  SIDE-EFFECTS, FURTHER INFORMATION Infusion-related reactions often occur, they can be managed by slowing the infusion rate or interrupting the infusion, and can be minimised by pre-treatment with an antihistamine and an antipyretic. Recurrent infusion-related reactions may require pre-treatment with a corticosteroid—consult product literature for details.

- **PREGNANCY** Manufacturer advises avoid unless essential—no information available.

- **BREAST FEEDING** Manufacturer advises avoid—no information available.

- **MONITORING REQUIREMENTS** Monitor immunoglobulin G (IgG) antibody concentration.

- **DIRECTIONS FOR ADMINISTRATION** For *intravenous infusion* (*Aldurazyme*®), manufacturer advises give intermittently in Sodium Chloride 0.9%; body-weight under 20 kg, use 100 mL infusion fluid; body-weight over 20 kg use 250 mL infusion fluid; withdraw volume of infusion fluid equivalent to volume of laronidase concentrate being added; give through in-line filter (0.2 micron) initially at a rate of 2 units/kg/hour then increase gradually every 15 minutes to max. 43 units/kg/hour.

- **MEDICINAL FORMS** There can be variation in the licensing of different medicines containing the same drug.
  Solution for infusion
  ELECTROLYTES: May contain Sodium
  ▶ Aldurazyme (Sanofi)
     Laronidase 100 unit per 1 ml Aldurazyme 500units/5ml concentrate for solution for infusion vials | 1 vial [PoM] £444.70

Vestronidase alfa
23-Sep-2024

- **DRUG ACTION** Vestronidase alfa is an enzyme produced by recombinant DNA technology used for long-term replacement therapy of non-neurological manifestations of mucopolysaccharidosis VII (Sly syndrome), a lysosomal storage disorder caused by deficiency of beta-glucuronidase.

- **INDICATIONS AND DOSE**
  Non-neurological manifestations of mucopolysaccharidosis VII (under expert supervision)
  ▶ BY INTRAVENOUS INFUSION
  ▶ Adult: 4 mg/kg every 2 weeks

- **CAUTIONS** Acute febrile illness (delay treatment) · acute respiratory illness (delay treatment) · hypersensitivity reactions

  CAUTIONS, FURTHER INFORMATION
  ‣ Hypersensitivity reactions [EvGr] Serious hypersensitivity reactions, including anaphylaxis, have been reported; these may be minimised by pre-treatment with a non-sedating antihistamine with or without an antipyretic, given 30–60 minutes before the start of the infusion. *Mepsevii*® should only be administered by appropriately trained staff, and patients should be observed for at least 1 hour after the infusion; manage hypersensitivity reactions by temporarily interrupting the infusion, reducing the rate of infusion and/or treatment with antihistamines, antipyretics, and/or corticosteroids. If a severe reaction occurs, stop infusion immediately and start appropriate medical treatment; caution is advised on re-administration. Ⓜ

- **SIDE-EFFECTS**
  ‣ **Common or very common** Diarrhoea · febrile seizure · hypersensitivity · skin reactions

- **PREGNANCY** [EvGr] Avoid unless potential benefit outweighs risk (no information available). Ⓜ

- **BREAST FEEDING** Specialist sources indicate use with caution (no information available). Large molecular weight suggests limited excretion into milk and drug molecule likely to be destroyed in the infant's gastro-intestinal tract; monitor breast-fed infants carefully.

- **DIRECTIONS FOR ADMINISTRATION** [EvGr] For *intravenous infusion* (*Mepsevii*®), dilute with Sodium Chloride 0.9%; give through a low-protein binding 0.2 micron in-line filter. Initially infuse 2.5% of the total volume in the first hour, then infuse remaining volume over the next 3 hours according to the recommended rate—consult product literature. Ⓜ

- **PRESCRIBING AND DISPENSING INFORMATION** Vestronidase alfa is a biological medicine. Biological medicines must be prescribed and dispensed by brand name, see *Biological medicines* and *Biosimilar medicines*, under Guidance on prescribing p. 1; record the brand name and batch number after each administration.

- **HANDLING AND STORAGE** Store in a refrigerator at 2–8°C and protect from light—consult product literature for storage conditions after dilution.

- **MEDICINAL FORMS** There can be variation in the licensing of different medicines containing the same drug.

  Solution for infusion
  EXCIPIENTS: May contain Polysorbates
  ELECTROLYTES: May contain Sodium
  ‣ **Mepsevii** (Ultragenyx UK Ltd) ▼
  Vestronidase alfa 2 mg per 1 ml Mepsevii 10mg/5ml concentrate for solution for infusion vials | 1 vial [PoM] £1,713.00 (Hospital only)

3.13 Niemann-Pick disease

ENZYME INHIBITORS › GLUCOSYLCERAMIDE SYNTHASE INHIBITORS

▌Miglustat

21-Oct-2024

- **DRUG ACTION**
  ‣ When used for Type 1 Gaucher's disease or Niemann-Pick type C disease Miglustat is an inhibitor of glucosylceramide synthase.
  ‣ When used for Pompe disease Miglustat is an enzyme stabiliser of cipaglucosidase alfa.

- **INDICATIONS AND DOSE**
  Mild to moderate type I Gaucher's disease for whom enzyme replacement therapy is unsuitable (under expert supervision)
  ‣ BY MOUTH
  ‣ Adult: 100 mg 3 times a day, reduced if not tolerated to 100 mg 1–2 times a day
  Treatment of progressive neurological manifestations of Niemann-Pick type C disease (under expert supervision)
  ‣ BY MOUTH
  ‣ Adult: 200 mg 3 times a day

  OPFOLDA®

  Pompe disease [in combination with cipaglucosidase alfa] (under expert supervision)
  ‣ BY MOUTH
  ‣ Adult (body-weight 40–49 kg): 195 mg every 2 weeks, dose to be taken 1 hour (but no more than 3 hours) before the start of cipaglucosidase alfa infusion
  ‣ Adult (body-weight 50 kg and above): 260 mg every 2 weeks, dose to be taken 1 hour (but no more than 3 hours) before the start of cipaglucosidase alfa infusion

> **IMPORTANT SAFETY INFORMATION**
> SAFE PRACTICE
> Miglustat could be confused with migalastat; care must be taken to ensure the correct drug is prescribed and dispensed.

- **SIDE-EFFECTS**
  ‣ **Common or very common** Appetite decreased · asthenia · chills · constipation · depression · diarrhoea · dizziness · flatulence · gastrointestinal discomfort · headache · insomnia · libido decreased · malaise · muscle spasms · muscle weakness · nausea · peripheral neuropathy · sensation abnormal · thrombocytopenia · tremor · vomiting · weight decreased
  ‣ **Uncommon** Feeling jittery

- **CONCEPTION AND CONTRACEPTION**
  ‣ When used for Type 1 Gaucher's disease or Niemann-Pick type C disease [EvGr] Effective contraception must be used during treatment. Male patients should avoid fathering a child during and for 3 months after treatment. Ⓜ

  OPFOLDA® [EvGr] Females of childbearing potential should use effective contraception during treatment and for 4 weeks after last treatment. Ⓜ

- **PREGNANCY** [EvGr] Avoid (toxicity in *animal* studies). Ⓜ
- **BREAST FEEDING** [EvGr] Avoid (no information available). Ⓜ
- **HEPATIC IMPAIRMENT**
  ‣ When used for Type 1 Gaucher's disease or Niemann-Pick type C disease Manufacturer advises caution (no information available).
- **RENAL IMPAIRMENT**
  ‣ When used for Type 1 Gaucher's disease or Niemann-Pick type C disease Avoid if eGFR less than 30 mL/minute/1.73 m^2.
  Dose adjustments For Gaucher's disease initially 100 mg twice daily if eGFR 50–70 mL/minute/1.73 m^2. Initially 100 mg once daily if eGFR 30–50 mL/minute/1.73 m^2.
  For Niemann-Pick type C disease, initially 200 mg twice daily if eGFR 50–70 mL/minute/1.73 m^2. Initially 100 mg twice daily if eGFR 30–50 mL/minute/1.73 m^2.
- **MONITORING REQUIREMENTS**
  ‣ When used for Type 1 Gaucher's disease or Niemann-Pick type C disease Monitor cognitive and neurological function. Monitor platelet count.

9
Blood and nutrition

● **DIRECTIONS FOR ADMINISTRATION**

OPFOLDA ® [EvGr] Food should not be consumed at least 2 hours before and 2 hours after taking *Opfolda*® capsules (minimum 4 hours fast).

   If the dose is missed, it should be given as soon as possible and the cipaglucosidase alfa infusion should not be started until 1 hour after *Opfolda*® is taken. ⓜ

● **PRESCRIBING AND DISPENSING INFORMATION**

OPFOLDA ® The manufacturer of *Opfolda*® has provided *Risk minimisation materials* documents for healthcare professionals.

● **PATIENT AND CARER ADVICE**

OPFOLDA ® Females of childbearing potential should be given a patient reminder card.

● **NATIONAL FUNDING/ACCESS DECISIONS**

For full details see funding body website

NICE decisions

▸ **Cipaglucosidase alfa with miglustat for treating late-onset Pompe disease (August 2023)** NICE TA912 Recommended

All Wales Medicines Strategy Group (AWMSG) decisions

▸ **Miglustat for the treatment of progressive neurological manifestations in adult patients and paediatric patients with Niemann-Pick type C disease (October 2024)** AWMSG No. 371 Recommended

● **MEDICINAL FORMS** There can be variation in the licensing of different medicines containing the same drug.

Oral capsule

▸ **Miglustat (Non-proprietary)**

Miglustat 100 mg Miglustat 100mg capsules | 84 capsule [PoM] £2,850.00–£3,934.00 (Hospital only) | 84 capsule [PoM] £3,442.00

▸ **Opfolda** (Amicus Therapeutics UK Operations Ltd)

Miglustat 65 mg Opfolda 65mg capsules | 4 capsule [PoM] £116.69 (Hospital only) | 24 capsule [PoM] £700.14 (Hospital only)

▸ **Yargesa** (Piramal Critical Care Ltd)

Miglustat 100 mg Yargesa 100mg capsules | 84 capsule [PoM] £3,500.00 (Hospital only)

▸ **Zavesca** (Janssen-Cilag Ltd)

Miglustat 100 mg Zavesca 100mg capsules | 84 capsule [PoM] £3,934.17 (Hospital only)

ENZYMES

Olipudase alfa

25-Apr-2025

● **DRUG ACTION** Olipudase alfa is an enzyme produced by recombinant DNA technology that is administered as enzyme replacement therapy for the treatment of acid sphingomyelinase deficiency (Niemann-Pick disease) type A/B or B, a lysosomal storage disorder affecting the normal function of tissues and organs such as the liver, spleen, lungs, heart, and brain.

● **INDICATIONS AND DOSE**

Non-neurological manifestations of acid sphingomyelinase deficiency (Niemann-Pick disease) type A/B or B (under expert supervision)

▸ BY INTRAVENOUS INFUSION

▸ Adult: Initially 100 micrograms/kg for 1 dose, subsequent doses to be administered every 2 weeks according to dose escalation regimen until maintenance phase is reached after 14 weeks—consult product literature; usual maintenance 3 mg/kg every 2 weeks

DOSES AT EXTREMES OF BODY-WEIGHT

▸ Doses should be calculated on the basis of optimal body-weight in patients with BMI > 30 kg/m² —consult product literature.

● **CAUTIONS** Infusion-related reactions

CAUTIONS, FURTHER INFORMATION

▸ Infusion-related reactions [EvGr] Serious infusion-related reactions can occur and olipudase alfa should only be administered when appropriately trained staff and resuscitation facilities are available; these reactions may be minimised by pre-medication with an antihistamine, antipyretic, and corticosteroid. Patients should be closely monitored for signs of infusion-related reactions during and after administration, and managed appropriately—consult product literature. ⓜ

● **SIDE-EFFECTS**

▸ **Common or very common** Angioedema · arthralgia · asthenia · chills · diarrhoea · dyspnoea · eye discomfort · eye erythema · fever · gastrointestinal discomfort · headache · hepatic pain · hypersensitivity · hypotension · myalgia · nausea · pain · palpitations · respiratory disorders · skin reactions · tachycardia · throat complaints · vasodilation · vomiting

● **PREGNANCY** [EvGr] Avoid unless potential benefit outweighs risk—toxicity in *animal* studies. ⓜ

● **BREAST FEEDING** Specialist sources indicate use with caution—no information available. Large molecular weight suggests limited excretion into milk and drug molecule likely to be partially destroyed in the infant's gastro-intestinal tract.

● **MONITORING REQUIREMENTS** [EvGr] Monitor hepatic transaminases (ALT and AST) within 1 month before treatment initiation, then within 72 hours before the next scheduled infusion during dose escalation or when resuming treatment, and as clinically indicated during maintenance phase—consult product literature. ⓜ

● **DIRECTIONS FOR ADMINISTRATION** [EvGr] For *intermittent intravenous infusion* (*Xenpozyme*®), reconstitute initially with Water for Injections then dilute requisite dose with Sodium Chloride 0.9%; give through a low-protein binding 0.2 micron in-line filter, preferably via an infusion pump, according to the recommended rate and duration—consult product literature. Patients stabilised on a maintenance dose may be considered for home infusion under the supervision of a healthcare professional—consult product literature. ⓜ

● **PRESCRIBING AND DISPENSING INFORMATION** Olipudase alfa is a biological medicine. Biological medicines must be prescribed and dispensed by brand name, see *Biological medicines* and *Biosimilar medicines*, under Guidance on prescribing p. 1; record the brand name and batch number after each administration.

● **HANDLING AND STORAGE** Store in a refrigerator (2–8°C)—consult product literature for storage conditions after reconstitution and dilution.

● **PATIENT AND CARER ADVICE**

Driving and skilled tasks Patients and carers should be cautioned on the effects on driving and performance of skilled tasks—increased risk of hypotension.

● **NATIONAL FUNDING/ACCESS DECISIONS**

For full details see funding body website

NICE decisions

▸ **Olipudase alfa for treating acid sphingomyelinase deficiency (Niemann–Pick disease) type AB and type B (April 2025)** NICE HST32 Not recommended

● **MEDICINAL FORMS** There can be variation in the licensing of different medicines containing the same drug.

Powder for solution for infusion

EXCIPIENTS: May contain Sucrose

ELECTROLYTES: May contain Sodium

▸ **Xenpozyme** (Sanofi) ▼

Olipudase alfa 20 mg Xenpozyme 20mg powder for concentrate for solution for infusion vials | 1 vial [PoM] £3,612.00 (Hospital only)

3.14 Pompe disease

> **Other drugs used for Pompe disease** Miglustat, p. 1217

ENZYMES

Alglucosidase alfa
28-May-2024

- **DRUG ACTION** Alglucosidase alfa is an enzyme produced by recombinant DNA technology licensed for long-term replacement therapy in Pompe disease, a lysosomal storage disorder caused by deficiency of acid alpha-glucosidase.

- **INDICATIONS AND DOSE**

Pompe disease (specialist use only)
  - ▸ BY INTRAVENOUS INFUSION
  - ▸ Adult: 20 mg/kg every 2 weeks

- **CAUTIONS** Cardiac dysfunction · infusion-related reactions—consult product literature · respiratory dysfunction

- **SIDE-EFFECTS**
  - ▸ **Common or very common** Anxiety · arrhythmias · chest discomfort · chills · cough · cyanosis · diarrhoea · dizziness · fever · flushing · hyperhidrosis · hypersensitivity · hypertension · irritability · local swelling · muscle complaints · nausea · oedema · pallor · paraesthesia · respiratory disorders · skin reactions · temperature sensation altered · throat complaints · tremor · vomiting
  - ▸ **Frequency not known** Angioedema · apnoea · arthralgia · asthenia · cardiac arrest · drowsiness · dysphagia · dyspnoea · excessive tearing · eye inflammation · gastrointestinal discomfort · headache · hypotension · hypoxia · influenza like illness · infusion related reaction · malaise · musculoskeletal chest pain · nephrotic syndrome · palpitations · peripheral coldness · proteinuria · skin ulcer · vasoconstriction

  SIDE-EFFECTS, FURTHER INFORMATION Infusion-related reactions are very common, calling for use of antihistamine, antipyretic, or corticosteroid; consult product literature for details.

- **PREGNANCY** Toxicity in *animal* studies, but treatment should not be withheld.

- **BREAST FEEDING** Manufacturer advises avoid—no information available.

- **MONITORING REQUIREMENTS**
  - ▸ Monitor closely if cardiac dysfunction.
  - ▸ Monitor closely if respiratory dysfunction.
  - ▸ Monitor immunoglobulin G (IgG) antibody concentration.

- **DIRECTIONS FOR ADMINISTRATION** For *intravenous infusion* (*Myozyme*®), manufacturer advises give intermittently *in* Sodium Chloride 0.9%; reconstitute 50 mg with 10.3 mL Water for Injections to produce 5 mg/mL solution; gently rotate vial without shaking; dilute requisite dose with infusion fluid to give a final concentration of 0.5–4 mg/mL; give through a low protein-binding in-line filter (0.2 micron) at an initial rate of 1 mg/kg/hour increased by 2 mg/kg/hour every 30 minutes to max. 7 mg/kg/hour.

- **NATIONAL FUNDING/ACCESS DECISIONS**
  For full details see funding body website
  All Wales Medicines Strategy Group (AWMSG) decisions
  - ▸ Alglucosidase alfa (*Myozyme*®) for long-term enzyme replacement therapy in patients with a confirmed diagnosis of Pompe disease (acid alpha-glucosidase deficiency) (May 2024) AWMSG No. 17 Recommended

- **MEDICINAL FORMS** There can be variation in the licensing of different medicines containing the same drug.
  Powder for solution for infusion
  - ▸ **Myozyme** (Sanofi)
    Alglucosidase alfa 50 mg Myozyme 50mg powder for concentrate for solution for infusion vials | 1 vial PoM £356.06 (Hospital only)

Avalglucosidase alfa
25-Jul-2023

- **DRUG ACTION** Avalglucosidase alfa, a modification of alglucosidase alfa, is an enzyme produced by recombinant DNA technology that is administered as enzyme replacement therapy in Pompe disease, a lysosomal storage disorder caused by deficiency of acid alpha-glucosidase.

- **INDICATIONS AND DOSE**

Pompe disease (under expert supervision)
  - ▸ BY INTRAVENOUS INFUSION
  - ▸ Adult: 20 mg/kg every 2 weeks

- **CAUTIONS** Cardiac dysfunction · infusion-related reactions · respiratory dysfunction · susceptibility to fluid volume overload

  CAUTIONS, FURTHER INFORMATION
  - ▸ Infusion-related reactions EvGr Infusion-related reactions can occur and avalglucosidase alfa should only be administered when appropriately trained staff are available; these reactions may be minimised by premedication with an antihistamine, antipyretic, and/or corticosteroid. Patients should be monitored for signs of infusion-related reactions during and after administration, and managed appropriately—consult product literature. M

- **SIDE-EFFECTS**
  - ▸ **Common or very common** Asthenia · chest discomfort · chills · cough · diarrhoea · dizziness · dyspnoea · eye disorders · headache · hypersensitivity · hypertension · influenza like illness · muscle complaints · nausea · oral disorders · pain · skin reactions · tremor · vomiting
  - ▸ **Uncommon** Angioedema · arrhythmias · conjunctivitis · drowsiness · dysphagia · eye pruritus · fever · flushing · gastrointestinal discomfort · hyperhidrosis · hyperthermia · hypotension · localised oedema · paraesthesia · peripheral swelling · respiratory disorders · throat irritation
  - ▸ **Frequency not known** Infusion related reaction

- **PREGNANCY** EvGr Use only if potential benefit outweighs risk—no information available. M

- **BREAST FEEDING** EvGr Use only if potential benefit outweighs risk—no information available. M

- **DIRECTIONS FOR ADMINISTRATION** EvGr For *intermittent intravenous infusion* (*Nexviadyme*®), reconstitute each 100-mg vial with 10 mL Water for Injections then dilute requisite dose to a concentration of 0.5–4 mg/mL with Glucose 5%; give through a low protein-binding 0.2 micron in-line filter, according to the recommended rate (initially 1 mg/kg/hour) and duration—consult product literature. Patients tolerating their infusions well may be considered for home infusion under the supervision of a healthcare professional—consult product literature. M

- **PRESCRIBING AND DISPENSING INFORMATION**
  Avalglucosidase alfa is a biological medicine. Biological medicines must be prescribed and dispensed by brand name, see *Biological medicines* and *Biosimilar medicines*, under Guidance on prescribing p. 1; record the brand name and batch number after each administration.

  The manufacturer of *Nexviadyme*® has provided *Risk minimisation materials* documents for healthcare professionals.

- **HANDLING AND STORAGE** Store in refrigerator (2–8°C)—consult product literature for storage conditions after reconstitution and dilution.

- **PATIENT AND CARER ADVICE**
Driving and skilled tasks Patients and carers should be counselled on the effects on driving and performance of skilled tasks—increased risk of dizziness.
- **NATIONAL FUNDING/ACCESS DECISIONS**
For full details see funding body website
NICE decisions
▸ Avalglucosidase alfa for treating Pompe disease (August 2022) NICE TA821 Recommended
Scottish Medicines Consortium (SMC) decisions
▸ Avalglucosidase alfa (*Nexviadyme*®) as a long-term enzyme replacement therapy for the treatment of patients with Pompe disease (acid alpha-glucosidase deficiency) (July 2023) SMC No. SMC2546 Recommended

---

- **MEDICINAL FORMS** There can be variation in the licensing of different medicines containing the same drug.
Powder for solution for infusion
EXCIPIENTS: May contain Polysorbates
▸ **Nexviadyme** (Sanofi) ▼
Avalglucosidase alfa 100 mg Nexviadyme 100mg powder for concentrate for solution for infusion vials | 1 vial [PoM] £783.33 (Hospital only)

Cipaglucosidase alfa
18-Dec-2023

- **DRUG ACTION** Cipaglucosidase alfa is an enzyme produced by recombinant DNA technology that is administered as enzyme replacement therapy in Pompe disease, a lysosomal storage disorder caused by deficiency of acid alpha-glucosidase.

- **INDICATIONS AND DOSE**
Pompe disease [in combination with miglustat] (under expert supervision)
▸ BY INTRAVENOUS INFUSION
▸ Adult: 20 mg/kg every 2 weeks, infusion to be started 1 hour (but no more than 3 hours) after taking miglustat

- **CAUTIONS** Cardiac dysfunction · infusion-related reactions · respiratory dysfunction
CAUTIONS, FURTHER INFORMATION
▸ Infusion-related reactions [EvGr] Infusion-related reactions can occur and cipaglucosidase alfa should only be administered when appropriately trained staff are available; these reactions may be minimised by premedication with an antihistamine, antipyretic, and/or corticosteroid. Patients should be monitored for signs of infusion-related reactions during and after administration, and managed appropriately—consult product literature. ◈

- **SIDE-EFFECTS**
▸ **Common or very common** Arrhythmias · asthenia · chest discomfort · chills · cough · diarrhoea · dizziness · drowsiness · dyspnoea · fever · flatulence · flushing · gastrointestinal discomfort · headaches · hyperhidrosis · hypersensitivity · hypertension · muscle complaints · muscle weakness · nausea · pain · skin reactions · taste altered · tremor · vomiting
▸ **Uncommon** Arthralgia · asthma · balance impaired · hypotension · malaise · musculoskeletal stiffness · oesophageal disorder · oral disorders · oropharyngeal discomfort · pallor · paraesthesia · peripheral swelling · throat oedema · wheezing

- **CONCEPTION AND CONTRACEPTION** [EvGr] Females of childbearing potential should use effective contraception during treatment and for 4 weeks after last treatment. ◈

- **PREGNANCY** [EvGr] Avoid (toxicity in animal studies). ◈

- **BREAST FEEDING** [EvGr] Avoid (present in milk in *animal* studies). ◈

- **DIRECTIONS FOR ADMINISTRATION** [EvGr] For *intermittent intravenous infusion* (*Pombiliti*®), reconstitute each 105-mg vial with 7.2 mL Water for Injections to give a 7 mg/mL solution; dilute requisite dose in Sodium Chloride 0.9% to a concentration of 0.5–4 mg/mL. Give through a low protein-binding 0.2 micron in-line filter, according to the recommended rate (initially 1 mg/kg/hour) and duration—consult product literature. If the infusion cannot be started within 3 hours of miglustat, reschedule administration of both cipaglucosidase alfa and miglustat for at least 24 hours later.
Patients tolerating their infusions may be considered for home infusion under the supervision of a healthcare professional—consult product literature. ◈

- **PRESCRIBING AND DISPENSING INFORMATION**
Cipaglucosidase alfa is a biological medicine. Biological medicines must be prescribed and dispensed by brand name, see *Biological medicines* and *Biosimilar medicines*, under Guidance on prescribing p. 1; record the brand name and batch number after each administration.
The manufacturer of *Pombiliti*® has provided *Risk minimisation materials* documents for healthcare professionals.

- **HANDLING AND STORAGE** Store in refrigerator (2–8°C)—consult product literature for storage conditions after reconstitution and dilution.

- **PATIENT AND CARER ADVICE** Females of childbearing potential should be given a patient reminder card. Patients receiving home infusions should be given a home infusion patient manual and infusion diary.
Driving and skilled tasks Patients and carers should be counselled on the effects on driving and performance of skilled tasks—increased risk of dizziness and somnolence.

- **NATIONAL FUNDING/ACCESS DECISIONS**
For full details see funding body website
NICE decisions
▸ Cipaglucosidase alfa with miglustat for treating late-onset Pompe disease (August 2023) NICE TA912 Recommended
Scottish Medicines Consortium (SMC) decisions
▸ Cipaglucosidase alfa (*Pombiliti*®) as a long-term enzyme replacement therapy used in combination with the enzyme stabiliser miglustat for the treatment of adults with late-onset Pompe disease (acid α-glucosidase [GAA] deficiency) (December 2023) SMC No. SMC2606 Recommended

---

- **MEDICINAL FORMS** There can be variation in the licensing of different medicines containing the same drug.
Powder for solution for infusion
EXCIPIENTS: May contain Polysorbates
▸ **Pombiliti** (Amicus Therapeutics UK Operations Ltd) ▼
Cipaglucosidase alfa 105 mg Pombiliti 105mg powder for concentrate for solution for infusion vials | 1 vial [PoM] £987.00 (Hospital only) | 10 vial [PoM] £9,870.00 (Hospital only)

3.15 Primary hyperoxaluria

DRUGS FOR METABOLIC DISORDERS > SMALL INTERFERING RIBONUCLEIC ACID

Lumasiran
04-Jul-2023

- **DRUG ACTION** Lumasiran is a double-stranded small interfering RNA, which reduces production of the enzyme glycolate oxidase involved in the synthesis of glyoxylate and oxalate, thereby reducing urinary and plasma oxalate levels.

- **INDICATIONS AND DOSE**

  Primary hyperoxaluria type 1 (under expert supervision)
  - ▸ BY SUBCUTANEOUS INJECTION
  - ▸ Adult: Loading dose 3 mg/kg once a month for 3 doses, then maintenance 3 mg/kg every 3 months, to be started 1 month after the last loading dose

- **SIDE-EFFECTS**
  - ▸ **Common or very common** Gastrointestinal discomfort

- **PREGNANCY** [EvGr] Use only if potential benefit outweighs risk (limited information available). ⓜ

- **BREAST FEEDING** [EvGr] Avoid (no information available). ⓜ

- **HEPATIC IMPAIRMENT** [EvGr] Caution in moderate or severe impairment (potential for decreased efficacy). ⓜ

- **RENAL IMPAIRMENT** Monitor for signs and symptoms of metabolic acidosis in severe impairment (increased plasma-glycolate levels caused by lumasiran therapy may increase the risk of, or worsen pre-existing, metabolic acidosis).

- **DIRECTIONS FOR ADMINISTRATION** Maximum 1.5 mL per injection site; inject into the abdomen, thigh, or upper arm and rotate injection site. Avoid injecting into scar tissue or skin that is reddened, inflamed, or swollen.

- **HANDLING AND STORAGE** Protect from light.

- **NATIONAL FUNDING/ACCESS DECISIONS** For full details see funding body website

  NICE decisions
  - ▸ Lumasiran for treating primary hyperoxaluria type 1 (April 2023) NICE HST25 Recommended

- **MEDICINAL FORMS** There can be variation in the licensing of different medicines containing the same drug.

  Solution for injection
  - ▸ **Oxlumo** (Alnylam UK Ltd) ▼
    Lumasiran (as Lumasiran sodium) 189 mg per 1 ml Oxlumo 94.5mg/0.5ml solution for injection vials | 1 vial [PoM] £61,068.98 (Hospital only)

3.16 Tyrosinaemia type I

ENZYME INHIBITORS > 4-HYDROXYPHENYLPYRUVATE DIOXYGENASE INHIBITORS

Nitisinone
19-Jul-2022

(NTBC)

- **DRUG ACTION** Nitisinone is a competitive inhibitor of 4-hydroxyphenylpyruvate dioxygenase which inhibits catabolism of tyrosine and thereby prevents accumulation of harmful metabolites.

- **INDICATIONS AND DOSE**

  Hereditary tyrosinaemia type I (in combination with dietary restriction of tyrosine and phenylalanine) (specialist use only)
  - ▸ BY MOUTH
  - ▸ Adult: Initially 1 mg/kg once daily, adjusted according to response; maximum 2 mg/kg per day

  ORFADIN ® CAPSULES

  Hereditary tyrosinaemia type I (in combination with dietary restriction of tyrosine and phenylalanine) (specialist use only)
  - ▸ BY MOUTH USING CAPSULES
  - ▸ Adult: Initially 1 mg/kg once daily, adjusted according to response; maximum 2 mg/kg per day

  Alkaptonuria (specialist use only)
  - ▸ BY MOUTH USING CAPSULES
  - ▸ Adult: 10 mg once daily

  ORFADIN ® ORAL SUSPENSION

  Hereditary tyrosinaemia type I (in combination with dietary restriction of tyrosine and phenylalanine) (specialist use only)
  - ▸ BY MOUTH USING ORAL SUSPENSION
  - ▸ Adult: Initially 1 mg/kg once daily, adjusted according to response; maximum 2 mg/kg per day

  Alkaptonuria (specialist use only)
  - ▸ BY MOUTH USING ORAL SUSPENSION
  - ▸ Adult: 10 mg once daily

- **INTERACTIONS** → Appendix 1: nitisinone

- **SIDE-EFFECTS**
  - ▸ **Common or very common** Corneal opacity · eye inflammation · eye pain · granulocytopenia · increased risk of infection · leucopenia · photophobia · skin reactions · thrombocytopenia
  - ▸ **Uncommon** Leucocytosis

- **PREGNANCY** Manufacturer advises avoid unless potential benefit outweighs risk—toxicity in *animal* studies.

- **BREAST FEEDING** Manufacturer advises avoid—adverse effects in *animal* studies.

- **MONITORING REQUIREMENTS**
  - ▸ When used for Hereditary tyrosinaemia type I (in combination with dietary restriction of tyrosine and phenylalanine) [EvGr] Slit-lamp examination of eyes is recommended before treatment and at least once a year thereafter. Monitor plasma tyrosine levels—consult product literature. Monitor platelet and white blood cell count every 6 months. Monitor liver function regularly. ⓜ

- **DIRECTIONS FOR ADMINISTRATION** Manufacturer advises capsules can be opened and the contents suspended in a small amount of water or formula diet and taken immediately.

- **HANDLING AND STORAGE** Store in a refrigerator (2−8°C).

- **PATIENT AND CARER ADVICE** Patients and carers should be advised to seek immediate medical attention if symptoms of visual disorders develop during treatment.
  Driving and skilled tasks Patients and carers should be cautioned on the effects on driving and performance of skilled tasks—increased risk of visual disorders.
  ORFADIN® ORAL SUSPENSION Patients or carers should be given advice on how to administer *Orfadin®* oral suspension.

- **NATIONAL FUNDING/ACCESS DECISIONS**
  For full details see funding body website
  All Wales Medicines Strategy Group (AWMSG) decisions
  ▸ Nitisinone 10 mg capsules (*Orfadin®*) for the treatment of adult patients with alkaptonuria (September 2021) AWMSG No. 2322 Recommended

- **MEDICINAL FORMS** There can be variation in the licensing of different medicines containing the same drug.
  Oral suspension
  CAUTIONARY AND ADVISORY LABELS 21
  EXCIPIENTS: May contain Polysorbates
  ELECTROLYTES: May contain Sodium
  ▸ Orfadin (Swedish Orphan Biovitrum Ltd)
    Nitisinone 4 mg per 1 ml Orfadin 4mg/1ml oral suspension | 90 ml PoM £1,692.00 (Hospital only) SF
  Oral capsule
  ▸ Nitisinone (Non-proprietary)
    Nitisinone 2 mg Nitisinone 2mg capsules | 60 capsule PoM £423.00
    Nitisinone 5 mg Nitisinone 5mg capsules | 60 capsule PoM £845.25
    Nitisinone 10 mg Nitisinone 10mg capsules | 60 capsule PoM £1,546.50
    Nitisinone 20 mg Nitisinone 20mg capsules | 60 capsule PoM £3,384.00
  ▸ Orfadin (Swedish Orphan Biovitrum Ltd)
    Nitisinone 2 mg Orfadin 2mg capsules | 60 capsule PoM £423.00 (Hospital only)
    Nitisinone 5 mg Orfadin 5mg capsules | 60 capsule PoM £845.25 (Hospital only)
    Nitisinone 10 mg Orfadin 10mg capsules | 60 capsule PoM £1,546.50 (Hospital only)
    Nitisinone 20 mg Orfadin 20mg capsules | 60 capsule PoM £3,384.00 (Hospital only)

3.17 Urea cycle disorders

AMINO ACIDS AND DERIVATIVES

Carglumic acid

24-Jul-2020

- **INDICATIONS AND DOSE**

Hyperammonaemia due to N-acetylglutamate synthase deficiency (under expert supervision)
▸ BY MOUTH
▸ Adult: Initially 50–125 mg/kg twice daily, to be taken immediately before food, dose adjusted according to plasma–ammonia concentration; maintenance 5–50 mg/kg twice daily, the total daily dose may alternatively be given in 3–4 divided doses

Hyperammonaemia due to organic acidaemia (under expert supervision)
▸ BY MOUTH
▸ Adult: Initially 50–125 mg/kg twice daily, to be taken immediately before food, dose adjusted according to plasma-ammonia concentration, the total daily dose may alternatively be given in 3–4 divided doses

IMPORTANT SAFETY INFORMATION
EMERGENCY MANAGEMENT OF UREA CYCLE DISORDERS
For further information on the emergency management of urea cycle disorders consult the British Inherited

Metabolic Disease Group (BIMDG) website at www.bimdg.org.uk.

- **SIDE-EFFECTS**
▸ **Common or very common** Hyperhidrosis
▸ **Uncommon** Bradycardia · diarrhoea · fever · vomiting
▸ **Frequency not known** Rash

- **PREGNANCY** Manufacturer advises avoid unless essential—no information available.

- **BREAST FEEDING** Manufacturer advises avoid—present in milk in *animal* studies.

- **DIRECTIONS FOR ADMINISTRATION** Manufacturer advises dispersible tablets must be dispersed in at least 5–10 mL of water and taken orally immediately, or administered via a nasogastric tube.

- **MEDICINAL FORMS** There can be variation in the licensing of different medicines containing the same drug.
  Dispersible tablet
  CAUTIONARY AND ADVISORY LABELS 13
  ▸ Carglumic acid (Non-proprietary)
    Carglumic acid 200 mg Carglumic acid 200mg dispersible tablets sugar free | 5 tablet PoM £218.69 SF | 15 tablet PoM £625.37 SF | 60 tablet PoM £2,624.30 SF
  ▸ Carbaglu (Recordati Rare Diseases UK Ltd)
    Carglumic acid 200 mg Carbaglu 200mg dispersible tablets | 5 tablet PoM £299.00 SF | 60 tablet PoM £3,499.00 SF
  ▸ Ucedane (Eurocept International bv)
    Carglumic acid 200 mg Ucedane 200mg dispersible tablets | 12 tablet PoM £660.00 SF | 60 tablet PoM £3,300.00 SF

BENZOATES

Sodium benzoate

16-Aug-2023

- **INDICATIONS AND DOSE**

Acute hyperammonaemia due to urea cycle disorders (initiated in hospital or under specialist supervision)
▸ BY CONTINUOUS INTRAVENOUS INFUSION
▸ Adult: 250 mg/kg/24 hours, dose to be given at an approximate rate of 10 mg/kg/hour

Maintenance treatment of hyperammonaemia due to urea cycle disorders (initiated by a specialist)
▸ BY MOUTH
▸ Adult: 250 mg/kg daily in 3–4 divided doses, dose to be taken with food; maximum 12 g per day

DOSES AT EXTREMES OF BODY-WEIGHT
▸ With intravenous use To avoid excessive dosage in obese patients, contact a specialist metabolic centre for advice.

- **UNLICENSED USE** Sodium benzoate is not licensed in the UK. It is used as detailed below:
  - EvGr Acute hyperammonaemia due to urea cycle disorders;
  - Maintenance treatment of hyperammonaemia due to urea cycle disorders. E

IMPORTANT SAFETY INFORMATION
EMERGENCY MANAGEMENT OF UREA CYCLE DISORDERS
For further information on the emergency management of urea cycle disorders, consult the British Inherited Metabolic Disease Group (BIMDG) website at: www.bimdg.org.uk.

- **CAUTIONS** Conditions involving sodium retention with oedema (preparations contain significant amounts of sodium) · congestive heart failure (preparations contain significant amounts of sodium)

- **SIDE-EFFECTS** Gastro-intestinal side-effects may be reduced by giving smaller doses more frequently.

- **PREGNANCY** No information available.

- **BREAST FEEDING** No information available.

- **RENAL IMPAIRMENT** Use with caution (preparations contain significant amounts of sodium).

- **DIRECTIONS FOR ADMINISTRATION** For administration *by mouth*, expert sources advise oral solution or powder may be administered in fruit drinks.
  For *intravenous infusion*, expert sources advise dilute to a max. concentration of 50 mg/mL with Glucose 10%.

- **MEDICINAL FORMS** There can be variation in the licensing of different medicines containing the same drug. Forms available from special-order manufacturers include: oral tablet, oral capsule, oral solution, solution for infusion
  Solution for infusion
  ELECTROLYTES: May contain Sodium

DRUGS FOR METABOLIC DISORDERS ›
AMMONIA LOWERING DRUGS

Glycerol phenylbutyrate
18-Nov-2020

- **DRUG ACTION** Glycerol phenylbutyrate is a nitrogen-binding agent that provides an alternative vehicle for waste nitrogen excretion.

- **INDICATIONS AND DOSE**

Urea cycle disorders (specialist use only)
▸ BY MOUTH, OR BY GASTROSTOMY TUBE, OR BY NASOGASTRIC TUBE
▸ Adult (body surface area up to 1.3 m^2): Initially 9.4 g/m^2 daily in divided doses, usual maintenance 5.3–12.4 g/m^2 daily in divided doses, each dose should be rounded up to the nearest 0.5 mL and given with each meal. For dose adjustments based on individual requirements—consult product literature
▸ Adult (body surface area 1.3 m^2 and above): Initially 8 g/m^2 daily in divided doses, usual maintenance 5.3–12.4 g/m^2 daily in divided doses, each dose should be rounded up to the nearest 0.5 mL and given with each meal. For dose adjustments based on individual requirements—consult product literature

DOSE EQUIVALENCE AND CONVERSION
▸ 1 mL of liquid contains 1.1 g of glycerol phenylbutyrate.
▸ For patients switching from sodium phenylbutyrate or sodium benzoate—consult product literature.

> **IMPORTANT SAFETY INFORMATION**
> **EMERGENCY MANAGEMENT OF UREA CYCLE DISORDERS**
> For further information on the emergency management of urea cycle disorders consult the British Inherited Metabolic Disease Group (BIMDG) website at www.bimdg.org.uk.

- **CONTRA-INDICATIONS** Treatment of acute hyperammonaemia

- **CAUTIONS** Elderly—limited information available · intestinal malabsorption · pancreatic insufficiency

- **INTERACTIONS** → Appendix 1: glycerol phenylbutyrate

- **SIDE-EFFECTS**
▸ **Common or very common** Appetite abnormal · constipation · diarrhoea · dizziness · fatigue · food aversion · gastrointestinal discomfort · gastrointestinal disorders · headache · menstrual cycle irregularities · nausea · oral disorders · peripheral oedema · skin reactions · tremor · vomiting
▸ **Uncommon** Akathisia · alopecia · biliary colic · bladder pain · burping · confusion · depressed mood · drowsiness · dry mouth · dysphonia · epistaxis · fever · gastrointestinal infection viral · hot flush · hyperhidrosis · hypoalbuminaemia · hypokalaemia · hypothyroidism · joint swelling · muscle spasms · nasal congestion · oropharyngeal pain · pain · paraesthesia · plantar fasciitis ·

speech disorder · taste altered · throat irritation · ventricular arrhythmia · weight changes

- **PREGNANCY** Manufacturer advises avoid unless essential—toxicity in *animal* studies.

- **BREAST FEEDING** Manufacturer advises avoid—no information available.

- **HEPATIC IMPAIRMENT** Manufacturer advises caution (risk of increased exposure).
  Dose adjustments Manufacturer advises use lowest possible dose—consult product literature.

- **RENAL IMPAIRMENT** Manufacturer advises use with caution in severe impairment—no information available.

- **DIRECTIONS FOR ADMINISTRATION** Manufacturer advises may be added to a small amount of apple sauce, ketchup, or squash puree and used within 2 hours. For administration advice via nasogastric or gastrostomy tube—consult product literature.

- **HANDLING AND STORAGE** Manufacturer advises discard contents of bottle 14 days after opening.

- **PATIENT AND CARER ADVICE**
  Driving and skilled tasks Manufacturer advises patients and carers should be counselled on the effects on driving and performance of skilled tasks—increased risk of dizziness.

- **NATIONAL FUNDING/ACCESS DECISIONS**
  For full details see funding body website

  Scottish Medicines Consortium (SMC) decisions
▸ Glycerol phenylbutyrate (*Ravicti*®) as adjunctive therapy for chronic management of adult and paediatric patients aged 2 months and older with urea cycle disorders who cannot be managed by dietary protein restriction and/or amino acid supplementation alone (August 2018) SMC No. 1342/18 Recommended

  All Wales Medicines Strategy Group (AWMSG) decisions
▸ Glycerol phenylbutyrate (*Ravicti*®) as adjunctive therapy for chronic management of patients with urea cycle disorders who cannot be managed by dietary protein restriction and/or amino acid supplementation alone (December 2019) AWMSG No. 2127 Recommended

- **MEDICINAL FORMS** There can be variation in the licensing of different medicines containing the same drug.
  Gastroenteral or oral liquid
▸ Ravicti (Immedica Pharma AB)
  Glycerol phenylbutyrate 1.1 gram per 1 ml Ravicti 1.1g/ml oral liquid | 25 ml PoM £161.00

Sodium phenylbutyrate
05-Oct-2021

- **INDICATIONS AND DOSE**

Long-term treatment of urea cycle disorders (as adjunctive therapy in all patients with neonatal-onset disease and in those with late-onset disease who have a history of hyperammonaemic encephalopathy) (under expert supervision)
▸ BY MOUTH
▸ Adult: 9.9–13 g/m^2 daily in divided doses, with meals; maximum 20 g per day

> **IMPORTANT SAFETY INFORMATION**
> **EMERGENCY MANAGEMENT OF UREA CYCLE DISORDERS**
> For further information on the emergency management of urea cycle disorders consult the British Inherited Metabolic Disease Group (BIMDG) website at www.bimdg.org.uk.

- **CAUTIONS** Conditions involving sodium retention with oedema (preparations contain significant amounts of sodium) · congestive heart failure (preparations contain significant amounts of sodium)

- INTERACTIONS → Appendix 1: sodium phenylbutyrate
- SIDE-EFFECTS
▶ **Common or very common** Abdominal pain · anaemia · appetite decreased · constipation · depression · headache · irritability · leucocytosis · leucopenia · menstrual cycle irregularities · metabolic acidosis · metabolic alkalosis · nausea · oedema · renal tubular acidosis · skin reactions · syncope · taste altered · thrombocytopenia · thrombocytosis · vomiting · weight increased
▶ **Uncommon** Anorectal haemorrhage · aplastic anaemia · arrhythmia · gastrointestinal disorders · pancreatitis
- CONCEPTION AND CONTRACEPTION Manufacturer advises adequate contraception during administration in women of child-bearing potential.
- PREGNANCY Avoid—toxicity in *animal* studies.
- BREAST FEEDING Manufacturer advises avoid—no information available.
- HEPATIC IMPAIRMENT Manufacturer advises caution.
- RENAL IMPAIRMENT Manufacturer advises use with caution (preparations contain significant amounts of sodium).
- DIRECTIONS FOR ADMINISTRATION EvGr *Pheburane*® granules may be directly swallowed with a drink or sprinkled on a spoonful of food, during feeds or mealtimes. Granules must not be administered by nasogastric or gastrostomy tubes. Ⓜ

- MEDICINAL FORMS There can be variation in the licensing of different medicines containing the same drug. Forms available from special-order manufacturers include: oral capsule, oral suspension, oral solution

Oral tablet
▶ Ammonaps (Immedica Pharma AB)
  Sodium phenylbutyrate 500 mg Ammonaps 500mg tablets | 250 tablet PoM £493.00 DT = £493.00

Oral granules
▶ Pheburane (Eurocept International bv)
  Sodium phenylbutyrate 483 mg per 1 gram Pheburane 483mg/g granules | 174 gram PoM £331.00

ENZYMES

Pegzilarginase

03-Dec-2024

- DRUG ACTION Pegzilarginase is an enzyme produced by recombinant DNA technology that is administered as enzyme replacement therapy for the treatment of arginase-1 deficiency (hyperargininaemia).

● **INDICATIONS AND DOSE**

Arginase-1 deficiency [hyperargininaemia] (under expert supervision)
▶ BY INTRAVENOUS INFUSION, OR BY SUBCUTANEOUS INJECTION
▶ Adult: Initially 0.1 mg/kg once weekly, dose should then be adjusted in steps of 0.05 mg/kg according to plasma-arginine concentrations—consult product literature, doses exceeding 0.2 mg/kg once weekly have not been studied

IMPORTANT SAFETY INFORMATION
EMERGENCY MANAGEMENT OF UREA CYCLE DISORDERS
For further information on the emergency management of urea cycle disorders consult the British Inherited Metabolic Disease Group (BIMDG) website at www.bimdg. org.uk.

- CAUTIONS Hypersensitivity reactions
CAUTIONS, FURTHER INFORMATION
▶ Hypersensitivity reactions
▶ With intravenous use EvGr Reactions, including facial swelling, rash, and flushing, have occurred usually with the first few doses; initial doses of pegzilarginase should be administered, under medical observation, by appropriately trained staff. These reactions may be managed by temporarily interrupting or reducing the rate of the infusion, and/or treatment with antihistamines and/or corticosteroids. Pre-medication with an antihistamine and/or corticosteroid should be considered on re-administration. Ⓜ

- SIDE-EFFECTS
▶ **Common or very common** Hypersensitivity
- PREGNANCY EvGr Avoid (toxicity in *animal* studies). Ⓜ
- BREAST FEEDING EvGr Avoid (no information available). Ⓜ
- DIRECTIONS FOR ADMINISTRATION For *intermittent intravenous infusion*, dilute requisite dose with Sodium Chloride 0.9% (up to a maximum concentration of 0.5 mg/mL) and give over at least 30 minutes.

  For *subcutaneous injection*, inject into the abdomen (except for area directly surrounding the navel), lateral part of the thigh, or side or back of the upper arm; if more than one injection is needed for a single dose, injection sites should be at least 3 cm apart. Rotate injection site and avoid skin that is scarred, red, inflamed, or swollen.

  After at least 8 weeks of treatment, *Loargys*® may be self-administered or administered by a carer if appropriate training in subcutaneous injection technique has been given.

- PRESCRIBING AND DISPENSING INFORMATION Pegzilarginase is a biological medicine. Biological medicines must be prescribed and dispensed by brand name, see *Biological medicines* and *Biosimilar medicines*, under Guidance on prescribing p. 1; record the brand name and batch number after each administration.
- HANDLING AND STORAGE Store in a refrigerator (2–8°C) and protect from light; may be stored at room temperature (below 25°C) for up to 2 hours—consult product literature for further information regarding storage after preparation.
- PATIENT AND CARER ADVICE
▶ With subcutaneous use Patients and their carers should be advised to stop administration and seek immediate medical attention if early signs of severe hypersensitivity reactions occur—consider prescribing medication for treatment of a potential severe hypersensitivity reaction.
Self-administration
▶ With subcutaneous use Patients or their carers should be given training in subcutaneous injection technique if appropriate. A patient guide on self-administration at home should be provided.
Missed doses If a dose is missed, it should be administered as soon as possible; there should be a minimum of 4 days between doses.

- MEDICINAL FORMS There can be variation in the licensing of different medicines containing the same drug.
Solution for injection
▶ Loargys (Immedica Pharma AB) ▼
  Pegzilarginase 5 mg per 1 ml Loargys 2mg/0.4ml solution for injection vials | 1 vial PoM £4,690.00 (Hospital only)

3.18 Wilson's disease

Other drugs used for Wilson's disease Penicillamine, p. 1255

ANTIDOTES AND CHELATORS › COPPER ABSORPTION INHIBITORS

Zinc acetate
23-Jul-2020

- **DRUG ACTION** Zinc prevents the absorption of copper in Wilson's disease.

- **INDICATIONS AND DOSE**

Wilson's disease (initiated under specialist supervision)
▸ BY MOUTH
▸ Adult: 50 mg 3 times a day (max. per dose 50 mg 5 times a day), adjusted according to response

DOSE EQUIVALENCE AND CONVERSION
▸ Doses expressed as elemental zinc.

PHARMACOKINETICS
▸ Symptomatic Wilson's disease patients should be treated initially with a chelating agent because zinc has a slow onset of action. When transferring from chelating treatment to zinc maintenance therapy, chelating treatment should be co-administered for 2–3 weeks until zinc produces its maximal effect.

- **CAUTIONS** Portal hypertension (risk of hepatic decompensation when switching from chelating agent)

- **INTERACTIONS** → Appendix 1: zinc

- **SIDE-EFFECTS**
▸ **Common or very common** Epigastric discomfort (usually transient)
▸ **Uncommon** Leucopenia · sideroblastic anaemia
▸ **Frequency not known** Condition aggravated

 SIDE-EFFECTS, FURTHER INFORMATION Transient gastric irritation may be reduced if first dose is taken mid-morning or with a little protein.

- **PREGNANCY**
Dose adjustments Reduce dose to 25 mg 3 times daily adjusted according to plasma-copper concentration and urinary copper excretion.

- **BREAST FEEDING** Manufacturer advises avoid; present in milk—may cause zinc-induced copper deficiency in infant.

- **MONITORING REQUIREMENTS** Monitor full blood count and serum cholesterol.

- **MEDICINAL FORMS** There can be variation in the licensing of different medicines containing the same drug.

Oral capsule
CAUTIONARY AND ADVISORY LABELS 23
▸ Wilzin (Recordati Rare Diseases UK Ltd)
Zinc (as Zinc acetate) 25 mg Wilzin 25mg capsules | 250 capsule PoM £132.00 DT = £132.00
Zinc (as Zinc acetate) 50 mg Wilzin 50mg capsules | 250 capsule PoM £242.00 DT = £242.00

ANTIDOTES AND CHELATORS › COPPER CHELATORS

Trientine
14-Jun-2023

- **DRUG ACTION** Trientine is a chelating agent that binds to copper, forming a complex that is readily excreted by the kidneys; it may also inhibit the absorption of copper from the gastro-intestinal tract.

- **INDICATIONS AND DOSE**

Wilson's disease in patients intolerant of penicillamine [using Tillomed generic capsules] (initiated by a specialist)
▸ BY MOUTH
▸ Adult: Initially 1000–2000 mg daily in 2–4 divided doses, dose should then be adjusted according to response and serum-copper concentrations

DOSE EQUIVALENCE AND CONVERSION
▸ For Tillomed generic: each capsule contains trientine base equivalent to 250 mg trientine dihydrochloride; doses expressed as trientine dihydrochloride.
▸ Preparations are not interchangeable on a milligram-for-milligram basis due to differences in bioavailability.

CUFENCE ®

Wilson's disease in patients intolerant of penicillamine (initiated by a specialist)
▸ BY MOUTH
▸ Adult: Initially 800–1600 mg daily in 2–4 divided doses, dose should then be adjusted according to response and serum-copper concentrations

DOSE EQUIVALENCE AND CONVERSION
▸ For *Cufence*®: each capsule contains trientine dihydrochloride equivalent to 200 mg trientine base; doses expressed as trientine base.
▸ Preparations are not interchangeable on a milligram-for-milligram basis due to differences in bioavailability.

CUPRIOR ®

Wilson's disease in patients intolerant of penicillamine (initiated by a specialist)
▸ BY MOUTH
▸ Adult: Initially 450–975 mg daily in 2–4 divided doses, dose should then be adjusted according to response and serum-copper concentrations

DOSE EQUIVALENCE AND CONVERSION
▸ For *Cuprior*®: each tablet contains trientine tetrahydrochloride equivalent to 150 mg of trientine base; doses expressed as trientine base.
▸ Preparations are not interchangeable on a milligram-for-milligram basis due to differences in bioavailability.

- **INTERACTIONS** → Appendix 1: trientine

- **SIDE-EFFECTS**
▸ **Common or very common** Nausea
▸ **Uncommon** Anaemia · aplastic anaemia · skin reactions
▸ **Frequency not known** Gastrointestinal disorders · neurological deterioration in Wilson's Disease

- **PREGNANCY** EvGr Teratogenic in *animal* studies—use only if benefit outweighs risk. Monitor maternal and neonatal serum-copper concentrations. Ⓜ

- **BREAST FEEDING** EvGr Specialist sources indicate caution—limited information available; effect on copper levels in milk conflicting and impact on infant unknown. ◇D◇

- **DIRECTIONS FOR ADMINISTRATION**
CUPRIOR ® Tablets can be divided into 2 equal halves.

- **PRESCRIBING AND DISPENSING INFORMATION** Trientine is **not** an alternative to penicillamine for rheumatoid arthritis or cystinuria. Penicillamine-induced systemic lupus erythematosus may not resolve on transfer to trientine.

- **NATIONAL FUNDING/ACCESS DECISIONS**
For full details see funding body website

Scottish Medicines Consortium (SMC) decisions
▸ Trientine tetrahydrochloride (*Cuprior*®) for the treatment of Wilson's disease in adults, adolescents and children aged 5 years and older, intolerant to D-penicillamine therapy (November 2019) SMC No. SMC2222 Recommended

- **MEDICINAL FORMS** There can be variation in the licensing of different medicines containing the same drug.
Oral tablet
CAUTIONARY AND ADVISORY LABELS 7, 23
▸ Cuprior (Orphalan UK Ltd)
Trientine (as Trientine tetrahydrochloride) 150 mg Cuprior 150mg tablets | 72 tablet PoM £2,725.00 (Hospital only)

Oral capsule
CAUTIONARY AND ADVISORY LABELS 7, 23, 25
- **Trientine (Non-proprietary)**
  Trientine (as Trientine dihydrochloride) 200 mg Trientine 200mg capsules | 100 capsule [PoM] £2,998.46–£5,577.12 DT = £3,075.13
  Trientine dihydrochloride 250 mg Metalite 250mg capsules | 100 capsule [PoM] [Ⓔ]
  Trientine dihydrochloride 250mg capsules | 100 capsule [PoM] £1,498.00 (Hospital only)
- **Cufence** (Univar Solutions B.V.)
  Trientine (as Trientine dihydrochloride) 100 mg Cufence 100mg capsules | 200 capsule [PoM] £3,075.13
  Trientine (as Trientine dihydrochloride) 200 mg Cufence 200mg capsules | 100 capsule [PoM] £3,075.13 DT = £3,075.13

4 Mineral and trace elements deficiencies

4.1 Selenium deficiency

Selenium deficiency

05-May-2021

Overview

Selenium deficiency can occur as a result of inadequate diet or prolonged parenteral nutrition. A selenium supplement should not be given unless there is good evidence of deficiency.

VITAMINS AND TRACE ELEMENTS

Selenium

- **INDICATIONS AND DOSE**

Selenium deficiency
- BY MOUTH, OR BY INTRAMUSCULAR INJECTION, OR BY INTRAVENOUS INJECTION
- Adult: 100–500 micrograms daily

- **INTERACTIONS** → Appendix 1: selenium

- **MEDICINAL FORMS** There can be variation in the licensing of different medicines containing the same drug. Forms available from special-order manufacturers include: solution for infusion

Oral tablet
- **Selenium (Non-proprietary)**
  L-Selenomethionine 200 microgram EN-Selenium 200microgram tablets | 30 tablet £88.60
- **200-SEL** (TriOn Pharma Ltd)
  L-Selenomethionine 200 microgram 200-SEL tablets | 30 tablet £2.31
- **Abselen** (Essential-Healthcare Ltd)
  L-Selenomethionine 200 microgram Abselen 200microgram tablets | 30 tablet £2.31
- **Bio-SelenoPrecise** (Pharma Nord (UK) Ltd)
  L-Selenomethionine 200 microgram Bio-SelenoPrecise 200microgram tablets | 60 tablet £4.85 | 150 tablet £8.84
- **SelenoPrecise** (Pharma Nord (UK) Ltd)
  Selenium (as L-Selenomethionine) 100 microgram SelenoPrecise 100microgram tablets | 60 tablet £4.29

Solution for injection
- **Selenase** (Kora Healthcare)
  Selenium (as Sodium selenite) 50 microgram per 1 ml Selenase 100micrograms/2ml solution for injection ampoules | 10 ampoule [PoM] £30.00
  Selenase 500micrograms/10ml solution for injection vials | 10 vial [PoM] £90.00

Oral capsule
- **Selenium (Non-proprietary)**
  L-Selenomethionine 200 microgram Selenium 200microgram capsules | 60 capsule £5.79

Solution for infusion
- **Selenium (Non-proprietary)**
  Selenium (as Sodium selenite) 10 microgram per 1 ml Selenium 100micrograms/10ml solution for infusion vials | 10 vial [PoM] £64.00

Oral solution
- **Selenase** (Kora Healthcare)
  Selenium (as Sodium selenite) 50 microgram per 1 ml Selenase 100micrograms/2ml oral solution 2ml unit dose ampoules | 20 unit dose [PoM] £26.00 DT = £26.00
  Selenase 500micrograms/10ml oral solution unit dose vials | 10 unit dose [PoM] £50.00

4.2 Zinc deficiency

Zinc deficiency

22-Mar-2021

Overview

Zinc is an essential trace element, involved in a number of body enzyme systems, and is found in a variety of foods. Patients with malnutrition, alcoholism, inflammatory bowel disease, and malabsorption syndromes are at an increased risk of zinc deficiency.

Zinc supplements can be given for zinc deficiency or in zinc-losing conditions. Continuous zinc supplementation is generally safe, however higher doses should be limited to short-term use due to an increased risk of gastro-intestinal adverse effects, copper deficiency, reduced immunity, anaemia, and genitourinary complications with long-term use.

Zinc is used in the treatment of Wilson's disease, and in acrodermatitis enteropathica—a rare inherited disorder characterised by impaired zinc absorption.

Parenteral nutrition regimens usually include trace amounts of zinc, see also Intravenous nutrition p. 1227. Further zinc can be added to intravenous feeding regimens if required.

ELECTROLYTES AND MINERALS ＞ ZINC

Zinc sulfate

23-Nov-2023

- **INDICATIONS AND DOSE**

Zinc deficiency or supplementation in zinc-losing conditions
- BY MOUTH USING EFFERVESCENT TABLETS
- Child (body-weight up to 10 kg): 22.5 mg daily, dose to be adjusted as necessary, to be dissolved in water and taken after food, dose expressed as elemental zinc
- Child (body-weight 10-30 kg): 22.5 mg 1–3 times a day, dose to be adjusted as necessary, to be dissolved in water and taken after food, dose expressed as elemental zinc
- Child (body-weight 31 kg and above): 45 mg 1–3 times a day, dose to be adjusted as necessary, to be dissolved in water and taken after food, dose expressed as elemental zinc
- Adult (body-weight 31 kg and above): 45 mg 1–3 times a day, dose to be adjusted as necessary, to be dissolved in water and taken after food, dose expressed as elemental zinc

Additional elemental zinc for intravenous nutrition
- BY INTRAVENOUS INJECTION
- Adult: 6.5 mg daily (Zn^{2+} 100 micromol)

IMPORTANT SAFETY INFORMATION
ZINC-INDUCED COPPER DEFICIENCY
Zinc inhibits the absorption of copper, thereby reducing copper levels and potentially causing copper deficiency. The risk of copper deficiency is greater with higher doses

of zinc and with long-term treatment, particularly if zinc deficiency is no longer present. Signs of copper deficiency include neurological and haematological symptoms.

- **CONTRA-INDICATIONS** Copper deficiency
- **INTERACTIONS** → Appendix 1: zinc
- **SIDE-EFFECTS** Copper deficiency · diarrhoea · gastritis · gastrointestinal discomfort · nausea · vomiting
- **PREGNANCY** Crosses placenta; risk theoretically minimal, but no information available.
- **BREAST FEEDING** Present in milk; risk theoretically minimal, but no information available.
- **RENAL IMPAIRMENT** EvGr Use with caution (accumulation may occur in renal failure). M
- **PRESCRIBING AND DISPENSING INFORMATION** Each *Solvazinc*® tablet contains zinc sulfate monohydrate 125 mg (45 mg zinc).

- **MEDICINAL FORMS** There can be variation in the licensing of different medicines containing the same drug. Forms available from special-order manufacturers include: oral solution, solution for injection

Effervescent tablet
CAUTIONARY AND ADVISORY LABELS 13, 21
EXCIPIENTS: May contain Sorbitol
ELECTROLYTES: May contain Sodium
▸ **Solvazinc** (Galen Ltd)
Zinc sulfate monohydrate 125 mg Solvazinc 125mg effervescent tablets | 90 tablet P £17.72 DT = £17.72 SF

5   Nutrition (intravenous)

Intravenous nutrition

Overview

When adequate feeding through the alimentary tract is not possible, nutrients may be given by intravenous infusion. This may be in addition to ordinary oral or tube feeding— **supplemental parenteral nutrition**, or may be the sole source of nutrition— **total parenteral nutrition** (TPN). Indications for this method include preparation of undernourished patients for surgery, chemotherapy, or radiation therapy; severe or prolonged disorders of the gastro-intestinal tract; major surgery, trauma, or burns; prolonged coma or refusal to eat; and some patients with renal or hepatic failure. The composition of proprietary preparations available is given under Proprietary Infusion Fluids for Parenteral Feeding p. 1228.

Parenteral nutrition requires the use of a solution containing amino acids, glucose, fat, electrolytes, trace elements, and vitamins. This is now commonly provided by the pharmacy in the form of a 3-litre bag. A single dose of vitamin B_{12}, as hydroxocobalamin p. 1162, is given by intramuscular injection; regular vitamin B_{12} injections are not usually required unless total parenteral nutrition continues for many months. Folic acid p. 1161 is given in a dose of 15 mg once or twice each week, usually in the nutrition solution. Other vitamins are usually given daily; they are generally introduced in the parenteral nutrition solution. Alternatively, if the patient is able to take small amounts by mouth, vitamins may be given orally.

The nutrition solution is infused through a central venous catheter inserted under full surgical precautions. Alternatively, infusion through a peripheral vein may be used for supplementary as well as total parenteral nutrition for periods of up to a month, depending on the availability of

peripheral veins; factors prolonging cannula life and preventing thrombophlebitis include the use of soft polyurethane paediatric cannulas and use of feeds of low osmolality and neutral pH. Only nutritional fluids should be given by the dedicated intravenous line.

Before starting, the patient should be well oxygenated with a near normal circulating blood volume and attention should be given to renal function and acid-base status. Appropriate biochemical tests should have been carried out beforehand and serious deficits corrected. Nutritional and electrolyte status must be monitored throughout treatment.

Complications of long-term parenteral nutrition include gall bladder sludging, gall stones, cholestasis and abnormal liver function tests. For details of the prevention and management of parenteral nutrition complications, specialist literature should be consulted.

Protein is given as mixtures of essential and non-essential synthetic L-amino acids. Ideally, all essential amino acids should be included with a wide variety of nonessential ones to provide sufficient nitrogen together with electrolytes. Solutions vary in their composition of amino acids; they often contain an energy source (usually glucose p. 1182) and electrolytes.

Energy is provided in a ratio of 0.6 to 1.1 megajoules (150–250 kcals) per gram of protein nitrogen. Energy requirements must be met if amino acids are to be utilised for tissue maintenance. A mixture of carbohydrate and fat energy sources (usually 30–50% as fat) gives better utilisation of amino acids than glucose alone.

Glucose is the preferred source of carbohydrate, but if more than 180 g is given per day frequent monitoring of blood glucose is required, and insulin may be necessary. Glucose in various strengths from 10 to 50% must be infused through a central venous catheter to avoid thrombosis.

In parenteral nutrition regimens, it is necessary to provide adequate **phosphate** in order to allow phosphorylation of glucose and to prevent hypophosphataemia; between 20 and 30 mmol of phosphate is required daily.

Fructose and sorbitol have been used in an attempt to avoid the problem of hyperosmolar hyperglycaemic non-ketotic acidosis but other metabolic problems may occur, as with xylitol and ethanol which are now rarely used.

Fat emulsions have the advantages of a high energy to fluid volume ratio, neutral pH, and iso-osmolarity with plasma, and provide essential fatty acids. Several days of adaptation may be required to attain maximal utilisation. Reactions include occasional febrile episodes (usually only with 20% emulsions) and rare anaphylactic responses. Interference with biochemical measurements such as those for blood gases and calcium may occur if samples are taken before fat has been cleared. Daily checks are necessary to ensure complete clearance from the plasma in conditions where fat metabolism may be disturbed. **Additives should not be mixed with fat emulsions unless compatibility is known.**

Administration

Because of the complex requirements relating to parenteral nutrition full details relating to administration have been omitted. In all cases *product literature and other specialist literature should be consulted.*

Proprietary Infusion Fluids for Parenteral Feeding

Preparation	Nitrogen g/litre	[1,2]Energy kJ/litre	Electrolytes mmol/litre					Other components/litre
			K⁺	Mg²⁺	Na⁺	Acet⁻	Cl⁻	
Aminoplasmal 10% (B.Braun Medical Ltd) Net price (10-bottle pack) 500 ml = £230.00; Net price (6-bottle pack) 1 litre = £320.00	15.8	–	–	–	–	28.0	–	citrate 1–2 mmol
Aminoplasmal 15% (B.Braun Medical Ltd) Net price (10-bottle pack) 500 ml = £230.00; Net price (6-bottle pack) 1 litre = £324.00	24.0	–	–	–	5.3	–	–	
Clinimix N14G30E (Baxter Healthcare Ltd) Net price (dual compartment bag of amino acids with electrolytes 1000 mL and glucose 30% with calcium 1000 mL) 2 litre = £31.52	7.0	2520	30.0	2.5	35.0	70.0	40.0	Ca²⁺ 2.3 mmol, phosphate 15 mmol, anhydrous glucose 150 g
ClinOleic 20% (Baxter Healthcare Ltd) Net price 100 ml = £6.28; Net price 250 ml = £10.08; Net price 500 ml = £13.88	–	8360	–	–	–	–	–	purified olive and soya oil 200 g, glycerol 22.5 g, egg phospholipids 12 g
Intralipid 10% (Fresenius Kabi Ltd) Net price (10-bag pack) 100 ml = £48.50; Net price (12-bag pack) 500 ml = £127.20	–	4600	–	–	–	–	–	soya oil 100 g, glycerol 22 g, purified egg phospholipids 12 g, phosphate 15 mmol
Intralipid 20% (Fresenius Kabi Ltd) Net price (10-bag pack) 100 ml = £73.00; Net price (10-bag pack) 250 ml = £119.50; Net price (12-bag pack) 500 ml = £190.80	–	8400	–	–	–	–	–	soya oil 200 g, glycerol 22 g, purified egg phospholipids 12 g, phosphate 15 mmol
Kabiven (Fresenius Kabi Ltd) Net price (triple compartment bag of amino acids and electrolytes 450 mL, glucose 790 mL, lipid emulsion 300 mL; 4-bag pack) 1.54 litre = £207.48; Net price (triple compartment bag of amino acids and electrolytes 600 mL, glucose 1053 mL, lipid emulsion 400 mL; 4-bag pack) 2.053 litre = £270.20; Net price (triple compartment bag of amino acids and electrolytes 750 mL, glucose 1316 mL, lipid emulsion 500 mL; 3-bag pack) 2.566 litre = £211.47	5.3	3275	23.0	4.0	31.0	38.0	45.0	Ca²⁺ 2 mmol, phosphate 9.7 mmol, anhydrous glucose 97 g, soya oil 39 g
Kabiven peripheral (Fresenius Kabi Ltd) Net price (triple compartment bag of amino acids and electrolytes 300 mL, glucose 885 mL, lipid emulsion 255 mL; 4-bag pack) 1.44 litre = £144.80; Net price (triple compartment bag of amino acids and electrolytes 400 mL, glucose 1180 mL, lipid emulsion 340 mL; 4-bag pack) 1.92 litre = £207.48; Net price (triple compartment bag of amino acids and electrolytes 500 mL, glucose 1475 mL, lipid emulsion 425 mL; 3-bag pack) 2.4 litre = £196.65	3.75	2625	17.0	2.8	22.0	27.0	33.0	Ca²⁺ 1.4 mmol, phosphate 7.5 mmol, anhydrous glucose 67.5 g, soya oil 35.4 g
Lipidem (B.Braun Medical Ltd) Net price 500 ml: no price available; Net price (6-bottle pack) 1 litre = £500.00	–	7900	–	–	–	–	–	omega-3-acid triglycerides 20 g, soya oil 80 g, medium chain triglycerides 100 g

1 1000 kcal = 4200 kJ; 1000 kJ = 238.8 kcal. All entries are Prescription-only medicines.

2 Excludes protein- or amino acid-derived energy

Preparation	Nitrogen g/litre	[1,2]Energy kJ/litre	Electrolytes mmol/litre						Other components/litre
			K+	Mg2+	Na+	Acet-	Cl-		
Lipoflex peri (B.Braun Medical Ltd) Net price (triple compartment bag of amino acids 500 mL, glucose 500 mL, lipid emulsion 250 mL) 1.25 litre: no price available; Net price (triple compartment bag of amino acids 750 mL, glucose 750 mL, lipid emulsion 375 mL) 1.875 litre: no price available; Net price (triple compartment bag of amino acids 1000 mL, glucose 1000 mL, lipid emulsion 500 mL) 2.5 litre: no price available	4.6	2665	24.0	2.4	40.0	32.0	38.0	Ca2+ 2.4 mmol, Zn2+ 24 micromol, phosphate 6 mmol, anhydrous glucose 64 g, soya oil 20 g, medium-chain triglycerides 20 g
Lipoflex plus (B.Braun Medical Ltd) Net price (triple compartment bag of amino acids 500 mL, glucose 500 mL, lipid emulsion 250 mL) 1.25 litre: no price available; Net price (triple compartment bag of amino acids 750 mL, glucose 750 mL, lipid emulsion 375 mL) 1.875 litre: no price available; Net price (triple compartment bag of amino acids 1000 mL, glucose 1000 mL, lipid emulsion 500 mL) 2.5 litre: no price available	5.4	3600	28.0	3.2	40.0	36.0	36.0	Ca2+ 3.2 mmol, Zn2+ 24 micromol, phosphate 12 mmol, anhydrous glucose 120 g, soya oil 20 g, medium-chain triglycerides 20 g
Lipoflex special (B.Braun Medical Ltd) Net price (triple compartment bag of amino acids 500 mL, glucose 500 mL, lipid emulsion 250 mL) 1.25 litre: no price available; Net price (triple compartment bag of amino acids 750 mL, glucose 750 mL, lipid emulsion 375 mL) 1.875 litre: no price available	8.0	4005	37.6	4.2	53.6	48.0	48.0	Ca2+ 4.2 mmol, Zn2+ 30 micromol, phosphate 16 mmol, anhydrous glucose 144 g, soya oil 20 g, medium-chain triglycerides 20 g
Lipoflex special without electrolytes (B.Braun Medical Ltd) Net price (triple compartment bag of amino acids 750 mL, glucose 750 mL, lipid emulsion 375 mL) 1.875 litre: no price available	8.0	4005	-	-	-	-	-	anhydrous glucose 144 g, soya oil 20 g, medium-chain triglycerides 20 g
Lipofundin MCT/LCT 20% (B.Braun Medical Ltd) Net price 500 ml: no price available	-	8095	-	-	-	-	-	soya oil 100 g, medium-chain triglycerides 100 g
Nutriflex basal (B.Braun Medical Ltd) Net price (dual compartment bag of amino acids 800 mL, glucose 1200 mL) 2 litre: no price available	4.6	2093	30.0	5.7	49.9	35.0	50.0	Ca2+ 3.6 mmol, phosphate 12.8 mmol, anhydrous glucose 125 g
Nutriflex peri (B.Braun Medical Ltd) Net price (dual compartment bag of amino acids 800 mL, glucose 1200 mL) 2 litre: no price available	5.7	1340	15.0	4.0	27.0	19.5	31.6	Ca2+ 2.5 mmol, phosphate 5.7 mmol, anhydrous glucose 80 g
Nutriflex plus (B.Braun Medical Ltd) Net price (dual compartment bag of amino acids 800 mL, glucose 1200 mL) 2 litre: no price available	6.8	2512	25.0	5.7	37.2	22.9	35.5	Ca2+ 3.6 mmol, phosphate 20 mmol, anhydrous glucose 150 g
Nutriflex special (B.Braun Medical Ltd) Net price (dual compartment bag of amino acids 750 mL, glucose 750 mL) 1.5 litre: no price available	10.0	4019	25.7	5.0	40.5	22.0	49.5	Ca2+ 4.1 mmol, phosphate 14.7 mmol, anhydrous glucose 240 g

1 1000 kcal = 4200kJ; 1000 kJ = 238.8 kcal. All entries are Prescription-only medicines.

2 Excludes protein- or amino acid-derived energy

Preparation	Nitrogen g/litre	[1,2]Energy kJ/litre	Electrolytes mmol/litre					Other components/litre
			K+	Mg2+	Na+	Acet-	Cl-	
Omeflex peri (B.Braun Medical Ltd) Net price (triple compartment bag of amino acids 500 mL, glucose 500 mL, lipid emulsion 250 mL) 1.25 litre: no price available; Net price (triple compartment bag of amino acids 750 mL, glucose 750 mL, lipid emulsion 375 mL) 1.875 litre: no price available; Net price (triple compartment bag of amino acids 1000 mL, glucose 1000 mL, lipid emulsion 500 mL) 2.5 litre: no price available	4.6	2665	24.0	2.4	40.0	32.0	38.0	Ca^{2+} 2.4 mmol, Zn^{2+} 24 micromol, phosphate 6 mmol, anhydrous glucose 64 g, soya oil 16 g, medium-chain triglycerides 20 g, omega-3-acid triglycerides 4 g
Omeflex plus (B.Braun Medical Ltd) Net price (triple compartment bag of amino acids 500 mL, glucose 500 mL, lipid emulsion 250 mL) 1.25 litre: no price available; Net price (triple compartment bag of amino acids 750 mL, glucose 750 mL, lipid emulsion 375 mL) 1.875 litre: no price available; Net price (triple compartment bag of amino acids 1000 mL, glucose 1000 mL, lipid emulsion 500 mL) 2.5 litre: no price available	5.4	3600	28.0	3.2	40.0	36.0	36.0	Ca^{2+} 3.2 mmol, Zn^{2+} 24 micromol, phosphate 12 mmol, anhydrous glucose 120 g, soya oil 16 g, medium-chain triglycerides 20 g, omega-3-acid triglycerides 4 g
Omeflex special (B.Braun Medical Ltd) Net price (triple compartment bag of amino acids 250 mL, glucose 250 mL, lipid emulsion 125 mL) 625 ml: no price available; Net price (triple compartment bag of amino acids 500 mL, glucose 500 mL, lipid emulsion 250 mL) 1.25 litre: no price available; Net price (triple compartment bag of amino acids 750 mL, glucose 750 mL, lipid emulsion 375 mL) 1.875 litre: no price available	8.0	4005	37.6	4.2	53.6	48.0	48.0	Ca^{2+} 4.2 mmol, Zn^{2+} 30 micromol, phosphate 16 mmol, anhydrous glucose 144 g, soya oil 16 g, medium-chain triglycerides 20 g, omega-3-acid triglycerides 4 g
Omeflex special without electrolytes (B.Braun Medical Ltd) Net price (triple compartment bag of amino acids 500 mL, glucose 500 mL, lipid emulsion 250 mL) 1.25 litre: no price available; Net price (triple compartment bag of amino acids 750 mL, glucose 750 mL, lipid emulsion 375 mL) 1.875 litre: no price available	8.0	4005	-	-	-	-	-	anhydrous glucose 144 g, soya oil 16 g, medium-chain triglycerides 20 g
Plasma-Lyte 148 (water) (Baxter Healthcare Ltd) Net price 500 ml = £1.46; Net price 1 litre = £1.83	-	-	5.0	1.5	140.0	27.0	98.0	gluconate 23 mmol
Plasma-Lyte 148 (dextrose 5%) (Baxter Healthcare Ltd) Net price 500 ml = £1.46; Net price 1 litre = £1.83	-	840	5.0	1.5	140.0	27.0	98.0	gluconate 23 mmol, glucose monohydrate 55 g

1 1000 kcal = 4200 kJ; 1000 kJ = 238.8 kcal. All entries are Prescription-only medicines.

2 Excludes protein- or amino acid-derived energy

Preparation	Nitrogen g/litre	1,2 Energy kJ/litre	Electrolytes mmol/litre						Other components/litre
			K⁺	Mg²⁺	Na⁺	Acet⁻	Cl⁻	
SmofKabiven (Fresenius Kabi Ltd) Net price (triple compartment bag of amino acids and electrolytes 250 mL, glucose 149 mL, lipid emulsion 94 mL; 6-bag pack) 493 ml = £348.00; Net price (triple compartment bag of amino acids and electrolytes 500 mL, glucose 298 mL, lipid emulsion 188 mL; 4-bag pack) 986 ml = £299.20; Net price (triple compartment bag of amino acids and electrolytes 750 mL, glucose 446 mL, lipid emulsion 281 mL; 4-bag pack) 1.477 litre = £301.40; Net price (triple compartment bag of amino acids and electrolytes 1000 mL, glucose 595 mL, lipid emulsion 375 mL; 4-bag pack) 1.97 litre = £318.72	8.0	3780	30.0	5.1	41.0	106.0	36.0	Ca²⁺ 2.5 mmol, phosphate 13 mmol, anhydrous glucose 127 g, fish oil 5.7 g, olive oil 9.5 g, soya oil 11.4 g, medium-chain triglycerides 11.4 g
SmofKabiven Electrolyte Free (Fresenius Kabi Ltd) Net price (triple compartment bag of amino acids 500 mL, glucose 298 mL, lipid emulsion 188 mL; 4-bag pack) 986 ml = £299.20; Net price (triple compartment bag of amino acids 750 mL, glucose 446 mL, lipid emulsion 281 mL; 4-bag pack) 1.477 litre = £301.40; Net price (triple compartment bag of amino acids 1000 mL, glucose 595 mL, lipid emulsion 375 mL; 4-bag pack) 1.97 litre = £318.72	8.0	3780	–	–	–	74.5	–	phosphate 2.8 mmol, anhydrous glucose 127 g, fish oil 5.7 g, olive oil 9.5 g, soya oil 11.4 g, medium-chain triglycerides 11.4 g
SmofKabiven extra Nitrogen (Fresenius Kabi Ltd) Net price (triple compartment bag of amino acids and electrolytes 662 mL, glucose 204 mL, lipid emulsion 146 mL; 4-bag pack) 1.012 litre = £300.00; Net price (triple compartment bag of amino acids and electrolytes 993 mL, glucose 306 mL, lipid emulsion 219 mL; 4-bag pack) 1.518 litre = £320.00; Net price (triple compartment bag of amino acids and electrolytes 1325 mL, glucose 408 mL, lipid emulsion 292 mL; 4-bag pack) 2.025 litre = £356.00	10.5	2633	30.5	5.1	40.8	125.0	35.6	Ca²⁺ 2.6 mmol, phosphate 12.7 mmol, anhydrous glucose 84.7 g, fish oil 4.3 g, olive oil 7.2 g, soya oil 8.7 g, medium-chain triglycerides 8.7 g
SmofKabiven extra Nitrogen Electrolyte free (Fresenius Kabi Ltd) Net price (triple compartment bag of amino acids 993 mL, glucose 306 mL, lipid emulsion 219 mL; 4-bag pack) 1.518 litre = £320.00; Net price (triple compartment bag of amino acids 1325 mL, glucose 408 mL, lipid emulsion 292 mL; 4-bag pack) 2.025 litre = £356.00	10.5	2633	–	–	–	96.0	–	phosphate 2.2 mmol, anhydrous glucose 84.7 g, fish oil 4.3 g, olive oil 7.2 g, soya oil 8.7 g, medium-chain triglycerides 8.7 g

1 1000 kcal = 4200 kJ; 1000 kJ = 238.8 kcal. All entries are Prescription-only medicines.

2 Excludes protein- or amino acid-derived energy

Preparation	Nitrogen g/litre	[1,2]Energy kJ/litre	Electrolytes mmol/litre					Other components/litre
			K+	Mg2+	Na+	Acet-	Cl-	
SmofKabiven Low Osmo Peripheral (Fresenius Kabi Ltd) Net price (triple compartment bag of amino acids and electrolytes 350 mL, glucose 805 mL, lipid emulsion 245 mL; 4-bag pack) 1.4 litre = £232.00; Net price (triple compartment bag of amino acids and electrolytes 488 mL, glucose 1121 mL, lipid emulsion 341 mL; 4-bag pack) 1.95 litre = £244.00; Net price (triple compartment bag of amino acids and electrolytes 625 mL, glucose 1438 mL, lipid emulsion 438 mL; 3-bag pack) 2.5 litre = £204.00	4.0	2617	15.0	2.5	20.0	52.0	18.0	Ca2+ 1.3 mmol, phosphate 7.5 mmol, anhydrous glucose 68 g, fish oil 5.3 g, olive oil 8.8 g, soya oil 11 g, medium-chain triglycerides 11 g
SmofKabiven Peripheral (Fresenius Kabi Ltd) Net price (triple compartment bag of amino acids and electrolytes 600 mL, glucose 1036 mL, lipid emulsion 268 mL; 4-bag pack) 1.904 litre = £255.36	5.1	2520	19.0	3.2	25.0	66.0	22.0	Ca2+ 1.6 mmol, phosphate 8.2 mmol, anhydrous glucose 71 g, fish oil 4.2 g, olive oil 7 g, soya oil 8.5 g, medium-chain triglycerides 8.5 g
SMOFlipid (Fresenius Kabi Ltd) Net price (10-bottle pack) 100 ml = £74.40; Net price (10-bottle pack) 250 ml = £119.00; Net price (10-bottle pack) 500 ml = £174.30	-	8400	-	-	-	-	-	fish oil 30 g, olive oil 50 g, soya oil 60 g, medium-chain triglycerides 60 g
Synthamin 9 EF (electrolyte-free) (Baxter Healthcare Ltd) Net price 500 ml = £6.97; Net price 1 litre = £12.92	9.1	-	-	-	-	44.0	22.0	
Synthamin 14 EF (electrolyte-free) (Baxter Healthcare Ltd) Net price 500 ml = £9.87; Net price 1 litre = £17.51	14.0	-	-	-	-	68.0	34.0	
Synthamin 17 EF (electrolyte-free) (Baxter Healthcare Ltd) Net price 500 ml = £12.66; Net price 3 litre = £55.00	16.5	-	-	-	-	82.0	40.0	
Vamin 14 (electrolyte-free) (Fresenius Kabi Ltd) Net price (10-bottle pack) 500 ml = £111.50; Net price (6-bottle pack) 1 litre = £113.10	13.5	-	-	-	-	90.0	-	
Vamin 18 (electrolyte-free) (Fresenius Kabi Ltd) Net price (10-bottle pack) 500 ml = £141.00; Net price (6-bottle pack) 1 litre = £165.00	18.0	-	-	-	-	110.0	-	

1 1000 kcal = 4200 kJ; 1000 kJ = 238.8 kcal. All entries are Prescription-only medicines.

2 Excludes protein- or amino acid-derived energy

Parenteral nutrition supplements

26-May-2021

● **INDICATIONS AND DOSE**

Supplement in intravenous nutrition

▶ BY INTRAVENOUS INFUSION, OR BY SLOW INTRAVENOUS INJECTION

▶ Adult: (consult product literature)

DIPEPTIVEN® 20G/100ML CONCENTRATE FOR SOLUTION FOR INFUSION BOTTLES

Amino acid supplement for hypercatabolic or hypermetabolic states

▶ BY INTRAVENOUS INFUSION

▶ Adult: 300–400 mg/kg daily, dose not to exceed 20% of total amino acid intake

● **DIRECTIONS FOR ADMINISTRATION** Because of the complex requirements relating to parenteral nutrition, full details relating to administration have been omitted. In all cases *specialist pharmacy advice, product literature, and other specialist literature should be consulted.* Compatibility with the infusion solution must be ascertained before adding supplementary preparations. **Additives should not be mixed with fat emulsions unless compatibility is known.**

ADDIPHOS® VIALS For addition to *Vamin®* solutions and glucose intravenous infusions.

ADDITRACE® SOLUTION FOR INFUSION 10ML AMPOULES For addition to *Vamin®* solutions and glucose intravenous infusions.

CERNEVIT® POWDER FOR SOLUTION FOR INJECTION VIALS Dissolve in 5 mL water for injections or Glucose 5% or Sodium Chloride 0.9% for adding to infusion solutions.

DECAN® CONCENTRATE FOR SOLUTION FOR INFUSION 40ML BOTTLES For addition to infusion solutions.

DIPEPTIVEN® 20G/100ML CONCENTRATE FOR SOLUTION FOR INFUSION BOTTLES For addition to infusion solutions containing amino acids.

SOLIVITO N® POWDER FOR SOLUTION FOR INFUSION VIALS Dissolve in water for injections or glucose intravenous infusion for adding to glucose intravenous infusion or *Intralipid®*; dissolve in *Vitlipid N®* or *Intralipid®* for adding to *Intralipid®* only.

TRACUTIL® AMPOULES For addition to infusion solutions.

● **PRESCRIBING AND DISPENSING INFORMATION**

ADDIPHOS® VIALS *Addiphos®* sterile solution contains phosphate 40 mmol, K$^+$ 30 mmol, Na$^+$ 30 mmol/20 mL.

ADDITRACE® SOLUTION FOR INFUSION 10ML AMPOULES For patients over 40 kg. *Additrace®* solution contains traces of Fe^{3+}, Zn^{2+}, Mn^{2+}, Cu^{2+}, Cr^{3+}, Se^{4+}, Mo^{6+}, F$^-$, I$^-$.

CERNEVIT® POWDER FOR SOLUTION FOR INJECTION VIALS *Cernevit®* powder for reconstitution contains *dl*-alpha tocopherol 10.2 mg, ascorbic acid 125 mg, biotin 69 micrograms, colecalciferol 220 units, cyanocobalamin 6 micrograms, folic acid 414 micrograms, nicotinamide 46 mg, pantothenic acid (as dexpanthenol) 17.25 mg, pyridoxine hydrochloride 5.5 mg, retinol (as palmitate) 3500 units, riboflavin (as dihydrated sodium phosphate) 4.14 mg, thiamine (as cocarboxylase tetrahydrate) 3.51 mg.

DECAN® CONCENTRATE FOR SOLUTION FOR INFUSION 40ML BOTTLES For patients over 40 kg. *Decan®* solution contains trace elements Fe^{2+}, Zn^{2+}, Cu^{2+}, Mn^{2+}, F$^-$, Co^{2+}, I$^-$, Se^{4+}, Mo^{6+}, Cr^{3+}.

DIPEPTIVEN® 20G/100ML CONCENTRATE FOR SOLUTION FOR INFUSION BOTTLES *Dipeptiven®* solution contains N(2)-L-alanyl-L-glutamine 200 mg/mL (providing L-alanine 82 mg, L-glutamine 134.6 mg).

SOLIVITO N® POWDER FOR SOLUTION FOR INFUSION VIALS *Solivito N®* powder for reconstitution contains biotin 60 micrograms, cyanocobalamin 5 micrograms, folic acid 400 micrograms, glycine 300 mg, nicotinamide 40 mg, pyridoxine hydrochloride 4.9 mg, riboflavin sodium phosphate 4.9 mg, sodium ascorbate 113 mg, sodium pantothenate 16.5 mg, thiamine mononitrate 3.1 mg.

TRACUTIL® AMPOULES *Tracutil®* solution contains trace elements Fe^{2+}, Zn^{2+}, Mn^{2+}, Cu^{2+}, Cr^{3+}, Se^{4+}, Mo^{6+}, I$^-$, F$^-$.

● **MEDICINAL FORMS** There can be variation in the licensing of different medicines containing the same drug. Forms available from special-order manufacturers include: solution for infusion

Solution for infusion

▶ **Parenteral nutrition supplements (Non-proprietary)**
Sodium glycerophosphate (as Sodium glycerophosphate pentahydrate) 216 mg per 1 ml Sodium glycerophosphate 4.32g/20ml concentrate for solution for infusion ampoules | 20 ampoule [PoM] £175.80

▶ **Dipeptiven** (Fresenius Kabi Ltd)
N(2)-L-alanyl-L-glutamine 200 mg per 1 ml Dipeptiven 20g/100ml concentrate for solution for infusion bottles | 10 bottle [PoM] £305.00

▶ **Peditrace** (Fresenius Kabi Ltd)
Manganese (as Manganese chloride) 1 microgram per 1 ml, Iodine (as Potassium iodide) 1 microgram per 1 ml, Selenium (as Sodium selenite) 2 microgram per 1 ml, Copper (as Copper chloride) 20 microgram per 1 ml, Fluoride (as Sodium fluoride) 57 microgram per 1 ml, Zinc (as Zinc chloride) 250 microgram per 1 ml Peditrace solution for infusion 10ml vials | 10 vial [PoM] £35.50

▶ **Tracutil** (B.Braun Medical Ltd)
Sodium molybdate dihydrate 2.42 microgram per 1 ml, Chromic chloride 5.3 microgram per 1 ml, Sodium selenite pentahydrate 7.89 microgram per 1 ml, Potassium iodide 16.6 microgram per 1 ml, Sodium fluoride 126 microgram per 1 ml, Manganese chloride 197.9 microgram per 1 ml, Copper chloride 204.6 microgram per 1 ml, Zinc chloride 681.5 microgram per 1 ml, Ferrous chloride 695.8 microgram per 1 ml Tracutil concentrate for solution for infusion 10ml ampoules | 5 ampoule [PoM] £9.50 (Hospital only)

Powder for solution for infusion

▶ **Solivito N** (Fresenius Kabi Ltd)
Cyanocobalamin 5 microgram, Biotin 60 microgram, Folic acid 400 microgram, Thiamine nitrate 3.1 mg, Pyridoxine hydrochloride 4.9 mg, Riboflavin sodium phosphate 4.9 mg, Sodium pantothenate 16.5 mg, Nicotinamide 40 mg, Sodium ascorbate 113 mg Solivito N powder for concentrate for solution for infusion vials | 10 vial [PoM] £23.20

Powder for solution for injection
EXCIPIENTS: May contain Glycocholic acid

▶ **Cernevit** (Baxter Healthcare Ltd)
Cyanocobalamin 6 microgram, Biotin 69 microgram, Folic acid 414 microgram, Thiamine 3.51 mg, Riboflavin (as Riboflavin sodium phosphate) 4.14 mg, Pyridoxine (as Pyridoxine hydrochloride) 4.53 mg, Pantothenic acid (as Dexpanthenol) 17.25 mg, Nicotinamide 46 mg, Ascorbic acid 125 mg, Alpha tocopherol 11.2 unit, Colecalciferol 220 unit, Retinol 3500 unit Cernevit powder for solution for injection vials | 10 vial [PoM] £50.50

6   Nutrition (oral)

Enteral nutrition

Overview

The body's reserves of protein rapidly become exhausted in severely ill patients, especially during chronic illness or in those with severe burns, extensive trauma, pancreatitis, or intestinal fistula. Much can be achieved by frequent meals and by persuading the patient to take supplementary snacks of ordinary food between the meals.

However, extra calories, protein, other nutrients, and vitamins are often best given by supplementing ordinary meals with enteral sip or tube feeds.

When patients cannot feed normally, for example, patients with severe facial injury, oesophageal obstruction, or coma, a nutritionally complete diet of enteral feeds must be given. The advice of a dietitian should be sought to determine the protein and total energy requirement of the patient and the form and relative contribution of carbohydrate and fat to the energy requirements.

Most enteral feeds contain protein derived from cows' milk or soya. Elemental feeds containing protein hydrolysates or free amino acids can be used for patients who have diminished ability to break down protein, for example in inflammatory bowel disease or pancreatic insufficiency.

Even when nutritionally complete feeds are given, water and electrolyte balance should be monitored. Haematological and biochemical parameters should also be monitored, particularly in clinically unstable patients. Extra minerals (e.g. magnesium and zinc) may be needed in patients where gastro-intestinal secretions are being lost. Additional vitamins may also be needed.

Enteral nutrition in children

Children have special requirements and in most situations liquid feeds prepared for adults are totally unsuitable—the advice of a paediatric dietitian should be sought.

6.1 Special diets

Nutrition in special diets
06-Apr-2021

Overview
In certain clinical conditions, some food preparations are regarded as drugs and can be prescribed within the NHS if they have been approved by the Advisory Committee on Borderline Substances (ACBS).

Coeliac disease
Coeliac disease is caused by an abnormal immune response to gluten. For further information, see Coeliac disease p. 39.

Phenylketonuria
Phenylketonuria results from the inability to metabolise phenylalanine. [EvGr] The treatment of phenylketonuria usually involves restricting dietary intake of phenylalanine to a small amount sufficient for tissue building and repair, in addition to phenylalanine-free L-amino acid supplementation.

A subset of patients with phenylketonuria may be responsive to sapropterin dihydrochloride below ⟨A⟩, a synthetic form of tetrahydrobiopterin. It is licensed as an adjunct to dietary restriction of phenylalanine in the management of patients with phenylketonuria and tetrahydrobiopterin deficiency.

Aspartame (used as a sweetener in some foods and medicines) contributes to phenylalanine intake and may affect control of phenylketonuria. Where the presence of aspartame in a preparation is specified in the product literature, it is listed as an excipient against the preparation in individual drug monographs. The patient should be informed the preparation contains aspartame.

6.1a Phenylketonuria

DRUGS FOR METABOLIC DISORDERS ›
TETRAHYDROBIOPTERIN AND DERIVATIVES

Sapropterin dihydrochloride
18-Oct-2021

- **DRUG ACTION** Sapropterin is synthetic 6R-tetrahydrobiopterin (6R-BH4), a cofactor for phenylalanine hydroxylase, and therefore restores the activity of phenylalanine hydroxylase and reduces phenylalanine concentration in the blood.

- **INDICATIONS AND DOSE**

  Phenylketonuria (adjunct to dietary restriction of phenylalanine) (specialist use only)
  ▸ BY MOUTH
  ▸ Adult: Initially 10 mg/kg once daily, adjusted according to response; usual dose 5–20 mg/kg once daily, dose to be taken preferably in the morning

  Tetrahydrobiopterin deficiency (adjunct to dietary restriction of phenylalanine) (specialist use only)
  ▸ BY MOUTH
  ▸ Adult: Initially 2–5 mg/kg daily in 2–3 divided doses, adjusted according to response; maximum 20 mg/kg per day

- **CAUTIONS** History of convulsions
- **INTERACTIONS** → Appendix 1: sapropterin
- **SIDE-EFFECTS**
▸ **Common or very common** Cough · diarrhoea · gastrointestinal discomfort · headache · laryngeal pain · nasal complaints · nausea · vomiting
▸ **Frequency not known** Gastrointestinal disorders · rash
- **PREGNANCY** Manufacturer advises caution—consider only if strict dietary management inadequate.
- **BREAST FEEDING** Manufacturer advises avoid—no information available.
- **HEPATIC IMPAIRMENT** Manufacturer advises caution (no information available).
- **RENAL IMPAIRMENT** Manufacturer advises caution—no information available.
- **MONITORING REQUIREMENTS**
▸ Monitor blood-phenylalanine concentration before and after first week of treatment—if unsatisfactory response increase dose at weekly intervals to max. dose and monitor blood-phenylalanine concentration weekly; discontinue treatment if unsatisfactory response after 1 month.
▸ Monitor blood-phenylalanine and tyrosine concentrations 1–2 weeks after dose adjustment and during treatment.
- **DIRECTIONS FOR ADMINISTRATION** Manufacturer advises tablets should be dissolved in water and taken within 20 minutes.
- **PATIENT AND CARER ADVICE** Patient or carers should be given advice on how to administer sapropterin dihydrochloride dispersible tablets.
- **NATIONAL FUNDING/ACCESS DECISIONS**
  For full details see funding body website
  NICE decisions
▸ Sapropterin for treating hyperphenylalaninaemia in phenylketonuria (September 2021) NICE TA729 Recommended with restrictions

  Scottish Medicines Consortium (SMC) decisions
▸ Sapropterin (*Kuvan*®) for the treatment of hyperphenylalaninaemia (HPA) in adults and paediatric patients of all ages with phenylketonuria (PKU) who have been shown to be responsive to such treatment (August 2018) SMC No. 558/09 Not recommended

● **MEDICINAL FORMS** There can be variation in the licensing of different medicines containing the same drug.

Soluble tablet

CAUTIONARY AND ADVISORY LABELS 13, 21

▸ **Sapropterin dihydrochloride (Non-proprietary)**
Sapropterin dihydrochloride 100 mg Sapropterin 100mg soluble tablets sugar free | 30 tablet [PoM] £537.50 [SF] | 30 tablet [PoM] £537.50 (Hospital only) [SF] | 120 tablet [PoM] £2,150.00 (Hospital only) [SF] | 120 tablet [PoM] £2,150.00 [SF]

7   Vitamin deficiency

Vitamins

03-Nov-2023

Overview

Vitamins are used for the prevention and treatment of specific deficiency states or where the diet is known to be inadequate; they may be prescribed in the NHS to prevent or treat deficiency but not as dietary supplements.

Their use as general 'pick-me-ups' is of unproven value and, in the case of preparations containing vitamin A or D, may actually be harmful if patients take more than the prescribed dose. The 'fad' for mega-vitamin therapy with water-soluble vitamins, such as ascorbic acid p. 1239 and pyridoxine hydrochloride p. 1237, is unscientific and can be harmful.

Dietary reference values for vitamins are available in the Department of Health publication:

Dietary Reference Values for Food Energy and Nutrients for the United Kingdom: Report of the Panel on Dietary Reference Values of the Committee on Medical Aspects of Food Policy. *Report on Health and Social Subjects* 41. London: HMSO, 1991.

Dental patients

It is unjustifiable to treat stomatitis or glossitis with mixtures of vitamin preparations; this delays diagnosis and correct treatment.

Most patients who develop a nutritional deficiency despite an adequate intake of vitamins have malabsorption and if this is suspected the patient should be referred to a medical practitioner.

Vitamin A

Deficiency of vitamin A p. 1237 (retinol) is associated with ocular defects (particularly xerophthalmia) and an increased susceptibility to infections, but deficiency is rare in the UK (even in disorders of fat absorption).

Vitamin B group

Deficiency of the B vitamins, other than vitamin B_{12}, is rare in the UK and is usually treated by preparations containing thiamine p. 1238 (B_1), riboflavin (B_2), and nicotinamide, which is used in preference to nicotinic acid p. 232, as it does not cause vasodilatation. Other members (or substances traditionally classified as members) of the vitamin B complex such as aminobenzoic acid, biotin, choline, inositol nicotinate p. 266, and pantothenic acid or panthenol may be included in vitamin B preparations but there is no evidence of their value.

The severe deficiency states Wernicke's encephalopathy and Korsakoff's psychosis, especially as seen in chronic alcoholism, are best treated initially by the parenteral administration of B vitamins (*Pabrinex®*), followed by oral administration of thiamine in the longer term. Anaphylaxis has been reported with parenteral B vitamins.

As with other vitamins of the B group, pyridoxine hydrochloride (B_6) deficiency is rare, but it may occur during isoniazid p. 679 therapy or penicillamine p. 1255 treatment in Wilson's disease and is characterised by peripheral neuritis. High doses of pyridoxine hydrochloride are given in some metabolic disorders, such as hyperoxaluria, and it is also used in sideroblastic anaemia. There is evidence to suggest that pyridoxine hydrochloride may provide some benefit in premenstrual syndrome. It has been tried for a wide variety of other disorders, but there is little sound evidence to support the claims of efficacy.

Nicotinic acid inhibits the synthesis of cholesterol and triglyceride. Folic acid p. 1161 and vitamin B_{12} are used in the treatment of megaloblastic anaemia. Folinic acid p. 1071 (available as calcium folinate) is used in association with cytotoxic therapy.

Vitamin C

Vitamin C (ascorbic acid) therapy is essential in scurvy, but less florid manifestations of vitamin C deficiency are commonly found, especially in the elderly.

Severe scurvy causes gingival swelling and bleeding margins as well as petechiae on the skin. This is, however, exceedingly rare and a patient with these signs is more likely to have leukaemia. Investigation should not be delayed by a trial period of vitamin treatment.

Claims that vitamin C ameliorates colds or promotes wound healing have not been proven.

Vitamin D

The term Vitamin D is used for a range of compounds which possess the property of preventing or curing rickets. They include ergocalciferol p. 1245 (calciferol, vitamin D_2), colecalciferol p. 1242 (vitamin D_3), dihydrotachysterol, alfacalcidol p. 1240 (1α-hydroxycholecalciferol), calcitriol p. 1241 (1,25-dihydroxycholecalciferol), and calcifediol monohydrate p. 1241 (25-hydroxycholecalciferol, calcidiol).

Vitamin D deficiency can occur in people whose exposure to sunlight is limited and in those whose diet is deficient in vitamin D. Specific populations at risk of vitamin D deficiency may include individuals with dark skin (such as those of African, African-Caribbean or South Asian origin) as their skin is less efficient at synthesising vitamin D, individuals aged over 65 years, individuals who have low or no exposure to the sun (such as those who are housebound or confined indoors, or who cover their skin for cultural reasons), pregnant and breastfeeding women (particularly teenagers and young women), and children aged under 4 years. Simple vitamin D deficiency can be prevented by taking an oral supplement of ergocalciferol (calciferol, vitamin D_2) or colecalciferol (vitamin D_3) daily. [EvGr] Supplements containing vitamin D (e.g. *Healthy Start*) should be considered for all pregnant and breastfeeding women, and children aged under 4 years, to prevent vitamin D deficiency (if clinically appropriate); Ⓐ information on the Healthy Start scheme can be found at: www.healthystart. nhs.uk/.

Ergocalciferol or colecalciferol by mouth may be given to treat vitamin D deficiency; higher doses may be necessary for *severe* deficiency. Patients who do not respond should be referred to a specialist.

Preparations containing colecalciferol with calcium carbonate p. 1244 are available for the management of combined calcium and vitamin D deficiency, or for those at high risk of deficiency.

Vitamin D deficiency caused by *intestinal malabsorption* or *chronic liver disease* usually requires vitamin D in pharmacological doses.

Vitamin D requires hydroxylation by the kidney to its active form, therefore the hydroxylated derivatives alfacalcidol or calcitriol should be prescribed if patients with *severe renal impairment* require vitamin D therapy. Calcitriol is also licensed for the management of postmenopausal osteoporosis.

Paricalcitol p. 1246, a synthetic vitamin D analogue, is licensed for the prevention and treatment of secondary hyperparathyroidism associated with chronic kidney disease.

Vitamin E

The daily requirement of vitamin E (tocopherol) has not been well defined but is probably 3 to 15 mg daily. There is little evidence that oral supplements of vitamin E are essential in adults, even where there is fat malabsorption secondary to cholestasis. In young children with congenital cholestasis, abnormally low vitamin E concentrations may be found in association with neuromuscular abnormalities, which usually respond only to the parenteral administration of vitamin E.

Vitamin E has been tried for various other conditions but there is little scientific evidence of its value.

Vitamin K

Vitamin K is necessary for the production of blood clotting factors and proteins necessary for the normal calcification of bone.

Because vitamin K is fat soluble, patients with fat malabsorption, especially in biliary obstruction or hepatic disease, may become deficient. Menadiol sodium phosphate p. 1248 is a water-soluble synthetic vitamin K derivative that can be given orally to prevent vitamin K deficiency in malabsorption syndromes.

Oral coumarin anticoagulants act by interfering with vitamin K metabolism in the hepatic cells and their effects can be antagonised by giving vitamin K.

Other compounds

Potassium aminobenzoate p. 1237 has been used in the treatment of various disorders associated with excessive fibrosis such as scleroderma and Peyronie's disease. In Peyronie's disease there is some evidence to support efficacy in reducing progression when given early in the disease; however, there is no evidence for reversal of the condition. The therapeutic value of potassium aminobenzoate in scleroderma is doubtful.

VITAMINS AND TRACE ELEMENTS ›
MULTIVITAMINS

Vitamins A and D
07-Sep-2021

The properties listed below are those particular to the combination only. For the properties of the components please consider, vitamin A p. 1237, colecalciferol p. 1242.

- **INDICATIONS AND DOSE**

Prevention of vitamin A and D deficiency (using 4500 units vitamin A/450 units vitamin D₃ capsules)

▸ BY MOUTH
▸ Child 7–17 years: 1 capsule daily, increased if necessary to 2 capsules daily, dose increase to be guided by serum values
▸ Adult: 1 capsule daily, increased if necessary to 2 capsules daily, dose increase to be guided by serum values

Prevention of vitamin A and D deficiency (using 4000 units vitamin A/400 units vitamin D capsules)

▸ BY MOUTH
▸ Child 1–17 years: 1 capsule daily
▸ Adult: (consult product literature or local protocols)

DOSE EQUIVALENCE AND CONVERSION
▸ Each 4500 units vitamin A/450 units vitamin D₃ capsule contains the equivalent of 11 micrograms vitamin D₃.
▸ Each 4000 units vitamin A/400 units vitamin D capsule (vitamins A and D capsules BPC 1973) contains the equivalent of 10 micrograms vitamin D.

- **INTERACTIONS** → Appendix 1: vitamin A · vitamin D substances

- **SIDE-EFFECTS**

Overdose Prolonged excessive ingestion of vitamins A and D can lead to hypervitaminosis.

- **BREAST FEEDING** Manufacturer advises avoid—present in milk.

- **PRESCRIBING AND DISPENSING INFORMATION** This drug contains vitamin D; consult individual vitamin D monographs.

- **MEDICINAL FORMS** There can be variation in the licensing of different medicines containing the same drug.

Oral capsule
EXCIPIENTS: May contain Gelatin
▸ **Vitamins a and d (Non-proprietary)**
   Vitamin D 400 unit, Vitamin A 4000 unit Vitamins A and D capsules BPC 1973 | 28 capsule GSL 🅧
   Colecalciferol 450 unit, Retinol palmitate 4500 unit Retinol 4,500unit / Colecalciferol 450unit capsules | 84 capsule P £25.95

Vitamins A, C and D
05-May-2020

The properties listed below are those particular to the combination only. For the properties of the components please consider, vitamin A p. 1237, ascorbic acid p. 1239.

- **INDICATIONS AND DOSE**

Prevention of vitamin deficiency
▸ BY MOUTH
▸ Child 1 month–4 years: 5 drops daily, 5 drops contain vitamin A approx. 700 units, vitamin D approx. 300 units (7.5 micrograms), ascorbic acid approx. 20 mg

- **INTERACTIONS** → Appendix 1: ascorbic acid · vitamin A
- **PRESCRIBING AND DISPENSING INFORMATION** This drug contains vitamin D; consult individual vitamin D monographs.

Available free of charge to children under 4 years in families on the Healthy Start Scheme, or alternatively may be available direct to the public—further information for healthcare professionals can be accessed at www.healthystart.nhs.uk. Beneficiaries can contact their midwife or health visitor for further information on where to obtain supplies.

Healthy Start Vitamins for women (containing ascorbic acid, vitamin D, and folic acid) are also available free of charge to women on the Healthy Start Scheme during pregnancy and until their baby is one year old, or alternatively may be available direct to the public—further information for healthcare professionals can be accessed at www.healthystart.nhs.uk. Beneficiaries can contact their midwife or health visitor for further information on where to obtain supplies.

- **MEDICINAL FORMS** There can be variation in the licensing of different medicines containing the same drug.

Oral drops
▸ **Healthy Start Children's Vitamin** (Secretary of State for Health)
   Vitamin A and D3 concentrate 0.55 mg per 1 ml, Sodium ascorbate 18.58 mg per 1 ml, Ascorbic acid 150 mg per 1 ml, Vitamin D 2000 unit per 1 ml, Vitamin A 5000 unit per 1 ml Healthy Start Children's Vitamin drops | 10 ml 🅧

VITAMINS AND TRACE ELEMENTS ›VITAMIN A

Vitamin A
(Retinol)

- **INDICATIONS AND DOSE**
Vitamin A deficiency
▸ BY MOUTH
▸ Child 1–11 months: 5000 units daily, to be taken with or after food, higher doses may be used initially for treatment of severe deficiency
▸ Child 1–17 years: 10 000 units daily, to be taken with or after food, higher doses may be used initially for treatment of severe deficiency

- **UNLICENSED USE** Preparations containing only vitamin A are not licensed.
- **INTERACTIONS** → Appendix 1: vitamin A
- **SIDE-EFFECTS**

Overdose Massive overdose can cause rough skin, dry hair, an enlarged liver, and increases in erythrocyte sedimentation rate, serum calcium and serum alkaline phosphatase concentration.

- **PREGNANCY** Excessive doses may be teratogenic. In view of evidence suggesting that high levels of vitamin A may cause birth defects, women who are (or may become) pregnant are advised not to take vitamin A supplements (including tablets and fish liver oil drops), except on the advice of a doctor or an antenatal clinic; nor should they eat liver or products such as liver paté or liver sausage.
- **BREAST FEEDING** Theoretical risk of toxicity in infants of mothers taking large doses.
- **MONITORING REQUIREMENTS** Treatment is sometimes initiated with very high doses of vitamin A and the child should be monitored closely; very high doses are associated with acute toxicity.

- **MEDICINAL FORMS** There can be variation in the licensing of different medicines containing the same drug. Forms available from special-order manufacturers include: oral drops
Oral drops
▸ Vitamin a (Non-proprietary)
  Vitamin A 150000 unit per 1 ml Arovit 150,000units/ml drops | 7.5 ml [PoM] [⅀]

Combinations available: *Vitamins A and D,* p. 1236 · *Vitamins A, C and D,* p. 1236

VITAMINS AND TRACE ELEMENTS ›VITAMIN B GROUP

Potassium aminobenzoate
09-Aug-2021

- **INDICATIONS AND DOSE**
Peyronie's disease | Scleroderma
▸ BY MOUTH
▸ Adult: 12 g daily in divided doses, to be taken after food

- **CONTRA-INDICATIONS** Hyperkalaemia · severe liver damage
- **CAUTIONS** Interrupt treatment during periods of low food intake (such as fasting, anorexia and nausea)—increased risk of hypoglycaemia
- **INTERACTIONS** → Appendix 1: potassium aminobenzoate
- **SIDE-EFFECTS** Hepatitis · hypoglycaemia
- **PREGNANCY** Manufacturer advises avoid—limited information available.
- **BREAST FEEDING** Manufacturer advises unknown if excreted in milk—risk to infant cannot be excluded.

- **RENAL IMPAIRMENT** [EvGr] Caution (increased risk of hyperkalaemia); avoid if eGFR less than 45 mL/minute/1.73 m^2. ⟨M⟩ See p. 21.
- **MONITORING REQUIREMENTS** Manufacturer advises liver function tests should be performed monthly—discontinue immediately if elevated.

- **MEDICINAL FORMS** There can be variation in the licensing of different medicines containing the same drug.
Powder for oral solution
CAUTIONARY AND ADVISORY LABELS 13, 21
▸ Potassium aminobenzoate (Non-proprietary)
  Potassium aminobenzoate 3 gram Potassium para-aminobenzoate 3g oral powder sachets | 40 sachet [P] £72.21 DT = £72.21

Pyridoxine hydrochloride
05-Oct-2021
(Vitamin B$_6$)

- **INDICATIONS AND DOSE**
Deficiency states
▸ BY MOUTH
▸ Adult: 20–50 mg 1–3 times a day
Isoniazid-induced neuropathy (prophylaxis)
▸ BY MOUTH
▸ Adult: 10–20 mg daily
Isoniazid-induced neuropathy (treatment)
▸ BY MOUTH
▸ Adult: 50 mg 3 times a day
Idiopathic sideroblastic anaemia
▸ BY MOUTH
▸ Adult: 100–400 mg daily in divided doses
Prevention of penicillamine-induced neuropathy in Wilson's disease
▸ BY MOUTH
▸ Adult: 20 mg daily
Premenstrual syndrome
▸ BY MOUTH
▸ Adult: 50–100 mg daily

- **UNLICENSED USE** Not licensed for prophylaxis of penicillamine-induced neuropathy in Wilson's disease. Not licensed for treatment of premenstrual syndrome.

> **IMPORTANT SAFETY INFORMATION**
> Prolonged use of pyridoxine in a dose of 10 mg daily is considered safe but the long-term use of pyridoxine in a dose of 200 mg or more daily has been associated with neuropathy. The safety of long-term pyridoxine supplementation with doses above 10 mg daily has not been established.

- **SIDE-EFFECTS** Peripheral neuritis

Overdose Overdosage induces toxic effects.

- **MEDICINAL FORMS** There can be variation in the licensing of different medicines containing the same drug. Forms available from special-order manufacturers include: oral capsule, oral suspension, oral solution
Oral tablet
▸ Pyridoxine hydrochloride (Non-proprietary)
  Pyridoxine hydrochloride 10 mg Pyridoxine 10mg tablets | 28 tablet [PoM] £17.64-£25.90 DT = £17.64
  Pyridoxine hydrochloride 20 mg Pyridoxine 20mg tablets | 500 tablet [GSL] [⅀]
  Pyridoxine hydrochloride 50 mg Pyridoxine 50mg tablets | 28 tablet [PoM] £16.91-£31.02 DT = £17.77
Oral capsule
▸ Pyridoxine hydrochloride (Non-proprietary)
  Pyridoxine hydrochloride 100 mg Solgar Vitamin B6 100mg capsules | 100 capsule [⅀]
  G & G Vitamin B6 100mg capsules | 120 capsule £5.00

Oral solution

▶ **Apyrid** (Essential-Healthcare Ltd)
Pyridoxine hydrochloride 20 mg per 1 ml Apyrid 100mg/5ml oral solution | 100 ml £23.97 DT = £22.80

▶ **PyriDose** (TriOn Pharma Ltd)
Pyridoxine hydrochloride 20 mg per 1 ml PyriDose 100mg/5ml oral solution | 100 ml £23.88 DT = £22.80

Thiamine
04-Feb-2021

(Vitamin B₁)

● **INDICATIONS AND DOSE**

Mild deficiency

▶ BY MOUTH

▶ Adult: 25–100 mg daily

Severe deficiency

▶ BY MOUTH

▶ Adult: 200–300 mg daily in divided doses

IMPORTANT SAFETY INFORMATION

MHRA/CHM ADVICE (SEPTEMBER 2007)

Although potentially serious allergic adverse reactions may rarely occur during, or shortly after, parenteral administration, the CHM has recommended that:

• This should not preclude the use of parenteral thiamine in patients where this route of administration is required, particularly in patients at risk of Wernicke-Korsakoff syndrome where treatment with thiamine is essential;

• Intravenous administration should be by infusion over 30 minutes;

• Facilities for treating anaphylaxis (including resuscitation facilities) should be available when parenteral thiamine is administered.

● **CAUTIONS** Anaphylaxis may occasionally follow injection, see *Important safety information*

● **BREAST FEEDING** Severely thiamine-deficient mothers should avoid breast-feeding as toxic methyl-glyoxal present in milk.

● **MEDICINAL FORMS** There can be variation in the licensing of different medicines containing the same drug. Forms available from special-order manufacturers include: oral suspension, oral solution

Oral tablet

▶ **Thiamine (Non-proprietary)**
Thiamine hydrochloride 50 mg Thiamine 50mg tablets | 28 tablet P £1.10-£24.00 | 100 tablet P £6.72 DT = £2.60
Thiamine hydrochloride 100 mg Thiamine 100mg tablets | 28 tablet P £1.35-£6.72 | 100 tablet P £11.55 DT = £3.26

Modified-release tablet

▶ **Athiam** (Essential-Healthcare Ltd)
Thiamine hydrochloride 100 mg Athiam 100mg sustained release tablets | 30 tablet £3.19

▶ **ThiaDose** (TriOn Pharma Ltd)
Thiamine hydrochloride 100 mg ThiaDose 100mg modified-release tablets | 30 tablet £3.19

Oral solution

▶ **Athiam** (Essential-Healthcare Ltd)
Thiamine hydrochloride 20 mg per 1 ml Athiam 100mg/5ml oral solution | 100 ml £23.97 SF

▶ **ThiaDose** (TriOn Pharma Ltd)
Thiamine hydrochloride 20 mg per 1 ml ThiaDose 100mg/5ml oral solution | 100 ml £22.90 SF

Vitamin B complex
21-May-2021

● **INDICATIONS AND DOSE**

Treatment of deficiency

▶ BY MOUTH USING TABLETS

▶ Adult: 1–2 tablets 3 times a day, this dose is for vitamin B compound **strong** tablets

Prophylaxis of deficiency

▶ BY MOUTH USING TABLETS

▶ Adult: 1–3 tablets daily, this dose is for vitamin B compound tablets

● **LESS SUITABLE FOR PRESCRIBING** Vitamin B compound tablets and vitamin B compound strong tablets are less suitable for prescribing.

● **MEDICINAL FORMS** There can be variation in the licensing of different medicines containing the same drug.

Oral tablet

▶ **Vitamin b complex (Non-proprietary)**
Riboflavin 1 mg, Thiamine hydrochloride 1 mg, Nicotinamide 15 mg Vitamin B compound tablets | 28 tablet P £26.63-£50.00 DT = £55.68
Pyridoxine hydrochloride 2 mg, Riboflavin 2 mg, Thiamine hydrochloride 5 mg, Nicotinamide 20 mg Vitamin B compound strong tablets | 28 tablet PoM £1.07 DT = £1.03

Vitamin B substances with ascorbic acid
29-Jul-2020

The properties listed below are those particular to the combination only. For the properties of the components please consider, thiamine above, ascorbic acid p. 1239.

● **INDICATIONS AND DOSE**

Severe depletion or malabsorption of vitamins B and C postoperatively

▶ BY INTRAVENOUS INFUSION, OR BY DEEP INTRAMUSCULAR INJECTION

▶ Adult: (consult product literature)

Treatment of suspected or established Wernicke's encephalopathy

▶ BY INTRAVENOUS INFUSION

▶ Adult: 2–3 pairs 3 times a day for 3–5 days, followed by 1 pair once daily for a further 3–5 days or for as long as improvement continues

Prophylaxis of Wernicke's encephalopathy [assisted alcohol withdrawal in an inpatient setting]

▶ BY DEEP INTRAMUSCULAR INJECTION

▶ Adult: 1 pair once daily for at least 5 days and up to 7 days if required, give into the gluteal muscle

Severe depletion or malabsorption of vitamins B and C in psychosis following narcosis or electroconvulsive therapy | Severe depletion or malabsorption of vitamins B and C following toxicity from acute infections

▶ BY INTRAVENOUS INFUSION, OR BY DEEP INTRAMUSCULAR INJECTION

▶ Adult: 1 pair twice daily for up to 7 days, give deep intramuscular injection into the gluteal muscle

Severe depletion or malabsorption of vitamins B and C in haemodialysis

▶ BY INTRAVENOUS INFUSION

▶ Adult: 1 pair every 2 weeks

DOSE EQUIVALENCE AND CONVERSION

▶ Dose is expressed in pairs of ampoules.

▶ For *intravenous* administration, 1 pair is one 5 mL ampoule containing thiamine 250 mg, riboflavin 4 mg and pyridoxine 50 mg, and one 5 mL ampoule containing ascorbic acid 500 mg, nicotinamide 160 mg and glucose 1000 mg.

▶ For *intramuscular* administration, 1 pair is one 5 mL ampoule containing thiamine 250 mg, riboflavin 4 mg and pyridoxine 50 mg, and one 2 mL ampoule containing ascorbic acid 500 mg and nicotinamide 160 mg.

● **UNLICENSED USE** Vitamin B substances with ascorbic acid may be used as detailed below, although these situations are considered outside the scope of its licence:
  ● EvGr durations and further dosing for treatment of suspected or established Wernicke's encephalopathy
  ● prophylaxis of Wernicke's encephalopathy ⓓ

● **INTERACTIONS** → Appendix 1: ascorbic acid

● **DIRECTIONS FOR ADMINISTRATION** Manufacturer advises give (*Pabrinex® I/V High Potency*) intermittently *or via* drip tubing *in* Glucose 5% *or* Sodium Chloride 0.9%. Manufacturer advises ampoules contents should be mixed, diluted, and administered without delay; give over 30 minutes. See MHRA/CHM advice in thiamine p. 1238.

● **PRESCRIBING AND DISPENSING INFORMATION** *Pabrinex®* I/M High Potency injection is for intramuscular use only. *Pabrinex®* I/V High Potency injection is for intravenous use only.

● **MEDICINAL FORMS** There can be variation in the licensing of different medicines containing the same drug.
Form unstated
EXCIPIENTS: May contain Benzyl alcohol
  ▶ **Vitamin b substances with ascorbic acid (Non-proprietary)**
    Vitamins B+C Intravenous High Potency concentrate for solution for infusion 5ml and 5ml ampoules | 12 ampoule PoM £138.04 (Hospital only)
  ▶ **Pabrinex Intramuscular High Potency** (Kyowa Kirin International UK NewCo Ltd)
    Pabrinex Intramuscular High Potency solution for injection 5ml and 2ml ampoules | 20 ampoule PoM £22.53 DT = £22.53
  ▶ **Pabrinex Intravenous High Potency** (Kyowa Kirin International UK NewCo Ltd)
    Pabrinex Intravenous High Potency concentrate for solution for infusion 5ml and 5ml ampoules | 12 ampoule PoM £16.23

Vitamins with minerals and trace elements

13-May-2020

● **INDICATIONS AND DOSE**
FORCEVAL® CAPSULES
Vitamin and mineral deficiency and as adjunct in synthetic diets
  ▶ BY MOUTH
  ▶ Adult: 1 capsule daily, one hour after a meal

KETOVITE® LIQUID
Prevention of vitamin deficiency in disorders of carbohydrate or amino-acid metabolism | Adjunct in restricted, specialised, or synthetic diets
  ▶ BY MOUTH
  ▶ Adult: 5 mL daily, use with *Ketovite® Tablets* for complete vitamin supplementation.

KETOVITE® TABLETS
Prevention of vitamin deficiency in disorders of carbohydrate or amino-acid metabolism | Adjunct in restricted, specialised, or synthetic diets
  ▶ BY MOUTH
  ▶ Adult: 1 tablet 3 times a day, use with *Ketovite® Liquid* for complete vitamin supplementation.

● **PRESCRIBING AND DISPENSING INFORMATION** To avoid potential toxicity, the content of all vitamin preparations, particularly vitamin A, should be considered when used together with other supplements.

● **PATIENT AND CARER ADVICE** *Ketovite®* liquid may be mixed with milk, cereal, or fruit juice.

KETOVITE® TABLETS Tablets may be crushed immediately before use.

● **MEDICINAL FORMS** There can be variation in the licensing of different medicines containing the same drug.
Oral emulsion
  ▶ **Vitamins with minerals and trace elements (Non-proprietary)**
    Cyanocobalamin 2.5 microgram per 1 ml, Choline chloride 30 mg per 1 ml, Ergocalciferol 80 unit per 1 ml, Vitamin A 500 unit per 1 ml Ketovite liquid | 150 ml P £119.10 SF
Oral tablet
  ▶ **Ketovite** (Essential Pharmaceuticals Ltd)
    Biotin 170 microgram, Folic acid 250 microgram, Pyridoxine hydrochloride 330 microgram, Acetomenaphthone 500 microgram, Riboflavin 1 mg, Thiamine hydrochloride 1 mg, Calcium pantothenate 1.16 mg, Nicotinamide 3.3 mg, Alpha tocopheryl acetate 5 mg, Ascorbic acid 16.6 mg, Inositol 50 mg Ketovite tablets | 100 tablet £28.19
Oral capsule
  ▶ **Forceval** (Alliance Pharmaceuticals Ltd)
    Cyanocobalamin 3 microgram, Selenium 50 microgram, Biotin 100 microgram, Iodine 140 microgram, Chromium 200 microgram, Molybdenum 250 microgram, Folic acid 400 microgram, Thiamine 1.2 mg, Riboflavin 1.6 mg, Copper 2 mg, Pyridoxine 2 mg, Manganese 3 mg, Pantothenic acid 4 mg, Potassium 4 mg, Tocopheryl acetate 10 mg, Iron 12 mg, Zinc 15 mg, Nicotinamide 18 mg, Magnesium 30 mg, Ascorbic acid 60 mg, Phosphorus 77 mg, Calcium 100 mg, Ergocalciferol 400 unit, Vitamin A 2500 unit Forceval capsules | 15 capsule P £6.28 | 30 capsule P £11.41 | 90 capsule P £33.09

VITAMINS AND TRACE ELEMENTS › VITAMIN C

Ascorbic acid

19-Feb-2021

(Vitamin C)

● **INDICATIONS AND DOSE**
Prevention of scurvy
  ▶ BY MOUTH
  ▶ Adult: 25–75 mg daily

Treatment of scurvy
  ▶ BY MOUTH
  ▶ Adult: Not less than 250 mg daily in divided doses

● **CONTRA-INDICATIONS** Hyperoxaluria

● **INTERACTIONS** → Appendix 1: ascorbic acid

● **SIDE-EFFECTS** Diarrhoea · gastrointestinal disorder · hyperoxaluria · oxalate nephrolithiasis · polyuria

● **PRESCRIBING AND DISPENSING INFORMATION** It is rarely necessary to prescribe more than 100 mg daily except early in the treatment of scurvy.

● **MEDICINAL FORMS** There can be variation in the licensing of different medicines containing the same drug. Forms available from special-order manufacturers include: oral tablet, oral suspension, oral solution
Oral tablet
EXCIPIENTS: May contain Aspartame
  ▶ **Ascorbic acid (Non-proprietary)**
    Ascorbic acid 50 mg Ascorbic acid 50mg tablets | 28 tablet GSL £60.00 DT = £69.55
    Ascorbic acid 100 mg Ascorbic acid 100mg tablets | 28 tablet GSL £44.00 DT = £26.71
    Ascorbic acid 200 mg Ascorbic acid 200mg tablets | 28 tablet GSL £84.00 DT = £59.86
    Ascorbic acid 250 mg Ascorbic acid 250mg tablets | 1000 tablet PoM Ⓢ
    Ascorbic acid 500 mg Ascorbic acid 500mg tablets | 28 tablet GSL £47.90 DT = £31.73
  ▶ **Vodexo** (Kent Pharma (UK) Ltd)
    Ascorbic acid 100 mg Vodexo 100mg tablets | 28 tablet GSL £2.48 DT = £26.71
    Ascorbic acid 200 mg Vodexo 200mg tablets | 28 tablet GSL £3.26 DT = £59.86

Ascorbic acid 500 mg Vodexo 500mg tablets | 28 tablet [GSL] £4.22 DT = £31.73

Oral capsule

▸ **Ascorbic acid (Non-proprietary)**

Ascorbic acid 500 mg BioCare Vitamin C 500mg capsules | 60 capsule £9.35 | 180 capsule £24.23

Chewable tablet

CAUTIONARY AND ADVISORY LABELS 24

EXCIPIENTS: May contain Aspartame

▸ **Ascorbic acid (Non-proprietary)**

Ascorbic acid 60 mg Tesco Vitamin C One A Day 60mg chewable tablets | 60 tablet 🅧

Ascorbic acid 500 mg Premier Vitamin C 500mg chewable tablets | 30 tablet £2.30 | 60 tablet £4.13

HealthAid Vitamin C 500mg chewable tablets | 60 tablet £5.58 | 100 tablet £7.25

Numark Vitamin C 500mg chewable tablets | 30 tablet £1.15

Tesco Vitamin C One A Day 500mg chewable tablets | 60 tablet 🅧

Ascorbic acid 1 gram HealthAid Vitamin C 1000mg chewable tablets | 30 tablet £5.58 | 60 tablet £8.37 | 100 tablet £11.16

Combinations available: *Vitamin B substances with ascorbic acid,* p. 1238 · *Vitamins A, C and D,* p. 1236

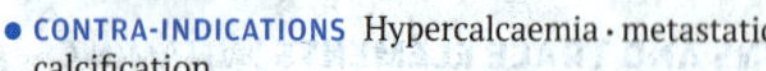

VITAMINS AND TRACE ELEMENTS > VITAMIN D AND ANALOGUES

Vitamin D and analogues (systemic) 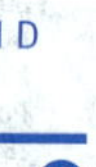

- **CONTRA-INDICATIONS** Hypercalcaemia · metastatic calcification

- **SIDE-EFFECTS**

▸ **Common or very common** Abdominal pain · headache · hypercalcaemia · hypercalciuria · nausea · skin reactions

▸ **Uncommon** Appetite decreased · arrhythmia · asthenia · constipation · diarrhoea · dry mouth · myalgia · vomiting · weight decreased

Overdose Symptoms of overdosage include anorexia, lassitude, nausea and vomiting, diarrhoea, constipation, weight loss, polyuria, sweating, headache, thirst, vertigo, and raised concentrations of calcium and phosphate in plasma and urine.

- **PREGNANCY** High doses teratogenic in *animals* but therapeutic doses unlikely to be harmful.

- **BREAST FEEDING** Caution with high doses; may cause hypercalcaemia in infant—monitor serum-calcium concentration.

- **MONITORING REQUIREMENTS Important**: all patients receiving pharmacological doses of vitamin D should have their plasma-calcium concentration checked at intervals as clinically indicated and whenever nausea or vomiting occur.

⌐ above

Alfacalcidol

15-Nov-2022

(1α-Hydroxycholecalciferol)

- **INDICATIONS AND DOSE**

Patients with severe renal impairment requiring vitamin D therapy

▸ BY MOUTH, OR BY INTRAVENOUS INJECTION

▸ Adult: Initially 1 microgram daily, dose to be adjusted to avoid hypercalcaemia; maintenance 0.25–1 microgram daily

▸ Elderly: Initially 500 nanograms daily, dose adjusted to avoid hypercalcaemia; maintenance 0.25–1 microgram daily

Hypophosphataemic rickets | Persistent hypocalcaemia due to hypoparathyroidism or pseudohypoparathyroidism

▸ BY MOUTH, OR BY INTRAVENOUS INJECTION

▸ Child 1 month–11 years: 25–50 nanograms/kg once daily, dose to be adjusted as necessary; maximum 1 microgram per day

▸ Child 12–17 years: 1 microgram once daily, dose to be adjusted as necessary

Prevention of vitamin D deficiency in renal or cholestatic liver disease

▸ BY MOUTH, OR BY INTRAVENOUS INJECTION

▸ Child 1 month–11 years (body-weight up to 20 kg): 15–30 nanograms/kg once daily (max. per dose 500 nanograms)

▸ Child 1 month–11 years (body-weight 20 kg and above): 250–500 nanograms once daily, dose to be adjusted as necessary

▸ Child 12–17 years: 250–500 nanograms once daily, dose to be adjusted as necessary

DOSE EQUIVALENCE AND CONVERSION

▸ One drop of alfacalcidol 2 microgram/mL oral drops contains approximately 100 nanograms alfacalcidol.

- **CAUTIONS** Granulomatous diseases (risk of increased sensitivity to vitamin D) · nephrolithiasis · take care to ensure correct dose in infants

- **INTERACTIONS** → Appendix 1: vitamin D substances

- **SIDE-EFFECTS**

▸ **Common or very common** Abdominal discomfort · hyperphosphataemia · rash pustular

▸ **Uncommon** Malaise · urolithiases

▸ **Rare or very rare** Dizziness

▸ **Frequency not known** Confusion · renal impairment

- **RENAL IMPAIRMENT** [EvGr] Monitor plasma-calcium and phosphate concentration closely in renal impairment. Ⓜ

- **MONITORING REQUIREMENTS** [EvGr] Monitor plasma-calcium concentration (ideally corrected for protein binding), especially in patients receiving high doses—if hypercalcaemia occurs, withhold treatment until calcium returns to normal, then restart at half the previous dose. Also monitor plasma-phosphate, parathyroid hormone, alkaline phosphatase and calcium phosphate. Measure parameters every week initially, then every 2–4 weeks when the dose is stabilised. Ⓜ

- **DIRECTIONS FOR ADMINISTRATION** For *injection*, manufacturer advises shake ampoule for at least 5 seconds before use, and give over 30 seconds.

- **HANDLING AND STORAGE**

▸ With intravenous use Store in a refrigerator (2–8°C) and protect from light.

- **MEDICINAL FORMS** There can be variation in the licensing of different medicines containing the same drug. Forms available from special-order manufacturers include: oral suspension, oral solution

Solution for injection

EXCIPIENTS: May contain Alcohol, propylene glycol

▸ **One-Alpha** (Neon Healthcare Ltd)

Alfacalcidol 2 microgram per 1 ml One-Alpha 2micrograms/1ml solution for injection ampoules | 10 ampoule [PoM] £41.13 DT = £41.13

One-Alpha 1micrograms/0.5ml solution for injection ampoules | 10 ampoule [PoM] £21.57 DT = £21.57

Oral capsule

EXCIPIENTS: May contain Potassium sorbate, sesame oil, vitamin e

▸ **Alfacalcidol (Non-proprietary)**

Alfacalcidol 250 nanogram Alfacalcidol 250nanogram capsules | 30 capsule [PoM] £4.94 DT = £2.28

Alfacalcidol 500 nanogram Alfacalcidol 500nanogram capsules | 30 capsule [PoM] £9.90 DT = £4.06

Alfacalcidol 1 microgram Alfacalcidol 1microgram capsules | 30 capsule [PoM] £8.75 DT = £8.75

> **AlfaD** (Theramex HQ UK Ltd)
> **Alfacalcidol 250 nanogram** AlfaD 0.25microgram capsules | 30 capsule [PoM] £5.00 DT = £2.28
> **Alfacalcidol 500 nanogram** AlfaD 0.5microgram capsules | 30 capsule [PoM] £10.00 DT = £4.06
> **Alfacalcidol 1 microgram** AlfaD 1microgram capsules | 30 capsule [PoM] £14.00 DT = £8.75
> **One-Alpha** (Neon Healthcare Ltd)
> **Alfacalcidol 250 nanogram** One-Alpha 250nanogram capsules | 30 capsule [PoM] £3.37 DT = £2.28
> **Alfacalcidol 500 nanogram** One-Alpha 0.5microgram capsules | 30 capsule [PoM] £6.27 DT = £4.06
> **Alfacalcidol 1 microgram** One-Alpha 1microgram capsules | 30 capsule [PoM] £8.75 DT = £8.75

Oral drops
EXCIPIENTS: May contain Alcohol, hydroxybenzoates (parabens), polyoxyl castor oils, sorbitol, vitamin e
> **One-Alpha** (Neon Healthcare Ltd)
> **Alfacalcidol 2 microgram per 1 ml** One-Alpha 2micrograms/ml oral drops | 10 ml [PoM] £21.30 DT = £21.30 [SF]

F 1240

Calcifediol monohydrate

31-Oct-2023

(25-Hydroxycholecalciferol; Calcidiol)

● **INDICATIONS AND DOSE**

Primary prevention of vitamin D deficiency
> BY MOUTH
> Adult: 266 micrograms once a month

Treatment of vitamin D deficiency
> BY MOUTH
> Adult: 266 micrograms once a month, increased if necessary up to 266 micrograms once weekly, dose to be adjusted according to plasma-25-hydroxyvitamin D concentration; maintenance 266 micrograms once a month

● **CAUTIONS** Granulomatous diseases (risk of increased sensitivity to vitamin D) · heart failure · nephrolithiasis · prolonged immobilisation (risk of hypercalcaemia—consider reducing dose)

CAUTIONS, FURTHER INFORMATION
> Heart failure [EvGr] Risk of hypercalcaemia and arrhythmias—monitor plasma-calcium concentration twice a week at start of treatment. ⟨M⟩

● **INTERACTIONS** → Appendix 1: vitamin D substances

● **SIDE-EFFECTS**
> **Rare or very rare** Conjunctivitis (with very high doses) · corneal calcification (with very high doses) · photophobia (with very high doses)
> **Frequency not known** Abdominal cramps · albuminuria · hypercholesterolaemia · soft tissue calcification · taste altered

● **RENAL IMPAIRMENT** [EvGr] Caution in mild to moderate impairment (risk of reduced efficacy—monitor plasma-calcium and plasma-phosphate concentration); avoid in severe impairment. ⟨M⟩

● **MONITORING REQUIREMENTS**
> [EvGr] Monitor calcium and phosphate levels in urine, plasma-calcium, plasma-phosphate, and plasma-alkaline phosphatase concentrations regularly. ⟨M⟩
> When used for Treatment of vitamin D deficiency [EvGr] Monitor plasma-25-hydroxyvitamin D concentration 3–4 months after starting maintenance dosing, then every 6 months thereafter. ⟨M⟩

● **MEDICINAL FORMS** There can be variation in the licensing of different medicines containing the same drug.

Oral capsule
EXCIPIENTS: May contain Ethanol, sorbitol
> **Domnisol** (Flynn Pharma Ltd)
> **Calcifediol monohydrate 266 microgram** Domnisol 266microgram capsules | 1 capsule [PoM] £1.99 DT = £1.99 | 3 capsule [PoM] £5.97 DT = £5.97

F 1240

Calcitriol

15-Nov-2022

(1,25-Dihydroxycholecalciferol)

● **INDICATIONS AND DOSE**

Renal osteodystrophy
> BY MOUTH
> Adult: Initially 250 nanograms daily, adjusted in steps of 250 nanograms every 2–4 weeks if required; usual dose 0.5–1 microgram daily

Renal osteodystrophy (in patients with normal or only slightly reduced plasma-calcium concentration)
> BY MOUTH
> Adult: Initially 250 nanograms once daily on alternate days, adjusted in steps of 250 nanograms every 2–4 weeks if required; usual dose 0.5–1 microgram daily

Established postmenopausal osteoporosis
> BY MOUTH
> Adult: 250 nanograms twice daily

● **INTERACTIONS** → Appendix 1: vitamin D substances

● **SIDE-EFFECTS**
> **Common or very common** Urinary tract infection
> **Frequency not known** Abdominal pain upper · apathy · dehydration · drowsiness · fever · growth retardation · muscle weakness · paralytic ileus · polydipsia · psychiatric disorder · sensory disorder · thirst · urinary disorders

● **RENAL IMPAIRMENT** Manufacturer advises avoid—no information available.

● **MONITORING REQUIREMENTS**
> [EvGr] Monitor plasma-calcium, phosphate, and creatinine concentrations regularly, particularly during dose titration. ⟨M⟩
> When used for Renal osteodystrophy [EvGr] Monitor plasma-calcium and creatinine concentrations at least twice weekly during dose titration—if calcium increases to 250 µmol/L above normal, or creatinine increases to >120 µmol/L, withhold treatment until calcium returns to normal. ⟨M⟩
> When used for Postmenopausal osteoporosis [EvGr] Monitor plasma-calcium and creatinine concentration at months 1, 3, and 6 and then at 6-monthly intervals thereafter—if calcium increases to 250 µmol/L above normal, or creatinine increases to >120 µmol/L, withhold treatment until calcium returns to normal. ⟨M⟩

● **MEDICINAL FORMS** There can be variation in the licensing of different medicines containing the same drug. Forms available from special-order manufacturers include: oral suspension, oral solution

Oral solution
> **Calcitriol** (Non-proprietary)
> **Calcitriol 1 microgram per 1 ml** Rocaltrol 1micrograms/ml oral solution | 10 ml [PoM] [▼] [SF]

Oral capsule
EXCIPIENTS: May contain Butylated hydroxyanisole, butylated hydroxytoluene, sorbitol
> **Calcitriol** (Non-proprietary)
> **Calcitriol 250 nanogram** Calcitriol 250nanogram capsules | 30 capsule [PoM] £18.04 (Hospital only) | 30 capsule [PoM] £5.41-£6.66

Calcitriol 500 nanogram Calcitriol 500nanogram capsules | 30 capsule [PoM] £32.25 (Hospital only) | 30 capsule [PoM] £9.68–£12.50

▶ **Rocaltrol** (Atnahs Pharma UK Ltd)
Calcitriol 250 nanogram Rocaltrol 250nanogram capsules | 100 capsule [PoM] £18.04 DT = £18.04
Calcitriol 500 nanogram Rocaltrol 500nanogram capsules | 100 capsule [PoM] £32.25 DT = £32.25

▶| 1240

Colecalciferol

20-Oct-2022

(Cholecalciferol; Vitamin D₃)

- **INDICATIONS AND DOSE**

Primary prevention of vitamin D deficiency
▶ BY MOUTH
▶ Adult: 400 units daily

Treatment of vitamin D deficiency [Loading dose]
▶ BY MOUTH
▶ Adult: 50 000 units once weekly for 6 weeks, alternatively 40 000 once weekly for 7 weeks, alternatively 4000 units daily for 10 weeks, different loading regimens can be used to achieve a cumulative total of approximately 300 000 units divided into daily or weekly doses over 6–10 weeks

Treatment of vitamin D deficiency [Maintenance dose]
▶ BY MOUTH
▶ Adult: 800–2000 units daily, maintenance dosing may be given daily or the equivalent dose given intermittently. Maintenance to be started one month after loading dose completed, or if correction of vitamin D deficiency is less urgent, maintenance may be started without the use of loading doses. Higher maintenance doses may be necessary in those at high risk of vitamin D deficiency; maximum 4000 units per day

DOSE EQUIVALENCE AND CONVERSION
▶ Colecalciferol 400 units is equivalent to 10 micrograms; dose expressed as units.

- **UNLICENSED USE** [EvGr] Colecalciferol is used in the doses provided in BNF publications, for the primary prevention and treatment of vitamin D deficiency, ⒶbutA these may differ from those licensed.

- **CAUTIONS** Sarcoidosis

- **INTERACTIONS** → Appendix 1: vitamin D substances

- **MONITORING REQUIREMENTS**
▶ When used for Treatment of vitamin D deficiency [EvGr] Monitor calcium concentration within 1 month after last loading dose or after starting maintenance dosing. Routine monitoring of plasma-25-hydroxyvitamin D concentration is not needed, but may be considered 3–6 months after starting treatment in some cases e.g. patients with symptomatic vitamin D deficiency or malabsorption, those taking antiresorptive therapy, or where poor compliance is suspected. Ⓐ

- **DIRECTIONS FOR ADMINISTRATION**
INVITA D3 ® ORAL SOLUTION Manufacturer advises may be mixed with a small amount of cold or lukewarm food immediately before administration.

- **MEDICINAL FORMS** There can be variation in the licensing of different medicines containing the same drug. Forms available from special-order manufacturers include: oral tablet, oral capsule, oral suspension, oral solution, oral drops

Oral tablet
▶ **Colecalciferol** (Non-proprietary)
Colecalciferol 400 unit FSC Vitamin D3 400unit tablets | 60 tablet £1.70
Prohealth Vitamin D3 10micrograms (400units) tablets | 120 tablet [S]
Dekristol 400unit tablets | 100 tablet [S]

Colecalciferol 800 unit Colecalciferol 800unit tablets | 30 tablet [PoM] £6.04 DT = £6.04
Colecalciferol 1000 unit Colecalciferol 1,000unit tablets | 30 tablet [PoM] £3.16–£5.30
Colecalciferol 2000 unit Colecalciferol 2,000unit tablets | 30 tablet [PoM] £13.50–£29.00
Colecalciferol 5000 unit Vitamin D3 High Strength 5,000unit tablets | 60 tablet £7.25

▶ **Aace D3** (Essential-Healthcare Ltd)
Colecalciferol 2200 unit Aace D3 2,200unit tablets | 28 tablet £7.03

▶ **Aactive D3** (TriOn Pharma Ltd)
Colecalciferol 2200 unit Aactive D3 2,200unit tablets | 30 tablet £7.49
Colecalciferol 3000 unit Aactive D3 3,000unit tablets | 30 tablet £3.89
Colecalciferol 10000 unit Aactive D3 10,000unit tablets | 30 tablet £5.19

▶ **AceCal D3** (Essential-Healthcare Ltd)
Colecalciferol 3000 unit AceCal D3 3,000unit tablets | 28 tablet £3.87
Colecalciferol 5000 unit AceCal D3 5,000unit tablets | 28 tablet £4.19
Colecalciferol 10000 unit AceCal D3 10,000unit tablets | 28 tablet £5.29
Colecalciferol 20000 unit AceCal D3 20,000unit tablets | 28 tablet £7.89

▶ **Aciferol D3** (Fontus Health Ltd)
Colecalciferol 400 unit Aciferol D3 400unit tablets | 90 tablet £12.95
Colecalciferol 2200 unit Aciferol D3 2,200unit tablets | 90 tablet £29.95
Colecalciferol 3000 unit Aciferol D3 3,000unit tablets | 60 tablet £16.99
Colecalciferol 5000 unit Aciferol D3 5,000unit tablets | 60 tablet £21.95
Colecalciferol 10000 unit Aciferol D3 10,000unit tablets | 30 tablet £15.99
Colecalciferol 20000 unit Aciferol D3 20,000unit tablets | 30 tablet £21.95

▶ **Actium D3** (MaN Pharma Ltd)
Colecalciferol 400 unit Actium D3 400unit tablets | 30 tablet £2.25

▶ **ColeDose D3** (TriOn Pharma Ltd)
Colecalciferol 5000 unit ColeDose D3 5,000unit tablets | 30 tablet £4.49
Colecalciferol 20000 unit ColeDose D3 20,000unit tablets | 30 tablet £7.45

▶ **ColeKal-D3** (Essential-Healthcare Ltd)
Colecalciferol 400 unit ColeKal-D3 400unit tablets | 30 tablet £2.23

▶ **Colextra-D3** (Synergy Biologics Ltd)
Colecalciferol 25000 unit Colextra-D3 25,000unit tablets | 12 tablet [PoM] £12.40 DT = £17.00

▶ **Cubicole D3** (Cubic Pharmaceuticals Ltd)
Colecalciferol 400 unit Cubicole D3 400unit tablets | 30 tablet £3.55

▶ **Desunin** (Viatris UK Healthcare Ltd)
Colecalciferol 800 unit Desunin 800unit tablets | 30 tablet [PoM] £3.60 DT = £6.04 | 90 tablet [PoM] £10.17
Colecalciferol 4000 unit Desunin 4,000unit tablets | 70 tablet [PoM] £15.90 DT = £15.90

▶ **E-D3** (Ennogen Healthcare International Ltd)
Colecalciferol 400 unit E-D3 400unit tablets | 30 tablet £78.50
Colecalciferol 10000 unit E-D3 10,000unit tablets | 30 tablet £95.00
Colecalciferol 20000 unit E-D3 20,000unit tablets | 30 tablet £95.90

▶ **Healthmarque** (Kinerva Ltd)
Colecalciferol 20000 unit Healthmarque D3 20,000unit tablets | 15 tablet £3.33

▶ **Pro D3** (Synergy Biologics Ltd)
Colecalciferol 400 unit Pro D3 400unit tablets | 30 tablet £1.90

▶ **Stexerol-D3** (Kyowa Kirin International UK NewCo Ltd)
Colecalciferol 1000 unit Stexerol-D3 1,000unit tablets | 28 tablet [PoM] £2.95 DT = £2.95
Colecalciferol 25000 unit Stexerol-D3 25,000unit tablets | 12 tablet [PoM] £17.00 DT = £17.00

▶ **SunVit D3** (SunVit-D3 Ltd)
Colecalciferol 400 unit SunVit-D3 400unit Vegan tablets | 60 tablet £4.72
SunVit-D3 400unit tablets | 28 tablet £2.89

Colecalciferol 3000 unit SunVit-D3 3,000unit tablets | 28 tablet £6.23

Colecalciferol 5000 unit SunVit-D3 5,000unit tablets | 28 tablet £5.66

Colecalciferol 10000 unit SunVit-D3 10,000unit tablets | 28 tablet £7.93

Colecalciferol 20000 unit SunVit-D3 20,000unit tablets | 28 tablet £4.99

Colecalciferol 50000 unit SunVit-D3 50,000unit tablets | 15 tablet £22.67

▸ **YPV Vitamin D3** (GlucoRx Ltd)

Colecalciferol 400 unit YPV Vitamin D3 400unit tablets | 180 tablet £4.95

Colecalciferol 20000 unit YPV Vitamin D3 20,000unit tablets | 14 tablet £4.95

Oral capsule
CAUTIONARY AND ADVISORY LABELS 25

▸ **Colecalciferol (Non-proprietary)**

Colecalciferol 400 unit Colecalciferol 400unit capsules | 30 capsule PoM 🅔

Colecalciferol 800 unit Colecalciferol 800unit capsules | 30 capsule PoM £3.60 DT = £3.60

Colecalciferol 1000 unit Colecalciferol 1,000unit capsules | 30 capsule PoM £10.00 DT = £5.69

Colecalciferol 3000 unit FSC High Strength Vitamin D3 3,000unit capsules | 60 capsule £1.95

Colecalciferol 3200 unit Colecalciferol 3,200unit capsules | 30 capsule PoM £13.32 DT = £13.32

Colecalciferol 5000 unit Colecalciferol 5,000unit capsules | 100 capsule PoM 🅔

Colecalciferol 10000 unit Colecalciferol 10,000unit capsules | 20 capsule PoM £14.06 DT = £14.06

Colecalciferol 20000 unit Colecalciferol 20,000unit capsules | 10 capsule PoM £9.67–£11.36 | 20 capsule PoM £13.15–£20.95 | 30 capsule PoM £29.00 DT = £29.00

▸ **Aace D3** (Essential-Healthcare Ltd)

Colecalciferol 600 unit Aace D3 600unit capsules | 28 capsule £4.17

Colecalciferol 2200 unit Aace D3 2,200unit capsules | 28 capsule £4.67

Colecalciferol 2500 unit Aace D3 2,500unit capsules | 28 capsule £4.59

Colecalciferol 3000 unit Aace D3 3,000unit capsules | 28 capsule £3.59

Colecalciferol 30000 unit Aace D3 30,000unit capsules | 10 capsule £7.43

▸ **Aactive D3** (TriOn Pharma Ltd)

Colecalciferol 600 unit Aactive D3 600unit capsules | 30 capsule £4.49

Colecalciferol 2200 unit Aactive D3 2,200unit capsules | 30 capsule £4.99

Colecalciferol 2500 unit Aactive D3 2,500unit capsules | 30 capsule £4.59

Colecalciferol 30000 unit Aactive D3 30,000unit capsules | 10 capsule £14.49

▸ **Aciferol D3** (Fontus Health Ltd)

Colecalciferol 30000 unit Aciferol D3 30,000unit capsules | 10 capsule £24.95

▸ **Actium D3** (MaN Pharma Ltd)

Colecalciferol 2500 unit Actium D3 2,500unit capsules | 30 capsule £5.00

▸ **Colextra-D3** (Synergy Biologics Ltd)

Colecalciferol 800 unit Colextra-D3 800unit capsules | 30 capsule PoM £2.40 DT = £3.60

Colecalciferol 20000 unit Colextra-D3 20,000unit capsules | 10 capsule PoM £5.90 | 30 capsule PoM £15.90 DT = £29.00

▸ **Cubicole D3** (Cubic Pharmaceuticals Ltd)

Colecalciferol 600 unit Cubicole D3 600unit capsules | 30 capsule £4.95

Colecalciferol 2200 unit Cubicole D3 2,200unit capsules | 30 capsule £5.55

Colecalciferol 3000 unit Cubicole D3 3,000unit capsules | 30 capsule £5.95

▸ **E-D3** (Ennogen Healthcare International Ltd)

Colecalciferol 600 unit E-D3 600unit capsules | 30 capsule £82.10

Colecalciferol 2200 unit E-D3 2,200unit capsules | 30 capsule £86.20

Colecalciferol 2500 unit E-D3 2,500unit capsules | 30 capsule £86.20

Colecalciferol 3000 unit E-D3 3,000unit capsules | 30 capsule £88.60

Colecalciferol 30000 unit E-D3 30,000unit capsules | 10 capsule £94.40

▸ **Fultium-D3** (Internis Pharmaceuticals Ltd)

Colecalciferol 800 unit Fultium-D3 800unit capsules | 30 capsule PoM £3.60 DT = £3.60 | 90 capsule PoM £8.85 DT = £8.85

Colecalciferol 3200 unit Fultium-D3 3,200unit capsules | 30 capsule PoM £13.32 DT = £13.32 | 90 capsule PoM £39.96

Colecalciferol 20000 unit Fultium-D3 20,000unit capsules | 15 capsule PoM £17.04 DT = £17.04 | 30 capsule PoM £29.00 DT = £29.00

▸ **InVita D3** (Consilient Health Ltd)

Colecalciferol 5600 unit InVita D3 5,600unit capsules | 4 capsule PoM £2.50 DT = £2.50

Colecalciferol 25000 unit InVita D3 25,000unit capsules | 3 capsule PoM £3.95 DT = £3.95

Colecalciferol 50000 unit InVita D3 50,000unit capsules | 3 capsule PoM £4.95 DT = £4.95

▸ **LipoSil (Colecalciferol)** (Silicon Pharma Ltd)

Colecalciferol 2000 unit LipoSil Liposomal D3 2,000unit capsules | 30 capsule £9.67

▸ **Plenachol** (Accord-UK Ltd)

Colecalciferol 20000 unit Plenachol D3 20,000unit capsules | 10 capsule PoM £9.00

Colecalciferol 40000 unit Plenachol D3 40,000unit capsules | 7 capsule PoM £10.50

▸ **Pro D3** (Synergy Biologics Ltd)

Colecalciferol 2500 unit Pro D3 2,500unit capsules | 30 capsule £9.99

Colecalciferol 30000 unit Pro D3 30,000unit capsules | 10 capsule £24.99

▸ **Strivit-D3** (Strides Pharma UK Ltd)

Colecalciferol 800 unit Strivit-D3 800unit capsules | 30 capsule PoM £2.50 DT = £3.60

Colecalciferol 3200 unit Strivit-D3 3,200unit capsules | 30 capsule PoM £9.32 DT = £13.32

Colecalciferol 20000 unit Strivit-D3 20,000unit capsules | 10 capsule PoM £9.60 | 20 capsule PoM £13.15

▸ **SunVit D3** (SunVit-D3 Ltd)

Colecalciferol 600 unit SunVit-D3 600unit capsules | 60 capsule £7.55

Colecalciferol 2200 unit SunVit-D3 2,200unit capsules | 28 capsule £5.66

Colecalciferol 2500 unit SunVit-D3 2,500unit capsules | 28 capsule £6.23

Oral drops

▸ **Colecalciferol (Non-proprietary)**

Colecalciferol 400 unit per 1 ml Life On Vitokid-D3 400unit oral drops sugar free | 30 ml £2.78 SF

Colecalciferol 20000 unit per 1 ml Vigantol 20,000units/ml oral drops | 10 ml 🅔

Colecalciferol 400 unit per 1 drop Prohealth Vitamin D3 10micrograms/drop (400units/drop) oral drops | 2.4 ml £2.49 SF

Colecalciferol 1000 unit per 1 drop Vitamin D3 1,000unit oral drops | 30 ml £8.93 SF

▸ **Aactive D3** (TriOn Pharma Ltd)

Colecalciferol 2000 unit per 1 ml Aactive D3 2,000units/ml oral drops | 20 ml £5.82 SF

Colecalciferol 200 unit per 1 drop Aactive D3 200units/drop oral drops | 15 ml £5.19 SF

▸ **E-D3** (Ennogen Healthcare International Ltd)

Colecalciferol 2000 unit per 1 ml E-D3 2,000units/ml oral drops | 20 ml 🅔 SF

▸ **Fultium-D3** (Internis Pharmaceuticals Ltd)

Colecalciferol 2740 unit per 1 ml Fultium-D3 2,740units/ml oral drops | 25 ml PoM £10.70 DT = £10.70 SF

▸ **Healthmarque** (Kinerva Ltd)

Colecalciferol 400 unit per 1 drop Healthmarque D3 400units/drop oral drops | 7.5 ml £5.83 SF

Colecalciferol 1000 unit per 1 drop Healthmarque D3 1,000unit oral drops | 20 ml £7.49 SF

▸ **InVita D3** (Consilient Health Ltd)

Colecalciferol 2400 unit per 1 ml InVita D3 2,400units/ml oral drops | 10 ml PoM £3.60 DT = £3.60 SF

▸ **Pro D3** (Synergy Biologics Ltd)

Colecalciferol 2000 unit per 1 ml Pro D3 2,000units/ml liquid drops | 20 ml £9.80 SF

Pro D3 2,000units/ml Vegan liquid drops | 20 ml £11.00 SF

- **Provitavit Vitamin D** (Cuttlefish Ltd)
  Colecalciferol 200 unit per 1 drop Provitavit Vitamin D 200units/drop oral drops | 7 ml £4.95 [SF]
- **SunVit D3** (SunVit-D3 Ltd)
  Colecalciferol 2000 unit per 1 ml SunVit-D3 2,000units/ml oral drops | 20 ml £7.03 [SF]
- **Thorens** (Galen Ltd)
  Colecalciferol 10000 unit per 1 ml Thorens 10,000units/ml oral drops | 10 ml [PoM] £5.85 DT = £5.85 [SF]

Oral solution

CAUTIONARY AND ADVISORY LABELS 21

- **Colecalciferol (Non-proprietary)**
  Colecalciferol 3000 unit per 1 ml Colecalciferol 3,000units/ml oral solution sugar free | 100 ml [PoM] £89.23-£144.00 DT = £99.14 [SF]
  E-D3 15,000units/5ml oral solution | 50 ml [Ⓧ]
  Colecalciferol 10000 unit per 1 ml ZymaD 10,000units/ml oral solution | 10 ml [PoM] [Ⓧ]
- **Aactive D3** (TriOn Pharma Ltd)
  Colecalciferol 2000 unit per 1 ml Aactive D3 2,000units/ml oral solution | 50 ml £8.96 [SF]
- **Aciferol D3** (Fontus Health Ltd)
  Colecalciferol 2000 unit per 1 ml Aciferol D3 2,000units/ml liquid | 100 ml £24.95
  Colecalciferol 3000 unit per 1 ml Aciferol D3 3,000units/ml liquid | 100 ml £65.99
- **Baby D** (Arok Healthcare)
  Colecalciferol 1000 unit per 1 ml BabyD 1,000units/ml oral solution | 30 ml £4.50
  Colecalciferol 1440 unit per 1 ml BabyD 1,440units/ml oral solution | 10 ml £2.77 [SF]
- **E-D3** (Ennogen Healthcare International Ltd)
  Colecalciferol 1000 unit per 1 ml E-D3 1,000units/ml oral solution | 15 ml [Ⓧ]
  Colecalciferol 3000 unit per 1 ml E-D3 3,000units/ml oral solution | 50 ml [Ⓧ]
- **InVita D3** (Consilient Health Ltd)
  Colecalciferol 25000 unit per 1 ml InVita D3 25,000units/1ml oral solution | 3 ampoule [PoM] £4.45 DT = £4.45 [SF]
  Colecalciferol 50000 unit per 1 ml InVita D3 50,000units/1ml oral solution | 3 ampoule [PoM] £6.25 DT = £6.25 [SF]
- **Pro D3** (Synergy Biologics Ltd)
  Colecalciferol 2000 unit per 1 ml Pro D3 2,000units/ml liquid | 50 ml £16.80 | 100 ml £22.50
  Pro D3 2,000units/ml Vegan liquid | 50 ml £17.80
  Colecalciferol 3000 unit per 1 ml Pro D3 forte 3,000units/ml liquid | 50 ml £18.90
- **SunVit D3** (SunVit-D3 Ltd)
  Colecalciferol 2000 unit per 1 ml SunVit-D3 10,000units/5ml oral solution | 50 ml £10.09 [SF]
  SunVit-D3 2,000units/ml oral solution | 50 ml £10.09 [SF]
- **Thorens** (Galen Ltd)
  Colecalciferol 10000 unit per 1 ml Thorens 25,000units/2.5ml oral solution | 2.5 ml [PoM] £1.55 DT = £1.55 [SF] | 10 ml [PoM] £5.85 DT = £5.85 [SF]

Chewable tablet

- **Urgent-D** (Vega Nutritionals Ltd)
  Colecalciferol 2000 unit Urgent-D 2,000unit chewable tablets | 60 tablet £4.31

Form unstated

- **Colecalciferol (Non-proprietary)**
  Colecalciferol 400 unit per 1 dose BetterYou D400 Junior Vitamin D 400units Daily oral spray | 15 ml £4.16 [SF]
  BetterYou Infant Vitamin D 400units Daily oral spray | 15 ml £4.16 [SF]
  Colecalciferol 1000 unit per 1 dose BetterYou D1000 Vitamin D 1,000units Daily oral spray | 15 ml £4.44 [SF]
  Colecalciferol 3000 unit per 1 dose BetterYou Vitamin D 3,000units Daily oral spray | 15 ml £5.28 [SF]
  Colecalciferol 4000 unit per 1 dose BetterYou D4000 Vitamin D 4,000units Daily oral spray | 15 ml £5.56 [SF]
- **DailyD** (Arok Healthcare)
  Colecalciferol 400 unit per 1 dose DailyD Vitamin D3 400units oral spray | 30 ml £4.99 [SF]
  Colecalciferol 1000 unit per 1 dose DailyD Vitamin D3 1,000units oral spray | 30 ml £8.88 [SF]
- **ToddlerD** (Arok Healthcare)
  Colecalciferol 200 unit per 1 dose ToddlerD Vitamin D3 200units oral spray | 30 ml £4.99 [SF]

Orodispersible tablet

- **Colecalciferol (Non-proprietary)**
  Colecalciferol 2000 unit Vitamin D3 Lemon Melts 2,000unit tablets | 120 tablet £7.25 [SF]

Combinations available: *Vitamins A and D,* p. 1236

Colecalciferol with calcium carbonate

The properties listed below are those particular to the combination only. For the properties of the components please consider, colecalciferol p. 1242, calcium carbonate p. 1188.

● INDICATIONS AND DOSE

Prevention and treatment of vitamin D and calcium deficiency

- ► BY MOUTH
- ► Adult: Dosed according to the deficit or daily maintenance requirements (consult product literature)

● INTERACTIONS → Appendix 1: calcium salts · vitamin D substances

● PRESCRIBING AND DISPENSING INFORMATION *Accrete D3* ® contains calcium carbonate 1.5 g (calcium 600 mg or Ca^{2+} 15 mmol), colecalciferol 10 micrograms (400 units); *Adcal-D3* ® tablets contain calcium carbonate 1.5 g (calcium 600 mg or Ca^{2+} 15 mmol), colecalciferol 10 micrograms (400 units); *Cacit* ® *D3* contains calcium carbonate 1.25 g (calcium 500 mg or Ca^{2+} 12.5 mmol), colecalciferol 11 micrograms (440 units)/sachet; *Calceos* ® contains calcium carbonate 1.25 g (calcium 500 mg or Ca^{2+} 12.5 mmol), colecalciferol 10 micrograms (400 units); *Calcichew-D3* ® tablets contain calcium carbonate 1.25 g (calcium 500 mg or Ca^{2+} 12.5 mmol), colecalciferol 5 micrograms (200 units); *Calcichew-D3* ® *Forte* tablets contain calcium carbonate 1.25 g (calcium 500 mg or Ca^{2+} 12.5 mmol), colecalciferol 10 micrograms (400 units); *Calcichew-D3* ® 500 mg/400 unit caplets contain calcium carbonate (calcium 500 mg or Ca^{2+} 12.5 mmol), colecalciferol 10 micrograms (400 units); *Kalcipos-D* ® contains calcium carbonate (calcium 500 mg or Ca^{2+} 12.5 mmol), colecalciferol 20 micrograms (800 units); *Natecal D3* ® contains calcium carbonate 1.5 g (calcium 600 mg or Ca^{2+} 15 mmol), colecalciferol 10 micrograms (400 units); consult product literature for details of other available products.

Flavours of chewable and soluble forms may include orange, lemon, aniseed, peppermint, molasses, or tutti-frutti.

● MEDICINAL FORMS There can be variation in the licensing of different medicines containing the same drug.

Oral tablet

EXCIPIENTS: May contain Propylene glycol

- **Accrete D3** (Thornton & Ross Ltd)
  Calcium carbonate 1.5 gram, Colecalciferol 400 unit Accrete D3 tablets | 60 tablet [P] £2.95 DT = £2.95
- **Adcal-D3** (Kyowa Kirin International UK NewCo Ltd)
  Calcium carbonate 750 mg, Colecalciferol 200 unit Adcal-D3 750mg/200unit caplets | 112 tablet [P] £4.25 DT = £4.25

Effervescent granules

CAUTIONARY AND ADVISORY LABELS 13

- **Colecalciferol with calcium carbonate (Non-proprietary)**
  Calcium carbonate 2.5 gram, Colecalciferol 880 unit Colecalciferol 880unit / Calcium carbonate 2.5g effervescent granules sachets | 24 sachet [PoM] [Ⓧ]
- **Cacit D3** (Theramex HQ UK Ltd)
  Calcium carbonate 1.25 gram, Colecalciferol 440 unit Cacit D3 effervescent granules sachets | 30 sachet [PoM] £4.06 DT = £4.06

Effervescent tablet

CAUTIONARY AND ADVISORY LABELS 13

- **Adcal-D3** (Kyowa Kirin International UK NewCo Ltd)
  Calcium carbonate 1.5 gram, Colecalciferol 400 unit Adcal-D3 Dissolve 1500mg/400unit effervescent tablets | 56 tablet [P] £6.74 DT = £6.74

Chewable tablet

CAUTIONARY AND ADVISORY LABELS 24

EXCIPIENTS: May contain Aspartame

▸ **Colecalciferol with calcium carbonate (Non-proprietary)**
 **Calcium carbonate 1.5 gram, Colecalciferol
 400 unit** Colecalciferol 400unit / Calcium carbonate 1.5g chewable
 tablets | 56 tablet P £5.12 DT = £5.12

▸ **A1-Cal D3** (TriOn Pharma Ltd)
 Calcium carbonate 1.25 gram, Colecalciferol 400 unit A1-Cal D3
 500mg/400unit chewable tablets | 60 tablet £3.49 SF | 100 tablet
 £4.98 SF

▸ **A1-Cal D3 Max** (TriOn Pharma Ltd)
 Calcium carbonate 1.5 gram, Colecalciferol 400 unit A1-Cal D3
 Max 600mg/400unit chewable tablets | 56 tablet £2.49 SF |
 112 tablet £4.89 SF

▸ **AaCa D3** (TriOn Pharma Ltd)
 Calcium carbonate 1.25 gram, Colecalciferol 200 unit AaCa D3
 1.25g/200unit chewable tablets | 100 tablet £6.99 SF

▸ **AaceCa D3** (Essential-Healthcare Ltd)
 Calcium carbonate 1.25 gram, Colecalciferol 400 unit AaceCa D3
 1250mg/400unit chewable tablets | 56 tablet £2.76 SF | 100 tablet
 £4.93 SF
 Calcium carbonate 1.5 gram, Colecalciferol 400 unit AaceCa D3
 1500mg/400unit chewable tablets | 56 tablet £2.49 SF

▸ **Accrete D3 One a Day** (Thornton & Ross Ltd)
 Calcium carbonate 2.5 gram, Colecalciferol 880 unit Accrete D3
 One a Day 1000mg/880unit chewable tablets | 30 tablet P £2.95 DT
 = £2.95

▸ **Adcal-D3** (Kyowa Kirin International UK NewCo Ltd)
 Calcium carbonate 1.5 gram, Colecalciferol 400 unit Adcal-D3
 Lemon chewable tablets | 56 tablet P £5.12 DT = £5.12 |
 112 tablet P £10.52
 Adcal-D3 chewable tablets tutti frutti | 56 tablet P £5.12 DT = £5.12
 | 112 tablet P £10.52

▸ **Calceos** (Galen Ltd)
 Calcium carbonate 1.25 gram, Colecalciferol 400 unit Calceos
 500mg/400unit chewable tablets | 60 tablet P £4.05 DT = £4.24

▸ **Calci-D** (Forum Health Products Ltd)
 Calcium carbonate 2.5 gram, Colecalciferol 1000 unit Calci-D
 1000mg/1,000unit chewable tablets | 28 tablet P £2.50 DT = £2.50

▸ **Calcichew D3** (Forum Health Products Ltd)
 Calcium carbonate 1.25 gram, Colecalciferol 200 unit Calcichew
 D3 chewable tablets | 100 tablet P £7.68 DT = £7.68
 Calcium carbonate 2.5 gram, Colecalciferol 800 unit Calcichew D3
 1000mg/800unit Once Daily chewable tablets | 30 tablet P £7.29 DT
 = £7.29

▸ **Calcichew D3 Forte** (Forum Health Products Ltd)
 Calcium carbonate 1.25 gram, Colecalciferol 400 unit Calcichew
 D3 Forte chewable tablets | 60 tablet P £4.24 DT = £4.24 |
 100 tablet P £7.08

▸ **Evacal D3** (Teva UK Ltd)
 Calcium carbonate 1.5 gram, Colecalciferol 400 unit Evacal D3
 1500mg/400unit chewable tablets | 56 tablet P £4.12 DT = £5.12 |
 112 tablet P £8.25

▸ **Kalcipos-D** (Ceuta Healthcare Ltd)
 Calcium carbonate 1.25 gram, Colecalciferol 800 unit Kalcipos-D
 500mg/800unit chewable tablets | 30 tablet PoM £4.21 DT = £4.21

▸ **Natecal** (Chiesi Ltd)
 Calcium carbonate 1.5 gram, Colecalciferol 400 unit Natecal D3
 600mg/400unit chewable tablets | 60 tablet P £3.63

▸ **TheiCal-D3** (Stirling Anglian Pharmaceuticals Ltd)
 Calcium carbonate 2.5 gram, Colecalciferol 880 unit TheiCal-D3
 1000mg/880unit chewable tablets | 30 tablet P £2.95 DT = £2.95

⚑ 1240

Ergocalciferol

20-Oct-2022

(Calciferol; Vitamin D₂)

● **INDICATIONS AND DOSE**

Primary prevention of vitamin D deficiency

▸ BY MOUTH

▸ Adult: 400 units daily

Treatment of vitamin D deficiency [Loading dose]

▸ BY MOUTH

▸ Adult: 50 000 units once weekly for 6 weeks,
 alternatively 40 000 units once weekly for 7 weeks,
 alternatively 4000 units daily for 10 weeks, different

loading regimens can be used to achieve a cumulative
total of approximately 300 000 units divided into daily
or weekly doses over 6–10 weeks

Treatment of vitamin D deficiency [Maintenance dose]

▸ BY MOUTH

▸ Adult: 800–2000 units daily, maintenance dosing may
 be given daily or the equivalent dose given
 intermittently. Maintenance to be started one month
 after loading dose completed, or if correction of
 vitamin D deficiency is less urgent, maintenance may
 be started without the use of loading doses. Higher
 maintenance doses may be necessary in those at high
 risk of vitamin D deficiency; maximum 4000 units per
 day

**Vitamin D deficiency caused by intestinal malabsorption
or chronic liver disease (under expert supervision)**

▸ BY INTRAMUSCULAR INJECTION

▸ Adult: 300 000 units every 3 to 6 months, dose to be
 adjusted as necessary

**Hypocalcaemia of hypoparathyroidism to achieve
normocalcaemia (under expert supervision)**

▸ BY MOUTH

▸ Adult: Up to 100 000 units daily

DOSE EQUIVALENCE AND CONVERSION

▸ Ergocalciferol 400 units is equivalent to 10 micrograms;
 dose expressed as units.

● **UNLICENSED USE**

▸ With oral use EvGr Ergocalciferol is used in the doses
 provided in BNF publications, for the primary prevention
 and treatment of vitamin D deficiency, Ⓐ but these may
 differ from those licensed.

● **INTERACTIONS** → Appendix 1: vitamin D substances

● **SIDE-EFFECTS**

▸ **Common or very common**

▸ With intramuscular use Hypoparathyroidism ·
 pseudohypoparathyroidism

▸ **Rare or very rare**

▸ With intramuscular use Psychosis

▸ **Frequency not known**

▸ With intramuscular use Acidosis · albuminuria · azotaemia ·
 bone pain · conjunctival deposit · drowsiness ·
 hypercholesterolaemia · hypertension · hyperthermia ·
 irritability · libido decreased · muscle weakness ·
 nephrocalcinosis · pancreatitis · photophobia · polydipsia ·
 rhinorrhoea · soft tissue calcification · taste metallic ·
 urinary disorders · vascular calcification

● **MONITORING REQUIREMENTS**

▸ When used for Treatment of vitamin D deficiency EvGr Monitor
 calcium concentration within 1 month after last loading
 dose or after starting maintenance dosing. Routine
 monitoring of plasma-25-hydroxyvitamin D concentration
 is not needed, but may be considered 3–6 months after
 starting treatment in some cases e.g. patients with
 symptomatic vitamin D deficiency or malabsorption, those
 taking antiresorptive therapy, or where poor compliance is
 suspected. Ⓐ

● **PRESCRIBING AND DISPENSING INFORMATION** The BP
 directs that when calciferol is prescribed or demanded,
 colecalciferol or ergocalciferol should be dispensed or
 supplied.
 When the strength of the tablets ordered or prescribed is
 not clear, the intention of the prescriber with respect to
 the strength (expressed in micrograms or milligrams per
 tablet) should be ascertained.

- **MEDICINAL FORMS** There can be variation in the licensing of different medicines containing the same drug. Forms available from special-order manufacturers include: oral tablet, oral capsule, oral suspension, oral solution, solution for injection

Oral tablet

▸ **Ergocalciferol (Non-proprietary)**
Ergocalciferol 12.5 microgram Ergo-D2 12.5microgram tablets | 30 tablet ⓧ

▸ **AacErgo** (Essential-Healthcare Ltd)
Ergocalciferol 12.5 microgram AacErgo 500unit tablets | 30 tablet £19.43
Ergocalciferol 250 microgram AacErgo 10,000unit tablets | 30 tablet £29.83

▸ **Ergoral** (Cubic Pharmaceuticals Ltd)
Ergocalciferol 250 microgram Ergoral D2 10,000unit tablets | 30 tablet £10.95

Solution for injection

▸ **Ergocalciferol (Non-proprietary)**
Ergocalciferol 300000 unit per 1 ml Ergocalciferol 300,000units/1ml solution for injection ampoules | 5 ampoule [PoM] £70.15 | 10 ampoule [PoM] £93.50 DT = £93.51
Ergocalciferol 400000 unit per 1 ml Sterogyl 15H 600,000units/1.5ml solution for injection ampoules | 1 ampoule [PoM] ⓧ

Oral capsule

▸ **Ergocalciferol (Non-proprietary)**
Ergocalciferol 1.25 mg Ergo-D2 1.25mg capsules | 30 capsule £96.80

▸ **AacErgo** (Essential-Healthcare Ltd)
Ergocalciferol 1.25 mg AacErgo 50,000unit capsules | 10 capsule £23.41

▸ **Eciferol** (Fontus Health Ltd)
Ergocalciferol 1.25 mg Eciferol D2 50,000unit capsules | 10 capsule £39.99

Oral solution

▸ **Ergocalciferol (Non-proprietary)**
Ergocalciferol 1500 unit per 1 ml Uvesterol D 1,500units/ml oral solution | 20 ml [PoM] ⓧ [SF]

▸ **Eciferol** (Fontus Health Ltd)
Ergocalciferol 3000 unit per 1 ml Eciferol D2 3,000units/ml liquid | 60 ml £95.00 DT = £41.14

Ergocalciferol with calcium lactate and calcium phosphate

28-Jun-2023

(Calcium and vitamin D)

The properties listed below are those particular to the combination only. For the properties of the components please consider, ergocalciferol p. 1245, calcium lactate p. 1190, calcium phosphate p. 1190.

- **INDICATIONS AND DOSE**

Prevention of calcium and vitamin D deficiency | Treatment of calcium and vitamin D deficiency

▸ BY MOUTH
▸ Adult: (consult product literature)

- **INTERACTIONS** → Appendix 1: calcium salts · vitamin D substances

- **DIRECTIONS FOR ADMINISTRATION** Manufacturer advises tablets may be crushed before administration, or may be chewed.

- **PRESCRIBING AND DISPENSING INFORMATION** Each tablet contains calcium lactate 300 mg, calcium phosphate 150 mg (calcium 97 mg or Ca^{2+} 2.4 mmol), ergocalciferol 10 micrograms (400 units).

- **PATIENT AND CARER ADVICE** Patient or carers should be given advice on how to administer calcium and ergocalciferol tablets.

- **MEDICINAL FORMS** There can be variation in the licensing of different medicines containing the same drug.

Oral tablet

▸ **Ergocalciferol with calcium lactate and calcium phosphate (Non-proprietary)**
Ergocalciferol 10 microgram, Calcium phosphate 150 mg, Calcium lactate 300 mg Calcium and Ergocalciferol tablets | 28 tablet [P] ⓧ DT = £5.93

⌖ 1240

Paricalcitol

27-Oct-2022

- **INDICATIONS AND DOSE**

Prevention and treatment of secondary hyperparathyroidism associated with chronic kidney disease

▸ BY MOUTH
▸ Adult: (consult product literature)

Prevention and treatment of secondary hyperparathyroidism associated with chronic renal failure in patients on haemodialysis

▸ Adult: To be administered via haemodialysis access (consult product literature)

- **INTERACTIONS** → Appendix 1: vitamin D substances

- **SIDE-EFFECTS**

GENERAL SIDE-EFFECTS

▸ **Common or very common** Electrolyte imbalance · hypoparathyroidism · taste altered
▸ **Uncommon** Dizziness · malaise · pain
▸ **Frequency not known** Angioedema · laryngeal oedema

SPECIFIC SIDE-EFFECTS

▸ **Uncommon**
▸ With oral use Breast tenderness · gastrointestinal discomfort · gastrooesophageal reflux disease · muscle spasms · palpitations · peripheral oedema · pneumonia
▸ With parenteral use Alopecia · anaemia · anxiety · asthma · atrial flutter · breast cancer · breast pain · cardiac arrest · cerebrovascular insufficiency · chest pain · coma · condition aggravated · confusion · conjunctivitis · cough · delirium · depersonalisation · dyspepsia · dysphagia · dyspnoea · ear disorder · erectile dysfunction · fever · gait abnormal · gastrointestinal disorders · glaucoma · haemorrhage · hirsutism · hyperhidrosis · hyperparathyroidism · hypertension · hypotension · increased risk of infection · insomnia · joint disorders · leucopenia · lymphadenopathy · muscle twitching · myoclonus · oedema · pulmonary oedema · sensation abnormal · sepsis · syncope · thirst

- **PREGNANCY** Manufacturer advises avoid—toxicity in *animal* studies.

- **BREAST FEEDING** Manufacturer advises avoid—no information available.

- **MONITORING REQUIREMENTS**
▸ With oral use [EvGr] Monitor plasma-calcium, phosphate and parathyroid hormone concentration regularly, particularly at initiation of treatment and during dose titration. Ⓜ

- **MEDICINAL FORMS** There can be variation in the licensing of different medicines containing the same drug.

Solution for injection
EXCIPIENTS: May contain Ethanol, propylene glycol

▸ **Zemplar** (AbbVie Ltd)
Paricalcitol 5 microgram per 1 ml Zemplar 5micrograms/1ml solution for injection vials | 5 vial [PoM] £62.00 (Hospital only)

Oral capsule
EXCIPIENTS: May contain Ethanol

▸ **Zemplar** (AbbVie Ltd)
Paricalcitol 1 microgram Zemplar 1microgram capsules | 28 capsule [PoM] £69.44 DT = £69.44
Paricalcitol 2 microgram Zemplar 2microgram capsules | 28 capsule [PoM] £138.88 DT = £138.88

Alpha tocopherol

04-Feb-2021

(Tocopherol)

- **INDICATIONS AND DOSE**

Vitamin E deficiency because of malabsorption in congenital or hereditary chronic cholestasis
- ▸ BY MOUTH USING ORAL SOLUTION
- ▸ Child: 17 mg/kg daily, dose to be adjusted as necessary

- **CAUTIONS** Predisposition to thrombosis
- **INTERACTIONS** → Appendix 1: vitamin E substances
- **SIDE-EFFECTS**
- ▸ **Common or very common** Diarrhoea
- ▸ **Uncommon** Alopecia · asthenia · headache · skin reactions
- ▸ **Frequency not known** Abdominal pain
- **PREGNANCY** Manufacturer advises caution, no evidence of harm in *animal* studies.
- **BREAST FEEDING** Manufacturer advises use only if potential benefit outweighs risk—no information available.
- **HEPATIC IMPAIRMENT** Manufacturer advises caution.
- **RENAL IMPAIRMENT** Manufacturer advises caution. Risk of renal toxicity due to polyethylene glycol content.
  Monitoring Manufacturer advises monitor closely in renal impairment.
- **PRESCRIBING AND DISPENSING INFORMATION**
  Tocofersolan is a water-soluble form of D-alpha tocopherol.

- **MEDICINAL FORMS** There can be variation in the licensing of different medicines containing the same drug.

Oral solution
- ▸ Vedrop (Recordati Rare Diseases UK Ltd) ▼
  D-alpha tocopherol (as Tocofersolan) 50 mg per 1 ml Vedrop 50mg/ml oral solution | 20 ml [PoM] £54.55 DT = £54.55 [SF] | 60 ml [PoM] £163.65 [SF]

Alpha tocopheryl acetate

04-Feb-2021

(Tocopherol)

- **INDICATIONS AND DOSE**

Vitamin E deficiency
- ▸ BY MOUTH
- ▸ Child: 2–10 mg/kg daily, increased if necessary up to 20 mg/kg daily

Malabsorption in cystic fibrosis
- ▸ BY MOUTH
- ▸ Child 1–11 months: 50 mg once daily, dose to be adjusted as necessary, to be taken with food and pancreatic enzymes
- ▸ Child 1–11 years: 100 mg once daily, dose to be adjusted as necessary, to be taken with food and pancreatic enzymes
- ▸ Child 12–17 years: 100–200 mg once daily, dose to be adjusted as necessary, to be taken with food and pancreatic enzymes
- ▸ Adult: 100–200 mg once daily, dose to be adjusted as necessary, to be taken with food and pancreatic enzymes

Vitamin E deficiency in cholestasis and severe liver disease
- ▸ BY MOUTH
- ▸ Child 1 month–11 years: Initially 100 mg daily, adjusted according to response, increased if necessary up to 200 mg/kg daily
- ▸ Child 12–17 years: Initially 200 mg daily, adjusted according to response, increased if necessary up to 200 mg/kg daily

Malabsorption in abetalipoproteinaemia
- ▸ BY MOUTH
- ▸ Adult: 50–100 mg/kg once daily

- **CAUTIONS** Predisposition to thrombosis
- **INTERACTIONS** → Appendix 1: vitamin E substances
- **SIDE-EFFECTS** Abdominal pain (more common at high doses) · bleeding tendency · diarrhoea (more common at high doses) · increased risk of thrombosis
- **PREGNANCY** No evidence of safety of high doses.
- **BREAST FEEDING** Excreted in milk; minimal risk, although caution with large doses.
- **MONITORING REQUIREMENTS** Increased bleeding tendency in vitamin-K deficient patients or those taking anticoagulants (prothrombin time and INR should be monitored).

- **MEDICINAL FORMS** There can be variation in the licensing of different medicines containing the same drug. Forms available from special-order manufacturers include: chewable tablet

Oral suspension
EXCIPIENTS: May contain Sucrose
- ▸ Alpha tocopheryl acetate (Non-proprietary)
  Alpha tocopheryl acetate 100 mg per 1 ml AlphaToc-E 500mg/5ml oral suspension | 100 ml £47.19 [SF]
  Alpha tocopheryl acetate 500mg/5ml oral suspension | 100 ml [GSL] £76.81–£84.49 DT = £76.81

Oral capsule
- ▸ AlphaToc-E (Essential-Healthcare Ltd)
  Alpha tocopherol 75 unit AlphaToc-E 75unit capsules | 100 capsule £5.83
  Alpha tocopherol 200 unit AlphaToc-E 200unit capsules | 100 capsule £12.93
  Alpha tocopherol 400 unit AlphaToc-E 400unit capsules | 100 capsule £19.82
- ▸ E-Caps (Ennogen Healthcare International Ltd)
  Alpha tocopherol 75 unit E-Caps 75unit capsules | 100 capsule £109.50
  Alpha tocopherol 100 unit E-Caps 100unit capsules | 30 capsule £84.40
  Alpha tocopherol 200 unit E-Caps 200unit capsules | 30 capsule £89.50
  Alpha tocopherol 400 unit E-Caps 400unit capsules | 30 capsule £128.50
  Alpha tocopherol 1000 unit E-Caps 1,000unit capsules | 30 capsule £130.20
- ▸ Nutra-E (TriOn Pharma Ltd)
  Alpha tocopherol 75 unit Nutra-E 75unit capsules | 100 capsule £5.86
  Alpha tocopherol 200 unit Nutra-E 200unit capsules | 100 capsule £12.88
  Alpha tocopherol 400 unit Nutra-E 400unit capsules | 100 capsule £19.82
- ▸ Vita-E (Typharm Ltd)
  Alpha tocopherol 75 unit Vita-E 75unit capsules | 100 capsule £9.65
  Alpha tocopherol 200 unit Vita-E 200unit capsules | 30 capsule £7.38 | 100 capsule £20.69
  Alpha tocopherol 400 unit Vita-E 400unit capsules | 30 capsule £11.03 | 100 capsule £30.16

Chewable tablet
- ▸ Alpha-E (TriOn Pharma Ltd)
  Alpha tocopheryl acetate 100 mg Alpha-E 100mg chewable tablets | 30 tablet £37.25
- ▸ AlphaToc-E (Essential-Healthcare Ltd)
  Alpha tocopheryl acetate 100 mg AlphaToc-E 100mg chewable tablets | 30 tablet £29.67
- ▸ E-Tabs (Ennogen Healthcare International Ltd)
  Alpha tocopheryl acetate 100 mg E-Tabs 100mg chewable tablets | 30 tablet £87.30
- ▸ Ephynal (Imported (Italy))
  Alpha tocopheryl acetate 100 mg Ephynal 100mg chewable tablets | 30 tablet [X]

Menadiol sodium phosphate
24-May-2021

- **INDICATIONS AND DOSE**

Prevention of Vitamin K deficiency in malabsorption syndromes
▸ BY MOUTH
▸ Adult: 10–40 mg daily, dose to be adjusted as necessary

- **CAUTIONS** G6PD deficiency (risk of haemolysis) · vitamin E deficiency (risk of haemolysis)

- **PREGNANCY** Avoid in late pregnancy and labour unless benefit outweighs risk of neonatal haemolytic anaemia, hyperbilirubinaemia, and kernicterus in neonate.

- **MEDICINAL FORMS** There can be variation in the licensing of different medicines containing the same drug.

Oral tablet
▸ Menadiol sodium phosphate (Non-proprietary)
Menadiol phosphate (as Menadiol sodium phosphate)
10 mg Menadiol 10mg tablets | 100 tablet P £273.42 DT = £248.56

Phytomenadione
04-Feb-2021

(Vitamin K₁)

- **INDICATIONS AND DOSE**

Major bleeding in patients on warfarin (in combination with dried prothrombin complex or fresh frozen plasma)
▸ BY SLOW INTRAVENOUS INJECTION
▸ Adult: 5 mg for 1 dose, stop warfarin treatment

INR > 8.0 with minor bleeding in patients on warfarin
▸ BY SLOW INTRAVENOUS INJECTION
▸ Adult: 1–3 mg for 1 dose, stop warfarin treatment, dose may be repeated if INR still too high after 24 hours, restart warfarin treatment when INR <5

INR > 8.0 with no bleeding in patients on warfarin
▸ BY MOUTH
▸ Adult: 1–5 mg for 1 dose, intravenous preparation to be used orally, stop warfarin treatment, repeat dose if INR still too high after 24 hours, restart warfarin treatment when INR <5

INR 5.0–8.0 with minor bleeding in patients on warfarin
▸ BY SLOW INTRAVENOUS INJECTION
▸ Adult: 1–3 mg for 1 dose, stop warfarin treatment, restart warfarin treatment when INR <5

Reversal of anticoagulation prior to elective surgery (after warfarin stopped)
▸ BY MOUTH
▸ Adult: 1–5 mg for 1 dose, intravenous preparation to be used orally, dose to be given the day before surgery if INR ≥1.5

Reversal of anticoagulation prior to emergency surgery (when surgery can be delayed 6–12 hours)
▸ BY INTRAVENOUS INJECTION
▸ Adult: 5 mg for 1 dose, if surgery cannot be delayed, dried prothrombin complex can be given in addition to phytomenadione and the INR checked before surgery

- **UNLICENSED USE** Oral use of intravenous preparations is unlicensed.

- **CAUTIONS** Intravenous injections should be given very slowly—reports of anaphylactoid reactions
KONAKION ® MM Reduce dose in elderly

- **PREGNANCY** Use if potential benefit outweighs risk.

- **BREAST FEEDING** Present in milk.

- **HEPATIC IMPAIRMENT**
KONAKION ® MM Manufacturer advises caution—monitor INR in patients with severe impairment (contains glycocholic acid which may displace bilirubin).

- **DIRECTIONS FOR ADMINISTRATION**
KONAKION ® MM *Konakion* ® *MM* may be administered *by slow intravenous injection* or *by intravenous infusion* in glucose 5%; **not** for intramuscular injection. For *intravenous infusion (Konakion* ® *MM)*, give intermittently in Glucose 5%; dilute with 55 mL; may be injected into lower part of infusion apparatus.
KONAKION ® MM PAEDIATRIC *Konakion* ® *MM Paediatric* may be administered *by mouth* or *by intramuscular injection* or *by intravenous injection*. For *intravenous injection*, expert sources advise may be diluted with Glucose 5% if necessary.

- **MEDICINAL FORMS** There can be variation in the licensing of different medicines containing the same drug. Forms available from special-order manufacturers include: oral suspension, oral solution

Solution for injection
EXCIPIENTS: May contain Glycocholic acid, lecithin
▸ Phytomenadione (Non-proprietary)
Phytomenadione 10 mg per 1 ml Phytomenadione 2mg/0.2ml solution for injection ampoules | 5 ampoule PoM £10.49–£11.01 DT = £11.01
Phytomenadione 10mg/1ml solution for injection ampoules | 10 ampoule PoM £11.01 DT = £11.01

7.1 Neural tube defects (prevention in pregnancy)

Neural tube defects (prevention in pregnancy)
01-Oct-2021

Description of condition

Neural tube defects represent a group of congenital defects, caused by incomplete closure of the neural tube within 28 days of conception. The most common forms are anencephaly, spina bifida and encephalocele.

The main risk factors are maternal folate deficiency, maternal vitamin B_{12} deficiency, previous history of having an infant with a neural tube defect, smoking, diabetes, obesity, and use of antiepileptic drugs. For information on smoking cessation see Smoking cessation p. 565.

Prevention in pregnancy

EvGr Pregnant women or women who wish to become pregnant should be advised to take supplementation with folic acid p. 1161 before conception and until week 12 of pregnancy.

A higher daily dose (see folic acid) is recommended for women at a high risk of conceiving a child with a neural tube defect, including women who have previously had an infant with a neural tube defect, who are receiving antiepileptic medication (see Epilepsy p. 349), or who have diabetes or sickle-cell disease. Ⓐ

Healthy Start vitamins for women (containing folic acid, ascorbic acid, and vitamin D) are available for pregnant women through the Healthy Start scheme. For further information, see www.healthystart.nhs.uk/. Vitamins for children are also available through the scheme.

Useful Resources

Fertility problems: assessment and treatment. National Institute for Health and Care Excellence. Clinical guideline 156. February 2013.
www.nice.org.uk/guidance/cg156

Chapter 10
Musculoskeletal system

CONTENTS

1   Arthritis

Osteoarthritis

09-Nov-2022

Overview

[EvGr] Patients diagnosed with osteoarthritis should receive an individualised management plan that may include self-care strategies and drug treatment options for symptom relief.

Non-drug measures, such as weight reduction (in overweight or obese patients, see Obesity p. 104) and exercise including local muscle strengthening and aerobic exercise, should be encouraged. Manual therapy such as manipulation, mobilisation, or soft tissue techniques, may be considered for people with hip or knee osteoarthritis if used alongside exercise.

If drug treatment is needed to manage osteoarthritis, it should be used alongside non-pharmacological treatments and to support exercise. The lowest effective dose should be used for the shortest possible time. For pain relief in osteoarthritis, a topical NSAID (particularly for knee involvement) is first-line treatment. If the topical NSAID is ineffective or unsuitable, consider an oral NSAID. Paracetamol p. 507 or weak opioids should only be used infrequently for short-term pain relief if all other pharmacological treatments are unsuitable, not tolerated, or ineffective.

Intra-articular corticosteroid injections can be considered to provide short-term relief when other pharmacological treatments are ineffective or unsuitable, or to support exercise. (A)

Topical capsaicin 0.025% p. 548 may provide relief of pain associated with osteoarthritis in some patients, particularly where there is knee involvement.

[EvGr] Strong opioids, glucosamine p. 1253, intra-articular injections of hyaluronic acid and its derivatives, chondroitin, and topical rubefacients (which may contain nicotinate compounds, salicylate compounds, essential oils, and camphor) are not recommended for the treatment of osteoarthritis.

If self-management and drug treatment strategies are ineffective or unsuitable, consider referral to a specialist multidisciplinary team. (A)

Useful resources

Osteoarthritis in over 16s: diagnosis and management. National Institute for Health and Care Excellence. NICE guideline 226. October 2022.

www.nice.org.uk/guidance/ng226

Rheumatoid arthritis

12-Nov-2021

Description of condition

Rheumatoid arthritis is a chronic systemic inflammatory disease that causes persistent symmetrical joint synovitis (inflammation of the synovial membrane) typically of the small joints of the hands and feet, although any synovial joint can be affected. Synovitis presents as pain and prolonged stiffness that tends to be worse at rest or following periods of inactivity, swelling, tenderness, and heat in the affected joints. Other symptoms of rheumatoid arthritis include rheumatoid nodules and non-specific symptoms such as malaise, fatigue, fever, and weight loss.

As the disease progresses, it can cause joint deformity and affect different organs of the body, such as the heart, lungs, and eyes; therefore early diagnosis and treatment of rheumatoid arthritis is essential to reduce the impact of the disease.

Palindromic rheumatism is a rare form of inflammatory arthritis which causes attacks of joint pain and swelling similar to rheumatoid arthritis, but the joints return to normal in between attacks. Patients with palindromic rheumatism may later develop rheumatoid arthritis.

Aims of treatment

The aims of treatment are to relieve the symptoms of rheumatoid arthritis, achieve disease remission or low disease activity if remission cannot be achieved, and to improve the patient's ability to perform daily activities.

Non-drug treatment

[EvGr] Patients with rheumatoid arthritis should have access to a multidisciplinary team, and may benefit from physiotherapy to encourage exercise, enhance flexibility of joints and strengthen muscles. Psychological interventions such as relaxation, stress management, and cognitive coping skills to support patients with their perception and management of their disease can also be offered. (A)

Drug treatment

[EvGr] All patients with suspected persistent synovitis of unknown cause should be referred to a specialist for advice as soon as possible to confirm diagnosis and evaluate disease activity.

In patients with newly diagnosed active rheumatoid arthritis, monotherapy with a conventional disease-modifying antirheumatic drug (DMARD) (oral methotrexate p. 1048, leflunomide p. 1254, or sulfasalazine p. 46) should be given as first-line treatment; hydroxychloroquine sulfate p. 1253, a weak conventional DMARD, is an alternative in patients with mild rheumatoid arthritis or those with palindromic rheumatism. Treatment should be started as soon as possible, ideally within 3 months of onset of persistent symptoms, and the dose should be titrated to the maximum tolerated effective dose. Ⓐ

Conventional DMARDs have a slow onset of action and can take 2–3 months to take effect. ｜EvGr｜ Consider short-term bridging treatment with a corticosteroid (by oral, intramuscular, or intra-articular administration) when starting treatment with a new conventional DMARD to provide rapid symptomatic control, while waiting for the new DMARD to take effect. Short-term corticosteroids should also be given to rapidly decrease inflammation during flare-ups.

If the treatment target (remission or low disease activity) has not been achieved despite dose escalation on conventional DMARD monotherapy, offer combination therapy with additional conventional DMARDs (oral methotrexate p. 1048, leflunomide p. 1254, sulfasalazine p. 46, or hydroxychloroquine sulfate p. 1253).

Treatment with a tumour necrosis factor (TNF) alpha inhibitor (adalimumab p. 1269, certolizumab pegol p. 1271, etanercept p. 1273, golimumab p. 1274, or infliximab p. 1275), other biological DMARD (abatacept p. 1269, sarilumab p. 1256, or tocilizumab p. 1258), or targeted synthetic DMARD (baricitinib p. 1262, filgotinib p. 1263, tofacitinib p. 1265, or upadacitinib p. 1267) is recommended if there has been an inadequate response to combination therapy with conventional DMARDs. Ⓐ For further information on their use, see NICE pathway: **Rheumatoid arthritis** (available at: pathways.nice.org.uk/pathways/ rheumatoid-arthritis).

｜EvGr｜ Rituximab p. 1019 in combination with methotrexate p. 1048 is an option for patients with severe active rheumatoid arthritis who have had an inadequate response to, or are intolerant of other DMARDs, including at least one TNF alpha inhibitor. Ⓐ For guidance on treatment options if rituximab is unsuitable, or there is an inadequate response to rituximab and other biological DMARDs, see NICE pathway: **Rheumatoid arthritis** (available at: pathways.nice. org.uk/pathways/rheumatoid-arthritis).

｜EvGr｜ In patients with established rheumatoid arthritis, the long-term use of corticosteroids should only be continued if all other treatments options (including biological and targeted synthetic DMARDs) have been offered.

Patients with active rheumatoid arthritis should be monitored monthly until the treatment target (either remission or low disease activity) has been achieved, and all patients with rheumatoid arthritis should be reviewed annually. In patients who have maintained the treatment target for at least 1 year without corticosteroids, cautiously reducing drug doses to the lowest that are clinically effective, or tapering and stopping at least one drug if the patient is being treated with two or more DMARDs should be considered. Ⓐ

Older conventional DMARDs such as sodium aurothiomalate (gold), azathioprine p. 965, ciclosporin p. 966 and penicillamine p. 1255 are no longer commonly used in practice due to the availability of newer, more effective drugs.

Pain relief

｜EvGr｜ Short-term use of an oral non-steroidal anti-inflammatory drug (NSAID) or a selective cyclo-oxygenase-2 inhibitor should be considered for additional control of pain and stiffness associated with rheumatoid arthritis. Patients should be offered a proton pump inhibitor to minimise associated gastrointestinal adverse effects. In patients already taking low-dose aspirin p. 142, other treatments should be considered before giving a NSAID. NSAIDs should be used at the lowest effective dose, and if possible, withdrawn when a good response to DMARDs is achieved. Ⓐ

Surgery

｜EvGr｜ Surgery may be an option for some patients if drug treatment has failed to adequately manage persistent pain due to joint damage or other identifiable soft tissue causes, if there is worsening of joint function, progressive deformity, or persistent localised synovitis. Ⓐ

Useful Resources

Rheumatoid arthritis in adults: management. National Institute for Health and Care Excellence. NICE guideline 100. October 2020.
www.nice.org.uk/guidance/ng100

Spondyloarthritis

11-Jan-2023

Description of condition

Spondyloarthritis refers to a group of inflammatory musculoskeletal conditions with shared features which affect both axial and peripheral joints. Most people with these conditions have either axial spondyloarthritis (which includes ankylosing spondylitis and non-radiographic axial spondyloarthritis) or psoriatic arthritis. Axial spondyloarthritis primarily affects the spine, in particular the sacroiliac joint.

Psoriatic arthritis may present in several forms, including involvement of small joints (in the hands and feet), large joints (particularly in the knees), or combinations of both. Psoriatic arthritis may also involve the axial joints, finger and toe joints, and inflammation of the connective tissue between tendon/ligament and bone.

Less common subgroups are enteropathic spondyloarthritis, which is associated with inflammatory bowel disease (Crohn's disease p. 40 and Ulcerative colitis p. 41), and reactive arthritis (a form of peripheral arthritis), which can occur following gastro-intestinal or genito-urinary infections.

Aims of treatment

The aims of treatment are to relieve symptoms, slow the progression of the condition, and improve quality of life.

Non-drug treatment

｜EvGr｜ Patients who have difficulties with everyday activities should be referred to a specialist therapist (such as a physiotherapist, occupational therapist, hand therapist, orthotist or podiatrist). Hydrotherapy can be considered as an adjunctive therapy to manage pain and maintain or improve function for people with axial spondyloarthritis. Ⓐ

Drug treatment

Axial spondyloarthritis

｜EvGr｜ For pain associated with axial spondyloarthritis, start one of the Non-steroidal anti-inflammatory drugs p. 1292 (NSAIDs) at the lowest effective dose. Clinical assessment, monitoring of risk factors, and the use of gastroprotective treatment should be considered. If an NSAID taken at the maximum tolerated dose for 2–4 weeks does not provide adequate pain relief, consider switching to a different NSAID.

Under specialist care, Janus kinase (JAK) inhibitors and biological drugs (such as interleukin inhibitors and tumor necrosis factor alpha (TNF-α) inhibitors) may be used for the treatment of **ankylosing spondylitis** or **non-radiographic axial spondyloarthritis**. Ⓐ

Psoriatic arthritis and other peripheral spondyloarthritides

｜EvGr｜ Monotherapy with local corticosteroid injections should be considered for non-progressive **monoarthritis** (see Corticosteroids, inflammatory disorders p. 1315).

Standard disease-modifying antirheumatic drugs (DMARDs), such as methotrexate p. 1048, leflunomide p. 1254 or sulfasalazine p. 46, can be used for patients with peripheral **polyarthritis**, **oligoarthritis**, or persistent or progressive **monoarthritis** associated with peripheral spondyloarthritis.

Standard DMARDs, such as methotrexate p. 1048 or leflunomide p. 1254 can also be used for patients with **psoriatic arthritis**.

The choice of DMARD will depend on numerous factors such as the patient's circumstances (such as pregnancy planning and alcohol consumption), comorbidities (such as uveitis, psoriasis and inflammatory bowel disease), and potential side-effects.

If a standard DMARD taken at the maximum tolerated dose for at least 3 months does not provide adequate relief from symptoms, a switch to, or the addition of, another standard DMARD can be considered.

An NSAID can be used as an adjunct to standard DMARDs or biological DMARDs to manage symptoms. If NSAIDs do not provide adequate relief from symptoms, consider corticosteroid injections or short-term oral corticosteroid therapy as an adjunct to standard DMARDs or biological DMARDs to manage symptoms.

If extra-articular disease is adequately controlled by an existing standard DMARD but peripheral spondyloarthritis is not, consider adding another standard DMARD. Ⓐ

Further options for psoriatic arthritis

[EvGr] Under specialist care, JAK inhibitors, phosphodiesterase type-4 (PDE4) inhibitors, and biological drugs (such as interleukin inhibitors and TNF-α inhibitors) may be used for the treatment of active or active and progressive psoriatic arthritis. Ⓐ

Reactive arthritis

[EvGr] After treating the initial infection, do not offer long-term (4 weeks or longer) treatment with an antibacterial solely to manage reactive arthritis caused by a gastro-intestinal or genito-urinary infection. Ⓐ

Useful Resources

Spondyloarthritis in over 16s: diagnosis and management. National Institute for Health and Care Excellence. Clinical Guideline NG65. February 2017.
www.nice.org.uk/guidance/ng65

Rheumatic disease, suppressing drugs

12-Nov-2021

Overview

Certain drugs such as those affecting the immune response can suppress the disease process in *rheumatoid arthritis* and *psoriatic arthritis*, see Rheumatoid arthritis p. 1249 or Spondyloarthritis p. 1250. *Systemic* and *discoid lupus erythematosus* are sometimes treated with chloroquine p. 710 or hydroxychloroquine sulfate p. 1253.

The choice of a disease-modifying antirheumatic drug (DMARD) should take into account co-morbidity and patient preference. Methotrexate p. 1048, sulfasalazine p. 46, intramuscular gold, and penicillamine p. 1255 are similar in efficacy. However, methotrexate or sulfasalazine may be better tolerated.

Gold

Gold, given as sodium aurothiomalate, is licensed for active progressive rheumatoid arthritis; it must be given by deep intramuscular injection and the area gently massaged. A test dose must be given followed by doses at weekly intervals until there is definite evidence of remission. In patients who do respond, the interval between injections is then gradually increased to 4 weeks and treatment is continued for up to 5 years after complete remission. If relapse occurs the dosage

frequency may be immediately increased and only once control has been obtained again should the dosage frequency be decreased; if no response is seen within 2 months, alternative treatment should be sought. It is important to avoid complete relapse since second courses of gold are not usually effective.

Penicillamine

Penicillamine has a similar action to gold. More patients are able to continue treatment than with gold but side-effects are common.

Patients should be warned not to expect improvement for at least 6 to 12 weeks after treatment is initiated. Penicillamine should be discontinued if there is no improvement within 1 year.

Sulfasalazine

Sulfasalazine has a beneficial effect in suppressing the inflammatory activity of rheumatoid arthritis. Sulfasalazine may also be used by specialists, in the management of psoriatic arthritis affecting peripheral joints [unlicensed]. Haematological abnormalities occur usually in the first 3 to 6 months of treatment and are reversible on cessation of treatment.

Antimalarials

The antimalarial hydroxychloroquine sulfate is used to treat rheumatoid arthritis of mild inflammatory activity; chloroquine is also licensed for treating inflammatory disorders but is used much less frequently and is generally reserved for use if other drugs have failed.

Chloroquine and hydroxychloroquine sulfate are effective for mild systemic lupus erythematosus, particularly involving the skin and joints. These drugs should not be used for psoriatic arthritis. Chloroquine and hydroxychloroquine sulfate are better tolerated than gold or penicillamine. Retinopathy rarely occurs provided that the recommended doses are not exceeded; in the elderly it is difficult to distinguish drug-induced retinopathy from changes of ageing.

Mepacrine hydrochloride p. 573 is sometimes used in discoid lupus erythematosus [unlicensed].

Drugs affecting the immune response

Methotrexate is a DMARD used in active rheumatoid arthritis. Methotrexate is usually given by mouth once a week, adjusted according to response. In patients who experience mucosal or gastro-intestinal side-effects with methotrexate, folic acid p. 1161 given every week [unlicensed], on a different day from the methotrexate, may help to reduce the frequency of such side-effects.

Leflunomide p. 1254 acts on the immune system as a DMARD. Its therapeutic effect starts after 4–6 weeks and improvement may continue for a further 4–6 months.

Drugs that affect the immune response are also used in the management of severe cases of *systemic lupus erythematosus* and other connective tissue disorders. They are often given in conjunction with corticosteroids for patients with severe or progressive renal disease. They may be used in cases of *polymyositis* that are resistant to corticosteroids. They are used for their corticosteroid-sparing effect in patients whose corticosteroid requirements are excessive. Azathioprine p. 965 is usually used.

In the specialist management of psoriatic arthritis affecting peripheral joints, leflunomide, methotrexate, or azathioprine [unlicensed] may be used.

Cytokine modulators

Cytokine modulators should be used under specialist supervision.

Adalimumab p. 1269, certolizumab pegol p. 1271, etanercept p. 1273, golimumab p. 1274, and infliximab p. 1275 inhibit the activity of tumour necrosis factor alpha (TNF-α).

Adalimumab is licensed for moderate to severe active *rheumatoid arthritis* when response to other DMARDs (including methotrexate) has been inadequate; it is also licensed for severe, active, and progressive disease in adults not previously treated with methotrexate. In the treatment of rheumatoid arthritis, adalimumab should be used in combination with methotrexate, but it can be given alone if methotrexate is inappropriate. Adalimumab is also licensed for the treatment of active and progressive *psoriatic arthritis* and severe active *ankylosing spondylitis* that have not responded adequately to other DMARDs. It is also licensed for the treatment of severe axial spondyloarthritis without radiographic evidence of ankylosing spondylitis but with objective signs of inflammation, in patients who have had an inadequate response to, or are intolerant of NSAIDs. Adalimumab also has a role in inflammatory bowel disease and plaque psoriasis.

Certolizumab pegol is licensed for use in patients with moderate to severe active *rheumatoid arthritis* when response to DMARDs (including methotrexate) has been inadequate. Certolizumab pegol can be used in combination with methotrexate, or as a monotherapy if methotrexate is not tolerated or is contra-indicated. Certolizumab pegol is also licensed for the treatment of severe active *ankylosing spondylitis* in patients who have had an inadequate response to, or are intolerant of NSAIDs. It is also licensed for the treatment of severe active *axial spondyloarthritis*, without radiographic evidence of ankylosing spondylitis but with objective signs of inflammation, in patients who have had an inadequate response to, or are intolerant of NSAIDs.

Etanercept is licensed for the treatment of moderate to severe active *rheumatoid arthritis* either alone or in combination with methotrexate when the response to other DMARDs is inadequate and in severe, active and progressive *rheumatoid arthritis* in patients not previously treated with methotrexate. It is also licensed for the treatment of active and progressive *psoriatic arthritis* inadequately responsive to other DMARDs, and for severe *ankylosing spondylitis* inadequately responsive to conventional therapy. Etanercept also has a role in plaque psoriasis.

Golimumab is licensed in combination with methotrexate for the treatment of moderate to severe active *rheumatoid arthritis* when response to DMARD therapy (including methotrexate) has been inadequate; it is also licensed in combination with methotrexate for patients with severe, active, and progressive rheumatoid arthritis not previously treated with methotrexate. Golimumab is also licensed for the treatment of active and progressive *psoriatic arthritis*, as monotherapy or in combination with methotrexate, when response to DMARD therapy has been inadequate; it is also licensed for the treatment of severe active *ankylosing spondylitis* when there is an inadequate response to conventional treatment.

Infliximab p. 1275 is licensed for the treatment of active *rheumatoid arthritis* in combination with methotrexate p. 1048 when the response to other DMARDs, including methotrexate, is inadequate; it is also licensed in combination with methotrexate for patients not previously treated with methotrexate or other DMARDs who have severe, active, and progressive rheumatoid arthritis. Infliximab is also licensed for the treatment of *ankylosing spondylitis*, in patients with severe axial symptoms who have not responded adequately to conventional therapy, and in combination with methotrexate (or alone if methotrexate is not tolerated or is contra-indicated) for the treatment of active and progressive *psoriatic arthritis* which has not responded adequately to DMARDs.

Rituximab p. 1019 is licensed in combination with methotrexate for the treatment of severe active *rheumatoid arthritis* in patients whose condition has not responded adequately to other DMARDs (including one or more tumour necrosis factor inhibitors) or who are intolerant of them. Rituximab has a role in malignant disease.

Abatacept p. 1269 prevents the full activation of T-lymphocytes. It is licensed for moderate to severe active *rheumatoid arthritis* in combination with methotrexate, in patients unresponsive to other DMARDs (including methotrexate or a tumour necrosis factor (TNF) inhibitor). Abatacept is not recommended for use in combination with TNF inhibitors.

Anakinra p. 1256 inhibits the activity of interleukin-1. Anakinra (in combination with methotrexate) is licensed for the treatment of *rheumatoid arthritis* which has not responded to methotrexate alone. Anakinra is not recommended for the treatment of rheumatoid arthritis except when used in a controlled long-term clinical study. Patients who are already receiving anakinra for rheumatoid arthritis should continue treatment until they and their specialist consider it appropriate to stop. Anakinra may also be appropriate for the treatment of systemic juvenile idiopathic arthritis and adult-onset Still's disease in certain individuals.

The Janus kinase inhibitors baricitinib p. 1262, filgotinib p. 1263, tofacitinib p. 1265, and upadacitinib p. 1267 are licensed for use as monotherapy or in combination with methotrexate for the treatment of moderate to severe active *rheumatoid arthritis* in patients who have had an inadequate response to, or who are intolerant to, one or more DMARDs.

Belimumab p. 976 inhibits the activity of B-lymphocyte stimulator. Belimumab is licensed as adjunctive therapy in patients with active, autoantibody-positive systemic lupus erythematosus with a high degree of disease activity despite standard therapy.

Sarilumab p. 1256 is a recombinant human monoclonal antibody that specifically binds to interleukin-6 receptors and blocks the activity of pro-inflammatory cytokines; it is licensed alone or in combination with methotrexate for the treatment of moderate to severe active rheumatoid arthritis in patients who have had an inadequate response to, or are intolerant to one or more DMARDs.

Secukinumab p. 1257 inhibits the activity of interleukin-17A. Secukinumab is licensed for the treatment of active *psoriatic arthritis*, in combination with methotrexate or alone, which has not responded adequately to DMARDs; it is also licensed for the treatment of *ankylosing spondylitis*, in patients who have not responded adequately to conventional therapy. Secukinumab also has a role in plaque psoriasis.

Tocilizumab p. 1258 antagonises the actions of interleukin-6. Tocilizumab is licensed for use in patients with moderate to severe active *rheumatoid arthritis* when response to at least one DMARD or tumour necrosis factor inhibitor has been inadequate, or in those who are intolerant of these drugs. Tocilizumab can be used in combination with methotrexate, or as monotherapy if methotrexate is not tolerated or is contra-indicated.

Ustekinumab p. 1260 inhibits the activity of interleukins 12 and 23. It is licensed for the treatment of active *psoriatic arthritis* (in combination with methotrexate or alone) in patients who have had an inadequate response to one or more DMARDs.

Juvenile idiopathic arthritis

Some children with *juvenile idiopathic arthritis* (juvenile chronic arthritis) do not require DMARDs. Methotrexate is effective; sulfasalazine [unlicensed] is an alternative but it should be avoided in *systemic-onset juvenile idiopathic arthritis*. Gold and penicillamine are no longer used. Cytokine modulators have a role in some forms of *juvenile idiopathic arthritis*.

Other drugs used for Arthritis Aceclofenac, p. 1294 · Bimekizumab, p. 1422 · Celecoxib, p. 1295 · Cyclophosphamide, p. 1032 · Diclofenac potassium, p. 1296 · Diclofenac sodium, p. 1297 · Etodolac, p. 1299 · Etoricoxib, p. 1300 · Flurbiprofen, p. 1301 · Guselkumab, p. 1425 · Ibuprofen, p. 1302 · Indometacin, p. 1305 · Ixekizumab, p. 1426 · Ketoprofen, p. 1306 · Mefenamic acid, p. 1308 · Meloxicam, p. 1309 · Nabumetone, p. 1309 · Naproxen, p. 1310 · Piroxicam, p. 1312 · Risankizumab, p. 1427 · Sulindac, p. 1313 · Tenoxicam, p. 1313 · Tiaprofenic acid, p. 1314

CHONDROPROTECTIVE DRUGS

Glucosamine
24-Nov-2020

- **DRUG ACTION** Glucosamine is a natural substance found in mucopolysaccharides, mucoproteins, and chitin.

- **INDICATIONS AND DOSE**

ALATERIS ®

Symptomatic relief of mild to moderate osteoarthritis of the knee
- ▸ BY MOUTH
- ▸ Adult: 1250 mg once daily, review treatment if no benefit after 2–3 months

DOLENIO ®

Symptomatic relief of mild to moderate osteoarthritis of the knee
- ▸ BY MOUTH
- ▸ Adult: 1500 mg once daily, review treatment if no benefit after 2–3 months

- **CAUTIONS** Asthma · impaired glucose tolerance · predisposition to cardiovascular disease

- **INTERACTIONS** → Appendix 1: glucosamine

- **SIDE-EFFECTS**
- ▸ **Common or very common** Constipation · diarrhoea · fatigue · gastrointestinal discomfort · headache · nausea
- ▸ **Uncommon** Flushing · skin reactions
- ▸ **Rare or very rare** Jaundice
- ▸ **Frequency not known** Angioedema · asthma · diabetes mellitus · dizziness · hypercholesterolaemia · oedema · vomiting

- **ALLERGY AND CROSS-SENSITIVITY** [EvGr] Contra-indicated if patient has a shellfish allergy. Ⓜ

- **PREGNANCY** Manufacturers advise avoid—no information available.

- **BREAST FEEDING** Manufacturers advise avoid—no information available.

- **MONITORING REQUIREMENTS**
- ▸ Monitor blood-glucose concentration before treatment and periodically thereafter in patients with impaired glucose tolerance.
- ▸ Monitor cholesterol in patients with predisposition to cardiovascular disease.

- **NATIONAL FUNDING/ACCESS DECISIONS**
  For full details see funding body website

  Scottish Medicines Consortium (SMC) decisions
- ▸ **Glucosamine (**_Alateris_ ®**) for relief of symptoms in mild to moderate osteoarthritis of the knee (June 2008)**
  SMC No. 471/08 Not recommended

- **LESS SUITABLE FOR PRESCRIBING** Less suitable for prescribing—the mechanism of action is not understood and there is limited evidence to show it is effective.

- **MEDICINAL FORMS** No licensed medicines listed.

DISEASE-MODIFYING ANTI-RHEUMATIC DRUGS

Hydroxychloroquine sulfate
16-Apr-2025

- **INDICATIONS AND DOSE**

Active rheumatoid arthritis (administered on expert advice) | Systemic and discoid lupus erythematosus (administered on expert advice) | Dermatological conditions caused or aggravated by sunlight (administered on expert advice)
- ▸ BY MOUTH
- ▸ Adult: 200–400 mg daily, daily maximum dose to be based on ideal body-weight; maximum 6.5 mg/kg per day

> **IMPORTANT SAFETY INFORMATION**
>
> MHRA/CHM ADVICE: HYDROXYCHLOROQUINE, CHLOROQUINE: INCREASED RISK OF CARDIOVASCULAR EVENTS WHEN USED WITH MACROLIDE ANTIBIOTICS; REMINDER OF PSYCHIATRIC REACTIONS (FEBRUARY 2022)
> An observational study has shown that co-administration of azithromycin with hydroxychloroquine in patients with rheumatoid arthritis was associated with an increased risk of cardiovascular events (including angina or chest pain and heart failure) and mortality. Healthcare professionals are reminded to consider the benefits and risks of co-prescribing systemic azithromycin, or other systemic macrolides, with hydroxychloroquine. If such use cannot be avoided, caution is recommended in patients with risk factors for cardiac events and they should be advised to seek urgent medical attention if any signs or symptoms develop.
>
> A European safety review has reported that psychiatric reactions associated with hydroxychloroquine (including rare cases of suicidal behaviour) typically occurred within the first month of treatment; events have been reported in patients with no history of psychiatric disorders. Healthcare professionals are reminded to be vigilant for psychiatric reactions, and counsel patients and carers to seek medical advice if any new or worsening mental health symptoms develop.

- **CAUTIONS** Acute porphyrias p. 1202 · diabetes (may lower blood glucose) · G6PD deficiency · maculopathy · may aggravate myasthenia gravis · may exacerbate psoriasis · neurological disorders (especially in those with a history of epilepsy—may lower seizure threshold) · severe gastro-intestinal disorders

- **INTERACTIONS** → Appendix 1: hydroxychloroquine

- **SIDE-EFFECTS**
- ▸ **Common or very common** Abdominal pain · appetite decreased · diarrhoea · headache · mood altered · nausea · skin reactions · vision disorders · vomiting
- ▸ **Uncommon** Alopecia · anxiety · corneal oedema · dizziness · eye disorders · hair colour changes · neuromuscular dysfunction · retinopathy · seizure · tinnitus · vertigo
- ▸ **Frequency not known** Acute hepatic failure · agranulocytosis · anaemia · angioedema · bone marrow disorders · bronchospasm · cardiac conduction disorders · cardiomyopathy · confusion · delusions · depression · hallucination · hearing loss · hypoglycaemia · leucopenia · movement disorders · muscle weakness · myopathy · photosensitivity reaction · psychiatric disorder · psychosis · QT interval prolongation · reflexes absent · severe cutaneous adverse reactions (SCARs) · sleep disorder · suicidal behaviour · thrombocytopenia · tremor · ventricular hypertrophy

Overdose Hydroxychloroquine is very toxic in overdosage; overdosage is extremely hazardous and difficult to treat. Urgent advice from the National Poisons Information

10

Musculoskeletal system

Service is essential. Life-threatening features include arrhythmias (which can have a very rapid onset) and convulsions (which can be intractable).

● PREGNANCY [EvGr] Hydroxychloroquine is the antimalarial drug of choice in females with rheumatic disease planning a pregnancy, and may be continued during pregnancy. ⟨A⟩

● BREAST FEEDING [EvGr] May be used during breast-feeding. ⟨A⟩[EvGr] Present in milk in very small amounts—very long plasma half-life increases risk of accumulation in the infant, however no adverse effects reported with longer term use. Although adverse effects are unlikely, monitor infant for irritability, insomnia, skin reactions, vomiting, diarrhoea, poor feeding, and adequate weight gain. Avoid in infants with G6PD deficiency, hyperbilirubinaemia, or jaundice (risk of haemolytic anaemia and kernicterus). ⟨E⟩

● HEPATIC IMPAIRMENT Manufacturer advises caution. **Dose adjustments** Manufacturer advises consider dose adjustment in severe impairment.

● RENAL IMPAIRMENT [EvGr] Caution—monitor plasma-hydroxychloroquine concentration in severe impairment. ⟨M⟩
Dose adjustments [EvGr] Consider dose adjustment in severe impairment. ⟨M⟩

● MONITORING REQUIREMENTS
▶ A review group convened by the Royal College of Ophthalmologists has updated guidelines on monitoring for chloroquine and hydroxychloroquine retinopathy (*Hydroxychloroquine and Chloroquine Retinopathy: Recommendations on Monitoring* 2020). Recent data has highlighted that hydroxychloroquine retinopathy is more common than previously reported. Annual monitoring (including fundus autofluorescence and spectral domain optical coherence tomography) is recommended in all patients who have taken hydroxychloroquine for longer than 5 years.
▶ Annual monitoring may be started before 5 years of treatment if additional risk factors for retinotoxicity exist, such as concomitant tamoxifen therapy, impaired renal function (eGFR less than 60 mL/minute/1.73 m^2), or high-dose therapy (more than 5 mg/kg/day of hydroxychloroquine sulfate).

● PRESCRIBING AND DISPENSING INFORMATION To avoid excessive dosage in obese patients, the dose of hydroxychloroquine should be calculated on the basis of ideal body-weight.

● MEDICINAL FORMS There can be variation in the licensing of different medicines containing the same drug. Forms available from special-order manufacturers include: oral suspension, oral solution

Oral tablet
CAUTIONARY AND ADVISORY LABELS 21
▶ Hydroxychloroquine sulfate (Non-proprietary)
  Hydroxychloroquine sulfate 200 mg Hydroxychloroquine 200mg tablets | 60 tablet [PoM] £8.64 DT = £2.73
  Hydroxychloroquine sulfate 300 mg Hydroxychloroquine 300mg tablets | 30 tablet [PoM] £14.95 DT = £14.95
▶ Quinoric (Bristol Laboratories Ltd)
  Hydroxychloroquine sulfate 200 mg Quinoric 200mg tablets | 60 tablet [PoM] [℥] DT = £2.73

Leflunomide

19-May-2021

● INDICATIONS AND DOSE
Moderate to severe active rheumatoid arthritis (specialist use only)
▶ BY MOUTH
▶ Adult: Initially 100 mg once daily for 3 days, then reduced to 10–20 mg once daily

Active psoriatic arthritis (specialist use only)
▶ BY MOUTH
▶ Adult: Initially 100 mg once daily for 3 days, then reduced to 20 mg once daily

● CONTRA-INDICATIONS Serious infection · severe hypoproteinaemia · severe immunodeficiency

● CAUTIONS Anaemia (avoid if significant and due to causes other than rheumatoid or psoriatic arthritis) · history of tuberculosis · impaired bone-marrow function (avoid if significant and due to causes other than rheumatoid or psoriatic arthritis) · leucopenia (avoid if significant and due to causes other than rheumatoid or psoriatic arthritis) · thrombocytopenia (avoid if significant and due to causes other than rheumatoid or psoriatic arthritis)

● INTERACTIONS → Appendix 1: leflunomide

● SIDE-EFFECTS
▶ **Common or very common** Abdominal pain · accelerated hair loss · appetite decreased · asthenia · diarrhoea · dizziness · gastrointestinal disorders · headache · hypersensitivity · hypertension · leucopenia · nausea · oral disorder · paraesthesia · peripheral neuropathy · skin reactions · tendon disorders · vomiting · weight decreased
▶ **Uncommon** Anaemia · anxiety · electrolyte imbalance · hyperlipidaemia · taste altered · thrombocytopenia
▶ **Rare or very rare** Agranulocytosis · eosinophilia · hepatic disorders · infection · interstitial lung disease · pancreatitis · pancytopenia · sepsis · severe cutaneous adverse reactions (SCARs) · vasculitis
▶ **Frequency not known** Cutaneous lupus erythematosus · hypouricaemia · progressive multifocal leukoencephalopathy (PML) · pulmonary hypertension · renal failure · skin ulcer

SIDE-EFFECTS, FURTHER INFORMATION Discontinue treatment and institute washout procedure in case of serious side-effect (consult product literature).
  Hepatotoxicity Potentially life-threatening hepatotoxicity reported usually in the first 6 months. Discontinue treatment (and institute washout procedure—consult product literature) or reduce dose according to liver-function abnormality; if liver-function abnormality persists after dose reduction, discontinue treatment and institute washout procedure.

● CONCEPTION AND CONTRACEPTION Effective contraception **essential** during treatment and for at least 2 years after treatment in women and at least 3 months after treatment in men (plasma concentration monitoring required; waiting time before conception may be reduced with washout procedure—consult product literature). The concentration of the active metabolite after washout should be less than 20 micrograms/litre (measured on 2 occasions 14 days apart) in men or women before conception—consult product literature.

● PREGNANCY Avoid—active metabolite teratogenic in *animal* studies.

● BREAST FEEDING Present in milk in *animal* studies—manufacturer advises avoid.

● HEPATIC IMPAIRMENT Manufacturer advises avoid—active metabolite may accumulate.

● RENAL IMPAIRMENT Manufacturer advises avoid in moderate or severe impairment—no information available.

● PRE-TREATMENT SCREENING Exclude pregnancy before treatment.

● MONITORING REQUIREMENTS
▶ Monitor full blood count (including differential white cell count and platelet count) before treatment and every 2 weeks for 6 months then every 8 weeks.
▶ Monitor liver function before treatment and every 2 weeks for first 6 months then every 8 weeks.
▶ Monitor blood pressure.

● **TREATMENT CESSATION**
Washout Procedure The active metabolite persists for a long period; to aid drug elimination in case of serious adverse effect, or before starting another disease-modifying antirheumatic drug, or before conception, stop treatment and give *either* colestyramine p. 229 *or* charcoal, activated p. 1561. Procedure may be repeated as necessary.

● **MEDICINAL FORMS** There can be variation in the licensing of different medicines containing the same drug.

Oral tablet
CAUTIONARY AND ADVISORY LABELS 4
▸ **Leflunomide (Non-proprietary)**
Leflunomide 10 mg Leflunomide 10mg tablets | 30 tablet [PoM] £46.02 DT = £1.91
Leflunomide 15 mg Leflunomide 15mg tablets | 30 tablet [PoM] £46.00 DT = £46.00
Leflunomide 20 mg Leflunomide 20mg tablets | 30 tablet [PoM] £55.22 DT = £2.38
▸ **Arava** (Sanofi)
Leflunomide 10 mg Arava 10mg tablets | 30 tablet [PoM] £51.13 DT = £1.91
Leflunomide 20 mg Arava 20mg tablets | 30 tablet [PoM] £61.36 DT = £2.38

Penicillamine　　　　　　　　　　19-May-2021

● **DRUG ACTION** Penicillamine aids the elimination of copper ions in Wilson's disease (hepatolenticular degeneration).

● **INDICATIONS AND DOSE**

Severe active rheumatoid arthritis (administered on expert advice)
▸ BY MOUTH
▸ Adult: Initially 125–250 mg daily for 1 month, then increased in steps of 125–250 mg, at intervals of not less than 4 weeks; maintenance 500–750 mg daily in divided doses, then reduced in steps of 125–250 mg every 12 weeks, dose reduction attempted only if remission sustained for 6 months; maximum 1.5 g per day
▸ Elderly: Initially up to 125 mg daily for 1 month, then increased in steps of up to 125 mg, at intervals of at least 4 weeks; maximum 1 g per day

Wilson's disease
▸ BY MOUTH
▸ Adult: 1.5–2 g daily in divided doses, adjusted according to response, to be taken before food; maintenance 0.75–1 g daily, a dose of 2 g daily should not be continued for more than one year; maximum 2 g per day
▸ Elderly: 20 mg/kg daily in divided doses, adjusted according to response

Autoimmune hepatitis (used rarely; after disease controlled with corticosteroids)
▸ BY MOUTH
▸ Adult: Initially 500 mg daily in divided doses, to be increased slowly over 3 months; maintenance 1.25 g daily

Cystinuria, therapeutic
▸ BY MOUTH
▸ Adult: 1–3 g daily in divided doses, to be adjusted to maintain urinary cystine below 200 mg/litre, to be taken before food

Cystinuria, prophylactic
▸ BY MOUTH
▸ Adult: 0.5–1 g daily, maintain urinary cystine below 300 mg/litre and adequate fluid intake (at least 3 litres daily), to be taken at bedtime
▸ Elderly: Minimum dose to maintain urinary cystine below 200 mg/litre is recommended

● **CONTRA-INDICATIONS** Lupus erythematosus

● **CAUTIONS** Neurological involvement in Wilson's disease

● **INTERACTIONS** → Appendix 1: penicillamine

● **SIDE-EFFECTS**
▸ **Common or very common** Proteinuria · thrombocytopenia
▸ **Rare or very rare** Alopecia · breast enlargement (males and females) · connective tissue disorders · haematuria (discontinue immediately if cause unknown) · hypersensitivity · oral disorders · skin reactions
▸ **Frequency not known** Agranulocytosis · aplastic anaemia · appetite decreased · fever · glomerulonephritis · Goodpasture's syndrome · haemolytic anaemia · increased risk of infection · jaundice cholestatic · leucopenia · lupus-like syndrome · myasthenia gravis · nausea · nephrotic syndrome · neurological deterioration in Wilson's Disease · neutropenia · pancreatitis · pneumonitis · polymyositis · pulmonary haemorrhage · rash (consider dose reduction) · respiratory tract inflammation · Stevens-Johnson syndrome · taste loss (mineral supplements not recommended) · vomiting · yellow nail syndrome

SIDE-EFFECTS, FURTHER INFORMATION Proteinuria occurs in up to 30% of patients—can be a sign of immune-mediated nephropathy. Discontinue immediately if nephrotoxicity occurs.
　Nausea and rash more common early in treatment if full dose used from initiation. Delayed rash can occur after months or years of treatment—manufacturer advises reduce dose.

● **ALLERGY AND CROSS-SENSITIVITY** Patients who are hypersensitive to penicillin may react rarely to penicillamine.

● **PREGNANCY** Fetal abnormalities reported rarely; avoid if possible.

● **BREAST FEEDING** Manufacturer advises avoid unless potential benefit outweighs risk—no information available.

● **RENAL IMPAIRMENT** [EvGr] Caution in mild impairment; avoid in moderate to severe impairment. ⓜ
Dose adjustments [EvGr] Dose reduction may be required in mild impairment depending on indication (consult product literature). ⓜ

● **MONITORING REQUIREMENTS**
▸ Consider withdrawal if platelet count falls below 120 000/mm^3 or white blood cells below 2500/mm^3 or if 3 successive falls within reference range (can restart at reduced dose when counts return to within reference range but permanent withdrawal necessary if recurrence of leucopenia or thrombocytopenia).
▸ Blood counts, including platelets, and urine examinations should be carried out before starting treatment and then every 1 or 2 weeks for the first 2 months then every 4 weeks to detect blood disorders and proteinuria (they should also be carried out in the week after any dose increase).
▸ A reduction in platelet count calls for discontinuation with subsequent re-introduction at a lower dosage and then, if possible, gradual increase.
▸ Longer intervals may be adequate in cystinuria and Wilson's disease.

● **PATIENT AND CARER ADVICE** Counselling on the symptoms of blood disorders is advised. Warn patient and carers to tell doctor immediately if sore throat, fever, infection, non-specific illness, unexplained bleeding and bruising, purpura, mouth ulcers, or rashes develop.

- **MEDICINAL FORMS** There can be variation in the licensing of different medicines containing the same drug. Forms available from special-order manufacturers include: oral solution

Oral tablet

CAUTIONARY AND ADVISORY LABELS 6, 22

▸ Penicillamine (Non-proprietary)
Penicillamine 125 mg Penicillamine 125mg tablets | 56 tablet [PoM] £111.60 DT = £93.11
Penicillamine 250 mg Penicillamine 250mg tablets | 56 tablet [PoM] £180.00 DT = £140.00

IMMUNOSUPPRESSANTS ⟩ INTERLEUKIN INHIBITORS

Anakinra
04-May-2021

- **INDICATIONS AND DOSE**

Rheumatoid arthritis (in combination with methotrexate) which has not responded to methotrexate alone (specialist use only)

▸ BY SUBCUTANEOUS INJECTION
▸ Adult: 100 mg once daily

Cryopyrin-associated periodic syndromes (specialist use only)

▸ BY SUBCUTANEOUS INJECTION
▸ Adult: 1–2 mg/kg daily, for severe cryopyrin-associated periodic syndromes, usual maintenance is 3–4 mg/kg daily, up to a maximum of 8 mg/kg daily

Still's disease (specialist use only)

▸ BY SUBCUTANEOUS INJECTION
▸ Adult (body-weight up to 49 kg): 1–2 mg/kg daily
▸ Adult (body-weight 50 kg and above): 100 mg daily

- **CONTRA-INDICATIONS** Active infection · neutropenia (absolute neutrophil count less than 1.5×10^9/litre)—do not initiate · pre-existing malignancy

- **CAUTIONS** Elderly · history of asthma (increased risk of serious infection) · history of recurrent infection · predisposition to infection

- **INTERACTIONS** → Appendix 1: anakinra

- **SIDE-EFFECTS**

▸ **Common or very common** Headache · infection · neutropenia · thrombocytopenia
▸ **Uncommon** Skin reactions
▸ **Frequency not known** Hepatitis

SIDE-EFFECTS, FURTHER INFORMATION Neutropenia reported commonly—discontinue if neutropenia develops.

- **PREGNANCY** Manufacturer advises avoid.

- **BREAST FEEDING** Manufacturer advises avoid—no information available.

- **HEPATIC IMPAIRMENT** Manufacturer advises caution in severe impairment.

- **RENAL IMPAIRMENT** Manufacturer advises caution in moderate impairment.
Dose adjustments Manufacturer advises consider alternate day dosing in severe impairment.

- **PRE-TREATMENT SCREENING** Manufacturer advises patients should be screened for latent tuberculosis and viral hepatitis prior to initiation of treatment.

- **MONITORING REQUIREMENTS**

▸ Manufacturer advises monitor neutrophil count before treatment, then every month for 6 months, then every 3 months thereafter.
▸ When used for Cryopyrin-associated periodic syndromes Manufacturer advises monitor for CNS inflammation (including ear and eye tests) 3 months after starting treatment, then every 6 months until effective treatment doses have been identified, then yearly thereafter.

▸ When used for Still's disease Manufacturer advises consider routine monitoring of hepatic enzymes during the first month of treatment.

- **PRESCRIBING AND DISPENSING INFORMATION**

▸ When used for Cryopyrin-associated periodic syndromes or Still's disease The manufacturer of *Kineret*® has provided a *Guide for Healthcare Professionals*.

- **PATIENT AND CARER ADVICE**

Blood disorders Patients should be instructed to seek medical advice if symptoms suggestive of neutropenia (such as fever, sore throat, bruising or, bleeding) develop.

▸ When used for Still's disease A patient card and patient booklet should be provided.
▸ When used for Cryopyrin-associated periodic syndromes A patient booklet should be provided.

- **NATIONAL FUNDING/ACCESS DECISIONS**

For full details see funding body website

NICE decisions

▸ Anakinra for treating Still's disease (March 2021) NICE TA685 Recommended with restrictions

Scottish Medicines Consortium (SMC) decisions

▸ Anakinra (*Kineret*®) for rheumatoid arthritis (November 2002) SMC No. 05/02 Not recommended
▸ Anakinra (*Kineret*®) for the treatment of Still's disease, as monotherapy or in combination with other anti-inflammatory drugs and disease-modifying antirheumatic drugs (October 2018) SMC No. SMC2104 Recommended

- **MEDICINAL FORMS** There can be variation in the licensing of different medicines containing the same drug.

Solution for injection

▸ Kineret (Swedish Orphan Biovitrum Ltd)
Anakinra 150 mg per 1 ml Kineret 100mg/0.67ml solution for injection pre-filled syringes | 7 pre-filled disposable injection [PoM] £183.61 DT = £183.61

Sarilumab
11-Nov-2020

- **DRUG ACTION** Sarilumab is a recombinant human monoclonal antibody that specifically binds to interleukin-6 receptors and blocks the activity of pro-inflammatory cytokines.

- **INDICATIONS AND DOSE**

Moderate-to-severe active rheumatoid arthritis in patients who have had an inadequate response to, or are intolerant to one or more disease-modifying anti-rheumatic drugs (as monotherapy or in combination with methotrexate) (specialist use only)

▸ BY SUBCUTANEOUS INJECTION
▸ Adult: 200 mg every 2 weeks, for dose adjustments due to neutropenia, thrombocytopenia, or liver enzyme elevations—consult product literature

- **CONTRA-INDICATIONS** Do not initiate if absolute neutrophil count less than 2×10^9/litre · do not initiate if platelet count less than 150×10^3/microlitre · do not initiate if serum transaminases (ALT or AST) greater than 1.5 times the upper limit of normal · severe active infection

- **CAUTIONS** Chronic or recurrent infection · elderly (increased risk of infection) · history of diverticulitis · history of intestinal ulceration · history of serious or opportunistic infection · predisposition to infection

CAUTIONS, FURTHER INFORMATION

▸ Infection Manufacturer advises caution in patients who have been exposed to tuberculosis, or who have lived in or travelled to areas of endemic tuberculosis or mycoses. Patients with latent tuberculosis should complete anti-tuberculosis therapy before initiation of sarilumab; consider anti-tuberculosis therapy before initiation of sarilumab in patients with a past history of latent or active tuberculosis in whom an adequate course of treatment cannot be confirmed, and for those with a negative test for latent tuberculosis but have risk factors for tuberculosis—consultation with a tuberculosis specialist may be appropriate.

Manufacturer advises patients should be brought up-to-date with current immunisation schedule before initiating treatment.

- **INTERACTIONS** → Appendix 1: monoclonal antibodies
- **SIDE-EFFECTS**
  - ▸ **Common or very common** Dyslipidaemia · increased risk of infection · leucopenia · neutropenia · thrombocytopenia
  - ▸ **Rare or very rare** Gastrointestinal perforation
  - ▸ **Frequency not known** Hypersensitivity (discontinue) · skin reactions
- **CONCEPTION AND CONTRACEPTION** Manufacturer advises effective contraception in women of childbearing potential during treatment and for up to 3 months after treatment.
- **PREGNANCY** Manufacturer advises avoid unless essential—limited information available.
- **BREAST FEEDING** Manufacturer advises avoid—no information available.
- **HEPATIC IMPAIRMENT** Manufacturer advises avoid (no information available).
- **PRE-TREATMENT SCREENING** Manufacturer advises that patients should be evaluated for tuberculosis before treatment.
- **MONITORING REQUIREMENTS**
  - ▸ Manufacturer advises monitor for signs and symptoms of infection; monitor neutrophil count 4 to 8 weeks after treatment initiation and according to clinical judgement thereafter—discontinue if absolute neutrophil count less than 0.5×10^9/litre.
  - ▸ Manufacturer advises monitor platelet count 4 to 8 weeks after treatment initiation and according to clinical judgement thereafter—discontinue if platelet count less than 50×10^3/microlitre.
  - ▸ Manufacturer advises monitor hepatic transaminases (ALT and AST) 4 to 8 weeks after treatment initiation and every 3 months thereafter, and consider other liver function tests if clinically indicated—discontinue if ALT is greater than 5 times the upper limit of normal.
  - ▸ Manufacturer advises monitor lipid profile approximately 4 to 8 weeks after treatment initiation and approximately every 6 months thereafter—hyperlipidaemia should be managed according to clinical guidelines.
- **DIRECTIONS FOR ADMINISTRATION** Manufacturer advises to avoid injecting into areas of the skin that are tender, damaged, or have bruises or scars; patients may self-administer *Kevzara*®, after appropriate training in subcutaneous injection technique.
- **PRESCRIBING AND DISPENSING INFORMATION** Sarilumab is a biological medicine. Biological medicines must be prescribed and dispensed by brand name, see *Biological medicines* and *Biosimilar medicines*, under Guidance on prescribing p. 1; manufacturer advises to record the brand name and batch number after each administration.
- **HANDLING AND STORAGE** Manufacturer advises store in a refrigerator (2–8°C) and protect from light—consult product literature for further information regarding storage outside refrigerator.
- **PATIENT AND CARER ADVICE** Manufacturer advises patients should be advised to seek immediate medical attention if symptoms of a hypersensitivity reaction occur. Self-administration Manufacturer advises patients and their carers should be given training in subcutaneous injection technique if appropriate.
  Alert card An alert card should be provided.

Missed doses Manufacturer advises if a dose is more than 3 days late, the missed dose should not be taken and the next dose should be taken at the normal time.

- **NATIONAL FUNDING/ACCESS DECISIONS** For full details see funding body website
  NICE decisions
  - ▸ Sarilumab for moderate-to-severe rheumatoid arthritis (November 2017) NICE TA485 Recommended with restrictions
  Scottish Medicines Consortium (SMC) decisions
  - ▸ Sarilumab (*Kevzara*®) in combination with methotrexate, or as monotherapy for the treatment of moderately to severely active rheumatoid arthritis in adult patients who have responded inadequately to, or who are intolerant to one or more disease modifying anti rheumatic drugs (April 2018) SMC No. 1314/18 Recommended with restrictions

- **MEDICINAL FORMS** There can be variation in the licensing of different medicines containing the same drug.
  Solution for injection
  CAUTIONARY AND ADVISORY LABELS 10
  - ▸ **Kevzara** (Sanofi)
    Sarilumab 131.6 mg per 1 ml Kevzara 150mg/1.14ml solution for injection pre-filled pens | 2 pre-filled disposable injection PoM £912.25
    Sarilumab 175 mg per 1 ml Kevzara 200mg/1.14ml solution for injection pre-filled syringes | 2 pre-filled disposable injection PoM £912.25
    Kevzara 200mg/1.14ml solution for injection pre-filled pens | 2 pre-filled disposable injection PoM £912.25

Secukinumab
05-Mar-2024

- **DRUG ACTION** Secukinumab is a recombinant human monoclonal antibody that selectively binds to cytokine interleukin-17A (IL-17A) and inhibits the release of proinflammatory cytokines and chemokines.

- **INDICATIONS AND DOSE**
  Ankylosing spondylitis (under expert supervision)
  - ▸ BY SUBCUTANEOUS INJECTION
  - ▸ Adult: 150 mg every week for 5 doses, then maintenance 150 mg every month, dose may be increased to 300 mg according to clinical response. Review treatment if no response within 16 weeks of initial dose

  Non-radiographic axial spondyloarthritis (under expert supervision)
  - ▸ BY SUBCUTANEOUS INJECTION
  - ▸ Adult: 150 mg every week for 5 doses, then maintenance 150 mg every month, review treatment if no response within 16 weeks of initial dose

  Psoriatic arthritis (under expert supervision)
  - ▸ BY SUBCUTANEOUS INJECTION
  - ▸ Adult: 150 mg every week for 5 doses, then maintenance 150 mg every month, dose may be increased to 300 mg according to clinical response. Review treatment if no response within 16 weeks of initial dose

  Psoriatic arthritis [with concomitant moderate to severe plaque psoriasis] (under expert supervision)
  - ▸ BY SUBCUTANEOUS INJECTION
  - ▸ Adult (body-weight up to 90 kg): 300 mg every week for 5 doses, then maintenance 300 mg every month, review treatment if no response within 16 weeks of initial dose
  - ▸ Adult (body-weight 90 kg and above): 300 mg every week for 5 doses, then maintenance 300 mg every month, review treatment if no response within 16 weeks of initial dose; increased if necessary to 300 mg every 2 weeks, review treatment if no response within 16 weeks of initial dose continued →

10

Musculoskeletal system

Psoriatic arthritis [if inadequate response to anti-TNFα treatment] (under expert supervision)
▶ BY SUBCUTANEOUS INJECTION
▶ Adult: 300 mg every week for 5 doses, then maintenance 300 mg every month, review treatment if no response within 16 weeks of initial dose

Plaque psoriasis (under expert supervision)
▶ BY SUBCUTANEOUS INJECTION
▶ Adult (body-weight up to 90 kg): 300 mg every week for 5 doses, then maintenance 300 mg every month, review treatment if no response within 16 weeks of initial dose
▶ Adult (body-weight 90 kg and above): 300 mg every week for 5 doses, then maintenance 300 mg every month, review treatment if no response within 16 weeks of initial dose; increased if necessary to 300 mg every 2 weeks, review treatment if no response within 16 weeks of initial dose

Hidradenitis suppurativa (under expert supervision)
▶ BY SUBCUTANEOUS INJECTION
▶ Adult: 300 mg every week for 5 doses, then maintenance 300 mg every month, review treatment if no response within 16 weeks of initial dose; increased if necessary to 300 mg every 2 weeks, review treatment if no response within 16 weeks of initial dose

● **CONTRA-INDICATIONS** Severe active infection
● **CAUTIONS** Chronic infection · history of recurrent infection · inflammatory bowel disease (discontinue if signs or symptoms develop, or an exacerbation occurs) · predisposition to infection (discontinue if new serious infection develops)
  CAUTIONS, FURTHER INFORMATION
  ▶ Tuberculosis [EvGr] Anti-tuberculosis therapy should be considered before starting secukinumab in patients with latent tuberculosis. Ⓜ
● **INTERACTIONS** → Appendix 1: monoclonal antibodies
● **SIDE-EFFECTS**
  ▶ **Common or very common** Diarrhoea · fatigue · headache · increased risk of infection · nausea · rhinorrhoea
  ▶ **Uncommon** Conjunctivitis · inflammatory bowel disease · neutropenia (usually mild and reversible) · skin reactions
  ▶ **Rare or very rare** Anaphylactic reaction · hypersensitivity vasculitis
  ▶ **Frequency not known** Pyoderma gangrenosum
● **CONCEPTION AND CONTRACEPTION** Manufacturer advises that women of childbearing potential should use effective contraception during treatment and for at least 20 weeks after stopping treatment.
● **PREGNANCY** Manufacturer advises avoid—no information available.
● **BREAST FEEDING** Manufacturer advises avoid during treatment and for up to 20 weeks after discontinuing treatment—no information available.
● **DIRECTIONS FOR ADMINISTRATION** Take syringe or pen out of the refrigerator and allow to reach room temperature before administration—consult product literature. Avoid injecting into areas of the skin that show psoriasis. Patients may self-administer *Cosentyx*® after appropriate training in subcutaneous injection technique.
● **PRESCRIBING AND DISPENSING INFORMATION** Secukinumab is a biological medicine. Biological medicines must be prescribed and dispensed by brand name, see *Biological medicines* and *Biosimilar medicines*, under Guidance on prescribing p. 1; [EvGr] record the brand name and batch number after each administration. Ⓜ
● **HANDLING AND STORAGE** Store in a refrigerator (2–8°C) and protect from light. Once removed from refrigerator, may be stored at room temperature (below 30°C) for up to 4 days.

● **PATIENT AND CARER ADVICE**
  Self-administration Patients and their carers should be given training in subcutaneous injection technique.
  Infection Patients and their carers should be advised to seek immediate medical attention if symptoms of infection develop during treatment with secukinumab.
● **NATIONAL FUNDING/ACCESS DECISIONS**
  For full details see funding body website
  NICE decisions
  ▶ Secukinumab for treating moderate to severe plaque psoriasis (July 2015) NICE TA350 Recommended with restrictions
  ▶ Secukinumab for active ankylosing spondylitis after treatment with non-steroidal anti-inflammatory drugs or TNF-alpha inhibitors (September 2016) NICE TA407 Recommended with restrictions
  ▶ Secukinumab for treating non-radiographic axial spondyloarthritis (July 2021) NICE TA719 Recommended with restrictions
  ▶ Certolizumab pegol and secukinumab for treating active psoriatic arthritis after inadequate response to DMARDs (May 2017) NICE TA445 Recommended with restrictions
  ▶ Secukinumab for treating moderate to severe hidradenitis suppurativa (December 2023) NICE TA935 Recommended with restrictions
  Scottish Medicines Consortium (SMC) decisions
  ▶ Secukinumab (*Cosentyx*®) for treatment of moderate to severe plaque psoriasis in adults who are candidates for systemic therapy (June 2015) SMC No. 1054/15 Recommended with restrictions
  ▶ Secukinumab (*Cosentyx*®) for the treatment of active non-radiographic axial spondyloarthritis with objective signs of inflammation as indicated by elevated C-reactive protein and/or magnetic resonance imaging evidence in adults who have responded inadequately to non-steroidal anti-inflammatory drugs (January 2021) SMC No. SMC2308 Recommended
  ▶ Secukinumab (*Cosentyx*®) for the treatment of active moderate to severe hidradenitis suppurativa (HS) in adults with an inadequate response to conventional systemic HS therapy (February 2024) SMC No. SMC2592 Recommended with restrictions

● **MEDICINAL FORMS** There can be variation in the licensing of different medicines containing the same drug.
  Solution for injection
  EXCIPIENTS: May contain Polysorbates
  ▶ **Cosentyx** (Novartis Pharmaceuticals UK Ltd)
    Secukinumab 150 mg per 1 ml Cosentyx 150mg/1ml solution for injection pre-filled pens | 2 pre-filled disposable injection [PoM] £1,218.78 (Hospital only)
    Cosentyx 150mg/1ml solution for injection pre-filled syringes | 2 pre-filled disposable injection [PoM] £1,218.78 (Hospital only)
    Cosentyx 300mg/2ml solution for injection pre-filled pens | 1 pre-filled disposable injection [PoM] £1,218.78 (Hospital only)
    Cosentyx 75mg/0.5ml solution for injection pre-filled syringes | 1 pre-filled disposable injection [PoM] £304.70 (Hospital only)

Tocilizumab

27-Mar-2024

● **DRUG ACTION** Tocilizumab is a recombinant humanised monoclonal antibody that binds to interleukin-6 receptors thereby blocking the activity of pro-inflammatory cytokines.

● **INDICATIONS AND DOSE**

Rheumatoid arthritis (initiated by a specialist)
▶ BY INTRAVENOUS INFUSION
▶ Adult: 8 mg/kg every 4 weeks (max. per dose 800 mg), for dose adjustments in patients with liver enzyme abnormalities, or low absolute neutrophil or platelet count—consult product literature

▸ BY SUBCUTANEOUS INJECTION

▸ **Adult:** 162 mg once weekly, administer to abdomen, thigh or upper arm, for dose adjustments in patients with liver enzyme abnormalities, or low absolute neutrophil or platelet count—consult product literature

Giant cell arteritis (initiated by a specialist)

▸ BY SUBCUTANEOUS INJECTION

▸ **Adult:** 162 mg once weekly, administer to abdomen, thigh or upper arm, for dose adjustments in patients with liver enzyme abnormalities, or low absolute neutrophil or platelet count—consult product literature, not to be used alone for acute relapses; review need for treatment beyond 52 weeks

COVID-19 in hospitalised patients who are receiving systemic corticosteroids and require oxygen supplementation or mechanical ventilation (initiated by a specialist)

▸ BY INTRAVENOUS INFUSION

▸ **Adult:** 8 mg/kg (max. per dose 800 mg) for 1 dose

Cytokine release syndrome (initiated by a specialist)

▸ BY INTRAVENOUS INFUSION

▸ **Adult (body-weight up to 30 kg):** 12 mg/kg (max. per dose 800 mg), if no improvement in symptoms after the first dose, up to 3 additional doses may be administered. The interval between the infusions should be at least 8 hours

▸ **Adult (body-weight 30 kg and above):** 8 mg/kg (max. per dose 800 mg), if no improvement in symptoms after the first dose, up to 3 additional doses may be administered. The interval between the infusions should be at least 8 hours

---

IMPORTANT SAFETY INFORMATION

MHRA/CHM ADVICE: TOCILIZUMAB (*ROACTEMRA*®): RARE RISK OF SERIOUS LIVER INJURY INCLUDING CASES REQUIRING TRANSPLANTATION (JULY 2019)

There have been reports of rare but serious cases of drug-induced liver injury, including acute liver failure and hepatitis, in patients treated with tocilizumab; some cases required liver transplantation. Serious liver injury was reported from 2 weeks to more than 5 years after initiation of tocilizumab. Healthcare professionals are advised to initiate tocilizumab treatment with caution in patients with active hepatic disease or hepatic impairment. Patients and their carers should be advised to seek immediate medical attention if signs and symptoms of liver injury, such as tiredness, abdominal pain, and jaundice, occur. For further information see *Cautions*, *Contra-indications* and *Monitoring requirements*.

● **CONTRA-INDICATIONS**

GENERAL CONTRA-INDICATIONS Severe active infection (unless used for the treatment of COVID-19)

SPECIFIC CONTRA-INDICATIONS

▸ When used for COVID-19 Do not initiate if absolute neutrophil count less than 1×10^9/litre · do not initiate if hepatic enzymes more than 10 times the upper limit of normal · do not initiate if platelet count less than 50×10^3/microlitre

▸ When used for Giant cell arteritis Do not initiate if hepatic enzymes more than 5 times the upper limit of normal · do not initiate in patients not previously treated with *RoActemra*® if absolute neutrophil count less than 2×10^9/litre

▸ When used for Rheumatoid arthritis Do not initiate if hepatic enzymes more than 5 times the upper limit of normal · do not initiate in patients not previously treated with *RoActemra*® if absolute neutrophil count less than 2×10^9/litre

● **CAUTIONS**

▸ When used for COVID-19 History of recurrent or chronic infection (interrupt treatment if serious infection occurs) · predisposition to infection (interrupt treatment if serious infection occurs)

▸ When used for Giant cell arteritis Hepatic enzymes more than 1.5 times the upper limit of normal · history of diverticulitis · history of intestinal ulceration · history of recurrent or chronic infection (interrupt treatment if serious infection occurs) · low absolute neutrophil count (discontinue treatment if neutrophil count less than 0.5×10^9/litre) · platelet count less than 100×10^3/microlitre (discontinue treatment if platelet count less than 50×10^3/microlitre) · predisposition to infection (interrupt treatment if serious infection occurs)

▸ When used for Rheumatoid arthritis Hepatic enzymes more than 1.5 times the upper limit of normal · history of diverticulitis · history of intestinal ulceration · history of recurrent or chronic infection (interrupt treatment if serious infection occurs) · low absolute neutrophil count (discontinue treatment if neutrophil count less than 0.5×10^9/litre) · platelet count less than 100×10^3/microlitre (discontinue treatment if platelet count less than 50×10^3/microlitre) · predisposition to infection (interrupt treatment if serious infection occurs)

CAUTIONS, FURTHER INFORMATION

▸ Tuberculosis

▸ When used for Rheumatoid arthritis or Giant cell arteritis [EvGr] Patients with latent tuberculosis should be treated with standard therapy before starting tocilizumab. [M]

● **INTERACTIONS** → Appendix 1: monoclonal antibodies

● **SIDE-EFFECTS**

▸ **Common or very common** Abdominal pain · anxiety · conjunctivitis · constipation · cough · diarrhoea · dizziness · dyslipidaemia · dyspnoea · gastrointestinal disorders · headache · hypersensitivity · hypertension · hypofibrinogenaemia · hypokalaemia · increased risk of infection · insomnia · leucopenia · nausea · neutropenia · oral disorders · peripheral oedema · skin reactions · weight increased

▸ **Uncommon** Hypothyroidism · nephrolithiasis

▸ **Rare or very rare** Hepatic disorders · Stevens-Johnson syndrome

▸ **Frequency not known** Infusion related reaction · interstitial lung disease · pancytopenia · pulmonary fibrosis · sepsis

● **CONCEPTION AND CONTRACEPTION** Effective contraception required during and for 3 months after treatment.

● **PREGNANCY** Manufacturer advises avoid unless essential—toxicity in *animal* studies.

● **BREAST FEEDING** Specialist sources indicate use with caution. Monitor breast-fed infants for adequate feeding, fever, frequent infections, diarrhoea, or unusual behaviour.

● **HEPATIC IMPAIRMENT** Manufacturer advises caution—consult product literature.

● **RENAL IMPAIRMENT**

▸ With intravenous use Manufacturer advises monitor renal function closely in moderate-to-severe impairment—no information available.

▸ With subcutaneous use Manufacturer advises monitor renal function closely in severe impairment—no information available.

● **PRE-TREATMENT SCREENING**

Tuberculosis

▸ When used for Rheumatoid arthritis or Giant cell arteritis Patients should be evaluated for tuberculosis before treatment.

10

Musculoskeletal system

- **MONITORING REQUIREMENTS**
  ▶ When used for Rheumatoid arthritis or Giant cell arteritis [EvGr] Monitor lipid profile 4–8 weeks after starting treatment and then as indicated. Monitor for demyelinating disorders. Monitor hepatic transaminases before starting treatment, every 4–8 weeks for first 6 months of treatment, then every 12 weeks thereafter. Monitor neutrophil and platelet count before starting treatment, 4–8 weeks after starting treatment and then as indicated. Ⓜ

- **DIRECTIONS FOR ADMINISTRATION** For *intravenous infusion*, manufacturer advises give intermittently in Sodium chloride 0.9%; dilute requisite dose to a volume of 100 mL with infusion fluid and give over 1 hour. For *subcutaneous injection*, manufacturer advises rotate injection site and avoid skin that is tender, damaged or scarred. Patients may self-administer *RoActemra*®, after appropriate training in subcutaneous injection technique.

- **PRESCRIBING AND DISPENSING INFORMATION** Tocilizumab is a biological medicine. Biological medicines must be prescribed and dispensed by brand name, see *Biological medicines* and *Biosimilar medicines*, under Guidance on prescribing p. 1; record the brand name and batch number after each administration.

- **HANDLING AND STORAGE** Manufacturer advises protect from light and store in a refrigerator (2–8 °C)—consult product literature for further information regarding storage conditions outside refrigerator and after preparation of the infusion.

- **PATIENT AND CARER ADVICE** Patients and carers should be advised to seek immediate medical attention if symptoms of infection occur, or if symptoms of diverticular perforation such as abdominal pain, haemorrhage, or fever accompanying change in bowel habits occur.
  An alert card and patient information brochure highlighting important safety information should be provided.
  Missed doses
  ▶ With subcutaneous use If an injection administered once every 2 weeks or once every 3 weeks is missed and it is within 7 days of the scheduled dose, it should be administered as soon as possible and the next dose taken at the normal time.
  Driving and skilled tasks Patients and carers should be counselled on the effects on driving and performance of skilled tasks—increased risk of dizziness.

- **NATIONAL FUNDING/ACCESS DECISIONS**
  For full details see funding body website
  NICE decisions
  ▶ **Adalimumab, etanercept, infliximab, certolizumab pegol, golimumab, tocilizumab and abatacept for rheumatoid arthritis not previously treated with DMARDs or after conventional DMARDs only have failed (January 2016)** NICE TA375 Recommended with restrictions
  ▶ **Tocilizumab for the treatment of rheumatoid arthritis (February 2012)** NICE TA247 Recommended with restrictions
  ▶ **Tocilizumab for treating giant cell arteritis (April 2018)** NICE TA518 Recommended with restrictions
  ▶ **Nirmatrelvir plus ritonavir, sotrovimab and tocilizumab for treating COVID-19 (updated March 2024)** NICE TA878 Recommended

  Scottish Medicines Consortium (SMC) decisions
  ▶ **Tocilizumab (*RoActemra*®) for the treatment of Giant Cell Arteritis (GCA) in adult patients (September 2018)** SMC No. SMC2014 Recommended with restrictions
  ▶ **Tocilizumab (*RoActemra*®) for the treatment of COVID-19 in adults who are receiving systemic corticosteroids and require supplemental oxygen or mechanical ventilation (March 2023)** SMC No. SMC2552 Recommended

- **MEDICINAL FORMS** There can be variation in the licensing of different medicines containing the same drug.
  Solution for injection
  EXCIPIENTS: May contain Polysorbates
  ▶ **RoActemra** (Roche Products Ltd)
    Tocilizumab 180 mg per 1 ml RoActemra 162mg/0.9ml solution for injection pre-filled syringes | 4 pre-filled disposable injection [PoM] £913.12 (Hospital only)
    RoActemra 162mg/0.9ml solution for injection pre-filled pens | 4 pre-filled disposable injection [PoM] £913.12 DT = £913.12
  ▶ **Tyenne** (Fresenius Kabi Ltd) ▼
    Tocilizumab 180 mg per 1 ml Tyenne 162mg/0.9ml solution for injection pre-filled pens | 4 pre-filled disposable injection [PoM] £821.81 DT = £913.12 (Hospital only)
    Tyenne 162mg/0.9ml solution for injection pre-filled syringes | 4 pre-filled disposable injection [PoM] £821.81 (Hospital only)
  Solution for infusion
  EXCIPIENTS: May contain Polysorbates
  ELECTROLYTES: May contain Sodium
  ▶ **RoActemra** (Roche Products Ltd)
    Tocilizumab 20 mg per 1 ml RoActemra 400mg/20ml concentrate for solution for infusion vials | 1 vial [PoM] £512.00 (Hospital only)
    RoActemra 200mg/10ml concentrate for solution for infusion vials | 1 vial [PoM] £256.00 (Hospital only)
    RoActemra 80mg/4ml concentrate for solution for infusion vials | 1 vial [PoM] £102.40 (Hospital only)
  ▶ **Tyenne** (Fresenius Kabi Ltd) ▼
    Tocilizumab 20 mg per 1 ml Tyenne 400mg/20ml concentrate for solution for infusion vials | 1 vial [PoM] £460.80 (Hospital only)
    Tyenne 200mg/10ml concentrate for solution for infusion vials | 1 vial [PoM] £230.40 (Hospital only)
    Tyenne 80mg/4ml concentrate for solution for infusion vials | 1 vial [PoM] £92.16 (Hospital only)

Ustekinumab

06-Apr-2023

- **INDICATIONS AND DOSE**

  Plaque psoriasis (under expert supervision)
  ▶ BY SUBCUTANEOUS INJECTION
  ▶ Adult (body-weight up to 101 kg): Initially 45 mg, then 45 mg after 4 weeks, then 45 mg every 12 weeks, consider discontinuation if no response within 28 weeks
  ▶ Adult (body-weight 101 kg and above): Initially 90 mg, then 90 mg after 4 weeks, then 90 mg every 12 weeks, consider discontinuation if no response within 28 weeks

  Psoriatic arthritis (under expert supervision)
  ▶ BY SUBCUTANEOUS INJECTION
  ▶ Adult: Initially 45 mg, then 45 mg after 4 weeks, then 45 mg every 12 weeks, higher doses of 90 mg may be used in patients with body-weight over 100 kg; consider discontinuation if no response within 28 weeks

  Crohn's disease (under expert supervision) | Ulcerative colitis (under expert supervision)
  ▶ INITIALLY BY INTRAVENOUS INFUSION
  ▶ Adult (body-weight up to 56 kg): 260 mg, then (by subcutaneous injection) 90 mg after 8 weeks, then (by subcutaneous injection) 90 mg every 12 weeks, if response is inadequate 8 weeks after first subcutaneous dose, or response is lost, dosing frequency may be increased—consult product literature; consider discontinuation if no response within 16 weeks of initial dose or increase in dosing frequency
  ▶ Adult (body-weight 56–85 kg): 390 mg, then (by subcutaneous injection) 90 mg after 8 weeks, then (by subcutaneous injection) 90 mg every 12 weeks, if response is inadequate 8 weeks after first subcutaneous dose, or response is lost, dosing frequency may be increased—consult product literature; consider discontinuation if no response within 16 weeks of initial dose or increase in dosing frequency

▸ **Adult (body-weight 86 kg and above):** 520 mg, then (by subcutaneous injection) 90 mg after 8 weeks, then (by subcutaneous injection) 90 mg every 12 weeks, if response is inadequate 8 weeks after first subcutaneous dose, or response is lost, dosing frequency may be increased—consult product literature; consider discontinuation if no response within 16 weeks of initial dose or increase in dosing frequency

● **CONTRA-INDICATIONS** Active infection

● **CAUTIONS** Development of malignancy · elderly · history of malignancy · predisposition to infection · start appropriate treatment if widespread erythema and skin exfoliation develop, and stop ustekinumab treatment if exfoliative dermatitis suspected

CAUTIONS, FURTHER INFORMATION

▸ **Tuberculosis** Active tuberculosis should be treated with standard treatment for at least 2 months before starting ustekinumab. Patients who have previously received adequate treatment for tuberculosis can start ustekinumab but should be monitored every 3 months for possible recurrence. In patients without active tuberculosis but who were previously not treated adequately, chemoprophylaxis should ideally be completed before starting ustekinumab. In patients at high risk of tuberculosis who cannot be assessed by tuberculin skin test, chemoprophylaxis can be given concurrently with ustekinumab.

● **INTERACTIONS** → Appendix 1: monoclonal antibodies

● **SIDE-EFFECTS**

▸ **Common or very common** Arthralgia · asthenia · back pain · diarrhoea · dizziness · headache · increased risk of infection · myalgia · nausea · oropharyngeal pain · skin reactions · vomiting

▸ **Uncommon** Depression · facial paralysis · hypersensitivity (may be delayed) · nasal congestion

▸ **Rare or very rare** Cutaneous lupus erythematosus · hypersensitivity vasculitis · interstitial lung disease · lupus-like syndrome · pneumonia eosinophilic

▸ **Frequency not known** Increased risk of cancer · meningitis listeria · tuberculosis reactivation

● **CONCEPTION AND CONTRACEPTION** Manufacturer advises effective contraception during treatment and for 15 weeks after stopping treatment.

● **PREGNANCY** Avoid.

● **BREAST FEEDING** Specialist sources indicate use with caution; negligible amounts present in milk which are likely to be destroyed in the infant's gastro-intestinal tract. In newborn or premature infants there may be greater intestinal absorption.

● **PRE-TREATMENT SCREENING**
Tuberculosis Patients should be evaluated for tuberculosis before treatment.

● **MONITORING REQUIREMENTS**

▸ Monitor for non-melanoma skin cancer, especially in patients with a history of PUVA treatment or prolonged immunosuppressant therapy, or those over 60 years of age.

▸ Monitor for signs and symptoms of exfoliative dermatitis or erythrodermic psoriasis.

● **DIRECTIONS FOR ADMINISTRATION** For *subcutaneous injection* (*Stelara*®), inject into the upper thigh or abdomen (except for the 5 cm around the navel), or upper arm (if not self-administered); avoid areas of the skin that show signs of psoriasis. Patients may self-administer *Stelara*®, after appropriate training in subcutaneous injection technique.

For *intravenous infusion* (*Stelara*®), give intermittently in Sodium Chloride 0.9%; dilute requisite dose with infusion fluid to final volume of 250 mL and give over at least 1 hour through an in-line low-protein binding filter (pore size 0.2 micron); use within 8 hours of dilution.

● **PRESCRIBING AND DISPENSING INFORMATION**
Ustekinumab is a biological medicine. Biological medicines must be prescribed and dispensed by brand name, see *Biological medicines* and *Biosimilar medicines*, under Guidance on prescribing p. 1; record the brand name and batch number after each administration.

● **HANDLING AND STORAGE** Store in a refrigerator (2–8°C) and protect from light—consult product literature for further information regarding storage outside refrigerator.

● **PATIENT AND CARER ADVICE**
Exfoliative dermatitis Patients and carers should be advised to seek prompt medical attention if symptoms suggestive of exfoliative dermatitis or erythrodermic psoriasis (such as increased redness and shedding of skin over a larger area of the body) develop.
Infection Patients and carers should be advised to seek medical attention if symptoms of infection develop.
Tuberculosis Patients and carers should be advised to seek medical attention if symptoms suggestive of tuberculosis (e.g. persistent cough, weight loss, and fever) develop.
Lupus-related conditions Patients and carers should be advised to seek prompt medical attention if symptoms suggestive of cutaneous lupus erythematosus or lupus-like syndrome (such as skin lesions in sun exposed areas, or that are accompanied by arthralgia) develop.

● **NATIONAL FUNDING/ACCESS DECISIONS**
For full details see funding body website
NICE decisions

▸ **Ustekinumab for the treatment of adults with moderate to severe psoriasis (updated March 2017)** NICE TA180 Recommended with restrictions

▸ **Ustekinumab for treating active psoriatic arthritis (updated March 2017)** NICE TA340 Recommended with restrictions

▸ **Ustekinumab for moderately to severely active Crohn's disease after previous treatment (July 2017)** NICE TA456 Recommended

▸ **Ustekinumab for treating moderately to severely active ulcerative colitis (June 2020)** NICE TA633 Recommended with restrictions

Scottish Medicines Consortium (SMC) decisions

▸ **Ustekinumab (*Stelara*®) alone or in combination with methotrexate, for the treatment of active psoriatic arthritis in adult patients when the response to previous non-biological disease-modifying anti-rheumatic drug therapy has been inadequate (March 2014)** SMC No. 944/14 Recommended with restrictions

▸ **Ustekinumab (*Stelara*®) for the treatment of adult patients with moderately to severely active Crohn's disease who have had an inadequate response with, lost response to, or were intolerant to either conventional therapy or a tumour necrosis factor-alpha antagonist or have medical contra-indications to such therapies (July 2017)** SMC No. 1250/17 Recommended

▸ **Ustekinumab (*Stelara*®) for the treatment of adult patients with moderately to severely active ulcerative colitis who have had an inadequate response with, lost response to, or were intolerant to either conventional therapy or a biologic or have medical contra-indications to such therapies (April 2020)** SMC No. SMC2250 Recommended

● **MEDICINAL FORMS** There can be variation in the licensing of different medicines containing the same drug.

Solution for injection
CAUTIONARY AND ADVISORY LABELS 10
EXCIPIENTS: May contain Polysorbates

▸ **Ustekinumab (non-proprietary)** ▼
Ustekinumab 90 mg per 1 ml Imuldosa 90mg/1ml solution for injection pre-filled syringes | 1 pre-filled disposable injection PoM £2,147.00 (Hospital only)
Otulfi 90mg/1ml solution for injection pre-filled syringes | 1 pre-filled disposable injection PoM £1,932.30 (Hospital only)
Otulfi 45mg/0.5ml solution for injection pre-filled syringes | 1 pre-filled disposable injection PoM £1,932.30 (Hospital only)

Imuldosa 45mg/0.5ml solution for injection pre-filled syringes | 1 pre-filled disposable injection [PoM] £2,147.00 (Hospital only)

▸ **Pyzchiva** (Sandoz Ltd) ▼
Ustekinumab 90 mg per 1 ml Pyzchiva 90mg/1ml solution for injection pre-filled syringes | 1 pre-filled disposable injection [PoM] £1,932.30 (Hospital only)
Pyzchiva 45mg/0.5ml solution for injection pre-filled syringes | 1 pre-filled disposable injection [PoM] £1,932.30 (Hospital only)

▸ **Stelara** (Janssen-Cilag Ltd)
Ustekinumab 90 mg per 1 ml Stelara 90mg/1ml solution for injection pre-filled syringes | 1 pre-filled disposable injection [PoM] £2,147.00 (Hospital only)
Stelara 45mg/0.5ml solution for injection pre-filled pens | 1 pre-filled disposable injection [PoM] £2,147.00 (Hospital only)
Stelara 90mg/1ml solution for injection pre-filled pens | 1 pre-filled disposable injection [PoM] £2,147.00 (Hospital only)
Stelara 45mg/0.5ml solution for injection vials | 1 vial [PoM] £2,147.00 (Hospital only)
Stelara 45mg/0.5ml solution for injection pre-filled syringes | 1 pre-filled disposable injection [PoM] £2,147.00 (Hospital only)

▸ **Steqeyma** (Celltrion Healthcare UK Ltd) ▼
Ustekinumab 90 mg per 1 ml Steqeyma 90mg/1ml solution for injection pre-filled syringes | 1 pre-filled disposable injection [PoM] £1,932.30 (Hospital only)
Steqeyma 45mg/0.5ml solution for injection pre-filled syringes | 1 pre-filled disposable injection [PoM] £1,932.30 (Hospital only)

▸ **Uzpruvo** (Genus Pharmaceuticals Holdings Ltd) ▼
Ustekinumab 90 mg per 1 ml Uzpruvo 45mg/0.5ml solution for injection pre-filled syringes | 1 pre-filled disposable injection [PoM] £1,932.30 (Hospital only)
Uzpruvo 90mg/1ml solution for injection pre-filled disposable injection [PoM] £1,932.30 (Hospital only)

▸ **Wezenla** (Amgen Ltd) ▼
Ustekinumab 90 mg per 1 ml Wezenla 90mg/1ml solution for injection pre-filled syringes | 1 pre-filled disposable injection [PoM] £2,147.00 (Hospital only)
Wezenla 45mg/0.5ml solution for injection vials | 1 vial [PoM] £2,147.00 (Hospital only)
Wezenla 45mg/0.5ml solution for injection pre-filled syringes | 1 pre-filled disposable injection [PoM] £2,147.00 (Hospital only)

Solution for infusion

CAUTIONARY AND ADVISORY LABELS 10
EXCIPIENTS: May contain Disodium edetate, polysorbates

▸ **Ustekinumab (non-proprietary)** ▼
Ustekinumab 5 mg per 1 ml Otulfi 130mg/26ml concentrate for solution for infusion vials | 1 vial [PoM] £1,932.30 (Hospital only)

▸ **Pyzchiva** (Sandoz Ltd) ▼
Ustekinumab 5 mg per 1 ml Pyzchiva 130mg/26ml concentrate for solution for infusion vials | 1 vial [PoM] £1,932.30 (Hospital only)

▸ **Stelara** (Janssen-Cilag Ltd)
Ustekinumab 5 mg per 1 ml Stelara 130mg/26ml concentrate for solution for infusion vials | 1 vial [PoM] £2,147.00 (Hospital only)

▸ **Steqeyma** (Celltrion Healthcare UK Ltd) ▼
Ustekinumab 5 mg per 1 ml Steqeyma 130mg/26ml concentrate for solution for infusion vials | 1 vial [PoM] £1,932.30 (Hospital only)

▸ **Uzpruvo** (Genus Pharmaceuticals Holdings Ltd) ▼
Ustekinumab 5 mg per 1 ml Uzpruvo 130mg/26ml concentrate for solution for infusion vials | 1 vial [PoM] £1,932.30 (Hospital only)

▸ **Wezenla** (Amgen Ltd) ▼
Ustekinumab 5 mg per 1 ml Wezenla 130mg/26ml concentrate for solution for infusion vials | 1 vial [PoM] £2,147.00 (Hospital only)

IMMUNOSUPPRESSANTS ⟩ JAK INHIBITORS

Baricitinib

09-Nov-2023

● **DRUG ACTION** Baricitinib selectively and reversibly inhibits the Janus-associated tyrosine kinases JAK1 and JAK2.

● **INDICATIONS AND DOSE**

Rheumatoid arthritis (initiated by a specialist)
▸ BY MOUTH
▸ **Adult:** 4 mg once daily, a reduced dose of 2 mg once daily is recommended for patients with certain risk factors—consult product literature, for dose adjustments due to clinical response or treatment

interruption due to side-effects—consult product literature
▸ **Elderly:** 2 mg once daily, for dose adjustments due to clinical response or treatment interruption due to side-effects—consult product literature

Atopic eczema (initiated by a specialist)
▸ BY MOUTH
▸ **Adult:** 4 mg once daily, a reduced dose of 2 mg once daily is recommended for patients with certain risk factors—consult product literature, consider discontinuation of treatment if no response after 8 weeks, for dose adjustments due to clinical response or treatment interruption due to side-effects—consult product literature
▸ **Elderly:** 2 mg once daily, consider discontinuation of treatment if no response after 8 weeks, for dose adjustments due to clinical response or treatment interruption due to side-effects—consult product literature

Alopecia areata (initiated by a specialist)
▸ BY MOUTH
▸ **Adult:** 4 mg once daily, a reduced dose of 2 mg once daily is recommended for patients with certain risk factors—consult product literature, consider discontinuation of treatment if no response after 36 weeks, for dose adjustments due to clinical response or treatment interruption due to side-effects—consult product literature
▸ **Elderly:** 2 mg once daily, consider discontinuation of treatment if no response after 36 weeks, for dose adjustments due to clinical response or treatment interruption due to side-effects—consult product literature

IMPORTANT SAFETY INFORMATION

MHRA/CHM ADVICE: BARICITINIB (*OLUMIANT*®): RISK OF VENOUS THROMBOEMBOLISM (MARCH 2020)
Clinical trial data have shown that baricitinib is associated with an increased frequency of venous thromboembolism (VTE) compared with placebo. Healthcare professionals are advised to use baricitinib with caution in patients with additional risk factors for VTE. Patients should be informed of the signs and symptoms of VTE before starting treatment and advised to seek urgent medical attention if these develop. Baricitinib should be permanently discontinued if clinical features of VTE occur.

MHRA/CHM ADVICE: BARICITINIB (*OLUMIANT*®): INCREASED RISK OF DIVERTICULITIS, PARTICULARLY IN PATIENTS WITH RISK FACTORS (AUGUST 2020)
A European review of worldwide data concluded that baricitinib is associated with an increased risk of diverticulitis. The MHRA recommends healthcare professionals use baricitinib with caution in patients with pre-existing diverticular disease, and in patients on long-term concomitant medicines associated with an increased risk of diverticulitis (including NSAIDs, corticosteroids, and opioids). Patients should be advised to seek immediate medical attention if they experience severe abdominal pain especially accompanied with fever, nausea and vomiting, or other symptoms of diverticulitis. Prompt evaluation is needed of any patients treated with baricitinib who present with new-onset abdominal signs and symptoms to identify early diverticulitis or gastro-intestinal perforation.

MHRA/CHM ADVICE: JANUS KINASE (JAK) INHIBITORS: NEW MEASURES TO REDUCE RISKS OF MAJOR CARDIOVASCULAR EVENTS, MALIGNANCY, VENOUS THROMBOEMBOLISM, SERIOUS INFECTIONS AND INCREASED MORTALITY (APRIL 2023)
In 2022, the EMA conducted a review of all JAK inhibitors indicated for chronic inflammatory diseases and concluded that the risks associated with the use of

tofacitinib could be considered a class effect (see *Important safety information* in tofacitinib p. 1265). Following a further review by the MHRA, some existing warnings for tofacitinib have been updated and implemented for all JAK inhibitors included in the review, such as baricitinib.

Healthcare professionals are advised to:
- avoid use in patients aged 65 years or older, in patients who are current or past long-time smokers, and in patients with other cardiovascular disease or malignancy risk factors, unless there are no suitable alternatives;
- use with caution in patients with risk factors for VTE;
- use lower doses in patients with risk factors, where applicable;
- periodically examine all patients' skin for malignancy;
- inform patients and their carers of these risks, and the signs and symptoms that warrant urgent medical attention.

● **CONTRA-INDICATIONS** Absolute lymphocyte count less than 0.5×10^9 cells/litre (do not initiate) · absolute neutrophil count less than 1×10^9 cells/litre (do not initiate) · haemoglobin less than 8 g/dL (do not initiate) · tuberculosis (active)

● **CAUTIONS** Active, chronic, or recurrent infection (interrupt treatment if no response to standard therapy) · elderly (65 years and older) · history of atherosclerotic cardiovascular disease or other cardiovascular risk factors · risk factors for deep-vein thrombosis or pulmonary embolism · risk factors for malignancy · risk of diverticulitis · risk of viral reactivation (consult product literature)

  CAUTIONS, FURTHER INFORMATION
▸ Tuberculosis EvGr Consider anti-tuberculosis therapy prior to initiation of baricitinib in patients with previously untreated latent tuberculosis. Ⓜ
▸ Immunisation EvGr Patients should receive all recommended vaccinations before starting treatment; live vaccines are not recommended immediately before, or during, treatment. Ⓜ

● **INTERACTIONS** → Appendix 1: baricitinib

● **SIDE-EFFECTS**
▸ **Common or very common** Abdominal pain · dyslipidaemia · headache · herpes zoster (interrupt treatment) · increased risk of infection · nausea · skin reactions · thrombocytosis
▸ **Uncommon** Deep vein thrombosis (discontinue permanently) · facial swelling · neutropenia · pulmonary embolism (discontinue permanently) · weight increased
▸ **Frequency not known** Cardiovascular event · gastrointestinal perforation · hypersensitivity (discontinue) · malignancy · neoplasms · reactivation of infections · venous thromboembolism (discontinue permanently)

● **CONCEPTION AND CONTRACEPTION** Manufacturer advises effective contraception during and for at least 1 week after treatment in women of child-bearing potential.

● **PREGNANCY** Manufacturer advises avoid—toxicity in *animal* studies.

● **BREAST FEEDING** Manufacturer advises avoid—present in milk in *animal* studies.

● **HEPATIC IMPAIRMENT** Manufacturer advises avoid in severe impairment (no information available).

● **RENAL IMPAIRMENT** Manufacturer advises avoid if creatinine clearance less than 30 mL/minute.
Dose adjustments Manufacturer advises reduce dose to 2 mg once daily if creatinine clearance 30–60 mL/minute. See p. 21.

● **PRE-TREATMENT SCREENING** Manufacturer advises patients should be evaluated for tuberculosis and viral hepatitis before treatment.

● **MONITORING REQUIREMENTS**
▸ EvGr Monitor patients with hepatitis B surface antibody and hepatitis B core antibody, without hepatitis B surface antigen, for expression of hepatitis B virus (HBV) DNA—if HBV DNA detected, consult liver specialist for advice.
▸ Monitor lipid profile 12 weeks after treatment initiation—hyperlipidaemia should be managed according to international clinical guidelines; monitor hepatic transaminases routinely—interrupt treatment if drug-induced liver injury suspected.
▸ Monitor for haematological abnormalities; interrupt treatment if absolute neutrophil count less than 1×10^9 cells/litre, absolute lymphocyte count less than 0.5×10^9 cells/litre, or haemoglobin less than 8 g/dL—treatment may be restarted when levels return above these values.
▸ Periodic skin examination is recommended in all patients, particularly those at increased risk of skin cancer. Ⓜ

● **PRESCRIBING AND DISPENSING INFORMATION** The manufacturer of *Olumiant*® has provided guides for healthcare professionals.

● **PATIENT AND CARER ADVICE**
Alert card A patient alert card should be provided.

● **NATIONAL FUNDING/ACCESS DECISIONS**
For full details see funding body website
NICE decisions
▸ **Baricitinib for moderate to severe rheumatoid arthritis (August 2017)** NICE TA466 Recommended with restrictions
▸ **Baricitinib for treating moderate to severe atopic dermatitis (March 2021)** NICE TA681 Recommended with restrictions
▸ **Baricitinib for treating severe alopecia areata (October 2023)** NICE TA926 Not recommended

Scottish Medicines Consortium (SMC) decisions
▸ **Baricitinib (*Olumiant*®) for treatment of moderate to severe active rheumatoid arthritis (RA) in adult patients who have responded inadequately to, or who are intolerant to one or more disease-modifying anti-rheumatic drugs (DMARDs). Baricitinib may be used as monotherapy or in combination with methotrexate (September 2017)** SMC No. 1265/17 Recommended with restrictions
▸ **Baricitinib (*Olumiant*®) for the treatment of moderate to severe atopic dermatitis in adult patients who are candidates for systemic therapy (June 2021)** SMC No. SMC2337 Recommended with restrictions
▸ **Baricitinib (*Olumiant*®) for the treatment of severe alopecia areata in adult patients (August 2023)** SMC No. SMC2572 Not recommended

● **MEDICINAL FORMS** There can be variation in the licensing of different medicines containing the same drug.
Oral tablet
▸ **Baricitinib (Non-proprietary)**
Baricitinib 2 mg Baricitinib 2mg tablets | 28 tablet PoM £805.56
DT = £805.56
Baricitinib 4 mg Baricitinib 4mg tablets | 28 tablet PoM £805.56
DT = £805.56

Filgotinib
15-Jun-2023

● **DRUG ACTION** Filgotinib is a selective inhibitor of the Janus-associated tyrosine kinase JAK1.

● **INDICATIONS AND DOSE**
Rheumatoid arthritis (initiated by a specialist)
▸ BY MOUTH
▸ Adult: 200 mg once daily, a reduced dose of 100 mg once daily is recommended for patients with certain risk factors—consult product literature, for treatment interruption due to side-effects—consult product literature

continued →

► Elderly: 100 mg once daily, for dose adjustments due to clinical response or treatment interruption due to side-effects—consult product literature

Ulcerative colitis (initiated by a specialist)
► BY MOUTH
► Adult: Initially 200 mg once daily for 10 weeks, if an adequate therapeutic response is not achieved after 10 weeks, the initial dose can be extended for an additional 12 weeks, discontinue treatment if no response after 22 weeks, for treatment interruption due to side-effects—consult product literature, then maintenance 200 mg once daily, a reduced maintenance dose of 100 mg once daily is recommended for patients with certain risk factors—consult product literature, for treatment interruption due to side-effects—consult product literature
► Adult 65-74 years: Initially 200 mg once daily for 10 weeks, if an adequate therapeutic response is not achieved after 10 weeks, the initial dose can be extended for an additional 12 weeks, discontinue treatment if no response after 22 weeks, for treatment interruption due to side-effects—consult product literature, then maintenance 100 mg once daily, for dose adjustments due to clinical response or treatment interruption due to side-effects—consult product literature

---

IMPORTANT SAFETY INFORMATION

MHRA/CHM ADVICE: JANUS KINASE (JAK) INHIBITORS: NEW MEASURES TO REDUCE RISKS OF MAJOR CARDIOVASCULAR EVENTS, MALIGNANCY, VENOUS THROMBOEMBOLISM, SERIOUS INFECTIONS AND INCREASED MORTALITY (APRIL 2023)

In 2022, the EMA conducted a review of all JAK inhibitors indicated for chronic inflammatory diseases and concluded that the risks associated with the use of tofacitinib could be considered a class effect (see *Important safety information* in tofacitinib p. 1265). Following a further review by the MHRA, some existing warnings for tofacitinib have been updated and implemented for all JAK inhibitors included in the review, such as filgotinib.

Healthcare professionals are advised to:
● avoid use in patients aged 65 years or older, in patients who are current or past long-time smokers, and in patients with other cardiovascular disease or malignancy risk factors, unless there are no suitable alternatives;
● use with caution in patients with risk factors for venous thromboembolism;
● use lower doses in patients with risk factors, where applicable;
● periodically examine all patients' skin for malignancy;
● inform patients and their carers of these risks, and the signs and symptoms that warrant urgent medical attention.

● **CONTRA-INDICATIONS** Absolute lymphocyte count less than 0.5×10^9 cells/litre · absolute neutrophil count less than 1×10^9 cells/litre · haemoglobin less than 8 g/dL · serious infection (active) · tuberculosis (active)
● **CAUTIONS** Elderly (65 years and older) · history of atherosclerotic cardiovascular disease or other cardiovascular risk factors · history of serious or opportunistic infection · infection (chronic or recurrent) · predisposition to infection · risk factors for malignancy · risk factors or venous thromboembolism (VTE) · risk of viral reactivation (consult product literature) · tuberculosis exposure

CAUTIONS, FURTHER INFORMATION
► Tuberculosis [EvGr] Anti-tuberculosis therapy should be initiated in patients with latent tuberculosis before

starting filgotinib. Use filgotinib with caution in patients who have travelled or resided in areas of endemic tuberculosis or endemic mycoses, or who have had previous exposure to tuberculosis. (M)
► Immunisation [EvGr] Patients should receive all recommended vaccinations before starting treatment; live vaccines are not recommended immediately before, or during, treatment. (M)
► Venous thromboembolism [EvGr] If signs and symptoms of VTE occur during treatment, prompt discontinuation of filgotinib is recommended. (M)

● **INTERACTIONS** → Appendix 1: filgotinib
● **SIDE-EFFECTS**
► **Common or very common** Dizziness · increased risk of infection · nausea
► **Uncommon** Hypercholesterolaemia · neutropenia
► **Frequency not known** Cardiovascular event · embolism and thrombosis · malignancy · non-melanoma skin cancer · reactivation of infections

● **CONCEPTION AND CONTRACEPTION** [EvGr] Females of childbearing potential should use effective contraception during and for at least 1 week after stopping treatment. (M)

● **PREGNANCY** [EvGr] Avoid—toxicity in *animal* studies. (M)
● **BREAST FEEDING** [EvGr] Avoid—no information available. (M)
● **HEPATIC IMPAIRMENT** [EvGr] Avoid in severe impairment (no information available). (M)
● **RENAL IMPAIRMENT** [EvGr] Caution in moderate or severe impairment; avoid in end-stage renal disease (no information available). (M)
Dose adjustments [EvGr] A dose of 100 mg once daily is recommended in moderate or severe impairment. (M)

● **PRE-TREATMENT SCREENING** [EvGr] Patients should be evaluated for tuberculosis and viral hepatitis before treatment. (M)

● **MONITORING REQUIREMENTS**
► [EvGr] Monitor for signs and symptoms of infections (including tuberculosis) during and after treatment—consider treatment interruption until the infection is controlled.
► Monitor for haematological abnormalities before and during treatment; interrupt treatment if absolute neutrophil count less than 1×10^9 cells/litre, absolute lymphocyte count less than 0.5×10^9 cells/litre, or haemoglobin less than 8 g/dL—treatment may be restarted when levels return above these values.
► Monitor lipid profile 12 weeks after treatment initiation and as needed thereafter—hyperlipidaemia should be managed according to international clinical guidelines.
► Monitor for viral reactivation (including viral hepatitis and herpes zoster) during treatment; interrupt treatment if herpes zoster infection develops and resume once resolved.
► Periodic skin examination is recommended in all patients, particularly those at increased risk of skin cancer. (M)

● **PRESCRIBING AND DISPENSING INFORMATION** The manufacturer of *Jyseleca*® has provided a guide for healthcare professionals.
● **PATIENT AND CARER ADVICE** For *Jyseleca*®, a patient alert card should be provided.

● **NATIONAL FUNDING/ACCESS DECISIONS**
For full details see funding body website
NICE decisions
► **Filgotinib for treating moderate to severe rheumatoid arthritis (February 2021)** NICE TA676 Recommended with restrictions
► **Filgotinib for treating moderately to severely active ulcerative colitis (June 2022)** NICE TA792 Recommended
Scottish Medicines Consortium (SMC) decisions
► Filgotinib (*Jyseleca*®) as monotherapy or in combination with methotrexate for the treatment of moderate to severe active

rheumatoid arthritis in adult patients who have responded inadequately to, or who are intolerant to one or more disease-modifying antirheumatic drugs (DMARDs) [in adults with severe disease] (September 2021) SMC No. SMC2365 Recommended with restrictions

▸ Filgotinib (*Jyseleca*®) as monotherapy or in combination with methotrexate for the treatment of moderate to severe active rheumatoid arthritis in adult patients who have responded inadequately to, or who are intolerant to one or more disease-modifying antirheumatic drugs (DMARDs) [in adults with moderate disease] (October 2022) SMC No. SMC2475 Recommended with restrictions

▸ Filgotinib (*Jyseleca*®) for the treatment of adult patients with moderately to severely active ulcerative colitis who have had an inadequate response with, lost response to, or were intolerant to either conventional therapy or a biologic agent (May 2022) SMC No. SMC2467 Recommended

● **MEDICINAL FORMS** There can be variation in the licensing of different medicines containing the same drug.

Oral tablet
CAUTIONARY AND ADVISORY LABELS 25
 ▸ Jyseleca (Alfasigma UK Ltd) ▼
  Filgotinib (as Filgotinib maleate) 100 mg Jyseleca 100mg tablets
  | 30 tablet [PoM] £863.10
  Filgotinib (as Filgotinib maleate) 200 mg Jyseleca 200mg tablets
  | 30 tablet [PoM] £863.10

Tofacitinib
10-Nov-2023

● **DRUG ACTION** Tofacitinib selectively inhibits the Janus-associated tyrosine kinases JAK1 and JAK3.

● **INDICATIONS AND DOSE**

Moderate to severe rheumatoid arthritis (specialist use only) | Psoriatic arthritis (specialist use only)
 ▸ BY MOUTH USING FILM-COATED TABLETS
 ▸ Adult: 5 mg twice daily, for dose interruption or treatment discontinuation due to side-effects—consult product literature
 ▸ BY MOUTH USING MODIFIED-RELEASE TABLETS
 ▸ Adult: 11 mg once daily, for dose interruption or treatment discontinuation due to side-effects—consult product literature

Moderate to severe ulcerative colitis (specialist use only)
 ▸ BY MOUTH USING FILM-COATED TABLETS
 ▸ Adult: Initially 10 mg twice daily for 8 weeks, then maintenance 5 mg twice daily, if an adequate therapeutic response is not achieved after 8 weeks, the initial dose can be extended for an additional 8 weeks, discontinue treatment if no response after 16 weeks, for dose adjustments due to side-effects, decreased response during maintenance treatment, or following treatment interruption—consult product literature

Ankylosing spondylitis (specialist use only)
 ▸ BY MOUTH USING FILM-COATED TABLETS
 ▸ Adult: 5 mg twice daily, consider treatment discontinuation if no response 16 weeks after initial dose, for dose interruption or treatment discontinuation due to side-effects—consult product literature

DOSE ADJUSTMENTS DUE TO INTERACTIONS
 ▸ [EvGr] Reduce total daily dose by half with concurrent use of potent CYP3A4 inhibitors, or concurrent use of a moderate CYP3A4 inhibitor and a potent CYP2C19 inhibitor, or concurrent use of drugs which are both moderate CYP3A4 and potent CYP2C19 inhibitors. Ⓜ

DOSE EQUIVALENCE AND CONVERSION
 ▸ When used for Rheumatoid arthritis or Psoriatic arthritis
 ▸ A twice-daily dose of *Xeljanz*® 5 mg film-coated tablets is equivalent to a once-daily dose of *Xeljanz*® 11 mg

modified-release tablets—they may be switched between each other on the day after the last dose of either tablet.

> **IMPORTANT SAFETY INFORMATION**
>
> MHRA/CHM ADVICE: TOFACITINIB (*XELJANZ*®): NEW MEASURES TO MINIMISE RISK OF VENOUS THROMBOEMBOLISM AND OF SERIOUS AND FATAL INFECTIONS (MARCH 2020)
> New recommendations have been issued following a European safety review that found a dose-dependent increased risk of serious venous thromboembolism (VTE) associated with tofacitinib. Healthcare professionals are advised to use tofacitinib with caution in any patients with known risk factors for VTE, in addition to the underlying disease. In patients with risk factors being treated for ulcerative colitis, the use of tofacitinib 10 mg twice daily as maintenance treatment is **not** recommended, unless no suitable alternative is available. In **all** patients being treated for rheumatoid or psoriatic arthritis, the recommended daily dose of tofacitinib should not be exceeded— *see Indications and dose*. Patients should be informed of the signs and symptoms of VTE before starting treatment and advised to seek urgent medical attention if these develop. Tofacitinib should be permanently discontinued if signs of VTE occur.
>
> Tofacitinib was also found to increase the risk of serious and fatal infections, with higher rates of infections in the elderly. Use of tofacitinib in patients older than 65 years is **not** recommended, unless no suitable alternative is available.
>
> MHRA/CHM ADVICE: TOFACITINIB (*XELJANZ*®): NEW MEASURES TO MINIMISE RISK OF MAJOR ADVERSE CARDIOVASCULAR EVENTS AND MALIGNANCIES (OCTOBER 2021)
> Data from a clinical trial of patients aged 50 years or older with rheumatoid arthritis and at least one cardiovascular risk factor showed an increased incidence of major adverse cardiovascular events and malignancies, particularly lung cancer and lymphoma (excluding non-melanoma skin cancer), when comparing tofacitinib with tumour necrosis factor alpha inhibitors. Healthcare professionals are advised to inform patients of the risks associated with tofacitinib treatment and should only use tofacitinib in patients over 65 years of age, in patients who are current or past smokers, patients with other cardiovascular risk factors (such as diabetes or coronary artery disease), and patients with other malignancy risk factors if no suitable alternatives are available.
>
> MHRA/CHM ADVICE: JANUS KINASE (JAK) INHIBITORS: NEW MEASURES TO REDUCE RISKS OF MAJOR CARDIOVASCULAR EVENTS, MALIGNANCY, VENOUS THROMBOEMBOLISM, SERIOUS INFECTIONS AND INCREASED MORTALITY (APRIL 2023)
> In 2022, the EMA conducted a review of all JAK inhibitors indicated for chronic inflammatory diseases and concluded that the risks associated with the use of tofacitinib could be considered a class effect. Following a further review by the MHRA, some existing warnings for tofacitinib have been updated and implemented for all JAK inhibitors included in the review.
> Healthcare professionals are advised to:
> ● avoid use in patients aged 65 years or older, in patients who are current or past long-time smokers, and in patients with other cardiovascular disease or malignancy risk factors, unless there are no suitable alternatives;
> ● use with caution in patients with risk factors for VTE;
> ● use lower doses in patients with risk factors, where applicable;
> ● periodically examine all patients' skin for malignancy;

- inform patients and their carers of these risks, and the signs and symptoms that warrant urgent medical attention.

- **CONTRA-INDICATIONS** Absolute lymphocyte count less than 750 cells/mm^3 (do not initiate) · absolute neutrophil count less than 1000 cells/mm^3 (do not initiate) · active infection including localised infection · active tuberculosis · haemoglobin less than 9 g/dL (do not initiate) · risk factors for venous thromboembolism (high doses)

- **CAUTIONS** Elderly (65 years and older) · history of atherosclerotic cardiovascular disease or other cardiovascular risk factors · known risk factors for fractures · patients at risk of gastro-intestinal perforation (new onset abdominal signs and symptoms should be evaluated promptly) · predisposition to infection · raised serum transaminases (particularly in combination with potentially hepatotoxic drugs) · recurrent infection or history of serious infection · risk factors for malignancy · risk factors for venous thromboembolism (VTE) · risk of diverticulitis · risk of viral reactivation (consult product literature) · tuberculosis exposure

CAUTIONS, FURTHER INFORMATION
- Immunisation [EvGr] Patients should receive all recommended vaccinations before starting treatment (consider prophylactic varicella zoster vaccination); live vaccines should be given at least 2 weeks, but preferably 4 weeks, before treatment initiation—consult product literature. Ⓜ
- Tuberculosis [EvGr] Anti-tuberculosis therapy should be initiated in patients with latent tuberculosis before starting tofacitinib. Consider anti-tuberculosis therapy prior to initiation of tofacitinib in patients with a history of previously untreated latent or active tuberculosis or in patients at risk of tuberculosis infection. Use tofacitinib with caution in patients who have travelled or resided in areas of endemic mycoses, or who have had previous exposure to tuberculosis. Ⓜ
- VTE
- When used for Rheumatoid arthritis [EvGr] In patients with known risk factors for VTE, consider measuring D-dimer levels after approximately 12 months of treatment. If D-dimer level is 2 times the upper limit of normal or more, consider treatment discontinuation unless potential benefit outweighs risk. Ⓜ

- **INTERACTIONS** → Appendix 1: tofacitinib

- **SIDE-EFFECTS**
- **Common or very common** Abdominal pain · anaemia · cough · diarrhoea · dyspepsia · fatigue · fever · gastrointestinal disorders · headache · hypertension · increased risk of infection · influenza · joint disorders · nausea · peripheral oedema · pharyngitis · sinusitis · skin reactions · vomiting
- **Uncommon** Decreased leucocytes · deep vein thrombosis (discontinue permanently) · dehydration · dyslipidaemia · dyspnoea · hepatic steatosis · insomnia · ligament sprain · muscle strain · musculoskeletal pain · myocardial infarction · neoplasms · neutropenia · paraesthesia · pulmonary embolism (discontinue permanently) · sinus congestion · tendinitis · venous thromboembolism (discontinue permanently) · viral infection · weight increased
- **Rare or very rare** Meningitis · sepsis
- **Frequency not known** Angioedema · BK virus infection · cardiovascular event · interstitial lung disease (including fatal cases) · malignancy · reactivation of infections · ulcerative colitis aggravated

- **CONCEPTION AND CONTRACEPTION** Manufacturer advises effective contraception during and for at least 4 weeks after treatment in women of child-bearing potential.

- **PREGNANCY** Manufacturer advises avoid—toxicity in *animal* studies.
- **BREAST FEEDING** Manufacturer advises avoid—present in milk in *animal* studies.
- **HEPATIC IMPAIRMENT** Manufacturer advises caution in moderate impairment; avoid in severe impairment. **Dose adjustments** Manufacturer advises dose reduction in moderate impairment—consult product literature.
- **RENAL IMPAIRMENT**
  Dose adjustments Manufacturer advises reduce dose in severe impairment—consult product literature.
- **PRE-TREATMENT SCREENING** Manufacturer advises patients should be evaluated for tuberculosis and viral hepatitis before treatment.
- **MONITORING REQUIREMENTS**
- [EvGr] Monitor for signs and symptoms of infection during and after treatment.
- Monitor liver function routinely; monitor lipid profile 8 weeks after treatment initiation.
- Monitor lymphocytes at baseline and every 3 months thereafter; neutrophils and haemoglobin should be monitored at baseline, after 4 to 8 weeks of treatment and every 3 months thereafter.
- Periodic skin examination is recommended in all patients, particularly those at increased risk of skin cancer. Ⓜ
- **DIRECTIONS FOR ADMINISTRATION** [EvGr] *Xeljanz*® film-coated tablets may be crushed and taken with water. Ⓜ
- **PRESCRIBING AND DISPENSING INFORMATION** The manufacturer of *Xeljanz*® has provided a *Prescriber Brochure, Initiation Checklist*, and *Maintenance Checklist*.
- **PATIENT AND CARER ADVICE**
  Alert card A patient alert card should be provided.
- **NATIONAL FUNDING/ACCESS DECISIONS**
  For full details see funding body website
  NICE decisions
- **Tofacitinib for moderate-to-severe rheumatoid arthritis (October 2017)** NICE TA480 Recommended with restrictions
- **Tofacitinib for treating active psoriatic arthritis after inadequate response to DMARDs (October 2018)** NICE TA543 Recommended with restrictions
- **Tofacitinib for treating active ankylosing spondylitis (October 2023)** NICE TA920 Recommended with restrictions
- **Tofacitinib for moderately to severely active ulcerative colitis (November 2018)** NICE TA547 Recommended with restrictions

Scottish Medicines Consortium (SMC) decisions
- **Tofacitinib citrate (*Xeljanz*®) in combination with methotrexate for the treatment of moderate to severe active rheumatoid arthritis in adult patients who have responded inadequately to, or who are intolerant to one or more disease-modifying anti-rheumatic drugs (DMARDs). Tofacitinib can be given as monotherapy in case of intolerance to methotrexate or when treatment with methotrexate is inappropriate (February 2018)** SMC No. 1298/18 Recommended with restrictions
- **Tofacitinib (*Xeljanz*®) in combination with methotrexate for the treatment of active psoriatic arthritis in adult patients who have had an inadequate response or who have been intolerant to a prior disease-modifying antirheumatic drug (DMARD) therapy (January 2019)** SMC No. SMC2116 Recommended with restrictions
- **Tofacitinib (*Xeljanz*®) for the treatment of adult patients with active ankylosing spondylitis who have responded inadequately to conventional therapy (September 2022)** SMC No. SMC2463 Recommended
- **Tofacitinib (*Xeljanz*®) for the treatment of adult patients with moderately to severely active ulcerative colitis who have had an inadequate response, lost response, or were intolerant to either conventional therapy or a biologic agent (February 2019)** SMC No. SMC2122 Recommended

● **MEDICINAL FORMS** There can be variation in the licensing of
different medicines containing the same drug.

Oral tablet
▶ **Xeljanz** (Pfizer Ltd)
Tofacitinib (as Tofacitinib citrate) 5 mg Xeljanz 5mg tablets |
56 tablet [PoM] £690.03 (Hospital only)
Tofacitinib (as Tofacitinib citrate) 10 mg Xeljanz 10mg tablets |
56 tablet [PoM] £1,380.06 (Hospital only)

Modified-release tablet
CAUTIONARY AND ADVISORY LABELS 25
EXCIPIENTS:　May contain Sorbitol
▶ **Xeljanz** (Pfizer Ltd)
Tofacitinib (as Tofacitinib citrate) 11 mg Xeljanz 11mg modified-
release tablets | 28 tablet [PoM] £690.03 (Hospital only)

Upadacitinib　　　　　　　　　　　　24-Apr-2025

● **DRUG ACTION** Upadacitinib is a selective and reversible
inhibitor of the Janus-associated tyrosine kinase JAK1.

● INDICATIONS AND DOSE

Rheumatoid arthritis (under expert supervision) | Psoriatic arthritis (under expert supervision)
▶ BY MOUTH
▶ Adult:　15 mg once daily, consider discontinuation of
treatment if no response after 12 weeks, for treatment
interruption due to side-effects—consult product
literature

Ankylosing spondylitis (under expert supervision) | Non-radiographic axial spondyloarthritis (under expert supervision)
▶ BY MOUTH
▶ Adult:　15 mg once daily, consider discontinuation of
treatment if no response after 16 weeks, for treatment
interruption due to side-effects—consult product
literature

Atopic eczema (under expert supervision)
▶ BY MOUTH
▶ Adult:　15 mg once daily, a higher dose of 30 mg once
daily may be appropriate for certain patients—consult
product literature, consider discontinuation of
treatment if no response after 12 weeks, for treatment
interruption due to side-effects—consult product
literature
▶ Elderly:　15 mg once daily, consider discontinuation of
treatment if no response after 12 weeks, for treatment
interruption due to side-effects—consult product
literature

Ulcerative colitis (under expert supervision)
▶ BY MOUTH
▶ Adult:　Initially 45 mg once daily for 8 weeks, if an
adequate therapeutic response is not achieved after
8 weeks, the initial dose can be extended for an
additional 8 weeks, discontinue treatment if no
response after 16 weeks, for treatment interruption
due to side-effects—consult product literature, then
maintenance 15 mg once daily, a higher maintenance
dose of 30 mg once daily may be appropriate for certain
patients—consult product literature, for treatment
interruption due to side-effects—consult product
literature
▶ Elderly:　Initially 45 mg once daily for 8 weeks, if an
adequate therapeutic response is not achieved after
8 weeks, the initial dose can be extended for an
additional 8 weeks, discontinue treatment if no
response after 16 weeks, for treatment interruption
due to side-effects—consult product literature, then
maintenance 15 mg once daily, for treatment
interruption due to side-effects—consult product
literature

Crohn's disease (under expert supervision)
▶ BY MOUTH
▶ Adult:　Initially 45 mg once daily for 12 weeks, if an
adequate therapeutic response is not achieved after
12 weeks, the dose may be decreased to 30 mg once
daily and given for an additional 12 weeks, discontinue
treatment if no response after 24 weeks, for treatment
interruption due to side-effects—consult product
literature, then maintenance 15 mg once daily, a higher
maintenance dose of 30 mg once daily may be
appropriate for certain patients—consult product
literature, for treatment interruption due to side-
effects—consult product literature
▶ Elderly:　Initially 45 mg once daily for 12 weeks, if an
adequate therapeutic response is not achieved after
12 weeks, the dose may be decreased to 30 mg once
daily and given for an additional 12 weeks, discontinue
treatment if no response after 24 weeks, for treatment
interruption due to side-effects—consult product
literature, then maintenance 15 mg once daily, for
treatment interruption due to side-effects—consult
product literature

DOSE ADJUSTMENTS DUE TO INTERACTIONS
▶ When used for Ulcerative colitis or Crohn's disease [EvGr] Use
an initial dose of 30 mg once daily, and a maintenance
dose of 15 mg once daily with concurrent use of potent
CYP3A4 inhibitors. ⓜ

IMPORTANT SAFETY INFORMATION

MHRA/CHM ADVICE: UPADACITINIB (*RINVOQ*®): ADVICE FOR VENOUS THROMBOEMBOLISM (MARCH 2020)
Cases of deep vein thrombosis and pulmonary embolism
have been reported in patients taking upadacitinib.
Healthcare professionals are advised to use upadacitinib
with caution in patients with risk factors for venous
thromboembolism (VTE). Patients should be informed of
the signs and symptoms of VTE before starting
treatment and advised to seek urgent medical attention
if these develop. Upadacitinib should be discontinued if
clinical features of VTE occur.

MHRA/CHM ADVICE: JANUS KINASE (JAK) INHIBITORS: NEW MEASURES TO REDUCE RISKS OF MAJOR CARDIOVASCULAR EVENTS, MALIGNANCY, VENOUS THROMBOEMBOLISM, SERIOUS INFECTIONS AND INCREASED MORTALITY (APRIL 2023)
In 2022, the EMA conducted a review of all JAK
inhibitors indicated for chronic inflammatory diseases
and concluded that the risks associated with the use of
tofacitinib could be considered a class effect (see
Important safety information in tofacitinib p. 1265).
Following a further review by the MHRA, some existing
warnings for tofacitinib have been updated and
implemented for all JAK inhibitors included in the
review, such as upadacitinib.
　Healthcare professionals are advised to:
● avoid use in patients aged 65 years or older, in patients
who are current or past long-time smokers, and in
patients with other cardiovascular disease or
malignancy risk factors, unless there are no suitable
alternatives;
● use with caution in patients with risk factors for VTE;
● use lower doses in patients with risk factors, where
applicable;
● periodically examine all patients' skin for malignancy;
● inform patients and their carers of these risks, and the
signs and symptoms that warrant urgent medical
attention.

● **CONTRA-INDICATIONS** Absolute lymphocyte count less
than 0.5×10^9 cells/litre · absolute neutrophil count less
than 1×10^9 cells/litre · active serious infection including
localised infection · active tuberculosis · haemoglobin less
than 8 g/dL

- **CAUTIONS** Chronic or recurrent infection · elderly (65 years and older) · history of atherosclerotic cardiovascular disease or other cardiovascular risk factors · history of serious or opportunistic infection · patients at risk of gastro-intestinal perforation (new onset abdominal signs and symptoms should be evaluated promptly) · predisposition to infection · risk factors for deep-vein thrombosis or pulmonary embolism · risk factors for malignancy · risk of viral reactivation (consult product literature) · tuberculosis exposure

CAUTIONS, FURTHER INFORMATION

▸ Immunisation [EvGr] Patients should receive all recommended vaccinations, including prophylactic varicella-zoster vaccination, before starting treatment; live vaccines are not recommended. Ⓜ

▸ Tuberculosis [EvGr] Consider anti-tuberculosis therapy prior to initiation of upadacitinib in patients with previously untreated latent tuberculosis or in patients at risk of tuberculosis infection. Use upadacitinib with caution in patients who have travelled or resided in areas of endemic tuberculosis or endemic mycoses. Ⓜ

- **INTERACTIONS** → Appendix 1: upadacitinib

- **SIDE-EFFECTS**
▸ **Common or very common** Abdominal pain · anaemia · cough · dyslipidaemia · fatigue · fever · headache · increased risk of infection · lymphopenia · nausea · neoplasms · neutropenia · skin reactions · weight increased
▸ **Uncommon** Sepsis
▸ **Frequency not known** Cardiovascular event · deep vein thrombosis (discontinue and initiate treatment promptly) · gastrointestinal perforation · malignancy · meningitis bacterial · pulmonary embolism (discontinue and initiate treatment promptly) · reactivation of infections · venous thromboembolism (discontinue and initiate treatment promptly)

- **CONCEPTION AND CONTRACEPTION** Manufacturer advises females of childbearing potential should use effective contraception during and for 4 weeks after treatment.

- **PREGNANCY** Manufacturer advises avoid—toxicity in *animal* studies.

- **BREAST FEEDING** Manufacturer advises avoid—present in milk in *animal* studies.

- **HEPATIC IMPAIRMENT** [EvGr] Avoid in severe impairment (no information available). Ⓜ

- **RENAL IMPAIRMENT** [EvGr] Caution in severe impairment (limited information available). Ⓜ
Dose adjustments
▸ When used for Atopic eczema [EvGr] A dose of 15 mg once daily should not be exceeded in severe impairment. Ⓜ
▸ When used for Ulcerative colitis or Crohn's disease [EvGr] An initial dose of 30 mg once daily and a maintenance dose of 15 mg once daily should not be exceeded in severe impairment. Ⓜ

- **PRE-TREATMENT SCREENING** Manufacturer advises patients should be evaluated for tuberculosis and viral hepatitis before treatment.

- **MONITORING REQUIREMENTS**
▸ [EvGr] Monitor for signs and symptoms of infection during and after treatment.
▸ Monitor neutrophils, lymphocytes, and haemoglobin before and during treatment (no later than 12 weeks after initiation), and as clinically indicated thereafter; interrupt treatment if absolute neutrophil count less than 1 × 10^9 cells/litre, absolute lymphocyte count less than 0.5 × 10^9 cells/litre, or haemoglobin less than 8 g/dL—treatment may be restarted when levels return above these values.
▸ Monitor hepatic transaminases before starting treatment, and as clinically indicated thereafter—interrupt treatment if drug-induced liver injury suspected; monitor lipids

12 weeks after starting treatment, and then as clinically indicated.

▸ Monitor for viral hepatitis reactivation during treatment; if hepatitis B virus DNA is detected, consult liver specialist for advice.

▸ Periodic skin examination is recommended in all patients, particularly those at increased risk of skin cancer. Ⓜ

- **PRESCRIBING AND DISPENSING INFORMATION** The manufacturer of *Rinvoq*® has provided a guide for healthcare professionals.

- **PATIENT AND CARER ADVICE** A patient alert card should be provided.

- **NATIONAL FUNDING/ACCESS DECISIONS**
For full details see funding body website

NICE decisions
▸ **Upadacitinib for treating severe rheumatoid arthritis (December 2020)** NICE TA665 Recommended with restrictions
▸ **Upadacitinib for treating moderate rheumatoid arthritis (November 2021)** NICE TA744 Recommended with restrictions
▸ **Upadacitinib for treating active psoriatic arthritis after inadequate response to DMARDs (February 2022)** NICE TA768 Recommended with restrictions
▸ **Upadacitinib for treating active ankylosing spondylitis (September 2022)** NICE TA829 Recommended with restrictions
▸ **Upadacitinib for treating active non-radiographic axial spondyloarthritis (February 2023)** NICE TA861 Recommended with restrictions
▸ **Abrocitinib, tralokinumab or upadacitinib for treating moderate to severe atopic dermatitis (August 2022)** NICE TA814 Recommended with restrictions
▸ **Upadacitinib for treating moderately to severely active ulcerative colitis (January 2023)** NICE TA856 Recommended
▸ **Upadacitinib for previously treated moderately to severely active Crohn's disease (June 2023)** NICE TA905 Recommended with restrictions

Scottish Medicines Consortium (SMC) decisions
▸ **Upadacitinib (*Rinvoq*®) for the treatment of moderate to severe active rheumatoid arthritis in adult patients who have responded inadequately to, or who are intolerant to one or more disease-modifying antirheumatic drugs [in adults with severe disease] (February 2021)** SMC No. SMC2315 Recommended with restrictions
▸ **Upadacitinib (*Rinvoq*®) for the treatment of moderate to severe active rheumatoid arthritis in adult patients who have responded inadequately to, or who are intolerant to one or more disease-modifying anti-rheumatic drugs. Upadacitinib may be used as monotherapy or in combination with methotrexate [in adults with moderate disease] (December 2022)** SMC No. SMC2495 Recommended with restrictions
▸ **Upadacitinib (*Rinvoq*®) for the treatment of active psoriatic arthritis in adult patients who have responded inadequately to, or who are intolerant to one or more disease-modifying antirheumatic drugs. Upadacitinib may be used as monotherapy or in combination with methotrexate (May 2021)** SMC No. SMC2361 Recommended with restrictions
▸ **Upadacitinib (*Rinvoq*®) for the treatment of active ankylosing spondylitis in adult patients who have responded inadequately to conventional therapy (November 2022)** SMC No. SMC2480 Recommended
▸ **Upadacitinib (*Rinvoq*®) for the treatment of active non-radiographic axial spondyloarthritis in adult patients with objective signs of inflammation as indicated by elevated C-reactive protein and/or magnetic resonance imaging, who have responded inadequately to non-steroidal anti-inflammatory drugs (February 2023)** SMC No. SMC2532 Recommended
▸ **Upadacitinib (*Rinvoq*®) for the treatment of moderate to severe atopic dermatitis in adults and adolescents 12 years**

and older who are candidates for systemic therapy (April 2022) SMC No. SMC2417 Recommended with restrictions

▸ Upadacitinib (*Rinvoq*®) for the treatment of adult patients with moderately to severely active ulcerative colitis who have had an inadequate response, loss of response or were intolerant to either conventional therapy or a biologic agent (October 2022) SMC No. SMC2510 Recommended

▸ Upadacitinib (*Rinvoq*®) for the treatment of adult patients with moderately to severely active Crohn's disease who have had an inadequate response or, lost response or were intolerant to either conventional therapy or a biologic agent, or for whom such therapies are not advisable (June 2023) SMC No. SMC2575 Recommended

● **MEDICINAL FORMS** There can be variation in the licensing of different medicines containing the same drug.

Modified-release tablet

CAUTIONARY AND ADVISORY LABELS 25

▸ Rinvoq (AbbVie Ltd)

Upadacitinib (as Upadacitinib hemihydrate) **15 mg** Rinvoq 15mg modified-release tablets | 28 tablet [PoM] £805.56 (Hospital only)
Upadacitinib (as Upadacitinib hemihydrate) **30 mg** Rinvoq 30mg modified-release tablets | 28 tablet [PoM] £1,281.54 (Hospital only)
Upadacitinib (as Upadacitinib hemihydrate) **45 mg** Rinvoq 45mg modified-release tablets | 28 tablet [PoM] £2,087.10 (Hospital only)

IMMUNOSUPPRESSANTS ›T-CELL ACTIVATION INHIBITORS

Abatacept
10-Aug-2021

● **INDICATIONS AND DOSE**

Moderate-to-severe active rheumatoid arthritis (specialist use only) | Active psoriatic arthritis (specialist use only)

▸ BY INTRAVENOUS INFUSION

▸ Adult (body-weight up to 60 kg): 500 mg every 2 weeks for 3 doses, then 500 mg every 4 weeks, review treatment if no response within 6 months

▸ Adult (body-weight 60–100 kg): 750 mg every 2 weeks for 3 doses, then 750 mg every 4 weeks, review treatment if no response within 6 months

▸ Adult (body-weight 101 kg and above): 1 g every 2 weeks for 3 doses, then 1 g every 4 weeks, review treatment if no response within 6 months

Moderate-to-severe active rheumatoid arthritis (specialist use only) | Active psoriatic arthritis (specialist use only)

▸ BY SUBCUTANEOUS INJECTION

▸ Adult: 125 mg once weekly, review treatment if no response within 6 months, subcutaneous dosing may be initiated with or without an intravenous loading dose—consult product literature

● **CONTRA-INDICATIONS** Severe infection

● **CAUTIONS** Do not initiate until active infections are controlled · elderly (increased risk of side-effects) · predisposition to infection (screen for latent tuberculosis and viral hepatitis) · progressive multifocal leucoencephalopathy (discontinue treatment if neurological symptoms present)

● **INTERACTIONS** → Appendix 1: abatacept

● **SIDE-EFFECTS**

▸ **Common or very common** Asthenia · cough · diarrhoea · dizziness · gastrointestinal discomfort · headaches · hypertension · increased risk of infection · nausea · oral ulceration · skin reactions · vomiting

▸ **Uncommon** Alopecia · anxiety · arrhythmias · arthralgia · bruising tendency · conjunctivitis · depression · dry eye · dyspnoea · gastritis · hyperhidrosis · hypotension · influenza like illness · leucopenia · menstrual cycle irregularities · neoplasms · pain in extremity · palpitations · paraesthesia · respiratory disorders · sepsis · sleep disorders · throat tightness · thrombocytopenia · vasculitis ·

vasodilation · vertigo · visual acuity decreased · weight increased

▸ **Rare or very rare** Pelvic inflammatory disease

● **CONCEPTION AND CONTRACEPTION** Effective contraception required during treatment and for 14 weeks after last dose.

● **PREGNANCY** Manufacturer advises avoid unless essential.

● **BREAST FEEDING** Present in milk in *animal* studies—manufacturer advises avoid breast-feeding during treatment and for 14 weeks after last dose.

● **DIRECTIONS FOR ADMINISTRATION** For *intravenous infusion*, manufacturer advises give intermittently *in* Sodium chloride 0.9%; reconstitute each vial with 10 mL water for injections using the silicone-free syringe provided; dilute requisite dose in Sodium Chloride 0.9% to 100 mL (using the same silicone-free syringe); give over 30 minutes through a low protein-binding filter (pore size 0.2–1.2 micron).

● **NATIONAL FUNDING/ACCESS DECISIONS** For full details see funding body website

NICE decisions

▸ Adalimumab, etanercept, infliximab, rituximab, and abatacept for the treatment of rheumatoid arthritis after the failure of a TNF inhibitor (August 2010) NICE TA195 Recommended

▸ Adalimumab, etanercept, infliximab, certolizumab pegol, golimumab, tocilizumab and abatacept for rheumatoid arthritis not previously treated with DMARDs or after conventional DMARDs only have failed (January 2016) NICE TA375 Recommended with restrictions

▸ Adalimumab, etanercept, infliximab and abatacept for treating moderate rheumatoid arthritis after conventional DMARDs have failed (July 2021) NICE TA715 Not recommended

● **MEDICINAL FORMS** There can be variation in the licensing of different medicines containing the same drug.

Solution for injection

▸ Orencia (Imported (Germany), Bristol-Myers Squibb Pharmaceuticals Ltd)

Abatacept **125 mg per 1 ml** Orencia 50mg/0.4ml solution for injection pre-filled syringes | 4 pre-filled disposable injection [PoM] [℥] (Hospital only)
Orencia 125mg/1ml solution for injection pre-filled syringes | 4 pre-filled disposable injection [PoM] £1,209.60 (Hospital only)
Orencia 87.5mg/0.7ml solution for injection pre-filled syringes | 4 pre-filled disposable injection [PoM] [℥] (Hospital only)

▸ Orencia ClickJect (Bristol-Myers Squibb Pharmaceuticals Ltd)

Abatacept **125 mg per 1 ml** Orencia ClickJect 125mg/1ml solution for injection pre-filled pens | 4 pre-filled disposable injection [PoM] £1,209.60 DT = £1,209.60

Powder for solution for infusion

ELECTROLYTES: May contain Sodium

▸ Orencia (Bristol-Myers Squibb Pharmaceuticals Ltd)

Abatacept **250 mg** Orencia 250mg powder for concentrate for solution for infusion vials | 1 vial [PoM] £302.40 (Hospital only)

IMMUNOSUPPRESSANTS ›TUMOR NECROSIS FACTOR ALPHA (TNF-α) INHIBITORS

Adalimumab
15-Jan-2024

● **INDICATIONS AND DOSE**

Plaque psoriasis (initiated by a specialist)

▸ BY SUBCUTANEOUS INJECTION

▸ Adult: Initially 80 mg, then 40 mg every 2 weeks, to be started 1 week after initial dose, review treatment if no response within 16 weeks—consult product literature

Rheumatoid arthritis (initiated by a specialist)

▸ BY SUBCUTANEOUS INJECTION

▸ Adult: 40 mg every 2 weeks, then increased if necessary to 40 mg once weekly, alternatively 80 mg every 2 weeks, dose to be increased only in

continued →

patients receiving adalimumab alone, review treatment if no response within 12 weeks

Psoriatic arthritis (initiated by a specialist) | Ankylosing spondylitis (initiated by a specialist) | Axial spondyloarthritis (initiated by a specialist)
▶ BY SUBCUTANEOUS INJECTION
▶ Adult: 40 mg every 2 weeks, review treatment if no response within 12 weeks

Crohn's disease (initiated by a specialist)
▶ BY SUBCUTANEOUS INJECTION
▶ Adult: Initially 80 mg, then 40 mg after 2 weeks; maintenance 40 mg every 2 weeks, increased if necessary to 40 mg once weekly, alternatively 80 mg every 2 weeks, review treatment if no response within 12 weeks

Crohn's disease (accelerated regimen) (initiated by a specialist)
▶ BY SUBCUTANEOUS INJECTION
▶ Adult: Initially 160 mg, dose can alternatively be given as divided injections over 2 days, then 80 mg after 2 weeks; maintenance 40 mg every 2 weeks, increased if necessary to 40 mg once weekly, alternatively 80 mg every 2 weeks, review treatment if no response within 12 weeks

Ulcerative colitis (initiated by a specialist)
▶ BY SUBCUTANEOUS INJECTION
▶ Adult: Initially 160 mg, dose can alternatively be given as divided injections over 2 days, then 80 mg after 2 weeks, then maintenance 40 mg every 2 weeks, increased if necessary to 40 mg once weekly, alternatively 80 mg every 2 weeks, review treatment if no response within 8 weeks

Hidradenitis suppurativa (initiated by a specialist)
▶ BY SUBCUTANEOUS INJECTION
▶ Adult: Initially 160 mg, dose can alternatively be given as divided injections over 2 days, followed by 80 mg after 2 weeks, then maintenance 40 mg once weekly, after 2 weeks, alternatively 80 mg every 2 weeks, after 2 weeks, review treatment if no response within 12 weeks; if treatment interrupted—consult product literature

Uveitis (initiated by a specialist)
▶ BY SUBCUTANEOUS INJECTION
▶ Adult: Initially 80 mg, then 40 mg after 1 week; maintenance 40 mg every 2 weeks

● **CONTRA-INDICATIONS** Moderate or severe heart failure · severe infections
● **CAUTIONS** Demyelinating disorders (risk of exacerbation) · development of malignancy · do not initiate until active infections are controlled (discontinue if new serious infection develops) · hepatitis B virus—monitor for active infection · history of malignancy · mild heart failure (discontinue if symptoms develop or worsen) · predisposition to infection
CAUTIONS, FURTHER INFORMATION
▶ Tuberculosis Active tuberculosis should be treated with standard treatment for at least 2 months before starting adalimumab. Patients who have previously received adequate treatment for tuberculosis can start adalimumab but should be monitored every 3 months for possible recurrence. In patients without active tuberculosis but who were previously not treated adequately, chemoprophylaxis should ideally be completed before starting adalimumab. In patients at high risk of tuberculosis who cannot be assessed by tuberculin skin test, chemoprophylaxis can be given concurrently with adalimumab.

● **INTERACTIONS** → Appendix 1: monoclonal antibodies

● **SIDE-EFFECTS**
▶ **Common or very common** Agranulocytosis · alopecia · anaemia · anxiety · arrhythmias · asthma · broken nails · chest pain · coagulation disorder · connective tissue disorders · cough · dehydration · depression · dyspnoea · electrolyte imbalance · eye inflammation · fever · flushing · gastrointestinal discomfort · gastrointestinal disorders · haemorrhage · headaches · healing impaired · hyperglycaemia · hypersensitivity · hypertension · increased risk of infection · insomnia · leucocytosis · leucopenia · mood altered · muscle spasms · musculoskeletal pain · nausea · neoplasms · nerve disorders · neutropenia · oedema · renal impairment · seasonal allergy · sensation abnormal · sepsis · skin reactions · sweat changes · thrombocytopenia · vertigo · vision disorders · vomiting
▶ **Uncommon** Aortic aneurysm · arterial occlusion · congestive heart failure · deafness · dysphagia · embolism and thrombosis · erectile dysfunction · gallbladder disorders · hepatic disorders · inflammation · interstitial lung disease · lupus erythematosus · meningitis viral · myocardial infarction · nocturia · pancreatitis · respiratory disorders · rhabdomyolysis · sarcoidosis · solid organ neoplasm · stroke · tinnitus · tremor · vasculitis
▶ **Rare or very rare** Bone marrow disorders · cardiac arrest · demyelinating disorders · pulmonary fibrosis · reactivation of infections · Stevens-Johnson syndrome
▶ **Frequency not known** Weight increased
SIDE-EFFECTS, FURTHER INFORMATION Associated with infections, sometimes severe, including tuberculosis, septicaemia, and hepatitis B reactivation.
● **CONCEPTION AND CONTRACEPTION** Manufacturer advises effective contraception required during treatment and for at least 5 months after last dose.
● **PREGNANCY** Manufacturer advises use only if potential benefit outweighs risk.
● **BREAST FEEDING** Manufacturer advises can be used—excreted in breast milk at very low concentrations (limited information available).
● **PRE-TREATMENT SCREENING**
Tuberculosis Manufacturer advises patients should be evaluated for active and latent tuberculosis before treatment.
● **MONITORING REQUIREMENTS**
▶ Manufacturer advises monitor for infection before, during, and for 4 months after treatment.
▶ Manufacturer advises monitor for non-melanoma skin cancer before and during treatment, especially in patients with a history of PUVA treatment for psoriasis or extensive immunosuppressant therapy.
▶ *For uveitis*, manufacturer advises patients should be assessed for pre-existing or developing central demyelinating disorders before and at regular intervals during treatment.
● **PRESCRIBING AND DISPENSING INFORMATION**
Adalimumab is a biological medicine. Biological medicines must be prescribed and dispensed by brand name, see *Biological medicines* and *Biosimilar medicines*, under Guidance on prescribing p. 1.
● **PATIENT AND CARER ADVICE** When used to treat *hidradenitis suppurativa*, patients and their carers should be advised to use a daily topical antiseptic wash on lesions during treatment with adalimumab.
Tuberculosis Patients and their carers should be advised to seek medical attention if symptoms suggestive of tuberculosis (e.g. persistent cough, weight loss, and fever) develop.
Blood disorders Patients and their carers should be advised to seek medical attention if symptoms suggestive of blood disorders (such as fever, sore throat, bruising, or bleeding) develop.

Alert card An alert card should be provided.

- **NATIONAL FUNDING/ACCESS DECISIONS**
  For full details see funding body website
  NICE decisions
- ▸ **Infliximab and adalimumab for Crohn's disease (May 2010)** NICE TA187 Recommended
- ▸ **Infliximab, adalimumab and golimumab for treating moderately to severely active ulcerative colitis after the failure of conventional therapy (February 2015)** NICE TA329 Recommended with restrictions
- ▸ **Etanercept, infliximab, and adalimumab for the treatment of psoriatic arthritis (August 2010)** NICE TA199 Recommended with restrictions
- ▸ **Adalimumab, etanercept, infliximab, rituximab, and abatacept for the treatment of rheumatoid arthritis after the failure of a TNF inhibitor (August 2010)** NICE TA195 Recommended with restrictions
- ▸ **Adalimumab, etanercept, infliximab, certolizumab pegol, golimumab, tocilizumab and abatacept for rheumatoid arthritis not previously treated with DMARDs or after conventional DMARDs only have failed (January 2016)** NICE TA375 Recommended with restrictions
- ▸ **Adalimumab, etanercept, infliximab and abatacept for treating moderate rheumatoid arthritis after conventional DMARDs have failed (July 2021)** NICE TA715 Recommended with restrictions
- ▸ **TNF-alpha inhibitors for ankylosing spondylitis and non-radiographic axial spondyloarthritis (February 2016)** NICE TA383 Recommended
- ▸ **Adalimumab for treating moderate-to-severe hidradenitis suppurativa (June 2016)** NICE TA392 Recommended with restrictions
- ▸ **Adalimumab for plaque psoriasis in adults (June 2008)** NICE TA146 Recommended with restrictions
- ▸ **Adalimumab and dexamethasone for treating non-infectious uveitis (July 2017)** NICE TA460 Recommended
  Scottish Medicines Consortium (SMC) decisions
- ▸ **Adalimumab (*Humira*®) for moderate to severe chronic plaque psoriasis in adult patients (June 2008)** SMC No. 468/08 Recommended with restrictions

- **MEDICINAL FORMS** There can be variation in the licensing of different medicines containing the same drug.
  Solution for injection
  CAUTIONARY AND ADVISORY LABELS 10
  - ▸ **Amgevita** (Amgen Ltd)
    Adalimumab 50 mg per 1 ml Amgevita 20mg/0.4ml solution for injection pre-filled syringes | 1 pre-filled disposable injection PoM £158.40 (Hospital only)
    Amgevita 40mg/0.8ml solution for injection pre-filled syringes | 2 pre-filled disposable injection PoM £633.60 (Hospital only)
    Amgevita 40mg/0.8ml solution for injection pre-filled pens | 2 pre-filled disposable injection PoM £633.60 (Hospital only)
    Adalimumab 100 mg per 1 ml Amgevita 80mg/0.8ml solution for injection pre-filled syringes | 1 pre-filled disposable injection PoM £633.60 (Hospital only)
    Amgevita 80mg/0.8ml solution for injection pre-filled pens | 1 pre-filled disposable injection PoM £633.60 (Hospital only) | 2 pre-filled disposable injection PoM £1,267.20 (Hospital only)
    Amgevita 20mg/0.2ml solution for injection pre-filled syringes | 1 pre-filled disposable injection PoM £158.40 (Hospital only)
    Amgevita 40mg/0.4ml solution for injection pre-filled syringes | 2 pre-filled disposable injection PoM £633.60 DT = £704.28 (Hospital only)
    Amgevita 40mg/0.4ml solution for injection pre-filled pens | 2 pre-filled disposable injection PoM £633.60 DT = £704.28 (Hospital only)
  - ▸ **Humira** (AbbVie Ltd)
    Adalimumab 100 mg per 1 ml Humira 40mg/0.4ml solution for injection pre-filled pens | 2 pre-filled disposable injection PoM £704.28 DT = £704.28
    Humira 80mg/0.8ml solution for injection pre-filled pens | 1 pre-filled disposable injection PoM £704.28
    Humira 20mg/0.2ml solution for injection pre-filled syringes | 2 pre-filled disposable injection PoM £352.14 DT = £352.14
    Humira 40mg/0.4ml solution for injection pre-filled syringes | 2 pre-filled disposable injection PoM £704.28 DT = £704.28

- ▸ **Hyrimoz** (Sandoz Ltd)
  Adalimumab 50 mg per 1 ml Hyrimoz 40mg/0.8ml solution for injection pre-filled syringes | 2 pre-filled disposable injection PoM £646.18
  Adalimumab 100 mg per 1 ml Hyrimoz 40mg/0.4ml solution for injection pre-filled syringes | 2 pre-filled disposable injection PoM £646.18 DT = £704.28
  Hyrimoz 40mg/0.4ml solution for injection pre-filled pens | 2 pre-filled disposable injection PoM £646.18 DT = £704.28 (Hospital only)
- ▸ **Idacio** (Fresenius Kabi Ltd)
  Adalimumab 50 mg per 1 ml Idacio 40mg/0.8ml solution for injection vials | 1 vial PoM £316.93 (Hospital only)
  Idacio 40mg/0.8ml solution for injection pre-filled syringes | 2 pre-filled disposable injection PoM £633.86
  Idacio 40mg/0.8ml solution for injection pre-filled pens | 2 pre-filled disposable injection PoM £633.86 (Hospital only)
- ▸ **Imraldi** (Biogen Idec Ltd)
  Adalimumab 50 mg per 1 ml Imraldi 40mg/0.8ml solution for injection pre-filled pens | 2 pre-filled disposable injection PoM £633.85
  Imraldi 40mg/0.8ml solution for injection pre-filled syringes | 2 pre-filled disposable injection PoM £633.85
  Adalimumab 100 mg per 1 ml Imraldi 40mg/0.4ml solution for injection pre-filled syringes | 2 pre-filled disposable injection PoM £633.85 DT = £704.28 (Hospital only)
  Imraldi 40mg/0.4ml solution for injection pre-filled pens | 2 pre-filled disposable injection PoM £633.85 DT = £704.28 (Hospital only)
- ▸ **Yuflyma** (Celltrion Healthcare UK Ltd) ▼
  Adalimumab 100 mg per 1 ml Yuflyma 40mg/0.4ml solution for injection pre-filled pens | 2 pre-filled disposable injection PoM £633.70 DT = £704.28
  Yuflyma 80mg/0.8ml solution for injection pre-filled pens | 1 pre-filled disposable injection PoM £633.70 (Hospital only)
  Yuflyma 20mg/0.2ml solution for injection pre-filled syringes | 2 pre-filled disposable injection PoM £316.93 DT = £352.14

Certolizumab pegol
12-Dec-2022

- **INDICATIONS AND DOSE**
  Moderate to severe active rheumatoid arthritis when response to disease-modifying antirheumatic drugs [including methotrexate] has been inadequate [as monotherapy or in combination with methotrexate] (initiated by a specialist) | Severe, active and progressive rheumatoid arthritis in patients not previously treated with methotrexate or other disease-modifying antirheumatic drugs [in combination with methotrexate] (initiated by a specialist) | Active psoriatic arthritis when response to disease-modifying antirheumatic drugs has been inadequate [as monotherapy or in combination with methotrexate] (initiated by a specialist)
  - ▸ BY SUBCUTANEOUS INJECTION
  - ▸ Adult: Loading dose 400 mg every 2 weeks for 3 doses, then maintenance 200 mg every 2 weeks, once clinical response is confirmed, an alternative maintenance dosing of 400 mg every 4 weeks can be considered, review treatment if no response within 12 weeks

  Severe active ankylosing spondylitis in patients who have had an inadequate response to, or are intolerant of NSAIDs (initiated by a specialist) | Severe active axial spondyloarthritis, without radiographic evidence of ankylosing spondylitis but with objective signs of inflammation, in patients who have had an inadequate response to, or are intolerant of NSAIDs (initiated by a specialist)
  - ▸ BY SUBCUTANEOUS INJECTION
  - ▸ Adult: Loading dose 400 mg every 2 weeks for 3 doses, then maintenance 200 mg every 2 weeks, alternatively maintenance 400 mg every 4 weeks, review treatment if no response within 12 weeks, after at least 1 year of treatment, an alternative maintenance dosing of 200 mg every 4 weeks can be considered in patients with sustained remission

continued →

Musculoskeletal system

Moderate to severe plaque psoriasis (initiated by a specialist)
▶ BY SUBCUTANEOUS INJECTION
▶ Adult: Loading dose 400 mg every 2 weeks for 3 doses, then maintenance 200 mg every 2 weeks, an alternative maintenance dosing of 400 mg every 2 weeks can be considered in patients with insufficient response, review treatment if no response within 16 weeks

● CONTRA-INDICATIONS Moderate to severe heart failure · severe active infection

● CAUTIONS Chronic obstructive pulmonary disease (risk of malignancy) · demyelinating CNS disorders (risk of exacerbation) · do not initiate until active infections are controlled (discontinue if new serious infection develops and until infection controlled) · elderly (risk of infections) · hepatitis B virus (monitor for active infection) · history or development of malignancy · mild heart failure (discontinue if symptoms develop or worsen) · predisposition to infection

CAUTIONS, FURTHER INFORMATION
▶ Tuberculosis Active tuberculosis should be treated with standard treatment for at least 2 months before starting certolizumab pegol. Patients who have previously received adequate treatment for tuberculosis can start certolizumab pegol but should be monitored every 3 months for possible recurrence. In patients without active tuberculosis but who were previously not treated adequately, chemoprophylaxis should ideally be completed before starting certolizumab pegol. In patients at high risk of tuberculosis who cannot be assessed by tuberculin skin test, chemoprophylaxis can be given concurrently with certolizumab pegol.

● INTERACTIONS → Appendix 1: monoclonal antibodies

● SIDE-EFFECTS
▶ Common or very common Abscess · asthenia · decreased leucocytes · eosinophilic disorders · fever · headaches · hepatic disorders · hypertension · increased risk of infection · nausea · neutropenia · pain · sensory disorder · skin reactions
▶ Uncommon Alopecia · anaemia · anxiety · appetite disorder · arrhythmias · ascites · asthma · breast disorder · cardiomyopathy · chills · coronary artery disease · cough · cyst · dizziness · dyslipidaemia · electrolyte imbalance · embolism and thrombosis · eye inflammation · flushing · gastrointestinal discomfort · gastrointestinal disorders · haemorrhage · healing impaired · heart failure · hypercoagulation · hypersensitivity · influenza like illness · lacrimation disorder · lupus erythematosus · lymphadenopathy · menstrual cycle irregularities · mood disorder · multi organ failure · muscle disorder · nail disorder · neoplasms · nerve disorders · oedema · oral disorders · oropharyngeal dryness · palpitations · photosensitivity reaction · renal impairment · respiratory disorders · sepsis · skin ulcer · solid organ neoplasm · sweat changes · syncope · temperature perception abnormal · thrombocytopenia · thrombocytosis · tinnitus · tremor · urinary tract disorder · vasculitides · vertigo · vision disorders · weight change
▶ Rare or very rare Angioedema · atherosclerosis · atrioventricular block · cholelithiasis · cognitive impairment · delirium · dermatomyositis exacerbated · fistula · haemosiderosis · hair texture abnormal · interstitial lung disease · movement disorders · nephritis · nephropathy · odynophagia · pancytopenia · panniculitis · pericarditis · polycythaemia · Raynaud's phenomenon · sarcoidosis · seizure · sexual dysfunction · splenomegaly · Stevens-Johnson syndrome · stroke · suicide attempt · telangiectasia · thyroid disorder
▶ Frequency not known Azoospermia · hepatitis B reactivation · multiple sclerosis

SIDE-EFFECTS, FURTHER INFORMATION Associated with infections, sometimes severe, including tuberculosis, septicaemia, and hepatitis B reactivation.

● CONCEPTION AND CONTRACEPTION Manufacturer advises adequate contraception in women of childbearing potential during treatment and for 5 months after last dose.

● PREGNANCY Manufacturer advises use only if potential benefit outweighs risk—limited information available.

● PRE-TREATMENT SCREENING
Tuberculosis Patients should be evaluated for tuberculosis before treatment.

● MONITORING REQUIREMENTS Monitor for infection before, during, and for 5 months after treatment.

● DIRECTIONS FOR ADMINISTRATION [EvGr] Allow the preparation to reach room temperature prior to administration. Inject into the thigh or abdomen (except for around the navel); rotate injection site and avoid skin that is red, bruised, or hard. ⓜ Patients may self-administer *Cimzia®* after appropriate training in preparation and administration.

● PRESCRIBING AND DISPENSING INFORMATION
Certolizumab pegol is a biological medicine. Biological medicines must be prescribed and dispensed by brand name, see *Biological medicines* and *Biosimilar medicines*, under Guidance on prescribing p. 1; record the brand name and batch number after each administration.

● HANDLING AND STORAGE Store in a refrigerator (2–8°C) and protect from light; may be stored at room temperature (below 25°C) for max. 10 days, then discarded.

● PATIENT AND CARER ADVICE
Blood disorders Patients should be advised to seek medical attention if symptoms suggestive of blood disorders (such as fever, sore throat, bruising, or bleeding) develop.
Tuberculosis Patients should be advised to seek medical attention if symptoms suggestive of tuberculosis (e.g. persistent cough, weight loss and fever) develop.
Self-administration Patients and their carers should be given training in subcutaneous injection technique.
Alert card An alert card should be provided.

● NATIONAL FUNDING/ACCESS DECISIONS
For full details see funding body website
NICE decisions
▶ Adalimumab, etanercept, infliximab, certolizumab pegol, golimumab, tocilizumab and abatacept for rheumatoid arthritis not previously treated with DMARDs or after conventional DMARDs only have failed (January 2016) NICE TA375 Recommended with restrictions
▶ TNF-alpha inhibitors for ankylosing spondylitis and non-radiographic axial spondyloarthritis (February 2016) NICE TA383 Recommended
▶ Certolizumab pegol for treating rheumatoid arthritis after inadequate response to a TNF-alpha inhibitor (October 2016) NICE TA415 Recommended with restrictions
▶ Certolizumab pegol and secukinumab for treating active psoriatic arthritis after inadequate response to DMARDs (May 2017) NICE TA445 Recommended with restrictions
▶ Certolizumab pegol for treating moderate to severe plaque psoriasis (April 2019) NICE TA574 Recommended with restrictions

Scottish Medicines Consortium (SMC) decisions
▶ Certolizumab pegol (*Cimzia®*) for the treatment of moderate to severe plaque psoriasis in adults who are candidates for systemic therapy (April 2019) SMC No. SMC2132 Recommended with restrictions

- **MEDICINAL FORMS** There can be variation in the licensing of different medicines containing the same drug.

Solution for injection

CAUTIONARY AND ADVISORY LABELS 10

▸ **Cimzia** (UCB Pharma Ltd)
Certolizumab pegol 200 mg per 1 ml Cimzia 200mg/1ml solution for injection in a dose-dispenser cartridge | 2 cartridge [PoM] £715.00 (Hospital only)
Cimzia 200mg/1ml solution for injection pre-filled syringes | 2 syringe [PoM] £715.00 (Hospital only)
Cimzia 200mg/1ml solution for injection pre-filled pens | 2 pre-filled disposable injection [PoM] £715.00 (Hospital only)

Etanercept

14-Mar-2022

- **INDICATIONS AND DOSE**

Rheumatoid arthritis (initiated by a specialist) | Psoriatic arthritis (initiated by a specialist) | Ankylosing spondylitis (initiated by a specialist) | Non-radiographic axial spondyloarthritis (initiated by a specialist)

▸ BY SUBCUTANEOUS INJECTION
▸ Adult: 25 mg twice weekly, alternatively 50 mg once weekly, review treatment if no response within 12 weeks of initial dose

Plaque psoriasis (initiated by a specialist)

▸ BY SUBCUTANEOUS INJECTION
▸ Adult: 25 mg twice weekly, alternatively 50 mg once weekly, alternatively 50 mg twice weekly for up to 12 weeks, followed by 25 mg twice weekly, alternatively 50 mg once weekly if required for up to 24 weeks—continuous therapy beyond 24 weeks may be appropriate in some patients (consult product literature), discontinue if no response after 12 weeks

- **CONTRA-INDICATIONS** Active infection
- **CAUTIONS** Development of malignancy · diabetes mellitus · heart failure (risk of exacerbation) · hepatitis B virus—monitor for active infection · hepatitis C infection (monitor for worsening infection) · history of blood disorders · history of malignancy · history or increased risk of demyelinating disorders · predisposition to infection (avoid if predisposition to septicaemia) · significant exposure to herpes zoster virus—interrupt treatment and consider varicella–zoster immunoglobulin

CAUTIONS, FURTHER INFORMATION

▸ Tuberculosis Active tuberculosis should be treated with standard treatment for at least 2 months before starting etanercept. Patients who have previously received adequate treatment for tuberculosis can start etanercept but should be monitored every 3 months for possible recurrence. In patients without active tuberculosis but who were previously not treated adequately, chemoprophylaxis should ideally be completed before starting etanercept. In patients at high risk of tuberculosis who cannot be assessed by tuberculin skin test, chemoprophylaxis can be given concurrently with etanercept.

- **INTERACTIONS** → Appendix 1: etanercept
- **SIDE-EFFECTS**

▸ **Common or very common** Cystitis · fever · headache · hypersensitivity · increased risk of infection · skin reactions
▸ **Uncommon** Abscess · anaemia · angioedema · bursitis · cholecystitis · diarrhoea · endocarditis · eye inflammation · gastritis · heart failure · hepatic disorders · inflammatory bowel disease · leucopenia · myositis · neoplasms · neutropenia · sepsis · skin ulcers · thrombocytopenia · vasculitis
▸ **Rare or very rare** Bone marrow disorders · cutaneous lupus erythematosus · demyelination · interstitial lung disease · lupus-like syndrome · nerve disorders · pulmonary fibrosis ·

sarcoidosis · seizure · severe cutaneous adverse reactions (SCARs) · transverse myelitis

▸ **Frequency not known** Dermatomyositis exacerbated · hepatitis B reactivation

SIDE-EFFECTS, FURTHER INFORMATION Associated with infections, sometimes severe, including tuberculosis, septicaemia, and hepatitis B reactivation.

- **CONCEPTION AND CONTRACEPTION** Manufacturer advises effective contraception required during treatment and for 3 weeks after last dose.
- **PREGNANCY** [EvGr] Use only if essential. ◈M◈
- **BREAST FEEDING** Manufacturer advises avoid—present in milk in *animal* studies.
- **HEPATIC IMPAIRMENT** Manufacturer advises caution in moderate to severe alcoholic hepatitis.
- **PRE-TREATMENT SCREENING**
Tuberculosis Patients should be evaluated for tuberculosis before treatment.
- **MONITORING REQUIREMENTS** [EvGr] Monitor for skin cancer during treatment, particularly in patients with risk factors or psoriasis. ◈M◈
- **PRESCRIBING AND DISPENSING INFORMATION** Etanercept is a biological medicine. Biological medicines must be prescribed and dispensed by brand name, see *Biological medicines* and *Biosimilar medicines*, under Guidance on prescribing p. 1.
- **HANDLING AND STORAGE** Store in a refrigerator (2–8°C)—consult product literature for further information regarding storage conditions outside refrigerator.
- **PATIENT AND CARER ADVICE**
Blood disorders Patients and their carers should be advised to seek medical attention if symptoms suggestive of blood disorders (such as fever, sore throat, bruising, or bleeding) develop.
Tuberculosis Patients and their carers should be advised to seek medical attention if symptoms suggestive of tuberculosis (e.g. persistent cough, weight loss, and fever) develop.
Patient card A patient card should be provided.
- **NATIONAL FUNDING/ACCESS DECISIONS**
For full details see funding body website

NICE decisions

▸ **Etanercept and efalizumab for plaque psoriasis (July 2006)** NICE TA103 Recommended with restrictions
▸ **Adalimumab, etanercept, infliximab, rituximab, and abatacept for the treatment of rheumatoid arthritis after the failure of a TNF inhibitor (August 2010)** NICE TA195 Recommended with restrictions
▸ **Adalimumab, etanercept, infliximab, certolizumab pegol, golimumab, tocilizumab and abatacept for rheumatoid arthritis not previously treated with DMARDs or after conventional DMARDs only have failed (January 2016)** NICE TA375 Recommended with restrictions
▸ **Adalimumab, etanercept, infliximab and abatacept for treating moderate rheumatoid arthritis after conventional DMARDs have failed (July 2021)** NICE TA715 Recommended with restrictions
▸ **Etanercept, infliximab, and adalimumab for the treatment of psoriatic arthritis (August 2010)** NICE TA199 Recommended with restrictions
▸ **TNF-alpha inhibitors for ankylosing spondylitis and non-radiographic axial spondyloarthritis (February 2016)** NICE TA383 Recommended

Musculoskeletal system

- **MEDICINAL FORMS** There can be variation in the licensing of different medicines containing the same drug.

Solution for injection

CAUTIONARY AND ADVISORY LABELS 10

▸ Benepali (Biogen Idec Ltd)

Etanercept 50 mg per 1 ml Benepali 25mg/0.5ml solution for injection pre-filled syringes | 4 pre-filled disposable injection [PoM] £328.00 (Hospital only)

Benepali 50mg/1ml solution for injection pre-filled pens | 4 pre-filled disposable injection [PoM] £656.00 (Hospital only)

Benepali 50mg/1ml solution for injection pre-filled syringes | 4 pre-filled disposable injection [PoM] £656.00 (Hospital only)

▸ Enbrel (Pfizer Ltd)

Etanercept 50 mg per 1 ml Enbrel 50mg/1ml solution for injection pre-filled syringes | 4 pre-filled disposable injection [PoM] £715.00 (Hospital only)

Enbrel 25mg/0.5ml solution for injection pre-filled syringes | 4 pre-filled disposable injection [PoM] £357.50 (Hospital only)

▸ Enbrel MyClic (Pfizer Ltd)

Etanercept 50 mg per 1 ml Enbrel 25mg/0.5ml solution for injection pre-filled MyClic pens | 4 pre-filled disposable injection [PoM] £357.50 (Hospital only)

Enbrel 50mg/1ml solution for injection pre-filled MyClic pens | 4 pre-filled disposable injection [PoM] £715.00 (Hospital only)

▸ Erelzi (Sandoz Ltd) ▼

Etanercept 50 mg per 1 ml Erelzi 50mg/1ml solution for injection pre-filled pens | 4 pre-filled disposable injection [PoM] £643.50 (Hospital only)

Erelzi 50mg/1ml solution for injection pre-filled syringes | 4 pre-filled disposable injection [PoM] £643.50 (Hospital only)

Erelzi 25mg/0.5ml solution for injection pre-filled syringes | 4 pre-filled disposable injection [PoM] £321.75 (Hospital only)

Powder and solvent for solution for injection

CAUTIONARY AND ADVISORY LABELS 10

▸ Enbrel (Pfizer Ltd)

Etanercept 10 mg Enbrel Paediatric 10mg powder and solvent for solution for injection vials | 4 vial [PoM] £143.00 (Hospital only)

Etanercept 25 mg Enbrel 25mg powder and solvent for solution for injection vials | 4 vial [PoM] £357.50 (Hospital only)

Golimumab

06-Nov-2020

- **INDICATIONS AND DOSE**

Ulcerative colitis (initiated by a specialist)

▸ BY SUBCUTANEOUS INJECTION

▸ Adult (body-weight up to 80 kg): Initially 200 mg, then 100 mg after 2 weeks; maintenance 50 mg every 4 weeks, alternatively maintenance 100 mg every 4 weeks, if inadequate response, review treatment if no response after 4 doses

▸ Adult (body-weight 80 kg and above): Initially 200 mg, then 100 mg after 2 weeks; maintenance 100 mg every 4 weeks, review treatment if no response after 4 doses

Rheumatoid arthritis (initiated by a specialist) | Psoriatic arthritis (initiated by a specialist) | Ankylosing spondylitis (initiated by a specialist) | Non-radiographic axial spondyloarthritis (initiated by a specialist)

▸ BY SUBCUTANEOUS INJECTION

▸ Adult (body-weight up to 100 kg): 50 mg once a month, on the same date each month, review treatment if no response after 3–4 doses

▸ Adult (body-weight 100 kg and above): Initially 50 mg once a month for 3–4 doses, on the same date each month, dose may be increased if inadequate response, increased to 100 mg once a month, review treatment if inadequate response to this higher dose after 3–4 doses

- **CONTRA-INDICATIONS** Moderate or severe heart failure · severe active arthinfection

- **CAUTIONS** Active infection (do not initiate until active infections are controlled; discontinue if new serious infection develops until infection controlled) · demyelinating disorders (risk of exacerbation) · hepatitis B virus—monitor for active infection · history or development of malignancy · mild heart failure (discontinue if symptoms develop or worsen) · predisposition to infection · risk factors for dysplasia or carcinoma of the colon—screen for dysplasia regularly

CAUTIONS, FURTHER INFORMATION

▸ Tuberculosis Active tuberculosis should be treated with standard treatment for at least 2 months before starting golimumab. Patients who have previously received adequate treatment for tuberculosis can start golimumab but should be monitored every 3 months for possible recurrence. In patients without active tuberculosis but who were previously not treated adequately, chemoprophylaxis should ideally be completed before starting golimumab. In patients at high risk of tuberculosis who cannot be assessed by tuberculin skin test, chemoprophylaxis can be given concurrently with golimumab. Patients who have tested negative for latent tuberculosis, and those who are receiving or who have completed treatment for latent tuberculosis, should be monitored closely for symptoms of active infection.

- **INTERACTIONS** → Appendix 1: monoclonal antibodies

- **SIDE-EFFECTS**

▸ **Common or very common** Abscess · alopecia · anaemia · asthenia · asthma · bone fracture · chest discomfort · depression · dizziness · fever · gastrointestinal discomfort · gastrointestinal disorders · gastrointestinal inflammatory disorders · headache · hypersensitivity · hypertension · increased risk of infection · insomnia · nausea · paraesthesia · respiratory disorders · skin reactions · stomatitis

▸ **Uncommon** Arrhythmia · balance impaired · bone marrow disorders · breast disorder · cholelithiasis · constipation · eye inflammation · eye irritation · flushing · goitre · hyperthyroidism · hypothyroidism · interstitial lung disease · leucopenia · liver disorder · menstrual disorder · myocardial ischaemia · neoplasms · sepsis · thrombocytopenia · thrombosis · thyroid disorder · vision disorders

▸ **Rare or very rare** Bladder disorder · congestive heart failure · demyelination · healing impaired · hepatitis B reactivation · lupus-like syndrome · Raynaud's phenomenon · renal disorder · sarcoidosis · taste altered · vasculitis

SIDE-EFFECTS, FURTHER INFORMATION Associated with infections, sometimes severe, including tuberculosis, septicaemia, and hepatitis B reactivation.

- **CONCEPTION AND CONTRACEPTION** Manufacturer advises adequate contraception during treatment and for at least 6 months after last dose.

- **PREGNANCY** Use only if essential.

- **BREAST FEEDING** Manufacturer advises avoid during and for at least 6 months after treatment—present in milk in *animal* studies.

- **HEPATIC IMPAIRMENT** Manufacturer advises caution (no information available).

- **PRE-TREATMENT SCREENING**

Tuberculosis Patients should be evaluated for tuberculosis before treatment.

- **MONITORING REQUIREMENTS** Monitor for infection before, during, and for 5 months after treatment.

- **DIRECTIONS FOR ADMINISTRATION** For doses requiring multiple injections, each injection should be administered at a different site.

Missed dose If dose administered more than 2 weeks late, manufacturer advises subsequent doses should be administered on the new monthly due date.

- **PATIENT AND CARER ADVICE**

Tuberculosis All patients and their carers should be advised to seek medical attention if symptoms suggestive of tuberculosis (e.g. persistent cough, weight loss, and fever) develop.

Blood disorders Patients and their carers should be advised to seek medical attention if symptoms suggestive of blood disorders (such as fever, sore throat, bruising, or bleeding) develop.

Alert card An alert card should be provided.

- ● NATIONAL FUNDING/ACCESS DECISIONS
  For full details see funding body website

  NICE decisions
  - ▸ Golimumab for the treatment of psoriatic arthritis (April 2011) NICE TA220 Recommended with restrictions
  - ▸ Adalimumab, etanercept, infliximab, certolizumab pegol, golimumab, tocilizumab and abatacept for rheumatoid arthritis not previously treated with DMARDs or after conventional DMARDs only have failed (January 2016) NICE TA375 Recommended with restrictions
  - ▸ Golimumab for the treatment of rheumatoid arthritis after the failure of previous disease-modifying anti-rheumatic drugs (June 2011) NICE TA225 Recommended with restrictions
  - ▸ TNF-alpha inhibitors for ankylosing spondylitis and non-radiographic axial spondyloarthritis (February 2016) NICE TA383 Recommended
  - ▸ Golimumab for treating non-radiographic axial spondyloarthritis (January 2018) NICE TA497 Recommended with restrictions
  - ▸ Infliximab, adalimumab and golimumab for treating moderately to severely active ulcerative colitis after the failure of conventional therapy (February 2015) NICE TA329 Recommended with restrictions

  Scottish Medicines Consortium (SMC) decisions
  - ▸ Golimumab 50 mg (*Simponi*®) for the treatment of active and progressive psoriatic arthritis in adult patients (July 2012) SMC No. 674/11 Recommended with restrictions
  - ▸ Golimumab (*Simponi*®) for the treatment of adults with severe non-radiographic axial spondyloarthritis with objective signs of inflammation as indicated by elevated C-reactive protein and/or magnetic resonance imaging (MRI) evidence, who have had an inadequate response to, or are intolerant to non-steroidal anti-inflammatory drugs (February 2016) SMC No. 1124/16 Recommended

- ● MEDICINAL FORMS There can be variation in the licensing of different medicines containing the same drug.

  Solution for injection
  CAUTIONARY AND ADVISORY LABELS 10
  - ▸ Simponi (Janssen-Cilag Ltd)
    Golimumab 100 mg per 1 ml Simponi 100mg/1ml solution for injection pre-filled pens | 1 pre-filled disposable injection [PoM] £1,525.94 DT = £1,525.94
    Simponi 50mg/0.5ml solution for injection pre-filled syringes | 1 pre-filled disposable injection [PoM] £762.97 DT = £762.97
    Simponi 50mg/0.5ml solution for injection pre-filled pens | 1 pre-filled disposable injection [PoM] £762.97 DT = £762.97

Infliximab

25-Feb-2022

- ● **INDICATIONS AND DOSE**

  Active Crohn's disease (under expert supervision)
  - ▸ BY INTRAVENOUS INFUSION
  - ▸ Adult: Initially 5 mg/kg, then 5 mg/kg after 2 weeks, then 5 mg/kg, to be taken at 6 weeks after initial dose if condition has responded; discontinue if no response within 6 weeks of initial infusion (after 2 doses), then maintenance 5 mg/kg every 8 weeks, maintenance treatment can be restarted after a drug-free interval if symptoms recur within 16 weeks of the last infusion. Consult product literature for dose escalation in selected patients

  - ▸ INITIALLY BY INTRAVENOUS INFUSION
  - ▸ Adult: Initially 5 mg/kg, then (by intravenous infusion) 5 mg/kg after 2 weeks; (by subcutaneous injection) maintenance 120 mg every 2 weeks, subcutaneous maintenance dosing to be started 4 weeks after the second of the initial intravenous infusions if a response has been seen. Discontinue if no response within 6 weeks of the initial infusion (after 2 doses). Treatment can be restarted after a drug-free interval if symptoms recur within 16 weeks of the last dose—consult product literature

  Fistulating Crohn's disease (under expert supervision)
  - ▸ BY INTRAVENOUS INFUSION
  - ▸ Adult: Initially 5 mg/kg, then 5 mg/kg, to be taken at week 2 and 6 after initial dose, discontinue if no response after initial 3 doses, then maintenance 5 mg/kg every 8 weeks, maintenance treatment can be restarted after a drug-free interval if symptoms recur within 16 weeks of the last infusion

  - ▸ INITIALLY BY INTRAVENOUS INFUSION
  - ▸ Adult: Initially 5 mg/kg, followed by (by intravenous infusion) 5 mg/kg after 2 weeks; (by subcutaneous injection) maintenance 120 mg every 2 weeks, subcutaneous maintenance dosing to be started 4 weeks after the second of the initial intravenous infusions. Discontinue if no response after 6 doses in total. Treatment can be restarted after a drug-free interval if symptoms recur within 16 weeks of the last dose—consult product literature

  Active ulcerative colitis (under expert supervision)
  - ▸ BY INTRAVENOUS INFUSION
  - ▸ Adult: Initially 5 mg/kg, then 5 mg/kg, to be taken at week 2 and 6 after initial dose, then 5 mg/kg every 8 weeks, consider discontinuation if no response within 14 weeks after initial infusion (3 doses)

  - ▸ INITIALLY BY INTRAVENOUS INFUSION
  - ▸ Adult: Initially 5 mg/kg, then (by intravenous infusion) 5 mg/kg after 2 weeks; (by subcutaneous injection) maintenance 120 mg every 2 weeks, subcutaneous maintenance dosing to be started 4 weeks after the second of the initial intravenous infusions. Consider discontinuation if no response within 14 weeks (after 6 doses in total)

  Rheumatoid arthritis (in combination with methotrexate) (under expert supervision)
  - ▸ BY INTRAVENOUS INFUSION
  - ▸ Adult: Initially 3 mg/kg, then 3 mg/kg, to be taken at week 2 and 6 after initial dose, then 3 mg/kg every 8 weeks, dose to be increased only if response is inadequate after 12 weeks of initial treatment; increased if necessary to 3 mg/kg every 4 weeks, alternatively increased in steps of 1.5 mg/kg every 8 weeks (max. per dose 7.5 mg/kg every 8 weeks), consider discontinuation if no response within 12 weeks of initial infusion (after 3 doses) or after dose adjustment. Maintenance treatment can be restarted after a drug-free interval if symptoms recur within 16 weeks of the last infusion

  - ▸ INITIALLY BY INTRAVENOUS INFUSION
  - ▸ Adult: Initially 3 mg/kg, then (by intravenous infusion) 3 mg/kg after 2 weeks; (by subcutaneous injection) maintenance 120 mg every 2 weeks, subcutaneous maintenance dosing to be started 4 weeks after the second of the initial intravenous infusions. Consider discontinuation if no response within 12 weeks of the initial infusion. Treatment can be restarted after a drug-free interval if symptoms recur within 16 weeks of the last dose—consult product literature continued →

Ankylosing spondylitis (under expert supervision)
▶ BY INTRAVENOUS INFUSION
▶ Adult: Initially 5 mg/kg, then 5 mg/kg, to be taken at week 2 and 6 after initial dose, then 5 mg/kg every 6–8 weeks, discontinue if no response by 6 weeks of initial infusion (after 2 doses)
▶ INITIALLY BY INTRAVENOUS INFUSION
▶ Adult: Initially 5 mg/kg, followed by (by intravenous infusion) 5 mg/kg after 2 weeks; (by subcutaneous injection) maintenance 120 mg every 2 weeks, subcutaneous maintenance dosing to be started 4 weeks after the second of the initial intravenous infusions. Discontinue if no response within 6 weeks of the initial infusion (after 2 doses)

Psoriatic arthritis (under expert supervision)
▶ BY INTRAVENOUS INFUSION
▶ Adult: Initially 5 mg/kg, then 5 mg/kg, to be taken at week 2 and 6 after initial dose, followed by 5 mg/kg every 8 weeks
▶ INITIALLY BY INTRAVENOUS INFUSION
▶ Adult: Initially 5 mg/kg, followed by (by intravenous infusion) 5 mg/kg after 2 weeks; (by subcutaneous injection) maintenance 120 mg every 2 weeks, subcutaneous maintenance dosing to be started 4 weeks after the second of the initial intravenous infusions

Plaque psoriasis (under expert supervision)
▶ BY INTRAVENOUS INFUSION
▶ Adult: Initially 5 mg/kg, then 5 mg/kg, to be taken at week 2 and 6 after initial dose, then 5 mg/kg every 8 weeks, discontinue if no response after 14 weeks of initial infusion (after 4 doses)
▶ INITIALLY BY INTRAVENOUS INFUSION
▶ Adult: Initially 5 mg/kg, followed by (by intravenous infusion) 5 mg/kg after 2 weeks; (by subcutaneous injection) maintenance 120 mg every 2 weeks, subcutaneous maintenance dosing to be started 4 weeks after the second of the initial intravenous infusions. Discontinue if no response after 14 weeks of the initial infusion (after 7 doses in total)

IMPORTANT SAFETY INFORMATION
Adequate resuscitation facilities must be available when infliximab is used.

● **CONTRA-INDICATIONS** Moderate or severe heart failure · severe infections
● **CAUTIONS** Demyelinating disorders (risk of exacerbation) · dermatomyositis · development of malignancy · hepatitis B virus—monitor for active infection · history of colon carcinoma (in inflammatory bowel disease) · history of dysplasia (in inflammatory bowel disease) · history of malignancy · history of prolonged immunosuppressant or PUVA treatment in patients with psoriasis · mild heart failure (discontinue if symptoms develop or worsen) · predisposition to infection (discontinue if new serious infection develops) · risk of delayed hypersensitivity reactions if drug-free interval exceeds 16 weeks (re-administration after interval exceeding 16 weeks not recommended)

CAUTIONS, FURTHER INFORMATION
▶ Infection Manufacturer advises patients should be up-to-date with current immunisation schedule before initiating treatment.
▶ Tuberculosis Manufacturer advises to evaluate patients for active and latent tuberculosis before treatment. Active tuberculosis should be treated with standard treatment for at least 2 months before starting infliximab. If latent tuberculosis is diagnosed, treatment should be started before commencing treatment with infliximab. Patients who have previously received adequate treatment for

tuberculosis can start infliximab but should be monitored every 3 months for possible recurrence. In patients without active tuberculosis but who were previously not treated adequately, chemoprophylaxis should ideally be completed before starting infliximab. In patients at high risk of tuberculosis who cannot be assessed by tuberculin skin test, chemoprophylaxis can be given concurrently with infliximab. Patients should be advised to seek medical attention if symptoms suggestive of tuberculosis develop (e.g. persistent cough, weight loss and fever).
▶ Hypersensitivity reactions Hypersensitivity reactions (including fever, chest pain, hypotension, hypertension, dyspnoea, transient visual loss, pruritus, urticaria, serum sickness-like reactions, angioedema, anaphylaxis) reported during or within 1–2 hours after infusion (risk greatest during first or second infusion or in patients who discontinue other immunosuppressants). Manufacturer advises prophylactic antipyretics, antihistamines, or hydrocortisone may be administered.

● **INTERACTIONS** → Appendix 1: monoclonal antibodies
● **SIDE-EFFECTS**
▶ **Common or very common** Abscess · alopecia · anaemia · arrhythmias · arthralgia · chest pain · chills · constipation · decreased leucocytes · depression · diarrhoea · dizziness · dyspnoea · eye inflammation · fatigue · fever · gastrointestinal discomfort · gastrointestinal disorders · haemorrhage · headache · hepatic disorders · hyperhidrosis · hypertension · hypotension · increased risk of infection · infusion related reaction · insomnia · lymphadenopathy · myalgia · nausea · neutropenia · oedema · pain · palpitations · respiratory disorders · sensation abnormal · sepsis · skin reactions · vasodilation · vertigo
▶ **Uncommon** Anxiety · cheilitis · cholecystitis · confusion · drowsiness · healing impaired · heart failure · hypersensitivity · lupus erythematosus · lymphocytosis · memory loss · neoplasms · nerve disorders · pancreatitis · peripheral ischaemia · pulmonary oedema · seborrhoea · seizure · syncope · thrombocytopenia · thrombophlebitis
▶ **Rare or very rare** Agranulocytosis · circulatory collapse · cyanosis · demyelinating disorders · granuloma · haemolytic anaemia · hepatitis B reactivation · interstitial lung disease · meningitis · pancytopenia · pericardial effusion · pulmonary fibrosis · sarcoid-like reaction · severe cutaneous adverse reactions (SCARs) · transverse myelitis · vasculitis · vasospasm
▶ **Frequency not known** Dermatomyositis exacerbated · hepatosplenic T-cell lymphoma (increased risk in inflammatory bowel disease) · myocardial infarction · myocardial ischaemia · sarcoidosis · stroke · vision loss
● **CONCEPTION AND CONTRACEPTION** Manufacturer advises adequate contraception during and for at least 6 months after last dose.
● **PREGNANCY** Use only if essential.
● **BREAST FEEDING** Specialist sources indicate amount present in milk probably too small to be harmful.
● **PRE-TREATMENT SCREENING**
Tuberculosis Manufacturer advises patients should be evaluated for tuberculosis before treatment.
● **MONITORING REQUIREMENTS**
▶ Monitor for infection before, during, and for 6 months after treatment.
▶ All patients should be observed carefully for 1–2 hours after infusion and resuscitation equipment should be available for immediate use (risk of hypersensitivity reactions).
▶ Monitor for symptoms of delayed hypersensitivity if re-administered after a prolonged period.
▶ Manufacturer advises periodic skin examination for non-melanoma skin cancer, particularly in patients with risk factors.

- **DIRECTIONS FOR ADMINISTRATION** [EvGr] For *intermittent intravenous infusion,* dilute reconstituted solution with Sodium Chloride 0.9%. Reconstitute each 100 mg vial with 10 mL Water for Injections using a 21-gauge or smaller needle and gently swirl vial without shaking to dissolve; allow to stand for 5 minutes. Dilute requisite dose with infusion fluid to a usual final volume of 250 mL (maximum concentration 4 mg/mL). Give over 2 hours through a low protein-binding filter (1.2 micron or less); adults who have tolerated 3 initial 2-hour infusions may be given subsequent infusions of up to 6 mg/kg over at least 1 hour. Start infusion within 3 hours of reconstitution. ⟨M⟩

- **PRESCRIBING AND DISPENSING INFORMATION** Infliximab is a biological medicine. Biological medicines must be prescribed and dispensed by brand name, see *Biological medicines* and *Biosimilar medicines*, under Guidance on prescribing p. 1.

- **HANDLING AND STORAGE** Store in a refrigerator (2–8°C)—consult product literature for further information regarding storage outside refrigerator.

- **PATIENT AND CARER ADVICE**
  Tuberculosis Patients and carers should be advised to seek medical attention if symptoms suggestive of tuberculosis (e.g. persistent cough, weight loss, and fever) develop.
  Blood disorders Patients and carers should be advised to seek medical attention if symptoms suggestive of blood disorders (such as fever, sore throat, bruising, or bleeding) develop.
  Hypersensitivity reactions Patients and carers should be advised to keep Alert card with them at all times and seek medical advice if symptoms of delayed hypersensitivity develop.
  Self-administration Manufacturer advises patients may self-administer *Remsima*® pre-filled syringes or pens following training in subcutaneous injection technique.
  Alert card An alert card should be provided.
  Driving and skilled tasks Manufacturer advises patients and carers should be counselled on the effects on driving and performance of skilled tasks—increased risk of dizziness.

- **NATIONAL FUNDING/ACCESS DECISIONS**
  For full details see funding body website
  NICE decisions
  ▸ Infliximab for plaque psoriasis in adults (January 2008) NICE TA134 Recommended with restrictions
  ▸ Adalimumab, etanercept, infliximab, rituximab, and abatacept for the treatment of rheumatoid arthritis after the failure of a **TNF** inhibitor (August 2010) NICE TA195 Recommended with restrictions
  ▸ Adalimumab, etanercept, infliximab, certolizumab pegol, golimumab, tocilizumab and abatacept for rheumatoid arthritis not previously treated with DMARDs or after conventional DMARDs only have failed (January 2016) NICE TA375 Recommended with restrictions
  ▸ Adalimumab, etanercept, infliximab and abatacept for treating moderate rheumatoid arthritis after conventional DMARDs have failed (July 2021) NICE TA715 Recommended with restrictions
  ▸ Etanercept, infliximab, and adalimumab for the treatment of psoriatic arthritis (August 2010) NICE TA199 Recommended with restrictions
  ▸ Infliximab and adalimumab for Crohn's disease (May 2010) NICE TA187 Recommended with restrictions
  ▸ Infliximab for acute exacerbations of ulcerative colitis (December 2008) NICE TA163 Recommended with restrictions
  ▸ Infliximab, adalimumab and golimumab for treating moderately to severely active ulcerative colitis after the failure of conventional therapy (February 2015) NICE TA329 Recommended with restrictions

▸ TNF-alpha inhibitors for ankylosing spondylitis and non-radiographic axial spondyloarthritis (February 2016) NICE TA383 Recommended

- **MEDICINAL FORMS** There can be variation in the licensing of different medicines containing the same drug.
  Solution for injection
  CAUTIONARY AND ADVISORY LABELS 10
  EXCIPIENTS: May contain Polysorbates
  ▸ Remsima (Celltrion Healthcare UK Ltd)
  Infliximab 120 mg per 1 ml Remsima 120mg/1ml solution for injection pre-filled pens | 2 pre-filled disposable injection [PoM] £755.32
  Powder for solution for infusion
  CAUTIONARY AND ADVISORY LABELS 10
  EXCIPIENTS: May contain Polysorbates
  ▸ Flixabi (Biogen Idec Ltd)
  Infliximab 100 mg Flixabi 100mg powder for concentrate for solution for infusion vials | 1 vial [PoM] £377.00 (Hospital only)
  ▸ Remicade (Janssen-Cilag Ltd)
  Infliximab 100 mg Remicade 100mg powder for concentrate for solution for infusion vials | 1 vial [PoM] £419.62 (Hospital only)
  ▸ Remsima (Celltrion Healthcare UK Ltd)
  Infliximab 100 mg Remsima 100mg powder for concentrate for solution for infusion vials | 1 vial [PoM] £377.66 (Hospital only)
  ▸ Zessly (Sandoz Ltd) ▼
  Infliximab 100 mg Zessly 100mg powder for concentrate for solution for infusion vials | 1 vial [PoM] £377.66 (Hospital only)

PHOSPHODIESTERASE TYPE-4 INHIBITORS

Apremilast
02-Aug-2021

- **DRUG ACTION** Apremilast inhibits the activity of phosphodiesterase type-4 (PDE4) which results in suppression of pro-inflammatory mediator synthesis and promotes anti-inflammatory mediators.

- **INDICATIONS AND DOSE**
  Active psoriatic arthritis (in combination with disease-modifying antirheumatic drugs or alone) in patients who have had an inadequate response or who have been intolerant to a prior disease-modifying antirheumatic drug therapy | Moderate to severe chronic plaque psoriasis that has not responded to standard systemic treatments or photochemotherapy, or when these treatments cannot be used because of intolerance or contra-indications
  ▸ BY MOUTH
  ▸ Adult: Initially 10 mg daily on day 1, then 10 mg twice daily on day 2, then 10 mg in the morning and 20 mg in the evening on day 3, then 20 mg twice daily on day 4, then 20 mg in the morning and 30 mg in the evening on day 5, then maintenance 30 mg twice daily, doses should be taken approximately 12 hours apart; review treatment if no response within 24 weeks of initiation

> **IMPORTANT SAFETY INFORMATION**
> MHRA/CHM ADVICE (JANUARY 2017): APREMILAST (*OTEZLA*®): RISK OF SUICIDAL THOUGHTS AND BEHAVIOUR
> A review of evidence from clinical trials and postmarketing cases has suggested a causal association between apremilast and suicidal thoughts and behaviour.

- **CAUTIONS** Concomitant use of drugs likely to cause psychiatric symptoms · history of psychiatric illness · low body-weight—consider discontinuation if weight loss is unexplained or clinically significant

- **INTERACTIONS** → Appendix 1: phosphodiesterase type-4 inhibitors

- **SIDE-EFFECTS**
  ▸ Common or very common Appetite decreased · back pain · cough · depression · diarrhoea · fatigue · gastrointestinal

10
Musculoskeletal system

discomfort · gastrointestinal disorders · headaches · increased risk of infection · insomnia · nausea · vomiting
► **Uncommon** Gastrointestinal haemorrhage · rash · suicidal behaviours · weight decreased

● **CONCEPTION AND CONTRACEPTION** Exclude pregnancy before treatment and ensure effective contraception during treatment.

● **PREGNANCY** Avoid—teratogenic in *animal* studies.

● **BREAST FEEDING** Manufacturer advises avoid—present in milk in *animal* studies.

● **RENAL IMPAIRMENT**
Dose adjustments EvGr Reduce dose if eGFR less than 30 mL/minute/1.73 m^2; consult product literature for initial dose titration. M See p. 21.

● **MONITORING REQUIREMENTS**
► Manufacturer advises monitor body-weight regularly in patients underweight at the start of treatment.
► Manufacturer advises monitor for psychiatric symptoms (including depression, suicidal ideation and behaviour)— discontinue treatment if new or worsening psychiatric symptoms are identified.

● **PATIENT AND CARER ADVICE** Manufacturer advises patients and carers should be instructed to notify the prescriber of any changes in behaviour or mood, and of any suicidal ideation.

● **NATIONAL FUNDING/ACCESS DECISIONS**
For full details see funding body website
NICE decisions
► **Apremilast for treating active psoriatic arthritis (February 2017)** NICE TA433 Recommended with restrictions
► **Apremilast for treating moderate to severe plaque psoriasis (November 2016)** NICE TA419 Recommended with restrictions

Scottish Medicines Consortium (SMC) decisions
► Apremilast (*Otezla*®) alone or in combination with disease modifying anti-rheumatic drugs (DMARDs), for the treatment of active psoriatic arthritis (PsA) in adult patients who have had an inadequate response or who have been intolerant to a prior DMARD therapy (June 2015) SMC No. 1053/15 Recommended with restrictions
► Apremilast (*Otezla*®) for the treatment of moderate to severe chronic plaque psoriasis in adult patients who have failed to respond to or who have a contra-indication to, or are intolerant to other systemic therapy including ciclosporin, methotrexate or psoralen and ultraviolet A light (PUVA) (June 2015) SMC No. 1052/15 Recommended

● **MEDICINAL FORMS** There can be variation in the licensing of different medicines containing the same drug.
Oral tablet
CAUTIONARY AND ADVISORY LABELS 25
► **Otezla** (Amgen Ltd)
Apremilast 10 mg Otezla 10mg tablets | 4 tablet PoM ⚠
Apremilast 20 mg Otezla 20mg tablets | 4 tablet PoM ⚠
Apremilast 30 mg Otezla 30mg tablets | 56 tablet PoM £550.00 DT = £550.00

Form unstated
CAUTIONARY AND ADVISORY LABELS 25
► **Otezla** (Amgen Ltd)
Otezla tablets treatment initiation pack | 27 tablet PoM £265.18

2   Hyperuricaemia and gout

Gout

21-Jul-2022

Overview

Gout is a common form of inflammatory arthritis characterised by raised uric acid concentration in the blood (hyperuricaemia) and the deposition of urate crystals in joints and other tissues. It occurs in distinct phases— asymptomatic hyperuricaemia, a period of acute attacks (flares) followed by variable intervals (months to years) of no attacks, and a final period of chronic tophaceous gout, where individuals have nodules affecting joints. EvGr Specialist referral or advice should be sought for the management of gout during pregnancy, in individuals aged under 30 years, or in those with complications (such as joint damage, renal stones). Ⓐ

Acute attacks of gout

EvGr Treatment for an acute attack of gout should be started as soon as possible. Acute attacks are usually treated with either colchicine p. 1279, high doses of an NSAID (excluding aspirin), or a short course of an oral corticosteroid. Consider prescribing a proton pump inhibitor for patients on NSAIDs. Ⓐ

Colchicine has a narrow therapeutic range and its use is limited by the development of toxicity at higher doses. However, unlike NSAIDs, it does not induce fluid retention; moreover, it can be co-administered with anticoagulants.
EvGr If NSAIDs or colchicine are unsuitable, an intra-articular [unlicensed use] or intramuscular injection of a corticosteroid can be considered. Joint aspiration may also be considered in certain patients with acute monoarticular gout (under specialist guidance).
Combination treatment can be considered for acute attacks of gout in patients with an inadequate response to monotherapy.
An interleukin-1 inhibitor can be considered for the treatment of acute attacks of gout in patients in whom NSAIDs, colchicine, and corticosteroids are unsuitable or ineffective (under specialist guidance). Ⓐ

Long-term control of gout

EvGr All patients with gout should be offered urate-lowering therapy, particularly those with multiple or troublesome acute attacks, chronic gouty arthritis, chronic kidney disease stages 3 to 5, large crystal deposits (tophi), or those on diuretic therapy. A treat-to-target strategy should be used when offering urate-lowering therapy, this involves starting with a low dose of therapy and using monthly serum urate levels to guide dose increases, as tolerated, until the target serum urate level is reached.
Aim for a target serum urate level below 360 micromol/litre. However, for patients with tophi, chronic gouty arthritis, or those who have frequent flares with a serum urate level below 360 micromol/litre, consider aiming for a target serum urate level below 300 micromol/litre.
For long-term control of gout, the formation of uric acid from purines may be reduced with the xanthine-oxidase inhibitors, allopurinol p. 1280 or febuxostat p. 1280. Either option may be offered as first-line treatment, taking into account the patient's preference and co-morbidities. Treatment should be started at least 2 to 4 weeks after a gout flare has settled, but if flares are more frequent, urate-lowering therapy can be started during a flare. Uricosuric drugs, such as sulfinpyrazone or benzbromarone (specialist use—available from 'special-order' manufacturers or specialist importing companies), may be used as urate-lowering therapy in patients who are resistant to or are intolerant of xanthine-oxidase inhibitors; they increase the excretion of uric acid in the urine. Uricosuric drugs may also be used in combination with xanthine-oxidase inhibitors in patients who have an inadequate response to monotherapy.
The initiation or up-titration of urate-lowering therapy may precipitate an acute attack, therefore colchicine should be offered as prophylaxis while the target serum urate level is being reached (treatment duration should be decided after factors such as flare frequency, gout duration, and the presence and size of tophi have been assessed). A low-dose

NSAID or a low-dose oral corticosteroid are alternative options if colchicine is unsuitable or ineffective. Consider co-prescribing a proton pump inhibitor with the NSAID or corticosteroid. An interleukin-1 inhibitor can be considered in patients in whom colchicine, NSAIDs, or corticosteroids are unsuitable or ineffective (under specialist guidance). If an acute attack develops during treatment, the urate-lowering therapy should continue at the same dosage and the acute attack treated separately.

Patients with gout and a history of urolithiasis should be advised to ensure adequate daily fluid intake and avoid dehydration. Alkalinisation of the urine with potassium citrate can be considered in recurrent stone formers. ⟨A⟩

Useful resources

Gout: diagnosis and management. National Institute for Health and Care Excellence. NICE guideline 219. June 2022.
www.nice.org.uk/guidance/ng219

The British Society for Rheumatology Guideline for the Management of Gout. British Society for Rheumatology. July 2017.
www.rheumatology.org.uk/practice-quality/guidelines

Other drugs used for Hyperuricaemia and gout
Canakinumab, p. 975 · Diclofenac potassium, p. 1296 · Diclofenac sodium, p. 1297 · Etoricoxib, p. 1300 · Indometacin, p. 1305 · Ketoprofen, p. 1306 · Naproxen, p. 1310 · Sulindac, p. 1313

ALKALOIDS ⟩ PLANT ALKALOIDS

Colchicine
04-Apr-2025

- ● **INDICATIONS AND DOSE**

Acute gout
▶ BY MOUTH
▸ Adult: 500 micrograms 2–4 times a day until symptoms relieved, total dose per course should not exceed 6 mg, do not repeat course within 3 days

Short-term prophylaxis of gout during initial therapy with allopurinol and uricosuric drugs
▶ BY MOUTH
▸ Adult: 500 micrograms twice daily

Prophylaxis of familial Mediterranean fever (recurrent polyserositis) (under expert supervision)
▶ BY MOUTH
▸ Adult: 1–3 mg daily in 1–2 divided doses, dose increased in increments up to maximum 3 mg per day; monitor closely for side-effects

DOSE ADJUSTMENTS DUE TO INTERACTIONS
▸ Manufacturer advises reduce dose by half with concurrent use of moderate inhibitors of CYP3A4.
▸ Manufacturer advises reduce dose by 75% (to one quarter of usual dose) with concurrent use of potent inhibitors of CYP3A4 or P-glycoprotein inhibitors; avoid concurrent use in patients with hepatic or renal impairment.

- ● **UNLICENSED USE** BNF doses may differ from those in the product literature.

IMPORTANT SAFETY INFORMATION
MHRA/CHM ADVICE: COLCHICINE: REMINDER ON RISK OF SERIOUS AND FATAL TOXICITY IN OVERDOSE (NOVEMBER 2009)
Colchicine has a narrow therapeutic window and a risk of serious and fatal toxicity in overdose. Patients at particular risk are those with renal or hepatic impairment, gastro-intestinal or cardiac disease, and patients at extremes of age. Colchicine overdose is complex and specialist advice should be promptly obtained. There is often a delay of up to 6 hours before

---

toxicity is apparent, and some features of toxicity may be delayed by 1 week or longer. Healthcare professionals are advised to refer all patients, even in the absence of early symptoms, for immediate medical assessment. Further information on the presentation and management of colchicine overdose is available from TOXBASE.

- ● **CONTRA-INDICATIONS** Blood disorders
- ● **CAUTIONS** Cardiac disease · elderly · gastro-intestinal disease

CAUTIONS, FURTHER INFORMATION
▸ Elderly Screening Tool of Older Persons' potentially inappropriate Prescriptions (STOPP) criteria to aid medication reviews (see Prescribing in the elderly p. 31 for information). Potentially inappropriate:
- ● if eGFR less than 10 mL/minute/1.73 m^2 (contra-indicated in severe renal impairment; risk of toxicity)
- ● for chronic treatment of gout where there is no contra-indication to a xanthine-oxidase inhibitor (xanthine-oxidase inhibitors are first choice prophylactic drugs in gout)

- ● **INTERACTIONS** → Appendix 1: colchicine
- ● **SIDE-EFFECTS**
▸ **Common or very common** Abdominal pain · diarrhoea · nausea · vomiting
▸ **Frequency not known** Agranulocytosis · alopecia · bone marrow disorders · gastrointestinal haemorrhage · kidney injury · liver injury · menstrual cycle irregularities · myopathy · nerve disorders · rash · sperm abnormalities · thrombocytopenia

Overdose Early signs of toxicity include abdominal pain, diarrhoea, nausea, and vomiting. Features after 1 to 7 days include arrhythmias, bone marrow depression, confusion, decreased cardiac output, hepatic impairment, hyperpyrexia, renal impairment, and respiratory distress.

- ● **PREGNANCY** Specialist sources indicate that, although teratogenicity was noted in *animal* studies, human data suggested risk to the fetus is low.
- ● **BREAST FEEDING** [EvGr] Present in milk. ⟨M⟩ Specialist sources indicate use with caution and note that no adverse effects have been reported in the breast-fed infant. Breast feeding can be delayed for 6–8 hours after a maternal dose to avoid peak milk concentrations.
- ● **HEPATIC IMPAIRMENT** [EvGr] Caution in mild to moderate impairment; avoid in severe impairment. ⟨M⟩
Dose adjustments
▸ When used for Prophylaxis of familial Mediterranean fever (recurrent polyserositis) [EvGr] Reduce initial dose to ≤1 mg once daily in mild to moderate impairment. ⟨M⟩
- ● **RENAL IMPAIRMENT** [EvGr] Caution in mild to moderate impairment; avoid in severe impairment. ⟨M⟩ See p. 21.
Dose adjustments [EvGr] Reduce dose or increase dosage interval if eGFR 10–50 mL/minute/1.73 m^2. ⟨A⟩
▸ When used for Prophylaxis of familial Mediterranean fever (recurrent polyserositis) [EvGr] Reduce initial dose to ≤1 mg once daily in mild to moderate impairment. ⟨M⟩
- ● **MONITORING REQUIREMENTS** [EvGr] Monitor full blood count periodically in patients on long-term therapy. ⟨M⟩
- ● **DIRECTIONS FOR ADMINISTRATION** [EvGr] Some tablet formulations may be dispersed in water and taken orally immediately, or administered via a nasogastric tube—consult product literature. ⟨M⟩
- ● **PATIENT AND CARER ADVICE** Patients and their carers should be instructed to stop treatment and seek urgent medical attention if signs or symptoms of toxicity or blood disorders occur.
▸ When used for Acute gout Patients and their carers should be counselled on how colchicine should be used, including when to stop treatment, total dose per course, and when the course can be repeated.

- **MEDICINAL FORMS** There can be variation in the licensing of different medicines containing the same drug.
  Oral tablet
  ▸ Colchicine (Non-proprietary)
    Colchicine 500 microgram Colchicine 500microgram tablets | 28 tablet [PoM] £2.54 | 100 tablet [PoM] £21.95 DT = £2.35

XANTHINE OXIDASE INHIBITORS

Allopurinol

12-Mar-2025

- ● **INDICATIONS AND DOSE**
  Prophylaxis of gout and of uric acid and calcium oxalate renal stones | Prophylaxis of hyperuricaemia associated with cancer chemotherapy
  ▸ BY MOUTH
  ▸ Adult: Initially 100 mg once daily, to be taken preferably after food, for maintenance adjust dose according to plasma- or urinary-uric acid concentration

  Prophylaxis of gout and of uric acid and calcium oxalate renal stones (usual maintenance in mild conditions) | Prophylaxis of hyperuricaemia associated with cancer chemotherapy (usual maintenance in mild conditions)
  ▸ BY MOUTH
  ▸ Adult: 100–200 mg once daily, to be taken preferably after food

  Prophylaxis of gout and of uric acid and calcium oxalate renal stones (usual maintenance in moderately severe conditions) | Prophylaxis of hyperuricaemia associated with cancer chemotherapy (usual maintenance in moderately severe conditions)
  ▸ BY MOUTH
  ▸ Adult: 300–600 mg once daily, to be taken preferably after food, if once-daily dose exceeds 300 mg consider dividing the dose to reduce gastro-intestinal intolerance

  Prophylaxis of gout and of uric acid and calcium oxalate renal stones (usual maintenance in severe conditions) | Prophylaxis of hyperuricaemia associated with cancer chemotherapy (usual maintenance in severe conditions)
  ▸ BY MOUTH
  ▸ Adult: 700–900 mg daily in 3 divided doses, to be taken preferably after food

- **CONTRA-INDICATIONS** Not a treatment for acute gout but continue if attack develops when already receiving allopurinol, and treat attack separately
- **CAUTIONS** Ensure adequate fluid intake (2–3 litres/day) · for hyperuricaemia associated with cancer therapy, allopurinol treatment should be started before cancer therapy · thyroid disorders
  CAUTIONS, FURTHER INFORMATION Initiation or up-titration of treatment may precipitate an acute attack of gout—for information on prophylaxis see Gout p. 1278
- **INTERACTIONS** → Appendix 1: allopurinol
- **SIDE-EFFECTS**
  ▸ **Common or very common** Rash (discontinue therapy; if rash mild re-introduce cautiously but discontinue immediately if recurrence)
  ▸ **Uncommon** Hypersensitivity · nausea · vomiting
  ▸ **Rare or very rare** Agranulocytosis · alopecia · angina pectoris · angioedema · angioimmunoblastic T-cell lymphoma · aplastic anaemia · asthenia · ataxia · boil · bradycardia · cataract · coma · depression · diabetes mellitus · drowsiness · erectile dysfunction · fever · gastrointestinal disorders · gynaecomastia · haemorrhage · hair colour changes · headache · hepatic disorders · hyperlipidaemia · hypertension · infertility male · maculopathy · malaise · oedema · paraesthesia · paralysis · peripheral neuropathy · severe cutaneous adverse

reactions (SCARs) · skin reactions · stomatitis · taste altered · thrombocytopenia · vertigo · visual impairment

- **PREGNANCY** Toxicity not reported. Manufacturer advises use only if no safer alternative and disease carries risk for mother or child.
- **BREAST FEEDING** Present in milk—not known to be harmful.
- **HEPATIC IMPAIRMENT** Manufacturer advises monitor liver function periodically during early stages of therapy.
  Dose adjustments Manufacturer advises reduce dose.
- **RENAL IMPAIRMENT** [EvGr] Use with caution (risk of accumulation). ⟨M⟩ Increased risk of hypersensitivity skin reactions.
  Dose adjustments [EvGr] Max. initial dose 100 mg daily, increased only if response inadequate; in severe impairment, reduce daily dose below 100 mg, or increase dose interval; if facilities available, adjust dose to maintain plasma-oxipurinol concentration below 100 micromol/litre. ⟨M⟩
- **MEDICINAL FORMS** There can be variation in the licensing of different medicines containing the same drug. Forms available from special-order manufacturers include: oral suspension, oral solution
  Oral tablet
  CAUTIONARY AND ADVISORY LABELS 8, 21, 27
  ▸ Allopurinol (Non-proprietary)
    Allopurinol 100 mg Allopurinol 100mg tablets | 28 tablet [PoM] £2.28 DT = £0.66
    Allopurinol 200 mg Allopurinol 200mg tablets | 28 tablet [PoM] [℞]
    Allopurinol 300 mg Allopurinol 300mg tablets | 28 tablet [PoM] £5.85 DT = £0.86
  ▸ Zyloric (Aspen Pharma Trading Ltd)
    Allopurinol 100 mg Zyloric 100mg tablets | 100 tablet [PoM] £10.19
    Allopurinol 300 mg Zyloric 300mg tablets | 28 tablet [PoM] £7.31 DT = £0.86

Febuxostat

12-Jul-2023

- ● **INDICATIONS AND DOSE**
  Treatment of chronic hyperuricaemia in gout
  ▸ BY MOUTH
  ▸ Adult: Initially 80 mg once daily, if after 2–4 weeks of initial dose, serum uric acid greater than 6 mg/100 mL then increase dose; increased if necessary to 120 mg once daily

  Prophylaxis and treatment of acute hyperuricaemia with initial chemotherapy for haematologic malignancies
  ▸ BY MOUTH
  ▸ Adult: 120 mg once daily, to be started 2 days before start of cytotoxic therapy and continued for 7–9 days, according to chemotherapy duration

---

IMPORTANT SAFETY INFORMATION

MHRA/CHM ADVICE: SERIOUS HYPERSENSITIVITY REACTIONS (JUNE 2012)

There have been rare but serious reports of hypersensitivity reactions, including Stevens-Johnson syndrome and acute anaphylactic shock with febuxostat. Patients should be advised of the signs and symptoms of severe hypersensitivity; febuxostat must be stopped immediately if these occur (early withdrawal is associated with a better prognosis), and must not be restarted in patients who have ever developed a hypersensitivity reaction to febuxostat. Most cases occur during the first month of treatment; a prior history of hypersensitivity to allopurinol and/or renal disease may indicate potential hypersensitivity to febuxostat.

MHRA/CHM ADVICE: FEBUXOSTAT: UPDATED ADVICE FOR THE TREATMENT OF PATIENTS WITH A HISTORY OF MAJOR CARDIOVASCULAR DISEASE (MAY 2023)
Two clinical studies have assessed the cardiovascular safety of febuxostat, compared with allopurinol, in patients with gout and a history of major cardiovascular disease (CARES) or with at least one cardiovascular risk factor (FAST). Whilst the CARES study found an increased risk of cardiovascular-related death and all-cause mortality associated with febuxostat, the FAST study did not find any such increased risk. However, differences in study populations and protocols between the two studies should be considered when comparing results.

Consequently, healthcare professionals are advised to:
- use febuxostat with caution in patients with pre-existing major cardiovascular disease (e.g. myocardial infarction, stroke, or unstable angina), especially those with high urate crystal and tophi burden or those initiating urate-lowering therapy;
- titrate the febuxostat dose, after initiation, to minimise gout flares and inflammation;
- note that clinical guidelines for gout recommend allopurinol as first-line treatment for patients with gout and major cardiovascular disease.

- **CONTRA-INDICATIONS** Not a treatment for acute gout but continue if attack develops when already receiving febuxostat, and treat attack separately
- **CAUTIONS** Major cardiovascular disease, see *Important safety information* · thyroid disorders · transplant recipients
  CAUTIONS, FURTHER INFORMATION EvGr Administer prophylactic NSAID (*not* aspirin or salicylates) or colchicine for at least 6 months after starting febuxostat to avoid precipitating an acute attack. ⟨M⟩
- **INTERACTIONS** → Appendix 1: febuxostat
- **SIDE-EFFECTS**
  - **Common or very common** Diarrhoea · dizziness · dyspnoea · fatigue · gout aggravated · headache · hepatic disorders · joint disorders · muscle complaints · nausea · oedema · pain · skin reactions
  - **Uncommon** Alopecia · altered smell sensation · appetite abnormal · arrhythmias · arthritis · bundle branch block · chest discomfort · constipation · cough · diabetes mellitus · drowsiness · dry mouth · gallbladder disorders · gastrointestinal discomfort · gastrointestinal disorders · haemorrhage · hemiparesis · hyperlipidaemia · hypertension · hypothyroidism · increased risk of infection · malaise · muscle weakness · musculoskeletal stiffness · nephrolithiasis · oral disorders · palpitations · pancreatitis · proteinuria · renal failure · rhinorrhoea · sensation abnormal · sexual dysfunction · sleep disorders · sweat changes · taste altered · tinnitus · urinary disorders · vasodilation · vision blurred · vomiting · weight changes
  - **Rare or very rare** Agranulocytosis · anaemia · angioedema · circulatory collapse · depressed mood · feeling hot · hypersensitivity · nephritis tubulointerstitial · nervousness · pancytopenia · polymyalgia rheumatica · retinal occlusion · rhabdomyolysis · severe cutaneous adverse reactions (SCARs) · sudden cardiac death · thirst · thrombocytopenia · vertigo
- **PREGNANCY** Manufacturer advises avoid—limited information available.
- **BREAST FEEDING** Manufacturer advises avoid—present in milk in *animal* studies.
- **HEPATIC IMPAIRMENT** Manufacturer advises caution.
  Dose adjustments Manufacturer advises max. 80 mg daily in mild impairment; no dose information available in moderate to severe impairment.

- **RENAL IMPAIRMENT** EvGr Use with caution if creatinine clearance less than 30 mL/minute (limited information available). ⟨M⟩ See p. 21.
- **PRE-TREATMENT SCREENING** Monitor liver function tests before treatment as indicated.
- **MONITORING REQUIREMENTS** Monitor liver function tests periodically during treatment as indicated.
- **NATIONAL FUNDING/ACCESS DECISIONS**
  For full details see funding body website
  NICE decisions
  ▸ **Febuxostat for the management of hyperuricaemia in patients with gout (December 2008)** NICE TA164 Recommended with restrictions
  Scottish Medicines Consortium (SMC) decisions
  ▸ **Febuxostat (*Adenuric*®) for the treatment of chronic hyperuricaemia (September 2010)** SMC No. 637/10 Recommended with restrictions
  ▸ **Febuxostat (*Adenuric*®) for the prevention and treatment of hyperuricaemia in adult patients undergoing chemotherapy for haematologic malignancies at intermediate to high risk of tumour lysis syndrome (TLS) (June 2016)** SMC No. 1153/16 Recommended with restrictions

- **MEDICINAL FORMS** There can be variation in the licensing of different medicines containing the same drug.
  Oral tablet
  ▸ **Febuxostat (Non-proprietary)**
  Febuxostat 80 mg Febuxostat 80mg tablets | 28 tablet PoM £24.36 DT = £2.19
  Febuxostat 120 mg Febuxostat 120mg tablets | 28 tablet PoM £24.36 DT = £5.57
  ▸ **Adenuric** (A. Menarini Farmaceutica Internazionale SRL)
  Febuxostat 80 mg Adenuric 80mg tablets | 28 tablet PoM £24.36 DT = £2.19
  Febuxostat 120 mg Adenuric 120mg tablets | 28 tablet PoM £24.36 DT = £5.57
  ▸ **Elstabya** (Amarox Ltd)
  Febuxostat 80 mg Elstabya 80mg tablets | 28 tablet PoM 🅂 DT = £2.19
  Febuxostat 120 mg Elstabya 120mg tablets | 28 tablet PoM 🅂 DT = £5.57

3   Neuromuscular disorders

Neuromuscular disorders   31-Aug-2022

Drugs that enhance neuromuscular transmission

Anticholinesterases are used as first-line treatment in *ocular myasthenia gravis* and as an adjunct to immunosuppressant therapy for *generalised myasthenia gravis*.

Corticosteroids are used when anticholinesterases do not control symptoms completely. A second-line immunosuppressant such as azathioprine p. 965 is frequently used to reduce the dose of corticosteroid.

Plasmapheresis or infusion of intravenous immunoglobulin [unlicensed indication] may induce temporary remission in severe relapses, particularly where bulbar or respiratory function is compromised or before thymectomy.

Anticholinesterases

Anticholinesterase drugs enhance neuromuscular transmission in voluntary and involuntary muscle in myasthenia gravis. Excessive dosage of these drugs can impair neuromuscular transmission and precipitate cholinergic crises by causing a depolarising block. This may be difficult to distinguish from a worsening myasthenic state.

Muscarinic side-effects of anticholinesterases include increased sweating, increased salivary and gastric secretions, increased gastro-intestinal and uterine motility, and bradycardia. These parasympathomimetic effects are antagonised by atropine sulfate p. 1526.

Neostigmine p. 1286 produces a therapeutic effect for up to 4 hours. Its pronounced muscarinic action is a disadvantage, and simultaneous administration of an antimuscarinic drug such as atropine sulfate or propantheline bromide p. 97 may be required to prevent colic, excessive salivation, or diarrhoea. In severe disease neostigmine can be given every 2 hours. The maximum that most patients can tolerate is 180 mg daily.

Pyridostigmine bromide p. 1286 is less powerful and slower in action than neostigmine but it has a longer duration of action. It is preferable to neostigmine because of its smoother action and the need for less frequent dosage. It is particularly preferred in patients whose muscles are weak on waking. It has a comparatively mild gastrointestinal effect but an antimuscarinic drug may still be required.

Neostigmine is also used to reverse the actions of the non-depolarising neuromuscular blocking drugs.

Immunosuppressant therapy
Corticosteroids are established as treatment for myasthenia gravis; although they are commonly given on alternate days there is little evidence of benefit over daily administration. Corticosteroid treatment is usually initiated under in-patient supervision and all patients should receive osteoporosis prophylaxis.

In *generalised myasthenia gravis* prednisolone p. 791 is given. About 10% of patients experience a transient but very serious worsening of symptoms in the first 2–3 weeks, especially if the corticosteroid is started at a high dose. Smaller doses of corticosteroid are usually required in *ocular myasthenia*. Once clinical remission has occurred (usually after 2–6 months), the dose of prednisolone should be reduced slowly to the minimum effective dose.

In generalised myasthenia gravis azathioprine is usually started at the same time as the corticosteroid and it allows a lower maintenance dose of the corticosteroid to be used. Ciclosporin p. 966, methotrexate p. 1048, or mycophenolate mofetil p. 977 can be used in patients unresponsive or intolerant to other treatments [unlicensed indications].

Acetylcholine-release enhancers
Amifampridine p. 1286 is licensed for the symptomatic treatment of Lambert-Eaton myasthenic syndrome (LEMS), a rare disorder of neuromuscular transmission.

Fampridine p. 981 is licensed for the improvement of walking in patients with Multiple sclerosis p. 979 who have a walking disability.

Skeletal muscle relaxants

The drugs described are used for the relief of chronic muscle spasm or spasticity associated with neurological damage; they are not indicated for spasm associated with minor injuries. Baclofen, diazepam, and tizanidine act principally on the central nervous system. Dantrolene has a peripheral site of action; cannabis extract has both a central and a peripheral action. Skeletal muscle relaxants differ in action from the muscle relaxants used in anaesthesia, which block transmission at the neuromuscular junction. For guidance on the use of skeletal muscle relaxants in multiple sclerosis, see Multiple sclerosis p. 979.

The underlying cause of spasticity should be treated and any aggravating factors (e.g. pressure sores, infection) remedied. Skeletal muscle relaxants are effective in most forms of spasticity except the rare alpha variety. The major disadvantage of treatment with these drugs is that reduction in muscle tone can cause a loss of splinting action of the spastic leg and trunk muscles and sometimes lead to an increase in disability.

Baclofen p. 1289 inhibits transmission at spinal level and also depresses the central nervous system. The dose should be increased slowly to avoid the major side-effects of

sedation and muscular hypotonia (other adverse events are uncommon).

Dantrolene sodium p. 1541 acts directly on skeletal muscle and produces fewer central adverse effects making it a drug of choice. The dose should be increased slowly.

Diazepam p. 398 can also be used. Sedation and occasionally extensor hypotonus are disadvantages. Other benzodiazepines also have muscle-relaxant properties. Muscle-relaxant doses of benzodiazepines are similar to anxiolytic doses.

Tizanidine p. 1291 is an alpha₂-adrenoceptor agonist licensed for spasticity associated with multiple sclerosis or spinal cord injury.

EvGr Cannabis extract p. 1288 can be trialled as an adjunct treatment for moderate to severe spasticity in multiple sclerosis if other pharmacological treatments are not effective. Treatment must be initiated and supervised by a specialist. For further information see Multiple sclerosis p. 979. Ⓐ

Other muscle relaxants
The clinical efficacy of methocarbamol p. 1290 and meprobamate as muscle relaxants is **not** well established, although they have been included in compound analgesic preparations.

NEUROPROTECTIVE DRUGS

| Riluzole
29-Feb-2024

● **INDICATIONS AND DOSE**

To extend life in patients with amyotrophic lateral sclerosis, initiated by specialist experienced in the management of motor neurone disease
▸ BY MOUTH
▸ Adult: 50 mg twice daily

● **CONTRA-INDICATIONS** Acute porphyrias p. 1202
● **CAUTIONS** Interstitial lung disease
CAUTIONS, FURTHER INFORMATION
▸ Interstitial lung disease EvGr Perform chest radiography if symptoms such as dry cough or dyspnoea develop; discontinue if interstitial lung disease is diagnosed. Ⓜ
● **INTERACTIONS** → Appendix 1: riluzole
● **SIDE-EFFECTS**
▸ **Common or very common** Abdominal pain · asthenia · diarrhoea · dizziness · drowsiness · headache · nausea · oral disorders · pain · tachycardia · vomiting
▸ **Uncommon** Anaemia · angioedema · interstitial lung disease · pancreatitis
▸ **Frequency not known** Hepatitis · neutropenia · rash
SIDE-EFFECTS, FURTHER INFORMATION White blood cell counts should be determined in febrile illness; neutropenia requires discontinuation of riluzole.
● **PREGNANCY** Avoid—no information available.
● **BREAST FEEDING** Avoid—no information available.
● **HEPATIC IMPAIRMENT** Avoid in hepatic disease or when baseline transaminases greater than 3 times the upper limit of normal. Caution in patients with a history of abnormal liver function or with slightly elevated transaminases (up to 3 times the upper limit of normal).
● **RENAL IMPAIRMENT** EvGr Avoid—no information available. Ⓜ
● **MONITORING REQUIREMENTS**
▸ EvGr Monitor hepatic transaminases, including ALT, at baseline and every month for the first 3 months of treatment, then every 3 months thereafter during the remainder of the first year, with subsequent monitoring as clinically indicated—stop treatment if ALT increases to more than 5 times the upper limit of normal. Ⓜ

- **DIRECTIONS FOR ADMINISTRATION** *Orodispersible films* should be placed on the tongue, allowed to disperse and swallowed. Mouth numbness can occur after the administration of an orodispersible film and may last for around 40 minutes; it is recommended to use caution if taking food until the symptom improves.

- **PATIENT AND CARER ADVICE**
Blood disorders Patients or their carers should be told how to recognise signs of neutropenia and advised to seek immediate medical attention if symptoms such as fever occur.
    Patients or their carers should be given advice on how to administer orodispersible films.
Driving and skilled tasks Dizziness or vertigo may affect performance of skilled tasks (e.g. driving).

- **NATIONAL FUNDING/ACCESS DECISIONS**
For full details see funding body website
    NICE decisions
    ‣ Guidance on the use of Riluzole (*Rilutek*®) for the treatment of Motor Neurone Disease (January 2001) NICE TA20 Recommended

- **MEDICINAL FORMS** There can be variation in the licensing of different medicines containing the same drug. Forms available from special-order manufacturers include: oral suspension, oral solution, oral powder
    Oral tablet
    ‣ **Riluzole (Non-proprietary)**
        Riluzole 50 mg Riluzole 50mg tablets | 56 tablet PoM £560.00 DT = £286.03
    Oral suspension
    ‣ **Teglutik** (Martindale Pharmaceuticals Ltd)
        Riluzole 5 mg per 1 ml Teglutik 5mg/1ml oral suspension | 300 ml PoM £100.00 DT = £100.00 SF
    Orodispersible film
    ‣ **Emylif** (Zambon UK Ltd)
        Riluzole 50 mg Emylif 50mg orodispersible films | 56 film PoM £168.00 DT = £168.00

3.1   Muscular dystrophy

CORTICOSTEROIDS

F 783

Vamorolone
03-Mar-2025

- **DRUG ACTION** Vamorolone is a dissociative corticosteroid that selectively binds to the glucocorticoid receptor and reduces inflammation by inhibiting cytokine production.

- **INDICATIONS AND DOSE**
Duchenne muscular dystrophy (initiated by a specialist)
    ‣ BY MOUTH
    ‣ Adult (body-weight up to 40 kg): 6 mg/kg once daily; reduced if not tolerated to 4 mg/kg once daily, reduced if not tolerated to 2 mg/kg once daily
    ‣ Adult (body-weight 40 kg and above): 240 mg once daily; reduced if not tolerated to 160 mg once daily, reduced if not tolerated to 80 mg once daily

- **INTERACTIONS** → Appendix 1: corticosteroids

- **SIDE-EFFECTS**
‣ **Common or very common** Diarrhoea · vomiting
‣ **Frequency not known** Suppression of the hypothalamic-pituitary-adrenal axis

- **PREGNANCY** EvGr Avoid unless potential benefit outweighs risk (no information available). M

- **BREAST FEEDING** EvGr Discontinue breast-feeding (no information available). M

- **HEPATIC IMPAIRMENT** EvGr Avoid in severe impairment; caution in moderate impairment. M

Dose adjustments EvGr Body-weight up to 40 kg, reduce dose to 2 mg/kg once daily in moderate impairment.
    Body-weight 40 kg and above, reduce dose to 80 mg once daily in moderate impairment. M

- **TREATMENT CESSATION** EvGr Avoid abrupt withdrawal if treatment duration more than 1 week—reduce dose by decrements of approx. 20% over weeks, according to tolerance. M

- **HANDLING AND STORAGE** Store in a refrigerator (2–8°C) after opening; discard any remaining suspension 3 months after opening.

- **PATIENT AND CARER ADVICE**
Alert card A patient alert card should be provided.

- **NATIONAL FUNDING/ACCESS DECISIONS**
For full details see funding body website
    NICE decisions
    ‣ Vamorolone for treating Duchenne muscular dystrophy in people 4 years and over (January 2025) NICE TA1031 Recommended
    Scottish Medicines Consortium (SMC) decisions
    ‣ Vamorolone (*Agamree*®) for the treatment of Duchenne muscular dystrophy (DMD) in patients aged 4 years and older (January 2025) SMC No. SMC2721 Recommended

- **MEDICINAL FORMS** There can be variation in the licensing of different medicines containing the same drug.
    Oral suspension
    ‣ **Agamree** (Santhera (UK) Ltd) ▼
        Vamorolone 40 mg per 1 ml Agamree 40mg/ml oral suspension | 100 ml PoM £4,585.87 (Hospital only) SF

DRUGS FOR NEUROMUSCULAR DISORDERS

Ataluren
28-Feb-2023

- **DRUG ACTION** Ataluren restores the synthesis of dystrophin by allowing ribosomes to read through premature stop codons that cause incomplete dystrophin synthesis in nonsense mutation Duchenne muscular dystrophy.

- **INDICATIONS AND DOSE**
Duchenne muscular dystrophy resulting from a nonsense mutation in the dystrophin gene, in ambulatory patients (initiated by a specialist)
    ‣ BY MOUTH
    ‣ Adult: (consult product literature)

- **INTERACTIONS** → Appendix 1: ataluren

- **SIDE-EFFECTS**
‣ **Common or very common** Appetite decreased · constipation · cough · enuresis · fever · flatulence · gastrointestinal discomfort · haemorrhage · headache · hypertension · hypertriglyceridaemia · nausea · pain · skin reactions · vomiting · weight decreased
‣ **Frequency not known** Ear infection · malaise

- **PREGNANCY** Manufacturer advises avoid—toxicity in *animal* studies.

- **BREAST FEEDING** Manufacturer advises discontinue breastfeeding—present in milk in *animal* studies.

- **RENAL IMPAIRMENT** Manufacturer advises close monitoring—safety and efficacy not established.

- **MONITORING REQUIREMENTS** Manufacturer advises monitor renal function at least every 6–12 months, and cholesterol and triglyceride concentrations at least annually.

- **DIRECTIONS FOR ADMINISTRATION** Manufacturer advises the contents of each sachet should be mixed with at least 30 mL of liquid (water, milk, fruit juice), or 3 tablespoons of semi-solid food (yoghurt or apple sauce).

- **PATIENT AND CARER ADVICE** Manufacturer advises patients should maintain adequate hydration during treatment.
  Missed doses Manufacturer advises if a morning or midday dose is more than 3 hours late, or an evening dose is more than 6 hours late, the missed dose should not be taken and the next dose should be taken at the normal time.

- **NATIONAL FUNDING/ACCESS DECISIONS** For full details see funding body website
  NICE decisions
  ▸ Ataluren for treating Duchenne muscular dystrophy with a nonsense mutation in the dystrophin gene (February 2023) NICE HST22 Recommended

  Scottish Medicines Consortium (SMC) decisions
  ▸ Ataluren (*Translarna®*) for the treatment of Duchenne muscular dystrophy resulting from a nonsense mutation in the dystrophin gene, in ambulatory patients aged 2 years and older (April 2021) SMC No. SMC2327 Recommended with restrictions

- **MEDICINAL FORMS** There can be variation in the licensing of different medicines containing the same drug.
  Granules for oral suspension
  ▸ Translarna (PTC Therapeutics Ltd) ▼
  Ataluren 125 mg Translarna 125mg granules for oral suspension sachets | 30 sachet [PoM] £2,532.00 (Hospital only)
  Ataluren 250 mg Translarna 250mg granules for oral suspension sachets | 30 sachet [PoM] £5,064.00 (Hospital only)
  Ataluren 1 gram Translarna 1,000mg granules for oral suspension sachets | 30 sachet [PoM] £20,256.00 (Hospital only)

Givinostat

25-Apr-2025

- **DRUG ACTION** Givinostat is a histone deacetylase inhibitor that reduces muscle loss and inflammation in dystrophic muscles, although its exact mechanism of action is unknown.

- **INDICATIONS AND DOSE**
  Duchenne muscular dystrophy
  ▸ BY MOUTH
  ▸ Adult (body-weight 20–39 kg): 31 mg twice daily, for dose adjustments, treatment interruption, or discontinuation due to side-effects—consult product literature
  ▸ Adult (body-weight 40–59 kg): 44.3 mg twice daily, for dose adjustments, treatment interruption, or discontinuation due to side-effects—consult product literature
  ▸ Adult (body-weight 60 kg and above): 53.2 mg twice daily, for dose adjustments, treatment interruption, or discontinuation due to side-effects—consult product literature

- **CONTRA-INDICATIONS** Platelet count less than 150 × 10^9 cells/litre (do not initiate) · QTc interval more than 500 milliseconds

- **CAUTIONS** Risk factors for ventricular arrhythmias (e.g congenital long QT syndrome, coronary artery disease, electrolyte disturbances, concomitant use with other drugs known to prolong the QT interval)
  CAUTIONS, FURTHER INFORMATION
  ▸ ECG monitoring [EvGr] In patients with underlying cardiac disease or using other drugs known to prolong the QT interval, an ECG should be obtained before starting treatment, during concomitant use, and as clinically indicated. ⟨M⟩

- **INTERACTIONS** → Appendix 1: givinostat

- **SIDE-EFFECTS**
  ▸ **Common or very common** Appetite decreased · arthralgia · constipation · diarrhoea · fatigue · fever · gastrointestinal discomfort · gastrointestinal disorders ·

hypertriglyceridaemia · myalgia · nausea · rash · thrombocytopenia · vomiting
▸ **Frequency not known** Hypothyroidism

- **PREGNANCY** [EvGr] Avoid (toxicity in *animal* studies). ⟨M⟩

- **BREAST FEEDING** Specialist sources indicate use with caution, especially if breast-feeding a newborn or pre-term infant (no information available). High plasma-protein binding suggests limited excretion into milk. Monitor breast-fed infant for side-effects.

- **MONITORING REQUIREMENTS**
  ▸ [EvGr] Obtain platelet count at baseline before starting treatment and monitor blood counts every 2 weeks for the first 2 months, then at month 3, and every 3 months thereafter during treatment. Reduce dose, withhold treatment, or permanently discontinue if thrombocytopenia occurs—consult product literature.
  ▸ Obtain triglycerides level at baseline before starting treatment and monitor at months 1, 3, and 6, then every 6 months thereafter during treatment. Reduce dose or permanently discontinue if triglycerides are elevated—consult product literature. ⟨M⟩

- **MEDICINAL FORMS** There can be variation in the licensing of different medicines containing the same drug.
  Oral suspension
  CAUTIONARY AND ADVISORY LABELS 21
  EXCIPIENTS: May contain Polysorbates, sorbitol
  ▸ Givinostat (non-proprietary) ▼
  Givinostat (as Givinostat hydrochloride monohydrate) 8.86 mg per 1 ml Duvyzat 8.86mg/ml oral suspension | 140 ml [PoM] £13,846.00 (Hospital only) [SF]

Nusinersen

11-Nov-2020

- **DRUG ACTION** Nusinersen is an antisense oligonucleotide that increases the production of survival motor neurone (SMN) protein, thereby helping to compensate for the defect in the SMN1 gene found in 5q spinal muscular atrophy.

- **INDICATIONS AND DOSE**
  5q spinal muscular atrophy (initiated by a specialist)
  ▸ BY INTRATHECAL INJECTION
  ▸ Adult: Initially 12 mg for 4 doses, on days 0, 14, 28 and 63, then 12 mg every 4 months, for advice on missed doses—consult product literature

> **IMPORTANT SAFETY INFORMATION**
>
> MHRA/CHM ADVICE: NUSINERSEN (*SPINRAZA®*): REPORTS OF COMMUNICATING HYDROCEPHALUS NOT RELATED TO MENINGITIS OR BLEEDING (JULY 2018)
> Communicating hydrocephalus not related to meningitis or bleeding has been reported in patients treated with *Spinraza®*. Patients and caregivers should be informed about the signs and symptoms of hydrocephalus before *Spinraza®* is started and should be instructed to seek medical attention in case of: persistent vomiting or headache, unexplained decrease in consciousness, and in children increase in head circumference. Patients with signs and symptoms suggestive of hydrocephalus should be further investigated by a physician with expertise in its management.

- **CAUTIONS** Risk factors for renal toxicity—monitor urine protein (preferably using a first morning urine specimen) · risk factors for thrombocytopenia and coagulation disorders—monitor platelet and coagulation profile before treatment

- **PREGNANCY** Manufacturer advises avoid—no information available.

- **BREAST FEEDING** Manufacturer advises avoid—no information available.
- **RENAL IMPAIRMENT** Manufacturer advises close monitoring—safety and efficacy not established.
- **HANDLING AND STORAGE** Manufacturer advises store in a refrigerator (2–8 °C); may be stored (in the original carton, protected from light) at or below 30 °C, for up to 14 days.
- **NATIONAL FUNDING/ACCESS DECISIONS** For full details see funding body website
  NICE decisions
  ▸ Nusinersen for treating spinal muscular atrophy (July 2019) NICE TA588 Recommended with restrictions
- **MEDICINAL FORMS** There can be variation in the licensing of different medicines containing the same drug.
  Solution for injection
  ▸ Spinraza (Biogen Idec Ltd)
    Nusinersen (as Nusinersen sodium) 2.4 mg per 1 ml Spinraza 12mg/5ml solution for injection vials | 1 vial [PoM] £75,000.00 (Hospital only)

Risdiplam
08-Oct-2024

- **DRUG ACTION** Risdiplam is a survival motor neurone 2 (SMN2) pre-mRNA splicing modifier that increases the production of SMN protein, thereby helping to compensate for the defect in the SMN1 gene found in 5q spinal muscular atrophy.

- **INDICATIONS AND DOSE**
  5q spinal muscular atrophy (initiated by a specialist)
  ▸ BY MOUTH
  ▸ Adult: 5 mg once daily, to be taken after a meal at the same time each day

- **INTERACTIONS** → Appendix 1: risdiplam
- **SIDE-EFFECTS**
  ▸ **Common or very common** Arthralgia · cystitis · diarrhoea · fever · headache · hyperpyrexia · increased risk of infection · nausea · oral ulceration · skin reactions
  ▸ **Frequency not known** Cutaneous vasculitis
- **CONCEPTION AND CONTRACEPTION** [EvGr] Females of childbearing potential should use highly effective contraception during treatment and for at least 1 month after last treatment; male patients should use highly effective contraception during treatment and for at least 4 months after last treatment if their partner is of childbearing potential. Male fertility may be impaired during treatment; sperm degeneration and reduced sperm numbers in *animal* studies. ⟨M⟩
- **PREGNANCY** [EvGr] Avoid—toxicity in *animal* studies. ⟨M⟩
- **BREAST FEEDING** [EvGr] Avoid—present in milk in *animal* studies. ⟨M⟩
- **DIRECTIONS FOR ADMINISTRATION** *Evrysdi*® must be reconstituted by a healthcare professional before dispensing. It should be administered orally with the reusable oral syringe provided; the patient should drink water after a dose to ensure that it has been completely swallowed. If a dose is not taken within 5 minutes of being drawn, it should be discarded and a new dose prepared. The solution can also be administered via nasogastric or gastrostomy tube.
- **PRESCRIBING AND DISPENSING INFORMATION** Patients or their carers should be counselled on the administration of the oral solution.
- **PATIENT AND CARER ADVICE** If *Evrysdi*® oral solution spills or gets on the skin, the area should be washed with soap and water. Store in a refrigerator (2–8°C); any unused portion must be discarded 64 days after reconstitution. **Vomiting** If a dose is not fully swallowed or vomiting occurs after taking a dose, no additional dose should be taken on that day and the next dose should be taken at the usual time.
  Missed doses If a dose is more than 6 hours late, the missed dose should not be taken and the next dose should be taken at the usual time.
- **NATIONAL FUNDING/ACCESS DECISIONS** For full details see funding body website
  NICE decisions
  ▸ Risdiplam for treating spinal muscular atrophy (updated December 2023) NICE TA755 Recommended with restrictions
  Scottish Medicines Consortium (SMC) decisions
  ▸ Risdiplam (*Evrysdi*®) for the treatment of 5q spinal muscular atrophy (SMA) in patients two months of age and older, with a clinical diagnosis of SMA type 1, type 2 or type 3 or with one to four survival of motor neuron 2 copies (February 2022) SMC No. SMC2401 Recommended
- **MEDICINAL FORMS** There can be variation in the licensing of different medicines containing the same drug.
  Oral solution
  CAUTIONARY AND ADVISORY LABELS 8
  EXCIPIENTS: May contain Disodium edetate
  ▸ Evrysdi (Roche Products Ltd) ▼
    Risdiplam 750 microgram per 1 ml Evrysdi 0.75mg/ml oral solution | 80 ml [PoM] £7,900.00 (Hospital only) [SF]

3.2 Myasthenia gravis and Lambert-Eaton myasthenic syndrome

> **Other drugs used for Myasthenia gravis and Lambert-Eaton myasthenic syndrome** Eculizumab, p. 1152

ANTICHOLINESTERASES

Anticholinesterases 

- **DRUG ACTION** They prolong the action of acetylcholine by inhibiting the action of the enzyme acetylcholinesterase.
- **CONTRA-INDICATIONS** Intestinal obstruction · urinary obstruction
- **CAUTIONS** Arrhythmias · asthma (extreme caution) · atropine or other antidote to muscarinic effects may be necessary (particularly when neostigmine is given by injection) but not given routinely because it may mask signs of overdosage · bradycardia · epilepsy · hyperthyroidism · hypotension · parkinsonism · peptic ulceration · recent myocardial infarction · vagotonia
  CAUTIONS, FURTHER INFORMATION
  ▸ **Elderly** Screening Tool of Older Persons' potentially inappropriate Prescriptions (STOPP) criteria to aid medication reviews (see Prescribing in the elderly p. 31 for information). Potentially inappropriate: in patients with a known history of persistent bradycardia (heart rate less than 60 beats per minute), heart block, or recurrent unexplained syncope, or concurrent treatment with drugs that reduce heart rate (risk of cardiac conduction failure, syncope, and injury).
- **SIDE-EFFECTS** Abdominal cramps · diarrhoea · excessive tearing · hypersalivation · nausea · vomiting
  Overdose Signs of overdosage include bronchoconstriction, increased bronchial secretions, lacrimation, excessive sweating, involuntary defaecation, involuntary micturition, miosis, nystagmus, bradycardia, heart block, arrhythmias, hypotension, agitation, excessive dreaming, and weakness eventually leading to fasciculation and paralysis.

10

Musculoskeletal system

- **PREGNANCY** Manufacturer advises use only if potential benefit outweighs risk.
- **BREAST FEEDING** Amount probably too small to be harmful.

⮞ 1285

Neostigmine

(Neostigmine methylsulfate)

- **INDICATIONS AND DOSE**

Treatment of myasthenia gravis
- ▶ BY MOUTH
- ▶ Adult: Initially 15–30 mg, dose repeated at suitable intervals throughout the day, total daily dose 75–300 mg, the maximum that most patients can tolerate is 180 mg daily
- ▶ BY SUBCUTANEOUS INJECTION, OR BY INTRAMUSCULAR INJECTION
- ▶ Adult: 1–2.5 mg, dose repeated at suitable intervals throughout the day (usual total daily dose 5–20 mg)

Reversal of non-depolarising (competitive) neuromuscular blockade
- ▶ BY INTRAVENOUS INJECTION
- ▶ Adult: 2.5 mg (max. per dose 5 mg), repeated if necessary after or with glycopyrronium or atropine, to be given over 1 minute

- **CAUTIONS** Glycopyrronium or atropine should also be given when reversing neuromuscular blockade
- **INTERACTIONS** → Appendix 1: neostigmine
- **SIDE-EFFECTS**
- ▶ With parenteral use Intestinal hypermotility · muscle spasms
- **RENAL IMPAIRMENT**
Dose adjustments May need dose reduction.

- **MEDICINAL FORMS** There can be variation in the licensing of different medicines containing the same drug. Forms available from special-order manufacturers include: oral solution

Solution for injection
- ▶ Neostigmine (Non-proprietary)
Neostigmine metilsulfate 2.5 mg per 1 ml Neostigmine 2.5mg/1ml solution for injection ampoules | 10 ampoule PoM £14.98-£15.00

⮞ 1285

Pyridostigmine bromide

05-Nov-2021

- **DRUG ACTION** Pyridostigmine bromide has weaker muscarinic action than neostigmine.

- **INDICATIONS AND DOSE**

Myasthenia gravis
- ▶ BY MOUTH
- ▶ Adult: 30–120 mg, doses to be given at suitable intervals throughout day; usual dose 0.3–1.2 g daily in divided doses, it is inadvisable to exceed a total daily dose of 450 mg in order to avoid acetylcholine receptor down-regulation; patients requiring doses exceeding 450 mg daily will usually require input from a specialised neuromuscular service.
Immunosuppressant therapy is usually considered if the dose of pyridostigmine exceeds 360 mg daily

- **INTERACTIONS** → Appendix 1: pyridostigmine
- **SIDE-EFFECTS** Gastrointestinal hypermotility · muscle cramps · rash
- **RENAL IMPAIRMENT**
Dose adjustments EvGr Consider dose reduction (excreted renally). Ⓜ

- **MEDICINAL FORMS** There can be variation in the licensing of different medicines containing the same drug. Forms available from special-order manufacturers include: oral tablet, oral suspension, oral solution

Oral tablet
- ▶ Pyridostigmine bromide (Non-proprietary)
Pyridostigmine bromide 60 mg Pyridostigmine bromide 60mg tablets | 200 tablet PoM £32.00 DT = £17.15
- ▶ Mestinon (Viatris UK Healthcare Ltd)
Pyridostigmine bromide 60 mg Mestinon 60mg tablets | 200 tablet PoM £45.57 DT = £17.15

Oral solution
EXCIPIENTS: May contain Propylene glycol, sorbitol
ELECTROLYTES: May contain Sodium
- ▶ Pyridostigmine bromide (Non-proprietary)
Pyridostigmine bromide 12 mg per 1 ml Pyridostigmine bromide 12mg/1ml oral solution sugar free | 150 ml PoM £90.00-£157.50 DT = £90.00 SF

CHOLINERGIC RECEPTOR STIMULATING DRUGS

Amifampridine

29-Nov-2022

- **INDICATIONS AND DOSE**

Symptomatic treatment of Lambert-Eaton myasthenic syndrome (specialist use only)
- ▶ BY MOUTH
- ▶ Adult: Initially 15 mg daily in 3 divided doses, then increased in steps of 5 mg every 4–5 days, increased to up to 60 mg daily in 3–4 divided doses (max. per dose 20 mg); maximum 60 mg per day

- **CONTRA-INDICATIONS** Congenital QT syndromes · epilepsy · uncontrolled asthma
- **CAUTIONS** Risk factors for schwannomas
- **INTERACTIONS** → Appendix 1: amifampridine
- **SIDE-EFFECTS**
- ▶ **Common or very common** Dizziness · gastrointestinal discomfort · nausea · oral disorders · peripheral coldness · sensation abnormal · sweat changes
- ▶ **Frequency not known** Anxiety · arrhythmia · asthenia · asthmatic attack · bronchial secretion increased · cough · diarrhoea · drowsiness · gastrointestinal disorder · headache · movement disorders · palpitations · Raynaud's phenomenon · seizures · sleep disorder · vision blurred
- **CONCEPTION AND CONTRACEPTION** Ensure effective contraception during treatment in men and women.
- **PREGNANCY** Manufacturer advises avoid.
- **BREAST FEEDING** Manufacturer advises avoid—no information available.
- **HEPATIC IMPAIRMENT** Manufacturer advises caution (risk of increased exposure).
Dose adjustments Manufacturer advises initial dose reduction to 5 mg twice daily in mild impairment, titrate in steps of 5 mg every 7 days.
   Manufacturer advises initial dose reduction to 5 mg once daily in moderate to severe impairment, titrate in steps of 5 mg every 7 days.
- **RENAL IMPAIRMENT** EvGr Use with caution (risk of increased exposure). Ⓜ
Dose adjustments EvGr Reduce initial dose to 5 mg twice daily in mild impairment, titrate in steps of 5 mg every 7 days.
   Reduce initial dose to 5 mg once daily in moderate to severe impairment, titrate in steps of 5 mg every 7 days. Ⓜ
- **MONITORING REQUIREMENTS** Clinical and ECG monitoring required at treatment initiation and yearly thereafter.

● **NATIONAL FUNDING/ACCESS DECISIONS**
For full details see funding body website
Scottish Medicines Consortium (SMC) decisions
▶ Amifampridine (*Firdapse*®) for the symptomatic treatment of Lambert-Eaton myasthenic syndrome (LEMS) in adults (August 2012) SMC No. 660/10 Not recommended

● **MEDICINAL FORMS** There can be variation in the licensing of different medicines containing the same drug. Forms available from special-order manufacturers include: oral tablet
Oral tablet
CAUTIONARY AND ADVISORY LABELS 3, 21
▶ **Firdapse** (SERB) ▼
Amifampridine (as Amifampridine phosphate) 10 mg Firdapse 10mg tablets | 100 tablet [PoM] £1,815.00 (Hospital only)

IMMUNOSUPPRESSANTS › COMPLEMENT INHIBITORS

Zilucoplan
28-Mar-2024

● **DRUG ACTION** Zilucoplan is a synthetic macrocyclic peptide that inhibits complement activation at the C5 protein, thereby reducing complement-mediated cell damage.

● **INDICATIONS AND DOSE**
Myasthenia gravis (under expert supervision)
▶ BY SUBCUTANEOUS INJECTION
▶ Adult (body-weight up to 56 kg): 16.6 mg once daily
▶ Adult (body-weight 56-76 kg): 23 mg once daily
▶ Adult (body-weight 77 kg and above): 32.4 mg once daily

● **CONTRA-INDICATIONS** Patients unvaccinated against *Neisseria meningitidis* · unresolved *Neisseria meningitidis* infection

● **CAUTIONS** *Neisseria* infection
CAUTIONS, FURTHER INFORMATION
▶ Meningococcal infection [EvGr] Vaccinate against *Neisseria meningitidis* at least 2 weeks before treatment (vaccines against serotypes A, C, Y, W135, and B where available, are recommended); revaccinate according to current medical guidelines. Patients receiving zilucoplan less than 2 weeks after receiving meningococcal vaccine must be given prophylactic antibiotics until 2 weeks after vaccination. Other immunisations should also be up to date. ⟨M⟩

● **SIDE-EFFECTS**
▶ **Common or very common** Diarrhoea · increased risk of infection · morphoea

● **PREGNANCY** [EvGr] Use only if potential benefit outweighs risk (no information available). ⟨M⟩

● **BREAST FEEDING** Specialist sources indicate probably compatible (no information available). Degradation into small peptides and amino acids via catabolic pathways in the maternal circulation and infant gastro-intestinal tract suggests unlikely to be absorbed by, or adversely affect the breast-fed infant.

● **DIRECTIONS FOR ADMINISTRATION** Inject into the abdomen, thigh, or upper arm (if not self-administered); rotate injection site and avoid skin that is tender, bruised, scarred, red, or hardened.
Patients may self-administer *Zilbrysq*® after appropriate training in subcutaneous injection technique.

● **HANDLING AND STORAGE** Store in a refrigerator (2–8°C) and protect from light—consult product literature for further information regarding storage outside refrigerator.

● **PATIENT AND CARER ADVICE** Patients or their carers should be advised to seek immediate medical attention if signs or symptoms of meningococcal infection occur. Advice about prevention of gonorrhoea should also be given.
Self administration Patients or their carers should be given training in subcutaneous injection technique.

Alert card and guide A patient alert card, and guide for patients and carers should be provided.

● **MEDICINAL FORMS** There can be variation in the licensing of different medicines containing the same drug.
Solution for injection
▶ **Zilbrysq** (UCB Pharma Ltd) ▼
Zilucoplan (as Zilucoplan sodium) 40 mg per 1 ml Zilbrysq 32.4mg/0.81ml solution for injection pre-filled syringes | 7 pre-filled disposable injection [PoM] £7,114.70 (Hospital only)
Zilbrysq 23mg/0.574ml solution for injection pre-filled syringes | 7 pre-filled disposable injection [PoM] £5,041.78 (Hospital only)
Zilbrysq 16.6mg/0.416ml solution for injection pre-filled syringes | 7 pre-filled disposable injection [PoM] £3,653.97 (Hospital only)

IMMUNOSUPPRESSANTS › IMMUNOMODULATING DRUGS

Efgartigimod alfa
16-Nov-2023

● **DRUG ACTION** Efgartigimod alfa is a human recombinant immunoglobulin G1 (IgG1) antibody fragment that binds to the neonatal Fc receptor (FcRn), thereby reducing the levels of circulating IgG, including pathogenic IgG autoantibodies, and improving neuromuscular transmission.

● **INDICATIONS AND DOSE**
Myasthenia gravis (under expert supervision)
▶ BY INTRAVENOUS INFUSION
▶ Adult: 10 mg/kg once weekly (max. per dose 1.2 g) for 4 weeks, subsequent 4-week cycles to be administered, according to response, at least 7 weeks from the start of the previous cycle, for advice on missed doses—consult product literature

● **CAUTIONS** Active infections · administration of vaccinations
CAUTIONS, FURTHER INFORMATION
▶ Vaccination [EvGr] Administer vaccinations at least 4 weeks before starting treatment. If vaccinations are required during treatment, administer them at least 2 weeks after the last infusion of a treatment cycle and 4 weeks before starting the next cycle—immunisation with vaccines during treatment has not been studied. Live or live attenuated vaccines should be avoided during treatment—safety is unknown. ⟨M⟩

● **INTERACTIONS** → Appendix 1: efgartigimod alfa

● **SIDE-EFFECTS**
▶ **Common or very common** Increased risk of infection · myalgia · procedural headache

● **PREGNANCY** [EvGr] Use only if potential benefit outweighs risk (no information available). ⟨M⟩

● **BREAST FEEDING** Specialist sources indicate use with caution (no information available). Large molecular weight suggests limited excretion into milk and drug molecule likely to be partially destroyed in the infant's gastro-intestinal tract.

● **DIRECTIONS FOR ADMINISTRATION** For *intermittent intravenous infusion* (*Vyvgart*®), dilute requisite dose with Sodium Chloride 0.9% to a final volume of 125 mL; give over 1 hour through an in-line filter (0.2 micron).

● **PRESCRIBING AND DISPENSING INFORMATION** Efgartigimod alfa is a biological medicine. Biological medicines must be prescribed and dispensed by brand name, see *Biological medicines* and *Biosimilar medicines*, under Guidance on prescribing p. 1; record the brand name and batch number after each administration.

● **HANDLING AND STORAGE** Store in a refrigerator (2–8°C) and protect from light—consult product literature for storage after dilution.

10 Musculoskeletal system

● **NATIONAL FUNDING/ACCESS DECISIONS**
For full details see funding body website
Scottish Medicines Consortium (SMC) decisions
▶ **Efgartigimod alfa (*Vyvgart*®) as an add-on to standard
therapy for the treatment of adult patients with generalised
myasthenia gravis who are anti-acetylcholine receptor
antibody positive (November 2023)** SMC No. SMC2561 Not
recommended

● **MEDICINAL FORMS** There can be variation in the licensing of
different medicines containing the same drug.
Solution for infusion
EXCIPIENTS: May contain Polysorbates
ELECTROLYTES: May contain Sodium
▶ Vyvgart (Argenx UK Ltd) ▼
Efgartigimod alfa 20 mg per 1 ml Vyvgart 400mg/20ml concentrate
for solution for infusion vials | 1 vial [PoM] [S] (Hospital only)

IMMUNOSUPPRESSANTS › MONOCLONAL ANTIBODIES

Rozanolixizumab

28-Jun-2024

● **DRUG ACTION** Rozanolixizumab is a humanised
recombinant immunoglobulin G4P (IgG4P) monoclonal
antibody that binds to the neonatal Fc receptor (FcRn),
thereby reducing the levels of circulating IgG, including
pathogenic IgG autoantibodies, and improving
neuromuscular transmission.

● **INDICATIONS AND DOSE**
Myasthenia gravis (under expert supervision)
▶ BY SUBCUTANEOUS INFUSION
▶ Adult (body-weight 35–49 kg): 280 mg once weekly for
6 weeks, subsequent 6-week treatment cycles to be
administered according to clinical evaluation
▶ Adult (body-weight 50–69 kg): 420 mg once weekly for
6 weeks, subsequent 6-week treatment cycles to be
administered according to clinical evaluation
▶ Adult (body-weight 70–99 kg): 560 mg once weekly for
6 weeks, subsequent 6-week treatment cycles to be
administered according to clinical evaluation
▶ Adult (body-weight 100 kg and above): 840 mg once
weekly for 6 weeks, subsequent 6-week treatment
cycles to be administered according to clinical
evaluation

● **CAUTIONS** Active infections · administration of
vaccinations
CAUTIONS, FURTHER INFORMATION
▶ Vaccination [EvGr] Administer vaccinations at least 4 weeks
before starting treatment. If vaccinations are required
during treatment, administer them at least 2 weeks after
the last infusion of a treatment cycle and 4 weeks before
starting the next cycle—immunisation with vaccines
during treatment has not been studied. Live or live
attenuated vaccines should be avoided during treatment—
safety is unknown. ⟨M⟩

● **INTERACTIONS** → Appendix 1: monoclonal antibodies

● **SIDE-EFFECTS**
▶ **Common or very common** Angioedema · arthralgia ·
diarrhoea · fever · headaches · skin reactions · tongue
swelling
▶ **Frequency not known** Increased risk of infection ·
meningitis aseptic

● **PREGNANCY** [EvGr] Use only if potential benefit outweighs
risk. ⟨M⟩

● **BREAST FEEDING** [EvGr] Avoid during first few days after
birth (possible risk from transfer of antibodies to infant).
After this time, use only if potential benefit outweighs
risk. ⟨M⟩

● **DIRECTIONS FOR ADMINISTRATION** To be administered via
an infusion pump at a constant rate of up to 20 mL/hour.
Administer into the lower left or lower right side of the
abdomen; avoid skin that is tender, bruised, scarred, red,
or hardened.
Missed doses If a scheduled dose is missed, the dose may be
administered up to 4 days after the scheduled time point,
and the next dose administered at the normal time.

● **PRESCRIBING AND DISPENSING INFORMATION**
Rozanolixizumab is a biological medicine. Biological
medicines must be prescribed and dispensed by brand
name, see *Biological medicines* and *Biosimilar medicines*,
under Guidance on prescribing p. 1; record the brand name
and batch number after each administration.

● **HANDLING AND STORAGE** Store in a refrigerator (2–8°C)
and protect from light.

● **MEDICINAL FORMS** There can be variation in the licensing of
different medicines containing the same drug.
Solution for infusion
EXCIPIENTS: May contain L-proline, polysorbates
▶ Rystiggo (UCB Pharma Ltd) ▼
Rozanolixizumab 140 mg per 1 ml Rystiggo 560mg/4ml solution for
injection vials | 1 vial [PoM] £17,883.19 (Hospital only)
Rystiggo 420mg/3ml solution for injection vials | 1 vial [PoM]
£13,412.39 (Hospital only)
Rystiggo 280mg/2ml solution for injection vials | 1 vial [PoM]
£8,941.59 (Hospital only)

3.3 Nocturnal leg cramps

Nocturnal leg cramps

03-May-2021

Quinine salts

Quinine salts p. 713, such as quinine sulfate, may reduce the
frequency of nocturnal leg cramps. [EvGr] However, because
of potential toxicity, quinine is not recommended for routine
treatment and should not be used unless cramps cause
regular disruption to sleep. Quinine should only be
considered when cramps are very painful or frequent, when
other treatable causes of cramp have been excluded, and
when non-pharmacological treatments have not worked (e.g.
passive stretching exercises). ⟨A⟩[EvGr] It may take up to
4 weeks for improvement to become apparent; if there is
benefit, quinine treatment can be continued. Treatment
should be interrupted at intervals of approximately 3 months
to assess the need for further quinine treatment. ⟨M⟩[EvGr] In
patients taking quinine long term, a trial discontinuation
may be considered. ⟨A⟩ Quinine is toxic in overdosage and
fatalities have occurred.

3.4 Spasticity

Other drugs used for Spasticity Dantrolene sodium, p. 1541
· Diazepam, p. 398

CANNABINOIDS

Cannabis extract

04-Oct-2022

The properties listed below are those particular to the
combination only. For the properties of the components
please consider, cannabidiol p. 355.

● **INDICATIONS AND DOSE**
**Adjunct in moderate to severe spasticity in multiple
sclerosis (specialist use only)**
▶ BY BUCCAL ADMINISTRATION
▶ Adult: (consult product literature)

- CONTRA-INDICATIONS Family history of psychosis · history of other severe psychiatric disorder · personal history of psychosis
- CAUTIONS History of epilepsy · significant cardiovascular disease
- INTERACTIONS → Appendix 1: cannabidiol · dronabinol
- SIDE-EFFECTS
  - **Common or very common** Appetite abnormal · balance impaired · concentration impaired · constipation · depression · diarrhoea · disorientation · dizziness · drowsiness · dry mouth · dysarthria · euphoric mood · feeling drunk · malaise · memory loss · nausea · oral disorders · perception altered · taste altered · vertigo · vision blurred · vomiting
  - **Uncommon** Abdominal pain upper · delusions · hallucinations · hypertension · palpitations · paranoia · pharyngitis · suicidal ideation · syncope · tachycardia · throat irritation · tooth discolouration
- CONCEPTION AND CONTRACEPTION Manufacturer recommends effective contraception during and for 3 months after treatment in men and women.
- PREGNANCY Manufacturer advises use only if potential benefit outweighs risks.
- BREAST FEEDING Avoid—present in milk.
- HEPATIC IMPAIRMENT Manufacturer advises avoid in moderate to severe impairment (risk of accumulation with chronic dosing)—no information available.
- RENAL IMPAIRMENT Manufacturer advises more frequent monitoring in significant impairment (no information available; possible risk of prolonged or enhanced effect).
- MONITORING REQUIREMENTS Monitor oral mucosa— interrupt treatment if lesions or persistent soreness.
- PATIENT AND CARER ADVICE
  Driving and skilled tasks For information on 2015 legislation regarding driving whilst taking certain controlled drugs, including cannabis, see Drugs and driving under Guidance on prescribing p. 1.
- NATIONAL FUNDING/ACCESS DECISIONS
  For full details see funding body website
  Scottish Medicines Consortium (SMC) decisions
  - Delta-9-tetrahydrocannabinol and cannabidiol (*Sativex®*) as treatment for symptom improvement in adult patients with moderate to severe spasticity due to multiple sclerosis who have not responded adequately to other anti-spasticity medication and who demonstrate clinically significant improvement in spasticity related symptoms during an initial trial of therapy (September 2022) SMC No. SMC2473 Recommended

- MEDICINAL FORMS There can be variation in the licensing of different medicines containing the same drug.
  Spray
  CAUTIONARY AND ADVISORY LABELS 2
  - Sativex (Jazz Pharmaceuticals Operations UK Ltd)
    Cannabidiol 2.5 mg per 1 dose, Dronabinol 2.7 mg per 1 dose Sativex oromucosal spray | 270 dose [PoM] £300.00 DT = £300.00 [CD4–1]

MUSCLE RELAXANTS › CENTRALLY ACTING

| Baclofen
08-Jan-2024

- **INDICATIONS AND DOSE**
  Pain of muscle spasm in palliative care
  - BY MOUTH
  - Adult: 5–10 mg 3 times a day
  Hiccup due to gastric distension in palliative care
  - BY MOUTH
  - Adult: 5 mg twice daily

Chronic severe spasticity resulting from disorders such as multiple sclerosis or traumatic partial section of spinal cord
  - BY MOUTH
  - Adult: Initially 5 mg 3 times a day, usual maintenance up to 20 mg 3 times a day, dose to be increased gradually to maintenance dose; dose can be increased if necessary up to maximum 100 mg per day, review treatment if no benefit within 6 weeks of achieving maximum dose

Severe chronic spasticity unresponsive to oral antispastic drugs (or where side-effects of oral therapy unacceptable) or as alternative to ablative neurosurgical procedures (specialist use only)
  - BY INTRATHECAL INJECTION
  - Adult: Test dose 25–50 micrograms, to be given over at least 1 minute via catheter or lumbar puncture, then increased in steps of 25 micrograms (max. per dose 100 micrograms), not given more often than every 24 hours to determine appropriate dose, then *dose-titration phase*, most often using infusion pump (implanted into chest wall or abdominal wall tissues) to establish maintenance dose (ranging from 12 micrograms to 2 mg daily for spasticity of spinal origin or 22 micrograms to 1.4 mg daily for spasticity of cerebral origin) retaining some spasticity to avoid sensation of paralysis

> **IMPORTANT SAFETY INFORMATION**
> Consult product literature for details on test dose and titration—important to monitor patients closely in appropriately equipped and staffed environment during screening and immediately after pump implantation. Resuscitation equipment must be available for immediate use. Treatment with continuous pump-administered intrathecal baclofen should be initiated within 3 months of a satisfactory response to intrathecal baclofen testing.

- CONTRA-INDICATIONS
  - With intrathecal use Local infection · systemic infection
  - With oral use Active peptic ulceration
- CAUTIONS
  GENERAL CAUTIONS Cerebrovascular disease · diabetes · elderly · epilepsy · history of peptic ulcer · history of substance abuse · hypertonic bladder sphincter · Parkinson's disease · psychiatric illness · respiratory impairment
  SPECIFIC CAUTIONS
  - With intrathecal use Coagulation disorders · malnutrition (increased risk of post-surgical complications) · previous spinal fusion procedure
- INTERACTIONS → Appendix 1: baclofen
- SIDE-EFFECTS
  GENERAL SIDE-EFFECTS
  - **Common or very common** Confusion · constipation · depression · diarrhoea · dizziness · drowsiness · dry mouth · euphoric mood · hallucination · headache · hyperhidrosis · hypotension · nausea · paraesthesia · skin reactions · urinary disorders · vision disorders · vomiting
  - **Uncommon** Bradycardia · hypothermia · suicidal behaviours
  - **Rare or very rare** Withdrawal syndrome
  SPECIFIC SIDE-EFFECTS
  - **Common or very common**
  - With intrathecal use Anxiety · appetite decreased · asthenia · chills · dyspnoea · fever · hypersalivation · insomnia · neuromuscular dysfunction · oedema · pain · pneumonia · respiratory disorders · seizure · sexual dysfunction

Musculoskeletal system

10

- With oral use Fatigue · gastrointestinal disorder · muscle weakness · myalgia · respiratory depression · sleep disorders
▶ **Uncommon**
▶ With intrathecal use Alopecia · deep vein thrombosis · dehydration · flushing · hypertension · hypogeusia · ileus · memory loss · pallor · paranoia
▶ **Rare or very rare**
▶ With oral use Abdominal pain · erectile dysfunction · hepatic function abnormal · taste altered
▶ **Frequency not known**
▶ With intrathecal use Scoliosis

● **PREGNANCY** Manufacturer advises use only if potential benefit outweighs risk (toxicity in *animal* studies).

● **BREAST FEEDING** Present in milk—amount probably too small to be harmful.

● **HEPATIC IMPAIRMENT**
▶ With oral use Manufacturer advises use with caution—no information available.

● **RENAL IMPAIRMENT** See p. 21. [EvGr] Use with caution. [M]
▶ With oral use [EvGr] Only use if potential benefit outweighs risk if eGFR less than 15 mL/minute/1.73 m². [M]
  Dose adjustments
  ▶ With oral use [EvGr] Use smaller doses (e.g. 5 mg daily) and if necessary increase dosage interval—monitor for signs and symptoms of toxicity. [M]

● **TREATMENT CESSATION** Avoid abrupt withdrawal (risk of hyperactive state, may exacerbate spasticity, and precipitate autonomic dysfunction including hyperthermia, psychiatric reactions and convulsions; to minimise risk, discontinue by gradual dose reduction over at least 1–2 weeks (longer if symptoms occur)).

● **PRESCRIBING AND DISPENSING INFORMATION** Flavours of oral liquid formulations may include raspberry.

  Palliative care For further information on the use of baclofen in palliative care, see www.medicinescomplete.com/#/content/palliative/baclofen.

● **PATIENT AND CARER ADVICE**
  Driving and skilled tasks Drowsiness may affect performance of skilled tasks (e.g. driving); effects of alcohol enhanced.

● **MEDICINAL FORMS** There can be variation in the licensing of different medicines containing the same drug. Forms available from special-order manufacturers include: oral suspension, oral solution, solution for injection

Oral tablet
CAUTIONARY AND ADVISORY LABELS 2, 8, 21
EXCIPIENTS: May contain Gluten
▶ Baclofen (Non-proprietary)
  Baclofen 5 mg Baclofen 5mg tablets | 84 tablet [PoM] £10.80–£19.44
  Baclofen 10 mg Baclofen 10mg tablets | 84 tablet [PoM] £2.33 DT = £1.70 | 250 tablet [PoM] £9.75
  Baclofen 20 mg Baclofen 20mg tablets | 84 tablet [PoM] £2.77–£4.98
▶ Lioresal (Novartis Pharmaceuticals UK Ltd)
  Baclofen 10 mg Lioresal 10mg tablets | 100 tablet [PoM] £14.86

Solution for injection
▶ Baclofen (Non-proprietary)
  Baclofen 50 microgram per 1 ml Baclofen 50micrograms/1ml solution for injection ampoules | 10 ampoule [PoM] £40.00
  Baclofen 1 mg per 1 ml Gablofen 20mg/20ml solution for injection pre-filled syringes | 1 pre-filled disposable injection [PoM] [⅀] (Hospital only)
  Gablofen 20mg/20ml solution for injection vials | 1 vial [PoM] [⅀] (Hospital only)
▶ Lioresal (Novartis Pharmaceuticals UK Ltd)
  Baclofen 50 microgram per 1 ml Lioresal Intrathecal 50micrograms/1ml solution for injection ampoules | 1 ampoule [PoM] £3.16 DT = £3.16

Solution for infusion
▶ Baclofen (Non-proprietary)
  Baclofen 500 microgram per 1 ml Baclofen 10mg/20ml solution for infusion ampoules | 1 ampoule [PoM] £80.00 DT = £70.01

  Baclofen 2 mg per 1 ml Baclofen 40mg/20ml solution for infusion ampoules | 1 ampoule [PoM] £600.00
  Baclofen 10mg/5ml solution for infusion ampoules | 10 ampoule [PoM] £650.00
▶ Lioresal (Novartis Pharmaceuticals UK Ltd)
  Baclofen 500 microgram per 1 ml Lioresal Intrathecal 10mg/20ml solution for infusion ampoules | 1 ampoule [PoM] £70.01 DT = £70.01
  Baclofen 2 mg per 1 ml Lioresal Intrathecal 10mg/5ml solution for infusion ampoules | 1 ampoule [PoM] £70.01 DT = £70.01

Oral solution
CAUTIONARY AND ADVISORY LABELS 2, 8, 21
▶ Baclofen (Non-proprietary)
  Baclofen 1 mg per 1 ml Baclofen 5mg/5ml oral solution sugar free | 300 ml [PoM] £10.29 DT = £3.25 [SF]
  Baclofen 2 mg per 1 ml Baclofen 10mg/5ml oral solution sugar free | 150 ml [PoM] £9.10 DT = £9.10 [SF]
▶ Lioresal (Novartis Pharmaceuticals UK Ltd)
  Baclofen 1 mg per 1 ml Lioresal 5mg/5ml liquid | 300 ml [PoM] £10.31 DT = £3.25 [SF]
▶ Lyflex (Rosemont Pharmaceuticals Ltd)
  Baclofen 1 mg per 1 ml Lyflex 5mg/5ml oral solution | 300 ml [PoM] £7.95 DT = £3.25 [SF]

Methocarbamol

11-Jun-2021

● **INDICATIONS AND DOSE**

Short-term symptomatic relief of muscle spasm
▶ BY MOUTH
▶ Adult: 1.5 g 4 times a day; reduced to 750 mg 3 times a day if required
▶ Elderly: Up to 750 mg 4 times a day, dose may be sufficient

● **CONTRA-INDICATIONS** Brain damage · coma · epilepsy · myasthenia gravis · pre-coma

● **INTERACTIONS** → Appendix 1: methocarbamol

● **SIDE-EFFECTS** Angioedema · anxiety · bradycardia · confusion · conjunctivitis · dizziness · drowsiness · dyspepsia · fever · flushing · headache · hepatic disorders · hypotension · insomnia · leucopenia · memory loss · nasal congestion · nausea · seizures · skin reactions · syncope · taste metallic · vertigo · vision disorders · vomiting

● **PREGNANCY** Manufacturer advises avoid unless potential benefit outweighs risk.

● **BREAST FEEDING** Present in milk in *animal studies*—manufacturer advises caution.

● **HEPATIC IMPAIRMENT** Manufacturer advises caution (risk of increased half-life).
  Dose adjustments Manufacturer advises consider increasing dose interval in chronic impairment.

● **RENAL IMPAIRMENT** Manufacturer advises caution.

● **PATIENT AND CARER ADVICE**
  Driving and skilled tasks Drowsiness may affect performance of skilled tasks (e.g. driving); effects of alcohol enhanced.

● **LESS SUITABLE FOR PRESCRIBING** Less suitable for prescribing.

● **MEDICINAL FORMS** There can be variation in the licensing of different medicines containing the same drug. Forms available from special-order manufacturers include: oral suspension

Oral tablet
CAUTIONARY AND ADVISORY LABELS 2
▶ Methocarbamol (Non-proprietary)
  Methocarbamol 750 mg Methocarbamol 750mg tablets | 100 tablet [PoM] £16.00 DT = £6.58
  Methocarbamol 1500 mg Methocarbamol 1500mg tablets | 96 tablet [PoM] £19.44–£33.00 DT = £19.44 | 100 tablet [PoM] £20.25 DT = £20.25
▶ Robaxin (Almirall Ltd)
  Methocarbamol 750 mg Robaxin 750 tablets | 100 tablet [PoM] £12.65 DT = £6.58

Pridinol

17-Nov-2020

- **DRUG ACTION** Pridinol is a centrally acting muscle relaxant.

  - **INDICATIONS AND DOSE**
  Central and peripheral muscle spasms
  ▶ BY MOUTH
  ▸ Adult: 1.5–3 mg 3 times a day

- **CONTRA-INDICATIONS** Arrhythmia · gastrointestinal obstruction · glaucoma · prostatic hypertrophy · urinary retention
- **CAUTIONS** Elderly (higher or longer-lasting blood levels expected) · hypotension (increased risk of circulatory problems)—take dose after meals
- **INTERACTIONS** → Appendix 1: pridinol
- **SIDE-EFFECTS**
▶ **Uncommon** Abdominal pain · anxiety · arrhythmias · asthenia · circulatory collapse · dizziness · dry mouth · headache · hypotension · nausea · speech disorder
▶ **Rare or very rare** Concentration impaired · coordination abnormal · depression · diarrhoea · taste altered · vision disorders · vomiting
▶ **Frequency not known** Constipation · feeling hot · hallucination · muscle weakness · mydriasis · paraesthesia · skin reactions · thirst · tremor · urinary disorder
- **PREGNANCY** EvGr Avoid in the first trimester; thereafter, use only if potential benefit outweighs risk (no information available). M
- **BREAST FEEDING** EvGr Avoid—no information available. M
- **HEPATIC IMPAIRMENT** EvGr Caution in severe impairment (no information available)—higher or longer-lasting blood levels expected. M
- **RENAL IMPAIRMENT** EvGr Caution in severe impairment (no information available)—higher or longer-lasting blood levels expected. M

- **MEDICINAL FORMS** No licensed medicines listed.

Tizanidine

09-Jul-2021

  - **INDICATIONS AND DOSE**
  Spasticity associated with multiple sclerosis or spinal cord injury or disease
  ▶ BY MOUTH
  ▸ Adult: Initially 2 mg daily, then increased in steps of 2 mg daily in divided doses, increased at intervals of at least 3–4 days and adjust according to response; usual dose up to 24 mg daily in 3–4 divided doses; maximum 36 mg per day

- **CAUTIONS** Elderly
- **INTERACTIONS** → Appendix 1: tizanidine
- **SIDE-EFFECTS**
▶ **Common or very common** Arrhythmias · dizziness · drowsiness · dry mouth · fatigue · hypotension · rebound hypertension
▶ **Rare or very rare** Gastrointestinal disorder · hallucination · hepatic disorders · muscle weakness · nausea · sleep disorders
▶ **Frequency not known** Abdominal pain · accommodation disorder · anxiety · appetite decreased · confusion · headache · QT interval prolongation · skin reactions · vomiting · withdrawal syndrome
  SIDE-EFFECTS, FURTHER INFORMATION Treatment should be discontinued if liver enzymes are persistently raised—consult product literature.
- **PREGNANCY** Avoid (toxicity in *animal* studies).
- **BREAST FEEDING** Avoid (present in milk in *animal* studies).

- **HEPATIC IMPAIRMENT** Manufacturer advises avoid in significant impairment.
- **RENAL IMPAIRMENT** EvGr Use with caution if creatinine clearance less than 25 mL/minute. M
  Dose adjustments EvGr Consider slower dose titration if creatinine clearance less than 25 mL/minute (consult product literature). M See p. 21.
- **MONITORING REQUIREMENTS** Monitor liver function monthly for first 4 months for daily doses of 12 mg or higher, and in those who develop unexplained nausea, anorexia or fatigue.
- **TREATMENT CESSATION** Avoid abrupt withdrawal (risk of rebound hypertension and tachycardia); to minimise risk, discontinue gradually and monitor blood pressure.
- **PATIENT AND CARER ADVICE**
  Driving and skilled tasks Drowsiness may affect performance of skilled tasks (e.g. driving); effects of alcohol enhanced.

- **MEDICINAL FORMS** There can be variation in the licensing of different medicines containing the same drug. Forms available from special-order manufacturers include: oral suspension, oral solution
  Oral tablet
  CAUTIONARY AND ADVISORY LABELS 2, 8
  ▶ Tizanidine (Non-proprietary)
    Tizanidine (as Tizanidine hydrochloride) 2 mg Tizagelan 2mg tablets | 120 tablet PoM £9.20 DT = £6.66
    Tizanidine 2mg tablets | 120 tablet PoM £10.54 DT = £6.66
    Tizanidine (as Tizanidine hydrochloride) 4 mg Tizanidine 4mg tablets | 120 tablet PoM £40.07 DT = £12.79
    Tizagelan 4mg tablets | 120 tablet PoM £13.90 DT = £12.79

4   Pain and inflammation in musculoskeletal disorders

Low back pain and sciatica

09-Aug-2021

Description of condition

Low back pain is pain in the lumbosacral area of the back. It can be described as *non-specific, mechanical, musculoskeletal,* or *simple* (if it is not associated with serious or potentially serious causes). Episodes of back pain do not usually last long, with rapid improvements in pain and disability seen within a few weeks to months.

Sciatica (*radicular pain* or *radiculopathy*) is neuropathic leg pain secondary to compressive lumbosacral nerve root pathology. Sciatica can also be present in about 5–10% of individuals with non-specific back pain, and where they coexist, the symptoms of sciatica tend to predominate.

Non-drug treatment

EvGr Exercise programmes, manual therapy (spinal manipulation, mobilisation, or soft-tissue techniques such as massage), and psychological therapies should be considered for managing low back pain with or without sciatica.

Spinal decompression may be considered in patients with sciatica when pain and function has not improved with non-surgical treatment (including drug treatment). A

Drug treatment

EvGr An oral NSAID (see Non-steroidal anti-inflammatory drugs p. 1292) should be considered for managing acute low back pain, taking into consideration the risks associated with NSAIDs, the need for continued monitoring, and the possible need for gastroprotective treatment (for further information, see Peptic ulcer disease p. 81).

A weak opioid, either alone or with paracetamol p. 507, can be used to manage acute low back pain only if an NSAID is contra-indicated, not tolerated or ineffective (see *Opioid analgesics* under Analgesics p. 505). Paracetamol alone is ineffective for managing low back pain. Ⓐ

EvGr Benzodiazepines are sometimes used to manage acute low back pain (particularly in loss of lordosis); however evidence to support their use is very weak. Ⓔ

EvGr In patients with chronic low back pain who have had an inadequate response to non-drug treatment, NSAIDs should be considered as first-line therapy. Opioids should be the last treatment option considered and should be considered only in patients for whom other therapies have failed and only if the potential benefits outweigh the risks for individual patients. If indicated, opioids should only be prescribed for a limited period of time. Long term opioid therapy should be avoided.

Selective serotonin re-uptake inhibitors (SSRIs), serotonin and noradrenaline re-uptake inhibitors (SNRIs), tricyclic antidepressants, gabapentinoids, and antiepileptic drugs should **not** be offered for managing low back pain.

When non-surgical treatment is ineffective in patients with moderate or severe localised back pain arising from structures supplied by the medial branch nerve, referral for radiofrequency denervation can be considered. Ⓐ

Sciatica

If prescribing NSAIDs for sciatica, take into consideration the limited evidence of benefit and the risks associated with their use.

EvGr Patients with acute and severe sciatica may benefit from treatment with epidural injections of a local anaesthetic and/or corticosteroid. Ⓐ

Useful Resources

Low back pain and sciatica. National Institute for Health and Care Excellence. Clinical guideline NG59. November 2016 (updated December 2020).
www.nice.org.uk/guidance/ng59

Non-steroidal anti-inflammatory drugs

01-Aug-2023

Therapeutic effects

In *single doses* non-steroidal anti-inflammatory drugs (NSAIDs) have analgesic activity comparable to that of paracetamol p. 507, but paracetamol is often preferred, particularly in the elderly.

In regular *full dosage* NSAIDs have both a lasting analgesic and an anti-inflammatory effect which makes them particularly useful for the treatment of continuous or regular pain associated with inflammation. NSAIDs are more appropriate than paracetamol or the opioid analgesics in the *inflammatory arthritides* (e.g. rheumatoid arthritis). NSAIDs can also be of benefit in the less well defined conditions of *back pain* and *soft-tissue disorders*.

Choice

Differences in anti-inflammatory activity between NSAIDs are small, but there is considerable variation in individual response and tolerance to these drugs. About 60% of patients will respond to any NSAID; of the others, those who do not respond to one may well respond to another. Pain relief starts soon after taking the first dose and a full analgesic effect should normally be obtained within a week, whereas an anti-inflammatory effect may not be achieved (or may not be clinically assessable) for up to 3 weeks. If appropriate responses are not obtained within these times, another NSAID should be tried.

NSAIDs reduce the production of prostaglandins by inhibiting the enzyme cyclo-oxygenase. They vary in their selectivity for inhibiting different types of cyclo-oxygenase; selective inhibition of cyclo-oxygenase-2 (COX-2) is associated with less gastro-intestinal intolerance. Several other factors also influence susceptibility to gastrointestinal effects, and a NSAID should be chosen on the basis of the incidence of gastro-intestinal and other side-effects.

Ibuprofen p. 1302 is a propionic acid derivative with anti-inflammatory, analgesic, and antipyretic properties. It has fewer side-effects than other non-selective NSAIDs but its anti-inflammatory properties are weaker. It is unsuitable for conditions where inflammation is prominent. Dexibuprofen is the active enantiomer of ibuprofen. It has similar properties to ibuprofen and is licensed for the relief of mild to moderate pain and inflammation.

Other propionic acid derivatives:

Naproxen p. 1310 is one of the first choices because it combines good efficacy with a low incidence of side-effects (but more than ibuprofen).

Flurbiprofen p. 1301 may be slightly more effective than naproxen, and is associated with slightly more gastro-intestinal side-effects than ibuprofen.

Ketoprofen p. 1306 has anti-inflammatory properties similar to ibuprofen and has more side-effects. Dexketoprofen p. 1295, an isomer of ketoprofen, has been introduced for the short-term relief of mild to moderate pain.

Tiaprofenic acid p. 1314 is as effective as naproxen; it has more side-effects than ibuprofen.

Drugs with properties similar to those of propionic acid derivatives:

Diclofenac sodium p. 1297 and aceclofenac p. 1294 are similar in efficacy to naproxen.

Etodolac p. 1299 is comparable in efficacy to naproxen; it is licensed for symptomatic relief of osteoarthritis and rheumatoid arthritis.

Indometacin p. 1305 has an action equal to or superior to that of naproxen, but with a high incidence of side-effects including headache, dizziness, and gastro-intestinal disturbances.

Mefenamic acid p. 1308 has minor anti-inflammatory properties. It has occasionally been associated with diarrhoea and haemolytic anaemia which require discontinuation of treatment.

Meloxicam p. 1309 is licensed for the short-term relief of pain in osteoarthritis and for long-term treatment of rheumatoid arthritis and ankylosing spondylitis.

Nabumetone p. 1309 is comparable in effect to naproxen.

Phenylbutazone is licensed for ankylosing spondylitis, but is not recommended because it is associated with serious side-effects, in particular haematological reactions; it should be used only by a specialist in severe cases where other treatments have been found unsuitable.

Piroxicam p. 1312 is as effective as naproxen and has a long duration of action which permits once-daily administration. However, it has more gastro-intestinal side-effects than most other NSAIDs, and is associated with more frequent serious skin reactions.

Sulindac p. 1313 is similar in tolerance to naproxen.

Tenoxicam p. 1313 is similar in activity and tolerance to naproxen. Its long duration of action allows once-daily administration.

Tolfenamic acid p. 539 is licensed for the treatment of migraine.

Ketorolac trometamol p. 1536 and the selective inhibitor of cyclo-oxygenase-2, parecoxib p. 1536, are licensed for the short-term management of postoperative pain.

The selective inhibitors of COX-2, etoricoxib p. 1300 and celecoxib p. 1295, are as effective as non-selective NSAIDs such as diclofenac sodium and naproxen. Although selective inhibitors can cause serious gastro-intestinal events, available evidence appears to indicate that the risk of serious upper gastro-intestinal events is lower with selective inhibitors compared to non-selective NSAIDs; this advantage may be lost in patients who require concomitant low-dose aspirin.

Celecoxib and etoricoxib are licensed for the relief of pain in osteoarthritis, rheumatoid arthritis, and ankylosing spondylitis; etoricoxib is also licensed for the relief of pain from acute gout.

Aspirin p. 142 has been used in high doses to treat rheumatoid arthritis, but other NSAIDs are now preferred.

Dental and orofacial pain

Most mild to moderate dental pain and inflammation is effectively relieved by NSAIDs. Those used for dental pain include ibuprofen, diclofenac sodium, and diclofenac potassium p. 1296.

Considerations in the elderly

The use of NSAIDs in elderly patients is potentially inappropriate (STOPP criteria) if prescribed:

- with a vitamin K antagonist, direct thrombin inhibitor or factor Xa inhibitor in combination (risk of major gastrointestinal bleeding);
- with concurrent antiplatelet agent(s) without proton pump inhibitor (PPI) prophylaxis (increased risk of peptic ulcer disease);
- in a history of peptic ulcer disease or gastrointestinal bleeding, unless with concurrent PPI or H$_2$-receptor antagonist (risk of peptic ulcer relapse)—not including COX-2 selective NSAIDs;
- with concurrent corticosteroids without PPI prophylaxis (increased risk of peptic ulcer disease);
- in patients with an eGFR less than 50 mL/minute/1.73 m^2 (risk of deterioration in renal function);
- in severe hypertension or severe heart failure (risk of exacerbation);
- for chronic treatment of gout where there is no contra-indication to a xanthine-oxidase inhibitor (xanthine-oxidase inhibitors are first choice prophylactic drugs in gout);
- a **COX-2 selective** NSAID in concurrent cardiovascular disease (increased risk of myocardial infarction and stroke).

For further information, see *STOPP/START criteria* in Prescribing in the elderly p. 31.

NSAIDs in pregnancy

MHRA/CHM advice: NSAIDs: potential risks following prolonged use after 20 weeks of pregnancy (June 2023)
A European review of data from a 2022 study identified that prolonged (more than a few days) use of systemic NSAIDs from week 20 of pregnancy onwards may be associated with an increased risk of:

- oligohydramnios resulting from fetal renal dysfunction—this may occur shortly after treatment initiation, although usually reversible upon discontinuation;
- constriction of the ductus arteriosus—most reported cases resolved after treatment cessation.

These risks are potentially serious as they can cause restriction of fetal growth and cardiac dysfunction.
Healthcare professionals are advised to:

- avoid prescribing systemic NSAIDs from week 20 of pregnancy (the EMA review advises to avoid during the first and second trimesters) unless clinically required, in which case the lowest dose should be prescribed for the shortest time;
- consider antenatal monitoring for oligohydramnios if the mother has been exposed to systemic NSAIDs for several days after week 20 of pregnancy—the NSAID should be discontinued if oligohydramnios is detected, or if the NSAID is no longer necessary;
- continue to follow clinical guidelines about recording current and recent medicines, including over-the-counter medicines, at each antenatal appointment.

Healthcare professionals are also reminded that systemic NSAIDs are contra-indicated during the third trimester (after 28 weeks) of pregnancy due to the risk of premature closure of the ductus arteriosus, fetal renal dysfunction, prolongation of maternal bleeding time, and inhibition of uterine contractions during labour.
In addition, patients or their carers should be advised that:

- systemic NSAIDs should be avoided altogether during the third trimester of pregnancy;
- systemic NSAIDs should also be avoided from week 20 of pregnancy onwards unless otherwise advised by a doctor;
- if a systemic NSAID is used for more than a few days during later pregnancy, additional monitoring such as ultrasound scans may be required;
- some non-prescription pain relief preparations contain more than one active drug and advice should be sought from a healthcare professional if there is any uncertainty—such preparations should be used at the lowest dose for the shortest possible time;
- it is vitally important to seek medical advice if pain persists for longer than 3 days, or if there is repeated pain during pregnancy.

This advice does not apply to aspirin, COX-2 selective inhibitors, and topical NSAIDs—separate advice on the use of these during pregnancy should be followed.

NSAIDs in asthma

Any degree of worsening of asthma may be related to the ingestion of NSAIDs, either prescribed or (in the case of ibuprofen **and** others) purchased over the counter.

NSAIDs and cardiovascular events

All NSAID use (including COX-2 selective inhibitors) can, to varying degrees, be associated with a small increased risk of thrombotic events (e.g. myocardial infarction and stroke) independent of baseline cardiovascular risk factors or duration of NSAID use; however, the greatest risk may be in those receiving high doses long term.

COX-2 selective inhibitors, diclofenac (150 mg daily) and ibuprofen p. 1302 (2.4 g daily) are associated with an increased risk of thrombotic events. Although there are limited data regarding the thrombotic effects of aceclofenac p. 1294, treatment advice has been updated in line with diclofenac, based on aceclofenac's structural similarity to diclofenac and its metabolism to diclofenac. The increased risk for diclofenac is similar to that of licensed doses of etoricoxib p. 1300. Naproxen p. 1310 (1 g daily) is associated with a lower thrombotic risk, and low doses of ibuprofen (1.2 g daily or less) have not been associated with an increased risk of myocardial infarction.

The lowest effective dose of NSAID should be prescribed for the shortest period of time to control symptoms and the need for long-term treatment should be reviewed periodically.

NSAIDs and gastro-intestinal events

All NSAIDs are associated with serious gastro-intestinal toxicity; the risk is higher in the elderly. Evidence on the relative safety of non-selective NSAIDs indicates differences in the risks of serious upper gastro-intestinal side-effects—piroxicam p. 1312, ketoprofen p. 1306, and ketorolac trometamol p. 1536 are associated with the highest risk; indometacin p. 1305, diclofenac, and naproxen are associated with intermediate risk, and ibuprofen with the lowest risk (although high doses of ibuprofen have been associated with intermediate risk). Selective inhibitors of COX-2 are associated with a *lower risk* of serious upper gastro-intestinal side-effects than non-selective NSAIDs.

Recommendations are that NSAIDs associated with a low risk e.g. ibuprofen are *generally preferred*, to start at the *lowest recommended dose* **and** not to use more than one oral NSAID at a time.

The combination of a NSAID **and** low-dose aspirin can increase the risk of gastro-intestinal side-effects; this combination should be used only if absolutely necessary **and** the patient should be monitored closely.

While it is preferable to avoid NSAIDs in patients with active or previous gastro-intestinal ulceration or bleeding, and to withdraw them if gastro-intestinal lesions develop, nevertheless patients with serious rheumatic diseases are usually dependent on NSAIDs for effective relief of pain and stiffness.

Patients at risk of gastro-intestinal ulceration (including the elderly), who need NSAID treatment should receive gastroprotective treatment.

Systemic as well as local effects of NSAIDs contribute to gastro–intestinal damage; taking oral formulations with milk or food, or using enteric-coated formulations, or changing the route of administration may only partially reduce symptoms such as dyspepsia.

NSAIDs and alcohol

Alcohol increases the risk of gastro-intestinal haemorrhage associated with NSAIDs. Specialist sources recommend that concurrent use need not be avoided with moderate alcohol intake, but greater caution is warranted in those who drink more than the recommended daily limits.

Some cases of acute kidney injury have been attributed to use of NSAIDs and acute excessive alcohol consumption.

> **Other drugs used for Pain and inflammation in musculoskeletal disorders** Tramadol with dexketoprofen, p. 536

ANALGESICS › NON-STEROIDAL ANTI-INFLAMMATORY DRUGS

Aceclofenac

01-Aug-2023

● **INDICATIONS AND DOSE**

Pain and inflammation in rheumatoid arthritis, osteoarthritis and ankylosing spondylitis

▶ BY MOUTH
▶ Adult: 100 mg twice daily

> **IMPORTANT SAFETY INFORMATION**
> MHRA/CHM ADVICE: NSAIDS: POTENTIAL RISKS FOLLOWING PROLONGED USE AFTER 20 WEEKS OF PREGNANCY (JUNE 2023)
> See Non-steroidal anti-inflammatory drugs p. 1292.

● **CONTRA-INDICATIONS** Active bleeding · active gastro-intestinal bleeding · active gastro-intestinal ulceration · bleeding disorders · cerebrovascular disease · history of gastro-intestinal bleeding related to previous NSAID therapy · history of gastro-intestinal perforation related to previous NSAID therapy · history of recurrent gastro-intestinal haemorrhage (two or more distinct episodes) · history of recurrent gastro-intestinal ulceration (two or more distinct episodes) · ischaemic heart disease · mild to severe heart failure · peripheral arterial disease · varicella infection

● **CAUTIONS** Allergic disorders · avoid in Acute porphyrias p. 1202 · cardiac impairment (NSAIDs may impair renal function) · connective-tissue disorders · dehydration (risk of renal impairment) · elderly (risk of serious side-effects and fatalities) · history of cardiac failure · history of cerebrovascular bleeding · history of gastro-intestinal disorders (e.g. ulcerative colitis, Crohn's disease) · hypertension · may mask symptoms of infection · oedema · risk factors for cardiovascular events

● **INTERACTIONS** → Appendix 1: NSAIDs

● **SIDE-EFFECTS**
▶ **Common or very common** Diarrhoea · dizziness · gastrointestinal discomfort · nausea
▶ **Uncommon** Constipation · gastrointestinal disorders · oral disorders · skin reactions · vomiting
▶ **Rare or very rare** Anaemia · angioedema · bone marrow disorders · depression · drowsiness · dyspnoea · fatigue · haemolytic anaemia · haemorrhage · headache · heart failure · hepatic disorders · hyperkalaemia · hypersensitivity · hypertension · inflammatory bowel disease · leg cramps · nephrotic syndrome · neutropenia · oedema · palpitations · pancreatitis · paraesthesia · renal failure (more common in patients with pre-existing renal impairment) · respiratory disorders · severe cutaneous adverse reactions (SCARs) · sleep disorders · taste altered · thrombocytopenia · tinnitus · tremor · vasculitis · vasodilation · vertigo · visual impairment · weight increased
▶ **Frequency not known** Acute coronary syndrome · agranulocytosis · asthma · confusion · hallucination · increased risk of arterial thromboembolism · increased risk of ischaemic stroke · malaise · meningitis aseptic (patients with connective-tissue disorders such as systemic lupus erythematosus may be especially susceptible) · nephritis tubulointerstitial · optic neuritis · photosensitivity reaction · platelet aggregation inhibition · respiratory tract reaction

SIDE-EFFECTS, FURTHER INFORMATION For information about cardiovascular and gastrointestinal side-effects, and a possible exacerbation of symptoms in asthma, see Non-steroidal anti-inflammatory drugs p. 1292

● **ALLERGY AND CROSS-SENSITIVITY** EvGr Contra-indicated in patients with a history of hypersensitivity to aspirin or any other NSAID—which includes those in whom attacks of asthma, angioedema, urticaria or rhinitis have been precipitated by aspirin or any other NSAID. Ⓜ

● **CONCEPTION AND CONTRACEPTION** EvGr Caution—long-term use of some NSAIDs is associated with reduced female fertility, which is reversible on stopping treatment. Ⓜ

● **PREGNANCY** Avoid use in first and second trimesters unless essential; the MHRA advises additional antenatal monitoring may be required if treatment is considered necessary by a doctor from week 20 of pregnancy onwards. Avoid use in third trimester. See *NSAIDs in Pregnancy* in Non-steroidal anti-inflammatory drugs p. 1292 for further details.

● **BREAST FEEDING** Use with caution during breast-feeding. Manufacturer advises avoid.

● **HEPATIC IMPAIRMENT** Manufacturer advises caution in mild to moderate impairment; avoid in hepatic failure.
Dose adjustments Manufacturer advises consider initial dose reduction to 100 mg daily in mild to moderate impairment.

● **RENAL IMPAIRMENT** In general, for *NSAIDs* the MHRA advises to avoid where possible; if necessary, use with caution (risk of fluid retention and further renal impairment, including renal failure). EvGr For *aceclofenac*, avoid in renal failure. Ⓜ

● **MEDICINAL FORMS** There can be variation in the licensing of different medicines containing the same drug.
Oral tablet
CAUTIONARY AND ADVISORY LABELS 21
▶ **Aceclofenac (Non-proprietary)**
  Aceclofenac 100 mg Aceclofenac 100mg tablets | 60 tablet PoM
  £8.67 DT = £8.67
▶ **Preservex** (Almirall Ltd)
  Aceclofenac 100 mg Preservex 100mg tablets | 60 tablet PoM
  £9.63 DT = £8.67

Celecoxib

12-Apr-2023

- **INDICATIONS AND DOSE**

Pain and inflammation in osteoarthritis
- BY MOUTH
  - Adult: 200 mg daily in 1–2 divided doses, then increased if necessary to 200 mg twice daily, discontinue if no improvement after 2 weeks on maximum dose

Pain and inflammation in rheumatoid arthritis
- BY MOUTH
  - Adult: 100 mg twice daily, then increased if necessary to 200 mg twice daily, discontinue if no improvement after 2 weeks on maximum dose

Ankylosing spondylitis
- BY MOUTH
  - Adult: 200 mg daily in 1–2 divided doses, then increased if necessary to 400 mg daily in 1–2 divided doses, discontinue if no improvement after 2 weeks on maximum dose

DOSE ADJUSTMENTS DUE TO INTERACTIONS
- Manufacturer advises reduce dose by half with concurrent use of fluconazole.

- **CONTRA-INDICATIONS** Active gastro-intestinal bleeding · active gastro-intestinal ulceration · cerebrovascular disease · inflammatory bowel disease · ischaemic heart disease · mild to severe heart failure · peripheral arterial disease

- **CAUTIONS** Allergic disorders · cardiac impairment (NSAIDs may impair renal function) · coagulation defects · connective-tissue disorders · dehydration (risk of renal impairment) · elderly (risk of serious side-effects and fatalities) · history of cardiac failure · history of gastro-intestinal disorders · hypertension · left ventricular dysfunction · may mask symptoms of infection · oedema · risk factors for cardiovascular events

- **INTERACTIONS** → Appendix 1: NSAIDs

- **SIDE-EFFECTS**
- **Common or very common** Angina pectoris · benign prostatic hyperplasia · cough · diarrhoea · dizziness · dysphagia · dyspnoea · fluid retention · gastrointestinal discomfort · gastrointestinal disorders · headache · hypersensitivity · hypertension · increased risk of infection · influenza like illness · injury · insomnia · irritable bowel syndrome · joint disorders · muscle tone increased · myocardial infarction · nausea · nephrolithiasis · oedema · skin reactions · vomiting · weight increased
- **Uncommon** Anaemia · anxiety · arrhythmias · breast tenderness · bronchospasm · burping · cerebral infarction · chest pain · conjunctivitis · constipation · depression · drowsiness · dysphonia · electrolyte imbalance · embolism and thrombosis · fatigue · haemorrhage · hearing impairment · heart failure · hepatic disorders · lipoma · lower limb fracture · muscle complaints · nocturia · oral disorders · palpitations · paraesthesia · tinnitus · vision blurred · vitreous floater
- **Rare or very rare** Acute kidney injury (more common in patients with pre-existing renal impairment) · alopecia · angioedema · anosmia · ataxia · confusion · flushing · hallucination · intracranial haemorrhage · leucopenia · meningitis aseptic · menstrual disorder · myositis · nephritis tubulointerstitial · nephropathy · pancreatitis · pancytopenia · photosensitivity reaction · pneumonitis · seizures · severe cutaneous adverse reactions (SCARs) · taste altered · thrombocytopenia · vasculitis
- **Frequency not known** Infertility

  SIDE-EFFECTS, FURTHER INFORMATION For information about cardiovascular and gastrointestinal side-effects, and a possible exacerbation of symptoms in asthma, see Non-steroidal anti-inflammatory drugs p. 1292

- **ALLERGY AND CROSS-SENSITIVITY** EvGr Contra-indicated in patients with a history of hypersensitivity to aspirin or any other NSAID—which includes those in whom attacks of asthma, angioedema, urticaria or rhinitis have been precipitated by aspirin or any other NSAID.
  Contra-indicated in patients with sulfonamide sensitivity. Ⓜ

- **CONCEPTION AND CONTRACEPTION** Caution—long-term use of some NSAIDs is associated with reduced female fertility, which is reversible on stopping treatment.

- **PREGNANCY** Avoid (teratogenic in *animal* studies).

- **BREAST FEEDING** Avoid—present in milk in *animal* studies.

- **HEPATIC IMPAIRMENT** Manufacturer advises caution in mild to moderate impairment; avoid in severe impairment (no information available).
  Dose adjustments Manufacturer advises initial dose reduction of 50% in moderate impairment.

- **RENAL IMPAIRMENT** In general, for *NSAIDs* the MHRA advises to avoid where possible; if necessary, use with caution (risk of fluid retention and further renal impairment, including renal failure). EvGr For *celecoxib*, avoid if creatinine clearance less than 30 mL/minute. Ⓜ See p. 21.

- **MONITORING REQUIREMENTS** Monitor blood pressure before and during treatment.

- **MEDICINAL FORMS** There can be variation in the licensing of different medicines containing the same drug.

  Oral capsule
  - **Celecoxib (Non-proprietary)**
    Celecoxib 100 mg Celecoxib 100mg capsules | 60 capsule [PoM] £25.86 DT = £2.47
    Celecoxib 200 mg Celecoxib 200mg capsules | 30 capsule [PoM] £25.86 DT = £2.55
  - **Celebrex** (Viatris UK Healthcare Ltd)
    Celecoxib 100 mg Celebrex 100mg capsules | 60 capsule [PoM] £21.55 DT = £2.47
    Celecoxib 200 mg Celebrex 200mg capsules | 30 capsule [PoM] £21.55 DT = £2.55

Dexketoprofen

01-Aug-2023

- **INDICATIONS AND DOSE**

Short-term treatment of mild to moderate pain including dysmenorrhoea
- BY MOUTH
  - Adult: 12.5 mg every 4–6 hours, alternatively 25 mg every 8 hours; maximum 75 mg per day
  - Elderly: 12.5 mg every 4–6 hours, alternatively 25 mg every 8 hours, initial max. 50 mg; maximum 75 mg daily

> **IMPORTANT SAFETY INFORMATION**
> MHRA/CHM ADVICE: NSAIDS: POTENTIAL RISKS FOLLOWING PROLONGED USE AFTER 20 WEEKS OF PREGNANCY (JUNE 2023)
> See Non-steroidal anti-inflammatory drugs p. 1292.

- **CONTRA-INDICATIONS** Active bleeding or bleeding disorders · active or recurrent gastro-intestinal haemorrhage · active or recurrent gastro-intestinal ulcer · chronic dyspepsia · Crohn's disease · history of NSAID-associated gastro-intestinal bleeding or perforation · known photoallergic or phototoxic reactions during treatment with ketoprofen or fibrates · severe dehydration · severe heart failure · ulcerative colitis · varicella infection

- **CAUTIONS** Allergic disorders · asthma · cerebrovascular disease · coagulation defects · congenital disorder of porphyrin metabolism · congestive heart failure · dehydration · elderly (risk of serious side-effects and fatalities) · following major surgery · haematopoietic disorders · history of cardiac disease (NSAIDs may cause fluid retention and oedema) · history of gastro-intestinal disease · history of gastro-intestinal toxicity · ischaemic heart disease · may mask symptoms of infection · mixed connective-tissue disorders · peripheral arterial disease · risk factors for cardiovascular events · systemic lupus erythematosus · uncontrolled hypertension

● **INTERACTIONS** → Appendix 1: NSAIDs

● **SIDE-EFFECTS**

▶ **Common or very common** Diarrhoea · gastrointestinal discomfort · nausea · vomiting

▶ **Uncommon** Anxiety · asthenia · chills · constipation · dizziness · drowsiness · dry mouth · flushing · gastrointestinal disorders · headache · insomnia · malaise · pain · palpitations · skin reactions · vertigo

▶ **Rare or very rare** Acute kidney injury (more common in patients with pre-existing renal impairment) · angioedema · appetite decreased · dyspnoea · haemorrhage · hepatocellular injury · hyperhidrosis · hypersensitivity · hypertension · hypotension · menstrual disorder · nephritis · nephrotic syndrome · neutropenia · oedema · pancreatitis · paraesthesia · photosensitivity reaction · polyuria · prostatic disorder · respiratory disorders · severe cutaneous adverse reactions (SCARs) · syncope · tachycardia · thrombocytopenia · tinnitus · vision blurred

▶ **Frequency not known** Oral ulceration

SIDE-EFFECTS, FURTHER INFORMATION For information about cardiovascular and gastrointestinal side-effects, and a possible exacerbation of symptoms in asthma, see Non-steroidal anti-inflammatory drugs p. 1292

● **ALLERGY AND CROSS-SENSITIVITY** [EvGr] Contra-indicated in patients with a history of hypersensitivity to aspirin or any other NSAID—which includes those in whom attacks of asthma, angioedema, urticaria or rhinitis have been precipitated by aspirin or any other NSAID. Ⓜ

● **CONCEPTION AND CONTRACEPTION** [EvGr] Caution—long-term use of some NSAIDs is associated with reduced female fertility, which is reversible on stopping treatment. Ⓜ

● **PREGNANCY** Avoid use in first and second trimesters unless essential; the MHRA advises additional antenatal monitoring may be required if treatment is considered necessary by a doctor from week 20 of pregnancy onwards. Avoid use in third trimester. See *NSAIDs in Pregnancy* in Non-steroidal anti-inflammatory drugs p. 1292 for further details.

● **BREAST FEEDING** Use with caution during breast-feeding. Manufacturer advises avoid—no information available.

● **HEPATIC IMPAIRMENT** Manufacturer advises caution in mild to moderate impairment; avoid in severe impairment. **Dose adjustments** Manufacturer advises initial dose reduction to max. 50 mg daily in mild to moderate impairment.

● **RENAL IMPAIRMENT** In general, for *NSAIDs* the MHRA advises to avoid where possible; if necessary, use with caution (risk of fluid retention and further renal impairment, including renal failure). [EvGr] For *dexketoprofen*, avoid if creatinine clearance 59 mL/minute or less. Ⓜ

Dose adjustments [EvGr] Reduce initial total daily dose to 50 mg if creatinine clearance 60–89 mL/minute. Ⓜ See p. 21.

● **MEDICINAL FORMS** There can be variation in the licensing of different medicines containing the same drug.

Oral tablet

CAUTIONARY AND ADVISORY LABELS 22

▶ Keral (A. Menarini Farmaceutica Internazionale SRL)
Dexketoprofen (as Dexketoprofen trometamol) 25 mg Keral 25mg tablets | 20 tablet [PoM] £3.67 | 50 tablet [PoM] £9.18 DT = £9.18

Combinations available: *Tramadol with dexketoprofen,* p. 536

Diclofenac potassium

01-Aug-2023

● **INDICATIONS AND DOSE**

Pain and inflammation in rheumatic disease and other musculoskeletal disorders

▶ BY MOUTH

▶ Child 14–17 years: 75–100 mg daily in 2–3 divided doses

▶ Adult: 75–150 mg daily in 2–3 divided doses

Acute gout

▶ BY MOUTH

▶ Adult: 75–150 mg daily in 2–3 divided doses

Postoperative pain

▶ BY MOUTH

▶ Child 9–13 years (body-weight 35 kg and above): Up to 2 mg/kg daily in 3 divided doses; maximum 100 mg per day

▶ Child 14–17 years: 75–100 mg daily in 2–3 divided doses

▶ Adult: 75–150 mg daily in 2–3 divided doses

Migraine

▶ BY MOUTH

▶ Adult: 50 mg, to be given at onset of migraine, then 50 mg after 2 hours if required, then 50 mg after 4–6 hours; maximum 200 mg per day

Fever in ear, nose, or throat infection

▶ BY MOUTH

▶ Child 9–17 years (body-weight 35 kg and above): Up to 2 mg/kg daily in 3 divided doses; maximum 100 mg per day

● **UNLICENSED USE** *Voltarol® Rapid* not licensed for use in children under 14 years or in fever.

> **IMPORTANT SAFETY INFORMATION**
> MHRA/CHM ADVICE: NSAIDS: POTENTIAL RISKS FOLLOWING PROLONGED USE AFTER 20 WEEKS OF PREGNANCY (JUNE 2023)
> See Non-steroidal anti-inflammatory drugs p. 1292.

● **CONTRA-INDICATIONS** Active gastro-intestinal bleeding · active gastro-intestinal ulceration · cerebrovascular disease · history of gastro-intestinal bleeding related to previous NSAID therapy · history of gastro-intestinal perforation related to previous NSAID therapy · history of recurrent gastro-intestinal haemorrhage (two or more distinct episodes) · history of recurrent gastro-intestinal ulceration (two or more distinct episodes) · ischaemic heart disease · mild to severe heart failure · peripheral arterial disease

● **CAUTIONS** Allergic disorders · cardiac impairment (NSAIDs may impair renal function) · coagulation defects · connective-tissue disorders · dehydration (risk of renal impairment) · elderly (risk of serious side-effects and fatalities) · history of cardiac failure · history of gastro-intestinal disorders (e.g. ulcerative colitis, Crohn's disease) · hypertension · may mask symptoms of infection · oedema · risk factors for cardiovascular events

● **INTERACTIONS** → Appendix 1: NSAIDs

● **SIDE-EFFECTS**

▶ **Common or very common** Appetite decreased · diarrhoea · dizziness · gastrointestinal discomfort · gastrointestinal disorders · headache · nausea · skin reactions · vertigo · vomiting

▶ **Uncommon** Chest pain · heart failure · myocardial infarction · palpitations

▶ **Rare or very rare** Acute kidney injury · agranulocytosis · alopecia · anaemia · angioedema · anxiety · aplastic anaemia · asthma · confusion · constipation · depression · drowsiness · dyspnoea · erectile dysfunction · fatigue · haemolytic anaemia · haemorrhage · hearing impairment · hepatic disorders · hypersensitivity · hypertension · hypotension · inflammatory bowel disease · irritability · leucopenia · memory loss · meningitis aseptic (patients with connective-tissue disorders such as systemic lupus erythematosus may be especially susceptible) · nephritis tubulointerstitial · nephrotic syndrome · oedema · oesophageal disorder · oral disorders · pancreatitis · photosensitivity reaction · pneumonitis · proteinuria · psychotic disorder · renal papillary necrosis · seizure · sensation abnormal · severe cutaneous adverse reactions (SCARs) · shock · sleep disorders · stroke · taste altered · thrombocytopenia · tinnitus · tremor · vasculitis · vision disorders

▶ **Frequency not known** Hallucination · malaise · optic neuritis

SIDE-EFFECTS, FURTHER INFORMATION For information about cardiovascular and gastrointestinal side-effects, and a possible exacerbation of symptoms in asthma, see Non-steroidal anti-inflammatory drugs p. 1292

● ALLERGY AND CROSS-SENSITIVITY [EvGr] Contra-indicated in patients with a history of hypersensitivity to aspirin or any other NSAID—which includes those in whom attacks of asthma, angioedema, urticaria or rhinitis have been precipitated by aspirin or any other NSAID. [M]

● CONCEPTION AND CONTRACEPTION [EvGr] Caution—long-term use of some NSAIDs is associated with reduced female fertility, which is reversible on stopping treatment. [M]

● PREGNANCY Avoid use in first and second trimesters unless essential; the MHRA advises additional antenatal monitoring may be required if treatment is considered necessary by a doctor from week 20 of pregnancy onwards. Avoid use in third trimester. See *NSAIDs in Pregnancy* in Non-steroidal anti-inflammatory drugs p. 1292 for further details.

● BREAST FEEDING Use with caution during breast-feeding. Amount in milk too small to be harmful.

● HEPATIC IMPAIRMENT Manufacturer advises caution in mild to moderate impairment; avoid in severe impairment.

● RENAL IMPAIRMENT In general, for *NSAIDs* the MHRA advises to avoid where possible; if necessary, use with caution (risk of fluid retention and further renal impairment, including renal failure). [EvGr] For *diclofenac potassium*, avoid in severe impairment. [M]

● PATIENT AND CARER ADVICE
Medicines for Children leaflet: Diclofenac for pain and inflammation www.medicinesforchildren.org.uk/medicines/diclofenac-for-pain-and-inflammation/

● MEDICINAL FORMS There can be variation in the licensing of different medicines containing the same drug.

Oral tablet
CAUTIONARY AND ADVISORY LABELS 21
▶ **Diclofenac potassium (Non-proprietary)**
Diclofenac potassium 50 mg Diclofenac potassium 50mg tablets | 28 tablet [PoM] [S] DT = £4.75
▶ **Voltarol Rapid** (Novartis Pharmaceuticals UK Ltd)
Diclofenac potassium 50 mg Voltarol Rapid 50mg tablets | 30 tablet [PoM] £7.94

Diclofenac sodium

14-Jun-2024

● **INDICATIONS AND DOSE**

Pain and inflammation in rheumatic disease and other musculoskeletal disorders | Acute gout | Postoperative pain
▶ BY MOUTH USING IMMEDIATE-RELEASE MEDICINES
▶ Adult: 75–150 mg daily in 2–3 divided doses
▶ BY MOUTH USING MODIFIED-RELEASE MEDICINES
▶ Adult: 75 mg 1–2 times a day, alternatively 100 mg once daily

▶ BY RECTUM
▶ Adult: 75–150 mg daily in 2–3 divided doses, alternatively 100 mg once daily

Actinic keratosis [using gel containing diclofenac sodium 3%]
▶ TO THE SKIN
▶ Adult: Apply twice daily usually for 60–90 days, maximum 8 g per day

Pain and inflammation in rheumatic disease and other musculoskeletal disorders [using gel containing diclofenac sodium 1%]
▶ TO THE SKIN
▶ Adult: Apply 3–4 times a day review after 14 days

Osteoarthritis of the knee or hand [using gel containing diclofenac sodium 1%]
▶ TO THE SKIN
▶ Adult: Apply 3–4 times a day review after 28 days

DOSE EQUIVALENCE AND CONVERSION
▶ *Voltarol*® 1.16% *Emulgel* contains 1.16% diclofenac diethylammonium equivalent to diclofenac sodium 1%.

VOLTAROL® SOLUTION FOR INJECTION

Postoperative pain
▶ BY DEEP INTRAMUSCULAR INJECTION
▶ Adult: 75 mg once daily for maximum 2 days, alternatively 75 mg twice daily for maximum 2 days, twice-daily administration to be used in severe cases

Acute exacerbations of pain
▶ BY DEEP INTRAMUSCULAR INJECTION
▶ Adult: 75 mg once daily for maximum 2 days, alternatively 75 mg twice daily for maximum 2 days, twice-daily administration to be used in severe cases

Ureteric colic
▶ BY DEEP INTRAMUSCULAR INJECTION
▶ Adult: 75 mg for 1 dose, dose can be repeated after 30 minutes if required; maximum 150 mg per day for maximum 2 days

Acute postoperative pain (in hospital setting)
▶ BY INTRAVENOUS INFUSION
▶ Adult: 75 mg for 1 dose, dose can be repeated after 4–6 hours if required; maximum 150 mg per day for maximum 2 days

Prevention of postoperative pain (in hospital setting)
▶ BY INTRAVENOUS INFUSION
▶ Adult: Initially 25–50 mg, to be given after surgery over 15–60 minutes, then 5 mg/hour for maximum 2 days; maximum 150 mg per day

---

IMPORTANT SAFETY INFORMATION

MHRA/CHM ADVICE: NSAIDS: POTENTIAL RISKS FOLLOWING PROLONGED USE AFTER 20 WEEKS OF PREGNANCY (JUNE 2023)
▶ With systemic use
See Non-steroidal anti-inflammatory drugs p. 1292.

● CONTRA-INDICATIONS
▶ With intravenous use Dehydration · history of asthma · history of confirmed or suspected cerebrovascular bleeding · history of haemorrhagic diathesis · hypovolaemia · operations with high risk of haemorrhage
▶ With systemic use Active gastro-intestinal bleeding · active gastro-intestinal ulceration · avoid suppositories in proctitis · cerebrovascular disease · history of gastro-intestinal bleeding related to previous NSAID therapy · history of gastro-intestinal perforation related to previous NSAID therapy · history of recurrent gastro-intestinal haemorrhage (two or more distinct episodes) · history of recurrent gastro-intestinal ulceration (two or more distinct episodes) · ischaemic heart disease · mild to severe heart failure · peripheral arterial disease

- **CAUTIONS**
  - With systemic use Allergic disorders · cardiac impairment (NSAIDs may impair renal function) · coagulation defects · connective-tissue disorders · dehydration (risk of renal impairment) · elderly (risk of serious side-effects and fatalities) · history of cardiac failure · history of gastro-intestinal disorders (e.g. ulcerative colitis, Crohn's disease) · hypertension · may mask symptoms of infection · oedema · risk factors for cardiovascular events
  - With topical use Avoid contact with eyes · avoid contact with inflamed or broken skin · avoid contact with mucous membranes · not for use with occlusive dressings · topical application of large amounts can result in systemic effects, including hypersensitivity and asthma (renal disease has also been reported)
- **INTERACTIONS** → Appendix 1: NSAIDs
- **SIDE-EFFECTS**
  - **GENERAL SIDE-EFFECTS**
  - **Common or very common** Diarrhoea · nausea · oedema · rash (discontinue) · sensation abnormal · skin reactions
  - **Uncommon** Alopecia · haemorrhage
  - **Rare or very rare** Acute kidney injury · angioedema · asthma · hypersensitivity · photosensitivity reaction
  - **SPECIFIC SIDE-EFFECTS**
  - **Common or very common**
  - With systemic use Appetite decreased · dizziness · gastrointestinal discomfort · gastrointestinal disorders · headache · vertigo · vomiting
  - With topical use Conjunctivitis · muscle tone increased · skin ulcer
  - **Uncommon**
  - With systemic use Chest pain · heart failure · myocardial infarction · palpitations
  - With topical use Abdominal pain · eye pain · lacrimation disorder · seborrhoea
  - **Rare or very rare**
  - With systemic use Agranulocytosis · anaemia · anxiety · aplastic anaemia · confusion · constipation · depression · drowsiness · dyspnoea · erectile dysfunction · haemolytic anaemia · hearing impairment · hepatic disorders · hypertension · hypotension · irritability · leucopenia · memory loss · meningitis aseptic (patients with connective-tissue disorders such as systemic lupus erythematosus may be especially susceptible) · nephritis tubulointerstitial · nephrotic syndrome · oesophageal disorder · oral disorders · pancreatitis · pneumonitis · proteinuria · psychotic disorder · renal papillary necrosis · seizure · severe cutaneous adverse reactions (SCARs) · shock · sleep disorders · stroke · taste altered · thrombocytopenia · tinnitus · tremor · vasculitis · vision disorders
  - With parenteral use Fatigue
  - With rectal use Fatigue · ulcerative colitis aggravated
  - With topical use Rash pustular
  - **Frequency not known**
  - With systemic use Fertility decreased female · hallucination · malaise · optic neuritis · platelet aggregation inhibition
  - With oral use Fluid retention
  - With parenteral use Fluid retention · injection site necrosis
  - With topical use Hair colour changes
  - **SIDE-EFFECTS, FURTHER INFORMATION** Topical application of large amounts of diclofenac can result in systemic effects.

    For information about cardiovascular and gastrointestinal side-effects, and a possible exacerbation of symptoms in asthma, see Non-steroidal anti-inflammatory drugs p. 1292
- **ALLERGY AND CROSS-SENSITIVITY** EvGr Contra-indicated in patients with a history of hypersensitivity to aspirin or any other NSAID—which includes those in whom attacks of asthma, angioedema, urticaria or rhinitis have been precipitated by aspirin or any other NSAID. M
- **CONCEPTION AND CONTRACEPTION**
  - With systemic use EvGr Caution—long-term use of some NSAIDs is associated with reduced female fertility, which is reversible on stopping treatment. M
- **PREGNANCY**
  - With systemic use Avoid use in first and second trimesters unless essential; the MHRA advises additional antenatal monitoring may be required if treatment is considered necessary by a doctor from week 20 of pregnancy onwards. Avoid use in third trimester. See *NSAIDs in Pregnancy* in Non-steroidal anti-inflammatory drugs p. 1292 for further details.
  - With topical use Patient packs for topical preparations carry a warning to avoid during pregnancy.
- **BREAST FEEDING**
  - With systemic use Use with caution during breast-feeding. Amount in milk too small to be harmful.
  - With topical use Patient packs for topical preparations carry a warning to avoid during breast-feeding.
- **HEPATIC IMPAIRMENT**
  - With systemic use Manufacturer advises caution in mild to moderate impairment; avoid in severe impairment.
- **RENAL IMPAIRMENT**
  - With systemic use In general, for *NSAIDs* the MHRA advises to avoid where possible; if necessary, use with caution (risk of fluid retention and further renal impairment, including renal failure). For *diclofenac sodium*, manufacturers advise avoid in severe impairment.
  - With intravenous use Manufacturers advise avoid in moderate to severe impairment.
  - With topical use In general, manufacturers advise caution (deterioration in renal function has also been reported after topical use).
- **DIRECTIONS FOR ADMINISTRATION** For *intravenous infusion* (*Voltarol®*), give continuously or intermittently in Glucose 5% or Sodium Chloride 0.9%. Dilute 75 mg with 100–500 mL infusion fluid (previously buffered with 0.5 mL Sodium Bicarbonate 8.4% solution *or* with 1 mL Sodium Bicarbonate 4.2% solution). For intermittent infusion give 25–50 mg over 15–60 minutes or 75 mg over 30–120 minutes. For continuous infusion give at a rate of 5 mg/hour.

  For *intramuscular injection*, inject into the gluteal muscle.
- **PRESCRIBING AND DISPENSING INFORMATION** *Voltarol®* dispersible tablets are more suitable for **short-term** use in acute conditions for which treatment required for no more than 3 months (no information on use beyond 3 months).
- **PATIENT AND CARER ADVICE**
  - With topical use For topical preparations, patients and their carers should be advised to wash hands immediately after use.

    Patients using topical gels such as *Solacutan®*, *Solaraze®*, or *Voltarol Emulgel®* should be instructed not to smoke or go near naked flames as clothing, bedding, dressings, and other fabrics that have been in contact with skin treated with these gels burn more easily and can rapidly ignite. Washing these materials may reduce build-up of these gels but not totally remove it.
    Photosensitivity Patients should be advised against excessive exposure to sunlight of area treated in order to avoid possibility of photosensitivity.
- **PROFESSION SPECIFIC INFORMATION**

  Dental practitioners' formulary Diclofenac Sodium Tablets may be prescribed.
- **EXCEPTIONS TO LEGAL CATEGORY**
  - With topical use for Pain and inflammation in rheumatic disease and other musculoskeletal disorders or Osteoarthritis of the knee

or hand Various pack sizes of gel preparations may be available on sale to the public.

- **MEDICINAL FORMS** There can be variation in the licensing of different medicines containing the same drug. Forms available from special-order manufacturers include: dispersible tablet, oral suspension, oral solution

Modified-release tablet

CAUTIONARY AND ADVISORY LABELS 21, 25

- ▸ Diclofenac sodium (Non-proprietary)

  Diclofenac sodium 75 mg Diclofenac sodium 75mg modified-release tablets | 28 tablet [PoM] £9.00 DT = £9.00 | 56 tablet [PoM] £17.56 DT = £17.56

  Diclofenac sodium 100 mg Diclofenac sodium 100mg modified-release tablets | 28 tablet [PoM] £11.33 DT = £11.33

- ▸ Diclo-SR (Strides Pharma UK Ltd)

  Diclofenac sodium 75 mg Diclo-SR 75mg tablets | 28 tablet [PoM] £6.50 DT = £9.00 | 56 tablet [PoM] £14.50 DT = £17.56

Gastro-resistant tablet

CAUTIONARY AND ADVISORY LABELS 5, 25

- ▸ Diclofenac sodium (Non-proprietary)

  Diclofenac sodium 25 mg Diclofenac sodium 25mg gastro-resistant tablets | 28 tablet [PoM] £4.13 DT = £4.13 | 84 tablet [PoM] £1.50–£12.39

  Diclofenac sodium 50 mg Diclofenac sodium 50mg gastro-resistant tablets | 28 tablet [PoM] £7.43 DT = £0.84 | 84 tablet [PoM] £2.49–£7.49

Suppository

- ▸ Econac (Advanz Pharma)

  Diclofenac sodium 100 mg Econac 100mg suppositories | 10 suppository [PoM] £3.04 DT = £3.64

- ▸ Voltarol (Novartis Pharmaceuticals UK Ltd)

  Diclofenac sodium 12.5 mg Voltarol 12.5mg suppositories | 10 suppository [PoM] £0.70 DT = £0.70

  Diclofenac sodium 25 mg Voltarol 25mg suppositories | 10 suppository [PoM] £1.24 DT = £1.24

  Diclofenac sodium 50 mg Voltarol 50mg suppositories | 10 suppository [PoM] £2.04 DT = £2.04

  Diclofenac sodium 100 mg Voltarol 100mg suppositories | 10 suppository [PoM] £3.64 DT = £3.64

Dispersible tablet

CAUTIONARY AND ADVISORY LABELS 13, 21

Solution for injection

EXCIPIENTS: May contain Benzyl alcohol, propylene glycol

- ▸ Akis (Flynn Pharma Ltd)

  Diclofenac sodium 75 mg per 1 ml Akis 75mg/1ml solution for injection ampoules | 5 ampoule [PoM] £24.00 DT = £24.00

- ▸ Voltarol (Novartis Pharmaceuticals UK Ltd)

  Diclofenac sodium 25 mg per 1 ml Voltarol 75mg/3ml solution for injection ampoules | 10 ampoule [PoM] £9.91 DT = £9.91

Modified-release capsule

CAUTIONARY AND ADVISORY LABELS 21(does not apply to Motifene® 75 mg), 25

EXCIPIENTS: May contain Propylene glycol

- ▸ Diclomax Retard (Galen Ltd)

  Diclofenac sodium 100 mg Diclomax Retard 100mg capsules | 28 capsule [PoM] £8.20 DT = £8.20

- ▸ Diclomax SR (Galen Ltd)

  Diclofenac sodium 75 mg Diclomax SR 75mg capsules | 56 capsule [PoM] £11.40 DT = £11.40

- ▸ Motifene (Glenwood GmbH)

  Diclofenac sodium 75 mg Motifene 75mg modified-release capsules | 56 capsule [PoM] £8.00 DT = £8.00

Cutaneous gel

CAUTIONARY AND ADVISORY LABELS 11, 15

EXCIPIENTS: May contain Benzyl alcohol, fragrances, propylene glycol

- ▸ Diclofenac sodium (Non-proprietary)

  Diclofenac sodium 10 mg per 1 gram Diclofenac 1% gel | 100 gram [PoM] £7.62 DT = £7.62

  Diclofenac diethylammonium 11.6 mg per 1 gram Diclofenac 1.16% gel | 30 gram [PoM] £3.50 | 50 gram [PoM] £4.85 | 100 gram [PoM] £7.82 DT = £4.63

  Diclofenac diethylammonium 23.2 mg per 1 gram Diclofenac 2.32% gel | 30 gram [PoM] £4.58–£7.30 DT = £5.40 | 50 gram [PoM] £6.47–£10.30 DT = £7.62 | 100 gram [PoM] £10.55 DT = £12.30

  Diclofenac sodium 30 mg per 1 gram Diclofenac sodium 3% gel | 50 gram [PoM] £36.38 DT = £38.30

- ▸ Solaraze (Almirall Ltd)

  Diclofenac sodium 30 mg per 1 gram Solaraze 3% gel | 50 gram [PoM] £38.30 DT = £38.30 | 100 gram [PoM] £76.60

- ▸ Voltarol Emulgel (Haleon UK Trading Ltd)

  Diclofenac diethylammonium 11.6 mg per 1 gram Voltarol 1.16% Emulgel | 100 gram [PoM] £4.63 DT = £4.63

Diclofenac sodium with misoprostol

05-Aug-2020

The properties listed below are those particular to the combination only. For the properties of the components please consider, diclofenac sodium p. 1297, misoprostol p. 85.

- **INDICATIONS AND DOSE**

ARTHROTEC® 50/200

Prophylaxis against NSAID-induced gastroduodenal ulceration in patients requiring diclofenac for rheumatoid arthritis or osteoarthritis

- ▸ BY MOUTH
- ▸ Adult: 1 tablet 2–3 times a day, take with food

ARTHROTEC® 75/200

Prophylaxis against NSAID-induced gastroduodenal ulceration in patients requiring diclofenac for rheumatoid arthritis or osteoarthritis

- ▸ BY MOUTH
- ▸ Adult: 1 tablet twice daily, take with food

MISOFEN® 50/200

Prophylaxis against NSAID-induced gastroduodenal ulceration in patients requiring diclofenac for rheumatoid arthritis or osteoarthritis

- ▸ BY MOUTH
- ▸ Adult: 1 tablet 2–3 times a day, take with food

MISOFEN® 75/200

Prophylaxis against NSAID-induced gastroduodenal ulceration in patients requiring diclofenac for rheumatoid arthritis or osteoarthritis

- ▸ BY MOUTH
- ▸ Adult: 1 tablet twice daily, take with food

- **INTERACTIONS** → Appendix 1: misoprostol · NSAIDs

- **MEDICINAL FORMS** There can be variation in the licensing of different medicines containing the same drug.

Gastro-resistant tablet

CAUTIONARY AND ADVISORY LABELS 21, 25

- ▸ Arthrotec (Pfizer Ltd)

  Misoprostol 200 microgram, Diclofenac sodium 50 mg Arthrotec 50 gastro-resistant tablets | 60 tablet [PoM] £11.98 DT = £11.98

  Misoprostol 200 microgram, Diclofenac sodium 75 mg Arthrotec 75 gastro-resistant tablets | 60 tablet [PoM] £15.83 DT = £15.83

Etodolac

01-Aug-2023

- **INDICATIONS AND DOSE**

Pain and inflammation in rheumatoid arthritis and osteoarthritis

- ▸ BY MOUTH USING MODIFIED-RELEASE MEDICINES
- ▸ Adult: 600 mg once daily

> **IMPORTANT SAFETY INFORMATION**
>
> MHRA/CHM ADVICE: NSAIDS: POTENTIAL RISKS FOLLOWING PROLONGED USE AFTER 20 WEEKS OF PREGNANCY (JUNE 2023)
> See Non-steroidal anti-inflammatory drugs p. 1292.

- **CONTRA-INDICATIONS** Active gastro-intestinal bleeding · active gastro-intestinal ulceration · history of gastro-intestinal bleeding related to previous NSAID therapy · history of gastro-intestinal perforation related to previous

NSAID therapy · history of recurrent gastro-intestinal haemorrhage (two or more distinct episodes) · history of recurrent gastro-intestinal ulceration (two or more distinct episodes) · severe heart failure

- **CAUTIONS** Allergic disorders · cardiac impairment (NSAIDs may impair renal function) · cerebrovascular disease · coagulation defects · connective-tissue disorders · dehydration (risk of renal impairment) · elderly (risk of serious side-effects and fatalities) · heart failure · history of gastro-intestinal disorders (e.g. ulcerative colitis, Crohn's disease) · ischaemic heart disease · may mask symptoms of infection · peripheral arterial disease · risk factors for cardiovascular events · uncontrolled hypertension

- **INTERACTIONS** → Appendix 1: NSAIDs

- **SIDE-EFFECTS** Agranulocytosis · angioedema · aplastic anaemia · asthenia · asthma · bilirubinuria · bronchospasm · chills · confusion · constipation · Crohn's disease aggravated · depression · diarrhoea · dizziness · drowsiness · dyspnoea · fever · gastrointestinal discomfort · gastrointestinal disorders · haemolytic anaemia · haemorrhage · hallucination · headache · heart failure · hepatic disorders · hypersensitivity · hypertension · insomnia · malaise · meningitis aseptic (patients with connective-tissue disorders such as systemic lupus erythematosus may be especially susceptible) · nausea · nephritic syndrome · nephritis tubulointerstitial · nephrotoxicity · nervousness · neutropenia · oedema · optic neuritis · oral ulceration · palpitations · pancreatitis · paraesthesia · photosensitivity reaction · renal failure (more common in patients with pre-existing renal impairment) · severe cutaneous adverse reactions (SCARs) · skin reactions · thrombocytopenia · tinnitus · tremor · urinary disorders · vasculitis · vertigo · visual impairment · vomiting

  SIDE-EFFECTS, FURTHER INFORMATION For information about cardiovascular and gastrointestinal side-effects, and a possible exacerbation of symptoms in asthma, see Non-steroidal anti-inflammatory drugs p. 1292

- **ALLERGY AND CROSS-SENSITIVITY** EvGr Contra-indicated in patients with a history of hypersensitivity to aspirin or any other NSAID—which includes those in whom attacks of asthma, angioedema, urticaria or rhinitis have been precipitated by aspirin or any other NSAID. Ⓜ

- **CONCEPTION AND CONTRACEPTION** EvGr Caution—long-term use of some NSAIDs is associated with reduced female fertility, which is reversible on stopping treatment. Ⓜ

- **PREGNANCY** Avoid use in first and second trimesters unless essential; the MHRA advises additional antenatal monitoring may be required if treatment is considered necessary by a doctor from week 20 of pregnancy onwards. Avoid use in third trimester. See *NSAIDs in Pregnancy* in Non-steroidal anti-inflammatory drugs p. 1292 for further details.

- **BREAST FEEDING** Use with caution during breast-feeding. Manufacturer advises avoid.

- **HEPATIC IMPAIRMENT** Manufacturer advises caution in mild to moderate impairment; avoid in severe impairment.

- **RENAL IMPAIRMENT** In general, for *NSAIDs* the MHRA advises to avoid where possible; if necessary, use with caution (risk of fluid retention and further renal impairment, including renal failure). EvGr For *etodolac*, avoid in severe impairment. Ⓜ

- **MEDICINAL FORMS** There can be variation in the licensing of different medicines containing the same drug.

  Modified-release tablet
  CAUTIONARY AND ADVISORY LABELS 25, 21

  ▶ **Etopan XL** (Sun Pharma UK Ltd)
  Etodolac 600 mg Etopan XL 600mg tablets | 30 tablet PoM £14.60
  DT = £15.50

▶ **Lodine SR** (Almirall Ltd)
Etodolac 600 mg Lodine SR 600mg tablets | 30 tablet PoM £15.50
DT = £15.50

Etoricoxib

22-Nov-2021

- **INDICATIONS AND DOSE**

Pain and inflammation in osteoarthritis
▶ BY MOUTH
- Child 16-17 years: 30 mg once daily, increased if necessary to 60 mg once daily
- Adult: 30 mg once daily, increased if necessary to 60 mg once daily

Pain and inflammation in rheumatoid arthritis | Ankylosing spondylitis
▶ BY MOUTH
- Child 16-17 years: 60 mg once daily, increased if necessary to 90 mg once daily
- Adult: 60 mg once daily, increased if necessary to 90 mg once daily

Acute gout
▶ BY MOUTH
- Child 16-17 years: 120 mg once daily for maximum 8 days
- Adult: 120 mg once daily for maximum 8 days

- **CONTRA-INDICATIONS** Active gastro-intestinal bleeding · active gastro-intestinal ulceration · cerebrovascular disease · inflammatory bowel disease · ischaemic heart disease · mild to severe heart failure · peripheral arterial disease · uncontrolled hypertension (persistently above 140/90 mmHg)

- **CAUTIONS** Allergic disorders · cardiac impairment (NSAIDs may impair renal function) · coagulation defects · connective-tissue disorders · dehydration (risk of renal impairment) · elderly (risk of serious side-effects and fatalities) · history of cardiac failure · history of gastro-intestinal disorders · hypertension · left ventricular dysfunction · may mask symptoms of infection · oedema · risk factors for cardiovascular events

- **INTERACTIONS** → Appendix 1: NSAIDs

- **SIDE-EFFECTS**
▶ **Common or very common** Arrhythmias · asthenia · bronchospasm · constipation · diarrhoea · dizziness · fluid retention · gastrointestinal discomfort · gastrointestinal disorders · headache · hypertension · increased risk of infection · influenza like illness · nausea · oedema · oral ulceration · palpitations · skin reactions · vomiting
▶ **Uncommon** Alertness decreased · anaemia · angina pectoris · anxiety · appetite abnormal · cerebrovascular insufficiency · chest pain · congestive heart failure · conjunctivitis · cough · depression · drowsiness · dry mouth · dyspnoea · flushing · haemorrhage · hallucination · hyperkalaemia · hypersensitivity · insomnia · irritable bowel syndrome · leucopenia · myocardial infarction · pancreatitis · proteinuria · renal failure (more common in patients with pre-existing renal impairment) · sensation abnormal · taste altered · thrombocytopenia · tinnitus · vasculitis · vertigo · vision blurred · weight increased
▶ **Rare or very rare** Angioedema · confusion · hepatic disorders · muscle complaints · severe cutaneous adverse reactions (SCARs) · shock
▶ **Frequency not known** Nephritis tubulointerstitial · nephropathy

  SIDE-EFFECTS, FURTHER INFORMATION For information about cardiovascular and gastrointestinal side-effects, and a possible exacerbation of symptoms in asthma, see Non-steroidal anti-inflammatory drugs p. 1292

- **ALLERGY AND CROSS-SENSITIVITY** EvGr Contra-indicated in patients with a history of hypersensitivity to aspirin or any other NSAID—which includes those in whom attacks of asthma, angioedema, urticaria or rhinitis have been precipitated by aspirin or any other NSAID. ◈

- **CONCEPTION AND CONTRACEPTION** Caution—long-term use of some NSAIDs is associated with reduced female fertility, which is reversible on stopping treatment.

- **PREGNANCY** Manufacturer advises avoid (teratogenic in *animal* studies). Avoid during the third trimester (risk of closure of fetal ductus arteriosus *in utero* and possibly persistent pulmonary hypertension of the newborn); onset of labour may be delayed and duration may be increased.

- **BREAST FEEDING** Use with caution during breast-feeding. Manufacturer advises avoid—present in milk in *animal* studies.

- **HEPATIC IMPAIRMENT** Manufacturer advises caution in mild to moderate impairment; avoid in severe impairment (no information available).
  Dose adjustments Manufacturer advises max. 60 mg once daily in mild impairment; max. 30 mg once daily in moderate impairment.

- **RENAL IMPAIRMENT** In general, for *NSAIDs* the MHRA advises to avoid where possible; if necessary, use with caution (risk of fluid retention and further renal impairment, including renal failure). [EvGr] For *etoricoxib*, avoid if creatinine clearance less than 30 mL/minute. ◈ See p. 21.

- **MONITORING REQUIREMENTS** Monitor blood pressure before treatment, 2 weeks after initiation and periodically during treatment.

- **MEDICINAL FORMS** There can be variation in the licensing of different medicines containing the same drug.

  Oral tablet
  - **Etoricoxib (Non-proprietary)**
    Etoricoxib 30 mg Etoricoxib 30mg tablets | 28 tablet [PoM] £13.99 DT = £2.67
    Etoricoxib 60 mg Etoricoxib 60mg tablets | 28 tablet [PoM] £20.11 DT = £4.40
    Etoricoxib 90 mg Etoricoxib 90mg tablets | 28 tablet [PoM] £22.96 DT = £4.58
    Etoricoxib 120 mg Etoricoxib 120mg tablets | 28 tablet [PoM] £24.11 DT = £9.32
  - **Arcoxia** (Organon Pharma (UK) Ltd)
    Etoricoxib 30 mg Arcoxia 30mg tablets | 28 tablet [PoM] £13.99 DT = £2.67
    Etoricoxib 60 mg Arcoxia 60mg tablets | 28 tablet [PoM] £20.11 DT = £4.40
    Etoricoxib 90 mg Arcoxia 90mg tablets | 28 tablet [PoM] £22.96 DT = £4.58
    Etoricoxib 120 mg Arcoxia 120mg tablets | 7 tablet [PoM] £6.03 | 28 tablet [PoM] £24.11 DT = £9.32

Felbinac

07-Dec-2020

- **DRUG ACTION** Felbinac is an active metabolite of the NSAID fenbufen.

- **INDICATIONS AND DOSE**

  Relief of pain in musculoskeletal conditions | Treatment in knee or hand osteoarthritis (adjunct)
  - TO THE SKIN
  - Adult: Apply 2–4 times a day, therapy should be reviewed after 14 days; maximum 25 g per day

- **CAUTIONS** Avoid contact with eyes · avoid contact with inflamed or broken skin · avoid contact with mucous membranes · not for use with occlusive dressings · topical application of large amounts can result in systemic effects, including hypersensitivity and asthma (renal disease has also been reported)

- **INTERACTIONS** → Appendix 1: NSAIDs

- **SIDE-EFFECTS** Bronchospasm · gastrointestinal disorder · hypersensitivity · paraesthesia · photosensitivity reaction · skin reactions

  SIDE-EFFECTS, FURTHER INFORMATION For information about cardiovascular and gastrointestinal side-effects, and a possible exacerbation of symptoms in asthma, see Non-steroidal anti-inflammatory drugs p. 1292

- **ALLERGY AND CROSS-SENSITIVITY** [EvGr] Contra-indicated in patients with a history of hypersensitivity to aspirin or any other NSAID—which includes those in whom attacks of asthma, angioedema, urticaria or rhinitis have been precipitated by aspirin or any other NSAID. ◈

- **PREGNANCY** Patient packs for topical preparations carry a warning to avoid during pregnancy.

- **BREAST FEEDING** Patient packs for topical preparations carry a warning to avoid during breast-feeding.

- **RENAL IMPAIRMENT** Deterioration in renal function has also been reported after topical use.

- **DIRECTIONS FOR ADMINISTRATION** Manufacturer advises for topical preparations, apply with gentle massage only.

- **PATIENT AND CARER ADVICE** For topical preparations patients and carers should be advised to wash hands immediately after use.
  Photosensitivity Patients should be advised against excessive exposure to sunlight of area treated in order to avoid possibility of photosensitivity.

- **MEDICINAL FORMS** No licensed medicines listed.

Flurbiprofen

01-Aug-2023

- **INDICATIONS AND DOSE**

  Pain and inflammation in rheumatic disease and other musculoskeletal disorders | Migraine | Postoperative analgesia | Mild to moderate pain
  - BY MOUTH
  - Child 12–17 years: 150–200 mg daily in 2–4 divided doses, then increased to 300 mg daily, dose to be increased only in acute conditions
  - Adult: 150–200 mg daily in 2–4 divided doses, then increased to 300 mg daily, dose to be increased only in acute conditions

  Dysmenorrhoea
  - BY MOUTH
  - Child 12–17 years: Initially 100 mg, then 50–100 mg every 4–6 hours; maximum 300 mg per day
  - Adult: Initially 100 mg, then 50–100 mg every 4–6 hours; maximum 300 mg per day

> **IMPORTANT SAFETY INFORMATION**
> MHRA/CHM ADVICE: NSAIDS: POTENTIAL RISKS FOLLOWING PROLONGED USE AFTER 20 WEEKS OF PREGNANCY (JUNE 2023)
> See Non-steroidal anti-inflammatory drugs p. 1292.

- **CONTRA-INDICATIONS** Active gastro-intestinal bleeding · active gastro-intestinal ulceration · Crohn's disease (may be exacerbated) · history of gastro-intestinal bleeding related to previous NSAID therapy · history of gastro-intestinal perforation related to previous NSAID therapy · history of recurrent gastro-intestinal haemorrhage (two or more distinct episodes) · history of recurrent gastro-intestinal ulceration (two or more distinct episodes) · severe heart failure · ulcerative colitis (may be exacerbated)

- **CAUTIONS** Allergic disorders · cardiac impairment (NSAIDs may impair renal function) · cerebrovascular disease · coagulation defects · connective-tissue disorders · dehydration (risk of renal impairment) · elderly (risk of serious side-effects and fatalities) · heart failure · history of gastro-intestinal disorders · ischaemic heart disease · may mask symptoms of infection · peripheral arterial disease · risk factors for cardiovascular events · uncontrolled hypertension

- **INTERACTIONS** → Appendix 1: NSAIDs
- **SIDE-EFFECTS** Agranulocytosis · angioedema · aplastic anaemia · asthma · bronchospasm · confusion · constipation · Crohn's disease · depression · diarrhoea · dizziness · drowsiness · dyspnoea · fatigue · fertility decreased female · gastrointestinal discomfort · gastrointestinal disorders · haemolytic anaemia · haemorrhage · hallucination · headache · heart failure · hepatic disorders · hypersensitivity · hypertension · malaise · meningitis aseptic (patients with connective-tissue disorders such as systemic lupus erythematosus may be especially susceptible) · nausea · nephritis tubulointerstitial · nephropathy · neutropenia · oedema · optic neuritis · oral ulceration · pancreatitis · paraesthesia · photosensitivity reaction · platelet aggregation inhibition · renal failure (more common in patients with pre-existing renal impairment) · respiratory tract reaction · severe cutaneous adverse reactions (SCARs) · skin reactions · stroke · thrombocytopenia · tinnitus · vertigo · visual impairment · vomiting

SIDE-EFFECTS, FURTHER INFORMATION For information about cardiovascular and gastrointestinal side-effects, and a possible exacerbation of symptoms in asthma, see Non-steroidal anti-inflammatory drugs p. 1292

- **ALLERGY AND CROSS-SENSITIVITY** EvGr Contra-indicated in patients with a history of hypersensitivity to aspirin or any other NSAID—which includes those in whom attacks of asthma, angioedema, urticaria or rhinitis have been precipitated by aspirin or any other NSAID. Ⓜ
- **CONCEPTION AND CONTRACEPTION** EvGr Caution—long-term use of some NSAIDs is associated with reduced female fertility, which is reversible on stopping treatment. Ⓜ
- **PREGNANCY** Avoid use in first and second trimesters unless essential; the MHRA advises additional antenatal monitoring may be required if treatment is considered necessary by a doctor from week 20 of pregnancy onwards. Avoid use in third trimester. See *NSAIDs in Pregnancy* in Non-steroidal anti-inflammatory drugs p. 1292 for further details.
- **BREAST FEEDING** Use with caution during breast-feeding. Small amount present in milk—manufacturer advises avoid.
- **HEPATIC IMPAIRMENT** Manufacturer advises caution in mild to moderate impairment; avoid in severe impairment.
- **RENAL IMPAIRMENT** In general, for *NSAIDs* the MHRA advises to avoid where possible; if necessary, use with caution (risk of fluid retention and further renal impairment, including renal failure). EvGr For *flurbiprofen*, avoid in severe impairment. Ⓜ
- **MEDICINAL FORMS** There can be variation in the licensing of different medicines containing the same drug.

Oral tablet

CAUTIONARY AND ADVISORY LABELS 21
- **Flurbiprofen (Non-proprietary)**
  Flurbiprofen 50 mg Flurbiprofen 50mg tablets | 100 tablet PoM £60.54-£69.08 DT = £60.54
  Flurbiprofen 100 mg Flurbiprofen 100mg tablets | 100 tablet PoM £123.52 DT = £107.00

Ibuprofen

18-Mar-2024

- **INDICATIONS AND DOSE**

Pain and inflammation in rheumatic disease and other musculoskeletal disorders | Mild to moderate pain including dysmenorrhoea | Postoperative analgesia | Dental pain
▶ BY MOUTH USING IMMEDIATE-RELEASE MEDICINES
▶ Adult: Initially 300–400 mg 3–4 times a day; maintenance 200–400 mg 3 times a day, increased if necessary up to 600 mg 4 times a day
▶ BY MOUTH USING MODIFIED-RELEASE MEDICINES
▶ Adult: 1.6 g once daily, dose to be taken in the early evening, increased if necessary to 2.4 g daily in 2 divided doses, dose to be increased only in severe cases

Acute migraine
▶ BY MOUTH USING IMMEDIATE-RELEASE MEDICINES
▶ Adult: 400–600 mg for 1 dose, to be taken as soon as migraine symptoms develop

Mild to moderate pain | Pain and inflammation of soft-tissue injuries | Pyrexia with discomfort
▶ BY MOUTH USING IMMEDIATE-RELEASE MEDICINES
▶ Child 3-5 months: 50 mg 3 times a day, maximum daily dose to be given in 3–4 divided doses; maximum 30 mg/kg per day
▶ Child 6-11 months: 50 mg 3–4 times a day, maximum daily dose to be given in 3–4 divided doses; maximum 30 mg/kg per day
▶ Child 1-3 years: 100 mg 3 times a day, maximum daily dose to be given in 3–4 divided doses; maximum 30 mg/kg per day
▶ Child 4-6 years: 150 mg 3 times a day, maximum daily dose to be given in 3–4 divided doses; maximum 30 mg/kg per day
▶ Child 7-9 years: 200 mg 3 times a day, maximum daily dose to be given in 3–4 divided doses; maximum 30 mg/kg per day; maximum 2.4 g per day
▶ Child 10-11 years: 300 mg 3 times a day, maximum daily dose to be given in 3–4 divided doses; maximum 30 mg/kg per day; maximum 2.4 g per day
▶ Child 12-17 years: Initially 300–400 mg 3–4 times a day; maintenance 200–400 mg 3 times a day, increased if necessary up to 600 mg 4 times a day

Pain and inflammation
▶ BY MOUTH USING MODIFIED-RELEASE MEDICINES
▶ Child 12-17 years: 1.6 g once daily, dose preferably taken in the early evening, increased to 2.4 g daily in 2 divided doses, dose to be increased only in severe cases

Pain and inflammation in rheumatic disease including juvenile idiopathic arthritis
▶ BY MOUTH USING IMMEDIATE-RELEASE MEDICINES
▶ Child 3 months-17 years: 30–40 mg/kg daily in 3 divided doses (max. per dose 800 mg), alternatively 30–40 mg/kg daily in 4 divided doses (max. per dose 600 mg)

Pain and inflammation in systemic juvenile idiopathic arthritis
▶ BY MOUTH USING IMMEDIATE-RELEASE MEDICINES
▶ Child 3 months-17 years (body-weight up to 40 kg): Up to 60 mg/kg daily in 4–6 divided doses
▶ Child 3 months-17 years (body-weight 40 kg and above): Up to 2.4 g daily in 4–6 divided doses

Post-immunisation pyrexia in infants (on doctor's advice only)
▶ BY MOUTH USING IMMEDIATE-RELEASE MEDICINES
▶ Child 2-3 months: 50 mg for 1 dose, followed by 50 mg for 1 dose, to be given 6 hours after first dose if required

Pain relief in musculoskeletal conditions | Treatment in knee or hand osteoarthritis (adjunct)
▶ TO THE SKIN
▶ Adult: Apply up to 3 times a day, ibuprofen 5% gel to be administered

Pain and inflammation in rheumatic disease and other musculoskeletal disorders (dose approved for use by community practitioner nurse prescribers) | Mild to moderate pain including dysmenorrhoea (dose approved for use by community practitioner nurse prescribers) | Migraine (dose approved for use by community practitioner nurse prescribers) | Dental pain (dose approved for use by community practitioner nurse prescribers) | Headache (dose approved for use by community practitioner nurse prescribers) | Fever (dose approved for use by community practitioner nurse prescribers) | Symptoms of colds and influenza (dose approved for use by community practitioner nurse prescribers) | Neuralgia (dose approved for use by community practitioner nurse prescribers)
▶ BY MOUTH USING IMMEDIATE-RELEASE MEDICINES
▶ Child 12-17 years: 200–400 mg 3 times a day, if symptoms worsen or persist for more than 3 days refer to doctor
▶ Adult: 200–400 mg 3 times a day, if symptoms worsen or persist for more than 10 days refer to doctor

Mild to moderate pain (dose approved for use by community practitioner nurse prescribers) | Pain and inflammation of soft-tissue injuries (dose approved for use by community practitioner nurse prescribers) | Pyrexia with discomfort (dose approved for use by community practitioner nurse prescribers)
▶ BY MOUTH USING IMMEDIATE-RELEASE MEDICINES
▶ Child 3-5 months (body-weight 5 kg and above): 20–30 mg/kg daily in divided doses, alternatively 50 mg 3 times a day for maximum of 24 hours, refer to doctor if symptoms persist for more than 24 hours
▶ Child 6-11 months: 50 mg 3–4 times a day, refer to doctor if symptoms persist for more than 3 days
▶ Child 1-3 years: 100 mg 3 times a day, refer to doctor if symptoms persist for more than 3 days
▶ Child 4-6 years: 150 mg 3 times a day, refer to doctor if symptoms persist for more than 3 days
▶ Child 7-9 years: 200 mg 3 times a day, refer to doctor if symptoms persist for more than 3 days
▶ Child 10-11 years: 300 mg 3 times a day, refer to doctor if symptoms persist for more than 3 days

Post-immunisation pyrexia in infants (dose approved for use by community practitioner nurse prescribers) (on doctor's advice only)
▶ BY MOUTH USING IMMEDIATE-RELEASE MEDICINES
▶ Child 3 months: 50 mg for 1 dose, followed by 50 mg for 1 dose, to be given 6 hours after first dose if required, if pyrexia persists refer to doctor

Acute moderate pain | Pyrexia
▶ BY INTRAVENOUS INFUSION
▶ Child 6-17 years (body-weight 20-29 kg): 200 mg 3 times a day as required for maximum 3 days, doses to be given at intervals of at least 6 hours; maximum 600 mg per day
▶ Child 6-17 years (body-weight 30-39 kg): 200 mg 4 times a day as required for maximum 3 days, doses to be given at intervals of at least 6 hours; maximum 800 mg per day
▶ Child 6-17 years (body-weight 40 kg and above): 200–400 mg 3 times a day as required for maximum 3 days, doses to be given at intervals of at least 6 hours; maximum 1.2 g per day

Acute moderate pain
▶ BY INTRAVENOUS INFUSION
▶ Adult: 400 mg 3 times a day as required for maximum 3 days, doses to be given at intervals of at least 6 hours, alternatively 600 mg twice daily as required for maximum 3 days, doses to be given at intervals of at least 6 hours; maximum 1.2 g per day

Pyrexia
▶ BY INTRAVENOUS INFUSION
▶ Adult: 400 mg 3 times a day as required for maximum 3 days, doses to be given at intervals of at least 6 hours; maximum 1.2 g per day

FENBID ® FORTE

Pain relief in musculoskeletal conditions | Treatment in knee or hand osteoarthritis (adjunct)
▶ TO THE SKIN
▶ Adult: Apply up to 4 times a day, therapy should be reviewed after 14 days

IBUGEL ® FORTE

Pain relief in musculoskeletal conditions | Treatment in knee or hand osteoarthritis (adjunct)
▶ TO THE SKIN
▶ Adult: Apply up to 3 times a day

● UNLICENSED USE
▶ With oral use in children Not licensed for use in children aged under 3 months or with body-weight under 5 kg. Maximum dose for systemic juvenile idiopathic arthritis is unlicensed.

> IMPORTANT SAFETY INFORMATION
> MHRA/CHM ADVICE: NSAIDS: POTENTIAL RISKS FOLLOWING PROLONGED USE AFTER 20 WEEKS OF PREGNANCY (JUNE 2023)
> ▶ With systemic use
> See Non-steroidal anti-inflammatory drugs p. 1292.

● CONTRA-INDICATIONS
▶ With intravenous use Active bleeding (especially intracranial or gastro-intestinal) · thrombocytopenia
▶ With systemic use Active gastro-intestinal bleeding · active gastro-intestinal ulceration · history of gastro-intestinal bleeding related to previous NSAID therapy · history of gastro-intestinal perforation related to previous NSAID therapy · history of recurrent gastro-intestinal haemorrhage (two or more distinct episodes) · history of recurrent gastro-intestinal ulceration (two or more distinct episodes) · severe heart failure · varicella infection

● CAUTIONS
▶ With systemic use Allergic disorders · cardiac impairment (NSAIDs may impair renal function) · cerebrovascular disease · coagulation defects · connective-tissue disorders · dehydration (risk of renal impairment) · elderly (risk of serious side-effects and fatalities) · heart failure · history of gastro-intestinal disorders (e.g. ulcerative colitis, Crohn's disease) · ischaemic heart disease · may mask symptoms of infection · peripheral arterial disease · risk factors for cardiovascular events · uncontrolled hypertension
▶ With topical use Avoid contact with eyes · avoid contact with inflamed or broken skin · avoid contact with mucous membranes · not for use with occlusive dressings · topical application of large amounts can result in systemic effects, including hypersensitivity and asthma (renal disease has also been reported)

CAUTIONS, FURTHER INFORMATION
▶ High-dose ibuprofen
▶ With oral use A small increase in cardiovascular risk, similar to the risk associated with cyclo-oxygenase-2 inhibitors and diclofenac, has been reported with high-dose ibuprofen ($\geq$ 2.4 g daily); use should be avoided in patients with established ischaemic heart disease, peripheral arterial disease, cerebrovascular disease, congestive heart

failure (New York Heart Association classification II-III), and uncontrolled hypertension.
▶ Masking of symptoms of underlying infections
▶ With systemic use Ibuprofen can mask symptoms of infection, which may lead to delayed initiation of appropriate treatment and thereby worsen infection outcome. This has been observed in bacterial community-acquired pneumonia and bacterial complications to varicella. When administered for fever or pain relief in relation to infection, monitoring of infection is advised.
● **INTERACTIONS** → Appendix 1: NSAIDs
● **SIDE-EFFECTS**
GENERAL SIDE-EFFECTS
▶ **Common or very common** Gastrointestinal discomfort · skin reactions
▶ **Uncommon** Asthma · hypersensitivity
▶ **Rare or very rare** Dyspnoea
SPECIFIC SIDE-EFFECTS
▶ **Common or very common**
▶ With systemic use Constipation · diarrhoea · gastrointestinal disorders · haemorrhage · headache · nausea · vomiting
▶ With intravenous use Dizziness · fatigue · inflammatory bowel disease · insomnia · oral disorders · vertigo
▶ **Uncommon**
▶ With systemic use Acute kidney injury · oedema
▶ With intravenous use Anxiety · irritability · nephritis tubulointerstitial · nephrotic syndrome · tinnitus · vasculitis · vision disorders
▶ With oral use Rash (discontinue)
▶ **Rare or very rare**
▶ With systemic use Agranulocytosis · anaemia · heart failure · hypertension · leucopenia · meningitis aseptic (patients with connective-tissue disorders such as systemic lupus erythematosus may be especially susceptible) · pancytopenia · renal papillary necrosis · respiratory disorders · severe cutaneous adverse reactions (SCARs) · shock · thrombocytopenia
▶ With intravenous use Alopecia · auditory disorder · confusion · depression · hepatic disorders · hypotension · infection exacerbated · myocardial infarction · neck stiffness · palpitations · pancreatitis · photosensitivity reaction · psychotic disorder · systemic lupus erythematosus (SLE)
▶ With oral use Angioedema · liver disorder · oral ulceration
▶ **Frequency not known**
▶ With systemic use Increased risk of arterial thromboembolism
▶ With oral use Crohn's disease · fertility decreased female · fluid retention · renal failure (more common in patients with pre-existing renal impairment) · respiratory tract reaction
▶ With topical use Angioedema · bronchospasm · rash (discontinue) · renal impairment · toxic epidermal necrolysis

SIDE-EFFECTS, FURTHER INFORMATION For information about cardiovascular and gastrointestinal side-effects, and a possible exacerbation of symptoms in asthma, see Non-steroidal anti-inflammatory drugs p. 1292

With topical use Topical application of large amounts can result in systemic effects, including hypersensitivity and asthma (renal disease has also been reported).

Overdose Overdosage with ibuprofen may cause nausea, vomiting, epigastric pain, and tinnitus, but more serious toxicity is very uncommon. Charcoal, activated followed by symptomatic measures are indicated if more than 100 mg/kg has been ingested within the preceding hour.

For details on the management of poisoning, see Emergency treatment of poisoning p. 1554.

● **ALLERGY AND CROSS-SENSITIVITY** EvGr Contra-indicated in patients with a history of hypersensitivity to aspirin or any other NSAID—which includes those in whom attacks of asthma, angioedema, urticaria or rhinitis have been precipitated by aspirin or any other NSAID. ⟨M⟩

● **CONCEPTION AND CONTRACEPTION**
▶ With systemic use EvGr Caution—long-term use of some NSAIDs is associated with reduced female fertility, which is reversible on stopping treatment. ⟨M⟩
● **PREGNANCY**
▶ With systemic use Avoid use in first and second trimesters unless essential; the MHRA advises additional antenatal monitoring may be required if treatment is considered necessary by a doctor from week 20 of pregnancy onwards. Avoid use in third trimester. See *NSAIDs in Pregnancy* in Non-steroidal anti-inflammatory drugs p. 1292 for further details.
▶ With topical use Patient packs for topical preparations carry a warning to avoid during pregnancy.
● **BREAST FEEDING** Specialist sources indicate suitable for use in breast-feeding—negligible amounts present in milk.
● **HEPATIC IMPAIRMENT**
▶ With systemic use for indications relating to Pain or Pyrexia EvGr Caution in mild to moderate impairment; avoid in severe impairment. ⟨M⟩
Dose adjustments
▶ With systemic use for indications relating to Pain or Pyrexia EvGr The lowest effective dose should be used for the shortest possible duration. ⟨M⟩
● **RENAL IMPAIRMENT**
▶ With systemic use for indications relating to Pain or Pyrexia In general, for *NSAIDs* the MHRA advises to avoid where possible; if necessary, use with caution (risk of fluid retention and further renal impairment, including renal failure). EvGr For *ibuprofen*, avoid in severe impairment. ⟨M⟩
▶ With topical use EvGr Caution (deterioration in renal function has also been reported after topical use). ⟨M⟩
Dose adjustments
▶ With systemic use for indications relating to Pain or Pyrexia EvGr The lowest effective dose should be used for the shortest possible duration. ⟨M⟩
● **DIRECTIONS FOR ADMINISTRATION** For *intravenous infusion*, give over 30 minutes.
▶ With topical use For topical preparations, apply with gentle massage only.
● **PRESCRIBING AND DISPENSING INFORMATION**
▶ With oral use Flavours of syrup may include orange.
● **PATIENT AND CARER ADVICE**
▶ With topical use For topical preparations, patients and their carers should be advised to wash hands immediately after use.
Photosensitivity For topical preparations, patients or their carers should be advised against excessive exposure to sunlight of area treated in order to avoid possibility of photosensitivity.
Medicines for Children leaflet: Ibuprofen for pain and inflammation www.medicinesforchildren.org.uk/medicines/ibuprofen-for-pain-and-inflammation/
● **PROFESSION SPECIFIC INFORMATION**
Dental practitioners' formulary Ibuprofen Oral Suspension Sugar-free may be prescribed. Ibuprofen Tablets may be prescribed.
● **EXCEPTIONS TO LEGAL CATEGORY**
▶ With topical use Smaller pack sizes of gel preparations may be available on sale to the public.
▶ With oral use Oral preparations can be sold to the public in certain circumstances.

- **MEDICINAL FORMS** There can be variation in the licensing of different medicines containing the same drug. Forms available from special-order manufacturers include: oral suspension

Oral tablet
CAUTIONARY AND ADVISORY LABELS 21
- Ibuprofen (Non-proprietary)
  Ibuprofen 200 mg Ibuprofen 200mg tablets | 84 tablet [PoM] [S] DT = £2.35 | 250 tablet [PoM] £9.30
  Ibuprofen sodium dihydrate 256 mg Ibuprofen sodium dihydrate 256mg tablets | 16 tablet [GSL] £4.19
  Ibuprofen 400 mg Ibuprofen 400mg tablets | 84 tablet [PoM] [S] DT = £2.59 | 250 tablet [PoM] £11.20
  Ibuprofen 600 mg Ibuprofen 600mg tablets | 84 tablet [PoM] £4.93 DT = £2.76
  Ibuprofen 600mg tablets film coated | 84 tablet [PoM] £2.76 DT = £2.76
- Brufen (Viatris UK Healthcare Ltd)
  Ibuprofen 400 mg Brufen 400mg tablets | 60 tablet [PoM] £4.90
- Feminax Express (Bayer Plc)
  Ibuprofen lysine 342 mg Feminax Express 342mg tablets | 8 tablet [GSL] £2.30 DT = £2.12 | 16 tablet [GSL] £3.62 DT = £3.37
- Nurofen Express (Ibuprofen sodium dihydrate) (Reckitt Benckiser Healthcare (UK) Ltd)
  Ibuprofen sodium dihydrate 256 mg Nurofen Express 256mg tablets | 16 tablet [GSL] £2.46
  Nurofen Express 256mg caplets | 16 tablet [GSL] £2.58
- Nurofen Maximum Strength Migraine Pain (Reckitt Benckiser Healthcare (UK) Ltd)
  Ibuprofen lysine 684 mg Nurofen Maximum Strength Migraine Pain 684mg caplets | 12 tablet [P] £4.04 DT = £4.04
- Nurofen Migraine Pain (Reckitt Benckiser Healthcare (UK) Ltd)
  Ibuprofen lysine 342 mg Nurofen Migraine Pain 342mg caplets | 12 tablet [GSL] £2.26
- Nurofen Pain Relief (Ibuprofen) (Reckitt Benckiser Healthcare (UK) Ltd)
  Ibuprofen sodium dihydrate 256 mg Nurofen Pain Relief 256mg tablets | 16 tablet [GSL] £2.46
  Nurofen Pain Relief 256mg caplets | 16 tablet [GSL] £2.58
  Ibuprofen sodium dihydrate 512 mg Nurofen Pain Relief Max Strength 512mg tablets | 24 tablet [P] £6.97

Effervescent granules
CAUTIONARY AND ADVISORY LABELS 13, 21
ELECTROLYTES: May contain Sodium
- Brufen (Viatris UK Healthcare Ltd)
  Ibuprofen 600 mg Brufen 600mg effervescent granules sachets | 20 sachet [PoM] £6.80 DT = £6.80

Modified-release tablet
CAUTIONARY AND ADVISORY LABELS 25, 27
- Brufen Retard (Viatris UK Healthcare Ltd)
  Ibuprofen 800 mg Brufen Retard 800mg tablets | 56 tablet [PoM] £7.74 DT = £7.74

Oral suspension
CAUTIONARY AND ADVISORY LABELS 21
- Ibuprofen (Non-proprietary)
  Ibuprofen 20 mg per 1 ml Ibuprofen 100mg/5ml oral suspension sugar free | 500 ml [PoM] [S] [SF]
  Ibuprofen 40 mg per 1 ml Ibuprofen Twelve Plus Pain Relief 200mg/5ml oral suspension | 100 ml [P] £3.49 DT = £3.49 [SF]
  Ibuprofen Seven Plus Pain Relief 200mg/5ml oral suspension | 100 ml [P] £3.49 DT = £3.49 [SF]
- Nurofen (Reckitt Benckiser Healthcare (UK) Ltd)
  Ibuprofen 40 mg per 1 ml Nurofen for Children 200mg/5ml oral suspension orange | 100 ml [P] £4.85 DT = £3.49 [SF]
  Nurofen for Children 200mg/5ml oral suspension strawberry | 100 ml [P] £4.85 DT = £3.49 [SF]

Modified-release capsule
- Galprofen Long Lasting (Galpharm International Ltd)
  Ibuprofen 200 mg Galprofen Long Lasting 200mg capsules | 8 capsule [GSL] £0.96
- Nurofen Long Lasting (Reckitt Benckiser Healthcare (UK) Ltd)
  Ibuprofen 300 mg Nurofen Long Lasting Pain Relief PR 300mg capsules | 24 capsule [P] £5.37 DT = £5.37

Oral capsule
- Ibuprofen (Non-proprietary)
  Ibuprofen 400 mg Ibuprofen 400mg capsules | 100 capsule [PoM] £26.00–£47.00
- Flarin (infirst Ltd)
  Ibuprofen 200 mg Flarin 200mg capsules | 12 capsule [P] £3.57 | 30 capsule [P] £7.38 DT = £5.22

- Nurofen Express (Reckitt Benckiser Healthcare (UK) Ltd)
  Ibuprofen 200 mg Nurofen Express 200mg liquid capsules | 30 capsule [P] £5.22 DT = £5.22

Solution for infusion
ELECTROLYTES: May contain Sodium
- Ibuprofen (Non-proprietary)
  Ibuprofen 4 mg per 1 ml Ibuprofen 400mg/100ml infusion polyethylene bottles | 10 bottle [PoM] £66.00 (Hospital only)
  Ibuprofen 200mg/50ml infusion polyethylene bottles | 10 bottle [PoM] £88.00 (Hospital only)
  Ibuprofen (as Ibuprofen lysine) 10 mg per 1 ml NeoProfen 20mg/2ml solution for infusion vials | 3 vial [PoM] [S] (Hospital only)
- Pedea (Recordati Rare Diseases UK Ltd)
  Ibuprofen 5 mg per 1 ml Pedea 10mg/2ml solution for infusion ampoules | 4 ampoule [PoM] £288.00 (Hospital only)

Chewable capsule
- Nurofen (Reckitt Benckiser Healthcare (UK) Ltd)
  Ibuprofen 100 mg Nurofen for Children 100mg chewable capsules | 12 capsule [P] £3.85 DT = £3.85

Cutaneous gel
EXCIPIENTS: May contain Benzyl alcohol
- Ibuprofen (Non-proprietary)
  Ibuprofen 50 mg per 1 gram Mentholatum Ibuprofen 5% gel | 100 gram [P] £5.69 DT = £2.44
  Ibuprofen 5% gel | 50 gram [P] £1.34 DT = £1.22 | 100 gram [P] £5.37 DT = £2.44
- Ibugel (Dermal Laboratories Ltd)
  Ibuprofen 50 mg per 1 gram Ibugel 5% gel | 100 gram [P] £4.87 DT = £2.44
  Ibuprofen 100 mg per 1 gram Ibugel Forte 10% gel | 100 gram [PoM] £5.79 DT = £5.79
- Ibuleve (Diomed Developments Ltd)
  Ibuprofen 50 mg per 1 gram Ibuleve 5% gel | 30 gram [P] £2.74 | 50 gram [P] £3.95 DT = £1.22 | 100 gram [P] £6.80 DT = £2.44
- Phorpain (Advanz Pharma)
  Ibuprofen 50 mg per 1 gram Phorpain 5% gel | 100 gram [P] £1.50 DT = £2.44

Orodispersible tablet
- Nurofen Meltlets (Reckitt Benckiser Healthcare (UK) Ltd)
  Ibuprofen 200 mg Nurofen Meltlets 200mg tablets | 12 tablet [GSL] £2.58 DT = £2.58 [SF]

Indometacin
(Indomethacin)

01-Aug-2023

- **INDICATIONS AND DOSE**

Pain and moderate to severe inflammation in rheumatic disease and other musculoskeletal disorders
- BY MOUTH USING IMMEDIATE-RELEASE MEDICINES
- Adult: 50–200 mg daily in divided doses
- BY RECTUM
- Adult: 100 mg 1–2 times a day, dose to be administered at night and in the morning if required, combined oral and rectal treatment maximum total daily dose 150–200 mg
- BY MOUTH USING MODIFIED-RELEASE MEDICINES
- Adult: 75 mg 1–2 times a day

Acute gout
- BY MOUTH USING IMMEDIATE-RELEASE MEDICINES
- Adult: 150–200 mg daily in divided doses
- BY RECTUM
- Adult: 100 mg 1–2 times a day, dose to be administered at night and in the morning if required, combined oral and rectal treatment maximum total daily dose 150–200 mg
- BY MOUTH USING MODIFIED-RELEASE MEDICINES
- Adult: 75 mg 1–2 times a day

Dysmenorrhoea
- BY MOUTH USING IMMEDIATE-RELEASE MEDICINES
- Adult: Up to 75 mg daily
- BY RECTUM
- Adult: 100 mg 1–2 times a day, dose to be administered at night and in the morning if required,   continued →

combined oral and rectal treatment maximum total daily dose 150–200 mg
▶ BY MOUTH USING MODIFIED-RELEASE MEDICINES
▶ Adult: 75 mg daily

IMPORTANT SAFETY INFORMATION

MHRA/CHM ADVICE: NSAIDS: POTENTIAL RISKS FOLLOWING PROLONGED USE AFTER 20 WEEKS OF PREGNANCY (JUNE 2023)
See Non-steroidal anti-inflammatory drugs p. 1292.

● **CONTRA-INDICATIONS** Active gastro-intestinal bleeding · active gastro-intestinal ulceration · history of gastro-intestinal bleeding related to previous NSAID therapy · history of gastro-intestinal perforation related to previous NSAID therapy · history of recurrent gastro-intestinal haemorrhage (two or more distinct episodes) · history of recurrent gastro-intestinal ulceration (two or more distinct episodes) · severe heart failure

● **CAUTIONS**

GENERAL CAUTIONS Allergic disorders · cardiac impairment (NSAIDs may impair renal function) · cerebrovascular disease · coagulation defects · connective-tissue disorders · dehydration (risk of renal impairment) · elderly (risk of serious side-effects and fatalities) · epilepsy · heart failure · history of gastro-intestinal disorders (e.g. ulcerative colitis, Crohn's disease) · ischaemic heart disease · may mask symptoms of infection · parkinsonism · peripheral arterial disease · psychiatric disturbances · risk factors for cardiovascular events · uncontrolled hypertension

SPECIFIC CAUTIONS
▶ With rectal use Avoid rectal administration in proctitis · avoid rectal administration in recent rectal bleeding

● **INTERACTIONS** → Appendix 1: NSAIDs

● **SIDE-EFFECTS**

GENERAL SIDE-EFFECTS Agranulocytosis · alopecia · anaphylactic reaction · angioedema · anxiety · appetite decreased · arrhythmias · asthma · blood disorder · bone marrow disorders · breast abnormalities · chest pain · coma · confusion · congestive heart failure · constipation · corneal deposits · depression · diarrhoea · disseminated intravascular coagulation · dizziness · drowsiness · dysarthria · erythema nodosum · eye disorder · eye pain · fatigue · fluid retention · flushing · gastrointestinal discomfort · gastrointestinal disorders · gynaecomastia · haemolytic anaemia · haemorrhage · hallucination · headache · hearing impairment · hepatic disorders · hyperglycaemia · hyperhidrosis · hyperkalaemia · hypotension · inflammatory bowel disease · insomnia · leucopenia · movement disorders · muscle weakness · nausea · nephritis tubulointerstitial · nephrotic syndrome · oedema · oral disorders · palpitations · pancreatitis · paraesthesia · peripheral neuropathy · photosensitivity reaction · platelet aggregation inhibition · psychiatric disorders · renal failure (more common in patients with pre-existing renal impairment) · respiratory disorders · seizures · severe cutaneous adverse reactions (SCARs) · skin reactions · syncope · thrombocytopenia · tinnitus · urine abnormalities · vasculitis · vertigo · vision disorders · vomiting

SPECIFIC SIDE-EFFECTS
▶ With oral use Dyspnoea · malaise · pulmonary oedema · sigmoid lesion perforation

SIDE-EFFECTS, FURTHER INFORMATION For information about cardiovascular and gastrointestinal side-effects, and a possible exacerbation of symptoms in asthma, see Non-steroidal anti-inflammatory drugs p. 1292

● **ALLERGY AND CROSS-SENSITIVITY** EvGr Contra-indicated in patients with a history of hypersensitivity to aspirin or any other NSAID—which includes those in whom attacks

of asthma, angioedema, urticaria or rhinitis have been precipitated by aspirin or any other NSAID. Ⓜ

● **CONCEPTION AND CONTRACEPTION** EvGr Caution—long-term use of some NSAIDs is associated with reduced female fertility, which is reversible on stopping treatment. Ⓜ

● **PREGNANCY** Avoid use in first and second trimesters unless essential; the MHRA advises additional antenatal monitoring may be required if treatment is considered necessary by a doctor from week 20 of pregnancy onwards. Avoid use in third trimester. See *NSAIDs in Pregnancy* in Non-steroidal anti-inflammatory drugs p. 1292 for further details.

● **BREAST FEEDING** Amount probably too small to be harmful—manufacturers advise avoid. Use with caution during breast-feeding.

● **HEPATIC IMPAIRMENT** Manufacturer advises caution in mild to moderate impairment; avoid in severe impairment (increased risk of gastro-intestinal bleeding and fluid retention).

● **RENAL IMPAIRMENT** In general, for *NSAIDs* the MHRA advises to avoid where possible; if necessary, use with caution (risk of fluid retention and further renal impairment, including renal failure). EvGr For *indometacin*, avoid in severe impairment. Ⓜ

● **MONITORING REQUIREMENTS** During prolonged therapy ophthalmic and blood examinations particularly advisable.

● **PATIENT AND CARER ADVICE**

Driving and skilled tasks Dizziness may affect performance of skilled tasks (e.g. driving).

● **MEDICINAL FORMS** There can be variation in the licensing of different medicines containing the same drug. Forms available from special-order manufacturers include: oral suspension, oral solution

Oral capsule
CAUTIONARY AND ADVISORY LABELS 21
▶ Indometacin (Non-proprietary)
  Indometacin 25 mg Indometacin 25mg capsules | 28 capsule PoM £2.03 DT = £1.59
  Indometacin 50 mg Indometacin 50mg capsules | 28 capsule PoM £2.29 DT = £2.05

Suppository
▶ Indometacin (Non-proprietary)
  Indometacin 100 mg Indometacin 100mg suppositories | 10 suppository PoM £17.61 DT = £17.61

Ketoprofen

01-Aug-2023

● **INDICATIONS AND DOSE**

Pain and mild inflammation in rheumatic disease and musculoskeletal conditions | Dysmenorrhoea | Acute gout
▶ BY MOUTH
▶ Adult: 100–200 mg once daily

Relief of pain in rheumatic disease and musculoskeletal conditions
▶ TO THE SKIN
▶ Adult: Apply 2–4 times a day for up to 7 days, ketoprofen 2.5% gel to be administered; maximum 15 g per day

POWERGEL®

Relief of pain in musculoskeletal conditions | Adjunctive treatment in knee or hand osteoarthritis
▶ TO THE SKIN
▶ Adult: Apply 2–3 times a day for up to max. 10 days

IMPORTANT SAFETY INFORMATION
MHRA/CHM ADVICE: NSAIDS: POTENTIAL RISKS FOLLOWING PROLONGED USE AFTER 20 WEEKS OF PREGNANCY (JUNE 2023)
▶ With systemic use
See Non-steroidal anti-inflammatory drugs p. 1292.

● **CONTRA-INDICATIONS**
▶ With systemic use Active gastro-intestinal bleeding · active gastro-intestinal ulceration · coagulation disorders · history of gastro-intestinal bleeding · history of gastro-intestinal perforation · history of gastro-intestinal ulceration · severe heart failure

● **CAUTIONS**
▶ With systemic use Allergic disorders · cardiac impairment (NSAIDs may impair renal function) · cerebrovascular disease · connective-tissue disorders · dehydration (risk of renal impairment) · elderly (risk of serious side-effects and fatalities) · heart failure · history of gastro-intestinal disorders (e.g. ulcerative colitis, Crohn's disease) · ischaemic heart disease · may mask symptoms of infection · peripheral arterial disease · risk factors for cardiovascular events · uncontrolled hypertension
▶ With topical use Avoid contact with eyes · avoid contact with inflamed or broken skin · avoid contact with mucous membranes · not for use with occlusive dressings · topical application of large amounts can result in systemic effects, including hypersensitivity and asthma (renal disease has also been reported)

CAUTIONS, FURTHER INFORMATION
▶ Masking of symptoms of underlying infections
▶ With systemic use Ketoprofen can mask symptoms of infection, which may lead to delayed initiation of appropriate treatment and thereby worsen infection outcome. This has been observed in bacterial community-acquired pneumonia and bacterial complications to varicella. When administered for fever or pain relief in relation to infection, monitoring of infection is advised.

● **INTERACTIONS** → Appendix 1: NSAIDs

● **SIDE-EFFECTS**

GENERAL SIDE-EFFECTS
▶ **Uncommon** Diarrhoea · paraesthesia · skin reactions
▶ **Rare or very rare** Hypersensitivity · photosensitivity reaction · renal impairment
▶ **Frequency not known** Angioedema

SPECIFIC SIDE-EFFECTS
▶ **Common or very common**
▶ With oral use Gastrointestinal discomfort · nausea · vomiting
▶ **Uncommon**
▶ With oral use Constipation · dizziness · drowsiness · fatigue · gastrointestinal disorders · headache · oedema · rash (discontinue)
▶ With topical use Increased risk of infection
▶ **Rare or very rare**
▶ With oral use Asthma · haemorrhagic anaemia · hepatic disorders · pancreatitis · shock · stomatitis · tinnitus · vision disorders · weight increased
▶ **Frequency not known**
▶ With oral use Acute kidney injury (more common in patients with pre-existing renal impairment) · agranulocytosis · alopecia · appetite decreased · bone marrow failure · bronchospasm · confusion · Crohn's disease aggravated · depression · dyspnoea · fertility decreased female · haemorrhage · hallucination · hearing

impairment · heart failure · hypertension · increased risk of arterial thromboembolism · increased risk of ischaemic stroke · increased risk of myocardial infarction · malaise · meningitis aseptic (patients with connective-tissue disorders such as systemic lupus erythematosus may be especially susceptible) · menometrorrhagia · mood altered · nephritic syndrome · nephritis tubulointerstitial · nephrotic syndrome · neutropenia · optic neuritis · rhinitis · seizure · severe cutaneous adverse reactions (SCARs) · taste altered · thrombocytopenia · vasodilation · vertigo
▶ With topical use Eosinophilia · eyelid oedema · fever · gastrointestinal haemorrhage · lip swelling · peptic ulcer · vasculitis · wound complications

SIDE-EFFECTS, FURTHER INFORMATION Topical application of large amounts can result in systemic effects, including hypersensitivity and asthma (renal disease has also been reported).
   For information about cardiovascular and gastrointestinal side-effects, and a possible exacerbation of symptoms in asthma, see Non-steroidal anti-inflammatory drugs p. 1292

● **ALLERGY AND CROSS-SENSITIVITY** [EvGr] Contra-indicated in patients with a history of hypersensitivity to aspirin or any other NSAID—which includes those in whom attacks of asthma, angioedema, urticaria or rhinitis have been precipitated by aspirin or any other NSAID. ⟨M⟩

● **CONCEPTION AND CONTRACEPTION**
▶ With systemic use [EvGr] Caution—long-term use of some NSAIDs is associated with reduced female fertility, which is reversible on stopping treatment. ⟨M⟩

● **PREGNANCY**
▶ With systemic use Avoid use in first and second trimesters unless essential; the MHRA advises additional antenatal monitoring may be required if treatment is considered necessary by a doctor from week 20 of pregnancy onwards. Avoid use in third trimester. See *NSAIDs in Pregnancy* in Non-steroidal anti-inflammatory drugs p. 1292 for further details.
▶ With topical use Patient packs for topical preparations carry a warning to avoid during pregnancy.

● **BREAST FEEDING**
▶ With systemic use Use with caution during breast-feeding. Amount probably too small to be harmful but manufacturers advise avoid.
▶ With topical use Patient packs for topical preparations carry a warning to avoid during breast-feeding.

● **HEPATIC IMPAIRMENT**
▶ With systemic use Manufacturer advises caution in mild to moderate impairment; avoid in severe impairment.
▶ With topical use Manufacturer advises caution.

● **RENAL IMPAIRMENT**
▶ With systemic use In general, for *NSAIDs* the MHRA advises to avoid where possible; if necessary, use with caution (risk of fluid retention and further renal impairment, including renal failure). [EvGr] For *ketoprofen*, avoid in severe renal insufficiency. ⟨M⟩
▶ With topical use [EvGr] Caution (deterioration in renal function has also been reported after topical use). ⟨M⟩

● **DIRECTIONS FOR ADMINISTRATION** For topical preparations, manufacturer advises apply with gentle massage only.

● **PATIENT AND CARER ADVICE**
▶ With topical use For topical preparations, patients and their carers should be advised to wash hands immediately after use.
Photosensitivity Patients should be advised against excessive exposure to sunlight of area treated in order to avoid possibility of photosensitivity. Patients should be advised not to expose area treated to sunbeds or sunlight (even on a bright but cloudy day) during, and for two

weeks after stopping treatment; treated areas should be protected with clothing.

- **EXCEPTIONS TO LEGAL CATEGORY** Smaller pack sizes of gel preparations may be available on sale to the public.

- **MEDICINAL FORMS** There can be variation in the licensing of different medicines containing the same drug.

Cutaneous gel

CAUTIONARY AND ADVISORY LABELS 11
EXCIPIENTS: May contain Ethanol, fragrances

▸ **Ketoprofen (Non-proprietary)**
Ketoprofen 25 mg per 1 gram Ketoprofen 2.5% gel | 50 gram [PoM]
£2.70 DT = £2.70 | 100 gram [PoM] £5.40

▸ **Powergel** (A. Menarini Farmaceutica Internazionale SRL)
Ketoprofen 25 mg per 1 gram Powergel 2.5% gel | 50 gram [PoM]
£3.06 DT = £2.70 | 100 gram [PoM] £5.89

▸ **Tiloket** (Tillomed Laboratories Ltd)
Ketoprofen 25 mg per 1 gram Tiloket 2.5% gel | 50 gram [PoM]
£3.00 DT = £2.70 | 100 gram [PoM] £6.00

Mefenamic acid

01-Aug-2023

- **INDICATIONS AND DOSE**

Pain and inflammation in rheumatoid arthritis and osteoarthritis | Postoperative pain | Mild to moderate pain
▸ BY MOUTH
▸ Adult: 500 mg 3 times a day

Acute pain including dysmenorrhoea | Menorrhagia
▸ BY MOUTH
▸ Child 12-17 years: 500 mg 3 times a day
▸ Adult: 500 mg 3 times a day

IMPORTANT SAFETY INFORMATION
MHRA/CHM ADVICE: NSAIDS: POTENTIAL RISKS FOLLOWING PROLONGED USE AFTER 20 WEEKS OF PREGNANCY (JUNE 2023)
See Non-steroidal anti-inflammatory drugs p. 1292.

- **CONTRA-INDICATIONS** Active gastro-intestinal bleeding · active gastro-intestinal ulceration · following coronary artery bypass graft (CABG) surgery · history of gastro-intestinal bleeding related to previous NSAID therapy · history of gastro-intestinal perforation related to previous NSAID therapy · history of recurrent gastro-intestinal haemorrhage (two or more distinct episodes) · history of recurrent gastro-intestinal ulceration (two or more distinct episodes) · inflammatory bowel disease · severe heart failure

- **CAUTIONS** Acute porphyrias p. 1202 · allergic disorders · cardiac impairment (NSAIDs may impair renal function) · cerebrovascular disease · coagulation defects · connective-tissue disorders · dehydration (risk of renal impairment) · elderly (risk of serious side-effects and fatalities) · epilepsy · heart failure · history of gastro-intestinal disorders (e.g. ulcerative colitis, Crohn's disease) · ischaemic heart disease · may mask symptoms of infection · peripheral arterial disease · risk factors for cardiovascular events · uncontrolled hypertension

- **INTERACTIONS** → Appendix 1: NSAIDs

- **SIDE-EFFECTS** Agranulocytosis · anaemia · angioedema · appetite decreased · asthma · bone marrow disorders · confusion · constipation · Crohn's disease · depression · diarrhoea (discontinue) · disseminated intravascular coagulation · dizziness · drowsiness · dyspnoea · dysuria · ear pain · eosinophilia · eye irritation · fatigue · fertility decreased female · gastrointestinal discomfort · gastrointestinal disorders · glomerulonephritis · glucose tolerance impaired · haemolytic anaemia · haemorrhage · hallucination · headache · heart failure · hepatic disorders · hyperhidrosis · hypersensitivity · hypertension · hyponatraemia · hypotension · insomnia · leucopenia ·

malaise · meningitis aseptic (patients with connective-tissue disorders such as systemic lupus erythematosus may be especially susceptible) · multi organ failure · nausea · nephritis acute interstitial · nephrotic syndrome · nervousness · neutropenia · oedema · optic neuritis · oral ulceration · palpitations · pancreatitis · paraesthesia · photosensitivity reaction · proteinuria · rash (discontinue) · renal failure (more common in patients with pre-existing renal impairment) · renal failure non-oliguric · renal papillary necrosis · respiratory disorders · seizure · sepsis · severe cutaneous adverse reactions (SCARs) · skin reactions · thrombocytopenia · tinnitus · vertigo · vision disorders · vomiting

SIDE-EFFECTS, FURTHER INFORMATION For information about cardiovascular and gastrointestinal side-effects, and a possible exacerbation of symptoms in asthma, see Non-steroidal anti-inflammatory drugs p. 1292

Overdose Mefenamic acid has important consequences in overdosage because it can cause convulsions, which if prolonged or recurrent, require treatment.
  For details on the management of poisoning, see Emergency treatment of poisoning p. 1554, in particular, Convulsions.

- **ALLERGY AND CROSS-SENSITIVITY** [EvGr] Contra-indicated in patients with a history of hypersensitivity to aspirin or any other NSAID—which includes those in whom attacks of asthma, angioedema, urticaria or rhinitis have been precipitated by aspirin or any other NSAID. [M]

- **CONCEPTION AND CONTRACEPTION** [EvGr] Caution—long-term use of some NSAIDs is associated with reduced female fertility, which is reversible on stopping treatment. [M]

- **PREGNANCY** Avoid use in first and second trimesters unless essential; the MHRA advises additional antenatal monitoring may be required if treatment is considered necessary by a doctor from week 20 of pregnancy onwards. Avoid use in third trimester. See *NSAIDs in Pregnancy* in Non-steroidal anti-inflammatory drugs p. 1292 for further details.

- **BREAST FEEDING** Use with caution during breast-feeding. Amount too small to be harmful but manufacturer advises avoid.

- **HEPATIC IMPAIRMENT** Manufacturer advises caution in mild to moderate impairment; avoid in severe impairment.

- **RENAL IMPAIRMENT** In general, for *NSAIDs* the MHRA advises to avoid where possible; if necessary, use with caution (risk of fluid retention and further renal impairment, including renal failure). [EvGr] For *mefenamic acid*, avoid in severe impairment. [M]

- **MEDICINAL FORMS** There can be variation in the licensing of different medicines containing the same drug. Forms available from special-order manufacturers include: oral suspension

Oral tablet
CAUTIONARY AND ADVISORY LABELS 21
▸ **Mefenamic acid (Non-proprietary)**
Mefenamic acid 250 mg Mefenamic acid 250mg tablets |
28 tablet [PoM] £5.69 DT = £5.69
Mefenamic acid 500 mg Mefenamic acid 500mg tablets |
28 tablet [PoM] £20.42 DT = £4.94 | 84 tablet [PoM] £24.32-£106.88

Oral suspension
CAUTIONARY AND ADVISORY LABELS 21
EXCIPIENTS: May contain Ethanol
▸ **Mefenamic acid (Non-proprietary)**
Mefenamic acid 10 mg per 1 ml Mefenamic acid 50mg/5ml oral suspension | 125 ml [PoM] £187.95 DT = £187.95

Oral capsule
CAUTIONARY AND ADVISORY LABELS 21
▸ **Mefenamic acid (Non-proprietary)**
Mefenamic acid 250 mg Mefenamic acid 250mg capsules |
100 capsule [PoM] £60.10 DT = £22.26

Meloxicam

01-Aug-2023

- **INDICATIONS AND DOSE**

Exacerbation of osteoarthritis (short-term)
▶ BY MOUTH
▸ Child 16–17 years: 7.5 mg once daily, then increased if necessary up to 15 mg once daily
▸ Adult: 7.5 mg once daily, then increased if necessary up to 15 mg once daily

Pain and inflammation in rheumatic disease | Ankylosing spondylitis
▶ BY MOUTH
▸ Child 16–17 years: 15 mg once daily, then reduced to 7.5 mg once daily if required
▸ Adult: 15 mg once daily, then reduced to 7.5 mg once daily if required
▸ Elderly: 7.5 mg once daily

Relief of pain and inflammation in juvenile idiopathic arthritis and other musculoskeletal disorders in children intolerant to other NSAIDs
▶ BY MOUTH
▸ Child 12–17 years (body-weight up to 50 kg): 7.5 mg once daily
▸ Child 12–17 years (body-weight 50 kg and above): 15 mg once daily

- **UNLICENSED USE** Expert sources advise that meloxicam may be used from the age of 12 years for the treatment of pain and inflammation in juvenile idiopathic arthritis and other musculoskeletal disorders in children intolerant to other NSAIDS, but it is not licensed for this age group.

> **IMPORTANT SAFETY INFORMATION**
> MHRA/CHM ADVICE: NSAIDS: POTENTIAL RISKS FOLLOWING PROLONGED USE AFTER 20 WEEKS OF PREGNANCY (JUNE 2023)
> See Non-steroidal anti-inflammatory drugs p. 1292.

- **CONTRA-INDICATIONS** Active gastro-intestinal bleeding · active gastro-intestinal ulceration · following coronary artery bypass graft surgery · history of gastro-intestinal bleeding related to previous NSAID therapy · history of gastro-intestinal perforation related to previous NSAID therapy · history of recurrent gastro-intestinal haemorrhage (two or more distinct episodes) · history of recurrent gastro-intestinal ulceration (two or more distinct episodes) · severe heart failure

- **CAUTIONS** Allergic disorders · cardiac impairment (NSAIDs may impair renal function) · cerebrovascular disease · coagulation defects · connective-tissue disorders · dehydration (risk of renal impairment) · elderly (risk of serious side-effects and fatalities) · heart failure · history of gastro-intestinal disorders (e.g. ulcerative colitis, Crohn's disease) · ischaemic heart disease · may mask symptoms of infection · peripheral arterial disease · risk factors for cardiovascular events · uncontrolled hypertension

- **INTERACTIONS** → Appendix 1: NSAIDs

- **SIDE-EFFECTS**
▶ **Common or very common** Constipation · diarrhoea · gastrointestinal discomfort · gastrointestinal disorders · headache · nausea · vomiting
▶ **Uncommon** Anaemia · angioedema · burping · dizziness · drowsiness · electrolyte imbalance · fluid retention · flushing · haemorrhage · hepatic disorders · hypersensitivity · oedema · skin reactions · stomatitis · vertigo
▶ **Rare or very rare** Acute kidney injury · asthma · conjunctivitis · leucopenia · mood altered · nightmare · palpitations · severe cutaneous adverse reactions (SCARs) · thrombocytopenia · tinnitus · vision disorders
▶ **Frequency not known** Agranulocytosis · confusion · fertility decreased female · heart failure · increased risk of arterial

thromboembolism · nephritis tubulointerstitial · nephrotic syndrome · photosensitivity reaction · renal necrosis

SIDE-EFFECTS, FURTHER INFORMATION For information about cardiovascular and gastrointestinal side-effects, and a possible exacerbation of symptoms in asthma, see Non-steroidal anti-inflammatory drugs p. 1292

- **ALLERGY AND CROSS-SENSITIVITY** [EvGr] Contra-indicated in patients with a history of hypersensitivity to aspirin or any other NSAID—which includes those in whom attacks of asthma, angioedema, urticaria or rhinitis have been precipitated by aspirin or any other NSAID. ⟨M⟩

- **CONCEPTION AND CONTRACEPTION** [EvGr] Caution—long-term use of some NSAIDs is associated with reduced female fertility, which is reversible on stopping treatment. ⟨M⟩

- **PREGNANCY** Avoid use in first and second trimesters unless essential; the MHRA advises additional antenatal monitoring may be required if treatment is considered necessary by a doctor from week 20 of pregnancy onwards. Avoid use in third trimester. See *NSAIDs in Pregnancy* in Non-steroidal anti-inflammatory drugs p. 1292 for further details.

- **BREAST FEEDING** Use with caution during breast-feeding. Present in milk in *animal* studies—manufacturer advises avoid.

- **HEPATIC IMPAIRMENT** Manufacturer advises caution in mild to moderate impairment; avoid in severe impairment.

- **RENAL IMPAIRMENT** In general, for *NSAIDs* the MHRA advises to avoid where possible; if necessary, use with caution (risk of fluid retention and further renal impairment, including renal failure). [EvGr] For *meloxicam*, avoid if creatinine clearance less than 25 mL/minute; ⟨M⟩ see p. 21.

- **MEDICINAL FORMS** There can be variation in the licensing of different medicines containing the same drug. Forms available from special-order manufacturers include: oral suspension

Oral tablet
CAUTIONARY AND ADVISORY LABELS 21
▸ Meloxicam (Non-proprietary)
  Meloxicam 7.5 mg Meloxicam 7.5mg tablets | 30 tablet [PoM] £3.00 DT = £0.90
  Meloxicam 15 mg Meloxicam 15mg tablets | 30 tablet [PoM] £13.00 DT = £0.91

Orodispersible tablet
▸ Meloxicam (Non-proprietary)
  Meloxicam 7.5 mg Meloxicam 7.5mg orodispersible tablets sugar free | 30 tablet [PoM] £49.99 DT = £49.99 [SF]
  Meloxicam 15 mg Meloxicam 15mg orodispersible tablets sugar free | 30 tablet [PoM] £49.99 DT = £49.99 [SF]

Nabumetone

01-Aug-2023

- **INDICATIONS AND DOSE**

Pain and inflammation in osteoarthritis and rheumatoid arthritis
▶ BY MOUTH
▸ Adult: 1 g once daily, dose to be taken at night
▸ Elderly: 0.5–1 g daily

Pain and inflammation in osteoarthritis and rheumatoid arthritis (severe and persistent symptoms)
▶ BY MOUTH
▸ Adult: 0.5–1 g, dose to be taken in the morning and 1 g, dose to be taken at night
▸ Elderly: 0.5–1 g daily

> **IMPORTANT SAFETY INFORMATION**
> MHRA/CHM ADVICE: NSAIDS: POTENTIAL RISKS FOLLOWING PROLONGED USE AFTER 20 WEEKS OF PREGNANCY (JUNE 2023)
> See Non-steroidal anti-inflammatory drugs p. 1292.

- **CONTRA-INDICATIONS** Active gastro-intestinal bleeding · active gastro-intestinal ulceration · history of gastro-intestinal bleeding related to previous NSAID therapy · history of gastro-intestinal perforation related to previous NSAID therapy · history of recurrent gastro-intestinal haemorrhage (two or more distinct episodes) · history of recurrent gastro-intestinal ulceration (two or more distinct episodes) · severe heart failure
- **CAUTIONS** Allergic disorders · cardiac impairment (NSAIDs may impair renal function) · cerebrovascular disease · coagulation defects · connective-tissue disorders · dehydration (risk of renal impairment) · elderly (risk of serious side-effects and fatalities) · heart failure · history of gastro-intestinal disorders (e.g. ulcerative colitis, Crohn's disease) · ischaemic heart disease · may mask symptoms of infection · peripheral arterial disease · risk factors for cardiovascular events · uncontrolled hypertension
- **INTERACTIONS** → Appendix 1: NSAIDs
- **SIDE-EFFECTS**
  - **Common or very common** Constipation · diarrhoea · ear disorder · gastrointestinal discomfort · gastrointestinal disorders · nausea · oedema · skin reactions · tinnitus
  - **Uncommon** Anxiety · asthenia · confusion · dizziness · drowsiness · dry mouth · dyspnoea · eye disorder · haemorrhage · headache · hyperhidrosis · insomnia · myopathy · oral disorders · paraesthesia · photosensitivity reaction · respiratory disorders · urinary tract disorder · visual impairment · vomiting
  - **Rare or very rare** Alopecia · angioedema · hepatic disorders · hypersensitivity · interstitial pneumonitis · menorrhagia · nephrotic syndrome · pancreatitis · renal failure (more common in patients with pre-existing renal impairment) · severe cutaneous adverse reactions (SCARs) · thrombocytopenia
  - **Frequency not known** Agranulocytosis · aplastic anaemia · asthma · Crohn's disease aggravated · depression · fertility decreased female · haemolytic anaemia · hallucination · heart failure · hypertension · increased risk of arterial thromboembolism · leucopenia · malaise · meningitis aseptic (patients with connective-tissue disorders such as systemic lupus erythematosus may be especially susceptible) · nephritis tubulointerstitial · neutropenia · optic neuritis · vertigo

  SIDE-EFFECTS, FURTHER INFORMATION For information about cardiovascular and gastrointestinal side-effects, and a possible exacerbation of symptoms in asthma, see Non-steroidal anti-inflammatory drugs p. 1292
- **ALLERGY AND CROSS-SENSITIVITY** [EvGr] Contra-indicated in patients with a history of hypersensitivity to aspirin or any other NSAID—which includes those in whom attacks of asthma, angioedema, urticaria or rhinitis have been precipitated by aspirin or any other NSAID. Ⓜ
- **CONCEPTION AND CONTRACEPTION** [EvGr] Caution—long-term use of some NSAIDs is associated with reduced female fertility, which is reversible on stopping treatment. Ⓜ
- **PREGNANCY** Avoid use in first and second trimesters unless essential; the MHRA advises additional antenatal monitoring may be required if treatment is considered necessary by a doctor from week 20 of pregnancy onwards. Avoid use in third trimester. See *NSAIDs in Pregnancy* in Non-steroidal anti-inflammatory drugs p. 1292 for further details.
- **BREAST FEEDING** Use with caution during breast-feeding. Manufacturer advises avoid.
- **HEPATIC IMPAIRMENT** Manufacturer advises caution in mild to moderate impairment; avoid in severe impairment.
- **RENAL IMPAIRMENT** In general, for *NSAIDs* the MHRA advises to avoid where possible; if necessary, use with caution (risk of fluid retention and further renal

impairment, including renal failure). [EvGr] For *nabumetone*, avoid in renal failure. Ⓜ

- **MEDICINAL FORMS** There can be variation in the licensing of different medicines containing the same drug.

Oral tablet
CAUTIONARY AND ADVISORY LABELS 21
► **Nabumetone (Non-proprietary)**
  Nabumetone 500 mg Nabumetone 500mg tablets | 56 tablet [PoM] £92.00 DT = £30.42

Naproxen
01-Aug-2023

- **INDICATIONS AND DOSE**

Pain and inflammation in rheumatic disease
► BY MOUTH
► Adult: 0.5–1 g daily in 1–2 divided doses

Pain and inflammation in musculoskeletal disorders | Dysmenorrhoea
► BY MOUTH
► Adult: Initially 500 mg for 1 dose, then 250 mg every 6–8 hours as required

Acute gout
► BY MOUTH
► Adult: Initially 750 mg for 1 dose, then 250 mg every 8 hours until attack has passed

Acute migraine
► BY MOUTH
► Adult: 500 mg for 1 dose, to be taken in combination with sumatriptan as soon as migraine symptoms develop

- **UNLICENSED USE** [EvGr] Naproxen is used for the treatment of acute migraine in combination with sumatriptan, Ⓐ but is not licensed for this indication.

> **IMPORTANT SAFETY INFORMATION**
> MHRA/CHM ADVICE: NSAIDS: POTENTIAL RISKS FOLLOWING PROLONGED USE AFTER 20 WEEKS OF PREGNANCY (JUNE 2023)
> See Non-steroidal anti-inflammatory drugs p. 1292.

- **CONTRA-INDICATIONS** Active gastro-intestinal bleeding · active gastro-intestinal ulceration · history of gastro-intestinal bleeding related to previous NSAID therapy · history of gastro-intestinal perforation related to previous NSAID therapy · history of recurrent gastro-intestinal haemorrhage (two or more distinct episodes) · history of recurrent gastro-intestinal ulceration (two or more distinct episodes) · severe heart failure
- **CAUTIONS** Allergic disorders · cardiac impairment (NSAIDs may impair renal function) · cerebrovascular disease · coagulation defects · connective-tissue disorders · dehydration (risk of renal impairment) · elderly (risk of serious side-effects and fatalities) · heart failure · history of gastro-intestinal disorders (e.g. ulcerative colitis, Crohn's disease) · ischaemic heart disease · may mask symptoms of infection · peripheral arterial disease · risk factors for cardiovascular events · uncontrolled hypertension
- **INTERACTIONS** → Appendix 1: NSAIDs
- **SIDE-EFFECTS** Agranulocytosis · alopecia · angioedema · aplastic anaemia · asthma · cognitive impairment · concentration impaired · confusion · constipation · corneal opacity · depression · diarrhoea · dizziness · drowsiness · drug cross-reactivity · dyspnoea · eosinophilia · erythema nodosum · fatigue · gastrointestinal discomfort · gastrointestinal disorders · glomerulonephritis · haemolytic anaemia · haemorrhage · hallucination · headache · hearing impairment · heart failure · hepatic disorders · hyperhidrosis · hyperkalaemia · hypertension · infertility female · inflammatory bowel disease · leucopenia · malaise · meningitis aseptic (patients with connective-

tissue disorders such as systemic lupus erythematosus may be especially susceptible) · muscle weakness · myalgia · nausea · nephritis tubulointerstitial · nephropathy · neutropenia · oedema · optic neuritis · palpitations · pancreatitis · papillitis · papilloedema · paraesthesia · photosensitivity reaction · pneumonia eosinophilic · proteinuria · pulmonary oedema · rash pustular · renal failure (more common in patients with pre-existing renal impairment) · renal impairment · renal papillary necrosis · seizure · severe cutaneous adverse reactions (SCARs) · skin reactions · sleep disorders · stomatitis · systemic lupus erythematosus (SLE) · thirst · thrombocytopenia · tinnitus · vasculitis · vertigo · visual impairment · vomiting

SIDE-EFFECTS, FURTHER INFORMATION For information about cardiovascular and gastrointestinal side-effects, and a possible exacerbation of symptoms in asthma, see Non-steroidal anti-inflammatory drugs p. 1292

- **ALLERGY AND CROSS-SENSITIVITY** [EvGr] Contra-indicated in patients with a history of hypersensitivity to aspirin or any other NSAID—which includes those in whom attacks of asthma, angioedema, urticaria or rhinitis have been precipitated by aspirin or any other NSAID. ◈M◈

- **CONCEPTION AND CONTRACEPTION** [EvGr] Caution—long-term use of some NSAIDs is associated with reduced female fertility, which is reversible on stopping treatment. ◈M◈

- **PREGNANCY** Avoid use in first and second trimesters unless essential; the MHRA advises additional antenatal monitoring may be required if treatment is considered necessary by a doctor from week 20 of pregnancy onwards. Avoid use in third trimester. See *NSAIDs in Pregnancy* in Non-steroidal anti-inflammatory drugs p. 1292 for further details.

- **BREAST FEEDING** Use with caution during breast-feeding. Amount too small to be harmful but manufacturer advises avoid.

- **HEPATIC IMPAIRMENT** Manufacturer advises caution in mild to moderate impairment; avoid in severe impairment. **Dose adjustments** Manufacturer advises consider dose reduction in mild to moderate impairment.

- **RENAL IMPAIRMENT** In general, for *NSAIDs* the MHRA advises to avoid where possible; if necessary, use with caution (risk of fluid retention and further renal impairment, including renal failure). [EvGr] For *naproxen*, avoid if creatinine clearance less than 30 mL/minute (risk of accumulation). ◈M◈
Dose adjustments [EvGr] Consider dose reduction if creatinine clearance 30 mL/minute or more. ◈M◈ See p. 21.

- **NATIONAL FUNDING/ACCESS DECISIONS** For full details see funding body website
Scottish Medicines Consortium (SMC) decisions
▶ Naproxen (*Stirlescent*®) for the treatment of rheumatoid arthritis, osteoarthritis, ankylosing spondylitis, acute musculoskeletal disorders, dysmenorrhoea and acute gout in adults (June 2016) SMC No. 1154/16 Recommended with restrictions

- **EXCEPTIONS TO LEGAL CATEGORY** Can be sold to the public for the treatment of primary dysmenorrhoea in women aged 15–50 years subject to max. single dose of 500 mg, max. daily dose of 750 mg for max. 3 days, and a max. pack size of 9 × 250 mg tablets.

- **MEDICINAL FORMS** There can be variation in the licensing of different medicines containing the same drug. Forms available from special-order manufacturers include: oral suspension
Oral tablet
CAUTIONARY AND ADVISORY LABELS 21
▶ Naproxen (Non-proprietary)
Naproxen 250 mg Naproxen 250mg tablets | 28 tablet [PoM] £1.71 DT = £0.87

Naproxen 500 mg Naproxen 500mg tablets | 28 tablet [PoM] £7.27 DT = £1.37 | 250 tablet [PoM] £11.88-£12.60 | 500 tablet [PoM] £21.00-£24.46
▶ Naprosyn (Atnahs Pharma UK Ltd)
Naproxen 250 mg Naprosyn 250mg tablets | 56 tablet [PoM] £4.29
Naproxen 500 mg Naprosyn 500mg tablets | 56 tablet [PoM] £8.56
Gastro-resistant tablet
CAUTIONARY AND ADVISORY LABELS 5, 25
▶ Naproxen (Non-proprietary)
Naproxen 250 mg Naproxen 250mg gastro-resistant tablets | 56 tablet [PoM] £18.65 DT = £9.14
Naproxen 375 mg Naproxen 375mg gastro-resistant tablets | 56 tablet [PoM] £19.98 DT = £14.14
Naproxen 500 mg Naproxen 500mg gastro-resistant tablets | 56 tablet [PoM] £34.50 DT = £18.74
▶ Naprosyn EC (Atnahs Pharma UK Ltd)
Naproxen 250 mg Naprosyn EC 250mg tablets | 56 tablet [PoM] £4.29 DT = £9.14
Naproxen 375 mg Naprosyn EC 375mg tablets | 56 tablet [PoM] £6.42 DT = £14.14
Naproxen 500 mg Naprosyn EC 500mg tablets | 56 tablet [PoM] £8.56 DT = £18.74
▶ Nexocin EC (Noumed Life Sciences Ltd)
Naproxen 250 mg Nexocin EC 250mg gastro-resistant tablets | 56 tablet [PoM] [Ⓧ] DT = £9.14
Naproxen 375 mg Nexocin EC 375mg gastro-resistant tablets | 56 tablet [PoM] [Ⓧ] DT = £14.14
Naproxen 500 mg Nexocin EC 500mg gastro-resistant tablets | 56 tablet [PoM] [Ⓧ] DT = £18.74
Oral suspension
▶ Naproxen (Non-proprietary)
Naproxen 25 mg per 1 ml Naproxen 25mg/ml oral suspension sugar free | 100 ml [PoM] £110.00 DT = £110.00 [SF]
Naproxen 125mg/5ml oral suspension sugar free | 100 ml [PoM] £110.00 DT = £110.00 [SF]
Naproxen 50 mg per 1 ml Naproxen 50mg/ml oral suspension | 100 ml [PoM] £45.00 DT = £45.00
Effervescent tablet
▶ Stirlescent (Stirling Anglian Pharmaceuticals Ltd)
Naproxen 250 mg Stirlescent 250mg effervescent tablets | 20 tablet [PoM] £52.72 DT = £52.72 [SF]

Naproxen with esomeprazole   17-Jul-2020

The properties listed below are those particular to the combination only. For the properties of the components please consider, naproxen p. 1310, esomeprazole p. 86.

- **INDICATIONS AND DOSE**
Patients requiring naproxen for osteoarthritis, rheumatoid arthritis, or ankylosing spondylitis, who are at risk of NSAID-associated duodenal or gastric ulcer and when treatment with lower doses of naproxen or other NSAIDs ineffective
▶ BY MOUTH
▶ Adult: 500/20 mg twice daily, dose expressed as *x/y* mg naproxen/esomeprazole

- **INTERACTIONS** → Appendix 1: NSAIDs · proton pump inhibitors

- **PRESCRIBING AND DISPENSING INFORMATION** Naproxen component is gastro-resistant.

- **MEDICINAL FORMS** There can be variation in the licensing of different medicines containing the same drug.
Modified-release tablet
CAUTIONARY AND ADVISORY LABELS 22, 25
▶ Vimovo (Grunenthal Ltd)
Esomeprazole (as Esomeprazole magnesium trihydrate) 20 mg, Naproxen 500 mg Vimovo 500mg/20mg modified-release tablets | 60 tablet [PoM] £14.95 DT = £14.95

Piroxicam

01-Aug-2023

● INDICATIONS AND DOSE

Rheumatoid arthritis (initiated by a specialist) | Osteoarthritis (initiated by a specialist) | Ankylosing spondylitis (initiated by a specialist)

▸ BY MOUTH
▸ Adult: Up to 20 mg once daily

Pain relief in musculoskeletal conditions | Treatment in knee or hand osteoarthritis (adjunct)

▸ TO THE SKIN
▸ Adult: Apply 3–4 times a day, 0.5% gel to be applied; review treatment after 4 weeks

---

IMPORTANT SAFETY INFORMATION

CHMP ADVICE—PIROXICAM (JUNE 2007)

▸ With systemic use

The CHMP has recommended restrictions on the use of piroxicam because of the increased risk of gastro-intestinal side-effects and serious skin reactions. The CHMP has advised that:

- piroxicam should be initiated only by physicians experienced in treating inflammatory or degenerative rheumatic diseases
- piroxicam should not be used as first-line treatment
- in adults, use of piroxicam should be limited to the symptomatic relief of osteoarthritis, rheumatoid arthritis, and ankylosing spondylitis
- piroxicam dose should not exceed 20 mg daily
- piroxicam should no longer be used for the treatment of acute painful and inflammatory conditions
- treatment should be reviewed 2 weeks after initiating piroxicam, and periodically thereafter
- concomitant administration of a gastro-protective agent should be considered.

Topical preparations containing piroxicam are not affected by these restrictions.

MHRA/CHM ADVICE: NSAIDS: POTENTIAL RISKS FOLLOWING PROLONGED USE AFTER 20 WEEKS OF PREGNANCY (JUNE 2023)

▸ With systemic use

See Non-steroidal anti-inflammatory drugs p. 1292.

● CONTRA-INDICATIONS

▸ With systemic use Active gastro-intestinal bleeding · active gastro-intestinal ulceration · history of gastro-intestinal bleeding · history of gastro-intestinal perforation · history of gastro-intestinal ulceration · inflammatory bowel disease · severe heart failure

● CAUTIONS

▸ With systemic use Allergic disorders · cardiac impairment (NSAIDs may impair renal function) · cerebrovascular disease · coagulation defects · connective-tissue disorders · dehydration (risk of renal impairment) · elderly (risk of serious side-effects and fatalities) · heart failure · history of gastro-intestinal disorders · ischaemic heart disease · may mask symptoms of infection · peripheral arterial disease · risk factors for cardiovascular events · uncontrolled hypertension

▸ With topical use Avoid contact with eyes · avoid contact with inflamed or broken skin · avoid contact with mucous membranes · not for use with occlusive dressings · topical application of large amounts can result in systemic effects, including hypersensitivity and asthma (renal disease has also been reported)

● INTERACTIONS → Appendix 1: NSAIDs

● SIDE-EFFECTS

GENERAL SIDE-EFFECTS

▸ **Common or very common** Gastrointestinal discomfort · gastrointestinal disorders · nausea · skin reactions

▸ **Rare or very rare** Severe cutaneous adverse reactions (SCARs)

▸ **Frequency not known** Bronchospasm · dyspnoea · photosensitivity reaction

SPECIFIC SIDE-EFFECTS

▸ **Common or very common**
▸ With oral use Anaemia · appetite decreased · constipation · diarrhoea · dizziness · drowsiness · eosinophilia · headache · hyperglycaemia · leucopenia · oedema · rash (discontinue) · thrombocytopenia · tinnitus · vertigo · vomiting · weight changes

▸ **Uncommon**
▸ With oral use Hypoglycaemia · palpitations · stomatitis · vision blurred

▸ **Rare or very rare**
▸ With oral use Nephritis tubulointerstitial · nephrotic syndrome · renal failure · renal papillary necrosis

▸ **Frequency not known**
▸ With oral use Alopecia · angioedema · aplastic anaemia · confusion · depression · embolism and thrombosis · eye irritation · eye swelling · fertility decreased female · fluid retention · haemolytic anaemia · haemorrhage · hallucination · hearing impairment · heart failure · hepatic disorders · hypersensitivity · hypertension · malaise · mood altered · nervousness · onycholysis · pancreatitis · paraesthesia · sleep disorders · vasculitis

SIDE-EFFECTS, FURTHER INFORMATION For information about cardiovascular and gastrointestinal side-effects, and a possible exacerbation of symptoms in asthma, see Non-steroidal anti-inflammatory drugs p. 1292

Topical application of large amounts can result in systemic effects.

● ALLERGY AND CROSS-SENSITIVITY [EvGr] Contra-indicated in patients with a history of hypersensitivity to aspirin or any other NSAID—which includes those in whom attacks of asthma, angioedema, urticaria or rhinitis have been precipitated by aspirin or any other NSAID. ◈

● CONCEPTION AND CONTRACEPTION

▸ With systemic use [EvGr] Caution—long-term use of some NSAIDs is associated with reduced female fertility, which is reversible on stopping treatment. ◈

● PREGNANCY

▸ With systemic use Avoid use in first and second trimesters unless essential; the MHRA advises additional antenatal monitoring may be required if treatment is considered necessary by a doctor from week 20 of pregnancy onwards. Avoid use in third trimester. See *NSAIDs in Pregnancy* in Non-steroidal anti-inflammatory drugs p. 1292 for further details.

▸ With topical use Patient packs for topical preparations carry a warning to avoid during pregnancy.

● BREAST FEEDING

▸ With systemic use Use with caution during breast-feeding. Amount too small to be harmful.

▸ With topical use Patient packs for topical preparations carry a warning to avoid during breast-feeding.

● HEPATIC IMPAIRMENT

▸ With oral use Manufacturer advises caution.

● RENAL IMPAIRMENT

▸ With systemic use In general, for *NSAIDs* the MHRA advises to avoid where possible; if necessary, use with caution (risk of fluid retention and further renal impairment, including renal failure).

▸ With topical use [EvGr] Caution (deterioration in renal function has also been reported after topical use). ◈

● DIRECTIONS FOR ADMINISTRATION

▸ With oral use Piroxicam orodispersible tablets can be taken by placing on the tongue and allowing to dissolve or by swallowing.

▸ With topical use For topical preparations, manufacturer advises apply with gentle massage only.

- **PATIENT AND CARER ADVICE**
  ▸ With topical use For topical preparations, patients and their carers should be advised to wash hands immediately after use.
  Photosensitivity Patients should be advised against excessive exposure to sunlight of area treated in order to avoid possibility of photosensitivity.
- **LESS SUITABLE FOR PRESCRIBING**
  ▸ With oral use Piroxicam is less suitable for prescribing.

- **MEDICINAL FORMS** There can be variation in the licensing of different medicines containing the same drug.

Orodispersible tablet
CAUTIONARY AND ADVISORY LABELS 10, 21
EXCIPIENTS: May contain Aspartame
  ▸ Feldene Melt (Pfizer Ltd)
  Piroxicam 20 mg Feldene Melt 20mg tablets | 30 tablet [PoM] £10.53 DT = £10.53 [SF]

Oral capsule
CAUTIONARY AND ADVISORY LABELS 21
  ▸ Piroxicam (Non-proprietary)
  Piroxicam 10 mg Piroxicam 10mg capsules | 56 capsule [PoM] £17.95 DT = £11.32
  Piroxicam 20 mg Piroxicam 20mg capsules | 28 capsule [PoM] £25.25 DT = £12.52
  ▸ Feldene (Pfizer Ltd)
  Piroxicam 10 mg Feldene 10mg capsules | 30 capsule [PoM] £3.86
  Piroxicam 20 mg Feldene 20 capsules | 30 capsule [PoM] £7.71

Cutaneous gel
EXCIPIENTS: May contain Benzyl alcohol, propylene glycol
  ▸ Piroxicam (Non-proprietary)
  Piroxicam 5 mg per 1 gram Piroxicam 0.5% gel | 60 gram [PoM] £2.20 DT = £2.01 | 112 gram [PoM] £5.00 DT = £3.75

Sulindac
01-Aug-2023

- **INDICATIONS AND DOSE**

Pain and inflammation in rheumatic disease and other musculoskeletal disorders | Acute gout
  ▸ BY MOUTH
  ▸ Adult: 200 mg twice daily for maximum duration 7–10 days in peri-articular disorders, dose may be reduced according to response; acute gout should respond within 7 days; maximum 400 mg per day

> **IMPORTANT SAFETY INFORMATION**
> MHRA/CHM ADVICE: NSAIDS: POTENTIAL RISKS FOLLOWING PROLONGED USE AFTER 20 WEEKS OF PREGNANCY (JUNE 2023)
> See Non-steroidal anti-inflammatory drugs p. 1292.

- **CONTRA-INDICATIONS** Active gastro-intestinal bleeding · active gastro-intestinal ulceration · history of gastro-intestinal bleeding related to previous NSAID therapy · history of gastro-intestinal perforation related to previous NSAID therapy · history of recurrent gastro-intestinal haemorrhage (two or more distinct episodes) · history of recurrent gastro-intestinal ulceration (two or more distinct episodes) · severe heart failure
- **CAUTIONS** Allergic disorders · cardiac impairment (NSAIDs may impair renal function) · cerebrovascular disease · coagulation defects · connective-tissue disorders · dehydration (risk of renal impairment) · elderly (risk of serious side-effects and fatalities) · heart failure · history of gastro-intestinal disorders (e.g. ulcerative colitis, Crohn's disease) · history of renal stones (ensure adequate hydration) · ischaemic heart disease · may mask symptoms of infection · peripheral arterial disease · risk factors for cardiovascular events · uncontrolled hypertension
- **INTERACTIONS** → Appendix 1: NSAIDs
- **SIDE-EFFECTS** Acute psychosis · agranulocytosis · alopecia · angioedema · appetite decreased · arrhythmia · asthenia · asthma · bone marrow disorders · cholecystitis · confusion ·

constipation · Crohn's disease aggravated · depression · diarrhoea · dizziness · drowsiness · dyspnoea · dysuria · eye disorder · fever · gastrointestinal discomfort · gastrointestinal disorders · gynaecomastia · haemolytic anaemia · haemorrhage · hallucination · headache · hearing loss · heart failure · hepatic disorders · hyperglycaemia · hyperhidrosis · hyperkalaemia · hypersensitivity · hypersensitivity vasculitis · hypertension · increased risk of arterial thromboembolism · increased risk of infection · insomnia · leucopenia · malaise · meningitis aseptic (patients with connective-tissue disorders such as systemic lupus erythematosus may be especially susceptible) · mucosal abnormalities · muscle weakness · nausea · nephritis tubulointerstitial · nephrotic syndrome · nerve disorders · nervousness · neutropenia · oedema · oral disorders · palpitations · pancreatitis · paraesthesia · photosensitivity reaction · psychiatric disorder · renal impairment · respiratory disorders · seizure · severe cutaneous adverse reactions (SCARs) · skin reactions · syncope · taste altered · thrombocytopenia · tinnitus · urine abnormalities · urine discolouration · vertigo · vision disorders · vomiting

SIDE-EFFECTS, FURTHER INFORMATION For information about cardiovascular and gastrointestinal side-effects, and a possible exacerbation of symptoms in asthma, see Non-steroidal anti-inflammatory drugs p. 1292

- **ALLERGY AND CROSS-SENSITIVITY** [EvGr] Contra-indicated in patients with a history of hypersensitivity to aspirin or any other NSAID—which includes those in whom attacks of asthma, angioedema, urticaria or rhinitis have been precipitated by aspirin or any other NSAID. ⟨M⟩
- **CONCEPTION AND CONTRACEPTION** [EvGr] Caution—long-term use of some NSAIDs is associated with reduced female fertility, which is reversible on stopping treatment. ⟨M⟩
- **PREGNANCY** Avoid use in first and second trimesters unless essential; the MHRA advises additional antenatal monitoring may be required if treatment is considered necessary by a doctor from week 20 of pregnancy onwards. Avoid use in third trimester. See *NSAIDs in Pregnancy* in Non-steroidal anti-inflammatory drugs p. 1292 for further details.
- **BREAST FEEDING** Use with caution during breast-feeding.
- **HEPATIC IMPAIRMENT** Manufacturer advises caution in mild to moderate impairment; avoid in severe impairment.
- **RENAL IMPAIRMENT** In general, for *NSAIDs* the MHRA advises to avoid where possible; if necessary, use with caution (risk of fluid retention and further renal impairment, including renal failure). [EvGr] For *sulindac*, avoid in severe impairment. ⟨M⟩

- **MEDICINAL FORMS** No licensed medicines listed.

Tenoxicam
01-Aug-2023

- **INDICATIONS AND DOSE**

Pain and inflammation in rheumatic disease
  ▸ BY MOUTH
  ▸ Adult: 20 mg once daily
  ▸ BY INTRAVENOUS INJECTION, OR BY INTRAMUSCULAR INJECTION
  ▸ Adult: 20 mg once daily as initial treatment for 1–2 days if oral administration not possible

Pain and inflammation in acute musculoskeletal disorders
  ▸ BY MOUTH
  ▸ Adult: 20 mg once daily for 7 days; maximum duration of treatment 14 days (including treatment by intravenous or intramuscular injection)   continued →

▶ BY INTRAVENOUS INJECTION, OR BY INTRAMUSCULAR
 INJECTION
▸ Adult: 20 mg once daily as initial treatment for
 1–2 days if oral administration not possible

IMPORTANT SAFETY INFORMATION

MHRA/CHM ADVICE: NSAIDS: POTENTIAL RISKS FOLLOWING
PROLONGED USE AFTER 20 WEEKS OF PREGNANCY (JUNE 2023)
See Non-steroidal anti-inflammatory drugs p. 1292.

● **CONTRA-INDICATIONS** Active gastro-intestinal bleeding ·
active gastro-intestinal ulceration · history of gastrointestinal bleeding related to previous NSAID therapy ·
history of gastro-intestinal perforation related to previous
NSAID therapy · history of recurrent gastro-intestinal
haemorrhage (two or more distinct episodes) · history of
recurrent gastro-intestinal ulceration (two or more
distinct episodes) · severe heart failure

● **CAUTIONS** Allergic disorders · cardiac impairment (NSAIDs
may impair renal function) · cerebrovascular disease ·
coagulation defects · connective-tissue disorders ·
dehydration (risk of renal impairment) · elderly (risk of
serious side-effects and fatalities) · heart failure · history of
gastro-intestinal disorders (e.g. ulcerative colitis, Crohn's
disease) · ischaemic heart disease · may mask symptoms of
infection · peripheral arterial disease · risk factors for
cardiovascular events · uncontrolled hypertension

● **INTERACTIONS** → Appendix 1: NSAIDs

● **SIDE-EFFECTS**

GENERAL SIDE-EFFECTS
▶ **Common or very common** Constipation · Crohn's disease
aggravated · diarrhoea · gastrointestinal discomfort ·
gastrointestinal disorders · haemorrhage · headache ·
nausea · vomiting
▶ **Uncommon** Fatigue · oedema · skin reactions
▶ **Rare or very rare** Asthma · bronchospasm · depression ·
dyspnoea · hyperglycaemia · nervousness · palpitations ·
pancreatitis · severe cutaneous adverse reactions (SCARs) ·
sleep disorders · vertigo · weight changes
▶ **Frequency not known** Agranulocytosis · alopecia · anaemia ·
angioedema · aplastic anaemia · confusion · eosinophilia ·
fertility decreased female · haemolytic anaemia ·
hallucination · heart failure · hepatic disorders ·
hypersensitivity · hypertension · leucopenia · malaise · nail
disorder · nephritis tubulointerstitial · nephropathy ·
paraesthesia · photosensitivity reaction · platelet
aggregation inhibition · purpura non-thrombocytopenic ·
renal failure (more common in patients with pre-existing
renal impairment) · thrombocytopenia · tinnitus · vasculitis
· vision disorders

SPECIFIC SIDE-EFFECTS
▶ **Common or very common**
▸ With oral use Dizziness · dry mouth · oral disorders
▶ **Rare or very rare**
▸ With oral use Embolism and thrombosis · metabolic
disorder
▶ **Frequency not known**
▸ With oral use Drowsiness · eye irritation · eye swelling
▸ With parenteral use Appetite decreased · increased risk of
arterial thromboembolism · increased risk of ischaemic
stroke · increased risk of myocardial infarction · meningitis
aseptic (patients with connective-tissue disorders such as
systemic lupus erythematosus may be especially
susceptible) · neutropenia · oral ulceration

SIDE-EFFECTS, FURTHER INFORMATION For information
about cardiovascular and gastrointestinal side-effects, and
a possible exacerbation of symptoms in asthma, see Non-
steroidal anti-inflammatory drugs p. 1292

● **ALLERGY AND CROSS-SENSITIVITY** [EvGr] Contra-indicated
in patients with a history of hypersensitivity to aspirin or

any other NSAID—which includes those in whom attacks
of asthma, angioedema, urticaria or rhinitis have been
precipitated by aspirin or any other NSAID. Ⓜ

● **CONCEPTION AND CONTRACEPTION** [EvGr] Caution—long-
term use of some NSAIDs is associated with reduced
female fertility, which is reversible on stopping treatment.
Ⓜ

● **PREGNANCY** Avoid use in first and second trimesters
unless essential; the MHRA advises additional antenatal
monitoring may be required if treatment is considered
necessary by a doctor from week 20 of pregnancy onwards.
Avoid use in third trimester. See *NSAIDs in Pregnancy* in
Non-steroidal anti-inflammatory drugs p. 1292 for further
details.

● **BREAST FEEDING** Use with caution during breast-feeding.
Present in milk in *animal* studies.

● **HEPATIC IMPAIRMENT** Manufacturer advises caution in
mild to moderate impairment; avoid in severe impairment.

● **RENAL IMPAIRMENT** In general, for *NSAIDs* the MHRA
advises to avoid where possible; if necessary, use with
caution (risk of fluid retention and further renal
impairment, including renal failure). [EvGr] For *tenoxicam*,
avoid in severe impairment. Ⓜ

● **MEDICINAL FORMS** No licensed medicines listed.

Tiaprofenic acid

01-Aug-2023

● **INDICATIONS AND DOSE**

**Pain and inflammation in rheumatic disease and other
musculoskeletal disorders**
▶ BY MOUTH
▸ Adult: 300 mg twice daily

IMPORTANT SAFETY INFORMATION

CSM ADVICE
Following reports of **severe cystitis** the CSM has
recommended that tiaprofenic acid should not be given
to patients with urinary-tract disorders and should be
stopped if urinary symptoms develop.

  Patients should be advised to stop taking tiaprofenic
acid and to report to their doctor promptly if they
develop urinary-tract symptoms (such as increased
frequency, nocturia, urgency, pain on urinating, or blood
in urine).

MHRA/CHM ADVICE: NSAIDS: POTENTIAL RISKS FOLLOWING
PROLONGED USE AFTER 20 WEEKS OF PREGNANCY (JUNE 2023)
See Non-steroidal anti-inflammatory drugs p. 1292.

● **CONTRA-INDICATIONS** Active bladder disease (or
symptoms) · active gastro-intestinal bleeding · active
gastro-intestinal ulceration · active prostate disease (or
symptoms) · history of gastro-intestinal bleeding related to
previous NSAID therapy · history of gastro-intestinal
perforation related to previous NSAID therapy · history of
recurrent gastro-intestinal haemorrhage (two or more
distinct episodes) · history of recurrent gastro-intestinal
ulceration (two or more distinct episodes) · history of
recurrent urinary-tract disorders (if urinary symptoms
develop discontinue immediately and perform urine tests
and culture) · severe heart failure

● **CAUTIONS** Allergic disorders · cardiac impairment (NSAIDs
may impair renal function) · cerebrovascular disease ·
coagulation defects · connective-tissue disorders ·
dehydration (risk of renal impairment) · elderly (risk of
serious side-effects and fatalities) · heart failure · history of
gastro-intestinal disorders (e.g. ulcerative colitis, Crohn's
disease) · ischaemic heart disease · may mask symptoms of
infection · peripheral arterial disease · risk factors for
cardiovascular events · uncontrolled hypertension

- **INTERACTIONS** → Appendix 1: NSAIDs
- **SIDE-EFFECTS** Agranulocytosis · alopecia · anaemia · angioedema · aplastic anaemia · appetite decreased · asthma · bladder pain · bronchospasm · confusion · constipation · Crohn's disease aggravated · cystitis · depression · diarrhoea · dizziness · drowsiness · dyspnoea · fatigue · fertility decreased female · fluid retention · gastrointestinal discomfort · gastrointestinal disorders · haemolytic anaemia · haemorrhage · hallucination · headache · heart failure · hepatic disorders · hypersensitivity · hypertension · increased risk of arterial thromboembolism · malaise · meningitis aseptic (patients with connective-tissue disorders such as systemic lupus erythematosus may be especially susceptible) · nausea · nephritis tubulointerstitial · nephropathy · neutropenia · oedema · optic neuritis · oral ulceration · pancreatitis · paraesthesia · photosensitivity reaction · renal failure (more common in patients with pre-existing renal impairment) · severe cutaneous adverse reactions (SCARs) · skin reactions · sodium retention · thrombocytopenia · tinnitus · urinary disorders · urinary tract inflammation · vertigo · visual impairment · vomiting

  SIDE-EFFECTS, FURTHER INFORMATION For information about cardiovascular and gastrointestinal side-effects, and a possible exacerbation of symptoms in asthma, see Non-steroidal anti-inflammatory drugs p. 1292

- **ALLERGY AND CROSS-SENSITIVITY** EvGr Contra-indicated in patients with a history of hypersensitivity to aspirin or any other NSAID—which includes those in whom attacks of asthma, angioedema, urticaria or rhinitis have been precipitated by aspirin or any other NSAID. M

- **CONCEPTION AND CONTRACEPTION** EvGr Caution—long-term use of some NSAIDs is associated with reduced female fertility, which is reversible on stopping treatment. M

- **PREGNANCY** Avoid use in first and second trimesters unless essential; the MHRA advises additional antenatal monitoring may be required if treatment is considered necessary by a doctor from week 20 of pregnancy onwards. Avoid use in third trimester. See *NSAIDs in Pregnancy* in Non-steroidal anti-inflammatory drugs p. 1292 for further details.

- **BREAST FEEDING** Use with caution during breast-feeding. Amount too small to be harmful.

- **HEPATIC IMPAIRMENT** Manufacturer advises caution in mild to moderate impairment; avoid in severe impairment. **Dose adjustments** In elderly patients, manufacturer advises dose reduction to 200 mg twice daily in mild to moderate impairment.

- **RENAL IMPAIRMENT** In general, for *NSAIDs* the MHRA advises to avoid where possible; if necessary, use with caution (risk of fluid retention and further renal impairment, including renal failure). EvGr For *tiaprofenic acid*, avoid in severe impairment. M **Dose adjustments** EvGr In elderly patients, reduce dose to 200 mg twice daily in mild to moderate impairment. M

- **MEDICINAL FORMS** There can be variation in the licensing of different medicines containing the same drug.
  Oral tablet
  CAUTIONARY AND ADVISORY LABELS 21
  ▸ Surgam (Beaumont Pharma Ltd)
   Tiaprofenic acid 300 mg Surgam 300mg tablets | 56 tablet PoM £14.95 DT = £14.95

5 Soft tissue and joint disorders

5.1 Local inflammation of joints and soft tissue

CORTICOSTEROIDS

Corticosteroids, inflammatory disorders

18-Sep-2020

Systemic corticosteroids

Short-term treatment with corticosteroids can help to rapidly decrease inflammatory symptoms of rheumatoid arthritis. EvGr Long-term treatment in patients with established rheumatoid arthritis should only be continued after evaluating the risks and all other treatments have been considered, see Rheumatoid arthritis p. 1249. A

Polymyalgia rheumatica and *giant cell (temporal) arteritis* are always treated with corticosteroids. Relapse is common if therapy is stopped prematurely. Many patients require treatment for at least 2 years and in some patients it may be necessary to continue long-term low-dose corticosteroid treatment.

Polyarteritis nodosa and *polymyositis* are usually treated with corticosteroids.

Systemic lupus erythematosus is treated with corticosteroids when necessary using a similar dosage regimen to that for polyarteritis nodosa and polymyositis. Patients with pleurisy, pericarditis, or other systemic manifestations will respond to corticosteroids. It may then be possible to reduce the dosage; alternate-day treatment is sometimes adequate, and the drug may be gradually withdrawn. In some mild cases corticosteroid treatment may be stopped after a few months. Many mild cases of systemic lupus erythematosus do not require corticosteroid treatment. Alternative treatment with anti-inflammatory analgesics, and possibly chloroquine p. 710 or hydroxychloroquine sulfate p. 1253, should be considered.

Ankylosing spondylitis should not be treated with long-term corticosteroids; rarely, pulse doses may be needed and may be useful in extremely active disease that does not respond to conventional treatment.

For further information on corticosteroid use, see Corticosteroids, general use p. 780.

Local corticosteroid injections

Corticosteroids are injected locally for an anti-inflammatory effect. In inflammatory conditions of the joints, particularly in rheumatoid arthritis, they are given by intra-articular injection to relieve pain, increase mobility, and reduce deformity in one or a few joints; they can also provide symptomatic relief while waiting for disease-modifying antirheumatic drugs (DMARDs) to take effect. Full aseptic precautions are essential; infected areas should be avoided. Occasionally an acute inflammatory reaction develops after an intra-articular or soft-tissue injection of a corticosteroid. This may be a reaction to the microcrystalline suspension of the corticosteroid used, but must be distinguished from sepsis introduced into the injection site.

Smaller amounts of corticosteroids may also be injected directly into soft tissues for the relief of inflammation in conditions such as *tennis* or *golfer's elbow* or *compression neuropathies*. In *tendinitis*, injections should be made into the tendon sheath and not directly into the tendon (due to the absence of a true tendon sheath and a high risk of rupture, the Achilles tendon should not be injected).

Hydrocortisone acetate or one of the synthetic analogues is generally used for local injection. Intra-articular corticosteroid injections can cause flushing and may affect the hyaline cartilage. Each joint should not usually be treated more than 4 times in one year.

Corticosteroid injections are also injected into soft tissues for the treatment of skin lesions.

For further information on corticosteroid use, see Corticosteroids, general use p. 780.

Dexamethasone
783 · 24-Jul-2024

- **DRUG ACTION** Dexamethasone has very high glucocorticoid activity and insignificant mineralocorticoid activity.

- **INDICATIONS AND DOSE**

Local inflammation of joints
▶ BY INTRA-ARTICULAR INJECTION
▶ Adult: 0.3–3.3 mg, where appropriate, dose may be repeated at intervals of 3–21 days according to response, dose given according to size—consult product literature

Local inflammation of soft tissues
▶ BY LOCAL INFILTRATION
▶ Adult: 1.7–5 mg, use the 3.3 mg/mL injection preparation for this dose, dose given according to size—consult product literature, where appropriate may be repeated at intervals of 3–21 days

DOSE EQUIVALENCE AND CONVERSION
▶ Doses expressed as dexamethasone base.
▶ Dexamethasone base 3.3 mg is equivalent to dexamethasone phosphate 4 mg.
▶ Dexamethasone base 3.3 mg is equivalent to dexamethasone sodium phosphate 4.3 mg.

- **INTERACTIONS** → Appendix 1: corticosteroids

- **PREGNANCY** Dexamethasone readily crosses the placenta.

- **PRESCRIBING AND DISPENSING INFORMATION** Dexamethasone 3.8 mg/mL Injection has replaced dexamethasone 4 mg/mL Injection.

- **MEDICINAL FORMS** There can be variation in the licensing of different medicines containing the same drug.

Solution for injection
CAUTIONARY AND ADVISORY LABELS 10
EXCIPIENTS: May contain Disodium edetate, propylene glycol
▶ Dexamethasone (Non-proprietary)
   Dexamethasone (as Dexamethasone sodium phosphate) 3.3 mg per 1 ml Dexamethasone (base) 6.6mg/2ml solution for injection ampoules | 10 ampoule [PoM] £24.59–£28.00
   Dexamethasone (base) 6.6mg/2ml solution for injection vials | 5 vial [PoM] £24.00 DT = £24.00
   Dexamethasone (base) 3.3mg/1ml solution for injection ampoules | 10 ampoule [PoM] £24.00 DT = £6.65 | 10 ampoule [PoM] £28.79 DT = £6.65 (Hospital only)
   Dexamethasone (as Dexamethasone sodium phosphate) 3.8 mg per 1 ml Dexamethasone (base) 3.8mg/1ml solution for injection vials | 10 vial [PoM] £19.99 DT = £19.99

Methylprednisolone
783 · 20-Jul-2023

- **DRUG ACTION** Methylprednisolone exerts predominantly glucocorticoid effects with minimal mineralcorticoid effects.

- **INDICATIONS AND DOSE**

DEPO-MEDRONE ®

Local inflammation of joints and soft tissues
▶ BY INTRA-ARTICULAR INJECTION
▶ Adult: 4–80 mg, select dose according to size; where appropriate dose may be repeated at intervals of 7–35 days, for details consult product literature

- **CAUTIONS** Systemic sclerosis (increased incidence of scleroderma renal crisis)

- **INTERACTIONS** → Appendix 1: corticosteroids

- **SIDE-EFFECTS** Angioedema · cataract · confusion · delusions · depressed mood · diarrhoea · dizziness · drug dependence · dyslipidaemia · embolism and thrombosis · epidural lipomatosis · fatigue · gastrointestinal disorders · glucose tolerance impaired · hallucination · hepatitis · hiccups · hypopituitarism · hypotension · increased insulin requirement · insomnia · intracranial pressure increased · malaise · memory loss · metabolic acidosis · muscle weakness · myalgia · neuropathic arthropathy · peripheral oedema · psychiatric disorder · schizophrenia exacerbated · sterile abscess · suicidal ideation · vision loss · withdrawal syndrome

- **MONITORING REQUIREMENTS** Manufacturer advises monitor blood pressure and renal function (s-creatinine) routinely in patients with systemic sclerosis—increased incidence of scleroderma renal crisis.

- **MEDICINAL FORMS** There can be variation in the licensing of different medicines containing the same drug.

Suspension for injection
CAUTIONARY AND ADVISORY LABELS 10
▶ Depo-Medrone (Pfizer Ltd)
   Methylprednisolone acetate 40 mg per 1 ml Depo-Medrone 40mg/1ml suspension for injection vials | 1 vial [PoM] £3.44 DT = £3.44 | 10 vial [PoM] £34.04
   Depo-Medrone 80mg/2ml suspension for injection vials | 1 vial [PoM] £6.18 DT = £6.18 | 10 vial [PoM] £61.39
   Depo-Medrone 120mg/3ml suspension for injection vials | 1 vial [PoM] £8.96 DT = £8.96 | 10 vial [PoM] £88.81

Methylprednisolone with lidocaine

The properties listed below are those particular to the combination only. For the properties of the components please consider, methylprednisolone above, lidocaine hydrochloride p. 117.

- **INDICATIONS AND DOSE**

Local inflammation of joints
▶ BY INTRA-ARTICULAR INJECTION
▶ Adult: 4–80 mg, dose adjusted according to size; where appropriate may be repeated at intervals of 7–35 days, for details consult product literature

- **INTERACTIONS** → Appendix 1: antiarrhythmics · corticosteroids

- **MEDICINAL FORMS** There can be variation in the licensing of different medicines containing the same drug.

Suspension for injection
▶ Depo-Medrone with Lidocaine (Pfizer Ltd)
   Lidocaine hydrochloride 10 mg per 1 ml, Methylprednisolone acetate 40 mg per 1 ml Depo-Medrone with Lidocaine suspension for injection 2ml vials | 1 vial [PoM] £7.06 DT = £7.06 | 10 vial [PoM] £70.13

Depo-Medrone with Lidocaine suspension for injection 1ml vials |
1 vial PoM £3.94 DT = £3.94 | 10 vial PoM £38.88

Triamcinolone acetonide
20-Jul-2023

● **DRUG ACTION** Triamcinolone exerts predominantly glucocorticoid effects with minimal mineralcorticoid effect.

● **INDICATIONS AND DOSE**

ADCORTYL® INTRA-ARTICULAR/INTRADERMAL

Local inflammation of joints and soft tissues
▸ BY INTRA-ARTICULAR INJECTION
▸ Adult: 2.5–15 mg, adjusted according to size (for larger doses use *Kenalog®*). Where appropriate dose may be repeated when relapse occurs, for details consult product literature.
▸ BY INTRADERMAL INJECTION
▸ Adult: 2–3 mg, max. 5 mg at any one site (total max. 30 mg). Where appropriate may be repeated at intervals of 1–2 weeks, for details consult product literature

KENALOG® VIALS

Local inflammation of joints and soft tissues
▸ BY INTRA-ARTICULAR INJECTION
▸ Adult: 5–40 mg (max. per dose 80 mg), for further details consult product literature, select dose according to size. For doses below 5 mg use *Adcortyl® Intra-articular/Intradermal* injection, where appropriate dose may be repeated when relapse occurs.

● **INTERACTIONS** → Appendix 1: corticosteroids

● **MEDICINAL FORMS** There can be variation in the licensing of different medicines containing the same drug.
Suspension for injection
CAUTIONARY AND ADVISORY LABELS 10
EXCIPIENTS: May contain Benzyl alcohol
▸ **Adcortyl Intra-articular / Intradermal** (Bristol-Myers Squibb Pharmaceuticals Ltd)
Triamcinolone acetonide 10 mg per 1 ml Adcortyl Intra-articular / Intradermal 50mg/5ml suspension for injection vials | 1 vial PoM £3.63 DT = £3.63
▸ **Kenalog** (Bristol-Myers Squibb Pharmaceuticals Ltd)
Triamcinolone acetonide 40 mg per 1 ml Kenalog Intra-articular / Intramuscular 40mg/1ml suspension for injection vials | 5 vial PoM £7.45 DT = £7.45

Triamcinolone hexacetonide
20-Jul-2023

● **DRUG ACTION** Triamcinolone exerts predominantly glucocorticoid effects with minimal mineralcorticoid effects.

● **INDICATIONS AND DOSE**

Local inflammation of joints and soft-tissues (for details, consult product literature)
▸ BY INTRA-ARTICULAR INJECTION
▸ Adult: 2–20 mg, adjusted according to size of joint, no more than 2 joints should be treated on any one day, where appropriate, may be repeated at intervals of 3–4 weeks
▸ BY PERI-ARTICULAR INJECTION
▸ Adult: 10–20 mg, adjusted according to size of joint, no more than 2 joints should be treated on any one day

● **CONTRA-INDICATIONS** Consult product literature

● **CAUTIONS** Consult product literature

● **INTERACTIONS** → Appendix 1: corticosteroids

● **SIDE-EFFECTS** Insomnia · protein catabolism

● **PRESCRIBING AND DISPENSING INFORMATION** Various strengths available from 'special order' manufacturers or specialist importing companies.

● **MEDICINAL FORMS** There can be variation in the licensing of different medicines containing the same drug.
Suspension for injection
EXCIPIENTS: May contain Benzyl alcohol
▸ **Triamcinolone hexacetonide (Non-proprietary)**
Triamcinolone hexacetonide 20 mg per 1 ml Triamcinolone hexacetonide 20mg/1ml suspension for injection ampoules | 10 ampoule PoM £120.00

5.2 Soft tissue disorders

Soft-tissue disorders
07-Jul-2020

Extravasation

Local guidelines for the management of extravasation should be followed where they exist or specialist advice sought.

Extravasation injury follows leakage of drugs or intravenous fluids from the veins or inadvertent administration into the subcutaneous or subdermal tissue. It must be dealt with **promptly** to prevent tissue necrosis.

Acidic or alkaline preparations and those with an osmolarity greater than that of plasma can cause extravasation injury; excipients including alcohol and polyethylene glycol have also been implicated. Cytotoxic drugs commonly cause extravasation injury. In addition, certain patients such as the very young and the elderly are at increased risk. Those receiving anticoagulants are more likely to lose blood into surrounding tissues if extravasation occurs, while those receiving sedatives or analgesics may not notice the early signs or symptoms of extravasation.

Extravasation prevention
Precautions should be taken to avoid extravasation; ideally, drugs likely to cause extravasation injury should be given through a central line and patients receiving repeated doses of hazardous drugs peripherally should have the cannula resited at regular intervals. Attention should be paid to the manufacturers' recommendations for administration. Placing a glyceryl trinitrate patch p. 252 distal to the cannula may improve the patency of the vessel in patients with small veins or in those whose veins are prone to collapse.

Patients should be asked to report any pain or burning at the site of injection immediately.

Extravasation management
If extravasation is suspected the infusion should be stopped immediately but the cannula should not be removed until after an attempt has been made to aspirate the area (through the cannula) in order to remove as much of the drug as possible. Aspiration is sometimes possible if the extravasation presents with a raised bleb or blister at the injection site and is surrounded by hardened tissue, but it is often unsuccessful if the tissue is soft or soggy.
Corticosteroids are usually given to treat inflammation, although there is little evidence to support their use in extravasation. Hydrocortisone p. 787 or dexamethasone p. 1316 can be given either locally by subcutaneous injection or intravenously at a site distant from the injury.
Antihistamines and **analgesics** may be required for symptom relief.

The management of extravasation beyond these measures is not well standardised and calls for specialist advice. Treatment depends on the nature of the offending substance; one approach is to localise and neutralise the substance whereas another is to spread and dilute it.

The first method may be appropriate following extravasation of vesicant drugs and involves administration of an antidote (if available) and the application of cold compresses 3–4 times a day (consult specialist literature for details of specific antidotes). Spreading and diluting the offending substance involves infiltrating the area with

Musculoskeletal system

physiological saline, applying warm compresses, elevating the affected limb, and administering hyaluronidase below. A saline flush-out technique (involving flushing the subcutaneous tissue with physiological saline) may be effective but requires specialist advice. Hyaluronidase should not be administered following extravasation of vesicant drugs (unless it is either specifically indicated or used in the saline flush-out technique). Dexrazoxane p. 1069 is licensed for the treatment of anthracycline-induced extravasation.

Enzymes used in soft-tissue disorders

Collagenase
Collagenases are proteolytic enzymes that are derived from the fermentation of *Clostridium histolyticum* and have the ability to break down collagen.

Hyaluronidase
Hyaluronidase is used to render the tissues more readily permeable to injected fluids, e.g. for introduction of fluids by subcutaneous infusion (termed hypodermoclysis).

Rubefacients

Rubefacients act by counter-irritation. Pain, whether superficial or deep-seated, is relieved by any method that itself produces irritation of the skin. Topical rubefacient preparations may contain nicotinate and salicylate compounds, essential oils, capsicum, and camphor.

Topical NSAIDs

The use of a NSAID by mouth is effective for relieving musculoskeletal pain. Topical NSAIDs (e.g. felbinac p. 1301, ibuprofen p. 1302, ketoprofen p. 1306, and piroxicam p. 1312) may provide some relief of pain in musculoskeletal conditions; they can be considered as an adjunctive treatment in knee or hand osteoarthritis.

ENZYMES

▌Hyaluronidase

24-Feb-2020

● **INDICATIONS AND DOSE**

Enhance permeation of subcutaneous or intramuscular injections
▸ BY SUBCUTANEOUS INJECTION, OR BY INTRAMUSCULAR INJECTION
▸ Adult: 1500 units, to be dissolved directly into the solution to be injected (ensure compatibility)

Enhance permeation of local anaesthetics
▸ BY LOCAL INFILTRATION
▸ Adult: 1500 units, to be mixed with the local anaesthetic solution

Enhance permeation of ophthalmic local anaesthetic
▸ TO THE EYE
▸ Adult: 15 units/mL, to be mixed with the local anaesthetic solution

Hypodermoclysis
▸ BY SUBCUTANEOUS INJECTION
▸ Adult: 1500 units, to be dissolved in 1 mL water for injections or 0.9% sodium chloride injection, administered before start of 500–1000 mL infusion fluid

Extravasation
▸ BY LOCAL INFILTRATION
▸ Adult: 1500 units, to be dissolved in 1 mL water for injections or 0.9% sodium chloride and infiltrated into affected area as soon as possible after extravasation

Haematoma
▸ BY LOCAL INFILTRATION
▸ Adult: 1500 units, to be dissolved in 1 mL water for injections or 0.9% sodium chloride and infiltrated into affected area

● **CONTRA-INDICATIONS** Avoid sites where infection is present · avoid sites where malignancy is present · do not apply direct to cornea · not for anaesthesia in unexplained premature labour · not for intravenous administration · not to be used to enhance the absorption and dispersion of dopamine and/or alpha-adrenoceptor agonists · not to be used to reduce swelling of bites · not to be used to reduce swelling of stings

● **CAUTIONS**
▸ When used for Hypodermoclysis Elderly (control speed and total volume and avoid overhydration especially in renal impairment)

● **SIDE-EFFECTS** Oedema · periorbital oedema

● **MEDICINAL FORMS** There can be variation in the licensing of different medicines containing the same drug.
Powder for solution for injection
▸ Hyaluronidase (Non-proprietary)
   Hyaluronidase 1500 unit Hyaluronidase 1,500unit powder for solution for injection ampoules | 10 ampoule [PoM] £218.51 (Hospital only)

Chapter 11
Eye

CONTENTS

11

Eye

Eye

30-Nov-2020

Eye treatment: drug administration

The structure of the eye is divided into two main parts: the anterior segment and the posterior segment. Drugs are most commonly administered to the anterior segment of the eye by topical application in the form of eye drops or ointments. When a higher drug concentration is required, and when wanting to achieve therapeutic drug concentrations to the posterior segment of the eye, administration by intravitreal injection, periocular injection, or by the systemic route may be necessary.

Eye drops and eye ointments

Eye drops are generally instilled into the pocket formed by gently pulling down the lower eyelid, blinking a few times to ensure even spread, and then closing the eye; in neonates and infants it may be more appropriate to administer the drop in the inner angle of the open eye. A small amount of eye ointment is applied similarly; blinking helps to spread it. [EvGr] Eye drops and ointments may cause temporary blurring of vision. If affected, patients should be warned not to drive or perform other skilled tasks until vision is clear.

When two different eye preparations are used at the same time of day, the patient should leave an interval of at least 5 minutes between the two, to allow the first to be fully absorbed; eye ointment should be applied after drops. (M)

Systemic effects may arise from absorption of drugs into the general circulation either directly from the conjunctival sac or after the excess preparation has drained down through the tear ducts into the nasal cavity. The extent of systemic absorption following ocular administration is highly variable due to a number of factors (e.g. drainage, blink rate, tear turnover). Nasal drainage of drugs is associated with eye drops much more often than with eye ointments. Applying pressure on the lacrimal punctum for at least a minute after administering eye drops reduces nasolacrimal drainage and therefore decreases systemic absorption from the nasal mucosa.

Eye-drop dispenser devices are available to aid the instillation of eye drops from plastic bottles and some are prescribable on the NHS (consult Drug Tariff—see Part IXA - Appliances). Product-specific devices may be supplied by manufacturers—consult individual manufacturers for information. They are particularly useful in patients with poor manual dexterity (e.g. due to arthritis) or reduced vision.

Eye irrigation solutions

These are solutions for the irrigation of the conjunctival sac. They act mechanically to flush out irritants or foreign bodies as a first-aid treatment. Sterile sodium chloride 0.9% solution p. 1330 is usually used. Clean water will suffice in an emergency.

Other preparations administered to the eye

The intravitreal route is used to administer drug into the posterior segment of the eye for conditions such as macular oedema and age-related macular degeneration. The intracameral route can be used to deliver certain drugs to the anterior chamber, for example antibacterials after cataract surgery. These injections should only be used under specialist supervision.

Ophthalmic Specials

The Royal College of Ophthalmologists and the UK Ophthalmic Pharmacy Group have produced the Ophthalmic Special Order Products guidance to help prescribers and pharmacists manage and restrict the use of unlicensed eye preparations. 'Specials' should only be prescribed in situations where a licensed product is not suitable for a patient's needs. The Ophthalmic Special Order Products guidance can be accessed on the Royal College of Ophthalmologists website (www.rcophth.ac.uk).

Preservatives and sensitisers

Information on preservatives and substances identified as skin sensitisers is provided under Excipients statements in Medicinal form entries—see individual drug monographs. Very rarely, cases of corneal calcification have been reported with the use of phosphate-containing eye drops in patients with significantly damaged corneas—consult product literature for further information.

Eye preparations: control of microbial contamination

Preparations for the eye should be sterile when issued. Care should be taken to avoid contamination of the contents during use.

Eye preparations in multiple-application containers for use by the patient *at home* are normally discarded 4 weeks after first opening (unless otherwise stated by the manufacturer).

Multiple application eye preparations for use in *hospital general wards* are also normally discarded 4 weeks after first opening (unless otherwise stated by the manufacturer)—local practice may vary. Individual containers should be provided for each patient. A separate container should be supplied for each eye only if there are special concerns about contamination. Patients admitted with an eye infection should be supplied with a fresh container on admission. On discharge from hospital, eye preparations used during the hospital stay should be assessed for suitability (e.g. period of use, risk of contamination); if unsuitable, a fresh supply should be provided.

During formal *eye examinations* and in *eye surgery*, single-application containers should be used if possible to reduce the risk of contamination. There is a high-risk of cross-contamination in areas such as operating theatres, eye disease clinics, and ophthalmic accident and emergency departments, therefore all containers should be discarded after single patient use whether they are single- or multiple-application containers.

Compared to eye preparations containing a preservative, unpreserved eye preparations may have a shorter period of safe use; consult packaging and see Guidance on the in-use shelf life for eye drops and ointments for more information (www.sps.nhs.uk/articles/guidance-on-in-use-shelf-life-for-eye-drops-and-ointments/).

Contact lenses

Contact lenses are usually worn for their visual corrective function (e.g. myopia, astigmatism). There are two main types of lenses; hard (rigid or gas-permeable rigid) lenses or soft (hydrogel or hydrophilic) lenses. Soft lenses are the most popular type because they tend to be more comfortable, but they may not give the best vision.

Lenses are usually worn for a specified number of hours each day and removed for sleeping unless specifically designed for overnight wear. The risk of infectious and non-infectious keratitis is increased by extended continuous contact lens wear, and poor compliance with directions for use, daily cleaning, and disinfection.

Acanthamoeba keratitis, a painful and severe sight-threatening infection of the cornea, can be associated with ineffective lens cleaning and disinfection, the use of contaminated lens cases, or tap water coming into contact with the lenses. The condition, which is treated promptly by specialists, is especially associated with the use of soft lenses (particularly reusable or extended wear lenses).

Contact lenses and drug treatment

Unless medically indicated, soft lenses should be removed before instillation of the eye preparation. Alternatively, unpreserved drops can be used, as preservatives accumulate in soft lenses and can cause irritation. Eye drops, however, may be instilled while patients are wearing hard contact lenses but removal prior to instillation is still generally advised. Ointment preparations should never be used in conjunction with contact lens wear; oily eye drops can cause lens deposits and should also be avoided.

Many drugs given systemically can also have adverse effects on contact lens wear. These include drugs which can cause corneal oedema (e.g. oral contraceptives–particularly those with a higher oestrogen content), drugs which reduce eye movement and blink reflex (e.g. anxiolytics, sedative hypnotics, antihistamines, and muscle relaxants), drugs which reduce lacrimation (e.g. older generation antihistamines, phenothiazines and related drugs, some beta-blockers, diuretics, and tricyclic antidepressants), and drugs which increase lacrimation (including ephedrine hydrochloride p. 311 and hydralazine hydrochloride p. 207). Other drugs that may affect contact lens wear include isotretinoin p. 1443 (can decrease tolerance to contact lens), aspirin p. 142 (can cause irritation), and rifampicin p. 674 and sulfasalazine p. 46 (can discolour lenses).

1 Allergic and inflammatory eye conditions

Eye, allergy and inflammation 05-Jun-2020

Corticosteroids

Corticosteroids administered locally to the eye or given by mouth are effective for treating anterior segment inflammation, including that which results from surgery.

Topical corticosteroids are applied frequently for the first 24–48 hours; once inflammation is controlled, the frequency of application is reduced. They should normally only be used under expert supervision; three main dangers are associated with their use:

- a 'red eye', when the diagnosis is unconfirmed, may be due to herpes simplex virus, and a corticosteroid may aggravate the condition, leading to corneal ulceration, with possible damage to vision and even loss of the eye. Bacterial, fungal, and amoebic infections pose a similar hazard;
- 'steroid glaucoma' can follow the use of corticosteroid eye preparations in susceptible individuals;
- a 'steroid cataract' can follow prolonged use.

Combination products containing a corticosteroid with an anti-infective drug are sometimes used after ocular surgery to reduce inflammation and prevent infection; use of combination products is otherwise rarely justified.

Systemic corticosteroids may be useful for ocular conditions. The risk of producing a 'steroid cataract' increases with the dose and duration of corticosteroid use.

Intravitreal corticosteroids

An intravitreal implant containing dexamethasone p. 1323 (*Ozurdex*®) is licensed for the treatment of adults with macular oedema following either branch retinal vein occlusion or central retinal vein occlusion; it is also licensed for the treatment of adult patients with inflammation of the posterior segment of the eye presenting as non-infectious uveitis.

An intravitreal implant containing fluocinolone acetonide p. 1355 (*Iluvien*®) is licensed for the treatment of visual impairment associated with chronic diabetic macular oedema which is insufficiently responsive to available therapies; it is also licensed for the prevention of relapse in recurrent non-infectious uveitis affecting the posterior segment of the eye. It should be administered by specialists experienced in the use of intravitreal injections.

Eye care, other anti-inflammatory preparations

Other preparations used for the topical treatment of inflammation and allergic conjunctivitis include antihistamines, lodoxamide p. 1322, and sodium cromoglicate p. 1322.

Eye drops containing antihistamines, such as antazoline with xylometazoline p. 1321, azelastine hydrochloride p. 1321, epinastine hydrochloride p. 1321, ketotifen p. 1321, and olopatadine p. 1322, can be used for allergic conjunctivitis.

Sodium cromoglicate (sodium cromoglycate) and nedocromil sodium eye drops can be useful for vernal keratoconjunctivitis and other allergic forms of conjunctivitis.

Lodoxamide eye drops are used for allergic conjunctival conditions including seasonal allergic conjunctivitis.

Diclofenac sodium eye drops p. 1339 are also licensed for seasonal allergic conjunctivitis.

Non-steroidal anti-inflammatory eye drops are used for the prophylaxis and treatment of inflammation of the eye following surgery or laser treatment.

Ciclosporin eye drops p. 1326 are licensed for severe keratitis in patients with dry eye disease, which has not improved despite treatment with tear substitutes.

1.1 Allergic conjunctivitis

ANTIHISTAMINES

Antazoline with xylometazoline

06-Apr-2020

● **INDICATIONS AND DOSE**

Allergic conjunctivitis
▸ TO THE EYE
▸ Child 12-17 years: Apply 2–3 times a day for maximum 7 days
▸ Adult: Apply 2–3 times a day for maximum 7 days

● **CAUTIONS** Angle-closure glaucoma · cardiovascular disease · diabetes mellitus · hypertension · hyperthyroidism · phaeochromocytoma · urinary retention

● **INTERACTIONS** → Appendix 1: antihistamines, sedating · sympathomimetics, vasoconstrictor

● **SIDE-EFFECTS** Drowsiness · eye irritation · headache · hyperhidrosis · hypertension · mydriasis · nausea · palpitations · vascular disorders · vision blurred

SIDE-EFFECTS, FURTHER INFORMATION Absorption of antazoline and xylometazoline may result in systemic side-effects.

● **MEDICINAL FORMS** There can be variation in the licensing of different medicines containing the same drug.
Eye drops
EXCIPIENTS: May contain Benzalkonium chloride, disodium edetate
▸ **Otrivine Antistin** (Thea Pharmaceuticals Ltd)
Xylometazoline hydrochloride 500 microgram per 1 ml, Antazoline sulfate 5 mg per 1 ml Otrivine Antistin 0.5%/0.05% eye drops | 10 ml P £3.35 DT = £3.35

Azelastine hydrochloride

03-Aug-2023

● **INDICATIONS AND DOSE**

Seasonal allergic conjunctivitis
▸ TO THE EYE
▸ Child 4-17 years: Apply twice daily, increased if necessary to 4 times a day
▸ Adult: Apply twice daily, increased if necessary to 4 times a day

Perennial conjunctivitis
▸ TO THE EYE
▸ Child 12-17 years: Apply twice daily for a maximum duration of 6 weeks, dose can be increased if necessary to 4 times a day
▸ Adult: Apply twice daily for a maximum duration of 6 weeks, dose can be increased if necessary to 4 times a day

● **INTERACTIONS** → Appendix 1: antihistamines, non-sedating

● **SIDE-EFFECTS**
▸ **Common or very common** Eye irritation
▸ **Uncommon** Taste bitter

SIDE-EFFECTS, FURTHER INFORMATION Altered taste may occur after administration, often due to incorrect application.

● **MEDICINAL FORMS** There can be variation in the licensing of different medicines containing the same drug.
Eye drops
EXCIPIENTS: May contain Benzalkonium chloride, disodium edetate
▸ **Azelastine hydrochloride (Non-proprietary)**
Azelastine hydrochloride 500 microgram per 1 ml Azelastine 0.05% eye drops | 8 ml PoM £6.40 DT = £6.40
▸ **Optilast** (Ceuta Healthcare Ltd)
Azelastine hydrochloride 500 microgram per 1 ml Optilast 0.05% eye drops | 8 ml PoM £6.40 DT = £6.40

Epinastine hydrochloride

26-Mar-2020

● **INDICATIONS AND DOSE**

Seasonal allergic conjunctivitis
▸ TO THE EYE
▸ Child 12-17 years: Apply twice daily for maximum 8 weeks
▸ Adult: Apply twice daily for maximum 8 weeks

● **SIDE-EFFECTS**
▸ **Common or very common** Eye discomfort
▸ **Uncommon** Dry eye · eye disorders · headache · nasal irritation · rhinitis · taste altered · visual impairment

● **MEDICINAL FORMS** There can be variation in the licensing of different medicines containing the same drug.
Eye drops
EXCIPIENTS: May contain Benzalkonium chloride, disodium edetate
▸ **Relestat** (AbbVie Ltd)
Epinastine hydrochloride 500 microgram per 1 ml Relestat 500micrograms/ml eye drops | 5 ml PoM £9.90 DT = £9.90

Ketotifen

14-Dec-2020

● **INDICATIONS AND DOSE**

Seasonal allergic conjunctivitis
▸ TO THE EYE
▸ Child 3-17 years: Apply twice daily
▸ Adult: Apply twice daily

● **INTERACTIONS** → Appendix 1: antihistamines, sedating

● **SIDE-EFFECTS**
▸ **Common or very common** Eye discomfort · eye disorders · eye inflammation
▸ **Uncommon** Conjunctival haemorrhage · drowsiness · dry eye · dry mouth · headache · skin reactions · vision disorders
▸ **Frequency not known** Asthma exacerbated · facial swelling · oedema

● **NATIONAL FUNDING/ACCESS DECISIONS**
For full details see funding body website

All Wales Medicines Strategy Group (AWMSG) decisions
▸ Ketotifen (*Ketofall*®) for symptomatic treatment of seasonal allergic conjunctivitis (June 2020) AWMSG No. 3930 Recommended with restrictions

● **MEDICINAL FORMS** There can be variation in the licensing of different medicines containing the same drug.
Eye drops
EXCIPIENTS: May contain Benzalkonium chloride
▸ **Ketofall** (Scope Ophthalmics Ltd)
Ketotifen (as Ketotifen hydrogen fumarate) 250 microgram per 1 ml Ketofall 0.25mg/ml eye drops 0.4ml unit dose | 30 unit dose PoM £6.95 DT = £6.95
▸ **Zaditen** (Thea Pharmaceuticals Ltd)
Ketotifen (as Ketotifen fumarate) 250 microgram per 1 ml Zaditen 250micrograms/ml eye drops | 5 ml PoM £7.80 DT = £7.80

Olopatadine

25-Mar-2020

- **INDICATIONS AND DOSE**

Seasonal allergic conjunctivitis
- ▶ TO THE EYE
- ▶ Child 3-17 years: Apply twice daily for maximum 4 months
- ▶ Adult: Apply twice daily for maximum 4 months

- **SIDE-EFFECTS**
- ▶ **Common or very common** Asthenia · dry eye · eye discomfort · headache · nasal dryness · taste altered
- ▶ **Uncommon** Dizziness · eye disorders · eye inflammation · increased risk of infection · numbness · skin reactions · vision disorders
- ▶ **Frequency not known** Drowsiness · dyspnoea · malaise · nausea · vomiting

- **MEDICINAL FORMS** There can be variation in the licensing of different medicines containing the same drug.

Eye drops
EXCIPIENTS: May contain Benzalkonium chloride
- ▶ **Olopatadine (Non-proprietary)**
  Olopatadine (as Olopatadine hydrochloride) 1 mg per 1 ml Olopatadine 1mg/ml eye drops | 5 ml [PoM] £8.12 DT = £7.30
- ▶ **Opatanol** (Novartis Pharmaceuticals UK Ltd)
  Olopatadine (as Olopatadine hydrochloride) 1 mg per 1 ml Opatanol 1mg/ml eye drops | 5 ml [PoM] £4.68 DT = £7.30

MAST-CELL STABILISERS

Lodoxamide

06-Apr-2020

- **INDICATIONS AND DOSE**

Allergic conjunctivitis
- ▶ TO THE EYE
- ▶ Child 4-17 years: Apply 4 times a day, improvement of symptoms may sometimes require treatment for up to 4 weeks
- ▶ Adult: Apply 4 times a day, improvement of symptoms may sometimes require treatment for up to 4 weeks

- **SIDE-EFFECTS**
- ▶ **Common or very common** Dry eye · eye discomfort · eye disorders · vision disorders
- ▶ **Uncommon** Corneal deposits · dizziness · eye inflammation · headache · nausea
- ▶ **Rare or very rare** Nasal complaints · rash · taste altered

- **EXCEPTIONS TO LEGAL CATEGORY** Lodoxamide 0.1% eye drops can be sold to the public for treatment of allergic conjunctivitis in adults and children over 4 years.

- **MEDICINAL FORMS** There can be variation in the licensing of different medicines containing the same drug.
Eye drops
EXCIPIENTS: May contain Benzalkonium chloride, disodium edetate
- ▶ **Alomide** (Novartis Pharmaceuticals UK Ltd)
  Lodoxamide (as Lodoxamide trometamol) 1 mg per 1 ml Alomide 0.1% eye drops | 10 ml [PoM] £5.21 DT = £5.21

Sodium cromoglicate

03-Aug-2023

(Sodium cromoglycate)

- **INDICATIONS AND DOSE**

Allergic conjunctivitis | Seasonal keratoconjunctivitis
- ▶ TO THE EYE
- ▶ Child: Apply 4 times a day
- ▶ Adult: Apply 4 times a day

- **SIDE-EFFECTS** Eye stinging

- **EXCEPTIONS TO LEGAL CATEGORY** Sodium cromoglicate 2% eye drops can be sold to the public (in max. pack size of 10 mL) for treatment of acute seasonal and perennial allergic conjunctivitis.

- **MEDICINAL FORMS** There can be variation in the licensing of different medicines containing the same drug.

Eye drops
- ▶ **Sodium cromoglicate (Non-proprietary)**
  Sodium cromoglicate 20 mg per 1 ml Sodium cromoglicate 2% eye drops | 13.5 ml [PoM] £8.03 DT = £3.60
  Vividrin 2% eye drops 0.5ml unit dose preservative free | 20 unit dose [PoM] [℞]
- ▶ **Catacrom** (Rayner Pharmaceuticals Ltd)
  Sodium cromoglicate 20 mg per 1 ml Catacrom 2% eye drops 0.3ml unit dose | 30 unit dose [P] £11.99 DT = £11.99
- ▶ **Eycrom** (Aspire Pharma Ltd)
  Sodium cromoglicate 20 mg per 1 ml Eycrom 2% eye drops | 13.5 ml [PoM] £8.03 DT = £8.03
- ▶ **Opticrom** (Thornton & Ross Ltd)
  Sodium cromoglicate 20 mg per 1 ml Opticrom Aqueous 2% eye drops | 13.5 ml [PoM] £8.03 DT = £3.60

1.2 Inflammatory eye conditions

Other drugs used for Inflammatory eye conditions
Adalimumab, p. 1269 · Fluocinolone acetonide, p. 1355

ANALGESICS › NON-STEROIDAL ANTI-INFLAMMATORY DRUGS

Nepafenac

26-Aug-2020

- **INDICATIONS AND DOSE**

Prophylaxis and treatment of postoperative pain and inflammation associated with cataract surgery | Reduction in the risk of postoperative macular oedema associated with cataract surgery in diabetic patients
- ▶ TO THE EYE
- ▶ Adult: (consult product literature)

- **CAUTIONS** Avoid sunlight · corneal epithelial breakdown (if evidence of, then discontinue immediately) · may mask symptoms of infection

- **INTERACTIONS** → Appendix 1: NSAIDs

- **SIDE-EFFECTS**
- ▶ **Uncommon** Eye discomfort · eye disorders · eye inflammation
- ▶ **Rare or very rare** Allergic dermatitis · corneal deposits · dizziness · dry eye · headache · nausea
- ▶ **Frequency not known** Cutis laxa · vision disorders · vomiting

- **NATIONAL FUNDING/ACCESS DECISIONS**
For full details see funding body website

Scottish Medicines Consortium (SMC) decisions
- ▶ Nepafenac (*Nevanac*®) 3 mg/mL eye drops for the reduction in risk of postoperative macular oedema associated with cataract surgery in diabetic patients (May 2017) SMC No. 1228/17 Recommended

- **MEDICINAL FORMS** There can be variation in the licensing of different medicines containing the same drug.
Eye drops
EXCIPIENTS: May contain Benzalkonium chloride, disodium edetate
- ▶ **Nevanac** (Novartis Pharmaceuticals UK Ltd)
  Nepafenac 1 mg per 1 ml Nevanac 1mg/ml eye drops | 5 ml [PoM] £14.92 DT = £14.92
  Nepafenac 3 mg per 1 ml Nevanac 3mg/ml eye drops | 3 ml [PoM] £14.92 DT = £14.92

CORTICOSTEROIDS

Betamethasone

F 783

08-Oct-2024

- **DRUG ACTION** Betamethasone has very high glucocorticoid activity and insignificant mineralocorticoid activity.

- **INDICATIONS AND DOSE**

Local treatment of inflammation (short-term)
▶ TO THE EYE USING EYE DROP
▶ Child: Apply every 1–2 hours until controlled then reduce frequency
▶ Adult: Apply every 1–2 hours until controlled then reduce frequency

- **INTERACTIONS** → Appendix 1: corticosteroids

- **SIDE-EFFECTS** Vision disorders

SIDE-EFFECTS, FURTHER INFORMATION Since systemic absorption can follow topical administration to the eye and ear, also consider the side-effects of systemic corticosteroids.

- **MEDICINAL FORMS** There can be variation in the licensing of different medicines containing the same drug.

Ear/eye/nose drops solution
EXCIPIENTS: May contain Benzalkonium chloride, disodium edetate
▶ Betamethasone (Non-proprietary)
Betamethasone sodium phosphate 1 mg per 1 ml Betamethasone 0.1% ear/eye/nose drops | 10 ml [PoM] £3.94–£7.00 DT = £2.32
▶ Betnesol (RPH Pharmaceuticals AB)
Betamethasone sodium phosphate 1 mg per 1 ml Betnesol 0.1% eye/ear/nose drops | 10 ml [PoM] £2.32 DT = £2.32
▶ Vistamethasone (Martindale Pharmaceuticals Ltd)
Betamethasone sodium phosphate 1 mg per 1 ml Vistamethasone 0.1% ear/eye/nose drops | 5 ml [PoM] £11.30

Combinations available: *Betamethasone with neomycin*, p. 1325

Dexamethasone

F 783

24-Jul-2024

- **DRUG ACTION** Dexamethasone has very high glucocorticoid activity and insignificant mineralocorticoid activity.

- **INDICATIONS AND DOSE**

Local treatment of inflammation (short-term)
▶ TO THE EYE USING EYE DROP
▶ Child: Apply 4–6 times a day
▶ Adult: Apply every 30–60 minutes until controlled, then reduced to 4–6 times a day

Short term local treatment of inflammation (severe conditions)
▶ TO THE EYE USING EYE DROP
▶ Child: Apply every 30–60 minutes until controlled, reduce frequency when control achieved

Macular oedema [following either branch retinal vein occlusion or central retinal vein occlusion] (specialist use only) | Diabetic macular oedema (specialist use only) | Inflammation of the posterior segment of the eye presenting as non-infectious uveitis (specialist use only)
▶ BY INTRAVITREAL INJECTION
▶ Adult: Specialist indication – access specialist resources for dosing information

ETACORTILEN ®

Local treatment of inflammation [short-term]
▶ TO THE EYE USING EYE DROP
▶ Child 13-17 years: Apply 1 drop 3–4 times a day, dose to be adjusted according to response
▶ Adult: Apply 1 drop 3–4 times a day, dose to be adjusted according to response

DOSE EQUIVALENCE AND CONVERSION
▶ *Etacortilen* ® eye drops contain dexamethasone sodium phosphate 1.5 mg/mL.

- **UNLICENSED USE** *Maxidex* ® not licensed for use in children under 2 years. *Dropodex* ® not licensed for use in children.

- **CONTRA-INDICATIONS**
▶ With intravitreal use Active ocular herpes simplex · active or suspected ocular infection · active or suspected periocular infection · rupture of the posterior lens capsule in patients with aphakia, iris or transscleral fixated intra-ocular lens or anterior chamber intra-ocular lens · uncontrolled advanced glaucoma

- **CAUTIONS**
▶ With intravitreal use History of ocular viral infection (including herpes simplex) · posterior capsule tear or iris defect (risk of implant migration into the anterior chamber which may cause corneal oedema and, in persistent severe cases, the need for corneal transplantation) · retinal vein occlusion with significant retinal ischaemia

- **INTERACTIONS** → Appendix 1: corticosteroids

- **SIDE-EFFECTS**
▶ **Common or very common** Eye discomfort
▶ **Uncommon**
▶ When used by eye (topical) Dry eye · taste altered · vision disorders
▶ With intravitreal use Necrotising retinitis
▶ **Frequency not known**
▶ When used by eye (topical) Dizziness · ulcerative keratitis

SIDE-EFFECTS, FURTHER INFORMATION Since systemic absorption can follow intravitreal use or topical administration to the eye, also consider the side-effects of systemic corticosteroids.

- **PREGNANCY** Dexamethasone readily crosses the placenta.
▶ With intravitreal use Manufacturer advises avoid unless potential benefit outweighs risk—no information available.

- **BREAST FEEDING**
▶ With intravitreal use Manufacturer advises avoid unless potential benefit outweighs risk—no information available.

- **MONITORING REQUIREMENTS**
▶ With intravitreal use Monitor intra-ocular pressure and for signs of ocular infection. In patients with posterior capsule tear or iris defect monitor for implant migration to allow for early diagnosis and management.

- **PRESCRIBING AND DISPENSING INFORMATION**
▶ When used by eye Although multi-dose dexamethasone eye drops commonly contain preservatives, preservative-free unit dose vials may be available.

- **NATIONAL FUNDING/ACCESS DECISIONS**
For full details see funding body website

NICE decisions
▶ Dexamethasone intravitreal implant for the treatment of macular oedema secondary to retinal vein occlusion (July 2011) NICE TA229 Recommended
▶ Dexamethasone intravitreal implant for treating diabetic macular oedema (September 2022) NICE TA824 Recommended
▶ Adalimumab and dexamethasone for treating non-infectious uveitis (July 2017) NICE TA460 Recommended

Scottish Medicines Consortium (SMC) decisions
▶ Dexamethasone intravitreal implant (*Ozurdex* ®) for the treatment of adult patients with macular oedema following either branch retinal vein occlusion (BRVO) or central retinal vein occlusion (CRVO) (June 2012) SMC No. 652/10 Recommended with restrictions

11

Eye

- **MEDICINAL FORMS** There can be variation in the licensing of different medicines containing the same drug. Forms available from special-order manufacturers include: eye drops

Eye drops

EXCIPIENTS: May contain Benzalkonium chloride, disodium edetate, polysorbates

▸ **Dexamethasone (Non-proprietary)**
Dexamethasone sodium phosphate 1 mg per 1 ml Minims dexamethasone 0.1% eye drops 0.5ml unit dose | 20 unit dose [PoM] £11.92 DT = £11.92
Dexamethasone 0.1% eye drops 0.3ml unit dose preservative free | 20 unit dose [PoM] £5.53–£9.75 | 30 unit dose [PoM] £8.30 (Hospital only)

▸ **Dexafree** (Thea Pharmaceuticals Ltd)
Dexamethasone sodium phosphate 1 mg per 1 ml Dexafree 1mg/1ml eye drops 0.4ml unit dose | 30 unit dose [PoM] £9.70

▸ **Dropodex** (Rayner Pharmaceuticals Ltd)
Dexamethasone sodium phosphate 1 mg per 1 ml Dropodex 0.1% eye drops 0.4ml unit dose | 20 unit dose [PoM] £11.53 DT = £11.53

▸ **Etacortilen** (Nordic Pharma Ltd)
Dexamethasone sodium phosphate 1.5 mg per 1 ml Etacortilen 1.5mg/ml eye drops 0.3ml unit dose | 20 unit dose [PoM] £11.53

▸ **Eythalm** (Aspire Pharma Ltd)
Dexamethasone phosphate (as Dexamethasone sodium phosphate) 1 mg per 1 ml Eythalm 1mg/ml eye drops | 6 ml [PoM] £9.75 DT = £9.75

▸ **Maxidex** (Novartis Pharmaceuticals UK Ltd)
Dexamethasone 1 mg per 1 ml Maxidex 0.1% eye drops | 5 ml [PoM] £1.42 DT = £1.42

▸ **Puradex** (Aspire Pharma Ltd)
Dexamethasone phosphate (as Dexamethasone sodium phosphate) 1 mg per 1 ml Puradex 1mg/ml eye drops | 6 ml [PoM] £9.75 DT = £9.75

Prolonged-release intravitreal implant

▸ **Ozurdex** (AbbVie Ltd)
Dexamethasone 700 microgram Ozurdex 700microgram intravitreal implant in applicator | 1 device [PoM] £870.00 (Hospital only)

Combinations available: *Dexamethasone with framycetin sulfate and gramicidin*, p. 1325 · *Dexamethasone with hypromellose, neomycin and polymyxin B sulfate*, p. 1325 · *Dexamethasone with netilmicin*, p. 1326 · *Dexamethasone with tobramycin*, p. 1326

Fluorometholone

20-Jul-2023

- **INDICATIONS AND DOSE**

Local treatment of inflammation (short-term)

▸ TO THE EYE
▸ Child 2-17 years: Apply every 1 hour for 24–48 hours, then reduced to 2–4 times a day
▸ Adult: Apply every 1 hour for 24–48 hours, then reduced to 2–4 times a day

IMPORTANT SAFETY INFORMATION

MHRA/CHM ADVICE: CORTICOSTEROIDS: RARE RISK OF CENTRAL SEROUS CHORIORETINOPATHY WITH LOCAL AS WELL AS SYSTEMIC ADMINISTRATION (AUGUST 2017)
See Corticosteroids, general use p. 780.

NHS IMPROVEMENT PATIENT SAFETY ALERT: STEROID EMERGENCY CARD TO SUPPORT EARLY RECOGNITION AND TREATMENT OF ADRENAL CRISIS IN ADULTS (AUGUST 2020)
See Adrenal insufficiency p. 781.

ADRENAL INSUFFICIENCY CARD (APRIL 2023)
The British Society for Paediatric Endocrinology and Diabetes (BSPED) has developed an Adrenal Insufficiency Card which should be issued to children with adrenal insufficiency and steroid dependence. The card includes a management summary for the emergency treatment of adrenal crisis and sick day dosing, and can be issued by any healthcare professional managing such patients. The BSPED Adrenal

Insufficiency Card is available at: www.bsped.org.uk/adrenal-insufficiency.

- **SIDE-EFFECTS** Cataract · eye discomfort · eye disorders · eye infection · eye inflammation · rash · taste altered · vision disorders

- **PATIENT AND CARER ADVICE**

▸ In adults If systemic absorption occurs following topical and local use, side-effects applicable to systemic corticosteroids may apply; a patient information leaflet should be supplied and the need for a Steroid Treatment Card and a Steroid Emergency Card considered, see Corticosteroids, general use p. 780.

▸ In children If systemic absorption occurs following topical and local use, side-effects applicable to systemic corticosteroids may apply; a patient information leaflet should be supplied and the need for a Steroid Treatment Card considered, see Corticosteroids, general use p. 780.

- **MEDICINAL FORMS** There can be variation in the licensing of different medicines containing the same drug.

Eye drops

EXCIPIENTS: May contain Benzalkonium chloride, disodium edetate, polysorbates

▸ **FML Liquifilm** (AbbVie Ltd)
Fluorometholone 1 mg per 1 ml FML Liquifilm 0.1% ophthalmic suspension | 5 ml [PoM] £1.71 DT = £1.71 | 10 ml [PoM] £2.95 DT = £2.95

⚑ 783

Hydrocortisone

08-Oct-2024

- **DRUG ACTION** Hydrocortisone has equal glucocorticoid and mineralocorticoid activity.

- **INDICATIONS AND DOSE**

Local treatment of conjunctival inflammation [short-term]

▸ TO THE EYE
▸ Adult: Apply 2 drops 2–4 times a day for up to 14 days, to avoid relapse, frequency may be gradually reduced to once every other day

- **INTERACTIONS** → Appendix 1: corticosteroids
- **SIDE-EFFECTS** Eye stinging

- **MEDICINAL FORMS** There can be variation in the licensing of different medicines containing the same drug.

Eye drops

EXCIPIENTS: May contain Disodium edetate

▸ **Softacort** (Thea Pharmaceuticals Ltd)
Hydrocortisone sodium phosphate 3.35 mg per 1 ml Softacort 3.35mg/ml eye drops 0.4ml unit dose | 30 unit dose [PoM] £10.99 DT = £10.99

⚑ 783

Prednisolone

24-Jun-2024

- **DRUG ACTION** Prednisolone exerts predominantly glucocorticoid effects with minimal mineralocorticoid effects.

- **INDICATIONS AND DOSE**

Local treatment of inflammation (short-term)

▸ TO THE EYE
▸ Child: Apply every 1–2 hours until controlled then reduce frequency
▸ Adult: Apply every 1–2 hours until controlled then reduce frequency

- **UNLICENSED USE** *Pred Forte* ® not licensed for use in children (age range not specified by manufacturer).

- **INTERACTIONS** → Appendix 1: corticosteroids

- **SIDE-EFFECTS** Eye discomfort · taste altered · visual impairment

SIDE-EFFECTS, FURTHER INFORMATION Since systemic absorption can follow rectal use or topical administration to the eye, also consider the side-effects of systemic corticosteroids.

- **PRESCRIBING AND DISPENSING INFORMATION** Although multi-dose prednisolone eye drops commonly contain preservatives, preservative-free unit dose vials may be available.

- **MEDICINAL FORMS** There can be variation in the licensing of different medicines containing the same drug. Forms available from special-order manufacturers include: eye drops

Eye drops
EXCIPIENTS: May contain Benzalkonium chloride, disodium edetate, polysorbates

- ▸ **Prednisolone (Non-proprietary)**
  Prednisolone sodium phosphate 5 mg per 1 ml Minims prednisolone sodium phosphate 0.5% eye drops 0.5ml unit dose | 20 unit dose [PoM] £14.04 DT = £14.04
- ▸ **Pred Forte** (AbbVie Ltd)
  Prednisolone acetate 10 mg per 1 ml Pred Forte 1% eye drops | 5 ml [PoM] £1.82 DT = £1.82 | 10 ml [PoM] £3.66 DT = £3.66

Ear/eye drops solution
EXCIPIENTS: May contain Benzalkonium chloride, disodium edetate

- ▸ **Prednisolone (Non-proprietary)**
  Prednisolone sodium phosphate 5 mg per 1 ml Prednisolone sodium phosphate 0.5% ear/eye drops | 10 ml [PoM] £2.57 DT = £2.57

CORTICOSTEROIDS › COMBINATIONS WITH ANTI-INFECTIVES

Betamethasone with neomycin   08-Oct-2024

The properties listed below are those particular to the combination only. For the properties of the components please consider, betamethasone p. 1323.

- **INDICATIONS AND DOSE**

Local treatment of eye inflammation and bacterial infection (short-term)
- ▸ TO THE EYE USING EYE DROP
- ▸ Adult: Apply up to 6 times a day

- **INTERACTIONS** → Appendix 1: corticosteroids · neomycin
- **SIDE-EFFECTS** Eye disorders · glaucoma · posterior subcapsular cataract · punctate keratitis · vision blurred
- **PRE-TREATMENT SCREENING** NHS England commissions genetic testing under the *National genomic test directory* indication: R65 - Aminoglycoside exposure posing risk to hearing. The testing criteria is significant exposure to aminoglycosides posing risk of ototoxicity. This testing is relevant to individuals with a predisposition to gram-negative infections or with hearing loss who have been exposed to aminoglycosides. For further information, see www.england.nhs.uk/publication/national-genomic-test-directories/.
- **LESS SUITABLE FOR PRESCRIBING** Betamethasone with neomycin eye-drops are less suitable for prescribing.

- **MEDICINAL FORMS** There can be variation in the licensing of different medicines containing the same drug.

Ear/eye/nose drops solution
EXCIPIENTS: May contain Benzalkonium chloride, disodium edetate

- ▸ **Betnesol-N** (RPH Pharmaceuticals AB)
  Betamethasone (as Betamethasone sodium phosphate) 1 mg per 1 ml, Neomycin sulfate 5 mg per 1 ml Betnesol-N ear/eye/nose drops | 10 ml [PoM] £2.39 DT = £2.39

Dexamethasone with framycetin sulfate and gramicidin   02-Mar-2021

The properties listed below are those particular to the combination only. For the properties of the components please consider, dexamethasone p. 1323, framycetin sulfate p. 1358.

- **INDICATIONS AND DOSE**

Local treatment of inflammation (short-term)
- ▸ TO THE EYE
- ▸ Child: Apply 4–6 times a day, may be administered every 30–60 minutes in severe conditions until controlled, then reduce frequency
- ▸ Adult: Apply 4–6 times a day, may be administered every 30–60 minutes in severe conditions until controlled, then reduce frequency

- **CAUTIONS** Avoid prolonged use
- **INTERACTIONS** → Appendix 1: corticosteroids
- **LESS SUITABLE FOR PRESCRIBING** *Sofradex*® is less suitable for prescribing.

- **MEDICINAL FORMS** There can be variation in the licensing of different medicines containing the same drug.

Ear/eye drops solution
EXCIPIENTS: May contain Polysorbates

- ▸ **Sofradex** (Neon Healthcare Ltd)
  Gramicidin 50 microgram per 1 ml, Dexamethasone (as Dexamethasone sodium metasulfobenzoate) 500 microgram per 1 ml, Framycetin sulfate 5 mg per 1 ml Sofradex ear/eye drops | 8 ml [PoM] £7.50

Dexamethasone with hypromellose, neomycin and polymyxin B sulfate

14-Dec-2020

The properties listed below are those particular to the combination only. For the properties of the components please consider, dexamethasone p. 1323, neomycin sulfate p. 597.

- **INDICATIONS AND DOSE**

Local treatment of inflammation (short-term)
- ▸ TO THE EYE USING EYE DROP
- ▸ Adult: Apply every 30–60 minutes until controlled, then reduced to 4–6 times a day
- ▸ TO THE EYE USING EYE OINTMENT
- ▸ Adult: Apply 3–4 times a day, alternatively apply once daily, to be applied at night, when used with eye drops

- **INTERACTIONS** → Appendix 1: corticosteroids · neomycin · polymyxin b
- **LESS SUITABLE FOR PRESCRIBING** Dexamethasone with neomycin and polymixin B sulfate is less suitable for prescribing.

- **MEDICINAL FORMS** There can be variation in the licensing of different medicines containing the same drug.

Eye ointment
EXCIPIENTS: May contain Hydroxybenzoates (parabens), woolfat and related substances (including lanolin)

- ▸ **Maxitrol** (Novartis Pharmaceuticals UK Ltd)
  Dexamethasone 1 mg per 1 gram, Neomycin (as Neomycin sulfate) 3500 unit per 1 gram, Polymyxin B sulfate 6000 unit per 1 gram Maxitrol eye ointment | 3.5 gram [PoM] £1.44

Eye drops
EXCIPIENTS: May contain Benzalkonium chloride, polysorbates

- ▸ **Maxitrol** (Novartis Pharmaceuticals UK Ltd)
  Dexamethasone 1 mg per 1 ml, Hypromellose 5 mg per 1 ml, Neomycin (as Neomycin sulfate) 3500 unit per 1 ml, Polymyxin B sulfate 6000 unit per 1 ml Maxitrol eye drops | 5 ml [PoM] £1.68

Dexamethasone with netilmicin

05-May-2025

The properties listed below are those particular to the combination only. For the properties of the components please consider, dexamethasone p. 1323, netilmicin p. 1332.

● **INDICATIONS AND DOSE**

NETILDEX ® EYE DROPS

Local treatment of inflammation and bacterial infection (short-term)
▸ TO THE EYE
▸ Adult: Apply 4 times a day

NETILDEX ® EYE GEL

Local treatment of inflammation and bacterial infection (short-term)
▸ TO THE EYE
▸ Adult: Apply twice daily

● **INTERACTIONS** → Appendix 1: aminoglycosides · corticosteroids

● **LESS SUITABLE FOR PRESCRIBING** Dexamethasone with netilmicin eye drops and eye gel are less suitable for prescribing.

● **MEDICINAL FORMS** There can be variation in the licensing of different medicines containing the same drug.
Eye gel
▸ Netildex (Nordic Pharma Ltd)
Dexamethasone (as Dexamethasone sodium phosphate) 1 mg per 1 ml, Netilmicin (as Netilmicin sulfate) 3 mg per 1 ml Netildex 3mg/ml / 1mg/ml eye gel 0.4ml unit dose | 15 dose PoM £14.96
Eye drops
EXCIPIENTS: May contain Benzalkonium chloride
▸ Netildex (Nordic Pharma Ltd)
Dexamethasone (as Dexamethasone sodium phosphate) 1 mg per 1 ml, Netilmicin (as Netilmicin sulfate) 3 mg per 1 ml Netildex 3mg/ml / 1mg/ml eye drops 0.3ml unit dose | 20 unit dose PoM £11.29 DT = £11.29

Dexamethasone with tobramycin

The properties listed below are those particular to the combination only. For the properties of the components please consider, dexamethasone p. 1323, tobramycin p. 1333.

● **INDICATIONS AND DOSE**

Local treatment of inflammation (short-term)
▸ TO THE EYE
▸ Adult: (consult product literature)

● **INTERACTIONS** → Appendix 1: aminoglycosides · corticosteroids

● **LESS SUITABLE FOR PRESCRIBING** Dexamethasone with tobramycin eye-drops are less suitable for prescribing.

● **MEDICINAL FORMS** There can be variation in the licensing of different medicines containing the same drug.
Eye drops
EXCIPIENTS: May contain Benzalkonium chloride, disodium edetate
▸ Dexamethasone with tobramycin (Non-proprietary)
Dexamethasone 1 mg per 1 ml, Tobramycin 3 mg per 1 ml Dexamethasone 0.1% / Tobramycin 0.3% eye drops | 5 ml PoM £5.37–£8.50 DT = £5.37
▸ Tobradex (Novartis Pharmaceuticals UK Ltd)
Dexamethasone 1 mg per 1 ml, Tobramycin 3 mg per 1 ml Tobradex 3mg/ml / 1mg/ml eye drops | 5 ml PoM £5.37 DT = £5.37

IMMUNOSUPPRESSANTS › CALCINEURIN INHIBITORS AND RELATED DRUGS

Ciclosporin

28-Jan-2025

(Cyclosporin)

● **DRUG ACTION** Ciclosporin inhibits production and release of lymphokines, thereby suppressing cell-mediated immune response.

● **INDICATIONS AND DOSE**

CEQUA ®

Moderate to severe dry eye disease that has not responded adequately to treatment with tear substitutes (initiated by a specialist)
▸ TO THE EYE
▸ Adult: Apply 1 drop twice daily, to be applied to the affected eye(s), review treatment at least every 3 months

IKERVIS ®

Severe keratitis in dry eye disease that has not responded to treatment with tear substitutes (initiated by a specialist)
▸ TO THE EYE
▸ Adult: Apply 1 drop once daily, to be applied to the affected eye(s) at bedtime, review treatment at least every 6 months

● **CONTRA-INDICATIONS** Active or suspected ocular or peri-ocular infection · ocular or peri-ocular malignancies or premalignant conditions

● **CAUTIONS** Contact lens wearers—consult product literature · glaucoma—limited information available · history of ocular herpes—no information available

● **INTERACTIONS** → Appendix 1: ciclosporin

● **SIDE-EFFECTS**
▸ **Common or very common** Eye discomfort · eye disorders · eye inflammation · vision blurred
▸ **Uncommon** Eye deposit · increased risk of infection

● **PREGNANCY** Manufacturer advises avoid unless potential benefit outweighs risk—no information available.

● **BREAST FEEDING** Manufacturer advises avoid—limited information.

● **MONITORING REQUIREMENTS** EvGr Regular eye examinations recommended—consult product literature. Ⓜ

● **DIRECTIONS FOR ADMINISTRATION** Keep eyes closed for 2 minutes after using eye drops to increase local drug action and reduce systemic absorption. If using other eye drops concomitantly, ciclosporin eye drops should be used at least 15 minutes after the other eye drops.

● **PATIENT AND CARER ADVICE**
Driving and skilled tasks Manufacturer advises patients and carers should be counselled on the effects on driving and performance of skilled tasks—increased risk of blurred vision.

● **NATIONAL FUNDING/ACCESS DECISIONS**
For full details see funding body website
NICE decisions
▸ **Ciclosporin for treating dry eye disease that has not improved despite treatment with artificial tears (December 2015)**
NICE TA369 Recommended

Scottish Medicines Consortium (SMC) decisions
▸ **Ciclosporin (Cequa ®) for the treatment of moderate-to-severe dry eye disease (keratoconjunctivitis sicca) in adult patients who have not responded adequately to artificial tears (January 2025)** SMC No. SMC2739 Recommended with restrictions

- **MEDICINAL FORMS** There can be variation in the licensing of different medicines containing the same drug.

Eye drops
- **Cequa** (Sun Pharma UK Ltd)
  Ciclosporin 900 microgram per 1 ml Cequa 0.9mg/ml eye drops 0.25ml unit dose | 60 unit dose [PoM] £64.80
- **Ikervis** (Santen UK Ltd)
  Ciclosporin 1 mg per 1 ml Ikervis 1mg/ml eye drops emulsion 0.3ml unit dose | 30 unit dose [PoM] £72.00 DT = £72.00

1.2a Anterior uveitis

ANTIMUSCARINICS

Antimuscarinics (eye)

- **CAUTIONS** Children under 3 months owing to the possible association between cycloplegia and the development of amblyopia · darkly pigmented iris is more resistant to pupillary dilatation and caution should be exercised to avoid overdosage · mydriasis can precipitate acute angle-closure glaucoma (usually in those aged over 60 years and hypermetropic (long-sighted), who are predisposed to the condition because of a shallow anterior chamber) (in adults) · mydriasis can precipitate acute angle-closure glaucoma (usually in those who are predisposed to the condition because of a shallow anterior chamber) (in children) · neonates at increased risk of systemic toxicity
- **SIDE-EFFECTS** Dizziness · photophobia · skin reactions · tachycardia
- **PATIENT AND CARER ADVICE** Patients may not be able to undertake skilled tasks until vision clears after mydriasis.

⚑ above

Atropine sulfate

22-Feb-2023

- **INDICATIONS AND DOSE**

Cycloplegia
- TO THE EYE USING EYE DROP
- Adult: (consult product literature)

Anterior uveitis
- TO THE EYE USING EYE DROP
- Adult: (consult product literature)

- **INTERACTIONS** → Appendix 1: atropine
- **SIDE-EFFECTS** Systemic side-effects can occur.
- **PRESCRIBING AND DISPENSING INFORMATION** Although multi-dose atropine sulphate eye drops commonly contain preservatives, preservative-free unit dose vials may be available.

- **MEDICINAL FORMS** There can be variation in the licensing of different medicines containing the same drug. Forms available from special-order manufacturers include: eye drops

Eye drops
- **Atropine sulfate (Non-proprietary)**
  Atropine sulfate 10 mg per 1 ml Atropine 1% eye drops | 5 ml [PoM] £85.97-£163.02 | 10 ml [PoM] £240.99 DT = £44.86
- **Atropine sulfate** (Bausch & Lomb UK Ltd)
  Atropine sulfate 10 mg per 1 ml Minims atropine sulfate 1% eye drops 0.5ml unit dose | 20 unit dose [PoM] £17.82 DT = £17.82

⚑ above

Cyclopentolate hydrochloride

- **INDICATIONS AND DOSE**

Cycloplegia
- TO THE EYE
- Child 3 months-11 years: Apply 1 drop, 30-60 minutes before examination, using 1% eye drops

- Child 12-17 years: Apply 1 drop, 30-60 minutes before examination, using 0.5% eye drops

Uveitis
- TO THE EYE
- Child 3 months-17 years: Apply 1 drop 2-4 times a day, using 0.5% eye drops (1% for deeply pigmented eyes)

Anterior uveitis | Cyclopegia
- TO THE EYE
- Adult: (consult product literature)

- **INTERACTIONS** → Appendix 1: cyclopentolate
- **SIDE-EFFECTS** Abdominal distension (in children) · arrhythmias · behaviour abnormal (in children) · cardio-respiratory distress (in children) · conjunctivitis (on prolonged administration) · constipation · dry mouth · eye oedema (on prolonged administration) · flushing · gastrointestinal disorders · hyperaemia (on prolonged administration) · mydriasis · palpitations · psychotic disorder (in children) · staggering · urinary disorders · vomiting

  SIDE-EFFECTS, FURTHER INFORMATION Systemic side-effects can occur, particularly in children and the elderly.
- **PRESCRIBING AND DISPENSING INFORMATION** Although multi-dose cyclopentolate eye drops commonly contain preservatives, preservative-free unit dose vials may be available.

- **MEDICINAL FORMS** There can be variation in the licensing of different medicines containing the same drug.

Eye drops
EXCIPIENTS: May contain Benzalkonium chloride
- **Cyclopentolate hydrochloride** (Bausch & Lomb UK Ltd)
  Cyclopentolate hydrochloride 5 mg per 1 ml Minims cyclopentolate hydrochloride 0.5% eye drops 0.5ml unit dose | 20 unit dose [PoM] £13.08 DT = £13.08
  Cyclopentolate hydrochloride 10 mg per 1 ml Minims cyclopentolate hydrochloride 1% eye drops 0.5ml unit dose | 20 unit dose [PoM] £13.38 DT = £13.38
- **Mydrilate** (Esteve Pharmaceuticals Ltd)
  Cyclopentolate hydrochloride 5 mg per 1 ml Mydrilate 0.5% solution | 5 ml [PoM] £8.08 DT = £8.08
  Cyclopentolate hydrochloride 10 mg per 1 ml Mydrilate 1% solution | 5 ml [PoM] £8.08 DT = £8.08

⚑ above

Homatropine hydrobromide

- **INDICATIONS AND DOSE**

Anterior uveitis
- TO THE EYE
- Adult: (consult product literature)

- **INTERACTIONS** → Appendix 1: homatropine

- **MEDICINAL FORMS** Forms available from special-order manufacturers include: eye drops

2 Dry eye conditions

Dry eye

08-Feb-2020

Description of condition

Dry eye presents as chronic soreness and inflammation of ocular surface associated with reduced or abnormal tear secretion (e.g. in Sjögren's syndrome). It often responds to tear replacement therapy in the form of eye drops (preferably preservative-free), eye ointment (used at night), or gels. Choice of preparation is based on the type of dry eye (e.g. aqueous-deficient or evaporative), symptoms, and patient preference.

Drug treatment

EvGr Hypromellose p. 1329 is the most frequently used treatment for tear deficiency in patients with mild dry eye. Ⓐ Initially, it may need to be instilled frequently (e.g. hourly) for adequate symptom relief, then at a reduced frequency. EvGr Carbomers below and polyvinyl alcohol p. 1330 are suitable alternatives. Ⓐ The ability of carbomers below and polyvinyl alcohol to cling to the eye surface and their higher viscosity may help reduce frequency of application to 4 times daily. Carbomers below can be less tolerated than hypromellose due to their impact on vision. EvGr Preservative-free tear replacement is preferred in cases of frequent and chronic application.

Ocular lubricants containing sodium hyaluronate p. 1331, hydroxypropyl guar, or carmellose sodium below can be used for moderate to severe dry eye following a suitable trial (6–8 weeks) of treatment options for mild dry eye.

Eye ointments containing a paraffin (e.g. liquid paraffin with white soft paraffin and wool alcohols p. 1329) can be used in addition to other options to lubricate the eye surface, especially in cases of recurrent corneal epithelial erosion. Ⓐ They may cause temporary visual disturbance and are best suited for application before sleep. Ointments should not be used during contact lens wear.

> **Other drugs used for Dry eye conditions** Pilocarpine, p. 1346

OCULAR LUBRICANTS

Acetylcysteine

01-Aug-2024

● **INDICATIONS AND DOSE**

Tear deficiency | Impaired or abnormal mucus production
▶ TO THE EYE
▶ Adult: Apply 3–4 times a day

● **INTERACTIONS** → Appendix 1: acetylcysteine

● **SIDE-EFFECTS** Eye discomfort · eye redness

● **MEDICINAL FORMS** There can be variation in the licensing of different medicines containing the same drug. Forms available from special-order manufacturers include: eye drops

Eye drops
EXCIPIENTS: May contain Benzalkonium chloride, disodium edetate
▶ **Ilube** (Rayner Pharmaceuticals Ltd)
Acetylcysteine 50 mg per 1 ml Ilube 5% eye drops | 10 ml PoM £92.75 DT = £92.75

Carbomers

09-Feb-2021

(Polyacrylic acid)

● **INDICATIONS AND DOSE**

Dry eyes including keratoconjunctivitis sicca, unstable tear film (using 0.2% preparation)
▶ TO THE EYE
▶ Child: Apply 3–4 times a day, alternatively apply as required
▶ Adult: Apply 3–4 times a day, alternatively apply as required

LIQUIVISC ® 0.25% EYE GEL

Dry eye conditions
▶ TO THE EYE
▶ Child: Apply 1–4 times a day
▶ Adult: Apply 1–4 times a day

● **PRESCRIBING AND DISPENSING INFORMATION** Synthetic high molecular weight polymers of acrylic acid cross-linked with either allyl ethers of sucrose or allyl ethers of pentaerithrityl.

● **MEDICINAL FORMS** There can be variation in the licensing of different medicines containing the same drug.

Eye gel
EXCIPIENTS: May contain Benzalkonium chloride, cetrimide, disodium edetate
▶ **Liquivisc** (Thea Pharmaceuticals Ltd)
Carbomer 974P 2.5 mg per 1 gram Liquivisc 0.25% eye gel | 10 gram P £4.50 DT = £4.50

Eye drops
▶ **GelTears** (Bausch & Lomb UK Ltd)
Carbomer 980 2 mg per 1 gram GelTears 0.2% gel | 10 gram P £2.80 DT = £2.80
▶ **Viscotears** (Bausch & Lomb UK Ltd)
Carbomer 980 2 mg per 1 gram Viscotears 2mg/g liquid gel | 10 gram P £1.59 DT = £2.80
Viscotears 2mg/g eye gel 0.6ml unit dose | 30 unit dose P £5.42 DT = £5.42

Carmellose sodium

04-Dec-2020

● **INDICATIONS AND DOSE**

Dry eye conditions
▶ TO THE EYE
▶ Child: Apply as required
▶ Adult: Apply as required

● **PRESCRIBING AND DISPENSING INFORMATION** Some preparations are contained units which are resealable and may be used for up to 12 hours.

● **MEDICINAL FORMS** There can be variation in the licensing of different medicines containing the same drug.

Eye drops
▶ **Carmellose sodium (Non-proprietary)**
Carmellose 0.5% eye drops | 10 ml £7.49
Evolve Carmellose 0.5% eye drops preservative free | 10 ml £5.25
VIZcellose 1% eye drops preservative free | 10 ml £1.82
VIZcellose 0.5% eye drops preservative free | 10 ml £2.88
▶ **AaqEye Carmellose** (Essential-Healthcare Ltd)
AaqEye Carmellose 0.5% eye drops | 10 ml £1.73
▶ **Aqualube** (TriOn Pharma Ltd)
Aqualube 0.5% eye drops | 10 ml £1.68
Aqualube Forte 1% eye drops | 10 ml £1.58
▶ **Carmellose** (Warneford Healthcare Ltd)
PF Drops Carmellose 0.5% eye drops preservative free | 10 ml £7.49
PF Drops Carmellose 1% eye drops preservative free | 10 ml £7.49
▶ **Carmize** (Aspire Pharma Ltd)
Carmize 1% eye drops | 10 ml £8.49
Carmize 0.5% eye drops | 10 ml £7.49
▶ **Cellusan** (Farmigea S.p.A.)
Cellusan 1% eye drops preservative free | 10 ml £4.92
Cellusan Light 0.5% eye drops preservative free | 10 ml £4.92
▶ **Celluvisc** (AbbVie Ltd)
Celluvisc 1% eye drops 0.4ml unit dose | 30 unit dose P £3.00 DT = £3.00 | 60 unit dose P £10.99
Carmellose sodium 5 mg per 1 ml Celluvisc 0.5% eye drops 0.4ml unit dose | 30 unit dose P £4.80 DT = £4.80 | 90 unit dose P £15.53
▶ **Eyeaze** (Ridge Pharma Ltd)
Eyeaze Carmellose 1% eye drops preservative free | 10 ml £1.81
Eyeaze Carmellose 0.5% eye drops preservative free | 10 ml £2.87
▶ **Ocu-Lube Carmellose** (Sai-Meds Ltd)
Ocu-Lube Carmellose 0.5% eye drops preservative free | 10 ml £7.49
Ocu-Lube Carmellose 1% eye drops preservative free | 10 ml £7.49
▶ **Ocufresh Comfort** (Blumont Healthcare Ltd)
Ocufresh Comfort Carmellose 0.5% eye drops preservative free | 10 ml £2.29
▶ **Ocufresh Comfort Plus** (Blumont Healthcare Ltd)
Ocufresh Comfort Plus 1% eye drops preservative free | 10 ml £1.70
▶ **Optho-Lique** (Essential-Healthcare Ltd)
Optho-Lique 0.5% eye drops | 10 ml £3.73
Optho-Lique Forte 1% eye drops | 10 ml £2.83
▶ **Optive** (Allergan Ltd)
Optive 0.5% eye drops | 10 ml £7.49
▶ **Optive Plus** (Allergan Ltd)
Optive Plus 0.5% eye drops | 10 ml £7.49
▶ **Tearvis** (Sai-Meds Ltd)
Tearvis 1% eye drops | 10 ml £8.49

Tearvis 0.5% eye drops | 10 ml £7.49
▸ **VisuXL** (Visufarma UK Ltd)
VisuXL Gel eye drops preservative free | 10 ml £7.49

Hydroxyethylcellulose　　　　　23-Mar-2020

● **INDICATIONS AND DOSE**
Tear deficiency
▸ TO THE EYE
▸ **Child:** Apply as required
▸ **Adult:** Apply as required

● **PRESCRIBING AND DISPENSING INFORMATION** Although multi-dose hydroxyethylcellulose eye drops commonly contain preservatives, preservative-free unit dose vials may be available.

● **MEDICINAL FORMS** There can be variation in the licensing of different medicines containing the same drug.
Eye drops
▸ **Artificial tears** (Bausch & Lomb UK Ltd)
Hydroxyethylcellulose 4.4 mg per 1 ml Minims artificial tears 0.44% eye drops 0.5ml unit dose | 20 unit dose P £9.33 DT = £9.33

Hydroxypropyl guar with polyethylene glycol and propylene glycol　09-May-2024

● **DRUG ACTION** Formulated as an ocular lubricant

● **INDICATIONS AND DOSE**
Dry eye conditions
▸ TO THE EYE
▸ **Child:** Apply as required
▸ **Adult:** Apply as required

● **MEDICINAL FORMS** No licensed medicines listed.

Hypromellose　　　　　　　　　23-Mar-2020

● **INDICATIONS AND DOSE**
Tear deficiency
▸ TO THE EYE
▸ **Child:** Apply as required
▸ **Adult:** Apply as required

● **PRESCRIBING AND DISPENSING INFORMATION** Although multi-dose hypromellose eye drops commonly contain preservatives, preservative-free unit dose vials may be available.

● **MEDICINAL FORMS** There can be variation in the licensing of different medicines containing the same drug. Forms available from special-order manufacturers include: eye drops
Eye drops
EXCIPIENTS: May contain Benzalkonium chloride, cetrimide, disodium edetate
▸ **Hypromellose (Non-proprietary)**
Hypromellose 3 mg per 1 ml Evolve Hypromellose 0.3% eye drops preservative free | 10 ml £2.03
Hypromellose 0.3% eye drops preservative free | 10 ml £5.75
Hypromellose 0.3% eye drops | 10 ml P £4.99
▸ **AacuLose** (TriOn Pharma Ltd)
Hypromellose 5 mg per 1 ml AacuLose Hypromellose 0.5% eye drops | 10 ml £0.95 DT = £0.00
▸ **AaproMel** (Essential-Healthcare Ltd)
Hypromellose 5 mg per 1 ml AaproMel 0.5% eye drops | 10 ml £0.97 DT = £0.00
▸ **AddTear** (TriOn Pharma Ltd)
Hypromellose 3 mg per 1 ml AddTear Hypromellose 0.3% eye drops preservative free | 10 ml £2.99

▸ **Hydromoor** (Rayner Pharmaceuticals Ltd)
Hydromoor 0.3% eye drops 0.4ml unit dose preservative free | 30 unit dose £5.99
▸ **Hypromellose** (Warneford Healthcare Ltd)
Hypromellose 3 mg per 1 ml PF Drops Hypromellose 0.3% eye drops preservative free | 10 ml £5.75
▸ **Hypromol** (Ennogen Healthcare Ltd)
Hypromellose 3 mg per 1 ml Hypromol 0.3% eye drops preservative free | 10 ml £4.55
▸ **Ocu-Lube** (Sai-Meds Ltd)
Hypromellose 3 mg per 1 ml Ocu-Lube 0.3% eye drops preservative free | 10 ml £5.75
▸ **Ocufresh (Hypromellose)** (Blumont Healthcare Ltd)
Hypromellose 3 mg per 1 ml Ocufresh Hypromellose 0.3% eye drops preservative free | 10 ml £2.99
▸ **Puroptics** (Biovantic Pharma Ltd)
Hypromellose 5 mg per 1 ml Puroptics Hypromellose 0.5% eye drops | 10 ml £0.95 DT = £0.00
▸ **Tear-Lac** (Scope Ophthalmics Ltd)
Hypromellose 3 mg per 1 ml Tear-Lac Hypromellose 0.3% eye drops preservative free | 10 ml £5.80
▸ **Teardew** (Sai-Meds Ltd)
Hypromellose 5 mg per 1 ml Teardew 0.5% eye drops | 10 ml £1.17 DT = £0.00

Hypromellose with dextran 70　07-Apr-2020

The properties listed below are those particular to the combination only. For the properties of the components please consider, hypromellose above.

● **INDICATIONS AND DOSE**
Tear deficiency
▸ TO THE EYE
▸ **Adult:** Apply as required

● **MEDICINAL FORMS** There can be variation in the licensing of different medicines containing the same drug.
Eye drops
EXCIPIENTS: May contain Benzalkonium chloride, disodium edetate
▸ **Tears Naturale II** (Alcon Eye Care UK Ltd)
Dextran 70 1 mg per 1 ml, Hypromellose 3 mg per 1 ml Tears Naturale II eye drops | 15 ml £2.78 DT = £0.00

Liquid paraffin with white soft paraffin and wool alcohols　26-Nov-2020

● **INDICATIONS AND DOSE**
Dry eye conditions
▸ TO THE EYE
▸ **Child:** Apply as required, best suited for application before sleep
▸ **Adult:** Apply as required, best suited for application before sleep

● **PATIENT AND CARER ADVICE** May cause temporary visual disturbance. Should not be used during contact lens wear.

● **MEDICINAL FORMS** There can be variation in the licensing of different medicines containing the same drug.
Eye ointment
▸ **Liquid paraffin with white soft paraffin and wool alcohols (Non-proprietary)**
Xailin Night eye ointment preservative free | 5 gram £2.74
▸ **Lacrilube** (AbbVie Ltd)
Wool alcohols 2 mg per 1 gram, Liquid paraffin 425 mg per 1 gram, White soft paraffin 573 mg per 1 gram Lacrilube eye ointment preservative free | 3.5 gram £2.05

Paraffin, yellow, soft

14-Jan-2025

● **INDICATIONS AND DOSE**

Eye surface lubrication
▸ TO THE EYE
▸ Child: Apply as required
▸ Adult: Apply as required

● **PATIENT AND CARER ADVICE** Ophthalmic preparations may cause temporary visual disturbance. Should not be used during contact lens wear.

● **MEDICINAL FORMS** There can be variation in the licensing of different medicines containing the same drug.
Eye ointment
▸ Paraffin, yellow, soft (Non-proprietary)
Liquid paraffin 100 mg per 1 gram, Wool fat 100 mg per 1 gram, Yellow soft paraffin 800 mg per 1 gram Simple eye ointment |
4 gram P £132.43 DT = £99.84

Polyvinyl alcohol

17-Apr-2020

● **INDICATIONS AND DOSE**

Tear deficiency
▸ TO THE EYE
▸ Child: Apply as required
▸ Adult: Apply as required

● **PRESCRIBING AND DISPENSING INFORMATION** Although multi-dose polyvinyl alcohol eye drops commonly contain preservatives, preservative-free unit dose vials may be available.

● **MEDICINAL FORMS** There can be variation in the licensing of different medicines containing the same drug. Forms available from special-order manufacturers include: eye drops
Eye drops
EXCIPIENTS: May contain Benzalkonium chloride, disodium edetate
▸ Liquifilm Tears (Allergan Ltd)
Polyvinyl alcohol 14 mg per 1 ml Liquifilm Tears 1.4% eye drops |
15 ml £1.93
Liquifilm Tears 1.4% eye drops 0.4ml unit dose preservative free |
30 unit dose £5.35
▸ Refresh Ophthalmic (Allergan Ltd)
Polyvinyl alcohol 14 mg per 1 ml Refresh Ophthalmic 1.4% eye drops 0.4ml unit dose | 30 unit dose £2.25
▸ Sno Tears (Bausch & Lomb UK Ltd)
Polyvinyl alcohol 14 mg per 1 ml Sno Tears 1.4% eye drops | 10 ml £1.06

Retinol palmitate with white soft paraffin, light liquid paraffin, liquid paraffin and wool fat

09-May-2024

● **DRUG ACTION** Formulated as an ocular lubricant

● **INDICATIONS AND DOSE**

Dry eye conditions
▸ TO THE EYE
▸ Adult: (consult product literature)

● **MEDICINAL FORMS** There can be variation in the licensing of different medicines containing the same drug.
Eye ointment
▸ Hylo Night (Scope Ophthalmics Ltd)
Hylo Night eye ointment preservative free | 5 gram £2.75

Sodium chloride

21-Jun-2023

● **INDICATIONS AND DOSE**

Tear deficiency | Ocular lubricants and astringents | Irrigation, including first-aid removal of harmful substances | Intra-ocular or topical irrigation during surgical procedures
▸ TO THE EYE
▸ Child: Apply as required, use 0.9% eye preparations
▸ Adult: Apply as required, use 0.9% eye preparations
Corneal oedema
▸ TO THE EYE
▸ Adult: Use 5% eye preparations (consult product literature)

● **PRESCRIBING AND DISPENSING INFORMATION** Although multi-dose sodium chloride eye drops commonly contain preservatives, preservative-free unit dose vials may be available.
▸ In adults Some sodium chloride 5% eye drop preparations may also contain sodium hyaluronate—consult product literature.

● **MEDICINAL FORMS** There can be variation in the licensing of different medicines containing the same drug. Forms available from special-order manufacturers include: eye drops, eye ointment
Eye drops
▸ Sodium chloride (Non-proprietary)
Sodium chloride 50 mg per 1 ml Sodium chloride 5% eye drops |
10 ml £25.25
▸ AabChlor (TriOn Pharma Ltd)
Sodium chloride 50 mg per 1 ml AabChlor Sodium Chloride 5% eye drops | 10 ml £7.97
▸ AacEdem (Essential-Healthcare Ltd)
Sodium chloride 50 mg per 1 ml AacEdem Sodium Chloride 5% eye drops | 10 ml £17.83
▸ AcuSal (Essential-Healthcare Ltd)
Sodium chloride 50 mg per 1 ml AcuSal 5% eye drops preservative free | 10 ml £15.98 DT = £0.00
▸ Aeon Sodium Chloride (Rayner Pharmaceuticals Ltd)
Sodium chloride 50 mg per 1 ml Aeon 5% eye drops preservative free | 10 ml £23.00 DT = £0.00
▸ DROPtonic (Kestrel Ophthalmics Ltd)
Sodium chloride 50 mg per 1 ml DROPtonic 5% eye drops preservative free | 10 ml £15.95 DT = £0.00
▸ Hypersal (Ennogen Healthcare Ltd)
Sodium chloride 50 mg per 1 ml Hypersal 5% eye drops | 10 ml £25.25
▸ Natklor (Blumont Healthcare Ltd)
Sodium chloride 50 mg per 1 ml Natklor 5% eye drops preservative free | 10 ml £7.99 DT = £0.00
▸ ODM5 (Kestrel Ophthalmics Ltd)
Sodium chloride 50 mg per 1 ml ODM5 5% eye drops preservative free | 10 ml £24.00 DT = £0.00
▸ Saline (Bausch & Lomb UK Ltd)
Sodium chloride 9 mg per 1 ml Minims saline 0.9% eye drops 0.5ml unit dose | 20 unit dose P £7.73 DT = £7.73
▸ SodiEye (TriOn Pharma Ltd)
SodiEye 5% eye drops 0.5ml unit dose preservative free | 20 unit dose £14.95
Sodium chloride 50 mg per 1 ml SodiEye 5% eye drops preservative free | 10 ml £15.98 DT = £0.00
▸ Sodium chloride (Essential Pharmaceuticals Ltd, Warneford Healthcare Ltd)
Sodium chloride 50 mg per 1 ml NaCl 5% eye drops 0.45ml unit dose preservative free | 20 unit dose £14.95
PF Drops Sodium Chloride 5% eye drops preservative free | 10 ml £25.20 DT = £0.00
Eye ointment
▸ Sodium chloride (Non-proprietary)
Sodium chloride 50 mg per 1 ml Sodium chloride 5% eye ointment preservative free | 5 gram £22.50
▸ SodiEye (TriOn Pharma Ltd)
SodiEye 6% eye ointment preservative free | 5 gram £18.92

Sodium hyaluronate

04-Dec-2020

● INDICATIONS AND DOSE

Dry eye conditions

▶ TO THE EYE

▶ Adult: Apply as required

● PRESCRIBING AND DISPENSING INFORMATION Some preparations are contained in units which are resealable and may be used for up to 12 hours.

Although multi-dose sodium hyaluronate eye drops commonly contain preservatives, preservative-free unit dose vials may be available.

● MEDICINAL FORMS There can be variation in the licensing of different medicines containing the same drug.

Eye drops

▶ **Sodium hyaluronate (Non-proprietary)**
VIZhyal 0.4% eye drops preservative free | 10 ml £4.10
ClinOptic HA 0.4% eye drops preservative free | 10 ml £4.15
PF Drops Sodium Hyaluronate 0.4% eye drops preservative free | 10 ml £6.99
Kent Pharma Sodium Hyaluronate 0.2% eye drops preservative free | 10 ml £3.40
VIZhyal 0.1% eye drops preservative free | 10 ml £4.10
PF Drops Sodium Hyaluronate 0.15% eye drops preservative free | 10 ml £6.99

▶ **Aactive HA** (TriOn Pharma Ltd)
Aactive HA 0.2% eye drops | 10 ml £3.36
Aactive HA PF 0.1% eye drops 0.4ml unit dose preservative free | 20 unit dose £3.99
Aactive HA 0.1% eye drops | 10 ml £3.93
Aactive HA PF 0.2% eye drops preservative free | 10 ml £3.46

▶ **AaqEye HA** (Essential-Healthcare Ltd)
AaqEye HA 0.2% eye drops | 10 ml £3.43
AaqEye HA 0.1% eye drops | 10 ml £3.91

▶ **Aeon Protect Plus** (Rayner Pharmaceuticals Ltd)
Aeon Protect Plus 0.3% eye drops preservative free | 10 ml £7.80

▶ **Aeon Repair** (Rayner Pharmaceuticals Ltd)
Aeon Repair 0.15% eye drops preservative free | 10 ml £4.00

▶ **Artelac Rebalance** (Bausch & Lomb UK Ltd)
Artelac Rebalance 0.15% eye drops | 10 ml £4.00

▶ **Artelac Splash** (Bausch & Lomb UK Ltd)
Artelac Splash 0.2% eye drops 0.5ml unit dose | 30 unit dose £7.00 | 60 unit dose £11.20

▶ **Blink Intensive** (AMO UK Ltd)
Blink Intensive Tears 0.2% eye drops 0.4ml unit dose | 20 unit dose £2.97
Blink Intensive Tears 0.2% eye drops | 10 ml £2.97

▶ **ClinOptic HA** (Warneford Healthcare Ltd)
ClinOptic HA 0.21% eye drops preservative free | 10 ml £4.15
ClinOptic HA 0.1% eye drops preservative free | 10 ml £4.15

▶ **Clinitas** (Altacor Ltd)
Clinitas Multi 0.4% eye drops preservative free | 10 ml £6.99
Clinitas 0.2% eye drops 0.5ml unit dose preservative free | 30 unit dose £5.59
Clinitas Multi 0.2% eye drops preservative free | 10 ml £5.99
Clinitas 0.4% eye drops 0.5ml unit dose preservative free | 30 unit dose £5.70

▶ **Evolve HA** (Medicom Healthcare Ltd)
Evolve HA 0.2% eye drops preservative free | 10 ml £6.05

▶ **Eyeaze** (Ridge Pharma Ltd)
Eyeaze 0.1% eye drops preservative free | 10 ml £4.15
Eyeaze 0.2% eye drops preservative free | 10 ml £4.15
Eyeaze 0.4% eye drops preservative free | 10 ml £4.15

▶ **Eyeaze Lyte** (Ridge Pharma Ltd)
Eyeaze Lyte 0.2% eye drops preservative free | 10 ml £4.15
Eyeaze Lyte 0.1% eye drops preservative free | 10 ml £4.15

▶ **Eyezin (sodium hyaluronate)** (Warneford Healthcare Ltd)
Eyezin XL 0.4% eye drops preservative free | 10 ml £6.99

▶ **Hy-Opti** (Alissa Healthcare Research Ltd)
Hy-Opti 0.1% eye drops preservative free | 12 ml £4.78
Hy-Opti 0.2% eye drops preservative free | 12 ml £4.78

▶ **Hyabak** (Thea Pharmaceuticals Ltd)
Hyabak 0.15% eye drops preservative free | 10 ml £7.99

▶ **Hycosan** (Scope Ophthalmics Ltd)
Hycosan Extra 0.2% eye drops | 7.5 ml 🅧
Hycosan 0.1% eye drops | 7.5 ml 🅧

▶ **HydraMed** (Farmigea S.p.A.)
HydraMed Forte 0.4% eye drops 0.5ml unit dose preservative free | 30 unit dose £5.74
HydraMed 0.2% eye drops preservative free | 10 ml £5.74
HydraMed Forte 0.4% eye drops preservative free | 10 ml £5.74
HydraMed 0.2% eye drops 0.5ml unit dose preservative free | 30 unit dose £5.74

▶ **Hylo Comod** (Ursapharm Arzneimittel GmbH)
Hylo Comod 0.1% eye drops | 10 ml 🅧

▶ **Hylo-Comod** (Scope Ophthalmics Ltd)
Hylo-Tear 0.1% eye drops preservative free | 10 ml £8.50
Hylo-Forte 0.2% eye drops preservative free | 10 ml £9.50

▶ **Hylo-fresh** (Scope Ophthalmics Ltd)
Hylo-Fresh 0.03% eye drops preservative free | 10 ml £4.95

▶ **Ocu-Lube HA** (Sai-Meds Ltd)
Ocu-Lube HA 0.1% eye drops preservative free | 10 ml £8.00
Ocu-Lube HA 0.2% eye drops preservative free | 10 ml £7.90

▶ **Ocufresh Everyday** (Blumont Healthcare Ltd)
Ocufresh Everyday 0.2% eye drops 0.5ml unit dose preservative free | 30 unit dose £4.70
Ocufresh Everyday 0.2% eye drops preservative free | 10 ml £3.49

▶ **Ocufresh Intense Relief** (Blumont Healthcare Ltd)
Ocufresh Intense Relief 0.4% eye drops preservative free | 10 ml £3.80
Ocufresh Intense Relief 0.4% eye drops 0.5ml unit dose preservative free | 30 unit dose £4.80

▶ **Ocusan** (Agepha Pharma s.r.o.)
Ocusan 0.2% eye drops 0.5ml unit dose | 20 unit dose £5.72

▶ **Oftaox** (Kestrel Ophthalmics Ltd)
Oftaox 0.25% eye drops | 8 ml £5.50

▶ **Optive Fusion** (Allergan Ltd)
Optive Fusion 0.1% eye drops | 10 ml £7.49

▶ **Oxyal** (Bausch & Lomb UK Ltd)
Oxyal 0.15% eye drops | 10 ml £4.15

▶ **VIZhyal** (East Midlands Pharma Ltd)
VIZhyal 0.2% eye drops preservative free | 10 ml £4.10

▶ **Viscotears HA** (Bausch & Lomb UK Ltd)
Viscotears HA 0.1% eye drops preservative free | 10 ml £5.10

▶ **Vismed** (TRB Chemidica (UK) Ltd)
Vismed Gel Multi 0.3% eye drops preservative free | 10 ml £8.37
Vismed Multi 0.18% eye drops preservative free | 10 ml £7.17
Vismed 0.18% eye drops 0.3ml unit dose preservative free | 20 unit dose £5.37

▶ **VisuXL** (Visufarma UK Ltd)
VisuXL eye drops preservative free | 10 ml £10.30

▶ **Xailin HA** (Visufarma UK Ltd)
Xailin HA 0.2% eye drops | 10 ml £7.85

▶ **Xailin Intense** (Visufarma UK Ltd)
Xailin Intense HA 0.3% eye drops preservative free | 10 ml £6.10

▶ **Xailin Plus** (Visufarma UK Ltd)
Xailin Plus HA 0.2% eye drops preservative free | 10 ml £4.15

▶ **Xailin Tears** (Visufarma UK Ltd)
Xailin Tears HA 0.1% eye drops preservative free | 10 ml £4.15

Eye gel

▶ **Vismed** (TRB Chemidica (UK) Ltd)
Vismed Gel 0.3% eye gel 0.45ml unit dose preservative free | 20 unit dose £6.29

Sodium hyaluronate with trehalose

28-Feb-2025

● INDICATIONS AND DOSE

Dry eye conditions

▶ TO THE EYE

▶ Adult: Apply as required

● PRESCRIBING AND DISPENSING INFORMATION Sodium hyaluronate and trehalose preparations do not contain preservatives; multi-dose preparation can be used for up to 3–6 months—consult product literature.

Preparations may contain additional active ingredients—consult product literature.

● MEDICINAL FORMS There can be variation in the licensing of different medicines containing the same drug.

Eye drops

▶ **Thealoz Duo** (Thea Pharmaceuticals Ltd)
Thealoz Duo eye drops preservative free | 10 ml £8.99

11

Eye

▸ **Trehapan** (Visufarma UK Ltd)
Trehapan eye drops preservative free | 10 ml £6.75
▸ **Viscotears Treha Duo** (Bausch & Lomb UK Ltd)
Viscotears Treha Duo eye drops preservative free | 10 ml £6.29
▸ **Viscotears Tri Action** (Bausch & Lomb UK Ltd)
Viscotears Tri Action eye drops preservative free | 10 ml £8.99

3 Eye infections

Eye, infections

07-Jun-2020

Overview

Most acute superficial eye infections can be treated topically with eye drops or ointment. Blepharitis is often caused by staphylococci. Bacterial conjunctivitis is commonly caused by *Streptococcus pneumoniae*, *Staphylococcus aureus*, or *Haemophilus influenzae*. Keratitis may be bacterial, viral, or fungal; it can also be caused by Acanthamoeba (parasite). Endophthalmitis is usually either bacterial or fungal; it can also be non-infective (retention of foreign material).

EvGr Anterior bacterial blepharitis is treated by application of an antibacterial eye ointment (such as chloramphenicol p. 1335) to the conjunctival sac or rubbed into the lid margins, if blepharitis is not controlled by eyelid hygiene alone. Systemic treatment (e.g. tetracyclines in patients over 12 years of age) may be required in patients with posterior blepharitis. Treatments can be intermittently stopped and restarted, based on the severity of the blepharitis and drug tolerance. Ⓐ

Most cases of acute bacterial conjunctivitis are self-limiting and resolve within 5–7 days without treatment. EvGr In severe infection or where rapid resolution is required, treatment with antibacterial eye drops or ointments are used. Ongoing symptoms despite treatment may indicate viral conjunctivitis or the need for a different antibacterial; cultures or referral to a specialist may be required.

Corneal ulcer and keratitis require specialist treatment and may call for hospital admission for intensive therapy.

Endophthalmitis is a medical emergency which also calls for specialist management and may require treatment with antibacterial drugs and steroids. Surgical intervention, such as vitrectomy, is sometimes indicated. Ⓐ

Trachoma which results from chronic infection with *Chlamydia trachomatis* can be treated with azithromycin p. 620 by mouth [unlicensed indication] as recommended by the World Health Organisation.

For information on the management of ocular herpes, see Herpesvirus infections p. 727.

Fungal infections of the cornea (e.g. fungal keratitis) are rare but can occur particularly in agricultural areas and tropical climates. Antifungal preparations for the eye are not generally available. For information about supply of preparations not commercially available, contact the local Clinical Commissioning Group (CCG), or equivalent in Scotland, Wales, or Northern Ireland, or the nearest hospital ophthalmology unit, or Moorfields Eye Hospital, 162 City Road, London EC1V 2PD (tel. (020) 7253 3411) or www.moorfields.nhs.uk.

3.1 Bacterial eye infection

ANTIBACTERIALS › AMINOGLYCOSIDES

⬥ 594

Gentamicin

10-Feb-2025

● **INDICATIONS AND DOSE**
Bacterial eye infections
▸ TO THE EYE
▸ Child: Apply 1 drop at least every 2 hours in severe infection, reduce frequency as infection is controlled and continue for 48 hours after healing, frequency of eye drops depends on the severity of the infection and the potential for irreversible ocular damage; for less severe infection 3–4 times daily is generally sufficient
▸ Adult: Apply 1 drop at least every 2 hours, reduce frequency as infection is controlled and continue for 48 hours after healing, frequency of eye drops depends on the severity of the infection and the potential for irreversible ocular damage; for less severe infection 3–4 times daily is generally sufficient

● **UNLICENSED USE** Gentamicin doses in BNF Publications may differ from those in product literature.

● **INTERACTIONS** → Appendix 1: aminoglycosides

● **SIDE-EFFECTS** Since systemic absorption can follow topical administration to the eye and ear, also consider the side-effects of systemic aminoglycosides.

● **PRE-TREATMENT SCREENING** NHS England commissions genetic testing under the *National genomic test directory* indication: R65 - Aminoglycoside exposure posing risk to hearing. The testing criteria is significant exposure to aminoglycosides posing risk of ototoxicity. This testing is relevant to individuals with a predisposition to gram-negative infections or with hearing loss who have been exposed to aminoglycosides. For further information, see www.england.nhs.uk/publication/national-genomic-test-directories/.

● **PRESCRIBING AND DISPENSING INFORMATION** Eye drops may be sourced as a manufactured special or from specialist importing companies.

● **MEDICINAL FORMS** There can be variation in the licensing of different medicines containing the same drug. Forms available from special-order manufacturers include: eye drops
Eye drops
EXCIPIENTS: May contain Benzalkonium chloride
Ear/eye drops solution
EXCIPIENTS: May contain Benzalkonium chloride
▸ **Gentamicin (Non-proprietary)**
Gentamicin (as Gentamicin sulfate) 3 mg per 1 ml Gentamicin 0.3% ear/eye drops | 10 ml PoM £20.00 DT = £20.00

Netilmicin

03-May-2024

● **INDICATIONS AND DOSE**
Local treatment of infections
▸ TO THE EYE
▸ Adult: Apply 3 times a day usually for 5 days

IMPORTANT SAFETY INFORMATION

MHRA/CHM ADVICE: AMINOGLYCOSIDES (GENTAMICIN, AMIKACIN, TOBRAMYCIN, AND NEOMYCIN): INCREASED RISK OF DEAFNESS IN PATIENTS WITH MITOCHONDRIAL MUTATIONS (JANUARY 2021)
The use of aminoglycosides is associated with rare cases of ototoxicity. A safety review found an increased risk of deafness in patients with mitochondrial mutations (particularly the m.1555A>G mutation), including cases where the patient's aminoglycoside serum levels were

within the recommended range. Nevertheless, these mitochondrial mutations are considered rare and penetrance is uncertain. No cases were identified with topical preparations but, based on a shared mechanism of effect, there is a potential risk with aminoglycosides administered at the site of toxicity i.e. the ear.

Healthcare professionals are advised to consider the need for aminoglycoside treatment versus alternative options in patients with susceptible mutations. The need for genetic testing especially in those requiring recurrent or long-term treatment with aminoglycosides should also be considered, however, urgent treatment should not be delayed. To minimise the risks of adverse effects, continuous monitoring of renal and auditory function, as well as hepatic and laboratory parameters, is recommended for all patients. Those with known mitochondrial mutations or a family history of ototoxicity are advised to inform their doctor or pharmacist before using an aminoglycoside.

- **INTERACTIONS** → Appendix 1: aminoglycosides
- **SIDE-EFFECTS** Eye discomfort · eye erythema · eyelid oedema · skin reactions
- **PREGNANCY** [EvGr] Use only if potential benefit outweighs risk, although systemic absorption is low and no evidence of toxicity in *animal* studies. ⟨M⟩
- **BREAST FEEDING** [EvGr] Avoid—limited information available. ⟨M⟩
- **PRE-TREATMENT SCREENING** NHS England commissions genetic testing under the *National genomic test directory* indication: R65 - Aminoglycoside exposure posing risk to hearing. The testing criteria is significant exposure to aminoglycosides posing risk of ototoxicity. This testing is relevant to individuals with a predisposition to gram-negative infections or with hearing loss who have been exposed to aminoglycosides. For further information, see www.england.nhs.uk/publication/national-genomic-test-directories/.

- **MEDICINAL FORMS** There can be variation in the licensing of different medicines containing the same drug.

Eye drops
- ▶ Nettacin (Nordic Pharma Ltd)
  Netilmicin (as Netilmicin sulfate) 3 mg per 1 ml Nettacin 3mg/ml eye drops | 5 ml [PoM] £10.92
  Nettacin 3mg/ml eye drops 0.3ml unit dose | 15 unit dose [PoM] £9.83 DT = £9.83

[F 594]

Tobramycin
13-May-2024

- **INDICATIONS AND DOSE**

Local treatment of infections
- ▶ TO THE EYE
- ▶ Child 1-17 years: Apply twice daily for 6–8 days
- ▶ Adult: Apply twice daily for 6–8 days

Local treatment of infections (severe infection)
- ▶ TO THE EYE
- ▶ Child 1-17 years: Apply 4 times a day for first day, then apply twice daily for 5–7 days
- ▶ Adult: Apply 4 times a day for first day, then apply twice daily for 5–7 days

- **INTERACTIONS** → Appendix 1: aminoglycosides
- **PRE-TREATMENT SCREENING** NHS England commissions genetic testing under the *National genomic test directory* indication: R65 - Aminoglycoside exposure posing risk to hearing. The testing criteria is significant exposure to aminoglycosides posing risk of ototoxicity. This testing is relevant to individuals with a predisposition to gram-negative infections or with hearing loss who have been exposed to aminoglycosides. For further information, see

www.england.nhs.uk/publication/national-genomic-test-directories/.

- **MEDICINAL FORMS** No licensed medicines listed.

ANTIBACTERIALS ⟩ CEPHALOSPORINS, SECOND-GENERATION

[F 603]

Cefuroxime
25-Oct-2021

- **INDICATIONS AND DOSE**

APROKAM® INTRACAMERAL INJECTION
Prophylaxis of endophthalmitis after cataract surgery
- ▶ BY INTRACAMERAL INJECTION
- ▶ Adult: 1 mg, dose to be injected into the anterior chamber of the eye at the end of cataract surgery

- **CAUTIONS**
  APROKAM® INTRACAMERAL INJECTION Combined operations with cataract surgery · complicated cataracts · reduced corneal endothelial cells (less than 2000) · severe risk of infection · severe thyroid disease
- **INTERACTIONS** → Appendix 1: cephalosporins
- **PREGNANCY** Not known to be harmful.
- **BREAST FEEDING** Present in milk in low concentration, but appropriate to use.
- **NATIONAL FUNDING/ACCESS DECISIONS**
  APROKAM® INTRACAMERAL INJECTION For full details see funding body website

  Scottish Medicines Consortium (SMC) decisions
- ▶ Cefuroxime (*Aprokam*®) for antibiotic prophylaxis of postoperative endophthalmitis after cataract surgery (December 2016) SMC No. 932/13 Recommended
  All Wales Medicines Strategy Group (AWMSG) decisions
- ▶ Cefuroxime (*Aprokam*®) for postoperative endophthalmitis after cataract surgery (August 2017) AWMSG No. 2224 Recommended

- **MEDICINAL FORMS** There can be variation in the licensing of different medicines containing the same drug.
  Powder for solution for injection
  ELECTROLYTES: May contain Sodium
- ▶ Aprokam (Thea Pharmaceuticals Ltd)
  Cefuroxime (as Cefuroxime sodium) 50 mg Aprokam 50mg powder for solution for injection vials | 10 vial [PoM] £49.95 (Hospital only)

ANTIBACTERIALS ⟩ MACROLIDES

[F 620]

Azithromycin
04-Dec-2023

- **INDICATIONS AND DOSE**

Trachomatous conjunctivitis caused by *Chlamydia trachomatis* | Purulent bacterial conjunctivitis
- ▶ TO THE EYE
- ▶ Child: Apply twice daily for 3 days, review if no improvement after 3 days of treatment
- ▶ Adult: Apply twice daily for 3 days, review if no improvement after 3 days of treatment

- **INTERACTIONS** → Appendix 1: macrolides
- **SIDE-EFFECTS**
- ▶ **Common or very common** Eye discomfort
- ▶ **Uncommon** Eye allergy

- **MEDICINAL FORMS** There can be variation in the licensing of different medicines containing the same drug.
  Eye drops
- ▶ Azyter (Thea Pharmaceuticals Ltd)
  Azithromycin dihydrate 15 mg per 1 gram Azyter 15mg/g eye drops 0.25g unit dose | 6 unit dose [PoM] £6.99 DT = £6.99

Ciprofloxacin

F 646

24-Jul-2024

● INDICATIONS AND DOSE

Superficial bacterial eye infection

▸ TO THE EYE USING EYE DROP
- Child: Apply 4 times a day for maximum duration of treatment 21 days
- Adult: Apply 4 times a day for maximum duration of treatment 21 days

▸ TO THE EYE USING EYE OINTMENT
- Child 1-17 years: Apply 1.25 centimetres 3 times a day for 2 days, then apply 1.25 centimetres twice daily for 5 days
- Adult: Apply 1.25 centimetres 3 times a day for 2 days, then apply 1.25 centimetres twice daily for 5 days

Superficial bacterial eye infection (severe infection)

▸ TO THE EYE USING EYE DROP
- Child: Apply every 2 hours during waking hours for 2 days, then apply 4 times a day for maximum duration of treatment 21 days
- Adult: Apply every 2 hours during waking hours for 2 days, then apply 4 times a day for maximum duration of treatment 21 days

Corneal ulcer

▸ TO THE EYE USING EYE DROP
- Child: Apply every 15 minutes for 6 hours, then apply every 30 minutes for the remainder of day 1, then apply every 1 hour on day 2, then apply every 4 hours on days 3–14, maximum duration of treatment 21 days, to be administered throughout the day and night
- Adult: Apply every 15 minutes for 6 hours, then apply every 30 minutes for the remainder of day 1, then apply every 1 hour on day 2, then apply every 4 hours on days 3–14, maximum duration of treatment 21 days, to be administered throughout the day and night

▸ TO THE EYE USING EYE OINTMENT
- Child 1-17 years: Apply 1.25 centimetres every 1–2 hours for 2 days, then apply 1.25 centimetres every 4 hours for the next 12 days, to be administered throughout the day and night
- Adult: Apply 1.25 centimetres every 1–2 hours for 2 days, then apply 1.25 centimetres every 4 hours for the next 12 days, to be administered throughout the day and night

● INTERACTIONS → Appendix 1: quinolones

● SIDE-EFFECTS
▸ **Common or very common** Corneal deposits (reversible after completion of treatment)
▸ **Rare or very rare** Ear pain · increased risk of infection · paranasal sinus hypersecretion

● PREGNANCY Manufacturer advises use only if potential benefit outweighs risk.

● BREAST FEEDING Manufacturer advises caution.

● MEDICINAL FORMS There can be variation in the licensing of different medicines containing the same drug. Forms available from special-order manufacturers include: eye drops, eye ointment

Eye drops
EXCIPIENTS: May contain Benzalkonium chloride
▸ **Ciloxan** (Novartis Pharmaceuticals UK Ltd)
Ciprofloxacin (as Ciprofloxacin hydrochloride) 3 mg per 1 ml Ciloxan 0.3% eye drops | 5 ml PoM £4.70 DT = £4.70

Levofloxacin

F 646

15-Jul-2021

● INDICATIONS AND DOSE

Local treatment of eye infections

▸ TO THE EYE
- Child 1-17 years: Apply every 2 hours for first 2 days, to be applied maximum 8 times a day, then apply 4 times a day for 3 days
- Adult: Apply every 2 hours for first 2 days, to be applied maximum 8 times a day, then apply 4 times a day for 3 days

● INTERACTIONS → Appendix 1: quinolones

● SIDE-EFFECTS
▸ **Uncommon** Rhinitis
▸ **Rare or very rare** Laryngeal oedema

● PREGNANCY Manufacturer advises use only if potential benefit outweighs risk.

● BREAST FEEDING Manufacturer advises use only if potential benefit outweighs risk.

● PRESCRIBING AND DISPENSING INFORMATION Although multi-dose levofloxacin eye drops commonly contain preservatives, preservative-free unit dose vials may be available.

● MEDICINAL FORMS There can be variation in the licensing of different medicines containing the same drug.

Eye drops
EXCIPIENTS: May contain Benzalkonium chloride
▸ **Levofloxacin (Non-proprietary)**
Levofloxacin (as Levofloxacin hemihydrate) 5 mg per 1 ml Levofloxacin 5mg/ml eye drops | 5 ml PoM £10.67 DT = £10.67 | 5 ml PoM £8.74 DT = £10.67 (Hospital only)
▸ **Eyflox** (Aspire Pharma Ltd)
Levofloxacin (as Levofloxacin hemihydrate) 5 mg per 1 ml Eyflox 5mg/ml eye drops | 5 ml PoM £13.46 DT = £13.46
▸ **Oftaquix** (Santen UK Ltd)
Levofloxacin (as Levofloxacin hemihydrate) 5 mg per 1 ml Oftaquix 5mg/ml eye drops 0.3ml unit dose | 30 unit dose PoM £17.95 DT = £17.95
Oftaquix 5mg/ml eye drops | 5 ml PoM £6.95 DT = £10.67
▸ **Oxalux** (Kestrel Ophthalmics Ltd)
Levofloxacin (as Levofloxacin hemihydrate) 5 mg per 1 ml Oxalux 5mg/ml eye drops 0.5ml unit dose | 20 unit dose PoM £9.90 DT = £9.90

Moxifloxacin

F 646

17-Apr-2020

● INDICATIONS AND DOSE

Local treatment of infections

▸ TO THE EYE
- Child: Apply 3 times a day continue treatment for 2–3 days after infection improves; review if no improvement within 5 days
- Adult: Apply 3 times a day continue treatment for 2–3 days after infection improves; review if no improvement within 5 days

● INTERACTIONS → Appendix 1: quinolones

● SIDE-EFFECTS
▸ **Uncommon** Conjunctival haemorrhage
▸ **Rare or very rare** Laryngeal pain · nasal discomfort
▸ **Frequency not known** Corneal deposits

● MEDICINAL FORMS There can be variation in the licensing of different medicines containing the same drug.

Eye drops
▸ **Moxifloxacin (Non-proprietary)**
Moxifloxacin (as Moxifloxacin hydrochloride) 5 mg per 1 ml Moxifloxacin 0.5% eye drops | 5 ml PoM £8.99–£9.80 DT = £9.80

▶ **Moxivig** (Novartis Pharmaceuticals UK Ltd)
**Moxifloxacin (as Moxifloxacin hydrochloride) 5 mg per
1 ml** Moxivig 0.5% eye drops | 5 ml [PoM] £9.80 DT = £9.80

⚑ 646

Ofloxacin
03-May-2024

● **INDICATIONS AND DOSE**
Local treatment of infections
▶ TO THE EYE
▶ Child 1-17 years: Apply every 2–4 hours for the first
2 days, then reduced to 4 times a day for maximum
10 days treatment
▶ Adult: Apply every 2–4 hours for the first 2 days, then
reduced to 4 times a day for maximum 10 days
treatment

● **CAUTIONS** Corneal ulcer (risk of corneal perforation) ·
epithelial defect (risk of corneal perforation)
● **INTERACTIONS** → Appendix 1: quinolones
● **SIDE-EFFECTS** Face oedema · oropharyngeal swelling ·
tongue swelling
● **PREGNANCY** Manufacturer advises use only if benefit
outweighs risk (systemic quinolones have caused
arthropathy in *animal* studies).
● **BREAST FEEDING** Manufacturer advises avoid.

● **MEDICINAL FORMS** There can be variation in the licensing of
different medicines containing the same drug.
Eye drops
EXCIPIENTS: May contain Benzalkonium chloride
▶ **Exocin** (AbbVie Ltd)
Ofloxacin 3 mg per 1 ml Exocin 0.3% eye drops | 5 ml [PoM] £2.17
DT = £2.17

ANTIBACTERIALS ⟩ OTHER

Chloramphenicol
24-Jul-2024

● **DRUG ACTION** Chloramphenicol is a potent broad-
spectrum antibiotic.

● **INDICATIONS AND DOSE**
Superficial eye infections
▶ TO THE EYE USING EYE DROP
▶ Child: Apply 1 drop every 2 hours, reduce frequency as
infection is controlled and continue for 48 hours after
healing, frequency is dependent on the severity of the
infection. For less severe infection 3–4 times daily is
generally sufficient
▶ Adult: Apply 1 drop every 2 hours, reduce frequency as
infection is controlled and continue for 48 hours after
healing, frequency is dependent on the severity of the
infection. For less severe infection 3–4 times daily is
generally sufficient
▶ TO THE EYE USING EYE OINTMENT
▶ Child: Apply once daily, to be applied at night, once
daily dosing to be used if eye drops are used during the
day, alternatively apply 3–4 times a day, multiple daily
dosing to be used if ointment is used alone
▶ Adult: Apply once daily, to be applied at night, once
daily dosing to be used if eye drops are used during the
day, alternatively apply 3–4 times a day, multiple daily
dosing to be used if ointment is used alone

IMPORTANT SAFETY INFORMATION
**MHRA/CHM ADVICE: CHLORAMPHENICOL EYE DROPS CONTAINING
BORAX OR BORIC ACID BUFFERS: USE IN CHILDREN YOUNGER
THAN 2 YEARS (JULY 2021)**
Some licences for chloramphenicol eye drops containing
borax or boric acid buffers were updated to restrict use in
children younger than 2 years of age to reflect warnings

on maximum daily limits for boron exposure. The MHRA
has reviewed the available evidence and consulted
independent expert advice and has concluded that the
benefits of chloramphenicol eye drops containing borax
or boric acid outweigh the potential risks, as the
potential exposure from topical application to both eyes,
in children aged 0 to 2 years old, was well below the
safety limit. Healthcare professionals should advise
parents and carers that these products can be safely used
in children younger than 2 years as advised by a doctor
or other prescriber.

● **INTERACTIONS** → Appendix 1: chloramphenicol
● **SIDE-EFFECTS** Angioedema · bone marrow disorders · eye
stinging · fever · paraesthesia · skin reactions
● **PREGNANCY** Avoid unless essential—no information on
topical use but risk of 'neonatal grey-baby syndrome' with
oral use in third trimester.
● **BREAST FEEDING** Avoid unless essential— *theoretical* risk
of bone-marrow toxicity.
● **PRESCRIBING AND DISPENSING INFORMATION** Although
multi-dose chloramphenicol eye drops commonly contain
preservatives, preservative-free unit dose vials may be
available.
● **PATIENT AND CARER ADVICE**
Medicines for Children leaflet: Chloramphenicol for eye infections
www.medicinesforchildren.org.uk/medicines/chloramphenicol-
for-eye-infections/
● **EXCEPTIONS TO LEGAL CATEGORY** Chloramphenicol 0.5%
eye drops (in max. pack size 10 mL) and 1% eye ointment
(in max. pack size 4 g) can be sold to the public for
treatment of acute bacterial conjunctivitis in adults and
children over 2 years; max. duration of treatment 5 days.

● **MEDICINAL FORMS** There can be variation in the licensing of
different medicines containing the same drug.
Eye drops
EXCIPIENTS: May contain Phenylmercuric acetate
▶ **Chloramphenicol (Non-proprietary)**
Chloramphenicol 5 mg per 1 ml Minims chloramphenicol 0.5% eye
drops 0.5ml unit dose | 20 unit dose [PoM] £11.89 DT = £11.89
Chloramphenicol 0.5% eye drops | 10 ml [PoM] £11.49 DT = £2.78
▶ **Eykappo** (Aspire Pharma Ltd)
Chloramphenicol 5 mg per 1 ml Eykappo 5mg/ml eye drops |
10 ml [PoM] £10.12 DT = £10.12
Eye ointment
▶ **Chloramphenicol (Non-proprietary)**
Chloramphenicol 10 mg per 1 gram Chloramphenicol 1% eye
ointment | 4 gram [PoM] £7.67 DT = £2.77

Fusidic acid
05-Oct-2021

● **DRUG ACTION** Fusidic acid and its salts are narrow-
spectrum antibiotics used for staphylococcal infections.

● **INDICATIONS AND DOSE**
Staphylococcal eye infections
▶ TO THE EYE
▶ Child: Apply twice daily
▶ Adult: Apply twice daily

● **INTERACTIONS** → Appendix 1: fusidate
● **SIDE-EFFECTS**
▶ **Common or very common** Dry eye · eye discomfort · vision
blurred
▶ **Uncommon** Crying on application · skin reactions ·
watering eye
▶ **Frequency not known** Angioedema · eye inflammation

• **MEDICINAL FORMS** There can be variation in the licensing of different medicines containing the same drug.
Modified-release drops
EXCIPIENTS: May contain Benzalkonium chloride, disodium edetate
▸ **Fusidic acid (Non-proprietary)**
Fusidic acid 10 mg per 1 gram Fusidic acid 1% modified-release eye drops | 5 gram [PoM] £66.00 DT = £14.58

ANTIPROTOZOALS

Propamidine isetionate

• **INDICATIONS AND DOSE**

***Acanthamoeba keratitis* infections (specialist use only) | Local treatment of eye infections**
▸ TO THE EYE USING EYE OINTMENT
▸ Adult: Apply 1–2 times a day
▸ TO THE EYE USING EYE DROP
▸ Adult: Apply up to 4 times a day

• **UNLICENSED USE** Not licensed for *acanthamoeba keratitis* infections.

• **SIDE-EFFECTS** Eye discomfort · vision blurred

• **PREGNANCY** Manufacturer advises avoid unless essential—no information available.

• **BREAST FEEDING** Manufacturer advises avoid unless essential—no information available.

• **MEDICINAL FORMS** There can be variation in the licensing of different medicines containing the same drug.
Eye drops
EXCIPIENTS: May contain Benzalkonium chloride
▸ **Brolene (Propamidine)** (Thornton & Ross Ltd)
Propamidine isetionate 1 mg per 1 ml Brolene 0.1% eye drops | 10 ml [P] £4.05 DT = £4.05
▸ **Golden Eye (propamidine)** (Cambridge Healthcare Supplies Ltd)
Propamidine isetionate 1 mg per 1 ml Golden Eye 0.1% drops | 10 ml [P] £5.25 DT = £4.05

3.2 Viral eye infection
3.2a Ophthalmic herpes simplex

ANTIVIRALS > NUCLEOSIDE ANALOGUES

Aciclovir

23-Sep-2022

(Acyclovir)

• **INDICATIONS AND DOSE**

Herpes simplex infection (local treatment)
▸ TO THE EYE USING EYE OINTMENT
▸ Adult: Apply 1 centimetre 5 times a day continue for at least 3 days after complete healing

• **INTERACTIONS** → Appendix 1: aciclovir

• **SIDE-EFFECTS**
▸ **Common or very common** Eye inflammation · eye pain

• **MEDICINAL FORMS** There can be variation in the licensing of different medicines containing the same drug.
Eye ointment
▸ **Aciclovir (Non-proprietary)**
Aciclovir 30 mg per 1 gram Aciclovir 30mg/g eye ointment | 4.5 gram [PoM] £45.00 DT = £45.00

Ganciclovir

15-Dec-2020

• **INDICATIONS AND DOSE**

Acute herpetic keratitis
▸ TO THE EYE
▸ Adult: Apply 5 times a day until healing complete, then apply 3 times a day for a further 7 days, treatment does not usually exceed 21 days

• **INTERACTIONS** → Appendix 1: ganciclovir
• **SIDE-EFFECTS**
▸ **Common or very common** Eye stinging · punctate keratitis
• **ALLERGY AND CROSS-SENSITIVITY** [EvGr] Contra-indicated in patients hypersensitive to valganciclovir.
Caution in patients hypersensitive to aciclovir, valaciclovir, or famciclovir. [M]
• **CONCEPTION AND CONTRACEPTION** As teratogenicity and impaired fertility observed in animal studies with *oral* and *intravenous* ganciclovir, manufacturer advises women of childbearing potential should use effective contraception during treatment; men with partners of childbearing potential should be advised to use barrier contraception during and for at least 90 days after treatment.
• **PREGNANCY** Manufacturer advises avoid unless no suitable alternative—limited information available.
• **BREAST FEEDING** Manufacturer advises avoid unless no suitable alternative—limited information available.

• **MEDICINAL FORMS** There can be variation in the licensing of different medicines containing the same drug.
Eye gel
EXCIPIENTS: May contain Benzalkonium chloride
▸ **Virgan** (Thea Pharmaceuticals Ltd)
Ganciclovir 1.5 mg per 1 gram Virgan 0.15% eye gel | 5 gram [PoM] £19.99 DT = £19.99

4 Eye procedures

Mydriatics and cycloplegics

25-Apr-2020

Overview

Antimuscarinics dilate the pupil and paralyse the ciliary muscle; they vary in potency and duration of action.
Short-acting, relatively weak mydriatics, such as tropicamide p. 1337 (action lasts for up to 6 hours), facilitate the examination of the fundus of the eye. Longer-acting options include cyclopentolate hydrochloride p. 1327 (complete recovery can take up to 24 hours) or atropine sulfate p. 1327 (action up to 7 days).
Phenylephrine hydrochloride p. 1337 is a sympathomimetic licensed for mydriasis in diagnostic or therapeutic procedures. Mydriasis occurs within 60–90 minutes and lasts up to 5–7 hours.
[EvGr] Mydriatics and cycloplegics are used in the treatment of anterior uveitis, usually as an adjunct to corticosteroids. Atropine sulfate or cyclopentolate hydrochloride can prevent posterior synechiae and relieve ciliary spasm when used for anterior uveitis. [A]

> **Other drugs used for Eye procedures** Apraclonidine, p. 1350

ANTIMUSCARINICS

▶ 1327

Tropicamide

- **INDICATIONS AND DOSE**

Funduscopy
▸ TO THE EYE
▸ Child: 0.5% eye drops to be applied 20 minutes before examination
▸ Adult: (consult product literature)

- **INTERACTIONS** → Appendix 1: tropicamide
- **SIDE-EFFECTS** Eye erythema · eye irritation (on prolonged administration) · eye pain · headache · hypotension · nausea · syncope · vision blurred
- **PRESCRIBING AND DISPENSING INFORMATION** Although multi-dose tropicamide eye drops commonly contain preservatives, preservative-free unit dose vials may be available.

- **MEDICINAL FORMS** There can be variation in the licensing of different medicines containing the same drug.

  Eye drops
  EXCIPIENTS: May contain Benzalkonium chloride, edetic acid (edta)
  ▸ Mydriacyl (Alcon Eye Care UK Ltd)
  Tropicamide 10 mg per 1 ml Mydriacyl 1% eye drops | 5 ml [PoM] £1.60 DT = £1.60
  ▸ Tropicamide (Bausch & Lomb UK Ltd)
  Tropicamide 5 mg per 1 ml Minims tropicamide 0.5% eye drops 0.5ml unit dose | 20 unit dose [PoM] £12.82 DT = £12.82
  Tropicamide 10 mg per 1 ml Minims tropicamide 1% eye drops 0.5ml unit dose | 20 unit dose [PoM] £12.97 DT = £12.97

  Combinations available: *Phenylephrine with tropicamide,* p. 1338 · *Tropicamide with phenylephrine and lidocaine,* p. 1338

ANTISEPTICS AND DISINFECTANTS > IODINE PRODUCTS

Povidone-iodine

08-Feb-2022

- **INDICATIONS AND DOSE**

Cutaneous peri-ocular and conjunctival antisepsis before ocular surgery
▸ TO THE EYE
▸ Adult: Apply, leave for 2 minutes, then irrigate thoroughly with sodium chloride 0.9%

- **CONTRA-INDICATIONS** Concomitant use of ocular antimicrobial drugs · concomitant use of ocular formulations containing mercury-based preservatives · preterm neonates
- **SIDE-EFFECTS**
▸ **Rare or very rare** Eye erythema · punctate keratitis
▸ **Frequency not known** Cytotoxicity · eye discolouration
- **BREAST FEEDING** Avoid regular or excessive use.
- **PRESCRIBING AND DISPENSING INFORMATION** Although multi-dose povidone iodine eye drops commonly contain preservatives, preservative-free unit dose vials may be available.

- **MEDICINAL FORMS** There can be variation in the licensing of different medicines containing the same drug. Forms available from special-order manufacturers include: eye lotion

  Eye drops
  ▸ Povidone-iodine (Non-proprietary)
  Povidone-Iodine 50 mg per 1 ml Povidone-Iodine 5% eye drops preservative free | 4 ml [PoM] £7.49 (Hospital only)
  ▸ Povidone iodine (Bausch & Lomb UK Ltd)
  Povidone-Iodine 50 mg per 1 ml Minims povidone iodine 5% eye drops 0.4ml unit dose | 20 unit dose [PoM] £17.47 DT = £17.47

DIAGNOSTIC AGENTS > DYES

Fluorescein sodium

- **INDICATIONS AND DOSE**

Detection of lesions and foreign bodies
▸ TO THE EYE
▸ Adult: Use sufficient amount to stain damaged areas

- **PRESCRIBING AND DISPENSING INFORMATION** Although multi-dose fluorescein eye drops commonly contain preservatives, preservative-free unit dose vials may be available.

- **MEDICINAL FORMS** There can be variation in the licensing of different medicines containing the same drug.

  Eye drops
  ▸ Fluorescein sodium (Bausch & Lomb UK Ltd)
  Fluorescein sodium 10 mg per 1 ml Minims fluorescein sodium 1% eye drops 0.5ml unit dose | 20 unit dose [P] £10.61 DT = £10.61
  Fluorescein sodium 20 mg per 1 ml Minims fluorescein sodium 2% eye drops 0.5ml unit dose | 20 unit dose [P] £10.81 DT = £10.81

MIOTICS > PARASYMPATHOMIMETICS

Acetylcholine chloride

22-Feb-2021

- **INDICATIONS AND DOSE**

Cataract surgery | Penetrating keratoplasty | Iridectomy | Anterior segment surgery requiring rapid complete miosis
▸ TO THE EYE
▸ Adult: (consult product literature)

- **SIDE-EFFECTS** Bradycardia · corneal decompensation · corneal oedema · dyspnoea · flushing · hyperhidrosis · hypotension
- **PREGNANCY** Avoid unless potential benefit outweighs risk—no information available.
- **BREAST FEEDING** Avoid unless potential benefit outweighs risk—no information available.

- **MEDICINAL FORMS** There can be variation in the licensing of different medicines containing the same drug.

  Powder and solvent for solution for intraocular irrigation
  ▸ Miphtel (Nordic Pharma Ltd)
  Acetylcholine chloride 20 mg Miphtel 20mg powder and solvent for solution for intraocular irrigation ampoules | 6 ampoule [PoM] £43.68 (Hospital only)

SYMPATHOMIMETICS > VASOCONSTRICTOR

Phenylephrine hydrochloride

- **INDICATIONS AND DOSE**

Mydriasis
▸ TO THE EYE
▸ Child: Apply 1 drop, to be administered before procedure, a drop of proxymetacaine topical anaesthetic may be applied to the eye a few minutes before using phenylephrine to prevent stinging
▸ Adult: Apply 1 drop, to be administered before procedure, then apply 1 drop after 60 minutes if required, a drop of topical anaesthetic may be applied to the eye a few minutes before using phenylephrine to prevent stinging

- **CONTRA-INDICATIONS** 10% strength eye drops in children · 10% strength eye drops in elderly · aneurysms · cardiovascular disease · hypertension · thyrotoxicosis
- **CAUTIONS** Asthma · cerebral arteriosclerosis (in adults) · corneal epithelial damage · darkly pigmented iris is more resistant to pupillary dilatation and caution should be

exercised to avoid overdosage · diabetes (avoid eye drops in long standing diabetes) · mydriasis can precipitate acute angle-closure glaucoma in a few patients, usually over 60 years and hypermetropic (long-sighted), who are predisposed to the condition because of a shallow anterior chamber · mydriasis can precipitate acute angle-closure glaucoma in the very few children who are predisposed to the condition because of a shallow anterior chamber · ocular hyperaemia · susceptibility to angle-closure glaucoma

● **INTERACTIONS** → Appendix 1: sympathomimetics, vasoconstrictor

● **SIDE-EFFECTS** Arrhythmias · conjunctivitis allergic · eye discomfort · hypertension · myocardial infarction (usually after use of 10% strength in patients with pre-existing cardiovascular disease) · palpitations · periorbital pallor (in children) · vision disorders

● **PREGNANCY** Use only if potential benefit outweighs risk.

● **BREAST FEEDING** Use only if potential benefit outweighs risk—no information available.

● **PRESCRIBING AND DISPENSING INFORMATION** Although multi-dose phenylephrine eye drops commonly contain preservatives, preservative-free unit dose vials may be available.

● **PATIENT AND CARER ADVICE**
Driving and skilled tasks Patients should be warned not to undertake skilled tasks (e.g. driving) until vision clears after mydriasis.

● **MEDICINAL FORMS** There can be variation in the licensing of different medicines containing the same drug. Forms available from special-order manufacturers include: eye drops
Eye drops
EXCIPIENTS: May contain Disodium edetate, sodium metabisulfite
▸ **Phenylephrine hydrochloride** (Bausch & Lomb UK Ltd)
Phenylephrine hydrochloride 25 mg per 1 ml Minims phenylephrine hydrochloride 2.5% eye drops 0.5ml unit dose | 20 unit dose ℗ £13.60 DT = £13.60
Phenylephrine hydrochloride 100 mg per 1 ml Minims phenylephrine hydrochloride 10% eye drops 0.5ml unit dose | 20 unit dose ℗ £14.00 DT = £14.00

Phenylephrine with tropicamide

12-Aug-2020

The properties listed below are those particular to the combination only. For the properties of the components please consider, phenylephrine hydrochloride p. 1337, tropicamide p. 1337.

● **INDICATIONS AND DOSE**

Pre-operative mydriasis | Diagnostic procedures when monotherapy insufficient
▸ TO THE EYE
▸ Adult: One insert to be applied into the lower conjunctival sac up to max. 2 hours before procedure; remove insert within 30 minutes of satisfactory mydriasis, and within 2 hours of application

● **INTERACTIONS** → Appendix 1: sympathomimetics, vasoconstrictor · tropicamide

● **DIRECTIONS FOR ADMINISTRATION** Manufacturer advises patients with severe dry eyes may require a drop of saline to improve insert tolerance.

● **MEDICINAL FORMS** There can be variation in the licensing of different medicines containing the same drug.
Ophthalmic insert
▸ **Mydriasert** (Thea Pharmaceuticals Ltd)
Tropicamide 280 microgram, Phenylephrine hydrochloride 5.4 mg Mydriasert 5.4mg/0.28mg ophthalmic inserts | 20 insert ℗ₒM £84.00

Tropicamide with phenylephrine and lidocaine

17-Aug-2017

● **INDICATIONS AND DOSE**

Mydriasis and intraocular anaesthesia during cataract surgery
▸ BY INTRACAMERAL INJECTION
▸ Adult: 0.2 mL for 1 dose, to be injected slowly at the start of the surgical procedure

DOSE EQUIVALENCE AND CONVERSION
▸ Each 0.2 mL dose of *Mydrane*® solution for injection contains 0.04 mg of tropicamide, 0.62 mg of phenylephrine hydrochloride and 2 mg of lidocaine hydrochloride.

● **CONTRA-INDICATIONS** Cataract surgery combined with vitrectomy · history of acute, narrow-angle glaucoma · shallow anterior chamber

● **CAUTIONS** Conditions where systemic exposure to phenylephrine or lidocaine could be harmful (consult product literature) · risk of floppy iris syndrome (consult product literature)

● **INTERACTIONS** → Appendix 1: antiarrhythmics · sympathomimetics, vasoconstrictor · tropicamide

● **SIDE-EFFECTS**
▸ **Uncommon** Headache · hyperaemia · hypertension · keratitis

● **ALLERGY AND CROSS-SENSITIVITY** Contra-indicated in patients with known hypersensitivity to amide-type anaesthetics or atropine derivatives.

● **PREGNANCY** Manufacturer advises avoid (systemic uptake after administration cannot be excluded)—insufficient data available for phenylephrine and tropicamide in pregnancy; lidocaine crosses the placenta but is not known to be harmful in *animal* studies.

● **BREAST FEEDING** Manufacturer advises avoid—no data available for phenylephrine or tropicamide; lidocaine present in milk in small amount.

● **PRE-TREATMENT SCREENING** Manufacturer advises patients must have demonstrated, at a previous visit, a satisfactory pupil dilation with topical mydriatic treatment.

● **PATIENT AND CARER ADVICE**
Driving and skilled tasks Manufacturer advises patients should be counselled about the effects on driving and skilled tasks.

● **MEDICINAL FORMS** There can be variation in the licensing of different medicines containing the same drug.
Solution for injection
EXCIPIENTS: May contain Disodium edetate
▸ **Mydrane** (Thea Pharmaceuticals Ltd)
Tropicamide 200 microgram per 1 ml, Phenylephrine hydrochloride 3.1 mg per 1 ml, Lidocaine hydrochloride 10 mg per 1 ml Mydrane 0.2mg/ml / 3.1mg/ml / 10mg/ml solution for injection 0.6ml ampoules | 20 ampoule ℗ₒM £119.95 (Hospital only)

4.1 Post-operative pain and inflammation

ANAESTHETICS, LOCAL

Fluorescein with lidocaine

● **INDICATIONS AND DOSE**

Local anaesthesia
▸ TO THE EYE
▸ Adult: Apply as required

● **PRESCRIBING AND DISPENSING INFORMATION** Although multi-dose lidocaine and fluorescein eye drops commonly contain preservatives, preservative-free unit dose vials may be available.

● **MEDICINAL FORMS** There can be variation in the licensing of different medicines containing the same drug.
Eye drops
▸ Lidocaine and Fluorescein (Bausch & Lomb UK Ltd)
Fluorescein sodium 2.5 mg per 1 ml, Lidocaine hydrochloride 40 mg per 1 ml Minims lidocaine and fluorescein eye drops 0.5ml unit dose | 20 unit dose [PoM] £13.40 DT = £13.40

Oxybuprocaine hydrochloride
(Benoxinate hydrochloride)

● **INDICATIONS AND DOSE**
Local anaesthetic
▸ TO THE EYE
▸ Adult: Apply as required

● **INTERACTIONS** → Appendix 1: anaesthetics, local

● **PRESCRIBING AND DISPENSING INFORMATION** Although multi-dose oxybuprocaine eye drops commonly contain preservatives, preservative-free unit dose vials may be available.

● **MEDICINAL FORMS** There can be variation in the licensing of different medicines containing the same drug.
Eye drops
▸ Oxybuprocaine hydrochloride (Bausch & Lomb UK Ltd)
Oxybuprocaine hydrochloride 4 mg per 1 ml Minims oxybuprocaine hydrochloride 0.4% eye drops 0.5ml unit dose | 20 unit dose [PoM] £12.45 DT = £12.45

Proxymetacaine hydrochloride

● **INDICATIONS AND DOSE**
Local anaesthetic
▸ TO THE EYE
▸ Adult: Apply as required

● **INTERACTIONS** → Appendix 1: anaesthetics, local

● **PRESCRIBING AND DISPENSING INFORMATION** Although multi-dose proxymetacaine eye drops commonly contain preservatives, preservative-free unit dose vials may be available.

● **MEDICINAL FORMS** There can be variation in the licensing of different medicines containing the same drug.
Eye drops
▸ Proxymetacaine (Bausch & Lomb UK Ltd)
Proxymetacaine hydrochloride 5 mg per 1 ml Minims proxymetacaine 0.5% eye drops 0.5ml unit dose | 20 unit dose [PoM] £14.29 DT = £14.29

Tetracaine
(Amethocaine)   11-Nov-2021

● **INDICATIONS AND DOSE**
Local anaesthetic
▸ TO THE EYE
▸ Adult: Apply as required

● **INTERACTIONS** → Appendix 1: anaesthetics, local

● **SIDE-EFFECTS** Dermatitis · eye disorders · eye inflammation · paraesthesia

● **PRESCRIBING AND DISPENSING INFORMATION** Although multi-dose tetracaine eye drops commonly contain

preservatives, preservative-free unit dose vials may be available.

● **MEDICINAL FORMS** There can be variation in the licensing of different medicines containing the same drug.
Eye drops
▸ Tetracaine (Non-proprietary)
Tetracaine hydrochloride 5 mg per 1 ml Minims tetracaine hydrochloride 0.5% eye drops 0.5ml unit dose | 20 unit dose [PoM] £12.13 DT = £12.13
Tetracaine hydrochloride 10 mg per 1 ml Minims tetracaine hydrochloride 1% eye drops 0.5ml unit dose | 20 unit dose [PoM] £12.13 DT = £12.13

ANALGESICS ⟩ NON-STEROIDAL ANTI-INFLAMMATORY DRUGS

11
Eye

Bromfenac   14-Jul-2020

● **INDICATIONS AND DOSE**
Postoperative inflammation following cataract surgery
▸ TO THE EYE
▸ Adult: (consult product literature)

● **INTERACTIONS** → Appendix 1: NSAIDs

● **MEDICINAL FORMS** There can be variation in the licensing of different medicines containing the same drug.
Eye drops
EXCIPIENTS: May contain Benzalkonium chloride, disodium edetate, sulfites
▸ Yellox (Bausch & Lomb UK Ltd)
Bromfenac (as Bromfenac sodium sesquihydrate) 900 microgram per 1 ml Yellox 900micrograms/ml eye drops | 5 ml [PoM] £8.50 DT = £8.50

Diclofenac sodium   14-Jun-2024

● **INDICATIONS AND DOSE**
Inhibition of intra-operative miosis during cataract surgery (but does not possess intrinsic mydriatic properties) | Postoperative inflammation in cataract surgery, strabismus surgery or argon laser trabeculoplasty | Pain in corneal epithelial defects after photorefractive keratectomy, radial keratotomy or accidental trauma | Seasonal allergic conjunctivitis
▸ TO THE EYE
▸ Adult: (consult product literature)

● **INTERACTIONS** → Appendix 1: NSAIDs

● **SIDE-EFFECTS**
▸ **Common or very common** Oedema · skin reactions
▸ **Rare or very rare** Asthma exacerbated · eye disorders · eye inflammation · hypersensitivity
▸ **Frequency not known** Dyspnoea · eye discomfort · rhinitis · vision blurred

● **ALLERGY AND CROSS-SENSITIVITY** [EvGr] Contra-indicated in patients with a history of hypersensitivity to aspirin or any other NSAID—which includes those in whom attacks of asthma, angioedema, urticaria or rhinitis have been precipitated by aspirin or any other NSAID. Ⓜ

● **PRESCRIBING AND DISPENSING INFORMATION** Although multi-dose diclofenac sodium eye drops commonly contain preservatives, preservative-free unit dose vials may be available.

● **MEDICINAL FORMS** There can be variation in the licensing of different medicines containing the same drug.
Eye drops
EXCIPIENTS: May contain Benzalkonium chloride, disodium edetate, propylene glycol
▸ Voltarol Ophtha (Thea Pharmaceuticals Ltd)
Diclofenac sodium 1 mg per 1 ml Voltarol Ophtha 0.1% eye drops 0.3ml unit dose | 40 unit dose [PoM] £32.00 DT = £32.00

▸ **Voltarol Ophtha Multidose** (Thea Pharmaceuticals Ltd)
Diclofenac sodium 1 mg per 1 ml Voltarol Ophtha Multidose 0.1%
eye drops | 5 ml [PoM] £6.68 DT = £6.68

Flurbiprofen

01-Aug-2023

● **INDICATIONS AND DOSE**

**Inhibition of intra-operative miosis (but does not possess
intrinsic mydriatic properties) | Control of anterior
segment inflammation following postoperative and post-
laser trabeculoplasty when corticosteroids contra-
indicated**

▸ TO THE EYE
▸ Adult: (consult product literature)

● **INTERACTIONS** → Appendix 1: NSAIDs

● **SIDE-EFFECTS**
▸ **Common or very common** Eye discomfort · haemorrhage
▸ **Frequency not known** Eye disorders

● **ALLERGY AND CROSS-SENSITIVITY** [EvGr] Contra-indicated
in patients with a history of hypersensitivity to aspirin or
any other NSAID—which includes those in whom attacks
of asthma, angioedema, urticaria or rhinitis have been
precipitated by aspirin or any other NSAID. Ⓜ

● **MEDICINAL FORMS** There can be variation in the licensing of
different medicines containing the same drug.
Eye drops
▸ **Ocufen** (AbbVie Ltd)
Flurbiprofen sodium 300 microgram per 1 ml Ocufen 0.03% eye
drops 0.4ml unit dose | 40 unit dose [PoM] £37.15 DT = £37.15

Ketorolac trometamol

01-Aug-2023

● **INDICATIONS AND DOSE**

**Prophylaxis and reduction of inflammation and
associated symptoms following ocular surgery**

▸ TO THE EYE
▸ Adult: (consult product literature)

● **CAUTIONS** May mask symptoms of infection

● **INTERACTIONS** → Appendix 1: NSAIDs

● **SIDE-EFFECTS**
▸ **Common or very common** Eye discomfort · eye disorders ·
eye infection · eye inflammation · headache ·
hypersensitivity · keratic deposits · paraesthesia · retinal
haemorrhage · vision disorders
▸ **Uncommon** Dry eye
▸ **Frequency not known** Asthma exacerbated · bronchospasm

● **ALLERGY AND CROSS-SENSITIVITY** [EvGr] Contra-indicated
in patients with a history of hypersensitivity to aspirin or
any other NSAID—which includes those in whom attacks
of asthma, angioedema, urticaria or rhinitis have been
precipitated by aspirin or any other NSAID. Ⓜ

● **MEDICINAL FORMS** There can be variation in the licensing of
different medicines containing the same drug.
Eye drops
EXCIPIENTS: May contain Benzalkonium chloride, disodium edetate
▸ **Ketorolac trometamol (Non-proprietary)**
Ketorolac trometamol 5 mg per 1 ml Ketorolac 0.5% eye drops |
5 ml [PoM] £9.99 DT = £5.35
▸ **Acular** (AbbVie Ltd)
Ketorolac trometamol 5 mg per 1 ml Acular 0.5% eye drops |
5 ml [PoM] £3.00 DT = £5.35

CORTICOSTEROIDS

Loteprednol etabonate

20-Jul-2023

● **INDICATIONS AND DOSE**

**Treatment of post-operative inflammation following
ocular surgery**

▸ TO THE EYE
▸ Adult: Apply 4 times a day for maximum duration of
treatment of 14 days, to be started 24 hours after
surgery

IMPORTANT SAFETY INFORMATION

MHRA/CHM ADVICE: CORTICOSTEROIDS: RARE RISK OF CENTRAL
SEROUS CHORIORETINOPATHY WITH LOCAL AS WELL AS SYSTEMIC
ADMINISTRATION (AUGUST 2017)
See Corticosteroids, general use p. 780.

NHS IMPROVEMENT PATIENT SAFETY ALERT: STEROID
EMERGENCY CARD TO SUPPORT EARLY RECOGNITION AND
TREATMENT OF ADRENAL CRISIS IN ADULTS (AUGUST 2020)
See Adrenal insufficiency p. 781.

● **SIDE-EFFECTS**
▸ **Common or very common** Dry eye · eye discomfort · eye
disorders · headaches
▸ **Uncommon** Conjunctival oedema · vision disorders
▸ **Rare or very rare** Breast neoplasm · face oedema · muscle
twitching · taste altered

● **PATIENT AND CARER ADVICE** If systemic absorption occurs
following topical and local use, side-effects applicable to
systemic corticosteroids may apply; a patient information
leaflet should be supplied and the need for a Steroid
Treatment Card and a Steroid Emergency Card considered,
see Corticosteroids, general use p. 780.

● **MEDICINAL FORMS** There can be variation in the licensing of
different medicines containing the same drug.
Eye drops
EXCIPIENTS: May contain Benzalkonium chloride, disodium edetate
▸ **Lotemax** (Bausch & Lomb UK Ltd)
Loteprednol etabonate 5 mg per 1 ml Lotemax 0.5% eye drops |
5 ml [PoM] £5.50 DT = £5.50

CORTICOSTEROIDS › COMBINATIONS WITH ANTI-INFECTIVES

Dexamethasone with levofloxacin

16-Nov-2022

The properties listed below are those particular to the
combination only. For the properties of the components
please consider, dexamethasone p. 1323, levofloxacin
p. 1334.

● **INDICATIONS AND DOSE**

**Prophylaxis and treatment of postoperative inflammation
following cataract surgery | Prevention of infection
following cataract surgery**

▸ TO THE EYE
▸ Adult: Apply every 6 hours for 7 days

● **INTERACTIONS** → Appendix 1: corticosteroids · quinolones

● **NATIONAL FUNDING/ACCESS DECISIONS**
For full details see funding body website

Scottish Medicines Consortium (SMC) decisions
▸ Levofloxacin plus dexamethasone (*Ducressa* ®) for prevention
and treatment of inflammation, and prevention of infection
associated with cataract surgery in adults (November 2022)
SMC No. SMC2511 Recommended

● **LESS SUITABLE FOR PRESCRIBING** Dexamethasone with
levofloxacin eye drops are less suitable for prescribing.

- **MEDICINAL FORMS** There can be variation in the licensing of different medicines containing the same drug.

Eye drops

EXCIPIENTS: May contain Benzalkonium chloride

▸ **Ducressa** (Santen UK Ltd)

Dexamethasone (as Dexamethasone sodium phosphate) 1 mg per 1 ml, Levofloxacin (as Levofloxacin hemihydrate) 5 mg per 1 ml　Ducressa 1mg/ml / 5mg/ml eye drops | 5 ml [PoM] £8.30 DT = £8.30

5　Glaucoma and ocular hypertension

Glaucoma and ocular hypertension

18-Feb-2022

Description of condition

Glaucoma is a group of eye disorders characterised by a loss of visual field associated with pathological cupping of the optic disc and optic nerve damage. While glaucoma is generally linked to raised intra-ocular pressure (IOP), which is the main treatable risk factor, it can also occur when the IOP is within the normal range. Other risk factors include age, family history, ethnicity, corticosteroid use, myopia, type 2 diabetes mellitus, cardiovascular disease, and hypertension.

The most common form of glaucoma is chronic open-angle glaucoma (also known as primary open-angle glaucoma) where drainage of the aqueous humour through the trabecular meshwork is restricted, and the angle between the iris and the cornea is normal. Initially, this condition tends to be asymptomatic, however, as glaucoma progresses, patients may present with irreversible sight loss or visual field defects. Patients with ocular hypertension (an IOP greater than 21 mmHg) are at high risk of developing chronic open-angle glaucoma. The diagnosis, monitoring, and management of patients with ocular hypertension, suspected chronic open-angle glaucoma, or chronic open-angle glaucoma should be carried out by a specialist; patients with suspected optic nerve damage or repeatable visual field defect, or both, should be referred to a consultant ophthalmologist.

Acute angle-closure glaucoma is less common and occurs when the outflow of aqueous humour from the eye is totally obstructed by bowing of the iris against the trabecular meshwork. It is characterised by its abrupt onset of symptoms, and is a sight-threatening medical emergency that requires urgent reduction of IOP to prevent loss of vision.

Aims of treatment

Treatment aims to control intra-ocular pressure to prevent the development or progression of glaucoma, and subsequent visual field damage or sight loss.

Ocular hypertension

[EvGr] Patients with ocular hypertension who are not at risk of visual impairment in their lifetime do not require treatment, but they should be monitored regularly.

Patients newly diagnosed with ocular hypertension with an intra-ocular pressure (IOP) of 24 mmHg or more and who are at risk of visual impairment within their lifetime (excluding cases associated with pigment dispersion syndrome), should be offered 360° selective laser trabeculoplasty (SLT) as first-line treatment. Patients suitable for 360° SLT should be referred to and discussed with a consultant ophthalmologist regarding the decision to offer it, and how it will be performed. A second 360° SLT procedure can be considered if the effect of an initial

successful SLT has subsequently reduced over time. Patients in whom 360° SLT does not reduce intra-ocular pressure to a satisfactory level, should be referred to a consultant ophthalmologist to discuss other treatment options.

A topical prostaglandin analogue, such as latanoprost p. 1346, tafluprost p. 1347, travoprost p. 1348, or bimatoprost p. 1349 (a synthetic prostamide), is recommended as first-line pharmacological treatment in patients who require treatment but choose not to have 360° SLT or it is unsuitable, or if they are waiting for 360° SLT and need interim treatment, or have previously had 360° SLT but need additional treatment to reduce their IOP sufficiently to prevent the risk of visual impairment.

If initial treatment with a topical prostaglandin analogue is not tolerated, an alternative prostaglandin analogue should be tried before switching to a topical beta-blocker such as betaxolol p. 1342, levobunolol hydrochloride p. 1342, or timolol maleate p. 1342. If treatment is still not tolerated, alternative options include carbonic anhydrase inhibitors such as brinzolamide p. 1344 or dorzolamide p. 1345, a topical sympathomimetic such as apraclonidine p. 1350 [unlicensed use] or brimonidine tartrate p. 1350, or a topical miotic such as pilocarpine p. 1346 [unlicensed use], given either as monotherapy or as combination therapy.

Alternative options as either monotherapy or combination therapy with drugs from different therapeutic classes (topical beta-blockers, carbonic anhydrase inhibitors, or topical sympathomimetics), should also be offered to patients with an IOP of 24 mmHg or more whose current treatment is not reducing IOP sufficiently to prevent the risk of progression to sight loss. The patient's adherence and drop instillation technique should also be checked. If drug treatment still does not reduce their IOP to a satisfactory level, patients should be referred to a consultant ophthalmologist to discuss other treatment options.

Preservative free eye drops should be used in patients who are allergic to preservatives, or in those who have clinically significant ocular surface disease and are at high risk of conversion to chronic open-angle glaucoma. Ⓐ

Note: based on cost-effective analysis, NICE guideline 81 *recommends generic prostaglandin analogues as first-line pharmacological treatment, and non-generic prostaglandin analogues as third-line pharmacological treatment if topical beta-blocker treatment is ineffective.*

Suspected chronic open-angle glaucoma

[EvGr] Patients with suspected chronic open-angle glaucoma and an intra-ocular pressure (IOP) below 24 mmHg do not require drug treatment unless they are at risk of visual impairment within their lifetime, but they should be regularly monitored for changes in IOP and visual impairment. Ⓐ

Chronic open-angle glaucoma

[EvGr] Patients with newly diagnosed chronic open-angle glaucoma (excluding cases associated with pigment dispersion syndrome), should be offered 360° selective laser trabeculoplasty (SLT) as first-line treatment. Patients suitable for 360° SLT should be referred to and discussed with a consultant ophthalmologist regarding the decision to offer it, and how it will be performed. A second 360° SLT procedure can be considered if the effect of an initial successful SLT has subsequently reduced over time.

Topical prostaglandin analogues such as latanoprost p. 1346, tafluprost p. 1347, travoprost p. 1348, or bimatoprost p. 1349 (a synthetic prostamide), are recommended as first-line pharmacological treatment options for patients who choose not to have 360° SLT or it is unsuitable, or if they are waiting for 360° SLT and need interim treatment, or have previously had 360° SLT but need additional treatment to reduce their intra-ocular pressure (IOP) sufficiently to prevent the risk of visual impairment.

If a topical prostaglandin analogue does not sufficiently reduce IOP and the patient's adherence to treatment and eye drop instillation technique are both satisfactory, treatment with either a topical beta-blocker such as betaxolol below, levobunolol hydrochloride below, or timolol maleate below, a carbonic anhydrase inhibitor such as brinzolamide p. 1344 or dorzolamide p. 1345, a topical sympathomimetic such as apraclonidine p. 1350 or brimonidine tartrate p. 1350, or a combination of these, should be offered. When a particular drug is not tolerated, another drug from a different therapeutic class can be tried. Preservative free eye drops should be used in patients who are allergic to preservatives, or those who have clinically significant ocular surface disease. Alternative treatment options are 360° SLT or glaucoma surgery with pharmacological augmentation (with mitomycin p. 1054 [unlicensed use]).

Patients with *advanced chronic open-angle glaucoma* should be offered glaucoma surgery with pharmacological augmentation (with mitomycin p. 1054 [unlicensed use]). Treatment with a topical prostaglandin analogue should be initiated and continued until surgery takes place.

If glaucoma surgery fails to adequately reduce the IOP in patients with chronic open-angle glaucoma, alternative options include pharmacological treatment (a combination of topical drugs from different therapeutic classes may be needed), further surgery, 360° SLT, or cyclodiode laser treatment.

Pharmacological treatment, 360° SLT, or cyclodiode laser treatment may also be offered to patients with chronic open-angle glaucoma (including advanced chronic open-angle glaucoma) who prefer not to have glaucoma surgery, or for whom surgery is unsuitable. Ⓐ

Useful Resources

Glaucoma: diagnosis and management. National Institute for Health and Care Excellence. NICE guideline 81. January 2022.
www.nice.org.uk/guidance/ng81

BETA-ADRENOCEPTOR BLOCKERS

Betaxolol

03-Apr-2020

● **INDICATIONS AND DOSE**

Chronic open-angle glaucoma | Ocular hypertension
▸ TO THE EYE
▸ Adult: Apply twice daily

● **CONTRA-INDICATIONS** Also consider contra-indications listed for systemically administered beta blockers · bradycardia · heart block
● **CAUTIONS** Patients with corneal disease
  CAUTIONS, FURTHER INFORMATION Systemic absorption can follow topical application to the eyes; consider cautions listed for systemically administered beta blockers.
● **INTERACTIONS** → Appendix 1: beta blockers, selective
● **SIDE-EFFECTS**
▸ **Common or very common** Eye discomfort · eye disorders · vision disorders
▸ **Uncommon** Dry eye · eye inflammation · rhinitis
▸ **Rare or very rare** Cataract · rhinorrhoea · skin reactions
▸ **Frequency not known** Angioedema · hypersensitivity
  SIDE-EFFECTS, FURTHER INFORMATION Systemic absorption can follow topical application to the eyes; consider side effects listed for systemically administered beta blockers.
● **PRESCRIBING AND DISPENSING INFORMATION** Although multi-dose bextaxolol eye drops commonly contain preservatives, preservative-free unit dose vials may be available.

● **MEDICINAL FORMS** There can be variation in the licensing of different medicines containing the same drug.
Eye drops
EXCIPIENTS: May contain Benzalkonium chloride, disodium edetate
▸ **Betaxolol (Non-proprietary)**
  Betaxolol (as Betaxolol hydrochloride) 5 mg per 1 ml Betaxolol 0.5% eye drops | 5 ml [PoM] Ⓢ DT = £1.90
▸ **Betoptic** (Immedica Pharma AB)
  Betaxolol (as Betaxolol hydrochloride) 2.5 mg per 1 ml Betoptic 0.25% suspension eye drops | 5 ml [PoM] £2.66 DT = £2.66
  Betoptic 0.25% eye drops suspension 0.25ml unit dose | 50 unit dose [PoM] £13.77 DT = £13.77
  Betaxolol (as Betaxolol hydrochloride) 5 mg per 1 ml Betoptic 0.5% eye drops | 5 ml [PoM] £1.90 DT = £1.90

Levobunolol hydrochloride

03-Apr-2020

● **INDICATIONS AND DOSE**

Chronic open-angle glaucoma | Ocular hypertension
▸ TO THE EYE
▸ Adult: Apply 1–2 times a day

● **CONTRA-INDICATIONS** Also consider contra-indications listed for systemically administered beta blockers · bradycardia · heart block
● **CAUTIONS** Patients with corneal disease
  CAUTIONS, FURTHER INFORMATION Systemic absorption can follow topical application to the eyes; consider cautions listed for systemically administered beta blockers.
● **INTERACTIONS** → Appendix 1: beta blockers, non-selective
● **SIDE-EFFECTS**
▸ **Common or very common** Eye discomfort · eye inflammation
▸ **Frequency not known** Dry eye · eye disorders · eyelid eczema · vision blurred
  SIDE-EFFECTS, FURTHER INFORMATION Systemic absorption can follow topical application to the eyes; consider side effects listed for systemically administered beta blockers.
● **PRESCRIBING AND DISPENSING INFORMATION** Although multi-dose levobunolol eye drops commonly contain preservatives, preservative-free unit dose vials may be available.

● **MEDICINAL FORMS** There can be variation in the licensing of different medicines containing the same drug.
Eye drops
EXCIPIENTS: May contain Disodium edetate
▸ **Betagan** (AbbVie Ltd)
  Levobunolol hydrochloride 5 mg per 1 ml Betagan Unit Dose 0.5% eye drops 0.4ml unit dose | 30 unit dose [PoM] £9.98 DT = £9.98

⚑ 175

Timolol maleate

05-May-2021

● **INDICATIONS AND DOSE**

Chronic open-angle glaucoma | Ocular hypertension
▸ TO THE EYE
▸ Adult: Apply twice daily

TIMOPTOL-LA ®

Reduction of intra-ocular pressure in primary open-angle glaucoma
▸ TO THE EYE
▸ Adult: Apply once daily

TIOPEX ®

Reduction of intra-ocular pressure in primary open-angle glaucoma
▸ TO THE EYE
▸ Adult: Apply once daily, to be applied in the morning

- **CONTRA-INDICATIONS** Also consider contra-indications listed for systemically administered beta blockers · bradycardia · heart block
- **CAUTIONS** Consider also cautions listed for systemically administered beta blockers · patients with corneal disease
- **INTERACTIONS** → Appendix 1: beta blockers, non-selective
- **SIDE-EFFECTS**
  ▶ **Common or very common** Eye discomfort · eye disorders · eye inflammation · vision disorders

  SIDE-EFFECTS, FURTHER INFORMATION Systemic absorption can follow topical application to the eyes; consider side-effects listed for systemically administered beta blockers.
- **BREAST FEEDING** Manufacturer advises avoidance.
- **PRESCRIBING AND DISPENSING INFORMATION** Although multi-dose timolol eye drops commonly contain preservatives, preservative-free unit dose vials may be available.
- **NATIONAL FUNDING/ACCESS DECISIONS**

  TIOPEX ® For full details see funding body website

  Scottish Medicines Consortium (SMC) decisions
  ▶ Timolol eye gel (*Tiopex*®) for the reduction of the elevated intra-ocular pressure in patients with ocular hypertension or chronic open angle glaucoma.(February 2014) SMC No. 941/14 Recommended with restrictions

- **MEDICINAL FORMS** There can be variation in the licensing of different medicines containing the same drug.

  Eye gel
  EXCIPIENTS: May contain Benzododecinium bromide
  ▶ Timoptol-LA (Santen UK Ltd)
    Timolol (as Timolol maleate) 2.5 mg per 1 ml Timoptol-LA 0.25% ophthalmic gel-forming solution | 2.5 ml PoM £3.12 DT = £3.12
    Timolol (as Timolol maleate) 5 mg per 1 ml Timoptol-LA 0.5% ophthalmic gel-forming solution | 2.5 ml PoM £3.12 DT = £3.12

  Eye drops
  EXCIPIENTS: May contain Benzalkonium chloride
  ▶ Timolol maleate (Non-proprietary)
    Timolol (as Timolol maleate) 2.5 mg per 1 ml Timolol 0.25% eye drops | 5 ml PoM £4.60 DT = £2.46
    Timolol (as Timolol maleate) 5 mg per 1 ml Timolol 0.5% eye drops | 5 ml PoM £5.60 DT = £1.88
  ▶ Eysano (Aspire Pharma Ltd)
    Timolol (as Timolol maleate) 2.5 mg per 1 ml Eysano 2.5mg/ml eye drops | 5 ml PoM £8.45 DT = £8.45
    Timolol (as Timolol maleate) 5 mg per 1 ml Eysano 5mg/ml eye drops | 5 ml PoM £9.65 DT = £9.65
  ▶ Timoptol (Santen UK Ltd)
    Timolol (as Timolol maleate) 2.5 mg per 1 ml Timoptol 0.25% eye drops | 5 ml PoM £3.12 DT = £2.46
    Timolol (as Timolol maleate) 5 mg per 1 ml Timoptol 0.5% eye drops | 5 ml PoM £3.12 DT = £1.88
  ▶ Tiopex (Thea Pharmaceuticals Ltd)
    Timolol (as Timolol maleate) 1 mg per 1 gram Tiopex 1mg/g eye gel 0.4g unit dose | 30 unit dose PoM £7.49 DT = £7.49

  Combinations available: *Bimatoprost with timolol*, p. 1349 · *Brimonidine with timolol*, p. 1351 · *Brinzolamide with timolol*, p. 1344 · *Dorzolamide with timolol*, p. 1345 · *Latanoprost with timolol*, p. 1347 · *Tafluprost with timolol*, p. 1348 · *Travoprost with timolol*, p. 1349

CARBONIC ANHYDRASE INHIBITORS

Acetazolamide
05-Feb-2021

- **INDICATIONS AND DOSE**

Reduction of intra-ocular pressure in open-angle glaucoma | Reduction of intra-ocular pressure in secondary glaucoma | Reduction of intra-ocular pressure perioperatively in angle-closure glaucoma
  ▶ BY MOUTH USING IMMEDIATE-RELEASE MEDICINES, OR BY INTRAVENOUS INJECTION, OR BY INTRAMUSCULAR INJECTION
  ▶ Adult: 0.25–1 g daily in divided doses, intramuscular injection preferably avoided because of alkalinity

Glaucoma
  ▶ BY MOUTH USING MODIFIED-RELEASE MEDICINES
  ▶ Adult: 250–500 mg daily

Epilepsy
  ▶ BY MOUTH USING IMMEDIATE-RELEASE MEDICINES, OR BY INTRAVENOUS INJECTION, OR BY INTRAMUSCULAR INJECTION
  ▶ Adult: 0.25–1 g daily in divided doses, intramuscular injection preferably avoided because of alkalinity

---

IMPORTANT SAFETY INFORMATION

MHRA/CHM ADVICE: ANTIEPILEPTICS: RISK OF SUICIDAL THOUGHTS AND BEHAVIOUR (AUGUST 2008)
See Epilepsy p. 349.

MHRA/CHM ADVICE: ANTIEPILEPTIC DRUGS: UPDATED ADVICE ON SWITCHING BETWEEN DIFFERENT MANUFACTURERS' PRODUCTS (NOVEMBER 2017)
See Epilepsy p. 349.

MHRA/CHM ADVICE: ANTIEPILEPTIC DRUGS IN PREGNANCY: UPDATED ADVICE FOLLOWING COMPREHENSIVE SAFETY REVIEW (JANUARY 2021)
See Epilepsy p. 349.

- **CONTRA-INDICATIONS** Adrenocortical insufficiency · hyperchloraemic acidosis · hypokalaemia · hyponatraemia · long-term administration in chronic angle-closure glaucoma
- **CAUTIONS** Avoid extravasation at injection site (risk of necrosis) · diabetes mellitus · elderly · impaired alveolar ventilation (risk of acidosis) · long-term use · pulmonary obstruction (risk of acidosis) · renal calculi
- **INTERACTIONS** → Appendix 1: acetazolamide
- **SIDE-EFFECTS**

  GENERAL SIDE-EFFECTS
  ▶ **Common or very common** Haemorrhage · metabolic acidosis · nephrolithiasis · sensation abnormal
  ▶ **Uncommon** Bone marrow disorders · depression · dizziness · electrolyte imbalance · hearing impairment · hepatic disorders · leucopenia · nausea · renal colic · renal impairment · renal lesions · severe cutaneous adverse reactions (SCARs) · skin reactions · thrombocytopenia · tinnitus · urinary tract discomfort · urine abnormalities · vomiting
  ▶ **Rare or very rare** Anaphylactic reaction · appetite disorder · confusion · diarrhoea · fatigue · fever · flushing · headache · irritability · libido decreased · paralysis · photosensitivity reaction · seizure
  ▶ **Frequency not known** Agranulocytosis · drowsiness · myopia · polyuria · suicidal behaviours · taste altered · thirst

  SPECIFIC SIDE-EFFECTS
  ▶ **Uncommon**
  ▶ With oral use Osteomalacia
  ▶ **Rare or very rare**
  ▶ With oral use Ataxia · hyperglycaemia · hypoglycaemia · renal tubular necrosis
  ▶ **Frequency not known**
  ▶ With oral use Agitation

11

Eye

SIDE-EFFECTS, FURTHER INFORMATION Acetazolamide is a sulfonamide derivative; blood disorders, rashes, and other sulfonamide-related side-effects occur occasionally — patients should be told to report any unusual skin rash.

If electrolyte disturbances and metabolic acidosis occur, these can be corrected by administering bicarbonate.

- **ALLERGY AND CROSS-SENSITIVITY** [EvGr] Contra-indicated if history of sulfonamide hypersensitivity. [M]
- **PREGNANCY** Manufacturer advises avoid, especially in first trimester (toxicity in *animal* studies). See also *Pregnancy* in Epilepsy p. 349.
- **BREAST FEEDING** Amount too small to be harmful.
- **HEPATIC IMPAIRMENT** Manufacturer advises avoid.
- **RENAL IMPAIRMENT** Avoid—risk of metabolic acidosis.
- **MONITORING REQUIREMENTS** Monitor blood count and plasma electrolyte concentrations with prolonged use.

- **MEDICINAL FORMS** There can be variation in the licensing of different medicines containing the same drug. Forms available from special-order manufacturers include: oral suspension, oral solution

Oral tablet
CAUTIONARY AND ADVISORY LABELS 3
▶ **Acetazolamide (Non-proprietary)**
  Acetazolamide 250 mg Acetazolamide 250mg tablets | 112 tablet [PoM] £75.40 DT = £5.18

Powder for solution for injection
▶ **Diamox** (Advanz Pharma)
  Acetazolamide 500 mg Diamox Sodium Parenteral 500mg powder for solution for injection vials | 1 vial [PoM] £14.76

Brinzolamide
23-Jul-2021

- **INDICATIONS AND DOSE**

  Reduction of intra-ocular pressure in ocular hypertension and open-angle glaucoma either as adjunct to beta-blockers or prostaglandin analogues or used alone in patients unresponsive to beta-blockers or if beta-blockers contra-indicated
  ▶ TO THE EYE
  ▶ Adult: Apply twice daily, then increased if necessary up to 3 times a day

- **CONTRA-INDICATIONS** Hyperchloraemic acidosis
- **CAUTIONS** Renal tubular immaturity or abnormality—risk of metabolic acidosis · systemic absorption follows topical application
- **INTERACTIONS** → Appendix 1: brinzolamide
- **SIDE-EFFECTS**
  ▶ **Common or very common** Eye discomfort · eye disorders · taste altered · vision disorders
  ▶ **Uncommon** Arrhythmias · asthenia · cardio-respiratory distress · chest discomfort · cough · depression · diarrhoea · dizziness · dry eye · dry mouth · dyspnoea · epistaxis · eye deposit · eye inflammation · feeling abnormal · foreign body in eye · gastrointestinal discomfort · gastrointestinal disorders · headache · increased risk of infection · memory impairment · motor dysfunction · muscle complaints · nasal complaints · nausea · nervousness · oral disorders · oropharyngeal pain · pain · palpitations · renal pain · scleral discolouration · sensation abnormal · sexual dysfunction · skin reactions · sleep disorders · throat complaints · vomiting
  ▶ **Rare or very rare** Alopecia · angina pectoris · drowsiness · irritability · respiratory disorders · tinnitus
  ▶ **Frequency not known** Appetite decreased · arthralgia · asthma · hypertension · malaise · peripheral oedema · severe cutaneous adverse reactions (SCARs) · tremor · urinary frequency increased · vertigo

SIDE-EFFECTS, FURTHER INFORMATION Systemic absorption can rarely cause sulfonamide-like side-effects and may require discontinuation if severe.

- **ALLERGY AND CROSS-SENSITIVITY** [EvGr] Contra-indicated if history of sulfonamide hypersensitivity. [M]
- **PREGNANCY** Avoid—toxicity in *animal* studies.
- **BREAST FEEDING** Use only if benefit outweighs risk.
- **HEPATIC IMPAIRMENT** Manufacturer advises avoid—no information available.
- **RENAL IMPAIRMENT** [EvGr] Avoid if creatinine clearance less than 30 mL/minute (no information available). [M] See p. 21.

- **MEDICINAL FORMS** There can be variation in the licensing of different medicines containing the same drug.
Eye drops
EXCIPIENTS: May contain Benzalkonium chloride, disodium edetate
▶ **Brinzolamide (Non-proprietary)**
  Brinzolamide 10 mg per 1 ml Brinzolamide 10mg/ml eye drops | 5 ml [PoM] £6.92 DT = £4.29
▶ **Azopt** (Novartis Pharmaceuticals UK Ltd)
  Brinzolamide 10 mg per 1 ml Azopt 10mg/ml eye drops | 5 ml [PoM] £6.92 DT = £4.29

Brinzolamide with brimonidine
11-May-2020

The properties listed below are those particular to the combination only. For the properties of the components please consider, brinzolamide above, brimonidine tartrate p. 1350.

- **INDICATIONS AND DOSE**

  Raised intra-ocular pressure in open-angle glaucoma and in ocular hypertension when monotherapy is inadequate
  ▶ TO THE EYE
  ▶ Adult: Apply 1 drop twice daily

- **INTERACTIONS** → Appendix 1: brimonidine · brinzolamide

- **MEDICINAL FORMS** There can be variation in the licensing of different medicines containing the same drug.
Eye drops
CAUTIONARY AND ADVISORY LABELS 3
EXCIPIENTS: May contain Benzalkonium chloride, propylene glycol
▶ **Brinzolamide with brimonidine (Non-proprietary)**
  Brimonidine tartrate 2 mg per 1 ml, Brinzolamide 10 mg per 1 ml Brinzolamide 10mg/ml / Brimonidine 2mg/ml eye drops | 5 ml [PoM] [℞] DT = £9.23
▶ **Simbrinza** (Novartis Pharmaceuticals UK Ltd)
  Brimonidine tartrate 2 mg per 1 ml, Brinzolamide 10 mg per 1 ml Simbrinza 10mg/ml / 2mg/ml eye drops | 5 ml [PoM] £9.23 DT = £9.23

Brinzolamide with timolol
11-May-2020

The properties listed below are those particular to the combination only. For the properties of the components please consider, brinzolamide above, timolol maleate p. 1342.

- **INDICATIONS AND DOSE**

  Raised intra-ocular pressure in open-angle glaucoma or ocular hypertension when beta-blocker alone not adequate
  ▶ TO THE EYE
  ▶ Adult: Apply twice daily

- **INTERACTIONS** → Appendix 1: beta blockers, non-selective · brinzolamide

- **MEDICINAL FORMS** There can be variation in the licensing of different medicines containing the same drug.
  Eye drops
  EXCIPIENTS: May contain Benzalkonium chloride, disodium edetate
  ► **Brinzolamide with timolol** (Non-proprietary)
    Timolol (as Timolol maleate) 5 mg per 1 ml, Brinzolamide 10 mg per 1 ml Brinzolamide 10mg/ml / Timolol 5mg/ml eye drops | 5 ml PoM £11.40 DT = £7.46
  ► **Azarga** (Novartis Pharmaceuticals UK Ltd)
    Timolol (as Timolol maleate) 5 mg per 1 ml, Brinzolamide 10 mg per 1 ml Azarga 10mg/ml / 5mg/ml eye drops | 5 ml PoM £11.05 DT = £7.46

Dorzolamide
29-Jul-2021

- **INDICATIONS AND DOSE**

Raised intra-ocular pressure in ocular hypertension used alone in patients unresponsive to beta-blockers or if beta-blockers contra-indicated | Open-angle glaucoma used alone in patients unresponsive to beta-blockers or if beta-blockers contra-indicated | Pseudo-exfoliative glaucoma used alone in patients unresponsive to beta-blockers or if beta-blockers contra-indicated
  ► TO THE EYE
  ► Adult: Apply 3 times a day

Raised intra-ocular pressure in ocular hypertension as adjunct to beta-blocker | Open-angle glaucoma as adjunct to beta-blocker | Pseudo-exfoliative glaucoma as adjunct to beta-blocker
  ► TO THE EYE
  ► Adult: Apply twice daily

- **CONTRA-INDICATIONS** Hyperchloraemic acidosis
- **CAUTIONS** Chronic corneal defects · history of intra-ocular surgery · history of renal calculi · low endothelial cell count · systemic absorption follows topical application
- **INTERACTIONS** → Appendix 1: dorzolamide
- **SIDE-EFFECTS**
  ► **Common or very common** Asthenia · eye discomfort · eye disorders · eye inflammation · headache · nausea · taste bitter · vision disorders
  ► **Rare or very rare** Angioedema · bronchospasm · dizziness · dry mouth · dyspnoea · epistaxis · local reaction · paraesthesia · severe cutaneous adverse reactions (SCARs) · skin reactions · throat irritation · urolithiasis
  ► **Frequency not known** Hypertension · palpitations · tachycardia

  SIDE-EFFECTS, FURTHER INFORMATION Systemic absorption can cause sulfonamide-like side-effects and may require discontinuation if severe.

- **ALLERGY AND CROSS-SENSITIVITY** EvGr Caution in patients with hypersensitivity to sulfonamides (systemic absorption occurs). ⟨M⟩
- **PREGNANCY** Manufacturer advises avoid—toxicity in *animal* studies.
- **BREAST FEEDING** Manufacturer advises avoid—no information available.
- **HEPATIC IMPAIRMENT** Manufacturer advises caution—no information available.
- **RENAL IMPAIRMENT** EvGr Avoid if creatinine clearance less than 30 mL/minute. ⟨M⟩ See p. 21.
- **PRESCRIBING AND DISPENSING INFORMATION** Although multi-dose dorzolamide eye drops commonly contain preservatives, preservative-free unit dose vials may be available.

- **MEDICINAL FORMS** There can be variation in the licensing of different medicines containing the same drug.
  Eye drops
  EXCIPIENTS: May contain Benzalkonium chloride
  ► **Dorzolamide** (Non-proprietary)
    Dorzolamide (as Dorzolamide hydrochloride) 20 mg per 1 ml Dorzolamide 20mg/ml eye drops | 5 ml PoM £6.30 DT = £3.37
  ► **Dimaz** (Scope Ophthalmics Ltd)
    Dorzolamide (as Dorzolamide hydrochloride) 20 mg per 1 ml Dimaz 20mg/ml eye drops | 5 ml PoM £6.98 DT = £7.08
  ► **Eydelto** (Aspire Pharma Ltd)
    Dorzolamide (as Dorzolamide hydrochloride) 20 mg per 1 ml Eydelto 20mg/ml eye drops | 5 ml PoM £7.08 DT = £7.08
  ► **Trusopt** (Santen UK Ltd)
    Dorzolamide (as Dorzolamide hydrochloride) 20 mg per 1 ml Trusopt 20mg/ml eye drops 0.2ml unit dose preservative free | 60 unit dose PoM £24.18 DT = £24.18
    Trusopt 20mg/ml eye drops | 5 ml PoM £6.33 DT = £3.37
  ► **Vizidor** (Bausch & Lomb UK Ltd)
    Dorzolamide (as Dorzolamide hydrochloride) 20 mg per 1 ml Vizidor 20mg/ml eye drops | 5 ml PoM £7.09 DT = £7.08

Dorzolamide with timolol

The properties listed below are those particular to the combination only. For the properties of the components please consider, dorzolamide above, timolol maleate p. 1342.

- **INDICATIONS AND DOSE**

Raised intra-ocular pressure in ocular hypertension when beta-blockers alone not adequate | Raised intra-ocular pressure in open-angle glaucoma when beta-blockers alone not adequate | Raised intra-ocular pressure in pseudo-exfoliative glaucoma when beta-blockers alone not adequate
  ► TO THE EYE
  ► Adult: Apply twice daily

- **INTERACTIONS** → Appendix 1: beta blockers, non-selective · dorzolamide
- **PRESCRIBING AND DISPENSING INFORMATION** Although multi-dose dorzolamide with timolol eye drops commonly contain preservatives, preservative-free unit dose vials may be available.

- **MEDICINAL FORMS** There can be variation in the licensing of different medicines containing the same drug.
  Eye drops
  EXCIPIENTS: May contain Benzalkonium chloride
  ► **Dorzolamide with timolol** (Non-proprietary)
    Timolol (as Timolol maleate) 5 mg per 1 ml, Dorzolamide (as Dorzolamide hydrochloride) 20 mg per 1 ml Dorzolamide 20mg/ml / Timolol 5mg/ml eye drops 0.2ml unit dose preservative free | 60 unit dose PoM £34.00 DT = £28.59
    Dorzolamide 20mg/ml / Timolol 5mg/ml eye drops | 5 ml PoM £27.16 DT = £9.85
  ► **Codimaz** (Scope Ophthalmics Ltd)
    Timolol (as Timolol maleate) 5 mg per 1 ml, Dorzolamide (as Dorzolamide hydrochloride) 20 mg per 1 ml Codimaz 20mg/ml / 5mg/ml eye drops | 5 ml PoM £8.03 DT = £8.13
  ► **Cosopt** (Santen UK Ltd)
    Timolol (as Timolol maleate) 5 mg per 1 ml, Dorzolamide (as Dorzolamide hydrochloride) 20 mg per 1 ml Cosopt 20mg/ml / 5mg/ml eye drops 0.2ml unit dose preservative free | 60 unit dose PoM £28.59 DT = £28.59
    Cosopt 20mg/ml / 5mg/ml eye drops | 5 ml PoM £10.05 DT = £9.85
  ► **Cosopt iMulti** (Santen UK Ltd)
    Timolol (as Timolol maleate) 5 mg per 1 ml, Dorzolamide (as Dorzolamide hydrochloride) 20 mg per 1 ml Cosopt iMulti 20mg/ml / 5mg/ml eye drops preservative free | 10 ml PoM £28.00
  ► **Eylamdo** (Aspire Pharma Ltd)
    Timolol (as Timolol maleate) 5 mg per 1 ml, Dorzolamide (as Dorzolamide hydrochloride) 20 mg per 1 ml Eylamdo 20mg/ml / 5mg/ml eye drops | 5 ml PoM £8.13 DT = £8.13

▶ **Glaucopt** (Visufarma UK Ltd)
Timolol (as Timolol maleate) 5 mg per 1 ml, Dorzolamide (as Dorzolamide hydrochloride) 20 mg per 1 ml Glaucopt 20mg/ml / 5mg/ml eye drops 0.166ml unit dose preservative free | 60 unit dose PoM £21.44 DT = £21.44

▶ **Vizidor Duo** (Bausch & Lomb UK Ltd)
Timolol (as Timolol maleate) 5 mg per 1 ml, Dorzolamide (as Dorzolamide hydrochloride) 20 mg per 1 ml Vizidor Duo 20mg/ml / 5mg/ml eye drops | 5 ml PoM £8.14 DT = £8.13

MIOTICS > PARASYMPATHOMIMETICS

Pilocarpine
11-May-2021

● **DRUG ACTION** Pilocarpine acts by opening the inefficient drainage channels in the trabecular meshwork.

● **INDICATIONS AND DOSE**

Primary angle-closure glaucoma | Some secondary glaucomas
▶ TO THE EYE
▶ Adult: Apply up to 4 times a day

● **CONTRA-INDICATIONS** Acute iritis · anterior uveitis · conditions where pupillary constriction is undesirable · some forms of secondary glaucoma (where pupillary constriction is undesirable)

● **CAUTIONS** A darkly pigmented iris may require a higher concentration of the miotic or more frequent administration and care should be taken to avoid overdosage · asthma · cardiac disease · care in conjunctival damage · care in corneal damage · epilepsy · gastro-intestinal spasm · hypertension · hyperthyroidism · hypotension · marked vasomotor instability · Parkinson's disease · peptic ulceration · retinal detachment has occurred in susceptible individuals and those with retinal disease · urinary-tract obstruction

● **INTERACTIONS** → Appendix 1: pilocarpine

● **SIDE-EFFECTS**
▶ **Common or very common** Diarrhoea · headache · hyperhidrosis · hypersalivation · nausea · skin reactions · vision disorders · vomiting
▶ **Frequency not known** Bradycardia · bronchospasm · conjunctival vascular congestion · eye disorder (long term use) · eye disorders · hypotension · lens changes (long term use) · pain · paraesthesia · pulmonary oedema · sensitisation · vitreous haemorrhage

● **PREGNANCY** Avoid unless the potential benefit outweighs risk—limited information available.

● **BREAST FEEDING** Avoid unless the potential benefit outweighs risk—no information available.

● **PRE-TREATMENT SCREENING** Fundus examination is advised before starting treatment with a miotic (retinal detachment has occurred).

● **MONITORING REQUIREMENTS** Intra-ocular pressure and visual fields should be monitored in those with chronic simple glaucoma and those receiving long-term treatment with a miotic.

● **PRESCRIBING AND DISPENSING INFORMATION** Although multi-dose pilocarpine eye drops commonly contain preservatives, preservative-free unit dose vials may be available.

● **PATIENT AND CARER ADVICE**
Driving and skilled tasks Blurred vision may affect performance of skilled tasks (e.g. driving) particularly at night or in reduced lighting.

● **MEDICINAL FORMS** There can be variation in the licensing of different medicines containing the same drug. Forms available from special-order manufacturers include: eye drops
Eye drops
EXCIPIENTS: May contain Benzalkonium chloride
▶ **Pilocarpine (Non-proprietary)**
Pilocarpine hydrochloride 10 mg per 1 ml Pilocarpine hydrochloride 1% eye drops | 10 ml PoM £26.75 DT = £26.75
Pilocarpine hydrochloride 20 mg per 1 ml Pilocarpine hydrochloride 2% eye drops | 10 ml PoM £57.01 DT = £57.01
Pilocarpine hydrochloride 40 mg per 1 ml Pilocarpine hydrochloride 4% eye drops | 10 ml PoM £34.21 DT = £34.21
▶ **Pilocarpine nitrate** (Bausch & Lomb UK Ltd)
Pilocarpine nitrate 20 mg per 1 ml Minims pilocarpine nitrate 2% eye drops 0.5ml unit dose | 20 unit dose PoM £14.29 DT = £14.29

PROSTAGLANDINS AND ANALOGUES

Latanoprost
16-Nov-2020

● **INDICATIONS AND DOSE**

Raised intra-ocular pressure in open-angle glaucoma | Ocular hypertension
▶ TO THE EYE
▶ Adult: Apply once daily, to be administered preferably in the evening

IMPORTANT SAFETY INFORMATION

MHRA/CHM ADVICE: LATANOPROST (*XALATAN*®): INCREASED REPORTING OF EYE IRRITATION SINCE REFORMULATION (JULY 2015)
Following reformulation of *Xalatan*®, to allow for long-term storage at room temperature, there has been an increase in the number of reports of eye irritation from across the EU. Patients should be advised to tell their health professional promptly (within a week) if they experience eye irritation (e.g. excessive watering) severe enough to make them consider stopping treatment. Review treatment and prescribe a different formulation if necessary.

● **CONTRA-INDICATIONS** Active herpes simplex keratitis · history of recurrent herpetic keratitis associated with prostaglandin analogues

● **CAUTIONS** Angle-closure glaucoma · aphakia · asthma · contact lens wearers · do not use within 5 minutes of thiomersal-containing preparations · history of significant ocular viral infections · inflammatory ocular conditions (no experience of use) · narrow-angle glaucoma (no experience of use) · neovascular glaucoma (no experience of use) · peri-operative period of cataract surgery · pseudophakia with torn posterior lens capsule or anterior chamber lenses · risk factors for cystoid macular oedema · risk factors for iritis · risk factors for uveitis

● **SIDE-EFFECTS**
▶ **Common or very common** Eye discolouration · eye discomfort · eye disorders · eye inflammation · vision disorders
▶ **Uncommon** Dry eye · rash
▶ **Rare or very rare** Asthma · chest pain · dyspnoea · unstable angina
▶ **Frequency not known** Arthralgia · dizziness · headache · myalgia · ophthalmic herpes simplex · palpitations

● **PREGNANCY** Manufacturer advises avoid.

● **BREAST FEEDING** May be present in milk—manufacturer advises avoid.

● **PRESCRIBING AND DISPENSING INFORMATION** Although multi-dose latanoprost eye drops commonly contain preservatives, preservative-free unit dose vials may be available.

- **PATIENT AND CARER ADVICE**
  Changes in eye colour Before initiating treatment, patients should be warned of a possible change in eye colour as an increase in the brown pigment in the iris can occur, which may be permanent; particular care is required in those with mixed coloured irides and those receiving treatment to one eye only. Changes in eyelashes and vellus hair can also occur, and patients should also be advised to avoid repeated contact of the eye drop solution with skin as this can lead to hair growth or skin pigmentation.

- **NATIONAL FUNDING/ACCESS DECISIONS**
  MONOPOST ® For full details see funding body website
  Scottish Medicines Consortium (SMC) decisions
  ▸ Latanoprost (*Monopost*®) for the reduction of elevated intraocular pressure in patients with open-angle glaucoma and ocular hypertension (July 2013) SMC No. 879/13 Recommended with restrictions

- **MEDICINAL FORMS** There can be variation in the licensing of different medicines containing the same drug.
  Eye drops
  EXCIPIENTS: May contain Benzalkonium chloride
  ▸ Latanoprost (Non-proprietary)
  Latanoprost 50 microgram per 1 ml Latanoprost 50micrograms/ml eye drops | 2.5 ml PoM £12.48 DT = £1.39
  Catiolanze 50micrograms/ml eye drops emulsion 0.3ml unit dose | 30 unit dose PoM £7.99
  ▸ Lotacryn (Scope Ophthalmics Ltd)
  Latanoprost 50 microgram per 1 ml Lotacryn 50micrograms/ml eye drops | 2.5 ml PoM £7.99 DT = £7.99
  ▸ Monopost (Thea Pharmaceuticals Ltd)
  Latanoprost 50 microgram per 1 ml Monopost 50micrograms/ml eye drops 0.2ml unit dose | 30 unit dose PoM £8.49 DT = £8.49 | 90 unit dose PoM £25.47 DT = £25.47
  ▸ Xalatan (Viatris UK Healthcare Ltd)
  Latanoprost 50 microgram per 1 ml Xalatan 50micrograms/ml eye drops | 2.5 ml PoM £12.48 DT = £1.39

Latanoprost with netarsudil
27-Feb-2025

The properties listed below are those particular to the combination only. For the properties of the components please consider, latanoprost p. 1346.

- **INDICATIONS AND DOSE**
  Raised intra-ocular pressure in open-angle glaucoma (initiated by a specialist) | Ocular hypertension (initiated by a specialist)
  ▸ TO THE EYE
  ▸ Adult: Apply once daily, to be administered preferably in the evening

- **SIDE-EFFECTS**
  ▸ **Common or very common** Dry eye · eye discomfort · eye disorders · eye inflammation · haemorrhage · skin reactions · vision disorders
  ▸ **Uncommon** Corneal deposits · device related eye complication · dizziness · eye discolouration · fatigue · headache · jaw pain · muscle contractions involuntary · muscle weakness · nasal congestion · Sjögren's syndrome · vomiting

- **NATIONAL FUNDING/ACCESS DECISIONS**
  For full details see funding body website
  NICE decisions
  ▸ Latanoprost–netarsudil for previously treated primary open-angle glaucoma or ocular hypertension (October 2024) NICE TA1009 Recommended with restrictions
  Scottish Medicines Consortium (SMC) decisions
  ▸ Netarsudil plus latanoprost (*Roclanda*®) for the reduction of elevated intraocular pressure (IOP) in adult patients with primary open-angle glaucoma or ocular hypertension (OHT) for whom monotherapy with a prostaglandin or netarsudil

provides insufficient IOP reduction (February 2025) SMC No. SMC2720 Recommended with restrictions

- **MEDICINAL FORMS** There can be variation in the licensing of different medicines containing the same drug.
  Eye drops
  EXCIPIENTS: May contain Benzalkonium chloride
  ▸ Roclanda (Santen UK Ltd) ▼
  Latanoprost 50 microgram per 1 ml, Netarsudil (as Netarsudil mesylate) 200 microgram per 1 ml Roclanda 50micrograms/ml + 200micrograms/ml eye drops | 2.5 ml PoM £10.00 DT = £10.00

Latanoprost with timolol
10-Nov-2020

The properties listed below are those particular to the combination only. For the properties of the components please consider, latanoprost p. 1346, timolol maleate p. 1342.

11
Eye

- **INDICATIONS AND DOSE**
  Raised intra-ocular pressure in patients with open-angle glaucoma and ocular hypertension when beta-blocker or prostaglandin analogue alone not adequate
  ▸ TO THE EYE
  ▸ Adult: Apply once daily

- **INTERACTIONS** → Appendix 1: beta blockers, non-selective
- **NATIONAL FUNDING/ACCESS DECISIONS**
  For full details see funding body website
  Scottish Medicines Consortium (SMC) decisions
  ▸ Latanoprost with timolol (*Fixapost*®) for the reduction of intraocular pressure (IOP) in patients with open-angle glaucoma and ocular hypertension who are insufficiently responsive to topical beta-blockers or prostaglandin analogues (May 2019) SMC No. SMC2159 Recommended with restrictions

- **MEDICINAL FORMS** There can be variation in the licensing of different medicines containing the same drug.
  Eye drops
  EXCIPIENTS: May contain Benzalkonium chloride
  ▸ Latanoprost with timolol (Non-proprietary)
  Latanoprost 50 microgram per 1 ml, Timolol (as Timolol maleate) 5 mg per 1 ml Latanoprost 50micrograms/ml / Timolol 5mg/ml eye drops | 2.5 ml PoM £14.32 DT = £3.73
  ▸ Fixapost (Thea Pharmaceuticals Ltd)
  Latanoprost 50 microgram per 1 ml, Timolol (as Timolol maleate) 5 mg per 1 ml Fixapost 50micrograms/ml / 5mg/ml eye drops 0.2ml unit dose | 30 unit dose PoM £13.49 DT = £13.49
  ▸ Vizilatan Duo (Bausch & Lomb UK Ltd)
  Latanoprost 50 microgram per 1 ml, Timolol (as Timolol maleate) 5 mg per 1 ml Vizilatan Duo eye drops | 2.5 ml PoM £13.49 DT = £13.49
  ▸ Xalacom (Viatris UK Healthcare Ltd)
  Latanoprost 50 microgram per 1 ml, Timolol (as Timolol maleate) 5 mg per 1 ml Xalacom eye drops | 2.5 ml PoM £14.32 DT = £3.73

Tafluprost
28-May-2021

- **INDICATIONS AND DOSE**
  Raised intra-ocular pressure in open-angle glaucoma | Ocular hypertension
  ▸ TO THE EYE
  ▸ Adult: Apply once daily, to be administered preferably in the evening

- **CAUTIONS** Angle-closure glaucoma (no experience of use) · aphakia · asthma · congenital glaucoma (no experience of use) · contact lens wearers · inflammatory ocular conditions (no experience of use) · narrow-angle glaucoma (no experience of use) · neovascular glaucoma (no experience of use) · pseudophakia with torn posterior lens capsule or anterior chamber lenses · risk factors for cystoid macular oedema · risk factors for iritis · risk factors for uveitis

- **SIDE-EFFECTS**
  - **Common or very common** Dry eye · eye discolouration · eye discomfort · eye disorders · eye inflammation · headache · vision disorders
  - **Uncommon** Hypertrichosis
  - **Frequency not known** Asthma exacerbated · dyspnoea
- **PREGNANCY** Manufacturer advises avoid unless potential benefit outweighs risk—toxicity in *animal* studies.
- **BREAST FEEDING** Manufacturer advises avoid—present in milk in *animal* studies.
- **HEPATIC IMPAIRMENT** Manufacturer advises caution (no information available).
- **RENAL IMPAIRMENT** [EvGr] Use with caution (no information available). ⟨M⟩
- **PRESCRIBING AND DISPENSING INFORMATION** Although multi-dose tafluprost eye drops commonly contain preservatives, preservative-free unit dose vials may be available.
- **PATIENT AND CARER ADVICE**
  Changes to eye colour Before initiating treatment, patients should be warned of a possible change in eye colour as an increase in the brown pigment in the iris can occur, which may be permanent; particular care is required in those with mixed coloured irides and those receiving treatment to one eye only. Changes in eyelashes and vellus hair can also occur, and patients should also be advised to avoid repeated contact of the eye drop solution with skin as this can lead to hair growth or skin pigmentation.

- **MEDICINAL FORMS** There can be variation in the licensing of different medicines containing the same drug.
  Eye drops
  EXCIPIENTS: May contain Disodium edetate
  - Tafluprost (Non-proprietary)
    Tafluprost 15 microgram per 1 ml Taflotan 15micrograms/ml eye drops | 2.5 ml [PoM] Ⓔ
  - Saflutan (Santen UK Ltd)
    Tafluprost 15 microgram per 1 ml Saflutan 15micrograms/ml eye drops 0.3ml unit dose | 30 unit dose [PoM] £12.20 DT = £12.20
    Saflutan 15micrograms/ml eye drops | 3 ml [PoM] £11.39 DT = £11.39

Tafluprost with timolol

16-Nov-2020

The properties listed below are those particular to the combination only. For the properties of the components please consider, tafluprost p. 1347, timolol maleate p. 1342.

- **INDICATIONS AND DOSE**

  Raised intra-ocular pressure in open-angle glaucoma and ocular hypertension when beta-blocker or prostaglandin analogue alone not adequate
  - TO THE EYE
  - Adult: Apply 1 drop once daily

- **INTERACTIONS** → Appendix 1: beta blockers, non-selective
- **PATIENT AND CARER ADVICE**
  Driving and skilled tasks Blurred vision may affect performance of skilled tasks (e.g. driving or operating machinery).
- **NATIONAL FUNDING/ACCESS DECISIONS**
  For full details see funding body website
  Scottish Medicines Consortium (SMC) decisions
  - Tafluprost with timolol (*Taptiqom*®) for reduction of intra-ocular pressure in adult patients with open angle glaucoma or ocular hypertension who are insufficiently responsive to topical monotherapy with beta-blockers or prostaglandin analogues and require a combination therapy, and who would benefit from preservative-free eye drops (September 2015) SMC No. 1085/15 Recommended with restrictions

- **MEDICINAL FORMS** There can be variation in the licensing of different medicines containing the same drug.
  Eye drops
  EXCIPIENTS: May contain Disodium edetate
  - Taptiqom (Santen UK Ltd)
    Tafluprost 15 microgram per 1 ml, Timolol (as Timolol maleate) 5 mg per 1 ml Taptiqom 15micrograms/ml / 5mg/ml eye drops 0.3ml unit dose | 30 unit dose [PoM] £14.50 DT = £14.50

Travoprost

03-Sep-2020

- **INDICATIONS AND DOSE**

  Raised intra-ocular pressure in open-angle glaucoma | Ocular hypertension
  - TO THE EYE
  - Adult: Apply once daily, to be administered preferably in the evening

- **CAUTIONS** Angle-closure glaucoma (no experience of use) · aphakia · asthma · congenital glaucoma (no experience of use) · contact lens wearers · inflammatory ocular conditions (no experience of use) · narrow-angle glaucoma (no experience of use) · neovascular glaucoma (no experience of use) · pseudophakia with torn posterior lens capsule or anterior chamber lenses · risk factors for cystoid macular oedema · risk factors for iritis · risk factors for uveitis
- **SIDE-EFFECTS**
  - **Common or very common** Dry eye · eye discolouration · eye discomfort · eye disorders
  - **Uncommon** Cataract · cough · eye inflammation · hair changes · headache · nasal complaints · palpitations · seasonal allergy · skin reactions · throat irritation · vision disorders
  - **Rare or very rare** Allergic rhinitis · arthralgia · asthenia · asthma · constipation · dizziness · dry mouth · dysphonia · dyspnoea · gastrointestinal disorders · hypertension · hypotension · madarosis · musculoskeletal pain · ophthalmic herpes simplex · oropharyngeal pain · respiratory disorder · taste altered
  - **Frequency not known** Abdominal pain · anxiety · arrhythmias · chest pain · depression · diarrhoea · epistaxis · insomnia · nausea · tinnitus · urinary disorders · vertigo · vomiting
- **PREGNANCY** Manufacturer advises avoid unless potential benefit outweighs risk—toxicity in *animal* studies.
- **BREAST FEEDING** Present in milk in *animal* studies; manufacturer advises avoid.
- **PATIENT AND CARER ADVICE**
  Changes to eye colour Before initiating treatment, patients should be warned of a possible change in eye colour as an increase in the brown pigment in the iris can occur, which may be permanent; particular care is required in those with mixed coloured irides and those receiving treatment to one eye only. Changes in eyelashes and vellus hair can also occur, and patients should also be advised to avoid repeated contact of the eye drop solution with skin as this can lead to hair growth or skin pigmentation.

- **MEDICINAL FORMS** There can be variation in the licensing of different medicines containing the same drug.
  Eye drops
  EXCIPIENTS: May contain Propylene glycol
  - Travoprost (Non-proprietary)
    Travoprost 40 microgram per 1 ml Travoprost 40micrograms/ml eye drops | 2.5 ml [PoM] £10.95 DT = £1.93
  - Travatan (Novartis Pharmaceuticals UK Ltd)
    Travoprost 40 microgram per 1 ml Travatan 40micrograms/ml eye drops | 2.5 ml [PoM] £10.95 DT = £1.93
  - Visutrax (Visufarma UK Ltd)
    Travoprost 40 microgram per 1 ml Visutrax 40micrograms/ml eye drops 0.1ml unit dose | 30 unit dose [PoM] £7.49 DT = £7.49

Travoprost with timolol
02-Jun-2020

The properties listed below are those particular to the combination only. For the properties of the components please consider, travoprost p. 1348, timolol maleate p. 1342.

- **INDICATIONS AND DOSE**
  Raised intra-ocular pressure in patients with open-angle glaucoma or ocular hypertension when beta-blocker or prostaglandin analogue alone not adequate
  ▸ TO THE EYE
  ▸ Adult: Apply once daily

- **INTERACTIONS** → Appendix 1: beta blockers, non-selective

- **MEDICINAL FORMS** There can be variation in the licensing of different medicines containing the same drug.
  Eye drops
  EXCIPIENTS: May contain Propylene glycol
  ▸ **Travoprost with timolol (Non-proprietary)**
    Travoprost 40 microgram per 1 ml, Timolol (as Timolol maleate) 5 mg per 1 ml Travoprost 40micrograms/ml / Timolol 5mg/ml eye drops | 2.5 ml PoM £17.90 DT = £16.66
  ▸ **DuoTrav** (Novartis Pharmaceuticals UK Ltd)
    Travoprost 40 microgram per 1 ml, Timolol (as Timolol maleate) 5 mg per 1 ml DuoTrav 40micrograms/ml / 5mg/ml eye drops | 2.5 ml PoM £13.95 DT = £16.66 | 7.5 ml PoM £39.68

PROSTAMIDES

Bimatoprost
03-Jun-2021

- **INDICATIONS AND DOSE**
  Raised intra-ocular pressure in open-angle glaucoma | Ocular hypertension
  ▸ TO THE EYE
  ▸ Adult: Apply once daily, to be administered preferably in the evening

- **CAUTIONS** Angle-closure glaucoma (no experience of use) · aphakia · asthma · chronic obstructive pulmonary disease · compromised respiratory function · congenital glaucoma (no experience of use) · contact lens wearers · history of significant ocular viral infections · inflammatory ocular conditions (no experience of use) · narrow-angle glaucoma (no experience of use) · neovascular glaucoma (no experience of use) · predisposition to bradycardia · predisposition to hypotension · pseudophakia with torn posterior lens capsule or anterior chamber lenses · risk factors for cystoid macular oedema · risk factors for iritis · risk factors for uveitis

- **SIDE-EFFECTS**
  ▸ **Common or very common** Dry eye · eye discolouration · eye discomfort · eye disorders · eye inflammation · headache · hypertension · hypertrichosis · skin reactions · vision disorders
  ▸ **Uncommon** Asthenia · dizziness · madarosis · nausea · retinal haemorrhage
  ▸ **Frequency not known** Asthma · bradycardia · dyspnoea · hypotension · reactivation of infection

- **PREGNANCY** Manufacturer advises use only if potential benefit outweighs risk.

- **BREAST FEEDING** Manufacturer advises avoid—present in milk in *animal* studies.

- **HEPATIC IMPAIRMENT** Manufacturer advises use with caution in moderate-to-severe impairment—no information available.

- **RENAL IMPAIRMENT** EvGr Use with caution (no information available). Ⓜ

- **PRESCRIBING AND DISPENSING INFORMATION** Although multi-dose bimatoprost eye drops commonly contain preservatives, preservative-free unit dose vials may be available.

- **PATIENT AND CARER ADVICE**
  Changes to eye colour Before initiating treatment, patients should be warned of a possible change in eye colour as an increase in the brown pigment in the iris can occur, which may be permanent; particular care is required in those with mixed coloured irides and those receiving treatment to one eye only. Changes in eyelashes and vellus hair can also occur, and patients should also be advised to avoid repeated contact of the eye drop solution with skin as this can lead to hair growth or skin pigmentation.

- **NATIONAL FUNDING/ACCESS DECISIONS**
  LUMIGAN ® For full details see funding body website
  Scottish Medicines Consortium (SMC) decisions
  ▸ Bimatoprost 300 micrograms/mL preservative-free eye drops (*Lumigan*® single-dose eye drops) for reduction of elevated intraocular pressure in chronic open-angle glaucoma and ocular hypertension in adults (as monotherapy or as adjunctive therapy to beta-blockers) (March 2013) SMC No. 839/13 Recommended with restrictions

- **MEDICINAL FORMS** There can be variation in the licensing of different medicines containing the same drug.
  Eye drops
  EXCIPIENTS: May contain Benzalkonium chloride
  ▸ **Bimatoprost (Non-proprietary)**
    Bimatoprost 100 microgram per 1 ml Bimatoprost 100micrograms/ml eye drops | 3 ml PoM £11.71 DT = £3.94 | 9 ml PoM £29.86-£35.13
    Bimatoprost 300 microgram per 1 ml Bimatoprost 300micrograms/ml eye drops 0.4ml unit dose preservative free | 30 unit dose PoM £9.98-£14.40 DT = £9.98
    Bimatoprost 300micrograms/ml eye drops | 3 ml PoM £12.16 DT = £13.47
  ▸ **Bimi** (Scope Ophthalmics Ltd)
    Bimatoprost 300 microgram per 1 ml Bimi 0.3mg/ml eye drops | 3 ml PoM £8.33 DT = £9.79 | 9 ml PoM £21.87
  ▸ **Eyreida** (Aspire Pharma Ltd)
    Bimatoprost 300 microgram per 1 ml Eyreida 0.3mg/ml eye drops | 3 ml PoM £9.79 DT = £9.79
  ▸ **Lumigan** (AbbVie Ltd)
    Bimatoprost 100 microgram per 1 ml Lumigan 100micrograms/ml eye drops | 3 ml PoM £11.71 DT = £3.94 | 9 ml PoM £35.13
    Bimatoprost 300 microgram per 1 ml Lumigan 300micrograms/ml eye drops 0.4ml unit dose | 30 unit dose PoM £13.75 DT = £9.98
  ▸ **Visuplain** (Visufarma UK Ltd)
    Bimatoprost 100 microgram per 1 ml Visuplain 0.1mg/ml eye drops | 3 ml PoM £7.49 DT = £3.94
  ▸ **Zimed** (Medicom Healthcare Ltd)
    Bimatoprost 300 microgram per 1 ml Zimed 0.3mg/ml eye drops preservative free | 3 ml PoM £7.99 DT = £9.79

Bimatoprost with timolol
02-Jun-2020

The properties listed below are those particular to the combination only. For the properties of the components please consider, bimatoprost above, timolol maleate p. 1342.

- **INDICATIONS AND DOSE**
  Raised intra-ocular pressure in patients with open-angle glaucoma or ocular hypertension when beta-blocker or prostaglandin analogue alone not adequate
  ▸ TO THE EYE
  ▸ Adult: Apply once daily

- **INTERACTIONS** → Appendix 1: beta blockers, non-selective

- **NATIONAL FUNDING/ACCESS DECISIONS**
  GANFORT ® SINGLE USE For full details see funding body website

  Scottish Medicines Consortium (SMC) decisions
  ▸ Bimatoprost with timolol (*Ganfort*®) unit dose eye drops for reduction of intraocular pressure (IOP) in adult patients with open-angle glaucoma or ocular hypertension who are insufficiently responsive to topical beta-blockers or

Eye

prostaglandin analogues (October 2013) SMC No. 906/13 Recommended with restrictions

- **MEDICINAL FORMS** There can be variation in the licensing of different medicines containing the same drug.

Eye drops
EXCIPIENTS: May contain Benzalkonium chloride
  - ▶ **Bimatoprost with timolol (Non-proprietary)**
    Bimatoprost 300 microgram per 1 ml, Timolol (as Timolol maleate) 5 mg per 1 ml Bimatoprost 300micrograms/ml / Timolol 5mg/ml eye drops | 3 ml [PoM] £15.00 DT = £8.35 | 9 ml [PoM] £26.49–£38.15
    Bimatoprost 300micrograms/ml / Timolol 5mg/ml eye drops 0.4ml unit dose preservative free | 30 unit dose [PoM] £17.50–£29.00 DT = £15.67
  - ▶ **Bimiduo** (Scope Ophthalmics Ltd)
    Bimatoprost 300 microgram per 1 ml, Timolol (as Timolol maleate) 5 mg per 1 ml Bimiduo 0.3mg/ml / 5mg/ml eye drops preservative free | 3 ml [PoM] £11.99 DT = £14.16
  - ▶ **Eyzeetan** (Aspire Pharma Ltd)
    Bimatoprost 300 microgram per 1 ml, Timolol (as Timolol maleate) 5 mg per 1 ml Eyzeetan 0.3mg/ml / 5mg/ml eye drops preservative free | 3 ml [PoM] £14.16 DT = £14.16
  - ▶ **Ganfort** (AbbVie Ltd)
    Bimatoprost 300 microgram per 1 ml, Timolol (as Timolol maleate) 5 mg per 1 ml Ganfort 0.3mg/ml / 5mg/ml eye drops | 3 ml [PoM] £14.16 DT = £8.35 | 9 ml [PoM] £38.15
    Ganfort 0.3mg/ml / 5mg/ml eye drops 0.4ml unit dose | 30 unit dose [PoM] £17.94 DT = £15.67
  - ▶ **Visublend** (Visufarma UK Ltd)
    Bimatoprost 300 microgram per 1 ml, Timolol (as Timolol maleate) 5 mg per 1 ml Visublend 0.3mg/ml / 5mg/ml eye drops | 3 ml [PoM] £9.93 DT = £8.35

SYMPATHOMIMETICS ▶ ALPHA₂-ADRENOCEPTOR AGONISTS

Apraclonidine
11-May-2021

- **DRUG ACTION** Apraclonidine is an alpha₂-adrenoceptor agonist that lowers intra-ocular pressure by reducing aqueous humour formation. It is a derivative of clonidine.

- **INDICATIONS AND DOSE**

Control or prevention of postoperative elevation of intra-ocular pressure after anterior segment laser surgery
  - ▶ TO THE EYE
  - ▶ Adult: Apply 1 drop, 1 hour before laser procedure, then 1 drop, immediately after completion of procedure, 1% eye drops to be administered

Short-term adjunctive treatment of chronic glaucoma in patients not adequately controlled by another drug
  - ▶ TO THE EYE
  - ▶ Adult: Apply 1 drop 3 times a day usually for maximum 1 month, 0.5% eye drops to be administered, may not provide additional benefit if patient already using two drugs that suppress the production of aqueous humour

- **CONTRA-INDICATIONS** History of severe or unstable and uncontrolled cardiovascular disease
- **CAUTIONS** Cerebrovascular disease · depression · heart failure · history of angina · hypertension · loss of effect may occur over time · Parkinson's syndrome · Raynaud's syndrome · recent myocardial infarction · reduction in vision in end-stage glaucoma (suspend treatment) · severe coronary insufficiency · thromboangiitis obliterans · vasovagal attack
- **INTERACTIONS** → Appendix 1: apraclonidine
- **SIDE-EFFECTS**
  - ▶ **Common or very common** Eye disorders
  - ▶ **Uncommon** Bradycardia · conjunctival haemorrhage · diarrhoea · dry eye · eye discomfort · eye inflammation · gastrointestinal discomfort · irritability · libido decreased · nasal dryness · palpitations · postural hypotension ·

sensation abnormal · sleep disorders · syncope · vision disorders · vomiting
  - ▶ **Rare or very rare** Chest pain · dry mouth · fatigue · headache · hyperhidrosis · pain in extremity · pruritus · taste altered · temperature sensation altered

SIDE-EFFECTS, FURTHER INFORMATION Since absorption may follow topical application, systemic effects may occur– see clonidine hydrochloride p. 172.
  Ocular intolerance Manufacturer advises withdrawal if eye pruritus, ocular hyperaemia, increased lacrimation, or oedema of the eyelids and conjunctiva occur.

- **PREGNANCY** Manufacturer advises avoid—no information available.
- **BREAST FEEDING** Manufacturer advises avoid—no information available.
- **HEPATIC IMPAIRMENT** Manufacturer advises use with caution and monitor, including close monitoring of cardiovascular parameters—no information available.
- **RENAL IMPAIRMENT** [EvGr] Use with caution in chronic renal failure. ⓜ
- **MONITORING REQUIREMENTS**
  - ▶ Monitor intra-ocular pressure and visual fields.
  - ▶ Monitor for excessive reduction in intra-ocular pressure following peri-operative use.
- **PATIENT AND CARER ADVICE**
  Driving and skilled tasks Drowsiness may affect performance of skilled tasks (e.g. driving).

- **MEDICINAL FORMS** There can be variation in the licensing of different medicines containing the same drug.

Eye drops
EXCIPIENTS: May contain Benzalkonium chloride
  - ▶ **Iopidine** (Essential Pharma Ltd)
    Apraclonidine (as Apraclonidine hydrochloride) 5 mg per 1 ml Iopidine 5mg/ml eye drops | 5 ml [PoM] £10.88 DT = £10.88
    Apraclonidine (as Apraclonidine hydrochloride) 10 mg per 1 ml Iopidine 1% eye drops 0.25ml unit dose | 24 unit dose [PoM] £110.69 DT = £110.69

Brimonidine tartrate
11-May-2021

- **DRUG ACTION** Brimonidine, an alpha₂-adrenoceptor agonist, is thought to lower intra-ocular pressure by reducing aqueous humour formation and increasing uveoscleral outflow.

- **INDICATIONS AND DOSE**

Raised intra-ocular pressure in open-angle glaucoma in patients for whom beta-blockers are inappropriate | Ocular hypertension in patients for whom beta-blockers are inappropriate | Adjunctive therapy when intra-ocular pressure is inadequately controlled by other antiglaucoma therapy
  - ▶ TO THE EYE
  - ▶ Adult: Apply twice daily

- **CAUTIONS** Cerebral insufficiency · coronary insufficiency · depression · postural hypotension · Raynaud's syndrome · severe cardiovascular disease · thromboangiitis obliterans
- **INTERACTIONS** → Appendix 1: brimonidine
- **SIDE-EFFECTS**
  - ▶ **Common or very common** Asthenia · dizziness · drowsiness · dry eye · dry mouth · eye discomfort · eye disorders · eye inflammation · gastrointestinal disorder · headache · hyperaemia · hypersensitivity · pulmonary reaction · sensation of foreign body · skin reactions · taste altered · vision disorders
  - ▶ **Uncommon** Arrhythmias · nasal dryness · palpitations
  - ▶ **Rare or very rare** Dyspnoea · hypertension · hypotension · insomnia · syncope
  - ▶ **Frequency not known** Face oedema · vasodilation

- **PREGNANCY** Manufacturer advises use only if benefit outweighs risk—limited information available.
- **BREAST FEEDING** Manufacturer advises avoid—no information available.
- **HEPATIC IMPAIRMENT** Manufacturer advises caution (no information available).
- **RENAL IMPAIRMENT** Manufacturer advises use with caution.
- **PATIENT AND CARER ADVICE**
  Driving and skilled tasks Drowsiness or blurred vision may affect performance of skilled tasks (e.g. driving).

- **MEDICINAL FORMS** There can be variation in the licensing of different medicines containing the same drug.
  Eye drops
  EXCIPIENTS: May contain Benzalkonium chloride
  ▸ **Brimonidine tartrate (Non-proprietary)**
    Brimonidine tartrate 2 mg per 1 ml Brimonidine 2mg/ml eye drops | 5 ml PoM £5.99 DT = £1.97
    Brimonidine 0.2% eye drops | 5 ml PoM £5.89 DT = £1.97
  ▸ **Alphagan** (AbbVie Ltd)
    Brimonidine tartrate 2 mg per 1 ml Alphagan 0.2% eye drops | 5 ml PoM £6.85 DT = £1.97

  Combinations available: _Brinzolamide with brimonidine,_ p. 1344

Brimonidine with timolol

02-Jun-2020

The properties listed below are those particular to the combination only. For the properties of the components please consider, brimonidine tartrate p. 1350, timolol maleate p. 1342.

- **INDICATIONS AND DOSE**
  Raised intra-ocular pressure in open-angle glaucoma and for ocular hypertension when beta-blocker alone not adequate
  ▸ TO THE EYE
  ▸ Adult: Apply twice daily

- **INTERACTIONS** → Appendix 1: beta blockers, non-selective · brimonidine

- **MEDICINAL FORMS** There can be variation in the licensing of different medicines containing the same drug.
  Eye drops
  EXCIPIENTS: May contain Benzalkonium chloride
  ▸ **Brimonidine with timolol (Non-proprietary)**
    Brimonidine tartrate 2 mg per 1 ml, Timolol (as Timolol maleate) 5 mg per 1 ml Brimonidine 2mg/ml / Timolol 5mg/ml eye drops | 5 ml PoM £8.50-£20.00 DT = £16.57
  ▸ **Combigan** (AbbVie Ltd)
    Brimonidine tartrate 2 mg per 1 ml, Timolol (as Timolol maleate) 5 mg per 1 ml Combigan eye drops | 5 ml PoM £10.00 DT = £16.57 | 15 ml PoM £27.00

6   Retinal disorders

6.1   Macular degeneration

Age-related macular degeneration

18-Jul-2022

Description of condition

Age-related macular degeneration is a progressive eye condition that affects the central area of the retina (macula). It occurs mainly in people aged 55 years and over and is a common cause of vision loss. The progressive loss of central vision affects the patient's ability to see well enough to recognise faces, drive, and to read and write. Although the exact cause is unknown, known risk factors in addition to increasing age include smoking and a family history of age-related macular degeneration.

There are two types of age-related macular degeneration—dry and wet. Dry (non-neovascular) age-related macular degeneration progresses slowly as extensive wasting of macula cells occurs. Whereas, with wet (neovascular) age-related macular degeneration, new blood vessels develop beneath and within the retina, and can lead to a rapid deterioration of vision. Wet age-related macular degeneration is further classified as _wet-active_ (neovascular lesions that may benefit from treatment) and _wet-inactive_ (neovascular disease with irreversible structural change).

Aims of treatment

The aim of treatment is to slow down the progression of age-related macular degeneration and central vision loss; treatment is initiated under specialist care.

Treatment

Treatment is dependent on the stage and type of age-related macular degeneration, with drug treatment only recommended in patients with _wet-active_ age-related macular degeneration. Counselling and support, advice on Smoking cessation p. 565, and use of visual aids is recommended in all patients with age related macular degeneration as appropriate.

EvGr An intravitreal anti vascular endothelial growth factor (anti-VEGF) is first-line treatment for certain patients with _wet-active_ age-related macular degeneration. Anti-VEGF treatment should only be administered by healthcare professionals experienced in the use of intravitreal injections.

Treatment should be stopped if the patient develops severe, progressive loss of visual acuity despite treatment, or if the patient's age-related macular degeneration develops into _wet-inactive_ with no prospect of visual function improvement. A treatment-free period can be considered in patients whose age-related macular degeneration appears to be stable.

Photodynamic therapy alone should not be given to patients with _wet-active_ age-related macular degeneration. It can be given as an adjunct to anti-VEGF treatment as a second-line option in the context of a randomised controlled trial. Intravitreal corticosteroids are not recommended in combination with anti-VEGF treatment because there is limited evidence of benefit to a patient's visual acuity.

Patients should be advised to attend routine sight tests, self-monitor, and to report any changes in vision such as appearance of grey patches or blurred vision, straight lines appearing distorted, and objects appearing smaller than normal. Ⓐ

Useful Resources

Age-related macular degeneration. National Institute for Health and Care Excellence. NICE guideline 82. January 2018.
www.nice.org.uk/guidance/ng82

ANTINEOVASCULARISATION DRUGS ›
VASCULAR ENDOTHELIAL GROWTH FACTOR INHIBITORS

Aflibercept [Specialist drug]
12-Mar-2024

● **INDICATIONS AND DOSE**

Neovascular (wet) age-related macular degeneration | Macular oedema secondary to retinal vein occlusion | Diabetic macular oedema | Myopic choroidal neovascularisation

▸ BY INTRAVITREAL INJECTION

▸ **Adult:** Specialist drug – access specialist resources for dosing information

IMPORTANT SAFETY INFORMATION

MHRA/CHM ADVICE: *EYLEA*® 40 MG/ML (AFLIBERCEPT SOLUTION FOR INTRAVITREAL INJECTION): HIGHER RISK OF INTRAOCULAR PRESSURE INCREASE WITH THE PRE-FILLED SYRINGE (APRIL 2021)

Cases of increased intra-ocular pressure in adults have been reported more frequently when using the *Eylea*® prefilled syringe compared with a luer-lock syringe used with *Eylea*® solution for injection in a vial. Incorrect handling in the preparation and injection is suspected as the cause of the observed cases of increased intra-ocular pressure with the *Eylea*® prefilled syringe. Injections should be performed by healthcare professionals familiar with the handling of this presentation; the manufacturer has provided educational materials which include a *Prescriber Guide* and a training video on how to prepare and administer the intravitreal injection. The patient's vision and intra-ocular pressure should be evaluated and monitored immediately after the intravitreal injection.

● **CONTRA-INDICATIONS** Clinical signs of irreversible ischaemic visual function loss · ocular or periocular infection · severe intra-ocular inflammation

● **INTERACTIONS** → Appendix 1: aflibercept

● **SIDE-EFFECTS**

▸ **Common or very common** Cataract · eye discomfort · eye disorders · eye inflammation · haemorrhage · retinal pigment epithelial tear · vision disorders

▸ **Uncommon** Lens opacity

SIDE-EFFECTS, FURTHER INFORMATION Discontinue treatment in the event of retinal break, rhegmatogenous retinal detachment, or if stage 3 or 4 macular holes develop.

● **CONCEPTION AND CONTRACEPTION** EvGr Females of childbearing potential should use effective contraception during and for at least 3 months after treatment. Ⓜ

● **NATIONAL FUNDING/ACCESS DECISIONS**
For full details see funding body website

NICE decisions

▸ **Aflibercept solution for injection for treating wet age-related macular degeneration (July 2013)** NICE TA294 Recommended with restrictions

▸ **Aflibercept for treating visual impairment caused by macular oedema secondary to central retinal vein occlusion (February 2014)** NICE TA305 Recommended

▸ **Aflibercept for treating diabetic macular oedema (July 2015)** NICE TA346 Recommended with restrictions

▸ **Aflibercept for treating visual impairment caused by macular oedema after branch retinal vein occlusion (September 2016)** NICE TA409 Recommended with restrictions

▸ **Aflibercept for treating choroidal neovascularisation (November 2017)** NICE TA486 Recommended with restrictions

Scottish Medicines Consortium (SMC) decisions

▸ **Aflibercept (*Eylea*®) for adults for the treatment of visual impairment due to myopic choroidal neovascularisation (myopic CNV) (October 2016)** SMC No. 1186/16 Recommended

● **MEDICINAL FORMS** There can be variation in the licensing of different medicines containing the same drug.

Solution for injection

EXCIPIENTS: May contain Polysorbates

▸ Eylea (Bayer Plc)
Aflibercept 40 mg per 1 ml Eylea 3.6mg/90microlitres solution for injection pre-filled syringes | 1 pre-filled disposable injection PoM £816.00 (Hospital only)
Eylea 4mg/100microlitres solution for injection vials | 1 vial PoM £816.00 (Hospital only)
Aflibercept 114.3 mg per 1 ml Eylea 21mg/184microlitres solution for injection pre-filled syringes | 1 pre-filled disposable injection PoM £998.00
Eylea 30.1mg/263microlitres solution for injection vials | 1 vial PoM £998.00 (Hospital only)

Bevacizumab [Specialist drug]
20-Mar-2025

● **INDICATIONS AND DOSE**

Neovascular (wet) age-related macular degeneration

▸ BY INTRAVITREAL INJECTION

▸ **Adult:** Specialist drug – access specialist resources for dosing information

DOSE EQUIVALENCE AND CONVERSION

▸ Bevacizumab for intravenous infusion and bevacizumab gamma for intravitreal injection are **not** interchangeable.

● **CONTRA-INDICATIONS** Intra-ocular inflammation (active) · ocular or peri-ocular infection

● **INTERACTIONS** → Appendix 1: monoclonal antibodies

● **SIDE-EFFECTS**

▸ **Common or very common** Eye discomfort · eye disorders · haemorrhage

▸ **Uncommon** Dry eye · eye inflammation · retinal pigment epithelial tear · vision disorders

▸ **Frequency not known** Arterial thromboembolism

SIDE-EFFECTS, FURTHER INFORMATION Discontinue treatment in the event of rhegmatogenous retinal detachment, or if stage 3 or 4 macular holes develop.

● **CONCEPTION AND CONTRACEPTION** EvGr Females of childbearing potential should use effective contraception during and for at least 3 months after treatment. Ⓜ

● **PATIENT AND CARER ADVICE** Patients or their carers should be counselled to immediately report any signs or symptoms suggestive of endophthalmitis, retinal detachment, retinal tear or intra-ocular inflammation.
Driving and skilled tasks Patients or their carers should be counselled on the effects on driving and performance of skilled tasks—avoid until visual function sufficiently recovered.

● **NATIONAL FUNDING/ACCESS DECISIONS**
For full details see funding body website

NICE decisions

▸ **Bevacizumab gamma for treating wet age-related macular degeneration (December 2024)** NICE TA1022 Recommended with restrictions

● **MEDICINAL FORMS** There can be variation in the licensing of different medicines containing the same drug. Forms available from special-order manufacturers include: solution for injection

Solution for injection

EXCIPIENTS: May contain Polysorbates

▸ Lytenava (Outlook Therapeutics Ltd) ▼
Bevacizumab gamma 25 mg per 1 ml Lytenava 7.5mg/0.3ml solution for injection vials | 1 vial PoM £470.00 (Hospital only)

Brolucizumab [Specialist drug]   19-Oct-2022

● **INDICATIONS AND DOSE**

Neovascular (wet) age-related macular degeneration | Diabetic macular oedema

▸ BY INTRAVITREAL INJECTION

▸ Adult: Specialist drug – access specialist resources for dosing information

---

IMPORTANT SAFETY INFORMATION

MHRA/CHM ADVICE: BROLUCIZUMAB (*BEOVU*®): RISK OF INTRAOCULAR INFLAMMATION AND RETINAL VASCULAR OCCLUSION INCREASED WITH SHORT DOSING INTERVALS (JANUARY 2022)

Cases of intra-ocular inflammation, including retinal vasculitis and/or retinal vascular occlusion have been reported during treatment with brolucizumab, occurring more frequently early on during treatment. Intra-ocular inflammation events were seen more frequently among patients who developed antibodies against brolucizumab during treatment; female sex and Japanese origin were also identified as additional risk factors. Healthcare professionals are reminded that maintenance doses of brolucizumab (after the initial loading doses) should not be administered at intervals of less than 8 weeks.

Brolucizumab should be discontinued if these events occur and patients with a medical history of intra-ocular inflammation and/or retinal vascular occlusion in the year prior to treatment should be closely monitored. Healthcare professionals should advise patients on how to identify early signs and symptoms of intra-ocular inflammation, retinal vasculitis and retinal vascular occlusion and to seek medical attention without delay, if these side-effects are suspected.

● **CONTRA-INDICATIONS** Active intra-ocular inflammation—see also *Important safety information* · active or suspected ocular or periocular infection

● **SIDE-EFFECTS**

▸ **Common or very common** Cataract · eye discomfort · eye disorders · haemorrhage · hypersensitivity · retinal pigment epithelial tear · skin reactions · vision disorders

▸ **Uncommon** Retinal occlusion (discontinue) · retinal vasculitis (discontinue)

▸ **Frequency not known** Arterial thromboembolism · myocardial infarction · stroke

SIDE-EFFECTS, FURTHER INFORMATION Eye inflammation, including retinal vasculitis and/or retinal occlusion, can occur at any time of treatment. These events were observed more frequently at the beginning of the treatment. Discontinue treatment if patients develop these side-effects. Treatment should also be discontinued if rhegmatogenous retinal detachment or stage 3 or 4 macular holes develop.

● **CONCEPTION AND CONTRACEPTION** Manufacturer advises females of childbearing potential to use effective contraception during treatment and for 1 month after treatment.

● **PATIENT AND CARER ADVICE** Patients or their carers should be counselled to immediately report any signs or symptoms suggestive of endophthalmitis, traumatic cataract, retinal detachment, retinal tear, intra-ocular inflammation, or retinal vascular occlusion.
Patient guide A patient guide should be provided.
Driving and skilled tasks Patients or their carers should be counselled on the effects on driving and performance of skilled tasks—avoid until visual function sufficiently recovered.

● **NATIONAL FUNDING/ACCESS DECISIONS**
For full details see funding body website

NICE decisions

▸ Brolucizumab for treating wet age-related macular degeneration (February 2021) NICE TA672 Recommended with restrictions

▸ Brolucizumab for treating diabetic macular oedema (August 2022) NICE TA820 Recommended with restrictions

Scottish Medicines Consortium (SMC) decisions

▸ Brolucizumab (*Beovu*®) for the treatment of neovascular (wet) age-related macular degeneration (wAMD) (September 2020) SMC No. SMC2272 Recommended

▸ Brolucizumab (*Beovu*®) in adults for the treatment of visual impairment due to diabetic macular oedema (October 2022) SMC No. SMC2508 Recommended with restrictions

● **MEDICINAL FORMS** There can be variation in the licensing of different medicines containing the same drug.

Solution for injection
EXCIPIENTS: May contain Polysorbates, sucrose

▸ Beovu (Novartis Pharmaceuticals UK Ltd)
Brolucizumab **120 mg per 1 ml** Beovu 19.8mg/0.165ml solution for injection pre-filled syringes | 1 pre-filled disposable injection [PoM] £816.00 (Hospital only)

Faricimab [Specialist drug]   21-Oct-2024

● **INDICATIONS AND DOSE**

Neovascular (wet) age-related macular degeneration | Diabetic macular oedema | Macular oedema secondary to retinal vein occlusion

▸ BY INTRAVITREAL INJECTION

▸ Adult: Specialist drug – access specialist resources for dosing information

● **CONTRA-INDICATIONS** Intra-ocular inflammation (active) · ocular or periocular infection

● **SIDE-EFFECTS**

▸ **Common or very common** Cataract · eye discomfort · eye disorders · haemorrhage · retinal pigment epithelial tear

▸ **Uncommon** Eye inflammation · procedural pain · sensation of foreign body · vision disorders

▸ **Frequency not known** Arterial thromboembolism

SIDE-EFFECTS, FURTHER INFORMATION Manufacturer advises discontinue treatment if rhegmatogenous retinal detachment, retinal break, or stage 3 or 4 macular holes develop; treatment should not be resumed until repaired.

● **CONCEPTION AND CONTRACEPTION** [EvGr] Females of childbearing potential should use effective contraception during treatment and for at least 3 months after last treatment. Ⓜ

● **PATIENT AND CARER ADVICE** Patients or their carers should be counselled to immediately report any signs or symptoms suggestive of endophthalmitis, rhegmatogenous retinal detachment, retinal tear or intra-ocular inflammation.
Patient guide A patient guide should be provided.
Driving and skilled tasks Patients or their carers should be counselled on the effects on driving and performance of skilled tasks—avoid until visual function sufficiently recovered.

● **NATIONAL FUNDING/ACCESS DECISIONS**
For full details see funding body website

NICE decisions

▸ Faricimab for treating diabetic macular oedema (June 2022) NICE TA799 Recommended with restrictions

▸ Faricimab for treating visual impairment caused by macular oedema after retinal vein occlusion (September 2024) NICE TA1004 Recommended

▸ Faricimab for treating wet age-related macular degeneration (June 2022) NICE TA800 Recommended with restrictions

Scottish Medicines Consortium (SMC) decisions

▶ Faricimab (*Vabysmo*®) for the treatment of adult patients with visual impairment due to diabetic macular oedema (DMO) (November 2022) SMC No. SMC2499 Recommended with restrictions

▶ Faricimab (*Vabysmo*®) for the treatment of adult patients with neovascular (wet) age-related macular degeneration (nAMD) (December 2022) SMC No. SMC2512 Recommended

▶ Faricimab (*Vabysmo*®) for the treatment of adult patients with visual impairment due to macular oedema secondary to branched and central retinal vein occlusion (BRVO and CRVO) (October 2024) SMC No. SMC2685 Recommended

● MEDICINAL FORMS There can be variation in the licensing of different medicines containing the same drug.

Solution for injection

EXCIPIENTS: May contain Polysorbates

▶ **Vabysmo** (Roche Products Ltd) ▼
Faricimab 120 mg per 1 ml Vabysmo 21mg/0.175ml solution for injection pre-filled syringes | 1 pre-filled disposable injection PoM £857.00 (Hospital only)
Vabysmo 28.8mg/0.24ml solution for injection vials | 1 vial PoM £857.00 (Hospital only)

Ranibizumab [Specialist drug]
28-May-2024

● **INDICATIONS AND DOSE**

Neovascular (wet) age-related macular degeneration | Diabetic macular oedema | Macular oedema secondary to retinal vein occlusion | Choroidal neovascularisation | Proliferative diabetic retinopathy

▶ BY INTRAVITREAL INJECTION

▶ Adult: Specialist drug – access specialist resources for dosing information

● CONTRA-INDICATIONS Ocular or periocular infection · severe intra-ocular inflammation · signs of irreversible ischaemic visual function loss in patients with retinal vein occlusion (no information available)

● INTERACTIONS → Appendix 1: ranibizumab

● SIDE-EFFECTS

▶ **Common or very common** Anaemia · anxiety · arthralgia · cataract · cough · dry eye · eye discomfort · eye disorders · eye inflammation · haemorrhage · headache · hypersensitivity · increased risk of infection · lens opacity · nausea · retinal pigment epithelial tear · vision disorders

▶ **Uncommon** Corneal deposits

▶ **Frequency not known** Arterial thromboembolism

SIDE-EFFECTS, FURTHER INFORMATION Discontinue treatment if rhegmatogenous retinal detachment, or stage 3 or 4 macular holes develop.

● CONCEPTION AND CONTRACEPTION EvGr Females of childbearing potential should use effective contraception during and for at least 3 months after treatment. Ⓜ

● PATIENT AND CARER ADVICE
Driving and skilled tasks Patients and carers should be counselled on the effects on driving and performance of skilled tasks—avoid until visual function sufficiently recovered.

● NATIONAL FUNDING/ACCESS DECISIONS
For full details see funding body website

NICE decisions

▶ Ranibizumab for treating choroidal neovascularisation associated with pathological myopia (updated May 2024) NICE TA298 Recommended

▶ Ranibizumab for treating diabetic macular oedema (updated October 2023) NICE TA274 Recommended with restrictions

▶ Ranibizumab for treating visual impairment caused by macular oedema secondary to retinal vein occlusion (updated May 2024) NICE TA283 Recommended with restrictions

▶ Ranibizumab and pegaptanib for the treatment of age-related macular degeneration (updated May 2024) NICE TA155 Recommended with restrictions

Scottish Medicines Consortium (SMC) decisions

▶ Ranibizumab (*Lucentis*®) for the treatment of visual impairment due to Diabetic Macular Oedema (December 2012) SMC No. 711/11 Recommended with restrictions

▶ Ranibizumab (*Lucentis*®) for the treatment of visual impairment due to macular oedema secondary to branch retinal vein occlusion (BRVO) in adults (May 2013) SMC No. 732/11 Recommended

▶ Ranibizumab (*Lucentis*®) for treatment of visual impairment due to choroidal neovascularisation secondary to pathologic myopia in adults (November 2013) SMC No. 907/13 Recommended

All Wales Medicines Strategy Group (AWMSG) decisions

▶ Ranibizumab (*Lucentis*®) for treatment of visual impairment in adults due to choroidal neovascularisation and not due to pathological myopia or wet age-related macular degeneration (June 2018) AWMSG No. 3233 Recommended

● MEDICINAL FORMS There can be variation in the licensing of different medicines containing the same drug.

Solution for injection

EXCIPIENTS: May contain Polysorbates

▶ **Byooviz** (Biogen Idec Ltd) ▼
Ranibizumab 10 mg per 1 ml Byooviz 2.3mg/0.23ml solution for injection vials | 1 vial PoM £523.45 (Hospital only)

▶ **Lucentis** (Novartis Pharmaceuticals UK Ltd)
Ranibizumab 10 mg per 1 ml Lucentis 2.3mg/0.23ml solution for injection vials | 1 vial PoM £551.00 (Hospital only)
Lucentis 1.65mg/0.165ml solution for injection pre-filled syringes | 1 pre-filled disposable injection PoM £551.00

▶ **Ongavia** (Teva UK Ltd) ▼
Ranibizumab 10 mg per 1 ml Ongavia 2.3mg/0.23ml solution for injection vials | 1 vial PoM £523.45 (Hospital only)

▶ **Rimmyrah** (Orion Pharma (UK) Ltd) ▼
Ranibizumab 10 mg per 1 ml Rimmyrah 2.3mg/0.23ml solution for injection vials | 1 vial PoM £523.45 (Hospital only)

▶ **Ximluci** (Genus Pharmaceuticals Ltd) ▼
Ranibizumab 10 mg per 1 ml Ximluci 2.3mg/0.23ml solution for injection vials | 1 vial PoM £495.90 (Hospital only)

PHOTOSENSITISERS

Verteporfin [Specialist drug]
02-Sep-2020

● **INDICATIONS AND DOSE**

Age-related macular degeneration

▶ BY INTRAVENOUS INFUSION

▶ Adult: Specialist drug – access specialist resources for dosing information

● CONTRA-INDICATIONS Acute porphyrias p. 1202

● INTERACTIONS → Appendix 1: verteporfin

● SIDE-EFFECTS

▶ **Common or very common** Asthenia · dizziness · dyspnoea · headache · hypercholesterolaemia · hypersensitivity · infusion related chest pain · infusion related reaction · nausea · photosensitivity reaction · syncope · vision disorders

▶ **Uncommon** Eye inflammation · fever · haemorrhage · hyperaesthesia · hypertension · pain · retinal detachment · skin reactions

▶ **Rare or very rare** Malaise · retinal ischaemia

▶ **Frequency not known** Myocardial infarction · retinal pigment epithelial tear

● PATIENT AND CARER ADVICE Photosensitivity—avoid exposure of unprotected skin and eyes to bright light during infusion and for 48 hours afterwards.

- **MEDICINAL FORMS** There can be variation in the licensing of different medicines containing the same drug.
  Powder for solution for infusion
  EXCIPIENTS: May contain Butylated hydroxytoluene
  ▸ **Verteporfin (Non-proprietary)**
  Verteporfin 15 mg Verteporfin 15mg powder for solution for infusion vials | 1 vial PoM £850.00 (Hospital only)

6.2 Macular oedema

> **Other drugs used for Macular oedema** Aflibercept, p. 1352 · Brolucizumab, p. 1353 · Dexamethasone, p. 1323 · Faricimab, p. 1353 · Ranibizumab, p. 1354

CORTICOSTEROIDS

Fluocinolone acetonide [Specialist drug]

08-Oct-2024

- **INDICATIONS AND DOSE**

Diabetic macular oedema | Prevention of relapse in recurrent non-infectious uveitis affecting the posterior segment of the eye
  ▸ BY INTRAVITREAL INJECTION
  ▸ Adult: Specialist drug – access specialist resources for dosing information

---

IMPORTANT SAFETY INFORMATION

MHRA/CHM ADVICE: CORTICOSTEROIDS: RARE RISK OF CENTRAL SEROUS CHORIORETINOPATHY WITH LOCAL AS WELL AS SYSTEMIC ADMINISTRATION (AUGUST 2017)
See Corticosteroids, general use p. 780.

NHS IMPROVEMENT PATIENT SAFETY ALERT: STEROID EMERGENCY CARD TO SUPPORT EARLY RECOGNITION AND TREATMENT OF ADRENAL CRISIS IN ADULTS (AUGUST 2020)
See Adrenal insufficiency p. 781.

- **CONTRA-INDICATIONS** Active or suspected ocular infection · active or suspected peri-ocular infection · pre-existing glaucoma
- **INTERACTIONS** → Appendix 1: fluocinolone
- **SIDE-EFFECTS**
  ▸ **Common or very common** Cataract · dry eye · eye discomfort · eye disorders · glaucoma · haemorrhage · vision disorders
  ▸ **Uncommon** Corneal deposits · eye inflammation · headache · optic nerve disorder
  ▸ **Frequency not known** Thromboembolism
- **NATIONAL FUNDING/ACCESS DECISIONS**
  For full details see funding body website
  NICE decisions
  ▸ **Fluocinolone acetonide intravitreal implant for treating recurrent non-infectious uveitis (July 2019)** NICE TA590
  Recommended with restrictions
  ▸ **Fluocinolone acetonide intravitreal implant for treating chronic diabetic macular oedema (March 2024)** NICE TA953
  Recommended
  Scottish Medicines Consortium (SMC) decisions
  ▸ **Fluocinolone acetonide (*Iluvien*®) for the treatment of vision impairment associated with chronic diabetic macular oedema, considered insufficiently responsive to available therapies (February 2014)** SMC No. 864/13 Recommended with restrictions
  ▸ **Fluocinolone acetonide (*Iluvien*®) for prevention of relapse in recurrent non-infectious uveitis affecting the posterior segment of the eye (September 2020)** SMC No. SMC2260 Recommended

- **MEDICINAL FORMS** There can be variation in the licensing of different medicines containing the same drug.
  Prolonged-release intravitreal implant
  ▸ **Iluvien** (Alimera Sciences Ltd)
  Fluocinolone acetonide 190 microgram ILUVIEN 190microgram intravitreal implant in applicator | 1 device PoM £5,500.00 (Hospital only)

6.3 Optic neuropathy

DRUGS FOR METABOLIC DISORDERS ›
ANTIOXIDANTS

Idebenone

30-Mar-2021

- **DRUG ACTION** Idebenone is a nootropic and antioxidant that is thought to act by restoring cellular ATP generation, thereby reactivating retinal ganglion cells.

- **INDICATIONS AND DOSE**

Leber's hereditary optic neuropathy (initiated by a specialist)
  ▸ BY MOUTH
  ▸ Adult: 300 mg 3 times a day

- **SIDE-EFFECTS**
  ▸ **Common or very common** Cough · diarrhoea · increased risk of infection · pain
  ▸ **Frequency not known** Agranulocytosis · anaemia · anxiety · appetite decreased · azotaemia · delirium · dizziness · dyspepsia · hallucination · headache · hepatitis · leucopenia · malaise · movement disorders · nausea · neutropenia · poriomania · seizure · skin reactions · stupor · thrombocytopenia · urine discolouration · vomiting

  SIDE-EFFECTS, FURTHER INFORMATION The metabolites of idebenone may cause red-brown discolouration of the urine. This effect is harmless, but the manufacturer advises caution as this may mask colour changes due to other causes (e.g. renal or blood disorders).

- **PREGNANCY** Manufacturer advises avoid unless potential benefit outweighs risk—no information available.
- **BREAST FEEDING** Manufacturer advises avoid—present in milk in *animal* studies.
- **HEPATIC IMPAIRMENT** Manufacturer advises caution (no information available).
- **RENAL IMPAIRMENT** Manufacturer advises use with caution—no information available.
- **NATIONAL FUNDING/ACCESS DECISIONS**
  For full details see funding body website
  Scottish Medicines Consortium (SMC) decisions
  ▸ **Idebenone (*Raxone*®) for the treatment of visual impairment in adolescent and adult patients with Leber's Hereditary Optic Neuropathy (LHON) (May 2017)** SMC No. 1226/17
  Recommended with restrictions
  All Wales Medicines Strategy Group (AWMSG) decisions
  ▸ **Idebenone (*Raxone*®) for the treatment of visual impairment in adolescent and adult patients with Leber's hereditary optic neuropathy (March 2021)** AWMSG No. 807 Recommended

- **MEDICINAL FORMS** There can be variation in the licensing of different medicines containing the same drug. Forms available from special-order manufacturers include: oral tablet
  Oral tablet
  CAUTIONARY AND ADVISORY LABELS 14, 21
  ▸ **Raxone** (Chiesi Ltd) ▼
  Idebenone 150 mg Raxone 150mg tablets | 180 tablet PoM £6,364.00 DT = £6,364.00

11

Eye

6.4 Vitreomacular traction

RECOMBINANT PROTEOLYTIC ENZYMES

Ocriplasmin [Specialist drug]

03-Aug-2020

● **INDICATIONS AND DOSE**

Vitreomacular traction

▸ BY INTRAVITREAL INJECTION

▸ **Adult:** Specialist drug – access specialist resources for dosing information

● **CONTRA-INDICATIONS** Active or suspected ocular or periocular infection · aphakia · exudative age-related macular degeneration · high myopia · history of rhegmatogenous retinal detachment · ischaemic retinopathies · large diameter macular hole (> 400 microns) · lens zonule instability · proliferative diabetic retinopathy · recent intra-ocular injection (including laser therapy) · recent ocular surgery · retinal vein occlusions · vitreous haemorrhage

● **SIDE-EFFECTS**

▸ **Common or very common** Dry eye · eye discomfort · eye disorders · eye inflammation · haemorrhage · retinal pigment epitheliopathy · vision disorders

● **NATIONAL FUNDING/ACCESS DECISIONS**
For full details see funding body website

NICE decisions

▸ Ocriplasmin for treating vitreomacular traction (October 2013) NICE TA297 Recommended with restrictions

Scottish Medicines Consortium (SMC) decisions

▸ Ocriplasmin (*Jetrea®*) in adults for the treatment of vitreomacular traction, including when associated with macular hole of diameter less than or equal to 400 microns (August 2014) SMC No. 892/13 Recommended with restrictions

● **MEDICINAL FORMS** No licensed medicines listed.

Chapter 12
Ear, nose and oropharynx

CONTENTS

Ear

Ear

17-May-2024

Otitis externa

Otitis externa refers to inflammation of the external ear canal which in some cases may involve oedema. It is primarily caused by bacterial infection. EvGr It is important to consider underlying otitis media as otitis externa may be secondary to otorrhoea from otitis media.

Any precipitating factors should be managed and cleaning the external ear canal should be considered (using dry swabbing, microsuction, or irrigation techniques) if ear wax or debris are blocking passage of topical medicine (may require specialist referral).

A solution of **acetic acid** 2% acts as an astringent in the external ear canal by reducing the pH and reducing bacterial and fungal cell growth. It may be used to treat mild otitis externa and is comparable to an anti-infective combined with a corticosteroid; efficacy is reduced if treatment extends beyond 1 week.

If infection is present, a topical anti-infective with or without a corticosteroid may be considered. These are used for a minimum of one week but if symptoms persist they can be used until they resolve, up to a maximum of 2 weeks. Prolonged and extensive use of topical anti-infective or corticosteroid treatment may affect the flora in the ear canal, increasing the risk of fungal infections. If a mild to moderate, uncomplicated fungal infection is suspected in the context of chronic otitis externa, a topical antifungal such as clotrimazole 1% solution p. 1361, acetic acid 2% spray [unlicensed indication], or clioquinol and a corticosteroid such as flumetasone pivalate with clioquinol p. 1361 can be offered. Sensitivity to topical ear preparations may also occur, especially with prolonged or recurrent use. Astringent agents such as aluminium acetate ear drops p. 1364 are also available. A

In view of reports of ototoxicity, treatment with topical **aminoglycosides** is contra-indicated in patients with a perforated tympanic membrane (eardrum). EvGr However, some specialists do use these drops cautiously in the presence of a perforation or patent grommet in patients with chronic suppurative otitis media and when other measures have failed for otitis externa; treatment should be considered only **by specialists** in the following circumstances:

- drops should only be used in the presence of obvious infection;
- treatment should be for no longer than 2 weeks;
- patients should be counselled on the risk of ototoxicity and given justification for the use of these topical antibiotics;
- baseline audiometry should be performed, if possible, before treatment is commenced.

Clinical expertise and judgement should be used to assess the risk of treatment versus the benefit to the patient in such circumstances. E

EvGr For severe pain associated with otitis externa, a simple analgesic, such as paracetamol p. 507 or ibuprofen p. 1302, is usually sufficient; codeine phosphate p. 517 may be used for severe pain. Oral antibacterials are rarely indicated but if they are required, consider seeking specialist advice. A systemic antibacterial may be considered if the infection is spreading outside the ear canal, the patient is systemically unwell, or in a high risk group (e.g. diabetics, immunocompromised patients, patients with severe infection or at high-risk of severe infection such as pseudomonal infections). Referral should be considered if there is extensive swelling of the auditory canal. A For further information, see *Otitis externa* in Ear infections, antibacterial therapy p. 582.

Otitis media

Acute otitis media

Acute otitis media is a self-limiting condition that mainly affects children. It is characterised by inflammation in the middle ear associated with effusion and accompanied by the rapid onset of signs and symptoms of an ear infection. The infection can be caused by viruses or bacteria; often both are present simultaneously.

Children with acute otitis media usually present with symptoms such as ear pain, rubbing of the ear, fever, irritability, crying, poor feeding, restlessness at night, cough, or rhinorrhoea. Symptoms usually resolve within 3 to 7 days without antibacterial drugs and they make little difference to the development of complications such as short-term hearing loss, perforated eardrum or recurrent infection. Acute complications such as mastoiditis, meningitis, intracranial abscess, sinus thrombosis, and facial nerve paralysis, are rare.

EvGr Children and their carers should be given advice about the usual duration of acute otitis media, self-care of symptoms such as pain and fever with paracetamol or ibuprofen p. 1302, and when to seek medical help. In addition to oral analgesics for pain relief, consider offering an ear drop containing an anaesthetic and an analgesic such as phenazone with lidocaine p. 1365, if immediate antibacterial treatment is not given and there is no eardrum perforation or otorrhoea. Children and their carers should be reassured that antibacterial drugs are usually not required.

An immediate antibacterial drug should be given if the child is systemically very unwell, has signs or symptoms of a more serious illness, or is at high risk of complications such as significant heart, lung, renal, liver or neuromuscular disease, immunosuppression, cystic fibrosis, or young children who were born prematurely. An immediate antibacterial drug can also be considered if otorrhoea (discharge following perforation of the eardrum) is present, or in children under 2 years of age with bilateral otitis media. (A) For further information, see *Otitis media* in Ear infections, antibacterial therapy p. 582.

[EvGr] Children with acute otitis media associated with a severe systemic infection or acute complications should be referred to hospital. (A)

Otitis media with effusion

Otitis media with effusion (OME), also known as glue ear, is characterised by the collection of fluid within the middle ear without any signs of inflammation or infection. It occurs most frequently in children, particularly in those aged between 6 months and 4 years, and is the most common cause of hearing impairment in children. It is more prevalent in children with cleft palate, Down's syndrome, primary ciliary dyskinesia, cystic fibrosis, and allergic rhinitis.

[EvGr] For children with OME without hearing loss, reassurance should be provided that it will often resolve on its own over time without treatment.

For children with suspected OME with hearing loss, referral to a specialist for a formal assessment should be made. If after 3 months, hearing loss is bilateral, or is impacting on daily living or communication, non-surgical or surgical interventions such as hearing aids or grommets, respectively, may be considered.

During grommet insertion, administration of a single dose of ciprofloxacin ear drops [unlicensed use] should be considered for prevention of otorrhoea and tube blockage. If there is otorrhoea after insertion, consider treatment with non-ototoxic antibacterial ear drops, such as ciprofloxacin [unlicensed use], for 5–7 days. For otorrhoea that persists and does not respond to antibacterial ear drops, consider grommet removal.

Oral or topical antibacterials, oral or nasal corticosteroids, antihistamines, leukotriene receptor antagonists, mucolytics, and decongestants are not recommended to treat OME due to a lack of evidence supporting their use. (A)

For further guidance on the management of OME, see NICE guideline: **Otitis media with effusion in under 12s** (see *Useful resources*).

Chronic suppurative otitis media

Chronic suppurative otitis media is a chronic inflammation of the middle ear and mastoid cavity, and is thought to be a complication of acute otitis media. The usual presentation is otorrhoea through a tympanic perforation and can involve infection due to a number of different bacteria or fungi. [EvGr] Referral to an ear, nose and throat specialist is required and treatment is likely to involve antibacterials, corticosteroids (usually topical), and intensive aural cleaning. (A)

Removal of ear wax

Ear wax (cerumen) is a normal bodily secretion which provides a protective film on the lining of the ear canal and need only be removed if it causes hearing loss or other symptoms (such as discomfort or tinnitus), or interferes with a proper view of the ear canal and/or ear drum, or in order to take an impression of the ear canal.

[EvGr] To soften ear wax and aid removal, ear drops can be used, such as olive oil ear drops p. 1365, almond oil ear drops p. 1365, sodium bicarbonate ear drops p. 1365, or sodium chloride 0.9% nasal drops p. 1180 [unlicensed use as ear drops]. (A) The drops can be used three to four times daily for several days. Lying down with the affected ear uppermost, ear drops are instilled before waiting for 5 minutes. Ear drops are not recommended for patients suspected of having a perforated tympanic membrane, active dermatitis, or active infection of the ear canal.

[EvGr] If necessary, ear wax may be removed by irrigation, microsuction, or another method of removal (such as removal using a probe). Pre-treatment wax softeners should be used, either immediately before ear irrigation or for up to 5 days beforehand. Pre-treatment and irrigation may need to be repeated once if unsuccessful after the first attempt; if unsuccessful after the second attempt, referral to a specialist ear care service or an ear, nose, and throat specialist is required. (A) Ear irrigation is not recommended in young children, in patients unable to co-operate with the procedure, in patients with acute otitis externa with an oedematous ear canal and painful pinna, or in those with a history of otitis media in the last six weeks, any ear surgery, or any previous problem with irrigation. It should also be avoided in patients with mucus discharge from the ear within the past 12 months, a foreign body in the ear, grommets in place, cleft palate, or factors that increase the risk of trauma, infection or haemorrhage (such as dermatitis, infection/abnormalities of the ear canal, or perforated tympanic membrane or history of perforated tympanic membrane). A person who has hearing in one ear only should not have that ear irrigated because even a very slight risk of damage may lead to permanent deafness. Irrigation should be used with caution and carried out on a low setting in patients with: tinnitus, vertigo, recurrent otitis externa, recurrent otitis media, a history of radiotherapy of the head or neck, and in patients who are immunocompromised or taking anticoagulants or high-dose steroids.

Useful resources

Otitis media with effusion in under 12s. National Institute for Health and Care Excellence. NICE guideline 233. August 2023.
www.nice.org.uk/guidance/ng233

1   Otitis externa

ANTIBACTERIALS > AMINOGLYCOSIDES

Framycetin sulfate

29-Mar-2023

● **INDICATIONS AND DOSE**

Bacterial infection in otitis externa

▶ TO THE EAR

▶ Adult: (consult product literature)

IMPORTANT SAFETY INFORMATION

MHRA/CHM ADVICE: AMINOGLYCOSIDES (GENTAMICIN, AMIKACIN, TOBRAMYCIN, AND NEOMYCIN): INCREASED RISK OF DEAFNESS IN PATIENTS WITH MITOCHONDRIAL MUTATIONS (JANUARY 2021)
The use of aminoglycosides is associated with rare cases of ototoxicity. A safety review found an increased risk of deafness in patients with mitochondrial mutations (particularly the m.1555A>G mutation), including cases where the patient's aminoglycoside serum levels were within the recommended range. Nevertheless, these mitochondrial mutations are considered rare and penetrance is uncertain. No cases were identified with topical preparations but, based on a shared mechanism of effect, there is a potential risk with aminoglycosides administered at the site of toxicity i.e. the ear.

Healthcare professionals are advised to consider the need for aminoglycoside treatment versus alternative options in patients with susceptible mutations. The need for genetic testing especially in those requiring recurrent or long-term treatment with aminoglycosides should also be considered, however, urgent treatment should not be delayed. To minimise the risks of adverse effects, continuous monitoring of renal and auditory function, as well as hepatic and laboratory parameters, is recommended for all patients. Those with known mitochondrial mutations or a family history of ototoxicity are advised to inform their doctor or pharmacist before using an aminoglycoside.

- **CONTRA-INDICATIONS** Perforated tympanic membrane
- **CAUTIONS** Avoid prolonged use
- **PRE-TREATMENT SCREENING** NHS England commissions genetic testing under the *National genomic test directory* indication: R65 - Aminoglycoside exposure posing risk to hearing. The testing criteria is significant exposure to aminoglycosides posing risk of ototoxicity. This testing is relevant to individuals with a predisposition to gram-negative infections or with hearing loss who have been exposed to aminoglycosides. For further information, see www.england.nhs.uk/publication/national-genomic-test-directories/.

- **MEDICINAL FORMS** No licensed medicines listed.

  Combinations available: *Dexamethasone with framycetin sulfate and gramicidin,* p. 1363

Gentamicin

☞ 594

10-Feb-2025

- **INDICATIONS AND DOSE**

Bacterial infection in otitis externa
- ▸ TO THE EAR
- ▸ Child: Apply 2–3 drops 4–5 times a day, (including a dose at bedtime)
- ▸ Adult: Apply 2–3 drops 4–5 times a day, (including a dose at bedtime)

- **UNLICENSED USE** Gentamicin doses in BNF Publications may differ from those in product literature.

IMPORTANT SAFETY INFORMATION

MHRA/CHM ADVICE: AMINOGLYCOSIDES (GENTAMICIN, AMIKACIN, TOBRAMYCIN, AND NEOMYCIN): INCREASED RISK OF DEAFNESS IN PATIENTS WITH MITOCHONDRIAL MUTATIONS (JANUARY 2021)

The use of aminoglycosides is associated with rare cases of ototoxicity. A safety review found an increased risk of deafness in patients with mitochondrial mutations (particularly the m.1555A>G mutation), including cases where the patient's aminoglycoside serum levels were within the recommended range. Nevertheless, these mitochondrial mutations are considered rare and penetrance is uncertain. No cases were identified with topical preparations but, based on a shared mechanism of effect, there is a potential risk with gentamicin and other aminoglycosides administered at the site of toxicity i.e. the ear.

Healthcare professionals are advised to consider the need for aminoglycoside treatment versus alternative options in patients with susceptible mutations. The need for genetic testing especially in those requiring recurrent or long-term treatment with aminoglycosides should also be considered, however, urgent treatment should not be delayed. To minimise the risks of adverse effects, continuous monitoring of renal and auditory function, as well as hepatic and laboratory parameters, is recommended for all patients. Those with known mitochondrial mutations or a family history of ototoxicity are advised to inform their doctor or pharmacist before using an aminoglycoside.

- **CONTRA-INDICATIONS** Patent grommet (although may be used by specialists, see Ear p. 1357) · perforated tympanic membrane (although may be used by specialists, see Ear p. 1357)
- **CAUTIONS** Avoid prolonged use
- **INTERACTIONS** → Appendix 1: aminoglycosides
- **SIDE-EFFECTS** Since systemic absorption can follow topical administration to the eye and ear, also consider the side-effects of systemic aminoglycosides.
- **PRE-TREATMENT SCREENING** NHS England commissions genetic testing under the *National genomic test directory* indication: R65 - Aminoglycoside exposure posing risk to hearing. The testing criteria is significant exposure to aminoglycosides posing risk of ototoxicity. This testing is relevant to individuals with a predisposition to gram-negative infections or with hearing loss who have been exposed to aminoglycosides. For further information, see www.england.nhs.uk/publication/national-genomic-test-directories/.

- **MEDICINAL FORMS** There can be variation in the licensing of different medicines containing the same drug.

  Ear/eye drops solution

  EXCIPIENTS: May contain Benzalkonium chloride

  ▸ **Gentamicin (Non-proprietary)**

    Gentamicin (as Gentamicin sulfate) 3 mg per 1 ml Gentamicin 0.3% ear/eye drops | 10 ml [PoM] £20.00 DT = £20.00

Gentamicin with hydrocortisone

20-Jul-2023

- **INDICATIONS AND DOSE**

Eczematous inflammation in otitis externa
- ▸ TO THE EAR
- ▸ Child: Apply 2–4 drops 4–5 times a day, (including a dose at bedtime)
- ▸ Adult: Apply 2–4 drops 4–5 times a day, (including a dose at bedtime)

IMPORTANT SAFETY INFORMATION

MHRA/CHM ADVICE: CORTICOSTEROIDS: RARE RISK OF CENTRAL SEROUS CHORIORETINOPATHY WITH LOCAL AS WELL AS SYSTEMIC ADMINISTRATION (AUGUST 2017)

See Corticosteroids, general use p. 780.

NHS IMPROVEMENT PATIENT SAFETY ALERT: STEROID EMERGENCY CARD TO SUPPORT EARLY RECOGNITION AND TREATMENT OF ADRENAL CRISIS IN ADULTS (AUGUST 2020)

See Adrenal insufficiency p. 781.

MHRA/CHM ADVICE: AMINOGLYCOSIDES (GENTAMICIN, AMIKACIN, TOBRAMYCIN, AND NEOMYCIN): INCREASED RISK OF DEAFNESS IN PATIENTS WITH MITOCHONDRIAL MUTATIONS (JANUARY 2021)

The use of aminoglycosides is associated with rare cases of ototoxicity. A safety review found an increased risk of deafness in patients with mitochondrial mutations (particularly the m.1555A>G mutation), including cases where the patient's aminoglycoside serum levels were within the recommended range. Nevertheless, these mitochondrial mutations are considered rare and penetrance is uncertain. No cases were identified with topical preparations but, based on a shared mechanism of effect, there is a potential risk with gentamicin and other aminoglycosides administered at the site of toxicity i.e. the ear.

Healthcare professionals are advised to consider the need for aminoglycoside treatment versus alternative options in patients with susceptible mutations. The need for genetic testing especially in those requiring recurrent or long-term treatment with aminoglycosides should also be considered, however, urgent treatment should not be delayed. To minimise the risks of adverse effects, continuous monitoring of renal and auditory function, as well as hepatic and laboratory parameters, is recommended for all patients. Those with known mitochondrial mutations or a family history of ototoxicity are advised to inform their doctor or pharmacist before using an aminoglycoside.

ADRENAL INSUFFICIENCY CARD (APRIL 2023)
The British Society for Paediatric Endocrinology and Diabetes (BSPED) has developed an Adrenal Insufficiency Card which should be issued to children with adrenal insufficiency and steroid dependence. The card includes a management summary for the emergency treatment of adrenal crisis and sick day dosing, and can be issued by any healthcare professional managing such patients. The BSPED Adrenal Insufficiency Card is available at: www.bsped.org.uk/adrenal-insufficiency.

● **CONTRA-INDICATIONS** Patent grommet (although may be used by specialists, see Ear p. 1357) · perforated tympanic membrane (although may be used by specialists, see Ear p. 1357)

● **CAUTIONS** Avoid prolonged use

● **SIDE-EFFECTS** Local reaction

● **PRE-TREATMENT SCREENING** NHS England commissions genetic testing under the *National genomic test directory* indication: R65 - Aminoglycoside exposure posing risk to hearing. The testing criteria is significant exposure to aminoglycosides posing risk of ototoxicity. This testing is relevant to individuals with a predisposition to gram-negative infections or with hearing loss who have been exposed to aminoglycosides. For further information, see www.england.nhs.uk/publication/national-genomic-test-directories/.

● **PATIENT AND CARER ADVICE**
▸ In adults If systemic absorption occurs following topical and local use, side-effects applicable to systemic corticosteroids may apply; a patient information leaflet should be supplied and the need for a Steroid Treatment Card and a Steroid Emergency Card considered, see Corticosteroids, general use p. 780.
▸ In children If systemic absorption occurs following topical and local use, side-effects applicable to systemic corticosteroids may apply; a patient information leaflet should be supplied and the need for a Steroid Treatment Card considered, see Corticosteroids, general use p. 780.
Medicines for Children leaflet: Gentamicin and hydrocortisone ear drops for inflammatory ear infections www.medicinesforchildren.org.uk/medicines/gentamicin-and-hydrocortisone-ear-drops-for-inflammatory-ear-infections/

● **MEDICINAL FORMS** There can be variation in the licensing of different medicines containing the same drug.
Ear drops
EXCIPIENTS: May contain Benzalkonium chloride, disodium edetate
▸ **Gentamicin with hydrocortisone (Non-proprietary)**
Gentamicin (as Gentamicin sulfate) 3 mg per 1 ml, Hydrocortisone acetate 10 mg per 1 ml Gentamicin 0.3% / Hydrocortisone acetate 1% ear drops | 10 ml PoM £33.26 DT = £33.26

ANTIBACTERIALS ❭ QUINOLONES

❧ 646

Ciprofloxacin

24-Jul-2024

● **INDICATIONS AND DOSE**

Acute otitis externa
▸ TO THE EAR USING EAR DROPS
▸ Child 1-17 years: Apply 0.25 mL twice daily for 7 days, each 0.25 mL dose contains 0.5 mg ciprofloxacin
▸ Adult: Apply 0.25 mL twice daily for 7 days, each 0.25 mL dose contains 0.5 mg ciprofloxacin

● **CAUTIONS** Known (or at risk of) perforated tympanic membrane

● **INTERACTIONS** → Appendix 1: quinolones

● **SIDE-EFFECTS**
▸ **Uncommon** Ear pruritus

● **PRESCRIBING AND DISPENSING INFORMATION** For choice of antibacterial therapy, see Ear infections, antibacterial therapy p. 582.

● **HANDLING AND STORAGE** Manufacturer advises discard any ampoules remaining 8 days after opening the pouch.

● **PATIENT AND CARER ADVICE**
Medicines for Children leaflet: Ciprofloxacin drops for infection www.medicinesforchildren.org.uk/medicines/ciprofloxacin-drops-for-infection/

● **NATIONAL FUNDING/ACCESS DECISIONS**
For full details see funding body website
Scottish Medicines Consortium (SMC) decisions
▸ Ciprofloxacin (*Cetraxal*®) for the treatment of acute otitis externa in adults and children older than 1 year with an intact tympanic membrane, caused by ciprofloxacin susceptible microorganisms (April 2018) SMC No. 1320/18 Recommended with restrictions
All Wales Medicines Strategy Group (AWMSG) decisions
▸ Ciprofloxacin (*Cetraxal*®) for the treatment of acute otitis externa in adults and children older than 1 year with an intact tympanic membrane, caused by ciprofloxacin susceptible microorganisms (July 2018) AWMSG No. 1343 Recommended

● **MEDICINAL FORMS** There can be variation in the licensing of different medicines containing the same drug. Forms available from special-order manufacturers include: ear drops
Ear drops
▸ **Cetraxal** (Aspire Pharma Ltd)
Ciprofloxacin (as Ciprofloxacin hydrochloride) 2 mg per 1 ml Cetraxal 2mg/ml ear drops 0.25ml unit dose | 15 unit dose PoM £6.01 DT = £6.01

Combinations available: *Ciprofloxacin with dexamethasone,* p. 1362 · *Ciprofloxacin with fluocinolone acetonide,* p. 1363

ANTIBACTERIALS ❭ OTHER

Chloramphenicol

24-Jul-2024

● **DRUG ACTION** Chloramphenicol is a potent broad-spectrum antibiotic.

● **INDICATIONS AND DOSE**

Bacterial infection in otitis externa
▸ TO THE EAR
▸ Child: Apply 2–3 drops 2–3 times a day
▸ Adult: Apply 2–3 drops 2–3 times a day

● **CAUTIONS** Avoid prolonged use

● **INTERACTIONS** → Appendix 1: chloramphenicol

● **SIDE-EFFECTS** Blood disorder · bone marrow depression

● **PATIENT AND CARER ADVICE**
Medicines for Children leaflet: Chloramphenicol ear drops for ear infections (otitis externa) www.medicinesforchildren.org.uk/medicines/chloramphenicol-ear-drops-for-ear-infections-otitis-externa/

● **LESS SUITABLE FOR PRESCRIBING** Chloramphenicol ear drops are less suitable for prescribing.

● **MEDICINAL FORMS** There can be variation in the licensing of different medicines containing the same drug.
Ear drops
EXCIPIENTS: May contain Propylene glycol
▸ **Chloramphenicol (Non-proprietary)**
Chloramphenicol 50 mg per 1 ml Chloramphenicol 5% ear drops | 10 ml PoM £132.44-£238.40 DT = £132.44
Chloramphenicol 100 mg per 1 ml Chloramphenicol 10% ear drops | 10 ml PoM £123.27-£221.88 DT = £123.27

ANTIFUNGALS > IMIDAZOLE ANTIFUNGALS

Clotrimazole

10-Nov-2021

- **INDICATIONS AND DOSE**

Fungal infection in otitis externa

▶ TO THE EAR
▸ Child: Apply 2–3 times a day continue for at least 14 days after disappearance of infection
▸ Adult: Apply 2–3 times a day continue for at least 14 days after disappearance of infection

- **INTERACTIONS** → Appendix 1: antifungals, azoles
- **SIDE-EFFECTS** Hypersensitivity · oedema · pain · paraesthesia · skin reactions
- **PATIENT AND CARER ADVICE**

Medicines for Children leaflet: Clotrimazole for fungal infections www.medicinesforchildren.org.uk/medicines/clotrimazole-for-fungal-infections/

- **MEDICINAL FORMS** There can be variation in the licensing of different medicines containing the same drug.

Cutaneous or ear solution

▸ Canesten (clotrimazole) (Bayer Plc)
Clotrimazole 10 mg per 1 ml Canesten 1% solution | 20 ml [P] £2.54 DT = £2.53

CORTICOSTEROIDS

F 1408

Betamethasone

08-Oct-2024

- **DRUG ACTION** Betamethasone has very high glucocorticoid activity and insignificant mineralocorticoid activity.

- **INDICATIONS AND DOSE**

BETNESOL ®

Eczematous inflammation in otitis externa

▶ TO THE EAR
▸ Adult: Apply 2–3 drops every 2–3 hours, reduce frequency when relief obtained

VISTAMETHASONE ®

Eczematous inflammation in otitis externa

▶ TO THE EAR
▸ Adult: Apply 2–3 drops every 3–4 hours, reduce frequency when relief obtained

- **CONTRA-INDICATIONS** Avoid alone in the presence of untreated infection (combine with suitable anti-infective)
- **CAUTIONS** Avoid prolonged use
- **INTERACTIONS** → Appendix 1: corticosteroids
- **SIDE-EFFECTS** Since systemic absorption can follow topical administration to the eye and ear, also consider the side-effects of systemic corticosteroids.

- **MEDICINAL FORMS** There can be variation in the licensing of different medicines containing the same drug.

Ear/eye/nose drops solution

EXCIPIENTS: May contain Benzalkonium chloride, disodium edetate

▸ Betnesol (RPH Pharmaceuticals AB)
Betamethasone sodium phosphate 1 mg per 1 ml Betnesol 0.1% eye/ear/nose drops | 10 ml [PoM] £2.32 DT = £2.32
▸ Vistamethasone (Martindale Pharmaceuticals Ltd)
Betamethasone sodium phosphate 1 mg per 1 ml Vistamethasone 0.1% ear/eye/nose drops | 5 ml [PoM] £11.30

Flumetasone pivalate with clioquinol

20-Jul-2023

- **INDICATIONS AND DOSE**

Eczematous inflammation in otitis externa | Mild bacterial or fungal infections in otitis externa

▶ TO THE EAR
▸ Child 2–17 years: 2–3 drops twice daily for 7–10 days
▸ Adult: 2–3 drops twice daily for 7–10 days

IMPORTANT SAFETY INFORMATION

MHRA/CHM ADVICE: CORTICOSTEROIDS: RARE RISK OF CENTRAL SEROUS CHORIORETINOPATHY WITH LOCAL AS WELL AS SYSTEMIC ADMINISTRATION (AUGUST 2017)
See Corticosteroids, general use p. 780.

NHS IMPROVEMENT PATIENT SAFETY ALERT: STEROID EMERGENCY CARD TO SUPPORT EARLY RECOGNITION AND TREATMENT OF ADRENAL CRISIS IN ADULTS (AUGUST 2020)
See Adrenal insufficiency p. 781.

ADRENAL INSUFFICIENCY CARD (APRIL 2023)
The British Society for Paediatric Endocrinology and Diabetes (BSPED) has developed an Adrenal Insufficiency Card which should be issued to children with adrenal insufficiency and steroid dependence. The card includes a management summary for the emergency treatment of adrenal crisis and sick day dosing, and can be issued by any healthcare professional managing such patients. The BSPED Adrenal Insufficiency Card is available at: www.bsped.org.uk/adrenal-insufficiency.

- **CONTRA-INDICATIONS** Iodine sensitivity
- **CAUTIONS** Avoid prolonged use · manufacturer advises avoid in perforated tympanic membrane (but used by specialists for short periods)
- **SIDE-EFFECTS** Paraesthesia · skin reactions
- **PATIENT AND CARER ADVICE** Clioquinol stains skin and clothing.
▸ In adults If systemic absorption occurs following topical and local use, side-effects applicable to systemic corticosteroids may apply; a patient information leaflet should be supplied and the need for a Steroid Treatment Card and a Steroid Emergency Card considered, see Corticosteroids, general use p. 780.
▸ In children If systemic absorption occurs following topical and local use, side-effects applicable to systemic corticosteroids may apply; a patient information leaflet should be supplied and the need for a Steroid Treatment Card considered, see Corticosteroids, general use p. 780.

- **MEDICINAL FORMS** There can be variation in the licensing of different medicines containing the same drug.

Ear drops

▸ Flumetasone pivalate with clioquinol (Non-proprietary)
Flumetasone pivalate 200 microgram per 1 ml, Clioquinol 10 mg per 1 ml Flumetasone 0.02% / Clioquinol 1% ear drops | 7.5 ml [PoM] £11.34 DT = £11.34

F 1408

Prednisolone

24-Jun-2024

- **DRUG ACTION** Prednisolone exerts predominantly glucocorticoid effects with minimal mineralocorticoid effects.

- **INDICATIONS AND DOSE**

Eczematous inflammation in otitis externa

▶ TO THE EAR
▸ Child: Apply 2–3 drops every 2–3 hours, frequency to be reduced when relief obtained
▸ Adult: Apply 2–3 drops every 2–3 hours, frequency to be reduced when relief obtained

- **CONTRA-INDICATIONS** Avoid alone in the presence of untreated infection (combine with suitable anti-infective)
- **CAUTIONS** Avoid prolonged use
- **INTERACTIONS** → Appendix 1: corticosteroids
- **SIDE-EFFECTS** Local reaction

- **MEDICINAL FORMS** There can be variation in the licensing of different medicines containing the same drug. Forms available from special-order manufacturers include: ear drops

Ear drops
EXCIPIENTS: May contain Benzalkonium chloride, disodium edetate

Ear/eye drops solution
EXCIPIENTS: May contain Benzalkonium chloride, disodium edetate
- ▶ **Prednisolone (Non-proprietary)**
  Prednisolone sodium phosphate 5 mg per 1 ml Prednisolone sodium phosphate 0.5% ear/eye drops | 10 ml [PoM] £2.57 DT = £2.57

CORTICOSTEROIDS > CORTICOSTEROID COMBINATIONS WITH ANTI-INFECTIVES

Betamethasone with neomycin   08-Oct-2024

The properties listed below are those particular to the combination only. For the properties of the components please consider, betamethasone p. 1361.

- **INDICATIONS AND DOSE**

Eczematous inflammation in otitis externa
- ▶ TO THE EAR USING EAR DROPS
- ▶ Child: Apply 2–3 drops 3–4 times a day
- ▶ Adult: Apply 2–3 drops 3–4 times a day

> **IMPORTANT SAFETY INFORMATION**
>
> MHRA/CHM ADVICE: AMINOGLYCOSIDES (GENTAMICIN, AMIKACIN, TOBRAMYCIN, AND NEOMYCIN): INCREASED RISK OF DEAFNESS IN PATIENTS WITH MITOCHONDRIAL MUTATIONS (JANUARY 2021)
>
> The use of aminoglycosides is associated with rare cases of ototoxicity. A safety review found an increased risk of deafness in patients with mitochondrial mutations (particularly the m.1555A>G mutation), including cases where the patient's aminoglycoside serum levels were within the recommended range. Nevertheless, these mitochondrial mutations are considered rare and penetrance is uncertain. No cases were identified with topical preparations but, based on a shared mechanism of effect, there is a potential risk with neomycin and other aminoglycosides administered at the site of toxicity i.e. the ear. Healthcare professionals are advised to consider the need for aminoglycoside treatment versus alternative options in patients with susceptible mutations. The need for genetic testing especially in those requiring recurrent or long-term treatment with aminoglycosides should also be considered, however, urgent treatment should not be delayed. To minimise the risks of adverse effects, continuous monitoring of renal and auditory function, as well as hepatic and laboratory parameters, is recommended for all patients. Those with known mitochondrial mutations or a family history of ototoxicity are advised to inform their doctor or pharmacist before using an aminoglycoside.

- **CONTRA-INDICATIONS** Patent grommet (although may be used by specialists, see Ear p. 1357) · perforated tympanic membrane (although may be used by specialists, see Ear p. 1357)
- **CAUTIONS** Avoid prolonged use
- **INTERACTIONS** → Appendix 1: corticosteroids · neomycin
- **PRE-TREATMENT SCREENING** NHS England commissions genetic testing under the *National genomic test directory* indication: R65 - Aminoglycoside exposure posing risk to hearing. The testing criteria is significant exposure to aminoglycosides posing risk of ototoxicity. This testing is relevant to individuals with a predisposition to gram-negative infections or with hearing loss who have been exposed to aminoglycosides. For further information, see www.england.nhs.uk/publication/national-genomic-test-directories/.

- **MEDICINAL FORMS** There can be variation in the licensing of different medicines containing the same drug.
Ear/eye/nose drops solution
EXCIPIENTS: May contain Benzalkonium chloride, disodium edetate
- ▶ **Betnesol-N** (RPH Pharmaceuticals AB)
  Betamethasone (as Betamethasone sodium phosphate) 1 mg per 1 ml, Neomycin sulfate 5 mg per 1 ml Betnesol-N ear/eye/nose drops | 10 ml [PoM] £2.39 DT = £2.39

Ciprofloxacin with dexamethasone

04-Nov-2020

The properties listed below are those particular to the combination only. For the properties of the components please consider, dexamethasone p. 786, ciprofloxacin p. 1360.

- **INDICATIONS AND DOSE**

Acute otitis media in patients with tympanostomy tubes
- ▶ TO THE EAR
- ▶ Adult: Apply 4 drops twice daily for 7 days
Acute otitis externa
- ▶ TO THE EAR
- ▶ Adult: Apply 4 drops twice daily for 7 days

- **CONTRA-INDICATIONS** Fungal ear infections · viral ear infections
- **CAUTIONS** Avoid prolonged use
- **INTERACTIONS** → Appendix 1: corticosteroids · quinolones
- **SIDE-EFFECTS**
- ▶ **Common or very common** Ear discomfort
- ▶ **Uncommon** Ear infection fungal · flushing · irritability · malaise · otorrhoea · paraesthesia · skin reactions · taste altered · vomiting
- ▶ **Rare or very rare** Dizziness · headache · hearing loss · tinnitus

  SIDE-EFFECTS, FURTHER INFORMATION Manufacturer advises further evaluation of underlying conditions if otorrhoea persists after a full course, or if at least two episodes of otorrhoea occur within 6 months.
- **PREGNANCY** Manufacturer advises use only if potential benefit outweighs risk—no information available.
- **BREAST FEEDING** Manufacturer advises caution—no information available.
- **PATIENT AND CARER ADVICE** Manufacturer advises counselling on administration.
- **NATIONAL FUNDING/ACCESS DECISIONS**
  For full details see funding body website

Scottish Medicines Consortium (SMC) decisions
- ▶ **Ciprofloxacin with dexamethasone (*Cilodex*®) for treatment of the following infections in adults and children: Acute otitis media in patients with tympanostomy tubes (AOMT) (July 2017)** SMC No. 1256/17 Recommended with restrictions

- **MEDICINAL FORMS** There can be variation in the licensing of different medicines containing the same drug.
Ear drops
EXCIPIENTS: May contain Benzalkonium chloride, disodium edetate
- ▶ **Ciprofloxacin with dexamethasone (Non-proprietary)**
  Dexamethasone 1 mg per 1 ml, Ciprofloxacin (as Ciprofloxacin hydrochloride) 3 mg per 1 ml Ciprofloxacin 0.3% / Dexamethasone 0.1% ear drops | 5 ml [PoM] £6.12 DT = £6.12

Ciprofloxacin with fluocinolone acetonide
20-Jul-2023

The properties listed below are those particular to the combination only. For the properties of the components please consider, ciprofloxacin p. 1360.

● INDICATIONS AND DOSE

Acute otitis externa | Acute otitis media in patients with tympanostomy tubes
▸ TO THE EAR
▸ Adult: Apply 0.25 mL twice daily for 7 days

DOSE EQUIVALENCE AND CONVERSION
▸ Each 0.25 mL dose contains 0.75 mg ciprofloxacin and 0.0625 mg of fluocinolone acetonide.

IMPORTANT SAFETY INFORMATION

MHRA/CHM ADVICE: CORTICOSTEROIDS: RARE RISK OF CENTRAL SEROUS CHORIORETINOPATHY WITH LOCAL AS WELL AS SYSTEMIC ADMINISTRATION (AUGUST 2017)
See Corticosteroids, general use p. 780.

NHS IMPROVEMENT PATIENT SAFETY ALERT: STEROID EMERGENCY CARD TO SUPPORT EARLY RECOGNITION AND TREATMENT OF ADRENAL CRISIS IN ADULTS (AUGUST 2020)
See Adrenal insufficiency p. 781.

● CONTRA-INDICATIONS Fungal ear infections · viral ear infections

● INTERACTIONS → Appendix 1: fluocinolone · quinolones

● SIDE-EFFECTS
▸ **Common or very common** Ear discomfort · taste altered
▸ **Uncommon** Crying · dizziness · fatigue · flushing · headache · hearing impairment · increased risk of infection · irritability · otorrhoea · paraesthesia · skin reactions · tinnitus · tympanic membrane disorder · vomiting

SIDE-EFFECTS, FURTHER INFORMATION Manufacturer advises further evaluation of underlying conditions if otorrhoea persists after a full course, or if at least two episodes of otorrhoea occur within 6 months.

● PREGNANCY Manufacturer advises use only if potential benefit outweighs risk—limited information available.

● BREAST FEEDING Manufacturer advises caution.

● PATIENT AND CARER ADVICE Manufacturer advises counselling on administration.

If systemic absorption occurs following topical and local use, side-effects applicable to systemic corticosteroids may apply; a patient information leaflet should be supplied and the need for a Steroid Treatment Card and a Steroid Emergency Card considered, see Corticosteroids, general use p. 780.

● MEDICINAL FORMS There can be variation in the licensing of different medicines containing the same drug.
Ear drops
EXCIPIENTS: May contain Polysorbates
▸ **Cetraxal Plus** (Aspire Pharma Ltd)
Fluocinolone acetonide 250 microgram per 1 ml, Ciprofloxacin (as Ciprofloxacin hydrochloride) 3 mg per 1 ml Cetraxal Plus 3mg/ml + 0.25mg/ml ear drops 0.25ml unit dose | 15 unit dose PoM £6.01 DT = £6.01

Dexamethasone with framycetin sulfate and gramicidin
02-Mar-2021

The properties listed below are those particular to the combination only. For the properties of the components please consider, dexamethasone p. 786, framycetin sulfate p. 1358.

● INDICATIONS AND DOSE

Eczematous inflammation in otitis externa
▸ TO THE EAR
▸ Child: 2–3 drops 3–4 times a day
▸ Adult: 2–3 drops 3–4 times a day

● CAUTIONS Avoid prolonged use

● INTERACTIONS → Appendix 1: corticosteroids

● LESS SUITABLE FOR PRESCRIBING *Sofradex*® is less suitable for prescribing.

● MEDICINAL FORMS There can be variation in the licensing of different medicines containing the same drug.
Ear/eye drops solution
EXCIPIENTS: May contain Polysorbates
▸ **Sofradex** (Neon Healthcare Ltd)
Gramicidin 50 microgram per 1 ml, Dexamethasone (as Dexamethasone sodium metasulfobenzoate) 500 microgram per 1 ml, Framycetin sulfate 5 mg per 1 ml Sofradex ear/eye drops | 8 ml PoM £7.50

Dexamethasone with glacial acetic acid and neomycin sulfate
29-Mar-2023

The properties listed below are those particular to the combination only. For the properties of the components please consider, dexamethasone p. 786.

● INDICATIONS AND DOSE

Eczematous inflammation in otitis externa
▸ TO THE EAR
▸ Child 2-17 years: Apply 1 spray 3 times a day
▸ Adult: Apply 1 spray 3 times a day

IMPORTANT SAFETY INFORMATION

MHRA/CHM ADVICE: AMINOGLYCOSIDES (GENTAMICIN, AMIKACIN, TOBRAMYCIN, AND NEOMYCIN): INCREASED RISK OF DEAFNESS IN PATIENTS WITH MITOCHONDRIAL MUTATIONS (JANUARY 2021)
The use of aminoglycosides is associated with rare cases of ototoxicity. A safety review found an increased risk of deafness in patients with mitochondrial mutations (particularly the m.1555A>G mutation), including cases where the patient's aminoglycoside serum levels were within the recommended range. Nevertheless, these mitochondrial mutations are considered rare and penetrance is uncertain. No cases were identified with topical preparations but, based on a shared mechanism of effect, there is a potential risk with neomycin and other aminoglycosides administered at the site of toxicity i.e. the ear.

Healthcare professionals are advised to consider the need for aminoglycoside treatment versus alternative options in patients with susceptible mutations. The need for genetic testing especially in those requiring recurrent or long-term treatment with aminoglycosides should also be considered, however, urgent treatment should not be delayed. To minimise the risks of adverse effects, continuous monitoring of renal and auditory function, as well as hepatic and laboratory parameters, is recommended for all patients. Those with known mitochondrial mutations or a family history of ototoxicity are advised to inform their doctor or pharmacist before using an aminoglycoside.

- **CONTRA-INDICATIONS** Patent grommet (although may be used by specialists, see Ear p. 1357) · perforated tympanic membrane (although may be used by specialists, see Ear p. 1357)
- **CAUTIONS** Avoid prolonged use
- **INTERACTIONS** → Appendix 1: corticosteroids · neomycin
- **SIDE-EFFECTS** Paraesthesia · skin reactions · vision blurred
- **PRE-TREATMENT SCREENING** NHS England commissions genetic testing under the *National genomic test directory* indication: R65 - Aminoglycoside exposure posing risk to hearing. The testing criteria is significant exposure to aminoglycosides posing risk of ototoxicity. This testing is relevant to individuals with a predisposition to gram-negative infections or with hearing loss who have been exposed to aminoglycosides. For further information, see www.england.nhs.uk/publication/national-genomic-test-directories/.

- **MEDICINAL FORMS** There can be variation in the licensing of different medicines containing the same drug.
  Spray
  EXCIPIENTS: May contain Hydroxybenzoates (parabens)
  - Otomize (Ennogen Healthcare International Ltd)
    Dexamethasone 1 mg per 1 gram, Neomycin sulfate 5 mg per 1 gram, Acetic acid glacial 20 mg per 1 gram Otomize ear spray | 5 ml PoM £3.27

Hydrocortisone with neomycin and polymyxin B sulfate

29-Mar-2023

The properties listed below are those particular to the combination only. For the properties of the components please consider, hydrocortisone p. 1413.

- **INDICATIONS AND DOSE**

  Bacterial infection in otitis externa
  - TO THE EAR
  - Child 3-17 years: Apply 3 drops 3–4 times a day for 7 days, review treatment if there is no clinical improvement
  - Adult: Apply 3 drops 3–4 times a day for 7 days, review treatment if there is no clinical improvement

---

IMPORTANT SAFETY INFORMATION

MHRA/CHM ADVICE: AMINOGLYCOSIDES (GENTAMICIN, AMIKACIN, TOBRAMYCIN, AND NEOMYCIN): INCREASED RISK OF DEAFNESS IN PATIENTS WITH MITOCHONDRIAL MUTATIONS (JANUARY 2021)

The use of aminoglycosides is associated with rare cases of ototoxicity. A safety review found an increased risk of deafness in patients with mitochondrial mutations (particularly the m.1555A>G mutation), including cases where the patient's aminoglycoside serum levels were within the recommended range. Nevertheless, these mitochondrial mutations are considered rare and penetrance is uncertain. No cases were identified with topical preparations but, based on a shared mechanism of effect, there is a potential risk with neomycin and other aminoglycosides administered at the site of toxicity i.e. the ear.

Healthcare professionals are advised to consider the need for aminoglycoside treatment versus alternative options in patients with susceptible mutations. The need for genetic testing especially in those requiring recurrent or long-term treatment with aminoglycosides should also be considered, however, urgent treatment should not be delayed. To minimise the risks of adverse effects, continuous monitoring of renal and auditory function, as well as hepatic and laboratory parameters, is recommended for all patients. Those with known mitochondrial mutations or a family history of

---

ototoxicity are advised to inform their doctor or pharmacist before using an aminoglycoside.

- **CONTRA-INDICATIONS** Patent grommet (although may be used by specialists, see Ear p. 1357) · perforated tympanic membrane (although may be used by specialists, see Ear p. 1357)
- **CAUTIONS** Avoid prolonged use
- **INTERACTIONS** → Appendix 1: corticosteroids · neomycin · polymyxin b
- **SIDE-EFFECTS**
  - **Rare or very rare** Headache · paraesthesia · skin reactions · telangiectasia
- **RENAL IMPAIRMENT** Manufacturer advises avoid prolonged, unsupervised use.
  Dose adjustments Manufacturer advises reduce dose.
- **PRE-TREATMENT SCREENING** NHS England commissions genetic testing under the *National genomic test directory* indication: R65 - Aminoglycoside exposure posing risk to hearing. The testing criteria is significant exposure to aminoglycosides posing risk of ototoxicity. This testing is relevant to individuals with a predisposition to gram-negative infections or with hearing loss who have been exposed to aminoglycosides. For further information, see www.england.nhs.uk/publication/national-genomic-test-directories/.

- **MEDICINAL FORMS** There can be variation in the licensing of different medicines containing the same drug.
  Ear drops
  EXCIPIENTS: May contain Cetostearyl alcohol (including cetyl and stearyl alcohol), hydroxybenzoates (parabens), polysorbates
  - Otosporin (Phoenix Labs Ltd)
    Hydrocortisone 10 mg per 1 ml, Neomycin sulfate 3400 unit per 1 ml, Polymyxin B sulfate 10000 unit per 1 ml Otosporin ear drops | 10 ml PoM £7.45

DERMATOLOGICAL DRUGS > ASTRINGENTS

Aluminium acetate

23-Nov-2023

- **INDICATIONS AND DOSE**

  OTINOVA ®

  Inflammation in otitis externa
  - TO THE EAR
  - Adult: Apply 1–2 sprays twice daily for max. 7 days, to be administered in the morning and evening

  DOSE EQUIVALENCE AND CONVERSION
  - *Otinova* ® contains aluminium acetate and aluminium acetotartrate equivalent to aluminium 1.8%, and acetic acid (Burow's solution BP).

- **MEDICINAL FORMS** There can be variation in the licensing of different medicines containing the same drug.
  Ear drops
  - Otinova (Kestrel Medical Ltd)
    Aluminium acetate 130 mg per 1 ml Otinova ear spray | 15 ml £8.96

2   Otitis media

Other drugs used for Otitis media Ciprofloxacin with dexamethasone, p. 1362 · Ciprofloxacin with fluocinolone acetonide, p. 1363

ANALGESICS > NON-STEROIDAL ANTI-INFLAMMATORY DRUGS

Phenazone with lidocaine
26-Nov-2020

The properties listed below are those particular to the combination only. For the properties of the components please consider, lidocaine hydrochloride p. 1547.

- **INDICATIONS AND DOSE**

Acute otitis media | Barotraumatic otitis
▸ TO THE EAR
▸ Child: Apply 4 drops 2–3 times a day, re-evaluate therapy if symptoms do not improve within 7 days or worsen at any time
▸ Adult: Apply 4 drops 2–3 times a day, re-evaluate therapy if symptoms do not improve within 7 days or worsen at any time

- **CONTRA-INDICATIONS** Perforated tympanic membrane (risk of ototoxicity)
- **INTERACTIONS** → Appendix 1: antiarrhythmics · NSAIDs
- **SIDE-EFFECTS**
▸ **Rare or very rare** Skin reactions · tympanic membrane hyperaemia
- **PREGNANCY** EvGr Use with caution—no information available but systemic absorption unlikely with intact tympanic membrane. Ⓜ
- **BREAST FEEDING** EvGr Use with caution—no information available but systemic absorption unlikely with intact tympanic membrane. Ⓜ

- **MEDICINAL FORMS** There can be variation in the licensing of different medicines containing the same drug.

Ear drops
EXCIPIENTS: May contain Ethanol
▸ Otigo (Renascience Pharma Ltd)
Lidocaine hydrochloride 10 mg per 1 gram, Phenazone 40 mg per 1 gram Otigo 40mg/g / 10mg/g ear drops | 15 ml PoM £8.92 DT = £8.92

3   Removal of earwax

BICARBONATE

Sodium bicarbonate
19-Apr-2022

- **INDICATIONS AND DOSE**

Removal of earwax (with 5% ear drop solution)
▸ TO THE EAR
▸ Child: (consult product literature)
▸ Adult: (consult product literature)

- **INTERACTIONS** → Appendix 1: sodium bicarbonate
- **SIDE-EFFECTS** Dry ear

- **MEDICINAL FORMS** There can be variation in the licensing of different medicines containing the same drug.

Ear drops
▸ Sodium bicarbonate (Non-proprietary)
Sodium bicarbonate 50 mg per 1 ml Sodium bicarbonate 5% ear drops | 10 ml £1.23–£1.25
▸ KliarVax Sodium Bicarbonate (Essential-Healthcare Ltd)
Sodium bicarbonate 50 mg per 1 ml KliarVax Sodium Bicarbonate ear drops | 10 ml £0.97
▸ Knoxzy (Biovantic Pharma Ltd)
Sodium bicarbonate 50 mg per 1 ml Knoxzy Sodium Bicarbonate 5% ear drops | 10 ml £0.95

SOFTENING DRUGS

Almond oil
04-Aug-2020

- **INDICATIONS AND DOSE**

Removal of earwax
▸ TO THE EAR
▸ Child: Allow drops to warm to room temperature before use (consult product literature)
▸ Adult: Allow drops to warm to room temperature before use (consult product literature)

- **DIRECTIONS FOR ADMINISTRATION** Expert sources advise the patient should lie with the affected ear uppermost for 5 to 10 minutes after a generous amount of the softening remedy has been introduced into the ear.

- **MEDICINAL FORMS** There can be variation in the licensing of different medicines containing the same drug.
Form unstated
▸ Almond oil (Non-proprietary)
Almond oil 1 ml per 1 ml Almond oil liquid | 70 ml £1.27 | 200 ml £2.52

Docusate sodium
12-Apr-2023

(Dioctyl sodium sulphosuccinate)

- **INDICATIONS AND DOSE**

Removal of ear wax
▸ TO THE EAR
▸ Adult: (consult product literature)

- **INTERACTIONS** → Appendix 1: docusates
- **SIDE-EFFECTS** Skin reactions
- **LESS SUITABLE FOR PRESCRIBING** Ear drops less suitable for prescribing.

- **MEDICINAL FORMS** There can be variation in the licensing of different medicines containing the same drug.
Ear drops
EXCIPIENTS: May contain Propylene glycol
▸ Molcer (Wallace Manufacturing Chemists Ltd)
Docusate sodium 50 mg per 1 ml Molcer ear drops | 15 ml P £5.60 DT = £5.60
▸ Waxsol (Ceuta Healthcare Ltd)
Docusate sodium 5 mg per 1 ml Waxsol ear drops | 10 ml P £1.95 DT = £1.95

Olive oil
04-Aug-2020

- **INDICATIONS AND DOSE**

Removal of earwax
▸ TO THE EAR
▸ Child: Apply twice daily for several days (if wax is hard and impacted)
▸ Adult: Apply twice daily for several days (if wax is hard and impacted)

Removal of earwax (dose approved for use by community practitioner nurse prescribers)
▸ TO THE EAR
▸ Child: (consult product literature)
▸ Adult: (consult product literature)

- **DIRECTIONS FOR ADMINISTRATION** Expert sources advise the patient should lie with the affected ear uppermost for 5 to 10 minutes after a generous amount of the softening remedy has been introduced into the ear. Allow ear drops to warm to room temperature before use.

- **MEDICINAL FORMS** There can be variation in the licensing of different medicines containing the same drug.

Ear drops

- ▸ **Olive oil (Non-proprietary)**
  Olive oil ear drops | 10 ml £1.35-£1.42
- ▸ **Arjun** (Arjun Products Ltd)
  Arjun ear drops | 10 ml £1.26
- ▸ **Cerumol (olive oil)** (Thornton & Ross Ltd)
  Cerumol olive oil ear drops | 10 ml Ⓔ
- ▸ **KliarVax** (Essential-Healthcare Ltd)
  KliarVax Olive Oil ear drops | 10 ml £0.97
- ▸ **Knoxzy** (Biovantic Pharma Ltd)
  Knoxzy Olive Oil ear drops | 10 ml £0.90
- ▸ **Olive oil** (Thornton & Ross Ltd)
  Care olive oil ear drops | 10 ml £1.42
- ▸ **Otadrop** (JFA Medical Ltd)
  Otadrop olive oil ear drops | 10 ml £0.80
- ▸ **St George's** (St Georges Medical Ltd)
  Olive oil ear drops | 10 ml £1.40 | 20 ml £2.70

Spray

- ▸ **Earol** (HL Healthcare Ltd)
  Earol olive oil ear spray | 10 ml Ⓔ

Urea hydrogen peroxide

02-Sep-2020

- ● **INDICATIONS AND DOSE**

Softening and removal of earwax
- ▸ TO THE EAR
- ▸ Adult: (consult product literature)

- ● **PATIENT AND CARER ADVICE** The patient should lie with the affected ear uppermost for 5 to 10 minutes after a generous amount of the softening remedy has been introduced into the ear.

- ● **LESS SUITABLE FOR PRESCRIBING** Urea-hydrogen peroxide ear drops are less suitable for prescribing.

- ● **MEDICINAL FORMS** There can be variation in the licensing of different medicines containing the same drug.

Ear drops

- ▸ **Otex** (Diomed Developments Ltd)
  Urea hydrogen peroxide 50 mg per 1 gram Otex 5% ear drops | 8 ml Ⓟ £3.41 DT = £3.41

Nose

Nose

04-Nov-2021

Rhinitis

Rhinitis may be acute or chronic, allergic or non-allergic. Nasal spray and drop preparations often carry indications for the management of allergic rhinitis and perennial rhinitis. Many nasal preparations contain sympathomimetic drugs which may irritate the nasal mucosa.

Patients with nasal congestion and obstructive sleep apnoea/hypopnoea syndrome or obesity hypoventilation syndrome may have underlying allergic or vasomotor rhinitis. For guidance on the management of rhinitis in these patients, see NICE guideline: **Obstructive sleep apnoea/hypopnoea syndrome and obesity hypoventilation syndrome in over 16s** (available at: www.nice.org.uk/guidance/ng202).

Drugs used in nasal allergy

[EvGr] Sodium chloride 0.9% solution p. 1180 may be used as nasal irrigation in allergic rhinitis for modest symptom reduction, and to reduce the need for other drug treatment.

Mild allergic rhinitis is controlled by **antihistamines** (see under Antihistamines, allergen immunotherapy and allergic emergencies p. 316) or topical **nasal corticosteroids**. Topical antihistamines (e.g. azelastine hydrochloride p. 1370) are faster acting than oral antihistamines and therefore useful for controlling breakthrough symptoms in allergic rhinitis; they are less effective than topical nasal corticosteroids. Topical nasal decongestants can be used for a short period to provide quick relief from congestion and allow penetration of a topical nasal corticosteroid. Systemic nasal decongestants are weakly effective in reducing nasal obstruction but have considerable potential for side-effects, and therefore are not recommended. Sodium cromoglicate is a weakly effective alternative in patients with mild symptoms, sporadic seasonal problems, or limited allergen exposure.

Moderate to severe allergic rhinitis can be relieved by topical **nasal corticosteroids** during periods of allergen exposure. Severe allergic rhinitis causing very disabling symptoms despite conventional treatment may justify the use of **oral corticosteroids** for short periods. In severe cases, oral corticosteroids may also be used in combination with nasal corticosteroids during treatment initiation to relieve severe mucosal oedema and allow the spray to penetrate the nasal cavity.

Nasal ipratropium bromide p. 1370 may be added to allergic rhinitis treatment when watery rhinorrhoea persists despite treatment with topical nasal corticosteroids and antihistamines; it has no effect on other nasal symptoms.

In seasonal allergic rhinitis (e.g. hay fever), treatment should begin 2 to 3 weeks before the season commences and/or exposure to the allergen.

Montelukast p. 310 is less effective than topical nasal corticosteroids but can be used in patients with seasonal allergic rhinitis and concomitant asthma. Ⓐ

Corticosteroids

[EvGr] Topical nasal corticosteroid preparations should be avoided in the presence of untreated nasal infections, after nasal surgery (until healing has occurred), and in pulmonary tuberculosis. Systemic absorption may follow nasal administration particularly if high doses are used or if treatment is prolonged. The extent of absorption varies between steroids; mometasone furoate p. 1373 and fluticasone p. 1372 have negligible systemic absorption, others have modest absorption, whilst betamethasone p. 1371 has high systemic absorption and should only be used short-term. The growth of children receiving treatment with corticosteroids should be monitored; especially in those receiving corticosteroids via multiple routes. Ⓐ

Nasal polyps

[EvGr] Patients presenting with nasal polyps should initially be reviewed by an ear, nose and throat specialist. Nasal polyps may be treated with topical nasal corticosteroids (drops or spray). There may be a higher risk of side-effects with use of nasal drops compared to nasal spray due to greater systemic absorption and incorrect administration of drops. To reduce the risk, the drops must be administered with the patient in the 'head down' position. A short course of a systemic corticosteroid can provide symptomatic relief but effects may be temporary and its use is rare due to concerns of systemic side-effects. If systemic corticosteroids are given, they should be used in combination with topical nasal corticosteroids. Ⓐ

Pregnancy

[EvGr] If a pregnant woman cannot tolerate the symptoms of allergic rhinitis, treatment may be given. Ⓐ Although the safety of nasal corticosteroids in pregnancy has not been established through clinical trials, only minimal amounts of nasal corticosteroids are systemically absorbed. Beclometasone dipropionate p. 1371, budesonide p. 1372, and fluticasone are widely used in asthmatic pregnant women; fluticasone has the lowest systemic absorption when used intra-nasally. [EvGr] Decongestants are not recommended however, some antihistamines and sodium cromoglicate may be used. Ⓐ

Topical nasal decongestants

The nasal mucosa is sensitive to changes in atmospheric temperature and humidity and these alone may cause slight nasal congestion. EvGr Sodium chloride 0.9% given as nasal drops, spray, or irrigation may relieve nasal congestion.

Steam inhalation may help to relieve congestion but care should be taken to avoid scalding (see under Aromatic inhalations, cough preparations and systemic nasal decongestants p. 339).

Symptoms of nasal congestion associated with allergic rhinitis, the common cold, and sinusitis may be relieved by the short-term use (usually not longer than 7 days) of decongestant nasal drops and sprays. A These all contain sympathomimetic drugs which exert their effect by vasoconstriction of the mucosal blood vessels which in turn reduces oedema of the nasal mucosa. Their use, especially with longer durations, can give rise to rebound congestion (rhinitis medicamentosa) on withdrawal, due to a secondary vasodilatation with a subsequent temporary increase in nasal congestion. This in turn tempts the further use of the decongestant, leading to a vicious cycle of events; tolerance with reduced effect may also be seen with excessive use.

EvGr Non-allergic watery rhinorrhoea often responds to treatment with nasal antimuscarinic ipratropium bromide. A

Nasal preparations for infection

Nasal staphylococci

EvGr Elimination of organisms such as staphylococci from the nasal vestibule can be achieved by the use of antimicrobial preparations such as chlorhexidine with neomycin cream p. 1369 (*Naseptin*®). A nasal ointment containing mupirocin p. 1369 is available if *Naseptin*® is unsuitable or ineffective.

In hospitals or in care establishments, mupirocin nasal ointment can be used for the eradication of nasal carriage of meticillin-resistant *Staphylococcus aureus* (MRSA). A

For information on eradication of MRSA, consult local infection control policy. See also management of MRSA p. 670.

1   Nasal congestion

SYMPATHOMIMETICS › VASOCONSTRICTOR

Ephedrine hydrochloride

29-Mar-2022

- **INDICATIONS AND DOSE**

Nasal congestion | Sinusitis affecting the maxillary antrum
- ▸ BY INTRANASAL ADMINISTRATION
- ▸ Child 12-17 years: Apply 1–2 drops up to 4 times a day as required for a maximum of 7 days, to be instilled into each nostril, administer ephedrine 0.5% nasal drops
- ▸ Adult: Apply 1–2 drops up to 4 times a day as required for a maximum of 7 days, to be instilled into each nostril

IMPORTANT SAFETY INFORMATION
CHM/MHRA ADVICE
The CHM/MHRA has stated that non-prescription cough and cold medicines containing ephedrine can be considered for up to 5 days' treatment in children aged 6–12 years after basic principles of best care have been tried; these medicines should not be used in children under 6 years of age.

- **CAUTIONS** Avoid excessive or prolonged use · cardiovascular disease (in children) · diabetes mellitus · elderly · hypertension · hyperthyroidism · ischaemic heart

disease (in adults) · prostatic hypertrophy (risk of acute urinary retention) (in adults)

- **INTERACTIONS** → Appendix 1: sympathomimetics, vasoconstrictor

- **SIDE-EFFECTS**
- ▸ **Common or very common** Anxiety · headache · insomnia · nausea
- ▸ **Frequency not known** Appetite decreased · arrhythmia · circulation impaired · dermatitis · dizziness · drug dependence · dry mouth · dyspnoea · hallucination · hyperglycaemia · hyperhidrosis · hypersalivation · hypertension · hypokalaemia · hypotension · irritability · muscle weakness · mydriasis · pain · palpitations · paranoia · piloerection · rebound congestion · syncope · thirst · tremor · urinary disorders · vasoconstriction · vasodilation · vomiting

- **PREGNANCY** Manufacturer advises avoid.

- **BREAST FEEDING** Present in milk; manufacturer advises avoid—irritability and disturbed sleep reported.

- **PRESCRIBING AND DISPENSING INFORMATION** For nasal drops, the BP directs that if no strength is specified 0.5% drops should be supplied.

- **PROFESSION SPECIFIC INFORMATION**

Dental practitioners' formulary Ephedrine nasal drops may be prescribed.

- **EXCEPTIONS TO LEGAL CATEGORY** Ephedrine nasal drops can be sold to the public provided no more than 180 mg of ephedrine base (or salts) are supplied at one time, and pseudoephedrine salts are not supplied at the same time; for conditions that apply to supplies made at the request of a patient, see *Medicines, Ethics and Practice*, London, Pharmaceutical Press (always consult latest edition).

- **MEDICINAL FORMS** Forms available from special-order manufacturers include: nasal drops

Pseudoephedrine hydrochloride

28-Mar-2024

- **INDICATIONS AND DOSE**

Congestion of mucous membranes of upper respiratory tract
- ▸ BY MOUTH
- ▸ Child 6-11 years: 30 mg 3–4 times a day
- ▸ Child 12-17 years: 60 mg 3–4 times a day
- ▸ Adult: 60 mg 3–4 times a day

IMPORTANT SAFETY INFORMATION
MHRA/CHM ADVICE: OVER-THE-COUNTER COUGH AND COLD MEDICINES FOR CHILDREN (APRIL 2009)
Children under 6 years should not be given over-the-counter cough and cold medicines containing pseudoephedrine.

MHRA/CHM ADVICE: PSEUDOEPHEDRINE: VERY RARE RISK OF POSTERIOR REVERSIBLE ENCEPHALOPATHY SYNDROME (PRES) AND REVERSIBLE CEREBRAL VASOCONSTRICTION SYNDROME (RCVS) (FEBRUARY 2024)
Healthcare professionals are reminded that PRES and RCVS are very rare side-effects of pseudoephedrine; affected patients typically recover fully within 3 months with early recognition and treatment. Pseudoephedrine-containing medicines are for short-term, symptomatic use only and are contra-indicated in patients with severe or uncontrolled hypertension, or severe renal disease. Patients and their carers should be advised on the symptoms of PRES and RCVS, and to stop taking pseudoephedrine-containing medicines and seek urgent medical attention if they develop a sudden severe headache or thunderclap headache, sudden onset of

nausea or vomiting, confusion, seizures, and/or visual disturbances. Healthcare professionals should ask about the patient's medication history when presented with these symptoms.

- **CONTRA-INDICATIONS** Severe or uncontrolled hypertension
- **CAUTIONS** Diabetes · heart disease · hyperthyroidism · ischaemic heart disease (in adults) · mild to moderate hypertension · prostatic hypertrophy (in adults) · raised intra-ocular pressure (in children) · susceptibility to angle-closure glaucoma (in adults)
- **INTERACTIONS** → Appendix 1: sympathomimetics, vasoconstrictor
- **SIDE-EFFECTS**
  - **Common or very common** Anxiety · dizziness · dry mouth · headache · nausea · sleep disorders
  - **Frequency not known** Akathisia · angioedema · angle closure glaucoma · arrhythmias · cerebrovascular insufficiency · circulation impaired · colitis ischaemic · drowsiness · hallucination · hypertension · mood altered · myocardial infarction · myocardial ischaemia · optic neuropathy · palpitations · paraesthesia · paranoid delusions · posterior reversible encephalopathy syndrome (PRES) · severe cutaneous adverse reactions (SCARs) · skin reactions · tremor · urinary disorders · vomiting
- **PREGNANCY** Defective closure of the abdominal wall (gastroschisis) reported very rarely in newborns after first trimester exposure.
- **BREAST FEEDING** May suppress lactation; avoid if lactation not well established or if milk production insufficient.
- **HEPATIC IMPAIRMENT** Manufacturer advises caution in severe impairment.
- **RENAL IMPAIRMENT** EvGr Use with caution in mild to moderate impairment; avoid in severe impairment. M
- **LESS SUITABLE FOR PRESCRIBING** Pseudoephedrine hydrochloride is less suitable for prescribing.
- **EXCEPTIONS TO LEGAL CATEGORY** *Galpseud*® and *Sudafed*® can be sold to the public provided no more than 720 mg of pseudoephedrine salts are supplied, and ephedrine base (or salts) are not supplied at the same time; for details see *Medicines, Ethics and Practice*, London, Pharmaceutical Press (always consult latest edition).

- **MEDICINAL FORMS** There can be variation in the licensing of different medicines containing the same drug.
  Oral tablet
  - Galpseud (Thornton & Ross Ltd)
    Pseudoephedrine hydrochloride 60 mg Galpseud 60mg tablets | 24 tablet PoM £2.25 DT = £2.25
  Oral solution
  EXCIPIENTS: May contain Alcohol
  - Galpseud (Thornton & Ross Ltd)
    Pseudoephedrine hydrochloride 6 mg per 1 ml Galpseud 30mg/5ml linctus | 2000 ml PoM £14.00 SF
  - Sudafed Non-Drowsy Decongestant (pseudoephedrine) (McNeil Products Ltd)
    Pseudoephedrine hydrochloride 6 mg per 1 ml Sudafed Decongestant 30mg/5ml liquid | 100 ml P £2.81 DT = £2.81

Xylometazoline hydrochloride

13-Feb-2020

- **DRUG ACTION** Xylometazoline is a sympathomimetic.

- **INDICATIONS AND DOSE**
  Nasal congestion
  - ▸ BY INTRANASAL ADMINISTRATION USING NASAL DROPS
  - ▸ Child 6-11 years: 1–2 drops 1–2 times a day as required for maximum duration of 5 days, 0.05% solution to be administered into each nostril

- ▸ Child 12-17 years: 2–3 drops 2–3 times a day as required for maximum duration of 7 days, 0.1% solution to be administered into each nostril
- ▸ Adult: 2–3 drops 2–3 times a day as required for maximum duration of 7 days, 0.1% solution to be administered into each nostril
- ▸ BY INTRANASAL ADMINISTRATION USING NASAL SPRAY
- ▸ Child 12-17 years: 1 spray 1–3 times a day as required for maximum duration of 7 days, to be administered into each nostril
- ▸ Adult: 1 spray 1–3 times a day as required for maximum duration of 7 days, to be administered into each nostril

> **IMPORTANT SAFETY INFORMATION**
> The CHM/MHRA has stated that non-prescription cough and cold medicines containing oxymetazoline or xylometazoline can be considered for up to 5 days' treatment in children aged 6–12 years after basic principles of best care have been tried; these medicines should not be used in children under 6 years of age.

- **CAUTIONS** Angle-closure glaucoma · avoid excessive or prolonged use · cardiovascular disease (in children) · diabetes mellitus · elderly · hypertension · hyperthyroidism · ischaemic heart disease (in adults) · prostatic hypertrophy (risk of acute retention) (in adults) · rebound congestion
  CAUTIONS, FURTHER INFORMATION
  - ▸ Rebound congestion Sympathomimetic drugs are of limited value in the treatment of nasal congestion because they can, following prolonged use (more than 7 days), give rise to a rebound congestion (rhinitis medicamentosa) on withdrawal, due to a secondary vasodilatation with a subsequent temporary increase in nasal congestion. This in turn tempts the further use of the decongestant, leading to a vicious cycle of events.
- **INTERACTIONS** → Appendix 1: sympathomimetics, vasoconstrictor
- **SIDE-EFFECTS** Cardiovascular effects · headache · hypersensitivity · nasal dryness · nausea · paraesthesia · visual impairment
  SIDE-EFFECTS, FURTHER INFORMATION Use of decongestants in infants and children under 6 years has been associated with agitated psychosis, ataxia, hallucinations, and even death—avoid.
- **PREGNANCY** Manufacturer advises avoid.
- **BREAST FEEDING** Manufacturer advises caution—no information available.

- **MEDICINAL FORMS** There can be variation in the licensing of different medicines containing the same drug.
  Spray
  - ▸ Xylometazoline hydrochloride (Non-proprietary)
    Xylometazoline hydrochloride 1 mg per 1 ml Xylometazoline 0.1% nasal spray | 10 ml GSL £ DT = £2.65
  Nasal drops
  - ▸ Otrivine (Haleon UK Trading Ltd)
    Xylometazoline hydrochloride 500 microgram per 1 ml Otrivine Child nasal drops | 10 ml P £2.80 DT = £2.80
    Xylometazoline hydrochloride 1 mg per 1 ml Otrivine Adult 0.1% nasal drops | 10 ml GSL £2.50 DT = £2.50

2 Nasal infection

Sinusitis (acute)

31-Oct-2017

Description of condition

Sinusitis is an inflammation of the mucosal lining of the paranasal sinuses. Acute sinusitis (rhinosinusitis) is a self-limiting condition usually triggered by a viral upper-respiratory tract infection such as the 'common cold'. Occasionally, acute sinusitis may become complicated by a bacterial infection (*see Antibacterial therapy for acute sinusitis* in Nose infections, antibacterial therapy p. 585).

Patients with acute sinusitis usually present with symptoms of nasal blockage or congestion, nasal discharge, dental or facial pain or pressure, and reduction or loss of the sense of smell.

Symptoms usually improve within 2 to 3 weeks without requiring treatment.

Rarely, acute sinusitis may lead to orbital, intracranial or skeletal complications (e.g. periorbital cellulitis, symptoms or signs of meningitis).

Aims of treatment

Treatment is aimed at managing symptoms including pain, fever, and nasal congestion as well as treatment of bacterial infection if present.

Treatment

[EvGr] Patients presenting with symptoms for around 10 *days or less*, should be given advice about the usual duration of acute sinusitis, self-care of pain or fever with paracetamol p. 507 or ibuprofen p. 1302, and when to seek medical help. Patients should be reassured that antibiotics are usually not required. Some patients may try nasal saline or nasal decongestants, however there is limited evidence to show they help to relieve nasal congestion.

Patients presenting with symptoms for around 10 *days or more* with no improvement could be considered for treatment with a high-dose nasal corticosteroid, such as mometasone furoate p. 1373 [unlicensed use] or fluticasone p. 1372 [unlicensed use] for 14 days. Supply of a back-up antibiotic prescription could be considered and used if symptoms do not improve within 7 days, or if they worsen rapidly or significantly.

If the patient is systemically very unwell, has signs and symptoms of a more serious illness or condition, or is at high-risk of complications, an immediate antibiotic should be given (A) (*see Antibacterial therapy for acute sinusitis* in Nose infections, antibacterial therapy p. 585).

[EvGr] Patients presenting with symptoms of acute sinusitis associated with a severe systemic infection or with orbital or intracranial complications should be referred to hospital. (A)

Useful Resources

Sinusitis (acute): antimicrobial prescribing. National Institute for Health and Care Excellence. NICE guideline 79. October 2017.
www.nice.org.uk/guidance/ng79

ANTIBACTERIALS › AMINOGLYCOSIDES

Chlorhexidine with neomycin
29-Mar-2023

- **INDICATIONS AND DOSE**

Eradication of nasal carriage of staphylococci
- ▸ BY INTRANASAL ADMINISTRATION
- ▸ Child: Apply 4 times a day for 10 days
- ▸ Adult: Apply 4 times a day for 10 days

Preventing nasal carriage of staphylococci
- ▸ BY INTRANASAL ADMINISTRATION
- ▸ Child: Apply twice daily
- ▸ Adult: Apply twice daily

- **PRE-TREATMENT SCREENING** NHS England commissions genetic testing under the *National genomic test directory* indication: R65 - Aminoglycoside exposure posing risk to hearing. The testing criteria is significant exposure to aminoglycosides posing risk of ototoxicity. This testing is relevant to individuals with a predisposition to gram-

negative infections or with hearing loss who have been exposed to aminoglycosides. For further information, see www.england.nhs.uk/publication/national-genomic-test-directories/.

- **MEDICINAL FORMS** There can be variation in the licensing of different medicines containing the same drug.
  Nasal cream
  EXCIPIENTS: May contain Arachis (peanut) oil, cetostearyl alcohol (including cetyl and stearyl alcohol)
  - ▸ Naseptin (Alliance Pharmaceuticals Ltd)
    Chlorhexidine hydrochloride 1 mg per 1 gram, Neomycin sulfate 5 mg per 1 gram Naseptin nasal cream | 15 gram [PoM] £1.99 DT = £1.99

ANTIBACTERIALS › OTHER

Mupirocin
07-May-2021

- **INDICATIONS AND DOSE**

BACTROBAN NASAL ®

For eradication of nasal carriage of staphylococci, including meticillin-resistant *Staphylococcus aureus* (MRSA)
- ▸ BY INTRANASAL ADMINISTRATION
- ▸ Child: Apply 2–3 times a day for 5 days, dose to be applied to the inner surface of each nostril, a sample should be taken 2 days after treatment to confirm eradication. Course may be repeated once if sample positive (and throat not colonised)
- ▸ Adult: Apply 2–3 times a day for 5 days, dose to be applied to the inner surface of each nostril, a sample should be taken 2 days after treatment to confirm eradication. Course may be repeated once if sample positive (and throat not colonised)

- **SIDE-EFFECTS**
- ▸ **Common or very common** Skin reactions
- ▸ **Uncommon** Nasal mucosal disorder

- **PREGNANCY** Manufacturer advises avoid unless potential benefit outweighs risk—no information available.

- **BREAST FEEDING** No information available.

- **MEDICINAL FORMS** There can be variation in the licensing of different medicines containing the same drug.
  Nasal ointment
  - ▸ Bactroban (GlaxoSmithKline UK Ltd)
    Mupirocin (as Mupirocin calcium) 20 mg per 1 gram Bactroban 2% nasal ointment | 3 gram [PoM] £4.24 DT = £4.24

CORTICOSTEROIDS › CORTICOSTEROID COMBINATIONS WITH ANTI-INFECTIVES

Betamethasone with neomycin
08-Oct-2024

The properties listed below are those particular to the combination only. For the properties of the components please consider, betamethasone p. 1371.

- **INDICATIONS AND DOSE**
Nasal infection
- ▸ BY INTRANASAL ADMINISTRATION USING NASAL DROPS
- ▸ Child: Apply 2–3 drops 2–3 times a day, to be applied into each nostril
- ▸ Adult: Apply 2–3 drops 2–3 times a day, to be applied into each nostril

- **INTERACTIONS** → Appendix 1: corticosteroids · neomycin

- **SIDE-EFFECTS** Asthma · dizziness · epistaxis · growth retardation (in children) · headache · nasal complaints · nausea · smell altered · taste altered · urticaria

- **PRE-TREATMENT SCREENING** NHS England commissions genetic testing under the *National genomic test directory* indication: R65 - Aminoglycoside exposure posing risk to hearing. The testing criteria is significant exposure to aminoglycosides posing risk of ototoxicity. This testing is relevant to individuals with a predisposition to gram-negative infections or with hearing loss who have been exposed to aminoglycosides. For further information, see www.england.nhs.uk/publication/national-genomic-test-directories/.

- **LESS SUITABLE FOR PRESCRIBING** Betamethasone with neomycin nasal-drops are less suitable for prescribing; there is no evidence that topical anti-infective nasal preparations have any therapeutic value in rhinitis or sinusitis.

- **MEDICINAL FORMS** There can be variation in the licensing of different medicines containing the same drug.
Ear/eye/nose drops solution
EXCIPIENTS: May contain Benzalkonium chloride, disodium edetate
▸ Betnesol-N (RPH Pharmaceuticals AB)
Betamethasone (as Betamethasone sodium phosphate) 1 mg per 1 ml, Neomycin sulfate 5 mg per 1 ml Betnesol-N ear/eye/nose drops | 10 ml PoM £2.39 DT = £2.39

3 Nasal inflammation, nasal polyps and rhinitis

Other drugs used for Nasal inflammation, nasal polyps and rhinitis Desloratadine, p. 319 · Dupilumab, p. 1423 · Fexofenadine hydrochloride, p. 320 · Ketotifen, p. 325 · Rupatadine, p. 322

ANTIHISTAMINES

Azelastine hydrochloride

03-Aug-2023

- **INDICATIONS AND DOSE**
AZELAIR®
Allergic rhinitis
▸ BY INTRANASAL ADMINISTRATION
▸ Child 6-11 years: 1 spray twice daily for a maximum duration of 4 weeks, to be administered into each nostril
▸ Child 12-17 years: 2 sprays once daily, to be administered into each nostril, increased if necessary up to 2 sprays twice daily, to be administered into each nostril
▸ Adult: 2 sprays once daily, to be administered into each nostril, increased if necessary up to 2 sprays twice daily, to be administered into each nostril

DOSE EQUIVALENCE AND CONVERSION
▸ For *Azelair*®: 1 spray equivalent to 210 micrograms.
RHINOLAST®
Allergic rhinitis
▸ BY INTRANASAL ADMINISTRATION
▸ Child 6-17 years: 1 spray twice daily, to be administered into each nostril
▸ Adult: 1 spray twice daily, to be administered into each nostril

DOSE EQUIVALENCE AND CONVERSION
▸ For *Rhinolast*®: 1 spray equivalent to 140 micrograms.

- **INTERACTIONS** → Appendix 1: antihistamines, non-sedating
- **SIDE-EFFECTS**
▸ **Common or very common** Taste altered
▸ **Uncommon** Epistaxis · nasal complaints
▸ **Rare or very rare** Asthenia · dizziness · drowsiness · skin reactions

SIDE-EFFECTS, FURTHER INFORMATION Altered taste may occur after administration, often due to incorrect application.

- **MEDICINAL FORMS** There can be variation in the licensing of different medicines containing the same drug.
Spray
▸ Azelair (Ceuta Healthcare Ltd)
Azelastine hydrochloride 210 microgram per 1 actuation Azelair 0.15% nasal spray | 20 ml PoM £9.90 DT = £9.90
▸ Rhinolast (Ceuta Healthcare Ltd)
Azelastine hydrochloride 140 microgram per 1 actuation Rhinolast 140micrograms/dose nasal spray | 22 ml PoM £10.50 DT = £10.50

Combinations available: *Fluticasone with azelastine*, p. 1373

ANTIMUSCARINICS

🝔 280

Ipratropium bromide

13-Mar-2025

- **INDICATIONS AND DOSE**
Rhinorrhoea associated with allergic and non-allergic rhinitis
▸ BY INTRANASAL ADMINISTRATION
▸ Child 12-17 years: 2 sprays 2–3 times a day, dose to be sprayed into each nostril
▸ Adult: 2 sprays 2–3 times a day, dose to be sprayed into each nostril

DOSE EQUIVALENCE AND CONVERSION
▸ 1 metered spray of nasal spray = 21 micrograms.

- **CAUTIONS** Avoid spraying near eyes · bladder outflow obstruction · cystic fibrosis · prostatic hyperplasia (in adults) · susceptibility to angle-closure glaucoma
- **INTERACTIONS** → Appendix 1: ipratropium
- **SIDE-EFFECTS**
▸ **Common or very common** Epistaxis · gastrointestinal motility disorder · headache · nasal complaints · throat complaints
▸ **Uncommon** Corneal oedema · eye disorders · eye pain · nausea · respiratory disorders · stomatitis · vision disorders
▸ **Rare or very rare** Palpitations

SIDE-EFFECTS, FURTHER INFORMATION For intranasal use, also consider the side-effects of inhaled antimuscarinics.

- **ALLERGY AND CROSS-SENSITIVITY** Contra-indicated in patients with hypersensitivity to atropine or its derivatives.
- **PREGNANCY** EvGr Use only if potential benefit outweighs the risk. Ⓜ
- **BREAST FEEDING** No information available—manufacturer advises only use if potential benefit outweighs risk.
- **PATIENT AND CARER ADVICE** Patients or carers should be counselled on appropriate administration technique and warned against accidental contact with the eye (due to risk of ocular complications).
Driving and skilled tasks Manufacturer advises patients and carers should be counselled on the effects on driving and performance of skilled tasks—increased risk of dizziness and vision disorders.

- **MEDICINAL FORMS** There can be variation in the licensing of different medicines containing the same drug.
Spray
EXCIPIENTS: May contain Benzalkonium chloride, disodium edetate
▸ Ipratropium bromide (Non-proprietary)
Ipratropium bromide 21 microgram per 1 dose Ipratropium bromide 21micrograms/dose nasal spray | 240 dose PoM £8.72-£14.82 DT = £8.72

CORTICOSTEROIDS

Corticosteroids (intranasal) 

IMPORTANT SAFETY INFORMATION

MHRA/CHM ADVICE: CORTICOSTEROIDS: RARE RISK OF CENTRAL SEROUS CHORIORETINOPATHY WITH LOCAL AS WELL AS SYSTEMIC ADMINISTRATION (AUGUST 2017)

Central serous chorioretinopathy is a retinal disorder that has been linked to the systemic use of corticosteroids. Recently, it has also been reported after local administration of corticosteroids via inhaled and intranasal, epidural, intra-articular, topical dermal, and periocular routes. The MHRA recommends that patients should be advised to report any blurred vision or other visual disturbances with corticosteroid treatment given by any route; consider referral to an ophthalmologist for evaluation of possible causes if a patient presents with vision problems.

NHS IMPROVEMENT PATIENT SAFETY ALERT: STEROID EMERGENCY CARD TO SUPPORT EARLY RECOGNITION AND TREATMENT OF ADRENAL CRISIS IN ADULTS (AUGUST 2020)

A patient-held **Steroid Emergency Card** has been developed for patients with adrenal insufficiency and steroid dependence who are at risk of adrenal crisis. It aims to support healthcare staff with the early recognition of patients at risk of adrenal crisis and the emergency treatment of adrenal crisis. All eligible patients should be issued a Steroid Emergency Card. Providers that treat patients with acute physical illness or trauma, or who may require emergency treatment, elective surgery, or other invasive procedures, should establish processes to check for risk of adrenal crisis and confirm if the patient has a Steroid Emergency Card.

ADRENAL INSUFFICIENCY CARD (APRIL 2023)

The British Society for Paediatric Endocrinology and Diabetes (BSPED) has developed an Adrenal Insufficiency Card which should be issued to children with adrenal insufficiency and steroid dependence. The card includes a management summary for the emergency treatment of adrenal crisis and sick day dosing, and can be issued by any healthcare professional managing such patients. The BSPED Adrenal Insufficiency Card is available at: www.bsped.org.uk/adrenal-insufficiency.

- **CAUTIONS** Avoid after nasal surgery (until healing has occurred) · avoid in pulmonary tuberculosis · avoid in the presence of untreated nasal infections · patients transferred from systemic corticosteroids may experience exacerbation of some symptoms

  CAUTIONS, FURTHER INFORMATION
  - Systemic absorption Systemic absorption may follow nasal administration particularly if high doses are used or if treatment is prolonged; therefore also consider the cautions and side-effects of systemic corticosteroids. The risk of systemic effects may be greater with nasal drops than with nasal sprays; drops are administered incorrectly more often than sprays.

- **SIDE-EFFECTS**
  - **Common or very common** Altered smell sensation · epistaxis · headache · nasal complaints · taste altered · throat irritation
  - **Rare or very rare** Glaucoma · nasal septum perforation (more common following nasal surgery) · vision blurred

  SIDE-EFFECTS, FURTHER INFORMATION Systemic absorption may follow nasal administration particularly if high doses are used or if treatment is prolonged. Therefore also consider the side-effects of systemic corticosteroids.

- **MONITORING REQUIREMENTS**
  - In children The height of children receiving prolonged treatment with nasal corticosteroids should be monitored; if growth is slowed, referral to a paediatrician should be considered.
- **PATIENT AND CARER ADVICE** If systemic absorption occurs following intranasal use, side-effects applicable to systemic corticosteroids may apply.

☛ above

Beclometasone dipropionate
08-Oct-2024

(Beclomethasone dipropionate)

- **INDICATIONS AND DOSE**

  Prophylaxis and treatment of allergic and vasomotor rhinitis
  - BY INTRANASAL ADMINISTRATION
  - Child 6–17 years: 100 micrograms twice daily, dose to be administered into each nostril, reduced to 50 micrograms twice daily, dose to be administered into each nostril, dose to be reduced when symptoms controlled
  - Adult: 100 micrograms twice daily, dose to be administered into each nostril, reduced to 50 micrograms twice daily, dose to be administered into each nostril, dose to be reduced when symptoms controlled

- **INTERACTIONS** → Appendix 1: corticosteroids
- **EXCEPTIONS TO LEGAL CATEGORY**
  - In adults Preparations of beclometasone dipropionate can be sold to the public for nasal administration as a nasal spray if supplied for the prevention and treatment of allergic rhinitis in adults over 18 years subject to max. single dose of 100 micrograms per nostril, max. daily dose of 200 micrograms per nostril for max. 3 months, and a pack size of 20 mg.

- **MEDICINAL FORMS** There can be variation in the licensing of different medicines containing the same drug.

  Spray
  EXCIPIENTS: May contain Benzalkonium chloride, polysorbates
  - **Beclometasone dipropionate (Non-proprietary)**
    Beclometasone dipropionate 50 microgram per 1 dose Beclometasone 50micrograms/dose nasal spray | 200 dose [PoM] [Ⓧ] DT = £2.63
  - **Beconase** (GlaxoSmithKline UK Ltd)
    Beclometasone dipropionate 50 microgram per 1 dose Beconase Aqueous 50micrograms/dose nasal spray | 200 dose [PoM] £2.63 DT = £2.63
  - **Nasobec** (Teva UK Ltd)
    Beclometasone dipropionate 50 microgram per 1 dose Nasobec Aqueous 50micrograms/dose nasal spray | 200 dose [PoM] £3.06 DT = £2.63

☛ above

Betamethasone
08-Oct-2024

- **DRUG ACTION** Betamethasone has very high glucocorticoid activity and insignificant mineralocorticoid activity.

- **INDICATIONS AND DOSE**

  BETNESOL®

  Non-infected inflammatory conditions of nose
  - BY INTRANASAL ADMINISTRATION
  - Adult: Apply 2–3 drops 2–3 times a day, dose to be applied into each nostril

  VISTAMETHASONE®

  Non-infected inflammatory conditions of nose
  - BY INTRANASAL ADMINISTRATION
  - Adult: Apply 2–3 drops twice daily, dose to be applied into each nostril

12

Ear, nose and oropharynx

- **INTERACTIONS** → Appendix 1: corticosteroids

- **MEDICINAL FORMS** There can be variation in the licensing of different medicines containing the same drug.

Ear/eye/nose drops solution

EXCIPIENTS: May contain Benzalkonium chloride, disodium edetate

- ▸ **Betnesol** (RPH Pharmaceuticals AB)
  Betamethasone sodium phosphate 1 mg per 1 ml Betnesol 0.1% eye/ear/nose drops | 10 ml PoM £2.32 DT = £2.32
- ▸ **Vistamethasone** (Martindale Pharmaceuticals Ltd)
  Betamethasone sodium phosphate 1 mg per 1 ml Vistamethasone 0.1% ear/eye/nose drops | 5 ml PoM £11.30

⚑ 1371

Budesonide

03-Apr-2024

- **DRUG ACTION** Budesonide is a glucocorticoid, which exerts significant local anti-inflammatory effects.

- **INDICATIONS AND DOSE**

Prophylaxis and treatment of allergic rhinitis | Nasal polyps

- ▸ BY INTRANASAL ADMINISTRATION
- ▸ Child 6-17 years: 256 micrograms once daily, to be administered as 2 sprays into each nostril in the morning, reduce dose when control achieved, alternatively 128 micrograms twice daily, to be administered as 1 spray into each nostril in the morning and in the evening, reduce dose when control achieved
- ▸ Adult: 256 micrograms once daily, to be administered as 2 sprays into each nostril in the morning, reduce dose when control achieved, alternatively 128 micrograms twice daily, to be administered as 1 spray into each nostril in the morning and in the evening, reduce dose when control achieved

- **INTERACTIONS** → Appendix 1: corticosteroids

- **SIDE-EFFECTS**
- ▸ **Rare or very rare** Adrenal suppression

- **EXCEPTIONS TO LEGAL CATEGORY**
- ▸ In adults Preparations of budesonide can be sold to the public for nasal administration as a nasal spray if supplied for the prevention and treatment of seasonal allergic rhinitis in adults over 18 years, subject to a max. single dose of 128 micrograms per nostril, max. daily dose of 256 micrograms for a max. period of 3 months, and a pack size of 120 actuations.

- **MEDICINAL FORMS** There can be variation in the licensing of different medicines containing the same drug.

Spray

EXCIPIENTS: May contain Disodium edetate, polysorbates, potassium sorbate

- ▸ **Budesonide (Non-proprietary)**
  Budesonide 64 microgram per 1 dose Budesonide 64micrograms/dose nasal spray | 120 dose PoM £15.24 DT = £15.24
  Budesonide 100 microgram per 1 dose Budeflam Aquanase 100micrograms/dose nasal spray | 150 dose PoM ⚠
  Aircort 100micrograms/dose nasal spray | 200 dose PoM ⚠

⚑ 1371

Fluticasone

08-Oct-2024

- **INDICATIONS AND DOSE**

Prophylaxis and treatment of allergic rhinitis and perennial rhinitis

- ▸ BY INTRANASAL ADMINISTRATION USING NASAL SPRAY
- ▸ Child 4-11 years: 50 micrograms once daily, dose to be administered into each nostril preferably in the morning, increased if necessary to 50 micrograms twice daily, dose to be administered into each nostril
- ▸ Child 12-17 years: 100 micrograms once daily, dose to be administered into each nostril preferably in the

morning, increased if necessary to 100 micrograms twice daily, dose to be administered into each nostril; reduced to 50 micrograms once daily, dose to be administered into each nostril, dose to be reduced when control achieved

- ▸ Adult: 100 micrograms once daily, dose to be administered into each nostril preferably in the morning, increased if necessary to 100 micrograms twice daily, dose to be administered into each nostril; reduced to 50 micrograms once daily, dose to be administered into each nostril, dose to be reduced when control achieved

Nasal polyps

- ▸ BY INTRANASAL ADMINISTRATION USING NASAL DROPS
- ▸ Child 16-17 years: 200 micrograms 1-2 times a day, dose to be administered into each nostril (200 micrograms is equivalent to approximately 6 drops), alternative treatment should be considered if no improvement after 4-6 weeks
- ▸ Adult: 200 micrograms 1-2 times a day, dose to be administered into each nostril (200 micrograms is equivalent to approximately 6 drops), alternative treatment should be considered if no improvement after 4-6 weeks

AVAMYS ® SPRAY

Prophylaxis and treatment of allergic rhinitis

- ▸ BY INTRANASAL ADMINISTRATION
- ▸ Child 6-11 years: 27.5 micrograms once daily, dose to be sprayed into each nostril, then increased if necessary to 55 micrograms once daily, dose to be sprayed into each nostril, reduced to 27.5 micrograms once daily, dose to be sprayed into each nostril, dose to be reduced once control achieved; use minimum effective dose
- ▸ Child 12-17 years: 55 micrograms once daily, dose to be sprayed into each nostril, reduced to 27.5 micrograms once daily, dose to be sprayed into each nostril, dose to be reduced once control achieved; use minimum effective dose
- ▸ Adult: 55 micrograms once daily, dose to be sprayed into each nostril, reduced to 27.5 micrograms once daily, dose to be sprayed into each nostril, dose to be reduced once control achieved; use minimum effective dose

DOSE EQUIVALENCE AND CONVERSION

- ▸ For *Avamys* ® spray: 1 spray equivalent to 27.5 micrograms.

- **INTERACTIONS** → Appendix 1: corticosteroids

- **SIDE-EFFECTS** Adrenal suppression

SIDE-EFFECTS, FURTHER INFORMATION Nasal ulceration occurs commonly with nasal preparations containing fluticasone furoate.

- **EXCEPTIONS TO LEGAL CATEGORY**
- ▸ In adults Preparations of fluticasone propionate can be sold to the public for nasal administration (other than by pressurised nasal spray) if supplied for the prevention and treatment of allergic rhinitis in adults over 18 years, subject to max. single dose of 100 micrograms per nostril, max. daily dose of 200 micrograms per nostril for max. 3 months, and a pack size of 3 mg.

- **MEDICINAL FORMS** There can be variation in the licensing of different medicines containing the same drug.

Spray

EXCIPIENTS: May contain Benzalkonium chloride, disodium edetate, polysorbates

- ▸ **Fluticasone (Non-proprietary)**
  Fluticasone propionate 50 microgram per 1 dose Fluticasone propionate 50micrograms/dose nasal spray | 150 dose PoM £11.01 DT = £11.01

▶ **Avamys** (GlaxoSmithKline UK Ltd)
Fluticasone furoate 27.5 microgram per 1 dose Avamys
27.5micrograms/dose nasal spray | 120 dose [PoM] £6.44 DT = £6.44

▶ **Coryen** (Alissa Healthcare Research Ltd)
Fluticasone furoate 27.5 microgram per 1 dose Coryen
27.5micrograms/dose nasal spray | 120 dose [PoM] £6.44 DT = £6.44

▶ **Flixonase** (GlaxoSmithKline UK Ltd)
Fluticasone propionate 50 microgram per 1 dose Flixonase
50micrograms/dose aqueous nasal spray | 150 dose [PoM] £11.01 DT
= £11.01

▶ **Nasofan** (Teva UK Ltd)
Fluticasone propionate 50 microgram per 1 dose Nasofan
50micrograms/dose aqueous nasal spray | 150 dose [PoM] £8.04 DT =
£11.01

Nasal drops
EXCIPIENTS: May contain Polysorbates

▶ **Fluticasone (Non-proprietary)**
Fluticasone propionate 400 microgram Fluticasone
400microgram/unit dose nasal drops | 30 unit dose [PoM] £15.99–
£29.42 DT = £15.99

Fluticasone with azelastine

The properties listed below are those particular to the
combination only. For the properties of the components
please consider, fluticasone p. 1372, azelastine
hydrochloride p. 1370.

● **INDICATIONS AND DOSE**

**Moderate to severe seasonal and perennial allergic
rhinitis, if monotherapy with antihistamine or
corticosteroid is inadequate**
▶ BY INTRANASAL ADMINISTRATION
▶ Child 12-17 years: 1 spray twice daily, dose to be
administered into each nostril
▶ Adult: 1 spray twice daily, dose to be administered into
each nostril

● INTERACTIONS → Appendix 1: antihistamines, non-
sedating · corticosteroids

● **MEDICINAL FORMS** There can be variation in the licensing of
different medicines containing the same drug.
Spray
EXCIPIENTS: May contain Benzalkonium chloride, polysorbates

▶ **Fluticasone with azelastine (Non-proprietary)**
**Fluticasone propionate 50 microgram per 1 dose, Azelastine
hydrochloride 137 microgram per 1 dose** Fluticasone propionate
50micrograms/dose / Azelastine 137micrograms/dose nasal spray |
120 dose [PoM] £12.58–£21.24 DT = £14.80

▶ **Dymista** (Viatris UK Healthcare Ltd)
**Fluticasone propionate 50 microgram per 1 dose, Azelastine
hydrochloride 137 microgram per 1 dose** Dymista
137micrograms/dose / 50micrograms/dose nasal spray |
120 dose [PoM] £14.80 DT = £14.80

▶ **Flomister** (Strides Pharma UK Ltd)
**Fluticasone propionate 50 microgram per 1 dose, Azelastine
hydrochloride 137 microgram per 1 dose** Flomister
137micrograms/dose / 50micrograms/dose nasal spray |
120 dose [PoM] £11.10 DT = £14.80

⚑ 1371

Mometasone furoate

08-Oct-2024

● **INDICATIONS AND DOSE**

**Prophylaxis and treatment of seasonal allergic or
perennial rhinitis**
▶ BY INTRANASAL ADMINISTRATION
▶ Child 3-11 years: 50 micrograms once daily, dose to be
sprayed into each nostril
▶ Child 12-17 years: 100 micrograms once daily, dose to be
sprayed into each nostril, increased if necessary up to
200 micrograms once daily, dose to be sprayed into
each nostril; reduced to 50 micrograms once daily, dose

to be sprayed into each nostril, dose to be reduced
when control achieved
▶ Adult: 100 micrograms once daily, dose to be sprayed
into each nostril, increased if necessary up to
200 micrograms once daily, dose to be sprayed into
each nostril; reduced to 50 micrograms once daily, dose
to be sprayed into each nostril, dose to be reduced
when control achieved

Nasal polyps
▶ BY INTRANASAL ADMINISTRATION
▶ Adult: Initially 100 micrograms once daily for
5–6 weeks, dose to be sprayed into each nostril, then
increased if necessary to 100 micrograms twice daily,
dose to be sprayed into each nostril, consider
alternative treatment if no improvement after further
5–6 weeks, reduce to the lowest effective dose when
control achieved

● INTERACTIONS → Appendix 1: corticosteroids

● SIDE-EFFECTS Nasal ulceration occurs commonly with
preparations containing mometasone furoate.

● **MEDICINAL FORMS** There can be variation in the licensing of
different medicines containing the same drug.
Spray
EXCIPIENTS: May contain Benzalkonium chloride, polysorbates

▶ **Mometasone furoate (Non-proprietary)**
Mometasone furoate 50 microgram per 1 dose Mometasone
50micrograms/dose nasal spray | 140 dose [PoM] £11.16 DT = £7.61

▶ **Nasonex** (Organon Pharma (UK) Ltd)
Mometasone furoate 50 microgram per 1 dose Nasonex
50micrograms/dose nasal spray | 140 dose [PoM] £7.68 DT = £7.61

Mometasone furoate with olopatadine

21-Jan-2022

The properties listed below are those particular to the
combination only. For the properties of the components
please consider, mometasone furoate above, olopatadine
p. 1322.

● **INDICATIONS AND DOSE**

Moderate to severe allergic rhinitis
▶ BY INTRANASAL ADMINISTRATION
▶ Child 12-17 years: 2 sprays twice daily into each nostril
in the morning and evening
▶ Adult: 2 sprays twice daily into each nostril in the
morning and evening

● INTERACTIONS → Appendix 1: corticosteroids

● SIDE-EFFECTS
▶ **Common or very common** Epistaxis · nasal complaints ·
taste altered
▶ **Uncommon** Abdominal pain · dizziness · drowsiness · dry
mouth · fatigue · headaches · nausea
▶ **Rare or very rare** Anxiety · constipation · depression · dry
eye · ear pain · eye discomfort · increased risk of infection ·
insomnia · laceration · oropharyngeal pain · throat
irritation · tongue pain · vision blurred
▶ **Frequency not known** Cataract · glaucoma

SIDE-EFFECTS, FURTHER INFORMATION Systemic
absorption can follow nasal administration particularly if
high doses are used or if treatment is prolonged; therefore,
also consider the side-effects of systemic corticosteroids.

● **PATIENT AND CARER ADVICE**
Driving and skilled tasks Patients and carers should be
cautioned on the effects on driving and performance of
skilled tasks—increased risk of dizziness, lethargy, fatigue,
and somnolence.

12

Ear, nose and oropharynx

- **NATIONAL FUNDING/ACCESS DECISIONS**
  For full details see funding body website
  Scottish Medicines Consortium (SMC) decisions
  ▶ Olopatadine hydrochloride and mometasone furoate monohydrate (*Ryaltris®*) for the treatment of moderate to severe nasal symptoms associated with allergic rhinitis in adults and adolescents 12 years of age and older (December 2021) SMC No. SMC2418 Recommended with restrictions

- **MEDICINAL FORMS** There can be variation in the licensing of different medicines containing the same drug.
  Spray
  EXCIPIENTS: May contain Benzalkonium chloride, disodium edetate, polysorbates
  ▶ **Ryaltris** (Glenmark Pharmaceuticals Europe Ltd)
  Mometasone furoate 25 microgram per 1 dose, Olopatadine (as Olopatadine hydrochloride) 600 microgram per 1 dose Ryaltris 25micrograms/dose / 600micrograms/dose nasal spray | 240 dose [PoM] £13.32 DT = £13.32

⚑ 1371

Triamcinolone acetonide

20-Jul-2023

- **DRUG ACTION** Triamcinolone exerts predominantly glucocorticoid effects with minimal mineralcorticoid effect.

- **INDICATIONS AND DOSE**
  Prophylaxis and treatment of allergic rhinitis
  ▶ BY INTRANASAL ADMINISTRATION
  ▶ Child 6-11 years: 55 micrograms once daily, dose to be sprayed into each nostril, increased if necessary to 110 micrograms once daily, dose to be sprayed into each nostril; reduced to 55 micrograms once daily, dose to be sprayed into each nostril, reduce dose when control achieved; maximum duration of treatment 3 months
  ▶ Child 12-17 years: 110 micrograms once daily, dose to be sprayed into each nostril, reduced to 55 micrograms once daily, dose to be sprayed into each nostril, reduce dose when control achieved
  ▶ Adult: 110 micrograms once daily, dose to be sprayed into each nostril, reduced to 55 micrograms once daily, dose to be sprayed into each nostril, reduce dose when control achieved

- **INTERACTIONS** → Appendix 1: corticosteroids

- **EXCEPTIONS TO LEGAL CATEGORY**
  ▶ In adults Preparations of triamcinolone acetonide can be sold to the public for nasal administration as a non-pressurised nasal spray if supplied for the symptomatic treatment of seasonal allergic rhinitis in adults over 18 years, subject to maximum daily dose of 110 micrograms per nostril for maximum 3 months, and a pack size of 3.575 mg.

- **MEDICINAL FORMS** There can be variation in the licensing of different medicines containing the same drug.
  Spray
  EXCIPIENTS: May contain Benzalkonium chloride, disodium edetate, polysorbates
  ▶ **Nasacort** (Opella Healthcare UK Ltd)
  Triamcinolone acetonide 55 microgram per 1 dose Nasacort 55micrograms/dose nasal spray | 120 dose [PoM] £7.39 DT = £7.39

Oropharynx

1 Dry mouth

Dry mouth

14-Dec-2020

Overview

Dry mouth (xerostomia) resulting from reduced saliva secretion may be caused by drugs such as antimuscarinics, antihistamines, tricyclic antidepressants, and some diuretics. It can also be caused by irradiation of the head and neck region, dehydration, anxiety, or Sjögren's syndrome. Patients with dry mouth may be at greater risk of developing dental caries, periodontal disease, and oral infections (particularly candidiasis).

[EvGr] Underlying causes of dry mouth such as dehydration, anxiety, infection, or drugs causing dry mouth should be managed if appropriate. Dry mouth may be relieved in many patients by simple measures that stimulate salivation such as frequent sips of cold unsweetened drinks, or sucking pieces of ice or sugar-free fruit pastilles, or chewing sugar-free gum.

An artificial saliva substitute can be considered if simple stimulatory measures are inadequate. Ⓐ The acidic pH of some artificial saliva products may be inappropriate for some patients as it may damage the enamel of natural teeth. Artificial saliva products below are available in oral lozenges, oral gel, oral spray, and pastille forms.

Pilocarpine tablets p. 1376 are licensed for the treatment of xerostomia following irradiation for head and neck cancer, and dry mouth and dry eyes (xerophthalmia) in Sjögren's syndrome. [EvGr] They may take up to 3 months to be effective; treatment should be withdrawn if there is no response within this time. Ⓐ

LUBRICANTS

Artificial saliva products

- **ARTIFICIAL SALIVA PRODUCTS**
  AS SALIVA ORTHANA ® LOZENGES
  Mucin 65 mg, xylitol 59 mg, in a sorbitol basis, pH neutral

- **INDICATIONS AND DOSE**
  Dry mouth as a result of having (or having undergone) radiotherapy (ACBS) | Dry mouth as a result of sicca syndrome (ACBS)
  ▶ BY MOUTH
  ▶ Adult: 1 lozenge as required, allow to dissolve slowly in the mouth

- **PRESCRIBING AND DISPENSING INFORMATION** *AS Saliva Orthana®* lozenges do not contain fluoride.

  AS SALIVA ORTHANA ® SPRAY
  Gastric mucin (porcine) 3.5%, xylitol 2%, sodium fluoride 4.2 mg/litre, with preservatives and flavouring agents, pH neutral.

- **INDICATIONS AND DOSE**
  Symptomatic treatment of dry mouth
  ▶ BY MOUTH
  ▶ Adult: Apply 2–3 sprays as required, spray onto oral and pharyngeal mucosa

- **PROFESSION SPECIFIC INFORMATION**
  Dental practitioners' formulary *AS Saliva Orthana®* Oral Spray may be prescribed.

AS Saliva Orthana spray (CCMed Ltd)
50 ml · NHS indicative price = £4.92 · Drug Tariff (Part IXa)

BIOXTRA ® DRY MOUTH GEL MOUTHSPRAY

Aqua, xylitol, hydrogenated starch hydrolysate, sorbitol, hydroxyethylcellulose, sodium monofluorophosphate, sodium saccharin, potassium chloride, sodium chloride, magnesium chloride, dipotassium phosphate, calcium chloride, colostrum whey, lactoperoxidase, citric acid, sodium benzoate, sodium methylparaben, sodium propylparaben, and potassium sorbate.

● **INDICATIONS AND DOSE**

Symptomatic treatment of dry mouth
▶ BY MOUTH
▶ Adult: Apply as required, spray onto gums, tongue, and lips

BIOXTRA ® DRY MOUTH ORAL GEL

Aqua, glycerin, sorbitol, hydrogenated starch hydrolysate, xylitol, hydroxyethylcellulose, glucose, butylene glycol, sodium polyacrylate, polyacrylic acid, colostrum whey, glucose oxidase, lactoperoxidase, lactoferrin, lysozyme, aloe barbadensis leaf juice, potassium thiocyanate and benzoic acid.

● **INDICATIONS AND DOSE**

Symptomatic treatment of dry mouth
▶ BY MOUTH
▶ Adult: Apply as required, particularly at night, to oral mucosa

● **PROFESSION SPECIFIC INFORMATION**

Dental practitioners' formulary *BioXtra* ® Dry Mouth Oral Gel may be prescribed as Artificial Saliva Gel.

BIOTENE ORALBALANCE ®

Lactoperoxidase, lactoferrin, lysozyme, glucose oxidase, xylitol in a gel basis

● **INDICATIONS AND DOSE**

Symptomatic treatment of dry mouth
▶ BY MOUTH
▶ Adult: Apply as required, apply to gums and tongue

● **PATIENT AND CARER ADVICE** Avoid use with toothpastes containing detergents (including foaming agents).

● **PROFESSION SPECIFIC INFORMATION**

Dental practitioners' formulary *Biotene Oralbalance* ® Saliva Replacement Gel may be prescribed as Artificial Saliva Gel.

Biotene Oralbalance dry mouth saliva replacement gel (Haleon UK Trading Ltd) **Glucose oxidase 12000 unit, Lactoferrin 12 mg, Lactoperoxidase 12000 unit, Muramidase 12 mg** 50 gram · NHS indicative price = £5.30 · Drug Tariff (Part IXa)

GLANDOSANE ®

Carmellose sodium 500 mg, sorbitol 1.5 g, potassium chloride 60 mg, sodium chloride 42.2 mg, magnesium chloride 2.6 mg, calcium chloride 7.3 mg, and dipotassium hydrogen phosphate 17.1 mg/50 g, pH 5.75.

● **INDICATIONS AND DOSE**

Dry mouth as a result of having (or having undergone) radiotherapy (ACBS) | Dry mouth as a result of sicca syndrome (ACBS)
▶ BY MOUTH
▶ Adult: Apply as required, spray onto oral and pharyngeal mucosa

● **PROFESSION SPECIFIC INFORMATION**

Dental practitioners' formulary *Glandosane* ® Aerosol Spray may be prescribed.

ORALIEVE ® MOISTURISING MOUTH GEL

Sorbitol, glycerin, aqua, xylitol, carbomer, sorbic acid, hydroxyethyl cellulose, whey protein, sodium hydroxide, benzoic acid, glucose, lactoferrin, lactoperoxidase, glucose oxidase, potassium thiocyanate, disodium phosphate and aloe vera.

● **INDICATIONS AND DOSE**

Symptomatic treatment of dry mouth
▶ BY MOUTH
▶ Adult: Apply as required, particularly at night, to oral mucosa

● **PROFESSION SPECIFIC INFORMATION**

Dental practitioners' formulary *Oralieve* ® Moisturising Mouth Gel may be prescribed as Artificial Saliva Gel.

Oralieve moisturising mouth gel (Oralieve UK)
50 ml · NHS indicative price = £3.16 · Drug Tariff (Part IXa)

ORALIEVE ® MOISTURISING MOUTH SPRAY

Aqua, glycerin, xylitol, poloxamer 407, sodium benzoate, sodium phosphate, xanthan gum, aroma, disodium phosphate, benzoic acid, whey protein, lactoferrin, lactoperoxidase, potassium thiocyanate, glucose oxidase, limonene, alcohol-free, detergent-free.

● **INDICATIONS AND DOSE**

Symptomatic treatment of dry mouth
▶ BY MOUTH
▶ Adult: 1 spray as required, on the inside of each cheek, gums and tongue

Oralieve moisturising mouth spray (Oralieve UK)
50 ml · NHS indicative price = £4.95 · Drug Tariff (Part IXa)

SST ®

Sugar-free, citric acid, malic acid and other ingredients in a sorbitol base.

● **INDICATIONS AND DOSE**

Symptomatic treatment of dry mouth in patients with impaired salivary gland function and patent salivary ducts
▶ BY MOUTH
▶ Adult: 1 tablet as required, allow tablet to dissolve slowly in the mouth

● **PROFESSION SPECIFIC INFORMATION**

Dental practitioners' formulary May be prescribed as Saliva Stimulating Tablets.

SST saliva stimulating tablets (Sinclair IS Pharma Plc)
100 tablet · NHS indicative price = £4.86 · Drug Tariff (Part IXa)

SALIVEZE ®

Carmellose sodium (sodium carboxymethylcellulose), calcium chloride, magnesium chloride, potassium chloride, sodium chloride, and dibasic sodium phosphate, pH neutral

● **INDICATIONS AND DOSE**

Dry mouth as a result of having (or having undergone) radiotherapy (ACBS) | Dry mouth as a result of sicca syndrome (ACBS)
▶ BY MOUTH
▶ Adult: Apply 1 spray as required, spray onto oral mucosa

● **PROFESSION SPECIFIC INFORMATION**

Dental practitioners' formulary *Saliveze* ® Oral Spray may be prescribed.

Saliveze mouth spray (Wyvern Medical Ltd)
50 ml · NHS indicative price = £3.70 · Drug Tariff (Part IXa)

12

Ear, nose and oropharynx

SALIVIX [®]

Sugar-free, reddish-amber, acacia, malic acid and other ingredients.

- **INDICATIONS AND DOSE**

Symptomatic treatment of dry mouth
▸ BY MOUTH USING PASTILLES
▸ Adult: 1 unit as required, suck pastille

- **PROFESSION SPECIFIC INFORMATION**

Dental practitioners' formulary *Salivix*[®] Pastilles may be prescribed as Artificial Saliva Pastilles.

Salivix pastilles (Galen Ltd)
50 pastille · NHS indicative price = £3.79 · Drug Tariff (Part IXa)

XEROTIN [®]

Sugar-free, water, sorbitol, carmellose (carboxymethylcellulose), potassium chloride, sodium chloride, potassium phosphate, magnesium chloride, calcium chloride and other ingredients, pH neutral.

- **INDICATIONS AND DOSE**

Symptomatic treatment of dry mouth
▸ BY MOUTH
▸ Adult: 1 spray as required

- **PROFESSION SPECIFIC INFORMATION**

Dental practitioners' formulary *Xerotin*[®] Oral Spray may be prescribed as Artificial Saliva Oral Spray.

Xerotin spray (SpePharm UK Ltd)
100 ml · NHS indicative price = £6.86 · Drug Tariff (Part IXa)

PARASYMPATHOMIMETICS

| Pilocarpine

11-May-2021

- **INDICATIONS AND DOSE**

Xerostomia following irradiation for head and neck cancer
▸ BY MOUTH
▸ Adult: 5 mg 3 times a day for 4 weeks, then increased if tolerated to up to 30 mg daily in divided doses if required, dose to be taken with or immediately after meals (last dose always with evening meal), maximum therapeutic effect normally within 4–8 weeks; discontinue if no improvement after 2–3 months

Dry mouth and dry eyes in Sjögren's syndrome
▸ BY MOUTH
▸ Adult: 5 mg 4 times a day; increased if tolerated to up to 30 mg daily in divided doses if required, dose to be taken with meals and at bedtime, discontinue if no improvement after 2–3 months

- **CONTRA-INDICATIONS** Acute iritis · uncontrolled asthma (increased bronchial secretions and increased airways resistance) · uncontrolled cardiorenal disease · uncontrolled chronic obstructive pulmonary disease (increased bronchial secretions and increased airways resistance)
- **CAUTIONS** Asthma (avoid if uncontrolled) · biliary-tract disease · cardiovascular disease (avoid if uncontrolled) · cholelithiasis · chronic obstructive pulmonary disease (avoid if uncontrolled) · cognitive disturbances · maintain adequate fluid intake to avoid dehydration associated with excessive sweating · peptic ulceration · psychiatric disturbances · risk of increased renal colic · risk of increased urethral smooth muscle tone · susceptibility to angle-closure glaucoma
- **INTERACTIONS** → Appendix 1: pilocarpine
- **SIDE-EFFECTS**
▸ **Common or very common** Asthenia · conjunctivitis · constipation · diarrhoea · dizziness · excessive tearing · eye pain · flushing · gastrointestinal discomfort · headache · hyperhidrosis · hypersalivation · hypersensitivity · hypertension · increased risk of infection · nausea · palpitations · skin reactions · urinary disorders · vision disorders · vomiting
▸ **Uncommon** Gastrointestinal disorders
▸ **Frequency not known** Affective disorder · agitation · arrhythmias · atrioventricular block · chills · confusion · hallucination · hypotension · memory loss · psychiatric disorder · respiratory distress · shock · tremor

- **PREGNANCY** Avoid—smooth muscle stimulant; toxicity in *animal* studies.
- **BREAST FEEDING** Manufacturer advises avoid—present in milk in *animal* studies.
- **HEPATIC IMPAIRMENT** Manufacturer advises caution in moderate to severe cirrhosis.
Dose adjustments Manufacturer advises initial dose reduction in moderate to severe cirrhosis.
- **RENAL IMPAIRMENT** Manufacturer advises caution with tablets.
- **PATIENT AND CARER ADVICE**
Driving and skilled tasks Blurred vision may affect performance of skilled tasks (e.g. driving) particularly at night or in reduced lighting.

- **MEDICINAL FORMS** There can be variation in the licensing of different medicines containing the same drug. Forms available from special-order manufacturers include: oral solution

Oral tablet
CAUTIONARY AND ADVISORY LABELS 21, 27
▸ Pilocarpine (Non-proprietary)
Pilocarpine hydrochloride 5 mg Pilocarpine 5mg tablets |
84 tablet [PoM] £41.14–£41.40 DT = £41.14
▸ Salagen (Norgine Pharmaceuticals Ltd)
Pilocarpine hydrochloride 5 mg Salagen 5mg tablets |
84 tablet [PoM] £41.14 DT = £41.14

2 Oral hygiene

Mouthwashes and other preparations for oropharyngeal use

01-Sep-2020

Lozenges and sprays

[EvGr] Lozenges containing either a local anaesthetic, an antiseptic, or a non-steroidal anti-inflammatory drug may be trialled but may only lead to a small reduction in pain. However, there is no evidence that non-medicated lozenges and local anaesthetic sprays have a beneficial action on their own in treating sore throat. [A]

Mouthwashes, gargles, and dentifrices

Expert sources advise that a saline mouthwash may be used for cleaning or freshening the mouth and can be prepared by dissolving half a teaspoonful of salt in a glassful of warm water.

[EvGr] Mouthwashes containing an oxidising agent, such as hydrogen peroxide p. 1377, may be useful in the treatment of acute ulcerative gingivitis whilst awaiting to be seen by a dentist. [A]

Chlorhexidine p. 1377 can be used as a mouthwash, spray, or gel and is licensed for the management of gingivitis and maintenance of oral hygiene, particularly where there is a painful periodontal condition or if the patient is unable to adequately brush their teeth (e.g. following dental procedures or due to disability). It is also licensed for the management of denture stomatitis, aphthous ulcers, oral candidiasis, and following post-periodontal treatment to promote healing. Chlorhexidine mouthwash should not be used for the prevention of endocarditis in patients undergoing dental procedures.

Chlorhexidine is an effective antiseptic which has the advantage of inhibiting plaque formation on the teeth but there is limited evidence to demonstrate efficacy in preventing dental caries. Public Health England advise to use other treatments for preventing dental caries, such as fluoride-based products.

Chlorhexidine is incompatible with anionic agents present in some toothpastes; it has therefore been suggested to wait 30 minutes between using these two preparations.

ANTISEPTICS AND DISINFECTANTS

Chlorhexidine
23-Feb-2022

● **INDICATIONS AND DOSE**

Oral hygiene and plaque inhibition | Oral candidiasis | Gingivitis | Management of aphthous ulcers
▸ BY OROMUCOSAL ADMINISTRATION USING MOUTHWASH
▸ Child: Rinse or gargle 10 mL twice daily, rinse or gargle for about 1 minute
▸ Adult: Rinse or gargle 10 mL twice daily, rinse or gargle for about 1 minute
▸ BY OROMUCOSAL ADMINISTRATION USING OROMUCOSAL SPRAY
▸ Child: Apply up to 12 sprays twice daily as required, to be applied on tooth, gingival, or ulcer surfaces
▸ Adult: Apply up to 12 sprays twice daily as required, to be applied on tooth, gingival, or ulcer surfaces

Denture stomatitis
▸ MOUTHWASH
▸ Adult: Cleanse and soak dentures in mouthwash solution for 15 minutes twice daily

Oral hygiene and plaque inhibition | Gingivitis
▸ BY OROMUCOSAL ADMINISTRATION USING DENTAL GEL
▸ Child: Apply 1–2 times a day, to be brushed on the teeth
▸ Adult: Apply 1–2 times a day, to be brushed on the teeth

Oral candidiasis | Management of aphthous ulcers
▸ BY OROMUCOSAL ADMINISTRATION USING DENTAL GEL
▸ Child: Apply 1–2 times a day, to affected areas
▸ Adult: Apply 1–2 times a day, to affected areas

DOSE EQUIVALENCE AND CONVERSION
▸ Mouthwashes and oromucosal sprays contain chlorhexidine gluconate 0.2% w/v.

● UNLICENSED USE *Corsodyl*® not licensed for use in children under 12 years (unless on the advice of a healthcare professional).

● SIDE-EFFECTS
▸ **Common or very common**
▸ With oromucosal use Dry mouth · hypersensitivity · oral disorders · taste altered · tongue discolouration · tooth discolouration

SIDE-EFFECTS, FURTHER INFORMATION If desquamation occurs with mucosal irritation, discontinue treatment.

● PRESCRIBING AND DISPENSING INFORMATION Chlorhexidine digluconate is a synonym for chlorhexidine gluconate.

● PATIENT AND CARER ADVICE Chlorhexidine gluconate may be incompatible with some ingredients in toothpaste; rinse the mouth thoroughly with water between using toothpaste and chlorhexidine-containing product.

● PROFESSION SPECIFIC INFORMATION
Dental practitioners' formulary *Corsodyl*® dental gel may be prescribed as Chlorhexidine Gluconate Gel; *Corsodyl*® mouthwash may be prescribed as Chlorhexidine

Mouthwash; *Corsodyl*® oral spray may be prescribed as Chlorhexidine Oral Spray.

● MEDICINAL FORMS There can be variation in the licensing of different medicines containing the same drug.
Dental gel
▸ Chlorhexidine (Non-proprietary)
Chlorhexidine gluconate 2 mg per 1 gram Perio-kin 0.2% gel | 30 ml ▣
▸ Corsodyl (Haleon UK Trading Ltd)
Chlorhexidine gluconate 10 mg per 1 gram Corsodyl 1% dental gel | 50 gram ℗ £3.24 DT = £3.24 SF
Mouthwash
▸ Chlorhexidine (Non-proprietary)
Chlorhexidine gluconate 2 mg per 1 ml Chlorhexidine gluconate 0.2% mouthwash original | 300 ml GSL ▣ DT = £3.16
Chlorhexidine gluconate 0.2% mouthwash aniseed | 300 ml GSL £2.64 DT = £3.16
Chlorhexidine gluconate 0.2% mouthwash peppermint | 300 ml GSL £3.16 DT = £3.16
Chlorhexidine gluconate 0.2% mouthwash plain | 300 ml GSL £3.16 DT = £3.16

Hexetidine
06-Aug-2018

● **INDICATIONS AND DOSE**

Oral hygiene
▸ BY OROMUCOSAL ADMINISTRATION USING MOUTHWASH
▸ Child 12-17 years: Rinse or gargle 15 mL 2–3 times a day, to be used undiluted
▸ Adult: Rinse or gargle 15 mL 2–3 times a day, to be used undiluted

● SIDE-EFFECTS
▸ **Rare or very rare** Anaesthesia · taste altered
▸ **Frequency not known** Cough · dry mouth · dysphagia · dyspnoea · nausea · salivary gland enlargement · vomiting

● MEDICINAL FORMS There can be variation in the licensing of different medicines containing the same drug.
Mouthwash
▸ Oraldene (McNeil Products Ltd)
Hexetidine 1 mg per 1 ml Oraldene 0.1% mouthwash peppermint | 200 ml GSL £2.92 DT = £2.92 SF

Hydrogen peroxide
14-May-2024

● DRUG ACTION Hydrogen peroxide is an oxidising agent.

● **INDICATIONS AND DOSE**

Oral hygiene (with hydrogen peroxide 6%)
▸ BY MOUTH USING MOUTHWASH
▸ Child: Rinse or gargle 15 mL 2–3 times a day for 2–3 minutes, to be diluted in half a tumblerful of warm water
▸ Adult: Rinse or gargle 15 mL 2–3 times a day for 2–3 minutes, to be diluted in half a tumblerful of warm water

PEROXYL®

Oral hygiene
▸ BY MOUTH USING MOUTHWASH
▸ Child 6-17 years: Rinse or gargle 10 mL 3 times a day for about 1 minute, for maximum 7 days, to be used after meals and at bedtime
▸ Adult: Rinse or gargle 10 mL up to 4 times a day for about 1 minute, to be used after meals and at bedtime

● PRESCRIBING AND DISPENSING INFORMATION When prepared extemporaneously, the BP states Hydrogen Peroxide Mouthwash, BP consists of hydrogen peroxide 6% solution (= approx. 20 volume) BP.

● HANDLING AND STORAGE Hydrogen peroxide bleaches fabric.

- **PROFESSION SPECIFIC INFORMATION**

Dental practitioners' formulary Hydrogen Peroxide Mouthwash may be prescribed.

- **MEDICINAL FORMS** There can be variation in the licensing of different medicines containing the same drug.

Cutaneous or oromucosal liquid

▶ Hydrogen peroxide (Non-proprietary)
Hydrogen peroxide 30 ml per 1 litre Hydrogen peroxide 3% solution | 100 ml [PoM] ⚠

Mouthwash

▶ Peroxyl (Colgate-Palmolive (UK) Ltd)
Hydrogen peroxide 15 mg per 1 ml Peroxyl 1.5% mouthwash | 300 ml [GSL] £2.94 DT = £2.94 [SF]

Sodium bicarbonate with sodium chloride

28-Nov-2022

- **INDICATIONS AND DOSE**

Oral hygiene

▶ BY OROMUCOSAL ADMINISTRATION USING MOUTHWASH
▶ Adult: Rinse or gargle as required

- **DIRECTIONS FOR ADMINISTRATION** To be diluted with an equal volume of warm water prior to use.

- **PRESCRIBING AND DISPENSING INFORMATION** Compound Sodium Chloride Mouthwash BP consists of sodium bicarbonate 1% and sodium chloride 1.5% in a suitable vehicle with peppermint flavour.

    Extemporaneous mouthwash preparations should be prepared according to the following formula: sodium chloride 1.5 g, sodium bicarbonate 1 g, concentrated peppermint emulsion 2.5 mL, double-strength chloroform water 50 mL, water to 100 mL.

- **PROFESSION SPECIFIC INFORMATION**

Dental practitioners' formulary Compound sodium chloride mouthwash may be prescribed.

- **MEDICINAL FORMS** Forms available from special-order manufacturers include: mouthwash

2.1 Dental caries

Fluoride

24-Apr-2020

Overview

Fluoride is a naturally occurring mineral found in water supplies in varying amounts and in some foods; it has beneficial topical effects on teeth. Public Health England advise that all adults and children brush their teeth with fluoridated toothpaste at least twice daily to help prevent tooth decay.

    Individuals who are either particularly caries prone or medically compromised may be given additional protection. Public Health England recommends the daily use of a fluoride mouthwash in adults and children aged 7 years and over who are causing concern to their dentist (e.g. those with active caries, dry mouth, or special needs). They should be used at a different time to brushing to avoid removal of the beneficial effects of fluoride in toothpaste.

    Fluoride varnish is also available and can be applied topically to both primary or permanent teeth. Public Health England recommends that all children aged 3 years and over have fluoride varnish applied (usually twice a year) regardless of their risk of caries. Application of fluoride varnish at least twice a year may also be considered in adults and children aged under 3 years who are causing concern to their dentist.

Useful resources

Delivering better oral health: an evidence-based toolkit for prevention. Public Health England. March 2017.
    www.gov.uk/government/publications/delivering-better-oral-health-an-evidence-based-toolkit-for-prevention

VITAMINS AND TRACE ELEMENTS

Sodium fluoride

25-Nov-2020

- **INDICATIONS AND DOSE**

Prophylaxis of dental caries for water content less than 300micrograms/litre (0.3 parts per million) of fluoride ion

▶ BY MOUTH USING TABLETS
▶ Child 6 months–2 years: 250 micrograms daily, doses expressed as fluoride ion (F⁻)
▶ Child 3–5 years: 500 micrograms daily, doses expressed as fluoride ion (F⁻)
▶ Child 6–17 years: 1 mg daily, doses expressed as fluoride ion (F⁻)
▶ Adult: 1 mg daily, doses expressed as fluoride ion (F⁻)

Prophylaxis of dental caries for water content between 300 and 700micrograms/litre (0.3–0.7 parts per million) of fluoride ion

▶ BY MOUTH USING TABLETS
▶ Child 3–5 years: 250 micrograms daily, doses expressed as fluoride ion (F⁻)
▶ Child 6–17 years: 500 micrograms daily, doses expressed as fluoride ion (F⁻)
▶ Adult: 500 micrograms daily, doses expressed as fluoride ion (F⁻)

Prophylaxis of dental caries

▶ BY MOUTH USING MOUTHWASH
▶ Adult: Rinse or gargle 5–10 mL daily

DOSE EQUIVALENCE AND CONVERSION

▶ Sodium fluoride 2.2 mg provides approx. 1 mg fluoride ion.

COLGATE DURAPHAT ® 2800PPM FLUORIDE TOOTHPASTE

Prophylaxis of dental caries

▶ BY MOUTH USING PASTE
▶ Child 10–17 years: Apply 1 centimetre twice daily, to be applied using a toothbrush
▶ Adult: Apply 1 centimetre twice daily, to be applied using a toothbrush

COLGATE DURAPHAT ® 5000PPM FLUORIDE TOOTHPASTE

Prophylaxis of dental caries

▶ BY MOUTH USING PASTE
▶ Child 16–17 years: Apply 2 centimetres 3 times a day, to be applied after meals using a toothbrush
▶ Adult: Apply 2 centimetres 3 times a day, to be applied after meals using a toothbrush

EN-DE-KAY ® FLUORINSE

Prophylaxis of dental caries

▶ BY MOUTH USING MOUTHWASH
▶ Adult: 5 drops daily, dilute 5 drops to 10 mL of water, alternatively 20 drops once weekly, dilute 20 drops to 10 mL

- **SIDE-EFFECTS** Dental fluorosis

- **DIRECTIONS FOR ADMINISTRATION**

▶ With oral use Manufacturer advises tablets should be sucked or dissolved in the mouth at a different time of day to tooth brushing.
▶ With oral (topical) use Manufacturer advises for mouthwash, rinse mouth for 1 minute and then spit out.

COLGATE DURAPHAT ® 2800PPM FLUORIDE TOOTHPASTE Manufacturer advises brush teeth for 1 minute before spitting out.

COLGATE DURAPHAT ® 5000PPM FLUORIDE TOOTHPASTE Manufacturer advises brush teeth for 3 minutes before spitting out.

- **PRESCRIBING AND DISPENSING INFORMATION** Flavours of oral tablet formulations may include orange.

- **PATIENT AND CARER ADVICE**

Mouthwash Avoid eating, drinking, or rinsing mouth for 15 minutes after use.

COLGATE DURAPHAT ® 2800PPM FLUORIDE TOOTHPASTE Patients or carers should be given advice on how to administer sodium fluoride toothpaste.

Avoid drinking or rinsing mouth for 30 minutes after use.

COLGATE DURAPHAT ® 5000PPM FLUORIDE TOOTHPASTE Patients or carers should be given advice on how to administer sodium fluoride toothpaste.

- **PROFESSION SPECIFIC INFORMATION**

Dental practitioners' formulary Tablets may be prescribed as Sodium Fluoride Tablets.

Oral drops may be prescribed as Sodium Fluoride Oral Drops.

Mouthwashes may be prescribed as Sodium Fluoride Mouthwash 0.05% or Sodium Fluoride Mouthwash 2%.

COLGATE DURAPHAT ® 2800PPM FLUORIDE TOOTHPASTE May be prescribed as Sodium Fluoride Toothpaste 0.619%.

COLGATE DURAPHAT ® 5000PPM FLUORIDE TOOTHPASTE May be prescribed as Sodium Fluoride Toothpaste 1.1%.

Dental information Fluoride mouthwash, oral drops, tablets and toothpaste are prescribable on form FP10D (GP14 in Scotland, WP10D in Wales).

There are also arrangements for health authorities to supply fluoride tablets in the course of pre-school dental schemes, and they may also be supplied in school dental schemes.

Fluoride gels are not prescribable on form FP10D (GP14 in Scotland, WP10D in Wales).

- **MEDICINAL FORMS** There can be variation in the licensing of different medicines containing the same drug.

Dental paste

▸ Colgate Duraphat (Colgate-Palmolive (UK) Ltd)

  Fluoride (as Sodium fluoride) 2.8 mg per 1 gram Colgate Duraphat 2800ppm fluoride toothpaste | 75 ml [PoM] £3.26 DT = £2.83 [SF]

  Fluoride (as Sodium fluoride) 5 mg per 1 gram Colgate Duraphat 5000ppm fluoride toothpaste | 51 gram [PoM] £6.50 DT = £8.81 [SF]

Mouthwash

▸ Colgate FluoriGard (Colgate-Palmolive (UK) Ltd)

  Sodium fluoride 500 microgram per 1 gram Colgate FluoriGard 0.05% daily dental rinse | 400 ml [GSL] £2.99 [SF]

▸ Endekay (Manx Healthcare Ltd)

  Sodium fluoride 500 microgram per 1 gram Endekay 0.05% daily fluoride mouthrinse | 250 ml [GSL] £2.13 DT = £2.13 [SF] | 500 ml [GSL] £2.94 [SF]

---

3   Oral ulceration and inflammation

Oral ulceration and inflammation

09-Dec-2020

Ulceration and inflammation

Ulceration of the oral mucosa is common and usually transient but may require treatment in some cases. Causes include mechanical trauma, infections, malignant lesions, inflammatory conditions, nutritional deficiencies (e.g. iron, folic acid, vitamin B_{12}), immunodeficiency states, gastro-intestinal disease, and drug therapy (see also *Chemotherapy induced mucositis and myelosuppression* under Cytotoxic drugs p. 1027).

Aphthous ulcers are often recurrent and are not associated with an underlying systemic disease; they are small, round or ovoid mouth ulcers with defined margins. Aphthous ulcers may be precipitated by triggers such as certain food and drinks, allergies, anxiety, or hormonal changes. It is important to consider and exclude any possible systemic disease; treatment may include correcting the underlying cause. Treatment aims to relieve pain, reduce ulcer duration, and reduce the frequency of recurrent episodes. Secondary bacterial infections may occur with mucosal ulceration; it can increase discomfort and delay healing.

[EvGr] Patients with an unexplained mouth ulcer of more than 3 weeks' duration should be referred urgently to a specialist to exclude oral cancer. ⟨A⟩

Treatment of aphthous ulcers

[EvGr] Advise patients to avoid known triggers for ulceration, such as oral trauma (e.g. biting during chewing, ill-fitting dentures) or certain food and drinks (e.g. coffee, gluten-containing products). If the ulcers are mild, infrequent, and do not interfere with daily activities (such as eating), treatment may not be required. ⟨A⟩

Corticosteroids

[EvGr] Topical corticosteroids are usually considered to be first-line treatment. ⟨A⟩ Expert sources advise that hydrocortisone oromucosal tablets p. 1382, beclometasone dipropionate inhaler p. 1381 [unlicensed indication] sprayed onto the oral mucosa, and betamethasone soluble tablets p. 1381 [unlicensed indication] used as a mouthwash are suitable options.

[EvGr] A short course of systemic corticosteroids may be prescribed for patients with severe recurrent aphthous ulcers. ⟨A⟩

Other therapies

[EvGr] Other therapies that may be used alone or in combination with topical corticosteroids include topical anaesthetics (e.g. lidocaine hydrochloride p. 1380), topical analgesics/anti-inflammatory agents (e.g. benzydamine hydrochloride p. 1380), and topical antimicrobial agents (e.g. chlorhexidine mouthwash p. 1377). ⟨A⟩[EvGr] Doxycycline p. 1383 [unlicensed indication], rinsed in the mouth and expelled, may be considered for recurrent aphthous ulceration when other treatments are unsuccessful or unsuitable. ⟨E⟩

Expert sources advise that a saline (with or without sodium bicarbonate) mouthwash may soothe ulcers, help to maintain oral hygiene, and prevent secondary infection. Tepid water appears to be more soothing than cold or warm water.

Expert sources advise that local anaesthetics have a short duration of action; there is limited evidence for their use in the management of oral ulceration. Lidocaine hydrochloride 5% ointment or lozenges containing the local anaesthetic may be applied to the ulcer. Lidocaine hydrochloride 10% solution [unlicensed indication] as spray can be applied thinly to the ulcer using a cotton bud. When local anaesthetics are used in the mouth, care must be taken to avoid causing anaesthesia of the pharynx before meals, as this might lead to choking.

Benzydamine hydrochloride and flurbiprofen p. 1381 are non-steroidal anti-inflammatory drugs (NSAIDs). Benzydamine hydrochloride mouthwash and spray are licensed for the relief of painful inflammatory conditions associated with a variety of ulcerative conditions, as well as for discomfort of tonsillectomy and post-irradiation mucositis. Benzydamine hydrochloride mouthwash should generally be used undiluted; it can be diluted with an equal volume of water if a stinging sensation occurs. Flurbiprofen lozenges are licensed for the relief of sore throat.

Choline salicylate p. 1382 is a derivative of salicylic acid and has some analgesic properties. The dental gel is licensed for pain relief in mouth ulcers including ulcers due to dentures and orthodontic devices.

[EvGr] Consider offering or advising the use of a vitamin B_{12} supplement regardless of serum vitamin B_{12} levels. ⒶΛ

ANAESTHETICS, LOCAL

Lidocaine hydrochloride
17-Aug-2020

(Lignocaine hydrochloride)

● **INDICATIONS AND DOSE**

Dental practice
▸ BY BUCCAL ADMINISTRATION USING OINTMENT
▸ Adult: Rub gently into dry gum

Relief of pain in oral lesions
▸ TO THE LESION USING OINTMENT
▸ Adult: Apply as required, rub sparingly and gently on affected areas

XYLOCAINE ®

Bronchoscopy | Laryngoscopy | Oesophagoscopy | Endotracheal intubation
▸ TO MUCOUS MEMBRANES
▸ Adult: Up to 20 doses

Dental practice
▸ TO MUCOUS MEMBRANES
▸ Adult: 1–5 doses

Maxillary sinus puncture
▸ TO MUCOUS MEMBRANES
▸ Adult: 3 doses

Relief of pain in oral lesions
▸ TO THE LESION
▸ Adult: Apply thinly to the ulcer using a cotton bud

● **UNLICENSED USE** Spray not licensed for the relief of pain in oral lesions.

● **CAUTIONS** Avoid anaesthesia of the pharynx before meals—risk of choking · can damage plastic cuffs of endotracheal tubes

● **INTERACTIONS** → Appendix 1: antiarrhythmics

● **ALLERGY AND CROSS-SENSITIVITY**
▸ Hypersensitivity and cross-sensitivity Hypersensitivity reactions occur mainly with the ester-type local anaesthetics, such as tetracaine; reactions are less frequent with the amide types, such as articaine, bupivacaine, levobupivacaine, lidocaine, mepivacaine, prilocaine, and ropivacaine. Cross-sensitivity reactions may be avoided by using the alternative chemical type.

● **PREGNANCY** Crosses the placenta but not known to be harmful in *animal* studies—use if benefit outweighs risk. When used as a local anaesthetic, large doses can cause fetal bradycardia; if given during delivery can also cause neonatal respiratory depression, hypotonia, or bradycardia after paracervical or epidural block.

● **BREAST FEEDING** Present in milk but amount too small to be harmful.

● **HEPATIC IMPAIRMENT** Manufacturer advises caution (risk of increased exposure).

● **RENAL IMPAIRMENT** Possible accumulation of lidocaine and active metabolite; caution in severe impairment.

● **PROFESSION SPECIFIC INFORMATION**

Dental practitioners' formulary Lidocaine ointment 5% may be prescribed.

Spray may be prescribed as Lidocaine Spray 10%

XYLOCAINE ® Dental practitioners' formulary May be prescribed as lidocaine spray 10%.

● **MEDICINAL FORMS** There can be variation in the licensing of different medicines containing the same drug. Forms available from special-order manufacturers include: ointment

Spray
▸ Xylocaine (Aspen Pharma Trading Ltd)
 Lidocaine 10 mg per 1 actuation Xylocaine 10mg/dose spray | 50 ml [P] £6.29 DT = £6.29 [SF]

Ointment
▸ Lidocaine hydrochloride (Non-proprietary)
 Lidocaine hydrochloride 50 mg per 1 gram Lidocaine 5% ointment | 15 gram [P] £18.75 DT = £15.00

ANALGESICS > NON-STEROIDAL ANTI-INFLAMMATORY DRUGS

Benzydamine hydrochloride
13-Jul-2023

● **INDICATIONS AND DOSE**

Painful inflammatory conditions of oropharynx [using 0.15% preparations]
▸ BY OROMUCOSAL ADMINISTRATION USING MOUTHWASH
▸ Child 13-17 years: Rinse or gargle 15 mL every 1.5–3 hours as required usually for not more than 7 days, dilute with an equal volume of water if stinging occurs
▸ Adult: Rinse or gargle 15 mL every 1.5–3 hours as required usually for not more than 7 days, dilute with an equal volume of water if stinging occurs
▸ BY OROMUCOSAL ADMINISTRATION USING OROMUCOSAL SPRAY
▸ Child 1 month–5 years (body-weight 4–7 kg): 1 spray every 1.5–3 hours, to be administered onto affected area
▸ Child 1 month–5 years (body-weight 8–11 kg): 2 sprays every 1.5–3 hours, to be administered onto affected area
▸ Child 1 month–5 years (body-weight 12–15 kg): 3 sprays every 1.5–3 hours, to be administered onto affected area
▸ Child 1 month–5 years (body-weight 16 kg and above): 4 sprays every 1.5–3 hours, to be administered onto affected area
▸ Child 6-11 years: 4 sprays every 1.5–3 hours, to be administered onto affected area
▸ Child 12-17 years: 4–8 sprays every 1.5–3 hours, to be administered onto affected area
▸ Adult: 4–8 sprays every 1.5–3 hours, to be administered onto affected area

Painful inflammatory conditions of oropharynx [using 0.3% preparations]
▸ BY OROMUCOSAL ADMINISTRATION USING OROMUCOSAL SPRAY
▸ Child 2–5 years (body-weight 8–15 kg): 1 spray every 1.5–3 hours, to be administered onto affected area
▸ Child 2–5 years (body-weight 16 kg and above): 2 sprays every 1.5–3 hours, to be administered onto affected area
▸ Child 6-11 years: 2 sprays every 1.5–3 hours, to be administered onto affected area
▸ Child 12-17 years: 2–4 sprays every 1.5–3 hours, to be administered onto affected area
▸ Adult: 2–4 sprays every 1.5–3 hours, to be administered onto affected area

● **CAUTIONS** Asthma

● **INTERACTIONS** → Appendix 1: NSAIDs

● **SIDE-EFFECTS**
▸ **Uncommon** Oral disorders · photosensitivity reaction
▸ **Rare or very rare** Angioedema · dry mouth · respiratory disorders · skin reactions
▸ **Frequency not known** Nausea · vomiting

● **PREGNANCY** [EvGr] Avoid unless essential (limited information available). ⓜ

- **BREAST FEEDING** EvGr Avoid unless essential (no information available). ◈M◈

- **PROFESSION SPECIFIC INFORMATION**

  Dental practitioners' formulary Benzydamine Oromucosal Spray 0.15% may be prescribed.

  Benzydamine mouthwash may be prescribed as Benzydamine Mouthwash 0.15%.

- **MEDICINAL FORMS** There can be variation in the licensing of different medicines containing the same drug.

  Spray

  EXCIPIENTS: May contain Benzyl alcohol, ethanol, hydroxybenzoates (parabens), polysorbates, propylene glycol

  ▸ Benzydamine hydrochloride (Non-proprietary)
    Benzydamine hydrochloride 1.5 mg per 1 ml Benzydamine 0.15% oromucosal spray sugar free | 30 ml P £4.73 DT = £1.80 SF
    Benzydamine hydrochloride 3 mg per 1 ml Benzydamine 0.30% oromucosal spray sugar free | 15 ml PoM £4.60-£7.82 DT = £4.60 SF
  ▸ Difflam (Ceuta Healthcare Ltd)
    Benzydamine hydrochloride 1.5 mg per 1 ml Difflam 0.15% spray | 30 ml P £4.74 DT = £1.80 SF

  Mouthwash

  ▸ Benzydamine hydrochloride (Non-proprietary)
    Benzydamine hydrochloride 1.5 mg per 1 ml Benzydamine 0.15% mouthwash sugar free | 300 ml P £7.60 DT = £4.44 SF
  ▸ Difflam (Ceuta Healthcare Ltd)
    Benzydamine hydrochloride 1.5 mg per 1 ml Difflam Oral Rinse 0.15% solution | 300 ml P £6.50 DT = £4.44 SF
    Difflam 0.15% Sore Throat Rinse | 200 ml P £5.03 SF

Diclofenac

28-Aug-2018

- **INDICATIONS AND DOSE**

  Painful inflammatory conditions of the oral cavity and throat and/or following dental treatment or dental extraction

  ▸ BY MOUTH USING MOUTHWASH
  ▸ Adult: Rinse or gargle 15 mL 2–3 times a day for 7 days, treatment may be extended to 6 weeks in mucositis caused by radiotherapy

- **INTERACTIONS** → Appendix 1: NSAIDs

- **PREGNANCY** Manufacturer advises avoid unless essential.

- **BREAST FEEDING** Manufacturer advises avoid unless essential.

- **DIRECTIONS FOR ADMINISTRATION** Manufacturer advises mouthwash may be diluted with a little water.

- **MEDICINAL FORMS** No licensed medicines listed.

Flurbiprofen

01-Aug-2023

- **INDICATIONS AND DOSE**

  Relief of sore throat

  ▸ BY MOUTH USING LOZENGES
  ▸ Child 12-17 years: 1 lozenge every 3–6 hours for maximum 3 days, allow lozenge to dissolve slowly in the mouth; maximum 5 lozenges per day
  ▸ Adult: 1 lozenge every 3–6 hours for maximum 3 days, allow lozenge to dissolve slowly in the mouth; maximum 5 lozenges per day

- **INTERACTIONS** → Appendix 1: NSAIDs

- **SIDE-EFFECTS** Oral ulceration (move lozenge around mouth) · taste altered

- **ALLERGY AND CROSS-SENSITIVITY** EvGr Contra-indicated in patients with a history of hypersensitivity to aspirin or any other NSAID—which includes those in whom attacks of asthma, angioedema, urticaria or rhinitis have been precipitated by aspirin or any other NSAID. ◈M◈

- **MEDICINAL FORMS** There can be variation in the licensing of different medicines containing the same drug.

  Lozenge

  ▸ Strefen (Reckitt Benckiser Healthcare (UK) Ltd)
    Flurbiprofen 8.75 mg Strefen Eucalyptus and Manuka Honey 8.75mg lozenges | 16 lozenge P £4.52 DT = £4.52
    Strefen Honey and Lemon 8.75mg lozenges | 16 lozenge P £4.52 DT = £4.52

CORTICOSTEROIDS

▶ 783

Beclometasone dipropionate

08-Oct-2024

(Beclomethasone dipropionate)

- **INDICATIONS AND DOSE**

  Management of oral ulceration

  ▸ BY OROMUCOSAL ADMINISTRATION
  ▸ Adult: 50–100 micrograms twice daily, administered to the affected area using an inhaler device

- **UNLICENSED USE** Use of inhaler is unlicensed for oral ulceration.

- **INTERACTIONS** → Appendix 1: corticosteroids

- **MEDICINAL FORMS** There can be variation in the licensing of different medicines containing the same drug.
  For preparations, see inhaled beclometasone, p. 292.

▶ 783

Betamethasone

08-Oct-2024

- **DRUG ACTION** Betamethasone has very high glucocorticoid activity and insignificant mineralocorticoid activity.

- **INDICATIONS AND DOSE**

  Oral ulceration

  ▸ BY OROMUCOSAL ADMINISTRATION USING SOLUBLE TABLETS
  ▸ Child 12-17 years: 500 micrograms 4 times a day, to be dissolved in 20 mL water and rinsed around the mouth; not to be swallowed
  ▸ Adult: 500 micrograms 4 times a day, to be dissolved in 20 mL water and rinsed around the mouth; not to be swallowed

- **UNLICENSED USE**
  ▸ In children Betamethasone soluble tablets not licensed for use as mouthwash or in oral ulceration.

- **CONTRA-INDICATIONS** Untreated local infection

- **INTERACTIONS** → Appendix 1: corticosteroids

- **PATIENT AND CARER ADVICE** Patient counselling is advised for betamethasone soluble tablets (administration).

- **PROFESSION SPECIFIC INFORMATION**

  Dental practitioners' formulary Betamethasone Soluble Tablets 500 micrograms may be prescribed.

- **MEDICINAL FORMS** There can be variation in the licensing of different medicines containing the same drug.

  Soluble tablet

  CAUTIONARY AND ADVISORY LABELS 10, 13, 21 (not for use as mouthwash for oral ulceration)

  ▸ Betamethasone (Non-proprietary)
    Betamethasone (as Betamethasone sodium phosphate)
    500 microgram Betamethasone 500microgram soluble tablets sugar free | 30 tablet PoM £7.00 SF | 100 tablet PoM £58.15 DT = £15.28 SF

Hydrocortisone

783

08-Oct-2024

- **DRUG ACTION** Hydrocortisone has equal glucocorticoid and mineralocorticoid activity.

- **INDICATIONS AND DOSE**

Aphthous ulcers
▸ BY OROMUCOSAL ADMINISTRATION USING BUCCAL TABLET
▸ Child 1 month–11 years: Only on medical advice
▸ Child 12–17 years: 2.5 mg 4 times a day, allow buccal tablet to dissolve slowly in the mouth in contact with the ulcer
▸ Adult: 2.5 mg 4 times a day, allow buccal tablet to dissolve slowly in the mouth in contact with the ulcer

- **UNLICENSED USE** *Hydrocortisone mucoadhesive buccal tablets* licensed for use in children (under 12 years—on medical advice only).

IMPORTANT SAFETY INFORMATION

MHRA/CHM ADVICE: HYDROCORTISONE MUCO-ADHESIVE BUCCAL TABLETS: SHOULD NOT BE USED OFF-LABEL FOR ADRENAL INSUFFICIENCY IN CHILDREN DUE TO SERIOUS RISKS (DECEMBER 2018)

The MHRA has received reports of off-label use of hydrocortisone muco-adhesive buccal tablets for adrenal insufficiency in children. Healthcare professionals are advised that:
- hydrocortisone muco-adhesive buccal tablets are indicated only for local use in the mouth for aphthous ulceration and should not be used to treat adrenal insufficiency;
- substitution of licensed oral hydrocortisone formulations with muco-adhesive buccal tablets can result in insufficient cortisol absorption and, in stress situations, life-threatening adrenal crisis;
- only hydrocortisone products licensed for adrenal replacement therapy should be used.

- **CONTRA-INDICATIONS** Untreated local infection
- **INTERACTIONS** → Appendix 1: corticosteroids
- **PROFESSION SPECIFIC INFORMATION**

Dental practitioners' formulary Mucoadhesive buccal tablets may be prescribed as Hydrocortisone Oromucosal Tablets.

- **MEDICINAL FORMS** There can be variation in the licensing of different medicines containing the same drug.

Muco-adhesive buccal tablet
▸ Hydrocortisone (Non-proprietary)
Hydrocortisone (as Hydrocortisone sodium succinate)
2.5 mg Hydrocortisone 2.5mg muco-adhesive buccal tablets sugar free | 20 tablet P £8.94 SF

SALICYLIC ACID AND DERIVATIVES

Choline salicylate

23-Nov-2020

- **INDICATIONS AND DOSE**

Mild oral and perioral lesions
▸ BY OROMUCOSAL ADMINISTRATION
▸ Child 16–17 years: Apply 0.5 inch, apply to the lesion with gentle massage, not more often than every 3 hours
▸ Adult: Apply 0.5 inch, apply to the lesion with gentle massage, not more often than every 3 hours

- **CONTRA-INDICATIONS** Children under 16 years
CONTRA-INDICATIONS, FURTHER INFORMATION
▸ Reye's syndrome The CHM has advised that topical oral pain relief products containing salicylate salts should not be used in children under 16 years, as a cautionary measure due to the theoretical risk of Reye's syndrome.

- **CAUTIONS** Frequent application, especially in children, may give rise to salicylate poisoning · not to be applied to dentures—leave at least 30 minutes before re-insertion of dentures (in adults)

- **INTERACTIONS** → Appendix 1: choline salicylate
- **SIDE-EFFECTS** Bronchospasm
- **PRESCRIBING AND DISPENSING INFORMATION** When prepared extemporaneously, the BP states Choline Salicylate Dental Gel, BP consists of choline salicylate 8.7% in a flavoured gel basis.
- **PROFESSION SPECIFIC INFORMATION**

Dental practitioners' formulary Choline Salicylate Dental Gel may be prescribed.

- **MEDICINAL FORMS** There can be variation in the licensing of different medicines containing the same drug.

Oromucosal gel
▸ Bonjela (Reckitt Benckiser Healthcare (UK) Ltd)
Choline salicylate 87 mg per 1 gram Bonjela Cool Mint gel | 15 gram GSL £3.82 DT = £3.82 SF
Bonjela Original gel | 15 gram GSL £3.82 DT = £3.82 SF

Salicylic acid with rhubarb extract

17-Feb-2023

- **INDICATIONS AND DOSE**

Mild oral and perioral lesions
▸ TO THE LESION
▸ Child 16–17 years: Apply 3–4 times a day maximum duration 7 days
▸ Adult: Apply 3–4 times a day maximum duration 7 days

- **CONTRA-INDICATIONS** Children under 16 years
CONTRA-INDICATIONS, FURTHER INFORMATION
▸ Reye's syndrome The CHM has advised that topical oral pain relief products containing salicylate salts should not be used in children under 16 years, as a cautionary measure due to the theoretical risk of Reye's syndrome.

- **CAUTIONS** Frequent application, especially in children, may give rise to salicylate poisoning · not to be applied to dentures—leave at least 30 minutes before re-insertion of dentures (in adults)

- **SIDE-EFFECTS**
▸ **Common or very common** Oral discolouration · tooth discolouration

- **DIRECTIONS FOR ADMINISTRATION** EvGr Apply using the brush provided and avoid rinsing the mouth or eating for 15 minutes after application. M

- **PATIENT AND CARER ADVICE** Patients or carers should be given advice on how to administer salicylic acid with rhubarb extract oromucosal solution. May cause temporary discolouration of teeth and oral mucosa.

- **MEDICINAL FORMS** No licensed medicines listed.

4   Oropharyngeal bacterial infections

Oropharyngeal infections, antibacterial therapy

24-Feb-2023

Pericoronitis

Public Health England advises antibacterial use only in the presence of systemic features of infection, or persistent swelling.

- Metronidazole p. 628, or *alternatively*, amoxicillin p. 635
- ▸ *Suggested duration of treatment* 3 days or until pain reduction allows for oral hygiene.

Gingivitis (acute necrotising ulcerative)

Public Health England advises antibacterial use only in the presence of systemic features of infection.

- Metronidazole
- ▸ *Suggested duration of treatment* 3 days.

[EvGr] If metronidazole is contra-indicated, use *alternative*, amoxicillin. Ⓐ

Abscess (periapical or periodontal)

Public Health England advises antibacterial use only if there are signs of severe infection, systemic symptoms, or a high risk of complications.

- Phenoxymethylpenicillin p. 634, or *alternatively*, amoxicillin
- ▸ Alternative in penicillin allergy: clarithromycin p. 621
- ▸ If signs of spreading infection (e.g. lymph node involvement, systemic signs), add metronidazole
- ▸ *Suggested duration of treatment* up to 5 days; review at 3 days.

Periodontitis

[EvGr] Antibacterials may be used as an adjunct to effective mechanical debridement in severe disease or disease unresponsive to local treatment alone on the advice of a specialist. Ⓐ

Sore throat (acute)

Acute sore throat is usually triggered by a viral infection and is self-limiting. Symptoms can last for around 1 week, and most people will improve within this time without treatment with antibacterials, regardless of the cause. [EvGr] A clinical scoring system should be used in combination with clinical judgement to identify individuals most likely to benefit from an antibacterial.

Patients who are systemically very unwell, or have signs and symptoms of a more serious illness or condition, or are at high risk of complications should be offered immediate antibacterial therapy. Patients with severe systemic infection or severe suppurative complications (such as peritonsillar abscess (quinsy) or cellulitis) should be referred to hospital.

- Phenoxymethylpenicillin p. 634
- ▸ *Suggested duration of treatment* 5 to 10 days.
- Alternative in penicillin allergy: clarithromycin p. 621 *or* erythromycin p. 624 (in pregnancy)
- ▸ *Suggested duration of treatment* 5 days. Ⓐ

For further guidance on the management of acute sore throat, see NICE guideline: **Sore throat (acute): antimicrobial prescribing** (see *Useful resources*).

Other infections

For further information on antibacterial treatment used in oropharyngeal infections, see Oral bacterial infections p. 585.

Useful resources

Sore throat (acute): antimicrobial prescribing. National Institute for Health and Care Excellence. NICE guideline 84. January 2018.
    www.nice.org.uk/guidance/ng84

ANTIBACTERIALS ⟩ TETRACYCLINES AND RELATED DRUGS

⚑ 655

Doxycycline

18-Apr-2025

● **INDICATIONS AND DOSE**

Treatment of recurrent aphthous ulceration
- ▸ BY OROMUCOSAL ADMINISTRATION USING DISPERSIBLE TABLETS
- ▸ Child 12–17 years: 100 mg 4 times a day usually for 3 days, dispersible tablet can be stirred into a small amount of water then rinsed around the mouth for 2–3 minutes, it should preferably not be swallowed
- ▸ Adult: 100 mg 4 times a day usually for 3 days, dispersible tablet can be stirred into a small amount of water then rinsed around the mouth for 2–3 minutes, it should preferably not be swallowed

● **UNLICENSED USE** Doxycycline may be used as detailed below, although considered outside the scope of its licence:
- recurrent aphthous ulceration.

● **CAUTIONS** Alcohol dependence

● **INTERACTIONS** → Appendix 1: tetracyclines

● **SIDE-EFFECTS**
- ▸ **Common or very common** Dyspnoea · hypotension · peripheral oedema · tachycardia
- ▸ **Uncommon** Gastrointestinal discomfort
- ▸ **Rare or very rare** Anxiety · arthralgia · Clostridioides difficile colitis · flushing · intracranial pressure increased with papilloedema · Jarisch-Herxheimer reaction · myalgia · photoonycholysis · severe cutaneous adverse reactions (SCARs) · skin hyperpigmentation (long term use) · stomatitis · tinnitus · vision disorders

● **PATIENT AND CARER ADVICE** Counselling on administration advised.
Photosensitivity Patients should be advised to avoid exposure to sunlight or sun lamps.

● **PROFESSION SPECIFIC INFORMATION**

Dental practitioners' formulary Dispersible tablets may be prescribed as Dispersible Doxycycline Tablets.

● **MEDICINAL FORMS** There can be variation in the licensing of different medicines containing the same drug.

Dispersible tablet
CAUTIONARY AND ADVISORY LABELS 6, 9, 11, 13
- ▸ **Vibramycin-D** (Pfizer Ltd)
   Doxycycline (as Doxycycline monohydrate) 100 mg Vibramycin-D 100mg dispersible tablets | 8 tablet [PoM] £4.91 DT = £4.91 [SF]

5 Oropharyngeal fungal infections

Oropharyngeal fungal infections

19-May-2022

Overview

Fungal infections of the mouth are usually caused by *Candida* spp. (candidiasis or candidosis). Different types of oropharyngeal candidiasis are managed as follows:

Thrush

Pseudomembranous candidiasis (thrush) is usually an acute infection but it may persist in chronic forms. Those at greater risk of candidal infections include patients receiving inhaled corticosteroids, chemotherapy, or broad-spectrum antibacterials, and in patients with serious systemic disease associated with reduced immunity such as leukaemia, other malignancies, and HIV infection. [EvGr] Any predisposing condition should be managed appropriately. [A] The risk of oral candidiasis associated with corticosteroid inhaler use can be reduced by rinsing the mouth with water (or cleaning teeth) immediately after using the inhaler, use of a spacer, or using an inhaler at its lowest effective dose.

[EvGr] For mild and localised infections, treatment with miconazole oral gel below is recommended; if this is unsuitable, oral nystatin p. 1385 may be given. Oral antifungal treatment with fluconazole p. 690 can be considered for patients that have extensive or severe infection, or when miconazole or nystatin treatment is unsuitable or ineffective. If the infection fails to respond to treatment after 1 week, consider extending the course for another week or referring to a specialist as appropriate.

Patients with moderate to severe infections may be considered for referral to a specialist; patients with evidence of a systemic disease or widespread infections should be admitted to hospital. For immunocompromised patients receiving treatment with ciclosporin, oral tacrolimus, or chemotherapy, seek specialist advice before starting antifungal treatment. [A]

Acute erythematous candidiasis

Acute erythematous (atrophic) candidiasis is usually associated with a burning sensation of the mouth or tongue and may be caused by corticosteroid or broad-spectrum antibacterial use. [EvGr] Treatment of acute erythematous candidiasis is the same as for pseudomembranous candidiasis [E]—for further information, see *Thrush*. Denture-related problems should be managed prior to antifungal treatment initiation.

Denture stomatitis

[EvGr] Patients with denture stomatitis (chronic atrophic candidiasis) should cleanse their dentures thoroughly, soak them overnight in disinfectant solution, and allow to air dry. Dentures should not be worn for 6 hours or more in each 24-hour period to promote gum healing. Refer to a dentist for ill-fitting dentures. Patients should also brush the mucosal surface regularly with a soft brush. [A]

Denture stomatitis is not always associated with candidiasis and other factors such as mechanical or chemical irritation, bacterial infection, or allergy to the denture material, may be the cause. [EvGr] Miconazole oral gel may be used as treatment if needed. [A]

Chronic hyperplastic candidiasis

[EvGr] Patients with chronic hyperplastic candidiasis (plaque-like candidiasis) should be referred to a specialist due to the increased risk of malignancy and potential need for a biopsy. The specialist may suggest treatment with a systemic antifungal to eliminate candidal overlay. [E]

Angular cheilitis

Angular cheilitis (angular stomatitis) is characterised by soreness, erythema, and fissuring at the angles of the mouth. It may be associated with ill-fitting dentures, nutritional deficiency, or immunosuppression. Both yeasts (*Candida* spp.) and bacteria (*Staphylococcus aureus* and streptococci) are commonly involved as interacting, infective factors. [EvGr] Angular cheilitis is normally self-limiting. While the underlying cause is being identified and treated, it may be helpful to apply topical emollients, miconazole cream or ointment for mild candida infection, or fusidic acid ointment p. 663 if there is evidence of bacterial infection. If the angular cheilitis is unresponsive to treatment, hydrocortisone with miconazole cream or ointment can be used. [E]

Drugs used in oropharyngeal candidiasis

Nystatin is not absorbed from the gastro-intestinal tract and is applied locally (as a suspension) to the mouth for treating local fungal infections. Miconazole is applied locally (as an oral gel) in the mouth but it is absorbed systemically so potential interactions need to be considered. Miconazole also has some activity against Gram-positive bacteria including streptococci and staphylococci. Oral itraconazole p. 692 is licensed for the treatment of fluconazole-resistant oral candidiasis.

For further information on systemic antifungal treatment, see Antifungals, systemic use p. 685.

ANTIFUNGALS > IMIDAZOLE ANTIFUNGALS

Miconazole

23-Jun-2023

● INDICATIONS AND DOSE

Oral candidiasis

▶ BY OROMUCOSAL ADMINISTRATION USING ORAL GEL

▶ Child 2–17 years: 2.5 mL 4 times a day treatment should be continued for at least 7 days after lesions have healed or symptoms have cleared, to be administered after meals, retain near oral lesions before swallowing (dental prostheses and orthodontic appliances should be removed at night and brushed with gel)

▶ Adult: 2.5 mL 4 times a day treatment should be continued for at least 7 days after lesions have healed or symptoms have cleared, to be administered after meals, retain near oral lesions before swallowing (dental prostheses and orthodontic appliances should be removed at night and brushed with gel)

Prevention and treatment of oral candidiasis (dose approved for use by community practitioner nurse prescribers)

▶ BY OROMUCOSAL ADMINISTRATION USING ORAL GEL

▶ Child 4–23 months: 1.25 mL 4 times a day treatment should be continued for at least 7 days after lesions have healed or symptoms have cleared, to be smeared around the inside of the mouth after feeds

▶ Child 2–17 years: 2.5 mL 4 times a day treatment should be continued for at least 7 days after lesions have healed or symptoms have cleared, to be administered after meals, retain near oral lesions before swallowing (dental prostheses and orthodontic appliances should be removed at night and brushed with gel)

▶ Adult: 2.5 mL 4 times a day treatment should be continued for at least 7 days after lesions have healed or symptoms have cleared, to be administered after meals, retain near oral lesions before swallowing (dental prostheses and orthodontic appliances should be removed at night and brushed with gel)

DOSE EQUIVALENCE AND CONVERSION

▶ One 5-mL spoonful of oral gel equivalent to 124 mg miconazole.

- **UNLICENSED USE** Not licensed for use in children under 4 months of age or during first 5–6 months of life of an infant born pre-term.
- **CONTRA-INDICATIONS** Infants with impaired swallowing reflex
- **CAUTIONS** Avoid in Acute porphyrias p. 1202
- **INTERACTIONS** → Appendix 1: antifungals, azoles
- **SIDE-EFFECTS**
  - **Common or very common** Dry mouth · nausea · oral disorders · vomiting
  - **Uncommon** Skin reactions · taste altered
  - **Frequency not known** Angioedema · choking (in children) · diarrhoea · hepatitis · severe cutaneous adverse reactions (SCARs) · tongue discolouration
- **PREGNANCY** Manufacturer advises avoid if possible— toxicity at high doses in *animal* studies.
- **BREAST FEEDING** Manufacturer advises caution—no information available.
- **HEPATIC IMPAIRMENT** Manufacturer advises avoid.
- **DIRECTIONS FOR ADMINISTRATION** Manufacturer advises oral gel should be held in mouth, after food.
- **PRESCRIBING AND DISPENSING INFORMATION** Flavours of oral gel may include orange.
- **PATIENT AND CARER ADVICE** Patients or carers should be given advice on how to administer miconazole oromucosal gel.
- **PROFESSION SPECIFIC INFORMATION**

  Dental practitioners' formulary Miconazole Oromucosal Gel may be prescribed.
- **EXCEPTIONS TO LEGAL CATEGORY** 15-g tube of oral gel can be sold to the public.

- **MEDICINAL FORMS** There can be variation in the licensing of different medicines containing the same drug.

  Oromucosal gel

  CAUTIONARY AND ADVISORY LABELS 9
  - Daktarin (Johnson & Johnson Ltd)
    Miconazole 20 mg per 1 gram Daktarin 20mg/g oromucosal gel | 15 gram P £5.26 DT = £5.26 SF

ANTIFUNGALS > POLYENE ANTIFUNGALS

Nystatin

10-Nov-2021

- **INDICATIONS AND DOSE**

Oral candidiasis

- BY OROMUCOSAL ADMINISTRATION
- Child: 100 000 units 4 times a day usually for 7 days, and continued for 48 hours after lesions have resolved
- Adult: 100 000 units 4 times a day usually for 7 days, and continued for 48 hours after lesions have resolved

Oral and perioral fungal infections (dose approved for use by community practitioner nurse prescribers)

- BY OROMUCOSAL ADMINISTRATION

- Neonate: 100 000 units 4 times a day usually for 7 days, and continued for 48 hours after lesions have resolved, to be given after feeds.

- Child: 100 000 units 4 times a day usually for 7 days, and continued for 48 hours after lesions have resolved
- Adult: 100 000 units 4 times a day usually for 7 days, and continued for 48 hours after lesions have resolved

- **UNLICENSED USE** Suspension not licensed for use in neonates for the treatment of candidiasis but the Department of Health has advised that a Community Practitioner Nurse Prescriber may prescribe nystatin oral suspension for a neonate, in the doses provided in BNF Publications, provided that there is a clear diagnosis of oral thrush. The nurse prescriber must only prescribe within their own competence and must accept clinical and medicolegal responsibility for prescribing.
- **SIDE-EFFECTS** Abdominal distress · angioedema · diarrhoea · face oedema · nausea · sensitisation · skin reactions · Stevens-Johnson syndrome · vomiting
- **PATIENT AND CARER ADVICE** Counselling advised with oral suspension (use of pipette, hold in mouth, after food). Medicines for Children leaflet: Nystatin for Candida infections www.medicinesforchildren.org.uk/medicines/nystatin-for-candida-infections/
- **PROFESSION SPECIFIC INFORMATION**

  Dental practitioners' formulary Nystatin Oral Suspension may be prescribed.

- **MEDICINAL FORMS** There can be variation in the licensing of different medicines containing the same drug. Forms available from special-order manufacturers include: oral suspension

  Oral suspension

  CAUTIONARY AND ADVISORY LABELS 9
  EXCIPIENTS: May contain Ethanol
  - Nystatin (Non-proprietary)
    Nystatin 100000 unit per 1 ml Nystatin 100,000units/ml oral suspension | 30 ml PoM £8.75 DT = £1.80

6 Oropharyngeal viral infections

Oropharyngeal viral infections

Management

Viral infections are the most common cause of a sore throat. They do not benefit from anti-infective treatment.

The management of primary herpetic gingivostomatitis is a soft diet, adequate fluid intake, and analgesics as required, including local use of benzydamine hydrochloride p. 1380. The use of chlorhexidine mouthwash p. 1377 will control plaque accumulation if toothbrushing is painful and will also help to control secondary infection in general.

In the case of severe herpetic stomatitis, a systemic antiviral such as aciclovir p. 729 is required. Valaciclovir p. 731 and famciclovir p. 730 are suitable alternatives for oral lesions associated with herpes zoster. Aciclovir and valaciclovir are also used for the prevention of frequently recurring herpes simplex lesions of the mouth, particularly when implicated in the initiation of erythema multiforme.

Chapter 13
Skin

CONTENTS

Skin conditions, management

21-Jul-2022

Vehicles

The British Association of Dermatologists list of preferred unlicensed dermatological preparations (specials) is available at www.bad.org.uk/guidelines-and-standards/access-to-medicines/.

Both vehicle and active ingredients are important in the treatment of skin conditions; the vehicle alone may have more than a mere placebo effect. The vehicle affects the degree of hydration of the skin, has a mild anti-inflammatory effect, and aids the penetration of active drug.

Applications are usually viscous solutions, emulsions, or suspensions for application to the skin (including the scalp) or nails.

Collodions are painted on the skin and allowed to dry to leave a flexible film over the site of application.

Creams are emulsions of oil and water and are generally well absorbed into the skin. They may contain an antimicrobial preservative unless the active ingredient or basis is intrinsically bactericidal and fungicidal. Generally, creams are cosmetically more acceptable than ointments because they are less greasy and easier to apply.

Gels consist of active ingredients in suitable hydrophilic or hydrophobic bases; they generally have a high water content. Gels are particularly suitable for application to the face and scalp.

Lotions have a cooling effect and may be preferred to ointments or creams for application over a hairy area. Lotions in alcoholic basis can sting if used on broken skin. *Shake lotions* (such as calamine lotion) contain insoluble powders which leave a deposit on the skin surface.

Ointments are greasy preparations which are normally anhydrous and insoluble in water, and are more occlusive than creams. They are particularly suitable for chronic, dry lesions. The most commonly used ointment bases consist of soft paraffin or a combination of soft, liquid, and hard paraffin. Some ointment bases have both *hydrophilic and lipophilic* properties; they may have occlusive properties on the skin surface, encourage hydration, and also be miscible with water; they often have a mild anti-inflammatory effect. *Water-soluble ointments* contain macrogols which are freely soluble in water and are therefore readily washed off; they have a limited but useful role where ready removal is desirable.

Pastes are stiff preparations containing a high proportion of finely powdered solids such as zinc oxide and starch suspended in an ointment. They are used for circumscribed lesions such as those which occur in lichen simplex, chronic eczema, or psoriasis. They are less occlusive than ointments and can be used to protect inflamed, lichenified, or excoriated skin.

Dusting powders are used only rarely. They reduce friction between opposing skin surfaces. Dusting powders should not be applied to moist areas because they can cake and abrade the skin. Talc is a lubricant but it does not absorb moisture; it can cause respiratory irritation. Starch is less lubricant but absorbs water.

Dilution

The BP directs that creams and ointments should **not** normally be diluted but that should dilution be necessary care should be taken, in particular, to prevent microbial contamination. The appropriate diluent should be used and heating should be avoided during mixing; excessive dilution may affect the stability of some creams. Diluted creams should normally be used within 2 weeks of preparation.

Suitable quantities for prescribing

Suitable quantities of dermatological preparations to be prescribed for specific areas of the body		
Area of body	Creams and Ointments	Lotions
Face	15–30 g	100 mL
Both hands	25–50 g	200 mL
Scalp	50–100 g	200 mL
Both arms or both legs	100–200 g	200 mL
Trunk	400 g	500 mL
Groins and genitalia	15–25 g	100 mL

These amounts are usually suitable for an adult for twice daily application for 1 week. The recommendations **do not apply to** corticosteroid preparations. For suitable quantities of corticosteroid preparations, see relevant table.

Excipients and sensitisation

Excipients in topical products rarely cause problems. If a patch test indicates allergy to an excipient, products containing the substance should be avoided. The following excipients in topical preparations are associated, rarely, with sensitisation; the presence of these excipients is indicated in the entries for topical products.

- Beeswax
- Benzyl alcohol
- Butylated hydroxyanisole
- Butylated hydroxytoluene
- Cetostearyl alcohol (including cetyl and stearyl alcohol)
- Chlorocresol
- Edetic acid (EDTA)
- Ethylenediamine
- Fragrances
- Hydroxybenzoates (parabens)
- Imidurea
- Isopropyl palmitate
- N-(3-Chloroallyl)hexaminium chloride (quaternium 15)
- Polysorbates
- Propylene glycol
- Sodium metabisulfite
- Sorbic acid
- Wool fat and related substances including lanolin (purified versions of wool fat have reduced the problem)

1   Benign neoplasms of skin

ANTINEOPLASTIC DRUGS > PROTEIN KINASE INHIBITORS

Sirolimus
19-Mar-2025

- **INDICATIONS AND DOSE**

Facial angiofibroma associated with tuberous sclerosis complex

▸ TO THE SKIN

▸ Adult: Apply a thin layer of gel twice daily to the affected areas, in the morning and at bedtime. A dose of sirolimus 0.25 mg (equivalent to 125 mg of gel or approximately 0.5 cm gel strand) should be administered per 50 cm^2 lesion, and applied twice daily; maximum total daily dose sirolimus 1.6 mg (equivalent to 800 mg of gel or approximately 2.5 cm gel strand), discontinue treatment if no response after 12 weeks

- **CAUTIONS** Hyperlipidaemia · immunosuppression · increased susceptibility to lymphoma and other malignancies, particularly of the skin (limit exposure to UV light)

- **INTERACTIONS** → Appendix 1: sirolimus

- **SIDE-EFFECTS**

▸ **Common or very common** Asteatosis · conjunctivitis · eye erythema · eye irritation · increased risk of infection · nasal discomfort · photosensitivity · skin haemorrhage · skin reactions · stomatitis

- **PREGNANCY** EvGr Avoid unless essential (toxicity in *animal* studies). M

- **BREAST FEEDING** Specialist sources suggest limited systemic absorption so unlikely to affect nursing infant.

- **HEPATIC IMPAIRMENT** EvGr Avoid in severe impairment (no information available, though in general blood concentrations are low following topical administration). M

- **DIRECTIONS FOR ADMINISTRATION** EvGr Apply a thin layer of gel to the affected area and rub in gently. Do not apply

on wounds, irritated, broken, or infected skin. Avoid contact with eyes and mucous membranes M.

- **HANDLING AND STORAGE** Protect from light. Topical gel: store in a refrigerator (2-8°C).

- **PATIENT AND CARER ADVICE** Advise patients to avoid excessive exposure to UV light including sunlight.

Patients and carers should be advised on the application of *Hyftor*® gel.

Missed doses If a morning dose is missed, it should be applied as soon as possible, provided it's before the evening dose. If the evening dose is missed, it should not be applied and the next dose should be applied at the normal time.

- **NATIONAL FUNDING/ACCESS DECISIONS**

For full details see funding body website

Scottish Medicines Consortium (SMC) decisions

▸ Sirolimus (*Hyftor*®) for the treatment of adult and paediatric patients aged 6 and above with facial angiofibroma associated with tuberous sclerosis complex (January 2025) SMC No. SMC2710 Recommended

- **MEDICINAL FORMS** There can be variation in the licensing of different medicines containing the same drug.

Cutaneous gel

CAUTIONARY AND ADVISORY LABELS 11
EXCIPIENTS: May contain Alcohol

▸ **Hyftor** (Plusultra Pharma UK Ltd)
Sirolimus 2 mg per 1 gram Hyftor 2mg/g gel | 10 gram PoM
£340.00 DT = £340.00

2   Dry and scaling skin disorders

Emollient and barrier preparations
04-Sep-2020

Borderline substances

The preparations marked 'ACBS' are regarded as drugs when prescribed in accordance with the advice of the Advisory Committee on Borderline Substances for the clinical conditions listed. Prescriptions issued in accordance with this advice and endorsed 'ACBS' will normally not be investigated (see *About Borderline Substances*).

Emollients

Emollients soothe, smooth and hydrate the skin and are indicated for all dry or scaling disorders. Their effects are short lived and they should be applied frequently even after improvement occurs. They are useful in dry and eczematous disorders, and to a lesser extent in psoriasis. The choice of an appropriate emollient will depend on the severity of the condition, patient preference, and the site of application. Some ingredients rarely cause sensitisation and this should be suspected if an eczematous reaction occurs. The use of aqueous cream as a leave-on emollient may increase the risk of skin reactions, particularly in eczema.

Preparations such as **aqueous cream** and **emulsifying ointment** can be used as soap substitutes for hand washing and in the bath; the preparation is rubbed on the skin before rinsing off completely. The addition of a bath oil may also be helpful.

Urea is occasionally used with other topical agents such as corticosteroids to enhance penetration of the skin.

Emollient bath and shower preparations

Emollient bath additives should be added to bath water; hydration can be improved by soaking in the bath for 10–20 minutes. Some bath emollients can be applied to wet skin undiluted and rinsed off. In dry skin conditions soap should be avoided.

The quantities of bath additives recommended for adults are suitable for an adult-size bath. Proportionately less should be used for a child-size bath or a washbasin; recommended bath additive quantities for children reflect this.

MHRA/CHM advice (updated December 2018): Emollients: new information about risk of severe and fatal burns with paraffin-containing and paraffin-free emollients
Emollients are an important and effective treatment for chronic dry skin disorders and people should continue to use these products. However, healthcare professionals must ensure that patients and their carers understand the fire risk associated with the build-up of residue on clothing and bedding and can take action to minimise the risk. There is a fire risk with all paraffin-containing emollients, regardless of paraffin concentration, and it cannot be excluded with paraffin-free emollients. A similar risk may apply to products that are applied to the skin over large body areas, or in large volumes for repeated use for more than a few days.

Healthcare professionals should advise patients not to smoke or go near naked flames because clothing, bedding, dressings, and other fabrics that have been in contact with an emollient or emollient-treated skin can rapidly ignite. Washing these materials at high temperature may reduce emollient build-up but not totally remove it.

The MHRA/CHM (August 2020) have released a toolkit of resources for health and social care professionals to support the safe use of emollients, available at: www.gov.uk/drug-safety-update/emollients-and-risk-of-severe-and-fatal-burns-new-resources-available.

Barrier preparations

Barrier preparations often contain water-repellent substances such as dimeticone (see barrier creams and ointments below) or other silicones. They are used on the skin around stomas, bedsores, and pressure areas in the elderly where the skin is intact. Where the skin has broken down, barrier preparations have a limited role in protecting adjacent skin. Barrier preparations are not a substitute for adequate nursing care.

Nappy rash
The first line of treatment is to ensure that nappies are changed frequently and that tightly fitting water-proof pants are avoided. The rash may clear when left exposed to the air and a barrier preparation, applied with each nappy change, can be helpful. A mild corticosteroid such as hydrocortisone 0.5% or 1% p. 1413 can be used if inflammation is causing discomfort, but it should be avoided in neonates. The barrier preparation should be applied after the corticosteroid preparation to prevent further damage. Preparations containing hydrocortisone should be applied for no more than a week; the hydrocortisone should be discontinued as soon as the inflammation subsides. The occlusive effect of nappies and waterproof pants may increase absorption of corticosteroids. If the rash is associated with candidal infection, a topical antifungal such as clotrimazole cream p. 1399 can be used. Topical antibacterial preparations can be used if bacterial infection is present; treatment with an oral antibacterial may occasionally be required in severe or recurrent infection. Hydrocortisone may be used in combination with antimicrobial preparations if there is considerable inflammation, erosion, and infection.

Barrier creams and ointments
13-Feb-2020

● **INDICATIONS AND DOSE**

For use as a barrier preparation
▸ TO THE SKIN
▸ Child: (consult product literature)
▸ Adult: (consult product literature)

● **MEDICINAL FORMS** There can be variation in the licensing of different medicines containing the same drug.

Cutaneous ointment
EXCIPIENTS: May contain Woolfat and related substances (including lanolin)
▸ Barrier creams and ointments (Non-proprietary)
Cetostearyl alcohol 20 mg per 1 gram, Zinc oxide 75 mg per 1 gram, Beeswax white 100 mg per 1 gram, Arachis oil 305 mg per 1 gram, Castor oil 500 mg per 1 gram Zinc and Castor oil ointment | 500 gram GSL £5.14 DT = £5.14

Cutaneous cream
EXCIPIENTS: May contain Beeswax, butylated hydroxyanisole, butylated hydroxytoluene, cetostearyl alcohol (including cetyl and stearyl alcohol), chlorocresol, fragrances, hydroxybenzoates (parabens), propylene glycol, woolfat and related substances (including lanolin)
▸ Conotrane (Evolan Pharma AB)
Benzalkonium chloride 1 mg per 1 gram, Dimeticone 220 mg per 1 gram Conotrane cream | 500 gram GSL £9.19
▸ Drapolene (Supra Enterprises Ltd)
Benzalkonium chloride 100 microgram per 1 gram, Cetrimide 2 mg per 1 gram Drapolene cream | 100 gram GSL £3.74 DT = £3.74 | 200 gram GSL £5.31 DT = £5.31 | 350 gram GSL £8.43 DT = £8.43
▸ Siopel (Derma UK Ltd)
Cetrimide 3 mg per 1 gram, Dimeticone 1000 100 mg per 1 gram Siopel cream | 50 gram GSL £4.73 DT = £4.73
▸ Sudocrem (Teva UK Ltd)
Benzyl cinnamate 1.5 mg per 1 gram, Benzyl alcohol 3.9 mg per 1 gram, Benzyl benzoate 10.1 mg per 1 gram, Wool fat hydrous 40 mg per 1 gram, Zinc oxide 152.5 mg per 1 gram Sudocrem antiseptic healing cream | 60 gram GSL £3.36 | 125 gram GSL £4.66 | 250 gram GSL £8.24 | 400 gram GSL £10.99

Emollient bath and shower products, antimicrobial-containing
15-Feb-2024

● **INDICATIONS AND DOSE**

DERMOL ® 200 SHOWER EMOLLIENT

Dry and pruritic skin conditions including eczema and dermatitis
▸ TO THE SKIN
▸ Child: To be applied to the skin or used as a soap substitute
▸ Adult: To be applied to the skin or used as a soap substitute

DERMOL ® 600 BATH EMOLLIENT

Dry and pruritic skin conditions including eczema and dermatitis
▸ TO THE SKIN
▸ Child 1-23 months: 5–15 mL/bath, not to be used undiluted
▸ Child 2-17 years: 15–30 mL/bath, not to be used undiluted
▸ Adult: Up to 30 mL/bath, not to be used undiluted

DERMOL ® WASH EMULSION

Dry and pruritic skin conditions including eczema and dermatitis
- ▸ TO THE SKIN
- ▸ Child: To be applied to the skin or used as a soap substitute
- ▸ Adult: To be applied to the skin or used as a soap substitute

EMULSIDERM ®

Dry skin conditions including eczema and ichthyosis
- ▸ TO THE SKIN
- ▸ Child 1-23 months: 5–10 mL/bath, alternatively, to be rubbed into dry skin until absorbed
- ▸ Child 2-17 years: 7–30 mL/bath, alternatively, to be rubbed into dry skin until absorbed
- ▸ Adult: 7–30 mL/bath, alternatively, to be rubbed into dry skin until absorbed

OILATUM ® PLUS

Topical treatment of eczema, including eczema at risk from infection
- ▸ TO THE SKIN
- ▸ Child 6-11 months: 1 mL/bath, not to be used undiluted
- ▸ Child 1-17 years: 1–2 capfuls/bath, not to be used undiluted
- ▸ Adult: 1–2 capfuls/bath, not to be used undiluted

IMPORTANT SAFETY INFORMATION

These preparations make skin and surfaces slippery—particular care is needed when bathing.

MHRA/CHM ADVICE (UPDATED DECEMBER 2018): EMOLLIENTS: NEW INFORMATION ABOUT RISK OF SEVERE AND FATAL BURNS WITH PARAFFIN-CONTAINING AND PARAFFIN-FREE EMOLLIENTS See Emollient and barrier preparations p. 1387.

- ● **DIRECTIONS FOR ADMINISTRATION** Emollient bath additives should be added to bath water; EvGr hydration can be improved by soaking in the bath for 5–20 minutes (consult product literature). Some bath emollients can be applied to wet skin undiluted and rinsed off. Ⓜ Emollient preparations contained in tubs should be removed with a clean spoon or spatula to reduce bacterial contamination of the emollient. Emollients should be applied in the direction of hair growth to reduce the risk of folliculitis.

- ● **PRESCRIBING AND DISPENSING INFORMATION** Preparations containing an antibacterial should be avoided unless infection is present or is a frequent complication.

- ● **MEDICINAL FORMS** There can be variation in the licensing of different medicines containing the same drug.

Bath additive

CAUTIONARY AND ADVISORY LABELS 15
EXCIPIENTS: May contain Acetylated lanolin alcohols, isopropyl palmitate, polysorbates

- ▸ Dermol 600 (Dermal Laboratories Ltd)
  Benzalkonium chloride 5 mg per 1 gram, Isopropyl myristate 250 mg per 1 gram, Liquid paraffin 250 mg per 1 gram Dermol 600 bath emollient | 600 ml Ⓟ £7.99
- ▸ Emulsiderm (Dermal Laboratories Ltd)
  Benzalkonium chloride 5 mg per 1 gram, Isopropyl myristate 250 mg per 1 gram, Liquid paraffin 250 mg per 1 gram Emulsiderm emollient | 300 ml Ⓟ £3.85 | 1000 ml Ⓟ £12.00
- ▸ Oilatum Plus (Thornton & Ross Ltd)
  Triclosan 20 mg per 1 gram, Benzalkonium chloride 60 mg per 1 gram, Liquid paraffin light 525 mg per 1 gram Oilatum Plus bath additive | 500 ml GSL £8.81

Cutaneous emulsion

CAUTIONARY AND ADVISORY LABELS 15
EXCIPIENTS: May contain Cetostearyl alcohol (including cetyl and stearyl alcohol)

- ▸ Dermol 200 (Dermal Laboratories Ltd)
  Benzalkonium chloride 1 mg per 1 gram, Chlorhexidine hydrochloride 1 mg per 1 gram, Isopropyl myristate 25 mg per 1 gram, Liquid paraffin 25 mg per 1 gram Dermol 200 shower emollient | 200 ml Ⓟ £3.76
- ▸ Dermol Wash (Dermal Laboratories Ltd)
  Benzalkonium chloride 1 mg per 1 gram, Chlorhexidine hydrochloride 1 mg per 1 gram, Isopropyl myristate 25 mg per 1 gram, Liquid paraffin 25 mg per 1 gram Dermol Wash cutaneous emulsion | 200 ml Ⓟ £3.76

Emollient bath and shower products, paraffin-containing
15-Aug-2024

- ● **INDICATIONS AND DOSE**

Dry skin conditions (using Aqueous Cream BP)
- ▸ TO THE SKIN
- ▸ Child: To be used as a soap substitute
- ▸ Adult: To be used as a soap substitute

AQUAMAX ® WASH

Dry skin conditions
- ▸ TO THE SKIN
- ▸ Child: To be applied to wet or dry skin and rinse
- ▸ Adult: To be applied to wet or dry skin and rinse

CETRABEN ® BATH

Dry skin conditions, including eczema
- ▸ TO THE SKIN
- ▸ Child 1 month-11 years: 0.5–1 capful/bath, alternatively, to be applied to wet skin and rinse
- ▸ Child 12-17 years: 1–2 capfuls/bath, alternatively, to be applied to wet skin and rinse
- ▸ Adult: 1–2 capfuls/bath, alternatively, to be applied to wet skin and rinse

DERMALO ®

Dermatitis | Dry skin conditions, including ichthyosis
- ▸ TO THE SKIN
- ▸ Child 1 month-11 years: 5–10 mL/bath, alternatively, to be applied to wet skin and rinse
- ▸ Child 12-17 years: 15–20 mL/bath, alternatively, to be applied to wet skin and rinse
- ▸ Adult: 15–20 mL/bath, alternatively, to be applied to wet skin and rinse

Pruritus of the elderly
- ▸ TO THE SKIN
- ▸ Elderly: 15–20 mL/bath, alternatively, to be applied to wet skin and rinse

DOUBLEBASE ® EMOLLIENT BATH ADDITIVE

Dry skin conditions including dermatitis and ichthyosis
- ▸ TO THE SKIN
- ▸ Child 1 month-11 years: 5–10 mL/bath
- ▸ Child 12-17 years: 15–20 mL/bath
- ▸ Adult: 15–20 mL/bath

Pruritus of the elderly
- ▸ TO THE SKIN
- ▸ Elderly: 15–20 mL/bath

DOUBLEBASE ® EMOLLIENT SHOWER GEL

Dry, chapped, or itchy skin conditions
- ▸ TO THE SKIN
- ▸ Child: To be applied to wet or dry skin and rinse, or apply to dry skin after showering
- ▸ Adult: To be applied to wet or dry skin and rinse, or apply to dry skin after showering

DOUBLEBASE ® EMOLLIENT WASH GEL

Dry, chapped, or itchy skin conditions
- ▸ TO THE SKIN
- ▸ Child: To be used as a soap substitute
- ▸ Adult: To be used as a soap substitute continued →

E45® BATH OIL

Endogenous and exogenous eczema, xeroderma, and ichthyosis
▸ TO THE SKIN
▸ Child 1 month-11 years: 5–10 mL/bath, alternatively, to be applied to wet skin and rinse
▸ Child 12-17 years: 15 mL/bath, alternatively, to be applied to wet skin and rinse
▸ Adult: 15 mL/bath, alternatively, to be applied to wet skin and rinse

Pruritus of the elderly associated with dry skin
▸ TO THE SKIN
▸ Elderly: 15 mL/bath, alternatively, to be applied to wet skin and rinse

E45® WASH CREAM

Endogenous and exogenous eczema, xeroderma, and ichthyosis
▸ TO THE SKIN
▸ Child: To be used as a soap substitute
▸ Adult: To be used as a soap substitute

Pruritus of the elderly associated with dry skin
▸ TO THE SKIN
▸ Elderly: To be used as a soap substitute

HYDROMOL® BATH AND SHOWER EMOLLIENT

Dry skin conditions | Eczema | Ichthyosis
▸ TO THE SKIN
▸ Child 1 month-11 years: 0.5–2 capfuls/bath, alternatively apply to wet skin and rinse
▸ Child 12-17 years: 1–3 capfuls/bath, alternatively apply to wet skin and rinse
▸ Adult: 1–3 capfuls/bath, alternatively apply to wet skin and rinse

Pruritus of the elderly
▸ TO THE SKIN
▸ Elderly: 1–3 capfuls/bath, alternatively apply to wet skin and rinse

LPL 63.4®

Dry skin conditions
▸ TO THE SKIN
▸ Child 1 month-11 years: 0.5–2 capfuls/bath, alternatively, to be applied to wet skin and rinse
▸ Child 12-17 years: 1–3 capfuls/bath, alternatively, to be applied to wet skin and rinse
▸ Adult: 1–3 capfuls/bath, alternatively, to be applied to wet skin and rinse

OILATUM® EMOLLIENT BATH ADDITIVE

Dry skin conditions including dermatitis and ichthyosis
▸ TO THE SKIN
▸ Child 1 month-11 years: 0.5–2 capfuls/bath, alternatively, to be applied to wet skin and rinse
▸ Child 12-17 years: 1–3 capfuls/bath, alternatively, to be applied to wet skin and rinse
▸ Adult: 1–3 capfuls/bath, alternatively, to be applied to wet skin and rinse

Pruritus of the elderly
▸ TO THE SKIN
▸ Elderly: 1–3 capfuls/bath, alternatively, to be applied to wet skin and rinse

OILATUM® JUNIOR BATH ADDITIVE

Dry skin conditions including dermatitis and ichthyosis
▸ TO THE SKIN
▸ Child 1 month-11 years: 0.5–2 capfuls/bath, alternatively, apply to wet skin and rinse
▸ Child 12-17 years: 1–3 capfuls/bath, alternatively, apply to wet skin and rinse
▸ Adult: 1–3 capfuls/bath, alternatively, apply to wet skin and rinse

Pruritus of the elderly
▸ TO THE SKIN
▸ Elderly: 1–3 capfuls/bath, alternatively, apply to wet skin and rinse

QV® BATH OIL

Dry skin conditions including eczema, psoriasis, ichthyosis, and pruritus
▸ TO THE SKIN
▸ Child 1-11 months: 5 mL/bath, alternatively, to be applied to wet skin and rinse
▸ Child 1-17 years: 10 mL/bath, alternatively, to be applied to wet skin and rinse
▸ Adult: 10 mL/bath, alternatively, to be applied to wet skin and rinse

QV® GENTLE WASH

Dry skin conditions including eczema, psoriasis, ichthyosis, and pruritus
▸ TO THE SKIN
▸ Child: To be used as a soap substitute
▸ Adult: To be used as a soap substitute

ZEROLATUM®

Dry skin conditions | Dermatitis | Ichthyosis
▸ TO THE SKIN
▸ Child 1 month-11 years: 5–10 mL/bath
▸ Child 12-17 years: 15–20 mL/bath
▸ Adult: 15–20 mL/bath

Pruritus of the elderly
▸ TO THE SKIN
▸ Elderly: 15–20 mL/bath

IMPORTANT SAFETY INFORMATION
These preparations make the skin and surfaces slippery—particular care is needed when bathing.

MHRA/CHM ADVICE (UPDATED DECEMBER 2018): EMOLLIENTS: NEW INFORMATION ABOUT RISK OF SEVERE AND FATAL BURNS WITH PARAFFIN-CONTAINING AND PARAFFIN-FREE EMOLLIENTS
See Emollient and barrier preparations p. 1387.

● **DIRECTIONS FOR ADMINISTRATION** Emollient bath additives should be added to bath water; EvGr hydration can be improved by soaking in the bath for 5–20 minutes (consult product literature). Some bath emollients can be applied to wet skin undiluted and rinsed off. ⟨M⟩Emollient preparations contained in tubs should be removed with a clean spoon or spatula to reduce bacterial contamination of the emollient. Emollients should be applied in the direction of hair growth to reduce the risk of folliculitis.

● **MEDICINAL FORMS** There can be variation in the licensing of different medicines containing the same drug.

Bath additive
CAUTIONARY AND ADVISORY LABELS 15
EXCIPIENTS: May contain Acetylated lanolin alcohols, cetostearyl alcohol (including cetyl and stearyl alcohol), fragrances, isopropyl palmitate
▸ Dermalo (Dermal Laboratories Ltd)
  Acetylated wool alcohols 50 mg per 1 gram, Liquid paraffin 650 mg per 1 gram Dermalo bath emollient | 500 ml GSL £3.44
▸ Doublebase (Dermal Laboratories Ltd)
  Liquid paraffin 650 mg per 1 gram Doublebase emollient bath additive | 500 ml GSL £5.45 DT = £5.45
▸ Hydromol (Alliance Pharmaceuticals Ltd)
  Isopropyl myristate 130 mg per 1 ml, Liquid paraffin light 378 mg per 1 ml Hydromol Bath & Shower emollient | 350 ml £4.17 | 500 ml £4.75 | 1000 ml £9.45
▸ LPL (Huxley Europe Ltd)
  Liquid paraffin light 634 mg per 1 ml LPL 63.4 bath additive and emollient | 500 ml £3.17 DT = £9.93
▸ Oilatum (Thornton & Ross Ltd)
  Liquid paraffin light 634 mg per 1 ml Oilatum Bath Formula | 150 ml GSL £3.89 DT = £3.89 | 300 ml GSL £6.42 DT = £6.42 Oilatum Emollient | 500 ml GSL £9.93 DT = £9.93

- **Oilatum junior** (Thornton & Ross Ltd)
  Liquid paraffin light 634 mg per 1 ml Oilatum Junior bath additive
  | 150 ml GSL £3.89 DT = £3.89 | 300 ml GSL £6.70 DT = £6.42 |
  600 ml GSL £9.54 DT = £9.54
- **Zerolatum** (Thornton & Ross Ltd)
  **Acetylated wool alcohols 50 mg per 1 gram, Liquid paraffin
  650 mg per 1 gram** Zerolatum Emollient bath additive | 500 ml
  £5.05

Cutaneous wash

CAUTIONARY AND ADVISORY LABELS 15
EXCIPIENTS: May contain Cetostearyl alcohol (including cetyl and
stearyl alcohol), polysorbates

- **Aquamax** (Esteve Pharmaceuticals Ltd)
  Aquamax wash | 250 gram £2.99
- **E45 emollient wash** (Karo Healthcare UK Ltd)
  E45 emollient wash cream | 250 ml £3.98

Cutaneous cream

CAUTIONARY AND ADVISORY LABELS 15
EXCIPIENTS: May contain Cetostearyl alcohol (including cetyl and
stearyl alcohol)

- **Emollient bath and shower products, paraffin-containing (Non-
  proprietary)**
  **Phenoxyethanol 10 mg per 1 gram, Liquid paraffin 60 mg per
  1 gram, Emulsifying wax 90 mg per 1 gram, White soft paraffin
  150 mg per 1 gram, Purified water 690 mg per 1 gram** Aqueous
  cream | 100 gram GSL £1.53 DT = £1.53 | 500 gram GSL £10.88
  DT = £7.65

Cutaneous gel

CAUTIONARY AND ADVISORY LABELS 15
EXCIPIENTS: May contain Cetostearyl alcohol (including cetyl and
stearyl alcohol), polysorbates

- **Doublebase** (Dermal Laboratories Ltd)
  **Isopropyl myristate 150 mg per 1 gram, Liquid paraffin 150 mg
  per 1 gram** Doublebase Dayleve gel | 100 gram P £2.65 DT = £2.65
  | 500 gram P £6.29 DT = £5.83
  Doublebase gel | 100 gram P £2.65 DT = £2.65 | 500 gram P
  £5.83 DT = £5.83 | 1000 gram P £10.98
  Doublebase emollient wash gel | 200 gram P £5.21
  Doublebase emollient shower gel | 200 gram P £5.21
- **Oilatum** (Thornton & Ross Ltd)
  Liquid paraffin light 700 mg per 1 gram Oilatum shower gel
  fragrance free | 150 gram GSL £6.62 DT = £6.62

Form unstated

CAUTIONARY AND ADVISORY LABELS 15

- **E45 emollient bath** (Karo Healthcare UK Ltd)
  E45 emollient bath oil | 500 ml £6.13

Products without form

CAUTIONARY AND ADVISORY LABELS 15
EXCIPIENTS: May contain Hydroxybenzoates (parabens)

- **QV Gentle** (Ego Pharmaceuticals)
  QV Gentle wash | 500 ml £5.55

Emollient bath and shower products, soya-bean oil-containing
19-Nov-2020

- ● **INDICATIONS AND DOSE**

BALNEUM ® BATH OIL

**Dry skin conditions including those associated with
dermatitis and eczema**
- ▸ TO THE SKIN
- ▸ Child 1-23 months: 5–15 mL/bath, not to be used
  undiluted
- ▸ Child 2-17 years: 20–60 mL/bath, not to be used
  undiluted
- ▸ Adult: 20–60 mL/bath, not to be used undiluted

BALNEUM ® PLUS BATH OIL

**Dry skin conditions including those associated with
dermatitis and eczema where pruritus also experienced**
- ▸ TO THE SKIN
- ▸ Child 1-23 months: 5 mL/bath, alternatively, to be
  applied to wet skin and rinse
- ▸ Child 2-17 years: 10–20 mL/bath, alternatively, to be
  applied to wet skin and rinse
- ▸ Adult: 20 mL/bath, alternatively, to be applied to wet
  skin and rinse

ZERONEUM ®

Dry skin conditions, including eczema
- ▸ TO THE SKIN
- ▸ Child 1 month-11 years: 5 mL/bath
- ▸ Child 12-17 years: 20 mL/bath
- ▸ Adult: 20 mL/bath

IMPORTANT SAFETY INFORMATION
These preparations make skin and surfaces slippery—
particular care is needed when bathing.

MHRA/CHM ADVICE (UPDATED DECEMBER 2018): EMOLLIENTS:
NEW INFORMATION ABOUT RISK OF SEVERE AND FATAL BURNS
WITH PARAFFIN-CONTAINING AND PARAFFIN-FREE EMOLLIENTS
See Emollient and barrier preparations p. 1387.

- ● **DIRECTIONS FOR ADMINISTRATION** Emollient bath
  additives should be added to bath water; EvGr hydration
  can be improved by soaking in the bath for 5–20 minutes
  (consult product literature). Some bath emollients can be
  applied to wet skin undiluted and rinsed off. M Emollient
  preparations contained in tubs should be removed with a
  clean spoon or spatula to reduce bacterial contamination
  of the emollient. Emollients should be applied in the
  direction of hair growth to reduce the risk of folliculitis.

- ● **MEDICINAL FORMS** There can be variation in the licensing of
  different medicines containing the same drug.

Bath additive

CAUTIONARY AND ADVISORY LABELS 15
EXCIPIENTS: May contain Butylated hydroxytoluene, fragrances,
propylene glycol

- **Balneum** (Almirall Ltd)
  **Lauromacrogols 150 mg per 1 gram, Soya oil 829.5 mg per
  1 gram** Balneum Plus bath oil | 500 ml GSL £6.66 DT = £6.66
  Soya oil 847.5 mg per 1 gram Balneum 84.75% bath oil |
  500 ml GSL £5.38 DT = £5.38
- **Zeroneum** (Thornton & Ross Ltd)
  Soya oil 833.5 mg per 1 gram Zeroneum 83.35% bath additive |
  500 ml £4.72

Emollient creams and ointments, antimicrobial-containing
19-Nov-2020

- ● **INDICATIONS AND DOSE**

**Dry and pruritic skin conditions including eczema and
dermatitis**
- ▸ TO THE SKIN
- ▸ Child: To be applied to the skin or used as a soap
  substitute
- ▸ Adult: To be applied to the skin or used as a soap
  substitute

IMPORTANT SAFETY INFORMATION
These preparations make skin and surfaces slippery—
particular care is needed when bathing.

MHRA/CHM ADVICE (UPDATED DECEMBER 2018): EMOLLIENTS:
NEW INFORMATION ABOUT RISK OF SEVERE AND FATAL BURNS
WITH PARAFFIN-CONTAINING AND PARAFFIN-FREE EMOLLIENTS
See Emollient and barrier preparations p. 1387.

- ● **DIRECTIONS FOR ADMINISTRATION** Emollients should be
  applied immediately after washing or bathing to maximise
  the effect of skin hydration. Emollient preparations
  contained in tubs should be removed with a clean spoon or
  spatula to reduce bacterial contamination of the emollient.
  Emollients should be applied in the direction of hair
  growth to reduce the risk of folliculitis.

- **PRESCRIBING AND DISPENSING INFORMATION**
Preparations containing an antibacterial should be avoided unless infection is present or is a frequent complication.

- **MEDICINAL FORMS** There can be variation in the licensing of different medicines containing the same drug.
Cutaneous cream
CAUTIONARY AND ADVISORY LABELS 15
EXCIPIENTS: May contain Cetostearyl alcohol (including cetyl and stearyl alcohol)
  ▸ Dermol (Dermal Laboratories Ltd)
  Benzalkonium chloride 1 mg per 1 gram, Chlorhexidine hydrochloride 1 mg per 1 gram, Isopropyl myristate 100 mg per 1 gram, Liquid paraffin 100 mg per 1 gram Dermol cream | 100 gram P £3.08 | 500 gram P £7.19
Cutaneous emulsion
CAUTIONARY AND ADVISORY LABELS 15
EXCIPIENTS: May contain Cetostearyl alcohol (including cetyl and stearyl alcohol)
  ▸ Dermol 500 (Dermal Laboratories Ltd)
  Benzalkonium chloride 1 mg per 1 gram, Chlorhexidine hydrochloride 1 mg per 1 gram, Isopropyl myristate 25 mg per 1 gram, Liquid paraffin 25 mg per 1 gram Dermol 500 lotion | 500 ml P £6.52

Emollient creams and ointments, colloidal oatmeal-containing
15-Aug-2024

- **INDICATIONS AND DOSE**

Dry skin conditions | Psoriasis | Eczema | Xeroderma | Ichthyosis
  ▸ TO THE SKIN
  ▸ Child: To be applied to the skin as an emollient
  ▸ Adult: To be applied to the skin as an emollient
Senile pruritus (pruritus of the elderly) associated with dry skin
  ▸ TO THE SKIN
  ▸ Elderly: To be applied to the skin as an emollient

> **IMPORTANT SAFETY INFORMATION**
> MHRA/CHM ADVICE (UPDATED DECEMBER 2018): EMOLLIENTS: NEW INFORMATION ABOUT RISK OF SEVERE AND FATAL BURNS WITH PARAFFIN-CONTAINING AND PARAFFIN-FREE EMOLLIENTS
> See Emollient and barrier preparations p. 1387.

- **DIRECTIONS FOR ADMINISTRATION** Emollients should be applied immediately after washing or bathing to maximise the effect of skin hydration. Emollient preparations contained in tubs should be removed with a clean spoon or spatula to reduce bacterial contamination of the emollient. Emollients should be applied in the direction of hair growth to reduce the risk of folliculitis.

- **MEDICINAL FORMS** There can be variation in the licensing of different medicines containing the same drug.
Form unstated
CAUTIONARY AND ADVISORY LABELS 15
EXCIPIENTS: May contain Benzyl alcohol, cetostearyl alcohol (including cetyl and stearyl alcohol), isopropyl palmitate
  ▸ Aveeno (Johnson & Johnson Ltd)
  Aveeno cream | 100 ml(ACBS) £4.85 | 300 ml(ACBS) £7.50 | 500 ml (ACBS) £6.72
Cream
CAUTIONARY AND ADVISORY LABELS 15
EXCIPIENTS: May contain Benzyl alcohol, cetostearyl alcohol (including cetyl and stearyl alcohol), isopropyl palmitate
  ▸ Emollient creams and ointments, colloidal oatmeal-containing (Non-proprietary)
  Epimax oatmeal cream | 100 gram £2.10 | 500 gram £3.16
Products without form
CAUTIONARY AND ADVISORY LABELS 15
EXCIPIENTS: May contain Benzyl alcohol, cetostearyl alcohol (including cetyl and stearyl alcohol), isopropyl palmitate

  ▸ Zeroveen (Thornton & Ross Ltd)
  Zeroveen cream | 100 gram £2.86 | 500 gram £6.13

Emollient creams and ointments, hydrogenated castor oil-containing
15-Aug-2024

- **INDICATIONS AND DOSE**

Dry skin conditions | Eczema | Psoriasis
  ▸ TO THE SKIN
  ▸ Child: To be applied to the skin as an emollient or used as a soap substitute
  ▸ Adult: To be applied to the skin as an emollient or used as a soap substitute

> **IMPORTANT SAFETY INFORMATION**
> MHRA/CHM ADVICE (UPDATED DECEMBER 2018): EMOLLIENTS: NEW INFORMATION ABOUT RISK OF SEVERE AND FATAL BURNS WITH PARAFFIN-CONTAINING AND PARAFFIN-FREE EMOLLIENTS
> See Emollient and barrier preparations p. 1387.
>
> MHRA/CHM ADVICE: *EPIMAX®* OINTMENT AND *EPIMAX®* PARAFFIN-FREE OINTMENT: REPORTS OF OCULAR SURFACE TOXICITY AND OCULAR CHEMICAL INJURY (JULY 2024)
> Following a cluster of reports of ocular surface toxicity associated with *Epimax®* ointment and *Epimax®* paraffin-free ointment, it is advised that these preparations should not be used on the face. If contact with the eyes occurs, patients may present with pain, swelling, redness or watering, sensitivity to light, blurred vision, burning, or grittiness. Symptoms should resolve with discontinuation of the product around the eyes and can be treated with topical lubricants, antibiotics or steroids as required—see advice in manufacturer's Field Safety Notice (available from: mhra-gov.filecamp.com/s/d/icXgbJO5IVPprV2f). Patients and carers should be advised to use *Epimax®* ointment or *Epimax®* paraffin-free ointment only on the body and not on the face, to wash their hands thoroughly after use, and to avoid contact with the eyes. They should also be counselled to rinse eyes well with water and seek medical advice if these preparations accidentally get into the eyes.

- **DIRECTIONS FOR ADMINISTRATION** Emollients should be applied immediately after washing or bathing to maximise the effect of skin hydration. Emollient preparations contained in tubs should be removed with a clean spoon or spatula to reduce bacterial contamination of the emollient. Emollients should be applied in the direction of hair growth to reduce the risk of folliculitis.

- **MEDICINAL FORMS** There can be variation in the licensing of different medicines containing the same drug.
Ointment
CAUTIONARY AND ADVISORY LABELS 15
EXCIPIENTS: May contain Cetostearyl alcohol (including cetyl and stearyl alcohol)
  ▸ Emollient creams and ointments, hydrogenated castor oil-containing (Non-proprietary)
  Epimax paraffin-free ointment | 500 gram £5.11

Emollient creams and ointments, paraffin-containing
15-Aug-2024

- **INDICATIONS AND DOSE**

Dry skin conditions | Eczema | Psoriasis | Ichthyosis | Pruritus
  ▸ TO THE SKIN
  ▸ Child: To be applied to the skin as an emollient

> ▸ **Adult:** To be applied to the skin as an emollient

IMPORTANT SAFETY INFORMATION

MHRA/CHM ADVICE (UPDATED DECEMBER 2018): EMOLLIENTS: NEW INFORMATION ABOUT RISK OF SEVERE AND FATAL BURNS WITH PARAFFIN-CONTAINING AND PARAFFIN-FREE EMOLLIENTS
See Emollient and barrier preparations p. 1387.

MHRA/CHM ADVICE: *EPIMAX*® OINTMENT AND *EPIMAX*® PARAFFIN-FREE OINTMENT: REPORTS OF OCULAR SURFACE TOXICITY AND OCULAR CHEMICAL INJURY (JULY 2024)
Following a cluster of reports of ocular surface toxicity associated with *Epimax*® ointment and *Epimax*® paraffin-free ointment, it is advised that these preparations should not be used on the face. If contact with the eyes occurs, patients may present with pain, swelling, redness or watering, sensitivity to light, blurred vision, burning, or grittiness. Symptoms should resolve with discontinuation of the product around the eyes and can be treated with topical lubricants, antibiotics or steroids as required—see advice in the manufacturer's Field Safety Notice (available from: mhra-gov.filecamp. com/s/d/icXgbJO5IVPprrV2f). Patients and carers should be advised to use *Epimax*® ointment or *Epimax*® paraffin-free ointment only on the body and not on the face, to wash their hands thoroughly after use, and to avoid contact with the eyes. They should also be counselled to rinse eyes well with water and seek medical advice if these preparations accidentally get into the eyes.

● **DIRECTIONS FOR ADMINISTRATION** Emollients should be applied immediately after washing or bathing to maximise the effect of skin hydration. Emollient preparations contained in tubs should be removed with a clean spoon or spatula to reduce bacterial contamination of the emollient. Emollients should be applied in the direction of hair growth to reduce the risk of folliculitis.

● **PRESCRIBING AND DISPENSING INFORMATION** Some preparations may contain other ingredients or additives—consult product literature.

● **MEDICINAL FORMS** There can be variation in the licensing of different medicines containing the same drug.

Cutaneous ointment
CAUTIONARY AND ADVISORY LABELS 15
EXCIPIENTS: May contain Cetostearyl alcohol (including cetyl and stearyl alcohol), polysorbates
▸ **Emollient creams and ointments, paraffin-containing (Non-proprietary)**
Cetraben ointment | 125 gram £3.68 | 450 gram £5.75
Liquid paraffin 200 mg per 1 gram, Emulsifying wax 300 mg per 1 gram, White soft paraffin 500 mg per 1 gram EmulsifEss ointment | 500 gram £3.97
Emulsifying ointment | 500 gram £4.15
Liquid paraffin 500 mg per 1 gram, White soft paraffin 500 mg per 1 gram White soft paraffin 50% / Liquid paraffin 50% ointment | 500 gram P £4.57 DT = £4.57
Magnesium sulfate dried 5 mg per 1 gram, Phenoxyethanol 10 mg per 1 gram, Wool alcohols ointment 500 mg per 1 gram Hydrous ointment | 500 gram GSL Ⓧ
Yellow soft paraffin 1 mg per 1 mg Yellow soft paraffin solid | 15 gram GSL £1.30
▸ **Emelpin** (Vitame Ltd)
Emulsifying wax 300 mg per 1 gram, Yellow soft paraffin 300 mg per 1 gram Emelpin ointment | 125 gram £3.08 | 500 gram £3.97
▸ **Epaderm** (Molnlycke Health Care Ltd)
Emulsifying wax 300 mg per 1 gram, Yellow soft paraffin 300 mg per 1 gram Epaderm ointment | 125 gram £4.07 | 500 gram £6.89 | 1000 gram £13.01
▸ **Epaderm Junior** (Molnlycke Health Care Ltd)
Emulsifying wax 300 mg per 1 gram, Yellow soft paraffin 300 mg per 1 gram Epaderm Junior ointment | 125 gram £4.03
▸ **Hydromol** (Alliance Pharmaceuticals Ltd)
Emulsifying wax 300 mg per 1 gram, Yellow soft paraffin 300 mg per 1 gram Hydromol ointment | 100 gram £3.30 | 125 gram £3.24 | 500 gram £5.50

▸ **Thirty:30** (Ennogen Healthcare Ltd)
Emulsifying wax 300 mg per 1 gram, Yellow soft paraffin 300 mg per 1 gram Thirty:30 ointment | 125 gram £4.08 | 250 gram £4.29 | 500 gram £6.93
▸ **Vaseline** (Unilever UK Home & Personal Care)
White soft paraffin 1 mg per 1 mg Vaseline Pure Petroleum jelly | 50 ml GSL Ⓧ
▸ **Zeroderm** (Thornton & Ross Ltd)
Zeroderm ointment | 125 gram £2.57 | 500 gram £4.35

Cutaneous emulsion
CAUTIONARY AND ADVISORY LABELS 15
EXCIPIENTS: May contain Hydroxybenzoates (parabens), isopropyl palmitate
▸ **E45** (Karo Healthcare UK Ltd)
E45 lotion | 200 ml £3.07 | 500 ml £6.13

Spray
CAUTIONARY AND ADVISORY LABELS 15
▸ **Emollin** (C D Medical Ltd)
Emollin aerosol spray | 240 ml £7.86

Cutaneous solution
CAUTIONARY AND ADVISORY LABELS 15
EXCIPIENTS: May contain Benzyl alcohol, cetostearyl alcohol (including cetyl and stearyl alcohol), hydroxybenzoates (parabens), isopropyl palmitate
▸ **QV** (Ego Pharmaceuticals)
White soft paraffin 50 mg per 1 gram QV 5% skin lotion | 500 ml £5.55

Cream
CAUTIONARY AND ADVISORY LABELS 15
EXCIPIENTS: May contain Cetostearyl alcohol (including cetyl and stearyl alcohol), polysorbates
▸ **Emollient creams and ointments, paraffin-containing (Non-proprietary)**
Epimax original cream | 100 gram £0.81 | 500 gram £2.72
▸ **Aquamax** (Esteve Pharmaceuticals Ltd)
Aquamax cream | 100 gram £1.89 | 500 gram £3.99
▸ **Epaderm** (Molnlycke Health Care Ltd)
Epaderm cream | 50 gram £1.79 | 150 gram £3.75 | 500 gram £7.34
▸ **Epimax intensive cream** (Aspire Pharma Ltd)
Epimax intensive cream | 500 gram £2.81
▸ **ZeroAQS** (Thornton & Ross Ltd)
ZeroAQS emollient cream | 500 gram £3.39

Cutaneous cream
CAUTIONARY AND ADVISORY LABELS 15
EXCIPIENTS: May contain Benzyl alcohol, cetostearyl alcohol (including cetyl and stearyl alcohol), chlorocresol, disodium edetate, fragrances, hydroxybenzoates (parabens), polysorbates, propylene glycol, sorbic acid, lanolin
▸ **Cetraben** (Thornton & Ross Ltd)
Liquid paraffin light 105 mg per 1 gram, White soft paraffin 132 mg per 1 gram Cetraben cream | 50 gram £1.50 | 150 gram £4.23 | 500 gram £6.38 | 1050 gram £12.41
▸ **E45** (Karo Healthcare UK Ltd)
Wool fat 10 mg per 1 gram, Liquid paraffin light 126 mg per 1 gram, White soft paraffin 145 mg per 1 gram E45 cream | 50 gram GSL £2.45 | 125 gram GSL £4.19 | 350 gram GSL £7.76 | 500 gram GSL £6.95
▸ **Enopen** (Ennogen Healthcare Ltd)
Liquid paraffin light 105 mg per 1 gram, White soft paraffin 132 mg per 1 gram Enopen cream | 50 gram £1.42 | 150 gram £4.03 | 500 gram £6.06 | 1050 gram £11.77
▸ **Epimax moisturising cream** (Aspire Pharma Ltd)
Liquid paraffin 126 mg per 1 gram, White soft paraffin 145 mg per 1 gram Epimax moisturising cream | 100 gram £2.02 | 500 gram £3.04
▸ **ExCetra** (Aspire Pharma Ltd)
Liquid paraffin light 105 mg per 1 gram, White soft paraffin 132 mg per 1 gram Epimax excetra cream | 100 gram £1.86 | 500 gram £3.15
▸ **Exmaben** (Ascot Laboratories Ltd)
Liquid paraffin light 105 mg per 1 gram, White soft paraffin 132 mg per 1 gram Exmaben cream | 500 gram £4.25
▸ **Hydromol** (Alliance Pharmaceuticals Ltd)
Sodium lactate 10 mg per 1 gram, Sodium pidolate 25 mg per 1 gram, Isopropyl myristate 50 mg per 1 gram, Liquid paraffin 100 mg per 1 gram Hydromol 2.5% cream | 50 gram £2.37 | 100 gram £4.42 | 500 gram £12.88
▸ **Lipobase** (Karo Healthcare UK Ltd)
Lipobase cream | 50 gram P £1.46

▶ **Oilatum** (Thornton & Ross Ltd)
Liquid paraffin light 60 mg per 1 gram, White soft paraffin 150 mg per 1 gram Oilatum cream | 150 gram GSL £4.18 DT = £4.18 | 500 ml GSL £8.57 DT = £8.57

▶ **Oilatum junior** (Thornton & Ross Ltd)
Liquid paraffin light 60 mg per 1 gram, White soft paraffin 150 mg per 1 gram Oilatum Junior cream | 150 gram GSL £4.19 DT = £4.18 | 350 ml GSL £6.66 DT = £6.66 | 500 ml GSL £7.81 DT = £8.57

▶ **QV** (Ego Pharmaceuticals)
White soft paraffin 50 mg per 1 gram, Glycerol 100 mg per 1 gram, Liquid paraffin light 100 mg per 1 gram QV cream | 100 gram £2.35 | 500 gram £6.69 | 1050 gram £12.58

▶ **Soffen** (Vitame Ltd)
Liquid paraffin light 105 mg per 1 gram, White soft paraffin 132 mg per 1 gram Soffen cream | 500 gram £4.79

▶ **Ultrabase** (Derma UK Ltd)
Ultrabase cream | 100 ml £2.85 | 500 ml £7.01

▶ **Unguentum M** (Almirall Ltd)
Unguentum M cream | 500 gram GSL £8.48

▶ **Zerobase** (Thornton & Ross Ltd)
Liquid paraffin 110 mg per 1 gram Zerobase 11% cream | 50 gram £1.12 | 500 gram £5.66

▶ **Zerocream** (Thornton & Ross Ltd)
Liquid paraffin 126 mg per 1 gram, White soft paraffin 145 mg per 1 gram Zerocream | 50 gram £1.25 | 500 gram £4.36

▶ **Zeroguent** (Thornton & Ross Ltd)
White soft paraffin 40 mg per 1 gram, Soya oil 50 mg per 1 gram, Liquid paraffin light 80 mg per 1 gram Zeroguent cream | 100 gram £2.44 | 500 gram £7.32

Cutaneous gel
CAUTIONARY AND ADVISORY LABELS 15
EXCIPIENTS: May contain Polysorbates

▶ **Doublebase** (Dermal Laboratories Ltd)
Isopropyl myristate 150 mg per 1 gram, Liquid paraffin 150 mg per 1 gram Doublebase Dayleve gel | 100 gram P £2.65 DT = £2.65 | 500 gram P £6.29 DT = £5.83
Doublebase gel | 100 gram P £2.65 DT = £2.65 | 500 gram P £5.83 DT = £5.83 | 1000 gram P £10.98
Doublebase emollient wash gel | 200 gram P £5.21
Doublebase emollient shower gel | 200 gram P £5.21

Ointment
CAUTIONARY AND ADVISORY LABELS 15
EXCIPIENTS: May contain Cetostearyl alcohol (including cetyl and stearyl alcohol)

▶ **Emollient creams and ointments, paraffin-containing (Non-proprietary)**
Epimax ointment | 125 gram £2.05 | 500 gram £3.19

Products without form
CAUTIONARY AND ADVISORY LABELS 15
EXCIPIENTS: May contain Cetostearyl alcohol (including cetyl and stearyl alcohol)

▶ **Emollient creams and ointments, paraffin-containing (Non-proprietary)**
Doublebase Once gel | 100 gram £2.69 | 500 gram £6.99
Cetraben lotion | 200 ml £4.00 | 500 ml £5.92

▶ **Adex** (Dermal Laboratories Ltd)
Adex gel | 100 gram £2.69 | 500 gram £5.99

▶ **QV intensive** (Ego Pharmaceuticals)
QV Intensive ointment | 450 gram £5.97

Emollients, urea-containing
19-Nov-2020

● **DRUG ACTION** Urea is a keratin softener and hydrating agent used in the treatment of dry, scaling conditions (including ichthyosis).

● **INDICATIONS AND DOSE**

AQUADRATE ®

Dry, scaling, and itching skin
▶ TO THE SKIN
▶ Child: Apply twice daily, to be applied thinly
▶ Adult: Apply twice daily, to be applied thinly

BALNEUM ® CREAM

Dry skin conditions
▶ TO THE SKIN
▶ Child: Apply twice daily
▶ Adult: Apply twice daily

BALNEUM ® PLUS CREAM

Dry, scaling, and itching skin
▶ TO THE SKIN
▶ Child: Apply twice daily
▶ Adult: Apply twice daily

CALMURID ®

Dry, scaling, and itching skin
▶ TO THE SKIN
▶ Child: Apply twice daily, apply a thick layer for 3–5 minutes, massage into area, and remove excess. Can be diluted with aqueous cream (life of diluted cream is 14 days). Half-strength cream can be used for 1 week if stinging occurs
▶ Adult: Apply twice daily, apply a thick layer for 3–5 minutes, massage into area, and remove excess. Can be diluted with aqueous cream (life of diluted cream is 14 days). Half-strength cream can be used for 1 week if stinging occurs

DERMATONICS ONCE HEEL BALM ®

Dry skin on soles of feet
▶ TO THE SKIN
▶ Child 12–17 years: Apply once daily
▶ Adult: Apply once daily

E45 ® ITCH RELIEF CREAM

Dry, scaling, and itching skin
▶ TO THE SKIN
▶ Child: Apply twice daily
▶ Adult: Apply twice daily

EUCERIN ® INTENSIVE CREAM

Dry skin conditions including eczema, ichthyosis, xeroderma, and hyperkeratosis
▶ TO THE SKIN
▶ Child: Apply twice daily, to be applied thinly and rubbed into area
▶ Adult: Apply twice daily, to be applied thinly and rubbed into area

FLEXITOL ®

Dry skin on soles of feet and heels
▶ TO THE SKIN
▶ Child 12–17 years: Apply 1–2 times a day
▶ Adult: Apply 1–2 times a day

HYDROMOL ® INTENSIVE

Dry, scaling, and itching skin
▶ TO THE SKIN
▶ Child: Apply twice daily, to be applied thinly
▶ Adult: Apply twice daily, to be applied thinly

IMUDERM ® EMOLLIENT

Dry skin conditions including eczema, psoriasis or dermatitis
▶ TO THE SKIN
▶ Adult: Apply to skin or use as a soap substitute

NUTRAPLUS ®

Dry, scaling, and itching skin
▶ TO THE SKIN
▶ Child: Apply 2–3 times a day

▸ Adult: Apply 2–3 times a day

> **IMPORTANT SAFETY INFORMATION**
>
> **MHRA/CHM ADVICE (UPDATED DECEMBER 2018): EMOLLIENTS: NEW INFORMATION ABOUT RISK OF SEVERE AND FATAL BURNS WITH PARAFFIN-CONTAINING AND PARAFFIN-FREE EMOLLIENTS**
> See Emollient and barrier preparations p. 1387.

● **DIRECTIONS FOR ADMINISTRATION** Emollients should be applied immediately after washing or bathing to maximise the effect of skin hydration. Emollient preparations contained in tubs should be removed with a clean spoon or spatula to reduce bacterial contamination of the emollient. Emollients should be applied in the direction of hair growth to reduce the risk of folliculitis.

● **MEDICINAL FORMS** There can be variation in the licensing of different medicines containing the same drug.

Cutaneous cream

CAUTIONARY AND ADVISORY LABELS 15
EXCIPIENTS: May contain Benzyl alcohol, cetostearyl alcohol (including cetyl and stearyl alcohol), hydroxybenzoates (parabens), isopropyl palmitate, polysorbates, propylene glycol, woolfat and related substances (including lanolin)

▸ **Aquadrate** (Alliance Pharmaceuticals Ltd)
Urea 100 mg per 1 gram Aquadrate 10% cream | 30 gram £1.64 | 100 gram £4.66

▸ **Balneum Plus** (Almirall Ltd)
Lauromacrogols 30 mg per 1 gram, Urea 50 mg per 1 gram Balneum Plus cream | 100 gram GSL £3.29 DT = £5.51 | 500 gram GSL £14.99 DT = £17.77

▸ **E45 Itch Relief** (Karo Healthcare UK Ltd)
Lauromacrogols 30 mg per 1 gram, Urea 50 mg per 1 gram E45 Itch Relief cream | 50 gram GSL £3.62 DT = £3.62 | 100 gram GSL £5.51 DT = £5.51 | 500 gram GSL £17.77 DT = £17.77

▸ **Hydromol Intensive** (Alliance Pharmaceuticals Ltd)
Urea 100 mg per 1 gram Hydromol Intensive 10% cream | 30 gram £1.75 | 100 gram £4.66

Products without form

CAUTIONARY AND ADVISORY LABELS 15
EXCIPIENTS: May contain Beeswax, benzyl alcohol, cetostearyl alcohol (including cetyl and stearyl alcohol), fragrances, lanolin

▸ **Emollients, urea-containing (Non-proprietary)**
imuDERM emollient | 500 gram £6.89

▸ **Dermatonics Once** (Dermatonics Ltd)
Dermatonics Once Heel Balm | 75 ml £3.83 | 200 ml £9.52

▸ **Flexitol** (Thornton & Ross Ltd)
Flexitol 25% Urea Heel Balm | 40 gram £2.92 | 75 gram £4.04 | 200 gram £9.99 | 500 gram £15.77

3   Epidermolysis bullosa

DERMATOLOGICAL DRUGS

Birch bark extract
26-Sep-2023

● **DRUG ACTION** Birch bark extract is thought to modulate inflammatory mediators and activate pathways involved in keratinocyte differentiation and migration, thereby promoting wound healing.

● **INDICATIONS AND DOSE**

Partial thickness wounds associated with dystrophic and junctional epidermolysis bullosa

▸ TO THE SKIN

▸ Adult: Apply to surface of cleansed wound at a thickness of approx. 1 mm and cover with a sterile non-adhesive dressing or apply directly to the dressing—do not rub in, reapply at each wound dressing change

● **CONTRA-INDICATIONS** Avoid application to mucous membranes · avoid contact with eyes

● **CAUTIONS** Squamous cell carcinoma or other skin malignancies (discontinue treatment of affected areas) ·

wound infection (interrupt treatment—may be restarted once infection has resolved)

● **SIDE-EFFECTS**

▸ **Common or very common** Hypersensitivity · skin reactions · wound complications · wound infection

▸ **Uncommon** Pain

● **PREGNANCY** [EvGr] Not known to be harmful (limited information available but systemic exposure is negligible). ⓜ

● **BREAST FEEDING** [EvGr] Avoid if the mother's chest area is being treated (no information available on presence in milk but systemic exposure is negligible). ⓜ

● **DIRECTIONS FOR ADMINISTRATION** Each tube is for single use only and should be used immediately once opened then discarded.

● **PRESCRIBING AND DISPENSING INFORMATION** In clinical studies, the maximum total wound area treated was 5 300 cm^2 (median of 735 cm^2).

● **PATIENT AND CARER ADVICE** Patients or their carers should be counselled on the application of *Filsuvez*® gel.

● **NATIONAL FUNDING/ACCESS DECISIONS**
For full details see funding body website

NICE decisions

▸ Birch bark extract for treating epidermolysis bullosa (September 2023) NICE HST28 Recommended

● **MEDICINAL FORMS** There can be variation in the licensing of different medicines containing the same drug.

Cutaneous gel

▸ **Filsuvez** (Chiesi Ltd)
Filsuvez gel | 702 gram PoM £8,259.90 (Hospital only)

4   Infections of the skin

Skin infections
22-Mar-2020

Antibacterial preparations for the skin

Cellulitis, erysipelas, and *leg ulcer* infections require systemic antibacterial treatment, see Skin infections, antibacterial therapy p. 589.

Impetigo requires topical antiseptic/antibacterial or systemic antibacterial treatment, see Skin infections, antibacterial therapy p. 589.

Although many antibacterial drugs are available in topical preparations, some are potentially hazardous and frequently their use is not necessary if adequate hygienic measures can be taken. Moreover, not all skin conditions that are oozing, crusted, or characterised by pustules are actually infected.

To minimise the development of resistant organisms it is advisable to limit the choice of antibacterials applied topically to those not used systemically. Unfortunately some of these, for example neomycin sulfate p. 1397, may cause sensitisation, and there is cross-sensitivity with other aminoglycoside antibiotics, such as gentamicin p. 596. If *large areas of skin* are being treated, ototoxicity may also be a hazard with aminoglycoside antibiotics, particularly in children, in the elderly, and in those with renal impairment. *Resistant organisms* are more common in hospitals, and whenever possible swabs should be taken for bacteriological examination before beginning treatment.

Mupirocin p. 1399 is not related to any other antibacterial in use; it is effective for skin infections, particularly those due to Gram-positive organisms but it is not indicated for pseudomonal infection. Although *Staphylococcus aureus* strains with low-level resistance to mupirocin are emerging, it is generally useful in infections resistant to other antibacterials. To avoid the development of resistance, mupirocin or fusidic acid p. 663 should not be used for longer than 10 days and local microbiology advice should be sought before using it in hospital. In the presence of mupirocin-resistant MRSA infection, a topical antiseptic such as povidone-iodine p. 1451, chlorhexidine p. 1452, or alcohol can be used; their use should be discussed with the local microbiologist.

Tedizolid p. 665 is licensed for the treatment of acute bacterial skin and skin structure infections.

Silver sulfadiazine p. 1398 is used in the treatment of infected burns.

Antibacterial preparations also used systemically

Fusidic acid is a narrow-spectrum antibacterial used for staphylococcal infections.

An ointment containing fusidic acid is used in the fissures of angular cheilitis when associated with staphylococcal infection. See Oropharyngeal fungal infections p. 1384 for further information on angular cheilitis.

Metronidazole p. 1398 is used topically for rosacea and to reduce the odour associated with anaerobic infections; oral metronidazole is used to treat wounds infected with anaerobic bacteria.

Antifungal preparations for the skin

Most localised fungal infections are treated with topical preparations. To prevent relapse, local antifungal treatment should be continued for 1–2 weeks after the disappearance of all signs of infection. Systemic therapy is necessary for scalp infection or if the skin infection is widespread, disseminated, or intractable; although topical therapy may be used to treat some nail infections, systemic therapy is more effective. Skin scrapings should be examined if systemic therapy is being considered or where there is doubt about the diagnosis.

Dermatophytoses

Ringworm infection can affect the scalp (tinea capitis), body (tinea corporis), groin (tinea cruris), hand (tinea manuum), foot (tinea pedis, athlete's foot), or nail (tinea unguium). Scalp infection requires systemic treatment; additional application of a topical antifungal, during the early stages of treatment, may reduce the risk of transmission. A topical antifungal can also be used to treat asymptomatic carriers of scalp ringworm. Most other local ringworm infections can be treated adequately with topical antifungal preparations (including shampoos). The imidazole antifungals clotrimazole p. 1399, econazole nitrate p. 1400, ketoconazole p. 1400, and miconazole p. 1400 are all effective. Terbinafine cream p. 1401 is also effective but it is more expensive. Other topical antifungals include griseofulvin p. 1401 and the **undecenoates**. **Compound benzoic acid ointment** (Whitfield's ointment) has been used for ringworm infections but it is cosmetically less acceptable than proprietary preparations. Topical preparations for athlete's foot containing **tolnaftate** are on sale to the public.

Antifungal dusting powders are of little therapeutic value in the treatment of fungal skin infections and may cause skin irritation; they may have some role in preventing re-infection.

Antifungal treatment may not be necessary in asymptomatic patients with tinea infection of the nails. If treatment is necessary, a systemic antifungal is more effective than topical therapy. However, topical application of amorolfine p. 1401 or tioconazole p. 1401 may be useful for treating early onychomycosis when involvement is limited to mild distal disease, or for superficial white onychomycosis, or where there are contra-indications to systemic therapy.

Pityriasis versicolor

Pityriasis (tinea) versicolor can be treated with ketoconazole shampoo. Alternatively, **selenium sulfide** shampoo [unlicensed indication] can be used as a lotion (diluting with a small amount of water can reduce irritation) and left on the affected area for 10 minutes before rinsing off; it should be applied once daily for 7 days, and the course repeated if necessary.

Topical imidazole antifungals such as clotrimazole, econazole nitrate, ketoconazole, and miconazole, or topical terbinafine are alternatives, but large quantities may be required.

If topical therapy fails, or if the infection is widespread, pityriasis versicolor is treated systemically with a triazole antifungal. Relapse is common, especially in the immunocompromised.

Candidiasis

Candidal skin infections can be treated with a topical imidazole antifungal, such as clotrimazole, econazole nitrate, ketoconazole, or miconazole; topical terbinafine is an alternative. Topical application of nystatin p. 1385 is also effective for candidiasis but it is ineffective against dermatophytosis. Refractory candidiasis requires systemic treatment generally with a triazole such as fluconazole p. 690; systemic treatment with terbinafine is **not appropriate** for refractory candidiasis.

Angular cheilitis

Miconazole cream is used in the fissures of angular cheilitis when associated with *Candida*.

Compound topical preparations

Combination of an imidazole and a mild corticosteroid (such as hydrocortisone 1% p. 1413) may be of value in the treatment of eczematous intertrigo and, in the first few days only, of a severely inflamed patch of ringworm.

Combination of a mild corticosteroid with either an imidazole or nystatin may be of use in the treatment of intertrigo associated with candida.

Antiviral preparations for the skin

Aciclovir cream p. 1405 is licensed for the treatment of initial and recurrent labial and genital *herpes simplex infections*; treatment should begin as early as possible. Systemic treatment is necessary for buccal or vaginal infections and for *herpes zoster (shingles)*.

Herpes labialis

Aciclovir cream can be used for the treatment of initial and recurrent labial herpes simplex infections (cold sores). It is best applied at the earliest possible stage, usually when prodromal changes of sensation are felt in the lip and before vesicles appear.

Penciclovir cream is also licensed for the treatment of herpes labialis; it needs to be applied more frequently than aciclovir cream p. 1405.

Systemic treatment is necessary if cold sores recur frequently or for infections in the mouth.

Parasiticidal preparations for the skin

Suitable quantities of parasiticidal preparations			
Area of body	Skin creams	Lotions	Cream rinses
Scalp (head lice)		50-100 mL	50-100 mL
Body (scabies)	30-60 g	100 mL	
Body (crab lice)	30-60 g	100 mL	
These amounts are usually suitable for an adult for single application.			

Scabies

Permethrin p. 1404 is used for the treatment of *scabies* (*Sarcoptes scabiei*); malathion p. 1404 can be used if permethrin is inappropriate.

Benzyl benzoate p. 1403 is an irritant and should be avoided in children; it is less effective than malathion and permethrin.

Ivermectin p. 700 (available on a named patient basis from 'special-order' manufacturers or specialist importing companies) by mouth has been used, in combination with topical drugs, for the treatment of hyperkeratotic (crusted or 'Norwegian') scabies that does not respond to topical treatment alone; further doses may be required.

Application

Although acaricides have traditionally been applied after a hot bath, this is **not** necessary and there is even evidence that a hot bath may increase absorption into the blood, removing them from their site of action on the skin.

All members of the affected household should be treated simultaneously. Treatment should be applied to the whole body including the scalp, neck, face, and ears. Particular attention should be paid to the webs of the fingers and toes and lotion brushed under the ends of nails. It is now recommended that malathion and permethrin should be applied twice, one week apart; in the case of benzyl benzoate in adults, up to 3 applications on consecutive days may be needed. It is important to warn users to reapply treatment to the hands if they are washed. Patients with hyperkeratotic scabies may require 2 or 3 applications of acaricide on consecutive days to ensure that enough penetrates the skin crusts to kill all the mites.

Itching

The *itch* and *eczema* of scabies persists for some weeks after the infestation has been eliminated and treatment for pruritus and eczema may be required. Application of crotamiton p. 1437 can be used to control itching after treatment with more effective acaricides. A topical corticosteroid may help to reduce itch and inflammation after scabies has been treated successfully; however, persistent symptoms suggest that scabies eradication was not successful. Oral administration of a **sedating antihistamine** at night may also be useful.

Head lice

Dimeticone p. 1403 is effective against head lice (*Pediculus humanus capitis*). It coats head lice and interferes with water balance in lice by preventing the excretion of water; it is less active against eggs and treatment should be repeated after 7 days. Malathion, an organophosphorus insecticide, is an alternative, but resistance has been reported. Benzyl benzoate is licensed for the treatment of head lice but it is less effective than other drugs and not recommended for use in children. Permethrin is active against head lice but the formulation and licensed methods of application of the current products make them unsuitable for the treatment of head lice.

Head lice infestation (pediculosis) should be treated using lotion or liquid formulations only if live lice are present. Shampoos are diluted too much in use to be effective. A contact time of 8–12 hours or overnight treatment is recommended for lotions and liquids; a 2-hour treatment is not sufficient to kill eggs.

In general, a course of treatment for head lice should be 2 applications of product 7 days apart to kill lice emerging from any eggs that survive the first application. All affected household members should be treated simultaneously.

MHRA/CHM advice: Head lice eradication products: risk of serious burns if treated hair is exposed to open flames or other sources of ignition (March 2018)

Some products for the eradication of head lice infestations are combustible/flammable when on the hair and can ignite and cause serious harm in the presence of an open flame or other source of ignition such as when lighting cigarettes.

Patients and carers should be advised on the safe and correct use of head lice eradication treatments and if appropriate, should be advised that they should not smoke around treated hair and that it should be kept away from open flames or other sources of ignition, including in the morning after overnight application until hair is washed.

Wet combing methods

Head lice can be mechanically removed by combing wet hair meticulously with a plastic detection comb (probably for at least 30 minutes each time) over the whole scalp at 4-day intervals for a minimum of 2 weeks, and continued until no lice are found on 3 consecutive sessions; hair conditioner or vegetable oil can be used to facilitate the process.

Several devices for the removal of head lice such as combs and topical solutions, are available and some are prescribable on the NHS.

The Drug Tariffs can be accessed online at:

- National Health Service Drug Tariff for England and Wales: www.ppa.org.uk/ppa/edt_intro.htm
- Health and Personal Social Services for Northern Ireland Drug Tariff: www.hscbusiness.hscni.net/services/2034.htm
- Scottish Drug Tariff: www.isdscotland.org/Health-topics/Prescribing-and-Medicines/Scottish-Drug-Tariff/

Crab lice

Permethrin and malathion are used to eliminate *crab lice* (*Pthirus pubis*). An aqueous preparation should be applied, allowed to dry naturally and washed off after 12 hours; a second treatment is needed after 7 days to kill lice emerging from surviving eggs. All surfaces of the body should be treated, including the scalp, neck, and face (paying particular attention to the eyebrows and other facial hair). A different insecticide should be used if a course of treatment fails.

4.1　Bacterial skin infections

ANTIBACTERIALS › AMINOGLYCOSIDES

Neomycin sulfate　　　　　　　　　29-Mar-2023

- **● INDICATIONS AND DOSE**

Bacterial skin infections
▸ TO THE SKIN
▸ Child: Apply up to 3 times a day, for short-term use only
▸ Adult: Apply up to 3 times a day, for short-term use only

- **● UNLICENSED USE**
▸ In children *Neomycin Cream BPC*—no information available.

- **● CONTRA-INDICATIONS** Neonates

- **● CAUTIONS**
▸ Large areas
▸ In adults If large areas of skin are being treated ototoxicity may be a hazard, particularly in the elderly, and in those with renal impairment.
▸ In children If large areas of skin are being treated ototoxicity may be a hazard in children, particularly in those with renal impairment.

- **● INTERACTIONS** → Appendix 1: neomycin

- **● SIDE-EFFECTS** Sensitisation (cross sensitivity with other aminoglycosides may occur)

- **● RENAL IMPAIRMENT** Ototoxicity may be a hazard if large areas of skin are treated.

- **● PRE-TREATMENT SCREENING** NHS England commissions genetic testing under the *National genomic test directory* indication: R65 - Aminoglycoside exposure posing risk to hearing. The testing criteria is significant exposure to aminoglycosides posing risk of ototoxicity. This testing is relevant to individuals with a predisposition to gram-negative infections or with hearing loss who have been exposed to aminoglycosides. For further information, see www.england.nhs.uk/publication/national-genomic-test-directories/.

- **LESS SUITABLE FOR PRESCRIBING** Neomycin sulfate cream is less suitable for prescribing.

- **MEDICINAL FORMS** There can be variation in the licensing of different medicines containing the same drug. Forms available from special-order manufacturers include: cutaneous cream

Cutaneous cream

EXCIPIENTS: May contain Cetostearyl alcohol (including cetyl and stearyl alcohol), edetic acid (edta)

ANTIBACTERIALS > NITROIMIDAZOLE DERIVATIVES

Metronidazole

10-Nov-2021

- **DRUG ACTION** Metronidazole is an antimicrobial drug with high activity against anaerobic bacteria and protozoa.

- **INDICATIONS AND DOSE**

ACEA ®

Acute inflammatory exacerbation of rosacea
- ▸ TO THE SKIN
- ▸ Adult: Apply twice daily for 8 weeks, to be applied thinly

ANABACT ®

Malodorous fungating tumours and malodorous gravitational and decubitus ulcers
- ▸ TO THE SKIN
- ▸ Adult: Apply 1–2 times a day, to be applied to clean wound and covered with non-adherent dressing

METROGEL ®

Acute inflammatory exacerbation of rosacea
- ▸ TO THE SKIN
- ▸ Adult: Apply twice daily for 8–9 weeks, to be applied thinly

Malodorous fungating tumours
- ▸ TO THE SKIN
- ▸ Adult: Apply 1–2 times a day, to be applied to clean wound and covered with non-adherent dressing

METROSA ®

Acute exacerbation of rosacea
- ▸ TO THE SKIN
- ▸ Adult: Apply twice daily for up to 8 weeks, to be applied thinly

ROSICED ®

Inflammatory papules and pustules of rosacea
- ▸ TO THE SKIN
- ▸ Adult: Apply twice daily for 6 weeks (longer if necessary)

ROZEX ® **CREAM**

Inflammatory papules, pustules and erythema of rosacea
- ▸ TO THE SKIN
- ▸ Adult: Apply twice daily for 3–4 months

ROZEX ® **GEL**

Inflammatory papules, pustules and erythema of rosacea
- ▸ TO THE SKIN
- ▸ Adult: Apply twice daily for 3–4 months

ZYOMET ®

Acute inflammatory exacerbation of rosacea
- ▸ TO THE SKIN
- ▸ Adult: Apply twice daily for 8–9 weeks, to be applied thinly

- **CAUTIONS** Avoid exposure to strong sunlight or UV light

- **INTERACTIONS** → Appendix 1: metronidazole

- **SIDE-EFFECTS**
- ▸ **Common or very common** Skin reactions

- **MEDICINAL FORMS** There can be variation in the licensing of different medicines containing the same drug.

Cutaneous cream

EXCIPIENTS: May contain Benzyl alcohol, isopropyl palmitate, propylene glycol
- ▸ **Rozex** (Galderma (UK) Ltd)
  Metronidazole 7.5 mg per 1 gram Rozex 0.75% cream |
  50 gram [PoM] £12.35 DT = £12.35

Cutaneous gel

EXCIPIENTS: May contain Benzyl alcohol, disodium edetate, hydroxybenzoates (parabens), propylene glycol
- ▸ **Acea** (Ferndale Pharmaceuticals Ltd)
  Metronidazole 7.5 mg per 1 gram Acea 0.75% gel | 40 gram [PoM]
  £9.95 DT = £22.63
- ▸ **Anabact** (Cambridge Healthcare Supplies Ltd)
  Metronidazole 7.5 mg per 1 gram Anabact 0.75% gel |
  15 gram [PoM] £5.98 DT = £5.98 | 30 gram [PoM] £7.89 |
  40 gram [PoM] £15.89 DT = £22.63
- ▸ **Metrogel** (Galderma (UK) Ltd)
  Metronidazole 7.5 mg per 1 gram Metrogel 0.75% gel |
  40 gram [PoM] £22.63 DT = £22.63
- ▸ **Metrosa** (Beaumont Pharma Ltd)
  Metronidazole 7.5 mg per 1 gram Metrosa 0.75% gel |
  30 gram [PoM] £12.00 | 40 gram [PoM] £19.90 DT = £22.63
- ▸ **Rozex** (Galderma (UK) Ltd)
  Metronidazole 7.5 mg per 1 gram Rozex 0.75% gel | 50 gram [PoM]
  £12.35

ANTIBACTERIALS > SULFONAMIDES

Silver sulfadiazine

14-Dec-2020

- **INDICATIONS AND DOSE**

Prophylaxis and treatment of infection in burn wounds
- ▸ TO THE SKIN
- ▸ Child: Apply daily, may be applied more frequently if very exudative
- ▸ Adult: Apply daily, may be applied more frequently if very exudative

For conservative management of finger-tip injuries
- ▸ TO THE SKIN
- ▸ Child: Apply every 2–3 days, consult product literature for details
- ▸ Adult: Apply every 2–3 days, consult product literature for details

Adjunct to prophylaxis of infection in skin graft donor sites and extensive abrasions
- ▸ TO THE SKIN
- ▸ Adult: (consult product literature)

Adjunct to short-term treatment of infection in pressure sores
- ▸ TO THE SKIN
- ▸ Adult: Apply once daily or on alternate days

As an adjunct to short-term treatment of infection in leg ulcers
- ▸ TO THE SKIN
- ▸ Adult: Apply once daily or on alternate days, not recommended if ulcer is very exudative

- **UNLICENSED USE**
- ▸ In children No age range specified by manufacturer.

- **CONTRA-INDICATIONS** Not recommended for neonates

- **CAUTIONS** G6PD deficiency

CAUTIONS, FURTHER INFORMATION
- ▸ Large areas Plasma-sulfadiazine concentrations may approach therapeutic levels with *side-effects* and *interactions* as for sulfonamides if large areas of skin are treated.

- **INTERACTIONS** → Appendix 1: silver sulfadiazine

- **SIDE-EFFECTS**
  ▶ **Common or very common** Leucopenia · skin reactions
  ▶ **Rare or very rare** Argyria (following treatment of large areas of skin or long term use) · renal failure

  SIDE-EFFECTS, FURTHER INFORMATION Leucopenia developing 2–3 days after starting treatment of burns patients is reported usually to be self-limiting and silver sulfadiazine need not usually be discontinued provided blood counts are monitored carefully to ensure return to normality within a few days.

- **ALLERGY AND CROSS-SENSITIVITY** [EvGr] Caution in patients with sensitivity to sulfonamides. ⓜ See, *Cautions, further information.*

- **PREGNANCY** Risk of neonatal haemolysis and methaemoglobinaemia in third trimester.

- **BREAST FEEDING** Small risk of kernicterus in jaundiced infants and of haemolysis in G6PD-deficient infants.

- **HEPATIC IMPAIRMENT** Manufacturer advises caution in significant hepatic impairment.

- **RENAL IMPAIRMENT** Manufacturer advises caution if significant impairment.

- **MONITORING REQUIREMENTS** Monitor for leucopenia.

- **DIRECTIONS FOR ADMINISTRATION** Manufacturer advises apply with sterile applicator.

- **MEDICINAL FORMS** There can be variation in the licensing of different medicines containing the same drug.

  Cutaneous cream
  EXCIPIENTS: May contain Cetostearyl alcohol (including cetyl and stearyl alcohol), polysorbates, propylene glycol
  ▶ **Flamazine** (Smith & Nephew Healthcare Ltd)
  Sulfadiazine silver 10 mg per 1 gram Flamazine 1% cream | 20 gram [PoM] £2.91 | 50 gram [PoM] £3.85 DT = £3.85 | 250 gram [PoM] £10.32 DT = £10.32 | 500 gram [PoM] £18.27 DT = £18.27

ANTIBACTERIALS 〉 OTHER

Mupirocin
07-May-2021

- **INDICATIONS AND DOSE**

  Bacterial skin infections, particularly those caused by Gram-positive organisms (except pseudomonal infection)
  ▶ TO THE SKIN
  ▶ Child: Apply up to 3 times a day for up to 10 days
  ▶ Adult: Apply up to 3 times a day for up to 10 days

  Non-bullous impetigo [in patients who are not systemically unwell or at high risk of complications]
  ▶ TO THE SKIN
  ▶ Child: Apply 3 times a day for 5–7 days
  ▶ Adult: Apply 3 times a day for 5–7 days

- **UNLICENSED USE** Mupirocin ointment licensed for use in children (age range not specified by manufacturer). *Bactroban*® cream not recommended for use in children under 1 year.

- **SIDE-EFFECTS**
  ▶ **Common or very common** Skin reactions

- **PREGNANCY** Manufacturer advises avoid unless potential benefit outweighs risk—no information available.

- **BREAST FEEDING** No information available.

- **RENAL IMPAIRMENT** [EvGr] Avoid using ointment in moderate to severe impairment when absorption of large quantities may occur (contains polyethylene glycol which is excreted renally). ⓜ

- **PRESCRIBING AND DISPENSING INFORMATION** For choice of antibacterial therapy, see Skin infections, antibacterial therapy p. 589.

- **MEDICINAL FORMS** There can be variation in the licensing of different medicines containing the same drug.

  Cutaneous ointment
  ▶ **Mupirocin (Non-proprietary)**
  Mupirocin 20 mg per 1 gram Mupirocin 2% ointment | 15 gram [PoM] £12.50 DT = £8.68
  ▶ **Bactroban** (GlaxoSmithKline UK Ltd)
  Mupirocin 20 mg per 1 gram Bactroban 2% ointment | 15 gram [PoM] £5.26 DT = £8.68

  Cutaneous cream
  EXCIPIENTS: May contain Benzyl alcohol, cetostearyl alcohol (including cetyl and stearyl alcohol)
  ▶ **Bactroban** (GlaxoSmithKline UK Ltd)
  Mupirocin (as Mupirocin calcium) 20 mg per 1 gram Bactroban 2% cream | 15 gram [PoM] £5.26 DT = £5.26

4.2 Fungal skin infections

> **Other drugs used for Fungal skin infections**
> Hydrocortisone with clotrimazole, p. 1417

ANTIFUNGALS 〉 IMIDAZOLE ANTIFUNGALS

Clotrimazole
10-Nov-2021

- **INDICATIONS AND DOSE**

  Fungal skin infections
  ▶ TO THE SKIN
  ▶ Child: Apply 2–3 times a day
  ▶ Adult: Apply 2–3 times a day

- **CAUTIONS** Contact with eyes and mucous membranes should be avoided

- **INTERACTIONS** → Appendix 1: antifungals, azoles

- **SIDE-EFFECTS** Oedema · pain · paraesthesia · skin reactions

- **PREGNANCY** Minimal absorption from skin; not known to be harmful.

- **PRESCRIBING AND DISPENSING INFORMATION** Spray may be useful for application of clotrimazole to large or hairy areas of the skin.

- **PATIENT AND CARER ADVICE**
  Medicines for Children leaflet: Clotrimazole for fungal infections
  www.medicinesforchildren.org.uk/medicines/clotrimazole-for-fungal-infections/

- **MEDICINAL FORMS** There can be variation in the licensing of different medicines containing the same drug. Forms available from special-order manufacturers include: cutaneous powder

  Cutaneous or ear solution
  ▶ **Canesten (clotrimazole)** (Bayer Plc)
  Clotrimazole 10 mg per 1 ml Canesten 1% solution | 20 ml [P] £2.54 DT = £2.53

  Cutaneous cream
  EXCIPIENTS: May contain Benzyl alcohol, cetostearyl alcohol (including cetyl and stearyl alcohol), polysorbates
  ▶ **Clotrimazole (Non-proprietary)**
  Clotrimazole 10 mg per 1 gram Clotrimazole 1% cream | 20 gram [P] £2.33 DT = £1.43 | 50 gram [P] £6.00 DT = £3.58
  ▶ **Canesten (clotrimazole)** (Bayer Plc)
  Clotrimazole 10 mg per 1 gram Canesten 1% cream | 20 gram [P] £2.89 DT = £1.43 | 50 gram [P] £4.71 DT = £3.58
  Canesten Antifungal cream | 20 gram [P] £2.22 DT = £1.43

  Spray
  CAUTIONARY AND ADVISORY LABELS 15
  EXCIPIENTS: May contain Propylene glycol
  ▶ **Canesten (clotrimazole)** (Bayer Plc)
  Clotrimazole 10 mg per 1 ml Canesten Dermatological 1% spray | 40 ml [P] £4.99 DT = £4.99

  Combinations available: *Hydrocortisone with clotrimazole,* p. 1417

Econazole nitrate
08-May-2020

- **INDICATIONS AND DOSE**

Fungal skin infections
- ▶ TO THE SKIN
- ▶ Child: Apply twice daily
- ▶ Adult: Apply twice daily

Fungal nail infections
- ▶ BY TRANSUNGUAL APPLICATION
- ▶ Child: Apply once daily, applied under occlusive dressing
- ▶ Adult: Apply once daily, applied under occlusive dressing

- **CAUTIONS** Avoid contact with eyes and mucous membranes
- **SIDE-EFFECTS**
- ▶ **Common or very common** Pain · skin reactions
- ▶ **Uncommon** Swelling
- ▶ **Frequency not known** Angioedema

  SIDE-EFFECTS, FURTHER INFORMATION Treatment should be discontinued if side-effects are severe.

- **PREGNANCY** Minimal absorption from skin; not known to be harmful.

- **PRESCRIBING AND DISPENSING INFORMATION** *Pevaryl* ® 1% cream should be used.

- **MEDICINAL FORMS** There can be variation in the licensing of different medicines containing the same drug.

  Cutaneous cream
  EXCIPIENTS: May contain Butylated hydroxyanisole, fragrances
  - ▶ **Pevaryl** (Karo Healthcare UK Ltd)
    Econazole nitrate 10 mg per 1 gram Pevaryl 1% cream | 30 gram P £3.71 DT = £3.71

Ketoconazole
30-May-2023

- **INDICATIONS AND DOSE**

Tinea pedis
- ▶ TO THE SKIN USING CREAM
- ▶ Adult: Apply twice daily

Fungal skin infection (not Tinea pedis)
- ▶ TO THE SKIN USING CREAM
- ▶ Adult: Apply 1–2 times a day

Treatment of seborrhoeic dermatitis and dandruff
- ▶ TO THE SKIN USING SHAMPOO
- ▶ Child 12-17 years: Apply twice weekly for 2–4 weeks, leave preparation on for 3–5 minutes before rinsing
- ▶ Adult: Apply twice weekly for 2–4 weeks, leave preparation on for 3–5 minutes before rinsing

Prophylaxis of seborrhoeic dermatitis and dandruff
- ▶ TO THE SKIN USING SHAMPOO
- ▶ Child 12-17 years: Apply every 1–2 weeks, leave preparation on for 3–5 minutes before rinsing
- ▶ Adult: Apply every 1–2 weeks, leave preparation on for 3–5 minutes before rinsing

Treatment of pityriasis versicolor
- ▶ TO THE SKIN USING SHAMPOO
- ▶ Child 12-17 years: Apply once daily for maximum 5 days, leave preparation on for 3–5 minutes before rinsing
- ▶ Adult: Apply once daily for maximum 5 days, leave preparation on for 3–5 minutes before rinsing

Prophylaxis of pityriasis versicolor
- ▶ TO THE SKIN USING SHAMPOO
- ▶ Child 12-17 years: Apply once daily for up to 3 days before sun exposure, leave preparation on for 3–5 minutes before rinsing
- ▶ Adult: Apply once daily for up to 3 days before sun exposure, leave preparation on for 3–5 minutes before rinsing

- **CONTRA-INDICATIONS** Acute porphyrias p. 1202
- **CAUTIONS** Avoid contact with eyes · avoid contact with mucous membranes
- **INTERACTIONS** → Appendix 1: antifungals, azoles
- **SIDE-EFFECTS**
- ▶ **Common or very common** Skin reactions
- ▶ **Uncommon** Alopecia · angioedema · excessive tearing · folliculitis · hair changes
- ▶ **Rare or very rare** Eye irritation · taste altered

- **NATIONAL FUNDING/ACCESS DECISIONS**
  NHS restrictions *Nizoral* ® cream is not prescribable in NHS primary care except for the treatment of seborrhoeic dermatitis and pityriasis versicolor; endorse prescription 'SLS'.

- **EXCEPTIONS TO LEGAL CATEGORY** A 15-g tube is available for sale to the public for the treatment of tinea pedis, tinea cruris, and candidal intertrigo.
  Can be sold to the public for the prevention and treatment of dandruff and seborrhoeic dermatitis of the scalp as a shampoo formulation containing ketoconazole maximum 2%, in a pack containing maximum 120 mL and labelled to show a maximum frequency of application of once every 3 days.

- **MEDICINAL FORMS** There can be variation in the licensing of different medicines containing the same drug.

  Cutaneous cream
  EXCIPIENTS: May contain Cetostearyl alcohol (including cetyl and stearyl alcohol), polysorbates, propylene glycol
  - ▶ **Nizoral** (Thornton & Ross Ltd)
    Ketoconazole 20 mg per 1 gram Nizoral 2% cream | 30 gram PoM £4.24 DT = £4.24

  Shampoo
  EXCIPIENTS: May contain Imidurea
  - ▶ **Ketoconazole (Non-proprietary)**
    Ketoconazole 20 mg per 1 gram Ketoconazole 2% shampoo | 120 ml PoM ⚠ DT = £31.77
  - ▶ **Dandrazol** (Crescent Pharma Ltd)
    Ketoconazole 20 mg per 1 gram Dandrazol 2% shampoo | 120 ml PoM £5.20 DT = £31.77
  - ▶ **Nizoral** (Thornton & Ross Ltd)
    Ketoconazole 20 mg per 1 gram Nizoral 2% shampoo | 120 ml PoM £3.59 DT = £31.77

Miconazole
23-Jun-2023

- **INDICATIONS AND DOSE**

Fungal skin infections
- ▶ TO THE SKIN
- ▶ Child: Apply twice daily continuing for 10 days after lesions have healed
- ▶ Adult: Apply twice daily continuing for 10 days after lesions have healed

Fungal nail infections
- ▶ BY TRANSUNGUAL APPLICATION
- ▶ Child: Apply 1–2 times a day
- ▶ Adult: Apply 1–2 times a day

- **UNLICENSED USE** Licensed for use in children (age range not specified by manufacturer).
- **CAUTIONS** Avoid in Acute porphyrias p. 1202 · contact with eyes and mucous membranes should be avoided
- **INTERACTIONS** → Appendix 1: antifungals, azoles
- **SIDE-EFFECTS**
- ▶ **Uncommon** Skin reactions
- ▶ **Frequency not known** Angioedema

- **PREGNANCY** Absorbed from the skin in small amounts; manufacturer advises caution.

- **BREAST FEEDING** Manufacturer advises caution—no information available.

● **PROFESSION SPECIFIC INFORMATION**

Dental practitioners' formulary Miconazole cream may be prescribed.

● **NATIONAL FUNDING/ACCESS DECISIONS**

NHS restrictions *Daktarin*® powder and *Daktarin*® cream 15 g are not prescribable in NHS primary care.

● **MEDICINAL FORMS** There can be variation in the licensing of different medicines containing the same drug.

Cutaneous powder
▸ Daktarin (McNeil Products Ltd)
  Miconazole nitrate 20 mg per 1 gram Daktarin 2% powder |
  20 gram [P] £4.19 DT = £4.19

Cutaneous cream
EXCIPIENTS: May contain Butylated hydroxyanisole
▸ Daktarin (McNeil Products Ltd)
  Miconazole nitrate 20 mg per 1 gram Daktarin 2% cream |
  15 gram [P] £3.42 | 30 gram [P] £5.05 DT = £5.05

Spray
CAUTIONARY AND ADVISORY LABELS 15
▸ Daktarin (Johnson & Johnson Ltd)
  Miconazole nitrate 1.6 mg per 1 gram Daktarin Aktiv 0.16% spray
  powder | 100 gram [GSL] £4.60 DT = £4.60

Tioconazole   03-Feb-2020

● **INDICATIONS AND DOSE**

Fungal nail infection
▸ BY TRANSUNGUAL APPLICATION
▸ Child: Apply twice daily usually for up to 6 months (may be extended to 12 months), apply to nails and surrounding skin
▸ Adult: Apply twice daily usually for up to 6 months (may be extended to 12 months), apply to nails and surrounding skin

● **UNLICENSED USE** Licensed for use in children (age range not specified by manufacturer).

● **CAUTIONS** Contact with eyes and mucous membranes should be avoided · use with caution if child likely to suck affected digits

● **SIDE-EFFECTS**
▸ **Common or very common** Peripheral oedema
▸ **Uncommon** Skin reactions
▸ **Frequency not known** Nail disorder · pain · paraesthesia · periorbital oedema

● **PREGNANCY** Manufacturer advises avoid.

● **MEDICINAL FORMS** There can be variation in the licensing of different medicines containing the same drug.

Medicated nail lacquer
▸ Tioconazole (Non-proprietary)
  Tioconazole 283 mg per 1 ml Tioconazole 283mg/ml medicated nail
  lacquer | 12 ml [PoM] £38.00 DT = £30.96
▸ Trosyl (Pfizer Ltd)
  Tioconazole 283 mg per 1 ml Trosyl 283mg/ml nail solution |
  12 ml [PoM] £27.38 DT = £30.96

ANTIFUNGALS 〉 OTHER

Amorolfine   06-Oct-2020

● **INDICATIONS AND DOSE**

Fungal nail infections
▸ BY TRANSUNGUAL APPLICATION
▸ Child 12-17 years: Apply 1–2 times a week for 6 months to treat finger nails and for toe nails 9–12 months (review at intervals of 3 months), apply to infected nails after filing and cleansing, allow to dry for approximately 3 minutes

▸ Adult: Apply 1–2 times a week for 6 months to treat finger nails and for toe nails 9–12 months (review at intervals of 3 months), apply to infected nails after filing and cleansing, allow to dry for approximately 3 minutes

● **CAUTIONS** Avoid contact with ears · avoid contact with eyes and mucous membranes · use with caution in child likely to suck affected digits

● **SIDE-EFFECTS**
▸ **Rare or very rare** Nail discolouration · skin reactions

● **PATIENT AND CARER ADVICE** Cosmetic nail varnish may be applied at least 10 minutes after amorolfine nail lacquer; the nail varnish should be removed before repeat application of amorolfine. Avoid artificial nails during treatment.

● **EXCEPTIONS TO LEGAL CATEGORY**
▸ In adults Amorolfine nail lacquer can be sold to the public if supplied for the treatment of mild cases of distal and lateral subungual onychomycoses caused by dermatophytes, yeasts and moulds; subject to treatment of max. 2 nails, max. strength of nail lacquer amorolfine 5% and a pack size of 3 mL.

● **MEDICINAL FORMS** There can be variation in the licensing of different medicines containing the same drug.

Medicated nail lacquer
CAUTIONARY AND ADVISORY LABELS 10
▸ Amorolfine (Non-proprietary)
  **Amorolfine (as Amorolfine hydrochloride) 50 mg per
  1 ml** Amorolfine 5% medicated nail lacquer | 5 ml [PoM] £16.21 DT =
  £8.31
▸ Loceryl (Galderma (UK) Ltd)
  Amorolfine (as Amorolfine hydrochloride) 50 mg per 1 ml Loceryl
  5% medicated nail lacquer | 5 ml [PoM] £9.08 DT = £8.31

Griseofulvin   16-Jan-2020

● **INDICATIONS AND DOSE**

Tinea pedis
▸ TO THE SKIN
▸ Adult: Apply 400 micrograms once daily, apply to an area approximately 13 cm^2; increased if necessary to 1.2 mg once daily for maximum treatment duration of 4 weeks, allow each spray to dry between application

● **CAUTIONS** Avoid contact with eyes and mucous membranes

● **INTERACTIONS** → Appendix 1: griseofulvin

● **SIDE-EFFECTS** Paraesthesia · skin irritation

● **PREGNANCY** Manufacturer advises avoid unless potential benefit outweighs risk.

● **BREAST FEEDING** Manufacturer advises avoid unless potential benefit outweighs risk.

● **MEDICINAL FORMS** No licensed medicines listed

Terbinafine   16-Aug-2021

● **INDICATIONS AND DOSE**

Tinea pedis
▸ TO THE SKIN USING CREAM
▸ Adult: Apply 1–2 times a day for up to 1 week, to be applied thinly
▸ BY MOUTH USING TABLETS
▸ Adult: 250 mg once daily for 2–6 weeks   continued →

13

Skin

Tinea corporis
▸ TO THE SKIN USING CREAM
▹ Adult: Apply 1–2 times a day for up to 1–2 weeks, to be applied thinly, review treatment after 2 weeks
▸ BY MOUTH USING TABLETS
▹ Adult: 250 mg once daily for 4 weeks

Tinea cruris
▸ TO THE SKIN USING CREAM
▹ Adult: Apply 1–2 times a day for up to 1–2 weeks, to be applied thinly, review treatment after 2 weeks
▸ BY MOUTH USING TABLETS
▹ Adult: 250 mg once daily for 2–4 weeks

Dermatophyte infections of the nails
▸ BY MOUTH USING TABLETS
▹ Adult: 250 mg once daily for 6 weeks–3 months (occasionally longer in toenail infections)

Cutaneous candidiasis | Pityriasis versicolor
▸ TO THE SKIN USING CREAM
▹ Adult: Apply 1–2 times a day for 2 weeks, to be applied thinly, review treatment after 2 weeks

● CAUTIONS
▹ With oral use Psoriasis (risk of exacerbation) · risk of lupus erythematosus
▹ With topical use Contact with eyes and mucous membranes should be avoided

● INTERACTIONS → Appendix 1: terbinafine

● SIDE-EFFECTS

GENERAL SIDE-EFFECTS
▹ **Common or very common** Skin reactions

SPECIFIC SIDE-EFFECTS
▹ **Common or very common**
▹ With oral use Appetite decreased · arthralgia · diarrhoea · gastrointestinal discomfort · gastrointestinal disorder · headache · myalgia · nausea
▹ **Uncommon**
▹ With oral use Taste altered
▹ With topical use Pain
▹ **Rare or very rare**
▹ With oral use Agranulocytosis · alopecia · cutaneous lupus erythematosus · dizziness · hepatic disorders · malaise · neutropenia · photosensitivity reaction · sensation abnormal · severe cutaneous adverse reactions (SCARs) · systemic lupus erythematosus (SLE) · thrombocytopenia · vertigo
▹ **Frequency not known**
▹ With oral use Anaemia · anxiety · depressive symptom · fatigue · fever · hearing impairment · influenza like illness · pancreatitis · pancytopenia · rhabdomyolysis · serum sickness-like reaction · smell altered · tinnitus · vasculitis · vision disorders
▹ With topical use Hypersensitivity

SIDE-EFFECTS, FURTHER INFORMATION **Liver toxicity**
With oral use; discontinue treatment if liver toxicity develops (including jaundice, cholestasis and hepatitis).
  Serious skin reactions With oral use; discontinue treatment in progressive skin rash (including Stevens-Johnson syndrome and toxic epidermal necrolysis).

● PREGNANCY
▹ With topical use Manufacturer advises use only if potential benefit outweighs risk—*animal* studies suggest no adverse effects.
▹ With oral use Manufacturer advises use only if potential benefit outweighs risk—no information available.

● BREAST FEEDING
▹ With topical use Manufacturer advises avoid—present in milk. Less than 5% of the dose is absorbed after topical application of terbinafine; avoid application to mother's chest.
▹ With oral use Avoid—present in milk.

● HEPATIC IMPAIRMENT
▹ With oral use Manufacturer advises avoid (risk of increased exposure).

● RENAL IMPAIRMENT
▹ With oral use EvGr Caution if creatinine clearance less than 50 mL/minute or serum creatinine concentration greater than 300 micromol/litre (limited information available). Ⓜ See p. 21.

● MONITORING REQUIREMENTS
▹ With oral use Monitor hepatic function before treatment and then periodically after 4–6 weeks of treatment—discontinue if abnormalities in liver function tests.

● PATIENT AND CARER ADVICE
▹ With oral use Manufacturer advises that patients should immediately report any signs or symptoms suggestive of liver dysfunction such as pruritus, unexplained persistent nausea, decreased appetite, anorexia, jaundice, vomiting, fatigue, right upper abdominal pain, dark urine, or pale stools. Patients with these symptoms should discontinue taking terbinafine and the patient's liver function should be immediately evaluated.

● EXCEPTIONS TO LEGAL CATEGORY Preparations of terbinafine hydrochloride (maximum 1%) can be sold to the public for use in those over 16 years for external use for the treatment of tinea pedis as a cream in a pack containing maximum 15 g, or for the treatment of tinea pedis and cruris as a cream in a pack containing maximum 15 g, or for the treatment of tinea pedis, cruris, and corporis as a spray in a pack containing maximum 30 mL spray or as a gel in a pack containing maximum 30 g gel.

● MEDICINAL FORMS There can be variation in the licensing of different medicines containing the same drug.

Oral tablet
CAUTIONARY AND ADVISORY LABELS 9
▸ Terbinafine (Non-proprietary)
  Terbinafine (as Terbinafine hydrochloride) 250 mg Terbinafine 250mg tablets | 14 tablet PoM £18.11 DT = £1.77 | 28 tablet PoM £3.00–£36.98
▸ Lamisil (Novartis Pharmaceuticals UK Ltd)
  Terbinafine (as Terbinafine hydrochloride) 250 mg Lamisil 250mg tablets | 14 tablet PoM £21.30 DT = £1.77 | 28 tablet PoM £41.09

Cutaneous cream
EXCIPIENTS: May contain Benzyl alcohol, cetostearyl alcohol (including cetyl and stearyl alcohol), polysorbates
▸ Terbinafine (Non-proprietary)
  Terbinafine hydrochloride 10 mg per 1 gram Terbinafine 1% cream | 15 gram PoM £4.37 DT = £3.16 | 30 gram PoM £6.84 DT = £6.32
▸ Lamisil (Karo Healthcare UK Ltd)
  Terbinafine hydrochloride 10 mg per 1 gram Lamisil 1% cream | 30 gram PoM £8.76 DT = £6.32

ANTISEPTICS AND DISINFECTANTS ›
UNDECENOATES

Undecenoic acid with zinc undecenoate

05-Oct-2021

● INDICATIONS AND DOSE

Treatment of athletes foot
▸ TO THE SKIN
▹ Child: Apply twice daily, continue use for 7 days after lesions have healed
▹ Adult: Apply twice daily, continue use for 7 days after lesions have healed

Prevention of athletes foot
▸ TO THE SKIN
▹ Child: Apply once daily
▹ Adult: Apply once daily

● UNLICENSED USE *Mycota*® licensed for use in children (age range not specified by manufacturer).

- **CAUTIONS** Avoid broken skin · contact with eyes should be avoided · contact with mucous membranes should be avoided

- **SIDE-EFFECTS**
▸ **Rare or very rare** Skin irritation
   SIDE-EFFECTS, FURTHER INFORMATION Treatment should be discontinued if irritation is severe.

- **MEDICINAL FORMS** There can be variation in the licensing of different medicines containing the same drug.
   Cutaneous cream
   EXCIPIENTS: May contain Cetostearyl alcohol (including cetyl and stearyl alcohol), fragrances
   ▸ Mycota (zinc undecenoate / undecenoic acid) (Thornton & Ross Ltd)
      Undecenoic acid 50 mg per 1 gram, Zinc undecenoate 200 mg per 1 gram Mycota cream | 25 gram [GSL] £3.07 DT = £3.07

ANTISEPTICS AND DISINFECTANTS ⟩ OTHER

Chlorhexidine with nystatin   01-Mar-2021

- **INDICATIONS AND DOSE**
   Skin infections due to *Candida* spp.
   ▸ TO THE SKIN
   ▸ Child: Apply 2–3 times a day continue for 7 days after lesions have healed
   ▸ Adult: Apply 2–3 times a day continue for 7 days after lesions have healed

- **UNLICENSED USE** Licensed for use in children (age range not specified by manufacturer).

- **CAUTIONS** Avoid contact with eyes and mucous membranes

- **SIDE-EFFECTS** Hypersensitivity · skin reactions

- **MEDICINAL FORMS** There can be variation in the licensing of different medicines containing the same drug.
   Cutaneous cream
   EXCIPIENTS: May contain Benzyl alcohol, cetostearyl alcohol (including cetyl and stearyl alcohol), polysorbates
   ▸ Nystaform (Typharm Ltd)
      Chlorhexidine hydrochloride 10 mg per 1 gram, Nystatin 100000 unit per 1 gram Nystaform cream | 30 gram [PoM] £9.50 DT = £9.50

BENZOATES

Benzoic acid with salicylic acid   22-Nov-2020

- **INDICATIONS AND DOSE**
   Ringworm (tinea)
   ▸ TO THE SKIN
   ▸ Child: Apply twice daily
   ▸ Adult: Apply twice daily

- **UNLICENSED USE** Licensed for use in children (age range not specified by manufacturer).

- **CAUTIONS** Avoid broken or inflamed skin · avoid contact with eyes · avoid contact with mucous membranes
   CAUTIONS, FURTHER INFORMATION
   ▸ Salicylate toxicity Salicylate toxicity may occur particularly if applied on large areas of skin.

- **SIDE-EFFECTS** Drug toxicity · eye irritation · mucosal irritation · skin reactions

- **PRESCRIBING AND DISPENSING INFORMATION** Benzoic Acid Ointment, Compound, BP has also been referred to as Whitfield's ointment.

- **MEDICINAL FORMS** There can be variation in the licensing of different medicines containing the same drug. Forms available from special-order manufacturers include: cutaneous cream, cutaneous ointment
   Cutaneous ointment
   EXCIPIENTS: May contain Cetostearyl alcohol (including cetyl and stearyl alcohol)

4.3 Parasitic skin infections

Other drugs used for Parasitic skin infections Ivermectin, p. 700

PARASITICIDES

Benzyl benzoate   19-May-2020

- **INDICATIONS AND DOSE**
   Scabies
   ▸ TO THE SKIN
   ▸ Adult: Apply over the whole body; repeat without bathing on the following day and wash off 24 hours later; a third application may be required in some cases

- **CAUTIONS** Avoid contact with eyes and mucous membranes · do not use on broken or secondarily infected skin

- **SIDE-EFFECTS** Eye irritation · mucosal irritation · skin irritation

- **BREAST FEEDING** Suspend feeding until product has been washed off.

- **PRESCRIBING AND DISPENSING INFORMATION** When prepared extemporaneously, the BP states Benzyl Benzoate Application, BP consists of benzyl benzoate 25% in an emulsion basis.
   Some manufacturers recommend application to the body but to exclude the head and neck. However, application should be extended to the scalp, neck, face, and ears. Note—dilution to reduce irritant effect also reduces efficacy.

- **LESS SUITABLE FOR PRESCRIBING** Benzyl benzoate is less suitable for prescribing.

- **MEDICINAL FORMS** No licensed medicines listed.

Dimeticone   04-Feb-2020

- **INDICATIONS AND DOSE**
   Head lice
   ▸ TO THE SKIN
   ▸ Child: Apply once weekly for 2 doses, rub into dry hair and scalp, allow to dry naturally, shampoo after minimum 8 hours (or overnight)
   ▸ Adult: Apply once weekly for 2 doses, rub into dry hair and scalp, allow to dry naturally, shampoo after minimum 8 hours (or overnight)

- **UNLICENSED USE** Not licensed for use in children under 6 months except under medical supervision.

> **IMPORTANT SAFETY INFORMATION**
> MHRA/CHM ADVICE: HEAD LICE ERADICATION PRODUCTS: RISK OF SERIOUS BURNS IF TREATED HAIR IS EXPOSED TO OPEN FLAMES OR OTHER SOURCES OF IGNITION (MARCH 2018)
> See Skin infections p. 1395.

- **CAUTIONS** Avoid contact with eyes · children under 6 months, medical supervision required

13

Skin

- **SIDE-EFFECTS** Alopecia · dyspnoea · eye irritation · hypersensitivity · scalp changes · skin reactions

- **MEDICINAL FORMS** There can be variation in the licensing of different medicines containing the same drug.
  Cutaneous solution
  ▸ Hedrin (Thornton & Ross Ltd)
  Dimeticone 40 mg per 1 gram Hedrin 4% lotion | 150 ml [P]
  £10.00 DT = £10.00
  Cutaneous spray solution
  ▸ Hedrin (Thornton & Ross Ltd)
  Dimeticone 40 mg per 1 gram Hedrin 4% spray | 120 ml [P] £10.30
  DT = £10.30

Malathion

04-Feb-2020

- **INDICATIONS AND DOSE**
  Head lice
  ▸ TO THE SKIN
  ▸ Child: Apply once weekly for 2 doses, rub preparation into dry hair and scalp, allow to dry naturally, remove by washing after 12 hours
  ▸ Adult: Apply once weekly for 2 doses, rub preparation into dry hair and scalp, allow to dry naturally, remove by washing after 12 hours

  Crab lice
  ▸ TO THE SKIN
  ▸ Child: Apply once weekly for 2 doses, apply preparation over whole body, allow to dry naturally, wash off after 12 hours or overnight
  ▸ Adult: Apply once weekly for 2 doses, apply preparation over whole body, allow to dry naturally, wash off after 12 hours or overnight

  Scabies
  ▸ TO THE SKIN
  ▸ Child: Apply once weekly for 2 doses, apply preparation over whole body, and wash off after 24 hours, if hands are washed with soap within 24 hours, they should be retreated
  ▸ Adult: Apply once weekly for 2 doses, apply preparation over whole body, and wash off after 24 hours, if hands are washed with soap within 24 hours, they should be retreated

- **UNLICENSED USE** Not licensed for use in children under 6 months except under medical supervision.

  IMPORTANT SAFETY INFORMATION
  MHRA/CHM ADVICE: HEAD LICE ERADICATION PRODUCTS: RISK OF SERIOUS BURNS IF TREATED HAIR IS EXPOSED TO OPEN FLAMES OR OTHER SOURCES OF IGNITION (MARCH 2018)
  See Skin infections p. 1395.

- **CAUTIONS** Alcoholic lotions **not** recommended for head lice in children with severe eczema or asthma, or for scabies or crab lice · avoid contact with eyes · children under 6 months, medical supervision required · do not use lotion more than once a week for 3 consecutive weeks · do not use on broken or secondarily infected skin

- **SIDE-EFFECTS** Angioedema · eye swelling · hypersensitivity · skin reactions

- **PRESCRIBING AND DISPENSING INFORMATION** For scabies, manufacturer recommends application to the body but not necessarily to the head and neck. However, application should be extended to the scalp, neck, face, and ears.

- **MEDICINAL FORMS** There can be variation in the licensing of different medicines containing the same drug.
  Cutaneous emulsion
  EXCIPIENTS: May contain Cetostearyl alcohol (including cetyl and stearyl alcohol), fragrances, hydroxybenzoates (parabens)

▸ Derbac-M (G.R. Lane Health Products Ltd)
Malathion 5 mg per 1 gram Derbac-M 0.5% liquid | 150 ml [P]
£15.96 DT = £15.96

Permethrin

04-Feb-2020

- **INDICATIONS AND DOSE**
  Scabies
  ▸ TO THE SKIN
  ▸ Child: Apply once weekly for 2 doses, apply 5% preparation over whole body including face, neck, scalp and ears then wash off after 8–12 hours. If hands are washed with soap within 8 hours of application, they should be treated again with cream
  ▸ Adult: Apply once weekly for 2 doses, apply 5% preparation over whole body including face, neck, scalp and ears then wash off after 8–12 hours. If hands are washed with soap within 8 hours of application, they should be treated again with cream

  Crab lice
  ▸ TO THE SKIN
  ▸ Adult: Apply once weekly for 2 doses, apply 5% cream over whole body, allow to dry naturally and wash off after 12 hours or after leaving on overnight

  Head lice
  ▸ TO THE SKIN
  ▸ Adult: Not recommended; no information given

- **UNLICENSED USE** *Dermal Cream* (scabies), not licensed for use in children under 2 months; not licensed for treatment of crab lice in children under 18 years.

  IMPORTANT SAFETY INFORMATION
  MHRA/CHM ADVICE: HEAD LICE ERADICATION PRODUCTS: RISK OF SERIOUS BURNS IF TREATED HAIR IS EXPOSED TO OPEN FLAMES OR OTHER SOURCES OF IGNITION (MARCH 2018)
  See Skin infections p. 1395.

- **CAUTIONS** Avoid contact with eyes · children aged 2 months–2 years, medical supervision required for dermal cream (scabies) · do not use on broken or secondarily infected skin

- **SIDE-EFFECTS** Scalp irritation · skin reactions

- **PRESCRIBING AND DISPENSING INFORMATION**
  Manufacturer recommends application to the body but to exclude head and neck. However, application should be extended to the scalp, neck, face, and ears.
  Larger patients may require up to two 30-g packs for adequate treatment.

- **LESS SUITABLE FOR PRESCRIBING** Lyclear® Creme Rinse is less suitable for prescribing.

- **MEDICINAL FORMS** There can be variation in the licensing of different medicines containing the same drug.
  Cutaneous cream
  CAUTIONARY AND ADVISORY LABELS 10 (Dermal cream only)
  EXCIPIENTS: May contain Butylated hydroxytoluene, woolfat and related substances (including lanolin)
  ▸ Permethrin (Non-proprietary)
  Permethrin 50 mg per 1 gram Permethrin 5% cream | 30 gram [P]
  £11.00 DT = £7.44
  ▸ Lyclear (Omega Pharma Ltd)
  Permethrin 50 mg per 1 gram Lyclear 5% dermal cream |
  30 gram [P] £6.82 DT = £7.44
  Cutaneous liquid
  EXCIPIENTS: May contain Cetostearyl alcohol (including cetyl and stearyl alcohol)
  ▸ Lyclear (Omega Pharma Ltd)
  Permethrin 10 mg per 1 gram Lyclear 1% creme rinse | 118 ml [P]
  £7.75 DT = £7.75

4.4 Viral skin infections

ANTIVIRALS > NUCLEOSIDE ANALOGUES

Aciclovir
(Acyclovir)

23-Sep-2022

- **INDICATIONS AND DOSE**

Herpes simplex infection (local treatment)
▶ TO THE SKIN
▶ **Adult:** Apply 5 times a day for 5–10 days, to be applied to lesions approximately every 4 hours, starting at first sign of attack

- **CAUTIONS** Avoid cream coming in to contact with eyes and mucous membranes
- **INTERACTIONS** → Appendix 1: aciclovir
- **SIDE-EFFECTS**
▶ **Uncommon** Skin reactions
- **PREGNANCY** Limited absorption from topical aciclovir preparations.
- **PROFESSION SPECIFIC INFORMATION**

  Dental practitioners' formulary Aciclovir Cream may be prescribed.
- **EXCEPTIONS TO LEGAL CATEGORY** A 2-g tube and a pump pack are on sale to the public for the treatment of cold sores.

- **MEDICINAL FORMS** There can be variation in the licensing of different medicines containing the same drug.

  Cutaneous cream
  EXCIPIENTS: May contain Cetostearyl alcohol (including cetyl and stearyl alcohol), propylene glycol
  ▶ **Aciclovir (Non-proprietary)**
  Aciclovir 50 mg per 1 gram Aciclovir 5% cream | 2 gram [PoM] £2.39 DT = £2.39 | 10 gram [PoM] £12.93 DT = £12.93
  ▶ **Zovirax** (GlaxoSmithKline UK Ltd)
  Aciclovir 50 mg per 1 gram Zovirax 5% cream | 2 gram [PoM] £4.63 DT = £2.39 | 10 gram [PoM] £13.96 DT = £12.93

5 Inflammatory skin conditions

5.1 Eczema and psoriasis

Eczema

06-May-2021

Types and management

Eczema (dermatitis) refers to a variety of skin conditions characterised by epidermal inflammation and itching. The main types of eczema are irritant, allergic contact, atopic, venous and discoid. Lichenification, due to scratching and rubbing, often presents in chronic eczema. *Atopic eczema* is one of the most common types and it usually involves itchy, red, dry skin which can become infected and lichenified.

[EvGr] Management of eczema involves the removal or treatment of contributory factors including occupational and domestic irritants. Known or suspected contact allergens should be avoided. (A) Rarely, ingredients in topical medicinal products may sensitise the skin; the BNF lists active ingredients together with excipients that have been associated with skin sensitisation.

[EvGr] Frequent and liberal use of emollients is advised for dry skin and itching associated with eczema. The choice of emollient is dependent on the dryness of the skin, and patient preference; this can be supplemented with bath or shower emollients. Emollients increase the efficacy of topical corticosteroids and have a steroid sparing action. The use of emollients should continue even if the eczema improves or if other treatment is being used. Aqueous cream is generally not recommended due to the high risk of developing skin reactions.

Topical corticosteroids are also often required in the management of eczema; the potency of the corticosteroid should be used in accordance to the severity and site of the condition. For eczema on the face, genitals, or axillae, consider a mild potency topical corticosteroid and only increase to a moderate potency topical corticosteroid if necessary. Moderate to potent topical corticosteroids are generally required for use in adults with moderate or severe eczema on the scalp, limbs, and trunk. Treatment should be reviewed regularly, especially if a potent topical corticosteroid is required. In patients with frequent flares, a topical corticosteroid can be applied to prevent further flares using various regimens (e.g. on 2 consecutive days each week). Emollient therapy should be continued during treatment with topical corticosteroids.

Under the care of a specialist, bandages (including those containing ichthammol with zinc oxide p. 1418) are sometimes applied over topical corticosteroids or emollients to treat eczema of the limbs. Dry-wrap dressings can be used to provide a physical barrier to help prevent scratching and improve retention of emollients. (A) See Wound management products and elasticated garments p. 1928 for details of elasticated viscose stockinette tubular bandages and garments, and silk clothing.

Topical pimecrolimus p. 1420 is licensed for the treatment of mild to moderate atopic eczema. Tacrolimus p. 1421 is licensed for topical use in the treatment of moderate to severe atopic eczema. [EvGr] Both are calcineurin inhibitors and should be considered as a second-line treatment option only, unless there is a specific reason to avoid or reduce the use of topical corticosteroids. Treatment of atopic eczema with topical pimecrolimus or topical tacrolimus should be initiated by a specialist.

Antihistamines are not recommended for routine use in the management of atopic eczema. However, if there is severe itching or urticaria, consider a non-sedating antihistamine. A sedating antihistamine can be considered if itching causes sleep disturbance. (A)

Infection

[EvGr] Breaks in the skin caused by eczema are susceptible to bacterial infection (commonly with *Staphylococcus aureus* and occasionally with *Streptococcus pyogenes*) and may require treatment with a topical or systemic antibacterial. For further information, see *Secondary bacterial infection of common skin conditions* in Skin infections, antibacterial therapy p. 589. Episodes of infected eczema usually co-exist with a flare and will require management with treatments such as emollients and topical corticosteroids. (A)

Eczema can also be infected with herpes simplex virus. [EvGr] Immediate referral to secondary care is required in patients presenting with suspected eczema herpeticum. (A)

Severe refractory eczema

[EvGr] Systemic drugs acting on the immune system (such as ciclosporin p. 966, azathioprine p. 965 [unlicensed indication], and mycophenolate mofetil p. 977 [unlicensed indication]) and phototherapy are available for the management of some cases of severe refractory eczema; they are used under specialist supervision. Dupilumab p. 1423 and baricitinib p. 1262 are options for the treatment of moderate to severe atopic eczema. (A)

Alitretinoin p. 1433 is licensed for the treatment of severe chronic hand eczema refractory to potent topical corticosteroids; patients with hyperkeratotic features are more likely to respond to alitretinoin than those with pompholyx.

Seborrhoeic dermatitis

Seborrhoeic dermatitis (seborrhoeic eczema) is associated with species of the yeast *Malassezia* and affects the scalp, paranasal areas, and eyebrows. EvGr Shampoos active against the yeast (including those containing ketoconazole p. 1400 or coal tar p. 1419) and combinations of mild topical corticosteroids with suitable antimicrobials are used. A

Psoriasis

25-Sep-2023

Overview

Psoriasis is an inflammatory skin disease that usually follows a relapsing and remitting course and may have nail or joint involvement. Different forms of psoriasis exist; chronic plaque psoriasis is the most common, and is characterised by epidermal thickening and scaling, usually affecting extensor surfaces and the scalp.

Occasionally, psoriasis is provoked or exacerbated by drugs such as lithium, chloroquine and hydroxychloroquine, beta-blockers, non-steroidal anti-inflammatory drugs, and ACE inhibitors. Psoriasis may not be seen until the drug has been taken for weeks or months.

Treatment

EvGr Offer topical treatment first-line to all patients with psoriasis. Topical treatment options include emollients, topical corticosteroids, coal tar preparations, and topical vitamin D or vitamin D analogues. When choosing topical treatment, consider patient preference, practical aspects of application, extent of psoriasis, and the variety of preparation forms available. A

Emollients are widely used in psoriasis; they moisturise dry skin, reduce scaling, and relieve itching. They also soften cracked areas and help other topical treatments absorb through the skin to work more effectively. Some cases of mild psoriasis may settle with the use of emollients alone. EvGr Emollients may also be useful adjuncts to other more specific treatment. A

Continuous long-term use of potent or very potent topical corticosteroids may cause psoriasis to become unstable, and lead to irreversible skin atrophy and striae. Widespread use (greater than 10% of body surface area affected) can also lead to systemic and local side-effects. EvGr Patients who have been on intermittent or short courses of potent or very potent topical corticosteroids should be offered a review of treatment at least annually.

Consecutive use of potent topical corticosteroids should not be used for more than 8 weeks at any one site; 4 weeks for very potent topical corticosteroids. Application may be restarted after a 4-week 'treatment break'; non-steroid treatments, such as topical vitamin D and vitamin D analogues, may be continued during this time. A

Coal tar p. 1419 has anti-inflammatory, antipruritic, and anti-scaling properties and is often combined with other topical treatments for psoriasis. Several coal tar preparations are available including ointments, shampoos, and bath additives. EvGr Newer products are preferred to older products containing crude coal tar (coal tar BP), which is malodorous and usually messier to apply. A

Topical vitamin D and vitamin D analogue preparations are available as ointments, gels, scalp solutions, and lotions. Tacalcitol p. 1435 and calcitriol p. 1435 may be less irritating than calcipotriol p. 1434.

Psoriasis of the trunk and limbs

EvGr Offer a potent topical corticosteroid and a topical vitamin D or vitamin D analogue applied once daily (at different times of the day) for up to 4 weeks as initial treatment. If satisfactory control is not achieved after a maximum of 8 weeks, offer a topical vitamin D or vitamin D analogue alone applied twice daily. If satisfactory control is

not achieved after 8–12 weeks of twice-daily topical vitamin D or vitamin D analogue, offer either a potent topical corticosteroid applied twice daily for up to 4 weeks, or a coal tar preparation. A combination product containing calcipotriol with betamethasone p. 1411 for up to 4 weeks is an alternative in patients unable to use twice-daily potent topical corticosteroids, a coal tar preparation, or in patients where a once-daily application would improve adherence. A very potent topical corticosteroid can be offered under specialist supervision for a maximum of 4 weeks when other topical treatments have failed.

In patients with treatment-resistant psoriasis of the trunk or limbs, consider treatment with short-contact dithranol p. 1418. Treatment should be given in a specialist setting or the patient should be provided with educational support for self-use. A

Scalp psoriasis

EvGr Offer a potent topical corticosteroid applied once daily for up to 4 weeks as initial treatment. If satisfactory control is not achieved after 4 weeks, consider a different formulation of the potent topical corticosteroid (e.g. a shampoo or mousse) and/or topical agents to remove or soften adherent scale (e.g. agents containing salicylic acid, emollients, oils). These agents should be used prior to applying the potent topical corticosteroid to allow effective penetration. If response to potent topical corticosteroid treatment remains unsatisfactory after a further 4 weeks of treatment, offer a combination product containing calcipotriol with betamethasone for up to 4 weeks. If treatment with calcipotriol with betamethasone for up to 4 weeks does not give a satisfactory response, offer either a very potent corticosteroid applied twice daily for 2 weeks, or a coal tar preparation, or refer the patient to a specialist.

In patients with mild to moderate scalp psoriasis who cannot use topical corticosteroids, offer treatment with a topical vitamin D or vitamin D analogue only. If treatment with a vitamin D or vitamin D analogue for up to 8 weeks does not give a satisfactory response, either offer a coal tar preparation or refer the patient to a specialist. The use of coal tar-based shampoos alone for the treatment of severe scalp psoriasis is not recommended. A

Facial, flexural, and genital psoriasis

EvGr Offer a mild or moderate potency topical corticosteroid as initial treatment. The face, flexures, and genitals are particularly vulnerable to steroid atrophy therefore topical corticosteroids should only be used short-term (e.g. 1–2 weeks per month). If response to a moderate potency topical corticosteroid is inadequate, or there is serious risk of side-effects from continuous use, offer a topical calcineurin inhibitor, such as pimecrolimus p. 1420 or tacrolimus p. 1421 [unlicensed indications], for up to 4 weeks (initiated under specialist supervision). A

Pustular or erythrodermic psoriasis

EvGr Widespread unstable psoriasis of erythrodermic or generalised pustular types requires urgent same-day specialist assessment and should be managed as a medical emergency. A

Phototherapy

Phototherapy is available under the supervision of an appropriately trained healthcare professional. EvGr Narrowband ultraviolet B (UVB) phototherapy can be offered to patients with plaque or guttate psoriasis in whom topical treatment has failed to achieve control. A

Photochemotherapy combining psoralen with ultraviolet A (PUVA) is available in specialist centres, given under the supervision of an appropriately trained healthcare professional. Psoralen enhances the effects of UVA and is administered either by mouth or topically. EvGr PUVA irradiation can be considered for the treatment of localised palmoplantar pustulosis and plaque-type psoriasis. A

Cumulative doses increase the risk of dysplastic and neoplastic skin lesions, especially squamous cell cancer.

[EvGr] Topical adjunctive therapy may be considered in patients receiving broadband or narrowband UVB phototherapy who have plaques that are resistant, or show an inadequate response to phototherapy alone, or are at difficult-to-treat sites, or in patients unable to take systemic treatment. Concomitant treatment of acitretin and PUVA is not routinely recommended. Ⓐ

Systemic treatment
Non-biological treatment

[EvGr] Under the supervision of a specialist, systemic non-biological treatment with methotrexate p. 1048 or ciclosporin p. 966 may be offered to some patients with psoriasis that cannot be controlled with topical treatment *and* if the psoriasis has a significant impact on physical, psychological or social well-being. In addition, the psoriasis would have to be extensive, or localised with significant distress or functional impairment, or have failed phototherapy treatment.

Ciclosporin can be considered first-line in patients who need rapid or short-term disease control, have palmoplantar pustulosis, or who are considering conception (both men and women).

Only consider acitretin p. 1432 in patients where methotrexate and ciclosporin are not appropriate or have failed, or in patients with pustular forms of psoriasis.

Under specialist care, apremilast p. 1277 or dimethyl fumarate p. 984 may be used for the treatment of severe chronic plaque psoriasis.

Under specialist care, certain Janus kinase inhibitors may be used for the treatment of moderate to severe plaque psoriasis. Ⓐ

Biological treatment

[EvGr] Biological drugs such as interleukin inhibitors and tumor necrosis factor alpha (TNF-α) inhibitors should be initiated and supervised only by specialists experienced in the diagnosis and management of psoriasis. Ⓐ

Other drugs used for Eczema and psoriasis Adalimumab, p. 1269 · Certolizumab pegol, p. 1271 · Etanercept, p. 1273 · Infliximab, p. 1275 · Secukinumab, p. 1257 · Upadacitinib, p. 1267 · Ustekinumab, p. 1260

CORTICOSTEROIDS

Topical corticosteroids

08-Oct-2024

Overview

Topical corticosteroids are used for the treatment of inflammatory conditions of the skin (other than those arising from an infection), in particular eczema, contact dermatitis, insect stings, and eczema of scabies. They are generally used to relieve symptoms and suppress signs of the disorder when other measures such as emollients are ineffective. Corticosteroids suppress the inflammatory reaction during use; they are not curative and on discontinuation a withdrawal reaction (rebound or flare) may occur. Withdrawal reactions are thought to occur after long-term continuous or inappropriate use of topical corticosteroids (particularly those of moderate to high potency). Signs and symptoms are reported to happen within days to weeks of stopping long-term topical corticosteroid treatment. A flare of the underlying skin disorder is the most common withdrawal reaction. Rarely, a specific type of withdrawal reaction may occur in which skin redness extends beyond the initial area of treatment, with burning or stinging that is worse than the original condition. For further information on topical corticosteroid withdrawal reactions,

see *Important safety information* in the individual drug monograph).

Topical corticosteroids are not recommended in the routine treatment of urticaria; treatment should only be initiated and supervised by a specialist. They should not be used indiscriminately in pruritus (where they will only benefit if inflammation is causing the itch) and are **not** recommended for acne vulgaris.

Systemic or very potent topical corticosteroids should be avoided or given only under specialist supervision in *psoriasis* because, although they may suppress the psoriasis in the short term, relapse or vigorous rebound occurs on withdrawal (sometimes precipitating severe pustular psoriasis). See the role of topical corticosteroids in the treatment of psoriasis.

In general, the most potent topical corticosteroids should be reserved for recalcitrant dermatoses such as *chronic discoid lupus erythematosus, lichen simplex chronicus, hypertrophic lichen planus,* and *palmoplantar pustulosis.* Potent corticosteroids should generally be avoided on the face and skin flexures, but specialists occasionally prescribe them for use on these areas in certain circumstances.

When topical treatment has failed, intralesional corticosteroid injections may be used. These are more effective than the very potent topical corticosteroid preparations and should be reserved for severe cases where there are localised lesions such as *keloid scars, hypertrophic lichen planus,* or *localised alopecia areata.*

Perioral lesions

Hydrocortisone cream 1% p. 1413 can be used for up to 7 days to treat uninfected inflammatory lesions on the lips. Hydrocortisone with miconazole cream or ointment p. 1418 is useful where infection by susceptible organisms and inflammation co-exist, particularly for initial treatment (up to 7 days) e.g. in angular cheilitis. Organisms susceptible to miconazole include *Candida* spp. and many Gram-positive bacteria including streptococci and staphylococci.

Choice of formulation

Water-miscible corticosteroid *creams* are suitable for moist or weeping lesions whereas *ointments* are generally chosen for dry, lichenified or scaly lesions or where a more occlusive effect is required. *Lotions* may be useful when minimal application to a large or hair-bearing area is required or for the treatment of exudative lesions. *Occlusive polythene* or *hydrocolloid dressings* increase absorption, but also increase the risk of side effects; they are therefore used only under supervision on a short-term basis for areas of very thick skin (such as the palms and soles). The inclusion of urea or salicylic acid also increases the penetration of the corticosteroid.

In the BNF publications topical corticosteroids for the skin are categorised as 'mild', 'moderately potent', 'potent' or 'very potent'; the **least potent** preparation which is effective should be chosen but dilution should be avoided whenever possible.

Absorption through the skin

Mild and *moderately potent* topical corticosteroids are associated with few side-effects but care is required in the use of *potent* and *very potent* corticosteroids. Absorption through the skin can rarely cause adrenal suppression and even Cushing's syndrome, depending on the area of the body being treated and the duration of treatment. Absorption is greatest where the skin is thin or raw, and from intertriginous areas; it is increased by occlusion.

For further information on side-effects that may occur from absorption through the skin, see Corticosteroids, general use p. 780.

Suitable quantities of corticosteroid preparations to be prescribed for specific areas of the body	
Area of body	Creams and Ointments
Face and neck	15 to 30 g
Both hands	15 to 30 g
Scalp	15 to 30 g
Both arms	30 to 60 g
Both legs	100 g
Trunk	100 g
Groins and genitalia	15 to 30 g
These amounts are usually suitable for an adult for a single daily application for 2 weeks	

Compound preparations

The advantages of including other substances (such as antibacterials or antifungals) with corticosteroids in topical preparations are uncertain, but such combinations may have a place where inflammatory skin conditions are associated with bacterial or fungal infection, such as infected eczema. In these cases the antimicrobial drug should be chosen according to the sensitivity of the infecting organism and used regularly for a short period (typically twice daily for 1 week). Longer use increases the likelihood of resistance and of sensitisation.

The keratolytic effect of salicylic acid p. 1460 facilitates the absorption of topical corticosteroids; however, excessive and prolonged use of topical preparations containing salicylic acid may cause salicylism.

Topical corticosteroid potencies

Potency of a topical corticosteroid preparation (including compound preparations) is based solely on the corticosteroid component, irrespective of the formulation and strength.
Mild
• Hydrocortisone p. 1413
Moderate
• Alclometasone dipropionate p. 1409
• Clobetasone butyrate p. 1412
• Hydrocortisone butyrate p. 1414
Potent
• Beclometasone dipropionate p. 1410
• Betamethasone p. 1410
• Fludroxycortide p. 1412
• Fluocinolone acetonide p. 1413
• Fluocinonide p. 1413
• Fluticasone p. 1413
• Mometasone furoate p. 1414
Very potent
• Clobetasol propionate p. 1411

Use in children

Children, especially infants, are particularly susceptible to side-effects. However, concern about the safety of topical corticosteroids in children should not result in the child being undertreated. The aim is to control the condition as well as possible; inadequate treatment will perpetuate the condition. A mild corticosteroid such as hydrocortisone 0.5% or 1% is useful for treating nappy rash and hydrocortisone 1% for atopic eczema in childhood. A moderately potent or potent corticosteroid may be appropriate for severe atopic eczema on the limbs, for 1–2 weeks only, switching to a less potent preparation as the condition improves. In an acute flare-up of atopic eczema, it may be appropriate to use more potent formulations of topical corticosteroids for a short period to regain control of the condition. A very potent

corticosteroid should be initiated under the supervision of a specialist. Carers of young children should be advised that treatment should **not** necessarily be reserved to 'treat only the worst areas' and they may need to be advised that patient information leaflets may contain inappropriate advice for the patient's condition.

Corticosteroids (topical) 

IMPORTANT SAFETY INFORMATION

MHRA/CHM ADVICE: CORTICOSTEROIDS: RARE RISK OF CENTRAL SEROUS CHORIORETINOPATHY WITH LOCAL AS WELL AS SYSTEMIC ADMINISTRATION (AUGUST 2017)
Central serous chorioretinopathy is a retinal disorder that has been linked to the systemic use of corticosteroids. Recently, it has also been reported after local administration of corticosteroids via inhaled and intranasal, epidural, intra-articular, topical dermal, and periocular routes. The MHRA recommends that patients should be advised to report any blurred vision or other visual disturbances with corticosteroid treatment given by any route; consider referral to an ophthalmologist for evaluation of possible causes if a patient presents with vision problems.

NHS IMPROVEMENT PATIENT SAFETY ALERT: STEROID EMERGENCY CARD TO SUPPORT EARLY RECOGNITION AND TREATMENT OF ADRENAL CRISIS IN ADULTS (AUGUST 2020)
A patient-held **Steroid Emergency Card** has been developed for patients with adrenal insufficiency and steroid dependence who are at risk of adrenal crisis. It aims to support healthcare staff with the early recognition of patients at risk of adrenal crisis and the emergency treatment of adrenal crisis. All eligible patients should be issued a Steroid Emergency Card. Providers that treat patients with acute physical illness or trauma, or who may require emergency treatment, elective surgery, or other invasive procedures, should establish processes to check for risk of adrenal crisis and confirm if the patient has a Steroid Emergency Card.

MHRA/CHM ADVICE: TOPICAL CORTICOSTEROIDS: INFORMATION ON THE RISK OF TOPICAL STEROID WITHDRAWAL REACTIONS (SEPTEMBER 2021)
Rarely, long-term continuous or inappropriate use of topical corticosteroids, particularly those of moderate to high potency, can result in the development of rebound flares, reported as dermatitis with intense redness, stinging, and burning that can spread beyond the initial treatment area.

The MHRA advises that the lowest potency topical corticosteroid needed should be used. For patients who are currently on long-term topical corticosteroid treatment, consider reducing potency or frequency of application (or both). Healthcare professionals should also be vigilant for the signs and symptoms of topical corticosteroid withdrawal reactions.

Healthcare professionals should inform patients:
• how much should be applied, as under-use can prolong treatment duration;
• how long they should use a topical corticosteroid for, especially on sensitive areas such as the face and genitals;
• to always apply topical corticosteroids as instructed and consult the patient information leaflet provided;
• to seek medical advice before using a topical corticosteroid on a new body area, as some areas of the body are more prone to side-effects;
• to return for medical advice if their skin condition worsens while using topical corticosteroid, and advise them when it would be appropriate to re-treat without a consultation and;

- if their skin worsens within 2 weeks of stopping a topical corticosteroid, treatment should not be started again without consulting their doctor unless they have previously been advised to do so

The MHRA advises healthcare professionals to report any suspected adverse effects, via the Yellow Card Scheme, even when the adverse affects occur after stopping corticosteroid treatment.

ADRENAL INSUFFICIENCY CARD (APRIL 2023)

The British Society for Paediatric Endocrinology and Diabetes (BSPED) has developed an Adrenal Insufficiency Card which should be issued to children with adrenal insufficiency and steroid dependence. The card includes a management summary for the emergency treatment of adrenal crisis and sick day dosing, and can be issued by any healthcare professional managing such patients. The BSPED Adrenal Insufficiency Card is available at: www.bsped.org.uk/adrenal-insufficiency.

MHRA/CHM ADVICE: TOPICAL STEROIDS: INTRODUCTION OF NEW LABELLING AND A REMINDER OF THE POSSIBILITY OF SEVERE SIDE EFFECTS, INCLUDING TOPICAL STEROID WITHDRAWAL REACTIONS (MAY 2024)

The risk of serious side-effects, such as Topical Steroid Withdrawal Reactions (TSW), thinning of the skin, and systemic effects, increases with prolonged use of higher potency topical corticosteroids. Regulatory action has resulted in new labelling for topical corticosteroids with information on their potency to assist with patient counselling and correct selection. The MHRA continue to receive reports regarding TSW, particularly associated with eczema treatment; healthcare professionals are reminded to continue to follow the advice issued in 2021 (see above). In addition, healthcare professionals are advised that alternative treatments should be considered if previous discontinuation of a topical corticosteroid was associated with a reaction suspicious of TSW, and that they should support patients living with symptoms of TSW and review treatment plans alongside them.

Healthcare professionals should review the position statement from the National Eczema Society, the British Dermatological Nursing Group, and the British Association of Dermatologists: www.bad.org.uk/topical-steroid-withdrawal-joint-statement/.

The MHRA Patient Safety Leaflet on topical corticosteroids and withdrawal reactions can be used to aid patient counselling: www.gov.uk/guidance/topical-corticosteroids-and-withdrawal-reactions.

- **CONTRA-INDICATIONS** Acne · perioral dermatitis · potent corticosteroids in widespread plaque psoriasis · rosacea · untreated bacterial, fungal or viral skin lesions
- **CAUTIONS** Avoid prolonged use (particularly on the face) · cautions applicable to systemic corticosteroids may also apply if absorption occurs following topical and local use · dermatoses of infancy, including nappy rash (extreme caution required—treatment should be limited to 5–7 days) · infection · keep away from eyes · use potent or very potent topical corticosteroids under specialist supervision (in children) · use potent or very potent topical corticosteroids under specialist supervision in psoriasis (can result in rebound relapse, development of generalised pustular psoriasis, and local and systemic toxicity) (in adults)

- **SIDE-EFFECTS**
- **Common or very common** Skin reactions · telangiectasia
- **Rare or very rare** Adrenal suppression · hypertrichosis · skin depigmentation (may be reversible)
- **Frequency not known** Local reaction · vasodilation

SIDE-EFFECTS, FURTHER INFORMATION Side-effects applicable to systemic corticosteroids may also apply if absorption occurs following topical and local use. In order to minimise the side-effects of a topical corticosteroid, it is important to apply it thinly to affected areas only, no more frequently than twice daily, and to use the least potent formulation which is fully effective.

- **DIRECTIONS FOR ADMINISTRATION** [EvGr] Topical corticosteroid preparations should be applied no more frequently than twice daily; once daily is often sufficient. [A] Topical corticosteroids should be applied in sufficient quantity to cover the affected areas. The length of cream or ointment expelled from a tube may be used to specify the quantity to be applied to a given area of skin. This length can be measured in terms of a *fingertip unit* (the distance from the tip of the adult index finger to the first crease). One fingertip unit (approximately 500 mg from a tube with a standard 5 mm diameter nozzle) is sufficient to cover an area that is twice that of the flat adult handprint (palm and fingers). [EvGr] Several minutes should elapse between application of topical corticosteroids and emollients. [A]
- In children 'Wet-wrap bandaging' increases absorption into the skin, but should be initiated under the supervision of a trained healthcare professional.

- **PRESCRIBING AND DISPENSING INFORMATION** The potency of each topical corticosteroid should be included on the label with the directions for use. The label should be attached to the container (for example, the tube) rather than the outer packaging.

- **PATIENT AND CARER ADVICE** Patients and their carers should be counselled on the terms used to describe the potency of topical corticosteroid preparations. For ease of understanding, *potent* and *very potent* corticosteroids may be referred to as *strong* and *very strong* corticosteroids, respectively. If a patient is using topical corticosteroids of different potencies, the patient should be told when to use each corticosteroid. Patients and their carers should be reassured that side-effects such as skin thinning and systemic effects rarely occur when topical corticosteroids are used appropriately.

If systemic absorption occurs following topical and local use, side-effects applicable to systemic corticosteroids may apply.

F 1408

Alclometasone dipropionate   08-Oct-2024

- **INDICATIONS AND DOSE**

Inflammatory skin disorders such as eczemas
- TO THE SKIN
- Child: Apply 1–2 times a day, to be applied thinly
- Adult: Apply 1–2 times a day, to be applied thinly

POTENCY
- Alclometasone dipropionate is a moderate corticosteroid.

- **UNLICENSED USE** Licensed for use in children (age range not specified by manufacturer).

- **PATIENT AND CARER ADVICE** Patients or carers should be counselled on the application of alclometasone dipropionate cream.

- **MEDICINAL FORMS** No licensed medicines listed.

Beclometasone dipropionate
F 1408
08-Oct-2024

(Beclomethasone dipropionate)

● **INDICATIONS AND DOSE**

Severe inflammatory skin disorders such as eczemas unresponsive to less potent corticosteroids | Psoriasis
▸ TO THE SKIN
▸ Child: Apply 1–2 times a day, to be applied thinly
▸ Adult: Apply 1–2 times a day, to be applied thinly
POTENCY
▸ Beclometasone dipropionate is a potent corticosteroid.

● **UNLICENSED USE** Not licensed for use in children under 1 year.

● **INTERACTIONS** → Appendix 1: corticosteroids

● **SIDE-EFFECTS** Vision blurred

● **MEDICINAL FORMS** There can be variation in the licensing of different medicines containing the same drug.
Cutaneous ointment
CAUTIONARY AND ADVISORY LABELS 28
▸ Beclometasone dipropionate (Non-proprietary)
Beclometasone dipropionate 250 microgram per
1 gram Beclometasone 0.025% ointment | 30 gram [PoM] £74.97 DT = £74.97
Cutaneous cream
CAUTIONARY AND ADVISORY LABELS 28
▸ Beclometasone dipropionate (Non-proprietary)
Beclometasone dipropionate 250 microgram per
1 gram Beclometasone 0.025% cream | 30 gram [PoM] £74.97 DT = £74.97

Betamethasone
F 1408
15-Jan-2025

● **DRUG ACTION** Betamethasone has very high glucocorticoid activity and insignificant mineralocorticoid activity.

● **INDICATIONS AND DOSE**

Severe inflammatory skin disorders such as eczemas unresponsive to less potent corticosteroids | Psoriasis
▸ TO THE SKIN
▸ Child: Apply 1–2 times a day, to be applied thinly
▸ Adult: Apply 1–2 times a day, to be applied thinly
POTENCY
▸ Betamethasone is a potent corticosteroid.

BETESIL ®

Inflammatory skin disorders [unresponsive to less potent corticosteroids]
▸ TO THE SKIN
▸ Adult: Apply every 24 hours for up to 30 days, wait at least 30 minutes between applications, up to 6 medicated plasters may be used per day
POTENCY
▸ Betamethasone is a potent corticosteroid.

● **UNLICENSED USE** *Betacap*®, *Betnovate*® and *Betnovate-RD*® are not licensed for use in children under 1 year. *Bettamousse*® is not licensed for use in children under 6 years.

● **CAUTIONS** Use of more than 100 g per week of 0.1% preparation likely to cause adrenal suppression

● **INTERACTIONS** → Appendix 1: corticosteroids

● **SIDE-EFFECTS** Colloid milia

● **DIRECTIONS FOR ADMINISTRATION**

BETESIL ® Manufacturer advises cleanse and dry skin prior to plaster application. Plaster may be cut to fit area to be treated.

● **PATIENT AND CARER ADVICE** Patient counselling is advised for betamethasone cream, ointment, scalp application and foam (application).

BETESIL ® Manufacturer advises avoid contact with water after plaster applied.

● **MEDICINAL FORMS** There can be variation in the licensing of different medicines containing the same drug.
Cutaneous ointment
CAUTIONARY AND ADVISORY LABELS 28
▸ Betamethasone (Non-proprietary)
Betamethasone (as Betamethasone valerate) 1 mg per
1 gram Betamethasone valerate 0.1% ointment | 30 gram [PoM] £1.76 DT = £1.76 | 100 gram [PoM] £5.87 DT = £5.87
▸ Betnovate (GlaxoSmithKline UK Ltd)
Betamethasone (as Betamethasone valerate) 250 microgram per
1 gram Betnovate RD 0.025% ointment | 100 gram [PoM] £3.15 DT = £3.15
Betamethasone (as Betamethasone valerate) 1 mg per
1 gram Betnovate 0.1% ointment | 30 gram [PoM] £1.43 DT = £1.76 | 100 gram [PoM] £4.05 DT = £5.87
▸ Diprosone (Organon Pharma (UK) Ltd)
Betamethasone (as Betamethasone dipropionate)
500 microgram per 1 gram Diprosone 0.05% ointment | 30 gram [PoM] £2.16 DT = £2.16
Cutaneous foam
CAUTIONARY AND ADVISORY LABELS 15, 28
EXCIPIENTS: May contain Cetostearyl alcohol (including cetyl and stearyl alcohol), polysorbates, propylene glycol
▸ Bettamousse (RPH Pharmaceuticals AB)
Betamethasone (as Betamethasone valerate) 1 mg per
1 gram Bettamousse 0.1% cutaneous foam | 100 gram [PoM] £11.62 DT = £11.62
Medicated plaster
▸ Betesil (Derma UK Ltd)
Betamethasone valerate 2.25 mg Betesil 2.25mg medicated plasters | 4 plaster [PoM] £13.98 DT = £13.98 | 8 plaster [PoM] £27.46
Cutaneous cream
CAUTIONARY AND ADVISORY LABELS 28
EXCIPIENTS: May contain Cetostearyl alcohol (including cetyl and stearyl alcohol), chlorocresol
▸ Betamethasone (Non-proprietary)
Betamethasone (as Betamethasone valerate) 1 mg per
1 gram Betamethasone valerate 0.1% cream | 30 gram [PoM] £3.60 DT = £3.39 | 100 gram [PoM] £8.41 DT = £8.41
▸ Audavate (Accord-UK Ltd)
Betamethasone (as Betamethasone valerate) 250 microgram per
1 gram Audavate RD 0.025% cream | 100 gram [PoM] £2.99 DT = £3.15
▸ Betnovate (GlaxoSmithKline UK Ltd)
Betamethasone (as Betamethasone valerate) 250 microgram per
1 gram Betnovate RD 0.025% cream | 100 gram [PoM] £3.15 DT = £3.15
Betamethasone (as Betamethasone valerate) 1 mg per
1 gram Betnovate 0.1% cream | 30 gram [PoM] £1.43 DT = £3.39 | 100 gram [PoM] £4.05 DT = £8.41
▸ Diprosone (Organon Pharma (UK) Ltd)
Betamethasone (as Betamethasone dipropionate)
500 microgram per 1 gram Diprosone 0.05% cream | 100 gram [PoM] £6.12 DT = £6.12
Cutaneous liquid
CAUTIONARY AND ADVISORY LABELS 15(scalp lotion only), 28
EXCIPIENTS: May contain Cetostearyl alcohol (including cetyl and stearyl alcohol), hydroxybenzoates (parabens)
▸ Betacap (Dermal Laboratories Ltd)
Betamethasone (as Betamethasone valerate) 1 mg per
1 gram Betacap 0.1% scalp application | 100 ml [PoM] £3.94 DT = £3.94
▸ Betnovate (GlaxoSmithKline UK Ltd)
Betamethasone (as Betamethasone valerate) 1 mg per
1 gram Betnovate 0.1% scalp application | 100 ml [PoM] £4.99 DT = £3.94
Betnovate 0.1% lotion | 100 ml [PoM] £4.58 DT = £4.58

▶ **Diprosone** (Organon Pharma (UK) Ltd)
Betamethasone (as Betamethasone dipropionate)
500 microgram per 1 ml Diprosone 0.05% lotion | 100 ml [PoM]
£7.80 DT = £7.80

Combinations available: *Betamethasone with clioquinol*,
p. 1415 · *Betamethasone with clotrimazole*, p. 1415 ·
Betamethasone with fusidic acid, p. 1415 · *Betamethasone
with neomycin*, p. 1415 · *Betamethasone with salicylic acid*,
p. 1416

Calcipotriol with betamethasone

15-Jan-2025

The properties listed below are those particular to the
combination only. For the properties of the components
please consider, calcipotriol p. 1434, betamethasone p. 1410.

● **INDICATIONS AND DOSE**
Psoriasis [using cream, gel, or ointment]
▶ TO THE SKIN
▶ Adult: Apply once daily usually for 4 to 8 weeks, if
necessary treatment may be continued for longer or
repeated on the advice of a specialist, when using
calcipotriol-containing preparations the maximum
total dose of calcipotriol is 5 mg (equivalent to 100 g
total amount of any formulation) in any 1 week,
applied to a maximum 30% of body surface

Scalp psoriasis [using cream or gel]
▶ TO THE SKIN
▶ Adult: Apply once daily usually for 4 to 8 weeks, if
necessary treatment may be continued for longer or
repeated on the advice of a specialist, when using
calcipotriol-containing preparations the maximum
total dose of calcipotriol is 5 mg (equivalent to 100 g
total amount of any formulation) in any 1 week,
applied to a maximum 30% of body surface

POTENCY
▶ Betamethasone is a potent corticosteroid.

ENSTILAR®
Psoriasis [flare treatment]
▶ TO THE SKIN USING FOAM
▶ Adult: Apply once daily for 4 weeks, if necessary
treatment may be continued for longer or repeated on
the advice of a specialist, when using calcipotriol-
containing preparations the maximum total dose of
calcipotriol is 5 mg (equivalent to 100 g total amount of
any formulation) in any 1 week, applied to a maximum
30% of body surface

Psoriasis [maintenance treatment]
▶ TO THE SKIN USING FOAM
▶ Adult: Apply twice weekly, maintenance treatment to
be started if adequate response is achieved after
4 weeks of once-daily treatment, apply on 2 non-
consecutive days to previously affected areas, when
using calcipotriol-containing preparations the
maximum total dose of calcipotriol is 5 mg (equivalent
to 100 g total amount of any formulation) in any
1 week, applied to a maximum 30% of body surface,
once-daily treatment should be restarted if relapse
occurs

POTENCY
▶ Betamethasone is a potent corticosteroid.

● **CONTRA-INDICATIONS** Erythrodermic psoriasis · pustular
psoriasis
● **INTERACTIONS** → Appendix 1: corticosteroids · vitamin D
substances
● **PATIENT AND CARER ADVICE** Patients or carers should be
advised to allow calcipotriol with betamethasone
preparations to remain on the scalp or skin overnight or

during the day, and not to shower or bathe immediately
after application.
  Hands should be washed thoroughly after application to
avoid inadvertent transfer to other body areas.
● **NATIONAL FUNDING/ACCESS DECISIONS**
ENSTILAR® For full details see funding body website
Scottish Medicines Consortium (SMC) decisions
▶ Calcipotriol and betamethasone cutaneous foam (*Enstilar*®)
for the topical treatment of psoriasis vulgaris in adults
(September 2016) SMC No. 1182/16 Recommended

● **MEDICINAL FORMS** There can be variation in the licensing of
different medicines containing the same drug.
Cutaneous foam
CAUTIONARY AND ADVISORY LABELS 15, 28
EXCIPIENTS: May contain Butylated hydroxytoluene
▶ **Enstilar** (LEO Pharma)
Calcipotriol (as Calcipotriol monohydrate) 50 microgram per
1 gram, Betamethasone (as Betamethasone dipropionate)
500 microgram per 1 gram Enstilar 50micrograms/g / 0.5 mg/g
cutaneous foam | 60 gram [PoM] £39.68 DT = £39.68 |
120 gram [PoM] £79.36
Cutaneous ointment
CAUTIONARY AND ADVISORY LABELS 28
EXCIPIENTS: May contain Butylated hydroxytoluene
▶ **Calcipotriol with betamethasone** (Non-proprietary)
Calcipotriol (as Calcipotriol monohydrate) 50 microgram per
1 gram, Betamethasone (as Betamethasone dipropionate)
500 microgram per 1 gram Calcipotriol 0.005% / Betamethasone
dipropionate 0.05% ointment | 30 gram [PoM] £19.84 DT = £19.84 |
60 gram [PoM] £31.74 | 120 gram [PoM] £59.09
▶ **Dovobet** (LEO Pharma)
Calcipotriol (as Calcipotriol monohydrate) 50 microgram per
1 gram, Betamethasone (as Betamethasone dipropionate)
500 microgram per 1 gram Dovobet ointment | 30 gram [PoM]
£19.84 DT = £19.84 | 60 gram [PoM] £39.68 | 120 gram [PoM] £73.86
Cutaneous cream
CAUTIONARY AND ADVISORY LABELS 28
EXCIPIENTS: May contain Butylated hydroxyanisole
▶ **Wynzora** (Almirall Ltd)
Calcipotriol 50 microgram per 1 gram, Betamethasone (as
Betamethasone dipropionate) 500 microgram per
1 gram Wynzora 50micrograms/g / 0.5mg/g cream | 60 gram [PoM]
£35.66 DT = £35.66
Cutaneous gel
CAUTIONARY AND ADVISORY LABELS 28
EXCIPIENTS: May contain Butylated hydroxytoluene
▶ **Calcipotriol with betamethasone** (Non-proprietary)
Calcipotriol (as Calcipotriol monohydrate) 50 microgram per
1 gram, Betamethasone (as Betamethasone dipropionate)
500 microgram per 1 gram Calcipotriol 0.005% / Betamethasone
dipropionate 0.05% gel | 60 gram [PoM] £37.20 DT = £37.21 |
120 gram [PoM] £47.40–£69.10
▶ **Dovobet** (LEO Pharma)
Calcipotriol (as Calcipotriol monohydrate) 50 microgram per
1 gram, Betamethasone (as Betamethasone dipropionate)
500 microgram per 1 gram Dovobet gel | 60 gram [PoM] £37.21 DT
= £37.21 | 120 gram [PoM] £69.11

⌖ 1408

Clobetasol propionate

15-Jan-2025

● **INDICATIONS AND DOSE**
**Short-term treatment only of severe resistant
inflammatory skin disorders such as recalcitrant
eczemas unresponsive to less potent corticosteroids |
Psoriasis**
▶ TO THE SKIN
▶ Child 1–17 years: Apply 1–2 times a day for up to
4 weeks, to be applied thinly
▶ Adult: Apply 1–2 times a day for up to 4 weeks, to be
applied thinly, maximum 50 g of 0.05% preparation per
week
POTENCY
▶ Clobetasol propionate is a very potent corticosteroid.

continued →

ETRIVEX ®

Moderate scalp psoriasis

▶ TO THE SKIN

▶ Adult: Apply once daily maximum duration of treatment 4 weeks, to be applied thinly then rinsed off after 15 minutes, frequency of application should be reduced after clinical improvement

POTENCY

▶ Clobetasol propionate is a very potent corticosteroid.

● **PATIENT AND CARER ADVICE** Patients or carers should be given advice on how to administer clobetasol propionate foam, liquid (scalp application), cream, ointment and shampoo.

Scalp application Patients or carers should be advised to apply foam directly to scalp lesions (foam begins to subside immediately on contact with skin).

● **MEDICINAL FORMS** There can be variation in the licensing of different medicines containing the same drug. Forms available from special-order manufacturers include: cutaneous cream, cutaneous ointment, cutaneous paste

Cutaneous ointment

CAUTIONARY AND ADVISORY LABELS 28

EXCIPIENTS: May contain Propylene glycol

▶ **Clobetasol propionate (Non-proprietary)**
Clobetasol propionate 500 microgram per 1 gram Clobetasol 0.05% ointment | 30 gram [PoM] £2.42–£4.30 DT = £2.69 | 100 gram [PoM] £7.11–£12.64 DT = £7.90

▶ **Dermovate** (GlaxoSmithKline UK Ltd)
Clobetasol propionate 500 microgram per 1 gram Dermovate 0.05% ointment | 30 gram [PoM] £2.69 DT = £2.69 | 100 gram [PoM] £7.90 DT = £7.90

Shampoo

CAUTIONARY AND ADVISORY LABELS 28

▶ **Etrivex** (Galderma (UK) Ltd)
Clobetasol propionate 500 microgram per 1 gram Etrivex 500micrograms/g shampoo | 125 ml [PoM] £9.15 DT = £9.15

Cutaneous cream

CAUTIONARY AND ADVISORY LABELS 28

EXCIPIENTS: May contain Beeswax, cetostearyl alcohol (including cetyl and stearyl alcohol), chlorocresol, propylene glycol

▶ **Clobetasol propionate (Non-proprietary)**
Clobetasol propionate 500 microgram per 1 gram Clobetasol 0.05% cream | 30 gram [PoM] £2.42 DT = £2.69 | 100 gram [PoM] £7.11 DT = £7.90

▶ **Dermovate** (GlaxoSmithKline UK Ltd)
Clobetasol propionate 500 microgram per 1 gram Dermovate 0.05% cream | 30 gram [PoM] £2.69 DT = £2.69 | 100 gram [PoM] £7.90 DT = £7.90

Cutaneous liquid

CAUTIONARY AND ADVISORY LABELS 15, 28

▶ **Dermovate** (GlaxoSmithKline UK Ltd)
Clobetasol propionate 500 microgram per 1 gram Dermovate 0.05% scalp application | 30 ml [PoM] £3.07 DT = £3.07 | 100 ml [PoM] £10.42 DT = £10.42

Combinations available: *Clobetasol propionate with neomycin sulfate and nystatin,* p. 1416

⚐ 1408

Clobetasone butyrate

08-Oct-2024

● **INDICATIONS AND DOSE**

Eczemas and dermatitis of all types | Maintenance between courses of more potent corticosteroids

▶ TO THE SKIN

▶ Child: Apply 1–2 times a day, to be applied thinly

▶ Adult: Apply 1–2 times a day, to be applied thinly

POTENCY

▶ Clobetasone butyrate is a moderate corticosteroid.

● **UNLICENSED USE** Licensed for use in children (age range not specified by manufacturer).

● **PATIENT AND CARER ADVICE** Patients or carers should be advised on the application of clobetasone butyrate containing preparations.

● **EXCEPTIONS TO LEGAL CATEGORY** Cream can be sold to the public for short-term symptomatic treatment and control of patches of eczema and dermatitis (but not seborrhoeic dermatitis) in adults and children over 12 years provided pack does not contain more than 15 g.

● **MEDICINAL FORMS** There can be variation in the licensing of different medicines containing the same drug.

Cutaneous ointment

CAUTIONARY AND ADVISORY LABELS 28

▶ **Clobavate** (Teva UK Ltd)
Clobetasone butyrate 500 microgram per 1 gram Clobavate 0.05% ointment | 30 gram [PoM] £1.49 DT = £1.86 | 100 gram [PoM] £4.35 DT = £5.44

▶ **Eumovate** (GlaxoSmithKline UK Ltd)
Clobetasone butyrate 500 microgram per 1 gram Eumovate 0.05% ointment | 30 gram [PoM] £1.86 DT = £1.86 | 100 gram [PoM] £5.44 DT = £5.44

Cutaneous cream

CAUTIONARY AND ADVISORY LABELS 28

EXCIPIENTS: May contain Cetostearyl alcohol (including cetyl and stearyl alcohol), chlorocresol

▶ **Eumovate** (GlaxoSmithKline UK Ltd)
Clobetasone butyrate 500 microgram per 1 gram Eumovate 0.05% cream | 30 gram [PoM] £1.86 DT = £1.86 | 100 gram [PoM] £5.44 DT = £5.44

Combinations available: *Clobetasone butyrate with nystatin and oxytetracycline,* p. 1416

⚐ 1408

Fludroxycortide

15-Jan-2025

(Flurandrenolone)

● **INDICATIONS AND DOSE**

Inflammatory skin disorders such as eczemas

▶ TO THE SKIN

▶ Child: Apply 1–2 times a day, to be applied thinly

▶ Adult: Apply 1–2 times a day, to be applied thinly

POTENCY

▶ Fludroxycortide is a potent corticosteroid.

HAELAN ® TAPE

Chronic localised recalcitrant dermatoses (but not acute or weeping)

▶ TO THE SKIN

▶ Child: Cut tape to fit lesion, apply to clean, dry skin shorn of hair, usually for 12 hours daily

▶ Adult: Cut tape to fit lesion, apply to clean, dry skin shorn of hair, usually for 12 hours daily

POTENCY

▶ Fludroxycortide is a potent corticosteroid.

● **UNLICENSED USE** Licensed for use in children (age range not specified by manufacturer).

● **SIDE-EFFECTS** Cushing's syndrome · increased risk of infection

● **PATIENT AND CARER ADVICE** Patients or carers should be counselled on application of fludroxycortide cream and ointment.

● **MEDICINAL FORMS** There can be variation in the licensing of different medicines containing the same drug.

Cutaneous cream

CAUTIONARY AND ADVISORY LABELS 28

EXCIPIENTS: May contain Cetostearyl alcohol (including cetyl and stearyl alcohol), propylene glycol

▶ **Fludroxycortide (Non-proprietary)**
Fludroxycortide 125 microgram per 1 gram Fludroxycortide 0.0125% cream | 60 gram [PoM] £12.49 DT = £12.49

Impregnated dressing

▸ **Fludroxycortide (Non-proprietary)**

Fludroxycortide 4 microgram per 1 square cm Fludroxycortide 4micrograms/square cm tape 7.5cm | 20 cm [PoM] £21.44-£34.64 DT = £34.64 | 50 cm [PoM] £37.49-£52.17 DT = £52.17

▣ 1408

Fluocinolone acetonide
08-Oct-2024

● **INDICATIONS AND DOSE**

Severe inflammatory skin disorders such as eczemas | Psoriasis

▸ TO THE SKIN

▸ **Child 1-17 years:** Apply 1–2 times a day, to be applied thinly, reduce strength as condition responds

▸ **Adult:** Apply 1–2 times a day, to be applied thinly, reduce strength as condition responds

POTENCY

▸ Fluocinolone acetonide is a potent corticosteroid.

● **INTERACTIONS** → Appendix 1: fluocinolone

● **PRESCRIBING AND DISPENSING INFORMATION** Gel is useful for application to the scalp and other hairy areas.

● **PATIENT AND CARER ADVICE** Patient counselling is advised for fluocinolone acetonide cream, gel and ointment (application).

● **MEDICINAL FORMS** There can be variation in the licensing of different medicines containing the same drug.

Cutaneous ointment

CAUTIONARY AND ADVISORY LABELS 28
EXCIPIENTS: May contain Propylene glycol, woolfat and related substances (including lanolin)

▸ **Synalar** (Reig Jofre UK Ltd)

Fluocinolone acetonide 62.5 microgram per 1 gram Synalar 1 in 4 Dilution 0.00625% ointment | 50 gram [PoM] £4.84 DT = £4.84

Fluocinolone acetonide 250 microgram per 1 gram Synalar 0.025% ointment | 30 gram [PoM] £4.14 DT = £4.14 | 100 gram [PoM] £11.75 DT = £11.75

Cutaneous cream

CAUTIONARY AND ADVISORY LABELS 28
EXCIPIENTS: May contain Benzyl alcohol, cetostearyl alcohol (including cetyl and stearyl alcohol), polysorbates, propylene glycol

▸ **Synalar** (Reig Jofre UK Ltd)

Fluocinolone acetonide 250 microgram per 1 gram Synalar 0.025% cream | 30 gram [PoM] £4.14 DT = £4.14 | 100 gram [PoM] £11.75 DT = £11.75

Cutaneous gel

CAUTIONARY AND ADVISORY LABELS 28
EXCIPIENTS: May contain Hydroxybenzoates (parabens), propylene glycol

▸ **Synalar** (Reig Jofre UK Ltd)

Fluocinolone acetonide 250 microgram per 1 gram Synalar 0.025% gel | 30 gram [PoM] £5.56 DT = £5.56 | 60 gram [PoM] £10.02 DT = £10.02

▣ 1408

Fluocinonide
08-Oct-2024

● **INDICATIONS AND DOSE**

Severe inflammatory skin disorders such as eczemas unresponsive to less potent corticosteroids | Psoriasis

▸ TO THE SKIN

▸ **Child:** Apply 1–2 times a day, to be applied thinly

▸ **Adult:** Apply 1–2 times a day, to be applied thinly

POTENCY

▸ Fluocinonide is a potent corticosteroid.

● **UNLICENSED USE** Not licensed for use in children under 1 year.

● **PATIENT AND CARER ADVICE** Patients or carers should be advised on the application of fluocinonide preparations.

● **MEDICINAL FORMS** There can be variation in the licensing of different medicines containing the same drug.

Cutaneous ointment

CAUTIONARY AND ADVISORY LABELS 28
EXCIPIENTS: May contain Propylene glycol, woolfat and related substances (including lanolin)

▸ **Metosyn** (Reig Jofre UK Ltd)

Fluocinonide 500 microgram per 1 gram Metosyn 0.05% ointment | 100 gram [PoM] £13.15 DT = £13.15

Cutaneous cream

CAUTIONARY AND ADVISORY LABELS 28
EXCIPIENTS: May contain Propylene glycol

▸ **Metosyn FAPG** (Reig Jofre UK Ltd)

Fluocinonide 500 microgram per 1 gram Metosyn FAPG 0.05% cream | 25 gram [PoM] £3.96 DT = £3.96 | 100 gram [PoM] £13.34 DT = £13.34

▣ 1408

Fluticasone
08-Oct-2024

● **INDICATIONS AND DOSE**

Severe inflammatory skin disorders such as dermatitis and eczemas unresponsive to less potent corticosteroids | Psoriasis

▸ TO THE SKIN

▸ **Child 3 months-17 years:** Apply 1–2 times a day, to be applied thinly

▸ **Adult:** Apply 1–2 times a day, to be applied thinly

POTENCY

▸ Fluticasone is a potent corticosteroid.

● **INTERACTIONS** → Appendix 1: corticosteroids

● **PATIENT AND CARER ADVICE** Patients or carers should be given advice on application of fluticasone creams and ointments.

● **MEDICINAL FORMS** There can be variation in the licensing of different medicines containing the same drug.

Cutaneous ointment

CAUTIONARY AND ADVISORY LABELS 28
EXCIPIENTS: May contain Propylene glycol

▸ **Cutivate** (GlaxoSmithKline UK Ltd)

Fluticasone propionate 50 microgram per 1 gram Cutivate 0.005% ointment | 30 gram [PoM] £4.24 DT = £4.24

Cutaneous cream

CAUTIONARY AND ADVISORY LABELS 28
EXCIPIENTS: May contain Cetostearyl alcohol (including cetyl and stearyl alcohol), imidurea, propylene glycol

▸ **Fluticasone (Non-proprietary)**

Fluticasone propionate 500 microgram per 1 gram Fluticasone 0.05% cream | 30 gram [PoM] £6.78 DT = £4.24

▣ 1408

Hydrocortisone
08-Oct-2024

● **DRUG ACTION** Hydrocortisone has equal glucocorticoid and mineralocorticoid activity.

● **INDICATIONS AND DOSE**

Mild inflammatory skin disorders such as eczemas

▸ TO THE SKIN

▸ **Child:** Apply 1–2 times a day, to be applied thinly

▸ **Adult:** Apply 1–2 times a day, to be applied thinly

Nappy rash

▸ TO THE SKIN

▸ **Child:** Apply 1–2 times a day for no longer than 1 week, to be discontinued as soon as the inflammation subsides

POTENCY

▸ Hydrocortisone is a mild corticosteroid.

● **INTERACTIONS** → Appendix 1: corticosteroids

● **PRESCRIBING AND DISPENSING INFORMATION** When hydrocortisone cream or ointment is prescribed and no strength is stated, the 1% strength should be supplied.

13

Skin

- **PATIENT AND CARER ADVICE** Patient counselling is advised for hydrocortisone cream and ointment (application).
- **PROFESSION SPECIFIC INFORMATION**
  Dental practitioners' formulary Hydrocortisone Cream 1% 15 g may be prescribed.
- **EXCEPTIONS TO LEGAL CATEGORY**
  Over-the-counter hydrocortisone preparations Skin creams and ointments containing hydrocortisone (alone or with other ingredients) can be sold to the public for the treatment of allergic contact dermatitis, irritant dermatitis, insect bite reactions and mild to moderate eczema in patients over 10 years, to be applied sparingly over the affected area 1–2 times daily for max. 1 week. Over-the-counter hydrocortisone preparations should not be sold without medical advice for children under 10 years or for pregnant women; they should **not** be sold for application to the face, anogenital region, broken or infected skin (including cold sores, acne, and athlete's foot).

- **MEDICINAL FORMS** There can be variation in the licensing of different medicines containing the same drug.
  Cutaneous ointment
  CAUTIONARY AND ADVISORY LABELS 28
  ▸ Hydrocortisone (Non-proprietary)
    Hydrocortisone 5 mg per 1 gram Hydrocortisone 0.5% ointment | 15 gram [PoM] £96.78 DT = £96.78 | 30 gram [PoM] £94.16–£160.42
    Hydrocortisone 10 mg per 1 gram Hydrocortisone 1% ointment | 15 gram [PoM] £2.86 DT = £2.04 | 30 gram [PoM] £5.93 DT = £5.21 | 50 gram [PoM] £9.98 DT = £8.20
    Hydrocortisone 25 mg per 1 gram Hydrocortisone 2.5% ointment | 15 gram [PoM] £52.27 DT = £52.27 | 30 gram [PoM] £95.04–£104.54
  Cutaneous cream
  CAUTIONARY AND ADVISORY LABELS 28
  EXCIPIENTS: May contain Benzyl alcohol, cetostearyl alcohol (including cetyl and stearyl alcohol), hydroxybenzoates (parabens), propylene glycol
  ▸ Hydrocortisone (Non-proprietary)
    Hydrocortisone 5 mg per 1 gram Hydrocortisone 0.5% cream | 30 gram [PoM] £88.00
    Hydrocortisone 10 mg per 1 gram Hydrocortisone 1% cream | 15 gram [PoM] £3.10 DT = £2.84 | 30 gram [PoM] £6.61 DT = £5.26 | 50 gram [PoM] £9.07 DT = £7.64
    Hydrocortisone 25 mg per 1 gram Hydrocortisone 2.5% cream | 15 gram [PoM] £96.74 DT = £96.74 | 30 gram [PoM] £95.04–£193.48
  ▸ Hc45 (Karo Healthcare UK Ltd)
    Hydrocortisone acetate 10 mg per 1 gram Hc45 Hydrocortisone 1% cream | 15 gram [P] £3.88 DT = £3.88

  Combinations available: *Hydrocortisone with benzalkonium chloride, dimeticone and nystatin*, p. 1417 · *Hydrocortisone with chlorhexidine hydrochloride and nystatin*, p. 1417 · *Hydrocortisone with clotrimazole*, p. 1417 · *Hydrocortisone with fusidic acid*, p. 1417 · *Hydrocortisone with miconazole*, p. 1418 · *Hydrocortisone with oxytetracycline*, p. 1418

▶ 1408

Hydrocortisone butyrate
08-Oct-2024

- **INDICATIONS AND DOSE**
  Severe inflammatory skin disorders such as eczemas unresponsive to less potent corticosteroids | Psoriasis
  ▸ TO THE SKIN
  ▸ Child 1–17 years: Apply 1–2 times a day, to be applied thinly
  ▸ Adult: Apply 1–2 times a day, to be applied thinly
  POTENCY
  ▸ Hydrocortisone butyrate is a moderate corticosteroid.

- **PATIENT AND CARER ADVICE** Patients or carers should be given advice on how to administer hydrocortisone butyrate lotion, cream, ointment and scalp lotion.
  Medicines for Children leaflet: Hydrocortisone (topical) for eczema www.medicinesforchildren.org.uk/medicines/hydrocortisone-topical-for-eczema/

- **MEDICINAL FORMS** There can be variation in the licensing of different medicines containing the same drug.
  Cutaneous ointment
  CAUTIONARY AND ADVISORY LABELS 28
  ▸ Locoid (Neon Healthcare Ltd)
    Hydrocortisone butyrate 1 mg per 1 gram Locoid 0.1% ointment | 100 gram [PoM] £4.93 DT = £4.93
  Cutaneous emulsion
  CAUTIONARY AND ADVISORY LABELS 15, 28
  EXCIPIENTS: May contain Butylated hydroxytoluene, cetostearyl alcohol (including cetyl and stearyl alcohol), hydroxybenzoates (parabens), propylene glycol
  ▸ Locoid Crelo (Neon Healthcare Ltd)
    Hydrocortisone butyrate 1 mg per 1 gram Locoid Crelo 0.1% topical emulsion | 100 gram [PoM] £5.91 DT = £5.91
  Cutaneous solution
  CAUTIONARY AND ADVISORY LABELS 15, 28
  EXCIPIENTS: May contain Butylated hydroxytoluene, cetostearyl alcohol (including cetyl and stearyl alcohol), hydroxybenzoates (parabens), propylene glycol
  ▸ Locoid (Neon Healthcare Ltd)
    Hydrocortisone butyrate 1 mg per 1 ml Locoid 0.1% scalp lotion | 100 ml [PoM] £6.83 DT = £6.83
  Cutaneous cream
  CAUTIONARY AND ADVISORY LABELS 28
  EXCIPIENTS: May contain Benzyl alcohol, cetostearyl alcohol (including cetyl and stearyl alcohol), hydroxybenzoates (parabens)
  ▸ Locoid (Neon Healthcare Ltd)
    Hydrocortisone butyrate 1 mg per 1 gram Locoid 0.1% cream | 100 gram [PoM] £4.93 DT = £4.93
  ▸ Locoid Lipocream (Neon Healthcare Ltd)
    Hydrocortisone butyrate 1 mg per 1 gram Locoid 0.1% Lipocream | 100 gram [PoM] £5.17 DT = £4.93

▶ 1408

Mometasone furoate
08-Oct-2024

- **INDICATIONS AND DOSE**
  Severe inflammatory skin disorders such as eczemas unresponsive to less potent corticosteroids | Psoriasis
  ▸ TO THE SKIN
  ▸ Child 2–17 years: Apply once daily, to be applied thinly (to scalp in case of lotion)
  ▸ Adult: Apply once daily, to be applied thinly (to scalp in case of lotion)
  POTENCY
  ▸ Mometasone furoate is a potent corticosteroid.

- **INTERACTIONS** → Appendix 1: corticosteroids

- **MEDICINAL FORMS** There can be variation in the licensing of different medicines containing the same drug.
  Cutaneous ointment
  CAUTIONARY AND ADVISORY LABELS 28
  EXCIPIENTS: May contain Beeswax, propylene glycol
  ▸ Mometasone furoate (Non-proprietary)
    Mometasone furoate 1 mg per 1 gram Mometasone 0.1% ointment | 15 gram [PoM] £4.32 | 30 gram [PoM] £5.60 DT = £2.78 | 50 gram [PoM] £12.44 | 100 gram [PoM] £18.00 DT = £9.27
  ▸ Elocon (Organon Pharma (UK) Ltd)
    Mometasone furoate 1 mg per 1 gram Elocon 0.1% ointment | 30 gram [PoM] £4.32 DT = £2.78 | 100 gram [PoM] £12.44 DT = £9.27
  Cutaneous cream
  CAUTIONARY AND ADVISORY LABELS 28
  EXCIPIENTS: May contain Beeswax
  ▸ Mometasone furoate (Non-proprietary)
    Mometasone furoate 1 mg per 1 gram Mometasone 0.1% cream | 30 gram [PoM] £5.00 DT = £2.73 | 100 gram [PoM] £13.90 DT = £9.10
  ▸ Elocon (Organon Pharma (UK) Ltd)
    Mometasone furoate 1 mg per 1 gram Elocon 0.1% cream | 30 gram [PoM] £4.80 DT = £2.73 | 100 gram [PoM] £15.10 DT = £9.10
  Cutaneous liquid
  CAUTIONARY AND ADVISORY LABELS 28
  EXCIPIENTS: May contain Propylene glycol
  ▸ Elocon (Organon Pharma (UK) Ltd)
    Mometasone furoate 1 mg per 1 gram Elocon 0.1% scalp lotion | 30 ml [PoM] £4.36 DT = £4.36

CORTICOSTEROIDS > CORTICOSTEROID COMBINATIONS WITH ANTI-INFECTIVES

Betamethasone with clioquinol   08-Oct-2024

The properties listed below are those particular to the combination only. For the properties of the components please consider, betamethasone p. 1410.

● **INDICATIONS AND DOSE**

Severe inflammatory skin disorders such as eczemas associated with infection and unresponsive to less potent corticosteroids | Psoriasis (excluding widespread plaque psoriasis)

▸ TO THE SKIN
▸ Child 1-17 years: (consult product literature)
▸ Adult: (consult product literature)

POTENCY
▸ Betamethasone is a potent corticosteroid.

● **INTERACTIONS** → Appendix 1: corticosteroids

● **PATIENT AND CARER ADVICE** Stains clothing. Patients or carers should be counselled on application of betamethasone with clioquinol preparations.

● **MEDICINAL FORMS** There can be variation in the licensing of different medicines containing the same drug.
Cutaneous ointment
CAUTIONARY AND ADVISORY LABELS 28
▸ **Betamethasone with clioquinol (Non-proprietary)**
Betamethasone (as Betamethasone valerate) 1 mg per 1 gram, Clioquinol 30 mg per 1 gram Betamethasone valerate 0.1% / Clioquinol 3% ointment | 30 gram [PoM] £49.21-£83.87 DT = £83.87
Cutaneous cream
CAUTIONARY AND ADVISORY LABELS 28
EXCIPIENTS: May contain Cetostearyl alcohol (including cetyl and stearyl alcohol), chlorocresol
▸ **Betamethasone with clioquinol (Non-proprietary)**
Betamethasone (as Betamethasone valerate) 1 mg per 1 gram, Clioquinol 30 mg per 1 gram Betamethasone valerate 0.1% / Clioquinol 3% cream | 30 gram [PoM] £72.86 DT = £72.86

Betamethasone with clotrimazole
08-Oct-2024

The properties listed below are those particular to the combination only. For the properties of the components please consider, betamethasone p. 1410, clotrimazole p. 1399.

● **INDICATIONS AND DOSE**

Short-term treatment of tinea infections and candidiasis

▸ TO THE SKIN
▸ Child 12-17 years: Apply twice daily for 2 weeks for tinea cruris, tinea corporis or candidiasis, or for 4 weeks for tinea pedis
▸ Adult: Apply twice daily for 2 weeks for tinea cruris, tinea corporis or candidiasis, or for 4 weeks for tinea pedis

POTENCY
▸ Betamethasone is a potent corticosteroid.

● **INTERACTIONS** → Appendix 1: antifungals, azoles · corticosteroids

● **PATIENT AND CARER ADVICE** Patients or carers should be given advice on how to administer betamethasone with clotrimazole cream.

● **MEDICINAL FORMS** There can be variation in the licensing of different medicines containing the same drug.
Cutaneous cream
CAUTIONARY AND ADVISORY LABELS 28
EXCIPIENTS: May contain Benzyl alcohol, cetostearyl alcohol (including cetyl and stearyl alcohol), propylene glycol

▸ Lotriderm (Organon Pharma (UK) Ltd)
Betamethasone dipropionate 640 microgram per 1 gram, Clotrimazole 10 mg per 1 gram Lotriderm cream | 30 gram [PoM] £6.34 DT = £6.34

Betamethasone with fusidic acid
08-Oct-2024

The properties listed below are those particular to the combination only. For the properties of the components please consider, betamethasone p. 1410, fusidic acid p. 663.

● **INDICATIONS AND DOSE**

Severe inflammatory skin disorders such as eczemas associated with infection and unresponsive to less potent corticosteroids

▸ TO THE SKIN
▸ Child: (consult product literature)
▸ Adult: (consult product literature)

POTENCY
▸ Betamethasone is a potent corticosteroid.

● **UNLICENSED USE** *Fucibet® Lipid Cream* is not licensed for use in children under 6 years.

● **INTERACTIONS** → Appendix 1: corticosteroids · fusidate

● **PATIENT AND CARER ADVICE** Patients or carers should be counselled on application of betamethasone with fusidic acid preparations.

● **MEDICINAL FORMS** There can be variation in the licensing of different medicines containing the same drug.
Cutaneous cream
CAUTIONARY AND ADVISORY LABELS 28
EXCIPIENTS: May contain Cetostearyl alcohol (including cetyl and stearyl alcohol), chlorocresol, hydroxybenzoates (parabens)
▸ **Betamethasone with fusidic acid (Non-proprietary)**
Betamethasone (as Betamethasone valerate) 1 mg per 1 gram, Fusidic acid 20 mg per 1 gram Betamethasone valerate 0.1% / Fusidic acid 2% cream | 30 gram [PoM] £5.80 DT = £6.38 | 60 gram [PoM] £12.15 DT = £12.76
▸ Fucibet (LEO Pharma)
Betamethasone (as Betamethasone valerate) 1 mg per 1 gram, Fusidic acid 20 mg per 1 gram Fucibet cream | 30 gram [PoM] £6.38 DT = £6.38 | 60 gram [PoM] £12.76 DT = £12.76
▸ Xemacort (Viatris UK Healthcare Ltd)
Betamethasone (as Betamethasone valerate) 1 mg per 1 gram, Fusidic acid 20 mg per 1 gram Xemacort 20mg/g / 1mg/g cream | 30 gram [PoM] £6.05 DT = £6.38 | 60 gram [PoM] £12.45 DT = £12.76

Betamethasone with neomycin   08-Oct-2024

The properties listed below are those particular to the combination only. For the properties of the components please consider, betamethasone p. 1410, neomycin sulfate p. 1397.

● **INDICATIONS AND DOSE**

Severe inflammatory skin disorders such as eczemas unresponsive to less potent corticosteroids | Psoriasis

▸ TO THE SKIN USING OINTMENT, OR TO THE SKIN USING CREAM
▸ Child 2-17 years: Apply 1–2 times a day, to be applied thinly
▸ Adult: Apply 1–2 times a day, to be applied thinly

POTENCY
▸ Betamethasone is a potent corticosteroid.

● **INTERACTIONS** → Appendix 1: corticosteroids · neomycin

● **PATIENT AND CARER ADVICE** Patient counselling is advised for betamethasone with neomycin cream and ointment (application).

- **MEDICINAL FORMS** There can be variation in the licensing of different medicines containing the same drug.
  Cutaneous ointment
  CAUTIONARY AND ADVISORY LABELS 28
  ▸ Betamethasone with neomycin (Non-proprietary)
    Betamethasone (as Betamethasone valerate) 1 mg per 1 gram, Neomycin sulfate 5 mg per 1 gram Betamethasone valerate 0.1% / Neomycin 0.5% ointment | 30 gram PoM £42.86 DT = £42.86 | 100 gram PoM £133.22 DT = £133.22
  Cutaneous cream
  CAUTIONARY AND ADVISORY LABELS 28
  EXCIPIENTS: May contain Cetostearyl alcohol (including cetyl and stearyl alcohol), chlorocresol
  ▸ Betamethasone with neomycin (Non-proprietary)
    Betamethasone (as Betamethasone valerate) 1 mg per 1 gram, Neomycin sulfate 5 mg per 1 gram Betamethasone valerate 0.1% / Neomycin 0.5% cream | 30 gram PoM £42.86 DT = £42.86 | 100 gram PoM £133.22 DT = £133.22

Betamethasone with salicylic acid

08-Oct-2024

The properties listed below are those particular to the combination only. For the properties of the components please consider, betamethasone p. 1410, salicylic acid p. 1460.

- **INDICATIONS AND DOSE**
  DIPROSALIC ® OINTMENT
  Severe inflammatory skin disorders such as eczemas unresponsive to less potent corticosteroids | Psoriasis
  ▸ TO THE SKIN
  ▸ Child: Apply 1–2 times a day, max. 60 g per week
  ▸ Adult: Apply 1–2 times a day, max. 60 g per week
  POTENCY
  ▸ Betamethasone is a potent corticosteroid.
  DIPROSALIC ® SCALP APPLICATION
  Severe inflammatory skin disorders such as eczemas unresponsive to less potent corticosteroids | Psoriasis
  ▸ TO THE SKIN
  ▸ Child: Apply 1–2 times a day, apply a few drops
  ▸ Adult: Apply 1–2 times a day, apply a few drops
  POTENCY
  ▸ Betamethasone is a potent corticosteroid.

- **INTERACTIONS** → Appendix 1: corticosteroids
- **PATIENT AND CARER ADVICE**
  DIPROSALIC ® OINTMENT Patients or carers should be counselled on application of betamethasone and salicylic acid preparations.
  DIPROSALIC ® SCALP APPLICATION Patients or carers should be counselled on application of betamethasone and salicylic acid scalp application.

- **MEDICINAL FORMS** There can be variation in the licensing of different medicines containing the same drug.
  Cutaneous solution
  CAUTIONARY AND ADVISORY LABELS 28
  EXCIPIENTS: May contain Disodium edetate
  ▸ Diprosalic (Organon Pharma (UK) Ltd)
    Betamethasone (as Betamethasone dipropionate) 500 microgram per 1 ml, Salicylic acid 20 mg per 1 ml Diprosalic 0.05%/2% scalp application | 100 ml PoM £10.10 DT = £10.10
  Cutaneous ointment
  CAUTIONARY AND ADVISORY LABELS 28
  ▸ Diprosalic (Organon Pharma (UK) Ltd)
    Betamethasone (as Betamethasone dipropionate) 500 microgram per 1 gram, Salicylic acid 30 mg per 1 gram Diprosalic 0.05%/3% ointment | 30 gram PoM £3.18 DT = £3.18 | 100 gram PoM £9.14 DT = £9.14

Clobetasol propionate with neomycin sulfate and nystatin

08-Oct-2024

The properties listed below are those particular to the combination only. For the properties of the components please consider, clobetasol propionate p. 1411, neomycin sulfate p. 1397.

- **INDICATIONS AND DOSE**
  Short-term treatment only of severe resistant inflammatory skin disorders such as recalcitrant eczemas associated with infection and unresponsive to less potent corticosteroids | Psoriasis associated with infection
  ▸ TO THE SKIN
  ▸ Adult: (consult product literature)
  POTENCY
  ▸ Clobetasol propionate is a very potent corticosteroid.

- **INTERACTIONS** → Appendix 1: neomycin
- **PATIENT AND CARER ADVICE** Patients or carers should be advised on application of clobetasol propionate, neomycin sulfate and nystatin containing preparations.

- **MEDICINAL FORMS** There can be variation in the licensing of different medicines containing the same drug.
  Cutaneous ointment
  CAUTIONARY AND ADVISORY LABELS 28
  ▸ Clobetasol propionate with neomycin sulfate and nystatin (Non-proprietary)
    Clobetasol propionate 500 microgram per 1 gram, Neomycin sulfate 5 mg per 1 gram, Nystatin 100000 unit per 1 gram Clobetasol 500microgram / Neomycin 5mg / Nystatin 100,000units/g ointment | 30 gram PoM £110.13 DT = £110.13
  Cutaneous cream
  CAUTIONARY AND ADVISORY LABELS 28
  ▸ Clobetasol propionate with neomycin sulfate and nystatin (Non-proprietary)
    Clobetasol propionate 500 microgram per 1 gram, Neomycin sulfate 5 mg per 1 gram, Nystatin 100000 unit per 1 gram Clobetasol 500microgram / Neomycin 5mg / Nystatin 100,000units/g cream | 30 gram PoM £110.13 DT = £110.13

Clobetasone butyrate with nystatin and oxytetracycline

08-Oct-2024

The properties listed below are those particular to the combination only. For the properties of the components please consider, clobetasone butyrate p. 1412, oxytetracycline p. 658.

- **INDICATIONS AND DOSE**
  Steroid-responsive dermatoses where candidal or bacterial infection is present
  ▸ TO THE SKIN
  ▸ Adult: (consult product literature)
  POTENCY
  ▸ Clobetasone butyrate is a moderate corticosteroid.

- **INTERACTIONS** → Appendix 1: tetracyclines
- **PATIENT AND CARER ADVICE** Stains clothing.

- **MEDICINAL FORMS** There can be variation in the licensing of different medicines containing the same drug.
  Cutaneous cream
  CAUTIONARY AND ADVISORY LABELS 28
  EXCIPIENTS: May contain Cetostearyl alcohol (including cetyl and stearyl alcohol), chlorocresol, sodium metabisulfite
  ▸ Trimovate (Ennogen Healthcare International Ltd)
    Clobetasone butyrate 500 microgram per 1 gram, Oxytetracycline (as Oxytetracycline calcium) 30 mg per 1 gram, Nystatin 100000 unit per 1 gram Trimovate cream | 30 gram PoM £14.99 DT = £14.99

Hydrocortisone with benzalkonium chloride, dimeticone and nystatin

08-Oct-2024

The properties listed below are those particular to the combination only. For the properties of the components please consider, hydrocortisone p. 1413, dimeticone p. 1403.

● **INDICATIONS AND DOSE**

Mild inflammatory skin disorders such as eczemas associated with infection

▸ TO THE SKIN
▸ Child: Apply 3 times a day until lesion has healed, to be applied thinly
▸ Adult: Apply 3 times a day until lesion has healed, to be applied thinly

POTENCY
▸ Hydrocortisone is a mild corticosteroid.

● INTERACTIONS → Appendix 1: corticosteroids

● **PATIENT AND CARER ADVICE** Patients or carers should be advised on application of hydrocortisone with benzalkonium chloride, dimeticone and nystatin preparations.

● **MEDICINAL FORMS** There can be variation in the licensing of different medicines containing the same drug.

Cutaneous cream
CAUTIONARY AND ADVISORY LABELS 28
EXCIPIENTS: May contain Butylated hydroxyanisole, cetostearyl alcohol (including cetyl and stearyl alcohol), hydroxybenzoates (parabens), sodium metabisulfite, sorbic acid
▸ **Timodine** (Alliance Pharmaceuticals Ltd)
Benzalkonium chloride 1 mg per 1 gram, Hydrocortisone 5 mg per 1 gram, Dimeticone 350 100 mg per 1 gram, Nystatin 100000 unit per 1 gram Timodine cream | 30 gram [PoM] £3.37

Hydrocortisone with chlorhexidine hydrochloride and nystatin

08-Oct-2024

The properties listed below are those particular to the combination only. For the properties of the components please consider, hydrocortisone p. 1413, chlorhexidine p. 1452.

● **INDICATIONS AND DOSE**

Mild inflammatory skin disorders such as eczemas associated with infection

▸ TO THE SKIN
▸ Child: (consult product literature)
▸ Adult: (consult product literature)

POTENCY
▸ Hydrocortisone is a mild corticosteroid.

● INTERACTIONS → Appendix 1: corticosteroids

● **PATIENT AND CARER ADVICE** Patients or carers should be given advice on application of hydrocortisone with chlorhexidine hydrochloride and nystatin preparations.

● **MEDICINAL FORMS** There can be variation in the licensing of different medicines containing the same drug.

Cutaneous ointment
CAUTIONARY AND ADVISORY LABELS 28
▸ **Nystaform HC** (Typharm Ltd)
Chlorhexidine acetate 10 mg per 1 gram, Hydrocortisone 10 mg per 1 gram, Nystatin 100000 unit per 1 gram Nystaform HC ointment | 30 gram [PoM] £9.66 DT = £9.66

Cutaneous cream
CAUTIONARY AND ADVISORY LABELS 28
EXCIPIENTS: May contain Benzyl alcohol, cetostearyl alcohol (including cetyl and stearyl alcohol), polysorbates

▸ **Nystaform HC** (Typharm Ltd)
Hydrocortisone 5 mg per 1 gram, Chlorhexidine hydrochloride 10 mg per 1 gram, Nystatin 100000 unit per 1 gram Nystaform HC cream | 30 gram [PoM] £9.66 DT = £9.66

Hydrocortisone with clotrimazole

08-Oct-2024

The properties listed below are those particular to the combination only. For the properties of the components please consider, hydrocortisone p. 1413, clotrimazole p. 1399.

● **INDICATIONS AND DOSE**

Mild inflammatory skin disorders such as eczemas (associated with fungal infection)

▸ TO THE SKIN
▸ Child: (consult product literature)
▸ Adult: (consult product literature)

POTENCY
▸ Hydrocortisone is a mild corticosteroid.

● INTERACTIONS → Appendix 1: antifungals, azoles · corticosteroids

● **PATIENT AND CARER ADVICE** Patients or carers should be given advice on how to administer hydrocortisone with clotrimazole cream.

● **EXCEPTIONS TO LEGAL CATEGORY** A 15-g tube is on sale to the public for the treatment of athlete's foot and fungal infection of skin folds with associated inflammation in patients 10 years and over.

● **MEDICINAL FORMS** There can be variation in the licensing of different medicines containing the same drug.

Cutaneous cream
CAUTIONARY AND ADVISORY LABELS 28
EXCIPIENTS: May contain Benzyl alcohol, cetostearyl alcohol (including cetyl and stearyl alcohol)
▸ **Canesten HC** (Bayer Plc)
Clotrimazole 10 mg per 1 gram, Hydrocortisone (as Hydrocortisone acetate) 10 mg per 1 gram Canesten HC cream | 30 gram [PoM] £2.42 DT = £2.42

Hydrocortisone with fusidic acid

08-Oct-2024

The properties listed below are those particular to the combination only. For the properties of the components please consider, hydrocortisone p. 1413, fusidic acid p. 663.

● **INDICATIONS AND DOSE**

Mild inflammatory skin disorders such as eczemas associated with infection

▸ TO THE SKIN
▸ Child: (consult product literature)
▸ Adult: (consult product literature)

POTENCY
▸ Hydrocortisone is a mild corticosteroid.

● INTERACTIONS → Appendix 1: corticosteroids · fusidate

● **PATIENT AND CARER ADVICE** Patients or carers should be advised on application of hydrocortisone with fusidic acid preparations.

● **MEDICINAL FORMS** There can be variation in the licensing of different medicines containing the same drug.

Cutaneous cream
CAUTIONARY AND ADVISORY LABELS 28
EXCIPIENTS: May contain Butylated hydroxyanisole, cetostearyl alcohol (including cetyl and stearyl alcohol), polysorbates, potassium sorbate
▸ **Fucidin H (Fusidic acid / Hydrocortisone)** (LEO Pharma)
Hydrocortisone acetate 10 mg per 1 gram, Fusidic acid 20 mg per 1 gram Fucidin H cream | 30 gram [PoM] £6.02 DT = £6.02 | 60 gram [PoM] £12.05 DT = £12.05

Hydrocortisone with miconazole

08-Oct-2024

The properties listed below are those particular to the combination only. For the properties of the components please consider, hydrocortisone p. 1413, miconazole p. 1400.

● **INDICATIONS AND DOSE**

Mild inflammatory skin disorders such as eczemas associated with infections
▶ TO THE SKIN
▶ Adult: (consult product literature)
POTENCY
▶ Hydrocortisone is a mild corticosteroid.

● INTERACTIONS → Appendix 1: antifungals, azoles · corticosteroids

● PATIENT AND CARER ADVICE Patients or carers should be advised on application of hydrocortisone with miconazole preparations.

● PROFESSION SPECIFIC INFORMATION

Dental practitioners' formulary May be prescribed as Miconazole and Hydrocortisone Cream or Ointment for max. 7 days.

● EXCEPTIONS TO LEGAL CATEGORY A 15-g tube of hydrocortisone with miconazole cream is on sale to the public for the treatment of athlete's foot and candidal intertrigo.

● MEDICINAL FORMS There can be variation in the licensing of different medicines containing the same drug.

Cutaneous cream

CAUTIONARY AND ADVISORY LABELS 28
EXCIPIENTS: May contain Butylated hydroxyanisole, disodium edetate
▶ Daktacort (McNeil Products Ltd)
Hydrocortisone 10 mg per 1 gram, Miconazole nitrate 20 mg per 1 gram Daktacort Hydrocortisone cream | 15 gram [P] £5.05 DT = £5.05

Hydrocortisone with oxytetracycline

08-Oct-2024

The properties listed below are those particular to the combination only. For the properties of the components please consider, hydrocortisone p. 1413, oxytetracycline p. 658.

● **INDICATIONS AND DOSE**

Mild inflammatory skin disorders such as eczemas
▶ TO THE SKIN
▶ Child 12-17 years: (consult product literature)
▶ Adult: (consult product literature)
POTENCY
▶ Hydrocortisone is a mild corticosteroid.

● INTERACTIONS → Appendix 1: corticosteroids · tetracyclines

● PREGNANCY Tetracyclines should not be given to pregnant women. Effects on skeletal development have been documented when tetracyclines have been used in the first trimester in animal studies. Administration during the second or third trimester may cause discoloration of the child's teeth.

● BREAST FEEDING Tetracyclines should not be given to women who are breast-feeding (although absorption and therefore discoloration of teeth in the infant is probably usually prevented by chelation with calcium in milk).

● PATIENT AND CARER ADVICE Patients should be given advice on the application of hydrocortisone with oxytetracycline ointment.

● MEDICINAL FORMS There can be variation in the licensing of different medicines containing the same drug.

Cutaneous ointment

CAUTIONARY AND ADVISORY LABELS 28
▶ Terra-Cortril (Esteve Pharmaceuticals Ltd)
Hydrocortisone 10 mg per 1 gram, Oxytetracycline (as Oxytetracycline hydrochloride) 30 mg per 1 gram Terra-Cortril ointment | 30 gram [PoM] £5.01 DT = £5.01

DERMATOLOGICAL DRUGS > ANTI-INFECTIVES

Ichthammol

● **INDICATIONS AND DOSE**

Chronic lichenified eczema
▶ TO THE SKIN
▶ Child 1–17 years: Apply 1–3 times a day
▶ Adult: Apply 1–3 times a day

● UNLICENSED USE
▶ In children No information available.

● SIDE-EFFECTS Skin irritation

● MEDICINAL FORMS Forms available from special-order manufacturers include: cutaneous ointment, cutaneous paste

Ichthammol with zinc oxide

The properties listed below are those particular to the combination only. For the properties of the components please consider, ichthammol above.

● **INDICATIONS AND DOSE**

Chronic lichenified eczema
▶ TO THE SKIN
▶ Adult: (consult product literature)

● MEDICINAL FORMS There can be variation in the licensing of different medicines containing the same drug. Forms available from special-order manufacturers include: cutaneous cream, cutaneous ointment

Impregnated dressing

▶ Ichthopaste (Evolan Pharma AB)
Ichthopaste bandage 7.5cm × 6m | 1 bandage £4.03

DERMATOLOGICAL DRUGS > ANTRACEN DERIVATIVES

Dithranol

23-Nov-2020

(Anthralin)

● **INDICATIONS AND DOSE**

Subacute and chronic psoriasis
▶ TO THE SKIN
▶ Adult: (consult product literature)

● CONTRA-INDICATIONS Acute and pustular psoriasis · hypersensitivity

● CAUTIONS Avoid sensitive areas of skin · avoid use near eyes

● SIDE-EFFECTS Skin reactions

● PREGNANCY No adverse effects reported.

● BREAST FEEDING No adverse effects reported.

● DIRECTIONS FOR ADMINISTRATION When applying dithranol, manufacturer advises hands should be protected by gloves or they should be washed thoroughly afterwards. Dithranol should be applied to chronic extensor plaques only, carefully avoiding normal skin.

● PRESCRIBING AND DISPENSING INFORMATION Treatment should be started with a low concentration such as dithranol 0.1%, and the strength increased gradually every few days up to 3%, according to tolerance.

- **PATIENT AND CARER ADVICE** Dithranol can stain the skin, hair and fabrics.

- **EXCEPTIONS TO LEGAL CATEGORY** Prescription only medicine if dithranol content more than 1%, otherwise may be sold to the public.

- **MEDICINAL FORMS** There can be variation in the licensing of different medicines containing the same drug. Forms available from special-order manufacturers include: cutaneous ointment

Cutaneous ointment
CAUTIONARY AND ADVISORY LABELS 28

Combinations available: *Coal tar with dithranol and salicylic acid*, p. 1420

Dithranol with salicylic acid and zinc oxide

The properties listed below are those particular to the combination only. For the properties of the components please consider, dithranol p. 1418, salicylic acid p. 1460.

- **INDICATIONS AND DOSE**

Subacute and chronic psoriasis
- ► TO THE SKIN
- ► Adult: (consult local protocol)

- **MEDICINAL FORMS** There can be variation in the licensing of different medicines containing the same drug. Forms available from special-order manufacturers include: cutaneous ointment, paste

Paste
CAUTIONARY AND ADVISORY LABELS 28

DERMATOLOGICAL DRUGS > TARS

Coal tar

01-Sep-2020

- **INDICATIONS AND DOSE**

Psoriasis | Scaly scalp disorders such as psoriasis, eczema, seborrhoeic dermatitis and dandruff
- ► TO THE SKIN
- ► Child: (consult product literature)
- ► Adult: (consult product literature)

- **CONTRA-INDICATIONS** Avoid broken or inflamed skin · avoid eye area · avoid genital area · avoid mucosal areas · avoid rectal area · infection · sore, acute, or pustular psoriasis

- **CAUTIONS**

GENERAL CAUTIONS Application to face

SPECIFIC CAUTIONS
- ► When used for Scaly scalp disorders, using shampoo Children under 12 years (consult product literature)

- **SIDE-EFFECTS** Photosensitivity reaction · skin reactions

- **PRESCRIBING AND DISPENSING INFORMATION** Coal Tar Solution BP contains coal tar 20%, Strong Coal Tar Solution BP contains coal tar 40%.

- **HANDLING AND STORAGE** Use suitable chemical protection gloves for extemporaneous preparation. May stain skin, hair and fabric.

- **PATIENT AND CARER ADVICE** May stain skin, hair and fabric.

- **MEDICINAL FORMS** There can be variation in the licensing of different medicines containing the same drug. Forms available from special-order manufacturers include: cutaneous cream, cutaneous ointment, paste

Cutaneous emulsion
EXCIPIENTS: May contain Hydroxybenzoates (parabens)
- ► **Exorex** (Teva UK Ltd)
  Coal tar solution 50 mg per 1 gram Exorex lotion | 100 ml GSL £8.11 DT = £8.11 | 250 ml GSL £16.24 DT = £16.24

Shampoo
EXCIPIENTS: May contain Fragrances, hydroxybenzoates (parabens)
- ► **Neutrogena T/Gel Therapeutic** (Johnson & Johnson Ltd)
  Coal tar extract 20 mg per 1 gram Neutrogena T/Gel Therapeutic shampoo | 125 ml GSL £4.36 DT = £4.36 | 250 ml GSL £6.61 DT = £6.61
- ► **Polytar Scalp** (Thornton & Ross Ltd)
  Coal tar solution 40 mg per 1 ml Polytar Scalp shampoo | 150 ml GSL £7.57 DT = £7.57
- ► **Psoriderm** (Dermal Laboratories Ltd)
  Coal tar distilled 25 mg per 1 ml Psoriderm scalp lotion | 250 ml P £4.74 DT = £4.74

Cutaneous cream
EXCIPIENTS: May contain Isopropyl palmitate, lecithin, propylene glycol
- ► **Psoriderm** (Dermal Laboratories Ltd)
  Coal tar distilled 60 mg per 1 gram Psoriderm cream | 225 ml P £9.42 DT = £9.42

Coal tar with calamine

15-Jan-2019

The properties listed below are those particular to the combination only. For the properties of the components please consider, coal tar above.

- **INDICATIONS AND DOSE**

Psoriasis | Chronic atopic eczema (occasionally)
- ► TO THE SKIN
- ► Adult: Apply 1–2 times a day

> **IMPORTANT SAFETY INFORMATION**
>
> MHRA/CHM ADVICE (UPDATED DECEMBER 2018): EMOLLIENTS: NEW INFORMATION ABOUT RISK OF SEVERE AND FATAL BURNS WITH PARAFFIN-CONTAINING AND PARAFFIN-FREE EMOLLIENTS See Emollient and barrier preparations p. 1387.

- **PRESCRIBING AND DISPENSING INFORMATION** When prepared extemporaneously, the BP states Calamine and Coal Tar Ointment BP, consists of calamine 12.5 g, strong coal tar solution 2.5 g, zinc oxide 12.5 g, hydrous wool fat 25 g, white soft paraffin 47.5 g.

- **MEDICINAL FORMS** No licensed medicines listed.

Coal tar with coconut oil and salicylic acid

19-Mar-2020

The properties listed below are those particular to the combination only. For the properties of the components please consider, coal tar above, salicylic acid p. 1460.

- **INDICATIONS AND DOSE**

Scaly scalp disorders | Psoriasis | Seborrhoeic dermatitis | Dandruff | Cradle cap
- ► TO THE SKIN USING SHAMPOO
- ► Child: Apply daily as required
- ► Adult: Apply daily as required

- **MEDICINAL FORMS** There can be variation in the licensing of different medicines containing the same drug.

Shampoo
- ► **Capasal** (Dermal Laboratories Ltd)
  Salicylic acid 5 mg per 1 gram, Coal tar distilled 10 mg per 1 gram, Coconut oil 10 mg per 1 gram Capasal Therapeutic shampoo | 250 ml P £5.29

Coal tar with dithranol and salicylic acid

The properties listed below are those particular to the combination only. For the properties of the components please consider, coal tar p. 1419, dithranol p. 1418, salicylic acid p. 1460.

● **INDICATIONS AND DOSE**

Subacute and chronic psoriasis
▸ TO THE SKIN
▸ Child: Apply up to twice daily
▸ Adult: Apply up to twice daily

● UNLICENSED USE *Psorin®* is licensed for use in children (age range not specified by manufacturer).

● MEDICINAL FORMS Forms available from special-order manufacturers include: cutaneous ointment

Coal tar with salicylic acid
16-Jan-2019

The properties listed below are those particular to the combination only. For the properties of the components please consider, coal tar p. 1419, salicylic acid p. 1460.

● **INDICATIONS AND DOSE**

Psoriasis | Chronic atopic eczema
▸ TO THE SKIN USING OINTMENT
▸ Adult: Apply 1–2 times a day

IMPORTANT SAFETY INFORMATION
MHRA/CHM ADVICE (UPDATED DECEMBER 2018): EMOLLIENTS: NEW INFORMATION ABOUT RISK OF SEVERE AND FATAL BURNS WITH PARAFFIN-CONTAINING AND PARAFFIN-FREE EMOLLIENTS
See Emollient and barrier preparations p. 1387.

● PRESCRIBING AND DISPENSING INFORMATION When prepared extemporaneously, the BP states Coal Tar and Salicylic Acid Ointment, BP consists of coal tar 2 g, salicylic acid 2 g, emulsifying wax 11.4 g, white soft paraffin 19 g, coconut oil 54 g, polysorbate '80' 4 g, liquid paraffin 7.6 g.

● MEDICINAL FORMS There can be variation in the licensing of different medicines containing the same drug. Forms available from special-order manufacturers include: cutaneous ointment
Cutaneous ointment
CAUTIONARY AND ADVISORY LABELS 15
EXCIPIENTS: May contain Cetostearyl alcohol (including cetyl and stearyl alcohol)

Coal tar with salicylic acid and precipitated sulfur
20-Mar-2020

The properties listed below are those particular to the combination only. For the properties of the components please consider, coal tar p. 1419, salicylic acid p. 1460.

● **INDICATIONS AND DOSE**

COCOIS® OINTMENT
Scaly scalp disorders including psoriasis, eczema, seborrhoeic dermatitis and dandruff
▸ TO THE SKIN USING SCALP OINTMENT
▸ Child 6-11 years: Medical supervision required
▸ Child 12-17 years: Apply once weekly as required, alternatively apply daily for the first 3–7 days (if severe), shampoo off after 1 hour
▸ Adult: Apply once weekly as required, alternatively apply daily for the first 3–7 days (if severe), shampoo off after 1 hour

SEBCO® OINTMENT
Scaly scalp disorders including psoriasis, eczema, seborrhoeic dermatitis and dandruff
▸ TO THE SKIN USING SCALP OINTMENT
▸ Child 6-11 years: Medical supervision required
▸ Child 12-17 years: Apply as required, alternatively apply daily for the first 3–7 days (if severe), shampoo off after 1 hour
▸ Adult: Apply as required, alternatively apply daily for the first 3–7 days (if severe), shampoo off after 1 hour

● MEDICINAL FORMS There can be variation in the licensing of different medicines containing the same drug.
Cutaneous ointment
EXCIPIENTS: May contain Cetostearyl alcohol (including cetyl and stearyl alcohol)
▸ Cocois (RPH Pharmaceuticals AB)
Salicylic acid 20 mg per 1 gram, Sulfur precipitated 40 mg per 1 gram, Coal tar solution 120 mg per 1 gram Cocois ointment | 40 gram GSL £9.35 | 100 gram GSL £14.50
▸ Sebco (Derma UK Ltd)
Salicylic acid 20 mg per 1 gram, Sulfur precipitated 40 mg per 1 gram, Coal tar solution 120 mg per 1 gram Sebco ointment | 40 gram GSL £10.41 | 100 gram GSL £15.88

Coal tar with zinc oxide
16-Jan-2019

The properties listed below are those particular to the combination only. For the properties of the components please consider, coal tar p. 1419.

● **INDICATIONS AND DOSE**

Psoriasis | Chronic atopic eczema
▸ TO THE SKIN
▸ Child: Apply 1–2 times a day
▸ Adult: Apply 1–2 times a day

IMPORTANT SAFETY INFORMATION
MHRA/CHM ADVICE (UPDATED DECEMBER 2018): EMOLLIENTS: NEW INFORMATION ABOUT RISK OF SEVERE AND FATAL BURNS WITH PARAFFIN-CONTAINING AND PARAFFIN-FREE EMOLLIENTS
See Emollient and barrier preparations p. 1387.

● PRESCRIBING AND DISPENSING INFORMATION No preparations available—when prepared extemporaneously, the BP states Zinc and Coal Tar Paste, BP consists of zinc oxide 6%, coal tar 6%, emulsifying wax 5%, starch 38%, yellow soft paraffin 45%.

● MEDICINAL FORMS There can be variation in the licensing of different medicines containing the same drug. Forms available from special-order manufacturers include: cutaneous ointment, cutaneous paste
Cutaneous ointment
CAUTIONARY AND ADVISORY LABELS 15
Cutaneous paste
CAUTIONARY AND ADVISORY LABELS 15

IMMUNOSUPPRESSANTS › CALCINEURIN INHIBITORS AND RELATED DRUGS

Pimecrolimus
20-Oct-2020

● **INDICATIONS AND DOSE**

Short-term treatment of mild to moderate atopic eczema (including flares) when topical corticosteroids cannot be used (initiated by a specialist)
▸ TO THE SKIN
▸ Adult: Apply twice daily until symptoms resolve (stop treatment if eczema worsens or no response after 6 weeks)

Short-term treatment of facial, flexural, or genital psoriasis in patients unresponsive to, or intolerant of other topical therapy (initiated by a specialist)
▸ TO THE SKIN
▸ Adult: Apply twice daily until symptoms resolve (maximum duration of treatment 4 weeks)

● UNLICENSED USE Pimecrolimus is not licensed for short-term treatment of facial, flexural, or genital psoriasis in patients unresponsive to, or intolerant of other topical therapy.

● CONTRA-INDICATIONS Application to malignant or potentially malignant skin lesions · application under occlusion · congenital epidermal barrier defects · contact with eyes · contact with mucous membranes · generalised erythroderma · immunodeficiency · infection at treatment site

● CAUTIONS Alcohol consumption (risk of facial flushing and skin irritation) · avoid other topical treatments except emollients at treatment site · UV light (avoid excessive exposure to sunlight and sunlamps)

● INTERACTIONS → Appendix 1: pimecrolimus

● SIDE-EFFECTS
▸ **Common or very common** Increased risk of infection
▸ **Uncommon** Neoplasms
▸ **Rare or very rare** Skin discolouration
▸ **Frequency not known** Lymphadenopathy · malignancy

● PREGNANCY Manufacturer advises avoid; toxicity in *animal* studies following systemic administration.

● BREAST FEEDING Manufacturer advises caution; ensure infant does not come in contact with treated areas.

● NATIONAL FUNDING/ACCESS DECISIONS
For full details see funding body website
NICE decisions
▸ Tacrolimus and pimecrolimus for atopic eczema [for patients with mild atopic eczema or as first-line treatment for atopic eczema of any severity] (August 2004) NICE TA82 Not recommended

● MEDICINAL FORMS There can be variation in the licensing of different medicines containing the same drug.
Cutaneous cream
CAUTIONARY AND ADVISORY LABELS 4, 11, 28
EXCIPIENTS: May contain Benzyl alcohol, cetostearyl alcohol (including cetyl and stearyl alcohol), propylene glycol
▸ **Elidel** (Viatris UK Healthcare Ltd)
Pimecrolimus 10 mg per 1 gram Elidel 1% cream | 30 gram PoM
£19.69 DT = £19.69 | 60 gram PoM £37.41 DT = £37.41 |
100 gram PoM £59.07 DT = £59.07

| Tacrolimus
　　　　　　　　　　　　　　　　　　　　　27-Sep-2024
● DRUG ACTION Tacrolimus is a calcineurin inhibitor.

● **INDICATIONS AND DOSE**
Short-term treatment of moderate to severe atopic eczema (including flares) in patients unresponsive to, or intolerant of conventional therapy (initiated by a specialist)
▸ TO THE SKIN
▸ Adult: Apply twice daily until lesion clears (consider other treatment if eczema worsens or no improvement after 2 weeks), initially 0.1% ointment to be applied thinly, reduce frequency to once daily or strength of ointment to 0.03% if condition allows

Prevention of flares in patients with moderate to severe atopic eczema and 4 or more flares a year who have responded to initial treatment with topical tacrolimus (initiated by a specialist)
▸ TO THE SKIN
▸ Adult: Apply twice weekly, 0.1% ointment to be applied thinly, with an interval of 2–3 days between applications, use short-term treatment regimen during an acute flare; review need for preventative therapy after 1 year

Short-term treatment of facial, flexural, or genital psoriasis in patients unresponsive to, or intolerant of other topical therapy (initiated under specialist supervision)
▸ TO THE SKIN
▸ Adult: Apply twice daily until symptoms resolve, 0.1% ointment to be applied thinly, reduce to once daily or switch to 0.03% ointment if condition allows, maximum duration of treatment 4 weeks

● UNLICENSED USE Short-term treatment of facial, flexural, or genital psoriasis is unlicensed.

● CONTRA-INDICATIONS Application to malignant or potentially malignant skin lesions · application under occlusion · avoid contact with eyes · avoid contact with mucous membranes · congenital epidermal barrier defects · generalised erythroderma · immunodeficiency · infection at treatment site

● CAUTIONS UV light (avoid excessive exposure to sunlight and sunlamps)

● INTERACTIONS → Appendix 1: tacrolimus

● SIDE-EFFECTS
▸ **Common or very common** Alcohol intolerance · increased risk of infection · sensation abnormal · skin reactions
▸ **Uncommon** Lymphadenopathy
▸ **Frequency not known** Malignancy · neoplasms

● ALLERGY AND CROSS-SENSITIVITY EvGr Contra-indicated if history of hypersensitivity to macrolides. Ⓜ

● PREGNANCY Specialist sources indicate that use can be considered if benefit outweighs potential risk—minimal systemic absorption; limited information available.

● BREAST FEEDING Specialist sources indicate present in milk (following systemic administration) but amount probably too small to be harmful—monitor exclusively breastfed infants, including blood concentrations, if there are concerns regarding toxicity.

● HEPATIC IMPAIRMENT Manufacturer advises caution in hepatic failure.

● PATIENT AND CARER ADVICE Advise patients to avoid excessive exposure to UV light including sunlight and to report symptoms of eye disorders for prompt evaluation by an ophthalmologist.

● NATIONAL FUNDING/ACCESS DECISIONS
For full details see funding body website
NICE decisions
▸ Tacrolimus and pimecrolimus for atopic eczema (August 2004) NICE TA82 Recommended
Scottish Medicines Consortium (SMC) decisions
▸ Tacrolimus 0.1% ointment (*Protopic*®) for moderate to severe atopic dermatitis in patients aged 16 years and over (April 2010) SMC No. 609/10 Recommended with restrictions

● **MEDICINAL FORMS** There can be variation in the licensing of different medicines containing the same drug.

Cutaneous ointment

CAUTIONARY AND ADVISORY LABELS 4, 11, 28
EXCIPIENTS: May contain Beeswax

▸ **Tacrolimus (Non-proprietary)**
Tacrolimus (as Tacrolimus monohydrate) 1 mg per 1 gram Tacrolimus 0.1% ointment | 30 gram PoM £25.46–£31.25 DT = £18.78 | 60 gram PoM £41.76–£47.27 DT = £37.56

▸ **Protopic** (LEO Pharma)
Tacrolimus (as Tacrolimus monohydrate) 300 microgram per 1 gram Protopic 0.03% ointment | 30 gram PoM £23.33 DT = £23.33 | 60 gram PoM £42.55 DT = £42.55
Tacrolimus (as Tacrolimus monohydrate) 1 mg per 1 gram Protopic 0.1% ointment | 30 gram PoM £25.92 DT = £18.78 | 60 gram PoM £47.28 DT = £37.56

IMMUNOSUPPRESSANTS ⟩ INTERLEUKIN INHIBITORS

Bimekizumab

30-Apr-2025

● **DRUG ACTION** Bimekizumab is a humanised monoclonal antibody that binds with high affinity to interleukin-17A, 17F and 17AF to block the activity of pro-inflammatory cytokines.

● **INDICATIONS AND DOSE**

Moderate-to-severe plaque psoriasis (under expert supervision)
▸ BY SUBCUTANEOUS INJECTION
▸ Adult: 320 mg every 4 weeks for 5 doses (at weeks 0, 4, 8, 12 and 16), followed by maintenance 320 mg every 8 weeks, patients weighing ≥ 120 kg who do not achieve completely clear skin after 16 weeks of treatment may be considered for maintenance dosing of 320 mg every 4 weeks

Psoriatic arthritis (under expert supervision) | Ankylosing spondylitis (under expert supervision) | Non-radiographic axial spondyloarthritis (under expert supervision)
▸ BY SUBCUTANEOUS INJECTION
▸ Adult: 160 mg every 4 weeks

Psoriatic arthritis with concomitant moderate-to-severe plaque psoriasis (under expert supervision)
▸ BY SUBCUTANEOUS INJECTION
▸ Adult: 320 mg every 4 weeks for 5 doses (at weeks 0, 4, 8, 12 and 16), followed by maintenance 320 mg every 8 weeks, if clinical response in joints cannot be maintained after 16 weeks of treatment, consider a dose of 160 mg every 4 weeks. Patients weighing ≥ 120 kg who do not achieve completely clear skin after 16 weeks of treatment may be considered for a dose of 320 mg every 4 weeks

Hidradenitis suppurativa (under expert supervision)
▸ BY SUBCUTANEOUS INJECTION
▸ Adult: 320 mg every 2 weeks up to week 16, followed by maintenance 320 mg every 4 weeks

● **CONTRA-INDICATIONS** Clinically significant active infection · inflammatory bowel disease

● **CAUTIONS** Chronic infection · history of recurrent infection

CAUTIONS, FURTHER INFORMATION
▸ Infection EvGr Consider anti-tuberculosis therapy before initiation of bimekizumab in patients with a history of tuberculosis in whom an adequate course of treatment cannot be confirmed.

  Consider completing appropriate immunisations according to current guidelines before starting. Ⓜ

● **INTERACTIONS** → Appendix 1: monoclonal antibodies

● **SIDE-EFFECTS**
▸ **Common or very common** Fatigue · headache · increased risk of infection · skin reactions
▸ **Uncommon** Conjunctivitis · inflammatory bowel disease · neutropenia

● **CONCEPTION AND CONTRACEPTION** EvGr Females of childbearing potential should use effective contraception during treatment and for at least 17 weeks after last treatment. Ⓜ

● **PREGNANCY** EvGr Avoid—no information available. Ⓜ

● **BREAST FEEDING** Specialist sources indicate use with caution, especially if breast-feeding a neonate or preterm infant (no information available). Large molecular weight suggests limited excretion into milk and drug molecule likely to be partially destroyed in the infant's gastro-intestinal tract.

● **PRE-TREATMENT SCREENING** EvGr Patients should be evaluated for tuberculosis infection before treatment. Ⓜ

● **MONITORING REQUIREMENTS** EvGr Monitor for signs and symptoms of infection (suspend treatment if infection is clinically significant or unresponsive to treatment). Ⓜ

● **DIRECTIONS FOR ADMINISTRATION** EvGr Inject into the thigh, abdomen or upper arm and rotate injection site; avoid injecting into areas of the skin that are tender, bruised, or affected by psoriasis. Patients may self-administer *Bimzelx®*, after appropriate training in subcutaneous injection technique. Ⓜ

● **PRESCRIBING AND DISPENSING INFORMATION** EvGr Consider discontinuing treatment if there is no response after 16 weeks. Ⓜ

  Bimekizumab is a biological medicine. Biological medicines must be prescribed and dispensed by brand name, see *Biological medicines* and *Biosimilar medicines*, under Guidance on prescribing p. 1; record the brand name and batch number after each administration.

● **HANDLING AND STORAGE** EvGr Store in a refrigerator (2–8°C) and protect from light. Once removed from refrigerator, may be stored at room temperature for 25 days, then discarded. Ⓜ

● **PATIENT AND CARER ADVICE** Patients and their carers should be advised to seek medical attention if signs or symptoms of infection occur.

● **NATIONAL FUNDING/ACCESS DECISIONS**
For full details see funding body website

NICE decisions
▸ **Bimekizumab for treating moderate to severe plaque psoriasis (September 2021)** NICE TA723 Recommended with restrictions
▸ **Bimekizumab for treating active psoriatic arthritis (October 2023)** NICE TA916 Recommended with restrictions
▸ **Bimekizumab for treating axial spondyloarthritis (October 2023)** NICE TA918 Recommended with restrictions

Scottish Medicines Consortium (SMC) decisions
▸ **Bimekizumab (*Bimzelx®*) for the treatment of moderate to severe plaque psoriasis in adults who are candidates for systemic therapy (November 2021)** SMC No. SMC2410 Recommended with restrictions
▸ **Bimekizumab (*Bimzelx®*), alone or in combination with methotrexate, for the treatment of active psoriatic arthritis in adults who have had an inadequate response or who have been intolerant to one or more disease-modifying antirheumatic drugs (November 2023)** SMC No. SMC2605 Recommended with restrictions
▸ **Bimekizumab (*Bimzelx®*) for the treatment of adults with active non-radiographic axial spondyloarthritis with objective signs of inflammation as indicated by elevated C-reactive protein and/or magnetic resonance imaging who have responded inadequately or are intolerant to NSAIDs, and adults with active ankylosing spondylitis who have responded

inadequately or are intolerant to conventional therapy (December 2023) SMC No. SMC2616 Recommended

▶ Bimekizumab (*Bimzelx*®) for the treatment of active moderate to severe hidradenitis suppurativa (HS) in adults with an inadequate response to conventional systemic HS therapy (April 2025) SMC No. SMC2698 Recommended with restrictions

● **MEDICINAL FORMS** There can be variation in the licensing of different medicines containing the same drug.

Solution for injection
EXCIPIENTS: May contain Polysorbates

▶ **Bimzelx** (UCB Pharma Ltd) ▼

Bimekizumab 160 mg per 1 ml Bimzelx 320mg/2ml solution for injection pre-filled syringes | 1 pre-filled disposable injection [PoM] £2,443.00 (Hospital only)
Bimzelx 160mg/1ml solution for injection pre-filled syringes | 2 pre-filled disposable injection [PoM] £2,443.00 (Hospital only)
Bimzelx 320mg/2ml solution for injection pre-filled pens | 1 pre-filled disposable injection [PoM] £2,443.00 (Hospital only)
Bimzelx 160mg/1ml solution for injection pre-filled pens | 2 pre-filled disposable injection [PoM] £2,443.00 (Hospital only)

Brodalumab
03-Nov-2020

● **DRUG ACTION** Brodalumab is a recombinant human monoclonal antibody that binds with high affinity to interleukin-17RA and blocks the activity of pro-inflammatory cytokines.

● **INDICATIONS AND DOSE**

Moderate-to-severe plaque psoriasis (under expert supervision)

▶ BY SUBCUTANEOUS INJECTION

▸ Adult: 210 mg every week for 3 doses, followed by 210 mg every 2 weeks, consider discontinuing treatment if no response after 16 weeks

● **CONTRA-INDICATIONS** Active Crohn's disease · clinically significant active infection

● **CAUTIONS** Chronic infection · history of Crohn's disease (monitor for exacerbations) · history of depressive disorders (discontinue if new or worsening symptoms develop) · history of recurrent infection · history of suicidal ideation or behaviour (discontinue if new or worsening symptoms develop)

CAUTIONS, FURTHER INFORMATION

▸ Infection Manufacturer advises to consider anti-tuberculosis therapy for patients with latent tuberculosis before starting treatment with brodalumab.
  Manufacturer advises patients should be brought up-to-date with current immunisation schedule before initiating treatment.

● **INTERACTIONS** → Appendix 1: monoclonal antibodies

● **SIDE-EFFECTS**

▸ **Common or very common** Arthralgia · diarrhoea · fatigue · headache · increased risk of infection · myalgia · nausea · oropharyngeal pain

▸ **Uncommon** Conjunctivitis

▸ **Rare or very rare** Anaphylactic reaction

▸ **Frequency not known** Meningitis cryptococcal · suicidal behaviours

● **CONCEPTION AND CONTRACEPTION** Manufacturer advises that women of childbearing potential should use effective contraception during treatment and for at least 12 weeks after stopping treatment.

● **PREGNANCY** Manufacturer advises avoid—limited information available.

● **BREAST FEEDING** Manufacturer advises avoid—no information available.

● **DIRECTIONS FOR ADMINISTRATION** Manufacturer advises to take the syringe out of the refrigerator at least

30 minutes before administration, and to avoid injecting into areas of the skin that are tender, bruised, or affected by psoriasis. Patients may self-administer *Kyntheum*®, after appropriate training in subcutaneous injection technique.

● **PRESCRIBING AND DISPENSING INFORMATION** Brodalumab is a biological medicine. Biological medicines must be prescribed and dispensed by brand name, see *Biological medicines* and *Biosimilar medicines*, under Guidance on prescribing p. 1; manufacturer advises to record the brand name and batch number after each administration.

● **HANDLING AND STORAGE** Manufacturer advises store in a refrigerator (2–8°C) and protect from light—consult product literature for further information regarding storage outside refrigerator.

● **PATIENT AND CARER ADVICE** Manufacturer advises patients and their carers should be given training in subcutaneous injection technique. Manufacturer advises patients and their carers should seek medical advice if new or worsening symptoms of depression, suicidal ideation, or behaviour occur; they should also be advised to report signs and symptoms of infection.

● **NATIONAL FUNDING/ACCESS DECISIONS**
For full details see funding body website

NICE decisions

▶ **Brodalumab for treating moderate to severe plaque psoriasis (March 2018)** NICE TA511 Recommended with restrictions

Scottish Medicines Consortium (SMC) decisions

▶ Brodalumab (*Kyntheum*®) for the treatment of moderate-to-severe plaque psoriasis in adult patients who are candidates for systemic therapy (May 2018) SMC No. 1283/17 Recommended with restrictions

● **MEDICINAL FORMS** There can be variation in the licensing of different medicines containing the same drug.

Solution for injection

▶ **Kyntheum** (LEO Pharma)
Brodalumab 140 mg per 1 ml Kyntheum 210mg/1.5ml solution for injection pre-filled syringes | 2 pre-filled disposable injection [PoM] £1,280.00 (Hospital only)

Dupilumab
24-Feb-2025

● **DRUG ACTION** Dupilumab is a recombinant human monoclonal antibody that inhibits interleukin-4 and interleukin-13 signaling.

● **INDICATIONS AND DOSE**

Moderate-to-severe atopic eczema (initiated by a specialist)

▶ BY SUBCUTANEOUS INJECTION

▸ Adult: Initially 600 mg, to be administered as two consecutive 300 mg injections at different injection sites, followed by 300 mg every 2 weeks, review treatment if no response after 16 weeks

Severe asthma with type 2 inflammation [add-on maintenance therapy] (initiated by a specialist)

▶ BY SUBCUTANEOUS INJECTION

▸ Adult: Initially 400 mg, to be administered as two consecutive 200 mg injections at different injection sites, followed by 200 mg every 2 weeks, review need for treatment yearly

continued →

Severe asthma with type 2 inflammation [add-on maintenance therapy for patients currently treated with oral corticosteroids or patients with co-morbid moderate-to-severe atopic eczema or patients with co-morbid severe chronic rhinosinusitis with nasal polyps] (initiated by a specialist)

▶ BY SUBCUTANEOUS INJECTION

▶ Adult: Initially 600 mg, to be administered as two consecutive 300 mg injections at different injection sites, followed by 300 mg every 2 weeks, review need for treatment yearly

Uncontrolled chronic obstructive pulmonary disease [add-on maintenance therapy] (initiated by a specialist)

▶ BY SUBCUTANEOUS INJECTION

▶ Adult: 300 mg every 2 weeks, review treatment if no response after 52 weeks

Severe chronic rhinosinusitis with nasal polyps [add-on therapy] (initiated by a specialist)

▶ BY SUBCUTANEOUS INJECTION

▶ Adult: Initially 300 mg, followed by 300 mg every 2 weeks, review treatment if no response after 24 weeks

Eosinophilic oesophagitis (initiated by a specialist)

▶ BY SUBCUTANEOUS INJECTION

▶ Adult (body-weight 40 kg and above): 300 mg once weekly

Moderate-to-severe prurigo nodularis (initiated by a specialist)

▶ BY SUBCUTANEOUS INJECTION

▶ Adult: Initially 600 mg, to be administered as two consecutive 300 mg injections at different injection sites, followed by 300 mg every 2 weeks, review treatment if no response after 24 weeks

---

IMPORTANT SAFETY INFORMATION

MHRA/CHM ADVICE: DUPILUMAB (*DUPIXENT*®): RISK OF OCULAR ADVERSE REACTIONS AND NEED FOR PROMPT MANAGEMENT (NOVEMBER 2022)

The MHRA, with input from independent advisers, has reviewed the risk of dry eye and serious ocular side-effects associated with dupilumab. In patients with atopic eczema especially, common ocular side-effects include conjunctivitis, allergic conjunctivitis, eye pruritus, blepharitis, and dry eye; infrequent cases of keratitis and ulcerative keratitis have also been reported. Most ocular reactions associated with dupilumab in the UK are mild and can be managed, but it is not currently possible to predict who may experience the rarer, severe reactions; early review and intervention in ocular reactions are therefore recommended.

Healthcare professionals are advised to:
- discuss with patients or their carers the possibility of ocular side-effects and the symptoms to look out for when initiating dupilumab;
- advise patients or their carers to report new-onset or worsening eye symptoms to a healthcare professional, rather than self-managing symptoms;
- promptly review new-onset or worsening ocular symptoms, and refer patients for ophthalmological examination if necessary (for example, cases of possible keratitis, and conjunctivitis or dry eye that does not resolve after treatment);
- urgently review patients with sudden changes in vision or significant eye pain that does not settle.

● CAUTIONS Helminth infection

CAUTIONS, FURTHER INFORMATION

▶ Risk of infection Dupilumab may influence the immune response to helminth infections. Resolve pre-existing infection before initiating treatment; suspend treatment if resistant infection develops during therapy.

Manufacturer advises patients should be brought up-to-date with live and live attenuated vaccines before initiating treatment.

● INTERACTIONS → Appendix 1: monoclonal antibodies

● SIDE-EFFECTS

▶ **Common or very common** Arthralgia · dry eye · eosinophilia · eye inflammation · eye pruritus · increased risk of infection

▶ **Uncommon** Angioedema · facial rash

▶ **Rare or very rare** Hypersensitivity

▶ **Frequency not known** Pneumonia eosinophilic · vasculitis

SIDE-EFFECTS, FURTHER INFORMATION **Eosinophilic granulomatosis with polyangiitis (Churg-Strauss syndrome)** Churg-Strauss syndrome has occurred in adult patients given dupilumab; the reaction may be associated with the reduction of oral corticosteroid therapy. Churg-Strauss syndrome can present as vasculitic rash, cardiac complications, worsening pulmonary symptoms, or peripheral neuropathy in patients with eosinophilia.

Hypersensitivity Anaphylactic reactions and angioedema have occurred from minutes to up to seven days after the dupilumab injection.

● PREGNANCY Manufacturer advises use only if potential benefit outweighs risk—limited information available.

● BREAST FEEDING Manufacturer advises avoid—no information available.

● DIRECTIONS FOR ADMINISTRATION Manufacturer advises to inject into the thigh or abdomen (except for the 5 cm around the navel), or upper arm (if not self-administered); rotate injection site and avoid skin that is tender, damaged or scarred. Patients may self-administer *Dupixent*® after appropriate training in preparation and administration.

● PRESCRIBING AND DISPENSING INFORMATION Dupilumab is a biological medicine. Biological medicines must be prescribed and dispensed by brand name, see *Biological medicines* and *Biosimilar medicines*, under Guidance on prescribing p. 1; record the brand name and batch number after each administration.

▶ When used for Asthma For choice of therapy, see Asthma, acute p. 274 and Asthma, chronic p. 271.

● HANDLING AND STORAGE Store in a refrigerator (2–8°C) and protect from light; may be kept at room temperature (max. 25°C) for max. 14 days.

● PATIENT AND CARER ADVICE

Missed doses If an injection administered *once weekly* is missed, it should be administered as soon as possible and a new schedule started based on this date.

If an injection administered *once every 2 weeks* is missed, it should be administered within 7 days of the missed dose and the next dose should be administered at the normal time. If more than 7 days has elapsed from the missed dose, it should not be administered and the next dose should be administered at the normal time.

● NATIONAL FUNDING/ACCESS DECISIONS

For full details see funding body website

NICE decisions

▶ **Dupilumab for treating moderate to severe atopic dermatitis (August 2018)** NICE TA534 Recommended with restrictions

▶ **Dupilumab for treating severe asthma with type 2 inflammation (December 2021)** NICE TA751 Recommended with restrictions

▶ **Dupilumab for treating moderate to severe prurigo nodularis (March 2024)** NICE TA955 Not recommended

Scottish Medicines Consortium (SMC) decisions

▶ **Dupilumab (*Dupixent*®) for treatment of moderate-to-severe atopic dermatitis (September 2018)** SMC No. SMC2011 Recommended with restrictions

▶ **Dupilumab (*Dupixent*®) as add-on maintenance treatment in adults and adolescents 12 years and older for severe asthma with type 2 inflammation, who are inadequately controlled

with high dose inhaled corticosteroids plus another medicinal product for maintenance treatment (April 2021) SMC No. SMC2317 Recommended with restrictions
▶ **Dupilumab (*Dupixent*®) for the treatment of adults with moderate-to-severe prurigo nodularis who are candidates for systemic therapy (February 2024)** SMC No. SMC2598 Recommended

● **MEDICINAL FORMS** There can be variation in the licensing of different medicines containing the same drug.

Solution for injection
EXCIPIENTS: May contain Polysorbates

▶ **Dupixent** (Sanofi)
Dupilumab 150 mg per 1 ml Dupixent 300mg/2ml solution for injection pre-filled syringes | 2 pre-filled disposable injection PoM £1,264.89 (Hospital only)
Dupixent 300mg/2ml solution for injection pre-filled pens | 2 pre-filled disposable injection PoM £1,264.89 (Hospital only)
Dupilumab 175 mg per 1 ml Dupixent 200mg/1.14ml solution for injection pre-filled syringes | 2 pre-filled disposable injection PoM £1,264.89 (Hospital only)
Dupixent 200mg/1.14ml solution for injection pre-filled pens | 2 pre-filled disposable injection PoM £1,264.89 (Hospital only)

| Guselkumab
13-Sep-2022

● **DRUG ACTION** Guselkumab is a recombinant human monoclonal antibody that binds selectively to interleukin-23 and blocks the activity of pro-inflammatory cytokines.

● **INDICATIONS AND DOSE**

Moderate-to-severe plaque psoriasis (specialist use only)
▶ BY SUBCUTANEOUS INJECTION
▶ Adult: Initially 100 mg, then 100 mg after 4 weeks, then maintenance 100 mg every 8 weeks, consider discontinuation of treatment if no response after 16 weeks

Psoriatic arthritis (specialist use only)
▶ BY SUBCUTANEOUS INJECTION
▶ Adult: Initially 100 mg, then 100 mg after 4 weeks, then maintenance 100 mg every 8 weeks, a maintenance dose of 100 mg every 4 weeks may be considered in patients at high risk for joint damage, consider discontinuation of treatment if no response after 24 weeks

● **CONTRA-INDICATIONS** Clinically significant active infection

● **CAUTIONS** Risk of infection
CAUTIONS, FURTHER INFORMATION
▶ Risk of infection Manufacturer advises consider anti-tuberculosis therapy before initiation of guselkumab in patients with a past history of latent or active tuberculosis in whom an adequate course of treatment cannot be confirmed.
　Manufacturer advises consider completion of appropriate immunisations according to current guidelines before initiating treatment (consult product literature for appropriate interval between vaccination and administration of guselkumab).

● **INTERACTIONS** → Appendix 1: monoclonal antibodies

● **SIDE-EFFECTS**
▶ **Common or very common** Arthralgia · diarrhoea · headache · increased risk of infection
▶ **Uncommon** Skin reactions

● **CONCEPTION AND CONTRACEPTION** Manufacturer advises effective contraception in women of childbearing potential during treatment and for at least 12 weeks after treatment.

● **PREGNANCY** Manufacturer advises avoid—no information available.

● **BREAST FEEDING** Manufacturer advises avoid during treatment and for up to 12 weeks after discontinuing treatment—no information available.

● **PRE-TREATMENT SCREENING** Manufacturer advises that patients should be evaluated for tuberculosis infection before treatment.

● **MONITORING REQUIREMENTS**
▶ EvGr Monitor for signs and symptoms of active tuberculosis during and after treatment. M
▶ When used for Psoriatic arthritis EvGr In patients receiving maintenance treatment every 4 weeks, monitor liver enzymes before starting treatment, and as clinically indicated thereafter—interrupt treatment if drug-induced liver injury suspected. M

● **DIRECTIONS FOR ADMINISTRATION** Manufacturer advises to avoid injecting into areas of the skin that show psoriasis. Patients may self-administer *Tremfya*®, after appropriate training in subcutaneous injection technique.

● **PRESCRIBING AND DISPENSING INFORMATION** Guselkumab is a biological medicine. Biological medicines must be prescribed and dispensed by brand name, see *Biological medicines* and *Biosimilar medicines*, under Guidance on prescribing p. 1; record the brand name and batch number after each administration.

● **HANDLING AND STORAGE** Manufacturer advises store in a refrigerator (2–8°C) and protect from light.

● **PATIENT AND CARER ADVICE** Manufacturer advises patients and their carers should be advised to seek medical attention if signs or symptoms of infection occur (monitor closely and suspend treatment if infection is clinically significant or unresponsive to treatment).
Self-administration Manufacturer advises patients may self-administer following training in subcutaneous injection technique.

● **NATIONAL FUNDING/ACCESS DECISIONS**
For full details see funding body website
NICE decisions
▶ **Guselkumab for treating moderate to severe plaque psoriasis (June 2018)** NICE TA521 Recommended with restrictions
▶ **Guselkumab for treating active psoriatic arthritis after inadequate response to DMARDs (August 2022)** NICE TA815 Recommended with restrictions
Scottish Medicines Consortium (SMC) decisions
▶ **Guselkumab (*Tremfya*®) for the treatment of moderate to severe plaque psoriasis in adults who are candidates for systemic therapy (June 2018)** SMC No. 1340/18 Recommended with restrictions
▶ **Guselkumab (*Tremfya*®) for the treatment of active psoriatic arthritis in adults who have had an inadequate response or who have been intolerant to a prior disease-modifying antirheumatic drug therapy, alone or in combination with methotrexate (August 2021)** SMC No. SMC2360 Recommended with restrictions

● **MEDICINAL FORMS** There can be variation in the licensing of different medicines containing the same drug.
Solution for injection
▶ **Tremfya** (Janssen-Cilag Ltd)
Guselkumab 100 mg per 1 ml Tremfya 100mg/1ml solution for injection pre-filled pens | 1 pre-filled disposable injection PoM £2,250.00

Ixekizumab
07-Jul-2022

- **DRUG ACTION** Ixekizumab is a human monoclonal antibody that binds to interleukin-17A and inhibits the release of pro-inflammatory cytokines and chemokines.

- **INDICATIONS AND DOSE**

Moderate-to-severe plaque psoriasis (under expert supervision) | Psoriatic arthritis with concomitant moderate-to-severe plaque psoriasis (under expert supervision)

▸ BY SUBCUTANEOUS INJECTION

▸ Adult: Initially 160 mg for 1 dose, followed by 80 mg after 2 weeks, then 80 mg every 2 weeks for 5 further doses (at weeks 4, 6, 8, 10 and 12), then maintenance 80 mg every 4 weeks, consider discontinuation of treatment if no response after 16–20 weeks

Psoriatic arthritis (under expert supervision) | Ankylosing spondylitis (under expert supervision) | Non-radiographic axial spondyloarthritis (under expert supervision)

▸ BY SUBCUTANEOUS INJECTION

▸ Adult: Initially 160 mg for 1 dose, then maintenance 80 mg every 4 weeks, consider discontinuation of treatment if no response after 16–20 weeks

- **CONTRA-INDICATIONS** Active infections (including active tuberculosis) · inflammatory bowel disease (discontinue if signs or symptoms develop, or an exacerbation occurs)

- **CAUTIONS** Chronic or recurrent infection—monitor carefully and discontinue if serious, unresponsive infection develops

CAUTIONS, FURTHER INFORMATION

▸ Latent tuberculosis [EvGr] Patients with latent tuberculosis should complete anti-tuberculosis therapy before starting ixekizumab. [M]

- **INTERACTIONS** → Appendix 1: monoclonal antibodies

- **SIDE-EFFECTS**

▸ **Common or very common** Conjunctivitis · increased risk of infection · nausea · oropharyngeal pain

▸ **Uncommon** Angioedema · inflammatory bowel disease · neutropenia · skin reactions · thrombocytopenia

▸ **Rare or very rare** Anaphylactic reaction

▸ **Frequency not known** Hypersensitivity (occasionally late-onset)

- **CONCEPTION AND CONTRACEPTION** Manufacturer advises effective contraception during treatment and for at least 10 weeks after treatment in women of childbearing potential.

- **PREGNANCY** Manufacturer advises avoid—limited information available.

- **BREAST FEEDING** Manufacturer advises avoid—present in milk in *animal* studies.

- **DIRECTIONS FOR ADMINISTRATION** [EvGr] Avoid injecting into areas of the skin that show psoriasis; injection sites may be alternated. [M] Patients may self-administer *Taltz*®, after appropriate training in subcutaneous injection technique; doses less than 80 mg must be prepared and administered by a healthcare professional.

- **PRESCRIBING AND DISPENSING INFORMATION** Ixekizumab is a biological medicine. Biological medicines must be prescribed and dispensed by brand name, see *Biological medicines* and *Biosimilar medicines*, under Guidance on prescribing p. 1; record the brand name and batch number after each administration.

- **HANDLING AND STORAGE** Manufacturer advises store in a refrigerator (2–8°C).

- **PATIENT AND CARER ADVICE** [EvGr] Patients and their carers should be advised to seek medical attention if symptoms of infection develop during treatment. [M]

Self-administration If appropriate, patients and their carers should be given training in subcutaneous injection technique.

A Patient Leaflet and User Manual should be provided.

- **NATIONAL FUNDING/ACCESS DECISIONS**
For full details see funding body website

NICE decisions

▸ **Ixekizumab for treating moderate to severe plaque psoriasis (April 2017)** NICE TA442 Recommended with restrictions

▸ **Ixekizumab for treating active psoriatic arthritis after inadequate response to DMARDs (August 2018)** NICE TA537 Recommended with restrictions

▸ **Ixekizumab for treating axial spondyloarthritis (July 2021)** NICE TA718 Recommended with restrictions

Scottish Medicines Consortium (SMC) decisions

▸ **Ixekizumab (*Taltz*®) for moderate to severe plaque psoriasis in adults who are candidates for systemic therapy (April 2017)** SMC No. 1223/17 Recommended with restrictions

▸ **Ixekizumab (*Taltz*®) alone or in combination with methotrexate for the treatment of active psoriatic arthritis in adult patients who have responded inadequately to, or who are intolerant to one or more disease-modifying anti-rheumatic drug therapies (October 2018)** SMC No. SMC2097 Recommended with restrictions

▸ **Ixekizumab (*Taltz*®) for the treatment of adults with active radiographic axial spondyloarthritis (also known as ankylosing spondylitis) who have responded inadequately to conventional therapy, and adults with active non-radiographic axial spondyloarthritis with objective signs of inflammation as indicated by elevated C-reactive protein and/or magnetic resonance imaging who have responded inadequately to NSAIDs (June 2022)** SMC No. SMC2440 Not recommended

- **MEDICINAL FORMS** There can be variation in the licensing of different medicines containing the same drug.

Solution for injection
EXCIPIENTS: May contain Polysorbates

▸ **Taltz** (Eli Lilly and Company Ltd)
Ixekizumab 80 mg per 1 ml Taltz 80mg/1ml solution for injection pre-filled pens | 1 pre-filled disposable injection [PoM] £1,125.00 (Hospital only)
Taltz 80mg/1ml solution for injection pre-filled syringes | 1 pre-filled disposable injection [PoM] £1,125.00 (Hospital only)

Lebrikizumab
26-Nov-2024

- **DRUG ACTION** Lebrikizumab is a recombinant humanised monoclonal antibody that inhibits interleukin-13 signaling.

- **INDICATIONS AND DOSE**

Moderate-to-severe atopic eczema (initiated by a specialist)

▸ BY SUBCUTANEOUS INJECTION

▸ Adult (body-weight 40 kg and above): Initially 500 mg every 2 weeks for 2 doses, to be administered as two consecutive 250 mg injections at different injection sites, followed by 250 mg every 2 weeks up to week 16, review after 16 weeks (consider discontinuing treatment if no response; if partial response consider continuing 250 mg every 2 weeks up to week 24), then maintenance 250 mg every 4 weeks

> **IMPORTANT SAFETY INFORMATION**
>
> MHRA/CHM ADVICE: DUPILUMAB (*DUPIXENT*®): RISK OF OCULAR ADVERSE REACTIONS AND NEED FOR PROMPT MANAGEMENT (NOVEMBER 2022)
>
> The MHRA has reviewed the risk of dry eye and serious ocular side-effects associated with dupilumab, an inhibitor of interleukin-4 and interleukin-13 signalling. Lebrikizumab, which similarly inhibits interleukin-13, is also associated with ocular side-effects; commonly,

conjunctivitis, allergic conjunctivitis, and dry eye, and less commonly, keratitis, and blepharitis. Patients who develop conjunctivitis that does not resolve following standard treatment should receive an ophthalmological examination. Healthcare professionals are advised to discuss with patients or their carers the potential for ocular side-effects and to manage any reactions promptly, especially in patients experiencing eye pain or changes to their vision.

- **CAUTIONS** Helminth infection
  CAUTIONS, FURTHER INFORMATION
- ► Risk of infection [EvGr] Lebrikizumab may influence the immune response to helminth infections. Resolve pre-existing infection before initiating treatment; suspend treatment if resistant infection develops during therapy.
  Patients should be brought up-to-date with live and live attenuated vaccines before initiating treatment. ⟨M⟩
- **INTERACTIONS** → Appendix 1: monoclonal antibodies
- **SIDE-EFFECTS**
- ► **Common or very common** Dry eye · eye inflammation
- ► **Uncommon** Eosinophilia · herpes zoster
- **PREGNANCY** [EvGr] Avoid as a precaution (limited information available). ⟨M⟩
- **BREAST FEEDING** [EvGr] Avoid—no information available. ⟨M⟩
- **DIRECTIONS FOR ADMINISTRATION** Take prefilled syringe or prefilled pen out of the refrigerator 45 minutes before administration. Inject into the thigh or abdomen (except for the 5 cm around the navel), or upper arm (if not self-administered); rotate injection site and avoid skin that is tender, damaged, bruised, or scarred. Patients may self-administer *Ebglyss*® after appropriate training in preparation and administration.
- **PRESCRIBING AND DISPENSING INFORMATION** Lebrikizumab is a biological medicine. Biological medicines must be prescribed and dispensed by brand name, see *Biological medicines* and *Biosimilar medicines*, under Guidance on prescribing p. 1; record the brand name and batch number after each administration.
- **HANDLING AND STORAGE** Store in a refrigerator (2–8°C) and protect from light; may be kept at room temperature (max. 30°C) for a maximum of 7 days.
- **PATIENT AND CARER ADVICE**
  Self-administration If appropriate, patients and their carers should be given training in subcutaneous injection technique.
- **NATIONAL FUNDING/ACCESS DECISIONS**
  For full details see funding body website
  NICE decisions
- ► **Lebrikizumab for treating moderate to severe atopic dermatitis in people 12 years and over (July 2024)** NICE TA986 Recommended with restrictions
  Scottish Medicines Consortium (SMC) decisions
- ► **Lebrikizumab (*Ebglyss*®) for the treatment of moderate-to-severe atopic dermatitis in adults and adolescents 12 years and older with a body weight of at least 40 kg who are candidates for systemic therapy (November 2024)** SMC No. SMC2707 Recommended with restrictions

- **MEDICINAL FORMS** There can be variation in the licensing of different medicines containing the same drug.
  Solution for injection
  EXCIPIENTS: May contain Polysorbates
  - ► **Ebglyss** (Almirall Ltd) ▼
    Lebrikizumab 125 mg per 1 ml Ebglyss 250mg/2ml solution for injection pre-filled pens | 2 pre-filled disposable injection [PoM] £2,271.26 (Hospital only)
    Ebglyss 250mg/2ml solution for injection pre-filled syringes | 2 pre-filled disposable injection [PoM] £2,271.26 (Hospital only)

Risankizumab

14-Jan-2025

- **DRUG ACTION** Risankizumab is a humanised monoclonal antibody that binds selectively to interleukin-23 and blocks the activity of pro-inflammatory cytokines.

- **INDICATIONS AND DOSE**
  Moderate-to-severe plaque psoriasis (specialist use only) | Psoriatic arthritis (specialist use only)
  - ► BY SUBCUTANEOUS INJECTION
  - ► Adult: Initially 150 mg, then 150 mg after 4 weeks, then maintenance 150 mg every 12 weeks, consider discontinuation if no response after 16 weeks
  Crohn's disease (under expert supervision)
  - ► INITIALLY BY INTRAVENOUS INFUSION
  - ► Adult: Initially 600 mg every 4 weeks for 3 doses, to be given on weeks 0, 4, and 8, then (by subcutaneous injection) maintenance 360 mg every 8 weeks, first subcutaneous dose to be given on week 12, consider discontinuation if no response after 24 weeks
  Ulcerative colitis (under expert supervision)
  - ► INITIALLY BY INTRAVENOUS INFUSION
  - ► Adult: Initially 1.2 g every 4 weeks for 3 doses, to be given on weeks 0, 4, and 8, then (by subcutaneous injection) maintenance 180 mg every 8 weeks, to be given if *adequate* disease improvement after induction regimen, first subcutaneous dose to be given on week 12, consider discontinuation if no response after 24 weeks, alternatively (by subcutaneous injection) maintenance 360 mg every 8 weeks, to be given if *inadequate* disease improvement after induction regimen, first subcutaneous dose to be given on week 12, consider discontinuation if no response after 24 weeks

- **CONTRA-INDICATIONS** Clinically significant active infection
- **CAUTIONS** Chronic infection · history of recurrent infection · risk of infection
  CAUTIONS, FURTHER INFORMATION
- ► Risk of infection Manufacturer advises consider anti-tuberculosis therapy before initiation of risankizumab in patients with a history of latent or active tuberculosis in whom an adequate course of treatment cannot be confirmed.
  Manufacturer advises consider completion of immunisations according to current guidelines before initiating treatment (consult product literature for appropriate interval between vaccination and administration of risankizumab).
- **INTERACTIONS** → Appendix 1: monoclonal antibodies
- **SIDE-EFFECTS**
- ► **Common or very common** Asthenia · headaches · increased risk of infection · malaise · skin reactions
- **CONCEPTION AND CONTRACEPTION** Manufacturer advises effective contraception in women of childbearing potential during treatment and for at least 21 weeks after treatment.
- **PREGNANCY** Manufacturer advises avoid (limited information available).
- **BREAST FEEDING** Manufacturer advises avoid (no information available).
- **PRE-TREATMENT SCREENING** Manufacturer advises patients should be evaluated for tuberculosis infection before treatment.
- **MONITORING REQUIREMENTS** Manufacturer advises monitor for signs and symptoms of active tuberculosis during treatment.
- **DIRECTIONS FOR ADMINISTRATION** For *prefilled syringe*, take carton out of the refrigerator at least 15 minutes

before administration. For *prefilled pen*, take carton out of the refrigerator at least 30 minutes before administration.

For *cartridge*, take carton out of the refrigerator at least 45 minutes before administration.

For *subcutaneous injection*, inject into the thigh or abdomen and avoid injecting into areas of the skin that are tender, bruised, erythematous, hardened, or affected by psoriasis. Patients may self-administer *Skyrizi*® after appropriate training in subcutaneous injection technique.

For *intermittent intravenous infusion*, dilute to a concentration of approximately 1.2–6 mg/mL with Glucose 5% and give over at least 1 hour.

- **PRESCRIBING AND DISPENSING INFORMATION** Risankizumab is a biological medicine. Biological medicines must be prescribed and dispensed by brand name, see *Biological medicines* and *Biosimilar medicines*, under Guidance on prescribing p. 1; manufacturer advises to record the brand name and batch number after each administration.

- **HANDLING AND STORAGE** Manufacturer advises store in a refrigerator (2–8°C) and protect from light.

- **PATIENT AND CARER ADVICE** Patients and their carers should be advised to seek medical attention if signs or symptoms of infection occur.
Self-administration If appropriate, patients and their carers should be given training in subcutaneous injection technique.

- **NATIONAL FUNDING/ACCESS DECISIONS** For full details see funding body website

NICE decisions
- **Risankizumab for treating moderate to severe plaque psoriasis (August 2019)** NICE TA596 Recommended with restrictions
- **Risankizumab for treating active psoriatic arthritis after inadequate response to DMARDs (July 2022)** NICE TA803 Recommended with restrictions
- **Risankizumab for previously treated moderately to severely active Crohn's disease (May 2023)** NICE TA888 Recommended with restrictions
- **Risankizumab for treating moderately to severely active ulcerative colitis (August 2024)** NICE TA998 Recommended with restrictions

Scottish Medicines Consortium (SMC) decisions
- **Risankizumab (*Skyrizi*®) for the treatment of moderate to severe plaque psoriasis in adults who are candidates for systemic therapy (October 2019)** SMC No. SMC2196 Recommended with restrictions
- **Risankizumab (*Skyrizi*®) alone or in combination with methotrexate for the treatment of active psoriatic arthritis in adults who have had an inadequate response or who have been intolerant to one or more disease-modifying antirheumatic drugs (April 2022)** SMC No. SMC2459 Recommended with restrictions
- **Risankizumab (*Skyrizi*®) for the treatment of patients 16 years and older with moderately to severely active Crohn's disease who have had an inadequate response to, lost response to, or were intolerant to conventional therapy or a biologic therapy, or if such therapies are not advisable (November 2023)** SMC No. SMC2534 Recommended
- **Risankizumab (*Skyrizi*®) for the treatment of adult patients with moderately to severely active ulcerative colitis who have had an inadequate response to, lost response to, or were intolerant to conventional therapy or a biologic therapy (January 2025)** SMC No. SMC2686 Recommended

- **MEDICINAL FORMS** There can be variation in the licensing of different medicines containing the same drug.

Solution for injection
EXCIPIENTS: May contain Polysorbates
- ▸ Skyrizi (AbbVie Ltd)
  Risankizumab 150 mg per 1 ml Skyrizi 180mg/1.2ml solution for injection cartridges | 1 cartridge [PoM] £3,326.09 (Hospital only)

Skyrizi 360mg/2.4ml solution for injection cartridges | 1 cartridge [PoM] £3,326.09
Skyrizi 150mg/1ml solution for injection pre-filled pens | 1 pre-filled disposable injection [PoM] £3,326.09 (Hospital only)
Skyrizi 150mg/1ml solution for injection pre-filled syringes | 1 pre-filled disposable injection [PoM] £3,326.09 (Hospital only)

Solution for infusion
EXCIPIENTS: May contain Polysorbates
- ▸ Skyrizi (AbbVie Ltd)
  Risankizumab 60 mg per 1 ml Skyrizi 600mg/10ml concentrate for solution for infusion vials | 1 vial [PoM] £3,326.09 (Hospital only)

Spesolimab
01-Apr-2025

- **DRUG ACTION** Spesolimab is a humanised recombinant monoclonal antibody that binds to interleukin-36R and blocks the activity of pro-inflammatory pathways.

- **INDICATIONS AND DOSE**

Generalised pustular psoriasis (under expert supervision)
- ▸ BY INTRAVENOUS INFUSION
- ▸ Adult: 900 mg for 1 dose, if flare symptoms persist, consider a further 900 mg dose after 1 week

- **CONTRA-INDICATIONS** Clinically significant active infection

- **CAUTIONS** Chronic infection · history of recurrent infection

CAUTIONS, FURTHER INFORMATION
- ▸ Immunisation [EvGr] Live vaccinations should be given at least 4 weeks before starting treatment, and should not be given during and for at least 16 weeks after treatment. [M]
- ▸ Tuberculosis [EvGr] Anti-tuberculosis therapy should be considered prior to initiating spesolimab treatment in patients with latent tuberculosis, a history of tuberculosis or possible previous exposure to tuberculosis in whom an adequate course of treatment cannot be confirmed. [M]

- **INTERACTIONS** → Appendix 1: monoclonal antibodies

- **SIDE-EFFECTS**
- ▸ Common or very common Fatigue · increased risk of infection · pruritus
- ▸ Frequency not known Peripheral neuropathy

- **PREGNANCY** [EvGr] Avoid (no information available). [M]

- **BREAST FEEDING** Specialist sources indicate use with caution, especially if breast-feeding a neonate or pre-term infant (no information available). Large molecular weight suggests limited excretion into milk and drug molecule likely to be partially destroyed in the infant's gastro-intestinal tract. [EvGr] If treatment has occurred in early pregnancy, breast-feeding may be started immediately after birth. [M]

- **PRE-TREATMENT SCREENING** [EvGr] Patients should be evaluated for tuberculosis infection before treatment. [M]

- **DIRECTIONS FOR ADMINISTRATION** For *intravenous infusion*, dilute the requisite dose in Sodium Chloride 0.9% to a final volume of 100 mL and give over 90 minutes using an in-line low-protein binding filter (0.2 micron). If the infusion is slowed or temporarily stopped, the total infusion time, including stop time, should not exceed 180 minutes.

- **PRESCRIBING AND DISPENSING INFORMATION** Spesolimab is a biological medicine. Biological medicines must be prescribed and dispensed by brand name, see *Biological medicines* and *Biosimilar medicines*, under Guidance on prescribing p. 1; record the brand name and batch number after each administration.

- **HANDLING AND STORAGE** Store in a refrigerator (2–8°C) and protect from light—consult product literature for further information regarding storage conditions outside refrigerator and after preparation of the infusion.

- **PATIENT AND CARER ADVICE** Patients and carers should be advised to seek medical attention if symptoms of infection develop.
- **NATIONAL FUNDING/ACCESS DECISIONS**
  For full details see funding body website
  Scottish Medicines Consortium (SMC) decisions
- ▸ Spesolimab (*Spevigo*®) for the treatment of flares in adult patients with generalised pustular psoriasis as monotherapy (March 2025) SMC No. SMC2729 Not recommended

- **MEDICINAL FORMS** There can be variation in the licensing of different medicines containing the same drug.
  Solution for infusion
  EXCIPIENTS: May contain Polysorbates, sucrose
  - ▸ **Spevigo** (Boehringer Ingelheim Ltd) ▼
    Spesolimab 60 mg per 1 ml Spevigo 450mg/7.5ml concentrate for solution for infusion vials | 2 vial [PoM] £15,000.00 (Hospital only)

Tildrakizumab
16-Nov-2020

- **DRUG ACTION** Tildrakizumab is a recombinant human monoclonal antibody that specifically binds to interleukin-23 and inhibits the release of pro-inflammatory cytokines and chemokines.

- ● **INDICATIONS AND DOSE**
  Moderate-to-severe plaque psoriasis (under expert supervision)
  - ▸ BY SUBCUTANEOUS INJECTION
  - ▸ Adult: Initially 100 mg, then 100 mg after 4 weeks, then maintenance 100 mg every 12 weeks, consider discontinuation if no response after 28 weeks, in patients with a high disease burden, or with a body weight ≥ 90kg, a dose of 200 mg may provide greater efficacy

- **CONTRA-INDICATIONS** Clinically significant active infection
- **CAUTIONS** Chronic infection · history of recurrent infection · recent serious infection
  CAUTIONS, FURTHER INFORMATION
  - ▸ Risk of infection Manufacturer advises consider anti-tuberculosis therapy before initiation of tildrakizumab in patients with a history of tuberculosis, in whom an adequate course of treatment cannot be confirmed.
    Manufacturer advises consider completion of immunisations according to current guidelines before initiating treatment (consult product literature for appropriate interval between vaccination and administration of tildrakizumab).
- **INTERACTIONS** → Appendix 1: monoclonal antibodies
- **SIDE-EFFECTS**
  - ▸ **Common or very common** Back pain · diarrhoea · headache · increased risk of infection · nausea
- **CONCEPTION AND CONTRACEPTION** Manufacturer advises that women of childbearing potential should use effective contraception during treatment and for at least 17 weeks after stopping treatment.
- **PREGNANCY** Manufacturer advises avoid—limited information available.
- **BREAST FEEDING** Manufacturer advises avoid—limited information available.
- **PRE-TREATMENT SCREENING** Manufacturer advises patients should be evaluated for tuberculosis infection before treatment.
- **MONITORING REQUIREMENTS** Manufacturer advises monitor for signs and symptoms of active tuberculosis during and after treatment
- **DIRECTIONS FOR ADMINISTRATION** Manufacturer advises to take the syringe out of the refrigerator at least

30 minutes before administration, and to avoid injecting into areas of the skin that are affected by psoriasis or are tender, bruised, red, hard, thick, or scaly. Patients may self-administer *Ilumetri*®, after appropriate training in subcutaneous injection technique.

- **PRESCRIBING AND DISPENSING INFORMATION** Tildrakizumab is a biological medicine. Biological medicines must be prescribed and dispensed by brand name, see *Biological medicines* and *Biosimilar medicines*, under Guidance on prescribing p. 1; manufacturer advises to record the brand name and batch number after each administration.
- **HANDLING AND STORAGE** Manufacturer advises store in a refrigerator (2–8°C) and protect from light—consult product literature for further information regarding storage outside refrigerator.
- **PATIENT AND CARER ADVICE** Manufacturer advises patients and their carers should be advised to seek medical advice if signs or symptoms of infection occur.
- **NATIONAL FUNDING/ACCESS DECISIONS**
  For full details see funding body website
  NICE decisions
  - ▸ **Tildrakizumab for treating moderate to severe plaque psoriasis (April 2019)** NICE TA575 Recommended with restrictions
  Scottish Medicines Consortium (SMC) decisions
  - ▸ **Tildrakizumab (*Ilumetri*®) for the treatment of adults with moderate to severe plaque psoriasis who are candidates for systemic therapy (August 2019)** SMC No. SMC2167 Recommended with restrictions

- **MEDICINAL FORMS** There can be variation in the licensing of different medicines containing the same drug.
  Solution for injection
  EXCIPIENTS: May contain Polysorbates
  - ▸ **Ilumetri** (Almirall Ltd)
    Tildrakizumab 100 mg per 1 ml Ilumetri 100mg/1ml solution for injection pre-filled syringes | 1 pre-filled disposable injection [PoM] £3,241.00 (Hospital only)
    Ilumetri 200mg/2ml solution for injection pre-filled syringes | 1 pre-filled disposable injection [PoM] £3,241.00 (Hospital only)

Tralokinumab
20-Jan-2023

- **DRUG ACTION** Tralokinumab is a human monoclonal antibody that inhibits the interleukin-13 pathway.

- ● **INDICATIONS AND DOSE**
  Moderate-to-severe atopic eczema (initiated by a specialist)
  - ▸ BY SUBCUTANEOUS INJECTION
  - ▸ Adult: Initially 600 mg, followed by maintenance 300 mg every 2 weeks, patients who achieve clear or almost clear skin after 16 weeks of treatment may be considered for maintenance dosing given every 4 weeks; this may not be appropriate in patients weighing over 100kg. Consider discontinuation of treatment if no response after 16 weeks

---

IMPORTANT SAFETY INFORMATION

MHRA/CHM ADVICE: DUPILUMAB (*DUPIXENT*®): RISK OF OCULAR ADVERSE REACTIONS AND NEED FOR PROMPT MANAGEMENT (NOVEMBER 2022)
The MHRA has reviewed the risk of dry eye and serious ocular side-effects associated with dupilumab, an inhibitor of interleukin-4 and interleukin-13 signalling. Tralokinumab, which similarly inhibits interleukin-13, is also associated with ocular side-effects; commonly, conjunctivitis and allergic conjunctivitis, and less commonly, keratitis. Patients who develop conjunctivitis that does not resolve following standard treatment

should receive an ophthalmological examination. Healthcare professionals are advised to discuss with patients or their carers the potential for ocular side-effects and to manage any reactions promptly, especially in patients experiencing eye pain or changes to their vision.

- **CAUTIONS** Helminth infection
  CAUTIONS, FURTHER INFORMATION
  ▸ Risk of infection [EvGr] Patients with pre-existing helminth infections should be treated before initiating treatment with tralokinumab. If patients become infected while receiving tralokinumab and do not respond to anthelminthic treatment, tralokinumab should be discontinued until infection resolves.

    Patients should be brought up-to-date with live and live attenuated vaccines before initiating treatment. (M)

- **INTERACTIONS** → Appendix 1: monoclonal antibodies

- **SIDE-EFFECTS**
  ▸ **Common or very common** Eosinophilia · eye inflammation · increased risk of infection

- **PREGNANCY** [EvGr] Avoid—limited information available. (M)

- **BREAST FEEDING** [EvGr] Avoid—no information available. (M)

- **DIRECTIONS FOR ADMINISTRATION** [EvGr] Remove syringe from the refrigerator 30 minutes before administration. Inject into the thigh or abdomen (except for the 5cm around the navel), or upper arm (if not self-administered); rotate injection site and avoid skin that is tender, damaged, or scarred. (M) Patients may self-administer *Adtralza*® after appropriate training in preparation and administration.

- **PRESCRIBING AND DISPENSING INFORMATION** Tralokinumab is a biological medicine. Biological medicines must be prescribed and dispensed by brand name, see *Biological medicines* and *Biosimilar medicines*, under Guidance on prescribing p. 1; record the brand name and batch number after each administration.

- **HANDLING AND STORAGE** Store in a refrigerator (2–8°C) and protect from light—consult product literature for further information regarding storage outside refrigerator.

- **PATIENT AND CARER ADVICE**
  Self-administration If appropriate, patients and their carers should be given training in subcutaneous injection technique.

- **NATIONAL FUNDING/ACCESS DECISIONS**
  For full details see funding body website
  NICE decisions
  ▸ Abrocitinib, tralokinumab or upadacitinib for treating moderate to severe atopic dermatitis (August 2022) NICE TA814 Recommended with restrictions
  Scottish Medicines Consortium (SMC) decisions
  ▸ Tralokinumab (*Adtralza*®) for the treatment of moderate-to-severe atopic dermatitis in adult patients who are candidates for systemic therapy (January 2022) SMC No. SMC2403 Recommended with restrictions

- **MEDICINAL FORMS** There can be variation in the licensing of different medicines containing the same drug.
  Solution for injection
  EXCIPIENTS: May contain Polysorbates
  ▸ **Adtralza** (LEO Pharma) ▼
    Tralokinumab 150 mg per 1 ml Adtralza 150mg/1ml solution for injection pre-filled syringes | 4 pre-filled disposable injection [PoM] £1,070.00 (Hospital only)
    Adtralza 300mg/2ml solution for injection pre-filled pens | 2 pre-filled disposable injection [PoM] £1,070.00 (Hospital only)

IMMUNOSUPPRESSANTS ⟩ JAK INHIBITORS

Abrocitinib

18-May-2023

- **DRUG ACTION** Abrocitinib is a selective inhibitor of the Janus-associated tyrosine kinase JAK1.

- **INDICATIONS AND DOSE**
  Moderate-to-severe atopic eczema (under expert supervision)
  ▸ BY MOUTH
  ▸ Adult: 200 mg once daily, a reduced initial dose of 100 mg once daily is recommended for patients less likely to tolerate treatment, consider discontinuation of treatment if no response after 12 weeks in all patients, for dose adjustments, interruption or discontinuation due to clinical response or side-effects—consult product literature; maximum 200 mg per day
  ▸ Elderly: Initially 100 mg once daily, increased to 200 mg once daily if necessary and if tolerated, consider discontinuation of treatment if no response after 12 weeks, for dose adjustments, interruption or discontinuation due to clinical response or side-effects—consult product literature; maximum 200 mg per day

  DOSE ADJUSTMENTS DUE TO INTERACTIONS
  ▸ [EvGr] Reduce initial dose by half with concurrent use of potent CYP2C19 inhibitors. (M)

IMPORTANT SAFETY INFORMATION
MHRA/CHM ADVICE: JANUS KINASE (JAK) INHIBITORS: NEW MEASURES TO REDUCE RISKS OF MAJOR CARDIOVASCULAR EVENTS, MALIGNANCY, VENOUS THROMBOEMBOLISM, SERIOUS INFECTIONS AND INCREASED MORTALITY (APRIL 2023)
In 2022, the EMA conducted a review of all JAK inhibitors indicated for chronic inflammatory diseases and concluded that the risks associated with the use of tofacitinib could be considered a class effect (see *Important safety information* in tofacitinib p. 1265). Following a further review by the MHRA, some existing warnings for tofacitinib have been updated and implemented for all JAK inhibitors included in the review, such as abrocitinib.
Healthcare professionals are advised to:
- avoid use in patients aged 65 years or older, in patients who are current or past long-time smokers, and in patients with other cardiovascular disease or malignancy risk factors, unless there are no suitable alternatives;
- use with caution in patients with risk factors for venous thromboembolism;
- use lower doses in patients with risk factors, where applicable;
- periodically examine all patients' skin for malignancy;
- inform patients and their carers of these risks, and the signs and symptoms that warrant urgent medical attention.

- **CONTRA-INDICATIONS** Absolute lymphocyte count less than 0.5×10^9 cells/litre (do not initiate) · absolute neutrophil count less than 1×10^9 cells/litre (do not initiate) · clinically significant active infection · haemoglobin less than 8 g/dL (do not initiate) · platelet count less than 150×10^9 cells/litre (do not initiate)

- **CAUTIONS** Chronic or recurrent infection · elderly (65 years and older) · history of atherosclerotic cardiovascular disease or other cardiovascular risk factors · history of serious or opportunistic infection · predisposition to infection · risk factors for deep-vein thrombosis or pulmonary embolism · risk factors for malignancy · risk of viral reactivation (consult product literature) · tuberculosis exposure

CAUTIONS, FURTHER INFORMATION

▶ Tuberculosis [EvGr] Consider anti-tuberculosis therapy prior to initiation of abrocitinib in patients with previously untreated latent tuberculosis. Use abrocitinib with caution in patients who have travelled or resided in areas of endemic tuberculosis or endemic mycoses. ⟨M⟩

▶ Immunisation [EvGr] Patients should receive all recommended vaccinations before starting treatment; live vaccines are not recommended immediately before, or during, treatment. ⟨M⟩

▶ Deep-vein thrombosis or pulmonary embolism [EvGr] If deep-vein thrombosis or pulmonary embolism occurs during treatment, discontinuation of abrocitinib is recommended. ⟨M⟩

- **INTERACTIONS** → Appendix 1: abrocitinib

- **SIDE-EFFECTS**

▶ **Common or very common** Abdominal pain upper · acne · dizziness · headache · increased risk of infection · nausea · vomiting

▶ **Uncommon** Dyslipidaemia · embolism and thrombosis · lymphopenia · thrombocytopenia

▶ **Frequency not known** Cardiovascular event · malignancy · neoplasms · reactivation of infections

- **CONCEPTION AND CONTRACEPTION** [EvGr] Females of childbearing potential should use effective contraception during treatment and for 1 month after last treatment. Female fertility may be temporarily reduced during treatment—studies in *animals* show that the effects on fertility are reversible 1 month after stopping treatment. ⟨M⟩

- **PREGNANCY** [EvGr] Avoid—toxicity in *animal* studies. ⟨M⟩

- **BREAST FEEDING** [EvGr] Avoid—present in milk in *animal* studies. ⟨M⟩

- **HEPATIC IMPAIRMENT** [EvGr] Avoid in severe impairment (no information available). ⟨M⟩

- **RENAL IMPAIRMENT** [EvGr] Caution in moderate and severe impairment. ⟨M⟩
  Dose adjustments [EvGr] Reduce dose by half in moderate impairment.
  Reduce initial dose to 50 mg once daily, and increase to maximum 100 mg once daily, in severe impairment. ⟨M⟩

- **PRE-TREATMENT SCREENING** [EvGr] Patients should be evaluated for tuberculosis and viral hepatitis before treatment. ⟨M⟩

- **MONITORING REQUIREMENTS**

▶ [EvGr] Monitor lipid profile at baseline, 4 weeks after treatment initiation, and then periodically—hyperlipidaemia should be managed according to clinical guidelines.

▶ Monitor for haematological abnormalities at baseline, 4 weeks after treatment initiation, and then periodically; interrupt treatment if absolute neutrophil count less than 1×10^9 cells/litre, absolute lymphocyte count less than 0.5×10^9 cells/litre, or haemoglobin less than 8 g/dL—treatment may be restarted when levels return above these values. Discontinue treatment if platelet count less than 50×10^9 cells/litre.

▶ Monitor for viral hepatitis during treatment. ⟨M⟩

▶ The MHRA recommends periodic skin examination in all patients, particularly those at increased risk of skin cancer.

- **PRESCRIBING AND DISPENSING INFORMATION** The manufacturer of *Cibinqo*® has provided a *Prescriber Brochure*.

- **PATIENT AND CARER ADVICE** Patients and carers should be advised that taking *Cibinqo*® with food may improve nausea.
  Risk minimisation materials A patient card should be provided.

Missed doses If a dose is more than 12 hours late, the missed dose should not be taken and the next dose should be taken at the normal time.
Driving and skilled tasks Patients and carers should be cautioned on the effects on driving and performance of skilled tasks—increased risk of dizziness.

- **NATIONAL FUNDING/ACCESS DECISIONS** For full details see funding body website

  NICE decisions
▶ **Abrocitinib, tralokinumab or upadacitinib for treating moderate to severe atopic dermatitis (August 2022)** NICE TA814 Recommended with restrictions

  Scottish Medicines Consortium (SMC) decisions
▶ **Abrocitinib (*Cibinqo*®) for the treatment of moderate-to-severe atopic dermatitis in adults and adolescents 12 years and older who are candidates for systemic therapy (June 2022)** SMC No. SMC2431 Recommended with restrictions

- **MEDICINAL FORMS** There can be variation in the licensing of different medicines containing the same drug.
  Oral tablet
▶ Cibinqo (Pfizer Ltd) ▼
  Abrocitinib 50 mg Cibinqo 50mg tablets | 28 tablet [PoM] £893.76
  Abrocitinib 100 mg Cibinqo 100mg tablets | 28 tablet [PoM] £893.76
  Abrocitinib 200 mg Cibinqo 200mg tablets | 28 tablet [PoM] £893.76

▎ Delgocitinib　　　　　　　　　　08-Apr-2025

- **DRUG ACTION** Delgocitinib is a pan Janus-associated tyrosine kinase inhibitor of JAK1, JAK2, JAK3, and tyrosine kinase 2 (TYK2).

- **INDICATIONS AND DOSE**

  Moderate-to-severe chronic hand eczema (under expert supervision)
  ▶ TO THE SKIN
  ▶ Adult: Apply twice daily until symptoms resolve, to be applied thinly to affected areas on the hands and wrists approx. every 12 hours, discontinue if no response after 12 weeks, treatment may be re-initiated if flares occur

- **CAUTIONS** Avoid contact with eyes · avoid contact with mouth · avoid contact with mucous membranes

- **SIDE-EFFECTS** Skin eruption localised

- **PREGNANCY** [EvGr] Avoid (limited information available). ⟨M⟩

- **BREAST FEEDING** [EvGr] Suitable for use in breast-feeding (negligible systemic exposure); avoid direct contact with breast or nipple area and infant's skin after application. ⟨M⟩

- **MONITORING REQUIREMENTS** [EvGr] Periodic skin examination of the application site is recommended in all patients, particularly those at increased risk of skin cancer. ⟨M⟩

- **PATIENT AND CARER ADVICE** Patients should be advised to avoid application of other topical preparations immediately before or after application of *Anzupgo*®. Carers should be instructed to wash their hands after application to the patient.

- **MEDICINAL FORMS** There can be variation in the licensing of different medicines containing the same drug.
  Cutaneous cream
  CAUTIONARY AND ADVISORY LABELS 15, 28
  EXCIPIENTS: May contain Benzyl alcohol, butylated hydroxyanisole, cetostearyl alcohol (including cetyl and stearyl alcohol), disodium edetate
▶ Anzupgo (LEO Pharma) ▼
  Delgocitinib 20 mg per 1 gram Anzupgo 20mg/g cream | 60 gram [PoM] £595.00

Deucravacitinib

18-Dec-2023

- **DRUG ACTION** Deucravacitinib selectively inhibits tyrosine kinase 2 (TYK2), which is a member of the Janus kinase (JAK) family; this inhibits the release of pro-inflammatory cytokines and chemokines.

- **INDICATIONS AND DOSE**

Plaque psoriasis (initiated by a specialist)
▶ BY MOUTH
- Adult: 6 mg once daily, consider discontinuation of treatment if no response after 24 weeks

> **IMPORTANT SAFETY INFORMATION**
> It is not known whether deucravacitinib, an inhibitor of tyrosine kinase 2 (TYK2), is associated with the adverse reactions of Janus kinase (JAK) inhibition. Risks that have been identified as a class effect of JAK inhibitors include major cardiovascular events, malignancy, venous thromboembolism, serious infections and increased mortality. See *Important safety information* in tofacitinib p. 1265 for MHRA/CHM safety advice relating to JAK inhibitors.

- **CONTRA-INDICATIONS** Active infection
- **CAUTIONS** Chronic infection · elderly (75 years and older) · history of recurrent infection
  CAUTIONS, FURTHER INFORMATION
▶ Tuberculosis [EvGr] Patients with latent tuberculosis should be started on anti-tuberculosis therapy before initiation of deucravacitinib. Consider anti-tuberculosis therapy before initiation of deucravacitinib in patients with a history of latent or active tuberculosis in whom an adequate course of treatment cannot be confirmed. [M]
▶ Immunisation [EvGr] Patients should receive all recommended vaccinations before initiating treatment; live vaccines are not recommended during treatment. [M]
- **INTERACTIONS** → Appendix 1: deucravacitinib
- **SIDE-EFFECTS**
▶ **Common or very common** Increased risk of infection · oral disorders · skin reactions
▶ **Frequency not known** Malignancy · neoplasms
- **PREGNANCY** [EvGr] Avoid (limited information available). [M]
- **BREAST FEEDING** [EvGr] Avoid (present in milk in *animal* studies). [M]
- **HEPATIC IMPAIRMENT** [EvGr] Avoid in severe impairment. [M]
- **PRE-TREATMENT SCREENING** [EvGr] Patients should be evaluated for tuberculosis prior to treatment. [M]
- **MONITORING REQUIREMENTS** [EvGr] Monitor for signs and symptoms of active tuberculosis during treatment. [M]
- **NATIONAL FUNDING/ACCESS DECISIONS**
  For full details see funding body website
  NICE decisions
▶ Deucravacitinib for treating moderate to severe plaque psoriasis (June 2023) NICE TA907 Recommended with restrictions
  Scottish Medicines Consortium (SMC) decisions
▶ Deucravacitinib (*Sotyktu*®) for the treatment of moderate to severe plaque psoriasis in adults who are candidates for systemic therapy (December 2023) SMC No. SMC2581 Recommended with restrictions

- **MEDICINAL FORMS** There can be variation in the licensing of different medicines containing the same drug.
  Oral tablet
  ▶ Sotyktu (Bristol-Myers Squibb Pharmaceuticals Ltd) ▼
  Deucravacitinib 6 mg Sotyktu 6mg tablets | 28 tablet [PoM] £690.00 | 84 tablet [PoM] £2,070.00

RETINOID AND RELATED DRUGS

Acitretin

06-Nov-2023

- **DRUG ACTION** Acitretin is a metabolite of etretinate.

- **INDICATIONS AND DOSE**

Severe extensive psoriasis resistant to other forms of therapy (under expert supervision) | Palmoplantar pustular psoriasis (under expert supervision) | Severe congenital ichthyosis (under expert supervision)
▶ BY MOUTH
- Adult: Initially 25–30 mg daily for 2–4 weeks, then adjusted according to response to 25–50 mg daily, increased to up to 75 mg daily, dose only increased to 75 mg daily for short periods in psoriasis

Severe Darier's disease (keratosis follicularis) (under expert supervision)
▶ BY MOUTH
- Adult: Initially 10 mg daily for 2–4 weeks, then adjusted according to response to 25–50 mg daily

> **IMPORTANT SAFETY INFORMATION**
> MHRA/CHM ADVICE: ORAL RETINOID MEDICINES: REVISED AND SIMPLIFIED PREGNANCY PREVENTION EDUCATIONAL MATERIALS FOR HEALTHCARE PROFESSIONALS AND WOMEN (JUNE 2019)
> New prescriber checklists, patient reminder cards, and pharmacy checklists are available to support the Pregnancy Prevention Programme in women and girls of childbearing potential taking oral acitretin, alitretinoin, or isotretinoin. Healthcare professionals are reminded that the use of oral retinoids is contra-indicated in pregnancy due to a high risk of serious congenital malformations, and any use in females must be within the conditions of the Pregnancy Prevention Programme (see *Conception and contraception* and *Prescribing and dispensing information*).
> Neuropsychiatric reactions have been reported in patients taking oral retinoids. Healthcare professionals are advised to monitor patients for signs of depression or suicidal ideation and refer for appropriate treatment, if necessary; particular care is needed in those with a history of depression. Patients should be advised to speak to their doctor if they experience any changes in mood or behaviour, and encouraged to ask family and friends to look out for any change in mood.

- **CONTRA-INDICATIONS** Hyperlipidaemia
- **CAUTIONS** Avoid excessive exposure to sunlight and unsupervised use of sunlamps · diabetes (can alter glucose tolerance—initial frequent blood glucose checks) · do not donate blood during and for 3 years after stopping therapy (teratogenic risk) · history of depression (risk of neuropsychiatric reactions) · investigate atypical musculoskeletal symptoms
- **INTERACTIONS** → Appendix 1: retinoids
- **SIDE-EFFECTS**
▶ **Common or very common** Abdominal pain · arthralgia · brittle nails · diarrhoea · dry mouth · eye inflammation · gastrointestinal disorder · haemorrhage · hair texture abnormal · headache · increased risk of infection · mucosal abnormalities · myalgia · nausea · oral disorders · peripheral oedema · skin reactions · thirst · vomiting · xerophthalmia
▶ **Uncommon** Dizziness · hepatic disorders · photosensitivity reaction · vision disorders
▶ **Rare or very rare** Bone pain · exostosis · idiopathic intracranial hypertension · peripheral neuropathy
▶ **Frequency not known** Angioedema · anxiety · capillary leak syndrome · depression · drowsiness · dysphonia · flushing · glucose tolerance impaired · granuloma · hearing impairment · hyperhidrosis · malaise · mood altered ·

psychiatric disorder · pyogenic granuloma · retinoic acid syndrome · taste altered · tinnitus

SIDE-EFFECTS, FURTHER INFORMATION **Exostosis** Skeletal hyperostosis and extra-osseous calcification reported following long-term treatment with etretinate (of which acitretin is a metabolite) and premature epiphyseal closure in children.

Benign intracranial hypertension Discontinue if severe headache, nausea, vomiting, or visual disturbances occur.

● **CONCEPTION AND CONTRACEPTION** The MHRA advises that women and girls of childbearing potential being treated with the oral retinoids acitretin, alitretinoin, or isotretinoin must be supported on a Pregnancy Prevention Programme with regular follow-up and pregnancy testing. **Pregnancy prevention** Effective contraception must be used.

In females of childbearing potential, exclude pregnancy up to 3 days before treatment, every month during treatment (unless there are compelling reasons to indicate that there is no risk of pregnancy), and every 1–3 months for 3 years after stopping treatment. Treatment should be started on day 2 or 3 of menstrual cycle. Females of childbearing age must practise effective contraception for at least 1 month before starting treatment, during treatment, and for at least 3 years after stopping treatment. Females should be advised to use at least 1 highly effective method of contraception (i.e. a user-independent form such as an intra-uterine device or implant) or 2 complementary user-dependent forms of contraception (e.g. oral contraceptives and barrier method). Females should be advised to seek medical attention immediately if they become pregnant during treatment or within 3 years of stopping treatment.

● **PREGNANCY** Manufacturer advises avoid—teratogenic.

● **BREAST FEEDING** Avoid.

● **HEPATIC IMPAIRMENT** Manufacturer advises avoid in severe impairment.

● **RENAL IMPAIRMENT** [EvGr] Avoid in severe impairment (increased risk of toxicity). ◈M◈

● **MONITORING REQUIREMENTS**
▸ Monitor serum-triglyceride and serum-cholesterol concentrations before treatment, 1 month after starting, then every 3 months.
▸ Check liver function at start, then every 2–4 weeks for first 2 months and then every 3 months.

● **PRESCRIBING AND DISPENSING INFORMATION**
Prescribing for females of childbearing potential The Pregnancy Prevention Programme is supported by the following materials provided by the manufacturer: *Checklists for prescribers and pharmacists*, and *Patient reminder cards*.

Each prescription for oral acitretin should be limited to a supply of up to 30 days' treatment. Pregnancy testing should ideally be carried out on the same day as prescription issuing and dispensing.

● **PATIENT AND CARER ADVICE** Females of childbearing potential should be advised to avoid alcohol during and for 2 months after stopping treatment (risk of formation of a highly teratogenic metabolite with a longer half-life).
Risk of neuropsychiatric reactions The MHRA advises patients and carers to seek medical attention if changes in mood or behaviour occur.
Pregnancy Prevention Programme Pharmacists must ensure that female patients have a patient card—see also *Important safety information*.

● **MEDICINAL FORMS** There can be variation in the licensing of different medicines containing the same drug. Forms available from special-order manufacturers include: oral suspension, oral solution

Oral capsule
CAUTIONARY AND ADVISORY LABELS 10, 11, 21
▸ **Acitretin (Non-proprietary)**
Acitretin 10 mg Acitretin 10mg capsules | 60 capsule [PoM] £23.80 DT = £21.13
Acitretin 25 mg Acitretin 25mg capsules | 60 capsule [PoM] £55.24 DT = £55.24
▸ **Neotigason** (Teva UK Ltd)
Acitretin 10 mg Neotigason 10mg capsules | 60 capsule [PoM] £17.30 DT = £21.13
Acitretin 25 mg Neotigason 25mg capsules | 60 capsule [PoM] £43.00 DT = £55.24

Alitretinoin
06-Nov-2023

● **INDICATIONS AND DOSE**

Severe chronic hand eczema refractory to potent topical corticosteroids
▸ BY MOUTH
▸ Adult (prescribed by or under supervision of a consultant dermatologist): 30 mg once daily; reduced if not tolerated to 10 mg once daily for 12–24 weeks total duration of treatment, discontinue if no response after 12 weeks, course may be repeated in those who relapse

DOSE ADJUSTMENTS DUE TO INTERACTIONS
▸ Manufacturer advises reduce dose to 10 mg once daily with concurrent use of potent inhibitors of CYP3A4, CYP2C8 and moderate inhibitors of CYP2C9.

IMPORTANT SAFETY INFORMATION
MHRA/CHM ADVICE: ORAL RETINOID MEDICINES: REVISED AND SIMPLIFIED PREGNANCY PREVENTION EDUCATIONAL MATERIALS FOR HEALTHCARE PROFESSIONALS AND WOMEN (JUNE 2019)
New prescriber checklists, patient reminder cards, and pharmacy checklists are available to support the Pregnancy Prevention Programme in women and girls of childbearing potential taking oral acitretin, alitretinoin, or isotretinoin. Healthcare professionals are reminded that the use of oral retinoids is contra-indicated in pregnancy due to a high risk of serious congenital malformations, and any use in females must be within the conditions of the Pregnancy Prevention Programme (see *Conception and contraception* and *Prescribing and dispensing information*).

Neuropsychiatric reactions have been reported in patients taking oral retinoids. Healthcare professionals are advised to monitor patients for signs of depression or suicidal ideation and refer for appropriate treatment, if necessary; particular care is needed in those with a history of depression. Patients should be advised to speak to their doctor if they experience any changes in mood or behaviour, and encouraged to ask family and friends to look out for any change in mood.

● **CONTRA-INDICATIONS** Hypervitaminosis A · uncontrolled hyperlipidaemia · uncontrolled hypothyroidism

● **CAUTIONS** Avoid blood donation during treatment and for at least 1 month after stopping treatment · dry eye syndrome · history of depression (risk of neuropsychiatric reactions)

● **INTERACTIONS** → Appendix 1: retinoids

● **SIDE-EFFECTS**
▸ **Common or very common** Alopecia · anaemia · conjunctivitis · dizziness · dry eye · dry mouth · eye irritation · fatigue · flushing · headache · hypercholesterolaemia · hypertension · hypertriglyceridaemia (risk of pancreatitis if triglycerides

above 9 mmol/litre) · joint disorders · myalgia · nausea · oral disorders · skin reactions · tinnitus · vomiting
▸ **Uncommon** Bone disorders · cataract · dyspepsia · epistaxis · vision disorders
▸ **Rare or very rare** Anxiety · behaviour abnormal · depression · hair texture abnormal · idiopathic intracranial hypertension · mood altered · nail disorder · photosensitivity reaction · psychotic disorder · suicidal behaviours · vasculitis
▸ **Frequency not known** Inflammatory bowel disease · peripheral oedema

SIDE-EFFECTS, FURTHER INFORMATION Dry eyes may respond to lubricating eye ointment or tear replacement therapy.

Discontinue treatment if signs or symptoms of idiopathic intracranial hypertension such as headache, nausea, vomiting, papilloedema, or visual disturbances occur.

Risk of pancreatitis if triglycerides above 9 mmol/litre— discontinue if uncontrolled hypertriglyceridaemia or pancreatitis.

● ALLERGY AND CROSS-SENSITIVITY [EvGr] Contra-indicated in patients with hypersensitivity to peanuts or soya (capsule filling contains soya-bean oil). ⓜ

● CONCEPTION AND CONTRACEPTION The MHRA advises that women and girls of childbearing potential being treated with the oral retinoids acitretin, alitretinoin, or isotretinoin must be supported on a Pregnancy Prevention Programme with regular follow-up and pregnancy testing. Pregnancy prevention Effective contraception must be used.

In females of childbearing potential, exclude pregnancy a few days before treatment, every month during treatment (unless there are compelling reasons to indicate that there is no risk of pregnancy), and 1 month after stopping treatment. Females of childbearing age must practise effective contraception for at least 1 month before starting treatment, during treatment, and for at least 1 month after stopping treatment. They should be advised to use at least 1 highly effective method of contraception (i.e. a user-independent form such as an intra-uterine device or implant) or 2 complementary user-dependent forms of contraception (e.g. oral contraceptives and barrier method). Females should be advised to discontinue treatment and to seek prompt medical attention if they become pregnant during treatment or within 1 month of stopping treatment.

● PREGNANCY Manufacturer advises avoid—teratogenic.

● BREAST FEEDING Manufacturer advises avoid.

● HEPATIC IMPAIRMENT Manufacturer advises avoid— limited information available.

● RENAL IMPAIRMENT [EvGr] Avoid in moderate to severe impairment (no information available). ⓜ

● MONITORING REQUIREMENTS Monitor serum lipids (more frequently in those with diabetes, history of hyperlipidaemia, or risk factors for cardiovascular disease)—discontinue if uncontrolled hyperlipidaemia.

● PRESCRIBING AND DISPENSING INFORMATION Prescribing for females of childbearing potential The Pregnancy Prevention Programme is supported by the following materials provided by the manufacturer: *Checklists for prescribers and pharmacists*, and *Patient reminder cards*.

Each prescription for oral alitretinoin should be limited to a supply of up to 30 days' treatment. Pregnancy testing should ideally be carried out on the same day as prescription issuing and dispensing.

● PATIENT AND CARER ADVICE Risk of neuropsychiatric reactions The MHRA advises patients and carers to seek medical attention if changes in mood or behaviour occur.

UV light Manufacturer advises patients to avoid excessive exposure to UV light (including sunlight, solariums)— sunscreen with a high protection factor should be applied. Pregnancy Prevention Programme Pharmacists must ensure that female patients have a patient card—see also *Important safety information*.

● NATIONAL FUNDING/ACCESS DECISIONS For full details see funding body website
NICE decisions
▸ **Alitretinoin for the treatment of severe chronic hand eczema (August 2009)** NICE TA177 Recommended

● MEDICINAL FORMS There can be variation in the licensing of different medicines containing the same drug.
Oral capsule
CAUTIONARY AND ADVISORY LABELS 10, 11, 21
EXCIPIENTS: May contain Sorbitol
▸ **Alitretinoin (Non-proprietary)**
Alitretinoin 10 mg Alitretinoin 10mg capsules | 30 capsule [PoM] £493.72-£868.94 DT = £493.72
Alitretinoin 30 mg Alitretinoin 30mg capsules | 30 capsule [PoM] £493.72-£868.94 DT = £493.72
▸ **Toctino** (Stiefel Laboratories (UK) Ltd)
Alitretinoin 10 mg Toctino 10mg capsules | 30 capsule [PoM] £493.72 DT = £493.72
Alitretinoin 30 mg Toctino 30mg capsules | 30 capsule [PoM] £493.72 DT = £493.72

SALICYLIC ACID AND DERIVATIVES

Salicylic acid with zinc oxide
23-Nov-2020

● **INDICATIONS AND DOSE**
Hyperkeratotic skin disorders
▸ TO THE SKIN
▸ Adult: Apply twice daily

● CAUTIONS Avoid broken skin · avoid inflamed skin
CAUTIONS, FURTHER INFORMATION
▸ Salicylate toxicity Salicylate toxicity may occur particularly if applied on large areas of skin.

● SIDE-EFFECTS Skin irritation

● PRESCRIBING AND DISPENSING INFORMATION Zinc and Salicylic Acid Paste BP is also referred to as Lassar's Paste. When prepared extemporaneously, the BP states Zinc and Salicylic Acid Paste, BP (Lassar's Paste) consists of zinc oxide 24%, salicylic acid 2%, starch 24%, white soft paraffin 50%.

● MEDICINAL FORMS Forms available from special-order manufacturers include: cutaneous paste

VITAMINS AND TRACE ELEMENTS 〉VITAMIN D AND ANALOGUES

Calcipotriol
28-Jun-2021

● **INDICATIONS AND DOSE**
Plaque psoriasis
▸ TO THE SKIN USING OINTMENT
▸ Adult: Apply 1–2 times a day, when preparations are used together maximum total calcipotriol 5 mg in any one week (e.g. scalp solution 60 mL with ointment 30 g or scalp solution 30 mL with ointment 60 g); maximum 100 g per week
Scalp psoriasis
▸ TO THE SKIN USING SCALP LOTION
▸ Adult: Apply twice daily, when preparations are used together maximum total calcipotriol 5 mg in any one week (e.g. scalp solution 60 mL with ointment 30 g or scalp solution 30 mL with ointment 60 g); maximum 60 mL per week

- **CONTRA-INDICATIONS** Calcium metabolism disorders
- **CAUTIONS** Avoid excessive exposure to sunlight and sunlamps · avoid use on face · erythrodermic exfoliative psoriasis (enhanced risk of hypercalcaemia) · generalised pustular psoriasis (enhanced risk of hypercalcaemia)
- **INTERACTIONS** → Appendix 1: vitamin D substances
- **SIDE-EFFECTS**
  - **Common or very common** Skin reactions
  - **Uncommon** Hypercalcaemia · increased risk of infection
  - **Rare or very rare** Hypercalciuria · photosensitivity reaction
- **PREGNANCY** Manufacturers advise avoid unless essential.
- **BREAST FEEDING** No information available.
- **HEPATIC IMPAIRMENT** Manufacturers advise avoid in severe impairment (no information available).
- **RENAL IMPAIRMENT** [EvGr] Avoid in severe impairment (no information available). ◈M
- **PATIENT AND CARER ADVICE**
  Advice on application Patient information leaflet for *Dovonex*® ointment advises liberal application. However, patients should be advised of maximum recommended weekly dose.
  Hands should be washed thoroughly after application to avoid inadvertent transfer to other body areas.

- **MEDICINAL FORMS** There can be variation in the licensing of different medicines containing the same drug.
  Cutaneous solution
  - Calcipotriol (Non-proprietary)
    Calcipotriol (as Calcipotriol monohydrate) 50 microgram per 1 ml Calcipotriol 50micrograms/ml scalp solution | 60 ml [PoM] £139.77 | 120 ml [PoM] £230.17
  Cutaneous ointment
  EXCIPIENTS: May contain Disodium edetate, propylene glycol
  - Calcipotriol (Non-proprietary)
    Calcipotriol 50 microgram per 1 gram Calcipotriol 50micrograms/g ointment | 30 gram [PoM] £9.82 DT = £8.35 | 60 gram [PoM] £9.83-£17.68 | 120 gram [PoM] £19.64-£35.12
  - Dovonex (LEO Pharma)
    Calcipotriol 50 microgram per 1 gram Dovonex 50micrograms/g ointment | 30 gram [PoM] £5.78 DT = £8.35 | 60 gram [PoM] £11.56

  Combinations available: *Calcipotriol with betamethasone,* p. 1411

⊩ 1240

Calcitriol
15-Nov-2022

(1,25-Dihydroxycholecalciferol)

- **INDICATIONS AND DOSE**
  Mild to moderate plaque psoriasis
  - TO THE SKIN
  - Adult: Apply twice daily, not more than 35% of body surface to be treated daily; maximum 30 g per day

- **CONTRA-INDICATIONS** Do not apply under occlusion · patients with calcium metabolism disorders
- **CAUTIONS** Erythrodermic exfoliative psoriasis (enhanced risk of hypercalcaemia) · generalised pustular psoriasis (enhanced risk of hypercalcaemia)
- **INTERACTIONS** → Appendix 1: vitamin D substances
- **SIDE-EFFECTS** Since systemic absorption might follow topical use, also consider the side-effects of systemic vitamin D and analogues.
- **PREGNANCY** Manufacturer advises use in restricted amounts only if clearly necessary.
  Monitoring [EvGr] Monitor plasma-calcium concentration in pregnancy. ◈M
- **BREAST FEEDING** Manufacturer advises avoid.
- **HEPATIC IMPAIRMENT** Manufacturer advises avoid.
- **RENAL IMPAIRMENT** Manufacturer advises avoid—no information available.

- **HANDLING AND STORAGE** Hands should be washed thoroughly after application to avoid inadvertent transfer to other body areas.

- **MEDICINAL FORMS** There can be variation in the licensing of different medicines containing the same drug.
  Cutaneous ointment
  - Silkis (Galderma (UK) Ltd)
    Calcitriol 3 microgram per 1 gram Silkis ointment | 100 gram [PoM] £18.06 DT = £18.06

Tacalcitol
16-Feb-2021

- **INDICATIONS AND DOSE**
  Plaque psoriasis
  - TO THE SKIN
  - Adult: Apply once daily, preferably at bedtime, maximum 10 g ointment or 10 mL lotion daily, when lotion and ointment used together, maximum total tacalcitol 280 micrograms in any one week (e.g. lotion 30 mL with ointment 40 g)

- **CONTRA-INDICATIONS** Calcium metabolism disorders
- **CAUTIONS** Avoid eyes · erythrodermic exfoliative psoriasis (enhanced risk of hypercalcaemia) · generalised pustular psoriasis (enhanced risk of hypercalcaemia) · if used in conjunction with UV treatment
  CAUTIONS, FURTHER INFORMATION
  - UV treatment [EvGr] If tacalcitol is used in conjunction with UV treatment, UV radiation should be given in the morning and tacalcitol applied at bedtime. ◈M
- **INTERACTIONS** → Appendix 1: vitamin D substances
- **SIDE-EFFECTS**
  - **Uncommon** Skin reactions
  - **Frequency not known** Hypercalcaemia
- **PREGNANCY** Manufacturer advises avoid unless no safer alternative—no information available.
- **BREAST FEEDING** Manufacturer advises avoid application to breast area; no information available on presence in milk.
- **MONITORING REQUIREMENTS** Monitor serum calcium if risk of hypercalcaemia.
- **PATIENT AND CARER ADVICE** Hands should be washed thoroughly after application to avoid inadvertent transfer to other body areas.

- **MEDICINAL FORMS** There can be variation in the licensing of different medicines containing the same drug.
  Cutaneous ointment
  - Curatoderm (Almirall Ltd)
    Tacalcitol (as Tacalcitol monohydrate) 4 microgram per 1 gram Curatoderm 4micrograms/g ointment | 100 gram [PoM] £30.86 DT = £30.86

6 Perspiration

6.1 Hyperhidrosis

Hyperhidrosis
08-Aug-2022

Overview

Hyperhidrosis is defined as sweating in excess of normal body temperature regulation. It can be localised (focal) or affect the entire skin area, and can be classified by the absence (primary) or presence (secondary) of an underlying cause.

[EvGr] Patients with primary focal hyperhidrosis affecting axillae, palmar, or plantar areas, should be offered a topical preparation containing 20% aluminium chloride hexahydrate below. ⒶThis is a more potent antiperspirant compared to commercially available preparations and is available as a spray, roll-on, or solution. [EvGr] If the response to treatment is inadequate or not tolerated after 6 weeks, consider referral to a specialist.

Specialist management may also be appropriate in more severe cases of hyperhidrosis. Topical glycopyrronium bromide as a 0.05% solution below, may be used in the iontophoretic treatment of hyperhidrosis of plantar and palmar areas. *Botox*® contains botulinum toxin type A complex p. 469 and is licensed for intradermal use for severe hyperhidrosis of the axillae unresponsive to topical antiperspirant or other antihidrotic treatment. Oral antimuscarinics (such as propantheline bromide p. 97, and oxybutynin hydrochloride p. 898 [unlicensed indication]) can cause a reduction in sweat secretion by effects on muscarinic receptors near the sweat glands; their use may be limited due to antimuscarinic adverse effects. Ⓐ

ANTIMUSCARINICS

☞ 896

Glycopyrronium bromide

17-Jan-2024

(Glycopyrrolate)

- **INDICATIONS AND DOSE**

Iontophoretic treatment of hyperhidrosis
▸ TO THE SKIN
▸ Adult: Only 1 site to be treated at a time, maximum 2 sites treated in any 24 hours, treatment not to be repeated within 7 days (consult product literature)

- **CONTRA-INDICATIONS** Infections affecting the treatment site

  CONTRA-INDICATIONS, FURTHER INFORMATION Contra-indications applicable to systemic use should be considered; however, glycopyrronium is poorly absorbed and systemic effects unlikely with topical use.

- **CAUTIONS** Cautions applicable to systemic use should be considered; however, glycopyrronium is poorly absorbed and systemic effects unlikely with topical use.

- **INTERACTIONS** → Appendix 1: glycopyrronium

- **SIDE-EFFECTS** Abdominal discomfort · eating disorder · pain · paraesthesia

  SIDE-EFFECTS, FURTHER INFORMATION The possibility of systemic side-effects should be considered; however, glycopyrronium is poorly absorbed and systemic effects are unlikely with topical use.

- **MEDICINAL FORMS** No licensed medicines listed.

DERMATOLOGICAL DRUGS > ASTRINGENTS

Aluminium chloride hexahydrate

21-Nov-2020

- **INDICATIONS AND DOSE**

Hyperhidrosis affecting axillae, hands or feet
▸ TO THE SKIN
▸ Adult: Apply once daily, apply liquid formulation at night to dry skin, wash off the following morning, reduce frequency as condition improves—do not bathe immediately before use

Hyperhidrosis | Bromidrosis | Intertrigo | Prevention of tinea pedis and related conditions
▸ TO THE SKIN
▸ Adult: Apply powder to dry skin

- **CAUTIONS** Avoid contact with eyes · avoid contact with mucous membranes · avoid use on broken or irritated skin ·

do not shave axillae or use depilatories within 12 hours of application

- **SIDE-EFFECTS** Skin reactions
- **PATIENT AND CARER ADVICE** Avoid contact with clothing.
- **EXCEPTIONS TO LEGAL CATEGORY** A 30 mL pack of aluminium chloride hexahydrate 20% is on sale to the public.

- **MEDICINAL FORMS** There can be variation in the licensing of different medicines containing the same drug.
  Cutaneous solution
  CAUTIONARY AND ADVISORY LABELS 15
  ▸ **Anhydrol** (Dermal Laboratories Ltd)
  Aluminium chloride hexahydrate 200 mg per 1 ml Anhydrol Forte 20% solution | 60 ml Ⓟ £2.99 DT = £2.99
  ▸ **Driclor** (Haleon UK Trading Ltd)
  Aluminium chloride hexahydrate 200 mg per 1 ml Driclor 20% solution | 75 ml Ⓟ £3.48

7 Pruritus

Topical local antipruritics

Overview

Pruritus may be caused by systemic disease (such as obstructive jaundice, endocrine disease, chronic renal disease, iron deficiency, and certain malignant diseases), skin disease (e.g. psoriasis, eczema, urticaria, and scabies), drug hypersensitivity, or as a side-effect of opioid analgesics. Where possible, the underlying causes should be treated. An **emollient** may be of value where the pruritus is associated with dry skin. Pruritus that occurs in otherwise healthy elderly people can also be treated with an emollient. Levomenthol **cream** p. 1438 can be used to relieve pruritus; it exerts a cooling effect on the skin. Local antipruritics have a role in the treatment of pruritus in palliative care.

Preparations containing crotamiton p. 1437 are sometimes used but are of uncertain value. Preparations containing calamine are often ineffective.

A topical preparation containing doxepin 5% p. 1437 is licensed for the relief of pruritus in eczema; it can cause drowsiness and there may be a risk of sensitisation.

Pruritus is common in biliary obstruction, especially in primary biliary cirrhosis and drug-induced cholestasis. Oral administration of colestyramine p. 229 is the treatment of choice.

Topical antihistamines and local anaesthetics are only marginally effective and occasionally cause hypersensitivity. For *insect stings* and *insect bites*, a short course of a topical corticosteroid is appropriate. Short-term treatment with a **sedating antihistamine** may help in insect stings and in intractable pruritus where sedation is desirable. Calamine preparations are of little value for the treatment of insect stings or bites.

Topical local anaesthetics are indicated for the relief of local pain. Preparations may be absorbed, especially through mucosal surfaces, therefore excessive application should be avoided and they should preferably not be used for more than 3 days; not generally suitable for young children and are less suitable for prescribing.

Topical antihistamines should be avoided in eczema and are not recommended for longer than 3 days. They are less suitable for prescribing.

Other drugs used for Pruritus Alimemazine tartrate, p. 322 · Cetirizine hydrochloride, p. 319 · Chlorphenamine maleate, p. 323 · Coal tar with calamine, p. 1419 · Dupilumab, p. 1423 · Hydroxyzine hydrochloride, p. 324 · Levocetirizine hydrochloride, p. 320

ANTIPRURITICS

Calamine with zinc oxide
11-Mar-2020

- **INDICATIONS AND DOSE**

Minor skin conditions
▸ TO THE SKIN
- Child: (consult product literature)
- Adult: (consult product literature)

IMPORTANT SAFETY INFORMATION
MHRA/CHM ADVICE (UPDATED DECEMBER 2018): EMOLLIENTS:
NEW INFORMATION ABOUT RISK OF SEVERE AND FATAL BURNS
WITH PARAFFIN-CONTAINING AND PARAFFIN-FREE EMOLLIENTS
See Emollient and barrier preparations p. 1387.

- **CONTRA-INDICATIONS** Avoid application of preparations containing zinc oxide prior to x-ray (zinc oxide may affect outcome of x-ray)

- **LESS SUITABLE FOR PRESCRIBING** Less suitable for prescribing.

- **MEDICINAL FORMS** There can be variation in the licensing of different medicines containing the same drug.

Cutaneous cream
CAUTIONARY AND ADVISORY LABELS 15
▸ Calamine with zinc oxide (Non-proprietary)
   Phenoxyethanol 5 mg per 1 gram, Zinc oxide 30 mg per 1 gram, Calamine 40 mg per 1 gram, Cetomacrogol emulsifying wax 50 mg per 1 gram, Self-emulsifying glyceryl monostearate 50 mg per 1 gram, Liquid paraffin 200 mg per 1 gram Aqueous calamine cream | 100 gram GSL £2.34 DT = £2.34

Cutaneous liquid
▸ Calamine with zinc oxide (Non-proprietary)
   Phenol liquefied 5 mg per 1 ml, Sodium citrate 5 mg per 1 ml, Bentonite 30 mg per 1 ml, Glycerol 50 mg per 1 ml, Zinc oxide 50 mg per 1 ml, Calamine 150 mg per 1 ml Calamine lotion | 200 ml GSL £1.73-£1.78 DT = £1.73

Crotamiton
29-Apr-2020

- **INDICATIONS AND DOSE**

Pruritus (including pruritus after scabies)
▸ TO THE SKIN
- Child 1 month-2 years (on doctor's advice only): Apply once daily
- Child 3-17 years: Apply 2–3 times a day
- Adult: Apply 2–3 times a day

- **CONTRA-INDICATIONS** Acute exudative dermatoses

- **CAUTIONS** Avoid use in buccal mucosa · avoid use near eyes · avoid use on broken skin · avoid use on very inflamed skin · use on doctor's advice for children under 3 years

- **PREGNANCY** Manufacturer advises avoid, especially during the first trimester—no information available.

- **BREAST FEEDING** No information available; avoid application to nipple area.

- **MEDICINAL FORMS** There can be variation in the licensing of different medicines containing the same drug.

Cutaneous cream
EXCIPIENTS: May contain Beeswax, cetostearyl alcohol (including cetyl and stearyl alcohol), fragrances, hydroxybenzoates (parabens)
▸ Eurax (Thornton & Ross Ltd)
   Crotamiton 100 mg per 1 gram Eurax 10% cream | 30 gram GSL £3.13 DT = £3.13 | 100 gram GSL £5.91 DT = £5.91

Difelikefalin
05-Mar-2024

- **DRUG ACTION** Difelikefalin is a selective kappa opioid-receptor agonist with low CNS penetration.

- **INDICATIONS AND DOSE**

Pruritus (associated with chronic kidney disease in patients on haemodialysis) (under expert supervision)
▸ BY INTRAVENOUS INJECTION
- Adult: 0.5 microgram/kg 3–4 times a week (max. per dose 100 micrograms), to be administered via haemodialysis access after dialysis session, for haemodialysis treatments less than 1 hour, administration of difelikefalin should be withheld until the next haemodialysis session, dose to be calculated using dry body weight

- **CAUTIONS** Disruptions to the blood-brain barrier (e.g. advanced Alzheimer's disease, active multiple sclerosis, primary brain malignancies)

- **INTERACTIONS** → Appendix 1: difelikefalin

- **SIDE-EFFECTS**
▸ **Common or very common** Drowsiness · oral disorders · sensation abnormal
▸ **Uncommon** Confusion · diarrhoea · dizziness · headache · nausea · psychiatric disorder · vomiting

- **PREGNANCY** EvGr Avoid unless potential benefit outweighs risk—no information available. ⟨M⟩

- **BREAST FEEDING** EvGr Avoid—present in milk in *animal* studies. ⟨M⟩

- **HEPATIC IMPAIRMENT** EvGr Avoid in severe impairment (no information available) ⟨M⟩

- **PATIENT AND CARER ADVICE**
Driving and skilled tasks Patients and carers should be cautioned on the effects on driving and performance of skilled tasks—increased risk of somnolence or dizziness.

- **NATIONAL FUNDING/ACCESS DECISIONS**
For full details see funding body website

NICE decisions
▸ Difelikefalin for treating pruritus in people having haemodialysis (May 2023) NICE TA890 Recommended

Scottish Medicines Consortium (SMC) decisions
▸ Difelikefalin (*Kapruvia*®) for the treatment of moderate-to-severe pruritus associated with chronic kidney disease in adult patients on haemodialysis (February 2024) SMC No. SMC2623 Recommended with restrictions

- **MEDICINAL FORMS** There can be variation in the licensing of different medicines containing the same drug.

Solution for injection
▸ Kapruvia (Vifor Fresenius Medical Care Renal Pharma UK Ltd) ▼
   Difelikefalin (as Difelikefalin acetate) 50 microgram per 1 ml Kapruvia 50micrograms/1ml solution for injection vials | 12 vial PoM £420.00 (Hospital only)

Doxepin
20-Apr-2021

- **INDICATIONS AND DOSE**

Pruritus in eczema
▸ TO THE SKIN
- Child 12-17 years: Apply up to 3 g 3–4 times a day, apply thinly; coverage should be less than 10% of body surface area; maximum 12 g per day
- Adult: Apply up to 3 g 3–4 times a day, apply thinly; coverage should be less than 10% of body surface area; maximum 12 g per day

- **CAUTIONS** Arrhythmias · avoid application to large areas · mania · severe heart disease · susceptibility to angle-closure glaucoma · urinary retention

- **INTERACTIONS** → Appendix 1: tricyclic antidepressants
- **SIDE-EFFECTS** Constipation · diarrhoea · dizziness · drowsiness · dry eye · dry mouth · dyspepsia · fever · headache · nausea · paraesthesia · skin reactions · suicidal behaviours · taste altered · urinary retention · vision blurred · vomiting
- **PREGNANCY** Manufacturer advises use only if potential benefit outweighs risk.
- **BREAST FEEDING** Manufacturer advises use only if potential benefit outweighs risk.
- **HEPATIC IMPAIRMENT** Manufacturer advises caution in severe impairment.
- **PATIENT AND CARER ADVICE** A patient information leaflet should be provided.
  Driving and skilled tasks Drowsiness may affect performance of skilled tasks (e.g. driving). Effects of alcohol enhanced.

- **MEDICINAL FORMS** There can be variation in the licensing of different medicines containing the same drug.
  Cutaneous cream
  CAUTIONARY AND ADVISORY LABELS 2, 10
  EXCIPIENTS: May contain Benzyl alcohol
  ▸ **Xepin** (Cambridge Healthcare Supplies Ltd)
  Doxepin hydrochloride 50 mg per 1 gram Xepin 5% cream | 30 gram [PoM] £13.66 DT = £13.66

MENTHOL AND DERIVATIVES

Levomenthol

- **INDICATIONS AND DOSE**
Pruritus
▸ TO THE SKIN
▸ Adult: Apply 1–2 times a day

- **MEDICINAL FORMS** There can be variation in the licensing of different medicines containing the same drug. Forms available from special-order manufacturers include: cutaneous cream
  Cutaneous cream
  ▸ **AquaSoothe** (Ennogen Healthcare Ltd)
  Menthol 10 mg per 1 gram AquaSoothe 1% cream | 100 gram £3.75 DT = £4.46 | 500 gram £15.62 DT = £18.64
  Menthol 20 mg per 1 gram AquaSoothe 2% cream | 50 gram £1.86 | 500 gram £15.62 DT = £19.07
  ▸ **Arjun** (Arjun Products Ltd)
  Menthol 5 mg per 1 gram Arjun 0.5% cream | 500 gram £15.68 DT = £18.05
  Menthol 10 mg per 1 gram Arjun 1% cream | 500 gram £15.68 DT = £18.64
  Menthol 20 mg per 1 gram Arjun 2% cream | 500 gram £15.68 DT = £19.07
  ▸ **Dermacool** (Pern Consumer Products Ltd)
  Menthol 5 mg per 1 gram Dermacool 0.5% cream | 100 gram £4.33 | 500 gram £18.05 DT = £18.05
  Menthol 10 mg per 1 gram Dermacool 1% cream | 100 gram £4.46 DT = £4.46 | 500 gram £18.64 DT = £18.64
  Menthol 20 mg per 1 gram Dermacool 2% cream | 100 gram £4.57 | 500 gram £19.07 DT = £19.07
  Menthol 50 mg per 1 gram Dermacool 5% cream | 100 gram £5.32 | 500 gram £19.83
  ▸ **Menthoderm** (Derma UK Ltd)
  Menthol 5 mg per 1 gram Menthoderm 0.5% cream | 500 gram £16.94 DT = £18.05
  Menthol 10 mg per 1 gram Menthoderm 1% cream | 100 gram £4.00 DT = £4.46 | 500 gram £17.50 DT = £18.64
  Menthol 20 mg per 1 gram Menthoderm 2% cream | 100 gram £4.10 | 500 gram £17.91 DT = £19.07
  Menthol 50 mg per 1 gram Menthoderm 5% cream | 500 gram £18.45

8 Rosacea and acne

Acne

18-Jun-2024

Description of condition

Acne is a common inflammatory skin condition that leads to lesions which consist of non-inflammatory comedones, and inflammatory papules, pustules, nodules and cysts. In patients with acne, lesions and/or scarring may be seen and severity can range from mild lesions to permanent disfiguration. It can also have a psychological and social impact on the patient.

Acne vulgaris is a common type of acne that primarily affects the face, back, and chest; it is most common in adolescence, but may affect those in any age group. Other types of acne include acne conglobata, a severe form of nodulo-cystic acne with interconnecting sinuses and abscesses; and acne fulminans, a very serious form of acne conglobata that is associated with systemic symptoms (such as fever and arthralgia).

The severity of acne varies along a continuum from mild to moderate to severe, that is characterised by the lesion type (s) and quantity. Patients with mild to moderate acne are those with 1 or more of the following: non-inflammatory lesions (of any number), up to 34 inflammatory lesions, up to 2 nodules. Patients with moderate to severe acne are those who have 35 or more inflammatory lesions and/or 3 or more nodules.

Aims of treatment

Treatment aims to reduce the severity of skin lesions and other complications, and to prevent recurrence and scarring.

Management of acne

Patients with acne fulminans should be urgently referred to hospital for assessment by the dermatology team within 24 hours.

Patients with acne conglobata, nodulo-cystic acne, or those with diagnostic uncertainty about their acne, should be referred to a consultant dermatologist-led team or a nationally accredited GP with an extended role (GPwER) working within a consultant dermatologist-agreed pathway.

For patients with acne vulgaris, referral to a consultant dermatologist-led team or a GPwER working within a consultant dermatologist-agreed pathway should be considered if they have scarring or persistent pigmentary changes, or if their acne or acne-related scarring is causing or contributing to persistent psychological distress or a mental health disorder.

Referral to a mental health service should also be considered for patients whose acne is contributing to psychological distress or a mental health disorder (including those who have a current or past history of suicidal ideation or self-harm, body morphic disorder, or a severe depressive or anxiety disorder).

[EvGr] Consider condition-specific management or specialist referral if a medication or medical disorder is contributing to the patient's acne. [A] Specialist referral should also be considered for individuals with acne and polycystic ovary syndrome (PCOS) with features of hyperandrogenism.

Non-drug treatment

[EvGr] Patients with acne vulgaris should be advised on appropriate skin care such as using a non-alkaline, synthetic detergent cleansing product twice daily on acne-prone areas, removing make up at the end of the day, and avoiding the use of oil-based or comedogenic skincare products, sunscreens, and make-up. They should also be advised to avoid persistent picking or scratching of lesions.

Photodynamic therapy should be considered for patients with moderate to severe acne vulgaris if other treatments are ineffective, contra-indicated, or not tolerated. ⒶⒷ

Drug treatment

EvGr Patients with mild to moderate and moderate to severe acne vulgaris should be offered a 12-week course of a first-line treatment option, taking into account the severity and distribution of their acne, their preferences, and that the risk of scarring increases with acne severity and duration. Any potential use of oral isotretinoin in the future for severe forms of acne will be dependent on the completion of adequate courses of first-line treatments including systemic antibacterials and topical therapy, and should also be taken into consideration when deciding on initial treatment options. The use of antibacterial monotherapy or a combination of a topical and oral antibacterial are not recommended. Patients should be informed that the benefits of treatment may take between 6–8 weeks to become noticeable and hence the importance of completing the course.

Females receiving acne treatment who wish to use hormonal contraception could consider using an oral combined hormonal contraceptive, Ⓐ as combined hormonal contraceptive use may be associated with improvement of acne.

EvGr When considering treatment options that include known teratogenic drugs or drugs with teratogenic potential (such as topical or oral retinoids, or oral tetracyclines), specific contraception requirements should be taken into consideration and discussed with patients, see individual drug monographs for further information. Ⓐ

First-line treatment options for acne vulgaris

- Acne of any severity:
  - ▸ EvGr Fixed combination topical adapalene with benzoyl peroxide p. 1443, or
  - ▸ Fixed combination topical tretinoin with clindamycin p. 1445. Ⓐ
- Mild to moderate acne:
  - ▸ EvGr Fixed combination topical benzoyl peroxide with clindamycin p. 1442. Ⓐ
- Moderate to severe acne:
  - ▸ EvGr Fixed combination topical adapalene with benzoyl peroxide **with** oral lymecycline p. 657 or doxycycline p. 655, or
  - ▸ Topical azelaic acid p. 1442 **with** oral lymecycline or doxycycline. Ⓐ
  - ▸ Alternative antibacterial options if lymecycline or doxycycline unsuitable: EvGr trimethoprim p. 665 [unlicensed] **or** a macrolide (such as erythromycin p. 624). Ⓐ
- Alternative if first-line options are contra-indicated, or the patient wishes to avoid antibacterials or topical retinoids: EvGr topical benzoyl peroxide p. 1442 monotherapy. Ⓐ

For further information on the management of acne vulgaris, such as the advantages and disadvantages of each treatment option, see NICE guideline: **Acne** (see *Useful resources*).

Reassessment and further treatment

EvGr Review first-line treatment after 12 weeks. For patients whose acne has cleared, maintenance options should also be considered Ⓐ (see *Maintenance*).

EvGr For patients whose treatment included an oral antibacterial and their acne has completely cleared, consider continuing their topical treatment and stopping the oral antibacterial. If their acne has improved but not cleared, consider continuing the course for up to a further 12 weeks. Treatment courses that include an antibacterial should only be continued for more than 6 months in exceptional circumstances, and should be reviewed every 3 months.

For patients with mild to moderate acne who have had an inadequate response to treatment after 12 weeks, offer another first-line option. Ⓐ For those who have mild to moderate acne unresponsive to 2 completed treatment courses, consider referral to a consultant dermatologist-led team or a GPwER working within a consultant dermatologist-agreed pathway.

EvGr For patients with moderate to severe acne who have had an inadequate response to treatment that did not include an oral antibacterial, offer another first-line option which includes an oral antibacterial. Ⓐ For those whose treatment included an oral antibacterial, consider referral to a consultant dermatologist-led team or a GPwER working within a consultant dermatologist-agreed pathway.

EvGr For females with PCOS that have not improved following treatment with a first-line option, consider adding ethinylestradiol with cyproterone (co-cyprindiol p. 1440) and review at 6 months, or an alternative combined oral contraceptive pill [unlicensed]. Ⓐ

For further information on the drug treatment of acne vulgaris, including the use of intralesional corticosteroids and the management of acne-related scarring, see NICE guideline: **Acne** (see *Useful resources*).

Isotretinoin

EvGr For patients with severe acne (such as acne conglobata or fulminans, nodulo-cystic acne, or acne at risk of permanent scarring) that is resistant to adequate courses of oral antibacterial-containing first-line treatments, consider oral isotretinoin p. 1443 (specialist use by a consultant dermatologist-led team or a GPwER working within a consultant dermatologist-agreed pathway). Take into account the patient's psychological wellbeing, and refer them to mental health services before starting treatment if appropriate. Ⓐ

Isotretinoin is a powerful teratogen; for females of childbearing potential isotretinoin must only be used if the conditions of the Pregnancy Prevention Programme are met. For further information, see *Important safety information*, *Conception and contraception*, and *Prescribing and dispensing information* in the isotretinoin monograph, and *Contraception in patients taking medication with teratogenic potential* in Contraceptives, hormonal p. 912.

EvGr For acne flares that occur after starting isotretinoin, a course of oral prednisolone p. 791 may be considered. Ⓐ For further information on acne flares, see NICE guideline: **Acne** (see *Useful resources*).

Relapse

EvGr For acne that responds adequately to a course of first-line treatment but then relapses, consider another 12-week course of either the same treatment or an alternative treatment option. Ⓐ For treatment options, see *First-line treatment options*.

EvGr If acne relapses after an adequate response to oral isotretinoin and is currently mild to moderate, offer an appropriate first-line treatment option. If acne relapses after an adequate response to oral isotretinoin and is currently moderate to severe, offer either a 12-week course of an appropriate first-line treatment option or re-referral if the patient is no longer under the care of a consultant dermatologist-led team or a GPwER working within a consultant dermatologist-agreed pathway. For individuals with moderate to severe acne that relapses after a second course of oral isotretinoin, further care should be provided by their dermatology team; offer re-referral if the patient is no longer under the care of the consultant dermatologist-led team or a GPwER working within a consultant dermatologist-agreed pathway. Ⓐ

Maintenance

EvGr On completion of treatment, the need for maintenance treatment is not always necessary; advise patients that appropriate skin care should be continued. In patients with a history of frequent relapse, consider maintenance treatment using a fixed combination of topical adapalene with benzoyl peroxide p. 1443. If this is not tolerated or one component of the combination is contra-indicated, consider topical monotherapy with either adapalene p. 1443, azelaic acid p. 1442, or benzoyl peroxide p. 1442. Maintenance treatments should be reviewed after 12 weeks and a decision made about continuation. Ⓐ

Useful Resources

Acne vulgaris: management. National Institute for Health and Care Excellence guideline NG198. June 2021, updated December 2023.
www.nice.org.uk/guidance/ng198

Rosacea
29-Sep-2020

Rosacea

Rosacea is not comedonal (but may exist with acne which may be comedonal). Brimonidine tartrate p. 1447 is licensed for the treatment of facial erythema in rosacea. The pustules and papules of rosacea respond to topical azelaic acid p. 1442, topical ivermectin p. 1446 or to topical metronidazole p. 1398. Alternatively oral administration of oxytetracycline p. 658 or tetracycline p. 659, or erythromycin p. 624, can be used; courses usually last 6–12 weeks and are repeated intermittently. Doxycycline p. 655 can be used [unlicensed indication] if oxytetracycline or tetracycline is inappropriate (e.g. in renal impairment). A modified-release preparation of doxycycline is licensed in low daily doses for the treatment of facial rosacea. Camouflages p. 1455 may be required for the redness.

8.1 Acne

> **Other drugs used for Acne** Minocycline, p. 658 · Oxytetracycline, p. 658

ANTI-ANDROGENS

Clascoterone
24-Mar-2025

- **DRUG ACTION** Clascoterone is an androgen receptor inhibitor.

- **INDICATIONS AND DOSE**

Acne vulgaris
▸ TO THE SKIN
▸ Child 12–17 years: Apply twice daily, 1 g of cream to be applied thinly in the morning and evening
▸ Adult: Apply twice daily, 1 g of cream to be applied thinly in the morning and evening

- **CAUTIONS** Avoid contact with broken skin · avoid contact with eczematous skin · avoid contact with eyes · avoid contact with mouth · avoid contact with mucous membranes · avoid contact with sunburned skin

- **SIDE-EFFECTS**
▸ **Common or very common** Hyperkalaemia · skin reactions · telangiectasia
▸ **Rare or very rare** Amenorrhoea · polycystic ovaries
▸ **Frequency not known** Hair colour changes · headache (in children) · suppression of the hypothalamic-pituitary-adrenal axis

- **PREGNANCY** EvGr Use with caution (limited information available). Ⓜ

- **BREAST FEEDING** Specialist sources indicate amounts in milk are probably low and unlikely to affect breast-fed

infants due to poor absorption and high plasma-protein binding (no information available); avoid application to nipple area and direct contact with treated skin.

- **MEDICINAL FORMS** There can be variation in the licensing of different medicines containing the same drug.
Cutaneous cream
EXCIPIENTS: May contain Cetostearyl alcohol (including cetyl and stearyl alcohol), disodium edetate, polysorbates, propylene glycol
▸ **Winlevi** (Glenmark Pharmaceuticals Europe Ltd) ▼
  Clascoterone 10 mg per 1 gram Winlevi 10mg/g cream | 60 gram PoM £19.43

Co-cyprindiol
23-Oct-2023

- **INDICATIONS AND DOSE**

Moderate to severe acne vulgaris related to hyperandrogenism caused by polycystic ovary syndrome [adjunct in refractory acne] | **Moderately severe hirsutism**
▸ BY MOUTH
▸ Females of childbearing potential: 1 tablet daily for 21 days, to be started on day 1 of menstrual cycle; subsequent courses repeated after a 7-day interval (during which withdrawal bleeding occurs), time to symptom remission, at least 3 months; review need for treatment regularly

> **IMPORTANT SAFETY INFORMATION**
>
> **MHRA/CHM ADVICE: CYPROTERONE ACETATE: NEW ADVICE TO MINIMISE RISK OF MENINGIOMA (JUNE 2020)**
> Cyproterone acetate has been associated with an overall rare, but cumulative dose-dependent, increased risk of meningioma (single and multiple), mainly at doses of 25 mg/day and higher. Healthcare professionals are advised to monitor patients for meningiomas, and to permanently discontinue treatment if diagnosed. Use of cyproterone acetate, including co-cyprindiol, for all indications is contra-indicated in those with meningioma or a history of meningioma.

- **CONTRA-INDICATIONS** Acute porphyrias p. 1202 · atrial fibrillation · Budd-Chiari syndrome · cardiomyopathy with impaired cardiac function · complicated congenital heart disease · complicated valvular heart disease · current breast cancer · history of stroke (including transient ischaemic attack) · hypertension (blood pressure systolic 160 mmHg or diastolic 100 mmHg or higher) · hypertensive retinopathy · ischaemic heart disease · known thrombogenic mutations (e.g. factor V Leiden, prothrombin mutation, protein S, protein C and antithrombin deficiencies) · less than 3 weeks postpartum in non-breastfeeding women with other risk factors for venous thromboembolism · major surgery with prolonged immobilisation · migraine with aura · peripheral vascular disease with intermittent claudication · positive antiphospholipid antibodies · presence or history of liver tumours (benign or malignant) · previous or current venous or arterial thrombosis · severe or multiple risk factors for arterial or venous thromboembolism · smoking in patients aged 35 years and over (15 or more cigarettes daily) · systemic lupus erythematosus with antiphospholipid antibodies

- **CAUTIONS** Cervical intraepithelial neoplasia or cancer · cholestasis with previous use of combined oral contraception—seek specialist advice before use · gallbladder disease—if medically treated or current, seek specialist advice before use · gene mutations associated with breast cancer (e.g. BRCA 1)—seek specialist advice before use · history of breast cancer—seek specialist advice before use · history of cholestasis during pregnancy ·

history of depression · inflammatory bowel disease · migraine · organ transplantation—when complicated, seek specialist advice before use · personal or family history of hypertriglyceridaemia (increased risk of pancreatitis) · prolactinoma—seek specialist advice before use · risk factors for arterial thromboembolism · risk factors for cardiovascular disease · risk factors for venous thromboembolism · sickle-cell disease · systemic lupus erythematosus · undiagnosed breast mass—seek specialist advice before use · undiagnosed vaginal bleeding

CAUTIONS, FURTHER INFORMATION

▸ Venous thromboembolism There is an increased risk of venous thromboembolism in females taking co-cyprindiol, particularly during the first year of use. The incidence of venous thromboembolism is 1.5–2 times higher in females using co-cyprindiol than in females using oral combined hormonal contraceptives containing levonorgestrel, but the risk may be similar to that associated with use of oral combined hormonal contraceptives containing third generation progestogens (desogestrel and gestodene) or drospirenone.

For more information about the risk factors for venous thromboembolism, see cautions for combined hormonal contraceptive preparations (e.g. ethinylestradiol with gestodene p. 924).

▸ Cardiovascular disease Co-cyprindiol also slightly increases the risk of cardiovascular disease, such as myocardial infarction and ischaemic stroke. Females requiring co-cyprindiol may have an inherently increased risk of cardiovascular disease such as that associated with polycystic ovary syndrome.

For more information about the risk factors for cardiovascular disease, see cautions for combined hormonal contraceptive preparations (e.g. ethinylestradiol with gestodene p. 924).

● INTERACTIONS → Appendix 1: anti-androgens · ethinylestradiol

● SIDE-EFFECTS

▸ **Common or very common** Abdominal pain · breast abnormalities · depression · headaches · mood altered · nausea · weight changes

▸ **Uncommon** Diarrhoea · fluid retention · sexual dysfunction · skin reactions · vomiting

▸ **Rare or very rare** Contact lens intolerance · erythema nodosum · thromboembolism · vaginal discharge

▸ **Frequency not known** Amenorrhoea (on discontinuation) · angioedema aggravated · chorea exacerbated · hepatic function abnormal · hepatic neoplasm · hypertension · hypertriglyceridaemia · inflammatory bowel disease · menstrual cycle irregularities · suicidal behaviours

● CONCEPTION AND CONTRACEPTION EvGr Co-cyprindiol contains an anti-androgen and is an effective hormonal contraceptive. However, it should not be used solely for contraception but reserved for females who require treatment for androgen-dependent skin conditions. Patients should not take other hormonal contraceptives while being treated with co-cyprindiol. Ⓜ

● PREGNANCY Avoid—risk of feminisation of male fetus with cyproterone.

● BREAST FEEDING Manufacturer advises avoid; possibility of anti-androgen effects in neonate with cyproterone.

● HEPATIC IMPAIRMENT Manufacturer advises caution; avoid in severe or active disease.

● PRESCRIBING AND DISPENSING INFORMATION A mixture of cyproterone acetate and ethinylestradiol in the mass proportions 2000 parts to 35 parts, respectively.

● MEDICINAL FORMS There can be variation in the licensing of different medicines containing the same drug.

Oral tablet

▸ Co-cyprindiol (Non-proprietary)

Ethinylestradiol 35 microgram, Cyproterone acetate 2 mg Co-cyprindiol 2000microgram/35microgram tablets | 63 tablet PoM £12.45 DT = £9.33

▸ Clairette (Kent Pharma (UK) Ltd)

Ethinylestradiol 35 microgram, Cyproterone acetate 2 mg Clairette 2000/35 tablets | 63 tablet PoM £5.90 DT = £9.33

▸ Dianette (Bayer Plc)

Ethinylestradiol 35 microgram, Cyproterone acetate 2 mg Dianette tablets | 63 tablet PoM £7.71 DT = £9.33

ANTIBACTERIALS › LINCOSAMIDES

Clindamycin   22-Mar-2024

● **INDICATIONS AND DOSE**

DALACIN T ® LOTION

Acne vulgaris

▸ TO THE SKIN

▸ Child: Apply twice daily, to be applied thinly

▸ Adult: Apply twice daily, to be applied thinly

ZINDACLIN ® GEL

Acne vulgaris

▸ TO THE SKIN

▸ Child 12–17 years: Apply once daily, to be applied thinly

▸ Adult: Apply once daily, to be applied thinly

● INTERACTIONS → Appendix 1: clindamycin

● SIDE-EFFECTS

▸ **Common or very common** Diarrhoea (discontinue) · skin reactions

▸ **Frequency not known** Abdominal pain · folliculitis gram-negative · gastrointestinal disorders · pseudomembranous enterocolitis

● PATIENT AND CARER ADVICE Patients and their carers should be advised to discontinue and contact a doctor immediately if severe, prolonged or bloody diarrhoea develops.

● MEDICINAL FORMS There can be variation in the licensing of different medicines containing the same drug.

Cutaneous emulsion

EXCIPIENTS: May contain Cetostearyl alcohol (including cetyl and stearyl alcohol), hydroxybenzoates (parabens)

▸ Dalacin T (Pfizer Ltd)

Clindamycin (as Clindamycin phosphate) 10 mg per 1 ml Dalacin T 1% topical lotion | 30 ml PoM £5.08 DT = £5.08 | 60 ml PoM £10.16

Cutaneous gel

EXCIPIENTS: May contain Propylene glycol

▸ Zindaclin (Aspire Pharma Ltd)

Clindamycin (as Clindamycin phosphate) 10 mg per 1 gram Zindaclin 1% gel | 30 gram PoM £9.95 DT = £9.95

Combinations available: *Benzoyl peroxide with clindamycin,* p. 1442 · *Tretinoin with clindamycin,* p. 1445

ANTIBACTERIALS › MACROLIDES

Erythromycin with zinc acetate   20-Apr-2020

The properties listed below are those particular to the combination only. For the properties of the components please consider, erythromycin p. 624.

● **INDICATIONS AND DOSE**

Acne vulgaris

▸ TO THE SKIN

▸ Child: Apply twice daily

▸ Adult: Apply twice daily

● **INTERACTIONS** → Appendix 1: macrolides

● **MEDICINAL FORMS** There can be variation in the licensing of different medicines containing the same drug.
Cutaneous solution
▸ **Erythromycin with zinc acetate (Non-proprietary)**
Zinc acetate 12 mg per 1 ml, Erythromycin 40 mg per 1 ml Erythromycin 40mg/ml / Zinc acetate 12mg/ml lotion | 30 ml PoM £9.25 DT = £9.25 | 90 ml PoM £20.02 DT = £20.02

ANTISEPTICS AND DISINFECTANTS › PEROXIDES

Benzoyl peroxide
01-Nov-2021

● **INDICATIONS AND DOSE**
Acne vulgaris
▸ TO THE SKIN
▸ **Child 12–17 years:** Apply 1–2 times a day, preferably apply after washing with soap and water
▸ **Adult:** Apply 1–2 times a day, preferably apply after washing with soap and water

● **CAUTIONS** Avoid contact with broken skin · avoid contact with eyes · avoid contact with mouth · avoid contact with mucous membranes · avoid excessive exposure to sunlight

● **SIDE-EFFECTS**
▸ **Common or very common** Skin reactions
▸ **Frequency not known** Facial swelling

● **PATIENT AND CARER ADVICE** May bleach fabrics and hair. If sun exposure is unavoidable, an appropriate sunscreen or protective clothing should be used. Patients and carers should be warned that some redness and skin peeling can occur initially but settles with time. To reduce the risk of skin irritation, treatment may be started with alternate-day or short-contact application (e.g. washing off after an hour) and progressed to standard application if tolerated. If severe irritation occurs, the frequency of application should be reduced, or treatment temporarily discontinued or stopped altogether.

● **MEDICINAL FORMS** There can be variation in the licensing of different medicines containing the same drug.
Cutaneous gel
EXCIPIENTS: May contain Fragrances, propylene glycol
▸ **Acnecide** (Galderma (UK) Ltd)
Benzoyl peroxide 50 mg per 1 gram Acnecide 5% gel | 30 gram P £6.26 DT = £6.26 | 60 gram P £12.28 DT = £12.28
Acnecide Wash 5% gel | 100 gram P £8.81

Combinations available: *Adapalene with benzoyl peroxide,* p. 1443

Benzoyl peroxide with clindamycin
09-Mar-2020

The properties listed below are those particular to the combination only. For the properties of the components please consider, benzoyl peroxide above, clindamycin p. 1441.

● **INDICATIONS AND DOSE**
Acne vulgaris
▸ TO THE SKIN
▸ **Child 12–17 years:** Apply once daily, dose to be applied in the evening
▸ **Adult:** Apply once daily, dose to be applied in the evening

● **INTERACTIONS** → Appendix 1: clindamycin

● **MEDICINAL FORMS** There can be variation in the licensing of different medicines containing the same drug.
Cutaneous gel
EXCIPIENTS: May contain Disodium edetate
▸ **Benzoyl peroxide with clindamycin (Non-proprietary)**
Clindamycin (as Clindamycin phosphate) 10 mg per 1 gram, Benzoyl peroxide 50 mg per 1 gram Benzoyl peroxide 5% / Clindamycin 1% gel | 30 gram PoM £21.02 DT = £13.14 | 60 gram PoM £42.04 DT = £26.28
▸ **Duac** (Stiefel Laboratories (UK) Ltd)
Clindamycin (as Clindamycin phosphate) 10 mg per 1 gram, Benzoyl peroxide 30 mg per 1 gram Duac Once Daily gel (3% and 1%) | 30 gram PoM £13.14 DT = £13.14 | 60 gram PoM £26.28
Clindamycin (as Clindamycin phosphate) 10 mg per 1 gram, Benzoyl peroxide 50 mg per 1 gram Duac Once Daily gel (5% and 1%) | 30 gram PoM £13.14 DT = £13.14 | 60 gram PoM £26.28 DT = £26.28

DERMATOLOGICAL DRUGS › ANTICOMEDONALS

Azelaic acid
04-Nov-2021

● **INDICATIONS AND DOSE**
FINACEA ®

Acne vulgaris
▸ TO THE SKIN
▸ **Child 12–17 years:** Apply twice daily
▸ **Adult:** Apply twice daily

Papulopustular rosacea
▸ TO THE SKIN
▸ **Adult:** Apply twice daily, discontinue if no improvement after 2 months

SKINOREN ®

Acne vulgaris
▸ TO THE SKIN
▸ **Child 12–17 years:** Apply twice daily
▸ **Adult:** Apply twice daily

● **CAUTIONS** Avoid contact with eyes · avoid contact with mouth · avoid contact with mucous membranes

● **SIDE-EFFECTS**
▸ **Uncommon** Skin reactions
▸ **Rare or very rare** Asthma exacerbated · cheilitis
▸ **Frequency not known** Angioedema · eye swelling

● **PATIENT AND CARER ADVICE** If severe skin irritation occurs, the amount of preparation applied or frequency of application should be reduced, or treatment temporarily discontinued. In patients with sensitive skin, treatment may be started with once-daily application (in the evening) and progressed to twice-daily application if tolerated.

● **MEDICINAL FORMS** There can be variation in the licensing of different medicines containing the same drug.
Cutaneous cream
EXCIPIENTS: May contain Propylene glycol
▸ **Skinoren** (LEO Pharma)
Azelaic acid 200 mg per 1 gram Skinoren 20% cream | 30 gram PoM £4.49 DT = £4.49
Cutaneous gel
EXCIPIENTS: May contain Disodium edetate, polysorbates, propylene glycol
▸ **Finacea** (LEO Pharma)
Azelaic acid 150 mg per 1 gram Finacea 15% gel | 30 gram PoM £7.48 DT = £7.48

RETINOID AND RELATED DRUGS

Adapalene
28-Jun-2023

- **INDICATIONS AND DOSE**

Mild to moderate acne vulgaris
▶ TO THE SKIN
▶ Child 12–17 years: Apply once daily, apply thinly in the evening
▶ Adult: Apply once daily, apply thinly in the evening

- **CAUTIONS** Avoid accumulation in angles of the nose · avoid contact with eyes, nostrils, mouth and mucous membranes, eczematous, broken or sunburned skin · avoid exposure to UV light (including sunlight, solariums) · avoid in severe acne involving large areas · caution in sensitive areas such as the neck

- **INTERACTIONS** → Appendix 1: retinoids

- **CONCEPTION AND CONTRACEPTION** The MHRA advises females of childbearing potential should use effective contraception.

- **PREGNANCY** The MHRA advises that systemic exposure is thought to be negligible following application of topical retinoids. However, since risk cannot be excluded, use of topical retinoids is contra-indicated during pregnancy as a precaution.

- **BREAST FEEDING** Amount of drug in milk probably too small to be harmful; ensure infant does not come in contact with treated areas.

- **PATIENT AND CARER ADVICE** If sun exposure is unavoidable, an appropriate sunscreen or protective clothing should be used. To reduce the risk of skin irritation, treatment may be started with alternate-day or short-contact application (e.g. washing off after an hour) and progressed to standard application if tolerated. If severe irritation occurs, the frequency of application should be reduced, or treatment temporarily discontinued or stopped altogether.

- **MEDICINAL FORMS** There can be variation in the licensing of different medicines containing the same drug.

Cutaneous cream
CAUTIONARY AND ADVISORY LABELS 11
EXCIPIENTS: May contain Disodium edetate, hydroxybenzoates (parabens)
▶ Differin (Galderma (UK) Ltd)
  Adapalene 1 mg per 1 gram Differin 0.1% cream | 45 gram PoM
  £16.43 DT = £16.43

Cutaneous gel
CAUTIONARY AND ADVISORY LABELS 11
EXCIPIENTS: May contain Disodium edetate, hydroxybenzoates (parabens), propylene glycol
▶ Differin (Galderma (UK) Ltd)
  Adapalene 1 mg per 1 gram Differin 0.1% gel | 45 gram PoM
  £16.43 DT = £16.43

Adapalene with benzoyl peroxide
28-Jun-2023

The properties listed below are those particular to the combination only. For the properties of the components please consider, adapalene above, benzoyl peroxide p. 1442.

- **INDICATIONS AND DOSE**

Acne vulgaris
▶ TO THE SKIN
▶ Child 9–17 years: Apply once daily, to be applied thinly in the evening
▶ Adult: Apply once daily, to be applied thinly in the evening

- **INTERACTIONS** → Appendix 1: retinoids

- **NATIONAL FUNDING/ACCESS DECISIONS**
For full details see funding body website
Scottish Medicines Consortium (SMC) decisions
▶ Adapalene 0.1% with benzoyl peroxide 2.5% gel (*Epiduo*®) for the cutaneous treatment of acne vulgaris when comedones, papules and pustules are present (April 2014) SMC No. 682/11 Recommended with restrictions

- **MEDICINAL FORMS** There can be variation in the licensing of different medicines containing the same drug.

Cutaneous gel
CAUTIONARY AND ADVISORY LABELS 11
EXCIPIENTS: May contain Disodium edetate, polysorbates, propylene glycol
▶ Adapalene with benzoyl peroxide (Non-proprietary)
  Adapalene 1 mg per 1 gram, Benzoyl peroxide 25 mg per 1 gram Adapalene 0.1% / Benzoyl peroxide 2.5% gel | 45 gram PoM £20.85
▶ Epiduo (Galderma (UK) Ltd)
  Adapalene 3 mg per 1 gram, Benzoyl peroxide 25 mg per 1 gram Epiduo 0.3%/2.5% gel | 60 gram PoM £27.80 DT = £27.80
  Adapalene 1 mg per 1 gram, Benzoyl peroxide 25 mg per 1 gram Epiduo 0.1%/2.5% gel | 60 gram PoM £27.80 DT = £27.80

Isotretinoin
06-Nov-2023

- **INDICATIONS AND DOSE**

Severe acne [(such as nodular or conglobate acne or acne at risk of permanent scarring) resistant to adequate courses of standard therapy with systemic antibacterials and topical therapy] (under expert supervision)
▶ BY MOUTH
▶ Adult: Initially 500 micrograms/kg daily in 1–2 divided doses, increased if necessary to 1 mg/kg daily and continued until a total cumulative dose of 120–150 mg/kg is reached—treatment may be discontinued sooner if there has been an adequate response and no new lesions for 4–8 weeks, treatment course may be repeated after a period of at least 8 weeks if relapse after first course, consider dose reduction to less than 500 micrograms/kg daily for patients at increased risk of, or experiencing, side-effects; maximum 150 mg/kg per course

IMPORTANT SAFETY INFORMATION
MHRA/CHM ADVICE: ISOTRETINOIN (*ROACCUTANE*®): RARE REPORTS OF ERECTILE DYSFUNCTION AND DECREASED LIBIDO (OCTOBER 2017)
An EU-wide review has concluded that on rare occasions, oral isotretinoin, indicated for severe acne, may cause sexual side-effects, including erectile dysfunction and decreased libido.

MHRA/CHM ADVICE: ORAL RETINOID MEDICINES: REVISED AND SIMPLIFIED PREGNANCY PREVENTION EDUCATIONAL MATERIALS FOR HEALTHCARE PROFESSIONALS AND WOMEN (JUNE 2019)
New prescriber checklists, patient reminder cards, and pharmacy checklists are available to support the Pregnancy Prevention Programme in women and girls of childbearing potential taking oral acitretin, alitretinoin, or isotretinoin. Healthcare professionals are reminded that the use of oral retinoids is contra-indicated in pregnancy due to a high risk of serious congenital malformations, and any use in females must be within the conditions of the Pregnancy Prevention Programme (see *Conception and contraception* and *Prescribing and dispensing information*).

Neuropsychiatric reactions have been reported in patients taking oral retinoids. Healthcare professionals are advised to monitor patients for signs of depression or suicidal ideation and refer for appropriate treatment, if necessary; particular care is needed in those with a history of depression. Patients should be advised to speak to their doctor if they experience any changes in mood or behaviour, and encouraged to ask family and friends to look out for any change in mood.

MHRA/CHM ADVICE: ISOTRETINOIN (*ROACCUTANE*®): REMINDER OF IMPORTANT RISKS AND PRECAUTIONS (AUGUST 2020)
The MHRA reminds healthcare professionals that isotretinoin should only be prescribed for the treatment of severe forms of acne resistant to adequate courses of standard therapy with systemic antibacterials and topical therapy. Isotretinoin should be given under the supervision of physicians with expertise in the use of systemic retinoids, and a complete understanding of the risks of therapy and monitoring requirements (including signs of depression).

Healthcare professionals are also advised to counsel patients on the potential risks of isotretinoin, including neuropsychiatric reactions and sexual dysfunction.

The MHRA further reminds healthcare professionals that isotretinoin is a powerful teratogen associated with a high frequency of severe and life-threatening birth defects if there is exposure *in utero*; females of childbearing potential must meet the conditions of the Pregnancy Prevention Programme (see *Conception and contraception* and *Prescribing and dispensing information*).

MHRA/CHM ADVICE: ISOTRETINOIN (*ROACCUTANE*®): INTRODUCTION OF NEW SAFETY MEASURES, INCLUDING ADDITIONAL OVERSIGHT OF THE INITIATION OF TREATMENT FOR PATIENTS UNDER 18 YEARS OF AGE (OCTOBER 2023)
Based on recommendations from the CHM after a review of the potential psychiatric and sexual side-effects of isotretinoin, the MHRA has introduced new safety measures that healthcare professionals are advised to follow:

- 2 independent prescribers must agree on treatment initiation in patients under 18 years old and only for severe acne resistant to adequate courses of standard therapy;
- all patients must be informed of the benefits and risks of treatment and have sufficient time to reflect and ask questions before starting treatment;
- additional counselling requirements about potential mental health and sexual function side-effects;
- improved assessment and monitoring of mental health and sexual function before starting and during treatment;
- new roles and responsibilities, such as the lead prescriber who initiates isotretinoin must have expertise in the use of systemic retinoids and a complete understanding of the risks of treatment and monitoring requirements, and patients should be reviewed face-to-face 1 month after treatment initiation;
- new compulsory regulatory risk minimisation materials, such as risk acknowledgement forms, patient reminder cards, and pharmacist checklists.

All healthcare professionals involved in the treatment of acne, particularly those who prescribe isotretinoin, are also advised to refer to the full details of the new requirements in the Report of the CHM Isotretinoin Implementation Advisory Expert Working Group, available at: www.gov.uk/government/publications/report-of-the-commission-on-human-medicines-isotretinoin-implementation-advisory-expert-working-group.

- **CONTRA-INDICATIONS** Hyperlipidaemia · hypervitaminosis A
- **CAUTIONS** Avoid blood donation during treatment and for at least 1 month after treatment · diabetes · dry eye syndrome (associated with risk of keratitis) · history of depression (risk of neuropsychiatric reactions)
- **INTERACTIONS** → Appendix 1: retinoids

- **SIDE-EFFECTS**
  - ▸ **Common or very common** Anaemia · arthralgia · back pain · cheilitis · dry eye · eye discomfort · eye inflammation · haemorrhage · headache · increased risk of infection · myalgia · nasal dryness · neutropenia · proteinuria · skin fragility (trauma may cause blistering) · skin reactions · thrombocytopenia · thrombocytosis
  - ▸ **Rare or very rare** Alopecia · anxiety · arthritis · behaviour abnormal · bronchospasm · cataract · corneal opacity · depression · diabetes mellitus · dizziness · drowsiness · dry throat · epiphyses premature fusion (following long-term use of high doses) · exostosis (following long-term use of high doses) · gastrointestinal disorders · glomerulonephritis · hair changes · hearing impairment · hepatitis · hoarseness · hyperhidrosis · hyperuricaemia · idiopathic intracranial hypertension · inflammatory bowel disease · ligament calcification (following long-term use of high doses) · lymphadenopathy · malaise · mood altered · nail dystrophy · nausea · pancreatitis · photosensitivity reaction · psychotic disorder · pyogenic granuloma · seizure · suicidal behaviours · tendinitis · tendon calcification (following long-term use of high doses) · vasculitis · vision disorders
  - ▸ **Frequency not known** Psychiatric disorder · rhabdomyolysis · severe cutaneous adverse reactions (SCARs) · sexual dysfunction · vulvovaginal dryness

  SIDE-EFFECTS, FURTHER INFORMATION Risk of pancreatitis if triglycerides above 9 mmol/litre—discontinue if uncontrolled hypertriglyceridaemia or pancreatitis.

  Discontinue treatment if skin peeling severe or haemorrhagic diarrhoea develops.

  Visual disturbances require expert referral and possible withdrawal.

  Psychiatric side-effects could require expert referral.

- **ALLERGY AND CROSS-SENSITIVITY** EvGr Contra-indicated in patients with hypersensitivity to peanuts or soya (capsule filling contains soya-bean oil). ⓜ
- **CONCEPTION AND CONTRACEPTION** The MHRA advises that women and girls of childbearing potential being treated with the oral retinoids acitretin, alitretinoin, or isotretinoin must be supported on a Pregnancy Prevention Programme with regular follow-up and pregnancy testing. Pregnancy prevention Effective contraception must be used.

  In females of childbearing potential, exclude pregnancy a few days before treatment, every month during treatment (unless there are compelling reasons to indicate that there is no risk of pregnancy), and 1 month after stopping treatment. Females of childbearing age must practise effective contraception for at least 1 month before starting treatment, during treatment, and for at least 1 month after stopping treatment. They should be advised to use at least 1 highly effective method of contraception (i.e. a user-independent form such as an intra-uterine device or implant) or 2 complementary user-dependent forms of contraception (e.g. oral contraceptives and barrier method). Females should be advised to discontinue treatment and to seek prompt medical attention if they become pregnant during treatment or within 1 month of stopping treatment.

- **PREGNANCY** Manufacturer advises avoid—teratogenic.
- **BREAST FEEDING** Avoid.
- **HEPATIC IMPAIRMENT** Manufacturer advises avoid—limited information available.
- **RENAL IMPAIRMENT**
  Dose adjustments EvGr In severe impairment, reduce initial dose (e.g. 10 mg daily) and increase gradually up to 1 mg/kg daily as tolerated. ⓜ
- **MONITORING REQUIREMENTS** Measure hepatic function and serum lipids before treatment, 1 month after starting and then every 3 months (reduce dose or discontinue if transaminase or serum lipids persistently raised).

- **PRESCRIBING AND DISPENSING INFORMATION** Isotretinoin is an isomer of tretinoin.

  The manufacturer has provided an *Acknowledgement of Risk Form* and *Pharmacist Checklist*.

  Applicability of the Pregnancy Prevention Programme to the patient's circumstances should be recorded on their prescription.

  Prescribing for females of childbearing potential Each prescription for oral isotretinoin should be limited to a supply of up to 30 days' treatment and dispensed within 7 days. Pregnancy testing should ideally be carried out on the same day as prescription issuing and dispensing.

- **PATIENT AND CARER ADVICE** Warn patient to avoid wax epilation (risk of epidermal stripping), dermabrasion, and laser skin treatments (risk of scarring) during treatment and for at least 6 months after stopping; patient should avoid exposure to UV light (including sunlight) and use sunscreen and emollient (including lip balm) preparations from the start of treatment.

  Risk of neuropsychiatric reactions The MHRA advises patients and carers to seek medical attention if changes in mood or behaviour occur.

  Patient Reminder Card Pharmacists must ensure that all patients have a patient reminder card—see also *Important safety information*.

- **MEDICINAL FORMS** There can be variation in the licensing of different medicines containing the same drug.

  Oral capsule

  CAUTIONARY AND ADVISORY LABELS 10, 11, 21

  ▸ **Isotretinoin (non-proprietary)** ▼

  Isotretinoin 5 mg Isotretinoin 5mg capsules | 56 capsule PoM £29.30 DT = £14.78

  Isotretinoin 10 mg Isotretinoin 10mg capsules | 30 capsule PoM £18.25 DT = £18.25

  Isotretinoin 20 mg Isotretinoin 20mg capsules | 30 capsule PoM £24.00 DT = £23.77 | 56 capsule PoM £23.80–£42.00

  ▸ **Roaccutane** (Neon Healthcare Ltd) ▼

  Isotretinoin 10 mg Roaccutane 10mg capsules | 30 capsule PoM £14.54 DT = £18.25

  Isotretinoin 20 mg Roaccutane 20mg capsules | 30 capsule PoM £20.02 DT = £23.77

Tretinoin with clindamycin

28-Jun-2023

The properties listed below are those particular to the combination only. For the properties of the components please consider, clindamycin p. 1441.

- **INDICATIONS AND DOSE**

  Acne vulgaris
  ▸ TO THE SKIN
  ▸ Child 12-17 years: Apply once daily, to be applied thinly at bedtime
  ▸ Adult: Apply once daily, to be applied thinly at bedtime

- **CONTRA-INDICATIONS** Perioral dermatitis · personal or familial history of skin cancer · rosacea

- **CAUTIONS** Allow peeling (resulting from other irritant treatments) to subside before using a topical retinoid · avoid accumulation in angles of the nose · avoid contact with eyes, nostrils, mouth and mucous membranes, eczematous, broken or sunburned skin · avoid exposure to UV light (including sunlight, solariums) · avoid use of topical retinoids with keratolytic agents, abrasive cleaners, comedogenic or astringent cosmetics · caution in sensitive areas such as the neck · severe acne

- **INTERACTIONS** → Appendix 1: clindamycin · retinoids

- **SIDE-EFFECTS** Dry skin (discontinue if severe) · eye irritation · oedema · photosensitivity reaction · skin pigmentation change (transient) · skin reactions

- **CONCEPTION AND CONTRACEPTION** The MHRA advises females of childbearing potential should use effective contraception.

- **PREGNANCY** The MHRA advises that systemic exposure is thought to be negligible following application of topical retinoids. However, since risk cannot be excluded, use of topical retinoids is contra-indicated during pregnancy as a precaution.

- **BREAST FEEDING** Amount of drug in milk after topical application probably too small to be harmful; ensure infant does not come in contact with treated areas.

- **PATIENT AND CARER ADVICE** If sun exposure is unavoidable, an appropriate sunscreen or protective clothing should be used.

  Patients and carers should be warned that some redness and skin peeling can occur initially but settles with time. To reduce the risk of skin irritation, treatment may be started with alternate-day or short-contact application (e.g. washing off after an hour) and progressed to standard application if tolerated. If severe irritation occurs, the frequency of application should be reduced or treatment suspended until the reaction subsides; if irritation persists, discontinue treatment. Several months of treatment may be needed to achieve an optimal response and the treatment should be continued until no new lesions develop.

- **MEDICINAL FORMS** There can be variation in the licensing of different medicines containing the same drug.

  Cutaneous gel

  CAUTIONARY AND ADVISORY LABELS 11
  EXCIPIENTS: May contain Butylated hydroxytoluene, hydroxybenzoates (parabens), polysorbates

  ▸ **Treclin** (Viatris UK Healthcare Ltd)

  Tretinoin 250 microgram per 1 gram, Clindamycin (as Clindamycin phosphate) 10 mg per 1 gram Treclin 1%/0.025% gel | 30 gram PoM £11.94 DT = £11.94

Tretinoin with erythromycin

28-Jun-2023

The properties listed below are those particular to the combination only. For the properties of the components please consider, erythromycin p. 624.

- **INDICATIONS AND DOSE**

  Acne
  ▸ TO THE SKIN
  ▸ Child: Apply 1–2 times a day, to be applied thinly
  ▸ Adult: Apply 1–2 times a day, to be applied thinly

- **CONTRA-INDICATIONS** Perioral dermatitis · personal or familial history of skin cancer · rosacea

- **CAUTIONS** Allow peeling (resulting from other irritant treatments) to subside before using a topical retinoid · avoid accumulation in angles of the nose · avoid contact with eyes, nostrils, mouth and mucous membranes, eczematous, broken or sunburned skin · avoid exposure to UV light (including sunlight, solariums) · avoid use of topical retinoids with keratolytic agents, abrasive cleaners, comedogenic or astringent cosmetics · caution in sensitive areas such as the neck · severe acne

- **INTERACTIONS** → Appendix 1: macrolides · retinoids

- **SIDE-EFFECTS** Dry skin (discontinue if severe) · eye irritation · oedema · photosensitivity reaction · skin eruption · skin pigmentation change (transient)

- **CONCEPTION AND CONTRACEPTION** The MHRA advises females of childbearing potential should use effective contraception.

- **PREGNANCY** The MHRA advises that systemic exposure is thought to be negligible following application of topical retinoids. However, since risk cannot be excluded, use of topical retinoids is contra-indicated during pregnancy as a precaution.

● **BREAST FEEDING** Amount of drug in milk after topical application probably too small to be harmful; ensure infant does not come in contact with treated areas.

● **PATIENT AND CARER ADVICE** If sun exposure is unavoidable, an appropriate sunscreen or protective clothing should be used.

  Patients and carers should be warned that some redness and skin peeling can occur initially but settles with time. To reduce the risk of skin irritation, treatment may be started with alternate-day or short-contact application (e.g. washing off after an hour) and progressed to standard application if tolerated. If severe irritation occurs, the frequency of application should be reduced or treatment suspended until the reaction subsides; if irritation persists, discontinue treatment. Several months of treatment may be needed to achieve an optimal response and the treatment should be continued until no new lesions develop.

● **MEDICINAL FORMS** There can be variation in the licensing of different medicines containing the same drug.
Cutaneous solution
CAUTIONARY AND ADVISORY LABELS 11
► **Aknemycin Plus** (Almirall Ltd)
  Tretinoin 250 microgram per 1 gram, Erythromycin 40 mg per 1 gram Aknemycin Plus solution | 25 ml [PoM] £7.05 DT = £7.05

Trifarotene
28-May-2024

● **INDICATIONS AND DOSE**
Acne vulgaris
► TO THE SKIN
► **Child 12–17 years:** Apply once daily, to be applied thinly in the evening
► **Adult:** Apply once daily, to be applied thinly in the evening

● **CAUTIONS** Avoid contact with eyes, nostrils, mouth and mucous membranes, eczematous, broken or sunburned skin · avoid exposure to UV light (including sunlight, sunlamps)

● **SIDE-EFFECTS**
► **Common or very common** Sunburn
► **Uncommon** Skin reactions
► **Rare or very rare** Cheilitis · eyelid exfoliation · eyelid oedema · flushing

● **CONCEPTION AND CONTRACEPTION** The MHRA advises females of childbearing potential should use effective contraception.

● **PREGNANCY** The MHRA advises that systemic exposure is thought to be negligible following application of topical retinoids. However, since risk cannot be excluded, use of topical retinoids is contra-indicated during pregnancy as a precaution.

● **BREAST FEEDING** Specialist sources indicate amount of drug in milk after topical application probably too small to be harmful; ensure infant does not come in contact with treated areas.

● **PATIENT AND CARER ADVICE** If sun exposure is unavoidable, an appropriate sunscreen or protective clothing should be used. To reduce the risk of skin irritation, patients should be instructed to use a moisturiser from the initiation of treatment, and if necessary the frequency of application should be reduced or treatment temporarily discontinued. If severe irritation occurs and persists despite these actions, treatment should be stopped altogether.

● **NATIONAL FUNDING/ACCESS DECISIONS**
For full details see funding body website
Scottish Medicines Consortium (SMC) decisions
► **Trifarotene** (*Aklief*®) for the cutaneous treatment of acne vulgaris of the face and/or the trunk in patients from 12 years of age and older, when many comedones, papules and pustules are present (September 2022) SMC No. SMC2441
Recommended

All Wales Medicines Strategy Group (AWMSG) decisions
► **Trifarotene** (*Aklief*®) for the cutaneous treatment of acne vulgaris of the face and/or the trunk in patients from 12 years of age and older, when many comedones, papules and pustules are present (April 2024) AWMSG No. 3153
Recommended

● **MEDICINAL FORMS** There can be variation in the licensing of different medicines containing the same drug.
Cutaneous cream
EXCIPIENTS: May contain Ethanol, polysorbates, propylene glycol
► **Aklief** (Galderma (UK) Ltd) ▼
  Trifarotene 50 microgram per 1 gram Aklief 50micrograms/g cream | 75 gram [PoM] £27.75 DT = £27.75

VITAMINS AND TRACE ELEMENTS › VITAMIN B GROUP

Nicotinamide
05-Oct-2021

● **INDICATIONS AND DOSE**
Inflammatory acne vulgaris
► TO THE SKIN
► **Adult:** Apply twice daily, reduced to once daily or on alternate days, dose reduced if irritation occurs

● **CAUTIONS** Avoid contact with eyes · avoid contact with mucous membranes (including nose and mouth) · reduce frequency of application if excessive dryness, irritation or peeling

● **SIDE-EFFECTS** Paraesthesia · skin reactions

● **MEDICINAL FORMS** There can be variation in the licensing of different medicines containing the same drug.
Cutaneous gel
► **Freederm** (Diomed Developments Ltd)
  Nicotinamide 40 mg per 1 gram Freederm Treatment 4% gel | 25 gram [P] £5.56 DT = £5.56

8.2 Rosacea

ANTHELMINTICS

Ivermectin
07-Jul-2024

● **INDICATIONS AND DOSE**
Papulopustular rosacea
► TO THE SKIN
► **Adult:** Apply once daily for up to 4 months, the treatment course may be repeated. Discontinue if no improvement after 3 months

● **INTERACTIONS** → Appendix 1: ivermectin

● **SIDE-EFFECTS**
► **Common or very common** Skin reactions

● **PREGNANCY** [EvGr] Use only if potential benefit outweighs risk—no adverse effects in limited human data (recommendation also supported by specialist sources). Ⓜ

● **HEPATIC IMPAIRMENT** [EvGr] Caution in severe impairment (no information available). Ⓜ

- **DIRECTIONS FOR ADMINISTRATION** [EvGr] Apply a pea-size amount thinly to each of the five areas of the face: forehead, chin, nose and each cheek, avoiding the eyes, lips and mucosa. Wash hands after use. Cosmetics may be applied after the cream has dried. ⓜ

- **NATIONAL FUNDING/ACCESS DECISIONS**
  For full details see funding body website
  Scottish Medicines Consortium (SMC) decisions
  ► Ivermectin (*Soolantra*®) for topical treatment of inflammatory lesions of rosacea (papulopustular) in adult patients (December 2015) SMC No. 1104/15 Recommended with restrictions
  All Wales Medicines Strategy Group (AWMSG) decisions
  ► Ivermectin (*Soolantra*®) for treatment of inflammatory lesions of rosacea (papulopustular) in adult patients (April 2016) AWMSG No. 1627 Recommended

- **MEDICINAL FORMS** There can be variation in the licensing of different medicines containing the same drug.
  Cutaneous cream
  CAUTIONARY AND ADVISORY LABELS 28
  EXCIPIENTS: May contain Cetostearyl alcohol (including cetyl and stearyl alcohol), disodium edetate, isopropyl palmitate, propylene glycol
  ► **Soolantra** (Galderma (UK) Ltd)
  Ivermectin 10 mg per 1 gram Soolantra 10mg/g cream | 60 gram [PoM] £36.58 DT = £36.58

SYMPATHOMIMETICS › ALPHA₂-ADRENOCEPTOR AGONISTS

Brimonidine tartrate
11-May-2021

- **DRUG ACTION** Brimonidine, an alpha₂-adrenoceptor agonist, is used to reduce erythema in rosacea by cutaneous vasoconstriction.

- **INDICATIONS AND DOSE**
  Facial erythema in rosacea
  ► TO THE SKIN
  ► Adult: Apply once daily until erythema subsides, apply thinly, divide dose over forehead, chin, nose, and cheeks, max. 1 g of gel per day

  DOSE EQUIVALENCE AND CONVERSION
  ► 1 g of gel contains 5 mg of brimonidine tartrate (equivalent to 3.3 mg of brimonidine).

IMPORTANT SAFETY INFORMATION
MHRA/CHM ADVICE: BRIMONIDINE GEL (*MIRVASO*®): RISK OF SYSTEMIC CARDIOVASCULAR EFFECTS (JUNE 2017)
Systemic cardiovascular effects including bradycardia, hypotension, and dizziness have been reported after application of brimonidine gel. To minimise the possibility of systemic absorption, it is important to avoid application to irritated or damaged skin, including after laser therapy.

MHRA/CHM ADVICE: BRIMONIDINE GEL (*MIRVASO*®): RISK OF EXACERBATION OF ROSACEA (NOVEMBER 2016)
Symptom exacerbation has been reported very commonly in patients treated with brimonidine gel. Treatment should be initiated with a small amount of gel (less than the maximum dose) for at least 1 week, then increased gradually, based on tolerability and response. Patients should be counselled on the importance of not exceeding the maximum daily dose, and advised to stop treatment and seek medical advice if symptoms worsen during treatment.

- **CAUTIONS** Cerebral insufficiency · coronary insufficiency · depression · postural hypotension · Raynaud's syndrome · severe cardiovascular disease · thromboangiitis obliterans

- **INTERACTIONS** → Appendix 1: brimonidine

- **SIDE-EFFECTS**
  ► **Common or very common** Dizziness · dry mouth · flushing · headache · skin reactions
  ► **Uncommon** Angioedema · eyelid oedema · feeling hot · nasal congestion · paraesthesia · peripheral coldness
  ► **Rare or very rare** Bradycardia · hypotension

- **PREGNANCY** Manufacturer advises avoid—limited information available.

- **BREAST FEEDING** Manufacturer advises avoid—no information available.

- **HEPATIC IMPAIRMENT** Manufacturer advises caution (no information available).

- **RENAL IMPAIRMENT** Manufacturer advises use with caution.

- **DIRECTIONS FOR ADMINISTRATION** Manufacturer advises avoid contact with eyes, mouth, and mucous membranes; avoid use on irritated or damaged skin or open wounds; apply other topical preparations (including cosmetics) only after brimonidine gel has dried on skin.

- **PATIENT AND CARER ADVICE** Patients should be advised on administration of gel.

- **NATIONAL FUNDING/ACCESS DECISIONS**
  For full details see funding body website
  Scottish Medicines Consortium (SMC) decisions
  ► Brimonidine (*Mirvaso*®) for the symptomatic treatment of facial erythema of rosacea in adult patients (January 2015) SMC No. 1016/14 Recommended with restrictions
  All Wales Medicines Strategy Group (AWMSG) decisions
  ► Brimonidine (*Mirvaso*®) for the symptomatic treatment of facial erythema of rosacea in adult patients (September 2015) AWMSG No. 2168 Recommended with restrictions

- **MEDICINAL FORMS** There can be variation in the licensing of different medicines containing the same drug.
  Cutaneous gel
  CAUTIONARY AND ADVISORY LABELS 28
  EXCIPIENTS: May contain Hydroxybenzoates (parabens), propylene glycol
  ► **Mirvaso** (Galderma (UK) Ltd)
  Brimonidine (as Brimonidine tartrate) 3 mg per 1 gram Mirvaso 3mg/g gel | 30 gram [PoM] £33.69 DT = £33.69

9   Scalp and hair conditions

Scalp and hair conditions
14-Aug-2020

Overview

Dandruff is considered to be a mild form of seborrhoeic dermatitis. Shampoos containing antimicrobial agents such as **pyrithione zinc** (which are widely available) and selenium p. 1448 may have beneficial effects. Shampoos containing **tar** extracts may be useful and they are also used in *psoriasis*. Ketoconazole shampoo p. 1400 should be considered for more persistent or severe dandruff or for seborrhoeic dermatitis of the scalp.

Corticosteroid gels and lotions can also be used.

Shampoos containing coal tar with salicylic acid p. 1420 may also be useful. A cream or an ointment containing coal tar with salicylic acid is very helpful in Psoriasis p. 1406 that affects the scalp. Patients who do not respond to these treatments may need to be referred to exclude the possibility of other skin conditions.

Cradle cap in infants may be treated with **coconut oil** or **olive oil** applications followed by shampooing.

13
Skin

Hirsutism

Hirsutism may result from hormonal disorders or as a side-effect of drugs such as minoxidil p. 1449, corticosteroids, anabolic steroids, androgens, danazol, and progestogens.

Weight loss can reduce hirsutism in obese women.

Women should be advised about local methods of hair removal, and in the mildest cases this may be all that is required.

Eflornithine p. 1450 an antiprotozoal drug, inhibits the enzyme ornithine decarboxylase in hair follicles. Topical eflornithine can be used as an adjunct to laser therapy for facial hirsutism in women.

Co-cyprindiol p. 1440 (cyproterone acetate with ethinylestradiol) may be effective for moderately severe hirsutism. Metformin hydrochloride p. 807 is an alternative in women with polycystic ovary syndrome [unlicensed indication]. Systemic treatment is required for 6–12 months before benefit is seen. The MHRA/CHM have released important safety information regarding the use of cyproterone acetate and the risk of meningioma. For further information, see *Important safety information* for co-cyprindiol. The Faculty of Sexual and Reproductive Healthcare have released a statement in response to the MHRA/CHM information (available at: www.fsrh.org/standards-and-guidance/documents/fsrh-ceu-statement-new-advice-from-the-mhra-regarding/).

Androgenetic alopecia

Finasteride p. 907 is licensed for the treatment of androgenetic alopecia in men. Continuous use for 3–6 months is required before benefit is seen, and effects are reversed 6–12 months after treatment is discontinued.

Topical application of minoxidil may stimulate limited hair growth in a small proportion of adults but only for as long as it is used.

> **Other drugs used for Scalp and hair conditions** Coal tar, p. 1419 · Coal tar with salicylic acid and precipitated sulfur, p. 1420

ANTISEPTICS AND DISINFECTANTS ❭ UNDECENOATES

Cetrimide with undecenoic acid

● **INDICATIONS AND DOSE**

Scalp psoriasis | Seborrhoeic dermatitis | Dandruff
▸ TO THE SKIN
▸ Child: Apply 3 times a week for 1 week, then apply twice weekly
▸ Adult: Apply 3 times a week for 1 week, then apply twice weekly

● **MEDICINAL FORMS** No licensed medicines listed.

ANTISEPTICS AND DISINFECTANTS ❭ OTHER

Benzalkonium chloride

26-Mar-2020

● **INDICATIONS AND DOSE**

Seborrhoeic scalp conditions associated with dandruff and scaling
▸ TO THE SKIN
▸ Child: Apply as required
▸ Adult: Apply as required

● **MEDICINAL FORMS** There can be variation in the licensing of different medicines containing the same drug.

Shampoo
▸ Dermax (Dermal Laboratories Ltd)
Benzalkonium chloride 5 mg per 1 ml Dermax Therapeutic 0.5% shampoo | 250 ml [P] £5.99 DT = £5.99

VITAMINS AND TRACE ELEMENTS

Selenium

● **INDICATIONS AND DOSE**

Seborrhoeic dermatitis | Dandruff
▸ TO THE SKIN USING SHAMPOO
▸ Child 5–17 years: Apply twice weekly for 2 weeks, then apply once weekly for 2 weeks, then apply as required
▸ Adult: Apply twice weekly for 2 weeks, then apply once weekly for 2 weeks, then apply as required

Pityriasis versicolor
▸ TO THE SKIN USING SHAMPOO
▸ Adult: Apply once daily for 7 days, apply to the affected area and leave on for 10 minutes before rinsing off. The course may be repeated if necessary. Diluting with a small amount of water prior to application can reduce irritation

● **UNLICENSED USE** The use of selenium sulfide shampoo as a lotion for the treatment of pityriasis (tinea) versicolor is an unlicensed indication.

● **INTERACTIONS** → Appendix 1: selenium

● **PATIENT AND CARER ADVICE** Avoid using 48 hours before or after applying hair colouring, straightening or waving preparations.

● **MEDICINAL FORMS** No licensed medicines listed

9.1 Alopecia

> **Other drugs used for Alopecia** Baricitinib, p. 1262

IMMUNOSUPPRESSANTS ❭ JAK INHIBITORS

Ritlecitinib

03-May-2024

● **DRUG ACTION** Ritlecitinib selectively and irreversibly inhibits the Janus-associated tyrosine kinase JAK3 and the tyrosine kinase TEC.

● **INDICATIONS AND DOSE**

Alopecia areata (under expert supervision)
▸ BY MOUTH
▸ Adult: 50 mg once daily, consider discontinuation of treatment if no response after 36 weeks

> **IMPORTANT SAFETY INFORMATION**
>
> MHRA/CHM ADVICE: JANUS KINASE (JAK) INHIBITORS: NEW MEASURES TO REDUCE RISKS OF MAJOR CARDIOVASCULAR EVENTS, MALIGNANCY, VENOUS THROMBOEMBOLISM, SERIOUS INFECTIONS AND INCREASED MORTALITY (APRIL 2023)
>
> In 2022, the EMA conducted a review of all JAK inhibitors indicated for chronic inflammatory diseases and concluded that the risks associated with the use of tofacitinib could be considered a class effect (see *Important safety information* in tofacitinib p. 1265). Following a further review by the MHRA, some existing warnings for tofacitinib have been updated and implemented for all JAK inhibitors included in the review.
>
> Healthcare professionals are advised to:

- avoid use in patients aged 65 years or older, in patients who are current or past long-time smokers, and in patients with other cardiovascular disease or malignancy risk factors, unless there are no suitable alternatives;
- use with caution in patients with risk factors for venous thromboembolism;
- use lower doses in patients with risk factors, where applicable;
- periodically examine all patients' skin for malignancy;
- inform patients and their carers of these risks, and the signs and symptoms that warrant urgent medical attention.

- **CONTRA-INDICATIONS** Absolute lymphocyte count less than 0.5×10^9 cells/litre (do not initiate) · platelet count less than 100×10^9 cells/litre (do not initiate) · serious infection (active) · tuberculosis (active)

- **CAUTIONS** Chronic or recurrent infection · elderly (65 years and older) · history of atherosclerotic cardiovascular disease or other cardiovascular risk factors · history of serious or opportunistic infection · predisposition to infection · risk factors for malignancy · risk factors for thromboembolism · risk of viral reactivation (consult product literature) · tuberculosis exposure

  CAUTIONS, FURTHER INFORMATION
  - Tuberculosis [EvGr] Consider anti-tuberculosis therapy prior to initiation of ritlecitinib in patients with previously untreated latent tuberculosis and those at high risk of tuberculosis infection. ⟨M⟩
  - Immunisation [EvGr] Patients should receive all recommended vaccinations before starting treatment; live vaccines are not recommended immediately before, or during, treatment. ⟨M⟩
  - Thromboembolism [EvGr] If a thromboembolic event occurs during treatment, discontinuation of ritlecitinib is recommended. ⟨M⟩

- **INTERACTIONS** → Appendix 1: ritlecitinib

- **SIDE-EFFECTS**
  - **Common or very common** Diarrhoea · dizziness · headache · increased risk of infection · skin reactions
  - **Frequency not known** Embolism and thrombosis · malignancy · non-melanoma skin cancer · reactivation of infections · sepsis

- **CONCEPTION AND CONTRACEPTION** [EvGr] Females of childbearing potential should use effective contraception during treatment and for 1 month after last treatment. ⟨M⟩

- **PREGNANCY** [EvGr] Avoid (toxicity in *animal* studies). ⟨M⟩

- **BREAST FEEDING** [EvGr] Avoid (present in milk in *animal* studies). ⟨M⟩

- **HEPATIC IMPAIRMENT** [EvGr] Avoid in severe impairment (no information available). ⟨M⟩

- **PRE-TREATMENT SCREENING** [EvGr] Patients should be evaluated for tuberculosis and viral hepatitis before treatment. ⟨M⟩

- **MONITORING REQUIREMENTS**
  - [EvGr] Monitor for signs and symptoms of infection during and after treatment—consider treatment interruption until the infection is controlled.
  - Monitor platelets and lymphocytes at baseline, 4 weeks after treatment initiation, and as clinically indicated thereafter. Interrupt treatment if absolute lymphocyte count less than 0.5×10^9 cells/litre; treatment may be restarted when levels return above this value. Discontinue treatment if platelet count less than 50×10^9 cells/litre.
  - Monitor for viral reactivation (including viral hepatitis and herpes zoster) during treatment; interrupt treatment if herpes zoster infection develops and resume once resolved. If there is evidence of hepatitis reactivation, consult a liver specialist for advice.

- Periodic skin examination is recommended in all patients, particularly those at increased risk of skin cancer. ⟨M⟩

- **PRESCRIBING AND DISPENSING INFORMATION** The manufacturer of *Litfulo*® has provided a *Prescriber Guide*, which includes a prescriber checklist.

- **HANDLING AND STORAGE** Protect from light.

- **PATIENT AND CARER ADVICE**
  Patient card A patient card should be provided.
  Missed doses If a dose is more than 16 hours late, the missed dose should not be taken and the next dose should be taken at the normal time.

- **NATIONAL FUNDING/ACCESS DECISIONS**
  For full details see funding body website
  NICE decisions
  - Ritlecitinib for treating severe alopecia areata in people 12 years and over (March 2024) NICE TA958 Recommended
  Scottish Medicines Consortium (SMC) decisions
  - Ritlecitinib (*Litfulo*®) for the treatment of severe alopecia areata in adults and adolescents aged 12 years and over (April 2024) SMC No. SMC2610 Recommended

- **MEDICINAL FORMS** There can be variation in the licensing of different medicines containing the same drug.
  Oral capsule
  - Litfulo (Pfizer Ltd) ▼
    Ritlecitinib (as Ritlecitinib tosylate) 50 mg Litfulo 50mg capsules | 30 capsule [PoM] £949.41 (Hospital only)

VASODILATORS › POTASSIUM-CHANNEL OPENERS

Minoxidil   08-Nov-2021

- **INDICATIONS AND DOSE**

  REGAINE® FOR MEN EXTRA STRENGTH FOAM

  Androgenetic alopecia
  - TO THE SKIN
  - Adult: Apply 0.5 capful twice daily, to be applied to the affected areas of scalp; discontinue if no improvement after 16 weeks

  REGAINE® FOR MEN EXTRA STRENGTH SOLUTION

  Androgenetic alopecia
  - TO THE SKIN
  - Adult: Apply 1 mL twice daily, to be applied to the affected areas of scalp; discontinue if no improvement after 1 year

  REGAINE® FOR WOMEN REGULAR STRENGTH

  Androgenetic alopecia
  - TO THE SKIN
  - Adult: Apply 1 mL twice daily, to be applied to the affected areas of scalp; discontinue if no improvement after 1 year

- **CONTRA-INDICATIONS** Phaeochromocytoma

- **CAUTIONS** Avoid contact with broken, infected, shaved, or inflamed skin · avoid contact with eyes · avoid contact with mouth · avoid contact with mucous membranes · avoid inhalation of spray mist · avoid occlusive dressings

- **INTERACTIONS** → Appendix 1: minoxidil

- **SIDE-EFFECTS**
  - **Common or very common** Hair changes
  - **Uncommon** Hypotension

  SIDE-EFFECTS, FURTHER INFORMATION When used topically systemic effects unlikely; only about 1–2% absorbed (greater absorption may occur with use on inflamed skin).

- **PREGNANCY** Avoid—possible toxicity including reduced placental perfusion. Neonatal hirsutism reported.

- **BREAST FEEDING** Present in milk but not known to be harmful.
- **PATIENT AND CARER ADVICE** Ensure hair and scalp dry before application. Patients and their carers should be advised to wash hands after application of liquid or foam.

- **MEDICINAL FORMS** There can be variation in the licensing of different medicines containing the same drug.

Cutaneous solution
CAUTIONARY AND ADVISORY LABELS 15
EXCIPIENTS: May contain Propylene glycol
▸ **Regaine** (McNeil Products Ltd, Johnson & Johnson Ltd)
  Minoxidil 20 mg per 1 ml Regaine for Women Regular Strength 2% solution | 60 ml GSL £16.24
  Minoxidil 50 mg per 1 ml Regaine for Men Extra Strength 5% scalp solution | 60 ml GSL £21.87 | 180 ml P £45.62

Cutaneous foam
CAUTIONARY AND ADVISORY LABELS 15
EXCIPIENTS: May contain Butylated hydroxytoluene, cetostearyl alcohol (including cetyl and stearyl alcohol), polysorbates
▸ **Regaine** (McNeil Products Ltd)
  Minoxidil 50 mg per 1 gram Regaine for Men Extra Strength 5% scalp foam | 60 gram GSL £21.87 DT = £21.87 | 180 gram GSL £45.62 DT = £45.62

9.2 Hirsutism

ANTIPROTOZOALS

Eflornithine
04-Nov-2020

- **DRUG ACTION** An antiprotozoal drug that inhibits the enzyme ornithine decarboxylase in hair follicles.

- **INDICATIONS AND DOSE**

Adjunct in the treatment of facial hirsutism in women
▸ TO THE SKIN
▸ Adult: Apply twice daily, to be applied thinly, discontinue use if no improvement after 4 months of treatment

- **SIDE-EFFECTS**
▸ **Common or very common** Alopecia · increased risk of infection · paraesthesia · skin reactions
▸ **Uncommon** Face oedema · flushing · hair changes · oral disorders · skin haemorrhage
▸ **Rare or very rare** Skin neoplasm

- **PREGNANCY** Toxicity in *animal* studies—manufacturer advises avoid.

- **BREAST FEEDING** Manufacturer advises avoid—no information available.

- **PATIENT AND CARER ADVICE** Medicines must be rubbed in thoroughly. Cosmetics may be applied over treated area 5 minutes after eflornithine, do not wash treated area for 4 hours after application.

- **NATIONAL FUNDING/ACCESS DECISIONS**
  For full details see funding body website
  Scottish Medicines Consortium (SMC) decisions
  ▸ Eflornithine (*Vaniqa*®) for facial hirsutism in women (September 2005) SMC No. 159/05 Recommended with restrictions

- **MEDICINAL FORMS** There can be variation in the licensing of different medicines containing the same drug.

Cutaneous cream
EXCIPIENTS: May contain Cetostearyl alcohol (including cetyl and stearyl alcohol), hydroxybenzoates (parabens)
▸ **Vaniqa** (Almirall Ltd)
  Eflornithine (as Eflornithine hydrochloride monohydrate) 115 mg per 1 gram Vaniqa 11.5% cream | 60 gram PoM £56.87 DT = £56.87

10 Skin cleansers, antiseptics and desloughing agents

Skin cleansers, antiseptics and desloughing agents
29-Nov-2023

Skin cleansers and antiseptics

Soap or detergent is used with water to cleanse intact skin; emollient preparations such as aqueous cream or emulsifying ointment can be used in place of soap or detergent for cleansing dry skin.

An antiseptic is used for skin that is infected or that is susceptible to recurrent infection. Detergent preparations containing chlorhexidine p. 1452 or povidone-iodine p. 1451, which should be thoroughly rinsed off, are used. Emollients may also contain antiseptics.

Antiseptics such as chlorhexidine or povidone-iodine are used on intact skin before surgical procedures; their antiseptic effect is enhanced by an alcoholic solvent. Antiseptic solutions containing cetrimide can be used if a detergent effect is also required.

Hydrogen peroxide p. 1453, an oxidising agent, can be used in solutions of up to 6% for skin disinfection, such as cleansing and deodorising wounds and ulcers. Hydrogen peroxide is also available as a cream for superficial bacterial skin infections.

For irrigating ulcers or wounds, lukewarm sterile sodium chloride 0.9% solution is used, but tap water is often appropriate.

Potassium permanganate solution 1 in 10 000 p. 1451, a mild antiseptic with astringent properties, can be used for exudative eczematous areas; treatment should be stopped when the skin becomes dry.

Borderline substances

Disinfectants (antiseptics) have ACBS approval (see *About Borderline Substances*) to be prescribed on an FP10 only when ordered in such quantities and with such directions as are appropriate for the treatment of patients, but not if ordered for general hygienic purposes.

Desloughing agents

Alginate, hydrogel and hydrocolloid dressings are effective at wound debridement. Sterile larvae (maggots) (available from BioMonde) are also used for managing sloughing wounds and are prescribable on the NHS.

Desloughing solutions and creams are of little clinical value. Substances applied to an open area are easily absorbed and perilesional skin is easily sensitised. Gravitational dermatitis may be complicated by superimposed contact sensitivity to substances such as neomycin sulfate p. 1397 or lanolin.

ANTISEPTICS AND DISINFECTANTS

Potassium permanganate

11-Jul-2022

- **INDICATIONS AND DOSE**

Cleansing and deodorising suppurating eczematous reactions and wounds
▸ TO THE SKIN
▸ Adult: For wet dressings or baths, use approximately 0.01% (1 in 10 000) solution

---

IMPORTANT SAFETY INFORMATION

NHS IMPROVEMENT PATIENT SAFETY ALERT: RISK OF DEATH OR SERIOUS HARM FROM ACCIDENTAL INGESTION OF POTASSIUM PERMANGANATE PREPARATIONS (DECEMBER 2014)

Potassium permanganate is for external use only. Oral ingestion can cause fatality due to local inflammatory reactions that block the airways or cause perforations of the gastrointestinal tract, or through toxicity and organ failure. Potassium permanganate is subject to the requirements of Control of Substances Hazardous to Health including: separate storage, additional hazard labelling, and issue only to staff and patients who have been educated to understand its safe use. Accidental ingestion should be treated as a medical emergency.

NHS IMPROVEMENT PATIENT SAFETY ALERT: INADVERTENT ORAL ADMINISTRATION OF POTASSIUM PERMANGANATE (APRIL 2022)

A review of reported incidents over a two-year period identified 35 cases of inadvertent ingestion of potassium permanganate. Of these, 15 cases were of healthcare staff administering potassium permanganate orally to patients and 9 cases, one fatal, of patients self-administering orally. To minimise the risk of harm from potassium permanganate, the British Association of Dermatologists (BAD) has issued advice on formulary management, prescribing, dispensing, storage, preparation and use, and waste: www.bad.org.uk/bad-and-nhs-england-nhs-improvement-guidance-on-the-safe-use-of-potassium-permanganate-soaks/.

The overall use of potassium permanganate should be reviewed locally and protocols for its use should be aligned with all BAD recommendations, including:
In primary care:
- patients are not on repeat prescriptions for potassium permanganate;
- prescriptions include clear instructions to dilute before use;
- dispensing label includes the warning 'harmful if swallowed'.
In secondary care:
- remove all stock supply (except for use within outpatient departments) and supply on a named patient basis only;
- potassium permanganate is prescribed as 'potassium permanganate 0.01% topical solution' and the dispensing label must include the warning 'harmful if swallowed';
- potassium permanganate is not stored with medicines for oral/internal use, including the ward drug trolley; dilution should occur away from the patient, and neither the concentrated form nor the diluted form should be left near the patient.
In all settings:
- prescriptions are only issued by an appropriate prescriber;
- if potassium permanganate is to be used in a patient's home, a risk assessment must be undertaken before prescribing;
- all patients must be supplied with a patient information leaflet, such as that produced by BAD:

www.bad.org.uk/pils/potassium-permanganate-solution-soaks/.

- **CAUTIONS** Irritant to mucous membranes
- **DIRECTIONS FOR ADMINISTRATION** With potassium permanganate tablets for solution, 1 tablet dissolved in 4 litres of water provides a 0.01% (1 in 10 000) solution.
- **PATIENT AND CARER ADVICE** Can stain clothing, skin and nails (especially with prolonged use).

- **MEDICINAL FORMS** There can be variation in the licensing of different medicines containing the same drug. Forms available from special-order manufacturers include: cutaneous solution

Tablet for cutaneous solution
CAUTIONARY AND ADVISORY LABELS 10
▸ **Potassium permanganate (Non-proprietary)**
   Potassium permanganate 400 mg EN-Potab 400mg tablets for cutaneous solution | 30 tablet 🛈 DT = £28.62
▸ **AnateP** (Essential-Healthcare Ltd)
   Potassium permanganate 400 mg AnateP 400mg tablets for cutaneous solution | 30 tablet £17.83 DT = £28.62
▸ **Permitabs** (Alliance Pharmaceuticals Ltd)
   Potassium permanganate 400 mg Permitabs 400mg tablets for cutaneous solution | 30 tablet £30.05 DT = £28.62

ANTISEPTICS AND DISINFECTANTS ⟩ ALCOHOL DISINFECTANTS

Alcohol

(Industrial methylated spirit)

- **INDICATIONS AND DOSE**

Skin preparation before injection
▸ TO THE SKIN
▸ Child: Apply as required
▸ Adult: Apply as required

- **CONTRA-INDICATIONS** Neonates
- **CAUTIONS** Avoid broken skin · flammable · patients have suffered severe burns when diathermy has been preceded by application of alcoholic skin disinfectants
- **INTERACTIONS** → Appendix 1: alcohol
- **SIDE-EFFECTS**

Overdose Features of acute alcohol intoxication include ataxia, dysarthria, nystagmus, and drowsiness, which may progress to coma, with hypotension and acidosis.
For details on the management of poisoning, see Alcohol, under Emergency treatment of poisoning p. 1554.
- **PRESCRIBING AND DISPENSING INFORMATION** Industrial methylated spirits defined by the BP as a mixture of 19 volumes of ethyl alcohol of an appropriate strength with 1 volume of approved wood naphtha.

- **MEDICINAL FORMS** No licensed medicines listed.

ANTISEPTICS AND DISINFECTANTS ⟩ IODINE PRODUCTS

Povidone-iodine

08-Feb-2022

- **INDICATIONS AND DOSE**

Skin disinfection
▸ TO THE SKIN
▸ Child: (consult product literature)
▸ Adult: (consult product literature)

VIDENE ® SOLUTION

Skin disinfection
▸ TO THE SKIN
▸ Child: Apply undiluted in pre-operative skin disinfection and general antisepsis

continued →

▶ Adult: Apply undiluted in pre-operative skin disinfection and general antisepsis

VIDENE ® SURGICAL SCRUB ®

Skin disinfection

▶ TO THE SKIN

▶ Child: Use as a pre-operative scrub for hand and skin disinfection

▶ Adult: Use as a pre-operative scrub for hand and skin disinfection

VIDENE ® TINCTURE

Skin disinfection

▶ TO THE SKIN

▶ Adult: Apply undiluted in pre-operative skin disinfection

● **CONTRA-INDICATIONS** Avoid regular use in patients with thyroid disorders (in adults) · concomitant use of lithium · corrected gestational age under 32 weeks · infants body-weight under 1.5 kg · regular use in neonates

● **CAUTIONS** Broken skin · large open wounds

CAUTIONS, FURTHER INFORMATION

▶ Large open wounds The application of povidone–iodine to large wounds or severe burns may produce systemic adverse effects such as metabolic acidosis, hypernatraemia and impairment of renal function.

▶ VIDENE ® TINCTURE Procedures involving hot wire cautery and diathermy

● **SIDE-EFFECTS** Acute kidney injury · goitre · hyperthyroidism · hypothyroidism · metabolic acidosis · skin burning sensation

● **PREGNANCY** Sufficient iodine may be absorbed to affect the fetal thyroid in the second and third trimester.

● **BREAST FEEDING** Avoid regular or excessive use.

● **RENAL IMPAIRMENT** EvGr Caution when applied to large wounds or severe burns (increased risk of systemic exposure). ⟨M⟩

● **EFFECT ON LABORATORY TESTS** May interfere with thyroid function tests.

● **MEDICINAL FORMS** There can be variation in the licensing of different medicines containing the same drug. Forms available from special-order manufacturers include: cutaneous solution

Cutaneous solution

CAUTIONARY AND ADVISORY LABELS 15 (Only for use with alcoholic solutions)

▶ Videne (Ecolab Healthcare Division)

Povidone-Iodine 75 mg per 1 ml Videne 7.5% surgical scrub solution | 500 ml P £8.61 DT = £8.61

Povidone-Iodine 100 mg per 1 ml Videne 10% antiseptic solution | 200 ml P £11.78

ANTISEPTICS AND DISINFECTANTS ❯ OTHER

Chlorhexidine

23-Feb-2022

● **INDICATIONS AND DOSE**

CEPTON ® LOTION

For skin disinfection in acne

▶ TO THE SKIN

▶ Child: (consult product literature)

▶ Adult: (consult product literature)

CEPTON ® SKIN WASH

For use as skin wash in acne

▶ TO THE SKIN

▶ Child: (consult product literature)

▶ Adult: (consult product literature)

HIBISCRUB ®

Pre-operative hand and skin disinfection | General hand and skin disinfection

▶ TO THE SKIN

▶ Child: Use as alternative to soap (consult product literature)

▶ Adult: Use as alternative to soap (consult product literature)

HIBITANE OBSTETRIC

For use in obstetrics and gynaecology as an antiseptic and lubricant

▶ TO THE SKIN

▶ Adult: To be applied to skin around vulva and perineum and to hands of midwife or doctor

HIBI ® LIQUID HAND RUB+

Hand and skin disinfection

▶ TO THE SKIN

▶ Child: To be used undiluted (consult product literature)

▶ Adult: To be used undiluted (consult product literature)

HYDREX ® SOLUTION

For pre-operative skin disinfection

▶ TO THE SKIN

▶ Child: (consult product literature)

▶ Adult: (consult product literature)

HYDREX ® SURGICAL SCRUB

For pre-operative hand and skin disinfection | General hand disinfection

▶ TO THE SKIN

▶ Child: (consult product literature)

▶ Adult: (consult product literature)

UNISEPT ®

For cleansing and disinfecting wounds and burns and swabbing in obstetrics

▶ TO THE SKIN

▶ Child: (consult product literature)

▶ Adult: (consult product literature)

IMPORTANT SAFETY INFORMATION

MHRA/CHM ADVICE: CHLORHEXIDINE SOLUTIONS: REMINDER OF THE RISK OF CHEMICAL BURNS IN PREMATURE INFANTS (NOVEMBER 2014)

In premature infants, use sparingly, monitor for skin reactions, and do not allow solution to pool—risk of severe chemical burns.

● **CONTRA-INDICATIONS** Not for use in body cavities

● **CAUTIONS** Avoid contact with brain · avoid contact with eyes · avoid contact with meninges · avoid contact with middle ear · use prior to diathermy (alcohol containing skin disinfectants)

● **SIDE-EFFECTS** Skin reactions

● **PRESCRIBING AND DISPENSING INFORMATION** Chlorhexidine digluconate is a synonym for chlorhexidine gluconate.

● **MEDICINAL FORMS** There can be variation in the licensing of different medicines containing the same drug.

Cutaneous solution

CAUTIONARY AND ADVISORY LABELS 15 (For ethanolic solutions (e.g. ChloraPrep ® and Hydrex ® only)

EXCIPIENTS: May contain Fragrances

▶ Cepton (Dendron Brands Ltd)

Chlorhexidine gluconate 10 mg per 1 ml Cepton 1% medicated skin wash | 150 ml GSL £37.13 DT = £37.13

▶ Hibi (Molnlycke Health Care Ltd)

Chlorhexidine gluconate 5 mg per 1 ml HiBi Liquid Hand Rub+ 0.5% solution | 500 ml £6.17 DT = £6.17

▸ **Hydrex** (Ecolab Healthcare Division)
Chlorhexidine gluconate 40 mg per 1 ml Hydrex 4% Surgical Scrub
| 250 ml GSL £4.83 DT = £5.26 | 500 ml GSL £5.36 DT = £8.28

Cutaneous cream

▸ **Hibitane Obstetric** (Derma UK Ltd)
Chlorhexidine gluconate 10 mg per 1 gram Hibitane Obstetric 1%
cream | 250 ml GSL £22.00 DT = £22.00 | 500 ml GSL £49.00
(Hospital only)

Chlorhexidine gluconate with isopropyl alcohol

The properties listed below are those particular to the
combination only. For the properties of the components
please consider, chlorhexidine p. 1452.

● **INDICATIONS AND DOSE**

Skin disinfection before invasive procedures
▸ TO THE SKIN
▸ Child 2 months–17 years: (consult product literature)
▸ Adult: (consult product literature)

● **MEDICINAL FORMS** There can be variation in the licensing of
different medicines containing the same drug. Forms available
from special-order manufacturers include: cutaneous solution

Cutaneous solution
CAUTIONARY AND ADVISORY LABELS 15

▸ **ChloraPrep** (Becton, Dickinson UK Ltd)
Chlorhexidine gluconate 20 mg per 1 ml, Isopropyl alcohol
700 ml per 1 litre ChloraPrep with Tint solution 10.5ml applicators |
25 applicator GSL £82.90 DT = £78.95
ChloraPrep solution 1ml applicators | 60 applicator GSL £20.82
ChloraPrep with Tint solution 26ml applicators | 25 applicator GSL
£184.75 DT = £175.75
ChloraPrep solution 3ml applicators | 25 applicator GSL £23.00 DT =
£23.00
ChloraPrep solution 1.5ml applicators | 20 applicator GSL £12.00 DT
= £12.00
ChloraPrep with Tint solution 3ml applicators | 25 applicator GSL
£24.25 DT = £23.00
ChloraPrep solution 10.5ml applicators | 25 applicator GSL £78.95
DT = £78.95
ChloraPrep solution 26ml applicators | 25 applicator GSL £175.75
DT = £175.75

Chlorhexidine with cetrimide

The properties listed below are those particular to the
combination only. For the properties of the components
please consider, chlorhexidine p. 1452.

● **INDICATIONS AND DOSE**

Skin disinfection such as wound cleansing and obstetrics
▸ TO THE SKIN
▸ Child: To be used undiluted
▸ Adult: To be used undiluted

● **MEDICINAL FORMS** There can be variation in the licensing of
different medicines containing the same drug.

Cutaneous cream

▸ **Chlorhexidine with cetrimide** (Non-proprietary)
Chlorhexidine gluconate 1 mg per 1 gram, Cetrimide 5 mg per
1 gram Savlon antiseptic cream | 15 gram GSL £1.27 DT = £1.27 |
30 gram GSL £1.70 DT = £1.70 | 60 gram GSL £2.54 DT = £2.54 |
100 gram GSL £3.67 DT = £3.67

Cutaneous irrigation solution

▸ **Chlorhexidine with cetrimide** (Non-proprietary)
Chlorhexidine acetate 150 microgram per 1 ml, Cetrimide 1.5 mg
per 1 ml Chlorhexidine acetate 0.015% / Cetrimide 0.15% irrigation
solution 1litre bottles | 1 bottle P ⊠

Diethyl phthalate with methyl salicylate

● **INDICATIONS AND DOSE**

Skin preparation before injection
▸ TO THE SKIN
▸ Adult: Apply to the area to be disinfected

● **MEDICINAL FORMS** There can be variation in the licensing of
different medicines containing the same drug.

Cutaneous solution
CAUTIONARY AND ADVISORY LABELS 15

▸ **Diethyl phthalate with methyl salicylate** (Non-proprietary)
Methyl salicylate 5 ml per 1 litre, Diethyl phthalate 20 ml per
1 litre, Castor oil 25 ml per 1 litre, Industrial methylated spirit
950 ml per 1 litre Surgical spirit | 200 ml GSL £1.89 DT = £1.89

Hydrogen peroxide

14-May-2024

● **DRUG ACTION** Hydrogen peroxide is an oxidising agent.

● **INDICATIONS AND DOSE**

**For skin disinfection, particularly cleansing and
deodorising wounds and ulcers**
▸ TO THE SKIN
▸ Adult: Use 3% and 6% solutions (consult product
literature)

CRYSTACIDE®

Superficial bacterial skin infection
▸ TO THE SKIN
▸ Child: Apply 2–3 times a day for up to 3 weeks
▸ Adult: Apply 2–3 times a day for up to 3 weeks

**Localised non-bullous impetigo [in patients who are not
systemically unwell or at high risk of complications]**
▸ TO THE SKIN
▸ Child: Apply 2–3 times a day for 5–7 days
▸ Adult: Apply 2–3 times a day for 5–7 days

● **CONTRA-INDICATIONS** Closed body cavities (in adults) ·
deep wounds · large wounds · use as disinfection agent for
surgical instruments (in adults) · use as enema (in adults) ·
use during surgery (in adults)

● **CAUTIONS** Avoid on eyes · avoid on healthy skin ·
incompatible with products containing iodine or
potassium permanganate

● **PRESCRIBING AND DISPENSING INFORMATION** The BP
directs that when hydrogen peroxide is prescribed,
hydrogen peroxide solution 6% (20 vols) should be
dispensed.
    Strong solutions of hydrogen peroxide which contain
27% (90 vols) and 30% (100 vols) are only for the
preparation of weaker solutions.
    CRYSTACIDE® For choice of therapy, see Skin infections,
antibacterial therapy p. 589.

● **HANDLING AND STORAGE** Hydrogen peroxide bleaches
fabric.

● **MEDICINAL FORMS** There can be variation in the licensing of
different medicines containing the same drug.

Cutaneous or oromucosal liquid

▸ Hydrogen peroxide (Non-proprietary)
Hydrogen peroxide 30 ml per 1 litre Hydrogen peroxide 3%
solution | 100 ml PoM ⊠

Cutaneous cream
EXCIPIENTS: May contain Edetic acid (edta), propylene glycol

▸ **Crystacide** (Reig Jofre UK Ltd)
Hydrogen peroxide 10 mg per 1 gram Crystacide 1% cream |
25 gram P £8.07 DT = £8.07 | 40 gram P £11.62 DT = £11.62

13

Skin

Irrigation solutions

- **INDICATIONS AND DOSE**

Skin cleansing
- ▶ TO THE SKIN
- ▶ Child: Use for topical irrigation of wounds
- ▶ Adult: Use for topical irrigation of wounds

- **IRRIGATION SOLUTIONS**

Flowfusor sodium chloride 0.9% irrigation solution 120ml bottles (Fresenius Kabi Ltd) **Sodium chloride 9 mg per 1 ml** 1 bottle · NHS indicative price = £2.88 · Drug Tariff (Part IXa)

Normasol sodium chloride 0.9% irrigation solution 100ml sachets (Molnlycke Health Care Ltd) **Sodium chloride 9 mg per 1 ml** 10 unit dose · NHS indicative price = £8.56 · Drug Tariff (Part IXa)

Normasol sodium chloride 0.9% irrigation solution 25ml sachets (Molnlycke Health Care Ltd) **Sodium chloride 9 mg per 1 ml** 25 unit dose · NHS indicative price = £6.93 · Drug Tariff (Part IXa)

Sodium chloride 0.9% irrigation solution 1litre bottles (Fresenius Kabi Ltd) **Sodium chloride 9 mg per 1 ml** 1 bottle · NHS indicative price = £2.57 · Drug Tariff (Part IXa)

Sodium chloride 0.9% irrigation solution 20ml AactiPod unit dose (Essential-Healthcare Ltd) **Sodium chloride 9 mg per 1 ml** 25 unit dose · NHS indicative price = £3.83 · Drug Tariff (Part IXa)

Sodium chloride 0.9% irrigation solution 20ml Alvita unit dose (Crest Medical Ltd) **Sodium chloride 9 mg per 1 ml** 25 unit dose · NHS indicative price = £4.80 · Drug Tariff (Part IXa)

Sodium chloride 0.9% irrigation solution 20ml Clinipod unit dose (Mayors Healthcare Ltd) **Sodium chloride 9 mg per 1 ml** 25 unit dose · NHS indicative price = £4.23 · Drug Tariff (Part IXa)

Sodium chloride 0.9% irrigation solution 20ml EasyPod unit dose (TriOn Pharma Ltd) **Sodium chloride 9 mg per 1 ml** 25 unit dose · NHS indicative price = £3.81 · Drug Tariff (Part IXa)

Sodium chloride 0.9% irrigation solution 20ml ISO-POD unit dose (St Georges Medical Ltd) **Sodium chloride 9 mg per 1 ml** 25 unit dose · NHS indicative price = £4.95 · Drug Tariff (Part IXa)

Sodium chloride 0.9% irrigation solution 20ml Irripod unit dose (Crest Medical Ltd) **Sodium chloride 9 mg per 1 ml** 25 unit dose · NHS indicative price = £6.10 · Drug Tariff (Part IXa)

Sodium chloride 0.9% irrigation solution 20ml Knoxzy unit dose (Biovantic Pharma Ltd) **Sodium chloride 9 mg per 1 ml** 25 unit dose · NHS indicative price = £4.35 · Drug Tariff (Part IXa)

Sodium chloride 0.9% irrigation solution 20ml Sal-e Pods unit dose (Ennogen Healthcare Ltd) **Sodium chloride 9 mg per 1 ml** 25 unit dose · NHS indicative price = £4.80 · Drug Tariff (Part IXa)

Sodium chloride 0.9% irrigation solution 20ml Salipod unit dose (Sai-Meds Ltd) **Sodium chloride 9 mg per 1 ml** 25 unit dose · NHS indicative price = £4.99 · Drug Tariff (Part IXa)

Sodium chloride 0.9% irrigation solution 20ml Sterowash unit dose (Steroplast Healthcare Ltd) **Sodium chloride 9 mg per 1 ml** 25 unit dose · NHS indicative price = £4.29 · Drug Tariff (Part IXa)

Sodium chloride 0.9% irrigation solution 20ml unit dose (Alissa Healthcare Research Ltd) **Sodium chloride 9 mg per 1 ml** 25 unit dose · NHS indicative price = £7.36 · Drug Tariff (Part IXa)

Sodium chloride 0.9% irrigation solution 20ml unit dose (Bell, Sons & Co (Druggists) Ltd) **Sodium chloride 9 mg per 1 ml** 25 unit dose · NHS indicative price = £6.76 · Drug Tariff (Part IXa)

Sodium chloride 0.9% irrigation solution 20ml unit dose (Crest Medical Ltd) **Sodium chloride 9 mg per 1 ml** 25 unit dose · NHS indicative price = £4.99 · Drug Tariff (Part IXa)

Sodium chloride 0.9% irrigation solution 20ml unit dose (Viatris UK Healthcare Ltd) **Sodium chloride 9 mg per 1 ml** 25 unit dose · NHS indicative price = £5.50 · Drug Tariff (Part IXa)

Stericlens sodium chloride 0.9% irrigation solution aerosol spray (Crest Medical Ltd) **Sodium chloride 9 mg per 1 ml** 100 ml · No NHS indicative price available 240 ml · NHS indicative price = £3.30 · Drug Tariff (Part IXa)

10.1 Minor cuts and abrasions

ANTISEPTICS AND DISINFECTANTS

Glycerol with magnesium sulfate and phenol

14-Dec-2020

- **INDICATIONS AND DOSE**

Treat carbuncles and boils
- ▶ TO THE SKIN
- ▶ Adult: To be applied under dressing

- **DIRECTIONS FOR ADMINISTRATION** Manufacturer advises paste should be stirred before use.

- **MEDICINAL FORMS** There can be variation in the licensing of different medicines containing the same drug.

Cutaneous paste
- ▶ Glycerol with magnesium sulfate and phenol (Non-proprietary) Phenol 5 mg per 1 gram, Magnesium sulfate dried 450 mg per 1 gram, Glycerol 550 mg per 1 gram Magnesium sulfate paste | 25 gram GSL £0.79 | 50 gram GSL £1.03–£2.69 DT = £2.69

DERMATOLOGICAL DRUGS > COLLODIONS

Castor oil with collodion and colophony

16-Dec-2020

- **INDICATIONS AND DOSE**

Used to seal minor cuts and wounds that have partially healed
- ▶ TO THE SKIN
- ▶ Child: (consult product literature)
- ▶ Adult: (consult product literature)

- **ALLERGY AND CROSS-SENSITIVITY** EvGr Contra-indicated if patient has an allergy to colophony in elastic adhesive plasters and tape. Ⓜ

- **MEDICINAL FORMS** No licensed medicines listed.

Skin adhesives

- **SKIN ADHESIVES**

Derma+Flex skin adhesive (Chemence Ltd)
0.5 ml · NHS indicative price = £5.36 · Drug Tariff (Part IXa)

Dermabond Advanced skin adhesive (Ethicon Ltd)
0.7 ml · NHS indicative price = £19.49 · Drug Tariff (Part IXa)

Dermabond Mini skin adhesive (Ethicon Ltd)
0.36 ml · NHS indicative price = £11.39 · Drug Tariff (Part IXa)

Dermabond ProPen skin adhesive (Ethicon Ltd)
0.5 ml · NHS indicative price = £19.95 · Drug Tariff (Part IXa)

Dermabond skin adhesive (Ethicon Ltd)
0.5 ml · NHS indicative price = £19.49 · Drug Tariff (Part IXa)

Histoacryl L skin adhesive (B.Braun Medical Ltd)
0.5 ml · NHS indicative price = £7.02 · Drug Tariff (Part IXa)

Histoacryl skin adhesive (B.Braun Medical Ltd)
0.5 ml · NHS indicative price = £6.79 · Drug Tariff (Part IXa)

Indermil skin adhesive (Covidien (UK) Commercial Ltd)
0.5 gram · NHS indicative price = £6.50 · Drug Tariff (Part IXa)

LiquiBand Optima skin adhesive (Advanced Medical Solutions Ltd)
0.5 gram · No NHS indicative price available · Drug Tariff (Part IXa)

LiquiBand flow control tissue adhesive (Advanced Medical Solutions Ltd)
0.5 gram · NHS indicative price = £5.50 · Drug Tariff (Part IXa)

LiquiBand tissue adhesive (Advanced Medical Solutions Ltd)
0.5 gram · NHS indicative price = £5.50 · Drug Tariff (Part IXa)

11   Skin disfigurement

Camouflages
30-Nov-2023

Overview

Disfigurement of the skin can be very distressing to patients and may have a marked psychological effect. In skilled hands, or with experience, camouflage cosmetics can be very effective in concealing scars and birthmarks. The depigmented patches in vitiligo are also very disfiguring and camouflage creams are of great cosmetic value.

Opaque cover foundation or cream is used to mask skin pigment abnormalities; careful application using a combination of dark- and light-coloured cover creams set with powder helps to minimise the appearance of skin deformities.

Borderline substances

Camouflages below marked 'ACBS' can be prescribed on the NHS (see *About Borderline Substances*) for postoperative scars and other deformities and as adjunctive therapy in the relief of emotional disturbances due to disfiguring skin disease, such as vitiligo. Cleansing creams, milks, and lotions are excluded.

Camouflages

- **CAMOUFLAGES**

Covermark classic foundation (Derma UK Ltd)
15 ml(ACBS) · NHS indicative price = £11.86

Covermark finishing powder (Derma UK Ltd)
25 gram(ACBS) · NHS indicative price = £11.86

Dermacolor fixing powder (Kryolan UK Ltd)
60 gram(ACBS) · NHS indicative price = £11.62

Keromask finishing powder (Bellava Ltd)
20 gram(ACBS) · NHS indicative price = £9.16

Keromask masking cream (Bellava Ltd)
15 ml(ACBS) · NHS indicative price = £9.16

Veil cover cream (Thomas Blake Cosmetic Creams Ltd)
19 gram(ACBS) · NHS indicative price = £24.66 44 gram(ACBS) · NHS indicative price = £36.68 70 gram(ACBS) · NHS indicative price = £46.31

Veil finishing powder (Thomas Blake Cosmetic Creams Ltd)
35 gram(ACBS) · NHS indicative price = £26.94

12   Sun protection and photodamage

Sunscreen
30-Nov-2023

Overview

Solar ultraviolet irradiation can be harmful to the skin. It is responsible for skin disorders such as *polymorphic light eruption*, *solar urticaria*, and it provokes the various *cutaneous porphyrias*. It may also trigger or aggravate skin lesions of *lupus erythematosus*, *rosacea*, and other *dermatoses*. Certain drugs, such as demeclocycline, phenothiazines, or amiodarone, can cause photosensitivity. Solar ultraviolet irradiation may also trigger attacks of recurrent herpes labialis.

The effects of exposure over longer periods include *ageing changes*, and more importantly the initiation of *skin cancer.*

Solar ultraviolet radiation is approximately 200–400 nm in wavelength. The medium wavelengths (290–320 nm, known as UVB) are the main cause of *sunburn*. The long wavelengths (320–400 nm, known as UVA) are responsible for many *photosensitivity reactions* and *photodermatoses*. Both UVA and UVB contribute to long-term *photodamage* and to the changes responsible for *skin cancer* and ageing.

Sunscreen preparations contain substances that protect the skin against UVA and UVB radiation, but they are not a substitute for covering the skin and avoiding sunlight. The sun protection factor (SPF, usually indicated in the preparation title) provides guidance on the degree of protection offered against UVB; it indicates the multiples of protection provided against burning, compared with unprotected skin; for example, an SPF of 8 should enable a person to remain 8 times longer in the sun without burning. However, in practice, most users do not apply sufficient sunscreen product. The amount of sunscreen needed to cover the body of an average adult to achieve the stated SPF is around 35 mL or 6–8 teaspoons of lotion.

The EU Commission (September 2006) has recommended that the UVA protection factor for a sunscreen should be at least one-third of the sun protection factor (SPF); products that achieve this requirement will be labelled with a UVA logo alongside the SPF classification. EvGr Sunscreens should meet the minimum standards for UVA protection and the label should state that it provides good UVA protection (e.g. at least '4-star UVA protection'). They should also provide a SPF of at least 15 for UVB protection. Ⓐ Preparations that also contain reflective substances, such as titanium dioxide, provide the most effective protection against UVA.

Sunscreen preparations may cause contact dermatitis as a result of an allergy to one of its ingredients.

For optimum photoprotection, sunscreen preparations should be applied **liberally** and **frequently** as per manufacturer instructions. As maximum protection from sunlight is desirable in patients with photodermatoses, sunscreen with the highest SPF is essential.

Borderline substances

Some sunscreen products have ACBS approval (see *About Borderline Substances*). They may be prescribed for skin protection against ultraviolet radiation and/or visible light in abnormal cutaneous photosensitivity causing severe cutaneous reactions in genetic disorders (including xeroderma pigmentosum and porphyrias), severe photodermatoses (both idiopathic and acquired) and in those with increased risk of ultraviolet radiation causing adverse effects due to chronic disease (such as haematological malignancies), medical therapies and/or procedures. Products with ACBS approval are *Anthelios*® Sunscreen Lotion SPF 50+, *Uvistat*® Lipscreen SPF 50, *Uvistat*® Suncream SPF 30, and *Uvistat*® Suncream SPF 50.

Photodamage
18-Nov-2020

Overview

EvGr Patients should be advised on the harms of prolonged sunlight exposure and how to adequately protect their skin from strong sunlight (e.g. use of topical sun protection preparations).

Topical treatments can be used for actinic (solar) keratoses. An emollient can be used as part of the management regimen for dry, sun-damaged elderly skin although the direct effect of emollient treatment is unclear; addition of urea or salicylic acid may provide benefit. Diclofenac sodium gel p. 1297 may be suitable for the treatment of superficial lesions in mild disease. Fluorouracil cream p. 1456 is effective against most types of non-hypertrophic actinic keratosis; a solution containing fluorouracil with salicylic acid p. 1456 can be used for the treatment of low or moderately thick hyperkeratotic actinic keratosis. Imiquimod p. 1459 can be used for lesions on the face and scalp when cryotherapy or other topical treatments cannot be used. Fluorouracil and imiquimod produce a more

13

Skin

marked inflammatory reaction than diclofenac sodium but lesions resolve faster. Photodynamic therapy in combination with methyl-5-aminolevulinate cream (*Metvix®*) or 5-aminolaevulinic acid gel (*Ameluz®*) is used in specialist centres for treating superficial and confluent, non-hypertrophic actinic keratosis when other treatments are inadequate or unsuitable; it is particularly suitable for multiple and large-area lesions, cosmetically sensitive sites, lesions located at sites of poor healing, or where pain is likely to be an issue. Ⓐ

Imiquimod and topical fluorouracil are licensed for treating superficial basal cell carcinomas. [EvGr] Patients with skin lesions suspected to be a basal cell carcinoma should be considered for routine referral; a suspected cancer pathway referral should only be considered if there are concerns that delay may have a significant impact (due to factors such as lesion size and site). Photodynamic therapy in combination with methyl-5-aminolevulinate cream is used in specialist centres for treating thin nodular basal cell carcinomas when other treatments are unsuitable. It may also be used for superficial basal cell carcinomas, particularly for multiple and large-area lesions, cosmetically sensitive sites, and lesions located at sites of poor healing. Ⓐ

ANTINEOPLASTIC DRUGS > ANTIMETABOLITES

Fluorouracil

19-Jan-2021

● **INDICATIONS AND DOSE**

Superficial malignant and pre-malignant skin lesions
▸ TO THE SKIN USING CREAM
▸ Adult: Apply 1–2 times a day for 3–4 weeks (usual duration of initial therapy), apply thinly to the affected area, maximum area of skin 500 cm² (e.g. 23 cm × 23 cm) treated at one time, alternative regimens may be used in some settings

● **CAUTIONS** Avoid contact with eyes and mucous membranes · dihydropyrimidine dehydrogenase deficiency · do not apply to bleeding lesions

● **INTERACTIONS** → Appendix 1: fluorouracil

● **SIDE-EFFECTS**
▸ **Common or very common** Alopecia · diarrhoea · mucositis · nausea · neutropenia · skin reactions · stomatitis · thrombocytopenia · vomiting
▸ **Uncommon** Dizziness · headache
▸ **Rare or very rare** Abdominal pain · chills · diarrhoea haemorrhagic · fever · leucocytosis · pancytopenia · skin irritation (use a topical corticosteroid for severe discomfort associated with inflammatory reactions) · skin ulcer
▸ **Frequency not known** Conjunctival irritation · excessive tearing · keratitis · taste altered

● **CONCEPTION AND CONTRACEPTION** Contraceptive advice required, see *Pregnancy and reproductive function* in Cytotoxic drugs p. 1027.

● **PREGNANCY** Manufacturers advise avoid (teratogenic).

● **BREAST FEEDING** Manufacturers advise avoid.

● **HANDLING AND STORAGE** Caution in handling—irritant to tissues.

● **MEDICINAL FORMS** There can be variation in the licensing of different medicines containing the same drug.
Cutaneous cream
CAUTIONARY AND ADVISORY LABELS 11
EXCIPIENTS: May contain Cetostearyl alcohol (including cetyl and stearyl alcohol), hydroxybenzoates (parabens), polysorbates, propylene glycol
▸ **Fluorouracil (Non-proprietary)**
Fluorouracil 5 mg per 1 gram Carac 0.5% cream | 30 gram [PoM] ⚠
Fluorouracil 50 mg per 1 gram Fluorouracil 5% cream | 1 gram [PoM] ⚠

▸ **Efudix** (Viatris UK Healthcare Ltd)
Fluorouracil 50 mg per 1 gram Efudix 5% cream | 40 gram [PoM] £32.90 DT = £32.90
▸ **Tolak** (Pierre Fabre Ltd)
Fluorouracil 40 mg per 1 gram Tolak 40mg/g cream | 20 gram [PoM] £28.00 DT = £28.00

Fluorouracil with salicylic acid

The properties listed below are those particular to the combination only. For the properties of the components please consider, fluorouracil above, salicylic acid p. 1460.

● **INDICATIONS AND DOSE**

Low or moderately thick hyperkeratotic actinic keratosis
▸ TO THE SKIN
▸ Adult: Apply once daily for up to 12 weeks, reduced to 3 times a week if severe side effects occur and until side-effects improve, to be applied to the affected area, if treating area with thin epidermis, reduce frequency of application and monitor response more often; maximum area of skin treated at one time, 25 cm² (e.g. 5 cm × 5 cm)

● **INTERACTIONS** → Appendix 1: fluorouracil

● **MEDICINAL FORMS** There can be variation in the licensing of different medicines containing the same drug.
Cutaneous solution
CAUTIONARY AND ADVISORY LABELS 15
▸ **Actikerall** (Almirall Ltd)
Fluorouracil 5 mg per 1 gram, Salicylic acid 100 mg per 1 gram Actikerall 5mg/g / 100mg/g cutaneous solution | 25 ml [PoM] £38.30 DT = £38.30

ANTINEOPLASTIC DRUGS > PROTEIN KINASE INHIBITORS

Tirbanibulin

12-Apr-2022

● **DRUG ACTION** Tirbanibulin is a tyrosine kinase inhibitor which binds to tubulin thereby inducing death of proliferating cells.

● **INDICATIONS AND DOSE**

Actinic keratosis on face or scalp
▸ TO THE SKIN
▸ Adult: Apply once daily for 5 consecutive days, consider other treatment options if treated area does not show complete clearance after about 8 weeks

● **CAUTIONS** Avoid contact with eyes · avoid contact with inside of ears · avoid contact with inside of nostrils · avoid contact with lips · avoid contact with open wounds or broken skin · avoid occlusive dressings on treated area · immunocompromised patients

● **SIDE-EFFECTS** Skin eruption localised

● **PREGNANCY** [EvGr] Avoid—toxicity in *animal* studies. Ⓜ

● **BREAST FEEDING** Specialist sources indicate use with caution—amount in milk is likely to be low. Do not apply to breast or nipple and avoid contact with infant's skin.

● **DIRECTIONS FOR ADMINISTRATION** [EvGr] Each sachet is for single use only and for a treatment area of up to 25 cm². Avoid applying on skin which has not healed from any previous treatment. Before applying, wash the treatment area with mild soap and water and dry. Avoid washing or touching the treated area for 8 hours after application; after this time, area may be washed with mild soap and water. Ⓜ

● **PATIENT AND CARER ADVICE** Patients and carers should be advised that excessive exposure to direct sunlight, including the use of sunlamps and sunbeds, are to be avoided. If sun exposure is unavoidable, protective clothing should be worn.

Patients and carers should be advised on the application of *Klisyri*® ointment.

Missed doses If a dose is missed, apply the ointment as soon as remembered and continue with the regular schedule. Avoid applying more than once a day.

● **NATIONAL FUNDING/ACCESS DECISIONS**
For full details see funding body website
Scottish Medicines Consortium (SMC) decisions
▶ Tirbanibulin (*Klisyri*®) for field treatment of non-hyperkeratotic, non-hypertrophic actinic keratosis (Olsen grade 1) of the face or scalp in adults (December 2021) SMC No. SMC2395 Recommended

All Wales Medicines Strategy Group (AWMSG) decisions
▶ Tirbanibulin (*Klisyri*®) for the field treatment of non-hyperkeratotic, non-hypertrophic actinic keratosis (Olsen grade 1) of the face or scalp in adults (February 2022) AWMSG No. 4076 Recommended

● **MEDICINAL FORMS** There can be variation in the licensing of different medicines containing the same drug.
Cutaneous ointment
CAUTIONARY AND ADVISORY LABELS 10, 11, 28
EXCIPIENTS: May contain Propylene glycol
▶ Klisyri (Almirall Ltd) ▼
Tirbanibulin 10 mg per 1 gram Klisyri 10mg/g ointment 250mg sachets | 5 sachet [PoM] £59.00 DT = £59.00

PROTEIN KINASE C ACTIVATORS

Ingenol mebutate

09-Mar-2020

● **INDICATIONS AND DOSE**
Actinic keratosis on face and scalp
▶ TO THE SKIN
▶ Adult: Apply once daily for 3 days, use the 150 microgram/g gel

Actinic keratosis on trunk and extremities
▶ TO THE SKIN
▶ Adult: Apply once daily for 2 days, use the 500 microgram/g gel

IMPORTANT SAFETY INFORMATION
MHRA/CHM ADVICE (UPDATED FEBRUARY 2020): INGENOL MEBUTATE GEL (*PICATO*®): SUSPENSION OF THE LICENCE DUE TO RISK OF SKIN MALIGNANCY
Clinical studies have shown an increased incidence of benign and malignant skin tumours (such as basal and squamous cell carcinoma, Bowen's disease, and keratoacanthoma) in patients using ingenol mebutate gel; cases of neuroendocrine carcinoma of the skin, and atypical fibroxanthoma have also been reported. Healthcare professionals are advised to stop prescribing ingenol mebutate gel and consider alternative treatment options for actinic keratosis. The licence of ingenol mebutate has been suspended as a precautionary measure while investigations are carried out. Healthcare professionals should advise patients to be vigilant for the development of any new skin lesions within the treatment area and to seek immediate medical advice if any occur.

● **CAUTIONS** Avoid contact with broken skin · avoid contact with eyes · avoid contact with inside of ears · avoid contact with inside of nostrils · avoid contact with lips · avoid occlusive dressings on treated area
● **SIDE-EFFECTS**
▶ **Common or very common** Headache
▶ **Frequency not known** Neoplasms · skin eruption localised

● **PREGNANCY** Not absorbed from skin, but manufacturer advises avoid.
● **BREAST FEEDING** Not absorbed from skin; ensure infant does not come in contact with treated area for 6 hours after application.
● **DIRECTIONS FOR ADMINISTRATION** One tube covers skin area of 25 cm². Allow gel to dry on treatment area for 15 minutes. Avoid washing or touching the treated area for 6 hours after application; after this time, area may be washed with mild soap and water. Avoid use immediately after shower or less than 2 hours before bedtime.

● **MEDICINAL FORMS** No licensed medicines listed.

13 Superficial soft-tissue injuries and superficial thrombophlebitis

13
Skin

HEPARINOIDS

Heparinoid

● **INDICATIONS AND DOSE**
Superficial thrombophlebitis | Bruising | Haematoma
▶ TO THE SKIN
▶ Adult: Apply up to 4 times a day

● **CONTRA-INDICATIONS** Should not be used on large areas of skin, broken or sensitive skin, or mucous membranes
● **LESS SUITABLE FOR PRESCRIBING** *Hirudoid*® is less suitable for prescribing.

● **MEDICINAL FORMS** There can be variation in the licensing of different medicines containing the same drug.
Cutaneous cream
EXCIPIENTS: May contain Cetostearyl alcohol (including cetyl and stearyl alcohol), hydroxybenzoates (parabens)
▶ Hirudoid (Thornton & Ross Ltd)
Heparinoid 3 mg per 1 gram Hirudoid 0.3% cream | 50 gram [P] £3.99 DT = £3.99
Cutaneous gel
EXCIPIENTS: May contain Fragrances, propylene glycol
▶ Hirudoid (Thornton & Ross Ltd)
Heparinoid 3 mg per 1 gram Hirudoid 0.3% gel | 50 gram [P] £3.99 DT = £3.99

14 Warts and calluses

Warts and calluses

08-Aug-2023

Cutaneous warts

Cutaneous warts are caused by infection of keratinocytes with the human papillomavirus (HPV). They can appear on any part of the body but commonly affect the feet (also known as plantar warts or verrucas) and hands. In most cases, warts resolve spontaneously usually within 2 years; sometimes within months. [EvGr] Treatment is required only if the warts are painful, unsightly, persistent, or are causing distress and the patient requests treatment.

Treatment choice is dependent on patient preference and response to previous treatments. Patients with facial warts should be referred to a specialist for treatment. Options for non-facial warts include either the topical keratolytic salicylic acid p. 1460 (or salicylic acid with lactic acid p. 1460), or cryotherapy using liquid nitrogen, or a combination of both. A shorter cryotherapy freeze or weaker salicylic acid preparation is recommended for warts on the back of the hands, as scarring is more likely to occur. Cryotherapy is unlikely to help in the treatment of plantar warts as they can be difficult to treat. When indicated, cryotherapy should be provided by an appropriately trained healthcare professional. Ⓐ

Preparations of formaldehyde p. 1459, and silver nitrate p. 1459 are also licensed for the treatment of warts on hands and feet.

Salicylic acid with lactic acid p. 1460 is also licensed for the removal of *corns and calluses*.

Anogenital warts

Anogenital warts (condylomata acuminata) are caused by the human papillomavirus. [EvGr] Patients with anogenital warts should be referred to a sexual health specialist where possible, and treatment should be accompanied by screening for other sexually transmitted infections. Treatment is not always required, as warts may resolve spontaneously, usually within 6 months.

Topical podophyllotoxin below (the major active ingredient of podophyllum) may be used to treat soft, non-keratinised external anogenital warts. Topical imiquimod cream p. 1459 may also be used to treat external anogenital warts; it is suitable for both keratinised and non-keratinised lesions. Cryotherapy or other forms of physical ablative therapy (e.g. surgery, laser treatment) may also be considered, particularly for patients with a small number of low-volume warts, irrespective of type. Ⓐ

Camellia sinensis ointment below is licensed for the treatment of external anogenital warts.

ANTINEOPLASTIC DRUGS > PLANT ALKALOIDS

Camellia sinensis

20-Aug-2020

- **DRUG ACTION** Camellia sinensis is an extract from green tea leaves. The exact mechanism of action is not known; non-clinical studies have shown inhibition of the growth of activated keratinocytes, and anti-oxidative effects at the site of application.

- **INDICATIONS AND DOSE**

Warts (external genital and perianal) in immunocompetent patients

▸ TO THE LESION
▸ Adult: Apply up to 250 mg 3 times a day until complete clearance of warts (maximum 16 weeks), do not exceed treatment period even if new warts develop; maximum 750 mg per day

DOSE EQUIVALENCE AND CONVERSION
▸ 250 mg is equivalent to 0.5 cm of ointment.

- **CAUTIONS** Avoid broken skin · avoid contact with eyes · avoid contact with lips · avoid contact with mouth · avoid contact with nostrils · avoid inflamed skin · uncircumcised males (risk of phimosis) · vulvar region

- **SIDE-EFFECTS**
▸ **Uncommon** Balanoposthitis · increased risk of infection · lymphatic abnormalities · necrosis · painful sexual intercourse · phimosis · skin reactions · urinary disorders
▸ **Frequency not known** Urinary tract stenosis · vaginal discharge

- **CONCEPTION AND CONTRACEPTION** Manufacturer advises *Catephen*® may weaken condoms and vaginal diaphragms—alternative methods of contraception should be considered.

- **PREGNANCY** Manufacturer advises avoid—toxicity in *animal* studies.

- **BREAST FEEDING** Manufacturer advises risk to infant cannot be excluded—no information available.

- **HEPATIC IMPAIRMENT** Manufacturer advises avoid in severe impairment (limited information available).

- **DIRECTIONS FOR ADMINISTRATION** Manufacturer advises apply to each wart, ensuring a thin layer is left on the wart. It is not necessary to wash off the ointment from the area before next application.

- **PATIENT AND CARER ADVICE** Manufacturer advises the ointment should be washed off before sexual activity. Manufacturer advises female patients using tampons should insert tampon before applying the ointment.

- **NATIONAL FUNDING/ACCESS DECISIONS**
For full details see funding body website

Scottish Medicines Consortium (SMC) decisions
▸ Camellia sinensis (green tea leaf) (*Catephen*®) for the cutaneous treatment of external genital and perianal warts (condylomata acuminata) in immunocompetent patients from the age of 18 years (April 2016) SMC No. 1133/16 Recommended with restrictions

All Wales Medicines Strategy Group (AWMSG) decisions
▸ Green tea leaf extract (*Catephen*®) for cutaneous treatment of external genital and perianal warts (condylomata acuminata) in immunocompetent patients from the age of 18 years (October 2016) AWMSG No. 2739 Recommended with restrictions

- **MEDICINAL FORMS** There can be variation in the licensing of different medicines containing the same drug.
Cutaneous ointment
▸ Catephen (Kora Healthcare)
Camellia sinensis extract 100 mg per 1 gram Catephen 10% ointment | 15 gram [PoM] £39.00 DT = £39.00

Podophyllotoxin

28-Jul-2020

- **INDICATIONS AND DOSE**
CONDYLINE®

Condylomata acuminata affecting the penis or the female external genitalia

▸ TO THE LESION
▸ Adult: Apply twice daily for 3 consecutive days, treatment may be repeated at weekly intervals if necessary for a total of five 3-day treatment courses, direct medical supervision for lesions in the female and for lesions greater than 4 cm^2 in the male, maximum 50 single applications ('loops') per session (consult product literature)

WARTICON® CREAM

Condylomata acuminata affecting the penis or the female external genitalia

▸ TO THE LESION
▸ Adult: Apply twice daily for 3 consecutive days, treatment may be repeated at weekly intervals if necessary for a total of four 3-day treatment courses, direct medical supervision for lesions greater than 4 cm^2

WARTICON® LIQUID

Condylomata acuminata affecting the penis or the female external genitalia

▸ TO THE LESION
▸ Adult: Apply twice daily for 3 consecutive days, treatment may be repeated at weekly intervals if necessary for a total of four 3-day treatment courses, direct medical supervision for lesions greater than 4 cm^2, maximum 50 single applications ('loops') per session (consult product literature)

- **CAUTIONS** Avoid normal skin · avoid open wounds · keep away from face · very irritant to eyes
- **SIDE-EFFECTS** Balanoposthitis · skin irritation
- **PREGNANCY** Avoid.
- **BREAST FEEDING** Avoid.

- **MEDICINAL FORMS** There can be variation in the licensing of different medicines containing the same drug.

Cutaneous solution

CAUTIONARY AND ADVISORY LABELS 15

▸ **Warticon** (Phoenix Labs Ltd)
Podophyllotoxin 5 mg per 1 ml Warticon 0.5% solution | 3 ml [PoM] £14.86 DT = £14.86

Cutaneous cream

EXCIPIENTS: May contain Butylated hydroxyanisole, cetostearyl alcohol (including cetyl and stearyl alcohol), hydroxybenzoates (parabens), sorbic acid

▸ **Warticon** (Phoenix Labs Ltd)
Podophyllotoxin 1.5 mg per 1 gram Warticon 0.15% cream | 5 gram [PoM] £17.83 DT = £17.83

ANTISEPTICS AND DISINFECTANTS ›
ALDEHYDES AND DERIVATIVES

Formaldehyde

- **INDICATIONS AND DOSE**

Warts, particularly plantar warts
▸ TO THE LESION
▸ Child: Apply twice daily
▸ Adult: Apply twice daily

- **UNLICENSED USE** Licensed for use in children (age range not specified by manufacturer).

- **CAUTIONS** Impaired peripheral circulation · not suitable for application to anogenital region · not suitable for application to face · not suitable for application to large areas · patients with diabetes at risk of neuropathic ulcers · protect surrounding skin and avoid broken skin · significant peripheral neuropathy

- **SIDE-EFFECTS** Asthma · cough · dysphagia · eye irritation · increased risk of infection · laryngospasm · skin reactions

- **MEDICINAL FORMS** There can be variation in the licensing of different medicines containing the same drug. Forms available from special-order manufacturers include: cutaneous solution

Cutaneous solution

▸ **Formaldehyde** (Non-proprietary)
Formaldehyde 40 mg per 1 ml Formaldehyde (Buffered) 4% solution | 1000 ml £4.91

ANTISEPTICS AND DISINFECTANTS › OTHER

Silver nitrate

- **INDICATIONS AND DOSE**

Common warts
▸ TO THE LESION
▸ Child: Apply every 24 hours for up to 3 applications, apply moistened caustic pencil tip for 1–2 minutes. Instructions in proprietary packs generally incorporate advice to remove dead skin before use by gentle filing and to cover with adhesive dressing after application
▸ Adult: Apply every 24 hours for up to 3 applications, apply moistened caustic pencil tip for 1–2 minutes. Instructions in proprietary packs generally incorporate advice to remove dead skin before use by gentle filing and to cover with adhesive dressing after application

Verrucas
▸ TO THE LESION
▸ Child: Apply every 24 hours for up to 6 applications, apply moistened caustic pencil tip for 1–2 minutes. Instructions in proprietary packs generally incorporate advice to remove dead skin before use by gentle filing and to cover with adhesive dressing after application
▸ Adult: Apply every 24 hours for up to 6 applications, apply moistened caustic pencil tip for 1–2 minutes. Instructions in proprietary packs generally incorporate

advice to remove dead skin before use by gentle filing and to cover with adhesive dressing after application

Umbilical granulomas
▸ TO THE SKIN
▸ Child: Apply moistened caustic pencil tip (usually containing silver nitrate 40%) for 1–2 minutes, protect surrounding skin with soft paraffin
▸ Adult: Apply moistened caustic pencil tip (usually containing silver nitrate 40%) for 1–2 minutes, protect surrounding skin with soft paraffin

- **UNLICENSED USE**
▸ In children No age range specified by manufacturer.

- **CAUTIONS** Avoid broken skin · not suitable for application to ano-genital region · not suitable for application to face · not suitable for application to large areas · protect surrounding skin

- **SIDE-EFFECTS**
▸ Rare or very rare Argyria · methaemoglobinaemia

- **PATIENT AND CARER ADVICE** Patients should be advised that silver nitrate may stain fabric.

- **MEDICINAL FORMS** There can be variation in the licensing of different medicines containing the same drug.

Stick

▸ **Avoca** (Bray Group Ltd)
Silver nitrate 400 mg per 1 gram Avoca 40% silver nitrate pencils | 1 applicator [P] £1.89 DT = £1.89
Silver nitrate 750 mg per 1 gram Avoca 75% silver nitrate applicators | 100 applicator [P] £79.71 DT = £79.71
Avoca 75% silver nitrate applicators with thick handles | 50 applicator [P] £78.64
Silver nitrate 950 mg per 1 gram Avoca 95% silver nitrate applicators | 100 applicator [P] £85.27 DT = £85.27
Avoca 95% silver nitrate pencils | 1 applicator [P] £4.28 DT = £5.00
Avoca wart and verruca treatment set | 1 applicator [P] £5.00 DT = £5.00

ANTIVIRALS › IMMUNE RESPONSE MODIFIERS

Imiquimod   09-Nov-2020

- **INDICATIONS AND DOSE**

ALDARA ®

Warts (external genital and perianal)
▸ TO THE LESION
▸ Adult: Apply 3 times a week until lesions resolve (maximum 16 weeks), to be applied thinly at night

Superficial basal cell carcinoma
▸ TO THE LESION
▸ Adult: Apply daily for 5 nights of each week for 6 weeks, to be applied to lesion and 1 cm beyond it, assess response 12 weeks after completing treatment

Actinic keratosis
▸ TO THE LESION
▸ Adult: Apply 3 times a week for 4 weeks, to be applied to lesion at night, assess response after a 4 week treatment-free interval; repeat 4-week course if lesions persist, maximum 2 courses

ZYCLARA ®

Actinic keratosis
▸ TO THE SKIN
▸ Adult: Apply once daily for 2 weeks, to be applied at bedtime to lesion on face or balding scalp, repeat course after a 2-week treatment-free interval, assess response 8 weeks after second course; maximum 2 sachets per day

- **CAUTIONS** Autoimmune disease · avoid broken skin · avoid contact with eyes · avoid contact with lips · avoid contact with nostrils · avoid open wounds · immunosuppressed patients · not suitable for internal genital warts ·

uncircumcised males (risk of phimosis or stricture of foreskin)

- **SIDE-EFFECTS**
- ▶ **Common or very common** Appetite decreased · arthralgia · asthenia · headaches · increased risk of infection · lymphadenopathy · myalgia · nausea · pain
- ▶ **Uncommon** Anorectal disorder · chills · conjunctival irritation · depression · diarrhoea · dizziness · drowsiness · dry mouth · dysuria · erectile dysfunction · eyelid oedema · face oedema · fever · flushing · gastrointestinal discomfort · genital pain · hyperhidrosis · inflammation · influenza like illness · insomnia · irritability · laryngeal pain · malaise · nasal congestion · painful sexual intercourse · paraesthesia · penis disorder · skin reactions · skin ulcer · tinnitus · uterovaginal prolapse · vomiting · vulvovaginal disorders
- ▶ **Rare or very rare** Autoimmune disorder exacerbated
- ▶ **Frequency not known** Alopecia · cutaneous lupus erythematosus · severe cutaneous adverse reactions (SCARs)
- **CONCEPTION AND CONTRACEPTION** May damage latex condoms and diaphragms.
- **PREGNANCY** No evidence of teratogenicity or toxicity in *animal* studies; manufacturer advises caution.
- **BREAST FEEDING** No information available.
- **DIRECTIONS FOR ADMINISTRATION**
 ALDARA ® ▶ **Important** Manufacturer advises cream should be rubbed in and allowed to stay on the treated area for 6–10 hours for warts or for 8 hours for basal cell carcinoma and actinic keratosis, then washed off with mild soap and water (uncircumcised males treating warts under foreskin should wash the area daily). The cream should be washed off before sexual contact.
 ZYCLARA ® ▶ **Important** Manufacturer advises cream should be rubbed in and allowed to stay on the treated area for 8 hours, then washed off with mild soap and water.
- **PATIENT AND CARER ADVICE** A patient information leaflet should be provided.
- **NATIONAL FUNDING/ACCESS DECISIONS**
 For full details see funding body website
 Scottish Medicines Consortium (SMC) decisions
- ▶ Imiquimod (*Zyclara*®) for the topical treatment of clinically typical, nonhyperkeratotic, nonhypertrophic, visible or palpable actinic keratosis (AK) of the full face or balding scalp in immunocompetent adults when other topical treatment options are contra-indicated or less appropriate (November 2019) SMC No. SMC2211 Recommended with restrictions
- **MEDICINAL FORMS** There can be variation in the licensing of different medicines containing the same drug.
 Cutaneous cream
 CAUTIONARY AND ADVISORY LABELS 10
 EXCIPIENTS: May contain Benzyl alcohol, cetostearyl alcohol (including cetyl and stearyl alcohol), hydroxybenzoates (parabens), polysorbates
- ▶ Aldara (Viatris UK Healthcare Ltd)
 Imiquimod 50 mg per 1 gram Aldara 5% cream 250mg sachets | 12 sachet [PoM] £48.60 DT = £48.60
- ▶ Zyclara (Viatris UK Healthcare Ltd)
 Imiquimod 37.5 mg per 1 gram Zyclara 3.75% cream 250mg sachets | 28 sachet [PoM] £54.75 DT = £54.75

SALICYLIC ACID AND DERIVATIVES

Salicylic acid
24-Nov-2020

- **INDICATIONS AND DOSE**
 OCCLUSAL ®
 Common and plantar warts
- ▶ TO THE LESION
- ▶ Child: Apply daily, treatment may need to be continued for up to 3 months
- ▶ Adult: Apply daily, treatment may need to be continued for up to 3 months
 VERRUGON ®
 For plantar warts
- ▶ TO THE LESION
- ▶ Child: Apply daily, treatment may need to be continued for up to 3 months
- ▶ Adult: Apply daily, treatment may need to be continued for up to 3 months

- **UNLICENSED USE** Not licensed for use in children under 2 years.
- **CAUTIONS** Application to large areas · avoid broken skin · impaired peripheral circulation · not suitable for application to anogenital region · not suitable for application to face · patients with diabetes at risk of neuropathic ulcers · severe peripheral neuropathy
 CAUTIONS, FURTHER INFORMATION
- ▶ Application to large areas and salicylate toxicity Salicylate toxicity may occur particularly if applied on large areas of skin or neonatal skin.
- **SIDE-EFFECTS** Skin irritation
- **PATIENT AND CARER ADVICE** Advise patient to apply carefully to wart and to protect surrounding skin (e.g. with soft paraffin or specially designed plaster); rub wart surface gently with file or pumice stone once weekly.

- **MEDICINAL FORMS** There can be variation in the licensing of different medicines containing the same drug.
 Cutaneous solution
 CAUTIONARY AND ADVISORY LABELS 15
- ▶ Occlusal (Alliance Pharmaceuticals Ltd)
 Salicylic acid 260 mg per 1 ml Occlusal 26% solution | 10 ml [P] £3.56 DT = £3.56

Salicylic acid with lactic acid
09-Aug-2023

The properties listed below are those particular to the combination only. For the properties of the components please consider, salicylic acid above.

- **INDICATIONS AND DOSE**
 DUOFILM ®
 Plantar and mosaic warts
- ▶ TO THE LESION
- ▶ Adult: Apply daily, treatment may need to be continued for up to 3 months
 SALACTOL ®
 Warts, particularly plantar warts | Verrucas | Corns | Calluses
- ▶ TO THE LESION
- ▶ Adult: Apply daily, treatment may need to be continued for up to 3 months
 SALATAC ®
 Warts | Verrucas | Corns | Calluses
- ▶ TO THE LESION
- ▶ Adult: Apply daily, treatment may need to be continued for up to 3 months

- **PRESCRIBING AND DISPENSING INFORMATION** Preparation of salicylic acid in a collodion basis (*Salactol*®) is available but some patients may develop an allergy to colophony in the formulation.

- **MEDICINAL FORMS** There can be variation in the licensing of different medicines containing the same drug.

Cutaneous gel
CAUTIONARY AND ADVISORY LABELS 15
- ▸ Salatac (Dermal Laboratories Ltd)
  Lactic acid 40 mg per 1 gram, Salicylic acid 120 mg per 1 gram Salatac gel | 8 gram Ⓟ £2.98 DT = £2.98

Cutaneous paint
CAUTIONARY AND ADVISORY LABELS 15
- ▸ Duofilm (Thornton & Ross Ltd)
  Lactic acid 150 mg per 1 gram, Salicylic acid 167 mg per 1 gram Duofilm paint | 15 ml Ⓟ £3.40 DT = £3.40
- ▸ Salactol (Dermal Laboratories Ltd)
  Lactic acid 167 mg per 1 gram, Salicylic acid 167 mg per 1 gram Salactol paint | 10 ml Ⓟ £2.09 DT = £2.09

Chapter 14
Vaccines

CONTENTS

1   Immunoglobulin therapy

IMMUNE SERA AND IMMUNOGLOBULINS ⟩
IMMUNOGLOBULINS

Immunoglobulins
20-May-2025

Passive immunity

Immunity with protection against certain infective organisms can be obtained by injecting preparations made from the plasma of immune individuals with adequate levels of antibody to the disease for which protection is sought. The duration of this passive immunity varies according to the dose and the type of immunoglobulin. Passive immunity may last only a few weeks; when necessary, passive immunisation can be repeated. Antibodies of human origin are usually termed immunoglobulins. The term antiserum is applied to material prepared in animals. Because of serum sickness and other allergic-type reactions that may follow injections of antisera, this therapy has been replaced wherever possible by the use of immunoglobulins. Reactions are theoretically possible after injection of human immunoglobulins but reports of such reactions are very rare.

Two types of human immunoglobulin preparation are available, normal immunoglobulin p. 1466 and **disease-specific immunoglobulins**.

Human normal immunoglobulin (HNIG) is prepared from pooled plasma obtained from donors outside the UK, tested and found non-reactive for hepatitis B surface antigen and for antibodies against hepatitis C virus and human immunodeficiency virus (types 1 and 2). A global shortage of human immunoglobulin and the rapidly increasing range of clinical indications for treatment with immunoglobulins has resulted in the need for a Demand Management plan in the UK, for further information consult the Department of Health and Social Care's **Demand Management Plan for Immunoglobulin Use** and NHS England's **Clinical Commissioning Policy for the use of therapeutic immunoglobulin** (both available at: igd.mdsas.com).

For further information on the use of immunoglobulins, see UKHSA guidance: **Immunoglobulin: when to use** (www.gov.uk/government/publications/immunoglobulin-when-to-use) and **Immunisation against Infectious Disease** (www.gov.uk/government/collections/immunisation-against-infectious-disease-the-green-book).

Availability

Human normal immunoglobulin for intramuscular administration is available from the Immunisation, Hepatitis and Blood Safety Department of PHE's Centre for Infectious Disease Surveillance and some regional PHE and NHS laboratories, for the protection of contacts and the control of outbreaks of hepatitis A, measles, and rubella only. For other indications, subcutaneous or intravenous normal immunoglobulin may be purchased from the manufacturer (see Index of manufacturers p. 1961).

Various **disease-specific immunoglobulins** for intramuscular use are available from either the Immunisation, Hepatitis and Blood Safety Department of PHE's Centre for Infectious Disease Surveillance; some regional PHE and NHS laboratories; PHE's Rabies and Immunoglobulin Service; and/or through Bio Products Laboratory (BPL). Tetanus immunoglobulin p. 1468 is available from BPL, hospital pharmacies, or blood transfusion departments. Hepatitis B immunoglobulin p. 1465 required by transplant centres should be obtained commercially.

In Scotland all immunoglobulins are available from the *Scottish National Blood Transfusion Service* (SNBTS).

In Wales all immunoglobulins are available from the *Welsh Blood Service* (WBS).

In Northern Ireland all immunoglobulins are available from the *Northern Ireland Blood Transfusion Service* (NIBTS).

Normal immunoglobulin

Human normal immunoglobulin is prepared from pools of at least 1000 donations of human plasma; it contains immunoglobulin G (IgG) and antibodies to hepatitis A, measles, mumps, rubella, varicella, and other viruses that are currently prevalent in the general population.

Uses

Normal immunoglobulin (containing 10%–18% protein) is administered by *intramuscular injection* for the protection of susceptible contacts against **hepatitis A** virus (infectious hepatitis), **measles** and, to a lesser extent, **rubella**. Injection of immunoglobulin produces immediate protection lasting several weeks.

Normal immunoglobulin (containing 3%–12% protein) for *intravenous administration* is used as *replacement therapy* for patients with congenital agammaglobulinaemia and hypogammaglobulinaemia, and for the short-term treatment of idiopathic thrombocytopenic purpura and Kawasaki disease; it is also used for the prophylaxis of infection following bone-marrow transplantation and in children with symptomatic HIV infection who have recurrent bacterial infections. Normal immunoglobulin for replacement therapy may also be given intramuscularly or subcutaneously, but intravenous formulations are normally preferred. Intravenous immunoglobulin is also used in the treatment of Guillain-Barré syndrome as an alternative to plasma exchange.

For information on the use of intravenous normal immunoglobulin and alternative therapies for certain conditions, see NHS England's: **Clinical Commissioning Policy for the use of therapeutic immunoglobulin** (available at: igd.mdsas.com).

Hepatitis A

For close contacts (of the index case) who have chronic liver disease (including chronic hepatitis B or C infection), HIV infection (with a CD4 count < 200 cells per microlitre), are immunosuppressed, or are aged 60 years or over, normal immunoglobulin in addition to the monovalent hepatitis A vaccine p. 1504 is recommended within 14 days of exposure to the index case (up to 28 days in those with chronic liver disease). Normal immunoglobulin and the monovalent hepatitis A vaccine can be given at the same time, but should be given at separate injection sites.

For further information on post-exposure prophylaxis and information on risk assessment, see Hepatitis A vaccine p. 1480.

Measles

Intravenous or subcutaneous normal immunoglobulin may be given to prevent or attenuate an attack of measles in individuals who do not have adequate immunity. Patients with compromised immunity who have come into contact with measles should receive intravenous or subcutaneous normal immunoglobulin as soon as possible after exposure. It is most effective if given within 72 hours but can be effective if given within 6 days.

Subcutaneous or intramuscular normal immunoglobulin should also be considered for the following individuals if they have been in contact with a confirmed case of measles or with a person associated with a local outbreak:

- non-immune pregnant women
- infants under 9 months

Further advice should be sought from the Centre for Infections, Public Health England (tel. (020) 8200 6868).

Individuals with normal immunity who are not in the above categories and who have not been fully immunised against measles, can be given measles, mumps and rubella vaccine p. 1516 for prophylaxis following exposure to measles.

Rubella

Intramuscular immunoglobulin after exposure to rubella does **not** prevent infection in non-immune contacts and is **not** recommended for protection of pregnant women exposed to rubella. It may, however, reduce the likelihood of a clinical attack which may possibly reduce the risk to the fetus. Risk of intra-uterine transmission is greatest in the first 11 weeks of pregnancy, between 16 and 20 weeks there is minimal risk of deafness only, after 20 weeks there is no increased risk. Intramuscular normal immunoglobulin should be used only if termination of pregnancy would be unacceptable to the pregnant woman—it should be given as soon as possible after exposure. Serological follow-up of recipients is essential to determine if the woman has become infected despite receiving immunoglobulin.

For routine prophylaxis against Rubella, see measles, mumps and rubella vaccine p. 1516.

Tetanus

Normal immunoglobulin [unlicensed] can be used an alternative when tetanus immunoglobulin is not available (see *Tetanus immunoglobulin* in *Disease-specific immunoglobulins*).

Disease-specific immunoglobulins

Specific immunoglobulins are prepared by pooling the plasma of selected human donors with high levels of the specific antibody required. For further information, see UKHSA guidance: **Immunoglobulin: when to use** (www.gov. uk/government/publications/immunoglobulin-when-to-use).

There are no specific immunoglobulins for hepatitis A, measles, or rubella— normal immunoglobulin p. 1466 is used in certain circumstances. There is no specific immunoglobulin for mumps; neither normal immunoglobulin nor measles, mumps and rubella vaccine is effective as post-exposure prophylaxis.

Hepatitis B immunoglobulin

Hepatitis B immunoglobulin p. 1465 (HBIG) in addition to the hepatitis B vaccine p. 1505 is recommended for post-exposure prophylaxis of individuals in certain high-risk groups to provide rapid protection against hepatitis B until the vaccine becomes effective. HBIG is also recommended in some known non-responders to the hepatitis B vaccine. The administration of HBIG at the same time as the vaccine will not inhibit the antibody response, but they should be given at different sites. For further information on high-risk groups and post-exposure management, see Hepatitis B vaccine p. 1481.

An intravenous and subcutaneous preparation of hepatitis B immunoglobulin is licensed for the prevention of hepatitis B recurrence in HBV-DNA negative patients who have undergone liver transplantation for liver failure caused by the virus.

Rabies immunoglobulin

Post-exposure prophylaxis with rabies immunoglobulin p. 1468 should be considered according to the risk assessment of rabies exposure. It provides rapid protection until rabies vaccine p. 1511 (administered at a separate site) becomes effective. When indicated, rabies immunoglobulin should be infiltrated around the site of the wound if possible, as it neutralises rabies virus before the immune system can respond. There is limited benefit of intramuscular administration away from the wound site. For further guidance on risk assessment and post-exposure treatment, see Rabies vaccine p. 1490, and for information about dosing and administration, see rabies immunoglobulin.

Tetanus immunoglobulin

Intravenous tetanus immunoglobulin is no longer available in the UK and the volume of intramuscular tetanus immunoglobulin required to reach a therapeutic dose would be too large in most individuals with tetanus. Therefore, for the management of suspected or confirmed tetanus infection (including localised tetanus), intravenous normal immunoglobulin [unlicensed] is recommended. For further guidance on the management of confirmed and suspected cases of tetanus (including localised tetanus), see Chapter 30, Tetanus, in *Immunisation against infectious disease- 'The Green Book'* (available at: **www.gov.uk/government/ publications/tetanus-the-green-book-chapter-30**) and UKHSA guidance: **Tetanus** (available at: **www.gov.uk/government/ publications/tetanus-advice-for-health-professionals**).

For the management of tetanus-prone wounds, tetanus immunoglobulin p. 1468 should be considered based on an individual's immunisation status and wound category. If tetanus immunoglobulin is not available, normal immunoglobulin [unlicensed] may be used. For further guidance on the management of tetanus-prone wounds, see UKHSA guidance: **Tetanus** (available at: **www.gov.uk/ government/publications/tetanus-advice-for-health-professionals**). When indicated for post-exposure prophylaxis, tetanus immunoglobulin should be used in addition to the other preventative measures of thorough wound cleansing and administration of a tetanus-containing vaccine (depending on immunisation status). Antibacterial therapy may also be warranted depending on clinical severity. For further information, see *Post-exposure management* in Tetanus vaccine p. 1493.

Varicella-zoster immunoglobulin

Varicella (chickenpox) infection in neonates, children aged under one year, immunosuppressed individuals, and pregnant females can lead to severe and even life-threatening varicella disease. Post-exposure prophylaxis is recommended to attenuate disease and to reduce the risk of complications. For further information on post-exposure prophylaxis, including risk assessment and the use of varicella-zoster immunoglobulin, see Herpesvirus infections p. 727.

Anti-D (Rh$_0$) immunoglobulin

Anti-D (Rh$_0$) immunoglobulin below is prepared from plasma taken from rhesus-negative donors who have been immunised against the anti-D-antigen. Anti-D (Rh$_0$) immunoglobulin is used to prevent a rhesus-negative mother from forming antibodies to fetal rhesus-positive cells which may pass into the maternal circulation. The objective is to protect any subsequent child from the hazard of haemolytic disease of the newborn.

Anti-D (Rh$_0$) immunoglobulin should be administered to the mother following any sensitising episode (e.g. abortion, miscarriage and birth); it should be injected within 72 hours of the episode but even if a longer period has elapsed it may still give protection and should be administered. Anti-D (Rh$_0$) immunoglobulin is also given when significant feto-maternal haemorrhage occurs in rhesus-negative women during delivery. The dose of anti-D (Rh$_0$) immunoglobulin is determined according to the level of exposure to rhesus-positive blood.

Use of routine *antenatal* anti-D prophylaxis should be given irrespective of previous anti-D prophylaxis for a sensitising event early in the same pregnancy. Similarly, *postpartum* anti-D prophylaxis should be given irrespective of previous routine antenatal anti-D prophylaxis or antenatal anti-D prophylaxis for a sensitising event in the same pregnancy.

Anti-D (Rh$_0$) immunoglobulin is also given to women of child-bearing potential after the inadvertent transfusion of rhesus-incompatible blood components and is used for the treatment of idiopathic thrombocytopenia purpura.

MMR vaccine

Measles, mumps and rubella vaccine may be given in the postpartum period with anti-D (Rh$_0$) immunoglobulin injection provided that separate syringes are used and the products are administered to different limbs. If blood is transfused, the antibody response to the vaccine may be inhibited—measure rubella antibodies after 6–8 weeks and revaccinate if necessary.

Anti-D (Rh$_0$) immunoglobulin

03-Mar-2020

● **INDICATIONS AND DOSE**

To rhesus-negative woman for prevention of Rh$_0$(D) sensitisation, following birth of rhesus-positive infant
▸ BY DEEP INTRAMUSCULAR INJECTION
▸ Females of childbearing potential: 500 units, dose to be administered immediately or within 72 hours; for transplacental bleed of over 4 mL fetal red cells, extra 100–125 units per mL fetal red cells, subcutaneous route used for patients with bleeding disorders

To rhesus-negative woman for prevention of Rh$_0$(D) sensitisation, following any potentially sensitising episode (e.g. stillbirth, abortion, amniocentesis) up to 20 weeks' gestation
▸ BY DEEP INTRAMUSCULAR INJECTION
▸ Females of childbearing potential: 250 units per episode, dose to be administered immediately or within 72 hours, subcutaneous route used for patients with bleeding disorders

To rhesus-negative woman for prevention of Rh$_0$(D) sensitisation, following any potentially sensitising episode (e.g. stillbirth, abortion, amniocentesis) after 20 weeks' gestation
▸ BY DEEP INTRAMUSCULAR INJECTION
▸ Females of childbearing potential: 500 units per episode, dose to be administered immediately or within 72 hours, subcutaneous route used for patients with bleeding disorders

To rhesus-negative woman for prevention of Rh$_0$(D) sensitisation, antenatal prophylaxis
▸ BY DEEP INTRAMUSCULAR INJECTION
▸ Females of childbearing potential: 500 units, dose to be given at weeks 28 and 34 of pregnancy, if infant rhesus-positive, a further dose is still needed immediately or within 72 hours of delivery, subcutaneous route used for patients with bleeding disorders

To rhesus-negative woman for prevention of Rh$_0$(D) sensitisation, antenatal prophylaxis (alternative NICE recommendation)
▸ BY DEEP INTRAMUSCULAR INJECTION
▸ Females of childbearing potential: 1000–1650 units, dose to be given at weeks 28 and 34 of pregnancy, alternatively 1500 units for 1 dose, dose to be given between 28 and 30 weeks gestation

To rhesus-negative woman for prevention of Rh$_0$(D) sensitisation, following Rh$_0$(D) incompatible blood transfusion
▸ BY DEEP INTRAMUSCULAR INJECTION
▸ Females of childbearing potential: 100–125 units per mL of transfused rhesus-positive red cells, subcutaneous route used for patients with bleeding disorders

RHOPHYLAC®

To rhesus-negative woman for prevention of Rh$_0$(D) sensitisation, following birth of rhesus-positive infant
▸ BY INTRAMUSCULAR INJECTION, OR BY INTRAVENOUS INJECTION
▸ Females of childbearing potential: 1000–1500 units, dose to administered immediately or within 72 hours; for large transplacental bleed, extra 100 units per mL fetal red cells (preferably by intravenous injection), intravenous route recommended for patients with bleeding disorders

To rhesus-negative woman for prevention of Rh$_0$(D) sensitisation, following any potentially sensitising episode (e.g. abortion, amniocentesis, chorionic villous sampling) up to 12 weeks' gestation
▸ BY INTRAMUSCULAR INJECTION, OR BY INTRAVENOUS INJECTION
▸ Females of childbearing potential: 1000 units per episode, dose to be administered immediately or within 72 hours, intravenous route recommended for patients with bleeding disorders, higher doses may be required after 12 weeks gestation

To rhesus-negative woman for prevention of Rh$_0$(D) sensitisation, antenatal prophylaxis
▸ BY INTRAMUSCULAR INJECTION, OR BY INTRAVENOUS INJECTION
▸ Females of childbearing potential: 1500 units, dose to be given between weeks 28–30 of pregnancy; if infant rhesus-positive, a further dose is still needed immediately or within 72 hours of delivery, intravenous route recommended for patients with bleeding disorders

To rhesus-negative woman for prevention of Rh$_0$(D) sensitisation, following Rh$_0$(D) incompatible blood transfusion
▸ BY INTRAVENOUS INJECTION
▸ Females of childbearing potential: 50 units per mL of transfused rhesus-positive blood, alternatively 100 units per of mL of erythrocyte concentrate, intravenous route recommended for patients with bleeding disorders

● **CAUTIONS** Immunoglobulin A deficiency · possible interference with live virus vaccines

CAUTIONS, FURTHER INFORMATION
▸ **MMR vaccine** MMR vaccine may be given in the postpartum

period with anti-D (Rh₀) immunoglobulin injection provided that separate syringes are used and the products are administered into different limbs. If blood is transfused, the antibody response to the vaccine may be inhibited—measure rubella antibodies after 6–8 weeks and revaccinate if necessary.

- **INTERACTIONS** → Appendix 1: immunoglobulins
- **SIDE-EFFECTS**
- ▸ **Uncommon** Chills · fever · headache · malaise · skin reactions
- ▸ **Rare or very rare** Arthralgia · dyspnoea · hypersensitivity · hypotension · nausea · tachycardia · vomiting
- ▸ **Frequency not known** Intravascular haemolysis
- **HANDLING AND STORAGE** Care must be taken to store all immunological products under the conditions recommended in the product literature, otherwise the preparation may become ineffective. **Refrigerated storage** is usually necessary; many immunoglobulins need to be stored at 2–8°C and not allowed to freeze. Immunoglobulins should be protected from light. Opened multidose vials must be used within the period recommended in the product literature.
- **NATIONAL FUNDING/ACCESS DECISIONS**
  For full details see funding body website
  NICE decisions
- ▸ **Routine antenatal anti-D prophylaxis for rhesus-negative women (August 2008)** NICE TA156 Recommended

- **MEDICINAL FORMS** There can be variation in the licensing of different medicines containing the same drug.
  Solution for injection
- ▸ **D-Gam** (Bio Products Laboratory Ltd)
  Anti-D (RHO) immunoglobulin 500 unit D-Gam Anti-D immunoglobulin 500unit solution for injection vials | 1 vial [PoM] £54.00
- ▸ **Rhophylac** (CSL Behring UK Ltd)
  Anti-D (RHO) immunoglobulin 750 unit per 1 ml Rhophylac 1,500units/2ml solution for injection pre-filled syringes | 1 pre-filled disposable injection [PoM] £85.00

Cytomegalovirus immunoglobulin

16-Apr-2020

- **INDICATIONS AND DOSE**
  Prophylaxis of cytomegalovirus infection in patients taking immunosuppressants, particularly transplant recipients (specialist use only)
- ▸ BY INTRAVENOUS INFUSION
- ▸ Adult: (consult product literature)

- **CONTRA-INDICATIONS** Selective IgA deficiency with IgA antibodies
- **CAUTIONS** Interference with live virus vaccines
  CAUTIONS, FURTHER INFORMATION
- ▸ Interference with live virus vaccines Cytomegalovirus immunoglobulin may impair the immune response to live virus vaccines; such vaccines should only be given 3 months after CMV immunoglobulin treatment. Patients receiving measles vaccines should have their antibody status checked as impairment of immune response may persist for up to 1 year.
- **INTERACTIONS** → Appendix 1: immunoglobulins
- **SIDE-EFFECTS** Arthralgia · back pain · chills · cutaneous lupus erythematosus · dizziness · embolism and thrombosis · fatigue · fever · haemolysis · haemolytic anaemia · headache · hypotension · infusion related reaction · meningitis aseptic · myocardial infarction · nausea · neutropenia · renal impairment · skin reactions · stroke · transfusion-related acute lung injury · vomiting

- **MONITORING REQUIREMENTS**
- ▸ Manufacturer advises monitor for signs of infusion-related reactions during and for at least one hour after each infusion in patients receiving cytomegalovirus immunoglobulin for the first time, or following a prolonged period between treatments, or when a different human immunoglobulin has been used previously; monitor all other patients for at least 20 minutes after each infusion—in case of reaction, reduce rate or stop infusion as clinically appropriate.
- ▸ Manufacturer advises monitor urine output and serum creatinine.
- **HANDLING AND STORAGE** Care must be taken to store all immunological products under the conditions recommended in the product literature, otherwise the preparation may become ineffective. **Refrigerated storage** is usually necessary; many immunoglobulins need to be stored at 2–8°C and not allowed to freeze. Immunoglobulins should be protected from light. Opened multidose vials must be used within the period recommended in the product literature.

- **MEDICINAL FORMS** There can be variation in the licensing of different medicines containing the same drug.
  Solution for infusion
- ▸ **Cytotect CP Biotest** (Grifols UK Ltd)
  Cytomegalovirus immunoglobulin human 100 unit per 1 ml Cytotect CP Biotest 5,000units/50ml solution for infusion vials | 1 vial [PoM] £917.70 (Hospital only)
  Cytotect CP Biotest 1,000units/10ml solution for infusion vials | 1 vial [PoM] £183.54 (Hospital only)

Hepatitis B immunoglobulin

05-Feb-2024

- **INDICATIONS AND DOSE**
  Post-exposure prophylaxis against hepatitis B infection
- ▸ BY INTRAMUSCULAR INJECTION
- ▸ Adult: 500 units for 1 dose, dose to be administered as soon as possible after exposure; ideally within 24–48 hours, but no later than 7 days after exposure
  Post-exposure prophylaxis against hepatitis B infection [after exposure to hepatitis B virus-contaminated material]
- ▸ BY INTRAVENOUS INFUSION
- ▸ Adult: Dose to be administered as soon as possible after exposure, but no later than 72 hours (consult product literature)
  Prevention of hepatitis B in haemodialysed patients
- ▸ BY INTRAVENOUS INFUSION
- ▸ Adult: (consult product literature)
  Prophylaxis against re-infection of transplanted liver
- ▸ BY INTRAVENOUS INFUSION
- ▸ Adult: (consult product literature)
  Prevention of hepatitis B re-infection more than 6 months after liver transplantation in stable HBV-DNA negative patients
- ▸ BY SUBCUTANEOUS INJECTION
- ▸ Adult (body-weight up to 75 kg): 500 units once weekly, increased if necessary up to 1000 units once weekly, dose to be started 2–3 weeks after last dose of intravenous hepatitis B immunoglobulin
- ▸ Adult (body-weight 75 kg and above): 1000 units once weekly, dose to be started 2–3 weeks after last dose of intravenous hepatitis B immunoglobulin

- **CAUTIONS** IgA deficiency · interference with live virus vaccines
- **INTERACTIONS** → Appendix 1: immunoglobulins
- **SIDE-EFFECTS**
- ▸ **Uncommon** Abdominal pain upper · headache

▶ **Rare or very rare** Cardiac discomfort · fatigue · hypersensitivity · hypertension · hypotension · muscle spasms · nasopharyngitis · oropharyngeal pain · palpitations · skin reactions

● **DIRECTIONS FOR ADMINISTRATION**
▶ With intramuscular use If more than 5 mL is to be given, give in divided doses at different sites.

● **PRESCRIBING AND DISPENSING INFORMATION** Vials containing 500 units (for intramuscular injection), are available from the UKHSA Rabies and Immunoglobulin Service, and are also available from Bio Products Laboratory (BPL).

● **HANDLING AND STORAGE** Care must be taken to store all immunological products under the conditions recommended in the product literature, otherwise the preparation may become ineffective. **Refrigerated storage** is usually necessary; many immunoglobulins need to be stored at 2–8°C and not allowed to freeze. Immunoglobulins should be protected from light. Opened multidose vials must be used within the period recommended in the product literature.

● **MEDICINAL FORMS** There can be variation in the licensing of different medicines containing the same drug.

Solution for injection
▶ **Hepatitis B immunoglobulin (Non-proprietary)**
Hepatitis B immunoglobulin human 100 unit per 1 ml Hepatitis B immunoglobulin human 500units/5ml solution for injection vials | 1 vial [PoM] £600.00
▶ **Zutectra** (Grifols UK Ltd)
Zutectra 500units/1ml solution for injection pre-filled syringes | 5 syringe [PoM] £1,500.00 (Hospital only)
Solution for infusion
▶ **Hepatect CP** (Grifols UK Ltd)
Hepatitis B immunoglobulin human 50 unit per 1 ml Hepatect CP 5000units/100ml solution for infusion vials | 1 vial [PoM] £2,750.00 (Hospital only)
▶ **Omri-Hep-B** (Imported (Israel))
Hepatitis B immunoglobulin human 50 unit per 1 ml Omri-Hep-B 5000units/100ml solution for infusion vials | 1 vial [PoM] [x] (Hospital only)

Normal immunoglobulin
02-Jul-2024

● **INDICATIONS AND DOSE**
Post-exposure prophylaxis against hepatitis A infection [using Subgam ®]
▶ BY DEEP INTRAMUSCULAR INJECTION
▶ Adult: 1000 mg for 1 dose
Rubella in pregnancy [post-exposure prophylaxis to prevent or attenuate clinical attack; only when termination of pregnancy is unacceptable]
▶ BY DEEP INTRAMUSCULAR INJECTION
▶ Females of childbearing potential: 750 mg for 1 dose
Replacement therapy in primary immunodeficiency disorders (specialist use only) | Replacement therapy in secondary immunodeficiency disorders (specialist use only)
▶ BY SUBCUTANEOUS INFUSION, OR BY INTRAVENOUS INFUSION
▶ Adult: (consult product literature)
Immune-mediated disorders (specialist use only)
▶ BY INTRAVENOUS INFUSION
▶ Adult: For some indications, subcutaneous infusion may be used for maintenance treatment (consult product literature)

● **UNLICENSED USE** PHE advises normal immunoglobulin (as *Subgam ®*) is used for post-exposure prophylaxis against hepatitis A infection, but it is not licensed for this indication. PHE advises normal immunoglobulin is used for rubella in pregnancy for prevention of clinical attack, but it is not licensed for this indication.

● **CONTRA-INDICATIONS** Patients with selective IgA deficiency who have known antibodies against IgA
CONTRA-INDICATIONS, FURTHER INFORMATION For full details on contra-indications, consult product literature.

● **CAUTIONS**
GENERAL CAUTIONS Agammaglobulinaemia with or without IgA deficiency · hypogammaglobulinaemia with or without IgA deficiency
SPECIFIC CAUTIONS
▶ With intravenous use Ensure adequate hydration · obesity · renal insufficiency · risk factors for arterial or venous thromboembolic events · thrombophilic disorders
CAUTIONS, FURTHER INFORMATION For full details on cautions, consult product literature.

● **INTERACTIONS** → Appendix 1: immunoglobulins

● **SIDE-EFFECTS**
GENERAL SIDE-EFFECTS
▶ **Common or very common** Diarrhoea · dizziness · fatigue · gastrointestinal discomfort · myalgia · nausea · pain · skin reactions
SPECIFIC SIDE-EFFECTS
▶ **Common or very common**
▶ With intravenous use Arthralgia · chills · embolism and thrombosis · feeling hot · fever · haemolysis · headache · hyperaemia · hypersensitivity · hypertension · infusion related reaction · palpitations · sensory disorder · taste altered · vomiting
▶ With subcutaneous use Drowsiness · headaches · hypotension · local reaction
▶ **Uncommon**
▶ With intravenous use Hypothermia
▶ With subcutaneous use Paraesthesia
▶ **Frequency not known**
▶ With intravenous use Acute kidney injury · angina pectoris · cutaneous lupus erythematosus · dyspnoea · leucopenia · meningitis aseptic · neutropenia · shock · transfusion-related acute lung injury

SIDE-EFFECTS, FURTHER INFORMATION Adverse reactions are more likely to occur in patients receiving normal immunoglobulin for the first time, or following a prolonged period between treatments, or when a different brand of normal immunoglobulin is administered.

● **MONITORING REQUIREMENTS** Monitor for acute renal failure; consider discontinuation if renal function deteriorates. Intravenous preparations with added sucrose have been associated with cases of renal dysfunction and acute renal failure.

● **DIRECTIONS FOR ADMINISTRATION** Administration advice (including licensed route of administration, recommended rate of infusion and reconstitution requirements) varies widely between normal immunoglobulin preparations from different manufacturers—formulations are **not interchangeable**; consult product literature.

● **PRESCRIBING AND DISPENSING INFORMATION** Antibody titres can vary widely between normal immunoglobulin preparations from different manufacturers—formulations are **not interchangeable**; patients should be maintained on the same formulation throughout long-term treatment to avoid adverse effects.

[EvGr] The brand name and batch number should be recorded after each administration (in case of transmission of infective agents). ◀Ⓜ

Indications, licensed age groups, and excipients differ between preparations. Some manufacturers also provide hyaluronidase to enhance the absorption of normal immunoglobulin. Further information can be found in the product literature for the individual preparations.
▶ With intramuscular use Available from ImmForm and from some Public Health England and NHS laboratories (for hepatitis A and rubella prophylaxis).

- **HANDLING AND STORAGE** Care must be taken to store all immunological products under the conditions recommended in the product literature, otherwise the preparation may become ineffective. **Refrigerated storage** is usually necessary; many immunoglobulins need to be stored at 2–8°C and not allowed to freeze. Immunoglobulins should be protected from light. Opened multidose vials must be used within the period recommended in the product literature.

- **MEDICINAL FORMS** There can be variation in the licensing of different medicines containing the same drug.

Solution for injection
EXCIPIENTS: May contain L-proline, polysorbates
ELECTROLYTES: May contain Sodium

▸ **Normal immunoglobulin (Non-proprietary)**
Normal immunoglobulin human 200 mg per 1 ml Hizentra 1g/5ml solution for injection pre-filled syringes | 1 pre-filled disposable injection [PoM] [Ⓑ]

▸ **Cutaquig** (Octapharma Ltd)
Normal immunoglobulin human 165 mg per 1 ml Cutaquig 1g/6ml solution for injection vials | 1 vial [PoM] £73.50 (Hospital only)
Cutaquig 2g/12ml solution for injection vials | 1 vial [PoM] £147.00 (Hospital only)
Cutaquig 8g/48ml solution for injection vials | 1 vial [PoM] £588.00 (Hospital only)
Cutaquig 4g/24ml solution for injection vials | 1 vial [PoM] £294.00 (Hospital only)

▸ **Hizentra** (CSL Behring UK Ltd)
Normal immunoglobulin human 200 mg per 1 ml Hizentra 4g/20ml solution for injection pre-filled syringes | 1 pre-filled disposable injection [PoM] £350.00 (Hospital only)
Hizentra 2g/10ml solution for injection pre-filled syringes | 1 pre-filled disposable injection [PoM] £175.00 (Hospital only)

▸ **Subgam** (Bio Products Laboratory Ltd)
Normal immunoglobulin human 160 mg per 1 ml Subgam 1g/6.25ml solution for injection vials | 1 vial [PoM] £80.00
Subgam 4g/25ml solution for injection vials | 1 vial [PoM] £321.00
Subgam 2g/12.5ml solution for injection vials | 1 vial [PoM] £161.00

▸ **Xembify** (Grifols UK Ltd) ▼
Normal immunoglobulin human 200 mg per 1 ml Xembify 4g/20ml solution for injection vials | 1 vial [PoM] £276.00 (Hospital only)
Xembify 2g/10ml solution for injection vials | 1 vial [PoM] £138.00 (Hospital only)
Xembify 1g/5ml solution for injection vials | 1 vial [PoM] £69.00 (Hospital only)
Xembify 10g/50ml solution for injection vials | 1 vial [PoM] £690.00 (Hospital only)

Solution for infusion
EXCIPIENTS: May contain Edetic acid (edta), glucose, l-proline, maltose, polysorbates, sorbitol, sucrose
ELECTROLYTES: May contain Sodium

▸ **Normal immunoglobulin (Non-proprietary)**
Normal immunoglobulin human 100 mg per 1 ml Normal immunoglobulin human 5g/50ml solution for infusion vials | 1 vial [PoM] [Ⓑ]
Normal immunoglobulin human 2.5g/25ml solution for infusion vials | 1 vial [PoM] [Ⓑ]
Normal immunoglobulin human 20g/200ml solution for infusion vials | 1 vial [PoM] [Ⓑ]
Normal immunoglobulin human 10g/100ml solution for infusion vials | 1 vial [PoM] [Ⓑ]
Normal immunoglobulin human 30g/300ml solution for infusion vials | 1 vial [PoM] [Ⓑ]

▸ **Cuvitru** (Takeda UK Ltd)
Normal immunoglobulin human 200 mg per 1 ml Cuvitru 4g/20ml solution for infusion vials | 1 vial [PoM] £276.00 (Hospital only)
Cuvitru 2g/10ml solution for infusion vials | 1 vial [PoM] £138.00 (Hospital only)
Cuvitru 1g/5ml solution for infusion vials | 1 vial [PoM] £69.00 (Hospital only)
Cuvitru 8g/40ml solution for infusion vials | 1 vial [PoM] £552.00 (Hospital only)
Cuvitru 10g/50ml solution for infusion vials | 1 vial [PoM] £690.00 (Hospital only)

▸ **Flebogammadif** (Grifols UK Ltd)
Normal immunoglobulin human 50 mg per 1 ml Flebogamma DIF 2.5g/50ml solution for infusion vials | 1 vial [PoM] £175.00

Flebogamma DIF 10g/200ml solution for infusion vials | 1 vial [PoM] £700.00
Flebogamma DIF 5g/100ml solution for infusion vials | 1 vial [PoM] £350.00
Flebogamma DIF 20g/400ml solution for infusion vials | 1 vial [PoM] £1,400.00

▸ **Gammaplex** (Bio Products Laboratory Ltd)
Normal immunoglobulin human 50 mg per 1 ml Gammaplex 10g/200ml solution for infusion vials | 1 vial [PoM] £721.00 (Hospital only)
Gammaplex 5g/100ml solution for infusion vials | 1 vial [PoM] £361.00 (Hospital only)
Gammaplex 20g/400ml solution for infusion vials | 1 vial [PoM] £1,442.00 (Hospital only)
Normal immunoglobulin human 100 mg per 1 ml Gammaplex 5g/50ml solution for infusion vials | 1 vial [PoM] £361.00 (Hospital only)
Gammaplex 10g/100ml solution for infusion vials | 1 vial [PoM] £721.00 (Hospital only)
Gammaplex 20g/200ml solution for infusion vials | 1 vial [PoM] £1,442.00 (Hospital only)

▸ **Gamten** (Octapharma Ltd)
Normal immunoglobulin human 100 mg per 1 ml Gamten 5g/50ml solution for infusion bottles | 1 bottle [PoM] £355.00 (Hospital only)
Gamten 20g/200ml solution for infusion bottles | 1 bottle [PoM] £1,420.00 (Hospital only)
Gamten 10g/100ml solution for infusion bottles | 1 bottle [PoM] £710.00 (Hospital only)

▸ **Gamunex** (Grifols UK Ltd)
Normal immunoglobulin human 100 mg per 1 ml Gamunex 10% 10g/100ml solution for infusion vials | 1 vial [PoM] £665.00 (Hospital only)
Gamunex 10% 20g/200ml solution for infusion vials | 1 vial [PoM] £1,330.00 (Hospital only)
Gamunex 10% 5g/50ml solution for infusion vials | 1 vial [PoM] £332.50 (Hospital only)

▸ **Hizentra** (CSL Behring UK Ltd)
Normal immunoglobulin human 200 mg per 1 ml Hizentra 2g/10ml solution for infusion vials | 1 vial [PoM] £175.00 (Hospital only)
Hizentra 1g/5ml solution for infusion vials | 1 vial [PoM] £87.50 (Hospital only)
Hizentra 4g/20ml solution for infusion vials | 1 vial [PoM] £350.00 (Hospital only)

▸ **Intratect** (Grifols UK Ltd)
Normal immunoglobulin human 50 mg per 1 ml Intratect 5g/100ml solution for infusion vials | 1 vial [PoM] £362.30 (Hospital only)
Intratect 2.5g/50ml solution for infusion vials | 1 vial [PoM] £181.15
Intratect 10g/200ml solution for infusion vials | 1 vial [PoM] £724.60 (Hospital only)
Normal immunoglobulin human 100 mg per 1 ml Intratect 10g/100ml solution for infusion vials | 1 vial [PoM] £724.60 (Hospital only)
Intratect 20g/200ml solution for infusion vials | 1 vial [PoM] £1,449.20 (Hospital only)
Intratect 5g/50ml solution for infusion vials | 1 vial [PoM] £362.30 (Hospital only)

▸ **Iqymune** (LFB Biopharmaceuticals Ltd)
Normal immunoglobulin human 100 mg per 1 ml Iqymune 10g/100ml solution for infusion vials | 1 vial [PoM] £700.00 (Hospital only)
Iqymune 2g/20ml solution for infusion vials | 1 vial [PoM] £140.00 (Hospital only)
Iqymune 20g/200ml solution for infusion vials | 1 vial [PoM] £1,400.00 (Hospital only)
Iqymune 5g/50ml solution for infusion vials | 1 vial [PoM] £350.00 (Hospital only)

▸ **Kiovig** (Takeda UK Ltd)
Normal immunoglobulin human 100 mg per 1 ml Kiovig 5g/50ml solution for infusion vials | 1 vial [PoM] £345.00 (Hospital only)
Kiovig 20g/200ml solution for infusion vials | 1 vial [PoM] £1,380.00 (Hospital only)
Kiovig 10g/100ml solution for infusion vials | 1 vial [PoM] £690.00 (Hospital only)
Kiovig 30g/300ml solution for infusion vials | 1 vial [PoM] £2,070.00
Kiovig 2.5g/25ml solution for infusion vials | 1 vial [PoM] £172.50
Kiovig 1g/10ml solution for infusion vials | 1 vial [PoM] £69.00

▸ **Octagam** (Octapharma Ltd)
Normal immunoglobulin human 50 mg per 1 ml Octagam 5% 10g/200ml solution for infusion bottles | 1 bottle [PoM] £690.00 (Hospital only)

Octagam 5% 5g/100ml solution for infusion bottles | 1 bottle [PoM] £345.00 (Hospital only)
Normal immunoglobulin human 100 mg per 1 ml Octagam 10% 10g/100ml solution for infusion bottles | 1 bottle [PoM] £710.00 (Hospital only)
Octagam 10% 5g/50ml solution for infusion bottles | 1 bottle [PoM] £355.00 (Hospital only)
Octagam 10% 20g/200ml solution for infusion bottles | 1 bottle [PoM] £1,420.00 (Hospital only)
Octagam 10% 2g/20ml solution for infusion vials | 1 vial [PoM] £142.00 (Hospital only)
▸ **Panzyga** (Octapharma Ltd)
Normal immunoglobulin human 100 mg per 1 ml Panzyga 20g/200ml solution for infusion bottles | 1 bottle [PoM] £1,380.00 (Hospital only)
Panzyga 10g/100ml solution for infusion bottles | 1 bottle [PoM] £690.00 (Hospital only)
Panzyga 5g/50ml solution for infusion bottles | 1 bottle [PoM] £345.00 (Hospital only)
▸ **Privigen** (CSL Behring UK Ltd)
Normal immunoglobulin human 100 mg per 1 ml Privigen 5g/50ml solution for infusion vials | 1 vial [PoM] £395.00 (Hospital only)
Privigen 20g/200ml solution for infusion vials | 1 vial [PoM] £1,580.00 (Hospital only)
Privigen 10g/100ml solution for infusion vials | 1 vial [PoM] £790.00 (Hospital only)
Privigen 2.5g/25ml solution for infusion vials | 1 vial [PoM] £197.50
▸ **Yimmugo** (Grifols UK Ltd) ▼
Normal immunoglobulin human 100 mg per 1 ml Yimmugo 20g/200ml solution for infusion vials | 1 vial [PoM] £1,444.00
Yimmugo 10g/100ml solution for infusion vials | 1 vial [PoM] £722.00
Yimmugo 5g/50ml solution for infusion vials | 1 vial [PoM] £361.00

Form unstated
EXCIPIENTS: May contain Edetic acid (edta)
▸ **HyQvia** (Takeda UK Ltd)
HyQvia 30g/300ml solution for infusion and 15ml vials | 1 pack [PoM] £2,070.00
HyQvia 20g/200ml solution for infusion and 10ml vials | 1 pack [PoM] £1,380.00
HyQvia 10g/100ml solution for infusion and 5ml vials | 1 pack [PoM] £690.00
HyQvia 5g/50ml solution for infusion and 2.5ml vials | 1 pack [PoM] £345.00
HyQvia 2.5g/25ml solution for infusion and 1.25ml vials | 1 pack [PoM] £172.50

Powder and solvent for solution for injection
EXCIPIENTS: May contain Glucose
▸ **Gammagard S/D** (Takeda UK Ltd)
Normal immunoglobulin human 10 gram Gammagard S/D 10g powder and solvent for solution for injection bottles | 1 bottle [PoM] £690.00

Rabies immunoglobulin

07-Feb-2023

● **INDICATIONS AND DOSE**
Post-exposure treatment against rabies infection
▸ BY LOCAL INFILTRATION, OR BY INTRAMUSCULAR INJECTION
▸ Child: 20 units/kg, dose administered by infiltration in and around the cleansed wound; if wound not visible or healed or if infiltration of whole volume not possible, give remainder by intramuscular injection into anterolateral thigh (remote from vaccination site). If more than 2 mL to be given by intramuscular injection then give in divided doses at different sites, to be given in combination with rabies vaccine, not required if more than 7 days have elapsed after the first dose of vaccine, or more than 1 day after the second dose of vaccine
▸ Adult: 20 units/kg, dose administered by infiltration in and around the cleansed wound; if wound not visible or healed or if infiltration of whole volume not possible, give remainder by intramuscular injection into anterolateral thigh (remote from vaccination site). If more than 5 mL to be given by intramuscular injection then give in divided doses at different sites, to be given in combination with rabies vaccine, not required if more than 7 days have elapsed after the first dose of vaccine, or more than 1 day after the second dose of vaccine

● **CAUTIONS** IgA deficiency · interference with live virus vaccines

● **INTERACTIONS** → Appendix 1: immunoglobulins

● **SIDE-EFFECTS**
▸ **Rare or very rare** Arthralgia · chills · fatigue · fever · headache · hypersensitivity · hypotension · influenza like illness · malaise · nausea · skin reactions · tachycardia · vomiting

● **PRESCRIBING AND DISPENSING INFORMATION** The potency of individual batches of rabies immunoglobulin from the manufacturer may vary. It is therefore critical to know the potency of the batch to be used and the weight of the patient in order to calculate the specific volume required to provide the necessary dose.
 Available from the Rabies and Immunoglobulin Service (RIgS) and/or Bio Products Laboratory (BPL).

● **HANDLING AND STORAGE** Care must be taken to store all immunological products under the conditions recommended in the product literature, otherwise the preparation may become ineffective. **Refrigerated storage** is usually necessary; many immunoglobulins need to be stored at 2–8°C and not allowed to freeze. Immunoglobulins should be protected from light. Opened multidose vials must be used within the period recommended in the product literature.

● **MEDICINAL FORMS** There can be variation in the licensing of different medicines containing the same drug.
Solution for injection
▸ **Rabies immunoglobulin (Non-proprietary)**
Rabies immunoglobulin human 500 unit Rabies immunoglobulin human 500unit solution for injection vials | 1 vial [PoM] £1,000.00

Tetanus immunoglobulin

18-Mar-2021

● **INDICATIONS AND DOSE**
Post-exposure prophylaxis
▸ BY INTRAMUSCULAR INJECTION
▸ Child: 250 units, alternatively 500 units, higher dose used if more than 24 hours have elapsed since injury, or there is risk of heavy contamination, or following burns
▸ Adult: 250 units, alternatively 500 units, higher dose used if more than 24 hours have elapsed since injury, or there is risk of heavy contamination, or following burns

● **CAUTIONS** IgA deficiency · interference with live virus vaccines

● **INTERACTIONS** → Appendix 1: immunoglobulins

● **SIDE-EFFECTS**
▸ **Rare or very rare** Anaphylactic reaction · hypotension
▸ **Frequency not known** Arthralgia · chest pain · dizziness · dyspnoea · face oedema · oral disorders · tremor

● **HANDLING AND STORAGE** Care must be taken to store all immunological products under the conditions recommended in the product literature, otherwise the preparation may become ineffective. **Refrigerated storage** is usually necessary; many immunoglobulins need to be stored at 2–8°C and not allowed to freeze. Immunoglobulins should be protected from light. Opened multidose vials must be used within the period recommended in the product literature.

- **MEDICINAL FORMS** There can be variation in the licensing of different medicines containing the same drug.
  ### Solution for injection
  ▸ **Tetanus immunoglobulin (Non-proprietary)**
    Tetanus immunoglobulin human 250 unit Tetanus immunoglobulin human 250unit solution for injection vials | 1 vial [PoM] £300.00 DT = £300.00

Varicella-zoster immunoglobulin

16-Oct-2020

(Antivaricella-zoster Immunoglobulin)

- **INDICATIONS AND DOSE**
  Prophylaxis against varicella infection
  ▸ BY INTRAMUSCULAR INJECTION
  ▸ Adult: 1 g, to be administered as soon as possible—not later than 10 days after exposure, second dose to be given if further exposure occurs more than 3 weeks after first dose

- **CAUTIONS** IgA deficiency · interference with live virus vaccines

- **INTERACTIONS** → Appendix 1: immunoglobulins

- **SIDE-EFFECTS** Arthralgia · chills · fever · headache · hypersensitivity · hypotension · malaise · nausea · skin reactions · tachycardia · vomiting

- **DIRECTIONS FOR ADMINISTRATION** Public Health England advises normal immunoglobulin for intravenous use may be used in those unable to receive intramuscular injections.
  Manufacturer advises if a large volume (>5 mL) is to be given by intramuscular injection then administer in divided doses at different sites.

- **PRESCRIBING AND DISPENSING INFORMATION** Available from selected Public Health England and NHS laboratories (also from Bio Products Laboratory).

- **HANDLING AND STORAGE** Care must be taken to store all immunological products under the conditions recommended in the product literature, otherwise the preparation may become ineffective. **Refrigerated storage** is usually necessary; many immunoglobulins need to be stored at 2–8°C and not allowed to freeze. Immunoglobulins should be protected from light. Opened multidose vials must be used within the period recommended in the product literature.

- **MEDICINAL FORMS** There can be variation in the licensing of different medicines containing the same drug.
  ### Solution for injection
  ▸ **Varicella-Zoster** (Bio Products Laboratory Ltd)
    Varicella-Zoster immunoglobulin human 250 mg Varicella-Zoster immunoglobulin human 250mg solution for injection vials | 1 vial [PoM] £750.00 DT = £750.00

2   Post-exposure prophylaxis

Botulism antitoxin

12-Jan-2021

Overview

Botulism antitoxin p. 1470 (botulinum antitoxin) [unlicensed] is a polyvalent preparation that contains equine-derived immune globulins against multiple *Clostridium botulinum* serotypes. It is used for the treatment of suspected cases of botulism, such as foodborne (pre-formed toxins ingested from contaminated food) and wound botulism (associated with parenteral drug abuse). Human-derived botulism immune globulin [unlicensed] is used for

the treatment of infant botulism as part of the Infant Botulism Treatment and Prevention Program. In infant botulism, neurotoxins are formed in the large intestine after ingestion of *Clostridium botulinum* spores, which are harmless to older children and adults.

Botulism is a notifiable disease in the UK, especially foodborne botulism, which is considered a public health emergency as contaminated food may be available to other individuals. For further information on reporting of suspected cases, see *Notifiable diseases* in Antibacterials, principles of therapy p. 573.

All cases of suspected botulism should be managed promptly—treatment should not be delayed while awaiting laboratory diagnosis. Supportive care (including artificial ventilation) and symptomatic treatment may also be necessary.

For individuals with wound botulism, surgical debridement and antibacterial therapy are recommended in addition to botulism antitoxin, to help reduce the organism load and toxin production.

For further information on the management of infant, foodborne and wound botulism, see Public Health England guidance: **Botulism: clinical and public health management** (see *Useful resources*).

Useful Resources

Recommendations reflect Botulism: clinical and public health management. Public Health England, December 2018. www.gov.uk/government/publications/botulism-clinical-and-public-health-management

IMMUNE SERA AND IMMUNOGLOBULINS ›
ANTITOXINS

Bezlotoxumab

18-Aug-2017

- **DRUG ACTION** Bezlotoxumab is a human monoclonal antitoxin antibody; it binds to *Clostridioides difficile* toxin B and neutralises its activity, preventing recurrence of *Clostridioides difficile* infection.

- **INDICATIONS AND DOSE**
  Prevention of recurrence of *Clostridioides difficile* infection in patients at high risk of reinfection
  ▸ BY INTRAVENOUS INFUSION
  ▸ Adult: 10 mg/kg for 1 dose, to be administered during the course of antibacterial therapy for *Clostridioides difficile* infection

- **SIDE-EFFECTS**
  ▸ **Common or very common** Fever · headache · infusion related reaction · nausea
  ▸ **Frequency not known** Dizziness · dyspnoea · fatigue · hypertension

- **PREGNANCY** Manufacturer advises avoid unless essential—limited information available.

- **BREAST FEEDING** Manufacturer advises avoid—no information available.

- **DIRECTIONS FOR ADMINISTRATION** Manufacturer advises for *intravenous infusion* (*Zinplava*®), give intermittently in Glucose 5 % *or* Sodium Chloride 0.9 %; dilute requisite dose to a concentration of 1–10 mg/mL with infusion fluid; give over 60 minutes via a central venous catheter or peripheral catheter using a low-protein binding filter (0.2–5 micron).

- **HANDLING AND STORAGE** Manufacturer advises store in a refrigerator (2–8 °C)—consult product literature for further information regarding storage conditions outside refrigerator and after preparation of the infusion.

- **MEDICINAL FORMS** No licensed medicines listed.

Botulism antitoxin

13-May-2021

● INDICATIONS AND DOSE
Treatment of botulism [suspected or confirmed]
▸ BY INTRAVENOUS INFUSION
▸ Adult: (consult product literature)

● **SIDE-EFFECTS** Hypersensitivity

SIDE-EFFECTS, FURTHER INFORMATION It is essential to read the contra-indications, warnings, and details of sensitivity tests on the package insert. Prior to treatment checks should be made regarding previous administration of any antitoxin and history of any allergic condition, e.g. asthma, hay fever, etc.

● **PRE-TREATMENT SCREENING** All patients should be tested for sensitivity (diluting the antitoxin if history of allergy).

● **PRESCRIBING AND DISPENSING INFORMATION** Available from designated centres after discussion with the on-call duty doctor at Colindale, Public Health England (during and outside of working hours) for risk assessment and further advice on treatment (Tel: (020) 8200 4400).
　For non-urgent queries, contact Botulism@phe.gov.uk.

● **MEDICINAL FORMS** No licensed medicines listed.

Diphtheria antitoxin

10-Nov-2023

(Dip/Ser)

● INDICATIONS AND DOSE
Treatment of diphtheria [confirmed or probable]
▸ BY INTRAVENOUS INFUSION
▸ Adult: Dose should be given without waiting for bacteriological confirmation (consult local protocol)

● **CAUTIONS**
▸ Hypersensitivity Hypersensitivity is common after administration; resuscitation facilities should be available.
　Diphtheria antitoxin is no longer used for prophylaxis because of the risk of hypersensitivity; unimmunised contacts should be promptly investigated and given antibacterial prophylaxis and vaccine.

● **SIDE-EFFECTS**
▸ **Common or very common** Hypersensitivity

● **PRE-TREATMENT SCREENING** Diphtheria antitoxin is derived from horse serum and reactions are common. Public Health England advises hypersensitivity testing should be carried out before use in certain individuals (e.g. those who have a positive history of animal allergy, or prior exposure to equine-derived immunoglobulin).

● **PRESCRIBING AND DISPENSING INFORMATION** Available from designated centres after discussion with the Duty Doctor at Colindale, Public Health England (during and outside of working hours) for risk assessment and further advice on treatment (Tel: (020) 8200 4400). In Northern Ireland, available from Public Health Laboratory, Belfast City Hospital (Tel (028) 9032 9241).

● **MEDICINAL FORMS** There can be variation in the licensing of different medicines containing the same drug.
Solution for injection
▸ Diphtheria antitoxin (Non-proprietary)
　Diphtheria antitoxin 1000 unit per 1 ml Antidiphtheria serum 10,000units/10ml solution for injection ampoules | 1 ampoule PoM ⚠ (Hospital only)

3　Tuberculosis diagnostic test

DIAGNOSTIC AGENTS

Tuberculin purified protein derivative
(Tuberculin PPD)

● INDICATIONS AND DOSE
Mantoux test
▸ BY INTRADERMAL INJECTION
▸ Child: 2 units for one dose
▸ Adult: 2 units for one dose

Mantoux test (if first test is negative and a further test is considered appropriate)
▸ BY INTRADERMAL INJECTION
▸ Child: 10 units for 1 dose
▸ Adult: 10 units for 1 dose

DOSE EQUIVALENCE AND CONVERSION
▸ 2 units is equivalent to 0.1 mL of 20 units/mL strength.
▸ 10 units is equivalent to 0.1 mL of 100 units/mL strength.

● **CAUTIONS**
▸ Mantoux test Response to tuberculin may be suppressed by viral infection, sarcoidosis, corticosteroid therapy, or immunosuppression due to disease or treatment and the MMR vaccine. If a tuberculin skin test has already been initiated, then the MMR should be delayed until the skin test has been read unless protection against measles is required urgently. If a child has had a recent MMR, and requires a tuberculin test, then a 4 week interval should be observed. Apart from tuberculin and MMR, all other live vaccines can be administered at any time before or after tuberculin.

● **PRESCRIBING AND DISPENSING INFORMATION** Available from ImmForm (SSI brand).
　The strength of tuberculin PPD in currently available products may be different to the strengths of products used previously for the Mantoux test; care is required to select the correct strength.

● **MEDICINAL FORMS** There can be variation in the licensing of different medicines containing the same drug. Forms available from special-order manufacturers include: solution for injection
Solution for injection
▸ Tuberculin purified protein derivative (Non-proprietary)
　Tuberculin purified protein derivative 20 tuberculin unit per 1 ml Tuberculin PPD RT 23 SSI 20 tuberculin units/ml solution for injection 1.5ml vials | 1 vial ⚠
　Tuberculin purified protein derivative 100 tuberculin unit per 1 ml Tuberculin PPD RT 23 SSI 100 tuberculin units/ml solution for injection 1.5ml vials | 1 vial ⚠

4　Vaccination

Vaccination, general principles

21-Dec-2023

Active immunity

Active immunity can be acquired by natural disease or by vaccination. Vaccines induce active immunity and provide immunological memory by stimulating the production of antibodies and cells involved in the immune response. As a result, the immune system is able to recognise and respond rapidly to natural infection at a later date. Antibodies can be detected in the patient's blood or serum, but even in the absence of detectable antibodies, immunological memory may still be present. Vaccines consist of either:

- a *live attenuated replicating* form of the virus (e.g. measles, mumps and rubella vaccine) or bacteria (e.g. Bacillus Calmette-Guérin vaccine);
- a *live attenuated non-replicating* form of the virus (e.g. smallpox and mpox vaccine);
- *inactivated* preparations of the virus (e.g. tick-borne encephalitis vaccine) or bacteria (e.g. meningococcal vaccine);
- *inactivated toxins (toxoids)* produced by a micro-organism (e.g. tetanus and diphtheria vaccines);
- *extracts of* a micro-organism which may be derived from the organism (e.g. pneumococcal vaccine), or produced by recombinant DNA technology (e.g. hepatitis B vaccine);
- *viral vectors of* replicating (attenuated or low pathogenicity viruses) or non-replicating viruses (e.g. *Vaxzevria*® COVID-19 vaccine), produced using recombinant technology; or
- *nucleic acid (DNA or RNA) of* an antigen derived from the virus (e.g. *Comirnaty*® or *Spikevax*® COVID-19 vaccines) or bacteria.

Live attenuated replicating viral vaccines and replicating viral vector vaccines usually promote a full, long-lasting antibody response. In rare cases, a mild form of the disease may occur with some vaccines, such as a rash following a measles-containing vaccine.

Inactivated or non-replicating vaccines (including toxoids and non-live vaccines) produce an antibody response following a primary course, which may last for months or years. In most cases booster (reinforcing) injections are required for long-term protection. To stimulate the immune system more broadly, some polysaccharide vaccines have been enhanced by conjugation (such as the *Haemophilus influenzae* type B and meningococcal group C vaccines), while some inactivated vaccines contain an adjuvant (such as aluminium hydroxide or aluminium phosphate) to enhance the antibody response. Inactivated and non-replicating vaccines cannot cause the disease that they are designed to prevent.

For further information on how vaccines are made and what they contain, see Chapter 1, Immunity and how vaccines work, in *Immunisation against infectious disease-* 'The Green Book' (see *Useful resources*).

Passive immunity

Passive immunity is acquired through the transfer of antibodies from immune individuals either across the placenta, or from the transfusion of blood or blood products including immunoglobulins (for further information, see Immunoglobulins p. 1462). Protection provided by the cross-placental transfer of antibodies provides the infant with temporary protection (commonly for a few weeks to months), and is more effective against some infections (e.g. tetanus and measles) than others (e.g. polio and pertussis).

Vaccination during pregnancy and breast-feeding

Live replicating vaccines should not be administered routinely to pregnant females due to the theoretical risk of fetal infection; these should generally be delayed until after delivery. The Immunisation and Vaccine Preventable Diseases Division at the UK Health Security Agency (UKHSA) run a UK-wide surveillance programme on the safety of certain vaccines (measles, mumps, rubella, varicella-zoster, and human papillomavirus) given inadvertently during pregnancy or shortly before conception. For advice on the reporting, risk assessment, and management of inadvertent vaccination in pregnancy, see UKHSA guidance: **Inadvertent vaccination in pregnancy (VIP)** (available at: www.gov.uk/guidance/vaccination-in-pregnancy-vip).

There is no evidence of risk from vaccinating pregnant females with inactivated viral or bacterial vaccines, or toxoids; they do not replicate so cannot harm the fetus. Some inactivated vaccines are actively recommended to prevent severe complications during pregnancy or to the new-born infant, such as the influenza vaccine, and diphtheria with tetanus, pertussis and poliomyelitis vaccine.

There is no evidence of risk from vaccinating females who are breast-feeding with inactivated viral or bacterial vaccines, or toxoids.

For further information on vaccination in pregnancy and breast-feeding, see individual vaccine treatment summaries.

Vaccines in immunosuppression and HIV infection

Almost all individuals can be safely vaccinated; in only a few individuals is vaccination either contra-indicated or should be deferred. Specialist advice should be sought when in doubt, if using live vaccines, or if there are queries about an individual's degree of immunosuppression. In some situations, the specialist may decide that the risk of a specific disease outweighs any potential risk from the vaccine. Antibody responses may be lower in immunosuppressed individuals, therefore additional vaccine doses may be required.

Live replicating vaccines can cause severe or fatal infections in some immunosuppressed individuals due to extensive replication of the vaccine strain. Live replicating vaccines are therefore not recommended for individuals with some types of severe primary or acquired immunodeficiency, or for those who are on or have recently received high doses of certain immunosuppressive or biological therapies.

Inactivated vaccines cannot replicate so may be given to immunosuppressed individuals.

Wherever possible, immunisation or additional booster doses for individuals with immunosuppression, should be carried out either before immunosuppression occurs or deferred until an improvement in immunity has been seen. The optimal timing for any vaccination should be based upon a judgement about the relative need for rapid protection and the likely response. For infants born to females taking immunosuppressive biological therapy during pregnancy, live replicating vaccines should be delayed by 6 months; therefore, the infant will not be eligible to receive the rotavirus vaccine, and if indicated, will need to have their Bacillus Calmette-Guérin vaccine deferred.

Most live vaccines used in the UK immunisation schedule can be safely given to close contacts of an immunosuppressed individual. They carry a low risk of transmission (or the risk can be minimised with simple precautions) from a recently vaccinated close contact to an immunosuppressed individual. Close contacts of immunosuppressed individuals should be fully immunised according to the national Immunisation schedule p. 1472 to reduce the risk of exposure to vaccine preventable conditions, and they should also be offered the annual Influenza vaccine p. 1484.

For further information on vaccines in immunosuppression, see Chapter 6, Contra-indications and special considerations, and Chapter 7, Immunisation of individuals with underlying medical conditions in *Immunisation against infectious disease-* 'The Green Book' (see *Useful resources*).

For further information on vaccines for individuals with HIV infection, see the British HIV Association guideline: **Use of vaccines in HIV-positive adults** (available at: www.bhiva.org/vaccination-guidelines), or the Children's HIV Association guidelines: **Vaccination of HIV infected children** and **Preparing HIV-infected children and adolescents for travel** (available at: www.chiva.org.uk).

Vaccines and asplenia, splenic dysfunction, or complement disorders

The following vaccines are recommended for individuals with asplenia, splenic dysfunction, or complement disorders (including those taking complement inhibitors) depending on the age at which their condition is diagnosed:

- Influenza vaccine (inactivated) p. 1508 or influenza vaccine (live) p. 1515;
- Meningococcal groups A with C and W135 and Y vaccine p. 1510 (MenACWY) and meningococcal group B vaccine (rDNA, component, adsorbed) p. 1509 (4CMenB);
- 13-valent or 15-valent pneumococcal polysaccharide conjugate vaccine (adsorbed) p. 1510 (PCV13 or PCV15) and/or 23-valent pneumococcal polysaccharide vaccine p. 1511 (PPV23). Patients on complement inhibitor therapy with eculizumab are not at increased risk of pneumococcal disease and do not require PPV23 or additional doses of PCV13 or PCV15.

Additional booster doses of other vaccines should be considered depending on the individual's underlying condition—specialist advice may be required. For information on specific indications for immunisation of vulnerable groups, see Chapter 7, Immunisation of individuals with underlying medical conditions, in *Immunisation against infectious disease*- 'The Green Book' (see *Useful resources*).

Children first diagnosed or presenting aged under 1 year should be immunised according to the Immunisation schedule below. During their first year they should also be given 2 doses of MenACWY at least 4 weeks apart, and a dose of PCV13 or PCV15 (in order to have received a total of 2 doses of PCV13 or PCV15 with an 8 week interval). 8 weeks following their routine 1 year booster vaccines, they should receive a booster dose of MenACWY. An additional dose of PCV13 or PCV15 should be given at least 8 weeks after the routine PCV13 or PCV15 booster scheduled at 1 year. After their second birthday, a dose of PPV23 should be given at least 8 weeks after the last dose of PCV13 or PCV15. The influenza vaccine should be given annually in children aged 6 months or older.

Children first diagnosed or presenting aged 1 year to under 2 years should be immunised according to the Immunisation schedule below, including any routine vaccines due at 1 year of age if not yet administered. 8 weeks following the routine 1 year booster vaccines a dose of MenACWY should be given. An additional dose of PCV13 or PCV15 should be given at least 8 weeks after the 1 year booster dose of PCV13 or PCV15. After their second birthday, a dose of PPV23 should be given at least 8 weeks after the last dose of PCV13 or PCV15. The influenza vaccine should be given annually.

Children first diagnosed or presenting aged 2 years to under 10 years should be immunised according to the Immunisation schedule below. Additionally, they should be given a dose of MenACWY and PPV23. For children who have not received the full routine immunisation for 4CMenB, ensure that 2 doses, 8 weeks apart have been given since their first birthday. For children who have not received any PCV13 or PCV15 previously, a single dose should be given, followed by a dose of PPV23 at least 8 weeks later. The influenza vaccine should be given annually.

Individuals first diagnosed aged 10 years and over regardless of previous immunisations, should be given a dose of PPV23, 4CMenB, and MenACWY. After 4 weeks, an additional dose of 4CMenB should be given. The influenza vaccine should be given annually. The PPV23 is not required if a dose has already been received within the previous 2 years, due to a theoretical risk of pneumococcal serotype-specific hypo-responsiveness with re-vaccination.

Vaccines and antitoxins availability

For information on availability of vaccines and antitoxins, see individual monographs.

For antivenom, see Poisoning, emergency treatment p. 1554.

Enquiries for vaccines not available commercially can also be made to:

Vaccines and Countermeasures Response Department
Public Health England
vaccinesupply@phe.gov.uk

In Northern Ireland, enquiries for vaccines not available commercially should be directed to Northern Health and Social Care Trust's Pharmacy Services (www.northerntrust. hscni.net/services/pharmaceutical-services/).

In Scotland, information about availability of vaccines can be obtained from a Specialist in Pharmaceutical Public Health.

In Wales, enquiries for vaccines not available commercially should be directed to the Welsh Medicines Information Centre (www.wmic.wales.nhs.uk/about/contactus/).

Useful Resources

Recommendations reflect advice from *Immunisation against infectious disease*- 'The Green Book'. UK Health Security Agency, 2013. Chapters from the handbook (including updates since 2013) are available at:
www.gov.uk/government/collections/immunisation-against-infectious-disease-the-green-book

Immunisation schedule

22-Jan-2025

Routine immunisations, sources of information

The following recommendations reflect advice from UKHSA. Recommendations specific to each vaccine can be found in *Immunisation against infectious disease*– 'The Green Book'. UKHSA at: www.gov.uk/government/collections/immunisation-against-infectious-disease-the-green-book.

The immunisation schedule reflects advice from 'The complete routine immunisation schedule' produced by UKHSA (2024). For the most up to date immunisation schedule, see: www.gov.uk/government/publications/the-complete-routine-immunisation-schedule.

The Influenza immunisation recommendations reflect advice from the 'National flu immunisation programme plan 2024/2025' produced by UKHSA, Department of Health and Social Care, and NHS England. For the most up to date letter, see: www.gov.uk/government/publications/national-flu-immunisation-programme-plan-2024-to-2025.

Vaccines for the immunisation schedule should be obtained from ImmForm at: portal.immform.ukhsa.gov.uk.

Preterm birth

Babies born preterm should receive all routine immunisations based on their actual date of birth. The risk of apnoea following vaccination is increased in preterm babies, particularly in those born at or before 28 weeks gestational age. If babies at risk of apnoea are in hospital at the time of their first immunisation, they should be monitored for respiratory complications for 48–72 hours after immunisation. If a baby develops apnoea, bradycardia, or desaturation after the first immunisation, the second immunisation should also be given in hospital with similar monitoring.

Individuals with unknown or incomplete immunisation history

For children born in the UK who present with an inadequate or unknown immunisation history, investigation into immunisations received should be carried out. Outstanding doses should be administered where the routine childhood immunisation schedule has not been completed.

For advice on dosing schedules for missed vaccinations, and the immunisation of individuals coming to the UK, consult Chapter 11, The UK immunisation schedule, in *Immunisation against infectious disease*– 'The Green Book'. UKHSA, available at: www.gov.uk/government/publications/immunisation-schedule-the-green-book-chapter-11, and UKHSA guidance: **Vaccination of individuals with uncertain or incomplete immunisation status**, available at: www.gov.uk/government/publications/vaccination-of-individuals-with-uncertain-or-incomplete-immunisation-status.

Immunisations for healthcare and laboratory staff

Vaccine-preventable diseases that can be transmitted from person to person are a risk for staff and patients in healthcare environments, and staff in laboratory environments. Therefore, all staff must be up-to-date with their routine immunisations. In addition, specific immunisations are recommended for certain staff groups due to the risk of acquiring or passing on infection. For

Routine immunisation schedule

When to immunise	Vaccine given and dose schedule (for details of dose, see under individual vaccines)
Neonates at risk only	▶ Bacillus Calmette-Guérin vaccine p. 1514 (around 4 weeks). Check severe combined immunodeficiency (SCID) screening outcome before giving, see Bacillus Calmette-Guérin vaccine p. 1474. ▶ Hepatitis B vaccine p. 1505 (at birth, 4 weeks, and 1 year, see Hepatitis B vaccine p. 1481).
8 weeks	▶ Diphtheria with tetanus, pertussis, hepatitis B, poliomyelitis and haemophilus influenzae type b vaccine p. 1502 (*Infanrix hexa*® or *Vaxelis*®). First dose. ▶ Meningococcal group B vaccine (rDNA, component, adsorbed) p. 1509 (*Bexsero*®). First dose. ▶ Rotavirus vaccine p. 1517 (*Rotarix*®). Check SCID screening outcome before giving. First dose.
12 weeks	▶ Diphtheria with tetanus, pertussis, hepatitis B, poliomyelitis and haemophilus influenzae type b vaccine (*Infanrix hexa*® or *Vaxelis*®). Second dose. ▶ Pneumococcal polysaccharide conjugate vaccine (adsorbed) p. 1510 (*Prevenar 13*® or *Vaxneuvance*®). Single dose. ▶ Rotavirus vaccine (*Rotarix*®). Check SCID screening outcome before giving. Second dose.
16 weeks	▶ Diphtheria with tetanus, pertussis, hepatitis B, poliomyelitis and haemophilus influenzae type b vaccine (*Infanrix hexa*® or *Vaxelis*®). Third dose. ▶ Meningococcal group B vaccine (rDNA, component, adsorbed) (*Bexsero*®). Second dose.
1 year (on or after first birthday)	▶ Measles, mumps and rubella vaccine p. 1516 (*MMR VaxPRO*® or *Priorix*®). First dose. ▶ Meningococcal group B vaccine (rDNA, component, adsorbed) (*Bexsero*®). Single booster dose. ▶ Pneumococcal polysaccharide conjugate vaccine (adsorbed) (*Prevenar 13*® or *Vaxneuvance*®). Single booster dose. ▶ Haemophilus influenzae type b with meningococcal group C vaccine p. 1503 (*Menitorix*®). Single booster dose.
2-3 years on 31st August 2024, primary school-aged children from reception to year 6, and secondary school-aged children in years 7-11	▶ Influenza vaccine (live) p. 1515. Each year from September. **Note:** live attenuated influenza nasal spray is recommended (*Fluenz*®); if contra-indicated or unsuitable, see Influenza vaccine p. 1484.
3 years and 4 months, or soon after	▶ Diphtheria with tetanus, pertussis and poliomyelitis vaccine p. 1502 (*Repevax*®). Single booster dose. ▶ Measles, mumps and rubella vaccine (*MMR VaxPRO*® or *Priorix*®). Second dose.
11-14 years. HPV vaccine will be offered to individuals aged 12-13 years in England and Wales, those aged 12-14 years in Northern Ireland, and those aged 11-13 years in Scotland.	▶ Human papillomavirus vaccine p. 1508 (*Gardasil*®*9*). 1 dose schedule. For individuals with immunosuppression or HIV infection, see Human papillomavirus vaccine p. 1483.
13-15 years	▶ Meningococcal groups A with C and W135 and Y vaccine p. 1510 (*MenQuadfi*®). Single dose.
13-18 years	▶ Diphtheria with tetanus and poliomyelitis vaccine p. 1501 (*Revaxis*®). Single booster dose. **Note:** Can be given at the same time as the dose of meningococcal groups A with C and W135 and Y vaccine at 13-15 years of age.
Females of child-bearing age susceptible to rubella	▶ Measles, mumps and rubella vaccine. Females of child-bearing age who have not received 2 doses of a rubella-containing vaccine or who do not have a positive antibody test for rubella should be offered rubella immunisation (using the MMR vaccine)—exclude pregnancy before immunisation, and avoid pregnancy for one month after vaccination.
Pregnant females	▶ Acellular pertussis-containing vaccine administered as diphtheria with tetanus and pertussis vaccine p. 1501 (*Adacel*®). 1 dose from the 16th week of pregnancy, usually around the time of the fetal anomaly scan (week 20). ▶ Influenza vaccine (inactivated) p. 1508. Single dose administered from September, regardless of the stage of pregnancy. For vaccine choice, see Influenza vaccine p. 1484.

Routine immunisations during adult life

For routine immunisations in pregnancy, see *Routine immunisation schedule*.

When to immunise	Vaccine given and dose schedule (for details of dose, see under individual vaccines)
Under 25 years, first time entrants to further or higher education	▸ Meningococcal groups A with C and W135 and Y vaccine (*Nimenrix*®, *MenQuadfi*®, or *Menveo*®). Single dose. **Note:** Should be offered to those aged under 25 years entering further or higher education who have not received the meningococcal groups A with C and W135 and Y vaccine over the age of 10 years.
During adult life, if not previously immunised or 5 dose course is incomplete	▸ Diphtheria with tetanus and poliomyelitis vaccine.
From 65 years	▸ Influenza vaccine (inactivated). Each year from October. For vaccine choice, see Influenza vaccine p. 1484.
65 years	▸ Pneumococcal polysaccharide vaccine p. 1511.
Individuals aged 65 years and 70-79 years	▸ Herpes-zoster vaccine. For guidance on immunisation and choice of vaccine, see Varicella-zoster vaccines p. 1495.

detailed recommendations, consult Chapter 12, Immunisation of healthcare and laboratory staff in *Immunisation against infectious disease*– 'The Green Book'. UKHSA, available at: www.gov.uk/government/publications/immunisation-of-healthcare-and-laboratory-staff-the-green-book-chapter-12.

Anthrax vaccine

04-May-2021

Overview

Anthrax vaccine p. 1499 is made from antigens from inactivated *Bacillus anthracis* adsorbed onto an adjuvant. Anthrax immunisation is indicated for individuals who handle infected animals or process infected animal products where there is a potential risk of occupational exposure to *B. anthracis*. It is also recommended for occupations where workers are at risk of one-off high level exposures to anthrax (e.g. following a deliberate or accidental release of spores).

A 4-dose regimen is used for primary immunisation; a single booster dose should be given at 10-year intervals on up to 3 occasions to workers at potential continuous low level risk of exposure to anthrax. In those with potential intermittent high level exposure, a single booster dose should be offered just before entering situations with a specific high exposure risk. If such opportunities do not arise, a single booster dose should be given at 10-year intervals on up to 3 occasions to sustain protection.

In the event of proven or high probability of exposure to anthrax spores, a single booster dose should be given, in addition to antibacterial prophylaxis, except when a dose has been given in the preceding 12 months.

Advice on the treatment of previously unvaccinated individuals with a proven or high probability of exposure to anthrax spores can be found at: www.gov.uk/government/publications/chemical-biological-radiological-and-nuclear-incidents-recognise-and-respond.

Anthrax is a notifiable disease in the UK. For further information, see *Notifiable diseases* in Antibacterials, principles of therapy p. 573.

Useful Resources

Recommendations reflect Chapter 13, Anthrax, in *Immunisation against infectious disease*– 'The Green Book'. Public Health England. February 2017. www.gov.uk/government/publications/anthrax-the-green-book-chapter-13

Bacillus Calmette-Guérin vaccine

08-Oct-2021

Overview

The Bacillus Calmette-Guérin vaccine p. 1514 (BCG vaccine) contains a live attenuated strain derived from *Mycobacterium bovis* and is indicated for the prevention of Tuberculosis p. 670.

BCG immunisation is recommended for the following individuals if immunisation has not previously been carried out and they are tuberculin-negative:

- all neonates and infants (aged 0–12 months) living in areas of the UK where the annual incidence of tuberculosis is 40 cases per 100 000 or greater;
- all neonates and infants (aged 0–12 months) with a parent or grandparent born in a country where the annual incidence of tuberculosis is 40 cases per 100 000 or greater;
- previously unvaccinated children (aged 1–5 years) with a parent or grandparent born in a country where the annual incidence of tuberculosis is 40 cases per 100 000 or greater (tuberculin testing is not usually required);
- previously unvaccinated children (aged 6–15 years) with a parent or grandparent born in a country where the annual incidence of tuberculosis is 40 cases per 100 000 or greater;
- previously unvaccinated children (aged under 16 years) with close contact to cases of sputum smear-positive pulmonary or laryngeal tuberculosis;
- previously unvaccinated children (aged under 16 years) who were born in, or lived for at least 3 months in a country where the annual incidence of tuberculosis is 40 cases per 100 000 or greater;
- previously unvaccinated individuals at occupational risk (irrespective of age). This includes healthcare workers or laboratory staff who have direct contact with patients with tuberculosis or potentially infectious clinical materials, and veterinary and abattoir staff handling animals or animal materials that could be infected with tuberculosis. BCG vaccination can also be considered for staff working with prisoners, homeless people, people with drug and alcohol misuse, and those who work with refugees and asylum seekers.

As part of the neonatal BCG immunisation programme, immunisation is recommended for eligible neonates at 28 days of age (or soon after), to ensure that the result of the severe combined immunodeficiency (SCID) screening is available and checked prior to it being given. Vaccination may be given earlier than 28 days of age, provided that the SCID screening result is available. For further information, see UKHSA guidance: **Changing the timing of the neonatal BCG immunisation programme to a 28 day immunisation programme: effective from 1 September 2021** (see *Useful resources*).

Although protection provided by BCG vaccine may decrease with time, there is no evidence that repeat vaccination offers significant additional protection and therefore repeat BCG vaccination is not recommended.

The Bacillus Calmette-Guérin vaccine is contra-indicated in all HIV-infected individuals. For advice on BCG vaccination in immunosuppressed individuals, consult Chapter 32: Tuberculosis - 'The Green Book', Public Health England (see *Useful resources*).

For advice on drug treatment, see Tuberculosis p. 670; for the treatment of infection following vaccination, seek expert advice.

Travel

The risk of a traveller acquiring tuberculosis infection depends on several factors including the incidence of tuberculosis in that country, the duration of travel, the degree of contact with the local population, the work setting of the traveller (if any), the reason for travel, and the susceptibility and age of the traveller.

BCG vaccine is recommended for previously unvaccinated, tuberculin-negative individuals aged under 16 years, or for healthcare workers at high risk of exposure to patients with tuberculosis, who intend to travel for 3 months or more in a country where the annual incidence of tuberculosis is 40 cases per 100 000 or greater, or where the risk of multi-drug resistant tuberculosis is high. The risk of tourists acquiring tuberculosis infection is low and BCG vaccine is not required if no other factors are present.

A list of countries where the annual incidence of tuberculosis is 40 cases per 100 000 or greater, is available at www.gov.uk/government/publications/tuberculosis-tb-by-country-rates-per-100000-people.

Tuberculin skin testing

The tuberculin skin test (*Mantoux test*) is used to assess an individual's sensitivity to tuberculin protein when BCG vaccination is being considered or as an aid to diagnosis of tuberculosis. A tuberculin skin test involves administration of tuberculin purified protein derivative p. 1470 by intradermal injection. It is necessary before BCG vaccination for:

- individuals aged 6 years and over;
- children aged under 6 years living in a country for more than 3 months with an annual tuberculosis incidence of 40 cases per 100 000 or greater;
- those who have had close contact with a person with known tuberculosis;
- those who have a family history of tuberculosis within the last 5 years.

BCG vaccination can be given up to three months following a negative tuberculin test.

The BCG vaccine should not be administered to an individual with a positive tuberculin test—it is unnecessary and may cause a more severe local reaction. Those with a *Mantoux test* induration of 5 mm and greater should be referred to a tuberculosis clinic for assessment of the need for further investigation and treatment.

Tuberculosis is a notifiable disease in the UK. For further information, see *Notifiable diseases* in Antibacterials, principles of therapy p. 573.

Useful Resources

Recommendations reflect Chapter 32, Tuberculosis, in *Immunisation against infectious disease*– 'The Green Book'. Public Health England, August 2018.
www.gov.uk/government/publications/tuberculosis-the-green-book-chapter-32

Changing the timing of the neonatal BCG immunisation programme to a 28 day immunisation programme: effective from 1 September 2021. UK Health Security Agency. October 2021.

www.gov.uk/government/publications/bcg-vaccine-information-on-the-28-day-immunisation-programme

---

Cholera vaccines   08-Aug-2024

Overview

Oral cholera vaccine (inactivated) p. 1499 contains inactivated Inaba (including El-Tor biotype) and Ogawa strains of *Vibrio cholerae* serotype O1, together with recombinant B-subunit of the cholera toxin produced in Inaba strains of *V. cholerae* serotype O1.

Oral cholera vaccine (live) p. 1515 contains live attenuated *V. cholerae* serotype O1 classical Inaba strain CVD 103-HgR produced by recombinant DNA technology.

Immunisation with either the inactivated or live vaccine (as appropriate) may be indicated for adults and children from 2 years of age who are travelling to endemic or epidemic areas on the basis of current recommendations; immunisation however is not a condition for entry into any country. Following a full risk assessment, immunisation can be considered for the following individuals:

- relief or disaster aid workers;
- persons with remote itineraries in areas where cholera epidemics are occurring and there is limited access to medical care;
- travellers to potential cholera risk areas, for whom vaccination is considered potentially beneficial;
- individuals at occupational risk, such as laboratory workers who may be regularly exposed to cholera.

Immunisation with the inactivated vaccine should be completed at least one week prior to potential exposure; re-immunisation or a booster dose may be required to provide continuous protection. Immunisation with the live vaccine should be completed at least 10 days prior to potential exposure; there are no data available on re-immunisation intervals. The live vaccine should not be used in certain individuals such as those with immunosuppression, for further information, see Chapter 14, Cholera, in *Immunisation against infectious diseases*- 'The Green Book' (see *Useful resources*). Protection from immunisation with cholera vaccines may be reduced in those living with HIV infection.

For dosing schedules, see cholera vaccine (inactivated) and cholera vaccine (live).

Immunisation with either vaccine does not provide complete protection and all travellers to a country where cholera exists should be warned that scrupulous attention to food, water, and personal hygiene is essential.

Cholera is a notifiable disease in the UK. For further information, see *Notifiable diseases* in Antibacterials, principles of therapy p. 573.

Contacts

Contacts of patients with cholera should maintain high standards of personal hygiene to avoid becoming infected. Cholera vaccines should not be used in the management of contacts of cases or in controlling the spread of infection.

There is a potential for transmission of the cholera vaccine (live) strain to unvaccinated close contacts caused by shedding in the stools.

Useful Resources

Recommendations reflect Chapter 14, Cholera, in *Immunisation against infectious disease*– 'The Green Book'. UK Health Security Agency. August 2024.
www.gov.uk/government/publications/cholera-the-green-book-chapter-14

COVID-19 vaccines

03-Apr-2023

Overview

Since the COVID-19 vaccination programme was initiated in December 2020, the majority of adults in the UK have been vaccinated, and most of the adult and child population have also been naturally infected. Vaccination against COVID-19 provides modest but short-term protection (lasting a few months) against infection and mild symptomatic disease, and transmission, however protection against severe disease and death appears to be greater and maintained over the medium term. The aim of the longer-term COVID-19 vaccination programme is therefore to reduce mortality and hospitalisation due to COVID-19 by providing ongoing protection for individuals considered to be at the highest risk of severe disease.

There are several COVID-19 vaccines authorised for use in the UK—the messenger RNA (mRNA) monovalent vaccines, *Comirnaty*® (Pfizer/BioNTech) and *Spikevax*® (Moderna); the mRNA bivalent vaccines, *Comirnaty*® Original/Omicron BA.1 and *Comirnaty*® Original/Omicron BA.4/5, and *Spikevax*® Original/Omicron BA.1 and *Spikevax*® Original/Omicron BA.4/5; the adenovirus vector monovalent vaccines, *Vaxzevria*® (AstraZeneca) and COVID-19 vaccine Janssen (Janssen-Cilag); and the recombinant, adjuvanted protein-based monovalent vaccines, *Nuvaxovid*® (Novavax) and *VidPrevtyn Beta*® (Sanofi Pasteur). The COVID-19 vaccine Janssen, *Nuvaxovid*®, and *Vaxzevria*® vaccines are currently not being supplied routinely in the UK, but *Nuvaxovid*® is available at specific vaccination centres.

There have been reports of a rare condition involving serious thromboembolic events with thrombocytopenia following vaccination with the COVID-19 vaccine Janssen and *Vaxzevria*® vaccines. This condition, known as vaccine-induced immune thrombocytopenia and thrombosis (VITT), is a syndrome that develops within 5 to 30 days of receiving vaccination. For further information on blood clotting following COVID-19 vaccination, see UKHSA guidance: **Information for healthcare professionals on blood clotting following COVID-19 vaccination** (available at: www.gov.uk/government/publications/covid-19-vaccination-blood-clotting-information-for-healthcare-professionals/information-for-healthcare-professionals-on-blood-clotting-following-covid-19-vaccination), and for guidance on the diagnosis and management of VITT, see NICE rapid guideline: **Vaccine-induced immune thrombocytopenia and thrombosis** (available at: www.nice.org.uk/guidance/ng200).

For guidance on inadvertent COVID-19 vaccine administration errors, and completing vaccination in individuals who received vaccine doses abroad, see UKHSA: **COVID-19 vaccination programme: Information for healthcare practitioners** (see *Useful resources*).

In individuals with confirmed COVID-19 infection, vaccination should ideally be deferred until clinical recovery. However, during care-home outbreaks, residents with confirmed COVID-19 infection may receive the vaccine provided they are clinically stable. In patients with prolonged COVID-19 symptoms, consider deferring the vaccine if the patient is seriously debilitated, under active investigation or has recently deteriorated, to avoid incorrect attribution of any change in symptoms to the vaccine.

COVID-19 vaccines are an area of ongoing research and recommendations may change as more data and other vaccines become available. For further information on the COVID-19 vaccination programme, see the UKHSA collection (available at: www.gov.uk/government/collections/covid-19-vaccination-programme).

Primary immunisation

All adults, and children who were aged 5 years and over on or before 31st August 2022, are eligible for a primary vaccination course. Children who reached the age of 5 years on or after 1st September 2022 are only eligible for vaccination if they are in a clinical at-risk group or are a household contact of an immunosuppressed individual. From spring 2023, children aged 6 months to 4 years are also eligible for a primary vaccination course if they are in a clinical at-risk group. For information on clinical at-risk groups, see Chapter 14a: COVID-19 - SARS-CoV-2, in *Immunisation against infectious disease*- 'The Green Book' (see *Useful resources*).

Most eligible individuals should receive 2 doses of COVID-19 vaccine p. 1500 for their primary course; 3 doses are required for individuals aged 6 months and over who were severely immunosuppressed at the time of their vaccination. For further information on vaccination in individuals with severe immunosuppression, see *Immunosuppression and HIV*. For most individuals, JCVI recommend a minimum 8 week interval between doses, unless rapid immunisation is required in specific circumstances (such as individuals about to receive immunosuppressive treatment). However, for healthy individuals aged under 18 years who are not health and social care workers, carers, or household contacts of immunosuppressed individuals, a minimum 12 week interval between doses is recommended.

The same COVID-19 vaccine should ideally be used for the entire primary course, where possible. If the same vaccine is not available or suitable, or if the first product received is unknown, a suitable available product should be given to complete the primary course. If the course is delayed, it should be resumed, but the previous dose should not be repeated. Individuals presenting for vaccination who have participated in a COVID-19 vaccine clinical trial should have written advice provided by their clinical trial investigators about vaccination in the routine programme.

Vaccine choice for the primary course

For children aged 6 months–4 years, the mRNA monovalent *Comirnaty*® COVID-19 vaccine is recommended.

For children aged 5–11 years, the mRNA monovalent *Comirnaty*® or bivalent paediatric *Comirnaty*® Original/Omicron BA.4/5 COVID-19 vaccine is recommended. Although the mRNA monovalent *Spikevax*® vaccine is licensed for use in children aged 6 years and over, *Comirnaty*® preparations are preferred due to a lower reported rate of myocarditis.

For children aged 12–17 years, the mRNA bivalent *Comirnaty*® Original/Omicron BA.4/5 COVID-19 vaccine is recommended. If this is unavailable, the bivalent *Comirnaty*® Original/Omicron BA.1 or monovalent *Comirnaty*® vaccine may be used. Although the mRNA *Spikevax*® vaccines are licensed for use in this age group, *Comirnaty*® preparations are preferred due to a lower reported rate of myocarditis.

For individuals aged 18 years and over, the mRNA bivalent *Comirnaty*® Original/Omicron BA.4/5 or *Spikevax*® Original/Omicron BA.4/5 COVID-19 vaccine is recommended. If these are unavailable, the bivalent *Comirnaty*® Original/Omicron BA.1 or *Spikevax*® Original/Omicron BA.1 vaccine, or the monovalent *Comirnaty*® or *Spikevax*® vaccine may be used; in those aged 65 years and over, *VidPrevtyn Beta*® may also be used.

When a mRNA vaccine is considered unsuitable, *Nuvaxovid*® may be used for primary vaccination of individuals aged 12 years and over, or in those aged 65 years and over, *VidPrevtyn Beta*® may be used.

Booster doses

From spring 2023, a booster dose will no longer be offered to individuals who are not in a clinical at-risk or other high-risk group.

During the spring 2023 booster programme, a booster dose should be offered provided that there has been an interval of at least 3 months from the previous dose, to the following individuals:

- residents in care homes for older adults;
- all individuals aged 75 years and over;
- individuals aged 5 years and over who are immunosuppressed.

For further information on eligible groups (including definition of immunosuppression), see Chapter 14a: COVID-19 - SARS-CoV-2, in *Immunisation against infectious disease-* 'The Green Book' (see *Useful resources*).

Vaccine choice for booster doses

For children aged 5–11 years, the mRNA monovalent *Comirnaty*® or bivalent paediatric *Comirnaty*® Original/Omicron BA.4/5 COVID-19 vaccine p. 1500 is recommended.

For children aged 12–17 years, the mRNA bivalent *Comirnaty*® Original/Omicron BA.4/5 COVID-19 vaccine is recommended. If this is unavailable, the bivalent *Comirnaty*® Original/Omicron BA.1 or monovalent *Comirnaty*® vaccine may be used. If a mRNA vaccine is unsuitable, *Nuvaxovid*® may be used.

For individuals aged 18 years–74 years, the mRNA bivalent *Comirnaty*® Original/Omicron BA.4/5 or *Spikevax*® Original/Omicron BA.4/5 COVID-19 vaccine is recommended. If these are unavailable, the bivalent *Comirnaty*® Original/Omicron BA.1 or *Spikevax*® Original/Omicron BA.1, or the monovalent *Comirnaty*® or *Spikevax*® vaccine may be used. Individuals aged 65–74 years in domiciliary settings may receive *VidPrevtyn Beta*® if that would facilitate operational delivery. If a mRNA vaccine is unsuitable, *Nuvaxovid*® may be used; in those aged 65 years and over, *VidPrevtyn Beta*® may also be used.

For individuals aged 75 years and over *and* for residents aged 65 years and over in care homes for the elderly, the mRNA bivalent *Comirnaty*® Original/Omicron BA.4/5 or *Spikevax*® Original/Omicron BA.4/5, or the *VidPrevtyn Beta*® COVID-19 vaccine is recommended. If these are unavailable, the bivalent *Comirnaty*® Original/Omicron BA.1 or *Spikevax*® Original/Omicron BA.1, or the monovalent *Comirnaty*® or *Spikevax*® vaccine may be used. If a mRNA vaccine is unsuitable, *Nuvaxovid*® or *VidPrevtyn Beta*® may be used.

Individuals who have participated in a COVID-19 vaccine clinical trial should have written advice provided by their clinical trial investigators about vaccination in the routine programme. For further information on booster doses (including dosing intervals for those about to receive immunosuppressive treatment), see Chapter 14a: COVID-19 - SARS-CoV-2, in *Immunisation against infectious disease-* 'The Green Book' (see *Useful resources*).

Pregnancy

Pregnant females should be offered immunisation against COVID-19 as pregnancy is a clinical risk factor for severe COVID-19 infection. Females who are planning a pregnancy or are immediately post-partum should also be offered vaccination with a suitable COVID-19 vaccine. For further guidance on COVID-19 vaccines, see *Primary immunisation* and *Booster doses*.

There is no longer a requirement to report inadvertent administration of COVID-19 vaccines in pregnancy to the UKHSA vaccination in pregnancy (VIP) surveillance programme.

For further information on COVID-19 vaccination in pregnancy, see UKHSA guidance: **COVID-19 vaccination: a guide on pregnancy and breastfeeding** (available at: www.gov.uk/government/publications/covid-19-vaccination-women-of-childbearing-age-currently-pregnant-planning-a-pregnancy-or-breastfeeding).

Immunosuppression and HIV

Individuals with immunosuppression and HIV infection (regardless of CD4 count) are considered at-risk and should be vaccinated against COVID-19 in accordance with JCVI recommendations (see *Primary immunisation* and *Booster doses*).

Individuals with severe immunosuppression may have an inadequate immune response to a primary course of vaccination and may therefore remain at high risk. JCVI advises that individuals aged 6 months and over who were severely immunosuppressed at the time of receiving their first or second dose of COVID-19 vaccine, should be offered a third dose as part of their primary course (ideally at least 8 weeks after the second dose). For vaccine choice, see *Vaccine choice for the primary course*, and for further information on the third primary dose (including the definition of severe immunosuppression), see Chapter 14a: COVID-19 - SARS-CoV-2, in *Immunisation against infectious disease-* 'The Green Book' (see *Useful resources*). Individuals aged 5 years and over with severe immunosuppression should also be offered booster doses to extend protection from their primary course. For further guidance, see *Booster doses*.

As there is limited evidence on response to immunisation in individuals with immunosuppression, specialists may advise their patients on optimal timing of vaccine delivery based on the patient's immune status, likely response to vaccination, risk of COVID-19 and of exposure. Post-vaccination testing for individuals with severe immunosuppression may be considered by specialists managing their care; advice on whether further precautions are required to reduce their risk can then be given if appropriate.

Refer to the British HIV Association for further information on the use of COVID-19 vaccine in HIV-positive individuals. See www.bhiva.org/Coronavirus-COVID-19 for further information.

Post-exposure management

COVID-19 is a notifiable disease in the UK. For further information, see *Notifiable diseases* in Antibacterials, principles of therapy p. 573.

There is limited evidence on the use of COVID-19 vaccines as post-exposure prophylaxis or to prevent transmission during outbreaks. For vulnerable individuals who require direct protection during prolonged community outbreaks, advice on post-exposure management can be sought from local health protection teams.

For the management of COVID-19 infection and links to other resources, see COVID-19 p. 714.

Useful Resources

Recommendations reflect Chapter 14a, COVID-19 - SARS-CoV-2, in *Immunisation against infectious disease-* 'The Green Book'. UK Health Security Agency. April 2023. www.gov.uk/government/publications/covid-19-the-green-book-chapter-14a

COVID-19 vaccination programme: Information for healthcare practitioners. UK Health Security Agency. October 2022. www.gov.uk/government/publications/covid-19-vaccination-programme-guidance-for-healthcare-practitioners

Diphtheria vaccine

18-Aug-2024

Overview

Diphtheria-containing vaccines are inactivated and prepared from a cell-free purified toxin of *Corynebacterium diphtheriae*, adsorbed on aluminium hydroxide or aluminium phosphate to improve immunogenicity. The diphtheria vaccine is only available as part of combination preparations containing other vaccines. The quantity of diphtheria toxoid in a preparation determines whether the vaccine is defined as 'high dose' or 'low dose', and this, as well as the need for protection against other infections, determines the choice of vaccine for each age group.

Prophylaxis

In most circumstances, the recommended vaccination schedule, comprising of a total of 5 doses of diphtheria-containing vaccine given at recommended intervals, is considered satisfactory in providing long-term protection against diphtheria infection.

Individuals due for their routine diphtheria immunisation may not require their routine dose if they have a history of vaccination (such as for a tetanus-prone wound) with the same diphtheria-containing vaccine that is due, and it was administered at an appropriate interval.

Laboratory and healthcare workers (including students and trainees) who may be exposed to diphtheria in the course of their work, such as in microbiology laboratories and clinical infectious disease units, are at risk and should be protected. For further information, see *Immunisations for healthcare and laboratory staff* in Immunisation schedule p. 1472.

For information on immunisation for individuals with neurological conditions, see Chapter 15, Diphtheria, in *Immunisation against infectious disease- 'The Green Book'.*

For information on immunisation in pregnancy, see *Pregnancy.*

Individuals with immunosuppression or HIV infection (regardless of CD4 count) should be given the recommended vaccination schedule of 5 doses of a diphtheria-containing vaccine (see *Primary Immunisation* and *Boosters*). Consider re-immunisation after treatment completion—specialist advice may be required. Refer to the British HIV Association or Children's HIV Association for further information on the use of diphtheria-containing vaccines in individuals with HIV infection. See www.bhiva.org or www.chiva.org.uk for further information.

Primary immunisation

Diphtheria vaccination is given as a component of the routine childhood immunisation programme for children aged under 10 years (see Immunisation schedule p. 1472). If the child's routine immunisation is delayed, children aged under 10 years should be immunised at the earliest opportunity.

Children aged under 10 years should be given a primary course consisting of 3 doses of the hexavalent diphtheria with tetanus, pertussis, hepatitis B, poliomyelitis and haemophilus influenzae type b vaccine p. 1502 at intervals of 4 weeks (it is the only suitable vaccine containing high dose diphtheria for priming children of this age). If interrupted, the primary course should be resumed but not repeated, allowing a 4 week interval between doses. For information on circumstances where early immunisation, or alternative dosing intervals for primary immunisation may be considered, see UKHSA guidance: **The hexavalent DTaP/IPV/Hib/HepB combination vaccine: information for healthcare practitioners** (see *Useful resources*).

If the primary course was commenced with the pentavalent diphtheria with tetanus, pertussis, poliomyelitis and haemophilus influenzae type b vaccine p. 1502, it can be completed with the hexavalent diphtheria with tetanus, pertussis, hepatitis B, poliomyelitis and haemophilus influenzae type b vaccine.

Individuals aged 10 years or over who have not been immunised previously, or have an unknown or incomplete history, should be given a primary course consisting of 3 doses of the 'low dose' diphtheria with tetanus and poliomyelitis vaccine p. 1501 at 4 week intervals. If interrupted, the primary course should be resumed but not repeated, allowing an interval of 4 weeks between doses.

For further information on vaccination of individuals with uncertain or incomplete immunisation status, see

Chapter 11, The UK immunisation schedule, in *Immunisation against infectious disease- 'The Green Book'.*

Boosters

Following a primary course, 2 doses of a suitable diphtheria-containing booster vaccine should be given at recommended intervals.

Children aged under 10 years should receive diphtheria with tetanus, pertussis and poliomyelitis vaccine p. 1502 for their first booster dose. This is usually given 3 years after completing the primary course (before school entry)—see Immunisation schedule p. 1472. However, when primary immunisation has been delayed, it may be given at the scheduled visit, provided it has been 1 year since the third dose of their primary course.

Individuals aged 10 years and over should be given the diphtheria with tetanus and poliomyelitis vaccine for their first booster dose. This should be at least 5 years after the third dose of their primary course.

All individuals should be given the diphtheria with tetanus and poliomyelitis vaccine for their second booster dose. This is usually given 10 years after the first booster (see Immunisation schedule p. 1472), but if previous doses have been delayed, it may be given at the school session or scheduled visit provided there has been at least a 5 year interval since the first booster dose.

Travel

All travellers to epidemic or endemic areas should ensure they are fully immunised (or are up-to-date) with their diphtheria vaccination (see *Primary Immunisation* and *Boosters*). Further doses may be required in some cases, such as for those intending to live or work with local people in epidemic or endemic areas. Where protection against diphtheria is required, and more than 10 years have elapsed since the final dose of diphtheria-containing vaccine was received, diphtheria with tetanus and poliomyelitis vaccine should be given.

Post-exposure management

Advice on the management of cases, carriers, contacts, and outbreaks must be sought from local health protection teams. The immunisation history of infected individuals and their contacts should be determined.

For further information on the management of possible cases, carriers, and close contacts, see UKHSA guidance: **Public health control and management of diphtheria in England** (see *Useful resources*). For information on diphtheria control for asylum seekers, see UKHSA guidance: **Infectious diseases in asylum seekers: actions for health professionals** (available at www.gov.uk/guidance/infectious-diseases-in-asylum-seekers-actions-for-health-professionals).

Cases

Diphtheria is a notifiable disease in the UK. For further information, see *Notifiable diseases* in Antibacterials, principles of therapy p. 573.

Diphtheria antitoxin p. 1470 should only be used for the treatment of confirmed or probable cases of diphtheria in a hospital setting. Treatment should proceed as soon as possible, as the effectiveness is strongly related to time since disease onset. For further information on the use of diphtheria antitoxin, see UKHSA guidance: **Diphtheria anti-toxin** (available at: www.gov.uk/government/publications/immunoglobulin-when-to-use/diphtheria-anti-toxin-clinical-guidance-issued-may-2022). All individuals with confirmed or probable diphtheria should also receive antibacterial therapy to eliminate the organism and prevent spread. Asymptomatic carriers of toxigenic strains should be treated with the same antibacterials as cases. Individuals identified with a non-toxigenic toxin gene-bearing (NTTB) strain should be given antibacterial therapy only if clinically indicated.

Diphtheria infection may not result in adequate levels of antitoxin, and vaccination of confirmed or probable cases is recommended once the patient is clinically stable. Asymptomatic carriers of toxigenic strains should also be vaccinated. Those who are unimmunised or partially immunised against diphtheria should complete their immunisation according to the routine schedule (see *Prophylaxis*). Fully immunised individuals should receive a reinforcing dose according to their age (see *Boosters*) unless a diphtheria-containing vaccine was given within the last 12 months.

Contacts

Close contacts of asymptomatic carriers or confirmed or probable cases should be investigated immediately, kept under surveillance, and be given antibacterial prophylaxis (see *Diphtheria: prevention of secondary cases* in Antibacterials, use for prophylaxis p. 574).

Unimmunised or partially immunised close contacts should complete their immunisation according to the routine schedule (see *Prophylaxis*). Fully immunised close contacts of asymptomatic carriers or confirmed or probable cases should receive a reinforcing dose according to their age (see *Boosters*) unless a diphtheria-containing vaccine was given within the last 12 months.

Pregnancy

Routine vaccination of pregnant females with diphtheria with tetanus and pertussis vaccine p. 1501 is recommended between 16 to 32 weeks of each pregnancy as part of the maternal pertussis programme, usually around the time of the fetal anomaly scan (20 weeks) for operational reasons. For further information, and for guidance for pregnant females with an incomplete or unknown vaccination history against diphtheria, tetanus and polio, see UKHSA guidance: **Pertussis (whooping cough) vaccination programme for pregnant women**, available at: www.gov.uk/government/ publications/vaccination-against-pertussis-whooping-cough-for-pregnant-women.

Pregnant females may be given diphtheria-containing vaccines where protection is needed without delay. For information on the management of cases, see *Post-exposure management*.

Useful Resources

Recommendations reflect Chapter 15, Diphtheria, in *Immunisation against infectious disease-* 'The Green Book'. UK Health Security Agency, April 2013. www.gov.uk/government/publications/diphtheria-the-green-book-chapter-15

Public health control and management of diphtheria in England. UK Health Security Agency, November 2023. www.gov.uk/government/publications/diphtheria-public-health-control-and-management-in-england-and-wales

The hexavalent DTaP/IPV/Hib/HepB combination vaccine: information for healthcare practitioners. UK Health Security Agency, May 2023. www.gov.uk/government/publications/hexavalent-combination-vaccine-programme-guidance

Haemophilus influenzae type b conjugate vaccine

15-Nov-2023

Overview

Haemophilus influenzae type b (Hib) containing vaccines are inactivated, and are made from capsular polysaccharide extracted from cultures of Hib bacteria. The polysaccharide is conjugated with a protein (such as tetanus toxoid) to increase immunogenicity, especially in young children. The Hib conjugate vaccine is only available as a combination preparation containing other vaccines.

Hib vaccination is given as a component of the routine childhood immunisation programme to provide protection against invasive Hib disease for children aged under 10 years (see Immunisation schedule p. 1472). If the child's routine immunisation is delayed, children aged under 10 years should be immunised at the earliest opportunity. Hib vaccination may also be given to individuals aged 10 years and over who are considered to be at increased risk of invasive Hib disease.

A primary course consists of 3 doses of the hexavalent diphtheria with tetanus, pertussis, hepatitis B, poliomyelitis and haemophilus influenzae type b vaccine p. 1502, given at 4 weekly intervals. For information on circumstances where early immunisation, or alternative dosing intervals for primary immunisation may be considered, see UKHSA guidance: **The hexavalent DTaP/IPV/Hib/HepB combination vaccine: information for healthcare practitioners** (see *Useful resources*).

Children aged under 1 year should be given a primary course, followed by a booster dose of the haemophilus influenzae type b with meningococcal group C vaccine p. 1503 at 1 year of age (usually on or after the child's first birthday). This should be given at least 4 weeks after the last dose of Hib-containing vaccine, and where there has been a delay, can be given up until 10 years of age.

If the primary course was commenced with the pentavalent diphtheria with tetanus, pertussis, poliomyelitis and haemophilus influenzae type b vaccine p. 1502, it can be completed with the hexavalent diphtheria with tetanus, pertussis, hepatitis B, poliomyelitis and haemophilus influenzae type b vaccine. If interrupted, the primary course should be resumed but not repeated, allowing a 4 week interval between doses.

Children aged 1 year to under 10 years who have not been immunised against Hib need to only receive 1 dose of the haemophilus influenzae type b with meningococcal group C vaccine. However, children who have not completed a primary course of diphtheria, tetanus, pertussis and polio, should be given 3 doses of the hexavalent diphtheria with tetanus, pertussis, hepatitis B, poliomyelitis and haemophilus influenzae type b vaccine at 4 weekly intervals, in order to be fully protected against diphtheria, tetanus, pertussis and polio.

For further information on vaccination of children with uncertain or incomplete immunisation status, see Chapter 11, The UK immunisation schedule, in *Immunisation against infectious disease-* 'The Green Book'.

For information on immunisation of individuals with neurological conditions, see Chapter 16, *Haemophilus influenzae* type b (Hib), in *Immunisation against infectious disease-* 'The Green Book'.

Children with immunosuppression and HIV infection (regardless of CD4 count) should be given Hib-containing vaccines according to the routine immunisation schedule (see Immunisation schedule p. 1472). Consider re-immunisation after treatment completion—specialist advice may be required. Refer to the British HIV Association and Children's HIV Association for further information on the use of Hib-containing vaccines in individuals with HIV infection. See www.bhiva.org/guidelines and www.chiva.org.uk/ for further information.

Post-exposure management of invasive *Haemophilus influenzae* type b disease

Acute meningitis caused by Hib is a notifiable disease in England, Northern Ireland and Wales. For further information, see *Notifiable diseases* in Antibacterials, principles of therapy p. 573.

To reduce the risk of secondary invasive Hib disease in the index case and their close contacts (such as contacts in a household, or a pre-school or primary school setting), antibacterial prophylaxis and vaccination may be required.

Individual risk is determined by factors such as age, health status, and immunisation history. For information on antibacterial prophylaxis, see *Haemophilus influenzae type b infection: prevention of secondary disease* in Antibacterials, use for prophylaxis p. 574.

Children aged under 10 years who are unimmunised or partially immunised against Hib disease and are either the index case, a household contact of the index case, or a contact of the index case in a pre-school or primary school setting, should complete their primary immunisation. Vaccination of the index case should occur after recovery from invasive Hib infection. For further information on primary immunisation, see *Overview*. Children aged under 10 years who have completed their age-specific primary immunisation, and individuals of any age with asplenia or splenic dysfunction, may need an additional dose of a Hib-containing vaccine. For further information on vaccination following a case of invasive Hib disease, see Public Health England guidance: ***Haemophilus influenzae* type b** (see *Useful resources*).

Useful Resources

Recommendations reflect Chapter 16, *Haemophilus influenzae* type b (Hib), in *Immunisation against infectious disease*- 'The Green Book'. Public Health England. March 2011.
www.gov.uk/government/publications/haemophilus-influenzae-type-hib-the-green-book-chapter-16

Revised recommendations for the prevention of secondary *Haemophilus influenzae* type b (Hib) disease. Public Health England. 2009, updated July 2013.
www.gov.uk/government/publications/haemophilus-influenzae-type-b-hib-revised-recommendations-for-the-prevention-of-secondary-cases

The hexavalent DTaP/IPV/Hib/HepB combination vaccine: information for healthcare practitioners. UK Health Security Agency, May 2023.
www.gov.uk/government/publications/hexavalent-combination-vaccine-programme-guidance

Hepatitis A vaccine

20-May-2022

Overview

The hepatitis A vaccine p. 1504 is prepared from different strains of the virus grown in human diploid cells. The inactivated vaccine is available as a monovalent vaccine (different monovalent vaccines can be used interchangeably), or in combination with hepatitis B or typhoid—vaccine choice is dependent on which infection(s) the individual requires protection from. Immunisation with normal immunoglobulin p. 1466 can be used to provide immediate but temporary protection against hepatitis A.

Pre-exposure prophylaxis

Immunisation against hepatitis A is recommended for individuals at high risk of hepatitis A exposure, those with certain underlying medical conditions, and those at risk of complications, as listed:

- laboratory staff who may be exposed to the virus;
- staff and residents of homes for those with severe learning difficulties, or where personal hygiene among patients may be poor;
- workers at risk of repeated exposure to untreated sewage;
- individuals who work with primates;
- patients with haemophilia being treated with plasma-derived clotting factors;
- patients with severe liver disease regardless of the cause (consider for those with chronic hepatitis B or C infection and for patients with milder liver disease);
- individuals travelling to or going to reside in areas of intermediate or high prevalence, see *Travel* below;
- individuals who are at risk due to their sexual behaviour (such as men who have sex with men);
- individuals who inject drugs.

Immunisation may be considered under certain circumstances for:

- food packagers and handlers where a case or outbreak occurs—advice should be sought from the local Health Protection Team;
- staff in day-care facilities where there is a community outbreak—advice should be sought from the local Health Protection Team;
- healthcare workers.

Immunisation against hepatitis A infection requires a primary pre-exposure course. The primary immunisation regimen for monovalent hepatitis A vaccine and hepatitis A with typhoid vaccine p. 1505 consists of a single dose. For immunisation using the combined hepatitis A and B vaccine, the primary course depends on the product used, see hepatitis A and B vaccine p. 1503 for dosing schedules (including accelerated course information).

Individuals with immunosuppression and HIV infection can be given hepatitis A-containing vaccines. Consider re-immunisation—specialist advice may be required. Refer to the British HIV Association or Children's HIV Association for further information on the use of hepatitis A vaccine in HIV-positive individuals. See www.bhiva.org or www.chiva.org.uk for further information.

Boosters

A booster dose is usually given 6–12 months after the initial dose of hepatitis A-containing vaccine, and ensures immunity beyond 10 years; however, successful boosting can occur even if the booster dose is delayed by several years. A further booster dose 25 years after full primary immunisation is only considered necessary if the risk of hepatitis A infection is still present.

Travel

Pre-exposure immunisation is recommended for individuals travelling to or going to reside in areas of high or intermediate prevalence. Immunisation should ideally be given 2 weeks prior to departure, but can be given up to the day of departure; the use of normal immunoglobulin for travel prophylaxis is no longer recommended. Care should also be taken to avoid hepatitis A exposure through food and water. Further information on country-specific hepatitis A risk is available from the National Travel Health Network and Centre (travelhealthpro.org.uk/) and Health Protection Scotland (www.travax.nhs.uk).

Post-exposure prophylaxis

Hepatitis A (acute infectious hepatitis) is a notifiable disease in the UK. For further information, see *Notifiable diseases* in Antibacterials, principles of therapy p. 573.

A risk assessment should be carried out for the index case (particularly if infection occurs in a non-household setting), and the national standard questionnaire also completed for all probable and confirmed cases. Verbal and written guidance on the importance of good hygiene practices (such as hand washing after using the toilet, changing nappies, and before preparing food) should be given to the index case, their family and other close contacts. If sexual transmission is the likely route (particularly between men who have sex with men), advice on prevention of hepatitis A spread during sex should also be given. For further information on the management of index cases and link to the national standard questionnaire, see PHE guidance: **Public Health control and management of hepatitis A** (see *Useful resources*).

Close contacts of the index case(s) should have a risk assessment as soon as possible within 14 days of exposure. Prophylactic treatment choice for close contacts depends on susceptibility (determined by age and health status) and time since exposure. There should be a low threshold for considering someone a close contact.

Close contacts should be considered immune if they have a documented history of either a completed course within the past 10 years, or a single dose of monovalent vaccine within the past year, or if they have previously had laboratory-confirmed hepatitis A.

Post-exposure prophylaxis is **not** required for healthy close contacts aged under 1 year not attending childcare; immunisation should be offered to all those who assist in the child's toileting to prevent tertiary infection. For close contacts aged 2–12 months attending childcare, a dose of monovalent hepatitis A vaccine [unlicensed use] should be given within 14 days of exposure. If the child contact cannot be immunised, appropriate advice should be given on enhanced hygiene in the childcare setting; if enhanced hygiene standards cannot be met, the child should be excluded from childcare for 30 days. If exclusion of the child is not possible, all carers and children aged 2 months and above in the childcare setting should be immunised. In these cases, any child that goes on to require long-term protection against hepatitis A after their first birthday, should be given the full course of two doses.

For healthy close contacts aged 1–59 years, a single dose of monovalent hepatitis A vaccine is recommended within 14 days of exposure. A risk assessment is required to determine any continued risk of hepatitis A infection. To ensure long term protection, a second dose of the vaccine should be given after 6–12 months.

For close contacts who have chronic liver disease (including chronic hepatitis B or C infection), HIV infection (with a CD4 count < 200 cells per microlitre), are immunosuppressed, or are aged 60 years or over, normal immunoglobulin in addition to monovalent hepatitis A vaccine is recommended within 14 days of exposure (up to 28 days in those with chronic liver disease). To provide long term protection, a second dose of the vaccine should be given after 6–12 months.

Refer to the British HIV Association or Children's HIV Association for further information on the use of hepatitis A vaccine p. 1504 in HIV-positive individuals. See www.bhiva. org or www.chiva.org.uk for further information.

In households with more than one close contact, all unvaccinated household contacts seen within 8 weeks of jaundice onset in the index case, should be given the monovalent hepatitis A vaccine to prevent tertiary spread within the household.

For further information on the management of susceptible close contacts and for information on outbreaks, see PHE guidance: **Public Health control and management of hepatitis A** (see *Useful resources*); and for further information on normal immunoglobulin, see Immunoglobulins p. 1462.

Useful Resources

Recommendations reflect Chapter 17, Hepatitis A, in *Immunisation against infectious disease- 'The Green Book'*. UK Health Security Agency. February 2022.
www.gov.uk/government/publications/hepatitis-a-the-green-book-chapter-17

Public health control and management of hepatitis A. Public Health England. June 2017.
www.gov.uk/government/publications/hepatitis-a-infection-prevention-and-control-guidance

Hepatitis B vaccine

19-Dec-2023

Overview

Hepatitis B vaccines contain inactivated hepatitis B surface antigen (HBsAg) prepared from yeast cells using recombinant DNA technology, which is adsorbed onto an adjuvant. The vaccine is available as a monovalent vaccine, a bivalent vaccine in combination with hepatitis A, and a hexavalent vaccine in combination with diphtheria, tetanus, acellular pertussis, inactivated poliomyelitis, and *Haemophilus influenzae* type b (Hib).

Pre-exposure prophylaxis

Hepatitis B vaccination is given as a component of the routine childhood immunisation programme to provide long-term protection against hepatitis B. Children aged under 1 year should be given a primary course consisting of 3 doses of the hexavalent diphtheria with tetanus, pertussis, hepatitis B, poliomyelitis and haemophilus influenzae type b vaccine p. 1502, given at 4 weekly intervals (see Immunisation schedule p. 1472). If interrupted, the primary course should be resumed but not repeated, allowing a 4 week interval between doses. For information on circumstances where early immunisation, or alternative dosing intervals may be considered, see UKHSA guidance: **The hexavalent DTaP/IPV/Hib/HepB combination vaccine: information for healthcare practitioners** (see *Useful resources*).

If the child's routine immunisation is delayed, children aged under 10 years should be immunised at the earliest opportunity.

If the primary course was commenced with the pentavalent diphtheria with tetanus, pertussis, poliomyelitis and haemophilus influenzae type b vaccine p. 1502, it can be completed with the hexavalent diphtheria with tetanus, pertussis, hepatitis B, poliomyelitis and haemophilus influenzae type b vaccine.

Children aged 1 year to under 10 years who have completed a primary course with the pentavalent vaccine but have not received any hepatitis B-containing vaccines, do not require a hepatitis B-containing vaccine unless they are in a high risk group (see below) or are exposed to hepatitis B (see *Post-exposure management*).

Immunisation against hepatitis B is also recommended for individuals in high risk groups (those at high risk of exposure or those at risk of complications), as listed:

- individuals who inject drugs and their sexual partners, other household and close family contacts;
- individuals who are likely to 'progress' to injecting drugs;
- close family, household, or sexual contacts of an individual with chronic hepatitis B infection;
- individuals who change sexual partners frequently (such as commercial sex workers);
- men who have sex with men;
- individuals receiving regular blood transfusions or blood products (such as those with haemophilia), and carers responsible for the administration of such products;
- patients with chronic renal failure who are on haemodialysis or a renal transplantation programme, and those predicted to require these interventions—use vaccines specifically formulated for patients with renal insufficiency;
- patients with severe liver disease regardless of the cause, or those with milder liver disease who may share risk factors for acquiring hepatitis B infection (such as individuals with chronic hepatitis C);
- healthcare workers (including students and trainees) who may have direct contact with patients' blood, blood-stained body fluids or tissues;
- laboratory staff who handle material that may contain the virus;
- other occupational risk groups (such as morticians and embalmers);
- staff and residents of homes for those with learning difficulties (consideration may also be given for those in day care, schools and centres for those with severe learning disability);

- staff and inmates of custodial institutions;
- individuals travelling to or going to reside in areas of high or intermediate prevalence of hepatitis B, see *Travel* below;
- families adopting children from countries with a high or intermediate prevalence of hepatitis B;
- some foster carers and their families.

Neonates born to a hepatitis B negative female but going home to a household with another individual who has hepatitis B infection may be at immediate risk of hepatitis B infection and should be given a dose of the monovalent hepatitis B vaccine p. 1505 before being discharged from the hospital. Routine childhood immunisation with the hexavalent diphtheria with tetanus, pertussis, hepatitis B, poliomyelitis and haemophilus influenzae type b vaccine should then be given as scheduled (see Immunisation schedule p. 1472).

For immunisation of other individuals in a high-risk group, the primary course dosing regimen depends on how rapidly protection is required, the likelihood of patient compliance, and the product used. For most individuals, an accelerated schedule should be given (particularly in individuals where compliance with immunisation is difficult). Alternative non-accelerated schedules are available, but should only be used when rapid protection is not required and there is a high likelihood of patient attendance for immunisation. In certain circumstances, a very rapid schedule may be given to individuals who are at immediate risk where a more rapid induction of protection is required. See hepatitis B vaccine and hepatitis A and B vaccine p. 1503 for information on dosing schedules.

During vaccination, advice should be provided on other preventative measures (such as condom use and needle exchange), and referral to specialist services arranged if appropriate.

Testing for response to vaccination is not routinely advised, but it is recommended for individuals at risk of occupational exposure and in patients with renal failure. For further information, see Chapter 18, Hepatitis B, in *Immunisation against infectious disease-* 'The Green Book' (see *Useful resources*).

Immunosuppressed individuals with HIV infection have higher rates of developing chronic infection; HIV-positive patients and those at risk of HIV infection should be offered vaccination. Refer to the British HIV Association and Children's HIV Association for further information on the use of hepatitis B-containing vaccines in individuals with HIV infection. See www.bhiva.org/guidelines and www.chiva. org.uk/ for further information.

Boosters

Following a primary course of immunisation, most individuals do not require a reinforcing dose of a hepatitis B-containing vaccine. For healthcare and laboratory workers, a single booster dose (once only) should be offered approximately 5 years after primary immunisation. For patients with renal failure and for individuals at the time of a subsequent significant exposure, a booster dose may be required. For further information, see Chapter 18, Hepatitis B, in *Immunisation against infectious disease-* 'The Green Book' (see *Useful resources*).

Travel

Pre-exposure immunisation is recommended for individuals travelling to or going to reside in areas of high or intermediate prevalence of hepatitis B and who, through their behaviour/activities may be at risk while abroad. These include sexual activity, injecting drug use, undertaking relief aid work, and/or playing contact sports. Travellers are also at risk of acquiring infection as a result of medical or dental procedures carried out in countries where unsafe therapeutic injections (e.g. the re-use of contaminated needles and syringes without sterilisation) are a risk factor for

hepatitis B. Individuals at high risk of requiring medical or dental procedures in such countries should therefore be immunised, including:

- those staying for lengthy periods;
- those with chronic medical conditions that may require hospitalisation;
- those travelling for medical or dental procedures.

Further information on country-specific hepatitis B risk is available from the National Travel Health Network and Centre (travelhealthpro.org.uk/) and Public Health Scotland (www.travax.nhs.uk).

Post-exposure prophylaxis

Hepatitis B (acute infectious hepatitis) is a notifiable disease in the UK. For further information, see *Notifiable diseases* in Antibacterials, principles of therapy p. 573.

Post-exposure prophylaxis should be given as soon as possible to neonates born to mothers infected with hepatitis B, see *Selective neonatal immunisation programme* below for further information. Immediate post-exposure prophylaxis should also be offered to any individual who has potentially been exposed to hepatitis B infected blood or bodily fluids, such as sexual contacts of an individual with acute hepatitis B or newly diagnosed chronic hepatitis B, or those exposed through a needle stick injury or bites from a known hepatitis B individual. Advice should be sought from the nearest public health laboratory, health protection team, or on-call virologist. The recommended vaccine course (including use of a booster dose) is dependent on the individual's vaccination history, source of exposure, and continued risk. For further information, see Chapter 18, Hepatitis B, in *Immunisation against infectious disease-* 'The Green Book' (see *Useful resources*).

Hepatitis B immunoglobulin p. 1465 may also be given to individuals at the same time as the hepatitis B vaccine following accidental exposure to hepatitis B-infected blood or bodily fluids through percutaneous inoculation, contamination of mucous membranes or non-intact skin. It is also recommended for use with the vaccine in sexual contacts of an individual with acute hepatitis B and may be considered in unprotected sexual contacts of an individual with newly diagnosed chronic hepatitis B, if seen within 1 week. Hepatitis B immunoglobulin is also recommended in some known non-responders to the hepatitis B vaccine. For further information, see UKHSA: **Hepatitis B immunoglobulin** (see *Useful resources*).

Selective neonatal immunisation programme

Neonates born to mothers who have chronic hepatitis B infection or who had acute hepatitis B during pregnancy, should be vaccinated with a dose of the monovalent hepatitis B vaccine p. 1505 as soon as possible (ideally within 24 hours of birth), followed by a second dose at 4 weeks. Routine childhood immunisation with the hexavalent diphtheria with tetanus, pertussis, hepatitis B, poliomyelitis and haemophilus influenzae type b vaccine p. 1502 should then be given as scheduled (see Immunisation schedule p. 1472), followed by a further dose of the monovalent hepatitis B vaccine and blood test (to exclude infection) at 1 year of age. For further information on the selective neonatal immunisation programme, see UKHSA guidance: **The hexavalent DTaP/IPV/Hib/HepB combination vaccine: information for healthcare practitioners**, and **Guidance on the hepatitis B antenatal screening and selective neonatal immunisation pathway** (see *Useful resources*).

For neonates with a birth weight below 1.5 kg born to an infected mother, or neonates born to a highly infectious mother, hepatitis B immunoglobulin should be given at the same time as the first dose of monovalent hepatitis B vaccine (administered at different sites) in order to provide rapid protection until the vaccine becomes effective. For further information on the use of hepatitis B immunoglobulin and which mothers are considered to be highly infectious, see

UKHSA guidance: **Hepatitis B immunoglobulin** (see *Useful resources*).

Useful Resources

Recommendations reflect Chapter 18, Hepatitis B, in *Immunisation against infectious disease*– 'The Green Book'. UK Health Security Agency. February 2022.
www.gov.uk/government/publications/hepatitis-b-the-green-book-chapter-18

The hexavalent DTaP/IPV/Hib/HepB combination vaccine: information for healthcare practitioners. UK Health Security Agency. May 2023.
www.gov.uk/government/publications/hexavalent-combination-vaccine-programme-guidance

Guidance on the hepatitis B antenatal screening and selective neonatal immunisation pathway. UK Health Security Agency. August 2023.
www.gov.uk/government/publications/hepatitis-b-antenatal-screening-and-selective-neonatal-immunisation-pathway

Hepatitis B immunoglobulin. UK Health Security Agency. November 2023.
www.gov.uk/government/publications/immunoglobulin-when-to-use

---

Human papillomavirus vaccine   19-Jul-2024

Overview

The human papillomavirus vaccine p. 1508 (HPV vaccine) consists of virus-like particles prepared from the major protein of the viral capsid that mimic the structure of the native virus, but does not contain any viral DNA. *Gardasil*® 9 is an adjuvanted nine-valent vaccine that contains HPV types 6, 11, 16, 18, 31, 33, 45, 52 and 58, and is the recommended vaccine for the national HPV vaccination programme.

It is used for the prevention of cervical and anal cancers, and pre-cancerous genital (cervical, vulvar, and vaginal) and anal lesions associated with HPV types 16 and 18. It is also effective at preventing genital warts, and may also provide some cross-protection against infection caused by other high-risk HPV types. As *Gardasil*® 9 does not protect against all strains of HPV, safe sex precautions should always be practiced; and for all females, routine cervical screening should continue at the scheduled age.

Children aged 9 to 10 years

The HPV vaccine is licensed for individuals from 9 years of age, however vaccination of children aged 9 to 10 years is not offered as part of the national vaccination programme.

Individuals aged 11 to 24 years

Immunisation is routinely recommended for children aged 11 to 14 years (the eligible age for vaccine administration varies within different countries within the UK, see Immunisation schedule p. 1472 for further guidance).

Under the national programme, individuals in eligible cohorts (all females aged under 25 years and males born after 1st September 2006) who did not receive the HPV vaccine when scheduled can still be offered the vaccine up until their 25th birthday. Where appropriate, immunisation should also be offered to individuals coming into the UK if they have not been offered protection in their country of origin.

A 1 dose schedule of HPV vaccine is recommended for all eligible individuals aged 11 to 24 years, except for those with immunosuppression or HIV infection. For guidance on the vaccination schedule for individuals with immunosuppression or HIV infection, see *Individuals with immunosuppression or HIV infection*.

Vaccination of gay, bisexual and other men who have sex with men, and other at risk individuals

Gay, bisexual and other men who have sex with men (GBMSM) who are aged up to 45 years and attend specialist sexual health services or HIV services, are eligible for vaccination if they have not previously been vaccinated.

There may be considerable benefit in offering HPV vaccination to other individuals who attend specialist sexual health services or HIV services who are not eligible under the national programme, but are deemed to have an equivalent risk of acquiring HPV to GBMSM. This includes some transgender individuals, sex workers, and males or females living with HIV infection.

For eligible individuals who do not have immunosuppression or HIV infection, a 1 dose schedule of HPV vaccine is recommended for those aged under 25 years, and a 2 dose schedule is recommended for those aged 25 to 45 years with the second dose given 6–24 months after the first dose. 2 doses of *Gardasil*® 9 given less than 5 months apart should not be considered adequate to provide long term protection. If the second dose was given early, it should be discounted and a third dose given once the recommended time period has elapsed and at least 4 weeks after the early dose that was given. If the 2 dose course has not been completed before the age of 46 years, it can still be completed provided the first dose was given as part of the pilot or national vaccination programme.

For guidance on the vaccination schedule for individuals with immunosuppression or HIV infection, see *Individuals with immunosuppression or HIV infection*.

Individuals with immunosuppression or HIV infection

A 3 dose schedule of HPV vaccine should be offered to eligible individuals who are known to be immunosuppressed at the time of immunisation. Re-immunisation may be considered after treatment is finished and/or recovery has occurred depending on the treatment received—specialist advice may be required.

A 3 dose schedule of HPV vaccine is also recommended for eligible individuals with HIV infection who attend HIV services, and should be given regardless of CD4 cell count, antiretroviral therapy use, or viral load.

The second dose in the 3 dose schedule should be given at least 1 month after the first dose, followed by a third dose at least 3 months after the second dose; ideally the course should be completed within a 12 month period. In cases where the second dose is given late and there is a high likelihood that the individual will not return, or if it is not practical for the third dose to be given after 3 months, then the third dose can be given at least 1 month after the second dose.

For eligible individuals of the GBMSM vaccination programme, variable administration intervals are possible in order to align administration of doses with existing clinic appointments, provided that for these individuals the course is completed within 24 months and the minimum interval between doses is followed where possible.

For further information on the use of the HPV vaccine in individuals with HIV infection, see British HIV Association guidance at: www.bhiva.org/guidelines.

Booster doses

Protection from the HPV vaccine is maintained for at least 10 years, although protection is expected to last longer. There is no recommendation for the need for booster doses.

Useful Resources

Recommendations reflect Chapter 18a, Human papillomavirus, in *Immunisation against infectious disease*- 'The Green Book'. UK Health Security Agency. June 2023.

www.gov.uk/government/publications/human-papillomavirus-hpv-the-green-book-chapter-18a

HPV vaccination: guidance for healthcare practitioners. UK Health Security Agency. June 2023.

www.gov.uk/government/publications/hpv-universal-vaccination-guidance-for-health-professionals

Influenza vaccine

30-Aug-2024

Overview

While most viruses are antigenically stable, the influenza viruses A and B (especially A) are constantly altering their antigenic structure as indicated by changes in the haemagglutinins (H) and neuraminidases (N) on the surface of the viruses. It is essential that influenza vaccines in use target the prevalent strain or strains as recommended each year by the WHO.

There are several types of influenza vaccine available (see influenza vaccine (inactivated) p. 1508 and influenza vaccine (live) p. 1515); the vaccines recommended for the 2024/2025 influenza season are the inactivated adjuvanted egg-grown quadrivalent influenza vaccine (aQIV), inactivated cell-based quadrivalent influenza vaccine (QIVc), inactivated egg-grown quadrivalent influenza vaccine (QIVe), inactivated high-dose egg-grown quadrivalent influenza vaccine (QIV-HD), and the live attenuated influenza vaccine (LAIV). The choice of vaccine is dependent on the person's age and contra-indications.

To provide optimal protection during the highest risk period (December to January), the ideal time for immunisation in adults is from the beginning of October to late November. Pregnant females, particularly those in the later stages of pregnancy, should be immunised from September. For children, the ideal time for immunisation is from the beginning of September to early December.

Immunisation is recommended for individuals at high risk of serious complications from influenza, and to reduce transmission of infection. In the national flu immunisation programme 2024/2025, influenza vaccination is recommended for the following eligible groups:

- Individuals aged 6 months and over in a clinical risk group, such as those with:
  - chronic respiratory disease;
  - chronic heart disease and vascular disease;
  - chronic liver disease;
  - chronic kidney disease;
  - chronic neurological disease;
  - diabetes mellitus;
  - adrenal insufficiency;
  - splenic dysfunction or asplenia;
  - immunosuppression because of disease or treatment (including prolonged systemic corticosteroid treatment [for over 1 month at dose equivalents of prednisolone p. 791: *adult and child over 20 kg*, 20 mg or more daily; *child under 20 kg*, 1 mg/kg or more daily], and chemotherapy);
  - HIV infection (regardless of immune status);
  - learning disability;
  - adults with class 3 obesity (BMI of 40 kg/m^2 and above).
- All children aged 2–3 years on 31st August 2024.
- All primary school-aged children (from reception to year 6).
- Secondary school-aged children in years 7–11.
- All pregnant females (including those who become pregnant during the flu season).
- All adults aged 65 years and over (including those who turn 65 by 31st March 2025).
- Residents of long-stay residential homes or other specific long-stay facilities, where rapid spread is likely to follow introduction of infection and cause high morbidity and mortality (this does not include, for instance, prisons, young offender institutions, or university halls of residence).
- Individuals who receive a carer's allowance, or who are the main carer of an older or disabled individual whose welfare may be at risk if the carer falls ill.
- Household contacts of immunocompromised individuals.
- Frontline health and social care workers.

Vaccine choice

Children aged 6 months to less than 2 years who are in a clinical risk group should be offered QIVc, if this is unavailable, QIVe may be offered.

Eligible children aged 2 to 17 years should be offered LAIV, as this has been shown to be more effective in children than inactivated influenza vaccines. Where parents decline LAIV for their child due to the porcine gelatine content, and for children in whom LAIV is contra-indicated or otherwise unsuitable, QIVc should be offered, if this is unavailable QIVe may be used. Children who have a very severely immunocompromised household contact should also be offered QIVc, or if unavailable QIVe, instead of LAIV.

Children aged 6 months to less than 9 years who are in a clinical risk group or who are household contacts of immunocompromised individuals, should be offered 2 doses of the appropriate influenza vaccine (at least 4 weeks apart) if they have never had the influenza vaccine previously.

Pregnant females (including those aged under 18 years) should be offered QIVc, if this is unavailable, QIVe may be offered.

Adults aged 18 to 59 years in a clinical risk group or other eligible group should be offered QIVc, if this is unavailable or unsuitable, QIVe may be offered.

Adults aged 60 to 64 years in a clinical risk group or other eligible group should be offered either QIVc or QIV-HD. If these are unavailable or unsuitable, QIVe may be offered.

Adults aged 65 years and over (including those who turn 65 by 31st March 2025) should be offered either aQIV or QIV-HD. If these are unavailable or unsuitable, QIVc may be offered.

For further information on the annual influenza programme, see UKHSA collection: **Annual flu programme** (available at: www.gov.uk/government/collections/annual-flu-programme).

For the management of influenza, see Influenza p. 757.

Useful Resources

Recommendations reflect the National flu immunisation programme plan 2024/2025. UK Health Security Agency, Department of Health and Social Care, and NHS England. June 2024.

www.gov.uk/government/publications/national-flu-immunisation-programme-plan-2024-to-2025

Chapter 19, Influenza, in *Immunisation against infectious disease*- 'The Green Book'. UK Health Security Agency. November 2023.

www.gov.uk/government/publications/influenza-the-green-book-chapter-19

Flu vaccination programme 2024 to 2025: information for healthcare practitioners. UK Health Security Agency. August 2024.

www.gov.uk/government/publications/flu-vaccination-programme-information-for-healthcare-practitioners/flu-vaccination-programme-2023-to-2024-information-for-healthcare-practitioners

Japanese encephalitis vaccine

14-Nov-2018

Overview

Japanese encephalitis is a mosquito-borne viral encephalitis caused by a *Flavivirus*.

Japanese encephalitis vaccine p. 1509 (*IXIARO*®) is an inactivated vaccine adsorbed onto an adjuvant. It is recommended for individuals who are going to reside in an area where Japanese encephalitis is endemic or epidemic. Travellers to South and South-East Asia and the Far East should be immunised if staying for a month or longer in endemic areas during the transmission season. Other travellers with shorter exposure periods should also be immunised if the risk is considered sufficient. Immunisation is also recommended for laboratory staff at risk of exposure to the virus.

The primary immunisation course of 2 doses should be completed at least one week before potential exposure to Japanese encephalitis virus.

In adults (aged under 65 years) and children (aged 2 months and over) at ongoing risk (including laboratory staff and long-term travellers), a single booster dose should be given 12 months after the primary immunisation course. A booster dose can be considered in adults aged 65 years and over, but the immune response is lower than in younger adults. For other travellers, a single booster dose should be given within 12–24 months after primary immunisation, before potential re-exposure to the Japanese encephalitis virus. Travellers aged 18–64 years should be offered a second booster dose at 10 years if they remain at risk.

Cases of Japanese encephalitis should be managed with supportive treatment.

Up-to-date information on the risk of Japanese encephalitis in specific countries can be obtained from the National Travel Health Network and Centre.

Useful Resources

Recommendations reflect Chapter 20, Japanese encephalitis, in *Immunisation against infectious disease*– 'The Green book'. Public Health England, June 2018.
www.gov.uk/government/publications/japanese-encephalitis-the-green-book-chapter-20

National Travel Health Network and Centre
nathnac.net

Measles, Mumps and Rubella vaccine

Overview

Measles vaccine has been replaced by a combined measles, mumps and rubella vaccine p. 1516 (MMR vaccine).

Measles, mumps and rubella vaccine aims to eliminate measles, mumps, and rubella (German measles) and congenital rubella syndrome. Every child should receive two doses of measles, mumps and rubella vaccine by entry to primary school, unless there is a valid contra-indication. Measles, mumps and rubella vaccine should be given irrespective of previous measles, mumps, or rubella infection or vaccination.

The first dose of measles, mumps and rubella vaccine is given to children at 1 year of age, on or after their first birthday. A second dose is given before starting school at 3 years and 4 months of age, or soon after (see Immunisation Schedule).

Children presenting for pre-school booster who have not received the first dose of measles, mumps and rubella vaccine should be given a dose of measles, mumps and rubella vaccine followed 3 months later by a second dose.

At school-leaving age or at entry into further education, measles, mumps and rubella vaccine immunisation should be offered to individuals of both sexes who have not received 2 doses during childhood. In those who have received only a single dose of measles, mumps and rubella vaccine in childhood, a second dose is recommended to achieve full protection. If 2 doses of measles, mumps and rubella vaccine are required, the second dose should be given one month after the initial dose. The decision on whether to vaccinate adults should take into consideration their vaccination history, the likelihood of the individual remaining susceptible, and the future risk of exposure and disease.

Measles, mumps and rubella vaccine should be used to protect against rubella in *seronegative women of child-bearing age* (see Immunisation Schedule); unimmunised healthcare workers who might put pregnant women and other vulnerable groups at risk of rubella or measles should be vaccinated. Measles, mumps and rubella vaccine may also be offered to previously *unimmunised and seronegative post-partum women* (see measles, mumps and rubella vaccine)— vaccination a few days after delivery is important because about 60% of congenital abnormalities from rubella infection occur in babies of women who have borne more than one child. Immigrants arriving after the age of school immunisation are particularly likely to require immunisation.

Contacts

Measles, mumps and rubella vaccine may also be used in the control of outbreaks of measles and should be offered to susceptible children aged over 6 months who are contacts of a case, within 3 days of exposure to infection. Children immunised before 12 months of age should still receive two doses of measles, mumps and rubella vaccine at the recommended ages. If one dose of measles, mumps and rubella vaccine has already been given to a child, then the second dose may be brought forward to at least one month after the first, to ensure complete protection. If the child is under 18 months of age and the second dose is given within 3 months of the first, then the routine dose before starting school at 3 years and 4 months of age (or soon after) should still be given. Children aged under 9 months for whom avoidance of measles infection is particularly important (such as those with history of recent severe illness) can be given normal immunoglobulin after exposure to measles; routine measles, mumps and rubella vaccine immunisation should then be given after at least 3 months at the appropriate age.

Measles, mumps and rubella vaccine is **not suitable** for prophylaxis following exposure to mumps or rubella since the antibody response to the mumps and rubella components is too slow for effective prophylaxis.

Children and adults with impaired immune response should not receive live vaccines (see advice on HIV). If they have been exposed to measles infection they should be given normal immunoglobulin.

Travel

Unimmunised travellers, including children over 6 months, to areas where measles is endemic or epidemic should receive measles, mumps and rubella vaccine. Children immunised before 12 months of age should still receive two doses of measles, mumps and rubella vaccine at the recommended ages. If one dose of measles, mumps and rubella vaccine has already been given to a child, then the second dose should be brought forward to at least one month after the first, to ensure complete protection. If the child is under 18 months of age and the second dose is given within 3 months of the first, then the routine dose before starting school at 3 years and 4 months of age (or soon after) should still be given.

Useful Resources

Advice reflects that in the handbook Immunisation against Infectious Disease (2013), which in turn reflects the guidance of the Joint Committee on Vaccination and Immunisation (JCVI). The advice also incorporates changes announced by the Chief Medical Officer and Health Department Updates. Chapters from the handbook (including updates since 2013) are available at:

www.gov.uk/government/collections/immunisation-against-infectious-disease-the-green-book

Meningococcal vaccines

20-Sep-2023

Overview

Meningococcal vaccines are inactivated and are available as either conjugated vaccines or as a multicomponent protein vaccine. The conjugate vaccines are made from capsular polysaccharides of serogroups A, C, W, and Y *Neisseria meningitidis* conjugated to a carrier protein (such as tetanus toxoid) to enhance immunogenicity. The conjugate vaccines are available as a combination preparation of haemophilus influenzae type b with meningococcal group C vaccine p. 1503 (**Hib/MenC**), or as a quadrivalent meningococcal groups A with C and W135 and Y vaccine p. 1510 (**MenACWY**). The multicomponent protein meningococcal group B vaccine (rDNA, component, adsorbed) p. 1509 (**4CMenB**) is made from 3 *N. meningitidis* proteins produced by recombinant DNA technology and a preparation of *N. meningitidis* group B outer membrane vesicles.

Pre-exposure prophylaxis

Routine childhood immunisation schedule

Meningococcal vaccinations are given as a component of the routine childhood immunisation programme (see Immunisation schedule p. 1472). Immunisation against infection by serogroup B of *Neisseria meningitidis* consists of a primary course of meningococcal group B vaccine (rDNA, component, adsorbed) p. 1509 (4CMenB) with 2 doses given 8 weeks apart, followed by a single booster dose of the 4CMenB vaccine at 1 year of age (usually on or after the child's first birthday). A single dose of the haemophilus influenzae type b with meningococcal group C vaccine p. 1503 (Hib/MenC) should also be given at 1 year of age to protect against infection by serogroup C of *N. meningitidis*; it is usually given at the same time as the 4CMenB booster dose.

The JCVI recommend prophylactic paracetamol p. 507 in children receiving 4CMenB with other routine immunisations under 1 year of age, to prevent fever following vaccination.

All individuals around the age of 13–15 years should be given a single dose of the conjugate meningococcal groups A with C and W135 and Y vaccine p. 1510 (MenACWY) (see Immunisation schedule p. 1472), including those who have already received a different meningococcal group C–containing vaccine over the age of 10 years. Individuals who have previously received the MenACWY conjugate vaccine under the age of 10 years (such as for travel reasons or because they were a close contact of a confirmed meningococcal case) will require an additional dose as scheduled. Individuals who have previously received the MenACWY conjugate vaccine at the age of 10 years or over (such as for travel reasons) do not require an additional dose as part of the routine immunisation programme.

First time entrants to further or higher education establishments, up to 25 years of age, who have not previously had a dose of MenACWY conjugate vaccine over the age of 10 years should be offered a single dose of the MenACWY conjugate vaccine. This includes both UK born and international students.

For further information on the MenACWY conjugate vaccine and the 4CMenB vaccine, see PHE guidance: **Meningococcal ACWY vaccination programme** and **Meningococcal B vaccination programme** (see *Useful resources*).

Individuals with unknown or incomplete vaccination history

Children under 1 year of age with unknown or incomplete vaccination histories should be given a primary course of 2 doses of the 4CMenB vaccine, ideally given 8 weeks apart. The 2 primary doses can be given 4 weeks apart if required to ensure the immunisation schedule is completed before the child's first birthday (i.e. if the schedule started at 10 months of age). The child should then be vaccinated according to the Immunisation schedule with a single booster dose of the 4CMenB vaccine and the Hib/MenC vaccine at 1 year of age, ideally ensuring at least an 8 week interval between the 4CMenB primary and booster doses (if primary doses have been given late, there should be a minimum 4 week interval between primary and booster doses). The Hib/MenC vaccine should be given at least 4 weeks after any previous Hib-containing vaccines.

Children 1 year to under 2 years of age with unknown or incomplete vaccination histories who have received less than 2 doses of 4CMenB within their first year of life, should receive 2 doses of 4CMenB given at least 8 weeks apart. However, they can be given 4 weeks apart if required to ensure the 2 dose schedule is completed before the child's second birthday (i.e. if the schedule started at 22 months of age). A single dose of the Hib/MenC vaccine should also be given.

Children 2 years to under 10 years of age with unknown or incomplete vaccination histories should receive a single dose of the Hib/MenC conjugate vaccine.

Individuals aged 10 years to under 25 years (including those attending further or higher education for the first time) who have an incomplete or uncertain vaccination history against meningococcal group C, should be offered a single dose of the MenACWY conjugate vaccine. No further meningococcal vaccinations are then required unless they are a close contact of a case of meningococcal infection, or for travel purposes.

For further information on the vaccination of individuals with uncertain or incomplete immunisation status, refer to Chapter 11, The UK immunisation schedule, in *Immunisation against infectious disease*- 'The Green Book' (available at: www.gov.uk/government/publications/immunisation-schedule-the-green-book-chapter-11) and UKHSA guidance: **Vaccination of individuals with uncertain or incomplete immunisation status** (available at: www.gov.uk/government/publications/vaccination-of-individuals-with-uncertain-or-incomplete-immunisation-status).

Immunosuppression and HIV

Individuals with asplenia, splenic dysfunction, complement disorders, or those who are taking monoclonal antibodies that inhibit the terminal complement pathway (such as eculizumab and ravulizumab) may be at increased risk of invasive meningococcal infection and require additional meningococcal vaccinations. Individuals who are taking monoclonal antibodies that inhibit the complement pathway should be vaccinated at least 2 weeks prior to starting therapy. For further information on immunising individuals at increased risk of meningococcal disease, see *Vaccines and asplenia, splenic dysfunction, or complement disorders* in Vaccination, general principles p. 1470.

Individuals with immunosuppression and HIV infection (regardless of CD4 count) should be given meningococcal vaccines according to the routine immunisation schedule (see Immunisation schedule p. 1472). Consider re-immunisation after treatment completion or recovery—specialist advice may be required. For further information on the use of meningococcal vaccines in individuals with HIV infection, refer to the British HIV Association guidelines (available at: www.bhiva.org/guidelines) and the Children's HIV Association guidelines (available at: www.chiva.org.uk/).

Travel

In some areas of the world, the risk of acquiring meningococcal infection is much higher than in the UK. For example, meningococcal infection is most common in sub-Saharan Africa, especially during the dry season (December to June). For travellers, the risk of acquiring meningococcal infection may be increased for those visiting areas prone to outbreaks or an area with a current outbreak. Travellers visiting those areas who are at greater risk include:

- long stay travellers in close contact with the local population;
- healthcare workers;
- those visiting friends and relatives;
- those who live or travel 'rough' (such as backpackers);
- individuals with asplenia, splenic dysfunction, or certain immune deficiencies.

All travellers should have a careful risk assessment prior to travel, taking into account their itinerary, duration of stay, and any planned activities. Travellers whose planned activities or medical conditions put them at an increased risk of meningococcal disease should consider vaccination with the MenACWY conjugate vaccine. Proof of vaccination against meningococcal capsular groups A, C, W, and Y is required for pilgrims and seasonal workers travelling to Saudi Arabia for Hajj and Umrah (where outbreaks of capsular groups A and W infections have occurred).

Further information on country-specific meningococcal risk is available from the National Travel Health Network and Centre (travelhealthpro.org.uk/) and Health Protection Scotland (www.travax.nhs.uk).

Laboratory staff

Any laboratory staff who handle strains of or clinical samples containing *Neisseria meningitidis* must receive a primary course of MenACWY conjugate vaccine and 4CMenB vaccine with booster doses of both vaccines every 5 years.

Post-exposure management

Meningitis (acute) and meningococcal septicaemia are notifiable diseases in the UK. For further information, see *Notifiable diseases* in Antibacterials, principles of therapy p. 573.

Advice on the management of cases, contacts, and outbreaks must be sought from health protection teams. For further advice on management (including antibacterial prophylaxis and vaccination) to prevent secondary infection, see PHE: **Guidance for public health management of meningococcal disease in the UK** (see *Useful resources*) and *Meningococcal meningitis: prevention of secondary cases* in Antibacterials, use for prophylaxis p. 574.

Useful Resources

Recommendations reflect Chapter 22, Meningococcal, in *Immunisation against infectious disease- 'The Green Book'.* UK Health Security Agency. May 2022.
www.gov.uk/government/publications/meningococcal-the-green-book-chapter-22

Meningococcal ACWY vaccination programme: Information for healthcare professionals. Public Health England. June 2020.
www.gov.uk/government/publications/menacwy-programme-information-for-healthcare-professionals

Meningococcal B vaccination: Information for healthcare professionals. Public Health England. July 2021.
www.gov.uk/government/publications/meningococcal-b-vaccine-information-for-healthcare-professionals

Guidance for public health management of meningococcal disease in the UK. Public Health England. August 2019.
www.gov.uk/government/publications/meningococcal-disease-guidance-on-public-health-management

Pertussis vaccine

18-Aug-2024

Overview

Acellular pertussis-containing vaccines are inactivated and are made from highly purified components of *Bordetella pertussis* adsorbed onto aluminium hydroxide or aluminium phosphate adjuvants to improve immunogenicity. The vaccines differ in source, number and amount of each component, and method of manufacture (resulting in differences in efficacy and frequency of side-effects), and are only available as part of combination preparations containing other vaccines. Pertussis-containing vaccines are recommended for primary immunisation, pre-school boosting, certain healthcare workers, and the maternal pertussis vaccination programme.

For guidance on vaccination of individuals with neurological conditions, refer to Chapter 24, Pertussis, in *Immunisation against infectious disease- 'The Green Book'* (see *Useful resources*).

Individuals with immunosuppression and HIV infection (regardless of CD4 count) should be vaccinated in accordance with the routine recommended immunisation schedule (see *Primary Immunisation* and *Booster dose*). Consider re-immunisation after treatment completion or recovery—specialist advice may be required. For further information on the use of pertussis-containing vaccines in individuals with HIV infection, refer to the British HIV Association guidelines (available at: www.bhiva.org/guidelines) and the Children's HIV Association guidelines (available at: www.chiva.org.uk/).

Primary immunisation

Pertussis vaccination is given as a component of the routine childhood immunisation programme for all children aged under 10 years (see Immunisation schedule p. 1472). If the child's routine immunisation is delayed, children aged under 10 years should be immunised at the earliest opportunity.

Immunisation consists of a primary course of 3 doses of the hexavalent diphtheria with tetanus, pertussis, hepatitis B, poliomyelitis and haemophilus influenzae type b vaccine p. 1502, given at intervals of 4 weeks from 2 months of age. If the course is interrupted it should be resumed but not repeated, allowing a 4 week interval between the remaining doses.

Early immunisation with the first dose can be given to infants from 6 weeks of age if required in certain circumstances, such as for travel to an endemic area. The course should then be completed with a minimum of 4 week intervals between the remaining doses.

For information on the vaccination of individuals with uncertain or incomplete immunisation status, refer to Chapter 11, The UK immunisation schedule, *in Immunisation against infectious disease- 'The Green Book'* (see *Useful resources*), and UKHSA guidance: **Vaccination of individuals with uncertain or incomplete immunisation status** (available at: www.gov.uk/government/publications/vaccination-of-individuals-with-uncertain-or-incomplete-immunisation-status).

Booster dose

A single booster dose of diphtheria with tetanus, pertussis and poliomyelitis vaccine p. 1502 is given 3 years after completion of the primary course, usually before school entry (see Immunisation schedule p. 1472). If the primary course was delayed, the booster dose can be given at the scheduled visit provided that it has been at least 1 year since the third primary dose.

Individuals aged 10 years or over who have only had three doses of pertussis vaccine do not need any further doses, except for occupational vaccination of certain healthcare workers, and during pregnancy.

Pregnancy

Routine vaccination of pregnant females with diphtheria with tetanus and pertussis vaccine p. 1501 is recommended between 16 to 32 weeks of each pregnancy as part of the maternal pertussis programme, usually around the time of the fetal anomaly scan (20 weeks) for operational reasons.

Females who miss the opportunity to be vaccinated may still be immunised after week 32 of pregnancy until delivery, however, this may not offer as high a level of passive protection to the infant, particularly if they are born pre-term. Females who have not received a pertussis-containing vaccine during pregnancy can be offered it in the 8 weeks following birth; this will protect the mother and may prevent them from becoming a source of infection for the infant, but it will not provide direct protection for the infant. For further information, see UKHSA guidance: **Pertussis (whooping cough) vaccination programme for pregnant women** (see *Useful resources*).

Healthcare workers

Healthcare workers can be an important source of infection for vulnerable infants and pregnant females. Occupational vaccination with a single dose of diphtheria with tetanus, pertussis and poliomyelitis vaccine should be offered to any healthcare worker who has not received a pertussis-containing vaccine in the previous 5 years and who has regular contact with pregnant females or young infants (under 3 months of age). Prioritisation of such healthcare workers for vaccination is based on their level of contact with infants and/or pregnant females. For further information on priority groups, see UKHSA guidance: **Occupational pertussis vaccination of healthcare workers** (see *Useful resources*).

Post-exposure management

Advice on the management of cases, contacts, and outbreaks should be sought from local health protection teams. The immunisation history of infected individuals and their contacts should be determined.

For further guidance on the definition of close contacts, priority groups for public health action, and the management of cases, see UKHSA **Guidance on the management of cases of pertussis in England during the re-emergence of pertussis in 2024** (see *Useful resources*).

Cases

Pertussis is a notifiable disease in the UK. For further information, see *Notifiable diseases* in Antibacterials, principles of therapy p. 573.

Based on clinical judgement, antibacterials may be offered to pertussis cases within 14 days from onset of cough. If the case has a household contact or other close contact who is in priority group 1 for public health action, or who is pregnant, then antibacterial treatment should be offered to the case, commencing within 21 days of onset of cough.

Unimmunised and partially immunised individuals aged up to 10 years should complete their primary and booster vaccination against pertussis once they have recovered. Routine immunisation against pertussis is not recommended for those aged 10 years and over, except for pregnant females and certain healthcare workers (see *Pregnancy* and *Healthcare workers*).

Contacts

Antibacterial prophylaxis should be offered to close contacts of the index case when coughing in the index case started within the preceding 14 days and if the close contact is in a priority group for public health action. For guidance on antibacterial prophylaxis in contacts, see *Pertussis: prevention of secondary cases* in Antibacterials, use for prophylaxis p. 574.

Unimmunised or partially immunised contacts under the age of 10 years should complete their primary and booster vaccination against pertussis. Any pregnant contacts who have reached or passed their 20th week of pregnancy and have not yet received a pertussis-containing vaccine, and females who have an infant under 8 weeks of age and who did not receive a pertussis-containing vaccine during that pregnancy should be vaccinated (see *Pregnancy*). Contacts who are healthcare workers who provide close, personal care

to infants in priority group 1 or to pregnant females, should be given a booster dose of a pertussis-containing vaccine if they have not received one in the last 5 years and have not received diphtheria with tetanus and poliomyelitis vaccine p. 1501 in the preceding month.

Useful Resources

Recommendations reflect Chapter 24, Pertussis, in *Immunisation against infectious disease-* 'The Green Book'. UK Health Security Agency. June 2024.
www.gov.uk/government/publications/pertussis-the-green-book-chapter-24

Guidance on the management of cases of pertussis in England during the re-emergence of pertussis in 2024. UK Health Security Agency. August 2024.
www.gov.uk/government/publications/pertussis-guidelines-for-public-health-management

Occupational pertussis vaccination of healthcare workers. UK Health Security Agency. August 2024.
www.gov.uk/government/publications/pertussis-occupational-vaccination-of-health-care-workers/occupational-pertussis-vaccination-of-healthcare-workers

Pertussis (whooping cough) vaccination programme for pregnant women. UK Health Security Agency. August 2024
www.gov.uk/government/publications/vaccination-against-pertussis-whooping-cough-for-pregnant-women

Pneumococcal vaccine
25-Feb-2025

Overview

The pneumococcal polysaccharide conjugate vaccine (adsorbed) p. 1510 and the pneumococcal polysaccharide vaccine p. 1511 protect against infection with *Streptococcus pneumoniae* (pneumococcus). Both types of vaccine are inactivated and contain polysaccharide from capsular pneumococci. The pneumococcal polysaccharide vaccine contains purified polysaccharide from 23 capsular types of pneumococcus (PPV23), whereas the pneumococcal polysaccharide conjugate vaccine (adsorbed) contains polysaccharide from either 13 capsular types (*Prevenar* 13® (PCV13)), 15 capsular types (*Vaxneuvance*® (PCV15)), or 20 capsular types (*Prevenar* 20® (PCV20)).

PCV13 or PCV15 are used for childhood immunisation, and are given as a 2-dose schedule at separate intervals (see Immunisation schedule p. 1472). Children who present late for vaccination should be immunised according to *Children with unknown or incomplete vaccination histories*. PCV20 is not currently recommended as part of the routine UK immunisation schedule.

For guidance for those with an at-risk condition, see *Individuals with an at-risk condition*.

PPV23 is recommended for all adults aged 65 years and over (including those immunised during the influenza season), and for adults and children aged 2 years and over in the following at-risk groups:

- asplenia or splenic dysfunction (including homozygous sickle cell disease and coeliac syndrome which could lead to splenic dysfunction);
- chronic respiratory disease (including severe asthma treated with continuous or frequent use of a systemic corticosteroid);
- chronic heart disease;
- chronic renal disease;
- chronic liver disease;
- chronic neurological disease;
- diabetes mellitus requiring insulin or anti-diabetic medication;
- immunosuppression because of disease (such as HIV infection regardless of immune status, and genetic disorders affecting the immune system) or treatment (such

as prolonged systemic corticosteroid treatment for over 1 month at dose equivalents of prednisolone: *adult and child 20 kg and over*, 20 mg or more daily; *child under 20 kg*, 1 mg/kg or more daily, and chemotherapy);

- presence of cochlear implant;
- conditions where leakage of cerebrospinal fluid may occur.

PPV23 should also be considered for those at risk of frequent or continuous occupational exposure to metal fume (such as welders).

Where possible, the vaccine should be given at least 2 weeks (ideally 4–6 weeks) before splenectomy, immunosuppressive treatment, chemotherapy or radiotherapy; patients should be given advice about the increased risk of pneumococcal infection. If it is not possible to vaccinate at least 2 weeks before splenectomy, chemotherapy or radiotherapy, the vaccine should be given at least 2 weeks after the splenectomy, and at least 3 months after completion of chemotherapy or radiotherapy. Vaccination advice for patients with leukaemia or those who have had a bone marrow transplant, and information on patient cards and leaflets for individuals with asplenia, is available in Chapter 25, Pneumococcal, in *Immunisation against infectious disease- 'The Green Book'* (see *Useful resources*).

Vaccination regimens may differ depending on the individual's age, risk of pneumococcal disease, vaccination history, and immune status. Individuals in at-risk groups may require additional protection.

For information on revaccination with PPV23 for individuals in whom the antibody concentration is likely to decline rapidly, see *Revaccination*.

Children with unknown or incomplete vaccination histories

Unimmunised or partially immunised children who present late for vaccination and before the age of 1 year should receive a single dose of PCV13 or PCV15, followed by a booster dose on or after their first birthday, at least 4 weeks after the 1st dose.

Children aged 1 year to under 2 years who are unimmunised or partially immunised should receive a single dose of PCV13 or PCV15.

Individuals with an at-risk condition

Children diagnosed with at-risk conditions aged under 1 year
Children in an at-risk group (excluding those with asplenia, splenic dysfunction or complement disorder, or who are severely immunocompromised) should receive the PCV13 or PCV15 according to the Immunisation schedule p. 1472. Those who present late for vaccination should be immunised according to *Children with unknown or incomplete vaccination histories*. A single dose of PPV23 should then be given at 2 years of age, at least 8 weeks after the last dose of PCV13 or PCV15.

Children who are severely immunocompromised, or those with asplenia, splenic dysfunction or complement disorders, should receive 2 doses of PCV13 or PCV15 at least 8 weeks apart (commencing no earlier than 6 weeks of age), followed by a single booster dose given on or after their first birthday. An additional dose of PCV13 or PCV15 should be given at least 8 weeks after the booster dose. A single dose of PPV23 should then be given at 2 years of age, at least 8 weeks after the last dose of PCV13 or PCV15.

For further information on vaccination in individuals with asplenia, splenic dysfunction, or complement disorders, see Vaccination, general principles p. 1470.

Children diagnosed with at-risk conditions aged 1 year to under 2 years
Children in an at-risk group (excluding those with asplenia, splenic dysfunction or complement disorder, or who are severely immunocompromised) should receive their PCV13 or PCV15 booster dose according to the Immunisation

schedule p. 1472. Those who present late for vaccination should be immunised according to *Children with unknown or incomplete vaccination histories*. A single dose of PPV23 should then be given at 2 years of age, at least 8 weeks after the last dose of PCV13 or PCV15.

Children who are severely immunocompromised, or those with asplenia, splenic dysfunction or complement disorders, should receive their PCV13 or PCV15 booster dose according to the Immunisation schedule p. 1472. Those who present late for vaccination should be immunised according to *Children with unknown or incomplete vaccination histories*. An additional dose of PCV13 or PCV15 should be given at least 8 weeks after the booster dose. A single dose of PPV23 should then be given at 2 years of age, at least 8 weeks after the last dose of PCV13 or PCV15.

For further information on vaccination in individuals with asplenia, splenic dysfunction, or complement disorders, see Vaccination, general principles p. 1470.

Children diagnosed with at-risk conditions aged 2 years to under 10 years
Children diagnosed or first presenting with an at-risk condition (excluding those severely immunocompromised) who have completed their routine immunisation schedule should receive a single dose of PPV23, at least 8 weeks after the last dose of PCV13 or PCV15.

Children diagnosed or first presenting with an at-risk condition (excluding those severely immunocompromised) who are previously unimmunised or partially immunised should receive a single dose of PCV13 or PCV15, followed by a single dose of PPV23 at least 8 weeks later.

For further information on vaccination in individuals with asplenia, splenic dysfunction, or complement disorders, see Vaccination, general principles p. 1470.

Severely immunocompromised children should be given a single dose of PCV13 or PCV15, regardless of immunisation status. This should be followed by a single dose of PPV23, at least 8 weeks after the last dose of PCV13 or PCV15.

Individuals diagnosed with at-risk conditions aged 10 years and over
Unimmunised or partially immunised individuals diagnosed or first presenting with an at-risk condition (excluding those with asplenia, splenic dysfunction, complement disorder, or who are severely immunocompromised) should receive a single dose of PCV13 or PCV15, followed by a single dose of PPV23 at least 8 weeks after.

Previously immunised individuals diagnosed or first presenting with an at-risk condition (excluding those who are severely immunocompromised) should be given a single dose of PPV23 at least 8 weeks after the last dose of PCV13 or PCV15. PPV23 is not required for individuals with asplenia, splenic dysfunction or complement disorders if they have already received a dose within the previous 2 years (due to a theoretical risk of pneumococcal serotype-specific hypo-responsiveness with revaccination).

For further information on vaccination in individuals with asplenia, splenic dysfunction, or complement disorders, see Vaccination, general principles p. 1470.

Severely immunocompromised individuals should be given a single dose of PCV13 or PCV15, followed by a single dose of PPV23 at least 8 weeks after. PCV13 or PCV15 or additional PPV23 are not required if PPV23 has already been received within the previous 2 years, due to a theoretical risk of pneumococcal serotype-specific hypo-responsiveness with re-vaccination.

Revaccination

Revaccination is not recommended for any clinical risk groups or age groups, except for individuals in whom the antibody concentration is likely to decline rapidly (e.g. asplenia, splenic dysfunction, or chronic renal disease), where revaccination is recommended every 5 years.

Management of cases

For the management of cases, contacts and outbreaks, refer to Chapter 25, Pneumococcal, in *Immunisation against infectious disease- 'The Green Book'* (see *Useful resources*).

Useful Resources

Recommendations reflect Chapter 25, Pneumococcal, in *Immunisation against infectious disease- 'The Green Book'*. UK Health Security Agency, August 2023.
www.gov.uk/government/publications/pneumococcal-the-green-book-chapter-25

Poliomyelitis vaccine

Overview

Two types of poliomyelitis vaccines (containing strains of poliovirus types 1, 2, and 3) are available, inactivated poliomyelitis vaccine (for injection) and live (oral) poliomyelitis vaccine. **Inactivated** poliomyelitis vaccines, only available in combined preparation, is recommended for routine immunisation.

A course of primary immunisation consists of 3 doses of a combined preparation containing inactivated poliomyelitis vaccines, starting at 2 months of age with intervals of 1 month between doses (see Immunisation schedule). A course of 3 doses should also be given to all unimmunised adults; no adult should remain unimmunised against poliomyelitis.

Two booster doses of a preparation containing inactivated poliomyelitis vaccines are recommended, the first before school entry and the second before leaving school (see Immunisation schedule). Further booster doses are only necessary for adults at special risk, such as travellers to endemic areas, or laboratory staff likely to be exposed to the viruses, or healthcare workers in possible contact with cases; booster doses should be given to such individuals every 10 years.

Live (oral) poliomyelitis vaccine is no longer available for routine use; its use may be considered during large outbreaks, but advice should be sought from Public Health England. The live (oral) vaccine poses a very rare risk of vaccine-associated paralytic polio because the attenuated strain of the virus can revert to a virulent form. For this reason the live (oral) vaccine must **not** be used for immunosuppressed individuals or their household contacts. The use of inactivated poliomyelitis vaccines removes the risk of vaccine-associated paralytic polio altogether.

Travel

Unimmunised travellers to areas with a high incidence of poliomyelitis should receive a full 3-dose course of a preparation containing inactivated poliomyelitis vaccines. Those who have not been vaccinated in the last 10 years should receive a booster dose of **adsorbed diphtheria [low dose], tetanus and poliomyelitis (inactivated) vaccine**. Information about countries with a high incidence of poliomyelitis can be obtained from www.travax.nhs.uk/ or from the National Travel Health Network and Centre (www.nathnac.org/).

Useful Resources

Advice reflects that in the handbook Immunisation against Infectious Disease (2013), which in turn reflects the guidance of the Joint Committee on Vaccination and Immunisation (JCVI). The advice also incorporates changes announced by the Chief Medical Officer and Health Department Updates. Chapters from the handbook (including updates since 2013) are available at:
www.gov.uk/government/collections/immunisation-against-infectious-disease-the-green-book

Rabies vaccine

09-Jun-2023

Overview

The rabies vaccine p. 1511 contains inactivated rabies virus cultured in purified chick embryo cells.

Pre-exposure prophylaxis

Immunisation with the rabies vaccine should be offered to individuals considered to be at risk of exposure to rabies within the UK, this includes:
- laboratory staff who routinely handle the rabies virus;
- workers at Defra-authorised quarantine premises and carriers;
- those who regularly handle bats, including on a voluntary basis;
- veterinary and technical staff who, by reason of their employment, encounter enhanced risk;
- recreational cavers.

Immunisation is also recommended for individuals considered to be at risk of exposure to rabies travelling outside the UK, including:
- animal control and wildlife workers, veterinary staff or zoologists who regularly work in rabies enzootic (high risk) areas;
- travellers to rabies enzootic areas, especially if:
  ‣ post-exposure medical care and rabies biologics at the destination are lacking or in short supply;
  ‣ they are undertaking higher risk activities such as cycling, running, or recreational caving;
  ‣ they are living or staying there for more than 1 month.

Immunisation against rabies requires a primary pre-exposure course of 3 doses administered over 21 or 28 days (preferred schedule if time allows), or an accelerated course of 3 doses over 7 days with an additional dose at 1 year. For dosing schedules, see rabies vaccine.

For further information on pre-exposure prophylaxis in individuals with immunosuppression and/or HIV infection, see *Immunosuppression and HIV infection*.

Boosters

The requirement for booster doses is dependent on an individual's indication for pre-exposure prophylaxis and the likely frequency of ongoing exposures.

For laboratory workers who handle lyssavirus containing material (includes the rabies virus) a single booster dose of rabies vaccine should be given 1 year after the primary course has been completed. Further booster doses should be given based on 6-monthly antibody levels.

For individuals who may have frequent unrecognised exposures to the virus (such as bat handlers) a single booster dose of rabies vaccine should be given 1 year after the primary course has been completed. Antibody levels 1 year after the last vaccine dose will determine the requirement for a further booster dose and/or further testing.

For individuals at infrequent risk of exposure but who are likely to have an unrecognised exposure (such as recreational cavers, veterinarians investigating suspected rabies cases and non-compliant imported pets, engineers maintaining rabies laboratory equipment, or those entering rabies laboratories but not directly working with the virus), antibody levels 1 year after the primary course will determine the requirement for a booster dose and/or further testing.

For further information on antibody testing and booster doses, see UKHSA guidance: **Guidelines on timing of rabies boosters based on antibody levels** (see *Useful resources*).

Travel

Routine booster doses are not recommended for most travellers. A single booster dose of rabies vaccine can be considered following a risk assessment in those who have completed a primary course over 1 year ago, and who are travelling to an enzootic area again. Only 1 booster is needed in a traveller's lifetime.

Further information on country-specific rabies travel risk is available from the National Travel Health Network and Centre (travelhealthpro.org.uk/) and, in Scotland, from Health Protection Scotland (www.hps.scot.nhs.uk).

Post-exposure management

Rabies is a notifiable disease in the UK. For further information, see *Notifiable diseases* in Antibacterials, principles of therapy p. 573.

Following potential exposure to rabies, the wound or site of exposure (e.g. mucous membrane) should be cleansed under running water and washed for several minutes with soapy water as soon as possible. Disinfectant and a simple dressing can be applied, but suturing should be delayed until post-exposure treatment has begun otherwise it may increase the risk of introducing rabies virus into the nerves. Antibacterial therapy may be required for some animal bites, see *Human and animal bites* in Skin infections, antibacterial therapy p. 589 for further guidance. For puncture wounds, tetanus risk should also be assessed, see Tetanus vaccine p. 1493 for information on the management of tetanus-prone wounds.

A full, rapid post-exposure risk assessment (based on detailed information about the circumstances of the potential exposure) is required so that post-exposure treatment, if indicated, can be started promptly. When post-exposure treatment is indicated, this should always be started without delay, even in the presence of other illness. If the exposure occurred many months or years previously, a full risk assessment should always be done and treatment considered as the incubation period for rabies can be prolonged.

The regimen used for post-exposure management depends on the composite rabies risk (assessed as a green, amber, or red rating using a combination of the country where the incident occurred and the type of animal involved, and the category of exposure), and the individual's past medical history (including immune status). For further information on risk assessment (including composite rabies risk) and the management of potential rabies exposure, see UKHSA guidance: **Guidelines on managing rabies post-exposure** (see *Useful resources*).

For individuals arriving in the UK who started post-exposure treatment via the intradermal route, the remaining doses should be given intramuscularly. If the regimen started was different to the UK regimen—seek specialist advice.

For post-exposure management in individuals with immunosuppression, see *Immunosuppression and HIV infection*; and for country-specific specialist contact details in England, Wales, Scotland and Northern Ireland, see Chapter 27: Rabies, in *Immunisation against infectious disease- 'The Green Book'*.

Post-exposure treatment of individuals who are fully immunised

Fully immunised individuals are those who have received at least 3 documented doses of rabies vaccine (on at least 2 separate days either as a primary pre-exposure prophylaxis course or as part of a previous post-exposure treatment course), or documented rabies virus neutralising antibody (VNA) titres of at least 0.5 IU/ml.

For *fully immunised* individuals with a *green* composite rabies risk or who have completed a rabies post-exposure treatment course in the last 3 months, no treatment is required.

For *fully immunised* individuals with an *amber* or *red* composite rabies risk, give 2 doses of rabies vaccine (first dose on day 0 and second dose between days 3–7). Rabies immunoglobulin is not needed for these individuals. If rabies immunoglobulin is inadvertently given, individuals will need

to complete a 4 dose course of rabies vaccine (on days 0, 3, 7 and 21).

Post-exposure treatment of individuals who are partially immunised

Partially immunised individuals are those who have had an incomplete/inadequate primary pre-exposure prophylaxis course or documented rabies virus neutralising antibody titres consistently less than 0.5 IU/mL.

For *partially immunised* individuals with a *green* composite rabies risk, no treatment is required.

For *partially immunised* individuals with an *amber* or *red* composite rabies risk, give 4 doses in total of rabies vaccine p. 1511 (on days 0, 3, 7 and 21). If the fourth dose of rabies vaccine is given before day 21, a fifth dose of vaccine should be administered 2 weeks after the fourth dose. Rabies immunoglobulin is not needed for these individuals.

Post-exposure treatment of individuals who are non-immunised

Non-immunised individuals are those who have never received rabies pre- or post-exposure immunisation.

For *non-immunised* individuals with a *green* composite rabies risk, no treatment is required.

For *non-immunised* individuals with an *amber* or *red* composite rabies risk, give 4 doses in total of rabies vaccine (on days 0, 3, 7 and 21). If the fourth dose of rabies vaccine is given before day 21, a fifth dose of vaccine should be administered 2 weeks after the fourth dose.

Individuals with a *red* composite rabies risk should also be given rabies immunoglobulin p. 1468. This is not required if more than 7 days has passed since the first dose of rabies vaccine or more than 1 day since the second dose, or if the exposure was more than 12 months ago.

Immunosuppression and HIV infection

Refer to the British HIV Association for further information on the use of *rabies vaccine* and *rabies immunoglobulin* in individuals with HIV infection. See www.bhiva.org/guidelines for further information.

Pre-exposure prophylaxis

Pre-exposure prophylaxis may be given to individuals with immunosuppression and/or HIV infection (regardless of CD4 count), but these individuals may not develop a full antibody response.

Individuals who are immunosuppressed or who become immunosuppressed at any point after receiving a primary course of immunisation, or after having an antibody test or booster, should be informed about the serious risks of continuing with activities that could potentially expose them to rabies as it is possible that they may not respond to post-exposure vaccine.

If immunisation is still required, antibody levels may be required 2 weeks after the last dose of vaccine to ensure an adequate immune response. For further information, see UKHSA guidance: **Guidelines on timing of rabies boosters based on antibody levels** (see *Useful resources*).

In individuals with immunosuppression and HIV infection, re-immunisation should be considered upon completion of treatment and recovery has occurred, or in those with HIV when there has been immune recovery following commencement of antiretroviral treatment (such as a CD4 count >200 per mm^3).

Post-exposure management

For *immunosuppressed* individuals with a *green* composite rabies risk, no treatment is required.

For *immunosuppressed* individuals with an *amber* or *red* composite rabies risk, give 5 doses of rabies vaccine (on days 0, 3, 7, 14, and 30) and rabies immunoglobulin—specialist advice should be sought for individuals who have commenced post-exposure vaccination without rabies immunoglobulin, or if the exposure was more than 12 months ago. Post-exposure treatment response should be confirmed using antibody testing at the same time as the fifth dose (day 30); further antibody tests may be required depending on the results.

Useful Resources

Recommendations reflect Chapter 27, Rabies, in *Immunisation against infectious disease-* 'The Green Book'. Public Health England, May 2023.
www.gov.uk/government/publications/rabies-the-green-book-chapter-27
  Guidelines on managing rabies post-exposure. UK Health Security Agency, January 2023.
www.gov.uk/government/publications/rabies-post-exposure-prophylaxis-management-guidelines
  Guidelines on timing of rabies boosters based on antibody levels. UK Health Security Agency, June 2022.
www.gov.uk/government/publications/rabies-post-exposure-treatment-timing-of-vaccine-booster

Rotavirus vaccine

11-Jan-2022

Overview

Rotavirus vaccine p. 1517 is a live, oral vaccine that protects young children against gastro-enteritis caused by rotavirus infection.
  Prior to vaccination with the rotavirus vaccine, the result of the severe combined immunodeficiency (SCID) screening should be checked. For further information, see PHE guidance: **The rotavirus vaccination programme: information for healthcare professionals** (see *Useful resources*).
  The recommended schedule consists of 2 doses, the first at 8 weeks of age, and the second at 12 weeks of age (see Immunisation schedule p. 1472). The first dose of rotavirus vaccine must be given between 6 weeks and under 15 weeks of age and the second dose should be given after an interval of at least 4 weeks; the vaccine should not be started in children 15 weeks of age or older. Ideally, the full course should be completed before 16 weeks of age to provide protection before the main burden of disease, and to avoid a temporal association between vaccination and intussusception; the course must be completed before 24 weeks of age.
  Children who inadvertently receive the first dose of rotavirus vaccine at 15 weeks of age or older should still receive a second dose after at least 4 weeks, providing that they will still be under 24 weeks of age at the time.
  The rotavirus vaccine virus is excreted in the stool and may be transmitted to close contacts; however, vaccination of children with *immunosuppressed* close contacts may protect the contacts from wild-type rotavirus disease and outweigh any risk from transmission of vaccine virus. Carers of a recently vaccinated child should be advised of the need to wash their hands after changing the child's nappies.

Useful Resources

Recommendations reflect Chapter 27b, Rotavirus, in *Immunisation against infectious disease–* 'The Green book'. UK Health Security Agency, August 2015.
www.gov.uk/government/publications/rotavirus-the-green-book-chapter-27b
  The rotavirus vaccination programme: information for healthcare professionals. Public Health England, September 2021.
www.gov.uk/government/publications/rotavirus-qas-for-healthcare-practitioners

Smallpox and mpox vaccine

06-Feb-2023

Overview

The smallpox and mpox (monkeypox) viruses belong to the genus *orthopoxvirus*, which also includes the vaccinia virus. The smallpox and mpox vaccine (*Imvanex®*, also known as MVA-BN) is prepared from the live vaccinia virus which has been modified so that it has very limited replication capability, and should be considered as an inactivated vaccine. When supplies of the vaccine are limited, its use should be prioritised according to whether it is for pre- or post-exposure use, the risk and timing of exposure, and the ability to benefit.
  Medical practitioners must notify the proper officer at their local council or local health protection team of all suspected cases of smallpox or mpox. For further information, see *Notifiable diseases* in Antibacterials, principles of therapy p. 573.
  For further guidance on smallpox and mpox, see Chapter 29: Smallpox and monkeypox, in *Immunisation against infectious disease-* 'The Green Book' (see *Useful resources*) and the UKHSA collection: **Mpox (monkeypox): guidance** (available at: www.gov.uk/government/collections/monkeypox-guidance).

Pre-exposure prophylaxis

Routine immunisation against smallpox and mpox is not indicated, however staff who work in specialist roles where exposure to mpox or other orthopoxviruses is likely to be more common may be offered vaccination following a risk assessment.
  During outbreaks or incidents of mpox, pre-exposure vaccination may be extended to other groups of staff, and to individuals at increased risk of exposure.

Pre-exposure vaccination regime

The primary course for individuals not previously vaccinated against smallpox or mpox consists of an initial dose of the smallpox and mpox vaccine, followed by a second dose after at least 28 days. For individuals who have previously received a single dose of the vaccine, completion of the primary course is recommended; there is no need to restart the course. Individuals who have previously been vaccinated against smallpox with a live smallpox vaccine only require a single dose of the smallpox and mpox vaccine. For information on vaccination in individuals with immunosuppression, see *Immunosuppression and HIV*.
  For further guidance on pre-exposure prophylaxis, see Chapter 29: Smallpox and monkeypox, in *Immunisation against infectious disease-* 'The Green Book' and UKHSA: **Recommendations for the use of pre- and post-exposure vaccination during a monkeypox incident** (see *Useful resources*).

Post-exposure management

Post-exposure immunisation may provide protection against mpox infection, and modify disease severity in individuals with recent exposure. Individuals should be risk assessed and if appropriate, vaccination should be given within 4 days of exposure. Vaccination may be offered up to 14 days following exposure in individuals at ongoing risk of exposure or in those who are at higher risk of severe disease.

Post-exposure vaccination regime

A single dose of the smallpox and mpox vaccine should be given. For individuals who are at risk of future exposure and who have not received pre-exposure immunisation previously, a second dose should be given after at least 28 days.
  For individuals who have previously received a single dose of the smallpox and mpox vaccine, completion of the primary course is recommended; there is no need to restart the course. Individuals who have previously received a

2-dose course of the vaccine, with the second dose given in the past 2 years, do not need a further dose following exposure. However, for those who are immunosuppressed and who may have had a reduced immune response, an additional dose can be considered—seek specialist advice.

For individuals with a history of receiving a single dose of a live smallpox vaccine, a single dose of the smallpox and mpox vaccine is recommended following exposure.

For individuals who have received a previous live smallpox vaccine and 1 dose of the smallpox and mpox vaccine, no further doses are recommended after exposure.

For further guidance on post-exposure vaccination, see Chapter 29: Smallpox and monkeypox, in *Immunisation against infectious disease- 'The Green Book'* and UKHSA: **Recommendations for the use of pre- and post-exposure vaccination during a monkeypox incident** (see *Useful resources*).

Antiviral treatment

Tecovirimat should be offered to patients who are hospitalised due to mpox if they meet the eligibility criteria. For further guidance, see NHS England Clinical Commissioning Rapid Policy Statement: **Tecovirimat as treatment for patients hospitalised due to monkeypox virus infection** (available at: www.england.nhs.uk/ commissioning/publication/tecovirimat-as-treatment-for-patients-hospitalised-due-to-monkeypox-virus-infection/).

Booster doses

Individuals who have received a primary course of the smallpox and mpox vaccine should be offered a single booster dose 2 years after the primary course if they are considered to be at on-going risk of exposure. If the primary course included a live smallpox vaccine, seek specialist advice regarding the need for a booster dose.

Immunosuppression and HIV

The smallpox and mpox vaccine contains a replication defective virus and is considered safe to use in individuals who are immunosuppressed or living with HIV infection. The recommendations above for pre-exposure prophylaxis or post-exposure immunisation therefore apply to individuals with immunosuppression or HIV. The immune response to the vaccine could be reduced in severely immunosuppressed individuals; specialist advice on other measures may be required and additional doses should be considered for those at ongoing-risk of exposure. Refer to the British HIV Association for further information on the use of smallpox and mpox vaccine in HIV-positive individuals (available at: www.bhiva.org/rapid-guidance-on-monkeypox-virus).

Useful Resources

Recommendations reflect Chapter 29, Smallpox and monkeypox, in *Immunisation against infectious disease- 'The Green Book'*. UK Health Security Agency. September 2022. www.gov.uk/government/publications/smallpox-and-vaccinia-the-green-book-chapter-29

Recommendations for the use of pre- and post-exposure vaccination during a monkeypox incident. UK Health Security Agency. August 2022. www.gov.uk/government/publications/monkeypox-vaccination

Tetanus vaccine

18-Aug-2024

Overview

Tetanus-containing vaccines are inactivated and are made from a cell-free purified toxin of *Clostridium tetani* adsorbed on aluminium hydroxide or aluminium phosphate to improve immunogenicity. The tetanus vaccine is only available as a combination preparation containing other vaccines.

Prophylaxis

In most circumstances, the recommended vaccination schedule, comprising of a total of 5 doses of tetanus-containing vaccine, is considered sufficient to provide long-term protection against tetanus infection.

Individuals due for their routine tetanus immunisation may not require their routine dose if they have a history of vaccination (such as for a tetanus-prone wound) with the same tetanus-containing vaccine that is due, and it was administered at an appropriate interval.

Parenteral drug misusers are at a greater risk of tetanus infection—every opportunity should be taken to ensure that they are fully vaccinated against tetanus.

For information on immunisation of individuals with neurological conditions, see Chapter 30, Tetanus, in *Immunisation against infectious disease- 'The Green Book'*.

For information on immunisation in pregnant females, see *Pregnancy*.

Individuals with immunosuppression or HIV infection (regardless of CD4 count) should be given the recommended vaccination schedule of 5 doses of a tetanus-containing vaccine (see *Primary Immunisation* and *Boosters*). Consider re-immunisation after treatment completion—specialist advice may be required. Refer to the British HIV Association and the Children's HIV Association for further information on the use of tetanus-containing vaccines in individuals with HIV infection. See www.bhiva.org/guidelines or www.chiva.org.uk/ for further information.

Primary immunisation

Tetanus vaccination is given as a component of the routine childhood immunisation programme for children aged under 10 years (see Immunisation schedule p. 1472). If the child's routine immunisation is delayed, children aged under 10 years should be immunised at the earliest opportunity.

Children aged under 10 years, should be given a primary course consisting of 3 doses of the hexavalent diphtheria with tetanus, pertussis, hepatitis B, poliomyelitis and haemophilus influenzae type b vaccine p. 1502 at intervals of 4 weeks (it is the only suitable vaccine containing high dose tetanus for priming children of this age). If interrupted, the primary course should be resumed but not repeated, allowing a 4 week interval between doses. For information on circumstances where early immunisation, or alternative dosing intervals for primary immunisation may be considered, see UKHSA guidance: **The hexavalent DTaP/IPV/Hib/HepB combination vaccine: information for healthcare practitioners** (see *Useful resources*).

If the primary course was commenced with the pentavalent diphtheria with tetanus, pertussis, poliomyelitis and haemophilus influenzae type b vaccine p. 1502, it can be completed with the hexavalent diphtheria with tetanus, pertussis, hepatitis B, poliomyelitis and haemophilus influenzae type b vaccine.

Individuals aged 10 years and over who have not been immunised previously or have an unknown or incomplete history, should be given a primary course consisting of 3 doses of the diphtheria with tetanus and poliomyelitis vaccine p. 1501 at 4 week intervals. If interrupted, the primary course should be resumed but not repeated, allowing an interval of 4 weeks between doses.

For further information on vaccination of individuals with uncertain or incomplete immunisation status, see Chapter 11, The UK immunisation schedule, in *Immunisation against infectious disease- 'The Green Book'*.

Boosters

Following a primary course, 2 doses of a tetanus-containing booster vaccine should be given. When an individual presents for a booster dose but has a history of being vaccinated following a tetanus-prone wound, the vaccine preparation administered at the time of injury should be determined. If this is not possible, or the vaccine administered was not the same as the vaccine due at the current visit or was not given after an appropriate interval, the scheduled booster should still be given to ensure long-term protection against all antigens.

Children aged under 10 years should be given the diphtheria with tetanus, pertussis and poliomyelitis vaccine p. 1502 for their first booster dose. This is usually given 3 years after completing the primary course (before school entry)—see Immunisation schedule p. 1472. However, when primary immunisation has been delayed, it may be given at the scheduled visit provided it has been 1 year since the third dose of their primary course.

Individuals aged 10 years and over should be given the diphtheria with tetanus and poliomyelitis vaccine for their first booster dose. This should be at least 5 years after the third dose of their primary course.

All individuals should be given the diphtheria with tetanus and poliomyelitis vaccine for their second booster dose. This is usually given 10 years after the first booster, but if previous doses have been delayed, it may be given at the school session or scheduled visit provided there has been at least a 5 year interval since the first booster dose.

Parenteral drug misusers should be given booster doses if there is any doubt about their immunisation status.

Travel

All travellers should ensure they are fully immunised (or are up-to-date) with their tetanus vaccination (see *Primary Immunisation* and *Boosters*). Travellers who last received a tetanus booster dose more than 10 years ago and are travelling to areas where medical attention may not be accessible, should be given a booster dose of tetanus-containing vaccine prior to travel, even if they have previously received 5 doses of tetanus-containing vaccines. This is a precautionary measure in case immunoglobulin is not available to the individual in the event of a tetanus-prone injury.

Post-exposure management

Cases

Tetanus is a notifiable disease in the UK. For further information, see *Notifiable diseases* in Antibacterials, principles of therapy p. 573.

Intravenous normal immunoglobulin [unlicensed] is used for the treatment of tetanus (for further information, see Immunoglobulins p. 1462). Antibacterials (such as benzylpenicillin sodium p. 633 and metronidazole p. 628) may also be required—discuss with the microbiology team. Tetanus infection may not result in immunity and vaccination is recommended following recovery (see *Prophylaxis*). For further guidance on the management of confirmed and suspected cases of tetanus (including localised tetanus), see Chapter 30, Tetanus, in *Immunisation against infectious disease*- 'The Green Book' and UKHSA guidance: **Tetanus** (see *Useful resources*).

Prophylaxis of tetanus-prone wounds

Any wound can give rise to tetanus. *Clean wounds* (less than 6 hours old, non-penetrating and have negligible tissue damage) are considered to have a low likelihood of harbouring tetanus spores and of developing conditions that promote spore germination. *Tetanus-prone* wounds include compound fractures, certain animal bites and scratches, puncture-type injuries acquired in a contaminated environment (these are likely to contain tetanus spores), wounds or burns with systemic sepsis, and wounds containing foreign bodies—this list is not exhaustive. *High-risk tetanus-prone* wounds include any *tetanus-prone* wounds or burns that either show extensive devitalised tissue or require surgical intervention that is delayed more than 6 hours, or wounds that are heavily contaminated with material likely to contain tetanus spores (such as soil or manure).

Post-exposure management of tetanus-prone wounds depends on the individual's immunisation status and wound category (*clean, tetanus-prone,* or *high-risk tetanus-prone*). For the risk-assessment of tetanus-prone wounds, an *adequate priming course* of tetanus vaccine is considered to be at least 3 doses of tetanus-containing vaccine at appropriate intervals.

All wounds should be thoroughly cleaned, and surgical debridement of devitalised tissue in *high-risk tetanus-prone* wounds is essential for the prevention of tetanus infection.

For individuals aged 11 years and over who have received an adequate priming course of tetanus vaccine with the last dose given within 10 years, for children aged 5–10 years whose tetanus immunisation is up to date, and for children aged under 5 years who have received an adequate priming course, no immediate treatment is required regardless of wound category.

For individuals who have received an adequate priming course of tetanus vaccine but the last dose was given more than 10 years ago (includes those born in the UK after 1961 with a history of accepting vaccinations), and for children aged 5–10 years who have received an adequate priming course but no booster, give an immediate booster dose of a suitable tetanus-containing vaccine to individuals with a wound that is *tetanus-prone* or *high-risk tetanus-prone*. In addition, for a *high-risk tetanus-prone* wound, give a single dose of tetanus immunoglobulin p. 1468 at a different site (or if unavailable, normal immunoglobulin [unlicensed] may be used—for further guidance, see UKHSA guidance: **Tetanus** (see *Useful resources*).

For individuals who have not received an adequate priming course of tetanus vaccine (includes those with uncertain immunisation status and/or born before 1961), give an immediate booster dose of a suitable tetanus-containing vaccine regardless of wound category. In addition, for a *tetanus-prone* or *high-risk tetanus-prone* wound, give a single dose of tetanus immunoglobulin at a different site (or if unavailable, normal immunoglobulin [unlicensed] may be used—for further guidance, see UKHSA guidance: **Tetanus** (see *Useful resources*).

Individuals who are severely immunosuppressed may not be adequately protected against tetanus, despite being fully immunised. An additional booster dose of a suitable tetanus-containing vaccine and/or immunoglobulin may be required.

To ensure immunity against future exposure, all individuals who are not completely immunised should be given further doses of a suitable tetanus-containing vaccine as required to complete their recommended schedule (see *Prophylaxis*).

Antibacterial therapy may also be considered for tetanus-prone wounds depending on clinical severity, to prevent tetanus. For further guidance on the management of tetanus-prone wounds, see Chapter 30, Tetanus, in *Immunisation against infectious disease*- 'The Green Book' and UKHSA guidance: **Tetanus** (see *Useful resources*).

Pregnancy

Routine vaccination of pregnant females with diphtheria with tetanus and pertussis vaccine p. 1501 is recommended between 16 to 32 weeks of each pregnancy as part of the maternal pertussis programme, usually around the time of the fetal anomaly scan (20 weeks) for operational reasons. For further information, and for guidance for pregnant females with an incomplete or unknown vaccination history against diphtheria, tetanus and polio, see UKHSA guidance: **Pertussis (whooping cough) vaccination programme for pregnant women**, available at: www.gov.uk/government/publications/vaccination-against-pertussis-whooping-cough-for-pregnant-women.

Pregnant females may be given tetanus-containing vaccines where protection is needed without delay. For information on the management of cases and prophylaxis of tetanus-prone wounds, see *Post-exposure management*.

Useful Resources

Recommendations reflect Chapter 30, Tetanus, in *Immunisation against infectious disease-* 'The Green Book'. UK Health Security Agency, June 2022.
www.gov.uk/government/publications/tetanus-the-green-book-chapter-30

Tetanus: Guidance on the management of suspected cases and on the assessment and management of tetanus-prone wounds. UK Health Security Agency, September 2023.
www.gov.uk/government/publications/tetanus-advice-for-health-professionals

The hexavalent DTaP/IPV/Hib/HepB combination vaccine: information for healthcare practitioners. UK Health Security Agency, May 2023.
www.gov.uk/government/publications/hexavalent-combination-vaccine-programme-guidance

Tick-borne encephalitis vaccine

08-Jul-2020

Overview

The tick-borne encephalitis (TBE) vaccine contains inactivated TBE virus (Neudörfl strain) grown in chick embryo cells. It is recommended for the protection of individuals at high risk of exposure to the TBE virus through their work or travel.

Immunisation with the tick-borne encephalitis vaccine p. 1513 is therefore recommended for:

- individuals who travel, particularly in spring and summer, to endemic forested areas where ticks are most prevalent (including those who hike, camp, hunt, and undertake fieldwork);
- individuals who will be residing in an area where TBE is endemic or epidemic, especially those working in forestry, woodcutting, farming, and the military;
- laboratory workers who may be exposed to the TBE virus.

A 3 dose schedule of the tick-borne encephalitis vaccine is recommended for children aged 1 year and over, and for adults. Sufficient protection can be expected for the ongoing tick season after the first 2 doses, and for at least 3 years after the 3rd dose. Booster doses are required every 3–5 years for those still at risk of TBE exposure. For dosing schedules, see tick-borne encephalitis vaccine.

Refer to the British HIV Association for information on the use of tick-borne encephalitis vaccine in individuals with HIV infection. See www.bhiva.org/guidelines for further information.

Further information on preventing or reducing the risk of TBE is available from the National Travel Health Network and Centre (nathnac.net/) and Health Protection Scotland (www.travax.nhs.uk/).

Post-exposure management

Unvaccinated individuals bitten by ticks in endemic areas should seek local medical advice. No specific therapy is available following exposure to tick-borne encephalitis; supportive treatment can significantly reduce morbidity and mortality. If tick-borne encephalitis is suspected, the referring clinician should discuss the case with a clinician at the Public Health England Rare and Imported Pathogens Laboratory (contact details are available at: www.gov.uk/guidance/tick-borne-encephalitis-epidemiology-diagnosis-and-prevention).

Medical practitioners must notify the proper officer at their local council or local health protection team of all suspected cases of acute encephalitis of any cause. For further information, see *Notifiable diseases* in Antibacterials, principles of therapy p. 573.

Useful Resources

Recommendations reflect Chapter 31, Tick-borne encephalitis, in *Immunisation against infectious disease-* 'The Green Book'. Public Health England, April 2013.
www.gov.uk/government/publications/tick-borne-encephalitis-the-green-book-chapter-31

Typhoid vaccine

20-Aug-2023

Overview

Typhoid vaccines are available as a Vi capsular polysaccharide (from *Salmonella typhi*) vaccine for injection and a live, attenuated *Salmonella typhi* vaccine for oral use.

Typhoid immunisation is advised for:

- travellers to areas where typhoid is endemic and whose planned activities put them at higher risk (country-by-country information is available from the National Travel Health Network and Centre);
- travellers to endemic areas where frequent or prolonged exposure to poor sanitation and poor food hygiene is likely;
- laboratory personnel who, in the course of their work, may be exposed to *Salmonella typhi*.

Capsular polysaccharide typhoid vaccine (inactivated) p. 1513 is given as a single dose, usually by intramuscular injection. Children under 2 years [unlicensed] may respond suboptimally to the vaccine, but children aged between 1–2 years should be immunised if the risk of typhoid fever is considered high (immunisation is not recommended for infants under 12 months). A single booster dose should be given at 3-year intervals in adults and children over 2 years of age who remain at risk from typhoid fever.

Oral typhoid vaccine (live) p. 1517 is a live, attenuated vaccine contained in an enteric-coated capsule recommended in individuals aged 5 years and over. One capsule taken on alternate days for a total of 3 doses, provides protection 7–10 days after the last dose. If travelling from a non-endemic area to an area where typhoid is endemic, a booster consisting of 3 doses is recommended every 3 years. The oral typhoid vaccine should be avoided in immunosuppressed and HIV-infected individuals.

Prevention of typhoid primarily depends on improving sanitation and water supplies in endemic areas and on scrupulous personal, food and water hygiene.

All suspected cases of typhoid fever must be notified to the local health protection unit. Where there is a community level outbreak, specialist advice should be sought from Public Health England (tel. 020 8200 4400) or, in Scotland, Health Protection Scotland (tel. 0140 300 1191).

Useful Resources

Recommendations reflect Chapter 33, Typhoid, in *Immunisation against infectious disease–* 'The Green Book'. Public Health England, May 2019.
www.gov.uk/government/publications/typhoid-the-green-book-chapter-33

National Travel Health Network and Centre nathnac.net

Varicella-zoster vaccines

13-Jan-2025

Overview

The vaccine preparations *Varilrix*® and *Varivax*® contain live, attenuated virus derived from the Oka strain of varicella-zoster virus, whereas *Shingrix*® is a recombinant, adjuvanted vaccine that contains varicella-zoster virus glycoprotein E antigen—it does not contain any live virus.

The *Varilrix®* and *Varivax®* vaccines provide protection against varicella (chickenpox).

The *Shingrix®* vaccine provides protection against herpes zoster (shingles).

Pre-exposure prophylaxis against varicella (chickenpox)

Varicella immunisation aims to protect individuals who are at most risk of serious illness from exposure to the varicella-zoster virus, by vaccinating specific individuals who are in regular or close contact with those at risk. Individuals with a definite history of chickenpox or shingles can be considered immune. However, for individuals born and raised overseas, a history of chickenpox is a less reliable predictor of immunity and routine testing should be considered.

Vaccination with the chickenpox varicella-zoster vaccine p. 1518 (*Varilrix®* or *Varivax®*) is recommended for:

- non-immune or varicella-zoster antibody-negative healthcare workers who have patient contact (including cleaners, catering staff, and receptionists);
- non-immune laboratory staff who may be exposed to varicella-zoster virus in the course of their work in virology laboratories and clinical infectious disease units;
- non-immune healthy susceptible contacts (aged 9 months and over) of immunocompromised patients where continuing close contact is unavoidable.

Children aged 9–11 months should receive 2 doses of the chickenpox varicella-zoster vaccine at least 3 months apart. Children aged 1 year and over and adults, should receive 2 doses at least 4–8 weeks apart.

Vaccination should be postponed in acutely unwell individuals until they have fully recovered, unless protection is urgently required. There is no data on interchangeability between the *Varilrix®* or *Varivax®* vaccines, but it is likely that a course can be completed effectively with the different vaccine.

Within 1 month of vaccination, some individuals may develop a localised rash at the injection site or a generalised rash (papular or vesicular). Healthcare workers who develop a post-vaccine rash should consult their occupational health department for assessment before commencing work. The vaccine virus strain can also establish latent infection and reactivate to cause shingles in some individuals (the risk is substantially lower than with wild chickenpox infection)—cases of shingles should be investigated. For further information on vaccine-related cutaneous rashes, see *Cautions, further information* in varicella-zoster vaccine, and Chapter 34, Varicella, in *Immunisation against infectious disease*- 'The Green Book' (see *Useful resources*).

The chickenpox vaccines are not recommended for individuals with immunosuppression—seek specialist advice for those who require protection against chickenpox. Refer to the British HIV Association or Children's HIV Association for guidance in individuals with HIV infection (available at: www.bhiva.org/guidelines and www.chiva.org.uk).

Post-exposure management of varicella (chickenpox)

Chickenpox is only a notifiable disease in Northern Ireland. For further information, see *Notifiable diseases* in Antibacterials, principles of therapy p. 573.

For guidance on post-exposure prophylaxis with an antiviral and/or varicella-zoster immunoglobulin for certain individuals who are at an increased risk of severe chickenpox, see *Post-exposure prophylaxis* in Herpesvirus infections p. 727.

During outbreaks where chickenpox is co-circulating with group A streptococcus infections (such as scarlet fever) in nurseries and pre-school settings, certain non-immune children aged 9 months and over and staff working in these

settings can be given 2 doses of the chickenpox varicella-zoster vaccine at least 4–8 weeks apart. The UKHSA health protection team should be contacted for advice. For further information, see UKHSA guidance: **Guidelines for the public health management of scarlet fever outbreaks in schools, nurseries and other childcare settings** (available at: www.gov.uk/government/publications/scarlet-fever-managing-outbreaks-in-schools-and-nurseries).

Immunisation against herpes zoster (shingles)

The risk of occurrence and the severity of shingles and its complications, such as subsequent post herpetic neuralgia (PHN), increases with age and is high in individuals who are severely immunosuppressed. The national shingles vaccination programme aims to lower the incidence and severity of shingles in older people and individuals with severe immunosuppression; severely immunosuppressed individuals represent the highest priority for vaccination given their risk of severe disease.

The herpes zoster (shingles) vaccine (*Shingrix®*) is not recommended for shingles post-exposure prophylaxis, or for the treatment of shingles or PHN, but it can be given to eligible individuals with a previous history of shingles or who experience residual nerve pain that may be permanent. For further information, see UKHSA guidance: **Shingles immunisation programme: information for healthcare professionals** (see *Useful resources*).

Immunocompetent (non-immunosuppressed) individuals

As part of the national shingles vaccination programme, immunisation is now recommended for immunocompetent individuals aged 60–79 years—the extension in age eligibility is being implemented in a 2-stage phased approach over a 10-year period. The herpes-zoster vaccine (recombinant, adjuvanted) p. 1507 (*Shingrix®*) has also replaced the herpes-zoster vaccine (live) (*Zostavax®*) in the vaccination programme. For information on shingles immunisation in individuals with immunosuppression and/or HIV infection, see *Immunosuppression and HIV*.

All immunocompetent individuals aged 70 to 79 years who have not previously received immunisation, should be offered 2 doses of *Shingrix®*.

During stage 1 of the age eligibility implementation period, 2 doses of *Shingrix®* will be offered to individuals aged 65 and 70 years of age. Further extension of the eligible vaccination age will occur in stage 2, with the aim to eventually offer routine vaccination to all immunocompetent individuals at 60 years of age.

All individuals remain eligible until their 80th birthday. Individuals who have turned 80 years of age following their first dose of *Shingrix®*, should be given a second dose to complete the 2-dose schedule before their 81st birthday. If the course is interrupted or delayed, it should be resumed but the first dose should not be repeated.

The 2 doses of *Shingrix®* vaccine should be given at least 8 weeks apart. However, a longer dose interval of 6–12 months in England, Wales, and Northern Ireland, and 2–6 months in Scotland may be used for operational reasons.

The need for a booster dose has not been established.

As *Shingrix®* is a non-live vaccine, there are no risks of developing a vesicular rash following administration. If a vesicular rash does develop, it is likely that the patient has developed shingles naturally and should be referred for assessment and management.

For further guidance, see Chapter 28a, Shingles (herpes zoster), in *Immunisation against infectious disease*- 'The Green Book'; UKHSA guidance: **Shingles immunisation programme: information for healthcare professionals** (see *Useful resources*), and the **Shingles Eligibility Calculator** available at: www.healthpublications.gov.uk/ViewArticle.html?sp=Sshingleseliligibiltycalculatorfromseptember2023.

For information on post-exposure management, see *Post-exposure prophylaxis* in Herpesvirus infections p. 727.

Immunosuppression and HIV

The decision to offer the shingles vaccine to individuals who are immunosuppressed should be based on a full clinical assessment. Seek specialist advice if there are doubts or concerns about an individual's immunosuppressive treatment, or degree of immunosuppression. Refer to the British HIV Association for guidance in individuals with HIV infection (available at: www.bhiva.org/guidelines).

Individuals with non-severe immunosuppression aged 60–79 years should be immunised in accordance with the guidance for immunocompetent individuals, see *Immunocompetent (non-immunosuppressed) individuals*.

Individuals with severe immunosuppression aged 50 years and over should be offered 2 doses of *Shingrix*®, given 8 weeks to 6 months apart. If the course of *Shingrix*® is interrupted or delayed, it should be resumed but the first dose should not be repeated.

Individuals aged 50 years and over who are anticipating treatment with immunosuppressive therapy should receive 2 doses of *Shingrix*®, given 8 weeks apart, at the earliest opportunity and at least 14 days before starting immunosuppressive therapy, although leaving 1 month would be preferable if a delay is possible.

The need for a booster dose has not been established.

Individuals who have received a stem cell transplant are at a particularly increased risk of developing severe shingles regardless of their age. For guidance on immunisation for individuals aged 18–49 years who are not otherwise eligible, and for further information on shingles immunisation in immunosuppressed individuals, including the definition of severe immunosuppression and eligibility for the vaccination programme, see Chapter 28a, Shingles (herpes zoster), in *Immunisation against infectious disease- 'The Green Book'*, and UKHSA guidance: **Shingles immunisation programme: information for healthcare professionals** (see Useful resources).

For information on post-exposure management, see *Post-exposure prophylaxis* in Herpesvirus infections p. 727.

Pregnancy

The live *Varilrix*® and *Varivax*® vaccines are not recommended during pregnancy. All exposure to live vaccines from 3 months before conception to any time during pregnancy, should be reported to the UKHSA vaccination in pregnancy (VIP) surveillance programme. Pregnant women should be advised to seek prompt medical advice if they develop a vesicular rash following inadvertent vaccination. For advice on the reporting, risk assessment, and management of inadvertent vaccination in pregnancy, see UKHSA guidance: **Inadvertent vaccination in pregnancy (VIP)** (available at: www.gov.uk/guidance/vaccination-in-pregnancy-vip).

There is no known risk associated with vaccinating pregnant females with inactivated recombinant vaccines. If indicated, *Shingrix*® can be considered in pregnancy after full discussion of the risks and benefits.

Useful Resources

Recommendations reflect Chapter 34, Varicella, in *Immunisation against infectious disease- 'The Green Book'*. UK Health Security Agency, August 2015.
www.gov.uk/government/publications/varicella-the-green-book-chapter-34

Recommendations reflect Chapter 28a, Shingles (herpes zoster), in *Immunisation against infectious disease- 'The Green Book'*. UK Health Security Agency, April 2024.
www.gov.uk/government/publications/shingles-herpes-zoster-the-green-book-chapter-28a

Shingles immunisation programme: information for healthcare professionals. UK Health Security Agency, November 2024.
www.gov.uk/government/publications/shingles-vaccination-guidance-for-healthcare-professionals

---

Yellow fever vaccine　　23-Jan-2020

MHRA/CHM advice: stronger precautions in people with weakened immunity and in those aged 60 years or older

The MHRA and CHM have released important safety information regarding the use of the live yellow fever vaccine in those with weakened immunity, and in those aged 60 years or older. For further information, see *Important safety information* for yellow fever vaccine p. 1518.

Overview

Yellow fever vaccine is an attenuated preparation of yellow fever virus grown in chick eggs. Yellow fever vaccine is recommended for:

- laboratory workers handling infected material;
- individuals aged 9 months or older who are travelling to, or living in areas or countries with a risk of yellow fever transmission;
- individuals aged 9 months or older who are travelling to, or living in countries that require an International Certificate of Vaccination or Prophylaxis (ICVP) for entry (information about countries at risk of yellow fever is available from the National Travel Health Network and Centre).

Children aged under 9 months are at higher risk of vaccine-associated encephalitis, with the risk being inversely proportional to age. Children aged under 6 months should **not** be vaccinated. Children aged 6–9 months should only be vaccinated following a detailed risk assessment, and vaccination is generally only recommended if the risk of yellow fever transmission is high (such as during epidemics/outbreaks). If travel is unavoidable, seek expert advice on whether to vaccinate.

Yellow fever vaccine should be avoided in individuals with primary or acquired immunodeficiency due to a congenital condition or disease process, and in individuals who are immunosuppressed as a result of treatment.

If the yellow fever risk is unavoidable in HIV-infected individuals, consult the British HIV Association (bhiva.org/vaccination-guidelines) or other specialist advice.

For additional guidance on the suitability of immunisation against yellow fever, standardised checklists are available from: National Travel Health Network and Centre (see *Useful resources*) or Health Protection Scotland (www.Travax.nhs.uk).

A single-dose of yellow fever vaccine confers life-long immunity against yellow fever disease. Immunisation should be performed at least 10 days before travelling to an endemic area to allow protective immunity to develop and for the ICVP (if required) to become valid.

Reinforcing immunisation is not needed, except for a small subset of individuals at continued risk who may not have developed long-term protection from their initial yellow fever vaccine vaccination–seek expert advice.

All suspected cases of yellow fever must be notified to the local health protection unit. Where there is a community level outbreak, specialist advice should be sought from Public Health England (tel. 020 8200 4400) or, in Scotland, Health Protection Scotland (tel. 0140 300 1191).

Useful Resources

Recommendations reflect Chapter 35, Yellow fever, in *Immunisation against infectious disease- 'The Green Book'*. Public Health England, January 2020.

www.gov.uk/government/publications/yellow-fever-the-green-book-chapter-35

National Travel Health Network and Centre travelhealthpro.org.uk

Travel vaccinations and precautions

20-Sep-2023

Immunisation for travel

The National Travel Health Network and Centre have issued guidance on how to manage interrupted vaccination schedules which includes general principles for consideration, such as keeping to the recommended schedules, lengthening and shortening schedules, off-label administration and re-starting courses. For further information, see travelhealthpro.org.uk/factsheet/100/interrupted-vaccination-schedules-general-principles.

No special immunisation is required for travellers to the United States, Europe, Australia, or New Zealand, although all travellers should have immunity to tetanus and poliomyelitis (and childhood immunisations should be up to date); the tick-borne encephalitis vaccine is recommended for immunisation of those working in, or visiting, high-risk areas. Certain special precautions are required in non-European areas surrounding the Mediterranean, in Africa, the Middle East, Asia, and South America.

Travellers to areas that have a high incidence of **poliomyelitis** should be immunised with the appropriate vaccine; previously immunised travellers may be given a booster dose of a preparation containing inactivated poliomyelitis vaccine.

Immunisation against **meningococcal meningitis** is recommended for a number of areas of the world.

For guidance on immunisation against the following infectious diseases, refer to the individual treatment summaries listed:

- Cholera (see Cholera vaccines p. 1475).
- Diphtheria (see Diphtheria vaccine p. 1477).
- Hepatitis A (see Hepatitis A vaccine p. 1480).
- Hepatitis B (see Hepatitis B vaccine p. 1481).
- Japanese encephalitis (see Japanese encephalitis vaccine p. 1484).
- Meningococcal meningitis (see Meningococcal vaccines p. 1486).
- Rabies (see Rabies vaccine p. 1490).
- Tetanus (see Tetanus vaccine p. 1493).
- Tick-borne encephalitis (see Tick-borne encephalitis vaccine p. 1495).
- Tuberculosis (see Bacillus Calmette-Guérin vaccine p. 1474).
- Typhoid (see Typhoid vaccine p. 1495).
- Yellow fever (see Yellow fever vaccine p. 1497).

Immunisation requirements change from time to time, and information on the current requirements for any particular country may be obtained from the embassy or legation of the appropriate country; or the National Travel Health Network and Centre, Health Protection Scotland, the Welsh Government, or the Department of Health Northern Ireland (see *Useful resources*).

Precautions for avoiding infectious disease

In areas where sanitation is poor, good food hygiene is important to help prevent hepatitis A, typhoid, cholera, and other diarrhoeal diseases (including travellers' diarrhoea). Food should be freshly prepared and hot, and uncooked vegetables (including green salads) should be avoided; only fruits which can be peeled should be eaten. Only suitable bottled water, or tap water that has been boiled or treated with sterilising tablets, should be used for drinking.

For guidance on malaria precautions, see Malaria, prophylaxis p. 702 and Malaria, treatment p. 708.

Further information on preventing or reducing the risk of infectious diseases when travelling, visiting, working, or living in high risk areas is available from the National Travel Health Network and Centre and Health Protection Scotland (see *Useful resources*).

Useful resources

Department of Health Northern Ireland.
www.health-ni.gov.uk/contact
Health Protection Scotland (free for NHS Scotland users (registration required); subscription fee may be payable for users outside NHS Scotland).
www.travax.nhs.uk
National Travel Health Network and Centre.
nathnac.net
Welsh Government.
www.gov.wales/contact-us

VACCINES

Vaccines, general

12-Sep-2023

- **CAUTIONS** Acute illness · minor illnesses
  CAUTIONS, FURTHER INFORMATION
  ▸ **Illness** UKHSA advises vaccination may be postponed if the individual is suffering from an acute illness; however, it is not necessary to postpone immunisation in patients with minor illnesses without fever or systemic upset.
  ▸ **Predisposition to neurological problems** UKHSA advises:
    - when there is a personal or family history of *febrile* convulsions, there is an increased risk of these occurring during fever from any cause including immunisation, but this is not a contra-indication to immunisation. In children who have had a seizure associated with fever without neurological deterioration, immunisation is *recommended*; advice on the *management of fever* should be given before immunisation. When a child has had a convulsion not associated with fever, and the neurological condition is not deteriorating, immunisation is *recommended*;
    - children with stable neurological disorders (e.g. spina bifida, congenital brain abnormality, and peri-natal hypoxic-ischaemic encephalopathy) should be immunised according to the recommended schedule;
    - when there is a *still evolving neurological problem*, including poorly controlled epilepsy, immunisation should be deferred and the child referred to a specialist. Immunisation is recommended if a cause for the neurological disorder is identified. If a cause is not identified, immunisation should be deferred until the condition is stable.
  ▸ **Impaired immune response and drugs affecting immune response** Immune response to vaccines may be reduced in immunosuppressed patients, UKHSA advises consider seeking specialist advice.

- **SIDE-EFFECTS**
  ▸ **Common or very common** Abdominal pain · appetite decreased · arthralgia · diarrhoea · fatigue · fever · headache · lymphadenopathy · malaise · myalgia · nausea · skin reactions · vomiting
  ▸ **Uncommon** Hypersensitivity

- **ALLERGY AND CROSS-SENSITIVITY** UKHSA advises contra-indicated in patients with a confirmed anaphylactic reaction to a preceding dose of a vaccine containing the same antigens or vaccine component (such as antibacterials in viral vaccines).

- **DIRECTIONS FOR ADMINISTRATION** UKHSA advises when 2 or more injections are required (and are not available as a combined preparation), they can be administered at any time before or after each other at different sites, preferably in a different limb; if more than one injection is to be given in the same limb, they should be administered at least 2.5 cm apart. See also Cautions, further information in Bacillus Calmette-Guérin vaccine p. 1514 and in measles, mumps and rubella vaccine p. 1516.

Vaccines should not be given intravenously. Most vaccines are given by the intramuscular route, although some are given by either the intradermal, deep subcutaneous, or oral route. UKHSA advises the intramuscular route is usually avoided in patients with **bleeding disorders** such as haemophilia or thrombocytopenia; vaccines usually given by the intramuscular route can be given by deep subcutaneous injection instead.

Particular attention must be paid to instructions on the use of diluents. Vaccines which are liquid suspensions or are reconstituted before use should be adequately mixed to ensure uniformity of the material to be injected.

- **HANDLING AND STORAGE** Care must be taken to store all vaccines under the conditions recommended in the product literature, otherwise the preparation may become ineffective. **Refrigerated storage** is usually necessary; many vaccines need to be stored at 2–8°C and not allowed to freeze. Vaccines should be protected from light. Reconstituted vaccines and opened multidose vials must be used within the period recommended in the product literature. Unused vaccines should be disposed of by incineration at a registered disposal contractor.

VACCINES › INACTIVATED AND NON-REPLICATING

Anthrax vaccine

F 1498

25-Aug-2023

- **DRUG ACTION** Anthrax vaccine is an inactivated vaccine containing antigens from *Bacillus anthracis* adsorbed onto an adjuvant.

- **INDICATIONS AND DOSE**

Immunisation against anthrax
- ▸ BY INTRAMUSCULAR INJECTION
- ▸ Adult: Initially 0.5 mL every 3 weeks for 3 doses, followed by 0.5 mL after 6 months, to be administered in the deltoid region

Booster
- ▸ BY INTRAMUSCULAR INJECTION
- ▸ Adult: 0.5 mL every 10 years for up to 3 doses, to be administered in deltoid region

- **SIDE-EFFECTS**
- ▸ **Common or very common** Febrile disorders · influenza like illness
- ▸ **Rare or very rare** Angioedema · asthenia · dizziness · hyperhidrosis · paraesthesia
- ▸ **Frequency not known** Bronchospasm · circulatory collapse · hypotension

- **PRESCRIBING AND DISPENSING INFORMATION** Available from Public Health England's Centre for Emergency Preparedness and Response (Porton Down).

- **MEDICINAL FORMS** There can be variation in the licensing of different medicines containing the same drug.
  ### Suspension for injection
  EXCIPIENTS: May contain Thiomersal
  - ▸ **Anthrax vaccine (Non-proprietary)**
    Anthrax vaccine (alum precipitated sterile filtrate) suspension for injection 0.5ml ampoules | 5 ampoule [PoM] [Ⓢ] (Hospital only)
  - ▸ **BioThrax** (Secretary of State for Health)
    BioThrax suspension for injection 5ml multidose vials | 1 vial [PoM] [Ⓢ] (Hospital only)

F 1498

Cholera vaccine (inactivated)

29-Aug-2024

- **DRUG ACTION** The inactivated cholera vaccine is an oral vaccine that contains inactivated *Vibrio cholerae* and recombinant cholera toxin B-subunit. For information on the live vaccine, see cholera vaccine (live) p. 1515.

- **INDICATIONS AND DOSE**

Immunisation against cholera [primary course]
- ▸ BY MOUTH
- ▸ Child 2–5 years: 1 dose every 1–6 weeks for 3 doses, if more than 6 weeks have elapsed between doses, the primary course should be restarted, immunisation should be completed at least one week before potential exposure
- ▸ Child 6–17 years: 1 dose every 1–6 weeks for 2 doses, if more than 6 weeks have elapsed between doses, the primary course should be restarted, immunisation should be completed at least one week before potential exposure
- ▸ Adult: 1 dose every 1–6 weeks for 2 doses, if more than 6 weeks have elapsed between doses, the primary course should be restarted, immunisation should be completed at least one week before potential exposure

Immunisation against cholera [booster dose]
- ▸ BY MOUTH
- ▸ Child 2–5 years: 1 dose, to be given within 6 months after primary course, if more than 6 months have elapsed since the last vaccination, the primary course should be repeated
- ▸ Child 6–17 years: 1 dose, to be given within 2 years after primary course, if more than 2 years have elapsed since the last vaccination, the primary course should be repeated
- ▸ Adult: 1 dose, to be given within 2 years after primary course, if more than 2 years have elapsed since the last vaccination, the primary course should be repeated

- **CONTRA-INDICATIONS** Acute gastro-intestinal illness

- **SIDE-EFFECTS**
- ▸ **Uncommon** Gastrointestinal discomfort · gastrointestinal disorders
- ▸ **Rare or very rare** Chills · cough · dehydration · dizziness · drowsiness · hyperhidrosis · increased risk of infection · insomnia · pulmonary reaction · syncope · taste altered · throat pain
- ▸ **Frequency not known** Angioedema · asthenia · dyspnoea · hypertension · influenza like illness · lymphadenitis · pain · paraesthesia · sputum increased

- **DIRECTIONS FOR ADMINISTRATION**
- ▸ In children Manufacturer advises dissolve effervescent sodium bicarbonate granules in a glassful of water *or* chlorinated water (approximately 150 mL). For children over 6 years, add vaccine suspension to make one dose. For child 2–5 years, discard half (approximately 75 mL) of the solution, then add vaccine suspension to make one dose. Drink within 2 hours. Food, drink, and other oral medicines should be avoided for 1 hour before and after vaccination.
- ▸ In adults Manufacturer advises dissolve effervescent sodium bicarbonate granules in a glassful of water *or* chlorinated water (approximately 150 mL). Add vaccine suspension to make one dose. Drink within 2 hours. Food, drink, and other oral medicines should be avoided for 1 hour before and after vaccination.

- **PATIENT AND CARER ADVICE** Counselling on administration advised. Immunisation with cholera vaccine does not provide complete protection and all travellers to a country where cholera exists should be warned that scrupulous attention to food, water, and personal hygiene is **essential**.

● **MEDICINAL FORMS** There can be variation in the licensing of different medicines containing the same drug.

Oral suspension

ELECTROLYTES: May contain Sodium

▸ **Dukoral** (Valneva UK Ltd)
Dukoral cholera vaccine effervescent powder and suspension for oral suspension | 2 dose [PoM] £52.19 DT = £52.19

⫟ 1498

COVID-19 vaccine

25-Aug-2023

● **DRUG ACTION** COVID-19 vaccines are inactivated vaccines that use the spike protein of the SARS-CoV-2 virus to act as an intracellular antigen and produce an antibody response, thereby protecting against COVID-19 infection. Pfizer/BioNTech (*Comirnaty*®) and Moderna (*Spikevax*®) are nucleoside-modified messenger RNA (mRNA) vaccines that deliver viral RNA into host cells to enable expression of the spike protein. Novavax (*Nuvaxovid*®) vaccine contains a recombinant spike protein with an adjuvant to strengthen the immune response. Sanofi Pasteur (*VidPrevtyn Beta*®) vaccine contains a soluble trimeric spike protein of the SARS-CoV-2 virus with an adjuvant to strengthen the immune response. AstraZeneca (*Vaxzevria*®) vaccine uses a chimpanzee-derived adenovirus vector to incorporate the spike protein into host cells; this vaccine is no longer routinely supplied in the UK.

Pfizer/BioNTech (*Comirnaty*®) vaccines contain tozinameran (rINN for the mRNA that encodes the viral spike protein of the original COVID-19 virus). The bivalent *Comirnaty*® Original/Omicron booster vaccine additionally contains either riltozinameran (rINN for the mRNA that encodes the viral spike protein of the Omicron BA.1 variant of the COVID-19 virus) or famtozinameran (rINN for the mRNA that encodes the viral spike protein of the Omicron BA.4-5 variant of the COVID-19 virus).

Moderna (*Spikevax*®) vaccines contain elasomeran (rINN for the mRNA that encodes the viral spike protein of the original COVID-19 virus). The bivalent *Spikevax*® Original/Omicron booster vaccines additionally contain either imelasomeran (rINN for the mRNA that encodes the viral spike protein of the Omicron B.1.1.529 variant of the COVID-19 virus) or davesomeran (rINN for the mRNA that encodes the viral spike protein of the Omicron BA.4-5 variant of the COVID-19 virus).

Pfizer/BioNTech (*Comirnaty*®) 30 micrograms/0.3 mL per dose vaccine may previously have been referred to as *Courageous* in practice.

AstraZeneca vaccine (*Vaxzevria*®) vaccine may previously have been referred to as *Talent* in practice.

● **INDICATIONS AND DOSE**

MODERNA VACCINES (SPIKEVAX ®**)**

Immunisation against COVID-19

▸ BY INTRAMUSCULAR INJECTION
▸ Adult: (consult local protocol)

NOVAVAX VACCINES (NUVAXOVID ®**)**

Immunisation against COVID-19

▸ BY INTRAMUSCULAR INJECTION
▸ Adult: (consult local protocol)

PFIZER/BIONTECH VACCINES (COMIRNATY ®**)**

Immunisation against COVID-19

▸ BY INTRAMUSCULAR INJECTION
▸ Adult: (consult local protocol)

● **CAUTIONS**

MODERNA VACCINES (SPIKEVAX ®**)** History of capillary leak syndrome (seek specialist advice)

● **SIDE-EFFECTS**

▸ **Common or very common** Axillary lymph node tenderness · chills · influenza like illness · pain in extremity · thrombocytopenia
▸ **Uncommon** Asthenia · dizziness · drowsiness · insomnia · sweat changes
▸ **Rare or very rare** Angioedema · cardiac inflammation · embolism and thrombosis · facial paralysis · Guillain-Barre syndrome · sensation abnormal · visceral venous thrombosis
▸ **Frequency not known** Capillary leak syndrome · extensive swelling of vaccinated limb · menorrhagia · transverse myelitis

● **ALLERGY AND CROSS-SENSITIVITY** UKHSA advises individuals with a history of anaphylaxis to food, an identified drug or vaccine, or an insect sting can receive any COVID-19 vaccine, as long as they are not allergic to any of its ingredients; consider observation for 15 minutes. Individuals who had a non-allergic reaction to a first dose of COVID-19 vaccine can receive a second dose, followed by an observation period of 15 minutes.

UKHSA advises individuals with a history of immediate onset anaphylaxis to multiple classes of drugs, or unexplained anaphylaxis, should not be vaccinated with Pfizer/BioNTech (*Comirnaty*®) or Moderna (*Spikevax*®) vaccines, except on advice of an allergy specialist or where at least one dose of the same vaccine has been tolerated previously. Novavax (*Nuvaxovid*®) or Sanofi Pasteur (*VidPrevtyn Beta*®) vaccines can be used as an alternative (if not otherwise contra-indicated); it should be administered in a setting with full resuscitation facilities, followed by an observation period of 30 minutes.

UKHSA advises individuals with a localised allergic reaction or with systemic symptoms, but not anaphylaxis, to the first dose of a COVID-19 vaccine can receive further doses with an observation period of 30 minutes. In these individuals, or if the reaction was delayed and self-limiting, or resolved with an oral antihistamine, consider pre-treatment with a non-sedating antihistamine 30 minutes before giving further doses. Seek advice from an allergy specialist if the reaction presented with anaphylaxis or required medical attention. If the anaphylactic reaction was to a previous dose of Novavax (*Nuvaxovid*®) or Sanofi Pasteur (*VidPrevtyn Beta*®) vaccine, complete vaccination with a different vaccine, which may include an mRNA vaccine; if the reaction was to an mRNA vaccine, either give the same or a different mRNA vaccine or Novavax (*Nuvaxovid*®) or Sanofi Pasteur (*VidPrevtyn Beta*®) vaccine in a hospital setting—an observation period of at least 30 minutes is recommended.

● **PREGNANCY** UKHSA advises COVID-19 vaccines should be offered—Pfizer/BioNTech (*Comirnaty*®) and Moderna (*Spikevax*®) vaccines preferred due to more clinical experience. Novavax (*Nuvaxovid*®) vaccine may be used if mRNA COVID-19 vaccines are not clinically suitable—limited information available.

● **BREAST FEEDING** UKHSA advises that COVID-19 vaccines are suitable.

● **MONITORING REQUIREMENTS**

▸ UKHSA advises healthcare professionals to monitor platelets 2 to 5 days after vaccination in patients with a history of immune thrombocytopenia.
▸ UKHSA advises healthcare professionals to be alert for signs and symptoms of myocarditis and pericarditis and inform vaccinated patients to seek immediate medical attention if they experience a new onset of chest pain, shortness of breath, palpitations or arrhythmias within 10 days of vaccination.
▸ For advice on further doses for those who have suspected Guillain-Barré syndrome, myocarditis, or pericarditis after vaccination, see Chapter 14a: COVID-19 - SARS-CoV-2, in *Immunisation against infectious disease*- 'The Green Book'.

- **DIRECTIONS FOR ADMINISTRATION** UKHSA advises that individuals with **bleeding disorders** may be vaccinated by the intramuscular route, on the advice of a doctor familiar with their bleeding risk. Patients treated with medicines to reduce bleeding (e.g. for haemophilia) are advised to administer their medicine shortly prior to intramuscular vaccination.

- **HANDLING AND STORAGE**

  MODERNA VACCINES (SPIKEVAX®) Store in a freezer at -50°C to -15°C—consult product literature about thawing and storage after thawing.

  PFIZER/BIONTECH VACCINES (COMIRNATY®) Store in a freezer at -90°C to -60°C—consult product literature about thawing and storage after thawing.

- **PATIENT AND CARER ADVICE**

  Driving and skilled tasks Healthcare professionals are advised to inform patients not to drive for 15 minutes after vaccination—increased risk of fainting.

- **MEDICINAL FORMS** There can be variation in the licensing of different medicines containing the same drug.

  Dispersion for injection
  EXCIPIENTS: May contain Polysorbates
  - ▶ Covid-19 vaccine (non-proprietary) ▼
    COVID-19 Vaccine Nuvaxovid (recombinant, adjuvanted) 5micrograms/0.5ml dose dispersion for injection multidose vials | 10 dose [PoM] 🅂
    Famtozinameran 50 microgram per 1 ml, Tozinameran 50 microgram per 1 ml Comirnaty Original/Omicron BA.4-5 COVID-19 mRNA Vaccine 15micrograms/15micrograms/0.3ml dose dispersion for injection multidose vials | 6 dose [PoM] 🅂
  - ▶ Comirnaty (Pfizer Ltd) ▼
    Tozinameran 100 microgram per 1 ml Comirnaty COVID-19 mRNA Vaccine ready to use 30micrograms/0.3ml dose dispersion for injection multidose vials | 6 dose [PoM] 🅂
  - ▶ Comirnaty Children (Pfizer Ltd) ▼
    Tozinameran 15 microgram per 1 ml Comirnaty Children 6 months - 4 years COVID-19 mRNA Vaccine 3micrograms/0.2ml dose concentrate for dispersion for injection multidose vials | 10 dose [PoM] 🅂
    Tozinameran 50 microgram per 1 ml Comirnaty Children 5-11 years COVID-19 mRNA Vaccine 10micrograms/0.2ml dose concentrate for dispersion for injection multidose vials | 10 dose [PoM] 🅂

⚑ 1498

Diphtheria with tetanus and pertussis vaccine

09-Sep-2024

- **DRUG ACTION** Diphtheria with tetanus and pertussis vaccine is a non-live, adsorbed, combination vaccine containing diphtheria and tetanus toxoids, and pertussis antigens.

- **INDICATIONS AND DOSE**

  Passive immunisation against pertussis [pregnant women in their second or third trimester]
  - ▶ BY INTRAMUSCULAR INJECTION
  - ▶ Females of childbearing potential: 0.5 mL for 1 dose

- **CONTRA-INDICATIONS** History of encephalopathy of unknown origin within 7 days of previous immunisation with a pertussis-containing vaccine

- **CAUTIONS** Guillain-Barre syndrome within 6 weeks of previous immunisation with a vaccine containing tetanus toxoid · progressive neurological disorders, uncontrolled epilepsy, or progressive encephalopathy (defer immunisation until condition has stabilised)

- **SIDE-EFFECTS**
- ▶ **Common or very common** Asthenia · axillary lymphadenopathy · chills · generalised pain · joint swelling · muscle weakness
- ▶ **Frequency not known** Extensive swelling of vaccinated limb · facial paralysis · myelitis · myocarditis · myositis · nerve disorders · seizure · sensation abnormal · syncope

- **PRESCRIBING AND DISPENSING INFORMATION** Details of routine immunisations are included in this monograph; for details of immunisation in other patient groups e.g. patients at high risk from infection, see Diphtheria vaccine p. 1477, Tetanus vaccine p. 1493, and Pertussis vaccine p. 1487 respectively.

- **MEDICINAL FORMS** There can be variation in the licensing of different medicines containing the same drug.
  Suspension for injection
  - ▶ Adacel (Sanofi)
    Adacel vaccine suspension for injection 0.5ml pre-filled syringes | 1 pre-filled disposable injection [PoM] £19.00

⚑ 1498

Diphtheria with tetanus and poliomyelitis vaccine

25-Aug-2023

- **DRUG ACTION** Diphtheria with tetanus and poliomyelitis vaccine is a non-live, adsorbed, combination vaccine containing diphtheria and tetanus toxoids, and inactivated poliomyelitis virus.

- **INDICATIONS AND DOSE**

  Primary immunisation
  - ▶ BY INTRAMUSCULAR INJECTION
  - ▶ Child 10-17 years: 0.5 mL every month for 3 doses
  - ▶ Adult: 0.5 mL every month for 3 doses

  Booster doses
  - ▶ BY INTRAMUSCULAR INJECTION
  - ▶ Child 10-17 years: 0.5 mL for 1 dose, first booster dose—should be given at least 5 years after primary course, then 0.5 mL for 1 dose, second booster dose—should be given 10 years after first booster dose (this interval can be reduced to a minimum of 5 years if previous doses were delayed)
  - ▶ Adult: 0.5 mL for 1 dose, first booster dose—should be given at least 5 years after primary course, then 0.5 mL for 1 dose, second booster dose—should be given 10 years after first booster dose (this interval can be reduced to a minimum of 5 years if previous doses were delayed)

- **SIDE-EFFECTS**
- ▶ **Common or very common** Vertigo
- ▶ **Frequency not known** Asthenia · chills · face oedema · influenza like illness · nerve disorders · pallor · seizure · shock · syncope · vaccination reactions

- **PRESCRIBING AND DISPENSING INFORMATION** Available as part of childhood schedule from health organisations or ImmForm.

- **MEDICINAL FORMS** There can be variation in the licensing of different medicines containing the same drug.
  Suspension for injection
  EXCIPIENTS: May contain Neomycin, polymyxin b, streptomycin
  - ▶ Revaxis (Sanofi)
    Revaxis vaccine suspension for injection 0.5ml pre-filled syringes | 1 pre-filled disposable injection [PoM] £7.80 DT = £7.80

⌐ 1498

Diphtheria with tetanus, pertussis and poliomyelitis vaccine
09-Sep-2024

- **DRUG ACTION** Diphtheria with tetanus, pertussis and poliomyelitis vaccine is a non-live, adsorbed, combination vaccine containing diphtheria and tetanus toxoids, pertussis antigens, and inactivated poliomyelitis virus.

- **INDICATIONS AND DOSE**

Immunisation against diphtheria, tetanus, pertussis and poliomyelitis [booster dose]
▶ BY INTRAMUSCULAR INJECTION
▸ Child 3-9 years: 0.5 mL for 1 dose, dose to be given 3 years after primary immunisation

- **SIDE-EFFECTS**
▶ **Common or very common** Asthenia · drowsiness · irritability · joint swelling · vaccination reactions
▶ **Uncommon** Apathy · dry throat · sleep disorder
▶ **Frequency not known** Angioedema · dizziness · facial paralysis · hypotonic-hyporesponsiveness episode · myelitis · nerve disorders · pallor · seizure

SIDE-EFFECTS, FURTHER INFORMATION The incidence of local and systemic reactions is lower with acellular pertussis vaccines than with whole-cell pertussis vaccines used previously.

Compared with primary vaccination, injection site reactions are more common with booster doses of vaccines containing acellular pertussis.

Public Health England has advised (2016) that the vaccine should not be withheld from children with a history to a preceding dose of: fever, irrespective of severity; hypotonic-hyporesonsive episodes; persistent crying or screaming for more than 3 hours; severe local reaction, irrespective of extent.

- **PREGNANCY** Contra-indicated in pregnant women with a history of encephalopathy of unknown origin within 7 days of previous immunisation with a pertussis-containing vaccine. Contra-indicated in pregnant women with a history of transient thrombocytopenia or neurological complications following previous immunisation against diphtheria or tetanus.

- **PRESCRIBING AND DISPENSING INFORMATION** Available as part of childhood immunisation schedule from health organisations or ImmForm.

Details of routine immunisations are included in this monograph; for details of immunisation in other patient groups e.g. patients at high risk from infection, see Diphtheria vaccine p. 1477, Tetanus vaccine p. 1493, Pertussis vaccine p. 1487, Poliomyelitis vaccine p. 1490, and Vaccination, general principles p. 1470.

- **MEDICINAL FORMS** There can be variation in the licensing of different medicines containing the same drug.

Suspension for injection
EXCIPIENTS: May contain Neomycin, polymyxin b, streptomycin
▸ **Boostrix-IPV** (GlaxoSmithKline UK Ltd)
Boostrix-IPV suspension for injection 0.5ml pre-filled syringes | 1 pre-filled disposable injection `PoM` £22.74 DT = £20.00
▸ **Repevax** (Sanofi)
Repevax vaccine suspension for injection 0.5ml pre-filled syringes | 1 pre-filled disposable injection `PoM` £20.00 DT = £20.00

⌐ 1498

Diphtheria with tetanus, pertussis, hepatitis B, poliomyelitis and haemophilus influenzae type b vaccine
09-Sep-2024

- **DRUG ACTION** Diphtheria with tetanus, pertussis, hepatitis B, poliomyelitis and *haemophilus influenzae* type b vaccine is a non-live combination vaccine.

- **INDICATIONS AND DOSE**

Primary immunisation against diphtheria, tetanus, pertussis, hepatitis B, poliomyelitis, and *Haemophilus influenzae* type b
▶ BY INTRAMUSCULAR INJECTION
▸ Child 2 months-9 years: 0.5 mL for 3 doses, doses to be separated by an interval of 4 weeks

- **SIDE-EFFECTS**
▶ **Common or very common** Anxiety · crying · drowsiness · irritability
▶ **Uncommon** Appetite increased · cough · extensive swelling of vaccinated limb · hyperhidrosis · increased risk of infection · neuromuscular dysfunction · pallor · sleep disorders
▶ **Rare or very rare** Angioedema · apnoea · seizure · swelling · thrombocytopenia

- **DIRECTIONS FOR ADMINISTRATION** Anterolateral thigh is the preferred site of injection in infants under 1 year of age; deltoid muscle is preferred in older children. Administer each dose at a different injection site to that of previous dose.

- **PRESCRIBING AND DISPENSING INFORMATION** Available as part of childhood schedule from health organisations or ImmForm.

Details of routine immunisations are included in this monograph; for details of immunisation in other patient groups e.g. patients at high risk from infection, see Diphtheria vaccine p. 1477, Tetanus vaccine p. 1493, Pertussis vaccine p. 1487, Hepatitis B vaccine p. 1481, Poliomyelitis vaccine p. 1490, Haemophilus influenzae type b conjugate vaccine p. 1479 and Vaccination, general principles p. 1470.

- **MEDICINAL FORMS** There can be variation in the licensing of different medicines containing the same drug.

Powder and suspension for suspension for injection
EXCIPIENTS: May contain Neomycin, polymyxin b
▸ **Infanrix Hexa** (GlaxoSmithKline UK Ltd)
Infanrix Hexa vaccine powder and suspension for suspension for injection 0.5ml pre-filled syringes | 1 pre-filled disposable injection `PoM` Ⓧ

Suspension for injection
EXCIPIENTS: May contain Neomycin, polymyxin b, streptomycin
▸ **Vaxelis** (Sanofi)
Vaxelis vaccine suspension for injection 0.5ml pre-filled syringes | 1 pre-filled disposable injection `PoM` £45.31

⌐ 1498

Diphtheria with tetanus, pertussis, poliomyelitis and haemophilus influenzae type b vaccine
09-Sep-2024

- **DRUG ACTION** Diphtheria with tetanus, pertussis, poliomyelitis and *haemophilus influenzae* type b vaccine is a non-live combination vaccine.

- **INDICATIONS AND DOSE**

Primary immunisation
▶ BY INTRAMUSCULAR INJECTION
▸ Child 2 months-9 years: 0.5 mL every month for 3 doses

● **SIDE-EFFECTS**
▸ **Common or very common** Crying abnormal · drowsiness · irritability · restlessness
▸ **Uncommon** Cough · extensive swelling of vaccinated limb · increased risk of infection · rhinorrhoea
▸ **Frequency not known** Angioedema · apnoea · hypotonic-hyporesponsiveness episode · seizure

  SIDE-EFFECTS, FURTHER INFORMATION The incidence of local and systemic reactions is lower with acellular pertussis vaccines than with whole-cell pertussis vaccines used previously.

  Compared with primary vaccination, injection site reactions are more common with booster doses of vaccines containing acellular pertussis.

  Public Health England has advised (2016) that the vaccine should not be withheld from children with a history to a preceding dose of: fever, irrespective of severity; hypotonic-hyporesonsive episodes; persistent crying or screaming for more than 3 hours; severe local reaction, irrespective of extent.

● **PRESCRIBING AND DISPENSING INFORMATION** UKHSA advises from Autumn 2017, all babies born on or after 1 August 2017 became eligible for the hexavalent vaccine, diphtheria with tetanus, pertussis, hepatitis B, poliomyelitis and haemophilus influenzae type b vaccine p. 1502, which replaces the pentavalent vaccine in the routine childhood immunisation schedule.

● **MEDICINAL FORMS** There can be variation in the licensing of different medicines containing the same drug.
  Powder and suspension for suspension for injection
▸ **Infanrix-IPV + Hib** (GlaxoSmithKline UK Ltd)
  Infanrix-IPV + Hib vaccine powder and suspension for suspension for injection 0.5ml pre-filled syringes | 1 pre-filled disposable injection [PoM] £27.86

  ℱ 1498

Haemophilus influenzae type b with meningococcal group C vaccine 28-Apr-2024

● **DRUG ACTION** *Haemophilus influenzae* type b with meningococcal group C vaccine is a non-live combination vaccine.

● **INDICATIONS AND DOSE**
  Primary immunisation against *Neisseria meningitidis* group C, and immunisation against *Haemophilus influenzae* type b (booster dose for infants who have received primary immunisation)
▸ BY INTRAMUSCULAR INJECTION
▸ Child 1 year: 0.5 mL for 1 dose

  Immunisation against *Neisseria meningitidis* group C and *Haemophilus influenzae* type b [patients with unknown or incomplete immunisation status]
▸ BY INTRAMUSCULAR INJECTION
▸ Child 1-9 years: 0.5 mL for 1 dose

● **UNLICENSED USE** Not licensed for use in patients over 2 years.

● **SIDE-EFFECTS**
▸ **Common or very common** Drowsiness · irritability
▸ **Uncommon** Crying
▸ **Rare or very rare** Insomnia
▸ **Frequency not known** Dizziness · febrile seizure · meningism (but no evidence that vaccine causes meningococcal C meningitis) · muscle tone decreased

● **PRESCRIBING AND DISPENSING INFORMATION** Details on routine immunisations are included in this monograph; for details of immunisation in other patient groups e.g. patients at high risk of infection, see Haemophilus influenzae type b conjugate vaccine p. 1479 and Vaccination, general principles p. 1470.

Available as part of the childhood immunisation schedule from ImmForm.

● **MEDICINAL FORMS** There can be variation in the licensing of different medicines containing the same drug.
  Powder and solvent for solution for injection
▸ **Menitorix** (GlaxoSmithKline UK Ltd)
  Menitorix vaccine powder and solvent for solution for injection 0.5ml vials | 1 vial [PoM] £37.76 DT = £37.76

Hepatitis A and B vaccine 25-Aug-2023

The properties listed below are those particular to the combination only. For the properties of the components please consider, hepatitis A vaccine p. 1504, hepatitis B vaccine p. 1505.

● **INDICATIONS AND DOSE**
  AMBIRIX ®
  Immunisation against hepatitis A and hepatitis B infection [primary course]
▸ BY INTRAMUSCULAR INJECTION
▸ Child 1-15 years: Initially 1 mL for 1 dose, then 1 mL after 6–12 months for 1 dose, the deltoid region is the preferred site of injection in older children; anterolateral thigh may be used in infants; not to be injected into the buttock (vaccine efficacy reduced), subcutaneous route used for patients with bleeding disorders (but immune response may be reduced)

  Post-exposure prophylaxis against hepatitis A infection [for rapid protection]
▸ BY INTRAMUSCULAR INJECTION
▸ Child 1-15 years: 1 mL for 1 dose, the deltoid region is the preferred site of injection in older children; anterolateral thigh may be used in infants; not to be injected into the buttock (vaccine efficacy reduced), subcutaneous route used for patients with bleeding disorders (but immune response may be reduced)

  TWINRIX ® ADULT
  Immunisation against hepatitis A and hepatitis B infection [primary course]
▸ BY INTRAMUSCULAR INJECTION
▸ Child 16-17 years: Initially 1 mL every month for 2 doses, then 1 mL after 5 months for 1 dose, the deltoid region is the preferred site of injection; not to be injected into the buttock (vaccine efficacy reduced), subcutaneous route used for patients with bleeding disorders (but immune response may be reduced)
▸ Adult: Initially 1 mL every month for 2 doses, then 1 mL after 5 months for 1 dose, the deltoid region is the preferred site of injection; not to be injected into the buttock (vaccine efficacy reduced), subcutaneous route used for patients with bleeding disorders (but immune response may be reduced)

  Immunisation against hepatitis A and hepatitis B infection [accelerated schedule for travellers departing within 1 month]
▸ BY INTRAMUSCULAR INJECTION
▸ Child 16-17 years: Initially 1 mL for 1 dose, then 1 mL after 7 days for 1 dose, then 1 mL after 14 days for 1 dose, then 1 mL for 1 dose given 12 months after the first dose, the deltoid region is the preferred site of injection; not to be injected into the buttock (vaccine efficacy reduced), subcutaneous route used for patients with bleeding disorders (but immune response may be reduced)
▸ Adult: Initially 1 mL for 1 dose, then 1 mL after 7 days for 1 dose, then 1 mL after 14 days for 1 dose, then 1 mL for 1 dose given 12 months after the first dose, the deltoid region is the preferred site of injection; not to be injected into the buttock (vaccine efficacy

continued →

reduced), subcutaneous route used for patients with bleeding disorders (but immune response may be reduced)

TWINRIX ® PAEDIATRIC

Immunisation against hepatitis A and hepatitis B infection [primary course]

▸ BY INTRAMUSCULAR INJECTION

▸ Child 1-15 years: Initially 0.5 mL every month for 2 doses, then 0.5 mL after 5 months for 1 dose, the deltoid region is the preferred site of injection in older children; anterolateral thigh is the preferred site in infants; not to be injected into the buttock (vaccine efficacy reduced), subcutaneous route used for patients with bleeding disorders (but immune response may be reduced)

● UNLICENSED USE

AMBIRIX ® Public Health England advises that *Ambirix* ® may be used for post-exposure prophylaxis against hepatitis A infection where rapid protection is required, but is not licensed for this indication.

> **IMPORTANT SAFETY INFORMATION**
> *Ambirix* ® and *Twinrix* ® are not recommended for post-exposure prophylaxis following percutaneous (needle-stick), ocular, or mucous membrane exposure to hepatitis B virus.

● PRESCRIBING AND DISPENSING INFORMATION

AMBIRIX ® Primary course should be completed with *Ambirix* ® (single component vaccines given at appropriate intervals may be used for booster dose).

TWINRIX ® ADULT Primary course should be completed with *Twinrix* ® (single component vaccines given at appropriate intervals may be used for booster dose).

TWINRIX ® PAEDIATRIC Primary course should be completed with *Twinrix* ® (single component vaccines given at appropriate intervals may be used for booster dose).

● MEDICINAL FORMS There can be variation in the licensing of different medicines containing the same drug.

Suspension for injection
EXCIPIENTS: May contain Neomycin

▸ Ambirix (GlaxoSmithKline UK Ltd)
Ambirix vaccine suspension for injection 1ml pre-filled syringes | 1 pre-filled disposable injection [PoM] £31.18 DT = £31.18

▸ Twinrix (GlaxoSmithKline UK Ltd)
Twinrix Paediatric vaccine suspension for injection 0.5ml pre-filled syringes | 1 pre-filled disposable injection [PoM] £20.79 DT = £20.79
Twinrix Adult vaccine suspension for injection 1ml pre-filled syringes | 1 pre-filled disposable injection [PoM] £33.31 DT = £31.18 | 10 pre-filled disposable injection [PoM] £333.13

⚑ 1498

Hepatitis A vaccine
25-Aug-2023

● DRUG ACTION Hepatitis A vaccine is an inactivated vaccine containing adsorbed hepatitis A virus.

● INDICATIONS AND DOSE

AVAXIM ®

Immunisation against hepatitis A infection

▸ BY INTRAMUSCULAR INJECTION

▸ Child 16-17 years: Initially 0.5 mL for 1 dose, then 0.5 mL after 6–12 months, dose given as booster; booster dose may be delayed by up to 3 years if not given after recommended interval following primary dose, the deltoid region is the preferred site of injection. The subcutaneous route may be used for patients with bleeding disorders; not to be injected into the buttock (vaccine efficacy reduced)

▸ Adult: Initially 0.5 mL for 1 dose, then 0.5 mL after 6–12 months, dose given as booster; booster dose may be delayed by up to 3 years if not given after recommended interval following primary dose, the deltoid region is the preferred site of injection. The subcutaneous route may be used for patients with bleeding disorders; not to be injected into the buttock (vaccine efficacy reduced)

HAVRIX JUNIOR MONODOSE ®

Immunisation against hepatitis A infection

▸ BY INTRAMUSCULAR INJECTION

▸ Child 1-15 years: Initially 0.5 mL for 1 dose, then 0.5 mL after 6–12 months, dose given as booster; booster dose may be delayed by up to 3 years if not given after recommended interval following primary dose, deltoid muscle is preferred site of injection in older children; anterolateral thigh is preferred site in infants and young children; not to be injected into the gluteal region. The subcutaneous route may be used for patients with bleeding disorders

HAVRIX MONODOSE ®

Immunisation against hepatitis A infection

▸ BY INTRAMUSCULAR INJECTION

▸ Child 16-17 years: Initially 1 mL for 1 dose, then 1 mL after 6–12 months, dose given as booster; booster dose may be delayed by up to 3 years if not given after recommended interval following primary dose, the deltoid region is the preferred site of injection; not to be injected into the gluteal region. The subcutaneous route may be used for patients with bleeding disorders

▸ Adult: Initially 1 mL for 1 dose, then 1 mL after 6–12 months, dose given as booster; booster dose may be delayed by up to 3 years if not given after recommended interval following primary dose, the deltoid region is the preferred site of injection; not to be injected into the gluteal region. The subcutaneous route may be used for patients with bleeding disorders

VAQTA ® ADULT

Immunisation against hepatitis A infection

▸ BY INTRAMUSCULAR INJECTION

▸ Adult: Initially 1 mL for 1 dose, then 1 mL after 6–18 months, dose given as booster, the deltoid region is the preferred site of injection. The subcutaneous route may be used for patients with bleeding disorders (but immune response may be delayed)

VAQTA ® PAEDIATRIC

Immunisation against hepatitis A infection

▸ BY INTRAMUSCULAR INJECTION

▸ Child 1-17 years: Initially 0.5 mL for 1 dose, then 0.5 mL after 6–18 months, dose given as booster, the deltoid region is the preferred site of injection. The subcutaneous route may be used for patients with bleeding disorders (but immune response may be reduced)

● SIDE-EFFECTS

▸ **Common or very common** Asthenia (uncommon in children) · pain (uncommon in children)

▸ **Uncommon** Anxiety (in children) · chills (in adults) · cough · crying (in children) · dizziness · ear pain (rare in children) · gastrointestinal disorders (rare in children) · increased risk of infection (in adults) · influenza like illness (rare in children) · muscle weakness (in adults) · musculoskeletal stiffness (rare in children) · nasal complaints · paraesthesia (rare in children) · respiratory disorders (rare in children) · sensation of tightness (rare in children) · temperature sensation altered (rare in children) · vasodilation (rare in children)

▸ **Rare or very rare** Allergic rhinitis (in children) · apathy (in adults) · asthma (in children) · ataxia (in children) · burping

(in children) · chest pain · constipation (in children) ·
dehydration (in children) · drowsiness (uncommon in
children) · dry mouth (in adults) · eye discomfort · gait
abnormal (in children) · gastrointestinal discomfort ·
infantile spitting up · irritability (very common in children)
· menstrual disorder (in adults) · migraine (in adults) ·
muscle complaints (in adults) · oral ulceration (in adults) ·
oropharyngeal pain (in children) · photophobia (in adults) ·
screaming (in children) · sleep disorders (uncommon in
children) · sweat changes · synovitis (in children) · throat
oedema (in adults) · tremor (in adults) · vertigo (in adults) ·
watering eye (in adults)
▶ **Frequency not known** Guillain-Barre syndrome ·
thrombocytopenia

● MEDICINAL FORMS There can be variation in the licensing of
different medicines containing the same drug.

Suspension for injection
EXCIPIENTS: May contain Neomycin
▶ Avaxim (Sanofi)
Avaxim vaccine suspension for injection 0.5ml pre-filled syringes |
1 pre-filled disposable injection PoM £21.72 | 10 pre-filled
disposable injection PoM £217.20
▶ Havrix (GlaxoSmithKline UK Ltd)
Havrix Monodose vaccine suspension for injection 1ml pre-filled
syringes | 1 pre-filled disposable injection PoM £22.14 DT = £22.14
| 10 pre-filled disposable injection PoM £221.43
Havrix Junior Monodose vaccine suspension for injection 0.5ml pre-
filled syringes | 1 pre-filled disposable injection PoM £16.77 |
10 pre-filled disposable injection PoM £167.68
▶ VAQTA (Merck Sharp & Dohme (UK) Ltd)
VAQTA Adult vaccine suspension for injection 1ml pre-filled syringes |
1 pre-filled disposable injection PoM £18.10 DT = £22.14
VAQTA Paediatric vaccine suspension for injection 0.5ml pre-filled
syringes | 1 pre-filled disposable injection PoM £14.74

Hepatitis A with typhoid vaccine

25-Aug-2023

The properties listed below are those particular to the
combination only. For the properties of the components
please consider, hepatitis A vaccine p. 1504, typhoid vaccine
(inactivated) p. 1513.

● INDICATIONS AND DOSE
VIATIM®

**Immunisation against hepatitis A and typhoid infection
[primary course]**
▶ BY INTRAMUSCULAR INJECTION
▶ Child 16-17 years: 1 mL for 1 dose, the deltoid region is
the preferred site of injection; not to be injected into
the buttock (vaccine efficacy reduced). The
subcutaneous route may be used for patients with
bleeding disorders, booster dose may be given using
single or multicomponent vaccines
▶ Adult: 1 mL for 1 dose, the deltoid region is the
preferred site of injection; not to be injected into the
buttock (vaccine efficacy reduced). The subcutaneous
route may be used for patients with bleeding disorders,
booster dose may be given using single or
multicomponent vaccines

**Immunisation against hepatitis A [booster dose for
individuals who have received primary immunisation
with monovalent hepatitis A vaccine, where protection
against typhoid is also required]**
▶ BY INTRAMUSCULAR INJECTION
▶ Child 16-17 years: 1 mL for 1 dose, within 36 months
(preferably 6–12 months) of primary immunisation,
the deltoid region is the preferred site of injection; not
to be injected into the buttock (vaccine efficacy
reduced). The subcutaneous route may be used for
patients with bleeding disorders

▶ Adult: 1 mL for 1 dose, within 36 months (preferably
6–12 months) of primary immunisation, the deltoid
region is the preferred site of injection; not to be
injected into the buttock (vaccine efficacy reduced).
The subcutaneous route may be used for patients with
bleeding disorders

**Immunisation against typhoid [booster dose for
individuals who have received primary immunisation
with hepatitis A and typhoid vaccine, where continued
protection against typhoid is required]**
▶ BY INTRAMUSCULAR INJECTION
▶ Child 16-17 years: 1 mL for 1 dose, 36 months after
primary immunisation, the deltoid region is the
preferred site of injection; not to be injected into the
buttock (vaccine efficacy reduced). The subcutaneous
route may be used for patients with bleeding disorders
▶ Adult: 1 mL for 1 dose, 36 months after primary
immunisation, the deltoid region is the preferred site
of injection; not to be injected into the buttock
(vaccine efficacy reduced). The subcutaneous route
may be used for patients with bleeding disorders

● MEDICINAL FORMS There can be variation in the licensing of
different medicines containing the same drug.

Suspension for injection
EXCIPIENTS: May contain Neomycin
▶ ViATIM (Sanofi)
ViATIM vaccine suspension for injection 1ml pre-filled syringes | 1 pre-
filled disposable injection PoM £35.76 DT = £35.76

F 1498

Hepatitis B vaccine

25-Aug-2023

● DRUG ACTION Hepatitis B vaccine is an inactivated vaccine
containing adsorbed hepatitis B surface antigen.

● INDICATIONS AND DOSE
ENGERIX B®

Immunisation against hepatitis B infection
▶ BY INTRAMUSCULAR INJECTION
▶ Child 1 month-15 years: 10 micrograms for 1 dose, then
10 micrograms after 1 month for 1 dose, followed by
10 micrograms after 5 months for 1 dose, deltoid
muscle is preferred site of injection in older children;
anterolateral thigh is preferred site in infants and
young children; not to be injected into the buttock
(vaccine efficacy reduced)
▶ Child 16-17 years: 20 micrograms for 1 dose, then
20 micrograms after 1 month for 1 dose, followed by
20 micrograms after 5 months for 1 dose, deltoid
muscle is preferred site of injection; not to be injected
into the buttock (vaccine efficacy reduced)
▶ Adult: 20 micrograms for 1 dose, then 20 micrograms
after 1 month for 1 dose, followed by 20 micrograms
after 5 months for 1 dose, deltoid muscle is preferred
site of injection; not to be injected into the buttock
(vaccine efficacy reduced)

**Immunisation against hepatitis B infection (accelerated
schedule for pre- and post-exposure prophylaxis)**
▶ BY INTRAMUSCULAR INJECTION

▶ Neonate: 10 micrograms every month for 3 doses,
followed by 10 micrograms after 10 months for 1 dose,
for post-exposure prophylaxis, PHE advises dose at
12 months not required if patient is at low risk,
anterolateral thigh is preferred site in neonates; not to
be injected into the buttock (vaccine efficacy reduced),
this dose should not be given to neonates born to
hepatitis B surface antigen-positive mothers.

▶ Child 1 month-15 years: 10 micrograms every month for
3 doses, followed by 10 micrograms after 10 months for
1 dose, for post-exposure prophylaxis,   continued →

PHE advises dose at 12 months not required if patient is at low risk, deltoid muscle is preferred site of injection in older children; anterolateral thigh is preferred site in infants and young children; not to be injected into the buttock (vaccine efficacy reduced)

▸ Child 16–17 years: 20 micrograms every month for 3 doses, followed by 20 micrograms after 10 months for 1 dose, for post-exposure prophylaxis, PHE advises dose at 12 months not required if patient is at low risk, deltoid muscle is preferred site of injection; not to be injected into the buttock (vaccine efficacy reduced)

▸ Adult: 20 micrograms every month for 3 doses, followed by 20 micrograms after 10 months for 1 dose, for post-exposure prophylaxis, PHE advises dose at 12 months not required if patient is at low risk, deltoid muscle is preferred site of injection; not to be injected into the buttock (vaccine efficacy reduced)

Immunisation against hepatitis B infection (alternative accelerated schedule)

▸ BY INTRAMUSCULAR INJECTION

▸ Child 11–15 years: 20 micrograms for 1 dose, followed by 20 micrograms after 6 months for 1 dose, this schedule is not suitable if high risk of infection between doses or if compliance with second dose uncertain, deltoid muscle is preferred site of injection; not to be injected into the buttock (vaccine efficacy reduced)

Immunisation against hepatitis B infection (very rapid schedule)

▸ BY INTRAMUSCULAR INJECTION

▸ Child 16–17 years: 20 micrograms for 1 dose, then 20 micrograms after 7 days for 1 dose, followed by 20 micrograms after 14 days for 1 dose, followed by 20 micrograms for 1 dose, to be given 12 months after the first dose, deltoid muscle is preferred site of injection; not to be injected into the buttock (vaccine efficacy reduced)

▸ Adult: 20 micrograms for 1 dose, then 20 micrograms after 7 days for 1 dose, followed by 20 micrograms after 14 days for 1 dose, followed by 20 micrograms for 1 dose, to be given 12 months after the first dose, deltoid muscle is preferred site of injection; not to be injected into the buttock (vaccine efficacy reduced)

Immunisation against hepatitis B infection (in renal insufficiency, including haemodialysis patients)

▸ BY INTRAMUSCULAR INJECTION

▸ Child 1 month–15 years: 10 micrograms every month for 2 doses, followed by 10 micrograms after 5 months for 1 dose, immunisation schedule and booster doses may need to be adjusted in those with low antibody concentration, deltoid muscle is preferred site of injection in older children; anterolateral thigh is preferred site in infants and young children; not to be injected into the buttock (vaccine efficacy reduced)

▸ Child 16–17 years: 40 micrograms every month for 3 doses, followed by 40 micrograms after 4 months for 1 dose, immunisation schedule and booster doses may need to be adjusted in those with low antibody concentration, deltoid muscle is preferred site of injection; not to be injected into the buttock (vaccine efficacy reduced)

▸ Adult: 40 micrograms every month for 3 doses, followed by 40 micrograms after 4 months for 1 dose, immunisation schedule and booster doses may need to be adjusted in those with low antibody concentration, deltoid muscle is preferred site of injection; not to be injected into the buttock (vaccine efficacy reduced)

Immunisation against hepatitis B infection (accelerated schedule for pre- and post-exposure prophylaxis in renal insufficiency, including haemodialysis patients)

▸ BY INTRAMUSCULAR INJECTION

▸ Child 1 month–15 years: 10 micrograms every month for 3 doses, followed by 10 micrograms after 10 months for 1 dose, for post-exposure prophylaxis, PHE advises dose at 12 months not required if patient is at low risk, immunisation schedule and booster doses may need to be adjusted in those with low antibody concentration, deltoid muscle is preferred site of injection in older children; anterolateral thigh is preferred site in infants and young children; not to be injected into the buttock (vaccine efficacy reduced)

FENDRIX ®

Immunisation against hepatitis B infection in renal insufficiency (including pre-haemodialysis and haemodialysis patients)

▸ BY INTRAMUSCULAR INJECTION

▸ Child 15–17 years: 20 micrograms every month for 3 doses, followed by 20 micrograms after 4 months for 1 dose, immunisation schedule and booster doses may need to be adjusted in those with low antibody concentration, deltoid muscle is preferred site of injection; not to be injected into the buttock (vaccine efficacy reduced)

▸ Adult: 20 micrograms every month for 3 doses, followed by 20 micrograms after 4 months for 1 dose, immunisation schedule and booster doses may need to be adjusted in those with low antibody concentration, deltoid muscle is preferred site of injection; not to be injected into the buttock (vaccine efficacy reduced)

HBVAXPRO ®

Immunisation against hepatitis B infection

▸ BY INTRAMUSCULAR INJECTION

▸ Neonate: 5 micrograms for 1 dose, followed by 5 micrograms after 1 month for 1 dose, then 5 micrograms after 5 months for 1 dose, booster doses may be required in immunocompromised patients with low antibody concentration, anterolateral thigh is preferred site in neonates; not to be injected into the buttock (vaccine efficacy reduced), dose not to be used in neonates born to hepatitis B surface antigen-positive mothers.

▸ Child 1 month–15 years: 5 micrograms for 1 dose, followed by 5 micrograms after 1 month for 1 dose, then 5 micrograms after 5 months for 1 dose, booster doses may be required in immunocompromised patients with low antibody concentration, deltoid muscle is preferred site of injection in adults and older children; anterolateral thigh is preferred site in infants; not to be injected into the buttock (vaccine efficacy reduced)

▸ Child 16–17 years: 10 micrograms for 1 dose, followed by 10 micrograms after 1 month for 1 dose, followed by 10 micrograms after 5 months for 1 dose, booster doses may be required in immunocompromised patients with low antibody concentration, deltoid muscle is preferred site of injection in adults and older children; not to be injected into the buttock (vaccine efficacy reduced)

▸ Adult: 10 micrograms for 1 dose, followed by 10 micrograms after 1 month for 1 dose, followed by 10 micrograms after 5 months for 1 dose, booster doses may be required in immunocompromised patients with low antibody concentration, deltoid muscle is preferred site of injection in adults and older children; not to be injected into the buttock (vaccine efficacy reduced)

Immunisation against hepatitis B infection (accelerated schedule for pre- and post-exposure prophylaxis)
▶ BY INTRAMUSCULAR INJECTION

▶ **Neonate:** 5 micrograms every month for 3 doses, followed by 5 micrograms after 10 months for 1 dose, for post-exposure prophylaxis, PHE advises dose at 12 months not required if patient is at low risk, booster doses may be required in immunocompromised patients with low antibody concentration, anterolateral thigh is preferred site in neonates; not to be injected into the buttock (vaccine efficacy reduced), dose not to be used in neonates born to hepatitis B surface antigen-positive mothers.

▶ **Child 1 month–15 years:** 5 micrograms every month for 3 doses, followed by 5 micrograms after 10 months for 1 dose, for post-exposure prophylaxis, PHE advises dose at 12 months not required if patient is at low risk, booster doses may be required in immunocompromised patients with low antibody concentration, deltoid muscle is preferred site of injection in older children; anterolateral thigh is preferred site in infants; not to be injected into the buttock (vaccine efficacy reduced)

▶ **Child 16–17 years:** 10 micrograms every month for 3 doses, followed by 10 micrograms after 10 months for 1 dose, for post-exposure prophylaxis, PHE advises dose at 12 months not required if patient is at low risk, booster doses may be required in immunocompromised patients with low antibody concentration, deltoid muscle is preferred site of injection in older children; not to be injected into the buttock (vaccine efficacy reduced)

▶ **Adult:** 10 micrograms every month for 3 doses, followed by 10 micrograms after 10 months for 1 dose, for post-exposure prophylaxis, PHE advises dose at 12 months not required if patient is at low risk, booster doses may be required in immunocompromised patients with low antibody concentration, deltoid muscle is preferred site of injection; not to be injected into the buttock (vaccine efficacy reduced)

Immunisation against hepatitis B infection (in chronic haemodialysis patients)
▶ BY INTRAMUSCULAR INJECTION

▶ **Child 16–17 years:** 40 micrograms every month for 2 doses, followed by 40 micrograms after 5 months for 1 dose, booster doses may be required in those with low antibody concentration, deltoid muscle is preferred site of injection in older children; not to be injected into the buttock (vaccine efficacy reduced)

▶ **Adult:** 40 micrograms every month for 2 doses, followed by 40 micrograms after 5 months for 1 dose, booster doses may be required in those with low antibody concentration, deltoid muscle is preferred site of injection; not to be injected into the buttock (vaccine efficacy reduced)

● **UNLICENSED USE**

ENGERIX B® PHE advises *Engerix B*® is used in the doses provided in BNF Publications for immunisation against hepatitis B infection (very rapid schedule) in children aged 16–17 years, but these are considered unlicensed.

● **SIDE-EFFECTS**
▶ **Common or very common** Drowsiness · gastrointestinal disorder · irritability
▶ **Uncommon** Dizziness · influenza like illness
▶ **Rare or very rare** Sensation abnormal
▶ **Frequency not known** Angioedema · apnoea · arthritis · encephalitis · encephalopathy · hypotension · meningitis · multiple sclerosis · muscle weakness · nerve disorders · paralysis · seizure · thrombocytopenia · vasculitis

● **PRESCRIBING AND DISPENSING INFORMATION** PHE advises different hepatitis B vaccine preparations can be used to complete a primary immunisation course, or to administer a booster dose.

● **MEDICINAL FORMS** There can be variation in the licensing of different medicines containing the same drug.
Suspension for injection
EXCIPIENTS: May contain Thiomersal
▶ Engerix B (GlaxoSmithKline UK Ltd)
Hepatitis B virus surface antigen 20 microgram per 1 ml Engerix B 10micrograms/0.5ml vaccine suspension for injection pre-filled syringes | 1 pre-filled disposable injection [PoM] £9.67 DT = £9.67
Engerix B 20micrograms/1ml vaccine suspension for injection pre-filled syringes | 1 pre-filled disposable injection [PoM] £12.99 DT = £12.99 | 10 pre-filled disposable injection [PoM] £129.92
▶ Fendrix (GlaxoSmithKline UK Ltd)
Hepatitis B virus surface antigen 40 microgram per 1 ml Fendrix 20micrograms/0.5ml vaccine suspension for injection pre-filled syringes | 1 pre-filled disposable injection [PoM] £38.10 DT = £38.10
▶ HBVAXPRO (Merck Sharp & Dohme (UK) Ltd)
Hepatitis B virus surface antigen 10 microgram per 1 ml HBVAXPRO 10micrograms/1ml vaccine suspension for injection pre-filled syringes | 1 pre-filled disposable injection [PoM] £12.20
HBVAXPRO 5micrograms/0.5ml vaccine suspension for injection pre-filled syringes | 1 pre-filled disposable injection [PoM] £8.95 DT = £8.95
Hepatitis B virus surface antigen 40 microgram per 1 ml HBvaxPRO 40micrograms/1ml vaccine suspension for injection vials | 1 vial [PoM] £27.60 DT = £27.60

▸ **1498**

Herpes-zoster vaccine (recombinant, adjuvanted)
17-Apr-2024

● **DRUG ACTION** *Shingrix*® is a non-live, recombinant, adjuvanted vaccine that protects against herpes zoster (shingles) caused by varicella-zoster virus infection.

● **INDICATIONS AND DOSE**

Immunisation against herpes zoster (shingles)
▶ BY INTRAMUSCULAR INJECTION
▶ **Adult 60-79 years:** 0.5 mL for 2 doses, doses to be separated by an interval of at least 8 weeks

Immunisation against herpes zoster (shingles) [in patients with severe immunosuppression]
▶ BY INTRAMUSCULAR INJECTION
▶ **Adult 50 years and over:** 0.5 mL for 2 doses, doses to be separated by an interval of 8 weeks to 6 months

● **SIDE-EFFECTS**
▶ **Common or very common** Chills · gastrointestinal disorder
▶ **Rare or very rare** Angioedema

● **DIRECTIONS FOR ADMINISTRATION** To be administered preferably into the deltoid region.

● **MEDICINAL FORMS** There can be variation in the licensing of different medicines containing the same drug.
Powder and suspension for suspension for injection
EXCIPIENTS: May contain Polysorbates
▶ Shingrix (GlaxoSmithKline UK Ltd)
Shingrix (Herpes Zoster) adjuvanted recombinant vaccine powder and suspension for suspension for injection 0.5ml vials | 1 vial [PoM] £160.00

F 1498

Human papillomavirus vaccine
19-Jul-2024

● **DRUG ACTION** Human papillomavirus vaccine is a non-live vaccine that contains adsorbed virus-like particles made from recombinant proteins.

● **INDICATIONS AND DOSE**

Primary immunisation against HPV-related premalignant lesions and cancer (cervical, vulvar, vaginal, and anal) and genital warts [1-dose schedule]
▸ BY INTRAMUSCULAR INJECTION
▸ Child 11-17 years: 0.5 mL for 1 dose
▸ Adult 18-24 years: 0.5 mL for 1 dose

Immunisation against HPV-related premalignant lesions and cancer (cervical, vulvar, vaginal, and anal) and genital warts [2-dose schedule for gay, bisexual and other men who have sex with men, and other at risk individuals]
▸ BY INTRAMUSCULAR INJECTION
▸ Adult 25-45 years: 0.5 mL for 1 dose, followed by 0.5 mL for 1 dose, second dose to be given 6–24 months after the first dose, if the 2-dose schedule is interrupted, it should be resumed but not repeated, even if more than 24 months have elapsed since the first dose

Immunisation against HPV-related premalignant lesions and cancer (cervical, vulvar, vaginal, and anal) and genital warts [3-dose schedule for immunocompromised or HIV-positive patients]
▸ BY INTRAMUSCULAR INJECTION
▸ Child 11-17 years: 0.5 mL for 1 dose, followed by 0.5 mL for 1 dose, second dose to be given at least 1 month after the first dose, then 0.5 mL for 1 dose, third dose to be given at least 3 months after the second dose, the 3-dose schedule should be completed within 12 months of the first dose, if the schedule is interrupted, it should be resumed but not repeated, allowing the appropriate interval between the remaining doses
▸ Adult: 0.5 mL for 1 dose, followed by 0.5 mL for 1 dose, second dose to be given at least 1 month after the first dose, then 0.5 mL for 1 dose, third dose to be given at least 3 months after the second dose, the 3-dose schedule should be completed within 12 months of the first dose, if the schedule is interrupted, it should be resumed but not repeated, allowing the appropriate interval between the remaining doses

● **UNLICENSED USE**
▸ In adults UKHSA advises that *Gardasil*® 9 may be used as detailed below, although these situations are considered unlicensed:
  ● 1-dose immunisation schedule;
  ● 2-dose immunisation schedule in individuals aged 25–45 years.
▸ In children UKHSA advises that *Gardasil*® 9 is used in a 1-dose immunisation schedule, but this is not licensed.

● **SIDE-EFFECTS**
▸ **Common or very common** Dizziness
▸ **Uncommon** Asthenia · chills · syncope
▸ **Frequency not known** Acute disseminated encephalomyelitis · bronchospasm · Guillain-Barre syndrome · immune thrombocytopenic purpura

● **PREGNANCY** Not known to be harmful, but vaccination should be postponed until completion of pregnancy.

● **DIRECTIONS FOR ADMINISTRATION** UKHSA advises that individuals with **bleeding disorders** may be vaccinated by the intramuscular route, on the advice of a doctor familiar with their bleeding risk. Patients treated with medicines to reduce bleeding (e.g. for haemophilia) are advised to administer their medicine shortly prior to intramuscular

vaccination. Deltoid region or higher anterolateral thigh are preferred sites of injection.

● **MEDICINAL FORMS** There can be variation in the licensing of different medicines containing the same drug.
Suspension for injection
EXCIPIENTS: May contain Polysorbates
▸ Gardasil 9 (Merck Sharp & Dohme (UK) Ltd)
  Gardasil 9 vaccine suspension for injection 0.5ml pre-filled syringes | 1 pre-filled disposable injection [PoM] £105.00 DT = £105.00

F 1498

Influenza vaccine (inactivated)
04-Jul-2024

● **DRUG ACTION** The inactivated influenza vaccines are injectable inactivated, or recombinant, vaccines that protect people at high risk from influenza and reduce transmission of infection. For information on the live vaccine, see influenza vaccine (live) p. 1515.

● **INDICATIONS AND DOSE**

Annual immunisation against seasonal influenza
▸ BY INTRAMUSCULAR INJECTION
▸ Child 6 months-17 years: 0.5 mL for 1 dose
▸ Adult: 0.5 mL for 1 dose

Annual immunisation against seasonal influenza (for children in clinical risk groups, or who are household contacts of others in clinical risk groups, and who have not received seasonal influenza vaccine previously)
▸ BY INTRAMUSCULAR INJECTION
▸ Child 6 months-8 years: 0.5 mL for 1 dose, followed by 0.5 mL for 1 dose, after at least 4 weeks

● **UNLICENSED USE** The Joint Committee on Vaccination and Immunisation advises offering a second dose of vaccine for annual immunisation against seasonal influenza to children in clinical risk groups only, but this differs from licensed advice.

● **SIDE-EFFECTS**
▸ **Common or very common** Appetite change (in children) · chills · drowsiness (in children) · hyperhidrosis · irritability (in children) · local reactions · pain
▸ **Frequency not known** Angioedema · encephalomyelitis · extensive swelling of vaccinated limb (in adults) · febrile seizure · nerve disorders · nervous system disorder · paraesthesia · thrombocytopenia · vasculitis

SIDE-EFFECTS, FURTHER INFORMATION Elderly patients might be more susceptible to side-effects.

● **ALLERGY AND CROSS-SENSITIVITY** UKHSA advises individuals with a history of egg allergy can be immunised with either an egg free influenza vaccine, if available, or an influenza vaccine with an ovalbumin content less than 120 nanograms/mL (facilities should be available to treat anaphylaxis). If an influenza vaccine containing ovalbumin is being considered in those with a history of severe anaphylaxis to egg which has previously required intensive care, these individuals should be referred to a specialist in hospital.

● **PREGNANCY** [EvGr] Inactivated vaccines not known to be harmful. ⟨M⟩

● **BREAST FEEDING** [EvGr] Inactivated vaccines not known to be harmful. ⟨M⟩

● **DIRECTIONS FOR ADMINISTRATION** UKHSA advises that individuals with **bleeding disorders** may be vaccinated by the intramuscular route, on the advice of a doctor familiar with their bleeding risk. Patients treated with medicines to reduce bleeding (e.g. for haemophilia) are advised to administer their medicine shortly prior to intramuscular vaccination.

● **PRESCRIBING AND DISPENSING INFORMATION** The available preparations are not licensed for use in all age-groups—further information can be found in the product

literature for the individual vaccines. For choice of vaccine, see Influenza vaccine p. 1484.
Ovalbumin content
Preparations with a very low ovalbumin content of less than 120 nanograms/mL: the quadrivalent influenza vaccine (split virion, inactivated) manufactured by Sanofi Pasteur and the quadrivalent influenza vaccine (surface antigen, inactivated) manufactured by Viatris. Preparations that are egg-free: the cell-based quadrivalent influenza vaccine manufactured by Seqirus.

● **MEDICINAL FORMS** There can be variation in the licensing of different medicines containing the same drug.
Suspension for injection
EXCIPIENTS: May contain Gentamicin, kanamycin, neomycin, polysorbates

▸ **Influenza vaccine (inactivated) (non-proprietary)** ▼
Quadrivalent influenza vaccine (split virion, inactivated) suspension for injection 0.5ml pre-filled syringes | 1 pre-filled disposable injection [PoM] £8.00 | 10 pre-filled disposable injection [PoM] £80.00
Quadrivalent influenza vaccine (split virion, inactivated) High-Dose suspension for injection 0.7ml pre-filled syringes | 10 pre-filled disposable injection [PoM] £240.00
Influenza Tetra MYL vaccine suspension for injection 0.5ml pre-filled syringes | 10 pre-filled disposable injection [PoM] £80.00
Adjuvanted quadrivalent influenza vaccine (surface antigen, inactivated) suspension for injection 0.5ml pre-filled syringes | 1 pre-filled disposable injection [PoM] £13.50 | 10 pre-filled disposable injection [PoM] £135.00
Cell-based quadrivalent influenza vaccine (surface antigen, inactivated) suspension for injection 0.5ml pre-filled syringes | 1 pre-filled disposable injection [PoM] £12.50 | 10 pre-filled disposable injection [PoM] £125.00

⚑ 1498

Japanese encephalitis vaccine
25-Aug-2023

● **DRUG ACTION** Japanese encephalitis vaccine is an inactivated vaccine containing adsorbed Japanese encephalitis virus.

● **INDICATIONS AND DOSE**
Immunisation against Japanese encephalitis
▸ BY INTRAMUSCULAR INJECTION
▸ Child 2–35 months: 0.25 mL every 28 days for 2 doses, alternatively 0.25 mL every 7 days for 2 doses, anterolateral thigh may be used as the injection site in infants; deltoid muscle is preferred site in older children, immunisation should be completed at least 1 week before potential exposure
▸ Child 3–17 years: 0.5 mL every 28 days for 2 doses, alternatively 0.5 mL every 7 days for 2 doses, deltoid muscle is preferred site in older children, immunisation should be completed at least 1 week before potential exposure
▸ Adult: 0.5 mL every 28 days for 2 doses, alternatively 0.5 mL every 7 days for 2 doses, deltoid muscle is preferred site of injection, immunisation should be completed at least 1 week before potential exposure

First booster
▸ BY INTRAMUSCULAR INJECTION
▸ Adult: 0.5 mL after 1–2 years, deltoid muscle is preferred site of injection, for those at continued risk, the booster dose should be given 1 year after completing the primary course
▸ Elderly: 0.5 mL after 1 year, for those at continued risk, deltoid muscle is preferred site of injection

Second booster
▸ BY INTRAMUSCULAR INJECTION
▸ Adult: 0.5 mL after 10 years, for those at continued risk, deltoid muscle is preferred site of injection

● **UNLICENSED USE** The rapid schedule administered at days 0 and 7 is not licensed in children or the elderly.

● **SIDE-EFFECTS**
▸ **Common or very common** Influenza like illness (frequency not known in children)
▸ **Uncommon** Asthenia (in adults) · chills (in adults) · dizziness (in adults) · hyperhidrosis (in adults) · migraine (in adults) · musculoskeletal stiffness (in adults) · vertigo (in adults)
▸ **Rare or very rare** Dyspnoea (in adults) · eyelid oedema (in adults) · neuritis (in adults) · pain in extremity (in adults) · palpitations (in adults) · paraesthesia (in adults) · peripheral oedema (in adults) · tachycardia (in adults) · taste altered (in adults) · thrombocytopenia (in adults)
▸ **Frequency not known** Cough (in children) · irritability (in children)

● **PREGNANCY** Although manufacturer advises avoid because of limited information, miscarriage has been associated with Japanese encephalitis virus infection acquired during the first 2 trimesters of pregnancy.

● **MEDICINAL FORMS** There can be variation in the licensing of different medicines containing the same drug.
Solution for injection
▸ **Japanese encephalitis vaccine (Non-proprietary)**
Japanese encephalitis GCVC vaccine solution for injection 1ml vials | 1 vial [℞]
Japanese encephalitis GCVC vaccine solution for injection 20ml vials | 1 vial [℞]
Japanese encephalitis GCVC vaccine solution for injection 10ml vials | 1 vial [℞]

Suspension for injection
▸ **Ixiaro** (Valneva UK Ltd)
Ixiaro vaccine suspension for injection 0.5ml pre-filled syringes | 1 pre-filled disposable injection [PoM] £62.48 DT = £62.48

⚑ 1498

Meningococcal group B vaccine (rDNA, component, adsorbed)
29-Apr-2024

● **DRUG ACTION** Meningococcal group B vaccine is a non-live vaccine that contains adsorbed recombinant *Neisseria meningitidis* serogroup B proteins.

● **INDICATIONS AND DOSE**
BEXSERO ®
Primary immunisation against *Neisseria meningitidis* group B
▸ BY INTRAMUSCULAR INJECTION
▸ Child 2–4 months: 0.5 mL for 2 doses, first dose to be given at 2 months of age and second dose to be given at 4 months of age

Immunisation against *Neisseria meningitidis* group B [booster dose]
▸ BY INTRAMUSCULAR INJECTION
▸ Child 12–23 months: 0.5 mL for 1 dose

Immunisation against *Neisseria meningitidis* group B [patients with unknown or incomplete immunisation status presenting before 1 year of age]
▸ BY INTRAMUSCULAR INJECTION
▸ Child 5–23 months: 0.5 mL for 3 doses, first and second doses separated by an interval of at least 8 weeks (or an interval of 4 weeks to ensure 2 doses given before the first birthday), then third dose to be given between 1 and 2 years of age and at least 4 weeks after the second dose

Immunisation against *Neisseria meningitidis* group B [patients with unknown or incomplete immunisation status presenting after 1 year of age]
▸ BY INTRAMUSCULAR INJECTION
▸ Child 12–23 months: 0.5 mL for 2 doses, doses to be separated by an interval of at least 8 weeks (or an interval of 4 weeks to ensure both doses are given before the second birthday)

continued →

Vaccines 14

TRUMENBA [®]

Immunisation against *Neisseria meningitidis*, primary immunisation

▶ BY INTRAMUSCULAR INJECTION

▶ Child 10–17 years: 0.5 mL for 2 doses, separated by an interval of 6 months, alternatively 0.5 mL for 2 doses, separated by an interval of at least 1 month, followed by 0.5 mL as a third dose, given at least 4 months after the second dose, injected preferably into deltoid region, a booster dose should be considered for individuals at continued risk—consult product literature

▶ Adult: 0.5 mL for 2 doses, separated by an interval of 6 months, alternatively 0.5 mL for 2 doses, separated by an interval of at least 1 month, followed by 0.5 mL as a third dose, given at least 4 months after the second dose, injected preferably into deltoid region, a booster dose should be considered for individuals at continued risk—consult product literature

● SIDE-EFFECTS

▶ **Common or very common** Crying abnormal (in children) · drowsiness (in children) · eating disorder (in children) · irritability (in children)

▶ **Uncommon** Seizures (in children) · vascular disorders (in children)

▶ **Frequency not known** Extensive swelling of vaccinated limb · hypotonic-hyporesponsiveness episode (in children) · meningism

● DIRECTIONS FOR ADMINISTRATION

BEXSERO [®] Anterolateral thigh is the preferred site of injection in infants under 1 year of age; deltoid muscle is preferred in older children and adults.

● PRESCRIBING AND DISPENSING INFORMATION Details on routine immunisations are included in this monograph; for details of immunisation in other patient groups e.g. patients at high risk of infection, see Meningococcal vaccines p. 1486 and Vaccination, general principles p. 1470.

BEXSERO [®] For information about the use of paracetamol for prophylaxis of post-immunisation pyrexia, see paracetamol p. 507.

● MEDICINAL FORMS There can be variation in the licensing of different medicines containing the same drug.

Suspension for injection

EXCIPIENTS: May contain Kanamycin

▶ Bexsero (GlaxoSmithKline UK Ltd)
Bexsero vaccine suspension for injection 0.5ml pre-filled syringes | 1 pre-filled disposable injection [PoM] £75.00

▶ Trumenba (Pfizer Ltd) ▼
Trumenba vaccine suspension for injection 0.5ml pre-filled syringes | 1 pre-filled disposable injection [PoM] £75.00

[F 1498]

Meningococcal groups A with C and W135 and Y vaccine

26-Mar-2024

● DRUG ACTION Meningococcal groups A with C and W135 and Y vaccine is a non-live conjugated vaccine.

● INDICATIONS AND DOSE

Primary immunisation against *Neisseria meningitidis* groups A, W135 and Y, and immunisation against *Neisseria meningitidis* group C (booster dose in those who have received primary immunisation)

▶ BY INTRAMUSCULAR INJECTION

▶ Child 13–15 years: 0.5 mL for 1 dose

Immunisation against *Neisseria meningitidis* groups A, C, W135 and Y [patients with unknown or incomplete immunisation status]

▶ BY INTRAMUSCULAR INJECTION

▶ Child 10–17 years: 0.5 mL for 1 dose

▶ Adult 18–24 years: 0.5 mL for 1 dose

● SIDE-EFFECTS

▶ **Common or very common** Drowsiness · irritability

▶ **Uncommon** Crying · dizziness · insomnia · numbness · pain in extremity

▶ **Frequency not known** Extensive swelling of vaccinated limb

● DIRECTIONS FOR ADMINISTRATION Deltoid muscle is preferred site of injection in older children and adults.

● PRESCRIBING AND DISPENSING INFORMATION Details on routine immunisations are included in this monograph; for details of immunisation in other patient groups e.g. patients at high risk of infection, see Meningococcal vaccines p. 1486 and Vaccination, general principles p. 1470.

● MEDICINAL FORMS There can be variation in the licensing of different medicines containing the same drug.

Solution for injection

▶ MenQuadfi (Sanofi) ▼
MenQuadfi vaccine solution for injection 0.5ml vials | 1 vial [PoM] £31.50

Powder and solvent for solution for injection

EXCIPIENTS: May contain Sucrose

▶ Menveo (GlaxoSmithKline UK Ltd)
Menveo vaccine powder and solvent for solution for injection 0.5ml vials | 1 vial [PoM] £30.00 DT = £30.00

▶ Nimenrix (Pfizer Ltd)
Nimenrix vaccine powder and solvent for solution for injection 0.5ml pre-filled syringes | 1 pre-filled disposable injection [PoM] £30.00 DT = £30.00

[F 1498]

Pneumococcal polysaccharide conjugate vaccine (adsorbed)

28-Jan-2025

● DRUG ACTION Pneumococcal polysaccharide conjugate vaccine is an inactivated vaccine that protects against infection caused by *Streptococcus pneumoniae*. The conjugate vaccine contains adsorbed pneumococcal polysaccharide from either 13 capsular types (13-valent *Prevenar* 13 [®]), 15 capsular types (15-valent *Vaxneuvance* [®]), or 20 capsular types (20-valent *Prevenar* 20 [®]). For information on the non-conjugate vaccine, see pneumococcal polysaccharide vaccine p. 1511.

● INDICATIONS AND DOSE

Primary immunisation against pneumococcal infection

▶ BY INTRAMUSCULAR INJECTION

▶ Child 12 weeks: 0.5 mL for 1 dose

Immunisation against pneumococcal infection [booster dose]

▶ BY INTRAMUSCULAR INJECTION

▶ Child 1 year: 0.5 mL for 1 dose

Immunisation against pneumococcal infection [in patients with unknown or incomplete immunisation status]

▶ BY INTRAMUSCULAR INJECTION

▶ Child 3–11 months: 0.5 mL for 1 dose, followed by 0.5 mL for 1 dose on or after their first birthday, to be given at least 4 weeks after the first dose

▶ Child 12–23 months: 0.5 mL for 1 dose

● SIDE-EFFECTS

▶ **Common or very common** Drowsiness · irritability · sleep disorder

▶ **Uncommon** Crying · seizures

▶ **Rare or very rare** Hypotonic-hyporesponsiveness episode

- **DIRECTIONS FOR ADMINISTRATION** Anterolateral thigh is preferred site of injection in infants under 1 year; deltoid muscle is preferred in older children and adults.
- **PRESCRIBING AND DISPENSING INFORMATION** Details on routine immunisations are included in this monograph; for details of immunisation in other patient groups e.g. patients at high risk of infection, see Pneumococcal vaccine p. 1488 and Vaccination, general principles p. 1470.

  Available as part of childhood immunisation schedule from ImmForm.

  The 20-valent vaccine *Prevenar 20* ® is not currently recommended as part of the routine UK immunisation schedule.

- **MEDICINAL FORMS** There can be variation in the licensing of different medicines containing the same drug.

Suspension for injection

- **Apexxnar** (Pfizer Ltd) ▼
  Prevenar 20 vaccine suspension for injection 0.5ml pre-filled syringes | 1 pre-filled disposable injection PoM £56.50 DT = £49.10
- **Prevenar** (Pfizer Ltd)
  Prevenar 13 vaccine suspension for injection 0.5ml pre-filled syringes | 1 pre-filled disposable injection PoM £49.10 DT = £49.10 | 10 pre-filled disposable injection PoM £491.00
- **Vaxneuvance** (Merck Sharp & Dohme (UK) Ltd) ▼
  Vaxneuvance vaccine suspension for injection 0.5ml pre-filled syringes | 1 pre-filled disposable injection PoM £50.30 DT = £49.10

☞ 1498

Pneumococcal polysaccharide vaccine

02-Jan-2024

- **DRUG ACTION** Pneumococcal polysaccharide vaccine is an inactivated, 23-valent vaccine that protects against pneumococcal disease caused by *Streptococcus pneumoniae*. For information on the conjugate vaccine, see pneumococcal polysaccharide conjugate vaccine (adsorbed) p. 1510.

- ● **INDICATIONS AND DOSE**

Primary immunisation against pneumococcal infection
- ▶ BY INTRAMUSCULAR INJECTION
- ▸ Elderly: 0.5 mL for 1 dose

- **SIDE-EFFECTS** Angioedema · arthritis · asthenia · chills · febrile seizure · haemolytic anaemia · injected limb mobility decreased · leucocytosis · lymphadenitis · nerve disorders · paraesthesia · peripheral oedema · thrombocytopenia

- **DIRECTIONS FOR ADMINISTRATION** Deltoid muscle is preferred site of injection in adults.

- **PRESCRIBING AND DISPENSING INFORMATION** Details on routine immunisations are included in this monograph; for details of immunisation in other patient groups e.g. patients at high risk of infection, see Pneumococcal vaccine p. 1488 and Vaccination, general principles p. 1470.

- **MEDICINAL FORMS** There can be variation in the licensing of different medicines containing the same drug.

Solution for injection

- **Pneumovax 23** (Merck Sharp & Dohme (UK) Ltd)
  Pneumovax 23 solution for injection 0.5ml pre-filled syringes | 1 pre-filled disposable injection PoM £16.80 DT = £16.80

☞ 1498

Rabies vaccine

19-Dec-2024

- **DRUG ACTION** Rabies vaccine is an inactivated vaccine containing rabies virus.

- ● **INDICATIONS AND DOSE**

RABIPUR ®

Primary pre-exposure immunisation against rabies infection
- ▶ BY INTRAMUSCULAR INJECTION
- ▸ Child: 1 mL for 3 doses (on days 0, 7, and 28), final dose may be given from day 21 if insufficient time before travel
- ▸ Adult: 1 mL for 3 doses (on days 0, 7, and 28), final dose may be given from day 21 if insufficient time before travel

Primary pre-exposure immunisation against rabies infection [accelerated course]
- ▶ BY INTRAMUSCULAR INJECTION
- ▸ Child: 1 mL for 3 doses (on days 0, 3, and 7), followed by 1 mL for 1 dose, to be given at 1 year if continued travel to high-risk areas
- ▸ Adult: 1 mL for 3 doses (on days 0, 3, and 7), followed by 1 mL for 1 dose, to be given at 1 year if continued travel to high-risk areas

Pre-exposure immunisation booster dose [patients at frequent risk of exposure e.g. laboratory workers who handle lyssavirus-containing material]
- ▶ BY INTRAMUSCULAR INJECTION
- ▸ Child: 1 mL for 1 dose, to be given 1 year after primary course is completed, then 1 mL, repeated if necessary, based on six-monthly antibody levels
- ▸ Adult: 1 mL for 1 dose, to be given 1 year after primary course is completed, then 1 mL, repeated if necessary, based on six-monthly antibody levels

Pre-exposure immunisation booster dose [patients who may have frequent, unrecognised exposures e.g. bat handlers]
- ▶ BY INTRAMUSCULAR INJECTION
- ▸ Child: 1 mL for 1 dose, to be given 1 year after primary course is completed, then 1 mL, repeated if necessary, based on antibody levels
- ▸ Adult: 1 mL for 1 dose, to be given 1 year after primary course is completed, then 1 mL, repeated if necessary, based on antibody levels

Pre-exposure immunisation booster dose [patients at infrequent risk of exposure]
- ▶ BY INTRAMUSCULAR INJECTION
- ▸ Child: 1 mL for 1 dose, to be given at least 1 year after primary course is completed based on antibody levels
- ▸ Adult: 1 mL for 1 dose, to be given at least 1 year after primary course is completed based on antibody levels

Post-exposure treatment [fully immunised patients with amber or red composite rabies risk] (administered on expert advice)
- ▶ BY INTRAMUSCULAR INJECTION
- ▸ Child: 1 mL for 1 dose, followed by 1 mL for 1 dose, to be given 3–7 days after the first dose, rabies immunoglobulin is not necessary
- ▸ Adult: 1 mL for 1 dose, followed by 1 mL for 1 dose, to be given 3–7 days after the first dose, rabies immunoglobulin is not necessary

Post-exposure treatment [partially immunised patients with amber or red composite rabies risk] (administered on expert advice)
- ▶ BY INTRAMUSCULAR INJECTION
- ▸ Child: 1 mL for 4 doses (on days 0, 3, 7, and 21), rabies immunoglobulin is not necessary

continued →

‣ **Adult:** 1 mL for 4 doses (on days 0, 3, 7, and 21), rabies immunoglobulin is not necessary

Post-exposure treatment [non-immunised patients with amber or red composite rabies risk] (administered on expert advice)
▸ BY INTRAMUSCULAR INJECTION
‣ **Child:** 1 mL for 4 doses (on days 0, 3, 7, and 21), rabies immunoglobulin also to be given to patients with red composite rabies risk (but is not required if more than 7 days have elapsed after the first dose of vaccine, or more than 1 day after the second dose of vaccine)
‣ **Adult:** 1 mL for 4 doses (on days 0, 3, 7, and 21), rabies immunoglobulin also to be given to patients with red composite rabies risk (but is not required if more than 7 days have elapsed after the first dose of vaccine, or more than 1 day after the second dose of vaccine)

Post-exposure treatment [immunosuppressed patients with amber or red composite rabies risk, regardless of immunisation status] (administered on expert advice)
▸ BY INTRAMUSCULAR INJECTION
‣ **Child:** 1 mL for 5 doses (on days 0, 3, 7, 14, and 30), rabies immunoglobulin also to be given
‣ **Adult:** 1 mL for 5 doses (on days 0, 3, 7, 14, and 30), rabies immunoglobulin also to be given

VERORAB®

Primary pre-exposure immunisation against rabies infection
▸ BY INTRAMUSCULAR INJECTION
‣ **Child:** 0.5 mL for 3 doses (on days 0, 7, and 28), final dose may be given from day 21 if insufficient time before travel
‣ **Adult:** 0.5 mL for 3 doses (on days 0, 7, and 28), final dose may be given from day 21 if insufficient time before travel

Primary pre-exposure immunisation against rabies infection [accelerated course]
▸ BY INTRAMUSCULAR INJECTION
‣ **Child:** 0.5 mL for 3 doses (on days 0, 3, and 7), followed by 0.5 mL for 1 dose, to be given at 1 year if continued travel to high-risk areas
‣ **Adult:** 0.5 mL for 3 doses (on days 0, 3, and 7), followed by 0.5 mL for 1 dose, to be given at 1 year if continued travel to high-risk areas

Pre-exposure immunisation booster dose [patients at frequent risk of exposure e.g. laboratory workers who handle lyssavirus-containing material]
▸ BY INTRAMUSCULAR INJECTION
‣ **Child:** 0.5 mL for 1 dose, to be given 1 year after primary course is completed, then 0.5 mL, repeated if necessary, based on six-monthly antibody levels
‣ **Adult:** 0.5 mL for 1 dose, to be given 1 year after primary course is completed, then 0.5 mL, repeated if necessary, based on six-monthly antibody levels

Pre-exposure immunisation booster dose [patients who may have frequent, unrecognised exposures e.g. bat handlers]
▸ BY INTRAMUSCULAR INJECTION
‣ **Child:** 0.5 mL for 1 dose, to be given 1 year after primary course is completed, then 0.5 mL, repeated if necessary, based on antibody levels
‣ **Adult:** 0.5 mL for 1 dose, to be given 1 year after primary course is completed, then 0.5 mL, repeated if necessary, based on antibody levels

Pre-exposure immunisation booster dose [patients at infrequent risk of exposure]
▸ BY INTRAMUSCULAR INJECTION
‣ **Child:** 0.5 mL for 1 dose, to be given at least 1 year after primary course is completed based on antibody levels
‣ **Adult:** 0.5 mL for 1 dose, to be given at least 1 year after primary course is completed based on antibody levels

Post-exposure treatment [fully immunised patients with amber or red composite rabies risk] (administered on expert advice)
▸ BY INTRAMUSCULAR INJECTION
‣ **Child:** 0.5 mL for 1 dose, followed by 0.5 mL for 1 dose, to be given 3–7 days after the first dose, rabies immunoglobulin is not necessary
‣ **Adult:** 0.5 mL for 1 dose, followed by 0.5 mL for 1 dose, to be given 3–7 days after the first dose, rabies immunoglobulin is not necessary

Post-exposure treatment [partially immunised patients with amber or red composite rabies risk] (administered on expert advice)
▸ BY INTRAMUSCULAR INJECTION
‣ **Child:** 0.5 mL for 4 doses (on days 0, 3, 7, and 21), rabies immunoglobulin is not necessary
‣ **Adult:** 0.5 mL for 4 doses (on days 0, 3, 7, and 21), rabies immunoglobulin is not necessary

Post-exposure treatment [non-immunised patients with amber or red composite rabies risk] (administered on expert advice)
▸ BY INTRAMUSCULAR INJECTION
‣ **Child:** 0.5 mL for 4 doses (on days 0, 3, 7, and 21), rabies immunoglobulin also to be given to patients with red composite rabies risk (but is not required if more than 7 days have elapsed after the first dose of vaccine, or more than 1 day after the second dose of vaccine)
‣ **Adult:** 0.5 mL for 4 doses (on days 0, 3, 7, and 21), rabies immunoglobulin also to be given to patients with red composite rabies risk (but is not required if more than 7 days have elapsed after the first dose of vaccine, or more than 1 day after the second dose of vaccine)

Post-exposure treatment [immunosuppressed patients with amber or red composite rabies risk, regardless of immunisation status] (administered on expert advice)
▸ BY INTRAMUSCULAR INJECTION
‣ **Child:** 0.5 mL for 5 doses (on days 0, 3, 7, 14, and 30), rabies immunoglobulin also to be given
‣ **Adult:** 0.5 mL for 5 doses (on days 0, 3, 7, 14, and 30), rabies immunoglobulin also to be given

● UNLICENSED USE Public Health England advises rabies vaccine may be used as detailed below, although these situations are considered unlicensed:
  ● dosing regimens for post-exposure treatment.

● INTERACTIONS → Appendix 1: rabies vaccine

● SIDE-EFFECTS
▸ **Common or very common** Abdominal discomfort · asthenia · dizziness
▸ **Rare or very rare** Angioedema · chills · encephalitis · Guillain-Barre syndrome · hyperhidrosis · paraesthesia · syncope · vertigo

● ALLERGY AND CROSS-SENSITIVITY
  RABIPUR®
▸ When used for Pre-exposure immunisation PHE advises to consider alternative rabies vaccine in individuals with a history of severe egg allergy.
▸ When used for Post-exposure treatment PHE advises it is not contra-indicated in individuals with severe egg allergies; if there is a history of hypersensitivity, specialist advice should be sought and further doses given under supervision.

● PREGNANCY Because of the potential consequences of untreated rabies exposure and because rabies vaccination has not been associated with fetal abnormalities, pregnancy is not considered a contra-indication to post-exposure prophylaxis. Immunisation against rabies is indicated during pregnancy if there is substantial risk of exposure to rabies and rapid access to post-exposure prophylaxis is likely to be limited.

- **DIRECTIONS FOR ADMINISTRATION** Anterolateral thigh is preferred site of injection in infants under 1 year of age; deltoid muscle is preferred in older children and adults.

- **PRESCRIBING AND DISPENSING INFORMATION** Ovalbumin content *Rabipur*® contains residues of chicken proteins, such as ovalbumin.

- **MEDICINAL FORMS** There can be variation in the licensing of different medicines containing the same drug.
  Powder and solvent for suspension for injection
  EXCIPIENTS: May contain Maltose, neomycin, phenylalanine, polymyxin b, streptomycin
  - **Verorab** (Sanofi)
    Verorab powder and solvent for suspension for injection 0.5ml vials | 1 vial [PoM] £75.00

  Powder and solvent for solution for injection
  EXCIPIENTS: May contain Neomycin, sucrose
  - **Rabipur** (Bavarian Nordic UK Ltd)
    Rabipur vaccine powder and solvent for solution for injection 1ml pre-filled syringes | 1 pre-filled disposable injection [PoM] £48.19

⚑ 1498

Tick-borne encephalitis vaccine   25-Aug-2023

- **DRUG ACTION** Tick-borne encephalitis vaccine is an inactivated vaccine containing adsorbed tick-borne encephalitis virus.

- **INDICATIONS AND DOSE**
  Initial immunisation against tick-borne encephalitis
  - BY INTRAMUSCULAR INJECTION
  - Child 1-15 years: 0.25 mL for 1 dose, followed by 0.25 mL after 1–3 months for 1 dose, then 0.25 mL after further 5–12 months for 1 dose, to achieve more rapid protection, second dose may be given 14 days after first dose, dose to be administered in deltoid region or anterolateral thigh in infants, in immunocompromised patients (including those receiving immunosuppressants), antibody concentration may be measured 4 weeks after second dose and dose repeated if protective levels not achieved
  - Child 16-17 years: 0.5 mL for 1 dose, followed by 0.5 mL after 1–3 months for 1 dose, then 0.5 mL after further 5–12 months for 1 dose, to achieve more rapid protection, second dose may be given 14 days after first dose, dose to be administered in deltoid region, in immunocompromised patients (including those receiving immunosuppressants), antibody concentration may be measured 4 weeks after second dose and dose repeated if protective levels not achieved
  - Adult: 0.5 mL for 1 dose, followed by 0.5 mL after 1–3 months for 1 dose, then 0.5 mL after further 5–12 months for 1 dose, to achieve more rapid protection, second dose may be given 14 days after first dose, dose to be administered in deltoid region, in immunocompromised patients (including those receiving immunosuppressants), antibody concentration may be measured 4 weeks after second dose and dose repeated if protective levels not achieved
  - Elderly: 0.5 mL for 1 dose, followed by 0.5 mL after 1–3 months for 1 dose, then 0.5 mL after further 5–12 months for 1 dose, to achieve more rapid protection, second dose may be given 14 days after first dose, dose to be administered in deltoid region, antibody concentration may be measured 4 weeks after second dose and dose repeated if protective levels not achieved

Immunisation against tick-borne encephalitis, booster doses
- BY INTRAMUSCULAR INJECTION
- Child 1-17 years: First dose to be given within 3 years after initial course completed and then every 3–5 years, dose to be administered in deltoid region or anterolateral thigh in infants (consult product literature)
- Adult: First dose to be given within 3 years after initial course completed and then every 3–5 years, dose to be administered in deltoid region (consult product literature)

- **SIDE-EFFECTS**
- **Common or very common** Restlessness (in children) · sleep disorder (in children)
- **Rare or very rare** Asthenia · autoimmune disorder (in adults) · chills (uncommon in children) · demyelination (in adults) · dizziness · drowsiness (in adults) · dyspepsia (in children) · dyspnoea · eye pain · gait abnormal · hyperhidrosis · increased risk of infection · influenza like illness · joint swelling (in adults) · meningism · meningitis aseptic (in adults) · motor dysfunction · musculoskeletal stiffness · nerve disorders · oedema · pain · seizures · sensory disorder · tachycardia (in adults) · tinnitus · vertigo · vision disorders

- **ALLERGY AND CROSS-SENSITIVITY** PHE advises individuals with evidence of previous anaphylactic reaction to egg should not be given tick-borne encephalitis vaccine.

- **MEDICINAL FORMS** There can be variation in the licensing of different medicines containing the same drug.
  Suspension for injection
  EXCIPIENTS: May contain Gentamicin, neomycin
  - **TicoVac** (Pfizer Ltd)
    TicoVac Junior vaccine suspension for injection 0.25ml pre-filled syringes | 1 pre-filled disposable injection [PoM] £28.00
    TicoVac vaccine suspension for injection 0.5ml pre-filled syringes | 1 pre-filled disposable injection [PoM] £32.00

⚑ 1498

Typhoid vaccine (inactivated)   12-Sep-2023

- **DRUG ACTION** The inactivated typhoid vaccine is an injectable polysaccharide vaccine that protects against typhoid fever caused by *Salmonella typhi* infection. For information on the live vaccine, see typhoid vaccine (live) p. 1517.

- **INDICATIONS AND DOSE**
  Immunisation against typhoid fever [in children at high risk of typhoid fever]
  - BY INTRAMUSCULAR INJECTION
  - Child 12-23 months: 0.5 mL for 1 dose, dose should be given at least 2 weeks before potential exposure to typhoid infection, response may be suboptimal

  Immunisation against typhoid fever
  - BY INTRAMUSCULAR INJECTION
  - Child 2-17 years: 0.5 mL for 1 dose, dose should be given at least 2 weeks before potential exposure to typhoid infection
  - Adult: 0.5 mL for 1 dose, dose should be given at least 2 weeks before potential exposure to typhoid infection

  Booster
  - BY INTRAMUSCULAR INJECTION
  - Child 2-17 years: 0.5 mL for 1 dose every 3 years
  - Adult: 0.5 mL for 1 dose every 3 years

- **UNLICENSED USE** UKHSA advises that inactivated typhoid vaccine may be used in children aged 12–23 months at high risk of typhoid fever, but it is not licensed for this age group.

- **SIDE-EFFECTS**
▸ **Common or very common** Asthenia
▸ **Frequency not known** Asthma · shock

- **MEDICINAL FORMS** There can be variation in the licensing of different medicines containing the same drug.

Solution for injection
▸ **Typhim Vi** (Sanofi)
Salmonella typhi Vi capsular polysaccharide 50 microgram per 1 ml Typhim Vi 25micrograms/0.5ml vaccine solution for injection pre-filled syringes | 1 pre-filled disposable injection [PoM] £11.16 DT = £11.16 | 10 pre-filled disposable injection [PoM] £111.60 DT = £111.60

VACCINES 〉 LIVE

Vaccines, live

12-Sep-2023 

> **IMPORTANT SAFETY INFORMATION**
> **MHRA/CHM ADVICE (UPDATED NOVEMBER 2017)**
> Following reports of death in neonates who received a live attenuated vaccine after exposure to a tumor necrosis factor alpha (TNF-a) inhibitor *in utero*, the MHRA has issued the following advice:
> - any infant who has been exposed to immunosuppressive treatment from the mother either *in utero* during pregnancy or via breastfeeding should have any live attenuated vaccination deferred for as long as a postnatal influence on the immune status of the infant remains possible;
> - in the case of infants who have been exposed to TNF-a inhibitors and other immunosuppressive biological medicines *in utero*, UKHSA advise that any live attenuated vaccination (e.g. BCG vaccine) should be deferred until the infant is age 6 months;
> - UKHSA advise if there is any doubt as to whether an infant due to receive a live attenuated vaccine may be immunosuppressed due to the mother's therapy, including exposure through breast-feeding, specialist advice should be sought.

- **CONTRA-INDICATIONS**
▸ Impaired immune response UKHSA advises severely immunosuppressed patients should not be given live vaccines (including those with severe primary immunodeficiency).

- **CAUTIONS**
▸ Impaired immune response and drugs affecting immune response There is a risk of generalised infection with live vaccines.
UKHSA advises seek specialist advice for immunosuppressed patients, including those who are:
- taking high doses of corticosteroids (dose equivalents of prednisolone: **adults**, at least 40 mg daily for more than 1 week or at least 20 mg daily for more than 14 days; **children**, 2 mg/kg (or more than 40 mg) daily for more than 1 week or 1 mg/kg (or more than 20 mg) daily for more than 14 days);
- taking immunosuppressive drugs;
- receiving treatment for malignant or non-malignant conditions with chemotherapy or generalised radiotherapy.
UKHSA advises live vaccines should be postponed until at least 3 months after stopping high-dose systemic corticosteroids, or non-biological oral immune modulating drugs; and at least 6 months after stopping other immunosuppressive drugs, or generalised radiotherapy; and at least 12 months after discontinuing immunosuppressive biological therapy.

- **SIDE-EFFECTS**
▸ **Common or very common** Abdominal pain · appetite decreased · arthralgia · diarrhoea · fever · headache ·

irritability · malaise · myalgia · nausea · skin reactions · vomiting
▸ **Uncommon** Dizziness
▸ **Rare or very rare** Anaphylactic reaction

- **PREGNANCY** UKHSA advises live vaccines should not be administered routinely to pregnant women because of the theoretical risk of fetal infection, but where there is a significant risk of exposure to disease the need for vaccination may outweigh any possible risk to the fetus. Termination of pregnancy following inadvertent immunisation is not recommended.

- **BREAST FEEDING** Although there is a theoretical risk of live vaccine being present in breast milk, vaccination is not contra-indicated for women who are breast-feeding when there is significant risk of exposure to disease.

- **DIRECTIONS FOR ADMINISTRATION** Manufacturer advises if alcohol or disinfectant is used for cleansing the skin it should be allowed to evaporate before vaccination to prevent possible inactivation of live vaccines.

⟋ above ⟋ 1498

Bacillus Calmette-Guérin vaccine

25-Aug-2023

(BCG vaccine)

- **DRUG ACTION** BCG (Bacillus Calmette-Guérin) vaccine is a live attenuated vaccine derived from *Mycobacterium bovis*.

- **INDICATIONS AND DOSE**

Immunisation against tuberculosis
▸ BY INTRADERMAL INJECTION
▸ Child 1–11 months: 0.05 mL, to be injected at insertion of deltoid muscle onto humerus (keloid formation more likely with sites higher on arm); tip of shoulder should be **avoided**
▸ Child 1–17 years: 0.1 mL, to be injected at insertion of deltoid muscle onto humerus (keloid formation more likely with sites higher on arm); tip of shoulder should be **avoided**
▸ Adult: 0.1 mL, to be injected at insertion of deltoid muscle onto humerus (keloid formation more likely with sites higher on arm); tip of shoulder should be **avoided**

- **CONTRA-INDICATIONS** Children less than 2 years of age in household contact with known or suspected case of active tuberculosis · generalised septic skin conditions · history of active or latent tuberculosis · severe combined immunodeficiency disorder

CONTRA-INDICATIONS, FURTHER INFORMATION
Manufacturer advises using a lesion-free site to administer BCG vaccine to patients with eczema.

- **CAUTIONS** When BCG is given to infants, there is no need to delay routine primary immunisations. No further vaccination should be given in the arm used for BCG vaccination for at least 3 months because of the risk of regional lymphadenitis.

- **INTERACTIONS** → Appendix 1: live vaccines

- **SIDE-EFFECTS**
▸ **Uncommon** Lymphadenitis suppurative
▸ **Rare or very rare** Osteitis · osteomyelitis
▸ **Frequency not known** Seizure · syncope

- **PRE-TREATMENT SCREENING** Apart from children under 6 years, any person being considered for BCG immunisation must first be given a skin test for hypersensitivity to tuberculoprotein (see tuberculin purified protein derivative p. 1470). A skin test is not necessary for a child under 6 years provided that the child has not stayed for longer than 3 months in a country with an incidence of tuberculosis greater than 40 per 100 000, the child has not had contact with a person with tuberculosis, and there is no family history of tuberculosis within the last 5 years.

- In children PHE advise that the results of the severe combined immunodeficiency (SCID) screening should be checked before administering BCG vaccine.

- **DIRECTIONS FOR ADMINISTRATION**
Intradermal injection technique Public Health England advises skin is stretched between thumb and forefinger and needle (size 26G) inserted (bevel upwards) for about 3 mm into superficial layers of dermis (almost parallel with surface). Needle should be short with short bevel (can usually be seen through epidermis during insertion). Tense raised blanched bleb is sign of correct injection; 7 mm bleb ≡ 0.1 mL injection, 3 mm bleb ≡ 0.05 mL injection; if considerable resistance not felt, needle too deep and should be removed and reinserted before giving more vaccine. Jet injectors and multiple puncture devices should not be used.
- **PRESCRIBING AND DISPENSING INFORMATION** Available from health organisations or direct from ImmForm.

- **MEDICINAL FORMS** There can be variation in the licensing of different medicines containing the same drug.

Powder for injection

- Bacillus calmette-guérin vaccine (Non-proprietary)
BCG Vaccine AJV powder for suspension for injection 1ml vials | 10 vial PoM

F 1514 F 1498

Cholera vaccine (live)

29-Aug-2024

- **DRUG ACTION** The live cholera vaccine is an oral vaccine that contains live attenuated *Vibrio cholerae*. For information on the inactivated vaccine, see cholera vaccine (inactivated) p. 1499.

- **INDICATIONS AND DOSE**

Immunisation against cholera

- BY MOUTH
- Child 2-17 years: 1 dose, immunisation should be completed at least 10 days before potential exposure
- Adult: 1 dose, immunisation should be completed at least 10 days before potential exposure

- **CONTRA-INDICATIONS** Acute gastro-intestinal illness
- **INTERACTIONS** → Appendix 1: live vaccines
- **SIDE-EFFECTS**
- **Uncommon** Burping · constipation · dry mouth · gastrointestinal discomfort · gastrointestinal disorders
- **Rare or very rare** Chills
- **DIRECTIONS FOR ADMINISTRATION** Administration of *Vaxchora*® and oral typhoid vaccine (live) should be separated by a 2-hour interval—transit of the capsules through the gastro-intestinal tract may be affected by the buffer administered with *Vaxchora*®.
- In children EvGr Mix buffer powder in 100 mL of cold or room temperature bottled water; for children aged 2–5 years, discard half (50 mL) of the buffer solution. Add active component to the buffer solution and stir for at least 30 seconds to make one dose. Drink within 15 minutes of reconstitution. Food and drink should be avoided for 1 hour before and after vaccination. ⟨M⟩
- In adults EvGr Mix buffer powder in 100 mL of cold or room temperature bottled water, then add active component and stir for at least 30 seconds to make one dose. Drink within 15 minutes of reconstitution. Food and drink should be avoided for 1 hour before and after vaccination. ⟨M⟩
- **PATIENT AND CARER ADVICE** Counselling on administration advised. Immunisation with cholera vaccine does not provide complete protection and all travellers to a country where cholera exists should be warned that scrupulous attention to food, water, and personal hygiene is **essential**. The live cholera vaccine virus may be excreted in the stool and could be transmitted to close contacts. UKHSA advises thorough handwashing after visiting the toilet and before preparing food for at least 14 days after immunisation.

- **MEDICINAL FORMS** There can be variation in the licensing of different medicines containing the same drug.

Effervescent powder and powder for oral suspension

EXCIPIENTS: May contain Sucrose
ELECTROLYTES: May contain Sodium

- Vaxchora (Bavarian Nordic UK Ltd)
Vaxchora vaccine effervescent powder and powder for oral suspension | 1 dose PoM £43.20

F 1514 F 1498

Dengue vaccine

24-Aug-2023

- **DRUG ACTION** Dengue vaccine is a live, attenuated vaccine that protects against dengue virus infection.

- **INDICATIONS AND DOSE**

Immunisation against dengue

- BY SUBCUTANEOUS INJECTION
- Child 4-17 years: 0.5 mL for 1 dose, then 0.5 mL for 1 dose, to be given 3 months after initial dose
- Adult: 0.5 mL for 1 dose, then 0.5 mL for 1 dose, to be given 3 months after initial dose

- **INTERACTIONS** → Appendix 1: live vaccines
- **SIDE-EFFECTS**
- **Common or very common** Asthenia · drowsiness (in children) · increased risk of infection · influenza like illness
- **Rare or very rare** Angioedema
- **CONCEPTION AND CONTRACEPTION** EvGr Avoid pregnancy for at least 1 month after vaccination. ⟨M⟩
- **DIRECTIONS FOR ADMINISTRATION** To be administered preferably into the deltoid region.
- **PATIENT AND CARER ADVICE** Immunisation with dengue vaccine does not provide complete protection and personal protective measures against mosquito bites are recommended.

- **MEDICINAL FORMS** There can be variation in the licensing of different medicines containing the same drug.

Powder and solvent for solution for injection

- Qdenga (Takeda UK Ltd) ▼
Qdenga vaccine powder and solvent for solution for injection 0.5ml pre-filled syringes | 1 pre-filled disposable injection PoM £68.75

F 1514 F 1498

Influenza vaccine (live)

16-Oct-2024

- **DRUG ACTION** The live influenza vaccine is a nasal spray containing live attenuated strains; it protects people at high risk from influenza and reduces transmission of infection. For information on the inactivated vaccines, see influenza vaccine (inactivated) p. 1508.

- **INDICATIONS AND DOSE**

Annual immunisation against seasonal influenza

- BY INTRANASAL ADMINISTRATION
- Child 2-17 years: 0.2 mL for 1 dose, to be administered as 0.1 mL into each nostril

Annual immunisation against seasonal influenza (for children in clinical risk groups, or who are household contacts of others in clinical risk groups, and who have not received seasonal influenza vaccine previously)

- BY INTRANASAL ADMINISTRATION
- Child 2-8 years: 0.2 mL for 1 dose, followed by 0.2 mL for 1 dose, after at least 4 weeks. Dose to be administered as 0.1 mL into each nostril

- **UNLICENSED USE** The Joint Committee on Vaccination and Immunisation advises offering a second dose of vaccine for annual immunisation against seasonal influenza to children in clinical risk groups only, but this differs from licensed advice.
- **CONTRA-INDICATIONS** Active wheezing · concomitant use with antiviral therapy for influenza · concomitant use with salicylates · severe asthma

CONTRA-INDICATIONS, FURTHER INFORMATION
- Concomitant use with antiviral therapy for influenza UKHSA advises avoid immunisation for at least 48 hours after stopping the influenza antiviral agent. Administration of influenza antiviral agents within two weeks of *Fluenz®* administration may reduce the effectiveness of the vaccine.

- **INTERACTIONS** → Appendix 1: live vaccines
- **SIDE-EFFECTS**
- **Common or very common** Nasal complaints
- **Uncommon** Epistaxis · face oedema
- **Frequency not known** Guillain-Barre syndrome
- **ALLERGY AND CROSS-SENSITIVITY** UKHSA advises individuals with a history of egg allergy can be immunised with either an egg free influenza vaccine, if available, or an influenza vaccine with an ovalbumin content less than 120 nanograms/mL (facilities should be available to treat anaphylaxis). If an influenza vaccine containing ovalbumin is being considered in those with a history of severe anaphylaxis to egg which has previously required intensive care, these individuals should be referred to a specialist in hospital.
- **PREGNANCY** [EvGr] Avoid—limited information available. ⟨M⟩
- **BREAST FEEDING** [EvGr] Avoid—limited information available. ⟨M⟩
- **PRESCRIBING AND DISPENSING INFORMATION** For choice of vaccine, see Influenza vaccine p. 1484.
  Ovalbumin content Preparations with a very low ovalbumin content of less than 120 nanograms/mL: *Fluenz®*.
- **PATIENT AND CARER ADVICE** Avoid close contact with severely immunocompromised patients for 1–2 weeks after vaccination.

- **MEDICINAL FORMS** There can be variation in the licensing of different medicines containing the same drug.
  Spray
  EXCIPIENTS: May contain Gelatin, gentamicin, sucrose
- **Fluenz** (AstraZeneca UK Ltd)
  Fluenz (trivalent) vaccine nasal suspension 0.2ml unit dose | 10 unit dose [PoM] £180.00

⏵ 1514 ⏵ 1498

Measles, mumps and rubella vaccine

25-Aug-2023

(MMR vaccine)

- **DRUG ACTION** Measles, mumps and rubella vaccine is a live, attenuated combination vaccine.

● INDICATIONS AND DOSE

Primary immunisation against measles, mumps, and rubella (first dose)
- BY INTRAMUSCULAR INJECTION, OR BY DEEP SUBCUTANEOUS INJECTION
- Child 12-13 months: 0.5 mL for 1 dose

Primary immunisation against measles, mumps, and rubella (second dose)
- BY INTRAMUSCULAR INJECTION, OR BY DEEP SUBCUTANEOUS INJECTION
- Child 40 months-5 years: 0.5 mL for 1 dose

Rubella immunisation (in seronegative women, susceptible to rubella and in unimmunised, seronegative women, post-partum)
- BY INTRAMUSCULAR INJECTION, OR BY DEEP SUBCUTANEOUS INJECTION
- Females of childbearing potential: (consult product literature or local protocols)

Children presenting for pre-school booster, who have not received the primary immunisation (first dose) | Immunisation for patients at school-leaving age or at entry into further education, who have not completed the primary immunisation course | Control of measles outbreak | Immunisation for patients travelling to areas where measles is endemic or epidemic, who have not completed the primary immunisation
- BY INTRAMUSCULAR INJECTION, OR BY DEEP SUBCUTANEOUS INJECTION
- Child 6 months-17 years: (consult product literature or local protocols)
- Adult: (consult product literature or local protocols)

- **UNLICENSED USE** Not licensed for use in children under 9 months.

IMPORTANT SAFETY INFORMATION
MMR VACCINATION AND BOWEL DISEASE OR AUTISM
Reviews undertaken on behalf of the CSM, the Medical Research Council, and the Cochrane Collaboration, have not found any evidence of a link between MMR vaccination and bowel disease or autism. Information (including fact sheets and a list of references) may be obtained from www.dh.gov.uk/immunisation.

- **CAUTIONS** Antibody response to measles component may be reduced after immunoglobulin administration or blood transfusion–leave an interval of at least 3 months before MMR immunisation

CAUTIONS, FURTHER INFORMATION
- Administration with other vaccines Public Health England advises MMR and yellow fever vaccines should not be administered on the same day; there should be a 4-week minimum interval between the vaccines. When protection is rapidly required, the vaccines can be given at any interval; an additional dose of MMR should be considered and re-vaccination with the yellow fever vaccine can also be considered in those at on-going risk.
  Public Health England advises MMR and varicella-zoster vaccines can be given on the same day or separated by a 4-week minimum interval. When protection is rapidly required, the vaccines can be given at any interval and an additional dose of the vaccine given second may be considered.

- **INTERACTIONS** → Appendix 1: live vaccines
- **SIDE-EFFECTS**
- **Uncommon** Increased risk of infection · rhinorrhoea
- **Frequency not known** Angioedema · arthritis · ataxia · bronchospasm · cough · encephalopathy · eye inflammation · meningitis aseptic · nerve deafness · nerve disorders · oculomotor nerve paralysis · oedema · panniculitis · papillitis · paraesthesia · pneumonitis · regional lymphadenopathy · seizures · Stevens-Johnson syndrome · subacute sclerosing panencephalitis · syncope · throat pain · thrombocytopenia · vasculitis

SIDE-EFFECTS, FURTHER INFORMATION Malaise, fever, or a rash can occur after the first dose of MMR vaccine–most commonly about a week after vaccination and lasting about 2 to 3 days.
  Febrile seizures occur rarely 6 to 11 days after MMR vaccination (the incidence is lower than that following measles infection).

Idiopathic thrombocytopenic purpura Idiopathic thrombocytopenic purpura has occurred rarely following MMR vaccination, usually within 6 weeks of the first dose. The risk of idiopathic thrombocytopenic purpura after MMR vaccine is much less than the risk after infection with wild measles or rubella virus. Children who develop idiopathic thrombocytopenic purpura within 6 weeks of the first dose of MMR should undergo serological testing before the second dose is due; if the results suggest incomplete immunity against measles, mumps or rubella then a second dose of MMR is recommended. Samples should be sent to the Virus Reference Laboratory of the Health Protection Agency.

Frequency of side effects Adverse reactions are considerably less frequent after the second dose of MMR vaccine than after the first.

- **ALLERGY AND CROSS-SENSITIVITY** PHE advises MMR vaccine can be given safely even when the child has had an anaphylactic reaction to food containing egg. Children with a confirmed anaphylactic reaction to the MMR vaccine should be assessed by a specialist. Dislike of eggs, refusal to eat egg, or confirmed anaphylactic reactions to egg-containing food is not a contra-indication to MMR vaccination.

- **CONCEPTION AND CONTRACEPTION** Exclude pregnancy before immunisation. Avoid pregnancy for at least 1 month after vaccination.

- **PRESCRIBING AND DISPENSING INFORMATION** Available as part of childhood immunisation schedule from health organisations or ImmForm.

- **MEDICINAL FORMS** There can be variation in the licensing of different medicines containing the same drug.

Powder and solvent for suspension for injection
EXCIPIENTS: May contain Gelatin, neomycin
- **M-M-RVAXPRO** (Merck Sharp & Dohme (UK) Ltd)
  M-M-RVAXPRO vaccine powder and solvent for suspension for injection 0.5ml pre-filled syringes | 1 pre-filled disposable injection [PoM] £11.00 DT = £11.00

Powder and solvent for solution for injection
EXCIPIENTS: May contain Neomycin
- **Priorix** (GlaxoSmithKline UK Ltd)
  Priorix vaccine powder and solvent for solution for injection 0.5ml pre-filled syringes | 1 pre-filled disposable injection [PoM] £7.64 DT = £7.64

🏷 1514   🏷 1498

Rotavirus vaccine
25-Aug-2023

- **DRUG ACTION** Rotavirus vaccine is a live, oral vaccine that protects against rotavirus gastro-enteritis.

- **INDICATIONS AND DOSE**

Immunisation against gastro-enteritis caused by rotavirus
- BY MOUTH
- Child 6-23 weeks: 1.5 mL for 2 doses separated by an interval of at least 4 weeks, first dose must be given between 6–14 weeks of age; course should be completed before 24 weeks of age (preferably before 16 weeks)

IMPORTANT SAFETY INFORMATION
PUBLIC HEALTH ENGLAND: UPDATE TO GREEN BOOK (OCTOBER 2017)
Public Health England advises that immunisation with live vaccines should be delayed until 6 months of age in children born to mothers who received immunosuppressive biological therapy during pregnancy. In practice, this means that children born to mothers who were on immunosuppressive biological therapy during pregnancy will not be eligible to receive rotavirus vaccine.

- **CONTRA-INDICATIONS** History of intussusception · predisposition to intussusception · severe combined immunodeficiency disorder

CONTRA-INDICATIONS, FURTHER INFORMATION
- Immunosuppression With the exception of severe combined immunodeficiency disorder (and children born to mothers who received immunosuppressive biological therapy during pregnancy, see *Important safety information*), rotavirus vaccine is not contra-indicated in immunosuppressed patients—benefit from vaccination is likely to outweigh the risk, if there is any doubt, Public Health England recommends seek specialist advice.

- **CAUTIONS** Diarrhoea (postpone vaccination) · immunosuppressed close contacts · vomiting (postpone vaccination)

CAUTIONS, FURTHER INFORMATION The rotavirus vaccine virus is excreted in the stool and may be transmitted to close contacts; however, Public Health England advises vaccination of those with immunosuppressed close contacts may protect the contacts from wild-type rotavirus disease and outweigh any risk from transmission of vaccine virus.

- **INTERACTIONS** → Appendix 1: live vaccines

- **SIDE-EFFECTS**
- **Uncommon** Gastrointestinal disorders
- **Frequency not known** Apnoea · haematochezia

- **PRE-TREATMENT SCREENING** PHE advise that the results of the severe combined immunodeficiency (SCID) screening should be checked before administering rotavirus vaccine.

- **PATIENT AND CARER ADVICE** The rotavirus vaccine virus is excreted in the stool and may be transmitted to close contacts; carers of a recently vaccinated baby should be advised of the need to wash their hands after changing the baby's nappies.

- **MEDICINAL FORMS** There can be variation in the licensing of different medicines containing the same drug.

Oral suspension
- **Rotarix** (GlaxoSmithKline UK Ltd)
  Rotarix vaccine live oral suspension 1.5ml tube | 1 tube [PoM] £34.76 DT = £34.76

🏷 1514   🏷 1498

Typhoid vaccine (live)
29-Aug-2024

- **DRUG ACTION** The live typhoid vaccine is an oral attenuated vaccine that protects against typhoid fever caused by *Salmonella typhi* infection. For information on the inactivated vaccine, see typhoid vaccine (inactivated) p. 1513.

- **INDICATIONS AND DOSE**

Immunisation against typhoid fever
- BY MOUTH
- Child 5-17 years: 1 capsule every 2 days for 3 doses (on days 1, 3, and 5), course should be completed at least 1 week before potential exposure to typhoid infection
- Adult: 1 capsule every 2 days for 3 doses (on days 1, 3, and 5), course should be completed at least 1 week before potential exposure to typhoid infection

Booster
- BY MOUTH
- Child 5-17 years: 1 capsule every 2 days for 3 doses (on days 1, 3, and 5) every 3 years
- Adult: 1 capsule every 2 days for 3 doses (on days 1, 3, and 5) every 3 years

- **CONTRA-INDICATIONS** Acute gastro-intestinal illness

- **INTERACTIONS** → Appendix 1: live vaccines

- **SIDE-EFFECTS** Abdominal distension · asthenia · back pain · chills · flatulence · influenza like illness · paraesthesia · shock

14
Vaccines

- **DIRECTIONS FOR ADMINISTRATION** Manufacturer advises capsule should be taken one hour before a meal. Swallow as soon as possible after placing in mouth with a cold or lukewarm drink.

  Administration of capsule and oral cholera vaccine (live) (*Vaxchora*®) should be separated by a 2-hour interval—transit of the capsules through the gastro-intestinal tract may be affected by the buffer administered with *Vaxchora*®.

- **HANDLING AND STORAGE** Store capsules in a refrigerator (2–8°C).

- **PATIENT AND CARER ADVICE** Patients or carers should be given advice on how to administer and store typhoid vaccine capsules.

- **MEDICINAL FORMS** There can be variation in the licensing of different medicines containing the same drug.

  Gastro-resistant capsule
  CAUTIONARY AND ADVISORY LABELS 25
  - Vivotif (Bavarian Nordic UK Ltd)
    Vivotif vaccine gastro-resistant capsules | 3 capsule [PoM] £14.77 DT = £14.77

⌐ 1514 ⌐ 1498

Varicella-zoster vaccine
25-Aug-2023

- **DRUG ACTION** Varicella-zoster vaccines are live attenuated vaccines that protect against varicella (chickenpox) caused by varicella-zoster virus infection.

- **INDICATIONS AND DOSE**

Immunisation against varicella infection (chickenpox)
- ▶ BY SUBCUTANEOUS INJECTION, OR BY INTRAMUSCULAR INJECTION
  - ▶ Child 9-11 months: 0.5 mL for 1 dose, then 0.5 mL for 1 dose, to be given at least 12 weeks after initial dose
  - ▶ Child 1-17 years: 0.5 mL for 1 dose, then 0.5 mL for 1 dose, to be given 4 to 8 weeks after initial dose
  - ▶ Adult: 0.5 mL for 1 dose, then 0.5 mL for 1 dose, to be given 4 to 8 weeks after initial dose

Post-exposure prophylaxis against varicella infection (chickenpox) during co-circulating group A streptococcal infection (e.g. scarlet fever)
- ▶ BY SUBCUTANEOUS INJECTION, OR BY INTRAMUSCULAR INJECTION
  - ▶ Child 9 months-17 years: 0.5 mL for 1 dose, then 0.5 mL for 1 dose, to be given 4 to 8 weeks after initial dose
  - ▶ Adult: 0.5 mL for 1 dose, then 0.5 mL for 1 dose, to be given 4 to 8 weeks after initial dose

- **CAUTIONS** Post-vaccination close contact with susceptible individuals

  CAUTIONS, FURTHER INFORMATION Rarely, the varicella–zoster vaccine virus has been transmitted from the vaccinated individual to close contacts. Therefore, manufacturer advises contact with the following should be avoided if a vaccine-related cutaneous rash develops within 4–6 weeks of the first or second dose:
  - varicella-susceptible pregnant women;
  - individuals at high risk of severe varicella, including those with immunodeficiency or those receiving immunosuppressive therapy.

  Public Health England advises healthcare workers who develop a generalised papular or vesicular rash on vaccination should avoid contact with patients until the lesions have crusted. Those who develop a localised rash after vaccination should cover the lesions and be allowed to continue working unless in contact with patients at high risk of severe varicella.
  - ▶ Administration with MMR vaccine Public Health England advises varicella–zoster and MMR vaccines can be given on the same day or separated by a 4-week minimum interval. When protection is rapidly required, the vaccines

can be given at any interval and an additional dose of the vaccine given second may be considered.

- **INTERACTIONS** → Appendix 1: live vaccines
- **SIDE-EFFECTS**
  - ▶ **Uncommon** Cough · drowsiness · increased risk of infection
  - ▶ **Rare or very rare** Conjunctivitis · Kawasaki disease · seizure · stroke · thrombocytopenia · vasculitis
- **CONCEPTION AND CONTRACEPTION** Manufacturer advises avoid pregnancy for 1 month after vaccination.
- **DIRECTIONS FOR ADMINISTRATION** To be administered into the deltoid region or anterolateral thigh (recommended in infants aged under 1 year).
- **PRESCRIBING AND DISPENSING INFORMATION** Advice in BNF Publications may differ from that in product literature.

- **MEDICINAL FORMS** There can be variation in the licensing of different medicines containing the same drug.

  Powder and solvent for suspension for injection
  EXCIPIENTS: May contain Gelatin, neomycin
  - Varivax (Merck Sharp & Dohme (UK) Ltd)
    Varivax vaccine powder and solvent for suspension for injection 0.5ml vials | 1 vial [PoM] £30.28 DT = £30.28

  Powder and solvent for solution for injection
  EXCIPIENTS: May contain Neomycin, phenylalanine
  - Varilrix (GlaxoSmithKline UK Ltd)
    Varilrix vaccine powder and solvent for solution for injection 0.5ml vials | 1 vial [PoM] £27.31 DT = £27.31

⌐ 1514 ⌐ 1498

Yellow fever vaccine
25-Aug-2023

- **DRUG ACTION** Yellow fever vaccine is a live attenuated vaccine.

- **INDICATIONS AND DOSE**

Immunisation against yellow fever
- ▶ BY DEEP SUBCUTANEOUS INJECTION
  - ▶ Child 6-8 months (administered on expert advice): Infants under 9 months should be vaccinated only if the risk of yellow fever is high and unavoidable (consult product literature or local protocols)
  - ▶ Child 9 months-17 years: 0.5 mL for 1 dose
  - ▶ Adult: 0.5 mL for 1 dose

IMPORTANT SAFETY INFORMATION

MHRA/CHM ADVICE (UPDATED NOVEMBER 2019): YELLOW FEVER VACCINE: STRONGER PRECAUTIONS IN PEOPLE WITH WEAKENED IMMUNITY AND IN THOSE AGED 60 YEARS OR OLDER

The yellow fever vaccine (*Stamaril*®) has been associated with the very rare, life-threatening reactions viscerotropic disease (YEL-AVD) and neurotropic disease (YEL-AND), which both resemble yellow fever infection. It must not be given to patients who have had a thymectomy, who are taking immunosuppressive or immunomodulating biological drugs, or who have a first-degree family history of YEL-AVD or YEL-AND following vaccination that was unrelated to a known medical risk factor. In patients aged 60 years and older, the vaccine should only be administered when there is a significant and unavoidable risk of acquiring yellow fever infection. It must only be administered by healthcare professionals specifically trained in the benefit-risk evaluation of yellow fever vaccine. Healthcare professionals must inform patients and carers about the early signs and symptoms of YEL-AVD and YEL-AND, and advise them to seek urgent medical attention if they occur; the manufacturer's patient information leaflet should also be provided. Healthcare professionals administering vaccines should consult information in the YF Vaccine Centre code of practice and strengthen protocols and checklists to avoid inappropriate administration.

● **CONTRA-INDICATIONS** Children under 6 months · history of thymus dysfunction · thymectomy

● **CAUTIONS** Individuals over 60 years—greater risk of vaccine-associated adverse effects

CAUTIONS, FURTHER INFORMATION

▸ **Administration with MMR vaccine** Public Health England advises yellow fever and MMR vaccines should not be administered on the same day; there should be a 4-week minimum interval between the vaccines. When protection is rapidly required, the vaccines can be given at any interval; an additional dose of MMR should be considered and re-vaccination with the yellow fever vaccine can also be considered in those at on-going risk.

● **INTERACTIONS** → Appendix 1: live vaccines

● **SIDE-EFFECTS**

▸ **Common or very common** Asthenia · crying (in children) · drowsiness (in children)

▸ **Rare or very rare** Rhinitis · yellow fever vaccine-associated neurotropic disease · yellow fever vaccine-associated viscerotropic disease

▸ **Frequency not known** Angioedema · influenza like illness · paraesthesia

SIDE-EFFECTS, FURTHER INFORMATION Very rare vaccine-associated adverse effects may occur, such as viscerotropic disease (yellow-fever vaccine-associated viscerotropic disease, YEL-AVD), a syndrome which may include metabolic acidosis, muscle and liver cirrhosis, and multi-organ failure. Neurological disorders (yellow fever vaccine-associated neurotropic disease, YEL-AND) such as encephalitis have also been reported. These very rare adverse effects usually occur after the first dose of yellow fever vaccine in those with no previous immunity. Increased risk of fatal reactions reported in patients aged 60 years and older and those who are immunosuppressed.

● **ALLERGY AND CROSS-SENSITIVITY** EvGr In individuals with a history of confirmed anaphylactic reaction to eggs and who are currently avoiding eggs due to ongoing hypersensitivity reactions, yellow fever vaccine should only be considered under the guidance of an allergy specialist. ⟨E⟩

● **PREGNANCY** Live yellow fever vaccine should not be given during pregnancy because there is a theoretical risk of fetal infection. Pregnant women should be advised not to travel to areas at high risk of yellow fever. If exposure cannot be avoided during pregnancy, then the vaccine should be given if the risk from disease in the mother outweighs the risk to the fetus from vaccination.

● **BREAST FEEDING** Avoid; seek specialist advice if exposure to virus cannot be avoided.

● **MEDICINAL FORMS** There can be variation in the licensing of different medicines containing the same drug.

Powder and solvent for suspension for injection

▸ **Stamaril** (Sanofi)
Stamaril vaccine powder and solvent for suspension for injection 0.5ml vials | 1 vial PoM £39.72 DT = £39.72

Chapter 15
Anaesthesia

CONTENTS

General anaesthesia

Anaesthesia (general)

Overview

Several different types of drug are given together during general anaesthesia. Anaesthesia is induced with either a volatile drug given by inhalation or with an intravenously administered drug; anaesthesia is maintained with an intravenous or inhalational anaesthetic. Analgesics, usually short-acting opioids, are also used. The use of neuromuscular blocking drugs necessitates intermittent positive-pressure ventilation. Following surgery, anticholinesterases can be given to reverse the effects of neuromuscular blocking drugs; specific antagonists can be used to reverse central and respiratory depression caused by some drugs used in surgery. A local topical anaesthetic can be used to reduce pain at the injection site.

Individual requirements vary considerably and the recommended doses are only a guide. Smaller doses are indicated in ill, shocked, or debilitated patients and in significant hepatic impairment, while robust individuals may require larger doses. The required dose of induction agent may be less if the patient has been premedicated with a sedative agent or if an opioid analgesic has been used.

Intravenous anaesthetics

Intravenous anaesthetics may be used either to induce anaesthesia or for maintenance of anaesthesia throughout surgery. Intravenous anaesthetics nearly all produce their effect in one arm-brain circulation time. Extreme care is required in surgery of the mouth, pharynx, or larynx where the airway may be difficult to maintain (e.g. in the presence of a tumour in the pharynx or larynx).

To facilitate tracheal intubation, induction is usually followed by a neuromuscular blocking drug or a short-acting opioid.

The doses of all intravenous anaesthetic drugs should be titrated to effect (except when using 'rapid sequence induction'); lower doses may be required in premedicated patients.

Total intravenous anaesthesia

This is a technique in which major surgery is carried out with all drugs given intravenously. Respiration can be spontaneous, or controlled with oxygen-enriched air. Neuromuscular blocking drugs can be used to provide relaxation and prevent reflex muscle movements. The main problem to be overcome is the assessment of depth of anaesthesia. Target Controlled Infusion (TCI) systems can be used to titrate intravenous anaesthetic infusions to predicted plasma-drug concentrations in ventilated adult patients.

Drugs used for intravenous anaesthesia

Propofol p. 1522, the most widely used intravenous anaesthetic, can be used for induction or maintenance of anaesthesia in adults and children, but it is not commonly used in neonates. Propofol is associated with rapid recovery and less hangover effect than other intravenous anaesthetics. Propofol can also be used for sedation during diagnostic procedures and sedation in adults in intensive care.

Thiopental sodium p. 392 is a barbiturate that is used for induction of anaesthesia, but has no analgesic properties. Induction is generally smooth and rapid, but dose-related cardiovascular and respiratory depression can occur. Awakening from a moderate dose of thiopental sodium is rapid because the drug redistributes into other tissues, particularly fat. However, metabolism is slow and sedative effects can persist for 24 hours. Repeated doses have a cumulative effect and recovery is much slower.

Etomidate p. 1522 is an intravenous agent associated with rapid recovery without a hangover effect. Etomidate causes less hypotension than thiopental sodium and propofol during induction. It produces a high incidence of extraneous muscle movements, which can be minimised by an opioid analgesic or a short-acting benzodiazepine given just before induction.

Ketamine p. 1539 is used rarely. Ketamine causes less hypotension than thiopental sodium and propofol during induction. It is used mainly for paediatric anaesthesia, particularly when repeated administration is required (such as for serial burns dressings); recovery is relatively slow and there is a high incidence of extraneous muscle movements. The main disadvantage of ketamine is the high incidence of hallucinations, nightmares, and other transient psychotic effects; these can be reduced by a benzodiazepine such as diazepam p. 398 or midazolam p. 394.

Inhalational anaesthetics

Inhalational anaesthetics include gases and volatile liquids. *Gaseous anaesthetics* require suitable equipment for storage and administration. *Volatile liquid anaesthetics* are administered using calibrated vaporisers, using air, oxygen, or nitrous oxide-oxygen mixtures as the carrier gas. To prevent hypoxia, the inspired gas mixture should contain a minimum of 25% oxygen at all times. Higher concentrations of oxygen (greater than 30%) are usually required during inhalational anaesthesia when nitrous oxide p. 1524 is being administered.

Volatile liquid anaesthetics

Volatile liquid anaesthetics can be used for induction and maintenance of anaesthesia, and following induction with an intravenous anaesthetic.

Isoflurane p. 1524 is a volatile liquid anaesthetic. Heart rhythm is generally stable during isoflurane anaesthesia, but heart-rate can rise, particularly in younger patients. Systemic arterial pressure and cardiac output can fall, owing to a decrease in systemic vascular resistance. Muscle relaxation occurs and the effects of muscle relaxant drugs are potentiated. Isoflurane is the preferred inhalational anaesthetic for use in obstetrics.

Desflurane p. 1524 is a rapid acting volatile liquid anaesthetic; it is reported to have about one-fifth the potency of isoflurane. Emergence and recovery from anaesthesia are particularly rapid because of its low solubility. Desflurane is not recommended for induction of anaesthesia as it is irritant to the upper respiratory tract.

Sevoflurane p. 1525 is a rapid acting volatile liquid anaesthetic and is more potent than desflurane. Emergence and recovery are particularly rapid, but slower than desflurane. Sevoflurane is non-irritant and is therefore often used for inhalational induction of anaesthesia; it has little effect on heart rhythm compared with other volatile liquid anaesthetics.

Nitrous oxide

Nitrous oxide is used for maintenance of anaesthesia and, in sub-anaesthetic concentrations, for analgesia. For *anaesthesia*, nitrous oxide is commonly used in a concentration of 50 to 66% in oxygen as part of a balanced technique in association with other inhalational or intravenous agents. Nitrous oxide is unsatisfactory as a sole anaesthetic owing to lack of potency, but is useful as part of a combination of drugs since it allows a significant reduction in dosage.

For analgesia (without loss of consciousness), a mixture of nitrous oxide and oxygen containing 50% of each gas (*Entonox*®, *Equanox*®) is used. Self-administration using a demand valve is popular in obstetric practice, for changing painful dressings, as an aid to postoperative physiotherapy, and in emergency ambulances.

Nitrous oxide may have a deleterious effect if used in patients with an air-containing closed space since nitrous oxide diffuses into such a space with a resulting increase in pressure. This effect may be dangerous in conditions such as pneumothorax, which may enlarge to compromise respiration, or in the presence of intracranial air after head injury, entrapped air following recent underwater dive, or recent intra-ocular gas injection.

Malignant hyperthermia

Malignant hyperthermia is a rare but potentially lethal complication of anaesthesia. It is characterised by a rapid rise in temperature, increased muscle rigidity, tachycardia, and acidosis. The most common triggers of malignant hyperthermia are the volatile anaesthetics. Suxamethonium chloride p. 1529 has also been implicated, but malignant hyperthermia is more likely if it is given following a volatile anaesthetic. Volatile anaesthetics and suxamethonium chloride should be avoided during anaesthesia in patients at high risk of malignant hyperthermia.

Dantrolene sodium p. 1541 is used in the treatment of malignant hyperthermia.

Sedation, anaesthesia, and resuscitation in dental practice

Overview

Sedation for dental procedures should be limited to conscious sedation. Diazepam p. 398 and temazepam p. 552 are effective anxiolytics for dental treatment in adults.

For details of sedation, anaesthesia, and resuscitation in dental practice see *A Conscious Decision: A review of the use of general anaesthesia and conscious sedation in primary dental care* ; report by a group chaired by the Chief Medical Officer and Chief Dental Officer, July 2000 and associated documents. Further details can also be found in *Standards for Conscious Sedation in the Provision of Dental Care*; report of an Intercollegiate Advisory Committee for Sedation in Dentistry, 2020 www.rcseng.ac.uk/dental-faculties/fds/publications-guidelines/standards-for-conscious-sedation-in-the-provision-of-dental-care-and-accreditation/.

Surgery and long-term medication

26-Mar-2021

Overview

The risk of losing disease control on stopping long-term medication before surgery is often greater than the risk posed by continuing it during surgery. It is vital that the anaesthetist knows about **all** drugs that a patient is (or has been) taking.

Patients with adrenal atrophy resulting from long-term corticosteroid use may suffer a precipitous fall in blood pressure unless corticosteroid cover is provided during anaesthesia and in the immediate postoperative period. Anaesthetists must therefore know whether a patient is, or has been, receiving corticosteroids (including high-dose inhaled corticosteroids). For further information, see *Glucocorticoid replacement during stress* in Adrenal insufficiency p. 781.

Other drugs that should normally not be stopped before surgery include antiepileptics, antiparkinsonian drugs, antipsychotics, anxiolytics, bronchodilators, cardiovascular drugs (but see potassium-sparing diuretics, angiotensin-converting enzyme inhibitors, and angiotensin-II receptor antagonists), glaucoma drugs, immunosuppressants, drugs of dependence, and thyroid or antithyroid drugs. Expert advice is required for patients receiving antivirals for HIV infection. See general advice on surgery in diabetic patients in Diabetes, surgery and medical illness p. 804.

Patients taking antiplatelet medication or an oral anticoagulant present an increased risk for surgery. In these circumstances, the anaesthetist and surgeon should assess the relative risks and decide jointly whether the antiplatelet or the anticoagulant drug should be stopped or replaced with heparin (unfractionated) p. 156 or low molecular weight heparin therapy. [EvGr] In patients with stable angina, perioperative aspirin p. 142 should be only continued where there is a high thrombotic risk (e.g. patients with a recent acute coronary syndrome, coronary artery stents, or an ischaemic stroke). ⟨A⟩

Drugs that should be stopped before surgery include combined hormonal contraceptives, see Contraceptives, hormonal p. 912; for advice on hormone replacement therapy, see Sex hormones p. 862. MAOIs can have important interactions with some drugs used during surgery, such as pethidine hydrochloride p. 531. Tricyclic antidepressants need not be stopped, but there may be an increased risk of arrhythmias and hypotension (and dangerous interactions with vasopressor drugs); therefore, the anaesthetist should be informed if they are not stopped. Lithium should be stopped 24 hours before major surgery but the normal dose can be continued for minor surgery (with careful monitoring of fluids and electrolytes). Potassium-sparing diuretics may need to be withheld on the morning of surgery because hyperkalaemia may develop if renal perfusion is impaired or if there is tissue damage. Angiotensin-converting enzyme (ACE) inhibitors and angiotensin-II receptor antagonists can be associated with severe hypotension after induction of anaesthesia; these drugs may need to be discontinued 24 hours before surgery. Herbal medicines may be associated with adverse effects when given with anaesthetic drugs and consideration should be given to stopping them before surgery.

ANAESTHETICS, GENERAL > INTRAVENOUS ANAESTHETICS

Etomidate
04-Sep-2020

● **INDICATIONS AND DOSE**

Induction of anaesthesia
▶ BY SLOW INTRAVENOUS INJECTION
▶ Adult: 150–300 micrograms/kg (max. per dose 60 mg), to be administered over 30-60 seconds (60 seconds in patients in whom hypotension might be hazardous)
▶ Elderly: 150–200 micrograms/kg (max. per dose 60 mg), to be administered over 30-60 seconds (60 seconds in patients in whom hypotension might be hazardous)

IMPORTANT SAFETY INFORMATION
Etomidate should only be administered by, or under the direct supervision of, personnel experienced in its use, with adequate training in anaesthesia and airway management, and when resuscitation equipment is available.

● CAUTIONS Acute circulatory failure (shock) · adrenal insufficiency · avoid in Acute porphyrias p. 1202 · cardiovascular disease · elderly · fixed cardiac output · hypovolaemia

CAUTIONS, FURTHER INFORMATION
▶ Adrenal insufficiency Etomidate suppresses adrenocortical function, particularly during continuous administration, and it should not be used for maintenance of anaesthesia. It should be used with caution in patients with underlying adrenal insufficiency, for example, those with sepsis.

● INTERACTIONS → Appendix 1: etomidate

● SIDE-EFFECTS
▶ **Common or very common** Apnoea · hypotension · movement disorders · nausea · respiratory disorders · skin reactions · vascular pain · vomiting
▶ **Uncommon** Arrhythmias · cough · hiccups · hypersalivation · hypertension · muscle rigidity · neuromuscular dysfunction · nystagmus · procedural complications
▶ **Frequency not known** Adrenal insufficiency · atrioventricular block · cardiac arrest · embolism and thrombosis · seizures · shock · Stevens-Johnson syndrome · trismus

SIDE-EFFECTS, FURTHER INFORMATION **Pain on injection** Can be reduced by injecting into a larger vein or by giving an opioid analgesic just before induction.

Extraneous muscle movements Extraneous muscle movements can be minimised by an opioid analgesic or a short-acting benzodiazepine given just before induction.

● PREGNANCY May depress neonatal respiration if used during delivery.

● BREAST FEEDING Breast-feeding can be resumed as soon as mother has recovered sufficiently from anaesthesia.

● HEPATIC IMPAIRMENT
Dose adjustments Manufacturer advises reduce dose in liver cirrhosis.

● DIRECTIONS FOR ADMINISTRATION Manufacturer advises give over 30–60 seconds (60 seconds in patients in whom hypotension might be hazardous).

● PATIENT AND CARER ADVICE
Driving and skilled tasks Patients given sedatives and analgesics during minor outpatient procedures should be very carefully warned about the risk of driving or undertaking skilled tasks afterwards. For a short general anaesthetic the risk extends to **at least 24 hours** after administration. Responsible persons should be available to take patients home. The dangers of taking **alcohol** should also be emphasised.

● MEDICINAL FORMS There can be variation in the licensing of different medicines containing the same drug.
Solution for injection
EXCIPIENTS: May contain Propylene glycol
▶ **Hypnomidate** (Piramal Critical Care Ltd)
Etomidate 2 mg per 1 ml Hypnomidate 20mg/10ml solution for injection ampoules | 5 ampoule [PoM] £6.90
Emulsion for injection
▶ **Etomidate (Non-proprietary)**
Etomidate 2 mg per 1 ml Etomidate 20mg/10ml emulsion for injection ampoules | 10 ampoule [PoM] £20.00 (Hospital only)

Propofol
13-Aug-2020

● **INDICATIONS AND DOSE**

Induction of anaesthesia using 0.5% or 1% injection
▶ BY SLOW INTRAVENOUS INJECTION, OR BY INTRAVENOUS INFUSION
▶ Adult 18-54 years: Usual dose 1.5–2.5 mg/kg, to be administered at a rate of 20–40 mg every 10 seconds until response, for debilitated patients use dose for 55 years and over
▶ Adult 55 years and over: Usual dose 1–1.5 mg/kg, to be administered at a rate of 20 mg every 10 seconds until response

Induction of anaesthesia using 2% injection
▶ BY INTRAVENOUS INFUSION
▶ Adult 18-54 years: Usual dose 1.5–2.5 mg/kg, to be administered at a rate of 20–40 mg every 10 seconds until response. For debilitated patients use dose for 55 years and over
▶ Adult 55 years and over: Usual dose 1–1.5 mg/kg, to be administered at a rate of 20 mg every 10 seconds until response

Maintenance of anaesthesia using 1% injection
▶ INITIALLY BY INTRAVENOUS INFUSION
▶ Adult: Usual dose 4–12 mg/kg/hour, alternatively (by slow intravenous injection) 25–50 mg, dose may be repeated according to response, for debilitated patients use dose for elderly
▶ Elderly: Usual dose 3–6 mg/kg/hour, alternatively (by slow intravenous injection) 25–50 mg, dose may be repeated according to response

Maintenance of anaesthesia using 2% injection
▶ BY INTRAVENOUS INFUSION
▶ Adult: Usual dose 4–12 mg/kg/hour, for debilitated patients use dose for elderly
▶ Elderly: Usual dose 3–6 mg/kg/hour

Sedation of ventilated patients in intensive care using 1% or 2% injection
▶ BY CONTINUOUS INTRAVENOUS INFUSION
▶ Adult: Usual dose 0.3–4 mg/kg/hour, adjusted according to response

Induction of sedation for surgical and diagnostic procedures using 0.5% or 1% injection
▶ BY SLOW INTRAVENOUS INJECTION
▶ Adult: Initially 0.5–1 mg/kg, to be administered over 1–5 minutes, dose and rate of administration adjusted according to desired level of sedation and response

Maintenance of sedation for surgical and diagnostic procedures using 0.5% injection
▶ INITIALLY BY INTRAVENOUS INFUSION
▶ Adult: Initially 1.5–4.5 mg/kg/hour, dose and rate of administration adjusted according to desired level of sedation and response, followed by (by slow intravenous injection) 10–20 mg, (if rapid increase in sedation required), patients over 55 years or debilitated may require lower initial dose and rate of administration

Maintenance of sedation for surgical and diagnostic procedures using 1% injection
▶ INITIALLY BY INTRAVENOUS INFUSION
▶ Adult: Initially 1.5–4.5 mg/kg/hour, dose and rate of administration adjusted according to desired level of sedation and response, followed by (by slow intravenous injection) 10–20 mg, (if rapid increase in sedation required), patients over 55 years or debilitated may require lower initial dose and rate of administration

Maintenance of sedation for surgical and diagnostic procedures using 2% injection
▶ INITIALLY BY INTRAVENOUS INFUSION
▶ Adult: Initially 1.5–4.5 mg/kg/hour, dose and rate of administration adjusted according to desired level of sedation and response, followed by (by slow intravenous injection) 10–20 mg, using 0.5% or 1% injection (if rapid increase in sedation required), patients over 55 years or debilitated may require lower initial dose and rate of administration

---

IMPORTANT SAFETY INFORMATION
Propofol should only be administered by, or under the direct supervision of, personnel experienced in its use, with adequate training in anaesthesia and airway management, and when resuscitation equipment is available.

● **CAUTIONS** Acute circulatory failure (shock) · cardiac impairment · cardiovascular disease · elderly · epilepsy · fixed cardiac output · hypotension · hypovolaemia · raised intracranial pressure · respiratory impairment

● **INTERACTIONS** → Appendix 1: propofol

● **SIDE-EFFECTS**
▶ **Common or very common** Apnoea · arrhythmias · headache · hypotension · localised pain · nausea · vomiting
▶ **Uncommon** Thrombosis
▶ **Rare or very rare** Epileptiform seizure (may be delayed) · movement disorders · pancreatitis · post procedural complications · pulmonary oedema · sexual dysfunction · urine discolouration
▶ **Frequency not known** Drug use disorders · euphoric mood · heart failure · hepatomegaly · hyperkalaemia · hyperlipidaemia · metabolic acidosis · renal failure · respiratory depression · rhabdomyolysis

SIDE-EFFECTS, FURTHER INFORMATION **Bradycardia** Bradycardia may be profound and may be treated with intravenous administration of an antimuscarinic drug.
　Pain on injection Pain on injection can be reduced by intravenous lidocaine.
　Propofol infusion syndrome Prolonged infusion of propofol doses exceeding 4mg/kg/hour may result in potentially fatal effects, including metabolic acidosis, arrhythmias, cardiac failure, rhabdomyolysis,

hyperlipidaemia, hyperkalaemia, hepatomegaly, and renal failure.

● **PREGNANCY** May depress neonatal respiration if used during delivery.
Dose adjustments Max. dose for maintenance of anaesthesia 6 mg/kg/hour.

● **BREAST FEEDING** Breast-feeding can be resumed as soon as mother has recovered sufficiently from anaesthesia.

● **HEPATIC IMPAIRMENT** Manufacturer advises caution.

● **RENAL IMPAIRMENT** Use with caution.

● **MONITORING REQUIREMENTS** Monitor blood-lipid concentration if risk of fat overload or if sedation longer than 3 days.

● **DIRECTIONS FOR ADMINISTRATION** Manufacturer advises shake before use; microbiological filter not recommended; may be administered via a Y-piece close to injection site co-administered with Glucose 5% *or* Sodium Chloride 0.9%. 0.5% **emulsion** for injection or intermittent infusion; manufacturer advises may be administered undiluted, or diluted with Glucose 5% *or* Sodium Chloride 0.9%; dilute to a concentration not less than 1 mg/mL. 1% **emulsion** for injection or infusion; manufacturer advises may be administered undiluted, or diluted with Glucose 5% (*Diprivan*®) or (*Propofol-Lipuro*®) *or* Sodium Chloride 0.9% (*Propofol-Lipuro*® only); dilute to a concentration not less than 2 mg/mL; use within 6 hours of preparation. 2% **emulsion** for infusion; manufacturer advises do not dilute.

● **PATIENT AND CARER ADVICE**
Driving and skilled tasks Patients given sedatives and analgesics during minor outpatient procedures should be very carefully warned about the risk of driving or undertaking skilled tasks afterwards. For a short general anaesthetic the risk extends to **at least 24 hours** after administration. Responsible persons should be available to take patients home. The dangers of taking **alcohol** should also be emphasised.

● **MEDICINAL FORMS** There can be variation in the licensing of different medicines containing the same drug.
Emulsion for infusion
▶ **Propofol (Non-proprietary)**
Propofol 10 mg per 1 ml Propofol 500mg/50ml emulsion for infusion vials | 1 vial [PoM] £13.20 (Hospital only) | 10 vial [PoM] £107.32 (Hospital only)
Propofol 500mg/50ml emulsion for infusion pre-filled syringes | 1 pre-filled disposable injection [PoM] £13.45 (Hospital only)
Propofol 1g/100ml emulsion for infusion vials | 1 vial [PoM] £26.40 (Hospital only) | 10 vial [PoM] £205.33 (Hospital only)
Propofol 20 mg per 1 ml Propofol 1g/50ml emulsion for infusion vials | 1 vial [PoM] £26.40 (Hospital only) | 10 vial [PoM] £205.30 (Hospital only)
Propofol 1g/50ml emulsion for infusion pre-filled syringes | 1 pre-filled disposable injection [PoM] £17.95 (Hospital only)
▶ **Propoven** (Fresenius Kabi Ltd)
Propofol 10 mg per 1 ml Propoven 1% emulsion for infusion 50ml vials | 10 vial [PoM] £264.00 (Hospital only)
Propoven 1% emulsion for infusion 100ml vials | 10 vial [PoM] £22.60 (Hospital only)
Propofol 20 mg per 1 ml Propoven 2% emulsion for infusion 50ml vials | 10 vial [PoM] £21.40 (Hospital only)
Emulsion for injection
▶ **Propofol (Non-proprietary)**
Propofol 10 mg per 1 ml Propofol 200mg/20ml emulsion for injection vials | 5 vial [PoM] £26.40 (Hospital only)
Propofol 200mg/20ml emulsion for injection ampoules | 5 ampoule [PoM] £15.36-£19.03 (Hospital only)
▶ **Propoven** (Fresenius Kabi Ltd)
Propofol 10 mg per 1 ml Propoven 1% emulsion for injection 20ml ampoules | 5 ampoule [PoM] £264.00 (Hospital only)

Volatile halogenated anaesthetics 

IMPORTANT SAFETY INFORMATION
Should only be administered by, or under the direct supervision of, personnel experienced in their use, with adequate training in anaesthesia and airway management, and when resuscitation equipment is available.

- **CONTRA-INDICATIONS** Susceptibility to malignant hyperthermia
- **CAUTIONS** Can trigger malignant hyperthermia · raised intracranial pressure (can increase cerebrospinal pressure)
- **SIDE-EFFECTS**
- **Common or very common** Agitation · apnoea · arrhythmias · chills · cough · dizziness · headache · hypersalivation · hypertension · hypotension · nausea · respiratory disorders · vomiting
- **Uncommon** Hypoxia
- **Frequency not known** Breath holding · cardiac arrest · haemorrhage · hepatic disorders · hyperkalaemia · malignant hyperthermia · QT interval prolongation · rhabdomyolysis · seizure
- **ALLERGY AND CROSS-SENSITIVITY** Can cause hepatotoxicity in those sensitised to halogenated anaesthetics.
- **DIRECTIONS FOR ADMINISTRATION** Volatile liquid anaesthetics are administered using calibrated vaporisers, using oxygen, oxygen-enriched air, or nitrous oxide-oxygen mixtures as the carrier gas (consult product literature).
- **PATIENT AND CARER ADVICE**
Driving and skilled tasks Patients given sedatives and analgesics during minor outpatient procedures should be very carefully warned about the risks of driving or undertaking skilled tasks afterwards. For a short general anaesthetic, the risk extends **to at least 24 hours** after administration. Responsible persons should be available to take patients home. The dangers of taking **alcohol** should also be emphasised.

⏵ above

Desflurane

- **INDICATIONS AND DOSE**

Induction of anaesthesia (but not recommended)
- BY INHALATION
- Adult: 4–11 %, to be inhaled through specifically calibrated vaporiser

Maintenance of anaesthesia (in nitrous oxide–oxygen)
- BY INHALATION
- Adult: 2–6 %, to be inhaled through a specifically calibrated vaporiser

Maintenance of anaesthesia (in oxygen or oxygen-enriched air)
- BY INHALATION
- Adult: 2.5–8.5 %, to be inhaled through a specifically calibrated vaporiser

- **INTERACTIONS** → Appendix 1: volatile halogenated anaesthetics
- **SIDE-EFFECTS**
- **Common or very common** Coagulation disorder · conjunctivitis

- **Uncommon** Myalgia · myocardial infarction · myocardial ischaemia · vasodilation
- **Frequency not known** Abdominal pain · asthenia · heart failure · hypokalaemia · malaise · metabolic acidosis · pancreatitis acute · shock · skin reactions · ventricular dysfunction · visual acuity decreased
- **PREGNANCY** May depress neonatal respiration if used during delivery.
- **BREAST FEEDING** Breast-feeding can be resumed as soon as mother has recovered sufficiently from anaesthesia.

- **MEDICINAL FORMS** There can be variation in the licensing of different medicines containing the same drug.
Inhalation vapour liquid
- Desflurane (Non-proprietary)
 Desflurane 1 ml per 1 ml Desflurane 100% inhalation vapour liquid | 240 ml PoM £120.00 (Hospital only) | 250 ml PoM £20.00 (Hospital only)

⏵ above

Isoflurane

12-Dec-2019

- **INDICATIONS AND DOSE**

Induction of anaesthesia (in oxygen or nitrous oxide-oxygen)
- BY INHALATION
- Adult: Initially 0.5 %, increased to 3 %, adjusted according to response, administered using specifically calibrated vaporiser

Maintenance of anaesthesia (in nitrous oxide–oxygen)
- BY INHALATION
- Adult: 1–2.5 %, to be administered using specifically calibrated vaporiser; an additional 0.5–1% may be required when given with oxygen alone

Maintenance of anaesthesia in caesarean section (in nitrous oxide–oxygen)
- BY INHALATION
- Adult: 0.5–0.75 %, to be administered using specifically calibrated vaporiser

- **INTERACTIONS** → Appendix 1: volatile halogenated anaesthetics
- **SIDE-EFFECTS** Carboxyhaemoglobinaemia · chest discomfort · cognitive impairment · delirium · dyspnoea · ileus · mood altered (that can last several days) · myoglobinuria · skin reactions
- **PREGNANCY** May depress neonatal respiration if used during delivery.
- **BREAST FEEDING** Breast-feeding can be resumed as soon as mother has recovered sufficiently from anaesthesia.

- **MEDICINAL FORMS** There can be variation in the licensing of different medicines containing the same drug.
Inhalation vapour liquid
- Isoflurane (Non-proprietary)
 Isoflurane 1 ml per 1 ml Isoflurane 100% inhalation vapour liquid | 250 ml PoM £120.00 (Hospital only)
- AErrane (Baxter Healthcare Ltd)
 Isoflurane 1 ml per 1 ml AErrane 100% inhalation vapour liquid | 250 ml PoM £27.00 (Hospital only)

Nitrous oxide

12-Aug-2020

- **INDICATIONS AND DOSE**

Maintenance of anaesthesia in conjunction with other anaesthetic agents
- BY INHALATION
- Adult: 50–66 %, to be administered using suitable anaesthetic apparatus in oxygen

Analgesia
▶ BY INHALATION
▶ Adult: Up to 50 %, to be administered using suitable anaesthetic apparatus in oxygen, adjusted according to the patient's needs

---

IMPORTANT SAFETY INFORMATION
Nitrous oxide should only be administered by, or under the direct supervision of, personnel experienced in its use, with adequate training in anaesthesia and airway management, and when resuscitation equipment is available.

● CAUTIONS Entrapped air following recent underwater dive · pneumothorax · presence of intracranial air after head injury · recent intra-ocular gas injection

CAUTIONS, FURTHER INFORMATION Nitrous oxide may have a deleterious effect if used in patients with an air-containing closed space since nitrous oxide diffuses into such a space with a resulting increase in pressure. This effect may be dangerous in conditions such as pneumothorax, which may enlarge to compromise respiration, or in the presence of intracranial air after head injury, entrapped air following recent underwater dive, or recent intra-ocular gas injection.

● INTERACTIONS → Appendix 1: nitrous oxide

● SIDE-EFFECTS Abdominal distension · addiction · agranulocytosis · disorientation · dizziness · euphoric mood · megaloblastic anaemia · middle ear damage · myeloneuropathy · nausea · paraesthesia · sedation · subacute combined cord degeneration · tympanic membrane perforation · vomiting

SIDE-EFFECTS, FURTHER INFORMATION Exposure of patients to nitrous oxide for prolonged periods, either by continuous or by intermittent administration, may result in megaloblastic anaemia owing to interference with the action of vitamin B_{12}; neurological toxic effects can occur without preceding overt haematological changes. Depression of white cell formation may also occur.

● PREGNANCY May depress neonatal respiration if used during delivery.

● BREAST FEEDING Breast-feeding can be resumed as soon as mother has recovered sufficiently from anaesthesia.

● MONITORING REQUIREMENTS
▶ Assessment of plasma-vitamin B_{12} concentration should be considered in those at risk of deficiency, including the elderly, those who have a poor, vegetarian, or vegan diet, and those with a history of anaemia.
▶ Nitrous oxide should **not** be given continuously for longer than 24 hours or more frequently than every 4 days without close supervision and haematological monitoring.

● DIRECTIONS FOR ADMINISTRATION For analgesia (without loss of consciousness), manufacturer advises a mixture of nitrous oxide and oxygen containing 50% of each gas (*Entonox*®) is used.

● HANDLING AND STORAGE Exposure of theatre staff to nitrous oxide should be minimised (risk of serious side-effects).

● MEDICINAL FORMS There can be variation in the licensing of different medicines containing the same drug.
Inhalation gas
▶ Nitrous oxide (Non-proprietary)
Nitrous oxide 1 ml per 1 ml Nitrous oxide cylinders size E | 1800 litre P ⚠ CD5
Nitrous oxide cylinders size F | 3600 litre P ⚠ CD5
Nitrous oxide cylinders size J | 18000 litre P ⚠ CD5
Nitrous oxide cylinders size G | 9000 litre P ⚠ CD5
Nitrous oxide cylinders size D | 900 litre P ⚠ CD5

◤ 1524

Sevoflurane

● INDICATIONS AND DOSE

Induction of anaesthesia (in oxygen or nitrous oxide–oxygen)
▶ BY INHALATION
▶ Adult: Initially 0.5–1 %, then increased to up to 8 %, increased gradually, according to response, to be administered using specifically calibrated vaporiser

Maintenance of anaesthesia (in oxygen or nitrous oxide–oxygen)
▶ BY INHALATION
▶ Adult: 0.5–3 %, adjusted according to response, to be administered using specifically calibrated vaporiser

● CAUTIONS Susceptibility to QT-interval prolongation

● INTERACTIONS → Appendix 1: volatile halogenated anaesthetics

● SIDE-EFFECTS
▶ **Common or very common** Drowsiness · fever · hypothermia
▶ **Uncommon** Asthma · atrioventricular block · confusion
▶ **Frequency not known** Dystonia · intracranial pressure increased · muscle rigidity · nephritis tubulointerstitial · oedema · pancreatitis

● PREGNANCY May depress neonatal respiration if used during delivery.

● BREAST FEEDING Breast-feeding can be resumed as soon as mother has recovered sufficiently from anaesthesia.

● RENAL IMPAIRMENT Use with caution.

● MEDICINAL FORMS There can be variation in the licensing of different medicines containing the same drug.
Inhalation vapour liquid
▶ Sevoflurane (Non-proprietary)
Sevoflurane 1 ml per 1 ml Sevoflurane 100% inhalation vapour liquid | 250 ml PoM £123.00 (Hospital only)

---

1   Anaesthesia adjuvants

Pre-medication and peri-operative drugs
01-Sep-2020

Drugs that affect gastric pH

Regurgitation and aspiration of gastric contents (Mendelson's syndrome) can be an important complication of general anaesthesia, particularly in obstetrics and during emergency surgery, and requires prophylaxis against acid aspiration. Prophylaxis is also needed in those with gastro-oesophageal reflux disease and in circumstances where gastric emptying may be delayed.

An **H_2-receptor antagonist** can be used before surgery to increase the pH and reduce the volume of gastric fluid. It does not affect the pH of fluid already in the stomach and this limits its value in emergency procedures; an oral H_2-receptor antagonist can be given 1–2 hours before the procedure. Antacids are frequently used to neutralise the acidity of the fluid already in the stomach; 'clear' (non-particulate) antacids such as sodium citrate p. 909 are preferred.

Antimuscarinic drugs

Antimuscarinic drugs are used (less commonly nowadays) as premedicants to dry bronchial and salivary secretions which are increased by intubation, upper airway surgery, or some inhalational anaesthetics. They are also used before or with neostigmine p. 1286 to prevent bradycardia, excessive salivation, and other muscarinic actions of neostigmine.

They also prevent bradycardia and hypotension associated with drugs such as propofol p. 1522 and suxamethonium chloride p. 1529.

Atropine sulfate below is now rarely used for premedication but still has an emergency role in the treatment of vagotonic side-effects. Atropine sulfate may have a role in acute arrhythmias after myocardial infarction.

Hyoscine hydrobromide p. 501 reduces secretions and also provides a degree of amnesia, sedation, and anti-emesis. Unlike atropine sulfate it may produce bradycardia rather than tachycardia.

Glycopyrronium bromide p. 1527 reduces salivary secretions. When given intravenously it produces less tachycardia than atropine sulfate. It is widely used with neostigmine for reversal of non-depolarising neuromuscular blocking drugs.

Phenothiazines do not effectively reduce secretions when used alone.

Sedative drugs

Fear and anxiety before a procedure (including the night before) can be minimised by using a sedative drug, usually a **benzodiazepine**. Premedication may also augment the action of anaesthetics and provide some degree of pre-operative amnesia. The choice of drug depends on the individual, the nature of the procedure, the anaesthetic to be used, and other prevailing circumstances such as outpatients, obstetrics, and availability of recovery facilities. The choice also varies between elective and emergency procedures.

Premedicants can be given the night before major surgery; a further, smaller dose may be required before surgery. Alternatively, the first dose may be given on the day of the procedure.

Benzodiazepines

Benzodiazepines possess useful properties for premedication including relief of anxiety, sedation, and amnesia; short-acting benzodiazepines taken by mouth are the most common premedicants. Benzodiazepines are also used in intensive care units for sedation, particularly in those receiving assisted ventilation. Flumazenil p. 1563 is used to antagonise the effects of benzodiazepines.

Diazepam p. 398 is used to produce mild sedation with amnesia. It is a long-acting drug with active metabolites and a second period of drowsiness can occur several hours after its administration. Peri-operative use of diazepam in children is not recommended; its effect and timing of response are unreliable and paradoxical effects may occur.

Diazepam is relatively insoluble in water and preparations formulated in organic solvents are painful on intravenous injection and give rise to a high incidence of venous thrombosis (which may not be noticed for several days after the injection). Intramuscular injection of diazepam is painful and absorption is erratic. An emulsion formulated for intravenous injection is less irritant and reduces the risk of venous thrombosis; it is not suitable for intramuscular injection.

Temazepam p. 552 is given by mouth for premedication and has a shorter duration of action and a more rapid onset than oral diazepam; anxiolytic and sedative effects last about 90 minutes although there may be residual drowsiness.

Lorazepam p. 393 produces more prolonged sedation than temazepam and it has marked amnesic effects.

Midazolam p. 394 is a water-soluble benzodiazepine that is often used in preference to intravenous diazepam; recovery is faster than from diazepam, but may be significantly longer in the elderly, in patients with a low cardiac output, or after repeated dosing. Midazolam is associated with profound sedation when high doses are given intravenously or when it is used with certain other drugs.

Other drugs for sedation

Dexmedetomidine p. 1540 and clonidine hydrochloride p. 172 are alpha$_2$-adrenergic agonists with sedative properties. Dexmedetomidine is licensed for the sedation of patients receiving intensive care who need to remain responsive to verbal stimulation. Clonidine hydrochloride [unlicensed indication] can be used by mouth or by intravenous injection as a sedative agent when adequate sedation cannot be achieved with standard treatment.

Analgesia

For guidance on the use of analgesics before, during, or after surgery, see Peri-operative analgesia p. 1532.

Antagonists for central and respiratory depression

Respiratory depression is a major concern with opioid analgesics and it may be treated by artificial ventilation or be reversed by naloxone hydrochloride p. 1564. Naloxone hydrochloride will immediately reverse opioid-induced respiratory depression but the dose may have to be repeated because of the short duration of action of naloxone hydrochloride; however, naloxone hydrochloride will also antagonise the analgesic effect.

Flumazenil is a benzodiazepine antagonist for the reversal of the central sedative effects of benzodiazepines after anaesthetic and similar procedures. Flumazenil has a shorter half-life and duration of action than diazepam or midazolam so patients may become resedated.

Doxapram hydrochloride p. 342 is a central and respiratory stimulant but is of limited value in anaesthesia.

ANTIMUSCARINICS

◣ 896

| Atropine sulfate

22-Feb-2023

● INDICATIONS AND DOSE

Symptomatic bradycardia due to acute overdosage of beta-blockers

▶ BY INTRAVENOUS INJECTION

▸ Child: 0.02 mg/kg (max. per dose 1.2 mg), repeat doses may be necessary

▸ Adult: 0.5–1.2 mg, repeat doses may be necessary

Treatment of poisoning by organophosphorus insecticide or nerve agent (in combination with pralidoxime chloride)

▶ BY INTRAVENOUS INJECTION

▸ Child: 20 micrograms/kg every 5–10 minutes (max. per dose 2 mg) until the skin becomes flushed and dry, the pupils dilate, and bradycardia is abolished, frequency of administration dependent on the severity of poisoning

▸ Adult: 2 mg every 5–10 minutes until the skin becomes flushed and dry, the pupils dilate, and bradycardia is abolished, frequency of administration dependent on the severity of poisoning

Symptomatic relief of gastro-intestinal disorders characterised by smooth muscle spasm

▶ BY MOUTH

▸ Adult: 0.6–1.2 mg daily, dose to be taken at night

Premedication

▶ BY INTRAVENOUS INJECTION

▸ Child 12–17 years: 300–600 micrograms, to be administered immediately before induction of anaesthesia

▸ Adult: 300–600 micrograms, to be administered immediately before induction of anaesthesia

▶ BY SUBCUTANEOUS INJECTION, OR BY INTRAMUSCULAR INJECTION
▸ Child 12-17 years: 300–600 micrograms, to be administered 30–60 minutes before induction of anaesthesia
▸ Adult: 300–600 micrograms, to be administered 30–60 minutes before induction of anaesthesia

Intra-operative bradycardia
▶ BY INTRAVENOUS INJECTION
▸ Child 12-17 years: 300–600 micrograms, larger doses may be used in emergencies
▸ Adult: 300–600 micrograms, larger doses may be used in emergencies

Control of muscarinic side-effects of neostigmine in reversal of competitive neuromuscular block
▶ BY INTRAVENOUS INJECTION
▸ Child 12-17 years: 0.6–1.2 mg
▸ Adult: 0.6–1.2 mg

Excessive bradycardia associated with beta-blocker use
▶ BY INTRAVENOUS INJECTION
▸ Adult: 0.6–2.4 mg in divided doses (max. per dose 600 micrograms)

Bradycardia following myocardial infarction (particularly if complicated by hypotension)
▶ BY INTRAVENOUS INJECTION
▸ Adult: 500 micrograms every 3–5 minutes; maximum 3 mg per course

● UNLICENSED USE TOXBASE advises atropine sulfate is used in the doses provided for the treatment of symptomatic bradycardia due to acute overdosage of beta-blockers, but these may vary from those licensed.

> **IMPORTANT SAFETY INFORMATION**
> Antimuscarinic drugs used for premedication to general anaesthesia should only be administered by, or under the direct supervision of, personnel experienced in their use.

● INTERACTIONS → Appendix 1: atropine

● SIDE-EFFECTS
▶ **Common or very common**
▸ With intramuscular use or intravenous use Abdominal distension · agitation · anhidrosis · dysphagia · hyperthermia · movement disorders · speech disorder · taste loss
▶ **Uncommon**
▸ With intramuscular use or intravenous use Psychotic disorder
▶ **Rare or very rare**
▸ With intramuscular use or intravenous use Angina pectoris · arrhythmias · hypertensive crisis · seizure
▶ **Frequency not known**
▸ With intramuscular use or intravenous use Insomnia
▸ With oral use Angle closure glaucoma · arrhythmias · bronchial secretion altered · chest pain · dysphagia · fever · gastrointestinal disorders · mydriasis · staggering · thirst
▸ With parenteral use Arrhythmias · atrioventricular block · bronchial secretion decreased · delirium · fever · gastrointestinal disorders · hallucination · mydriasis · restlessness · thirst

● PREGNANCY Not known to be harmful; manufacturer advises caution.

● BREAST FEEDING May suppress lactation; small amount present in milk—manufacturer advises caution.

● MONITORING REQUIREMENTS
▶ Control of muscarinic side-effects of neostigmine in reversal of competitive neuromuscular block Since atropine has a shorter duration of action than neostigmine, late unopposed bradycardia may result; close monitoring of the patient is necessary.

● LESS SUITABLE FOR PRESCRIBING Atropine tablets less suitable for prescribing. Any clinical benefit as a gastro-intestinal antispasmodic is outweighed by atropinic side-effects.

● EXCEPTIONS TO LEGAL CATEGORY
▶ With parenteral use Prescription only medicine restriction does not apply where administration is for saving life in emergency.

● MEDICINAL FORMS There can be variation in the licensing of different medicines containing the same drug. Forms available from special-order manufacturers include: oral suspension, oral solution, solution for injection, solution for infusion

Solution for injection
▶ Atropine sulfate (Non-proprietary)
  Atropine sulfate 100 microgram per 1 ml Atropine 1mg/10ml solution for injection pre-filled syringes | 1 pre-filled disposable injection [PoM] £12.35
  Atropine 500micrograms/5ml solution for injection pre-filled syringes | 1 pre-filled disposable injection [PoM] £13.00 | 10 pre-filled disposable injection [PoM] £130.00
  Atropine sulfate 200 microgram per 1 ml Atropine 1mg/5ml solution for injection pre-filled syringes | 1 pre-filled disposable injection [PoM] £13.00 | 10 pre-filled disposable injection [PoM] £130.00
  Atropine sulfate 300 microgram per 1 ml Atropine 3mg/10ml solution for injection pre-filled syringes | 1 pre-filled disposable injection [PoM] £13.00 DT = £13.00 | 10 pre-filled disposable injection [PoM] £130.00
  Atropine sulfate 600 microgram per 1 ml Atropine 600micrograms/1ml solution for injection ampoules | 10 ampoule [PoM] £11.71-£14.30
  Atropine sulfate 1 mg per 1 ml Atropine 1mg/1ml solution for injection ampoules | 10 ampoule [PoM] £168.05-£285.68

◢ 896

Glycopyrronium bromide
(Glycopyrrolate)
    17-Jan-2024

● INDICATIONS AND DOSE
Premedication at induction
▶ BY INTRAMUSCULAR INJECTION, OR BY INTRAVENOUS INJECTION
▸ Adult: 200–400 micrograms, alternatively 4–5 micrograms/kg (max. per dose 400 micrograms)

Intra-operative bradycardia
▶ BY INTRAVENOUS INJECTION
▸ Adult: 200–400 micrograms, alternatively 4–5 micrograms/kg (max. per dose 400 micrograms), repeated if necessary

Control of muscarinic side-effects of neostigmine in reversal of non-depolarising neuromuscular block
▶ BY INTRAVENOUS INJECTION
▸ Adult: 10–15 micrograms/kg, alternatively, 200 micrograms per 1 mg of neostigmine to be administered

Bowel colic in palliative care | Excessive respiratory secretions in palliative care
▶ BY SUBCUTANEOUS INJECTION
▸ Adult: 200 micrograms every 4 hours and when required, hourly use is occasionally necessary, particularly in excessive respiratory secretions
▶ BY SUBCUTANEOUS INFUSION
▸ Adult: 0.6–1.2 mg/24 hours

> **IMPORTANT SAFETY INFORMATION**
> Antimuscarinic drugs used for premedication to general anaesthesia should only be administered by, or under the direct supervision of, personnel experienced in their use.

● INTERACTIONS → Appendix 1: glycopyrronium

- **SIDE-EFFECTS** Anhidrosis · bronchial secretion decreased · mydriasis
- **RENAL IMPAIRMENT** See p. 21. EvGr Caution in renal impairment—duration of action may be prolonged. Repeated or large doses should be avoided in patients with uraemia due to risk of accumulation. M
- **PRESCRIBING AND DISPENSING INFORMATION**

  Palliative care For further information on the use of glycopyrronium bromide in palliative care, see www.medicinescomplete.com/#/content/palliative/glycopyrronium.

- **MEDICINAL FORMS** There can be variation in the licensing of different medicines containing the same drug.
  Solution for injection
  ▸ Glycopyrronium bromide (Non-proprietary)
  Glycopyrronium bromide 200 microgram per 1 ml Glycopyrronium bromide 200micrograms/1ml solution for injection ampoules | 10 ampoule PoM £10.50 DT = £21.40 (Hospital only) | 10 ampoule PoM £22.07 DT = £21.40
  Glycopyrronium bromide 600micrograms/3ml solution for injection ampoules | 3 ampoule PoM £8.00 | 10 ampoule PoM £21.12-£21.20 DT = £21.12 | 10 ampoule PoM £14.99 DT = £21.12 (Hospital only)

1.1 Neuromuscular blockade

Neuromuscular blockade

Neuromuscular blocking drugs

Neuromuscular blocking drugs used in anaesthesia are also known as **muscle relaxants**. By specific blockade of the neuromuscular junction they enable light anaesthesia to be used with adequate relaxation of the muscles of the abdomen and diaphragm. They also relax the vocal cords and allow the passage of a tracheal tube. Their action differs from the muscle relaxants used in musculoskeletal disorders that act on the spinal cord or brain.

Patients who have received a neuromuscular blocking drug should **always** have their respiration assisted or controlled until the drug has been inactivated or antagonised. They should also receive sufficient concomitant inhalational or intravenous anaesthetic or sedative drugs to prevent awareness.

Non-depolarising neuromuscular blocking drugs

Non-depolarising neuromuscular blocking drugs (also known as competitive muscle relaxants) compete with acetylcholine for receptor sites at the neuromuscular junction and their action can be reversed with anticholinesterases such as neostigmine p. 1286. Non-depolarising neuromuscular blocking drugs can be divided into the **aminosteroid** group, comprising pancuronium bromide p. 1530, rocuronium bromide p. 1531, and vecuronium bromide p. 1531, and the **benzylisoquinolinium** group, comprising atracurium besilate p. 1529, cisatracurium p. 1530, and mivacurium p. 1530.

Non-depolarising neuromuscular blocking drugs have a slower onset of action than suxamethonium chloride p. 1529. These drugs can be classified by their duration of action as short-acting (15–30 minutes), intermediate-acting (30–40 minutes), and long-acting (60–120 minutes), although duration of action is dose-dependent. Drugs with a shorter or intermediate duration of action, such as atracurium besilate and vecuronium bromide p. 1531, are more widely used than those with a longer duration of action, such as pancuronium bromide.

Non-depolarising neuromuscular blocking drugs have no sedative or analgesic effects and are not considered to trigger malignant hyperthermia.

For patients receiving intensive care and who require tracheal intubation and mechanical ventilation, a non-depolarising neuromuscular blocking drug is chosen according to its onset of effect, duration of action, and side-effects. Rocuronium bromide, with a rapid onset of effect, may facilitate intubation. Atracurium besilate or cisatracurium may be suitable for long-term neuromuscular blockade since their duration of action is not dependent on elimination by the liver or the kidneys.

Atracurium besilate, a mixture of 10 isomers, is a benzylisoquinolinium neuromuscular blocking drug with an intermediate duration of action. It undergoes non-enzymatic metabolism which is independent of liver and kidney function, thus allowing its use in patients with hepatic or renal impairment. Cardiovascular effects are associated with significant histamine release; histamine release can be minimised by administering slowly or in divided doses over at least 1 minute.

Cisatracurium is a single isomer of atracurium besilate. It is more potent and has a slightly longer duration of action than atracurium besilate and provides greater cardiovascular stability because cisatracurium lacks histamine-releasing effects.

Mivacurium, a benzylisoquinolinium neuromuscular blocking drug, has a short duration of action. It is metabolised by plasma cholinesterase and muscle paralysis is prolonged in individuals deficient in this enzyme. It is not associated with vagolytic activity or ganglionic blockade although histamine release can occur, particularly with rapid injection.

Pancuronium bromide, an aminosteroid neuromuscular blocking drug, has a long duration of action and is often used in patients receiving long-term mechanical ventilation in intensive care units. It lacks a histamine-releasing effect, but vagolytic and sympathomimetic effects can cause tachycardia and hypertension.

Rocuronium bromide exerts an effect within 2 minutes and has the most rapid onset of any of the non-depolarising neuromuscular blocking drugs. It is an aminosteroid neuromuscular blocking drug with an intermediate duration of action. It is reported to have minimal cardiovascular effects; high doses produce mild vagolytic activity.

Vecuronium bromide p. 1531, an aminosteroid neuromuscular blocking drug, has an intermediate duration of action. It does not generally produce histamine release and lacks cardiovascular effects.

Depolarising neuromuscular blocking drugs

Suxamethonium chloride has the most rapid onset of action of any of the neuromuscular blocking drugs and is ideal if fast onset and brief duration of action are required, e.g. with tracheal intubation. Unlike the non-depolarising neuromuscular blocking drugs, its action cannot be reversed and recovery is spontaneous; anticholinesterases such as neostigmine potentiate the neuromuscular block.

Suxamethonium chloride should be given after anaesthetic induction because paralysis is usually preceded by painful muscle fasciculations. While tachycardia occurs with single use, bradycardia may occur with repeated doses in adults and with the first dose in children. Premedication with atropine reduces bradycardia as well as the excessive salivation associated with suxamethonium chloride use.

Prolonged paralysis may occur in **dual block**, which occurs with high or repeated doses of suxamethonium chloride and is caused by the development of a non-depolarising block following the initial depolarising block. Individuals with myasthenia gravis are resistant to suxamethonium chloride but can develop dual block resulting in delayed recovery. Prolonged paralysis may also occur in those with low or atypical plasma cholinesterase. Assisted ventilation should be continued until muscle function is restored.

Suxamethonium chloride
02-Dec-2020

(Succinylcholine chloride)

- **DRUG ACTION** Suxamethonium acts by mimicking acetylcholine at the neuromuscular junction but hydrolysis is much slower than for acetylcholine; depolarisation is therefore prolonged, resulting in neuromuscular blockade.

- ● **INDICATIONS AND DOSE**

Neuromuscular blockade (short duration) during surgery and intubation
- ► BY INTRAVENOUS INJECTION
- ► Adult: 1–1.5 mg/kg

- **UNLICENSED USE** Doses of suxamethonium in BNF may differ from those in product literature.

> **IMPORTANT SAFETY INFORMATION**
> Should only be administered by, or under the direct supervision of, personnel experienced in its use.

- **CONTRA-INDICATIONS** Hyperkalaemia · low plasma-cholinesterase activity (including severe liver disease) · major trauma · neurological disease involving acute wasting of major muscle · personal or family history of congenital myotonic disease · personal or family history of malignant hyperthermia · prolonged immobilisation (risk of hyperkalaemia) · severe burns · skeletal muscle myopathies (e.g. Duchenne muscular dystrophy)

- **CAUTIONS** Cardiac disease · neuromuscular disease · raised intra-ocular pressure (avoid in penetrating eye injury) · respiratory disease · severe sepsis (risk of hyperkalaemia)

- **INTERACTIONS** → Appendix 1: suxamethonium

- **SIDE-EFFECTS**
- ► **Common or very common** Arrhythmias · bradycardia (may occur with repeated doses) · flushing · muscle contractions involuntary · myoglobinuria · myopathy · post procedural muscle pain · rash
- ► **Rare or very rare** Apnoea · cardiac arrest · hypersensitivity · malignant hyperthermia · respiratory disorders · trismus
  SIDE-EFFECTS, FURTHER INFORMATION Premedication with atropine reduces bradycardia associated with suxamethonium use.

- **ALLERGY AND CROSS-SENSITIVITY** EvGr Allergic cross-reactivity between neuromuscular blocking drugs has been reported; caution is advised in cases of hypersensitivity to these drugs. ⓜ

- **PREGNANCY** Mildly prolonged maternal neuromuscular blockade may occur.

- **BREAST FEEDING** Unlikely to be present in breast milk in significant amounts (ionised at physiological pH). Breast-feeding may be resumed once the mother recovered from neuromuscular block.

- **HEPATIC IMPAIRMENT** Manufacturer advises caution, particularly in end stage hepatic failure (increased risk of prolonged apnoea due to reduced hepatic synthesis of plasma cholinesterase).

- **MEDICINAL FORMS** There can be variation in the licensing of different medicines containing the same drug. Forms available from special-order manufacturers include: solution for injection

Solution for injection
- ► Suxamethonium chloride (Non-proprietary)
  Suxamethonium chloride 50 mg per 1 ml Suxamethonium chloride 100mg/2ml solution for injection ampoules | 10 ampoule PoM £28.80–£50.00

Non-depolarising neuromuscular blocking drugs

> **IMPORTANT SAFETY INFORMATION**
> Non-depolarising neuromuscular blocking drugs should only be administered by, or under direct supervision of, personnel experienced in their use, with adequate training in anaesthesia and airway management.

- **CAUTIONS** Burns (resistance can develop, increased doses may be required) · cardiovascular disease (reduce rate of administration) · electrolyte disturbances (response unpredictable) · fluid disturbances (response unpredictable) · hypothermia (activity prolonged, lower doses required) · myasthenia gravis (activity prolonged, lower doses required) · neuromuscular disorders (response unpredictable)

- **SIDE-EFFECTS**
- ► **Common or very common** Flushing · hypotension
- ► **Uncommon** Bronchospasm · hypersensitivity · skin reactions · tachycardia
- ► **Rare or very rare** Circulatory collapse · muscle weakness (after prolonged use in intensive care) · myopathy (after prolonged use in intensive care) · shock

- **ALLERGY AND CROSS-SENSITIVITY** Allergic cross-reactivity between neuromuscular blocking drugs has been reported; caution is advised in cases of hypersensitivity to these drugs.

- **PREGNANCY** Non-depolarising neuromuscular blocking drugs are highly ionised at physiological pH and are therefore unlikely to cross the placenta in significant amounts.

- **BREAST FEEDING** Non-depolarising neuromuscular blocking drugs are ionised at physiological pH and are unlikely to be present in milk in significant amounts. Breast-feeding may be resumed once the mother has recovered from neuromuscular block.

▸ **above**

Atracurium besilate

(Atracurium besylate)

- ● **INDICATIONS AND DOSE**

Neuromuscular blockade (short to intermediate duration) for surgery and intubation
- ► INITIALLY BY INTRAVENOUS INJECTION
- ► Adult: Initially 300–600 micrograms/kg, then (by intravenous injection) 100–200 micrograms/kg as required, alternatively (by intravenous injection) initially 300–600 micrograms/kg, followed by (by intravenous infusion) 300–600 micrograms/kg/hour

Neuromuscular blockade during intensive care
- ► INITIALLY BY INTRAVENOUS INJECTION
- ► Adult: Initially 300–600 micrograms/kg, initial dose is optional, then (by intravenous infusion) 270–1770 micrograms/kg/hour; (by intravenous infusion) usual dose 650–780 micrograms/kg/hour

DOSES AT EXTREMES OF BODY-WEIGHT
- ► To avoid excessive dosage in obese patients, dose should be calculated on the basis of ideal body-weight.

- **INTERACTIONS** → Appendix 1: neuromuscular blocking drugs, non-depolarising

- **SIDE-EFFECTS**
- ► **Rare or very rare** Cardiac arrest
- ► **Frequency not known** Seizure

SIDE-EFFECTS, FURTHER INFORMATION Hypotension, skin flushing, and bronchospasm is associated with histamine release. Manufacturer advises minimising effects of histamine release by administering over 1 minute in patients with cardiovascular disease or sensitivity to hypotension.

- **DIRECTIONS FOR ADMINISTRATION** For *intravenous infusion* (*Tracrium®*; Atracurium besilate injection, Hospira; Atracurium injection/infusion, Genus), give continuously in Glucose 5% or Sodium Chloride 0.9%; stability varies with diluent; dilute requisite dose with infusion fluid to a concentration of 0.5–5 mg/mL.

- **MEDICINAL FORMS** There can be variation in the licensing of different medicines containing the same drug. Forms available from special-order manufacturers include: solution for injection

Solution for injection

- Atracurium besilate (Non-proprietary)
  Atracurium besilate 10 mg per 1 ml Atracurium besilate 250mg/25ml solution for injection vials | 1 vial PoM £16.50 (Hospital only) | 2 vial PoM £25.81 (Hospital only)
  Atracurium besilate 25mg/2.5ml solution for injection ampoules | 5 ampoule PoM £8.28 (Hospital only) | 10 ampoule PoM £27.50 | 10 ampoule PoM £16.56 (Hospital only)
  Atracurium besilate 50mg/5ml solution for injection ampoules | 5 ampoule PoM £15.02 (Hospital only) | 10 ampoule PoM £42.35 | 10 ampoule PoM £30.04 (Hospital only)

Cisatracurium

⚑ 1529
24-Jul-2020

- **INDICATIONS AND DOSE**

Neuromuscular blockade (intermediate duration) during surgery and intubation

- INITIALLY BY INTRAVENOUS INJECTION
- Adult: Initially 150 micrograms/kg, then (by intravenous injection) maintenance 30 micrograms/kg every 20 minutes, alternatively (by intravenous infusion) initially 180 micrograms/kg/hour, then (by intravenous infusion) maintenance 60–120 micrograms/kg/hour, maintenance dose administered after stabilisation

Neuromuscular blockade (intermediate duration) during intensive care

- INITIALLY BY INTRAVENOUS INJECTION
- Adult: Initially 150 micrograms/kg, initial dose is optional, then (by intravenous infusion) 180 micrograms/kg/hour, adjusted according to response; (by intravenous infusion) usual dose 30–600 micrograms/kg/hour

DOSES AT EXTREMES OF BODY-WEIGHT

- To avoid excessive dosage in obese patients, dose should be calculated on the basis of ideal body-weight.

- **INTERACTIONS** → Appendix 1: neuromuscular blocking drugs, non-depolarising

- **SIDE-EFFECTS**
- **Common or very common** Bradycardia

- **DIRECTIONS FOR ADMINISTRATION** For *intravenous infusion* (*Nimbex®*, *Nimbex Forte®*), manufacturer advises give continuously in Glucose 5% or Sodium Chloride 0.9%; solutions of 2 mg/mL and 5 mg/mL may be infused undiluted; alternatively dilute with infusion fluid to a concentration of 0.1–2 mg/mL.

- **MEDICINAL FORMS** There can be variation in the licensing of different medicines containing the same drug.
Solution for injection

- Cisatracurium (Non-proprietary)
  Cisatracurium (as Cisatracurium besilate) 2 mg per 1 ml Cisatracurium besilate 10mg/5ml solution for injection ampoules | 5 ampoule PoM ⊠ (Hospital only)

Cisatracurium besilate 20mg/10ml solution for injection ampoules | 5 ampoule PoM £32.09–£37.75 (Hospital only)
Cisatracurium besilate 10mg/5ml solution for injection vials | 1 vial PoM £30.00 (Hospital only)
Cisatracurium (as Cisatracurium besilate) 5 mg per 1 ml Cisatracurium besilate 150mg/30ml solution for injection vials | 1 vial PoM £26.43–£31.09 (Hospital only) | 5 vial PoM £132.15 (Hospital only)

Mivacurium

⚑ 1529
10-May-2021

- **INDICATIONS AND DOSE**

Neuromuscular blockade (short duration) during surgery and intubation

- INITIALLY BY INTRAVENOUS INJECTION
- Adult: 70–250 micrograms/kg; (by intravenous injection) maintenance 100 micrograms/kg every 15 minutes, alternatively (by intravenous infusion) maintenance 8–10 micrograms/kg/minute, (by intravenous infusion) adjusted in steps of 1 microgram/kg/minute every 3 minutes if required; (by intravenous infusion) usual dose 6–7 micrograms/kg/minute

DOSES AT EXTREMES OF BODY-WEIGHT

- To avoid excessive dosage in obese patients, dose should be calculated on the basis of ideal body-weight.

- **CAUTIONS** Burns (low plasma cholinesterase activity; dose titration required) · elderly

- **INTERACTIONS** → Appendix 1: neuromuscular blocking drugs, non-depolarising

- **HEPATIC IMPAIRMENT** Manufacturer advises caution in hepatic failure (increased duration of action).
Dose adjustments Manufacturer advises dose reduction in hepatic failure.

- **RENAL IMPAIRMENT** EvGr Use with caution. Ⓜ
Dose adjustments EvGr Reduce dose according to response in end-stage renal disease (clinical effect prolonged). Ⓜ

- **DIRECTIONS FOR ADMINISTRATION** For *intravenous infusion*, give continuously in Glucose 5% or Sodium Chloride 0.9%. Dilute to a concentration of 500 micrograms/mL; may also be given undiluted. Doses up to 150 micrograms/kg may be given over 5–15 seconds, higher doses should be given over 30 seconds. In asthma, cardiovascular disease or in those sensitive to reduced arterial blood pressure, give over 60 seconds.

- **MEDICINAL FORMS** There can be variation in the licensing of different medicines containing the same drug.
Solution for injection

- Mivacurium (Non-proprietary)
  Mivacurium (as Mivacurium chloride) 2 mg per 1 ml Mivacurium chloride 20mg/10ml solution for injection ampoules | 5 ampoule PoM £22.57 (Hospital only)
  Mivacurium chloride 10mg/5ml solution for injection ampoules | 5 ampoule PoM £13.95 (Hospital only)

Pancuronium bromide

⚑ 1529
10-May-2021

- **INDICATIONS AND DOSE**

Neuromuscular blockade (long duration) during surgery and intubation

- BY INTRAVENOUS INJECTION
- Adult: Initially 100 micrograms/kg, then 20 micrograms/kg as required

Neuromuscular blockade (long duration) during intensive care

- BY INTRAVENOUS INJECTION
- Adult: Initially 100 micrograms/kg, initial dose is optional, then 60 micrograms/kg every 60–90 minutes

DOSES AT EXTREMES OF BODY-WEIGHT
‣ To avoid excessive dosage in obese patients, dose should be calculated on the basis of ideal body-weight.

● INTERACTIONS → Appendix 1: neuromuscular blocking drugs, non-depolarising

● SIDE-EFFECTS Apnoea · arrhythmia · hypersalivation · increased cardiac output · miosis

SIDE-EFFECTS, FURTHER INFORMATION Pancuronium lacks histamine-releasing effect, but vagolytic and sympathomimetic effects can cause tachycardia.

● HEPATIC IMPAIRMENT Manufacturer advises caution (possibly slower onset and higher dose requirements due to resistance to neuromuscular blocking action which may lead to a prolonged recovery time).

● RENAL IMPAIRMENT [EvGr] Use with caution (may prolong duration of block). ⟨M⟩

● MEDICINAL FORMS No licensed medicines listed.

⚑ 1529

Rocuronium bromide
10-May-2021

● INDICATIONS AND DOSE

Neuromuscular blockade (intermediate duration) during surgery and intubation
‣ INITIALLY BY INTRAVENOUS INJECTION
‣ Adult: Initially 600 micrograms/kg; (by intravenous injection) maintenance 150 micrograms/kg, alternatively (by intravenous infusion) maintenance 300–600 micrograms/kg/hour, adjusted according to response
‣ Elderly: Initially 600 micrograms/kg; (by intravenous injection) maintenance 75–100 micrograms/kg, alternatively (by intravenous infusion) maintenance up to 400 micrograms/kg/hour, adjusted according to response

Neuromuscular blockade (intermediate duration) during intensive care
‣ INITIALLY BY INTRAVENOUS INJECTION
‣ Adult: Initially 600 micrograms/kg, initial dose is optional; (by intravenous infusion) maintenance 300–600 micrograms/kg/hour for first hour, then (by intravenous infusion), adjusted according to response

DOSES AT EXTREMES OF BODY-WEIGHT
‣ To avoid excessive dosage in obese patients, dose should be calculated on the basis of ideal body-weight.

● INTERACTIONS → Appendix 1: neuromuscular blocking drugs, non-depolarising

● SIDE-EFFECTS
‣ **Uncommon** Procedural complications
‣ **Rare or very rare** Angioedema · face oedema · paralysis
‣ **Frequency not known** Malignant hyperthermia

● HEPATIC IMPAIRMENT Manufacturer advises caution (may prolong duration of action).
Dose adjustments Manufacturer advises consider dose reduction—consult product literature.

● RENAL IMPAIRMENT [EvGr] Use with caution (may prolong duration of block). ⟨M⟩
Dose adjustments [EvGr] Reduce maintenance dose (consult product literature). ⟨M⟩

● DIRECTIONS FOR ADMINISTRATION [EvGr] For *continuous intravenous infusion* or via drip tubing, may be diluted with Glucose 5% or Sodium Chloride 0.9%. ⟨M⟩

● MEDICINAL FORMS There can be variation in the licensing of different medicines containing the same drug. Forms available from special-order manufacturers include: solution for injection
Solution for injection
‣ Rocuronium bromide (Non-proprietary)
Rocuronium bromide 10 mg per 1 ml Rocuronium bromide 100mg/10ml solution for injection vials | 10 vial [PoM] £57.00–£102.90 (Hospital only)
Rocuronium bromide 50mg/5ml solution for injection ampoules | 10 ampoule [PoM] £28.00 | 10 ampoule [PoM] £28.00 (Hospital only) | 20 ampoule [PoM] £95.00 (Hospital only)
Rocuronium bromide 100mg/10ml solution for injection ampoules | 10 ampoule [PoM] £57.00
Rocuronium bromide 50mg/5ml solution for injection pre-filled syringes | 10 pre-filled disposable injection [PoM] £190.00 (Hospital only)
Rocuronium bromide 50mg/5ml solution for injection vials | 10 vial [PoM] £28.00–£50.90 (Hospital only)

⚑ 1529

Vecuronium bromide
10-May-2021

● INDICATIONS AND DOSE

Neuromuscular blockade (intermediate duration) during surgery and intubation
‣ INITIALLY BY INTRAVENOUS INJECTION
‣ Adult: 80–100 micrograms/kg; (by intravenous injection) maintenance 20–30 micrograms/kg, adjusted according to response, max. 100 micrograms/kg in caesarean section, alternatively (by intravenous infusion) maintenance 0.8–1.4 micrograms/kg/minute, adjusted according to response

DOSES AT EXTREMES OF BODY-WEIGHT
‣ To avoid excessive dosage in obese patients, dose should be calculated on the basis of ideal body-weight.

● INTERACTIONS → Appendix 1: neuromuscular blocking drugs, non-depolarising

● SIDE-EFFECTS
‣ **Uncommon** Procedural complications
‣ **Rare or very rare** Angioedema · face oedema · paralysis

● HEPATIC IMPAIRMENT Manufacturer advises caution in significant impairment.

● RENAL IMPAIRMENT [EvGr] Use with caution. ⟨M⟩

● DIRECTIONS FOR ADMINISTRATION Manufacturer advises reconstitute each vial with 5 mL Water for Injections to give 2 mg/mL solution; *alternatively* reconstitute with up to 10 mL Glucose 5% *or* Sodium Chloride 0.9% *or* Water for Injections—unsuitable for further dilution if not reconstituted with Water for Injections. For *continuous intravenous infusion*, manufacturer advises dilute reconstituted solution to a concentration up to 40 micrograms/mL with Glucose 5% or Sodium Chloride 0.9%; reconstituted solution can also be given via drip tubing.

● MEDICINAL FORMS There can be variation in the licensing of different medicines containing the same drug.
Powder for solution for injection
‣ Vecuronium bromide (Non-proprietary)
Vecuronium bromide 10 mg Vecuronium bromide 10mg powder for solution for injection vials | 10 vial [PoM] Ⓢ (Hospital only)

1.2 Neuromuscular blockade reversal

Neuromuscular blockade reversal

Neuromuscular blockade reversal

Anticholinesterases

Anticholinesterases reverse the effects of the non-depolarising (competitive) neuromuscular blocking drugs such as pancuronium bromide p. 1530 but they prolong the action of the depolarising neuromuscular blocking drug suxamethonium chloride p. 1529.

Neostigmine p. 1286 is used specifically for reversal of non-depolarising (competitive) blockade. It acts within one minute of intravenous injection and its effects last for 20 to 30 minutes; a second dose may then be necessary. Glycopyrronium bromide p. 1527 or alternatively atropine sulfate p. 1526, given before or with neostigmine, prevent bradycardia, excessive salivation, and other muscarinic effects of neostigmine.

Other drugs for reversal of neuromuscular blockade

Sugammadex below is a modified gamma cyclodextrin that can be used for rapid reversal of neuromuscular blockade induced by rocuronium bromide p. 1531 or vecuronium bromide p. 1531. In practice, sugammadex is used mainly for rapid reversal of neuromuscular blockade in an emergency.

ANTICHOLINESTERASES

Neostigmine with glycopyrronium bromide

17-Jul-2020

The properties listed below are those particular to the combination only. For the properties of the components please consider, neostigmine p. 1286, glycopyrronium bromide p. 1527.

- **INDICATIONS AND DOSE**

Reversal of non-depolarising neuromuscular blockade
- ▸ BY INTRAVENOUS INJECTION
- ▸ Adult: 1–2 mL, repeated if necessary, alternatively 0.02 mL/kilogram, repeated if necessary; maximum 2 mL per course

- **INTERACTIONS** → Appendix 1: glycopyrronium · neostigmine

- **DIRECTIONS FOR ADMINISTRATION** For *intravenous injection*, manufacturer advises give over 10–30 seconds.

- **MEDICINAL FORMS** There can be variation in the licensing of different medicines containing the same drug.

Solution for injection
- ▸ Neostigmine with glycopyrronium bromide (Non-proprietary)
  Glycopyrronium bromide 500 microgram per 1 ml, Neostigmine metilsulfate 2.5 mg per 1 ml Neostigmine 2.5mg/1ml / Glycopyrronium bromide 500micrograms/1ml solution for injection ampoules | 10 ampoule [PoM] £11.50–£13.03

ANTIDOTES AND CHELATORS

Sugammadex

10-Aug-2021

- **INDICATIONS AND DOSE**

Routine reversal of neuromuscular blockade induced by rocuronium or vecuronium
- ▸ BY INTRAVENOUS INJECTION
- ▸ Adult: Initially 2–4 mg/kg, then 4 mg/kg if required, administered if recurrence of neuromuscular blockade occurs; consult product literature for further details

Immediate reversal of neuromuscular blockade induced by rocuronium
- ▸ BY INTRAVENOUS INJECTION
- ▸ Adult: 16 mg/kg (consult product literature)

IMPORTANT SAFETY INFORMATION
Should only be administered by, or under the direct supervision of, personnel experienced in its use.

- **CAUTIONS** Cardiovascular disease (recovery may be delayed) · elderly (recovery may be delayed) · pre-existing coagulation disorders · recurrence of neuromuscular blockade—monitor respiratory function until fully recovered · use of anticoagulants (unrelated to surgery) · wait 24 hours before re-administering rocuronium · wait 24 hours before re-administering vecuronium

- **INTERACTIONS** → Appendix 1: sugammadex

- **SIDE-EFFECTS**
- ▸ **Common or very common** Abdominal pain · cough · dizziness · headache · nausea · procedural complications · skin reactions · taste altered · vomiting
- ▸ **Frequency not known** Arrhythmias

- **PREGNANCY** Use with caution—no information available.

- **RENAL IMPAIRMENT** [EvGr] Avoid if creatinine clearance less than 30 mL/minute. Ⓜ See p. 21.

- **NATIONAL FUNDING/ACCESS DECISIONS** For full details see funding body website

Scottish Medicines Consortium (SMC) decisions
- ▸ Sugammadex (*Bridion*®) for the routine reversal of neuromuscular blockade induced by rocuronium or vecuronium in adults and rocuronium in paediatric patients (March 2013) SMC No. 527/09 Recommended with restrictions

- **MEDICINAL FORMS** There can be variation in the licensing of different medicines containing the same drug.

Solution for injection
ELECTROLYTES: May contain Sodium
- ▸ Sugammadex (Non-proprietary)
  Sugammadex (as Sugammadex sodium) 100 mg per 1 ml Sugammadex 500mg/5ml solution for injection vials | 10 vial [PoM] £1,192.80–£1,491.00 (Hospital only)
  Sugammadex 200mg/2ml solution for injection vials | 10 vial [PoM] £418.00–£596.40 (Hospital only)
- ▸ Bridion (Merck Sharp & Dohme (UK) Ltd)
  Sugammadex (as Sugammadex sodium) 100 mg per 1 ml Bridion 500mg/5ml solution for injection vials | 10 vial [PoM] £1,491.00 (Hospital only)
  Bridion 200mg/2ml solution for injection vials | 10 vial [PoM] £596.40 (Hospital only)

1.3 Peri-operative analgesia

Peri-operative analgesia

01-Sep-2020

Overview

[EvGr] Postoperative pain management options should be discussed with patients prior to surgery. Take into account the patient's clinical features and the type of surgery, and discuss the patient's pain history, preferences and expectations, likely impact of the procedure on their pain, potential benefits and risks of treatment, and discharge plan. A multimodal approach using a combination of analgesics from different classes to manage postoperative pain should be offered.

Consider prescribing pre-emptive analgesia to ensure that the patient's pain is managed when the effects of local anaesthesia wears off. Ⓐ

Non-opioid analgesics

[EvGr] Oral paracetamol p. 507 should be offered before and after surgery irrespective of pain severity, with intravenous paracetamol reserved for patients unable to take oral medication.

Offer oral ibuprofen p. 1302 to manage immediate postoperative pain (pain during the first 24 hours after surgery) of all severities, except for patients who have had surgery for a hip fracture—see NICE guideline: **Hip fractures: management** for guidance, available at: www.nice.org.uk/guidance/cg124. Intravenous NSAIDs should be reserved for patients unable to take oral medication; if offering intravenous NSAIDs, choose a traditional NSAID rather than a COX-2 (cyclo-oxygenase-2) inhibitor. Ⓐ

Intramuscular injections of diclofenac sodium p. 1297 and ketoprofen p. 1306 are rarely used; they are given deep into the gluteal muscle to minimise pain and tissue damage. Ketorolac trometamol p. 1536 is less irritant on intramuscular injection but pain has been reported; it can also be given by intravenous injection. Suppositories of diclofenac sodium and ketoprofen may be effective alternatives to the parenteral use of these drugs.

Since non-steroidal anti-inflammatory drugs (NSAIDs) do not depress respiration, do not impair gastro-intestinal motility, and do not cause dependence, they may be useful alternatives or adjuncts to opioids for the relief of postoperative pain.

Opioid analgesics

Opioid analgesics are now rarely used as premedicants; they are more likely to be administered at induction. Pre-operative use of opioid analgesics is generally limited to those patients who require control of existing pain.

[EvGr] An oral opioid should only be offered if immediate postoperative pain is expected to be moderate to severe. It should be given as soon as the patient can eat and drink after surgery, and the dose adjusted to help achieve functional recovery (such as coughing and mobilising) as soon as possible. Patients unable to take oral opioids should be offered either a patient-controlled analgesia (PCA) or continuous epidural. The benefit of a continuous epidural should be taken into consideration for patients who are having major or complex open-torso surgery, are expected to have severe pain, or those who have cognitive impairment. If opioids are used, see NICE guideline: **Controlled drugs: safe use and management** (available at: www.nice.org.uk/guidance/ng46) for information on prescribing controlled drugs. Ⓐ

For guidance on the management of opioid-induced respiratory depression, see Pre-medication and peri-operative drugs p. 1525.

Intra-operative analgesia

Opioid analgesics given in small doses before or with induction reduce the dose requirement of some drugs used during anaesthesia.

Alfentanil p. 1537, fentanyl p. 520, and remifentanil p. 1538 are particularly useful because they act within 1–2 minutes and have short durations of action. The initial doses of alfentanil or fentanyl are followed either by successive intravenous injections or by an intravenous infusion; prolonged infusions increase the duration of effect. Repeated intra-operative doses of alfentanil or fentanyl

should be given with care since the resulting respiratory depression can persist postoperatively and occasionally it may become apparent for the first time postoperatively when monitoring of the patient might be less intensive. Alfentanil, fentanyl, and remifentanil can cause muscle rigidity, particularly of the chest wall or jaw; this can be managed by the use of neuromuscular blocking drugs.

In contrast to other opioids which are metabolised in the liver, remifentanil undergoes rapid metabolism by nonspecific blood and tissue esterases; its short duration of action allows prolonged administration at high dosage, without accumulation, and with little risk of residual postoperative respiratory depression. Remifentanil should not be given by intravenous injection intraoperatively, but it is well suited to continuous infusion; a supplementary analgesic is given before stopping the infusion of remifentanil.

[EvGr] A single dose of intravenous ketamine p. 1539 [unlicensed] should be considered either during or immediately after surgery to supplement other types of pain relief if, the patient's pain is expected to be moderate to severe and an intravenous opioid alone does not provide adequate pain relief, or the patient has opioid sensitivity. Ⓐ

Useful resources

Perioperative care in adults. National Institute for Health and Care Excellence. NICE guideline 180. August 2020. www.nice.org.uk/guidance/ng180

ANAESTHETICS, GENERAL › NMDA RECEPTOR ANTAGONISTS

Esketamine
05-Jan-2023

- **DRUG ACTION** Esketamine is an isomer of ketamine that blocks N-methyl-D-aspartate (NMDA) receptors and interrupts the association pathways of the brain, resulting in dissociative anaesthesia and analgesia and in restoration of neural pathways regulating mood and emotional behaviour.

- **INDICATIONS AND DOSE**

Induction and maintenance of anaesthesia (specialist use only)
▸ BY SLOW INTRAVENOUS INJECTION
▸ Adult: 0.5–1 mg/kg, then maintenance 0.25–0.5 mg/kg every 10–15 minutes, adjusted according to response
▸ BY INTRAMUSCULAR INJECTION
▸ Adult: 2–4 mg/kg, then maintenance 1–2 mg/kg every 10–15 minutes, adjusted according to response
▸ BY CONTINUOUS INTRAVENOUS INFUSION
▸ Adult: 0.5–3 mg/kg/hour, adjusted according to response

Analgesic supplementation of regional and local anaesthesia (specialist use only)
▸ BY CONTINUOUS INTRAVENOUS INFUSION
▸ Adult: 0.125–0.25 mg/kg/hour, adjusted according to response

Analgesia in emergency medicine (specialist use only)
▸ BY INTRAMUSCULAR INJECTION
▸ Adult: 0.25–0.5 mg/kg, adjusted according to response
▸ BY SLOW INTRAVENOUS INJECTION
▸ Adult: 0.125–0.25 mg/kg, adjusted according to response

Major depressive disorder (specialist use only)
▸ BY INTRANASAL ADMINISTRATION
▸ Adult: Initially 56 mg on day 1, then 56–84 mg twice weekly for weeks 1–4, then 56–84 mg once weekly for weeks 5–8, then 56–84 mg every 1–2 weeks from week 9 onwards, review continued treatment periodically, treatment is recommended for at least   continued →

15

Anaesthesia

- 6 months after depressive symptoms improve, all dose adjustments to be made in 28 mg increments
- ▸ Elderly: Initially 28 mg on day 1, then 28–84 mg twice weekly for weeks 1–4, then 28–84 mg once weekly for weeks 5–8, then 28–84 mg every 1–2 weeks from week 9 onwards, review continued treatment periodically, treatment is recommended for at least 6 months after depressive symptoms improve, all dose adjustments to be made in 28 mg increments

Major depressive disorder (patients of Japanese origin) (specialist use only)

- ▸ BY INTRANASAL ADMINISTRATION
- ▸ Adult: Initially 28 mg on day 1, then 28–84 mg twice weekly for weeks 1–4, then 28–84 mg once weekly for weeks 5–8, then 28–84 mg every 1–2 weeks from week 9 onwards, review continued treatment periodically, treatment is recommended for at least 6 months after depressive symptoms improve, all dose adjustments to be made in 28 mg increments

DOSE EQUIVALENCE AND CONVERSION
- ▸ With intranasal use
- ▸ 28 mg equivalent to 2 sprays (1 spray administered into each nostril).

IMPORTANT SAFETY INFORMATION
Esketamine should only be administered by, or under the direct supervision of, personnel experienced in its use, with adequate training in anaesthesia and airway management, and when resuscitation equipment is available.

● CONTRA-INDICATIONS
GENERAL CONTRA-INDICATIONS Acute porphyrias p. 1202 · patients in whom hypertension or raised intracranial pressure forms a serious risk
SPECIFIC CONTRA-INDICATIONS
- ▸ When used for Induction and maintenance of anaesthesia or Analgesic supplementation of regional and local anaesthesia or Analgesia in emergency medicine Eclampsia · ischaemic cardiac disorders (when used as sole anaesthetic agent) · pre-eclampsia
- ▸ When used for Major depressive disorder Aneurysmal vascular disease · cardiovascular events, including myocardial infarction (within 6 weeks) · intracerebral haemorrhage

● CAUTIONS
GENERAL CAUTIONS History of drug abuse · hypertension · raised intracranial pressure · thyroid dysfunction
SPECIFIC CAUTIONS
- ▸ When used for Induction and maintenance of anaesthesia or Analgesic supplementation of regional and local anaesthesia or Analgesia in emergency medicine Chronic or acute alcohol consumption · decompensated cardiac failure · increased cerebrospinal fluid pressure · patients with multiple injuries or in poor condition—consult product literature · prolapsed umbilical cord · raised intra-ocular pressure · severe psychotic disorders · unstable angina pectoris · uterine rupture
- ▸ When used for Major depressive disorder Bipolar disorder (active or previous history) · cardiovascular conditions (clinically significant or unstable) · mania (active or previous history) · psychosis (active or previous history) · respiratory conditions (clinically significant or unstable)
CAUTIONS, FURTHER INFORMATION
- ▸ History of drug abuse
- ▸ When used for Major depressive disorder EvGr Patients should be assessed for the risk of drug abuse prior to starting treatment, and monitored for signs of this during therapy.

Ⓜ

- ▸ Cardiovascular or respiratory conditions
- ▸ When used for Major depressive disorder Esketamine should be administered where appropriately trained staff and resuscitation facilities are available.

● INTERACTIONS → Appendix 1: esketamine

● SIDE-EFFECTS
GENERAL SIDE-EFFECTS
- ▸ **Common or very common** Anxiety · dizziness · nausea · vomiting
SPECIFIC SIDE-EFFECTS
- ▸ **Common or very common**
- ▸ With intranasal use Drowsiness · dry mouth · dysarthria · feeling abnormal · feeling of body temperature change · hallucinations · headache · hyperacusia · hyperhidrosis · hypertension · mood altered · nasal complaints · oral disorders · perception altered · psychiatric disorders · sensation abnormal · tachycardia · taste altered · tinnitus · tremor · urinary disorders · vertigo · vision blurred
- ▸ With parenteral use Arrhythmias · hypersalivation · movement disorders · respiratory disorders · respiratory secretion increased · sleep disorders · vision disorders
- ▸ **Uncommon**
- ▸ With parenteral use Muscle tone increased · nystagmus · skin reactions
- ▸ **Rare or very rare**
- ▸ With parenteral use Hypotension
- ▸ **Frequency not known**
- ▸ With intranasal use Cystitis
- ▸ With parenteral use Disorientation · drug-induced liver injury · dysphoria · hallucination

● PREGNANCY
- ▸ When used for Induction and maintenance of anaesthesia or Analgesic supplementation of regional and local anaesthesia or Analgesia in emergency medicine Manufacturer advises use only if potential benefit outweighs risk—may depress neonatal respiration if used during delivery.
- ▸ When used for Major depressive disorder Manufacturer advises avoid—no information available.

● BREAST FEEDING
- ▸ When used for Induction and maintenance of anaesthesia or Analgesic supplementation of regional and local anaesthesia or Analgesia in emergency medicine Manufacturer advises present in milk—not thought to be harmful at therapeutic doses.
- ▸ When used for Major depressive disorder Manufacturer advises avoid—present in milk in *animal* studies.

● HEPATIC IMPAIRMENT
- ▸ When used for Induction and maintenance of anaesthesia or Analgesic supplementation of regional and local anaesthesia or Analgesia in emergency medicine Manufacturer advises caution (risk of prolonged action).
- ▸ When used for Major depressive disorder Manufacturer advises caution in moderate impairment when using maximum dose (84 mg); avoid in severe impairment—no information available.
Dose adjustments
- ▸ When used for Induction and maintenance of anaesthesia or Analgesic supplementation of regional and local anaesthesia or Analgesia in emergency medicine Manufacturer advises consider dose reduction.

● MONITORING REQUIREMENTS
- ▸ When used for Major depressive disorder Manufacturer advises monitor blood pressure at baseline, approximately 40 minutes after treatment, and as clinically indicated thereafter. Manufacturer advises monitor for urinary tract and bladder symptoms during treatment and refer to an appropriate healthcare provider if symptoms persist.

● DIRECTIONS FOR ADMINISTRATION
- ▸ With intramuscular use or intravenous use Manufacturer advises solution can be diluted with Glucose 5% *or* Sodium Chloride 0.9%.

► With intranasal use Manufacturer advises dose is administered via a single-use device delivering 28 mg as 2 sprays (1 spray per nostril). A second device is required for a 56 mg dose, and a third device is required for an 84 mg dose. Allow a break of 5 minutes between use of each device.

● **PRESCRIBING AND DISPENSING INFORMATION**
► When used for Major depressive disorder The manufacturer of *Spravato*® has provided the following materials: *Guide for Healthcare Professionals, Checklist for Healthcare Professionals* and *Patient Guide*. Patients must be enrolled onto the *Spravato*® Register and Alert System (available at: spravatoregister.clinpal.com) before first prescription or within 24 hours of the first administration for new patients, or before the next prescription for existing patients.

● **PATIENT AND CARER ADVICE**
► When used for Major depressive disorder Manufacturer advises patients should be informed not to eat for at least 2 hours before and not to drink liquids for at least 30 minutes before treatment. Manufacturer advises patients who require a nasal corticosteroid or nasal decongestant on a dosing day should be informed not to administer these within 1 hour prior to treatment. Manufacturer advises patients and carers should seek immediate medical advice if symptoms worsen, or if suicidal behaviour or thoughts and unusual changes in behaviour occur.
   A patient guide should be provided.

Missed doses
► When used for Major depressive disorder Manufacturer advises if more than 2 treatment sessions are missed, adjustment of the dose or frequency of treatment may be clinically appropriate.

Driving and skilled tasks
► When used for Induction and maintenance of anaesthesia or Analgesic supplementation of regional and local anaesthesia or Analgesia in emergency medicine Patients given sedatives and analgesics during minor outpatient procedures should be very carefully warned about the risk of driving or undertaking skilled tasks afterwards. For a short general anaesthetic the risk extends to **at least 24 hours** after administration. Responsible persons should be available to take patients home. The dangers of taking **alcohol** should also be emphasised. For information on 2015 legislation regarding driving whilst taking certain controlled drugs, including ketamine which has similar pharmacokinetic properties to esketamine, see *Drugs and driving* under Guidance on prescribing p. 1.
► When used for Major depressive disorder Manufacturer advises patients and carers should be counselled on the effects on driving and performance of skilled tasks— increased risk of somnolence, sedation, dissociative symptoms, perception disturbances, dizziness, vertigo and anxiety. For information on 2015 legislation regarding driving whilst taking certain controlled drugs, including ketamine which has similar pharmacokinetic properties to esketamine, see *Drugs and driving* under Guidance on prescribing p. 1.

● **NATIONAL FUNDING/ACCESS DECISIONS**
For full details see funding body website

NICE decisions
► Esketamine nasal spray for treatment-resistant depression (December 2022) NICE TA854 Not recommended

Scottish Medicines Consortium (SMC) decisions
► Esketamine nasal spray (*Spravato*®) in combination with a selective serotonin reuptake inhibitor (SSRI) or serotonin-norepinephrine reuptake inhibitor (SNRI), for adults with treatment-resistant Major Depressive Disorder, who have not responded to at least two different treatments with antidepressants in the current moderate to severe depressive episode (September 2020) SMC No. SMC2258 Recommended

● **MEDICINAL FORMS** There can be variation in the licensing of different medicines containing the same drug.

Solution for injection
► **Esketamine** (Non-proprietary)
   Esketamine (as Esketamine hydrochloride) 5 mg per 1 ml Esketamine 25mg/5ml solution for injection ampoules | 10 ampoule [PoM] £18.98 (Hospital only) [CD2]
   Esketamine (as Esketamine hydrochloride) 25 mg per 1 ml Esketamine 250mg/10ml solution for injection ampoules | 5 ampoule [PoM] [⅀] (Hospital only) [CD2]
   Esketamine 50mg/2ml solution for injection ampoules | 10 ampoule [PoM] £26.31 (Hospital only) [CD2]

Spray
CAUTIONARY AND ADVISORY LABELS 2, 10
► **Spravato** (Janssen-Cilag Ltd) ▼
   Esketamine (as Esketamine hydrochloride) 140 mg per 1 ml Spravato 28mg/0.2ml nasal spray unit dose | 1 unit dose [PoM] £163.00 (Hospital only) [CD2] | 2 unit dose [PoM] £326.00 (Hospital only) [CD2] | 3 unit dose [PoM] £489.00 (Hospital only) [CD2]

ANAESTHETICS, LOCAL

Bupivacaine with fentanyl

The properties listed below are those particular to the combination only. For the properties of the components please consider, bupivacaine hydrochloride p. 1544, fentanyl p. 520.

● **INDICATIONS AND DOSE**
During labour (once epidural block established)
► BY CONTINUOUS LUMBAR EPIDURAL INFUSION
► Adult: 10–18.75 mg/hour, dose of bupivacaine to be administered, maximum 400 mg bupivacaine in 24 hours and 16–30 micrograms/hour, dose of fentanyl to be administered, maximum 720 micrograms fentanyl in 24 hours

Postoperative pain (once epidural block established)
► BY CONTINUOUS EPIDURAL INFUSION
► Adult: 4–18.75 mg/hour, dose of bupivacaine to be administered, maximum 400 mg bupivacaine in 24 hours and 8–30 micrograms/hour, dose of fentanyl to be administered, maximum 720 micrograms fentanyl in 24 hours, to be administered by thoracic, upper abdominal or lower abdominal epidural infusion

● **INTERACTIONS** → Appendix 1: opioids

● **MEDICINAL FORMS** There can be variation in the licensing of different medicines containing the same drug. Forms available from special-order manufacturers include: infusion, solution for infusion

Infusion
► **Bufyl** (Sandoz Ltd)
   Fentanyl 2 microgram per 1 ml, Bupivacaine hydrochloride 1 mg per 1 ml Bufyl 1mg/ml and 2micrograms/ml 250ml infusion bags | 5 bag [PoM] £42.50 (Hospital only) [CD2]
   Bufyl 1mg/ml and 2micrograms/ml 500ml infusion bags | 5 bag [PoM] £46.00 (Hospital only) [CD2]
   Fentanyl (as Fentanyl citrate) 2 microgram per 1 ml, Bupivacaine hydrochloride 1.25 mg per 1 ml Bufyl 1.25mg/ml and 2micrograms/ml 250ml infusion bags | 5 bag [PoM] £45.25 (Hospital only) [CD2]
   Bufyl 1.25mg/ml and 2micrograms/ml 500ml infusion bags | 5 bag [PoM] £46.00 (Hospital only) [CD2]

ANALGESICS > NON-STEROIDAL ANTI-INFLAMMATORY DRUGS

Ketorolac trometamol

01-Aug-2023

● INDICATIONS AND DOSE

Short-term management of moderate to severe acute postoperative pain only

▶ BY INTRAMUSCULAR INJECTION, OR BY INTRAVENOUS INJECTION

▶ Adult (body-weight up to 50 kg): Initially 10 mg, then 10–30 mg every 4–6 hours as required for maximum duration of treatment 2 days, frequency may be increased to up to every 2 hours during initial postoperative period; maximum 60 mg per day

▶ Adult (body-weight 50 kg and above): Initially 10 mg, then 10–30 mg every 4–6 hours as required for maximum duration of treatment 2 days, frequency may be increased to up to every 2 hours during initial postoperative period; maximum 90 mg per day

▶ Elderly: Initially 10 mg, then 10–30 mg every 4–6 hours as required for maximum duration of treatment 2 days, frequency may be increased to up to every 2 hours during initial postoperative period; maximum 60 mg per day

IMPORTANT SAFETY INFORMATION

MHRA/CHM ADVICE: NSAIDS: POTENTIAL RISKS FOLLOWING PROLONGED USE AFTER 20 WEEKS OF PREGNANCY (JUNE 2023)

See Non-steroidal anti-inflammatory drugs p. 1292.

● **CONTRA-INDICATIONS** Active or history of gastro-intestinal bleeding · active or history of gastro-intestinal ulceration · coagulation disorders · complete or partial syndrome of nasal polyps · confirmed or suspected cerebrovascular bleeding · dehydration · following operations with high risk of haemorrhage or incomplete haemostasis · haemorrhagic diatheses · history of gastro-intestinal bleeding related to previous NSAID therapy · history of gastro-intestinal perforation related to previous NSAID therapy · hypovolaemia · severe heart failure

● **CAUTIONS** Allergic disorders · cardiac impairment (NSAIDs may impair renal function) · cerebrovascular disease · connective-tissue disorders · elderly (risk of serious side-effects and fatalities) · heart failure · history of gastro-intestinal disorders (e.g. ulcerative colitis, Crohn's disease) · ischaemic heart disease · may mask symptoms of infection · peripheral arterial disease · risk factors for cardiovascular events · uncontrolled hypertension

● **INTERACTIONS** → Appendix 1: NSAIDs

● **SIDE-EFFECTS** Agranulocytosis · angioedema · anxiety · aplastic anaemia · appetite decreased · asthenia · asthma · azotaemia · bradycardia · burping · chest pain · concentration impaired · confusion · constipation · Crohn's disease aggravated · depression · diarrhoea · dizziness · drowsiness · dry mouth · dyspnoea · electrolyte imbalance · embolism and thrombosis · euphoric mood · fever · flank pain · fluid retention · flushing · gastrointestinal discomfort · gastrointestinal disorders · haemolytic anaemia · haemorrhage · hallucination · headache · hearing loss · heart failure · hepatic disorders · hyperhidrosis · hyperkinesia · hypersensitivity · hypertension · hypotension · infertility female · malaise · meningitis aseptic (patients with connective-tissue disorders such as systemic lupus erythematosus may be especially susceptible) · musculoskeletal disorder · myalgia · myocardial infarction · nausea · nephritis tubulointerstitial · nephropathy · neutropenia · oedema · optic neuritis · oral disorders · pallor · palpitations · pancreatitis · paraesthesia · perforation · photosensitivity reaction · platelet aggregation inhibition · psychotic disorder · pulmonary

oedema · renal impairment · respiratory disorders · seizure · severe cutaneous adverse reactions (SCARs) · skin reactions · sleep disorders · stroke · taste altered · thinking abnormal · thirst · thrombocytopenia · tinnitus · ulcer · urinary disorders · vertigo · visual impairment · vomiting · weight increased · wound haemorrhage

SIDE-EFFECTS, FURTHER INFORMATION For information about cardiovascular and gastrointestinal side-effects, and a possible exacerbation of symptoms in asthma, see Non-steroidal anti-inflammatory drugs. p. 1292

● **ALLERGY AND CROSS-SENSITIVITY** EvGr Contra-indicated in patients with a history of hypersensitivity to aspirin or any other NSAID—which includes those in whom attacks of asthma, angioedema, urticaria or rhinitis have been precipitated by aspirin or any other NSAID. ◈M◈

● **CONCEPTION AND CONTRACEPTION** EvGr Caution—long-term use of some NSAIDs is associated with reduced female fertility, which is reversible on stopping treatment. ◈M◈

● **PREGNANCY** Avoid use in first and second trimesters unless essential; the MHRA advises additional antenatal monitoring may be required if treatment is considered necessary by a doctor from week 20 of pregnancy onwards. Avoid use in third trimester. See *NSAIDs in Pregnancy* in Non-steroidal anti-inflammatory drugs p. 1292 for further details.

● **BREAST FEEDING** Amount too small to be harmful.

● **HEPATIC IMPAIRMENT** Manufacturer advises caution—may increase risk of renal impairment; avoid in hepatic failure.

● **RENAL IMPAIRMENT** In general, for *NSAIDs* the MHRA advises to avoid where possible; if necessary, use with caution (risk of fluid retention and further renal impairment, including renal failure). EvGr For *ketorolac*, avoid if serum creatinine greater than 160 micromol/litre. ◈M◈

Dose adjustments EvGr Max. 60 mg daily if serum creatinine 160 micromol/litre or less. ◈M◈

● **DIRECTIONS FOR ADMINISTRATION** For *intravenous injection*, manufacturer advises give over at least 15 seconds.

● **MEDICINAL FORMS** There can be variation in the licensing of different medicines containing the same drug.

Solution for injection

▶ **Ketorolac trometamol (Non-proprietary)**
  Ketorolac trometamol 30 mg per 1 ml Ketorolac 30mg/1ml solution for injection ampoules | 5 ampoule PoM £5.50 DT = £5.36 (Hospital only)

▶ **Toradol** (Atnahs Pharma UK Ltd)
  Ketorolac trometamol 30 mg per 1 ml Toradol 30mg/1ml solution for injection ampoules | 5 ampoule PoM £5.36 DT = £5.36 (Hospital only)

Parecoxib

22-Nov-2021

● **DRUG ACTION** Parecoxib is a selective inhibitor of cyclo-oxygenase-2.

● INDICATIONS AND DOSE

Short-term management of acute postoperative pain

▶ BY DEEP INTRAMUSCULAR INJECTION, OR BY INTRAVENOUS INJECTION

▶ Adult: Initially 40 mg, then 20–40 mg every 6–12 hours as required for up to 3 days; maximum 80 mg per day

▶ Elderly (body-weight up to 50 kg): Initially 20 mg; maximum 40 mg per day

● **CONTRA-INDICATIONS** Active gastro-intestinal bleeding · active gastro-intestinal ulceration · cerebrovascular disease · following coronary artery bypass graft surgery · inflammatory bowel disease · ischaemic heart disease · mild to severe heart failure · peripheral arterial disease

- **CAUTIONS** Allergic disorders · cardiac impairment (NSAIDs may impair renal function) · coagulation defects · connective-tissue disorders · dehydration (risk of renal impairment) · elderly (risk of serious side-effects and fatalities) · history of cardiac failure · history of gastro-intestinal disorders · hypertension · may mask symptoms of infection · oedema · risk factors for cardiovascular events

- **INTERACTIONS** → Appendix 1: NSAIDs

- **SIDE-EFFECTS**

  ▸ **Common or very common** Agitation · back pain · constipation · dizziness · gastrointestinal discomfort · gastrointestinal disorders · hyperhidrosis · hypertension · hypokalaemia · hypotension · increased risk of infection · insomnia · nausea · numbness · peripheral oedema · post procedural complications · renal impairment · respiratory disorders · skin reactions · vomiting

  ▸ **Uncommon** Appetite decreased · arrhythmias · arthralgia · asthenia · cerebrovascular insufficiency · dry mouth · ear pain · embolism and thrombosis · hyperglycaemia · myocardial infarction · thrombocytopenia

  ▸ **Rare or very rare** Hypersensitivity · pancreatitis · perioral swelling

  ▸ **Frequency not known** Angioedema · cardiovascular event · circulatory collapse · congestive heart failure · dyspnoea · fluid retention · hepatitis · renal failure (more common in patients with pre-existing renal impairment) · severe cutaneous adverse reactions (SCARs)

  SIDE-EFFECTS, FURTHER INFORMATION For information about cardiovascular and gastrointestinal side-effects, and a possible exacerbation of symptoms in asthma, see Non-steroidal anti-inflammatory drugs. p. 1292

- **ALLERGY AND CROSS-SENSITIVITY** [EvGr] Contra-indicated in patients with a history of hypersensitivity to aspirin or any other NSAID—which includes those in whom attacks of asthma, angioedema, urticaria or rhinitis have been precipitated by aspirin or any other NSAID. Contra-indicated in patients with a history of allergic drug reactions including sulfonamide hypersensitivity. ⬥

- **CONCEPTION AND CONTRACEPTION** Caution—long-term use of some NSAIDs is associated with reduced female fertility, which is reversible on stopping treatment.

- **PREGNANCY** Avoid unless the potential benefit outweighs the risk. Avoid during the third trimester (risk of closure of fetal ductus arteriosus *in utero* and possibly persistent pulmonary hypertension of the newborn); onset of labour may be delayed and duration may be increased.

- **BREAST FEEDING** Avoid—present in milk.

- **HEPATIC IMPAIRMENT** Manufacturer advises caution in moderate impairment (risk of increased exposure); avoid in severe impairment (no information available).
  Dose adjustments Manufacturer advises dose reduction to half the usual recommended dose in moderate impairment; maximum 40 mg daily.

- **RENAL IMPAIRMENT** In general, for *NSAIDs* the MHRA advises to avoid where possible; if necessary, use with caution (risk of fluid retention and further renal impairment, including renal failure).
  Dose adjustments [EvGr] Reduce initial dose to 20 mg if creatinine clearance less than 30 mL/minute. ⬥ See p. 21.

- **NATIONAL FUNDING/ACCESS DECISIONS**
  For full details see funding body website
  Scottish Medicines Consortium (SMC) decisions
  ▸ Parecoxib (*Dynastat*®) for the short-term treatment of postoperative pain (January 2003) SMC No. 27/02 Not recommended

- **MEDICINAL FORMS** There can be variation in the licensing of different medicines containing the same drug.

  Powder and solvent for solution for injection
  ▸ Parecoxib (Non-proprietary)
    Parecoxib (as Parecoxib sodium) 40 mg Parecoxib 40mg powder and solvent for solution for injection vials | 5 vial [PoM] £28.34 DT = £28.34 | 5 vial [PoM] £28.34 DT = £28.34 (Hospital only)
  ▸ Dynastat (Pfizer Ltd)
    Parecoxib (as Parecoxib sodium) 40 mg Dynastat 40mg powder and solvent for solution for injection vials | 5 vial [PoM] £28.34 DT = £28.34

  Powder for solution for injection
  ▸ Parecoxib (Non-proprietary)
    Parecoxib (as Parecoxib sodium) 40 mg Parecoxib 40mg powder for solution for injection vials | 10 vial [PoM] £49.60 DT = £49.60 (Hospital only) | 10 vial [PoM] £49.60 DT = £49.60
  ▸ Dynastat (Pfizer Ltd)
    Parecoxib (as Parecoxib sodium) 40 mg Dynastat 40mg powder for solution for injection vials | 10 vial [PoM] £49.60 DT = £49.60

ANALGESICS › OPIOIDS

▸ **F** 510

Alfentanil

10-May-2021

- **INDICATIONS AND DOSE**

  Spontaneous respiration: analgesia and enhancement of anaesthesia for short procedures
  ▸ BY INTRAVENOUS INJECTION
  ▸ Adult: Initially up to 500 micrograms, dose to be administered over 30 seconds; supplemental doses 250 micrograms

  Assisted ventilation: analgesia and enhancement of anaesthesia for short procedures
  ▸ BY INTRAVENOUS INJECTION
  ▸ Adult: Initially 30–50 micrograms/kg, supplemental doses 15 micrograms/kg

  Assisted ventilation: analgesia and enhancement of anaesthesia during maintenance of anaesthesia for longer procedures
  ▸ BY INTRAVENOUS INFUSION
  ▸ Adult: Initially 50–100 micrograms/kg, dose to be administered over 10 minutes or as a bolus, followed by maintenance 30–60 micrograms/kg/hour

  Assisted ventilation: analgesia and suppression of respiratory activity during intensive care for up to 4 days
  ▸ BY INTRAVENOUS INFUSION
  ▸ Adult: Initially 2 mg/hour, adjusted according to response; usual dose 0.5–10 mg/hour, alternatively initially 5 mg in divided doses, to be administered over 10 minutes; dose used for more rapid initial control, reduce rate of administration if hypotension or bradycardia occur; additional doses of 0.5–1 mg may be given by intravenous injection during short painful procedures

  DOSES AT EXTREMES OF BODY-WEIGHT
  ▸ To avoid excessive dosage in obese patients, dose should be calculated on the basis of ideal body-weight.

- **CAUTIONS** [EvGr] Repeated intra-operative doses of alfentanil should be given with care since the resulting respiratory depression can persist postoperatively and occasionally it may become apparent for the first time postoperatively when monitoring of the patient might be less intensive. ⬥

- **INTERACTIONS** → Appendix 1: opioids

- **SIDE-EFFECTS**
  ▸ **Common or very common** Apnoea · chills · fatigue · hypertension · movement disorders · muscle rigidity · procedural complications
  ▸ **Uncommon** Coma · hiccups · hypercapnia · pain · post procedural complications · respiratory disorders

- **Rare or very rare** Agitation · crying · epistaxis · vascular pain
- **Frequency not known** Cardiac arrest · cough · fever · loss of consciousness

  SIDE-EFFECTS, FURTHER INFORMATION Alfentanil can cause muscle rigidity, particularly of the chest wall or jaw; this can be managed by the use of neuromuscular blocking drugs.

- **BREAST FEEDING** Present in milk—withhold breast-feeding for 24 hours.

- **HEPATIC IMPAIRMENT** Manufacturer advises caution. **Dose adjustments** Manufacturer advises dose reduction and cautious titration.

- **RENAL IMPAIRMENT** [EvGr] Use with caution and titrate carefully (risk of increased and prolonged effects). ⓜ **Dose adjustments** [EvGr] Dose reduction may be required in renal failure. ⓜ

- **DIRECTIONS FOR ADMINISTRATION** Manufacturer advises 5 mg/mL injection should be diluted in Glucose 5% *or* Sodium Chloride 0.9% before use.

- **MEDICINAL FORMS** There can be variation in the licensing of different medicines containing the same drug. Forms available from special-order manufacturers include: solution for injection

  Solution for injection
  - **Alfentanil (Non-proprietary)**
    Alfentanil (as Alfentanil hydrochloride) 500 microgram per 1 ml Alfentanil 1mg/2ml solution for injection ampoules | 10 ampoule [PoM] £27.80 DT = £6.34 (Hospital only) [CD2] | 10 ampoule [PoM] £9.00 DT = £6.34 [CD2]
    Alfentanil 25mg/50ml solution for injection vials | 1 vial [PoM] £31.00 [CD2]
    Alfentanil 5mg/10ml solution for injection ampoules | 5 ampoule [PoM] £16.00 DT = £16.00 (Hospital only) [CD2] | 10 ampoule [PoM] £31.00 DT = £31.00 [CD2]
    Alfentanil (as Alfentanil hydrochloride) 5 mg per 1 ml Alfentanil 5mg/1ml solution for injection ampoules | 10 ampoule [PoM] £25.00 DT = £23.19 [CD2]
  - **Rapifen** (Piramal Critical Care Ltd)
    Alfentanil (as Alfentanil hydrochloride) 500 microgram per 1 ml Rapifen 5mg/10ml solution for injection ampoules | 5 ampoule [PoM] £16.00 DT = £16.00 [CD2]
    Rapifen 1mg/2ml solution for injection ampoules | 10 ampoule [PoM] £6.34 DT = £6.34 [CD2]
    Alfentanil (as Alfentanil hydrochloride) 5 mg per 1 ml Rapifen Intensive Care 5mg/1ml solution for injection ampoules | 10 ampoule [PoM] £23.19 DT = £23.19 (Hospital only) [CD2]

[F 510]

Remifentanil

12-May-2021

- **INDICATIONS AND DOSE**

Analgesia and enhancement of anaesthesia at induction (initial bolus injection)
- ▸ BY INTRAVENOUS INJECTION
- ▸ Adult: Initially 0.25–1 microgram/kg, dose to be administered over at least 30 seconds, if patient is to be intubated more than 8 minutes after start of intravenous infusion, initial bolus intravenous injection dose is not necessary

Analgesia and enhancement of anaesthesia at induction with or without initial bolus dose
- ▸ BY INTRAVENOUS INFUSION
- ▸ Adult: 30–60 micrograms/kg/hour, if patient is to be intubated more than 8 minutes after start of intravenous infusion, initial bolus intravenous injection dose is not necessary

Assisted ventilation: analgesia and enhancement of anaesthesia during maintenance of anaesthesia (initial bolus injection)
- ▸ BY INTRAVENOUS INJECTION
- ▸ Adult: Initially 0.25–1 microgram/kg, dose to be administered over at least 30 seconds

Assisted ventilation: analgesia and enhancement of anaesthesia during maintenance of anaesthesia with or without initial bolus dose
- ▸ BY INTRAVENOUS INFUSION
- ▸ Adult: 3–120 micrograms/kg/hour, dose to be administered according to anaesthetic technique and adjusted according to response, in light anaesthesia additional doses can be given *by intravenous injection* every 2–5 minutes during the intravenous infusion

Spontaneous respiration: analgesia and enhancement of anaesthesia during maintenance of anaesthesia
- ▸ BY INTRAVENOUS INFUSION
- ▸ Adult: Initially 2.4 micrograms/kg/hour, adjusted according to response; usual dose 1.5–6 micrograms/kg/hour

Assisted ventilation: analgesia and sedation in intensive-care patients (for max 3 days)
- ▸ BY INTRAVENOUS INFUSION
- ▸ Adult: Initially 6–9 micrograms/kg/hour, then adjusted in steps of 1.5 micrograms/kg/hour, allow at least 5 minutes between dose adjustments; usual dose 0.36–44.4 micrograms/kg/hour, if an infusion rate of 12 micrograms/kg/hour does not produce adequate sedation add another sedative (consult product literature for details)

Assisted ventilation: additional analgesia during stimulating or painful procedures in intensive-care patients
- ▸ BY INTRAVENOUS INFUSION
- ▸ Adult: Usual dose 15–45 micrograms/kg/hour, maintain infusion rate of at least 6 micrograms/kg/hour for at least 5 minutes before procedure and adjust every 2–5 minutes according to requirements

Cardiac surgery
- ▸ Adult: (consult product literature)

DOSES AT EXTREMES OF BODY-WEIGHT
- ▸ To avoid excessive dosage in obese patients, dose should be calculated on the basis of ideal body-weight.

- **UNLICENSED USE** Remifentanil doses in BNF may differ from those in product literature.

- **CONTRA-INDICATIONS** Analgesia in conscious patients

- **INTERACTIONS** → Appendix 1: opioids

- **SIDE-EFFECTS**
- ▸ **Common or very common** Apnoea · muscle rigidity · post procedural complications
- ▸ **Uncommon** Hypoxia
- ▸ **Rare or very rare** Cardiac arrest
- ▸ **Frequency not known** Agitation · atrioventricular block · hypertension

  SIDE-EFFECTS, FURTHER INFORMATION In contrast to other opioids which are metabolised in the liver, remifentanil undergoes rapid metabolism by plasma esterases; it has short duration of action which is independent of dose and duration of infusion.

  Muscle rigidity Remifentanil can cause muscle rigidity that can be managed by the use of neuromuscular blocking drugs.

- **PREGNANCY** No information available.

- **BREAST FEEDING** Avoid breast-feeding for 24 hours after administration—present in milk in *animal* studies.

- **HEPATIC IMPAIRMENT** Manufacturer advises caution in severe impairment (limited information available).

- **RENAL IMPAIRMENT**
Dose adjustments EvGr No dose adjustment necessary in renal impairment. ⟨M⟩

- **DIRECTIONS FOR ADMINISTRATION** For *intravenous infusion* (*Ultiva* ®), manufacturer advises give continuously in Glucose 5% or Sodium Chloride 0.9% or Water for Injections; reconstitute with infusion fluid to a concentration of 1 mg/mL then dilute further to a concentration of 20–250 micrograms/mL (50 micrograms/mL recommended for general anaesthesia, 20–50 micrograms/mL recommended when used with target controlled infusion (TCI) device).

- **PRESCRIBING AND DISPENSING INFORMATION**
Remifentanil should not be given by intravenous injection intra-operatively, but it is well suited to continuous infusion; a supplementary analgesic is given before stopping the infusion of remifentanil.

- **MEDICINAL FORMS** There can be variation in the licensing of different medicines containing the same drug.
Powder for solution for injection
  ▸ Remifentanil (Non-proprietary)
  Remifentanil (as Remifentanyl hydrochloride) 1 mg Remifentanil 1mg powder for concentrate for solution for injection vials | 5 vial PoM £25.58-£33.70 (Hospital only) CD2 | 5 vial PoM £25.50 CD2
  Remifentanil (as Remifentanyl hydrochloride) 2 mg Remifentanil 2mg powder for concentrate for solution for injection vials | 5 vial PoM £51.13-£67.40 (Hospital only) CD2 | 5 vial PoM £51.00-£51.15 CD2
  Remifentanil (as Remifentanyl hydrochloride) 5 mg Remifentanil 5mg powder for concentrate for solution for injection vials | 5 vial PoM £127.88-£171.26 (Hospital only) CD2 | 5 vial PoM £127.50 CD2

1.4   Peri-operative sedation

Conscious sedation for clinical procedures

Overview

Sedation of patients during diagnostic and therapeutic procedures is used to reduce fear and anxiety, to control pain, and to minimise excessive movement. The choice of sedative drug will depend upon the intended procedure; some procedures are safer and more successful under anaesthesia. The patient should be *monitored carefully*; monitoring should begin as soon as the sedative is given or when the patient becomes drowsy, and should be continued until the patient wakes up.

ANAESTHETICS, GENERAL ⟩ NMDA RECEPTOR ANTAGONISTS

▎Ketamine

04-Dec-2019

- **INDICATIONS AND DOSE**
Induction and maintenance of anaesthesia for short procedures
  ▸ BY INTRAMUSCULAR INJECTION
  ▸ Adult: Initially 6.5–13 mg/kg, adjusted according to response, a dose of 10 mg/kg usually produces 12–25 minutes of surgical anaesthesia
  ▸ BY INTRAVENOUS INJECTION
  ▸ Adult: Initially 1–4.5 mg/kg, adjusted according to response, to be administered over at least 60 seconds, a dose of 2 mg/kg usually produces 5–10 minutes of surgical anaesthesia

Diagnostic manoeuvres and procedures not involving intense pain
  ▸ BY INTRAMUSCULAR INJECTION
  ▸ Adult: Initially 4 mg/kg
Induction and maintenance of anaesthesia for long procedures
  ▸ BY INTRAVENOUS INFUSION
  ▸ Adult: Initially 0.5–2 mg/kg, using an infusion solution containing 1 mg/mL; maintenance 10–45 micrograms/kg/minute, adjusted according to response

> **IMPORTANT SAFETY INFORMATION**
> Ketamine should only be administered by, or under the direct supervision of, personnel experienced in its use, with adequate training in anaesthesia and airway management, and when resuscitation equipment is available.

- **CONTRA-INDICATIONS** Acute porphyrias p. 1202 · eclampsia · head trauma · hypertension · pre-eclampsia · raised intracranial pressure · severe cardiac disease · stroke

- **CAUTIONS** Acute circulatory failure (shock) · cardiovascular disease · dehydration · elderly · fixed cardiac output · hallucinations · head injury · hypertension · hypovolaemia · increased cerebrospinal fluid pressure · intracranial mass lesions · nightmares · predisposition to seizures · psychotic disorders · raised intra-ocular pressure · respiratory tract infection · thyroid dysfunction

- **INTERACTIONS** → Appendix 1: ketamine

- **SIDE-EFFECTS**
  ▸ **Common or very common** Anxiety · behaviour abnormal · confusion · diplopia · hallucination · muscle tone increased · nausea · nystagmus · skin reactions · sleep disorders · tonic clonic movements · vomiting
  ▸ **Uncommon** Appetite decreased · arrhythmias · hypotension · respiratory disorders
  ▸ **Rare or very rare** Apnoea · cystitis · cystitis haemorrhagic · delirium · dysphoria · flashback · hypersalivation
  ▸ **Frequency not known** Drug-induced liver injury
  SIDE-EFFECTS, FURTHER INFORMATION Incidence of hallucinations can be reduced by premedicaton with a benzodiazepine (such as midazolam).

- **PREGNANCY** May depress neonatal respiration if used during delivery.

- **BREAST FEEDING** Avoid for at least 12 hours after last dose.

- **HEPATIC IMPAIRMENT** Manufacturer advises caution (risk of prolonged duration of action).
Dose adjustments Manufacturer advises consider dose reduction.

- **DIRECTIONS FOR ADMINISTRATION** For *continuous intravenous infusion*, dilute to a concentration of 1 mg/mL with Glucose 5% *or* Sodium Chloride 0.9%; use microdrip infusion for maintenance of anaesthesia. For *intravenous injection*, dilute 100 mg/mL strength to a concentration of not more than 50 mg/mL with Glucose 5% *or* Sodium Chloride 0.9% *or* Water for Injections.

- **PATIENT AND CARER ADVICE**
Driving and skilled tasks Patients given sedatives and analgesics during minor outpatient procedures should be very carefully warned about the risk of driving or undertaking skilled tasks afterwards. For a short general anaesthetic the risk extends to **at least 24 hours** after administration. Responsible persons should be available to take patients home. The dangers of taking **alcohol** should also be emphasised.

For information on 2015 legislation regarding driving whilst taking certain controlled drugs, including ketamine, see *Drugs and driving* under Guidance on prescribing p. 1.

● **MEDICINAL FORMS** There can be variation in the licensing of different medicines containing the same drug. Forms available from special-order manufacturers include: solution for injection

Solution for injection

▸ **Ketamine (Non-proprietary)**
Ketamine (as Ketamine hydrochloride) 10 mg per 1 ml Ketamin 10 Curamed 50mg/5ml solution for injection ampoules | 10 ampoule [PoM] [🏥] [CD2]
Ketamine 200mg/20ml solution for injection vials | 1 vial [PoM] £6.04 DT = £5.06 (Hospital only) [CD2]
Ketamine (as Ketamine hydrochloride) 50 mg per 1 ml Ketamine 500mg/10ml solution for injection vials | 10 vial [PoM] £70.00 [CD2] | 10 vial [PoM] £70.00 (Hospital only) [CD2]
Ketamin 100mg/2ml solution for injection ampoules | 10 ampoule [PoM] [🏥] [CD2]
Ketamine (as Ketamine hydrochloride) 100 mg per 1 ml Ketalar 200mg/2ml solution for injection vials | 5 vial [PoM] [🏥] (Hospital only) [CD2]

▸ **Ketalar (Pfizer Ltd)**
Ketamine (as Ketamine hydrochloride) 10 mg per 1 ml Ketalar 200mg/20ml solution for injection vials | 1 vial [PoM] £5.06 DT = £5.06 (Hospital only) [CD2]
Ketamine (as Ketamine hydrochloride) 50 mg per 1 ml Ketalar 500mg/10ml solution for injection vials | 1 vial [PoM] £8.77 DT = £8.77 (Hospital only) [CD2]

HYPNOTICS, SEDATIVES AND ANXIOLYTICS ⟩ BENZODIAZEPINES

⚑ 397

Remimazolam

14-Sep-2022

● **INDICATIONS AND DOSE**

Conscious sedation for procedures
▸ BY INTRAVENOUS INJECTION
▸ Adult: (consult product literature)

IMPORTANT SAFETY INFORMATION
ANAESTHESIA
Benzodiazepines should only be administered for anaesthesia by, or under the direct supervision of, personnel experienced in their use, with adequate training in anaesthesia and airway management.

● **CAUTIONS** Cardiac disease
CAUTIONS, FURTHER INFORMATION
▸ Recovery when used for sedation Remimazolam has a fast onset of action, recovery is faster than for other benzodiazepines such as diazepam, but may be significantly longer in the elderly, in patients with severe hepatic impairment, or with body weight less than 50 kg.

● **INTERACTIONS** → Appendix 1: benzodiazepines

● **SIDE-EFFECTS**
▸ **Common or very common** Arrhythmias · dyspnoea · gas exchange abnormal · respiratory disorders · vomiting
▸ **Uncommon** Chills · feeling cold · hiccups

● **PREGNANCY** [EvGr] Avoid—limited information available. Ⓜ

● **BREAST FEEDING** [EvGr] Avoid breast feeding for 24 hours after administration—present in milk in *animal* studies. Ⓜ

● **HEPATIC IMPAIRMENT** [EvGr] Caution in severe impairment (more pronounced and prolonged effects). Ⓜ
Dose adjustments [EvGr] Titrate doses with caution in severe impairment. Ⓜ

● **PATIENT AND CARER ADVICE** Patients should be advised to avoid alcohol intake for 24 hours before the procedure.
Driving and skilled tasks Patients given sedatives and analgesics during minor outpatient procedures should be very carefully warned about the risks of undertaking skilled tasks (e.g. driving) afterwards. For intravenous benzodiazepines the risk extends to **at least 24 hours**

after administration. Responsible persons should be available to take patients home afterwards. The dangers of taking **alcohol** should be emphasised.

● **NATIONAL FUNDING/ACCESS DECISIONS**
For full details see funding body website
Scottish Medicines Consortium (SMC) decisions
▸ Remimazolam (*Byfavo*®) in adults for procedural sedation (August 2022) SMC No. SMC2454 Not recommended

● **MEDICINAL FORMS** There can be variation in the licensing of different medicines containing the same drug.

Powder for solution for injection
▸ **Byfavo** (PAION Deutschland GmbH) ▼
Remimazolam (as Remimazolam besylate) 20 mg Byfavo 20mg powder for solution for injection vials | 10 vial [PoM] £187.50 (Hospital only)
Remimazolam (as Remimazolam besylate) 50 mg Byfavo 50mg powder for concentrate for solution for injection vials | 10 vial [PoM] £470.00 (Hospital only)

HYPNOTICS, SEDATIVES AND ANXIOLYTICS ⟩ NON-BENZODIAZEPINE HYPNOTICS AND SEDATIVES

Dexmedetomidine

01-Nov-2022

● **INDICATIONS AND DOSE**

Maintenance of sedation during intensive care
▸ BY INTRAVENOUS INFUSION
▸ Adult: 0.7 microgram/kg/hour, adjusted according to response; usual dose 0.2–1.4 micrograms/kg/hour

IMPORTANT SAFETY INFORMATION
Dexmedetomidine should only be administered by, or under the direct supervision of, personnel experienced in its use, with adequate training in anaesthesia and airway management.

MHRA/CHM ADVICE: DEXMEDETOMIDINE: CLINICAL TRIAL FINDS INCREASED RISK OF MORTALITY IN INTENSIVE CARE UNIT (ICU) PATIENTS AGED 65 YEARS OR YOUNGER (JUNE 2022)
A randomised controlled trial (SPICE III) in ventilated adult ICU patients found an increased risk of mortality in those aged 65 years or younger (median: 63.7 years) given dexmedetomidine when compared with usual standard of care. This effect was most prominent in patients admitted for reasons other than postoperative care, and increased with increasing APACHE II scores and with decreasing age; the mechanism is unknown. Healthcare professionals are advised to weigh these findings against the potential benefit of using dexmedetomidine compared with alternative sedatives in younger patients.

● **CONTRA-INDICATIONS** Acute cerebrovascular disorders · second- or third-degree AV block (unless pacemaker fitted) · uncontrolled hypotension

● **CAUTIONS** Abrupt withdrawal after prolonged use · bradycardia · elderly (risk of hypotension) · ischaemic heart disease (especially at higher doses) · malignant hyperthermia · severe cerebrovascular disease (especially at higher doses) · severe neurological disorders · spinal cord injury

● **INTERACTIONS** → Appendix 1: dexmedetomidine

● **SIDE-EFFECTS**
▸ **Common or very common** Agitation · arrhythmias · dry mouth · hyperglycaemia · hypertension · hyperthermia · hypoglycaemia · hypotension · myocardial infarction · myocardial ischaemia · nausea · respiratory depression · vomiting

▶ **Uncommon** Abdominal distension · apnoea · atrioventricular block · dyspnoea · hallucination · hypoalbuminaemia · metabolic acidosis · thirst

● **PREGNANCY** Manufacturer advises avoid unless potential benefit outweighs risk—toxicity in *animal* studies.

● **BREAST FEEDING** Manufacturer advises avoid unless potential benefit outweighs risk—present in milk in *animal* studies.

● **HEPATIC IMPAIRMENT** Manufacturer advises caution (increased risk of toxicity due to decreased clearance). **Dose adjustments** Manufacturer advises consider dose reduction.

● **MONITORING REQUIREMENTS**
▶ Monitor cardiac function.
▶ Monitor respiratory function in non-intubated patients.

● **DIRECTIONS FOR ADMINISTRATION** [EvGr] For *intravenous infusion*, give continuously in Glucose 5% or Sodium Chloride 0.9%; dilute concentrate for solution for infusion to 4 micrograms/mL or 8 micrograms/mL. Ⓜ

● **MEDICINAL FORMS** There can be variation in the licensing of different medicines containing the same drug.

Infusion
▶ **Dexmedetomidine (Non-proprietary)**
Dexmedetomidine (as Dexmedetomidine hydrochloride)
4 microgram per 1 ml Dexmedetomidine 400micrograms/100ml infusion bags | 4 bag [PoM] £101.52 (Hospital only)

Solution for infusion
▶ **Dexmedetomidine (Non-proprietary)**
Dexmedetomidine (as Dexmedetomidine hydrochloride)
100 microgram per 1 ml Dexmedetomidine 1mg/10ml concentrate for solution for infusion ampoules | 4 ampoule [PoM] £313.10 (Hospital only)
Dexmedetomidine 200micrograms/2ml concentrate for solution for infusion ampoules | 5 ampoule [PoM] £78.30 (Hospital only) | 10 ampoule [PoM] £164.43 (Hospital only)
Dexmedetomidine 1mg/10ml concentrate for solution for infusion vials | 4 vial [PoM] £313.10 (Hospital only)
Dexmedetomidine 400micrograms/4ml concentrate for solution for infusion vials | 4 vial [PoM] £125.28 (Hospital only) | 10 vial [PoM] £421.40 (Hospital only)
Dexmedetomidine 400micrograms/4ml concentrate for solution for infusion ampoules | 4 ampoule [PoM] £125.30 (Hospital only) | 5 ampoule [PoM] £156.63 (Hospital only)
▶ **Dexdor** (Orion Pharma (UK) Ltd)
Dexmedetomidine (as Dexmedetomidine hydrochloride)
100 microgram per 1 ml Dexdor 1mg/10ml concentrate for solution for infusion vials | 4 vial [PoM] £313.20 (Hospital only)
Dexdor 400micrograms/4ml concentrate for solution for infusion vials | 4 vial [PoM] £125.28 (Hospital only)
Dexdor 200micrograms/2ml concentrate for solution for infusion ampoules | 5 ampoule [PoM] £78.30 (Hospital only)

2   Malignant hyperthermia

MUSCLE RELAXANTS 〉 DIRECTLY ACTING

| Dantrolene sodium
08-Mar-2021

● **DRUG ACTION** Acts on skeletal muscle cells by interfering with calcium efflux, thereby stopping the contractile process.

● **INDICATIONS AND DOSE**
Malignant hyperthermia
▶ BY RAPID INTRAVENOUS INJECTION
▶ Adult: Initially 2–3 mg/kg, then 1 mg/kg, repeated if necessary; maximum 10 mg/kg per course

Chronic severe spasticity of voluntary muscle
▶ BY MOUTH
▶ Adult: Initially 25 mg daily, then increased to up to 100 mg 4 times a day, dose increased at weekly intervals; usual dose 75 mg 3 times a day

Muscle cramps in motor neurone disease (specialist use only)
▶ BY MOUTH
▶ Adult: Initially 25 mg daily, then increased to up to 100 mg 4 times a day, dose increased at weekly intervals

● **UNLICENSED USE** [EvGr] Dantrolene sodium is used for the treatment of muscle cramps in motor neurone disease, Ⓔ but is not licensed for this indication.

IMPORTANT SAFETY INFORMATION
Should only be administered by, or under the direct supervision of, personnel experienced in the use of dantrolene when used for malignant hyperthermia.

● **CONTRA-INDICATIONS**
▶ With oral use Acute muscle spasm · avoid when spasticity is useful, for example, locomotion

● **CAUTIONS**
▶ With intravenous use Avoid extravasation (risk of tissue necrosis)
▶ With oral use Females (hepatotoxicity) · history of liver disorders (hepatotoxicity) · if doses greater than 400 mg daily (hepatotoxicity) · impaired cardiac function · impaired pulmonary function · patients over 30 years (hepatotoxicity) · therapeutic effect may take a few weeks to develop— discontinue if no response within 6–8 weeks

● **INTERACTIONS** → Appendix 1: dantrolene

● **SIDE-EFFECTS**
GENERAL SIDE-EFFECTS
▶ **Common or very common** Asthenia · diarrhoea · dizziness · drowsiness · gastrointestinal discomfort · headache · hepatic disorders · muscle weakness · nausea · respiratory disorders · seizure · skin reactions · speech disorder · vomiting
▶ **Uncommon** Arrhythmias · crystalluria · heart failure · hyperhidrosis
SPECIFIC SIDE-EFFECTS
▶ **Common or very common**
▶ With oral use Appetite decreased · cardiac inflammation · chills · confusion · depression · fever · insomnia · malaise · nervousness · vision disorders
▶ **Uncommon**
▶ With oral use Anaemia · aplastic anaemia · back pain · constipation · dysphagia · dyspnoea · excessive tearing · haemorrhage · hair growth abnormal · hallucination · hypersalivation · leucopenia · myalgia · neoplasms · photosensitivity reaction · taste altered · thrombocytopenia · urinary disorders
▶ **Rare or very rare**
▶ With oral use Erectile dysfunction
▶ **Frequency not known**
▶ With intravenous use Gastrointestinal haemorrhage · hyperkalaemia · muscle fatigue · pulmonary oedema · thrombophlebitis
▶ With oral use Dry mouth · muscle tone decreased · pericardial effusion · urine discolouration

● **PREGNANCY**
▶ With intravenous use Use only if potential benefit outweighs risk.
▶ With oral use Although teratological studies in *animals* have proved satisfactory, dantrolene sodium does cross the placenta, therefore manufacturer advises avoid.

15

Anaesthesia

- **BREAST FEEDING**
  ▸ With intravenous use Present in milk—use only if potential benefit outweighs risk.
  ▸ With oral use Present in milk—manufacturer advises avoid.
- **HEPATIC IMPAIRMENT**
  ▸ With oral use Manufacturer advises avoid in hepatic impairment.
- **MONITORING REQUIREMENTS**
  ▸ With oral use Test liver function before and at intervals during therapy.
- **PATIENT AND CARER ADVICE**
  Hepatotoxicity
  ▸ With oral use Patients should be told how to recognise signs of liver disorder and advised to seek prompt medical attention if symptoms such as anorexia, nausea, vomiting, fatigue, abdominal pain, dark urine, or pruritus develop.
  Driving and skilled tasks
  ▸ With oral use Drowsiness may affect performance of skilled tasks (e.g. driving); effects of alcohol enhanced.

- **MEDICINAL FORMS** There can be variation in the licensing of different medicines containing the same drug. Forms available from special-order manufacturers include: oral suspension, oral solution

  Oral capsule
  CAUTIONARY AND ADVISORY LABELS 2
  ▸ Dantrium (Forum Health Products Ltd)
  Dantrolene sodium 25 mg Dantrium 25mg capsules |
  100 capsule PoM £16.87 DT = £16.87
  Dantrolene sodium 100 mg Dantrium 100mg capsules |
  100 capsule PoM £43.07 DT = £43.07
  Powder for solution for injection
  ▸ Agilus (Forum Health Products Ltd)
  Dantrolene sodium 120 mg Agilus 120mg powder for solution for injection vials | 6 vial PoM £2,184.85 (Hospital only)
  ▸ Dantrium (Forum Health Products Ltd)
  Dantrolene sodium 20 mg Dantrium Intravenous 20mg powder for solution for injection vials | 12 vial PoM £612.00 (Hospital only)

Local anaesthesia

Anaesthesia (local)

18-Sep-2023

Local anaesthetic drugs

The use of local anaesthetics by injection or by application to mucous membranes to produce local analgesia is discussed in this section.

Local anaesthetic drugs act by causing a reversible block to conduction along nerve fibres. They vary widely in their potency, toxicity, duration of action, stability, solubility in water, and ability to penetrate mucous membranes. These factors determine their application, e.g. topical (surface), infiltration, peripheral nerve block, intravenous regional anaesthesia (Bier's block), plexus, epidural (extradural), or spinal (intrathecal or subarachnoid) block. Local anaesthetics may also be used for postoperative pain relief, thereby reducing the need for analgesics such as opioids.

Bupivacaine hydrochloride p. 1544 has a longer duration of action than other local anaesthetics. It has a slow onset of action, taking up to 30 minutes for full effect. It is often used in lumbar epidural blockade and is particularly suitable for continuous epidural analgesia in labour, or for postoperative pain relief. It is the principal drug used for spinal anaesthesia. Hyperbaric solutions containing glucose may be used for spinal block.

Levobupivacaine p. 1546, an isomer of bupivacaine, has anaesthetic and analgesic properties similar to bupivacaine hydrochloride, but is thought to have fewer adverse effects.

Lidocaine hydrochloride p. 1380 is effectively absorbed from mucous membranes and is a useful surface anaesthetic in concentrations up to 10%. Except for surface anaesthesia

and dental anaesthesia, solutions used do not usually exceed 1% in strength. The duration of the block (with adrenaline/epinephrine p. 256) is about 90 minutes.

Prilocaine hydrochloride p. 1551 is a local anaesthetic of low toxicity which is similar to lidocaine hydrochloride. A hyperbaric solution of prilocaine hydrochloride (containing glucose) may be used for spinal anaesthesia.

Ropivacaine hydrochloride p. 1552 is an amide-type local anaesthetic agent similar to bupivacaine hydrochloride. It is less cardiotoxic than bupivacaine hydrochloride, but also less potent.

Tetracaine p. 1553, a para-aminobenzoic acid ester, is an effective local anaesthetic for topical application; a 4% gel is indicated for anaesthesia before venepuncture or venous cannulation. It is rapidly absorbed from mucous membranes and should **never** be applied to inflamed, traumatised, or highly vascular surfaces. It should never be used to provide anaesthesia for bronchoscopy or cystoscopy because lidocaine hydrochloride is a safer alternative.

Administration by injection

The dose of local anaesthetic depends on the injection site and the procedure used. In determining the safe dosage, it is important to take account of the rate of absorption and excretion, and of the potency. The patient's age, weight, physique, and clinical condition, and the vascularity of the administration site and the duration of administration, must also be considered.

Uptake of local anaesthetics into the systemic circulation determines their duration of action and produces toxicity.

NHS Improvement has advised (September 2016) that, prior to administration, all injectable medicines must be drawn directly from their original ampoule or container into a syringe and should **never** be decanted into gallipots or open containers. This is to avoid the risk of medicines being confused with other substances, e.g. skin disinfectants, and to reduce the risk of contamination.

Great care must be taken to avoid accidental intravascular injection; local anaesthetic injections should be given slowly in order to detect inadvertent intravascular administration. When prolonged analgesia is required, a long-acting local anaesthetic is preferred to minimise the likelihood of cumulative systemic toxicity. Local anaesthesia around the oral cavity may impair swallowing and therefore increases the risk of aspiration.

Epidural anaesthesia is commonly used during surgery, often combined with general anaesthesia, because of its protective effect against the stress response of surgery. It is often used when good postoperative pain relief is essential.

Vasoconstrictors in combination with local anaesthetics

Local anaesthetics cause dilatation of blood vessels. The addition of a vasoconstrictor such as adrenaline/epinephrine to the local anaesthetic preparation diminishes local blood flow, slowing the rate of absorption and thereby prolonging the anaesthetic effect. Great care should be taken to avoid inadvertent intravenous administration of a preparation containing adrenaline/epinephrine. The use of adrenaline/epinephrine with a local anaesthetic injection in digits or appendages [unlicensed use] may be associated with a risk of ischaemic necrosis though the combination is used in some circumstances (such as hand surgery that uses the Wide-awake Local Anaesthesia No Tourniquet (WALANT) technique).

Adrenaline/epinephrine must be used in a low concentration when administered with a local anaesthetic. Care must also be taken to calculate a safe maximum dose of local anaesthetic when using combination products.

In patients with severe hypertension or unstable cardiac rhythm, the use of adrenaline/epinephrine with a local anaesthetic may be hazardous. For these patients an anaesthetic without adrenaline/epinephrine should be used.

Dental anaesthesia

Lidocaine hydrochloride is widely used in dental procedures; it is most often used in combination with adrenaline/epinephrine. Lidocaine hydrochloride 2% combined with adrenaline/epinephrine 1 in 80 000 (12.5 micrograms/mL) is a safe and effective preparation; there is no justification for using higher concentrations of adrenaline/epinephrine.

The amide-type local anaesthetics **articaine** and mepivacaine hydrochloride p. 1550 are also used in dentistry; they are available in cartridges suitable for dental use. Mepivacaine hydrochloride is available with or without adrenaline/epinephrine and articaine is available with adrenaline.

In patients with severe hypertension or unstable cardiac rhythm, mepivacaine hydrochloride without adrenaline/epinephrine may be used. Alternatively, prilocaine hydrochloride with or without felypressin can be used but there is no evidence that it is any safer. Felypressin can cause coronary vasoconstriction when used at high doses; limit dose in patients with coronary artery disease.

Toxicity induced by local anaesthesia

For management of toxicity see Severe local anaesthetic-induced cardiovascular toxicity below.

Severe local anaesthetic-induced cardiovascular toxicity

Overview

After injection of a bolus of local anaesthetic, toxicity may develop at any time in the following hour. In the event of signs of toxicity during injection, the administration of the local anaesthetic must be stopped immediately.

Cardiovascular status must be assessed and cardiopulmonary resuscitation procedures must be followed.

In the event of local anaesthetic-induced cardiac arrest, standard cardiopulmonary resuscitation should be initiated immediately. Lidocaine must not be used as anti-arrhythmic therapy.

If the patient does not respond rapidly to standard procedures, 20% lipid emulsion such as *Intralipid®* [unlicensed indication] should be given intravenously at an initial bolus dose of 1.5 mL/kg over 1 minute, followed by an infusion of 15 mL/kg/hour. After 5 minutes, if cardiovascular stability has not been restored or circulation deteriorates, give a maximum of two further bolus doses of 1.5 mL/kg over 1 minute, 5 minutes apart, and increase the infusion rate to 30 mL/kg/hour. Continue infusion until cardiovascular stability and adequate circulation are restored or maximum cumulative dose of 12 mL/kg is given.

Standard cardiopulmonary resuscitation must be maintained throughout lipid emulsion treatment.

Propofol is not a suitable alternative to lipid emulsion.

Further advice on ongoing treatment should be obtained from the National Poisons Information Service.

Detailed treatment algorithms and accompanying notes are available at www.toxbase.org *or* can be found in the Association of Anaesthetists of Great Britain and Ireland safety guideline, Management of Severe Local Anaesthetic Toxicity and Management of Severe Local Anaesthetic Toxicity – Accompanying notes.

ANAESTHETICS, LOCAL

Adrenaline with articaine hydrochloride

19-Dec-2019

(Carticaine hydrochloride with epinephrine)

● **INDICATIONS AND DOSE**

Infiltration anaesthesia in dentistry
▶ BY REGIONAL ADMINISTRATION
▸ Adult: Consult expert dental sources

DOSES AT EXTREMES OF BODY-WEIGHT
▸ To avoid excessive dosage in obese patients, dose should be calculated on the basis of ideal body-weight.

IMPORTANT SAFETY INFORMATION
Should only be administered by, or under the direct supervision of, personnel experienced in their use, with adequate training in anaesthesia and airway management, and should not be administered parenterally unless adequate resuscitation equipment is available.

● **CONTRA-INDICATIONS** Injection into infected tissues · injection into inflamed tissues · preparations containing preservatives should not be used for caudal, epidural, or spinal block

CONTRA-INDICATIONS, FURTHER INFORMATION
▸ Injection site Manufacturer advises the local anaesthetic effect may be reduced when injected into an inflamed or infected area, due to altered local pH. Increased absorption into the blood also increases the possibility of systemic side-effects.

● **CAUTIONS** Arrhythmias · arteriosclerosis · cardiovascular disease · cerebrovascular disease · cor pulmonale · debilitated patients (consider dose reduction) · diabetes mellitus · elderly (consider dose reduction) · epilepsy · hypercalcaemia · hyperreflexia · hypertension · hyperthyroidism · hypokalaemia · hypovolaemia · impaired cardiac conduction · impaired respiratory function · ischaemic heart disease · myasthenia gravis · obstructive cardiomyopathy · occlusive vascular disease · organic brain damage · phaeochromocytoma · prostate disorders · psychoneurosis · severe angina · shock · susceptibility to angle-closure glaucoma

CAUTIONS, FURTHER INFORMATION
▸ Use of vasoconstrictors In patients with severe hypertension or unstable cardiac rhythm, the use of adrenaline with a local anaesthetic may be hazardous. For these patients an anaesthetic without adrenaline should be used.

● **INTERACTIONS** → Appendix 1: sympathomimetics, vasoconstrictor

● **SIDE-EFFECTS** Face oedema · gingivitis · headache · nausea · sensation abnormal

SIDE-EFFECTS, FURTHER INFORMATION Toxic effects after administration of local anaesthetics are a result of excessively high plasma concentrations; severe toxicity usually results from inadvertent intravascular injection. The toxicity mainly involves the central nervous and cardiovascular systems. The onset of toxicity can be unpredictable and delayed. Monitor as per local protocol for at least 30 minutes after administration.

● **ALLERGY AND CROSS-SENSITIVITY**
▸ Hypersensitivity and cross-sensitivity Hypersensitivity reactions occur mainly with the ester-type local anaesthetics, such as tetracaine; reactions are less frequent with the amide types, such as articaine, bupivacaine, levobupivacaine, lidocaine, mepivacaine, prilocaine, and ropivacaine. Cross-sensitivity reactions may be avoided by using the alternative chemical type.

- PREGNANCY Use only if potential benefit outweighs risk—no information available.
- BREAST FEEDING Avoid breast-feeding for 48 hours after administration.
- HEPATIC IMPAIRMENT Manufacturer advises caution (increased risk of toxicity in severe impairment).
- RENAL IMPAIRMENT Manufacturers advise use with caution in severe impairment.
- MONITORING REQUIREMENTS Consider monitoring blood pressure and ECG (advised with systemic adrenaline/epinephrine).

- MEDICINAL FORMS There can be variation in the licensing of different medicines containing the same drug.

Solution for injection
EXCIPIENTS: May contain Sulfites
- Anestadent (Dentsply Ltd)
  Adrenaline (as Adrenaline acid tartrate) 10 microgram per 1 ml, Articaine hydrochloride 40 mg per 1 ml Anestadent 4% and 1:100,000 solution for injection 2.2ml cartridges | 50 cartridge PoM ⚠ (Hospital only)
- Septanest (Septodont Ltd)
  Adrenaline (as Adrenaline acid tartrate) 10 microgram per 1 ml, Articaine hydrochloride 40 mg per 1 ml Septanest 1 in 100,000 solution for injection 2.2ml cartridges | 50 cartridge PoM £38.95 (Hospital only)
  Adrenaline (as Adrenaline acid tartrate) 5 microgram per 1 ml, Articaine hydrochloride 40 mg per 1 ml Septanest 1 in 200,000 solution for injection 2.2ml cartridges | 50 cartridge PoM £38.95 (Hospital only)

Bupivacaine hydrochloride

09-Dec-2019

- INDICATIONS AND DOSE

Surgical anaesthesia, lumbar epidural block
- BY REGIONAL ADMINISTRATION
- Adult: 75–150 mg, dose administered using a 5 mg/mL (0.5%) solution

Surgical anaesthesia, field block
- BY REGIONAL ADMINISTRATION
- Adult: Up to 150 mg, dose administered using a 2.5 mg/mL (0.25%) or 5 mg/mL (0.5%) solution

Surgical anaesthesia, thoracic epidural block
- BY THORACIC EPIDURAL
- Adult: 12.5–50 mg, dose administered using a 2.5 mg/mL (0.25%) or 5 mg/mL (0.5%) solution

Surgical anaesthesia, caudal epidural block
- BY REGIONAL ADMINISTRATION
- Adult: 50–150 mg, dose administered using a 2.5 mg/mL (0.25%) or 5 mg/mL (0.5%) solution

Surgical anaesthesia, major nerve block
- BY REGIONAL ADMINISTRATION
- Adult: 50–175 mg, dose administered using 5 mg/mL (0.5%) solution

Acute pain, intra-articular block
- BY INTRA-ARTICULAR INJECTION
- Adult: Up to 100 mg, dose administered using a 2.5 mg/mL (0.25%) solution; when co-administered with bupivacaine by another route, total max. 150 mg

Acute pain, thoracic epidural block
- BY CONTINUOUS EPIDURAL INFUSION
- Adult: 6.3–18.8 mg/hour, dose administered using a 1.25 mg/mL (0.125%) or 2.5 mg/mL (0.25%) solution; maximum 400 mg per day

Acute pain, labour
- BY CONTINUOUS EPIDURAL INFUSION
- Adult: 6.25–12.5 mg/hour, dose administered using a 1.25 mg/mL (0.125%) solution; maximum 400 mg per day

Acute pain, lumbar epidural block
- INITIALLY BY LUMBAR EPIDURAL
- Adult: 15–37.5 mg, then (by lumbar epidural) 15–37.5 mg, repeated when required at intervals of at least 30 minutes, dose administered by intermittent injection using a 2.5 mg/mL (0.25%) solution, alternatively (by continuous epidural infusion) 12.5–18.8 mg/hour, dose administered using a 1.25 mg/mL (0.125%) or 2.5 mg/mL (0.25%) solution; maximum 400 mg per day

Acute pain, field block
- BY REGIONAL ADMINISTRATION
- Adult: Up to 150 mg, dose administered using a 2.5 mg/mL (0.25%) solution

DOSES AT EXTREMES OF BODY-WEIGHT
- To avoid excessive dosage in obese patients, dose should be calculated on the basis of ideal body-weight.

MARCAIN HEAVY ®

Intrathecal anaesthesia for surgery
- BY INTRATHECAL INJECTION
- Adult: 10–20 mg

IMPORTANT SAFETY INFORMATION
The licensed doses stated may not be appropriate in some settings and expert advice should be sought.
   Should only be administered by, or under the direct supervision of, personnel experienced in their use, with adequate training in anaesthesia and airway management, and should not be administered parenterally unless adequate resuscitation equipment is available.

- CONTRA-INDICATIONS Avoid injection into infected tissues · avoid injection into inflamed tissues · intravenous regional anaesthesia (Bier's block) · preparations containing preservatives should not be used for caudal, epidural, or spinal block

CONTRA-INDICATIONS, FURTHER INFORMATION
- Injection site Manufacturer advises local anaesthetics should not be injected into inflamed or infected tissues. Increased absorption into the blood increases the possibility of systemic side-effects, and the local anaesthetic effect may also be reduced by altered local pH.

- CAUTIONS Cardiovascular disease · cerebral atheroma · complete heart block · debilitated patients (consider dose reduction) · elderly (consider dose reduction) · epilepsy · hypertension · hypotension · hypovolaemia · impaired cardiac conduction · impaired respiratory function · myasthenia gravis · myocardial depression may be more severe and more resistant to treatment · shock

- SIDE-EFFECTS
- **Common or very common** Arrhythmias · dizziness · hypertension · hypotension · nausea · paraesthesia · urinary retention · vomiting
- **Uncommon** Neurotoxicity
- **Rare or very rare** Arachnoiditis · cardiac arrest · diplopia · nerve disorders · paraplegia · paresis · respiratory depression

SIDE-EFFECTS, FURTHER INFORMATION Toxic effects after administration of local anaesthetics are a result of excessively high plasma concentrations; severe toxicity usually results from inadvertent intravascular injection. The systemic toxicity of local anaesthetics mainly involves the central nervous and cardiovascular systems. The onset of toxicity can be unpredictable and delayed. Monitor as per local protocol for at least 30 minutes after administration.

- ALLERGY AND CROSS-SENSITIVITY
- **Hypersensitivity and cross-sensitivity** Hypersensitivity reactions occur mainly with the ester-type local

anaesthetics, such as tetracaine; reactions are less frequent with the amide types, such as articaine, bupivacaine, levobupivacaine, lidocaine, mepivacaine, prilocaine, and ropivacaine. Cross-sensitivity reactions may be avoided by using the alternative chemical type.

● PREGNANCY Large doses during delivery can cause neonatal respiratory depression, hypotonia, and bradycardia after epidural block.
Dose adjustments Use lower doses for intrathecal use during late pregnancy.

● BREAST FEEDING Amount too small to be harmful.

● HEPATIC IMPAIRMENT Manufacturer advises use with caution in advanced liver dysfunction.

● RENAL IMPAIRMENT Use with caution in severe impairment.

● MEDICINAL FORMS There can be variation in the licensing of different medicines containing the same drug. Forms available from special-order manufacturers include: solution for injection, infusion, solution for infusion
Solution for injection
▸ Bupivacaine hydrochloride (Non-proprietary)
　Bupivacaine hydrochloride 2.5 mg per 1 ml Bupivacaine 25mg/10ml (0.25%) solution for injection ampoules │ 5 ampoule PoM £9.99 DT = £9.99 (Hospital only) │ 10 ampoule PoM £15.84–£18.30 (Hospital only)
　Bupivacaine 25mg/10ml (0.25%) solution for injection vials │ 10 vial PoM 🅢 (Hospital only)
　Bupivacaine 0.25% solution for injection 10ml Sure-Amp ampoules │ 20 ampoule PoM £17.50 DT = £17.50
　Bupivacaine hydrochloride 5 mg per 1 ml Bupivacaine 0.5% solution for injection 10ml Sure-Amp ampoules │ 20 ampoule PoM £18.30 DT = £18.30 (Hospital only)
　Bupivacaine 100mg/20ml (0.5%) solution for injection vials │ 10 vial PoM 🅢 (Hospital only)
　Bupivacaine 50mg/10ml (0.5%) solution for injection ampoules │ 5 ampoule PoM £11.25 DT = £11.25 (Hospital only) │ 10 ampoule PoM £7.56–£80.30 DT = £7.56 (Hospital only)
　Bupivacaine hydrochloride anhydrous 40 mg per 1 ml Bupivacain Sintetica 40mg/ml (4%) solution for injection ampoules │ 10 ampoule PoM 🅢 (Hospital only)
Infusion
▸ Bupivacaine hydrochloride (Non-proprietary)
　Bupivacaine hydrochloride 1 mg per 1 ml Bupivacaine 250mg/250ml (0.1%) infusion bags │ 5 bag PoM £60.87
　Bupivacaine hydrochloride 1.25 mg per 1 ml Bupivacaine 312.5mg/250ml (0.125%) infusion bags │ 5 bag PoM £62.12

Bupivacaine with adrenaline　　19-Dec-2019

The properties listed below are those particular to the combination only. For the properties of the components please consider, bupivacaine hydrochloride p. 1544, adrenaline/epinephrine p. 256.

● **INDICATIONS AND DOSE**
Surgical anaesthesia
▸ BY LUMBAR EPIDURAL, OR BY LOCAL INFILTRATION, OR BY CAUDAL EPIDURAL
▸ Adult: (consult product literature)
Acute pain management
▸ BY LUMBAR EPIDURAL, OR BY LOCAL INFILTRATION
▸ Adult: (consult product literature)

● CAUTIONS In patients with severe hypertension or unstable cardiac rhythm, the use of adrenaline with a local anaesthetic may be hazardous. For these patients an anaesthetic without adrenaline should be used.

● INTERACTIONS → Appendix 1: sympathomimetics, vasoconstrictor

● MEDICINAL FORMS There can be variation in the licensing of different medicines containing the same drug.
Solution for injection
▸ Bupivacaine with adrenaline (Non-proprietary)
　Adrenaline (as Adrenaline acid tartrate) 5 microgram per 1 ml, Bupivacaine hydrochloride 2.5 mg per 1 ml Bupivacaine 25mg/10ml (0.25%) / Adrenaline (base) 50micrograms/10ml (1 in 200,000) solution for injection ampoules │ 10 ampoule PoM £46.00 DT = £46.00
　Adrenaline (as Adrenaline acid tartrate) 5 microgram per 1 ml, Bupivacaine hydrochloride anhydrous 2.5 mg per 1 ml Carbostesin-adrenaline 0.25% / 100micrograms/20ml (1 in 200,000) solution for injection ampoules │ 1 ampoule PoM 🅢 (Hospital only)
　Carbostesin-adrenaline 0.25% / 25micrograms/5ml (1 in 200,000) solution for injection ampoules │ 1 ampoule PoM 🅢 (Hospital only)
　Adrenaline (as Adrenaline acid tartrate) 5 microgram per 1 ml, Bupivacaine hydrochloride 5 mg per 1 ml Bupivacaine 50mg/10ml (0.5%) / Adrenaline (base) 50micrograms/10ml (1 in 200,000) solution for injection ampoules │ 10 ampoule PoM £51.75 DT = £51.75
　Adrenaline (as Adrenaline acid tartrate) 5 microgram per 1 ml, Bupivacaine hydrochloride anhydrous 5 mg per 1 ml Carbostesin-adrenaline 0.5% / 25micrograms/5ml (1 in 200,000) solution for injection ampoules │ 1 ampoule PoM 🅢 (Hospital only)
　Carbostesin-adrenaline 0.5% / 100micrograms/20ml (1 in 200,000) solution for injection ampoules │ 1 ampoule PoM 🅢 (Hospital only)

Chloroprocaine hydrochloride　　07-Nov-2021

● DRUG ACTION Chloroprocaine is an ester-type local anaesthetic that blocks the generation and conduction of nerve impulses.

● **INDICATIONS AND DOSE**
Spinal anaesthesia for surgical procedures lasting 40 minutes or less (using 10 mg/ml solution) (specialist use only)
▸ BY SLOW INTRATHECAL INJECTION
▸ Adult: 40–50 mg (max. per dose 50 mg), dose depends on desired length of block
Surgical anaesthesia for procedures lasting 60 minutes or less, peripheral nerve block (using 20 mg/ml solution) (specialist use only)
▸ BY REGIONAL ADMINISTRATION
▸ Adult: (consult product literature)

IMPORTANT SAFETY INFORMATION
The licensed doses stated above may not be appropriate in some settings and expert advice should be sought.
　Should only be administered by, or under the direct supervision of, personnel experienced in their use, with adequate training in anaesthesia and airway management, and should not be administered parenterally unless adequate resuscitation equipment is available.

● CONTRA-INDICATIONS Avoid injection into infected tissues · avoid injection into inflamed tissues · hypovolaemia · impaired cardiac conduction · intravenous regional anaesthesia (Bier's block) · severe anaemia

CONTRA-INDICATIONS, FURTHER INFORMATION
▸ Injection site Local anaesthetics should not be injected into inflamed or infected tissues nor should they be applied to damaged skin. Increased absorption into the blood increases the possibility of systemic side-effects, and the local anaesthetic effect may also be reduced by altered local pH.

● CAUTIONS Acute porphyrias p. 1202 · cardiovascular disease · complete heart block · debilitated patients (consider dose reduction) · elderly (consider dose reduction) · low plasma-cholinesterase activity (including severe liver disease) · neurological disorders · neuromuscular disorders · partial heart block

- **INTERACTIONS** → Appendix 1: chloroprocaine
- **SIDE-EFFECTS**
GENERAL SIDE-EFFECTS
▶ **Common or very common** Anxiety · dizziness · hypotension · nausea · vomiting
▶ **Uncommon** Arrhythmias · hearing impairment · hypertension · loss of consciousness · neurotoxicity · oral disorders · seizure · speech disorder · tinnitus · tremor · vision disorders
▶ **Rare or very rare** Cardiac arrest · drowsiness · faecal incontinence · myocardial contractility decreased · nerve disorders · neurological injury · perineal numbness · sexual dysfunction · urinary incontinence
SPECIFIC SIDE-EFFECTS
▶ **Common or very common**
▶ With intrathecal use Sensation abnormal
▶ When used by regional administration Anaesthetic complication · paraesthesia
▶ **Uncommon**
▶ With intrathecal use Headache · pain
▶ **Rare or very rare**
▶ With intrathecal use Motor dysfunction · respiratory disorders · spinal block
▶ When used by regional administration Dyspnoea · respiratory arrest

SIDE-EFFECTS, FURTHER INFORMATION Toxic effects after administration of local anaesthetics are a result of excessively high plasma concentrations; severe toxicity usually results from inadvertent intravascular injection. The systemic toxicity of local anaesthetics mainly involves the central nervous and cardiovascular systems. The onset of toxicity can be unpredictable and delayed. Monitor as per local protocol for at least 30 minutes after administration.

- **ALLERGY AND CROSS-SENSITIVITY**
▶ Hypersensitivity and cross-sensitivity Hypersensitivity reactions occur mainly with the ester-type local anaesthetics, such as tetracaine and chloroprocaine; reactions are less frequent with the amide types, such as articaine, bupivacaine, levobupivacaine, lidocaine, mepivacaine, prilocaine, and ropivacaine. Cross-sensitivity reactions may be avoided by using the alternative chemical type.

- **PREGNANCY** Manufacturer advises use only if potential benefit outweighs risk (limited information available); this does not preclude use at term for obstetrical anaesthesia.

- **HEPATIC IMPAIRMENT** Manufacturer advises caution in severe impairment.

- **RENAL IMPAIRMENT** Manufacturer advises use with caution.

- **HANDLING AND STORAGE** Manufacturer advises protect from light.

- **NATIONAL FUNDING/ACCESS DECISIONS**
For full details see funding body website
Scottish Medicines Consortium (SMC) decisions
▶ Chloroprocaine hydrochloride (*Ampres*®) for spinal anaesthesia in adults where the planned surgical procedure should not exceed 40 minutes (October 2021) SMC No. SMC2373 Recommended with restrictions

- **MEDICINAL FORMS** There can be variation in the licensing of different medicines containing the same drug.
Solution for injection
▶ Ampres (B.Braun Medical Ltd)
Chloroprocaine hydrochloride 10 mg per 1 ml Ampres 50mg/5ml solution for injection ampoules | 10 ampoule PoM £87.50 (Hospital only)

Levobupivacaine

08-Sep-2020

- **INDICATIONS AND DOSE**
Acute postoperative pain
▶ BY CONTINUOUS EPIDURAL INFUSION
▶ Adult: 12.5–18.75 mg/hour, dose administered using a 1.25 mg/mL (0.125%) or 2.5 mg/mL (0.25%) solution; maximum 400 mg per day
Acute labour pain
▶ BY LUMBAR EPIDURAL
▶ Adult: 15–25 mg, repeated at intervals of at least 15 minutes, dose administered using a 2.5 mg/mL (0.25%) solution; maximum 400 mg per day
▶ BY CONTINUOUS EPIDURAL INFUSION
▶ Adult: 5–12.5 mg/hour, dose administered using a 1.25 mg/mL (0.125%) solution; maximum 400 mg per day
Surgical anaesthesia, peripheral nerve block
▶ BY REGIONAL ADMINISTRATION
▶ Adult: 2.5–150 mg, dose administered using a 2.5 mg/mL (0.25%) or 5 mg/mL (0.5%) solution
Surgical anaesthesia, peribulbular nerve block
▶ BY REGIONAL ADMINISTRATION
▶ Adult: 37.5–112.5 mg, dose administered using a 7.5 mg/mL (0.75%) solution
Surgical anaesthesia for caesarean section
▶ BY LUMBAR EPIDURAL
▶ Adult: 75–150 mg, to be given over 15 –20 minutes, dose administered using a 5 mg/mL (0.5%) solution
Surgical anaesthesia
▶ BY LUMBAR EPIDURAL
▶ Adult: 50–150 mg, to be given over 5 minutes, dose administered using a 5 mg/mL (0.5%) or 7.5 mg/mL (0.75%) solution
▶ BY INTRATHECAL INJECTION
▶ Adult: 15 mg, dose administered using a 5 mg/mL (0.5%) solution
▶ BY LOCAL INFILTRATION
▶ Adult: 2.5–150 mg, dose administered using a 2.5 mg/mL (0.25%) solution
DOSES AT EXTREMES OF BODY-WEIGHT
▶ To avoid excessive dosage in obese patients, dose should be calculated on the basis of ideal body-weight.

IMPORTANT SAFETY INFORMATION
The licensed doses stated may not be appropriate in some settings and expert advice should be sought.
  Should only be administered by, or under the direct supervision of, personnel experienced in their use, with adequate training in anaesthesia and airway management, and should not be administered parenterally unless adequate resuscitation equipment is available.

- **CONTRA-INDICATIONS** Avoid injection into infected tissues · avoid injection into inflamed tissues · intravenous regional anaesthesia (Bier's block) · preparations containing preservatives should not be used for caudal, epidural, or spinal block
CONTRA-INDICATIONS, FURTHER INFORMATION
▶ Injection site Manufacturer advises local anaesthetics should not be injected into inflamed or infected tissues. Increased absorption into the blood increases the possibility of systemic side-effects, and the local anaesthetic effect may also be reduced by altered local pH.

- **CAUTIONS** Cardiovascular disease · complete heart block · debilitated patients (consider dose reduction) · elderly (consider dose reduction) · epilepsy · hypovolaemia · impaired cardiac conduction · impaired respiratory function · myasthenia gravis · shock

- **INTERACTIONS** → Appendix 1: anaesthetics, local
- **SIDE-EFFECTS**
▶ **Common or very common** Anaemia·back pain·dizziness· fever·headache·hypotension·nausea·procedural pain· vomiting
▶ **Frequency not known** Angioedema·apnoea·arrhythmias· asthenia·atrioventricular block·bladder disorder·cardiac arrest·drowsiness·eye disorders·faecal incontinence· flushing·loss of consciousness·muscle twitching·muscle weakness·nerve disorders·neurological injury·oral hypoaesthesia·paralysis·priapism·respiratory disorders· seizure·sensation abnormal·skin reactions·sneezing· sweat changes·syncope·vision blurred

SIDE-EFFECTS, FURTHER INFORMATION The systemic toxicity of local anaesthetics mainly involves the central nervous and cardiovascular systems. Systemic toxicity can occur due to inadvertent intravascular injection. The onset of toxicity can be unpredictable and delayed. Monitor as per local protocol for at least 30 minutes after administration.

- **ALLERGY AND CROSS-SENSITIVITY**
▶ Hypersensitivity and cross-sensitivity Hypersensitivity reactions occur mainly with the ester-type local anaesthetics, such as tetracaine; reactions are less frequent with the amide types, such as articaine, bupivacaine, levobupivacaine, lidocaine, mepivacaine, prilocaine, and ropivacaine. Cross-sensitivity reactions may be avoided by using the alternative chemical type.

- **PREGNANCY** Large doses during delivery can cause neonatal respiratory depression, hypotonia, and bradycardia after epidural block. Avoid if possible in the first trimester—toxicity in *animal* studies. May cause fetal distress syndrome. Do not use for paracervical block in obstetrics. Do not use 7.5 mg/mL strength in obstetrics.

- **BREAST FEEDING** Amount too small to be harmful.

- **HEPATIC IMPAIRMENT** Manufacturer advises caution in impairment or patients with reduced hepatic blood flow (no information available).

- **PRESCRIBING AND DISPENSING INFORMATION** Levobupivacaine is an isomer of bupivacaine.

- **MEDICINAL FORMS** There can be variation in the licensing of different medicines containing the same drug.

Solution for injection
▶ Levobupivacaine (Non-proprietary)
Levobupivacaine (as Levobupivacaine hydrochloride) 2.5 mg per 1 ml Levobupivacaine 25mg/10ml solution for injection ampoules | 5 ampoule [PoM] £12.45-£13.50 (Hospital only)
Levobupivacaine (as Levobupivacaine hydrochloride) 5 mg per 1 ml Levobupivacaine 50mg/10ml solution for injection ampoules | 5 ampoule [PoM] £14.35-£22.89 (Hospital only)
Levobupivacaine (as Levobupivacaine hydrochloride) 7.5 mg per 1 ml Levobupivacaine 75mg/10ml solution for injection ampoules | 5 ampoule [PoM] £21.40-£21.78 (Hospital only)

Infusion
▶ Levobupivacaine (Non-proprietary)
Levobupivacaine (as Levobupivacaine hydrochloride) 625 microgram per 1 ml Levobupivacaine 125mg/200ml infusion bags | 5 bag [PoM] £83.25 (Hospital only)
Levobupivacaine (as Levobupivacaine hydrochloride) 1.25 mg per 1 ml Levobupivacaine 125mg/100ml infusion bags | 5 bag [PoM] £51.85-£63.30 (Hospital only)
Levobupivacaine 250mg/200ml infusion bags | 12 bag [PoM] £143.55 (Hospital only)

Lidocaine hydrochloride
10-Nov-2020
(Lignocaine hydrochloride)

- **INDICATIONS AND DOSE**
Infiltration anaesthesia
▶ BY LOCAL INFILTRATION
▶ Adult: Dose to be given according to patient's weight and nature of procedure; max. 200 mg, maximum dose 500 mg if given in solutions containing adrenaline

DOSES AT EXTREMES OF BODY-WEIGHT
▶ When used by local infiltration To avoid excessive dosage in obese patients, weight-based doses for non-emergency indications may need to be calculated on the basis of ideal body-weight.

Intravenous regional anaesthesia and nerve block
▶ BY REGIONAL ADMINISTRATION
▶ Adult: Seek expert advice

Pain relief (in anal fissures, haemorrhoids, pruritus ani, pruritus vulvae, herpes zoster, or herpes labialis) | Lubricant in cystoscopy | Lubricant in proctoscopy
▶ TO THE SKIN USING OINTMENT
▶ Adult: Apply 1–2 mL as required, avoid long-term use

Sore nipples from breast-feeding
▶ TO THE SKIN USING OINTMENT
▶ Adult: Apply using gauze and wash off immediately before next feed

LMX 4 ®
Anaesthesia before venous cannulation or venepuncture
▶ TO THE SKIN
▶ Child 1-2 months: Apply up to 1 g, apply thick layer to small area (2.5 cm × 2.5 cm) of non-irritated skin at least 30 minutes before procedure; may be applied under an occlusive dressing; max. application time 60 minutes, remove cream with gauze and perform procedure after approximately 5 minutes
▶ Child 3-11 months: Apply up to 1 g, apply thick layer to small area (2.5 cm × 2.5 cm) of non-irritated skin at least 30 minutes before procedure; may be applied under an occlusive dressing; max. application time 4 hours, remove cream with gauze and perform procedure after approximately 5 minutes
▶ Child 1-17 years: Apply 1–2.5 g, apply thick layer to small area (2.5 cm × 2.5 cm) of non-irritated skin at least 30 minutes before procedure; may be applied under an occlusive dressing; max. application time 5 hours, remove cream with gauze and perform procedure after approximately 5 minutes
▶ Adult: Apply 1–2.5 g, apply thick layer to small area (2.5 cm × 2.5 cm) of non-irritated skin at least 30 minutes before procedure; may be applied under an occlusive dressing; max. application time 5 hours, remove cream with gauze and perform procedure after approximately 5 minutes

VERSATIS ®
Postherpetic neuralgia
▶ TO THE SKIN
▶ Adult: Apply once daily for up to 12 hours, followed by a 12-hour plaster-free period; discontinue if no response after 4 weeks, to be applied to intact, dry, non-hairy, non-irritated skin, up to 3 plasters may be used to cover large areas; plasters may be cut

continued →

XYLOCAINE ®

During delivery in obstetrics
▸ TO THE SKIN
▸ Adult: Up to 20 doses

IMPORTANT SAFETY INFORMATION
▸ When used by local infiltration
The licensed doses stated may not be appropriate in
some settings and expert advice should be sought.
Should only be administered by, or under the direct
supervision of, personnel experienced in their use, with
adequate training in anaesthesia and airway
management, and should not be administered
parenterally unless adequate resuscitation equipment is
available.

● **CONTRA-INDICATIONS**
▸ When used by regional administration Avoid injection into
infected tissues · avoid injection into inflamed tissues ·
complete heart block · preparations containing
preservatives should not be used for caudal, epidural, or
spinal block, or for intravenous regional anaesthesia
(Bier's block)
▸ With topical use Application to the middle ear (can cause
ototoxicity) · should not be applied to damaged skin
CONTRA-INDICATIONS, FURTHER INFORMATION
▸ Administration site
▸ With topical use or when used by regional administration
Manufacturer advises local anaesthetics should not be
injected into inflamed or infected tissues nor should they
be applied to damaged skin. Increased absorption into the
blood increases the possibility of systemic side-effects,
and the local anaesthetic effect may also be reduced by
altered local pH.

● **CAUTIONS**
▸ When used by regional administration Acute porphyrias
p. 1202 (consider infusion with glucose for its anti-
porphyrinogenic effects) · congestive cardiac failure
(consider lower dose) · debilitated patients (consider dose
reduction) · elderly (consider dose reduction) · epilepsy ·
hypovolaemia · impaired cardiac conduction · impaired
respiratory function · myasthenia gravis · post cardiac
surgery (consider lower dose) · shock

● **INTERACTIONS** → Appendix 1: antiarrhythmics

● **SIDE-EFFECTS**
▸ With parenteral use Anxiety · arrhythmias · atrioventricular
block · cardiac arrest · circulatory collapse · confusion ·
dizziness · drowsiness · euphoric mood · headache ·
hypotension (may lead to cardiac arrest) · loss of
consciousness · methaemoglobinaemia · muscle twitching ·
myocardial contractility decreased · nausea · neurological
effects · nystagmus · pain · psychosis · respiratory disorders
· seizure · sensation abnormal · temperature sensation
altered · tinnitus · tremor · vision blurred · vomiting

SIDE-EFFECTS, FURTHER INFORMATION **Toxic effects** The
systemic toxicity of local anaesthetics mainly involves the
central nervous and cardiovascular systems.

   Methaemoglobinaemia Methylthioninium chloride is
licensed for the acute symptomatic treatment of drug-
induced methaemoglobinaemia.

● **ALLERGY AND CROSS-SENSITIVITY**
▸ Hypersensitivity and cross-sensitivity Hypersensitivity
reactions occur mainly with the ester-type local
anaesthetics, such as tetracaine; reactions are less
frequent with the amide types, such as articaine,
bupivacaine, levobupivacaine, lidocaine, mepivacaine,
prilocaine, and ropivacaine. Cross-sensitivity reactions
may be avoided by using the alternative chemical type.

● **PREGNANCY** Crosses the placenta but not known to be
harmful in *animal* studies—use if benefit outweighs risk.

When used as a local anaesthetic, large doses can cause
fetal bradycardia; if given during delivery can also cause
neonatal respiratory depression, hypotonia, or bradycardia
after paracervical or epidural block.

● **BREAST FEEDING** Present in milk but amount too small to
be harmful.

● **HEPATIC IMPAIRMENT** Manufacturer advises caution (risk
of increased exposure).

● **RENAL IMPAIRMENT** Possible accumulation of lidocaine
and active metabolite; caution in severe impairment.

● **MONITORING REQUIREMENTS**
▸ With systemic use Monitor ECG and have resuscitation
facilities available.

● **NATIONAL FUNDING/ACCESS DECISIONS**
VERSATIS ® For full details see funding body website
Scottish Medicines Consortium (SMC) decisions
▸ Lidocaine hydrochloride (*Versatis* ®) for the treatment of
neuropathic pain associated with previous herpes zoster
infection (post-herpetic neuralgia, PHN) (August 2008)
SMC No. 334/06 Recommended with restrictions

● **MEDICINAL FORMS** There can be variation in the licensing of
different medicines containing the same drug. Forms available
from special-order manufacturers include: solution for
injection

Solution for injection
▸ **Lidocaine hydrochloride (Non-proprietary)**
Lidocaine hydrochloride 5 mg per 1 ml Lidocaine 50mg/10ml
(0.5%) solution for injection ampoules | 10 ampoule PoM £10.00 DT
= £10.00
Lidocaine hydrochloride 10 mg per 1 ml Lidocaine 100mg/10ml
(1%) solution for injection Mini-Plasco ampoules | 20 ampoule PoM
£13.80
Lidocaine 100mg/10ml (1%) solution for injection ampoules |
10 ampoule PoM £5.00–£7.00 DT = £7.00 | 20 ampoule PoM
£14.00–£234.00 (Hospital only)
Lidocaine 200mg/20ml (1%) solution for injection vials | 10 vial PoM
£26.40 DT = £26.40
Lidocaine 200mg/20ml (1%) solution for injection ampoules |
1 ampoule PoM £25.07 (Hospital only) | 10 ampoule PoM £10.00–
£14.00 DT = £14.00 | 20 ampoule PoM £19.00–£501.40 (Hospital
only)
Lidocaine 50mg/5ml (1%) solution for injection ampoules |
1 ampoule PoM £8.28 (Hospital only) | 10 ampoule PoM £3.10–
£6.23 DT = £6.23 | 20 ampoule PoM £12.40–£165.60 (Hospital only)
Lidocaine 20mg/2ml (1%) solution for injection ampoules |
10 ampoule PoM £5.03 DT = £5.03
Lidocaine 50mg/5ml (1%) solution for injection Mini-Plasco ampoules
| 20 ampoule PoM £8.05
Lidocaine hydrochloride 20 mg per 1 ml Lidocaine 100mg/5ml
(2%) solution for injection ampoules | 10 ampoule PoM £3.80–£6.00
DT = £6.00 | 20 ampoule PoM £15.60–£165.00 (Hospital only)
Lidocaine 400mg/20ml (2%) solution for injection vials | 10 vial PoM
£27.50 DT = £27.50
Lidocaine 40mg/2ml (2%) solution for injection ampoules |
10 ampoule PoM £5.20 DT = £5.20
Lidocaine 100mg/5ml (2%) solution for injection Mini-Plasco ampoules
| 20 ampoule PoM £12.00
Lidocaine 200mg/10ml (2%) solution for injection ampoules |
20 ampoule PoM £14.95–£382.80 (Hospital only)
Lidocaine 400mg/20ml (2%) solution for injection ampoules |
10 ampoule PoM £11.00–£15.00 DT = £15.00 | 20 ampoule PoM
£31.00–£521.80 (Hospital only)

Medicated plaster
EXCIPIENTS: May contain Hydroxybenzoates (parabens), propylene
glycol
▸ **Versatis** (Grunenthal Ltd)
Lidocaine 50 mg per 1 gram Versatis 700mg medicated plasters |
30 plaster PoM £72.40 DT = £72.40

Cutaneous cream
EXCIPIENTS: May contain Benzyl alcohol, propylene glycol
▸ **LMX 4** (Ferndale Pharmaceuticals Ltd)
Lidocaine 40 mg per 1 gram LMX 4 cream | 5 gram P £2.98 DT =
£2.98 | 30 gram P £14.90 DT = £14.90

Ointment

▸ Lidocaine hydrochloride (Non-proprietary)

Lidocaine hydrochloride 50 mg per 1 gram Lidocaine 5% ointment | 15 gram [P] £18.75 DT = £15.00

Spray

▸ Xylocaine (Aspen Pharma Trading Ltd)

Lidocaine 10 mg per 1 actuation Xylocaine 10mg/dose spray sugar free | 50 ml [P] £6.29 DT = £6.29 [SF]

Lidocaine with adrenaline   19-Dec-2019

The properties listed below are those particular to the combination only. For the properties of the components please consider, lidocaine hydrochloride p. 1547, adrenaline/epinephrine p. 256.

● **INDICATIONS AND DOSE**

Local anaesthesia

▸ BY LOCAL INFILTRATION

▸ Adult: Dosed according to the type of nerve block required (consult product literature)

● INTERACTIONS → Appendix 1: antiarrhythmics · sympathomimetics, vasoconstrictor

● **PROFESSION SPECIFIC INFORMATION**

Dental information A variety of lidocaine injections with adrenaline is available in dental cartridges.

Consult expert dental sources for specific advice in relation to dose of lidocaine for dental anaesthesia.

● MEDICINAL FORMS There can be variation in the licensing of different medicines containing the same drug. Forms available from special-order manufacturers include: solution for injection

Solution for injection

EXCIPIENTS: May contain Sulfites

▸ Lidocaine with adrenaline (Non-proprietary)

Adrenaline (as Adrenaline acid tartrate) 5 microgram per 1 ml, Lidocaine hydrochloride 10 mg per 1 ml Lidocaine 200mg/20ml (1%) / Adrenaline (base) 100micrograms/20ml (1 in 200,000) solution for injection vials | 5 vial [PoM] £9.66 DT = £9.66 (Hospital only)

Adrenaline (as Adrenaline acid tartrate) 5 microgram per 1 ml, Lidocaine hydrochloride 20 mg per 1 ml Lidocaine 400mg/20ml (2%) / Adrenaline (base) 100micrograms/20ml (1 in 200,000) solution for injection vials | 5 vial [PoM] £8.85 DT = £8.85

▸ Lignospan Special (Septodont Ltd)

Adrenaline (as Adrenaline acid tartrate) 12.5 microgram per 1 ml, Lidocaine hydrochloride 20 mg per 1 ml Lignospan Special 20mg/ml / 12.5micrograms/ml solution for injection 2.2ml cartridges | 50 cartridge [PoM] £32.95 DT = £32.95

Lignospan Special 20mg/ml / 12.5micrograms/ml solution for injection 1.8ml cartridges | 50 cartridge [PoM] £32.95 DT = £32.95

▸ Rexocaine (Henry Schein Ltd)

Adrenaline (as Adrenaline acid tartrate) 12.5 microgram per 1 ml, Lidocaine hydrochloride 20 mg per 1 ml Rexocaine 2% injection 2.2ml cartridges | 50 cartridge [PoM] £24.75 DT = £32.95

▸ Xylocaine with Adrenaline (Dentsply Ltd)

Adrenaline (as Adrenaline acid tartrate) 12.5 microgram per 1 ml, Lidocaine hydrochloride 20 mg per 1 ml Xylocaine 2% with Adrenaline 1 in 80,000 Dental injection 2.2ml cartridges | 50 cartridge [PoM] [£] DT = £32.95

Lidocaine with cetrimide   27-Apr-2018

The properties listed below are those particular to the combination only. For the properties of the components please consider, lidocaine hydrochloride p. 1547.

● **INDICATIONS AND DOSE**

Anaesthesia and disinfection in dental practice

▸ TO MUCOUS MEMBRANES USING OROMUCOSAL SPRAY

▸ Adult: 10–20 mg, no more than 30 mg should be applied to the same quadrant of the buccal cavity— consult product literature, dose expressed as lidocaine

Anaesthesia in dental practice

▸ TO MUCOUS MEMBRANES USING DENTAL GEL

▸ Adult: Apply 100–500 mg, use cotton pellet for application to dried mucosa, dose expressed as weight of gel

DOSE EQUIVALENCE AND CONVERSION

▸ 1 metered dose of *Xylonor*® spray is equivalent to 10 mg of lidocaine.

▸ 2 millimetres of *Xylonor*® gel is approximately equivalent to 100 mg of gel (approximately equivalent to 5 mg of lidocaine).

● CAUTIONS Sepsis (risk of rapid systemic absorption) · traumatised mucosa (risk of rapid systemic absorption)

● INTERACTIONS → Appendix 1: antiarrhythmics

● MEDICINAL FORMS There can be variation in the licensing of different medicines containing the same drug.

Oromucosal gel

▸ Xylonor (Septodont Ltd)

Cetrimide 1.5 mg per 1 gram, Lidocaine 50 mg per 1 gram Xylonor 50mg/g / 1.5mg/g gel | 15 gram [P] £13.75 [SF]

Spray

▸ Xylonor (Septodont Ltd)

Cetrimide 1.5 mg per 1 gram, Lidocaine 150 mg per 1 gram Xylonor 150mg/g / 1.5mg/g oromucosal spray | 36 gram [PoM] £35.90 [SF]

Lidocaine with phenylephrine

The properties listed below are those particular to the combination only. For the properties of the components please consider, lidocaine hydrochloride p. 1547, phenylephrine hydrochloride p. 218.

● **INDICATIONS AND DOSE**

Anaesthesia before nasal surgery, endoscopy, laryngoscopy, or removal of foreign bodies from the nose

▸ BY INTRANASAL ADMINISTRATION

▸ Adult: Up to 8 sprays

● INTERACTIONS → Appendix 1: antiarrhythmics · sympathomimetics, vasoconstrictor

● MEDICINAL FORMS There can be variation in the licensing of different medicines containing the same drug.

Spray

▸ Lidocaine with phenylephrine (Non-proprietary)

Phenylephrine hydrochloride 5 mg per 1 ml, Lidocaine hydrochloride 50 mg per 1 ml Lidocaine 5% / Phenylephrine 0.5% nasal spray | 2.5 ml [PoM] £16.39–£20.01 DT = £20.01

Lidocaine with prilocaine   10-Nov-2021

The properties listed below are those particular to the combination only. For the properties of the components please consider, lidocaine hydrochloride p. 1547, prilocaine hydrochloride p. 1551.

● **INDICATIONS AND DOSE**

Anaesthesia before minor skin procedures including venepuncture

▸ TO THE SKIN

▸ Child 1–2 months: Apply up to 1 g for maximum 1 hour before procedure, to be applied under occlusive dressing, shorter application time of 15–30 minutes is recommended for children with atopic dermatitis (30 minutes before removal of mollusca); maximum 1 dose per day

▸ Child 3–11 months: Apply up to 2 g for maximum 1 hour before procedure, to be applied under occlusive dressing, shorter application time of 15–30 minutes   continued →

is recommended for children with atopic dermatitis (30 minutes before removal of mollusca); maximum 2 doses per day
- **Child 1-11 years:** Apply 1–5 hours before procedure, a thick layer should be applied under occlusive dressing, shorter application time of 15–30 minutes is recommended for children with atopic dermatitis (30 minutes before removal of mollusca); maximum 2 doses per day
- **Child 12-17 years:** Apply 1–5 hours before procedure (2–5 hours before procedures on large areas e.g. split skin grafting), a thick layer should be applied under occlusive dressing, shorter application time of 15–30 minutes is recommended for children with atopic dermatitis (30 minutes before removal of mollusca)
- **Adult:** Apply 1–5 hours before procedure (2–5 hours before procedures on large areas e.g. split skin grafting), a thick layer should be applied under occlusive dressing

Anaesthesia on genital skin before injection of local anaesthetics
- TO THE SKIN
- **Adult:** Apply under occlusive dressing for 15 minutes (males) or 60 minutes (females) before procedure

Anaesthesia before surgical treatment of lesions on genital mucosa
- TO THE SKIN
- **Adult:** Apply up to 10 g, to be applied 5–10 minutes before procedure

Anaesthesia before cervical curettage
- TO THE SKIN
- **Adult:** Apply 10 g in lateral vaginal fornices for 10 minutes

Anaesthesia before mechanical cleansing or debridement of leg ulcer
- TO THE SKIN
- **Adult:** Apply up to 10 g for 30–60 minutes, to be applied under occlusive dressing

- **CONTRA-INDICATIONS** Use in child less than 37 weeks corrected gestational age
- **INTERACTIONS** → Appendix 1: anaesthetics, local · antiarrhythmics
- **SIDE-EFFECTS**
- **Common or very common** Sexual dysfunction (in adults)
- **Uncommon** Fever (in adults) · headache (in adults) · penis disorder (in adults)
- **Rare or very rare** Methaemoglobinaemia · skin reactions
  SIDE-EFFECTS, FURTHER INFORMATION When applied to the glans penis, side-effects for sexual partners should be considered. Side-effects reported in female partners include vaginal candidiasis and dysuria.

- **PATIENT AND CARER ADVICE**
  Medicines for Children leaflet: EMLA cream for local anaesthesia
  www.medicinesforchildren.org.uk/medicines/emla-cream-for-local-anaesthesia/

- **MEDICINAL FORMS** There can be variation in the licensing of different medicines containing the same drug.
  Cutaneous cream
  - Emla (Aspen Pharma Trading Ltd)
    Lidocaine 25 mg per 1 gram, Prilocaine 25 mg per 1 gram Emla 5% cream | 5 gram Ⓟ £2.25-£2.99 | 25 gram Ⓟ £11.70 | 30 gram Ⓟ £12.30 DT = £12.30
  - Nulbia (Glenmark Pharmaceuticals Europe Ltd)
    Lidocaine 25 mg per 1 gram, Prilocaine 25 mg per 1 gram Nulbia 5% cream | 5 gram Ⓟ £1.69 | 25 gram Ⓟ £8.44 | 30 gram Ⓟ £9.23 DT = £12.30

Mepivacaine hydrochloride

04-Dec-2019

- **INDICATIONS AND DOSE**

Infiltration anaesthesia and nerve block in dentistry
- **Child 3-17 years:** Consult expert dental sources
- **Adult:** Consult expert dental sources
DOSES AT EXTREMES OF BODY-WEIGHT
- To avoid excessive dosage in obese patients, dose should be calculated on the basis of ideal body-weight.

IMPORTANT SAFETY INFORMATION
Should only be administered by, or under the direct supervision of, personnel experienced in their use, with adequate training in anaesthesia and airway management, and should not be administered parenterally unless adequate resuscitation equipment is available.

- **CONTRA-INDICATIONS** Avoid injection into infected tissues · avoid injection into inflamed tissues · intravenous regional anaesthesia (Bier's block) · preparations containing preservatives should not be used for caudal, epidural, or spinal block · severe atrio-ventricular conduction disorders not controlled by a pacemaker
  CONTRA-INDICATIONS, FURTHER INFORMATION
- Injection site Manufacturer advises the local anaesthetic effect may be reduced when injected into an inflamed or infected area, due to altered local pH. Increased absorption into the blood also increases the possibility of systemic side-effects.
- **CAUTIONS** Cardiovascular disease · children (consider dose reduction) · debilitated patients (consider dose reduction) · elderly (consider dose reduction) · epilepsy · hypovolaemia · impaired cardiac conduction · impaired respiratory function · myasthenia gravis · shock
- **SIDE-EFFECTS**
- **Common or very common** Arrhythmias · dizziness · hypertension · hypotension · nausea · paraesthesia · vomiting
- **Uncommon** Neurotoxicity
- **Rare or very rare** Arachnoiditis · cardiac arrest · diplopia · nerve disorders · respiratory depression
  SIDE-EFFECTS, FURTHER INFORMATION Toxic effects after administration of local anaesthetics are a result of excessively high plasma concentrations; severe toxicity usually results from inadvertent intravascular injection or too rapid injection. The systemic toxicity of local anaesthetics mainly involves the central nervous and cardiovascular systems. The onset of toxicity can be unpredictable and delayed. Monitor as per local protocol for at least 30 minutes after administration.
- **ALLERGY AND CROSS-SENSITIVITY**
- Hypersensitivity and cross-sensitivity Hypersensitivity reactions occur mainly with the ester-type local anaesthetics, such as tetracaine; reactions are less frequent with the amide types, such as articaine, bupivacaine, levobupivacaine, lidocaine, mepivacaine, prilocaine, and ropivacaine. Cross-sensitivity reactions may be avoided by using the alternative chemical type.
- **PREGNANCY** Use with caution in early pregnancy.
- **BREAST FEEDING** Use with caution.
- **HEPATIC IMPAIRMENT** Manufacturer advises caution; increased risk of toxic plasma concentrations in severe impairment.
- **RENAL IMPAIRMENT** Use with caution; increased risk of side-effects.

● **MEDICINAL FORMS** There can be variation in the licensing of different medicines containing the same drug.
Solution for injection
▸ Scandonest plain (Septodont Ltd)
  Mepivacaine hydrochloride 30 mg per 1 ml Scandonest plain 3% solution for injection 2.2ml cartridges | 50 cartridge [PoM] £34.05

Mepivacaine with adrenaline   19-Dec-2019

The properties listed below are those particular to the combination only. For the properties of the components please consider, mepivacaine hydrochloride p. 1550, adrenaline/epinephrine p. 256.

● **INDICATIONS AND DOSE**
Infiltration anaesthesia and nerve block in dentistry
▸ BY LOCAL INFILTRATION
▸ Adult: (consult product literature)

● **INTERACTIONS** → Appendix 1: sympathomimetics, vasoconstrictor

● **MEDICINAL FORMS** No licensed medicines listed.

Prilocaine hydrochloride   12-Nov-2020

● **INDICATIONS AND DOSE**
CITANEST 1% ®
Infiltration anaesthesia | Nerve block
▸ BY REGIONAL ADMINISTRATION
▸ Adult: 100–200 mg/minute, alternatively may be given in incremental doses; dose adjusted according to site of administration and response, and in elderly and debilitated patients (smaller doses may be required); maximum 400 mg per course
PRILOTEKAL ®
Spinal anaesthesia
▸ BY INTRATHECAL INJECTION
▸ Adult: Usual dose 40–60 mg (max. per dose 80 mg), dose may need to be reduced in elderly or debilitated patients, or in late pregnancy
DOSES AT EXTREMES OF BODY-WEIGHT
▸ To avoid excessive dosage in obese patients, dose should be calculated on the basis of ideal body-weight.

IMPORTANT SAFETY INFORMATION
Should only be administered by, or under the direct supervision of, personnel experienced in their use, with adequate training in anaesthesia and airway management, and should not be administered parenterally unless adequate resuscitation equipment is available.

● **CONTRA-INDICATIONS**
GENERAL CONTRA-INDICATIONS Acquired methaemoglobinaemia · anaemia · avoid injection into infected tissues · avoid injection into inflamed tissues · congenital methaemoglobinaemia · preparations containing preservatives should not be used for caudal, epidural, or spinal block
SPECIFIC CONTRA-INDICATIONS
▸ With intrathecal use Serious cardiac conduction disorders
CONTRA-INDICATIONS, FURTHER INFORMATION
▸ Injection site Manufacturer advises local anaesthetics should not be injected into inflamed or infected tissues. Increased absorption into the blood increases the possibility of systemic side-effects, and the local anaesthetic effect may also be reduced by altered local pH.

● **CAUTIONS** Cardiovascular disease · debilitated patients (consider dose reduction) · elderly (consider dose reduction) · epilepsy · hypovolaemia · impaired cardiac conduction · impaired respiratory function · myasthenia gravis · severe or untreated hypertension · shock

● **SIDE-EFFECTS**
▸ **Common or very common** Arrhythmias · dizziness · hypertension · hypotension · nausea · paraesthesia · vomiting
▸ **Uncommon** Neurotoxicity
▸ **Rare or very rare** Cardiac arrest · methaemoglobinaemia · nerve disorders
▸ **Frequency not known** Diplopia · respiratory depression
SIDE-EFFECTS, FURTHER INFORMATION **Toxic effects**
Toxic effects after administration of local anaesthetics are a result of excessively high plasma concentrations; severe toxicity usually results from inadvertent intravascular injection or too rapid injection. The systemic toxicity of local anaesthetics mainly involves the central nervous and cardiovascular systems. The onset of toxicity can be unpredictable and delayed. Monitor as per local protocol for at least 30 minutes after administration.
  Methaemoglobinaemia Methaemoglobinaemia can be treated with an intravenous injection of methylthioninium chloride.

● **ALLERGY AND CROSS-SENSITIVITY**
▸ Hypersensitivity and cross-sensitivity Hypersensitivity reactions occur mainly with the ester-type local anaesthetics, such as tetracaine; reactions are less frequent with the amide types, such as articaine, bupivacaine, levobupivacaine, lidocaine, mepivacaine, prilocaine, and ropivacaine. Cross-sensitivity reactions may be avoided by using the alternative chemical type.

● **PREGNANCY** Large doses during delivery can cause neonatal respiratory depression, hypotonia, and bradycardia after epidural block. Avoid paracervical or pudendal block in obstetrics (neonatal methaemoglobinaemia reported).
Dose adjustments Use lower doses for intrathecal use during late pregnancy.

● **BREAST FEEDING** Present in milk but not known to be harmful.

● **HEPATIC IMPAIRMENT** Manufacturer advises caution.
Dose adjustments
▸ With intrathecal use Manufacturer advises consider dose reduction.

● **RENAL IMPAIRMENT** Use with caution.
Dose adjustments Lower doses may be required for intrathecal anaesthesia.

● **NATIONAL FUNDING/ACCESS DECISIONS**
PRILOTEKAL ® For full details see funding body website
Scottish Medicines Consortium (SMC) decisions
▸ **Prilocaine hydrochloride (*Prilotekal*®) for spinal anaesthesia (January 2011) SMC No. 665/10 Recommended with restrictions**

● **MEDICINAL FORMS** There can be variation in the licensing of different medicines containing the same drug.
Solution for injection
▸ Prilotekal (B.Braun Medical Ltd)
  Prilocaine hydrochloride 20 mg per 1 ml Prilotekal 100mg/5ml solution for injection ampoules | 10 ampoule [PoM] £78.75 (Hospital only)

Prilocaine with felypressin

The properties listed below are those particular to the combination only. For the properties of the components please consider, prilocaine hydrochloride p. 1551.

- **INDICATIONS AND DOSE**

Dental anaesthesia
- ▶ BY REGIONAL ADMINISTRATION
- ▶ Adult: Consult expert dental sources for specific advice

- **SIDE-EFFECTS** Bradycardia · cardiac arrest · dizziness · drowsiness · hypotension · loss of consciousness · methaemoglobinaemia · myocardial contractility decreased · nervousness · respiratory arrest · seizure · tremor · vision blurred

- **MEDICINAL FORMS** There can be variation in the licensing of different medicines containing the same drug.

Solution for injection
- ▶ Citanest with Octapressin (Dentsply Ltd)
  Felypressin 540 nanogram per 1 ml, Prilocaine hydrochloride 30 mg per 1 ml Citanest 3% with Octapressin Dental 1.19micrograms/2.2ml solution for injection cartridges | 50 cartridge PoM ⓢ

Ropivacaine hydrochloride

09-Dec-2019

- **INDICATIONS AND DOSE**

Acute pain, peripheral nerve block
- ▶ BY REGIONAL ADMINISTRATION
- ▶ Adult: 10–20 mg/hour, dose administered as a continuous infusion or by intermittent injection using a 2 mg/mL (0.2%) solution

Acute pain, field block
- ▶ BY REGIONAL ADMINISTRATION
- ▶ Adult: 2–200 mg, dose administered using a 2 mg/mL (0.2%) solution

Acute pain, lumbar epidural block
- ▶ BY LUMBAR EPIDURAL
- ▶ Adult: 20–40 mg, followed by 20–30 mg at least every 30 minutes, dose administered using a 2 mg/mL (0.2%) solution

Acute labour pain
- ▶ BY CONTINUOUS EPIDURAL INFUSION
- ▶ Adult: 12–20 mg/hour, dose administered using a 2 mg/mL (0.2%) solution

Acute postoperative pain
- ▶ BY CONTINUOUS EPIDURAL INFUSION
- ▶ Adult: Up to 28 mg/hour, dose administered using a 2 mg/mL (0.2%) solution

Postoperative pain, thoracic epidural block
- ▶ BY CONTINUOUS EPIDURAL INFUSION
- ▶ Adult: 12–28 mg/hour, dose administered using a 2 mg/mL (0.2%) solution

Surgical anaesthesia, field block
- ▶ BY REGIONAL ADMINISTRATION
- ▶ Adult: 7.5–225 mg, dose administered using a 7.5 mg/mL (0.75%) solution

Surgical anaesthesia, major nerve block (brachial plexus block)
- ▶ BY REGIONAL ADMINISTRATION
- ▶ Adult: 225–300 mg, dose administered using a 7.5 mg/mL (0.75%) solution

Surgical anaesthesia, thoracic epidural block (to establish block for postoperative pain)
- ▶ BY THORACIC EPIDURAL
- ▶ Adult: 38–113 mg, dose administered using a 7.5 mg/mL (0.75%) solution

Surgical anaesthesia for caesarean section
- ▶ BY LUMBAR EPIDURAL
- ▶ Adult: 113–150 mg, to be administered in incremental doses using a 7.5 mg/mL (0.75%) solution

Surgical anaesthesia, lumbar epidural block
- ▶ BY LUMBAR EPIDURAL
- ▶ Adult: 113–200 mg, dose administered using a 7.5 mg/mL (0.75%) or 10 mg/mL (1%) solution

DOSES AT EXTREMES OF BODY-WEIGHT
- ▶ To avoid excessive dosage in obese patients, dose may need to be calculated on the basis of ideal bodyweight.

IMPORTANT SAFETY INFORMATION
Should only be administered by, or under the direct supervision of, personnel experienced in their use, with adequate training in anaesthesia and airway management, and should not be administered parenterally unless adequate resuscitation equipment is available.

- **CONTRA-INDICATIONS** Avoid injection into infected tissues · avoid injection into inflamed tissues · intravenous regional anaesthesia (Bier's block) · preparations containing preservatives should not be used for caudal, epidural, or spinal block

CONTRA-INDICATIONS, FURTHER INFORMATION
- ▶ Injection site Manufacturer advises local anaesthetics should not be injected into inflamed or infected tissues. Increased absorption into the blood increases the possibility of systemic side-effects, and the local anaesthetic effect may also be reduced by altered local pH.

- **CAUTIONS** Acute porphyrias p. 1202 · cardiovascular disease · complete heart block · debilitated patients (consider dose reduction) · elderly (consider dose reduction) · epilepsy · hypovolaemia · impaired cardiac conduction · impaired respiratory function · myasthenia gravis · shock

- **INTERACTIONS** → Appendix 1: anaesthetics, local

- **SIDE-EFFECTS**
- ▶ **Common or very common** Arrhythmias · back pain · chills · dizziness · headache · hypertension · hypotension · nausea · sensation abnormal · urinary retention · vomiting
- ▶ **Uncommon** Anxiety · dyspnoea · hypothermia · neurotoxicity · syncope
- ▶ **Rare or very rare** Cardiac arrest
- ▶ **Frequency not known** Dyskinesia

SIDE-EFFECTS, FURTHER INFORMATION Toxic effects after administration of local anaesthetics are a result of excessively high plasma concentrations; severe toxicity usually results from inadvertent intravascular injection. The systemic toxicity of local anaesthetics mainly involves the central nervous and cardiovascular systems. The onset of toxicity can be unpredictable and delayed. Monitor as per local protocol for at least 30 minutes after administration.

- **ALLERGY AND CROSS-SENSITIVITY**
- ▶ Hypersensitivity and cross-sensitivity Hypersensitivity reactions occur mainly with the ester-type local anaesthetics, such as tetracaine; reactions are less frequent with the amide types, such as articaine, bupivacaine, levobupivacaine, lidocaine, mepivacaine, prilocaine, and ropivacaine. Cross-sensitivity reactions may be avoided by using the alternative chemical type.

- **PREGNANCY** Not known to be harmful. Do not use for paracervical block in obstetrics.

- **BREAST FEEDING** Not known to be harmful.

- **HEPATIC IMPAIRMENT** Manufacturer advises caution in severe impairment.

Dose adjustments Manufacturer advises consider dose reduction for repeat doses in severe impairment.

● **RENAL IMPAIRMENT** Caution in severe impairment. Increased risk of systemic toxicity in chronic renal failure.

● **MEDICINAL FORMS** There can be variation in the licensing of different medicines containing the same drug.

Solution for injection

ELECTROLYTES: May contain Sodium

▸ **Ropivacaine hydrochloride (Non-proprietary)**

Ropivacaine hydrochloride 2 mg per 1 ml Ropivacaine 20mg/10ml solution for injection ampoules | 5 ampoule [PoM] £13.10–£27.84 (Hospital only)

Ropivacaine hydrochloride 7.5 mg per 1 ml Ropivacaine 75mg/10ml solution for injection ampoules | 5 ampoule [PoM] £15.90–£20.40 (Hospital only)

Ropivacaine hydrochloride 10 mg per 1 ml Ropivacaine 100mg/10ml solution for injection ampoules | 5 ampoule [PoM] £15.87–£22.70 (Hospital only)

▸ **Naropin** (Aspen Pharma Trading Ltd)

Ropivacaine hydrochloride 2 mg per 1 ml Naropin 20mg/10ml solution for injection ampoules | 5 ampoule [PoM] £12.79 (Hospital only)

Infusion

ELECTROLYTES: May contain Sodium

▸ **Ropivacaine hydrochloride (Non-proprietary)**

Ropivacaine hydrochloride 2 mg per 1 ml Ropivacaine 400mg/200ml infusion bags | 5 bag [PoM] £78.50–£108.50 (Hospital only)

Tetracaine

(Amethocaine)

11-Nov-2021

● **INDICATIONS AND DOSE**

Anaesthesia before venepuncture or venous cannulation

▸ TO THE SKIN

▸ Child 1 month–4 years: Apply contents of up to 1 tube (applied at separate sites at a single time or appropriate proportion) to site of venepuncture or venous cannulation and cover with occlusive dressing; remove gel and dressing after 30 minutes for venepuncture and after 45 minutes for venous cannulation

▸ Child 5–17 years: Apply contents of up to 5 tubes (applied at separate sites at a single time or appropriate proportion) to site of venepuncture or venous cannulation and cover with occlusive dressing; remove gel and dressing after 30 minutes for venepuncture and after 45 minutes for venous cannulation

▸ Adult: Apply contents of up to 5 tubes (applied at separate sites at a single time or appropriate proportion) to site of venepuncture or venous cannulation and cover with occlusive dressing; remove gel and dressing after 30 minutes for venepuncture and after 45 minutes for venous cannulation

● **CONTRA-INDICATIONS** Should not be applied to damaged skin

● **INTERACTIONS** → Appendix 1: anaesthetics, local

● **SIDE-EFFECTS** Oedema · skin reactions

SIDE-EFFECTS, FURTHER INFORMATION The systemic toxicity of local anaesthetics mainly involves the central nervous system; systemic side effects unlikely as minimal absorption following topical application.

● **ALLERGY AND CROSS-SENSITIVITY**

▸ Hypersensitivity and cross-sensitivity Hypersensitivity reactions occur mainly with the ester-type local anaesthetics, such as tetracaine; reactions are less frequent with the amide types, such as articaine, bupivacaine, levobupivacaine, lidocaine, mepivacaine, prilocaine, and ropivacaine. Cross-sensitivity reactions may be avoided by using the alternative chemical type.

● **BREAST FEEDING** Not known to be harmful.

● **PATIENT AND CARER ADVICE**

Medicines for Children leaflet: Tetracaine gel for local anaesthesia www.medicinesforchildren.org.uk/medicines/tetracaine-gel-for-local-anaesthesia/

● **MEDICINAL FORMS** There can be variation in the licensing of different medicines containing the same drug.

Cutaneous gel

EXCIPIENTS: May contain Hydroxybenzoates (parabens)

▸ **Ametop** (Alliance Pharmaceuticals Ltd)

Tetracaine 40 mg per 1 gram Ametop 4% gel | 1.5 gram [P] £1.20 DT = £1.20

Chapter 16
Emergency treatment of poisoning

CONTENTS

Poisoning, emergency treatment

01-Mar-2024

Overview

These notes provide only an overview of the treatment of poisoning, and it is strongly recommended that either **TOXBASE** or the **UK National Poisons Information Service** be consulted when there is doubt about the degree of risk or about management.

Hospital admission

Patients who have features of poisoning should generally be admitted to hospital. Patients who have taken poisons with delayed action should also be admitted, even if they appear well. Delayed-action poisons include aspirin p. 142, iron, paracetamol p. 507, tricyclic antidepressants, and co-phenotrope p. 73 (diphenoxylate with atropine, *Lomotil*®); the effects of modified-release preparations are also delayed. A note of all relevant information, including what treatment has been given, should accompany the patient to hospital.

Further information

TOXBASE, the primary clinical toxicology database of the National Poisons Information Service, is available on the internet to registered users at www.toxbase.org (a backup site is available at www.toxbasebackup.org if the main site cannot be accessed). It provides information about routine diagnosis, treatment, and management of patients exposed to drugs, household products, and industrial and agricultural chemicals.

Specialist information and advice on the treatment of poisoning is available day and night from the **UK National Poisons Information Service** on the following number: Tel: 0344 892 0111.

Advice on laboratory analytical services can be obtained from TOXBASE or from the National Poisons Information Service. Help with identifying capsules or tablets may be available from a regional medicines information centre or from the National Poisons Information Service (out of hours).

Storage of specialist antidotes

Due to the risk of unintended administration, NHS England advises emergency departments and pharmacies to ensure that 'specialist antidotes' are stored either in automatic dispensing cabinets/systems, or in a separate area specifically designated for antidotes. Those requiring refrigeration should be separated from other medicines in the medication fridge and clearly identified as antidotes. If 'specialist antidotes' are kept in the emergency/out-of-hours medicine cupboards, they should be separated from other medicines and clearly identified as antidotes.

'Specialist antidotes' are defined as those on the **Royal College of Emergency Medicine/ UK National Poisons Information Service** list (available at www.npis.org/Publications.html) and only used in emergency departments as a specific antidote.

General care

It is often impossible to establish with certainty the identity of the poison and the size of the dose. This is not usually important because only a few poisons (such as opioids, paracetamol, and iron) have specific antidotes; few patients require active removal of the poison. In most patients, treatment is directed at managing symptoms as they arise. Nevertheless, knowledge of the type and timing of poisoning can help in anticipating the course of events. All relevant information should be sought from the poisoned individual and from carers or parents. However, such information should be interpreted with care because it may not be complete or entirely reliable. Sometimes symptoms arise from other illnesses and patients should be assessed carefully. Accidents may involve domestic and industrial products (the contents of which are not generally known). The **National Poisons Information Service** should be consulted when there is doubt about any aspect of suspected poisoning.

Respiration

Respiration is often impaired in unconscious patients. An obstructed airway requires immediate attention. In the absence of trauma, the airway should be opened with simple measures such as chin lift or jaw thrust. An oropharyngeal or nasopharyngeal airway may be useful in patients with reduced consciousness to prevent obstruction, provided ventilation is adequate. Intubation and ventilation should be considered in patients whose airway cannot be protected or who have respiratory acidosis because of inadequate ventilation; such patients should be monitored in a critical care area.

Most poisons that impair consciousness also depress respiration. Assisted ventilation (either mouth-to-mouth or using a bag-valve-mask device) may be needed. Oxygen is not a substitute for adequate ventilation, although it should be given in the highest concentration possible in poisoning with carbon monoxide and irritant gases.

Blood pressure

Hypotension is common in severe poisoning with central nervous system depressants. A systolic blood pressure of less than 70 mmHg may lead to irreversible brain damage or renal tubular necrosis. Hypotension should be corrected initially by raising the foot of the bed and administration of an infusion of either sodium chloride p. 1180 or a colloid. Vasoconstrictor sympathomimetics are rarely required and their use may be discussed with the National Poisons Information Service.

Fluid depletion without hypotension is common after prolonged coma and after aspirin poisoning due to vomiting, sweating, and hyperpnoea.

Hypertension, often transient, occurs less frequently than hypotension in poisoning; it may be associated with sympathomimetic drugs such as amfetamines, phencyclidine, and cocaine.

Heart

Cardiac conduction defects and arrhythmias can occur in acute poisoning, notably with tricyclic antidepressants, some antipsychotics, and some antihistamines. Arrhythmias often respond to correction of underlying hypoxia, acidosis, or other biochemical abnormalities, but ventricular arrhythmias that cause serious hypotension require treatment. If the QT interval is prolonged, specialist advice should be sought because the use of some anti-arrhythmic drugs may be inappropriate. Supraventricular arrhythmias are seldom life-threatening and drug treatment is best withheld until the patient reaches hospital.

Body temperature

Hypothermia may develop in patients of any age who have been deeply unconscious for some hours, particularly following overdose with barbiturates or phenothiazines. It may be missed unless core temperature is measured using a low-reading rectal thermometer or by some other means. Hypothermia should be managed by prevention of further heat loss and appropriate re-warming as clinically indicated.

Hyperthermia can develop in patients taking CNS stimulants; children and the elderly are also at risk when taking therapeutic doses of drugs with antimuscarinic properties. Hyperthermia is initially managed by removing all unnecessary clothing and using a fan. Sponging with **tepid** water will promote evaporation. Advice should be sought from the National Poisons Information Service on the management of severe hyperthermia resulting from conditions such as the serotonin syndrome.

Both hypothermia and hyperthermia require **urgent** hospitalisation for assessment and supportive treatment.

Convulsions during poisoning

Single short-lived convulsions (lasting less than 5 minutes) do not require treatment. If convulsions are protracted or recur frequently, lorazepam p. 393 or diazepam p. 398 (preferably as emulsion) should be given by slow intravenous injection into a large vein. Benzodiazepines should not be given by the intramuscular route for convulsions. If the intravenous route is not readily available, midazolam p. 394 oromucosal solution [unlicensed use in adults and children under 3 months] can be given by the buccal route or diazepam p. 398 can be administered as a rectal solution.

Methaemoglobinaemia

Drug- or chemical-induced methaemoglobinaemia should be treated with methylthioninium chloride p. 1567 if the methaemoglobin concentration is 30% or higher, *or* if symptoms of tissue hypoxia are present despite oxygen therapy. Methylthioninium chloride reduces the ferric iron of methaemoglobin back to the ferrous iron of haemoglobin; in high doses, methylthioninium chloride can itself cause methaemoglobinaemia.

Poison removal and elimination

Prevention of absorption

Given by mouth, charcoal, activated p. 1561 can bind many poisons in the gastro-intestinal system, thereby reducing their absorption. The **sooner** it is given the **more effective** it is, but it may still be effective up to 1 hour after ingestion of the poison—longer in the case of modified-release preparations or of drugs with antimuscarinic (anticholinergic) properties. It is particularly useful for the prevention of absorption of poisons that are toxic in small amounts, such as antidepressants.

Active elimination techniques

Repeated doses of charcoal, activated by mouth *enhance the elimination* of some drugs after they have been absorbed; repeated doses are given after overdosage with:

- Carbamazepine
- Dapsone
- Phenobarbital
- Quinine
- Theophylline

If vomiting occurs after dosing it should be treated (e.g. with an antiemetic drug) since it may reduce the efficacy of charcoal treatment. In cases of intolerance, the dose may be reduced and the frequency increased but this may compromise efficacy.

Charcoal, activated should **not** be used for poisoning with petroleum distillates, corrosive substances, alcohols, malathion, cyanides and metal salts including iron and lithium salts.

Other techniques intended to enhance the elimination of poisons after absorption are only practicable in hospital and are only suitable for a small number of severely poisoned patients. Moreover, they only apply to a limited number of poisons. Examples include:

- haemodialysis for ethylene glycol, lithium, methanol, phenobarbital, salicylates, and sodium valproate;
- alkalinisation of the urine for salicylates.

Removal from the gastro-intestinal tract

Gastric lavage is rarely required; for substances that cannot be removed effectively by other means (e.g. iron), it should be considered only if a life-threatening amount has been ingested within the previous hour. It should be carried out only if the airway can be protected adequately. Gastric lavage is contra-indicated if a corrosive substance or a petroleum distillate has been ingested, but it may occasionally be considered in patients who have ingested drugs that are not adsorbed by charcoal, such as iron or lithium. Induction of *emesis* (e.g. with ipecacuanha) is **not** recommended because there is no evidence that it affects absorption and it may increase the risk of aspiration.

Whole bowel irrigation (by means of a bowel cleansing preparation) has been used in poisoning with certain modified-release or enteric-coated formulations, in severe poisoning with iron and lithium salts, and if illicit drugs are carried in the gastro-intestinal tract ('body-packing'). However, it is not clear that the procedure improves outcome and advice should be sought from the National Poisons Information Service.

Alcohol, acute intoxication

Acute intoxication with alcohol (ethanol) is common in adults but also occurs in children. The features include ataxia, dysarthria, nystagmus, and drowsiness, which may progress to coma, with hypotension and acidosis. Aspiration of vomit is a special hazard and hypoglycaemia may occur in children and some adults. Patients are managed supportively, with particular attention to maintaining a clear airway and measures to reduce the risk of aspiration of gastric contents. The blood glucose is measured and glucose given if indicated.

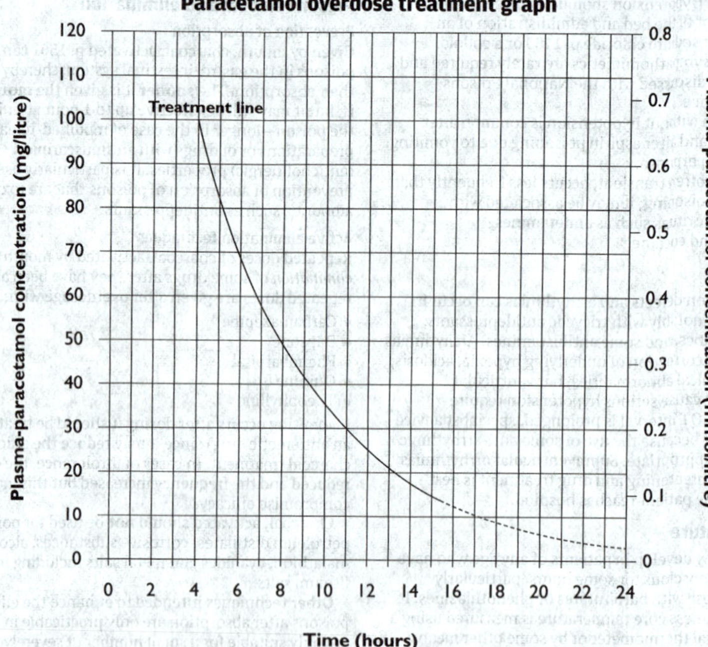

Paracetamol overdose treatment graph

Patients whose plasma-paracetamol concentrations are on or above the **treatment line** should be treated with acetylcysteine by intravenous infusion.

The prognostic accuracy after 15 hours is uncertain, but a plasma-paracetamol concentration on or above the treatment line should be regarded as carrying a serious risk of liver damage.

Graph reproduced courtesy of Medicines and Healthcare products Regulatory Agency

Aspirin poisoning

The main features of salicylate poisoning are hyperventilation, tinnitus, deafness, vasodilatation, and sweating. Coma is uncommon but indicates very severe poisoning. The associated acid-base disturbances are complex.

Treatment must be in hospital, where plasma salicylate, pH, and electrolytes can be measured; absorption of aspirin may be slow and the plasma-salicylate concentration may continue to rise for several hours, requiring repeated measurement. Plasma-salicylate concentration may not correlate with clinical severity in the young and the elderly, and clinical and biochemical assessment is necessary. Generally, the clinical severity of poisoning is less below a plasma-salicylate concentration of 500 mg/litre (3.6 mmol/litre), unless there is evidence of metabolic acidosis. Activated charcoal can be given within 1 hour of ingesting more than 125 mg/kg of aspirin. Fluid losses should be replaced and intravenous sodium bicarbonate may be given (ensuring plasma-potassium concentration is within the reference range) to enhance urinary salicylate excretion (optimum urinary pH 7.5–8.5).

Plasma-potassium concentration should be corrected before giving sodium bicarbonate as hypokalaemia may complicate alkalinisation of the urine.

Haemodialysis is the treatment of choice for severe salicylate poisoning and should be considered when the plasma-salicylate concentration exceeds 700 mg/litre (5.1 mmol/litre) or in the presence of severe metabolic acidosis.

Opioid poisoning

Opioids (narcotic analgesics) cause coma, respiratory depression, and pinpoint pupils. The specific antidote naloxone hydrochloride p. 1564 is indicated if there is coma or bradypnoea. Since naloxone has a shorter duration of action than many opioids, close monitoring and repeated injections are necessary according to the respiratory rate and depth of coma. When repeated administration of naloxone is required, it can be given by continuous intravenous infusion instead and the rate of infusion adjusted according to vital signs. The effects of some opioids, such as buprenorphine, are only partially reversed by naloxone. Dextropropoxyphene and methadone have very long durations of action; patients may need to be monitored for long periods following large overdoses.

Naloxone reverses the opioid effects of dextropropoxyphene. The long duration of action of dextropropoxyphene calls for prolonged monitoring and further doses of naloxone may be required. Norpropoxyphene, a metabolite of dextropropoxyphene, also has cardiotoxic effects which may require treatment with sodium bicarbonate p. 1178 or magnesium sulfate p. 1193, or both. Arrhythmias may occur for up to 12 hours.

Paracetamol poisoning

In all cases of **intravenous paracetamol poisoning** clinicians are encouraged to contact the National Poisons Information Service for advice on risk assessment and management.

Toxic doses of paracetamol p. 507 may cause severe hepatocellular necrosis and, much less frequently, renal tubular necrosis. Nausea and vomiting, the early features of poisoning, usually settle within 24 hours. The recurrence of nausea and vomiting after 2–3 days, often associated with the onset of right subcostal pain and tenderness, usually indicates development of hepatic necrosis. Liver damage is maximal 3–4 days after paracetamol overdose and may lead to liver failure, encephalopathy, coma, and death.

The following guidance provides only an overview of the management of paracetamol overdosage from the *National Poisons Information Service TOXBASE* database.

To avoid underestimating the potentially toxic paracetamol dose ingested by obese patients who weigh more than 110 kg, use a body-weight of 110 kg (rather than their actual body-weight) when calculating the total dose of paracetamol ingested (in mg/kg).

For pregnant patients the potentially toxic paracetamol dose should be calculated using the patient's pre-pregnancy weight.

Acetylcysteine p. 1566 prevents or reduces the severity of liver damage if given up to, and possibly beyond (in patients at risk of severe liver disease) 24 hours of ingesting paracetamol. It is most effective if given within 8 hours of paracetamol ingestion, after which effectiveness declines. Very rarely, giving acetylcysteine by mouth [unlicensed] is an alternative if intravenous access is not possible (for further information, see **Acetylcysteine—oral doses**, available from TOXBASE).

Acute overdose

Acute overdose involves ingestion of a potentially toxic dose of paracetamol p. 507 in 1 hour or less.

For **adults and children aged 6 years and over**, serious toxicity is unlikely to occur from a single ingestion of less than 75 mg/kg of paracetamol taken in less than 1 hour. Refer patients to hospital for medical assessment if they meet any of the following criteria:

- have ingested paracetamol in the context of self-harm,
- are symptomatic,
- have ingested 75 mg/kg or more of paracetamol in 1 hour or less, or
- where the time of ingestion is uncertain but the dose ingested is 75 mg/kg or more.

For **children aged under 6 years**, serious toxicity is unlikely to occur from a single ingestion of less than 150 mg/kg of paracetamol taken in less than 1 hour. Refer children to hospital for medical assessment if they meet any of the following criteria:

- are symptomatic,
- have ingested 150 mg/kg or more of paracetamol in 1 hour or less, or
- where there is uncertainty about the dose ingested or circumstance of ingestion.

Although the benefit of gastric decontamination is uncertain, charcoal, activated p. 1561 should be considered if the patient presents within 1 hour of ingesting paracetamol in excess of 150 mg/kg.

Patients at risk of liver damage and therefore requiring acetylcysteine, can be identified from a single measurement of the plasma-paracetamol concentration related to the time from ingestion, provided this time interval is not less than 4 hours; earlier samples cannot be interpreted. The concentration is plotted on a paracetamol treatment graph, with a reference line ('treatment line') joining plots of 100 mg/litre (0.66 mmol/litre) at 4 hours and 3.13 mg/litre (0.02 mmol/litre) at 24 hours, see *Paracetamol overdose treatment graph*.

Acetylcysteine treatment should commence in patients:

- whose plasma-paracetamol concentration falls on or above the *treatment line* on the paracetamol treatment graph;
- who present within 8 hours of ingestion of more than 150 mg/kg of paracetamol if there is going to be a delay of

8 hours or more in obtaining the paracetamol concentration after the overdose;

- who present 8–24 hours after ingestion of an acute overdose of more than 150 mg/kg of paracetamol or the amount ingested is unknown, or if the patient is symptomatic with jaundice or hepatic tenderness, even if the plasma-paracetamol concentration is not yet available;
- who present more than 24 hours after ingestion of an overdose of more than 150 mg/kg of paracetamol or the amount ingested is unknown, or if they are clearly jaundiced or have hepatic tenderness, or the paracetamol concentration is detectable.
- whose biochemical tests suggest acute liver injury, such as ALT above the upper limit of normal (patients with chronically elevated ALT should be discussed with the National Poisons Information Service), or INR greater than 1.3 (in the absence of another cause), even if the plasma paracetamol concentration is below the treatment line on the paracetamol overdose treatment graph.

If the patient is not at risk of liver toxicity (i.e. the paracetamol concentration is below the treatment line or undetectable; the INR and ALT are normal; and the patient is asymptomatic) no treatment with an antidote is indicated; acetylcysteine may be discontinued if it has been started.

Where the time of ingestion is unknown, patients should be managed as a *staggered overdose*.

Therapeutic excess or staggered overdose

Patients who have ingested more than 150 mg/kg of paracetamol in any 24-hour period are at risk of serious toxicity. Toxicity rarely occurs with paracetamol doses between 75–150 mg/kg in any 24-hour period. Doses consistently less than 75 mg/kg in any 24-hour period are very unlikely to be toxic; however risk may be increased if this dose is repeatedly ingested over 2 or more days. Ingestion of a licensed dose of paracetamol is not considered an overdose.

Therapeutic excess is the ingestion of a potentially toxic dose of paracetamol with intent to treat pain or fever and without self-harm intent during its clinical use. All patients should be referred to hospital for medical assessment if they meet any of the following criteria:

- are symptomatic,
- have ingested more than a licensed dose and more than or equal to 75 mg/kg in any 24-hour period, or
- have ingested more than the licensed dose but less than 75 mg/kg/24 hours on each day of the last 72 hours.

Patients with clinical features of hepatic injury such as jaundice or hepatic tenderness should be treated urgently with acetylcysteine. For other patients, management is determined by the maximum dose of paracetamol ingested in any 24-hour period (for further information, see **Paracetamol—therapeutic excess**, available from TOXBASE).

Asymptomatic patients who present more than 7 days after the last dose of paracetamol was ingested, who have had no new symptoms since the time of ingestion, and who have no history of chronic kidney or liver disease, will not normally require further assessment, providing the timing of ingestion is certain.

When there is uncertainty about whether the presentation was due to therapeutic excess, the patient should be managed as a *staggered overdose*.

A **staggered overdose** involves ingestion of a potentially toxic dose of paracetamol over more than 1 hour, with the possible intention of causing self-harm. All patients who have taken a staggered overdose should be referred to hospital for medical assessment. The MHRA advises that all patients who have ingested a staggered overdose should be treated with acetylcysteine without delay.

Clinically significant hepatotoxicity is unlikely and the patient is not considered to be at risk if, after at least 4 hours or more since the last paracetamol ingestion, the patient has no symptoms suggesting liver damage, the paracetamol concentration is less than 10 mg/L, their ALT is within the normal range, and their INR is 1.3 or less. Acetylcysteine can be discontinued in patients not considered to be at risk of clinically significant liver damage. If there is uncertainty about a patient's risk of toxicity after paracetamol overdose, advice should be sought from the National Poisons Information Service.

Acetylcysteine dose and administration
For paracetamol overdosage, there are two intravenous acetylcysteine regimens: the standard 21-hour regimen and the modified 12-hour regimen (also known as the Scottish and Newcastle Acetylcysteine Protocol (SNAP)). The SNAP regimen [unlicensed] is not endorsed by the MHRA, but it is recommended by the Royal College of Emergency Medicine and the National Poisons Information Service. For further information, see acetylcysteine p. 1566, **Acetylcysteine SNAP Doses—Adult**, **Acetylcysteine SNAP Doses—Children** and **Paracetamol - Guidance for the end of the modified 12-hour IV acetylcysteine regimen (SNAP)**, available from TOXBASE.

For the standard 21-hour regimen, acetylcysteine is given in a total dose that is divided into 3 consecutive intravenous infusions over a total of 21 hours. For information on dosing/administration for adults and children, see acetylcysteine, **Acetylcysteine Doses** and **Paracetamol - Guidance for the end of the standard 21-hour IV acetylcysteine regimen**, available from TOXBASE.

Antidepressant poisoning

Tricyclic and related antidepressants
Tricyclic and related antidepressants cause dry mouth, coma of varying degree, hypotension, hypothermia, hyperreflexia, extensor plantar responses, convulsions, respiratory failure, cardiac conduction defects, and arrhythmias. Dilated pupils and urinary retention also occur. Metabolic acidosis may complicate severe poisoning; delirium with confusion, agitation, and visual and auditory hallucinations are common during recovery.

Assessment in hospital is strongly advised in case of poisoning by tricyclic and related antidepressants but symptomatic treatment can be given before transfer. Supportive measures to ensure a clear airway and adequate ventilation during transfer are mandatory. Intravenous lorazepam or intravenous diazepam (preferably in emulsion form) may be required to treat convulsions. Activated charcoal given within 1 hour of the overdose reduces absorption of the drug. Although arrhythmias are worrying, some will respond to correction of hypoxia and acidosis. The use of anti-arrhythmic drugs is best avoided, but intravenous infusion of sodium bicarbonate can arrest arrhythmias or prevent them in those with an extended QRS duration. Diazepam given by mouth is usually adequate to sedate delirious patients but large doses may be required.

Selective serotonin re-uptake inhibitors (SSRIs)
Symptoms of poisoning by selective serotonin re-uptake inhibitors include nausea, vomiting, agitation, tremor, nystagmus, drowsiness, and sinus tachycardia; convulsions may occur. Rarely, severe poisoning results in the serotonin syndrome, with marked neuropsychiatric effects, neuromuscular hyperactivity, and autonomic instability; hyperthermia, rhabdomyolysis, renal failure, and coagulopathies may develop.

Management of SSRI poisoning is supportive. Activated charcoal given within 1 hour of the overdose reduces absorption of the drug. Convulsions can be treated with lorazepam, diazepam, or midazolam oromucosal solution [unlicensed use in adults and children under 3 months] (see *Convulsions*). Contact the National Poisons Information Service for the management of hyperthermia or the serotonin syndrome.

Antimalarial poisoning
Overdosage with quinine, chloroquine, or hydroxychloroquine is extremely hazardous and difficult to treat. Urgent advice from the National Poisons Information Service is essential. Life-threatening features include arrhythmias (which can have a very rapid onset) and convulsions (which can be intractable).

Antipsychotic poisoning

Phenothiazines and related drugs
Phenothiazines cause less depression of consciousness and respiration than other sedatives. Hypotension, hypothermia, sinus tachycardia, and arrhythmias may complicate poisoning. Dystonic reactions can occur with therapeutic doses (particularly with prochlorperazine and trifluoperazine), and convulsions may occur in severe cases. Arrhythmias may respond to correction of hypoxia, acidosis, and other biochemical abnormalities, but specialist advice should be sought if arrhythmias result from a prolonged QT interval; the use of some anti-arrhythmic drugs can worsen such arrhythmias. Dystonic reactions are rapidly abolished by injection of drugs such as procyclidine hydrochloride p. 472 or diazepam p. 398 (emulsion preferred).

Second-generation antipsychotic drugs
Features of poisoning by second-generation antipsychotic drugs include drowsiness, convulsions, extrapyramidal symptoms, hypotension, and ECG abnormalities (including prolongation of the QT interval). Management is supportive. Charcoal, activated p. 1561 can be given within 1 hour of ingesting a significant quantity of a second-generation antipsychotic drug.

Benzodiazepine poisoning
Benzodiazepines taken alone cause drowsiness, ataxia, dysarthria, nystagmus, and occasionally respiratory depression, and coma. Charcoal, activated can be given within 1 hour of ingesting a significant quantity of benzodiazepine, provided the patient is awake and the airway is protected. Benzodiazepines potentiate the effects of other central nervous system depressants taken concomitantly. Use of the benzodiazepine antagonist flumazenil p. 1563 [unlicensed indication] can be hazardous, particularly in mixed overdoses involving tricyclic antidepressants or in benzodiazepine-dependent patients. Flumazenil may prevent the need for ventilation, particularly in patients with severe respiratory disorders; it should be used on expert advice only and not as a diagnostic test in patients with a reduced level of consciousness.

Beta-blockers poisoning
Overdosages with beta-blockers may cause cardiac effects such as bradycardia, hypotension, syncope, conduction abnormalities, and heart failure. Bradycardia is the most common arrhythmia, but some beta-blockers may induce ventricular tachyarrhythmias secondary to prolongation of QT interval (e.g. sotalol) or QRS duration (e.g. propranolol). Although the predominant effects of beta-blocker overdose are on the heart, other features may also occur, such as central nervous system effects (including drowsiness, confusion, convulsions, hallucinations, and in severe cases coma), respiratory depression, and bronchospasm. The effects of overdosage can vary from one beta-blocker to another; propranolol overdosage in particular may cause coma and convulsions.

The following guidance provides only an overview of the management of beta-blocker overdosage from the *National Poisons Information Service TOXBASE database*.

All patients who have been exposed to beta-blockers as a result of self-harm should be referred for assessment. Medical assessment is recommended for all patients who are symptomatic or have ingested more than a toxic dose; and in those who are treatment naive or have taken more than their therapeutic dose, and have a significant cardiac history, asthma, chronic obstructive pulmonary disease, or are elderly. All patients who have exceeded their prescribed daily dose of 2 or more cardiotoxic agents should also be referred for medical assessment irrespective of the dose ingested. Hospital clinicians are encouraged to discuss all serious cases with the UK National Poisons Information Service.

For patients presenting with overdose, maintain a clear airway and adequate ventilation. Although the benefit of gastric decontamination is uncertain, charcoal, activated p. 1561 can be considered if the patient presents within 1 hour of ingestion of more than a potentially toxic dose.

For the management of hypotension, ensure adequate fluid resuscitation; in an emergency, vasopressors and inotropes can be initiated under the advice of an experienced physician. Intravenous glucagon p. 845 [unlicensed] is a treatment option for severe hypotension, heart failure, or cardiogenic shock. In severe cases, an insulin and glucose infusion can improve myocardial contractility and systemic perfusion, especially in the presence of acidosis. Consider intravenous sodium bicarbonate p. 1178 for correction of metabolic acidosis that persists despite correction of hypoxia and adequate fluid resuscitation—rapid correction is particularly important if QRS duration is prolonged. For symptomatic bradycardia, give intravenous atropine sulfate p. 1526; dobutamine p. 215 [unlicensed] or isoprenaline [unlicensed] (available from 'special-order' manufacturers or specialist importing companies) may be considered if bradycardia is associated with hypotension. A temporary cardiac pacemaker can be used to increase the heart rate.

Treat bronchospasm with nebulised bronchodilators and corticosteroids.

If convulsions occur give oxygen, and correct acid-base and metabolic disturbances as required. Prolonged or frequent convulsions should be controlled with intravenous diazepam p. 398, lorazepam p. 393, or midazolam p. 394. If convulsions are unresponsive to treatment, the patient should be referred urgently to critical care.

Calcium-channel blockers poisoning

Features of calcium-channel blocker poisoning include nausea, vomiting, dizziness, agitation, confusion, and coma in severe poisoning. Metabolic acidosis and hyperglycaemia may occur. Verapamil and diltiazem have a profound cardiac depressant effect causing hypotension and arrhythmias, including complete heart block and asystole. The dihydropyridine calcium-channel blockers cause severe hypotension secondary to profound peripheral vasodilatation.

Charcoal, activated should be considered if the patient presents within 1 hour of overdosage with a calcium-channel blocker; repeated doses of activated charcoal are considered if a modified-release preparation is involved. In patients with significant features of poisoning, calcium chloride p. 1188 or calcium gluconate p. 1189 is given by injection; atropine sulfate is given to correct symptomatic bradycardia. In severe cases, an insulin and glucose infusion may be required in the management of hypotension and myocardial failure. For the management of hypotension, the choice of inotropic sympathomimetic depends on whether hypotension is secondary to vasodilatation or to myocardial depression—advice should be sought from the National Poisons Information Service.

Iron salts poisoning

Iron poisoning in childhood is usually accidental. The symptoms are nausea, vomiting, abdominal pain, diarrhoea, haematemesis, and rectal bleeding. Hypotension and hepatocellular necrosis can occur later. Coma, shock, and metabolic acidosis indicate severe poisoning.

Advice should be sought from the National Poisons Information Service if a significant quantity of iron has been ingested within the previous hour.

Mortality is reduced by intensive and specific therapy with desferrioxamine mesilate p. 1165, which chelates iron. The serum-iron concentration is measured as an emergency and intravenous desferrioxamine mesilate given to chelate absorbed iron in excess of the expected iron binding capacity. In severe toxicity intravenous desferrioxamine mesilate should be given immediately without waiting for the result of the serum-iron measurement.

Lithium poisoning

Most cases of lithium intoxication occur as a complication of long-term therapy and are caused by reduced excretion of the drug because of a variety of factors including dehydration, deterioration of renal function, infections, and co-administration of diuretics or NSAIDs (or other drugs that interact). Acute deliberate overdoses may also occur with delayed onset of symptoms (12 hours or more) owing to slow entry of lithium into the tissues and continuing absorption from modified-release formulations.

The early clinical features are non-specific and may include apathy and restlessness which could be confused with mental changes arising from the patient's depressive illness. Vomiting, diarrhoea, ataxia, weakness, dysarthria, muscle twitching, and tremor may follow. Severe poisoning is associated with convulsions, coma, renal failure, electrolyte imbalance, dehydration, and hypotension.

Therapeutic serum-lithium concentrations are within the range of 0.4–1 mmol/litre; concentrations in excess of 2 mmol/litre are usually associated with serious toxicity and such cases may need treatment with haemodialysis if neurological symptoms or renal failure are present. In acute overdosage much higher serum-lithium concentrations may be present without features of toxicity and all that is usually necessary is to take measures to increase urine output (e.g. by increasing fluid intake but avoiding diuretics). Otherwise, treatment is supportive with special regard to electrolyte balance, renal function, and control of convulsions. Gastric lavage may be considered if it can be performed within 1 hour of ingesting significant quantities of lithium. Whole-bowel irrigation should be considered for significant ingestion, but advice should be sought from the National Poisons Information Service.

Stimulant-drug poisoning

Amfetamines cause wakefulness, excessive activity, paranoia, hallucinations, and hypertension followed by exhaustion, convulsions, hyperthermia, and coma. The early stages can be controlled by diazepam or lorazepam; advice should be sought from the National Poisons Information Service on the management of hypertension. Later, tepid sponging, anticonvulsants, and artificial respiration may be needed.

Cocaine

Cocaine stimulates the central nervous system, causing agitation, dilated pupils, tachycardia, hypertension, hallucinations, hyperthermia, hypertonia, and hyperreflexia; cardiac effects include chest pain, myocardial infarction, and arrhythmias.

Initial treatment of cocaine poisoning involves intravenous administration of diazepam to control agitation and cooling measures for hyperthermia (see *Body temperature*); hypertension and cardiac effects require specific treatment and expert advice should be sought.

Ecstasy

Ecstasy (methylenedioxymethamfetamine, MDMA) may cause severe reactions, even at doses that were previously tolerated. The most serious effects are delirium, coma, convulsions, ventricular arrhythmias, hyperthermia, rhabdomyolysis, acute renal failure, acute hepatitis, disseminated intravascular coagulation, adult respiratory distress syndrome, hyperreflexia, hypotension and intracerebral haemorrhage; hyponatraemia has also been associated with ecstasy use.

Treatment of methylenedioxymethamfetamine poisoning is supportive, with diazepam to control severe agitation or persistent convulsions and close monitoring including ECG. Self-induced water intoxication should be considered in patients with ecstasy poisoning.

'Liquid ecstasy' is a term used for sodium oxybate (gamma-hydroxybutyrate, GHB), which is a sedative.

Theophylline poisoning

Theophylline and related drugs are often prescribed as modified-release formulations and toxicity can therefore be delayed. They cause vomiting (which may be severe and intractable), agitation, restlessness, dilated pupils, sinus tachycardia, and hyperglycaemia. More serious effects are haematemesis, convulsions, and supraventricular and ventricular arrhythmias. Severe hypokalaemia may develop rapidly.

Repeated doses of activated charcoal can be used to eliminate theophylline even if more than 1 hour has elapsed after ingestion and especially if a modified-release preparation has been taken (see also under *Active Elimination Techniques*). Ondansetron p. 497 may be effective for severe vomiting that is resistant to other antiemetics [unlicensed indication]. Hypokalaemia is corrected by intravenous infusion of potassium chloride p. 1201 and may be so severe as to require 60 mmol/hour (high doses require ECG monitoring). Convulsions should be controlled by intravenous administration of lorazepam p. 393 or diazepam p. 398 (see *Convulsions*). Sedation with diazepam may be necessary in agitated patients.

Provided the patient does not suffer from asthma, a short-acting beta-blocker can be administered intravenously to reverse severe tachycardia, hypokalaemia, and hyperglycaemia.

Cyanide poisoning

Oxygen should be administered to patients with cyanide poisoning. The choice of antidote depends on the severity of poisoning, certainty of diagnosis, and the cause. Dicobalt edetate p. 1562 is the antidote of choice when there is a strong clinical suspicion of severe cyanide poisoning, but it should **not** be used as a precautionary measure. Dicobalt edetate itself is toxic, associated with anaphylactoid reactions, and is potentially fatal if administered in the absence of cyanide poisoning. A regimen of sodium nitrite p. 1562 followed by sodium thiosulfate p. 1562 is an alternative if dicobalt edetate is not available.

Hydroxocobalamin p. 1162 (*Cyanokit*®—no other preparation of hydroxocobalamin is suitable) can be considered for use in victims of smoke inhalation who show signs of significant cyanide poisoning.

Ethylene glycol and methanol poisoning

Fomepizole (available from 'special-order' manufacturers or specialist importing companies) is the treatment of choice for ethylene glycol and methanol (methyl alcohol) poisoning. If necessary, **ethanol** (by mouth or by intravenous infusion) can be used, but with caution. Advice on the treatment of ethylene glycol and methanol poisoning should be obtained from the National Poisons Information Service. It is important to start antidote treatment promptly in cases of suspected poisoning with these agents.

Heavy metal poisoning

Heavy metal antidotes include succimer (DMSA) [unlicensed], unithiol (DMPS) [unlicensed], sodium calcium edetate [unlicensed], and dimercaprol. Dimercaprol in the management of heavy metal poisoning has been superseded by other chelating agents. In all cases of heavy metal poisoning, the advice of the National Poisons Information Service should be sought.

Noxious gases poisoning

Carbon monoxide

Carbon monoxide poisoning is usually due to inhalation of smoke, car exhaust, or fumes caused by blocked flues or incomplete combustion of fuel gases in confined spaces.

Immediate treatment of carbon monoxide poisoning is essential. The person should be moved to fresh air, the airway cleared, and high-flow **oxygen** 100% administered through a tight-fitting mask with an inflated face seal. Artificial respiration should be given as necessary and continued until adequate spontaneous breathing starts, or stopped only after persistent and efficient treatment of cardiac arrest has failed. The patient should be admitted to hospital because complications may arise after a delay of hours or days. Cerebral oedema may occur in severe poisoning and is treated with an intravenous infusion of mannitol p. 262. Referral for hyperbaric oxygen treatment should be discussed with the National Poisons Information Service if the patient is pregnant or in cases of severe poisoning, such as if the patient is or has been unconscious, or has psychiatric or neurological features other than a headache, or has myocardial ischaemia or an arrhythmia, or has a blood carboxyhaemoglobin concentration of more than 20%.

Sulfur dioxide, chlorine, phosgene, and ammonia

All of these gases can cause upper respiratory tract and conjunctival irritation. Pulmonary oedema, with severe breathlessness and cyanosis may develop suddenly up to 36 hours after exposure. Death may occur. Patients are kept under observation and those who develop pulmonary oedema are given oxygen. Assisted ventilation may be necessary in the most serious cases.

CS Spray poisoning

CS spray, which is used for riot control, irritates the eyes (hence 'tear gas') and the respiratory tract; symptoms normally settle spontaneously within 15 minutes. If symptoms persist, the patient should be removed to a well-ventilated area, and the exposed skin washed with soap and water after removal of contaminated clothing. Contact lenses should be removed and rigid ones washed (soft ones should be discarded). Eye symptoms should be treated by irrigating the eyes with physiological saline (or water if saline is not available) and advice sought from an ophthalmologist. Patients with features of severe poisoning, particularly respiratory complications, should be admitted to hospital for symptomatic treatment.

Pesticide poisoning

Organophosphorus insecticides

Organophosphorus insecticides are usually supplied as powders or dissolved in organic solvents. All are absorbed through the bronchi and intact skin as well as through the gut and inhibit cholinesterase activity, thereby prolonging and intensifying the effects of acetylcholine. Toxicity between different compounds varies considerably, and onset may be delayed after skin exposure.

Anxiety, restlessness, dizziness, headache, miosis, nausea, hypersalivation, vomiting, abdominal colic, diarrhoea, bradycardia, and sweating are common features of organophosphorus poisoning. Muscle weakness and fasciculation may develop and progress to generalised flaccid paralysis, including the ocular and respiratory muscles. Convulsions, coma, pulmonary oedema with copious bronchial secretions, hypoxia, and arrhythmias occur in severe cases. Hyperglycaemia and glycosuria without ketonuria may also be present.

Further absorption of the organophosphorus insecticide should be prevented by moving the patient to fresh air, removing soiled clothing, and washing contaminated skin. In severe poisoning it is vital to ensure a clear airway, frequent removal of bronchial secretions, and adequate ventilation and oxygenation; gastric lavage may be considered provided that the airway is protected. Atropine sulfate p. 1526 will reverse the muscarinic effects of acetylcholine and is given by intravenous injection until the skin becomes flushed and dry, the pupils dilate, and bradycardia is abolished.

Pralidoxime chloride p. 1563, a cholinesterase reactivator, is used as an adjunct to atropine sulfate in moderate or severe poisoning. It improves muscle tone within 30 minutes of administration. Pralidoxime chloride is continued until the patient has not required atropine sulfate for 12 hours. Pralidoxime chloride can be obtained from designated centres, the names of which are held by the National Poisons Information Service.

Snake bites and animal stings

Snake bites

Envenoming from snake bite is uncommon in the UK. Many exotic snakes are kept, some illegally, but the only indigenous venomous snake is the adder (*Vipera berus*). The bite may cause local and systemic effects. Local effects include pain, swelling, bruising, and tender enlargement of regional lymph nodes. Systemic effects include early anaphylactic symptoms (transient hypotension with syncope, angioedema, urticaria, abdominal colic, diarrhoea, and vomiting), with later persistent or recurrent hypotension, ECG abnormalities, spontaneous systemic bleeding, coagulopathy, adult respiratory distress syndrome, and acute renal failure. Fatal envenoming is rare but the potential for severe envenoming must not be underestimated.

Early anaphylactic symptoms should be treated with intramuscular adrenaline/epinephrine p. 256, see Antihistamines, allergen immunotherapy and allergic emergencies p. 316 for further guidance on anaphylaxis management. Indications for european viper snake venom antiserum p. 1568 treatment include *systemic envenoming*, especially hypotension, ECG abnormalities, vomiting, haemostatic abnormalities, and marked local envenoming such that after bites on the hand or foot, swelling extends beyond the wrist or ankle within 4 hours of the bite. For those patients who present with clinical features of *severe envenoming* (e.g. shock, ECG abnormalities, or local swelling that has advanced from the foot to above the knee or from the hand to above the elbow within 2 hours of the bite), a higher initial dose of the european viper snake venom antiserum is recommended; if symptoms of *systemic envenoming* persist contact the National Poisons Information Service. Adrenaline/epinephrine injection must be immediately to hand for treatment of anaphylactic reactions to the european viper snake venom antiserum.

Antivenom is available for bites by certain foreign snakes and spiders, stings by scorpions and fish. For information on identification, management, and for supply in an emergency, telephone the National Poisons Information Service. Whenever possible the TOXBASE entry should be read, and relevant information collected, before telephoning the National Poisons Information Service.

Insect stings

Stings from ants, wasps, hornets, and bees cause local pain and swelling but seldom cause severe direct toxicity unless many stings are inflicted at the same time. If the sting is in the mouth or on the tongue local swelling may threaten the upper airway. The stings from these insects are usually treated by cleaning the area with a topical antiseptic. Bee stings should be removed as quickly as possible. Anaphylactic reactions require immediate treatment with intramuscular **adrenaline/epinephrine**; self-administered

intramuscular adrenaline/epinephrine is the best first-aid treatment for patients with severe hypersensitivity. An inhaled bronchodilator may also be considered for patients with persisting respiratory problems, see Antihistamines, allergen immunotherapy and allergic emergencies p. 316 for further guidance on anaphylaxis management. A short course of an **oral antihistamine** or a **topical corticosteroid** may help to reduce inflammation and relieve itching. A vaccine containing extracts of bee and wasp venom can be used to reduce the risk of anaphylaxis and systemic reactions in patients with systemic hypersensitivity to bee or wasp stings.

Marine stings

The severe pain of weeverfish (*Trachinus vipera*) and Portuguese man-o'-war stings can be relieved by immersing the stung area immediately in uncomfortably hot, but not scalding, water (not more than 45° C). People stung by jellyfish and Portuguese man-o'-war around the UK coast should be removed from the sea as soon as possible. Adherent tentacles should be lifted off carefully (wearing gloves or using tweezers) or washed off with seawater. Alcoholic solutions, including suntan lotions, should **not** be applied because they can cause further discharge of stinging hairs. Ice packs can be used to reduce pain.

Other poisons

Consult either the National Poisons Information Service day and night or TOXBASE.

The **National Poisons Information Service** (Tel: 0344 892 0111) will provide specialist advice on all aspects of poisoning day and night.

1   Active elimination from the gastro-intestinal tract

ANTIDOTES AND CHELATORS ⟩ INTESTINAL ADSORBENTS

Charcoal, activated
23-Jul-2020

● **INDICATIONS AND DOSE**

Reduction of absorption of poisons in the gastro-intestinal system

▶ BY MOUTH

▹ Neonate: 1 g/kg.

▹ Child 1 month–11 years: 1 g/kg (max. per dose 50 g)
▹ Child 12–17 years: 50 g
▹ Adult: 50 g

Active elimination of poisons

▶ BY MOUTH

▹ Neonate: 1 g/kg every 4 hours, dose may be reduced and the frequency increased if not tolerated, reduced dose may compromise efficacy.

▹ Child 1 month–11 years: 1 g/kg every 4 hours (max. per dose 50 g), dose may be reduced and the frequency increased if not tolerated, reduced dose may compromise efficacy
▹ Child 12–17 years: Initially 50 g, then 50 g every 4 hours, reduced if not tolerated to 25 g every 2 hours, alternatively 12.5 g every 1 hour, reduced dose may compromise efficacy
▹ Adult: Initially 50 g, then 50 g every 4 hours, reduced if not tolerated to 25 g every 2 hours, alternatively 12.5 g every 1 hour, reduced dose may compromise efficacy
continued →

16

Emergency treatment of poisoning

Accelerated elimination of teriflunomide
▶ BY MOUTH USING GRANULES
▶ Adult: 50 g every 12 hours for 11 days

Accelerated elimination of leflunomide (washout procedure)
▶ BY MOUTH USING GRANULES
▶ Adult: 50 g 4 times a day for 11 days

● UNLICENSED USE
▶ In adults Activated charcoal doses in BNF may differ from those in product literature.

● CAUTIONS Comatose patient (risk of aspiration—ensure airway is protected) · drowsy patient (risk of aspiration—ensure airway protected) · reduced gastrointestinal motility (risk of obstruction)

● SIDE-EFFECTS Bezoar · constipation · diarrhoea · gastrointestinal disorders

● DIRECTIONS FOR ADMINISTRATION TOXBASE advises suspension or reconstituted powder may be mixed with soft drinks (e.g. caffeine-free diet cola) or fruit juices to mask the taste.

● MEDICINAL FORMS There can be variation in the licensing of different medicines containing the same drug.

Oral suspension
▶ Charcodote (Teva UK Ltd)
  Activated charcoal 200 mg per 1 ml Charcodote 200mg/ml oral suspension | 250 ml Ⓟ £14.25 DT = £14.25 ⓢⓕ

Granules for gastroenteral or oral suspension
▶ Carbomix (Kent Pharma (UK) Ltd)
  Activated charcoal 813 mg per 1 gram Carbomix 81.3% granules for oral suspension | 50 gram Ⓟ £11.90 DT = £11.90 ⓢⓕ

2 Chemical toxicity

2.1 Cyanide toxicity

ANTIDOTES AND CHELATORS

Dicobalt edetate

07-Oct-2021

● INDICATIONS AND DOSE

Severe poisoning with cyanides
▶ BY INTRAVENOUS INJECTION
▶ Child: Consult the National Poisons Information Service
▶ Adult: 300 mg, to be given over 1 minute (or 5 minutes if condition less serious), dose to be followed immediately by 50 mL of glucose intravenous infusion 50%; if response inadequate a second dose of both may be given, but risk of cobalt toxicity

● CAUTIONS Owing to toxicity to be used only for definite cyanide poisoning when patient tending to lose, or has lost, consciousness

● SIDE-EFFECTS Reflex tachycardia · vomiting

● EXCEPTIONS TO LEGAL CATEGORY Prescription only medicine restriction does not apply where administration is for saving life in emergency.

● MEDICINAL FORMS No licensed medicines listed.

Sodium nitrite

05-May-2021

● INDICATIONS AND DOSE

Poisoning with cyanides (used in conjunction with sodium thiosulfate)
▶ BY INTRAVENOUS INJECTION
▶ Child: Consult the National Poisons Information Service
▶ Adult: 300 mg

> **IMPORTANT SAFETY INFORMATION**
>
> NHS IMPROVEMENT PATIENT SAFETY ALERT: RISK OF DEATH FROM UNINTENDED ADMINISTRATION OF SODIUM NITRITE (AUGUST 2020)
>
> Cases of unintended administration of sodium nitrite have been reported, including 2 fatalities. Sodium nitrite can cause significant side-effects such as methaemoglobinaemia and nitric oxide-induced vasodilation.
>
> Acute trusts are advised to check all clinical areas to ensure that sodium nitrite injection has not been inadvertently supplied, and to only retain stock in emergency departments. Unlicensed sodium nitrite ampoules in emergency departments should also be destroyed appropriately and replaced with licensed vials.
>
> For information on the storage of 'specialist antidotes', see Poisoning, emergency treatment p. 1554.

● SIDE-EFFECTS Arrhythmias · dizziness · headache · hypotension · methaemoglobinaemia · palpitations

● EXCEPTIONS TO LEGAL CATEGORY Prescription only medicine restriction does not apply where administration is for saving life in emergency.

● MEDICINAL FORMS There can be variation in the licensing of different medicines containing the same drug.

Solution for injection
▶ Sodium nitrite (Non-proprietary)
  Sodium nitrite 30 mg per 1 ml Sodium nitrite 300mg/10ml solution for injection vials | 1 vial ⓅⓄⓂ Ⓢ (Hospital only)

Sodium thiosulfate

16-Mar-2018

● INDICATIONS AND DOSE

Poisoning with cyanides
▶ BY INTRAVENOUS INJECTION
▶ Child: Consult the National Poisons Information Service
▶ Adult: 12.5 g, to be given over 10 minutes, dose may be repeated in severe cyanide poisoning

DOSE EQUIVALENCE AND CONVERSION
▶ 12.5 g equates to 50 mL of a 25% solution *or* 25 mL of a 50% solution.

● SIDE-EFFECTS
▶ **Common or very common** Electrolyte imbalance (in children) · hypersensitivity (in children) · hypertension (in children) · metabolic acidosis (in children)
▶ **Frequency not known** Disorientation · feeling hot · headache · hypotension (very common in children) · nausea (very common in children) · taste salty · vomiting (very common in children)

● EXCEPTIONS TO LEGAL CATEGORY Prescription only medicine restriction does not apply where administration is for saving life in emergency.

- **MEDICINAL FORMS** There can be variation in the licensing of different medicines containing the same drug. Forms available from special-order manufacturers include: solution for injection

Solution for injection

▸ **Sodium thiosulfate (Non-proprietary)**
  Sodium thiosulfate 250 mg per 1 ml　Sodium thiosulfate 12.5g/50ml solution for injection vials | 1 vial [PoM] [S] (Hospital only)

2.2　Organophosphorus toxicity

> **Other drugs used for Organophosphorus toxicity** Atropine sulfate, p. 1526

ANTIDOTES AND CHELATORS

Pralidoxime chloride　　　　　　　31-Jan-2022

- **INDICATIONS AND DOSE**

Adjunct to atropine in the treatment of poisoning by organophosphorus insecticide or nerve agent

▸ BY INTRAVENOUS INFUSION

▸ Child: Initially 30 mg/kg, to be given over 20 minutes, followed by 8 mg/kg/hour; maximum 12 g per day

▸ Adult: Initially 30 mg/kg, to be given over 20 minutes, followed by 8 mg/kg/hour; maximum 12 g per day

- **UNLICENSED USE** Pralidoxime chloride doses may differ from those in product literature. Licensed for use in children (age range not specified by manufacturer).

- **CONTRA-INDICATIONS** Poisoning with carbamates · poisoning with organophosphorus compounds without anticholinesterase activity

- **CAUTIONS** Myasthenia gravis

- **SIDE-EFFECTS** Dizziness · drowsiness · headache · hyperventilation · muscle weakness · nausea · tachycardia · vision disorders

- **RENAL IMPAIRMENT** [EvGr] Use with caution. ⟨M⟩

- **DIRECTIONS FOR ADMINISTRATION** Manufacturer advises the loading dose may be administered by intravenous injection (diluted to a concentration of 50 mg/mL with water for injections) over at least 5 minutes if pulmonary oedema is present or if it is not practical to administer an intravenous infusion.

▸ In children For *intravenous infusion*, manufacturer advises reconstitute each vial with 20 mL Water for Injections, then dilute to a concentration of 10–20 mg/mL with Sodium Chloride 0.9%.

- **PRESCRIBING AND DISPENSING INFORMATION** Available from designated centres for organophosphorus insecticide poisoning—see TOXBASE for list of holding centres.

- **EXCEPTIONS TO LEGAL CATEGORY** Prescription only medicine restriction does not apply where administration is for saving life in emergency.

- **MEDICINAL FORMS** There can be variation in the licensing of different medicines containing the same drug.

Powder for solution for injection

▸ **Pralidoxime chloride (Non-proprietary)**
  Pralidoxime chloride 1 gram　Protopam Chloride 1g powder for solution for injection vials | 6 vial [PoM] [S] (Hospital only)

3　Drug toxicity

3.1　Benzodiazepine toxicity

ANTIDOTES AND CHELATORS ⟩
BENZODIAZEPINE ANTAGONISTS

Flumazenil　　　　　　　　　　　24-Jul-2020

- **INDICATIONS AND DOSE**

Reversal of sedative effects of benzodiazepines in anaesthesia and clinical procedures

▸ BY INTRAVENOUS INJECTION

▸ Adult: 200 micrograms, dose to be administered over 15 seconds, then 100 micrograms every 1 minute if required; usual dose 300–600 micrograms; maximum 1 mg per course

Reversal of sedative effects of benzodiazepines in intensive care

▸ BY INTRAVENOUS INJECTION

▸ Adult: 300 micrograms, dose to be administered over 15 seconds, then 100 micrograms every 1 minute if required; maximum 2 mg per course

Reversal of sedative effects of benzodiazepines in intensive care (if drowsiness recurs after injection)

▸ INITIALLY BY INTRAVENOUS INFUSION

▸ Adult: 100–400 micrograms/hour, adjusted according to response, alternatively (by intravenous injection) 300 micrograms, adjusted according to response

> **IMPORTANT SAFETY INFORMATION**
> Flumazenil should only be administered by, or under the direct supervision of, personnel experienced in its use.

- **CONTRA-INDICATIONS** Life-threatening condition (e.g. raised intracranial pressure, status epilepticus) controlled by benzodiazepines

- **CAUTIONS** Avoid rapid injection following major surgery · avoid rapid injection in high-risk or anxious patients · benzodiazepine dependence (may precipitate withdrawal symptoms) · elderly · ensure neuromuscular blockade cleared before giving · head injury (rapid reversal of benzodiazepine sedation may cause convulsions) · history of panic disorders (risk of recurrence) · prolonged benzodiazepine therapy for epilepsy (risk of convulsions) · short-acting (repeat doses may be necessary— benzodiazepine effects may persist for at least 24 hours)

- **SIDE-EFFECTS**

▸ **Common or very common** Anxiety · diplopia · dry mouth · eye disorders · flushing · headache · hiccups · hyperhidrosis · hyperventilation · hypotension · insomnia · nausea · palpitations · paraesthesia · speech disorder · tremor · vertigo · vomiting

▸ **Uncommon** Abnormal hearing · arrhythmias · chest pain · chills · cough · dyspnoea · nasal congestion · seizure (more common in patients with epilepsy)

▸ **Frequency not known** Withdrawal syndrome

- **PREGNANCY** Not known to be harmful.

- **BREAST FEEDING** Avoid breast-feeding for 24 hours.

- **HEPATIC IMPAIRMENT** Manufacturer advises caution (risk of increased half-life).
  Dose adjustments Manufacturer advises cautious dose titration.

- **DIRECTIONS FOR ADMINISTRATION** For *continuous intravenous infusion*, manufacturer advises dilute with Glucose 5% or Sodium Chloride 0.9%.

- **MEDICINAL FORMS** There can be variation in the licensing of different medicines containing the same drug.

  Solution for injection
  - **Flumazenil (Non-proprietary)**
    Flumazenil 100 microgram per 1 ml Flumazenil 500micrograms/5ml solution for injection ampoules | 5 ampoule [PoM] £72.46 (Hospital only) | 10 ampoule [PoM] £150.00 | 10 ampoule [PoM] £150.00 (Hospital only)

3.2 Digoxin toxicity

ANTIDOTES AND CHELATORS > ANTIBODIES

Digoxin-specific antibody

20-Jul-2020

- **INDICATIONS AND DOSE**

  Treatment of known or strongly suspected life-threatening digoxin toxicity associated with ventricular arrhythmias or bradyarrhythmias unresponsive to atropine and when measures beyond the withdrawal of digoxin and correction of any electrolyte abnormalities are considered necessary
  - BY INTRAVENOUS INFUSION
  - Child: Serious cases of digoxin toxicity should be discussed with the National Poisons Information Service (consult product literature)
  - Adult: Serious cases of digoxin toxicity should be discussed with the National Poisons Information Service (consult product literature)

- **DIRECTIONS FOR ADMINISTRATION**
  - In adults For *intravenous infusion (DigiFab®)*, manufacturer advises give intermittently in Sodium chloride 0.9%. Reconstitute with water for injections (4 mL/vial), then dilute with infusion fluid and give over 30 minutes.

- **MEDICINAL FORMS** There can be variation in the licensing of different medicines containing the same drug.

  Powder for solution for infusion
  - **DigiFab** (Protherics Medicines Development Ltd)
    Digoxin-specific antibody fragments 40 mg DigiFab 40mg powder for solution for infusion vials | 1 vial [PoM] £750.00 (Hospital only)

3.3 Heparin toxicity

ANTIDOTES AND CHELATORS

Protamine sulfate

02-Dec-2020

- **INDICATIONS AND DOSE**

  Overdosage with intravenous injection of unfractionated heparin
  - BY INTRAVENOUS INJECTION
  - Adult: Dose to be administered at a rate not exceeding 5 mg/minute, 1 mg neutralises 80–100 units heparin when given within 15 minutes; if longer than 15 minute since heparin, less protamine required (consult product literature for details) as heparin rapidly excreted; maximum 50 mg

  Overdosage with intravenous infusion of unfractionated heparin
  - BY INTRAVENOUS INJECTION
  - Adult: 25–50 mg, to be administered once heparin infusion stopped at a rate not exceeding 5 mg/minute

  Overdosage with subcutaneous injection of unfractionated heparin
  - INITIALLY BY INTRAVENOUS INJECTION
  - Adult: Initially 25–50 mg, to be administered at a rate not exceeding 5 mg/minute, 1 mg neutralises 100 units

heparin, then (by intravenous infusion), any remaining dose to be administered over 8–16 hours; maximum 50 mg per course

Overdosage with subcutaneous injection of low molecular weight heparin
- BY INTRAVENOUS INJECTION, OR BY CONTINUOUS INTRAVENOUS INFUSION
- Adult: Dose to be administered by intermittent intravenous injection at a rate not exceeding 5 mg/minute, 1 mg neutralises approx. 100 units low molecular weight heparin (consult product literature of low molecular weight heparin for details); maximum 50 mg

- **CAUTIONS** Excessive doses can have an anticoagulant effect

- **SIDE-EFFECTS**
  - **Rare or very rare** Pulmonary oedema non-cardiogenic
  - **Frequency not known** Acute pulmonary vasoconstriction · back pain · bradycardia · circulatory collapse · dyspnoea · fatigue · feeling hot · flushing · hypertension · hypotension · nausea · pulmonary hypertension · vomiting

- **ALLERGY AND CROSS-SENSITIVITY** [EvGr] Caution if increased risk of allergic reaction to protamine (includes previous treatment with protamine or protamine insulin, allergy to fish, men who are infertile or who have had a vasectomy and who may have antibodies to protamine). ◇M◇

- **MONITORING REQUIREMENTS** Monitor activated partial thromboplastin time or other appropriate blood clotting parameters.

- **PRESCRIBING AND DISPENSING INFORMATION** The long half-life of low molecular weight heparins should be taken into consideration when determining the dose of protamine sulfate; the effects of low molecular weight heparins can persist for up to 24 hours after administration.

- **MEDICINAL FORMS** There can be variation in the licensing of different medicines containing the same drug.

  Solution for injection
  - **Protamine sulfate (Non-proprietary)**
    Protamine sulfate 10 mg per 1 ml Protamine sulfate 50mg/5ml solution for injection ampoules | 10 ampoule [PoM] £66.89

3.4 Opioid toxicity

OPIOID RECEPTOR ANTAGONISTS

Naloxone hydrochloride

03-Aug-2023

- **INDICATIONS AND DOSE**

  Acute opioid overdose–high-dose regimen [when rapid titration with naloxone is necessary to reverse potentially life-threatening effects]
  - BY INTRAVENOUS INJECTION
  - Neonate: Initially 100 micrograms/kg, if no response, repeat at intervals of 1 minute to a total max. of 2 mg, then review diagnosis; further doses may be required if respiratory function deteriorates following initial response, intravenous administration has more rapid onset of action, doses may be given by intramuscular route but only if intravenous route is not feasible.

  - Child 1 month–11 years: Initially 100 micrograms/kg (max. per dose 2 mg), if no response, repeat at intervals of 1 minute to a total max. of 2 mg, then review diagnosis; further doses may be required if respiratory function deteriorates following initial response, intravenous administration has more rapid onset of action, doses may be given by intramuscular route but only if intravenous route is not feasible

‣ Child 12-17 years: Initially 400 micrograms for 1 dose, then 800 micrograms for up to 2 doses at 1 minute intervals if no response to preceding dose, then increased to 2 mg for 1 dose if still no response (4 mg dose may be required in seriously poisoned patients), then review diagnosis; further doses may be required if respiratory function deteriorates following initial response, intravenous administration has more rapid onset of action, doses may be given by intramuscular route but only if intravenous route is not feasible

‣ Adult: Initially 400 micrograms for 1 dose, then 800 micrograms for up to 2 doses at 1 minute intervals if no response to preceding dose, then increased to 2 mg for 1 dose if still no response (4 mg dose may be required in seriously poisoned patients), then review diagnosis; further doses may be required if respiratory function deteriorates following initial response, intravenous administration has more rapid onset of action, doses may be given by intramuscular route but only if intravenous route is not feasible

‣ BY CONTINUOUS INTRAVENOUS INFUSION

‣ Neonate: Using an infusion pump, adjust rate according to response, initially, rate may be set at 60% of the initial resuscitative intravenous injection dose per hour. The initial resuscitative *intravenous injection* dose is that which maintained satisfactory respiratory effort for at least 15 minutes.

‣ Child: Using an infusion pump, adjust rate according to response, initially, rate may be set at 60% of the initial resuscitative intravenous injection dose per hour. The initial resuscitative *intravenous injection* dose is that which maintained satisfactory respiratory effort for at least 15 minutes

‣ Adult: Using an infusion pump, adjust rate according to response, initially, rate may be set at 60% of the initial resuscitative intravenous injection dose per hour. The initial resuscitative *intravenous injection* dose is that which maintained satisfactory respiratory effort for at least 15 minutes

Opioid overdose–low-dose regimen [when there is risk of acute withdrawal, or when a continued therapeutic effect is required (e.g. postoperative use, palliative care)]

‣ BY INTRAVENOUS INJECTION

‣ Neonate: Initially 1–10 micrograms/kg, if no response, repeat at intervals of 1 minute up to 5 times, if no response then give a single dose of 100 micrograms/kg then review diagnosis if still no response, further doses may be required if respiratory function deteriorates following initial response, intravenous administration has a more rapid onset of action, doses may be given by intramuscular route but only if intravenous route is not feasible.

‣ Child 1 month-11 years: Initially 1–10 micrograms/kg (max. per dose 200 micrograms), if no response, repeat at intervals of 1 minute up to 5 times, if no response then give a single dose of 100 micrograms/kg (max. dose 2 mg) then review diagnosis if still no response, further doses may be required if respiratory function deteriorates following initial response, intravenous administration has a more rapid onset of action, doses may be given by intramuscular route but only if intravenous route is not feasible

‣ Child 12-17 years: Initially 100–200 micrograms for 1 dose, then 100 micrograms for up to 2 doses at 1 minute intervals if no response to preceding dose, continue titrating up to a max. of 2 mg until adequate response achieved. If still no response, give a further 2 mg dose (4 mg dose may be required in seriously poisoned patients), then review diagnosis; further doses may be required if respiratory function deteriorates following initial response, intravenous administration has a more rapid onset of action, doses may be given by intramuscular route but only if intravenous route is not feasible

‣ Adult: Initially 100–200 micrograms for 1 dose, then 100 micrograms for up to 2 doses at 1 minute intervals if no response to preceding dose, continue titrating up to a max. of 2 mg until adequate response achieved. If still no response, give a further 2 mg dose (4 mg dose may be required in seriously poisoned patients), then review diagnosis; further doses may be required if respiratory function deteriorates following initial response, intravenous administration has a more rapid onset of action, doses may be given by intramuscular route but only if intravenous route is not feasible

Opioid overdose in non-medical and medical settings

‣ BY INTRANASAL ADMINISTRATION

‣ Child 14-17 years: 1.8 mg, administered into one nostril, if no response, give a second dose after 2–3 minutes. If the patient responds to the first dose then relapses into respiratory depression, give the second dose immediately. Further doses should be administered into alternate nostrils

‣ Adult: 1.8 mg, administered into one nostril, if no response, give a second dose after 2–3 minutes. If the patient responds to the first dose then relapses into respiratory depression, give the second dose immediately. Further doses should be administered into alternate nostrils

Opioid overdose in non-medical and medical settings [in opioid-dependent patients when there is risk of acute withdrawal]

‣ BY INTRANASAL ADMINISTRATION

‣ Adult: 1.26 mg, administered into one nostril, if no response, give a second dose after 2–3 minutes. If the patient responds to the first dose then relapses into respiratory depression, give the second dose immediately. Further doses should be administered into alternate nostrils

Opioid overdose in a non-medical setting

‣ BY INTRAMUSCULAR INJECTION

‣ Adult: 400 micrograms every 2–3 minutes, each dose given in subsequent resuscitation cycles if patient not breathing normally, continue until consciousness regained, breathing normally, medical assistance available, or contents of syringe used up; to be injected into deltoid region or anterolateral thigh

DOSE EQUIVALENCE AND CONVERSION

‣ With intranasal use

‣ For *Nyxoid* ® nasal spray, 1 spray is equivalent to naloxone 1.8 mg. For *naloxone 1.26 mg nasal spray*, 1 spray is equivalent to naloxone 1.26 mg.

PHARMACOKINETICS

‣ Naloxone has a short duration of action; repeated doses or infusion may be necessary to reverse effects of opioids with longer duration of action.

● UNLICENSED USE TOXBASE advises naloxone is used in both high- and low-dose regimens for the management of opioid overdose, but these may differ from those licensed.

> **IMPORTANT SAFETY INFORMATION**
> SAFE PRACTICE
> Doses used in acute opioid overdose may not be appropriate when there is risk of acute withdrawal (e.g. chronic opioid use), or when a continued therapeutic effect is required (e.g. postoperative use, palliative care).

- **CAUTIONS** Cardiovascular disease or those receiving cardiotoxic drugs (serious adverse cardiovascular effects reported) · chronic opioid use (risk of acute withdrawal) · maternal chronic opioid use (risk of acute withdrawal in newborn) · palliative care (risk of returning pain and acute withdrawal) · postoperative use (risk of returning pain)

  CAUTIONS, FURTHER INFORMATION
- Titration of dose [EvGr] In postoperative use, the dose should be titrated for each patient in order to obtain sufficient respiratory response; however, naloxone antagonises analgesia. (M)

- **SIDE-EFFECTS**

  GENERAL SIDE-EFFECTS
- **Common or very common** Arrhythmias · dizziness · headache · hypertension · hypotension · nausea · vomiting
- **Uncommon** Diarrhoea · dry mouth · hyperhidrosis · hyperventilation · tremor
- **Rare or very rare** Cardiac arrest · erythema multiforme · pulmonary oedema

  SPECIFIC SIDE-EFFECTS
- **Uncommon**
- With parenteral use Inflammation localised · pain · vascular irritation
- **Rare or very rare**
- With parenteral use Anxiety · seizure
- **Frequency not known**
- With parenteral use Analgesia reversed · asthenia · chills · death · dyspnoea · fever · irritability · nasal complaints · piloerection · yawning

- **PREGNANCY** Use only if potential benefit outweighs risk.

- **BREAST FEEDING** Not orally bioavailable.

- **MONITORING REQUIREMENTS** Specialist sources indicate that blood gases, oxygen saturation and respiratory rate should be monitored once breathing is restored. Patients should be monitored for recurrence of signs and symptoms of opioid toxicity, such as relapse in respiratory or CNS symptoms.

- **DIRECTIONS FOR ADMINISTRATION**
- In children For *continuous intravenous infusion*, dilute to a concentration of up to 200 micrograms/mL with Glucose 5% or Sodium Chloride 0.9%.
- In adults For *intravenous infusion* (*Minijet* ® Naloxone Hydrochloride), give continuously in Glucose 5% or Sodium Chloride 0.9%. Dilute to a concentration of up to 200 micrograms/mL and administer via an infusion pump.

- **PRESCRIBING AND DISPENSING INFORMATION**
- With intranasal use The manufacturer has provided a *Healthcare Professional Guidance Document*.

- **PATIENT AND CARER ADVICE**
- With intranasal use Patients and carers should be given advice on how to administer naloxone nasal spray.
  Patient training and information cards should be provided.

- **MEDICINAL FORMS** There can be variation in the licensing of different medicines containing the same drug.

  Solution for injection
- Naloxone hydrochloride (Non-proprietary)
  Naloxone hydrochloride (as Naloxone hydrochloride dihydrate) 400 microgram per 1 ml Naloxone 400micrograms/1ml solution for injection ampoules | 10 ampoule [PoM] £41.00–£49.00 | 10 ampoule [PoM] £43.00 (Hospital only)
  Naloxone hydrochloride 1 mg per 1 ml Naloxone 2mg/2ml solution for injection pre-filled syringes | 1 pre-filled disposable injection [PoM] £18.00 DT = £18.00
- Prenoxad (Martindale Pharmaceuticals Ltd)
  Naloxone hydrochloride 1 mg per 1 ml Prenoxad 2mg/2ml solution for injection pre-filled syringes | 1 pre-filled disposable injection [PoM] £18.00 DT = £18.00

Spray
- Naloxone hydrochloride (Non-proprietary)
  Naloxone (as Naloxone hydrochloride dihydrate) 12.6 mg per 1 ml Naloxone 1.26mg/0.1ml nasal spray unit dose | 2 unit dose [PoM] £25.00 DT = £25.00
- Nyxoid (Napp Pharmaceuticals Ltd)
  Naloxone (as Naloxone hydrochloride dihydrate) 18 mg per 1 ml Nyxoid 1.8mg/0.1ml nasal spray 0.1ml unit dose | 2 unit dose [PoM] £26.00 DT = £26.00

3.5 Paracetamol toxicity

ANTIDOTES AND CHELATORS

Acetylcysteine

01-Aug-2024

- **INDICATIONS AND DOSE**

Paracetamol overdose [12-hour SNAP regimen]
- BY INTRAVENOUS INFUSION
- Child (body-weight up to 40 kg): 100 mg/kg over 2 hours, dose to be administered as a 50 mg/mL solution in glucose 5% or sodium chloride 0.9%, then 200 mg/kg over 10 hours, dose to be administered as a 10 mg/mL solution in glucose 5% or sodium chloride 0.9%, and started immediately after completion of first infusion
- Child (body-weight 40 kg and above): 100 mg/kg over 2 hours, dose to be administered in 200 mL glucose 5% or sodium chloride 0.9%, then 200 mg/kg over 10 hours, dose to be administered in 1 litre glucose 5% or sodium chloride 0.9%, and started immediately after completion of first infusion
- Adult (body-weight up to 40 kg): 100 mg/kg over 2 hours, dose to be administered as a 50 mg/mL solution in glucose 5% or sodium chloride 0.9%, then 200 mg/kg over 10 hours, dose to be administered as a 10 mg/mL solution in glucose 5% or sodium chloride 0.9%, and started immediately after completion of first infusion
- Adult (body-weight 40 kg and above): 100 mg/kg over 2 hours, dose to be administered in 200 mL glucose 5% or sodium chloride 0.9%, then 200 mg/kg over 10 hours, dose to be administered in 1 litre glucose 5% or sodium chloride 0.9%, and started immediately after completion of first infusion

Paracetamol overdose [21-hour regimen]
- BY INTRAVENOUS INFUSION
- Child (body-weight up to 40 kg): 150 mg/kg over 1 hour, dose to be administered as a 50 mg/mL solution in glucose 5% or sodium chloride 0.9%, then 50 mg/kg over 4 hours, dose to be administered as a 6.25 mg/mL solution in glucose 5% or sodium chloride 0.9%, and started immediately after completion of first infusion, then 100 mg/kg over 16 hours, dose to be administered as a 6.25 mg/mL solution in glucose 5% or sodium chloride 0.9%, and started immediately after completion of second infusion
- Child (body-weight 40 kg and above): 150 mg/kg over 1 hour, dose to be administered in 200 mL glucose 5% or sodium chloride 0.9%, then 50 mg/kg over 4 hours, dose to be administered in 500 mL glucose 5% or sodium chloride 0.9%, and started immediately after completion of first infusion, then 100 mg/kg over 16 hours, dose to be administered in 1 litre glucose 5% or sodium chloride 0.9%, and started immediately after completion of second infusion
- Adult (body-weight 40 kg and above): 150 mg/kg over 1 hour, dose to be administered in 200 mL glucose 5% or sodium chloride 0.9%, then 50 mg/kg over 4 hours, dose to be administered in 500 mL glucose 5% or sodium chloride 0.9%, and started immediately after completion of first infusion, then 100 mg/kg over

16 hours, dose to be administered in 1 litre glucose 5% or sodium chloride 0.9%, and started immediately after completion of second infusion

DOSES AT EXTREMES OF BODY-WEIGHT
► To avoid excessive dosage in obese patients, a ceiling weight of 110 kg should be used when calculating the dose for paracetamol overdosage.

● **UNLICENSED USE** TOXBASE advises acetylcysteine is used in the 12-hour SNAP regimen for paracetamol overdose, although it is considered unlicensed.

IMPORTANT SAFETY INFORMATION
PARACETAMOL OVERDOSE
There are two intravenous regimens for paracetamol overdose: the standard 21-hour regimen and the modified 12-hour regimen (also known as the Scottish and Newcastle Acetylcysteine Protocol (SNAP)).

The SNAP regimen is not endorsed by the MHRA but is recommended by the Royal College of Emergency Medicine and the National Poisons Information Service. Continued treatment after the second infusion may be necessary depending on the clinical evaluation of the individual patient—for further information, see TOXBASE.

MHRA/CHM ADVICE: INTRAVENOUS ACETYLCYSTEINE FOR PARACETAMOL OVERDOSE: REMINDER OF AUTHORISED DOSE REGIMEN; POSSIBLE NEED FOR CONTINUED TREATMENT (JANUARY 2017)
The authorised dose regimen for acetylcysteine in paracetamol overdose is 3 consecutive intravenous infusions given over a total of 21 hours.

Continued treatment (given at the dose and rate as used in the third infusion) may be necessary depending on the clinical evaluation of the individual patient.

● **CAUTIONS** Asthma · atopy · may slightly increase INR · may slightly increase prothrombin time

● **INTERACTIONS** → Appendix 1: acetylcysteine

● **SIDE-EFFECTS**
► **Frequency not known** Acidosis · anaphylactoid reaction · angioedema · anxiety · arrhythmias · cardiac arrest · chest discomfort · cough · cyanosis · eye pain · eye swelling · generalised seizure · hyperhidrosis · hypertension · hypotension · joint disorders · malaise · nausea · pain facial · respiratory disorders · skin reactions · syncope · thrombocytopenia · vasodilation · vision blurred · vomiting

SIDE-EFFECTS, FURTHER INFORMATION Anaphylactoid reactions can be managed by suspending treatment and initiating appropriate management. Treatment may then be restarted at lower rate.

● **PREGNANCY**
Dose adjustments TOXBASE advises that the toxic dose of *paracetamol* ingested should be calculated using the patient's pre-pregnancy body-weight and the *acetylcysteine* dose (for both regimens) should be calculated using the patient's actual pregnant body-weight.

● **DIRECTIONS FOR ADMINISTRATION** [EvGr] For *intravenous infusion*, Glucose 5% is the preferred infusion fluid; if unsuitable then Sodium Chloride 0.9% can be used as an alternative. ⓜ For further information on administration, see TOXBASE.

● **MEDICINAL FORMS** There can be variation in the licensing of different medicines containing the same drug. Forms available from special-order manufacturers include: solution for infusion
Solution for infusion
ELECTROLYTES: May contain Sodium
► **Acetylcysteine (Non-proprietary)**
Acetylcysteine 200 mg per 1 ml Acetylcysteine 6g/30ml solution for infusion vials | 4 vial [PoM] [Ⓢ] (Hospital only)
Acetadote 6g/30ml solution for infusion vials | 4 vial [PoM] [Ⓢ] (Hospital only)
Acetylcysteine 2g/10ml solution for infusion ampoules | 10 ampoule [PoM] £21.26–£34.02 DT = £21.26
► **Parvolex** (Phoenix Labs Ltd)
Acetylcysteine 200 mg per 1 ml Parvolex 2g/10ml concentrate for solution for infusion ampoules | 10 ampoule [PoM] £22.50 DT = £21.26

---

4   Methaemoglobinaemia

ANTIDOTES AND CHELATORS

Methylthioninium chloride   11-Feb-2022
(Methylene blue)

● **INDICATIONS AND DOSE**
Drug- or chemical-induced methaemoglobinaemia
► BY SLOW INTRAVENOUS INJECTION
► **Child 3 months–17 years:** Initially 1–2 mg/kg, then 1–2 mg/kg after 30–60 minutes if required, to be given over 5 minutes, seek advice from National Poisons Information Service if further repeat doses are required; maximum 7 mg/kg per course
► **Adult:** Initially 1–2 mg/kg, then 1–2 mg/kg after 30–60 minutes if required, to be given over 5 minutes, seek advice from National Poisons Information Service if further repeat doses are required; maximum 7 mg/kg per course

Aniline- or dapsone-induced methaemoglobinaemia
► BY SLOW INTRAVENOUS INJECTION
► **Child 3 months–17 years:** Initially 1–2 mg/kg, then 1–2 mg/kg after 30–60 minutes if required, to be given over 5 minutes, seek advice from National Poisons Information Service if further repeat doses are required; maximum 4 mg/kg per course
► **Adult:** Initially 1–2 mg/kg, then 1–2 mg/kg after 30–60 minutes if required, to be given over 5 minutes, seek advice from National Poisons Information Service if further repeat doses are required; maximum 4 mg/kg per course

● **CAUTIONS** Chlorate poisoning (reduces efficacy of methylthioninium) · G6PD deficiency (seek advice from National Poisons Information Service) · methaemoglobinaemia due to treatment of cyanide poisoning with sodium nitrite (seek advice from National Poisons Information Service) · pulse oximetry may give false estimation of oxygen saturation

● **INTERACTIONS** → Appendix 1: methylthioninium chloride
● **SIDE-EFFECTS**
► **Common or very common** Abdominal pain · anxiety · chest pain · dizziness · headache · hyperhidrosis · nausea · pain in extremity · paraesthesia · skin reactions · taste altered · urine discolouration · vomiting
► **Frequency not known** Aphasia · arrhythmias · confusion · faeces discoloured · fever · haemolytic anaemia · hyperbilirubinaemia (in infants) · hypertension · hypotension · injection site necrosis · mydriasis · tremor

● **PREGNANCY** No information available, but risk to fetus of untreated methaemoglobinaemia likely to be significantly higher than risk of treatment.

- **BREAST FEEDING** Manufacturer advises avoid breastfeeding for up to 6 days after administration—no information available.
- **RENAL IMPAIRMENT** National Poisons Information Service advises caution in severe impairment.
  Dose adjustments Manufacturer advises lower doses may be required (consult product literature).
- **DIRECTIONS FOR ADMINISTRATION**
- ▸ In children For *intravenous injection*, manufacturer advises may be diluted with Glucose 5% to minimise injection-site pain; not compatible with Sodium Chloride 0.9%.

- **MEDICINAL FORMS** There can be variation in the licensing of different medicines containing the same drug. Forms available from special-order manufacturers include: solution for injection

Solution for injection

- ▸ Methylthioninium chloride (Non-proprietary)
  Methylthioninium chloride 5 mg per 1 ml Methylthioninium chloride Proveblue 50mg/10ml solution for injection ampoules | 5 ampoule [PoM] £196.89 (Hospital only)
  Methylthioninium chloride 10 mg per 1 ml Methylthioninium chloride (methylene blue) 50mg/5ml concentrate for solution for injection vials | 5 vial [PoM] £150.00 (Hospital only)

---

5 Snake bites

IMMUNE SERA AND IMMUNOGLOBULINS ⟩ ANTITOXINS

European viper snake venom antiserum

05-Feb-2021

- **INDICATIONS AND DOSE**

VIPERATAB ®

Envenoming from *Vipera berus* bites (under expert supervision)

- ▸ BY INTRAVENOUS INFUSION
- ▸ Child: Initially 8 mL for 1 dose, then 8 mL if required, the second and subsequent doses should only be given if signs and symptoms of envenomation persist or recur, if signs and symptoms of envenoming progress or persist contact the National Poisons Information Service
- ▸ Adult: Initially 8 mL for 1 dose, then 8 mL if required, the second and subsequent doses should only be given if signs and symptoms of envenomation persist or recur, if signs and symptoms of envenoming progress or persist contact the National Poisons Information Service

- **DIRECTIONS FOR ADMINISTRATION**
  VIPERATAB ® [EvGr] For *intravenous infusion*, dilute with 100 mL of Sodium Chloride 0.9%; give over 30 minutes. 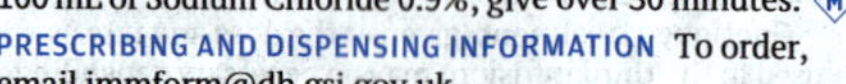
- **PRESCRIBING AND DISPENSING INFORMATION** To order, email immform@dh.gsi.gov.uk.

- **MEDICINAL FORMS** There can be variation in the licensing of different medicines containing the same drug. Forms available from special-order manufacturers include: solution for infusion

Appendix 1
Interactions

Two or more drugs given at the same time can exert their effects independently or they can interact. Interactions may be beneficial and exploited therapeutically; this type of interaction is not within the scope of this appendix. Many interactions are harmless, and even those that are potentially harmful can often be managed, allowing the drugs to be used safely together. Nevertheless, adverse drug interactions should be reported to the Medicines and Healthcare products Regulatory Agency (MHRA), through the Yellow Card Scheme (see Adverse reactions to drugs p. 11), as for other adverse drug reactions.

Potentially harmful drug interactions may occur in only a small number of patients, but the true incidence is often hard to establish. Furthermore the severity of a harmful interaction is likely to vary from one patient to another. Patients at increased risk from drug interactions include the elderly and those with impaired renal or hepatic function.

Interactions can result in the potentiation or antagonism of one drug by another, or result in another effect, such as renal impairment. Drug interactions may develop either through pharmacokinetic or pharmacodynamic mechanisms.

Pharmacodynamic interactions

These are interactions between drugs which have similar or antagonistic pharmacological effects or side-effects. They might be due to competition at receptor sites, or occur between drugs acting on the same physiological system. They are usually predictable from a knowledge of the pharmacology of the interacting drugs; in general, those demonstrated with one drug are likely to occur with related drugs.

Pharmacokinetic interactions

These occur when one drug alters the absorption, distribution, metabolism, or excretion of another, thus increasing or decreasing the amount of drug available to produce its pharmacological effects. Pharmacokinetic interactions occurring with one drug do not necessarily occur uniformly across a group of related drugs.

Affecting absorption The rate of absorption and the total amount absorbed can both be altered by drug interactions. Delayed absorption is rarely of clinical importance unless a rapid effect is required (e.g. when giving an analgesic). Reduction in the total amount absorbed, however, can result in ineffective therapy.

Affecting distribution *Due to changes in protein binding*: To a variable extent most drugs are loosely bound to plasma proteins. Protein-binding sites are non-specific and one drug can displace another thereby increasing the proportion free to diffuse from plasma to its site of action. This only produces a detectable increase in effect if it is an extensively bound drug (more than 90%) that is not widely distributed throughout the body. Even so displacement rarely produces more than transient potentiation because this increased concentration of free drug will usually be eliminated.

Displacement from protein binding plays a part in the potentiation of warfarin by sulfonamides but these interactions become clinically relevant mainly because warfarin metabolism is also inhibited.

Induction or inhibition of drug transporter proteins: Drug transporter proteins, such as P-glycoprotein, actively transport drugs across biological membranes. Transporters can be induced or inhibited, resulting in changes in the concentrations of drugs that are substrates for the transporter. For example, rifampicin induces P-glycoprotein, particularly in the gut wall, resulting in decreased plasma concentrations of digoxin, a P-glycoprotein substrate.

Affecting metabolism Many drugs are metabolised in the liver. Drugs are either metabolised by phase I reactions (oxidation, reduction, or hydrolysis) or by phase II reactions (e.g. glucoronidation).

Phase I reactions are mainly carried out by the cytochrome P450 family of isoenzymes, of which CYP3A4 is the most important isoenzyme involved in the metabolism of drugs. Induction of cytochrome P450 isoenzymes by one drug can increase the rate of metabolism of another, resulting in lower plasma concentrations and a reduced effect. On withdrawal of the inducing drug, plasma concentrations increase and toxicity can occur.

Conversely when one drug inhibits cytochrome P450 isoenzymes, it can decrease the metabolism of another, leading to higher plasma concentrations, resulting in an increased effect with a risk of toxicity.

Isoenzymes of the hepatic cytochrome P450 system interact with a wide range of drugs. With knowledge of which isoenzymes are involved in a drug's metabolism, it is possible to predict whether certain pharmacokinetic interactions will occur. For example, carbamazepine is a potent inducer of CYP3A4, ketoconazole is potent inhibitor of CYP3A4, and midazolam is a substrate of CYP3A4. Carbamazepine reduces midazolam concentrations, and it is therefore likely that other drugs that are potent inducers of CYP3A4 will interact similarly with midazolam. Ketoconazole, however, increases midazolam concentrations, and it can be predicted that other drugs that are potent inhibitors of CYP3A4 will interact similarly.

Less is known about the enzymes involved in phase II reactions. These include UDP-glucuronyltransferases which, for example, might be induced by rifampicin, resulting in decreased metabolism of mycophenolate (a substrate for this enzyme) to its active form, mycophenolic acid.

Affecting renal excretion Drugs are eliminated through the kidney both by glomerular filtration and by active tubular secretion. Competition occurs between those which share active transport mechanisms in the proximal tubule. For example, salicylates and some other NSAIDs delay the excretion of methotrexate; serious methotrexate toxicity is possible. Changes in urinary pH can also affect the reabsorption of a small number of drugs, including methenamine.

Relative importance of interactions

Levels of severity: Most interactions have been assigned a severity; this describes the likely effect of an unmanaged interaction on the patient.

Severe—the result may be a life-threatening event or have a permanent detrimental effect.

Moderate—the result could cause considerable distress or partially incapacitate a patient; they are unlikely to be life-threatening or result in long-term effects.

Mild—the result is unlikely to cause concern or incapacitate the majority of patients.

Unknown—used for those interactions that are predicted, but there is insufficient evidence to hazard a guess at the outcome.

Levels of evidence: Most interactions have been assigned a rating to indicate the weight of evidence behind the interaction.

Study—for interactions where the information is based on formal study including those for other drugs with same mechanism (e.g. known inducers, inhibitors, or substrates of cytochrome P450 isoenzymes or P-glycoprotein).

Anecdotal—interactions based on either a single case report or a limited number of case reports.

Theoretical—interactions that are predicted based on sound theoretical considerations. The information may have been derived from *in vitro* studies or based on the way other members in the same class act.

Action messages: Each interaction describes the effect that occurs, and the action to be taken, either based on manufacturer's advice from the relevant Summary of Product Characteristics or advice from a relevant authority (e.g. MHRA). An action message is only included where the combination is to be avoided, where a dose adjustment is required, or where specific administration requirements (e.g timing of doses) are recommended. **Pharmacodynamic interactions**, with the exception of interactions with drugs that may prolong the QT interval, do not have an action message included as these will depend on individual patient circumstances.

Appendix 1 structure

❶ Drugs

Drugs are listed alphabetically. If a drug is a member of a drug class, all interactions for that drug will be listed under the drug class entry; in this case the drug entry provides direction to the relevant drug class where its interactions can be found.

Within a drug or drug class entry, interactions are listed alphabetically by the interacting drug or drug class. The interactions describe the effect that occurs, and the action to be taken, either based on manufacturer's advice from the relevant Summary of Product Characteristics or advice from a relevant authority (e.g. MHRA). An action message is only included where the combination is to be avoided, where a dose adjustment is required, or where specific administration requirements (e.g. timing of doses) are recommended. If two drugs have a pharmacodynamic effect in addition to a pharmacokinetic interaction, a cross-reference to the relevant pharmacodynamic effect table is included at the end of the pharmacokinetic message.

❷ Drug classes

The drugs that are members of a drug class are listed underneath the drug class entry in a blue box. Interactions for the class are then listed alphabetically by the interacting drug or drug class. If the interaction only applies to certain drugs in the class, these drugs will be shown in brackets after the drug class name.

❸ Supplementary information

If a drug has additional important information to be considered, this is shown in a blue box underneath the drug or drug class entry. This information might be food and lifestyle advice (including smoking and alcohol consumption), relate to the pharmacology of the drug or applicability of interactions to certain routes of administration, or it might be advice about separating administration times.

❹ Pharmacodynamic effects

Tables at the beginning of Appendix 1 cover pharmacodynamic effects. If a drug is included in one or more of these tables, this will be indicated at the top of the

---

❶ **Drug entry**
- ► Details of interaction between **drug entry** and another **drug** or **drug class**. Action statement. [Severity] Evidence
- ► Details of interaction between **drug entry** and another **drug** or **drug class**. Action statement. [Severity] Evidence
  → Also see TABLE 1

Drug entry → see Drug class entry

❷ **Drug class entry**

Drug A · Drug B · Drug C · Drug D

- ► Details of interaction between **drug class entry** and another **drug** or **drug class**. Action statement. [Severity] Evidence

❸ **Drug entry or Drug class entry**

Supplementary information

❹ **Drug entry or Drug class entry** → see TABLE 1

TABLE 1

Name of pharmacodynamic effect

Explanation of the effect

Drug	Drug	Drug
Drug	Drug	Drug

---

list of interactions for the drug or drug class. In addition to the list of interactions for a drug or drug class, these tables should always be consulted.

Each table describes the relevant pharmacodynamic effect and lists those drugs that are commonly associated with the effect. Concurrent use of two or more drugs from the same table is expected to increase the risk of the pharmacodynamic effect occurring. Please note these tables are not exhaustive.

TABLE 1
Drugs that cause hepatotoxicity

The following is a list of some drugs that cause hepatotoxicity (note that this list is not exhaustive). Concurrent use of two or more drugs from the list might increase this risk.

acitretin	dactinomycin	isotretinoin	oxandrolone	streptozocin
alectinib	decitabine	itraconazole	oxymetholone	testosterone
amiodarone	demeclocycline	lenalidomide	oxytetracycline	tetracycline
anidulafungin	doxycycline	lomitapide	paracetamol	thalidomide
asparaginase	eravacycline	lymecycline	pegaspargase	tigecycline
atorvastatin	fluconazole	mercaptopurine	pemetrexed	tioguanine
bexarotene	fludarabine	methotrexate	pomalidomide	trabectedin
capecitabine	fluorouracil	micafungin	pravastatin	valproate
carmustine	flutamide	minocycline	pyrazinamide	vitamin A
caspofungin	fluvastatin	nelarabine	ritonavir	voriconazole
clofarabine	gemcitabine	neratinib	rosuvastatin	zidovudine
crisantaspase	heparin	nevirapine	simvastatin	
cytarabine	isoniazid	nicotinic acid	sotorasib	

TABLE 2
Drugs that cause nephrotoxicity

The following is a list of some drugs that cause nephrotoxicity (note that this list is not exhaustive). Concurrent use of two or more drugs from the list might increase this risk.

aceclofenac	ceftaroline	flurbiprofen	methotrexate	streptozocin
aciclovir	ceftazidime	foscarnet	nabumetone	sulfasalazine
adefovir	ceftobiprole	fosinopril	naproxen	sulindac
amikacin	ceftolozane	ganciclovir	neomycin	tacrolimus
amphotericin B	ceftriaxone	gentamicin	netilmicin	tenofovir disoproxil
aspirin	cefuroxime	ibuprofen	oxaliplatin	tenoxicam
captopril	celecoxib	ifosfamide	pamidronate	tiaprofenic acid
carboplatin	ciclosporin	imidapril	parecoxib	tobramycin
cefaclor	cidofovir	indometacin	pemetrexed	tolfenamic acid
cefadroxil	cisplatin	inotersen	pentamidine	trandolapril
cefalexin	colistimethate	ketoprofen	perindopril	trimethoprim
cefazolin	deferasirox	ketorolac	phenazone	valaciclovir
cefepime	dexketoprofen	lisinopril	piroxicam	valganciclovir
cefixime	diclofenac	lithium	quinapril	vancomycin
cefotaxime	enalapril	mefenamic acid	ramipril	voclosporin
cefoxitin	etodolac	meloxicam	rifampicin	zoledronate
cefradine	etoricoxib	mesalazine	streptomycin	

TABLE 3
Drugs with anticoagulant effects

The following is a list of drugs that have anticoagulant effects. Concurrent use of two or more drugs from this list might increase the risk of bleeding; concurrent use of drugs with antiplatelet effects (see table of drugs with antiplatelet effects) might also increase this risk.

acenocoumarol	bivalirudin	enoxaparin	pentosan	tirofiban
alteplase	crisantaspase	eptifibatide	phenindione	urokinase
apixaban	dabigatran	fondaparinux	rivaroxaban	warfarin
argatroban	dalteparin	heparin	streptokinase	
asparaginase	danaparoid	nicotinic acid	tenecteplase	
bemiparin	edoxaban	pegaspargase	tinzaparin	

TABLE 4
Drugs with antiplatelet effects

The following is a list of drugs that have antiplatelet effects (note that this list is not exhaustive). Concurrent use of two or more drugs from this list might increase the risk of bleeding; concurrent use of drugs with anticoagulant effects (see table of drugs with anticoagulant effects) might also increase this risk.

acalabrutinib	clopidogrel	flurbiprofen	naproxen	sulindac
aceclofenac	dapoxetine	fluvoxamine	nintedanib	sunitinib
alprostadil	dasatinib	ibrutinib	omega-3-acid ethyl esters	tenoxicam
anagrelide	dexketoprofen	ibuprofen	parecoxib	tiaprofenic acid
aspirin	diclofenac	iloprost	paroxetine	ticagrelor
axitinib	dipyridamole	imatinib	pazopanib	tolfenamic acid
benzydamine	duloxetine	indometacin	phenazone	treprostinil
bosutinib	eicosapentaenoic acid	ketoprofen	piroxicam	venlafaxine
bromfenac	epoprostenol	ketorolac	ponatinib	vortioxetine
cangrelor	escitalopram	lenvatinib	prasugrel	zanubrutinib
celecoxib	etodolac	mefenamic acid	regorafenib	
cilostazol	etoricoxib	meloxicam	sertraline	
citalopram	fluoxetine	nabumetone	sorafenib	

TABLE 5
Drugs that cause bradycardia

The following is a list of drugs that cause bradycardia (note that this list is not exhaustive). Concurrent use of two or more drugs from the list might increase this risk.

acebutolol	celiprolol	fingolimod	ozanimod	siponimod
alectinib	ceritinib	flecainide	pasireotide	sotalol
alfentanil	clonidine	galantamine	pindolol	sufentanil
amiodarone	crizotinib	ivabradine	ponesimod	suxamethonium
apraclonidine	digoxin	labetalol	propafenone	thalidomide
atenolol	diltiazem	landiolol	propofol	ticagrelor
betaxolol	donepezil	levobunolol	propranolol	timolol
bisoprolol	dronedarone	metoprolol	pyridostigmine	tizanidine
brigatinib	esmolol	nadolol	remifentanil	verapamil
brimonidine	etrasimod	nebivolol	rivastigmine	
carvedilol	fentanyl	neostigmine	selegiline	

TABLE 6
Drugs that cause first dose hypotension

The following is a list of some drugs that can cause first-dose hypotension (note that this list is not exhaustive). Concurrent use of two or more drugs from the list might increase this risk.

alfuzosin	enalapril	indoramin	prazosin	tamsulosin
captopril	fosinopril	lisinopril	quinapril	terazosin
doxazosin	imidapril	perindopril	ramipril	trandolapril

TABLE 7
Drugs that cause hypotension

The following is a list of some drugs that cause hypotension (note that this list is not exhaustive). Concurrent use of two or more drugs from the list might increase this risk.

acebutolol	chlorpromazine	hydralazine	moxonidine	sacubitril
alcohol	chlortalidone	hydrochlorothiazide	nadolol	sapropterin
alfuzosin	clomipramine	hydroflumethiazide	nebivolol	selegiline
aliskiren	clonidine	iloprost	nicardipine	sevoflurane
alprostadil	clozapine	imidapril	nicorandil	sildenafil
amantadine	dapagliflozin	imipramine	nifedipine	sodium oxybate
amitriptyline	desflurane	indapamide	nimodipine	sotalol
amlodipine	diazoxide	indoramin	nitroprusside	spironolactone
apomorphine	diltiazem	irbesartan	nitrous oxide	sulpiride
apraclonidine	dipyridamole	isocarboxazid	nortriptyline	tadalafil
aripiprazole	dosulepin	isoflurane	olanzapine	tamsulosin
asenapine	doxazosin	isosorbide dinitrate	olmesartan	telmisartan
atenolol	doxepin	isosorbide mononitrate	paliperidone	terazosin
avanafil	droperidol	ketamine	pericyazine	thiopental
azilsartan	empagliflozin	labetalol	perindopril	timolol
baclofen	enalapril	lacidipine	phenelzine	tizanidine
bendroflumethiazide	eplerenone	landiolol	pimozide	torasemide
benperidol	epoprostenol	lercanidipine	pindolol	trandolapril
betaxolol	eprosartan	levobunolol	pramipexole	tranylcypromine
bisoprolol	ertugliflozin	levodopa	prazosin	treprostinil
bortezomib	esketamine	levomepromazine	prochlorperazine	trifluoperazine
brimonidine	esmolol	lisinopril	promazine	trimipramine
bromocriptine	etomidate	lofepramine	propofol	valsartan
bumetanide	felodipine	lofexidine	propranolol	vardenafil
cabergoline	finerenone	losartan	quetiapine	verapamil
canagliflozin	flupentixol	loxapine	quinagolide	vericiguat
candesartan	fosinopril	lurasidone	quinapril	vernakalant
captopril	foslevodopa	methoxyflurane	ramipril	xipamide
cariprazine	furosemide	methyldopa	riociguat	zuclopenthixol
carvedilol	glyceryl trinitrate	metolazone	risperidone	
celiprolol	guanfacine	metoprolol	ropinirole	
chlorothiazide	haloperidol	minoxidil	rotigotine	

TABLE 8
Drugs that prolong the QT interval

The following is a list of some drugs that prolong the QT-interval (note that this list is not exhaustive). In general, manufacturers advise that the use of two or more drugs that are associated with QT prolongation should be avoided. Increasing age, female sex, cardiac disease, and some metabolic disturbances (notably hypokalaemia) predispose to QT prolongation—concurrent use of drugs that reduce serum potassium might further increase this risk (see table of drugs that reduce serum potassium).

Drugs that are not known to prolong the QT interval but are predicted (by the manufacturer) to increase the risk of QT prolongation include: domperidone, etrasimod, fingolimod, granisetron, ivabradine, mefloquine, mizolastine, ozanimod, palonosetron, intravenous or intramuscular pentamidine, ponesimod, and siponimod. Most manufacturers advise avoiding concurrent use with drugs that prolong the QT interval.

amifampridine	clomipramine	glasdegib	osilodrostat	sotalol
amiodarone	crizotinib	haloperidol	osimertinib	sunitinib
amisulpride	dasatinib	hydroxychloroquine	paliperidone	tetrabenazine
anagrelide	delamanid	hydroxyzine	panobinostat	tolterodine
apalutamide	desflurane	inotuzumab ozogamicin	pasireotide	toremifene
apomorphine	disopyramide	isoflurane	pazopanib	vandetanib
aripiprazole	dronedarone	ivosidenib	pimozide	vardenafil
arsenic trioxide	droperidol	lapatinib	promethazine	vemurafenib
artemether	efavirenz	lenvatinib	quinine	vernakalant
bedaquiline	encorafenib	levomepromazine	quizartinib	voclosporin
bosutinib	entrectinib	methadone	ranolazine	voriconazole
cabozantinib	eribulin	mobocertinib	ribociclib	
ceritinib	erythromycin	moxifloxacin	selpercatinib	
chlorpromazine	escitalopram	nilotinib	sevoflurane	
citalopram	fluconazole	ondansetron	sorafenib	

TABLE 9
Drugs with antimuscarinic effects

The following is a list of some drugs that have antimuscarinic effects (note that this list is not exhaustive). Concurrent use of two or more drugs from this list might increase the risk of these effects occurring.

aclidinium	cyproheptadine	haloperidol	orphenadrine	propiverine
amantadine	darifenacin	homatropine	oxybutynin	solifenacin
amitriptyline	dicycloverine	hydroxyzine	pericyazine	tiotropium
atropine	dimenhydrinate	hyoscine	pimozide	tolterodine
baclofen	disopyramide	imipramine	pridinol	trifluoperazine
chlorphenamine	dosulepin	ipratropium	prochlorperazine	trihexyphenidyl
chlorpromazine	doxepin	levomepromazine	procyclidine	trimipramine
clomipramine	fesoterodine	lofepramine	promazine	tropicamide
clozapine	flavoxate	loxapine	promethazine	trospium
cyclizine	flupentixol	nortriptyline	propafenone	umeclidinium
cyclopentolate	glycopyrronium	olanzapine	propantheline	zuclopenthixol

TABLE 10

Drugs with effects on the CNS

The following is a list of some drugs that have effects on the CNS (note that this list is not exhaustive). Concurrent use of two or more drugs from this list might increase the risk of sedation, which might affect the ability to perform skilled tasks (see 'Drugs and Driving' in Guidance on Prescribing p. 1). In some cases, concurrent use of two or more drugs from this list might also increase the risk of CNS depressant effects (which could range from sedation to unconsciousness, coma, respiratory depression, and/or cardiovascular depression).

agomelatine	clonazepam	fluvoxamine	mirtazapine	quinagolide
alcohol	clonidine	foslevodopa	morphine	remifentanil
alfentanil	clozapine	fosphenytoin	moxonidine	remimazolam
alimemazine	codeine	gabapentin	nabilone	risperidone
alprazolam	cyclizine	guanfacine	nitrazepam	ropinirole
amisulpride	cyproheptadine	haloperidol	nitrous oxide	rotigotine
amitriptyline	dapoxetine	hydromorphone	nortriptyline	rufinamide
apomorphine	daridorexant	hydroxyzine	olanzapine	sertraline
apraclonidine	desflurane	imipramine	orphenadrine	sevoflurane
aripiprazole	dexmedetomidine	isoflurane	oxazepam	sodium oxybate
asenapine	diamorphine	ketamine	oxycodone	sufentanil
baclofen	diazepam	ketotifen	paliperidone	sulpiride
benperidol	difelikefalin	lamotrigine	paroxetine	tapentadol
brimonidine	dihydrocodeine	levetiracetam	pentazocine	temazepam
bromocriptine	dimenhydrinate	levodopa	perampanel	tetrabenazine
buclizine	dipipanone	levomepromazine	pericyazine	thalidomide
buprenorphine	dosulepin	lofepramine	pethidine	thiopental
cabergoline	doxepin	lofexidine	phenobarbital	tizanidine
cannabidiol	doxylamine	loprazolam	phenytoin	tramadol
cariprazine	dronabinol	lorazepam	pimozide	trazodone
cenobamate	droperidol	lormetazepam	pizotifen	trifluoperazine
chloral hydrate	duloxetine	loxapine	pramipexole	trihexyphenidyl
chlordiazepoxide	escitalopram	lurasidone	pregabalin	trimipramine
chlorphenamine	esketamine	melatonin	primidone	venlafaxine
chlorpromazine	eszopiclone	meptazinol	prochlorperazine	vigabatrin
cinnarizine	etomidate	methadone	procyclidine	zolpidem
citalopram	fentanyl	methocarbamol	promazine	zopiclone
clobazam	fluoxetine	methoxyflurane	promethazine	zuclopenthixol
clomethiazole	flupentixol	mianserin	propofol	
clomipramine	flurazepam	midazolam	quetiapine	

TABLE 11

Drugs that cause peripheral neuropathy

The following is a list of some drugs that cause peripheral neuropathy (note that this list is not exhaustive). Concurrent use of two or more drugs from the list might increase this risk.

amiodarone	cytarabine	leflunomide	phenytoin	vindesine
bortezomib	docetaxel	lenalidomide	pomalidomide	vinorelbine
brentuximab vedotin	enfuvirtide	metronidazole	teriflunomide	
cabazitaxel	eribulin	nitrofurantoin	thalidomide	
carboplatin	isoniazid	oxaliplatin	vinblastine	
cisplatin	lamivudine	paclitaxel	vincristine	

TABLE 12

Drugs that cause serotonin syndrome

The following is a list of some drugs that cause serotonin syndrome (note that this list is not exhaustive). See 'Serotonin Syndrome' and 'Monoamine-Oxidase Inhibitors' under Antidepressant drugs, p. 417 for more information and for specific advice on avoiding monoamine-oxidase inhibitors during and after administration of other serotonergic drugs.

almotriptan	fentanyl	lithium	pentazocine	sumatriptan
citalopram	fluoxetine	methadone	pethidine	tramadol
clomipramine	fluvoxamine	methylthioninium chloride	phenelzine	tranylcypromine
dapoxetine	frovatriptan	mirtazapine	rasagiline	trazodone
dexamfetamine	granisetron	moclobemide	rizatriptan	tryptophan
duloxetine	imipramine	naratriptan	safinamide	venlafaxine
eletriptan	isocarboxazid	ondansetron	selegiline	vortioxetine
escitalopram	linezolid	palonosetron	sertraline	zolmitriptan
fenfluramine	lisdexamfetamine	paroxetine	St John's wort	

TABLE 13
Antidiabetic drugs

The following is a list of antidiabetic drugs (note that this list is not exhaustive). Concurrent use of two or more drugs from the list might increase the risk of hypoglycaemia.

acarbose	empagliflozin	glimepiride	lixisenatide	semaglutide
alogliptin	ertugliflozin	glipizide	metformin	sitagliptin
canagliflozin	exenatide	insulin	pioglitazone	tirzepatide
dapagliflozin	glibenclamide	linagliptin	repaglinide	tolbutamide
dulaglutide	gliclazide	liraglutide	saxagliptin	vildagliptin

TABLE 14
Drugs that cause myelosuppression

The following is a list of some drugs that cause myelosuppression (note that this list is not exhaustive). Concurrent use of two or more drugs from the list might increase this risk.

adalimumab	carmustine	fluorouracil	nelarabine	ruxolitinib
aldesleukin	ceritinib	ganciclovir	nilotinib	sorafenib
alemtuzumab	certolizumab pegol	gemcitabine	niraparib	streptozocin
amsacrine	chlorambucil	gemtuzumab ozogamicin	nivolumab	sulfasalazine
arsenic trioxide	cisplatin	golimumab	obinutuzumab	sunitinib
asparaginase	cladribine	hydroxycarbamide	olaparib	talazoparib
axitinib	clofarabine	ibrutinib	oxaliplatin	tegafur
azacitidine	crisantaspase	idarubicin	paclitaxel	temozolomide
azathioprine	cyclophosphamide	ifosfamide	palbociclib	temsirolimus
belatacept	cytarabine	imatinib	panobinostat	thalidomide
bendamustine	dacarbazine	infliximab	pegaspargase	thiotepa
bevacizumab	dactinomycin	inotuzumab ozogamicin	peginterferon alfa	tioguanine
bexarotene	daratumumab	ipilimumab	pembrolizumab	topotecan
bleomycin	dasatinib	irinotecan	pemetrexed	trabectedin
blinatumomab	daunorubicin	leflunomide	pentostatin	trastuzumab
bortezomib	decitabine	lenalidomide	pixantrone	trastuzumab deruxtecan
bosutinib	dexrazoxane	lomustine	pomalidomide	trastuzumab emtansine
brentuximab vedotin	dinutuximab	melphalan	procarbazine	treosulfan
busulfan	docetaxel	mercaptopurine	raltitrexed	valganciclovir
cabazitaxel	doxorubicin	methotrexate	ramucirumab	vinblastine
cabozantinib	epirubicin	mifamurtide	regorafenib	vincristine
canakinumab	eribulin	mitomycin	ribociclib	vindesine
capecitabine	estramustine	mitotane	rituximab	vinorelbine
carboplatin	etoposide	mitoxantrone	ropeginterferon alfa	
carfilzomib	fludarabine	mogamulizumab	rucaparib	

TABLE 15
Drugs that increase serum potassium

The following is a list of some drugs that increase serum potassium concentrations (note that this list is not exhaustive). Concurrent use of two or more drugs from this list might increase the risk of hyperkalaemia (hyperkalaemia is particularly notable when ACE inhibitors or angiotensin-II receptor antagonists are given with spironolactone or eplerenone).

aceclofenac	drospirenone	indometacin	pentamidine	telmisartan
aliskiren	enalapril	irbesartan	perindopril	tenoxicam
amiloride	enoxaparin	ketoprofen	phenazone	tiaprofenic acid
azilsartan	eplerenone	ketorolac	piroxicam	tinzaparin
bemiparin	eprosartan	labetalol	potassium aminobenzoate	tolfenamic acid
bromfenac	etodolac	lisinopril	potassium canrenoate	tolvaptan
candesartan	etoricoxib	losartan	potassium chloride	trandolapril
captopril	finerenone	mefenamic acid	quinapril	triamterene
celecoxib	flurbiprofen	meloxicam	ramipril	trimethoprim
ciclosporin	fosinopril	nabumetone	spironolactone	valsartan
dalteparin	heparin	naproxen	sulindac	voclosporin
dexketoprofen	ibuprofen	olmesartan	suxamethonium	
diclofenac	imidapril	parecoxib	tacrolimus	

TABLE 16
Drugs that reduce serum potassium

The following is a list of some drugs that reduce serum potassium concentrations (note that this list is not exhaustive and that other drugs can cause hypokalaemia in overdose). Concurrent use of two or more drugs from this list might increase the risk of hypokalaemia. Hypokalaemia can increase the risk of torsade de pointes, which might be additive with the effects of drugs that prolong the QT interval (see table of drugs that prolong the QT interval).

aminophylline	chlorothiazide	hydrochlorothiazide	metolazone	torasemide
amphotericin B	chlortalidone	hydrocortisone	olodaterol	triamcinolone
beclometasone	deflazacort	hydroflumethiazide	prednisolone	vamorolone
bendroflumethiazide	dexamethasone	indacaterol	salbutamol	vilanterol
betamethasone	fludrocortisone	indapamide	salmeterol	xipamide
budesonide	formoterol	isoprenaline	terbutaline	
bumetanide	furosemide	methylprednisolone	theophylline	

TABLE 17
Drugs that cause hyponatraemia

The following is a list of some drugs that reduce sodium concentrations (note that this list is not exhaustive). Concurrent use of two or more drugs from this list might increase the risk of hyponatraemia.

aceclofenac	clomipramine	furosemide	mirtazapine	sertraline
amiloride	clozapine	haloperidol	nabumetone	sulindac
amisulpride	cyclophosphamide	hydrochlorothiazide	naproxen	sulpiride
amitriptyline	desmopressin	hydroflumethiazide	nortriptyline	tenoxicam
aripiprazole	dexketoprofen	ibuprofen	olanzapine	tiaprofenic acid
asenapine	diclofenac	imipramine	oxcarbazepine	tolfenamic acid
bendroflumethiazide	dosulepin	indapamide	oxytocin	torasemide
benperidol	doxepin	indometacin	paliperidone	tramadol
bumetanide	droperidol	ketoprofen	parecoxib	trazodone
carbamazepine	duloxetine	ketorolac	paroxetine	trifluoperazine
carboplatin	escitalopram	levomepromazine	pericyazine	trimipramine
cariprazine	eslicarbazepine	lofepramine	phenazone	valproate
celecoxib	etodolac	loxapine	pimozide	venlafaxine
chlorothiazide	etoricoxib	lurasidone	piroxicam	vinblastine
chlorpromazine	fluoxetine	mannitol	prochlorperazine	vincristine
chlortalidone	flupentixol	mefenamic acid	promazine	vinorelbine
cisplatin	flurbiprofen	meloxicam	quetiapine	xipamide
citalopram	fluvoxamine	metolazone	risperidone	zuclopenthixol

TABLE 18
Drugs that cause ototoxicity

The following is a list of some drugs that cause ototoxicity (note that this list is not exhaustive). Concurrent use of two or more drugs from the list might increase this risk.

amikacin	cisplatin	mefloquine	streptomycin	vincristine
amphotericin B	colistimethate	neomycin	tobramycin	vindesine
bumetanide	furosemide	netilmicin	torasemide	vinorelbine
carboplatin	gentamicin	oxaliplatin	vancomycin	
chloroquine	hydroxychloroquine	quinine	vinblastine	

TABLE 19
Drugs with neuromuscular blocking effects

The following is a list of some drugs with neuromuscular blocking effects (note that this list is not exhaustive). Concurrent use of two or more drugs from the list might increase this risk.

amikacin	colistimethate	netilmicin	streptomycin
atracurium	gentamicin	pancuronium	suxamethonium
botulinum toxin type A	mivacurium	polymyxin b	tobramycin
cisatracurium	neomycin	rocuronium	vecuronium

List of drug interactions

The following is an alphabetical list of drugs and their interactions; to avoid excessive cross-referencing each drug or group is listed twice: in the alphabetical list and also against the drug or group with which it interacts.

5-HT3-receptor antagonists → see TABLE 12 p. 1574 (serotonin syndrome), TABLE 8 p. 1573 (QT-interval prolongation)

granisetron · ondansetron · palonosetron

▶ Anti-androgens (apalutamide, enzalutamide) are predicted to decrease the exposure to ondansetron. Moderate Study → Also see TABLE 8 p. 1573

▶ Antiepileptics (carbamazepine, fosphenytoin, phenobarbital, phenytoin, primidone) are predicted to decrease the exposure to ondansetron. Moderate Study

▶ Dopamine receptor agonists (apomorphine) increase the risk of severe hypotension when given with ondansetron. Avoid. Severe Study → Also see TABLE 8 p. 1573

▶ Dopamine receptor agonists (apomorphine) are predicted to increase the risk of severe hypotension when given with 5-HT3-receptor antagonists (granisetron, palonosetron). Severe Theoretical

▶ Encorafenib is predicted to decrease the exposure to ondansetron. Moderate Study → Also see TABLE 8 p. 1573

▶ Ivosidenib is predicted to decrease the exposure to ondansetron. Moderate Study → Also see TABLE 8 p. 1573

▶ Lumacaftor is predicted to decrease the exposure to ondansetron. Moderate Study

▶ Mitotane is predicted to decrease the exposure to ondansetron. Moderate Study

▶ Rifamycins (rifampicin) are predicted to decrease the exposure to ondansetron. Moderate Study

Abacavir → see NRTIs

Abatacept

▶ Anakinra is predicted to increase the risk of generalised infection (possibly life-threatening) when given with abatacept. Severe Theoretical

▶ Abatacept is predicted to increase the risk of generalised infection (possibly life-threatening) when given with etanercept. Avoid. Severe Theoretical

▶ Filgotinib is predicted to increase the risk of immunosuppression when given with abatacept. Avoid. Severe Theoretical

▶ Live vaccines are predicted to increase the risk of generalised infection (possibly life-threatening) when given with abatacept. UKHSA advises avoid (refer to Green Book). Severe Theoretical

▶ Monoclonal antibodies (certolizumab pegol) are predicted to increase the risk of generalised infection (possibly life-threatening) when given with abatacept. Avoid. Severe Theoretical

▶ Monoclonal antibodies (rozanolixizumab) might decrease the concentration of abatacept. Avoid and for 2 weeks after stopping rozanolixizumab. Moderate Theoretical

▶ Abatacept is predicted to increase the risk of generalised infection (possibly life-threatening) when given with monoclonal antibodies (adalimumab, golimumab, infliximab). Avoid. Severe Theoretical

Abemaciclib

▶ Anti-androgens (apalutamide, enzalutamide) are predicted to markedly decrease the exposure to abemaciclib. Avoid. Severe Study

▶ Antiarrhythmics (dronedarone) are predicted to increase the exposure to abemaciclib. Moderate Study

▶ Antiepileptics (carbamazepine, fosphenytoin, phenobarbital, phenytoin, primidone) are predicted to markedly decrease the exposure to abemaciclib. Avoid. Severe Study

▶ Antifungals, azoles (fluconazole, isavuconazole) are predicted to increase the exposure to abemaciclib. Moderate Study

▶ Antifungals, azoles (itraconazole, ketoconazole, posaconazole, voriconazole) are predicted to increase the exposure to abemaciclib. Avoid or adjust dose—consult product literature. Severe Study

▶ Berotralstat is predicted to increase the exposure to abemaciclib. Moderate Study

▶ Calcium channel blockers (diltiazem, verapamil) are predicted to increase the exposure to abemaciclib. Moderate Study

▶ Ceritinib is predicted to increase the exposure to abemaciclib. Avoid or adjust dose—consult product literature. Severe Study

▶ Cobicistat is predicted to increase the exposure to abemaciclib. Avoid or adjust dose—consult product literature. Severe Study

▶ Crizotinib is predicted to increase the exposure to abemaciclib. Moderate Study

▶ Encorafenib is predicted to markedly decrease the exposure to abemaciclib. Avoid. Severe Study

▶ Fedratinib is predicted to increase the exposure to abemaciclib. Moderate Study

▶ Grapefruit juice is predicted to increase the exposure to abemaciclib. Avoid. Moderate Theoretical

▶ HIV-protease inhibitors are predicted to increase the exposure to abemaciclib. Avoid or adjust dose—consult product literature. Severe Study

▶ Idelalisib is predicted to increase the exposure to abemaciclib. Avoid or adjust dose—consult product literature. Severe Study

▶ Imatinib is predicted to increase the exposure to abemaciclib. Moderate Study

▶ Ivosidenib is predicted to markedly decrease the exposure to abemaciclib. Avoid. Severe Study

▶ Letermovir is predicted to increase the exposure to abemaciclib. Moderate Study

▶ Lumacaftor is predicted to markedly decrease the exposure to abemaciclib. Avoid. Severe Study

▶ Macrolides (clarithromycin) are predicted to increase the exposure to abemaciclib. Avoid or adjust dose—consult product literature. Severe Study

▶ Macrolides (erythromycin) are predicted to increase the exposure to abemaciclib. Moderate Study

▶ Mitotane is predicted to markedly decrease the exposure to abemaciclib. Avoid. Severe Study

▶ Neurokinin-1 receptor antagonists (aprepitant, netupitant) are predicted to increase the exposure to abemaciclib. Moderate Study

▶ Nilotinib is predicted to increase the exposure to abemaciclib. Moderate Study

▶ Nirmatrelvir boosted with ritonavir is predicted to increase the concentration of abemaciclib. Avoid or adjust dose—consult product literature. Severe Theoretical

▶ Rifamycins (rifampicin) are predicted to markedly decrease the exposure to abemaciclib. Avoid. Severe Study

▶ St John's wort is predicted to decrease the exposure to abemaciclib. Avoid. Severe Study

▶ Tucatinib is predicted to increase the exposure to abemaciclib. Avoid or adjust dose—consult product literature. Severe Study

Abiraterone → see anti-androgens

Abrocitinib

▶ Anti-androgens (apalutamide, enzalutamide) are predicted to decrease the exposure to abrocitinib. Avoid. Moderate Study

▶ Antiepileptics (fosphenytoin, phenytoin) are predicted to decrease the exposure to abrocitinib. Avoid. Moderate Theoretical

▶ Antifungals, azoles (fluconazole) are predicted to increase the exposure to abrocitinib. Adjust abrocitinib dose, p. 1430. Severe Study

▶ Abrocitinib might increase the exposure to ciclosporin. Moderate Theoretical

▶ Abrocitinib might increase the exposure to digoxin. Moderate Theoretical

▶ Abrocitinib might increase the exposure to everolimus. Moderate Theoretical

▶ Abrocitinib might increase the exposure to factor XA inhibitors (edoxaban). Moderate Theoretical

▶ Live vaccines are predicted to increase the risk of generalised infection (possibly life-threatening) when given with abrocitinib. Avoid. Severe Theoretical

▶ NNRTIs (efavirenz) are predicted to decrease the exposure to abrocitinib. Avoid. Moderate Theoretical

▶ Rifamycins (rifampicin) are predicted to decrease the exposure to abrocitinib. Avoid. Moderate Study

Abrocitinib (continued)

▶ **Abrocitinib** might increase the exposure to sirolimus. Moderate Theoretical

▶ SSRIs (fluoxetine, fluvoxamine) are predicted to increase the exposure to **abrocitinib**. Adjust **abrocitinib** dose, p. 1430. Severe Study

▶ **Abrocitinib** slightly increases the exposure to thrombin inhibitors (dabigatran). Moderate Study

Acalabrutinib → see TABLE 4 p. 1571 (antiplatelet effects)

▶ Anti-androgens (apalutamide, enzalutamide) are predicted to decrease the exposure to **acalabrutinib**. Avoid. Severe Study

▶ Antiarrhythmics (dronedarone) are predicted to increase the exposure to **acalabrutinib**. Avoid or monitor. Severe Study

▶ Antiepileptics (carbamazepine, fosphenytoin, phenobarbital, phenytoin, primidone) are predicted to decrease the exposure to **acalabrutinib**. Avoid. Severe Study

▶ Antifungals, azoles (fluconazole, isavuconazole) are predicted to increase the exposure to **acalabrutinib**. Avoid or monitor. Severe Study

▶ Antifungals, azoles (itraconazole, ketoconazole, posaconazole, voriconazole) are predicted to increase the exposure to **acalabrutinib**. Avoid. Severe Study

▶ Berotralstat is predicted to increase the exposure to **acalabrutinib**. Avoid or monitor. Severe Study

▶ Calcium channel blockers (diltiazem, verapamil) are predicted to increase the exposure to **acalabrutinib**. Avoid or monitor. Severe Study

▶ Cenobamate is predicted to decrease the exposure to **acalabrutinib**. Adjust dose. Moderate Theoretical

▶ Ceritinib is predicted to increase the exposure to **acalabrutinib**. Avoid. Severe Study

▶ Cobicistat is predicted to increase the exposure to **acalabrutinib**. Avoid. Severe Study

▶ Crizotinib is predicted to increase the exposure to **acalabrutinib**. Avoid or monitor. Severe Study

▶ Dabrafenib is predicted to decrease the exposure to **acalabrutinib**. Severe Study

▶ Encorafenib is predicted to decrease the exposure to **acalabrutinib**. Avoid. Severe Study

▶ Endothelin receptor antagonists (bosentan) are predicted to decrease the exposure to **acalabrutinib**. Severe Study

▶ Fedratinib is predicted to increase the exposure to **acalabrutinib**. Avoid or monitor. Severe Study

▶ HIV-protease inhibitors are predicted to increase the exposure to **acalabrutinib**. Avoid. Severe Study

▶ Idelalisib is predicted to increase the exposure to **acalabrutinib**. Avoid. Severe Study

▶ Imatinib is predicted to increase the exposure to **acalabrutinib**. Avoid or monitor. Severe Study → Also see TABLE 4 p. 1571

▶ Ivosidenib is predicted to decrease the exposure to **acalabrutinib**. Avoid. Severe Study

▶ Letermovir is predicted to increase the exposure to **acalabrutinib**. Avoid or monitor. Severe Study

▶ Lumacaftor is predicted to decrease the exposure to **acalabrutinib**. Avoid. Severe Study

▶ Macrolides (clarithromycin) are predicted to increase the exposure to **acalabrutinib**. Avoid. Severe Study

▶ Macrolides (erythromycin) are predicted to increase the exposure to **acalabrutinib**. Avoid or monitor. Severe Study

▶ Mitotane is predicted to decrease the exposure to **acalabrutinib**. Avoid. Severe Study

▶ Neurokinin-1 receptor antagonists (aprepitant, netupitant) are predicted to increase the exposure to **acalabrutinib**. Avoid or monitor. Severe Study

▶ Nilotinib is predicted to increase the exposure to **acalabrutinib**. Avoid or monitor. Severe Study

▶ NNRTIs (efavirenz, nevirapine) are predicted to decrease the exposure to **acalabrutinib**. Severe Study

▶ Rifamycins (rifampicin) are predicted to decrease the exposure to **acalabrutinib**. Avoid. Severe Study

▶ St John's wort is predicted to decrease the exposure to **acalabrutinib**. Avoid. Severe Study

▶ Tucatinib is predicted to increase the exposure to **acalabrutinib**. Avoid. Severe Study

Acarbose → see TABLE 13 p. 1575 (antidiabetic drugs)

▶ **Acarbose** decreases the concentration of digoxin. Moderate Study

▶ Fenfluramine might decrease blood glucose concentrations when given with **acarbose**. Moderate Theoretical

▶ Pancreatin is predicted to decrease the effects of **acarbose**. Avoid. Moderate Theoretical

▶ Somapacitan might increase blood glucose concentrations, opposing the blood glucose-lowering effects of **acarbose**. Adjust dose. Moderate Theoretical

▶ Somatrogon might increase blood glucose concentrations, opposing the blood glucose-lowering effects of **acarbose**. Adjust dose. Moderate Theoretical

ACE inhibitors → see TABLE 6 p. 1572 (first-dose hypotension), TABLE 7 p. 1572 (hypotension), TABLE 2 p. 1571 (nephrotoxicity), TABLE 15 p. 1575 (increased serum potassium)

captopril · enalapril · fosinopril · imidapril · lisinopril · perindopril · quinapril · ramipril · trandolapril

▶ **ACE inhibitors** increase the risk of renal impairment when given with aliskiren. Use with caution or avoid aliskiren in selected patients, p. 207. Severe Study → Also see TABLE 7 p. 1572 → Also see TABLE 15 p. 1575

▶ **ACE inhibitors** are predicted to increase the risk of hypersensitivity and haematological reactions when given with allopurinol. Severe Anecdotal

▶ **ACE inhibitors** are predicted to increase the risk of anaemia and/or leucopenia when given with azathioprine. Severe Anecdotal

▶ Everolimus potentially increases the risk of angioedema when given with **ACE inhibitors**. Severe Anecdotal

▶ Captopril is predicted to increase the exposure to gilteritinib. Moderate Theoretical

▶ **ACE inhibitors** are predicted to decrease the efficacy of icatibant and icatibant is predicted to decrease the efficacy of **ACE inhibitors**. Avoid. Moderate Theoretical

▶ **ACE inhibitors** are predicted to increase the concentration of lithium. Monitor and adjust dose. Severe Anecdotal → Also see TABLE 2 p. 1571

▶ **ACE inhibitors** are predicted to increase the risk of angioedema when given with temsirolimus. Moderate Theoretical

▶ Oral **quinapril** (magnesium carbonate-containing forms) might decrease the absorption of oral tetracyclines. Avoid. Moderate Study

▶ Enalapril might enhance the antidiuretic and hypertensive effects of vasopressin. Moderate Theoretical

Acebutolol → see beta blockers, selective

Aceclofenac → see NSAIDs

Acenocoumarol → see coumarins

Acetazolamide

▶ **Acetazolamide** potentially increases the risk of toxicity when given with antiepileptics (valproate). Severe Study

▶ **Acetazolamide** potentially increases the risk of overheating and dehydration when given with antiepileptics (zonisamide). Avoid in children. Severe Theoretical

▶ **Acetazolamide** increases the risk of severe toxic reaction when given with aspirin (high-dose). Severe Study

▶ **Acetazolamide** alters the concentration of lithium. Severe Anecdotal

▶ **Acetazolamide** is predicted to decrease the efficacy of methenamine. Avoid. Moderate Theoretical

▶ **Acetazolamide** increases the urinary excretion of methotrexate. Moderate Study

▶ **Acetazolamide** might decrease the efficacy of nitrofurantoin. Unknown Theoretical

Acetylcysteine

▶ **Acetylcysteine** might increase the vasodilatory effects of nitrates (glyceryl trinitrate). Moderate Theoretical

Aciclovir → see TABLE 2 p. 1571 (nephrotoxicity)

ROUTE-SPECIFIC INFORMATION Since systemic absorption can follow topical application, the possibility of interactions should be borne in mind.

▶ **Aciclovir** increases the exposure to aminophylline. Monitor and adjust dose. Severe Anecdotal

- **Mycophenolate** is predicted to increase the risk of haematological toxicity when given with **aciclovir**. Moderate Theoretical
- **Aciclovir** is predicted to increase the exposure to **theophylline**. Monitor and adjust dose. Severe Theoretical

Acipimox
- **Acipimox** is predicted to increase the risk of rhabdomyolysis when given with **fibrates**. Severe Theoretical
- **Acipimox** is predicted to increase the risk of rhabdomyolysis when given with **statins**. Severe Theoretical

Acitretin → see retinoids

Aclidinium → see TABLE 9 p. 1573 (antimuscarinics)
- **Antipsychotics, second generation (clozapine)** can cause constipation, as can **aclidinium**; concurrent use might increase the risk of developing intestinal obstruction. Severe Theoretical → Also see TABLE 9 p. 1573

Acrivastine → see antihistamines, non-sedating

Adalimumab → see monoclonal antibodies

Adapalene → see retinoids

Adefovir → see TABLE 2 p. 1571 (nephrotoxicity)
- **Ivosidenib** is predicted to increase the exposure to **adefovir**. Use with caution or avoid. Moderate Theoretical
- **Leflunomide** is predicted to increase the exposure to **adefovir**. Moderate Study
- **Nitisinone** is predicted to increase the exposure to **adefovir**. Moderate Study
- **Teriflunomide** is predicted to increase the exposure to **adefovir**. Moderate Study

Adenosine → see antiarrhythmics

Adrenaline/epinephrine → see sympathomimetics, vasoconstrictor

Afatinib
- **Antiarrhythmics (amiodarone, dronedarone)** are predicted to increase the exposure to **afatinib**. Moderate Study
- **Antiepileptics (carbamazepine)** are predicted to decrease the exposure to **afatinib**. Moderate Study
- **Antiepileptics (phenobarbital, phenytoin)** are predicted to decrease the exposure to **afatinib**. Moderate Theoretical
- **Antifungals, azoles (itraconazole, ketoconazole)** are predicted to increase the exposure to **afatinib**. Moderate Study
- **Calcium channel blockers (verapamil)** are predicted to increase the exposure to **afatinib**. Moderate Study
- **Ciclosporin** is predicted to increase the exposure to **afatinib**. Moderate Study
- **Cobicistat** is predicted to increase the exposure to **afatinib**. Moderate Study
- **Glecaprevir** is predicted to increase the exposure to **afatinib**. Moderate Study
- **HIV-protease inhibitors (lopinavir, ritonavir)** are predicted to increase the exposure to **afatinib**. Moderate Study
- **Lapatinib** is predicted to increase the exposure to **afatinib**. Moderate Study
- **Lorlatinib** is predicted to decrease the exposure to **afatinib**. Moderate Study
- **Macrolides** are predicted to increase the exposure to **afatinib**. Moderate Study
- **Nirmatrelvir** boosted with ritonavir is predicted to increase the concentration of **afatinib**. Moderate Theoretical
- **Pibrentasvir** is predicted to increase the exposure to **afatinib**. Moderate Study
- **Ranolazine** is predicted to increase the exposure to **afatinib**. Moderate Study
- **Rifamycins (rifampicin)** are predicted to decrease the exposure to **afatinib**. Moderate Study
- **Afatinib** is predicted to increase the exposure to the active component of **sacituzumab govitecan**. Severe Theoretical
- **St John's wort** is predicted to decrease the exposure to **afatinib**. Moderate Study
- **Tacrolimus** is predicted to increase the exposure to **afatinib**. Moderate Theoretical
- **Velpatasvir** is predicted to increase the exposure to **afatinib**. Moderate Study
- **Vemurafenib** is predicted to increase the exposure to **afatinib**. Moderate Study
- **Voxilaprevir** is predicted to increase the exposure to **afatinib**. Moderate Study

Aflibercept
ROUTE-SPECIFIC INFORMATION Interactions do not generally apply to topical use unless specified.
- **Monoclonal antibodies (rozanolixizumab)** might decrease the concentration of **aflibercept**. Avoid and for 2 weeks after stopping **rozanolixizumab**. Moderate Theoretical

Agalsidase alfa
- **Aminoglycosides** are predicted to decrease the effects of **agalsidase alfa**. Avoid. Moderate Theoretical
- **Antiarrhythmics (amiodarone)** are predicted to decrease the effects of **agalsidase alfa**. Avoid. Moderate Theoretical
- **Antimalarials (chloroquine)** are predicted to decrease the effects of **agalsidase alfa**. Avoid. Moderate Theoretical
- **Hydroxychloroquine** is predicted to decrease the effects of **agalsidase alfa**. Moderate Theoretical

Agalsidase beta
- **Aminoglycosides** are predicted to decrease the effects of **agalsidase beta**. Avoid. Moderate Theoretical
- **Antiarrhythmics (amiodarone)** are predicted to decrease the effects of **agalsidase beta**. Avoid. Moderate Theoretical
- **Antimalarials (chloroquine)** are predicted to decrease the effects of **agalsidase beta**. Avoid. Moderate Theoretical
- **Hydroxychloroquine** is predicted to decrease the exposure to **agalsidase beta**. Moderate Theoretical

Agomelatine → see TABLE 10 p. 1574 (CNS effects)

- Dose adjustment might be necessary if smoking started or stopped during treatment.
- Caution with concurrent use of drugs associated with hepatic injury.

- **Antiepileptics (fosphenytoin, phenytoin)** are predicted to decrease the exposure to **agomelatine**. Moderate Theoretical → Also see TABLE 10 p. 1574
- **Axitinib** is predicted to increase the exposure to **agomelatine**. Moderate Theoretical
- **Combined hormonal contraceptives** is predicted to increase the exposure to **agomelatine**. Moderate Study
- **Givosiran** is predicted to increase the exposure to **agomelatine**. Moderate Study
- **HIV-protease inhibitors (ritonavir)** are predicted to decrease the exposure to **agomelatine**. Moderate Theoretical
- **Leflunomide** is predicted to decrease the exposure to **agomelatine**. Moderate Theoretical
- **Mexiletine** is predicted to increase the exposure to **agomelatine**. Moderate Study
- **Osilodrostat** is predicted to increase the exposure to **agomelatine**. Moderate Study
- **Quinolones (ciprofloxacin)** are predicted to increase the exposure to **agomelatine**. Moderate Study
- **Rifamycins (rifampicin)** are predicted to decrease the exposure to **agomelatine**. Moderate Theoretical
- **Rucaparib** is predicted to increase the exposure to **agomelatine**. Moderate Study
- **SSRIs (fluvoxamine)** very markedly increase the exposure to **agomelatine**. Avoid. Severe Study → Also see TABLE 10 p. 1574
- **Teriflunomide** is predicted to decrease the exposure to **agomelatine**. Moderate Theoretical
- **Vemurafenib** is predicted to increase the exposure to **agomelatine**. Moderate Study

Albendazole
- **Antiepileptics (carbamazepine, fosphenytoin, phenobarbital, phenytoin, primidone)** decrease the concentration of **albendazole**. Moderate Study
- **H_2 receptor antagonists (cimetidine)** decrease the clearance of **albendazole**. Moderate Study
- **HIV-protease inhibitors (ritonavir)** decrease the exposure to **albendazole**. Moderate Study
- **Albendazole** slightly decreases the exposure to **levamisole** and **levamisole** moderately decreases the exposure to **albendazole**. Moderate Study

Alcohol → see TABLE 7 p. 1572 (hypotension), TABLE 10 p. 1574 (CNS effects)

ROUTE-SPECIFIC INFORMATION Interactions do not generally apply to alcohol used for topical action unless specified.

Alcohol (continued)

▶ Antiepileptics **(sultiame)** might cause a disulfiram-like reaction when given with **alcohol**. Avoid. Moderate Theoretical

▶ **Alcohol** potentially increases the risk of visual disturbances when given with antiepileptics **(retigabine)**. Moderate Study

▶ **Alcohol** potentially causes a disulfiram-like reaction when given with antifungals, azoles **(ketoconazole)**. Avoid. Moderate Anecdotal

▶ **Alcohol** causes serious, potentially fatal, CNS depression when given with **clomethiazole**. Avoid. Severe Study → Also see TABLE 10 p. 1574

▶ **Alcohol** (in those who drink heavily) potentially decreases the anticoagulant effect of **coumarins**. Severe Study

▶ **Alcohol** (excessive consumption) potentially increases the risk of gastrointestinal adverse effects when given with **dimethyl fumarate**. Avoid. Moderate Theoretical

▶ **Alcohol** causes an extremely unpleasant systemic reaction when given with **disulfiram**. Avoid for at least 24 hours before and up to 14 days after stopping treatment. Severe Study

▶ **Alcohol**-induced liver disease increases the risk of hepatotoxicity in those taking **drugs that cause hepatotoxicity** (see TABLE 1 p. 1571). Severe Theoretical

▶ **Alcohol** potentially causes a disulfiram-like reaction when given with **griseofulvin**. Moderate Anecdotal

▶ **Alcohol** potentially causes a disulfiram-like reaction when given with **levamisole**. Moderate Study

▶ **Alcohol** (excessive consumption) potentially increases the risk of lactic acidosis when given with **metformin**. Avoid excessive alcohol consumption. Moderate Theoretical

▶ **Alcohol** might increase the concentration of **methylphenidate**. Avoid. Moderate Study

▶ **Alcohol** potentially causes a disulfiram-like reaction when given with **metronidazole**. Avoid for at least 48 hours after stopping treatment. Moderate Study

▶ **Alcohol** causes rapid release of opioids **(hydromorphone, morphine)** from extended-release preparations. Avoid. Severe Study → Also see TABLE 10 p. 1574

▶ **Alcohol** (in those who drink heavily) causes severe liver damage when given with **paracetamol**. Severe Study

▶ **Alcohol** increases the risk of facial flushing and skin irritation when given with topical **pimecrolimus**. Moderate Study

▶ **Alcohol** potentially causes a disulfiram-like reaction when given with **procarbazine**. Moderate Anecdotal

▶ **Alcohol** potentially increases the concentration of retinoids **(acitretin)**. Avoid and for 2 months after stopping **acitretin**. Moderate Study

▶ **Alcohol** increases the risk of facial flushing and skin irritation when given with topical **tacrolimus**. Moderate Study

▶ **Alcohol** might decrease the antidiuretic effect of **vasopressin**. Moderate Theoretical

Aldesleukin → see TABLE 14 p. 1575 (myelosuppression)

Alectinib → see TABLE 5 p. 1572 (bradycardia), TABLE 1 p. 1571 (hepatotoxicity)

Alemtuzumab → see monoclonal antibodies

Alendronate → see bisphosphonates

Alfacalcidol → see vitamin D substances

Alfentanil → see opioids

Alfuzosin → see alpha blockers

Alimemazine → see antihistamines, sedating

Aliskiren → see TABLE 7 p. 1572 (hypotension), TABLE 15 p. 1575 (increased serum potassium)

FOOD AND LIFESTYLE Avoid apple juice and orange juice as they greatly decrease aliskiren concentrations and plasma renin activity.

▶ ACE inhibitors increase the risk of renal impairment when given with **aliskiren**. Use with caution or avoid **aliskiren** in selected patients, p. 207. Severe Study → Also see TABLE 7 p. 1572 → Also see TABLE 15 p. 1575

▶ Angiotensin-II receptor antagonists increase the risk of renal impairment when given with **aliskiren**. Use with caution or avoid **aliskiren** in selected patients, p. 207. Severe Study → Also see TABLE 7 p. 1572 → Also see TABLE 15 p. 1575

▶ Anti-androgens **(apalutamide)** are predicted to decrease the exposure to **aliskiren**. Monitor and adjust dose. Moderate Study

▶ Antiarrhythmics **(amiodarone, dronedarone)** are predicted to increase the exposure to **aliskiren**. Severe Study

▶ Antiepileptics **(carbamazepine)** decrease the exposure to **aliskiren**. Moderate Study

▶ Antifungals, azoles **(itraconazole)** markedly increase the exposure to **aliskiren**. Avoid. Severe Study

▶ Antifungals, azoles **(ketoconazole)** moderately increase the exposure to **aliskiren**. Moderate Study

▶ Calcium channel blockers **(verapamil)** moderately increase the exposure to **aliskiren**. Moderate Study → Also see TABLE 7 p. 1572

▶ **Ceritinib** is predicted to increase the exposure to **aliskiren**. Moderate Theoretical

▶ **Ciclosporin** markedly increases the exposure to **aliskiren**. Avoid. Severe Study → Also see TABLE 15 p. 1575

▶ **Cobicistat** is predicted to increase the exposure to **aliskiren**. Moderate Theoretical

▶ **Danicopan** is predicted to increase the exposure to **aliskiren**. Moderate Study

▶ **Eliglustat** is predicted to increase the exposure to **aliskiren**. Adjust dose. Moderate Study

▶ **Glecaprevir** is predicted to increase the exposure to **aliskiren**. Severe Theoretical

▶ **Grapefruit** juice moderately decreases the exposure to **aliskiren**. Avoid. Severe Study

▶ HIV-protease inhibitors **(ritonavir)** are predicted to increase the exposure to **aliskiren**. Moderate Theoretical

▶ **Ivosidenib** is predicted to alter the exposure to **aliskiren**. Moderate Theoretical

▶ **Lapatinib** is predicted to increase the exposure to **aliskiren**. Moderate Theoretical

▶ **Aliskiren** slightly decreases the exposure to loop diuretics **(furosemide)**. Moderate Study → Also see TABLE 7 p. 1572

▶ **Lorlatinib** decreases the exposure to **aliskiren**. Moderate Study

▶ Macrolides **(azithromycin)** are predicted to increase the exposure to **aliskiren**. Moderate Theoretical

▶ Macrolides **(clarithromycin, erythromycin)** are predicted to increase the exposure to **aliskiren**. Moderate Study

▶ **Mirabegron** is predicted to increase the exposure to **aliskiren**. Mild Theoretical

▶ **Nirmatrelvir** boosted with ritonavir is predicted to increase the concentration of **aliskiren**. Avoid. Severe Theoretical

▶ **Olaparib** might increase the exposure to **aliskiren**. Moderate Theoretical

▶ **Osimertinib** is predicted to increase the exposure to **aliskiren**. Moderate Study

▶ **Pibrentasvir** with glecaprevir is predicted to increase the exposure to **aliskiren**. Moderate Study

▶ **Pitolisant** is predicted to decrease the exposure to **aliskiren**. Mild Theoretical

▶ **Ranolazine** is predicted to increase the exposure to **aliskiren**. Moderate Theoretical

▶ Rifamycins **(rifampicin)** decrease the exposure to **aliskiren**. Moderate Study

▶ **St John's wort** decreases the exposure to **aliskiren**. Moderate Study

▶ Statins **(atorvastatin)** slightly to moderately increase the exposure to **aliskiren**. Moderate Study

▶ **Tepotinib** is predicted to increase the concentration of **aliskiren**. Severe Study

▶ **Velpatasvir** is predicted to increase the exposure to **aliskiren**. Severe Theoretical

▶ **Vemurafenib** is predicted to increase the exposure to **aliskiren**. Use with caution and adjust dose. Moderate Theoretical

▶ **Voxilaprevir** with sofosbuvir and velpatasvir is predicted to increase the exposure to **aliskiren**. Severe Theoretical

Alitretinoin → see retinoids

Alkylating agents → see TABLE 1 p. 1571 (hepatotoxicity), TABLE 17 p. 1576 (hyponatraemia), TABLE 14 p. 1575 (myelosuppression), TABLE 2 p. 1571 (nephrotoxicity)

bendamustine · busulfan · carmustine · chlorambucil · cyclophosphamide · dacarbazine · estramustine · ifosfamide · lomustine · melphalan · temozolomide · thiotepa · treosulfan

▶ Oral **antacids** are predicted to decrease the absorption of oral **estramustine**. Avoid. Moderate Study

▸ Antifungals, azoles **(isavuconazole)** are predicted to increase the exposure to **cyclophosphamide**. [Moderate] Study

▸ Antifungals, azoles **(itraconazole)** increase the risk of busulfan toxicity when given with **busulfan**. Monitor and adjust dose. [Moderate] Study

▸ Antifungals, azoles **(miconazole)** are predicted to increase the concentration of **busulfan**. Use with caution and adjust dose. [Moderate] Theoretical

▸ Oral **calcium salts** decrease the absorption of oral **estramustine**. [Severe] Study

▸ Iron chelators **(deferasirox)** have been reported to increase the exposure to **busulfan**. Monitor and adjust dose. [Unknown] Anecdotal

▸ **Ivosidenib** might decrease the exposure to alkylating agents **(cyclophosphamide, ifosfamide)**. Avoid or monitor efficacy. [Unknown] Theoretical

▸ **Live vaccines** are predicted to increase the risk of generalised infection (possibly life-threatening) when given with **alkylating agents**. UKHSA advises avoid (refer to Green Book). [Severe] Theoretical

▸ **Metronidazole** increases the risk of toxicity when given with **busulfan**. [Severe] Study

▸ **Neurokinin-1 receptor antagonists (aprepitant, fosaprepitant)** are predicted to increase the exposure to **ifosfamide**. [Severe] Theoretical

▸ **Neurokinin-1 receptor antagonists (netupitant)** very slightly increase the exposure to **cyclophosphamide**. [Moderate] Study

▸ **Neurokinin-1 receptor antagonists (netupitant)** are predicted to increase the exposure to **ifosfamide**. [Moderate] Study

▸ **Paracetamol** is predicted to decrease the clearance of **busulfan**. [Moderate] Theoretical

▸ **Pemigatinib** might increase the exposure to the active metabolite of **cyclophosphamide**. [Moderate] Theoretical

▸ **Pemigatinib** might decrease the exposure to **ifosfamide**. [Moderate] Theoretical

▸ **Cyclophosphamide** (high-dose) increases the risk of toxicity when given with **pentostatin**. Avoid. [Severe] Anecdotal → Also see **TABLE 14** p. 1575

▸ **Cyclophosphamide** increases the risk of prolonged neuromuscular blockade when given with **suxamethonium**. [Moderate] Study

▸ Alkylating agents **(cyclophosphamide, ifosfamide)** might enhance the antidiuretic and hypertensive effects of **vasopressin**. [Moderate] Theoretical

Allopurinol

▸ **ACE inhibitors** are predicted to increase the risk of hypersensitivity and haematological reactions when given with **allopurinol**. [Severe] Anecdotal

▸ **Allopurinol** potentially increases the risk of haematological toxicity when given with **azathioprine**. Adjust **azathioprine** dose, p. 965. [Severe] Study

▸ **Allopurinol** is predicted to decrease the effects of **capecitabine**. Avoid. [Severe] Study

▸ **Allopurinol** potentially increases the risk of haematological toxicity when given with **mercaptopurine**. Adjust **mercaptopurine** dose, p. 1047. [Severe] Study

▸ **Allopurinol** increases the risk of skin rash when given with **penicillins (amoxicillin, ampicillin)**. [Moderate] Study

▸ **Allopurinol** is predicted to increase the risk of hyperuricaemia when given with **pyrazinamide**. [Moderate] Theoretical

▸ **Thiazide diuretics** are predicted to increase the risk of hypersensitivity reactions when given with **allopurinol**. [Severe] Theoretical

Almotriptan → see triptans

Alogliptin → see dipeptidylpeptidase-4 inhibitors

Alpelisib

▸ **Anti-androgens (apalutamide, enzalutamide)** are predicted to decrease the exposure to **alpelisib**. Avoid. [Moderate] Study

▸ **Anti-androgens (darolutamide)** are predicted to increase the exposure to **alpelisib**. [Moderate] Theoretical

▸ **Antiepileptics (carbamazepine, fosphenytoin, phenobarbital, phenytoin, primidone)** are predicted to decrease the exposure to **alpelisib**. Avoid. [Moderate] Study

▸ **Ciclosporin** is predicted to increase the exposure to **alpelisib**. [Moderate] Theoretical

▸ **Eltrombopag** is predicted to increase the exposure to **alpelisib**. [Moderate] Theoretical

▸ **Encorafenib** is predicted to decrease the exposure to **alpelisib**. Avoid. [Moderate] Study

▸ **Febuxostat** is predicted to increase the exposure to **alpelisib**. [Moderate] Theoretical

▸ **Fostamatinib** is predicted to increase the exposure to **alpelisib**. [Moderate] Theoretical

▸ **Ivosidenib** is predicted to decrease the exposure to **alpelisib**. Avoid. [Moderate] Study

▸ **Lapatinib** is predicted to increase the exposure to **alpelisib**. [Moderate] Theoretical

▸ **Leflunomide** is predicted to increase the exposure to **alpelisib**. [Moderate] Theoretical

▸ **Lumacaftor** is predicted to decrease the exposure to **alpelisib**. Avoid. [Moderate] Study

▸ **Mitotane** is predicted to decrease the exposure to **alpelisib**. Avoid. [Moderate] Study

▸ **Proton pump inhibitors (pantoprazole)** are predicted to increase the exposure to **alpelisib**. [Moderate] Theoretical

▸ **Rifamycins (rifampicin)** are predicted to decrease the exposure to **alpelisib**. Avoid. [Moderate] Study

▸ **Teriflunomide** is predicted to increase the exposure to **alpelisib**. [Moderate] Theoretical

▸ **Velpatasvir** is predicted to increase the exposure to **alpelisib**. [Moderate] Theoretical

▸ **Voxilaprevir** is predicted to increase the exposure to **alpelisib**. [Moderate] Theoretical

Alpha blockers → see **TABLE 6** p. 1572 (first-dose hypotension), **TABLE 7** p. 1572 (hypotension)

alfuzosin · doxazosin · indoramin · prazosin · tamsulosin · terazosin

▸ **Antiarrhythmics (dronedarone)** are predicted to increase the exposure to **tamsulosin**. [Moderate] Theoretical

▸ **Antifungals, azoles (fluconazole, isavuconazole)** are predicted to increase the exposure to **tamsulosin**. [Moderate] Theoretical

▸ **Antifungals, azoles (itraconazole, ketoconazole, posaconazole, voriconazole)** are predicted to increase the exposure to **doxazosin**. [Moderate] Study

▸ **Antifungals, azoles (itraconazole, ketoconazole, posaconazole, voriconazole)** are predicted to moderately increase the exposure to alpha blockers **(alfuzosin, tamsulosin)**. Use with caution or avoid. [Moderate] Study

▸ **Berotralstat** is predicted to increase the exposure to **tamsulosin**. [Moderate] Theoretical

▸ **Calcium channel blockers (diltiazem, verapamil)** are predicted to increase the exposure to **tamsulosin**. [Moderate] Theoretical → Also see **TABLE 7** p. 1572

▸ **Ceritinib** is predicted to moderately increase the exposure to alpha blockers **(alfuzosin, tamsulosin)**. Use with caution or avoid. [Moderate] Study

▸ **Ceritinib** is predicted to increase the exposure to **doxazosin**. [Moderate] Study

▸ **Cobicistat** is predicted to moderately increase the exposure to alpha blockers **(alfuzosin, tamsulosin)**. Use with caution or avoid. [Moderate] Study

▸ **Cobicistat** is predicted to increase the exposure to **doxazosin**. [Moderate] Study

▸ **Crizotinib** is predicted to increase the exposure to **tamsulosin**. [Moderate] Theoretical

▸ **Fedratinib** is predicted to increase the exposure to **tamsulosin**. [Moderate] Theoretical

▸ **HIV-protease inhibitors** are predicted to moderately increase the exposure to alpha blockers **(alfuzosin, tamsulosin)**. Use with caution or avoid. [Moderate] Study

▸ **HIV-protease inhibitors** are predicted to increase the exposure to **doxazosin**. [Moderate] Study

▸ **Idelalisib** is predicted to moderately increase the exposure to alpha blockers **(alfuzosin, tamsulosin)**. Use with caution or avoid. [Moderate] Study

▸ **Idelalisib** is predicted to increase the exposure to **doxazosin**. [Moderate] Study

▸ **Imatinib** is predicted to increase the exposure to **tamsulosin**. [Moderate] Theoretical

▸ **Letermovir** is predicted to increase the exposure to **tamsulosin**. [Moderate] Theoretical

Alpha blockers (continued)

▶ Macrolides (clarithromycin) are predicted to increase the exposure to **doxazosin**. Moderate Study

▶ Macrolides (erythromycin) are predicted to increase the exposure to **tamsulosin**. Moderate Theoretical

▶ Macrolides (clarithromycin) are predicted to moderately increase the exposure to alpha blockers (alfuzosin, tamsulosin). Use with caution or avoid. Moderate Study

▶ MAOIs, irreversible are predicted to increase the effects of **indoramin**. Avoid. Severe Theoretical → Also see TABLE 7 p. 1572

▶ Neurokinin-1 receptor antagonists (aprepitant, netupitant) are predicted to increase the exposure to **tamsulosin**. Moderate Theoretical

▶ Nilotinib is predicted to increase the exposure to **tamsulosin**. Moderate Theoretical

▶ Nirmatrelvir boosted with ritonavir is predicted to increase the concentration of alpha blockers (alfuzosin, tamsulosin). Avoid. Severe Theoretical

▶ Alpha blockers cause significant hypotensive effects when given with phosphodiesterase type-5 inhibitors. Patient should be stabilised on first drug then second drug should be added at the lowest recommended dose. Severe Study → Also see TABLE 7 p. 1572

▶ Ribociclib (high-dose) is predicted to increase the exposure to **alfuzosin**. Avoid. Moderate Theoretical

▶ Tucatinib is predicted to moderately increase the exposure to alpha blockers (alfuzosin, tamsulosin). Use with caution or avoid. Moderate Study

▶ Tucatinib is predicted to increase the exposure to **doxazosin**. Moderate Study

Alprazolam → see benzodiazepines

Alprostadil → see TABLE 7 p. 1572 (hypotension), TABLE 4 p. 1571 (antiplatelet effects)

Alteplase → see TABLE 3 p. 1571 (anticoagulant effects)

Aluminium hydroxide

SEPARATION OF ADMINISTRATION **Aluminium-containing antacids** should preferably not be taken at the same time as other drugs since they might impair absorption. **Aluminium-containing antacids** might damage enteric coatings designed to prevent dissolution in the stomach.

▶ Oral **aluminium hydroxide** might decrease the concentration of the active metabolite of oral baloxavir marboxil. Severe Theoretical

▶ Oral **aluminium hydroxide** decreases the absorption of chenodeoxycholic acid. Moderate Study

▶ **Aluminium hydroxide** increases the risk of blocked enteral or nasogastric tubes when given with enteral feeds. Moderate Study

▶ **Aluminium hydroxide** is predicted to decrease the exposure to iron chelators (deferasirox). Avoid. Moderate Theoretical

▶ **Aluminium hydroxide** is predicted to decrease the absorption of iron chelators (deferiprone). Avoid. Moderate Theoretical

▶ **Aluminium hydroxide** might decrease the exposure to roxadustat. Manufacturer advises take at least 1 hour after aluminium-containing products. Moderate Theoretical

▶ Oral **aluminium hydroxide** is predicted to decrease the exposure to oral vadadustat. Manufacturer advises take 1 hour before or 2 hours after aluminium-containing products. Moderate Theoretical

Amantadine → see dopamine receptor agonists

Ambrisentan → see endothelin receptor antagonists

Amfetamines → see TABLE 12 p. 1574 (serotonin syndrome)

dexamfetamine · lisdexamfetamine

▶ **Amfetamines** are predicted to decrease the effects of apraclonidine. Avoid. Severe Theoretical

▶ **Amfetamines** are predicted to increase the risk of adverse effects when given with atomoxetine. Severe Theoretical

▶ **Dexamfetamine** might increase the anticoagulant effect of coumarins. Monitor INR and adjust dose. Moderate Theoretical

▶ HIV-protease inhibitors (ritonavir) are predicted to increase the exposure to **amfetamines**. Severe Theoretical

▶ MAO-B inhibitors (rasagiline, selegiline) are predicted to increase the risk of severe hypertension when given with **amfetamines**. Avoid. Severe Theoretical → Also see TABLE 12 p. 1574

▶ MAO-B inhibitors (safinamide) are predicted to increase the risk of severe hypertension when given with **amfetamines**. Severe Theoretical → Also see TABLE 12 p. 1574

▶ **Amfetamines** are predicted to increase the risk of a hypertensive crisis when given with MAOIs, irreversible. Avoid and for 14 days after stopping the MAOI. Severe Anecdotal → Also see TABLE 12 p. 1574

▶ **Amfetamines** are predicted to increase the risk of a hypertensive crisis when given with moclobemide. Avoid. Severe Theoretical → Also see TABLE 12 p. 1574

▶ Nabilone is predicted to increase the risk of cardiovascular adverse effects when given with **amfetamines**. Severe Theoretical

▶ Nirmatrelvir boosted with ritonavir is predicted to increase the concentration of **amfetamines**. Severe Theoretical

▶ Phenothiazines are predicted to decrease the effects of **amfetamines** and **amfetamines** are predicted to decrease the effects of phenothiazines. Moderate Study

▶ SSRIs (fluoxetine, paroxetine) are predicted to increase the exposure to **amfetamines**. Severe Theoretical → Also see TABLE 12 p. 1574

▶ Volatile halogenated anaesthetics (sevoflurane) can cause hypertension, as can **amfetamines**. Avoid **amfetamines** for several days before surgery. Severe Theoretical

Amifampridine → see TABLE 8 p. 1573 (QT-interval prolongation)

Amikacin → see aminoglycosides

Amiloride → see potassium-sparing diuretics

Aminoglycosides → see TABLE 2 p. 1571 (nephrotoxicity), TABLE 18 p. 1576 (ototoxicity), TABLE 19 p. 1576 (neuromuscular blocking effects)

amikacin · gentamicin · netilmicin · streptomycin · tobramycin

ROUTE-SPECIFIC INFORMATION Since systemic absorption can follow topical application, the possibility of interactions with topical **gentamicin**, **netilmicin** and **tobramycin** should be borne in mind.

▶ **Aminoglycosides** are predicted to decrease the effects of agalsidase alfa. Avoid. Moderate Theoretical

▶ **Aminoglycosides** are predicted to decrease the effects of agalsidase beta. Avoid. Moderate Theoretical

▶ Antifungals, azoles (miconazole) potentially decrease the exposure to **tobramycin**. Moderate Anecdotal

▶ Ataluren is predicted to increase the risk of nephrotoxicity when given with intravenous **aminoglycosides**. Avoid. Severe Study

▶ **Aminoglycosides** increase the risk of hypocalcaemia when given with bisphosphonates. Moderate Anecdotal → Also see TABLE 2 p. 1571

▶ **Aminoglycosides** potentially increase the concentration of digoxin. Monitor and adjust dose. Mild Study

▶ Loop diuretics increase the risk of nephrotoxicity when given with **aminoglycosides**. Avoid. Moderate Study → Also see TABLE 18 p. 1576

▶ **Aminoglycosides** are predicted to decrease the effects of neostigmine. Moderate Theoretical

▶ **Aminoglycosides** are predicted to decrease the effects of pyridostigmine. Moderate Theoretical

▶ Gentamicin is predicted to increase the exposure to relugolix. Avoid or take relugolix first and separate administration by at least 6 hours. Moderate Theoretical

Aminophylline → see TABLE 16 p. 1575 (reduced serum potassium)

FOOD AND LIFESTYLE Smoking can increase aminophylline clearance and increased doses of aminophylline are therefore required; dose adjustments are likely to be necessary if smoking started or stopped during treatment.

▶ Aciclovir increases the exposure to **aminophylline**. Monitor and adjust dose. Severe Anecdotal

▶ **Aminophylline** is predicted to decrease the efficacy of antiarrhythmics (adenosine). Separate administration by 24 hours. Mild Theoretical

▶ Antiepileptics (fosphenytoin) are predicted to decrease the exposure to **aminophylline**. Adjust dose. Moderate Study

▶ Antiepileptics (phenobarbital) are predicted to decrease the exposure to **aminophylline**. Adjust dose. Moderate Theoretical

▶ Antiepileptics **(phenytoin)** decrease the exposure to aminophylline. Adjust dose. Moderate Study

▶ Antiepileptics **(primidone)** are predicted to increase the clearance of aminophylline. Adjust dose. Moderate Theoretical

▶ Antiepileptics **(stiripentol)** are predicted to increase the exposure to aminophylline. Avoid. Moderate Theoretical

▶ **Axitinib** is predicted to increase the exposure to aminophylline. Moderate Theoretical

▶ **Beta blockers, non-selective** are predicted to increase the risk of bronchospasm when given with aminophylline. Avoid. Severe Theoretical

▶ **Beta blockers, selective** are predicted to increase the risk of bronchospasm when given with aminophylline. Avoid. Severe Theoretical

▶ **Combined hormonal contraceptives** is predicted to increase the exposure to aminophylline. Adjust dose. Moderate Theoretical

▶ **Aminophylline** increases the risk of agitation when given with **doxapram**. Moderate Study

▶ **Esketamine** is predicted to increase the risk of seizures when given with aminophylline. Avoid. Severe Theoretical

▶ **Givosiran** is predicted to increase the exposure to aminophylline. Adjust dose. Moderate Theoretical

▶ H_2 **receptor antagonists (cimetidine)** increase the concentration of aminophylline. Adjust dose. Severe Study

▶ **HIV-protease inhibitors (ritonavir)** decrease the exposure to aminophylline. Adjust dose. Moderate Study

▶ **Interferons** are predicted to slightly increase the exposure to aminophylline. Adjust dose. Moderate Theoretical

▶ **Iron chelators (deferasirox)** are predicted to increase the exposure to aminophylline. Avoid. Moderate Theoretical

▶ **Isoniazid** is predicted to affect the clearance of aminophylline. Severe Theoretical

▶ **Leflunomide** decreases the exposure to aminophylline. Adjust dose. Moderate Study

▶ **Aminophylline** is predicted to decrease the concentration of **lithium**. Moderate Theoretical

▶ **Macrolides (azithromycin)** are predicted to increase the exposure to aminophylline. Moderate Theoretical

▶ **Macrolides (clarithromycin)** are predicted to increase the exposure to aminophylline. Adjust dose. Moderate Theoretical

▶ **Aminophylline** is predicted to decrease the exposure to macrolides **(erythromycin)**. Adjust dose. Severe Study

▶ **Methotrexate** is predicted to decrease the clearance of aminophylline. Moderate Theoretical

▶ **Metreleptin** might alter the exposure to aminophylline. Severe Theoretical

▶ **Mexiletine** is predicted to increase the exposure to aminophylline. Adjust dose. Moderate Theoretical

▶ **Monoclonal antibodies (blinatumomab)** are predicted to transiently increase the exposure to aminophylline. Monitor and adjust dose. Moderate Theoretical

▶ **Monoclonal antibodies (sarilumab)** potentially affect the exposure to aminophylline. Monitor and adjust dose. Moderate Theoretical

▶ **Monoclonal antibodies (tocilizumab)** are predicted to decrease the exposure to aminophylline. Monitor and adjust dose. Moderate Theoretical

▶ **Nirmatrelvir** boosted with ritonavir is predicted to decrease the concentration of aminophylline. Adjust dose. Moderate Theoretical

▶ **Osilodrostat** is predicted to increase the exposure to aminophylline. Adjust dose. Moderate Theoretical

▶ **Pentoxifylline** is predicted to increase the concentration of aminophylline. Use with caution or avoid. Severe Theoretical

▶ **Aminophylline** is predicted to slightly increase the exposure to phosphodiesterase type-4 inhibitors **(roflumilast)**. Avoid. Moderate Theoretical

▶ **Quinolones (ciprofloxacin)** are predicted to increase the exposure to aminophylline. Adjust dose. Moderate Theoretical

▶ **Rifamycins (rifampicin)** decrease the exposure to aminophylline. Adjust dose. Moderate Study

▶ **Rucaparib** is predicted to increase the exposure to aminophylline. Adjust dose. Moderate Theoretical

▶ **SSRIs (fluvoxamine)** moderately to markedly increase the exposure to aminophylline. Avoid. Severe Study

▶ **St John's wort** is predicted to decrease the concentration of aminophylline. Severe Theoretical

▶ **Sympathomimetics, vasoconstrictor (ephedrine)** increase the risk of adverse effects when given with aminophylline. Avoid in children. Moderate Study

▶ **Teriflunomide** decreases the exposure to aminophylline. Adjust dose. Moderate Study

▶ **Valaciclovir** is predicted to increase the exposure to aminophylline. Severe Anecdotal

▶ **Vemurafenib** is predicted to increase the exposure to aminophylline. Adjust dose. Moderate Theoretical

Amiodarone → see antiarrhythmics

Amisulpride → see antipsychotics, second generation

Amitriptyline → see tricyclic antidepressants

Amlodipine → see calcium channel blockers

Amoxicillin → see penicillins

Amphotericin B → see TABLE 2 p. 1571 (nephrotoxicity), TABLE 18 p. 1576 (ototoxicity), TABLE 16 p. 1575 (reduced serum potassium)

▶ **Amphotericin B** increases the risk of toxicity when given with **flucytosine**. Severe Study

▶ **Micafungin** slightly increases the exposure to amphotericin B. Avoid or monitor toxicity. Moderate Study

Ampicillin → see penicillins

Amsacrine → see TABLE 14 p. 1575 (myelosuppression)

▶ **Live vaccines** are predicted to increase the risk of generalised infection (possibly life-threatening) when given with amsacrine. UKHSA advises avoid (refer to Green Book). Severe Theoretical

Anaesthetics, local

> bupivacaine · levobupivacaine · mepivacaine · oxybuprocaine · prilocaine · proxymetacaine · ropivacaine · tetracaine

> **ROUTE-SPECIFIC INFORMATION** Since systemic absorption can follow topical application, the possibility of interactions should be borne in mind.

▶ **Antiepileptics (phenytoin)** are predicted to decrease the exposure to ropivacaine. Moderate Theoretical

▶ **Axitinib** is predicted to increase the exposure to ropivacaine. Moderate Theoretical

▶ **Combined hormonal contraceptives** is predicted to increase the exposure to ropivacaine. Moderate Theoretical

▶ **Givosiran** is predicted to increase the exposure to ropivacaine. Moderate Theoretical

▶ **HIV-protease inhibitors (ritonavir)** are predicted to decrease the exposure to ropivacaine. Moderate Theoretical

▶ **Leflunomide** is predicted to decrease the exposure to ropivacaine. Moderate Theoretical

▶ **Mexiletine** is predicted to increase the exposure to ropivacaine. Moderate Theoretical

▶ **Osilodrostat** is predicted to increase the exposure to ropivacaine. Moderate Theoretical

▶ **Quinolones (ciprofloxacin)** are predicted to increase the exposure to ropivacaine. Moderate Theoretical

▶ **Rifamycins (rifampicin)** are predicted to decrease the exposure to ropivacaine. Moderate Theoretical

▶ **Rucaparib** is predicted to increase the exposure to ropivacaine. Moderate Theoretical

▶ **SSRIs (fluvoxamine)** decrease the clearance of ropivacaine. Avoid prolonged use. Moderate Study

▶ **Teriflunomide** is predicted to decrease the exposure to ropivacaine. Moderate Theoretical

▶ **Vemurafenib** is predicted to increase the exposure to ropivacaine. Moderate Theoretical

Anagrelide → see TABLE 8 p. 1573 (QT-interval prolongation), TABLE 4 p. 1571 (antiplatelet effects)

▶ **Combined hormonal contraceptives** is predicted to increase the exposure to anagrelide. Moderate Theoretical

▶ **Givosiran** is predicted to increase the exposure to anagrelide. Moderate Theoretical

▶ **Mexiletine** is predicted to increase the exposure to anagrelide. Moderate Theoretical

▶ **Osilodrostat** is predicted to increase the exposure to anagrelide. Moderate Theoretical → Also see TABLE 8 p. 1573

▶ **Quinolones (ciprofloxacin)** are predicted to increase the exposure to anagrelide. Moderate Theoretical

Anagrelide (continued)

▸ **Rucaparib** is predicted to increase the exposure to **anagrelide**. Moderate Theoretical

▸ **SSRIs (fluvoxamine)** are predicted to increase the exposure to **anagrelide**. Moderate Theoretical → Also see **TABLE 4** p. 1571

▸ **Vemurafenib** is predicted to increase the exposure to **anagrelide**. Moderate Theoretical → Also see **TABLE 8** p. 1573

Anakinra

▸ **Anakinra** is predicted to increase the risk of generalised infection (possibly life-threatening) when given with **abatacept**. Severe Theoretical

▸ **Anakinra** is predicted to increase the risk of generalised infection (possibly life-threatening) when given with **etanercept**. Avoid. Severe Theoretical

▸ **Filgotinib** is predicted to increase the risk of immunosuppression when given with **anakinra**. Avoid. Severe Theoretical

▸ **Live vaccines** are predicted to increase the risk of generalised infection (possibly life-threatening) when given with **anakinra**. UKHSA advises avoid (refer to Green Book). Severe Theoretical

▸ **Monoclonal antibodies (certolizumab pegol)** are predicted to increase the risk of generalised infection (possibly life-threatening) when given with **anakinra**. Avoid. Severe Theoretical

▸ **Anakinra** is predicted to increase the risk of generalised infection (possibly life-threatening) when given with **monoclonal antibodies (golimumab)**. Avoid. Severe Theoretical

Andexanet alfa

▸ **Andexanet alfa** has been reported to affect the anticoagulant effect of **heparin**. Avoid. Severe Anecdotal

▸ **Andexanet alfa** is predicted to affect the anticoagulant effect of **low molecular-weight heparins**. Avoid. Severe Theoretical

Angiotensin-II receptor antagonists → see **TABLE 7** p. 1572 (hypotension), **TABLE 15** p. 1575 (increased serum potassium)

> azilsartan · candesartan · eprosartan · irbesartan · losartan · olmesartan · telmisartan · valsartan

▸ **Angiotensin-II receptor antagonists** increase the risk of renal impairment when given with **aliskiren**. Use with caution or avoid **aliskiren** in selected patients, p. 207. Severe Study → Also see **TABLE 7** p. 1572 → Also see **TABLE 15** p. 1575

▸ **Telmisartan** is predicted to increase the exposure to **atogepant**. Adjust **atogepant** dose, p. 540. Moderate Theoretical

▸ **Bulevirtide** is predicted to increase the exposure to angiotensin-II receptor antagonists **(olmesartan, telmisartan, valsartan)**. Avoid or monitor. Moderate Theoretical

▸ **Irbesartan** is predicted to affect the efficacy of **bulevirtide**. Avoid. Severe Theoretical

▸ **Angiotensin-II receptor antagonists** might increase the risk of first dose hypotension when given with **drugs that cause first dose hypotension** (see **TABLE 6** p. 1572) particularly in those with volume and/or salt depletion. Mild Theoretical

▸ **Angiotensin-II receptor antagonists** potentially increase the concentration of **lithium**. Avoid or monitor. Severe Anecdotal

▸ **Taxanes (cabazitaxel)** are predicted to affect the exposure to **valsartan**. Manufacturer advises take 12 hours before or 3 hours after **cabazitaxel**. Moderate Theoretical

▸ **Vadadustat** is predicted to increase the exposure to **olmesartan**. Monitor and adjust dose. Moderate Study

Anidulafungin → see **TABLE 1** p. 1571 (hepatotoxicity)

Antacids

> **SEPARATION OF ADMINISTRATION** Aluminium- and magnesium-containing antacids should preferably not be taken at the same time as other drugs since they might impair absorption. Aluminium- and magnesium-containing antacids might damage enteric coatings designed to prevent dissolution in the stomach.

▸ Oral **antacids** are predicted to decrease the absorption of oral alkylating agents **(estramustine)**. Avoid. Moderate Study

▸ Oral **antacids** decrease the absorption of oral antiepileptics **(gabapentin)**. Manufacturer advises take 2 hours after antacids. Moderate Study

▸ Oral **antacids** decrease the absorption of oral antifungals, azoles **(itraconazole)** capsules. Manufacturer advises take 2 hours before or 1 hour after antacids. Moderate Study

▸ Oral **antacids** decrease the absorption of oral antifungals, azoles **(ketoconazole)**. Separate administration by at least 2 hours. Moderate Study

▸ Oral **antacids** decrease the absorption of oral antihistamines, non-sedating **(fexofenadine)**. Separate administration by 2 hours. Mild Study

▸ Oral **antacids** are predicted to decrease the absorption of oral antimalarials **(chloroquine)**. Separate administration by at least 4 hours. Moderate Theoretical

▸ Oral **antacids** are predicted to decrease the absorption of oral antimalarials **(proguanil)**. Separate administration by at least 2 hours. Moderate Study

▸ Oral **antacids** decrease the absorption of oral **aspirin** (high-dose). Moderate Study

▸ Oral **antacids** might decrease the concentration of the active metabolite of oral **baloxavir marboxil**. Avoid. Severe Theoretical

▸ **Antacids** is predicted to decrease the exposure to **belumosudil**. Separate administration by 12 hours. Moderate Theoretical

▸ Oral **antacids** decrease the exposure to oral **bictegravir**. Separate administration by at least 2 hours. Moderate Study

▸ Oral **antacids** decrease the absorption of oral bisphosphonates **(alendronate)**. Manufacturer advises take at least 30 minutes before antacids. Moderate Study

▸ Oral **antacids** decrease the absorption of oral bisphosphonates **(clodronate)**. Avoid antacids for 2 hours before or 1 hour after **clodronate**. Moderate Study

▸ Oral **antacids** are predicted to decrease the absorption of oral bisphosphonates **(ibandronate)**. Avoid antacids for at least 6 hours before or 1 hour after **ibandronate**. Moderate Theoretical

▸ Oral **antacids** decrease the absorption of oral bisphosphonates **(risedronate)**. Separate administration by at least 2 hours. Moderate Study

▸ Oral **antacids** are predicted to decrease the absorption of oral **bosutinib**. Manufacturer advises take at least 12 hours before antacids. Moderate Theoretical

▸ Oral **antacids** are predicted to decrease the concentration of oral **cabotegravir**. Manufacturer advises take 4 hours before or 2 hours after antacids. Moderate Theoretical

▸ Oral **antacids** are predicted to decrease the absorption of oral **ceritinib**. Separate administration by 2 hours. Moderate Theoretical

▸ Oral **antacids** are predicted to decrease the absorption of oral **cholic acid**. Separate administration by 5 hours. Mild Theoretical

▸ Oral **antacids** are predicted to decrease the absorption of oral corticosteroids **(deflazacort)**. Separate administration by 2 hours. Moderate Theoretical

▸ Oral **antacids** decrease the absorption of oral corticosteroids **(dexamethasone)**. Moderate Study

▸ Oral **antacids** decrease the absorption of oral **dasatinib**. Separate administration by at least 2 hours. Moderate Study

▸ Oral **antacids** decrease the absorption of oral **digoxin**. Separate administration by 2 hours. Mild Study

▸ Oral **antacids** are predicted to decrease the absorption of oral **dipyridamole** (immediate release tablets). Moderate Theoretical

▸ Oral **antacids** decrease the exposure to oral **dolutegravir**. Manufacturer advises take 2 hours before or 6 hours after antacids. Moderate Study

▸ Oral **antacids** decrease the absorption of oral **eltrombopag**. Manufacturer advises take 2 hours before or 4 hours after antacids. Severe Study

▸ Oral **antacids** decrease the exposure to oral **elvitegravir**. Separate administration by at least 4 hours. Moderate Study

▸ Oral **antacids** are predicted to decrease the absorption of oral **erlotinib**. Manufacturer advises take 2 hours before or 4 hours after antacids. Moderate Theoretical

▸ Oral **antacids** decrease the exposure to oral fibrates **(gemfibrozil)**. Moderate Study

▸ Oral **antacids** are predicted to decrease the exposure to oral **gefitinib**. Moderate Theoretical

▸ Oral **antacids** are predicted to decrease the absorption of oral HIV-protease inhibitors **(atazanavir)**. Manufacturer advises take 2 hours before or 1 hour after antacids. Severe Theoretical

- Oral **antacids** are predicted to decrease the absorption of oral hydroxychloroquine. Separate administration by at least 4 hours. Moderate Theoretical
- Oral **antacids** decrease the absorption of oral iron. Manufacturer advises iron should be taken 1 hour before or 2 hours after antacids. Moderate Study
- Oral **antacids** is predicted to decrease the absorption of oral lapatinib. Avoid. Moderate Theoretical
- Oral **antacids** are predicted to decrease the exposure to oral ledipasvir. Separate administration by 4 hours. Moderate Theoretical
- Oral **antacids** decrease the exposure to oral mycophenolate. Moderate Study
- Oral **antacids** are predicted to decrease the exposure to oral neratinib. Separate administration by at least 3 hours. Mild Theoretical
- Oral **antacids** might affect the absorption of oral nilotinib. Separate administration by at least 2 hours. Moderate Theoretical
- Oral **antacids** are predicted to decrease the exposure to oral NNRTIs (rilpivirine). Manufacturer advises take 4 hours before or 2 hours after antacids. Severe Theoretical
- Oral **antacids** are predicted to decrease the absorption of oral pazopanib. Manufacturer advises take 1 hour before or 2 hours after antacids. Moderate Theoretical
- Oral **antacids** decrease the absorption of oral penicillamine. Separate administration by 2 hours. Mild Study
- Oral **antacids** decrease the absorption of oral phenothiazines. Moderate Anecdotal
- Oral **antacids** increase the risk of metabolic alkalosis when given with oral polystyrene sulfonate. Severe Anecdotal
- Oral **antacids** decrease the absorption of oral quinolones. Manufacturer advises take 2 hours before or 4 hours after antacids. Moderate Study
- Oral **antacids** decrease the exposure to oral raltegravir. Avoid. Moderate Study
- Oral **antacids** decrease the absorption of oral rifamycins (rifampicin). Manufacturer advises take 1 hour before antacids. Moderate Study
- Oral **antacids** decrease the exposure to oral riociguat. Manufacturer advises take 1 hour before or 2 hours after antacids. Mild Study
- **Antacids** might decrease the exposure to roxadustat. Manufacturer advises take at least 1 hour after antacids. Moderate Theoretical
- **Antacids** are predicted to decrease the exposure to selpercatinib. Moderate Theoretical
- Oral **antacids** are predicted to decrease the exposure to oral sotorasib. Manufacturer advises take 4 hours before or 10 hours after antacids. Moderate Theoretical
- Oral **antacids** decrease the absorption of oral statins (rosuvastatin). Separate administration by 2 hours. Moderate Study
- Oral **antacids** decrease the absorption of oral strontium. Separate administration by 2 hours. Moderate Study
- Oral **antacids** decrease the absorption of oral sulpiride. Separate administration by 2 hours. Moderate Study
- Oral **antacids** greatly decrease the absorption of oral tetracyclines. Separate administration by 2 to 3 hours. Moderate Study
- Oral **antacids** are predicted to decrease the absorption of oral thyroid hormones (levothyroxine). Separate administration by at least 4 hours. Moderate Anecdotal
- **Antacids** might decrease the efficacy of ulipristal for emergency hormonal contraception. For FSRH guidance, see Contraceptives, interactions p. 917. Unknown Theoretical
- Oral **antacids** are predicted to decrease the absorption of oral ursodeoxycholic acid. Separate administration by 2 hours. Moderate Theoretical
- Oral **antacids** are predicted to decrease the concentration of oral velpatasvir. Separate administration by 4 hours. Moderate Theoretical

Antazoline → see antihistamines, sedating

Anthracyclines → see TABLE 14 p. 1575 (myelosuppression)

daunorubicin · doxorubicin · epirubicin · idarubicin · mitoxantrone · pixantrone

GENERAL INFORMATION Caution is necessary with concurrent use of **anthracyclines** with cardiotoxic drugs, or drugs that reduce cardiac contractility.

- Calcium channel blockers (verapamil) moderately increase the exposure to doxorubicin. Moderate Study
- Ciclosporin increases the concentration of anthracyclines (daunorubicin, doxorubicin, epirubicin, idarubicin, mitoxantrone). Severe Study
- H₂ receptor antagonists (cimetidine) slightly increase the exposure to epirubicin. Avoid. Moderate Study
- Leflunomide is predicted to increase the exposure to anthracyclines (daunorubicin, doxorubicin, mitoxantrone). Moderate Theoretical → Also see TABLE 14 p. 1575
- Live vaccines are predicted to increase the risk of generalised infection (possibly life-threatening) when given with **anthracyclines**. UKHSA advises avoid (refer to Green Book). Severe Theoretical
- **Anthracyclines** are predicted to increase the risk of cardiotoxicity when given with monoclonal antibodies (trastuzumab, trastuzumab emtansine). Avoid. Severe Theoretical → Also see TABLE 14 p. 1575
- **Anthracyclines** are predicted to increase the risk of cardiotoxicity when given with monoclonal antibodies (trastuzumab deruxtecan). Severe Theoretical → Also see TABLE 14 p. 1575
- Teriflunomide is predicted to increase the exposure to anthracyclines (daunorubicin, doxorubicin, mitoxantrone). Moderate Theoretical

Anti-androgens → see TABLE 1 p. 1571 (hepatotoxicity), TABLE 8 p. 1573 (QT-interval prolongation)

abiraterone · apalutamide · bicalutamide · cyproterone · darolutamide · enzalutamide · flutamide

GENERAL INFORMATION Caution with concurrent chemotherapy—safety and efficacy with **abiraterone** and **enzalutamide** not established.

- Anti-androgens (apalutamide, enzalutamide) are predicted to decrease the exposure to 5-HT3-receptor antagonists (ondansetron). Moderate Study → Also see TABLE 8 p. 1573
- Anti-androgens (apalutamide, enzalutamide) are predicted to markedly decrease the exposure to abemaciclib. Avoid. Severe Study
- Anti-androgens (apalutamide, enzalutamide) are predicted to decrease the exposure to abrocitinib. Avoid. Moderate Study
- Anti-androgens (apalutamide, enzalutamide) are predicted to decrease the exposure to acalabrutinib. Avoid. Severe Study
- **Apalutamide** is predicted to decrease the exposure to aliskiren. Monitor and adjust dose. Moderate Study
- Anti-androgens (apalutamide, enzalutamide) are predicted to decrease the exposure to alpelisib. Avoid. Moderate Study
- **Darolutamide** is predicted to increase the exposure to alpelisib. Moderate Theoretical
- Anti-androgens (apalutamide, enzalutamide) are predicted to decrease the exposure to anti-androgens (abiraterone). Avoid. Severe Study
- Anti-androgens (apalutamide) are predicted to decrease the exposure to anti-androgens (darolutamide). Avoid. Moderate Study
- Anti-androgens (enzalutamide) are predicted to decrease the exposure to anti-androgens (darolutamide). Avoid. Moderate Study
- Anti-androgens (apalutamide, enzalutamide) are predicted to decrease the exposure to antiarrhythmics (disopyramide, dronedarone). Avoid. Severe Study → Also see TABLE 8 p. 1573
- Anti-androgens (apalutamide, enzalutamide) are predicted to decrease the efficacy of antiarrhythmics (propafenone). Moderate Study
- Anti-androgens (apalutamide, enzalutamide) are predicted to decrease the exposure to anticholinesterases, centrally acting (donepezil). Mild Study
- Antiepileptics (carbamazepine, eslicarbazepine, fosphenytoin, oxcarbazepine, perampanel, phenobarbital, phenytoin,

Anti-androgens (continued)
primidone, rufinamide, topiramate) are predicted to decrease the efficacy of **cyproterone** with ethinylestradiol (co-cyprindiol). Use alternative methods during treatment with, and for 28 days after, the enzyme inducing drug is stopped. Severe Study

▶ Antiepileptics (carbamazepine, fosphenytoin, phenobarbital, phenytoin, primidone) are predicted to decrease the exposure to **abiraterone**. Avoid. Severe Study

▶ Antiepileptics (carbamazepine, fosphenytoin, phenobarbital, phenytoin, primidone) are predicted to decrease the exposure to **darolutamide**. Avoid. Moderate Study

▶ **Enzalutamide** is predicted to slightly decrease the exposure to antiepileptics (brivaracetam). Moderate Theoretical

▶ Anti-androgens (apalutamide, enzalutamide) are predicted to decrease the exposure to antiepileptics (perampanel). Monitor and adjust dose. Moderate Study

▶ **Apalutamide** potentially decreases the exposure to antiepileptics (valproate). Mild Theoretical

▶ **Enzalutamide** is predicted to affect the exposure to antiepileptics (valproate). Use with caution or avoid. Moderate Theoretical

▶ Antifungals, azoles (itraconazole) slightly increase the exposure to **darolutamide**. Monitor and adjust dose. Moderate Study

▶ Antifungals, azoles (itraconazole, ketoconazole, posaconazole, voriconazole) are predicted to increase the exposure to **apalutamide**. Monitor and adjust dose. Mild Study → Also see TABLE 8 p. 1573

▶ Antifungals, azoles (ketoconazole) are predicted to increase the exposure to **darolutamide**. Monitor and adjust dose. Moderate Theoretical

▶ Anti-androgens (apalutamide, enzalutamide) are predicted to decrease the exposure to antifungals, azoles (isavuconazole). Avoid. Severe Study

▶ **Apalutamide** slightly decreases the exposure to antihistamines, non-sedating (fexofenadine). Mild Study

▶ **Darolutamide** is predicted to increase the concentration of antihistamines, non-sedating (fexofenadine). Moderate Theoretical

▶ Anti-androgens (apalutamide, enzalutamide) are predicted to decrease the exposure to antimalarials (artemether) with lumefantrine. Avoid. Severe Study → Also see TABLE 8 p. 1573

▶ Anti-androgens (apalutamide, enzalutamide) are predicted to moderately decrease the exposure to antipsychotics, second generation (aripiprazole). Adjust **aripiprazole** dose, p. 454. Moderate Study → Also see TABLE 8 p. 1573

▶ Anti-androgens (apalutamide, enzalutamide) are predicted to decrease the exposure to antipsychotics, second generation (cariprazine). Avoid. Severe Theoretical

▶ **Enzalutamide** is predicted to decrease the exposure to antipsychotics, second generation (clozapine). Moderate Theoretical

▶ Anti-androgens (apalutamide, enzalutamide) are predicted to decrease the exposure to antipsychotics, second generation (lurasidone). Avoid. Moderate Study

▶ Anti-androgens (apalutamide, enzalutamide) are predicted to decrease the exposure to antipsychotics, second generation (paliperidone). Monitor and adjust dose. Severe Study → Also see TABLE 8 p. 1573

▶ Anti-androgens (apalutamide, enzalutamide) are predicted to decrease the exposure to antipsychotics, second generation (quetiapine). Moderate Study

▶ Anti-androgens (apalutamide, enzalutamide) are predicted to decrease the exposure to antipsychotics, second generation (risperidone). Adjust dose. Moderate Study

▶ Anti-androgens (apalutamide, enzalutamide) are predicted to decrease the exposure to avacopan. Avoid or monitor. Severe Study

▶ Anti-androgens (apalutamide, enzalutamide) are predicted to decrease the exposure to avapritinib. Avoid. Severe Study

▶ **Enzalutamide** is predicted to decrease the exposure to avatrombopag. Adjust **avatrombopag** dose with moderate CYP2C9 inducers in chronic immune thrombocytopenia, p. 1169. Moderate Study

▶ Anti-androgens (apalutamide, enzalutamide) are predicted to decrease the exposure to axitinib. Avoid or adjust dose. Moderate Study

▶ Anti-androgens (apalutamide, enzalutamide) decrease the exposure to bedaquiline. Avoid. Severe Study → Also see TABLE 8 p. 1573

▶ Anti-androgens (apalutamide, enzalutamide) are predicted to decrease the exposure to belumosudil. Adjust **belumosudil** dose, p. 979. Severe Study

▶ Anti-androgens (apalutamide, enzalutamide) are predicted to decrease the exposure to benzodiazepines (alprazolam). Adjust dose. Moderate Theoretical

▶ **Enzalutamide** is predicted to affect the exposure to benzodiazepines (clonazepam). Use with caution or avoid. Moderate Theoretical

▶ **Apalutamide** is predicted to decrease the exposure to benzodiazepines (diazepam). Avoid or monitor. Mild Study

▶ Anti-androgens (apalutamide, enzalutamide) are predicted to decrease the exposure to benzodiazepines (midazolam). Monitor and adjust dose. Severe Study

▶ **Enzalutamide** is predicted to affect the exposure to beta blockers, non-selective (propranolol). Use with caution or avoid. Moderate Theoretical

▶ **Enzalutamide** is predicted to affect the exposure to beta blockers, selective (bisoprolol). Use with caution or avoid. Moderate Theoretical

▶ **Abiraterone** is predicted to increase the exposure to beta blockers, selective (metoprolol). Moderate Study

▶ **Apalutamide** is predicted to decrease the exposure to beta₂ agonists (salmeterol). Avoid or monitor. Moderate Study

▶ Anti-androgens (apalutamide, enzalutamide) are predicted to decrease the exposure to bictegravir. Avoid. Moderate Study

▶ Anti-androgens (apalutamide, enzalutamide) slightly decrease the exposure to bortezomib. Avoid. Severe Study

▶ Anti-androgens (apalutamide, enzalutamide) are predicted to very markedly decrease the exposure to bosutinib. Avoid. Severe Study → Also see TABLE 8 p. 1573

▶ Anti-androgens (apalutamide, enzalutamide) are predicted to decrease the exposure to brigatinib. Avoid. Severe Study

▶ Anti-androgens (apalutamide, enzalutamide) are predicted to decrease the exposure to buspirone. Use with caution and adjust dose. Severe Study

▶ Anti-androgens (apalutamide, enzalutamide) moderately decrease the exposure to cabozantinib. Avoid. Moderate Study → Also see TABLE 8 p. 1573

▶ Anti-androgens (apalutamide, enzalutamide) are predicted to decrease the exposure to calcium channel blockers (amlodipine, felodipine, lacidipine, lercanidipine, nicardipine, nifedipine, nimodipine). Monitor and adjust dose. Moderate Study

▶ **Enzalutamide** is predicted to decrease the exposure to calcium channel blockers (diltiazem, verapamil). Severe Study

▶ Anti-androgens (apalutamide, enzalutamide) are predicted to decrease the exposure to cannabidiol. Adjust dose. Moderate Study

▶ Anti-androgens (apalutamide, enzalutamide) are predicted to decrease the exposure to capivasertib. Avoid. Moderate Study

▶ **Cenobamate** is predicted to decrease the exposure to **darolutamide**. Avoid. Moderate Theoretical

▶ Anti-androgens (apalutamide, enzalutamide) are predicted to decrease the exposure to ceritinib. Avoid. Severe Study → Also see TABLE 8 p. 1573

▶ **Ceritinib** is predicted to increase the exposure to **apalutamide**. Monitor and adjust dose. Mild Study → Also see TABLE 8 p. 1573

▶ Anti-androgens (apalutamide, enzalutamide) decrease the concentration of ciclosporin. Severe Study

▶ Anti-androgens (apalutamide, enzalutamide) are predicted to alter the effects of cilostazol. Moderate Theoretical

▶ Anti-androgens (apalutamide, enzalutamide) are predicted to decrease the exposure to cinacalcet. Monitor and adjust dose. Moderate Study

▶ **Darolutamide** is predicted to increase the exposure to cladribine. Avoid or adjust dose. Moderate Theoretical

▶ Anti-androgens (apalutamide, enzalutamide) decrease the exposure to clomethiazole. Monitor and adjust dose. Moderate Study

▶ **Clopidogrel** is predicted to increase the exposure to **apalutamide** and apalutamide is predicted to increase the exposure to the active metabolite of clopidogrel. Avoid or monitor. [Moderate] Study

▸ Clopidogrel moderately increases the exposure to enzalutamide. Avoid or adjust **enzalutamide** dose, p. 1078. [Severe] Study

▸ Anti-androgens **(apalutamide, enzalutamide)** are predicted to decrease the exposure to cobicistat. Avoid. [Severe] Study

▸ Cobicistat is predicted to increase the exposure to apalutamide. Monitor and adjust dose. [Mild] Study

▸ Anti-androgens **(apalutamide, enzalutamide)** are predicted to decrease the exposure to cobimetinib. Avoid. [Severe] Theoretical

▸ **Apalutamide** is predicted to decrease the exposure to colchicine. [Mild] Study

▸ Anti-androgens **(apalutamide, enzalutamide)** are predicted to decrease the exposure to corticosteroids (budesonide, deflazacort, dexamethasone, fludrocortisone, hydrocortisone, methylprednisolone, prednisolone, triamcinolone). Monitor and adjust dose. [Moderate] Study

▸ Anti-androgens **(apalutamide, enzalutamide)** are predicted to decrease the exposure to corticosteroids (fluticasone). [Unknown] Theoretical

▸ **Apalutamide** is predicted to decrease the exposure to coumarins. Avoid or monitor. [Mild] Study

▸ **Enzalutamide** potentially decreases the exposure to coumarins. Avoid or adjust dose and monitor INR. [Severe] Study

▸ Anti-androgens **(apalutamide, enzalutamide)** are predicted to markedly decrease the exposure to crizotinib. Avoid. [Severe] Study → Also see **TABLE 8** p. 1573

▸ Anti-androgens **(apalutamide, enzalutamide)** are predicted to decrease the exposure to dabrafenib. Avoid. [Moderate] Theoretical

▸ Dabrafenib is predicted to decrease the exposure to darolutamide. Avoid. [Moderate] Theoretical

▸ Anti-androgens **(apalutamide, enzalutamide)** are predicted to decrease the exposure to daridorexant. [Severe] Study

▸ Anti-androgens **(apalutamide, enzalutamide)** are predicted to decrease the exposure to darifenacin. [Moderate] Theoretical

▸ Anti-androgens **(apalutamide, enzalutamide)** are predicted to markedly decrease the exposure to dasatinib. Avoid. [Severe] Study → Also see **TABLE 8** p. 1573

▸ Anti-androgens **(apalutamide, enzalutamide)** are predicted to slightly decrease the exposure to delamanid. Avoid. [Moderate] Study → Also see **TABLE 8** p. 1573

▸ Anti-androgens **(apalutamide, enzalutamide)** are predicted to markedly decrease the exposure to dienogest. [Severe] Study

▸ **Apalutamide** is predicted to decrease the exposure to digoxin. [Mild] Study

▸ **Enzalutamide** is predicted to increase the exposure to digoxin. Use with caution or avoid. [Moderate] Theoretical

▸ Anti-androgens **(apalutamide, enzalutamide)** are predicted to decrease the exposure to dipeptidylpeptidase-4 inhibitors (linagliptin). [Moderate] Study

▸ Anti-androgens **(apalutamide, enzalutamide)** are predicted to moderately decrease the exposure to dipeptidylpeptidase-4 inhibitors (saxagliptin). [Moderate] Study

▸ Anti-androgens **(apalutamide, enzalutamide)** are predicted to decrease the exposure to dolutegravir. [Severe] Study

▸ Anti-androgens **(apalutamide, enzalutamide)** are predicted to decrease the exposure to dronabinol. Avoid or adjust dose. [Mild] Study

▸ Anti-androgens **(apalutamide, enzalutamide)** are predicted to decrease the exposure to elacestrant. Avoid or adjust dose depending on duration—consult product literature. [Severe] Study

▸ Anti-androgens **(apalutamide, enzalutamide)** are predicted to decrease the exposure to elbasvir. Avoid. [Severe] Study

▸ Anti-androgens **(apalutamide, enzalutamide)** is predicted to decrease the exposure to elexacaftor. Avoid. [Severe] Theoretical

▸ **Abiraterone** is predicted to increase the exposure to eliglustat. Avoid or adjust dose—consult product literature. [Severe] Study

▸ Anti-androgens **(apalutamide, enzalutamide)** are predicted to decrease the exposure to eliglustat. Avoid. [Severe] Study

▸ Anti-androgens **(apalutamide, enzalutamide)** are predicted to decrease the concentration of elvitegravir. Avoid. [Severe] Study

▸ Encorafenib is predicted to decrease the exposure to abiraterone. Avoid. [Severe] Study

▸ Anti-androgens **(apalutamide, enzalutamide)** are predicted to decrease the exposure to encorafenib. [Severe] Theoretical → Also see **TABLE 8** p. 1573

▸ Encorafenib is predicted to decrease the exposure to darolutamide. Avoid. [Moderate] Study

▸ Endothelin receptor antagonists (bosentan) are predicted to decrease the efficacy of **cyproterone** with ethinylestradiol (co-cyprindiol). Use alternative methods during treatment with, and for 28 days after, the enzyme inducing drug is stopped. [Severe] Study

▸ Endothelin receptor antagonists (bosentan) are predicted to decrease the exposure to **darolutamide**. Avoid. [Moderate] Theoretical

▸ Anti-androgens **(apalutamide, enzalutamide)** affect the exposure to endothelin receptor antagonists (bosentan). Avoid. [Severe] Study

▸ Anti-androgens **(apalutamide, enzalutamide)** are predicted to decrease the exposure to endothelin receptor antagonists (macitentan). Avoid. [Severe] Study

▸ Anti-androgens **(apalutamide, enzalutamide)** are predicted to decrease the exposure to the cytotoxic component of enfortumab vedotin. [Moderate] Theoretical

▸ Anti-androgens **(apalutamide, enzalutamide)** are predicted to decrease the exposure to entrectinib. Avoid. [Severe] Study → Also see **TABLE 8** p. 1573

▸ Anti-androgens **(apalutamide, enzalutamide)** are predicted to decrease the exposure to erdafitinib. Avoid. [Severe] Study

▸ Anti-androgens **(apalutamide, enzalutamide)** are predicted to decrease the exposure to erlotinib. Avoid or adjust dose—consult product literature. [Severe] Study

▸ Anti-androgens **(apalutamide, enzalutamide)** are predicted to decrease the exposure to esketamine. Adjust dose. [Mild] Theoretical

▸ Anti-androgens **(apalutamide, enzalutamide)** are predicted to decrease the exposure to eszopiclone. Adjust dose. [Moderate] Theoretical

▸ **Enzalutamide** is predicted to decrease the exposure to etrasimod. Avoid. [Severe] Theoretical

▸ Anti-androgens **(apalutamide, enzalutamide)** are predicted to decrease the concentration of everolimus. Avoid or adjust dose. [Severe] Study

▸ Anti-androgens **(apalutamide, enzalutamide)** moderately decrease the exposure to exemestane. [Moderate] Study

▸ Anti-androgens **(apalutamide, enzalutamide)** are predicted to decrease the exposure to factor XA inhibitors (apixaban). [Moderate] Study

▸ **Apalutamide** is predicted to decrease the exposure to factor XA inhibitors (edoxaban). Monitor and adjust dose. [Moderate] Study

▸ Anti-androgens **(apalutamide, enzalutamide)** are predicted to decrease the exposure to factor XA inhibitors (rivaroxaban). Avoid unless patient can be monitored for signs of thrombosis. [Severe] Study

▸ Anti-androgens **(apalutamide, enzalutamide)** are predicted to decrease the exposure to fedratinib. Avoid. [Moderate] Study

▸ Anti-androgens **(apalutamide, enzalutamide)** are predicted to decrease the exposure to fenfluramine. [Moderate] Theoretical

▸ Anti-androgens **(apalutamide, enzalutamide)** are predicted to decrease the exposure to fesoterodine. Avoid. [Moderate] Study

▸ Fibrates (gemfibrozil) slightly increase the exposure to apalutamide. [Mild] Study

▸ Fibrates (gemfibrozil) moderately increase the exposure to enzalutamide. Avoid or adjust **enzalutamide** dose, p. 1078. [Severe] Study

▸ Anti-androgens **(apalutamide, enzalutamide)** are predicted to decrease the exposure to fostamatinib. Avoid. [Severe] Study

▸ Anti-androgens **(apalutamide, enzalutamide)** are predicted to decrease the exposure to the active metabolite of fostemsavir. Avoid. [Severe] Study

▸ Anti-androgens **(apalutamide, enzalutamide)** are predicted to decrease the exposure to fruquintinib. Avoid. [Moderate] Study

▸ Anti-androgens **(apalutamide, enzalutamide)** are predicted to decrease the exposure to gefitinib. Avoid. [Severe] Study

Anti-androgens (continued)

▶ **Enzalutamide** is predicted to increase the exposure to gilteritinib. [Moderate] Theoretical

▶ Anti-androgens **(apalutamide, enzalutamide)** are predicted to decrease the exposure to glasdegib. Avoid. [Severe] Study → Also see **TABLE 8** p. 1573

▶ **Enzalutamide** is predicted to greatly decrease the concentration of glecaprevir. Avoid. [Severe] Study

▶ Anti-androgens **(apalutamide, enzalutamide)** are predicted to decrease the exposure to grazoprevir. Avoid. [Severe] Study

▶ Anti-androgens **(apalutamide, enzalutamide)** are predicted to decrease the concentration of guanfacine. Adjust **guanfacine** dose, p. 407. [Moderate] Study

▶ Anti-androgens **(apalutamide, enzalutamide)** decrease the concentration of haloperidol. Adjust dose. [Moderate] Study → Also see **TABLE 8** p. 1573

▶ **HIV-protease inhibitors** are predicted to increase the exposure to **apalutamide**. Monitor and adjust dose. [Mild] Study

▶ HIV-protease inhibitors **(lopinavir, ritonavir)** are predicted to increase the exposure to **darolutamide**. Monitor and adjust dose. [Moderate] Theoretical

▶ HIV-protease inhibitors **(ritonavir)** are predicted to decrease the efficacy of **cyproterone** with ethinylestradiol (co-cyprindiol). Use alternative methods during treatment with, and for 28 days after, the enzyme inducing drug is stopped. [Severe] Study

▶ **Enzalutamide** is predicted to affect the exposure to HIV-protease inhibitors **(ritonavir)**. Use with caution or avoid. [Moderate] Theoretical

▶ Anti-androgens **(apalutamide, enzalutamide)** are predicted to decrease the exposure to ibrutinib. Avoid or monitor. [Severe] Study

▶ Anti-androgens **(apalutamide, enzalutamide)** are predicted to decrease the exposure to idelalisib. Avoid. [Severe] Study

▶ **Idelalisib** is predicted to increase the exposure to **apalutamide**. Monitor and adjust dose. [Mild] Study

▶ Anti-androgens **(apalutamide, enzalutamide)** are predicted to decrease the exposure to imatinib. Avoid. [Moderate] Study

▶ Anti-androgens **(apalutamide, enzalutamide)** are predicted to decrease the exposure to irinotecan. Avoid. [Severe] Study

▶ Anti-androgens **(apalutamide, enzalutamide)** are predicted to decrease the exposure to ivabradine. Adjust dose. [Moderate] Theoretical

▶ Anti-androgens **(apalutamide, enzalutamide)** are predicted to decrease the exposure to ivacaftor. Avoid. [Severe] Study

▶ **Ivosidenib** is predicted to decrease the exposure to **abiraterone**. Avoid. [Severe] Study

▶ Anti-androgens **(apalutamide, enzalutamide)** are predicted to decrease the exposure to ivosidenib. Avoid. [Severe] Theoretical → Also see **TABLE 8** p. 1573

▶ **Ivosidenib** is predicted to decrease the exposure to **darolutamide**. Avoid. [Moderate] Study

▶ Anti-androgens **(apalutamide, enzalutamide)** are predicted to decrease the exposure to ixazomib. Avoid. [Severe] Study

▶ Anti-androgens **(apalutamide, enzalutamide)** are predicted to decrease the exposure to lapatinib. Avoid. [Severe] Study → Also see **TABLE 8** p. 1573

▶ Anti-androgens **(apalutamide, enzalutamide)** are predicted to moderately decrease the exposure to larotrectinib. Avoid. [Moderate] Study

▶ Anti-androgens **(apalutamide, enzalutamide)** are predicted to decrease the exposure to leniolisib. Avoid. [Severe] Theoretical

▶ Anti-androgens **(apalutamide, enzalutamide)** are predicted to decrease the exposure to lomitapide. Monitor and adjust dose. [Moderate] Theoretical

▶ **Bicalutamide** is predicted to increase the exposure to lomitapide. Separate administration by 12 hours. [Moderate] Theoretical

▶ **Apalutamide** is predicted to decrease the exposure to loperamide. Monitor and adjust dose. [Moderate] Study

▶ Anti-androgens **(apalutamide, enzalutamide)** are predicted to decrease the exposure to lorlatinib. Avoid. [Severe] Study

▶ **Lorlatinib** is predicted to decrease the exposure to **darolutamide**. Avoid. [Moderate] Theoretical

▶ **Lumacaftor** is predicted to decrease the exposure to **abiraterone**. Avoid. [Severe] Study

▶ **Lumacaftor** is predicted to decrease the exposure to **darolutamide**. Avoid. [Moderate] Study

▶ Macrolides **(clarithromycin)** are predicted to increase the exposure to **apalutamide**. Monitor and adjust dose. [Mild] Study

▶ Macrolides **(clarithromycin)** are predicted to increase the exposure to **darolutamide**. Monitor and adjust dose. [Moderate] Theoretical

▶ **Enzalutamide** is predicted to affect the exposure to macrolides **(clarithromycin)**. Use with caution or avoid. [Moderate] Theoretical

▶ Anti-androgens **(apalutamide, enzalutamide)** are predicted to decrease the exposure to maraviroc. Adjust dose. [Severe] Study

▶ Anti-androgens **(apalutamide, enzalutamide)** are predicted to decrease the exposure to maribavir. Avoid or adjust **maribavir** dose, p. 735. [Severe] Study

▶ Anti-androgens **(apalutamide, enzalutamide)** are predicted to decrease the exposure to mavacamten. Monitor and adjust dose—consult product literature. [Severe] Theoretical

▶ **Abiraterone** is predicted to increase the exposure to meglitinides **(repaglinide)**. [Moderate] Anecdotal

▶ **Darolutamide** is predicted to increase the concentration of meglitinides **(repaglinide)**. [Moderate] Theoretical

▶ Anti-androgens **(apalutamide, enzalutamide)** are predicted to decrease the exposure to meglitinides **(repaglinide)**. Monitor blood glucose and adjust dose. [Moderate] Study

▶ **Apalutamide** is predicted to decrease the exposure to methotrexate. [Mild] Study

▶ **Darolutamide** is predicted to increase the concentration of methotrexate. [Moderate] Theoretical

▶ Anti-androgens **(apalutamide, enzalutamide)** are predicted to decrease the exposure to midostaurin. Avoid. [Severe] Study

▶ Anti-androgens **(apalutamide, enzalutamide)** are predicted to decrease the exposure to mifepristone. Adjust **mifepristone** dose, p. 954. [Severe] Study

▶ Mineralocorticoid receptor antagonists **(spironolactone)** might oppose the effects of **abiraterone**. Avoid. [Severe] Anecdotal

▶ Anti-androgens **(apalutamide, enzalutamide)** are predicted to decrease the exposure to mineralocorticoid receptor antagonists **(eplerenone)**. Avoid. [Moderate] Theoretical

▶ Anti-androgens **(apalutamide, enzalutamide)** are predicted to decrease the exposure to mineralocorticoid receptor antagonists **(finerenone)**. Avoid. [Severe] Study

▶ Anti-androgens **(apalutamide, enzalutamide)** are predicted to decrease the exposure to mirtazapine. Adjust dose. [Moderate] Study

▶ **Mitotane** is predicted to decrease the exposure to **abiraterone**. Avoid. [Severe] Study

▶ **Mitotane** is predicted to decrease the exposure to **darolutamide**. Avoid. [Moderate] Study

▶ Anti-androgens **(apalutamide, enzalutamide)** are predicted to decrease the exposure to mobocertinib. Avoid. [Severe] Study → Also see **TABLE 8** p. 1573

▶ **Apalutamide** is predicted to decrease the exposure to moclobemide. Avoid or monitor. [Mild] Study

▶ **Modafinil** is predicted to decrease the efficacy of **cyproterone** with ethinylestradiol (co-cyprindiol). Use alternative methods during treatment with, and for 28 days after, the enzyme inducing drug is stopped. [Severe] Study

▶ **Darolutamide** is predicted to increase the exposure to momelotinib. [Moderate] Study

▶ Anti-androgens **(apalutamide, enzalutamide)** are predicted to decrease the exposure to monoclonal antibodies **(polatuzumab vedotin)**. [Moderate] Theoretical

▶ Anti-androgens **(apalutamide, enzalutamide)** are predicted to decrease the exposure to the cytotoxic component of monoclonal antibodies **(trastuzumab emtansine)**. [Severe] Theoretical

▶ Anti-androgens **(apalutamide, enzalutamide)** are predicted to decrease the exposure to montelukast. [Mild] Study

▶ Anti-androgens **(apalutamide, enzalutamide)** are predicted to markedly decrease the exposure to naldemedine. Avoid. [Severe] Study

- Anti-androgens **(apalutamide, enzalutamide)** are predicted to markedly decrease the exposure to naloxegol. Avoid. Moderate Study
- Anti-androgens **(apalutamide, enzalutamide)** are predicted to decrease the exposure to neratinib. Avoid. Severe Study
- Neurokinin-1 receptor antagonists **(aprepitant, fosaprepitant)** are predicted to decrease the efficacy of **cyproterone** with ethinylestradiol (co-cyprindiol). Use alternative methods during treatment with, and for 28 days after, the enzyme inducing drug is stopped. Severe Study
- Anti-androgens **(apalutamide, enzalutamide)** are predicted to markedly decrease the exposure to neurokinin-1 receptor antagonists **(aprepitant)**. Avoid. Moderate Study
- Anti-androgens **(apalutamide, enzalutamide)** are predicted to decrease the exposure to neurokinin-1 receptor antagonists **(fosaprepitant)**. Avoid. Moderate Theoretical
- Anti-androgens **(apalutamide, enzalutamide)** are predicted to decrease the exposure to neurokinin-1 receptor antagonists **(netupitant)**. Avoid. Severe Study
- Anti-androgens **(apalutamide, enzalutamide)** are predicted to moderately decrease the exposure to nilotinib. Avoid. Severe Study → Also see **TABLE 8** p. 1573
- Anti-androgens **(apalutamide, enzalutamide)** are predicted to decrease the exposure to nirmatrelvir boosted with ritonavir. Avoid. Severe Study
- Anti-androgens **(apalutamide, enzalutamide)** are predicted to decrease the exposure to nitisinone. Adjust dose. Moderate Theoretical
- NNRTIs **(efavirenz, etravirine, nevirapine)** are predicted to decrease the exposure to **darolutamide**. Avoid. Moderate Theoretical
- NNRTIs **(efavirenz, nevirapine)** are predicted to decrease the efficacy of **cyproterone** with ethinylestradiol (co-cyprindiol). Use alternative methods during treatment with, and for 28 days after, the enzyme inducing drug is stopped. Severe Study
- Anti-androgens **(apalutamide, enzalutamide)** are predicted to decrease the exposure to NNRTIs **(doravirine)**. Avoid. Severe Study
- Anti-androgens **(apalutamide, enzalutamide)** are predicted to decrease the exposure to NNRTIs **(etravirine)**. Avoid. Severe Theoretical
- Anti-androgens **(apalutamide, enzalutamide)** are predicted to decrease the exposure to NNRTIs **(nevirapine)**. Severe Study
- Anti-androgens **(apalutamide, enzalutamide)** markedly decrease the exposure to NNRTIs **(rilpivirine)**. Avoid. Severe Study
- Anti-androgens **(apalutamide, enzalutamide)** are predicted to decrease the exposure to olaparib. Avoid. Moderate Theoretical
- Anti-androgens **(apalutamide, enzalutamide)** are predicted to decrease the exposure to opioids **(alfentanil, fentanyl)**. Moderate Study
- Anti-androgens **(apalutamide, enzalutamide)** are predicted to decrease the exposure to opioids **(buprenorphine)**. Monitor and adjust dose. Moderate Theoretical
- Anti-androgens **(apalutamide, enzalutamide)** decrease the exposure to opioids **(methadone)**. Monitor and adjust dose. Severe Study → Also see **TABLE 8** p. 1573
- Anti-androgens **(apalutamide, enzalutamide)** are predicted to decrease the exposure to opioids **(oxycodone)**. Monitor and adjust dose. Moderate Study
- **Enzalutamide** is predicted to affect the exposure to opioids **(tramadol)**. Use with caution or avoid. Moderate Theoretical
- Anti-androgens **(apalutamide, enzalutamide)** are predicted to decrease the exposure to osilodrostat. Moderate Theoretical → Also see **TABLE 8** p. 1573
- Anti-androgens **(apalutamide, enzalutamide)** are predicted to moderately decrease the exposure to osimertinib. Avoid. Moderate Study → Also see **TABLE 8** p. 1573
- Anti-androgens **(apalutamide, enzalutamide)** are predicted to moderately decrease the exposure to ospemifene. Moderate Study
- Anti-androgens **(apalutamide, enzalutamide)** are predicted to decrease the exposure to palbociclib. Avoid. Severe Study

- Anti-androgens **(apalutamide, enzalutamide)** are predicted to decrease the exposure to panobinostat. Avoid. Moderate Theoretical → Also see **TABLE 8** p. 1573
- Anti-androgens **(apalutamide, enzalutamide)** are predicted to decrease the exposure to pazopanib. Avoid. Severe Theoretical → Also see **TABLE 8** p. 1573
- Anti-androgens **(apalutamide, enzalutamide)** are predicted to decrease the exposure to pemigatinib. Avoid. Severe Study
- Anti-androgens **(apalutamide, enzalutamide)** moderately decrease the exposure to phosphodiesterase type-4 inhibitors **(apremilast)**. Avoid. Severe Study
- Anti-androgens **(apalutamide, enzalutamide)** are predicted to decrease the exposure to phosphodiesterase type-4 inhibitors **(roflumilast)**. Avoid. Moderate Study
- Anti-androgens **(apalutamide, enzalutamide)** are predicted to decrease the exposure to phosphodiesterase type-5 inhibitors **(avanafil, tadalafil)**. Avoid. Severe Study
- Anti-androgens **(apalutamide, enzalutamide)** are predicted to decrease the exposure to phosphodiesterase type-5 inhibitors **(sildenafil, vardenafil)**. Moderate Theoretical → Also see **TABLE 8** p. 1573
- Anti-androgens **(apalutamide, enzalutamide)** are predicted to moderately to markedly decrease the exposure to pibrentasvir. Avoid. Severe Study
- **Abiraterone** slightly increases the exposure to pioglitazone. Moderate Study
- Anti-androgens **(apalutamide, enzalutamide)** are predicted to moderately decrease the exposure to pitolisant. Moderate Study
- Anti-androgens **(apalutamide, enzalutamide)** are predicted to decrease the exposure to ponatinib. Avoid. Moderate Theoretical
- Anti-androgens **(apalutamide, enzalutamide)** are predicted to decrease the exposure to pralsetinib. Avoid or adjust dose with potent CYP3A4 inducers—consult product literature. Moderate Study
- Anti-androgens **(apalutamide, enzalutamide)** are predicted to markedly decrease the exposure to praziquantel. Avoid. Moderate Study
- **Apalutamide** is predicted to decrease the exposure to proton pump inhibitors **(lansoprazole, rabeprazole)**. Avoid or monitor. Mild Study
- **Apalutamide** markedly decreases the exposure to proton pump inhibitors **(omeprazole)**. Avoid or monitor. Moderate Study
- Anti-androgens **(apalutamide, enzalutamide)** are predicted to decrease the exposure to quizartinib. Avoid. Severe Study → Also see **TABLE 8** p. 1573
- Anti-androgens **(apalutamide, enzalutamide)** are predicted to decrease the exposure to ranolazine. Avoid. Severe Study → Also see **TABLE 8** p. 1573
- Anti-androgens **(apalutamide, enzalutamide)** are predicted to decrease the exposure to reboxetine. Moderate Anecdotal
- Anti-androgens **(apalutamide, enzalutamide)** are predicted to decrease the exposure to regorafenib. Avoid. Moderate Study
- **Apalutamide** is predicted to decrease the exposure to relugolix. Avoid or adjust dose depending on indication—consult product literature. Moderate Study
- Anti-androgens **(apalutamide, enzalutamide)** are predicted to markedly decrease the exposure to ribociclib. Avoid. Severe Study → Also see **TABLE 8** p. 1573
- Rifamycins **(rifampicin)** are predicted to decrease the exposure to **abiraterone**. Avoid. Severe Study
- Rifamycins are predicted to decrease the efficacy of **cyproterone** with ethinylestradiol (co-cyprindiol). Use alternative methods during treatment with, and for 28 days after, the enzyme inducing drug is stopped. Severe Study
- Rifamycins **(rifampicin)** are predicted to decrease the exposure to **darolutamide**. Avoid. Moderate Study
- Anti-androgens **(apalutamide, enzalutamide)** are predicted to decrease the exposure to rimegepant. Avoid. Moderate Theoretical
- Anti-androgens **(apalutamide, enzalutamide)** are predicted to decrease the exposure to ripretinib. Avoid or adjust dose— consult product literature. Severe Study
- Anti-androgens **(apalutamide, enzalutamide)** are predicted to decrease the exposure to ruxolitinib. Monitor and adjust dose. Moderate Study

Anti-androgens (continued)

▶ Anti-androgens **(apalutamide, enzalutamide)** are predicted to decrease the exposure to selpercatinib. Avoid. Moderate Study → Also see **TABLE 8** p. 1573

▶ Anti-androgens **(apalutamide, enzalutamide)** are predicted to decrease the exposure to selumetinib. Avoid. Severe Study

▶ Anti-androgens **(apalutamide, enzalutamide)** are predicted to decrease the exposure to siponimod. Manufacturer advises caution depending on genotype—consult product literature. Severe Study

▶ Anti-androgens **(apalutamide, enzalutamide)** are predicted to decrease the concentration of sirolimus. Avoid or monitor and adjust dose. Severe Study

▶ Anti-androgens **(apalutamide, enzalutamide)** are predicted to decrease the exposure to solifenacin. Moderate Theoretical

▶ Anti-androgens **(apalutamide, enzalutamide)** are predicted to decrease the exposure to sorafenib. Moderate Theoretical → Also see **TABLE 8** p. 1573

▶ Anti-androgens **(apalutamide, enzalutamide)** are predicted to decrease the exposure to sotorasib. Avoid. Severe Study

▶ **Sotorasib** is predicted to decrease the exposure to darolutamide. Avoid. Moderate Theoretical

▶ **Apalutamide** is predicted to decrease the exposure to SSRIs **(citalopram)**. Avoid or monitor. Mild Study → Also see **TABLE 8** p. 1573

▶ **St John's wort** is predicted to decrease the efficacy of cyproterone with ethinylestradiol (co-cyprindiol). Use alternative methods during treatment with, and for 28 days after, the enzyme inducing drug is stopped. Severe Study

▶ **St John's wort** is predicted to decrease the exposure to darolutamide. Avoid. Moderate Theoretical

▶ **Apalutamide** is predicted to decrease the exposure to statins **(atorvastatin)**. Moderate Study

▶ **Darolutamide** is predicted to increase the exposure to statins **(atorvastatin, fluvastatin)**. Avoid. Severe Theoretical

▶ **Enzalutamide** is predicted to decrease the exposure to statins **(atorvastatin, simvastatin)**. Moderate Study

▶ **Apalutamide** is predicted to decrease the exposure to statins **(fluvastatin)**. Monitor and adjust dose. Mild Theoretical

▶ **Apalutamide** is predicted to decrease the exposure to statins **(pravastatin)**. Mild Study

▶ **Darolutamide** is predicted to increase the concentration of statins **(pravastatin, simvastatin)**. Moderate Theoretical

▶ **Apalutamide** slightly decreases the exposure to statins **(rosuvastatin)**. Mild Study

▶ **Darolutamide** markedly increases the exposure to statins **(rosuvastatin)**. Avoid or adjust **rosuvastatin** dose, p. 235. Severe Study

▶ **Apalutamide** is predicted to decrease the exposure to statins **(simvastatin)**. Avoid or monitor. Moderate Study

▶ **Apalutamide** is predicted to decrease the exposure to sulfasalazine. Mild Study

▶ **Darolutamide** is predicted to increase the exposure to sulfasalazine. Avoid. Severe Theoretical

▶ **Apalutamide** is predicted to decrease the exposure to sulfonylureas **(glibenclamide)**. Monitor and adjust dose. Mild Theoretical

▶ **Darolutamide** is predicted to increase the concentration of sulfonylureas **(glibenclamide)**. Moderate Theoretical

▶ Anti-androgens **(apalutamide, enzalutamide)** are predicted to decrease the exposure to sunitinib. Avoid or adjust dose—consult product literature. Moderate Study → Also see **TABLE 8** p. 1573

▶ Anti-androgens **(apalutamide, enzalutamide)** decrease the concentration of tacrolimus. Avoid or monitor and adjust dose. Severe Study

▶ **Apalutamide** is predicted to decrease the exposure to talazoparib. Monitor and adjust dose. Moderate Study

▶ **Enzalutamide** moderately increases the exposure to talazoparib. Adjust starting dose. Moderate Study

▶ Anti-androgens **(apalutamide, enzalutamide)** are predicted to decrease the exposure to taxanes **(cabazitaxel)**. Avoid. Moderate Study

▶ Anti-androgens **(apalutamide, enzalutamide)** are predicted to decrease the exposure to taxanes **(docetaxel)**. Severe Theoretical

▶ **Darolutamide** is predicted to increase the exposure to taxanes **(paclitaxel)**. Severe Theoretical

▶ Anti-androgens **(apalutamide, enzalutamide)** are predicted to decrease the exposure to taxanes **(paclitaxel)**. Avoid. Severe Study

▶ Anti-androgens **(apalutamide, enzalutamide)** are predicted to decrease the concentration of temsirolimus. Avoid. Severe Study

▶ **Darolutamide** is predicted to increase the exposure to tenofovir alafenamide. Moderate Theoretical

▶ **Darolutamide** is predicted to increase the exposure to tenofovir disoproxil. Moderate Theoretical

▶ Anti-androgens **(apalutamide, enzalutamide)** might decrease the exposure to tepotinib. Avoid. Severe Theoretical

▶ **Enzalutamide** is predicted to affect the exposure to tetracyclines **(doxycycline)**. Use with caution or avoid. Moderate Theoretical

▶ Anti-androgens **(apalutamide, enzalutamide)** are predicted to decrease the exposure to tetracyclines **(eravacycline)**. Adjust **eravacycline** dose, p. 657. Moderate Study

▶ Anti-androgens **(apalutamide, enzalutamide)** are predicted to decrease the exposure to tezacaftor. Avoid. Severe Theoretical

▶ **Apalutamide** is predicted to decrease the exposure to thrombin inhibitors **(dabigatran)**. Mild Study

▶ **Apalutamide** potentially decreases the exposure to thyroid hormones **(levothyroxine)**. Mild Theoretical

▶ **Enzalutamide** is predicted to affect the exposure to thyroid hormones **(levothyroxine)**. Use with caution or avoid. Moderate Theoretical

▶ Anti-androgens **(apalutamide, enzalutamide)** are predicted to markedly decrease the exposure to ticagrelor. Avoid. Severe Study

▶ Anti-androgens **(apalutamide, enzalutamide)** are predicted to decrease the exposure to tivozanib. Severe Study

▶ Anti-androgens **(apalutamide, enzalutamide)** are predicted to decrease the exposure to tofacitinib. Avoid. Severe Study

▶ Anti-androgens **(apalutamide, enzalutamide)** are predicted to decrease the exposure to tolvaptan. Use with caution or avoid depending on indication. Severe Study

▶ **Apalutamide** is predicted to decrease the exposure to topotecan. Monitor and adjust dose. Moderate Theoretical

▶ **Darolutamide** is predicted to increase the exposure to topotecan. Avoid. Severe Theoretical

▶ Anti-androgens **(apalutamide, enzalutamide)** are predicted to decrease the exposure to toremifene. Adjust dose. Moderate Study → Also see **TABLE 8** p. 1573

▶ Anti-androgens **(apalutamide, enzalutamide)** are predicted to decrease the exposure to trabectedin. Avoid. Severe Theoretical

▶ **Enzalutamide** is predicted to decrease the exposure to triptans **(eletriptan)**. Severe Study

▶ Anti-androgens **(apalutamide, enzalutamide)** are predicted to decrease the exposure to tucatinib. Avoid. Severe Study

▶ **Tucatinib** is predicted to increase the exposure to **apalutamide**. Monitor and adjust dose. Mild Study

▶ **Apalutamide** is predicted to decrease the efficacy of ulipristal. Avoid and for 4 weeks after stopping **apalutamide**. Severe Theoretical

▶ **Enzalutamide** is predicted to decrease the efficacy of ulipristal. Avoid and for 4 weeks after stopping **enzalutamide**. Severe Theoretical

▶ Anti-androgens **(apalutamide, enzalutamide)** are predicted to decrease the exposure to upadacitinib. Moderate Study

▶ Anti-androgens **(apalutamide, enzalutamide)** are predicted to decrease the exposure to vandetanib. Avoid. Moderate Study → Also see **TABLE 8** p. 1573

▶ Anti-androgens **(apalutamide, enzalutamide)** are predicted to moderately decrease the exposure to velpatasvir. Avoid. Severe Study

▶ Anti-androgens **(apalutamide, enzalutamide)** are predicted to decrease the exposure to vemurafenib. Avoid. Severe Study → Also see **TABLE 8** p. 1573

▶ Anti-androgens **(apalutamide, enzalutamide)** are predicted to decrease the exposure to venetoclax. Avoid. Severe Study

► Anti-androgens **(apalutamide, enzalutamide)** are predicted to decrease the exposure to vinca alkaloids **(vinblastine, vincristine, vindesine).** Severe Theoretical

► Anti-androgens **(apalutamide, enzalutamide)** are predicted to decrease the exposure to vinca alkaloids **(vinorelbine).** Use with caution or avoid. Severe Theoretical

► Anti-androgens **(apalutamide, enzalutamide)** are predicted to decrease the exposure to vismodegib. Avoid. Moderate Theoretical

► Anti-androgens **(apalutamide, enzalutamide)** are predicted to decrease the exposure to voclosporin. Avoid. Severe Study → Also see **TABLE 8** p. 1573

► Anti-androgens **(apalutamide, enzalutamide)** are predicted to decrease the exposure to vortioxetine. Monitor and adjust dose. Moderate Study

► Anti-androgens **(apalutamide, enzalutamide)** are predicted to decrease the concentration of voxilaprevir. Avoid. Severe Study

► Anti-androgens **(apalutamide, enzalutamide)** are predicted to decrease the exposure to zanubrutinib. Avoid. Severe Study

► **Enzalutamide** is predicted to affect the exposure to zolpidem. Use with caution or avoid. Moderate Theoretical

► Anti-androgens **(apalutamide, enzalutamide)** are predicted to decrease the exposure to zopiclone. Adjust dose. Moderate Study

Anti-D (Rh$_0$) immunoglobulin → see immunoglobulins

Antiarrhythmics → see **TABLE 5** p. 1572 (bradycardia), **TABLE 1** p. 1571 (hepatotoxicity), **TABLE 7** p. 1572 (hypotension), **TABLE 11** p. 1574 (peripheral neuropathy), **TABLE 8** p. 1573 (QT-interval prolongation), **TABLE 9** p. 1573 (antimuscarinics)

adenosine · amiodarone · disopyramide · dronedarone · flecainide · lidocaine · propafenone · vernakalant

> ► **Amiodarone** has a long half-life; there is potential for drug interactions to occur for several weeks (or even months) after treatment with it has been stopped.
> ► Since systemic absorption can follow topical application of **lidocaine**, the possibility of interactions should be borne in mind.
> ► Avoid intravenous class I and class III antiarrhythmics for 4 hours before and after **vernakalant.**

► **Dronedarone** is predicted to increase the exposure to abemaciclib. Moderate Study

► **Dronedarone** is predicted to increase the exposure to acalabrutinib. Avoid or monitor. Severe Study

► Antiarrhythmics **(amiodarone, dronedarone)** are predicted to increase the exposure to afatinib. Moderate Study

► **Amiodarone** is predicted to decrease the effects of agalsidase alfa. Avoid. Moderate Theoretical

► **Amiodarone** is predicted to decrease the effects of agalsidase beta. Avoid. Moderate Theoretical

► Antiarrhythmics **(amiodarone, dronedarone)** are predicted to increase the exposure to aliskiren. Severe Study

► **Dronedarone** is predicted to increase the exposure to alpha blockers **(tamsulosin).** Moderate Theoretical

► **Aminophylline** is predicted to decrease the efficacy of **adenosine.** Separate administration by 24 hours. Mild Theoretical

► Anti-androgens (apalutamide, enzalutamide) are predicted to decrease the efficacy of **propafenone.** Moderate Study

► Anti-androgens (apalutamide, enzalutamide) are predicted to decrease the exposure to antiarrhythmics **(disopyramide, dronedarone).** Avoid. Severe Study → Also see **TABLE 8** p. 1573

► Antiarrhythmics **(propafenone)** are predicted to increase the risk of cardiodepression when given with antiarrhythmics **(amiodarone).** Monitor and adjust dose. Severe Theoretical → Also see **TABLE 5** p. 1572

► Antiarrhythmics **(amiodarone)** increase the concentration of antiarrhythmics **(flecainide).** Adjust **flecainide** dose and monitor adverse effects. Severe Study → Also see **TABLE 5** p. 1572

► Antiarrhythmics **(propafenone)** are predicted to increase the risk of cardiodepression when given with antiarrhythmics **(lidocaine).** Moderate Study

► Antiarrhythmics **(dronedarone)** are predicted to increase the exposure to antiarrhythmics **(propafenone).** Monitor and adjust dose. Moderate Study → Also see **TABLE 5** p. 1572

► Antiepileptics **(carbamazepine, fosphenytoin, phenobarbital, phenytoin, primidone)** are predicted to decrease the efficacy of **propafenone.** Moderate Study

► Antiepileptics **(fosphenytoin, phenytoin)** are predicted to decrease the exposure to **lidocaine.** Severe Anecdotal

► Antiepileptics **(carbamazepine, fosphenytoin, phenobarbital, phenytoin, primidone)** are predicted to decrease the exposure to antiarrhythmics **(disopyramide, dronedarone).** Avoid. Severe Study

► **Amiodarone** is predicted to slightly increase the concentration of antiepileptics **(fosphenytoin, phenytoin).** Monitor and adjust dose. Severe Study → Also see **TABLE 11** p. 1574

► Antifungals, azoles **(fluconazole)** are predicted to increase the exposure to **dronedarone.** Severe Theoretical → Also see **TABLE 8** p. 1573

► Antifungals, azoles **(fluconazole, isavuconazole)** are predicted to increase the exposure to **propafenone.** Monitor and adjust dose. Moderate Study

► Antifungals, azoles **(itraconazole)** are predicted to increase the exposure to **amiodarone.** Avoid. Severe Anecdotal → Also see **TABLE 1** p. 1571

► Antifungals, azoles **(itraconazole, ketoconazole, posaconazole, voriconazole)** are predicted to increase the exposure to **disopyramide.** Avoid. Severe Theoretical → Also see **TABLE 8** p. 1573

► Antifungals, azoles **(itraconazole, ketoconazole, posaconazole, voriconazole)** very markedly increase the exposure to **dronedarone.** Avoid. Severe Study → Also see **TABLE 8** p. 1573

► Antifungals, azoles **(itraconazole, ketoconazole, posaconazole, voriconazole)** are predicted to increase the exposure to **propafenone.** Monitor and adjust dose. Severe Study

► Antifungals, azoles **(ketoconazole, voriconazole)** are predicted to increase the exposure to **amiodarone.** Avoid. Moderate Theoretical → Also see **TABLE 1** p. 1571 → Also see **TABLE 8** p. 1573

► Antifungals, azoles **(miconazole)** are predicted to increase the exposure to **disopyramide.** Use with caution and adjust dose. Severe Theoretical

► **Dronedarone** is predicted to increase the exposure to antifungals, azoles **(isavuconazole).** Moderate Theoretical

► **Amiodarone** is predicted to increase the exposure to antihistamines, non-sedating **(fexofenadine).** Moderate Study

► **Dronedarone** is predicted to increase the exposure to antihistamines, non-sedating **(fexofenadine, mizolastine).** Severe Theoretical

► **Dronedarone** is predicted to increase the exposure to antihistamines, non-sedating **(rupatadine).** Avoid. Moderate Study

► **Dronedarone** is predicted to increase the exposure to antipsychotics, second generation **(cariprazine).** Avoid. Severe Study

► Antipsychotics, second generation **(clozapine)** can cause constipation, as can antiarrhythmics **(disopyramide, propafenone)**; concurrent use might increase the risk of developing intestinal obstruction. Severe Theoretical → Also see **TABLE 9** p. 1573

► **Dronedarone** is predicted to increase the exposure to antipsychotics, second generation **(lurasidone).** Adjust **lurasidone** dose. Moderate Study

► **Dronedarone** is predicted to increase the exposure to antipsychotics, second generation **(quetiapine).** Avoid. Moderate Study

► **Dronedarone** is predicted to increase the exposure to avapritinib. Avoid or adjust dose—consult product literature. Moderate Study

► **Amiodarone** is predicted to increase the exposure to avatrombopag. Adjust **avatrombopag** dose with moderate CYP2C9 inhibitors in chronic immune thrombocytopenia, p. 1169. Moderate Study

► **Dronedarone** is predicted to increase the exposure to axitinib. Moderate Study

► **Dronedarone** might increases the exposure to bedaquiline. Mild Theoretical → Also see **TABLE 8** p. 1573

► **Dronedarone** is predicted to increase the exposure to benzodiazepines **(alprazolam).** Severe Study

► **Dronedarone** is predicted to increase the exposure to benzodiazepines **(midazolam).** Monitor adverse effects and adjust dose. Severe Study

Antiarrhythmics (continued)

▸ Berotralstat is predicted to increase the exposure to propafenone. Monitor and adjust dose. [Moderate] Study
▸ Antiarrhythmics (amiodarone, disopyramide, dronedarone, flecainide, lidocaine) are predicted to increase the risk of cardiovascular adverse effects when given with beta blockers, non-selective. Use with caution or avoid. [Severe] Study → Also see TABLE 5 p. 1572 → Also see TABLE 8 p. 1573
▸ Propafenone is predicted to increase the risk of cardiovascular adverse effects when given with beta blockers, non-selective (labetalol, levobunolol, nadolol, pindolol, sotalol). Use with caution or avoid. [Severe] Study → Also see TABLE 5 p. 1572
▸ Propafenone increases the risk of cardiovascular adverse effects when given with beta blockers, non-selective (propranolol). Use with caution or avoid. [Severe] Study → Also see TABLE 5 p. 1572
▸ Propafenone is predicted to increase the exposure to beta blockers, non-selective (timolol) and beta blockers, non-selective (timolol) are predicted to increase the risk of cardiodepression when given with propafenone. [Severe] Anecdotal → Also see TABLE 5 p. 1572
▸ Antiarrhythmics (amiodarone, disopyramide, dronedarone, flecainide, lidocaine) are predicted to increase the risk of cardiovascular adverse effects when given with beta blockers, selective. Use with caution or avoid. [Severe] Study → Also see TABLE 5 p. 1572
▸ Propafenone is predicted to increase the risk of cardiovascular adverse effects when given with beta blockers, selective (acebutolol, atenolol, betaxolol, bisoprolol, celiprolol, esmolol). Use with caution or avoid. [Severe] Study → Also see TABLE 5 p. 1572
▸ Propafenone is predicted to increase the exposure to beta blockers, selective (metoprolol). [Moderate] Study → Also see TABLE 5 p. 1572
▸ Propafenone is predicted to increase the exposure to beta blockers, selective (nebivolol) and beta blockers, selective (nebivolol) are predicted to increase the risk of cardiodepression when given with propafenone. Avoid. [Severe] Theoretical → Also see TABLE 5 p. 1572
▸ Antiarrhythmics (amiodarone, dronedarone) are predicted to increase the exposure to bictegravir. Use with caution or avoid. [Moderate] Theoretical
▸ Dronedarone is predicted to increase the exposure to bosutinib. Avoid or adjust dose. [Severe] Study → Also see TABLE 8 p. 1573
▸ Dronedarone is predicted to increase the exposure to brigatinib. [Moderate] Study → Also see TABLE 5 p. 1572
▸ Dronedarone is predicted to increase the exposure to buspirone. Use with caution and adjust dose. [Moderate] Study
▸ Dronedarone is predicted to increase the exposure to cabozantinib. [Moderate] Study → Also see TABLE 8 p. 1573
▸ Caffeine citrate decreases the efficacy of adenosine. Separate administration by 24 hours. [Mild] Study
▸ Calcium channel blockers (diltiazem, verapamil) increase the exposure to dronedarone and dronedarone increases the exposure to calcium channel blockers (diltiazem, verapamil). [Moderate] Study → Also see TABLE 5 p. 1572
▸ Calcium channel blockers (diltiazem, verapamil) are predicted to increase the exposure to propafenone. Monitor and adjust dose. [Moderate] Study → Also see TABLE 5 p. 1572
▸ Calcium channel blockers (verapamil) increase the risk of cardiodepression when given with flecainide. [Severe] Anecdotal → Also see TABLE 5 p. 1572
▸ Dronedarone is predicted to increase the exposure to calcium channel blockers (amlodipine, felodipine, lacidipine, lercanidipine, nicardipine, nifedipine, nimodipine). Monitor and adjust dose. [Moderate] Study
▸ Amiodarone is predicted to increase the risk of cardiodepression when given with calcium channel blockers (diltiazem, verapamil). Avoid. [Severe] Theoretical → Also see TABLE 5 p. 1572
▸ Disopyramide is predicted to increase the risk of cardiodepression when given with calcium channel blockers (verapamil). [Severe] Theoretical
▸ Dronedarone is predicted to increase the exposure to capivasertib. Adjust dose. [Moderate] Study

▸ Ceritinib very markedly increases the exposure to dronedarone. Avoid. [Severe] Study → Also see TABLE 5 p. 1572 → Also see TABLE 8 p. 1573
▸ Dronedarone is predicted to increase the exposure to ceritinib. [Moderate] Study → Also see TABLE 5 p. 1572 → Also see TABLE 8 p. 1573
▸ Ceritinib is predicted to increase the exposure to propafenone. Monitor and adjust dose. [Severe] Study → Also see TABLE 5 p. 1572
▸ Chloroprocaine is predicted to increase the risk of cardiovascular adverse effects when given with antiarrhythmics (amiodarone, dronedarone, vernakalant). [Severe] Theoretical
▸ Amiodarone increases the concentration of ciclosporin. Monitor concentration and adjust dose. [Severe] Study
▸ Dronedarone is predicted to increase the concentration of ciclosporin. [Severe] Study
▸ Cobicistat potentially increases the concentration of antiarrhythmics (amiodarone, disopyramide, flecainide, lidocaine). [Severe] Theoretical
▸ Cobicistat very markedly increases the exposure to dronedarone. Avoid. [Severe] Study
▸ Cobicistat is predicted to increase the exposure to propafenone. Monitor and adjust dose. [Severe] Study
▸ Dronedarone is predicted to increase the exposure to cobimetinib. [Severe] Study
▸ Amiodarone is predicted to increase the exposure to colchicine. Avoid P-glycoprotein inhibitors or adjust colchicine dose, p. 1279. [Severe] Theoretical
▸ Dronedarone is predicted to increase the exposure to colchicine. Adjust colchicine dose with moderate CYP3A4 inhibitors, p. 1279. [Severe] Study
▸ Dronedarone is predicted to increase the exposure to corticosteroids (methylprednisolone). Monitor and adjust dose. [Moderate] Study
▸ Amiodarone increases the anticoagulant effect of coumarins. [Severe] Study
▸ Dronedarone might increase the anticoagulant effect of coumarins. [Moderate] Anecdotal
▸ Propafenone increases the anticoagulant effect of coumarins. Monitor INR and adjust dose. [Moderate] Study
▸ Dronedarone is predicted to increase the exposure to crizotinib. [Moderate] Study → Also see TABLE 5 p. 1572 → Also see TABLE 8 p. 1573
▸ Crizotinib is predicted to increase the exposure to propafenone. Monitor and adjust dose. [Moderate] Study → Also see TABLE 5 p. 1572
▸ Dronedarone is predicted to increase the exposure to dabrafenib. [Moderate] Study
▸ Dronedarone is predicted to increase the exposure to daridorexant. Adjust daridorexant dose, p. 554. [Severe] Study
▸ Dronedarone is predicted to increase the exposure to darifenacin. [Moderate] Study
▸ Darifenacin is predicted to increase the concentration of flecainide. [Moderate] Theoretical
▸ Dronedarone is predicted to increase the exposure to dasatinib. [Severe] Study → Also see TABLE 8 p. 1573
▸ Dronedarone is predicted to slightly increase the exposure to dienogest. [Moderate] Study
▸ Antiarrhythmics (amiodarone, dronedarone) are predicted to moderately increase the exposure to digoxin. Monitor and adjust digoxin dose, p. 125. [Severe] Study → Also see TABLE 5 p. 1572
▸ Propafenone increases the concentration of digoxin. Monitor and adjust dose. [Severe] Study → Also see TABLE 5 p. 1572
▸ Dronedarone is predicted to increase the exposure to dipeptidylpeptidase-4 inhibitors (saxagliptin). [Mild] Study
▸ Dipyridamole increases the exposure to adenosine. Avoid or adjust dose. [Severe] Study
▸ Dronedarone is predicted to increase the exposure to domperidone. Avoid. [Severe] Study
▸ Dronedarone is predicted to increase the exposure to dopamine receptor agonists (bromocriptine). [Severe] Theoretical
▸ Dronedarone is predicted to increase the concentration of dopamine receptor agonists (cabergoline). [Severe] Anecdotal
▸ Dronedarone is predicted to increase the exposure to drospirenone. [Severe] Study
▸ Dronedarone is predicted to moderately increase the exposure to dutasteride. [Mild] Study

▸ **Dronedarone** is predicted to increase the exposure to elacestrant. Avoid moderate CYP3A4 inhibitors or adjust elacestrant dose, p. 1084. Severe Theoretical

▸ **Dronedarone** is predicted to increase the exposure to elexacaftor. Adjust ivacaftor with tezacaftor and elexacaftor p. 337 dose with moderate CYP3A4 inhibitors. Severe Theoretical

▸ Antiarrhythmics **(dronedarone, propafenone)** are predicted to increase the exposure to eliglustat. Avoid or adjust dose—consult product literature. Severe Study

▸ Encorafenib is predicted to decrease the exposure to antiarrhythmics **(disopyramide, dronedarone)**. Avoid. Severe Study → Also see **TABLE 8** p. 1573

▸ **Dronedarone** is predicted to moderately increase the exposure to encorafenib. Moderate Study → Also see **TABLE 8** p. 1573

▸ Encorafenib is predicted to decrease the efficacy of **propafenone**. Moderate Study

▸ Endothelin receptor antagonists (bosentan) are predicted to decrease the exposure to **dronedarone**. Severe Theoretical

▸ Antiarrhythmics **(amiodarone, dronedarone)** are predicted to increase the exposure to endothelin receptor antagonists (macitentan). Manufacturer advises caution depending on other drugs taken—consult product literature. Moderate Theoretical

▸ **Dronedarone** is predicted to increase the exposure to entrectinib. Avoid or adjust dose with moderate CYP3A4 inhibitors—consult product literature. Severe Theoretical → Also see **TABLE 8** p. 1573

▸ **Amiodarone** is predicted to increase the exposure to erdafitinib. Adjust dose. Severe Study

▸ **Dronedarone** is predicted to increase the risk of ergotism when given with **ergometrine**. Severe Theoretical

▸ **Amiodarone** is predicted to increase the exposure to erlotinib. Moderate Theoretical

▸ **Dronedarone** is predicted to increase the exposure to erlotinib. Moderate Study

▸ **Dronedarone** is predicted to increase the exposure to etrasimod. Avoid in poor CYP2C9 metabolisers. Severe Theoretical → Also see **TABLE 5** p. 1572

▸ **Amiodarone** is predicted to increase the exposure to everolimus. Monitor and adjust dose. Severe Study

▸ **Dronedarone** is predicted to increase the concentration of everolimus. Avoid or adjust dose. Moderate Study

▸ Antiarrhythmics **(amiodarone, dronedarone)** are predicted to increase the exposure to factor XA inhibitors (apixaban). Moderate Theoretical

▸ **Amiodarone** slightly increases the exposure to factor XA inhibitors (edoxaban). Severe Study

▸ **Dronedarone** slightly increases the exposure to factor XA inhibitors (edoxaban). Adjust **edoxaban** dose, p. 147. Severe Study

▸ **Amiodarone** might increase the exposure to factor XA inhibitors (rivaroxaban). Moderate Study

▸ **Dronedarone** might increase the exposure to factor XA inhibitors (rivaroxaban). Avoid. Moderate Study

▸ **Dronedarone** is predicted to increase the exposure to fedratinib. Monitor and adjust dose. Moderate Study

▸ Fedratinib is predicted to increase the exposure to **propafenone**. Monitor and adjust dose. Moderate Study

▸ **Dronedarone** is predicted to increase the exposure to fesoterodine. Adjust **fesoterodine** dose with moderate CYP3A4 inhibitors in hepatic and renal impairment, p. 897. Mild Study

▸ Antiarrhythmics **(amiodarone, dronedarone)** are predicted to increase the exposure to fidaxomicin. Avoid. Moderate Study

▸ **Dronedarone** is predicted to increase the exposure to gefitinib. Moderate Study

▸ Antiarrhythmics **(amiodarone, dronedarone)** are predicted to increase the exposure to gilteritinib. Moderate Theoretical

▸ **Dronedarone** potentially increases the exposure to glecaprevir. Moderate Theoretical

▸ Grapefruit juice increases the exposure to **amiodarone**. Avoid. Moderate Study

▸ Grapefruit juice moderately increases the exposure to **dronedarone**. Avoid. Severe Study

▸ Grapefruit juice increases the exposure to **propafenone**. Monitor and adjust dose. Moderate Study

▸ **Dronedarone** is predicted to increase the concentration of guanfacine. Adjust **guanfacine** dose, p. 407. Moderate Theoretical

▸ H₂ receptor antagonists **(cimetidine)** increase the exposure to amiodarone. Moderate Study

▸ H₂ receptor antagonists **(cimetidine)** slightly increase the exposure to **flecainide**. Monitor and adjust dose. Mild Study

▸ H₂ receptor antagonists **(cimetidine)** increase the exposure to **lidocaine**. Monitor and adjust dose. Moderate Study

▸ H₂ receptor antagonists **(cimetidine)** are predicted to increase the exposure to **propafenone**. Monitor and adjust dose. Moderate Theoretical

▸ HIV-protease inhibitors are predicted to increase the exposure to **amiodarone**. Avoid. Severe Theoretical → Also see **TABLE 1** p. 1571

▸ HIV-protease inhibitors are predicted to increase the exposure to **disopyramide**. Severe Theoretical

▸ HIV-protease inhibitors very markedly increase the exposure to **dronedarone**. Avoid. Severe Study

▸ HIV-protease inhibitors (ritonavir) are predicted to increase the exposure to **flecainide**. Avoid or monitor adverse effects. Severe Theoretical

▸ HIV-protease inhibitors are predicted to increase the exposure to **lidocaine**. Avoid. Severe Study

▸ HIV-protease inhibitors are predicted to increase the exposure to **propafenone**. Monitor and adjust dose. Severe Study

▸ **Amiodarone** is predicted to increase the exposure to ibrutinib. Adjust dose—consult product literature. Severe Theoretical

▸ **Dronedarone** is predicted to increase the exposure to ibrutinib. Adjust dose with moderate CYP3A4 inhibitors—consult product literature. Severe Study

▸ Idelalisib is predicted to increase the exposure to **amiodarone**. Avoid. Moderate Theoretical

▸ Idelalisib very markedly increases the exposure to **dronedarone**. Avoid. Severe Study

▸ Idelalisib is predicted to increase the exposure to **propafenone**. Monitor and adjust dose. Severe Study

▸ Imatinib is predicted to increase the exposure to **dronedarone**. Severe Theoretical

▸ Imatinib is predicted to increase the exposure to **propafenone**. Monitor and adjust dose. Moderate Study

▸ **Dronedarone** is predicted to increase the exposure to ivabradine. Adjust **ivabradine** dose, p. 245. Severe Theoretical → Also see **TABLE 5** p. 1572

▸ **Dronedarone** is predicted to increase the exposure to ivacaftor. Adjust dose with moderate CYP3A4 inhibitors, see ivacaftor p. 336, tezacaftor with ivacaftor p. 339, and ivacaftor with tezacaftor and elexacaftor p. 337. Moderate Study

▸ Ivosidenib is predicted to decrease the exposure to antiarrhythmics **(disopyramide, dronedarone)**. Avoid. Severe Study → Also see **TABLE 8** p. 1573

▸ **Dronedarone** is predicted to increase the exposure to ivosidenib. Monitor and adjust dose—consult product literature. Severe Study → Also see **TABLE 8** p. 1573

▸ Ivosidenib is predicted to decrease the efficacy of **propafenone**. Moderate Study

▸ **Dronedarone** is predicted to increase the exposure to lapatinib. Moderate Study → Also see **TABLE 8** p. 1573

▸ **Dronedarone** is predicted to increase the exposure to larotrectinib. Monitor and adjust dose. Moderate Theoretical

▸ Ledipasvir increases the risk of severe bradycardia or heart block when given with **amiodarone**. Refer to specialist literature. Severe Anecdotal

▸ **Dronedarone** is predicted to increase the exposure to leniolisib. Avoid. Moderate Study

▸ Letermovir is predicted to increase the concentration of **amiodarone**. Moderate Theoretical

▸ Letermovir is predicted to increase the exposure to **propafenone**. Monitor and adjust dose. Moderate Study

▸ **Amiodarone** is predicted to increase the exposure to lomitapide. Separate administration by 12 hours. Moderate Theoretical → Also see **TABLE 1** p. 1571

▸ **Dronedarone** is predicted to increase the exposure to lomitapide. Avoid. Moderate Theoretical

▸ **Dronedarone** is predicted to increase the exposure to loperamide. Severe Theoretical

Antiarrhythmics (continued)

▸ Lumacaftor is predicted to decrease the exposure to antiarrhythmics (**disopyramide, dronedarone**). Avoid. [Severe] Study

▸ Lumacaftor is predicted to decrease the efficacy of **propafenone**. [Moderate] Study

▸ Macrolides (**clarithromycin**) are predicted to increase the exposure to **amiodarone**. Avoid. [Moderate] Theoretical

▸ Macrolides (**clarithromycin**) very markedly increase the exposure to **dronedarone**. Avoid. [Severe] Study

▸ Macrolides (**clarithromycin**) are predicted to increase the exposure to **propafenone**. Monitor and adjust dose. [Severe] Study

▸ Macrolides (**clarithromycin, erythromycin**) are predicted to increase the exposure to **lidocaine**. [Moderate] Theoretical

▸ Macrolides (**erythromycin**) are predicted to moderately increase the exposure to **dronedarone**. Avoid. [Severe] Theoretical → Also see **TABLE 8** p. 1573

▸ Macrolides (**erythromycin**) are predicted to increase the exposure to **propafenone**. Monitor and adjust dose. [Moderate] Study

▸ **Amiodarone** is predicted to increase the exposure to mavacamten. Monitor and adjust dose—consult product literature. [Moderate] Theoretical

▸ **Dronedarone** is predicted to increase the exposure to mavacamten. Adjust dose—consult product literature. [Moderate] Study

▸ Mexiletine is predicted to increase the risk of torsade de pointes when given with **antiarrhythmics**. Avoid. [Severe] Theoretical

▸ **Dronedarone** is predicted to increase the exposure to midostaurin. [Moderate] Theoretical

▸ **Amiodarone** is predicted to increase the exposure to mineralocorticoid receptor antagonists (**eplerenone**). Adjust **eplerenone** dose, p. 223. [Severe] Theoretical

▸ **Dronedarone** is predicted to increase the exposure to mineralocorticoid receptor antagonists (**eplerenone**). Adjust **eplerenone** dose, p. 223. [Severe] Study

▸ **Dronedarone** is predicted to increase the exposure to mineralocorticoid receptor antagonists (**finerenone**). [Severe] Study

▸ Mitotane is predicted to decrease the exposure to antiarrhythmics (**disopyramide, dronedarone**). Avoid. [Severe] Study

▸ Mitotane is predicted to decrease the efficacy of **propafenone**. [Moderate] Study

▸ **Dronedarone** is predicted to increase the exposure to mobocertinib. Avoid or adjust dose and monitor ECG—consult product literature. [Severe] Study → Also see **TABLE 8** p. 1573

▸ **Amiodarone** is predicted to increase the risk of neutropenia when given with monoclonal antibodies (**brentuximab vedotin**). Monitor and adjust dose. [Severe] Theoretical → Also see **TABLE 11** p. 1574

▸ **Dronedarone** increases the risk of neutropenia when given with monoclonal antibodies (**brentuximab vedotin**). Monitor and adjust dose. [Severe] Theoretical

▸ Antiarrhythmics (**amiodarone, dronedarone**) are predicted to increase the exposure to naldemedine. [Moderate] Study

▸ **Dronedarone** is predicted to increase the exposure to naloxegol. Adjust **naloxegol** dose and monitor adverse effects, p. 72. [Moderate] Study

▸ **Amiodarone** is predicted to increase the exposure to neratinib. Avoid or adjust dose and monitor for gastrointestinal adverse effects—consult product literature. [Severe] Study → Also see **TABLE 1** p. 1571

▸ **Dronedarone** is predicted to increase the exposure to neratinib. Avoid moderate CYP3A4 inhibitors or adjust dose and monitor for gastrointestinal adverse effects—consult product literature. [Severe] Study

▸ Neurokinin-1 receptor antagonists (**aprepitant**) increase the exposure to **dronedarone**. [Severe] Theoretical

▸ Neurokinin-1 receptor antagonists (**aprepitant, netupitant**) are predicted to increase the exposure to **propafenone**. Monitor and adjust dose. [Moderate] Study

▸ Nilotinib is predicted to increase the exposure to **propafenone**. Monitor and adjust dose. [Moderate] Study

▸ Antiarrhythmics (**amiodarone, dronedarone**) are predicted to increase the exposure to nintedanib. [Moderate] Study

▸ Nirmatrelvir boosted with ritonavir is predicted to increase the concentration of antiarrhythmics (**amiodarone, dronedarone, flecainide, propafenone**). Avoid. [Severe] Theoretical

▸ Nirmatrelvir boosted with ritonavir is predicted to increase the concentration of antiarrhythmics (**disopyramide, lidocaine**). [Severe] Theoretical

▹ NNRTIs (**efavirenz, etravirine, nevirapine**) are predicted to decrease the exposure to **dronedarone**. [Severe] Theoretical → Also see **TABLE 8** p. 1573

▹ NSAIDs (**celecoxib**) are predicted to increase the exposure to antiarrhythmics (**flecainide, propafenone**). Monitor and adjust dose. [Moderate] Theoretical

▸ **Dronedarone** is predicted to increase the exposure to olaparib. Avoid or adjust dose with moderate CYP3A4 inhibitors—consult product literature. [Moderate] Theoretical

▸ **Dronedarone** is predicted to increase the exposure to opioids (**alfentanil, buprenorphine, fentanyl, oxycodone**). Monitor and adjust dose. [Moderate] Study → Also see **TABLE 5** p. 1572

▸ **Amiodarone** is predicted to increase the concentration of opioids (**fentanyl**). Monitor and adjust dose. [Moderate] Theoretical → Also see **TABLE 5** p. 1572

▸ **Dronedarone** is predicted to increase the exposure to opioids (**methadone, sufentanil**). [Moderate] Theoretical → Also see **TABLE 5** p. 1572 → Also see **TABLE 8** p. 1573

▸ Antiarrhythmics (**amiodarone, dronedarone**) are predicted to increase the exposure to panobinostat. Adjust dose. [Moderate] Theoretical → Also see **TABLE 8** p. 1573

▸ **Dronedarone** is predicted to increase the exposure to pazopanib. [Moderate] Study → Also see **TABLE 8** p. 1573

▸ **Dronedarone** is predicted to increase the exposure to pemigatinib. [Severe] Study

▸ **Dronedarone** might increase the anticoagulant effect of phenindione. [Moderate] Anecdotal

▸ **Propafenone** is predicted to increase the anticoagulant effect of phenindione. Monitor and adjust dose. [Moderate] Theoretical

▸ **Dronedarone** is predicted to increase the exposure to phosphodiesterase type-5 inhibitors (**avanafil**). Adjust **avanafil** dose, p. 939. [Moderate] Theoretical

▸ **Dronedarone** is predicted to increase the exposure to phosphodiesterase type-5 inhibitors (**sildenafil**). Monitor or adjust **sildenafil** dose with moderate CYP3A4 inhibitors, p. 940. [Moderate] Study

▸ **Dronedarone** is predicted to increase the exposure to phosphodiesterase type-5 inhibitors (**tadalafil**). [Severe] Theoretical

▸ **Dronedarone** is predicted to increase the exposure to phosphodiesterase type-5 inhibitors (**vardenafil**). Adjust dose. [Severe] Theoretical → Also see **TABLE 8** p. 1573

▸ **Amiodarone** is predicted to increase the exposure to pibrentasvir. [Moderate] Theoretical

▸ **Dronedarone** potentially increases the exposure to pibrentasvir. [Moderate] Theoretical

▸ **Dronedarone** is predicted to increase the exposure to pimozide. Avoid. [Severe] Theoretical → Also see **TABLE 8** p. 1573

▸ **Dronedarone** is predicted to increase the exposure to ponatinib. [Moderate] Study

▸ Antiarrhythmics (**amiodarone, dronedarone**) are predicted to increase the exposure to pralsetinib. [Moderate] Theoretical

▹ Quinolones (**ciprofloxacin**) slightly increase the exposure to **lidocaine**. [Mild] Study

▸ **Dronedarone** is predicted to increase the exposure to ranolazine. [Severe] Study → Also see **TABLE 8** p. 1573

▸ **Dronedarone** is predicted to increase the exposure to regorafenib. [Moderate] Study

▸ Antiarrhythmics (**amiodarone, dronedarone**) are predicted to increase the exposure to relugolix. Avoid or take relugolix first and separate administration by at least 6 hours. [Moderate] Study

▸ **Propafenone** is predicted to increase the exposure to relugolix. Avoid or take relugolix first and separate administration by at least 6 hours. [Moderate] Theoretical

▸ **Amiodarone** is predicted to increase the exposure to retinoids (**alitretinoin**). Adjust **alitretinoin** dose, p. 1433. [Moderate] Theoretical

- **Ribociclib** (high-dose) is predicted to increase the exposure to amiodarone. Avoid. Moderate Theoretical → Also see **TABLE 8** p. 1573
- **Dronedarone** is predicted to increase the exposure to ribociclib. Moderate Study → Also see **TABLE 8** p. 1573
- **Rifamycins (rifampicin)** are predicted to decrease the efficacy of **propafenone**. Moderate Study
- **Rifamycins (rifampicin)** are predicted to decrease the exposure to antiarrhythmics **(disopyramide, dronedarone)**. Avoid. Severe Study
- **Amiodarone** is predicted to increase the exposure to rimegepant. Avoid another dose of rimegepant within 48 hours of concurrent use. Moderate Theoretical
- **Dronedarone** is predicted to increase the exposure to rimegepant. Avoid another dose of rimegepant within 48 hours of concurrent use. Moderate Study
- **Dronedarone** is predicted to increase the exposure to ruxolitinib. Moderate Study
- **Dronedarone** is predicted to increase the exposure to selpercatinib. Moderate Study → Also see **TABLE 8** p. 1573
- **Dronedarone** is predicted to increase the exposure to selumetinib. Avoid or adjust dose—consult product literature. Severe Study
- Antiarrhythmics **(amiodarone, dronedarone)** are predicted to increase the exposure to siponimod. Avoid depending on other drugs taken—consult product literature. Severe Study → Also see **TABLE 5** p. 1572
- **Amiodarone** is predicted to increase the concentration of sirolimus. Severe Anecdotal
- **Dronedarone** increases the concentration of sirolimus. Monitor and adjust dose. Moderate Study
- **Sofosbuvir** is predicted to increase the risk of severe bradycardia or heart block when given with **amiodarone**. Refer to specialist literature. Severe Anecdotal
- **SSRIs (fluvoxamine)** are predicted to increase the exposure to **propafenone**. Monitor and adjust dose. Moderate Study
- **Dronedarone** is predicted to increase the exposure to SSRIs **(citalopram, escitalopram, fluoxetine, fluvoxamine, paroxetine, sertraline)**. Severe Theoretical → Also see **TABLE 8** p. 1573
- **Dronedarone** is predicted to increase the exposure to SSRIs **(dapoxetine)**. Adjust **dapoxetine** dose with moderate CYP3A4 inhibitors, p. 947. Moderate Theoretical
- **St John's wort** is predicted to decrease the exposure to **dronedarone**. Avoid. Severe Theoretical
- **Amiodarone** is predicted to increase the exposure to statins **(atorvastatin)**. Monitor and adjust dose. Moderate Theoretical → Also see **TABLE 1** p. 1571
- **Dronedarone** slightly increases the exposure to statins **(atorvastatin)**. Monitor and adjust dose. Severe Study
- **Amiodarone** is predicted to increase the exposure to statins **(fluvastatin)**. Moderate Study → Also see **TABLE 1** p. 1571
- **Dronedarone** slightly increases the exposure to statins **(rosuvastatin)**. Adjust dose. Severe Study
- **Amiodarone** increases the exposure to statins **(simvastatin)**. Adjust **simvastatin** dose, p. 237. Severe Study → Also see **TABLE 1** p. 1571
- **Dronedarone** moderately increases the exposure to statins **(simvastatin)**. Monitor and adjust dose. Severe Study
- **Amiodarone** is predicted to increase the exposure to sulfonylureas. Use with caution and adjust dose. Moderate Study
- **Dronedarone** is predicted to increase the exposure to sunitinib. Moderate Study → Also see **TABLE 8** p. 1573
- **Lidocaine** is predicted to increase the effects of suxamethonium. Moderate Study
- **Amiodarone** is predicted to increase the concentration of tacrolimus. Severe Anecdotal
- **Dronedarone** is predicted to increase the concentration of tacrolimus. Severe Study
- Antiarrhythmics **(amiodarone, dronedarone)** are predicted to slightly increase the exposure to talazoparib. Avoid or adjust dose—consult product literature. Severe Study
- **Propafenone** is predicted to increase the exposure to talazoparib. Avoid or adjust dose—consult product literature. Moderate Theoretical

- **Dronedarone** is predicted to increase the exposure to taxanes **(cabazitaxel)**. Moderate Theoretical
- **Dronedarone** is predicted to increase the exposure to taxanes **(docetaxel)**. Severe Study
- **Amiodarone** is predicted to increase the exposure to taxanes **(paclitaxel)**. Severe Theoretical → Also see **TABLE 11** p. 1574
- **Dronedarone** is predicted to increase the exposure to taxanes **(paclitaxel)**. Moderate Anecdotal
- **Dronedarone** is predicted to increase the concentration of temsirolimus. Use with caution or avoid. Moderate Theoretical
- **Dronedarone** is predicted to increase the exposure to tezacaftor. Adjust dose with moderate CYP3A4 inhibitors, see tezacaftor with ivacaftor p. 339 and ivacaftor with tezacaftor and elexacaftor p. 337. Severe Study
- **Theophylline** decreases the efficacy of **adenosine**. Separate administration by 24 hours. Mild Study
- **Amiodarone** increases the exposure to thrombin inhibitors **(dabigatran)**. Monitor and adjust dose. Severe Study
- **Dronedarone** moderately increases the exposure to thrombin inhibitors **(dabigatran)**. Avoid. Severe Study
- **Amiodarone** is predicted to increase the risk of thyroid dysfunction when given with **thyroid hormones**. Avoid. Moderate Study
- **Amiodarone** is predicted to increase the exposure to ticagrelor. Use with caution or avoid. Severe Study → Also see **TABLE 5** p. 1572
- Antiarrhythmics **(amiodarone, dronedarone)** might increase the exposure to tigecycline. Mild Anecdotal → Also see **TABLE 1** p. 1571
- **Dronedarone** given with a potent CYP2C19 inhibitor is predicted to increase the exposure to tofacitinib. Adjust **tofacitinib** dose, p. 1265. Moderate Study
- **Dronedarone** is predicted to increase the exposure to tolvaptan. Manufacturer advises caution or adjust **tolvaptan** dose with moderate CYP3A4 inhibitors, p. 767. Moderate Study
- Antiarrhythmics **(amiodarone, dronedarone)** are predicted to increase the exposure to topotecan. Severe Study
- Antiarrhythmics **(amiodarone, dronedarone)** are predicted to increase the concentration of trametinib. Moderate Theoretical
- **Dronedarone** is predicted to increase the exposure to trazodone. Moderate Theoretical
- **Dronedarone** is predicted to increase the exposure to tricyclic antidepressants. Avoid. Severe Theoretical → Also see **TABLE 8** p. 1573
- **Propafenone** is predicted to increase the concentration of tricyclic antidepressants. Moderate Theoretical → Also see **TABLE 9** p. 1573
- **Tucatinib** very markedly increases the exposure to **dronedarone**. Avoid. Severe Study
- **Tucatinib** is predicted to increase the exposure to **propafenone**. Monitor and adjust dose. Severe Study
- **Dronedarone** is predicted to increase the exposure to ulipristal. Avoid if used for uterine fibroids. Moderate Study
- **Amiodarone** is predicted to increase the concentration of velpatasvir. Avoid or monitor. Moderate Theoretical
- **Dronedarone** is predicted to increase the exposure to vemurafenib. Severe Theoretical → Also see **TABLE 8** p. 1573
- **Amiodarone** is predicted to increase the exposure to venetoclax. Avoid or monitor for toxicity. Severe Theoretical
- **Dronedarone** is predicted to increase the exposure to venetoclax. Avoid or adjust dose—consult product literature. Severe Study
- **Amiodarone** might increase the exposure to vinca alkaloids. Severe Theoretical → Also see **TABLE 11** p. 1574
- **Dronedarone** is predicted to increase the exposure to vinca alkaloids. Severe Theoretical
- **Dronedarone** is predicted to increase the exposure to voclosporin. Adjust **voclosporin** dose, p. 973. Severe Study → Also see **TABLE 8** p. 1573
- **Dronedarone** is predicted to increase the exposure to zanubrutinib. Avoid or adjust dose with moderate CYP3A4 inhibitors—consult product literature. Severe Study
- **Dronedarone** is predicted to increase the exposure to zopiclone. Adjust dose. Moderate Study

Anticholinesterases, centrally acting → see **TABLE 5** p. 1572 (bradycardia)

donepezil · galantamine · rivastigmine

▸ Anti-androgens (apalutamide, enzalutamide) are predicted to decrease the exposure to **donepezil**. [Mild] Study

▸ Antiepileptics (carbamazepine, fosphenytoin, phenobarbital, phenytoin, primidone) are predicted to decrease the exposure to **donepezil**. [Mild] Study

▸ Antifungals, azoles (itraconazole, ketoconazole, posaconazole, voriconazole) are predicted to increase the exposure to **galantamine**. Monitor and adjust dose. [Moderate] Study

▸ Bupropion is predicted to increase the exposure to **galantamine**. Monitor and adjust dose. [Moderate] Study

▸ Ceritinib is predicted to increase the exposure to **galantamine**. Monitor and adjust dose. [Moderate] Study → Also see TABLE 5 p. 1572

▸ Cinacalcet is predicted to increase the exposure to **galantamine**. Monitor and adjust dose. [Moderate] Study

▸ Cobicistat is predicted to increase the exposure to **galantamine**. Monitor and adjust dose. [Moderate] Study

▸ Dacomitinib is predicted to increase the exposure to **galantamine**. Monitor and adjust dose. [Moderate] Study

▸ Encorafenib is predicted to decrease the exposure to **donepezil**. [Mild] Study

▸ HIV-protease inhibitors are predicted to increase the exposure to **galantamine**. Monitor and adjust dose. [Moderate] Study

▸ Idelalisib is predicted to increase the exposure to **galantamine**. Monitor and adjust dose. [Moderate] Study

▸ Ivosidenib is predicted to decrease the exposure to **donepezil**. [Mild] Study

▸ Lumacaftor is predicted to decrease the exposure to **donepezil**. [Mild] Study

▸ Macrolides (clarithromycin) are predicted to increase the exposure to **galantamine**. Monitor and adjust dose. [Moderate] Study

▸ Mitotane is predicted to decrease the exposure to **donepezil**. [Mild] Study

▸ **Anticholinesterases, centrally acting** are predicted to decrease the effects of neuromuscular blocking drugs, non-depolarising. [Moderate] Theoretical

▸ Rifamycins (rifampicin) are predicted to decrease the exposure to **donepezil**. [Mild] Study

▸ SSRIs (fluoxetine, paroxetine) are predicted to increase the exposure to **galantamine**. Monitor and adjust dose. [Moderate] Study

▸ **Anticholinesterases, centrally acting** increase the effects of suxamethonium. [Moderate] Theoretical → Also see TABLE 5 p. 1572

▸ Terbinafine is predicted to increase the exposure to **galantamine**. Monitor and adjust dose. [Moderate] Study

▸ Tucatinib is predicted to increase the exposure to **galantamine**. Monitor and adjust dose. [Moderate] Study

Antiepileptics → see TABLE 1 p. 1571 (hepatotoxicity), TABLE 17 p. 1576 (hyponatraemia), TABLE 11 p. 1574 (peripheral neuropathy), TABLE 10 p. 1574 (CNS effects)

brivaracetam · carbamazepine · eslicarbazepine · ethosuximide · fosphenytoin · gabapentin · lacosamide · lamotrigine · levetiracetam · oxcarbazepine · paraldehyde · perampanel · phenobarbital · phenytoin · pregabalin · primidone · retigabine · rufinamide · stiripentol · sultiame · tiagabine · topiramate · valproate · vigabatrin · zonisamide

▸ Manufacturer advises caution on concurrent use of **eslicarbazepine** or **lacosamide** with drugs that prolong the PR interval

▸ Avoid taking milk, dairy products, carbonated drinks, fruit juices, or caffeine-containing food and drinks at the same time as **stiripentol**.

▸ Antiepileptics (carbamazepine, fosphenytoin, phenobarbital, phenytoin, primidone) are predicted to decrease the exposure to 5-HT3-receptor antagonists (ondansetron). [Moderate] Study

▸ Antiepileptics (carbamazepine, fosphenytoin, phenobarbital, phenytoin, primidone) are predicted to markedly decrease the exposure to abemaciclib. Avoid. [Severe] Study

▸ Antiepileptics (fosphenytoin, phenytoin) are predicted to decrease the exposure to abrocitinib. Avoid. [Moderate] Theoretical

▸ Antiepileptics (carbamazepine, fosphenytoin, phenobarbital, phenytoin, primidone) are predicted to decrease the exposure to acalabrutinib. Avoid. [Severe] Study

▸ Acetazolamide potentially increases the risk of toxicity when given with **valproate**. [Severe] Study

▸ Acetazolamide potentially increases the risk of overheating and dehydration when given with zonisamide. Avoid in children. [Severe] Theoretical

▸ Antiepileptics (phenobarbital, phenytoin) are predicted to decrease the exposure to afatinib. [Moderate] Theoretical

▸ **Carbamazepine** is predicted to decrease the exposure to afatinib. [Moderate] Study

▸ Antiepileptics (fosphenytoin, phenytoin) are predicted to decrease the exposure to agomelatine. [Moderate] Theoretical → Also see TABLE 10 p. 1574

▸ Antiepileptics (carbamazepine, fosphenytoin, phenobarbital, phenytoin, primidone) decrease the concentration of albendazole. [Moderate] Study

▸ Alcohol potentially increases the risk of visual disturbances when given with retigabine. [Moderate] Study

▸ **Sultiame** might cause a disulfiram-like reaction when given with alcohol. Avoid. [Moderate] Theoretical

▸ **Carbamazepine** decreases the exposure to aliskiren. [Moderate] Study

▸ Antiepileptics (carbamazepine, fosphenytoin, phenobarbital, phenytoin, primidone) are predicted to decrease the exposure to alpelisib. Avoid. [Moderate] Study

▸ **Fosphenytoin** is predicted to decrease the exposure to aminophylline. Adjust dose. [Moderate] Study

▸ **Phenobarbital** is predicted to decrease the exposure to aminophylline. Adjust dose. [Moderate] Theoretical

▸ **Phenytoin** decreases the exposure to aminophylline. Adjust dose. [Moderate] Study

▸ **Primidone** is predicted to increase the clearance of aminophylline. Adjust dose. [Moderate] Theoretical

▸ **Stiripentol** is predicted to increase the exposure to aminophylline. Avoid. [Moderate] Theoretical

▸ **Phenytoin** is predicted to decrease the exposure to anaesthetics, local (ropivacaine). [Moderate] Theoretical

▸ Oral antacids decrease the absorption of oral **gabapentin**. Manufacturer advises take 2 hours after antacids. [Moderate] Study

▸ Anti-androgens (apalutamide) potentially decrease the exposure to **valproate**. [Mild] Theoretical

▸ Anti-androgens (apalutamide, enzalutamide) are predicted to decrease the exposure to **perampanel**. Monitor and adjust dose. [Moderate] Study

▸ Anti-androgens (enzalutamide) are predicted to slightly decrease the exposure to **brivaracetam**. [Moderate] Theoretical

▸ Anti-androgens (enzalutamide) are predicted to affect the exposure to **valproate**. Use with caution or avoid. [Moderate] Theoretical

▸ Antiepileptics (carbamazepine, fosphenytoin, phenobarbital, phenytoin, primidone) are predicted to decrease the exposure to anti-androgens (abiraterone). Avoid. [Severe] Study

▸ Antiepileptics (carbamazepine, eslicarbazepine, fosphenytoin, oxcarbazepine, perampanel, phenobarbital, phenytoin, primidone, rufinamide, topiramate) are predicted to decrease the efficacy of anti-androgens (cyproterone) with ethinylestradiol (co-cyprindiol). Use alternative methods during treatment with, and for 28 days after, the enzyme inducing drug is stopped. [Severe] Study

▸ Antiepileptics (carbamazepine, fosphenytoin, phenobarbital, phenytoin, primidone) are predicted to decrease the exposure to anti-androgens (darolutamide). Avoid. [Moderate] Study

▸ Antiepileptics (carbamazepine, fosphenytoin, phenobarbital, phenytoin, primidone) are predicted to decrease the exposure to antiarrhythmics (disopyramide, dronedarone). Avoid. [Severe] Study

▸ Antiarrhythmics (amiodarone) are predicted to slightly increase the concentration of antiepileptics (fosphenytoin, phenytoin). Monitor and adjust dose. [Severe] Study → Also see TABLE 11 p. 1574

▸ Antiepileptics (fosphenytoin, phenytoin) are predicted to decrease the exposure to antiarrhythmics (lidocaine). [Severe] Anecdotal

▶ Antiepileptics (carbamazepine, fosphenytoin, phenobarbital, phenytoin, primidone) are predicted to decrease the efficacy of antiarrhythmics (propafenone). Moderate Study

▶ Antiepileptics (carbamazepine, fosphenytoin, phenobarbital, phenytoin, primidone) are predicted to decrease the exposure to anticholinesterases, centrally acting (donepezil). Mild Study

▶ Antiepileptics (carbamazepine) decrease the concentration of antiepileptics (brivaracetam). Moderate Study

▶ Antiepileptics (fosphenytoin, phenytoin) decrease the concentration of antiepileptics (brivaracetam). Moderate Study

▶ Antiepileptics (lamotrigine) potentially increase the concentration of antiepileptics (carbamazepine) and antiepileptics (carbamazepine) decrease the concentration of antiepileptics (lamotrigine). Adjust lamotrigine dose and monitor carbamazepine concentration, p. 366, p. 355. Moderate Study

▶ Antiepileptics (phenobarbital) affect the concentration of antiepileptics (carbamazepine) and antiepileptics (carbamazepine) increase the concentration of antiepileptics (phenobarbital). Adjust dose. Moderate Study

▶ Antiepileptics (topiramate) increase the risk of carbamazepine toxicity when given with antiepileptics (carbamazepine). Moderate Study

▶ Antiepileptics (stiripentol) increase the concentration of antiepileptics (carbamazepine, phenobarbital). Avoid in Dravet syndrome. Severe Study

▶ Antiepileptics (carbamazepine) slightly decrease the exposure to antiepileptics (eslicarbazepine, oxcarbazepine). Monitor and adjust dose. Moderate Study → Also see TABLE 17 p. 1576

▶ Antiepileptics (oxcarbazepine) are predicted to increase the concentration of antiepileptics (fosphenytoin). Monitor concentration and adjust dose. Moderate Study

▶ Antiepileptics (stiripentol) are predicted to increase the concentration of antiepileptics (fosphenytoin). Severe Study

▶ Antiepileptics (sultiame) might increase the concentration of antiepileptics (fosphenytoin). Monitor phenytoin concentration. Severe Theoretical

▶ Antiepileptics (carbamazepine) affect the concentration of antiepileptics (fosphenytoin, phenytoin) and antiepileptics (fosphenytoin, phenytoin) decrease the concentration of antiepileptics (carbamazepine). Monitor and adjust dose. Severe Study

▶ Antiepileptics (eslicarbazepine) increase the exposure to antiepileptics (fosphenytoin, phenytoin) and antiepileptics (fosphenytoin, phenytoin) decrease the exposure to antiepileptics (eslicarbazepine). Monitor and adjust dose. Moderate Study

▶ Antiepileptics (valproate) affect the concentration of antiepileptics (fosphenytoin, phenytoin) and antiepileptics (fosphenytoin, phenytoin) decrease the concentration of antiepileptics (valproate). Severe Study

▶ Antiepileptics (vigabatrin) decrease the concentration of antiepileptics (fosphenytoin, phenytoin). Mild Study → Also see TABLE 10 p. 1574

▶ Antiepileptics (fosphenytoin) decrease the concentration of antiepileptics (lamotrigine). Monitor and adjust lamotrigine dose, p. 366. Moderate Study → Also see TABLE 10 p. 1574

▶ Antiepileptics (phenobarbital, phenytoin, primidone) decrease the concentration of antiepileptics (lamotrigine). Monitor and adjust lamotrigine dose, p. 366. Moderate Study → Also see TABLE 10 p. 1574

▶ Antiepileptics (valproate) increase the exposure to antiepileptics (lamotrigine). Adjust lamotrigine dose and monitor rash, p. 366. Severe Study

▶ Antiepileptics (lamotrigine) are predicted to increase the concentration of antiepileptics (oxcarbazepine) and antiepileptics (oxcarbazepine) are predicted to decrease the concentration of antiepileptics (lamotrigine). Monitor adverse effects and adjust dose. Moderate Study

▶ Antiepileptics (carbamazepine, fosphenytoin) are predicted to decrease the exposure to antiepileptics (perampanel). Monitor and adjust dose. Moderate Study → Also see TABLE 10 p. 1574

▶ Antiepileptics (oxcarbazepine) decrease the concentration of antiepileptics (perampanel) and antiepileptics (perampanel)

increase the concentration of antiepileptics (oxcarbazepine). Monitor and adjust dose. Moderate Study

▶ Antiepileptics (phenobarbital, phenytoin, primidone) are predicted to decrease the exposure to antiepileptics (perampanel). Monitor and adjust dose. Moderate Study → Also see TABLE 10 p. 1574

▶ Antiepileptics (phenytoin) increase the concentration of antiepileptics (phenobarbital) and antiepileptics (phenobarbital) affect the concentration of antiepileptics (phenytoin). Moderate Study → Also see TABLE 10 p. 1574

▶ Antiepileptics (fosphenytoin) increase the concentration of antiepileptics (phenobarbital, primidone) and antiepileptics (phenobarbital, primidone) affect the concentration of antiepileptics (fosphenytoin). Moderate Study → Also see TABLE 10 p. 1574

▶ Antiepileptics (oxcarbazepine) are predicted to increase the concentration of antiepileptics (phenytoin). Monitor concentration and adjust dose. Moderate Study

▶ Antiepileptics (stiripentol) are predicted to increase the concentration of antiepileptics (phenytoin). Avoid in Dravet syndrome. Severe Study

▶ Antiepileptics (sultiame) might increase the concentration of antiepileptics (phenytoin). Severe Study

▶ Antiepileptics (carbamazepine) potentially decrease the concentration of antiepileptics (primidone) and antiepileptics (primidone) potentially decrease the concentration of antiepileptics (carbamazepine). Adjust dose. Moderate Anecdotal

▶ Antiepileptics (phenytoin) increase the concentration of antiepileptics (primidone) and antiepileptics (primidone) affect the concentration of antiepileptics (phenytoin). Moderate Study → Also see TABLE 10 p. 1574

▶ Antiepileptics (stiripentol) are predicted to increase the concentration of antiepileptics (primidone). Severe Theoretical

▶ Antiepileptics (valproate) affect the concentration of antiepileptics (primidone). Monitor and adjust dose. Severe Study

▶ Antiepileptics (carbamazepine) slightly increase the clearance of antiepileptics (retigabine). Moderate Study

▶ Antiepileptics (fosphenytoin, phenytoin) are predicted to slightly increase the clearance of antiepileptics (retigabine). Moderate Study

▶ Antiepileptics (valproate) increase the exposure to antiepileptics (rufinamide). Adjust rufinamide dose, p. 376. Moderate Study

▶ Antiepileptics (primidone) might increase the adverse effects of antiepileptics (sultiame). Moderate Theoretical

▶ Antiepileptics (carbamazepine, fosphenytoin, phenobarbital, phenytoin, primidone) decrease the exposure to antiepileptics (tiagabine). Monitor and adjust tiagabine dose, p. 383. Moderate Study

▶ Antiepileptics (fosphenytoin, phenytoin) decrease the concentration of antiepileptics (topiramate) and antiepileptics (topiramate) increase the concentration of antiepileptics (fosphenytoin, phenytoin). Monitor and adjust dose. Moderate Study

▶ Antiepileptics (phenobarbital, primidone) are predicted to decrease the concentration of antiepileptics (topiramate). Mild Study

▶ Antiepileptics (phenobarbital) decrease the concentration of antiepileptics (valproate) and antiepileptics (valproate) increase the concentration of antiepileptics (phenobarbital). Monitor and adjust dose. Moderate Study

▶ Antiepileptics (topiramate) increase the risk of toxicity when given with antiepileptics (valproate). Severe Study

▶ Antiepileptics (carbamazepine) slightly to moderately decrease the concentration of antiepileptics (zonisamide) and antiepileptics (zonisamide) affect the concentration of antiepileptics (carbamazepine). Monitor and adjust dose. Moderate Study

▶ Antiepileptics (fosphenytoin, phenytoin) slightly to moderately decrease the concentration of antiepileptics (zonisamide). Monitor and adjust dose. Moderate Study

▶ Antiepileptics (phenobarbital, primidone) are predicted to decrease the concentration of antiepileptics (zonisamide). Monitor and adjust dose. Moderate Study

Antiepileptics (continued)

▸ Antiepileptics (**topiramate**) potentially increase the risk of overheating and dehydration when given with antiepileptics (**zonisamide**). Avoid in children. Severe Theoretical

▸ Antifungals, azoles (**itraconazole, ketoconazole, posaconazole, voriconazole**) are predicted to very slightly increase the exposure to **perampanel**. Mild Study

▸ Antifungals, azoles (**miconazole**) increase the risk of carbamazepine toxicity when given with **carbamazepine**. Monitor and adjust dose. Severe Anecdotal

▸ Antifungals, azoles (**miconazole**) increase the risk of phenytoin toxicity when given with **fosphenytoin**. Monitor and adjust dose. Severe Anecdotal

▸ Antifungals, azoles (**miconazole**) increase the risk of phenytoin toxicity when given with **phenytoin**. Monitor and adjust dose. Severe Anecdotal

▸ **Carbamazepine** is predicted to decrease the efficacy of antifungals, azoles (**fluconazole**) and antifungals, azoles (**fluconazole**) increase the concentration of **carbamazepine**. Avoid or monitor **carbamazepine** concentration and adjust dose accordingly, p. 355. Severe Theoretical

▸ Antifungals, azoles (**fluconazole**) increase the concentration of antiepileptics (**fosphenytoin, phenytoin**). Monitor concentration and adjust dose. Moderate Study

▸ Antiepileptics (**carbamazepine, fosphenytoin, phenobarbital, phenytoin, primidone**) are predicted to decrease the exposure to antifungals, azoles (**isavuconazole**). Avoid. Severe Study

▸ **Fosphenytoin** very markedly decreases the exposure to antifungals, azoles (**itraconazole**). Avoid and for 14 days after stopping **fosphenytoin**. Moderate Study

▸ **Phenobarbital** decreases the concentration of antifungals, azoles (**itraconazole**). Avoid and for 14 days after stopping **phenobarbital**. Moderate Study

▸ **Phenytoin** very markedly decreases the exposure to antifungals, azoles (**itraconazole**). Avoid and for 14 days after stopping **phenytoin**. Moderate Study

▸ **Primidone** is predicted to decrease the concentration of antifungals, azoles (**itraconazole**). Moderate Theoretical

▸ **Carbamazepine** is predicted to decrease the efficacy of antifungals, azoles (**itraconazole, voriconazole**) and antifungals, azoles (**itraconazole, voriconazole**) increase the concentration of **carbamazepine**. Avoid or adjust dose. Moderate Theoretical

▸ **Carbamazepine** is predicted to decrease the efficacy of antifungals, azoles (**ketoconazole**) and antifungals, azoles (**ketoconazole**) slightly increase the concentration of **carbamazepine**. Avoid or monitor **carbamazepine** concentration and adjust dose accordingly, p. 355. Moderate Study

▸ **Phenobarbital** is predicted to decrease the concentration of antifungals, azoles (**ketoconazole**). Avoid. Moderate Study

▸ Antiepileptics (**fosphenytoin, phenytoin**) decrease the exposure to antifungals, azoles (**ketoconazole**). Avoid. Moderate Study

▸ **Primidone** is predicted to decrease the concentration of antifungals, azoles (**ketoconazole, posaconazole**). Avoid. Moderate Study

▸ **Carbamazepine** is predicted to decrease the efficacy of antifungals, azoles (**posaconazole**) and antifungals, azoles (**posaconazole**) increase the concentration of **carbamazepine**. Avoid. Moderate Theoretical

▸ **Phenobarbital** is predicted to decrease the concentration of antifungals, azoles (**posaconazole**). Avoid. Moderate Study

▸ Antiepileptics (**fosphenytoin, phenytoin**) are predicted to decrease the exposure to antifungals, azoles (**posaconazole**). Avoid. Moderate Study

▸ **Fosphenytoin** decreases the exposure to antifungals, azoles (**voriconazole**) and antifungals, azoles (**voriconazole**) increase the exposure to **fosphenytoin**. Avoid or adjust **voriconazole** dose and monitor phenytoin concentration, p. 695. Moderate Study

▸ **Phenytoin** decreases the exposure to antifungals, azoles (**voriconazole**) and antifungals, azoles (**voriconazole**) increase the exposure to **phenytoin**. Avoid or adjust **voriconazole** dose and monitor **phenytoin** concentration, p. 695, p. 372. Moderate Study

▸ Antiepileptics (**phenobarbital, primidone**) are predicted to decrease the concentration of antifungals, azoles (**voriconazole**). Avoid. Moderate Theoretical

▸ Antihistamines, sedating (**hydroxyzine**) potentially increase the risk of overheating and dehydration when given with **zonisamide**. Avoid in children. Severe Theoretical

▸ Antiepileptics (**carbamazepine, fosphenytoin, phenobarbital, phenytoin, primidone**) are predicted to decrease the exposure to antimalarials (**artemether**) with lumefantrine. Avoid. Severe Study

▸ Antimalarials (**pyrimethamine**) increase the risk of haematological toxicity when given with antiepileptics (**fosphenytoin, phenytoin**). Severe Study

▸ Antimalarials (**pyrimethamine**) are predicted to increase the risk of haematological toxicity when given with antiepileptics (**phenobarbital, primidone**). Severe Theoretical

▸ Antiepileptics (**carbamazepine, phenobarbital, primidone**) potentially increase the risk of toxicity when given with antimalarials (**quinine**). Unknown Study

▸ Antiepileptics (**carbamazepine, fosphenytoin, phenobarbital, phenytoin, primidone**) are predicted to moderately decrease the exposure to antipsychotics, second generation (**aripiprazole**). Adjust **aripiprazole** dose, p. 454. Moderate Study → Also see TABLE 17 p. 1576 → Also see TABLE 10 p. 1574

▸ Antiepileptics (**carbamazepine, fosphenytoin, phenobarbital, phenytoin, primidone**) are predicted to decrease the exposure to antipsychotics, second generation (**cariprazine**). Avoid. Severe Theoretical → Also see TABLE 17 p. 1576 → Also see TABLE 10 p. 1574

▸ **Carbamazepine** is predicted to increase the risk of myelosuppression when given with antipsychotics, second generation (**clozapine**). Avoid. Severe Anecdotal → Also see TABLE 17 p. 1576

▸ Antiepileptics (**fosphenytoin, phenobarbital, phenytoin, primidone**) are predicted to decrease the exposure to antipsychotics, second generation (**clozapine**). Moderate Anecdotal → Also see TABLE 10 p. 1574

▸ Antiepileptics (**carbamazepine, fosphenytoin, phenobarbital, phenytoin, primidone**) are predicted to decrease the exposure to antipsychotics, second generation (**lurasidone**). Avoid. Moderate Study → Also see TABLE 17 p. 1576 → Also see TABLE 10 p. 1574

▸ **Carbamazepine** potentially decreases the exposure to antipsychotics, second generation (**olanzapine**). Monitor and adjust dose. Moderate Study → Also see TABLE 17 p. 1576

▸ **Phenytoin** is predicted to decrease the exposure to antipsychotics, second generation (**olanzapine**). Monitor and adjust dose. Moderate Study → Also see TABLE 10 p. 1574

▸ **Valproate** increases the risk of adverse effects when given with antipsychotics, second generation (**olanzapine**). Severe Study → Also see TABLE 17 p. 1576

▸ **Valproate** slightly increases the exposure to antipsychotics, second generation (**paliperidone**). Adjust dose. Moderate Study → Also see TABLE 17 p. 1576

▸ Antiepileptics (**carbamazepine, fosphenytoin, phenobarbital, phenytoin, primidone**) are predicted to decrease the exposure to antipsychotics, second generation (**paliperidone**). Monitor and adjust dose. Severe Study → Also see TABLE 17 p. 1576 → Also see TABLE 10 p. 1574

▸ **Valproate** potentially increases the risk of neutropenia when given with antipsychotics, second generation (**quetiapine**). Moderate Study → Also see TABLE 17 p. 1576

▸ Antiepileptics (**carbamazepine, fosphenytoin, phenobarbital, phenytoin, primidone**) are predicted to decrease the exposure to antipsychotics, second generation (**quetiapine**). Moderate Study → Also see TABLE 17 p. 1576 → Also see TABLE 10 p. 1574

▸ Antiepileptics (**carbamazepine, fosphenytoin, phenobarbital, phenytoin, primidone**) are predicted to decrease the exposure to antipsychotics, second generation (**risperidone**). Adjust dose. Moderate Study → Also see TABLE 17 p. 1576 → Also see TABLE 10 p. 1574

▸ Antiepileptics (**carbamazepine, fosphenytoin, phenobarbital, phenytoin, primidone**) are predicted to decrease the exposure to **avacopan**. Avoid or monitor. Severe Study

► Antiepileptics **(carbamazepine, fosphenytoin, phenobarbital, phenytoin, primidone)** are predicted to decrease the exposure to avapritinib. Avoid. Severe Study

► Antiepileptics **(carbamazepine, fosphenytoin, phenobarbital, phenytoin, primidone)** are predicted to decrease the exposure to axitinib. Avoid or adjust dose. Moderate Study

► Antiepileptics **(carbamazepine, fosphenytoin, phenobarbital, phenytoin, primidone)** are predicted to decrease the exposure to bazedoxifene. Moderate Theoretical

► Antiepileptics **(carbamazepine, fosphenytoin, phenobarbital, phenytoin, primidone)** decrease the exposure to bedaquiline. Avoid. Severe Study

► Antiepileptics **(carbamazepine, fosphenytoin, phenobarbital, phenytoin, primidone)** are predicted to decrease the exposure to belumosudil. Adjust **belumosudil** dose, p. 979. Severe Study

► Antiepileptics **(carbamazepine, fosphenytoin, phenobarbital, phenytoin, primidone)** are predicted to decrease the exposure to benzodiazepines **(alprazolam)**. Adjust dose. Moderate Theoretical → Also see TABLE 10 p. 1574

► **Stiripentol** increases the concentration of benzodiazepines **(clobazam)**. Severe Study

► Benzodiazepines **(chlordiazepoxide)** affect the concentration of antiepileptics **(fosphenytoin, phenytoin)**. Severe Study → Also see TABLE 10 p. 1574

► Benzodiazepines **(clobazam, clonazepam)** potentially affect the concentration of antiepileptics **(fosphenytoin, phenytoin)**. Severe Anecdotal → Also see TABLE 10 p. 1574

► Benzodiazepines **(diazepam)** potentially affect the concentration of antiepileptics **(fosphenytoin, phenytoin)**. Monitor concentration and adjust dose. Severe Study → Also see TABLE 10 p. 1574

► Antiepileptics **(carbamazepine, fosphenytoin, phenobarbital, phenytoin, primidone)** are predicted to decrease the exposure to benzodiazepines **(midazolam)**. Monitor and adjust dose. Severe Study → Also see TABLE 10 p. 1574

► **Carbamazepine** is predicted to decrease the concentration of berotralstat. Avoid. Severe Theoretical

► Antiepileptics **(phenobarbital, primidone)** are predicted to decrease the exposure to beta blockers, non-selective **(carvedilol, labetalol)**. Moderate Theoretical

► Antiepileptics **(phenobarbital, primidone)** are predicted to decrease the exposure to beta blockers, non-selective **(propranolol)**. Moderate Study

► Antiepileptics **(phenobarbital, primidone)** are predicted to decrease the exposure to beta blockers, selective **(acebutolol, bisoprolol, metoprolol, nebivolol)**. Moderate Study

► Antiepileptics **(carbamazepine, fosphenytoin, phenobarbital, phenytoin, primidone)** are predicted to decrease the exposure to bictegravir. Avoid. Moderate Study

► **Oxcarbazepine** is predicted to decrease the exposure to bictegravir. Avoid. Moderate Theoretical

► **Bleomycin** -containing cytotoxic regimens might affect the concentration of antiepileptics **(fosphenytoin, phenytoin)**. Avoid. Severe Anecdotal

► Antiepileptics **(carbamazepine, fosphenytoin, phenobarbital, phenytoin, primidone)** slightly decrease the exposure to bortezomib. Avoid. Severe Study → Also see TABLE 11 p. 1574

► Antiepileptics **(carbamazepine, fosphenytoin, phenobarbital, phenytoin, primidone)** are predicted to very markedly decrease the exposure to bosutinib. Avoid. Severe Study

► Antiepileptics **(carbamazepine, fosphenytoin, phenobarbital, phenytoin, primidone)** are predicted to decrease the exposure to brigatinib. Avoid. Severe Study

► **Bulevirtide** is predicted to increase the exposure to carbamazepine. Moderate Theoretical

► Antiepileptics **(carbamazepine, fosphenytoin, phenobarbital, phenytoin, primidone)** are predicted to markedly decrease the exposure to bupropion. Severe Study

► **Valproate** increases the exposure to bupropion. Severe Study

► Antiepileptics **(carbamazepine, fosphenytoin, phenobarbital, phenytoin, primidone)** are predicted to decrease the exposure to buspirone. Use with caution and adjust dose. Severe Study

► Antiepileptics **(carbamazepine, fosphenytoin, oxcarbazepine, phenobarbital, phenytoin, primidone)** might decrease the concentration of cabotegravir. Avoid. Severe Theoretical

► Antiepileptics **(carbamazepine, fosphenytoin, phenobarbital, phenytoin, primidone)** moderately decrease the exposure to cabozantinib. Avoid. Moderate Study

► Antiepileptics **(fosphenytoin, phenytoin)** are predicted to moderately increase the clearance of caffeine citrate. Monitor and adjust dose. Moderate Study

► Calcium channel blockers **(diltiazem)** increase the concentration of **carbamazepine** and **carbamazepine** is predicted to decrease the exposure to calcium channel blockers **(diltiazem)**. Monitor concentration and adjust dose. Severe Anecdotal

► Calcium channel blockers **(verapamil)** increase the concentration of **carbamazepine** and **carbamazepine** is predicted to decrease the exposure to calcium channel blockers **(verapamil)**. Severe Anecdotal

► Antiepileptics **(carbamazepine, fosphenytoin, phenobarbital, phenytoin, primidone)** are predicted to decrease the exposure to calcium channel blockers **(amlodipine, felodipine, lacidipine, lercanidipine, nicardipine, nifedipine, nimodipine)**. Monitor and adjust dose. Moderate Study

► Antiepileptics **(phenobarbital, primidone)** are predicted to decrease the exposure to calcium channel blockers **(diltiazem, verapamil)**. Severe Study

► Calcium channel blockers **(diltiazem, verapamil)** potentially increase the concentration of antiepileptics **(fosphenytoin, phenytoin)** and antiepileptics **(fosphenytoin, phenytoin)** are predicted to decrease the exposure to calcium channel blockers **(diltiazem, verapamil)**. Severe Study

► **Valproate** increases the exposure to calcium channel blockers **(nimodipine)**. Adjust dose. Moderate Study

► Antiepileptics **(carbamazepine, fosphenytoin, phenobarbital, phenytoin, primidone)** are predicted to decrease the exposure to cannabidiol. Adjust dose. Moderate Study → Also see TABLE 10 p. 1574

► **Cannabidiol** increases the risk of increased ALT concentrations when given with **valproate**. Avoid or adjust dose. Severe Study

► **Capecitabine** increases the concentration of antiepileptics **(fosphenytoin, phenytoin)**. Severe Anecdotal

► Antiepileptics **(carbamazepine, fosphenytoin, phenobarbital, phenytoin, primidone)** are predicted to decrease the exposure to capivasertib. Avoid. Moderate Study

► **Carbapenems** decrease the concentration of **valproate**. Avoid. Severe Anecdotal

► Antiepileptics **(carbamazepine, fosphenytoin, phenytoin)** are predicted to decrease the concentration of caspofungin. Adjust **caspofungin** dose, p. 687. Moderate Theoretical

► **Cenobamate** might increase the exposure to antiepileptics **(fosphenytoin, primidone)**. Moderate Theoretical → Also see TABLE 10 p. 1574

► **Cenobamate** slightly increases the exposure to antiepileptics **(phenobarbital, phenytoin)**. Monitor and adjust dose. Moderate Study → Also see TABLE 10 p. 1574

► **Cenobamate** is predicted to decrease the concentration of **lamotrigine** and **lamotrigine** might affect the efficacy of cenobamate. Adjust dose. Moderate Study → Also see TABLE 10 p. 1574

► Antiepileptics **(carbamazepine, fosphenytoin, phenobarbital, phenytoin, primidone)** are predicted to decrease the exposure to ceritinib. Avoid. Severe Study

► **Ceritinib** is predicted to very slightly increase the exposure to **perampanel**. Mild Study

► Antiepileptics **(phenobarbital, primidone)** are predicted to affect the efficacy of chenodeoxycholic acid. Monitor and adjust dose. Moderate Theoretical

► Antiepileptics **(phenobarbital, primidone)** decrease the concentration of chloramphenicol. Moderate Study

► Intravenous **chloramphenicol** increases the concentration of antiepileptics **(fosphenytoin, phenytoin)** and antiepileptics **(fosphenytoin, phenytoin)** affect the concentration of intravenous **chloramphenicol**. Monitor concentration and adjust dose. Severe Study

► **Phenobarbital** decreases the effects of cholic acid. Avoid. Moderate Study

► Antiepileptics **(carbamazepine, fosphenytoin, phenobarbital, phenytoin, primidone)** decrease the concentration of ciclosporin. Severe Study

Antiepileptics (continued)
▸ Oxcarbazepine decreases the concentration of ciclosporin. Severe Anecdotal
▸ Antiepileptics (carbamazepine, fosphenytoin, phenobarbital, phenytoin, primidone) are predicted to alter the effects of cilostazol. Moderate Theoretical
▸ Antiepileptics (carbamazepine, fosphenytoin, phenobarbital, phenytoin, primidone) are predicted to decrease the exposure to cinacalcet. Monitor and adjust dose. Moderate Study
▸ Carbamazepine is predicted to increase the risk of haematological toxicity when given with oral cladribine. Moderate Theoretical
▸ Antiepileptics (carbamazepine, fosphenytoin, phenobarbital, phenytoin, primidone) decrease the exposure to clomethiazole. Monitor and adjust dose. Moderate Study → Also see TABLE 10 p. 1574
▸ Antiepileptics (carbamazepine, fosphenytoin, phenobarbital, phenytoin, primidone) are predicted to decrease the exposure to cobicistat. Avoid. Severe Study
▸ Antiepileptics (eslicarbazepine, oxcarbazepine) are predicted to decrease the concentration of cobicistat. Severe Theoretical
▸ Cobicistat is predicted to very slightly increase the exposure to perampanel. Mild Study
▸ Antiepileptics (carbamazepine, fosphenytoin, phenobarbital, phenytoin, primidone) are predicted to decrease the exposure to cobimetinib. Avoid. Severe Theoretical
▸ Carbamazepine is predicted to decrease the exposure to colchicine. Moderate Theoretical
▸ Antiepileptics (carbamazepine, eslicarbazepine, fosphenytoin, oxcarbazepine, perampanel, phenobarbital, phenytoin, primidone, rufinamide, topiramate) are predicted to decrease the efficacy of combined hormonal contraceptives. For FSRH guidance, see Contraceptives, interactions p. 917. Severe Study
▸ Combined hormonal contraceptives alter the exposure to lamotrigine and lamotrigine might decrease the efficacy of combined hormonal contraceptives. Adjust dose. Moderate Study
▸ Antiepileptics (carbamazepine, fosphenytoin, phenobarbital, phenytoin, primidone) are predicted to decrease the exposure to corticosteroids (budesonide, deflazacort, dexamethasone, fludrocortisone, hydrocortisone, methylprednisolone, prednisolone, triamcinolone). Monitor and adjust dose. Moderate Study
▸ Antiepileptics (carbamazepine, fosphenytoin, phenobarbital, phenytoin, primidone) are predicted to decrease the exposure to corticosteroids (fluticasone). Unknown Theoretical
▸ Antiepileptics (fosphenytoin, phenytoin) are predicted to alter the anticoagulant effect of coumarins. Moderate Anecdotal
▸ Antiepileptics (phenobarbital, primidone) decrease the anticoagulant effect of coumarins. Monitor INR and adjust dose. Moderate Study
▸ Carbamazepine decreases the effects of coumarins. Monitor and adjust dose. Severe Study
▸ Antiepileptics (carbamazepine, fosphenytoin, phenobarbital, phenytoin, primidone) are predicted to markedly decrease the exposure to crizotinib. Avoid. Severe Study
▸ Antiepileptics (carbamazepine, fosphenytoin, phenobarbital, phenytoin, primidone) are predicted to decrease the exposure to dabrafenib. Avoid. Moderate Theoretical
▸ Antiepileptics (carbamazepine, fosphenytoin, phenobarbital, phenytoin, primidone) are predicted to decrease the exposure to daridorexant. Severe Study → Also see TABLE 10 p. 1574
▸ Antiepileptics (carbamazepine, fosphenytoin, phenobarbital, phenytoin, primidone) are predicted to decrease the exposure to darifenacin. Moderate Theoretical
▸ Antiepileptics (carbamazepine, fosphenytoin, phenobarbital, phenytoin, primidone) are predicted to markedly decrease the exposure to dasatinib. Avoid. Severe Study
▸ Antiepileptics (carbamazepine, fosphenytoin, phenobarbital, phenytoin, primidone) are predicted to slightly decrease the exposure to delamanid. Avoid. Moderate Study
▸ Lamotrigine is predicted to increase the risk of hyponatraemia when given with desmopressin. Severe Theoretical
▸ Antiepileptics (carbamazepine, eslicarbazepine, fosphenytoin, oxcarbazepine, perampanel, phenobarbital, phenytoin, primidone, rufinamide, topiramate) are predicted to decrease

the efficacy of desogestrel. For FSRH guidance, see Contraceptives, interactions p. 917. Severe Theoretical
▸ Desogestrel is predicted to increase the exposure to lamotrigine and lamotrigine might decrease the effects of desogestrel. For FSRH guidance, see Contraceptives, interactions p. 917. Moderate Study
▸ Diazoxide decreases the concentration of antiepileptics (fosphenytoin, phenytoin) and antiepileptics (fosphenytoin, phenytoin) are predicted to decrease the effects of diazoxide. Monitor concentration and adjust dose. Moderate Anecdotal
▸ Antiepileptics (carbamazepine, fosphenytoin, phenobarbital, phenytoin, primidone) are predicted to markedly decrease the exposure to dienogest. Severe Study
▸ Antiepileptics (fosphenytoin, phenytoin) are predicted to decrease the concentration of digoxin. Moderate Anecdotal
▸ Antiepileptics (carbamazepine, fosphenytoin, phenobarbital, phenytoin, primidone) are predicted to decrease the exposure to dipeptidylpeptidase-4 inhibitors (linagliptin). Moderate Study
▸ Antiepileptics (carbamazepine, fosphenytoin, phenobarbital, phenytoin, primidone) are predicted to moderately decrease the exposure to dipeptidylpeptidase-4 inhibitors (saxagliptin). Moderate Study
▸ Disulfiram increases the concentration of antiepileptics (fosphenytoin, phenytoin). Monitor concentration and adjust dose. Severe Study
▸ Antiepileptics (fosphenytoin, phenobarbital, phenytoin, primidone) are predicted to decrease the exposure to dolutegravir. Adjust dolutegravir dose, p. 739. Severe Study
▸ Carbamazepine decreases the exposure to dolutegravir. Adjust dolutegravir dose, p. 739. Severe Study
▸ Oxcarbazepine is predicted to decrease the exposure to dolutegravir. Adjust dolutegravir dose, p. 739. Severe Theoretical
▸ Antiepileptics (carbamazepine, fosphenytoin, phenobarbital, phenytoin, primidone) are predicted to decrease the exposure to dronabinol. Avoid or adjust dose. Mild Study → Also see TABLE 10 p. 1574
▸ Antiepileptics (carbamazepine, eslicarbazepine, fosphenytoin, oxcarbazepine, perampanel, phenobarbital, phenytoin, primidone, rufinamide, topiramate) are predicted to decrease the efficacy of drospirenone. For FSRH guidance, see Contraceptives, interactions p. 917. Severe Theoretical
▸ Lamotrigine might decreases the effects of drospirenone. For FSRH guidance, see Contraceptives, interactions p. 917. Severe Theoretical
▸ Antiepileptics (carbamazepine, fosphenytoin, phenobarbital, phenytoin, primidone) are predicted to decrease the exposure to elacestrant. Avoid or adjust dose depending on duration— consult product literature. Severe Study
▸ Antiepileptics (carbamazepine, fosphenytoin, phenobarbital, phenytoin, primidone) are predicted to decrease the exposure to elbasvir. Avoid. Severe Study
▸ Antiepileptics (carbamazepine, fosphenytoin, phenobarbital, phenytoin, primidone) is predicted to decrease the exposure to elexacaftor. Avoid. Severe Theoretical
▸ Antiepileptics (carbamazepine, fosphenytoin, phenobarbital, phenytoin, primidone) are predicted to decrease the exposure to eliglustat. Avoid. Severe Study
▸ Antiepileptics (carbamazepine, fosphenytoin, phenobarbital, phenytoin, primidone) are predicted to decrease the concentration of elvitegravir. Avoid. Severe Study
▸ Antiepileptics (carbamazepine, fosphenytoin, phenobarbital, phenytoin, primidone) are predicted to decrease the exposure to encorafenib. Severe Theoretical
▸ Encorafenib is predicted to decrease the exposure to perampanel. Monitor and adjust dose. Moderate Study
▸ Antiepileptics (carbamazepine, fosphenytoin, phenobarbital, phenytoin, primidone) affect the exposure to endothelin receptor antagonists (bosentan). Avoid. Severe Study
▸ Antiepileptics (carbamazepine, fosphenytoin, phenobarbital, phenytoin, primidone) are predicted to decrease the exposure to endothelin receptor antagonists (macitentan). Avoid. Severe Study
▸ Antiepileptics (carbamazepine, fosphenytoin, phenobarbital, phenytoin, primidone) are predicted to decrease the exposure

to the cytotoxic component of enfortumab vedotin. Moderate Theoretical

▸ **Enteral feeds** decrease the absorption of **phenytoin**. Severe Study

▸ Antiepileptics (carbamazepine, fosphenytoin, phenobarbital, phenytoin, primidone) are predicted to decrease the exposure to entrectinib. Avoid. Severe Study

▸ Antiepileptics (carbamazepine, fosphenytoin, phenobarbital, phenytoin, primidone) are predicted to decrease the exposure to erdafitinib. Avoid. Severe Study

▸ Antiepileptics (carbamazepine, fosphenytoin, phenobarbital, phenytoin, primidone) are predicted to decrease the exposure to erlotinib. Avoid or adjust dose—consult product literature. Severe Study

▸ **Eslicarbazepine** is predicted to decrease the exposure to erlotinib. Severe Theoretical

▸ **Oxcarbazepine** decreases the exposure to erlotinib. Severe Study

▸ Antiepileptics (carbamazepine, fosphenytoin, phenobarbital, phenytoin, primidone) are predicted to decrease the exposure to esketamine. Adjust dose. Mild Theoretical → Also see **TABLE 10** p. 1574

▸ Antiepileptics (carbamazepine, eslicarbazepine, fosphenytoin, oxcarbazepine, perampanel, phenobarbital, phenytoin, primidone, rufinamide, topiramate) are predicted to decrease the efficacy of estradiol. Moderate Theoretical

▸ Antiepileptics (carbamazepine, fosphenytoin, phenobarbital, phenytoin, primidone) are predicted to decrease the exposure to eszopiclone. Adjust dose. Moderate Theoretical → Also see **TABLE 10** p. 1574

▸ Antiepileptics (carbamazepine, eslicarbazepine, fosphenytoin, oxcarbazepine, perampanel, phenobarbital, phenytoin, primidone, rufinamide, topiramate) are predicted to decrease the efficacy of etonogestrel. For FSRH guidance, see Contraceptives, interactions p. 917. Severe Theoretical

▸ **Lamotrigine** might decrease the effects of etonogestrel. For FSRH guidance, see Contraceptives, interactions p. 917. Moderate Theoretical

▸ Antiepileptics (carbamazepine, fosphenytoin, phenobarbital, phenytoin, primidone) are predicted to decrease the efficacy of etoposide. Moderate Study

▸ Antiepileptics (carbamazepine, fosphenytoin, phenobarbital, phenytoin, primidone) are predicted to decrease the concentration of everolimus. Avoid or adjust dose. Severe Study

▸ Antiepileptics (carbamazepine, fosphenytoin, phenobarbital, phenytoin, primidone) moderately decrease the exposure to exemestane. Moderate Study

▸ **Phenobarbital** is predicted to decrease the exposure to factor XA inhibitors (apixaban). Use with caution or avoid. Severe Anecdotal

▸ Antiepileptics (carbamazepine, phenytoin) are predicted to decrease the exposure to factor XA inhibitors (apixaban). Use with caution or avoid. Severe Study

▸ Antiepileptics (fosphenytoin, primidone) are predicted to decrease the exposure to factor XA inhibitors (apixaban). Severe Study

▸ **Carbamazepine** is predicted to decrease the exposure to factor XA inhibitors (edoxaban). Moderate Study

▸ Antiepileptics (fosphenytoin, phenobarbital, phenytoin, primidone) are predicted to decrease the exposure to factor XA inhibitors (edoxaban). Severe Theoretical

▸ **Fosphenytoin** is predicted to decrease the exposure to factor XA inhibitors (rivaroxaban). Avoid unless patient can be monitored for signs of thrombosis. Severe Theoretical

▸ **Oxcarbazepine** is predicted to decrease the exposure to factor XA inhibitors (rivaroxaban). Severe Study

▸ Antiepileptics (carbamazepine, phenobarbital, phenytoin, primidone) are predicted to decrease the exposure to factor XA inhibitors (rivaroxaban). Avoid unless patient can be monitored for signs of thrombosis. Severe Study

▸ Antiepileptics (carbamazepine, fosphenytoin, phenobarbital, phenytoin, primidone) are predicted to decrease the exposure to fedratinib. Avoid. Moderate Study

▸ Antiepileptics (fosphenytoin, phenobarbital, phenytoin, primidone) are predicted to decrease the exposure to fenfluramine. Moderate Theoretical

▸ **Carbamazepine** is predicted to decrease the concentration of fenfluramine. Adjust dose. Moderate Theoretical

▸ **Stiripentol** (given with clobazam, and with or without valproate) modestly increases the exposure to fenfluramine. Adjust **fenfluramine** dose, p. 361. Severe Study

▸ Antiepileptics (carbamazepine, fosphenytoin, phenobarbital, phenytoin, primidone) are predicted to decrease the exposure to fesoterodine. Avoid. Moderate Study

▸ **Fluorouracil** increases the concentration of antiepileptics (fosphenytoin, phenytoin). Monitor concentration and adjust dose. Severe Anecdotal

▸ **Folates** are predicted to decrease the concentration of antiepileptics (fosphenytoin, phenobarbital, phenytoin, primidone). Monitor concentration and adjust dose. Severe Study

▸ **Phenytoin** might decrease the effects of foslevodopa. Moderate Theoretical → Also see **TABLE 10** p. 1574

▸ Antiepileptics (carbamazepine, fosphenytoin, phenobarbital, phenytoin, primidone) are predicted to decrease the exposure to fostamatinib. Avoid. Severe Study

▸ Antiepileptics (carbamazepine, fosphenytoin, phenobarbital, phenytoin, primidone) are predicted to decrease the exposure to the active metabolite of fostemsavir. Avoid. Severe Study

▸ Antiepileptics (carbamazepine, fosphenytoin, phenobarbital, phenytoin, primidone) are predicted to decrease the exposure to fruquintinib. Avoid. Moderate Study

▸ Antiepileptics (carbamazepine, fosphenytoin, phenobarbital, phenytoin, primidone) are predicted to decrease the exposure to gefitinib. Avoid. Severe Study

▸ **Eslicarbazepine** is predicted to decrease the exposure to gefitinib. Moderate Theoretical

▸ **Oxcarbazepine** decreases the exposure to gefitinib. Severe Study

▸ Antiepileptics (carbamazepine, phenytoin) are predicted to decrease the exposure to gilteritinib. Avoid. Severe Study

▸ Antiepileptics (carbamazepine, fosphenytoin, phenobarbital, phenytoin, primidone) are predicted to decrease the exposure to glasdegib. Avoid. Severe Study

▸ Antiepileptics (carbamazepine, fosphenytoin, phenobarbital, phenytoin, primidone) are predicted to moderately decrease the exposure to glecaprevir. Avoid. Severe Study

▸ Antiepileptics (eslicarbazepine, oxcarbazepine) potentially decrease the exposure to glecaprevir. Avoid. Severe Theoretical

▸ **Valproate** potentially opposes the effects of glycerol phenylbutyrate. Moderate Theoretical

▸ **Grapefruit** juice slightly increases the exposure to carbamazepine. Monitor and adjust dose. Moderate Study

▸ Antiepileptics (carbamazepine, fosphenytoin, phenobarbital, phenytoin, primidone) are predicted to decrease the exposure to grazoprevir. Avoid. Severe Study

▸ Antiepileptics (phenobarbital, primidone) decrease the effects of griseofulvin. Moderate Study

▸ Antiepileptics (carbamazepine, fosphenytoin, phenobarbital, phenytoin, primidone) are predicted to decrease the concentration of guanfacine. Adjust **guanfacine** dose, p. 407. Moderate Study → Also see **TABLE 10** p. 1574

▸ **Oxcarbazepine** is predicted to decrease the concentration of guanfacine. Monitor and adjust **guanfacine** dose, p. 407. Moderate Theoretical

▸ **Guanfacine** increases the concentration of **valproate**. Monitor and adjust dose. Moderate Study

▸ H_2 receptor antagonists (cimetidine) transiently increase the concentration of **carbamazepine**. Monitor concentration and adjust dose. Moderate Study

▸ H_2 receptor antagonists (cimetidine) increase the concentration of antiepileptics (fosphenytoin, phenytoin). Monitor concentration and adjust dose. Severe Study

▸ Antiepileptics (carbamazepine, fosphenytoin, phenobarbital, phenytoin, primidone) decrease the concentration of haloperidol. Adjust dose. Moderate Study → Also see **TABLE 17** p. 1576 → Also see **TABLE 10** p. 1574

▸ **Haloperidol** potentially increases the risk of overheating and dehydration when given with **zonisamide**. Avoid in children. Severe Theoretical

▸ **HIV-protease inhibitors** are predicted to increase the exposure to **carbamazepine** and **carbamazepine** is predicted to decrease

A1

Interactions | Appendix 1

Antiepileptics (continued)

the exposure to **HIV-protease inhibitors**. Monitor and adjust dose. [Severe] Theoretical

▸ HIV-protease inhibitors (ritonavir) decrease the exposure to **lamotrigine**. [Severe] Study

▸ HIV-protease inhibitors (ritonavir) are predicted to decrease the concentration of **valproate**. [Severe] Anecdotal → Also see **TABLE 1** p. 1571

▸ **HIV-protease inhibitors** are predicted to affect the exposure to antiepileptics (**fosphenytoin, phenytoin**) and antiepileptics (**fosphenytoin, phenytoin**) decrease the concentration of **HIV-protease inhibitors**. [Severe] Theoretical

▸ **HIV-protease inhibitors** are predicted to affect the concentration of antiepileptics (**phenobarbital, primidone**) and antiepileptics (**phenobarbital, primidone**) are predicted to decrease the concentration of **HIV-protease inhibitors**. [Severe] Theoretical

▸ **HIV-protease inhibitors** are predicted to very slightly increase the exposure to **perampanel**. [Mild] Study

▸ Antiepileptics (**carbamazepine, eslicarbazepine, fosphenytoin, oxcarbazepine, perampanel, phenobarbital, phenytoin, primidone, rufinamide, topiramate**) are predicted to decrease the effects of **hormone replacement therapy**. [Moderate] Anecdotal

▸ **Hormone replacement therapy** is predicted to alter the exposure to **lamotrigine**. [Moderate] Theoretical

▸ Antiepileptics (**carbamazepine, fosphenytoin, phenobarbital, phenytoin, primidone**) are predicted to decrease the exposure to **ibrutinib**. Avoid or monitor. [Severe] Study

▸ Antiepileptics (**carbamazepine, fosphenytoin, phenobarbital, phenytoin, primidone**) are predicted to decrease the exposure to **idelalisib**. Avoid. [Severe] Study

▸ **Idelalisib** is predicted to very slightly increase the exposure to **perampanel**. [Mild] Study

▸ Antiepileptics (**carbamazepine, fosphenytoin, oxcarbazepine, phenobarbital, phenytoin, primidone**) are predicted to decrease the exposure to **imatinib**. Avoid. [Moderate] Study

▸ **Eslicarbazepine** is predicted to decrease the exposure to **imatinib**. [Moderate] Theoretical

▸ **Topiramate** is predicted to decrease the exposure to **imatinib**. [Moderate] Study

▸ Antiepileptics (**carbamazepine, fosphenytoin, phenobarbital, phenytoin, primidone**) are predicted to decrease the exposure to **irinotecan**. Avoid. [Severe] Study

▸ Antiepileptics (**carbamazepine, fosphenytoin, phenobarbital, phenytoin, primidone**) are predicted to decrease the exposure to iron chelators (deferasirox). Monitor serum ferritin and adjust dose. [Moderate] Theoretical

▸ Iron chelators (dexrazoxane) might decrease the absorption of antiepileptics (**fosphenytoin, phenytoin**). Avoid. [Severe] Theoretical

▸ **Isoniazid** increases the concentration of antiepileptics (**fosphenytoin, phenytoin**). [Moderate] Study → Also see **TABLE 11** p. 1574

▸ **Isoniazid** markedly increases the concentration of **carbamazepine** and **carbamazepine** increases the risk of hepatotoxicity when given with **isoniazid**. Monitor concentration and adjust dose. [Severe] Study

▸ Antiepileptics (**carbamazepine, fosphenytoin, phenobarbital, phenytoin, primidone**) are predicted to decrease the exposure to **ivabradine**. Adjust dose. [Moderate] Theoretical

▸ Antiepileptics (**carbamazepine, fosphenytoin, phenobarbital, phenytoin, primidone**) are predicted to decrease the exposure to **ivacaftor**. Avoid. [Severe] Study

▸ Antiepileptics (**carbamazepine, fosphenytoin, phenobarbital, primidone**) are predicted to decrease the exposure to **ivosidenib**. Avoid. [Severe] Theoretical

▸ **Ivosidenib** might decrease the exposure to **lamotrigine**. Avoid or monitor efficacy. [Unknown] Theoretical

▸ **Ivosidenib** is predicted to decrease the exposure to **perampanel**. Monitor and adjust dose. [Moderate] Study

▸ **Phenytoin** is predicted to decrease the exposure to **ivosidenib** and **ivosidenib** might decrease the exposure to **phenytoin**. Avoid. [Severe] Study

▸ Antiepileptics (**carbamazepine, fosphenytoin, phenobarbital, phenytoin, primidone**) are predicted to decrease the exposure to **ixazomib**. Avoid. [Severe] Study

▸ Antiepileptics (**carbamazepine, fosphenytoin, phenobarbital, phenytoin, primidone**) are predicted to decrease the exposure to **lapatinib**. Avoid. [Severe] Study

▸ Antiepileptics (**carbamazepine, fosphenytoin, phenobarbital, phenytoin, primidone**) are predicted to moderately decrease the exposure to **larotrectinib**. Avoid. [Moderate] Study

▸ Antiepileptics (**fosphenytoin, oxcarbazepine, phenobarbital, phenytoin, primidone**) are predicted to decrease the exposure to **ledipasvir**. Avoid. [Severe] Theoretical

▸ **Carbamazepine** is predicted to decrease the exposure to **ledipasvir**. Avoid. [Severe] Study

▸ Antiepileptics (**carbamazepine, fosphenytoin, phenobarbital, phenytoin, primidone**) are predicted to decrease the exposure to **leniolisib**. Avoid. [Severe] Theoretical

▸ Antiepileptics (**carbamazepine, phenobarbital, primidone**) are predicted to decrease the concentration of **letermovir**. [Moderate] Theoretical

▸ **Letermovir** is predicted to decrease the concentration of antiepileptics (**fosphenytoin, phenytoin**) and antiepileptics (**fosphenytoin, phenytoin**) are predicted to decrease the concentration of **letermovir**. [Moderate] Theoretical

▸ Antiepileptics (**fosphenytoin, phenytoin**) decrease the effects of **levodopa**. [Moderate] Study → Also see **TABLE 10** p. 1574

▸ Antiepileptics (**carbamazepine, eslicarbazepine, fosphenytoin, oxcarbazepine, perampanel, phenobarbital, phenytoin, primidone, rufinamide, topiramate**) are predicted to decrease the efficacy of some contraceptive methods containing **levonorgestrel**. For FSRH guidance, see Contraceptives, interactions p. 917. [Severe] Theoretical

▸ **Lamotrigine** might decrease the effects of **levonorgestrel**. For FSRH guidance, see Contraceptives, interactions p. 917. [Moderate] Theoretical

▸ Antiepileptics (**carbamazepine, oxcarbazepine**) are predicted to increase the risk of neurotoxicity when given with **lithium**. [Severe] Anecdotal

▸ Antiepileptics (**carbamazepine, fosphenytoin, phenobarbital, phenytoin, primidone**) are predicted to decrease the exposure to **lomitapide**. Monitor and adjust dose. [Moderate] Theoretical

▸ Antiepileptics (**fosphenytoin, phenytoin**) decrease the effects of loop diuretics (furosemide). [Moderate] Study

▸ Antiepileptics (**carbamazepine, fosphenytoin, phenobarbital, phenytoin, primidone**) are predicted to decrease the exposure to **lorlatinib**. Avoid. [Severe] Study

▸ **Lumacaftor** is predicted to decrease the exposure to antiepileptics (**carbamazepine, fosphenytoin, phenobarbital, phenytoin, primidone**). Avoid. [Severe] Theoretical

▸ **Lumacaftor** is predicted to decrease the exposure to **perampanel**. Monitor and adjust dose. [Moderate] Study

▸ Macrolides (clarithromycin) slightly increase the concentration of **carbamazepine**. Monitor concentration and adjust dose. [Severe] Study

▸ Macrolides (clarithromycin) are predicted to very slightly increase the exposure to **perampanel**. [Mild] Study

▸ Macrolides (erythromycin) markedly increase the concentration of **carbamazepine**. Monitor concentration and adjust dose. [Severe] Study

▸ Antiepileptics (**phenobarbital, primidone**) are predicted to increase the effects of **MAOIs, irreversible**. [Severe] Theoretical

▸ **Carbamazepine** is predicted to increase the risk of severe toxic reaction when given with **MAOIs, irreversible**. Avoid and for 14 days after stopping the MAOI. [Severe] Theoretical

▸ Antiepileptics (**carbamazepine, fosphenytoin, phenobarbital, phenytoin, primidone**) are predicted to decrease the exposure to **maraviroc**. Adjust dose. [Severe] Study

▸ Antiepileptics (**carbamazepine, fosphenytoin, phenobarbital, phenytoin, primidone**) are predicted to decrease the exposure to **maribavir**. Avoid or adjust **maribavir** dose, p. 735. [Severe] Study

▸ Antiepileptics (**carbamazepine, fosphenytoin, phenobarbital, phenytoin, primidone**) are predicted to decrease the exposure to **mavacamten**. Monitor and adjust dose—consult product literature. [Severe] Theoretical

▸ Antiepileptics (**carbamazepine, fosphenytoin, phenobarbital, phenytoin, primidone**) are predicted to decrease the exposure

to meglitinides (repaglinide). Monitor blood glucose and adjust dose. Moderate Study
‣ **Phenytoin** is predicted to decrease the exposure to melatonin. Moderate Theoretical → Also see **TABLE 10** p. 1574
‣ **Sultiame** might increase the risk of lactic acidosis when given with metformin. Severe Theoretical
‣ **Levetiracetam** decreases the clearance of methotrexate. Severe Anecdotal
‣ **Carbamazepine** might decrease the concentration of methylphenidate. Moderate Anecdotal
‣ **Valproate** might enhance the effects of methylphenidate. Severe Anecdotal
‣ Antiepileptics (**phenobarbital, primidone**) are predicted to decrease the exposure to metronidazole. Moderate Study
‣ Antiepileptics (**fosphenytoin, phenobarbital, phenytoin, primidone**) are predicted to decrease the effects of metyrapone. Avoid. Moderate Study
‣ **Phenytoin** is predicted to increase the clearance of mexiletine. Monitor and adjust dose. Moderate Study
‣ Antiepileptics (**phenobarbital, primidone**) are predicted to decrease the exposure to mianserin. Moderate Study → Also see **TABLE 10** p. 1574
‣ **Carbamazepine** markedly decreases the exposure to mianserin. Adjust dose. Moderate Study
‣ Antiepileptics (**carbamazepine, fosphenytoin, phenobarbital, phenytoin, primidone**) are predicted to decrease the exposure to midostaurin. Avoid. Severe Study
‣ Antiepileptics (**carbamazepine, fosphenytoin, phenobarbital, phenytoin, primidone**) are predicted to decrease the exposure to mifepristone. Adjust **mifepristone** dose, p. 954. Severe Study
‣ Antiepileptics (**carbamazepine, fosphenytoin, phenobarbital, phenytoin, primidone**) are predicted to decrease the exposure to mineralocorticoid receptor antagonists (**eplerenone**). Avoid. Moderate Theoretical
‣ Antiepileptics (**carbamazepine, fosphenytoin, phenobarbital, phenytoin, primidone**) are predicted to decrease the exposure to mineralocorticoid receptor antagonists (**finerenone**). Avoid. Severe Study
‣ Antiepileptics (**carbamazepine, fosphenytoin, phenobarbital, phenytoin, primidone**) are predicted to decrease the exposure to mirtazapine. Adjust dose. Moderate Study → Also see **TABLE 17** p. 1576 → Also see **TABLE 10** p. 1574
‣ **Mitotane** is predicted to decrease the exposure to **perampanel**. Monitor and adjust dose. Moderate Study
‣ Antiepileptics (**carbamazepine, fosphenytoin, phenobarbital, phenytoin, primidone**) are predicted to decrease the exposure to mobocertinib. Avoid. Severe Study
‣ Antiepileptics (**carbamazepine, phenobarbital, primidone**) are predicted to decrease the exposure to modafinil. Mild Theoretical
‣ Antiepileptics (**fosphenytoin, phenytoin**) are predicted to decrease the exposure to modafinil and modafinil is predicted to increase the concentration of antiepileptics (**fosphenytoin, phenytoin**). Monitor concentration and adjust dose. Moderate Theoretical
‣ Monoclonal antibodies (**elranatamab**) might affect the exposure to **phenytoin**. Monitor and adjust dose. Moderate Theoretical
‣ **Carbamazepine** is predicted to decrease the effects of monoclonal antibodies (**brentuximab vedotin**). Severe Theoretical
‣ Monoclonal antibodies (**tocilizumab**) are predicted to decrease the exposure to antiepileptics (**fosphenytoin, phenytoin**). Monitor and adjust dose. Moderate Theoretical
‣ Antiepileptics (**carbamazepine, fosphenytoin, phenobarbital, phenytoin, primidone**) are predicted to decrease the exposure to monoclonal antibodies (**polatuzumab vedotin**). Moderate Theoretical
‣ Antiepileptics (**carbamazepine, fosphenytoin, phenobarbital, phenytoin, primidone**) are predicted to decrease the exposure to the cytotoxic component of monoclonal antibodies (**trastuzumab emtansine**). Severe Theoretical
‣ Antiepileptics (**carbamazepine, fosphenytoin, phenobarbital, phenytoin, primidone**) are predicted to decrease the exposure to montelukast. Mild Study

‣ Antiepileptics (**carbamazepine, fosphenytoin, phenobarbital, phenytoin, primidone**) are predicted to markedly decrease the exposure to naldemedine. Avoid. Severe Study
‣ Antiepileptics (**carbamazepine, fosphenytoin, phenobarbital, phenytoin, primidone**) are predicted to markedly decrease the exposure to naloxegol. Avoid. Moderate Study
‣ Antiepileptics (**carbamazepine, fosphenytoin, phenobarbital, phenytoin, primidone**) are predicted to decrease the exposure to neratinib. Avoid. Severe Study
‣ Antiepileptics (**carbamazepine, fosphenytoin, phenobarbital, phenytoin, primidone**) are predicted to markedly decrease the exposure to neurokinin-1 receptor antagonists (**aprepitant**). Avoid. Moderate Study
‣ Antiepileptics (**carbamazepine, fosphenytoin, phenobarbital, phenytoin, primidone**) are predicted to decrease the exposure to neurokinin-1 receptor antagonists (**fosaprepitant**). Avoid. Moderate Theoretical
‣ Antiepileptics (**carbamazepine, fosphenytoin, phenobarbital, phenytoin, primidone**) are predicted to decrease the exposure to neurokinin-1 receptor antagonists (**netupitant**). Avoid. Severe Study
‣ **Carbamazepine** is predicted to decrease the effects of (but acute use increases the effects of) neuromuscular blocking drugs, non-depolarising (**atracurium, cisatracurium, pancuronium, rocuronium, vecuronium**). Monitor and adjust dose. Moderate Study
‣ Antiepileptics (**fosphenytoin, phenytoin**) decrease the effects of (but acute use increases the effects of) neuromuscular blocking drugs, non-depolarising (**atracurium, cisatracurium, pancuronium, rocuronium, vecuronium**). Moderate Study
‣ Antiepileptics (**carbamazepine, fosphenytoin, phenobarbital, phenytoin, primidone**) are predicted to moderately decrease the exposure to nilotinib. Avoid. Severe Study
‣ Antiepileptics (**phenobarbital, phenytoin**) are predicted to decrease the exposure to nintedanib. Severe Theoretical
‣ **Carbamazepine** is predicted to decrease the exposure to nintedanib. Moderate Study
‣ Antiepileptics (**carbamazepine, fosphenytoin, phenobarbital, phenytoin, primidone**) are predicted to decrease the exposure to nirmatrelvir boosted with ritonavir. Avoid. Severe Study
‣ **Nirmatrelvir** boosted with ritonavir is predicted to decrease the concentration of antiepileptics (**lamotrigine, valproate**). Severe Theoretical
‣ Antiepileptics (**carbamazepine, fosphenytoin, phenobarbital, phenytoin, primidone**) are predicted to decrease the exposure to nitisinone. Adjust dose. Moderate Theoretical
‣ NNRTIs (**efavirenz**) are predicted to affect the efficacy of **primidone** and **primidone** is predicted to slightly decrease the exposure to NNRTIs (**efavirenz**). Severe Theoretical
‣ NNRTIs (**nevirapine**) are predicted to decrease the concentration of antiepileptics (**carbamazepine, fosphenytoin, phenobarbital, phenytoin, primidone**) and antiepileptics (**carbamazepine, fosphenytoin, phenobarbital, phenytoin, primidone**) are predicted to decrease the concentration of NNRTIs (**nevirapine**). Severe Study
‣ **Oxcarbazepine** is predicted to decrease the exposure to NNRTIs (**doravirine**). Avoid. Severe Theoretical
‣ Antiepileptics (**carbamazepine, fosphenytoin, phenobarbital, phenytoin, primidone**) are predicted to decrease the exposure to NNRTIs (**doravirine**). Avoid. Severe Study
‣ **Carbamazepine** slightly decreases the exposure to NNRTIs (**efavirenz**) and NNRTIs (**efavirenz**) slightly decrease the exposure to **carbamazepine**. Severe Study
‣ **Phenobarbital** is predicted to decrease the exposure to NNRTIs (**efavirenz**) and NNRTIs (**efavirenz**) affect the concentration of **phenobarbital**. Severe Theoretical
‣ Antiepileptics (**fosphenytoin, phenytoin**) slightly decrease the exposure to NNRTIs (**efavirenz**) and NNRTIs (**efavirenz**) affect the concentration of antiepileptics (**fosphenytoin, phenytoin**). Severe Theoretical
‣ Antiepileptics (**carbamazepine, fosphenytoin, phenobarbital, phenytoin, primidone**) are predicted to decrease the exposure to NNRTIs (**etravirine**). Avoid. Severe Theoretical
‣ **Oxcarbazepine** is predicted to decrease the concentration of NNRTIs (**rilpivirine**). Avoid. Severe Theoretical

Antiepileptics (continued)

▸ Antiepileptics **(carbamazepine, fosphenytoin, phenobarbital, phenytoin, primidone)** markedly decrease the exposure to NNRTIs **(rilpivirine)**. Avoid. Severe Study

▸ Antiepileptics **(carbamazepine, eslicarbazepine, fosphenytoin, oxcarbazepine, perampanel, phenobarbital, phenytoin, primidone, rufinamide, topiramate)** are predicted to decrease the efficacy of some contraceptive methods containing norethisterone. For FSRH guidance, see Contraceptives, interactions p. 917. Severe Anecdotal

▸ **Lamotrigine** might decrease the effects of norethisterone. For FSRH guidance, see Contraceptives, interactions p. 917. Moderate Theoretical

▸ Antiepileptics **(carbamazepine, fosphenytoin, phenobarbital, phenytoin, primidone)** are predicted to decrease the exposure to NRTIs **(abacavir)**. Moderate Theoretical

▸ **Valproate** slightly increases the exposure to NRTIs **(zidovudine)**. Moderate Study → Also see **TABLE 1** p. 1571

▸ Antiepileptics **(carbamazepine, fosphenytoin, phenobarbital, phenytoin, primidone)** are predicted to decrease the exposure to olaparib. Avoid. Moderate Theoretical

▸ Antiepileptics **(carbamazepine, fosphenytoin, phenobarbital, phenytoin, primidone)** are predicted to decrease the exposure to opioids **(alfentanil, fentanyl)**. Moderate Study → Also see **TABLE 10** p. 1574

▸ Antiepileptics **(carbamazepine, fosphenytoin, phenobarbital, phenytoin, primidone)** are predicted to decrease the exposure to opioids **(buprenorphine)**. Monitor and adjust dose. Moderate Theoretical → Also see **TABLE 10** p. 1574

▸ Antiepileptics **(carbamazepine, fosphenytoin, phenobarbital, phenytoin, primidone)** decrease the exposure to opioids **(methadone)**. Monitor and adjust dose. Severe Study → Also see **TABLE 10** p. 1574

▸ Antiepileptics **(carbamazepine, fosphenytoin, phenobarbital, phenytoin, primidone)** are predicted to decrease the exposure to opioids **(oxycodone)**. Monitor and adjust dose. Moderate Study → Also see **TABLE 10** p. 1574

▸ **Carbamazepine** decreases the concentration of opioids **(tramadol)**. Adjust dose. Severe Study → Also see **TABLE 17** p. 1576

▸ Antiepileptics **(carbamazepine, fosphenytoin, phenobarbital, phenytoin, primidone)** are predicted to decrease the exposure to osilodrostat. Moderate Theoretical

▸ Antiepileptics **(carbamazepine, fosphenytoin, phenobarbital, phenytoin, primidone)** are predicted to moderately decrease the exposure to osimertinib. Avoid. Moderate Study

▸ Antiepileptics **(carbamazepine, fosphenytoin, phenobarbital, phenytoin, primidone)** are predicted to moderately decrease the exposure to ospemifene. Moderate Study

▸ **Oxybutynin** potentially increases the risk of overheating and dehydration when given with **zonisamide**. Avoid in children. Severe Theoretical

▸ Antiepileptics **(carbamazepine, fosphenytoin, phenobarbital, phenytoin, primidone)** are predicted to decrease the exposure to palbociclib. Avoid. Severe Study

▸ Antiepileptics **(carbamazepine, fosphenytoin, phenobarbital, phenytoin, primidone)** are predicted to decrease the exposure to panobinostat. Avoid. Moderate Theoretical

▸ Antiepileptics **(carbamazepine, fosphenytoin, phenobarbital, phenytoin, primidone)** decrease the exposure to paracetamol. Moderate Study

▸ Antiepileptics **(carbamazepine, fosphenytoin, phenobarbital, phenytoin, primidone)** are predicted to decrease the exposure to pazopanib. Avoid. Severe Theoretical

▸ Antiepileptics **(carbamazepine, fosphenytoin, phenobarbital, phenytoin, primidone)** are predicted to decrease the exposure to pemigatinib. Avoid. Severe Study

▸ **Valproate** increases the risk of adverse effects when given with penicillins **(pivmecillinam)**. Avoid. Severe Anecdotal

▸ Phenothiazines **(chlorpromazine)** decrease the concentration of antiepileptics **(phenobarbital, primidone)** and antiepileptics **(phenobarbital, primidone)** decrease the concentration of phenothiazines **(chlorpromazine)**. Moderate Study → Also see **TABLE 10** p. 1574

▸ Antiepileptics **(carbamazepine, fosphenytoin, phenobarbital, phenytoin, primidone)** moderately decrease the exposure to

phosphodiesterase type-4 inhibitors **(apremilast)**. Avoid. Severe Study

▸ Antiepileptics **(carbamazepine, fosphenytoin, phenobarbital, phenytoin, primidone)** are predicted to decrease the exposure to phosphodiesterase type-4 inhibitors **(roflumilast)**. Avoid. Moderate Study

▸ Antiepileptics **(carbamazepine, fosphenytoin, phenobarbital, phenytoin, primidone)** are predicted to decrease the exposure to phosphodiesterase type-5 inhibitors **(avanafil, tadalafil)**. Avoid. Severe Study

▸ Antiepileptics **(carbamazepine, fosphenytoin, phenobarbital, phenytoin, primidone)** are predicted to decrease the exposure to phosphodiesterase type-5 inhibitors **(sildenafil, vardenafil)**. Moderate Theoretical

▸ Antiepileptics **(carbamazepine, fosphenytoin, phenobarbital, phenytoin, primidone)** are predicted to moderately to markedly decrease the exposure to pibrentasvir. Avoid. Severe Study

▸ Antiepileptics **(eslicarbazepine, oxcarbazepine)** potentially decrease the exposure to pibrentasvir. Avoid. Severe Theoretical

▸ Antiepileptics **(fosphenytoin, phenytoin)** are predicted to decrease the exposure to pirfenidone. Moderate Theoretical

▸ Antiepileptics **(carbamazepine, fosphenytoin, phenobarbital, phenytoin, primidone)** are predicted to moderately decrease the exposure to pitolisant. Moderate Study

▸ Antiepileptics **(carbamazepine, fosphenytoin, phenobarbital, phenytoin, primidone)** are predicted to decrease the exposure to ponatinib. Avoid. Moderate Theoretical

▸ Antiepileptics **(carbamazepine, fosphenytoin, phenobarbital, phenytoin, primidone)** are predicted to decrease the exposure to pralsetinib. Avoid or adjust dose with potent CYP3A4 inducers—consult product literature. Moderate Study

▸ Antiepileptics **(carbamazepine, fosphenytoin, phenobarbital, phenytoin, primidone)** are predicted to markedly decrease the exposure to praziquantel. Avoid. Moderate Study

▸ Antiepileptics **(carbamazepine, phenobarbital, phenytoin, primidone)** are predicted to increase the risk of hypersensitivity reactions when given with procarbazine. Severe Anecdotal

▸ **Fosphenytoin** is predicted to increase the risk of hypersensitivity when given with procarbazine. Severe Anecdotal

▸ **Valproate** potentially increases the concentration of propofol. Adjust dose. Severe Theoretical

▸ Quinolones **(ciprofloxacin)** affect the concentration of antiepileptics **(fosphenytoin, phenytoin)**. Monitor concentration and adjust dose. Severe Study

▸ Antiepileptics **(carbamazepine, fosphenytoin, phenobarbital, phenytoin, primidone)** are predicted to decrease the exposure to quizartinib. Avoid. Severe Study

▸ Antiepileptics **(fosphenytoin, phenobarbital, phenytoin, primidone)** are predicted to affect the exposure to raltegravir. Use with caution or avoid. Moderate Theoretical

▸ **Carbamazepine** is predicted to affect the exposure to raltegravir. Moderate Theoretical

▸ Antiepileptics **(carbamazepine, fosphenytoin, phenobarbital, phenytoin, primidone)** are predicted to decrease the exposure to ranolazine. Avoid. Severe Study

▸ Antiepileptics **(carbamazepine, fosphenytoin, phenobarbital, phenytoin, primidone)** are predicted to decrease the exposure to reboxetine. Moderate Anecdotal

▸ Antiepileptics **(carbamazepine, fosphenytoin, phenobarbital, phenytoin, primidone)** are predicted to decrease the exposure to regorafenib. Avoid. Moderate Study

▸ Antiepileptics **(carbamazepine, phenobarbital, phenytoin)** are predicted to decrease the exposure to relugolix. Avoid or adjust dose depending on indication—consult product literature. Moderate Study

▸ Antiepileptics **(oxcarbazepine, topiramate)** are predicted to decrease the exposure to relugolix. Avoid. Moderate Theoretical

▸ Antiepileptics **(carbamazepine, fosphenytoin, phenobarbital, phenytoin, primidone)** are predicted to markedly decrease the exposure to ribociclib. Avoid. Severe Study

▸ Rifamycins **(rifampicin)** slightly decrease the exposure to brivaracetam. Adjust dose. Moderate Study

- **Rifamycins (rifampicin)** markedly increase the clearance of **lamotrigine**. Adjust **lamotrigine** dose, p. 366. [Moderate] Study
- **Rifamycins (rifampicin)** are predicted to decrease the exposure to **perampanel**. Monitor and adjust dose. [Moderate] Study
- **Rifamycins (rifampicin)** are predicted to decrease the concentration of **zonisamide**. Monitor and adjust dose. [Moderate] Theoretical
- **Rifamycins (rifampicin)** decrease the concentration of antiepileptics (**fosphenytoin, phenytoin**). Use with caution and adjust dose. [Moderate] Study
- Antiepileptics (**phenobarbital, primidone**) are predicted to decrease the exposure to **rifamycins (rifampicin)** and **rifamycins (rifampicin)** are predicted to decrease the exposure to antiepileptics (**phenobarbital, primidone**). Use with caution and adjust dose. [Moderate] Study
- Antiepileptics (**carbamazepine, fosphenytoin, phenobarbital, phenytoin, primidone**) are predicted to decrease the exposure to **rimegepant**. Avoid. [Moderate] Theoretical
- Antiepileptics (**carbamazepine, fosphenytoin, phenobarbital, phenytoin, primidone**) are predicted to decrease the exposure to **ripretinib**. Avoid or adjust dose—consult product literature. [Severe] Study
- **Rucaparib** is predicted to increase the exposure to **phenytoin**. Monitor and adjust dose. [Moderate] Study
- Antiepileptics (**carbamazepine, fosphenytoin, phenobarbital, phenytoin, primidone**) are predicted to decrease the exposure to **ruxolitinib**. Monitor and adjust dose. [Moderate] Study
- Antiepileptics (**carbamazepine, fosphenytoin, phenytoin**) are predicted to decrease the exposure to the active component of **sacituzumab govitecan**. [Severe] Theoretical
- Antiepileptics (**carbamazepine, fosphenytoin, phenytoin**) are predicted to decrease the exposure to the active metabolite of **selexipag**. Adjust dose. [Moderate] Study
- **Valproate** is predicted to increase the exposure to **selexipag**. [Unknown] Theoretical
- Antiepileptics (**carbamazepine, fosphenytoin, phenobarbital, phenytoin, primidone**) are predicted to decrease the exposure to **selpercatinib**. Avoid. [Moderate] Study
- Antiepileptics (**carbamazepine, fosphenytoin, phenobarbital, phenytoin, primidone**) are predicted to decrease the exposure to **selumetinib**. Avoid. [Severe] Study
- Antiepileptics (**carbamazepine, fosphenytoin, phenobarbital, phenytoin, primidone**) are predicted to decrease the exposure to **siponimod**. Manufacturer advises caution depending on genotype—consult product literature. [Severe] Study
- Antiepileptics (**carbamazepine, fosphenytoin, phenobarbital, phenytoin, primidone**) are predicted to decrease the concentration of **sirolimus**. Avoid or monitor and adjust dose. [Severe] Study
- **Phenytoin** is predicted to decrease the exposure to SNRIs (**duloxetine**). [Moderate] Theoretical → Also see **TABLE 10** p. 1574
- Antiepileptics (**carbamazepine, phenobarbital, phenytoin, primidone**) are predicted to decrease the exposure to sodium glucose co-transporter 2 inhibitors (**canagliflozin**). Adjust **canagliflozin** dose, p. 824. [Moderate] Study
- **Fosphenytoin** is predicted to decrease the exposure to sodium glucose co-transporter 2 inhibitors (**empagliflozin**). Avoid or monitor diabetic control. [Moderate] Theoretical
- **Phenytoin** might decrease the exposure to sodium glucose co-transporter 2 inhibitors (**empagliflozin**). Avoid or monitor diabetic control. [Moderate] Theoretical
- **Valproate** increases the exposure to sodium oxybate. Adjust sodium oxybate dose, p. 558. [Moderate] Study
- **Valproate** potentially decreases the effects of sodium phenylbutyrate. [Moderate] Anecdotal
- Antiepileptics (**fosphenytoin, oxcarbazepine, phenobarbital, phenytoin, primidone**) are predicted to decrease the exposure to **sofosbuvir**. Avoid. [Severe] Theoretical
- **Carbamazepine** is predicted to decrease the exposure to **sofosbuvir**. Avoid. [Severe] Study
- Antiepileptics (**carbamazepine, fosphenytoin, phenobarbital, phenytoin, primidone**) are predicted to decrease the exposure to **solifenacin**. [Moderate] Theoretical
- **Somapacitan** might decrease the exposure to **carbamazepine**. [Moderate] Theoretical

- **Somatrogon** might decreases the exposure to **carbamazepine**. [Moderate] Theoretical
- Antiepileptics (**carbamazepine, eslicarbazepine, fosphenytoin, phenobarbital, phenytoin, primidone**) are predicted to decrease the exposure to **sorafenib**. [Moderate] Theoretical
- **Oxcarbazepine** is predicted to decrease the exposure to **sorafenib**. [Moderate] Study
- Antiepileptics (**carbamazepine, fosphenytoin, phenobarbital, phenytoin, primidone**) are predicted to decrease the exposure to **sotorasib**. Avoid. [Severe] Study
- SSRIs (**fluoxetine, fluvoxamine**) are predicted to increase the concentration of antiepileptics (**fosphenytoin, phenytoin**). Monitor and adjust dose. [Severe] Anecdotal → Also see **TABLE 10** p. 1574
- SSRIs (**sertraline**) potentially increase the risk of toxicity when given with antiepileptics (**fosphenytoin, phenytoin**). Monitor concentration and adjust dose. [Severe] Anecdotal → Also see **TABLE 10** p. 1574
- Antiepileptics (**fosphenytoin, phenytoin**) decrease the concentration of SSRIs (**paroxetine**). [Moderate] Study → Also see **TABLE 10** p. 1574
- **St John's wort** is predicted to decrease the concentration of antiepileptics (**fosphenytoin, phenobarbital, phenytoin, primidone**). Avoid. [Severe] Theoretical
- **St John's wort** is predicted to decrease the exposure to **brivaracetam**. [Moderate] Theoretical
- **St John's wort** is predicted to decrease the concentration of **carbamazepine**. Monitor and adjust dose. [Moderate] Theoretical
- **St John's wort** is predicted to decrease the exposure to **perampanel**. Monitor and adjust dose. [Moderate] Theoretical
- **St John's wort** is predicted to decrease the exposure to **tiagabine**. Avoid. [Mild] Theoretical
- **Carbamazepine** is predicted to decrease the exposure to statins (**atorvastatin**). Monitor and adjust dose. [Moderate] Study
- **Eslicarbazepine** is predicted to decrease the exposure to statins (**atorvastatin**). Monitor and adjust dose. [Moderate] Theoretical
- **Phenytoin** moderately decreases the exposure to statins (**atorvastatin**). [Moderate] Study
- **Oxcarbazepine** is predicted to decrease the exposure to statins (**atorvastatin, simvastatin**). [Moderate] Theoretical
- Antiepileptics (**fosphenytoin, phenobarbital, primidone**) are predicted to decrease the exposure to statins (**atorvastatin, simvastatin**). [Moderate] Study
- **Eslicarbazepine** decreases the exposure to statins (**rosuvastatin**). [Moderate] Study
- **Phenytoin** is predicted to decrease the exposure to statins (**simvastatin**). [Moderate] Study
- Antiepileptics (**carbamazepine, eslicarbazepine**) moderately decrease the exposure to statins (**simvastatin**). Monitor and adjust dose. [Moderate] Study
- Sulfonamides (**sulfadiazine**) are predicted to increase the concentration of **fosphenytoin**. Monitor and adjust dose. [Moderate] Study
- Sulfonamides (**sulfadiazine**) increase the concentration of **phenytoin**. Monitor and adjust dose. [Moderate] Study
- Antiepileptics (**carbamazepine, fosphenytoin, phenobarbital, phenytoin, primidone**) are predicted to decrease the exposure to **sunitinib**. Avoid or adjust dose—consult product literature. [Moderate] Study
- Antiepileptics (**fosphenytoin, phenytoin**) increase the effects of **suxamethonium**. [Moderate] Study
- **Carbamazepine** increases the risk of prolonged neuromuscular blockade when given with **suxamethonium**. [Moderate] Study
- Antiepileptics (**carbamazepine, fosphenytoin, phenobarbital, phenytoin, primidone**) decrease the concentration of **tacrolimus**. Avoid or monitor and adjust dose. [Severe] Study
- **Tamoxifen** (high-dose) might increase the concentration of **fosphenytoin** and **fosphenytoin** might decrease the concentration of **tamoxifen** (high-dose). [Severe] Theoretical
- **Tamoxifen** (high-dose) might increase the concentration of **phenytoin** and **phenytoin** might decrease the concentration of **tamoxifen** (high-dose). [Severe] Anecdotal
- Antiepileptics (**carbamazepine, fosphenytoin, phenobarbital, phenytoin, primidone**) are predicted to decrease the exposure

Antiepileptics (continued)
- to taxanes **(cabazitaxel)**. Avoid. [Moderate] Study → Also see **TABLE 11** p. 1574
▸ Antiepileptics **(carbamazepine, fosphenytoin, phenobarbital, phenytoin, primidone)** are predicted to decrease the exposure to taxanes **(docetaxel)**. [Severe] Theoretical → Also see **TABLE 11** p. 1574
▸ Antiepileptics **(carbamazepine, fosphenytoin, phenobarbital, phenytoin, primidone)** are predicted to decrease the exposure to taxanes **(paclitaxel)**. Avoid. [Severe] Study → Also see **TABLE 11** p. 1574
▸ **Tegafur** potentially increases the concentration of antiepileptics **(fosphenytoin, phenytoin)**. Monitor concentration and adjust dose. [Severe] Anecdotal
▸ Antiepileptics **(carbamazepine, fosphenytoin, phenobarbital, phenytoin, primidone)** are predicted to decrease the concentration of **temsirolimus**. Avoid. [Severe] Study
▸ Antiepileptics **(carbamazepine, fosphenytoin, oxcarbazepine, phenobarbital, phenytoin, primidone)** are predicted to decrease the exposure to **tenofovir alafenamide**. Avoid. [Moderate] Theoretical
▸ Antiepileptics **(carbamazepine, fosphenytoin, phenobarbital, phenytoin, primidone)** might decrease the exposure to **tepotinib**. Avoid. [Severe] Theoretical
▸ **Fosphenytoin** is predicted to decrease the concentration of tetracyclines **(doxycycline)**. Adjust dose. [Moderate] Theoretical
▸ Antiepileptics **(carbamazepine, phenobarbital, phenytoin, primidone)** decrease the concentration of tetracyclines **(doxycycline)**. Adjust dose. [Moderate] Study
▸ Antiepileptics **(carbamazepine, fosphenytoin, phenobarbital, phenytoin, primidone)** are predicted to decrease the exposure to tetracyclines **(eravacycline)**. Adjust **eravacycline** dose, p. 657. [Moderate] Study
▸ Antiepileptics **(carbamazepine, fosphenytoin, phenobarbital, phenytoin, primidone)** are predicted to decrease the exposure to **tezacaftor**. Avoid. [Severe] Theoretical
▸ Antiepileptics **(fosphenytoin, phenytoin)** are predicted to decrease the exposure to **theophylline**. Adjust dose. [Moderate] Study
▸ Antiepileptics **(phenobarbital, primidone)** are predicted to increase the clearance of **theophylline**. Adjust dose. [Moderate] Theoretical
▸ **Carbamazepine** potentially increases the clearance of **theophylline** and **theophylline** decreases the exposure to carbamazepine. Adjust dose. [Moderate] Anecdotal
▸ **Stiripentol** is predicted to increase the exposure to **theophylline**. Avoid. [Moderate] Theoretical
▸ **Carbamazepine** is predicted to decrease the exposure to thrombin inhibitors **(dabigatran)**. Avoid. [Severe] Study
▸ Antiepileptics **(fosphenytoin, phenytoin)** are predicted to decrease the exposure to thrombin inhibitors **(dabigatran)**. Avoid. [Severe] Theoretical
▸ Antiepileptics **(fosphenytoin, phenytoin)** are predicted to increase the risk of hypothyroidism when given with **thyroid hormones**. [Moderate] Study
▸ Antiepileptics **(phenobarbital, primidone)** are predicted to decrease the effects of **thyroid hormones**. [Moderate] Theoretical
▸ **Carbamazepine** is predicted to increase the risk of hypothyroidism when given with **thyroid hormones**. Monitor and adjust dose. [Moderate] Study
▸ Antiepileptics **(carbamazepine, fosphenytoin, phenobarbital, phenytoin, primidone)** are predicted to markedly decrease the exposure to **ticagrelor**. Avoid. [Severe] Study
▸ **Carbamazepine** might decrease the exposure to **tigecycline**. [Mild] Theoretical
▸ Antiepileptics **(carbamazepine, fosphenytoin, phenobarbital, phenytoin, primidone)** are predicted to decrease the exposure to **tivozanib**. [Severe] Study
▸ Antiepileptics **(fosphenytoin, phenytoin)** moderately decrease the exposure to **tizanidine**. [Mild] Study → Also see **TABLE 10** p. 1574
▸ Antiepileptics **(carbamazepine, fosphenytoin, phenobarbital, phenytoin, primidone)** are predicted to decrease the exposure to **tofacitinib**. Avoid. [Severe] Study
▸ Antiepileptics **(carbamazepine, fosphenytoin, phenobarbital, phenytoin, primidone)** are predicted to decrease the exposure

to **tolvaptan**. Use with caution or avoid depending on indication. [Severe] Study
▸ Antiepileptics **(fosphenytoin, phenytoin)** increase the clearance of **topotecan**. [Moderate] Study
▸ Antiepileptics **(carbamazepine, fosphenytoin, phenobarbital, phenytoin, primidone)** are predicted to decrease the exposure to **toremifene**. Adjust dose. [Moderate] Study
▸ Antiepileptics **(carbamazepine, fosphenytoin, phenobarbital, phenytoin, primidone)** are predicted to decrease the exposure to **trabectedin**. Avoid. [Severe] Theoretical
▸ **Carbamazepine** decreases the concentration of **trazodone**. Adjust dose. [Moderate] Anecdotal → Also see **TABLE 17** p. 1576
▸ Antiepileptics **(carbamazepine, phenobarbital, phenytoin)** are predicted to decrease the exposure to **treprostinil**. Adjust dose. [Mild] Theoretical
▸ Antiepileptics **(phenobarbital, primidone)** are predicted to decrease the exposure to **tricyclic antidepressants**. [Moderate] Study → Also see **TABLE 10** p. 1574
▸ **Carbamazepine** decreases the exposure to tricyclic **antidepressants**. Adjust dose. [Moderate] Study → Also see **TABLE 17** p. 1576
▸ Tricyclic antidepressants **(clomipramine, imipramine)** potentially increase the risk of overheating and dehydration when given with **zonisamide**. Avoid in children. [Severe] Theoretical
▸ **Valproate** increases the concentration of tricyclic antidepressants **(nortriptyline)**. [Severe] Study → Also see **TABLE 17** p. 1576
▸ **Trimethoprim** increases the concentration of antiepileptics **(fosphenytoin, phenytoin)**. [Moderate] Study
▸ Antiepileptics **(carbamazepine, fosphenytoin, phenobarbital, phenytoin, primidone)** are predicted to decrease the exposure to **tucatinib**. Avoid. [Severe] Study
▸ **Tucatinib** is predicted to very slightly increase the exposure to **perampanel**. [Mild] Study
▸ Antiepileptics **(carbamazepine, eslicarbazepine, fosphenytoin, oxcarbazepine, perampanel, phenobarbital, phenytoin, primidone, rufinamide, topiramate)** decrease the efficacy of **ulipristal**. Avoid and for 4 weeks after stopping the enzyme inducing drug. For FSRH guidance, see Contraceptives, interactions p. 917. [Severe] Anecdotal
▸ Antiepileptics **(carbamazepine, fosphenytoin, phenobarbital, phenytoin, primidone)** are predicted to decrease the exposure to **upadacitinib**. [Moderate] Study
▸ Antiepileptics **(carbamazepine, fosphenytoin, phenobarbital, phenytoin, primidone)** are predicted to decrease the exposure to **vandetanib**. Avoid. [Moderate] Study
▸ **Carbamazepine** might enhance the antidiuretic effect of **vasopressin**. [Moderate] Theoretical
▸ Antiepileptics **(carbamazepine, fosphenytoin, phenobarbital, phenytoin, primidone)** are predicted to moderately decrease the exposure to **velpatasvir**. Avoid. [Severe] Study
▸ **Oxcarbazepine** is predicted to decrease the exposure to **velpatasvir**. Avoid. [Severe] Theoretical
▸ Antiepileptics **(carbamazepine, fosphenytoin, phenobarbital, phenytoin, primidone)** are predicted to decrease the exposure to **vemurafenib**. Avoid. [Severe] Study
▸ Antiepileptics **(carbamazepine, fosphenytoin, phenobarbital, phenytoin, primidone)** are predicted to decrease the exposure to **venetoclax**. Avoid. [Severe] Study
▸ Antiepileptics **(carbamazepine, fosphenytoin, phenobarbital, phenytoin, primidone)** are predicted to decrease the exposure to vinca alkaloids **(vinblastine, vincristine, vindesine)**. [Severe] Theoretical → Also see **TABLE 17** p. 1576 → Also see **TABLE 11** p. 1574
▸ Antiepileptics **(carbamazepine, fosphenytoin, phenobarbital, phenytoin, primidone)** are predicted to decrease the exposure to vinca alkaloids **(vinorelbine)**. Use with caution or avoid. [Severe] Theoretical → Also see **TABLE 17** p. 1576 → Also see **TABLE 11** p. 1574
▸ Antiepileptics **(carbamazepine, fosphenytoin, phenobarbital, phenytoin, primidone)** are predicted to decrease the exposure to **vismodegib**. Avoid. [Moderate] Theoretical
▸ Antiepileptics **(fosphenytoin, phenytoin)** decrease the effects of **vitamin D substances**. [Moderate] Study

▶ Antiepileptics **(phenobarbital, primidone)** are predicted to decrease the effects of vitamin D substances. Moderate Theoretical

▶ **Carbamazepine** is predicted to decrease the effects of vitamin D substances. Moderate Study

▶ Antiepileptics **(carbamazepine, fosphenytoin, phenobarbital, phenytoin, primidone)** are predicted to decrease the exposure to voclosporin. Avoid. Severe Study

▶ Antiepileptics **(phenobarbital, primidone)** potentially increase the risk of nephrotoxicity when given with volatile halogenated anaesthetics (methoxyflurane). Avoid. Severe Theoretical → Also see **TABLE 10** p. 1574

▶ Antiepileptics **(carbamazepine, fosphenytoin, phenobarbital, phenytoin, primidone)** are predicted to decrease the exposure to vortioxetine. Monitor and adjust dose. Moderate Study

▶ Antiepileptics **(carbamazepine, fosphenytoin, phenobarbital, phenytoin, primidone)** are predicted to decrease the concentration of voxilaprevir. Avoid. Severe Study

▶ **Oxcarbazepine** is predicted to decrease the concentration of voxilaprevir. Avoid. Severe Theoretical

▶ Antiepileptics **(carbamazepine, fosphenytoin, phenobarbital, phenytoin, primidone)** are predicted to decrease the exposure to zanubrutinib. Avoid. Severe Study

▶ **Carbamazepine** moderately decreases the exposure to zolpidem. Moderate Study

▶ Antiepileptics **(carbamazepine, fosphenytoin, phenobarbital, phenytoin, primidone)** are predicted to decrease the exposure to zopiclone. Adjust dose. Moderate Study → Also see **TABLE 10** p. 1574

Antifungals, azoles → see **TABLE 1** p. 1571 (hepatotoxicity), **TABLE 8** p. 1573 (QT-interval prolongation)

clotrimazole · fluconazole · isavuconazole · itraconazole · ketoconazole · miconazole · posaconazole · voriconazole

▶ Since systemic absorption can follow topical application, the possibility of interactions with topical **clotrimazole** and topical **ketoconazole** should be borne in mind.

▶ In general, **fluconazole** interactions relate to multiple-dose treatment.

▶ The use of carbonated drinks, such as cola, improves **itraconazole**, **ketoconazole**, and **posaconazole** bioavailability.

▶ Interactions of **miconazole** apply to the oral gel formulation, as a sufficient quantity can be absorbed to cause systemic effects. Systemic absorption from intravaginal and topical formulations might also occur.

▶ Antifungals, azoles **(fluconazole, isavuconazole)** are predicted to increase the exposure to abemaciclib. Moderate Study

▶ Antifungals, azoles **(itraconazole, ketoconazole, posaconazole, voriconazole)** are predicted to increase the exposure to abemaciclib. Avoid or adjust dose—consult product literature. Severe Study

▶ **Fluconazole** is predicted to increase the exposure to abrocitinib. Adjust **abrocitinib** dose, p. 1430. Severe Study

▶ Antifungals, azoles **(fluconazole, isavuconazole)** are predicted to increase the exposure to acalabrutinib. Avoid or monitor. Severe Study

▶ Antifungals, azoles **(itraconazole, ketoconazole, posaconazole, voriconazole)** are predicted to increase the exposure to acalabrutinib. Avoid. Severe Study

▶ Antifungals, azoles **(itraconazole, ketoconazole)** are predicted to increase the exposure to afatinib. Moderate Study

▶ Alcohol potentially causes a disulfiram-like reaction when given with **ketoconazole**. Avoid. Moderate Anecdotal

▶ **Itraconazole** markedly increases the exposure to aliskiren. Avoid. Severe Study

▶ **Ketoconazole** moderately increases the exposure to aliskiren. Moderate Study

▶ **Itraconazole** increases the risk of busulfan toxicity when given with alkylating agents (busulfan). Monitor and adjust dose. Moderate Study

▶ **Miconazole** is predicted to increase the concentration of alkylating agents (busulfan). Use with caution and adjust dose. Moderate Theoretical

▶ **Isavuconazole** is predicted to increase the exposure to alkylating agents (cyclophosphamide). Moderate Study

▶ Antifungals, azoles **(itraconazole, ketoconazole, posaconazole, voriconazole)** are predicted to moderately increase the exposure to alpha blockers (alfuzosin, tamsulosin). Use with caution or avoid. Moderate Study

▶ Antifungals, azoles **(itraconazole, ketoconazole, posaconazole, voriconazole)** are predicted to increase the exposure to alpha blockers (doxazosin). Moderate Study

▶ Antifungals, azoles **(fluconazole, isavuconazole)** are predicted to increase the exposure to alpha blockers (tamsulosin). Moderate Theoretical

▶ **Miconazole** potentially decreases the exposure to aminoglycosides (tobramycin). Moderate Anecdotal

▶ Oral antacids decrease the absorption of oral **itraconazole** capsules. Manufacturer advises take 2 hours before or 1 hour after antacids. Moderate Study

▶ Oral antacids decrease the absorption of oral **ketoconazole**. Separate administration by at least 2 hours. Moderate Study

▶ Anti-androgens (apalutamide, enzalutamide) are predicted to decrease the exposure to **isavuconazole**. Avoid. Severe Study

▶ Antifungals, azoles **(itraconazole, ketoconazole, posaconazole, voriconazole)** are predicted to increase the exposure to anti-androgens (apalutamide). Monitor and adjust dose. Mild Study → Also see **TABLE 8** p. 1573

▶ **Itraconazole** slightly increases the exposure to anti-androgens (darolutamide). Monitor and adjust dose. Moderate Study

▶ **Ketoconazole** is predicted to increase the exposure to anti-androgens (darolutamide). Monitor and adjust dose. Moderate Theoretical

▶ Antiarrhythmics (dronedarone) are predicted to increase the exposure to **isavuconazole**. Moderate Theoretical

▶ **Itraconazole** is predicted to increase the exposure to antiarrhythmics (amiodarone). Avoid. Severe Anecdotal → Also see **TABLE 1** p. 1571

▶ Antifungals, azoles **(ketoconazole, voriconazole)** are predicted to increase the exposure to antiarrhythmics (amiodarone). Avoid. Moderate Theoretical → Also see **TABLE 1** p. 1571 → Also see **TABLE 8** p. 1573

▶ **Miconazole** is predicted to increase the exposure to antiarrhythmics (disopyramide). Use with caution and adjust dose. Severe Theoretical

▶ Antifungals, azoles **(itraconazole, ketoconazole, posaconazole, voriconazole)** are predicted to increase the exposure to antiarrhythmics (disopyramide). Avoid. Severe Theoretical → Also see **TABLE 8** p. 1573

▶ **Fluconazole** is predicted to increase the exposure to antiarrhythmics (dronedarone). Severe Theoretical → Also see **TABLE 8** p. 1573

▶ Antifungals, azoles **(itraconazole, ketoconazole, posaconazole, voriconazole)** very markedly increase the exposure to antiarrhythmics (dronedarone). Avoid. Severe Study → Also see **TABLE 8** p. 1573

▶ Antifungals, azoles **(fluconazole, isavuconazole)** are predicted to increase the exposure to antiarrhythmics (propafenone). Monitor and adjust dose. Moderate Study

▶ Antifungals, azoles **(itraconazole, ketoconazole, posaconazole, voriconazole)** are predicted to increase the exposure to antiarrhythmics (propafenone). Monitor and adjust dose. Severe Study

▶ Antifungals, azoles **(itraconazole, ketoconazole, posaconazole, voriconazole)** are predicted to increase the exposure to anticholinesterases, centrally acting (galantamine). Monitor and adjust dose. Moderate Study

▶ Antiepileptics (carbamazepine) are predicted to decrease the efficacy of **fluconazole** and **fluconazole** increases the concentration of antiepileptics (carbamazepine). Avoid or monitor **carbamazepine** concentration and adjust dose accordingly, p. 355. Severe Theoretical

▶ Antiepileptics (carbamazepine) are predicted to decrease the efficacy of **ketoconazole** and **ketoconazole** slightly increases the concentration of antiepileptics (carbamazepine). Avoid or monitor **carbamazepine** concentration and adjust dose accordingly, p. 355. Moderate Study

Antifungals, azoles (continued)

▸ Antiepileptics (carbamazepine) are predicted to decrease the efficacy of **posaconazole** and **posaconazole** increases the concentration of antiepileptics (carbamazepine). Avoid. Moderate Theoretical

▸ Antiepileptics (carbamazepine, fosphenytoin, phenobarbital, phenytoin, primidone) are predicted to decrease the exposure to **isavuconazole**. Avoid. Severe Study

▸ Antiepileptics (fosphenytoin) very markedly decrease the exposure to **itraconazole**. Avoid and for 14 days after stopping **fosphenytoin**. Moderate Study

▸ Antiepileptics (fosphenytoin) decrease the exposure to **voriconazole** and **voriconazole** increases the exposure to antiepileptics (fosphenytoin). Avoid or adjust **voriconazole** dose and monitor phenytoin concentration, p. 695. Moderate Study

▸ Antiepileptics (fosphenytoin, phenytoin) decrease the exposure to **ketoconazole**. Avoid. Moderate Study

▸ Antiepileptics (fosphenytoin, phenytoin) are predicted to decrease the exposure to **posaconazole**. Avoid. Moderate Study

▸ Antiepileptics (phenobarbital) decrease the concentration of **itraconazole**. Avoid and for 14 days after stopping **phenobarbital**. Moderate Study

▸ Antiepileptics (phenobarbital) are predicted to decrease the concentration of **ketoconazole**. Avoid. Moderate Study

▸ Antiepileptics (phenobarbital) are predicted to decrease the concentration of **posaconazole**. Avoid. Moderate Study

▸ Antiepileptics (phenobarbital, primidone) are predicted to decrease the concentration of **voriconazole**. Avoid. Moderate Theoretical

▸ Antiepileptics (phenytoin) very markedly decrease the exposure to **itraconazole**. Avoid and for 14 days after stopping **phenytoin**. Moderate Study

▸ Antiepileptics (phenytoin) decrease the exposure to **voriconazole** and **voriconazole** increases the exposure to antiepileptics (phenytoin). Avoid or adjust **voriconazole** dose and monitor **phenytoin** concentration, p. 695, p. 372. Moderate Study

▸ Antiepileptics (primidone) are predicted to decrease the concentration of **itraconazole**. Moderate Theoretical

▸ **Miconazole** increases the risk of carbamazepine toxicity when given with antiepileptics (carbamazepine). Monitor and adjust dose. Severe Anecdotal

▸ **Miconazole** increases the risk of phenytoin toxicity when given with antiepileptics (fosphenytoin). Monitor and adjust dose. Severe Anecdotal

▸ **Fluconazole** increases the concentration of antiepileptics (fosphenytoin, phenytoin). Monitor concentration and adjust dose. Moderate Study

▸ Antiepileptics (carbamazepine) are predicted to decrease the efficacy of antifungals, azoles (itraconazole, voriconazole) and antifungals, azoles (itraconazole, voriconazole) increase the concentration of antiepileptics (carbamazepine). Avoid or adjust dose. Moderate Theoretical

▸ Antiepileptics (primidone) are predicted to decrease the concentration of antifungals, azoles (**ketoconazole, posaconazole**). Avoid. Moderate Study

▸ Antifungals, azoles (itraconazole, ketoconazole, posaconazole, voriconazole) are predicted to very slightly increase the exposure to antiepileptics (perampanel). Mild Study

▸ **Miconazole** increases the risk of phenytoin toxicity when given with antiepileptics (phenytoin). Monitor and adjust dose. Severe Anecdotal

▸ Antifungals, azoles (fluconazole) are predicted to increase the exposure to antifungals, azoles (isavuconazole). Severe Theoretical

▸ Antifungals, azoles (itraconazole, ketoconazole, posaconazole, voriconazole) are predicted to increase the exposure to antifungals, azoles (isavuconazole). Avoid or monitor adverse effects. Severe Study

▸ **Miconazole** is predicted to increase the exposure to antihistamines, non-sedating (mizolastine). Avoid. Moderate Theoretical

▸ Antifungals, azoles (fluconazole, isavuconazole) are predicted to increase the exposure to antihistamines, non-sedating (mizolastine). Severe Theoretical

▸ Antifungals, azoles (itraconazole, ketoconazole, posaconazole, voriconazole) are predicted to increase the exposure to antihistamines, non-sedating (mizolastine). Avoid. Severe Study

▸ Antifungals, azoles (fluconazole, isavuconazole, itraconazole, ketoconazole, posaconazole, voriconazole) are predicted to increase the exposure to antihistamines, non-sedating (rupatadine). Avoid. Moderate Study

▸ **Ketoconazole** increases the exposure to antimalarials (mefloquine). Moderate Study

▸ Antifungals, azoles (fluconazole, itraconazole, posaconazole, voriconazole) are predicted to increase the exposure to antimalarials (mefloquine). Moderate Theoretical

▸ Antifungals, azoles (itraconazole, ketoconazole, posaconazole, voriconazole) are predicted to slightly increase the exposure to antipsychotics, second generation (aripiprazole). Adjust **aripiprazole** dose, p. 454. Moderate Study → Also see TABLE 8 p. 1573

▸ Antifungals, azoles (fluconazole, isavuconazole) are predicted to increase the exposure to antipsychotics, second generation (cariprazine). Avoid. Severe Study

▸ Antifungals, azoles (itraconazole, ketoconazole, posaconazole, voriconazole) are predicted to moderately increase the exposure to antipsychotics, second generation (cariprazine). Avoid. Severe Study

▸ Antifungals, azoles (fluconazole, isavuconazole) are predicted to increase the exposure to antipsychotics, second generation (lurasidone). Adjust **lurasidone** dose. Moderate Study

▸ Antifungals, azoles (itraconazole, ketoconazole, posaconazole, voriconazole) are predicted to increase the exposure to antipsychotics, second generation (lurasidone, quetiapine). Avoid. Severe Study

▸ Antifungals, azoles (fluconazole, isavuconazole) are predicted to increase the exposure to antipsychotics, second generation (quetiapine). Avoid. Moderate Study

▸ Antifungals, azoles (itraconazole, ketoconazole, posaconazole, voriconazole) are predicted to increase the exposure to antipsychotics, second generation (risperidone). Adjust dose. Moderate Study

▸ Antifungals, azoles (itraconazole, ketoconazole, posaconazole, voriconazole) are predicted to increase the exposure to **atogepant**. Adjust **atogepant** dose, p. 540. Moderate Study

▸ Antifungals, azoles (itraconazole, ketoconazole, posaconazole, voriconazole) are predicted to increase the exposure to avacopan. Severe Study

▸ Antifungals, azoles (fluconazole, isavuconazole) are predicted to increase the exposure to avapritinib. Avoid or adjust dose— consult product literature. Moderate Study

▸ Antifungals, azoles (itraconazole, ketoconazole, posaconazole, voriconazole) are predicted to increase the exposure to avapritinib. Avoid. Moderate Study

▸ Antifungals, azoles (fluconazole, miconazole) are predicted to increase the exposure to avatrombopag. Adjust **avatrombopag** dose with moderate CYP2C9 inhibitors in chronic immune thrombocytopenia, p. 1169. Moderate Study

▸ Antifungals, azoles (fluconazole, isavuconazole) are predicted to increase the exposure to axitinib. Moderate Study

▸ Antifungals, azoles (itraconazole, ketoconazole, posaconazole, voriconazole) are predicted to increase the exposure to axitinib. Avoid or adjust dose. Moderate Study

▸ Antifungals, azoles (fluconazole, isavuconazole) might increase the exposure to bedaquiline. Mild Theoretical → Also see TABLE 8 p. 1573

▸ Antifungals, azoles (itraconazole, ketoconazole, posaconazole, voriconazole) might increase the exposure to bedaquiline. Mild Study → Also see TABLE 8 p. 1573

▸ Antifungals, azoles (fluconazole, voriconazole) are predicted to increase the exposure to belzutifan. Monitor and adjust dose. Severe Theoretical

▸ **Miconazole** is predicted to increase the exposure to benzodiazepines (alprazolam). Use with caution and adjust dose. Moderate Theoretical

▸ Antifungals, azoles (fluconazole, isavuconazole) are predicted to increase the exposure to benzodiazepines (alprazolam). Severe Study

- Antifungals, azoles **(itraconazole, ketoconazole, posaconazole, voriconazole)** moderately increase the exposure to benzodiazepines **(alprazolam)**. Avoid. Moderate Study
- Antifungals, azoles **(fluconazole, voriconazole)** potentially increase the exposure to benzodiazepines **(clobazam)**. Adjust dose. Moderate Theoretical
- Antifungals, azoles **(fluconazole, voriconazole)** moderately increase the exposure to benzodiazepines **(diazepam)**. Monitor and adjust dose. Moderate Study
- **Miconazole** is predicted to increase the exposure to intravenous benzodiazepines **(midazolam)**. Use with caution and adjust dose. Moderate Theoretical
- **Miconazole** is predicted to increase the exposure to oral benzodiazepines **(midazolam)**. Avoid. Moderate Theoretical
- Antifungals, azoles **(fluconazole, isavuconazole)** are predicted to increase the exposure to benzodiazepines **(midazolam)**. Monitor adverse effects and adjust dose. Severe Study
- Antifungals, azoles **(itraconazole, ketoconazole, posaconazole, voriconazole)** are predicted to markedly to very markedly increase the exposure to benzodiazepines **(midazolam)**. Avoid or adjust dose. Severe Study
- **Berotralstat** is predicted to increase the exposure to isavuconazole. Moderate Theoretical
- Antifungals, azoles **(itraconazole, ketoconazole)** are predicted to increase the exposure to beta blockers, non-selective **(nadolol)**. Moderate Study
- Antifungals, azoles **(itraconazole, ketoconazole, posaconazole, voriconazole)** are predicted to increase the exposure to beta$_2$ agonists **(salmeterol)**. Avoid. Severe Study
- Antifungals, azoles **(itraconazole, ketoconazole)** are predicted to increase the exposure to bictegravir. Use with caution or avoid. Moderate Theoretical
- Antifungals, azoles **(itraconazole, ketoconazole, posaconazole, voriconazole)** slightly increase the exposure to bortezomib. Moderate Study
- Antifungals, azoles **(fluconazole, isavuconazole, itraconazole, ketoconazole, posaconazole, voriconazole)** are predicted to increase the exposure to bosutinib. Avoid or adjust dose. Severe Study → Also see **TABLE 8** p. 1573
- Antifungals, azoles **(fluconazole, isavuconazole)** are predicted to increase the exposure to brigatinib. Moderate Study
- Antifungals, azoles **(itraconazole, ketoconazole, posaconazole, voriconazole)** are predicted to increase the exposure to brigatinib. Avoid or adjust dose—consult product literature. Severe Study
- **Isavuconazole** slightly increases the exposure to bupropion. Adjust dose. Moderate Study
- Antifungals, azoles **(fluconazole, isavuconazole)** are predicted to increase the exposure to buspirone. Use with caution and adjust dose. Moderate Study
- Antifungals, azoles **(itraconazole, ketoconazole, posaconazole, voriconazole)** are predicted to increase the exposure to buspirone. Adjust **buspirone** dose, p. 396. Severe Study
- **Miconazole** is predicted to increase the concentration of buspirone. Use with caution and adjust dose. Moderate Theoretical
- Antifungals, azoles **(fluconazole, isavuconazole, itraconazole, ketoconazole, posaconazole, voriconazole)** are predicted to increase the exposure to cabozantinib. Moderate Study → Also see **TABLE 8** p. 1573
- Calcium channel blockers **(diltiazem, verapamil)** are predicted to increase the exposure to **isavuconazole**. Moderate Theoretical
- Antifungals, azoles **(fluconazole, isavuconazole)** are predicted to increase the exposure to calcium channel blockers **(amlodipine, felodipine, lacidipine, lercanidipine, nicardipine, nifedipine, nimodipine)**. Monitor and adjust dose. Moderate Study
- **Miconazole** is predicted to increase the exposure to calcium channel blockers **(amlodipine, felodipine, lacidipine, lercanidipine, nicardipine, nifedipine, nimodipine, verapamil)**. Use with caution and adjust dose. Moderate Theoretical
- Antifungals, azoles **(itraconazole, ketoconazole, posaconazole, voriconazole)** are predicted to increase the exposure to calcium channel blockers **(amlodipine, felodipine, lacidipine, nicardipine, nifedipine, nimodipine)**. Monitor and adjust dose. Moderate Study

- **Miconazole** is predicted to increase the exposure to calcium channel blockers **(diltiazem)**. Moderate Theoretical
- **Fluconazole** (high-dose) is predicted to increase the exposure to calcium channel blockers **(diltiazem, verapamil)**. Moderate Theoretical
- Antifungals, azoles **(itraconazole, ketoconazole, posaconazole, voriconazole)** are predicted to increase the exposure to calcium channel blockers **(diltiazem, verapamil)**. Severe Study
- Antifungals, azoles **(itraconazole, ketoconazole, posaconazole, voriconazole)** are predicted to markedly increase the exposure to calcium channel blockers **(lercanidipine)**. Avoid. Severe Study
- Antifungals, azoles **(itraconazole, ketoconazole, posaconazole, voriconazole)** are predicted to increase the exposure to cannabidiol. Avoid or adjust dose. Mild Study
- **Fluconazole** is predicted to increase the exposure to cannabidiol. Moderate Theoretical
- Antifungals, azoles **(fluconazole, isavuconazole, itraconazole, ketoconazole, posaconazole, voriconazole)** are predicted to increase the exposure to capivasertib. Adjust dose. Moderate Study
- **Cenobamate** is predicted to decrease the exposure to isavuconazole. Avoid. Severe Theoretical
- Antifungals, azoles **(fluconazole, isavuconazole)** are predicted to increase the exposure to ceritinib. Moderate Study → Also see **TABLE 8** p. 1573
- Antifungals, azoles **(itraconazole, voriconazole)** are predicted to increase the exposure to ceritinib. Avoid or adjust dose—consult product literature. Severe Study → Also see **TABLE 8** p. 1573
- **Ceritinib** is predicted to increase the exposure to isavuconazole. Avoid or monitor adverse effects. Severe Study
- **Ketoconazole** moderately increases the exposure to ceritinib. Avoid or adjust dose—consult product literature. Severe Study
- Antifungals, azoles **(fluconazole, isavuconazole)** are predicted to increase the concentration of ciclosporin. Severe Study
- Antifungals, azoles **(itraconazole, ketoconazole, posaconazole, voriconazole)** increase the concentration of ciclosporin. Severe Study
- **Miconazole** increases the concentration of ciclosporin. Monitor and adjust dose. Severe Anecdotal
- Antifungals, azoles **(itraconazole, ketoconazole, posaconazole, voriconazole)** are predicted to moderately increase the exposure to cilostazol. Adjust **cilostazol** dose, p. 266. Moderate Study
- **Fluconazole** is predicted to increase the exposure to cilostazol. Adjust **cilostazol** dose, p. 266. Moderate Theoretical
- **Miconazole** is predicted to increase the exposure to cilostazol. Use with caution and adjust dose. Moderate Theoretical
- Antifungals, azoles **(itraconazole, ketoconazole, posaconazole, voriconazole)** are predicted to moderately increase the exposure to cinacalcet. Adjust dose. Moderate Study
- **Fluconazole** is predicted to decrease the efficacy of clopidogrel. Avoid. Severe Theoretical
- **Voriconazole** is predicted to decrease the efficacy of clopidogrel. Avoid. Moderate Study
- **Cobicistat** is predicted to increase the exposure to antifungals, azoles **(fluconazole, posaconazole)**. Moderate Theoretical
- **Cobicistat** is predicted to increase the exposure to isavuconazole. Avoid or monitor adverse effects. Severe Study
- **Cobicistat** is predicted to increase the exposure to itraconazole. Adjust **itraconazole** dose, p. 692. Moderate Theoretical
- **Cobicistat** is predicted to increase the exposure to ketoconazole. Adjust **ketoconazole** dose, p. 794. Moderate Theoretical
- **Cobicistat** is predicted to affect the exposure to **voriconazole**. Avoid. Moderate Theoretical
- Antifungals, azoles **(fluconazole, isavuconazole)** are predicted to increase the exposure to cobimetinib. Severe Study
- Antifungals, azoles **(itraconazole, ketoconazole, posaconazole, voriconazole)** are predicted to increase the exposure to cobimetinib. Avoid or monitor for toxicity. Severe Study
- **Miconazole** is predicted to increase the exposure to cobimetinib. Severe Theoretical

Antifungals, azoles (continued)

▸ Antifungals, azoles **(fluconazole, isavuconazole)** are predicted to increase the exposure to colchicine. Adjust **colchicine** dose with moderate CYP3A4 inhibitors, p. 1279. Severe Study

▸ Antifungals, azoles **(itraconazole, ketoconazole, posaconazole, voriconazole)** are predicted to increase the exposure to colchicine. Avoid potent CYP3A4 inhibitors or adjust **colchicine** dose, p. 1279. Severe Study

▸ Antifungals, azoles **(itraconazole, ketoconazole, posaconazole, voriconazole)** are predicted to increase the exposure to corticosteroids (beclometasone) (risk with beclometasone is likely to be lower than with other corticosteroids). Moderate Theoretical

▸ Antifungals, azoles **(itraconazole, ketoconazole, posaconazole, voriconazole)** are predicted to increase the exposure to corticosteroids (betamethasone, budesonide, ciclesonide, deflazacort, dexamethasone, fludrocortisone, fluticasone, hydrocortisone, methylprednisolone, mometasone, prednisolone, triamcinolone). Avoid or monitor adverse effects. Severe Study

▸ **Miconazole** is predicted to increase the concentration of corticosteroids (methylprednisolone). Monitor and adjust dose. Moderate Theoretical

▸ Antifungals, azoles **(fluconazole, isavuconazole)** are predicted to increase the exposure to corticosteroids (methylprednisolone). Monitor and adjust dose. Moderate Study

▸ Antifungals, azoles **(itraconazole, ketoconazole, posaconazole, voriconazole)** are predicted to increase the exposure to corticosteroids (vamorolone). Adjust dose. Severe Study

▸ **Fluconazole** increases the anticoagulant effect of coumarins. Monitor INR and adjust dose. Severe Study

▸ **Itraconazole** potentially increases the anticoagulant effect of coumarins. Severe Anecdotal

▸ **Ketoconazole** potentially increases the anticoagulant effect of coumarins (warfarin). Monitor INR and adjust dose. Severe Anecdotal

▸ **Miconazole** greatly increases the anticoagulant effect of coumarins. MHRA advises avoid unless INR can be monitored closely; monitor for signs of bleeding. Severe Study

▸ **Voriconazole** increases the anticoagulant effect of coumarins. Monitor INR and adjust dose. Moderate Study

▸ Antifungals, azoles **(fluconazole, isavuconazole)** are predicted to increase the exposure to crizotinib. Moderate Study → Also see **TABLE 8** p. 1573

▸ Antifungals, azoles **(itraconazole, ketoconazole, posaconazole, voriconazole)** are predicted to increase the exposure to crizotinib. Avoid. Moderate Study → Also see **TABLE 8** p. 1573

▸ Antifungals, azoles **(fluconazole, isavuconazole)** are predicted to increase the exposure to dabrafenib. Moderate Study

▸ Antifungals, azoles **(itraconazole, ketoconazole, posaconazole, voriconazole)** are predicted to increase the exposure to dabrafenib. Use with caution or avoid. Moderate Study

▸ **Dabrafenib** is predicted to decrease the exposure to isavuconazole. Avoid. Severe Theoretical

▸ Antifungals, azoles **(fluconazole, isavuconazole)** are predicted to increase the exposure to daridorexant. Adjust **daridorexant** dose, p. 554. Severe Study

▸ Antifungals, azoles **(itraconazole, ketoconazole, posaconazole, voriconazole)** are predicted to increase the exposure to daridorexant. Avoid. Severe Study

▸ Antifungals, azoles **(itraconazole, ketoconazole, posaconazole, voriconazole)** are predicted to markedly to very markedly increase the exposure to darifenacin. Avoid. Severe Study

▸ **Fluconazole** slightly increases the exposure to darifenacin. Moderate Study

▸ **Isavuconazole** is predicted to increase the exposure to darifenacin. Moderate Study

▸ Antifungals, azoles **(fluconazole, isavuconazole)** are predicted to increase the exposure to dasatinib. Severe Study → Also see **TABLE 8** p. 1573

▸ Antifungals, azoles **(itraconazole, ketoconazole, posaconazole, voriconazole)** are predicted to increase the exposure to dasatinib. Avoid or adjust dose—consult product literature. Severe Study → Also see **TABLE 8** p. 1573

▸ Antifungals, azoles **(itraconazole, ketoconazole, posaconazole, voriconazole)** very slightly increase the exposure to delamanid. Severe Study → Also see **TABLE 8** p. 1573

▸ Antifungals, azoles **(fluconazole, isavuconazole)** are predicted to slightly increase the exposure to dienogest. Moderate Study

▸ Antifungals, azoles **(itraconazole, ketoconazole, posaconazole, voriconazole)** are predicted to moderately increase the exposure to dienogest. Moderate Study

▸ **Isavuconazole** slightly increases the exposure to digoxin. Monitor and adjust dose. Moderate Study

▸ **Itraconazole** increases the concentration of digoxin. Monitor and adjust dose. Severe Study

▸ **Ketoconazole** is predicted to markedly increase the concentration of digoxin. Severe Study

▸ **Posaconazole** is predicted to increase the concentration of digoxin. Severe Study

▸ Antifungals, azoles **(fluconazole, isavuconazole)** are predicted to increase the exposure to dipeptidylpeptidase-4 inhibitors (saxagliptin). Mild Study

▸ Antifungals, azoles **(itraconazole, ketoconazole, posaconazole, voriconazole)** are predicted to increase the exposure to dipeptidylpeptidase-4 inhibitors (saxagliptin). Moderate Study

▸ Antifungals, azoles **(fluconazole, isavuconazole, itraconazole, ketoconazole, posaconazole, voriconazole)** are predicted to increase the exposure to domperidone. Avoid. Severe Study

▸ Antifungals, azoles **(fluconazole, isavuconazole)** are predicted to increase the exposure to dopamine receptor agonists (bromocriptine). Severe Theoretical

▸ Antifungals, azoles **(itraconazole, ketoconazole, posaconazole, voriconazole)** increase the exposure to dopamine receptor agonists (bromocriptine). Severe Study

▸ Antifungals, azoles **(fluconazole, isavuconazole, itraconazole, ketoconazole, posaconazole, voriconazole)** are predicted to increase the concentration of dopamine receptor agonists (cabergoline). Moderate Anecdotal

▸ **Isavuconazole** is predicted to increase the exposure to dopamine receptor agonists (pramipexole). Adjust dose. Moderate Study

▸ Antifungals, azoles **(itraconazole, ketoconazole, posaconazole, voriconazole)** are predicted to increase the exposure to dronabinol. Adjust dose. Mild Study

▸ Antifungals, azoles **(fluconazole, isavuconazole, itraconazole, posaconazole, voriconazole)** are predicted to increase the exposure to drospirenone. Severe Study

▸ **Ketoconazole** moderately increases the exposure to drospirenone. Severe Study

▸ Antifungals, azoles **(fluconazole, isavuconazole)** are predicted to moderately increase the exposure to dutasteride. Mild Study

▸ Antifungals, azoles **(itraconazole, ketoconazole, posaconazole, voriconazole)** are predicted to increase the exposure to dutasteride. Monitor adverse effects and adjust dose. Moderate Theoretical

▸ Antifungals, azoles **(fluconazole, isavuconazole)** are predicted to increase the exposure to elacestrant. Avoid moderate CYP3A4 inhibitors or adjust **elacestrant** dose, p. 1084. Severe Theoretical

▸ Antifungals, azoles **(itraconazole, ketoconazole, posaconazole, voriconazole)** are predicted to increase the exposure to elacestrant. Avoid potent CYP3A4 inhibitors or adjust **elacestrant** dose, p. 1084. Severe Study

▸ Antifungals, azoles **(fluconazole, isavuconazole)** are predicted to increase the exposure to elexacaftor. Adjust ivacaftor with tezacaftor and elexacaftor p. 337 dose with moderate CYP3A4 inhibitors. Severe Theoretical

▸ Antifungals, azoles **(itraconazole, ketoconazole, posaconazole, voriconazole)** are predicted to increase the exposure to elexacaftor. Adjust ivacaftor with tezacaftor and elexacaftor p. 337 dose with potent CYP3A4 inhibitors. Severe Study

▸ Antifungals, azoles **(fluconazole, isavuconazole, itraconazole, ketoconazole, posaconazole, voriconazole)** are predicted to increase the exposure to eliglustat. Avoid or adjust dose— consult product literature. Severe Study

▸ Antifungals, azoles **(fluconazole, isavuconazole)** are predicted to moderately increase the exposure to encorafenib. Moderate Study → Also see **TABLE 8** p. 1573

- Antifungals, azoles (itraconazole, ketoconazole, posaconazole, voriconazole) are predicted to increase the exposure to encorafenib. Avoid or monitor. Severe Study → Also see TABLE 8 p. 1573
- Encorafenib is predicted to decrease the exposure to isavuconazole. Avoid. Severe Study
- Endothelin receptor antagonists (bosentan) are predicted to decrease the exposure to isavuconazole. Avoid. Severe Theoretical
- Fluconazole is predicted to increase the exposure to endothelin receptor antagonists (bosentan). Avoid. Severe Study
- Itraconazole is predicted to increase the exposure to endothelin receptor antagonists (bosentan). Moderate Theoretical
- Ketoconazole moderately increases the exposure to endothelin receptor antagonists (bosentan). Moderate Study
- Voriconazole is predicted to increase the exposure to endothelin receptor antagonists (bosentan). Avoid. Severe Theoretical
- Antifungals, azoles (fluconazole, isavuconazole, miconazole) are predicted to increase the exposure to endothelin receptor antagonists (macitentan). Manufacturer advises caution depending on other drugs taken—consult product literature. Moderate Theoretical
- Antifungals, azoles (itraconazole, ketoconazole, posaconazole, voriconazole) are predicted to increase the exposure to endothelin receptor antagonists (macitentan). Moderate Study
- Antifungals, azoles (itraconazole, ketoconazole, posaconazole, voriconazole) are predicted to increase the exposure to the cytotoxic component of enfortumab vedotin. Severe Theoretical
- Antifungals, azoles (fluconazole, isavuconazole) are predicted to increase the exposure to entrectinib. Avoid or adjust dose with moderate CYP3A4 inhibitors—consult product literature. Severe Theoretical → Also see TABLE 8 p. 1573
- Antifungals, azoles (itraconazole, ketoconazole, posaconazole, voriconazole) are predicted to increase the exposure to entrectinib. Avoid or adjust dose with potent CYP3A4 inhibitors—consult product literature. Severe Study → Also see TABLE 8 p. 1573
- Antifungals, azoles (fluconazole, itraconazole, ketoconazole, miconazole, posaconazole, voriconazole) are predicted to increase the exposure to erdafitinib. Adjust dose. Severe Study
- Antifungals, azoles (fluconazole, isavuconazole) are predicted to increase the risk of ergotism when given with ergometrine. Severe Theoretical
- Antifungals, azoles (itraconazole, ketoconazole, posaconazole, voriconazole) are predicted to increase the risk of ergotism when given with ergometrine. Avoid. Severe Theoretical
- Miconazole is predicted to increase the exposure to ergometrine. Avoid. Moderate Theoretical
- Antifungals, azoles (fluconazole, isavuconazole) are predicted to increase the exposure to erlotinib. Moderate Study
- Antifungals, azoles (itraconazole, ketoconazole, posaconazole, voriconazole) are predicted to increase the exposure to erlotinib. Use with caution and adjust dose. Severe Study
- Antifungals, azoles (itraconazole, ketoconazole, posaconazole, voriconazole) are predicted to increase the exposure to esketamine. Adjust dose. Moderate Study
- Antifungals, azoles (itraconazole, ketoconazole, posaconazole, voriconazole) are predicted to increase the exposure to eszopiclone. Adjust eszopiclone dose; avoid in the elderly, p. 554. Moderate Study
- Antifungals, azoles (itraconazole, ketoconazole, posaconazole, voriconazole) are predicted to increase the concentration of subdermal etonogestrel. Moderate Theoretical
- Antifungals, azoles (isavuconazole, itraconazole, ketoconazole, posaconazole, voriconazole) are predicted to increase the exposure to etrasimod. Avoid in poor CYP2C9 metabolisers. Severe Theoretical
- Fluconazole slightly increases the exposure to etrasimod. Avoid. Severe Study
- Antifungals, azoles (fluconazole, isavuconazole) are predicted to increase the concentration of everolimus. Avoid or adjust dose. Moderate Study
- Antifungals, azoles (itraconazole, ketoconazole, posaconazole, voriconazole) are predicted to increase the exposure to everolimus. Avoid. Severe Study
- Fluconazole might increase the risk of bleeding when given with factor XA inhibitors (apixaban). Moderate Study
- Antifungals, azoles (posaconazole, voriconazole) are predicted to increase the exposure to factor XA inhibitors (apixaban). Avoid. Moderate Theoretical
- Itraconazole is predicted to increase the exposure to factor XA inhibitors (apixaban, rivaroxaban). Avoid. Severe Theoretical
- Ketoconazole moderately increases the exposure to factor XA inhibitors (apixaban, rivaroxaban). Avoid. Severe Study
- Itraconazole is predicted to increase the exposure to factor XA inhibitors (edoxaban). Severe Theoretical
- Ketoconazole slightly increases the exposure to factor XA inhibitors (edoxaban). Adjust edoxaban dose, p. 147. Severe Study
- Antifungals, azoles (posaconazole, voriconazole) are predicted to increase the exposure to factor XA inhibitors (rivaroxaban). Avoid. Severe Theoretical
- Antifungals, azoles (itraconazole, ketoconazole, posaconazole, voriconazole) are predicted to increase the exposure to fedratinib. Adjust dose, but avoid depending on other drugs taken—consult product literature. Moderate Study
- Fluconazole is predicted to increase the exposure to fedratinib. Avoid. Moderate Theoretical
- Isavuconazole is predicted to increase the exposure to fedratinib. Monitor and adjust dose. Moderate Study
- Antifungals, azoles (fluconazole, isavuconazole) are predicted to increase the exposure to fesoterodine. Adjust fesoterodine dose with moderate CYP3A4 inhibitors in hepatic and renal impairment, p. 897. Mild Study
- Antifungals, azoles (itraconazole, ketoconazole, posaconazole, voriconazole) are predicted to moderately increase the exposure to fesoterodine. Adjust fesoterodine dose with potent CYP3A4 inhibitors; avoid in hepatic and renal impairment, p. 897. Severe Study
- Antifungals, azoles (itraconazole, ketoconazole) are predicted to increase the exposure to fidaxomicin. Avoid. Moderate Study
- Antifungals, azoles (itraconazole, ketoconazole, posaconazole, voriconazole) are predicted to increase the exposure to fostamatinib. Monitor adverse effects and adjust dose. Moderate Study
- Antifungals, azoles (fluconazole, isavuconazole) are predicted to increase the exposure to gefitinib. Moderate Study
- Antifungals, azoles (itraconazole, ketoconazole, posaconazole, voriconazole) are predicted to increase the exposure to gefitinib. Severe Study
- Antifungals, azoles (itraconazole, ketoconazole, posaconazole, voriconazole) are predicted to increase the exposure to gilteritinib. Moderate Study
- Antifungals, azoles (itraconazole, ketoconazole, posaconazole, voriconazole) are predicted to increase the exposure to glasdegib. Use with caution or avoid. Severe Study → Also see TABLE 8 p. 1573
- Antifungals, azoles (itraconazole, ketoconazole) potentially increase the exposure to glecaprevir. Moderate Theoretical
- Antifungals, azoles (itraconazole, ketoconazole, posaconazole, voriconazole) are predicted to moderately to markedly increase the exposure to grazoprevir. Avoid. Severe Study
- Antifungals, azoles (fluconazole, isavuconazole) are predicted to increase the concentration of guanfacine. Adjust guanfacine dose, p. 407. Moderate Theoretical
- Antifungals, azoles (itraconazole, ketoconazole, posaconazole, voriconazole) are predicted to increase the exposure to guanfacine. Adjust guanfacine dose, p. 407. Moderate Study
- H$_2$ receptor antagonists are predicted to decrease the absorption of itraconazole. Administer itraconazole capsules with an acidic beverage. Moderate Study
- H$_2$ receptor antagonists are predicted to decrease the absorption of ketoconazole. Administer ketoconazole with an acidic beverage. Moderate Study
- H$_2$ receptor antagonists are predicted to decrease the exposure to posaconazole. Avoid use of posaconazole oral suspension. Moderate Study

Antifungals, azoles (continued)

▸ **Itraconazole** increases the concentration of haloperidol. Moderate Study

▸ **HIV-protease inhibitors** are predicted to increase the exposure to **isavuconazole**. Avoid or monitor adverse effects. Severe Study

▸ **HIV-protease inhibitors** are predicted to increase the exposure to **itraconazole**. Use with caution and adjust dose. Severe Study → Also see **TABLE 1** p. 1571

▸ **HIV-protease inhibitors** are predicted to increase the exposure to **ketoconazole**. Use with caution and adjust dose. Moderate Study

▸ **Miconazole** is predicted to increase the concentration of HIV-protease inhibitors. Use with caution and adjust dose. Moderate Theoretical

▸ **Posaconazole** is predicted to increase the exposure to HIV-protease inhibitors. Moderate Study

▸ **HIV-protease inhibitors** are predicted to affect the exposure to **voriconazole** and **voriconazole** potentially affects the exposure to HIV-protease inhibitors. Severe Study → Also see **TABLE 1** p. 1571

▸ Antifungals, azoles (fluconazole, isavuconazole) are predicted to increase the exposure to ibrutinib. Adjust dose with moderate CYP3A4 inhibitors—consult product literature. Severe Study

▸ Antifungals, azoles (itraconazole, ketoconazole, posaconazole, voriconazole) are predicted to increase the exposure to ibrutinib. Avoid or adjust dose with potent CYP3A4 inhibitors—consult product literature. Severe Study

▸ Antifungals, azoles (itraconazole, voriconazole) are predicted to increase the exposure to idelalisib. Moderate Theoretical

▸ **Idelalisib** is predicted to increase the exposure to **isavuconazole**. Avoid or monitor adverse effects. Severe Study

▸ **Ketoconazole** slightly increases the exposure to idelalisib. Moderate Study

▸ Antifungals, azoles (itraconazole, ketoconazole, posaconazole, voriconazole) are predicted to increase the exposure to imatinib. Moderate Study

▸ **Fluconazole** is predicted to increase the exposure to imatinib. Moderate Theoretical

▸ **Imatinib** is predicted to increase the exposure to **isavuconazole**. Moderate Theoretical

▸ Antifungals, azoles (itraconazole, ketoconazole, posaconazole, voriconazole) are predicted to increase the risk of toxicity when given with irinotecan. Avoid. Severe Study

▸ Antifungals, azoles (fluconazole, isavuconazole) are predicted to increase the exposure to ivabradine. Adjust **ivabradine** dose, p. 245. Severe Theoretical

▸ Antifungals, azoles (itraconazole, ketoconazole, posaconazole, voriconazole) are predicted to increase the exposure to ivabradine. Avoid. Severe Study

▸ Antifungals, azoles (fluconazole, isavuconazole) are predicted to increase the exposure to ivacaftor. Adjust dose with moderate CYP3A4 inhibitors, see ivacaftor p. 336, tezacaftor with ivacaftor p. 339, and ivacaftor with tezacaftor and elexacaftor p. 337. Moderate Study

▸ Antifungals, azoles (itraconazole, ketoconazole, posaconazole, voriconazole) are predicted to increase the exposure to ivacaftor. Adjust dose with potent CYP3A4 inhibitors, see ivacaftor p. 336, lumacaftor with ivacaftor p. 338, tezacaftor with ivacaftor p. 339, and ivacaftor with tezacaftor and elexacaftor p. 337. Severe Study

▸ Antifungals, azoles (fluconazole, isavuconazole, voriconazole) are predicted to increase the exposure to ivosidenib. Monitor and adjust dose—consult product literature. Severe Study → Also see **TABLE 8** p. 1573

▸ **Ivosidenib** is predicted to decrease the exposure to **isavuconazole**. Avoid. Severe Study

▸ **Itraconazole** moderately increases the exposure to ivosidenib and **ivosidenib** is predicted to decrease the exposure to **itraconazole**. Avoid or adjust dose—consult product literature. Severe Study

▸ **Ketoconazole** is predicted to increase the exposure to ivosidenib and **ivosidenib** is predicted to decrease the exposure to **ketoconazole**. Avoid or adjust dose—consult product literature. Severe Study

▸ **Lanthanum** is predicted to decrease the absorption of **ketoconazole**. Separate administration by at least 2 hours. Moderate Theoretical

▸ Antifungals, azoles (fluconazole, isavuconazole) are predicted to increase the exposure to lapatinib. Moderate Study → Also see **TABLE 8** p. 1573

▸ Antifungals, azoles (itraconazole, ketoconazole, posaconazole, voriconazole) are predicted to increase the exposure to lapatinib. Avoid. Moderate Study → Also see **TABLE 8** p. 1573

▸ Antifungals, azoles (fluconazole, isavuconazole) are predicted to increase the exposure to larotrectinib. Monitor and adjust dose. Moderate Theoretical

▸ Antifungals, azoles (itraconazole, ketoconazole, posaconazole, voriconazole) are predicted to moderately increase the exposure to larotrectinib. Avoid or adjust dose—consult product literature. Moderate Study

▸ Antifungals, azoles (fluconazole, isavuconazole, itraconazole, ketoconazole, posaconazole, voriconazole) are predicted to increase the exposure to leniolisib. Avoid. Moderate Study

▸ **Letermovir** is predicted to increase the exposure to **isavuconazole**. Moderate Theoretical

▸ **Letermovir** slightly decreases the exposure to **voriconazole**. Moderate Study

▸ Antifungals, azoles (fluconazole, isavuconazole) are predicted to increase the exposure to lomitapide. Avoid. Moderate Theoretical → Also see **TABLE 1** p. 1571

▸ Antifungals, azoles (itraconazole, ketoconazole, posaconazole, voriconazole) are predicted to markedly increase the exposure to lomitapide. Avoid. Severe Study → Also see **TABLE 1** p. 1571

▸ **Clotrimazole** is predicted to increase the exposure to lomitapide. Separate administration by 12 hours. Moderate Theoretical

▸ Antifungals, azoles (itraconazole, ketoconazole, posaconazole, voriconazole) are predicted to increase the exposure to lorlatinib. Avoid or adjust dose—consult product literature. Severe Study

▸ **Fluconazole** is predicted to increase the exposure to lorlatinib. Moderate Theoretical

▸ **Lorlatinib** is predicted to decrease the exposure to **isavuconazole**. Avoid. Severe Theoretical

▸ **Lumacaftor** is predicted to decrease the exposure to antifungals, azoles (itraconazole, ketoconazole, posaconazole, voriconazole). Avoid or monitor efficacy. Moderate Theoretical

▸ **Lumacaftor** is predicted to decrease the exposure to **isavuconazole**. Avoid. Severe Study

▸ Macrolides (clarithromycin) are predicted to increase the exposure to **isavuconazole**. Avoid or monitor adverse effects. Severe Study

▸ Macrolides (erythromycin) are predicted to increase the exposure to **isavuconazole**. Moderate Theoretical

▸ Antifungals, azoles (itraconazole, ketoconazole, voriconazole) are predicted to markedly increase the exposure to maraviroc. Adjust dose. Severe Study

▸ Antifungals, azoles (fluconazole, isavuconazole) are predicted to increase the exposure to mavacamten. Adjust dose—consult product literature. Moderate Study

▸ Antifungals, azoles (itraconazole, ketoconazole, posaconazole, voriconazole) are predicted to increase the exposure to mavacamten. Avoid or monitor—consult product literature. Severe Study

▸ Antifungals, azoles (itraconazole, ketoconazole, posaconazole, voriconazole) are predicted to increase the concentration of intramuscular medroxyprogesterone. Moderate Theoretical

▸ **Isavuconazole** is predicted to increase the exposure to metformin. Use with caution and adjust dose. Moderate Study

▸ **Metoclopramide** potentially decreases the absorption of **posaconazole** oral suspension. Moderate Study

▸ Antifungals, azoles (fluconazole, isavuconazole) are predicted to increase the exposure to midostaurin. Moderate Theoretical

▸ Antifungals, azoles (itraconazole, ketoconazole, posaconazole, voriconazole) are predicted to increase the exposure to midostaurin. Avoid or monitor for toxicity. Severe Study

▸ **Posaconazole** is predicted to increase the exposure to mifepristone. Moderate Theoretical

▸ Antifungals, azoles **(fluconazole, isavuconazole)** are predicted to increase the exposure to mineralocorticoid receptor antagonists **(eplerenone)**. Adjust **eplerenone** dose, p. 223. Severe Study

▸ Antifungals, azoles **(itraconazole, ketoconazole, posaconazole, voriconazole)** are predicted to markedly increase the exposure to mineralocorticoid receptor antagonists **(eplerenone)**. Avoid. Severe Study

▸ Antifungals, azoles **(fluconazole, isavuconazole)** are predicted to increase the exposure to mineralocorticoid receptor antagonists **(finerenone)**. Severe Study

▸ Antifungals, azoles **(itraconazole, ketoconazole, posaconazole, voriconazole)** are predicted to increase the exposure to mineralocorticoid receptor antagonists **(finerenone)**. Avoid. Severe Study

▸ Antifungals, azoles **(itraconazole, ketoconazole, posaconazole, voriconazole)** are predicted to increase the exposure to **mirabegron**. Adjust **mirabegron** dose in hepatic and renal impairment, p. 901. Moderate Study

▸ Antifungals, azoles **(itraconazole, ketoconazole, posaconazole, voriconazole)** are predicted to increase the exposure to **mirtazapine**. Moderate Study

▸ **Mitotane** is predicted to decrease the exposure to **isavuconazole**. Avoid. Severe Study

▸ Antifungals, azoles **(fluconazole, isavuconazole)** are predicted to increase the exposure to **mobocertinib**. Avoid or adjust dose and monitor ECG—consult product literature. Severe Study → Also see **TABLE 8** p. 1573

▸ Antifungals, azoles **(itraconazole, ketoconazole, posaconazole, voriconazole)** are predicted to increase the exposure to **mobocertinib**. Avoid. Severe Study → Also see **TABLE 8** p. 1573

▸ Antifungals, azoles **(itraconazole, ketoconazole, posaconazole, voriconazole)** are predicted to increase the exposure to **modafinil**. Mild Theoretical

▸ Monoclonal antibodies **(mosunetuzumab)** are predicted to transiently increase the exposure to **voriconazole**. Monitor and adjust dose. Moderate Theoretical

▸ Antifungals, azoles **(itraconazole, ketoconazole, posaconazole, voriconazole)** are predicted to increase the risk of neutropenia when given with monoclonal antibodies **(brentuximab vedotin)**. Monitor and adjust dose. Severe Study

▸ Antifungals, azoles **(itraconazole, ketoconazole, posaconazole, voriconazole)** are predicted to increase the exposure to monoclonal antibodies **(polatuzumab vedotin)**. Moderate Theoretical

▸ Antifungals, azoles **(itraconazole, ketoconazole, posaconazole, voriconazole)** are predicted to increase the exposure to the cytotoxic component of monoclonal antibodies **(trastuzumab emtansine)**. Avoid or monitor. Severe Theoretical

▸ **Isavuconazole** increases the exposure to **mycophenolate**. Moderate Study

▸ Antifungals, azoles **(fluconazole, isavuconazole)** are predicted to increase the exposure to **naldemedine**. Moderate Study

▸ Antifungals, azoles **(itraconazole, ketoconazole, posaconazole, voriconazole)** are predicted to increase the exposure to **naldemedine**. Avoid or monitor. Moderate Study

▸ Antifungals, azoles **(fluconazole, isavuconazole)** are predicted to increase the exposure to **naloxegol**. Adjust **naloxegol** dose and monitor adverse effects, p. 72. Moderate Study

▸ Antifungals, azoles **(itraconazole, ketoconazole, posaconazole, voriconazole)** are predicted to markedly increase the exposure to **naloxegol**. Avoid. Severe Study

▸ Antifungals, azoles **(fluconazole, isavuconazole)** are predicted to increase the exposure to **neratinib**. Avoid moderate CYP3A4 inhibitors or adjust dose and monitor for gastrointestinal adverse effects—consult product literature. Severe Study → Also see **TABLE 1** p. 1571

▸ Antifungals, azoles **(itraconazole, ketoconazole, posaconazole, voriconazole)** are predicted to increase the exposure to **neratinib**. Avoid or adjust dose with potent CYP3A4 inhibitors—consult product literature. Severe Study → Also see **TABLE 1** p. 1571

▸ Neurokinin-1 receptor antagonists **(aprepitant)** are predicted to increase the exposure to **isavuconazole**. Moderate Theoretical

▸ Neurokinin-1 receptor antagonists **(netupitant)** are predicted to decrease the exposure to **isavuconazole**. Moderate Theoretical

▸ **Fluconazole** is predicted to increase the exposure to neurokinin-1 receptor antagonists **(aprepitant)**. Moderate Theoretical

▸ Antifungals, azoles **(itraconazole, ketoconazole, posaconazole, voriconazole)** are predicted to markedly increase the exposure to neurokinin-1 receptor antagonists **(aprepitant)**. Moderate Study

▸ Antifungals, azoles **(itraconazole, ketoconazole, posaconazole, voriconazole)** are predicted to increase the exposure to neurokinin-1 receptor antagonists **(fosaprepitant)**. Moderate Theoretical

▸ Antifungals, azoles **(itraconazole, ketoconazole, posaconazole, voriconazole)** are predicted to increase the exposure to neurokinin-1 receptor antagonists **(netupitant)**. Moderate Study

▸ Antifungals, azoles **(fluconazole, isavuconazole)** are predicted to increase the exposure to **nilotinib**. Moderate Study → Also see **TABLE 8** p. 1573

▸ Antifungals, azoles **(itraconazole, ketoconazole, posaconazole, voriconazole)** are predicted to increase the exposure to **nilotinib**. Avoid. Severe Study → Also see **TABLE 8** p. 1573

▸ Antifungals, azoles **(itraconazole, ketoconazole)** are predicted to increase the exposure to **nintedanib**. Moderate Study

▸ **Voriconazole** is predicted to increase the exposure to **nintedanib**. Moderate Theoretical

▸ **Nirmatrelvir** boosted with ritonavir is predicted to increase the concentration of **isavuconazole**. Severe Theoretical

▸ **Nirmatrelvir** boosted with ritonavir increases the exposure to **itraconazole**. Severe Study

▸ **Nirmatrelvir** boosted with ritonavir is predicted to increase the concentration of **ketoconazole**. Adjust dose. Moderate Theoretical

▸ **Nirmatrelvir** boosted with ritonavir is predicted to decrease the concentration of **voriconazole**. Avoid. Severe Theoretical

▸ Antifungals, azoles **(itraconazole, ketoconazole, posaconazole, voriconazole)** are predicted to increase the exposure to **nitisinone**. Adjust dose. Moderate Theoretical

▸ NNRTIs **(efavirenz)** slightly decrease the exposure to **itraconazole**. Avoid and for 14 days after stopping **efavirenz**. Moderate Study

▸ NNRTIs **(efavirenz)** moderately decrease the exposure to **ketoconazole**. Severe Study

▸ NNRTIs **(efavirenz)** slightly decrease the exposure to **posaconazole**. Avoid. Moderate Study

▸ NNRTIs **(efavirenz)** moderately decrease the exposure to **voriconazole** and **voriconazole** slightly increases the exposure to NNRTIs **(efavirenz)**. Adjust dose. Severe Study → Also see **TABLE 8** p. 1573

▸ NNRTIs **(efavirenz, etravirine, nevirapine)** are predicted to decrease the exposure to **isavuconazole**. Avoid. Severe Theoretical

▸ NNRTIs **(nevirapine)** moderately decrease the exposure to **itraconazole**. Avoid and for 14 days after stopping **nevirapine**. Moderate Study → Also see **TABLE 1** p. 1571

▸ NNRTIs **(nevirapine)** moderately decrease the exposure to **ketoconazole**. Avoid. Severe Study

▸ NNRTIs **(nevirapine)** are predicted to decrease the exposure to **voriconazole** and **voriconazole** increases the exposure to NNRTIs **(nevirapine)**. Monitor and adjust dose. Severe Theoretical → Also see **TABLE 1** p. 1571

▸ **Fluconazole** slightly to moderately increases the exposure to NNRTIs **(nevirapine)**. Moderate Study → Also see **TABLE 1** p. 1571

▸ **Fluconazole** slightly increases the exposure to NRTIs **(zidovudine)**. Moderate Study → Also see **TABLE 1** p. 1571

▸ **Fluconazole** moderately increases the exposure to NSAIDs **(celecoxib)**. Adjust **celecoxib** dose, p. 1295. Moderate Study

▸ **Voriconazole** slightly increases the exposure to NSAIDs **(diclofenac)**. Monitor and adjust dose. Moderate Study

▸ **Voriconazole** moderately increases the exposure to NSAIDs **(ibuprofen)**. Adjust dose. Moderate Study

▸ **Fluconazole** increases the exposure to NSAIDs **(parecoxib)**. Monitor and adjust dose. Moderate Study

▸ Antifungals, azoles **(fluconazole, isavuconazole)** are predicted to increase the exposure to **olaparib**. Avoid or adjust dose with moderate CYP3A4 inhibitors—consult product literature. Moderate Theoretical

▸ Antifungals, azoles **(itraconazole, ketoconazole, posaconazole, voriconazole)** are predicted to increase the exposure to

Antifungals, azoles (continued)

olaparib. Avoid or adjust dose with potent CYP3A4 inhibitors—consult product literature. Moderate Study

▶ **Miconazole** is predicted to increase the exposure to opioids (alfentanil). Use with caution and adjust dose. Moderate Theoretical

▶ Antifungals, azoles **(fluconazole, isavuconazole)** are predicted to increase the exposure to opioids (alfentanil, buprenorphine, fentanyl, oxycodone). Monitor and adjust dose. Moderate Study

▶ Antifungals, azoles **(itraconazole, ketoconazole, posaconazole, voriconazole)** are predicted to increase the exposure to opioids (alfentanil, buprenorphine, fentanyl, oxycodone). Monitor and adjust dose. Severe Study

▶ Antifungals, azoles **(itraconazole, ketoconazole, voriconazole)** are predicted to increase the exposure to opioids (methadone). Adjust dose. Severe Theoretical → Also see TABLE 8 p. 1573

▶ Antifungals, azoles **(fluconazole, isavuconazole)** are predicted to increase the exposure to opioids (methadone, sufentanil). Moderate Theoretical → Also see TABLE 8 p. 1573

▶ Antifungals, azoles **(itraconazole, ketoconazole, posaconazole, voriconazole)** are predicted to increase the exposure to opioids (sufentanil). Moderate Study

▶ Antifungals, azoles **(itraconazole, ketoconazole, posaconazole, voriconazole)** are predicted to increase the exposure to osilodrostat. Moderate Theoretical → Also see TABLE 8 p. 1573

▶ Antifungals, azoles **(itraconazole, ketoconazole, posaconazole, voriconazole)** are predicted to increase the exposure to ospemifene. Avoid in poor CYP2C9 metabolisers. Moderate Study

▶ **Fluconazole** increases the exposure to ospemifene. Use with caution or avoid. Moderate Study

▶ Antifungals, azoles **(itraconazole, ketoconazole, posaconazole, voriconazole)** are predicted to increase the exposure to oxybutynin. Mild Study

▶ Antifungals, azoles **(itraconazole, ketoconazole, posaconazole, voriconazole)** are predicted to increase the exposure to palbociclib. Avoid or adjust dose—consult product literature. Severe Study

▶ Antifungals, azoles **(itraconazole, ketoconazole, posaconazole, voriconazole)** are predicted to increase the exposure to panobinostat. Adjust dose—consult product literature; in hepatic impairment avoid. Moderate Study → Also see TABLE 8 p. 1573

▶ Antifungals, azoles **(fluconazole, isavuconazole)** are predicted to increase the exposure to pazopanib. Moderate Study → Also see TABLE 8 p. 1573

▶ Antifungals, azoles **(itraconazole, ketoconazole, posaconazole, voriconazole)** are predicted to increase the exposure to pazopanib. Avoid or adjust dose—consult product literature. Moderate Study → Also see TABLE 8 p. 1573

▶ Antifungals, azoles **(fluconazole, isavuconazole)** are predicted to increase the exposure to pemigatinib. Severe Study

▶ Antifungals, azoles **(itraconazole, ketoconazole, posaconazole, voriconazole)** are predicted to increase the exposure to pemigatinib. Avoid or adjust dose—consult product literature. Severe Study

▶ Penicillins **(flucloxacillin)** (particularly high-dose) might greatly decrease the concentration of **isavuconazole**. Moderate Anecdotal

▶ Penicillins **(flucloxacillin)** (particularly high-dose) might greatly decrease the concentration of **posaconazole**. Moderate Study

▶ Penicillins **(flucloxacillin)** (particularly high-dose) might greatly decrease the concentration of **voriconazole**. Avoid or monitor. Moderate Study

▶ **Miconazole** greatly increases the anticoagulant effect of phenindione. Severe Theoretical

▶ Antifungals, azoles **(fluconazole, isavuconazole)** are predicted to increase the exposure to phosphodiesterase type-5 inhibitors (avanafil). Adjust **avanafil** dose, p. 939. Moderate Theoretical

▶ Antifungals, azoles **(itraconazole, ketoconazole, posaconazole, voriconazole)** are predicted to increase the exposure to phosphodiesterase type-5 inhibitors (avanafil, vardenafil). Avoid. Severe Study → Also see TABLE 8 p. 1573

▶ **Miconazole** is predicted to increase the exposure to phosphodiesterase type-5 inhibitors (sildenafil). Use with caution and adjust dose. Severe Theoretical

▶ Antifungals, azoles **(fluconazole, isavuconazole)** are predicted to increase the exposure to phosphodiesterase type-5 inhibitors (sildenafil). Monitor or adjust **sildenafil** dose with moderate CYP3A4 inhibitors, p. 940. Moderate Study

▶ Antifungals, azoles **(itraconazole, ketoconazole, posaconazole, voriconazole)** are predicted to increase the exposure to phosphodiesterase type-5 inhibitors (sildenafil). Avoid potent CYP3A4 inhibitors or adjust **sildenafil** dose, p. 940. Severe Study

▶ Antifungals, azoles **(fluconazole, isavuconazole)** are predicted to increase the exposure to phosphodiesterase type-5 inhibitors (tadalafil). Severe Theoretical

▶ Antifungals, azoles **(itraconazole, ketoconazole, posaconazole, voriconazole)** are predicted to increase the exposure to phosphodiesterase type-5 inhibitors (tadalafil). Use with caution or avoid. Severe Study

▶ Antifungals, azoles **(fluconazole, isavuconazole)** are predicted to increase the exposure to phosphodiesterase type-5 inhibitors (vardenafil). Adjust dose. Severe Theoretical → Also see TABLE 8 p. 1573

▶ Antifungals, azoles **(itraconazole, ketoconazole)** are predicted to increase the exposure to pibrentasvir. Moderate Theoretical

▶ Antifungals, azoles **(fluconazole, isavuconazole)** are predicted to increase the exposure to pimozide. Avoid. Severe Theoretical → Also see TABLE 8 p. 1573

▶ Antifungals, azoles **(itraconazole, ketoconazole, posaconazole, voriconazole)** are predicted to increase the exposure to pimozide. Avoid. Severe Study → Also see TABLE 8 p. 1573

▶ **Miconazole** is predicted to increase the exposure to pimozide. Avoid. Moderate Theoretical

▶ **Pioglitazone** potentially decreases the exposure to **isavuconazole**. Use with caution or avoid. Moderate Theoretical

▶ Antifungals, azoles **(fluconazole, isavuconazole)** are predicted to increase the exposure to ponatinib. Moderate Study

▶ Antifungals, azoles **(itraconazole, ketoconazole, posaconazole, voriconazole)** are predicted to slightly increase the exposure to ponatinib. Monitor and adjust dose—consult product literature. Moderate Study

▶ Antifungals, azoles **(fluconazole, isavuconazole)** are predicted to increase the exposure to pralsetinib. Moderate Theoretical

▶ Antifungals, azoles **(itraconazole, ketoconazole, posaconazole, voriconazole)** are predicted to increase the exposure to pralsetinib. Avoid or adjust dose with potent CYP3A4 inhibitors—consult product literature. Moderate Study

▶ Antifungals, azoles **(itraconazole, ketoconazole, posaconazole, voriconazole)** are predicted to moderately increase the exposure to praziquantel. Mild Study

▶ Antifungals, azoles **(itraconazole, ketoconazole, posaconazole, voriconazole)** given with carbimazole are predicted to increase the exposure to propiverine. Adjust starting dose. Moderate Theoretical

▶ **Proton pump inhibitors** decrease the absorption of **itraconazole**. Administer itraconazole capsules with an acidic beverage. Moderate Study

▶ **Proton pump inhibitors** decrease the absorption of **ketoconazole**. Administer ketoconazole with an acidic beverage. Moderate Study

▶ **Proton pump inhibitors** decrease the absorption of **posaconazole** oral suspension. Avoid. Moderate Study

▶ **Voriconazole** increases the exposure to proton pump inhibitors (esomeprazole, omeprazole). Adjust dose. Moderate Study

▶ Antifungals, azoles **(itraconazole, ketoconazole, posaconazole, voriconazole)** are predicted to increase the exposure to quizartinib. Adjust dose—consult product literature. Severe Study → Also see TABLE 8 p. 1573

▶ Antifungals, azoles **(fluconazole, isavuconazole)** are predicted to increase the exposure to ranolazine. Severe Study → Also see TABLE 8 p. 1573

▶ Antifungals, azoles **(itraconazole, ketoconazole, posaconazole, voriconazole)** are predicted to increase the exposure to ranolazine. Avoid. Severe Study → Also see TABLE 8 p. 1573

▶ Antifungals, azoles **(itraconazole, ketoconazole, posaconazole, voriconazole)** are predicted to increase the exposure to reboxetine. Avoid. Moderate Study

▶ **Miconazole** is predicted to increase the concentration of reboxetine. Use with caution and adjust dose. Moderate Theoretical

▶ Antifungals, azoles **(fluconazole, isavuconazole)** are predicted to increase the exposure to regorafenib. Moderate Study

▶ Antifungals, azoles **(itraconazole, ketoconazole, posaconazole, voriconazole)** are predicted to increase the exposure to regorafenib. Avoid. Moderate Study

▶ Antifungals, azoles **(itraconazole, ketoconazole)** are predicted to increase the exposure to relugolix. Avoid or take relugolix first and separate administration by at least 6 hours. Moderate Study

▶ Antifungals, azoles **(fluconazole, itraconazole, ketoconazole, miconazole, posaconazole, voriconazole)** are predicted to increase the exposure to retinoids (alitretinoin). Adjust **alitretinoin** dose, p. 1433. Moderate Theoretical

▶ **Posaconazole** is predicted to increase the risk of tretinoin toxicity when given with retinoids (tretinoin). Monitor and adjust dose. Severe Theoretical

▶ Antifungals, azoles **(fluconazole, ketoconazole, voriconazole)** are predicted to increase the risk of tretinoin toxicity when given with retinoids (tretinoin). Moderate Study

▶ Antifungals, azoles **(fluconazole, isavuconazole)** are predicted to increase the exposure to ribociclib. Moderate Study → Also see **TABLE 8** p. 1573

▶ Antifungals, azoles **(itraconazole, ketoconazole, posaconazole, voriconazole)** are predicted to increase the exposure to ribociclib. Avoid or adjust dose—consult product literature. Moderate Study → Also see **TABLE 8** p. 1573

▶ Rifamycins (rifabutin) are predicted to decrease the exposure to **isavuconazole**. Avoid. Severe Theoretical

▶ Rifamycins (rifabutin) decrease the concentration of **voriconazole** and **voriconazole** increases the concentration of rifamycins (rifabutin). Avoid or adjust **voriconazole** dose, p. 695. Severe Study

▶ Rifamycins (rifampicin) slightly decrease the exposure to **fluconazole**. Adjust dose. Moderate Study

▶ Rifamycins (rifampicin) are predicted to decrease the exposure to **isavuconazole**. Avoid. Severe Study

▶ Rifamycins (rifampicin) markedly decrease the exposure to **itraconazole**. Avoid and for 14 days after stopping **rifampicin**. Moderate Study

▶ Rifamycins (rifampicin) markedly decrease the exposure to **ketoconazole** and **ketoconazole** potentially decreases the exposure to rifamycins (rifampicin). Avoid. Moderate Study

▶ Rifamycins (rifampicin) are predicted to decrease the exposure to **posaconazole**. Avoid. Moderate Anecdotal

▶ Rifamycins (rifampicin) very markedly decrease the exposure to **voriconazole**. Avoid. Moderate Study

▶ **Fluconazole** increases the risk of uveitis when given with rifamycins (rifabutin). Adjust dose. Severe Study

▶ **Ketoconazole** is predicted to increase the concentration of rifamycins (rifabutin) and rifamycins (rifabutin) are predicted to decrease the concentration of **ketoconazole**. Avoid. Severe Theoretical

▶ **Miconazole** is predicted to increase the concentration of rifamycins (rifabutin). Use with caution and adjust dose. Moderate Theoretical

▶ Antifungals, azoles **(itraconazole, posaconazole)** increase the concentration of rifamycins (rifabutin) and rifamycins (rifabutin) decrease the concentration of antifungals, azoles **(itraconazole, posaconazole)**. Avoid. Severe Study

▶ Antifungals, azoles **(fluconazole, isavuconazole)** are predicted to increase the exposure to rimegepant. Avoid another dose of rimegepant within 48 hours of concurrent use. Moderate Study

▶ Antifungals, azoles **(itraconazole, ketoconazole, posaconazole, voriconazole)** are predicted to increase the exposure to rimegepant. Avoid. Moderate Study

▶ Antifungals, azoles **(itraconazole, posaconazole)** are predicted to increase the exposure to riociguat. Adjust **riociguat** dose and monitor blood pressure, p. 212. Moderate Theoretical

▶ **Ketoconazole** moderately increases the exposure to riociguat. Adjust **riociguat** dose and monitor blood pressure, p. 212. Moderate Study

▶ Antifungals, azoles **(itraconazole, ketoconazole, posaconazole, voriconazole)** are predicted to increase the exposure to ripretinib. Moderate Theoretical

▶ Antifungals, azoles **(itraconazole, ketoconazole, posaconazole, voriconazole)** are predicted to increase the exposure to ruxolitinib. Adjust dose and monitor adverse effects. Moderate Study

▶ **Fluconazole** is predicted to increase the exposure to ruxolitinib. Avoid or adjust dose. Moderate Theoretical

▶ **Isavuconazole** is predicted to increase the exposure to ruxolitinib. Moderate Study

▶ **Ketoconazole** is predicted to increase the exposure to the active component of sacituzumab govitecan. Severe Theoretical

▶ **Fluconazole** is predicted to increase the exposure to selexipag. Unknown Theoretical

▶ Antifungals, azoles **(fluconazole, isavuconazole)** are predicted to increase the exposure to selpercatinib. Moderate Study → Also see **TABLE 8** p. 1573

▶ Antifungals, azoles **(itraconazole, ketoconazole, posaconazole, voriconazole)** are predicted to increase the exposure to selpercatinib. Adjust dose—consult product literature. Moderate Study → Also see **TABLE 8** p. 1573

▶ Antifungals, azoles **(fluconazole, isavuconazole, itraconazole, ketoconazole, posaconazole, voriconazole)** are predicted to increase the exposure to selumetinib. Avoid or adjust dose—consult product literature. Severe Study

▶ Antifungals, azoles **(fluconazole, isavuconazole, miconazole)** are predicted to increase the exposure to siponimod. Avoid depending on other drugs taken—consult product literature. Severe Study

▶ Antifungals, azoles **(itraconazole, ketoconazole, posaconazole, voriconazole)** are predicted to increase the exposure to siponimod. Avoid depending on other drugs taken—consult product literature. Severe Theoretical

▶ Antifungals, azoles **(fluconazole, isavuconazole)** increase the concentration of sirolimus. Monitor and adjust dose. Moderate Study

▶ Antifungals, azoles **(itraconazole, ketoconazole, posaconazole, voriconazole)** are predicted to increase the concentration of sirolimus. Avoid or monitor and adjust dose. Severe Study

▶ **Miconazole** is predicted to increase the concentration of sirolimus. Monitor and adjust dose. Moderate Study

▶ Antifungals, azoles **(itraconazole, ketoconazole, posaconazole, voriconazole)** are predicted to increase the exposure to SNRIs (venlafaxine). Moderate Study

▶ Oral sodium bicarbonate decreases the absorption of oral **ketoconazole**. Moderate Study

▶ Sodium zirconium cyclosilicate is predicted to decrease the exposure to **antifungals, azoles**. Separate administration by at least 2 hours. Moderate Theoretical

▶ Antifungals, azoles **(itraconazole, ketoconazole, posaconazole, voriconazole)** are predicted to increase the exposure to solifenacin. Adjust solifenacin p. 899 or tamsulosin with solifenacin p. 906 dose; avoid in hepatic and renal impairment. Severe Study

▶ Sotorasib is predicted to decrease the exposure to **isavuconazole**. Avoid. Severe Theoretical

▶ **Voriconazole** is predicted to increase the exposure to SSRIs (citalopram). Severe Theoretical → Also see **TABLE 8** p. 1573

▶ Antifungals, azoles **(fluconazole, isavuconazole)** are predicted to increase the exposure to SSRIs (dapoxetine). Adjust **dapoxetine** dose with moderate CYP3A4 inhibitors, p. 947. Moderate Theoretical

▶ Antifungals, azoles **(itraconazole, ketoconazole, posaconazole, voriconazole)** are predicted to moderately increase the exposure to SSRIs (dapoxetine). Avoid potent CYP3A4 inhibitors or adjust **dapoxetine** dose, p. 947. Severe Study

▶ Antifungals, azoles **(fluconazole, voriconazole)** are predicted to increase the exposure to SSRIs (escitalopram). Use with caution and adjust dose. Severe Study → Also see **TABLE 8** p. 1573

▶ St John's wort is predicted to decrease the exposure to **isavuconazole**. Avoid. Severe Theoretical

Antifungals, azoles (continued)

▶ **St John's wort** moderately decreases the exposure to **voriconazole**. Avoid. Moderate Study

▶ **Isavuconazole** slightly increases the exposure to statins (atorvastatin). Moderate Study

▶ **Miconazole** (including the oral gel) might increase the exposure to statins (atorvastatin). Moderate Theoretical

▶ Antifungals, azoles (**itraconazole, ketoconazole, posaconazole, voriconazole**) are predicted to increase the exposure to statins (atorvastatin). Avoid or adjust dose and monitor rhabdomyolysis. Severe Study → Also see **TABLE 1** p. 1571

▶ **Fluconazole** is predicted to increase the exposure to statins (atorvastatin, simvastatin). Monitor and adjust dose. Severe Anecdotal → Also see **TABLE 1** p. 1571

▶ Antifungals, azoles (**fluconazole, miconazole**) are predicted to increase the exposure to statins (fluvastatin). Moderate Study → Also see **TABLE 1** p. 1571

▶ **Isavuconazole** is predicted to increase the exposure to statins (fluvastatin, rosuvastatin). Moderate Theoretical

▶ **Isavuconazole** is predicted to increase the exposure to statins (simvastatin). Monitor and adjust dose. Severe Theoretical

▶ **Miconazole** (including the oral gel) is predicted to increase the exposure to statins (simvastatin). Avoid. Severe Anecdotal

▶ Antifungals, azoles (**itraconazole, ketoconazole, posaconazole, voriconazole**) are predicted to increase the exposure to statins (simvastatin). Avoid. Severe Study → Also see **TABLE 1** p. 1571

▶ **Isavuconazole** is predicted to increase the exposure to sulfasalazine. Moderate Theoretical

▶ Antifungals, azoles (**fluconazole, miconazole**) are predicted to increase the exposure to sulfonylureas. Use with caution and adjust dose. Moderate Study

▶ **Voriconazole** is predicted to increase the concentration of sulfonylureas. Use with caution and adjust dose. Moderate Study

▶ Antifungals, azoles (**fluconazole, isavuconazole**) are predicted to increase the exposure to sunitinib. Moderate Study → Also see **TABLE 8** p. 1573

▶ Antifungals, azoles (**itraconazole, ketoconazole, posaconazole, voriconazole**) are predicted to increase the exposure to sunitinib. Avoid or adjust dose—consult product literature. Moderate Study → Also see **TABLE 8** p. 1573

▶ Antifungals, azoles (**fluconazole, isavuconazole**) are predicted to increase the concentration of tacrolimus. Severe Study

▶ Antifungals, azoles (**itraconazole, ketoconazole, posaconazole, voriconazole**) are predicted to increase the concentration of tacrolimus. Monitor and adjust dose. Severe Study

▶ **Miconazole** is predicted to increase the concentration of tacrolimus. Monitor and adjust dose. Severe Theoretical

▶ Antifungals, azoles (**itraconazole, ketoconazole**) are predicted to slightly increase the exposure to talazoparib. Avoid or adjust dose—consult product literature. Severe Study

▶ Antifungals, azoles (**fluconazole, isavuconazole**) are predicted to increase the exposure to taxanes (cabazitaxel). Moderate Theoretical

▶ Antifungals, azoles (**itraconazole, ketoconazole, posaconazole, voriconazole**) are predicted to increase the exposure to taxanes (cabazitaxel). Avoid or adjust dose—consult product literature. Severe Study

▶ **Miconazole** is predicted to increase the concentration of taxanes (docetaxel). Use with caution and adjust dose. Moderate Theoretical

▶ Antifungals, azoles (**fluconazole, isavuconazole**) are predicted to increase the exposure to taxanes (docetaxel). Severe Study

▶ Antifungals, azoles (**itraconazole, ketoconazole, posaconazole, voriconazole**) are predicted to increase the exposure to taxanes (docetaxel). Avoid or adjust dose. Severe Study

▶ Antifungals, azoles (**fluconazole, isavuconazole, itraconazole, ketoconazole, posaconazole, voriconazole**) are predicted to increase the exposure to taxanes (paclitaxel). Moderate Anecdotal

▶ Antifungals, azoles (**fluconazole, isavuconazole**) are predicted to increase the concentration of temsirolimus. Use with caution or avoid. Moderate Theoretical

▶ Antifungals, azoles (**itraconazole, ketoconazole, posaconazole, voriconazole**) are predicted to increase the concentration of temsirolimus. Avoid. Severe Theoretical

▶ Antifungals, azoles (**itraconazole, ketoconazole**) might increase the exposure to tepotinib. Avoid. Severe Theoretical

▶ Antifungals, azoles (**fluconazole, isavuconazole**) are predicted to increase the exposure to tezacaftor. Adjust dose with moderate CYP3A4 inhibitors, see tezacaftor with ivacaftor p. 339 and ivacaftor with tezacaftor and elexacaftor p. 337. Severe Study

▶ Antifungals, azoles (**itraconazole, ketoconazole, posaconazole, voriconazole**) are predicted to increase the exposure to tezacaftor. Adjust dose with potent CYP3A4 inhibitors, see tezacaftor with ivacaftor p. 339 and ivacaftor with tezacaftor and elexacaftor p. 337. Severe Study

▶ **Isavuconazole** is predicted to increase the exposure to thrombin inhibitors (dabigatran). Monitor and adjust dose. Moderate Study

▶ Antifungals, azoles (**fluconazole, posaconazole**) are predicted to increase the exposure to thrombin inhibitors (dabigatran). Severe Study

▶ Antifungals, azoles (**itraconazole, ketoconazole**) are predicted to increase the exposure to thrombin inhibitors (dabigatran). Avoid. Severe Study

▶ Antifungals, azoles (**itraconazole, ketoconazole, posaconazole, voriconazole**) are predicted to markedly increase the exposure to ticagrelor. Avoid. Severe Study

▶ Antifungals, azoles (**itraconazole, ketoconazole**) might increase the exposure to tigecycline. Mild Anecdotal → Also see **TABLE 1** p. 1571

▶ Antifungals, azoles (**itraconazole, ketoconazole, posaconazole, voriconazole**) are predicted to increase the exposure to tofacitinib. Adjust **tofacitinib** dose, p. 1265. Moderate Study

▶ **Fluconazole** increases the exposure to tofacitinib. Adjust **tofacitinib** dose, p. 1265. Moderate Study

▶ **Isavuconazole** given with a potent CYP2C19 inhibitor is predicted to increase the exposure to tofacitinib. Adjust **tofacitinib** dose, p. 1265. Moderate Study

▶ Antifungals, azoles (**itraconazole, ketoconazole, posaconazole, voriconazole**) are predicted to increase the exposure to tolterodine. Avoid. Severe Study → Also see **TABLE 8** p. 1573

▶ Antifungals, azoles (**fluconazole, isavuconazole**) are predicted to increase the exposure to tolvaptan. Manufacturer advises caution or adjust **tolvaptan** dose with moderate CYP3A4 inhibitors, p. 767. Moderate Study

▶ Antifungals, azoles (**itraconazole, ketoconazole, posaconazole, voriconazole**) are predicted to increase the exposure to tolvaptan. Manufacturer advises caution or adjust **tolvaptan** dose with potent CYP3A4 inhibitors, p. 767. Severe Study

▶ Antifungals, azoles (**itraconazole, ketoconazole**) are predicted to increase the exposure to topotecan. Severe Study

▶ **Isavuconazole** is predicted to increase the exposure to topotecan. Moderate Theoretical

▶ Antifungals, azoles (**itraconazole, ketoconazole, posaconazole, voriconazole**) are predicted to increase the exposure to toremifene. Moderate Theoretical → Also see **TABLE 8** p. 1573

▶ Antifungals, azoles (**itraconazole, ketoconazole, posaconazole, voriconazole**) are predicted to increase the exposure to trabectedin. Avoid or adjust dose. Severe Theoretical → Also see **TABLE 1** p. 1571

▶ Antifungals, azoles (**itraconazole, ketoconazole**) are predicted to increase the concentration of trametinib. Moderate Theoretical

▶ Antifungals, azoles (**fluconazole, isavuconazole**) are predicted to increase the exposure to trazodone. Moderate Theoretical

▶ Antifungals, azoles (**itraconazole, ketoconazole, posaconazole, voriconazole**) are predicted to moderately increase the exposure to trazodone. Avoid or adjust dose. Moderate Study

▶ Antifungals, azoles (**itraconazole, ketoconazole, posaconazole, voriconazole**) increase the exposure to triptans (almotriptan). Mild Study

▶ Antifungals, azoles (**itraconazole, ketoconazole, posaconazole, voriconazole**) are predicted to markedly increase the exposure to triptans (eletriptan). Avoid. Severe Study

▶ **Tucatinib** is predicted to increase the exposure to isavuconazole. Avoid or monitor adverse effects. Severe Study

▶ Antifungals, azoles (**fluconazole, isavuconazole, posaconazole**) are predicted to increase the exposure to ulipristal. Avoid if used for uterine fibroids. Moderate Study

▸ Antifungals, azoles (itraconazole, ketoconazole, voriconazole) are predicted to increase the exposure to uliprista. Avoid if used for uterine fibroids. [Severe] Study

▸ Antifungals, azoles (itraconazole, ketoconazole, posaconazole, voriconazole) are predicted to increase the exposure to upadacitinib. Manufacturer advises caution or avoid, or adjust upadacitinib dose depending on indication, p. 1267. [Severe] Study

▸ Antifungals, azoles (fluconazole, isavuconazole, itraconazole, ketoconazole, posaconazole, voriconazole) are predicted to increase the exposure to vemurafenib. [Severe] Theoretical → Also see TABLE 8 p. 1573

▸ Antifungals, azoles (fluconazole, isavuconazole, itraconazole, ketoconazole, posaconazole, voriconazole) are predicted to increase the exposure to venetoclax. Avoid or adjust dose— consult product literature. [Severe] Study

▸ Antifungals, azoles (fluconazole, isavuconazole, itraconazole, ketoconazole, posaconazole, voriconazole) are predicted to increase the exposure to vinca alkaloids. [Severe] Theoretical

▸ **Miconazole** is predicted to increase the concentration of vinca alkaloids. Use with caution and adjust dose. [Moderate] Theoretical

▸ Antifungals, azoles (clotrimazole, ketoconazole) are predicted to decrease the exposure to vitamin D substances (colecalciferol). [Moderate] Theoretical

▸ Antifungals, azoles (itraconazole, ketoconazole, posaconazole, voriconazole) are predicted to increase the exposure to vitamin D substances (paricalcitol). [Moderate] Study

▸ Antifungals, azoles (fluconazole, isavuconazole) are predicted to increase the exposure to voclosporin. Adjust voclosporin dose, p. 973. [Severe] Study → Also see TABLE 8 p. 1573

▸ Antifungals, azoles (itraconazole, ketoconazole, posaconazole, voriconazole) are predicted to increase the exposure to voclosporin. Avoid. [Severe] Study → Also see TABLE 8 p. 1573

▸ Antifungals, azoles (fluconazole, isavuconazole) are predicted to increase the exposure to zanubrutinib. Avoid or adjust dose with moderate CYP3A4 inhibitors—consult product literature. [Severe] Study

▸ Antifungals, azoles (itraconazole, ketoconazole, posaconazole, voriconazole) are predicted to increase the exposure to zanubrutinib. Avoid or adjust dose with potent CYP3A4 inhibitors—consult product literature. [Moderate] Study

▸ Antifungals, azoles (fluconazole, isavuconazole) are predicted to increase the exposure to zopiclone. Adjust dose. [Moderate] Study

▸ Antifungals, azoles (itraconazole, ketoconazole, posaconazole, voriconazole) are predicted to increase the exposure to zopiclone. Adjust dose. [Moderate] Theoretical

Antihistamines, non-sedating → see TABLE 8 p. 1573 (QT-interval prolongation)

acrivastine · azelastine · bilastine · cetirizine · desloratadine · fexofenadine · levocetirizine · loratadine · mizolastine · rupatadine

▸ Since systemic absorption can follow topical application, the possibility of interactions with topical **azelastine** should be borne in mind.

▸ Apple juice and orange juice decrease the exposure to **fexofenadine**.

▸ Oral antacids decrease the absorption of oral **fexofenadine**. Separate administration by 2 hours. [Mild] Study

▸ Anti-androgens (apalutamide) slightly decrease the exposure to **fexofenadine**. [Mild] Study

▸ Anti-androgens (darolutamide) are predicted to increase the concentration of **fexofenadine**. [Moderate] Theoretical

▸ Antiarrhythmics (amiodarone) are predicted to increase the exposure to **fexofenadine**. [Moderate] Study

▸ Antiarrhythmics (dronedarone) are predicted to increase the exposure to **rupatadine**. Avoid. [Moderate] Study

▸ Antiarrhythmics (dronedarone) are predicted to increase the exposure to antihistamines, non-sedating (**fexofenadine, mizolastine**). [Severe] Theoretical

▸ Antifungals, azoles (fluconazole, isavuconazole) are predicted to increase the exposure to **mizolastine**. [Severe] Theoretical

▸ Antifungals, azoles (fluconazole, isavuconazole, itraconazole, ketoconazole, posaconazole, voriconazole) are predicted to increase the exposure to **rupatadine**. Avoid. [Moderate] Study

▸ Antifungals, azoles (itraconazole, ketoconazole, posaconazole, voriconazole) are predicted to increase the exposure to **mizolastine**. Avoid. [Severe] Study

▸ Antifungals, azoles (miconazole) are predicted to increase the exposure to **mizolastine**. Avoid. [Moderate] Theoretical

▸ **Belumosudil** is predicted to increase the exposure to **fexofenadine**. Avoid or adjust dose. [Moderate] Study

▸ **Berotralstat** is predicted to increase the exposure to **mizolastine**. [Severe] Theoretical

▸ **Berotralstat** is predicted to increase the exposure to **rupatadine**. Avoid. [Moderate] Study

▸ **Antihistamines, non-sedating** are predicted to decrease the effects of betahistine. [Moderate] Theoretical

▸ **Bulevirtide** is predicted to increase the exposure to **fexofenadine**. Avoid or monitor. [Moderate] Theoretical

▸ Calcium channel blockers (diltiazem, verapamil) are predicted to increase the exposure to **mizolastine**. [Severe] Theoretical

▸ Calcium channel blockers (diltiazem, verapamil) are predicted to increase the exposure to **rupatadine**. Avoid. [Moderate] Study

▸ **Ceritinib** is predicted to increase the exposure to **fexofenadine**. [Moderate] Theoretical

▸ **Ceritinib** is predicted to increase the exposure to **mizolastine**. Avoid. [Severe] Study

▸ **Ceritinib** is predicted to increase the exposure to **rupatadine**. Avoid. [Moderate] Study

▸ **Ciclosporin** is predicted to increase the exposure to **fexofenadine**. [Moderate] Theoretical

▸ **Cobicistat** is predicted to increase the exposure to **fexofenadine**. [Moderate] Theoretical

▸ **Cobicistat** is predicted to increase the exposure to **mizolastine**. Avoid. [Severe] Study

▸ **Cobicistat** is predicted to increase the exposure to **rupatadine**. Avoid. [Moderate] Study

▸ **Crizotinib** is predicted to increase the exposure to **mizolastine**. [Severe] Theoretical

▸ **Crizotinib** is predicted to increase the exposure to **rupatadine**. Avoid. [Moderate] Study

▸ **Danicopan** is predicted to increase the exposure to **fexofenadine**. [Moderate] Study

▸ **Elexacaftor** is predicted to increase the exposure to **fexofenadine**. [Moderate] Theoretical

▸ **Eliglustat** is predicted to increase the exposure to **fexofenadine**. Adjust dose. [Moderate] Study

▸ **Encorafenib** is predicted to increase the exposure to **fexofenadine**. [Mild] Study

▸ **Fedratinib** is predicted to increase the exposure to **mizolastine**. [Severe] Theoretical

▸ **Fedratinib** is predicted to increase the exposure to **rupatadine**. Avoid. [Moderate] Study

▸ Fibrates (gemfibrozil) are predicted to increase the exposure to **fexofenadine**. [Moderate] Theoretical

▸ **Glecaprevir** is predicted to increase the exposure to **fexofenadine**. [Severe] Theoretical

▸ **Grapefruit** juice slightly decreases the exposure to **bilastine**. **Bilastine** should be taken 1 hour before or 2 hours after grapefruit. [Moderate] Study

▸ **Grapefruit** juice increases the exposure to **rupatadine**. Avoid. [Moderate] Study

▸ HIV-protease inhibitors (atazanavir) boosted with ritonavir are predicted to increase the exposure to **fexofenadine**. [Moderate] Theoretical

▸ HIV-protease inhibitors are predicted to increase the exposure to **mizolastine**. Avoid. [Severe] Study

▸ HIV-protease inhibitors are predicted to increase the exposure to **rupatadine**. Avoid. [Moderate] Study

▸ **Idelalisib** is predicted to increase the exposure to **mizolastine**. Avoid. [Severe] Study

▸ **Idelalisib** is predicted to increase the exposure to **rupatadine**. Avoid. [Moderate] Study

▸ **Imatinib** is predicted to increase the exposure to **mizolastine**. [Severe] Theoretical

▸ **Imatinib** is predicted to increase the exposure to **rupatadine**. Avoid. [Moderate] Study

▸ **Ivosidenib** is predicted to alter the exposure to **fexofenadine**. [Moderate] Theoretical

Antihistamines, non-sedating (continued)
- **Lapatinib** is predicted to increase the exposure to **fexofenadine**. Moderate Theoretical
- **Leflunomide** is predicted to increase the exposure to **fexofenadine**. Moderate Study
- **Leniolisib** is predicted to increase the exposure to **fexofenadine**. Avoid. Moderate Theoretical
- **Letermovir** is predicted to increase the concentration of **fexofenadine**. Moderate Theoretical
- **Letermovir** is predicted to increase the exposure to **mizolastine**. Severe Theoretical
- **Letermovir** is predicted to increase the exposure to **rupatadine**. Avoid. Moderate Study
- **Lorlatinib** decreases the exposure to **fexofenadine**. Moderate Study
- **Macrolides (clarithromycin)** are predicted to increase the exposure to **fexofenadine**. Moderate Theoretical
- **Macrolides (clarithromycin)** are predicted to increase the exposure to **mizolastine**. Avoid. Severe Study
- **Macrolides (clarithromycin, erythromycin)** are predicted to increase the exposure to **rupatadine**. Avoid. Moderate Study
- **Macrolides (erythromycin)** are predicted to increase the exposure to **mizolastine**. Severe Theoretical
- **MAOIs, irreversible** are predicted to increase the risk of antimuscarinic adverse effects when given with **antihistamines, non-sedating**. Avoid. Severe Theoretical
- **Mirabegron** is predicted to increase the exposure to **fexofenadine**. Mild Theoretical
- **Neurokinin-1 receptor antagonists (aprepitant, netupitant)** are predicted to increase the exposure to **mizolastine**. Severe Theoretical
- **Neurokinin-1 receptor antagonists (aprepitant, netupitant)** are predicted to increase the exposure to **rupatadine**. Avoid. Moderate Study
- **Nilotinib** is predicted to increase the exposure to **mizolastine**. Severe Theoretical
- **Nilotinib** is predicted to increase the exposure to **rupatadine**. Avoid. Moderate Study
- **Olaparib** might increase the exposure to **fexofenadine**. Moderate Theoretical
- **Osimertinib** is predicted to increase the exposure to **fexofenadine**. Moderate Study
- **Pibrentasvir** with glecaprevir is predicted to increase the exposure to **fexofenadine**. Moderate Study
- **Pitolisant** is predicted to decrease the exposure to **fexofenadine**. Mild Theoretical
- **Ranolazine** is predicted to increase the exposure to **fexofenadine**. Moderate Theoretical
- **Rifamycins (rifampicin)** are predicted to decrease the exposure to **bilastine**. Moderate Theoretical
- **Rifamycins (rifampicin)** increase the clearance of **fexofenadine**. Moderate Study
- **Roxadustat** is predicted to increase the exposure to **fexofenadine**. Monitor adverse effects and adjust dose. Moderate Study
- **Taxanes (cabazitaxel)** are predicted to affect the exposure to **fexofenadine**. Manufacturer advises take 12 hours before or 3 hours after **cabazitaxel**. Moderate Theoretical
- **Tepotinib** is predicted to increase the concentration of **fexofenadine**. Severe Study
- **Teriflunomide** is predicted to increase the exposure to **fexofenadine**. Moderate Study
- **Tucatinib** is predicted to increase the exposure to **mizolastine**. Avoid. Severe Study
- **Tucatinib** is predicted to increase the exposure to **rupatadine**. Avoid. Moderate Study
- **Velpatasvir** is predicted to increase the exposure to **fexofenadine**. Severe Theoretical
- **Vemurafenib** is predicted to increase the exposure to **fexofenadine**. Use with caution and adjust dose. Severe Theoretical
- **Venetoclax** is predicted to increase the exposure to **fexofenadine**. Moderate Theoretical
- **Voclosporin** is predicted to increase the exposure to **fexofenadine**. Mild Theoretical
- **Voxilaprevir** with sofosbuvir and velpatasvir is predicted to increase the exposure to **fexofenadine**. Moderate Study

Antihistamines, sedating → see TABLE 8 p. 1573 (QT-interval prolongation), TABLE 9 p. 1573 (antimuscarinics), TABLE 10 p. 1574 (CNS effects)

alimemazine · antazoline · buclizine · chlorphenamine · cinnarizine · cyclizine · cyproheptadine · doxylamine · hydroxyzine · ketotifen · pizotifen · promethazine

ROUTE-SPECIFIC INFORMATION Since systemic absorption can follow topical application of **ketotifen**, the possibility of interactions should be borne in mind.

- **Hydroxyzine** potentially increases the risk of overheating and dehydration when given with antiepileptics (zonisamide). Avoid in children. Severe Theoretical
- Antipsychotics, second generation (clozapine) can cause constipation, as can antihistamines, sedating (chlorphenamine, cyclizine, cyproheptadine, hydroxyzine, promethazine); concurrent use might increase the risk of developing intestinal obstruction. Severe Theoretical → Also see TABLE 9 p. 1573 → Also see TABLE 10 p. 1574
- **Antihistamines, sedating** are predicted to decrease the effects of betahistine. Moderate Theoretical
- **Cyproheptadine** might decrease the efficacy of fenfluramine. Severe Theoretical
- **MAOIs, irreversible** are predicted to increase the risk of antimuscarinic adverse effects when given with **antihistamines, sedating**. Avoid. Severe Theoretical
- **Cyproheptadine** decreases the effects of metyrapone. Avoid. Moderate Study
- **Antihistamines, sedating** are predicted to decrease the efficacy of pitolisant. Moderate Theoretical
- **Cyproheptadine** potentially decreases the effects of SSRIs. Moderate Anecdotal → Also see TABLE 10 p. 1574

Antimalarials → see TABLE 18 p. 1576 (ototoxicity), TABLE 8 p. 1573 (QT-interval prolongation)

artemether · atovaquone · chloroquine · lumefantrine · mefloquine · primaquine · proguanil · pyrimethamine · quinine

- **Chloroquine** is predicted to decrease the effects of agalsidase alfa. Avoid. Moderate Theoretical
- **Chloroquine** is predicted to decrease the effects of agalsidase beta. Avoid. Moderate Theoretical
- Oral antacids are predicted to decrease the absorption of oral **chloroquine**. Separate administration by at least 4 hours. Moderate Theoretical
- Oral antacids are predicted to decrease the absorption of oral **proguanil**. Separate administration by at least 2 hours. Moderate Study
- Anti-androgens (apalutamide, enzalutamide) are predicted to decrease the exposure to **artemether** with lumefantrine. Avoid. Severe Study → Also see TABLE 8 p. 1573
- Antiepileptics (carbamazepine, fosphenytoin, phenobarbital, phenytoin, primidone) are predicted to decrease the exposure to **artemether** with lumefantrine. Avoid. Severe Study
- Antiepileptics (carbamazepine, phenobarbital, primidone) potentially increase the risk of toxicity when given with **quinine**. Unknown Study
- **Pyrimethamine** increases the risk of haematological toxicity when given with antiepileptics (fosphenytoin, phenytoin). Severe Study
- **Pyrimethamine** is predicted to increase the risk of haematological toxicity when given with antiepileptics (phenobarbital, primidone). Severe Theoretical
- Antifungals, azoles (fluconazole, itraconazole, posaconazole, voriconazole) are predicted to increase the exposure to **mefloquine**. Moderate Theoretical
- Antifungals, azoles (ketoconazole) increase the exposure to **mefloquine**. Moderate Study
- Antimalarials (proguanil) are predicted to increase the risk of adverse effects when given with antimalarials (pyrimethamine). Severe Theoretical
- **Mefloquine** is predicted to increase the risk of bradycardia when given with beta blockers, non-selective. Severe Theoretical

▸ **Mefloquine** is predicted to increase the risk of bradycardia when given with beta blockers, selective. Severe Theoretical
▸ **Mefloquine** is predicted to increase the risk of bradycardia when given with calcium channel blockers. Severe Theoretical
▸ Oral calcium salts (calcium carbonate) might decrease the absorption of oral **chloroquine**. Separate administration by at least 4 hours. Moderate Study
▸ **Mefloquine** is predicted to increase the risk of bradycardia when given with digoxin. Severe Theoretical
▸ **Quinine** increases the concentration of digoxin. Monitor and adjust **digoxin** dose, p. 125. Severe Anecdotal
▸ Encorafenib is predicted to decrease the exposure to **artemether** with lumefantrine. Avoid. Severe Study → Also see TABLE 8 p. 1573
▸ Grapefruit juice increases the exposure to **artemether**. Unknown Study
▸ H₂ receptor antagonists (cimetidine) decrease the clearance of **chloroquine**. Moderate Study
▸ H₂ receptor antagonists (cimetidine) slightly increase the exposure to **quinine**. Moderate Study
▸ HIV-protease inhibitors decrease the exposure to **atovaquone**. Avoid if boosted with ritonavir. Moderate Study
▸ HIV-protease inhibitors are predicted to decrease the exposure to **proguanil**. Avoid. Moderate Study
▸ HIV-protease inhibitors are predicted to affect the exposure to **quinine**. Severe Study
▸ Ivosidenib is predicted to decrease the exposure to **artemether** with lumefantrine. Avoid. Severe Study → Also see TABLE 8 p. 1573
▸ Oral kaolin decreases the absorption of oral **chloroquine**. Separate administration by at least 4 hours. Moderate Study
▸ Lanthanum is predicted to decrease the absorption of **chloroquine**. Separate administration by at least 2 hours. Moderate Theoretical
▸ **Chloroquine** is predicted to decrease the exposure to laronidase. Avoid simultaneous administration. Severe Theoretical
▸ **Chloroquine** might decrease the efficacy of live vaccines (cholera vaccine (live)). Avoid for at least 10 days before **chloroquine**. Moderate Study
▸ Lumacaftor is predicted to decrease the exposure to **artemether** with lumefantrine. Avoid. Severe Study
▸ Macrolides might increase the risk of serious cardiovascular adverse effects when given with **chloroquine**. Severe Theoretical
▸ Oral magnesium trisilicate decreases the absorption of oral **chloroquine**. Separate administration by at least 4 hours. Moderate Study
▸ Mepacrine is predicted to increase the concentration of **primaquine**. Avoid. Moderate Theoretical
▸ **Pyrimethamine** is predicted to increase the exposure to metformin. Use with caution and adjust dose. Moderate Study
▸ **Pyrimethamine** is predicted to increase the risk of adverse effects when given with methotrexate. Severe Theoretical
▸ Metoclopramide decreases the concentration of **atovaquone**. Avoid. Moderate Study
▸ Mitotane is predicted to decrease the exposure to **artemether** with lumefantrine. Avoid. Severe Study
▸ Nirmatrelvir boosted with ritonavir is predicted to decrease the concentration of **atovaquone**. Moderate Theoretical
▸ NNRTIs (efavirenz) decrease the concentration of **artemether**. Severe Study → Also see TABLE 8 p. 1573
▸ NNRTIs (efavirenz) moderately decrease the exposure to **atovaquone**. Avoid. Moderate Study
▸ NNRTIs (efavirenz) affect the exposure to **proguanil**. Avoid. Moderate Study
▸ NNRTIs (etravirine) decrease the exposure to **artemether**. Moderate Study
▸ **Pyrimethamine** is predicted to increase the risk of adverse effects when given with NRTIs (zidovudine). Severe Theoretical
▸ **Pyrimethamine** is predicted to increase the risk of adverse effects when given with pemetrexed. Severe Theoretical
▸ **Chloroquine** is predicted to increase the risk of haematological toxicity when given with penicillamine. Avoid. Severe Theoretical
▸ **Chloroquine** moderately decreases the exposure to praziquantel. Use with caution and adjust dose. Moderate Study

▸ **Chloroquine** decreases the efficacy of rabies vaccine (intradermal). Avoid. Moderate Study
▸ **Chloroquine** might decrease the effects of remdesivir. Avoid. Moderate Theoretical
▸ Rifamycins (rifabutin) slightly decrease the exposure to **atovaquone**. Avoid. Moderate Study
▸ Rifamycins (rifampicin) are predicted to decrease the exposure to **artemether** with lumefantrine. Avoid. Severe Study
▸ Rifamycins (rifampicin) moderately decrease the exposure to **atovaquone** and **atovaquone** slightly increases the exposure to rifamycins (rifampicin). Avoid. Moderate Study
▸ Rifamycins (rifampicin) moderately decrease the exposure to **mefloquine**. Severe Study
▸ Rifamycins (rifampicin) decrease the exposure to **quinine**. Severe Study
▸ **Pyrimethamine** increases the risk of adverse effects when given with sulfonamides. Severe Study
▸ Tamoxifen increases the risk of retinopathy when given with **chloroquine**. RCOphth guidance advises monitor. Severe Study
▸ Tetracyclines (tetracycline) decrease the concentration of **atovaquone**. Moderate Study
▸ **Pyrimethamine** increases the risk of adverse effects when given with trimethoprim. Severe Study

Antipsychotics, second generation → see TABLE 17 p. 1576 (hyponatraemia), TABLE 7 p. 1572 (hypotension), TABLE 8 p. 1573 (QT-interval prolongation), TABLE 9 p. 1573 (antimuscarinics), TABLE 10 p. 1574 (CNS effects)

amisulpride · aripiprazole · asenapine · cariprazine · clozapine · lurasidone · olanzapine · paliperidone · quetiapine · risperidone

▸ **Clozapine** and **olanzapine** dose adjustment might be necessary if smoking started or stopped during treatment.
▸ Avoid concomitant use of **clozapine** with drugs that have a substantial potential for causing agranulocytosis or a substantial potential to depress bone marrow function.

▸ **Clozapine** can cause constipation, as can aclidinium; concurrent use might increase the risk of developing intestinal obstruction. Severe Theoretical → Also see TABLE 9 p. 1573
▸ Anti-androgens (apalutamide, enzalutamide) are predicted to moderately decrease the exposure to **aripiprazole**. Adjust **aripiprazole** dose, p. 454. Moderate Study → Also see TABLE 8 p. 1573
▸ Anti-androgens (apalutamide, enzalutamide) are predicted to decrease the exposure to **cariprazine**. Avoid. Severe Theoretical
▸ Anti-androgens (apalutamide, enzalutamide) are predicted to decrease the exposure to **lurasidone**. Avoid. Moderate Study
▸ Anti-androgens (apalutamide, enzalutamide) are predicted to decrease the exposure to **paliperidone**. Monitor and adjust dose. Severe Study → Also see TABLE 8 p. 1573
▸ Anti-androgens (apalutamide, enzalutamide) are predicted to decrease the exposure to **quetiapine**. Moderate Study
▸ Anti-androgens (apalutamide, enzalutamide) are predicted to decrease the exposure to **risperidone**. Adjust dose. Moderate Study
▸ Anti-androgens (enzalutamide) are predicted to decrease the exposure to **clozapine**. Moderate Theoretical
▸ Antiarrhythmics (dronedarone) are predicted to increase the exposure to **cariprazine**. Avoid. Severe Study
▸ Antiarrhythmics (dronedarone) are predicted to increase the exposure to **lurasidone**. Adjust **lurasidone** dose, p. 458. Moderate Study
▸ Antiarrhythmics (dronedarone) are predicted to increase the exposure to **quetiapine**. Avoid. Moderate Study
▸ **Clozapine** can cause constipation, as can antiarrhythmics (disopyramide, propafenone); concurrent use might increase the risk of developing intestinal obstruction. Severe Theoretical → Also see TABLE 9 p. 1573
▸ Antiepileptics (carbamazepine) are predicted to increase the risk of myelosuppression when given with **clozapine**. Avoid. Severe Anecdotal → Also see TABLE 17 p. 1576
▸ Antiepileptics (carbamazepine) potentially decrease the exposure to **olanzapine**. Monitor and adjust dose. Moderate Study → Also see TABLE 17 p. 1576

Antipsychotics, second generation (continued)

▶ Antiepileptics (carbamazepine, fosphenytoin, phenobarbital, phenytoin, primidone) are predicted to moderately decrease the exposure to **aripiprazole**. Adjust **aripiprazole** dose, p. 454. Moderate Study → Also see TABLE 17 p. 1576 → Also see TABLE 10 p. 1574

▶ Antiepileptics (carbamazepine, fosphenytoin, phenobarbital, phenytoin, primidone) are predicted to decrease the exposure to **cariprazine**. Avoid. Severe Theoretical → Also see TABLE 17 p. 1576 → Also see TABLE 10 p. 1574

▶ Antiepileptics (carbamazepine, fosphenytoin, phenobarbital, phenytoin, primidone) are predicted to decrease the exposure to **lurasidone**. Avoid. Moderate Study → Also see TABLE 17 p. 1576 → Also see TABLE 10 p. 1574

▶ Antiepileptics (carbamazepine, fosphenytoin, phenobarbital, phenytoin, primidone) are predicted to decrease the exposure to **paliperidone**. Monitor and adjust dose. Severe Study → Also see TABLE 17 p. 1576 → Also see TABLE 10 p. 1574

▶ Antiepileptics (carbamazepine, fosphenytoin, phenobarbital, phenytoin, primidone) are predicted to decrease the exposure to **quetiapine**. Moderate Study → Also see TABLE 17 p. 1576 → Also see TABLE 10 p. 1574

▶ Antiepileptics (carbamazepine, fosphenytoin, phenobarbital, phenytoin, primidone) are predicted to decrease the exposure to **risperidone**. Adjust dose. Moderate Study → Also see TABLE 17 p. 1576 → Also see TABLE 10 p. 1574

▶ Antiepileptics (fosphenytoin, phenobarbital, phenytoin, primidone) are predicted to decrease the exposure to **clozapine**. Moderate Anecdotal → Also see TABLE 10 p. 1574

▶ Antiepileptics (phenytoin) are predicted to decrease the exposure to **olanzapine**. Monitor and adjust dose. Moderate Study → Also see TABLE 10 p. 1574

▶ Antiepileptics (valproate) increase the risk of adverse effects when given with **olanzapine**. Severe Study → Also see TABLE 17 p. 1576

▶ Antiepileptics (valproate) slightly increase the exposure to **paliperidone**. Adjust dose. Moderate Study → Also see TABLE 17 p. 1576

▶ Antiepileptics (valproate) potentially increase the risk of neutropenia when given with **quetiapine**. Moderate Study → Also see TABLE 17 p. 1576

▶ Antifungals, azoles (fluconazole, isavuconazole) are predicted to increase the exposure to **cariprazine**. Avoid. Severe Study

▶ Antifungals, azoles (fluconazole, isavuconazole) are predicted to increase the exposure to **lurasidone**. Adjust **lurasidone** dose, p. 458. Moderate Study

▶ Antifungals, azoles (fluconazole, isavuconazole) are predicted to increase the exposure to **quetiapine**. Avoid. Moderate Study

▶ Antifungals, azoles (itraconazole, ketoconazole, posaconazole, voriconazole) are predicted to slightly increase the exposure to **aripiprazole**. Adjust **aripiprazole** dose, p. 454. Moderate Study → Also see TABLE 8 p. 1573

▶ Antifungals, azoles (itraconazole, ketoconazole, posaconazole, voriconazole) are predicted to moderately increase the exposure to **cariprazine**. Avoid. Severe Study

▶ Antifungals, azoles (itraconazole, ketoconazole, posaconazole, voriconazole) are predicted to increase the exposure to **risperidone**. Adjust dose. Moderate Study

▶ Antifungals, azoles (itraconazole, ketoconazole, posaconazole, voriconazole) are predicted to increase the exposure to antipsychotics, second generation (**lurasidone, quetiapine**). Avoid. Severe Study

▶ **Clozapine** can cause constipation, as can antihistamines, sedating (chlorphenamine, cyclizine, cyproheptadine, hydroxyzine, promethazine); concurrent use might increase the risk of developing intestinal obstruction. Severe Theoretical → Also see TABLE 9 p. 1573 → Also see TABLE 10 p. 1574

▶ Antipsychotics, second generation (clozapine) can cause constipation, as can antipsychotics, second generation (olanzapine, quetiapine); concurrent use might increase the risk of developing intestinal obstruction. Severe Anecdotal → Also see TABLE 17 p. 1576 → Also see TABLE 7 p. 1572 → Also see TABLE 9 p. 1573 → Also see TABLE 10 p. 1574

▶ **Clozapine** can cause constipation, as can **atropine**; concurrent use might increase the risk of developing intestinal obstruction. Severe Theoretical → Also see TABLE 9 p. 1573

▶ **Axitinib** is predicted to increase the exposure to antipsychotics, second generation (**clozapine, olanzapine**). Moderate Theoretical

▶ **Clozapine** can cause constipation, as can **baclofen**; concurrent use might increase the risk of developing intestinal obstruction. Severe Theoretical → Also see TABLE 7 p. 1572 → Also see TABLE 9 p. 1573 → Also see TABLE 10 p. 1574

▶ **Clozapine** might increase the risk of respiratory depression and circulatory collapse when given with **benzodiazepines**. Severe Anecdotal → Also see TABLE 10 p. 1574

▶ **Berotralstat** is predicted to increase the exposure to **cariprazine**. Avoid. Severe Study

▶ **Berotralstat** is predicted to increase the exposure to **quetiapine**. Avoid. Moderate Study

▶ **Bupropion** is predicted to moderately increase the exposure to **aripiprazole**. Adjust **aripiprazole** dose, p. 454. Moderate Study

▶ **Bupropion** is predicted to increase the exposure to **clozapine**. Use with caution and adjust dose. Severe Study

▶ **Bupropion** is predicted to increase the exposure to **risperidone**. Adjust dose. Moderate Study

▶ Calcium channel blockers (diltiazem, verapamil) are predicted to increase the exposure to **cariprazine**. Avoid. Severe Study → Also see TABLE 7 p. 1572

▶ Calcium channel blockers (diltiazem, verapamil) are predicted to increase the exposure to **lurasidone**. Adjust **lurasidone** dose, p. 458. Moderate Study → Also see TABLE 7 p. 1572

▶ Calcium channel blockers (diltiazem, verapamil) are predicted to increase the exposure to **quetiapine**. Avoid. Moderate Study → Also see TABLE 7 p. 1572

▶ **Cenobamate** is predicted to decrease the exposure to **cariprazine**. Avoid. Severe Theoretical → Also see TABLE 10 p. 1574

▶ **Cenobamate** is predicted to decrease the exposure to **lurasidone**. Monitor and adjust dose. Moderate Theoretical → Also see TABLE 10 p. 1574

▶ **Cenobamate** is predicted to decrease the exposure to **quetiapine**. Moderate Study → Also see TABLE 10 p. 1574

▶ **Ceritinib** is predicted to increase the exposure to antipsychotics, second generation (**lurasidone, quetiapine**). Avoid. Severe Study

▶ **Ceritinib** is predicted to slightly increase the exposure to **aripiprazole**. Adjust **aripiprazole** dose, p. 454. Moderate Study → Also see TABLE 8 p. 1573

▶ **Ceritinib** is predicted to moderately increase the exposure to **cariprazine**. Avoid. Severe Study

▶ **Ceritinib** is predicted to increase the exposure to **risperidone**. Adjust dose. Moderate Study

▶ **Cinacalcet** is predicted to moderately increase the exposure to **aripiprazole**. Adjust **aripiprazole** dose, p. 454. Moderate Study

▶ **Cinacalcet** is predicted to increase the exposure to **clozapine**. Use with caution and adjust dose. Severe Study

▶ **Cinacalcet** is predicted to increase the exposure to **risperidone**. Adjust dose. Moderate Study

▶ **Cobicistat** is predicted to increase the exposure to antipsychotics, second generation (**lurasidone, quetiapine**). Avoid. Severe Study

▶ **Cobicistat** is predicted to slightly increase the exposure to **aripiprazole**. Adjust **aripiprazole** dose, p. 454. Moderate Study

▶ **Cobicistat** is predicted to moderately increase the exposure to **cariprazine**. Avoid. Severe Study

▶ **Cobicistat** is predicted to increase the exposure to **risperidone**. Adjust dose. Moderate Study

▶ **Combined hormonal contraceptives** increases the concentration of **clozapine**. Monitor adverse effects and adjust dose. Severe Study

▶ **Combined hormonal contraceptives** is predicted to increase the exposure to **olanzapine**. Adjust dose. Moderate Anecdotal

▶ **Crizotinib** is predicted to increase the exposure to **cariprazine**. Avoid. Severe Study

▶ **Crizotinib** is predicted to increase the exposure to **lurasidone**. Adjust **lurasidone** dose, p. 458. Moderate Study

▶ **Crizotinib** is predicted to increase the exposure to **quetiapine**. Avoid. Moderate Study

▶ **Clozapine** can cause constipation, as can **cyclopentolate**; concurrent use might increase the risk of developing intestinal obstruction. [Severe] Theoretical → Also see **TABLE 9** p. 1573

► **Dabrafenib** is predicted to decrease the exposure to cariprazine. Avoid. [Severe] Theoretical

► **Dabrafenib** is predicted to decrease the exposure to **lurasidone**. Monitor and adjust dose. [Moderate] Theoretical

► **Dabrafenib** is predicted to decrease the exposure to **quetiapine**. [Moderate] Study

► **Dacomitinib** is predicted to moderately increase the exposure to **aripiprazole**. Adjust **aripiprazole** dose, p. 454. [Moderate] Study

► **Dacomitinib** is predicted to increase the exposure to **clozapine**. Use with caution and adjust dose. [Severe] Study

► **Dacomitinib** is predicted to increase the exposure to **risperidone**. Adjust dose. [Moderate] Study

► **Clozapine** can cause constipation, as can **darifenacin**; concurrent use might increase the risk of developing intestinal obstruction. [Severe] Theoretical → Also see **TABLE 9** p. 1573

► **Clozapine** can cause constipation, as can **dicycloverine**; concurrent use might increase the risk of developing intestinal obstruction. [Severe] Theoretical → Also see **TABLE 9** p. 1573

► **Clozapine** can cause constipation, as can **dimenhydrinate**; concurrent use might increase the risk of developing intestinal obstruction. [Severe] Theoretical → Also see **TABLE 9** p. 1573 → Also see **TABLE 10** p. 1574

► Antipsychotics, second generation **(amisulpride, olanzapine, paliperidone, quetiapine, risperidone)** are predicted to decrease the effects of **dopamine receptor agonists**. Avoid. [Moderate] Theoretical → Also see **TABLE 7** p. 1572 → Also see **TABLE 8** p. 1573 → Also see **TABLE 9** p. 1573 → Also see **TABLE 10** p. 1574

► Antipsychotics, second generation **(aripiprazole, clozapine)** are predicted to decrease the effects of **dopamine receptor agonists**. [Moderate] Theoretical → Also see **TABLE 7** p. 1572 → Also see **TABLE 8** p. 1573 → Also see **TABLE 9** p. 1573 → Also see **TABLE 10** p. 1574

► **Asenapine** is predicted to decrease the effects of **dopamine receptor agonists**. Adjust dose. [Moderate] Theoretical → Also see **TABLE 7** p. 1572 → Also see **TABLE 10** p. 1574

► **Encorafenib** is predicted to moderately decrease the exposure to **aripiprazole**. Adjust **aripiprazole** dose, p. 454. [Moderate] Study → Also see **TABLE 8** p. 1573

► **Encorafenib** is predicted to decrease the exposure to **cariprazine**. Avoid. [Severe] Theoretical

► **Encorafenib** is predicted to decrease the exposure to **lurasidone**. Avoid. [Moderate] Study

► **Encorafenib** is predicted to decrease the exposure to **paliperidone**. Monitor and adjust dose. [Severe] Study → Also see **TABLE 8** p. 1573

► **Encorafenib** is predicted to decrease the exposure to **quetiapine**. [Moderate] Study

► **Encorafenib** is predicted to decrease the exposure to **risperidone**. Adjust dose. [Moderate] Study

► **Endothelin receptor antagonists (bosentan)** are predicted to decrease the exposure to **cariprazine**. Avoid. [Severe] Theoretical

► **Endothelin receptor antagonists (bosentan)** are predicted to decrease the exposure to **lurasidone**. Monitor and adjust dose. [Moderate] Theoretical

► **Endothelin receptor antagonists (bosentan)** are predicted to decrease the exposure to **quetiapine**. [Moderate] Study

► **Fedratinib** is predicted to increase the exposure to **cariprazine**. Avoid. [Severe] Study

► **Fedratinib** is predicted to increase the exposure to **quetiapine**. Avoid. [Moderate] Study

► **Clozapine** can cause constipation, as can **fesoterodine**; concurrent use might increase the risk of developing intestinal obstruction. [Severe] Theoretical → Also see **TABLE 9** p. 1573

► **Clozapine** can cause constipation, as can **flavoxate**; concurrent use might increase the risk of developing intestinal obstruction. [Severe] Theoretical → Also see **TABLE 9** p. 1573

► **Clozapine** can cause constipation, as can **flupentixol**; concurrent use might increase the risk of developing intestinal obstruction. [Severe] Theoretical → Also see **TABLE 17**

p. 1576 → Also see **TABLE 7** p. 1572 → Also see **TABLE 9** p. 1573 → Also see **TABLE 10** p. 1574

► **Antipsychotics, second generation** might decrease the effects of the active metabolite of **foslevodopa**. [Severe] Theoretical → Also see **TABLE 7** p. 1572 → Also see **TABLE 10** p. 1574

► **Givosiran** increases the concentration of **clozapine**. Monitor adverse effects and adjust dose. [Severe] Study

► **Givosiran** is predicted to increase the exposure to **olanzapine**. Adjust dose. [Moderate] Anecdotal

► **Clozapine** can cause constipation, as can **glycopyrronium**; concurrent use might increase the risk of developing intestinal obstruction. [Severe] Theoretical → Also see **TABLE 9** p. 1573

► **Grapefruit** juice is predicted to increase the exposure to antipsychotics, second generation **(lurasidone, quetiapine)**. Avoid. [Severe] Theoretical

► **Grapefruit** juice is predicted to increase the exposure to **cariprazine**. Avoid. [Moderate] Study

► **Clozapine** can cause constipation, as can **haloperidol**; concurrent use might increase the risk of developing intestinal obstruction. [Severe] Theoretical → Also see **TABLE 17** p. 1576 → Also see **TABLE 7** p. 1572 → Also see **TABLE 9** p. 1573 → Also see **TABLE 10** p. 1574

► **HIV-protease inhibitors** are predicted to slightly increase the exposure to **aripiprazole**. Adjust **aripiprazole** dose, p. 454. [Moderate] Study

► **HIV-protease inhibitors** are predicted to moderately increase the exposure to **cariprazine**. Avoid. [Severe] Study

► HIV-protease inhibitors **(ritonavir)** are predicted to affect the exposure to **clozapine**. Avoid. [Severe] Theoretical

► HIV-protease inhibitors **(ritonavir)** are predicted to decrease the exposure to **olanzapine**. Monitor and adjust dose. [Moderate] Study

► **HIV-protease inhibitors** are predicted to increase the exposure to antipsychotics, second generation **(lurasidone, quetiapine)**. Avoid. [Severe] Study

► **HIV-protease inhibitors** are predicted to increase the exposure to **risperidone**. Adjust dose. [Moderate] Study

► **Clozapine** can cause constipation, as can **homatropine**; concurrent use might increase the risk of developing intestinal obstruction. [Severe] Theoretical → Also see **TABLE 9** p. 1573

► **Clozapine** can cause constipation, as can **hyoscine**; concurrent use might increase the risk of developing intestinal obstruction. [Severe] Theoretical → Also see **TABLE 9** p. 1573

► **Idelalisib** is predicted to increase the exposure to antipsychotics, second generation **(lurasidone, quetiapine)**. Avoid. [Severe] Study

► **Idelalisib** is predicted to slightly increase the exposure to **aripiprazole**. Adjust **aripiprazole** dose, p. 454. [Moderate] Study

► **Idelalisib** is predicted to moderately increase the exposure to **cariprazine**. Avoid. [Severe] Study

► **Idelalisib** is predicted to increase the exposure to **risperidone**. Adjust dose. [Moderate] Study

► **Imatinib** is predicted to increase the exposure to **cariprazine**. Avoid. [Severe] Study

► **Imatinib** is predicted to increase the exposure to **lurasidone**. Adjust **lurasidone** dose, p. 458. [Moderate] Study

► **Imatinib** is predicted to increase the exposure to **quetiapine**. Avoid. [Moderate] Study

► **Interferons (ropeginterferon alfa)** are predicted to increase the exposure to **risperidone**. [Moderate] Theoretical

► **Clozapine** can cause constipation, as can **ipratropium**; concurrent use might increase the risk of developing intestinal obstruction. [Severe] Theoretical → Also see **TABLE 9** p. 1573

► **Clozapine** can cause constipation, as can **iron**; concurrent use might increase the risk of developing intestinal obstruction. [Severe] Anecdotal

► **Iron chelators (deferasirox)** are predicted to increase the exposure to **clozapine**. Avoid. [Moderate] Theoretical

► **Ivosidenib** is predicted to moderately decrease the exposure to **aripiprazole**. Adjust **aripiprazole** dose, p. 454. [Moderate] Study → Also see **TABLE 8** p. 1573

Antipsychotics, second generation (continued)

▶ **Ivosidenib** is predicted to decrease the exposure to **cariprazine**. Avoid. Severe Theoretical

▶ **Ivosidenib** is predicted to decrease the exposure to **lurasidone**. Avoid. Moderate Study

▶ **Ivosidenib** is predicted to decrease the exposure to **paliperidone**. Monitor and adjust dose. Severe Study → Also see **TABLE 8** p. 1573

▶ **Ivosidenib** is predicted to decrease the exposure to **quetiapine**. Moderate Study

▶ **Ivosidenib** is predicted to decrease the exposure to **risperidone**. Adjust dose. Moderate Study

▶ **Leflunomide** is predicted to decrease the exposure to **clozapine**. Moderate Theoretical

▶ **Leflunomide** is predicted to decrease the exposure to **olanzapine**. Monitor and adjust dose. Moderate Study

▶ **Leniolisib** is predicted to increase the exposure to **clozapine**. Avoid. Moderate Theoretical

▶ **Letermovir** is predicted to increase the exposure to **cariprazine**. Avoid. Severe Study

▶ **Letermovir** is predicted to increase the exposure to **quetiapine**. Avoid. Moderate Study

▶ **Amisulpride** is predicted to decrease the effects of **levodopa**. Avoid. Severe Theoretical → Also see **TABLE 10** p. 1574

▶ Antipsychotics, second generation (**aripiprazole, clozapine, lurasidone, paliperidone**) are predicted to decrease the effects of **levodopa**. Severe Theoretical → Also see **TABLE 7** p. 1572 → Also see **TABLE 10** p. 1574

▶ **Asenapine** is predicted to decrease the effects of **levodopa**. Adjust dose. Severe Theoretical → Also see **TABLE 7** p. 1572 → Also see **TABLE 10** p. 1574

▶ **Olanzapine** decreases the effects of **levodopa**. Avoid or monitor worsening parkinsonian symptoms. Severe Anecdotal → Also see **TABLE 7** p. 1572 → Also see **TABLE 10** p. 1574

▶ **Quetiapine** decreases the effects of **levodopa**. Severe Anecdotal → Also see **TABLE 7** p. 1572 → Also see **TABLE 10** p. 1574

▶ **Risperidone** is predicted to decrease the effects of **levodopa**. Avoid or adjust dose. Severe Anecdotal → Also see **TABLE 7** p. 1572 → Also see **TABLE 10** p. 1574

▶ Antipsychotics, second generation (**quetiapine, risperidone**) potentially increase the risk of neurotoxicity when given with **lithium**. Severe Anecdotal

▶ **Clozapine** can cause constipation, as can **loperamide**; concurrent use might increase the risk of developing intestinal obstruction. Severe Anecdotal

▶ **Lorlatinib** is predicted to decrease the exposure to **cariprazine**. Avoid. Severe Theoretical

▶ **Lorlatinib** is predicted to decrease the exposure to **lurasidone**. Monitor and adjust dose. Moderate Theoretical

▶ **Lorlatinib** is predicted to decrease the exposure to **quetiapine**. Moderate Study

▶ **Clozapine** can cause constipation, as can **loxapine**; concurrent use might increase the risk of developing intestinal obstruction. Severe Theoretical → Also see **TABLE 17** p. 1576 → Also see **TABLE 7** p. 1572 → Also see **TABLE 9** p. 1573 → Also see **TABLE 10** p. 1574

▶ **Lumacaftor** is predicted to moderately decrease the exposure to **aripiprazole**. Adjust **aripiprazole** dose, p. 454. Moderate Study

▶ **Lumacaftor** is predicted to decrease the exposure to **cariprazine**. Avoid. Severe Theoretical

▶ **Lumacaftor** is predicted to decrease the exposure to **lurasidone**. Avoid. Moderate Study

▶ **Lumacaftor** is predicted to decrease the exposure to **paliperidone**. Monitor and adjust dose. Severe Study

▶ **Lumacaftor** is predicted to decrease the exposure to **quetiapine**. Moderate Study

▶ **Lumacaftor** is predicted to decrease the exposure to **risperidone**. Adjust dose. Moderate Study

▶ **Macrolides (clarithromycin)** are predicted to slightly increase the exposure to **aripiprazole**. Adjust **aripiprazole** dose, p. 454. Moderate Study

▶ **Macrolides (clarithromycin)** are predicted to moderately increase the exposure to **cariprazine**. Avoid. Severe Study

▶ **Macrolides (clarithromycin)** are predicted to increase the exposure to **risperidone**. Adjust dose. Moderate Study

▶ **Macrolides (erythromycin)** are predicted to increase the exposure to **cariprazine**. Avoid. Severe Study

▶ **Macrolides (erythromycin)** potentially increase the risk of toxicity when given with **clozapine**. Severe Anecdotal

▶ **Macrolides (erythromycin)** are predicted to increase the exposure to **lurasidone**. Adjust **lurasidone** dose, p. 458. Moderate Study

▶ **Macrolides (erythromycin)** are predicted to increase the exposure to **quetiapine**. Avoid. Moderate Study

▶ **Macrolides (clarithromycin)** are predicted to increase the exposure to antipsychotics, second generation (**lurasidone, quetiapine**). Avoid. Severe Study

▶ **Methylphenidate** might increase the risk of dyskinesias when given with **paliperidone**. Severe Theoretical

▶ **Methylphenidate** increases the risk of dyskinesias when given with **risperidone**. Severe Anecdotal

▶ **Mexiletine** increases the concentration of **clozapine**. Monitor adverse effects and adjust dose. Severe Study

▶ **Mexiletine** is predicted to increase the exposure to **olanzapine**. Adjust dose. Moderate Anecdotal

▶ **Mitotane** is predicted to moderately decrease the exposure to **aripiprazole**. Adjust **aripiprazole** dose, p. 454. Moderate Study

▶ **Mitotane** is predicted to decrease the exposure to **cariprazine**. Avoid. Severe Theoretical

▶ **Mitotane** is predicted to decrease the exposure to **lurasidone**. Avoid. Moderate Study

▶ **Mitotane** is predicted to decrease the exposure to **paliperidone**. Monitor and adjust dose. Severe Study

▶ **Mitotane** is predicted to decrease the exposure to **quetiapine**. Moderate Study

▶ **Mitotane** is predicted to decrease the exposure to **risperidone**. Adjust dose. Moderate Study

▶ **Neurokinin-1 receptor antagonists (aprepitant, netupitant)** are predicted to increase the exposure to **cariprazine**. Avoid. Severe Study

▶ **Neurokinin-1 receptor antagonists (aprepitant, netupitant)** are predicted to increase the exposure to **lurasidone**. Adjust **lurasidone** dose, p. 458. Moderate Study

▶ **Neurokinin-1 receptor antagonists (aprepitant, netupitant)** are predicted to increase the exposure to **quetiapine**. Avoid. Moderate Study

▶ **Nilotinib** is predicted to increase the exposure to **cariprazine**. Avoid. Severe Study

▶ **Nilotinib** is predicted to increase the exposure to **lurasidone**. Adjust **lurasidone** dose, p. 458. Moderate Study

▶ **Nilotinib** is predicted to increase the exposure to **quetiapine**. Avoid. Moderate Study

▶ **Nirmatrelvir** boosted with ritonavir is predicted to increase the concentration of antipsychotics, second generation (**lurasidone, quetiapine**). Avoid. Severe Theoretical

▶ **Nirmatrelvir** boosted with ritonavir is predicted to increase the concentration of **aripiprazole**. Adjust dose. Moderate Theoretical

▶ **Nirmatrelvir** boosted with ritonavir is predicted to increase the concentration of **cariprazine**. Avoid. Moderate Theoretical

▶ **Nirmatrelvir** boosted with ritonavir is predicted to increase the concentration of **clozapine**. Avoid or adjust dose. Severe Theoretical

▶ **Nirmatrelvir** boosted with ritonavir is predicted to increase the concentration of **risperidone**. Severe Theoretical

▶ **NNRTIs (efavirenz, etravirine, nevirapine)** are predicted to decrease the exposure to **cariprazine**. Avoid. Severe Theoretical

▶ **NNRTIs (efavirenz, etravirine, nevirapine)** are predicted to decrease the exposure to **lurasidone**. Monitor and adjust dose. Moderate Theoretical

▶ **NNRTIs (efavirenz, etravirine, nevirapine)** are predicted to decrease the exposure to **quetiapine**. Moderate Study

▶ **Olaparib** might alter the exposure to **quetiapine**. Moderate Theoretical

▶ **Clozapine** can cause constipation, as can **opioids**; concurrent use might increase the risk of developing intestinal obstruction. Severe Anecdotal → Also see **TABLE 17** p. 1576 → Also see **TABLE 10** p. 1574

▶ **Clozapine** can cause constipation, as can **orphenadrine**; concurrent use might increase the risk of developing intestinal obstruction. Severe Theoretical → Also see **TABLE 9** p. 1573 → Also see **TABLE 10** p. 1574

▸ **Osilodrostat** increases the concentration of **clozapine**. Monitor adverse effects and adjust dose. Severe Study

▸ **Osilodrostat** is predicted to increase the exposure to **olanzapine**. Adjust dose. Moderate Anecdotal

▸ **Clozapine** can cause constipation, as can **oxybutynin**; concurrent use might increase the risk of developing intestinal obstruction. Severe Theoretical → Also see **TABLE 9** p. 1573

▸ **Clozapine** can cause constipation, as can **phenothiazines**; concurrent use might increase the risk of developing intestinal obstruction. Severe Theoretical → Also see **TABLE 17** p. 1576 → Also see **TABLE 7** p. 1572 → Also see **TABLE 9** p. 1573 → Also see **TABLE 10** p. 1574

▸ **Clozapine** can cause constipation, as can **pimozide**; concurrent use might increase the risk of developing intestinal obstruction. Severe Theoretical → Also see **TABLE 17** p. 1576 → Also see **TABLE 7** p. 1572 → Also see **TABLE 9** p. 1573 → Also see **TABLE 10** p. 1574

▸ **Clozapine** can cause constipation, as can **pridinol**; concurrent use might increase the risk of developing intestinal obstruction. Severe Theoretical → Also see **TABLE 9** p. 1573

▸ **Clozapine** can cause constipation, as can **procyclidine**; concurrent use might increase the risk of developing intestinal obstruction. Severe Theoretical → Also see **TABLE 9** p. 1573 → Also see **TABLE 10** p. 1574

▸ **Clozapine** can cause constipation, as can **propantheline**; concurrent use might increase the risk of developing intestinal obstruction. Severe Theoretical → Also see **TABLE 9** p. 1573

▸ **Clozapine** can cause constipation, as can **propiverine**; concurrent use might increase the risk of developing intestinal obstruction. Severe Theoretical → Also see **TABLE 9** p. 1573

▸ **Quinolones (ciprofloxacin)** increase the concentration of **clozapine**. Monitor adverse effects and adjust dose. Severe Study

▸ **Quinolones (ciprofloxacin)** are predicted to increase the exposure to **olanzapine**. Adjust dose. Moderate Anecdotal

▸ **Ribociclib** (high-dose) is predicted to increase the exposure to **quetiapine**. Avoid. Moderate Theoretical

▸ **Rifamycins (rifampicin)** are predicted to moderately decrease the exposure to **aripiprazole**. Adjust **aripiprazole** dose, p. 454. Moderate Study

▸ **Rifamycins (rifampicin)** are predicted to decrease the exposure to **cariprazine**. Avoid. Severe Theoretical

▸ **Rifamycins (rifampicin)** decrease the exposure to **clozapine**. Severe Anecdotal

▸ **Rifamycins (rifampicin)** are predicted to decrease the exposure to **lurasidone**. Avoid. Moderate Study

▸ **Rifamycins (rifampicin)** are predicted to decrease the exposure to **olanzapine**. Monitor and adjust dose. Moderate Study

▸ **Rifamycins (rifampicin)** are predicted to decrease the exposure to **paliperidone**. Monitor and adjust dose. Severe Study

▸ **Rifamycins (rifampicin)** are predicted to decrease the exposure to **quetiapine**. Moderate Study

▸ **Rifamycins (rifampicin)** are predicted to decrease the exposure to **risperidone**. Adjust dose. Moderate Study

▸ **Rucaparib** increases the concentration of **clozapine**. Monitor adverse effects and adjust dose. Severe Study

▸ **Rucaparib** is predicted to increase the exposure to **olanzapine**. Adjust dose. Moderate Anecdotal

▸ **Clozapine** can cause constipation, as can **solifenacin**; concurrent use might increase the risk of developing intestinal obstruction. Severe Theoretical → Also see **TABLE 9** p. 1573

▸ **Sotorasib** is predicted to decrease the exposure to **cariprazine**. Avoid. Severe Theoretical

▸ **Sotorasib** is predicted to decrease the exposure to **lurasidone**. Monitor and adjust dose. Moderate Theoretical

▸ **Sotorasib** is predicted to decrease the exposure to **quetiapine**. Moderate Study

▸ **SSRIs (fluoxetine, paroxetine)** are predicted to moderately increase the exposure to **aripiprazole**. Adjust **aripiprazole** dose, p. 454. Moderate Study → Also see **TABLE 17** p. 1576 → Also see **TABLE 10** p. 1574

▸ **SSRIs (fluoxetine, paroxetine)** are predicted to increase the exposure to **clozapine**. Use with caution and adjust dose. Severe Study → Also see **TABLE 17** p. 1576 → Also see **TABLE 10** p. 1574

▸ **SSRIs (fluoxetine, paroxetine)** are predicted to increase the exposure to **risperidone**. Adjust dose. Moderate Study → Also see **TABLE 17** p. 1576 → Also see **TABLE 10** p. 1574

▸ **SSRIs (fluvoxamine)** increase the exposure to **asenapine**. Moderate Study → Also see **TABLE 17** p. 1576 → Also see **TABLE 10** p. 1574

▸ **SSRIs (fluvoxamine)** increase the concentration of **clozapine**. Monitor adverse effects and adjust dose. Severe Study → Also see **TABLE 17** p. 1576 → Also see **TABLE 10** p. 1574

▸ **SSRIs (fluvoxamine)** moderately increase the exposure to **olanzapine**. Adjust dose. Severe Anecdotal → Also see **TABLE 17** p. 1576 → Also see **TABLE 10** p. 1574

▸ **SSRIs (paroxetine)** moderately increase the exposure to **asenapine**. Moderate Study → Also see **TABLE 17** p. 1576 → Also see **TABLE 10** p. 1574

▸ **St John's wort** is predicted to decrease the exposure to **cariprazine**. Avoid. Severe Theoretical

▸ **St John's wort** is predicted to decrease the exposure to **lurasidone**. Monitor and adjust dose. Moderate Theoretical

▸ **St John's wort** is predicted to decrease the exposure to **paliperidone**. Severe Theoretical

▸ **St John's wort** is predicted to decrease the exposure to **quetiapine**. Moderate Study

▸ **Sulfonamides** might increase the risk of neutropenia when given with **clozapine**. Avoid. Severe Theoretical

▸ **Terbinafine** is predicted to moderately increase the exposure to **aripiprazole**. Adjust **aripiprazole** dose, p. 454. Moderate Study

▸ **Terbinafine** is predicted to increase the exposure to **clozapine**. Use with caution and adjust dose. Severe Study

▸ **Terbinafine** is predicted to increase the exposure to **risperidone**. Adjust dose. Moderate Study

▸ **Teriflunomide** is predicted to decrease the exposure to **clozapine**. Moderate Theoretical

▸ **Teriflunomide** is predicted to decrease the exposure to **olanzapine**. Monitor and adjust dose. Moderate Study

▸ **Clozapine** can cause constipation, as can **tiotropium**; concurrent use might increase the risk of developing intestinal obstruction. Severe Theoretical → Also see **TABLE 9** p. 1573

▸ **Clozapine** can cause constipation, as can **tolterodine**; concurrent use might increase the risk of developing intestinal obstruction. Severe Theoretical → Also see **TABLE 9** p. 1573

▸ **Clozapine** can cause constipation, as can **tricyclic antidepressants** ; concurrent use might increase the risk of developing intestinal obstruction. Severe Theoretical → Also see **TABLE 17** p. 1576 → Also see **TABLE 7** p. 1572 → Also see **TABLE 9** p. 1573 → Also see **TABLE 10** p. 1574

▸ **Clozapine** can cause constipation, as can **trihexyphenidyl**; concurrent use might increase the risk of developing intestinal obstruction. Severe Theoretical → Also see **TABLE 9** p. 1573 → Also see **TABLE 10** p. 1574

▸ **Trimethoprim** might increase the risk of neutropenia when given with **clozapine**. Avoid. Severe Theoretical

▸ **Clozapine** can cause constipation, as can **tropicamide**; concurrent use might increase the risk of developing intestinal obstruction. Severe Theoretical → Also see **TABLE 9** p. 1573

▸ **Clozapine** can cause constipation, as can **trospium**; concurrent use might increase the risk of developing intestinal obstruction. Severe Theoretical → Also see **TABLE 9** p. 1573

▸ **Tucatinib** is predicted to increase the exposure to antipsychotics, second generation (**lurasidone, quetiapine**). Avoid. Severe Study

▸ **Tucatinib** is predicted to slightly increase the exposure to **aripiprazole**. Adjust **aripiprazole** dose, p. 454. Moderate Study

▸ **Tucatinib** is predicted to moderately increase the exposure to **cariprazine**. Avoid. Severe Study

▸ **Tucatinib** is predicted to increase the exposure to **risperidone**. Adjust dose. Moderate Study

Antipsychotics, second generation (continued)

▶ **Clozapine** can cause constipation, as can umeclidinium; concurrent use might increase the risk of developing intestinal obstruction. Severe Theoretical → Also see TABLE 9 p. 1573

▶ **Clozapine** might decrease the antidiuretic and hypertensive effects of vasopressin. Moderate Theoretical

▶ **Vemurafenib** increases the concentration of **clozapine**. Monitor adverse effects and adjust dose. Severe Study

▶ **Vemurafenib** is predicted to increase the exposure to olanzapine. Adjust dose. Moderate Anecdotal

▶ **Clozapine** can cause constipation, as can zuclopenthixol; concurrent use might increase the risk of developing intestinal obstruction. Severe Theoretical → Also see TABLE 17 p. 1576 → Also see TABLE 7 p. 1572 → Also see TABLE 9 p. 1573 → Also see TABLE 10 p. 1574

Antithymocyte immunoglobulin (rabbit) → see immunoglobulins

Apalutamide → see anti-androgens

Apixaban → see factor XA inhibitors

Apomorphine → see dopamine receptor agonists

Apraclonidine → see TABLE 5 p. 1572 (bradycardia), TABLE 7 p. 1572 (hypotension), TABLE 10 p. 1574 (CNS effects)

▶ **Amfetamines** are predicted to decrease the effects of apraclonidine. Avoid. Severe Theoretical

▶ **Methylphenidate** is predicted to decrease the effects of apraclonidine. Avoid. Severe Theoretical

▶ **Sympathomimetics, inotropic** are predicted to decrease the effects of apraclonidine. Avoid. Severe Theoretical

▶ **Sympathomimetics, vasoconstrictor** are predicted to decrease the effects of apraclonidine. Avoid. Severe Theoretical

Apremilast → see phosphodiesterase type-4 inhibitors

Aprepitant → see neurokinin-1 receptor antagonists

Argatroban → see thrombin inhibitors

Aripiprazole → see antipsychotics, second generation

Arsenic trioxide → see TABLE 14 p. 1575 (myelosuppression), TABLE 8 p. 1573 (QT-interval prolongation)

Artemether → see antimalarials

Asciminib

▶ **Asciminib** slightly to moderately increases the exposure to coumarins (warfarin). Severe Theoretical

▶ **Asciminib** is predicted to increase the exposure to digoxin. Severe Theoretical

▶ **Asciminib** is predicted to increase the exposure to everolimus. Severe Theoretical

▶ **Asciminib** is predicted to increase the exposure to factor XA inhibitors (edoxaban). Severe Theoretical

▶ **Asciminib** is predicted to increase the exposure to opioids (alfentanil). Severe Theoretical

▶ **Asciminib** is predicted to increase the exposure to sirolimus. Severe Theoretical

▶ **Asciminib** is predicted to increase the exposure to temsirolimus. Severe Theoretical

▶ **Asciminib** is predicted to increase the exposure to thrombin inhibitors (dabigatran). Severe Theoretical

Ascorbic acid

▶ **Ascorbic acid** is predicted to increase the risk of cardiovascular adverse effects when given with iron chelators (deferiprone). Severe Theoretical

▶ **Ascorbic acid** might increase the risk of cardiovascular adverse effects when given with iron chelators (desferrioxamine). Manufacturer advises caution or adjust ascorbic acid dose; monitor cardiac function and avoid concurrent use in those with cardiac failure. Severe Theoretical

Asenapine → see antipsychotics, second generation

Asparaginase → see TABLE 1 p. 1571 (hepatotoxicity), TABLE 14 p. 1575 (myelosuppression), TABLE 3 p. 1571 (anticoagulant effects)

▶ **Asparaginase** is predicted to increase the risk of hepatotoxicity when given with imatinib. Severe Theoretical → Also see TABLE 14 p. 1575

▶ **Asparaginase** affects the efficacy of methotrexate. Severe Anecdotal → Also see TABLE 1 p. 1571 → Also see TABLE 14 p. 1575

▶ **Asparaginase** potentially increases the risk of neurotoxicity when given with vinca alkaloids (vincristine). **Vincristine** should

be taken 3 to 24 hours before **asparaginase**. Severe Anecdotal → Also see TABLE 14 p. 1575

Aspirin → see TABLE 2 p. 1571 (nephrotoxicity), TABLE 4 p. 1571 (antiplatelet effects)

▶ **Acetazolamide** increases the risk of severe toxic reaction when given with **aspirin** (high-dose). Severe Study

▶ Oral **antacids** decrease the absorption of oral **aspirin** (high-dose). Moderate Study

▶ **Bismuth** subsalicylate is predicted to increase the risk of adverse effects when given with **aspirin**. Avoid. Moderate Theoretical

▶ **Aspirin** (high-dose) is predicted to increase the risk of gastrointestinal irritation when given with bisphosphonates (alendronate, ibandronate). Moderate Study

▶ **Aspirin** (high-dose) is predicted to increase the risk of renal impairment when given with bisphosphonates (clodronate). Severe Theoretical

▶ **Corticosteroids** are predicted to decrease the concentration of **aspirin** (high-dose) and **aspirin** (high-dose) increases the risk of gastrointestinal bleeding when given with corticosteroids. Moderate Study

▶ **Aspirin** (high-dose) increases the risk of renal impairment when given with daptomycin. Moderate Theoretical

▶ **Erlotinib** is predicted to increase the risk of gastrointestinal perforation when given with **aspirin** (high-dose). Severe Theoretical

▶ **Aspirin** (high-dose) increases the exposure to factor XA inhibitors (edoxaban). Avoid. Severe Study

▶ **Aspirin** (high-dose) is predicted to increase the risk of gastrointestinal bleeds when given with iron chelators (deferasirox). Severe Theoretical → Also see TABLE 2 p. 1571

▶ **Live vaccines (influenza vaccine (live))** might increase the risk of Reye's syndrome when given with **aspirin**. Avoid **aspirin** for 4 weeks after vaccination. Severe Theoretical

▶ **Live vaccines (varicella-zoster vaccine)** might increase the risk of Reye's syndrome when given with **aspirin**. Avoid **aspirin** for 6 weeks after vaccination. Severe Theoretical

▶ **Aspirin** (high-dose) is predicted to increase the risk of toxicity when given with methotrexate. Severe Study → Also see TABLE 2 p. 1571

▶ **Aspirin** is predicted to increase the risk of gastrointestinal perforation when given with nicorandil. Severe Theoretical

▶ **NRTIs (zidovudine)** increase the risk of haematological toxicity when given with **aspirin** (high-dose). Severe Study

▶ **Aspirin** (high-dose) potentially increases the exposure to pemetrexed. Use with caution or avoid. Severe Theoretical → Also see TABLE 2 p. 1571

▶ **Selumetinib** might increase the risk of bleeding when given with **aspirin**. Severe Theoretical

▶ **Aspirin** (high-dose) increases the risk of acute renal failure when given with thiazide diuretics. Severe Theoretical

Ataluren

▶ **Ataluren** is predicted to increase the risk of nephrotoxicity when given with intravenous aminoglycosides. Avoid. Severe Study

▶ **Rifamycins (rifampicin)** decrease the exposure to **ataluren**. Moderate Study

Atazanavir → see HIV-protease inhibitors

Atenolol → see beta blockers, selective

Atezolizumab → see monoclonal antibodies

Atogepant

▶ **Angiotensin-II receptor antagonists (telmisartan)** are predicted to increase the exposure to **atogepant**. Adjust **atogepant** dose, p. 540. Moderate Theoretical

▶ **Antifungals, azoles (itraconazole, ketoconazole, posaconazole, voriconazole)** are predicted to increase the exposure to **atogepant**. Adjust **atogepant** dose, p. 540. Moderate Study

▶ **Cenobamate** is predicted to decrease the exposure to **atogepant**. Adjust dose. Moderate Theoretical

▶ **Ceritinib** is predicted to increase the exposure to **atogepant**. Adjust **atogepant** dose, p. 540. Moderate Study

▶ **Ciclosporin** is predicted to increase the exposure to **atogepant**. Adjust **atogepant** dose, p. 540. Moderate Theoretical

▶ **Cobicistat** is predicted to increase the exposure to **atogepant**. Adjust **atogepant** dose, p. 540. Moderate Study

▶ **Eltrombopag** is predicted to increase the exposure to atogepant. Adjust **atogepant** dose, p. 540. Moderate Theoretical

▶ **Fibrates (gemfibrozil)** are predicted to increase the exposure to atogepant. Adjust **atogepant** dose, p. 540. Moderate Theoretical

▶ **HIV-protease inhibitors** are predicted to increase the exposure to atogepant. Adjust **atogepant** dose, p. 540. Moderate Study

▶ **Idelalisib** is predicted to increase the exposure to atogepant. Adjust **atogepant** dose, p. 540. Moderate Study

▶ **Leflunomide** is predicted to increase the exposure to atogepant. Adjust **atogepant** dose, p. 540. Moderate Theoretical

▶ **Macrolides (clarithromycin)** are predicted to increase the exposure to atogepant. Adjust **atogepant** dose, p. 540. Moderate Study

▶ **Macrolides (erythromycin)** are predicted to increase the exposure to atogepant. Adjust **atogepant** dose, p. 540. Moderate Theoretical

▶ **Rifamycins (rifampicin)** (single-dose) increase the exposure to atogepant. Adjust **atogepant** dose, p. 540. Moderate Study

▶ **Teriflunomide** is predicted to increase the exposure to atogepant. Adjust **atogepant** dose, p. 540. Moderate Theoretical

▶ **Tucatinib** is predicted to increase the exposure to **atogepant**. Adjust **atogepant** dose, p. 540. Moderate Study

Atomoxetine

▶ **Amfetamines** are predicted to increase the risk of adverse effects when given with **atomoxetine**. Severe Theoretical

▶ **Berotralstat** is predicted to increase the exposure to atomoxetine. Adjust dose. Moderate Study

▶ **Atomoxetine** is predicted to increase the risk of cardiovascular adverse effects when given with **beta₂ agonists** (high-dose). Moderate Study

▶ **Bupropion** is predicted to markedly increase the exposure to atomoxetine. Adjust dose. Severe Study

▶ **Cinacalcet** is predicted to markedly increase the exposure to atomoxetine. Adjust dose. Severe Study

▶ **Dacomitinib** is predicted to markedly increase the exposure to atomoxetine. Adjust dose. Severe Study

▶ **Eliglustat** is predicted to increase the exposure to **atomoxetine**. Adjust dose. Moderate Theoretical

▶ **Givosiran** is predicted to increase the exposure to **atomoxetine**. Use with caution and adjust dose. Moderate Study

▶ **Interferons (ropeginterferon alfa)** are predicted to increase the exposure to **atomoxetine**. Moderate Theoretical

▶ **MAOIs, irreversible** are predicted to increase the risk of adverse effects when given with **atomoxetine**. Avoid and for 2 weeks after stopping the MAOI. Severe Theoretical

▶ **Panobinostat** is predicted to increase the exposure to atomoxetine. Monitor and adjust dose. Severe Theoretical

▶ **SSRIs (fluoxetine, paroxetine)** are predicted to markedly increase the exposure to **atomoxetine**. Adjust dose. Severe Study

▶ **Terbinafine** is predicted to markedly increase the exposure to atomoxetine. Adjust dose. Severe Study

Atorvastatin → see statins

Atovaquone → see antimalarials

Atracurium → see neuromuscular blocking drugs, non-depolarising

Atropine → see TABLE 9 p. 1573 (antimuscarinics)

ROUTE-SPECIFIC INFORMATION Since systemic absorption can follow topical application of **atropine**, the possibility of interactions should be borne in mind.

▶ **Antipsychotics, second generation (clozapine)** can cause constipation, as can **atropine**; concurrent use might increase the risk of developing intestinal obstruction. Severe Theoretical → Also see TABLE 9 p. 1573

▶ **Atropine** increases the risk of severe hypertension when given with **sympathomimetics, vasoconstrictor (phenylephrine)**. Severe Study

Avacopan

▶ **Anti-androgens (apalutamide, enzalutamide)** are predicted to decrease the exposure to **avacopan**. Avoid or monitor. Severe Study

▶ **Antiepileptics (carbamazepine, fosphenytoin, phenobarbital, phenytoin, primidone)** are predicted to decrease the exposure to **avacopan**. Avoid or monitor. Severe Study

▶ **Antifungals, azoles (itraconazole, ketoconazole, posaconazole, voriconazole)** are predicted to increase the exposure to avacopan. Severe Study

▶ **Cenobamate** is predicted to decrease the exposure to avacopan. Severe Theoretical

▶ **Ceritinib** is predicted to increase the exposure to **avacopan**. Severe Study

▶ **Cobicistat** is predicted to increase the exposure to **avacopan**. Severe Study

▶ **Dabrafenib** is predicted to decrease the exposure to **avacopan**. Severe Theoretical

▶ **Encorafenib** is predicted to decrease the exposure to **avacopan**. Avoid or monitor. Severe Study

▶ **Endothelin receptor antagonists (bosentan)** are predicted to decrease the exposure to **avacopan**. Severe Theoretical

▶ **Grapefruit** and grapefruit juice is predicted to increase the exposure to avacopan. Avoid. Moderate Theoretical

▶ **HIV-protease inhibitors** are predicted to increase the exposure to avacopan. Severe Study

▶ **Idelalisib** is predicted to increase the exposure to **avacopan**. Severe Study

▶ **Ivosidenib** is predicted to decrease the exposure to **avacopan**. Avoid or monitor. Severe Study

▶ **Lorlatinib** is predicted to decrease the exposure to **avacopan**. Severe Theoretical

▶ **Lumacaftor** is predicted to decrease the exposure to **avacopan**. Avoid or monitor. Severe Study

▶ **Macrolides (clarithromycin)** are predicted to increase the exposure to avacopan. Severe Study

▶ **Mitotane** is predicted to decrease the exposure to **avacopan**. Avoid or monitor. Severe Study

▶ **Modafinil** is predicted to decrease the exposure to **avacopan**. Severe Theoretical

▶ **NNRTIs (efavirenz, etravirine, nevirapine)** are predicted to decrease the exposure to **avacopan**. Severe Theoretical

▶ **Rifamycins (rifampicin)** are predicted to decrease the exposure to avacopan. Avoid or monitor. Severe Study

▶ **Sotorasib** is predicted to decrease the exposure to **avacopan**. Severe Theoretical

▶ **St John's wort** is predicted to decrease the exposure to avacopan. Severe Theoretical

▶ **Tucatinib** is predicted to increase the exposure to **avacopan**. Severe Study

Avanafil → see phosphodiesterase type-5 inhibitors

Avapritinib

▶ **Anti-androgens (apalutamide, enzalutamide)** are predicted to decrease the exposure to **avapritinib**. Avoid. Severe Study

▶ **Antiarrhythmics (dronedarone)** are predicted to increase the exposure to **avapritinib**. Avoid or adjust dose—consult product literature. Moderate Study

▶ **Antiepileptics (carbamazepine, fosphenytoin, phenobarbital, phenytoin, primidone)** are predicted to decrease the exposure to **avapritinib**. Avoid. Severe Study

▶ **Antifungals, azoles (fluconazole, isavuconazole)** are predicted to increase the exposure to **avapritinib**. Avoid or adjust dose—consult product literature. Moderate Study

▶ **Antifungals, azoles (itraconazole, ketoconazole, posaconazole, voriconazole)** are predicted to increase the exposure to **avapritinib**. Avoid. Moderate Study

▶ **Berotralstat** is predicted to increase the exposure to **avapritinib**. Avoid or adjust dose—consult product literature. Moderate Study

▶ **Calcium channel blockers (diltiazem, verapamil)** are predicted to increase the exposure to **avapritinib**. Avoid or adjust dose—consult product literature. Moderate Study

▶ **Cenobamate** is predicted to decrease the exposure to **avapritinib**. Avoid. Severe Study

▶ **Ceritinib** is predicted to increase the exposure to **avapritinib**. Avoid. Moderate Study

▶ **Cobicistat** is predicted to increase the exposure to **avapritinib**. Avoid. Moderate Study

▶ **Corticosteroids (dexamethasone)** are predicted to decrease the exposure to **avapritinib**. Avoid. Severe Theoretical

Avapritinib (continued)

▸ **Crizotinib** is predicted to increase the exposure to **avapritinib**. Avoid or adjust dose—consult product literature. [Moderate] Study

▸ **Dabrafenib** is predicted to decrease the exposure to **avapritinib**. Avoid. [Severe] Study

▸ **Drugs with anticoagulant effects** (see TABLE 3 p. 1571) might increase the risk of bleeding when given with **avapritinib**. [Severe] Theoretical

▸ **Drugs with antiplatelet effects** (see TABLE 4 p. 1571) might increase the risk of bleeding when given with **avapritinib**. [Severe] Theoretical

▸ **Encorafenib** is predicted to decrease the exposure to **avapritinib**. Avoid. [Severe] Study

▸ **Endothelin receptor antagonists (bosentan)** are predicted to decrease the exposure to **avapritinib**. Avoid. [Severe] Study

▸ **Fedratinib** is predicted to increase the exposure to **avapritinib**. Avoid or adjust dose—consult product literature. [Moderate] Study

▸ **Grapefruit** juice is predicted to increase the exposure to **avapritinib**. Avoid. [Moderate] Theoretical

▸ **HIV-protease inhibitors** are predicted to increase the exposure to **avapritinib**. Avoid. [Moderate] Study

▸ **Idelalisib** is predicted to increase the exposure to **avapritinib**. Avoid. [Moderate] Study

▸ **Imatinib** is predicted to increase the exposure to **avapritinib**. Avoid or adjust dose—consult product literature. [Moderate] Study

▸ **Ivosidenib** is predicted to decrease the exposure to **avapritinib**. Avoid. [Severe] Study

▸ **Letermovir** is predicted to increase the exposure to **avapritinib**. Avoid or adjust dose—consult product literature. [Moderate] Study

▸ **Lorlatinib** is predicted to decrease the exposure to **avapritinib**. Avoid. [Severe] Study

▸ **Lumacaftor** is predicted to decrease the exposure to **avapritinib**. Avoid. [Severe] Study

▸ **Macrolides (clarithromycin)** are predicted to increase the exposure to **avapritinib**. Avoid. [Moderate] Study

▸ **Macrolides (erythromycin)** are predicted to increase the exposure to **avapritinib**. Avoid or adjust dose—consult product literature. [Moderate] Study

▸ **Mitotane** is predicted to decrease the exposure to **avapritinib**. Avoid. [Severe] Study

▸ **Modafinil** is predicted to decrease the exposure to **avapritinib**. Avoid. [Severe] Theoretical

▸ **Neurokinin-1 receptor antagonists (aprepitant, netupitant)** are predicted to increase the exposure to **avapritinib**. Avoid or adjust dose—consult product literature. [Moderate] Study

▸ **Nilotinib** is predicted to increase the exposure to **avapritinib**. Avoid or adjust dose—consult product literature. [Moderate] Study

▸ **NNRTIs (efavirenz, etravirine, nevirapine)** are predicted to decrease the exposure to **avapritinib**. Avoid. [Severe] Study

▸ **Rifamycins (rifampicin)** are predicted to decrease the exposure to **avapritinib**. Avoid. [Severe] Study

▸ **Sotorasib** is predicted to decrease the exposure to **avapritinib**. Avoid. [Severe] Study

▸ **St John's wort** is predicted to decrease the exposure to **avapritinib**. Avoid. [Severe] Study

▸ **Tucatinib** is predicted to increase the exposure to **avapritinib**. Avoid. [Moderate] Study

Avatrombopag

▸ **Anti-androgens (enzalutamide)** are predicted to decrease the exposure to **avatrombopag**. Adjust **avatrombopag** dose with moderate CYP2C9 inducers in chronic immune thrombocytopenia, p. 1169. [Moderate] Study

▸ **Antiarrhythmics (amiodarone)** are predicted to increase the exposure to **avatrombopag**. Adjust **avatrombopag** dose with moderate CYP2C9 inhibitors in chronic immune thrombocytopenia, p. 1169. [Moderate] Study

▸ **Antifungals, azoles (fluconazole, miconazole)** are predicted to increase the exposure to **avatrombopag**. Adjust **avatrombopag** dose with moderate CYP2C9 inhibitors in chronic immune thrombocytopenia, p. 1169. [Moderate] Study

▸ **Mifepristone** is predicted to increase the exposure to **avatrombopag**. [Moderate] Theoretical

▸ **Rifamycins (rifampicin)** are predicted to decrease the exposure to **avatrombopag**. Adjust **avatrombopag** dose with moderate CYP2C9 inducers in chronic immune thrombocytopenia, p. 1169. [Moderate] Study

Avelumab → see monoclonal antibodies

Axitinib → see TABLE 14 p. 1575 (myelosuppression), TABLE 4 p. 1571 (antiplatelet effects)

▸ **Axitinib** is predicted to increase the exposure to **agomelatine**. [Moderate] Theoretical

▸ **Axitinib** is predicted to increase the exposure to **aminophylline**. [Moderate] Theoretical

▸ **Axitinib** is predicted to increase the exposure to **anaesthetics, local (ropivacaine)**. [Moderate] Theoretical

▸ **Anti-androgens (apalutamide, enzalutamide)** are predicted to decrease the exposure to **axitinib**. Avoid or adjust dose. [Moderate] Study

▸ **Antiarrhythmics (dronedarone)** are predicted to increase the exposure to **axitinib**. [Moderate] Study

▸ **Antiepileptics (carbamazepine, fosphenytoin, phenobarbital, phenytoin, primidone)** are predicted to decrease the exposure to **axitinib**. Avoid or adjust dose. [Moderate] Study

▸ **Antifungals, azoles (fluconazole, isavuconazole)** are predicted to increase the exposure to **axitinib**. [Moderate] Study

▸ **Antifungals, azoles (itraconazole, ketoconazole, posaconazole, voriconazole)** are predicted to increase the exposure to **axitinib**. Avoid or adjust dose. [Moderate] Study

▸ **Axitinib** is predicted to increase the exposure to antipsychotics, second generation **(clozapine, olanzapine)**. [Moderate] Theoretical

▸ **Berotralstat** is predicted to increase the exposure to **axitinib**. [Moderate] Study

▸ **Calcium channel blockers (diltiazem, verapamil)** are predicted to increase the exposure to **axitinib**. [Moderate] Study

▸ **Ceritinib** is predicted to increase the exposure to **axitinib**. Avoid or adjust dose. [Moderate] Study → Also see TABLE 14 p. 1575

▸ **Cobicistat** is predicted to increase the exposure to **axitinib**. Avoid or adjust dose. [Moderate] Study

▸ **Crizotinib** is predicted to increase the exposure to **axitinib**. [Moderate] Study

▸ **Dabrafenib** is predicted to decrease the exposure to **axitinib**. [Moderate] Study

▸ **Axitinib** is predicted to increase the exposure to dopamine receptor agonists **(ropinirole)**. [Moderate] Theoretical

▸ **Encorafenib** is predicted to decrease the exposure to **axitinib**. Avoid or adjust dose. [Moderate] Study

▸ **Endothelin receptor antagonists (bosentan)** are predicted to decrease the exposure to **axitinib**. [Moderate] Study

▸ **Fedratinib** is predicted to increase the exposure to **axitinib**. [Moderate] Study

▸ **Grapefruit** juice is predicted to increase the exposure to **axitinib**. [Moderate] Theoretical

▸ **HIV-protease inhibitors** are predicted to increase the exposure to **axitinib**. Avoid or adjust dose. [Moderate] Study

▸ **Idelalisib** is predicted to increase the exposure to **axitinib**. Avoid or adjust dose. [Moderate] Study

▸ **Imatinib** is predicted to increase the exposure to **axitinib**. [Moderate] Study → Also see TABLE 14 p. 1575 → Also see TABLE 4 p. 1571

▸ **Ivosidenib** is predicted to decrease the exposure to **axitinib**. Avoid or adjust dose. [Moderate] Study

▸ **Letermovir** is predicted to increase the exposure to **axitinib**. [Moderate] Study

▸ **Lumacaftor** is predicted to decrease the exposure to **axitinib**. Avoid or adjust dose. [Moderate] Study

▸ **Macrolides (clarithromycin)** are predicted to increase the exposure to **axitinib**. Avoid or adjust dose. [Moderate] Study

▸ **Macrolides (erythromycin)** are predicted to increase the exposure to **axitinib**. [Moderate] Study

▸ **Axitinib** is predicted to increase the exposure to MAO-B inhibitors **(rasagiline)**. [Moderate] Theoretical

▸ **Axitinib** is predicted to increase the exposure to melatonin. [Moderate] Theoretical

▸ **Mitotane** is predicted to decrease the exposure to **axitinib**. Avoid or adjust dose. [Moderate] Study → Also see TABLE 14 p. 1575

- Neurokinin-1 receptor antagonists (aprepitant, netupitant) are predicted to increase the exposure to axitinib. [Moderate] Study
- Nilotinib is predicted to increase the exposure to axitinib. [Moderate] Study → Also see TABLE 14 p. 1575
- NNRTIs (efavirenz, nevirapine) are predicted to decrease the exposure to axitinib. [Moderate] Study
- Axitinib is predicted to increase the exposure to pirfenidone. [Moderate] Theoretical
- Rifamycins (rifampicin) are predicted to decrease the exposure to axitinib. Avoid or adjust dose. [Moderate] Study
- Axitinib is predicted to increase the exposure to SNRIs (duloxetine). [Moderate] Theoretical → Also see TABLE 4 p. 1571
- St John's wort is predicted to decrease the exposure to axitinib. Avoid or adjust dose. [Moderate] Study
- Axitinib is predicted to increase the exposure to theophylline. [Moderate] Theoretical
- Axitinib is predicted to increase the exposure to tizanidine. [Moderate] Theoretical
- Tucatinib is predicted to increase the exposure to axitinib. Avoid or adjust dose. [Moderate] Study

Azacitidine → see TABLE 14 p. 1575 (myelosuppression)
- Cedazuridine is predicted to increase the exposure to azacitidine. Avoid. [Moderate] Theoretical

Azathioprine → see TABLE 14 p. 1575 (myelosuppression)
- ACE inhibitors are predicted to increase the risk of anaemia and/or leucopenia when given with azathioprine. [Severe] Anecdotal
- Allopurinol potentially increases the risk of haematological toxicity when given with azathioprine. Adjust azathioprine dose, p. 965. [Severe] Study
- Baricitinib is predicted to enhance the risk of immunosuppression when given with azathioprine. [Severe] Theoretical
- Azathioprine decreases the anticoagulant effect of coumarins. [Moderate] Study
- Febuxostat is predicted to increase the exposure to azathioprine. Avoid. [Severe] Theoretical
- Live vaccines are predicted to increase the risk of generalised infection (possibly life-threatening) when given with azathioprine (high-dose). UKHSA advises avoid (refer to Green Book). [Severe] Theoretical
- Trimethoprim might increase the risk of haematological toxicity when given with azathioprine in renal transplant patients. [Severe] Anecdotal

Azelastine → see antihistamines, non-sedating
Azilsartan → see angiotensin-II receptor antagonists
Azithromycin → see macrolides
Bacillus Calmette-Guérin vaccine → see live vaccines
Baclofen → see TABLE 7 p. 1572 (hypotension), TABLE 9 p. 1573 (antimuscarinics), TABLE 10 p. 1574 (CNS effects)
- Antipsychotics, second generation (clozapine) can cause constipation, as can baclofen; concurrent use might increase the risk of developing intestinal obstruction. [Severe] Theoretical → Also see TABLE 7 p. 1572 → Also see TABLE 9 p. 1573 → Also see TABLE 10 p. 1574
- Baclofen is predicted to increase the risk of adverse effects when given with levodopa. [Severe] Anecdotal → Also see TABLE 7 p. 1572 → Also see TABLE 10 p. 1574

Baloxavir marboxil
- Oral aluminium hydroxide might decrease the concentration of the active metabolite of oral baloxavir marboxil. [Severe] Theoretical
- Oral antacids might decrease the concentration of the active metabolite of oral baloxavir marboxil. Avoid. [Severe] Theoretical
- Oral calcium salts might decrease the concentration of the active metabolite of oral baloxavir marboxil. Avoid. [Severe] Theoretical
- Oral docusates might decrease the concentration of the active metabolite of oral baloxavir marboxil. [Severe] Theoretical
- Oral iron might decrease the concentration of the active metabolite of oral baloxavir marboxil. Avoid. [Severe] Theoretical
- Baloxavir marboxil might decrease the efficacy of live vaccines (influenza vaccine (live)). [Moderate] Theoretical

- Oral magnesium might decrease the concentration of the active metabolite of oral baloxavir marboxil. Avoid. [Severe] Theoretical
- Oral selenium might decrease the concentration of the active metabolite of oral baloxavir marboxil. Avoid. [Severe] Theoretical
- Oral sodium picosulfate might decrease the concentration of the active metabolite of oral baloxavir marboxil. [Severe] Theoretical
- Oral zinc might decrease the concentration of the active metabolite of oral baloxavir marboxil. Avoid. [Severe] Theoretical

Balsalazide
- Balsalazide is predicted to decrease the concentration of digoxin. [Moderate] Theoretical

Baricitinib
- Baricitinib is predicted to enhance the risk of immunosuppression when given with azathioprine. [Severe] Theoretical
- Baricitinib is predicted to enhance the risk of immunosuppression when given with ciclosporin. Manufacturer advises caution or avoid—consult product literature. [Severe] Theoretical
- Filgotinib is predicted to increase the risk of immunosuppression when given with baricitinib. Avoid. [Severe] Theoretical
- Leflunomide is predicted to increase the exposure to baricitinib. [Moderate] Study
- Live vaccines are predicted to increase the risk of generalised infection (possibly life-threatening) when given with baricitinib. Avoid. [Severe] Theoretical
- Baricitinib is predicted to enhance the risk of immunosuppression when given with methotrexate. [Severe] Study
- Nitisinone is predicted to increase the exposure to baricitinib. [Moderate] Study
- Baricitinib is predicted to enhance the risk of immunosuppression when given with tacrolimus. [Severe] Theoretical
- Teriflunomide is predicted to increase the exposure to baricitinib. [Moderate] Study
- Vadadustat is predicted to increase the exposure to baricitinib. Monitor and adjust dose. [Moderate] Study

Basiliximab → see monoclonal antibodies
Bazedoxifene
- Antiepileptics (carbamazepine, fosphenytoin, phenobarbital, phenytoin, primidone) are predicted to decrease the exposure to bazedoxifene. [Moderate] Theoretical
- Rifamycins (rifampicin) are predicted to decrease the exposure to bazedoxifene. [Moderate] Theoretical

Beclometasone → see corticosteroids
Bedaquiline → see TABLE 8 p. 1573 (QT-interval prolongation)
- Anti-androgens (apalutamide, enzalutamide) decrease the exposure to bedaquiline. Avoid. [Severe] Study → Also see TABLE 8 p. 1573
- Antiarrhythmics (dronedarone) might increase the exposure to bedaquiline. [Mild] Theoretical → Also see TABLE 8 p. 1573
- Antiepileptics (carbamazepine, fosphenytoin, phenobarbital, phenytoin, primidone) decrease the exposure to bedaquiline. Avoid. [Severe] Study
- Antifungals, azoles (fluconazole, isavuconazole) might increase the exposure to bedaquiline. [Mild] Theoretical → Also see TABLE 8 p. 1573
- Antifungals, azoles (itraconazole, ketoconazole, posaconazole, voriconazole) might increase the exposure to bedaquiline. [Mild] Study → Also see TABLE 8 p. 1573
- Berotralstat might increases the exposure to bedaquiline. [Mild] Theoretical
- Calcium channel blockers (diltiazem, verapamil) might increase the exposure to bedaquiline. [Mild] Theoretical
- Cenobamate is predicted to decrease the exposure to bedaquiline. Avoid. [Severe] Study
- Ceritinib might increases the exposure to bedaquiline. [Mild] Study → Also see TABLE 8 p. 1573
- Clofazimine potentially increases the risk of QT-prolongation when given with bedaquiline. [Severe] Study

Bedaquiline (continued)

▸ **Cobicistat** might increases the exposure to **bedaquiline**. Mild Study

▸ **Crizotinib** might increases the exposure to **bedaquiline**. Mild Theoretical → Also see TABLE 8 p. 1573

▸ **Dabrafenib** is predicted to decrease the exposure to **bedaquiline**. Avoid. Severe Study

▸ **Encorafenib** decreases the exposure to **bedaquiline**. Avoid. Severe Study → Also see TABLE 8 p. 1573

▸ **Endothelin receptor antagonists (bosentan)** are predicted to decrease the exposure to **bedaquiline**. Avoid. Severe Study

▸ **Fedratinib** might increases the exposure to **bedaquiline**. Mild Theoretical

▸ **HIV-protease inhibitors** might increase the exposure to **bedaquiline**. Mild Study

▸ **Idelalisib** might increases the exposure to **bedaquiline**. Mild Study

▸ **Imatinib** might increases the exposure to **bedaquiline**. Mild Theoretical

▸ **Ivosidenib** decreases the exposure to **bedaquiline**. Avoid. Severe Study → Also see TABLE 8 p. 1573

▸ **Letermovir** might increases the exposure to **bedaquiline**. Mild Theoretical

▸ **Lorlatinib** is predicted to decrease the exposure to **bedaquiline**. Avoid. Severe Study

▸ **Lumacaftor** decreases the exposure to **bedaquiline**. Avoid. Severe Study

▸ **Macrolides (clarithromycin)** might increase the exposure to **bedaquiline**. Mild Study

▸ **Macrolides (erythromycin)** might increase the exposure to **bedaquiline**. Mild Theoretical → Also see TABLE 8 p. 1573

▸ **Mitotane** decreases the exposure to **bedaquiline**. Avoid. Severe Study

▸ **Neurokinin-1 receptor antagonists (aprepitant, netupitant)** might increase the exposure to **bedaquiline**. Mild Theoretical

▸ **Nilotinib** might increases the exposure to **bedaquiline**. Mild Theoretical → Also see TABLE 8 p. 1573

▸ **Nirmatrelvir** boosted with ritonavir is predicted to increase the concentration of **bedaquiline**. Avoid or monitor. Moderate Theoretical

▸ **NNRTIs (efavirenz, etravirine, nevirapine)** are predicted to decrease the exposure to **bedaquiline**. Avoid. Severe Study → Also see TABLE 8 p. 1573

▸ **Quinolones (ciprofloxacin)** might increase the exposure to **bedaquiline**. Mild Theoretical

▸ **Rifamycins (rifampicin)** decrease the exposure to **bedaquiline**. Avoid. Severe Study

▸ **Sotorasib** is predicted to decrease the exposure to **bedaquiline**. Avoid. Severe Study

▸ **St John's wort** is predicted to decrease the exposure to **bedaquiline**. Avoid. Severe Study

▸ **Tucatinib** might increases the exposure to **bedaquiline**. Mild Study

Bee venom extract

GENERAL INFORMATION Desensitising vaccines should be avoided in patients taking beta-blockers (adrenaline might be ineffective in case of a hypersensitivity reaction) or ACE inhibitors (risk of severe anaphylactoid reactions).

Belatacept → see TABLE 14 p. 1575 (myelosuppression)

▸ **Live vaccines** are predicted to increase the risk of generalised infection (possibly life-threatening) when given with **belatacept**. UKHSA advises avoid (refer to Green Book). Severe Theoretical

▸ **Monoclonal antibodies (rozanolixizumab)** might decrease the concentration of **belatacept**. Avoid and for 2 weeks after stopping **rozanolixizumab**. Moderate Theoretical

Belimumab → see monoclonal antibodies

Belumosudil

▸ **Antacids** is predicted to decrease the exposure to **belumosudil**. Separate administration by 12 hours. Moderate Theoretical

▸ **Anti-androgens (apalutamide, enzalutamide)** are predicted to decrease the exposure to **belumosudil**. Adjust **belumosudil** dose, p. 979. Severe Study

▸ **Antiepileptics (carbamazepine, fosphenytoin, phenobarbital, phenytoin, primidone)** are predicted to decrease the exposure to **belumosudil**. Adjust **belumosudil** dose, p. 979. Severe Study

▸ **Belumosudil** is predicted to increase the exposure to antihistamines, non-sedating **(fexofenadine)**. Avoid or adjust dose. Moderate Study

▸ **Calcium salts (calcium carbonate)** -containing antacids are predicted to decrease the exposure to **belumosudil**. Separate administration by 12 hours. Moderate Theoretical

▸ **Belumosudil** might increase the exposure to digoxin. Avoid or adjust dose. Moderate Theoretical

▸ **Encorafenib** is predicted to decrease the exposure to **belumosudil**. Adjust **belumosudil** dose, p. 979. Severe Study

▸ **Belumosudil** is predicted to increase the exposure to endothelin receptor antagonists **(bosentan)**. Avoid or adjust dose. Moderate Study

▸ **Belumosudil** might increase the exposure to everolimus. Avoid or adjust dose. Moderate Theoretical

▸ **H₂ receptor antagonists** are predicted to decrease the exposure to **belumosudil**. Separate administration by 12 hours. Moderate Theoretical

▸ **Ivosidenib** is predicted to decrease the exposure to **belumosudil**. Adjust **belumosudil** dose, p. 979. Severe Study

▸ **Lumacaftor** is predicted to decrease the exposure to **belumosudil**. Adjust **belumosudil** dose, p. 979. Severe Study

▸ **Belumosudil** is predicted to increase the exposure to meglitinides **(repaglinide)**. Avoid or adjust dose. Moderate Study

▸ **Mitotane** is predicted to decrease the exposure to **belumosudil**. Adjust **belumosudil** dose, p. 979. Severe Study

▸ **Proton pump inhibitors** are predicted to decrease the exposure to **belumosudil**. Adjust **belumosudil** dose, p. 979. Severe Study

▸ **Belumosudil** is predicted to affect the exposure to raltegravir. Moderate Theoretical

▸ **Rifamycins (rifampicin)** are predicted to decrease the exposure to **belumosudil**. Adjust **belumosudil** dose, p. 979. Severe Study

▸ **Belumosudil** might increase the exposure to sirolimus. Avoid or adjust dose. Moderate Theoretical

▸ **Belumosudil** is predicted to increase the exposure to statins **(atorvastatin, pravastatin, rosuvastatin, simvastatin)**. Avoid or adjust dose. Moderate Study

▸ **Belumosudil** is predicted to increase the exposure to statins **(fluvastatin)**. Avoid or adjust dose. Moderate Theoretical

▸ **Belumosudil** is predicted to increase the exposure to sulfasalazine. Avoid or adjust dose. Moderate Theoretical

▸ **Belumosudil** is predicted to increase the exposure to sulfonylureas **(glibenclamide)**. Avoid or adjust dose. Moderate Study

▸ **Belumosudil** might increase the exposure to talazoparib. Avoid or adjust dose. Moderate Theoretical

▸ **Belumosudil** is predicted to increase the exposure to taxanes **(docetaxel, paclitaxel)**. Avoid or adjust dose. Moderate Study

▸ **Belumosudil** increases the exposure to thrombin inhibitors **(dabigatran)**. Avoid or adjust dose. Moderate Study

▸ **Belumosudil** is predicted to increase the exposure to topotecan. Avoid or adjust dose. Moderate Theoretical

Belzutifan

▸ **Antifungals, azoles (fluconazole, voriconazole)** are predicted to increase the exposure to **belzutifan**. Monitor and adjust dose. Severe Theoretical

▸ **Belzutifan** is predicted to decrease the exposure to bosutinib. Avoid or adjust dose. Severe Theoretical

▸ **Cenobamate** is predicted to increase the exposure to **belzutifan**. Monitor and adjust dose. Severe Theoretical

▸ **Belzutifan** is predicted to decrease the exposure to cobimetinib. Avoid or adjust dose. Severe Theoretical

▸ **Belzutifan** might decrease the efficacy of combined hormonal contraceptives. Use additional contraceptive precautions. Severe Theoretical

▸ **Belzutifan** is predicted to decrease the exposure to dasatinib. Avoid or adjust dose. Severe Theoretical

▸ **Belzutifan** is predicted to decrease the exposure to everolimus. Avoid or adjust dose. Severe Theoretical

▸ **Fedratinib** is predicted to increase the exposure to **belzutifan**. Monitor and adjust dose. Severe Theoretical

▸ **Belzutifan** is predicted to decrease the exposure to ibrutinib. Avoid or adjust dose. [Severe] Theoretical

▸ **Belzutifan** is predicted to decrease the exposure to maraviroc. Avoid or adjust dose. [Severe] Theoretical

▸ Moclobemide is predicted to increase the exposure to **belzutifan**. Monitor and adjust dose. [Severe] Theoretical

▸ Proton pump inhibitors (esomeprazole, omeprazole) are predicted to increase the exposure to **belzutifan**. Monitor and adjust dose. [Severe] Theoretical

▸ **Belzutifan** is predicted to decrease the exposure to sirolimus. Avoid or adjust dose. [Severe] Theoretical

▸ SSRIs (fluoxetine, fluvoxamine) are predicted to increase the exposure to **belzutifan**. Monitor and adjust dose. [Severe] Theoretical

▸ **Belzutifan** is predicted to decrease the exposure to temsirolimus. Avoid or adjust dose. [Severe] Theoretical

Bemiparin → see low molecular-weight heparins

Bempedoic acid

▸ **Bempedoic acid** increases the exposure to statins (pravastatin). [Moderate] Study

▸ **Bempedoic acid** increases the exposure to statins (simvastatin). Adjust **simvastatin** dose, p. 237. [Moderate] Study

Bendamustine → see alkylating agents

Bendroflumethiazide → see thiazide diuretics

Benperidol → see TABLE 17 p. 1576 (hyponatraemia), TABLE 7 p. 1572 (hypotension), TABLE 10 p. 1574 (CNS effects)

▸ **Benperidol** is predicted to decrease the effects of dopamine receptor agonists. Avoid. [Moderate] Theoretical → Also see TABLE 7 p. 1572 → Also see TABLE 10 p. 1574

▸ **Benperidol** opposes the effects of the active metabolite of foslevodopa. [Severe] Theoretical → Also see TABLE 7 p. 1572 → Also see TABLE 10 p. 1574

▸ **Benperidol** is predicted to decrease the effects of levodopa. [Severe] Study → Also see TABLE 7 p. 1572 → Also see TABLE 10 p. 1574

Benzathine benzylpenicillin → see penicillins

Benzodiazepines → see TABLE 10 p. 1574 (CNS effects)

> alprazolam · chlordiazepoxide · clobazam · clonazepam · diazepam · flurazepam · loprazolam · lorazepam · lormetazepam · midazolam · nitrazepam · oxazepam · remimazolam · temazepam

▸ Anti-androgens (apalutamide) are predicted to decrease the exposure to **diazepam**. Avoid or monitor. [Mild] Study

▸ Anti-androgens (apalutamide, enzalutamide) are predicted to decrease the exposure to **alprazolam**. Adjust dose. [Moderate] Theoretical

▸ Anti-androgens (apalutamide, enzalutamide) are predicted to decrease the exposure to **midazolam**. Monitor and adjust dose. [Severe] Study

▸ Anti-androgens (enzalutamide) are predicted to affect the exposure to **clonazepam**. Use with caution or avoid. [Moderate] Theoretical

▸ Antiarrhythmics (dronedarone) are predicted to increase the exposure to **alprazolam**. [Severe] Study

▸ Antiarrhythmics (dronedarone) are predicted to increase the exposure to **midazolam**. Monitor adverse effects and adjust dose. [Severe] Study

▸ Antiepileptics (carbamazepine, fosphenytoin, phenobarbital, phenytoin, primidone) are predicted to decrease the exposure to **alprazolam**. Adjust dose. [Moderate] Theoretical → Also see TABLE 10 p. 1574

▸ Antiepileptics (carbamazepine, fosphenytoin, phenobarbital, phenytoin, primidone) are predicted to decrease the exposure to **midazolam**. Monitor and adjust dose. [Severe] Study → Also see TABLE 10 p. 1574

▸ Antiepileptics (stiripentol) increase the concentration of **clobazam**. [Severe] Study

▸ **Chlordiazepoxide** affects the concentration of antiepileptics (fosphenytoin, phenytoin). [Severe] Study → Also see TABLE 10 p. 1574

▸ **Diazepam** potentially affects the concentration of antiepileptics (fosphenytoin, phenytoin). Monitor concentration and adjust dose. [Severe] Study → Also see TABLE 10 p. 1574

▸ Benzodiazepines (clobazam, clonazepam) potentially affect the concentration of antiepileptics (fosphenytoin, phenytoin). [Severe] Anecdotal → Also see TABLE 10 p. 1574

▸ Antifungals, azoles (fluconazole, isavuconazole) are predicted to increase the exposure to **alprazolam**. [Severe] Study

▸ Antifungals, azoles (fluconazole, isavuconazole) are predicted to increase the exposure to **midazolam**. Monitor adverse effects and adjust dose. [Severe] Study

▸ Antifungals, azoles (fluconazole, voriconazole) potentially increase the exposure to **clobazam**. Adjust dose. [Moderate] Theoretical

▸ Antifungals, azoles (fluconazole, voriconazole) moderately increase the exposure to **diazepam**. Monitor and adjust dose. [Moderate] Study

▸ Antifungals, azoles (itraconazole, ketoconazole, posaconazole, voriconazole) moderately increase the exposure to **alprazolam**. Avoid. [Moderate] Study

▸ Antifungals, azoles (itraconazole, ketoconazole, posaconazole, voriconazole) are predicted to markedly to very markedly increase the exposure to **midazolam**. Avoid or adjust dose. [Severe] Study

▸ Antifungals, azoles (miconazole) are predicted to increase the exposure to **alprazolam**. Use with caution and adjust dose. [Moderate] Theoretical

▸ Antifungals, azoles (miconazole) are predicted to increase the exposure to intravenous **midazolam**. Use with caution and adjust dose. [Moderate] Theoretical

▸ Antifungals, azoles (miconazole) are predicted to increase the exposure to oral **midazolam**. Avoid. [Moderate] Theoretical

▸ Antipsychotics, second generation (clozapine) might increase the risk of respiratory depression and circulatory collapse when given with **benzodiazepines**. [Severe] Anecdotal → Also see TABLE 10 p. 1574

▸ Berotralstat is predicted to increase the exposure to **alprazolam**. [Severe] Study

▸ Berotralstat is predicted to increase the exposure to **midazolam**. Monitor adverse effects and adjust dose. [Severe] Study

▸ Bulevirtide slightly increases the exposure to **midazolam**. [Moderate] Theoretical

▸ Cabozantinib is predicted to increase the exposure to **midazolam**. [Moderate] Theoretical

▸ Calcium channel blockers (diltiazem, verapamil) are predicted to increase the exposure to **alprazolam**. [Severe] Study

▸ Calcium channel blockers (diltiazem, verapamil) are predicted to increase the exposure to **midazolam**. Monitor adverse effects and adjust dose. [Severe] Study

▸ Cannabidiol increases the exposure to the active metabolite of **clobazam** and **clobazam** increases the exposure to the active metabolite of cannabidiol. Adjust dose. [Moderate] Study → Also see TABLE 10 p. 1574

▸ Cenobamate potentially increases the exposure to **clobazam**. Adjust dose. [Moderate] Theoretical → Also see TABLE 10 p. 1574

▸ Cenobamate moderately decreases the exposure to **midazolam**. Adjust dose. [Moderate] Study → Also see TABLE 10 p. 1574

▸ Ceritinib moderately increases the exposure to **alprazolam**. Avoid. [Moderate] Study

▸ Ceritinib is predicted to markedly to very markedly increase the exposure to **midazolam**. Avoid or adjust dose. [Severe] Study

▸ Cobicistat moderately increases the exposure to **alprazolam**. Avoid. [Moderate] Study

▸ Cobicistat is predicted to markedly to very markedly increase the exposure to **midazolam**. Avoid or adjust dose. [Severe] Study

▸ Crizotinib is predicted to increase the exposure to **alprazolam**. [Severe] Study

▸ Crizotinib is predicted to increase the exposure to **midazolam**. Monitor adverse effects and adjust dose. [Severe] Study

▸ Dabrafenib decreases the exposure to **midazolam**. Monitor and adjust dose. [Moderate] Study

▸ Encorafenib is predicted to decrease the exposure to **alprazolam**. Adjust dose. [Moderate] Theoretical

▸ Encorafenib is predicted to decrease the exposure to **midazolam**. Monitor and adjust dose. [Severe] Study

▸ Endothelin receptor antagonists (bosentan) are predicted to decrease the concentration of **midazolam**. Monitor and adjust dose. [Moderate] Theoretical

▸ Fedratinib is predicted to increase the exposure to **alprazolam**. [Severe] Study

Benzodiazepines (continued)

▶ **Fedratinib** potentially increases the exposure to **clobazam**. Adjust dose. Moderate Theoretical

▶ **Fedratinib** is predicted to increase the exposure to **midazolam**. Monitor adverse effects and adjust dose. Severe Study

▶ **Benzodiazepines** might decrease the effects of **foslevodopa**. Moderate Theoretical → Also see **TABLE 10** p. 1574

▶ **Givinostat** increases the exposure to **midazolam**. Moderate Study

▶ **HIV-protease inhibitors** moderately increase the exposure to **alprazolam**. Avoid. Moderate Study

▶ **HIV-protease inhibitors (ritonavir)** are predicted to increase the exposure to benzodiazepines (**diazepam, flurazepam**). Avoid. Moderate Theoretical

▶ **HIV-protease inhibitors** are predicted to markedly to very markedly increase the exposure to **midazolam**. Avoid or adjust dose. Severe Study

▶ **Idelalisib** moderately increases the exposure to **alprazolam**. Avoid. Moderate Study

▶ **Idelalisib** is predicted to increase the exposure to benzodiazepines (**diazepam, flurazepam**). Monitor and adjust dose. Moderate Theoretical

▶ **Idelalisib** is predicted to markedly to very markedly increase the exposure to **midazolam**. Avoid or adjust dose. Severe Study

▶ **Imatinib** is predicted to increase the exposure to **alprazolam**. Severe Study

▶ **Imatinib** is predicted to increase the exposure to **midazolam**. Monitor adverse effects and adjust dose. Severe Study

▶ **Ivosidenib** is predicted to decrease the exposure to **alprazolam**. Adjust dose. Moderate Theoretical

▶ **Ivosidenib** is predicted to decrease the exposure to **midazolam**. Monitor and adjust dose. Severe Study

▶ **Larotrectinib** slightly increases the exposure to **midazolam**. Use with caution and adjust dose. Mild Study

▶ **Letermovir** is predicted to increase the exposure to **alprazolam**. Severe Study

▶ **Letermovir** is predicted to increase the exposure to **midazolam**. Monitor adverse effects and adjust dose. Severe Study

▶ **Alprazolam** is predicted to increase the exposure to **lomitapide**. Separate administration by 12 hours. Moderate Theoretical

▶ **Lorlatinib** moderately decreases the exposure to **midazolam**. Avoid. Moderate Study

▶ **Lumacaftor** is predicted to decrease the exposure to **alprazolam**. Adjust dose. Moderate Theoretical

▶ **Lumacaftor** is predicted to decrease the exposure to **midazolam**. Monitor and adjust dose. Severe Study

▶ **Macrolides (clarithromycin)** moderately increase the exposure to **alprazolam**. Avoid. Moderate Study

▶ **Macrolides (clarithromycin)** are predicted to markedly to very markedly increase the exposure to **midazolam**. Avoid or adjust dose. Severe Study

▶ **Macrolides (erythromycin)** are predicted to increase the exposure to **alprazolam**. Severe Study

▶ **Macrolides (erythromycin)** are predicted to increase the exposure to **midazolam**. Monitor adverse effects and adjust dose. Severe Study

▶ **Mitotane** is predicted to decrease the exposure to **alprazolam**. Adjust dose. Moderate Theoretical

▶ **Mitotane** is predicted to decrease the exposure to **midazolam**. Monitor and adjust dose. Severe Study

▶ **Moclobemide** potentially increases the exposure to **clobazam**. Adjust dose. Moderate Theoretical

▶ **Monoclonal antibodies (tocilizumab)** are predicted to decrease the exposure to benzodiazepines (**alprazolam, diazepam, midazolam**). Monitor and adjust dose. Moderate Theoretical

▶ **Neurokinin-1 receptor antagonists (aprepitant, netupitant)** are predicted to increase the exposure to **alprazolam**. Severe Study

▶ **Neurokinin-1 receptor antagonists (aprepitant, netupitant)** are predicted to increase the exposure to **midazolam**. Monitor adverse effects and adjust dose. Severe Study

▶ **Neurokinin-1 receptor antagonists (fosaprepitant)** are predicted to increase the exposure to **alprazolam**. Moderate Study

▶ **Neurokinin-1 receptor antagonists (fosaprepitant)** slightly increase the exposure to **midazolam**. Moderate Study

▶ **Nilotinib** is predicted to increase the exposure to **alprazolam**. Severe Study

▶ **Nilotinib** is predicted to increase the exposure to **midazolam**. Monitor adverse effects and adjust dose. Severe Study

▶ **Nirmatrelvir** boosted with ritonavir is predicted to increase the concentration of **alprazolam**. Moderate Theoretical

▶ **Nirmatrelvir** boosted with ritonavir is predicted to increase the concentration of benzodiazepines (**clonazepam, diazepam, flurazepam**). Monitor and adjust dose. Severe Theoretical

▶ **Nirmatrelvir** boosted with ritonavir very markedly increases the exposure to **midazolam**. Avoid or adjust dose. Severe Study

▶ **NNRTIs (efavirenz)** are predicted to alter the effects of **midazolam**. Avoid. Moderate Theoretical

▶ **NNRTIs (efavirenz, nevirapine)** are predicted to decrease the concentration of **alprazolam**. Moderate Theoretical

▶ **NNRTIs (etravirine)** have been reported to increase the concentration of **clobazam**. Moderate Anecdotal

▶ **NNRTIs (etravirine)** are predicted to increase the exposure to **diazepam**. Avoid. Severe Theoretical

▶ **NNRTIs (nevirapine)** are predicted to decrease the concentration of **clonazepam** and **clonazepam** is predicted to decrease the concentration of **NNRTIs (nevirapine)**. Moderate Theoretical

▶ **NNRTIs (nevirapine)** decrease the concentration of **midazolam**. Monitor and adjust dose. Moderate Study

▶ **Palbociclib** increases the exposure to **midazolam**. Moderate Study

▶ **Proton pump inhibitors (esomeprazole, omeprazole)** potentially increase the exposure to **clobazam**. Adjust dose. Moderate Theoretical

▶ **Ribociclib** moderately increases the exposure to **midazolam**. Avoid. Moderate Study

▶ **Rifamycins (rifampicin)** are predicted to decrease the exposure to **alprazolam**. Adjust dose. Moderate Theoretical

▶ **Rifamycins (rifampicin)** are predicted to decrease the exposure to **chlordiazepoxide**. Moderate Theoretical

▶ **Rifamycins (rifampicin)** moderately decrease the exposure to **diazepam**. Avoid. Moderate Study

▶ **Rifamycins (rifampicin)** are predicted to decrease the exposure to **midazolam**. Monitor and adjust dose. Severe Study

▶ **Rifamycins (rifampicin)** increase the clearance of benzodiazepines (**lorazepam, nitrazepam**). Moderate Study

▶ **Ritlecitinib** moderately increases the exposure to **midazolam**. Moderate Study

▶ **Rucaparib** slightly increases the exposure to **midazolam**. Monitor and adjust dose. Severe Study

▶ **Sotorasib** moderately decreases the exposure to **midazolam**. Moderate Study

▶ **SSRIs (fluoxetine, fluvoxamine)** potentially increase the exposure to **clobazam**. Adjust dose. Moderate Theoretical → Also see **TABLE 10** p. 1574

▶ **SSRIs (fluvoxamine)** moderately increase the exposure to **alprazolam**. Adjust dose. Moderate Study → Also see **TABLE 10** p. 1574

▶ **SSRIs (fluvoxamine)** moderately increase the exposure to **diazepam**. Moderate Study → Also see **TABLE 10** p. 1574

▶ **St John's wort** moderately decreases the exposure to **alprazolam**. Moderate Study

▶ **St John's wort** moderately decreases the exposure to **midazolam**. Monitor and adjust dose. Moderate Study

▶ **Telotristat ethyl** decreases the exposure to **midazolam**. Moderate Study

▶ **Tucatinib** moderately increases the exposure to **alprazolam**. Avoid. Moderate Study

▶ **Tucatinib** is predicted to markedly to very markedly increase the exposure to **midazolam**. Avoid or adjust dose. Severe Study

▶ **Vemurafenib** slightly to moderately decreases the exposure to **midazolam**. Moderate Study

Benzydamine → see NSAIDs

Benzylpenicillin → see penicillins

Berotralstat

▶ **Berotralstat** is predicted to increase the exposure to **abemaciclib**. Moderate Study

▶ **Berotralstat** is predicted to increase the exposure to **acalabrutinib**. Avoid or monitor. Severe Study

▶ **Berotralstat** is predicted to increase the exposure to alpha blockers (**tamsulosin**). Moderate Theoretical

- **Berotralstat** is predicted to increase the exposure to antiarrhythmics (propafenone). Monitor and adjust dose. Moderate Study
- Antiepileptics (carbamazepine) are predicted to decrease the concentration of **berotralstat**. Avoid. Severe Theoretical
- **Berotralstat** is predicted to increase the exposure to antifungals, azoles (isavuconazole). Moderate Theoretical
- **Berotralstat** is predicted to increase the exposure to antihistamines, non-sedating (mizolastine). Severe Theoretical
- **Berotralstat** is predicted to increase the exposure to antihistamines, non-sedating (rupatadine). Avoid. Moderate Study
- **Berotralstat** is predicted to increase the exposure to antipsychotics, second generation (cariprazine). Avoid. Severe Study
- **Berotralstat** is predicted to increase the exposure to antipsychotics, second generation (quetiapine). Avoid. Moderate Study
- **Berotralstat** is predicted to increase the exposure to atomoxetine. Adjust dose. Moderate Study
- **Berotralstat** is predicted to increase the exposure to avapritinib. Avoid or adjust dose—consult product literature. Moderate Study
- **Berotralstat** is predicted to increase the exposure to axitinib. Moderate Study
- **Berotralstat** might increases the exposure to bedaquiline. Mild Theoretical
- **Berotralstat** is predicted to increase the exposure to benzodiazepines (alprazolam). Severe Study
- **Berotralstat** is predicted to increase the exposure to benzodiazepines (midazolam). Monitor adverse effects and adjust dose. Severe Study
- **Berotralstat** is predicted to increase the exposure to beta blockers, selective (metoprolol). Moderate Study
- **Berotralstat** is predicted to increase the exposure to beta blockers, selective (nebivolol). Adjust dose. Moderate Study
- **Berotralstat** is predicted to increase the exposure to bosutinib. Avoid or adjust dose. Severe Study
- **Berotralstat** is predicted to increase the exposure to brigatinib. Moderate Study
- **Berotralstat** is predicted to increase the exposure to buspirone. Use with caution and adjust dose. Moderate Study
- **Berotralstat** is predicted to increase the exposure to cabozantinib. Moderate Study
- **Berotralstat** is predicted to increase the exposure to calcium channel blockers (amlodipine, felodipine, lacidipine, lercanidipine, nicardipine, nifedipine, nimodipine). Monitor and adjust dose. Moderate Study
- **Berotralstat** is predicted to increase the exposure to capivasertib. Adjust dose. Moderate Study
- **Berotralstat** is predicted to increase the exposure to ceritinib. Moderate Study
- **Berotralstat** is predicted to increase the exposure to cobimetinib. Severe Study
- **Berotralstat** is predicted to increase the exposure to colchicine. Adjust **colchicine** dose with moderate CYP3A4 inhibitors, p. 1279. Severe Study
- **Berotralstat** is predicted to increase the exposure to corticosteroids (methylprednisolone). Monitor and adjust dose. Moderate Study
- **Berotralstat** is predicted to increase the exposure to dabrafenib. Moderate Study
- **Berotralstat** is predicted to increase the exposure to daridorexant. Adjust **daridorexant** dose, p. 554. Severe Study
- **Berotralstat** is predicted to increase the exposure to dasatinib. Severe Study
- **Berotralstat** is predicted to slightly increase the exposure to dienogest. Moderate Study
- **Berotralstat** is predicted to increase the concentration of digoxin. Monitor and adjust dose. Moderate Study
- **Berotralstat** is predicted to increase the exposure to dipeptidylpeptidase-4 inhibitors (saxagliptin). Mild Study
- **Berotralstat** is predicted to increase the exposure to domperidone. Avoid. Severe Study
- **Berotralstat** is predicted to increase the exposure to dopamine receptor agonists (bromocriptine). Severe Theoretical

- **Berotralstat** is predicted to increase the exposure to drospirenone. Severe Study
- **Berotralstat** is predicted to moderately increase the exposure to dutasteride. Mild Study
- **Berotralstat** is predicted to increase the exposure to elacestrant. Avoid moderate CYP3A4 inhibitors or adjust **elacestrant** dose, p. 1084. Severe Theoretical
- **Berotralstat** is predicted to increase the exposure to elexacaftor. Adjust ivacaftor with tezacaftor and elexacaftor p. 337 dose with moderate CYP3A4 inhibitors. Severe Theoretical
- **Berotralstat** is predicted to increase the exposure to eliglustat. Avoid or adjust dose—consult product literature. Severe Study
- **Berotralstat** is predicted to moderately increase the exposure to encorafenib. Moderate Study
- **Berotralstat** is predicted to increase the exposure to endothelin receptor antagonists (macitentan). Manufacturer advises caution depending on other drugs taken—consult product literature. Moderate Theoretical
- **Berotralstat** is predicted to increase the exposure to entrectinib. Avoid or adjust dose with moderate CYP3A4 inhibitors—consult product literature. Severe Theoretical
- **Berotralstat** is predicted to increase the risk of ergotism when given with ergometrine. Severe Theoretical
- **Berotralstat** is predicted to increase the exposure to erlotinib. Moderate Study
- **Berotralstat** is predicted to increase the exposure to etrasimod. Avoid in poor CYP2C9 metabolisers. Severe Theoretical
- **Berotralstat** is predicted to increase the concentration of everolimus. Avoid or adjust dose. Moderate Study
- **Berotralstat** is predicted to increase the exposure to fedratinib. Monitor and adjust dose. Moderate Study
- **Berotralstat** is predicted to increase the exposure to fesoterodine. Adjust **fesoterodine** dose with moderate CYP3A4 inhibitors in hepatic and renal impairment, p. 897. Mild Study
- **Berotralstat** is predicted to increase the exposure to gefitinib. Moderate Study
- Grapefruit juice is predicted to increase the exposure to **berotralstat**. Moderate Theoretical
- **Berotralstat** is predicted to increase the concentration of guanfacine. Adjust **guanfacine** dose, p. 407. Moderate Theoretical
- **Berotralstat** is predicted to increase the exposure to ibrutinib. Adjust dose with moderate CYP3A4 inhibitors—consult product literature. Severe Study
- **Berotralstat** is predicted to increase the exposure to ivacaftor. Adjust dose with moderate CYP3A4 inhibitors, see ivacaftor p. 336, tezacaftor with ivacaftor p. 339, and ivacaftor with tezacaftor and elexacaftor p. 337. Moderate Study
- **Berotralstat** is predicted to increase the exposure to ivosidenib. Monitor and adjust dose—consult product literature. Severe Study
- **Berotralstat** is predicted to increase the exposure to lapatinib. Moderate Study
- **Berotralstat** is predicted to increase the exposure to larotrectinib. Monitor and adjust dose. Moderate Theoretical
- **Berotralstat** is predicted to increase the exposure to leniolisib. Avoid. Moderate Study
- **Berotralstat** is predicted to increase the exposure to lomitapide. Avoid. Moderate Theoretical
- Lorlatinib is predicted to decrease the concentration of **berotralstat**. Avoid. Severe Theoretical
- **Berotralstat** is predicted to increase the exposure to mavacamten. Adjust dose—consult product literature. Moderate Study
- **Berotralstat** is predicted to increase the exposure to midostaurin. Moderate Theoretical
- **Berotralstat** is predicted to increase the exposure to mineralocorticoid receptor antagonists (eplerenone). Adjust **eplerenone** dose, p. 223. Severe Study
- **Berotralstat** is predicted to increase the exposure to mineralocorticoid receptor antagonists (finerenone). Severe Study
- **Berotralstat** is predicted to increase the exposure to mobocertinib. Avoid or adjust dose and monitor ECG—consult product literature. Severe Study

Berotralstat (continued)

▶ **Berotralstat** is predicted to increase the exposure to naldemedine. [Moderate] Study
▶ **Berotralstat** is predicted to increase the exposure to naloxegol. Adjust **naloxegol** dose and monitor adverse effects, p. 72. [Moderate] Study
▶ **Berotralstat** is predicted to increase the exposure to neratinib. Avoid moderate CYP3A4 inhibitors or adjust dose and monitor for gastrointestinal adverse effects—consult product literature. [Severe] Study
▶ **Berotralstat** is predicted to increase the exposure to olaparib. Avoid or adjust dose with moderate CYP3A4 inhibitors—consult product literature. [Moderate] Theoretical
▶ **Berotralstat** is predicted to increase the exposure to opioids (alfentanil, buprenorphine, fentanyl, oxycodone). Monitor and adjust dose. [Moderate] Study
▶ **Berotralstat** is predicted to increase the exposure to opioids (methadone, sufentanil). [Moderate] Theoretical
▶ **Berotralstat** is predicted to increase the exposure to pazopanib. [Moderate] Study
▶ **Berotralstat** is predicted to increase the exposure to pemigatinib. [Severe] Study
▶ **Berotralstat** is predicted to increase the exposure to phosphodiesterase type-5 inhibitors (avanafil). Adjust **avanafil** dose, p. 939. [Moderate] Theoretical
▶ **Berotralstat** is predicted to increase the exposure to phosphodiesterase type-5 inhibitors (sildenafil). Monitor or adjust **sildenafil** dose with moderate CYP3A4 inhibitors, p. 940. [Moderate] Study
▶ **Berotralstat** is predicted to increase the exposure to phosphodiesterase type-5 inhibitors (tadalafil). [Severe] Theoretical
▶ **Berotralstat** is predicted to increase the exposure to phosphodiesterase type-5 inhibitors (vardenafil). Adjust dose. [Severe] Theoretical
▶ **Berotralstat** is predicted to increase the exposure to pimozide. Avoid. [Severe] Theoretical
▶ **Berotralstat** is predicted to increase the exposure to ponatinib. [Moderate] Study
▶ **Berotralstat** is predicted to increase the exposure to pralsetinib. [Moderate] Theoretical
▶ **Berotralstat** is predicted to increase the exposure to ranolazine. [Severe] Study
▶ **Berotralstat** is predicted to increase the exposure to regorafenib. [Moderate] Study
▶ **Berotralstat** is predicted to increase the exposure to ribociclib. [Moderate] Study
▶ Rifamycins (rifampicin) are predicted to decrease the concentration of **berotralstat**. Avoid. [Severe] Theoretical
▶ **Berotralstat** is predicted to increase the exposure to rimegepant. Avoid another dose of rimegepant within 48 hours of concurrent use. [Moderate] Study
▶ **Berotralstat** is predicted to increase the exposure to selpercatinib. [Moderate] Study
▶ **Berotralstat** is predicted to increase the exposure to selumetinib. Avoid or adjust dose—consult product literature. [Severe] Study
▶ **Berotralstat** is predicted to increase the exposure to siponimod. Avoid depending on other drugs taken—consult product literature. [Severe] Study
▶ **Berotralstat** increases the concentration of sirolimus. Monitor and adjust dose. [Moderate] Study
▶ **Berotralstat** is predicted to increase the exposure to SSRIs (dapoxetine). Adjust **dapoxetine** dose with moderate CYP3A4 inhibitors, p. 947. [Moderate] Theoretical
▶ St John's wort is predicted to decrease the concentration of berotralstat. Avoid. [Severe] Theoretical
▶ **Berotralstat** is predicted to increase the exposure to sunitinib. [Moderate] Study
▶ **Berotralstat** is predicted to increase the concentration of tacrolimus. [Severe] Study
▶ **Berotralstat** is predicted to increase the concentration of talazoparib. Monitor and adjust dose. [Moderate] Study
▶ **Berotralstat** is predicted to increase the exposure to taxanes (cabazitaxel). [Moderate] Theoretical

▶ **Berotralstat** is predicted to increase the exposure to taxanes (docetaxel). [Severe] Study
▶ **Berotralstat** is predicted to increase the exposure to taxanes (paclitaxel). [Moderate] Anecdotal
▶ **Berotralstat** is predicted to increase the exposure to temsirolimus. Use with caution or avoid. [Moderate] Study
▶ **Berotralstat** is predicted to increase the exposure to tezacaftor. Adjust dose with moderate CYP3A4 inhibitors, see tezacaftor with ivacaftor p. 339 and ivacaftor with tezacaftor and elexacaftor p. 337. [Severe] Study
▶ **Berotralstat** is predicted to increase the exposure to tolvaptan. Manufacturer advises caution or adjust **tolvaptan** dose with moderate CYP3A4 inhibitors, p. 767. [Moderate] Study
▶ **Berotralstat** is predicted to increase the exposure to trazodone. [Moderate] Theoretical
▶ **Berotralstat** is predicted to increase the exposure to tricyclic antidepressants. Monitor and adjust dose. [Moderate] Theoretical
▶ **Berotralstat** is predicted to increase the exposure to vemurafenib. [Severe] Theoretical
▶ **Berotralstat** is predicted to increase the exposure to venetoclax. Avoid or adjust dose—consult product literature. [Severe] Study
▶ **Berotralstat** is predicted to increase the exposure to vinca alkaloids. [Severe] Theoretical
▶ **Berotralstat** is predicted to increase the exposure to voclosporin. Adjust **voclosporin** dose, p. 973. [Severe] Study
▶ **Berotralstat** is predicted to increase the exposure to zanubrutinib. Avoid or adjust dose with moderate CYP3A4 inhibitors—consult product literature. [Severe] Study
▶ **Berotralstat** is predicted to increase the exposure to zopiclone. Adjust dose. [Moderate] Study

Beta blockers, non-selective → see TABLE 5 p. 1572 (bradycardia), TABLE 7 p. 1572 (hypotension), TABLE 15 p. 1575 (increased serum potassium), TABLE 8 p. 1573 (QT-interval prolongation)

carvedilol · labetalol · levobunolol · nadolol · pindolol · propranolol · sotalol · timolol

ROUTE-SPECIFIC INFORMATION Since systemic absorption can follow topical application of **levobunolol** or **timolol** the possibility of interactions should be borne in mind.

▶ **Beta blockers, non-selective** are predicted to increase the risk of bronchospasm when given with aminophylline. Avoid. [Severe] Theoretical
▶ Anti-androgens (enzalutamide) are predicted to affect the exposure to **propranolol**. Use with caution or avoid. [Moderate] Theoretical
▶ Antiarrhythmics (amiodarone, disopyramide, dronedarone, flecainide, lidocaine) are predicted to increase the risk of cardiovascular adverse effects when given with **beta blockers, non-selective**. Use with caution or avoid. [Severe] Study → Also see TABLE 5 p. 1572 → Also see TABLE 8 p. 1573
▶ Antiarrhythmics (propafenone) increase the risk of cardiovascular adverse effects when given with **propranolol**. Use with caution or avoid. [Severe] Study → Also see TABLE 5 p. 1572
▶ Antiarrhythmics (propafenone) are predicted to increase the exposure to **timolol** and **timolol** is predicted to increase the risk of cardiodepression when given with antiarrhythmics (propafenone). [Severe] Anecdotal → Also see TABLE 5 p. 1572
▶ Antiarrhythmics (propafenone) are predicted to increase the risk of cardiovascular adverse effects when given with beta blockers, non-selective (labetalol, levobunolol, nadolol, pindolol, sotalol). Use with caution or avoid. [Severe] Study → Also see TABLE 5 p. 1572
▶ Antiepileptics (phenobarbital, primidone) are predicted to decrease the exposure to **propranolol**. [Moderate] Study
▶ Antiepileptics (phenobarbital, primidone) are predicted to decrease the exposure to beta blockers, non-selective (carvedilol, labetalol). [Moderate] Theoretical
▶ Antifungals, azoles (itraconazole, ketoconazole) are predicted to increase the exposure to nadolol. [Moderate] Study
▶ Antimalarials (mefloquine) are predicted to increase the risk of bradycardia when given with **beta blockers, non-selective**. [Severe] Theoretical
▶ Calcium channel blockers (diltiazem) are predicted to increase the risk of cardiodepression when given with **beta blockers,**

non-selective. [Severe] Study → Also see **TABLE 5** p. 1572 → Also see **TABLE 7** p. 1572

▸ Calcium channel blockers **(verapamil)** increase the risk of cardiovascular adverse effects when given with **beta blockers, non-selective**. Avoid intravenous **verapamil**. [Severe] Study → Also see **TABLE 5** p. 1572 → Also see **TABLE 7** p. 1572

▸ Chloroprocaine is predicted to increase the risk of cardiovascular adverse effects when given with **sotalol**. [Severe] Theoretical

▸ Ciclosporin is predicted to increase the exposure to **nadolol**. [Moderate] Study

▸ Dacomitinib is predicted to markedly increase the exposure to **propranolol**. Avoid. [Severe] Study

▸ Eliglustat is predicted to increase the exposure to **propranolol**. Adjust dose. [Moderate] Study

▸ **Beta blockers, non-selective** are predicted to increase the risk of peripheral vasoconstriction when given with ergometrine. [Severe] Study

▸ **Carvedilol** is predicted to increase the exposure to gilteritinib. [Moderate] Theoretical

▸ HIV-protease inhibitors **(lopinavir, ritonavir)** are predicted to increase the exposure to **nadolol**. [Moderate] Study

▸ **Beta blockers, non-selective** are predicted to increase the risk of bradycardia when given with lanreotide. [Moderate] Theoretical

▸ Lapatinib is predicted to increase the exposure to **nadolol**. [Moderate] Study

▸ Macrolides are predicted to increase the exposure to **nadolol**. [Moderate] Study

▸ Mavacamten can cause negative inotropic effects, as can **beta blockers, non-selective**. [Severe] Theoretical

▸ Mexiletine potentially increases the risk of cardiovascular adverse effects when given with **beta blockers, non-selective**. Avoid or monitor. [Severe] Theoretical

▸ Omega-3-acid ethyl esters might enhance the blood pressure-lowering effects of **beta blockers, non-selective**. [Moderate] Study

▸ Ranolazine is predicted to increase the exposure to **nadolol**. [Moderate] Study

▸ **Carvedilol** is predicted to increase the exposure to relugolix. Avoid or take relugolix first and separate administration by at least 6 hours. [Moderate] Theoretical

▸ Rifamycins **(rifampicin)** moderately decrease the exposure to carvedilol. [Moderate] Study

▸ Rifamycins **(rifampicin)** decrease the exposure to **propranolol**. Monitor and adjust dose. [Moderate] Study

▸ SSRIs **(fluvoxamine)** moderately increase the concentration of **propranolol**. [Moderate] Study

▸ **Beta blockers, non-selective** increase the risk of hypertension and bradycardia when given with sympathomimetics, inotropic **(dobutamine)**. [Severe] Theoretical

▸ **Beta blockers, non-selective** are predicted to increase the risk of hypertension and bradycardia when given with sympathomimetics, vasoconstrictor **(adrenaline/epinephrine, noradrenaline/norepinephrine)**. [Severe] Study

▸ **Carvedilol** causes a small increase in the bioavailability of talazoparib. Avoid or adjust dose—consult product literature. [Moderate] Study

▸ **Beta blockers, non-selective** are predicted to increase the risk of bronchospasm when given with theophylline. Avoid. [Severe] Theoretical

▸ **Propranolol** slightly to moderately increases the exposure to triptans **(rizatriptan)**. Adjust **rizatriptan** dose and separate administration by at least 2 hours, p. 545. [Moderate] Study

▸ Vemurafenib is predicted to increase the exposure to **nadolol**. [Moderate] Study

Beta blockers, selective → see **TABLE 5** p. 1572 (bradycardia), **TABLE 7** p. 1572 (hypotension)

acebutolol · atenolol · betaxolol · bisoprolol · celiprolol · esmolol · landiolol · metoprolol · nebivolol

▸ Since systemic absorption can follow topical application of **betaxolol**, the possibility of interactions should be borne in mind.

▸ Orange juice greatly decreases the exposure to **celiprolol**.

▸ **Beta blockers, selective** are predicted to increase the risk of bronchospasm when given with aminophylline. Avoid. [Severe] Theoretical

▸ Anti-androgens **(abiraterone)** are predicted to increase the exposure to **metoprolol**. [Moderate] Study

▸ Anti-androgens **(enzalutamide)** are predicted to affect the exposure to **bisoprolol**. Use with caution or avoid. [Moderate] Theoretical

▸ Antiarrhythmics **(amiodarone, disopyramide, dronedarone, flecainide, lidocaine)** are predicted to increase the risk of cardiovascular adverse effects when given with **beta blockers, selective**. Use with caution or avoid. [Severe] Study → Also see **TABLE 5** p. 1572

▸ Antiarrhythmics **(propafenone)** are predicted to increase the exposure to **metoprolol**. [Moderate] Study → Also see **TABLE 5** p. 1572

▸ Antiarrhythmics **(propafenone)** are predicted to increase the exposure to **nebivolol** and **nebivolol** is predicted to increase the risk of cardiodepression when given with antiarrhythmics **(propafenone)**. Avoid. [Severe] Theoretical → Also see **TABLE 5** p. 1572

▸ Antiarrhythmics **(propafenone)** are predicted to increase the risk of cardiovascular adverse effects when given with beta blockers, selective **(acebutolol, atenolol, betaxolol, bisoprolol, celiprolol, esmolol)**. Use with caution or avoid. [Severe] Study → Also see **TABLE 5** p. 1572

▸ Antiepileptics **(phenobarbital, primidone)** are predicted to decrease the exposure to beta blockers, selective **(acebutolol, bisoprolol, metoprolol, nebivolol)**. [Moderate] Study

▸ Antimalarials **(mefloquine)** are predicted to increase the risk of bradycardia when given with **beta blockers, selective**. [Severe] Theoretical

▸ Berotralstat is predicted to increase the exposure to **metoprolol**. [Moderate] Study

▸ Berotralstat is predicted to increase the exposure to **nebivolol**. Adjust dose. [Moderate] Study

▸ Bupropion is predicted to increase the exposure to beta blockers, selective **(metoprolol, nebivolol)**. [Moderate] Study

▸ Calcium channel blockers **(diltiazem)** are predicted to increase the risk of cardiodepression when given with **beta blockers, selective**. Avoid or monitor. [Severe] Study → Also see **TABLE 5** p. 1572 → Also see **TABLE 7** p. 1572

▸ Calcium channel blockers **(verapamil)** increase the risk of cardiovascular adverse effects when given with **beta blockers, selective**. Use with caution or avoid. [Severe] Study → Also see **TABLE 5** p. 1572 → Also see **TABLE 7** p. 1572

▸ Cinacalcet is predicted to increase the exposure to beta blockers, selective **(metoprolol, nebivolol)**. [Moderate] Study

▸ Dacomitinib is predicted to increase the exposure to beta blockers, selective **(metoprolol, nebivolol)**. [Moderate] Study

▸ Eliglustat is predicted to increase the exposure to **metoprolol**. Adjust dose. [Moderate] Study

▸ **Beta blockers, selective** are predicted to increase the risk of peripheral vasoconstriction when given with ergometrine. [Severe] Study

▸ Givosiran is predicted to increase the exposure to **metoprolol**. [Moderate] Study

▸ Givosiran is predicted to increase the exposure to **nebivolol**. Use with caution and adjust dose. [Moderate] Study

▸ Grapefruit juice greatly decreases the exposure to **celiprolol**. [Moderate] Study

▸ HIV-protease inhibitors **(ritonavir)** are predicted to increase the exposure to **metoprolol**. [Moderate] Study

▸ Interferons **(ropeginterferon alfa)** are predicted to increase the exposure to **nebivolol**. [Moderate] Theoretical

▸ **Beta blockers, selective** are predicted to increase the risk of bradycardia when given with lanreotide. [Moderate] Theoretical

▸ Mavacamten can cause negative inotropic effects, as can **beta blockers, selective**. [Severe] Theoretical

▸ Mexiletine potentially increases the risk of cardiovascular adverse effects when given with **beta blockers, selective**. Avoid or monitor. [Severe] Theoretical

▸ Mirabegron is predicted to increase the exposure to **metoprolol**. [Moderate] Study

▸ Omega-3-acid ethyl esters might enhance the blood pressure-lowering effects of **beta blockers, selective**. [Moderate] Study

Beta blockers, selective (continued)

- ▶ **Panobinostat** is predicted to increase the exposure to **metoprolol**. Monitor and adjust dose. [Moderate] Theoretical
- ▶ **Panobinostat** is predicted to increase the exposure to **nebivolol**. Monitor and adjust dose. [Mild] Theoretical
- ▶ **Rifamycins (rifampicin)** moderately decrease the exposure to **celiprolol**. [Moderate] Study
- ▶ **Rifamycins (rifampicin)** slightly decrease the exposure to beta blockers, selective **(bisoprolol, metoprolol)**. [Mild] Study
- ▶ **SNRIs (duloxetine)** are predicted to increase the exposure to **metoprolol**. [Moderate] Study
- ▶ **SSRIs (fluoxetine, paroxetine)** are predicted to increase the exposure to beta blockers, selective **(metoprolol, nebivolol)**. [Moderate] Study
- ▶ **Suxamethonium** might increase the concentration of **landiolol** and **landiolol** might prolong the effects of **suxamethonium**. [Moderate] Study → Also see **TABLE 5** p. 1572
- ▶ **Beta blockers, selective** increase the risk of hypertension and bradycardia when given with **sympathomimetics, inotropic (dobutamine)**. [Moderate] Theoretical
- ▶ **Beta blockers, selective** are predicted to increase the risk of hypertension and bradycardia when given with **sympathomimetics, vasoconstrictor (adrenaline/epinephrine, noradrenaline/norepinephrine)**. [Severe] Study
- ▶ **Terbinafine** is predicted to increase the exposure to beta blockers, selective **(metoprolol, nebivolol)**. [Moderate] Study
- ▶ **Beta blockers, selective** are predicted to increase the risk of bronchospasm when given with **theophylline**. Avoid. [Severe] Theoretical
- ▶ **Vaborbactam** is predicted to increase the concentration of **metoprolol**. [Unknown] Theoretical

Beta₂ agonists → see **TABLE 16** p. 1575 (reduced serum potassium)

> formoterol · indacaterol · olodaterol · salbutamol · salmeterol · terbutaline · vilanterol

- ▶ **Anti-androgens (apalutamide)** are predicted to decrease the exposure to **salmeterol**. Avoid or monitor. [Moderate] Study
- ▶ **Antifungals, azoles (itraconazole, ketoconazole, posaconazole, voriconazole)** are predicted to increase the exposure to **salmeterol**. Avoid. [Severe] Study
- ▶ **Atomoxetine** is predicted to increase the risk of cardiovascular adverse effects when given with **beta₂ agonists** (high-dose). [Moderate] Study
- ▶ **Cenobamate** is predicted to decrease the exposure to **salmeterol**. Adjust dose. [Moderate] Theoretical
- ▶ **Ceritinib** is predicted to increase the exposure to **salmeterol**. Avoid. [Severe] Study
- ▶ **Cobicistat** is predicted to increase the exposure to **salmeterol**. Avoid. [Severe] Study
- ▶ **HIV-protease inhibitors** are predicted to increase the exposure to **salmeterol**. Avoid. [Severe] Study
- ▶ **Idelalisib** is predicted to increase the exposure to **salmeterol**. Avoid. [Severe] Study
- ▶ **Beta₂ agonists** are predicted to increase the risk of glaucoma when given with **ipratropium**. [Moderate] Anecdotal
- ▶ **Ivosidenib** might decrease the exposure to **salmeterol**. Avoid or monitor. [Moderate] Theoretical
- ▶ **Beta₂ agonists** are predicted to increase the risk of elevated blood pressure when given with **linezolid**. Avoid. [Severe] Theoretical
- ▶ **Macrolides (clarithromycin)** are predicted to increase the exposure to **salmeterol**. Avoid. [Severe] Study
- ▶ **MAO-B inhibitors (rasagiline, selegiline)** are predicted to increase the risk of severe hypertension when given with **beta₂ agonists**. Avoid. [Severe] Theoretical
- ▶ **MAO-B inhibitors (safinamide)** are predicted to increase the risk of severe hypertension when given with **beta₂ agonists**. [Severe] Theoretical
- ▶ **MAOIs, irreversible** are predicted to increase the risk of cardiovascular adverse effects when given with **beta₂ agonists**. [Moderate] Anecdotal
- ▶ **Neurokinin-1 receptor antagonists (aprepitant, netupitant)** are predicted to increase the exposure to **salmeterol**. [Moderate] Study
- ▶ **Nirmatrelvir** boosted with ritonavir is predicted to increase the concentration of **salmeterol**. Avoid. [Severe] Theoretical

- ▶ **Tucatinib** is predicted to increase the exposure to **salmeterol**. Avoid. [Severe] Study

Betahistine

- ▶ **Antihistamines, non-sedating** are predicted to decrease the effects of **betahistine**. [Moderate] Theoretical
- ▶ **Antihistamines, sedating** are predicted to decrease the effects of **betahistine**. [Moderate] Theoretical

Betamethasone → see corticosteroids

Betaxolol → see beta blockers, selective

Bevacizumab → see monoclonal antibodies

Bexarotene → see retinoids

Bezafibrate → see fibrates

Bicalutamide → see anti-androgens

Bictegravir

- ▶ Oral **antacids** decrease the exposure to oral **bictegravir**. Separate administration by at least 2 hours. [Moderate] Study
- ▶ **Anti-androgens (apalutamide, enzalutamide)** are predicted to decrease the exposure to **bictegravir**. Avoid. [Moderate] Study
- ▶ **Antiarrhythmics (amiodarone, dronedarone)** are predicted to increase the exposure to **bictegravir**. Use with caution or avoid. [Moderate] Theoretical
- ▶ **Antiepileptics (carbamazepine, fosphenytoin, phenobarbital, phenytoin, primidone)** are predicted to decrease the exposure to **bictegravir**. Avoid. [Moderate] Study
- ▶ **Antiepileptics (oxcarbazepine)** are predicted to decrease the exposure to **bictegravir**. Avoid. [Moderate] Theoretical
- ▶ **Antifungals, azoles (itraconazole, ketoconazole)** are predicted to increase the exposure to **bictegravir**. Use with caution or avoid. [Moderate] Theoretical
- ▶ **Calcium channel blockers (verapamil)** are predicted to increase the exposure to **bictegravir**. Use with caution or avoid. [Moderate] Theoretical
- ▶ **Ciclosporin** is predicted to increase the exposure to **bictegravir**. Use with caution or avoid. [Moderate] Theoretical
- ▶ **Cobicistat** is predicted to increase the exposure to **bictegravir**. Use with caution or avoid. [Moderate] Theoretical
- ▶ **Encorafenib** is predicted to decrease the exposure to **bictegravir**. Avoid. [Moderate] Study
- ▶ **Glecaprevir** is predicted to increase the exposure to **bictegravir**. Use with caution or avoid. [Moderate] Theoretical
- ▶ **HIV-protease inhibitors (atazanavir)** moderately increase the exposure to **bictegravir**. Avoid. [Moderate] Study
- ▶ **HIV-protease inhibitors (lopinavir, ritonavir)** are predicted to increase the exposure to **bictegravir**. Use with caution or avoid. [Moderate] Theoretical
- ▶ Oral **iron** decreases the exposure to oral **bictegravir**. Manufacturer advises bictegravir should be taken 2 hours before iron. [Moderate] Study
- ▶ **Ivosidenib** is predicted to decrease the exposure to **bictegravir**. Avoid. [Moderate] Study
- ▶ **Lapatinib** is predicted to increase the exposure to **bictegravir**. Use with caution or avoid. [Moderate] Theoretical
- ▶ **Lumacaftor** is predicted to decrease the exposure to **bictegravir**. Avoid. [Moderate] Study
- ▶ **Macrolides** are predicted to increase the exposure to **bictegravir**. Use with caution or avoid. [Moderate] Theoretical
- ▶ **Bictegravir** slightly increases the exposure to **metformin**. [Moderate] Study
- ▶ **Mitotane** is predicted to decrease the exposure to **bictegravir**. Avoid. [Moderate] Study
- ▶ **Pibrentasvir** is predicted to increase the exposure to **bictegravir**. Use with caution or avoid. [Moderate] Theoretical
- ▶ **Ranolazine** is predicted to increase the exposure to **bictegravir**. Use with caution or avoid. [Moderate] Theoretical
- ▶ **Rifamycins (rifabutin)** slightly decrease the exposure to **bictegravir**. Avoid. [Mild] Study
- ▶ **Rifamycins (rifampicin)** are predicted to decrease the exposure to **bictegravir**. Avoid. [Moderate] Study
- ▶ **St John's wort** is predicted to decrease the exposure to **bictegravir**. Avoid. [Moderate] Theoretical
- ▶ **Sucralfate** is predicted to decrease the exposure to **bictegravir**. Avoid. [Moderate] Theoretical
- ▶ **Velpatasvir** is predicted to increase the exposure to **bictegravir**. Use with caution or avoid. [Moderate] Theoretical

▸ **Vemurafenib** is predicted to increase the exposure to bictegravir. Use with caution or avoid. [Moderate] Theoretical
▸ **Voxilaprevir** is predicted to increase the exposure to bictegravir. Use with caution or avoid. [Moderate] Theoretical

Bilastine → see antihistamines, non-sedating
Bimekizumab → see monoclonal antibodies
Bismuth
▸ **Bismuth** subsalicylate is predicted to increase the risk of adverse effects when given with aspirin. Avoid. [Moderate] Theoretical
▸ **Bismuth** subsalicylate is predicted to increase the risk of bleeding events when given with drugs with anticoagulant effects (see TABLE 3 p. 1571). [Moderate] Theoretical
▸ Oral **bismuth** greatly decreases the absorption of oral tetracyclines. Separate administration by at least 2 to 3 hours. [Moderate] Study

Bisoprolol → see beta blockers, selective
Bisphosphonates → see TABLE 2 p. 1571 (nephrotoxicity)

alendronate · clodronate · ibandronate · pamidronate · risedronate · zoledronate

▸ **Aminoglycosides** increase the risk of hypocalcaemia when given with **bisphosphonates**. [Moderate] Anecdotal → Also see TABLE 2 p. 1571
▸ Oral **antacids** decrease the absorption of oral **alendronate**. Manufacturer advises take at least 30 minutes before antacids. [Moderate] Study
▸ Oral **antacids** decrease the absorption of oral **clodronate**. Avoid antacids for 2 hours before or 1 hour after **clodronate**. [Moderate] Study
▸ Oral **antacids** are predicted to decrease the absorption of oral **ibandronate**. Avoid antacids for at least 6 hours before or 1 hour after **ibandronate**. [Moderate] Theoretical
▸ Oral **antacids** decrease the absorption of oral **risedronate**. Separate administration by at least 2 hours. [Moderate] Study
▸ **Aspirin** (high-dose) is predicted to increase the risk of gastrointestinal irritation when given with bisphosphonates (alendronate, ibandronate). [Moderate] Study
▸ **Aspirin** (high-dose) is predicted to increase the risk of renal impairment when given with **clodronate**. [Severe] Theoretical
▸ Oral **calcium salts** decrease the absorption of oral **alendronate**. Alendronate should be taken at least 30 minutes before calcium. [Moderate] Study
▸ Oral **calcium salts** decrease the absorption of oral **clodronate**. Avoid **calcium salts** for 2 hours before or 1 hour after **clodronate**. [Moderate] Study
▸ Oral **calcium salts** are predicted to decrease the absorption of oral **ibandronate**. Avoid **calcium salts** for at least 6 hours before or 1 hour after **ibandronate**. [Moderate] Theoretical
▸ Oral **calcium salts** decrease the absorption of oral **risedronate**. Separate administration by at least 2 hours. [Moderate] Study
▸ Oral **iron** decreases the absorption of oral **clodronate**. **Clodronate** should be taken 1 hour before or 2 hours after iron. [Moderate] Study
▸ Oral **iron** is predicted to decrease the absorption of oral **ibandronate**. **Ibandronate** should be taken 1 hour before or 6 hours after iron. [Moderate] Theoretical
▸ Oral **iron** decreases the absorption of oral **risedronate**. Separate administration by at least 2 hours. [Moderate] Study
▸ **Bisphosphonates** are predicted to increase the risk of gastrointestinal bleeding when given with iron chelators (deferasirox). [Severe] Theoretical → Also see TABLE 2 p. 1571
▸ Oral **magnesium** decreases the absorption of oral **alendronate**. Manufacturer advises take at least 30 minutes before magnesium. [Moderate] Study
▸ Oral **magnesium** decreases the absorption of oral **clodronate**. Avoid magnesium for 2 hours before or 1 hour after **clodronate**. [Moderate] Study
▸ Oral **magnesium** is predicted to decrease the absorption of oral **ibandronate**. Avoid for at least 6 hours before or 1 hour after **ibandronate**. [Moderate] Theoretical
▸ Oral **magnesium** decreases the absorption of oral **risedronate**. Separate administration by at least 2 hours. [Moderate] Study
▸ **NSAIDs** are predicted to increase the risk of gastrointestinal irritation when given with bisphosphonates (alendronate, ibandronate). [Moderate] Study

▸ **NSAIDs** are predicted to increase the risk of renal impairment when given with **clodronate**. [Moderate] Study
▸ **Bisphosphonates** are predicted to decrease the effects of parathyroid hormone. Avoid. [Moderate] Study
▸ Oral **zinc** decreases the absorption of oral **alendronate**. **Alendronate** should be taken at least 30 minutes before zinc. [Moderate] Study
▸ Oral **zinc** decreases the absorption of oral **clodronate**. Avoid zinc for 2 hours before or 1 hour after **clodronate**. [Moderate] Study
▸ Oral **zinc** is predicted to decrease the absorption of oral **ibandronate**. Avoid zinc for at least 6 hours before or 1 hour after **ibandronate**, p. 1226, p. 771. [Moderate] Theoretical
▸ Oral **zinc** decreases the absorption of oral **risedronate**. Separate administration by at least 2 hours. [Moderate] Study

Bivalirudin → see thrombin inhibitors
Bleomycin → see TABLE 14 p. 1575 (myelosuppression)
▸ **Bleomycin** -containing cytotoxic regimens might affect the concentration of antiepileptics (fosphenytoin, phenytoin). Avoid. [Severe] Anecdotal
▸ **Filgrastim** might increase the risk of pulmonary toxicity when given with **bleomycin**. [Severe] Theoretical
▸ **Lenograstim** might increase the risk of pulmonary toxicity when given with **bleomycin**. [Severe] Theoretical
▸ **Lipegfilgrastim** might increase the risk of pulmonary toxicity when given with **bleomycin**. [Severe] Theoretical
▸ **Live vaccines** are predicted to increase the risk of generalised infection (possibly life-threatening) when given with **bleomycin**. UKHSA advises avoid (refer to Green Book). [Severe] Theoretical
▸ Monoclonal antibodies (brentuximab vedotin) increase the risk of pulmonary toxicity when given with **bleomycin**. Avoid. [Severe] Study → Also see TABLE 14 p. 1575
▸ **Pegfilgrastim** might increase the risk of pulmonary toxicity when given with **bleomycin**. [Severe] Theoretical
▸ Platinum compounds (cisplatin) increase the risk of pulmonary toxicity when given with **bleomycin**. [Severe] Study → Also see TABLE 14 p. 1575

Blinatumomab → see monoclonal antibodies
Bortezomib → see TABLE 7 p. 1572 (hypotension), TABLE 14 p. 1575 (myelosuppression), TABLE 11 p. 1574 (peripheral neuropathy)
▸ Anti-androgens (apalutamide, enzalutamide) slightly decrease the exposure to **bortezomib**. Avoid. [Severe] Study
▸ Antiepileptics (carbamazepine, fosphenytoin, phenobarbital, phenytoin, primidone) slightly decrease the exposure to **bortezomib**. Avoid. [Severe] Study → Also see TABLE 11 p. 1574
▸ Antifungals, azoles (itraconazole, ketoconazole, posaconazole, voriconazole) slightly increase the exposure to **bortezomib**. [Moderate] Study
▸ **Ceritinib** slightly increases the exposure to **bortezomib**. [Moderate] Study → Also see TABLE 14 p. 1575
▸ **Cobicistat** slightly increases the exposure to **bortezomib**. [Moderate] Study
▸ **Encorafenib** slightly decreases the exposure to **bortezomib**. Avoid. [Severe] Study
▸ **HIV-protease inhibitors** slightly increase the exposure to **bortezomib**. [Moderate] Study
▸ **Idelalisib** slightly increases the exposure to **bortezomib**. [Moderate] Study
▸ **Ivosidenib** slightly decreases the exposure to **bortezomib**. Avoid. [Severe] Study
▸ **Lumacaftor** slightly decreases the exposure to **bortezomib**. Avoid. [Severe] Study
▸ **Macrolides** (clarithromycin) slightly increase the exposure to **bortezomib**. [Moderate] Study
▸ **Mitotane** slightly decreases the exposure to **bortezomib**. Avoid. [Severe] Study → Also see TABLE 14 p. 1575
▸ Rifamycins (rifampicin) slightly decrease the exposure to **bortezomib**. Avoid. [Severe] Study
▸ **Tucatinib** slightly increases the exposure to **bortezomib**. [Moderate] Study

Bosentan → see endothelin receptor antagonists
Bosutinib → see TABLE 14 p. 1575 (myelosuppression), TABLE 8 p. 1573 (QT-interval prolongation), TABLE 4 p. 1571 (antiplatelet effects)

Bosutinib (continued)

▶ Oral antacids are predicted to decrease the absorption of oral **bosutinib**. Manufacturer advises take at least 12 hours before antacids. Moderate Theoretical

▶ Anti-androgens (apalutamide, enzalutamide) are predicted to very markedly decrease the exposure to **bosutinib**. Avoid. Severe Study → Also see TABLE 8 p. 1573

▶ Antiarrhythmics (dronedarone) are predicted to increase the exposure to **bosutinib**. Avoid or adjust dose. Severe Study → Also see TABLE 8 p. 1573

▶ Antiepileptics (carbamazepine, fosphenytoin, phenobarbital, phenytoin, primidone) are predicted to very markedly decrease the exposure to **bosutinib**. Avoid. Severe Study

▶ Antifungals, azoles (fluconazole, isavuconazole, itraconazole, ketoconazole, posaconazole, voriconazole) are predicted to increase the exposure to **bosutinib**. Avoid or adjust dose. Severe Study → Also see TABLE 8 p. 1573

▶ Belzutifan is predicted to decrease the exposure to **bosutinib**. Avoid or adjust dose. Severe Theoretical

▶ Berotralstat is predicted to increase the exposure to **bosutinib**. Avoid or adjust dose. Severe Study

▶ Calcium channel blockers (diltiazem, verapamil) are predicted to increase the exposure to **bosutinib**. Avoid or adjust dose. Severe Study

▶ Oral calcium salts (calcium carbonate) -containing antacids are predicted to decrease the absorption of oral **bosutinib**. Manufacturer advises take at least 12 hours before antacids. Moderate Theoretical

▶ Cenobamate is predicted to decrease the exposure to **bosutinib**. Avoid. Severe Study

▶ Ceritinib is predicted to increase the exposure to **bosutinib**. Avoid or adjust dose. Severe Study → Also see TABLE 14 p. 1575 → Also see TABLE 8 p. 1573

▶ Cobicistat is predicted to increase the exposure to **bosutinib**. Avoid or adjust dose. Severe Study

▶ Crizotinib is predicted to increase the exposure to **bosutinib**. Avoid or adjust dose. Severe Study → Also see TABLE 8 p. 1573

▶ Dabrafenib is predicted to decrease the exposure to **bosutinib**. Avoid. Severe Study

▶ Encorafenib is predicted to very markedly decrease the exposure to **bosutinib**. Avoid. Severe Study → Also see TABLE 8 p. 1573

▶ Endothelin receptor antagonists (bosentan) are predicted to decrease the exposure to **bosutinib**. Avoid. Severe Study

▶ Fedratinib is predicted to increase the exposure to **bosutinib**. Avoid or adjust dose. Severe Study

▶ Grapefruit juice is predicted to increase the exposure to **bosutinib**. Avoid. Moderate Theoretical

▶ H₂ receptor antagonists are predicted to decrease the absorption of **bosutinib**. Moderate Theoretical

▶ HIV-protease inhibitors are predicted to increase the exposure to **bosutinib**. Avoid or adjust dose. Severe Study

▶ Idelalisib is predicted to increase the exposure to **bosutinib**. Avoid or adjust dose. Severe Study

▶ Imatinib is predicted to increase the exposure to **bosutinib**. Avoid or adjust dose. Severe Study → Also see TABLE 14 p. 1575 → Also see TABLE 4 p. 1571

▶ Ivosidenib is predicted to very markedly decrease the exposure to **bosutinib**. Avoid. Severe Study → Also see TABLE 8 p. 1573

▶ Letermovir is predicted to increase the exposure to **bosutinib**. Avoid or adjust dose. Severe Study

▶ Lorlatinib is predicted to decrease the exposure to **bosutinib**. Avoid. Severe Study

▶ Lumacaftor is predicted to very markedly decrease the exposure to **bosutinib**. Avoid. Severe Study

▶ Macrolides (clarithromycin, erythromycin) are predicted to increase the exposure to **bosutinib**. Avoid or adjust dose. Severe Study → Also see TABLE 8 p. 1573

▶ Mitotane is predicted to very markedly decrease the exposure to **bosutinib**. Avoid. Severe Study → Also see TABLE 14 p. 1575

▶ Modafinil is predicted to decrease the exposure to **bosutinib**. Avoid. Severe Theoretical

▶ Neurokinin-1 receptor antagonists (aprepitant, netupitant) are predicted to increase the exposure to **bosutinib**. Avoid or adjust dose. Severe Study

▶ Neurokinin-1 receptor antagonists (fosaprepitant) are predicted to increase the exposure to **bosutinib**. Severe Theoretical

▶ Nilotinib is predicted to increase the exposure to **bosutinib**. Avoid or adjust dose. Severe Study → Also see TABLE 14 p. 1575 → Also see TABLE 8 p. 1573

▶ NNRTIs (efavirenz, etravirine, nevirapine) are predicted to decrease the exposure to **bosutinib**. Avoid. Severe Study → Also see TABLE 8 p. 1573

▶ Pitolisant is predicted to decrease the exposure to **bosutinib**. Avoid. Severe Theoretical

▶ Proton pump inhibitors are predicted to decrease the absorption of **bosutinib**. Moderate Study

▶ Rifamycins (rifampicin) are predicted to very markedly decrease the exposure to **bosutinib**. Avoid. Severe Study

▶ Oral sodium bicarbonate-containing antacids are predicted to decrease the absorption of oral **bosutinib**. Manufacturer advises take at least 12 hours before antacids. Moderate Theoretical

▶ Sotorasib is predicted to decrease the exposure to **bosutinib**. Avoid. Severe Study

▶ St John's wort is predicted to decrease the exposure to **bosutinib**. Avoid. Severe Study

▶ Tucatinib is predicted to increase the exposure to **bosutinib**. Avoid or adjust dose. Severe Study

Botulinum toxin type A → see botulinum toxins

Botulinum toxins → see TABLE 19 p. 1576 (neuromuscular blocking effects)

> botulinum toxin type A

Bowel cleansing preparations

SEPARATION OF ADMINISTRATION Other oral drugs should not be taken 1 hour before, or after, administration of bowel cleansing preparations because absorption might be impaired. Consider withholding ACE inhibitors, angiotensin-II receptor antagonists, and NSAIDs on the day that bowel cleansing preparations are given and for up to 72 hours after the procedure. Also consider withholding diuretics on the day that bowel cleansing preparations are given.

Brentuximab vedotin → see monoclonal antibodies

Brigatinib → see TABLE 5 p. 1572 (bradycardia)

▶ Anti-androgens (apalutamide, enzalutamide) are predicted to decrease the exposure to **brigatinib**. Avoid. Severe Study

▶ Antiarrhythmics (dronedarone) are predicted to increase the exposure to **brigatinib**. Moderate Study → Also see TABLE 5 p. 1572

▶ Antiepileptics (carbamazepine, fosphenytoin, phenobarbital, phenytoin, primidone) are predicted to decrease the exposure to **brigatinib**. Avoid. Severe Study

▶ Antifungals, azoles (fluconazole, isavuconazole) are predicted to increase the exposure to **brigatinib**. Moderate Study

▶ Antifungals, azoles (itraconazole, ketoconazole, posaconazole, voriconazole) are predicted to increase the exposure to **brigatinib**. Avoid or adjust dose—consult product literature. Severe Study

▶ Berotralstat is predicted to increase the exposure to **brigatinib**. Moderate Study

▶ Calcium channel blockers (diltiazem, verapamil) are predicted to increase the exposure to **brigatinib**. Moderate Study → Also see TABLE 5 p. 1572

▶ Cenobamate is predicted to decrease the exposure to **brigatinib**. Avoid or adjust dose—consult product literature. Moderate Study

▶ Ceritinib is predicted to increase the exposure to **brigatinib**. Avoid or adjust dose—consult product literature. Severe Study → Also see TABLE 5 p. 1572

▶ **Brigatinib** might decrease the exposure to ciclosporin. Avoid. Moderate Theoretical

▶ Cobicistat is predicted to increase the exposure to **brigatinib**. Avoid or adjust dose—consult product literature. Severe Study

▶ **Brigatinib** is predicted to decrease the exposure to combined hormonal contraceptives. Use additional contraceptive precautions. Severe Theoretical

▶ Crizotinib is predicted to increase the exposure to **brigatinib**. Moderate Study → Also see TABLE 5 p. 1572

▸ **Dabrafenib** is predicted to decrease the exposure to **brigatinib**. Avoid or adjust dose—consult product literature. Moderate Study

▸ **Encorafenib** is predicted to decrease the exposure to **brigatinib**. Avoid. Severe Study

▸ **Endothelin receptor antagonists (bosentan)** are predicted to decrease the exposure to **brigatinib**. Avoid or adjust dose—consult product literature. Moderate Study

▸ **Fedratinib** is predicted to increase the exposure to **brigatinib**. Moderate Study

▸ **Grapefruit** juice is predicted to increase the concentration of **brigatinib**. Avoid. Severe Study

▸ **HIV-protease inhibitors** are predicted to increase the exposure to **brigatinib**. Avoid or adjust dose—consult product literature. Severe Study

▸ **Idelalisib** is predicted to increase the exposure to **brigatinib**. Avoid or adjust dose—consult product literature. Severe Study

▸ **Imatinib** is predicted to increase the exposure to **brigatinib**. Moderate Study

▸ **Ivosidenib** is predicted to decrease the exposure to **brigatinib**. Avoid. Severe Study

▸ **Letermovir** is predicted to increase the exposure to **brigatinib**. Moderate Study

▸ **Lorlatinib** is predicted to decrease the exposure to **brigatinib**. Avoid or adjust dose—consult product literature. Moderate Study

▸ **Lumacaftor** is predicted to decrease the exposure to **brigatinib**. Avoid. Severe Study

▸ **Macrolides (clarithromycin)** are predicted to increase the exposure to **brigatinib**. Avoid or adjust dose—consult product literature. Severe Study

▸ **Macrolides (erythromycin)** are predicted to increase the exposure to **brigatinib**. Moderate Study

▸ **Mitotane** is predicted to decrease the exposure to **brigatinib**. Avoid. Severe Study

▸ **Modafinil** is predicted to decrease the exposure to **brigatinib**. Avoid or adjust dose—consult product literature. Moderate Theoretical

▸ **Neurokinin-1 receptor antagonists (aprepitant, netupitant)** are predicted to increase the exposure to **brigatinib**. Moderate Study

▸ **Nilotinib** is predicted to increase the exposure to **brigatinib**. Moderate Study

▸ **NNRTIs (efavirenz, etravirine, nevirapine)** are predicted to decrease the exposure to **brigatinib**. Avoid or adjust dose—consult product literature. Moderate Study

▸ **Brigatinib** potentially decreases the concentration of opioids **(alfentanil, fentanyl)**. Avoid. Moderate Theoretical → Also see **TABLE 5** p. 1572

▸ **Rifamycins (rifampicin)** are predicted to decrease the exposure to **brigatinib**. Avoid. Severe Study

▸ **Brigatinib** potentially decreases the concentration of **sirolimus**. Avoid. Moderate Theoretical

▸ **Sotorasib** is predicted to decrease the exposure to **brigatinib**. Avoid or adjust dose—consult product literature. Moderate Study

▸ **St John's wort** is predicted to decrease the exposure to **brigatinib**. Avoid or adjust dose—consult product literature. Moderate Study

▸ **Brigatinib** potentially decreases the concentration of **tacrolimus**. Avoid. Moderate Theoretical

▸ **Tucatinib** is predicted to increase the exposure to **brigatinib**. Avoid or adjust dose—consult product literature. Severe Study

Brimonidine → see **TABLE 5** p. 1572 (bradycardia), **TABLE 7** p. 1572 (hypotension), **TABLE 10** p. 1574 (CNS effects)

Brinzolamide

> **ROUTE-SPECIFIC INFORMATION** Since systemic absorption can follow topical application of **brinzolamide**, the possibility of interactions should be borne in mind.

Brivaracetam → see antiepileptics
Brodalumab → see monoclonal antibodies
Bromfenac → see NSAIDs
Bromocriptine → see dopamine receptor agonists
Buclizine → see antihistamines, sedating
Budesonide → see corticosteroids

Bulevirtide

▸ **Angiotensin-II receptor antagonists (irbesartan)** are predicted to affect the efficacy of **bulevirtide**. Avoid. Severe Theoretical

▸ **Bulevirtide** is predicted to increase the exposure to angiotensin-II receptor antagonists **(olmesartan, telmisartan, valsartan)**. Avoid or monitor. Moderate Theoretical

▸ **Bulevirtide** is predicted to increase the exposure to antiepileptics **(carbamazepine)**. Moderate Theoretical

▸ **Bulevirtide** is predicted to increase the exposure to antihistamines, non-sedating **(fexofenadine)**. Avoid or monitor. Moderate Theoretical

▸ **Bulevirtide** slightly increases the exposure to benzodiazepines **(midazolam)**. Moderate Theoretical

▸ **Ciclosporin** is predicted to affect the efficacy of **bulevirtide** and **bulevirtide** is predicted to increase the exposure to ciclosporin. Avoid. Severe Theoretical

▸ **Bulevirtide** is predicted to increase the exposure to endothelin receptor antagonists **(bosentan)**. Avoid or monitor. Moderate Theoretical

▸ **Bulevirtide** is predicted to increase the exposure to everolimus. Moderate Theoretical

▸ **Ezetimibe** is predicted to affect the efficacy of **bulevirtide**. Avoid. Severe Theoretical

▸ **Bulevirtide** is predicted to increase the exposure to glecaprevir. Avoid or monitor. Moderate Theoretical

▸ **Bulevirtide** is predicted to increase the exposure to grazoprevir. Avoid or monitor. Moderate Theoretical

▸ **HIV-protease inhibitors (ritonavir)** are predicted to affect the efficacy of **bulevirtide**. Avoid. Severe Theoretical

▸ **Bulevirtide** is predicted to increase the exposure to meglitinides **(repaglinide)**. Avoid or monitor. Moderate Theoretical

▸ **Bulevirtide** is predicted to increase the exposure to opioids **(alfentanil)**. Moderate Theoretical

▸ **Bulevirtide** is predicted to increase the exposure to sirolimus. Moderate Theoretical

▸ **Bulevirtide** is predicted to increase the exposure to statins. Avoid or monitor. Moderate Theoretical

▸ **Sulfasalazine** is predicted to affect the efficacy of **bulevirtide**. Avoid. Severe Theoretical

▸ **Bulevirtide** is predicted to increase the exposure to sulfonylureas **(glibenclamide)**. Avoid or monitor. Moderate Theoretical

▸ **Bulevirtide** is predicted to increase the exposure to tacrolimus. Moderate Theoretical

▸ **Bulevirtide** is predicted to increase the exposure to taxanes **(docetaxel, paclitaxel)**. Avoid or monitor. Moderate Theoretical

▸ **Bulevirtide** is predicted to increase the exposure to temsirolimus. Moderate Theoretical

▸ **Bulevirtide** is predicted to increase the exposure to thyroid hormones. Avoid or monitor. Moderate Theoretical

▸ **Bulevirtide** is predicted to increase the exposure to voxilaprevir. Avoid or monitor. Moderate Theoretical

Bumetanide → see loop diuretics
Bupivacaine → see anaesthetics, local
Buprenorphine → see opioids
Bupropion

▸ **Bupropion** is predicted to increase the exposure to anticholinesterases, centrally acting **(galantamine)**. Monitor and adjust dose. Moderate Study

▸ Antiepileptics **(carbamazepine, fosphenytoin, phenobarbital, phenytoin, primidone)** are predicted to markedly decrease the exposure to **bupropion**. Severe Study

▸ Antiepileptics **(valproate)** increase the exposure to **bupropion**. Severe Study

▸ Antifungals, azoles **(isavuconazole)** slightly increase the exposure to **bupropion**. Adjust dose. Moderate Study

▸ **Bupropion** is predicted to moderately increase the exposure to antipsychotics, second generation **(aripiprazole)**. Adjust **aripiprazole** dose, p. 454. Moderate Study

▸ **Bupropion** is predicted to increase the exposure to antipsychotics, second generation **(clozapine)**. Use with caution and adjust dose. Severe Study

▸ **Bupropion** is predicted to increase the exposure to antipsychotics, second generation **(risperidone)**. Adjust dose. Moderate Study

Interactions | Appendix 1   A1

Bupropion (continued)

▶ **Bupropion** is predicted to markedly increase the exposure to **atomoxetine**. Adjust dose. [Severe] Study
▶ **Bupropion** is predicted to increase the exposure to beta blockers, selective **(metoprolol, nebivolol)**. [Moderate] Study
▶ **Clopidogrel** slightly increases the exposure to **bupropion**. [Moderate] Study
▶ **Bupropion** is predicted to slightly increase the exposure to darifenacin. [Mild] Study
▶ **Bupropion** might decrease the exposure to digoxin. [Severe] Study
▶ **Bupropion** increases the risk of adverse effects when given with dopamine receptor agonists **(amantadine)**. [Moderate] Study
▶ **Bupropion** might enhance the risk of serotonin syndrome when given with drugs that cause serotonin syndrome (see **TABLE 12** p. 1574). [Severe] Anecdotal
▶ **Bupropion** is predicted to increase the exposure to eliglustat. Avoid or adjust dose—consult product literature. [Severe] Study
▶ **Bupropion** is predicted to increase the exposure to fenfluramine. [Moderate] Study
▶ **Bupropion** is predicted to increase the exposure to fesoterodine. Use with caution and adjust dose. [Mild] Theoretical
▶ **Bupropion** is predicted to increase the exposure to gefitinib. [Moderate] Theoretical
▶ HIV-protease inhibitors are predicted to decrease the exposure to **bupropion**. [Moderate] Study
▶ **Bupropion** increases the risk of adverse effects when given with levodopa. [Moderate] Study
▶ **Bupropion** is predicted to increase the risk of intraoperative hypertension when given with linezolid. [Severe] Anecdotal
▶ **Lumacaftor** is predicted to decrease the exposure to bupropion. Adjust dose. [Moderate] Theoretical
▶ **Bupropion** is predicted to increase the risk of severe hypertension when given with **MAO-B inhibitors**. Avoid. [Moderate] Theoretical
▶ **Bupropion** is predicted to increase the risk of severe hypertension when given with **MAOIs, irreversible**. Avoid and for 14 days after stopping the MAOI. [Severe] Theoretical
▶ Methylthioninium chloride is predicted to increase the risk of severe hypertension when given with **bupropion**. Avoid. [Severe] Theoretical
▶ **Bupropion** is predicted to increase the exposure to mexiletine. [Moderate] Study
▶ Midostaurin moderately decreases the exposure to the active metabolite of **bupropion**. [Moderate] Study
▶ **Bupropion** is predicted to increase the risk of severe hypertension when given with moclobemide. Avoid. [Severe] Theoretical
▶ Nirmatrelvir boosted with ritonavir is predicted to decrease the concentration of **bupropion**. [Moderate] Theoretical
▶ NNRTIs **(efavirenz)** are predicted to decrease the exposure to **bupropion**. [Moderate] Study
▶ **Bupropion** is predicted to decrease the efficacy of opioids **(codeine)**. [Moderate] Theoretical
▶ **Bupropion** is predicted to decrease the efficacy of opioids **(tramadol)**. [Severe] Study
▶ **Bupropion** is predicted to moderately increase the exposure to pitolisant. Use with caution and adjust dose. [Moderate] Study
▶ Rifamycins **(rifampicin)** are predicted to decrease the exposure to **bupropion**. [Moderate] Study
▶ **Bupropion** is predicted to increase the exposure to SSRIs **(dapoxetine)**. [Moderate] Theoretical
▶ **Bupropion** is predicted to decrease the efficacy of tamoxifen. Avoid. [Severe] Study
▶ **Bupropion** is predicted to increase the exposure to the active metabolite of tetrabenazine. [Moderate] Study
▶ **Bupropion** is predicted to increase the exposure to tricyclic antidepressants. Monitor for toxicity and adjust dose. [Severe] Study
▶ Vemurafenib is predicted to decrease the concentration of **bupropion**. [Moderate] Theoretical
▶ **Bupropion** is predicted to increase the exposure to vortioxetine. Monitor and adjust dose. [Moderate] Study

Buspirone

▶ Anti-androgens **(apalutamide, enzalutamide)** are predicted to decrease the exposure to **buspirone**. Use with caution and adjust dose. [Severe] Study
▶ Antiarrhythmics **(dronedarone)** are predicted to increase the exposure to **buspirone**. Use with caution and adjust dose. [Moderate] Study
▶ Antiepileptics **(carbamazepine, fosphenytoin, phenobarbital, phenytoin, primidone)** are predicted to decrease the exposure to **buspirone**. Use with caution and adjust dose. [Severe] Study
▶ Antifungals, azoles **(fluconazole, isavuconazole)** are predicted to increase the exposure to **buspirone**. Use with caution and adjust dose. [Moderate] Study
▶ Antifungals, azoles **(itraconazole, ketoconazole, posaconazole, voriconazole)** are predicted to increase the exposure to **buspirone**. Adjust **buspirone** dose, p. 396. [Severe] Study
▶ Antifungals, azoles **(miconazole)** are predicted to increase the concentration of **buspirone**. Use with caution and adjust dose. [Moderate] Theoretical
▶ **Berotralstat** is predicted to increase the exposure to **buspirone**. Use with caution and adjust dose. [Moderate] Study
▶ Calcium channel blockers **(diltiazem, verapamil)** are predicted to increase the exposure to **buspirone**. Use with caution and adjust dose. [Moderate] Study
▶ **Cenobamate** is predicted to decrease the exposure to **buspirone**. Adjust dose. [Moderate] Theoretical
▶ **Ceritinib** is predicted to increase the exposure to **buspirone**. Adjust **buspirone** dose, p. 396. [Severe] Study
▶ **Cobicistat** is predicted to increase the exposure to **buspirone**. Adjust **buspirone** dose, p. 396. [Severe] Study
▶ **Crizotinib** is predicted to increase the exposure to **buspirone**. Use with caution and adjust dose. [Moderate] Study
▶ **Encorafenib** is predicted to decrease the exposure to **buspirone**. Use with caution and adjust dose. [Severe] Study
▶ **Fedratinib** is predicted to increase the exposure to **buspirone**. Use with caution and adjust dose. [Moderate] Study
▶ **Grapefruit** juice increases the exposure to **buspirone**. Avoid. [Mild] Study
▶ HIV-protease inhibitors are predicted to increase the exposure to **buspirone**. Adjust **buspirone** dose, p. 396. [Severe] Study
▶ **Idelalisib** is predicted to increase the exposure to **buspirone**. Adjust **buspirone** dose, p. 396. [Severe] Study
▶ **Imatinib** is predicted to increase the exposure to **buspirone**. Use with caution and adjust dose. [Moderate] Study
▶ **Ivosidenib** is predicted to decrease the exposure to **buspirone**. Use with caution and adjust dose. [Severe] Study
▶ **Letermovir** is predicted to increase the exposure to **buspirone**. Use with caution and adjust dose. [Moderate] Study
▶ **Buspirone** is predicted to increase the risk of elevated blood pressure when given with linezolid. Avoid. [Severe] Theoretical
▶ **Lumacaftor** is predicted to decrease the exposure to **buspirone**. Use with caution and adjust dose. [Severe] Study
▶ Macrolides **(clarithromycin)** are predicted to increase the exposure to **buspirone**. Adjust **buspirone** dose, p. 396. [Severe] Study
▶ Macrolides **(erythromycin)** are predicted to increase the exposure to **buspirone**. Use with caution and adjust dose. [Moderate] Study
▶ **Buspirone** is predicted to increase the risk of elevated blood pressure when given with **MAOIs, irreversible**. Avoid. [Severe] Anecdotal
▶ **Mitotane** is predicted to decrease the exposure to **buspirone**. Use with caution and adjust dose. [Severe] Study
▶ Neurokinin-1 receptor antagonists **(aprepitant, netupitant)** are predicted to increase the exposure to **buspirone**. Use with caution and adjust dose. [Moderate] Study
▶ **Nilotinib** is predicted to increase the exposure to **buspirone**. Use with caution and adjust dose. [Moderate] Study
▶ **Nirmatrelvir** boosted with ritonavir is predicted to increase the concentration of **buspirone**. Monitor and adjust dose. [Moderate] Theoretical
▶ Rifamycins **(rifampicin)** are predicted to decrease the exposure to **buspirone**. Use with caution and adjust dose. [Severe] Study
▶ **Tucatinib** is predicted to increase the exposure to **buspirone**. Adjust **buspirone** dose, p. 396. [Severe] Study

Busulfan → see alkylating agents
Cabazitaxel → see taxanes
Cabergoline → see dopamine receptor agonists
Cabotegravir
▸ Oral antacids are predicted to decrease the concentration of oral **cabotegravir**. Manufacturer advises take 4 hours before or 2 hours after antacids. Moderate Theoretical
▸ Antiepileptics (carbamazepine, fosphenytoin, oxcarbazepine, phenobarbital, phenytoin, primidone) might decrease the concentration of **cabotegravir**. Avoid. Severe Theoretical
▸ Rifamycins (rifabutin) have been reported to cause a small decrease in the exposure to **cabotegravir**. Avoid intramuscular **cabotegravir**, p. 737. Moderate Study
▸ Rifamycins (rifampicin) modestly decrease the exposure to **cabotegravir**. Avoid. Severe Study
Cabozantinib → see TABLE 14 p. 1575 (myelosuppression), TABLE 8 p. 1573 (QT-interval prolongation)
▸ Anti-androgens (apalutamide, enzalutamide) moderately decrease the exposure to **cabozantinib**. Avoid. Moderate Study → Also see TABLE 8 p. 1573
▸ Antiarrhythmics (dronedarone) are predicted to increase the exposure to **cabozantinib**. Moderate Study → Also see TABLE 8 p. 1573
▸ Antiepileptics (carbamazepine, fosphenytoin, phenobarbital, phenytoin, primidone) moderately decrease the exposure to **cabozantinib**. Avoid. Moderate Study
▸ Antifungals, azoles (fluconazole, isavuconazole, itraconazole, ketoconazole, posaconazole, voriconazole) are predicted to increase the exposure to **cabozantinib**. Moderate Study → Also see TABLE 8 p. 1573
▸ **Cabozantinib** is predicted to increase the exposure to benzodiazepines (midazolam). Moderate Theoretical
▸ **Berotralstat** is predicted to increase the exposure to **cabozantinib**. Moderate Study
▸ Calcium channel blockers (diltiazem, verapamil) are predicted to increase the exposure to **cabozantinib**. Moderate Study
▸ **Cenobamate** is predicted to decrease the exposure to **cabozantinib**. Moderate Study
▸ **Ceritinib** is predicted to increase the exposure to **cabozantinib**. Moderate Study → Also see TABLE 14 p. 1575 → Also see TABLE 8 p. 1573
▸ **Cobicistat** is predicted to increase the exposure to **cabozantinib**. Moderate Study
▸ **Cabozantinib** might affect the effects of combined hormonal contraceptives. Use additional contraceptive precautions. Severe Theoretical
▸ **Crizotinib** is predicted to increase the exposure to **cabozantinib**. Moderate Study → Also see TABLE 8 p. 1573
▸ **Dabrafenib** is predicted to decrease the exposure to **cabozantinib**. Moderate Study
▸ Drugs with anticoagulant effects (see TABLE 3 p. 1571) cause bleeding, as can **cabozantinib**; concurrent use might increase the risk of developing this effect. Severe Theoretical
▸ Drugs with antiplatelet effects (see TABLE 4 p. 1571) cause bleeding, as can **cabozantinib**; concurrent use might increase the risk of developing this effect. Severe Theoretical
▸ **Encorafenib** moderately decreases the exposure to **cabozantinib**. Avoid. Moderate Study → Also see TABLE 8 p. 1573
▸ Endothelin receptor antagonists (bosentan) are predicted to decrease the exposure to **cabozantinib**. Moderate Study
▸ **Fedratinib** is predicted to increase the exposure to **cabozantinib**. Moderate Study
▸ **Grapefruit** juice is predicted to increase the exposure to **cabozantinib**. Moderate Theoretical
▸ HIV-protease inhibitors are predicted to increase the exposure to **cabozantinib**. Moderate Study
▸ **Idelalisib** is predicted to increase the exposure to **cabozantinib**. Moderate Study
▸ **Imatinib** is predicted to increase the exposure to **cabozantinib**. Moderate Study → Also see TABLE 14 p. 1575
▸ **Ivosidenib** moderately decreases the exposure to **cabozantinib**. Avoid. Moderate Study → Also see TABLE 8 p. 1573
▸ **Letermovir** is predicted to increase the exposure to **cabozantinib**. Moderate Study

▸ **Lorlatinib** is predicted to decrease the exposure to **cabozantinib**. Moderate Study
▸ **Lumacaftor** moderately decreases the exposure to **cabozantinib**. Avoid. Moderate Study
▸ Macrolides (clarithromycin, erythromycin) are predicted to increase the exposure to **cabozantinib**. Moderate Study → Also see TABLE 8 p. 1573
▸ **Mitotane** moderately decreases the exposure to **cabozantinib**. Avoid. Moderate Study → Also see TABLE 14 p. 1575
▸ Neurokinin-1 receptor antagonists (aprepitant, netupitant) are predicted to increase the exposure to **cabozantinib**. Moderate Study
▸ **Nilotinib** is predicted to increase the exposure to **cabozantinib**. Moderate Study → Also see TABLE 14 p. 1575 → Also see TABLE 8 p. 1573
▸ NNRTIs (efavirenz, etravirine, nevirapine) are predicted to decrease the exposure to **cabozantinib**. Moderate Study → Also see TABLE 8 p. 1573
▸ Rifamycins (rifampicin) moderately decrease the exposure to **cabozantinib**. Avoid. Moderate Study
▸ **Sotorasib** is predicted to decrease the exposure to **cabozantinib**. Moderate Study
▸ St John's wort is predicted to decrease the exposure to **cabozantinib**. Moderate Study
▸ **Tucatinib** is predicted to increase the exposure to **cabozantinib**. Moderate Study
Caffeine citrate
▸ **Caffeine citrate** decreases the efficacy of antiarrhythmics (adenosine). Separate administration by 24 hours. Mild Study
▸ Antiepileptics (fosphenytoin, phenytoin) are predicted to moderately increase the clearance of **caffeine citrate**. Monitor and adjust dose. Moderate Study
▸ HIV-protease inhibitors (ritonavir) are predicted to moderately increase the clearance of **caffeine citrate**. Monitor and adjust dose. Moderate Study
▸ **Leflunomide** is predicted to moderately increase the clearance of **caffeine citrate**. Monitor and adjust dose. Moderate Study
▸ Rifamycins (rifampicin) are predicted to moderately increase the clearance of **caffeine citrate**. Monitor and adjust dose. Moderate Study
▸ SSRIs (fluvoxamine) markedly decrease the clearance of **caffeine citrate**. Monitor and adjust dose. Severe Study
▸ **Teriflunomide** is predicted to moderately increase the clearance of **caffeine citrate**. Monitor and adjust dose. Moderate Study
▸ **Caffeine citrate** decreases the clearance of theophylline. Moderate Study
Calcifediol → see vitamin D substances
Calcipotriol → see vitamin D substances
Calcitonins
▸ **Calcitonins** decrease the concentration of lithium. Adjust dose. Moderate Study
Calcitriol → see vitamin D substances
Calcium acetate → see calcium salts
Calcium carbonate → see calcium salts
Calcium channel blockers → see TABLE 5 p. 1572 (bradycardia), TABLE 7 p. 1572 (hypotension)

> amlodipine · diltiazem · felodipine · lacidipine · lercanidipine · nicardipine · nifedipine · nimodipine · verapamil

▸ Calcium channel blockers (diltiazem, verapamil) are predicted to increase the exposure to abemaciclib. Moderate Study
▸ Calcium channel blockers (diltiazem, verapamil) are predicted to increase the exposure to acalabrutinib. Avoid or monitor. Severe Study
▸ **Verapamil** is predicted to increase the exposure to afatinib. Moderate Study
▸ **Verapamil** moderately increases the exposure to aliskiren. Moderate Study → Also see TABLE 7 p. 1572
▸ Calcium channel blockers (diltiazem, verapamil) are predicted to increase the exposure to alpha blockers (tamsulosin). Moderate Theoretical → Also see TABLE 7 p. 1572
▸ **Verapamil** moderately increases the exposure to anthracyclines (doxorubicin). Moderate Study
▸ Anti-androgens (apalutamide, enzalutamide) are predicted to decrease the exposure to calcium channel blockers (amlodipine,

Calcium channel blockers (continued)
felodipine, lacidipine, lercanidipine, nicardipine, nifedipine, nimodipine). Monitor and adjust dose. Moderate Study

▸ Anti-androgens (enzalutamide) are predicted to decrease the exposure to calcium channel blockers (diltiazem, verapamil). Severe Study

▸ Antiarrhythmics (disopyramide) are predicted to increase the risk of cardiodepression when given with verapamil. Severe Theoretical

▸ Antiarrhythmics (dronedarone) are predicted to increase the exposure to calcium channel blockers (amlodipine, felodipine, lacidipine, lercanidipine, nicardipine, nifedipine, nimodipine). Monitor and adjust dose. Moderate Study

▸ Antiarrhythmics (amiodarone) are predicted to increase the risk of cardiodepression when given with calcium channel blockers (diltiazem, verapamil). Avoid. Severe Theoretical → Also see **TABLE 5** p. 1572

▸ Calcium channel blockers (diltiazem, verapamil) increase the exposure to antiarrhythmics (dronedarone) and antiarrhythmics (dronedarone) increase the exposure to calcium channel blockers (diltiazem, verapamil). Moderate Study → Also see **TABLE 5** p. 1572

▸ **Verapamil** increases the risk of cardiodepression when given with antiarrhythmics (flecainide). Severe Anecdotal → Also see **TABLE 5** p. 1572

▸ Calcium channel blockers (diltiazem, verapamil) are predicted to increase the exposure to antiarrhythmics (propafenone). Monitor and adjust dose. Moderate Study → Also see **TABLE 5** p. 1572

▸ Antiepileptics (valproate) increase the exposure to **nimodipine**. Adjust dose. Moderate Study

▸ Antiepileptics (carbamazepine, fosphenytoin, phenobarbital, phenytoin, primidone) are predicted to decrease the exposure to calcium channel blockers (amlodipine, felodipine, lacidipine, lercanidipine, nicardipine, nifedipine, nimodipine). Monitor and adjust dose. Moderate Study

▸ **Diltiazem** increases the concentration of antiepileptics (carbamazepine) and antiepileptics (carbamazepine) are predicted to decrease the exposure to **diltiazem**. Monitor concentration and adjust dose. Severe Anecdotal

▸ **Verapamil** increases the concentration of antiepileptics (carbamazepine) and antiepileptics (carbamazepine) are predicted to decrease the exposure to **verapamil**. Severe Anecdotal

▸ Antiepileptics (phenobarbital, primidone) are predicted to decrease the exposure to calcium channel blockers (diltiazem, verapamil). Severe Study

▸ Calcium channel blockers (diltiazem, verapamil) potentially increase the concentration of antiepileptics (fosphenytoin, phenytoin) and antiepileptics (fosphenytoin, phenytoin) are predicted to decrease the exposure to calcium channel blockers (diltiazem, verapamil). Severe Study

▸ Antifungals, azoles (itraconazole, ketoconazole, posaconazole, voriconazole) are predicted to markedly increase the exposure to **lercanidipine**. Avoid. Severe Study

▸ Antifungals, azoles (miconazole) are predicted to increase the exposure to **diltiazem**. Moderate Theoretical

▸ Antifungals, azoles (fluconazole, isavuconazole) are predicted to increase the exposure to calcium channel blockers (amlodipine, felodipine, lacidipine, lercanidipine, nicardipine, nifedipine, nimodipine). Monitor and adjust dose. Moderate Study

▸ Antifungals, azoles (miconazole) are predicted to increase the exposure to calcium channel blockers (amlodipine, felodipine, lacidipine, lercanidipine, nicardipine, nifedipine, nimodipine, verapamil). Use with caution and adjust dose. Moderate Theoretical

▸ Antifungals, azoles (itraconazole, ketoconazole, posaconazole, voriconazole) are predicted to increase the exposure to calcium channel blockers (amlodipine, felodipine, lacidipine, nicardipine, nifedipine, nimodipine). Monitor and adjust dose. Moderate Study

▸ Antifungals, azoles (fluconazole) (high-dose) are predicted to increase the exposure to calcium channel blockers (diltiazem, verapamil). Moderate Theoretical

▸ Antifungals, azoles (itraconazole, ketoconazole, posaconazole, voriconazole) are predicted to increase the exposure to calcium channel blockers (diltiazem, verapamil). Severe Study

▸ Calcium channel blockers (diltiazem, verapamil) are predicted to increase the exposure to antifungals, azoles (isavuconazole). Moderate Theoretical

▸ Calcium channel blockers (diltiazem, verapamil) are predicted to increase the exposure to antihistamines, non-sedating (mizolastine). Severe Theoretical

▸ Calcium channel blockers (diltiazem, verapamil) are predicted to increase the exposure to antihistamines, non-sedating (rupatadine). Avoid. Moderate Study

▸ Antimalarials (mefloquine) are predicted to increase the risk of bradycardia when given with **calcium channel blockers**. Severe Theoretical

▸ Calcium channel blockers (diltiazem, verapamil) are predicted to increase the exposure to antipsychotics, second generation (cariprazine). Avoid. Severe Study → Also see **TABLE 7** p. 1572

▸ Calcium channel blockers (diltiazem, verapamil) are predicted to increase the exposure to antipsychotics, second generation (lurasidone). Adjust **lurasidone** dose. Moderate Study → Also see **TABLE 7** p. 1572

▸ Calcium channel blockers (diltiazem, verapamil) are predicted to increase the exposure to antipsychotics, second generation (quetiapine). Avoid. Moderate Study → Also see **TABLE 7** p. 1572

▸ Calcium channel blockers (diltiazem, verapamil) are predicted to increase the exposure to avapritinib. Avoid or adjust dose—consult product literature. Moderate Study

▸ Calcium channel blockers (diltiazem, verapamil) are predicted to increase the exposure to axitinib. Moderate Study

▸ Calcium channel blockers (diltiazem, verapamil) might increase the exposure to bedaquiline. Mild Theoretical

▸ Calcium channel blockers (diltiazem, verapamil) are predicted to increase the exposure to benzodiazepines (alprazolam). Severe Study

▸ Calcium channel blockers (diltiazem, verapamil) are predicted to increase the exposure to benzodiazepines (midazolam). Monitor adverse effects and adjust dose. Severe Study

▸ Berotralstat is predicted to increase the exposure to calcium channel blockers (amlodipine, felodipine, lacidipine, lercanidipine, nicardipine, nifedipine, nimodipine). Monitor and adjust dose. Moderate Study

▸ **Diltiazem** is predicted to increase the risk of cardiodepression when given with beta blockers, non-selective. Severe Study → Also see **TABLE 5** p. 1572 → Also see **TABLE 7** p. 1572

▸ **Verapamil** increases the risk of cardiovascular adverse effects when given with beta blockers, non-selective. Avoid intravenous verapamil, p. 191. Severe Study → Also see **TABLE 5** p. 1572 → Also see **TABLE 7** p. 1572

▸ **Diltiazem** is predicted to increase the risk of cardiodepression when given with beta blockers, selective. Avoid or monitor. Severe Study → Also see **TABLE 5** p. 1572 → Also see **TABLE 7** p. 1572

▸ **Verapamil** increases the risk of cardiovascular adverse effects when given with beta blockers, selective. Use with caution or avoid. Severe Study → Also see **TABLE 5** p. 1572 → Also see **TABLE 7** p. 1572

▸ **Verapamil** is predicted to increase the exposure to bictegravir. Use with caution or avoid. Moderate Theoretical

▸ Calcium channel blockers (diltiazem, verapamil) are predicted to increase the exposure to bosutinib. Avoid or adjust dose. Severe Study

▸ Calcium channel blockers (diltiazem, verapamil) are predicted to increase the exposure to brigatinib. Moderate Study → Also see **TABLE 5** p. 1572

▸ Calcium channel blockers (diltiazem, verapamil) are predicted to increase the exposure to buspirone. Use with caution and adjust dose. Moderate Study

▸ Calcium channel blockers (diltiazem, verapamil) are predicted to increase the exposure to cabozantinib. Moderate Study

▸ Calcium channel blockers (diltiazem) are predicted to increase the exposure to calcium channel blockers (amlodipine). Monitor and adjust dose. Moderate Study → Also see **TABLE 7** p. 1572

▸ Calcium channel blockers (verapamil) are predicted to increase the exposure to calcium channel blockers (amlodipine, felodipine, lacidipine, lercanidipine, nicardipine, nifedipine,

nimodipine). Monitor and adjust dose. Moderate Study → Also see TABLE 7 p. 1572
- Calcium channel blockers (diltiazem) are predicted to increase the exposure to calcium channel blockers (felodipine, lacidipine, lercanidipine, nicardipine, nifedipine, nimodipine). Monitor and adjust dose. Moderate Study → Also see TABLE 7 p. 1572
- Calcium channel blockers (diltiazem, verapamil) are predicted to increase the exposure to capivasertib. Adjust dose. Moderate Study
- Cenobamate is predicted to decrease the exposure to calcium channel blockers (amlodipine, felodipine, lacidipine, lercanidipine, nicardipine, nifedipine, nimodipine). Monitor and adjust dose. Moderate Theoretical
- Cenobamate is predicted to decrease the exposure to calcium channel blockers (diltiazem, verapamil). Moderate Theoretical
- Calcium channel blockers (diltiazem, verapamil) are predicted to increase the exposure to ceritinib. Moderate Study → Also see TABLE 5 p. 1572
- Ceritinib is predicted to increase the exposure to calcium channel blockers (amlodipine, felodipine, lacidipine, nicardipine, nifedipine, nimodipine). Monitor and adjust dose. Moderate Study
- Ceritinib is predicted to increase the exposure to calcium channel blockers (diltiazem, verapamil). Severe Study → Also see TABLE 5 p. 1572
- Ceritinib is predicted to markedly increase the exposure to lercanidipine. Avoid. Severe Study
- Calcium channel blockers (diltiazem, verapamil) are predicted to increase the concentration of ciclosporin. Severe Study
- Ciclosporin moderately increases the exposure to lercanidipine. Use with caution or avoid. Severe Study
- Nicardipine increases the concentration of ciclosporin. Severe Study
- Calcium channel blockers (nifedipine, nimodipine) might increase the exposure to cladribine. Avoid or adjust dose. Moderate Theoretical
- Cobicistat is predicted to increase the exposure to calcium channel blockers (amlodipine, felodipine, lacidipine, nicardipine, nifedipine, nimodipine). Monitor and adjust dose. Moderate Study
- Cobicistat is predicted to increase the exposure to calcium channel blockers (diltiazem, verapamil). Severe Study
- Cobicistat is predicted to markedly increase the exposure to lercanidipine. Avoid. Severe Study
- Calcium channel blockers (diltiazem, verapamil) are predicted to increase the exposure to cobimetinib. Severe Study
- Calcium channel blockers (diltiazem, verapamil) are predicted to increase the exposure to colchicine. Adjust colchicine dose with moderate CYP3A4 inhibitors, p. 1279. Severe Study
- Calcium channel blockers (diltiazem, verapamil) are predicted to increase the exposure to corticosteroids (methylprednisolone). Monitor and adjust dose. Moderate Study
- Calcium channel blockers (diltiazem, verapamil) are predicted to increase the exposure to crizotinib. Avoid. Moderate Study → Also see TABLE 5 p. 1572
- Crizotinib is predicted to increase the exposure to calcium channel blockers (amlodipine, felodipine, lacidipine, lercanidipine, nicardipine, nifedipine, nimodipine). Monitor and adjust dose. Moderate Study
- Calcium channel blockers (diltiazem, verapamil) are predicted to increase the exposure to dabrafenib. Moderate Study
- Dabrafenib is predicted to decrease the exposure to calcium channel blockers (amlodipine, felodipine, lacidipine, lercanidipine, nicardipine, nifedipine, nimodipine). Monitor and adjust dose. Moderate Theoretical
- Dabrafenib is predicted to decrease the exposure to calcium channel blockers (diltiazem, verapamil). Moderate Theoretical
- Intravenous dantrolene potentially increases the risk of acute hyperkalaemia and cardiovascular collapse when given with calcium channel blockers (diltiazem, verapamil). Avoid. Severe Anecdotal
- Calcium channel blockers (diltiazem, verapamil) are predicted to increase the exposure to daridorexant. Adjust daridorexant dose, p. 554. Severe Study

- Diltiazem is predicted to increase the exposure to darifenacin. Moderate Study
- Verapamil is predicted to increase the exposure to darifenacin. Avoid. Moderate Study
- Calcium channel blockers (diltiazem, verapamil) are predicted to increase the exposure to dasatinib. Severe Study
- Calcium channel blockers (diltiazem, verapamil) are predicted to slightly increase the exposure to dienogest. Moderate Study
- Calcium channel blockers (diltiazem, verapamil) increase the concentration of digoxin. Monitor and adjust dose. Severe Study → Also see TABLE 5 p. 1572
- Calcium channel blockers (diltiazem, verapamil) are predicted to increase the exposure to dipeptidylpeptidase-4 inhibitors (saxagliptin). Mild Study
- Calcium channel blockers (diltiazem, verapamil) are predicted to increase the exposure to domperidone. Avoid. Severe Study
- Calcium channel blockers (diltiazem, verapamil) are predicted to increase the exposure to dopamine receptor agonists (bromocriptine). Severe Theoretical → Also see TABLE 7 p. 1572
- Calcium channel blockers (diltiazem, verapamil) are predicted to increase the concentration of dopamine receptor agonists (cabergoline). Moderate Anecdotal → Also see TABLE 7 p. 1572
- Calcium channel blockers (diltiazem, verapamil) are predicted to increase the exposure to drospirenone. Severe Study
- Calcium channel blockers (diltiazem, verapamil) are predicted to moderately increase the exposure to dutasteride. Mild Study
- Calcium channel blockers (diltiazem, verapamil) are predicted to increase the exposure to elacestrant. Avoid moderate CYP3A4 inhibitors or adjust elacestrant dose, p. 1084. Severe Theoretical
- Calcium channel blockers (diltiazem, verapamil) are predicted to increase the exposure to elexacaftor. Adjust ivacaftor with tezacaftor and elexacaftor p. 337 dose with moderate CYP3A4 inhibitors. Severe Theoretical
- Calcium channel blockers (diltiazem, verapamil) are predicted to increase the exposure to eliglustat. Avoid or adjust dose— consult product literature. Severe Study
- Calcium channel blockers (diltiazem, verapamil) are predicted to moderately increase the exposure to encorafenib. Moderate Study
- Encorafenib is predicted to decrease the exposure to calcium channel blockers (amlodipine, felodipine, lacidipine, lercanidipine, nicardipine, nifedipine, nimodipine). Monitor and adjust dose. Moderate Study
- Endothelin receptor antagonists (bosentan) are predicted to decrease the exposure to calcium channel blockers (amlodipine, felodipine, lacidipine, lercanidipine, nicardipine, nifedipine, nimodipine). Monitor and adjust dose. Moderate Theoretical
- Endothelin receptor antagonists (bosentan) are predicted to decrease the exposure to calcium channel blockers (diltiazem, verapamil). Moderate Theoretical
- Calcium channel blockers (diltiazem, verapamil) are predicted to increase the exposure to endothelin receptor antagonists (macitentan). Manufacturer advises caution depending on other drugs taken—consult product literature. Moderate Theoretical
- Calcium channel blockers (diltiazem, verapamil) are predicted to increase the exposure to entrectinib. Avoid or adjust dose with moderate CYP3A4 inhibitors—consult product literature. Severe Theoretical
- Calcium channel blockers (diltiazem, verapamil) are predicted to increase the risk of ergotism when given with ergometrine. Severe Theoretical
- Calcium channel blockers (diltiazem, verapamil) are predicted to increase the exposure to erlotinib. Moderate Study
- Calcium channel blockers (diltiazem, verapamil) are predicted to increase the exposure to etrasimod. Avoid in poor CYP2C9 metabolisers. Severe Theoretical → Also see TABLE 5 p. 1572
- Calcium channel blockers (diltiazem, verapamil) are predicted to increase the concentration of everolimus. Avoid or adjust dose. Moderate Study
- Verapamil is predicted to increase the exposure to factor XA inhibitors (apixaban). Moderate Theoretical
- Verapamil slightly increases the exposure to factor XA inhibitors (edoxaban). Severe Study

Calcium channel blockers (continued)

▶ Calcium channel blockers (**diltiazem, verapamil**) are predicted to increase the exposure to **fedratinib**. Monitor and adjust dose. Moderate Study

▶ **Fedratinib** is predicted to increase the exposure to calcium channel blockers (**amlodipine, felodipine, lacidipine, lercanidipine, nicardipine, nifedipine, nimodipine**). Monitor and adjust dose. Moderate Study

▶ Calcium channel blockers (**diltiazem, verapamil**) are predicted to increase the exposure to **fesoterodine**. Adjust **fesoterodine** dose with moderate CYP3A4 inhibitors in hepatic and renal impairment, p. 897. Mild Study

▶ **Verapamil** is predicted to increase the exposure to **fidaxomicin**. Avoid. Moderate Study

▶ **Diltiazem** is predicted to increase the exposure to **fostamatinib**. Monitor adverse effects and adjust dose. Moderate Theoretical

▶ Calcium channel blockers (**diltiazem, verapamil**) are predicted to increase the exposure to **gefitinib**. Moderate Study

▶ **Verapamil** is predicted to increase the exposure to **gilteritinib**. Moderate Theoretical

▶ **Grapefruit** juice very slightly increases the exposure to **amlodipine**. Avoid. Mild Study

▶ **Grapefruit** juice increases the exposure to calcium channel blockers (**nifedipine, verapamil**). Avoid. Mild Study

▶ **Grapefruit** juice increases the exposure to **felodipine**. Avoid. Moderate Study

▶ **Grapefruit** juice is predicted to increase the exposure to **lercanidipine**. Avoid. Moderate Theoretical

▶ **Grapefruit** juice increases the exposure to **nicardipine**. Mild Study

▶ **Grazoprevir** is predicted to increase the concentration of **calcium channel blockers**. Moderate Theoretical

▶ Calcium channel blockers (**diltiazem, verapamil**) are predicted to increase the concentration of **guanfacine**. Adjust **guanfacine** dose, p. 407. Moderate Theoretical → Also see **TABLE 7** p. 1572

▶ H₂ receptor antagonists (**cimetidine**) (high-dose) are predicted to increase the exposure to **lercanidipine**. Moderate Theoretical

▶ H₂ receptor antagonists (**cimetidine**) moderately increase the exposure to **nifedipine**. Monitor and adjust dose. Severe Study

▶ H₂ receptor antagonists (**cimetidine**) increase the exposure to **verapamil**. Moderate Study

▶ H₂ receptor antagonists (**cimetidine**) slightly increase the exposure to calcium channel blockers (**diltiazem, nimodipine**). Monitor and adjust dose. Moderate Study

▶ **HIV-protease inhibitors** are predicted to increase the exposure to calcium channel blockers (**amlodipine, felodipine, lacidipine, nicardipine, nifedipine, nimodipine**). Monitor and adjust dose. Moderate Study

▶ **HIV-protease inhibitors** are predicted to increase the exposure to calcium channel blockers (**diltiazem, verapamil**). Severe Study

▶ **HIV-protease inhibitors** are predicted to markedly increase the exposure to **lercanidipine**. Avoid. Severe Study

▶ Calcium channel blockers (**diltiazem, verapamil**) are predicted to increase the exposure to **ibrutinib**. Adjust dose with moderate CYP3A4 inhibitors—consult product literature. Severe Study

▶ **Idelalisib** is predicted to increase the exposure to calcium channel blockers (**amlodipine, felodipine, lacidipine, nicardipine, nifedipine, nimodipine**). Monitor and adjust dose. Moderate Study

▶ **Idelalisib** is predicted to increase the exposure to calcium channel blockers (**diltiazem, verapamil**). Severe Study

▶ **Idelalisib** is predicted to markedly increase the exposure to **lercanidipine**. Avoid. Severe Study

▶ Calcium channel blockers (**diltiazem, verapamil**) are predicted to increase the exposure to **imatinib**. Moderate Theoretical

▶ **Imatinib** is predicted to increase the exposure to calcium channel blockers (**amlodipine, felodipine, lacidipine, lercanidipine, nicardipine, nifedipine, nimodipine**). Monitor and adjust dose. Moderate Study

▶ Calcium channel blockers (**diltiazem, verapamil**) are predicted to increase the exposure to **ivabradine**. Avoid. Moderate Study → Also see **TABLE 5** p. 1572

▶ Calcium channel blockers (**diltiazem, verapamil**) are predicted to increase the exposure to **ivacaftor**. Adjust dose with moderate CYP3A4 inhibitors, see ivacaftor p. 336, tezacaftor with

ivacaftor p. 339, and ivacaftor with tezacaftor and elexacaftor p. 337. Moderate Study

▶ Calcium channel blockers (**diltiazem, verapamil**) are predicted to increase the exposure to **ivosidenib**. Monitor and adjust dose—consult product literature. Severe Study

▶ **Ivosidenib** is predicted to decrease the exposure to calcium channel blockers (**amlodipine, felodipine, lacidipine, lercanidipine, nicardipine, nifedipine, nimodipine**). Monitor and adjust dose. Moderate Study

▶ Calcium channel blockers (**diltiazem, verapamil**) are predicted to increase the exposure to **lapatinib**. Moderate Study

▶ Calcium channel blockers (**diltiazem, verapamil**) are predicted to increase the exposure to **larotrectinib**. Monitor and adjust dose. Moderate Theoretical

▶ Calcium channel blockers (**diltiazem, verapamil**) are predicted to increase the exposure to **leniolisib**. Avoid. Moderate Study

▶ **Letermovir** is predicted to increase the exposure to calcium channel blockers (**amlodipine, felodipine, lacidipine, lercanidipine, nicardipine, nifedipine, nimodipine**). Monitor and adjust dose. Moderate Study

▶ Calcium channel blockers (**diltiazem, verapamil**) are predicted to increase the risk of neurotoxicity when given with **lithium**. Severe Anecdotal

▶ Calcium channel blockers (**amlodipine, lacidipine**) are predicted to increase the exposure to **lomitapide**. Separate administration by 12 hours. Moderate Theoretical

▶ Calcium channel blockers (**diltiazem, verapamil**) are predicted to increase the exposure to **lomitapide**. Avoid. Moderate Theoretical

▶ **Lorlatinib** is predicted to decrease the exposure to calcium channel blockers (**amlodipine, felodipine, lacidipine, lercanidipine, nicardipine, nifedipine, nimodipine**). Monitor and adjust dose. Moderate Theoretical

▶ **Lorlatinib** is predicted to decrease the exposure to calcium channel blockers (**diltiazem, verapamil**). Moderate Theoretical

▶ **Lumacaftor** is predicted to decrease the exposure to calcium channel blockers (**amlodipine, felodipine, lacidipine, lercanidipine, nicardipine, nifedipine, nimodipine**). Monitor and adjust dose. Moderate Study

▶ Macrolides (**clarithromycin**) are predicted to markedly increase the exposure to **lercanidipine**. Avoid. Severe Study

▶ Macrolides (**erythromycin**) are predicted to increase the exposure to **diltiazem**. Severe Theoretical

▶ Macrolides (**erythromycin**) are predicted to increase the exposure to **verapamil**. Severe Study

▶ Macrolides (**erythromycin**) are predicted to increase the exposure to calcium channel blockers (**amlodipine, felodipine, lacidipine, lercanidipine, nicardipine, nifedipine, nimodipine**). Monitor and adjust dose. Moderate Study

▶ Macrolides (**clarithromycin**) are predicted to increase the exposure to calcium channel blockers (**amlodipine, felodipine, lacidipine, nicardipine, nifedipine, nimodipine**). Monitor and adjust dose. Moderate Study

▶ Macrolides (**clarithromycin**) are predicted to increase the exposure to calcium channel blockers (**diltiazem, verapamil**). Severe Study

▶ Intravenous **magnesium** potentially increases the risk of hypotension when given with calcium channel blockers (**amlodipine, felodipine, lacidipine, lercanidipine, nicardipine, nifedipine, nimodipine, verapamil**) in pregnant women. Severe Anecdotal

▶ Calcium channel blockers (**diltiazem, verapamil**) are predicted to increase the exposure to **mavacamten**. Adjust dose—consult product literature. Moderate Study

▶ **Mexiletine** increases the risk of cardiovascular adverse effects when given with **diltiazem**. Avoid or monitor. Severe Theoretical

▶ **Mexiletine** potentially increases the risk of cardiovascular adverse effects when given with **verapamil**. Avoid or monitor. Severe Theoretical

▶ Calcium channel blockers (**diltiazem, verapamil**) are predicted to increase the exposure to **midostaurin**. Moderate Theoretical

▶ Calcium channel blockers (**diltiazem, verapamil**) are predicted to increase the exposure to **mineralocorticoid receptor antagonists (eplerenone)**. Adjust **eplerenone** dose, p. 223. Severe Study → Also see **TABLE 7** p. 1572

▶ Calcium channel blockers **(diltiazem, verapamil)** are predicted to increase the exposure to mineralocorticoid receptor antagonists **(finerenone)**. Severe Study → Also see **TABLE 7** p. 1572

▶ **Mitotane** is predicted to decrease the exposure to calcium channel blockers **(amlodipine, felodipine, lacidipine, lercanidipine, nicardipine, nifedipine, nimodipine)**. Monitor and adjust dose. Moderate Study

▶ **Mitotane** is predicted to decrease the exposure to **diltiazem**. Severe Study

▶ Calcium channel blockers **(diltiazem, verapamil)** are predicted to increase the exposure to mobocertinib. Avoid or adjust dose and monitor ECG—consult product literature. Severe Study

▶ Monoclonal antibodies **(tocilizumab)** are predicted to decrease the exposure to **calcium channel blockers**. Monitor and adjust dose. Moderate Theoretical

▶ **Verapamil** increases the risk of neutropenia when given with monoclonal antibodies **(brentuximab vedotin)**. Monitor and adjust dose. Severe Theoretical

▶ Calcium channel blockers **(diltiazem, verapamil)** are predicted to increase the exposure to naldemedine. Moderate Study

▶ Calcium channel blockers **(diltiazem, verapamil)** are predicted to increase the exposure to naloxegol. Adjust **naloxegol** dose and monitor adverse effects, p. 72. Moderate Study

▶ Calcium channel blockers **(diltiazem, verapamil)** are predicted to increase the exposure to neratinib. Avoid moderate CYP3A4 inhibitors or adjust dose and monitor for gastrointestinal adverse effects—consult product literature. Severe Study

▶ Neurokinin-1 receptor antagonists **(aprepitant, netupitant)** are predicted to increase the exposure to calcium channel blockers **(amlodipine, felodipine, lacidipine, lercanidipine, nicardipine, nifedipine, nimodipine)**. Monitor and adjust dose. Moderate Study

▶ Calcium channel blockers **(diltiazem, verapamil)** are predicted to increase the exposure to neurokinin-1 receptor antagonists **(aprepitant)** and neurokinin-1 receptor antagonists **(aprepitant)** are predicted to increase the exposure to calcium channel blockers **(diltiazem, verapamil)**. Moderate Study

▶ Calcium channel blockers **(diltiazem, verapamil)** are predicted to increase the exposure to nilotinib. Moderate Theoretical

▶ **Nilotinib** is predicted to increase the exposure to calcium channel blockers **(amlodipine, felodipine, lacidipine, lercanidipine, nicardipine, nifedipine, nimodipine)**. Monitor and adjust dose. Moderate Study

▶ **Verapamil** is predicted to increase the exposure to nintedanib. Moderate Study

▶ **Nirmatrelvir** boosted with ritonavir is predicted to increase the concentration of **calcium channel blockers**. Severe Theoretical

▶ NNRTIs **(efavirenz, etravirine, nevirapine)** are predicted to decrease the exposure to calcium channel blockers **(amlodipine, felodipine, lacidipine, lercanidipine, nicardipine, nifedipine, nimodipine)**. Monitor and adjust dose. Moderate Theoretical

▶ NNRTIs **(efavirenz, etravirine, nevirapine)** are predicted to decrease the exposure to calcium channel blockers **(diltiazem, verapamil)**. Moderate Theoretical

▶ Calcium channel blockers **(diltiazem, verapamil)** are predicted to increase the exposure to olaparib. Avoid or adjust dose with moderate CYP3A4 inhibitors—consult product literature. Moderate Theoretical

▶ Calcium channel blockers **(diltiazem, verapamil)** are predicted to increase the exposure to opioids **(alfentanil, buprenorphine, fentanyl, oxycodone)**. Monitor and adjust dose. Moderate Study → Also see **TABLE 5** p. 1572

▶ **Nicardipine** is predicted to increase the exposure to opioids **(fentanyl)**. Monitor and adjust dose. Moderate Theoretical

▶ Calcium channel blockers **(diltiazem, verapamil)** are predicted to increase the exposure to opioids **(methadone, sufentanil)**. Moderate Theoretical → Also see **TABLE 5** p. 1572

▶ **Verapamil** is predicted to increase the exposure to panobinostat. Adjust dose. Moderate Theoretical

▶ Calcium channel blockers **(diltiazem, verapamil)** are predicted to increase the exposure to pazopanib. Moderate Study

▶ Calcium channel blockers **(diltiazem, verapamil)** are predicted to increase the exposure to pemigatinib. Severe Study

▶ Calcium channel blockers **(diltiazem, verapamil)** are predicted to increase the exposure to phosphodiesterase type-5 inhibitors **(avanafil)**. Adjust **avanafil** dose, p. 939. Moderate Theoretical → Also see **TABLE 7** p. 1572

▶ Calcium channel blockers **(diltiazem, verapamil)** are predicted to increase the exposure to phosphodiesterase type-5 inhibitors **(sildenafil)**. Monitor or adjust **sildenafil** dose with moderate CYP3A4 inhibitors, p. 940. Moderate Study → Also see **TABLE 7** p. 1572

▶ Calcium channel blockers **(diltiazem, verapamil)** are predicted to increase the exposure to phosphodiesterase type-5 inhibitors **(tadalafil)**. Severe Theoretical → Also see **TABLE 7** p. 1572

▶ Calcium channel blockers **(diltiazem, verapamil)** are predicted to increase the exposure to phosphodiesterase type-5 inhibitors **(vardenafil)**. Adjust dose. Severe Theoretical → Also see **TABLE 7** p. 1572

▶ **Verapamil** is predicted to increase the exposure to pibrentasvir. Moderate Theoretical

▶ Calcium channel blockers **(diltiazem, verapamil)** are predicted to increase the exposure to pimozide. Avoid. Severe Theoretical → Also see **TABLE 7** p. 1572

▶ Calcium channel blockers **(diltiazem, verapamil)** are predicted to increase the exposure to ponatinib. Moderate Study

▶ Calcium channel blockers **(diltiazem, verapamil)** are predicted to increase the exposure to pralsetinib. Moderate Theoretical

▶ Calcium channel blockers **(diltiazem, verapamil)** are predicted to increase the exposure to ranolazine. Severe Study

▶ Calcium channel blockers **(diltiazem, verapamil)** are predicted to increase the exposure to regorafenib. Moderate Study

▶ **Verapamil** is predicted to increase the exposure to relugolix. Avoid or take relugolix first and separate administration by at least 6 hours. Moderate Study

▶ Calcium channel blockers **(diltiazem, verapamil)** are predicted to increase the exposure to ribociclib. Moderate Study

▶ Rifamycins **(rifampicin)** greatly decrease the exposure to **nifedipine**. Avoid. Severe Study

▶ Rifamycins **(rifampicin)** are predicted to decrease the exposure to calcium channel blockers **(amlodipine, felodipine, lacidipine, lercanidipine, nicardipine, nimodipine)**. Monitor and adjust dose. Moderate Study

▶ Rifamycins **(rifampicin)** greatly decrease the exposure to calcium channel blockers **(diltiazem, verapamil)**. Severe Study

▶ Calcium channel blockers **(diltiazem, verapamil)** are predicted to increase the exposure to rimegepant. Avoid another dose of rimegepant within 48 hours of concurrent use. Moderate Study

▶ Calcium channel blockers **(diltiazem, verapamil)** are predicted to increase the exposure to ruxolitinib. Moderate Study

▶ Calcium channel blockers **(diltiazem, verapamil)** are predicted to increase the exposure to selpercatinib. Moderate Study

▶ Calcium channel blockers **(diltiazem, verapamil)** are predicted to increase the exposure to selumetinib. Avoid or adjust dose—consult product literature. Severe Study

▶ Calcium channel blockers **(diltiazem, verapamil)** are predicted to increase the exposure to siponimod. Avoid depending on other drugs taken—consult product literature. Severe Study → Also see **TABLE 5** p. 1572

▶ Calcium channel blockers **(diltiazem, verapamil)** increase the concentration of sirolimus. Monitor and adjust dose. Moderate Study

▶ **Sotorasib** is predicted to decrease the exposure to calcium channel blockers **(amlodipine, felodipine, lacidipine, lercanidipine, nicardipine, nifedipine, nimodipine)**. Monitor and adjust dose. Moderate Theoretical

▶ **Sotorasib** is predicted to decrease the exposure to calcium channel blockers **(diltiazem, verapamil)**. Moderate Theoretical

▶ Calcium channel blockers **(diltiazem, verapamil)** are predicted to increase the exposure to SSRIs **(dapoxetine)**. Adjust **dapoxetine** dose with moderate CYP3A4 inhibitors, p. 947. Moderate Theoretical

▶ **St John's wort** is predicted to decrease the exposure to calcium channel blockers **(amlodipine, felodipine, lacidipine, lercanidipine, nicardipine, nifedipine, nimodipine)**. Monitor and adjust dose. Moderate Theoretical

▶ **St John's wort** is predicted to decrease the exposure to calcium channel blockers **(diltiazem, verapamil)**. Moderate Theoretical

▶ **Diltiazem** slightly increases the exposure to statins **(atorvastatin)**. Monitor and adjust dose. Severe Study

Calcium channel blockers (continued)

▶ **Verapamil** is predicted to slightly to moderately increase the exposure to statins (atorvastatin). Monitor and adjust dose. Severe Theoretical

▶ **Amlodipine** causes a small increase in the exposure to statins (simvastatin). Adjust **simvastatin** dose, p. 237. Moderate Study

▶ Calcium channel blockers (diltiazem, verapamil) moderately increase the exposure to statins (simvastatin). Monitor and adjust dose. Severe Study

▶ Calcium channel blockers (diltiazem, verapamil) are predicted to increase the exposure to sunitinib. Moderate Study

▶ Calcium channel blockers (diltiazem, verapamil) are predicted to increase the concentration of tacrolimus. Severe Study

▶ **Nicardipine** potentially increases the concentration of tacrolimus. Monitor concentration and adjust dose. Severe Anecdotal

▶ Calcium channel blockers (diltiazem, felodipine) very slightly increase the exposure to talazoparib. Moderate Study

▶ **Verapamil** is predicted to slightly increase the exposure to talazoparib. Avoid or adjust dose—consult product literature. Severe Study

▶ Calcium channel blockers (diltiazem, verapamil) are predicted to increase the exposure to taxanes (cabazitaxel). Moderate Theoretical

▶ Calcium channel blockers (diltiazem, verapamil) are predicted to increase the exposure to taxanes (docetaxel). Severe Study

▶ Calcium channel blockers (diltiazem, verapamil) are predicted to increase the exposure to taxanes (paclitaxel). Moderate Anecdotal

▶ Calcium channel blockers (diltiazem, verapamil) are predicted to increase the concentration of and the risk of angioedema when given with temsirolimus. Use with caution or avoid. Moderate Theoretical

▶ **Temsirolimus** is predicted to increase the risk of angioedema when given with calcium channel blockers (amlodipine, felodipine, lacidipine, lercanidipine, nicardipine, nifedipine, nimodipine). Moderate Theoretical

▶ Calcium channel blockers (diltiazem, verapamil) are predicted to increase the exposure to tezacaftor. Adjust dose with moderate CYP3A4 inhibitors, see tezacaftor with ivacaftor p. 339 and ivacaftor with tezacaftor and elexacaftor p. 337. Severe Study

▶ **Verapamil** increases the exposure to thrombin inhibitors (dabigatran). Monitor and adjust dose. Severe Study

▶ **Verapamil** might increase the exposure to tigecycline. Mild Anecdotal

▶ Calcium channel blockers (diltiazem, verapamil) given with a potent CYP2C19 inhibitor are predicted to increase the exposure to tofacitinib. Adjust **tofacitinib** dose, p. 1265. Moderate Study

▶ Calcium channel blockers (diltiazem, verapamil) are predicted to increase the exposure to tolvaptan. Manufacturer advises caution or adjust **tolvaptan** dose with moderate CYP3A4 inhibitors, p. 767. Moderate Study

▶ **Verapamil** is predicted to increase the exposure to topotecan. Severe Study

▶ **Verapamil** is predicted to increase the concentration of trametinib. Moderate Theoretical

▶ Calcium channel blockers (diltiazem, verapamil) are predicted to increase the exposure to trazodone. Moderate Theoretical

▶ **Tucatinib** is predicted to increase the exposure to calcium channel blockers (amlodipine, felodipine, lacidipine, nicardipine, nifedipine, nimodipine). Monitor and adjust dose. Moderate Study

▶ **Tucatinib** is predicted to increase the exposure to calcium channel blockers (diltiazem, verapamil). Severe Study

▶ **Tucatinib** is predicted to markedly increase the exposure to lercanidipine. Avoid. Severe Study

▶ Calcium channel blockers (diltiazem, verapamil) are predicted to increase the exposure to ulipristal. Avoid if used for uterine fibroids. Moderate Study

▶ Calcium channel blockers (diltiazem, verapamil) are predicted to increase the exposure to vemurafenib. Severe Theoretical

▶ Calcium channel blockers (diltiazem, verapamil) are predicted to increase the exposure to venetoclax. Avoid or adjust dose—consult product literature. Severe Study

▶ Calcium channel blockers (diltiazem, verapamil) are predicted to increase the exposure to vinca alkaloids. Severe Theoretical

▶ Calcium channel blockers (diltiazem, verapamil) are predicted to increase the exposure to voclosporin. Adjust **voclosporin** dose, p. 973. Severe Study

▶ Calcium channel blockers (diltiazem, verapamil) are predicted to increase the exposure to zanubrutinib. Avoid or adjust dose with moderate CYP3A4 inhibitors—consult product literature. Severe Study

▶ Calcium channel blockers (diltiazem, verapamil) are predicted to increase the exposure to zopiclone. Adjust dose. Moderate Study

Calcium chloride → see calcium salts

Calcium gluconate → see calcium salts

Calcium lactate → see calcium salts

Calcium phosphate → see calcium salts

Calcium salts

calcium acetate · calcium carbonate · calcium chloride · calcium gluconate · calcium lactate · calcium phosphate

SEPARATION OF ADMINISTRATION **Calcium carbonate-containing antacids** should preferably not be taken at the same time as other drugs since they might impair absorption. **Antacids** might damage enteric coatings designed to prevent dissolution in the stomach.

▶ Oral **calcium salts** decrease the absorption of oral alkylating agents (estramustine). Severe Study

▶ Oral **calcium carbonate** might decreases the absorption of oral antimalarials (chloroquine). Separate administration by at least 4 hours. Moderate Study

▶ Oral **calcium salts** might decrease the concentration of the active metabolite of oral baloxavir marboxil. Avoid. Severe Theoretical

▶ **Calcium carbonate** -containing antacids is predicted to decrease the exposure to belumosudil. Separate administration by 12 hours. Moderate Theoretical

▶ Oral **calcium salts** decrease the absorption of oral bisphosphonates (alendronate). **Alendronate** should be taken at least 30 minutes before calcium. Moderate Study

▶ Oral **calcium salts** decrease the absorption of oral bisphosphonates (clodronate). Avoid **calcium salts** for 2 hours before or 1 hour after clodronate. Moderate Study

▶ Oral **calcium salts** are predicted to decrease the absorption of oral bisphosphonates (ibandronate). Avoid **calcium salts** for at least 6 hours before or 1 hour after ibandronate. Moderate Theoretical

▶ Oral **calcium salts** decrease the absorption of oral bisphosphonates (risedronate). Separate administration by at least 2 hours. Moderate Study

▶ Oral **calcium carbonate**-containing antacids are predicted to decrease the absorption of oral bosutinib. Manufacturer advises take at least 12 hours before antacids. Moderate Theoretical

▶ Intravenous cephalosporins (ceftriaxone) increase the risk of cardio-respiratory arrest when given with intravenous **calcium salts**. Avoid. Severe Anecdotal

▶ Oral **calcium carbonate** -containing antacids are predicted to decrease the exposure to oral dasatinib. Separate administration by at least 2 hours. Moderate Study

▶ Intravenous **calcium salts** increase the effects of digoxin. Avoid. Moderate Anecdotal

▶ Oral **calcium salts** decrease the absorption of oral dolutegravir. **Dolutegravir** should be taken 2 hours before or 6 hours after calcium. Moderate Study

▶ Oral **calcium salts** decrease the absorption of oral eltrombopag. **Eltrombopag** should be taken 2 hours before or 4 hours after calcium. Severe Study

▶ Oral **calcium carbonate**-containing antacids are predicted to decrease the absorption of oral erlotinib. Manufacturer advises take 2 hours before or 4 hours after antacids. Moderate Theoretical

▶ Oral **calcium carbonate** -containing antacids are predicted to decrease the exposure to oral gefitinib. Moderate Theoretical

▶ Oral **calcium carbonate** might decreases the absorption of oral hydroxychloroquine. Moderate Theoretical

► Oral **calcium carbonate** decreases the absorption of oral iron. **Calcium carbonate** should be taken 1 hour before or 2 hours after iron. Moderate Study

► Oral **calcium carbonate**-containing antacids are predicted to decrease the absorption of oral lapatinib. Avoid. Moderate Theoretical

► Oral **calcium carbonate** -containing antacids are predicted to decrease the exposure to oral ledipasvir. Separate administration by 4 hours. Moderate Theoretical

► Oral **calcium carbonate** -containing antacids are predicted to decrease the exposure to oral neratinib. Separate administration by at least 3 hours. Mild Theoretical

► Oral **calcium carbonate** -containing antacids might affect the exposure to oral nilotinib. Separate administration by at least 2 hours. Moderate Study

► Oral **calcium carbonate** -containing antacids are predicted to decrease the exposure to oral NNRTIs (rilpivirine). Manufacturer advises take 4 hours before or 2 hours after antacids. Severe Theoretical

► Oral **calcium carbonate** -containing antacids might decrease the absorption of oral pazopanib. Manufacturer advises take 1 hour before or 2 hours after antacids. Moderate Theoretical

► Oral **calcium salts** decrease the absorption of oral quinolones (ciprofloxacin). Separate administration by 2 hours. Moderate Study

► Oral **calcium carbonate** -containing antacids greatly decrease the exposure to oral raltegravir (high-dose). Avoid. Severe Study

► Oral **calcium salts** minimally decrease the exposure to oral roxadustat. **Roxadustat** should be taken at least 1 hour after calcium. Moderate Study

► Oral **calcium carbonate** is predicted to decrease the exposure to oral sotorasib. Manufacturer advises take 4 hours before or 10 hours after antacids. Moderate Theoretical

► Oral **calcium salts** decrease the absorption of oral strontium. Separate administration by 2 hours. Moderate Study

► Oral **calcium salts** are predicted to decrease the absorption of oral tetracyclines. Separate administration by 2 to 3 hours. Moderate Theoretical

► Thiazide diuretics increase the risk of hypercalcaemia when given with **calcium salts**. Severe Anecdotal

► Oral **calcium salts** are predicted to decrease the absorption of oral thyroid hormones (levothyroxine). Separate administration by at least 4 hours. Moderate Anecdotal

► **Calcium carbonate** -containing antacids might decrease the efficacy of ulipristal for emergency hormonal contraception. For FSRH guidance, see Contraceptives, interactions p. 917. Unknown Theoretical

► Oral **calcium acetate** decreases the exposure to oral vadadustat. Manufacturer advises take 1 hour before or 2 hours after **calcium acetate**. Moderate Study

► Oral **calcium carbonate** is predicted to decrease the exposure to oral vadadustat. Manufacturer advises take 1 hour before or 2 hours after **calcium carbonate**. Moderate Theoretical

► Oral **calcium carbonate**-containing antacids are predicted to decrease the concentration of oral velpatasvir. Separate administration by 4 hours. Moderate Theoretical

► Oral **calcium salts** decrease the absorption of oral zinc. Moderate Study

Canagliflozin → see sodium glucose co-transporter 2 inhibitors

Canakinumab → see monoclonal antibodies

Candesartan → see angiotensin-II receptor antagonists

Cangrelor → see TABLE 4 p. 1571 (antiplatelet effects)

► Selumetinib might increase the risk of bleeding when given with **cangrelor**. Severe Theoretical

Cannabidiol → see TABLE 10 p. 1574 (CNS effects)

► Anti-androgens (apalutamide, enzalutamide) are predicted to decrease the exposure to **cannabidiol**. Adjust dose. Moderate Study

► Antiepileptics (carbamazepine, fosphenytoin, phenobarbital, phenytoin, primidone) are predicted to decrease the exposure to **cannabidiol**. Adjust dose. Moderate Study → Also see TABLE 10 p. 1574

► **Cannabidiol** increases the risk of increased ALT concentrations when given with antiepileptics (valproate). Avoid or adjust dose. Severe Study

► Antifungals, azoles (fluconazole) are predicted to increase the exposure to **cannabidiol**. Moderate Theoretical

► Antifungals, azoles (itraconazole, ketoconazole, posaconazole, voriconazole) are predicted to increase the exposure to **cannabidiol**. Avoid or adjust dose. Mild Study

► **Cannabidiol** increases the exposure to the active metabolite of benzodiazepines (clobazam) and benzodiazepines (clobazam) increase the exposure to the active metabolite of **cannabidiol**. Adjust dose. Moderate Study → Also see TABLE 10 p. 1574

► Ceritinib is predicted to increase the exposure to **cannabidiol**. Avoid or adjust dose. Mild Study

► **Cannabidiol** is predicted to increase the concentration of ciclosporin. Monitor and adjust dose. Severe Theoretical

► Cobicistat is predicted to increase the exposure to **cannabidiol**. Avoid or adjust dose. Mild Study

► **Cannabidiol** is predicted to increase the exposure to digoxin. Monitor and adjust dose. Moderate Study

► Encorafenib is predicted to decrease the exposure to **cannabidiol**. Adjust dose. Moderate Study

► **Cannabidiol** moderately increases the exposure to everolimus. Monitor and adjust dose. Moderate Study

► HIV-protease inhibitors are predicted to increase the exposure to **cannabidiol**. Avoid or adjust dose. Mild Study

► Idelalisib is predicted to increase the exposure to **cannabidiol**. Avoid or adjust dose. Mild Study

► Ivosidenib is predicted to decrease the exposure to **cannabidiol**. Adjust dose. Moderate Study

► Lumacaftor is predicted to decrease the exposure to **cannabidiol**. Adjust dose. Moderate Study

► Macrolides (clarithromycin) are predicted to increase the exposure to **cannabidiol**. Avoid or adjust dose. Mild Study

► Mitotane is predicted to decrease the exposure to **cannabidiol**. Adjust dose. Moderate Study

► Moclobemide is predicted to increase the exposure to **cannabidiol**. Moderate Theoretical

► Proton pump inhibitors (esomeprazole) are predicted to increase the exposure to **cannabidiol**. Moderate Theoretical

► Rifamycins (rifampicin) are predicted to decrease the exposure to **cannabidiol**. Adjust dose. Moderate Study

► **Cannabidiol** is predicted to increase the exposure to sirolimus. Monitor and adjust dose. Moderate Study

► SSRIs (fluoxetine, fluvoxamine) are predicted to increase the exposure to **cannabidiol**. Moderate Theoretical → Also see TABLE 10 p. 1574

► St John's wort is predicted to decrease the exposure to **cannabidiol**. Adjust dose. Mild Study

► **Cannabidiol** is predicted to increase the concentration of tacrolimus. Monitor and adjust dose. Moderate Theoretical

► **Cannabidiol** is predicted to increase the exposure to talazoparib. Monitor and adjust dose. Moderate Study

► **Cannabidiol** is predicted to increase the exposure to taxanes (paclitaxel). Monitor and adjust dose. Moderate Study

► Tucatinib is predicted to increase the exposure to **cannabidiol**. Avoid or adjust dose. Mild Study

Capecitabine → see TABLE 1 p. 1571 (hepatotoxicity), TABLE 14 p. 1575 (myelosuppression)

► Allopurinol is predicted to decrease the effects of **capecitabine**. Avoid. Severe Study

► **Capecitabine** increases the concentration of antiepileptics (fosphenytoin, phenytoin). Severe Anecdotal

► **Capecitabine** increases the effects of coumarins. Monitor INR and adjust dose. Moderate Anecdotal

► Folates are predicted to increase the risk of toxicity when given with **capecitabine**. Severe Anecdotal

► H₂ receptor antagonists (cimetidine) are predicted to slightly increase the exposure to **capecitabine**. Severe Theoretical

► Live vaccines are predicted to increase the risk of generalised infection (possibly life-threatening) when given with **capecitabine**. UKHSA advises avoid (refer to Green Book). Severe Theoretical

► Metronidazole is predicted to increase the risk of capecitabine toxicity when given with **capecitabine**. Severe Theoretical

Capivasertib

▸ Anti-androgens (apalutamide, enzalutamide) are predicted to decrease the exposure to **capivasertib**. Avoid. Moderate Study
▸ Antiarrhythmics (dronedarone) are predicted to increase the exposure to **capivasertib**. Adjust dose. Moderate Study
▸ Antiepileptics (carbamazepine, fosphenytoin, phenobarbital, phenytoin, primidone) are predicted to decrease the exposure to **capivasertib**. Avoid. Moderate Study
▸ Antifungals, azoles (fluconazole, isavuconazole, itraconazole, ketoconazole, posaconazole, voriconazole) are predicted to increase the exposure to **capivasertib**. Adjust dose. Moderate Study
▸ Berotralstat is predicted to increase the exposure to **capivasertib**. Adjust dose. Moderate Study
▸ Calcium channel blockers (diltiazem, verapamil) are predicted to increase the exposure to **capivasertib**. Adjust dose. Moderate Study
▸ Cenobamate is predicted to decrease the exposure to **capivasertib**. Avoid. Moderate Study
▸ Ceritinib is predicted to increase the exposure to capivasertib. Adjust dose. Moderate Study
▸ Ciclosporin is predicted to increase the exposure to **capivasertib**. Adjust dose. Moderate Theoretical
▸ Cobicistat is predicted to increase the exposure to **capivasertib**. Adjust dose. Moderate Study
▸ Crizotinib is predicted to increase the exposure to **capivasertib**. Adjust dose. Moderate Study
▸ Dabrafenib is predicted to decrease the exposure to **capivasertib**. Avoid. Moderate Study
▸ Encorafenib is predicted to decrease the exposure to **capivasertib**. Avoid. Moderate Study
▸ Endothelin receptor antagonists (bosentan) are predicted to decrease the exposure to **capivasertib**. Avoid. Moderate Study
▸ Fedratinib is predicted to increase the exposure to **capivasertib**. Adjust dose. Moderate Study
▸ Grapefruit and grapefruit juice is predicted to increase the exposure to **capivasertib**. Adjust dose. Moderate Theoretical
▸ HIV-protease inhibitors are predicted to increase the exposure to **capivasertib**. Adjust dose. Moderate Study
▸ Idelalisib is predicted to increase the exposure to **capivasertib**. Adjust dose. Moderate Study
▸ Imatinib is predicted to increase the exposure to **capivasertib**. Adjust dose. Moderate Study
▸ Ivosidenib is predicted to decrease the exposure to **capivasertib**. Avoid. Moderate Study
▸ Letermovir is predicted to increase the exposure to **capivasertib**. Adjust dose. Moderate Study
▸ Lorlatinib is predicted to decrease the exposure to **capivasertib**. Avoid. Moderate Study
▸ Lumacaftor is predicted to decrease the exposure to **capivasertib**. Avoid. Moderate Study
▸ Macrolides (clarithromycin, erythromycin) are predicted to increase the exposure to **capivasertib**. Adjust dose. Moderate Study
▸ Mifepristone is predicted to increase the exposure to **capivasertib**. Adjust dose. Moderate Theoretical
▸ Mitotane is predicted to decrease the exposure to **capivasertib**. Avoid. Moderate Study
▸ Modafinil is predicted to decrease the exposure to **capivasertib**. Avoid. Moderate Theoretical
▸ Neurokinin-1 receptor antagonists (aprepitant, netupitant) are predicted to increase the exposure to **capivasertib**. Adjust dose. Moderate Study
▸ Nilotinib is predicted to increase the exposure to **capivasertib**. Adjust dose. Moderate Study
▸ NNRTIs (efavirenz, etravirine, nevirapine) are predicted to decrease the exposure to **capivasertib**. Avoid. Moderate Study
▸ Quinolones (ciprofloxacin) are predicted to increase the exposure to **capivasertib**. Adjust dose. Moderate Theoretical
▸ Ribociclib is predicted to increase the exposure to **capivasertib**. Adjust dose. Moderate Theoretical
▸ Rifamycins (rifabutin) are predicted to decrease the exposure to **capivasertib**. Avoid. Moderate Theoretical
▸ Rifamycins (rifampicin) are predicted to decrease the exposure to **capivasertib**. Avoid. Moderate Study

▸ Sotorasib is predicted to decrease the exposure to **capivasertib**. Avoid. Moderate Study
▸ SSRIs (fluvoxamine) are predicted to increase the exposure to **capivasertib**. Adjust dose. Moderate Theoretical
▸ St John's wort is predicted to decrease the exposure to **capivasertib**. Avoid. Moderate Study
▸ Telotristat ethyl is predicted to decrease the exposure to **capivasertib**. Avoid. Moderate Theoretical
▸ Tucatinib is predicted to increase the exposure to **capivasertib**. Adjust dose. Moderate Study

Caplacizumab

▸ Drugs with anticoagulant effects (see TABLE 3 p. 1571) cause bleeding, as can **caplacizumab**; concurrent use might increase the risk of developing this effect. Severe Theoretical
▸ Drugs with antiplatelet effects (see TABLE 4 p. 1571) cause bleeding, as can **caplacizumab**; concurrent use might increase the risk of developing this effect. Severe Theoretical

Captopril → see ACE inhibitors
Carbamazepine → see antiepileptics
Carbapenems

ertapenem · imipenem · meropenem

▸ **Carbapenems** decrease the concentration of antiepileptics (valproate). Avoid. Severe Anecdotal
▸ Ganciclovir is predicted to increase the risk of seizures when given with **imipenem**. Avoid. Severe Anecdotal
▸ Valganciclovir is predicted to increase the risk of seizures when given with **imipenem**. Avoid. Severe Anecdotal

Carbidopa

▸ Oral iron is predicted to decrease the exposure to oral **carbidopa**. Moderate Theoretical

Carbimazole

▸ **Carbimazole** affects the concentration of digoxin. Monitor and adjust dose. Moderate Theoretical
▸ **Carbimazole** decreases the effects of metyrapone. Avoid. Moderate Theoretical
▸ **Carbimazole** given with a potent CYP3A4 inhibitor is predicted to increase the exposure to propiverine. Adjust starting dose. Moderate Theoretical

Carboplatin → see platinum compounds
Carfilzomib → see TABLE 14 p. 1575 (myelosuppression)
▸ **Carfilzomib** potentially decreases the efficacy of combined hormonal contraceptives. Use additional contraceptive precautions. Severe Theoretical

Cariprazine → see antipsychotics, second generation
Carmustine → see alkylating agents
Carvedilol → see beta blockers, non-selective
Caspofungin → see TABLE 1 p. 1571 (hepatotoxicity)
▸ Antiepileptics (carbamazepine, fosphenytoin, phenytoin) are predicted to decrease the concentration of **caspofungin**. Adjust **caspofungin** dose, p. 687. Moderate Theoretical
▸ Ciclosporin slightly increases the exposure to **caspofungin**. Severe Study
▸ Corticosteroids (dexamethasone) are predicted to decrease the concentration of **caspofungin**. Adjust **caspofungin** dose, p. 687. Moderate Theoretical
▸ NNRTIs (efavirenz) are predicted to decrease the concentration of **caspofungin**. Adjust dose. Moderate Study
▸ NNRTIs (nevirapine) are predicted to decrease the concentration of **caspofungin**. Adjust dose. Moderate Theoretical → Also see TABLE 1 p. 1571
▸ Rifamycins (rifampicin) decrease the concentration of **caspofungin**. Adjust **caspofungin** dose, p. 687. Moderate Study

Cedazuridine

▸ **Cedazuridine** is predicted to increase the exposure to azacitidine. Avoid. Moderate Theoretical
▸ **Cedazuridine** is predicted to increase the exposure to cytarabine. Avoid. Moderate Theoretical
▸ **Cedazuridine** is predicted to increase the exposure to gemcitabine. Avoid. Moderate Theoretical

Cefaclor → see cephalosporins
Cefadroxil → see cephalosporins
Cefalexin → see cephalosporins
Cefazolin → see cephalosporins
Cefepime → see cephalosporins
Cefiderocol → see cephalosporins

Cefixime → see cephalosporins
Cefotaxime → see cephalosporins
Cefoxitin → see cephalosporins
Cefradine → see cephalosporins
Ceftaroline → see cephalosporins
Ceftazidime → see cephalosporins
Ceftobiprole → see cephalosporins
Ceftolozane → see cephalosporins
Ceftriaxone → see cephalosporins
Cefuroxime → see cephalosporins
Celecoxib → see NSAIDs
Celiprolol → see beta blockers, selective
Cemiplimab → see monoclonal antibodies
Cenobamate → see TABLE 10 p. 1574 (CNS effects)

▶ **Cenobamate** is predicted to decrease the exposure to acalabrutinib. Adjust dose. Moderate Theoretical
▶ **Cenobamate** is predicted to decrease the exposure to anti-androgens (darolutamide). Avoid. Moderate Theoretical
▶ **Cenobamate** might increase the exposure to antiepileptics (fosphenytoin, primidone). Moderate Theoretical → Also see TABLE 10 p. 1574
▶ **Cenobamate** is predicted to decrease the concentration of antiepileptics (lamotrigine) and antiepileptics (lamotrigine) might affect the efficacy of **cenobamate**. Adjust dose. Moderate Study → Also see TABLE 10 p. 1574
▶ **Cenobamate** slightly increases the exposure to antiepileptics (phenobarbital, phenytoin). Monitor and adjust dose. Moderate Study → Also see TABLE 10 p. 1574
▶ **Cenobamate** is predicted to decrease the exposure to antifungals, azoles (isavuconazole). Avoid. Severe Theoretical
▶ **Cenobamate** is predicted to decrease the exposure to antipsychotics, second generation (cariprazine). Avoid. Severe Theoretical → Also see TABLE 10 p. 1574
▶ **Cenobamate** is predicted to decrease the exposure to antipsychotics, second generation (lurasidone). Monitor and adjust dose. Moderate Theoretical → Also see TABLE 10 p. 1574
▶ **Cenobamate** is predicted to decrease the exposure to antipsychotics, second generation (quetiapine). Moderate Study → Also see TABLE 10 p. 1574
▶ **Cenobamate** is predicted to decrease the exposure to atogepant. Adjust dose. Moderate Theoretical
▶ **Cenobamate** is predicted to decrease the exposure to avacopan. Severe Theoretical
▶ **Cenobamate** is predicted to decrease the exposure to avapritinib. Avoid. Severe Study
▶ **Cenobamate** is predicted to decrease the exposure to bedaquiline. Avoid. Severe Study
▶ **Cenobamate** is predicted to increase the exposure to belzutifan. Monitor and adjust dose. Severe Theoretical
▶ **Cenobamate** potentially increases the exposure to benzodiazepines (clobazam). Adjust dose. Moderate Theoretical → Also see TABLE 10 p. 1574
▶ **Cenobamate** moderately decreases the exposure to benzodiazepines (midazolam). Adjust dose. Moderate Study → Also see TABLE 10 p. 1574
▶ **Cenobamate** is predicted to decrease the exposure to beta₂ agonists (salmeterol). Adjust dose. Moderate Theoretical
▶ **Cenobamate** is predicted to decrease the exposure to bosutinib. Avoid. Severe Study
▶ **Cenobamate** is predicted to decrease the exposure to brigatinib. Avoid or adjust dose—consult product literature. Moderate Study
▶ **Cenobamate** is predicted to decrease the exposure to buspirone. Adjust dose. Moderate Theoretical
▶ **Cenobamate** is predicted to decrease the exposure to cabozantinib. Moderate Study
▶ **Cenobamate** is predicted to decrease the exposure to calcium channel blockers (amlodipine, felodipine, lacidipine, lercanidipine, nicardipine, nifedipine, nimodipine). Monitor and adjust dose. Moderate Theoretical
▶ **Cenobamate** is predicted to decrease the exposure to calcium channel blockers (diltiazem, verapamil). Moderate Theoretical
▶ **Cenobamate** is predicted to decrease the exposure to capivasertib. Avoid. Moderate Study

▶ **Cenobamate** is predicted to decrease the efficacy of clopidogrel. Avoid. Moderate Study
▶ **Cenobamate** is predicted to decrease the exposure to cobicistat. Avoid. Severe Theoretical
▶ **Cenobamate** is predicted to decrease the exposure to cobimetinib. Avoid. Severe Theoretical
▶ **Cenobamate** might decrease the efficacy of oral combined hormonal contraceptives. Use additional contraceptive precautions. Severe Theoretical
▶ **Cenobamate** is predicted to decrease the exposure to oral corticosteroids (budesonide). Adjust dose. Moderate Theoretical
▶ **Cenobamate** is predicted to decrease the exposure to corticosteroids (fluticasone). Adjust dose. Moderate Theoretical
▶ **Cenobamate** is predicted to decrease the exposure to crizotinib. Avoid. Severe Study
▶ **Cenobamate** is predicted to decrease the exposure to daridorexant. Severe Study → Also see TABLE 10 p. 1574
▶ **Cenobamate** is predicted to decrease the exposure to darifenacin. Adjust dose. Moderate Theoretical
▶ **Cenobamate** is predicted to decrease the exposure to dasatinib. Severe Study
▶ **Cenobamate** is predicted to decrease the exposure to elacestrant. Avoid or adjust dose depending on duration—consult product literature. Severe Theoretical
▶ **Cenobamate** is predicted to moderately decrease the exposure to elbasvir. Avoid. Severe Study
▶ **Cenobamate** is predicted to decrease the concentration of elvitegravir. Avoid. Severe Theoretical
▶ **Cenobamate** is predicted to decrease the exposure to encorafenib. Moderate Study
▶ **Cenobamate** is predicted to decrease the exposure to entrectinib. Avoid. Moderate Theoretical
▶ **Cenobamate** is predicted to decrease the exposure to erdafitinib. Adjust dose. Moderate Theoretical
▶ **Cenobamate** is predicted to decrease the exposure to erlotinib. Severe Study
▶ **Cenobamate** is predicted to decrease the concentration of everolimus. Avoid or adjust dose. Severe Study
▶ **Cenobamate** is predicted to decrease the exposure to fedratinib. Avoid. Moderate Study
▶ **Cenobamate** is predicted to decrease the exposure to fruquintinib. Avoid. Moderate Study
▶ **Cenobamate** is predicted to decrease the exposure to gefitinib. Avoid. Severe Study
▶ **Cenobamate** is predicted to decrease the exposure to glasdegib. Avoid or adjust dose—consult product literature. Moderate Theoretical
▶ **Cenobamate** is predicted to decrease the exposure to glecaprevir. Avoid. Severe Study
▶ **Cenobamate** is predicted to markedly decrease the exposure to grazoprevir. Avoid. Severe Study
▶ **Cenobamate** is predicted to decrease the concentration of guanfacine. Adjust dose. Moderate Theoretical → Also see TABLE 10 p. 1574
▶ **Cenobamate** is predicted to decrease the exposure to ibrutinib. Adjust dose. Moderate Theoretical
▶ **Cenobamate** is predicted to decrease the exposure to idelalisib. Avoid. Moderate Theoretical
▶ **Cenobamate** is predicted to decrease the exposure to imatinib. Moderate Study
▶ **Cenobamate** is predicted to decrease the exposure to ivacaftor. Adjust dose. Moderate Theoretical
▶ **Cenobamate** is predicted to decrease the exposure to ixazomib. Moderate Theoretical
▶ **Cenobamate** is predicted to decrease the exposure to lapatinib. Avoid. Severe Study
▶ **Cenobamate** is predicted to decrease the exposure to larotrectinib. Avoid. Moderate Study
▶ **Cenobamate** is predicted to decrease the exposure to leniolisib. Avoid. Severe Theoretical
▶ **Cenobamate** is predicted to decrease the exposure to lomitapide. Adjust dose. Moderate Theoretical
▶ **Cenobamate** is predicted to decrease the exposure to maraviroc. Adjust dose. Moderate Theoretical

Cenobamate (continued)
- **Cenobamate** is predicted to decrease the exposure to mavacamten. Monitor and adjust dose—consult product literature. Severe Theoretical
- **Cenobamate** is predicted to decrease the exposure to mifepristone. Adjust **mifepristone** dose, p. 954. Severe Study
- **Cenobamate** is predicted to decrease the exposure to mineralocorticoid receptor antagonists (eplerenone). Adjust dose. Moderate Theoretical
- **Cenobamate** is predicted to decrease the exposure to mineralocorticoid receptor antagonists (finerenone). Avoid. Severe Study
- **Cenobamate** is predicted to decrease the exposure to mobocertinib. Avoid. Severe Study
- **Cenobamate** is predicted to decrease the exposure to naloxegol. Adjust dose. Moderate Theoretical
- **Cenobamate** is predicted to decrease the exposure to neratinib. Avoid. Severe Theoretical
- **Cenobamate** is predicted to decrease the exposure to neurokinin-1 receptor antagonists (netupitant). Moderate Theoretical
- **Cenobamate** is predicted to decrease the exposure to nilotinib. Avoid. Severe Theoretical
- **Cenobamate** is predicted to decrease the exposure to NNRTIs (rilpivirine). Avoid. Severe Theoretical
- **Cenobamate** is predicted to decrease the exposure to olaparib. Avoid. Moderate Theoretical
- **Cenobamate** is predicted to decrease the exposure to opioids (alfentanil). Adjust dose. Moderate Theoretical → Also see TABLE 10 p. 1574
- **Cenobamate** decreases the exposure to opioids (methadone). Monitor and adjust dose. Severe Study → Also see TABLE 10 p. 1574
- **Cenobamate** is predicted to decrease the exposure to ospemifene. Moderate Study
- **Cenobamate** is predicted to decrease the exposure to pazopanib. Severe Study
- **Cenobamate** is predicted to decrease the exposure to phosphodiesterase type-5 inhibitors (avanafil, sildenafil, vardenafil). Adjust dose. Moderate Theoretical
- **Cenobamate** is predicted to decrease the exposure to pibrentasvir. Avoid. Severe Study
- **Cenobamate** is predicted to decrease the exposure to ponatinib. Severe Study
- **Cenobamate** is predicted to decrease the exposure to pralsetinib. Moderate Theoretical
- **Cenobamate** moderately increases the exposure to proton pump inhibitors (omeprazole). Adjust dose. Moderate Study
- **Cenobamate** is predicted to decrease the exposure to quizartinib. Avoid. Severe Study
- **Cenobamate** is predicted to decrease the exposure to rimegepant. Avoid. Moderate Theoretical
- **Cenobamate** is predicted to decrease the exposure to ripretinib. Avoid or adjust dose—consult product literature. Moderate Theoretical
- **Cenobamate** is predicted to decrease the exposure to ruxolitinib. Monitor and adjust dose. Moderate Study
- **Cenobamate** is predicted to decrease the exposure to selumetinib. Avoid. Severe Study
- **Cenobamate** is predicted to decrease the exposure to siponimod. Manufacturer advises caution depending on genotype—consult product literature. Moderate Theoretical
- **Cenobamate** is predicted to decrease the exposure to sirolimus. Adjust dose. Moderate Theoretical
- **Cenobamate** is predicted to decrease the exposure to sorafenib. Moderate Study
- **Cenobamate** is predicted to increase the exposure to SSRIs (escitalopram). Use with caution and adjust dose. Severe Study → Also see TABLE 10 p. 1574
- **Cenobamate** is predicted to decrease the exposure to statins (atorvastatin, simvastatin). Moderate Study
- **Cenobamate** is predicted to decrease the exposure to sunitinib. Moderate Study
- **Cenobamate** is predicted to decrease the exposure to taxanes (docetaxel). Severe Theoretical

- **Cenobamate** is predicted to decrease the exposure to taxanes (paclitaxel). Avoid. Severe Study
- **Cenobamate** is predicted to decrease the concentration of temsirolimus. Avoid. Moderate Theoretical
- **Cenobamate** is predicted to decrease the exposure to ticagrelor. Moderate Theoretical
- **Cenobamate** is predicted to decrease the exposure to tofacitinib. Severe Study
- **Cenobamate** is predicted to decrease the exposure to tolvaptan. Adjust dose. Moderate Theoretical
- **Cenobamate** is predicted to decrease the exposure to triptans (eletriptan). Adjust dose. Moderate Theoretical
- **Cenobamate** is predicted to decrease the exposure to velpatasvir. Avoid. Moderate Theoretical
- **Cenobamate** is predicted to decrease the exposure to venetoclax. Avoid. Severe Study
- **Cenobamate** is predicted to decrease the exposure to voclosporin. Adjust dose. Moderate Theoretical
- **Cenobamate** is predicted to decrease the concentration of voxilaprevir. Avoid. Severe Theoretical
- **Cenobamate** is predicted to decrease the exposure to zanubrutinib. Avoid or adjust dose with moderate CYP3A4 inducers—consult product literature. Severe Theoretical

Cephalosporins → see TABLE 2 p. 1571 (nephrotoxicity)

cefaclor · cefadroxil · cefalexin · cefazolin · cefepime · cefiderocol · cefixime · cefotaxime · cefoxitin · cefradine · ceftaroline · ceftazidime · ceftobiprole · ceftolozane · ceftriaxone · cefuroxime

ROUTE-SPECIFIC INFORMATION Interactions do not generally apply to topical use of **cefuroxime** unless specified.

- Intravenous **ceftriaxone** increases the risk of cardio-respiratory arrest when given with intravenous calcium salts. Avoid. Severe Anecdotal
- Cephalosporins (cefazolin, ceftriaxone) potentially increase the risk of bleeding events when given with coumarins. Severe Anecdotal
- **Ceftobiprole** is predicted to increase the exposure to endothelin receptor antagonists (bosentan). Moderate Theoretical
- **Ivosidenib** is predicted to increase the exposure to **cefaclor**. Use with caution or avoid. Moderate Theoretical
- **Leflunomide** is predicted to increase the exposure to **cefaclor**. Moderate Study
- **Nitisinone** is predicted to increase the exposure to **cefaclor**. Moderate Study
- Cephalosporins (cefazolin, ceftriaxone) potentially increase the risk of bleeding events when given with phenindione. Severe Anecdotal
- **Ceftobiprole** is predicted to increase the concentration of statins. Moderate Theoretical
- **Ceftobiprole** is predicted to increase the concentration of sulfonylureas (glibenclamide). Moderate Theoretical
- **Teriflunomide** is predicted to increase the exposure to **cefaclor**. Moderate Study
- **Vadadustat** is predicted to increase the exposure to **cefaclor**. Monitor and adjust dose. Moderate Study

Ceritinib → see TABLE 5 p. 1572 (bradycardia), TABLE 14 p. 1575 (myelosuppression), TABLE 8 p. 1573 (QT-interval prolongation)
- **Ceritinib** is predicted to increase the exposure to abemaciclib. Avoid or adjust dose—consult product literature. Severe Study
- **Ceritinib** is predicted to increase the exposure to acalabrutinib. Avoid. Severe Study
- **Ceritinib** is predicted to increase the exposure to aliskiren. Moderate Theoretical
- **Ceritinib** is predicted to moderately increase the exposure to alpha blockers (alfuzosin, tamsulosin). Use with caution or avoid. Moderate Study
- **Ceritinib** is predicted to increase the exposure to alpha blockers (doxazosin). Moderate Study
- Oral antacids are predicted to decrease the absorption of oral **ceritinib**. Separate administration by 2 hours. Moderate Theoretical
- Anti-androgens (apalutamide, enzalutamide) are predicted to decrease the exposure to **ceritinib**. Avoid. Severe Study → Also see TABLE 8 p. 1573

▸ **Ceritinib** is predicted to increase the exposure to anti-androgens **(apalutamide)**. Monitor and adjust dose. Mild Study → Also see **TABLE 8** p. 1573

▸ Antiarrhythmics **(dronedarone)** are predicted to increase the exposure to **ceritinib**. Moderate Study → Also see **TABLE 5** p. 1572 → Also see **TABLE 8** p. 1573

▸ **Ceritinib** very markedly increases the exposure to antiarrhythmics **(dronedarone)**. Avoid. Severe Study → Also see **TABLE 5** p. 1572 → Also see **TABLE 8** p. 1573

▸ **Ceritinib** is predicted to increase the exposure to antiarrhythmics **(propafenone)**. Monitor and adjust dose. Severe Study → Also see **TABLE 5** p. 1572

▸ **Ceritinib** is predicted to increase the exposure to anticholinesterases, centrally acting **(galantamine)**. Monitor and adjust dose. Moderate Study → Also see **TABLE 5** p. 1572

▸ Antiepileptics **(carbamazepine, fosphenytoin, phenobarbital, phenytoin, primidone)** are predicted to decrease the exposure to **ceritinib**. Avoid. Severe Study

▸ **Ceritinib** is predicted to very slightly increase the exposure to antiepileptics **(perampanel)**. Mild Study

▸ Antifungals, azoles **(fluconazole, isavuconazole)** are predicted to increase the exposure to **ceritinib**. Moderate Study → Also see **TABLE 8** p. 1573

▸ Antifungals, azoles **(itraconazole, voriconazole)** are predicted to increase the exposure to **ceritinib**. Avoid or adjust dose—consult product literature. Severe Study → Also see **TABLE 8** p. 1573

▸ Antifungals, azoles **(ketoconazole)** moderately increase the exposure to **ceritinib**. Avoid or adjust dose—consult product literature. Severe Study

▸ **Ceritinib** is predicted to increase the exposure to antifungals, azoles **(isavuconazole)**. Avoid or monitor adverse effects. Severe Study

▸ **Ceritinib** is predicted to increase the exposure to antihistamines, non-sedating **(fexofenadine)**. Moderate Theoretical

▸ **Ceritinib** is predicted to increase the exposure to antihistamines, non-sedating **(mizolastine)**. Avoid. Severe Study

▸ **Ceritinib** is predicted to increase the exposure to antihistamines, non-sedating **(rupatadine)**. Avoid. Moderate Study

▸ **Ceritinib** is predicted to slightly increase the exposure to antipsychotics, second generation **(aripiprazole)**. Adjust **aripiprazole** dose, p. 454. Moderate Study → Also see **TABLE 8** p. 1573

▸ **Ceritinib** is predicted to moderately increase the exposure to antipsychotics, second generation **(cariprazine)**. Avoid. Severe Study

▸ **Ceritinib** is predicted to increase the exposure to antipsychotics, second generation **(lurasidone, quetiapine)**. Avoid. Severe Study

▸ **Ceritinib** is predicted to increase the exposure to antipsychotics, second generation **(risperidone)**. Adjust dose. Moderate Study

▸ **Ceritinib** is predicted to increase the exposure to **atogepant**. Adjust **atogepant** dose, p. 540. Moderate Study

▸ **Ceritinib** is predicted to increase the exposure to **avacopan**. Severe Study

▸ **Ceritinib** is predicted to increase the exposure to **avapritinib**. Avoid. Moderate Study

▸ **Ceritinib** is predicted to increase the exposure to **axitinib**. Avoid or adjust dose. Moderate Study → Also see **TABLE 14** p. 1575

▸ **Ceritinib** might increases the exposure to **bedaquiline**. Mild Study → Also see **TABLE 8** p. 1573

▸ **Ceritinib** moderately increases the exposure to benzodiazepines **(alprazolam)**. Avoid. Moderate Study

▸ **Ceritinib** is predicted to markedly to very markedly increase the exposure to benzodiazepines **(midazolam)**. Avoid or adjust dose. Severe Study

▸ **Berotralstat** is predicted to increase the exposure to **ceritinib**. Moderate Study

▸ **Ceritinib** is predicted to increase the exposure to beta$_2$ agonists **(salmeterol)**. Avoid. Severe Study

▸ **Ceritinib** slightly increases the exposure to **bortezomib**. Moderate Study → Also see **TABLE 14** p. 1575

▸ **Ceritinib** is predicted to increase the exposure to **bosutinib**. Avoid or adjust dose. Severe Study → Also see **TABLE 14** p. 1575 → Also see **TABLE 8** p. 1573

▸ **Ceritinib** is predicted to increase the exposure to **brigatinib**. Avoid or adjust dose—consult product literature. Severe Study → Also see **TABLE 5** p. 1572

▸ **Ceritinib** is predicted to increase the exposure to **buspirone**. Adjust **buspirone** dose, p. 396. Severe Study

▸ **Ceritinib** is predicted to increase the exposure to **cabozantinib**. Moderate Study → Also see **TABLE 14** p. 1575 → Also see **TABLE 8** p. 1573

▸ Calcium channel blockers **(diltiazem, verapamil)** are predicted to increase the exposure to **ceritinib**. Moderate Study → Also see **TABLE 5** p. 1572

▸ **Ceritinib** is predicted to increase the exposure to calcium channel blockers **(amlodipine, felodipine, lacidipine, nicardipine, nifedipine, nimodipine)**. Monitor and adjust dose. Moderate Study

▸ **Ceritinib** is predicted to increase the exposure to calcium channel blockers **(diltiazem, verapamil)**. Severe Study → Also see **TABLE 5** p. 1572

▸ **Ceritinib** is predicted to markedly increase the exposure to calcium channel blockers **(lercanidipine)**. Avoid. Severe Study

▸ **Ceritinib** is predicted to increase the exposure to **cannabidiol**. Avoid or adjust dose. Mild Study

▸ **Ceritinib** is predicted to increase the exposure to **capivasertib**. Adjust dose. Moderate Study

▸ **Ceritinib** increases the concentration of **ciclosporin**. Severe Study

▸ **Ceritinib** is predicted to moderately increase the exposure to **cilostazol**. Adjust **cilostazol** dose, p. 266. Moderate Study

▸ **Ceritinib** is predicted to moderately increase the exposure to **cinacalcet**. Adjust dose. Moderate Study

▸ **Cobicistat** is predicted to increase the exposure to **ceritinib**. Avoid or adjust dose—consult product literature. Severe Study

▸ **Ceritinib** is predicted to increase the exposure to **cobimetinib**. Avoid or monitor for toxicity. Severe Study

▸ **Ceritinib** is predicted to increase the exposure to **colchicine**. Avoid potent CYP3A4 inhibitors or adjust **colchicine** dose, p. 1279. Severe Study

▸ **Ceritinib** is predicted to increase the exposure to corticosteroids **(beclometasone)** (risk with beclometasone is likely to be lower than with other corticosteroids). Moderate Theoretical

▸ **Ceritinib** is predicted to increase the exposure to corticosteroids **(betamethasone, budesonide, ciclesonide, deflazacort, dexamethasone, fludrocortisone, fluticasone, hydrocortisone, methylprednisolone, mometasone, prednisolone, triamcinolone)**. Avoid or monitor adverse effects. Severe Study

▸ **Ceritinib** is predicted to increase the exposure to corticosteroids **(vamorolone)**. Adjust dose. Severe Study

▸ **Ceritinib** is predicted to increase the exposure to coumarins **(acenocoumarol)**. Severe Theoretical

▸ **Ceritinib** increases the exposure to coumarins **(warfarin)**. Avoid or monitor INR. Severe Study

▸ **Ceritinib** is predicted to increase the exposure to **crizotinib**. Avoid. Moderate Study → Also see **TABLE 5** p. 1572 → Also see **TABLE 8** p. 1573

▸ **Crizotinib** is predicted to increase the exposure to **ceritinib**. Moderate Study → Also see **TABLE 5** p. 1572 → Also see **TABLE 8** p. 1573

▸ **Dabrafenib** is predicted to decrease the exposure to **ceritinib**. Severe Study

▸ **Ceritinib** is predicted to increase the exposure to **dabrafenib**. Use with caution or avoid. Moderate Study

▸ **Ceritinib** is predicted to increase the exposure to **daridorexant**. Avoid. Severe Study

▸ **Ceritinib** is predicted to markedly to very markedly increase the exposure to **darifenacin**. Avoid. Severe Study

▸ **Ceritinib** is predicted to increase the exposure to **dasatinib**. Avoid or adjust dose—consult product literature. Severe Study → Also see **TABLE 14** p. 1575 → Also see **TABLE 8** p. 1573

▸ **Ceritinib** very slightly increases the exposure to **delamanid**. Severe Study → Also see **TABLE 8** p. 1573

▸ **Ceritinib** is predicted to moderately increase the exposure to **dienogest**. Moderate Study

▸ **Ceritinib** is predicted to increase the risk of bradycardia when given with **digoxin**. Avoid. Severe Theoretical → Also see **TABLE 5** p. 1572

Ceritinib (continued)

▶ **Ceritinib** is predicted to increase the exposure to dipeptidylpeptidase-4 inhibitors (saxagliptin). Moderate Study

▶ **Ceritinib** is predicted to increase the exposure to domperidone. Avoid. Severe Study

▶ **Ceritinib** increases the exposure to dopamine receptor agonists (bromocriptine). Severe Study

▶ **Ceritinib** is predicted to increase the exposure to dronabinol. Adjust dose. Mild Study

▶ **Ceritinib** is predicted to increase the exposure to dutasteride. Monitor adverse effects and adjust dose. Moderate Theoretical

▶ **Ceritinib** is predicted to increase the exposure to elacestrant. Avoid potent CYP3A4 inhibitors or adjust **elacestrant** dose, p. 1084. Severe Study

▶ **Ceritinib** is predicted to increase the exposure to elexacaftor. Adjust ivacaftor with tezacaftor and elexacaftor p. 337 dose with potent CYP3A4 inhibitors. Severe Study

▶ **Ceritinib** is predicted to increase the exposure to eliglustat. Avoid or adjust dose—consult product literature. Severe Study

▶ **Encorafenib** is predicted to decrease the exposure to **ceritinib**. Avoid. Severe Study → Also see TABLE 8 p. 1573

▶ **Ceritinib** is predicted to increase the exposure to encorafenib. Avoid or monitor. Severe Study → Also see TABLE 8 p. 1573

▶ Endothelin receptor antagonists (bosentan) are predicted to decrease the exposure to **ceritinib**. Severe Study

▶ **Ceritinib** is predicted to increase the exposure to endothelin receptor antagonists (macitentan). Moderate Study

▶ **Ceritinib** is predicted to increase the exposure to the cytotoxic component of enfortumab vedotin. Severe Theoretical

▶ **Ceritinib** is predicted to increase the exposure to entrectinib. Avoid or adjust dose with potent CYP3A4 inhibitors—consult product literature. Severe Study → Also see TABLE 8 p. 1573

▶ **Ceritinib** is predicted to increase the exposure to erdafitinib. Adjust dose. Severe Study

▶ **Ceritinib** is predicted to increase the risk of ergotism when given with ergometrine. Avoid. Severe Theoretical

▶ **Ceritinib** is predicted to increase the exposure to erlotinib. Use with caution and adjust dose. Severe Study

▶ **Ceritinib** is predicted to increase the exposure to esketamine. Adjust dose. Moderate Study

▶ **Ceritinib** is predicted to increase the exposure to eszopiclone. Adjust **eszopiclone** dose; avoid in the elderly, p. 554. Moderate Study

▶ **Ceritinib** is predicted to increase the concentration of subdermal etonogestrel. Moderate Theoretical

▶ **Ceritinib** is predicted to increase the exposure to etrasimod. Avoid in poor CYP2C9 metabolisers. Severe Theoretical → Also see TABLE 5 p. 1572

▶ **Ceritinib** is predicted to increase the exposure to everolimus. Avoid. Severe Study

▶ **Ceritinib** is predicted to increase the exposure to factor XA inhibitors (edoxaban). Moderate Theoretical

▶ **Ceritinib** is predicted to increase the exposure to fedratinib. Adjust dose, but avoid depending on other drugs taken— consult product literature. Moderate Study

▶ **Fedratinib** is predicted to increase the exposure to **ceritinib**. Moderate Study

▶ **Ceritinib** is predicted to moderately increase the exposure to fesoterodine. Adjust **fesoterodine** dose with potent CYP3A4 inhibitors; avoid in hepatic and renal impairment, p. 897. Severe Study

▶ **Ceritinib** is predicted to increase the exposure to fostamatinib. Monitor adverse effects and adjust dose. Moderate Study

▶ **Ceritinib** is predicted to increase the exposure to gefitinib. Severe Study

▶ **Ceritinib** is predicted to increase the exposure to gilteritinib. Moderate Study

▶ **Ceritinib** is predicted to increase the exposure to glasdegib. Use with caution or avoid. Severe Study → Also see TABLE 8 p. 1573

▶ **Grapefruit** juice is predicted to increase the exposure to **ceritinib**. Avoid. Severe Theoretical

▶ **Ceritinib** is predicted to moderately to markedly increase the exposure to grazoprevir. Avoid. Severe Study

▶ **Ceritinib** is predicted to increase the exposure to guanfacine. Adjust **guanfacine** dose, p. 407. Moderate Study

▶ H₂ receptor antagonists are predicted to decrease the absorption of **ceritinib**. Moderate Theoretical

▶ HIV-protease inhibitors (atazanavir, darunavir, lopinavir) boosted with ritonavir are predicted to increase the exposure to **ceritinib**. Avoid or adjust dose—consult product literature. Severe Study

▶ HIV-protease inhibitors (fosamprenavir, ritonavir) are predicted to increase the exposure to **ceritinib**. Avoid or adjust dose— consult product literature. Severe Study

▶ **Ceritinib** is predicted to increase the exposure to ibrutinib. Avoid or adjust dose with potent CYP3A4 inhibitors—consult product literature. Severe Study → Also see TABLE 14 p. 1575

▶ **Idelalisib** is predicted to increase the exposure to **ceritinib**. Avoid or adjust dose—consult product literature. Severe Study

▶ **Ceritinib** is predicted to increase the exposure to imatinib. Moderate Study → Also see TABLE 14 p. 1575

▶ **Imatinib** is predicted to increase the exposure to **ceritinib**. Moderate Study → Also see TABLE 14 p. 1575

▶ **Ceritinib** is predicted to increase the risk of toxicity when given with irinotecan. Avoid. Severe Study → Also see TABLE 14 p. 1575

▶ **Ceritinib** is predicted to increase the exposure to ivabradine. Avoid. Severe Study → Also see TABLE 5 p. 1572

▶ **Ceritinib** is predicted to increase the exposure to ivacaftor. Adjust dose with potent CYP3A4 inhibitors, see ivacaftor p. 336, lumacaftor with ivacaftor p. 338, tezacaftor with ivacaftor p. 339, and ivacaftor with tezacaftor and elexacaftor p. 337. Severe Study

▶ **Ivosidenib** is predicted to decrease the exposure to **ceritinib**. Avoid. Severe Study → Also see TABLE 8 p. 1573

▶ **Lapatinib** is predicted to increase the exposure to **ceritinib**. Moderate Theoretical → Also see TABLE 8 p. 1573

▶ **Ceritinib** is predicted to increase the exposure to lapatinib. Avoid. Moderate Study → Also see TABLE 8 p. 1573

▶ **Ceritinib** is predicted to moderately increase the exposure to larotrectinib. Avoid or adjust dose—consult product literature. Moderate Study

▶ **Ceritinib** is predicted to increase the exposure to leniolisib. Avoid. Moderate Study

▶ **Letermovir** is predicted to increase the exposure to **ceritinib**. Moderate Study

▶ **Ceritinib** is predicted to markedly increase the exposure to lomitapide. Avoid. Severe Study

▶ **Ceritinib** is predicted to increase the exposure to loperamide. Moderate Theoretical

▶ **Ceritinib** is predicted to increase the exposure to lorlatinib. Avoid or adjust dose—consult product literature. Severe Study

▶ **Lumacaftor** is predicted to decrease the exposure to **ceritinib**. Avoid. Severe Study

▶ Macrolides (clarithromycin) are predicted to increase the exposure to **ceritinib**. Avoid or adjust dose—consult product literature. Severe Study

▶ Macrolides (erythromycin) are predicted to increase the exposure to **ceritinib**. Moderate Study → Also see TABLE 8 p. 1573

▶ **Ceritinib** is predicted to increase the exposure to mavacamten. Avoid or monitor—consult product literature. Severe Study

▶ **Ceritinib** is predicted to increase the concentration of intramuscular medroxyprogesterone. Moderate Theoretical

▶ **Ceritinib** is predicted to increase the exposure to midostaurin. Avoid or monitor for toxicity. Severe Study

▶ **Ceritinib** is predicted to markedly increase the exposure to mineralocorticoid receptor antagonists (eplerenone). Avoid. Severe Study

▶ **Ceritinib** is predicted to increase the exposure to mineralocorticoid receptor antagonists (finerenone). Avoid. Severe Study

▶ **Ceritinib** is predicted to increase the exposure to mirabegron. Adjust **mirabegron** dose in hepatic and renal impairment, p. 901. Moderate Study

▶ **Ceritinib** is predicted to increase the exposure to mirtazapine. Moderate Study

▶ **Mitotane** is predicted to decrease the exposure to **ceritinib**. Avoid. Severe Study → Also see TABLE 14 p. 1575

▶ **Ceritinib** is predicted to increase the exposure to mobocertinib. Avoid. Severe Study → Also see TABLE 8 p. 1573

▶ **Ceritinib** is predicted to increase the exposure to modafinil. Mild Theoretical

▶ **Ceritinib** is predicted to increase the risk of neutropenia when given with monoclonal antibodies (brentuximab vedotin). Monitor and adjust dose. Severe Study → Also see **TABLE 14** p. 1575

▶ **Ceritinib** is predicted to increase the exposure to monoclonal antibodies (polatuzumab vedotin). Moderate Theoretical

▶ **Ceritinib** is predicted to increase the exposure to the cytotoxic component of monoclonal antibodies (trastuzumab emtansine). Avoid or monitor. Severe Theoretical → Also see **TABLE 14** p. 1575

▶ **Ceritinib** is predicted to increase the exposure to naldemedine. Avoid or monitor. Moderate Study

▶ **Ceritinib** is predicted to markedly increase the exposure to naloxegol. Avoid. Severe Study

▶ **Ceritinib** is predicted to increase the exposure to neratinib. Avoid or adjust dose with potent CYP3A4 inhibitors—consult product literature. Severe Study

▶ Neurokinin-1 receptor antagonists (aprepitant, netupitant) are predicted to increase the exposure to **ceritinib**. Moderate Study

▶ Neurokinin-1 receptor antagonists (fosaprepitant) are predicted to increase the exposure to **ceritinib**. Severe Theoretical

▶ **Ceritinib** is predicted to markedly increase the exposure to neurokinin-1 receptor antagonists (aprepitant). Moderate Study

▶ **Ceritinib** is predicted to increase the exposure to neurokinin-1 receptor antagonists (fosaprepitant). Moderate Theoretical

▶ **Ceritinib** is predicted to increase the exposure to neurokinin-1 receptor antagonists (netupitant). Moderate Study

▶ **Ceritinib** is predicted to increase the exposure to nilotinib. Avoid. Severe Study → Also see **TABLE 14** p. 1575 → Also see **TABLE 8** p. 1573

▶ Nilotinib is predicted to increase the exposure to **ceritinib**. Moderate Study → Also see **TABLE 14** p. 1575 → Also see **TABLE 8** p. 1573

▶ Nirmatrelvir boosted with ritonavir is predicted to increase the concentration of **ceritinib**. Avoid or adjust dose—consult product literature. Severe Theoretical

▶ **Ceritinib** is predicted to increase the exposure to nitisinone. Adjust dose. Moderate Theoretical

▶ NNRTIs (efavirenz, nevirapine) are predicted to decrease the exposure to **ceritinib**. Severe Study → Also see **TABLE 8** p. 1573

▶ NNRTIs (etravirine) are predicted to decrease the exposure to **ceritinib**. Severe Theoretical

▶ **Ceritinib** is predicted to increase the exposure to NSAIDs (celecoxib, diclofenac). Adjust dose. Moderate Theoretical

▶ **Ceritinib** is predicted to increase the exposure to olaparib. Avoid or adjust dose with potent CYP3A4 inhibitors—consult product literature. Moderate Study → Also see **TABLE 14** p. 1575

▶ **Ceritinib** is predicted to increase the exposure to opioids (alfentanil, buprenorphine, fentanyl, oxycodone). Monitor and adjust dose. Severe Study → Also see **TABLE 5** p. 1572

▶ **Ceritinib** is predicted to increase the exposure to opioids (sufentanil). Moderate Study → Also see **TABLE 5** p. 1572

▶ **Ceritinib** is predicted to increase the exposure to osilodrostat. Moderate Theoretical → Also see **TABLE 8** p. 1573

▶ **Ceritinib** is predicted to increase the exposure to ospemifene. Avoid in poor CYP2C9 metabolisers. Moderate Study

▶ **Ceritinib** is predicted to increase the exposure to oxybutynin. Mild Study

▶ **Ceritinib** is predicted to increase the exposure to palbociclib. Avoid or adjust dose—consult product literature. Severe Study → Also see **TABLE 14** p. 1575

▶ **Ceritinib** is predicted to increase the exposure to panobinostat. Adjust dose—consult product literature; in hepatic impairment avoid. Moderate Study → Also see **TABLE 14** p. 1575 → Also see **TABLE 8** p. 1573

▶ **Ceritinib** is predicted to increase the exposure to pazopanib. Avoid or adjust dose—consult product literature. Moderate Study → Also see **TABLE 8** p. 1573

▶ **Ceritinib** is predicted to increase the exposure to pemigatinib. Avoid or adjust dose—consult product literature. Severe Study

▶ **Ceritinib** is predicted to increase the exposure to phenindione. Severe Theoretical

▶ **Ceritinib** is predicted to increase the exposure to phosphodiesterase type-5 inhibitors (avanafil, vardenafil). Avoid. Severe Study → Also see **TABLE 8** p. 1573

▶ **Ceritinib** is predicted to increase the exposure to phosphodiesterase type-5 inhibitors (sildenafil). Avoid potent CYP3A4 inhibitors or adjust **sildenafil** dose, p. 940. Severe Study

▶ **Ceritinib** is predicted to increase the exposure to phosphodiesterase type-5 inhibitors (tadalafil). Use with caution or avoid. Severe Study

▶ **Ceritinib** is predicted to increase the exposure to pimozide. Avoid. Severe Study → Also see **TABLE 8** p. 1573

▶ **Ceritinib** is predicted to slightly increase the exposure to ponatinib. Monitor and adjust dose—consult product literature. Moderate Study

▶ **Ceritinib** is predicted to increase the exposure to pralsetinib. Avoid or adjust dose with potent CYP3A4 inhibitors—consult product literature. Moderate Study

▶ **Ceritinib** is predicted to moderately increase the exposure to praziquantel. Mild Study

▶ **Ceritinib** given with carbimazole is predicted to increase the exposure to propiverine. Adjust starting dose. Moderate Theoretical

▶ Proton pump inhibitors are predicted to decrease the absorption of **ceritinib**. Moderate Theoretical

▶ **Ceritinib** is predicted to increase the exposure to quizartinib. Adjust dose—consult product literature. Severe Study → Also see **TABLE 8** p. 1573

▶ **Ceritinib** is predicted to increase the exposure to ranolazine. Avoid. Severe Study → Also see **TABLE 8** p. 1573

▶ **Ceritinib** is predicted to increase the exposure to reboxetine. Avoid. Moderate Study

▶ **Ceritinib** is predicted to increase the exposure to regorafenib. Avoid. Moderate Study → Also see **TABLE 14** p. 1575

▶ **Ceritinib** is predicted to increase the exposure to retinoids (alitretinoin). Adjust **alitretinoin** dose, p. 1433. Moderate Theoretical

▶ **Ceritinib** is predicted to increase the exposure to ribociclib. Avoid or adjust dose—consult product literature. Moderate Study → Also see **TABLE 14** p. 1575 → Also see **TABLE 8** p. 1573

▶ Rifamycins (rifampicin) are predicted to decrease the exposure to **ceritinib**. Avoid. Severe Study

▶ **Ceritinib** is predicted to increase the exposure to rimegepant. Avoid. Moderate Study

▶ **Ceritinib** is predicted to increase the exposure to ripretinib. Moderate Theoretical

▶ **Ceritinib** is predicted to increase the exposure to ruxolitinib. Adjust dose and monitor adverse effects. Moderate Study → Also see **TABLE 14** p. 1575

▶ **Ceritinib** is predicted to increase the exposure to selpercatinib. Adjust dose—consult product literature. Moderate Study → Also see **TABLE 8** p. 1573

▶ **Ceritinib** is predicted to increase the exposure to selumetinib. Avoid or adjust dose—consult product literature. Severe Study

▶ **Ceritinib** is predicted to increase the exposure to siponimod. Avoid depending on other drugs taken—consult product literature. Severe Theoretical → Also see **TABLE 5** p. 1572

▶ **Ceritinib** is predicted to increase the concentration of sirolimus. Avoid or monitor and adjust dose. Severe Study

▶ **Ceritinib** is predicted to increase the exposure to SNRIs (venlafaxine). Moderate Study

▶ **Ceritinib** is predicted to increase the exposure to solifenacin. Adjust solifenacin p. 899 or tamsulosin with solifenacin p. 906 dose; avoid in hepatic and renal impairment. Severe Study

▶ **Ceritinib** is predicted to moderately increase the exposure to SSRIs (dapoxetine). Avoid potent CYP3A4 inhibitors or adjust **dapoxetine** dose, p. 947. Severe Study

▶ St John's wort is predicted to decrease the exposure to **ceritinib**. Avoid. Severe Theoretical

▶ **Ceritinib** is predicted to increase the exposure to statins (atorvastatin). Avoid or adjust dose and monitor rhabdomyolysis. Severe Study

▶ **Ceritinib** is predicted to increase the exposure to statins (simvastatin). Avoid. Severe Study

▶ **Ceritinib** is predicted to increase the exposure to sulfonylureas (glimepiride). Adjust dose. Moderate Theoretical

▶ **Ceritinib** is predicted to increase the exposure to sunitinib. Avoid or adjust dose—consult product literature. Moderate Study → Also see **TABLE 14** p. 1575 → Also see **TABLE 8** p. 1573

Ceritinib (continued)

▶ **Ceritinib** is predicted to increase the concentration of tacrolimus. Monitor and adjust dose. [Severe] Study
▶ **Ceritinib** is predicted to increase the exposure to taxanes (cabazitaxel). Avoid or adjust dose—consult product literature. [Severe] Study → Also see **TABLE 14** p. 1575
▶ **Ceritinib** is predicted to increase the exposure to taxanes (docetaxel). Avoid or adjust dose. [Severe] Study → Also see **TABLE 14** p. 1575
▶ **Ceritinib** is predicted to increase the exposure to taxanes (paclitaxel). [Moderate] Anecdotal → Also see **TABLE 14** p. 1575
▶ **Ceritinib** is predicted to increase the concentration of temsirolimus. Avoid. [Severe] Theoretical → Also see **TABLE 14** p. 1575
▶ **Ceritinib** is predicted to increase the exposure to tezacaftor. Adjust dose with potent CYP3A4 inhibitors, see tezacaftor with ivacaftor p. 339 and ivacaftor with tezacaftor and elexacaftor p. 337. [Severe] Study
▶ **Ceritinib** is predicted to increase the exposure to thrombin inhibitors (dabigatran). [Moderate] Theoretical
▶ **Ceritinib** is predicted to markedly increase the exposure to ticagrelor. Avoid. [Severe] Study → Also see **TABLE 5** p. 1572
▶ **Ceritinib** is predicted to increase the exposure to tofacitinib. Adjust **tofacitinib** dose, p. 1265. [Moderate] Study
▶ **Ceritinib** is predicted to increase the exposure to tolterodine. Avoid. [Severe] Study → Also see **TABLE 8** p. 1573
▶ **Ceritinib** is predicted to increase the exposure to tolvaptan. Manufacturer advises caution or adjust **tolvaptan** dose with potent CYP3A4 inhibitors, p. 767. [Severe] Study
▶ **Ceritinib** is predicted to increase the exposure to topotecan. [Moderate] Theoretical → Also see **TABLE 14** p. 1575
▶ **Ceritinib** is predicted to increase the exposure to toremifene. [Moderate] Theoretical → Also see **TABLE 8** p. 1573
▶ **Ceritinib** is predicted to increase the exposure to trabectedin. Avoid or adjust dose. [Severe] Theoretical → Also see **TABLE 14** p. 1575
▶ **Ceritinib** is predicted to moderately increase the exposure to trazodone. Avoid or adjust dose. [Moderate] Study
▶ **Ceritinib** increases the exposure to triptans (almotriptan). [Mild] Study
▶ **Ceritinib** is predicted to markedly increase the exposure to triptans (eletriptan). Avoid. [Severe] Study
▶ **Tucatinib** is predicted to increase the exposure to **ceritinib**. Avoid or adjust dose—consult product literature. [Severe] Study
▶ **Ceritinib** is predicted to increase the exposure to upadacitinib. Manufacturer advises caution or avoid, or adjust **upadacitinib** dose depending on indication, p. 1267. [Severe] Study
▶ **Ceritinib** is predicted to increase the exposure to vemurafenib. [Severe] Theoretical → Also see **TABLE 8** p. 1573
▶ **Ceritinib** is predicted to increase the exposure to venetoclax. Avoid or adjust dose—consult product literature. [Severe] Study
▶ **Ceritinib** is predicted to increase the exposure to vinca alkaloids. [Severe] Theoretical → Also see **TABLE 14** p. 1575
▶ **Ceritinib** is predicted to increase the exposure to vitamin D substances (paricalcitol). [Moderate] Study
▶ **Ceritinib** is predicted to increase the exposure to voclosporin. Avoid. [Severe] Study → Also see **TABLE 8** p. 1573
▶ **Ceritinib** is predicted to increase the exposure to zanubrutinib. Avoid or adjust dose with potent CYP3A4 inhibitors—consult product literature. [Moderate] Study
▶ **Ceritinib** is predicted to increase the exposure to zopiclone. Adjust dose. [Moderate] Theoretical

Certolizumab pegol → see monoclonal antibodies
Cetirizine → see antihistamines, non-sedating
Cetuximab → see monoclonal antibodies

Chenodeoxycholic acid

▶ Oral aluminium hydroxide decreases the absorption of chenodeoxycholic acid. [Moderate] Study
▶ Antiepileptics (phenobarbital, primidone) are predicted to affect the efficacy of **chenodeoxycholic acid**. Monitor and adjust dose. [Moderate] Theoretical
▶ Ciclosporin is predicted to affect the efficacy of **chenodeoxycholic acid**. Monitor and adjust dose. [Moderate] Theoretical

▶ Oral combined hormonal contraceptives potentially decrease the efficacy of oral **chenodeoxycholic acid**. Avoid. [Moderate] Theoretical
▶ Sirolimus is predicted to affect the efficacy of **chenodeoxycholic acid**. Monitor and adjust dose. [Moderate] Theoretical

Chloral hydrate → see **TABLE 10** p. 1574 (CNS effects)

▶ Intravenous loop diuretics (furosemide) potentially increase the risk of sweating, variable blood pressure, and tachycardia when given after **chloral hydrate**. [Moderate] Anecdotal

Chlorambucil → see alkylating agents

Chloramphenicol

> **ROUTE-SPECIFIC INFORMATION** Since systemic absorption can follow topical application, the possibility of interactions should be borne in mind.

▶ Antiepileptics (phenobarbital, primidone) decrease the concentration of **chloramphenicol**. [Moderate] Study
▶ Intravenous **chloramphenicol** increases the concentration of antiepileptics (fosphenytoin, phenytoin) and antiepileptics (fosphenytoin, phenytoin) affect the concentration of intravenous **chloramphenicol**. Monitor concentration and adjust dose. [Severe] Study
▶ **Chloramphenicol** potentially increases the anticoagulant effect of coumarins. [Moderate] Anecdotal
▶ **Chloramphenicol** is predicted to increase the exposure to guanfacine. Adjust **guanfacine** dose, p. 407. [Moderate] Theoretical
▶ **Chloramphenicol** decreases the efficacy of iron. [Moderate] Anecdotal
▶ Rifamycins (rifampicin) decrease the concentration of **chloramphenicol**. [Moderate] Study
▶ **Chloramphenicol** is predicted to increase the exposure to sulfonylureas. [Severe] Study
▶ **Chloramphenicol** increases the concentration of tacrolimus. [Severe] Study

Chlordiazepoxide → see benzodiazepines

Chlormethine

> **ROUTE-SPECIFIC INFORMATION** Since systemic absorption can follow topical application, the possibility of interactions should be borne in mind.

Chloroprocaine

▶ **Chloroprocaine** is predicted to increase the risk of cardiovascular adverse effects when given with antiarrhythmics (amiodarone, dronedarone, vernakalant). [Severe] Theoretical
▶ **Chloroprocaine** is predicted to increase the risk of cardiovascular adverse effects when given with beta blockers, non-selective (sotalol). [Severe] Theoretical
▶ **Chloroprocaine** is predicted to decrease the effects of sulfonamides. Avoid. [Severe] Theoretical

Chloroquine → see antimalarials
Chlorothiazide → see thiazide diuretics
Chlorphenamine → see antihistamines, sedating
Chlorpromazine → see phenothiazines
Chlortalidone → see thiazide diuretics
Cholera vaccine (live) → see live vaccines

Cholic acid

▶ Oral antacids are predicted to decrease the absorption of oral cholic acid. Separate administration by 5 hours. [Mild] Theoretical
▶ Antiepileptics (phenobarbital) decrease the effects of **cholic acid**. Avoid. [Moderate] Study
▶ Ciclosporin affects the concentration of **cholic acid**. Avoid. [Moderate] Study

Choline salicylate

▶ Corticosteroids are predicted to decrease the concentration of choline salicylate. [Moderate] Study

Ciclesonide → see corticosteroids

Ciclosporin → see **TABLE 2** p. 1571 (nephrotoxicity), **TABLE 15** p. 1575 (increased serum potassium)

> ▶ Pomelo juice is predicted to increase ciclosporin exposure, and purple grape juice is predicted to decrease ciclosporin exposure.
> ▶ Since systemic absorption can follow topical application, the possibility of interactions should be borne in mind.

▶ Abrocitinib might increase the exposure to **ciclosporin**. [Moderate] Theoretical

▸ **Ciclosporin** is predicted to increase the exposure to afatinib. Moderate Study

▸ **Ciclosporin** markedly increases the exposure to aliskiren. Avoid. Severe Study → Also see **TABLE 15** p. 1575

▸ **Ciclosporin** is predicted to increase the exposure to alpelisib. Moderate Theoretical

▸ **Ciclosporin** increases the concentration of anthracyclines (daunorubicin, doxorubicin, epirubicin, idarubicin, mitoxantrone). Severe Study

▸ Anti-androgens (apalutamide, enzalutamide) decrease the concentration of **ciclosporin**. Severe Study

▸ Antiarrhythmics (amiodarone) increase the concentration of **ciclosporin**. Monitor concentration and adjust dose. Severe Study

▸ Antiarrhythmics (dronedarone) are predicted to increase the concentration of **ciclosporin**. Severe Study

▸ Antiepileptics (carbamazepine, fosphenytoin, phenobarbital, phenytoin, primidone) decrease the concentration of **ciclosporin**. Severe Study

▸ Antiepileptics (oxcarbazepine) decrease the concentration of **ciclosporin**. Severe Anecdotal

▸ Antifungals, azoles (fluconazole, isavuconazole) are predicted to increase the concentration of **ciclosporin**. Severe Study

▸ Antifungals, azoles (itraconazole, ketoconazole, posaconazole, voriconazole) increase the concentration of **ciclosporin**. Severe Study

▸ Antifungals, azoles (miconazole) increase the concentration of **ciclosporin**. Monitor and adjust dose. Severe Anecdotal

▸ **Ciclosporin** is predicted to increase the exposure to antihistamines, non-sedating (fexofenadine). Moderate Theoretical

▸ **Ciclosporin** is predicted to increase the exposure to atogepant. Adjust **atogepant** dose, p. 540. Moderate Theoretical

▸ Baricitinib is predicted to enhance the risk of immunosuppression when given with **ciclosporin**. Manufacturer advises caution or avoid—consult product literature. Severe Theoretical

▸ **Ciclosporin** is predicted to increase the exposure to beta blockers, non-selective (nadolol). Moderate Study

▸ **Ciclosporin** is predicted to increase the exposure to bictegravir. Use with caution or avoid. Moderate Theoretical

▸ Brigatinib might decrease the exposure to **ciclosporin**. Avoid. Moderate Theoretical

▸ **Ciclosporin** is predicted to affect the efficacy of bulevirtide and bulevirtide is predicted to increase the exposure to **ciclosporin**. Avoid. Severe Theoretical

▸ Calcium channel blockers (diltiazem, verapamil) are predicted to increase the concentration of **ciclosporin**. Severe Study

▸ Calcium channel blockers (nicardipine) increase the concentration of **ciclosporin**. Severe Study

▸ **Ciclosporin** moderately increases the exposure to calcium channel blockers (lercanidipine). Use with caution or avoid. Severe Study

▸ Cannabidiol is predicted to increase the concentration of **ciclosporin**. Monitor and adjust dose. Severe Theoretical

▸ **Ciclosporin** is predicted to increase the exposure to capivasertib. Adjust dose. Moderate Theoretical

▸ **Ciclosporin** slightly increases the exposure to caspofungin. Severe Study

▸ Ceritinib increases the concentration of **ciclosporin**. Severe Study

▸ **Ciclosporin** is predicted to affect the efficacy of chenodeoxycholic acid. Monitor and adjust dose. Moderate Theoretical

▸ **Ciclosporin** affects the concentration of cholic acid. Avoid. Moderate Study

▸ **Ciclosporin** is predicted to increase the exposure to cladribine. Avoid or adjust dose. Moderate Theoretical

▸ Cobicistat increases the concentration of **ciclosporin**. Severe Study

▸ **Ciclosporin** increases the exposure to colchicine. Avoid P-glycoprotein inhibitors or adjust **colchicine** dose, p. 1279. Severe Study

▸ Crizotinib is predicted to increase the concentration of **ciclosporin**. Severe Study

▸ **Ciclosporin** is predicted to increase the risk of rhabdomyolysis when given with daptomycin. Severe Theoretical

▸ **Ciclosporin** is predicted to increase the exposure to daridorexant. Adjust **daridorexant** dose, p. 554. Unknown Theoretical

▸ **Ciclosporin** is predicted to increase the exposure to darifenacin. Avoid. Moderate Theoretical

▸ **Ciclosporin** increases the concentration of digoxin. Monitor and adjust dose. Severe Theoretical

▸ **Ciclosporin** is predicted to increase the exposure to elacestrant. Avoid or adjust **elacestrant** dose, p. 1084. Severe Theoretical

▸ **Ciclosporin** causes a small decrease in the exposure to eltrombopag. Monitor platelet count and adjust dose. Moderate Study

▸ Encorafenib decreases the concentration of **ciclosporin**. Severe Study

▸ Endothelin receptor antagonists (bosentan) moderately decrease the exposure to **ciclosporin** and **ciclosporin** moderately increases the exposure to endothelin receptor antagonists (bosentan). Avoid. Severe Study

▸ **Ciclosporin** moderately increases the exposure to endothelin receptor antagonists (ambrisentan). Adjust **ambrisentan** dose and monitor, p. 210. Moderate Study

▸ **Ciclosporin** is predicted to increase the exposure to erlotinib. Moderate Theoretical

▸ **Ciclosporin** increases the exposure to etoposide. Monitor and adjust dose. Severe Study

▸ **Ciclosporin** moderately increases the exposure to everolimus. Avoid or adjust dose. Severe Study

▸ **Ciclosporin** moderately increases the exposure to ezetimibe and ezetimibe slightly increases the exposure to **ciclosporin**. Moderate Study

▸ **Ciclosporin** is predicted to increase the exposure to factor XA inhibitors (apixaban). Moderate Theoretical

▸ **Ciclosporin** slightly increases the exposure to factor XA inhibitors (edoxaban). Adjust **edoxaban** dose, p. 147. Severe Study

▸ **Ciclosporin** slightly increases the exposure to factor XA inhibitors (rivaroxaban). Moderate Study

▸ Fibrates (bezafibrate) are predicted to increase the risk of nephrotoxicity when given with **ciclosporin**. Severe Theoretical

▸ Fibrates (fenofibrate) increase the risk of nephrotoxicity when given with **ciclosporin**. Severe Study

▸ **Ciclosporin** is predicted to increase the exposure to fidaxomicin. Avoid. Moderate Study

▸ Filgotinib is predicted to increase the risk of immunosuppression when given with **ciclosporin**. Avoid. Severe Theoretical

▸ **Ciclosporin** is predicted to increase the exposure to gilteritinib. Moderate Theoretical

▸ **Ciclosporin** increases the exposure to glecaprevir. Avoid or monitor. Severe Study

▸ Glofitamab might affect the exposure to **ciclosporin**. Moderate Theoretical

▸ Grapefruit juice increases the concentration of **ciclosporin**. Avoid. Severe Study

▸ **Ciclosporin** greatly increases the exposure to grazoprevir. Avoid. Severe Study

▸ H₂ receptor antagonists (cimetidine) increase the concentration of **ciclosporin**. Mild Study

▸ HIV-protease inhibitors increase the concentration of **ciclosporin**. Severe Study

▸ Idelalisib increases the concentration of **ciclosporin**. Severe Study

▸ Imatinib is predicted to increase the concentration of **ciclosporin**. Severe Study

▸ Iron chelators (dexrazoxane) might increase the risk of immunosuppression when given with **ciclosporin**. Severe Theoretical

▸ Ivacaftor is predicted to increase the exposure to **ciclosporin**. Moderate Theoretical

▸ Ivosidenib decreases the concentration of **ciclosporin**. Severe Study

▸ **Ciclosporin** is predicted to increase the exposure to ivosidenib and ivosidenib might decrease the exposure to **ciclosporin**.

Ciclosporin (continued)

Monitor and adjust dose—consult product literature. [Severe] Study

▸ **Lanreotide** is predicted to decrease the absorption of oral **ciclosporin**. Adjust dose. [Severe] Theoretical

▸ **Ciclosporin** might increase the concentration of **lapatinib**. [Severe] Theoretical

▸ **Larotrectinib** is predicted to increase the exposure to **ciclosporin**. Use with caution and adjust dose. [Mild] Theoretical

▸ **Letermovir** increases the exposure to **ciclosporin** and **ciclosporin** increases the exposure to **letermovir**. Monitor and adjust **letermovir** dose, p. 735. [Severe] Study

▸ **Live vaccines** are predicted to increase the risk of generalised infection (possibly life-threatening) when given with **ciclosporin**. UKHSA advises avoid (refer to Green Book). [Severe] Theoretical

▸ **Ciclosporin** is predicted to increase the exposure to **lomitapide**. Separate administration by 12 hours. [Moderate] Theoretical

▸ **Lorlatinib** is predicted to decrease the exposure to **ciclosporin**. Avoid. [Moderate] Theoretical

▸ **Lumacaftor** decreases the concentration of **ciclosporin**. [Severe] Study

▸ **Macrolides (clarithromycin)** increase the concentration of **ciclosporin**. [Severe] Study

▸ **Macrolides (erythromycin)** greatly increase the exposure to **ciclosporin**. Avoid or monitor. [Severe] Study

▸ **Maribavir** is predicted to increase the exposure to **ciclosporin**. Monitor and adjust dose. [Severe] Theoretical

▸ **Ciclosporin** moderately increases the exposure to **meglitinides (repaglinide)**. [Moderate] Study

▸ **Metreleptin** might alter the exposure to **ciclosporin**. Monitor concentration and adjust dose. [Severe] Theoretical

▸ **Midostaurin** might increase the concentration of **ciclosporin**. [Severe] Anecdotal

▸ **Ciclosporin** is predicted to decrease the efficacy of **mifamurtide**. Avoid. [Severe] Theoretical

▸ **Mitotane** decreases the concentration of **ciclosporin**. [Severe] Study

▸ **Ciclosporin** is predicted to increase the exposure to **momelotinib**. [Moderate] Study

▸ **Monoclonal antibodies (blinatumomab, mosunetuzumab)** are predicted to transiently increase the exposure to **ciclosporin**. Monitor and adjust dose. [Moderate] Theoretical

▸ **Monoclonal antibodies (elranatamab)** might affect the exposure to **ciclosporin**. Monitor and adjust dose. [Moderate] Theoretical

▸ **Monoclonal antibodies (sarilumab)** potentially affect the exposure to **ciclosporin**. Monitor and adjust dose. [Moderate] Theoretical

▸ **Monoclonal antibodies (teclistamab)** might affect the exposure to **ciclosporin**. [Moderate] Theoretical

▸ **Monoclonal antibodies (tocilizumab)** are predicted to decrease the exposure to **ciclosporin**. Monitor and adjust dose. [Moderate] Theoretical

▸ **Ciclosporin** increases the risk of neutropenia when given with **monoclonal antibodies (brentuximab vedotin)**. Monitor and adjust dose. [Severe] Theoretical

▸ **Ciclosporin** is predicted to increase the exposure to **naldemedine**. [Moderate] Study

▸ **Ciclosporin** is predicted to increase the exposure to **neratinib**. Avoid or adjust dose and monitor for gastrointestinal adverse effects—consult product literature. [Severe] Study

▸ **Neurokinin-1 receptor antagonists (aprepitant, netupitant)** are predicted to increase the concentration of **ciclosporin**. [Severe] Study

▸ **Nilotinib** is predicted to increase the concentration of **ciclosporin**. [Severe] Study

▸ **Ciclosporin** is predicted to increase the exposure to **nintedanib**. [Moderate] Study

▸ **Nirmatrelvir** boosted with ritonavir is predicted to increase the concentration of **ciclosporin**. Avoid. [Severe] Theoretical

▸ **NNRTIs (efavirenz)** decrease the concentration of **ciclosporin**. Monitor concentration and adjust dose. [Moderate] Study

▸ **NNRTIs (etravirine)** are predicted to decrease the exposure to **ciclosporin**. [Moderate] Theoretical

▸ **NNRTIs (nevirapine)** are predicted to decrease the concentration of **ciclosporin**. [Moderate] Study

▸ **Ciclosporin** increases the concentration of **NSAIDs (diclofenac)**. [Severe] Study → Also see **TABLE 2** p. 1571 → Also see **TABLE 15** p. 1575

▸ **Octreotide** decreases the absorption of oral **ciclosporin**. Adjust **ciclosporin** dose, p. 966. [Severe] Anecdotal

▸ **Olaparib** might alter the exposure to **ciclosporin**. [Moderate] Theoretical

▸ **Palbociclib** is predicted to increase the exposure to **ciclosporin**. Adjust dose. [Moderate] Theoretical

▸ **Ciclosporin** is predicted to increase the exposure to **panobinostat**. Adjust dose. [Moderate] Theoretical

▸ **Pasireotide** is predicted to decrease the absorption of oral **ciclosporin**. Adjust dose. [Severe] Theoretical

▸ **Pitolisant** is predicted to decrease the exposure to **ciclosporin**. Avoid. [Severe] Theoretical

▸ **Pralsetinib** might affect the exposure to **ciclosporin** and **ciclosporin** is predicted to increase the exposure to **pralsetinib**. Avoid. [Moderate] Theoretical

▸ **Ciclosporin** is predicted to increase the concentration of **ranolazine** and **ranolazine** is predicted to increase the concentration of **ciclosporin**. [Moderate] Theoretical

▸ **Ciclosporin** is predicted to increase the exposure to **relugolix**. Avoid or take relugolix first and separate administration by at least 6 hours. [Moderate] Study

▸ **Ribociclib** is predicted to increase the exposure to **ciclosporin**. Use with caution and adjust dose. [Moderate] Theoretical

▸ **Rifamycins (rifampicin)** decrease the concentration of **ciclosporin**. [Severe] Study → Also see **TABLE 2** p. 1571

▸ **Ciclosporin** very markedly increases the exposure to **rifaximin**. [Severe] Study

▸ **Ciclosporin** slightly increases the exposure to **rimegepant**. Avoid another dose of rimegepant within 48 hours of concurrent use. [Moderate] Study

▸ **Ciclosporin** is predicted to increase the exposure to **riociguat**. [Moderate] Theoretical

▸ **Ritlecitinib** is predicted to increase the exposure to **ciclosporin** and **ciclosporin** is predicted to increase the risk of generalised infection (possibly life-threatening) when given with **ritlecitinib**. Avoid. [Severe] Theoretical

▸ **Rucaparib** is predicted to increase the exposure to **ciclosporin**. Monitor and adjust dose. [Moderate] Study

▸ **Ciclosporin** moderately increases the exposure to **sirolimus**. Separate administration by 4 hours. [Severe] Study

▸ **Somapacitan** might decrease the exposure to **ciclosporin**. [Severe] Theoretical

▸ **Somatrogon** might decrease the exposure to **ciclosporin**. [Severe] Theoretical

▸ **St John's wort** decreases the concentration of **ciclosporin**. Avoid. [Moderate] Study

▸ **Ciclosporin** markedly to very markedly increases the exposure to statins **(atorvastatin)**. Avoid or adjust **atorvastatin** dose, p. 234. [Severe] Study

▸ **Ciclosporin** moderately increases the exposure to statins **(fluvastatin)**. [Severe] Study

▸ **Ciclosporin** markedly to very markedly increases the exposure to statins **(pravastatin)**. Adjust dose. [Severe] Study

▸ **Ciclosporin** markedly increases the exposure to statins **(rosuvastatin)**. Avoid. [Severe] Study

▸ **Ciclosporin** markedly to very markedly increases the exposure to statins **(simvastatin)**. Avoid. [Severe] Study

▸ **Ciclosporin** is predicted to increase the exposure to **sulfonylureas (glibenclamide)** and **sulfonylureas (glibenclamide)** might increase the exposure to **ciclosporin**. Monitor and adjust **ciclosporin** dose, p. 966. [Moderate] Study

▸ **Ciclosporin** increases the concentration of **tacrolimus**. Avoid. [Severe] Study → Also see **TABLE 2** p. 1571 → Also see **TABLE 15** p. 1575

▸ **Ciclosporin** is predicted to slightly increase the exposure to **talazoparib**. Avoid or adjust dose—consult product literature. [Severe] Study

▸ **Ciclosporin** increases the concentration of **taxanes (docetaxel)** (oral). [Unknown] Study

▸ **Ciclosporin** increases the concentration of **taxanes (paclitaxel)**. [Severe] Study

- **Tebentafusp** is predicted to transiently increase the exposure to **ciclosporin**. Monitor and adjust dose. Moderate Theoretical
- **Ciclosporin** is predicted to increase the exposure to tenofovir alafenamide. Moderate Theoretical
- **Ciclosporin** is predicted to increase the exposure to tenofovir disoproxil. Moderate Theoretical → Also see TABLE 2 p. 1571
- **Tetracyclines (doxycycline)** are predicted to increase the concentration of **ciclosporin**. Severe Theoretical
- **Ciclosporin** is predicted to increase the exposure to thrombin inhibitors (dabigatran). Avoid. Severe Study
- **Ciclosporin** is predicted to increase the exposure to ticagrelor. Use with caution or avoid. Severe Study
- **Ciclosporin** might increase the exposure to tigecycline and tigecycline has been reported to increase the concentration of **ciclosporin**. Severe Anecdotal
- **Ciclosporin** increases the exposure to tofacitinib. Avoid. Severe Study
- **Ciclosporin** is predicted to increase the exposure to topotecan. Severe Study
- **Ciclosporin** is predicted to increase the concentration of trametinib. Moderate Theoretical
- **Tucatinib** increases the concentration of **ciclosporin**. Severe Study
- **Ursodeoxycholic acid** affects the concentration of **ciclosporin**. Use with caution and adjust dose. Severe Anecdotal
- **Ciclosporin** might affect the exposure to vemurafenib. Severe Theoretical
- **Ciclosporin** is predicted to increase the exposure to venetoclax. Avoid or monitor for toxicity. Severe Theoretical
- **Ciclosporin** might increase the exposure to vinca alkaloids. Severe Theoretical
- **Vitamin E substances** affect the exposure to **ciclosporin**. Moderate Study
- **Ciclosporin** increases the concentration of voxilaprevir. Avoid. Severe Study

Cidofovir → see TABLE 2 p. 1571 (nephrotoxicity)
Cilostazol → see TABLE 4 p. 1571 (antiplatelet effects)

GENERAL INFORMATION Concurrent use with 2 or more antiplatelets or anticoagulants is contra-indicated.

- **Anti-androgens (apalutamide, enzalutamide)** are predicted to alter the effects of **cilostazol**. Moderate Theoretical
- **Antiepileptics (carbamazepine, fosphenytoin, phenobarbital, phenytoin, primidone)** are predicted to alter the effects of **cilostazol**. Moderate Theoretical
- **Antifungals, azoles (fluconazole)** are predicted to increase the exposure to **cilostazol**. Adjust **cilostazol** dose, p. 266. Moderate Theoretical
- **Antifungals, azoles (itraconazole, ketoconazole, posaconazole, voriconazole)** are predicted to moderately increase the exposure to **cilostazol**. Adjust **cilostazol** dose, p. 266. Moderate Study
- **Antifungals, azoles (miconazole)** are predicted to increase the exposure to **cilostazol**. Use with caution and adjust dose. Moderate Theoretical
- **Ceritinib** is predicted to moderately increase the exposure to **cilostazol**. Adjust **cilostazol** dose, p. 266. Moderate Study
- **Cilostazol** might increases the exposure to cladribine. Avoid or adjust dose. Moderate Theoretical
- **Cobicistat** is predicted to moderately increase the exposure to **cilostazol**. Adjust **cilostazol** dose, p. 266. Moderate Study
- **Encorafenib** is predicted to alter the effects of **cilostazol**. Moderate Theoretical
- **HIV-protease inhibitors** are predicted to moderately increase the exposure to **cilostazol**. Adjust **cilostazol** dose, p. 266. Moderate Study
- **Idelalisib** is predicted to moderately increase the exposure to **cilostazol**. Adjust **cilostazol** dose, p. 266. Moderate Study
- **Ivosidenib** is predicted to alter the effects of **cilostazol**. Moderate Theoretical
- **Cilostazol** is predicted to increase the exposure to lomitapide. Separate administration by 12 hours. Moderate Theoretical
- **Lumacaftor** is predicted to alter the effects of **cilostazol**. Moderate Theoretical

- **Macrolides (clarithromycin)** are predicted to moderately increase the exposure to **cilostazol**. Adjust **cilostazol** dose, p. 266. Moderate Study
- **Macrolides (erythromycin)** slightly increase the exposure to **cilostazol**. Adjust **cilostazol** dose, p. 266. Moderate Study
- **Cilostazol** might increase the exposure to metoclopramide. Moderate Study
- **Mitotane** is predicted to alter the effects of **cilostazol**. Moderate Theoretical
- **Moclobemide** is predicted to increase the exposure to **cilostazol**. Moderate Theoretical
- **Nirmatrelvir** boosted with ritonavir is predicted to increase the concentration of **cilostazol**. Adjust dose. Moderate Theoretical
- **Proton pump inhibitors (esomeprazole)** are predicted to increase the exposure to **cilostazol**. Moderate Theoretical
- **Proton pump inhibitors (omeprazole)** are predicted to increase the exposure to **cilostazol**. Adjust **cilostazol** dose, p. 266. Moderate Study
- **Rifamycins (rifampicin)** are predicted to alter the effects of **cilostazol**. Moderate Theoretical
- **Selumetinib** might increase the risk of bleeding when given with **cilostazol**. Severe Theoretical
- **SSRIs (fluoxetine, fluvoxamine)** are predicted to increase the exposure to **cilostazol**. Adjust **cilostazol** dose, p. 266. Moderate Theoretical → Also see TABLE 4 p. 1571
- **St John's wort** is predicted to alter the effects of **cilostazol**. Moderate Theoretical
- **Cilostazol** is predicted to increase the exposure to statins (atorvastatin). Moderate Theoretical
- **Cilostazol** slightly increases the exposure to statins (simvastatin). Moderate Study
- **Tucatinib** is predicted to moderately increase the exposure to **cilostazol**. Adjust **cilostazol** dose, p. 266. Moderate Study

Cimetidine → see H₂ receptor antagonists
Cinacalcet

FOOD AND LIFESTYLE Dose adjustment might be necessary if smoking started or stopped during treatment.

- **Anti-androgens (apalutamide, enzalutamide)** are predicted to decrease the exposure to **cinacalcet**. Monitor and adjust dose. Moderate Study
- **Cinacalcet** is predicted to increase the exposure to anticholinesterases, centrally acting (galantamine). Monitor and adjust dose. Moderate Study
- **Antiepileptics (carbamazepine, fosphenytoin, phenobarbital, phenytoin, primidone)** are predicted to decrease the exposure to **cinacalcet**. Monitor and adjust dose. Moderate Study
- **Antifungals, azoles (itraconazole, ketoconazole, posaconazole, voriconazole)** are predicted to moderately increase the exposure to **cinacalcet**. Adjust dose. Moderate Study
- **Cinacalcet** is predicted to moderately increase the exposure to antipsychotics, second generation (aripiprazole). Adjust **aripiprazole** dose, p. 454. Moderate Study
- **Cinacalcet** is predicted to increase the exposure to antipsychotics, second generation (clozapine). Use with caution and adjust dose. Severe Study
- **Cinacalcet** is predicted to increase the exposure to antipsychotics, second generation (risperidone). Adjust dose. Moderate Study
- **Cinacalcet** is predicted to markedly increase the exposure to atomoxetine. Adjust dose. Severe Study
- **Cinacalcet** is predicted to increase the exposure to beta blockers, selective (metoprolol, nebivolol). Moderate Study
- **Ceritinib** is predicted to moderately increase the exposure to **cinacalcet**. Adjust dose. Moderate Study
- **Cobicistat** is predicted to moderately increase the exposure to **cinacalcet**. Adjust dose. Moderate Study
- **Cinacalcet** is predicted to slightly increase the exposure to darifenacin. Mild Study
- **Cinacalcet** might increase the risk of hypocalcaemia when given with denosumab. Severe Theoretical
- **Cinacalcet** is predicted to increase the exposure to eliglustat. Avoid or adjust dose—consult product literature. Severe Study
- **Encorafenib** is predicted to decrease the exposure to **cinacalcet**. Monitor and adjust dose. Moderate Study

Cinacalcet (continued)

▸ **Cinacalcet** increases the risk of hypocalcaemia when given with etelcalcetide. Avoid. [Severe] Theoretical

▸ **Cinacalcet** is predicted to increase the exposure to fenfluramine. [Moderate] Study

▸ **Cinacalcet** is predicted to increase the exposure to fesoterodine. Use with caution and adjust dose. [Mild] Theoretical

▸ **Cinacalcet** is predicted to increase the exposure to gefitinib. [Moderate] Theoretical

▸ HIV-protease inhibitors are predicted to moderately increase the exposure to **cinacalcet**. Adjust dose. [Moderate] Study

▸ Idelalisib is predicted to moderately increase the exposure to **cinacalcet**. Adjust dose. [Moderate] Study

▸ Ivosidenib is predicted to decrease the exposure to **cinacalcet**. Monitor and adjust dose. [Moderate] Study

▸ Lumacaftor is predicted to decrease the exposure to **cinacalcet**. Monitor and adjust dose. [Moderate] Study

▸ Macrolides (clarithromycin) are predicted to moderately increase the exposure to **cinacalcet**. Adjust dose. [Moderate] Study

▸ **Cinacalcet** is predicted to increase the exposure to mexiletine. [Moderate] Study

▸ Mitotane is predicted to decrease the exposure to **cinacalcet**. Monitor and adjust dose. [Moderate] Study

▸ **Cinacalcet** is predicted to decrease the efficacy of opioids (codeine). [Moderate] Theoretical

▸ **Cinacalcet** is predicted to decrease the efficacy of opioids (tramadol). [Severe] Study

▸ **Cinacalcet** is predicted to moderately increase the exposure to pitolisant. Use with caution and adjust dose. [Moderate] Study

▸ Rifamycins (rifampicin) are predicted to decrease the exposure to **cinacalcet**. Monitor and adjust dose. [Moderate] Study

▸ SSRIs (fluvoxamine) are predicted to increase the exposure to **cinacalcet**. Adjust dose. [Moderate] Theoretical

▸ **Cinacalcet** is predicted to increase the exposure to SSRIs (dapoxetine). [Moderate] Theoretical

▸ **Cinacalcet** is predicted to decrease the efficacy of tamoxifen. Avoid. [Severe] Study

▸ **Cinacalcet** is predicted to increase the exposure to the active metabolite of tetrabenazine. [Moderate] Study

▸ **Cinacalcet** is predicted to increase the exposure to tricyclic antidepressants. Monitor for toxicity and adjust dose. [Severe] Study

▸ Tucatinib is predicted to moderately increase the exposure to **cinacalcet**. Adjust dose. [Moderate] Study

▸ **Cinacalcet** is predicted to increase the exposure to vortioxetine. Monitor and adjust dose. [Moderate] Study

Cinnarizine → see antihistamines, sedating

Ciprofibrate → see fibrates

Ciprofloxacin → see quinolones

Cisatracurium → see neuromuscular blocking drugs, non-depolarising

Cisplatin → see platinum compounds

Citalopram → see SSRIs

Cladribine → see TABLE 14 p. 1575 (myelosuppression)

SEPARATION OF ADMINISTRATION Oral cladribine might affect the absorption of concurrently administered drugs—consider separating administration by at least 3 hours.

▸ Anti-androgens (darolutamide) are predicted to increase the exposure to **cladribine**. Avoid or adjust dose. [Moderate] Theoretical

▸ Antiepileptics (carbamazepine) are predicted to increase the risk of haematological toxicity when given with oral **cladribine**. [Moderate] Theoretical

▸ Calcium channel blockers (nifedipine, nimodipine) might increase the exposure to **cladribine**. Avoid or adjust dose. [Moderate] Theoretical

▸ Ciclosporin is predicted to increase the exposure to **cladribine**. Avoid or adjust dose. [Moderate] Theoretical

▸ Cilostazol might increases the exposure to **cladribine**. Avoid or adjust dose. [Moderate] Theoretical

▸ Dipyridamole might increases the exposure to **cladribine**. [Moderate] Theoretical

▸ Eltrombopag is predicted to increase the exposure to **cladribine**. Avoid or adjust dose. [Moderate] Theoretical

▸ Febuxostat is predicted to increase the exposure to **cladribine**. Avoid or adjust dose. [Moderate] Theoretical

▸ Fostamatinib is predicted to increase the exposure to **cladribine**. Avoid or adjust dose. [Moderate] Theoretical

▸ HIV-protease inhibitors (ritonavir) might increase the exposure to **cladribine**. [Moderate] Theoretical

▸ Leflunomide is predicted to increase the exposure to **cladribine**. Avoid or adjust dose. [Moderate] Theoretical → Also see TABLE 14 p. 1575

▸ Live vaccines are predicted to increase the risk of generalised infection (possibly life-threatening) when given with **cladribine**. UKHSA advises avoid (refer to Green Book). [Severe] Theoretical

▸ NSAIDs (sulindac) might increase the exposure to **cladribine**. Avoid or adjust dose. [Moderate] Theoretical

▸ Teriflunomide is predicted to increase the exposure to **cladribine**. Avoid or adjust dose. [Moderate] Theoretical

▸ Velpatasvir is predicted to increase the exposure to **cladribine**. Avoid or adjust dose. [Moderate] Theoretical

▸ Voxilaprevir is predicted to increase the exposure to **cladribine**. Avoid or adjust dose. [Moderate] Theoretical

Clarithromycin → see macrolides

Clindamycin

ROUTE-SPECIFIC INFORMATION Since systemic absorption can follow topical application of **clindamycin**, the possibility of interactions should be borne in mind.

▸ **Clindamycin** increases the effects of neuromuscular blocking drugs, non-depolarising. [Severe] Anecdotal

▸ **Clindamycin** increases the effects of suxamethonium. [Severe] Anecdotal

Clobazam → see benzodiazepines

Clodronate → see bisphosphonates

Clofarabine → see TABLE 1 p. 1571 (hepatotoxicity), TABLE 14 p. 1575 (myelosuppression)

▸ Live vaccines are predicted to increase the risk of generalised infection (possibly life-threatening) when given with **clofarabine**. UKHSA advises avoid (refer to Green Book). [Severe] Theoretical

Clofazimine

▸ **Clofazimine** potentially increases the risk of QT-prolongation when given with bedaquiline. [Severe] Study

Clomethiazole → see TABLE 10 p. 1574 (CNS effects)

▸ Alcohol causes serious, potentially fatal, CNS depression when given with **clomethiazole**. Avoid. [Severe] Study → Also see TABLE 10 p. 1574

▸ Anti-androgens (apalutamide, enzalutamide) decrease the exposure to **clomethiazole**. Monitor and adjust dose. [Moderate] Study

▸ Antiepileptics (carbamazepine, fosphenytoin, phenobarbital, phenytoin, primidone) decrease the exposure to **clomethiazole**. Monitor and adjust dose. [Moderate] Study → Also see TABLE 10 p. 1574

▸ Encorafenib decreases the exposure to **clomethiazole**. Monitor and adjust dose. [Moderate] Study

▸ Ivosidenib decreases the exposure to **clomethiazole**. Monitor and adjust dose. [Moderate] Study

▸ Lumacaftor decreases the exposure to **clomethiazole**. Monitor and adjust dose. [Moderate] Study

▸ Mitotane decreases the exposure to **clomethiazole**. Monitor and adjust dose. [Moderate] Study

▸ Rifamycins (rifampicin) decrease the exposure to **clomethiazole**. Monitor and adjust dose. [Moderate] Study

Clomipramine → see tricyclic antidepressants

Clonazepam → see benzodiazepines

Clonidine → see TABLE 5 p. 1572 (bradycardia), TABLE 7 p. 1572 (hypotension), TABLE 10 p. 1574 (CNS effects)

▸ Tricyclic antidepressants decrease the antihypertensive effects of **clonidine**. Monitor and adjust dose. [Moderate] Anecdotal → Also see TABLE 7 p. 1572 → Also see TABLE 10 p. 1574

Clopidogrel → see TABLE 4 p. 1571 (antiplatelet effects)

▸ **Clopidogrel** is predicted to increase the exposure to anti-androgens (apalutamide) and anti-androgens (apalutamide) are predicted to increase the exposure to the active metabolite of **clopidogrel**. Avoid or monitor. [Moderate] Study

▸ **Clopidogrel** moderately increases the exposure to anti-androgens **(enzalutamide)**. Avoid or adjust **enzalutamide** dose, p. 1078. [Severe] Study

▸ Antifungals, azoles **(fluconazole)** are predicted to decrease the efficacy of **clopidogrel**. Avoid. [Severe] Theoretical

▸ Antifungals, azoles **(voriconazole)** are predicted to decrease the efficacy of **clopidogrel**. Avoid. [Moderate] Study

▸ **Clopidogrel** slightly increases the exposure to bupropion. [Moderate] Study

▸ Cenobamate is predicted to decrease the efficacy of **clopidogrel**. Avoid. [Moderate] Study

▸ Cobicistat is predicted to decrease the concentration of the active metabolite of **clopidogrel**. Avoid. [Severe] Theoretical

▸ **Clopidogrel** is predicted to increase the exposure to dabrafenib. [Moderate] Theoretical

▸ **Clopidogrel** are predicted to increases the exposure to etrasimod. Avoid in poor CYP2C9 metabolisers. [Severe] Theoretical

▸ Fedratinib is predicted to decrease the efficacy of **clopidogrel**. Avoid. [Moderate] Study

▸ Grapefruit juice markedly decreases the exposure to **clopidogrel**. [Severe] Study

▸ HIV-protease inhibitors **(ritonavir)** might decrease the efficacy of **clopidogrel**. Avoid. [Moderate] Theoretical

▸ **Clopidogrel** increases the exposure to meglitinides **(repaglinide)**. Avoid. [Severe] Study

▸ Moclobemide is predicted to decrease the efficacy of **clopidogrel**. Avoid. [Moderate] Study

▸ **Clopidogrel** is predicted to moderately increase the exposure to montelukast. [Moderate] Study

▸ Nirmatrelvir boosted with ritonavir is predicted to decrease the concentration of **clopidogrel**. [Severe] Theoretical

▸ **Clopidogrel** is predicted to increase the exposure to the active metabolites of ozanimod. [Moderate] Study

▸ **Clopidogrel** increases the exposure to pioglitazone. Monitor blood glucose and adjust dose. [Severe] Study

▸ Proton pump inhibitors **(esomeprazole, omeprazole)** are predicted to decrease the efficacy of **clopidogrel**. Avoid. [Moderate] Study

▸ **Clopidogrel** is predicted to increase the exposure to retinoids **(alitretinoin)**. Adjust **alitretinoin** dose, p. 1433. [Moderate] Theoretical

▸ Rifamycins **(rifampicin)** moderately increase the exposure to the active metabolite of **clopidogrel**. Avoid. [Moderate] Study

▸ **Clopidogrel** is predicted to increase the exposure to selexipag. Adjust **selexipag** dose, p. 209. [Moderate] Study

▸ Selumetinib might increase the risk of bleeding when given with **clopidogrel**. [Severe] Theoretical

▸ SSRIs **(fluoxetine, fluvoxamine)** are predicted to decrease the efficacy of **clopidogrel**. Avoid. [Severe] Theoretical → Also see **TABLE 4** p. 1571

▸ **Clopidogrel** increases the exposure to statins **(rosuvastatin)**. Adjust **rosuvastatin** dose, p. 235. [Moderate] Study

▸ **Clopidogrel** is predicted to increase the concentration of taxanes **(paclitaxel)**. [Severe] Anecdotal

▸ **Clopidogrel** is predicted to increase the exposure to treprostinil. Adjust dose. [Moderate] Theoretical → Also see **TABLE 4** p. 1571

▸ **Clopidogrel** is predicted to increase the exposure to tucatinib. Avoid or adjust dose—consult product literature. [Severe] Study

Clotrimazole → see antifungals, azoles

Clozapine → see antipsychotics, second generation

Cobicistat

▸ **Cobicistat** is predicted to increase the exposure to abemaciclib. Avoid or adjust dose—consult product literature. [Severe] Study

▸ **Cobicistat** is predicted to increase the exposure to acalabrutinib. Avoid. [Severe] Study

▸ **Cobicistat** is predicted to increase the exposure to afatinib. [Moderate] Study

▸ **Cobicistat** is predicted to increase the exposure to aliskiren. [Moderate] Study

▸ **Cobicistat** is predicted to moderately increase the exposure to alpha blockers **(alfuzosin, tamsulosin)**. Use with caution or avoid. [Moderate] Study

▸ **Cobicistat** is predicted to increase the exposure to alpha blockers **(doxazosin)**. [Moderate] Study

▸ Anti-androgens **(apalutamide, enzalutamide)** are predicted to decrease the exposure to **cobicistat**. Avoid. [Severe] Study

▸ **Cobicistat** is predicted to increase the exposure to anti-androgens **(apalutamide)**. Monitor and adjust dose. [Mild] Study

▸ **Cobicistat** potentially increases the concentration of antiarrhythmics **(amiodarone, disopyramide, flecainide, lidocaine)**. [Severe] Theoretical

▸ **Cobicistat** very markedly increases the exposure to antiarrhythmics **(dronedarone)**. Avoid. [Severe] Study

▸ **Cobicistat** is predicted to increase the exposure to antiarrhythmics **(propafenone)**. Monitor and adjust dose. [Severe] Study

▸ **Cobicistat** is predicted to increase the exposure to anticholinesterases, centrally acting **(galantamine)**. Monitor and adjust dose. [Moderate] Study

▸ Antiepileptics **(carbamazepine, fosphenytoin, phenobarbital, phenytoin, primidone)** are predicted to decrease the exposure to **cobicistat**. Avoid. [Severe] Study

▸ Antiepileptics **(eslicarbazepine, oxcarbazepine)** are predicted to decrease the concentration of **cobicistat**. [Severe] Theoretical

▸ **Cobicistat** is predicted to very slightly increase the exposure to antiepileptics **(perampanel)**. [Mild] Study

▸ **Cobicistat** is predicted to increase the exposure to antifungals, azoles **(fluconazole, posaconazole)**. [Moderate] Theoretical

▸ **Cobicistat** is predicted to increase the exposure to antifungals, azoles **(isavuconazole)**. Avoid or monitor adverse effects. [Severe] Study

▸ **Cobicistat** is predicted to increase the exposure to antifungals, azoles **(itraconazole)**. Adjust **itraconazole** dose, p. 692. [Moderate] Theoretical

▸ **Cobicistat** is predicted to increase the exposure to antifungals, azoles **(ketoconazole)**. Adjust **ketoconazole** dose, p. 794. [Moderate] Theoretical

▸ **Cobicistat** is predicted to affect the exposure to antifungals, azoles **(voriconazole)**. Avoid. [Moderate] Theoretical

▸ **Cobicistat** is predicted to increase the exposure to antihistamines, non-sedating **(fexofenadine)**. [Moderate] Theoretical

▸ **Cobicistat** is predicted to increase the exposure to antihistamines, non-sedating **(mizolastine)**. Avoid. [Severe] Study

▸ **Cobicistat** is predicted to increase the exposure to antihistamines, non-sedating **(rupatadine)**. Avoid. [Moderate] Study

▸ **Cobicistat** is predicted to slightly increase the exposure to antipsychotics, second generation **(aripiprazole)**. Adjust **aripiprazole** dose, p. 454. [Moderate] Study

▸ **Cobicistat** is predicted to moderately increase the exposure to antipsychotics, second generation **(cariprazine)**. Avoid. [Severe] Study

▸ **Cobicistat** is predicted to increase the exposure to antipsychotics, second generation **(lurasidone, quetiapine)**. Avoid. [Severe] Study

▸ **Cobicistat** is predicted to increase the exposure to antipsychotics, second generation **(risperidone)**. Adjust dose. [Moderate] Study

▸ **Cobicistat** is predicted to increase the exposure to atogepant. Adjust **atogepant** dose, p. 540. [Moderate] Study

▸ **Cobicistat** is predicted to increase the exposure to avacopan. [Severe] Study

▸ **Cobicistat** is predicted to increase the exposure to avapritinib. Avoid. [Moderate] Study

▸ **Cobicistat** is predicted to increase the exposure to axitinib. Avoid or adjust dose. [Moderate] Study

▸ **Cobicistat** might increases the exposure to bedaquiline. [Mild] Study

▸ **Cobicistat** moderately increases the exposure to benzodiazepines **(alprazolam)**. Avoid. [Moderate] Study

▸ **Cobicistat** is predicted to markedly to very markedly increase the exposure to benzodiazepines **(midazolam)**. Avoid or adjust dose. [Severe] Study

▸ **Cobicistat** is predicted to increase the exposure to beta$_2$ agonists **(salmeterol)**. Avoid. [Severe] Study

▸ **Cobicistat** is predicted to increase the exposure to bictegravir. Use with caution or avoid. [Moderate] Theoretical

Cobicistat (continued)

▶ **Cobicistat** slightly increases the exposure to bortezomib. Moderate Study

▶ **Cobicistat** is predicted to increase the exposure to bosutinib. Avoid or adjust dose. Severe Study

▶ **Cobicistat** is predicted to increase the exposure to brigatinib. Avoid or adjust dose—consult product literature. Severe Study

▶ **Cobicistat** is predicted to increase the exposure to buspirone. Adjust **buspirone** dose, p. 396. Severe Study

▶ **Cobicistat** is predicted to increase the exposure to cabozantinib. Moderate Study

▶ **Cobicistat** is predicted to increase the exposure to calcium channel blockers (amlodipine, felodipine, lacidipine, nicardipine, nifedipine, nimodipine). Monitor and adjust dose. Moderate Study

▶ **Cobicistat** is predicted to increase the exposure to calcium channel blockers (diltiazem, verapamil). Severe Study

▶ **Cobicistat** is predicted to markedly increase the exposure to calcium channel blockers (lercanidipine). Avoid. Severe Study

▶ **Cobicistat** is predicted to increase the exposure to cannabidiol. Avoid or adjust dose. Mild Study

▶ **Cobicistat** is predicted to increase the exposure to capivasertib. Adjust dose. Moderate Study

▶ Cenobamate is predicted to decrease the exposure to cobicistat. Avoid. Severe Theoretical

▶ **Cobicistat** is predicted to increase the exposure to ceritinib. Avoid or adjust dose—consult product literature. Severe Study

▶ **Cobicistat** increases the concentration of ciclosporin. Severe Study

▶ **Cobicistat** is predicted to moderately increase the exposure to cilostazol. Adjust **cilostazol** dose, p. 266. Moderate Study

▶ **Cobicistat** is predicted to moderately increase the exposure to cinacalcet. Adjust dose. Moderate Study

▶ **Cobicistat** is predicted to decrease the concentration of the active metabolite of clopidogrel. Avoid. Severe Theoretical

▶ **Cobicistat** is predicted to increase the exposure to cobimetinib. Avoid or monitor for toxicity. Severe Study

▶ **Cobicistat** is predicted to increase the exposure to colchicine. Avoid potent CYP3A4 inhibitors or adjust **colchicine** dose, p. 1279. Severe Study

▶ **Cobicistat** is predicted to decrease the efficacy of combined hormonal contraceptives. Avoid. Severe Study

▶ **Cobicistat** is predicted to increase the exposure to corticosteroids (beclometasone) (risk with beclometasone is likely to be lower than with other corticosteroids). Moderate Theoretical

▶ **Cobicistat** is predicted to increase the exposure to corticosteroids (betamethasone, budesonide, ciclesonide, deflazacort, dexamethasone, fludrocortisone, fluticasone, hydrocortisone, methylprednisolone, mometasone, prednisolone, triamcinolone). Avoid or monitor adverse effects. Severe Study

▶ **Cobicistat** is predicted to increase the exposure to corticosteroids (vamorolone). Adjust dose. Severe Study

▶ **Cobicistat** is predicted to affect the exposure to coumarins (warfarin). Moderate Theoretical

▶ **Cobicistat** is predicted to increase the exposure to crizotinib. Avoid. Moderate Study

▶ Dabrafenib is predicted to decrease the exposure to cobicistat. Avoid. Severe Theoretical

▶ **Cobicistat** is predicted to increase the exposure to dabrafenib. Use with caution or avoid. Moderate Study

▶ **Cobicistat** is predicted to increase the exposure to daridorexant. Avoid. Severe Study

▶ **Cobicistat** is predicted to markedly to very markedly increase the exposure to darifenacin. Avoid. Severe Study

▶ **Cobicistat** is predicted to increase the exposure to dasatinib. Avoid or adjust dose—consult product literature. Severe Study

▶ **Cobicistat** very slightly increases the exposure to delamanid. Severe Study

▶ **Cobicistat** is predicted to moderately increase the exposure to dienogest. Moderate Study

▶ **Cobicistat** is predicted to increase the exposure to dipeptidylpeptidase-4 inhibitors (saxagliptin). Moderate Study

▶ **Cobicistat** is predicted to increase the exposure to domperidone. Avoid. Severe Study

▶ **Cobicistat** increases the exposure to dopamine receptor agonists (bromocriptine). Severe Study

▶ **Cobicistat** is predicted to increase the concentration of dopamine receptor agonists (cabergoline). Moderate Anecdotal

▶ **Cobicistat** is predicted to increase the exposure to dronabinol. Adjust dose. Mild Study

▶ **Cobicistat** is predicted to increase the exposure to drospirenone. Severe Study

▶ **Cobicistat** is predicted to increase the exposure to dutasteride. Monitor adverse effects and adjust dose. Moderate Theoretical

▶ **Cobicistat** is predicted to increase the exposure to elacestrant. Avoid potent CYP3A4 inhibitors or adjust **elacestrant** dose, p. 1084. Severe Study

▶ **Cobicistat** is predicted to increase the exposure to elexacaftor. Adjust ivacaftor with tezacaftor and elexacaftor p. 337 dose with potent CYP3A4 inhibitors. Severe Study

▶ **Cobicistat** is predicted to increase the exposure to eliglustat. Avoid or adjust dose—consult product literature. Severe Study

▶ Encorafenib is predicted to decrease the exposure to cobicistat. Avoid. Severe Study

▶ **Cobicistat** is predicted to increase the exposure to encorafenib. Avoid or monitor. Severe Study

▶ Endothelin receptor antagonists (bosentan) are predicted to decrease the exposure to cobicistat. Avoid. Severe Theoretical

▶ **Cobicistat** is predicted to increase the exposure to endothelin receptor antagonists (macitentan). Moderate Study

▶ **Cobicistat** is predicted to increase the exposure to the cytotoxic component of enfortumab vedotin. Severe Theoretical

▶ **Cobicistat** is predicted to increase the exposure to entrectinib. Avoid or adjust dose with potent CYP3A4 inhibitors—consult product literature. Severe Study

▶ **Cobicistat** is predicted to increase the exposure to erdafitinib. Adjust dose. Severe Study

▶ **Cobicistat** is predicted to increase the risk of ergotism when given with ergometrine. Avoid. Severe Theoretical

▶ **Cobicistat** is predicted to increase the exposure to erlotinib. Use with caution and adjust dose. Severe Study

▶ **Cobicistat** is predicted to increase the exposure to esketamine. Adjust dose. Moderate Study

▶ **Cobicistat** is predicted to increase the exposure to eszopiclone. Adjust **eszopiclone** dose; avoid in the elderly, p. 554. Moderate Study

▶ **Cobicistat** is predicted to increase the concentration of subdermal etonogestrel. Moderate Theoretical

▶ **Cobicistat** is predicted to increase the exposure to etrasimod. Avoid in poor CYP2C9 metabolisers. Severe Theoretical

▶ **Cobicistat** is predicted to increase the exposure to everolimus. Avoid. Severe Study

▶ **Cobicistat** is predicted to increase the exposure to factor XA inhibitors (apixaban, edoxaban, rivaroxaban). Avoid. Severe Theoretical

▶ **Cobicistat** is predicted to increase the exposure to fedratinib. Adjust dose, but avoid depending on other drugs taken—consult product literature. Moderate Study

▶ **Cobicistat** is predicted to moderately increase the exposure to fesoterodine. Adjust **fesoterodine** dose with potent CYP3A4 inhibitors; avoid in hepatic and renal impairment, p. 897. Severe Study

▶ **Cobicistat** is predicted to increase the exposure to fidaxomicin. Avoid. Moderate Study

▶ **Cobicistat** is predicted to increase the exposure to fostamatinib. Monitor adverse effects and adjust dose. Moderate Study

▶ **Cobicistat** is predicted to increase the exposure to gefitinib. Severe Study

▶ **Cobicistat** is predicted to increase the exposure to gilteritinib. Moderate Study

▶ **Cobicistat** is predicted to increase the exposure to glasdegib. Use with caution or avoid. Severe Study

▶ **Cobicistat** potentially increases the exposure to glecaprevir. Moderate Theoretical

▶ **Cobicistat** is predicted to moderately to markedly increase the exposure to grazoprevir. Avoid. Severe Study

- **Cobicistat** is predicted to increase the exposure to guanfacine. Adjust **guanfacine** dose, p. 407. [Moderate] Study
- **Cobicistat** is predicted to increase the exposure to ibrutinib. Avoid or adjust dose with potent CYP3A4 inhibitors—consult product literature. [Severe] Study
- **Cobicistat** is predicted to increase the exposure to idelalisib. [Moderate] Theoretical
- **Cobicistat** is predicted to increase the exposure to imatinib. [Moderate] Study
- **Cobicistat** is predicted to increase the risk of toxicity when given with irinotecan. Avoid. [Severe] Study
- **Cobicistat** is predicted to increase the exposure to ivabradine. Avoid. [Severe] Study
- **Cobicistat** is predicted to increase the exposure to ivacaftor. Adjust dose with potent CYP3A4 inhibitors, see ivacaftor p. 336, lumacaftor with ivacaftor p. 338, tezacaftor with ivacaftor p. 339, and ivacaftor with tezacaftor and elexacaftor p. 337. [Severe] Study
- Ivosidenib is predicted to decrease the exposure to **cobicistat**. Avoid. [Severe] Study
- **Cobicistat** is predicted to increase the exposure to ivosidenib. Monitor and adjust dose—consult product literature. [Severe] Study
- **Cobicistat** is predicted to increase the exposure to lapatinib. Avoid. [Moderate] Study
- **Cobicistat** is predicted to moderately increase the exposure to larotrectinib. Avoid or adjust dose—consult product literature. [Moderate] Study
- **Cobicistat** is predicted to increase the exposure to leniolisib. Avoid. [Moderate] Study
- **Cobicistat** is predicted to markedly increase the exposure to lomitapide. Avoid. [Severe] Study
- **Cobicistat** is predicted to increase the exposure to lorlatinib. Avoid or adjust dose—consult product literature. [Severe] Study
- Lorlatinib is predicted to decrease the exposure to **cobicistat**. Avoid. [Severe] Theoretical
- Lumacaftor is predicted to decrease the exposure to **cobicistat**. Avoid. [Severe] Study
- **Cobicistat** is predicted to increase the concentration of macrolides (erythromycin). [Moderate] Theoretical
- **Cobicistat** markedly increases the exposure to maraviroc. Refer to specialist literature. [Severe] Study
- **Cobicistat** is predicted to increase the exposure to mavacamten. Avoid or monitor—consult product literature. [Severe] Study
- **Cobicistat** is predicted to increase the concentration of intramuscular medroxyprogesterone. [Moderate] Theoretical
- **Cobicistat** potentially increases the exposure to mexiletine. [Severe] Theoretical
- **Cobicistat** is predicted to increase the exposure to midostaurin. Avoid or monitor for toxicity. [Severe] Study
- **Cobicistat** is predicted to markedly increase the exposure to mineralocorticoid receptor antagonists (eplerenone). Avoid. [Severe] Study
- **Cobicistat** is predicted to increase the exposure to mineralocorticoid receptor antagonists (finerenone). Avoid. [Severe] Study
- **Cobicistat** is predicted to increase the exposure to mirabegron. Adjust **mirabegron** dose in hepatic and renal impairment, p. 901. [Moderate] Study
- **Cobicistat** is predicted to increase the exposure to mirtazapine. [Moderate] Study
- Mitotane is predicted to decrease the exposure to **cobicistat**. Avoid. [Severe] Study
- **Cobicistat** is predicted to increase the exposure to mobocertinib. Avoid. [Severe] Study
- **Cobicistat** is predicted to increase the exposure to modafinil. [Mild] Theoretical
- **Cobicistat** is predicted to increase the risk of neutropenia when given with monoclonal antibodies (brentuximab vedotin). Monitor and adjust dose. [Severe] Study
- **Cobicistat** is predicted to increase the exposure to monoclonal antibodies (polatuzumab vedotin). [Moderate] Theoretical

- **Cobicistat** is predicted to increase the exposure to the cytotoxic component of monoclonal antibodies (trastuzumab emtansine). Avoid or monitor. [Severe] Theoretical
- **Cobicistat** is predicted to increase the exposure to naldemedine. Avoid or monitor. [Moderate] Study
- **Cobicistat** is predicted to markedly increase the exposure to naloxegol. Avoid. [Severe] Study
- **Cobicistat** is predicted to increase the exposure to neratinib. Avoid or adjust dose with potent CYP3A4 inhibitors—consult product literature. [Severe] Study
- **Cobicistat** is predicted to markedly increase the exposure to neurokinin-1 receptor antagonists (aprepitant). [Moderate] Study
- **Cobicistat** is predicted to increase the exposure to neurokinin-1 receptor antagonists (fosaprepitant). [Moderate] Theoretical
- **Cobicistat** is predicted to increase the exposure to neurokinin-1 receptor antagonists (netupitant). [Moderate] Study
- **Cobicistat** is predicted to increase the exposure to nilotinib. Avoid. [Severe] Study
- **Cobicistat** is predicted to increase the exposure to nintedanib. [Moderate] Study
- **Cobicistat** is predicted to increase the exposure to nitisinone. Adjust dose. [Moderate] Theoretical
- NNRTIs (efavirenz, etravirine, nevirapine) are predicted to decrease the exposure to **cobicistat**. Avoid. [Severe] Theoretical
- **Cobicistat** is predicted to increase the exposure to olaparib. Avoid or adjust dose with potent CYP3A4 inhibitors—consult product literature. [Moderate] Study
- **Cobicistat** is predicted to increase the exposure to opioids (alfentanil, buprenorphine, fentanyl, oxycodone). Monitor and adjust dose. [Severe] Study
- **Cobicistat** is predicted to increase the exposure to opioids (sufentanil). [Moderate] Study
- **Cobicistat** is predicted to increase the exposure to osilodrostat. [Moderate] Theoretical
- **Cobicistat** is predicted to increase the exposure to ospemifene. Avoid in poor CYP2C9 metabolisers. [Moderate] Study
- **Cobicistat** is predicted to increase the exposure to oxybutynin. [Mild] Study
- **Cobicistat** is predicted to increase the exposure to palbociclib. Avoid or adjust dose—consult product literature. [Severe] Study
- **Cobicistat** is predicted to increase the exposure to panobinostat. Adjust dose—consult product literature; in hepatic impairment avoid. [Moderate] Study
- **Cobicistat** is predicted to increase the exposure to pazopanib. Avoid or adjust dose—consult product literature. [Moderate] Study
- **Cobicistat** is predicted to increase the exposure to pemigatinib. Avoid or adjust dose—consult product literature. [Severe] Study
- **Cobicistat** is predicted to increase the exposure to phosphodiesterase type-5 inhibitors (avanafil, vardenafil). Avoid. [Severe] Study
- **Cobicistat** is predicted to increase the exposure to phosphodiesterase type-5 inhibitors (sildenafil). Avoid potent CYP3A4 inhibitors or adjust **sildenafil** dose, p. 940. [Severe] Study
- **Cobicistat** is predicted to increase the exposure to phosphodiesterase type-5 inhibitors (tadalafil). Use with caution or avoid. [Severe] Study
- **Cobicistat** is predicted to increase the exposure to pimozide. Avoid. [Severe] Study
- **Cobicistat** is predicted to slightly increase the exposure to ponatinib. Monitor and adjust dose—consult product literature. [Moderate] Study
- **Cobicistat** is predicted to increase the exposure to pralsetinib. Avoid or adjust dose with potent CYP3A4 inhibitors—consult product literature. [Moderate] Study
- **Cobicistat** is predicted to moderately increase the exposure to praziquantel. [Mild] Study
- **Cobicistat** given with carbimazole is predicted to increase the exposure to propiverine. Adjust starting dose. [Moderate] Theoretical
- **Cobicistat** is predicted to increase the exposure to quizartinib. Adjust dose—consult product literature. [Severe] Study
- **Cobicistat** is predicted to increase the exposure to ranolazine. Avoid. [Severe] Study

Cobicistat (continued)

▶ **Cobicistat** is predicted to increase the exposure to reboxetine. Avoid. [Moderate] Study

▶ **Cobicistat** is predicted to increase the exposure to regorafenib. Avoid. [Moderate] Study

▶ **Cobicistat** is predicted to increase the exposure to relugolix. Avoid or take relugolix first and separate administration by at least 6 hours. [Moderate] Study

▶ **Cobicistat** is predicted to increase the exposure to retinoids (alitretinoin). Adjust **alitretinoin** dose, p. 1433. [Moderate] Theoretical

▶ **Cobicistat** is predicted to increase the exposure to ribociclib. Avoid or adjust dose—consult product literature. [Moderate] Study

▶ Rifamycins (rifabutin) decrease the concentration of **cobicistat** and **cobicistat** increases the exposure to rifamycins (rifabutin). Avoid or adjust dose. [Severe] Study

▶ Rifamycins (rifampicin) are predicted to decrease the exposure to **cobicistat**. Avoid. [Severe] Study

▶ **Cobicistat** is predicted to increase the exposure to rimegepant. Avoid. [Moderate] Study

▶ **Cobicistat** is predicted to increase the exposure to ripretinib. [Moderate] Theoretical

▶ **Cobicistat** is predicted to increase the exposure to ruxolitinib. Adjust dose and monitor adverse effects. [Moderate] Study

▶ **Cobicistat** is predicted to increase the exposure to selpercatinib. Adjust dose—consult product literature. [Moderate] Study

▶ **Cobicistat** is predicted to increase the exposure to selumetinib. Avoid or adjust dose—consult product literature. [Severe] Study

▶ **Cobicistat** is predicted to increase the exposure to siponimod. Avoid depending on other drugs taken—consult product literature. [Severe] Theoretical

▶ **Cobicistat** is predicted to increase the concentration of sirolimus. Avoid or monitor and adjust dose. [Severe] Study

▶ **Cobicistat** is predicted to increase the exposure to SNRIs (venlafaxine). [Moderate] Study

▶ **Cobicistat** is predicted to increase the exposure to solifenacin. Adjust solifenacin p. 899 or tamsulosin with solifenacin p. 906 dose; avoid in hepatic and renal impairment. [Severe] Study

▶ Sotorasib is predicted to decrease the exposure to **cobicistat**. Avoid. [Severe] Theoretical

▶ **Cobicistat** is predicted to increase the exposure to SSRIs (citalopram, escitalopram, fluoxetine, fluvoxamine, paroxetine, sertraline). Monitor and adjust dose. [Moderate] Theoretical

▶ **Cobicistat** is predicted to moderately increase the exposure to SSRIs (dapoxetine). Avoid potent CYP3A4 inhibitors or adjust **dapoxetine** dose, p. 947. [Severe] Study

▶ St John's wort is predicted to decrease the exposure to **cobicistat**. Avoid. [Severe] Theoretical

▶ **Cobicistat** is predicted to increase the exposure to statins (atorvastatin). Avoid or adjust dose and monitor rhabdomyolysis. [Severe] Study

▶ **Cobicistat** is predicted to increase the exposure to statins (simvastatin). Avoid. [Severe] Study

▶ **Cobicistat** is predicted to increase the exposure to sunitinib. Avoid or adjust dose—consult product literature. [Moderate] Study

▶ **Cobicistat** is predicted to increase the concentration of tacrolimus. Monitor and adjust dose. [Severe] Study

▶ **Cobicistat** is predicted to slightly increase the exposure to talazoparib. Avoid or adjust dose—consult product literature. [Severe] Study

▶ **Cobicistat** is predicted to increase the exposure to taxanes (cabazitaxel). Avoid or adjust dose—consult product literature. [Severe] Study

▶ **Cobicistat** is predicted to increase the exposure to taxanes (docetaxel). Avoid or adjust dose. [Severe] Study

▶ **Cobicistat** is predicted to increase the exposure to taxanes (paclitaxel). [Moderate] Anecdotal

▶ **Cobicistat** is predicted to increase the concentration of temsirolimus. Avoid. [Severe] Theoretical

▶ **Cobicistat** is predicted to increase the exposure to tezacaftor. Adjust dose with potent CYP3A4 inhibitors, see tezacaftor with ivacaftor p. 339 and ivacaftor with tezacaftor and elexacaftor p. 337. [Severe] Study

▶ **Cobicistat** moderately increases the exposure to thrombin inhibitors (dabigatran). Avoid. [Severe] Study

▶ **Cobicistat** is predicted to markedly increase the exposure to ticagrelor. Avoid. [Severe] Study

▶ **Cobicistat** is predicted to increase the exposure to tofacitinib. Adjust **tofacitinib** dose, p. 1265. [Moderate] Study

▶ **Cobicistat** is predicted to increase the exposure to tolterodine. Avoid. [Severe] Study

▶ **Cobicistat** is predicted to increase the exposure to tolvaptan. Manufacturer advises caution or adjust **tolvaptan** dose with potent CYP3A4 inhibitors, p. 767. [Severe] Study

▶ **Cobicistat** is predicted to increase the exposure to topotecan. [Severe] Study

▶ **Cobicistat** is predicted to increase the exposure to toremifene. [Moderate] Theoretical

▶ **Cobicistat** is predicted to increase the exposure to trabectedin. Avoid or adjust dose. [Severe] Theoretical

▶ **Cobicistat** is predicted to increase the concentration of trametinib. [Moderate] Theoretical

▶ **Cobicistat** is predicted to moderately increase the exposure to trazodone. Avoid or adjust dose. [Moderate] Study

▶ **Cobicistat** is predicted to slightly increase the exposure to tricyclic antidepressants. [Mild] Study

▶ **Cobicistat** increases the exposure to triptans (almotriptan). [Mild] Study

▶ **Cobicistat** is predicted to markedly increase the exposure to triptans (eletriptan). Avoid. [Severe] Study

▶ **Cobicistat** is predicted to increase the exposure to ulipristal. Avoid if used for uterine fibroids. [Severe] Study

▶ **Cobicistat** is predicted to increase the exposure to upadacitinib. Manufacturer advises caution or avoid, or adjust **upadacitinib** dose depending on indication, p. 1267. [Severe] Study

▶ **Cobicistat** is predicted to increase the exposure to vemurafenib. [Severe] Theoretical

▶ **Cobicistat** is predicted to increase the exposure to venetoclax. Avoid or adjust dose—consult product literature. [Severe] Study

▶ **Cobicistat** is predicted to increase the exposure to vinca alkaloids. [Severe] Theoretical

▶ **Cobicistat** is predicted to increase the exposure to vitamin D substances (paricalcitol). [Moderate] Study

▶ **Cobicistat** is predicted to increase the exposure to voclosporin. Avoid. [Severe] Study

▶ **Cobicistat** is predicted to increase the exposure to zanubrutinib. Avoid or adjust dose with potent CYP3A4 inhibitors—consult product literature. [Moderate] Study

▶ **Cobicistat** is predicted to increase the exposure to zopiclone. Adjust dose. [Moderate] Theoretical

Cobimetinib

▶ Anti-androgens (apalutamide, enzalutamide) are predicted to decrease the exposure to **cobimetinib**. Avoid. [Severe] Theoretical

▶ Antiarrhythmics (dronedarone) are predicted to increase the exposure to **cobimetinib**. [Severe] Study

▶ Antiepileptics (carbamazepine, fosphenytoin, phenobarbital, phenytoin, primidone) are predicted to decrease the exposure to **cobimetinib**. Avoid. [Severe] Theoretical

▶ Antifungals, azoles (fluconazole, isavuconazole) are predicted to increase the exposure to **cobimetinib**. [Severe] Study

▶ Antifungals, azoles (itraconazole, ketoconazole, posaconazole, voriconazole) are predicted to increase the exposure to **cobimetinib**. Avoid or monitor for toxicity. [Severe] Study

▶ Antifungals, azoles (miconazole) are predicted to increase the exposure to **cobimetinib**. [Severe] Theoretical

▶ Belzutifan is predicted to decrease the exposure to **cobimetinib**. Avoid or adjust dose. [Severe] Theoretical

▶ Berotralstat is predicted to increase the exposure to **cobimetinib**. [Severe] Study

▶ Calcium channel blockers (diltiazem, verapamil) are predicted to increase the exposure to **cobimetinib**. [Severe] Study

▶ Cenobamate is predicted to decrease the exposure to **cobimetinib**. Avoid. [Severe] Theoretical

▶ Ceritinib is predicted to increase the exposure to **cobimetinib**. Avoid or monitor for toxicity. [Severe] Study

▸ **Cobicistat** is predicted to increase the exposure to **cobimetinib**. Avoid or monitor for toxicity. ⟨Severe⟩ Study

▸ **Crizotinib** is predicted to increase the exposure to **cobimetinib**. ⟨Severe⟩ Study

▸ **Dabrafenib** is predicted to decrease the exposure to **cobimetinib**. Avoid. ⟨Severe⟩ Theoretical

▸ **Drugs with anticoagulant effects** (see TABLE 3 p. 1571) cause bleeding, as can **cobimetinib**; concurrent use might increase the risk of developing this effect. ⟨Severe⟩ Theoretical

▸ **Drugs with antiplatelet effects** (see TABLE 4 p. 1571) cause bleeding, as can **cobimetinib**; concurrent use might increase the risk of developing this effect. ⟨Severe⟩ Theoretical

▸ **Encorafenib** is predicted to decrease the exposure to **cobimetinib**. Avoid. ⟨Severe⟩ Theoretical

▸ **Endothelin receptor antagonists (bosentan)** are predicted to decrease the exposure to **cobimetinib**. Avoid. ⟨Severe⟩ Theoretical

▸ **Fedratinib** is predicted to increase the exposure to **cobimetinib**. ⟨Severe⟩ Study

▸ **Grapefruit** juice is predicted to increase the exposure to **cobimetinib**. Avoid. ⟨Severe⟩ Theoretical

▸ **HIV-protease inhibitors** are predicted to increase the exposure to **cobimetinib**. Avoid or monitor for toxicity. ⟨Severe⟩ Study

▸ **Idelalisib** is predicted to increase the exposure to **cobimetinib**. Avoid or monitor for toxicity. ⟨Severe⟩ Study

▸ **Imatinib** is predicted to increase the exposure to **cobimetinib**. ⟨Severe⟩ Study

▸ **Ivosidenib** is predicted to decrease the exposure to **cobimetinib**. Avoid. ⟨Severe⟩ Theoretical

▸ **Letermovir** is predicted to increase the exposure to **cobimetinib**. ⟨Severe⟩ Study

▸ **Lorlatinib** is predicted to decrease the exposure to **cobimetinib**. Avoid. ⟨Severe⟩ Theoretical

▸ **Lumacaftor** is predicted to decrease the exposure to **cobimetinib**. Avoid. ⟨Severe⟩ Theoretical

▸ **Macrolides (clarithromycin)** are predicted to increase the exposure to **cobimetinib**. Avoid or monitor for toxicity. ⟨Severe⟩ Study

▸ **Macrolides (erythromycin)** are predicted to increase the exposure to **cobimetinib**. ⟨Severe⟩ Study

▸ **Mitotane** is predicted to decrease the exposure to **cobimetinib**. Avoid. ⟨Severe⟩ Theoretical

▸ **Neurokinin-1 receptor antagonists (aprepitant, netupitant)** are predicted to increase the exposure to **cobimetinib**. ⟨Severe⟩ Study

▸ **Nilotinib** is predicted to increase the exposure to **cobimetinib**. ⟨Severe⟩ Study

▸ **NNRTIs (efavirenz, etravirine, nevirapine)** are predicted to decrease the exposure to **cobimetinib**. Avoid. ⟨Severe⟩ Theoretical

▸ **Rifamycins (rifampicin)** are predicted to decrease the exposure to **cobimetinib**. Avoid. ⟨Severe⟩ Theoretical

▸ **Sotorasib** is predicted to decrease the exposure to **cobimetinib**. Avoid. ⟨Severe⟩ Theoretical

▸ **St John's wort** is predicted to decrease the exposure to **cobimetinib**. Avoid. ⟨Severe⟩ Theoretical

▸ **Tucatinib** is predicted to increase the exposure to **cobimetinib**. Avoid or monitor for toxicity. ⟨Severe⟩ Study

Codeine → see opioids

Colchicine

▸ **Anti-androgens (apalutamide)** are predicted to decrease the exposure to **colchicine**. ⟨Mild⟩ Study

▸ **Antiarrhythmics (amiodarone)** are predicted to increase the exposure to **colchicine**. Avoid P-glycoprotein inhibitors or adjust **colchicine** dose, p. 1279. ⟨Severe⟩ Theoretical

▸ **Antiarrhythmics (dronedarone)** are predicted to increase the exposure to **colchicine**. Adjust **colchicine** dose with moderate CYP3A4 inhibitors, p. 1279. ⟨Severe⟩ Study

▸ **Antiepileptics (carbamazepine)** are predicted to decrease the exposure to **colchicine**. ⟨Moderate⟩ Theoretical

▸ **Antifungals, azoles (fluconazole, isavuconazole)** are predicted to increase the exposure to **colchicine**. Adjust **colchicine** dose with moderate CYP3A4 inhibitors, p. 1279. ⟨Severe⟩ Study

▸ **Antifungals, azoles (itraconazole, ketoconazole, posaconazole, voriconazole)** are predicted to increase the exposure to **colchicine**. Avoid potent CYP3A4 inhibitors or adjust **colchicine** dose, p. 1279. ⟨Severe⟩ Study

▸ **Berotralstat** is predicted to increase the exposure to **colchicine**. Adjust **colchicine** dose with moderate CYP3A4 inhibitors, p. 1279. ⟨Severe⟩ Study

▸ **Calcium channel blockers (diltiazem, verapamil)** are predicted to increase the exposure to **colchicine**. Adjust **colchicine** dose with moderate CYP3A4 inhibitors, p. 1279. ⟨Severe⟩ Study

▸ **Ceritinib** is predicted to increase the exposure to **colchicine**. Avoid potent CYP3A4 inhibitors or adjust **colchicine** dose, p. 1279. ⟨Severe⟩ Study

▸ **Ciclosporin** increases the exposure to **colchicine**. Avoid P-glycoprotein inhibitors or adjust **colchicine** dose, p. 1279. ⟨Severe⟩ Study

▸ **Cobicistat** is predicted to increase the exposure to **colchicine**. Avoid potent CYP3A4 inhibitors or adjust **colchicine** dose, p. 1279. ⟨Severe⟩ Study

▸ **Crizotinib** is predicted to increase the exposure to **colchicine**. Adjust **colchicine** dose with moderate CYP3A4 inhibitors, p. 1279. ⟨Severe⟩ Study

▸ **Danicopan** is predicted to increase the exposure to **colchicine**. ⟨Moderate⟩ Study

▸ **Eliglustat** is predicted to increase the exposure to **colchicine**. Avoid or adjust **colchicine** dose, p. 1279. ⟨Severe⟩ Theoretical

▸ **Erdafitinib** is predicted to increase the exposure to **colchicine**. Separate administration by at least 6 hours. ⟨Moderate⟩ Theoretical

▸ **Fedratinib** is predicted to increase the exposure to **colchicine**. Adjust **colchicine** dose with moderate CYP3A4 inhibitors, p. 1279. ⟨Severe⟩ Study

▸ **Colchicine** increases the risk of rhabdomyolysis when given with **fibrates**. ⟨Severe⟩ Anecdotal

▸ **Glecaprevir** is predicted to increase the exposure to **colchicine**. Avoid P-glycoprotein inhibitors or adjust **colchicine** dose, p. 1279. ⟨Severe⟩ Theoretical

▸ **HIV-protease inhibitors** are predicted to increase the exposure to **colchicine**. Avoid potent CYP3A4 inhibitors or adjust **colchicine** dose, p. 1279. ⟨Severe⟩ Study

▸ **Idelalisib** is predicted to increase the exposure to **colchicine**. Avoid potent CYP3A4 inhibitors or adjust **colchicine** dose, p. 1279. ⟨Severe⟩ Study

▸ **Imatinib** is predicted to increase the exposure to **colchicine**. Adjust **colchicine** dose with moderate CYP3A4 inhibitors, p. 1279. ⟨Severe⟩ Study

▸ **Ivosidenib** is predicted to alter the exposure to **colchicine**. ⟨Moderate⟩ Theoretical

▸ **Lapatinib** is predicted to increase the exposure to **colchicine**. Avoid P-glycoprotein inhibitors or adjust **colchicine** dose, p. 1279. ⟨Moderate⟩ Theoretical

▸ **Letermovir** is predicted to increase the exposure to **colchicine**. Adjust **colchicine** dose with moderate CYP3A4 inhibitors, p. 1279. ⟨Severe⟩ Study

▸ **Lorlatinib** is predicted to decrease the exposure to **colchicine**. ⟨Moderate⟩ Theoretical

▸ **Macrolides (azithromycin)** are predicted to increase the exposure to **colchicine**. Avoid P-glycoprotein inhibitors or adjust **colchicine** dose, p. 1279. ⟨Severe⟩ Theoretical

▸ **Macrolides (clarithromycin)** are predicted to increase the exposure to **colchicine**. Avoid potent CYP3A4 inhibitors or adjust **colchicine** dose, p. 1279. ⟨Severe⟩ Study

▸ **Macrolides (erythromycin)** are predicted to increase the exposure to **colchicine**. Adjust **colchicine** dose with moderate CYP3A4 inhibitors, p. 1279. ⟨Severe⟩ Study

▸ **Mirabegron** is predicted to increase the exposure to **colchicine**. ⟨Mild⟩ Theoretical

▸ **Neurokinin-1 receptor antagonists (aprepitant, netupitant)** are predicted to increase the exposure to **colchicine**. Adjust **colchicine** dose with moderate CYP3A4 inhibitors, p. 1279. ⟨Severe⟩ Study

▸ **Nilotinib** is predicted to increase the exposure to **colchicine**. Adjust **colchicine** dose with moderate CYP3A4 inhibitors, p. 1279. ⟨Severe⟩ Study

▸ **Nirmatrelvir** boosted with ritonavir is predicted to increase the concentration of **colchicine**. Avoid. ⟨Severe⟩ Theoretical

▸ **Olaparib** might increase the exposure to **colchicine**. ⟨Moderate⟩ Theoretical

Colchicine (continued)

▸ **Osimertinib** is predicted to increase the exposure to **colchicine**. Moderate Study

▸ **Pibrentasvir** with glecaprevir is predicted to increase the exposure to **colchicine**. Moderate Study

▸ **Pitolisant** is predicted to decrease the exposure to **colchicine**. Mild Theoretical

▸ **Ranolazine** is predicted to increase the exposure to **colchicine**. Avoid P-glycoprotein inhibitors or adjust **colchicine** dose, p. 1279. Severe Theoretical

▸ **Rifamycins (rifampicin)** are predicted to decrease the exposure to **colchicine**. Moderate Theoretical

▸ **Ritlecitinib** is predicted to increase the exposure to **colchicine**. Adjust dose. Moderate Theoretical

▸ **St John's wort** is predicted to decrease the exposure to **colchicine**. Moderate Theoretical

▸ **Colchicine** has been reported to cause rhabdomyolysis when given with **statins**. Severe Anecdotal

▸ **Tepotinib** is predicted to increase the concentration of **colchicine**. Severe Study

▸ **Tucatinib** is predicted to increase the exposure to **colchicine**. Avoid potent CYP3A4 inhibitors or adjust **colchicine** dose, p. 1279. Severe Study

▸ **Velpatasvir** is predicted to increase the exposure to **colchicine**. Severe Theoretical

▸ **Vemurafenib** is predicted to increase the exposure to **colchicine**. Avoid P-glycoprotein inhibitors or adjust **colchicine** dose, p. 1279. Severe Theoretical

▸ **Venetoclax** is predicted to increase the exposure to **colchicine**. Avoid or adjust dose. Severe Study

▸ **Voxilaprevir** with sofosbuvir and velpatasvir is predicted to increase the exposure to **colchicine**. Avoid P-glycoprotein inhibitors or adjust **colchicine** dose, p. 1279. Severe Theoretical

Colecalciferol → see vitamin D substances

Colesevelam

SEPARATION OF ADMINISTRATION Manufacturer advises take 4 hours before, or after, other drugs.

Colestipol

SEPARATION OF ADMINISTRATION Manufacturer advises take other drugs at least 1 hour before, or 4 hours after, colestipol.

Colestyramine

SEPARATION OF ADMINISTRATION Manufacturer advises take other drugs at least 1 hour before, or 4 to 6 hours after, colestyramine.

Colistimethate → see TABLE 2 p. 1571 (nephrotoxicity), TABLE 18 p. 1576 (ototoxicity), TABLE 19 p. 1576 (neuromuscular blocking effects)

Combined hormonal contraceptives

▸ **Combined hormonal contraceptives** is predicted to increase the exposure to **agomelatine**. Moderate Study

▸ **Combined hormonal contraceptives** is predicted to increase the exposure to **aminophylline**. Adjust dose. Moderate Theoretical

▸ **Combined hormonal contraceptives** is predicted to increase the exposure to **anaesthetics, local (ropivacaine)**. Moderate Theoretical

▸ **Combined hormonal contraceptives** is predicted to increase the exposure to **anagrelide**. Moderate Theoretical

▸ **Antiepileptics (carbamazepine, eslicarbazepine, fosphenytoin, oxcarbazepine, perampanel, phenobarbital, phenytoin, primidone, rufinamide, topiramate)** are predicted to decrease the efficacy of **combined hormonal contraceptives**. For FSRH guidance, see Contraceptives, interactions p. 917. Severe Study

▸ **Combined hormonal contraceptives** alter the exposure to **antiepileptics (lamotrigine)** and **antiepileptics (lamotrigine)** might decrease the efficacy of **combined hormonal contraceptives**. Adjust dose. Moderate Study

▸ **Combined hormonal contraceptives** increases the concentration of **antipsychotics, second generation (clozapine)**. Monitor adverse effects and adjust dose. Severe Study

▸ **Combined hormonal contraceptives** is predicted to increase the exposure to **antipsychotics, second generation (olanzapine)**. Adjust dose. Moderate Anecdotal

▸ **Belzutifan** might decrease the efficacy of **combined hormonal contraceptives**. Use additional contraceptive precautions. Severe Theoretical

▸ **Brigatinib** is predicted to decrease the exposure to **combined hormonal contraceptives**. Use additional contraceptive precautions. Severe Theoretical

▸ **Cabozantinib** might affect the effects of **combined hormonal contraceptives**. Use additional contraceptive precautions. Severe Theoretical

▸ **Carfilzomib** potentially decreases the efficacy of **combined hormonal contraceptives**. Use additional contraceptive precautions. Severe Theoretical

▸ **Cenobamate** might decrease the efficacy of oral **combined hormonal contraceptives**. Use additional contraceptive precautions. Severe Theoretical

▸ Oral **combined hormonal contraceptives** potentially decrease the efficacy of oral **chenodeoxycholic acid**. Avoid. Moderate Theoretical

▸ **Cobicistat** is predicted to decrease the efficacy of **combined hormonal contraceptives**. Avoid. Severe Study

▸ **Cytisinicline** might decrease the efficacy of **combined hormonal contraceptives**. Use additional contraceptive precautions. Severe Theoretical

▸ **Dabrafenib** is predicted to decrease the efficacy of **combined hormonal contraceptives**. Use additional contraceptive precautions. Severe Theoretical

▸ **Combined hormonal contraceptives** is predicted to increase the exposure to **dopamine receptor agonists (ropinirole)**. Adjust dose. Moderate Study

▸ **Encorafenib** might decrease the efficacy of **combined hormonal contraceptives**. Use additional contraceptive precautions or alternative methods. Severe Theoretical

▸ **Endothelin receptor antagonists (bosentan)** are predicted to decrease the efficacy of **combined hormonal contraceptives**. For FSRH guidance, see Contraceptives, interactions p. 917. Severe Study

▸ **Erdafitinib** might decrease the efficacy of **combined hormonal contraceptives**. Use alternative methods during treatment with, and for at least 28 days after stopping, **erdafitinib**. Severe Theoretical

▸ **Combined hormonal contraceptives** are predicted to increases the exposure to **erlotinib**. Monitor adverse effects and adjust dose. Moderate Study

▸ **Combined hormonal contraceptives** is predicted to increase the exposure to **fezolinetant**. Avoid. Moderate Study

▸ **Combined hormonal contraceptives** (containing ethinylestradiol) are predicted to increase the risk of increased ALT concentrations when given with **glecaprevir**. Avoid. Severe Study

▸ **Glucagon-like peptide-1 receptor agonists (tirzepatide)** might affect the absorption of oral **combined hormonal contraceptives**. Manufacturer advises precautions for those who are overweight or obese—see Conception and contraception p. 822. Moderate Study

▸ **HIV-protease inhibitors (atazanavir)** affect the exposure to **combined hormonal contraceptives**. Adjust dose. Severe Study

▸ **HIV-protease inhibitors (ritonavir)** are predicted to decrease the efficacy of **combined hormonal contraceptives**. For FSRH guidance, see Contraceptives, interactions p. 917. Severe Study

▸ **Ivosidenib** might decrease the concentration of **combined hormonal contraceptives**. Use alternative methods during treatment with, and for at least 28 days after stopping, **ivosidenib**. Severe Theoretical

▸ **Larotrectinib** potentially decreases the efficacy of **combined hormonal contraceptives**. Use additional contraceptive precautions. Severe Theoretical

▸ **Combined hormonal contraceptives** are predicted to increase the risk of venous thromboembolism when given with **lenalidomide**. Avoid. Severe Theoretical

▸ Oral **combined hormonal contraceptives** slightly increase the exposure to **lomitapide**. Separate administration by 12 hours. Moderate Theoretical

▸ **Lorlatinib** is predicted to decrease the exposure to **combined hormonal contraceptives**. Avoid. Moderate Theoretical

▶ **Combined hormonal contraceptives** is predicted to increase the exposure to loxapine. Avoid. [Unknown] Theoretical

▶ Lumacaftor is predicted to decrease the exposure to **combined hormonal contraceptives**. Use additional contraceptive precautions. [Severe] Theoretical

▶ **Combined hormonal contraceptives** slightly increases the exposure to MAO-B inhibitors (rasagiline). [Moderate] Study

▶ **Combined hormonal contraceptives** increase the exposure to MAO-B inhibitors (selegiline). Avoid. [Severe] Study

▶ Mavacamten is predicted to affect the efficacy of some **combined hormonal contraceptives**. Use additional contraceptive precautions. [Severe] Theoretical

▶ **Combined hormonal contraceptives** is predicted to increase the exposure to melatonin. [Moderate] Theoretical

▶ Metreleptin might decrease the efficacy of **combined hormonal contraceptives**. Use additional contraceptive precautions. [Severe] Theoretical

▶ **Combined hormonal contraceptives** decrease the effects of metyrapone. Avoid. [Moderate] Theoretical

▶ Mitotane might decrease the efficacy of **combined hormonal contraceptives**. Use alternative methods with, and until concentrations are undetectable after stopping, **mitotane**. [Severe] Theoretical

▶ Mobocertinib is predicted to decrease the exposure to **combined hormonal contraceptives**. Use alternative methods during treatment with, and for at least 28 days after stopping, mobocertinib. [Moderate] Theoretical

▶ Modafinil is predicted to decrease the efficacy of **combined hormonal contraceptives**. For FSRH guidance, see Contraceptives, interactions p. 917. [Severe] Study

▶ Momelotinib might decrease the efficacy of **combined hormonal contraceptives**. Additional non-hormonal contraception should be used for 7 days following administration. [Severe] Theoretical

▶ Monoclonal antibodies (sarilumab) potentially decrease the exposure to **combined hormonal contraceptives**. [Severe] Theoretical

▶ Neratinib might affect the efficacy of **combined hormonal contraceptives**. Use additional contraceptive precautions. [Severe] Theoretical

▶ Neurokinin-1 receptor antagonists (aprepitant, fosaprepitant) are predicted to decrease the efficacy of **combined hormonal contraceptives**. For FSRH guidance, see Contraceptives, interactions p. 917. [Severe] Study

▶ Nirmatrelvir boosted with ritonavir is predicted to decrease the concentration of **combined hormonal contraceptives** (containing ethinylestradiol). Use additional contraceptive precautions. [Moderate] Theoretical

▶ NNRTIs (efavirenz, nevirapine) are predicted to decrease the efficacy of **combined hormonal contraceptives**. For FSRH guidance, see Contraceptives, interactions p. 917. [Severe] Study

▶ NNRTIs (etravirine) might decrease the efficacy of **combined hormonal contraceptives**. Follow FSRH guidance for enzyme inducers, see Contraceptives, interactions p. 917. [Severe] Theoretical

▶ NSAIDs (etoricoxib) increase the exposure to **combined hormonal contraceptives**. [Moderate] Study

▶ Olaparib potentially affects the efficacy of **combined hormonal contraceptives**. Use additional contraceptive precautions. [Moderate] Theoretical

▶ **Combined hormonal contraceptives** potentially oppose the effects of ospemifene. Avoid. [Severe] Theoretical

▶ **Combined hormonal contraceptives** is predicted to increase the exposure to phenothiazines (chlorpromazine). [Moderate] Theoretical

▶ **Combined hormonal contraceptives** is predicted to increase the exposure to phosphodiesterase type-4 inhibitors (roflumilast). [Moderate] Theoretical

▶ **Combined hormonal contraceptives** (containing ethinylestradiol) are predicted to increase the risk of increased ALT concentrations when given with pibrentasvir. Avoid. [Severe] Study

▶ **Combined hormonal contraceptives** is predicted to increase the exposure to pirfenidone. Use with caution and adjust dose. [Moderate] Study

▶ Pitolisant is predicted to decrease the efficacy of **combined hormonal contraceptives**. Avoid. [Severe] Theoretical

▶ **Combined hormonal contraceptives** are predicted to increase the risk of venous thromboembolism when given with pomalidomide. Avoid. [Severe] Theoretical

▶ Ponatinib might affect the effects of **combined hormonal contraceptives**. Avoid or use additional contraceptive precautions. [Severe] Theoretical

▶ Pralsetinib might decrease the efficacy of **combined hormonal contraceptives**. Avoid or use additional contraceptive precautions. [Severe] Theoretical

▶ **Combined hormonal contraceptives** potentially oppose the effects of raloxifene. Avoid. [Severe] Theoretical

▶ Rifamycins are predicted to decrease the efficacy of **combined hormonal contraceptives**. For FSRH guidance, see Contraceptives, interactions p. 917. [Severe] Study

▶ **Combined hormonal contraceptives** is predicted to increase the exposure to riluzole. [Moderate] Theoretical

▶ St John's wort decreases the efficacy of **combined hormonal contraceptives**. MHRA advises avoid. For FSRH guidance, see Contraceptives, interactions p. 917. [Severe] Anecdotal

▶ Sugammadex is predicted to decrease the exposure to **combined hormonal contraceptives**. Refer to patient information leaflet for missed pill advice. [Severe] Theoretical

▶ **Combined hormonal contraceptives** might exacerbate skin pigmentation when given with tetracyclines (minocycline). [Moderate] Anecdotal

▶ **Combined hormonal contraceptives** are predicted to increase the risk of venous thromboembolism when given with thalidomide. Avoid. [Severe] Study

▶ **Combined hormonal contraceptives** is predicted to increase the exposure to theophylline. Monitor and adjust dose. [Moderate] Theoretical

▶ **Combined hormonal contraceptives** increases the exposure to tizanidine. Avoid. [Moderate] Study

▶ **Combined hormonal contraceptives** is predicted to increase the exposure to triptans (zolmitriptan). Adjust **zolmitriptan** dose, p. 546. [Moderate] Theoretical

▶ **Combined hormonal contraceptives** might decrease the efficacy of ulipristal and ulipristal might decrease the efficacy of **combined hormonal contraceptives**. Avoid or use additional contraceptive precautions. [Severe] Theoretical

▶ Vemurafenib might decrease the efficacy of **combined hormonal contraceptives**. Use additional contraceptive precautions. [Severe] Theoretical

▶ **Combined hormonal contraceptives** (containing ethinylestradiol) are predicted to increase the risk of increased ALT concentrations when given with voxilaprevir with sofosbuvir and velpatasvir. Avoid. [Severe] Study

Corticosteroids → see TABLE 16 p. 1575 (reduced serum potassium)

beclometasone · betamethasone · budesonide · ciclesonide · deflazacort · dexamethasone · fludrocortisone · fluticasone · hydrocortisone · methylprednisolone · mometasone · prednisolone · triamcinolone · vamorolone

▶ With intravitreal use of **dexamethasone** in adults: caution with concurrent administration of anticoagulant or antiplatelet drugs—increased risk of haemorrhagic events.

▶ Interactions do not generally apply to corticosteroids (except **budesonide** and **fluticasone**) used for topical action (including inhalation) unless specified. However, as systemic absorption might occur with **hydrocortisone** *eye drops*, the possibility of interactions should be borne in mind.

▶ Oral antacids are predicted to decrease the absorption of oral **deflazacort**. Separate administration by 2 hours. [Moderate] Theoretical

▶ Oral antacids decrease the absorption of oral **dexamethasone**. [Moderate] Study

▶ Anti-androgens (apalutamide, enzalutamide) are predicted to decrease the exposure to **fluticasone**. [Unknown] Theoretical

▶ Anti-androgens (apalutamide, enzalutamide) are predicted to decrease the exposure to corticosteroids (budesonide, deflazacort, dexamethasone, fludrocortisone, hydrocortisone,

Corticosteroids (continued)
methylprednisolone, prednisolone, triamcinolone). Monitor and adjust dose. Moderate Study

▸ Antiarrhythmics (dronedarone) are predicted to increase the exposure to **methylprednisolone**. Monitor and adjust dose. Moderate Study

▸ Antiepileptics (carbamazepine, fosphenytoin, phenobarbital, phenytoin, primidone) are predicted to decrease the exposure to **fluticasone**. Unknown Theoretical

▸ Antiepileptics (carbamazepine, fosphenytoin, phenobarbital, phenytoin, primidone) are predicted to decrease the exposure to corticosteroids (**budesonide, deflazacort, dexamethasone, fludrocortisone, hydrocortisone, methylprednisolone, prednisolone, triamcinolone**). Monitor and adjust dose. Moderate Study

▸ Antifungals, azoles (fluconazole, isavuconazole) are predicted to increase the exposure to **methylprednisolone**. Monitor and adjust dose. Moderate Study

▸ Antifungals, azoles (itraconazole, ketoconazole, posaconazole, voriconazole) are predicted to increase the exposure to **beclometasone** (risk with beclometasone is likely to be lower than with other corticosteroids). Moderate Theoretical

▸ Antifungals, azoles (itraconazole, ketoconazole, posaconazole, voriconazole) are predicted to increase the exposure to **vamorolone**. Adjust dose. Severe Study

▸ Antifungals, azoles (miconazole) are predicted to increase the concentration of **methylprednisolone**. Monitor and adjust dose. Moderate Theoretical

▸ Antifungals, azoles (itraconazole, ketoconazole, posaconazole, voriconazole) are predicted to increase the exposure to corticosteroids (**betamethasone, budesonide, ciclesonide, deflazacort, dexamethasone, fludrocortisone, fluticasone, hydrocortisone, methylprednisolone, mometasone, prednisolone, triamcinolone**). Avoid or monitor adverse effects. Severe Study

▸ **Corticosteroids** are predicted to decrease the concentration of aspirin (high-dose) and aspirin (high-dose) increases the risk of gastrointestinal bleeding when given with **corticosteroids**. Moderate Study

▸ **Dexamethasone** is predicted to decrease the exposure to avapritinib. Avoid. Severe Theoretical

▸ Berotralstat is predicted to increase the exposure to **methylprednisolone**. Monitor and adjust dose. Moderate Study

▸ Calcium channel blockers (diltiazem, verapamil) are predicted to increase the exposure to **methylprednisolone**. Monitor and adjust dose. Moderate Study

▸ **Dexamethasone** is predicted to decrease the concentration of caspofungin. Adjust **caspofungin** dose, p. 687. Moderate Theoretical

▸ Cenobamate is predicted to decrease the exposure to oral **budesonide**. Adjust dose. Moderate Theoretical

▸ Cenobamate is predicted to decrease the exposure to **fluticasone**. Adjust dose. Moderate Theoretical

▸ Ceritinib is predicted to increase the exposure to **beclometasone** (risk with beclometasone is likely to be lower than with other corticosteroids). Moderate Theoretical

▸ Ceritinib is predicted to increase the exposure to corticosteroids (**betamethasone, budesonide, ciclesonide, deflazacort, dexamethasone, fludrocortisone, fluticasone, hydrocortisone, methylprednisolone, mometasone, prednisolone, triamcinolone**). Avoid or monitor adverse effects. Severe Study

▸ Ceritinib is predicted to increase the exposure to **vamorolone**. Adjust dose. Severe Study

▸ **Corticosteroids** are predicted to decrease the concentration of choline salicylate. Moderate Study

▸ Cobicistat is predicted to increase the exposure to **beclometasone** (risk with beclometasone is likely to be lower than with other corticosteroids). Moderate Theoretical

▸ Cobicistat is predicted to increase the exposure to corticosteroids (**betamethasone, budesonide, ciclesonide, deflazacort, dexamethasone, fludrocortisone, fluticasone, hydrocortisone, methylprednisolone, mometasone, prednisolone, triamcinolone**). Avoid or monitor adverse effects. Severe Study

▸ Cobicistat is predicted to increase the exposure to **vamorolone**. Adjust dose. Severe Study

▸ **Corticosteroids** are predicted to increase the effects of coumarins. Moderate Study

▸ Crizotinib is predicted to increase the exposure to **methylprednisolone**. Monitor and adjust dose. Moderate Study

▸ **Corticosteroids** are predicted to increase the risk of digoxin toxicity when given with **digoxin**. Avoid. Severe Theoretical

▸ Encorafenib is predicted to decrease the exposure to corticosteroids (**budesonide, deflazacort, dexamethasone, fludrocortisone, hydrocortisone, methylprednisolone, prednisolone, triamcinolone**). Monitor and adjust dose. Moderate Study

▸ Encorafenib is predicted to decrease the exposure to **fluticasone**. Unknown Theoretical

▸ Erlotinib is predicted to increase the risk of gastrointestinal perforation when given with **corticosteroids**. Severe Theoretical

▸ Fedratinib is predicted to increase the exposure to **methylprednisolone**. Monitor and adjust dose. Moderate Study

▸ **Corticosteroids** potentially oppose the effects of glycerol phenylbutyrate. Moderate Theoretical

▸ Grapefruit juice moderately increases the exposure to oral **budesonide**. Avoid. Moderate Study

▸ HIV-protease inhibitors are predicted to increase the exposure to **beclometasone** (risk with beclometasone is likely to be lower than with other corticosteroids). Moderate Theoretical

▸ HIV-protease inhibitors are predicted to increase the exposure to corticosteroids (**betamethasone, budesonide, ciclesonide, deflazacort, dexamethasone, fludrocortisone, fluticasone, hydrocortisone, methylprednisolone, mometasone, prednisolone, triamcinolone**). Avoid or monitor adverse effects. Severe Study

▸ HIV-protease inhibitors are predicted to increase the exposure to **vamorolone**. Adjust dose. Severe Study

▸ Idelalisib is predicted to increase the exposure to **beclometasone** (risk with beclometasone is likely to be lower than with other corticosteroids). Moderate Theoretical

▸ Idelalisib is predicted to increase the exposure to corticosteroids (**betamethasone, budesonide, ciclesonide, deflazacort, dexamethasone, fludrocortisone, fluticasone, hydrocortisone, methylprednisolone, mometasone, prednisolone, triamcinolone**). Avoid or monitor adverse effects. Severe Study

▸ Idelalisib is predicted to increase the exposure to **vamorolone**. Adjust dose. Severe Study

▸ Imatinib is predicted to increase the exposure to **methylprednisolone**. Monitor and adjust dose. Moderate Study

▸ **Corticosteroids** are predicted to increase the risk of gastrointestinal bleeding when given with iron chelators (deferasirox). Severe Theoretical

▸ Ivosidenib is predicted to decrease the exposure to corticosteroids (**budesonide, deflazacort, dexamethasone, fludrocortisone, hydrocortisone, methylprednisolone, prednisolone, triamcinolone**). Monitor and adjust dose. Moderate Study

▸ Ivosidenib is predicted to decrease the exposure to **fluticasone**. Unknown Theoretical

▸ Letermovir is predicted to increase the exposure to **methylprednisolone**. Monitor and adjust dose. Moderate Study

▸ Live vaccines are predicted to increase the risk of generalised infection (possibly life-threatening) when given with **corticosteroids** (high-dose). UKHSA advises avoid (refer to Green Book). Severe Theoretical

▸ Lumacaftor is predicted to decrease the exposure to corticosteroids (**budesonide, deflazacort, dexamethasone, fludrocortisone, hydrocortisone, methylprednisolone, prednisolone, triamcinolone**). Monitor and adjust dose. Moderate Study

▸ Lumacaftor is predicted to decrease the exposure to **fluticasone**. Unknown Theoretical

▸ Macrolides (clarithromycin) are predicted to increase the exposure to **beclometasone** (risk with beclometasone is likely to be lower than with other corticosteroids). Moderate Theoretical

- Macrolides (clarithromycin) are predicted to increase the exposure to **vamorolone**. Adjust dose. [Severe] Study
- Macrolides (erythromycin) are predicted to increase the exposure to **methylprednisolone**. Monitor and adjust dose. [Moderate] Study
- Macrolides (clarithromycin) are predicted to increase the exposure to corticosteroids (**betamethasone, budesonide, ciclesonide, deflazacort, dexamethasone, fludrocortisone, fluticasone, hydrocortisone, methylprednisolone, mometasone, prednisolone, triamcinolone**). Avoid or monitor adverse effects. [Severe] Study
- **Corticosteroids** are predicted to decrease the efficacy of mifamurtide. Avoid. [Severe] Theoretical
- Mifepristone is predicted to decrease the efficacy of **corticosteroids**. Use with caution and adjust dose. [Moderate] Theoretical
- Mitotane is predicted to decrease the exposure to corticosteroids (**budesonide, deflazacort, dexamethasone, fludrocortisone, hydrocortisone, methylprednisolone, prednisolone, triamcinolone**). Monitor and adjust dose. [Moderate] Study
- Mitotane is predicted to decrease the exposure to **fluticasone**. [Unknown] Theoretical
- **Corticosteroids** might affect the efficacy of monoclonal antibodies (atezolizumab, pembrolizumab). Use with caution or avoid. [Severe] Theoretical
- Monoclonal antibodies (tocilizumab) are predicted to decrease the exposure to corticosteroids (**dexamethasone, methylprednisolone**). Monitor and adjust dose. [Moderate] Theoretical
- **Corticosteroids** are predicted to increase the risk of immunosuppression when given with monoclonal antibodies (dinutuximab). Avoid except in life-threatening situations. [Severe] Theoretical
- **Corticosteroids** might affect the efficacy of monoclonal antibodies (ipilimumab, nivolumab). Use with caution or avoid. [Severe] Theoretical
- **Corticosteroids** might increase the risk of generalised infection (possibly life-threatening) when given with monoclonal antibodies (natalizumab). Manufacturer advises short courses of corticosteroids can be taken. [Severe] Theoretical
- Neurokinin-1 receptor antagonists (aprepitant) moderately increase the exposure to **dexamethasone**. Monitor and adjust dose. [Moderate] Study
- Neurokinin-1 receptor antagonists (aprepitant, netupitant) are predicted to increase the exposure to oral **budesonide**. [Moderate] Study
- Neurokinin-1 receptor antagonists (aprepitant, netupitant) are predicted to increase the exposure to **fluticasone**. [Moderate] Study
- Neurokinin-1 receptor antagonists (aprepitant, netupitant) are predicted to increase the exposure to **methylprednisolone**. Monitor and adjust dose. [Moderate] Study
- Neurokinin-1 receptor antagonists (netupitant) moderately increase the exposure to **dexamethasone**. Adjust dose. [Moderate] Study
- **Corticosteroids** are predicted to decrease the effects of neuromuscular blocking drugs, non-depolarising. [Severe] Anecdotal
- **Corticosteroids** increase the risk of gastrointestinal perforation when given with nicorandil. [Severe] Anecdotal
- Nilotinib is predicted to increase the exposure to **methylprednisolone**. Monitor and adjust dose. [Moderate] Study
- Nirmatrelvir boosted with ritonavir is predicted to increase the concentration of **beclometasone** (risk with beclometasone is likely to be lower than with other corticosteroids). [Moderate] Theoretical
- Nirmatrelvir boosted with ritonavir is predicted to increase the concentration of corticosteroids (**betamethasone, budesonide, ciclesonide, deflazacort, dexamethasone, fluticasone, hydrocortisone, methylprednisolone, mometasone, prednisolone, triamcinolone**). Avoid or monitor adverse effects and consider beclometasone as an alternative. [Severe] Theoretical

- Nirmatrelvir boosted with ritonavir is predicted to increase the concentration of corticosteroids (**fludrocortisone, vamorolone**). Avoid or monitor adverse effects. [Severe] Theoretical
- **Dexamethasone** is predicted to decrease the concentration of NNRTIs (rilpivirine). Avoid multiple-dose dexamethasone. [Severe] Theoretical
- NSAIDs increase the risk of gastrointestinal bleeding when given with **corticosteroids**. [Severe] Study
- **Corticosteroids** are predicted to increase the effects of phenindione. [Moderate] Anecdotal
- **Dexamethasone** decreases the exposure to praziquantel. [Moderate] Study
- Rifamycins (rifampicin) are predicted to decrease the exposure to **fluticasone**. [Unknown] Theoretical
- Rifamycins (rifampicin) are predicted to decrease the exposure to corticosteroids (**budesonide, deflazacort, dexamethasone, fludrocortisone, hydrocortisone, methylprednisolone, prednisolone, triamcinolone**). Monitor and adjust dose. [Moderate] Study
- **Corticosteroids** potentially decrease the effects of sodium phenylbutyrate. [Moderate] Theoretical
- **Corticosteroids** might decrease the efficacy of somapacitan. Monitor and adjust dose. [Moderate] Theoretical
- **Corticosteroids** might decrease the efficacy of somatrogon. Monitor and adjust dose. [Moderate] Theoretical
- **Corticosteroids** are predicted to decrease the effects of somatropin. [Moderate] Theoretical
- **Corticosteroids** are predicted to decrease the effects of suxamethonium. [Severe] Anecdotal
- Tucatinib is predicted to increase the exposure to **beclometasone** (risk with beclometasone is likely to be lower than with other corticosteroids). [Moderate] Theoretical
- Tucatinib is predicted to increase the exposure to corticosteroids (**betamethasone, budesonide, ciclesonide, deflazacort, dexamethasone, fludrocortisone, fluticasone, hydrocortisone, methylprednisolone, mometasone, prednisolone, triamcinolone**). Avoid or monitor adverse effects. [Severe] Study
- Tucatinib is predicted to increase the exposure to **vamorolone**. Adjust dose. [Severe] Study
- **Fludrocortisone** might enhance the antidiuretic effect of vasopressin. [Moderate] Theoretical

Coumarins → see **TABLE 3** p. 1571 (anticoagulant effects)

acenocoumarol · warfarin

FOOD AND LIFESTYLE The effects of coumarins can be reduced or abolished by vitamin K, including that found in health foods, food supplements, enteral feeds, or large amounts of some green vegetables or green tea. Major changes in diet (especially involving salads and vegetables) and in alcohol consumption can affect anticoagulant control. Pomegranate juice is predicted to increase the INR in response to **acenocoumarol** and **warfarin**.

- Alcohol (in those who drink heavily) potentially decreases the anticoagulant effect of **coumarins**. [Severe] Study
- Amfetamines (dexamfetamine) might increase the anticoagulant effect of **coumarins**. Monitor INR and adjust dose. [Moderate] Theoretical
- Anti-androgens (apalutamide) are predicted to decrease the exposure to **coumarins**. Avoid or monitor. [Mild] Study
- Anti-androgens (enzalutamide) potentially decrease the exposure to **coumarins**. Avoid or adjust dose and monitor INR. [Severe] Study
- Antiarrhythmics (amiodarone) increase the anticoagulant effect of **coumarins**. [Severe] Study
- Antiarrhythmics (dronedarone) might increase the anticoagulant effect of **coumarins**. [Moderate] Anecdotal
- Antiarrhythmics (propafenone) increase the anticoagulant effect of **coumarins**. Monitor INR and adjust dose. [Moderate] Study
- Antiepileptics (carbamazepine) decrease the effects of **coumarins**. Monitor and adjust dose. [Severe] Study
- Antiepileptics (fosphenytoin, phenytoin) are predicted to alter the anticoagulant effect of **coumarins**. [Moderate] Anecdotal

Coumarins (continued)

▶ **Antiepileptics (phenobarbital, primidone)** decrease the anticoagulant effect of **coumarins**. Monitor INR and adjust dose. Moderate Study

▶ **Antifungals, azoles (fluconazole)** increase the anticoagulant effect of **coumarins**. Monitor INR and adjust dose. Severe Study

▶ **Antifungals, azoles (itraconazole)** potentially increase the anticoagulant effect of **coumarins**. Severe Anecdotal

▶ **Antifungals, azoles (ketoconazole)** potentially increase the anticoagulant effect of **warfarin**. Monitor INR and adjust dose. Severe Anecdotal

▶ **Antifungals, azoles (miconazole)** greatly increase the anticoagulant effect of **coumarins**. MHRA advises avoid unless INR can be monitored closely; monitor for signs of bleeding. Severe Study

▶ **Antifungals, azoles (voriconazole)** increase the anticoagulant effect of **coumarins**. Monitor INR and adjust dose. Moderate Study

▶ **Asciminib** slightly to moderately increases the exposure to **warfarin**. Severe Theoretical

▶ **Azathioprine** decreases the anticoagulant effect of **coumarins**. Moderate Study

▶ **Capecitabine** increases the effects of **coumarins**. Monitor INR and adjust dose. Moderate Anecdotal

▶ **Cephalosporins (cefazolin, ceftriaxone)** potentially increase the risk of bleeding events when given with **coumarins**. Severe Anecdotal

▶ **Ceritinib** is predicted to increase the exposure to **acenocoumarol**. Severe Theoretical

▶ **Ceritinib** increases the exposure to **warfarin**. Avoid or monitor INR. Severe Study

▶ **Chloramphenicol** potentially increases the anticoagulant effect of **coumarins**. Moderate Anecdotal

▶ **Cobicistat** is predicted to affect the exposure to **warfarin**. Moderate Theoretical

▶ **Corticosteroids** are predicted to increase the effects of **coumarins**. Moderate Study

▶ **Cranberry** juice potentially increases the anticoagulant effect of **warfarin**. Avoid. Severe Anecdotal

▶ **Crizotinib** is predicted to increase the risk of bleeding events when given with **coumarins**. Severe Theoretical

▶ **Dabrafenib** is predicted to decrease the anticoagulant effect of **coumarins**. Severe Theoretical

▶ **Disulfiram** increases the anticoagulant effect of **coumarins**. Monitor and adjust dose. Severe Study

▶ **Elvitegravir** is predicted to decrease the anticoagulant effect of **coumarins**. Moderate Anecdotal

▶ **Endothelin receptor antagonists (bosentan)** decrease the anticoagulant effect of **coumarins**. Moderate Study

▶ **Enteral feeds** (vitamin-K containing) potentially decrease the anticoagulant effect of **coumarins**. Severe Anecdotal

▶ **Erlotinib** increases the anticoagulant effect of **coumarins**. Severe Anecdotal

▶ **Fibrates** are predicted to increase the anticoagulant effect of **coumarins**. Monitor INR and adjust dose. Severe Study

▶ **Fluorouracil** increases the anticoagulant effect of **coumarins**. Severe Anecdotal

▶ **Fostamatinib** might cause bleeding when given with **acenocoumarol**. Moderate Theoretical

▶ **Fostamatinib** might causes bleeding when given with **warfarin**. Moderate Theoretical

▶ **Gefitinib** is predicted to increase the anticoagulant effect of **coumarins**. Severe Anecdotal

▶ **Glofitamab** might affect the exposure to **warfarin**. Moderate Theoretical

▶ **Glucagon** increases the anticoagulant effect of **warfarin**. Severe Study

▶ **Glucagon-like peptide-1 receptor agonists (semaglutide)** might decrease the anticoagulant effect of **acenocoumarol**. Severe Anecdotal

▶ **Glucagon-like peptide-1 receptor agonists (tirzepatide)** might affect the absorption of **warfarin**. Severe Theoretical

▶ **Glucosamine** potentially decreases the anticoagulant effect of **acenocoumarol**. Moderate Anecdotal

▶ **Glucosamine** potentially increases the anticoagulant effect of **warfarin**. Avoid. Moderate Anecdotal

▶ **Griseofulvin** potentially decreases the anticoagulant effect of **coumarins**. Moderate Anecdotal

▶ **H₂ receptor antagonists (cimetidine)** increase the anticoagulant effect of **coumarins**. Severe Study

▶ **HIV-protease inhibitors** are predicted to affect the anticoagulant effect of **coumarins**. Moderate Study

▶ **Imatinib** is predicted to increase the risk of bleeding events when given with **coumarins**. Severe Theoretical

▶ **Ivacaftor** is predicted to increase the exposure to **warfarin**. Moderate Theoretical

▶ **Ivermectin** potentially increases the anticoagulant effect of **coumarins**. Severe Anecdotal

▶ **Ivosidenib** might decrease the exposure to **warfarin**. Avoid or monitor efficacy. Unknown Study

▶ **Lapatinib** is predicted to increase the risk of bleeding events when given with **coumarins**. Severe Theoretical

▶ **Leflunomide** increases the anticoagulant effect of **coumarins**. Severe Anecdotal

▶ **Letermovir** is predicted to decrease the concentration of **warfarin**. Monitor and adjust dose. Moderate Theoretical

▶ **Lomitapide** increases the exposure to **warfarin**. Monitor INR and adjust dose. Severe Study

▶ **Lorlatinib** is predicted to decrease the exposure to **coumarins**. Moderate Theoretical

▶ **Macrolides (azithromycin)** might increase the risk of bleeding events when given with **coumarins**. Severe Anecdotal

▶ **Macrolides (clarithromycin, erythromycin)** increase the anticoagulant effect of **coumarins**. Monitor INR and adjust dose. Severe Anecdotal

▶ **Mercaptopurine** decreases the anticoagulant effect of **coumarins**. Moderate Anecdotal

▶ **Metreleptin** might alter the exposure to **warfarin**. Monitor INR and adjust dose. Severe Theoretical

▶ **Metronidazole** increases the anticoagulant effect of **coumarins**. Monitor INR and adjust dose. Severe Study

▶ **Mexiletine** potentially affects the exposure to **warfarin**. Avoid. Unknown Theoretical

▶ **Mifepristone** is predicted to increase the exposure to **warfarin**. Moderate Theoretical

▶ **Monoclonal antibodies (bimekizumab)** might affect the exposure to **warfarin**. Moderate Theoretical

▶ **Monoclonal antibodies (blinatumomab, mosunetuzumab)** are predicted to transiently increase the exposure to **warfarin**. Monitor and adjust dose. Moderate Theoretical

▶ **Monoclonal antibodies (elranatamab)** might affect the exposure to **warfarin**. Monitor and adjust dose. Moderate Theoretical

▶ **Monoclonal antibodies (sarilumab)** potentially affect the exposure to **warfarin**. Monitor and adjust dose. Severe Theoretical

▶ **Monoclonal antibodies (tocilizumab)** are predicted to decrease the exposure to **warfarin**. Monitor and adjust dose. Moderate Theoretical

▶ **Neurokinin-1 receptor antagonists (aprepitant)** decrease the anticoagulant effect of **coumarins**. Moderate Study

▶ **Neurokinin-1 receptor antagonists (fosaprepitant)** are predicted to decrease the anticoagulant effect of **coumarins**. Moderate Theoretical

▶ **Nilotinib** is predicted to increase the risk of bleeding events when given with **coumarins**. Severe Theoretical

▶ **Nirmatrelvir** boosted with ritonavir is predicted to affect the concentration of **warfarin**. Moderate Theoretical

▶ **Nitisinone** is predicted to increase the exposure to **warfarin**. Moderate Study

▶ **NNRTIs (efavirenz)** are predicted to affect the concentration of **coumarins**. Adjust dose. Moderate Theoretical

▶ **NNRTIs (etravirine)** increase the anticoagulant effect of **coumarins**. Moderate Theoretical

▶ **NNRTIs (nevirapine)** potentially alter the anticoagulant effect of **coumarins**. Severe Anecdotal

▶ **Obeticholic acid** decreases the anticoagulant effect of **warfarin**. Severe Study

▶ **Opioids (tramadol)** might increase the anticoagulant effect of **acenocoumarol**. Severe Study

▸ Opioids **(tramadol)** have been reported to increase the anticoagulant effect of **warfarin**. Severe Anecdotal

▸ Oritavancin might increase the exposure to **warfarin**. Moderate Theoretical

▸ Oxymetholone increases the anticoagulant effect of **coumarins**. Severe Anecdotal

▸ Paracetamol increases the anticoagulant effect of **coumarins**. Moderate Study

▸ Penicillins potentially alter the anticoagulant effect of **coumarins**. Monitor INR and adjust dose. Severe Anecdotal

▸ Pitolisant is predicted to decrease the exposure to **warfarin**. Mild Theoretical

▸ Pralsetinib might affect the exposure to **warfarin**. Avoid. Moderate Theoretical

▸ Quinolones increase the anticoagulant effect of **coumarins**. Severe Anecdotal

▸ Rifamycins **(rifabutin)** might decrease the anticoagulant effect of **coumarins**. Moderate Theoretical

▸ Rifamycins **(rifampicin)** decrease the anticoagulant effect of **coumarins**. Severe Study

▸ Rifaximin has been reported to decrease the anticoagulant effect of **warfarin**. Monitor INR and adjust dose. Severe Anecdotal

▸ Rucaparib slightly increases the exposure to **warfarin**. Monitor and adjust dose. Severe Study

▸ Selumetinib might increase the risk of bleeding when given with **coumarins**. Severe Theoretical

▸ St John's wort decreases the anticoagulant effect of **coumarins**. Avoid. Severe Anecdotal

▸ Statins **(fluvastatin, rosuvastatin)** increase the anticoagulant effect of **coumarins**. Monitor INR and adjust dose. Severe Study

▸ Sucralfate potentially decreases the effects of **warfarin**. Separate administration by 2 hours. Moderate Anecdotal

▸ Sulfonamides **(sulfadiazine)** are predicted to increase the anticoagulant effect of **coumarins**. Severe Theoretical

▸ Sulfonamides **(sulfamethoxazole)** increase the anticoagulant effect of **coumarins**. Severe Study

▸ Tamoxifen increases the anticoagulant effect of **coumarins**. Severe Study

▸ Tebentafusp is predicted to transiently increase the exposure to **warfarin**. Monitor and adjust dose. Moderate Theoretical

▸ Tegafur increases the anticoagulant effect of **coumarins**. Moderate Theoretical

▸ Teriflunomide affects the anticoagulant effect of **coumarins**. Severe Study

▸ Tetracyclines increase the anticoagulant effect of **coumarins**. Severe Anecdotal

▸ Tigecycline is predicted to alter the anticoagulant effect of **coumarins**. Moderate Anecdotal

▸ Tofacitinib is predicted to increase the risk of bleeding when given with **coumarins**. Severe Theoretical

▸ Toremifene is predicted to increase the anticoagulant effect of **coumarins**. Severe Theoretical

▸ Trimethoprim is predicted to increase the anticoagulant effect of **coumarins**. Severe Study

▸ Vemurafenib is predicted to increase the exposure to **coumarins**. Moderate Study

▸ Venetoclax slightly increases the exposure to **warfarin**. Moderate Study

Cranberry

▸ **Cranberry** juice potentially increases the anticoagulant effect of coumarins **(warfarin)**. Avoid. Severe Anecdotal

Crisantaspase → see TABLE 1 p. 1571 (hepatotoxicity), TABLE 14 p. 1575 (myelosuppression), TABLE 3 p. 1571 (anticoagulant effects)

▸ **Crisantaspase** is predicted to increase the risk of hepatotoxicity when given with imatinib. Severe Theoretical → Also see TABLE 14 p. 1575

▸ **Crisantaspase** affects the efficacy of methotrexate. Severe Anecdotal → Also see TABLE 1 p. 1571 → Also see TABLE 14 p. 1575

▸ **Crisantaspase** potentially increases the risk of neurotoxicity when given with vinca alkaloids **(vincristine)**. **Vincristine** should be taken 3 to 24 hours before **crisantaspase**. Severe Anecdotal → Also see TABLE 14 p. 1575

Crizotinib → see TABLE 5 p. 1572 (bradycardia), TABLE 8 p. 1573 (QT-interval prolongation)

GENERAL INFORMATION   Caution with concurrent use of drugs that cause gastrointestinal perforation—discontinue treatment if gastrointestinal perforation occurs.

▸ **Crizotinib** is predicted to increase the exposure to abemaciclib. Moderate Study

▸ **Crizotinib** is predicted to increase the exposure to acalabrutinib. Avoid or monitor. Severe Study

▸ **Crizotinib** is predicted to increase the exposure to alpha blockers **(tamsulosin)**. Moderate Theoretical

▸ Anti-androgens **(apalutamide, enzalutamide)** are predicted to markedly decrease the exposure to **crizotinib**. Avoid. Severe Study → Also see TABLE 8 p. 1573

▸ Antiarrhythmics **(dronedarone)** are predicted to increase the exposure to **crizotinib**. Moderate Study → Also see TABLE 5 p. 1572 → Also see TABLE 8 p. 1573

▸ **Crizotinib** is predicted to increase the exposure to antiarrhythmics **(propafenone)**. Monitor and adjust dose. Moderate Study → Also see TABLE 5 p. 1572

▸ Antiepileptics **(carbamazepine, fosphenytoin, phenobarbital, phenytoin, primidone)** are predicted to markedly decrease the exposure to **crizotinib**. Avoid. Severe Study

▸ Antifungals, azoles **(fluconazole, isavuconazole)** are predicted to increase the exposure to **crizotinib**. Moderate Study → Also see TABLE 8 p. 1573

▸ Antifungals, azoles **(itraconazole, ketoconazole, posaconazole, voriconazole)** are predicted to increase the exposure to **crizotinib**. Avoid. Moderate Study → Also see TABLE 8 p. 1573

▸ **Crizotinib** is predicted to increase the exposure to antihistamines, non-sedating **(mizolastine)**. Severe Theoretical

▸ **Crizotinib** is predicted to increase the exposure to antihistamines, non-sedating **(rupatadine)**. Avoid. Moderate Study

▸ **Crizotinib** is predicted to increase the exposure to antipsychotics, second generation **(cariprazine)**. Avoid. Severe Study

▸ **Crizotinib** is predicted to increase the exposure to antipsychotics, second generation **(lurasidone)**. Adjust **lurasidone** dose. Moderate Study

▸ **Crizotinib** is predicted to increase the exposure to antipsychotics, second generation **(quetiapine)**. Avoid. Moderate Study

▸ **Crizotinib** is predicted to increase the exposure to avapritinib. Avoid or adjust dose—consult product literature. Moderate Study

▸ **Crizotinib** is predicted to increase the exposure to axitinib. Moderate Study

▸ **Crizotinib** might increases the exposure to bedaquiline. Mild Theoretical → Also see TABLE 8 p. 1573

▸ **Crizotinib** is predicted to increase the exposure to benzodiazepines **(alprazolam)**. Severe Study

▸ **Crizotinib** is predicted to increase the exposure to benzodiazepines **(midazolam)**. Monitor adverse effects and adjust dose. Severe Study

▸ **Crizotinib** is predicted to increase the exposure to bosutinib. Avoid or adjust dose. Severe Study → Also see TABLE 8 p. 1573

▸ **Crizotinib** is predicted to increase the exposure to brigatinib. Moderate Study → Also see TABLE 5 p. 1572

▸ **Crizotinib** is predicted to increase the exposure to buspirone. Use with caution and adjust dose. Moderate Study

▸ **Crizotinib** is predicted to increase the exposure to cabozantinib. Moderate Study → Also see TABLE 8 p. 1573

▸ Calcium channel blockers **(diltiazem, verapamil)** are predicted to increase the exposure to **crizotinib**. Avoid. Moderate Study → Also see TABLE 5 p. 1572

▸ **Crizotinib** is predicted to increase the exposure to calcium channel blockers **(amlodipine, felodipine, lacidipine, lercanidipine, nicardipine, nifedipine, nimodipine)**. Monitor and adjust dose. Moderate Study

▸ **Crizotinib** is predicted to increase the exposure to capivasertib. Adjust dose. Moderate Study

▸ Cenobamate is predicted to decrease the exposure to **crizotinib**. Avoid. Severe Study

Crizotinib (continued)

▸ **Ceritinib** is predicted to increase the exposure to **crizotinib**. Avoid. Moderate Study → Also see TABLE 5 p. 1572 → Also see TABLE 8 p. 1573

▸ **Crizotinib** is predicted to increase the exposure to ceritinib. Moderate Study → Also see TABLE 5 p. 1572 → Also see TABLE 8 p. 1573

▸ **Crizotinib** is predicted to increase the concentration of ciclosporin. Severe Study

▸ **Cobicistat** is predicted to increase the exposure to **crizotinib**. Avoid. Moderate Study

▸ **Crizotinib** is predicted to increase the exposure to cobimetinib. Severe Study

▸ **Crizotinib** is predicted to increase the exposure to colchicine. Adjust **colchicine** dose with moderate CYP3A4 inhibitors, p. 1279. Severe Study

▸ **Crizotinib** is predicted to increase the exposure to corticosteroids (methylprednisolone). Monitor and adjust dose. Moderate Study

▸ **Crizotinib** is predicted to increase the risk of bleeding events when given with coumarins. Severe Theoretical

▸ **Dabrafenib** is predicted to decrease the exposure to **crizotinib**. Avoid. Severe Study

▸ **Crizotinib** is predicted to increase the exposure to dabrafenib. Moderate Study

▸ **Crizotinib** is predicted to increase the exposure to daridorexant. Adjust **daridorexant** dose, p. 554. Severe Study

▸ **Crizotinib** is predicted to increase the exposure to darifenacin. Moderate Study

▸ **Crizotinib** is predicted to increase the exposure to dasatinib. Severe Study → Also see TABLE 8 p. 1573

▸ **Crizotinib** is predicted to slightly increase the exposure to dienogest. Moderate Study

▸ **Crizotinib** is predicted to increase the exposure to dipeptidylpeptidase-4 inhibitors (saxagliptin). Mild Study

▸ **Crizotinib** is predicted to increase the exposure to domperidone. Avoid. Severe Study

▸ **Crizotinib** is predicted to increase the exposure to dopamine receptor agonists (bromocriptine). Severe Theoretical

▸ **Crizotinib** is predicted to increase the concentration of dopamine receptor agonists (cabergoline). Moderate Anecdotal

▸ **Crizotinib** is predicted to increase the exposure to drospirenone. Severe Study

▸ **Crizotinib** is predicted to moderately increase the exposure to dutasteride. Mild Study

▸ **Crizotinib** is predicted to increase the exposure to elacestrant. Avoid moderate CYP3A4 inhibitors or adjust **elacestrant** dose, p. 1084. Severe Theoretical

▸ **Crizotinib** is predicted to increase the exposure to elexacaftor. Adjust ivacaftor with tezacaftor and elexacaftor p. 337 dose with moderate CYP3A4 inhibitors. Severe Theoretical

▸ **Crizotinib** is predicted to increase the exposure to eliglustat. Avoid or adjust dose—consult product literature. Severe Study

▸ **Encorafenib** is predicted to markedly decrease the exposure to **crizotinib**. Avoid. Severe Study → Also see TABLE 8 p. 1573

▸ **Crizotinib** is predicted to moderately increase the exposure to encorafenib. Moderate Study → Also see TABLE 8 p. 1573

▸ Endothelin receptor antagonists (bosentan) are predicted to decrease the exposure to **crizotinib**. Avoid. Severe Study

▸ **Crizotinib** is predicted to increase the exposure to endothelin receptor antagonists (macitentan). Manufacturer advises caution depending on other drugs taken—consult product literature. Moderate Theoretical

▸ **Crizotinib** is predicted to increase the exposure to entrectinib. Avoid or adjust dose with moderate CYP3A4 inhibitors—consult product literature. Severe Theoretical → Also see TABLE 8 p. 1573

▸ **Crizotinib** is predicted to increase the risk of ergotism when given with ergometrine. Severe Theoretical

▸ **Crizotinib** is predicted to increase the exposure to erlotinib. Moderate Study

▸ **Crizotinib** is predicted to increase the exposure to etrasimod. Avoid in poor CYP2C9 metabolisers. Severe Theoretical → Also see TABLE 5 p. 1572

▸ **Crizotinib** is predicted to increase the concentration of everolimus. Avoid or adjust dose. Moderate Study

▸ **Crizotinib** is predicted to increase the exposure to fedratinib. Monitor and adjust dose. Moderate Study

▸ **Crizotinib** is predicted to increase the exposure to fesoterodine. Adjust **fesoterodine** dose with moderate CYP3A4 inhibitors in hepatic and renal impairment, p. 897. Mild Study

▸ **Crizotinib** is predicted to increase the exposure to gefitinib. Moderate Study

▸ **Crizotinib** potentially decreases the exposure to glecaprevir. Avoid. Severe Theoretical

▸ **Grapefruit** juice is predicted to increase the exposure to crizotinib. Avoid. Moderate Theoretical

▸ **Crizotinib** is predicted to increase the concentration of guanfacine. Adjust **guanfacine** dose, p. 407. Moderate Theoretical

▸ **HIV-protease inhibitors** are predicted to increase the exposure to **crizotinib**. Avoid. Moderate Study

▸ **Crizotinib** is predicted to increase the exposure to ibrutinib. Adjust dose with moderate CYP3A4 inhibitors—consult product literature. Severe Study

▸ **Idelalisib** is predicted to increase the exposure to **crizotinib**. Avoid. Moderate Study

▸ **Imatinib** is predicted to increase the exposure to **crizotinib**. Moderate Study

▸ **Crizotinib** is predicted to increase the exposure to ivabradine. Adjust **ivabradine** dose, p. 245. Severe Theoretical → Also see TABLE 5 p. 1572

▸ **Crizotinib** is predicted to increase the exposure to ivacaftor. Adjust dose with moderate CYP3A4 inhibitors, see ivacaftor p. 336, tezacaftor with ivacaftor p. 339, and ivacaftor with tezacaftor and elexacaftor p. 337. Moderate Study

▸ **Crizotinib** is predicted to increase the exposure to ivosidenib. Monitor and adjust dose—consult product literature. Severe Study → Also see TABLE 8 p. 1573

▸ **Ivosidenib** is predicted to markedly decrease the exposure to **crizotinib**. Avoid. Severe Study → Also see TABLE 8 p. 1573

▸ **Crizotinib** is predicted to increase the exposure to lapatinib. Moderate Study → Also see TABLE 8 p. 1573

▸ **Crizotinib** is predicted to increase the exposure to larotrectinib. Monitor and adjust dose. Moderate Theoretical

▸ **Crizotinib** is predicted to increase the exposure to leniolisib. Avoid. Moderate Study

▸ **Letermovir** is predicted to increase the exposure to **crizotinib**. Moderate Study

▸ **Crizotinib** is predicted to increase the exposure to lomitapide. Avoid. Moderate Theoretical

▸ **Lorlatinib** is predicted to decrease the exposure to **crizotinib**. Avoid. Severe Study

▸ **Lumacaftor** is predicted to markedly decrease the exposure to **crizotinib**. Avoid. Severe Study

▸ **Macrolides (clarithromycin, erythromycin)** are predicted to increase the exposure to **crizotinib**. Avoid. Moderate Study → Also see TABLE 8 p. 1573

▸ **Crizotinib** is predicted to increase the exposure to mavacamten. Adjust dose—consult product literature. Moderate Study

▸ **Crizotinib** is predicted to increase the exposure to midostaurin. Moderate Theoretical

▸ **Crizotinib** is predicted to increase the exposure to mineralocorticoid receptor antagonists (eplerenone). Adjust eplerenone dose, p. 223. Severe Study

▸ **Crizotinib** is predicted to increase the exposure to mineralocorticoid receptor antagonists (finerenone). Severe Study

▸ **Mitotane** is predicted to markedly decrease the exposure to **crizotinib**. Avoid. Severe Study

▸ **Crizotinib** is predicted to increase the exposure to mobocertinib. Avoid or adjust dose and monitor ECG—consult product literature. Severe Study → Also see TABLE 8 p. 1573

▸ **Crizotinib** is predicted to increase the exposure to naldemedine. Moderate Study

▸ **Crizotinib** is predicted to increase the exposure to naloxegol. Adjust **naloxegol** dose and monitor adverse effects, p. 72. Moderate Study

▸ **Crizotinib** is predicted to increase the exposure to neratinib. Avoid moderate CYP3A4 inhibitors or adjust dose and monitor for gastrointestinal adverse effects—consult product literature. Severe Study

- ▸ Neurokinin-1 receptor antagonists (**netupitant**) are predicted to increase the exposure to **crizotinib**. Moderate Study
- ▸ NNRTIs (**efavirenz, etravirine, nevirapine**) are predicted to decrease the exposure to **crizotinib**. Avoid. Severe Study → Also see TABLE 8 p. 1573
- ▸ **Crizotinib** is predicted to increase the exposure to olaparib. Avoid or adjust dose with moderate CYP3A4 inhibitors—consult product literature. Moderate Theoretical
- ▸ **Crizotinib** is predicted to increase the exposure to opioids (**alfentanil, buprenorphine, fentanyl, oxycodone**). Monitor and adjust dose. Moderate Study → Also see TABLE 5 p. 1572
- ▸ **Crizotinib** is predicted to increase the exposure to opioids (**methadone, sufentanil**). Moderate Theoretical → Also see TABLE 5 p. 1572 → Also see TABLE 8 p. 1573
- ▸ **Crizotinib** is predicted to increase the exposure to pazopanib. Moderate Study → Also see TABLE 8 p. 1573
- ▸ **Crizotinib** is predicted to increase the exposure to pemigatinib. Severe Study
- ▸ **Crizotinib** is predicted to increase the risk of bleeding events when given with phenindione. Severe Theoretical
- ▸ **Crizotinib** is predicted to increase the exposure to phosphodiesterase type-5 inhibitors (**avanafil**). Adjust **avanafil** dose, p. 939. Moderate Theoretical
- ▸ **Crizotinib** is predicted to increase the exposure to phosphodiesterase type-5 inhibitors (**sildenafil**). Monitor or adjust **sildenafil** dose with moderate CYP3A4 inhibitors, p. 940. Moderate Study
- ▸ **Crizotinib** is predicted to increase the exposure to phosphodiesterase type-5 inhibitors (**tadalafil**). Severe Theoretical
- ▸ **Crizotinib** is predicted to increase the exposure to phosphodiesterase type-5 inhibitors (**vardenafil**). Adjust dose. Severe Theoretical → Also see TABLE 8 p. 1573
- ▸ **Crizotinib** potentially decreases the exposure to pibrentasvir. Avoid. Severe Theoretical
- ▸ **Crizotinib** is predicted to increase the exposure to pimozide. Avoid. Severe Theoretical → Also see TABLE 8 p. 1573
- ▸ Pitolisant is predicted to decrease the exposure to **crizotinib**. Avoid. Severe Theoretical
- ▸ **Crizotinib** is predicted to increase the exposure to ponatinib. Moderate Study
- ▸ **Crizotinib** is predicted to increase the exposure to pralsetinib. Moderate Theoretical
- ▸ **Crizotinib** is predicted to increase the exposure to ranolazine. Severe Study → Also see TABLE 8 p. 1573
- ▸ **Crizotinib** is predicted to increase the exposure to regorafenib. Moderate Study
- ▸ **Crizotinib** is predicted to increase the exposure to ribociclib. Moderate Study → Also see TABLE 8 p. 1573
- ▸ Rifamycins (**rifampicin**) are predicted to markedly decrease the exposure to **crizotinib**. Avoid. Severe Study
- ▸ **Crizotinib** is predicted to increase the exposure to rimegepant. Avoid another dose of rimegepant within 48 hours of concurrent use. Moderate Study
- ▸ **Crizotinib** is predicted to increase the exposure to ruxolitinib. Moderate Study
- ▸ **Crizotinib** is predicted to increase the exposure to selpercatinib. Moderate Study → Also see TABLE 8 p. 1573
- ▸ **Crizotinib** is predicted to increase the exposure to selumetinib. Avoid or adjust dose—consult product literature. Severe Study
- ▸ **Crizotinib** is predicted to increase the exposure to siponimod. Avoid depending on other drugs taken—consult product literature. Severe Study → Also see TABLE 5 p. 1572
- ▸ **Crizotinib** increases the concentration of sirolimus. Monitor and adjust dose. Moderate Study
- ▸ Sotorasib is predicted to decrease the exposure to **crizotinib**. Avoid. Severe Study
- ▸ **Crizotinib** is predicted to increase the exposure to SSRIs (**dapoxetine**). Adjust **dapoxetine** dose with moderate CYP3A4 inhibitors, p. 947. Moderate Theoretical
- ▸ St John's wort is predicted to decrease the exposure to **crizotinib**. Avoid. Severe Study
- ▸ **Crizotinib** is predicted to increase the exposure to statins (**atorvastatin**). Monitor and adjust dose. Moderate Theoretical
- ▸ **Crizotinib** is predicted to increase the exposure to statins (**pravastatin**). Moderate Theoretical

- ▸ **Crizotinib** is predicted to increase the exposure to statins (**simvastatin**). Monitor and adjust dose. Severe Theoretical
- ▸ **Crizotinib** is predicted to increase the exposure to sunitinib. Moderate Study → Also see TABLE 8 p. 1573
- ▸ **Crizotinib** is predicted to increase the concentration of tacrolimus. Severe Study
- ▸ **Crizotinib** is predicted to increase the exposure to taxanes (**cabazitaxel**). Moderate Theoretical
- ▸ **Crizotinib** is predicted to increase the exposure to taxanes (**docetaxel**). Severe Study
- ▸ **Crizotinib** is predicted to increase the exposure to taxanes (**paclitaxel**). Moderate Anecdotal
- ▸ **Crizotinib** is predicted to increase the concentration of temsirolimus. Use with caution or avoid. Moderate Theoretical
- ▸ **Crizotinib** is predicted to increase the exposure to tezacaftor. Adjust dose with moderate CYP3A4 inhibitors, see tezacaftor with ivacaftor p. 339 and ivacaftor with tezacaftor and elexacaftor p. 337. Severe Study
- ▸ **Crizotinib** given with a potent CYP2C19 inhibitor is predicted to increase the exposure to tofacitinib. Adjust **tofacitinib** dose, p. 1265. Moderate Study
- ▸ **Crizotinib** is predicted to increase the exposure to tolvaptan. Manufacturer advises caution or adjust **tolvaptan** dose with moderate CYP3A4 inhibitors, p. 767. Moderate Study
- ▸ **Crizotinib** is predicted to increase the exposure to trazodone. Moderate Theoretical
- ▸ Tucatinib is predicted to increase the exposure to **crizotinib**. Avoid. Moderate Study
- ▸ **Crizotinib** is predicted to increase the exposure to ulipristal. Avoid if used for uterine fibroids. Moderate Study
- ▸ **Crizotinib** is predicted to increase the exposure to vemurafenib. Severe Theoretical → Also see TABLE 8 p. 1573
- ▸ **Crizotinib** is predicted to increase the exposure to venetoclax. Avoid or adjust dose—consult product literature. Severe Study
- ▸ **Crizotinib** is predicted to increase the exposure to vinca alkaloids. Severe Theoretical
- ▸ **Crizotinib** is predicted to increase the exposure to voclosporin. Adjust **voclosporin** dose, p. 973. Severe Study → Also see TABLE 8 p. 1573
- ▸ **Crizotinib** is predicted to increase the exposure to zanubrutinib. Avoid or adjust dose with moderate CYP3A4 inhibitors—consult product literature. Severe Study
- ▸ **Crizotinib** is predicted to increase the exposure to zopiclone. Adjust dose. Moderate Study

Crovalimab
- ▸ **Crovalimab** increases the risk of hypersensitivity reactions when given with monoclonal antibodies (**eculizumab**). Severe Study
- ▸ **Crovalimab** increases the risk of hypersensitivity reactions when given with ravulizumab. Severe Study

Cyclizine → see antihistamines, sedating

Cyclopentolate → see TABLE 9 p. 1573 (antimuscarinics)
- ▸ Antipsychotics, second generation (**clozapine**) can cause constipation, as can **cyclopentolate**; concurrent use might increase the risk of developing intestinal obstruction. Severe Theoretical → Also see TABLE 9 p. 1573

Cyclophosphamide → see alkylating agents

Cycloserine
- ▸ **Cycloserine** increases the risk of CNS toxicity when given with isoniazid. Monitor and adjust dose. Moderate Study

Cyproheptadine → see antihistamines, sedating

Cyproterone → see anti-androgens

Cytarabine → see TABLE 1 p. 1571 (hepatotoxicity), TABLE 14 p. 1575 (myelosuppression), TABLE 11 p. 1574 (peripheral neuropathy)
- ▸ Cedazuridine is predicted to increase the exposure to **cytarabine**. Avoid. Moderate Theoretical
- ▸ **Cytarabine** decreases the concentration of flucytosine. Avoid. Severe Study
- ▸ Live vaccines are predicted to increase the risk of generalised infection (possibly life-threatening) when given with **cytarabine**. UKHSA advises avoid (refer to Green Book). Severe Theoretical

Cytisinicline
- Cytisinicline might decrease the efficacy of combined hormonal contraceptives. Use additional contraceptive precautions. Severe Theoretical

Cytomegalovirus immunoglobulin → see immunoglobulins

Dabigatran → see thrombin inhibitors

Dabrafenib
- Dabrafenib is predicted to decrease the exposure to acalabrutinib. Severe Study
- Anti-androgens (apalutamide, enzalutamide) are predicted to decrease the exposure to dabrafenib. Avoid. Moderate Theoretical
- Dabrafenib is predicted to decrease the exposure to anti-androgens (darolutamide). Avoid. Moderate Theoretical
- Antiarrhythmics (dronedarone) are predicted to increase the exposure to dabrafenib. Moderate Study
- Antiepileptics (carbamazepine, fosphenytoin, phenobarbital, phenytoin, primidone) are predicted to decrease the exposure to dabrafenib. Avoid. Moderate Theoretical
- Antifungals, azoles (fluconazole, isavuconazole) are predicted to increase the exposure to dabrafenib. Moderate Study
- Antifungals, azoles (itraconazole, ketoconazole, posaconazole, voriconazole) are predicted to increase the exposure to dabrafenib. Use with caution or avoid. Moderate Study
- Dabrafenib is predicted to decrease the exposure to antifungals, azoles (isavuconazole). Avoid. Severe Theoretical
- Dabrafenib is predicted to decrease the exposure to antipsychotics, second generation (cariprazine). Avoid. Severe Theoretical
- Dabrafenib is predicted to decrease the exposure to antipsychotics, second generation (lurasidone). Monitor and adjust dose. Moderate Theoretical
- Dabrafenib is predicted to decrease the exposure to antipsychotics, second generation (quetiapine). Moderate Study
- Dabrafenib is predicted to decrease the exposure to avacopan. Severe Theoretical
- Dabrafenib is predicted to decrease the exposure to avapritinib. Avoid. Severe Study
- Dabrafenib is predicted to decrease the exposure to axitinib. Moderate Study
- Dabrafenib is predicted to decrease the exposure to bedaquiline. Avoid. Severe Study
- Dabrafenib decreases the exposure to benzodiazepines (midazolam). Monitor and adjust dose. Moderate Study
- Berotralstat is predicted to increase the exposure to dabrafenib. Moderate Study
- Dabrafenib is predicted to decrease the exposure to bosutinib. Avoid. Severe Study
- Dabrafenib is predicted to decrease the exposure to brigatinib. Avoid or adjust dose—consult product literature. Moderate Study
- Dabrafenib is predicted to decrease the exposure to cabozantinib. Moderate Study
- Calcium channel blockers (diltiazem, verapamil) are predicted to increase the exposure to dabrafenib. Moderate Study
- Dabrafenib is predicted to decrease the exposure to calcium channel blockers (amlodipine, felodipine, lacidipine, lercanidipine, nicardipine, nifedipine, nimodipine). Monitor and adjust dose. Moderate Theoretical
- Dabrafenib is predicted to decrease the exposure to calcium channel blockers (diltiazem, verapamil). Moderate Theoretical
- Dabrafenib is predicted to decrease the exposure to capivasertib. Avoid. Moderate Study
- Dabrafenib is predicted to decrease the exposure to ceritinib. Severe Study
- Ceritinib is predicted to increase the exposure to dabrafenib. Use with caution or avoid. Moderate Study
- Clopidogrel is predicted to increase the exposure to dabrafenib. Moderate Theoretical
- Dabrafenib is predicted to decrease the exposure to cobicistat. Avoid. Severe Theoretical
- Cobicistat is predicted to increase the exposure to dabrafenib. Use with caution or avoid. Moderate Study
- Dabrafenib is predicted to decrease the exposure to cobimetinib. Avoid. Severe Theoretical

- Dabrafenib is predicted to decrease the efficacy of combined hormonal contraceptives. Use additional contraceptive precautions. Severe Theoretical
- Dabrafenib is predicted to decrease the anticoagulant effect of coumarins. Severe Theoretical
- Dabrafenib is predicted to decrease the exposure to crizotinib. Avoid. Severe Study
- Crizotinib is predicted to increase the exposure to dabrafenib. Moderate Study
- Dabrafenib is predicted to decrease the exposure to daridorexant. Severe Study
- Dabrafenib is predicted to decrease the exposure to dasatinib. Severe Study
- Dabrafenib is predicted to decrease the exposure to digoxin. Moderate Theoretical
- Dabrafenib is predicted to decrease the exposure to dolutegravir. Severe Study
- Dabrafenib is predicted to decrease the exposure to elacestrant. Avoid or adjust dose depending on duration—consult product literature. Severe Theoretical
- Dabrafenib is predicted to moderately decrease the exposure to elbasvir. Avoid. Severe Study
- Dabrafenib is predicted to decrease the concentration of elvitegravir. Avoid. Severe Theoretical
- Dabrafenib is predicted to decrease the exposure to encorafenib. Moderate Study
- Encorafenib is predicted to decrease the exposure to dabrafenib. Avoid. Moderate Theoretical
- Endothelin receptor antagonists (bosentan) are predicted to decrease the exposure to dabrafenib. Moderate Study
- Dabrafenib is predicted to decrease the exposure to entrectinib. Avoid. Moderate Theoretical
- Dabrafenib is predicted to decrease the exposure to erdafitinib. Adjust dose. Moderate Theoretical
- Dabrafenib is predicted to decrease the exposure to erlotinib. Severe Study
- Dabrafenib is predicted to decrease the concentration of everolimus. Avoid or adjust dose. Severe Study
- Fedratinib is predicted to increase the exposure to dabrafenib. Moderate Study
- Dabrafenib is predicted to decrease the exposure to fedratinib. Avoid. Moderate Study
- Fibrates (gemfibrozil) are predicted to increase the exposure to dabrafenib. Moderate Theoretical
- Dabrafenib is predicted to decrease the exposure to fruquintinib. Avoid. Moderate Study
- Dabrafenib is predicted to decrease the exposure to gefitinib. Avoid. Severe Study
- Dabrafenib is predicted to decrease the exposure to glasdegib. Avoid or adjust dose—consult product literature. Moderate Theoretical
- Dabrafenib is predicted to decrease the exposure to glecaprevir. Avoid. Severe Study
- Dabrafenib is predicted to markedly decrease the exposure to grazoprevir. Avoid. Severe Study
- Dabrafenib is predicted to decrease the concentration of guanfacine. Adjust dose. Moderate Theoretical
- HIV-protease inhibitors are predicted to increase the exposure to dabrafenib. Use with caution or avoid. Moderate Study
- Dabrafenib is predicted to decrease the exposure to ibrutinib. Avoid or monitor. Severe Study
- Idelalisib is predicted to increase the exposure to dabrafenib. Use with caution or avoid. Moderate Study
- Dabrafenib is predicted to decrease the exposure to idelalisib. Avoid. Moderate Theoretical
- Imatinib is predicted to increase the exposure to dabrafenib. Moderate Study
- Dabrafenib is predicted to decrease the exposure to imatinib. Moderate Study
- Dabrafenib is predicted to decrease the exposure to ivacaftor. Moderate Study
- Ivosidenib is predicted to decrease the exposure to dabrafenib. Avoid. Moderate Theoretical
- Dabrafenib is predicted to decrease the exposure to ixazomib. Moderate Theoretical

- **Dabrafenib** is predicted to decrease the exposure to lapatinib. Avoid. [Severe] Study
- **Dabrafenib** is predicted to decrease the exposure to larotrectinib. Avoid. [Moderate] Study
- **Dabrafenib** is predicted to decrease the exposure to leniolisib. Avoid. [Severe] Theoretical
- Letermovir is predicted to increase the exposure to **dabrafenib**. [Moderate] Study
- Lumacaftor is predicted to decrease the exposure to **dabrafenib**. Avoid. [Moderate] Theoretical
- Macrolides (clarithromycin) are predicted to increase the exposure to **dabrafenib**. Use with caution or avoid. [Moderate] Study
- Macrolides (erythromycin) are predicted to increase the exposure to **dabrafenib**. [Moderate] Study
- **Dabrafenib** is predicted to decrease the exposure to maribavir. Avoid or adjust **maribavir** dose, p. 735. [Severe] Study
- **Dabrafenib** is predicted to decrease the exposure to mavacamten. Monitor and adjust dose—consult product literature. [Severe] Theoretical
- **Dabrafenib** is predicted to decrease the exposure to midostaurin. [Severe] Study
- **Dabrafenib** is predicted to decrease the exposure to mifepristone. Adjust **mifepristone** dose, p. 954. [Severe] Study
- **Dabrafenib** is predicted to decrease the exposure to mineralocorticoid receptor antagonists (finerenone). Avoid. [Severe] Study
- Mitotane is predicted to decrease the exposure to **dabrafenib**. Avoid. [Moderate] Theoretical
- **Dabrafenib** is predicted to decrease the exposure to mobocertinib. Avoid. [Severe] Study
- **Dabrafenib** is predicted to decrease the exposure to naloxegol. [Moderate] Theoretical
- **Dabrafenib** is predicted to decrease the exposure to neratinib. Avoid. [Severe] Theoretical
- Neurokinin-1 receptor antagonists (aprepitant, netupitant) are predicted to increase the exposure to **dabrafenib**. [Moderate] Study
- **Dabrafenib** is predicted to decrease the exposure to neurokinin-1 receptor antagonists (netupitant). [Moderate] Theoretical
- **Dabrafenib** is predicted to decrease the exposure to nilotinib. Avoid. [Severe] Theoretical
- Nilotinib is predicted to increase the exposure to **dabrafenib**. [Moderate] Study
- NNRTIs (efavirenz, nevirapine) are predicted to decrease the exposure to **dabrafenib**. [Moderate] Study
- **Dabrafenib** is predicted to decrease the exposure to NNRTIs (doravirine). Avoid or adjust doravirine p. 741 or lamivudine with tenofovir disoproxil and doravirine p. 751 dose. [Severe] Theoretical
- **Dabrafenib** is predicted to decrease the exposure to NNRTIs (rilpivirine). Avoid. [Severe] Theoretical
- **Dabrafenib** is predicted to decrease the exposure to olaparib. Avoid. [Moderate] Theoretical
- **Dabrafenib** decreases the exposure to opioids (methadone). Monitor and adjust dose. [Severe] Study
- **Dabrafenib** is predicted to decrease the exposure to osimertinib. Use with caution or avoid. [Severe] Study
- **Dabrafenib** is predicted to decrease the exposure to ospemifene. [Moderate] Study
- **Dabrafenib** is predicted to decrease the exposure to pazopanib. [Severe] Study
- **Dabrafenib** is predicted to decrease the exposure to pemigatinib. Avoid or monitor. [Severe] Study
- **Dabrafenib** is predicted to decrease the exposure to phenindione. [Moderate] Study
- **Dabrafenib** is predicted to decrease the exposure to pibrentasvir. Avoid. [Severe] Study
- **Dabrafenib** is predicted to decrease the exposure to ponatinib. [Severe] Study
- **Dabrafenib** is predicted to decrease the exposure to pralsetinib. [Moderate] Theoretical
- **Dabrafenib** is predicted to decrease the exposure to quizartinib. Avoid. [Severe] Study

- **Dabrafenib** is predicted to decrease the exposure to regorafenib. [Severe] Study
- Rifamycins (rifampicin) are predicted to decrease the exposure to **dabrafenib**. Avoid. [Moderate] Theoretical
- **Dabrafenib** is predicted to decrease the exposure to rimegepant. Avoid. [Moderate] Theoretical
- **Dabrafenib** is predicted to decrease the exposure to ripretinib. Avoid or adjust dose—consult product literature. [Moderate] Theoretical
- **Dabrafenib** is predicted to decrease the exposure to ruxolitinib. Monitor and adjust dose. [Moderate] Study
- **Dabrafenib** is predicted to decrease the exposure to selpercatinib. [Moderate] Study
- **Dabrafenib** is predicted to decrease the exposure to selumetinib. Avoid. [Severe] Study
- **Dabrafenib** is predicted to decrease the exposure to siponimod. Manufacturer advises caution depending on genotype—consult product literature. [Moderate] Theoretical
- **Dabrafenib** is predicted to decrease the exposure to sorafenib. [Moderate] Study
- St John's wort is predicted to decrease the exposure to **dabrafenib**. Avoid. [Moderate] Study
- **Dabrafenib** is predicted to decrease the exposure to statins (atorvastatin, simvastatin). [Moderate] Study
- **Dabrafenib** is predicted to decrease the exposure to sunitinib. [Moderate] Study
- **Dabrafenib** is predicted to decrease the exposure to tacrolimus. Monitor and adjust dose. [Moderate] Theoretical
- **Dabrafenib** is predicted to decrease the exposure to taxanes (cabazitaxel). [Moderate] Theoretical
- **Dabrafenib** is predicted to decrease the exposure to taxanes (docetaxel). [Severe] Theoretical
- **Dabrafenib** is predicted to decrease the exposure to taxanes (paclitaxel). Avoid. [Severe] Study
- **Dabrafenib** is predicted to decrease the concentration of temsirolimus. Avoid. [Moderate] Theoretical
- **Dabrafenib** is predicted to decrease the exposure to ticagrelor. [Moderate] Theoretical
- **Dabrafenib** is predicted to decrease the exposure to tofacitinib. [Severe] Study
- Tucatinib is predicted to increase the exposure to **dabrafenib**. Use with caution or avoid. [Moderate] Study
- **Dabrafenib** is predicted to decrease the efficacy of ulipristal. Avoid and for 4 weeks after stopping **dabrafenib**. [Severe] Theoretical
- **Dabrafenib** is predicted to decrease the exposure to vandetanib. [Moderate] Study
- **Dabrafenib** is predicted to decrease the exposure to velpatasvir. Avoid. [Moderate] Theoretical
- **Dabrafenib** is predicted to decrease the exposure to vemurafenib. [Severe] Study
- **Dabrafenib** is predicted to decrease the exposure to venetoclax. Avoid. [Severe] Study
- **Dabrafenib** is predicted to decrease the exposure to voclosporin. Avoid. [Severe] Theoretical
- **Dabrafenib** is predicted to decrease the concentration of voxilaprevir. Avoid. [Severe] Theoretical
- **Dabrafenib** is predicted to decrease the exposure to zanubrutinib. Avoid or adjust dose with moderate CYP3A4 inducers—consult product literature. [Severe] Theoretical

Dacarbazine → see alkylating agents

Dacomitinib
- **Dacomitinib** is predicted to increase the exposure to anticholinesterases, centrally acting (galantamine). Monitor and adjust dose. [Moderate] Study
- **Dacomitinib** is predicted to moderately increase the exposure to antipsychotics, second generation (aripiprazole). Adjust **aripiprazole** dose, p. 454. [Moderate] Study
- **Dacomitinib** is predicted to increase the exposure to antipsychotics, second generation (clozapine). Use with caution and adjust dose. [Severe] Study
- **Dacomitinib** is predicted to increase the exposure to antipsychotics, second generation (risperidone). Adjust dose. [Moderate] Study

Dacomitinib (continued)
- **Dacomitinib** is predicted to markedly increase the exposure to atomoxetine. Adjust dose. Severe Study
- **Dacomitinib** is predicted to markedly increase the exposure to beta blockers, non-selective (propranolol). Avoid. Severe Study
- **Dacomitinib** is predicted to increase the exposure to beta blockers, selective (metoprolol, nebivolol). Moderate Study
- **Dacomitinib** is predicted to slightly increase the exposure to darifenacin. Mild Study
- **Dacomitinib** is predicted to increase the exposure to eliglustat. Avoid or adjust dose—consult product literature. Severe Study
- **Dacomitinib** is predicted to increase the exposure to fenfluramine. Moderate Study
- **Dacomitinib** is predicted to increase the exposure to fesoterodine. Use with caution and adjust dose. Mild Theoretical
- **Dacomitinib** is predicted to increase the exposure to gefitinib. Moderate Theoretical
- **H₂ receptor antagonists** are predicted to decrease the concentration of **dacomitinib**. **Dacomitinib** should be taken 2 hours before or 10 hours after **H₂ receptor antagonists**. Unknown Theoretical
- **Dacomitinib** is predicted to increase the exposure to mexiletine. Moderate Study
- **Dacomitinib** is predicted to decrease the efficacy of opioids (codeine). Moderate Theoretical
- **Dacomitinib** is predicted to decrease the efficacy of opioids (tramadol). Severe Study
- **Dacomitinib** is predicted to moderately increase the exposure to pitolisant. Use with caution and adjust dose. Moderate Study
- **Proton pump inhibitors** are predicted to decrease the exposure to **dacomitinib**. Avoid. Moderate Study
- **Dacomitinib** is predicted to increase the exposure to the active component of sacituzumab govitecan. Severe Theoretical
- **Dacomitinib** is predicted to increase the exposure to SSRIs (dapoxetine). Moderate Theoretical
- **Dacomitinib** is predicted to decrease the efficacy of tamoxifen. Avoid. Severe Study
- **Dacomitinib** is predicted to increase the exposure to the active metabolite of tetrabenazine. Moderate Study
- **Dacomitinib** is predicted to markedly increase the exposure to tolterodine. Avoid. Severe Study
- **Dacomitinib** is predicted to increase the exposure to tricyclic antidepressants. Monitor for toxicity and adjust dose. Severe Study
- **Dacomitinib** is predicted to increase the exposure to vortioxetine. Monitor and adjust dose. Moderate Study

Dactinomycin → see TABLE 1 p. 1571 (hepatotoxicity), TABLE 14 p. 1575 (myelosuppression)
- Live vaccines are predicted to increase the risk of generalised infection (possibly life-threatening) when given with **dactinomycin**. UKHSA advises avoid (refer to Green Book). Severe Theoretical

Dalteparin → see low molecular-weight heparins
Danaparoid → see TABLE 3 p. 1571 (anticoagulant effects)
Danicopan
- **Danicopan** is predicted to increase the exposure to aliskiren. Moderate Study
- **Danicopan** is predicted to increase the exposure to antihistamines, non-sedating (fexofenadine). Moderate Study
- **Danicopan** is predicted to increase the exposure to colchicine. Moderate Study
- **Danicopan** is predicted to increase the exposure to digoxin. Moderate Study
- **Danicopan** is predicted to increase the exposure to everolimus. Moderate Study
- **Danicopan** is predicted to increase the exposure to factor XA inhibitors (edoxaban). Moderate Study
- **Danicopan** is predicted to increase the exposure to loperamide. Moderate Study
- **Danicopan** is predicted to increase the exposure to pralsetinib. Moderate Study
- **Danicopan** is predicted to increase the exposure to ranolazine. Moderate Study
- **Danicopan** is predicted to increase the exposure to rimegepant. Moderate Study

- **Danicopan** is predicted to increase the exposure to sirolimus. Moderate Study
- **Danicopan** is predicted to increase the exposure to statins (atorvastatin, fluvastatin, rosuvastatin). Moderate Study
- **Danicopan** is predicted to increase the exposure to sulfasalazine. Moderate Study
- **Danicopan** is predicted to increase the exposure to tacrolimus. Moderate Theoretical
- **Danicopan** is predicted to increase the exposure to talazoparib. Moderate Study
- **Danicopan** is predicted to increase the exposure to taxanes (paclitaxel). Moderate Study
- **Danicopan** is predicted to increase the exposure to thrombin inhibitors (dabigatran). Moderate Study
- **Danicopan** is predicted to increase the exposure to topotecan. Moderate Study

Dantrolene
- Intravenous **dantrolene** potentially increases the risk of acute hyperkalaemia and cardiovascular collapse when given with calcium channel blockers (diltiazem, verapamil). Avoid. Severe Anecdotal

Dapagliflozin → see sodium glucose co-transporter 2 inhibitors
Dapoxetine → see SSRIs
Dapsone
- Rifamycins decrease the exposure to **dapsone**. Moderate Study
- **Dapsone** increases the exposure to trimethoprim and trimethoprim increases the exposure to **dapsone**. Severe Study

Daptomycin
- Aspirin (high-dose) increases the risk of renal impairment when given with **daptomycin**. Moderate Theoretical
- Ciclosporin is predicted to increase the risk of rhabdomyolysis when given with **daptomycin**. Severe Theoretical
- Fibrates are predicted to increase the risk of rhabdomyolysis when given with **daptomycin**. Severe Theoretical
- NSAIDs increase the risk of renal impairment when given with **daptomycin**. Moderate Theoretical
- Statins are predicted to increase the risk of rhabdomyolysis when given with **daptomycin**. Severe Theoretical

Daratumumab → see monoclonal antibodies
Daridorexant → see TABLE 10 p. 1574 (CNS effects)
- Anti-androgens (apalutamide, enzalutamide) are predicted to decrease the exposure to **daridorexant**. Severe Study
- Antiarrhythmics (dronedarone) are predicted to increase the exposure to **daridorexant**. Adjust **daridorexant** dose, p. 554. Severe Study
- Antiepileptics (carbamazepine, fosphenytoin, phenobarbital, phenytoin, primidone) are predicted to decrease the exposure to **daridorexant**. Severe Study → Also see TABLE 10 p. 1574
- Antifungals, azoles (fluconazole, isavuconazole) are predicted to increase the exposure to **daridorexant**. Adjust **daridorexant** dose, p. 554. Severe Study
- Antifungals, azoles (itraconazole, ketoconazole, posaconazole, voriconazole) are predicted to increase the exposure to **daridorexant**. Avoid. Severe Study
- Berotralstat is predicted to increase the exposure to **daridorexant**. Adjust **daridorexant** dose, p. 554. Severe Study
- Calcium channel blockers (diltiazem, verapamil) are predicted to increase the exposure to **daridorexant**. Adjust **daridorexant** dose, p. 554. Severe Study
- Cenobamate is predicted to decrease the exposure to **daridorexant**. Severe Study → Also see TABLE 10 p. 1574
- Ceritinib is predicted to increase the exposure to **daridorexant**. Avoid. Severe Study
- Ciclosporin is predicted to increase the exposure to **daridorexant**. Adjust **daridorexant** dose, p. 554. Unknown Theoretical
- Cobicistat is predicted to increase the exposure to **daridorexant**. Avoid. Severe Study
- Crizotinib is predicted to increase the exposure to **daridorexant**. Adjust **daridorexant** dose, p. 554. Severe Study
- Dabrafenib is predicted to decrease the exposure to **daridorexant**. Severe Study
- **Daridorexant** is predicted to increase the exposure to digoxin. Moderate Study

- **Encorafenib** is predicted to decrease the exposure to **daridorexant**. [Severe] Study
- **Endothelin receptor antagonists (bosentan)** are predicted to decrease the exposure to **daridorexant**. [Severe] Study
- **Daridorexant** is predicted to increase the exposure to **everolimus**. [Moderate] Study
- **Fedratinib** is predicted to increase the exposure to **daridorexant**. Adjust **daridorexant** dose, p. 554. [Severe] Study
- **Grapefruit** and grapefruit juice is predicted to increase the exposure to **daridorexant**. Avoid **grapefruit** in the evening. [Moderate] Theoretical
- **HIV-protease inhibitors** are predicted to increase the exposure to **daridorexant**. Avoid. [Severe] Study
- **Idelalisib** is predicted to increase the exposure to **daridorexant**. Avoid. [Severe] Study
- **Imatinib** is predicted to increase the exposure to **daridorexant**. Adjust **daridorexant** dose, p. 554. [Severe] Study
- **Ivosidenib** is predicted to decrease the exposure to **daridorexant**. [Severe] Study
- **Letermovir** is predicted to increase the exposure to **daridorexant**. Adjust **daridorexant** dose, p. 554. [Severe] Study
- **Lorlatinib** is predicted to decrease the exposure to **daridorexant**. [Severe] Study
- **Lumacaftor** is predicted to decrease the exposure to **daridorexant**. [Severe] Study
- **Macrolides (clarithromycin)** are predicted to increase the exposure to **daridorexant**. Avoid. [Severe] Study
- **Macrolides (erythromycin)** are predicted to increase the exposure to **daridorexant**. Adjust **daridorexant** dose, p. 554. [Severe] Study
- **Mitotane** is predicted to decrease the exposure to **daridorexant**. [Severe] Study
- **Neurokinin-1 receptor antagonists (aprepitant, netupitant)** are predicted to increase the exposure to **daridorexant**. Adjust **daridorexant** dose, p. 554. [Severe] Study
- **Nilotinib** is predicted to increase the exposure to **daridorexant**. Adjust **daridorexant** dose, p. 554. [Severe] Study
- **NNRTIs (efavirenz, etravirine, nevirapine)** are predicted to decrease the exposure to **daridorexant**. [Severe] Study
- **Quinolones (ciprofloxacin)** are predicted to increase the exposure to **daridorexant**. Adjust **daridorexant** dose, p. 554. [Moderate] Theoretical
- **Rifamycins (rifampicin)** are predicted to decrease the exposure to **daridorexant**. [Severe] Study
- **Daridorexant** is predicted to increase the exposure to **sirolimus**. [Moderate] Study
- **Sotorasib** is predicted to decrease the exposure to **daridorexant**. [Severe] Study
- **St John's wort** is predicted to decrease the exposure to **daridorexant**. [Severe] Study
- **Daridorexant** is predicted to increase the exposure to **talazoparib**. [Moderate] Study
- **Daridorexant** is predicted to increase the exposure to taxanes **(paclitaxel)**. [Moderate] Study
- **Tucatinib** is predicted to increase the exposure to **daridorexant**. Avoid. [Severe] Study

Darifenacin → see TABLE 9 p. 1573 (antimuscarinics)

- **Anti-androgens (apalutamide, enzalutamide)** are predicted to decrease the exposure to **darifenacin**. [Moderate] Theoretical
- **Antiarrhythmics (dronedarone)** are predicted to increase the exposure to **darifenacin**. [Moderate] Study
- **Darifenacin** is predicted to increase the concentration of antiarrhythmics **(flecainide)**. [Moderate] Theoretical
- **Antiepileptics (carbamazepine, fosphenytoin, phenobarbital, phenytoin, primidone)** are predicted to decrease the exposure to **darifenacin**. [Moderate] Theoretical
- **Antifungals, azoles (fluconazole)** slightly increase the exposure to **darifenacin**. [Moderate] Study
- **Antifungals, azoles (isavuconazole)** are predicted to increase the exposure to **darifenacin**. [Moderate] Study
- **Antifungals, azoles (itraconazole, ketoconazole, posaconazole, voriconazole)** are predicted to markedly to very markedly increase the exposure to **darifenacin**. Avoid. [Severe] Study
- **Antipsychotics, second generation (clozapine)** can cause constipation, as can **darifenacin**; concurrent use might increase the risk of developing intestinal obstruction. [Severe] Theoretical → Also see TABLE 9 p. 1573

- **Bupropion** is predicted to slightly increase the exposure to **darifenacin**. [Mild] Study
- **Calcium channel blockers (diltiazem)** are predicted to increase the exposure to **darifenacin**. [Moderate] Study
- **Calcium channel blockers (verapamil)** are predicted to increase the exposure to **darifenacin**. Avoid. [Moderate] Study
- **Cenobamate** is predicted to decrease the exposure to **darifenacin**. Adjust dose. [Moderate] Theoretical
- **Ceritinib** is predicted to markedly to very markedly increase the exposure to **darifenacin**. Avoid. [Severe] Study
- **Ciclosporin** is predicted to increase the exposure to **darifenacin**. Avoid. [Moderate] Theoretical
- **Cinacalcet** is predicted to slightly increase the exposure to **darifenacin**. [Mild] Study
- **Cobicistat** is predicted to markedly to very markedly increase the exposure to **darifenacin**. Avoid. [Severe] Study
- **Crizotinib** is predicted to increase the exposure to **darifenacin**. [Moderate] Study
- **Dacomitinib** is predicted to slightly increase the exposure to **darifenacin**. [Mild] Study
- **Encorafenib** is predicted to decrease the exposure to **darifenacin**. [Moderate] Theoretical
- **Grapefruit** juice is predicted to increase the exposure to **darifenacin**. [Moderate] Study
- **H$_2$ receptor antagonists (cimetidine)** increase the exposure to **darifenacin**. [Mild] Study
- **HIV-protease inhibitors** are predicted to markedly to very markedly increase the exposure to **darifenacin**. Avoid. [Severe] Study
- **Idelalisib** is predicted to markedly to very markedly increase the exposure to **darifenacin**. Avoid. [Severe] Study
- **Imatinib** is predicted to increase the exposure to **darifenacin**. [Moderate] Study
- **Ivosidenib** is predicted to decrease the exposure to **darifenacin**. [Moderate] Theoretical
- **Letermovir** is predicted to increase the exposure to **darifenacin**. [Moderate] Study
- **Lumacaftor** is predicted to decrease the exposure to **darifenacin**. [Moderate] Theoretical
- **Macrolides (clarithromycin)** are predicted to markedly to very markedly increase the exposure to **darifenacin**. Avoid. [Severe] Study
- **Macrolides (erythromycin)** slightly increase the exposure to **darifenacin**. [Moderate] Study
- **Mitotane** is predicted to decrease the exposure to **darifenacin**. [Moderate] Theoretical
- **Neurokinin-1 receptor antagonists (aprepitant, netupitant)** are predicted to increase the exposure to **darifenacin**. [Moderate] Study
- **Nilotinib** is predicted to increase the exposure to **darifenacin**. [Moderate] Study
- **Nirmatrelvir** boosted with ritonavir is predicted to increase the concentration of **darifenacin**. Adjust dose. [Severe] Theoretical
- **Rifamycins (rifampicin)** are predicted to decrease the exposure to **darifenacin**. [Moderate] Theoretical
- **SSRIs (fluoxetine, paroxetine)** are predicted to slightly increase the exposure to **darifenacin**. [Mild] Study
- **St John's wort** is predicted to decrease the exposure to **darifenacin**. [Moderate] Theoretical
- **Terbinafine** is predicted to slightly increase the exposure to **darifenacin**. [Mild] Study
- **Darifenacin** (high-dose) is predicted to increase the exposure to tricyclic antidepressants. [Moderate] Study → Also see TABLE 9 p. 1573
- **Tucatinib** is predicted to markedly to very markedly increase the exposure to **darifenacin**. Avoid. [Severe] Study

Darolutamide → see anti-androgens

Darunavir → see HIV-protease inhibitors

Dasatinib → see TABLE 14 p. 1575 (myelosuppression), TABLE 8 p. 1573 (QT-interval prolongation), TABLE 4 p. 1571 (antiplatelet effects)

- Oral antacids decrease the absorption of oral **dasatinib**. Separate administration by at least 2 hours. [Moderate] Study

Dasatinib (continued)

▸ Anti-androgens (apalutamide, enzalutamide) are predicted to markedly decrease the exposure to **dasatinib**. Avoid. Severe Study → Also see **TABLE 8** p. 1573

▸ Antiarrhythmics (dronedarone) are predicted to increase the exposure to **dasatinib**. Severe Study → Also see **TABLE 8** p. 1573

▸ Antiepileptics (carbamazepine, fosphenytoin, phenobarbital, phenytoin, primidone) are predicted to markedly decrease the exposure to **dasatinib**. Avoid. Severe Study

▸ Antifungals, azoles (fluconazole, isavuconazole) are predicted to increase the exposure to **dasatinib**. Severe Study → Also see **TABLE 8** p. 1573

▸ Antifungals, azoles (itraconazole, ketoconazole, posaconazole, voriconazole) are predicted to increase the exposure to **dasatinib**. Avoid or adjust dose—consult product literature. Severe Study → Also see **TABLE 8** p. 1573

▸ Belzutifan is predicted to decrease the exposure to **dasatinib**. Avoid or adjust dose. Severe Theoretical

▸ Berotralstat is predicted to increase the exposure to **dasatinib**. Severe Study

▸ Calcium channel blockers (diltiazem, verapamil) are predicted to increase the exposure to **dasatinib**. Severe Study

▸ Oral calcium salts (calcium carbonate) -containing antacids are predicted to decrease the exposure to oral **dasatinib**. Separate administration by at least 2 hours. Moderate Study

▸ Cenobamate is predicted to decrease the exposure to **dasatinib**. Severe Study

▸ Ceritinib is predicted to increase the exposure to **dasatinib**. Avoid or adjust dose—consult product literature. Severe Study → Also see **TABLE 14** p. 1575 → Also see **TABLE 8** p. 1573

▸ Cobicistat is predicted to increase the exposure to **dasatinib**. Avoid or adjust dose—consult product literature. Severe Study

▸ Crizotinib is predicted to increase the exposure to **dasatinib**. Severe Study → Also see **TABLE 8** p. 1573

▸ Dabrafenib is predicted to decrease the exposure to **dasatinib**. Severe Study

▸ Encorafenib is predicted to markedly decrease the exposure to **dasatinib**. Avoid. Severe Study → Also see **TABLE 8** p. 1573

▸ Endothelin receptor antagonists (bosentan) are predicted to decrease the exposure to **dasatinib**. Severe Study

▸ Fedratinib is predicted to increase the exposure to **dasatinib**. Severe Study

▸ Grapefruit juice is predicted to increase the exposure to **dasatinib**. Avoid. Moderate Theoretical

▸ H₂ receptor antagonists are predicted to decrease the exposure to **dasatinib**. Avoid. Moderate Study

▸ HIV-protease inhibitors are predicted to increase the exposure to **dasatinib**. Avoid or adjust dose—consult product literature. Severe Study

▸ Idelalisib is predicted to increase the exposure to **dasatinib**. Avoid or adjust dose—consult product literature. Severe Study

▸ Imatinib is predicted to increase the exposure to **dasatinib**. Severe Study → Also see **TABLE 14** p. 1575 → Also see **TABLE 4** p. 1571

▸ Ivosidenib is predicted to markedly decrease the exposure to **dasatinib**. Avoid. Severe Study → Also see **TABLE 8** p. 1573

▸ Letermovir is predicted to increase the exposure to **dasatinib**. Severe Study

▸ Lorlatinib is predicted to decrease the exposure to **dasatinib**. Severe Study

▸ Lumacaftor is predicted to markedly decrease the exposure to **dasatinib**. Avoid. Severe Study

▸ Macrolides (clarithromycin) are predicted to increase the exposure to **dasatinib**. Avoid or adjust dose—consult product literature. Severe Study

▸ Macrolides (erythromycin) are predicted to increase the exposure to **dasatinib**. Severe Study → Also see **TABLE 8** p. 1573

▸ Mitotane is predicted to markedly decrease the exposure to **dasatinib**. Avoid. Severe Study → Also see **TABLE 14** p. 1575

▸ Neurokinin-1 receptor antagonists (aprepitant, netupitant) are predicted to increase the exposure to **dasatinib**. Severe Study

▸ Nilotinib is predicted to increase the exposure to **dasatinib**. Severe Study → Also see **TABLE 14** p. 1575 → Also see **TABLE 8** p. 1573

▸ Nirmatrelvir boosted with ritonavir is predicted to increase the concentration of **dasatinib**. Avoid. Severe Theoretical

▸ NNRTIs (efavirenz, etravirine, nevirapine) are predicted to decrease the exposure to **dasatinib**. Severe Study → Also see **TABLE 8** p. 1573

▸ Pitolisant is predicted to decrease the exposure to **dasatinib**. Avoid. Severe Theoretical

▸ Proton pump inhibitors are predicted to decrease the exposure to **dasatinib**. Avoid. Severe Study

▸ Rifamycins (rifampicin) are predicted to markedly decrease the exposure to **dasatinib**. Avoid. Severe Study

▸ Oral sodium bicarbonate -containing antacids are predicted to decrease the exposure to oral **dasatinib**. Separate administration by at least 2 hours. Moderate Study

▸ Sodium zirconium cyclosilicate is predicted to decrease the exposure to **dasatinib**. Separate administration by at least 2 hours. Moderate Theoretical

▸ Sotorasib is predicted to decrease the exposure to **dasatinib**. Severe Study

▸ St John's wort is predicted to decrease the exposure to **dasatinib**. Severe Study

▸ **Dasatinib** is predicted to increase the exposure to statins (simvastatin). Moderate Theoretical

▸ Tucatinib is predicted to increase the exposure to **dasatinib**. Avoid or adjust dose—consult product literature. Severe Study

Daunorubicin → see anthracyclines

Decitabine → see **TABLE 1** p. 1571 (hepatotoxicity), **TABLE 14** p. 1575 (myelosuppression)

Deferasirox → see iron chelators

Deferiprone → see iron chelators

Deflazacort → see corticosteroids

Delafloxacin → see quinolones

Delamanid → see **TABLE 8** p. 1573 (QT-interval prolongation)

▸ Anti-androgens (apalutamide, enzalutamide) are predicted to slightly decrease the exposure to **delamanid**. Avoid. Moderate Study → Also see **TABLE 8** p. 1573

▸ Antiepileptics (carbamazepine, fosphenytoin, phenobarbital, phenytoin, primidone) are predicted to slightly decrease the exposure to **delamanid**. Avoid. Moderate Study

▸ Antifungals, azoles (itraconazole, ketoconazole, posaconazole, voriconazole) very slightly increase the exposure to **delamanid**. Severe Study → Also see **TABLE 8** p. 1573

▸ Ceritinib very slightly increases the exposure to **delamanid**. Severe Study → Also see **TABLE 8** p. 1573

▸ Cobicistat very slightly increases the exposure to **delamanid**. Severe Study

▸ Encorafenib is predicted to slightly decrease the exposure to **delamanid**. Avoid. Moderate Study → Also see **TABLE 8** p. 1573

▸ HIV-protease inhibitors very slightly increase the exposure to **delamanid**. Severe Study

▸ Idelalisib very slightly increases the exposure to **delamanid**. Severe Study

▸ Ivosidenib is predicted to slightly decrease the exposure to **delamanid**. Avoid. Moderate Study → Also see **TABLE 8** p. 1573

▸ Lumacaftor is predicted to slightly decrease the exposure to **delamanid**. Avoid. Moderate Study

▸ Macrolides (clarithromycin) very slightly increase the exposure to **delamanid**. Severe Study

▸ Mitotane is predicted to slightly decrease the exposure to **delamanid**. Avoid. Moderate Study

▸ Nirmatrelvir boosted with ritonavir is predicted to increase the concentration of **delamanid**. Severe Theoretical

▸ Rifamycins (rifampicin) are predicted to slightly decrease the exposure to **delamanid**. Avoid. Moderate Study

▸ Tucatinib very slightly increases the exposure to **delamanid**. Severe Study

Demeclocycline → see tetracyclines

Dengue vaccine → see live vaccines

Denosumab

▸ Cinacalcet might increase the risk of hypocalcaemia when given with **denosumab**. Severe Theoretical

▸ Etelcalcetide might increase the risk of hypocalcaemia when given with **denosumab**. Severe Theoretical

Desferrioxamine → see iron chelators

Desflurane → see volatile halogenated anaesthetics

Desloratadine → see antihistamines, non-sedating

Desmopressin → see **TABLE 17** p. 1576 (hyponatraemia)

▸ Antiepileptics **(lamotrigine)** are predicted to increase the risk of hyponatraemia when given with **desmopressin**. [Severe] Theoretical

▸ **Loperamide** greatly increases the absorption of oral **desmopressin** (and possibly sublingual). [Moderate] Study

▸ Phenothiazines **(chlorpromazine)** are predicted to increase the risk of hyponatraemia when given with **desmopressin**. [Severe] Theoretical → Also see **TABLE 17** p. 1576

Desogestrel

▸ Antiepileptics **(carbamazepine, eslicarbazepine, fosphenytoin, oxcarbazepine, perampanel, phenobarbital, phenytoin, primidone, rufinamide, topiramate)** are predicted to decrease the efficacy of **desogestrel**. For FSRH guidance, see Contraceptives, interactions p. 917. [Severe] Theoretical

▸ **Desogestrel** is predicted to increase the exposure to antiepileptics **(lamotrigine)** and antiepileptics **(lamotrigine)** might decrease the effects of **desogestrel**. For FSRH guidance, see Contraceptives, interactions p. 917. [Moderate] Study

▸ Endothelin receptor antagonists **(bosentan)** are predicted to decrease the efficacy of **desogestrel**. For FSRH guidance, see Contraceptives, interactions p. 917. [Severe] Theoretical

▸ Glucagon-like peptide-1 receptor agonists **(tirzepatide)** might affect the absorption of **desogestrel**. Manufacturer advises precautions for those who are overweight or obese—see Conception and contraception p. 822. [Moderate] Study

▸ HIV-protease inhibitors **(ritonavir)** are predicted to decrease the efficacy of **desogestrel**. For FSRH guidance, see Contraceptives, interactions p. 917. [Severe] Theoretical

▸ **Lumacaftor** might decrease the efficacy of **desogestrel**. Use additional contraceptive precautions. [Severe] Theoretical

▸ **Modafinil** is predicted to decrease the efficacy of **desogestrel**. For FSRH guidance, see Contraceptives, interactions p. 917. [Severe] Theoretical

▸ Neurokinin-1 receptor antagonists **(aprepitant, fosaprepitant)** are predicted to decrease the efficacy of **desogestrel**. For FSRH guidance, see Contraceptives, interactions p. 917. [Severe] Theoretical

▸ NNRTIs **(efavirenz, nevirapine)** are predicted to decrease the efficacy of **desogestrel**. For FSRH guidance, see Contraceptives, interactions p. 917. [Severe] Theoretical

▸ NNRTIs **(etravirine)** might decrease the efficacy of **desogestrel**. Follow FSRH guidance for enzyme inducers, see Contraceptives, interactions p. 917. [Severe] Theoretical

▸ Rifamycins are predicted to decrease the efficacy of **desogestrel**. For FSRH guidance, see Contraceptives, interactions p. 917. [Severe] Theoretical

▸ **St John's wort** is predicted to decrease the efficacy of **desogestrel**. MHRA advises avoid. For FSRH guidance, see Contraceptives, interactions p. 917. [Severe] Theoretical

▸ **Sugammadex** is predicted to decrease the exposure to **desogestrel**. Refer to patient information leaflet for missed pill advice. [Severe] Theoretical

▸ **Desogestrel** might decrease the efficacy of ulipristal and ulipristal might decrease the efficacy of **desogestrel**. Avoid or use additional contraceptive precautions. [Severe] Theoretical

Deucravacitinib

▸ Live vaccines are predicted to increase the risk of generalised infection (possibly life-threatening) when given with **deucravacitinib**. Avoid. [Severe] Theoretical

Dexamethasone → see corticosteroids

Dexamfetamine → see amfetamines

Dexketoprofen → see NSAIDs

Dexmedetomidine → see **TABLE 10** p. 1574 (CNS effects)

Dexrazoxane → see iron chelators

Diamorphine → see opioids

Diazepam → see benzodiazepines

Diazoxide → see **TABLE 7** p. 1572 (hypotension)

▸ **Diazoxide** decreases the concentration of antiepileptics **(fosphenytoin, phenytoin)** and antiepileptics **(fosphenytoin, phenytoin)** are predicted to decrease the effects of **diazoxide**. Monitor concentration and adjust dose. [Moderate] Anecdotal

▸ **Diazoxide** increases the risk of severe hypotension when given with hydralazine. [Severe] Study → Also see **TABLE 7** p. 1572

Diclofenac → see NSAIDs

Dicycloverine → see **TABLE 9** p. 1573 (antimuscarinics)

▸ Antipsychotics, second generation **(clozapine)** can cause constipation, as can **dicycloverine**; concurrent use might increase the risk of developing intestinal obstruction. [Severe] Theoretical → Also see **TABLE 9** p. 1573

Dienogest

▸ Anti-androgens **(apalutamide, enzalutamide)** are predicted to markedly decrease the exposure to **dienogest**. [Severe] Study

▸ Antiarrhythmics **(dronedarone)** are predicted to slightly increase the exposure to **dienogest**. [Moderate] Study

▸ Antiepileptics **(carbamazepine, fosphenytoin, phenobarbital, phenytoin, primidone)** are predicted to markedly decrease the exposure to **dienogest**. [Severe] Study

▸ Antifungals, azoles **(fluconazole, isavuconazole)** are predicted to slightly increase the exposure to **dienogest**. [Moderate] Study

▸ Antifungals, azoles **(itraconazole, ketoconazole, posaconazole, voriconazole)** are predicted to moderately increase the exposure to **dienogest**. [Moderate] Study

▸ **Berotralstat** is predicted to slightly increase the exposure to **dienogest**. [Moderate] Study

▸ Calcium channel blockers **(diltiazem, verapamil)** are predicted to slightly increase the exposure to **dienogest**. [Moderate] Study

▸ **Ceritinib** is predicted to moderately increase the exposure to **dienogest**. [Moderate] Study

▸ **Cobicistat** is predicted to moderately increase the exposure to **dienogest**. [Moderate] Study

▸ **Crizotinib** is predicted to slightly increase the exposure to **dienogest**. [Moderate] Study

▸ **Encorafenib** is predicted to markedly decrease the exposure to **dienogest**. [Severe] Study

▸ **Fedratinib** is predicted to slightly increase the exposure to **dienogest**. [Moderate] Study

▸ HIV-protease inhibitors are predicted to moderately increase the exposure to **dienogest**. [Moderate] Study

▸ **Idelalisib** is predicted to moderately increase the exposure to **dienogest**. [Moderate] Study

▸ **Imatinib** is predicted to slightly increase the exposure to **dienogest**. [Moderate] Study

▸ **Ivosidenib** is predicted to markedly decrease the exposure to **dienogest**. [Severe] Study

▸ **Letermovir** is predicted to slightly increase the exposure to **dienogest**. [Moderate] Study

▸ **Lumacaftor** is predicted to markedly decrease the exposure to **dienogest**. [Severe] Study

▸ Macrolides **(clarithromycin)** are predicted to moderately increase the exposure to **dienogest**. [Moderate] Study

▸ Macrolides **(erythromycin)** are predicted to slightly increase the exposure to **dienogest**. [Moderate] Study

▸ **Mitotane** is predicted to markedly decrease the exposure to **dienogest**. [Severe] Study

▸ Neurokinin-1 receptor antagonists **(aprepitant, netupitant)** are predicted to slightly increase the exposure to **dienogest**. [Moderate] Study

▸ **Nilotinib** is predicted to slightly increase the exposure to **dienogest**. [Moderate] Study

▸ Rifamycins **(rifampicin)** are predicted to markedly decrease the exposure to **dienogest**. [Severe] Study

▸ **Tucatinib** is predicted to moderately increase the exposure to **dienogest**. [Moderate] Study

Difelikefalin → see **TABLE 10** p. 1574 (CNS effects)

Digoxin → see **TABLE 5** p. 1572 (bradycardia)

▸ **Abrocitinib** might increase the exposure to **digoxin**. [Moderate] Theoretical

▸ **Acarbose** decreases the concentration of **digoxin**. [Moderate] Study

▸ **Aminoglycosides** potentially increase the concentration of **digoxin**. Monitor and adjust dose. [Mild] Study

▸ Oral antacids decrease the absorption of oral **digoxin**. Separate administration by 2 hours. [Mild] Study

▸ Anti-androgens **(apalutamide)** are predicted to decrease the exposure to **digoxin**. [Mild] Study

▸ Anti-androgens **(enzalutamide)** are predicted to increase the exposure to **digoxin**. Use with caution or avoid. [Moderate] Theoretical

Digoxin (continued)

▶ Antiarrhythmics **(amiodarone, dronedarone)** are predicted to moderately increase the exposure to **digoxin**. Monitor and adjust **digoxin** dose, p. 125. Severe Study → Also see **TABLE 5** p. 1572

▶ Antiarrhythmics **(propafenone)** increase the concentration of **digoxin**. Monitor and adjust dose. Severe Study → Also see **TABLE 5** p. 1572

▶ Antiepileptics **(fosphenytoin, phenytoin)** are predicted to decrease the concentration of **digoxin**. Moderate Anecdotal

▶ Antifungals, azoles **(isavuconazole)** slightly increase the exposure to **digoxin**. Monitor and adjust dose. Moderate Study

▶ Antifungals, azoles **(itraconazole)** increase the concentration of **digoxin**. Monitor and adjust dose. Severe Study

▶ Antifungals, azoles **(ketoconazole)** are predicted to markedly increase the concentration of **digoxin**. Severe Study

▶ Antifungals, azoles **(posaconazole)** are predicted to increase the concentration of **digoxin**. Severe Study

▶ Antimalarials **(mefloquine)** are predicted to increase the risk of bradycardia when given with **digoxin**. Severe Theoretical

▶ Antimalarials **(quinine)** increase the concentration of **digoxin**. Monitor and adjust **digoxin** dose, p. 125. Severe Anecdotal

▶ Asciminib is predicted to increase the exposure to **digoxin**. Severe Theoretical

▶ Balsalazide is predicted to decrease the concentration of **digoxin**. Moderate Theoretical

▶ Belumosudil might increase the exposure to **digoxin**. Avoid or adjust dose. Moderate Theoretical

▶ Berotralstat is predicted to increase the concentration of **digoxin**. Monitor and adjust dose. Moderate Study

▶ Bupropion might decrease the exposure to **digoxin**. Severe Study

▶ Calcium channel blockers **(diltiazem, verapamil)** increase the concentration of **digoxin**. Monitor and adjust dose. Severe Study → Also see **TABLE 5** p. 1572

▶ Intravenous **calcium salts** increase the effects of **digoxin**. Avoid. Moderate Anecdotal

▶ Cannabidiol is predicted to increase the exposure to **digoxin**. Monitor and adjust dose. Moderate Study

▶ Carbimazole affects the concentration of **digoxin**. Monitor and adjust dose. Moderate Theoretical

▶ Ceritinib is predicted to increase the risk of bradycardia when given with **digoxin**. Avoid. Severe Theoretical → Also see **TABLE 5** p. 1572

▶ Ciclosporin increases the concentration of **digoxin**. Monitor and adjust dose. Severe Theoretical

▶ Corticosteroids are predicted to increase the risk of digoxin toxicity when given with **digoxin**. Avoid. Severe Theoretical

▶ Dabrafenib is predicted to decrease the exposure to **digoxin**. Moderate Theoretical

▶ Danicopan is predicted to increase the exposure to **digoxin**. Moderate Study

▶ Daridorexant is predicted to increase the exposure to **digoxin**. Moderate Study

▶ Drugs that reduce serum potassium (see **TABLE 16** p. 1575) are predicted to increase the risk of digoxin toxicity when given with **digoxin**. Severe Study

▶ Eliglustat increases the exposure to **digoxin**. Adjust dose. Moderate Study

▶ Erdafitinib is predicted to increase the exposure to **digoxin**. Separate administration by at least 6 hours. Moderate Theoretical

▶ Glecaprevir with pibrentasvir increases the exposure to **digoxin**. Moderate Study

▶ Glucagon-like peptide-1 receptor agonists **(tirzepatide)** might affect the absorption of **digoxin**. Moderate Theoretical

▶ HIV-protease inhibitors **(lopinavir)** boosted with ritonavir are predicted to increase the exposure to **digoxin**. Severe Theoretical

▶ HIV-protease inhibitors **(ritonavir)** increase the concentration of **digoxin**. Adjust dose and monitor concentration. Severe Study

▶ Ibrutinib might increase the exposure to **digoxin**. Separate administration by at least 6 hours. Moderate Theoretical

▶ Ivacaftor slightly increases the exposure to **digoxin**. Moderate Study

▶ Ivosidenib is predicted to alter the exposure to **digoxin**. Moderate Theoretical

▶ Lapatinib slightly increases the exposure to **digoxin**. Moderate Study

▶ Ledipasvir is predicted to increase the exposure to **digoxin**. Monitor and adjust dose. Moderate Theoretical

▶ Lomitapide might increase the exposure to **digoxin**. Adjust dose. Moderate Theoretical

▶ Lorlatinib is predicted to decrease the exposure to **digoxin**. Moderate Study

▶ Macrolides increase the concentration of **digoxin**. Severe Anecdotal

▶ Maribavir very slightly increases the exposure to **digoxin**. Monitor and adjust dose. Moderate Study

▶ Mineralocorticoid receptor antagonists **(eplerenone)** very slightly increase the exposure to **digoxin**. Mild Study

▶ Mineralocorticoid receptor antagonists **(spironolactone)** increase the concentration of **digoxin**. Monitor and adjust dose. Moderate Study

▶ Mirabegron slightly increases the exposure to **digoxin**. Monitor concentration and adjust dose. Severe Study

▶ Neomycin decreases the absorption of **digoxin**. Moderate Study

▶ Neratinib slightly increases the exposure to **digoxin**. Moderate Study

▶ Neuromuscular blocking drugs, non-depolarising **(pancuronium)** are predicted to increase the risk of cardiovascular adverse effects when given with **digoxin**. Severe Anecdotal

▶ Nirmatrelvir boosted with ritonavir is predicted to increase the concentration of **digoxin**. Severe Theoretical

▶ NSAIDs **(indometacin)** increase the concentration of **digoxin**. Severe Study

▶ Olaparib might increase the exposure to **digoxin**. Moderate Theoretical

▶ Osimertinib is predicted to increase the exposure to **digoxin**. Moderate Study

▶ Pemigatinib might increase the exposure to **digoxin**. Separate administration by at least 6 hours. Moderate Theoretical

▶ Penicillamine potentially decreases the concentration of **digoxin**. Separate administration by 2 hours. Severe Anecdotal

▶ Pibrentasvir with glecaprevir increases the exposure to **digoxin**. Moderate Study

▶ Pitolisant is predicted to decrease the exposure to **digoxin**. Mild Theoretical

▶ Ranolazine increases the concentration of **digoxin**. Moderate Study

▶ Ribociclib is predicted to increase the exposure to **digoxin**. Moderate Theoretical

▶ Rifamycins **(rifampicin)** decrease the concentration of **digoxin**. Moderate Study

▶ Selpercatinib is predicted to increase the exposure to **digoxin**. Moderate Study

▶ Sotorasib very slightly increases the exposure to **digoxin**. Avoid or adjust dose. Moderate Study

▶ St John's wort decreases the concentration of **digoxin**. Avoid. Severe Anecdotal

▶ Sucralfate decreases the absorption of **digoxin**. Separate administration by 2 hours. Severe Anecdotal

▶ Sulfasalazine decreases the concentration of **digoxin**. Moderate Study

▶ Suxamethonium is predicted to increase the risk of cardiovascular adverse effects when given with **digoxin**. Severe Anecdotal → Also see **TABLE 5** p. 1572

▶ Tepotinib is predicted to increase the concentration of **digoxin**. Severe Study

▶ Thyroid hormones are predicted to affect the concentration of **digoxin**. Monitor and adjust dose. Moderate Theoretical

▶ Ticagrelor increases the concentration of **digoxin**. Moderate Study → Also see **TABLE 5** p. 1572

▶ Tolvaptan slightly increases the exposure to **digoxin**. Moderate Study

▶ Trimethoprim increases the concentration of **digoxin**. Moderate Study

▶ Tucatinib slightly increases the exposure to **digoxin**. Use with caution and adjust dose. Moderate Study

▶ Vandetanib very slightly increases the exposure to **digoxin**. Moderate Study

- **Velpatasvir** is predicted to increase the exposure to **digoxin**. Severe Study
- **Vemurafenib** slightly increases the exposure to **digoxin**. Use with caution and adjust dose. Severe Study
- **Venetoclax** increases the exposure to **digoxin**. Avoid or adjust dose. Severe Study
- **Vitamin D substances** are predicted to increase the risk of toxicity when given with **digoxin**. Severe Theoretical
- **Voclosporin** slightly increases the exposure to **digoxin**. Moderate Study
- **Voxilaprevir** with sofosbuvir and velpatasvir is predicted to increase the exposure to **digoxin**. Monitor and adjust dose. Severe Theoretical

Dihydrocodeine → see opioids

Diltiazem → see calcium channel blockers

Dimenhydrinate → see TABLE 9 p. 1573 (antimuscarinics), TABLE 10 p. 1574 (CNS effects)

- **Antipsychotics, second generation (clozapine)** can cause constipation, as can **dimenhydrinate**; concurrent use might increase the risk of developing intestinal obstruction. Severe Theoretical → Also see TABLE 9 p. 1573 → Also see TABLE 10 p. 1574

Dimethyl fumarate

- **Alcohol** (excessive consumption) potentially increases the risk of gastrointestinal adverse effects when given with **dimethyl fumarate**. Avoid. Moderate Theoretical
- **Live vaccines** are predicted to increase the risk of generalised infection (possibly life-threatening) when given with **dimethyl fumarate**. UKHSA advises avoid (refer to Green Book). Severe Theoretical

Dinutuximab → see monoclonal antibodies

Dipeptidylpeptidase-4 inhibitors → see TABLE 13 p. 1575 (antidiabetic drugs)

alogliptin · linagliptin · saxagliptin · sitagliptin · vildagliptin

- **Anti-androgens (apalutamide, enzalutamide)** are predicted to decrease the exposure to **linagliptin**. Moderate Study
- **Anti-androgens (apalutamide, enzalutamide)** are predicted to moderately decrease the exposure to **saxagliptin**. Moderate Study
- **Antiarrhythmics (dronedarone)** are predicted to increase the exposure to **saxagliptin**. Mild Study
- **Antiepileptics (carbamazepine, fosphenytoin, phenobarbital, phenytoin, primidone)** are predicted to decrease the exposure to **linagliptin**. Moderate Study
- **Antiepileptics (carbamazepine, fosphenytoin, phenobarbital, phenytoin, primidone)** are predicted to moderately decrease the exposure to **saxagliptin**. Moderate Study
- **Antifungals, azoles (fluconazole, isavuconazole)** are predicted to increase the exposure to **saxagliptin**. Mild Study
- **Antifungals, azoles (itraconazole, ketoconazole, posaconazole, voriconazole)** are predicted to increase the exposure to **saxagliptin**. Moderate Study
- **Berotralstat** is predicted to increase the exposure to **saxagliptin**. Mild Study
- **Calcium channel blockers (diltiazem, verapamil)** are predicted to increase the exposure to **saxagliptin**. Mild Study
- **Ceritinib** is predicted to increase the exposure to **saxagliptin**. Moderate Study
- **Cobicistat** is predicted to increase the exposure to **saxagliptin**. Moderate Study
- **Crizotinib** is predicted to increase the exposure to **saxagliptin**. Mild Study
- **Encorafenib** is predicted to decrease the exposure to **linagliptin**. Moderate Study
- **Encorafenib** is predicted to moderately decrease the exposure to **saxagliptin**. Moderate Study
- **Fedratinib** is predicted to increase the exposure to **saxagliptin**. Mild Study
- **Fenfluramine** might decrease blood glucose concentrations when given with **dipeptidylpeptidase-4 inhibitors**. Moderate Theoretical
- **Grapefruit** juice is predicted to increase the exposure to **saxagliptin**. Mild Theoretical
- **HIV-protease inhibitors** are predicted to increase the exposure to **saxagliptin**. Moderate Study

- **Idelalisib** is predicted to increase the exposure to **saxagliptin**. Moderate Study
- **Imatinib** is predicted to increase the exposure to **saxagliptin**. Mild Study
- **Ivosidenib** is predicted to decrease the exposure to **linagliptin**. Moderate Study
- **Ivosidenib** is predicted to moderately decrease the exposure to **saxagliptin**. Moderate Study
- **Letermovir** is predicted to increase the exposure to **saxagliptin**. Mild Study
- **Linagliptin** is predicted to increase the exposure to **lomitapide**. Separate administration by 12 hours. Moderate Theoretical
- **Lumacaftor** is predicted to decrease the exposure to **linagliptin**. Moderate Study
- **Lumacaftor** is predicted to moderately decrease the exposure to **saxagliptin**. Moderate Study
- **Macrolides (clarithromycin)** are predicted to increase the exposure to **saxagliptin**. Moderate Study
- **Macrolides (erythromycin)** are predicted to increase the exposure to **saxagliptin**. Mild Study
- **Mitotane** is predicted to decrease the exposure to **linagliptin**. Moderate Study
- **Mitotane** is predicted to moderately decrease the exposure to **saxagliptin**. Moderate Study
- **Neurokinin-1 receptor antagonists (aprepitant, netupitant)** are predicted to increase the exposure to **saxagliptin**. Mild Study
- **Nilotinib** is predicted to increase the exposure to **saxagliptin**. Mild Study
- **Nirmatrelvir** boosted with ritonavir is predicted to increase the concentration of **saxagliptin**. Adjust dose. Moderate Theoretical
- **Rifamycins (rifampicin)** are predicted to decrease the exposure to **linagliptin**. Moderate Study
- **Rifamycins (rifampicin)** are predicted to moderately decrease the exposure to **saxagliptin**. Moderate Study
- **Selpercatinib** is predicted to increase the exposure to **saxagliptin**. Moderate Study
- **Somapacitan** might increase blood glucose concentrations, opposing the blood glucose-lowering effects of **dipeptidylpeptidase-4 inhibitors**. Adjust dose. Moderate Theoretical
- **Somatrogon** might increase blood glucose concentrations, opposing the blood glucose-lowering effects of **dipeptidylpeptidase-4 inhibitors**. Adjust dose. Moderate Theoretical
- **Tucatinib** is predicted to increase the exposure to **saxagliptin**. Moderate Study
- **Vadadustat** is predicted to increase the exposure to **sitagliptin**. Monitor and adjust dose. Moderate Study
- **Vemurafenib** is predicted to increase the exposure to **sitagliptin**. Use with caution or avoid. Moderate Theoretical

Diphenoxylate → see opioids

Dipipanone → see opioids

Dipyridamole → see TABLE 7 p. 1572 (hypotension), TABLE 4 p. 1571 (antiplatelet effects)

- **Oral antacids** are predicted to decrease the absorption of oral **dipyridamole** (immediate release tablets). Moderate Theoretical
- **Dipyridamole** increases the exposure to **antiarrhythmics (adenosine)**. Avoid or adjust dose. Severe Study
- **Dipyridamole** might increases the exposure to **cladribine**. Moderate Theoretical
- **H$_2$ receptor antagonists** are predicted to decrease the absorption of **dipyridamole** (immediate release tablets). Moderate Theoretical
- **Proton pump inhibitors** are predicted to decrease the absorption of **dipyridamole** (immediate release tablets). Moderate Theoretical
- **Selumetinib** might increase the risk of bleeding when given with **dipyridamole**. Moderate Theoretical

Diroximel fumarate

- **Live vaccines** are predicted to increase the risk of generalised infection (possibly life-threatening) when given with **diroximel fumarate**. Use with caution or avoid. Severe Theoretical

Disopyramide → see antiarrhythmics

Disulfiram
▸ Alcohol causes an extremely unpleasant systemic reaction when given with **disulfiram**. Avoid for at least 24 hours before and up to 14 days after stopping treatment. Severe Study
▸ **Disulfiram** increases the concentration of antiepileptics (fosphenytoin, phenytoin). Monitor concentration and adjust dose. Severe Study
▸ **Disulfiram** increases the anticoagulant effect of coumarins. Monitor and adjust dose. Severe Study
▸ Methylphenidate has been reported to cause psychotic symptoms when given with **disulfiram**. Severe Anecdotal
▸ **Disulfiram** increases the risk of acute psychoses when given with metronidazole. Severe Study
▸ **Disulfiram** is predicted to increase the anticoagulant effect of phenindione. Severe Theoretical

Dobutamine → see sympathomimetics, inotropic
Docetaxel → see taxanes
Docusates

> **ROUTE-SPECIFIC INFORMATION** Interactions do not generally apply to topical use of **docusates** unless specified.

▸ Oral **docusates** might decrease the concentration of the active metabolite of oral baloxavir marboxil. Severe Theoretical

Dolutegravir
▸ Oral antacids decrease the exposure to oral **dolutegravir**. Manufacturer advises take 2 hours before or 6 hours after antacids. Moderate Study
▸ Anti-androgens (apalutamide, enzalutamide) are predicted to decrease the exposure to **dolutegravir**. Severe Study
▸ Antiepileptics (carbamazepine) decrease the exposure to **dolutegravir**. Adjust **dolutegravir** dose, p. 739. Severe Study
▸ Antiepileptics (fosphenytoin, phenobarbital, phenytoin, primidone) are predicted to decrease the exposure to **dolutegravir**. Adjust **dolutegravir** dose, p. 739. Severe Study
▸ Antiepileptics (oxcarbazepine) are predicted to decrease the exposure to **dolutegravir**. Adjust **dolutegravir** dose, p. 739. Severe Theoretical
▸ Oral calcium salts decrease the absorption of oral **dolutegravir**. **Dolutegravir** should be taken 2 hours before or 6 hours after calcium. Moderate Study
▸ Dabrafenib is predicted to decrease the exposure to **dolutegravir**. Severe Study
▸ **Dolutegravir** is predicted to increase the exposure to dopamine receptor agonists (pramipexole). Adjust dose. Moderate Study
▸ Encorafenib is predicted to increase the exposure to **dolutegravir**. Moderate Theoretical
▸ Endothelin receptor antagonists (bosentan) are predicted to decrease the exposure to **dolutegravir**. Severe Study
▸ **Dolutegravir** might increase the concentration of fampridine. Avoid. Severe Theoretical
▸ HIV-protease inhibitors (atazanavir) (alone or boosted with ritonavir) slightly increase the exposure to **dolutegravir**. Adjust dose—consult product literature. Moderate Study
▸ HIV-protease inhibitors (fosamprenavir) boosted with ritonavir slightly decrease the exposure to **dolutegravir**. Avoid if resistant to HIV-integrase inhibitors. Severe Study
▸ Oral iron decreases the absorption of oral **dolutegravir**. **Dolutegravir** should be taken 2 hours before or 6 hours after iron. Moderate Study
▸ **Dolutegravir** is predicted to increase the exposure to metformin. Use with caution and adjust dose. Moderate Study
▸ Mitotane is predicted to decrease the exposure to **dolutegravir**. Severe Study
▸ NNRTIs (efavirenz) moderately decrease the exposure to **dolutegravir**. Adjust **dolutegravir** dose, p. 739. Severe Study
▸ NNRTIs (etravirine) moderately decrease the exposure to **dolutegravir**. Adjust **dolutegravir** dose unless given with atazanavir, darunavir, or lopinavir (all boosted with ritonavir), p. 739. Severe Study
▸ NNRTIs (nevirapine) are predicted to decrease the exposure to **dolutegravir**. Adjust **dolutegravir** dose, p. 739. Severe Study
▸ Rifamycins (rifampicin) moderately decrease the exposure to **dolutegravir**. Adjust **dolutegravir** dose, p. 739. Severe Study
▸ St John's wort is predicted to decrease the exposure to **dolutegravir**. Adjust **dolutegravir** dose, p. 739. Severe Study

▸ Sucralfate decreases the absorption of **dolutegravir**. Moderate Study

Domperidone → see TABLE 8 p. 1573 (QT-interval prolongation)
▸ Antiarrhythmics (dronedarone) are predicted to increase the exposure to **domperidone**. Avoid. Severe Study
▸ Antifungals, azoles (fluconazole, isavuconazole, itraconazole, ketoconazole, posaconazole, voriconazole) are predicted to increase the exposure to **domperidone**. Avoid. Severe Study
▸ Berotralstat is predicted to increase the exposure to **domperidone**. Avoid. Severe Study
▸ Calcium channel blockers (diltiazem, verapamil) are predicted to increase the exposure to **domperidone**. Avoid. Severe Study
▸ Ceritinib is predicted to increase the exposure to **domperidone**. Avoid. Severe Study
▸ Cobicistat is predicted to increase the exposure to **domperidone**. Avoid. Severe Study
▸ Crizotinib is predicted to increase the exposure to **domperidone**. Avoid. Severe Study
▸ **Domperidone** is predicted to decrease the prolactin-lowering effect of dopamine receptor agonists (bromocriptine, cabergoline). Moderate Theoretical
▸ Fedratinib is predicted to increase the exposure to **domperidone**. Avoid. Severe Study
▸ HIV-protease inhibitors are predicted to increase the exposure to **domperidone**. Avoid. Severe Study
▸ Idelalisib is predicted to increase the exposure to **domperidone**. Avoid. Severe Study
▸ Imatinib is predicted to increase the exposure to **domperidone**. Avoid. Severe Study
▸ Letermovir is predicted to increase the exposure to **domperidone**. Avoid. Severe Study
▸ Macrolides (clarithromycin, erythromycin) are predicted to increase the exposure to **domperidone**. Avoid. Severe Study
▸ Neurokinin-1 receptor antagonists (aprepitant, netupitant) are predicted to increase the exposure to **domperidone**. Avoid. Severe Study
▸ Nilotinib is predicted to increase the exposure to **domperidone**. Avoid. Severe Study
▸ Tucatinib is predicted to increase the exposure to **domperidone**. Avoid. Severe Study

Donanemab
▸ **Donanemab** can increase the risk of brain haemorrhage when given with drugs with anticoagulant effects (see TABLE 3 p. 1571). Avoid. Severe Anecdotal
▸ **Donanemab** can increase the risk of bleeding when given with drugs with antiplatelet effects (see TABLE 4 p. 1571). Severe Theoretical

Donepezil → see anticholinesterases, centrally acting
Dopamine → see sympathomimetics, inotropic
Dopamine receptor agonists → see TABLE 7 p. 1572 (hypotension), TABLE 8 p. 1573 (QT-interval prolongation), TABLE 9 p. 1573 (antimuscarinics), TABLE 10 p. 1574 (CNS effects)

> amantadine · apomorphine · bromocriptine · cabergoline · pramipexole · quinagolide · ropinirole · rotigotine

> **FOOD AND LIFESTYLE** Dose adjustment might be necessary if smoking started or stopped during treatment with **ropinirole**.

▸ **Apomorphine** is predicted to increase the risk of severe hypotension when given with 5-HT3-receptor antagonists (granisetron, palonosetron). Severe Theoretical
▸ **Apomorphine** increases the risk of severe hypotension when given with 5-HT3-receptor antagonists (ondansetron). Avoid. Severe Study → Also see TABLE 8 p. 1573
▸ Antiarrhythmics (dronedarone) are predicted to increase the exposure to **bromocriptine**. Severe Theoretical
▸ Antiarrhythmics (dronedarone) are predicted to increase the concentration of **cabergoline**. Severe Anecdotal
▸ Antifungals, azoles (fluconazole, isavuconazole) are predicted to increase the exposure to **bromocriptine**. Severe Theoretical
▸ Antifungals, azoles (fluconazole, isavuconazole, itraconazole, ketoconazole, posaconazole, voriconazole) are predicted to increase the concentration of **cabergoline**. Moderate Anecdotal
▸ Antifungals, azoles (isavuconazole) are predicted to increase the exposure to **pramipexole**. Adjust dose. Moderate Study

▶ Antifungals, azoles **(itraconazole, ketoconazole, posaconazole, voriconazole)** increase the exposure to **bromocriptine**. [Severe] Study

▶ Antipsychotics, second generation **(amisulpride, olanzapine, paliperidone, quetiapine, risperidone)** are predicted to decrease the effects of **dopamine receptor agonists**. Avoid. [Moderate] Theoretical → Also see **TABLE 7** p. 1572 → Also see **TABLE 8** p. 1573 → Also see **TABLE 9** p. 1573 → Also see **TABLE 10** p. 1574

▶ Antipsychotics, second generation **(aripiprazole, clozapine)** are predicted to decrease the effects of **dopamine receptor agonists**. [Moderate] Theoretical → Also see **TABLE 7** p. 1572 → Also see **TABLE 8** p. 1573 → Also see **TABLE 9** p. 1573 → Also see **TABLE 10** p. 1574

▶ Antipsychotics, second generation **(asenapine)** are predicted to decrease the effects of **dopamine receptor agonists**. Adjust dose. [Moderate] Theoretical → Also see **TABLE 7** p. 1572 → Also see **TABLE 10** p. 1574

▶ **Axitinib** is predicted to increase the exposure to **ropinirole**. [Moderate] Theoretical

▶ **Benperidol** is predicted to decrease the effects of **dopamine receptor agonists**. Avoid. [Moderate] Theoretical → Also see **TABLE 7** p. 1572 → Also see **TABLE 10** p. 1574

▶ **Berotralstat** is predicted to increase the exposure to **bromocriptine**. [Severe] Theoretical

▶ **Bupropion** increases the risk of adverse effects when given with **amantadine**. [Moderate] Study

▶ Calcium channel blockers **(diltiazem, verapamil)** are predicted to increase the exposure to **bromocriptine**. [Severe] Theoretical → Also see **TABLE 7** p. 1572

▶ Calcium channel blockers **(diltiazem, verapamil)** are predicted to increase the concentration of **cabergoline**. [Moderate] Anecdotal → Also see **TABLE 7** p. 1572

▶ **Ceritinib** increases the exposure to **bromocriptine**. [Severe] Study

▶ **Cobicistat** increases the exposure to **bromocriptine**. [Severe] Study

▶ **Cobicistat** is predicted to increase the concentration of **cabergoline**. [Moderate] Anecdotal

▶ **Combined hormonal contraceptives** is predicted to increase the exposure to **ropinirole**. Adjust dose. [Moderate] Study

▶ **Crizotinib** is predicted to increase the exposure to **bromocriptine**. [Severe] Theoretical

▶ **Crizotinib** is predicted to increase the concentration of **cabergoline**. [Moderate] Anecdotal

▶ **Dolutegravir** is predicted to increase the exposure to **pramipexole**. Adjust dose. [Moderate] Study

▶ **Domperidone** is predicted to decrease the prolactin-lowering effect of dopamine receptor agonists **(bromocriptine, cabergoline)**. [Moderate] Theoretical

▶ Dopamine receptor agonists **(cabergoline)** are predicted to increase the risk of ergotism when given with dopamine receptor agonists **(bromocriptine)**. Avoid. [Moderate] Theoretical → Also see **TABLE 7** p. 1572 → Also see **TABLE 10** p. 1574

▶ Dopamine receptor agonists **(amantadine)** are predicted to increase the exposure to dopamine receptor agonists **(pramipexole)**. Adjust dose. [Moderate] Theoretical → Also see **TABLE 7** p. 1572

▶ **Droperidol** is predicted to decrease the effects of **dopamine receptor agonists**. Avoid. [Moderate] Theoretical → Also see **TABLE 7** p. 1572 → Also see **TABLE 8** p. 1573 → Also see **TABLE 10** p. 1574

▶ **Ergometrine** is predicted to increase the risk of ergotism when given with **cabergoline**. Avoid. [Moderate] Theoretical

▶ **Fedratinib** is predicted to increase the exposure to **bromocriptine**. [Severe] Theoretical

▶ **Flupentixol** is predicted to decrease the effects of **dopamine receptor agonists**. Avoid. [Moderate] Theoretical → Also see **TABLE 7** p. 1572 → Also see **TABLE 9** p. 1573 → Also see **TABLE 10** p. 1574

▶ **Amantadine** might increase the adverse effects of **foslevodopa**. Adjust dose. [Moderate] Theoretical → Also see **TABLE 7** p. 1572

▶ **Givosiran** is predicted to increase the exposure to **ropinirole**. Adjust dose. [Moderate] Study

▶ H_2 receptor antagonists **(cimetidine)** are predicted to increase the exposure to **pramipexole**. Adjust dose. [Moderate] Study

▶ **Haloperidol** is predicted to decrease the effects of **dopamine receptor agonists**. Avoid. [Moderate] Theoretical → Also see **TABLE 7**

p. 1572 → Also see **TABLE 8** p. 1573 → Also see **TABLE 9** p. 1573 → Also see **TABLE 10** p. 1574

▶ **HIV-protease inhibitors** increase the exposure to **bromocriptine**. [Severe] Study

▶ **HIV-protease inhibitors** are predicted to increase the concentration of **cabergoline**. [Moderate] Anecdotal

▶ **Hormone replacement therapy** decreases the clearance of **ropinirole**. Monitor and adjust dose. [Moderate] Study

▶ **Idelalisib** increases the exposure to **bromocriptine**. [Severe] Study

▶ **Idelalisib** is predicted to increase the concentration of **cabergoline**. [Moderate] Anecdotal

▶ **Imatinib** is predicted to increase the exposure to **bromocriptine**. [Severe] Theoretical

▶ **Imatinib** is predicted to increase the concentration of **cabergoline**. [Moderate] Anecdotal

▶ **Letermovir** is predicted to increase the exposure to **bromocriptine**. [Severe] Theoretical

▶ **Loxapine** is predicted to decrease the effects of **dopamine receptor agonists**. [Moderate] Theoretical → Also see **TABLE 7** p. 1572 → Also see **TABLE 9** p. 1573 → Also see **TABLE 10** p. 1574

▶ Macrolides **(clarithromycin)** increase the exposure to **bromocriptine**. [Severe] Study

▶ Macrolides **(clarithromycin, erythromycin)** are predicted to increase the concentration of **cabergoline**. Avoid. [Severe] Study

▶ Macrolides **(erythromycin)** are predicted to increase the exposure to **bromocriptine**. [Severe] Theoretical

▶ **Amantadine** increases the risk of CNS toxicity when given with **memantine**. Use with caution or avoid. [Severe] Theoretical

▶ **Memantine** is predicted to increase the effects of dopamine receptor agonists **(apomorphine, bromocriptine, cabergoline, pramipexole, quinagolide, ropinirole, rotigotine)**. [Moderate] Theoretical

▶ **Metoclopramide** is predicted to decrease the effects of dopamine receptor agonists **(apomorphine, bromocriptine, cabergoline, pramipexole, quinagolide, ropinirole, rotigotine)**. Avoid. [Moderate] Study

▶ **Mexiletine** is predicted to increase the exposure to **ropinirole**. Adjust dose. [Moderate] Study

▶ Neurokinin-1 receptor antagonists **(aprepitant, netupitant)** are predicted to increase the exposure to **bromocriptine**. [Severe] Theoretical

▶ Neurokinin-1 receptor antagonists **(aprepitant, netupitant)** are predicted to increase the concentration of **cabergoline**. [Moderate] Anecdotal

▶ **Nilotinib** is predicted to increase the exposure to **bromocriptine**. [Severe] Theoretical

▶ **Nilotinib** is predicted to increase the concentration of **cabergoline**. [Moderate] Anecdotal

▶ **Osilodrostat** is predicted to increase the exposure to **ropinirole**. Adjust dose. [Moderate] Study

▶ **Phenothiazines** are predicted to decrease the effects of **dopamine receptor agonists**. Avoid. [Moderate] Theoretical → Also see **TABLE 7** p. 1572 → Also see **TABLE 8** p. 1573 → Also see **TABLE 9** p. 1573 → Also see **TABLE 10** p. 1574

▶ **Pimozide** is predicted to decrease the effects of **dopamine receptor agonists**. Avoid. [Moderate] Theoretical → Also see **TABLE 7** p. 1572 → Also see **TABLE 8** p. 1573 → Also see **TABLE 9** p. 1573 → Also see **TABLE 10** p. 1574

▶ Quinolones **(ciprofloxacin)** are predicted to increase the exposure to **ropinirole**. Adjust dose. [Moderate] Study

▶ **Ranolazine** is predicted to increase the exposure to **pramipexole**. Adjust dose. [Moderate] Study

▶ **Rucaparib** is predicted to increase the exposure to **ropinirole**. Adjust dose. [Moderate] Study

▶ SSRIs **(fluvoxamine)** are predicted to increase the exposure to **ropinirole**. Adjust dose. [Moderate] Study → Also see **TABLE 10** p. 1574

▶ **Sulpiride** is predicted to decrease the effects of **dopamine receptor agonists**. Avoid. [Moderate] Theoretical → Also see **TABLE 7** p. 1572 → Also see **TABLE 10** p. 1574

▶ Sympathomimetics, vasoconstrictor **(isometheptene)** potentially increase the risk of adverse effects when given with **bromocriptine**. Avoid. [Severe] Anecdotal

▶ **Trimethoprim** is predicted to increase the exposure to **pramipexole**. Adjust dose. [Moderate] Study

Dopamine receptor agonists (continued)

▸ **Tucatinib** increases the exposure to **bromocriptine**. [Severe] Study

▸ **Vandetanib** is predicted to increase the exposure to **pramipexole**. Adjust dose. [Moderate] Study

▸ **Vemurafenib** is predicted to increase the exposure to **ropinirole**. Adjust dose. [Moderate] Study

▸ **Zuclopenthixol** is predicted to decrease the effects of **dopamine receptor agonists**. Avoid. [Moderate] Theoretical → Also see TABLE 7 p. 1572 → Also see TABLE 9 p. 1573 → Also see TABLE 10 p. 1574

Doravirine → see NNRTIs

Dorzolamide

ROUTE-SPECIFIC INFORMATION Since systemic absorption can follow topical application of **dorzolamide**, the possibility of interactions should be borne in mind.

Dostarlimab → see monoclonal antibodies

Dosulepin → see tricyclic antidepressants

Doxapram

▸ **Aminophylline** increases the risk of agitation when given with doxapram. [Moderate] Study

▸ **MAOIs, irreversible** are predicted to increase the effects of doxapram. [Moderate] Theoretical

▸ **Theophylline** increases the risk of agitation when given with doxapram. [Moderate] Study

Doxazosin → see alpha blockers

Doxepin → see tricyclic antidepressants

Doxorubicin → see anthracyclines

Doxycycline → see tetracyclines

Doxylamine → see antihistamines, sedating

Dronabinol → see TABLE 10 p. 1574 (CNS effects)

▸ **Anti-androgens (apalutamide, enzalutamide)** are predicted to decrease the exposure to **dronabinol**. Avoid or adjust dose. [Mild] Study

▸ **Antiepileptics (carbamazepine, fosphenytoin, phenobarbital, phenytoin, primidone)** are predicted to decrease the exposure to **dronabinol**. Avoid or adjust dose. [Mild] Study → Also see TABLE 10 p. 1574

▸ **Antifungals, azoles (itraconazole, ketoconazole, posaconazole, voriconazole)** are predicted to increase the exposure to **dronabinol**. Adjust dose. [Mild] Study

▸ **Ceritinib** is predicted to increase the exposure to **dronabinol**. Adjust dose. [Mild] Study

▸ **Cobicistat** is predicted to increase the exposure to **dronabinol**. Adjust dose. [Mild] Study

▸ **Encorafenib** is predicted to decrease the exposure to **dronabinol**. Avoid or adjust dose. [Mild] Study

▸ **HIV-protease inhibitors** are predicted to increase the exposure to **dronabinol**. Adjust dose. [Mild] Study

▸ **Idelalisib** is predicted to increase the exposure to **dronabinol**. Adjust dose. [Mild] Study

▸ **Ivosidenib** is predicted to decrease the exposure to **dronabinol**. Avoid or adjust dose. [Mild] Study

▸ **Lumacaftor** is predicted to decrease the exposure to **dronabinol**. Avoid or adjust dose. [Mild] Study

▸ **Macrolides (clarithromycin)** are predicted to increase the exposure to **dronabinol**. Adjust dose. [Mild] Study

▸ **Mitotane** is predicted to decrease the exposure to **dronabinol**. Avoid or adjust dose. [Mild] Study

▸ **Rifamycins (rifampicin)** are predicted to decrease the exposure to **dronabinol**. Avoid or adjust dose. [Mild] Study

▸ **St John's wort** is predicted to decrease the exposure to **dronabinol**. Avoid or adjust dose. [Mild] Study

▸ **Tucatinib** is predicted to increase the exposure to **dronabinol**. Adjust dose. [Mild] Study

Dronedarone → see antiarrhythmics

Droperidol → see TABLE 17 p. 1576 (hyponatraemia), TABLE 7 p. 1572 (hypotension), TABLE 8 p. 1573 (QT-interval prolongation), TABLE 10 p. 1574 (CNS effects)

▸ **Droperidol** is predicted to decrease the effects of dopamine receptor agonists. Avoid. [Moderate] Theoretical → Also see TABLE 7 p. 1572 → Also see TABLE 8 p. 1573 → Also see TABLE 10 p. 1574

▸ **Droperidol** opposes the effects of the active metabolite of foslevodopa. [Severe] Theoretical → Also see TABLE 7 p. 1572 → Also see TABLE 10 p. 1574

▸ **Droperidol** decreases the effects of levodopa. [Severe] Study → Also see TABLE 7 p. 1572 → Also see TABLE 10 p. 1574

Drospirenone → see TABLE 15 p. 1575 (increased serum potassium)

▸ **Antiarrhythmics (dronedarone)** are predicted to increase the exposure to **drospirenone**. [Severe] Study

▸ **Antiepileptics (carbamazepine, eslicarbazepine, fosphenytoin, oxcarbazepine, perampanel, phenobarbital, phenytoin, primidone, rufinamide, topiramate)** are predicted to decrease the efficacy of **drospirenone**. For FSRH guidance, see Contraceptives, interactions p. 917. [Severe] Theoretical

▸ **Antiepileptics (lamotrigine)** might decrease the effects of **drospirenone**. For FSRH guidance, see Contraceptives, interactions p. 917. [Severe] Theoretical

▸ **Antifungals, azoles (fluconazole, isavuconazole, itraconazole, posaconazole, voriconazole)** are predicted to increase the exposure to **drospirenone**. [Severe] Study

▸ **Antifungals, azoles (ketoconazole)** moderately increase the exposure to **drospirenone**. [Severe] Study

▸ **Berotralstat** is predicted to increase the exposure to **drospirenone**. [Severe] Study

▸ **Calcium channel blockers (diltiazem, verapamil)** are predicted to increase the exposure to **drospirenone**. [Severe] Study

▸ **Cobicistat** is predicted to increase the exposure to **drospirenone**. [Severe] Study

▸ **Crizotinib** is predicted to increase the exposure to **drospirenone**. [Severe] Study

▸ **Endothelin receptor antagonists (bosentan)** are predicted to decrease the efficacy of **drospirenone**. For FSRH guidance, see Contraceptives, interactions p. 917. [Severe] Theoretical

▸ **Fedratinib** is predicted to increase the exposure to **drospirenone**. [Severe] Study

▸ **Glucagon-like peptide-1 receptor agonists (tirzepatide)** might affect the absorption of **drospirenone**. Manufacturer advises precautions for those who are overweight or obese—see Conception and contraception p. 822. [Moderate] Study

▸ **HIV-protease inhibitors (atazanavir, darunavir, fosamprenavir, lopinavir)** are predicted to increase the exposure to **drospirenone**. [Severe] Study

▸ **HIV-protease inhibitors (ritonavir)** are predicted to decrease the efficacy of **drospirenone**. For FSRH guidance, see Contraceptives, interactions p. 917. [Severe] Theoretical

▸ **Idelalisib** is predicted to increase the exposure to **drospirenone**. [Severe] Study

▸ **Imatinib** is predicted to increase the exposure to **drospirenone**. [Severe] Study

▸ **Letermovir** is predicted to increase the exposure to **drospirenone**. [Severe] Study

▸ **Lumacaftor** is predicted to decrease the efficacy of **drospirenone**. Use additional contraceptive precautions. [Severe] Theoretical

▸ **Macrolides (clarithromycin, erythromycin)** are predicted to increase the exposure to **drospirenone**. [Severe] Study

▸ **Modafinil** is predicted to decrease the efficacy of **drospirenone**. For FSRH guidance, see Contraceptives, interactions p. 917. [Severe] Theoretical

▸ **Neurokinin-1 receptor antagonists (aprepitant, fosaprepitant)** are predicted to decrease the efficacy of **drospirenone**. For FSRH guidance, see Contraceptives, interactions p. 917. [Severe] Theoretical

▸ **Neurokinin-1 receptor antagonists (netupitant)** are predicted to increase the exposure to **drospirenone**. [Severe] Study

▸ **Nilotinib** is predicted to increase the exposure to **drospirenone**. [Severe] Study

▸ **NNRTIs (efavirenz, nevirapine)** are predicted to decrease the efficacy of **drospirenone**. For FSRH guidance, see Contraceptives, interactions p. 917. [Severe] Theoretical

▸ **NNRTIs (etravirine)** might decrease the efficacy of **drospirenone**. Follow FSRH guidance for enzyme inducers, see Contraceptives, interactions p. 917. [Severe] Theoretical

▸ **Rifamycins** are predicted to decrease the efficacy of **drospirenone**. For FSRH guidance, see Contraceptives, interactions p. 917. [Severe] Theoretical

▸ **St John's wort** is predicted to decrease the efficacy of **drospirenone**. For FSRH guidance, see Contraceptives, interactions p. 917. [Severe] Theoretical

▶ **Sugammadex** is predicted to decrease the exposure to **drospirenone**. Use additional contraceptive precautions. Severe Theoretical

▶ **Drospirenone** might decreases the efficacy of **ulipristal** and **ulipristal** might decreases the efficacy of **drospirenone**. Avoid. Severe Theoretical

Drugs that cause first dose hypotension

▶ **Angiotensin-II receptor antagonists** might increase the risk of first dose hypotension when given with **drugs that cause first dose hypotension** (see TABLE 6 p. 1572) particularly in those with volume and/or salt depletion. Mild Theoretical

Drugs that cause hepatotoxicity

▶ **Alcohol**-induced liver disease increases the risk of hepatotoxicity in those taking **drugs that cause hepatotoxicity** (see TABLE 1 p. 1571). Severe Theoretical

▶ **Drugs that cause hepatotoxicity** (see TABLE 1 p. 1571) might increase the risk of hepatotoxicity when given with **low molecular-weight heparins** (high-dose). Severe Theoretical

Drugs that cause serotonin syndrome

▶ **Bupropion** might enhance the risk of serotonin syndrome when given with **drugs that cause serotonin syndrome** (see TABLE 12 p. 1574). Severe Anecdotal

▶ **Opioids (tapentadol)** are predicted to increase the risk of serotonin syndrome when given with **drugs that cause serotonin syndrome** (see TABLE 12 p. 1574). Severe Theoretical

Drugs that reduce serum potassium

▶ **Drugs that reduce serum potassium** (see TABLE 16 p. 1575) are predicted to increase the risk of digoxin toxicity when given with **digoxin**. Severe Study

Drugs with anticoagulant effects

▶ **Drugs with anticoagulant effects** (see TABLE 3 p. 1571) might increase the risk of bleeding when given with **avapritinib**. Severe Theoretical

▶ **Bismuth** subsalicylate is predicted to increase the risk of bleeding events when given with **drugs with anticoagulant effects** (see TABLE 3 p. 1571). Moderate Theoretical

▶ **Drugs with anticoagulant effects** (see TABLE 3 p. 1571) cause bleeding, as can **cabozantinib**; concurrent use might increase the risk of developing this effect. Severe Theoretical

▶ **Drugs with anticoagulant effects** (see TABLE 3 p. 1571) cause bleeding, as can **caplacizumab**; concurrent use might increase the risk of developing this effect. Severe Theoretical

▶ **Drugs with anticoagulant effects** (see TABLE 3 p. 1571) cause bleeding, as can **cobimetinib**; concurrent use might increase the risk of developing this effect. Severe Theoretical

▶ **Donanemab** can increase the risk of brain haemorrhage when given with **drugs with anticoagulant effects** (see TABLE 3 p. 1571). Avoid. Severe Anecdotal

▶ **Drugs with anticoagulant effects** (see TABLE 3 p. 1571) cause bleeding, as can **inotersen**; concurrent use might increase the risk of developing this effect. Severe Theoretical

▶ **Lecanemab** can increase the risk of brain haemorrhage when given with **drugs with anticoagulant effects** (see TABLE 3 p. 1571). Avoid. Severe Anecdotal

▶ **Drugs with anticoagulant effects** (see TABLE 3 p. 1571) cause bleeding, as can **monoclonal antibodies (bevacizumab, trastuzumab emtansine)**; concurrent use might increase the risk of developing this effect. Severe Theoretical

▶ **Drugs with anticoagulant effects** (see TABLE 3 p. 1571) might increase the risk of gastrointestinal bleeding when given with **monoclonal antibodies (ipilimumab)**. Severe Theoretical

▶ **Drugs with anticoagulant effects** (see TABLE 3 p. 1571) cause bleeding, as can **ranibizumab**; concurrent use might increase the risk of developing this effect. Severe Theoretical

▶ **Drugs with anticoagulant effects** (see TABLE 3 p. 1571) cause bleeding, as can **ruxolitinib**; concurrent use might increase the risk of developing this effect. Severe Theoretical

▶ **Drugs with anticoagulant effects** (see TABLE 3 p. 1571) cause bleeding, as can **trametinib**; concurrent use might increase the risk of developing this effect. Severe Theoretical

▶ **Drugs with anticoagulant effects** (see TABLE 3 p. 1571) cause bleeding, as can **volanesorsen**; concurrent use might increase the risk of developing this effect. Avoid depending on platelet count—consult product literature. Severe Theoretical

Drugs with antimuscarinic effects

▶ **Drugs with antimuscarinic effects** (see TABLE 9 p. 1573) might decrease the absorption of **levodopa**. Moderate Theoretical

Drugs with antiplatelet effects

▶ **Drugs with antiplatelet effects** (see TABLE 4 p. 1571) might increase the risk of bleeding when given with **avapritinib**. Severe Theoretical

▶ **Drugs with antiplatelet effects** (see TABLE 4 p. 1571) cause bleeding, as can **cabozantinib**; concurrent use might increase the risk of developing this effect. Severe Theoretical

▶ **Drugs with antiplatelet effects** (see TABLE 4 p. 1571) cause bleeding, as can **caplacizumab**; concurrent use might increase the risk of developing this effect. Severe Theoretical

▶ **Drugs with antiplatelet effects** (see TABLE 4 p. 1571) cause bleeding, as can **cobimetinib**; concurrent use might increase the risk of developing this effect. Severe Theoretical

▶ **Donanemab** can increase the risk of bleeding when given with **drugs with antiplatelet effects** (see TABLE 4 p. 1571). Severe Theoretical

▶ **Drugs with antiplatelet effects** (see TABLE 4 p. 1571) cause bleeding, as can **inotersen**; concurrent use might increase the risk of developing this effect. Severe Theoretical

▶ **Lecanemab** can increase the risk of bleeding when given with **drugs with antiplatelet effects** (see TABLE 4 p. 1571). Severe Theoretical

▶ **Drugs with antiplatelet effects** (see TABLE 4 p. 1571) cause bleeding, as can **monoclonal antibodies (bevacizumab, trastuzumab emtansine)**; concurrent use might increase the risk of developing this effect. Severe Theoretical

▶ **Drugs with antiplatelet effects** (see TABLE 4 p. 1571) cause bleeding, as can **ranibizumab**; concurrent use might increase the risk of developing this effect. Severe Theoretical

▶ **Drugs with antiplatelet effects** (see TABLE 4 p. 1571) cause bleeding, as can **ruxolitinib**; concurrent use might increase the risk of developing this effect. Severe Theoretical

▶ **Drugs with antiplatelet effects** (see TABLE 4 p. 1571) cause bleeding, as can **trametinib**; concurrent use might increase the risk of developing this effect. Severe Theoretical

▶ **Drugs with antiplatelet effects** (see TABLE 4 p. 1571) cause bleeding, as can **volanesorsen**; concurrent use might increase the risk of developing this effect. Avoid depending on platelet count—consult product literature. Severe Theoretical

Dulaglutide → see glucagon-like peptide-1 receptor agonists

Duloxetine → see SNRIs

Dupilumab → see monoclonal antibodies

Dutasteride

▶ **Antiarrhythmics (dronedarone)** are predicted to moderately increase the exposure to **dutasteride**. Mild Study

▶ **Antifungals, azoles (fluconazole, isavuconazole)** are predicted to moderately increase the exposure to **dutasteride**. Mild Study

▶ **Antifungals, azoles (itraconazole, ketoconazole, posaconazole, voriconazole)** are predicted to increase the exposure to **dutasteride**. Monitor adverse effects and adjust dose. Moderate Theoretical

▶ **Berotralstat** is predicted to moderately increase the exposure to **dutasteride**. Mild Study

▶ **Calcium channel blockers (diltiazem, verapamil)** are predicted to moderately increase the exposure to **dutasteride**. Mild Study

▶ **Ceritinib** is predicted to increase the exposure to **dutasteride**. Monitor adverse effects and adjust dose. Moderate Theoretical

▶ **Cobicistat** is predicted to increase the exposure to **dutasteride**. Monitor adverse effects and adjust dose. Moderate Theoretical

▶ **Crizotinib** is predicted to moderately increase the exposure to **dutasteride**. Mild Study

▶ **Fedratinib** is predicted to moderately increase the exposure to **dutasteride**. Mild Study

▶ **HIV-protease inhibitors** are predicted to increase the exposure to **dutasteride**. Monitor adverse effects and adjust dose. Moderate Theoretical

▶ **Idelalisib** is predicted to increase the exposure to **dutasteride**. Monitor adverse effects and adjust dose. Moderate Theoretical

▶ **Imatinib** is predicted to moderately increase the exposure to **dutasteride**. Mild Study

▶ **Letermovir** is predicted to moderately increase the exposure to **dutasteride**. Mild Study

Dutasteride (continued)

▶ Macrolides **(clarithromycin)** are predicted to increase the exposure to **dutasteride**. Monitor adverse effects and adjust dose. Moderate Theoretical

▶ Macrolides **(erythromycin)** are predicted to moderately increase the exposure to **dutasteride**. Mild Study

▶ Neurokinin-1 receptor antagonists **(aprepitant, netupitant)** are predicted to moderately increase the exposure to **dutasteride**. Mild Study

▶ Nilotinib is predicted to moderately increase the exposure to **dutasteride**. Mild Study

▶ Tucatinib is predicted to increase the exposure to **dutasteride**. Monitor adverse effects and adjust dose. Moderate Theoretical

Eculizumab → see monoclonal antibodies

Edoxaban → see factor XA inhibitors

Efavirenz → see NNRTIs

Efgartigimod alfa

▶ Live vaccines might increase the risk of generalised infection (possibly life-threatening) when given with **efgartigimod alfa**. Avoid. Severe Theoretical

Eicosapentaenoic acid → see TABLE 4 p. 1571 (antiplatelet effects)

Elacestrant

▶ Anti-androgens **(apalutamide, enzalutamide)** are predicted to decrease the exposure to **elacestrant**. Avoid or adjust dose depending on duration—consult product literature. Severe Study

▶ Antiarrhythmics **(dronedarone)** are predicted to increase the exposure to **elacestrant**. Avoid moderate CYP3A4 inhibitors or adjust **elacestrant** dose, p. 1084. Severe Theoretical

▶ Antiepileptics **(carbamazepine, fosphenytoin, phenobarbital, phenytoin, primidone)** are predicted to decrease the exposure to **elacestrant**. Avoid or adjust dose depending on duration—consult product literature. Severe Study

▶ Antifungals, azoles **(fluconazole, isavuconazole)** are predicted to increase the exposure to **elacestrant**. Avoid moderate CYP3A4 inhibitors or adjust **elacestrant** dose, p. 1084. Severe Theoretical

▶ Antifungals, azoles **(itraconazole, ketoconazole, posaconazole, voriconazole)** are predicted to increase the exposure to **elacestrant**. Avoid potent CYP3A4 inhibitors or adjust **elacestrant** dose, p. 1084. Severe Study

▶ Berotralstat is predicted to increase the exposure to **elacestrant**. Avoid moderate CYP3A4 inhibitors or adjust **elacestrant** dose, p. 1084. Severe Theoretical

▶ Calcium channel blockers **(diltiazem, verapamil)** are predicted to increase the exposure to **elacestrant**. Avoid moderate CYP3A4 inhibitors or adjust **elacestrant** dose, p. 1084. Severe Theoretical

▶ Cenobamate is predicted to decrease the exposure to **elacestrant**. Avoid or adjust dose depending on duration—consult product literature. Severe Theoretical

▶ Ceritinib is predicted to increase the exposure to **elacestrant**. Avoid potent CYP3A4 inhibitors or adjust **elacestrant** dose, p. 1084. Severe Study

▶ Ciclosporin is predicted to increase the exposure to **elacestrant**. Avoid or adjust **elacestrant** dose, p. 1084. Severe Theoretical

▶ Cobicistat is predicted to increase the exposure to **elacestrant**. Avoid potent CYP3A4 inhibitors or adjust **elacestrant** dose, p. 1084. Severe Study

▶ Crizotinib is predicted to increase the exposure to **elacestrant**. Avoid moderate CYP3A4 inhibitors or adjust **elacestrant** dose, p. 1084. Severe Theoretical

▶ Dabrafenib is predicted to decrease the exposure to **elacestrant**. Avoid or adjust dose depending on duration—consult product literature. Severe Theoretical

▶ Encorafenib is predicted to decrease the exposure to **elacestrant**. Avoid or adjust dose depending on duration—consult product literature. Severe Study

▶ Endothelin receptor antagonists **(bosentan)** are predicted to decrease the exposure to **elacestrant**. Avoid or adjust dose depending on duration—consult product literature. Severe Theoretical

▶ Fedratinib is predicted to increase the exposure to **elacestrant**. Avoid moderate CYP3A4 inhibitors or adjust **elacestrant** dose, p. 1084. Severe Theoretical

▶ Grapefruit is predicted to increase the exposure to **elacestrant**. Avoid. Moderate Theoretical

▶ HIV-protease inhibitors are predicted to increase the exposure to **elacestrant**. Avoid potent CYP3A4 inhibitors or adjust **elacestrant** dose, p. 1084. Severe Study

▶ Idelalisib is predicted to increase the exposure to **elacestrant**. Avoid potent CYP3A4 inhibitors or adjust **elacestrant** dose, p. 1084. Severe Study

▶ Imatinib is predicted to increase the exposure to **elacestrant**. Avoid moderate CYP3A4 inhibitors or adjust **elacestrant** dose, p. 1084. Severe Theoretical

▶ Ivosidenib is predicted to decrease the exposure to **elacestrant**. Avoid or adjust dose depending on duration—consult product literature. Severe Study

▶ Letermovir is predicted to increase the exposure to **elacestrant**. Avoid moderate CYP3A4 inhibitors or adjust **elacestrant** dose, p. 1084. Severe Theoretical

▶ Lorlatinib is predicted to decrease the exposure to **elacestrant**. Avoid or adjust dose depending on duration—consult product literature. Severe Theoretical

▶ Lumacaftor is predicted to decrease the exposure to **elacestrant**. Avoid or adjust dose depending on duration—consult product literature. Severe Study

▶ Macrolides **(clarithromycin)** are predicted to increase the exposure to **elacestrant**. Avoid potent CYP3A4 inhibitors or adjust **elacestrant** dose, p. 1084. Severe Study

▶ Macrolides **(erythromycin)** are predicted to increase the exposure to **elacestrant**. Avoid moderate CYP3A4 inhibitors or adjust **elacestrant** dose, p. 1084. Severe Theoretical

▶ Mitotane is predicted to decrease the exposure to **elacestrant**. Avoid or adjust dose depending on duration—consult product literature. Severe Study

▶ Neurokinin-1 receptor antagonists **(aprepitant, netupitant)** are predicted to increase the exposure to **elacestrant**. Avoid moderate CYP3A4 inhibitors or adjust **elacestrant** dose, p. 1084. Severe Theoretical

▶ Nilotinib is predicted to increase the exposure to **elacestrant**. Avoid moderate CYP3A4 inhibitors or adjust **elacestrant** dose, p. 1084. Severe Theoretical

▶ NNRTIs **(efavirenz, etravirine, nevirapine)** are predicted to decrease the exposure to **elacestrant**. Avoid or adjust dose depending on duration—consult product literature. Severe Theoretical

▶ Quinolones **(ciprofloxacin)** are predicted to increase the exposure to **elacestrant**. Avoid or adjust **elacestrant** dose, p. 1084. Severe Theoretical

▶ Rifamycins **(rifampicin)** are predicted to decrease the exposure to **elacestrant**. Avoid or adjust dose depending on duration—consult product literature. Severe Study

▶ Sotorasib is predicted to decrease the exposure to **elacestrant**. Avoid or adjust dose depending on duration—consult product literature. Severe Theoretical

▶ SSRIs **(fluvoxamine)** are predicted to increase the exposure to **elacestrant**. Avoid or adjust **elacestrant** dose, p. 1084. Severe Theoretical

▶ St John's wort is predicted to decrease the exposure to **elacestrant**. Avoid or adjust dose depending on duration—consult product literature. Severe Theoretical

▶ Tucatinib is predicted to increase the exposure to **elacestrant**. Avoid potent CYP3A4 inhibitors or adjust **elacestrant** dose, p. 1084. Severe Study

Elafibranor

▶ Elafibranor might increase the risk of muscle effects when given with statins. Severe Theoretical

Elbasvir

▶ Anti-androgens **(apalutamide, enzalutamide)** are predicted to decrease the exposure to **elbasvir**. Avoid. Severe Study

▶ Antiepileptics **(carbamazepine, fosphenytoin, phenobarbital, phenytoin, primidone)** are predicted to decrease the exposure to **elbasvir**. Avoid. Severe Study

▶ Cenobamate is predicted to moderately decrease the exposure to **elbasvir**. Avoid. Severe Study

▶ Dabrafenib is predicted to moderately decrease the exposure to **elbasvir**. Avoid. Severe Study

- ▸ **Encorafenib** is predicted to decrease the exposure to **elbasvir**. Avoid. Severe Study
- ▸ **Endothelin receptor antagonists (bosentan)** are predicted to moderately decrease the exposure to **elbasvir**. Avoid. Severe Study
- ▸ **Ivosidenib** is predicted to decrease the exposure to **elbasvir**. Avoid. Severe Study
- ▸ **Lorlatinib** is predicted to moderately decrease the exposure to **elbasvir**. Avoid. Severe Study
- ▸ **Lumacaftor** is predicted to decrease the exposure to **elbasvir**. Avoid. Severe Study
- ▸ **Mitotane** is predicted to decrease the exposure to **elbasvir**. Avoid. Severe Study
- ▸ **Modafinil** is predicted to decrease the exposure to **elbasvir**. Avoid. Unknown Theoretical
- ▸ **NNRTIs (efavirenz, etravirine, nevirapine)** are predicted to moderately decrease the exposure to **elbasvir**. Avoid. Severe Study
- ▸ **Rifamycins (rifampicin)** are predicted to decrease the exposure to **elbasvir**. Avoid. Severe Study
- ▸ **Sotorasib** is predicted to moderately decrease the exposure to **elbasvir**. Avoid. Severe Study
- ▸ **St John's wort** is predicted to moderately decrease the exposure to **elbasvir**. Avoid. Severe Study
- ▸ **Elbasvir** with grazoprevir slightly increases the exposure to statins (atorvastatin). Adjust **atorvastatin** dose, p. 234. Moderate Study
- ▸ **Elbasvir** with grazoprevir is predicted to increase the exposure to statins (fluvastatin). Adjust **fluvastatin** dose, p. 234. Moderate Theoretical
- ▸ **Elbasvir** with grazoprevir moderately increases the exposure to statins (rosuvastatin). Adjust **rosuvastatin** dose, p. 235. Moderate Study
- ▸ **Elbasvir** with grazoprevir is predicted to increase the exposure to statins (simvastatin). Adjust **simvastatin** dose, p. 237. Moderate Theoretical
- ▸ **Elbasvir** is predicted to increase the concentration of sunitinib. Use with caution and adjust dose. Moderate Theoretical
- ▸ **Elbasvir** is predicted to increase the concentration of thrombin inhibitors (dabigatran). Moderate Theoretical

Eletriptan → see triptans

Elexacaftor
- ▸ **Anti-androgens (apalutamide, enzalutamide)** is predicted to decrease the exposure to **elexacaftor**. Avoid. Severe Theoretical
- ▸ **Antiarrhythmics (dronedarone)** are predicted to increase the exposure to **elexacaftor**. Adjust ivacaftor with tezacaftor and elexacaftor p. 337 dose with moderate CYP3A4 inhibitors. Severe Theoretical
- ▸ **Antiepileptics (carbamazepine, fosphenytoin, phenobarbital, phenytoin, primidone)** is predicted to decrease the exposure to **elexacaftor**. Avoid. Severe Theoretical
- ▸ **Antifungals, azoles (fluconazole, isavuconazole)** are predicted to increase the exposure to **elexacaftor**. Adjust ivacaftor with tezacaftor and elexacaftor p. 337 dose with moderate CYP3A4 inhibitors. Severe Theoretical
- ▸ **Antifungals, azoles (itraconazole, ketoconazole, posaconazole, voriconazole)** are predicted to increase the exposure to **elexacaftor**. Adjust ivacaftor with tezacaftor and elexacaftor p. 337 dose with potent CYP3A4 inhibitors. Severe Study
- ▸ **Elexacaftor** is predicted to increase the exposure to antihistamines, non-sedating (fexofenadine). Moderate Theoretical
- ▸ **Berotralstat** is predicted to increase the exposure to **elexacaftor**. Adjust ivacaftor with tezacaftor and elexacaftor p. 337 dose with moderate CYP3A4 inhibitors. Severe Theoretical
- ▸ **Calcium channel blockers (diltiazem, verapamil)** are predicted to increase the exposure to **elexacaftor**. Adjust ivacaftor with tezacaftor and elexacaftor p. 337 dose with moderate CYP3A4 inhibitors. Severe Theoretical
- ▸ **Ceritinib** is predicted to increase the exposure to **elexacaftor**. Adjust ivacaftor with tezacaftor and elexacaftor p. 337 dose with potent CYP3A4 inhibitors. Severe Study
- ▸ **Cobicistat** is predicted to increase the exposure to **elexacaftor**. Adjust ivacaftor with tezacaftor and elexacaftor p. 337 dose with potent CYP3A4 inhibitors. Severe Study

- ▸ **Crizotinib** is predicted to increase the exposure to **elexacaftor**. Adjust ivacaftor with tezacaftor and elexacaftor p. 337 dose with moderate CYP3A4 inhibitors. Severe Theoretical
- ▸ **Encorafenib** is predicted to decreases the exposure to **elexacaftor**. Avoid. Severe Theoretical
- ▸ **Elexacaftor** is predicted to increase the exposure to endothelin receptor antagonists (bosentan). Moderate Theoretical
- ▸ **Fedratinib** is predicted to increase the exposure to **elexacaftor**. Adjust ivacaftor with tezacaftor and elexacaftor p. 337 dose with moderate CYP3A4 inhibitors. Severe Theoretical
- ▸ **Grapefruit** juice is predicted to increase the exposure to **elexacaftor**. Avoid. Moderate Theoretical
- ▸ **HIV-protease inhibitors** are predicted to increase the exposure to **elexacaftor**. Adjust ivacaftor with tezacaftor and elexacaftor p. 337 dose with potent CYP3A4 inhibitors. Severe Study
- ▸ **Idelalisib** is predicted to increase the exposure to **elexacaftor**. Adjust ivacaftor with tezacaftor and elexacaftor p. 337 dose with potent CYP3A4 inhibitors. Severe Study
- ▸ **Imatinib** is predicted to increase the exposure to **elexacaftor**. Adjust ivacaftor with tezacaftor and elexacaftor p. 337 dose with moderate CYP3A4 inhibitors. Severe Theoretical
- ▸ **Ivosidenib** is predicted to decreases the exposure to **elexacaftor**. Avoid. Severe Theoretical
- ▸ **Letermovir** is predicted to increase the exposure to **elexacaftor**. Adjust ivacaftor with tezacaftor and elexacaftor p. 337 dose with moderate CYP3A4 inhibitors. Severe Theoretical
- ▸ **Lumacaftor** is predicted to decreases the exposure to **elexacaftor**. Avoid. Severe Theoretical
- ▸ **Macrolides (clarithromycin)** are predicted to increase the exposure to **elexacaftor**. Adjust ivacaftor with tezacaftor and elexacaftor p. 337 dose with potent CYP3A4 inhibitors. Severe Study
- ▸ **Macrolides (erythromycin)** are predicted to increase the exposure to **elexacaftor**. Adjust ivacaftor with tezacaftor and elexacaftor p. 337 dose with moderate CYP3A4 inhibitors. Severe Theoretical
- ▸ **Elexacaftor** is predicted to increase the exposure to meglitinides (repaglinide). Moderate Theoretical
- ▸ **Mitotane** is predicted to decreases the exposure to **elexacaftor**. Avoid. Severe Theoretical
- ▸ **Neurokinin-1 receptor antagonists (aprepitant, netupitant)** are predicted to increase the exposure to **elexacaftor**. Adjust ivacaftor with tezacaftor and elexacaftor p. 337 dose with moderate CYP3A4 inhibitors. Severe Theoretical
- ▸ **Nilotinib** is predicted to increase the exposure to **elexacaftor**. Adjust ivacaftor with tezacaftor and elexacaftor p. 337 dose with moderate CYP3A4 inhibitors. Severe Theoretical
- ▸ **Nirmatrelvir** boosted with ritonavir is predicted to increase the concentration of **elexacaftor** with tezacaftor and ivacaftor. Adjust dose. Severe Theoretical
- ▸ **Rifamycins (rifabutin)** are predicted to decrease the exposure to **elexacaftor**. Avoid. Severe Theoretical
- ▸ **Rifamycins (rifampicin)** is predicted to decrease the exposure to **elexacaftor**. Avoid. Severe Theoretical
- ▸ **St John's wort** is predicted to decrease the exposure to **elexacaftor**. Avoid. Severe Theoretical
- ▸ **Elexacaftor** is predicted to increase the exposure to statins (atorvastatin, pravastatin, rosuvastatin, simvastatin). Moderate Theoretical
- ▸ **Elexacaftor** is predicted to increase the exposure to sulfonylureas (glibenclamide). Moderate Theoretical
- ▸ **Elexacaftor** is predicted to increase the exposure to taxanes (docetaxel, paclitaxel). Moderate Theoretical
- ▸ **Tucatinib** is predicted to increase the exposure to **elexacaftor**. Adjust ivacaftor with tezacaftor and elexacaftor p. 337 dose with potent CYP3A4 inhibitors. Severe Study

Eliglustat
- ▸ **Eliglustat** is predicted to increase the exposure to aliskiren. Adjust dose. Moderate Study
- ▸ **Anti-androgens (abiraterone)** are predicted to increase the exposure to **eliglustat**. Avoid or adjust dose—consult product literature. Severe Study
- ▸ **Anti-androgens (apalutamide, enzalutamide)** are predicted to decrease the exposure to **eliglustat**. Avoid. Severe Study

Eliglustat (continued)

▶ Antiarrhythmics (dronedarone, propafenone) are predicted to increase the exposure to **eliglustat**. Avoid or adjust dose—consult product literature. Severe Study

▶ Antiepileptics (carbamazepine, fosphenytoin, phenobarbital, phenytoin, primidone) are predicted to decrease the exposure to **eliglustat**. Avoid. Severe Study

▶ Antifungals, azoles (fluconazole, isavuconazole, itraconazole, ketoconazole, posaconazole, voriconazole) are predicted to increase the exposure to **eliglustat**. Avoid or adjust dose—consult product literature. Severe Study

▶ **Eliglustat** is predicted to increase the exposure to antihistamines, non-sedating (fexofenadine). Adjust dose. Moderate Study

▶ **Eliglustat** is predicted to increase the exposure to atomoxetine. Adjust dose. Moderate Theoretical

▶ Berotralstat is predicted to increase the exposure to **eliglustat**. Avoid or adjust dose—consult product literature. Severe Study

▶ **Eliglustat** is predicted to increase the exposure to beta blockers, non-selective (propranolol). Adjust dose. Moderate Study

▶ **Eliglustat** is predicted to increase the exposure to beta blockers, selective (metoprolol). Adjust dose. Moderate Study

▶ Bupropion is predicted to increase the exposure to **eliglustat**. Avoid or adjust dose—consult product literature. Severe Study

▶ Calcium channel blockers (diltiazem, verapamil) are predicted to increase the exposure to **eliglustat**. Avoid or adjust dose—consult product literature. Severe Study

▶ Ceritinib is predicted to increase the exposure to **eliglustat**. Avoid or adjust dose—consult product literature. Severe Study

▶ Cinacalcet is predicted to increase the exposure to **eliglustat**. Avoid or adjust dose—consult product literature. Severe Study

▶ Cobicistat is predicted to increase the exposure to **eliglustat**. Avoid or adjust dose—consult product literature. Severe Study

▶ **Eliglustat** is predicted to increase the exposure to colchicine. Avoid or adjust **colchicine** dose, p. 1279. Severe Theoretical

▶ Crizotinib is predicted to increase the exposure to **eliglustat**. Avoid or adjust dose—consult product literature. Severe Study

▶ Dacomitinib is predicted to increase the exposure to **eliglustat**. Avoid or adjust dose—consult product literature. Severe Study

▶ **Eliglustat** increases the exposure to digoxin. Adjust dose. Moderate Study

▶ Encorafenib is predicted to decrease the exposure to **eliglustat**. Avoid. Severe Study

▶ Endothelin receptor antagonists (bosentan) are predicted to decrease the exposure to **eliglustat**. Moderate Theoretical

▶ **Eliglustat** is predicted to increase the exposure to everolimus. Adjust dose. Moderate Study

▶ **Eliglustat** is predicted to increase the exposure to factor XA inhibitors (edoxaban). Adjust dose. Moderate Study

▶ Fedratinib is predicted to increase the exposure to **eliglustat**. Avoid or adjust dose—consult product literature. Severe Study

▶ Givosiran is predicted to increase the exposure to **eliglustat**. Use with caution and adjust dose. Moderate Study

▶ Grapefruit juice is predicted to increase the exposure to **eliglustat**. Avoid. Severe Theoretical

▶ HIV-protease inhibitors are predicted to increase the exposure to **eliglustat**. Avoid or adjust dose—consult product literature. Severe Study

▶ Idelalisib is predicted to increase the exposure to **eliglustat**. Avoid or adjust dose—consult product literature. Severe Study

▶ Imatinib is predicted to increase the exposure to **eliglustat**. Avoid or adjust dose—consult product literature. Severe Study

▶ Interferons (ropeginterferon alfa) are predicted to increase the exposure to **eliglustat**. Moderate Theoretical

▶ Ivosidenib is predicted to decrease the exposure to **eliglustat**. Avoid. Severe Study

▶ Letermovir is predicted to increase the exposure to **eliglustat**. Avoid or adjust dose—consult product literature. Severe Study

▶ **Eliglustat** is predicted to increase the exposure to loperamide. Adjust dose. Moderate Study

▶ Lumacaftor is predicted to decrease the exposure to **eliglustat**. Avoid. Severe Study

▶ Macrolides (clarithromycin, erythromycin) are predicted to increase the exposure to **eliglustat**. Avoid or adjust dose—consult product literature. Severe Study

▶ Mirabegron is predicted to increase the exposure to **eliglustat**. Avoid or adjust dose—consult product literature. Severe Study

▶ Mitotane is predicted to decrease the exposure to **eliglustat**. Avoid. Severe Study

▶ Moclobemide is predicted to increase the exposure to **eliglustat**. Avoid or adjust dose—consult product literature. Severe Theoretical

▶ Neurokinin-1 receptor antagonists (aprepitant, netupitant) are predicted to increase the exposure to **eliglustat**. Avoid or adjust dose—consult product literature. Severe Study

▶ Nilotinib is predicted to increase the exposure to **eliglustat**. Avoid or adjust dose—consult product literature. Severe Study

▶ NNRTIs (efavirenz, etravirine, nevirapine) are predicted to decrease the exposure to **eliglustat**. Moderate Theoretical

▶ **Eliglustat** is predicted to increase the exposure to pralsetinib. Adjust dose. Moderate Study

▶ Quinolones (ciprofloxacin) are predicted to increase the exposure to **eliglustat**. Avoid or adjust dose—consult product literature. Severe Theoretical

▶ **Eliglustat** is predicted to increase the exposure to ranolazine. Adjust dose. Moderate Study

▶ Rifamycins (rifampicin) are predicted to decrease the exposure to **eliglustat**. Avoid. Severe Study

▶ **Eliglustat** is predicted to increase the exposure to rimegepant. Adjust dose. Moderate Study

▶ **Eliglustat** is predicted to increase the exposure to sirolimus. Adjust dose. Moderate Study

▶ SNRIs (duloxetine) are predicted to increase the exposure to **eliglustat**. Avoid or adjust dose—consult product literature. Severe Study

▶ SSRIs (fluoxetine, paroxetine) are predicted to increase the exposure to **eliglustat**. Avoid or adjust dose—consult product literature. Severe Study

▶ St John's wort is predicted to increase the exposure to **eliglustat**. Avoid. Severe Study

▶ **Eliglustat** is predicted to increase the exposure to statins (pravastatin). Adjust dose. Moderate Study

▶ **Eliglustat** is predicted to increase the exposure to talazoparib. Adjust dose. Moderate Study

▶ **Eliglustat** is predicted to increase the exposure to taxanes (paclitaxel). Adjust dose. Moderate Study

▶ Terbinafine is predicted to increase the exposure to **eliglustat**. Avoid or adjust dose—consult product literature. Severe Study

▶ **Eliglustat** is predicted to increase the exposure to thrombin inhibitors (dabigatran). Adjust dose. Moderate Study

▶ **Eliglustat** is predicted to increase the exposure to tolterodine. Adjust dose. Moderate Theoretical

▶ **Eliglustat** is predicted to increase the exposure to tricyclic antidepressants (nortriptyline). Adjust dose. Moderate Theoretical

▶ Tucatinib is predicted to increase the exposure to **eliglustat**. Avoid or adjust dose—consult product literature. Severe Study

Elotuzumab → see monoclonal antibodies

Elranatamab → see monoclonal antibodies

Eltrombopag

▶ **Eltrombopag** is predicted to increase the exposure to alpelisib. Moderate Theoretical

▶ Oral antacids decrease the absorption of oral **eltrombopag**. Manufacturer advises take 2 hours before or 4 hours after antacids. Severe Study

▶ **Eltrombopag** is predicted to increase the exposure to atogepant. Adjust **atogepant** dose, p. 540. Moderate Theoretical

▶ Oral calcium salts decrease the absorption of oral **eltrombopag**. **Eltrombopag** should be taken 2 hours before or 4 hours after calcium. Severe Study

▶ Ciclosporin causes a small decrease in the exposure to **eltrombopag**. Monitor platelet count and adjust dose. Moderate Study

▶ **Eltrombopag** is predicted to increase the exposure to cladribine. Avoid or adjust dose. Moderate Theoretical

▶ Oral iron is predicted to decrease the absorption of oral **eltrombopag**. **Eltrombopag** should be taken 2 hours before or 4 hours after iron. Severe Theoretical

▶ **Eltrombopag** is predicted to increase the concentration of letermovir. Moderate Study

▶ **Eltrombopag** is predicted to increase the concentration of methotrexate. Moderate Theoretical

▶ **Eltrombopag** is predicted to increase the exposure to momelotinib. Moderate Study

▶ Rifamycins (rifampicin) are predicted to decrease the exposure to **eltrombopag** and **eltrombopag** is predicted to increase the concentration of rifamycins (rifampicin). Moderate Theoretical

▶ Oral selenium is predicted to decrease the absorption of **eltrombopag**. **Eltrombopag** should be taken 2 hours before or 4 hours after **selenium**. Severe Theoretical

▶ SSRIs (fluvoxamine) are predicted to increase the exposure to **eltrombopag**. Moderate Theoretical

▶ **Eltrombopag** is predicted to increase the exposure to statins. Monitor and adjust dose. Moderate Study

▶ **Eltrombopag** is predicted to increase the exposure to talazoparib. Avoid or monitor. Moderate Theoretical

▶ **Eltrombopag** is predicted to increase the exposure to taxanes (docetaxel, paclitaxel). Moderate Theoretical

▶ **Eltrombopag** is predicted to increase the exposure to tenofovir alafenamide. Moderate Theoretical

▶ **Eltrombopag** is predicted to increase the exposure to tenofovir disoproxil. Moderate Theoretical

▶ **Eltrombopag** is predicted to increase the exposure to topotecan. Moderate Theoretical

▶ **Eltrombopag** is predicted to increase the exposure to venetoclax. Avoid or monitor for toxicity. Severe Theoretical

▶ Oral zinc is predicted to decrease the absorption of **eltrombopag**. **Eltrombopag** should be taken 2 hours before or 4 hours after **zinc**. Severe Theoretical

Elvitegravir

▶ Oral antacids decrease the exposure to oral **elvitegravir**. Separate administration by at least 4 hours. Moderate Study

▶ Anti-androgens (apalutamide, enzalutamide) are predicted to decrease the concentration of **elvitegravir**. Avoid. Severe Study

▶ Antiepileptics (carbamazepine, fosphenytoin, phenobarbital, phenytoin, primidone) are predicted to decrease the concentration of **elvitegravir**. Avoid. Severe Study

▶ Cenobamate is predicted to decrease the concentration of **elvitegravir**. Avoid. Severe Theoretical

▶ **Elvitegravir** is predicted to decrease the anticoagulant effect of coumarins. Moderate Anecdotal

▶ Dabrafenib is predicted to decrease the concentration of **elvitegravir**. Avoid. Severe Theoretical

▶ Encorafenib is predicted to decrease the concentration of **elvitegravir**. Avoid. Severe Study

▶ Endothelin receptor antagonists (bosentan) are predicted to decrease the concentration of **elvitegravir**. Avoid. Severe Theoretical

▶ **Elvitegravir** markedly increases the exposure to grazoprevir. Avoid. Severe Study

▶ HIV-protease inhibitors (atazanavir, lopinavir) boosted with ritonavir increase the concentration of **elvitegravir**. Refer to specialist literature. Moderate Study

▶ Ivosidenib is predicted to decrease the concentration of **elvitegravir**. Avoid. Severe Study

▶ Lorlatinib is predicted to decrease the concentration of **elvitegravir**. Avoid. Severe Theoretical

▶ Lumacaftor is predicted to decrease the concentration of **elvitegravir**. Avoid. Severe Study

▶ **Elvitegravir** boosted with ritonavir is predicted to increase the exposure to midostaurin. Severe Theoretical

▶ Mitotane is predicted to decrease the concentration of **elvitegravir**. Avoid. Severe Study

▶ NNRTIs (efavirenz, etravirine, nevirapine) are predicted to decrease the concentration of **elvitegravir**. Avoid. Severe Theoretical

▶ Rifamycins (rifampicin) are predicted to decrease the concentration of **elvitegravir**. Avoid. Severe Study

▶ Sotorasib is predicted to decrease the concentration of **elvitegravir**. Avoid. Severe Theoretical

▶ St John's wort is predicted to decrease the concentration of **elvitegravir**. Avoid. Severe Theoretical

Empagliflozin → see sodium glucose co-transporter 2 inhibitors

Emtricitabine → see NRTIs

Enalapril → see ACE inhibitors

Encorafenib → see TABLE 8 p. 1573 (QT-interval prolongation)

▶ **Encorafenib** is predicted to decrease the exposure to 5-HT3-receptor antagonists (ondansetron). Moderate Study → Also see TABLE 8 p. 1573

▶ **Encorafenib** is predicted to markedly decrease the exposure to abemaciclib. Avoid. Severe Study

▶ **Encorafenib** is predicted to decrease the exposure to acalabrutinib. Avoid. Severe Study

▶ **Encorafenib** is predicted to decrease the exposure to alpelisib. Avoid. Moderate Study

▶ Anti-androgens (apalutamide, enzalutamide) are predicted to decrease the exposure to **encorafenib**. Severe Theoretical → Also see TABLE 8 p. 1573

▶ **Encorafenib** is predicted to decrease the exposure to anti-androgens (abiraterone). Avoid. Severe Study

▶ **Encorafenib** is predicted to decrease the exposure to anti-androgens (darolutamide). Avoid. Moderate Study

▶ Antiarrhythmics (dronedarone) are predicted to moderately increase the exposure to **encorafenib**. Moderate Study → Also see TABLE 8 p. 1573

▶ **Encorafenib** is predicted to decrease the exposure to antiarrhythmics (disopyramide, dronedarone). Avoid. Severe Study → Also see TABLE 8 p. 1573

▶ **Encorafenib** is predicted to decrease the efficacy of antiarrhythmics (propafenone). Moderate Study

▶ **Encorafenib** is predicted to decrease the exposure to anticholinesterases, centrally acting (donepezil). Mild Study

▶ Antiepileptics (carbamazepine, fosphenytoin, phenobarbital, phenytoin, primidone) are predicted to decrease the exposure to **encorafenib**. Severe Theoretical

▶ **Encorafenib** is predicted to decrease the exposure to antiepileptics (perampanel). Monitor and adjust dose. Moderate Study

▶ Antifungals, azoles (fluconazole, isavuconazole) are predicted to moderately increase the exposure to **encorafenib**. Moderate Study → Also see TABLE 8 p. 1573

▶ Antifungals, azoles (itraconazole, ketoconazole, posaconazole, voriconazole) are predicted to increase the exposure to **encorafenib**. Avoid or monitor. Severe Study → Also see TABLE 8 p. 1573

▶ **Encorafenib** is predicted to decrease the exposure to antifungals, azoles (isavuconazole). Avoid. Severe Study

▶ **Encorafenib** is predicted to increase the exposure to antihistamines, non-sedating (fexofenadine). Mild Study

▶ **Encorafenib** is predicted to decrease the exposure to antimalarials (artemether) with lumefantrine. Avoid. Severe Study → Also see TABLE 8 p. 1573

▶ **Encorafenib** is predicted to moderately decrease the exposure to antipsychotics, second generation (aripiprazole). Adjust **aripiprazole** dose, p. 454. Moderate Study → Also see TABLE 8 p. 1573

▶ **Encorafenib** is predicted to decrease the exposure to antipsychotics, second generation (cariprazine). Avoid. Severe Theoretical

▶ **Encorafenib** is predicted to decrease the exposure to antipsychotics, second generation (lurasidone). Avoid. Moderate Study

▶ **Encorafenib** is predicted to decrease the exposure to antipsychotics, second generation (paliperidone). Monitor and adjust dose. Severe Study → Also see TABLE 8 p. 1573

▶ **Encorafenib** is predicted to decrease the exposure to antipsychotics, second generation (quetiapine). Moderate Study

▶ **Encorafenib** is predicted to decrease the exposure to antipsychotics, second generation (risperidone). Adjust dose. Moderate Study

▶ **Encorafenib** is predicted to decrease the exposure to avacopan. Avoid or monitor. Severe Study

▶ **Encorafenib** is predicted to decrease the exposure to avapritinib. Avoid. Severe Study

▶ **Encorafenib** is predicted to decrease the exposure to axitinib. Avoid or adjust dose. Moderate Study

▶ **Encorafenib** decreases the exposure to bedaquiline. Avoid. Severe Study → Also see TABLE 8 p. 1573

▶ **Encorafenib** is predicted to decrease the exposure to belumosudil. Adjust **belumosudil** dose, p. 979. Severe Study

Encorafenib (continued)

▶ **Encorafenib** is predicted to decrease the exposure to benzodiazepines (alprazolam). Adjust dose. Moderate Theoretical

▶ **Encorafenib** is predicted to decrease the exposure to benzodiazepines (midazolam). Monitor and adjust dose. Severe Study

▶ Berotralstat is predicted to moderately increase the exposure to **encorafenib**. Moderate Study

▶ **Encorafenib** is predicted to decrease the exposure to bictegravir. Avoid. Moderate Study

▶ **Encorafenib** slightly decreases the exposure to bortezomib. Avoid. Severe Study

▶ **Encorafenib** is predicted to very markedly decrease the exposure to bosutinib. Avoid. Severe Study → Also see TABLE 8 p. 1573

▶ **Encorafenib** is predicted to decrease the exposure to brigatinib. Avoid. Severe Study

▶ **Encorafenib** is predicted to decrease the exposure to buspirone. Use with caution and adjust dose. Severe Study

▶ **Encorafenib** moderately decreases the exposure to cabozantinib. Avoid. Moderate Study → Also see TABLE 8 p. 1573

▶ Calcium channel blockers (diltiazem, verapamil) are predicted to moderately increase the exposure to **encorafenib**. Moderate Study

▶ **Encorafenib** is predicted to decrease the exposure to calcium channel blockers (amlodipine, felodipine, lacidipine, lercanidipine, nicardipine, nifedipine, nimodipine). Monitor and adjust dose. Moderate Study

▶ **Encorafenib** is predicted to decrease the exposure to cannabidiol. Adjust dose. Moderate Study

▶ **Encorafenib** is predicted to decrease the exposure to capivasertib. Avoid. Moderate Study

▶ Cenobamate is predicted to decrease the exposure to **encorafenib**. Moderate Study

▶ **Encorafenib** is predicted to decrease the exposure to ceritinib. Avoid. Severe Study → Also see TABLE 8 p. 1573

▶ Ceritinib is predicted to increase the exposure to **encorafenib**. Avoid or monitor. Severe Study → Also see TABLE 8 p. 1573

▶ **Encorafenib** decreases the concentration of ciclosporin. Severe Study

▶ **Encorafenib** is predicted to alter the effects of cilostazol. Moderate Theoretical

▶ **Encorafenib** is predicted to decrease the exposure to cinacalcet. Monitor and adjust dose. Moderate Study

▶ **Encorafenib** decreases the exposure to clomethiazole. Monitor and adjust dose. Moderate Study

▶ **Encorafenib** is predicted to decrease the exposure to cobicistat. Avoid. Severe Study

▶ Cobicistat is predicted to increase the exposure to **encorafenib**. Avoid or monitor. Severe Study

▶ **Encorafenib** is predicted to decrease the exposure to cobimetinib. Avoid. Severe Theoretical

▶ **Encorafenib** might decrease the efficacy of combined hormonal contraceptives. Use additional contraceptive precautions or alternative methods. Severe Theoretical

▶ **Encorafenib** is predicted to decrease the exposure to corticosteroids (budesonide, deflazacort, dexamethasone, fludrocortisone, hydrocortisone, methylprednisolone, prednisolone, triamcinolone). Monitor and adjust dose. Moderate Study

▶ **Encorafenib** is predicted to decrease the exposure to corticosteroids (fluticasone). Unknown Theoretical

▶ **Encorafenib** is predicted to markedly decrease the exposure to crizotinib. Avoid. Severe Study → Also see TABLE 8 p. 1573

▶ Crizotinib is predicted to moderately increase the exposure to **encorafenib**. Moderate Study → Also see TABLE 8 p. 1573

▶ Dabrafenib is predicted to decrease the exposure to **encorafenib**. Moderate Study

▶ **Encorafenib** is predicted to decrease the exposure to dabrafenib. Avoid. Moderate Theoretical

▶ **Encorafenib** is predicted to decrease the exposure to daridorexant. Severe Study

▶ **Encorafenib** is predicted to decrease the exposure to darifenacin. Moderate Theoretical

▶ **Encorafenib** is predicted to markedly decrease the exposure to dasatinib. Avoid. Severe Study → Also see TABLE 8 p. 1573

▶ **Encorafenib** is predicted to slightly decrease the exposure to delamanid. Avoid. Moderate Study → Also see TABLE 8 p. 1573

▶ **Encorafenib** is predicted to markedly decrease the exposure to dienogest. Severe Study

▶ **Encorafenib** is predicted to decrease the exposure to dipeptidylpeptidase-4 inhibitors (linagliptin). Moderate Study

▶ **Encorafenib** is predicted to moderately decrease the exposure to dipeptidylpeptidase-4 inhibitors (saxagliptin). Moderate Study

▶ **Encorafenib** is predicted to increase the exposure to dolutegravir. Moderate Theoretical

▶ **Encorafenib** is predicted to decrease the exposure to dronabinol. Avoid or adjust dose. Mild Study

▶ **Encorafenib** is predicted to decrease the exposure to elacestrant. Avoid or adjust dose depending on duration— consult product literature. Severe Study

▶ **Encorafenib** is predicted to decrease the exposure to elbasvir. Avoid. Severe Study

▶ **Encorafenib** is predicted to decreases the exposure to elexacaftor. Avoid. Severe Theoretical

▶ **Encorafenib** is predicted to decrease the exposure to eliglustat. Avoid. Severe Study

▶ **Encorafenib** is predicted to decrease the concentration of elvitegravir. Avoid. Severe Study

▶ Endothelin receptor antagonists (bosentan) are predicted to decrease the exposure to **encorafenib**. Moderate Study

▶ **Encorafenib** affects the exposure to endothelin receptor antagonists (bosentan). Avoid. Severe Study

▶ **Encorafenib** is predicted to decrease the exposure to endothelin receptor antagonists (macitentan). Avoid. Severe Study

▶ **Encorafenib** is predicted to decrease the exposure to the cytotoxic component of enfortumab vedotin. Moderate Theoretical

▶ **Encorafenib** is predicted to decrease the exposure to entrectinib. Avoid. Severe Study → Also see TABLE 8 p. 1573

▶ **Encorafenib** is predicted to decrease the exposure to erdafitinib. Avoid. Severe Study

▶ **Encorafenib** is predicted to decrease the exposure to erlotinib. Avoid or adjust dose—consult product literature. Severe Study

▶ **Encorafenib** is predicted to decrease the exposure to esketamine. Adjust dose. Mild Theoretical

▶ **Encorafenib** is predicted to decrease the exposure to eszopiclone. Adjust dose. Moderate Theoretical

▶ **Encorafenib** is predicted to decrease the concentration of everolimus. Avoid or adjust dose. Severe Study

▶ **Encorafenib** moderately decreases the exposure to exemestane. Moderate Study

▶ Fedratinib is predicted to moderately increase the exposure to **encorafenib**. Moderate Study

▶ **Encorafenib** is predicted to decrease the exposure to fedratinib. Avoid. Moderate Study

▶ **Encorafenib** is predicted to decrease the exposure to fesoterodine. Avoid. Moderate Study

▶ **Encorafenib** is predicted to decrease the exposure to fostamatinib. Avoid. Severe Study

▶ **Encorafenib** is predicted to decrease the exposure to the active metabolite of fostemsavir. Avoid. Severe Study

▶ **Encorafenib** is predicted to decrease the exposure to fruquintinib. Avoid. Moderate Study

▶ **Encorafenib** is predicted to decrease the exposure to gefitinib. Avoid. Severe Study

▶ **Encorafenib** is predicted to decrease the exposure to glasdegib. Avoid. Severe Study → Also see TABLE 8 p. 1573

▶ Grapefruit juice is predicted to increase the exposure to **encorafenib**. Avoid. Moderate Study

▶ **Encorafenib** is predicted to decrease the exposure to grazoprevir. Avoid. Severe Study

▶ **Encorafenib** is predicted to decrease the concentration of guanfacine. Adjust **guanfacine** dose, p. 407. Moderate Study

▶ **Encorafenib** decreases the concentration of haloperidol. Adjust dose. Moderate Study → Also see TABLE 8 p. 1573

▶ HIV-protease inhibitors are predicted to increase the exposure to **encorafenib**. Avoid or monitor. Severe Study

▸ **Encorafenib** is predicted to decrease the exposure to ibrutinib. Avoid or monitor. [Severe] Study

▸ Idelalisib is predicted to increase the exposure to **encorafenib**. Avoid or monitor. [Severe] Study

▸ **Encorafenib** is predicted to decrease the exposure to idelalisib. Avoid. [Severe] Study

▸ **Encorafenib** is predicted to decrease the exposure to imatinib. Avoid. [Moderate] Study

▸ Imatinib is predicted to moderately increase the exposure to **encorafenib**. [Moderate] Study

▸ **Encorafenib** is predicted to decrease the exposure to irinotecan. Avoid. [Severe] Study

▸ **Encorafenib** is predicted to decrease the exposure to ivabradine. Adjust dose. [Moderate] Theoretical

▸ **Encorafenib** is predicted to decrease the exposure to ivacaftor. Avoid. [Severe] Study

▸ Ivosidenib is predicted to decrease the exposure to **encorafenib**. [Severe] Theoretical → Also see **TABLE 8** p. 1573

▸ **Encorafenib** is predicted to decrease the exposure to ixazomib. Avoid. [Severe] Study

▸ **Encorafenib** is predicted to decrease the exposure to lapatinib. Avoid. [Severe] Study → Also see **TABLE 8** p. 1573

▸ **Encorafenib** is predicted to moderately decrease the exposure to larotrectinib. Avoid. [Moderate] Study

▸ **Encorafenib** is predicted to decrease the exposure to leniolisib. Avoid. [Severe] Theoretical

▸ Letermovir is predicted to moderately increase the exposure to **encorafenib**. [Moderate] Study

▸ **Encorafenib** is predicted to decrease the exposure to lomitapide. Monitor and adjust dose. [Moderate] Theoretical

▸ **Encorafenib** is predicted to decrease the exposure to lorlatinib. Avoid. [Severe] Study

▸ Lorlatinib is predicted to decrease the exposure to **encorafenib**. [Moderate] Study

▸ Lumacaftor is predicted to decrease the exposure to **encorafenib**. [Severe] Theoretical

▸ Macrolides (clarithromycin) are predicted to increase the exposure to **encorafenib**. Avoid or monitor. [Severe] Study

▸ Macrolides (erythromycin) are predicted to moderately increase the exposure to **encorafenib**. [Moderate] Study → Also see **TABLE 8** p. 1573

▸ **Encorafenib** is predicted to decrease the exposure to maraviroc. Adjust dose. [Severe] Study

▸ **Encorafenib** is predicted to decrease the exposure to mavacamten. Monitor and adjust dose—consult product literature. [Severe] Theoretical

▸ **Encorafenib** is predicted to decrease the exposure to meglitinides (repaglinide). Monitor blood glucose and adjust dose. [Moderate] Study

▸ **Encorafenib** is predicted to decrease the exposure to midostaurin. Avoid. [Severe] Study

▸ **Encorafenib** is predicted to decrease the exposure to mifepristone. Adjust **mifepristone** dose, p. 954. [Severe] Study

▸ **Encorafenib** is predicted to decrease the exposure to mineralocorticoid receptor antagonists (eplerenone). Avoid. [Moderate] Theoretical

▸ **Encorafenib** is predicted to decrease the exposure to mineralocorticoid receptor antagonists (finerenone). Avoid. [Severe] Study

▸ **Encorafenib** is predicted to decrease the exposure to mirtazapine. Adjust dose. [Moderate] Study

▸ Mitotane is predicted to decrease the exposure to **encorafenib**. [Severe] Theoretical

▸ **Encorafenib** is predicted to decrease the exposure to mobocertinib. Avoid. [Severe] Study → Also see **TABLE 8** p. 1573

▸ Modafinil slightly decreases the exposure to **encorafenib**. [Moderate] Study

▸ **Encorafenib** is predicted to decrease the exposure to monoclonal antibodies (polatuzumab vedotin). [Moderate] Theoretical

▸ **Encorafenib** is predicted to decrease the exposure to the cytotoxic component of monoclonal antibodies (trastuzumab emtansine). [Severe] Theoretical

▸ **Encorafenib** is predicted to decrease the exposure to montelukast. [Mild] Study

▸ **Encorafenib** is predicted to markedly decrease the exposure to naldemedine. Avoid. [Severe] Study

▸ **Encorafenib** is predicted to markedly decrease the exposure to naloxegol. Avoid. [Moderate] Study

▸ **Encorafenib** is predicted to decrease the exposure to neratinib. Avoid. [Severe] Study

▸ Neurokinin-1 receptor antagonists (aprepitant, netupitant) are predicted to moderately increase the exposure to **encorafenib**. [Moderate] Study

▸ **Encorafenib** is predicted to markedly decrease the exposure to neurokinin-1 receptor antagonists (aprepitant). Avoid. [Moderate] Study

▸ **Encorafenib** is predicted to decrease the exposure to neurokinin-1 receptor antagonists (fosaprepitant). Avoid. [Moderate] Theoretical

▸ **Encorafenib** is predicted to decrease the exposure to neurokinin-1 receptor antagonists (netupitant). Avoid. [Severe] Study

▸ **Encorafenib** is predicted to moderately decrease the exposure to nilotinib. Avoid. [Severe] Study → Also see **TABLE 8** p. 1573

▸ Nilotinib is predicted to moderately increase the exposure to **encorafenib**. [Moderate] Study → Also see **TABLE 8** p. 1573

▸ Nirmatrelvir boosted with ritonavir is predicted to increase the concentration of **encorafenib**. Avoid or monitor. [Severe] Theoretical

▸ **Encorafenib** is predicted to decrease the exposure to nirmatrelvir boosted with ritonavir. Avoid. [Severe] Study

▸ **Encorafenib** is predicted to decrease the exposure to nitisinone. Adjust dose. [Moderate] Theoretical

▸ NNRTIs (efavirenz, etravirine, nevirapine) are predicted to decrease the exposure to **encorafenib**. [Moderate] Study → Also see **TABLE 8** p. 1573

▸ **Encorafenib** is predicted to decrease the exposure to NNRTIs (doravirine). Avoid. [Severe] Study

▸ **Encorafenib** is predicted to decrease the exposure to NNRTIs (etravirine). Avoid. [Severe] Theoretical

▸ **Encorafenib** markedly decreases the exposure to NNRTIs (rilpivirine). Avoid. [Severe] Study

▸ **Encorafenib** is predicted to decrease the exposure to olaparib. Avoid. [Moderate] Theoretical

▸ **Encorafenib** is predicted to decrease the exposure to opioids (alfentanil, fentanyl). [Moderate] Study

▸ **Encorafenib** is predicted to decrease the exposure to opioids (buprenorphine). Monitor and adjust dose. [Moderate] Theoretical

▸ **Encorafenib** decreases the exposure to opioids (methadone). Monitor and adjust dose. [Severe] Study → Also see **TABLE 8** p. 1573

▸ **Encorafenib** is predicted to decrease the exposure to opioids (oxycodone). Monitor and adjust dose. [Moderate] Study

▸ **Encorafenib** is predicted to decrease the exposure to osilodrostat. [Moderate] Theoretical → Also see **TABLE 8** p. 1573

▸ **Encorafenib** is predicted to moderately decrease the exposure to osimertinib. Avoid. [Moderate] Study → Also see **TABLE 8** p. 1573

▸ **Encorafenib** is predicted to moderately decrease the exposure to ospemifene. [Moderate] Study

▸ **Encorafenib** is predicted to decrease the exposure to palbociclib. Avoid. [Severe] Study

▸ **Encorafenib** is predicted to decrease the exposure to panobinostat. Avoid. [Moderate] Theoretical → Also see **TABLE 8** p. 1573

▸ **Encorafenib** is predicted to decrease the exposure to pazopanib. Avoid. [Severe] Theoretical → Also see **TABLE 8** p. 1573

▸ **Encorafenib** is predicted to decrease the exposure to pemigatinib. Avoid. [Severe] Study

▸ **Encorafenib** moderately decreases the exposure to phosphodiesterase type-4 inhibitors (apremilast). Avoid. [Severe] Study

▸ **Encorafenib** is predicted to decrease the exposure to phosphodiesterase type-4 inhibitors (roflumilast). Avoid. [Moderate] Study

▸ **Encorafenib** is predicted to decrease the exposure to phosphodiesterase type-5 inhibitors (avanafil, tadalafil). Avoid. [Severe] Study

▸ **Encorafenib** is predicted to decrease the exposure to phosphodiesterase type-5 inhibitors (sildenafil, vardenafil). [Moderate] Theoretical → Also see **TABLE 8** p. 1573

Encorafenib (continued)

▶ **Encorafenib** is predicted to moderately to markedly decrease the exposure to pibrentasvir. Avoid. [Severe] Study
▶ **Encorafenib** is predicted to moderately decrease the exposure to pitolisant. [Moderate] Study
▶ **Encorafenib** is predicted to decrease the exposure to ponatinib. Avoid. [Moderate] Theoretical
▶ **Encorafenib** is predicted to decrease the exposure to pralsetinib. Avoid or adjust dose with potent CYP3A4 inducers—consult product literature. [Moderate] Study
▶ **Encorafenib** is predicted to markedly decrease the exposure to praziquantel. Avoid. [Moderate] Study
▶ **Encorafenib** is predicted to decrease the exposure to quizartinib. Avoid. [Severe] Study → Also see **TABLE 8** p. 1573
▶ **Encorafenib** is predicted to increase the exposure to raltegravir. [Moderate] Theoretical
▶ **Encorafenib** is predicted to decrease the exposure to ranolazine. Avoid. [Severe] Study → Also see **TABLE 8** p. 1573
▶ **Encorafenib** is predicted to decrease the exposure to reboxetine. [Moderate] Anecdotal
▶ **Encorafenib** is predicted to decrease the exposure to regorafenib. Avoid. [Moderate] Study
▶ **Encorafenib** is predicted to markedly decrease the exposure to ribociclib. Avoid. [Severe] Study → Also see **TABLE 8** p. 1573
▶ Rifamycins (rifampicin) are predicted to decrease the exposure to **encorafenib**. [Severe] Theoretical
▶ **Encorafenib** is predicted to decrease the exposure to rimegepant. Avoid. [Moderate] Theoretical
▶ **Encorafenib** is predicted to decrease the exposure to ripretinib. Avoid or adjust dose—consult product literature. [Severe] Study
▶ **Encorafenib** is predicted to decrease the exposure to ruxolitinib. Monitor and adjust dose. [Moderate] Study
▶ **Encorafenib** is predicted to decrease the exposure to selpercatinib. Avoid. [Moderate] Study → Also see **TABLE 8** p. 1573
▶ **Encorafenib** is predicted to decrease the exposure to selumetinib. Avoid. [Severe] Study
▶ **Encorafenib** is predicted to decrease the exposure to siponimod. Manufacturer advises caution depending on genotype—consult product literature. [Severe] Study
▶ **Encorafenib** is predicted to decrease the concentration of sirolimus. Avoid or monitor and adjust dose. [Severe] Study
▶ **Encorafenib** is predicted to decrease the exposure to solifenacin. [Moderate] Theoretical
▶ **Encorafenib** is predicted to decrease the exposure to sorafenib. [Moderate] Theoretical → Also see **TABLE 8** p. 1573
▶ **Encorafenib** is predicted to decrease the exposure to sotorasib. Avoid. [Severe] Study
▶ Sotorasib is predicted to decrease the exposure to **encorafenib**. [Moderate] Study
▶ St John's wort is predicted to decrease the exposure to **encorafenib**. [Severe] Theoretical
▶ **Encorafenib** is predicted to increase the exposure to statins (atorvastatin). [Mild] Theoretical
▶ **Encorafenib** is predicted to increase the exposure to statins (fluvastatin, pravastatin). [Mild] Study
▶ **Encorafenib** is predicted to affect the exposure to statins (simvastatin). [Mild] Theoretical
▶ **Encorafenib** is predicted to increase the exposure to sulfasalazine. [Mild] Study
▶ **Encorafenib** is predicted to increase the exposure to sulfonylureas (glibenclamide). [Mild] Study
▶ **Encorafenib** is predicted to decrease the exposure to sunitinib. Avoid or adjust dose—consult product literature. [Moderate] Study → Also see **TABLE 8** p. 1573
▶ **Encorafenib** decreases the concentration of tacrolimus. Avoid or monitor and adjust dose. [Severe] Study
▶ **Encorafenib** is predicted to decrease the exposure to taxanes (cabazitaxel). Avoid. [Moderate] Study
▶ **Encorafenib** is predicted to decrease the exposure to taxanes (docetaxel). [Severe] Theoretical
▶ **Encorafenib** is predicted to decrease the exposure to taxanes (paclitaxel). Avoid. [Severe] Study
▶ **Encorafenib** is predicted to decrease the concentration of temsirolimus. Avoid. [Severe] Study

▶ **Encorafenib** might decrease the exposure to tepotinib. Avoid. [Severe] Theoretical
▶ **Encorafenib** is predicted to decrease the exposure to tetracyclines (eravacycline). Adjust **eravacycline** dose, p. 657. [Moderate] Study
▶ **Encorafenib** is predicted to decrease the exposure to tezacaftor. Avoid. [Severe] Theoretical
▶ **Encorafenib** is predicted to markedly decrease the exposure to ticagrelor. Avoid. [Severe] Study
▶ **Encorafenib** is predicted to decrease the exposure to tivozanib. [Severe] Study
▶ **Encorafenib** is predicted to decrease the exposure to tofacitinib. Avoid. [Severe] Study
▶ **Encorafenib** is predicted to decrease the exposure to tolvaptan. Use with caution or avoid depending on indication. [Severe] Study
▶ **Encorafenib** is predicted to increase the effects of topotecan. [Mild] Study
▶ **Encorafenib** is predicted to decrease the exposure to toremifene. Adjust dose. [Moderate] Study → Also see **TABLE 8** p. 1573
▶ **Encorafenib** is predicted to decrease the exposure to trabectedin. Avoid. [Severe] Theoretical
▶ **Encorafenib** is predicted to decrease the exposure to tucatinib. Avoid. [Severe] Study
▶ Tucatinib is predicted to increase the exposure to **encorafenib**. Avoid or monitor. [Severe] Study
▶ **Encorafenib** is predicted to decrease the exposure to upadacitinib. [Moderate] Study
▶ **Encorafenib** is predicted to decrease the exposure to vandetanib. Avoid. [Moderate] Study → Also see **TABLE 8** p. 1573
▶ **Encorafenib** is predicted to moderately decrease the exposure to velpatasvir. Avoid. [Severe] Study
▶ **Encorafenib** is predicted to decrease the exposure to vemurafenib. Avoid. [Severe] Study → Also see **TABLE 8** p. 1573
▶ **Encorafenib** is predicted to decrease the exposure to venetoclax. Avoid. [Severe] Study
▶ **Encorafenib** is predicted to decrease the exposure to vinca alkaloids (vinblastine, vincristine, vindesine). [Severe] Theoretical
▶ **Encorafenib** is predicted to decrease the exposure to vinca alkaloids (vinorelbine). Use with caution or avoid. [Severe] Theoretical
▶ **Encorafenib** is predicted to decrease the exposure to vismodegib. Avoid. [Moderate] Theoretical
▶ **Encorafenib** is predicted to decrease the exposure to voclosporin. Avoid. [Severe] Study → Also see **TABLE 8** p. 1573
▶ **Encorafenib** is predicted to decrease the exposure to vortioxetine. Monitor and adjust dose. [Moderate] Study
▶ **Encorafenib** is predicted to decrease the concentration of voxilaprevir. Avoid. [Severe] Study
▶ **Encorafenib** is predicted to decrease the exposure to zanubrutinib. Avoid. [Severe] Study
▶ **Encorafenib** is predicted to decrease the exposure to zopiclone. Adjust dose. [Moderate] Study

Endothelin receptor antagonists

ambrisentan · bosentan · macitentan

▶ **Bosentan** is predicted to decrease the exposure to acalabrutinib. [Severe] Study
▶ Anti-androgens (apalutamide, enzalutamide) affect the exposure to **bosentan**. Avoid. [Severe] Study
▶ Anti-androgens (apalutamide, enzalutamide) are predicted to decrease the exposure to **macitentan**. Avoid. [Severe] Study
▶ **Bosentan** is predicted to decrease the efficacy of anti-androgens (cyproterone) with ethinylestradiol (co-cyprindiol). Use alternative methods during treatment with, and for 28 days after, the enzyme inducing drug is stopped. [Severe] Study
▶ **Bosentan** is predicted to decrease the exposure to anti-androgens (darolutamide). Avoid. [Moderate] Theoretical
▶ Antiarrhythmics (amiodarone, dronedarone) are predicted to increase the exposure to **macitentan**. Manufacturer advises caution depending on other drugs taken—consult product literature. [Moderate] Theoretical
▶ **Bosentan** is predicted to decrease the exposure to antiarrhythmics (dronedarone). [Severe] Theoretical

- ▸ **Antiepileptics (carbamazepine, fosphenytoin, phenobarbital, phenytoin, primidone)** affect the exposure to **bosentan**. Avoid. Severe Study
- ▸ **Antiepileptics (carbamazepine, fosphenytoin, phenobarbital, phenytoin, primidone)** are predicted to decrease the exposure to **macitentan**. Avoid. Severe Study
- ▸ **Antifungals, azoles (fluconazole)** are predicted to increase the exposure to **bosentan**. Avoid. Severe Study
- ▸ **Antifungals, azoles (fluconazole, isavuconazole, miconazole)** are predicted to increase the exposure to **macitentan**. Manufacturer advises caution depending on other drugs taken—consult product literature. Moderate Theoretical
- ▸ **Antifungals, azoles (itraconazole)** are predicted to increase the exposure to **bosentan**. Moderate Theoretical
- ▸ **Antifungals, azoles (itraconazole, ketoconazole, posaconazole, voriconazole)** are predicted to increase the exposure to **macitentan**. Moderate Study
- ▸ **Antifungals, azoles (ketoconazole)** moderately increase the exposure to **bosentan**. Moderate Study
- ▸ **Antifungals, azoles (voriconazole)** are predicted to increase the exposure to **bosentan**. Avoid. Severe Theoretical
- ▸ **Bosentan** is predicted to decrease the exposure to **antifungals, azoles (isavuconazole)**. Avoid. Severe Theoretical
- ▸ **Bosentan** is predicted to decrease the exposure to **antipsychotics, second generation (cariprazine)**. Avoid. Severe Theoretical
- ▸ **Bosentan** is predicted to decrease the exposure to **antipsychotics, second generation (lurasidone)**. Monitor and adjust dose. Moderate Theoretical
- ▸ **Bosentan** is predicted to decrease the exposure to **antipsychotics, second generation (quetiapine)**. Moderate Study
- ▸ **Bosentan** is predicted to decrease the exposure to **avacopan**. Severe Theoretical
- ▸ **Bosentan** is predicted to decrease the exposure to **avapritinib**. Avoid. Severe Study
- ▸ **Bosentan** is predicted to decrease the exposure to **axitinib**. Moderate Study
- ▸ **Bosentan** is predicted to decrease the exposure to **bedaquiline**. Avoid. Severe Study
- ▸ **Belumosudil** is predicted to increase the exposure to **bosentan**. Avoid or adjust dose. Moderate Study
- ▸ **Bosentan** is predicted to decrease the concentration of **benzodiazepines (midazolam)**. Monitor and adjust dose. Moderate Theoretical
- ▸ **Berotralstat** is predicted to increase the exposure to **macitentan**. Manufacturer advises caution depending on other drugs taken—consult product literature. Moderate Theoretical
- ▸ **Bosentan** is predicted to decrease the exposure to **bosutinib**. Avoid. Severe Study
- ▸ **Bosentan** is predicted to decrease the exposure to **brigatinib**. Avoid or adjust dose—consult product literature. Moderate Study
- ▸ **Bulevirtide** is predicted to increase the exposure to **bosentan**. Avoid or monitor. Moderate Theoretical
- ▸ **Bosentan** is predicted to decrease the exposure to **cabozantinib**. Moderate Study
- ▸ **Calcium channel blockers (diltiazem, verapamil)** are predicted to increase the exposure to **macitentan**. Manufacturer advises caution depending on other drugs taken—consult product literature. Moderate Theoretical
- ▸ **Bosentan** is predicted to decrease the exposure to **calcium channel blockers (amlodipine, felodipine, lacidipine, lercanidipine, nicardipine, nifedipine, nimodipine)**. Monitor and adjust dose. Moderate Theoretical
- ▸ **Bosentan** is predicted to decrease the exposure to **calcium channel blockers (diltiazem, verapamil)**. Moderate Theoretical
- ▸ **Bosentan** is predicted to decrease the exposure to **capivasertib**. Avoid. Moderate Study
- ▸ **Cephalosporins (ceftobiprole)** are predicted to increase the exposure to **bosentan**. Moderate Theoretical
- ▸ **Bosentan** is predicted to decrease the exposure to **ceritinib**. Severe Study
- ▸ **Ceritinib** is predicted to increase the exposure to **macitentan**. Moderate Study

- ▸ **Ciclosporin** moderately increases the exposure to **ambrisentan**. Adjust **ambrisentan** dose and monitor, p. 210. Moderate Study
- ▸ **Bosentan** moderately decreases the exposure to **ciclosporin** and **ciclosporin** moderately increases the exposure to **bosentan**. Avoid. Severe Study
- ▸ **Bosentan** is predicted to decrease the exposure to **cobicistat**. Avoid. Severe Theoretical
- ▸ **Cobicistat** is predicted to increase the exposure to **macitentan**. Moderate Study
- ▸ **Bosentan** is predicted to decrease the exposure to **cobimetinib**. Avoid. Severe Theoretical
- ▸ **Bosentan** is predicted to decrease the efficacy of **combined hormonal contraceptives**. For FSRH guidance, see Contraceptives, interactions p. 917. Severe Study
- ▸ **Bosentan** decreases the anticoagulant effect of **coumarins**. Moderate Study
- ▸ **Bosentan** is predicted to decrease the exposure to **crizotinib**. Avoid. Severe Study
- ▸ **Crizotinib** is predicted to increase the exposure to **macitentan**. Manufacturer advises caution depending on other drugs taken—consult product literature. Moderate Theoretical
- ▸ **Bosentan** is predicted to decrease the exposure to **dabrafenib**. Moderate Study
- ▸ **Bosentan** is predicted to decrease the exposure to **daridorexant**. Severe Study
- ▸ **Bosentan** is predicted to decrease the exposure to **dasatinib**. Severe Study
- ▸ **Bosentan** is predicted to decrease the efficacy of **desogestrel**. For FSRH guidance, see Contraceptives, interactions p. 917. Severe Theoretical
- ▸ **Bosentan** is predicted to decrease the exposure to **dolutegravir**. Severe Study
- ▸ **Bosentan** is predicted to decrease the efficacy of **drospirenone**. For FSRH guidance, see Contraceptives, interactions p. 917. Severe Theoretical
- ▸ **Bosentan** is predicted to decrease the exposure to **elacestrant**. Avoid or adjust dose depending on duration—consult product literature. Severe Theoretical
- ▸ **Bosentan** is predicted to moderately decrease the exposure to **elbasvir**. Avoid. Severe Study
- ▸ **Elexacaftor** is predicted to increase the exposure to **bosentan**. Moderate Theoretical
- ▸ **Bosentan** is predicted to decrease the exposure to **eliglustat**. Moderate Theoretical
- ▸ **Bosentan** is predicted to decrease the concentration of **elvitegravir**. Avoid. Severe Theoretical
- ▸ **Encorafenib** affects the exposure to **bosentan**. Avoid. Severe Study
- ▸ **Bosentan** is predicted to decrease the exposure to **encorafenib**. Moderate Study
- ▸ **Encorafenib** is predicted to decrease the exposure to **macitentan**. Avoid. Severe Study
- ▸ **Bosentan** is predicted to decrease the exposure to **entrectinib**. Avoid. Moderate Theoretical
- ▸ **Bosentan** is predicted to decrease the exposure to **erdafitinib**. Adjust dose. Moderate Theoretical
- ▸ **Bosentan** is predicted to decrease the exposure to **erlotinib**. Severe Study
- ▸ **Bosentan** is predicted to decrease the efficacy of **estradiol**. Moderate Theoretical
- ▸ **Bosentan** is predicted to decrease the efficacy of **etonogestrel**. For FSRH guidance, see Contraceptives, interactions p. 917. Severe Theoretical
- ▸ **Bosentan** is predicted to decrease the concentration of **everolimus**. Avoid or adjust dose. Severe Study
- ▸ **Bosentan** is predicted to decrease the exposure to **fedratinib**. Avoid. Moderate Study
- ▸ **Fedratinib** is predicted to increase the exposure to **macitentan**. Manufacturer advises caution depending on other drugs taken—consult product literature. Moderate Theoretical
- ▸ **Bosentan** is predicted to decrease the exposure to **fruquintinib**. Avoid. Moderate Study
- ▸ **Bosentan** is predicted to decrease the exposure to **gefitinib**. Avoid. Severe Study

Endothelin receptor antagonists (continued)

▶ **Bosentan** is predicted to decrease the exposure to glasdegib. Avoid or adjust dose—consult product literature. [Moderate] Theoretical

▶ **Bosentan** is predicted to decrease the exposure to glecaprevir. Avoid. [Severe] Study

▶ **Bosentan** is predicted to markedly decrease the exposure to grazoprevir. Avoid. [Severe] Study

▶ **Bosentan** is predicted to decrease the concentration of guanfacine. Adjust dose. [Moderate] Theoretical

▶ HIV-protease inhibitors are predicted to increase the exposure to bosentan. [Severe] Study

▶ HIV-protease inhibitors are predicted to increase the exposure to macitentan. [Moderate] Study

▶ **Bosentan** is predicted to decrease the effects of hormone replacement therapy. [Moderate] Anecdotal

▶ **Bosentan** is predicted to decrease the exposure to ibrutinib. Avoid or monitor. [Severe] Study

▶ **Bosentan** is predicted to decrease the exposure to idelalisib. Avoid. [Moderate] Theoretical

▶ Idelalisib is predicted to increase the exposure to macitentan. [Moderate] Study

▶ **Bosentan** is predicted to decrease the exposure to imatinib. [Moderate] Study

▶ Imatinib is predicted to increase the exposure to macitentan. Manufacturer advises caution depending on other drugs taken—consult product literature. [Moderate] Theoretical

▶ **Bosentan** is predicted to decrease the exposure to ivacaftor. [Moderate] Study

▶ Ivosidenib affects the exposure to bosentan. Avoid. [Severe] Study

▶ Ivosidenib is predicted to decrease the exposure to macitentan. Avoid. [Severe] Study

▶ **Bosentan** is predicted to decrease the exposure to ixazomib. [Moderate] Theoretical

▶ **Bosentan** is predicted to decrease the exposure to lapatinib. Avoid. [Severe] Study

▶ **Bosentan** is predicted to decrease the exposure to larotrectinib. Avoid. [Moderate] Study

▶ Leflunomide is predicted to increase the exposure to bosentan. [Moderate] Study

▶ **Bosentan** is predicted to decrease the exposure to leniolisib. Avoid. [Severe] Theoretical

▶ Leniolisib is predicted to increase the exposure to bosentan. Avoid. [Moderate] Theoretical

▶ Letermovir is predicted to increase the concentration of bosentan. [Moderate] Theoretical

▶ Letermovir is predicted to increase the exposure to macitentan. Manufacturer advises caution depending on other drugs taken—consult product literature. [Moderate] Theoretical

▶ **Bosentan** is predicted to decrease the efficacy of some contraceptive methods containing levonorgestrel. For FSRH guidance, see Contraceptives, interactions p. 917. [Severe] Theoretical

▶ Lumacaftor affects the exposure to bosentan. Avoid. [Severe] Study

▶ Lumacaftor is predicted to decrease the exposure to macitentan. Avoid. [Severe] Study

▶ Macrolides (clarithromycin) are predicted to increase the exposure to bosentan. [Moderate] Theoretical

▶ Macrolides (clarithromycin) are predicted to increase the exposure to macitentan. [Moderate] Study

▶ Macrolides (erythromycin) are predicted to increase the exposure to macitentan. Manufacturer advises caution depending on other drugs taken—consult product literature. [Moderate] Theoretical

▶ **Bosentan** is predicted to decrease the exposure to maraviroc. Avoid. [Moderate] Theoretical

▶ **Bosentan** is predicted to decrease the exposure to maribavir. Avoid or adjust maribavir dose, p. 735. [Severe] Study

▶ **Bosentan** is predicted to decrease the exposure to mavacamten. Monitor and adjust dose—consult product literature. [Severe] Theoretical

▶ **Bosentan** is predicted to decrease the exposure to midostaurin and midostaurin is predicted to increase the exposure to bosentan. [Severe] Study

▶ **Bosentan** is predicted to decrease the exposure to mifepristone. Adjust mifepristone dose, p. 954. [Severe] Study

▶ **Bosentan** is predicted to decrease the exposure to mineralocorticoid receptor antagonists (finerenone). Avoid. [Severe] Study

▶ Mitotane affects the exposure to bosentan. Avoid. [Severe] Study

▶ Mitotane is predicted to decrease the exposure to macitentan. Avoid. [Severe] Study

▶ **Bosentan** is predicted to decrease the exposure to mobocertinib. Avoid. [Severe] Study

▶ **Bosentan** is predicted to decrease the exposure to naloxegol. [Moderate] Theoretical

▶ **Bosentan** is predicted to decrease the exposure to neratinib. Avoid. [Severe] Theoretical

▶ Neurokinin-1 receptor antagonists (aprepitant, netupitant) are predicted to increase the exposure to macitentan. Manufacturer advises caution depending on other drugs taken—consult product literature. [Moderate] Theoretical

▶ **Bosentan** is predicted to decrease the exposure to neurokinin-1 receptor antagonists (aprepitant). [Moderate] Study

▶ **Bosentan** is predicted to decrease the exposure to neurokinin-1 receptor antagonists (fosaprepitant, netupitant). [Moderate] Theoretical

▶ **Bosentan** is predicted to decrease the exposure to nilotinib. Avoid. [Severe] Theoretical

▶ Nilotinib is predicted to increase the exposure to macitentan. Manufacturer advises caution depending on other drugs taken—consult product literature. [Moderate] Theoretical

▶ Nirmatrelvir boosted with ritonavir is predicted to increase the concentration of bosentan. [Severe] Theoretical

▶ **Bosentan** is predicted to decrease the exposure to NNRTIs (doravirine). Avoid or adjust doravirine p. 741 or lamivudine with tenofovir disoproxil and doravirine p. 751 dose. [Severe] Theoretical

▶ **Bosentan** is predicted to decrease the exposure to NNRTIs (nevirapine). [Severe] Theoretical

▶ **Bosentan** is predicted to decrease the exposure to NNRTIs (rilpivirine). Avoid. [Severe] Theoretical

▶ **Bosentan** is predicted to decrease the efficacy of some contraceptive methods containing norethisterone. For FSRH guidance, see Contraceptives, interactions p. 917. [Severe] Anecdotal

▶ **Bosentan** is predicted to decrease the exposure to olaparib. Avoid. [Moderate] Theoretical

▶ **Bosentan** decreases the exposure to opioids (methadone). Monitor and adjust dose. [Severe] Study

▶ **Bosentan** is predicted to decrease the exposure to osimertinib. Use with caution or avoid. [Severe] Study

▶ **Bosentan** is predicted to decrease the exposure to ospemifene. [Moderate] Study

▶ **Bosentan** is predicted to decrease the exposure to pazopanib. [Severe] Study

▶ **Bosentan** is predicted to decrease the exposure to pemigatinib. Avoid or monitor. [Severe] Study

▶ **Bosentan** decreases the exposure to phosphodiesterase type-5 inhibitors. [Moderate] Study

▶ **Bosentan** is predicted to decrease the exposure to pibrentasvir. Avoid. [Severe] Study

▶ **Bosentan** is predicted to decrease the exposure to ponatinib. [Severe] Study

▶ **Bosentan** is predicted to decrease the exposure to pralsetinib. [Moderate] Theoretical

▶ **Bosentan** is predicted to decrease the exposure to quizartinib. Avoid. [Severe] Study

▶ **Bosentan** is predicted to decrease the exposure to regorafenib. [Severe] Study

▶ **Bosentan** is predicted to decrease the exposure to ribociclib. [Moderate] Study

▶ Rifamycins (rifampicin) transiently increase the exposure to ambrisentan. [Moderate] Study

▶ Rifamycins (rifampicin) affect the exposure to bosentan. Avoid. [Severe] Study

▸ Rifamycins **(rifampicin)** are predicted to decrease the exposure to **macitentan**. Avoid. [Severe] Study

▸ **Bosentan** is predicted to decrease the exposure to **rimegepant**. Avoid. [Moderate] Theoretical

▸ **Bosentan** is predicted to decrease the exposure to **ripretinib**. Avoid or adjust dose—consult product literature. [Moderate] Theoretical

▸ **Roxadustat** is predicted to increase the exposure to **bosentan**. Monitor adverse effects and adjust dose. [Moderate] Study

▸ **Bosentan** is predicted to decrease the exposure to **ruxolitinib**. Monitor and adjust dose. [Moderate] Study

▸ **Bosentan** is predicted to decrease the exposure to **selpercatinib**. [Moderate] Study

▸ **Bosentan** is predicted to decrease the exposure to **selumetinib**. Avoid. [Severe] Study

▸ **Bosentan** is predicted to decrease the exposure to **siponimod**. Manufacturer advises caution depending on genotype—consult product literature. [Moderate] Theoretical

▸ **Bosentan** is predicted to decrease the concentration of **sirolimus** and **sirolimus** potentially increases the concentration of **bosentan**. Avoid. [Severe] Theoretical

▸ **Bosentan** is predicted to decrease the exposure to **sorafenib**. [Moderate] Study

▸ **St John's wort** is predicted to decrease the exposure to **bosentan**. Avoid. [Moderate] Theoretical

▸ **St John's wort** is predicted to decrease the exposure to **macitentan**. Avoid. [Severe] Theoretical

▸ **Bosentan** is predicted to decrease the exposure to **statins (atorvastatin, simvastatin)**. [Moderate] Study

▸ **Bosentan** increases the risk of hepatotoxicity when given with **sulfonylureas (glibenclamide)**. Avoid. [Severe] Study

▸ **Bosentan** is predicted to decrease the exposure to **sunitinib**. [Moderate] Study

▸ **Bosentan** is predicted to decrease the concentration of **tacrolimus** and **tacrolimus** potentially increases the concentration of **bosentan**. Avoid. [Severe] Theoretical

▸ **Bosentan** is predicted to decrease the exposure to **taxanes (cabazitaxel)**. [Moderate] Theoretical

▸ **Bosentan** is predicted to decrease the exposure to **taxanes (docetaxel)**. [Severe] Theoretical

▸ **Bosentan** is predicted to decrease the exposure to **taxanes (paclitaxel)**. Avoid. [Severe] Study

▸ **Bosentan** is predicted to decrease the concentration of **temsirolimus**. Avoid. [Moderate] Theoretical

▸ **Teriflunomide** is predicted to increase the exposure to **bosentan**. [Moderate] Study

▸ **Bosentan** is predicted to decrease the exposure to **ticagrelor**. [Moderate] Theoretical

▸ **Bosentan** is predicted to decrease the exposure to **tofacitinib**. [Severe] Study

▸ **Tucatinib** is predicted to increase the exposure to **macitentan**. [Moderate] Study

▸ **Bosentan** decreases the efficacy of **ulipristal**. Avoid and for 4 weeks after stopping the enzyme inducing drug. For FSRH guidance, see Contraceptives, interactions p. 917. [Severe] Anecdotal

▸ **Bosentan** is predicted to decrease the exposure to **vandetanib**. [Moderate] Study

▸ **Bosentan** is predicted to decrease the exposure to **velpatasvir**. Avoid. [Moderate] Theoretical

▸ **Vemurafenib** is predicted to increase the exposure to **ambrisentan**. Use with caution or avoid. [Moderate] Theoretical

▸ **Bosentan** is predicted to decrease the exposure to **vemurafenib**. [Severe] Study

▸ **Bosentan** is predicted to decrease the exposure to **venetoclax**. Avoid. [Severe] Study

▸ **Venetoclax** is predicted to increase the exposure to **bosentan**. [Moderate] Theoretical

▸ **Bosentan** is predicted to decrease the exposure to **voclosporin** and **voclosporin** is predicted to increase the concentration of **bosentan**. Avoid. [Severe] Theoretical

▸ **Bosentan** is predicted to decrease the concentration of **voxilaprevir**. Avoid. [Severe] Theoretical

▸ **Bosentan** is predicted to decrease the exposure to **zanubrutinib**. Avoid or adjust dose with moderate CYP3A4 inducers—consult product literature. [Severe] Theoretical

Enfortumab vedotin

▸ **Anti-androgens (apalutamide, enzalutamide)** are predicted to decrease the exposure to the cytotoxic component of **enfortumab vedotin**. [Moderate] Theoretical

▸ **Antiepileptics (carbamazepine, fosphenytoin, phenobarbital, phenytoin, primidone)** are predicted to decrease the exposure to the cytotoxic component of **enfortumab vedotin**. [Moderate] Theoretical

▸ **Antifungals, azoles (itraconazole, ketoconazole, posaconazole, voriconazole)** are predicted to increase the exposure to the cytotoxic component of **enfortumab vedotin**. [Severe] Theoretical

▸ **Ceritinib** is predicted to increase the exposure to the cytotoxic component of **enfortumab vedotin**. [Severe] Theoretical

▸ **Cobicistat** is predicted to increase the exposure to the cytotoxic component of **enfortumab vedotin**. [Severe] Theoretical

▸ **Encorafenib** is predicted to decrease the exposure to the cytotoxic component of **enfortumab vedotin**. [Moderate] Theoretical

▸ **HIV-protease inhibitors** are predicted to increase the exposure to the cytotoxic component of **enfortumab vedotin**. [Severe] Theoretical

▸ **Idelalisib** is predicted to increase the exposure to the cytotoxic component of **enfortumab vedotin**. [Severe] Theoretical

▸ **Ivosidenib** is predicted to decrease the exposure to the cytotoxic component of **enfortumab vedotin**. [Moderate] Theoretical

▸ **Lumacaftor** is predicted to decrease the exposure to the cytotoxic component of **enfortumab vedotin**. [Moderate] Theoretical

▸ **Macrolides (clarithromycin)** are predicted to increase the exposure to the cytotoxic component of **enfortumab vedotin**. [Severe] Theoretical

▸ **Mitotane** is predicted to decrease the exposure to the cytotoxic component of **enfortumab vedotin**. [Moderate] Theoretical

▸ **Rifamycins (rifampicin)** are predicted to decrease the exposure to the cytotoxic component of **enfortumab vedotin**. [Moderate] Theoretical

▸ **St John's wort** is predicted to decrease the exposure to the cytotoxic component of **enfortumab vedotin**. [Moderate] Theoretical

▸ **Tucatinib** is predicted to increase the exposure to the cytotoxic component of **enfortumab vedotin**. [Severe] Theoretical

Enfuvirtide → see TABLE 11 p. 1574 (peripheral neuropathy)

Enoxaparin → see low molecular-weight heparins

Entacapone

▸ **Entacapone** might increase the exposure to the active metabolite of **foslevodopa**. Adjust dose. [Moderate] Theoretical

▸ Oral **entacapone** is predicted to decrease the absorption of oral **iron**. Separate administration by at least 2 hours. [Moderate] Theoretical

▸ **Entacapone** is predicted to increase the risk of cardiovascular adverse effects when given with **isoprenaline**. [Moderate] Study

▸ **Entacapone** increases the exposure to **levodopa**. Monitor adverse effects and adjust dose. [Moderate] Study

▸ **Entacapone** is predicted to increase the risk of elevated blood pressure when given with **MAOIs, irreversible**. Avoid. [Severe] Theoretical

▸ **Entacapone** is predicted to increase the exposure to **methyldopa**. [Moderate] Theoretical

▸ **Entacapone** is predicted to increase the risk of cardiovascular adverse effects when given with **sympathomimetics, inotropic**. [Moderate] Theoretical

▸ **Entacapone** is predicted to increase the risk of cardiovascular adverse effects when given with **sympathomimetics, vasoconstrictor (adrenaline/epinephrine, noradrenaline/norepinephrine)**. [Moderate] Study

Enteral feeds

▸ **Aluminium hydroxide** increases the risk of blocked enteral or nasogastric tubes when given with **enteral feeds**. [Moderate] Study

▸ **Enteral feeds** decrease the absorption of **antiepileptics (phenytoin)**. [Severe] Study

Enteral feeds (continued)
- **Enteral feeds** (vitamin-K containing) potentially decrease the anticoagulant effect of coumarins. [Severe] Anecdotal
- **Enteral feeds** (vitamin-K containing) potentially decrease the effects of phenindione. [Severe] Theoretical
- **Enteral feeds** decrease the exposure to quinolones (ciprofloxacin). [Moderate] Study
- Sucralfate increases the risk of blocked enteral or nasogastric tubes when given with **enteral feeds**. Separate administration by 1 hour. [Moderate] Study
- **Enteral feeds** decrease the exposure to theophylline. [Moderate] Study

Entrectinib → see TABLE 8 p. 1573 (QT-interval prolongation)

FOOD AND LIFESTYLE Bitter (Seville) orange is predicted to increase the exposure to entrectinib; manufacturer advises avoid.

- Anti-androgens (apalutamide, enzalutamide) are predicted to decrease the exposure to **entrectinib**. Avoid. [Severe] Study → Also see TABLE 8 p. 1573
- Antiarrhythmics (dronedarone) are predicted to increase the exposure to **entrectinib**. Avoid or adjust dose with moderate CYP3A4 inhibitors—consult product literature. [Severe] Theoretical → Also see TABLE 8 p. 1573
- Antiepileptics (carbamazepine, fosphenytoin, phenobarbital, phenytoin, primidone) are predicted to decrease the exposure to **entrectinib**. Avoid. [Severe] Study
- Antifungals, azoles (fluconazole, isavuconazole) are predicted to increase the exposure to **entrectinib**. Avoid or adjust dose with moderate CYP3A4 inhibitors—consult product literature. [Severe] Theoretical → Also see TABLE 8 p. 1573
- Antifungals, azoles (itraconazole, ketoconazole, posaconazole, voriconazole) are predicted to increase the exposure to **entrectinib**. Avoid or adjust dose with potent CYP3A4 inhibitors—consult product literature. [Severe] Study → Also see TABLE 8 p. 1573
- Berotralstat is predicted to increase the exposure to **entrectinib**. Avoid or adjust dose with moderate CYP3A4 inhibitors—consult product literature. [Severe] Theoretical
- Calcium channel blockers (diltiazem, verapamil) are predicted to increase the exposure to **entrectinib**. Avoid or adjust dose with moderate CYP3A4 inhibitors—consult product literature. [Severe] Theoretical
- Cenobamate is predicted to decrease the exposure to **entrectinib**. Avoid. [Moderate] Theoretical
- Ceritinib is predicted to increase the exposure to **entrectinib**. Avoid or adjust dose with potent CYP3A4 inhibitors—consult product literature. [Severe] Study → Also see TABLE 8 p. 1573
- Cobicistat is predicted to increase the exposure to **entrectinib**. Avoid or adjust dose with potent CYP3A4 inhibitors—consult product literature. [Severe] Study
- Crizotinib is predicted to increase the exposure to **entrectinib**. Avoid or adjust dose with moderate CYP3A4 inhibitors—consult product literature. [Severe] Theoretical → Also see TABLE 8 p. 1573
- Dabrafenib is predicted to decrease the exposure to **entrectinib**. Avoid. [Moderate] Theoretical
- Encorafenib is predicted to decrease the exposure to **entrectinib**. Avoid. [Severe] Study → Also see TABLE 8 p. 1573
- Endothelin receptor antagonists (bosentan) are predicted to decrease the exposure to **entrectinib**. Avoid. [Moderate] Theoretical
- Fedratinib is predicted to increase the exposure to **entrectinib**. Avoid or adjust dose with moderate CYP3A4 inhibitors—consult product literature. [Severe] Theoretical
- Grapefruit is predicted to increase the exposure to **entrectinib**. Avoid. [Severe] Theoretical
- HIV-protease inhibitors are predicted to increase the exposure to **entrectinib**. Avoid or adjust dose with potent CYP3A4 inhibitors—consult product literature. [Severe] Study
- Idelalisib is predicted to increase the exposure to **entrectinib**. Avoid or adjust dose with potent CYP3A4 inhibitors—consult product literature. [Severe] Study
- Imatinib is predicted to increase the exposure to **entrectinib**. Avoid or adjust dose with moderate CYP3A4 inhibitors—consult product literature. [Severe] Theoretical

- Ivosidenib is predicted to decrease the exposure to **entrectinib**. Avoid. [Severe] Study → Also see TABLE 8 p. 1573
- Letermovir is predicted to increase the exposure to **entrectinib**. Avoid or adjust dose with moderate CYP3A4 inhibitors—consult product literature. [Severe] Theoretical
- Lorlatinib is predicted to decrease the exposure to **entrectinib**. Avoid. [Moderate] Theoretical
- Lumacaftor is predicted to decrease the exposure to **entrectinib**. Avoid. [Severe] Study
- Macrolides (clarithromycin) are predicted to increase the exposure to **entrectinib**. Avoid or adjust dose with potent CYP3A4 inhibitors—consult product literature. [Severe] Study
- Macrolides (erythromycin) are predicted to increase the exposure to **entrectinib**. Avoid or adjust dose with moderate CYP3A4 inhibitors—consult product literature. [Severe] Theoretical → Also see TABLE 8 p. 1573
- **Entrectinib** is predicted to increase the exposure to mavacamten. Monitor and adjust dose—consult product literature. [Moderate] Theoretical
- Mitotane is predicted to decrease the exposure to **entrectinib**. Avoid. [Severe] Study
- Neurokinin-1 receptor antagonists (aprepitant, netupitant) are predicted to increase the exposure to **entrectinib**. Avoid or adjust dose with moderate CYP3A4 inhibitors—consult product literature. [Severe] Theoretical
- Nilotinib is predicted to increase the exposure to **entrectinib**. Avoid or adjust dose with moderate CYP3A4 inhibitors—consult product literature. [Severe] Theoretical → Also see TABLE 8 p. 1573
- NNRTIs (efavirenz, etravirine, nevirapine) are predicted to decrease the exposure to **entrectinib**. Avoid. [Moderate] Theoretical → Also see TABLE 8 p. 1573
- Rifamycins (rifampicin) are predicted to decrease the exposure to **entrectinib**. Avoid. [Severe] Study
- Sotorasib is predicted to decrease the exposure to **entrectinib**. Avoid. [Moderate] Theoretical
- St John's wort is predicted to decrease the exposure to **entrectinib**. Avoid. [Moderate] Theoretical
- Tucatinib is predicted to increase the exposure to **entrectinib**. Avoid or adjust dose with potent CYP3A4 inhibitors—consult product literature. [Severe] Study

Enzalutamide → see anti-androgens

Ephedrine → see sympathomimetics, vasoconstrictor

Epirubicin → see anthracyclines

Eplerenone → see mineralocorticoid receptor antagonists

Epoprostenol → see TABLE 7 p. 1572 (hypotension), TABLE 4 p. 1571 (antiplatelet effects)

Eprosartan → see angiotensin-II receptor antagonists

Eptifibatide → see TABLE 3 p. 1571 (anticoagulant effects)

Eravacycline → see tetracyclines

Erdafitinib

FOOD AND LIFESTYLE Avoid bitter (Seville) oranges as they might increase the exposure to erdafitinib.

- Anti-androgens (apalutamide, enzalutamide) are predicted to decrease the exposure to **erdafitinib**. Avoid. [Severe] Study
- Antiarrhythmics (amiodarone) are predicted to increase the exposure to **erdafitinib**. Adjust dose. [Severe] Study
- Antiepileptics (carbamazepine, fosphenytoin, phenobarbital, phenytoin, primidone) are predicted to decrease the exposure to **erdafitinib**. Avoid. [Severe] Study
- Antifungals, azoles (fluconazole, itraconazole, ketoconazole, miconazole, posaconazole, voriconazole) are predicted to increase the exposure to **erdafitinib**. Adjust dose. [Severe] Study
- Cenobamate is predicted to decrease the exposure to **erdafitinib**. Adjust dose. [Moderate] Theoretical
- Ceritinib is predicted to increase the exposure to **erdafitinib**. Adjust dose. [Severe] Study
- Cobicistat is predicted to increase the exposure to **erdafitinib**. Adjust dose. [Severe] Study
- **Erdafitinib** is predicted to increase the exposure to colchicine. Separate administration by at least 6 hours. [Moderate] Theoretical
- **Erdafitinib** might decrease the efficacy of combined hormonal contraceptives. Use alternative methods during treatment

with, and for at least 28 days after stopping, **erdafitinib**. Severe Theoretical

▶ **Dabrafenib** is predicted to decrease the exposure to **erdafitinib**. Adjust dose. Moderate Theoretical

▶ **Erdafitinib** is predicted to increase the exposure to digoxin. Separate administration by at least 6 hours. Moderate Theoretical

▶ **Encorafenib** is predicted to decrease the exposure to erdafitinib. Avoid. Severe Study

▶ Endothelin receptor antagonists (bosentan) are predicted to decrease the exposure to **erdafitinib**. Adjust dose. Moderate Theoretical

▶ **Erdafitinib** is predicted to increase the exposure to everolimus. Separate administration by at least 6 hours. Moderate Theoretical

▶ **Erdafitinib** is predicted to increase the exposure to factor XA inhibitors (apixaban). Separate administration by at least 6 hours. Moderate Theoretical

▶ Grapefruit is predicted to increase the exposure to **erdafitinib**. Avoid. Moderate Theoretical

▶ HIV-protease inhibitors are predicted to increase the exposure to **erdafitinib**. Adjust dose. Severe Study

▶ Idelalisib is predicted to increase the exposure to **erdafitinib**. Adjust dose. Severe Study

▶ Ivosidenib is predicted to decrease the exposure to **erdafitinib**. Avoid. Severe Study

▶ Lorlatinib is predicted to decrease the exposure to **erdafitinib**. Adjust dose. Moderate Theoretical

▶ Lumacaftor is predicted to decrease the exposure to erdafitinib. Avoid. Severe Study

▶ Macrolides (clarithromycin) are predicted to increase the exposure to **erdafitinib**. Adjust dose. Severe Study

▶ Mitotane is predicted to decrease the exposure to **erdafitinib**. Avoid. Severe Study

▶ Modafinil is predicted to decrease the exposure to **erdafitinib**. Adjust dose. Moderate Theoretical

▶ NNRTIs (efavirenz, etravirine, nevirapine) are predicted to decrease the exposure to **erdafitinib**. Adjust dose. Moderate Theoretical

▶ Rifamycins (rifabutin) are predicted to decrease the exposure to **erdafitinib**. Adjust dose. Moderate Theoretical

▶ Rifamycins (rifampicin) are predicted to decrease the exposure to **erdafitinib**. Avoid. Severe Study

▶ **Erdafitinib** is predicted to increase the exposure to sirolimus. Separate administration by at least 6 hours. Moderate Theoretical

▶ Sotorasib is predicted to decrease the exposure to **erdafitinib**. Adjust dose. Moderate Theoretical

▶ St John's wort is predicted to decrease the exposure to **erdafitinib**. Avoid. Moderate Study

▶ **Erdafitinib** is predicted to increase the exposure to talazoparib. Separate administration by at least 6 hours. Moderate Theoretical

▶ **Erdafitinib** is predicted to increase the exposure to taxanes (paclitaxel). Separate administration by at least 6 hours. Moderate Theoretical

▶ Telotristat ethyl is predicted to decrease the exposure to **erdafitinib**. Adjust dose. Moderate Theoretical

▶ **Erdafitinib** is predicted to increase the exposure to thrombin inhibitors (dabigatran). Separate administration by at least 6 hours. Moderate Theoretical

▶ Tucatinib is predicted to increase the exposure to **erdafitinib**. Adjust dose. Severe Study

Erenumab

GENERAL INFORMATION Caution on concurrent use of **erenumab** with drugs that cause constipation.

Ergocalciferol → see vitamin D substances

Ergometrine

▶ Antiarrhythmics (dronedarone) are predicted to increase the risk of ergotism when given with **ergometrine**. Severe Theoretical

▶ Antifungals, azoles (fluconazole, isavuconazole) are predicted to increase the risk of ergotism when given with **ergometrine**. Severe Theoretical

▶ Antifungals, azoles (itraconazole, ketoconazole, posaconazole, voriconazole) are predicted to increase the risk of ergotism when given with **ergometrine**. Avoid. Severe Theoretical

▶ Antifungals, azoles (miconazole) are predicted to increase the exposure to **ergometrine**. Avoid. Moderate Theoretical

▶ Berotralstat is predicted to increase the risk of ergotism when given with **ergometrine**. Severe Theoretical

▶ Beta blockers, non-selective are predicted to increase the risk of peripheral vasoconstriction when given with **ergometrine**. Severe Study

▶ Beta blockers, selective are predicted to increase the risk of peripheral vasoconstriction when given with **ergometrine**. Severe Study

▶ Calcium channel blockers (diltiazem, verapamil) are predicted to increase the risk of ergotism when given with **ergometrine**. Severe Theoretical

▶ Ceritinib is predicted to increase the risk of ergotism when given with **ergometrine**. Avoid. Severe Theoretical

▶ Cobicistat is predicted to increase the risk of ergotism when given with **ergometrine**. Avoid. Severe Theoretical

▶ Crizotinib is predicted to increase the risk of ergotism when given with **ergometrine**. Severe Theoretical

▶ **Ergometrine** is predicted to increase the risk of ergotism when given with dopamine receptor agonists (cabergoline). Avoid. Moderate Theoretical

▶ Esketamine is predicted to increase the risk of elevated blood pressure when given with **ergometrine**. Avoid. Severe Theoretical

▶ Fedratinib is predicted to increase the risk of ergotism when given with **ergometrine**. Severe Theoretical

▶ Grapefruit juice is predicted to increase the exposure to **ergometrine**. Severe Theoretical

▶ HIV-protease inhibitors are predicted to increase the risk of ergotism when given with **ergometrine**. Avoid. Severe Theoretical

▶ Idelalisib is predicted to increase the risk of ergotism when given with **ergometrine**. Avoid. Severe Theoretical

▶ Imatinib is predicted to increase the risk of ergotism when given with **ergometrine**. Severe Theoretical

▶ Ketamine is predicted to increase the risk of elevated blood pressure when given with **ergometrine**. Severe Theoretical

▶ Letermovir is predicted to increase the risk of ergotism when given with **ergometrine**. Severe Theoretical

▶ Macrolides (clarithromycin) are predicted to increase the risk of ergotism when given with **ergometrine**. Avoid. Severe Theoretical

▶ Macrolides (erythromycin) are predicted to increase the risk of ergotism when given with **ergometrine**. Severe Theoretical

▶ Neurokinin-1 receptor antagonists (aprepitant, netupitant) are predicted to increase the risk of ergotism when given with **ergometrine**. Severe Theoretical

▶ Nilotinib is predicted to increase the risk of ergotism when given with **ergometrine**. Severe Theoretical

▶ Nirmatrelvir boosted with ritonavir is predicted to increase the concentration of **ergometrine**. Avoid. Severe Theoretical

▶ Olaparib might alter the exposure to **ergometrine**. Moderate Theoretical

▶ **Ergometrine** potentially increases the risk of peripheral vasoconstriction when given with sympathomimetics, inotropic (dopamine). Avoid. Severe Anecdotal

▶ **Ergometrine** is predicted to increase the risk of peripheral vasoconstriction when given with sympathomimetics, vasoconstrictor (noradrenaline/norepinephrine). Severe Anecdotal

▶ Tucatinib is predicted to increase the risk of ergotism when given with **ergometrine**. Avoid. Severe Theoretical

Eribulin → see TABLE 14 p. 1575 (myelosuppression), TABLE 11 p. 1574 (peripheral neuropathy), TABLE 8 p. 1573 (QT-interval prolongation)

Erlotinib

FOOD AND LIFESTYLE Dose adjustment may be necessary if smoking started or stopped during treatment.

▶ Oral antacids are predicted to decrease the absorption of oral **erlotinib**. Manufacturer advises take 2 hours before or 4 hours after antacids. Moderate Theoretical

Erlotinib (continued)

- Anti-androgens (apalutamide, enzalutamide) are predicted to decrease the exposure to **erlotinib**. Avoid or adjust dose—consult product literature. [Severe] Study
- Antiarrhythmics (amiodarone) are predicted to increase the exposure to **erlotinib**. [Moderate] Theoretical
- Antiarrhythmics (dronedarone) are predicted to increase the exposure to **erlotinib**. [Moderate] Study
- Antiepileptics (carbamazepine, fosphenytoin, phenobarbital, phenytoin, primidone) are predicted to decrease the exposure to **erlotinib**. Avoid or adjust dose—consult product literature. [Severe] Study
- Antiepileptics (eslicarbazepine) are predicted to decrease the exposure to **erlotinib**. [Severe] Theoretical
- Antiepileptics (oxcarbazepine) decrease the exposure to **erlotinib**. [Severe] Study
- Antifungals, azoles (fluconazole, isavuconazole) are predicted to increase the exposure to **erlotinib**. [Moderate] Study
- Antifungals, azoles (itraconazole, ketoconazole, posaconazole, voriconazole) are predicted to increase the exposure to **erlotinib**. Use with caution and adjust dose. [Severe] Study
- **Erlotinib** is predicted to increase the risk of gastrointestinal perforation when given with aspirin (high-dose). [Severe] Theoretical
- Berotralstat is predicted to increase the exposure to **erlotinib**. [Moderate] Study
- Calcium channel blockers (diltiazem, verapamil) are predicted to increase the exposure to **erlotinib**. [Moderate] Study
- Oral calcium salts (calcium carbonate) -containing antacids are predicted to decrease the absorption of oral **erlotinib**. Manufacturer advises take 2 hours before or 4 hours after antacids. [Moderate] Theoretical
- Cenobamate is predicted to decrease the exposure to **erlotinib**. [Severe] Study
- Ceritinib is predicted to increase the exposure to **erlotinib**. Use with caution and adjust dose. [Severe] Study
- Ciclosporin is predicted to increase the exposure to **erlotinib**. [Moderate] Theoretical
- Cobicistat is predicted to increase the exposure to **erlotinib**. Use with caution and adjust dose. [Severe] Study
- Combined hormonal contraceptives are predicted to increases the exposure to **erlotinib**. Monitor adverse effects and adjust dose. [Moderate] Study
- **Erlotinib** is predicted to increase the risk of gastrointestinal perforation when given with corticosteroids. [Severe] Theoretical
- **Erlotinib** increases the anticoagulant effect of coumarins. [Severe] Anecdotal
- Crizotinib is predicted to increase the exposure to **erlotinib**. [Moderate] Study
- Dabrafenib is predicted to decrease the exposure to **erlotinib**. [Severe] Study
- Encorafenib is predicted to decrease the exposure to **erlotinib**. Avoid or adjust dose—consult product literature. [Severe] Study
- Endothelin receptor antagonists (bosentan) are predicted to decrease the exposure to **erlotinib**. [Severe] Study
- Fedratinib is predicted to increase the exposure to **erlotinib**. [Moderate] Study
- Givosiran are predicted to increases the exposure to **erlotinib**. Monitor adverse effects and adjust dose. [Moderate] Study
- Grapefruit juice is predicted to increase the exposure to **erlotinib**. [Moderate] Theoretical
- H₂ receptor antagonists are predicted to decrease the exposure to **erlotinib**. Manufacturer advises take 2 hours before or 10 hours after H₂ receptor antagonists. [Moderate] Study
- HIV-protease inhibitors are predicted to increase the exposure to **erlotinib**. Use with caution and adjust dose. [Severe] Study
- Idelalisib is predicted to increase the exposure to **erlotinib**. Use with caution and adjust dose. [Severe] Study
- Imatinib is predicted to increase the exposure to **erlotinib**. [Moderate] Study
- Ivacaftor is predicted to increase the exposure to **erlotinib**. [Moderate] Theoretical
- Ivosidenib is predicted to decrease the exposure to **erlotinib**. Avoid or adjust dose—consult product literature. [Severe] Study

- Lapatinib is predicted to increase the exposure to **erlotinib**. [Moderate] Theoretical
- Letermovir is predicted to increase the exposure to **erlotinib**. [Moderate] Study
- Lorlatinib is predicted to decrease the exposure to **erlotinib**. [Severe] Study
- Lumacaftor is predicted to decrease the exposure to **erlotinib**. Avoid or adjust dose—consult product literature. [Severe] Study
- Macrolides (azithromycin) are predicted to increase the exposure to **erlotinib**. [Moderate] Theoretical
- Macrolides (clarithromycin) are predicted to increase the exposure to **erlotinib**. Use with caution and adjust dose. [Severe] Study
- Macrolides (erythromycin) are predicted to increase the exposure to **erlotinib**. [Moderate] Study
- Mexiletine are predicted to increases the exposure to **erlotinib**. Monitor adverse effects and adjust dose. [Moderate] Study
- Mitotane is predicted to decrease the exposure to **erlotinib**. Avoid or adjust dose—consult product literature. [Severe] Study
- Neratinib is predicted to increase the exposure to **erlotinib**. [Moderate] Theoretical
- Neurokinin-1 receptor antagonists (aprepitant, netupitant) are predicted to increase the exposure to **erlotinib**. [Moderate] Study
- Nilotinib is predicted to increase the exposure to **erlotinib**. [Moderate] Study
- NNRTIs (efavirenz, etravirine, nevirapine) are predicted to decrease the exposure to **erlotinib**. [Severe] Study
- **Erlotinib** is predicted to increase the risk of gastrointestinal perforation when given with NSAIDs. [Severe] Theoretical
- Osilodrostat are predicted to increases the exposure to **erlotinib**. Monitor adverse effects and adjust dose. [Moderate] Study
- **Erlotinib** is predicted to increase the risk of bleeding events when given with phenindione. [Severe] Theoretical
- Proton pump inhibitors are predicted to decrease the exposure to **erlotinib**. Avoid. [Moderate] Study
- Quinolones (ciprofloxacin) are predicted to increase the exposure to **erlotinib**. Monitor adverse effects and adjust dose. [Moderate] Study
- Ranolazine is predicted to increase the exposure to **erlotinib**. [Moderate] Theoretical
- Rifamycins (rifampicin) are predicted to decrease the exposure to **erlotinib**. Avoid or adjust dose—consult product literature. [Severe] Study
- Rucaparib are predicted to increases the exposure to **erlotinib**. Monitor adverse effects and adjust dose. [Moderate] Study
- **Erlotinib** is predicted to increase the exposure to the active component of sacituzumab govitecan. [Severe] Theoretical
- Oral sodium bicarbonate-containing antacids are predicted to decrease the absorption of oral **erlotinib**. Manufacturer advises take 2 hours before or 4 hours after antacids. [Moderate] Theoretical
- Sodium zirconium cyclosilicate is predicted to decrease the exposure to **erlotinib**. Separate administration by at least 2 hours. [Moderate] Theoretical
- Sotorasib is predicted to decrease the exposure to **erlotinib**. [Severe] Study
- SSRIs (fluvoxamine) are predicted to increase the exposure to **erlotinib**. Monitor adverse effects and adjust dose. [Moderate] Theoretical
- St John's wort is predicted to decrease the exposure to **erlotinib**. [Severe] Study
- Tucatinib is predicted to increase the exposure to **erlotinib**. Use with caution and adjust dose. [Severe] Study
- Vandetanib is predicted to increase the exposure to **erlotinib**. [Moderate] Theoretical
- Vemurafenib are predicted to increases the exposure to **erlotinib**. Monitor adverse effects and adjust dose. [Moderate] Study

Ertapenem → see carbapenems

Ertugliflozin → see sodium glucose co-transporter 2 inhibitors

Erythromycin → see macrolides

Escitalopram → see SSRIs

Esketamine → see TABLE 7 p. 1572 (hypotension), TABLE 10 p. 1574 (CNS effects)

▶ **Esketamine** is predicted to increase the risk of seizures when given with aminophylline. Avoid. Severe Theoretical

▶ Anti-androgens (apalutamide, enzalutamide) are predicted to decrease the exposure to **esketamine**. Adjust dose. Mild Theoretical

▶ Antiepileptics (carbamazepine, fosphenytoin, phenobarbital, phenytoin, primidone) are predicted to decrease the exposure to **esketamine**. Adjust dose. Mild Theoretical → Also see TABLE 10 p. 1574

▶ Antifungals, azoles (itraconazole, ketoconazole, posaconazole, voriconazole) are predicted to increase the exposure to **esketamine**. Adjust dose. Moderate Study

▶ Ceritinib is predicted to increase the exposure to **esketamine**. Adjust dose. Moderate Study

▶ Cobicistat is predicted to increase the exposure to **esketamine**. Adjust dose. Moderate Study

▶ Encorafenib is predicted to decrease the exposure to **esketamine**. Adjust dose. Mild Theoretical

▶ **Esketamine** is predicted to increase the risk of elevated blood pressure when given with ergometrine. Avoid. Severe Theoretical

▶ HIV-protease inhibitors are predicted to increase the exposure to **esketamine**. Adjust dose. Moderate Study

▶ Idelalisib is predicted to increase the exposure to **esketamine**. Adjust dose. Moderate Study

▶ Ivosidenib is predicted to decrease the exposure to **esketamine**. Adjust dose. Mild Theoretical

▶ Lumacaftor is predicted to decrease the exposure to **esketamine**. Adjust dose. Mild Theoretical

▶ Macrolides (clarithromycin) are predicted to increase the exposure to **esketamine**. Adjust dose. Moderate Study

▶ Mitotane is predicted to decrease the exposure to **esketamine**. Adjust dose. Mild Theoretical

▶ Rifamycins (rifampicin) are predicted to decrease the exposure to **esketamine**. Adjust dose. Mild Theoretical

▶ **Esketamine** is predicted to increase the risk of seizures when given with theophylline. Avoid. Severe Theoretical

▶ Tucatinib is predicted to increase the exposure to **esketamine**. Adjust dose. Moderate Study

Eslicarbazepine → see antiepileptics

Esmolol → see beta blockers, selective

Esomeprazole → see proton pump inhibitors

Estradiol

▶ Antiepileptics (carbamazepine, eslicarbazepine, fosphenytoin, oxcarbazepine, perampanel, phenobarbital, phenytoin, primidone, rufinamide, topiramate) are predicted to decrease the efficacy of **estradiol**. Moderate Theoretical

▶ Endothelin receptor antagonists (bosentan) are predicted to decrease the efficacy of **estradiol**. Moderate Theoretical

▶ HIV-protease inhibitors (ritonavir) are predicted to decrease the efficacy of **estradiol**. Moderate Theoretical

▶ Modafinil is predicted to decrease the efficacy of **estradiol**. Moderate Theoretical

▶ Neurokinin-1 receptor antagonists (aprepitant, fosaprepitant) are predicted to decrease the efficacy of **estradiol**. Moderate Theoretical

▶ NNRTIs (efavirenz, nevirapine) are predicted to decrease the efficacy of **estradiol**. Moderate Theoretical

▶ Rifamycins are predicted to decrease the efficacy of **estradiol**. Moderate Theoretical

▶ St John's wort is predicted to decrease the efficacy of **estradiol**. Moderate Theoretical

Estramustine → see alkylating agents

Eszopiclone → see TABLE 10 p. 1574 (CNS effects)

▶ Anti-androgens (apalutamide, enzalutamide) are predicted to decrease the exposure to **eszopiclone**. Adjust dose. Moderate Theoretical

▶ Antiepileptics (carbamazepine, fosphenytoin, phenobarbital, phenytoin, primidone) are predicted to decrease the exposure to **eszopiclone**. Adjust dose. Moderate Theoretical → Also see TABLE 10 p. 1574

▶ Antifungals, azoles (itraconazole, ketoconazole, posaconazole, voriconazole) are predicted to increase the exposure to **eszopiclone**. Adjust **eszopiclone** dose; avoid in the elderly, p. 554. Moderate Study

▶ Ceritinib is predicted to increase the exposure to **eszopiclone**. Adjust **eszopiclone** dose; avoid in the elderly, p. 554. Moderate Study

▶ Cobicistat is predicted to increase the exposure to **eszopiclone**. Adjust **eszopiclone** dose; avoid in the elderly, p. 554. Moderate Study

▶ Encorafenib is predicted to decrease the exposure to **eszopiclone**. Adjust dose. Moderate Theoretical

▶ HIV-protease inhibitors are predicted to increase the exposure to **eszopiclone**. Adjust **eszopiclone** dose; avoid in the elderly, p. 554. Moderate Study

▶ Idelalisib is predicted to increase the exposure to **eszopiclone**. Adjust **eszopiclone** dose; avoid in the elderly, p. 554. Moderate Study

▶ Ivosidenib is predicted to decrease the exposure to **eszopiclone**. Adjust dose. Moderate Theoretical

▶ Lumacaftor is predicted to decrease the exposure to **eszopiclone**. Adjust dose. Moderate Theoretical

▶ Macrolides (clarithromycin) are predicted to increase the exposure to **eszopiclone**. Adjust **eszopiclone** dose; avoid in the elderly, p. 554. Moderate Study

▶ Mitotane is predicted to decrease the exposure to **eszopiclone**. Adjust dose. Moderate Theoretical

▶ Rifamycins (rifampicin) are predicted to decrease the exposure to **eszopiclone**. Adjust dose. Moderate Theoretical

▶ St John's wort is predicted to decrease the exposure to **eszopiclone**. Adjust dose. Moderate Theoretical

▶ Tucatinib is predicted to increase the exposure to **eszopiclone**. Adjust **eszopiclone** dose; avoid in the elderly, p. 554. Moderate Study

Etanercept

▶ Abatacept is predicted to increase the risk of generalised infection (possibly life-threatening) when given with **etanercept**. Avoid. Severe Theoretical

▶ Anakinra is predicted to increase the risk of generalised infection (possibly life-threatening) when given with **etanercept**. Avoid. Severe Theoretical

▶ Filgotinib is predicted to increase the risk of immunosuppression when given with **etanercept**. Avoid. Severe Theoretical

▶ Live vaccines are predicted to increase the risk of generalised infection (possibly life-threatening) when given with **etanercept**. UKHSA advises avoid (refer to Green Book). Severe Theoretical

▶ Monoclonal antibodies (rozanolixizumab) might decrease the concentration of **etanercept**. Avoid and for 2 weeks after stopping rozanolixizumab. Moderate Theoretical

▶ Monoclonal antibodies (sarilumab) might cause severe infection and neutropenia when given with **etanercept**. Severe Theoretical

Etelcalcetide

▶ Cinacalcet increases the risk of hypocalcaemia when given with **etelcalcetide**. Avoid. Severe Theoretical

▶ **Etelcalcetide** might increase the risk of hypocalcaemia when given with denosumab. Severe Theoretical

Ethambutol

▶ Isoniazid increases the risk of optic neuropathy when given with **ethambutol**. Severe Anecdotal

Ethinylestradiol

▶ Fostemsavir increases the concentration of **ethinylestradiol** from a combined hormonal contraceptive. Adjust dose— consult product literature. Severe Study

Ethosuximide → see antiepileptics

Etodolac → see NSAIDs

Etomidate → see TABLE 7 p. 1572 (hypotension), TABLE 10 p. 1574 (CNS effects)

Etonogestrel

▶ Antiepileptics (carbamazepine, eslicarbazepine, fosphenytoin, oxcarbazepine, perampanel, phenobarbital, phenytoin, primidone, rufinamide, topiramate) are predicted to decrease the efficacy of **etonogestrel**. For FSRH guidance, see Contraceptives, interactions p. 917. Severe Theoretical

▶ Antiepileptics (lamotrigine) might decrease the effects of **etonogestrel**. For FSRH guidance, see Contraceptives, interactions p. 917. Moderate Theoretical

Etonogestrel (continued)

▸ Antifungals, azoles (itraconazole, ketoconazole, posaconazole, voriconazole) are predicted to increase the concentration of subdermal **etonogestrel**. Moderate Theoretical

▸ Ceritinib is predicted to increase the concentration of subdermal **etonogestrel**. Moderate Theoretical

▸ Cobicistat is predicted to increase the concentration of subdermal **etonogestrel**. Moderate Theoretical

▸ Endothelin receptor antagonists (bosentan) are predicted to decrease the efficacy of **etonogestrel**. For FSRH guidance, see Contraceptives, interactions p. 917. Severe Theoretical

▸ HIV-protease inhibitors (ritonavir) are predicted to decrease the efficacy of **etonogestrel**. For FSRH guidance, see Contraceptives, interactions p. 917. Severe Theoretical

▸ HIV-protease inhibitors are predicted to increase the concentration of subdermal **etonogestrel**. Moderate Theoretical

▸ Idelalisib is predicted to increase the concentration of subdermal **etonogestrel**. Moderate Theoretical

▸ Lumacaftor might decrease the efficacy of subdermal **etonogestrel**. Use additional contraceptive precautions. Severe Theoretical

▸ Macrolides (clarithromycin) are predicted to increase the concentration of subdermal **etonogestrel**. Moderate Theoretical

▸ Modafinil is predicted to decrease the efficacy of **etonogestrel**. For FSRH guidance, see Contraceptives, interactions p. 917. Severe Theoretical

▸ Neurokinin-1 receptor antagonists (aprepitant, fosaprepitant) are predicted to decrease the efficacy of **etonogestrel**. For FSRH guidance, see Contraceptives, interactions p. 917. Severe Theoretical

▸ NNRTIs (efavirenz, nevirapine) are predicted to decrease the efficacy of **etonogestrel**. For FSRH guidance, see Contraceptives, interactions p. 917. Severe Theoretical

▸ NNRTIs (etravirine) might decrease the efficacy of **etonogestrel**. Follow FSRH guidance for enzyme inducers, see Contraceptives, interactions p. 917. Severe Theoretical

▸ Rifamycins are predicted to decrease the efficacy of **etonogestrel**. For FSRH guidance, see Contraceptives, interactions p. 917. Severe Theoretical

▸ St John's wort is predicted to decrease the efficacy of **etonogestrel**. MHRA advises avoid. For FSRH guidance, see Contraceptives, interactions p. 917. Severe Theoretical

▸ Sugammadex is predicted to decrease the efficacy of **etonogestrel**. Use additional contraceptive precautions. Severe Theoretical

▸ Tucatinib is predicted to increase the concentration of subdermal **etonogestrel**. Moderate Theoretical

▸ **Etonogestrel** might decrease the efficacy of ulipristal and ulipristal might decrease the efficacy of **etonogestrel**. Avoid. Severe Theoretical

Etoposide → see TABLE 14 p. 1575 (myelosuppression)

▸ Antiepileptics (carbamazepine, fosphenytoin, phenobarbital, phenytoin, primidone) are predicted to decrease the efficacy of **etoposide**. Moderate Study

▸ Ciclosporin increases the exposure to **etoposide**. Monitor and adjust dose. Severe Study

▸ Live vaccines are predicted to increase the risk of generalised infection (possibly life-threatening) when given with **etoposide**. UKHSA advises avoid (refer to Green Book). Severe Theoretical

▸ Neurokinin-1 receptor antagonists (netupitant) slightly increase the exposure to **etoposide**. Moderate Study

Etoricoxib → see NSAIDs

Etrasimod → see TABLE 5 p. 1572 (bradycardia), TABLE 8 p. 1573 (QT-interval prolongation)

▸ Anti-androgens (enzalutamide) are predicted to decrease the exposure to **etrasimod**. Avoid. Severe Theoretical

▸ Antiarrhythmics (dronedarone) are predicted to increase the exposure to **etrasimod**. Avoid in poor CYP2C9 metabolisers. Severe Theoretical → Also see TABLE 5 p. 1572

▸ Antifungals, azoles (fluconazole) slightly increase the exposure to **etrasimod**. Avoid. Severe Study

▸ Antifungals, azoles (isavuconazole, itraconazole, ketoconazole, posaconazole, voriconazole) are predicted to increase the

exposure to **etrasimod**. Avoid in poor CYP2C9 metabolisers. Severe Theoretical

▸ Berotralstat is predicted to increase the exposure to **etrasimod**. Avoid in poor CYP2C9 metabolisers. Severe Theoretical

▸ Calcium channel blockers (diltiazem, verapamil) are predicted to increase the exposure to **etrasimod**. Avoid in poor CYP2C9 metabolisers. Severe Theoretical → Also see TABLE 5 p. 1572

▸ Ceritinib is predicted to increase the exposure to **etrasimod**. Avoid in poor CYP2C9 metabolisers. Severe Theoretical → Also see TABLE 5 p. 1572

▸ Clopidogrel are predicted to increases the exposure to **etrasimod**. Avoid in poor CYP2C9 metabolisers. Severe Theoretical

▸ Cobicistat is predicted to increase the exposure to **etrasimod**. Avoid in poor CYP2C9 metabolisers. Severe Theoretical

▸ Crizotinib is predicted to increase the exposure to **etrasimod**. Avoid in poor CYP2C9 metabolisers. Severe Theoretical → Also see TABLE 5 p. 1572

▸ Fedratinib is predicted to increase the exposure to **etrasimod**. Avoid in poor CYP2C9 metabolisers. Severe Theoretical

▸ Fibrates (gemfibrozil) are predicted to increase the exposure to **etrasimod**. Avoid in poor CYP2C9 metabolisers. Severe Theoretical

▸ HIV-protease inhibitors are predicted to increase the exposure to **etrasimod**. Avoid in poor CYP2C9 metabolisers. Severe Theoretical

▸ Idelalisib is predicted to increase the exposure to **etrasimod**. Avoid in poor CYP2C9 metabolisers. Severe Theoretical

▸ Imatinib is predicted to increase the exposure to **etrasimod**. Avoid in poor CYP2C9 metabolisers. Severe Theoretical

▸ Iron chelators (deferasirox) are predicted to increase the exposure to **etrasimod**. Avoid in poor CYP2C9 metabolisers. Severe Theoretical

▸ Leflunomide are predicted to increases the exposure to **etrasimod**. Avoid in poor CYP2C9 metabolisers. Severe Theoretical

▸ Letermovir is predicted to increase the exposure to **etrasimod**. Avoid in poor CYP2C9 metabolisers. Severe Theoretical

▸ Live vaccines might increase the risk of generalised infection (possibly life-threatening) when given with **etrasimod**. Avoid and for at least 4 weeks before and 2 weeks after stopping **etrasimod**. Severe Theoretical

▸ Macrolides (clarithromycin, erythromycin) are predicted to increase the exposure to **etrasimod**. Avoid in poor CYP2C9 metabolisers. Severe Theoretical

▸ Neurokinin-1 receptor antagonists (aprepitant, netupitant) are predicted to increase the exposure to **etrasimod**. Avoid in poor CYP2C9 metabolisers. Severe Theoretical

▸ Nilotinib is predicted to increase the exposure to **etrasimod**. Avoid in poor CYP2C9 metabolisers. Severe Theoretical

▸ Rifamycins (rifampicin) slightly decrease the exposure to **etrasimod**. Avoid. Severe Study

▸ Teriflunomide are predicted to increases the exposure to **etrasimod**. Avoid in poor CYP2C9 metabolisers. Severe Theoretical

▸ Tucatinib is predicted to increase the exposure to **etrasimod**. Avoid in poor CYP2C9 metabolisers. Severe Theoretical

Etravirine → see NNRTIs

Everolimus

▸ Abrocitinib might increase the exposure to **everolimus**. Moderate Theoretical

▸ **Everolimus** potentially increases the risk of angioedema when given with ACE inhibitors. Severe Anecdotal

▸ Anti-androgens (apalutamide, enzalutamide) are predicted to decrease the concentration of **everolimus**. Avoid or adjust dose. Severe Study

▸ Antiarrhythmics (amiodarone) are predicted to increase the exposure to **everolimus**. Monitor and adjust dose. Severe Study

▸ Antiarrhythmics (dronedarone) are predicted to increase the concentration of **everolimus**. Avoid or adjust dose. Moderate Study

▸ Antiepileptics (carbamazepine, fosphenytoin, phenobarbital, phenytoin, primidone) are predicted to decrease the concentration of **everolimus**. Avoid or adjust dose. Severe Study

▸ Antifungals, azoles (**fluconazole, isavuconazole**) are predicted to increase the concentration of **everolimus**. Avoid or adjust dose. [Moderate] Study

▸ Antifungals, azoles (**itraconazole, ketoconazole, posaconazole, voriconazole**) are predicted to increase the exposure to **everolimus**. Avoid. [Severe] Study

▸ Asciminib is predicted to increase the exposure to **everolimus**. [Severe] Theoretical

▸ Belumosudil might increase the exposure to **everolimus**. Avoid or adjust dose. [Moderate] Theoretical

▸ Belzutifan is predicted to decrease the exposure to **everolimus**. Avoid or adjust dose. [Severe] Theoretical

▸ Berotralstat is predicted to increase the concentration of **everolimus**. Avoid or adjust dose. [Moderate] Study

▸ Bulevirtide is predicted to increase the exposure to **everolimus**. [Moderate] Theoretical

▸ Calcium channel blockers (**diltiazem, verapamil**) are predicted to increase the concentration of **everolimus**. Avoid or adjust dose. [Moderate] Study

▸ Cannabidiol moderately increases the exposure to **everolimus**. Monitor and adjust dose. [Moderate] Study

▸ Cenobamate is predicted to decrease the concentration of **everolimus**. Avoid or adjust dose. [Severe] Study

▸ Ceritinib is predicted to increase the exposure to **everolimus**. Avoid. [Severe] Study

▸ Ciclosporin moderately increases the exposure to **everolimus**. Avoid or adjust dose. [Severe] Study

▸ Cobicistat is predicted to increase the exposure to **everolimus**. Avoid. [Severe] Study

▸ Crizotinib is predicted to increase the concentration of **everolimus**. Avoid or adjust dose. [Moderate] Study

▸ Dabrafenib is predicted to decrease the concentration of **everolimus**. Avoid or adjust dose. [Severe] Study

▸ Danicopan is predicted to increase the exposure to **everolimus**. [Moderate] Study

▸ Daridorexant is predicted to increase the exposure to **everolimus**. [Moderate] Study

▸ Eliglustat is predicted to increase the exposure to **everolimus**. Adjust dose. [Moderate] Study

▸ Encorafenib is predicted to decrease the concentration of **everolimus**. Avoid or adjust dose. [Severe] Study

▸ Endothelin receptor antagonists (**bosentan**) are predicted to decrease the concentration of **everolimus**. Avoid or adjust dose. [Severe] Study

▸ Erdafitinib is predicted to increase the exposure to **everolimus**. Separate administration by at least 6 hours. [Moderate] Theoretical

▸ Fedratinib is predicted to increase the concentration of **everolimus**. Avoid or adjust dose. [Moderate] Study

▸ Fostamatinib is predicted to increase the exposure to **everolimus**. Monitor and adjust dose. [Moderate] Theoretical

▸ Givinostat might increase the exposure to **everolimus**. [Moderate] Study

▸ Glecaprevir is predicted to increase the exposure to **everolimus**. [Moderate] Study

▸ Grapefruit juice is predicted to increase the exposure to **everolimus**. Avoid. [Severe] Theoretical

▸ HIV-protease inhibitors are predicted to increase the exposure to **everolimus**. Avoid. [Severe] Study

▸ Ibrutinib might increase the exposure to **everolimus**. Separate administration by at least 6 hours. [Moderate] Theoretical

▸ Idelalisib is predicted to increase the exposure to **everolimus**. Avoid. [Severe] Study

▸ Imatinib is predicted to increase the concentration of **everolimus**. Avoid or adjust dose. [Moderate] Study

▸ Ivacaftor is predicted to increase the exposure to **everolimus**. [Moderate] Study

▸ Ivosidenib is predicted to decrease the concentration of **everolimus**. Avoid or adjust dose. [Severe] Study

▸ Lapatinib is predicted to increase the exposure to **everolimus**. [Moderate] Theoretical

▸ Larotrectinib is predicted to increase the exposure to **everolimus**. Use with caution and adjust dose. [Mild] Theoretical

▸ Letermovir is predicted to increase the concentration of **everolimus**. Avoid or adjust dose. [Moderate] Study

▸ Live vaccines are predicted to increase the risk of generalised infection (possibly life-threatening) when given with **everolimus**. UKHSA advises avoid (refer to Green Book). [Severe] Theoretical

▸ **Everolimus** is predicted to increase the exposure to lomitapide and lomitapide might increase the exposure to **everolimus**. Adjust **everolimus** dose and separate administration by 12 hours, p. 1109. [Moderate] Theoretical

▸ Lorlatinib is predicted to decrease the concentration of **everolimus**. Avoid or adjust dose. [Severe] Study

▸ Lumacaftor is predicted to decrease the concentration of **everolimus**. Avoid or adjust dose. [Severe] Study

▸ Macrolides (**clarithromycin**) are predicted to increase the exposure to **everolimus**. Avoid. [Severe] Study

▸ Macrolides (**erythromycin**) are predicted to increase the concentration of **everolimus**. Avoid or adjust dose. [Moderate] Study

▸ Maribavir increases the exposure to **everolimus**. Monitor and adjust dose. [Severe] Study

▸ **Everolimus** is predicted to increase the exposure to mavacamten. Monitor and adjust dose—consult product literature. [Moderate] Theoretical

▸ Mifepristone is predicted to increase the exposure to **everolimus**. [Severe] Theoretical

▸ Mirabegron is predicted to increase the exposure to **everolimus**. [Mild] Theoretical

▸ Mitotane is predicted to decrease the concentration of **everolimus**. Avoid or adjust dose. [Severe] Study

▸ Mobocertinib is predicted to decrease the exposure to **everolimus**. [Severe] Theoretical

▸ Neratinib is predicted to increase the exposure to **everolimus**. [Moderate] Study

▸ Neurokinin-1 receptor antagonists (**aprepitant, netupitant**) are predicted to increase the concentration of **everolimus**. Avoid or adjust dose. [Moderate] Study

▸ Nilotinib is predicted to increase the concentration of **everolimus**. Avoid or adjust dose. [Moderate] Study

▸ Nirmatrelvir boosted with ritonavir is predicted to increase the concentration of **everolimus**. Avoid. [Severe] Theoretical

▸ NNRTIs (**efavirenz, etravirine, nevirapine**) are predicted to decrease the concentration of **everolimus**. Avoid or adjust dose. [Severe] Study

▸ Olaparib might increase the exposure to **everolimus**. [Moderate] Theoretical

▸ Osimertinib is predicted to increase the exposure to **everolimus**. [Moderate] Study

▸ Palbociclib is predicted to increase the exposure to **everolimus**. Adjust dose. [Moderate] Theoretical

▸ Pemigatinib might increase the exposure to **everolimus**. Separate administration by at least 6 hours. [Moderate] Theoretical

▸ Penicillins (**flucloxacillin**) (high-dose) might decrease the exposure to **everolimus**. [Moderate] Study

▸ Pibrentasvir with glecaprevir is predicted to increase the exposure to **everolimus**. [Moderate] Study

▸ Pitolisant is predicted to decrease the exposure to **everolimus**. Avoid. [Severe] Theoretical

▸ Ribociclib is predicted to increase the exposure to **everolimus**. Use with caution and adjust dose. [Moderate] Theoretical

▸ Rifamycins (**rifampicin**) are predicted to decrease the concentration of **everolimus**. Avoid or adjust dose. [Severe] Study

▸ Ritlecitinib is predicted to increase the exposure to **everolimus**. Adjust dose. [Moderate] Theoretical

▸ Selpercatinib is predicted to increase the exposure to **everolimus**. Avoid. [Moderate] Study

▸ Sotorasib is predicted to decrease the concentration of **everolimus**. Avoid or adjust dose. [Severe] Study

▸ St John's wort is predicted to decrease the concentration of **everolimus**. Avoid or adjust dose. [Severe] Study

▸ Tepotinib is predicted to increase the concentration of **everolimus**. [Severe] Study

▸ Tucatinib is predicted to increase the exposure to **everolimus**. Avoid. [Severe] Study

▸ Velpatasvir is predicted to increase the exposure to **everolimus**. [Severe] Theoretical

Everolimus (continued)

- ▶ **Vemurafenib** is predicted to increase the exposure to **everolimus**. Use with caution and adjust dose. Severe Theoretical
- ▶ **Venetoclax** is predicted to increase the exposure to **everolimus**. Avoid or adjust dose. Severe Study
- ▶ **Voclosporin** is predicted to increase the exposure to **everolimus**. Moderate Study
- ▶ **Voxilaprevir** with sofosbuvir and velpatasvir is predicted to increase the exposure to **everolimus**. Severe Theoretical

Exemestane

- ▶ Anti-androgens (apalutamide, enzalutamide) moderately decrease the exposure to **exemestane**. Moderate Study
- ▶ Antiepileptics (carbamazepine, fosphenytoin, phenobarbital, phenytoin, primidone) moderately decrease the exposure to **exemestane**. Moderate Study
- ▶ **Encorafenib** moderately decreases the exposure to **exemestane**. Moderate Study
- ▶ **Ivosidenib** moderately decreases the exposure to **exemestane**. Moderate Study
- ▶ **Lumacaftor** moderately decreases the exposure to **exemestane**. Moderate Study
- ▶ **Mitotane** moderately decreases the exposure to **exemestane**. Moderate Study
- ▶ Rifamycins (rifampicin) moderately decrease the exposure to **exemestane**. Moderate Study
- ▶ St John's wort is predicted to decrease the exposure to **exemestane**. Moderate Theoretical

Exenatide → see glucagon-like peptide-1 receptor agonists

Ezetimibe

- ▶ **Ezetimibe** is predicted to affect the efficacy of bulevirtide. Avoid. Severe Theoretical
- ▶ **Ciclosporin** moderately increases the exposure to **ezetimibe** and **ezetimibe** slightly increases the exposure to ciclosporin. Moderate Study
- ▶ Fibrates are predicted to increase the risk of gallstones when given with **ezetimibe**. Severe Theoretical

Factor XA inhibitors → see TABLE 3 p. 1571 (anticoagulant effects)

apixaban · edoxaban · fondaparinux · rivaroxaban

- ▶ **Abrocitinib** might increase the exposure to **edoxaban**. Moderate Theoretical
- ▶ Anti-androgens (apalutamide) are predicted to decrease the exposure to **edoxaban**. Monitor and adjust dose. Moderate Study
- ▶ Anti-androgens (apalutamide, enzalutamide) are predicted to decrease the exposure to **apixaban**. Moderate Study
- ▶ Anti-androgens (apalutamide, enzalutamide) are predicted to decrease the exposure to **rivaroxaban**. Avoid unless patient can be monitored for signs of thrombosis. Severe Study
- ▶ Antiarrhythmics (amiodarone) slightly increase the exposure to **edoxaban**. Severe Study
- ▶ Antiarrhythmics (amiodarone) might increase the exposure to **rivaroxaban**. Moderate Study
- ▶ Antiarrhythmics (amiodarone, dronedarone) are predicted to increase the exposure to **apixaban**. Moderate Theoretical
- ▶ Antiarrhythmics (dronedarone) slightly increase the exposure to **edoxaban**. Adjust **edoxaban** dose, p. 147. Severe Study
- ▶ Antiarrhythmics (dronedarone) might increase the exposure to **rivaroxaban**. Avoid. Moderate Study
- ▶ Antiepileptics (carbamazepine) are predicted to decrease the exposure to **edoxaban**. Moderate Study
- ▶ Antiepileptics (carbamazepine, phenobarbital, phenytoin, primidone) are predicted to decrease the exposure to **rivaroxaban**. Avoid unless patient can be monitored for signs of thrombosis. Severe Study
- ▶ Antiepileptics (carbamazepine, phenytoin) are predicted to decrease the exposure to **apixaban**. Use with caution or avoid. Severe Study
- ▶ Antiepileptics (fosphenytoin) are predicted to decrease the exposure to **rivaroxaban**. Avoid unless patient can be monitored for signs of thrombosis. Severe Theoretical
- ▶ Antiepileptics (fosphenytoin, phenobarbital, phenytoin, primidone) are predicted to decrease the exposure to **edoxaban**. Severe Theoretical
- ▶ Antiepileptics (fosphenytoin, primidone) are predicted to decrease the exposure to **apixaban**. Severe Study

- ▶ Antiepileptics (oxcarbazepine) are predicted to decrease the exposure to **rivaroxaban**. Severe Study
- ▶ Antiepileptics (phenobarbital) are predicted to decrease the exposure to **apixaban**. Use with caution or avoid. Severe Anecdotal
- ▶ Antifungals, azoles (fluconazole) might increase the risk of bleeding when given with **apixaban**. Moderate Study
- ▶ Antifungals, azoles (itraconazole) are predicted to increase the exposure to **edoxaban**. Severe Theoretical
- ▶ Antifungals, azoles (ketoconazole) slightly increase the exposure to **edoxaban**. Adjust **edoxaban** dose, p. 147. Severe Study
- ▶ Antifungals, azoles (posaconazole, voriconazole) are predicted to increase the exposure to **apixaban**. Avoid. Moderate Theoretical
- ▶ Antifungals, azoles (posaconazole, voriconazole) are predicted to increase the exposure to **rivaroxaban**. Avoid. Severe Theoretical
- ▶ Antifungals, azoles (itraconazole) are predicted to increase the exposure to factor XA inhibitors (**apixaban, rivaroxaban**). Avoid. Severe Theoretical
- ▶ Antifungals, azoles (ketoconazole) moderately increase the exposure to factor XA inhibitors (**apixaban, rivaroxaban**). Avoid. Severe Study
- ▶ **Asciminib** is predicted to increase the exposure to **edoxaban**. Severe Theoretical
- ▶ **Aspirin** (high-dose) increases the exposure to **edoxaban**. Avoid. Severe Study
- ▶ Calcium channel blockers (verapamil) are predicted to increase the exposure to **apixaban**. Moderate Theoretical
- ▶ Calcium channel blockers (verapamil) slightly increase the exposure to **edoxaban**. Severe Study
- ▶ **Ceritinib** is predicted to increase the exposure to **edoxaban**. Moderate Theoretical
- ▶ **Ciclosporin** is predicted to increase the exposure to **apixaban**. Moderate Theoretical
- ▶ **Ciclosporin** slightly increases the exposure to **edoxaban**. Adjust **edoxaban** dose, p. 147. Severe Study
- ▶ **Ciclosporin** slightly increases the exposure to **rivaroxaban**. Moderate Study
- ▶ **Cobicistat** is predicted to increase the exposure to factor XA inhibitors (**apixaban, edoxaban, rivaroxaban**). Avoid. Severe Theoretical
- ▶ **Danicopan** is predicted to increase the exposure to **edoxaban**. Moderate Study
- ▶ **Eliglustat** is predicted to increase the exposure to **edoxaban**. Adjust dose. Moderate Study
- ▶ **Erdafitinib** is predicted to increase the exposure to **apixaban**. Separate administration by at least 6 hours. Moderate Theoretical
- ▶ **Glecaprevir** is predicted to increase the exposure to **edoxaban**. Severe Theoretical
- ▶ HIV-protease inhibitors (atazanavir) boosted with ritonavir are predicted to increase the exposure to **apixaban**. Severe Theoretical
- ▶ HIV-protease inhibitors (atazanavir, fosamprenavir) boosted with ritonavir are predicted to increase the exposure to **rivaroxaban**. Avoid. Severe Theoretical
- ▶ HIV-protease inhibitors (darunavir) boosted with ritonavir or cobicistat are predicted to increase the exposure to **apixaban**. Avoid. Severe Theoretical
- ▶ HIV-protease inhibitors (darunavir) boosted with ritonavir are predicted to increase the exposure to **rivaroxaban**. Avoid. Severe Anecdotal
- ▶ HIV-protease inhibitors (fosamprenavir) boosted with ritonavir are predicted to increase the exposure to **apixaban**. Moderate Theoretical
- ▶ HIV-protease inhibitors (lopinavir) boosted with ritonavir are predicted to slightly increase the exposure to **edoxaban**. Severe Theoretical
- ▶ HIV-protease inhibitors (ritonavir) are predicted to increase the exposure to **apixaban**. Avoid. Severe Theoretical
- ▶ HIV-protease inhibitors (ritonavir) are predicted to slightly increase the exposure to **edoxaban**. Severe Theoretical
- ▶ HIV-protease inhibitors (ritonavir) moderately increase the exposure to **rivaroxaban**. Avoid. Severe Study

▶ HIV-protease inhibitors **(lopinavir)** boosted with ritonavir are predicted to increase the exposure to factor XA inhibitors **(apixaban, rivaroxaban)**. Avoid. Severe Theoretical

▶ **Idelalisib** is predicted to increase the exposure to **apixaban**. Moderate Theoretical

▶ **Ivosidenib** is predicted to alter the exposure to **edoxaban**. Moderate Theoretical

▶ **Lapatinib** is predicted to increase the exposure to **apixaban**. Moderate Theoretical

▶ **Lapatinib** is predicted to slightly increase the exposure to **edoxaban**. Severe Theoretical

▶ **Lorlatinib** is predicted to decrease the exposure to **apixaban**. Use with caution or avoid. Severe Study

▶ **Lorlatinib** is predicted to decrease the exposure to **edoxaban**. Moderate Study

▶ **Lorlatinib** is predicted to decrease the exposure to **rivaroxaban**. Avoid unless patient can be monitored for signs of thrombosis. Severe Study

▶ Macrolides **(azithromycin, clarithromycin)** are predicted to increase the exposure to **edoxaban**. Severe Theoretical

▶ Macrolides **(azithromycin, erythromycin)** are predicted to increase the exposure to **apixaban**. Moderate Theoretical

▶ Macrolides **(clarithromycin)** slightly increase the exposure to **apixaban**. Moderate Study

▶ Macrolides **(erythromycin)** slightly increase the exposure to **edoxaban**. Adjust **edoxaban** dose, p. 147. Severe Study

▶ Macrolides **(erythromycin)** slightly increase the exposure to **rivaroxaban**. Mild Study

▶ **Mirabegron** is predicted to increase the exposure to **edoxaban**. Mild Theoretical

▶ **Mitotane** is predicted to decrease the exposure to **apixaban**. Moderate Study

▶ **Mitotane** is predicted to decrease the exposure to **rivaroxaban**. Avoid unless patient can be monitored for signs of thrombosis. Severe Study

▶ **Neratinib** is predicted to increase the exposure to **apixaban**. Moderate Theoretical

▶ **Nirmatrelvir** boosted with ritonavir is predicted to increase the concentration of factor XA inhibitors **(apixaban, rivaroxaban)**. Avoid. Severe Theoretical

▶ NNRTIs **(nevirapine)** are predicted to decrease the exposure to **rivaroxaban**. Severe Anecdotal

▶ **Olaparib** might increase the exposure to **edoxaban**. Moderate Theoretical

▶ **Osimertinib** is predicted to increase the exposure to **edoxaban**. Moderate Study

▶ **Pibrentasvir** with glecaprevir is predicted to increase the exposure to **edoxaban**. Moderate Study

▶ **Pitolisant** is predicted to decrease the exposure to **edoxaban**. Mild Theoretical

▶ **Ranolazine** is predicted to increase the exposure to **apixaban**. Moderate Theoretical

▶ **Ranolazine** is predicted to slightly increase the exposure to **edoxaban**. Severe Theoretical

▶ Rifamycins **(rifampicin)** are predicted to decrease the exposure to **apixaban**. Use with caution or avoid. Severe Study

▶ Rifamycins **(rifampicin)** are predicted to decrease the exposure to **edoxaban**. Moderate Study

▶ Rifamycins **(rifampicin)** are predicted to decrease the exposure to **rivaroxaban**. Avoid unless patient can be monitored for signs of thrombosis. Severe Study

▶ **St John's wort** is predicted to decrease the exposure to **apixaban**. Use with caution or avoid. Severe Study

▶ **St John's wort** is predicted to decrease the exposure to **edoxaban**. Moderate Study

▶ **St John's wort** is predicted to decrease the exposure to **rivaroxaban**. Avoid unless patient can be monitored for signs of thrombosis. Severe Study

▶ **Tepotinib** is predicted to increase the concentration of **edoxaban**. Severe Study

▶ **Vandetanib** is predicted to increase the exposure to **apixaban**. Moderate Theoretical

▶ **Velpatasvir** is predicted to increase the exposure to **edoxaban**. Severe Theoretical

▶ **Vemurafenib** is predicted to increase the exposure to **apixaban**. Moderate Theoretical

▶ **Vemurafenib** is predicted to slightly increase the exposure to **edoxaban**. Severe Theoretical

▶ **Venetoclax** is predicted to increase the exposure to factor XA inhibitors **(edoxaban, rivaroxaban)**. Avoid or adjust dose. Severe Study

▶ **Voxilaprevir** with sofosbuvir and velpatasvir is predicted to increase the concentration of **edoxaban**. Avoid. Severe Theoretical

Famotidine → see H₂ receptor antagonists

Fampridine

▶ **Dolutegravir** might increase the concentration of **fampridine**. Avoid. Severe Theoretical

▶ H₂ receptor antagonists **(cimetidine)** increase the concentration of **fampridine**. Avoid. Severe Theoretical

Febuxostat

▶ **Febuxostat** is predicted to increase the exposure to **alpelisib**. Moderate Theoretical

▶ **Febuxostat** is predicted to increase the exposure to **azathioprine**. Avoid. Severe Theoretical

▶ **Febuxostat** is predicted to increase the exposure to **cladribine**. Avoid or adjust dose. Moderate Theoretical

▶ **Febuxostat** is predicted to increase the exposure to **mercaptopurine**. Avoid. Severe Theoretical

▶ **Febuxostat** increases the exposure to statins **(rosuvastatin)**. Adjust **rosuvastatin** dose, p. 235. Moderate Study

▶ **Febuxostat** is predicted to increase the exposure to **tenofovir alafenamide**. Moderate Theoretical

▶ **Febuxostat** is predicted to increase the exposure to **tenofovir disoproxil**. Moderate Theoretical

▶ **Febuxostat** is predicted to increase the exposure to **topotecan**. Moderate Theoretical

Fedratinib

▶ **Fedratinib** is predicted to increase the exposure to **abemaciclib**. Moderate Study

▶ **Fedratinib** is predicted to increase the exposure to **acalabrutinib**. Avoid or monitor. Severe Study

▶ **Fedratinib** is predicted to increase the exposure to alpha blockers **(tamsulosin)**. Moderate Theoretical

▶ Anti-androgens **(apalutamide, enzalutamide)** are predicted to decrease the exposure to **fedratinib**. Avoid. Moderate Study

▶ Antiarrhythmics **(dronedarone)** are predicted to increase the exposure to **fedratinib**. Monitor and adjust dose. Moderate Study

▶ **Fedratinib** is predicted to increase the exposure to antiarrhythmics **(propafenone)**. Monitor and adjust dose. Moderate Study

▶ Antiepileptics **(carbamazepine, fosphenytoin, phenobarbital, phenytoin, primidone)** are predicted to decrease the exposure to **fedratinib**. Avoid. Moderate Study

▶ Antifungals, azoles **(fluconazole)** are predicted to increase the exposure to **fedratinib**. Avoid. Moderate Theoretical

▶ Antifungals, azoles **(isavuconazole)** are predicted to increase the exposure to **fedratinib**. Monitor and adjust dose. Moderate Study

▶ Antifungals, azoles **(itraconazole, ketoconazole, posaconazole, voriconazole)** are predicted to increase the exposure to **fedratinib**. Adjust dose, but avoid depending on other drugs taken—consult product literature. Moderate Study

▶ **Fedratinib** is predicted to increase the exposure to antihistamines, non-sedating **(mizolastine)**. Severe Theoretical

▶ **Fedratinib** is predicted to increase the exposure to antihistamines, non-sedating **(rupatadine)**. Avoid. Moderate Study

▶ **Fedratinib** is predicted to increase the exposure to antipsychotics, second generation **(cariprazine)**. Avoid. Severe Study

▶ **Fedratinib** is predicted to increase the exposure to antipsychotics, second generation **(quetiapine)**. Avoid. Moderate Study

▶ **Fedratinib** is predicted to increase the exposure to **avapritinib**. Avoid or adjust dose—consult product literature. Moderate Study

▶ **Fedratinib** is predicted to increase the exposure to **axitinib**. Moderate Study

Fedratinib (continued)

▸ **Fedratinib** might increases the exposure to bedaquiline. Mild Theoretical

▸ **Fedratinib** is predicted to increase the exposure to belzutifan. Monitor and adjust dose. Severe Theoretical

▸ **Fedratinib** is predicted to increase the exposure to benzodiazepines (alprazolam). Severe Study

▸ **Fedratinib** potentially increases the exposure to benzodiazepines (clobazam). Adjust dose. Moderate Theoretical

▸ **Fedratinib** is predicted to increase the exposure to benzodiazepines (midazolam). Monitor adverse effects and adjust dose. Severe Study

▸ Berotralstat is predicted to increase the exposure to **fedratinib**. Monitor and adjust dose. Moderate Study

▸ **Fedratinib** is predicted to increase the exposure to bosutinib. Avoid or adjust dose. Severe Study

▸ **Fedratinib** is predicted to increase the exposure to brigatinib. Moderate Study

▸ **Fedratinib** is predicted to increase the exposure to buspirone. Use with caution and adjust dose. Moderate Study

▸ **Fedratinib** is predicted to increase the exposure to cabozantinib. Moderate Study

▸ Calcium channel blockers (diltiazem, verapamil) are predicted to increase the exposure to **fedratinib**. Monitor and adjust dose. Moderate Study

▸ **Fedratinib** is predicted to increase the exposure to calcium channel blockers (amlodipine, felodipine, lacidipine, lercanidipine, nicardipine, nifedipine, nimodipine). Monitor and adjust dose. Moderate Study

▸ **Fedratinib** is predicted to increase the exposure to capivasertib. Adjust dose. Moderate Study

▸ Cenobamate is predicted to decrease the exposure to **fedratinib**. Avoid. Moderate Study

▸ Ceritinib is predicted to increase the exposure to **fedratinib**. Adjust dose, but avoid depending on other drugs taken— consult product literature. Moderate Study

▸ **Fedratinib** is predicted to increase the exposure to ceritinib. Moderate Study

▸ **Fedratinib** is predicted to decrease the efficacy of clopidogrel. Avoid. Moderate Study

▸ Cobicistat is predicted to increase the exposure to **fedratinib**. Adjust dose, but avoid depending on other drugs taken— consult product literature. Moderate Study

▸ **Fedratinib** is predicted to increase the exposure to cobimetinib. Severe Study

▸ **Fedratinib** is predicted to increase the exposure to colchicine. Adjust **colchicine** dose with moderate CYP3A4 inhibitors, p. 1279. Severe Study

▸ **Fedratinib** is predicted to increase the exposure to corticosteroids (methylprednisolone). Monitor and adjust dose. Moderate Study

▸ Crizotinib is predicted to increase the exposure to **fedratinib**. Monitor and adjust dose. Moderate Study

▸ **Fedratinib** is predicted to increase the exposure to dabrafenib. Moderate Study

▸ Dabrafenib is predicted to decrease the exposure to **fedratinib**. Avoid. Moderate Study

▸ **Fedratinib** is predicted to increase the exposure to daridorexant. Adjust **daridorexant** dose, p. 554. Severe Study

▸ **Fedratinib** is predicted to increase the exposure to dasatinib. Severe Study

▸ **Fedratinib** is predicted to slightly increase the exposure to dienogest. Moderate Study

▸ **Fedratinib** is predicted to increase the exposure to dipeptidylpeptidase-4 inhibitors (saxagliptin). Mild Study

▸ **Fedratinib** is predicted to increase the exposure to domperidone. Avoid. Severe Study

▸ **Fedratinib** is predicted to increase the exposure to dopamine receptor agonists (bromocriptine). Severe Theoretical

▸ **Fedratinib** is predicted to increase the exposure to drospirenone. Severe Study

▸ **Fedratinib** is predicted to moderately increase the exposure to dutasteride. Mild Study

▸ **Fedratinib** is predicted to increase the exposure to elacestrant. Avoid moderate CYP3A4 inhibitors or adjust **elacestrant** dose, p. 1084. Severe Theoretical

▸ **Fedratinib** is predicted to increase the exposure to elexacaftor. Adjust ivacaftor with tezacaftor and elexacaftor p. 337 dose with moderate CYP3A4 inhibitors. Severe Theoretical

▸ **Fedratinib** is predicted to increase the exposure to eliglustat. Avoid or adjust dose—consult product literature. Severe Study

▸ **Fedratinib** is predicted to moderately increase the exposure to encorafenib. Moderate Study

▸ Encorafenib is predicted to decrease the exposure to **fedratinib**. Avoid. Moderate Study

▸ Endothelin receptor antagonists (bosentan) are predicted to decrease the exposure to **fedratinib**. Avoid. Moderate Study

▸ **Fedratinib** is predicted to increase the exposure to endothelin receptor antagonists (macitentan). Manufacturer advises caution depending on other drugs taken—consult product literature. Moderate Theoretical

▸ **Fedratinib** is predicted to increase the exposure to entrectinib. Avoid or adjust dose with moderate CYP3A4 inhibitors— consult product literature. Severe Theoretical

▸ **Fedratinib** is predicted to increase the risk of ergotism when given with ergometrine. Severe Theoretical

▸ **Fedratinib** is predicted to increase the exposure to erlotinib. Moderate Study

▸ **Fedratinib** is predicted to increase the exposure to etrasimod. Avoid in poor CYP2C9 metabolisers. Severe Theoretical

▸ **Fedratinib** is predicted to increase the concentration of everolimus. Avoid or adjust dose. Moderate Study

▸ **Fedratinib** is predicted to increase the exposure to fesoterodine. Adjust **fesoterodine** dose with moderate CYP3A4 inhibitors in hepatic and renal impairment, p. 897. Mild Study

▸ **Fedratinib** is predicted to increase the exposure to gefitinib. Moderate Study

▸ Grapefruit and grapefruit juice is predicted to increase the exposure to **fedratinib**. Avoid. Moderate Theoretical

▸ **Fedratinib** is predicted to increase the concentration of guanfacine. Adjust **guanfacine** dose, p. 407. Moderate Theoretical

▸ HIV-protease inhibitors are predicted to increase the exposure to **fedratinib**. Adjust dose, but avoid depending on other drugs taken—consult product literature. Moderate Study

▸ **Fedratinib** is predicted to increase the exposure to ibrutinib. Adjust dose with moderate CYP3A4 inhibitors—consult product literature. Severe Study

▸ Idelalisib is predicted to increase the exposure to **fedratinib**. Adjust dose, but avoid depending on other drugs taken— consult product literature. Moderate Study

▸ Imatinib is predicted to increase the exposure to **fedratinib**. Monitor and adjust dose. Moderate Study

▸ **Fedratinib** is predicted to increase the exposure to ivacaftor. Adjust dose with moderate CYP3A4 inhibitors, see ivacaftor p. 336, tezacaftor with ivacaftor p. 339, and ivacaftor with tezacaftor and elexacaftor p. 337. Moderate Study

▸ **Fedratinib** is predicted to increase the exposure to ivosidenib. Monitor and adjust dose—consult product literature. Severe Study

▸ Ivosidenib is predicted to decrease the exposure to **fedratinib**. Avoid. Moderate Study

▸ **Fedratinib** is predicted to increase the exposure to lapatinib. Moderate Study

▸ **Fedratinib** is predicted to increase the exposure to larotrectinib. Monitor and adjust dose. Moderate Theoretical

▸ **Fedratinib** is predicted to increase the exposure to leniolisib. Avoid. Moderate Study

▸ Letermovir is predicted to increase the exposure to **fedratinib**. Monitor and adjust dose. Moderate Study

▸ **Fedratinib** is predicted to increase the exposure to lomitapide. Avoid. Moderate Theoretical

▸ Lorlatinib is predicted to decrease the exposure to **fedratinib**. Avoid. Moderate Study

▸ Lumacaftor is predicted to decrease the exposure to **fedratinib**. Avoid. Moderate Study

▸ Macrolides (clarithromycin) are predicted to increase the exposure to **fedratinib**. Adjust dose, but avoid depending on other drugs taken—consult product literature. Moderate Study

- Macrolides **(erythromycin)** are predicted to increase the exposure to **fedratinib**. Monitor and adjust dose. [Moderate] Study
- **Fedratinib** is predicted to increase the exposure to mavacamten. Adjust dose—consult product literature. [Moderate] Study
- **Fedratinib** is predicted to increase the exposure to midostaurin. [Moderate] Theoretical
- **Fedratinib** is predicted to increase the exposure to mineralocorticoid receptor antagonists **(eplerenone)**. Adjust **eplerenone** dose, p. 223. [Severe] Study
- **Fedratinib** is predicted to increase the exposure to mineralocorticoid receptor antagonists **(finerenone)**. [Severe] Study
- Mitotane is predicted to decrease the exposure to **fedratinib**. Avoid. [Moderate] Study
- **Fedratinib** is predicted to increase the exposure to mobocertinib. Avoid or adjust dose and monitor ECG—consult product literature. [Severe] Study
- **Fedratinib** is predicted to increase the exposure to naldemedine. [Moderate] Study
- **Fedratinib** is predicted to increase the exposure to naloxegol. Adjust **naloxegol** dose and monitor adverse effects, p. 72. [Moderate] Study
- **Fedratinib** is predicted to increase the exposure to neratinib. Avoid moderate CYP3A4 inhibitors or adjust dose and monitor for gastrointestinal adverse effects—consult product literature. [Severe] Study
- Neurokinin-1 receptor antagonists **(aprepitant, netupitant)** are predicted to increase the exposure to **fedratinib**. Monitor and adjust dose. [Moderate] Study
- Nilotinib is predicted to increase the exposure to **fedratinib**. Monitor and adjust dose. [Moderate] Study
- NNRTIs **(efavirenz, etravirine, nevirapine)** are predicted to decrease the exposure to **fedratinib**. Avoid. [Moderate] Study
- **Fedratinib** is predicted to increase the exposure to olaparib. Avoid or adjust dose with moderate CYP3A4 inhibitors—consult product literature. [Moderate] Theoretical
- **Fedratinib** is predicted to increase the exposure to opioids **(alfentanil, buprenorphine, fentanyl, oxycodone)**. Monitor and adjust dose. [Moderate] Study
- **Fedratinib** is predicted to increase the exposure to opioids **(methadone, sufentanil)**. [Moderate] Theoretical
- **Fedratinib** is predicted to increase the exposure to pazopanib. [Moderate] Study
- **Fedratinib** is predicted to increase the exposure to pemigatinib. [Severe] Study
- **Fedratinib** is predicted to increase the exposure to phosphodiesterase type-5 inhibitors **(avanafil)**. Adjust **avanafil** dose, p. 939. [Moderate] Theoretical
- **Fedratinib** is predicted to increase the exposure to phosphodiesterase type-5 inhibitors **(sildenafil)**. Monitor or adjust **sildenafil** dose with moderate CYP3A4 inhibitors, p. 940. [Moderate] Study
- **Fedratinib** is predicted to increase the exposure to phosphodiesterase type-5 inhibitors **(tadalafil)**. [Severe] Theoretical
- **Fedratinib** is predicted to increase the exposure to phosphodiesterase type-5 inhibitors **(vardenafil)**. Adjust dose. [Severe] Theoretical
- **Fedratinib** is predicted to increase the exposure to pimozide. Avoid. [Severe] Theoretical
- **Fedratinib** is predicted to increase the exposure to ponatinib. [Moderate] Study
- **Fedratinib** is predicted to increase the exposure to pralsetinib. [Moderate] Theoretical
- **Fedratinib** moderately increases the exposure to proton pump inhibitors **(omeprazole)**. Monitor and adjust dose. [Moderate] Study
- **Fedratinib** is predicted to increase the exposure to ranolazine. [Severe] Study
- **Fedratinib** is predicted to increase the exposure to regorafenib. [Moderate] Study
- **Fedratinib** is predicted to increase the exposure to ribociclib. [Moderate] Study
- Rifamycins **(rifampicin)** are predicted to decrease the exposure to **fedratinib**. Avoid. [Moderate] Study

- **Fedratinib** is predicted to increase the exposure to rimegepant. Avoid another dose of rimegepant within 48 hours of concurrent use. [Moderate] Study
- **Fedratinib** is predicted to increase the exposure to selpercatinib. [Moderate] Study
- **Fedratinib** is predicted to increase the exposure to selumetinib. Avoid or adjust dose—consult product literature. [Severe] Study
- **Fedratinib** is predicted to increase the exposure to siponimod. Avoid depending on other drugs taken—consult product literature. [Severe] Study
- **Fedratinib** increases the concentration of sirolimus. Monitor and adjust dose. [Moderate] Study
- Sotorasib is predicted to decrease the exposure to **fedratinib**. Avoid. [Moderate] Study
- SSRIs **(fluoxetine)** are predicted to increase the exposure to **fedratinib**. Avoid depending on other drugs taken—consult product literature. [Moderate] Theoretical
- SSRIs **(fluvoxamine)** are predicted to increase the exposure to **fedratinib**. Avoid. [Moderate] Theoretical
- **Fedratinib** is predicted to increase the exposure to SSRIs **(dapoxetine)**. Adjust **dapoxetine** dose with moderate CYP3A4 inhibitors, p. 947. [Moderate] Theoretical
- **Fedratinib** is predicted to increase the exposure to SSRIs **(escitalopram)**. Use with caution and adjust dose. [Severe] Study
- St John's wort is predicted to decrease the exposure to **fedratinib**. Avoid. [Moderate] Study
- **Fedratinib** is predicted to increase the exposure to sunitinib. [Moderate] Study
- **Fedratinib** is predicted to increase the concentration of tacrolimus. [Severe] Study
- **Fedratinib** is predicted to increase the exposure to taxanes **(cabazitaxel)**. [Moderate] Theoretical
- **Fedratinib** is predicted to increase the exposure to taxanes **(docetaxel)**. [Severe] Study
- **Fedratinib** is predicted to increase the exposure to taxanes **(paclitaxel)**. [Moderate] Anecdotal
- **Fedratinib** is predicted to increase the exposure to temsirolimus (oral). Monitor and adjust dose. [Moderate] Theoretical
- **Fedratinib** is predicted to increase the exposure to tezacaftor. Adjust dose with moderate CYP3A4 inhibitors, see tezacaftor with ivacaftor p. 339 and ivacaftor with tezacaftor and elexacaftor p. 337. [Severe] Study
- **Fedratinib** is predicted to increase the exposure to tolvaptan. Manufacturer advises caution or adjust **tolvaptan** dose with moderate CYP3A4 inhibitors, p. 767. [Moderate] Study
- **Fedratinib** is predicted to increase the exposure to trazodone. [Moderate] Theoretical
- Tucatinib is predicted to increase the exposure to **fedratinib**. Adjust dose, but avoid depending on other drugs taken—consult product literature. [Moderate] Study
- **Fedratinib** is predicted to increase the exposure to vemurafenib. [Severe] Theoretical
- **Fedratinib** is predicted to increase the exposure to venetoclax. Avoid or adjust dose—consult product literature. [Severe] Study
- **Fedratinib** is predicted to increase the exposure to vinca alkaloids. [Severe] Theoretical
- **Fedratinib** is predicted to increase the exposure to voclosporin. Adjust **voclosporin** dose, p. 973. [Severe] Study
- **Fedratinib** is predicted to increase the exposure to zanubrutinib. Avoid or adjust dose with moderate CYP3A4 inhibitors—consult product literature. [Severe] Study
- **Fedratinib** is predicted to increase the exposure to zopiclone. Adjust dose. [Moderate] Study

Felbinac → see NSAIDs

Felodipine → see calcium channel blockers

Fenfluramine → see TABLE 12 p. 1574 (serotonin syndrome)

- **Fenfluramine** might decrease blood glucose concentrations when given with acarbose. [Moderate] Theoretical
- Anti-androgens **(apalutamide, enzalutamide)** are predicted to decrease the exposure to **fenfluramine**. [Moderate] Theoretical
- Antiepileptics **(carbamazepine)** are predicted to decrease the concentration of **fenfluramine**. Adjust dose. [Moderate] Theoretical

Fenfluramine (continued)

▸ Antiepileptics (fosphenytoin, phenobarbital, phenytoin, primidone) are predicted to decrease the exposure to fenfluramine. Moderate Theoretical

▸ Antiepileptics (stiripentol) (given with clobazam, and with or without valproate) modestly increase the exposure to fenfluramine. Adjust fenfluramine dose, p. 361. Severe Study

▸ Antihistamines, sedating (cyproheptadine) might decrease the efficacy of fenfluramine. Severe Theoretical

▸ Bupropion is predicted to increase the exposure to fenfluramine. Moderate Study

▸ Cinacalcet is predicted to increase the exposure to fenfluramine. Moderate Study

▸ Dacomitinib is predicted to increase the exposure to fenfluramine. Moderate Study

▸ Fenfluramine might decrease blood glucose concentrations when given with dipeptidylpeptidase-4 inhibitors. Moderate Theoretical

▸ Fenfluramine might decrease blood glucose concentrations when given with glucagon-like peptide-1 receptor agonists. Moderate Theoretical

▸ Fenfluramine might decrease blood glucose concentrations when given with insulin. Moderate Theoretical

▸ Fenfluramine might decrease blood glucose concentrations when given with meglitinides. Moderate Theoretical

▸ Fenfluramine might decrease blood glucose concentrations when given with metformin. Moderate Theoretical

▸ Mitotane is predicted to decrease the exposure to fenfluramine. Moderate Theoretical

▸ Fenfluramine might decrease blood glucose concentrations when given with pioglitazone. Moderate Theoretical

▸ Rifamycins (rifampicin) are predicted to decrease the concentration of fenfluramine. Moderate Theoretical

▸ Fenfluramine might decrease blood glucose concentrations when given with sodium glucose co-transporter 2 inhibitors. Moderate Theoretical

▸ SSRIs (fluoxetine, paroxetine) are predicted to increase the exposure to fenfluramine. Moderate Study → Also see **TABLE 12** p. 1574

▸ SSRIs (fluvoxamine) moderately increase the exposure to fenfluramine. Moderate Study → Also see **TABLE 12** p. 1574

▸ Fenfluramine might decrease blood glucose concentrations when given with sulfonylureas. Moderate Theoretical

▸ Terbinafine is predicted to increase the exposure to fenfluramine. Moderate Study

Fenofibrate → see fibrates

Fentanyl → see opioids

Fesoterodine → see **TABLE 9** p. 1573 (antimuscarinics)

▸ Anti-androgens (apalutamide, enzalutamide) are predicted to decrease the exposure to fesoterodine. Avoid. Moderate Study

▸ Antiarrhythmics (dronedarone) are predicted to increase the exposure to fesoterodine. Adjust fesoterodine dose with moderate CYP3A4 inhibitors in hepatic and renal impairment, p. 897. Mild Study

▸ Antiepileptics (carbamazepine, fosphenytoin, phenobarbital, phenytoin, primidone) are predicted to decrease the exposure to fesoterodine. Avoid. Moderate Study

▸ Antifungals, azoles (fluconazole, isavuconazole) are predicted to increase the exposure to fesoterodine. Adjust fesoterodine dose with moderate CYP3A4 inhibitors in hepatic and renal impairment, p. 897. Mild Study

▸ Antifungals, azoles (itraconazole, ketoconazole, posaconazole, voriconazole) are predicted to moderately increase the exposure to fesoterodine. Adjust fesoterodine dose with potent CYP3A4 inhibitors; avoid in hepatic and renal impairment, p. 897. Severe Study

▸ Antipsychotics, second generation (clozapine) can cause constipation, as can fesoterodine; concurrent use might increase the risk of developing intestinal obstruction. Severe Theoretical → Also see **TABLE 9** p. 1573

▸ Berotralstat is predicted to increase the exposure to fesoterodine. Adjust fesoterodine dose with moderate CYP3A4 inhibitors in hepatic and renal impairment, p. 897. Mild Study

▸ Bupropion is predicted to increase the exposure to fesoterodine. Use with caution and adjust dose. Mild Theoretical

▸ Calcium channel blockers (diltiazem, verapamil) are predicted to increase the exposure to fesoterodine. Adjust fesoterodine dose with moderate CYP3A4 inhibitors in hepatic and renal impairment, p. 897. Mild Study

▸ Ceritinib is predicted to moderately increase the exposure to fesoterodine. Adjust fesoterodine dose with potent CYP3A4 inhibitors; avoid in hepatic and renal impairment, p. 897. Severe Study

▸ Cinacalcet is predicted to increase the exposure to fesoterodine. Use with caution and adjust dose. Mild Theoretical

▸ Cobicistat is predicted to moderately increase the exposure to fesoterodine. Adjust fesoterodine dose with potent CYP3A4 inhibitors; avoid in hepatic and renal impairment, p. 897. Severe Study

▸ Crizotinib is predicted to increase the exposure to fesoterodine. Adjust fesoterodine dose with moderate CYP3A4 inhibitors in hepatic and renal impairment, p. 897. Mild Study

▸ Dacomitinib is predicted to increase the exposure to fesoterodine. Use with caution and adjust dose. Mild Theoretical

▸ Encorafenib is predicted to decrease the exposure to fesoterodine. Avoid. Moderate Study

▸ Fedratinib is predicted to increase the exposure to fesoterodine. Adjust fesoterodine dose with moderate CYP3A4 inhibitors in hepatic and renal impairment, p. 897. Mild Study

▸ HIV-protease inhibitors are predicted to moderately increase the exposure to fesoterodine. Adjust fesoterodine dose with potent CYP3A4 inhibitors; avoid in hepatic and renal impairment, p. 897. Severe Study

▸ Idelalisib is predicted to moderately increase the exposure to fesoterodine. Adjust fesoterodine dose with potent CYP3A4 inhibitors; avoid in hepatic and renal impairment, p. 897. Severe Study

▸ Imatinib is predicted to increase the exposure to fesoterodine. Adjust fesoterodine dose with moderate CYP3A4 inhibitors in hepatic and renal impairment, p. 897. Mild Study

▸ Ivosidenib is predicted to decrease the exposure to fesoterodine. Avoid. Moderate Study

▸ Letermovir is predicted to increase the exposure to fesoterodine. Adjust fesoterodine dose with moderate CYP3A4 inhibitors in hepatic and renal impairment, p. 897. Mild Study

▸ Lumacaftor is predicted to decrease the exposure to fesoterodine. Avoid. Moderate Study

▸ Macrolides (clarithromycin) are predicted to moderately increase the exposure to fesoterodine. Adjust fesoterodine dose with potent CYP3A4 inhibitors; avoid in hepatic and renal impairment, p. 897. Severe Study

▸ Macrolides (erythromycin) are predicted to increase the exposure to fesoterodine. Adjust fesoterodine dose with moderate CYP3A4 inhibitors in hepatic and renal impairment, p. 897. Mild Study

▸ Mitotane is predicted to decrease the exposure to fesoterodine. Avoid. Moderate Study

▸ Neurokinin-1 receptor antagonists (aprepitant, netupitant) are predicted to increase the exposure to fesoterodine. Adjust fesoterodine dose with moderate CYP3A4 inhibitors in hepatic and renal impairment, p. 897. Mild Study

▸ Nilotinib is predicted to increase the exposure to fesoterodine. Adjust fesoterodine dose with moderate CYP3A4 inhibitors in hepatic and renal impairment, p. 897. Mild Study

▸ Rifamycins (rifampicin) are predicted to decrease the exposure to fesoterodine. Avoid. Moderate Study

▸ SSRIs (fluoxetine, paroxetine) are predicted to increase the exposure to fesoterodine. Use with caution and adjust dose. Mild Theoretical

▸ St John's wort is predicted to decrease the exposure to fesoterodine. Avoid. Severe Theoretical

▸ Terbinafine is predicted to increase the exposure to fesoterodine. Use with caution and adjust dose. Mild Theoretical

▸ Tucatinib is predicted to moderately increase the exposure to fesoterodine. Adjust fesoterodine dose with potent CYP3A4 inhibitors; avoid in hepatic and renal impairment, p. 897. Severe Study

Fexofenadine → see antihistamines, non-sedating

Fezolinetant

- **Combined hormonal contraceptives** is predicted to increase the exposure to **fezolinetant**. Avoid. [Moderate] Study
- **Givosiran** is predicted to increase the exposure to **fezolinetant**. Avoid. [Moderate] Study
- **Mexiletine** is predicted to increase the exposure to **fezolinetant**. Avoid. [Moderate] Study
- **Osilodrostat** is predicted to increase the exposure to **fezolinetant**. Avoid. [Moderate] Study
- **Quinolones (ciprofloxacin)** are predicted to increase the exposure to **fezolinetant**. Avoid. [Moderate] Study
- **Rucaparib** is predicted to increase the exposure to **fezolinetant**. Avoid. [Moderate] Study
- **SSRIs (fluvoxamine)** are predicted to increase the exposure to **fezolinetant**. Avoid. [Moderate] Study
- **Vemurafenib** is predicted to increase the exposure to **fezolinetant**. Avoid. [Moderate] Study

Fibrates

bezafibrate · ciprofibrate · fenofibrate · gemfibrozil

- **Acipimox** is predicted to increase the risk of rhabdomyolysis when given with **fibrates**. [Severe] Theoretical
- Oral **antacids** decrease the exposure to oral **gemfibrozil**. [Moderate] Study
- **Gemfibrozil** slightly increases the exposure to anti-androgens (apalutamide). [Mild] Study
- **Gemfibrozil** moderately increases the exposure to anti-androgens (enzalutamide). Avoid or adjust **enzalutamide** dose, p. 1078. [Severe] Study
- **Gemfibrozil** is predicted to increase the exposure to antihistamines, non-sedating (fexofenadine). [Moderate] Theoretical
- **Gemfibrozil** is predicted to increase the exposure to atogepant. Adjust **atogepant** dose, p. 540. [Moderate] Theoretical
- **Bezafibrate** is predicted to increase the risk of nephrotoxicity when given with ciclosporin. [Severe] Theoretical
- **Fenofibrate** increases the risk of nephrotoxicity when given with ciclosporin. [Severe] Study
- **Colchicine** increases the risk of rhabdomyolysis when given with **fibrates**. [Severe] Anecdotal
- **Fibrates** are predicted to increase the anticoagulant effect of coumarins. Monitor INR and adjust dose. [Severe] Study
- **Gemfibrozil** is predicted to increase the exposure to dabrafenib. [Moderate] Theoretical
- **Fibrates** are predicted to increase the risk of rhabdomyolysis when given with daptomycin. [Severe] Theoretical
- **Gemfibrozil** are predicted to increases the exposure to etrasimod. Avoid in poor CYP2C9 metabolisers. [Severe] Theoretical
- **Fibrates** are predicted to increase the risk of gallstones when given with ezetimibe. [Severe] Theoretical
- **Fibrates** are predicted to increase the risk of hypoglycaemia when given with insulin. [Moderate] Theoretical
- **Gemfibrozil** is predicted to increase the exposure to irinotecan. Avoid. [Moderate] Theoretical
- **Gemfibrozil** is predicted to increase the concentration of letermovir. [Moderate] Study
- **Gemfibrozil** increases the exposure to meglitinides (repaglinide). Avoid. [Severe] Study
- **Gemfibrozil** is predicted to increase the exposure to momelotinib. [Moderate] Study
- **Gemfibrozil** is predicted to moderately increase the exposure to montelukast. [Moderate] Study
- **Gemfibrozil** is predicted to increase the exposure to the active metabolites of ozanimod. [Moderate] Study
- **Fibrates** are predicted to increase the anticoagulant effect of phenindione. Monitor INR and adjust dose. [Severe] Study
- **Gemfibrozil** increases the exposure to pioglitazone. Monitor blood glucose and adjust dose. [Severe] Study
- **Gemfibrozil** is predicted to increase the exposure to retinoids (alitretinoin). Adjust **alitretinoin** dose, p. 1433. [Moderate] Theoretical
- **Gemfibrozil** increases the concentration of retinoids (bexarotene). Avoid. [Severe] Study
- **Gemfibrozil** moderately increases the exposure to roxadustat. Monitor haemoglobin and adjust dose. [Moderate] Study
- **Gemfibrozil** increases the exposure to selexipag. Avoid. [Severe] Study
- **Ciprofibrate** increases the risk of rhabdomyolysis when given with statins (atorvastatin). Avoid or adjust dose. [Severe] Study
- **Fenofibrate** increases the risk of rhabdomyolysis when given with statins (atorvastatin). Monitor and adjust **fenofibrate** dose, p. 231. [Severe] Anecdotal
- **Gemfibrozil** causes a small increase in the exposure to statins (atorvastatin). Avoid. [Severe] Study
- **Bezafibrate** increases the risk of rhabdomyolysis when given with statins (atorvastatin, fluvastatin). [Severe] Study
- **Ciprofibrate** increases the risk of rhabdomyolysis when given with statins (fluvastatin). [Severe] Study
- **Fenofibrate** is predicted to increase the risk of rhabdomyolysis when given with statins (fluvastatin). Use with caution and adjust **fenofibrate** dose, p. 231. [Severe] Theoretical
- **Gemfibrozil** increases the risk of rhabdomyolysis when given with statins (fluvastatin). [Severe] Anecdotal
- **Fenofibrate** is predicted to increase the risk of rhabdomyolysis when given with statins (pravastatin). Avoid. [Severe] Theoretical
- **Gemfibrozil** modestly increases the exposure to statins (pravastatin). Avoid or monitor. [Severe] Study
- **Fibrates (bezafibrate, ciprofibrate)** increase the risk of rhabdomyolysis when given with statins (pravastatin). Avoid. [Severe] Study
- **Fenofibrate** increases the risk of rhabdomyolysis when given with statins (rosuvastatin). Adjust **fenofibrate** and **rosuvastatin** doses, p. 231, p. 235. [Severe] Anecdotal
- **Gemfibrozil** causes a small increase in the exposure to statins (rosuvastatin). Avoid or adjust **rosuvastatin** dose, p. 235. [Severe] Study
- **Fibrates (bezafibrate, ciprofibrate)** increase the risk of rhabdomyolysis when given with statins (rosuvastatin). Adjust **rosuvastatin** dose, p. 235. [Severe] Study
- **Fenofibrate** increases the risk of rhabdomyolysis when given with statins (simvastatin). Adjust **fenofibrate** dose, p. 231. [Severe] Anecdotal
- **Gemfibrozil** modestly increases the exposure to statins (simvastatin). Avoid. [Severe] Anecdotal
- **Fibrates (bezafibrate, ciprofibrate)** increase the risk of rhabdomyolysis when given with statins (simvastatin). Adjust **simvastatin** dose, p. 237. [Severe] Study
- **Fibrates** are predicted to increase the risk of hypoglycaemia when given with sulfonylureas. [Moderate] Theoretical
- **Gemfibrozil** is predicted to increase the exposure to taxanes (docetaxel). [Moderate] Theoretical
- **Gemfibrozil** is predicted to increase the concentration of taxanes (paclitaxel). [Severe] Anecdotal
- **Gemfibrozil** increases the exposure to treprostinil. Adjust dose. [Moderate] Study
- **Gemfibrozil** is predicted to increase the exposure to tucatinib. Avoid or adjust dose—consult product literature. [Severe] Study
- **Fibrates** are predicted to decrease the efficacy of ursodeoxycholic acid. Avoid. [Severe] Theoretical

Fidaxomicin

- **Antiarrhythmics (amiodarone, dronedarone)** are predicted to increase the exposure to **fidaxomicin**. Avoid. [Moderate] Study
- **Antifungals, azoles (itraconazole, ketoconazole)** are predicted to increase the exposure to **fidaxomicin**. Avoid. [Moderate] Study
- **Calcium channel blockers (verapamil)** are predicted to increase the exposure to **fidaxomicin**. Avoid. [Moderate] Study
- **Ciclosporin** is predicted to increase the exposure to **fidaxomicin**. Avoid. [Moderate] Study
- **Cobicistat** is predicted to increase the exposure to **fidaxomicin**. Avoid. [Moderate] Study
- **Glecaprevir** is predicted to increase the exposure to **fidaxomicin**. Avoid. [Moderate] Study
- **HIV-protease inhibitors (lopinavir, ritonavir)** are predicted to increase the exposure to **fidaxomicin**. Avoid. [Moderate] Study
- **Lapatinib** is predicted to increase the exposure to **fidaxomicin**. Avoid. [Moderate] Study
- **Macrolides** are predicted to increase the exposure to **fidaxomicin**. Avoid. [Moderate] Study
- **Pibrentasvir** is predicted to increase the exposure to **fidaxomicin**. Avoid. [Moderate] Study

Fidaxomicin (continued)

▸ **Ranolazine** is predicted to increase the exposure to fidaxomicin. Avoid. [Moderate] Study
▸ **Velpatasvir** is predicted to increase the exposure to fidaxomicin. Avoid. [Moderate] Study
▸ **Vemurafenib** is predicted to increase the exposure to fidaxomicin. Avoid. [Moderate] Study
▸ **Voxilaprevir** is predicted to increase the exposure to fidaxomicin. Avoid. [Moderate] Study

Filgotinib

▸ **Filgotinib** is predicted to increase the risk of immunosuppression when given with **abatacept**. Avoid. [Severe] Theoretical
▸ **Filgotinib** is predicted to increase the risk of immunosuppression when given with **anakinra**. Avoid. [Severe] Theoretical
▸ **Filgotinib** is predicted to increase the risk of immunosuppression when given with **baricitinib**. Avoid. [Severe] Theoretical
▸ **Filgotinib** is predicted to increase the risk of immunosuppression when given with **ciclosporin**. Avoid. [Severe] Theoretical
▸ **Filgotinib** is predicted to increase the risk of immunosuppression when given with **etanercept**. Avoid. [Severe] Theoretical
▸ **Live vaccines** are predicted to increase the risk of generalised infection (possibly life-threatening) when given with filgotinib. Avoid. [Severe] Theoretical
▸ **Filgotinib** is predicted to increase the risk of immunosuppression when given with **monoclonal antibodies (adalimumab, certolizumab pegol, golimumab, infliximab, rituximab, sarilumab, secukinumab, tocilizumab)**. Avoid. [Severe] Theoretical
▸ **Filgotinib** is predicted to increase the risk of immunosuppression when given with **tacrolimus**. Avoid. [Severe] Theoretical
▸ **Filgotinib** is predicted to increase the risk of immunosuppression when given with **tofacitinib**. Avoid. [Severe] Theoretical
▸ **Filgotinib** is predicted to increase the risk of immunosuppression when given with **upadacitinib**. Avoid. [Severe] Theoretical

Filgrastim

▸ **Filgrastim** might increase the risk of pulmonary toxicity when given with **bleomycin**. [Severe] Theoretical

Finerenone → see mineralocorticoid receptor antagonists

Fingolimod → see TABLE 5 p. 1572 (bradycardia), TABLE 8 p. 1573 (QT-interval prolongation)

▸ **Live vaccines** might increase the risk of generalised infection (possibly life-threatening) when given with **fingolimod**. UKHSA advises avoid (refer to Green Book). [Severe] Theoretical
▸ **Monoclonal antibodies (alemtuzumab)** are predicted to increase the risk of generalised infection (possibly life-threatening) when given with **fingolimod**. Avoid. [Severe] Theoretical
▸ **St John's wort** is predicted to decrease the exposure to **fingolimod**. Avoid. [Moderate] Theoretical

Flavoxate → see TABLE 9 p. 1573 (antimuscarinics)

▸ **Antipsychotics, second generation (clozapine)** can cause constipation, as can **flavoxate**; concurrent use might increase the risk of developing intestinal obstruction. [Severe] Theoretical → Also see TABLE 9 p. 1573

Flecainide → see antiarrhythmics
Flucloxacillin → see penicillins
Fluconazole → see antifungals, azoles

Flucytosine

▸ **Amphotericin B** increases the risk of toxicity when given with **flucytosine**. [Severe] Study
▸ **Cytarabine** decreases the concentration of **flucytosine**. Avoid. [Severe] Study
▸ **NRTIs (zidovudine)** increase the risk of haematological toxicity when given with **flucytosine**. Monitor and adjust dose. [Severe] Theoretical

Fludarabine → see TABLE 1 p. 1571 (hepatotoxicity), TABLE 14 p. 1575 (myelosuppression)

▸ **Live vaccines** are predicted to increase the risk of generalised infection (possibly life-threatening) when given with **fludarabine**. UKHSA advises avoid (refer to Green Book). [Severe] Theoretical
▸ **Fludarabine** increases the risk of pulmonary toxicity when given with **pentostatin**. Avoid. [Severe] Study → Also see TABLE 14 p. 1575

Fludrocortisone → see corticosteroids

Fluocinolone

ROUTE-SPECIFIC INFORMATION With intravitreal use of **fluocinolone** in adults: caution with concurrent administration of anticoagulant or antiplatelet drugs (higher incidence of conjunctival haemorrhage). Interactions do not generally apply to corticosteroids used for topical action unless specified.

Fluorouracil → see TABLE 1 p. 1571 (hepatotoxicity), TABLE 14 p. 1575 (myelosuppression)

ROUTE-SPECIFIC INFORMATION Since systemic absorption can follow topical application of **fluorouracil**, the possibility of interactions should be borne in mind.

▸ **Fluorouracil** increases the concentration of **antiepileptics (fosphenytoin, phenytoin)**. Monitor concentration and adjust dose. [Severe] Anecdotal
▸ **Fluorouracil** increases the anticoagulant effect of **coumarins**. [Severe] Anecdotal
▸ **Folates (folic acid)** are predicted to increase the risk of toxicity when given with **fluorouracil**. Avoid. [Severe] Theoretical
▸ **Folates (folinic acid)** are predicted to increase the risk of toxicity when given with **fluorouracil**. Monitor and adjust dose. [Severe] Theoretical
▸ **H₂ receptor antagonists (cimetidine)** slightly increase the exposure to **fluorouracil**. [Severe] Study
▸ **Live vaccines** are predicted to increase the risk of generalised infection (possibly life-threatening) when given with **fluorouracil**. UKHSA advises avoid (refer to Green Book). [Severe] Theoretical
▸ **Methotrexate** potentially increases the risk of severe skin reaction when given with topical **fluorouracil**. [Severe] Anecdotal → Also see TABLE 1 p. 1571 → Also see TABLE 14 p. 1575
▸ **Metronidazole** increases the risk of toxicity when given with **fluorouracil**. [Severe] Study

Fluoxetine → see SSRIs

Flupentixol → see TABLE 17 p. 1576 (hyponatraemia), TABLE 7 p. 1572 (hypotension), TABLE 9 p. 1573 (antimuscarinics), TABLE 10 p. 1574 (CNS effects)

▸ **Antipsychotics, second generation (clozapine)** can cause constipation, as can **flupentixol**; concurrent use might increase the risk of developing intestinal obstruction. [Severe] Theoretical → Also see TABLE 17 p. 1576 → Also see TABLE 7 p. 1572 → Also see TABLE 9 p. 1573 → Also see TABLE 10 p. 1574
▸ **Flupentixol** is predicted to decrease the effects of **dopamine receptor agonists**. Avoid. [Moderate] Theoretical → Also see TABLE 7 p. 1572 → Also see TABLE 9 p. 1573 → Also see TABLE 10 p. 1574
▸ **Flupentixol** opposes the effects of the active metabolite of **foslevodopa**. [Severe] Theoretical → Also see TABLE 7 p. 1572 → Also see TABLE 10 p. 1574
▸ **Flupentixol** decreases the effects of **levodopa**. Avoid or monitor worsening parkinsonian symptoms. [Severe] Theoretical → Also see TABLE 7 p. 1572 → Also see TABLE 10 p. 1574

Flurazepam → see benzodiazepines
Flurbiprofen → see NSAIDs
Flutamide → see anti-androgens
Fluticasone → see corticosteroids
Fluvastatin → see statins
Fluvoxamine → see SSRIs

Folates

folic acid · folinic acid · levofolinic acid

▸ **Folates** are predicted to decrease the concentration of **antiepileptics (fosphenytoin, phenobarbital, phenytoin, primidone)**. Monitor concentration and adjust dose. [Severe] Study
▸ **Folates** are predicted to increase the risk of toxicity when given with **capecitabine**. [Severe] Anecdotal

- **Folic acid** is predicted to increase the risk of toxicity when given with **fluorouracil**. Avoid. Severe Theoretical
- **Folinic acid** is predicted to increase the risk of toxicity when given with **fluorouracil**. Monitor and adjust dose. Severe Theoretical
- **Glucarpidase** decreases the exposure to **folinic acid**. Separate administration by at least 2 hours. Moderate Study
- **Glucarpidase** might decrease the exposure to **levofolinic acid**. Separate administration by at least 2 hours. Moderate Theoretical
- **Folates** are predicted to alter the effects of **raltitrexed**. Avoid. Moderate Study
- **Sulfasalazine** is predicted to decrease the absorption of **folates**. Moderate Study
- **Folates** are predicted to increase the risk of toxicity when given with **tegafur**. Severe Theoretical

Folic acid → see folates
Folinic acid → see folates
Fondaparinux → see factor XA inhibitors
Formoterol → see beta₂ agonists
Fosamprenavir → see HIV-protease inhibitors
Fosaprepitant → see neurokinin-1 receptor antagonists
Foscarnet → see TABLE 2 p. 1571 (nephrotoxicity)

- **Foscarnet** increases the risk of hypocalcaemia when given with **pentamidine**. Severe Anecdotal → Also see TABLE 2 p. 1571
- **Foscarnet** might decrease the antidiuretic and hypertensive effects of **vasopressin**. Moderate Theoretical

Fosinopril → see ACE inhibitors
Foslevodopa → see TABLE 7 p. 1572 (hypotension), TABLE 10 p. 1574 (CNS effects)

- **Antiepileptics (phenytoin)** might decrease the effects of **foslevodopa**. Moderate Theoretical → Also see TABLE 10 p. 1574
- **Antipsychotics, second generation** might decrease the effects of the active metabolite of **foslevodopa**. Severe Theoretical → Also see TABLE 7 p. 1572 → Also see TABLE 10 p. 1574
- **Benperidol** opposes the effects of the active metabolite of **foslevodopa**. Severe Theoretical → Also see TABLE 7 p. 1572 → Also see TABLE 10 p. 1574
- **Benzodiazepines** might decrease the effects of **foslevodopa**. Moderate Theoretical → Also see TABLE 10 p. 1574
- **Dopamine receptor agonists (amantadine)** might increase the adverse effects of **foslevodopa**. Adjust dose. Moderate Theoretical → Also see TABLE 7 p. 1572
- **Droperidol** opposes the effects of the active metabolite of **foslevodopa**. Severe Theoretical → Also see TABLE 7 p. 1572 → Also see TABLE 10 p. 1574
- **Entacapone** might increase the exposure to the active metabolite of **foslevodopa**. Adjust dose. Moderate Theoretical
- **Flupentixol** opposes the effects of the active metabolite of **foslevodopa**. Severe Theoretical → Also see TABLE 7 p. 1572 → Also see TABLE 10 p. 1574
- **Haloperidol** opposes the effects of the active metabolite of **foslevodopa**. Severe Theoretical → Also see TABLE 7 p. 1572 → Also see TABLE 10 p. 1574
- **Isoniazid** might decrease the effects of **foslevodopa**. Moderate Theoretical
- **Loxapine** opposes the effects of the active metabolite of **foslevodopa**. Severe Theoretical → Also see TABLE 7 p. 1572 → Also see TABLE 10 p. 1574
- **MAO-B inhibitors** are predicted to increase the dopaminergic effects of **foslevodopa**. Adjust dose. Mild Theoretical → Also see TABLE 7 p. 1572
- **MAOIs, irreversible** might cause a hypertensive crisis when given with **foslevodopa**. Avoid and for 14 days after stopping the MAOI. Severe Theoretical → Also see TABLE 7 p. 1572
- **Metoclopramide** might decrease the effects of **foslevodopa**. Moderate Theoretical
- **Moclobemide** might increase the adverse effects of **foslevodopa**. Moderate Theoretical
- **Opicapone** might increase the exposure to the active metabolite of **foslevodopa**. Adjust dose. Moderate Theoretical
- **Phenothiazines** oppose the effects of the active metabolite of **foslevodopa**. Severe Theoretical → Also see TABLE 7 p. 1572 → Also see TABLE 10 p. 1574

- **Pimozide** opposes the effects of the active metabolite of **foslevodopa**. Severe Theoretical → Also see TABLE 7 p. 1572 → Also see TABLE 10 p. 1574
- **Sulpiride** opposes the effects of the active metabolite of **foslevodopa**. Severe Theoretical → Also see TABLE 7 p. 1572 → Also see TABLE 10 p. 1574
- **Sympathomimetics, vasoconstrictor (adrenaline/epinephrine, noradrenaline/norepinephrine)** might increase the cardiovascular adverse effects of the active metabolite of **foslevodopa**. Moderate Theoretical
- **Tolcapone** might increase the exposure to the active metabolite of **foslevodopa**. Adjust dose. Moderate Theoretical
- **Zuclopenthixol** opposes the effects of the active metabolite of **foslevodopa**. Severe Theoretical → Also see TABLE 7 p. 1572 → Also see TABLE 10 p. 1574

Fosphenytoin → see antiepileptics
Fostamatinib

- **Fostamatinib** is predicted to increase the exposure to **alpelisib**. Moderate Theoretical
- **Anti-androgens (apalutamide, enzalutamide)** are predicted to decrease the exposure to **fostamatinib**. Avoid. Severe Study
- **Antiepileptics (carbamazepine, fosphenytoin, phenobarbital, phenytoin, primidone)** are predicted to decrease the exposure to **fostamatinib**. Avoid. Severe Study
- **Antifungals, azoles (itraconazole, ketoconazole, posaconazole, voriconazole)** are predicted to increase the exposure to **fostamatinib**. Monitor adverse effects and adjust dose. Moderate Study
- **Calcium channel blockers (diltiazem)** are predicted to increase the exposure to **fostamatinib**. Monitor adverse effects and adjust dose. Moderate Theoretical
- **Ceritinib** is predicted to increase the exposure to **fostamatinib**. Monitor adverse effects and adjust dose. Moderate Study
- **Fostamatinib** is predicted to increase the exposure to **cladribine**. Avoid or adjust dose. Moderate Theoretical
- **Cobicistat** is predicted to increase the exposure to **fostamatinib**. Monitor adverse effects and adjust dose. Moderate Study
- **Fostamatinib** might cause bleeding when given with **coumarins (acenocoumarol)**. Moderate Theoretical
- **Fostamatinib** might causes bleeding when given with **coumarins (warfarin)**. Moderate Theoretical
- **Encorafenib** is predicted to decrease the exposure to **fostamatinib**. Avoid. Severe Study
- **Fostamatinib** is predicted to increase the exposure to **everolimus**. Monitor and adjust dose. Moderate Theoretical
- **Grapefruit** juice is predicted to increase the exposure to **fostamatinib**. Monitor adverse effects and adjust dose. Moderate Theoretical
- **HIV-protease inhibitors** are predicted to increase the exposure to **fostamatinib**. Monitor adverse effects and adjust dose. Moderate Study
- **Idelalisib** is predicted to increase the exposure to **fostamatinib**. Monitor adverse effects and adjust dose. Moderate Study
- **Ivosidenib** is predicted to decrease the exposure to **fostamatinib**. Avoid. Severe Study
- **Lumacaftor** is predicted to decrease the exposure to **fostamatinib**. Avoid. Severe Study
- **Macrolides (clarithromycin)** are predicted to increase the exposure to **fostamatinib**. Monitor adverse effects and adjust dose. Moderate Study
- **Mitotane** is predicted to decrease the exposure to **fostamatinib**. Avoid. Severe Study
- **Nirmatrelvir** boosted with ritonavir is predicted to increase the concentration of **fostamatinib**. Monitor adverse effects and adjust dose. Moderate Theoretical
- **Fostamatinib** is predicted to increase the exposure to **opioids (alfentanil)**. Monitor and adjust dose. Moderate Theoretical
- **Fostamatinib** might cause bleeding when given with **phenindione**. Moderate Theoretical
- **Rifamycins (rifampicin)** are predicted to decrease the exposure to **fostamatinib**. Avoid. Severe Study
- **Fostamatinib** is predicted to increase the exposure to **sirolimus**. Monitor and adjust dose. Moderate Theoretical

Fostamatinib (continued)

▶ **Fostamatinib** is predicted to increase the exposure to statins (atorvastatin, fluvastatin). Monitor and adjust dose. Moderate Theoretical

▶ **Fostamatinib** moderately increases the exposure to statins (rosuvastatin). Avoid or adjust **rosuvastatin** dose, p. 235. Moderate Study

▶ **Fostamatinib** slightly increases the exposure to statins (simvastatin). Monitor adverse effects and adjust dose. Moderate Study

▶ **Fostamatinib** is predicted to increase the exposure to sulfasalazine. Monitor and adjust dose. Moderate Theoretical

▶ **Fostamatinib** is predicted to increase the exposure to temsirolimus. Monitor and adjust dose. Moderate Theoretical

▶ **Fostamatinib** is predicted to increase the exposure to tenofovir alafenamide. Moderate Theoretical

▶ **Fostamatinib** is predicted to increase the exposure to tenofovir disoproxil. Moderate Theoretical

▶ **Fostamatinib** is predicted to increase the exposure to topotecan. Monitor and adjust dose. Moderate Theoretical

▶ Tucatinib is predicted to increase the exposure to **fostamatinib**. Monitor adverse effects and adjust dose. Moderate Study

Fostemsavir

▶ Anti-androgens (apalutamide, enzalutamide) are predicted to decrease the exposure to the active metabolite of **fostemsavir**. Avoid. Severe Study

▶ Antiepileptics (carbamazepine, fosphenytoin, phenobarbital, phenytoin, primidone) are predicted to decrease the exposure to the active metabolite of **fostemsavir**. Avoid. Severe Study

▶ Encorafenib is predicted to decrease the exposure to the active metabolite of **fostemsavir**. Avoid. Severe Study

▶ **Fostemsavir** increases the concentration of ethinylestradiol from a combined hormonal contraceptive. Adjust dose—consult product literature. Severe Study

▶ **Fostemsavir** is predicted to increase the exposure to grazoprevir. Avoid. Severe Theoretical

▶ Ivosidenib is predicted to decrease the exposure to the active metabolite of **fostemsavir**. Avoid. Severe Study

▶ Lumacaftor is predicted to decrease the exposure to the active metabolite of **fostemsavir**. Avoid. Severe Study

▶ Mitotane is predicted to decrease the exposure to the active metabolite of **fostemsavir**. Avoid. Severe Study

▶ Rifamycins (rifampicin) are predicted to decrease the exposure to the active metabolite of **fostemsavir**. Avoid. Severe Study

▶ St John's wort is predicted to decrease the exposure to the active metabolite of **fostemsavir**. Avoid. Severe Study

▶ **Fostemsavir** is predicted to increase the exposure to statins (atorvastatin, fluvastatin, simvastatin). Adjust starting dose and monitor. Severe Theoretical

▶ **Fostemsavir** increases the exposure to statins (rosuvastatin). Adjust starting dose and monitor. Severe Study

▶ **Fostemsavir** is predicted to increase the exposure to tenofovir alafenamide. Adjust dose—consult product literature. Moderate Theoretical

Frovatriptan → see triptans

Fruquintinib

▶ Anti-androgens (apalutamide, enzalutamide) are predicted to decrease the exposure to **fruquintinib**. Avoid. Moderate Study

▶ Antiepileptics (carbamazepine, fosphenytoin, phenobarbital, phenytoin, primidone) are predicted to decrease the exposure to **fruquintinib**. Avoid. Moderate Study

▶ Cenobamate is predicted to decrease the exposure to **fruquintinib**. Avoid. Moderate Study

▶ Dabrafenib is predicted to decrease the exposure to **fruquintinib**. Avoid. Moderate Study

▶ Encorafenib is predicted to decrease the exposure to **fruquintinib**. Avoid. Moderate Study

▶ Endothelin receptor antagonists (bosentan) are predicted to decrease the exposure to **fruquintinib**. Avoid. Moderate Study

▶ Ivosidenib is predicted to decrease the exposure to **fruquintinib**. Avoid. Moderate Study

▶ Lorlatinib is predicted to decrease the exposure to **fruquintinib**. Avoid. Moderate Study

▶ Lumacaftor is predicted to decrease the exposure to **fruquintinib**. Avoid. Moderate Study

▶ Mitotane is predicted to decrease the exposure to **fruquintinib**. Avoid. Moderate Study

▶ NNRTIs (efavirenz, etravirine, nevirapine) are predicted to decrease the exposure to **fruquintinib**. Avoid. Moderate Study

▶ Rifamycins (rifampicin) are predicted to decrease the exposure to **fruquintinib**. Avoid. Moderate Study

▶ Sotorasib is predicted to decrease the exposure to **fruquintinib**. Avoid. Moderate Study

▶ St John's wort is predicted to decrease the exposure to **fruquintinib**. Avoid. Moderate Study

Furosemide → see loop diuretics

Fusidate

▶ Nirmatrelvir boosted with ritonavir is predicted to increase the concentration of **fusidate**. Avoid. Moderate Theoretical

▶ **Fusidate** has been reported to cause rhabdomyolysis when given with statins. Avoid. Severe Anecdotal

Gabapentin → see antiepileptics

Galantamine → see anticholinesterases, centrally acting

Ganciclovir → see TABLE 14 p. 1575 (myelosuppression), TABLE 2 p. 1571 (nephrotoxicity)

ROUTE-SPECIFIC INFORMATION Since systemic absorption can follow topical application, the possibility of interactions should be borne in mind.

▶ **Ganciclovir** is predicted to increase the risk of seizures when given with carbapenems (imipenem). Avoid. Severe Anecdotal

▶ Ivosidenib is predicted to increase the exposure to **ganciclovir**. Use with caution or avoid. Moderate Theoretical

▶ Leflunomide is predicted to increase the exposure to **ganciclovir**. Moderate Study → Also see TABLE 14 p. 1575

▶ Maribavir might decrease the efficacy of **ganciclovir**. Avoid. Severe Theoretical

▶ Mycophenolate is predicted to increase the risk of haematological toxicity when given with **ganciclovir**. Moderate Theoretical

▶ Nitisinone is predicted to increase the exposure to **ganciclovir**. Moderate Study

▶ Teriflunomide is predicted to increase the exposure to **ganciclovir**. Moderate Study

▶ Vadadustat is predicted to increase the exposure to **ganciclovir**. Monitor and adjust dose. Moderate Study

Gefitinib

▶ Oral antacids are predicted to decrease the exposure to oral **gefitinib**. Moderate Theoretical

▶ Anti-androgens (apalutamide, enzalutamide) are predicted to decrease the exposure to **gefitinib**. Avoid. Severe Study

▶ Antiarrhythmics (dronedarone) are predicted to increase the exposure to **gefitinib**. Moderate Study

▶ Antiepileptics (carbamazepine, fosphenytoin, phenobarbital, phenytoin, primidone) are predicted to decrease the exposure to **gefitinib**. Avoid. Severe Study

▶ Antiepileptics (eslicarbazepine) are predicted to decrease the exposure to **gefitinib**. Moderate Theoretical

▶ Antiepileptics (oxcarbazepine) decrease the exposure to **gefitinib**. Severe Study

▶ Antifungals, azoles (fluconazole, isavuconazole) are predicted to increase the exposure to **gefitinib**. Moderate Study

▶ Antifungals, azoles (itraconazole, ketoconazole, posaconazole, voriconazole) are predicted to increase the exposure to **gefitinib**. Severe Study

▶ Berotralstat is predicted to increase the exposure to **gefitinib**. Moderate Study

▶ Bupropion is predicted to increase the exposure to **gefitinib**. Moderate Theoretical

▶ Calcium channel blockers (diltiazem, verapamil) are predicted to increase the exposure to **gefitinib**. Moderate Study

▶ Oral calcium salts (calcium carbonate) -containing antacids are predicted to decrease the exposure to oral **gefitinib**. Moderate Theoretical

▶ Cenobamate is predicted to decrease the exposure to **gefitinib**. Avoid. Severe Study

▶ Ceritinib is predicted to increase the exposure to **gefitinib**. Severe Study

▶ Cinacalcet is predicted to increase the exposure to **gefitinib**. Moderate Theoretical

▸ **Cobicistat** is predicted to increase the exposure to **gefitinib**. Severe Study

▸ **Gefitinib** is predicted to increase the anticoagulant effect of **coumarins**. Severe Anecdotal

▸ **Crizotinib** is predicted to increase the exposure to **gefitinib**. Moderate Study

▸ **Dabrafenib** is predicted to decrease the exposure to **gefitinib**. Avoid. Severe Study

▸ **Dacomitinib** is predicted to increase the exposure to **gefitinib**. Moderate Theoretical

▸ **Encorafenib** is predicted to decrease the exposure to **gefitinib**. Avoid. Severe Study

▸ Endothelin receptor antagonists **(bosentan)** are predicted to decrease the exposure to **gefitinib**. Avoid. Severe Study

▸ **Fedratinib** is predicted to increase the exposure to **gefitinib**. Moderate Study

▸ **H₂ receptor antagonists** are predicted to slightly to moderately decrease the exposure to **gefitinib**. Moderate Study

▸ **HIV-protease inhibitors** are predicted to increase the exposure to **gefitinib**. Severe Study

▸ **Idelalisib** is predicted to increase the exposure to **gefitinib**. Severe Study

▸ **Imatinib** is predicted to increase the exposure to **gefitinib**. Moderate Study

▸ **Ivosidenib** is predicted to decrease the exposure to **gefitinib**. Avoid. Severe Study

▸ **Letermovir** is predicted to increase the exposure to **gefitinib**. Moderate Study

▸ **Lorlatinib** is predicted to decrease the exposure to **gefitinib**. Avoid. Severe Study

▸ **Lumacaftor** is predicted to decrease the exposure to **gefitinib**. Avoid. Severe Study

▸ Macrolides **(clarithromycin)** are predicted to increase the exposure to **gefitinib**. Severe Study

▸ Macrolides **(erythromycin)** are predicted to increase the exposure to **gefitinib**. Moderate Study

▸ **Mitotane** is predicted to decrease the exposure to **gefitinib**. Avoid. Severe Study

▸ Neurokinin-1 receptor antagonists **(aprepitant, netupitant)** are predicted to increase the exposure to **gefitinib**. Moderate Study

▸ **Nilotinib** is predicted to increase the exposure to **gefitinib**. Moderate Study

▸ NNRTIs **(efavirenz, etravirine, nevirapine)** are predicted to decrease the exposure to **gefitinib**. Avoid. Severe Study

▸ **Gefitinib** is predicted to increase the risk of bleeding events when given with **phenindione**. Severe Theoretical

▸ **Proton pump inhibitors** are predicted to decrease the exposure to **gefitinib**. Severe Theoretical

▸ Rifamycins **(rifampicin)** are predicted to decrease the exposure to **gefitinib**. Avoid. Severe Study

▸ **Gefitinib** is predicted to increase the exposure to the active component of **sacituzumab govitecan**. Severe Theoretical

▸ Oral **sodium bicarbonate** -containing antacids are predicted to decrease the exposure to oral **gefitinib**. Moderate Theoretical

▸ **Sotorasib** is predicted to decrease the exposure to **gefitinib**. Avoid. Severe Study

▸ SSRIs **(fluoxetine, paroxetine)** are predicted to increase the exposure to **gefitinib**. Moderate Theoretical

▸ **St John's wort** is predicted to decrease the exposure to **gefitinib**. Avoid. Severe Study

▸ **Terbinafine** is predicted to increase the exposure to **gefitinib**. Moderate Theoretical

▸ **Tucatinib** is predicted to increase the exposure to **gefitinib**. Severe Study

▸ **Gefitinib** might affect the exposure to **vemurafenib**. Moderate Theoretical

Gemcitabine → see TABLE 1 p. 1571 (hepatotoxicity), TABLE 14 p. 1575 (myelosuppression)

▸ **Cedazuridine** is predicted to increase the exposure to **gemcitabine**. Avoid. Moderate Theoretical

▸ **Live vaccines** are predicted to increase the risk of generalised infection (possibly life-threatening) when given with **gemcitabine**. UKHSA advises avoid (refer to Green Book). Severe Theoretical

Gemfibrozil → see fibrates

Gemtuzumab ozogamicin → see TABLE 14 p. 1575 (myelosuppression)

Gentamicin → see aminoglycosides

Gilteritinib

▸ ACE inhibitors **(captopril)** are predicted to increase the exposure to **gilteritinib**. Moderate Theoretical

▸ Anti-androgens **(enzalutamide)** are predicted to increase the exposure to **gilteritinib**. Moderate Theoretical

▸ Antiarrhythmics **(amiodarone, dronedarone)** are predicted to increase the exposure to **gilteritinib**. Moderate Theoretical

▸ Antiepileptics **(carbamazepine, phenytoin)** are predicted to decrease the exposure to **gilteritinib**. Avoid. Severe Study

▸ Antifungals, azoles **(itraconazole, ketoconazole, posaconazole, voriconazole)** are predicted to increase the exposure to **gilteritinib**. Moderate Study

▸ Beta blockers, non-selective **(carvedilol)** are predicted to increase the exposure to **gilteritinib**. Moderate Theoretical

▸ Calcium channel blockers **(verapamil)** are predicted to increase the exposure to **gilteritinib**. Moderate Theoretical

▸ **Ceritinib** is predicted to increase the exposure to **gilteritinib**. Moderate Study

▸ **Ciclosporin** is predicted to increase the exposure to **gilteritinib**. Moderate Theoretical

▸ **Cobicistat** is predicted to increase the exposure to **gilteritinib**. Moderate Study

▸ **HIV-protease inhibitors** are predicted to increase the exposure to **gilteritinib**. Moderate Study

▸ **Idelalisib** is predicted to increase the exposure to **gilteritinib**. Moderate Study

▸ **Ivacaftor** is predicted to increase the exposure to **gilteritinib**. Moderate Theoretical

▸ **Lapatinib** is predicted to increase the exposure to **gilteritinib**. Moderate Theoretical

▸ Macrolides **(azithromycin, erythromycin)** are predicted to increase the exposure to **gilteritinib**. Moderate Theoretical

▸ Macrolides **(clarithromycin)** are predicted to increase the exposure to **gilteritinib**. Moderate Study

▸ **Maribavir** is predicted to increase the exposure to **gilteritinib**. Moderate Theoretical

▸ **Neratinib** is predicted to increase the exposure to **gilteritinib**. Moderate Theoretical

▸ **Ranolazine** is predicted to increase the exposure to **gilteritinib**. Moderate Theoretical

▸ Rifamycins **(rifampicin)** moderately decrease the exposure to **gilteritinib**. Avoid. Severe Study

▸ **Rucaparib** is predicted to increase the exposure to **gilteritinib**. Moderate Theoretical

▸ **Gilteritinib** is predicted to decrease the efficacy of SSRIs **(escitalopram, fluoxetine, sertraline)**. Avoid. Moderate Theoretical

▸ **St John's wort** is predicted to decrease the exposure to **gilteritinib**. Avoid. Severe Study

▸ **Tucatinib** is predicted to increase the exposure to **gilteritinib**. Moderate Study

▸ **Vandetanib** is predicted to increase the exposure to **gilteritinib**. Moderate Theoretical

▸ **Vemurafenib** is predicted to increase the exposure to **gilteritinib**. Moderate Theoretical

▸ **Voclosporin** is predicted to increase the exposure to **gilteritinib**. Moderate Theoretical

Givinostat

▸ **Givinostat** increases the exposure to benzodiazepines **(midazolam)**. Moderate Study

▸ **Givinostat** might increase the exposure to **everolimus**. Moderate Study

▸ **Givinostat** might increase the exposure to **metformin**. Moderate Theoretical

▸ **Givinostat** might increase the exposure to opioids **(alfentanil)**. Moderate Study

▸ **Givinostat** might increase the exposure to phosphodiesterase type-5 inhibitors **(sildenafil)**. Moderate Study

▸ **Givinostat** might increase the exposure to **sirolimus**. Moderate Study

▸ **Givinostat** might increase the exposure to statins **(simvastatin)**. Moderate Study

Givinostat (continued)
▶ **Givinostat** might increase the exposure to **tacrolimus**. Moderate Study
▶ **Givinostat** might increase the exposure to **temsirolimus**. Moderate Study
▶ **Givinostat** might increase the exposure to **triptans (eletriptan)**. Moderate Study

Givosiran
▶ **Givosiran** is predicted to increase the exposure to **agomelatine**. Moderate Study
▶ **Givosiran** is predicted to increase the exposure to **aminophylline**. Adjust dose. Moderate Theoretical
▶ **Givosiran** is predicted to increase the exposure to **anaesthetics, local (ropivacaine)**. Moderate Theoretical
▶ **Givosiran** is predicted to increase the exposure to **anagrelide**. Moderate Theoretical
▶ **Givosiran** increases the concentration of **antipsychotics, second generation (clozapine)**. Monitor adverse effects and adjust dose. Severe Study
▶ **Givosiran** is predicted to increase the exposure to **antipsychotics, second generation (olanzapine)**. Adjust dose. Moderate Anecdotal
▶ **Givosiran** is predicted to increase the exposure to **atomoxetine**. Use with caution and adjust dose. Moderate Study
▶ **Givosiran** is predicted to increase the exposure to **beta blockers, selective (metoprolol)**. Moderate Study
▶ **Givosiran** is predicted to increase the exposure to **beta blockers, selective (nebivolol)**. Use with caution and adjust dose. Moderate Study
▶ **Givosiran** is predicted to increase the exposure to **dopamine receptor agonists (ropinirole)**. Adjust dose. Moderate Study
▶ **Givosiran** is predicted to increase the exposure to **eliglustat**. Use with caution and adjust dose. Moderate Study
▶ **Givosiran** are predicted to increases the exposure to **erlotinib**. Monitor adverse effects and adjust dose. Moderate Study
▶ **Givosiran** is predicted to increase the exposure to **fezolinetant**. Avoid. Moderate Study
▶ **Givosiran** is predicted to increase the exposure to **loxapine**. Avoid. Unknown Theoretical
▶ **Givosiran** slightly increases the exposure to **MAO-B inhibitors (rasagiline)**. Moderate Study
▶ **Givosiran** is predicted to increase the exposure to **mavacamten**. Monitor and adjust dose—consult product literature. Moderate Theoretical
▶ **Givosiran** is predicted to increase the exposure to **melatonin**. Moderate Theoretical
▶ **Givosiran** is predicted to increase the exposure to **phenothiazines (chlorpromazine)**. Moderate Theoretical
▶ **Givosiran** is predicted to increase the exposure to **phosphodiesterase type-4 inhibitors (roflumilast)**. Moderate Theoretical
▶ **Givosiran** is predicted to increase the exposure to **pirfenidone**. Use with caution and adjust dose. Moderate Study
▶ **Givosiran** is predicted to increase the exposure to **riluzole**. Moderate Theoretical
▶ **Givosiran** is predicted to increase the exposure to **SNRIs (duloxetine)**. Use with caution and adjust dose. Moderate Study
▶ **Givosiran** is predicted to increase the exposure to **theophylline**. Monitor and adjust dose. Moderate Theoretical
▶ **Givosiran** increases the exposure to **tizanidine**. Avoid. Moderate Study
▶ **Givosiran** is predicted to increase the exposure to **triptans (zolmitriptan)**. Adjust **zolmitriptan** dose, p. 546. Moderate Theoretical

Glasdegib → see TABLE 8 p. 1573 (QT-interval prolongation)
▶ **Anti-androgens (apalutamide, enzalutamide)** are predicted to decrease the exposure to **glasdegib**. Avoid. Severe Study → Also see TABLE 8 p. 1573
▶ **Antiepileptics (carbamazepine, fosphenytoin, phenobarbital, phenytoin, primidone)** are predicted to decrease the exposure to **glasdegib**. Avoid. Severe Study
▶ **Antifungals, azoles (itraconazole, ketoconazole, posaconazole, voriconazole)** are predicted to increase the exposure to **glasdegib**. Use with caution or avoid. Severe Study → Also see TABLE 8 p. 1573

▶ **Cenobamate** is predicted to decrease the exposure to **glasdegib**. Avoid or adjust dose—consult product literature. Moderate Theoretical
▶ **Ceritinib** is predicted to increase the exposure to **glasdegib**. Use with caution or avoid. Severe Study → Also see TABLE 8 p. 1573
▶ **Cobicistat** is predicted to increase the exposure to **glasdegib**. Use with caution or avoid. Severe Study
▶ **Dabrafenib** is predicted to decrease the exposure to **glasdegib**. Avoid or adjust dose—consult product literature. Moderate Theoretical
▶ **Encorafenib** is predicted to decrease the exposure to **glasdegib**. Avoid. Severe Study → Also see TABLE 8 p. 1573
▶ **Endothelin receptor antagonists (bosentan)** are predicted to decrease the exposure to **glasdegib**. Avoid or adjust dose—consult product literature. Moderate Theoretical
▶ **Grapefruit** juice is predicted to increase the exposure to **glasdegib**. Use with caution or avoid. Moderate Theoretical
▶ **HIV-protease inhibitors** are predicted to increase the exposure to **glasdegib**. Use with caution or avoid. Severe Study
▶ **Idelalisib** is predicted to increase the exposure to **glasdegib**. Use with caution or avoid. Severe Study
▶ **Ivosidenib** is predicted to decrease the exposure to **glasdegib**. Avoid. Severe Study → Also see TABLE 8 p. 1573
▶ **Lorlatinib** is predicted to decrease the exposure to **glasdegib**. Avoid or adjust dose—consult product literature. Moderate Theoretical
▶ **Lumacaftor** is predicted to decrease the exposure to **glasdegib**. Avoid. Severe Study
▶ **Macrolides (clarithromycin)** are predicted to increase the exposure to **glasdegib**. Use with caution or avoid. Severe Study
▶ **Mitotane** is predicted to decrease the exposure to **glasdegib**. Avoid. Severe Study
▶ **Modafinil** is predicted to decrease the exposure to **glasdegib**. Avoid or adjust dose—consult product literature. Moderate Theoretical
▶ **NNRTIs (efavirenz, etravirine, nevirapine)** are predicted to decrease the exposure to **glasdegib**. Avoid or adjust dose—consult product literature. Moderate Theoretical → Also see TABLE 8 p. 1573
▶ **Rifamycins (rifampicin)** are predicted to decrease the exposure to **glasdegib**. Avoid. Severe Study
▶ **Sotorasib** is predicted to decrease the exposure to **glasdegib**. Avoid or adjust dose—consult product literature. Moderate Theoretical
▶ **St John's wort** is predicted to decrease the exposure to **glasdegib**. Avoid or adjust dose—consult product literature. Moderate Theoretical
▶ **Tucatinib** is predicted to increase the exposure to **glasdegib**. Use with caution or avoid. Severe Study

Glecaprevir
▶ **Glecaprevir** is predicted to increase the exposure to **afatinib**. Moderate Study
▶ **Glecaprevir** is predicted to increase the exposure to **aliskiren**. Severe Theoretical
▶ **Anti-androgens (enzalutamide)** are predicted to greatly decrease the concentration of **glecaprevir**. Avoid. Severe Study
▶ **Antiarrhythmics (dronedarone)** potentially increase the exposure to **glecaprevir**. Moderate Theoretical
▶ **Antiepileptics (carbamazepine, fosphenytoin, phenobarbital, phenytoin, primidone)** are predicted to moderately decrease the exposure to **glecaprevir**. Avoid. Severe Study
▶ **Antiepileptics (eslicarbazepine, oxcarbazepine)** potentially decrease the exposure to **glecaprevir**. Avoid. Severe Theoretical
▶ **Antifungals, azoles (itraconazole, ketoconazole)** potentially increase the exposure to **glecaprevir**. Moderate Theoretical
▶ **Glecaprevir** is predicted to increase the exposure to **antihistamines, non-sedating (fexofenadine)**. Severe Theoretical
▶ **Glecaprevir** is predicted to increase the exposure to **bictegravir**. Use with caution or avoid. Moderate Theoretical
▶ **Bulevirtide** is predicted to increase the exposure to **glecaprevir**. Avoid or monitor. Moderate Theoretical
▶ **Cenobamate** is predicted to decrease the exposure to **glecaprevir**. Avoid. Severe Study
▶ **Ciclosporin** increases the exposure to **glecaprevir**. Avoid or monitor. Severe Study

▸ **Cobicistat** potentially increases the exposure to **glecaprevir**. Moderate Theoretical
▸ **Glecaprevir** is predicted to increase the exposure to colchicine. Avoid P-glycoprotein inhibitors or adjust **colchicine** dose, p. 1279. Severe Theoretical
▸ **Combined hormonal contraceptives** (containing ethinylestradiol) are predicted to increase the risk of increased ALT concentrations when given with **glecaprevir**. Avoid. Severe Study
▸ **Crizotinib** potentially decreases the exposure to **glecaprevir**. Avoid. Severe Theoretical
▸ **Dabrafenib** is predicted to decrease the exposure to **glecaprevir**. Avoid. Severe Study
▸ **Glecaprevir** with pibrentasvir increases the exposure to digoxin. Moderate Study
▸ **Endothelin receptor antagonists (bosentan)** are predicted to decrease the exposure to **glecaprevir**. Avoid. Severe Study
▸ **Glecaprevir** is predicted to increase the exposure to everolimus. Moderate Study
▸ **Glecaprevir** is predicted to increase the exposure to factor XA inhibitors (edoxaban). Severe Theoretical
▸ **Glecaprevir** is predicted to increase the exposure to fidaxomicin. Avoid. Moderate Study
▸ **HIV-protease inhibitors (atazanavir, darunavir, lopinavir)** boosted with ritonavir increase the exposure to **glecaprevir**. Avoid. Severe Study
▸ **HIV-protease inhibitors (ritonavir)** increase the exposure to **glecaprevir**. Avoid. Severe Study
▸ **Glecaprevir** is predicted to increase the exposure to loperamide. Severe Theoretical
▸ **Lorlatinib** is predicted to decrease the exposure to **glecaprevir**. Avoid. Severe Study
▸ **Lumacaftor** potentially decreases the exposure to **glecaprevir**. Avoid. Severe Theoretical
▸ **Mitotane** is predicted to greatly decrease the concentration of **glecaprevir**. Avoid. Severe Study
▸ **Glecaprevir** is predicted to increase the risk of neutropenia when given with monoclonal antibodies (brentuximab vedotin). Monitor and adjust dose. Severe Theoretical
▸ **Glecaprevir** is predicted to increase the exposure to neratinib. Avoid or adjust dose and monitor for gastrointestinal adverse effects—consult product literature. Severe Study
▸ **Glecaprevir** is predicted to increase the exposure to nintedanib. Moderate Study
▸ **Nirmatrelvir** boosted with ritonavir is predicted to increase the concentration of **glecaprevir**. Avoid. Severe Theoretical
▸ **NNRTIs (efavirenz, etravirine, nevirapine)** are predicted to decrease the exposure to **glecaprevir**. Avoid. Severe Study
▸ **Glecaprevir** is predicted to increase the exposure to pralsetinib. Moderate Theoretical
▸ **Glecaprevir** is predicted to increase the exposure to ranolazine. Adjust dose. Severe Theoretical
▸ **Glecaprevir** is predicted to increase the exposure to relugolix. Avoid or take relugolix first and separate administration by at least 6 hours. Moderate Study
▸ **Rifamycins (rifampicin)** markedly affect the exposure to **glecaprevir**. Avoid. Severe Study
▸ **Glecaprevir** is predicted to increase the exposure to rimegepant. Avoid another dose of rimegepant within 48 hours of concurrent use. Moderate Theoretical
▸ **Glecaprevir** is predicted to increase the exposure to sirolimus. Severe Theoretical
▸ **Sotorasib** is predicted to decrease the exposure to **glecaprevir**. Avoid. Severe Study
▸ **St John's wort** is predicted to decrease the exposure to **glecaprevir**. Avoid. Severe Study
▸ **Glecaprevir** with pibrentasvir markedly increases the exposure to statins (atorvastatin). Avoid. Severe Study
▸ **Glecaprevir** with pibrentasvir is predicted to increase the exposure to statins (fluvastatin). Moderate Theoretical
▸ **Glecaprevir** with pibrentasvir moderately increases the exposure to statins (pravastatin). Use with caution and adjust **pravastatin** dose. Moderate Study

▸ **Glecaprevir** with pibrentasvir moderately increases the exposure to statins (rosuvastatin). Use with caution and adjust **rosuvastatin** dose, p. 235. Moderate Study
▸ **Glecaprevir** with pibrentasvir moderately increases the exposure to statins (simvastatin). Avoid. Moderate Study
▸ **Glecaprevir** with pibrentasvir slightly increases the exposure to tacrolimus. Monitor and adjust dose. Mild Study
▸ **Glecaprevir** is predicted to slightly increase the exposure to talazoparib. Avoid or adjust dose—consult product literature. Severe Study
▸ **Glecaprevir** is predicted to increase the exposure to taxanes (paclitaxel). Severe Theoretical
▸ **Glecaprevir** with pibrentasvir increases the exposure to thrombin inhibitors (dabigatran). Avoid. Moderate Study
▸ **Glecaprevir** is predicted to increase the exposure to topotecan. Severe Study
▸ **Glecaprevir** is predicted to increase the concentration of trametinib. Moderate Theoretical

Glibenclamide → see sulfonylureas
Gliclazide → see sulfonylureas
Glimepiride → see sulfonylureas
Glipizide → see sulfonylureas

Glofitamab
▸ **Glofitamab** might affect the exposure to ciclosporin. Moderate Theoretical
▸ **Glofitamab** might affect the exposure to coumarins (warfarin). Moderate Theoretical

Glucagon
▸ **Glucagon** increases the anticoagulant effect of coumarins (warfarin). Severe Study

Glucagon-like peptide-1 receptor agonists → see TABLE 13 p. 1575 (antidiabetic drugs)

dulaglutide · exenatide · liraglutide · lixisenatide · semaglutide · tirzepatide

▸ With standard-release **exenatide**: some orally administered drugs should be taken at least 1 hour before, or 4 hours after, exenatide injection.
▸ Some orally administered drugs should be taken at least 1 hour before, or 4 hours after, **lixisenatide** injection.

▸ **Tirzepatide** might affect the absorption of oral combined hormonal contraceptives. Manufacturer advises precautions for those who are overweight or obese—see Conception and contraception p. 822. Moderate Study
▸ **Semaglutide** might decrease the anticoagulant effect of coumarins (acenocoumarol). Severe Anecdotal
▸ **Tirzepatide** might affect the absorption of coumarins (warfarin). Severe Theoretical
▸ **Tirzepatide** might affect the absorption of desogestrel. Manufacturer advises precautions for those who are overweight or obese—see Conception and contraception p. 822. Moderate Study
▸ **Tirzepatide** might affect the absorption of digoxin. Moderate Theoretical
▸ **Tirzepatide** might affect the absorption of drospirenone. Manufacturer advises precautions for those who are overweight or obese—see Conception and contraception p. 822. Moderate Study
▸ **Fenfluramine** might decrease blood glucose concentrations when given with **glucagon-like peptide-1 receptor agonists**. Moderate Theoretical
▸ **Tirzepatide** might affect the absorption of oral levonorgestrel. Manufacturer advises precautions for those who are overweight or obese—see Conception and contraception p. 822. Moderate Study
▸ **Monoclonal antibodies (rozanolixizumab)** might decrease the concentration of **dulaglutide**. Avoid and for 2 weeks after stopping **rozanolixizumab**. Moderate Theoretical
▸ **Tirzepatide** might affect the absorption of oral norethisterone. Manufacturer advises precautions for those who are overweight or obese—see Conception and contraception p. 822. Moderate Study
▸ **Somapacitan** might increase blood glucose concentrations, opposing the blood glucose-lowering effects of **glucagon-like peptide-1 receptor agonists**. Adjust dose. Moderate Theoretical

Glucagon-like peptide-1 receptor agonists (continued)
▶ **Somatrogon** might increase blood glucose concentrations, opposing the blood glucose-lowering effects of **glucagon-like peptide-1 receptor agonists**. Adjust dose. Moderate Theoretical
▶ **Semaglutide** slightly increases the exposure to thyroid hormones **(levothyroxine)**. Moderate Study

Glucarpidase
▶ **Glucarpidase** decreases the exposure to folates **(folinic acid)**. Separate administration by at least 2 hours. Moderate Study
▶ **Glucarpidase** might decrease the exposure to folates **(levofolinic acid)**. Separate administration by at least 2 hours. Moderate Theoretical

Glucosamine
▶ **Glucosamine** potentially decreases the anticoagulant effect of coumarins **(acenocoumarol)**. Moderate Anecdotal
▶ **Glucosamine** potentially increases the anticoagulant effect of coumarins **(warfarin)**. Avoid. Moderate Anecdotal

Glycerol phenylbutyrate
▶ **Antiepileptics (valproate)** potentially oppose the effects of glycerol phenylbutyrate. Moderate Theoretical
▶ **Corticosteroids** potentially oppose the effects of **glycerol phenylbutyrate**. Moderate Theoretical
▶ **Haloperidol** potentially opposes the effects of **glycerol phenylbutyrate**. Moderate Theoretical

Glyceryl trinitrate → see nitrates
Glycopyrronium → see TABLE 9 p. 1573 (antimuscarinics)

> ROUTE-SPECIFIC INFORMATION Since systemic absorption can follow topical application of **glycopyrronium**, the possibility of interactions should be borne in mind.

▶ **Antipsychotics, second generation (clozapine)** can cause constipation, as can **glycopyrronium**; concurrent use might increase the risk of developing intestinal obstruction. Severe Theoretical → Also see TABLE 9 p. 1573

Golimumab → see monoclonal antibodies
Granisetron → see 5-HT3-receptor antagonists
Grapefruit
▶ **Grapefruit** juice is predicted to increase the exposure to abemaciclib. Avoid. Moderate Theoretical
▶ **Grapefruit** juice moderately decreases the exposure to aliskiren. Avoid. Severe Study
▶ **Grapefruit** juice increases the exposure to antiarrhythmics **(amiodarone)**. Avoid. Moderate Study
▶ **Grapefruit** juice moderately increases the exposure to antiarrhythmics **(dronedarone)**. Avoid. Severe Study
▶ **Grapefruit** juice increases the exposure to antiarrhythmics **(propafenone)**. Monitor and adjust dose. Moderate Study
▶ **Grapefruit** juice slightly increases the exposure to antiepileptics **(carbamazepine)**. Monitor and adjust dose. Moderate Study
▶ **Grapefruit** juice slightly decreases the exposure to antihistamines, non-sedating **(bilastine)**. **Bilastine** should be taken 1 hour before or 2 hours after **grapefruit**. Moderate Study
▶ **Grapefruit** juice increases the exposure to antihistamines, non-sedating **(rupatadine)**. Avoid. Moderate Study
▶ **Grapefruit** juice increases the exposure to antimalarials **(artemether)**. Unknown Study
▶ **Grapefruit** juice is predicted to increase the exposure to antipsychotics, second generation **(cariprazine)**. Avoid. Moderate Study
▶ **Grapefruit** juice is predicted to increase the exposure to antipsychotics, second generation **(lurasidone, quetiapine)**. Avoid. Severe Theoretical
▶ **Grapefruit** and grapefruit juice is predicted to increase the exposure to avacopan. Avoid. Moderate Theoretical
▶ **Grapefruit** juice is predicted to increase the exposure to avapritinib. Avoid. Moderate Theoretical
▶ **Grapefruit** juice is predicted to increase the exposure to axitinib. Moderate Theoretical
▶ **Grapefruit** juice is predicted to increase the exposure to berotralstat. Moderate Theoretical
▶ **Grapefruit** juice greatly decreases the exposure to beta blockers, selective **(celiprolol)**. Moderate Study
▶ **Grapefruit** juice is predicted to increase the exposure to bosutinib. Avoid. Moderate Theoretical
▶ **Grapefruit** juice is predicted to increase the concentration of brigatinib. Avoid. Severe Study

▶ **Grapefruit** juice increases the exposure to buspirone. Avoid. Mild Study
▶ **Grapefruit** juice is predicted to increase the exposure to cabozantinib. Moderate Theoretical
▶ **Grapefruit** juice very slightly increases the exposure to calcium channel blockers **(amlodipine)**. Avoid. Mild Study
▶ **Grapefruit** juice increases the exposure to calcium channel blockers **(felodipine)**. Avoid. Moderate Study
▶ **Grapefruit** juice is predicted to increase the exposure to calcium channel blockers **(lercanidipine)**. Avoid. Moderate Theoretical
▶ **Grapefruit** juice increases the exposure to calcium channel blockers **(nicardipine)**. Mild Study
▶ **Grapefruit** juice increases the exposure to calcium channel blockers **(nifedipine, verapamil)**. Avoid. Mild Study
▶ **Grapefruit** and grapefruit juice is predicted to increase the exposure to capivasertib. Adjust dose. Moderate Theoretical
▶ **Grapefruit** juice is predicted to increase the exposure to ceritinib. Avoid. Severe Theoretical
▶ **Grapefruit** juice increases the concentration of ciclosporin. Avoid. Severe Study
▶ **Grapefruit** juice markedly decreases the exposure to clopidogrel. Severe Study
▶ **Grapefruit** juice is predicted to increase the exposure to cobimetinib. Avoid. Severe Theoretical
▶ **Grapefruit** juice moderately increases the exposure to oral corticosteroids **(budesonide)**. Avoid. Moderate Study
▶ **Grapefruit** juice is predicted to increase the exposure to crizotinib. Avoid. Moderate Theoretical
▶ **Grapefruit** and grapefruit juice is predicted to increase the exposure to daridorexant. Avoid **grapefruit** in the evening. Moderate Theoretical
▶ **Grapefruit** juice is predicted to increase the exposure to darifenacin. Moderate Study
▶ **Grapefruit** juice is predicted to increase the exposure to dasatinib. Avoid. Moderate Theoretical
▶ **Grapefruit** juice is predicted to increase the exposure to dipeptidylpeptidase-4 inhibitors **(saxagliptin)**. Mild Theoretical
▶ **Grapefruit** is predicted to increase the exposure to elacestrant. Avoid. Moderate Theoretical
▶ **Grapefruit** juice is predicted to increase the exposure to elexacaftor. Avoid. Moderate Theoretical
▶ **Grapefruit** juice is predicted to increase the exposure to eliglustat. Avoid. Severe Theoretical
▶ **Grapefruit** juice is predicted to increase the exposure to encorafenib. Avoid. Moderate Study
▶ **Grapefruit** is predicted to increase the exposure to entrectinib. Avoid. Severe Theoretical
▶ **Grapefruit** is predicted to increase the exposure to erdafitinib. Avoid. Moderate Theoretical
▶ **Grapefruit** juice is predicted to increase the exposure to ergometrine. Severe Theoretical
▶ **Grapefruit** juice is predicted to increase the exposure to erlotinib. Moderate Theoretical
▶ **Grapefruit** juice is predicted to increase the exposure to everolimus. Avoid. Severe Theoretical
▶ **Grapefruit** and grapefruit juice is predicted to increase the exposure to fedratinib. Avoid. Moderate Theoretical
▶ **Grapefruit** juice is predicted to increase the exposure to fostamatinib. Monitor adverse effects and adjust dose. Moderate Theoretical
▶ **Grapefruit** juice is predicted to increase the exposure to glasdegib. Use with caution or avoid. Moderate Theoretical
▶ **Grapefruit** juice is predicted to increase the exposure to guanfacine. Avoid. Moderate Theoretical
▶ **Grapefruit** juice is predicted to increase the exposure to ibrutinib. Avoid. Moderate Theoretical
▶ **Grapefruit** juice is predicted to increase the exposure to imatinib. Moderate Theoretical
▶ **Grapefruit** juice is predicted to increase the exposure to ivabradine. Avoid. Moderate Study
▶ **Grapefruit** juice is predicted to increase the exposure to ivacaftor. Avoid. Moderate Theoretical
▶ **Grapefruit** and grapefruit juice are predicted to increase the exposure to ivosidenib. Avoid. Moderate Study

- **Grapefruit** juice is predicted to increase the exposure to lapatinib. Avoid. [Moderate] Theoretical
- **Grapefruit** juice is predicted to increase the exposure to larotrectinib. Avoid. [Moderate] Theoretical
- **Grapefruit** juice is predicted to increase the exposure to leniolisib. Avoid. [Moderate] Theoretical
- **Grapefruit** juice is predicted to increase the exposure to lomitapide. Avoid. [Mild] Theoretical
- **Grapefruit** juice is predicted to increase the concentration of lorlatinib. Avoid. [Moderate] Theoretical
- **Grapefruit** is predicted to increase the exposure to mavacamten. Monitor and adjust dose—consult product literature. [Moderate] Theoretical
- **Grapefruit** juice is predicted to increase the exposure to midostaurin. [Moderate] Theoretical
- **Grapefruit** juice is predicted to increase the exposure to mifepristone. [Moderate] Theoretical
- **Grapefruit** and grapefruit juice is predicted to increase the exposure to mineralocorticoid receptor antagonists (finerenone). Avoid. [Moderate] Theoretical
- **Grapefruit** and grapefruit juice are predicted to increase the exposure to mobocertinib. Avoid. [Severe] Theoretical
- **Grapefruit** juice is predicted to increase the exposure to naldemedine. Avoid or monitor. [Moderate] Theoretical
- **Grapefruit** juice is predicted to increase the exposure to naloxegol. Avoid. [Moderate] Theoretical
- **Grapefruit** juice is predicted to increase the exposure to neratinib. Avoid. [Severe] Theoretical
- **Grapefruit** juice is predicted to increase the exposure to nilotinib. Avoid. [Severe] Theoretical
- **Grapefruit** juice is predicted to increase the exposure to olaparib. Avoid. [Moderate] Theoretical
- **Grapefruit** juice is predicted to increase the exposure to palbociclib. Avoid. [Severe] Theoretical
- **Grapefruit** and grapefruit juice is predicted to increase the exposure to panobinostat. Avoid. [Moderate] Theoretical
- **Grapefruit** juice is predicted to increase the exposure to pazopanib. Avoid. [Severe] Theoretical
- **Grapefruit** and grapefruit juice is predicted to increase the exposure to pemigatinib. Avoid. [Severe] Study
- **Grapefruit** juice is predicted to increase the exposure to phosphodiesterase type-5 inhibitors. Use with caution or avoid. [Moderate] Study
- **Grapefruit** juice increases the exposure to pimozide. Avoid. [Severe] Theoretical
- **Grapefruit** juice is predicted to increase the exposure to ponatinib. [Moderate] Theoretical
- **Grapefruit** juice is predicted to increase the exposure to pralsetinib. Avoid. [Moderate] Study
- **Grapefruit** juice is predicted to increase the exposure to praziquantel. [Moderate] Study
- **Grapefruit** juice is predicted to increase the concentration of ranolazine. Avoid. [Severe] Theoretical
- **Grapefruit** juice is predicted to increase the exposure to regorafenib. Avoid. [Moderate] Theoretical
- **Grapefruit** juice is predicted to increase the exposure to ribociclib. Avoid. [Moderate] Theoretical
- **Grapefruit** juice is predicted to increase the exposure to ripretinib. Avoid. [Mild] Theoretical
- **Grapefruit** juice is predicted to increase the exposure to ruxolitinib. [Severe] Theoretical
- **Grapefruit** juice is predicted to increase the exposure to selumetinib. Avoid. [Moderate] Theoretical
- **Grapefruit** juice increases the concentration of sirolimus. Avoid. [Moderate] Study
- **Grapefruit** juice moderately increases the exposure to SSRIs (sertraline). Avoid. [Moderate] Study
- **Grapefruit** juice increases the exposure to statins (atorvastatin). [Mild] Study
- **Grapefruit** juice increases the exposure to statins (simvastatin). Avoid. [Severe] Study
- **Grapefruit** juice is predicted to increase the exposure to sunitinib. Avoid. [Moderate] Theoretical
- **Grapefruit** juice greatly increases the concentration of tacrolimus. Avoid. [Severe] Study

- **Grapefruit** juice is predicted to increase the concentration of temsirolimus. Use with caution or avoid. [Moderate] Theoretical
- **Grapefruit** juice is predicted to increase the exposure to tezacaftor. Avoid. [Severe] Study
- **Grapefruit** juice moderately increases the exposure to ticagrelor. [Moderate] Study
- **Grapefruit** juice increases the exposure to tolvaptan. Avoid. [Moderate] Study
- **Grapefruit** juice is predicted to increase the exposure to ulipristal. Avoid if used for uterine fibroids. [Moderate] Theoretical
- **Grapefruit** is predicted to increase the exposure to upadacitinib. Avoid. [Moderate] Theoretical
- **Grapefruit** juice is predicted to increase the exposure to venetoclax. Avoid. [Severe] Theoretical
- **Grapefruit** and grapefruit juice are predicted to increase the exposure to voclosporin. Avoid. [Moderate] Theoretical
- **Grapefruit** juice is predicted to increase the exposure to zanubrutinib. [Moderate] Theoretical

Grass pollen extract

GENERAL INFORMATION Desensitising vaccines should be avoided in patients taking beta-blockers (adrenaline might be ineffective in case of a hypersensitivity reaction) or ACE inhibitors (risk of severe anaphylactoid reactions).

Grazoprevir

- Anti-androgens (apalutamide, enzalutamide) are predicted to decrease the exposure to **grazoprevir**. Avoid. [Severe] Study
- Antiepileptics (carbamazepine, fosphenytoin, phenobarbital, phenytoin, primidone) are predicted to decrease the exposure to **grazoprevir**. Avoid. [Severe] Study
- Antifungals, azoles (itraconazole, ketoconazole, posaconazole, voriconazole) are predicted to moderately to markedly increase the exposure to **grazoprevir**. Avoid. [Severe] Study
- Bulevirtide is predicted to increase the exposure to **grazoprevir**. Avoid or monitor. [Moderate] Theoretical
- **Grazoprevir** is predicted to increase the concentration of calcium channel blockers. [Moderate] Theoretical
- Cenobamate is predicted to markedly decrease the exposure to **grazoprevir**. Avoid. [Severe] Study
- Ceritinib is predicted to moderately to markedly increase the exposure to **grazoprevir**. Avoid. [Severe] Study
- Ciclosporin greatly increases the exposure to **grazoprevir**. Avoid. [Severe] Study
- Cobicistat is predicted to moderately to markedly increase the exposure to **grazoprevir**. Avoid. [Severe] Study
- Dabrafenib is predicted to markedly decrease the exposure to **grazoprevir**. Avoid. [Severe] Study
- Elvitegravir markedly increases the exposure to **grazoprevir**. Avoid. [Severe] Study
- Encorafenib is predicted to decrease the exposure to **grazoprevir**. Avoid. [Severe] Study
- Endothelin receptor antagonists (bosentan) are predicted to markedly decrease the exposure to **grazoprevir**. Avoid. [Severe] Study
- Fostemsavir is predicted to increase the exposure to **grazoprevir**. Avoid. [Severe] Theoretical
- HIV-protease inhibitors are predicted to moderately to markedly increase the exposure to **grazoprevir**. Avoid. [Severe] Study
- Idelalisib is predicted to moderately to markedly increase the exposure to **grazoprevir**. Avoid. [Severe] Study
- Ivosidenib is predicted to decrease the exposure to **grazoprevir**. Avoid. [Severe] Study
- Lorlatinib is predicted to markedly decrease the exposure to **grazoprevir**. Avoid. [Severe] Study
- Lumacaftor is predicted to decrease the exposure to **grazoprevir**. Avoid. [Severe] Study
- Macrolides (clarithromycin) are predicted to moderately to markedly increase the exposure to **grazoprevir**. Avoid. [Severe] Study
- Mitotane is predicted to decrease the exposure to **grazoprevir**. Avoid. [Severe] Study
- Modafinil is predicted to decrease the exposure to **grazoprevir**. Avoid. [Severe] Theoretical
- Nirmatrelvir boosted with ritonavir is predicted to increase the concentration of **grazoprevir**. [Severe] Theoretical

Grazoprevir (continued)

▸ **NNRTIs (efavirenz, etravirine, nevirapine)** are predicted to markedly decrease the exposure to **grazoprevir**. Avoid. Severe Study

▸ **Rifamycins (rifampicin)** are predicted to decrease the exposure to **grazoprevir**. Avoid. Severe Study

▸ **Sotorasib** is predicted to markedly decrease the exposure to **grazoprevir**. Avoid. Severe Study

▸ **St John's wort** is predicted to markedly decrease the exposure to **grazoprevir**. Avoid. Severe Study

▸ **Grazoprevir** moderately increases the exposure to statins (atorvastatin). Adjust **atorvastatin** dose, p. 234. Moderate Study

▸ **Grazoprevir** with elbasvir is predicted to increase the exposure to statins (fluvastatin). Adjust **fluvastatin** dose, p. 234. Moderate Theoretical

▸ **Grazoprevir** with elbasvir moderately increases the exposure to statins (rosuvastatin). Adjust **rosuvastatin** dose, p. 235. Moderate Study

▸ **Grazoprevir** with elbasvir is predicted to increase the exposure to statins (simvastatin). Adjust **simvastatin** dose, p. 237. Moderate Theoretical

▸ **Grazoprevir** is predicted to increase the concentration of sunitinib. Use with caution and adjust dose. Moderate Theoretical

▸ **Grazoprevir** increases the exposure to tacrolimus. Moderate Study

▸ **Tucatinib** is predicted to moderately to markedly increase the exposure to **grazoprevir**. Avoid. Severe Study

Griseofulvin

ROUTE-SPECIFIC INFORMATION Interactions do not generally apply to topical use unless specified.

▸ **Alcohol** potentially causes a disulfiram-like reaction when given with **griseofulvin**. Moderate Anecdotal

▸ **Antiepileptics (phenobarbital, primidone)** decrease the effects of **griseofulvin**. Moderate Study

▸ **Griseofulvin** potentially decreases the anticoagulant effect of coumarins. Moderate Anecdotal

Guanfacine → see TABLE 7 p. 1572 (hypotension), TABLE 10 p. 1574 (CNS effects)

▸ **Anti-androgens (apalutamide, enzalutamide)** are predicted to decrease the concentration of **guanfacine**. Adjust **guanfacine** dose, p. 407. Moderate Study

▸ **Antiarrhythmics (dronedarone)** are predicted to increase the concentration of **guanfacine**. Adjust **guanfacine** dose, p. 407. Moderate Theoretical

▸ **Antiepileptics (carbamazepine, fosphenytoin, phenobarbital, phenytoin, primidone)** are predicted to decrease the concentration of **guanfacine**. Adjust **guanfacine** dose, p. 407. Moderate Study → Also see TABLE 10 p. 1574

▸ **Antiepileptics (oxcarbazepine)** are predicted to decrease the concentration of **guanfacine**. Monitor and adjust **guanfacine** dose, p. 407. Moderate Theoretical

▸ **Guanfacine** increases the concentration of antiepileptics (valproate). Monitor and adjust dose. Moderate Study

▸ **Antifungals, azoles (fluconazole, isavuconazole)** are predicted to increase the concentration of **guanfacine**. Adjust **guanfacine** dose, p. 407. Moderate Theoretical

▸ **Antifungals, azoles (itraconazole, ketoconazole, posaconazole, voriconazole)** are predicted to increase the exposure to **guanfacine**. Adjust **guanfacine** dose, p. 407. Moderate Study

▸ **Berotralstat** is predicted to increase the concentration of **guanfacine**. Adjust **guanfacine** dose, p. 407. Moderate Theoretical

▸ **Calcium channel blockers (diltiazem, verapamil)** are predicted to increase the concentration of **guanfacine**. Adjust **guanfacine** dose, p. 407. Moderate Theoretical → Also see TABLE 7 p. 1572

▸ **Cenobamate** is predicted to decrease the concentration of **guanfacine**. Adjust dose. Moderate Theoretical → Also see TABLE 10 p. 1574

▸ **Ceritinib** is predicted to increase the exposure to **guanfacine**. Adjust **guanfacine** dose, p. 407. Moderate Study

▸ **Chloramphenicol** is predicted to increase the exposure to **guanfacine**. Adjust **guanfacine** dose, p. 407. Moderate Theoretical

▸ **Cobicistat** is predicted to increase the exposure to **guanfacine**. Adjust **guanfacine** dose, p. 407. Moderate Study

▸ **Crizotinib** is predicted to increase the concentration of guanfacine. Adjust **guanfacine** dose, p. 407. Moderate Theoretical

▸ **Dabrafenib** is predicted to decrease the concentration of guanfacine. Adjust dose. Moderate Theoretical

▸ **Encorafenib** is predicted to decrease the concentration of guanfacine. Adjust **guanfacine** dose, p. 407. Moderate Study

▸ **Endothelin receptor antagonists (bosentan)** are predicted to decrease the concentration of **guanfacine**. Adjust dose. Moderate Theoretical

▸ **Fedratinib** is predicted to increase the concentration of guanfacine. Adjust **guanfacine** dose, p. 407. Moderate Theoretical

▸ **Grapefruit** juice is predicted to increase the exposure to guanfacine. Avoid. Moderate Theoretical

▸ **HIV-protease inhibitors** are predicted to increase the exposure to **guanfacine**. Adjust **guanfacine** dose, p. 407. Moderate Study

▸ **Idelalisib** is predicted to increase the exposure to **guanfacine**. Adjust **guanfacine** dose, p. 407. Moderate Study

▸ **Imatinib** is predicted to increase the concentration of guanfacine. Adjust **guanfacine** dose, p. 407. Moderate Theoretical

▸ **Ivosidenib** is predicted to decrease the concentration of guanfacine. Adjust **guanfacine** dose, p. 407. Moderate Study

▸ **Letermovir** is predicted to increase the concentration of guanfacine. Adjust **guanfacine** dose, p. 407. Moderate Theoretical

▸ **Lorlatinib** is predicted to decrease the concentration of guanfacine. Adjust dose. Moderate Theoretical

▸ **Lumacaftor** is predicted to decrease the concentration of guanfacine. Adjust **guanfacine** dose, p. 407. Moderate Study

▸ **Macrolides (clarithromycin)** are predicted to increase the exposure to **guanfacine**. Adjust **guanfacine** dose, p. 407. Moderate Study

▸ **Macrolides (erythromycin)** are predicted to increase the concentration of **guanfacine**. Adjust **guanfacine** dose, p. 407. Moderate Theoretical

▸ **Guanfacine** is predicted to increase the concentration of metformin. Moderate Theoretical

▸ **Mitotane** is predicted to decrease the concentration of guanfacine. Adjust **guanfacine** dose, p. 407. Moderate Study

▸ **Neurokinin-1 receptor antagonists (aprepitant, netupitant)** are predicted to increase the concentration of **guanfacine**. Adjust **guanfacine** dose, p. 407. Moderate Theoretical

▸ **Neurokinin-1 receptor antagonists (fosaprepitant)** are predicted to increase the concentration of **guanfacine**. Moderate Theoretical

▸ **Nilotinib** is predicted to increase the concentration of guanfacine. Adjust **guanfacine** dose, p. 407. Moderate Theoretical

▸ **NNRTIs (efavirenz, etravirine, nevirapine)** are predicted to decrease the concentration of **guanfacine**. Adjust dose. Moderate Theoretical

▸ **Quinolones (ciprofloxacin)** are predicted to increase the concentration of **guanfacine**. Adjust **guanfacine** dose, p. 407. Moderate Theoretical

▸ **Rifamycins (rifampicin)** are predicted to decrease the concentration of **guanfacine**. Adjust **guanfacine** dose, p. 407. Moderate Study

▸ **Sotorasib** is predicted to decrease the concentration of guanfacine. Adjust dose. Moderate Theoretical

▸ **St John's wort** is predicted to decrease the concentration of guanfacine. Adjust dose. Moderate Theoretical

▸ **Tucatinib** is predicted to increase the exposure to **guanfacine**. Adjust **guanfacine** dose, p. 407. Moderate Study

Guselkumab → see monoclonal antibodies

H₂ receptor antagonists

cimetidine · famotidine · nizatidine · ranitidine

▸ **Cimetidine** decreases the clearance of albendazole. Moderate Study

▸ **Cimetidine** increases the concentration of aminophylline. Adjust dose. Severe Study

▸ **Cimetidine** slightly increases the exposure to anthracyclines (epirubicin). Avoid. Moderate Study

▸ **Cimetidine** increases the exposure to antiarrhythmics (amiodarone). Moderate Study

▸ **Cimetidine** slightly increases the exposure to antiarrhythmics (flecainide). Monitor and adjust dose. Mild Study

▸ **Cimetidine** increases the exposure to antiarrhythmics (lidocaine). Monitor and adjust dose. Moderate Study

- **Cimetidine** is predicted to increase the exposure to antiarrhythmics **(propafenone)**. Monitor and adjust dose. Moderate Theoretical
- **Cimetidine** transiently increases the concentration of antiepileptics **(carbamazepine)**. Monitor concentration and adjust dose. Moderate Study
- **Cimetidine** increases the concentration of antiepileptics **(fosphenytoin, phenytoin)**. Monitor concentration and adjust dose. Severe Study
- **H₂ receptor antagonists** are predicted to decrease the absorption of antifungals, azoles **(itraconazole)**. Administer **itraconazole** capsules with an acidic beverage. Moderate Study
- **H₂ receptor antagonists** are predicted to decrease the absorption of antifungals, azoles **(ketoconazole)**. Administer **ketoconazole** with an acidic beverage. Moderate Study
- **H₂ receptor antagonists** are predicted to decrease the exposure to antifungals, azoles **(posaconazole)**. Avoid use of posaconazole oral suspension. Moderate Study
- **Cimetidine** decreases the clearance of antimalarials **(chloroquine)**. Moderate Study
- **Cimetidine** slightly increases the exposure to antimalarials **(quinine)**. Moderate Study
- **H₂ receptor antagonists** are predicted to decrease the exposure to **belumosudil**. Separate administration by 12 hours. Moderate Theoretical
- **H₂ receptor antagonists** are predicted to decrease the absorption of **bosutinib**. Moderate Theoretical
- **Cimetidine** slightly increases the exposure to calcium channel blockers **(diltiazem, nimodipine)**. Monitor and adjust dose. Moderate Study
- **Cimetidine** (high-dose) is predicted to increase the exposure to calcium channel blockers **(lercanidipine)**. Moderate Theoretical
- **Cimetidine** moderately increases the exposure to calcium channel blockers **(nifedipine)**. Monitor and adjust dose. Severe Study
- **Cimetidine** increases the exposure to calcium channel blockers **(verapamil)**. Moderate Study
- **Cimetidine** is predicted to slightly increase the exposure to **capecitabine**. Severe Theoretical
- **H₂ receptor antagonists** are predicted to decrease the absorption of **ceritinib**. Moderate Theoretical
- **Cimetidine** increases the concentration of **ciclosporin**. Mild Study
- **Cimetidine** increases the anticoagulant effect of **coumarins**. Severe Study
- **H₂ receptor antagonists** are predicted to decrease the concentration of **dacomitinib**. **Dacomitinib** should be taken 2 hours before or 10 hours after **H₂ receptor antagonists**. Unknown Theoretical
- **Cimetidine** increases the exposure to **darifenacin**. Mild Study
- **H₂ receptor antagonists** are predicted to decrease the exposure to **dasatinib**. Avoid. Moderate Study
- **H₂ receptor antagonists** are predicted to decrease the absorption of **dipyridamole** (immediate release tablets). Moderate Theoretical
- **Cimetidine** is predicted to increase the exposure to dopamine receptor agonists **(pramipexole)**. Adjust dose. Moderate Study
- **H₂ receptor antagonists** are predicted to decrease the exposure to **erlotinib**. Manufacturer advises take 2 hours before or 10 hours after **H₂ receptor antagonists**. Moderate Study
- **Cimetidine** increases the concentration of **fampridine**. Avoid. Severe Theoretical
- **Cimetidine** slightly increases the exposure to **fluorouracil**. Severe Study
- **H₂ receptor antagonists** are predicted to slightly to moderately decrease the exposure to **gefitinib**. Moderate Study
- **H₂ receptor antagonists** decrease the exposure to HIV-protease inhibitors **(atazanavir)**. Monitor and adjust dose. Moderate Study
- **Cimetidine** is predicted to decrease the clearance of **hydroxychloroquine**. Moderate Theoretical
- **Ivosidenib** is predicted to increase the exposure to H₂ receptor antagonists **(cimetidine, famotidine)**. Use with caution or avoid. Moderate Theoretical
- **H₂ receptor antagonists** are predicted to decrease the absorption of **lapatinib**. Avoid. Moderate Theoretical

- **H₂ receptor antagonists** are predicted to decrease the exposure to **ledipasvir**. Adjust dose, see ledipasvir with sofosbuvir p. 724. Moderate Study
- **Leflunomide** is predicted to increase the exposure to **famotidine**. Moderate Study
- **Cimetidine** is predicted to increase the exposure to **lomitapide**. Separate administration by 12 hours. Mild Theoretical
- **Ranitidine** is predicted to increase the exposure to **lomitapide**. Separate administration by 12 hours. Moderate Theoretical
- **Cimetidine** slightly increases the exposure to macrolides **(erythromycin)**. Moderate Study
- **Cimetidine** is predicted to increase the exposure to **mavacamten**. Monitor and adjust dose—consult product literature. Moderate Theoretical
- **Cimetidine** increases the concentration of **mebendazole**. Moderate Study
- **Cimetidine** is predicted to increase the exposure to **metformin**. Use with caution and adjust dose. Moderate Study
- **Cimetidine** slightly increases the exposure to **mirtazapine**. Use with caution and adjust dose. Moderate Theoretical
- **Cimetidine** increases the exposure to **moclobemide**. Adjust **moclobemide** dose, p. 420. Mild Study
- **H₂ receptor antagonists** are predicted to decrease the exposure to **neratinib**. Manufacturer advises take 2 hours before or 10 hours after **H₂ receptor antagonists**. Severe Study
- **H₂ receptor antagonists** might affect the absorption of **nilotinib**. **H₂ receptor antagonists** should be taken 10 hours before or 2 hours after **nilotinib**. Mild Theoretical
- **Nitisinone** is predicted to increase the exposure to **famotidine**. Moderate Study
- **H₂ receptor antagonists** are predicted to decrease the exposure to NNRTIs **(rilpivirine)**. **H₂ receptor antagonists** should be taken 12 hours before or 4 hours after **rilpivirine**. Severe Study
- **Cimetidine** increases the concentration of opioids **(alfentanil)**. Use with caution and adjust dose. Severe Study
- **Cimetidine** might increase the exposure to opioids **(fentanyl)**. Monitor and adjust dose. Moderate Study
- **H₂ receptor antagonists** are predicted to decrease the exposure to **pazopanib**. Manufacturer advises take 2 hours before or 10 hours after **H₂ receptor antagonists**. Moderate Theoretical
- **Cimetidine** increases the exposure to **phenindione**. Severe Anecdotal
- **Cimetidine** slightly increases the exposure to phosphodiesterase type-4 inhibitors **(roflumilast)**. Moderate Study
- **Cimetidine** moderately increases the exposure to **praziquantel**. Moderate Study
- **H₂ receptor antagonists** are predicted to decrease the exposure to **selpercatinib**. Manufacturer advises take 2 hours before or 10 hours after **H₂ receptor antagonists**. Moderate Study
- **Cimetidine** slightly increases the exposure to SNRIs **(venlafaxine)**. Mild Study
- **H₂ receptor antagonists** potentially decrease the exposure to **sofosbuvir**. Adjust dose, see ledipasvir with sofosbuvir p. 724, sofosbuvir with velpatasvir p. 725, and sofosbuvir with velpatasvir and voxilaprevir p. 726. Moderate Study
- **H₂ receptor antagonists** are predicted to decrease the exposure to **sotorasib**. Manufacturer advises give **sotorasib** with an acidic beverage or use an antacid. Moderate Study
- **Cimetidine** slightly increases the exposure to SSRIs **(citalopram, escitalopram)**. Adjust dose. Moderate Study
- **Cimetidine** slightly increases the exposure to SSRIs **(paroxetine, sertraline)**. Moderate Study
- **Cimetidine** is predicted to increase the risk of toxicity when given with **tegafur**. Severe Theoretical
- **Teriflunomide** is predicted to increase the exposure to **famotidine**. Moderate Study
- **Cimetidine** increases the concentration of **theophylline**. Adjust dose. Severe Study
- **Cimetidine** increases the exposure to **tricyclic antidepressants**. Moderate Study
- **Cimetidine** slightly increases the exposure to triptans **(zolmitriptan)**. Adjust **zolmitriptan** dose, p. 546. Mild Study
- **H₂ receptor antagonists** might decrease the efficacy of **ulipristal** for emergency hormonal contraception. For FSRH guidance, see Contraceptives, interactions p. 917. Unknown Theoretical

H$_2$ receptor antagonists (continued)
- **Vadadustat** is predicted to increase the exposure to **famotidine**. Monitor and adjust dose. [Moderate] Study
- **H$_2$ receptor antagonists** are predicted to decrease the concentration of **velpatasvir**. Adjust dose, see sofosbuvir with velpatasvir p. 725. [Moderate] Study

Haloperidol → see TABLE 17 p. 1576 (hyponatraemia), TABLE 7 p. 1572 (hypotension), TABLE 8 p. 1573 (QT-interval prolongation), TABLE 9 p. 1573 (antimuscarinics), TABLE 10 p. 1574 (CNS effects)

FOOD AND LIFESTYLE Dose adjustment might be necessary if smoking started or stopped during treatment.

- Anti-androgens (apalutamide, enzalutamide) decrease the concentration of **haloperidol**. Adjust dose. [Moderate] Study → Also see TABLE 8 p. 1573
- Antiepileptics (carbamazepine, fosphenytoin, phenobarbital, phenytoin, primidone) decrease the concentration of **haloperidol**. Adjust dose. [Moderate] Study → Also see TABLE 17 p. 1576 → Also see TABLE 10 p. 1574
- **Haloperidol** potentially increases the risk of overheating and dehydration when given with antiepileptics (zonisamide). Avoid in children. [Severe] Theoretical
- Antifungals, azoles (itraconazole) increase the concentration of **haloperidol**. [Moderate] Study
- Antipsychotics, second generation (clozapine) can cause constipation, as can **haloperidol**; concurrent use might increase the risk of developing intestinal obstruction. [Severe] Theoretical → Also see TABLE 17 p. 1576 → Also see TABLE 7 p. 1572 → Also see TABLE 9 p. 1573 → Also see TABLE 10 p. 1574
- **Haloperidol** is predicted to decrease the effects of dopamine receptor agonists. Avoid. [Moderate] Theoretical → Also see TABLE 7 p. 1572 → Also see TABLE 8 p. 1573 → Also see TABLE 9 p. 1573 → Also see TABLE 10 p. 1574
- **Encorafenib** decreases the concentration of **haloperidol**. Adjust dose. [Moderate] Study → Also see TABLE 8 p. 1573
- **Haloperidol** opposes the effects of the active metabolite of foslevodopa. [Severe] Theoretical → Also see TABLE 7 p. 1572 → Also see TABLE 10 p. 1574
- **Haloperidol** potentially opposes the effects of glycerol phenylbutyrate. [Moderate] Theoretical
- HIV-protease inhibitors (ritonavir) are predicted to increase the exposure to **haloperidol**. [Severe] Theoretical
- **Ivosidenib** decreases the concentration of **haloperidol**. Adjust dose. [Moderate] Study → Also see TABLE 8 p. 1573
- **Haloperidol** decreases the effects of levodopa. [Severe] Study → Also see TABLE 7 p. 1572 → Also see TABLE 10 p. 1574
- **Lumacaftor** decreases the concentration of **haloperidol**. Adjust dose. [Moderate] Study
- **Mitotane** decreases the concentration of **haloperidol**. Adjust dose. [Moderate] Study
- **Nirmatrelvir** boosted with ritonavir is predicted to increase the concentration of **haloperidol**. [Severe] Theoretical
- Rifamycins (rifampicin) decrease the concentration of **haloperidol**. Adjust dose. [Moderate] Study
- SNRIs (venlafaxine) slightly increase the exposure to **haloperidol**. [Severe] Study → Also see TABLE 17 p. 1576 → Also see TABLE 10 p. 1574
- **Haloperidol** potentially decreases the effects of sodium phenylbutyrate. [Moderate] Anecdotal
- SSRIs (fluoxetine) increase the concentration of **haloperidol**. Adjust dose. [Moderate] Anecdotal → Also see TABLE 17 p. 1576 → Also see TABLE 10 p. 1574
- SSRIs (fluvoxamine) increase the concentration of **haloperidol**. Adjust dose. [Moderate] Study → Also see TABLE 17 p. 1576 → Also see TABLE 10 p. 1574
- **Haloperidol** might enhance the antidiuretic and hypertensive effects of vasopressin. [Moderate] Theoretical

Heparin → see TABLE 1 p. 1571 (hepatotoxicity), TABLE 15 p. 1575 (increased serum potassium), TABLE 3 p. 1571 (anticoagulant effects)

- **Andexanet alfa** has been reported to affect the anticoagulant effect of **heparin**. Avoid. [Severe] Anecdotal
- **Oritavancin** might cause a falsely elevated aPTT when given with **heparin**. Avoid and for 120 hours after stopping oritavancin. [Severe] Theoretical

- **Heparin** might decrease the antidiuretic effect of vasopressin. [Moderate] Theoretical

Hepatitis B immunoglobulin → see immunoglobulins

HIV-protease inhibitors → see TABLE 1 p. 1571 (hepatotoxicity)

atazanavir · darunavir · fosamprenavir · lopinavir · ritonavir

GENERAL INFORMATION Caution on concurrent use of **atazanavir**, **lopinavir with ritonavir**, or **ritonavir** with drugs that prolong the PR interval.

- **HIV-protease inhibitors** are predicted to increase the exposure to abemaciclib. Avoid or adjust dose—consult product literature. [Severe] Study
- **HIV-protease inhibitors** are predicted to increase the exposure to acalabrutinib. Avoid. [Severe] Study
- HIV-protease inhibitors (lopinavir, ritonavir) are predicted to increase the exposure to afatinib. [Moderate] Study
- **Ritonavir** is predicted to decrease the exposure to agomelatine. [Moderate] Theoretical
- **Ritonavir** decreases the exposure to albendazole. [Moderate] Study
- **Ritonavir** is predicted to increase the exposure to aliskiren. [Moderate] Theoretical
- **HIV-protease inhibitors** are predicted to moderately increase the exposure to alpha blockers (alfuzosin, tamsulosin). Use with caution or avoid. [Moderate] Study
- **HIV-protease inhibitors** are predicted to increase the exposure to alpha blockers (doxazosin). [Moderate] Study
- **Ritonavir** is predicted to increase the exposure to amfetamines. [Severe] Theoretical
- **Ritonavir** decreases the exposure to aminophylline. Adjust dose. [Moderate] Study
- **Ritonavir** is predicted to decrease the exposure to anaesthetics, local (ropivacaine). [Moderate] Theoretical
- Oral antacids are predicted to decrease the absorption of oral atazanavir. Manufacturer advises take 2 hours before or 1 hour after antacids. [Severe] Theoretical
- Anti-androgens (enzalutamide) are predicted to affect the exposure to **ritonavir**. Use with caution or avoid. [Moderate] Theoretical
- **HIV-protease inhibitors** are predicted to increase the exposure to anti-androgens (apalutamide). Monitor and adjust dose. [Mild] Study
- **Ritonavir** is predicted to decrease the efficacy of anti-androgens (cyproterone) with ethinylestradiol (co-cyprindiol). Use alternative methods during treatment with, and for 28 days after, the enzyme inducing drug is stopped. [Severe] Study
- HIV-protease inhibitors (lopinavir, ritonavir) are predicted to increase the exposure to anti-androgens (darolutamide). Monitor and adjust dose. [Moderate] Theoretical
- **HIV-protease inhibitors** are predicted to increase the exposure to antiarrhythmics (amiodarone). Avoid. [Severe] Theoretical → Also see TABLE 1 p. 1571
- **HIV-protease inhibitors** are predicted to increase the exposure to antiarrhythmics (disopyramide). [Severe] Theoretical
- **HIV-protease inhibitors** very markedly increase the exposure to antiarrhythmics (dronedarone). Avoid. [Severe] Study
- **Ritonavir** is predicted to increase the exposure to antiarrhythmics (flecainide). Avoid or monitor adverse effects. [Severe] Theoretical
- **HIV-protease inhibitors** are predicted to increase the exposure to antiarrhythmics (lidocaine). Avoid. [Severe] Study
- **HIV-protease inhibitors** are predicted to increase the exposure to antiarrhythmics (propafenone). Monitor and adjust dose. [Severe] Study
- **HIV-protease inhibitors** are predicted to increase the exposure to anticholinesterases, centrally acting (galantamine). Monitor and adjust dose. [Moderate] Study
- **HIV-protease inhibitors** are predicted to increase the exposure to antiepileptics (carbamazepine) and antiepileptics (carbamazepine) are predicted to decrease the exposure to **HIV-protease inhibitors**. Monitor and adjust dose. [Severe] Theoretical
- **HIV-protease inhibitors** are predicted to affect the exposure to antiepileptics (fosphenytoin, phenytoin) and antiepileptics

(fosphenytoin, phenytoin) decrease the concentration of **HIV-protease inhibitors**. Severe Theoretical

▸ **Ritonavir** decreases the exposure to antiepileptics (lamotrigine). Severe Study

▸ **HIV-protease inhibitors** are predicted to very slightly increase the exposure to antiepileptics (perampanel). Mild Study

▸ **HIV-protease inhibitors** are predicted to affect the concentration of antiepileptics (phenobarbital, primidone) and antiepileptics (phenobarbital, primidone) are predicted to decrease the concentration of **HIV-protease inhibitors**. Severe Theoretical

▸ **Ritonavir** is predicted to decrease the concentration of antiepileptics (valproate). Severe Anecdotal → Also see **TABLE 1** p. 1571

▸ Antifungals, azoles (miconazole) are predicted to increase the concentration of **HIV-protease inhibitors**. Use with caution and adjust dose. Moderate Theoretical

▸ Antifungals, azoles (posaconazole) are predicted to increase the exposure to **HIV-protease inhibitors**. Moderate Study

▸ **HIV-protease inhibitors** are predicted to increase the exposure to antifungals, azoles (isavuconazole). Avoid or monitor adverse effects. Severe Study

▸ **HIV-protease inhibitors** are predicted to increase the exposure to antifungals, azoles (itraconazole). Use with caution and adjust dose. Severe Study → Also see **TABLE 1** p. 1571

▸ **HIV-protease inhibitors** are predicted to increase the exposure to antifungals, azoles (ketoconazole). Use with caution and adjust dose. Moderate Study

▸ **HIV-protease inhibitors** are predicted to affect the exposure to antifungals, azoles (voriconazole) and antifungals, azoles (voriconazole) potentially affect the exposure to **HIV-protease inhibitors**. Severe Study → Also see **TABLE 1** p. 1571

▸ **Atazanavir** boosted with ritonavir is predicted to increase the exposure to antihistamines, non-sedating (fexofenadine). Moderate Theoretical

▸ **HIV-protease inhibitors** are predicted to increase the exposure to antihistamines, non-sedating (mizolastine). Avoid. Severe Study

▸ **HIV-protease inhibitors** are predicted to increase the exposure to antihistamines, non-sedating (rupatadine). Avoid. Moderate Study

▸ **HIV-protease inhibitors** decrease the exposure to antimalarials (atovaquone). Avoid if boosted with ritonavir. Moderate Study

▸ **HIV-protease inhibitors** are predicted to decrease the exposure to antimalarials (proguanil). Avoid. Moderate Study

▸ **HIV-protease inhibitors** are predicted to affect the exposure to antimalarials (quinine). Severe Study

▸ **HIV-protease inhibitors** are predicted to slightly increase the exposure to antipsychotics, second generation (aripiprazole). Adjust **aripiprazole** dose, p. 454. Moderate Study

▸ **HIV-protease inhibitors** are predicted to moderately increase the exposure to antipsychotics, second generation (cariprazine). Avoid. Severe Study

▸ **Ritonavir** is predicted to affect the exposure to antipsychotics, second generation (clozapine). Avoid. Severe Theoretical

▸ **HIV-protease inhibitors** are predicted to increase the exposure to antipsychotics, second generation (lurasidone, quetiapine). Avoid. Severe Study

▸ **Ritonavir** is predicted to decrease the exposure to antipsychotics, second generation (olanzapine). Monitor and adjust dose. Moderate Study

▸ **HIV-protease inhibitors** are predicted to increase the exposure to antipsychotics, second generation (risperidone). Adjust dose. Moderate Study

▸ **HIV-protease inhibitors** are predicted to increase the exposure to atogepant. Adjust **atogepant** dose, p. 540. Moderate Study

▸ **HIV-protease inhibitors** are predicted to increase the exposure to avacopan. Severe Study

▸ **HIV-protease inhibitors** are predicted to increase the exposure to avapritinib. Avoid. Moderate Study

▸ **HIV-protease inhibitors** are predicted to increase the exposure to axitinib. Avoid or adjust dose. Moderate Study

▸ **HIV-protease inhibitors** might increase the exposure to bedaquiline. Mild Study

▸ **HIV-protease inhibitors** moderately increase the exposure to benzodiazepines (alprazolam). Avoid. Moderate Study

▸ **Ritonavir** is predicted to increase the exposure to benzodiazepines (diazepam, flurazepam). Avoid. Moderate Theoretical

▸ **HIV-protease inhibitors** are predicted to markedly to very markedly increase the exposure to benzodiazepines (midazolam). Avoid or adjust dose. Severe Study

▸ HIV-protease inhibitors (lopinavir, ritonavir) are predicted to increase the exposure to beta blockers, non-selective (nadolol). Moderate Study

▸ **Ritonavir** is predicted to increase the exposure to beta blockers, selective (metoprolol). Moderate Study

▸ **HIV-protease inhibitors** are predicted to increase the exposure to beta$_2$ agonists (salmeterol). Avoid. Severe Study

▸ **Atazanavir** moderately increases the exposure to bictegravir. Avoid. Moderate Study

▸ HIV-protease inhibitors (lopinavir, ritonavir) are predicted to increase the exposure to bictegravir. Use with caution or avoid. Moderate Theoretical

▸ **HIV-protease inhibitors** slightly increase the exposure to bortezomib. Moderate Study

▸ **HIV-protease inhibitors** are predicted to increase the exposure to bosutinib. Avoid or adjust dose. Severe Study

▸ **HIV-protease inhibitors** are predicted to increase the exposure to brigatinib. Avoid or adjust dose—consult product literature. Severe Study

▸ **Ritonavir** is predicted to affect the efficacy of bulevirtide. Avoid. Severe Theoretical

▸ **HIV-protease inhibitors** are predicted to decrease the exposure to bupropion. Moderate Study

▸ **HIV-protease inhibitors** are predicted to increase the exposure to buspirone. Adjust **buspirone** dose, p. 396. Severe Study

▸ **HIV-protease inhibitors** are predicted to increase the exposure to cabozantinib. Moderate Study

▸ **Ritonavir** is predicted to moderately increase the clearance of caffeine citrate. Monitor and adjust dose. Moderate Study

▸ **HIV-protease inhibitors** are predicted to increase the exposure to calcium channel blockers (amlodipine, felodipine, lacidipine, nicardipine, nifedipine, nimodipine). Monitor and adjust dose. Moderate Study

▸ **HIV-protease inhibitors** are predicted to increase the exposure to calcium channel blockers (diltiazem, verapamil). Severe Study

▸ **HIV-protease inhibitors** are predicted to markedly increase the exposure to calcium channel blockers (lercanidipine). Avoid. Severe Study

▸ **HIV-protease inhibitors** are predicted to increase the exposure to cannabidiol. Avoid or adjust dose. Mild Study

▸ **HIV-protease inhibitors** are predicted to increase the exposure to capivasertib. Adjust dose. Moderate Study

▸ HIV-protease inhibitors (atazanavir, darunavir, lopinavir) boosted with ritonavir are predicted to increase the exposure to ceritinib. Avoid or adjust dose—consult product literature. Severe Study

▸ HIV-protease inhibitors (fosamprenavir, ritonavir) are predicted to increase the exposure to ceritinib. Avoid or adjust dose—consult product literature. Severe Study

▸ **HIV-protease inhibitors** increase the concentration of ciclosporin. Severe Study

▸ **HIV-protease inhibitors** are predicted to moderately increase the exposure to cilostazol. Adjust **cilostazol** dose, p. 266. Moderate Study

▸ **HIV-protease inhibitors** are predicted to moderately increase the exposure to cinacalcet. Adjust dose. Moderate Study

▸ **Ritonavir** might increases the exposure to cladribine. Moderate Theoretical

▸ **Ritonavir** might decrease the efficacy of clopidogrel. Avoid. Moderate Theoretical

▸ **HIV-protease inhibitors** are predicted to increase the exposure to cobimetinib. Avoid or monitor for toxicity. Severe Study

▸ **HIV-protease inhibitors** are predicted to increase the exposure to colchicine. Avoid potent CYP3A4 inhibitors or adjust **colchicine** dose, p. 1279. Severe Study

▸ **Atazanavir** affects the exposure to combined hormonal contraceptives. Adjust dose. Severe Study

HIV-protease inhibitors (continued)

► **Ritonavir** is predicted to decrease the efficacy of combined hormonal contraceptives. For FSRH guidance, see Contraceptives, interactions p. 917. [Severe] Study

► **HIV-protease inhibitors** are predicted to increase the exposure to corticosteroids (beclometasone) (risk with beclometasone is likely to be lower than with other corticosteroids). [Moderate] Theoretical

► **HIV-protease inhibitors** are predicted to increase the exposure to corticosteroids (betamethasone, budesonide, ciclesonide, deflazacort, dexamethasone, fludrocortisone, fluticasone, hydrocortisone, methylprednisolone, mometasone, prednisolone, triamcinolone). Avoid or monitor adverse effects. [Severe] Study

► **HIV-protease inhibitors** are predicted to increase the exposure to corticosteroids (vamorolone). Adjust dose. [Severe] Study

► **HIV-protease inhibitors** are predicted to affect the anticoagulant effect of coumarins. [Moderate] Study

► **HIV-protease inhibitors** are predicted to increase the exposure to crizotinib. Avoid. [Moderate] Study

► **HIV-protease inhibitors** are predicted to increase the exposure to dabrafenib. Use with caution or avoid. [Moderate] Study

► **HIV-protease inhibitors** are predicted to increase the exposure to daridorexant. Avoid. [Severe] Study

► **HIV-protease inhibitors** are predicted to markedly to very markedly increase the exposure to darifenacin. Avoid. [Severe] Study

► **HIV-protease inhibitors** are predicted to increase the exposure to dasatinib. Avoid or adjust dose—consult product literature. [Severe] Study

► **HIV-protease inhibitors** very slightly increase the exposure to delamanid. [Severe] Study

► **Ritonavir** is predicted to decrease the efficacy of desogestrel. For FSRH guidance, see Contraceptives, interactions p. 917. [Severe] Theoretical

► **HIV-protease inhibitors** are predicted to moderately increase the exposure to dienogest. [Moderate] Study

► **Lopinavir** boosted with ritonavir is predicted to increase the exposure to digoxin. [Severe] Theoretical

► **Ritonavir** increases the concentration of digoxin. Adjust dose and monitor concentration. [Severe] Study

► **HIV-protease inhibitors** are predicted to increase the exposure to dipeptidylpeptidase-4 inhibitors (saxagliptin). [Moderate] Study

► **Atazanavir** (alone or boosted with ritonavir) slightly increases the exposure to dolutegravir. Adjust dose—consult product literature. [Moderate] Study

► **Fosamprenavir** boosted with ritonavir slightly decreases the exposure to dolutegravir. Avoid if resistant to HIV-integrase inhibitors. [Severe] Study

► **HIV-protease inhibitors** are predicted to increase the exposure to domperidone. Avoid. [Severe] Study

► **HIV-protease inhibitors** increase the exposure to dopamine receptor agonists (bromocriptine). [Severe] Study

► **HIV-protease inhibitors** are predicted to increase the concentration of dopamine receptor agonists (cabergoline). [Moderate] Anecdotal

► **HIV-protease inhibitors** are predicted to increase the exposure to dronabinol. Adjust dose. [Mild] Study

► HIV-protease inhibitors (atazanavir, darunavir, fosamprenavir, lopinavir) are predicted to increase the exposure to drospirenone. [Severe] Study

► **Ritonavir** is predicted to decrease the efficacy of drospirenone. For FSRH guidance, see Contraceptives, interactions p. 917. [Severe] Theoretical

► **HIV-protease inhibitors** are predicted to increase the exposure to dutasteride. Monitor adverse effects and adjust dose. [Moderate] Theoretical

► **HIV-protease inhibitors** are predicted to increase the exposure to elacestrant. Avoid potent CYP3A4 inhibitors or adjust **elacestrant** dose, p. 1084. [Severe] Study

► **HIV-protease inhibitors** are predicted to increase the exposure to elexacaftor. Adjust ivacaftor with tezacaftor and elexacaftor p. 337 dose with potent CYP3A4 inhibitors. [Severe] Study

► **HIV-protease inhibitors** are predicted to increase the exposure to eliglustat. Avoid or adjust dose—consult product literature. [Severe] Study

► HIV-protease inhibitors (atazanavir, lopinavir) boosted with ritonavir increase the concentration of elvitegravir. Refer to specialist literature. [Moderate] Study

► **HIV-protease inhibitors** are predicted to increase the exposure to encorafenib. Avoid or monitor. [Severe] Study

► **HIV-protease inhibitors** are predicted to increase the exposure to endothelin receptor antagonists (bosentan). [Severe] Study

► **HIV-protease inhibitors** are predicted to increase the exposure to endothelin receptor antagonists (macitentan). [Moderate] Study

► **HIV-protease inhibitors** are predicted to increase the exposure to the cytotoxic component of enfortumab vedotin. [Severe] Theoretical

► **HIV-protease inhibitors** are predicted to increase the exposure to entrectinib. Avoid or adjust dose with potent CYP3A4 inhibitors—consult product literature. [Severe] Study

► **HIV-protease inhibitors** are predicted to increase the exposure to erdafitinib. Adjust dose. [Severe] Study

► **HIV-protease inhibitors** are predicted to increase the risk of ergotism when given with ergometrine. Avoid. [Severe] Theoretical

► **HIV-protease inhibitors** are predicted to increase the exposure to erlotinib. Use with caution and adjust dose. [Severe] Study

► **HIV-protease inhibitors** are predicted to increase the exposure to esketamine. Adjust dose. [Moderate] Study

► **Ritonavir** is predicted to decrease the efficacy of estradiol. [Moderate] Theoretical

► **HIV-protease inhibitors** are predicted to increase the exposure to eszopiclone. Adjust **eszopiclone** dose; avoid in the elderly, p. 554. [Moderate] Study

► **HIV-protease inhibitors** are predicted to increase the concentration of subdermal etonogestrel. [Moderate] Theoretical

► **Ritonavir** is predicted to decrease the efficacy of etonogestrel. For FSRH guidance, see Contraceptives, interactions p. 917. [Severe] Theoretical

► **HIV-protease inhibitors** are predicted to increase the exposure to etrasimod. Avoid in poor CYP2C9 metabolisers. [Severe] Theoretical

► **HIV-protease inhibitors** are predicted to increase the exposure to everolimus. Avoid. [Severe] Study

► **Atazanavir** boosted with ritonavir is predicted to increase the exposure to factor XA inhibitors (apixaban). [Severe] Theoretical

► **Darunavir** boosted with ritonavir or cobicistat is predicted to increase the exposure to factor XA inhibitors (apixaban). Avoid. [Severe] Theoretical

► **Fosamprenavir** boosted with ritonavir is predicted to increase the exposure to factor XA inhibitors (apixaban). [Moderate] Theoretical

► **Ritonavir** is predicted to increase the exposure to factor XA inhibitors (apixaban). Avoid. [Severe] Theoretical

► **Lopinavir** boosted with ritonavir is predicted to increase the exposure to factor XA inhibitors (apixaban, rivaroxaban). Avoid. [Severe] Theoretical

► **Lopinavir** boosted with ritonavir is predicted to slightly increase the exposure to factor XA inhibitors (edoxaban). [Severe] Theoretical

► **Ritonavir** is predicted to slightly increase the exposure to factor XA inhibitors (edoxaban). [Severe] Theoretical

► **Darunavir** boosted with ritonavir is predicted to increase the exposure to factor XA inhibitors (rivaroxaban). Avoid. [Severe] Anecdotal

► **Ritonavir** moderately increases the exposure to factor XA inhibitors (rivaroxaban). Avoid. [Severe] Study

► HIV-protease inhibitors (atazanavir, fosamprenavir) boosted with ritonavir are predicted to increase the exposure to factor XA inhibitors (rivaroxaban). Avoid. [Severe] Theoretical

► **HIV-protease inhibitors** are predicted to increase the exposure to fedratinib. Adjust dose, but avoid depending on other drugs taken—consult product literature. [Moderate] Study

► **HIV-protease inhibitors** are predicted to moderately increase the exposure to fesoterodine. Adjust **fesoterodine** dose with potent CYP3A4 inhibitors; avoid in hepatic and renal impairment, p. 897. [Severe] Study

- HIV-protease inhibitors **(lopinavir, ritonavir)** are predicted to increase the exposure to fidaxomicin. Avoid. Moderate Study
- **HIV-protease inhibitors** are predicted to increase the exposure to fostamatinib. Monitor adverse effects and adjust dose. Moderate Study
- **HIV-protease inhibitors** are predicted to increase the exposure to gefitinib. Severe Study
- **HIV-protease inhibitors** are predicted to increase the exposure to gilteritinib. Moderate Study
- **HIV-protease inhibitors** are predicted to increase the exposure to glasdegib. Use with caution or avoid. Severe Study
- **HIV-protease inhibitors (atazanavir, darunavir, lopinavir)** boosted with ritonavir increase the exposure to glecaprevir. Avoid. Severe Study
- **Ritonavir** increases the exposure to glecaprevir. Avoid. Severe Study
- **HIV-protease inhibitors** are predicted to moderately to markedly increase the exposure to grazoprevir. Avoid. Severe Study
- **HIV-protease inhibitors** are predicted to increase the exposure to guanfacine. Adjust **guanfacine** dose, p. 407. Moderate Study
- **H₂ receptor antagonists** decrease the exposure to **atazanavir**. Monitor and adjust dose. Moderate Study
- **Ritonavir** is predicted to increase the exposure to haloperidol. Severe Theoretical
- **Ritonavir** is predicted to decrease the effects of hormone replacement therapy. Moderate Anecdotal
- **HIV-protease inhibitors** are predicted to increase the exposure to ibrutinib. Avoid or adjust dose with potent CYP3A4 inhibitors—consult product literature. Severe Study
- **HIV-protease inhibitors (atazanavir, darunavir, fosamprenavir, lopinavir)** boosted with ritonavir are predicted to increase the exposure to idelalisib. Moderate Theoretical
- **Ritonavir** is predicted to increase the exposure to idelalisib. Moderate Theoretical
- **HIV-protease inhibitors** are predicted to increase the exposure to imatinib. Moderate Study
- **HIV-protease inhibitors** are predicted to increase the risk of toxicity when given with irinotecan. Avoid. Severe Study
- **Ritonavir** is predicted to decrease the exposure to iron chelators (deferasirox). Monitor serum ferritin and adjust dose. Moderate Theoretical
- **HIV-protease inhibitors** are predicted to increase the exposure to ivabradine. Avoid. Severe Study
- **HIV-protease inhibitors** are predicted to increase the exposure to ivacaftor. Adjust dose with potent CYP3A4 inhibitors, see ivacaftor p. 336, lumacaftor with ivacaftor p. 338, tezacaftor with ivacaftor p. 339, and ivacaftor with tezacaftor and elexacaftor p. 337. Severe Study
- **HIV-protease inhibitors** are predicted to increase the exposure to ivosidenib. Monitor and adjust dose—consult product literature. Severe Study
- **HIV-protease inhibitors** are predicted to increase the exposure to lapatinib. Avoid. Moderate Study
- **HIV-protease inhibitors** are predicted to moderately increase the exposure to larotrectinib. Avoid or adjust dose—consult product literature. Moderate Study
- **HIV-protease inhibitors** are predicted to increase the exposure to leniolisib. Avoid. Moderate Study
- HIV-protease inhibitors **(atazanavir, lopinavir)** boosted with ritonavir are predicted to increase the concentration of letermovir. Moderate Study
- **Ritonavir** is predicted to decrease the concentration of letermovir. Moderate Theoretical
- **Ritonavir** is predicted to decrease the efficacy of some contraceptive methods containing levonorgestrel. For FSRH guidance, see Contraceptives, interactions p. 917. Severe Theoretical
- **HIV-protease inhibitors** are predicted to markedly increase the exposure to lomitapide. Avoid. Severe Study → Also see **TABLE 1** p. 1571
- **HIV-protease inhibitors** are predicted to increase the exposure to lorlatinib. Avoid or adjust dose—consult product literature. Severe Study

- **Atazanavir** is predicted to increase the exposure to macrolides (clarithromycin). Adjust dose in renal impairment. Severe Study
- **Ritonavir** increases the exposure to macrolides (clarithromycin). Adjust dose in renal impairment. Severe Study
- HIV-protease inhibitors **(darunavir, fosamprenavir, lopinavir)** boosted with ritonavir are predicted to increase the exposure to macrolides (clarithromycin). Adjust dose in renal impairment. Severe Study
- **HIV-protease inhibitors** are predicted to increase the exposure to macrolides (erythromycin). Severe Theoretical
- **Atazanavir** moderately to markedly increases the exposure to maraviroc. Refer to specialist literature. Severe Study
- **Darunavir** boosted with ritonavir markedly increases the exposure to maraviroc. Refer to specialist literature. Severe Study
- **Maraviroc** potentially decreases the exposure to **fosamprenavir** and **fosamprenavir** potentially decreases the exposure to maraviroc. Avoid. Severe Study
- **Lopinavir** boosted with ritonavir moderately increases the exposure to maraviroc. Refer to specialist literature. Severe Study
- **Ritonavir** markedly increases the exposure to maraviroc. Refer to specialist literature. Severe Study
- **HIV-protease inhibitors** are predicted to increase the exposure to mavacamten. Avoid or monitor—consult product literature. Severe Study
- **HIV-protease inhibitors** are predicted to increase the concentration of intramuscular medroxyprogesterone. Moderate Theoretical
- **Ritonavir** is predicted to decrease the exposure to melatonin. Moderate Theoretical
- **Ritonavir** is predicted to increase the clearance of mexiletine. Monitor and adjust dose. Moderate Study
- **HIV-protease inhibitors** are predicted to increase the exposure to midostaurin. Avoid or monitor for toxicity. Severe Study
- **HIV-protease inhibitors** are predicted to markedly increase the exposure to mineralocorticoid receptor antagonists (eplerenone). Avoid. Severe Study
- **HIV-protease inhibitors** are predicted to increase the exposure to mineralocorticoid receptor antagonists (finerenone). Avoid. Severe Study
- **HIV-protease inhibitors** are predicted to increase the exposure to mirabegron. Adjust **mirabegron** dose in hepatic and renal impairment, p. 901. Moderate Study
- **HIV-protease inhibitors** are predicted to increase the exposure to mirtazapine. Moderate Study
- **HIV-protease inhibitors** are predicted to increase the exposure to mobocertinib. Avoid. Severe Study
- **HIV-protease inhibitors** are predicted to increase the exposure to modafinil. Mild Theoretical
- HIV-protease inhibitors **(atazanavir, lopinavir)** are predicted to increase the exposure to momelotinib. Moderate Study
- **HIV-protease inhibitors** are predicted to increase the risk of neutropenia when given with monoclonal antibodies (brentuximab vedotin). Monitor and adjust dose. Severe Study
- **HIV-protease inhibitors** are predicted to increase the exposure to monoclonal antibodies (polatuzumab vedotin). Moderate Theoretical
- **HIV-protease inhibitors** are predicted to increase the exposure to the cytotoxic component of monoclonal antibodies (trastuzumab emtansine). Avoid or monitor. Severe Theoretical
- **HIV-protease inhibitors** are predicted to increase the exposure to naldemedine. Avoid or monitor. Moderate Study
- **HIV-protease inhibitors** are predicted to markedly increase the exposure to naloxegol. Avoid. Severe Study
- **HIV-protease inhibitors** are predicted to increase the exposure to neratinib. Avoid or adjust dose with potent CYP3A4 inhibitors—consult product literature. Severe Study → Also see **TABLE 1** p. 1571
- **HIV-protease inhibitors** are predicted to markedly increase the exposure to neurokinin-1 receptor antagonists (aprepitant). Moderate Study
- **HIV-protease inhibitors** are predicted to increase the exposure to neurokinin-1 receptor antagonists (fosaprepitant). Moderate Theoretical

HIV-protease inhibitors (continued)

▸ **HIV-protease inhibitors** are predicted to increase the exposure to neurokinin-1 receptor antagonists (netupitant). Moderate Study

▸ **HIV-protease inhibitors** are predicted to increase the exposure to nilotinib. Avoid. Severe Study

▸ HIV-protease inhibitors (atazanavir, darunavir, fosamprenavir) boosted with ritonavir are predicted to increase the exposure to nintedanib. Moderate Theoretical

▸ HIV-protease inhibitors (lopinavir, ritonavir) are predicted to increase the exposure to nintedanib. Moderate Study

▸ Nirmatrelvir boosted with ritonavir is predicted to increase the concentration of HIV-protease inhibitors (atazanavir, darunavir, fosamprenavir, lopinavir). Moderate Theoretical

▸ **HIV-protease inhibitors** are predicted to increase the exposure to nitisinone. Adjust dose. Moderate Theoretical

▸ NNRTIs (efavirenz) decrease the exposure to **HIV-protease inhibitors**. Refer to specialist literature. Severe Study

▸ NNRTIs (etravirine) increase the exposure to **fosamprenavir** boosted with ritonavir. Refer to specialist literature. Moderate Study

▸ NNRTIs (nevirapine) decrease the exposure to **HIV-protease inhibitors**. Refer to specialist literature. Moderate Study → Also see **TABLE 1** p. 1571

▸ **Ritonavir** is predicted to decrease the efficacy of some contraceptive methods containing norethisterone. For FSRH guidance, see Contraceptives, interactions p. 917. Severe Anecdotal

▸ **HIV-protease inhibitors** are predicted to increase the exposure to olaparib. Avoid or adjust dose with potent CYP3A4 inhibitors—consult product literature. Moderate Study

▸ **HIV-protease inhibitors** are predicted to increase the exposure to opioids (alfentanil, buprenorphine, fentanyl, oxycodone). Monitor and adjust dose. Severe Study

▸ **HIV-protease inhibitors** boosted with ritonavir are predicted to decrease the exposure to opioids (methadone). Moderate Study

▸ **Ritonavir** is predicted to decrease the concentration of opioids (morphine). Moderate Theoretical

▸ **Ritonavir** increases the risk of CNS toxicity when given with opioids (pethidine). Avoid. Severe Study

▸ **HIV-protease inhibitors** are predicted to increase the exposure to opioids (sufentanil). Moderate Study

▸ **HIV-protease inhibitors** are predicted to increase the exposure to osilodrostat. Moderate Theoretical

▸ **HIV-protease inhibitors** are predicted to increase the exposure to ospemifene. Avoid in poor CYP2C9 metabolisers. Moderate Study

▸ **HIV-protease inhibitors** are predicted to increase the exposure to oxybutynin. Mild Study

▸ **HIV-protease inhibitors** are predicted to increase the exposure to palbociclib. Avoid or adjust dose—consult product literature. Severe Study

▸ **HIV-protease inhibitors** are predicted to increase the exposure to panobinostat. Adjust dose—consult product literature; in hepatic impairment avoid. Moderate Study

▸ **HIV-protease inhibitors** are predicted to increase the exposure to pazopanib. Avoid or adjust dose—consult product literature. Moderate Study

▸ **HIV-protease inhibitors** are predicted to increase the exposure to pemigatinib. Avoid or adjust dose—consult product literature. Severe Study

▸ **HIV-protease inhibitors** are predicted to increase the exposure to phosphodiesterase type-5 inhibitors (avanafil, vardenafil). Avoid. Severe Study

▸ **HIV-protease inhibitors** are predicted to increase the exposure to phosphodiesterase type-5 inhibitors (sildenafil). Avoid potent CYP3A4 inhibitors or adjust **sildenafil** dose, p. 940. Severe Study

▸ **HIV-protease inhibitors** are predicted to increase the exposure to phosphodiesterase type-5 inhibitors (tadalafil). Use with caution or avoid. Severe Study

▸ HIV-protease inhibitors (atazanavir, lopinavir) boosted with ritonavir increase the exposure to pibrentasvir. Avoid. Severe Study

▸ **Ritonavir** potentially increases the exposure to pibrentasvir. Severe Theoretical

▸ **HIV-protease inhibitors** are predicted to increase the exposure to pimozide. Avoid. Severe Study

▸ **Ritonavir** is predicted to decrease the exposure to pirfenidone. Moderate Theoretical

▸ **HIV-protease inhibitors** are predicted to slightly increase the exposure to ponatinib. Monitor and adjust dose—consult product literature. Moderate Study

▸ **HIV-protease inhibitors** are predicted to increase the exposure to pralsetinib. Avoid or adjust dose with potent CYP3A4 inhibitors—consult product literature. Moderate Study

▸ **HIV-protease inhibitors** are predicted to moderately increase the exposure to praziquantel. Mild Study

▸ **HIV-protease inhibitors** given with carbimazole are predicted to increase the exposure to propiverine. Adjust starting dose. Moderate Theoretical

▸ Proton pump inhibitors decrease the exposure to **atazanavir**. Avoid or adjust dose. Severe Study

▸ **HIV-protease inhibitors** are predicted to increase the exposure to quizartinib. Adjust dose—consult product literature. Severe Study

▸ **Atazanavir** increases the exposure to raltegravir (high-dose). Avoid. Moderate Study

▸ **Darunavir** increases the risk of rash when given with raltegravir. Moderate Study

▸ **Fosamprenavir** boosted with ritonavir decreases the exposure to raltegravir and raltegravir decreases the exposure to fosamprenavir boosted with ritonavir. Avoid. Severe Study

▸ **HIV-protease inhibitors** are predicted to increase the exposure to ranolazine. Avoid. Severe Study

▸ **HIV-protease inhibitors** are predicted to increase the exposure to reboxetine. Avoid. Moderate Study

▸ **HIV-protease inhibitors** are predicted to increase the exposure to regorafenib. Avoid. Moderate Study

▸ HIV-protease inhibitors (lopinavir, ritonavir) are predicted to increase the exposure to relugolix. Avoid or take relugolix first and separate administration by at least 6 hours. Moderate Study

▸ **HIV-protease inhibitors** are predicted to increase the exposure to retinoids (alitretinoin). Adjust **alitretinoin** dose, p. 1433. Moderate Theoretical

▸ **HIV-protease inhibitors** are predicted to increase the exposure to ribociclib. Avoid or adjust dose—consult product literature. Moderate Study

▸ Rifamycins (rifampicin) slightly decrease the exposure to ritonavir. Severe Study

▸ Rifamycins (rifampicin) are predicted to moderately to markedly decrease the exposure to HIV-protease inhibitors (atazanavir, darunavir, fosamprenavir, lopinavir). Avoid. Severe Study

▸ **Ritonavir** markedly increases the exposure to rifamycins (rifabutin). Avoid or adjust dose. Severe Study

▸ HIV-protease inhibitors (atazanavir, darunavir, fosamprenavir, lopinavir) boosted with ritonavir increase the exposure to rifamycins (rifabutin). Monitor and adjust dose. Severe Study

▸ **HIV-protease inhibitors** are predicted to increase the exposure to rimegepant. Avoid. Moderate Study

▸ **Ritonavir** is predicted to increase the exposure to riociguat. Adjust dose and monitor blood pressure. Moderate Theoretical

▸ **HIV-protease inhibitors** are predicted to increase the exposure to ripretinib. Moderate Theoretical

▸ **HIV-protease inhibitors** are predicted to increase the exposure to ruxolitinib. Adjust dose and monitor adverse effects. Moderate Study

▸ **HIV-protease inhibitors** are predicted to decrease the exposure to the active component of sacituzumab govitecan. Severe Theoretical

▸ **HIV-protease inhibitors** are predicted to increase the exposure to selpercatinib. Adjust dose—consult product literature. Moderate Study

▸ **HIV-protease inhibitors** are predicted to increase the exposure to selumetinib. Avoid or adjust dose—consult product literature. Severe Study

▸ **HIV-protease inhibitors** are predicted to increase the exposure to siponimod. Avoid depending on other drugs taken—consult product literature. Severe Theoretical

▸ **HIV-protease inhibitors** are predicted to increase the concentration of sirolimus. Avoid or monitor and adjust dose. Severe Study

▸ **Ritonavir** is predicted to decrease the exposure to SNRIs (duloxetine). Moderate Theoretical

▸ **HIV-protease inhibitors** are predicted to increase the exposure to SNRIs (venlafaxine). Moderate Study

▸ **Ritonavir** is predicted to decrease the exposure to sodium glucose co-transporter 2 inhibitors (canagliflozin). Adjust **canagliflozin** dose, p. 824. Moderate Study

▸ Sodium zirconium cyclosilicate is predicted to decrease the exposure to **HIV-protease inhibitors**. Separate administration by at least 2 hours. Moderate Theoretical

▸ **HIV-protease inhibitors** are predicted to increase the exposure to solifenacin. Adjust solifenacin p. 899 or tamsulosin with solifenacin p. 906 dose; avoid in hepatic and renal impairment. Severe Study

▸ **HIV-protease inhibitors** are predicted to moderately increase the exposure to SSRIs (dapoxetine). Avoid potent CYP3A4 inhibitors or adjust **dapoxetine** dose, p. 947. Severe Study

▸ St John's wort is predicted to decrease the exposure to **HIV-protease inhibitors**. Avoid. Severe Study

▸ **HIV-protease inhibitors** are predicted to increase the exposure to statins (atorvastatin). Avoid or adjust dose and monitor rhabdomyolysis. Severe Study → Also see **TABLE 1** p. 1571

▸ **HIV-protease inhibitors** might affect the exposure to statins (pravastatin). Moderate Study → Also see **TABLE 1** p. 1571

▸ **Fosamprenavir** is predicted to increase the exposure to statins (rosuvastatin). Use with caution and adjust dose. Severe Study

▸ HIV-protease inhibitors (**atazanavir, lopinavir**) boosted with ritonavir moderately increase the exposure to statins (rosuvastatin). Avoid or adjust **rosuvastatin** dose, p. 235. Severe Study

▸ HIV-protease inhibitors (**darunavir, ritonavir**) are predicted to increase the exposure to statins (rosuvastatin). Avoid or adjust dose. Severe Study → Also see **TABLE 1** p. 1571

▸ **HIV-protease inhibitors** are predicted to increase the exposure to statins (simvastatin). Avoid. Severe Study → Also see **TABLE 1** p. 1571

▸ HIV-protease inhibitors (**atazanavir, lopinavir**) boosted with ritonavir are predicted to increase the exposure to sulfonylureas (glibenclamide). Moderate Theoretical

▸ **HIV-protease inhibitors** are predicted to increase the exposure to sunitinib. Avoid or adjust dose—consult product literature. Moderate Study

▸ **HIV-protease inhibitors** are predicted to increase the concentration of tacrolimus. Monitor and adjust dose. Severe Study

▸ **Darunavir** is predicted to increase the exposure to talazoparib. Avoid or adjust dose—consult product literature. Moderate Theoretical

▸ HIV-protease inhibitors (**lopinavir, ritonavir**) are predicted to slightly increase the exposure to talazoparib. Avoid or adjust dose—consult product literature. Severe Study

▸ **HIV-protease inhibitors** are predicted to increase the exposure to taxanes (cabazitaxel). Avoid or adjust dose—consult product literature. Severe Study

▸ **HIV-protease inhibitors** are predicted to increase the exposure to taxanes (docetaxel). Avoid or adjust dose. Severe Study

▸ **HIV-protease inhibitors** are predicted to increase the exposure to taxanes (paclitaxel). Moderate Anecdotal

▸ **HIV-protease inhibitors** are predicted to increase the concentration of temsirolimus. Avoid. Severe Theoretical

▸ HIV-protease inhibitors (**atazanavir, darunavir, lopinavir**) increase the exposure to tenofovir alafenamide. Avoid or adjust dose. Moderate Study

▸ HIV-protease inhibitors (**atazanavir, darunavir, lopinavir**) are predicted to increase the risk of renal impairment when given with tenofovir disoproxil. Severe Anecdotal

▸ **Lopinavir** boosted with ritonavir might increase the exposure to tepotinib. Avoid. Severe Theoretical

▸ **Ritonavir** might increase the exposure to tepotinib. Avoid. Severe Theoretical

▸ **HIV-protease inhibitors** are predicted to increase the exposure to tezacaftor. Adjust dose with potent CYP3A4 inhibitors, see

tezacaftor with ivacaftor p. 339 and ivacaftor with tezacaftor and elexacaftor p. 337. Severe Study

▸ **Ritonavir** is predicted to decrease the exposure to theophylline. Adjust dose. Moderate Study

▸ **Fosamprenavir** boosted with ritonavir is predicted to increase the exposure to thrombin inhibitors (dabigatran). Avoid. Severe Theoretical

▸ **Ritonavir** is predicted to increase the exposure to thrombin inhibitors (dabigatran). Avoid. Severe Study

▸ HIV-protease inhibitors (**atazanavir, darunavir, lopinavir**) boosted with ritonavir are predicted to increase the exposure to thrombin inhibitors (dabigatran). Avoid. Severe Anecdotal

▸ **Ritonavir** decreases the concentration of thyroid hormones (levothyroxine). MHRA advises monitor TSH for at least one month after starting or stopping ritonavir. Moderate Anecdotal

▸ **HIV-protease inhibitors** are predicted to markedly increase the exposure to ticagrelor. Avoid. Severe Study

▸ HIV-protease inhibitors (**lopinavir, ritonavir**) might increase the exposure to tigecycline. Mild Anecdotal → Also see **TABLE 1** p. 1571

▸ **Ritonavir** moderately decreases the exposure to tizanidine. Mild Study

▸ **HIV-protease inhibitors** are predicted to increase the exposure to tofacitinib. Adjust **tofacitinib** dose, p. 1265. Moderate Study

▸ **HIV-protease inhibitors** are predicted to increase the exposure to tolterodine. Avoid. Severe Study

▸ **HIV-protease inhibitors** are predicted to increase the exposure to tolvaptan. Manufacturer advises caution or adjust **tolvaptan** dose with potent CYP3A4 inhibitors, p. 767. Severe Study

▸ HIV-protease inhibitors (**lopinavir, ritonavir**) are predicted to increase the exposure to topotecan. Severe Study

▸ **HIV-protease inhibitors** are predicted to increase the exposure to toremifene. Moderate Theoretical

▸ **HIV-protease inhibitors** are predicted to increase the exposure to trabectedin. Avoid or adjust dose. Severe Theoretical → Also see **TABLE 1** p. 1571

▸ HIV-protease inhibitors (**lopinavir, ritonavir**) are predicted to increase the concentration of trametinib. Moderate Theoretical

▸ **HIV-protease inhibitors** are predicted to moderately increase the exposure to trazodone. Avoid or adjust dose. Moderate Study

▸ **Ritonavir** is predicted to increase the exposure to tricyclic antidepressants. Moderate Theoretical

▸ **HIV-protease inhibitors** increase the exposure to triptans (almotriptan). Mild Study

▸ **HIV-protease inhibitors** are predicted to markedly increase the exposure to triptans (eletriptan). Avoid. Severe Study

▸ HIV-protease inhibitors (**atazanavir, darunavir, fosamprenavir, lopinavir**) boosted with ritonavir are predicted to increase the exposure to ulipristal. Avoid if used for uterine fibroids. Severe Study

▸ **Ritonavir** decreases the efficacy of ulipristal. Avoid and for 4 weeks after stopping the enzyme inducing drug. For FSRH guidance, see Contraceptives, interactions p. 917. Severe Anecdotal

▸ **HIV-protease inhibitors** are predicted to increase the exposure to upadacitinib. Manufacturer advises caution or avoid, or adjust **upadacitinib** dose depending on indication, p. 1267. Severe Study

▸ **HIV-protease inhibitors** are predicted to increase the exposure to vemurafenib. Severe Theoretical

▸ **HIV-protease inhibitors** are predicted to increase the exposure to venetoclax. Avoid or adjust dose—consult product literature. Severe Study

▸ **HIV-protease inhibitors** are predicted to increase the exposure to vinca alkaloids. Severe Theoretical

▸ **HIV-protease inhibitors** are predicted to increase the exposure to vitamin D substances (paricalcitol). Moderate Study

▸ **HIV-protease inhibitors** are predicted to increase the exposure to voclosporin. Avoid. Severe Study

▸ **Atazanavir** boosted with ritonavir increases the concentration of voxilaprevir. Avoid. Severe Study

▸ **Lopinavir** boosted with ritonavir is predicted to increase the concentration of voxilaprevir. Avoid. Severe Theoretical

HIV-protease inhibitors (continued)

▸ **HIV-protease inhibitors** are predicted to increase the exposure to zanubrutinib. Avoid or adjust dose with potent CYP3A4 inhibitors—consult product literature. Moderate Study

▸ **HIV-protease inhibitors** are predicted to increase the exposure to zopiclone. Adjust dose. Moderate Theoretical

Homatropine → see TABLE 9 p. 1573 (antimuscarinics)

▸ Antipsychotics, second generation (clozapine) can cause constipation, as can **homatropine**; concurrent use might increase the risk of developing intestinal obstruction. Severe Theoretical → Also see TABLE 9 p. 1573

Hormone replacement therapy

▸ Antiepileptics (carbamazepine, eslicarbazepine, fosphenytoin, oxcarbazepine, perampanel, phenobarbital, phenytoin, primidone, rufinamide, topiramate) are predicted to decrease the effects of **hormone replacement therapy**. Moderate Anecdotal

▸ **Hormone replacement therapy** is predicted to alter the exposure to antiepileptics (lamotrigine). Moderate Theoretical

▸ **Hormone replacement therapy** decreases the clearance of dopamine receptor agonists (ropinirole). Monitor and adjust dose. Moderate Study

▸ Endothelin receptor antagonists (bosentan) are predicted to decrease the effects of **hormone replacement therapy**. Moderate Anecdotal

▸ HIV-protease inhibitors (ritonavir) are predicted to decrease the effects of **hormone replacement therapy**. Moderate Anecdotal

▸ **Hormone replacement therapy** is predicted to increase the risk of venous thromboembolism when given with lenalidomide. Moderate Theoretical

▸ **Hormone replacement therapy** is predicted to increase the exposure to MAO-B inhibitors (selegiline). Avoid. Moderate Study

▸ Modafinil is predicted to decrease the effects of **hormone replacement therapy**. Moderate Anecdotal

▸ Neurokinin-1 receptor antagonists (aprepitant, fosaprepitant) are predicted to decrease the effects of **hormone replacement therapy**. Moderate Anecdotal

▸ NNRTIs (efavirenz, nevirapine) are predicted to decrease the effects of **hormone replacement therapy**. Moderate Anecdotal

▸ NSAIDs (etoricoxib) increase the exposure to **hormone replacement therapy**. Moderate Study

▸ **Hormone replacement therapy** potentially opposes the effects of ospemifene. Avoid. Severe Theoretical

▸ **Hormone replacement therapy** is predicted to increase the risk of venous thromboembolism when given with pomalidomide. Severe Theoretical

▸ **Hormone replacement therapy** potentially opposes the effects of raloxifene. Avoid. Severe Theoretical

▸ Rifamycins are predicted to decrease the effects of **hormone replacement therapy**. Moderate Anecdotal

▸ St John's wort is predicted to decrease the efficacy of **hormone replacement therapy**. Moderate Theoretical

▸ **Hormone replacement therapy** is predicted to increase the risk of venous thromboembolism when given with thalidomide. Severe Theoretical

▸ Oral **hormone replacement therapy** is predicted to decrease the effects of thyroid hormones. Moderate Theoretical

Hydralazine → see TABLE 7 p. 1572 (hypotension)

▸ Diazoxide increases the risk of severe hypotension when given with **hydralazine**. Severe Study → Also see TABLE 7 p. 1572

Hydrochlorothiazide → see thiazide diuretics

Hydrocortisone → see corticosteroids

Hydroflumethiazide → see thiazide diuretics

Hydromorphone → see opioids

Hydroxycarbamide → see TABLE 14 p. 1575 (myelosuppression)

▸ Live vaccines are predicted to increase the risk of generalised infection (possibly life-threatening) when given with **hydroxycarbamide**. UKHSA advises avoid (refer to Green Book). Severe Theoretical

Hydroxychloroquine → see TABLE 18 p. 1576 (ototoxicity), TABLE 8 p. 1573 (QT-interval prolongation)

▸ **Hydroxychloroquine** is predicted to decrease the effects of agalsidase alfa. Moderate Theoretical

▸ **Hydroxychloroquine** is predicted to decrease the exposure to agalsidase beta. Moderate Theoretical

▸ Oral antacids are predicted to decrease the absorption of oral **hydroxychloroquine**. Separate administration by at least 4 hours. Moderate Theoretical

▸ Oral calcium salts (calcium carbonate) might decrease the absorption of oral **hydroxychloroquine**. Moderate Theoretical

▸ H$_2$ receptor antagonists (cimetidine) are predicted to decrease the clearance of **hydroxychloroquine**. Moderate Theoretical

▸ Oral kaolin is predicted to decrease the absorption of oral **hydroxychloroquine**. Moderate Theoretical

▸ Lanthanum is predicted to decrease the absorption of **hydroxychloroquine**. Separate administration by at least 2 hours. Moderate Theoretical

▸ **Hydroxychloroquine** is predicted to decrease the exposure to laronidase. Avoid simultaneous administration. Severe Theoretical

▸ Macrolides might increase the risk of serious cardiovascular adverse effects when given with **hydroxychloroquine**. Severe Theoretical → Also see TABLE 8 p. 1573

▸ Oral magnesium trisilicate is predicted to decrease the absorption of oral **hydroxychloroquine**. Moderate Theoretical

▸ **Hydroxychloroquine** is predicted to increase the risk of haematological toxicity when given with penicillamine. Avoid. Severe Theoretical

▸ **Hydroxychloroquine** is predicted to decrease efficacy rabies vaccine. Moderate Theoretical

▸ **Hydroxychloroquine** might decrease the effects of remdesivir. Avoid. Moderate Theoretical

▸ Tamoxifen increases the risk of retinopathy when given with **hydroxychloroquine**. RCOphth guidance advises monitor. Severe Study

Hydroxyzine → see antihistamines, sedating

Hyoscine → see TABLE 9 p. 1573 (antimuscarinics)

▸ Antipsychotics, second generation (clozapine) can cause constipation, as can **hyoscine**; concurrent use might increase the risk of developing intestinal obstruction. Severe Theoretical → Also see TABLE 9 p. 1573

Ibandronate → see bisphosphonates

Ibrutinib → see TABLE 14 p. 1575 (myelosuppression), TABLE 4 p. 1571 (antiplatelet effects)

FOOD AND LIFESTYLE Avoid food or drink containing bitter (Seville) oranges as they are predicted to increase the exposure to ibrutinib.

▸ Anti-androgens (apalutamide, enzalutamide) are predicted to decrease the exposure to **ibrutinib**. Avoid or monitor. Severe Study

▸ Antiarrhythmics (amiodarone) are predicted to increase the exposure to **ibrutinib**. Adjust dose—consult product literature. Severe Theoretical

▸ Antiarrhythmics (dronedarone) are predicted to increase the exposure to **ibrutinib**. Adjust dose with moderate CYP3A4 inhibitors—consult product literature. Severe Study

▸ Antiepileptics (carbamazepine, fosphenytoin, phenobarbital, phenytoin, primidone) are predicted to decrease the exposure to **ibrutinib**. Avoid or monitor. Severe Study

▸ Antifungals, azoles (fluconazole, isavuconazole) are predicted to increase the exposure to **ibrutinib**. Adjust dose with moderate CYP3A4 inhibitors—consult product literature. Severe Study

▸ Antifungals, azoles (itraconazole, ketoconazole, posaconazole, voriconazole) are predicted to increase the exposure to **ibrutinib**. Avoid or adjust dose with potent CYP3A4 inhibitors—consult product literature. Severe Study

▸ Belzutifan is predicted to decrease the exposure to **ibrutinib**. Avoid or adjust dose. Severe Theoretical

▸ Berotralstat is predicted to increase the exposure to **ibrutinib**. Adjust dose with moderate CYP3A4 inhibitors—consult product literature. Severe Study

▸ Calcium channel blockers (diltiazem, verapamil) are predicted to increase the exposure to **ibrutinib**. Adjust dose with moderate CYP3A4 inhibitors—consult product literature. Severe Study

▸ Cenobamate is predicted to decrease the exposure to **ibrutinib**. Adjust dose. Moderate Theoretical

▸ Ceritinib is predicted to increase the exposure to **ibrutinib**. Avoid or adjust dose with potent CYP3A4 inhibitors—consult product literature. Severe Study → Also see TABLE 14 p. 1575

▶ **Cobicistat** is predicted to increase the exposure to **ibrutinib**. Avoid or adjust dose with potent CYP3A4 inhibitors—consult product literature. Severe Study

▶ **Crizotinib** is predicted to increase the exposure to **ibrutinib**. Adjust dose with moderate CYP3A4 inhibitors—consult product literature. Severe Study

▶ **Dabrafenib** is predicted to decrease the exposure to **ibrutinib**. Avoid or monitor. Severe Study

▶ **Ibrutinib** might increase the exposure to digoxin. Separate administration by at least 6 hours. Moderate Theoretical

▶ **Encorafenib** is predicted to decrease the exposure to **ibrutinib**. Avoid or monitor. Severe Study

▶ Endothelin receptor antagonists (bosentan) are predicted to decrease the exposure to **ibrutinib**. Avoid or monitor. Severe Study

▶ **Ibrutinib** might increase the exposure to everolimus. Separate administration by at least 6 hours. Moderate Theoretical

▶ **Fedratinib** is predicted to increase the exposure to **ibrutinib**. Adjust dose with moderate CYP3A4 inhibitors—consult product literature. Severe Study

▶ **Grapefruit** juice is predicted to increase the exposure to **ibrutinib**. Avoid. Moderate Theoretical

▶ **HIV-protease inhibitors** are predicted to increase the exposure to **ibrutinib**. Avoid or adjust dose with potent CYP3A4 inhibitors—consult product literature. Severe Study

▶ **Idelalisib** is predicted to increase the exposure to **ibrutinib**. Avoid or adjust dose with potent CYP3A4 inhibitors—consult product literature. Severe Study

▶ **Imatinib** is predicted to increase the exposure to **ibrutinib**. Adjust dose with moderate CYP3A4 inhibitors—consult product literature. Severe Study → Also see **TABLE 14** p. 1575 → Also see **TABLE 4** p. 1571

▶ **Ivosidenib** is predicted to decrease the exposure to **ibrutinib**. Avoid or monitor. Severe Study

▶ **Letermovir** is predicted to increase the exposure to **ibrutinib**. Adjust dose with moderate CYP3A4 inhibitors—consult product literature. Severe Study

▶ **Lumacaftor** is predicted to decrease the exposure to **ibrutinib**. Avoid or monitor. Severe Study

▶ Macrolides (clarithromycin) are predicted to increase the exposure to **ibrutinib**. Avoid or adjust dose with potent CYP3A4 inhibitors—consult product literature. Severe Study

▶ Macrolides (erythromycin) are predicted to increase the exposure to **ibrutinib**. Adjust dose with moderate CYP3A4 inhibitors—consult product literature. Severe Study

▶ **Mitotane** is predicted to decrease the exposure to **ibrutinib**. Avoid or monitor. Severe Study → Also see **TABLE 14** p. 1575

▶ Neurokinin-1 receptor antagonists (aprepitant, netupitant) are predicted to increase the exposure to **ibrutinib**. Adjust dose with moderate CYP3A4 inhibitors—consult product literature. Severe Study

▶ Neurokinin-1 receptor antagonists (fosaprepitant) are predicted to slightly increase the exposure to **ibrutinib**. Moderate Theoretical

▶ **Nilotinib** is predicted to increase the exposure to **ibrutinib**. Adjust dose with moderate CYP3A4 inhibitors—consult product literature. Severe Study → Also see **TABLE 14** p. 1575

▶ **Nirmatrelvir** boosted with ritonavir is predicted to increase the concentration of **ibrutinib**. Avoid or adjust dose—consult product literature. Severe Theoretical

▶ NNRTIs (efavirenz, etravirine, nevirapine) are predicted to decrease the exposure to **ibrutinib**. Avoid or monitor. Severe Study

▶ Quinolones (ciprofloxacin) are predicted to increase the exposure to **ibrutinib**. Adjust dose—consult product literature. Severe Theoretical

▶ Rifamycins (rifampicin) are predicted to decrease the exposure to **ibrutinib**. Avoid or monitor. Severe Study

▶ **Ibrutinib** might increase the exposure to sirolimus. Separate administration by at least 6 hours. Moderate Theoretical

▶ **St John's wort** is predicted to decrease the exposure to **ibrutinib**. Avoid. Severe Theoretical

▶ **Ibrutinib** might increase the exposure to talazoparib. Separate administration by at least 6 hours. Moderate Theoretical → Also see **TABLE 14** p. 1575

▶ **Ibrutinib** might increase the exposure to taxanes (paclitaxel). Separate administration by at least 6 hours. Moderate Theoretical → Also see **TABLE 14** p. 1575

▶ **Tucatinib** is predicted to increase the exposure to **ibrutinib**. Avoid or adjust dose with potent CYP3A4 inhibitors—consult product literature. Severe Study

Ibuprofen → see NSAIDs

Icatibant

▶ **ACE inhibitors** are predicted to decrease the efficacy of **icatibant** and **icatibant** is predicted to decrease the efficacy of **ACE inhibitors**. Avoid. Moderate Theoretical

Idarubicin → see anthracyclines

Idelalisib

▶ **Idelalisib** is predicted to increase the exposure to abemaciclib. Avoid or adjust dose—consult product literature. Severe Study

▶ **Idelalisib** is predicted to increase the exposure to acalabrutinib. Avoid. Severe Study

▶ **Idelalisib** is predicted to moderately increase the exposure to alpha blockers (alfuzosin, tamsulosin). Use with caution or avoid. Moderate Study

▶ **Idelalisib** is predicted to increase the exposure to alpha blockers (doxazosin). Moderate Study

▶ Anti-androgens (apalutamide, enzalutamide) are predicted to decrease the exposure to **idelalisib**. Avoid. Severe Study

▶ **Idelalisib** is predicted to increase the exposure to anti-androgens (apalutamide). Monitor and adjust dose. Mild Study

▶ **Idelalisib** is predicted to increase the exposure to antiarrhythmics (amiodarone). Avoid. Moderate Theoretical

▶ **Idelalisib** very markedly increases the exposure to antiarrhythmics (dronedarone). Avoid. Severe Study

▶ **Idelalisib** is predicted to increase the exposure to antiarrhythmics (propafenone). Monitor and adjust dose. Severe Study

▶ **Idelalisib** is predicted to increase the exposure to anticholinesterases, centrally acting (galantamine). Monitor and adjust dose. Moderate Study

▶ Antiepileptics (carbamazepine, fosphenytoin, phenobarbital, phenytoin, primidone) are predicted to decrease the exposure to **idelalisib**. Avoid. Severe Study

▶ **Idelalisib** is predicted to very slightly increase the exposure to antiepileptics (perampanel). Mild Study

▶ Antifungals, azoles (itraconazole, voriconazole) are predicted to increase the exposure to **idelalisib**. Moderate Theoretical

▶ Antifungals, azoles (ketoconazole) slightly increase the exposure to **idelalisib**. Moderate Study

▶ **Idelalisib** is predicted to increase the exposure to antifungals, azoles (isavuconazole). Avoid or monitor adverse effects. Severe Study

▶ **Idelalisib** is predicted to increase the exposure to antihistamines, non-sedating (mizolastine). Avoid. Severe Study

▶ **Idelalisib** is predicted to increase the exposure to antihistamines, non-sedating (rupatadine). Avoid. Moderate Study

▶ **Idelalisib** is predicted to slightly increase the exposure to antipsychotics, second generation (aripiprazole). Adjust **aripiprazole** dose, p. 454. Moderate Study

▶ **Idelalisib** is predicted to moderately increase the exposure to antipsychotics, second generation (cariprazine). Avoid. Severe Study

▶ **Idelalisib** is predicted to increase the exposure to antipsychotics, second generation (lurasidone, quetiapine). Avoid. Severe Study

▶ **Idelalisib** is predicted to increase the exposure to antipsychotics, second generation (risperidone). Adjust dose. Moderate Study

▶ **Idelalisib** is predicted to increase the exposure to atogepant. Adjust **atogepant** dose, p. 540. Moderate Study

▶ **Idelalisib** is predicted to increase the exposure to avacopan. Severe Study

▶ **Idelalisib** is predicted to increase the exposure to avapritinib. Avoid. Moderate Study

▶ **Idelalisib** is predicted to increase the exposure to axitinib. Avoid or adjust dose. Moderate Study

▶ **Idelalisib** might increases the exposure to bedaquiline. Mild Study

Idelalisib (continued)

▶ **Idelalisib** moderately increases the exposure to benzodiazepines (alprazolam). Avoid. Moderate Study

▶ **Idelalisib** is predicted to increase the exposure to benzodiazepines (diazepam, flurazepam). Monitor and adjust dose. Moderate Theoretical

▶ **Idelalisib** is predicted to markedly to very markedly increase the exposure to benzodiazepines (midazolam). Avoid or adjust dose. Severe Study

▶ **Idelalisib** is predicted to increase the exposure to beta₂ agonists (salmeterol). Avoid. Severe Study

▶ **Idelalisib** slightly increases the exposure to bortezomib. Moderate Study

▶ **Idelalisib** is predicted to increase the exposure to bosutinib. Avoid or adjust dose. Severe Study

▶ **Idelalisib** is predicted to increase the exposure to brigatinib. Avoid or adjust dose—consult product literature. Severe Study

▶ **Idelalisib** is predicted to increase the exposure to buspirone. Adjust **buspirone** dose, p. 396. Severe Study

▶ **Idelalisib** is predicted to increase the exposure to cabozantinib. Moderate Study

▶ **Idelalisib** is predicted to increase the exposure to calcium channel blockers (amlodipine, felodipine, lacidipine, nicardipine, nifedipine, nimodipine). Monitor and adjust dose. Moderate Study

▶ **Idelalisib** is predicted to increase the exposure to calcium channel blockers (diltiazem, verapamil). Severe Study

▶ **Idelalisib** is predicted to markedly increase the exposure to calcium channel blockers (lercanidipine). Avoid. Severe Study

▶ **Idelalisib** is predicted to increase the exposure to cannabidiol. Avoid or adjust dose. Mild Study

▶ **Idelalisib** is predicted to increase the exposure to capivasertib. Adjust dose. Moderate Study

▶ Cenobamate is predicted to decrease the exposure to **idelalisib**. Avoid. Moderate Theoretical

▶ **Idelalisib** is predicted to increase the exposure to ceritinib. Avoid or adjust dose—consult product literature. Severe Study

▶ **Idelalisib** increases the concentration of ciclosporin. Severe Study

▶ **Idelalisib** is predicted to moderately increase the exposure to cilostazol. Adjust **cilostazol** dose, p. 266. Moderate Study

▶ **Idelalisib** is predicted to moderately increase the exposure to cinacalcet. Adjust dose. Moderate Study

▶ Cobicistat is predicted to increase the exposure to **idelalisib**. Moderate Theoretical

▶ **Idelalisib** is predicted to increase the exposure to cobimetinib. Avoid or monitor for toxicity. Severe Study

▶ **Idelalisib** is predicted to increase the exposure to colchicine. Avoid potent CYP3A4 inhibitors or adjust **colchicine** dose, p. 1279. Severe Study

▶ **Idelalisib** is predicted to increase the exposure to corticosteroids (beclometasone) (risk with beclometasone is likely to be lower than with other corticosteroids). Moderate Theoretical

▶ **Idelalisib** is predicted to increase the exposure to corticosteroids (betamethasone, budesonide, ciclesonide, deflazacort, dexamethasone, fludrocortisone, fluticasone, hydrocortisone, methylprednisolone, mometasone, prednisolone, triamcinolone). Avoid or monitor adverse effects. Severe Study

▶ **Idelalisib** is predicted to increase the exposure to corticosteroids (vamorolone). Adjust dose. Severe Study

▶ **Idelalisib** is predicted to increase the exposure to crizotinib. Avoid. Moderate Study

▶ **Idelalisib** is predicted to increase the exposure to dabrafenib. Use with caution or avoid. Moderate Study

▶ Dabrafenib is predicted to decrease the exposure to **idelalisib**. Avoid. Moderate Theoretical

▶ **Idelalisib** is predicted to increase the exposure to daridorexant. Avoid. Severe Study

▶ **Idelalisib** is predicted to markedly to very markedly increase the exposure to darifenacin. Avoid. Severe Study

▶ **Idelalisib** is predicted to increase the exposure to dasatinib. Avoid or adjust dose—consult product literature. Severe Study

▶ **Idelalisib** very slightly increases the exposure to delamanid. Severe Study

▶ **Idelalisib** is predicted to moderately increase the exposure to dienogest. Moderate Study

▶ **Idelalisib** is predicted to increase the exposure to dipeptidylpeptidase-4 inhibitors (saxagliptin). Moderate Study

▶ **Idelalisib** is predicted to increase the exposure to domperidone. Avoid. Severe Study

▶ **Idelalisib** increases the exposure to dopamine receptor agonists (bromocriptine). Severe Study

▶ **Idelalisib** is predicted to increase the concentration of dopamine receptor agonists (cabergoline). Moderate Anecdotal

▶ **Idelalisib** is predicted to increase the exposure to dronabinol. Adjust dose. Mild Study

▶ **Idelalisib** is predicted to increase the exposure to drospirenone. Severe Study

▶ **Idelalisib** is predicted to increase the exposure to dutasteride. Monitor adverse effects and adjust dose. Moderate Theoretical

▶ **Idelalisib** is predicted to increase the exposure to elacestrant. Avoid potent CYP3A4 inhibitors or adjust **elacestrant** dose, p. 1084. Severe Study

▶ **Idelalisib** is predicted to increase the exposure to elexacaftor. Adjust ivacaftor with tezacaftor and elexacaftor p. 337 dose with potent CYP3A4 inhibitors. Severe Study

▶ **Idelalisib** is predicted to increase the exposure to eliglustat. Avoid or adjust dose—consult product literature. Severe Study

▶ **Idelalisib** is predicted to increase the exposure to encorafenib. Avoid or monitor. Severe Study

▶ Encorafenib is predicted to decrease the exposure to **idelalisib**. Avoid. Severe Study

▶ Endothelin receptor antagonists (bosentan) are predicted to decrease the exposure to **idelalisib**. Avoid. Moderate Theoretical

▶ **Idelalisib** is predicted to increase the exposure to endothelin receptor antagonists (macitentan). Moderate Study

▶ **Idelalisib** is predicted to increase the exposure to the cytotoxic component of enfortumab vedotin. Severe Theoretical

▶ **Idelalisib** is predicted to increase the exposure to entrectinib. Avoid or adjust dose with potent CYP3A4 inhibitors—consult product literature. Severe Study

▶ **Idelalisib** is predicted to increase the exposure to erdafitinib. Adjust dose. Severe Study

▶ **Idelalisib** is predicted to increase the risk of ergotism when given with ergometrine. Avoid. Severe Theoretical

▶ **Idelalisib** is predicted to increase the exposure to erlotinib. Use with caution and adjust dose. Severe Study

▶ **Idelalisib** is predicted to increase the exposure to esketamine. Adjust dose. Moderate Study

▶ **Idelalisib** is predicted to increase the exposure to eszopiclone. Adjust **eszopiclone** dose; avoid in the elderly, p. 554. Moderate Study

▶ **Idelalisib** is predicted to increase the concentration of subdermal etonogestrel. Moderate Theoretical

▶ **Idelalisib** is predicted to increase the exposure to etrasimod. Avoid in poor CYP2C9 metabolisers. Severe Theoretical

▶ **Idelalisib** is predicted to increase the exposure to everolimus. Avoid. Severe Study

▶ **Idelalisib** is predicted to increase the exposure to factor XA inhibitors (apixaban). Moderate Theoretical

▶ **Idelalisib** is predicted to increase the exposure to fedratinib. Adjust dose, but avoid depending on other drugs taken—consult product literature. Moderate Study

▶ **Idelalisib** is predicted to moderately increase the exposure to fesoterodine. Adjust **fesoterodine** dose with potent CYP3A4 inhibitors; avoid in hepatic and renal impairment, p. 897. Severe Study

▶ **Idelalisib** is predicted to increase the exposure to fostamatinib. Monitor adverse effects and adjust dose. Moderate Study

▶ **Idelalisib** is predicted to increase the exposure to gefitinib. Severe Study

▶ **Idelalisib** is predicted to increase the exposure to gilteritinib. Moderate Study

▶ **Idelalisib** is predicted to increase the exposure to glasdegib. Use with caution or avoid. Severe Study

▶ **Idelalisib** is predicted to moderately to markedly increase the exposure to grazoprevir. Avoid. Severe Study

- **Idelalisib** is predicted to increase the exposure to guanfacine. Adjust **guanfacine** dose, p. 407. Moderate Study
- HIV-protease inhibitors (atazanavir, darunavir, fosamprenavir, lopinavir) boosted with ritonavir are predicted to increase the exposure to **idelalisib**. Moderate Theoretical
- HIV-protease inhibitors (ritonavir) are predicted to increase the exposure to **idelalisib**. Moderate Theoretical
- **Idelalisib** is predicted to increase the exposure to ibrutinib. Avoid or adjust dose with potent CYP3A4 inhibitors—consult product literature. Severe Study
- **Idelalisib** is predicted to increase the exposure to imatinib. Moderate Study
- **Idelalisib** is predicted to increase the risk of toxicity when given with irinotecan. Avoid. Severe Study
- **Idelalisib** is predicted to increase the exposure to ivabradine. Avoid. Severe Study
- **Idelalisib** is predicted to increase the exposure to ivacaftor. Adjust dose with potent CYP3A4 inhibitors, see ivacaftor p. 336, lumacaftor with ivacaftor p. 338, tezacaftor with ivacaftor p. 339, and ivacaftor with tezacaftor and elexacaftor p. 337. Severe Study
- **Idelalisib** is predicted to increase the exposure to ivosidenib. Monitor and adjust dose—consult product literature. Severe Study
- Ivosidenib is predicted to decrease the exposure to **idelalisib**. Avoid. Severe Study
- **Idelalisib** is predicted to increase the exposure to lapatinib. Avoid. Moderate Study
- **Idelalisib** is predicted to moderately increase the exposure to larotrectinib. Avoid or adjust dose—consult product literature. Moderate Study
- **Idelalisib** is predicted to increase the exposure to leniolisib. Avoid. Moderate Study
- **Idelalisib** is predicted to markedly increase the exposure to lomitapide. Avoid. Severe Study
- **Idelalisib** is predicted to increase the exposure to lorlatinib. Avoid or adjust dose—consult product literature. Severe Study
- Lorlatinib is predicted to decrease the exposure to **idelalisib**. Avoid. Moderate Theoretical
- Lumacaftor is predicted to decrease the exposure to **idelalisib**. Avoid. Severe Study
- Macrolides are predicted to increase the exposure to **idelalisib**. Moderate Theoretical
- **Idelalisib** markedly increases the exposure to maraviroc. Adjust dose. Severe Theoretical
- Maribavir is predicted to increase the exposure to **idelalisib**. Moderate Theoretical
- **Idelalisib** is predicted to increase the exposure to mavacamten. Avoid or monitor—consult product literature. Severe Study
- **Idelalisib** is predicted to increase the concentration of intramuscular medroxyprogesterone. Moderate Theoretical
- **Idelalisib** is predicted to increase the exposure to midostaurin. Avoid or monitor for toxicity. Severe Study
- **Idelalisib** is predicted to markedly increase the exposure to mineralocorticoid receptor antagonists (eplerenone). Avoid. Severe Study
- **Idelalisib** is predicted to increase the exposure to mineralocorticoid receptor antagonists (finerenone). Avoid. Severe Study
- **Idelalisib** is predicted to increase the exposure to mirabegron. Adjust **mirabegron** dose in hepatic and renal impairment, p. 901. Moderate Study
- **Idelalisib** is predicted to increase the exposure to mirtazapine. Moderate Study
- Mitotane is predicted to decrease the exposure to **idelalisib**. Avoid. Severe Study
- **Idelalisib** is predicted to increase the exposure to mobocertinib. Avoid. Severe Study
- **Idelalisib** is predicted to increase the exposure to modafinil. Mild Theoretical
- **Idelalisib** is predicted to increase the risk of neutropenia when given with monoclonal antibodies (brentuximab vedotin). Monitor and adjust dose. Severe Study
- **Idelalisib** is predicted to increase the exposure to monoclonal antibodies (polatuzumab vedotin). Moderate Theoretical

- **Idelalisib** is predicted to increase the exposure to the cytotoxic component of monoclonal antibodies (trastuzumab emtansine). Avoid or monitor. Severe Theoretical
- **Idelalisib** is predicted to increase the exposure to naldemedine. Avoid or monitor. Moderate Study
- **Idelalisib** is predicted to markedly increase the exposure to naloxegol. Avoid. Severe Study
- **Idelalisib** is predicted to increase the exposure to neratinib. Avoid or adjust dose with potent CYP3A4 inhibitors—consult product literature. Severe Study
- **Idelalisib** is predicted to markedly increase the exposure to neurokinin-1 receptor antagonists (aprepitant). Moderate Study
- **Idelalisib** is predicted to increase the exposure to neurokinin-1 receptor antagonists (fosaprepitant). Moderate Theoretical
- **Idelalisib** is predicted to increase the exposure to neurokinin-1 receptor antagonists (netupitant). Moderate Study
- **Idelalisib** is predicted to increase the exposure to nilotinib. Avoid. Severe Study
- **Idelalisib** is predicted to increase the exposure to nitisinone. Adjust dose. Moderate Theoretical
- NNRTIs (efavirenz, etravirine, nevirapine) are predicted to decrease the exposure to **idelalisib**. Avoid. Moderate Theoretical
- **Idelalisib** is predicted to increase the exposure to olaparib. Avoid or adjust dose with potent CYP3A4 inhibitors—consult product literature. Moderate Study
- **Idelalisib** is predicted to increase the exposure to opioids (alfentanil, buprenorphine, fentanyl, oxycodone). Monitor and adjust dose. Severe Study
- **Idelalisib** is predicted to increase the exposure to opioids (methadone). Severe Theoretical
- **Idelalisib** is predicted to increase the exposure to opioids (sufentanil). Moderate Study
- **Idelalisib** is predicted to increase the exposure to osilodrostat. Moderate Theoretical
- **Idelalisib** is predicted to increase the exposure to ospemifene. Avoid in poor CYP2C9 metabolisers. Moderate Study
- **Idelalisib** is predicted to increase the exposure to oxybutynin. Mild Study
- **Idelalisib** is predicted to increase the exposure to palbociclib. Avoid or adjust dose—consult product literature. Severe Study
- **Idelalisib** is predicted to increase the exposure to panobinostat. Adjust dose—consult product literature; in hepatic impairment avoid. Moderate Study
- **Idelalisib** is predicted to increase the exposure to pazopanib. Avoid or adjust dose—consult product literature. Moderate Study
- **Idelalisib** is predicted to increase the exposure to pemigatinib. Avoid or adjust dose—consult product literature. Severe Study
- **Idelalisib** is predicted to increase the exposure to phosphodiesterase type-5 inhibitors (avanafil, vardenafil). Avoid. Severe Study
- **Idelalisib** is predicted to increase the exposure to phosphodiesterase type-5 inhibitors (sildenafil). Avoid potent CYP3A4 inhibitors or adjust **sildenafil** dose, p. 940. Severe Study
- **Idelalisib** is predicted to increase the exposure to phosphodiesterase type-5 inhibitors (tadalafil). Use with caution or avoid. Severe Study
- **Idelalisib** is predicted to increase the exposure to pimozide. Avoid. Severe Study
- **Idelalisib** is predicted to slightly increase the exposure to ponatinib. Monitor and adjust dose—consult product literature. Moderate Study
- **Idelalisib** is predicted to increase the exposure to pralsetinib. Avoid or adjust dose with potent CYP3A4 inhibitors—consult product literature. Moderate Study
- **Idelalisib** is predicted to moderately increase the exposure to praziquantel. Mild Study
- **Idelalisib** given with carbimazole is predicted to increase the exposure to propiverine. Adjust starting dose. Moderate Theoretical
- **Idelalisib** is predicted to increase the exposure to quizartinib. Adjust dose—consult product literature. Severe Study
- **Idelalisib** is predicted to increase the exposure to ranolazine. Avoid. Severe Study

Idelalisib (continued)
▸ **Idelalisib** is predicted to increase the exposure to reboxetine. Avoid. Moderate Study
▸ **Idelalisib** is predicted to increase the exposure to regorafenib. Avoid. Moderate Study
▸ **Idelalisib** is predicted to increase the exposure to retinoids (alitretinoin). Adjust **alitretinoin** dose, p. 1433. Moderate Theoretical
▸ **Idelalisib** is predicted to increase the exposure to ribociclib. Avoid or adjust dose—consult product literature. Moderate Study
▸ Rifamycins (rifampicin) are predicted to decrease the exposure to **idelalisib**. Avoid. Severe Study
▸ **Idelalisib** is predicted to increase the exposure to rimegepant. Avoid. Moderate Study
▸ **Idelalisib** is predicted to increase the exposure to ripretinib. Moderate Theoretical
▸ Rucaparib is predicted to increase the exposure to **idelalisib**. Moderate Theoretical
▸ **Idelalisib** is predicted to increase the exposure to ruxolitinib. Adjust dose and monitor adverse effects. Moderate Study
▸ **Idelalisib** is predicted to increase the exposure to selpercatinib. Adjust dose—consult product literature. Moderate Study
▸ **Idelalisib** is predicted to increase the exposure to selumetinib. Avoid or adjust dose—consult product literature. Severe Study
▸ **Idelalisib** is predicted to increase the exposure to siponimod. Avoid depending on other drugs taken—consult product literature. Severe Theoretical
▸ **Idelalisib** is predicted to increase the concentration of sirolimus. Avoid or monitor and adjust dose. Severe Study
▸ **Idelalisib** is predicted to increase the exposure to SNRIs (venlafaxine). Moderate Study
▸ **Idelalisib** is predicted to increase the exposure to solifenacin. Adjust solifenacin p. 899 or tamsulosin with solifenacin p. 906 dose; avoid in hepatic and renal impairment. Severe Study
▸ Sotorasib is predicted to decrease the exposure to **idelalisib**. Avoid. Moderate Theoretical
▸ **Idelalisib** is predicted to moderately increase the exposure to SSRIs (dapoxetine). Avoid potent CYP3A4 inhibitors or adjust dapoxetine dose, p. 947. Severe Study
▸ St John's wort is predicted to decrease the exposure to **idelalisib**. Avoid. Moderate Theoretical
▸ **Idelalisib** is predicted to increase the exposure to statins (atorvastatin). Avoid or adjust dose and monitor rhabdomyolysis. Severe Study
▸ **Idelalisib** is predicted to increase the exposure to statins (simvastatin). Avoid. Severe Study
▸ **Idelalisib** is predicted to increase the exposure to sunitinib. Avoid or adjust dose—consult product literature. Moderate Study
▸ **Idelalisib** is predicted to increase the concentration of tacrolimus. Monitor and adjust dose. Severe Study
▸ **Idelalisib** is predicted to increase the exposure to taxanes (cabazitaxel). Avoid or adjust dose—consult product literature. Severe Study
▸ **Idelalisib** is predicted to increase the exposure to taxanes (docetaxel). Avoid or adjust dose. Severe Study
▸ **Idelalisib** is predicted to increase the exposure to taxanes (paclitaxel). Moderate Anecdotal
▸ **Idelalisib** is predicted to increase the concentration of temsirolimus. Avoid. Severe Theoretical
▸ **Idelalisib** is predicted to increase the exposure to tezacaftor. Adjust dose with potent CYP3A4 inhibitors, see tezacaftor with ivacaftor p. 339 and ivacaftor with tezacaftor and elexacaftor p. 337. Severe Study
▸ **Idelalisib** is predicted to markedly increase the exposure to ticagrelor. Avoid. Severe Study
▸ **Idelalisib** is predicted to increase the exposure to tofacitinib. Adjust **tofacitinib** dose, p. 1265. Moderate Study
▸ **Idelalisib** is predicted to increase the exposure to tolterodine. Avoid. Severe Study
▸ **Idelalisib** is predicted to increase the exposure to tolvaptan. Manufacturer advises caution or adjust **tolvaptan** dose with potent CYP3A4 inhibitors, p. 767. Severe Study

▸ **Idelalisib** is predicted to increase the exposure to toremifene. Moderate Theoretical
▸ **Idelalisib** is predicted to increase the exposure to trabectedin. Avoid or adjust dose. Severe Theoretical
▸ **Idelalisib** is predicted to moderately increase the exposure to trazodone. Avoid or adjust dose. Moderate Study
▸ **Idelalisib** increases the exposure to triptans (almotriptan). Mild Study
▸ **Idelalisib** is predicted to markedly increase the exposure to triptans (eletriptan). Avoid. Severe Study
▸ Tucatinib is predicted to increase the exposure to **idelalisib**. Moderate Theoretical
▸ **Idelalisib** is predicted to increase the exposure to ulipristal. Avoid if used for uterine fibroids. Severe Study
▸ **Idelalisib** is predicted to increase the exposure to upadacitinib. Manufacturer advises caution or avoid, or adjust **upadacitinib** dose depending on indication, p. 1267. Severe Study
▸ Vandetanib is predicted to increase the exposure to **idelalisib**. Moderate Theoretical
▸ **Idelalisib** is predicted to increase the exposure to vemurafenib. Severe Theoretical
▸ **Idelalisib** is predicted to increase the exposure to venetoclax. Avoid or adjust dose—consult product literature. Severe Study
▸ **Idelalisib** is predicted to increase the exposure to vinca alkaloids. Severe Theoretical
▸ **Idelalisib** is predicted to increase the exposure to vitamin D substances (paricalcitol). Moderate Study
▸ **Idelalisib** is predicted to increase the exposure to voclosporin. Avoid. Severe Study
▸ **Idelalisib** is predicted to increase the exposure to zanubrutinib. Avoid or adjust dose with potent CYP3A4 inhibitors—consult product literature. Moderate Study
▸ **Idelalisib** is predicted to increase the exposure to zolpidem. Monitor and adjust dose. Moderate Theoretical
▸ **Idelalisib** is predicted to increase the exposure to zopiclone. Adjust dose. Moderate Theoretical

Ifosfamide → see alkylating agents

Iloprost → see TABLE 7 p. 1572 (hypotension), TABLE 4 p. 1571 (antiplatelet effects)

Imatinib → see TABLE 14 p. 1575 (myelosuppression), TABLE 4 p. 1571 (antiplatelet effects)
▸ **Imatinib** is predicted to increase the exposure to abemaciclib. Moderate Study
▸ **Imatinib** is predicted to increase the exposure to acalabrutinib. Avoid or monitor. Severe Study → Also see TABLE 4 p. 1571
▸ **Imatinib** is predicted to increase the exposure to alpha blockers (tamsulosin). Moderate Theoretical
▸ Anti-androgens (apalutamide, enzalutamide) are predicted to decrease the exposure to **imatinib**. Avoid. Moderate Study
▸ **Imatinib** is predicted to increase the exposure to antiarrhythmics (dronedarone). Severe Theoretical
▸ **Imatinib** is predicted to increase the exposure to antiarrhythmics (propafenone). Monitor and adjust dose. Moderate Study
▸ Antiepileptics (carbamazepine, fosphenytoin, oxcarbazepine, phenobarbital, phenytoin, primidone) are predicted to decrease the exposure to **imatinib**. Avoid. Moderate Study
▸ Antiepileptics (eslicarbazepine) are predicted to decrease the exposure to **imatinib**. Moderate Theoretical
▸ Antiepileptics (topiramate) are predicted to decrease the exposure to **imatinib**. Moderate Study
▸ Antifungals, azoles (fluconazole) are predicted to increase the exposure to **imatinib**. Moderate Theoretical
▸ Antifungals, azoles (itraconazole, ketoconazole, posaconazole, voriconazole) are predicted to increase the exposure to **imatinib**. Moderate Study
▸ **Imatinib** is predicted to increase the exposure to antifungals, azoles (isavuconazole). Moderate Theoretical
▸ **Imatinib** is predicted to increase the exposure to antihistamines, non-sedating (mizolastine). Severe Theoretical
▸ **Imatinib** is predicted to increase the exposure to antihistamines, non-sedating (rupatadine). Avoid. Moderate Study
▸ **Imatinib** is predicted to increase the exposure to antipsychotics, second generation (cariprazine). Avoid. Severe Study

▶ **Imatinib** is predicted to increase the exposure to antipsychotics, second generation (lurasidone). Adjust **lurasidone** dose. Moderate Study

▶ **Imatinib** is predicted to increase the exposure to antipsychotics, second generation (quetiapine). Avoid. Moderate Study

▶ Asparaginase is predicted to increase the risk of hepatotoxicity when given with **imatinib**. Severe Theoretical → Also see **TABLE 14** p. 1575

▶ **Imatinib** is predicted to increase the exposure to avapritinib. Avoid or adjust dose—consult product literature. Moderate Study

▶ **Imatinib** is predicted to increase the exposure to axitinib. Moderate Study → Also see **TABLE 14** p. 1575 → Also see **TABLE 4** p. 1571

▶ **Imatinib** might increases the exposure to bedaquiline. Mild Theoretical

▶ **Imatinib** is predicted to increase the exposure to benzodiazepines (alprazolam). Severe Study

▶ **Imatinib** is predicted to increase the exposure to benzodiazepines (midazolam). Monitor adverse effects and adjust dose. Severe Study

▶ **Imatinib** is predicted to increase the exposure to bosutinib. Avoid or adjust dose. Severe Study → Also see **TABLE 14** p. 1575 → Also see **TABLE 4** p. 1571

▶ **Imatinib** is predicted to increase the exposure to brigatinib. Moderate Study

▶ **Imatinib** is predicted to increase the exposure to buspirone. Use with caution and adjust dose. Moderate Study

▶ **Imatinib** is predicted to increase the exposure to cabozantinib. Moderate Study → Also see **TABLE 14** p. 1575

▶ Calcium channel blockers (diltiazem, verapamil) are predicted to increase the exposure to **imatinib**. Moderate Theoretical

▶ **Imatinib** is predicted to increase the exposure to calcium channel blockers (amlodipine, felodipine, lacidipine, lercanidipine, nicardipine, nifedipine, nimodipine). Monitor and adjust dose. Moderate Study

▶ **Imatinib** is predicted to increase the exposure to capivasertib. Adjust dose. Moderate Study

▶ Cenobamate is predicted to decrease the exposure to **imatinib**. Moderate Study

▶ Ceritinib is predicted to increase the exposure to **imatinib**. Moderate Study → Also see **TABLE 14** p. 1575

▶ **Imatinib** is predicted to increase the exposure to ceritinib. Moderate Study → Also see **TABLE 14** p. 1575

▶ **Imatinib** is predicted to increase the concentration of ciclosporin. Severe Study

▶ Cobicistat is predicted to increase the exposure to **imatinib**. Moderate Study

▶ **Imatinib** is predicted to increase the exposure to cobimetinib. Severe Study

▶ **Imatinib** is predicted to increase the exposure to colchicine. Adjust **colchicine** dose with moderate CYP3A4 inhibitors, p. 1279. Severe Study

▶ **Imatinib** is predicted to increase the exposure to corticosteroids (methylprednisolone). Monitor and adjust dose. Moderate Study

▶ **Imatinib** is predicted to increase the risk of bleeding events when given with coumarins. Severe Theoretical

▶ Crisantaspase is predicted to increase the risk of hepatotoxicity when given with **imatinib**. Severe Theoretical → Also see **TABLE 14** p. 1575

▶ **Imatinib** is predicted to increase the exposure to crizotinib. Moderate Study

▶ **Imatinib** is predicted to increase the exposure to dabrafenib. Moderate Study

▶ Dabrafenib is predicted to decrease the exposure to **imatinib**. Moderate Study

▶ **Imatinib** is predicted to increase the exposure to daridorexant. Adjust **daridorexant** dose, p. 554. Severe Study

▶ **Imatinib** is predicted to increase the exposure to darifenacin. Moderate Study

▶ **Imatinib** is predicted to increase the exposure to dasatinib. Severe Study → Also see **TABLE 14** p. 1575 → Also see **TABLE 4** p. 1571

▶ **Imatinib** is predicted to slightly increase the exposure to dienogest. Moderate Study

▶ **Imatinib** is predicted to increase the exposure to dipeptidylpeptidase-4 inhibitors (saxagliptin). Mild Study

▶ **Imatinib** is predicted to increase the exposure to domperidone. Avoid. Severe Study

▶ **Imatinib** is predicted to increase the exposure to dopamine receptor agonists (bromocriptine). Severe Theoretical

▶ **Imatinib** is predicted to increase the concentration of dopamine receptor agonists (cabergoline). Moderate Anecdotal

▶ **Imatinib** is predicted to increase the exposure to drospirenone. Severe Study

▶ **Imatinib** is predicted to moderately increase the exposure to dutasteride. Mild Study

▶ **Imatinib** is predicted to increase the exposure to elacestrant. Avoid moderate CYP3A4 inhibitors or adjust **elacestrant** dose, p. 1084. Severe Theoretical

▶ **Imatinib** is predicted to increase the exposure to elexacaftor. Adjust ivacaftor with tezacaftor and elexacaftor p. 337 dose with moderate CYP3A4 inhibitors. Severe Theoretical

▶ **Imatinib** is predicted to increase the exposure to eliglustat. Avoid or adjust dose—consult product literature. Severe Study

▶ Encorafenib is predicted to decrease the exposure to **imatinib**. Avoid. Moderate Study

▶ **Imatinib** is predicted to moderately increase the exposure to encorafenib. Moderate Study

▶ Endothelin receptor antagonists (bosentan) are predicted to decrease the exposure to **imatinib**. Moderate Study

▶ **Imatinib** is predicted to increase the exposure to endothelin receptor antagonists (macitentan). Manufacturer advises caution depending on other drugs taken—consult product literature. Moderate Theoretical

▶ **Imatinib** is predicted to increase the exposure to entrectinib. Avoid or adjust dose with moderate CYP3A4 inhibitors— consult product literature. Severe Theoretical

▶ **Imatinib** is predicted to increase the risk of ergotism when given with ergometrine. Severe Theoretical

▶ **Imatinib** is predicted to increase the exposure to erlotinib. Moderate Study

▶ **Imatinib** is predicted to increase the exposure to etrasimod. Avoid in poor CYP2C9 metabolisers. Severe Theoretical

▶ **Imatinib** is predicted to increase the concentration of everolimus. Avoid or adjust dose. Moderate Study

▶ **Imatinib** is predicted to increase the exposure to fedratinib. Monitor and adjust dose. Moderate Study

▶ **Imatinib** is predicted to increase the exposure to fesoterodine. Adjust **fesoterodine** dose with moderate CYP3A4 inhibitors in hepatic and renal impairment, p. 897. Mild Study

▶ **Imatinib** is predicted to increase the exposure to gefitinib. Moderate Study

▶ Grapefruit juice is predicted to increase the exposure to **imatinib**. Moderate Theoretical

▶ **Imatinib** is predicted to increase the concentration of guanfacine. Adjust **guanfacine** dose, p. 407. Moderate Theoretical

▶ HIV-protease inhibitors are predicted to increase the exposure to **imatinib**. Moderate Study

▶ **Imatinib** is predicted to increase the exposure to ibrutinib. Adjust dose with moderate CYP3A4 inhibitors—consult product literature. Severe Study → Also see **TABLE 14** p. 1575 → Also see **TABLE 4** p. 1571

▶ Idelalisib is predicted to increase the exposure to **imatinib**. Moderate Study

▶ **Imatinib** is predicted to increase the exposure to ivabradine. Adjust **ivabradine** dose, p. 245. Severe Theoretical

▶ **Imatinib** is predicted to increase the exposure to ivacaftor. Adjust dose with moderate CYP3A4 inhibitors, see ivacaftor p. 336, tezacaftor with ivacaftor p. 339, and ivacaftor with tezacaftor and elexacaftor p. 337. Moderate Study

▶ **Imatinib** is predicted to increase the exposure to ivosidenib. Monitor and adjust dose—consult product literature. Severe Study

▶ Ivosidenib is predicted to decrease the exposure to **imatinib**. Avoid. Moderate Study

▶ **Imatinib** is predicted to increase the exposure to lapatinib. Moderate Study

▶ **Imatinib** is predicted to increase the exposure to larotrectinib. Monitor and adjust dose. Moderate Theoretical

Imatinib (continued)

▶ **Imatinib** is predicted to increase the exposure to leniolisib. Avoid. Moderate Study

▶ Letermovir is predicted to increase the exposure to **imatinib**. Moderate Study

▶ **Imatinib** is predicted to increase the exposure to lomitapide. Avoid. Moderate Theoretical

▶ Lorlatinib is predicted to decrease the exposure to **imatinib**. Moderate Study

▶ Lumacaftor is predicted to decrease the exposure to **imatinib**. Avoid. Moderate Study

▶ Macrolides (clarithromycin) are predicted to increase the exposure to **imatinib**. Moderate Study

▶ Macrolides (erythromycin) are predicted to increase the exposure to **imatinib**. Moderate Theoretical

▶ **Imatinib** is predicted to increase the exposure to mavacamten. Adjust dose—consult product literature. Moderate Study

▶ **Imatinib** is predicted to increase the exposure to midostaurin. Moderate Theoretical

▶ **Imatinib** is predicted to increase the exposure to mineralocorticoid receptor antagonists (eplerenone). Adjust eplerenone dose, p. 223. Severe Study

▶ **Imatinib** is predicted to increase the exposure to mineralocorticoid receptor antagonists (finerenone). Severe Study

▶ Mitotane is predicted to decrease the exposure to **imatinib**. Avoid. Moderate Study → Also see TABLE 14 p. 1575

▶ **Imatinib** is predicted to increase the exposure to mobocertinib. Avoid or adjust dose and monitor ECG—consult product literature. Severe Study

▶ **Imatinib** is predicted to increase the exposure to naldemedine. Moderate Study

▶ **Imatinib** is predicted to increase the exposure to naloxegol. Adjust naloxegol dose and monitor adverse effects, p. 72. Moderate Study

▶ **Imatinib** is predicted to increase the exposure to neratinib. Avoid moderate CYP3A4 inhibitors or adjust dose and monitor for gastrointestinal adverse effects—consult product literature. Severe Study

▶ Neurokinin-1 receptor antagonists (aprepitant, netupitant) are predicted to increase the exposure to **imatinib**. Moderate Theoretical

▶ Nilotinib is predicted to increase the exposure to **imatinib**. Moderate Study → Also see TABLE 14 p. 1575

▶ NNRTIs (efavirenz, etravirine, nevirapine) are predicted to decrease the exposure to **imatinib**. Moderate Study

▶ **Imatinib** is predicted to increase the exposure to olaparib. Avoid or adjust dose with moderate CYP3A4 inhibitors—consult product literature. Moderate Theoretical → Also see TABLE 14 p. 1575

▶ **Imatinib** is predicted to increase the exposure to opioids (alfentanil, buprenorphine, fentanyl, oxycodone). Monitor and adjust dose. Moderate Study

▶ **Imatinib** is predicted to increase the exposure to opioids (methadone, sufentanil). Moderate Theoretical

▶ **Imatinib** increases the risk of hepatotoxicity when given with paracetamol. Severe Anecdotal

▶ **Imatinib** is predicted to increase the exposure to pazopanib. Moderate Study → Also see TABLE 4 p. 1571

▶ Pegaspargase is predicted to increase the risk of hepatotoxicity when given with **imatinib**. Severe Theoretical → Also see TABLE 14 p. 1575

▶ **Imatinib** is predicted to increase the exposure to pemigatinib. Severe Study

▶ **Imatinib** is predicted to increase the risk of bleeding events when given with phenindione. Severe Theoretical

▶ **Imatinib** is predicted to increase the exposure to phosphodiesterase type-5 inhibitors (avanafil). Adjust avanafil dose, p. 939. Moderate Theoretical

▶ **Imatinib** is predicted to increase the exposure to phosphodiesterase type-5 inhibitors (sildenafil). Monitor or adjust sildenafil dose with moderate CYP3A4 inhibitors, p. 940. Moderate Study

▶ **Imatinib** is predicted to increase the exposure to phosphodiesterase type-5 inhibitors (tadalafil). Severe Theoretical

▶ **Imatinib** is predicted to increase the exposure to phosphodiesterase type-5 inhibitors (vardenafil). Adjust dose. Severe Theoretical

▶ **Imatinib** is predicted to increase the exposure to pimozide. Avoid. Severe Theoretical

▶ **Imatinib** is predicted to increase the exposure to ponatinib. Moderate Study → Also see TABLE 4 p. 1571

▶ **Imatinib** is predicted to increase the exposure to pralsetinib. Moderate Theoretical

▶ **Imatinib** is predicted to increase the exposure to ranolazine. Severe Study

▶ **Imatinib** is predicted to increase the exposure to regorafenib. Moderate Study → Also see TABLE 14 p. 1575 → Also see TABLE 4 p. 1571

▶ **Imatinib** is predicted to increase the exposure to ribociclib. Moderate Study → Also see TABLE 14 p. 1575

▶ Rifamycins (rifampicin) are predicted to decrease the exposure to **imatinib**. Avoid. Moderate Study

▶ **Imatinib** is predicted to increase the exposure to rimegepant. Avoid another dose of rimegepant within 48 hours of concurrent use. Moderate Study

▶ **Imatinib** is predicted to increase the exposure to ruxolitinib. Moderate Study → Also see TABLE 14 p. 1575

▶ **Imatinib** is predicted to increase the exposure to selpercatinib. Moderate Study

▶ **Imatinib** is predicted to increase the exposure to selumetinib. Avoid or adjust dose—consult product literature. Severe Study

▶ **Imatinib** is predicted to increase the exposure to siponimod. Avoid depending on other drugs taken—consult product literature. Severe Study

▶ **Imatinib** increases the concentration of sirolimus. Monitor and adjust dose. Moderate Study

▶ Sotorasib is predicted to decrease the exposure to **imatinib**. Moderate Study

▶ **Imatinib** is predicted to increase the exposure to SSRIs (dapoxetine). Adjust dapoxetine dose with moderate CYP3A4 inhibitors, p. 947. Moderate Theoretical → Also see TABLE 4 p. 1571

▶ St John's wort is predicted to decrease the exposure to **imatinib**. Moderate Study

▶ **Imatinib** is predicted to increase the exposure to statins (atorvastatin). Monitor and adjust dose. Severe Theoretical

▶ **Imatinib** moderately increases the exposure to statins (simvastatin). Monitor and adjust dose. Severe Study

▶ **Imatinib** is predicted to increase the exposure to sunitinib. Moderate Study → Also see TABLE 14 p. 1575 → Also see TABLE 4 p. 1571

▶ **Imatinib** is predicted to increase the concentration of tacrolimus. Severe Study

▶ **Imatinib** is predicted to increase the exposure to taxanes (cabazitaxel). Moderate Theoretical → Also see TABLE 14 p. 1575

▶ **Imatinib** is predicted to increase the exposure to taxanes (docetaxel). Severe Study → Also see TABLE 14 p. 1575

▶ **Imatinib** is predicted to increase the exposure to taxanes (paclitaxel). Moderate Anecdotal → Also see TABLE 14 p. 1575

▶ Tedizolid is predicted to increase the exposure to **imatinib**. Avoid. Moderate Theoretical

▶ **Imatinib** is predicted to increase the concentration of temsirolimus. Use with caution or avoid. Moderate Theoretical → Also see TABLE 14 p. 1575

▶ **Imatinib** is predicted to increase the exposure to tezacaftor. Adjust dose with moderate CYP3A4 inhibitors, see tezacaftor with ivacaftor p. 339 and ivacaftor with tezacaftor and elexacaftor p. 337. Severe Study

▶ **Imatinib** causes hypothyroidism when given with thyroid hormones (levothyroxine) in thyroidectomy patients. Moderate Study

▶ **Imatinib** given with a potent CYP2C19 inhibitor is predicted to increase the exposure to tofacitinib. Adjust tofacitinib dose, p. 1265. Moderate Study

▶ **Imatinib** is predicted to increase the exposure to tolvaptan. Manufacturer advises caution or adjust tolvaptan dose with moderate CYP3A4 inhibitors, p. 767. Moderate Study

▶ **Imatinib** is predicted to increase the exposure to trazodone. Moderate Theoretical

▶ **Tucatinib** is predicted to increase the exposure to **imatinib**. Moderate Study
▶ **Imatinib** is predicted to increase the exposure to **ulipristal**. Avoid if used for uterine fibroids. Moderate Study
▶ **Imatinib** is predicted to increase the exposure to **vemurafenib**. Severe Theoretical
▶ **Imatinib** is predicted to increase the exposure to **venetoclax**. Avoid or adjust dose—consult product literature. Severe Study
▶ **Imatinib** is predicted to increase the exposure to **vinca alkaloids**. Severe Theoretical → Also see TABLE 14 p. 1575
▶ **Imatinib** is predicted to increase the exposure to **voclosporin**. Adjust **voclosporin** dose, p. 973. Severe Study
▶ **Imatinib** is predicted to increase the exposure to **zanubrutinib**. Avoid or adjust dose with moderate CYP3A4 inhibitors—consult product literature. Severe Study → Also see TABLE 4 p. 1571
▶ **Imatinib** is predicted to increase the exposure to **zopiclone**. Adjust dose. Moderate Study

Imidapril → see ACE inhibitors
Imipenem → see carbapenems
Imipramine → see tricyclic antidepressants
Immunoglobulins

Anti-D (Rh₀) immunoglobulin · antithymocyte immunoglobulin (rabbit) · cytomegalovirus immunoglobulin · hepatitis B immunoglobulin · normal immunoglobulin · rabies immunoglobulin · tetanus immunoglobulin · varicella-zoster immunoglobulin

▶ **Immunoglobulins** are predicted to decrease the efficacy of live vaccines (cholera vaccine (live), dengue vaccine, influenza vaccine (live), measles, mumps and rubella vaccine, rotavirus vaccine, typhoid vaccine (live), varicella-zoster vaccine). Avoid and for 3 months after stopping **immunoglobulins**. Moderate Theoretical
▶ **Loop diuretics** are predicted to increase the risk of adverse effects when given with **cytomegalovirus immunoglobulin**. Avoid. Moderate Theoretical
▶ **Loop diuretics** might increase the risk of adverse effects when given with **hepatitis B immunoglobulin**. Avoid. Moderate Theoretical
▶ **Loop diuretics** might increase the risk of adverse effects when given with **normal immunoglobulin**. Avoid. Moderate Theoretical
▶ Monoclonal antibodies (rozanolixizumab) might decrease the concentration of **immunoglobulins**. Avoid and for 2 weeks after stopping **rozanolixizumab**. Moderate Theoretical
▶ **Normal immunoglobulin** is predicted to alter the effects of monoclonal antibodies (dinutuximab). Avoid. Severe Theoretical

Indacaterol → see beta₂ agonists
Indapamide → see thiazide diuretics
Indometacin → see NSAIDs
Indoramin → see alpha blockers
Infliximab → see monoclonal antibodies
Influenza vaccine (live) → see live vaccines
Inotersen → see TABLE 2 p. 1571 (nephrotoxicity)
▶ Drugs with anticoagulant effects (see TABLE 3 p. 1571) cause bleeding, as can **inotersen**; concurrent use might increase the risk of developing this effect. Severe Theoretical
▶ Drugs with antiplatelet effects (see TABLE 4 p. 1571) cause bleeding, as can **inotersen**; concurrent use might increase the risk of developing this effect. Severe Theoretical
Inotuzumab ozogamicin → see monoclonal antibodies
Insulin → see TABLE 13 p. 1575 (antidiabetic drugs)
▶ **Fenfluramine** might decrease blood glucose concentrations when given with **insulin**. Moderate Theoretical
▶ **Fibrates** are predicted to increase the risk of hypoglycaemia when given with **insulin**. Moderate Theoretical
▶ **Macrolides (clarithromycin)** have been reported to cause hypoglycaemia when given with **insulin**. Severe Anecdotal
▶ **Metreleptin** is predicted to increase the risk of hypoglycaemia when given with **insulin**. Monitor blood glucose and adjust dose. Severe Theoretical
▶ **Somapacitan** might increase blood glucose concentrations, opposing the blood glucose-lowering effects of **insulin**. Adjust dose. Moderate Theoretical
▶ **Somatrogon** might increase blood glucose concentrations, opposing the blood glucose-lowering effects of **insulin**. Adjust dose. Moderate Theoretical

Interferon beta → see interferons
Interferons → see TABLE 14 p. 1575 (myelosuppression)

interferon beta · peginterferon alfa · ropeginterferon alfa

▶ **Interferons** are predicted to slightly increase the exposure to **aminophylline**. Adjust dose. Moderate Theoretical
▶ **Ropeginterferon alfa** is predicted to increase the exposure to antipsychotics, second generation (risperidone). Moderate Theoretical
▶ **Ropeginterferon alfa** is predicted to increase the exposure to **atomoxetine**. Moderate Theoretical
▶ **Ropeginterferon alfa** is predicted to increase the exposure to beta blockers, selective (nebivolol). Moderate Theoretical
▶ **Ropeginterferon alfa** is predicted to increase the exposure to **eliglustat**. Moderate Theoretical
▶ **Ropeginterferon alfa** is predicted to increase the exposure to opioids (methadone). Moderate Theoretical
▶ **Interferons** slightly increase the exposure to theophylline. Adjust dose. Moderate Study
▶ **Ropeginterferon alfa** is predicted to increase the exposure to **vortioxetine**. Moderate Theoretical

Ipilimumab → see monoclonal antibodies
Ipratropium → see TABLE 9 p. 1573 (antimuscarinics)
▶ Antipsychotics, second generation (clozapine) can cause constipation, as can **ipratropium**; concurrent use might increase the risk of developing intestinal obstruction. Severe Theoretical → Also see TABLE 9 p. 1573
▶ **Beta₂ agonists** are predicted to increase the risk of glaucoma when given with **ipratropium**. Moderate Anecdotal
Iptacopan
▶ Rifamycins (rifampicin) are predicted to decrease the exposure to **iptacopan**. Avoid or monitor. Moderate Theoretical
Irbesartan → see angiotensin-II receptor antagonists
Irinotecan → see TABLE 14 p. 1575 (myelosuppression)
▶ Anti-androgens (apalutamide, enzalutamide) are predicted to decrease the exposure to **irinotecan**. Avoid. Severe Study
▶ Antiepileptics (carbamazepine, fosphenytoin, phenobarbital, phenytoin, primidone) are predicted to decrease the exposure to **irinotecan**. Avoid. Severe Study
▶ Antifungals, azoles (itraconazole, ketoconazole, posaconazole, voriconazole) are predicted to increase the risk of toxicity when given with **irinotecan**. Avoid. Severe Study
▶ **Ceritinib** is predicted to increase the risk of toxicity when given with **irinotecan**. Avoid. Severe Study → Also see TABLE 14 p. 1575
▶ **Cobicistat** is predicted to increase the risk of toxicity when given with **irinotecan**. Avoid. Severe Study
▶ **Encorafenib** is predicted to decrease the exposure to **irinotecan**. Avoid. Severe Study
▶ Fibrates (gemfibrozil) are predicted to increase the exposure to **irinotecan**. Avoid. Moderate Theoretical
▶ **HIV-protease inhibitors** are predicted to increase the risk of toxicity when given with **irinotecan**. Avoid. Severe Study
▶ **Idelalisib** is predicted to increase the risk of toxicity when given with **irinotecan**. Avoid. Severe Study
▶ **Ivosidenib** is predicted to decrease the exposure to **irinotecan**. Avoid. Severe Study
▶ **Lapatinib** increases the exposure to the active metabolite of **irinotecan**. Monitor adverse effects and adjust dose. Severe Study
▶ **Live vaccines** are predicted to increase the risk of generalised infection (possibly life-threatening) when given with **irinotecan**. UKHSA advises avoid (refer to Green Book). Severe Theoretical
▶ **Lumacaftor** is predicted to decrease the exposure to **irinotecan**. Avoid. Severe Study
▶ **Macrolides (clarithromycin)** are predicted to increase the risk of toxicity when given with **irinotecan**. Avoid. Severe Study
▶ **Mitotane** is predicted to decrease the exposure to **irinotecan**. Avoid. Severe Study → Also see TABLE 14 p. 1575
▶ Neurokinin-1 receptor antagonists (aprepitant, fosaprepitant) are predicted to increase the exposure to intravenous **irinotecan**. Severe Theoretical
▶ Neurokinin-1 receptor antagonists (netupitant) are predicted to increase the exposure to **irinotecan**. Moderate Study

Irinotecan (continued)
▸ **Irinotecan** is predicted to decrease the effects of **neuromuscular blocking drugs, non-depolarising**. Moderate Theoretical
▸ **Pitolisant** is predicted to decrease the exposure to **irinotecan**. Mild Theoretical
▸ **Rifamycins (rifampicin)** are predicted to decrease the exposure to **irinotecan**. Avoid. Severe Study
▸ **St John's wort** slightly decreases the exposure to **irinotecan**. Avoid. Severe Study
▸ **Irinotecan** is predicted to increase the risk of prolonged neuromuscular blockade when given with **suxamethonium**. Moderate Theoretical
▸ **Tucatinib** is predicted to increase the risk of toxicity when given with **irinotecan**. Avoid. Severe Study

Iron
▸ Oral **antacids** decrease the absorption of oral **iron**. Manufacturer advises iron should be taken 1 hour before or 2 hours after antacids. Moderate Study
▸ **Antipsychotics, second generation (clozapine)** can cause constipation, as can **iron**; concurrent use might increase the risk of developing intestinal obstruction. Severe Anecdotal
▸ Oral **iron** might decrease the concentration of the active metabolite of oral **baloxavir marboxil**. Avoid. Severe Theoretical
▸ Oral **iron** decreases the exposure to oral **bictegravir**. Manufacturer advises bictegravir should be taken 2 hours before iron. Moderate Study
▸ Oral **iron** decreases the absorption of oral **bisphosphonates (clodronate)**. **Clodronate** should be taken 1 hour before or 2 hours after iron. Moderate Study
▸ Oral **iron** is predicted to decrease the absorption of oral **bisphosphonates (ibandronate)**. **Ibandronate** should be taken 1 hour before or 6 hours after iron. Moderate Theoretical
▸ Oral **iron** decreases the absorption of oral **bisphosphonates (risedronate)**. Separate administration by at least 2 hours. Moderate Study
▸ Oral **calcium salts (calcium carbonate)** decrease the absorption of oral **iron**. **Calcium carbonate** should be taken 1 hour before or 2 hours after iron. Moderate Study
▸ Oral **iron** is predicted to decrease the exposure to oral **carbidopa**. Moderate Theoretical
▸ **Chloramphenicol** decreases the efficacy of **iron**. Moderate Anecdotal
▸ Oral **iron** decreases the absorption of oral **dolutegravir**. **Dolutegravir** should be taken 2 hours before or 6 hours after iron. Moderate Study
▸ Oral **iron** is predicted to decrease the absorption of oral **eltrombopag**. **Eltrombopag** should be taken 2 hours before or 4 hours after iron. Severe Theoretical
▸ Oral **entacapone** is predicted to decrease the absorption of oral **iron**. Separate administration by at least 2 hours. Moderate Theoretical
▸ Oral **iron** is predicted to decrease the absorption of oral **iron chelators (deferiprone)**. Moderate Theoretical
▸ Oral **iron** decreases the absorption of oral **levodopa**. Moderate Study
▸ Oral **iron** decreases the effects of oral **methyldopa**. Moderate Study
▸ Oral **iron** is predicted to decrease the absorption of oral **penicillamine**. Separate administration by at least 2 hours. Mild Study
▸ Oral **iron** decreases the exposure to oral **quinolones**. Separate administration by at least 2 hours. Moderate Study
▸ Oral **iron** is predicted to decrease the exposure to oral **raltegravir**. Separate administration by at least 2 hours. Moderate Theoretical
▸ **Iron** might decrease the exposure to **roxadustat**. **Roxadustat** should be taken at least 1 hour after iron. Moderate Theoretical
▸ Oral **iron** decreases the absorption of oral **tetracyclines**. **Tetracyclines** should be taken 2 to 3 hours after iron. Moderate Study
▸ Oral **iron** decreases the absorption of oral **thyroid hormones (levothyroxine)**. Separate administration by at least 4 hours. Moderate Study

▸ Oral **trientine** potentially decreases the absorption of oral **iron**. Moderate Theoretical
▸ Oral **iron** decreases the exposure to oral **vadadustat**. Manufacturer advises take 1 hour before vadadustat. Moderate Study
▸ Oral **zinc** is predicted to decrease the efficacy of oral **iron** and oral **iron** is predicted to decrease the efficacy of oral **zinc**. Moderate Study

Iron chelators → see TABLE 14 p. 1575 (myelosuppression), TABLE 2 p. 1571 (nephrotoxicity)

deferasirox · deferiprone · desferrioxamine · dexrazoxane

▸ **Deferasirox** has been reported to increase the exposure to **alkylating agents (busulfan)**. Monitor and adjust dose. Unknown Anecdotal
▸ **Aluminium hydroxide** is predicted to decrease the exposure to **deferasirox**. Avoid. Moderate Theoretical
▸ **Aluminium hydroxide** is predicted to decrease the absorption of **deferiprone**. Avoid. Moderate Theoretical
▸ **Deferasirox** is predicted to increase the exposure to **aminophylline**. Avoid. Moderate Theoretical
▸ **Antiepileptics (carbamazepine, fosphenytoin, phenobarbital, phenytoin, primidone)** are predicted to decrease the exposure to **deferasirox**. Monitor serum ferritin and adjust dose. Moderate Theoretical
▸ **Dexrazoxane** might decrease the absorption of **antiepileptics (fosphenytoin, phenytoin)**. Avoid. Severe Theoretical
▸ **Deferasirox** is predicted to increase the exposure to **antipsychotics, second generation (clozapine)**. Avoid. Moderate Theoretical
▸ **Ascorbic acid** is predicted to increase the risk of cardiovascular adverse effects when given with **deferiprone**. Severe Theoretical
▸ **Ascorbic acid** might increase the risk of cardiovascular adverse effects when given with **desferrioxamine**. Manufacturer advises caution or adjust ascorbic acid dose; monitor cardiac function and avoid concurrent use in those with cardiac failure. Severe Theoretical
▸ **Aspirin** (high-dose) is predicted to increase the risk of gastrointestinal bleeds when given with **deferasirox**. Severe Theoretical → Also see TABLE 2 p. 1571
▸ **Bisphosphonates** are predicted to increase the risk of gastrointestinal bleeding when given with **deferasirox**. Severe Theoretical → Also see TABLE 2 p. 1571
▸ **Dexrazoxane** might increase the risk of immunosuppression when given with **ciclosporin**. Severe Theoretical
▸ **Corticosteroids** are predicted to increase the risk of gastrointestinal bleeding when given with **deferasirox**. Severe Theoretical
▸ **Deferasirox** are predicted to increases the exposure to **etrasimod**. Avoid in poor CYP2C9 metabolisers. Severe Theoretical
▸ **HIV-protease inhibitors (ritonavir)** are predicted to decrease the exposure to **deferasirox**. Monitor serum ferritin and adjust dose. Moderate Theoretical
▸ Oral **iron** is predicted to decrease the absorption of oral **deferiprone**. Moderate Theoretical
▸ **Live vaccines** are predicted to increase the risk of generalised infection (possibly life-threatening) when given with **dexrazoxane**. Avoid. Severe Theoretical
▸ **Deferasirox** moderately increases the exposure to **meglitinides (repaglinide)**. Avoid. Moderate Study
▸ **Deferasirox** is predicted to increase the exposure to **montelukast**. Moderate Theoretical
▸ **NSAIDs** are predicted to increase the risk of gastrointestinal bleeding when given with **deferasirox**. Severe Theoretical → Also see TABLE 2 p. 1571
▸ **NSAIDs (diclofenac)** are predicted to increase the exposure to **deferiprone**. Moderate Theoretical
▸ **Deferasirox** is predicted to increase the exposure to **pioglitazone**. Moderate Study
▸ **Rifamycins (rifampicin)** are predicted to decrease the exposure to **deferasirox**. Monitor serum ferritin and adjust dose. Moderate Study → Also see TABLE 2 p. 1571
▸ **Deferasirox** is predicted to increase the exposure to **selexipag**. Adjust **selexipag** dose, p. 209. Moderate Study

- **Dexrazoxane** might increase the risk of immunosuppression when given with tacrolimus. [Severe] Theoretical
- **Deferasirox** is predicted to increase the concentration of taxanes (paclitaxel). [Severe] Anecdotal
- **Deferasirox** increases the exposure to theophylline. Avoid. [Moderate] Study
- **Deferasirox** is predicted to increase the exposure to tizanidine. Avoid. [Moderate] Theoretical
- **Deferasirox** is predicted to increase the exposure to treprostinil. Adjust dose. [Moderate] Theoretical
- **Deferasirox** is predicted to increase the exposure to tucatinib. [Moderate] Theoretical
- Oral zinc is predicted to decrease the absorption of oral **deferiprone**. [Moderate] Theoretical

Isavuconazole → see antifungals, azoles

Isocarboxazid → see MAOIs, irreversible

Isoflurane → see volatile halogenated anaesthetics

Isometheptene → see sympathomimetics, vasoconstrictor

Isoniazid → see TABLE 1 p. 1571 (hepatotoxicity), TABLE 11 p. 1574 (peripheral neuropathy)

FOOD AND LIFESTYLE Avoid tyramine-rich foods (such as mature cheeses, salami, pickled herring, *Bovril®*, *Oxo®*, *Marmite®* or any similar meat or yeast extract or fermented soya bean extract, and some beers, lagers or wines) or histamine-rich foods (such as very mature cheese or fish from the scromboid family (e.g. tuna, mackerel, salmon)) with **isoniazid**, as tachycardia, palpitation, hypotension, flushing, headache, dizziness, and sweating reported.

- **Isoniazid** is predicted to affect the clearance of aminophylline. [Severe] Theoretical
- **Isoniazid** markedly increases the concentration of antiepileptics (carbamazepine) and antiepileptics (carbamazepine) increase the risk of hepatotoxicity when given with **isoniazid**. Monitor concentration and adjust dose. [Severe] Study
- **Isoniazid** increases the concentration of antiepileptics (fosphenytoin, phenytoin). [Moderate] Study → Also see TABLE 11 p. 1574
- Cycloserine increases the risk of CNS toxicity when given with **isoniazid**. Monitor and adjust dose. [Moderate] Study
- **Isoniazid** increases the risk of optic neuropathy when given with ethambutol. [Severe] Anecdotal
- **Isoniazid** might decrease the effects of foslevodopa. [Moderate] Theoretical
- **Isoniazid** decreases the effects of levodopa. [Moderate] Study
- **Isoniazid** is predicted to increase the exposure to lomitapide. Separate administration by 12 hours. [Unknown] Theoretical → Also see TABLE 1 p. 1571
- **Isoniazid** is predicted to increase the exposure to mavacamten. Monitor and adjust dose—consult product literature. [Moderate] Theoretical
- **Isoniazid** is predicted to affect the clearance of theophylline. [Severe] Anecdotal
- **Isoniazid** potentially increases the risk of nephrotoxicity when given with volatile halogenated anaesthetics (methoxyflurane). Avoid. [Severe] Theoretical
- **Isoniazid** might increase the risk of sevoflurane toxicity when given with volatile halogenated anaesthetics (sevoflurane). Avoid **isoniazid** from 1 week before, until 15 days after, surgery. [Moderate] Theoretical

Isoprenaline → see TABLE 16 p. 1575 (reduced serum potassium)

- Entacapone is predicted to increase the risk of cardiovascular adverse effects when given with **isoprenaline**. [Moderate] Study
- Opicapone is predicted to increase the risk of cardiovascular adverse effects when given with **isoprenaline**. [Moderate] Theoretical
- Tolcapone is predicted to increase the risk of cardiovascular adverse effects when given with **isoprenaline**. [Moderate] Theoretical

Isosorbide dinitrate → see nitrates

Isosorbide mononitrate → see nitrates

Isotretinoin → see retinoids

Itraconazole → see antifungals, azoles

Ivabradine → see TABLE 5 p. 1572 (bradycardia), TABLE 8 p. 1573 (QT-interval prolongation)

- Anti-androgens (apalutamide, enzalutamide) are predicted to decrease the exposure to **ivabradine**. Adjust dose. [Moderate] Theoretical
- Antiarrhythmics (dronedarone) are predicted to increase the exposure to **ivabradine**. Adjust **ivabradine** dose, p. 245. [Severe] Theoretical → Also see TABLE 5 p. 1572
- Antiepileptics (carbamazepine, fosphenytoin, phenobarbital, phenytoin, primidone) are predicted to decrease the exposure to **ivabradine**. Adjust dose. [Moderate] Theoretical
- Antifungals, azoles (fluconazole, isavuconazole) are predicted to increase the exposure to **ivabradine**. Adjust **ivabradine** dose, p. 245. [Severe] Theoretical
- Antifungals, azoles (itraconazole, ketoconazole, posaconazole, voriconazole) are predicted to increase the exposure to **ivabradine**. Avoid. [Severe] Study
- Calcium channel blockers (diltiazem, verapamil) are predicted to increase the exposure to **ivabradine**. Avoid. [Moderate] Study → Also see TABLE 5 p. 1572
- Ceritinib is predicted to increase the exposure to **ivabradine**. Avoid. [Severe] Study → Also see TABLE 5 p. 1572
- Cobicistat is predicted to increase the exposure to **ivabradine**. Avoid. [Severe] Study
- Crizotinib is predicted to increase the exposure to **ivabradine**. Adjust **ivabradine** dose, p. 245. [Severe] Theoretical → Also see TABLE 5 p. 1572
- Encorafenib is predicted to decrease the exposure to **ivabradine**. Adjust dose. [Moderate] Theoretical
- Grapefruit juice is predicted to increase the exposure to **ivabradine**. Avoid. [Moderate] Study
- HIV-protease inhibitors are predicted to increase the exposure to **ivabradine**. Avoid. [Severe] Study
- Idelalisib is predicted to increase the exposure to **ivabradine**. Avoid. [Severe] Study
- Imatinib is predicted to increase the exposure to **ivabradine**. Adjust **ivabradine** dose, p. 245. [Severe] Theoretical
- Ivosidenib is predicted to decrease the exposure to **ivabradine**. Adjust dose. [Moderate] Theoretical
- **Lumacaftor** is predicted to decrease the exposure to **ivabradine**. Adjust dose. [Moderate] Theoretical
- Macrolides (clarithromycin) are predicted to increase the exposure to **ivabradine**. Avoid. [Severe] Study
- Macrolides (erythromycin) are predicted to increase the exposure to **ivabradine**. Avoid. [Severe] Theoretical
- **Mitotane** is predicted to decrease the exposure to **ivabradine**. Adjust dose. [Moderate] Theoretical
- Neurokinin-1 receptor antagonists (aprepitant, netupitant) are predicted to increase the exposure to **ivabradine**. Adjust **ivabradine** dose, p. 245. [Severe] Theoretical
- Nilotinib is predicted to increase the exposure to **ivabradine**. Adjust **ivabradine** dose, p. 245. [Severe] Theoretical
- Nirmatrelvir boosted with ritonavir is predicted to increase the concentration of **ivabradine**. Avoid. [Severe] Theoretical
- Rifamycins (rifampicin) are predicted to decrease the exposure to **ivabradine**. Adjust dose. [Moderate] Theoretical
- St John's wort decreases the exposure to **ivabradine**. Avoid. [Moderate] Study
- Tucatinib is predicted to increase the exposure to **ivabradine**. Avoid. [Severe] Study

Ivacaftor

FOOD AND LIFESTYLE Food or drinks containing bitter (Seville) oranges are predicted to increase the exposure to ivacaftor.

- Anti-androgens (apalutamide, enzalutamide) are predicted to decrease the exposure to **ivacaftor**. Avoid. [Severe] Study
- Antiarrhythmics (dronedarone) are predicted to increase the exposure to **ivacaftor**. Adjust dose with moderate CYP3A4 inhibitors, see ivacaftor p. 336, tezacaftor with ivacaftor p. 339, and ivacaftor with tezacaftor and elexacaftor p. 337. [Moderate] Study
- Antiepileptics (carbamazepine, fosphenytoin, phenobarbital, phenytoin, primidone) are predicted to decrease the exposure to **ivacaftor**. Avoid. [Severe] Study
- Antifungals, azoles (fluconazole, isavuconazole) are predicted to increase the exposure to **ivacaftor**. Adjust dose with moderate CYP3A4 inhibitors, see ivacaftor p. 336, tezacaftor with

Ivacaftor (continued)
ivacaftor p. 339, and ivacaftor with tezacaftor and elexacaftor p. 337. Moderate Study

▸ **Antifungals, azoles (itraconazole, ketoconazole, posaconazole, voriconazole)** are predicted to increase the exposure to **ivacaftor**. Adjust dose with potent CYP3A4 inhibitors, see ivacaftor p. 336, lumacaftor with ivacaftor p. 338, tezacaftor with ivacaftor p. 339, and ivacaftor with tezacaftor and elexacaftor p. 337. Severe Study

▸ **Berotralstat** is predicted to increase the exposure to **ivacaftor**. Adjust dose with moderate CYP3A4 inhibitors, see ivacaftor p. 336, tezacaftor with ivacaftor p. 339, and ivacaftor with tezacaftor and elexacaftor p. 337. Moderate Study

▸ **Calcium channel blockers (diltiazem, verapamil)** are predicted to increase the exposure to **ivacaftor**. Adjust dose with moderate CYP3A4 inhibitors, see ivacaftor p. 336, tezacaftor with ivacaftor p. 339, and ivacaftor with tezacaftor and elexacaftor p. 337. Moderate Study

▸ **Cenobamate** is predicted to decrease the exposure to **ivacaftor**. Adjust dose. Moderate Theoretical

▸ **Ceritinib** is predicted to increase the exposure to **ivacaftor**. Adjust dose with potent CYP3A4 inhibitors, see ivacaftor p. 336, lumacaftor with ivacaftor p. 338, tezacaftor with ivacaftor p. 339, and ivacaftor with tezacaftor and elexacaftor p. 337. Severe Study

▸ **Ivacaftor** is predicted to increase the exposure to **ciclosporin**. Moderate Theoretical

▸ **Cobicistat** is predicted to increase the exposure to **ivacaftor**. Adjust dose with potent CYP3A4 inhibitors, see ivacaftor p. 336, lumacaftor with ivacaftor p. 338, tezacaftor with ivacaftor p. 339, and ivacaftor with tezacaftor and elexacaftor p. 337. Severe Study

▸ **Ivacaftor** is predicted to increase the exposure to **coumarins (warfarin)**. Moderate Theoretical

▸ **Crizotinib** is predicted to increase the exposure to **ivacaftor**. Adjust dose with moderate CYP3A4 inhibitors, see ivacaftor p. 336, tezacaftor with ivacaftor p. 339, and ivacaftor with tezacaftor and elexacaftor p. 337. Moderate Study

▸ **Dabrafenib** is predicted to decrease the exposure to **ivacaftor**. Moderate Study

▸ **Ivacaftor** slightly increases the exposure to **digoxin**. Moderate Study

▸ **Encorafenib** is predicted to decrease the exposure to **ivacaftor**. Avoid. Severe Study

▸ **Endothelin receptor antagonists (bosentan)** are predicted to decrease the exposure to **ivacaftor**. Moderate Study

▸ **Ivacaftor** is predicted to increase the exposure to **erlotinib**. Moderate Theoretical

▸ **Ivacaftor** is predicted to increase the exposure to **everolimus**. Moderate Study

▸ **Fedratinib** is predicted to increase the exposure to **ivacaftor**. Adjust dose with moderate CYP3A4 inhibitors, see ivacaftor p. 336, tezacaftor with ivacaftor p. 339, and ivacaftor with tezacaftor and elexacaftor p. 337. Moderate Study

▸ **Ivacaftor** is predicted to increase the exposure to **gilteritinib**. Moderate Theoretical

▸ **Grapefruit** juice is predicted to increase the exposure to **ivacaftor**. Avoid. Moderate Theoretical

▸ **HIV-protease inhibitors** are predicted to increase the exposure to **ivacaftor**. Adjust dose with potent CYP3A4 inhibitors, see ivacaftor p. 336, lumacaftor with ivacaftor p. 338, tezacaftor with ivacaftor p. 339, and ivacaftor with tezacaftor and elexacaftor p. 337. Severe Study

▸ **Idelalisib** is predicted to increase the exposure to **ivacaftor**. Adjust dose with potent CYP3A4 inhibitors, see ivacaftor p. 336, lumacaftor with ivacaftor p. 338, tezacaftor with ivacaftor p. 339, and ivacaftor with tezacaftor and elexacaftor p. 337. Severe Study

▸ **Imatinib** is predicted to increase the exposure to **ivacaftor**. Adjust dose with moderate CYP3A4 inhibitors, see ivacaftor p. 336, tezacaftor with ivacaftor p. 339, and ivacaftor with tezacaftor and elexacaftor p. 337. Moderate Study

▸ **Ivosidenib** is predicted to decrease the exposure to **ivacaftor**. Avoid. Severe Study

▸ **Letermovir** is predicted to increase the exposure to **ivacaftor**. Adjust dose with moderate CYP3A4 inhibitors, see ivacaftor p. 336, tezacaftor with ivacaftor p. 339, and ivacaftor with tezacaftor and elexacaftor p. 337. Moderate Study

▸ **Ivacaftor** is predicted to increase the exposure to **lomitapide**. Separate administration by 12 hours. Moderate Theoretical

▸ **Lumacaftor** is predicted to decrease the exposure to **ivacaftor**. Avoid. Severe Study

▸ **Macrolides (clarithromycin)** are predicted to increase the exposure to **ivacaftor**. Adjust dose with potent CYP3A4 inhibitors, see ivacaftor p. 336, lumacaftor with ivacaftor p. 338, tezacaftor with ivacaftor p. 339, and ivacaftor with tezacaftor and elexacaftor p. 337. Severe Study

▸ **Macrolides (erythromycin)** are predicted to increase the exposure to **ivacaftor**. Adjust dose with moderate CYP3A4 inhibitors, see ivacaftor p. 336, tezacaftor with ivacaftor p. 339, and ivacaftor with tezacaftor and elexacaftor p. 337. Moderate Study

▸ **Mitotane** is predicted to decrease the exposure to **ivacaftor**. Avoid. Severe Study

▸ **Neurokinin-1 receptor antagonists (aprepitant, netupitant)** are predicted to increase the exposure to **ivacaftor**. Adjust dose with moderate CYP3A4 inhibitors, see ivacaftor p. 336, tezacaftor with ivacaftor p. 339, and ivacaftor with tezacaftor and elexacaftor p. 337. Moderate Study

▸ **Nilotinib** is predicted to increase the exposure to **ivacaftor**. Adjust dose with moderate CYP3A4 inhibitors, see ivacaftor p. 336, tezacaftor with ivacaftor p. 339, and ivacaftor with tezacaftor and elexacaftor p. 337. Moderate Study

▸ **Nirmatrelvir** boosted with ritonavir is predicted to increase the concentration of **ivacaftor**. Adjust dose. Severe Theoretical

▸ **NNRTIs (efavirenz, nevirapine)** are predicted to decrease the exposure to **ivacaftor**. Moderate Study

▸ **Rifamycins (rifampicin)** are predicted to decrease the exposure to **ivacaftor**. Avoid. Severe Study

▸ **Ivacaftor** is predicted to increase the exposure to **sirolimus**. Moderate Study

▸ **St John's wort** is predicted to decrease the exposure to **ivacaftor**. Avoid. Severe Study

▸ **Ivacaftor** is predicted to increase the exposure to **tacrolimus**. Moderate Theoretical

▸ **Ivacaftor** is predicted to increase the exposure to **talazoparib**. Moderate Study

▸ **Ivacaftor** is predicted to increase the exposure to **taxanes (paclitaxel)**. Moderate Study

▸ **Ivacaftor** might increase the exposure to **tigecycline**. Mild Anecdotal

▸ **Tucatinib** is predicted to increase the exposure to **ivacaftor**. Adjust dose with potent CYP3A4 inhibitors, see ivacaftor p. 336, lumacaftor with ivacaftor p. 338, tezacaftor with ivacaftor p. 339, and ivacaftor with tezacaftor and elexacaftor p. 337. Severe Study

▸ **Ivacaftor** is predicted to increase the exposure to **venetoclax**. Avoid or monitor for toxicity. Severe Theoretical

▸ **Ivacaftor** might increase the exposure to **vinca alkaloids**. Severe Theoretical

Ivermectin

ROUTE-SPECIFIC INFORMATION Since systemic absorption can follow topical application, the possibility of interactions should be borne in mind.

▸ **Ivermectin** potentially increases the anticoagulant effect of **coumarins**. Severe Anecdotal

▸ **Levamisole** increases the exposure to **ivermectin**. Moderate Study

Ivosidenib → see TABLE 8 p. 1573 (QT-interval prolongation)

▸ **Ivosidenib** is predicted to decrease the exposure to **5-HT3-receptor antagonists (ondansetron)**. Moderate Study → Also see TABLE 8 p. 1573

▸ **Ivosidenib** is predicted to markedly decrease the exposure to **abemaciclib**. Avoid. Severe Study

▸ **Ivosidenib** is predicted to decrease the exposure to **acalabrutinib**. Avoid. Severe Study

▸ **Ivosidenib** is predicted to increase the exposure to **adefovir**. Use with caution or avoid. Moderate Theoretical

▶ **Ivosidenib** is predicted to alter the exposure to aliskiren. Moderate Theoretical

▶ **Ivosidenib** might decrease the exposure to alkylating agents (cyclophosphamide, ifosfamide). Avoid or monitor efficacy. Unknown Theoretical

▶ **Ivosidenib** is predicted to decrease the exposure to alpelisib. Avoid. Moderate Study

▶ Anti-androgens (apalutamide, enzalutamide) are predicted to decrease the exposure to **ivosidenib**. Avoid. Severe Theoretical → Also see TABLE 8 p. 1573

▶ **Ivosidenib** is predicted to decrease the exposure to anti-androgens (abiraterone). Avoid. Severe Study

▶ **Ivosidenib** is predicted to decrease the exposure to anti-androgens (darolutamide). Avoid. Moderate Study

▶ Antiarrhythmics (dronedarone) are predicted to increase the exposure to **ivosidenib**. Monitor and adjust dose—consult product literature. Severe Study → Also see TABLE 8 p. 1573

▶ **Ivosidenib** is predicted to decrease the exposure to antiarrhythmics (disopyramide, dronedarone). Avoid. Severe Study → Also see TABLE 8 p. 1573

▶ **Ivosidenib** is predicted to decrease the efficacy of antiarrhythmics (propafenone). Moderate Study

▶ **Ivosidenib** is predicted to decrease the exposure to anticholinesterases, centrally acting (donepezil). Mild Study

▶ Antiepileptics (carbamazepine, fosphenytoin, phenobarbital, primidone) are predicted to decrease the exposure to **ivosidenib**. Avoid. Severe Theoretical

▶ Antiepileptics (phenytoin) are predicted to decrease the exposure to **ivosidenib** and **ivosidenib** might decrease the exposure to antiepileptics (phenytoin). Avoid. Severe Study

▶ **Ivosidenib** might decrease the exposure to antiepileptics (lamotrigine). Avoid or monitor efficacy. Unknown Theoretical

▶ **Ivosidenib** is predicted to decrease the exposure to antiepileptics (perampanel). Monitor and adjust dose. Moderate Study

▶ Antifungals, azoles (fluconazole, isavuconazole, voriconazole) are predicted to increase the exposure to **ivosidenib**. Monitor and adjust dose—consult product literature. Severe Study → Also see TABLE 8 p. 1573

▶ Antifungals, azoles (itraconazole) moderately increase the exposure to **ivosidenib** and **ivosidenib** is predicted to decrease the exposure to antifungals, azoles (itraconazole). Avoid or adjust dose—consult product literature. Severe Study

▶ Antifungals, azoles (ketoconazole) are predicted to increase the exposure to **ivosidenib** and **ivosidenib** is predicted to decrease the exposure to antifungals, azoles (ketoconazole). Avoid or adjust dose—consult product literature. Severe Study

▶ **Ivosidenib** is predicted to decrease the exposure to antifungals, azoles (isavuconazole). Avoid. Severe Study

▶ **Ivosidenib** is predicted to alter the exposure to antihistamines, non-sedating (fexofenadine). Moderate Theoretical

▶ **Ivosidenib** is predicted to decrease the exposure to antimalarials (artemether) with lumefantrine. Avoid. Severe Study → Also see TABLE 8 p. 1573

▶ **Ivosidenib** is predicted to moderately decrease the exposure to antipsychotics, second generation (aripiprazole). Adjust **aripiprazole** dose, p. 454. Moderate Study → Also see TABLE 8 p. 1573

▶ **Ivosidenib** is predicted to decrease the exposure to antipsychotics, second generation (cariprazine). Avoid. Severe Theoretical

▶ **Ivosidenib** is predicted to decrease the exposure to antipsychotics, second generation (lurasidone). Avoid. Moderate Study

▶ **Ivosidenib** is predicted to decrease the exposure to antipsychotics, second generation (paliperidone). Monitor and adjust dose. Severe Study → Also see TABLE 8 p. 1573

▶ **Ivosidenib** is predicted to decrease the exposure to antipsychotics, second generation (quetiapine). Moderate Study

▶ **Ivosidenib** is predicted to decrease the exposure to antipsychotics, second generation (risperidone). Adjust dose. Moderate Study

▶ **Ivosidenib** is predicted to decrease the exposure to avacopan. Avoid or monitor. Severe Study

▶ **Ivosidenib** is predicted to decrease the exposure to avapritinib. Avoid. Severe Study

▶ **Ivosidenib** is predicted to decrease the exposure to axitinib. Avoid or adjust dose. Moderate Study

▶ **Ivosidenib** decreases the exposure to bedaquiline. Avoid. Severe Study → Also see TABLE 8 p. 1573

▶ **Ivosidenib** is predicted to decrease the exposure to belumosudil. Adjust **belumosudil** dose, p. 979. Severe Study

▶ **Ivosidenib** is predicted to decrease the exposure to benzodiazepines (alprazolam). Adjust dose. Moderate Theoretical

▶ **Ivosidenib** is predicted to decrease the exposure to benzodiazepines (midazolam). Monitor and adjust dose. Severe Study

▶ Berotralstat is predicted to increase the exposure to **ivosidenib**. Monitor and adjust dose—consult product literature. Severe Study

▶ **Ivosidenib** might decrease the exposure to beta$_2$ agonists (salmeterol). Avoid or monitor. Moderate Theoretical

▶ **Ivosidenib** is predicted to decrease the exposure to bictegravir. Avoid. Moderate Study

▶ **Ivosidenib** slightly decreases the exposure to bortezomib. Avoid. Severe Study

▶ **Ivosidenib** is predicted to very markedly decrease the exposure to bosutinib. Avoid. Severe Study → Also see TABLE 8 p. 1573

▶ **Ivosidenib** is predicted to decrease the exposure to brigatinib. Avoid. Severe Study

▶ **Ivosidenib** is predicted to decrease the exposure to buspirone. Use with caution and adjust dose. Severe Study

▶ **Ivosidenib** moderately decreases the exposure to cabozantinib. Avoid. Moderate Study → Also see TABLE 8 p. 1573

▶ Calcium channel blockers (diltiazem, verapamil) are predicted to increase the exposure to **ivosidenib**. Monitor and adjust dose—consult product literature. Severe Study

▶ **Ivosidenib** is predicted to decrease the exposure to calcium channel blockers (amlodipine, felodipine, lacidipine, lercanidipine, nicardipine, nifedipine, nimodipine). Monitor and adjust dose. Moderate Study

▶ **Ivosidenib** is predicted to decrease the exposure to cannabidiol. Adjust dose. Moderate Study

▶ **Ivosidenib** is predicted to decrease the exposure to capivasertib. Avoid. Moderate Study

▶ **Ivosidenib** is predicted to increase the exposure to cephalosporins (cefaclor). Use with caution or avoid. Moderate Theoretical

▶ **Ivosidenib** is predicted to decrease the exposure to ceritinib. Avoid. Severe Study → Also see TABLE 8 p. 1573

▶ **Ivosidenib** decreases the concentration of ciclosporin. Severe Study

▶ Ciclosporin is predicted to increase the exposure to **ivosidenib** and **ivosidenib** might decrease the exposure to ciclosporin. Monitor and adjust dose—consult product literature. Severe Study

▶ **Ivosidenib** is predicted to alter the effects of cilostazol. Moderate Theoretical

▶ **Ivosidenib** is predicted to decrease the exposure to cinacalcet. Monitor and adjust dose. Moderate Study

▶ **Ivosidenib** decreases the exposure to clomethiazole. Monitor and adjust dose. Moderate Study

▶ **Ivosidenib** is predicted to decrease the exposure to cobicistat. Avoid. Severe Study

▶ Cobicistat is predicted to increase the exposure to **ivosidenib**. Monitor and adjust dose—consult product literature. Severe Study

▶ **Ivosidenib** is predicted to decrease the exposure to cobimetinib. Avoid. Severe Theoretical

▶ **Ivosidenib** is predicted to alter the exposure to colchicine. Moderate Theoretical

▶ **Ivosidenib** might decrease the concentration of combined hormonal contraceptives. Use alternative methods during treatment with, and for at least 28 days after stopping, **ivosidenib**. Severe Theoretical

▶ **Ivosidenib** is predicted to decrease the exposure to corticosteroids (budesonide, deflazacort, dexamethasone, fludrocortisone, hydrocortisone, methylprednisolone,

A1

Ivosidenib (continued)
prednisolone, triamcinolone). Monitor and adjust dose. Moderate Study

▸ **Ivosidenib** is predicted to decrease the exposure to corticosteroids **(fluticasone)**. Unknown Theoretical

▸ **Ivosidenib** might decrease the exposure to coumarins **(warfarin)**. Avoid or monitor efficacy. Unknown Study

▸ Crizotinib is predicted to increase the exposure to **ivosidenib**. Monitor and adjust dose—consult product literature. Severe Study → Also see **TABLE 8** p. 1573

▸ **Ivosidenib** is predicted to markedly decrease the exposure to crizotinib. Avoid. Severe Study → Also see **TABLE 8** p. 1573

▸ **Ivosidenib** is predicted to decrease the exposure to dabrafenib. Avoid. Moderate Theoretical

▸ **Ivosidenib** is predicted to decrease the exposure to daridorexant. Severe Study

▸ **Ivosidenib** is predicted to decrease the exposure to darifenacin. Moderate Theoretical

▸ **Ivosidenib** is predicted to markedly decrease the exposure to dasatinib. Avoid. Severe Study → Also see **TABLE 8** p. 1573

▸ **Ivosidenib** is predicted to slightly decrease the exposure to delamanid. Avoid. Moderate Study → Also see **TABLE 8** p. 1573

▸ **Ivosidenib** is predicted to markedly decrease the exposure to dienogest. Severe Study

▸ **Ivosidenib** is predicted to alter the exposure to digoxin. Moderate Theoretical

▸ **Ivosidenib** is predicted to decrease the exposure to dipeptidylpeptidase-4 inhibitors **(linagliptin)**. Moderate Study

▸ **Ivosidenib** is predicted to moderately decrease the exposure to dipeptidylpeptidase-4 inhibitors **(saxagliptin)**. Moderate Study

▸ **Ivosidenib** is predicted to decrease the exposure to dronabinol. Avoid or adjust dose. Mild Study

▸ **Ivosidenib** is predicted to decrease the exposure to elacestrant. Avoid or adjust dose depending on duration—consult product literature. Severe Study

▸ **Ivosidenib** is predicted to decrease the exposure to elbasvir. Avoid. Severe Study

▸ **Ivosidenib** is predicted to decreases the exposure to elexacaftor. Avoid. Severe Theoretical

▸ **Ivosidenib** is predicted to decrease the exposure to eliglustat. Avoid. Severe Study

▸ **Ivosidenib** is predicted to decrease the concentration of elvitegravir. Avoid. Severe Study

▸ **Ivosidenib** is predicted to decrease the exposure to encorafenib. Severe Theoretical → Also see **TABLE 8** p. 1573

▸ **Ivosidenib** affects the exposure to endothelin receptor antagonists **(bosentan)**. Avoid. Severe Study

▸ **Ivosidenib** is predicted to decrease the exposure to endothelin receptor antagonists **(macitentan)**. Avoid. Severe Study

▸ **Ivosidenib** is predicted to decrease the exposure to the cytotoxic component of enfortumab vedotin. Moderate Theoretical

▸ **Ivosidenib** is predicted to decrease the exposure to entrectinib. Avoid. Severe Study → Also see **TABLE 8** p. 1573

▸ **Ivosidenib** is predicted to decrease the exposure to erdafitinib. Avoid. Severe Study

▸ **Ivosidenib** is predicted to decrease the exposure to erlotinib. Avoid or adjust dose—consult product literature. Severe Study

▸ **Ivosidenib** is predicted to decrease the exposure to esketamine. Adjust dose. Mild Theoretical

▸ **Ivosidenib** is predicted to decrease the exposure to eszopiclone. Adjust dose. Moderate Theoretical

▸ **Ivosidenib** is predicted to decrease the concentration of everolimus. Avoid or adjust dose. Severe Study

▸ **Ivosidenib** moderately decreases the exposure to exemestane. Moderate Study

▸ **Ivosidenib** is predicted to alter the exposure to factor XA inhibitors **(edoxaban)**. Moderate Theoretical

▸ Fedratinib is predicted to increase the exposure to **ivosidenib**. Monitor and adjust dose—consult product literature. Severe Study

▸ **Ivosidenib** is predicted to decrease the exposure to fedratinib. Avoid. Moderate Study

▸ **Ivosidenib** is predicted to decrease the exposure to fesoterodine. Avoid. Moderate Study

▸ **Ivosidenib** is predicted to decrease the exposure to fostamatinib. Avoid. Severe Study

▸ **Ivosidenib** is predicted to decrease the exposure to the active metabolite of fostemsavir. Avoid. Severe Study

▸ **Ivosidenib** is predicted to decrease the exposure to fruquintinib. Avoid. Moderate Study

▸ **Ivosidenib** is predicted to increase the exposure to ganciclovir. Use with caution or avoid. Moderate Theoretical

▸ **Ivosidenib** is predicted to decrease the exposure to gefitinib. Avoid. Severe Study

▸ **Ivosidenib** is predicted to decrease the exposure to glasdegib. Avoid. Severe Study → Also see **TABLE 8** p. 1573

▸ Grapefruit and grapefruit juice are predicted to increase the exposure to **ivosidenib**. Avoid. Moderate Study

▸ **Ivosidenib** is predicted to decrease the exposure to grazoprevir. Avoid. Severe Study

▸ **Ivosidenib** is predicted to decrease the concentration of guanfacine. Adjust **guanfacine** dose, p. 407. Moderate Study

▸ **Ivosidenib** is predicted to increase the exposure to H_2 receptor antagonists **(cimetidine, famotidine)**. Use with caution or avoid. Moderate Theoretical

▸ **Ivosidenib** decreases the concentration of haloperidol. Adjust dose. Moderate Study → Also see **TABLE 8** p. 1573

▸ HIV-protease inhibitors are predicted to increase the exposure to **ivosidenib**. Monitor and adjust dose—consult product literature. Severe Study

▸ **Ivosidenib** is predicted to decrease the exposure to ibrutinib. Avoid or monitor. Severe Study

▸ Idelalisib is predicted to increase the exposure to **ivosidenib**. Monitor and adjust dose—consult product literature. Severe Study

▸ **Ivosidenib** is predicted to decrease the exposure to idelalisib. Avoid. Severe Study

▸ Imatinib is predicted to increase the exposure to **ivosidenib**. Monitor and adjust dose—consult product literature. Severe Study

▸ **Ivosidenib** is predicted to decrease the exposure to imatinib. Avoid. Moderate Study

▸ **Ivosidenib** is predicted to decrease the exposure to irinotecan. Avoid. Severe Study

▸ **Ivosidenib** is predicted to decrease the exposure to ivabradine. Adjust dose. Moderate Theoretical

▸ **Ivosidenib** is predicted to decrease the exposure to ivacaftor. Avoid. Severe Study

▸ **Ivosidenib** is predicted to decrease the exposure to ixazomib. Avoid. Severe Study

▸ **Ivosidenib** is predicted to decrease the exposure to lapatinib. Avoid. Severe Study → Also see **TABLE 8** p. 1573

▸ **Ivosidenib** is predicted to moderately decrease the exposure to larotrectinib. Avoid. Moderate Study

▸ **Ivosidenib** is predicted to decrease the exposure to leniolisib. Avoid. Severe Theoretical

▸ Letermovir is predicted to increase the exposure to **ivosidenib**. Monitor and adjust dose—consult product literature. Severe Study

▸ **Ivosidenib** is predicted to decrease the exposure to lomitapide. Monitor and adjust dose. Moderate Theoretical

▸ **Ivosidenib** is predicted to increase the exposure to loop diuretics **(furosemide)**. Manufacturer advises caution or avoid—consult product literature. Moderate Theoretical

▸ **Ivosidenib** is predicted to alter the exposure to loperamide. Moderate Theoretical

▸ **Ivosidenib** is predicted to decrease the exposure to lorlatinib. Avoid. Severe Study

▸ Macrolides **(clarithromycin, erythromycin)** are predicted to increase the exposure to **ivosidenib**. Monitor and adjust dose—consult product literature. Severe Study → Also see **TABLE 8** p. 1573

▸ **Ivosidenib** is predicted to decrease the exposure to maraviroc. Adjust dose. Severe Study

▸ **Ivosidenib** is predicted to decrease the exposure to mavacamten. Monitor and adjust dose—consult product literature. Severe Theoretical

- **Ivosidenib** is predicted to decrease the exposure to meglitinides (repaglinide). Monitor blood glucose and adjust dose. Moderate Study
- **Ivosidenib** is predicted to increase the exposure to methotrexate. Use with caution or avoid. Moderate Theoretical
- **Ivosidenib** is predicted to decrease the exposure to midostaurin. Avoid. Severe Study
- **Ivosidenib** is predicted to decrease the exposure to mifepristone. Adjust **mifepristone** dose, p. 954. Severe Study
- **Ivosidenib** is predicted to decrease the exposure to mineralocorticoid receptor antagonists (eplerenone). Avoid. Moderate Theoretical
- **Ivosidenib** is predicted to decrease the exposure to mineralocorticoid receptor antagonists (finerenone). Avoid. Severe Study
- **Ivosidenib** is predicted to decrease the exposure to mirtazapine. Adjust dose. Moderate Study
- **Mitotane** is predicted to decrease the exposure to **ivosidenib**. Avoid. Severe Theoretical
- **Ivosidenib** is predicted to decrease the exposure to mobocertinib. Avoid. Severe Study → Also see **TABLE 8** p. 1573
- **Ivosidenib** is predicted to decrease the exposure to monoclonal antibodies (polatuzumab vedotin). Moderate Theoretical
- **Ivosidenib** is predicted to decrease the exposure to the cytotoxic component of monoclonal antibodies (trastuzumab emtansine). Severe Theoretical
- **Ivosidenib** is predicted to decrease the exposure to montelukast. Mild Study
- **Ivosidenib** is predicted to markedly decrease the exposure to naldemedine. Avoid. Severe Study
- **Ivosidenib** is predicted to markedly decrease the exposure to naloxegol. Avoid. Moderate Study
- **Ivosidenib** is predicted to decrease the exposure to neratinib. Avoid. Severe Study
- Neurokinin-1 receptor antagonists (aprepitant, netupitant) are predicted to increase the exposure to **ivosidenib**. Monitor and adjust dose—consult product literature. Severe Study
- **Ivosidenib** is predicted to markedly decrease the exposure to neurokinin-1 receptor antagonists (aprepitant). Avoid. Moderate Study
- **Ivosidenib** is predicted to decrease the exposure to neurokinin-1 receptor antagonists (fosaprepitant). Avoid. Moderate Theoretical
- **Ivosidenib** is predicted to decrease the exposure to neurokinin-1 receptor antagonists (netupitant). Avoid. Severe Study
- **Nilotinib** is predicted to increase the exposure to **ivosidenib**. Monitor and adjust dose—consult product literature. Severe Study → Also see **TABLE 8** p. 1573
- **Ivosidenib** is predicted to moderately decrease the exposure to nilotinib. Avoid. Severe Study → Also see **TABLE 8** p. 1573
- **Nirmatrelvir** boosted with ritonavir is predicted to increase the concentration of **ivosidenib**. Monitor and adjust dose—consult product literature. Severe Theoretical
- **Ivosidenib** is predicted to decrease the exposure to nirmatrelvir boosted with ritonavir. Avoid. Severe Study
- **Ivosidenib** is predicted to decrease the exposure to nitisinone. Adjust dose. Moderate Theoretical
- **Ivosidenib** is predicted to decrease the exposure to NNRTIs (doravirine). Avoid. Severe Study
- **Ivosidenib** is predicted to decrease the exposure to NNRTIs (etravirine). Avoid. Severe Theoretical
- **Ivosidenib** markedly decreases the exposure to NNRTIs (rilpivirine). Avoid. Severe Study
- **Ivosidenib** is predicted to decrease the exposure to olaparib. Avoid. Moderate Theoretical
- **Ivosidenib** is predicted to decrease the exposure to opioids (alfentanil, fentanyl). Moderate Study
- **Ivosidenib** is predicted to decrease the exposure to opioids (buprenorphine). Monitor and adjust dose. Moderate Theoretical
- **Ivosidenib** decreases the exposure to opioids (methadone). Monitor and adjust dose. Severe Study → Also see **TABLE 8** p. 1573
- **Ivosidenib** is predicted to decrease the exposure to opioids (oxycodone). Monitor and adjust dose. Moderate Study
- **Ivosidenib** is predicted to increase the exposure to the active metabolite of oseltamivir. Use with caution or avoid. Moderate Theoretical

- **Ivosidenib** is predicted to decrease the exposure to osilodrostat. Moderate Theoretical → Also see **TABLE 8** p. 1573
- **Ivosidenib** is predicted to moderately decrease the exposure to osimertinib. Avoid. Moderate Study → Also see **TABLE 8** p. 1573
- **Ivosidenib** is predicted to moderately decrease the exposure to ospemifene. Moderate Study
- **Ivosidenib** is predicted to decrease the exposure to palbociclib. Avoid. Severe Study
- **Ivosidenib** is predicted to decrease the exposure to panobinostat. Avoid. Moderate Theoretical → Also see **TABLE 8** p. 1573
- **Ivosidenib** is predicted to decrease the exposure to pazopanib. Avoid. Severe Theoretical → Also see **TABLE 8** p. 1573
- **Ivosidenib** is predicted to decrease the exposure to pemigatinib. Avoid. Severe Study
- **Ivosidenib** is predicted to increase the exposure to penicillins (benzylpenicillin). Use with caution or avoid. Moderate Theoretical
- **Ivosidenib** moderately decreases the exposure to phosphodiesterase type-4 inhibitors (apremilast). Avoid. Severe Study
- **Ivosidenib** is predicted to decrease the exposure to phosphodiesterase type-4 inhibitors (roflumilast). Avoid. Moderate Study
- **Ivosidenib** is predicted to decrease the exposure to phosphodiesterase type-5 inhibitors (avanafil, tadalafil). Avoid. Severe Study
- **Ivosidenib** is predicted to decrease the exposure to phosphodiesterase type-5 inhibitors (sildenafil, vardenafil). Moderate Theoretical → Also see **TABLE 8** p. 1573
- **Ivosidenib** is predicted to moderately to markedly decrease the exposure to pibrentasvir. Avoid. Severe Study
- **Ivosidenib** might decrease the exposure to pimozide. Avoid or monitor efficacy. Moderate Theoretical → Also see **TABLE 8** p. 1573
- **Ivosidenib** might decrease the exposure to pioglitazone. Avoid or monitor efficacy. Unknown Study
- **Ivosidenib** is predicted to moderately decrease the exposure to pitolisant. Moderate Study
- **Ivosidenib** is predicted to decrease the exposure to ponatinib. Avoid. Moderate Theoretical
- **Ivosidenib** is predicted to decrease the exposure to pralsetinib. Avoid or adjust dose with potent CYP3A4 inducers—consult product literature. Moderate Study
- **Ivosidenib** is predicted to markedly decrease the exposure to praziquantel. Avoid. Moderate Study
- **Ivosidenib** might decrease the exposure to proton pump inhibitors (omeprazole). Avoid or monitor efficacy. Unknown Theoretical
- **Ivosidenib** is predicted to decrease the exposure to quizartinib. Avoid. Severe Study → Also see **TABLE 8** p. 1573
- **Ivosidenib** might decrease the exposure to raltegravir. Avoid or monitor efficacy. Unknown Theoretical
- **Ivosidenib** is predicted to decrease the exposure to ranolazine. Avoid. Severe Study → Also see **TABLE 8** p. 1573
- **Ivosidenib** is predicted to decrease the exposure to reboxetine. Moderate Anecdotal
- **Ivosidenib** is predicted to decrease the exposure to regorafenib. Avoid. Moderate Study
- **Ivosidenib** is predicted to markedly decrease the exposure to ribociclib. Avoid. Severe Study → Also see **TABLE 8** p. 1573
- **Rifamycins (rifampicin)** are predicted to decrease the exposure to **ivosidenib**. Avoid. Severe Theoretical
- **Ivosidenib** is predicted to decrease the exposure to rimegepant. Avoid. Moderate Theoretical
- **Ivosidenib** is predicted to decrease the exposure to ripretinib. Avoid or adjust dose—consult product literature. Severe Study
- **Ivosidenib** is predicted to decrease the exposure to ruxolitinib. Monitor and adjust dose. Moderate Study
- **Ivosidenib** is predicted to decrease the exposure to selpercatinib. Avoid. Moderate Study → Also see **TABLE 8** p. 1573
- **Ivosidenib** is predicted to decrease the exposure to selumetinib. Avoid. Severe Study
- **Ivosidenib** is predicted to decrease the exposure to siponimod. Manufacturer advises caution depending on genotype—consult product literature. Severe Study

Ivosidenib (continued)

- **Ivosidenib** is predicted to decrease the concentration of sirolimus. Avoid or monitor and adjust dose. Severe Study
- **Ivosidenib** is predicted to decrease the exposure to solifenacin. Moderate Theoretical
- **Ivosidenib** is predicted to decrease the exposure to sorafenib. Moderate Theoretical → Also see **TABLE 8** p. 1573
- **Ivosidenib** is predicted to decrease the exposure to sotorasib. Avoid. Severe Study
- **St John's wort** is predicted to decreases the exposure to ivosidenib. Avoid. Moderate Theoretical
- **Ivosidenib** is predicted to increase the exposure to statins (atorvastatin, pravastatin, rosuvastatin). Use with caution or avoid. Unknown Theoretical
- **Ivosidenib** might affect the exposure to statins (simvastatin). Avoid or monitor. Moderate Theoretical
- **Ivosidenib** is predicted to decrease the exposure to sunitinib. Avoid or adjust dose—consult product literature. Moderate Study → Also see **TABLE 8** p. 1573
- **Ivosidenib** decreases the concentration of tacrolimus. Avoid or monitor and adjust dose. Severe Study
- **Ivosidenib** is predicted to alter the exposure to talazoparib. Moderate Theoretical
- **Ivosidenib** is predicted to decrease the exposure to taxanes (cabazitaxel). Avoid. Moderate Study
- **Ivosidenib** is predicted to decrease the exposure to taxanes (docetaxel). Severe Theoretical
- **Ivosidenib** is predicted to decrease the exposure to taxanes (paclitaxel). Avoid. Severe Study
- **Ivosidenib** is predicted to decrease the concentration of temsirolimus. Avoid. Severe Study
- **Ivosidenib** might decrease the exposure to tepotinib. Avoid. Severe Theoretical
- **Ivosidenib** is predicted to decrease the exposure to tetracyclines (eravacycline). Adjust **eravacycline** dose, p. 657. Moderate Study
- **Ivosidenib** is predicted to decrease the exposure to tezacaftor. Avoid. Severe Theoretical
- **Ivosidenib** is predicted to alter the exposure to thrombin inhibitors (dabigatran). Avoid. Moderate Theoretical
- **Ivosidenib** is predicted to markedly decrease the exposure to ticagrelor. Avoid. Severe Study
- **Ivosidenib** is predicted to decrease the exposure to tivozanib. Severe Study
- **Ivosidenib** is predicted to decrease the exposure to tofacitinib. Avoid. Severe Study
- **Ivosidenib** is predicted to decrease the exposure to tolvaptan. Use with caution or avoid depending on indication. Severe Study
- **Ivosidenib** is predicted to decrease the exposure to toremifene. Adjust dose. Moderate Study → Also see **TABLE 8** p. 1573
- **Ivosidenib** is predicted to decrease the exposure to trabectedin. Avoid. Severe Theoretical
- **Ivosidenib** might decrease the exposure to triptans (eletriptan). Avoid or monitor. Moderate Theoretical
- **Ivosidenib** is predicted to decrease the exposure to tucatinib. Avoid. Severe Study
- **Ivosidenib** is predicted to decrease the exposure to upadacitinib. Moderate Study
- **Ivosidenib** is predicted to decrease the exposure to vandetanib. Avoid. Moderate Study → Also see **TABLE 8** p. 1573
- **Ivosidenib** is predicted to moderately decrease the exposure to velpatasvir. Avoid. Severe Study
- **Ivosidenib** is predicted to decrease the exposure to vemurafenib. Avoid. Severe Study → Also see **TABLE 8** p. 1573
- **Ivosidenib** is predicted to decrease the exposure to venetoclax. Avoid. Severe Study
- **Ivosidenib** ivosidenib to decrease the exposure to vinca alkaloids (vinblastine, vincristine, vindesine). Severe Theoretical
- **Ivosidenib** is predicted to decrease the exposure to vinca alkaloids (vinorelbine). Use with caution or avoid. Severe Theoretical
- **Ivosidenib** is predicted to decrease the exposure to vismodegib. Avoid. Moderate Theoretical
- **Ivosidenib** is predicted to decrease the exposure to voclosporin. Avoid. Severe Study → Also see **TABLE 8** p. 1573

- **Ivosidenib** is predicted to decrease the exposure to vortioxetine. Monitor and adjust dose. Moderate Study
- **Ivosidenib** is predicted to decrease the concentration of voxilaprevir. Avoid. Severe Study
- **Ivosidenib** is predicted to decrease the exposure to zanubrutinib. Avoid. Severe Study
- **Ivosidenib** is predicted to decrease the exposure to zopiclone. Adjust dose. Moderate Study

Ixazomib

- **Anti-androgens (apalutamide, enzalutamide)** are predicted to decrease the exposure to ixazomib. Avoid. Severe Study
- **Antiepileptics (carbamazepine, fosphenytoin, phenobarbital, phenytoin, primidone)** are predicted to decrease the exposure to ixazomib. Avoid. Severe Study
- **Cenobamate** is predicted to decrease the exposure to ixazomib. Moderate Theoretical
- **Dabrafenib** is predicted to decrease the exposure to ixazomib. Moderate Theoretical
- **Encorafenib** is predicted to decrease the exposure to ixazomib. Avoid. Severe Study
- **Endothelin receptor antagonists (bosentan)** are predicted to decrease the exposure to ixazomib. Moderate Theoretical
- **Ivosidenib** is predicted to decrease the exposure to ixazomib. Avoid. Severe Study
- **Lorlatinib** is predicted to decrease the exposure to ixazomib. Moderate Theoretical
- **Lumacaftor** is predicted to decrease the exposure to ixazomib. Avoid. Severe Study
- **Mitotane** is predicted to decrease the exposure to ixazomib. Avoid. Severe Study
- **NNRTIs (efavirenz, etravirine, nevirapine)** are predicted to decrease the exposure to ixazomib. Moderate Theoretical
- **Rifamycins (rifampicin)** are predicted to decrease the exposure to ixazomib. Avoid. Severe Study
- **Sotorasib** is predicted to decrease the exposure to ixazomib. Moderate Theoretical
- **St John's wort** is predicted to decrease the exposure to ixazomib. Avoid. Severe Theoretical

Ixekizumab → see monoclonal antibodies

Kaolin

- **Oral kaolin** decreases the absorption of oral antimalarials (chloroquine). Separate administration by at least 4 hours. Moderate Study
- **Oral kaolin** is predicted to decrease the absorption of oral hydroxychloroquine. Moderate Theoretical
- **Oral kaolin** is predicted to decrease the absorption of oral tetracyclines. Moderate Theoretical

Ketamine → see **TABLE 7** p. 1572 (hypotension), **TABLE 10** p. 1574 (CNS effects)

- **Ketamine** is predicted to increase the risk of elevated blood pressure when given with ergometrine. Severe Theoretical
- **Memantine** is predicted to increase the risk of CNS adverse effects when given with ketamine. Avoid. Severe Theoretical

Ketoconazole → see antifungals, azoles

Ketoprofen → see NSAIDs

Ketorolac → see NSAIDs

Ketotifen → see antihistamines, sedating

Labetalol → see beta blockers, non-selective

Lacidipine → see calcium channel blockers

Lacosamide → see antiepileptics

Lamivudine → see NRTIs

Lamotrigine → see antiepileptics

Landiolol → see beta blockers, selective

Lanreotide

- **Beta blockers, non-selective** are predicted to increase the risk of bradycardia when given with lanreotide. Moderate Theoretical
- **Beta blockers, selective** are predicted to increase the risk of bradycardia when given with lanreotide. Moderate Theoretical
- **Lanreotide** is predicted to decrease the absorption of oral ciclosporin. Adjust dose. Severe Theoretical

Lansoprazole → see proton pump inhibitors

Lanthanum

- **Lanthanum** is predicted to decrease the absorption of antifungals, azoles (ketoconazole). Separate administration by at least 2 hours. Moderate Theoretical

- **Lanthanum** is predicted to decrease the absorption of antimalarials **(chloroquine)**. Separate administration by at least 2 hours. Moderate Theoretical
- **Lanthanum** is predicted to decrease the absorption of hydroxychloroquine. Separate administration by at least 2 hours. Moderate Theoretical
- **Lanthanum** moderately decreases the exposure to quinolones. **Quinolones** should be taken 2 hours before or 4 hours after **lanthanum**. Moderate Study
- Oral **lanthanum** might decrease the absorption of oral tetracyclines. Separate administration by 2 hours. Moderate Theoretical
- **Lanthanum** decreases the absorption of thyroid hormones. Separate administration by 2 hours. Moderate Study
- Oral **lanthanum** is predicted to decrease the exposure to oral vadadustat. Manufacturer advises take 1 hour before or 2 hours after **lanthanum**. Moderate Theoretical

Lapatinib → see TABLE 8 p. 1573 (QT-interval prolongation)
- **Lapatinib** is predicted to increase the exposure to afatinib. Moderate Study
- **Lapatinib** is predicted to increase the exposure to aliskiren. Moderate Theoretical
- **Lapatinib** is predicted to increase the exposure to alpelisib. Moderate Theoretical
- Oral antacids is predicted to decrease the absorption of oral **lapatinib**. Avoid. Moderate Theoretical
- Anti-androgens **(apalutamide, enzalutamide)** are predicted to decrease the exposure to **lapatinib**. Avoid. Severe Study → Also see TABLE 8 p. 1573
- Antiarrhythmics **(dronedarone)** are predicted to increase the exposure to **lapatinib**. Moderate Study → Also see TABLE 8 p. 1573
- Antiepileptics **(carbamazepine, fosphenytoin, phenobarbital, phenytoin, primidone)** are predicted to decrease the exposure to **lapatinib**. Avoid. Severe Study
- Antifungals, azoles **(fluconazole, isavuconazole)** are predicted to increase the exposure to **lapatinib**. Moderate Study → Also see TABLE 8 p. 1573
- Antifungals, azoles **(itraconazole, ketoconazole, posaconazole, voriconazole)** are predicted to increase the exposure to **lapatinib**. Avoid. Moderate Study → Also see TABLE 8 p. 1573
- **Lapatinib** is predicted to increase the exposure to antihistamines, non-sedating **(fexofenadine)**. Moderate Theoretical
- Berotralstat is predicted to increase the exposure to **lapatinib**. Moderate Study
- **Lapatinib** is predicted to increase the exposure to beta blockers, non-selective **(nadolol)**. Moderate Study
- **Lapatinib** is predicted to increase the exposure to bictegravir. Use with caution or avoid. Moderate Theoretical
- Calcium channel blockers **(diltiazem, verapamil)** are predicted to increase the exposure to **lapatinib**. Moderate Study
- Oral calcium salts **(calcium carbonate)** -containing antacids are predicted to decrease the absorption of oral **lapatinib**. Avoid. Moderate Theoretical
- Cenobamate is predicted to decrease the exposure to **lapatinib**. Avoid. Severe Study
- **Lapatinib** is predicted to increase the exposure to ceritinib. Moderate Theoretical → Also see TABLE 8 p. 1573
- Ceritinib is predicted to increase the exposure to **lapatinib**. Avoid. Moderate Study → Also see TABLE 8 p. 1573
- Ciclosporin might increase the concentration of **lapatinib**. Severe Theoretical
- Cobicistat is predicted to increase the exposure to **lapatinib**. Avoid. Moderate Study
- **Lapatinib** is predicted to increase the exposure to colchicine. Avoid P-glycoprotein inhibitors or adjust **colchicine** dose, p. 1279. Moderate Theoretical
- **Lapatinib** is predicted to increase the risk of bleeding events when given with coumarins. Severe Theoretical
- Crizotinib is predicted to increase the exposure to **lapatinib**. Moderate Study → Also see TABLE 8 p. 1573
- Dabrafenib is predicted to decrease the exposure to **lapatinib**. Avoid. Severe Study
- **Lapatinib** slightly increases the exposure to digoxin. Moderate Study

- Encorafenib is predicted to decrease the exposure to **lapatinib**. Avoid. Severe Study → Also see TABLE 8 p. 1573
- Endothelin receptor antagonists **(bosentan)** are predicted to decrease the exposure to **lapatinib**. Avoid. Severe Study
- **Lapatinib** is predicted to increase the exposure to erlotinib. Moderate Theoretical
- **Lapatinib** is predicted to increase the exposure to everolimus. Moderate Theoretical
- **Lapatinib** is predicted to increase the exposure to factor XA inhibitors **(apixaban)**. Moderate Theoretical
- **Lapatinib** is predicted to slightly increase the exposure to factor XA inhibitors **(edoxaban)**. Severe Theoretical
- Fedratinib is predicted to increase the exposure to **lapatinib**. Moderate Study
- **Lapatinib** is predicted to increase the exposure to fidaxomicin. Avoid. Moderate Study
- **Lapatinib** is predicted to increase the exposure to gilteritinib. Moderate Theoretical
- Grapefruit juice is predicted to increase the exposure to **lapatinib**. Avoid. Moderate Theoretical
- H₂ receptor antagonists are predicted to decrease the absorption of **lapatinib**. Avoid. Moderate Theoretical
- HIV-protease inhibitors are predicted to increase the exposure to **lapatinib**. Avoid. Moderate Study
- Idelalisib is predicted to increase the exposure to **lapatinib**. Avoid. Moderate Study
- Imatinib is predicted to increase the exposure to **lapatinib**. Moderate Study
- **Lapatinib** increases the exposure to the active metabolite of irinotecan. Monitor adverse effects and adjust dose. Severe Study
- Ivosidenib is predicted to decrease the exposure to **lapatinib**. Avoid. Severe Study → Also see TABLE 8 p. 1573
- Letermovir is predicted to increase the exposure to **lapatinib**. Moderate Study
- **Lapatinib** is predicted to increase the exposure to lomitapide. Separate administration by 12 hours. Mild Theoretical
- **Lapatinib** is predicted to increase the exposure to loperamide. Moderate Theoretical
- Lorlatinib is predicted to decrease the exposure to **lapatinib**. Avoid. Severe Study
- Lumacaftor is predicted to decrease the exposure to **lapatinib**. Avoid. Severe Study
- Macrolides **(clarithromycin)** are predicted to increase the exposure to **lapatinib**. Avoid. Moderate Study
- Macrolides **(erythromycin)** are predicted to increase the exposure to **lapatinib**. Moderate Study → Also see TABLE 8 p. 1573
- **Lapatinib** is predicted to increase the exposure to mavacamten. Monitor and adjust dose—consult product literature. Moderate Theoretical
- Mitotane is predicted to decrease the exposure to **lapatinib**. Avoid. Severe Study
- **Lapatinib** increases the risk of neutropenia when given with monoclonal antibodies **(brentuximab vedotin)**. Monitor and adjust dose. Severe Theoretical
- Neurokinin-1 receptor antagonists **(aprepitant, netupitant)** are predicted to increase the exposure to **lapatinib**. Moderate Study
- Nilotinib is predicted to increase the exposure to **lapatinib**. Moderate Study → Also see TABLE 8 p. 1573
- **Lapatinib** is predicted to increase the exposure to nintedanib. Moderate Study
- NNRTIs **(efavirenz, etravirine, nevirapine)** are predicted to decrease the exposure to **lapatinib**. Avoid. Severe Study → Also see TABLE 8 p. 1573
- **Lapatinib** is predicted to increase the exposure to panobinostat. Adjust dose. Moderate Theoretical → Also see TABLE 8 p. 1573
- **Lapatinib** increases the exposure to pazopanib. Avoid. Severe Study → Also see TABLE 8 p. 1573
- **Lapatinib** is predicted to increase the risk of bleeding events when given with phenindione. Severe Theoretical
- **Lapatinib** is predicted to increase the exposure to pibrentasvir. Moderate Theoretical
- Pitolisant is predicted to decrease the exposure to **lapatinib**. Avoid. Severe Theoretical

Lapatinib (continued)
▸ **Lapatinib** is predicted to increase the exposure to pralsetinib. [Moderate] Theoretical
▸ **Lapatinib** is predicted to increase the exposure to ranolazine. [Moderate] Theoretical → Also see **TABLE 8** p. 1573
▸ **Lapatinib** is predicted to increase the exposure to relugolix. Avoid or take relugolix first and separate administration by at least 6 hours. [Moderate] Study
▸ Rifamycins (rifampicin) are predicted to decrease the exposure to **lapatinib**. Avoid. [Severe] Study
▸ **Lapatinib** is predicted to increase the exposure to rimegepant. Avoid another dose of rimegepant within 48 hours of concurrent use. [Moderate] Theoretical
▸ **Lapatinib** is predicted to increase the exposure to the active component of sacituzumab govitecan. [Severe] Theoretical
▸ **Lapatinib** is predicted to increase the exposure to sirolimus. [Moderate] Theoretical
▸ Oral sodium bicarbonate-containing antacids are predicted to decrease the absorption of oral **lapatinib**. Avoid. [Moderate] Theoretical
▸ Sotorasib is predicted to decrease the exposure to **lapatinib**. Avoid. [Severe] Study
▸ St John's wort is predicted to decrease the exposure to **lapatinib**. Avoid. [Severe] Study
▸ **Lapatinib** is predicted to slightly increase the exposure to talazoparib. Avoid or adjust dose—consult product literature. [Severe] Study
▸ **Lapatinib** slightly increases the exposure to taxanes (paclitaxel). [Severe] Study
▸ Tedizolid is predicted to increase the exposure to **lapatinib**. Avoid. [Moderate] Theoretical
▸ **Lapatinib** is predicted to increase the exposure to thrombin inhibitors (dabigatran). [Severe] Theoretical
▸ **Lapatinib** might increase the exposure to tigecycline. [Mild] Anecdotal
▸ **Lapatinib** is predicted to increase the exposure to topotecan. [Severe] Study
▸ **Lapatinib** is predicted to increase the concentration of trametinib. [Moderate] Theoretical
▸ Tucatinib is predicted to increase the exposure to **lapatinib**. Avoid. [Moderate] Study
▸ **Lapatinib** is predicted to increase the exposure to venetoclax. Avoid or monitor for toxicity. [Severe] Theoretical
▸ **Lapatinib** might increase the exposure to vinca alkaloids. [Severe] Theoretical

Laronidase
▸ Antimalarials (chloroquine) are predicted to decrease the exposure to **laronidase**. Avoid simultaneous administration. [Severe] Theoretical
▸ Hydroxychloroquine is predicted to decrease the exposure to **laronidase**. Avoid simultaneous administration. [Severe] Theoretical

Larotrectinib
▸ Anti-androgens (apalutamide, enzalutamide) are predicted to moderately decrease the exposure to **larotrectinib**. Avoid. [Moderate] Study
▸ Antiarrhythmics (dronedarone) are predicted to increase the exposure to **larotrectinib**. Monitor and adjust dose. [Moderate] Theoretical
▸ Antiepileptics (carbamazepine, fosphenytoin, phenobarbital, phenytoin, primidone) are predicted to moderately decrease the exposure to **larotrectinib**. Avoid. [Moderate] Study
▸ Antifungals, azoles (fluconazole, isavuconazole) are predicted to increase the exposure to **larotrectinib**. Monitor and adjust dose. [Moderate] Theoretical
▸ Antifungals, azoles (itraconazole, ketoconazole, posaconazole, voriconazole) are predicted to moderately increase the exposure to **larotrectinib**. Avoid or adjust dose—consult product literature. [Moderate] Study
▸ **Larotrectinib** slightly increases the exposure to benzodiazepines (midazolam). Use with caution and adjust dose. [Mild] Study
▸ Berotralstat is predicted to increase the exposure to **larotrectinib**. Monitor and adjust dose. [Moderate] Theoretical

▸ Calcium channel blockers (diltiazem, verapamil) are predicted to increase the exposure to **larotrectinib**. Monitor and adjust dose. [Moderate] Theoretical
▸ Cenobamate is predicted to decrease the exposure to **larotrectinib**. Avoid. [Moderate] Study
▸ Ceritinib is predicted to moderately increase the exposure to **larotrectinib**. Avoid or adjust dose—consult product literature. [Moderate] Study
▸ **Larotrectinib** is predicted to increase the exposure to ciclosporin. Use with caution and adjust dose. [Mild] Theoretical
▸ Cobicistat is predicted to moderately increase the exposure to **larotrectinib**. Avoid or adjust dose—consult product literature. [Moderate] Study
▸ **Larotrectinib** potentially decreases the efficacy of combined hormonal contraceptives. Use additional contraceptive precautions. [Severe] Theoretical
▸ Crizotinib is predicted to increase the exposure to **larotrectinib**. Monitor and adjust dose. [Moderate] Theoretical
▸ Dabrafenib is predicted to decrease the exposure to **larotrectinib**. Avoid. [Moderate] Study
▸ Encorafenib is predicted to moderately decrease the exposure to **larotrectinib**. Avoid. [Moderate] Study
▸ Endothelin receptor antagonists (bosentan) are predicted to decrease the exposure to **larotrectinib**. Avoid. [Moderate] Study
▸ **Larotrectinib** is predicted to increase the exposure to everolimus. Use with caution and adjust dose. [Mild] Theoretical
▸ Fedratinib is predicted to increase the exposure to **larotrectinib**. Monitor and adjust dose. [Moderate] Theoretical
▸ Grapefruit juice is predicted to increase the exposure to **larotrectinib**. Avoid. [Moderate] Theoretical
▸ HIV-protease inhibitors are predicted to moderately increase the exposure to **larotrectinib**. Avoid or adjust dose—consult product literature. [Moderate] Study
▸ Idelalisib is predicted to moderately increase the exposure to **larotrectinib**. Avoid or adjust dose—consult product literature. [Moderate] Study
▸ Imatinib is predicted to increase the exposure to **larotrectinib**. Monitor and adjust dose. [Moderate] Theoretical
▸ Ivosidenib is predicted to moderately decrease the exposure to **larotrectinib**. Avoid. [Moderate] Study
▸ Letermovir is predicted to increase the exposure to **larotrectinib**. Monitor and adjust dose. [Moderate] Theoretical
▸ Lorlatinib is predicted to decrease the exposure to **larotrectinib**. Avoid. [Moderate] Study
▸ Lumacaftor is predicted to moderately decrease the exposure to **larotrectinib**. Avoid. [Moderate] Study
▸ Macrolides (clarithromycin) are predicted to moderately increase the exposure to **larotrectinib**. Avoid or adjust dose—consult product literature. [Moderate] Study
▸ Macrolides (erythromycin) are predicted to increase the exposure to **larotrectinib**. Monitor and adjust dose. [Moderate] Theoretical
▸ **Larotrectinib** is predicted to increase the exposure to mavacamten. Monitor and adjust dose—consult product literature. [Moderate] Theoretical
▸ Mitotane is predicted to moderately decrease the exposure to **larotrectinib**. Avoid. [Moderate] Study
▸ Neurokinin-1 receptor antagonists (aprepitant, netupitant) are predicted to increase the exposure to **larotrectinib**. Monitor and adjust dose. [Moderate] Theoretical
▸ Nilotinib is predicted to increase the exposure to **larotrectinib**. Monitor and adjust dose. [Moderate] Theoretical
▸ NNRTIs (efavirenz, etravirine, nevirapine) are predicted to decrease the exposure to **larotrectinib**. Avoid. [Moderate] Study
▸ **Larotrectinib** is predicted to increase the exposure to opioids (alfentanil, fentanyl). Use with caution and adjust dose. [Mild] Theoretical
▸ **Larotrectinib** is predicted to increase the exposure to pimozide. Use with caution and adjust dose. [Mild] Theoretical
▸ Rifamycins (rifampicin) are predicted to moderately decrease the exposure to **larotrectinib**. Avoid. [Moderate] Study
▸ **Larotrectinib** is predicted to increase the exposure to sirolimus. Use with caution and adjust dose. [Mild] Theoretical
▸ Sotorasib is predicted to decrease the exposure to **larotrectinib**. Avoid. [Moderate] Study

- **St John's wort** is predicted to decrease the exposure to larotrectinib. Avoid. [Moderate] Study
- **Larotrectinib** is predicted to increase the exposure to tacrolimus. Use with caution and adjust dose. [Mild] Theoretical
- **Larotrectinib** is predicted to increase the exposure to temsirolimus. Use with caution and adjust dose. [Mild] Theoretical
- **Tucatinib** is predicted to moderately increase the exposure to larotrectinib. Avoid or adjust dose—consult product literature. [Moderate] Study

Lebrikizumab → see monoclonal antibodies

Lecanemab
- **Lecanemab** can increase the risk of brain haemorrhage when given with drugs with anticoagulant effects (see **TABLE 3** p. 1571). Avoid. [Severe] Anecdotal
- **Lecanemab** can increase the risk of bleeding when given with drugs with antiplatelet effects (see **TABLE 4** p. 1571). [Severe] Theoretical

Ledipasvir
- Oral antacids are predicted to decrease the exposure to oral ledipasvir. Separate administration by 4 hours. [Moderate] Theoretical
- **Ledipasvir** increases the risk of severe bradycardia or heart block when given with antiarrhythmics (amiodarone). Refer to specialist literature. [Severe] Anecdotal
- Antiepileptics (carbamazepine) are predicted to decrease the exposure to **ledipasvir**. Avoid. [Severe] Study
- Antiepileptics (fosphenytoin, oxcarbazepine, phenobarbital, phenytoin, primidone) are predicted to decrease the exposure to **ledipasvir**. Avoid. [Severe] Theoretical
- Oral calcium salts (calcium carbonate) -containing antacids are predicted to decrease the exposure to oral **ledipasvir**. Separate administration by 4 hours. [Moderate] Theoretical
- **Ledipasvir** is predicted to increase the exposure to digoxin. Monitor and adjust dose. [Moderate] Theoretical
- H$_2$ receptor antagonists are predicted to decrease the exposure to **ledipasvir**. Adjust dose, see ledipasvir with sofosbuvir p. 724. [Moderate] Study
- **Lorlatinib** is predicted to decrease the exposure to ledipasvir. Avoid. [Severe] Study
- **Proton pump inhibitors** are predicted to decrease the exposure to **ledipasvir**. Adjust dose, see ledipasvir with sofosbuvir p. 724. [Moderate] Theoretical
- Rifamycins (rifabutin) are predicted to decrease the exposure to ledipasvir. Avoid. [Severe] Theoretical
- Rifamycins (rifampicin) are predicted to decrease the exposure to **ledipasvir**. Avoid. [Severe] Study
- **Sodium zirconium cyclosilicate** is predicted to decrease the exposure to ledipasvir. Separate administration by at least 2 hours. [Moderate] Theoretical
- **St John's wort** is predicted to decrease the exposure to ledipasvir. Avoid. [Severe] Study
- **Ledipasvir** with sofosbuvir is predicted to increase the exposure to statins (atorvastatin). Monitor and adjust dose. [Moderate] Anecdotal
- **Ledipasvir** with sofosbuvir is predicted to increase the exposure to statins (fluvastatin, pravastatin, simvastatin). Monitor and adjust dose. [Moderate] Theoretical
- **Ledipasvir** with sofosbuvir is predicted to increase the exposure to statins (rosuvastatin). Avoid. [Severe] Theoretical
- **Ledipasvir** with sofosbuvir slightly increases the exposure to tenofovir disoproxil. [Moderate] Study
- **Ledipasvir** is predicted to increase the exposure to thrombin inhibitors (dabigatran). [Moderate] Theoretical

Leflunomide → see **TABLE 14** p. 1575 (myelosuppression), **TABLE 11** p. 1574 (peripheral neuropathy)

PHARMACOLOGY Leflunomide has a long half-life; washout procedure recommended before switching to other DMARDs (consult product literature).

- **Leflunomide** is predicted to increase the exposure to adefovir. [Moderate] Study
- **Leflunomide** is predicted to decrease the exposure to agomelatine. [Moderate] Theoretical
- **Leflunomide** is predicted to increase the exposure to alpelisib. [Moderate] Theoretical
- **Leflunomide** decreases the exposure to aminophylline. Adjust dose. [Moderate] Study
- **Leflunomide** is predicted to decrease the exposure to anaesthetics, local (ropivacaine). [Moderate] Theoretical
- **Leflunomide** is predicted to increase the exposure to anthracyclines (daunorubicin, doxorubicin, mitoxantrone). [Moderate] Theoretical → Also see **TABLE 14** p. 1575
- **Leflunomide** is predicted to increase the exposure to antihistamines, non-sedating (fexofenadine). [Moderate] Study
- **Leflunomide** is predicted to decrease the exposure to antipsychotics, second generation (clozapine). [Moderate] Theoretical
- **Leflunomide** is predicted to decrease the exposure to antipsychotics, second generation (olanzapine). Monitor and adjust dose. [Moderate] Study
- **Leflunomide** is predicted to increase the exposure to atogepant. Adjust **atogepant** dose, p. 540. [Moderate] Theoretical
- **Leflunomide** is predicted to increase the exposure to baricitinib. [Moderate] Study
- **Leflunomide** is predicted to moderately increase the clearance of caffeine citrate. Monitor and adjust dose. [Moderate] Study
- **Leflunomide** is predicted to increase the exposure to cephalosporins (cefaclor). [Moderate] Study
- **Leflunomide** is predicted to increase the exposure to cladribine. Avoid or adjust dose. [Moderate] Theoretical → Also see **TABLE 14** p. 1575
- **Leflunomide** increases the anticoagulant effect of coumarins. [Severe] Anecdotal
- **Leflunomide** is predicted to increase the exposure to endothelin receptor antagonists (bosentan). [Moderate] Study
- **Leflunomide** are predicted to increases the exposure to etrasimod. Avoid in poor CYP2C9 metabolisers. [Severe] Theoretical
- **Leflunomide** is predicted to increase the exposure to ganciclovir. [Moderate] Study → Also see **TABLE 14** p. 1575
- **Leflunomide** is predicted to increase the exposure to H$_2$ receptor antagonists (famotidine). [Moderate] Study
- **Leflunomide** is predicted to increase the concentration of letermovir. [Moderate] Study
- **Live vaccines** are predicted to increase the risk of generalised infection (possibly life-threatening) when given with **leflunomide**. UKHSA advises avoid (refer to Green Book). [Severe] Theoretical
- **Leflunomide** is predicted to increase the exposure to loop diuretics (furosemide). [Moderate] Study
- **Leflunomide** is predicted to increase the exposure to meglitinides (repaglinide). [Moderate] Study
- **Leflunomide** is predicted to decrease the exposure to melatonin. [Moderate] Theoretical
- **Leflunomide** is predicted to increase the exposure to methotrexate. Avoid. [Severe] Study → Also see **TABLE 14** p. 1575
- **Leflunomide** is predicted to increase the clearance of mexiletine. Monitor and adjust dose. [Moderate] Study
- **Leflunomide** is predicted to increase the exposure to momelotinib. [Moderate] Study
- **Leflunomide** is predicted to increase the exposure to montelukast. [Moderate] Theoretical
- **Leflunomide** is predicted to increase the exposure to NRTIs (zidovudine). [Moderate] Theoretical
- **Leflunomide** is predicted to increase the exposure to NSAIDs (indometacin, ketoprofen). [Moderate] Theoretical
- **Leflunomide** is predicted to increase the exposure to oseltamivir. [Moderate] Study
- **Leflunomide** is predicted to increase the exposure to penicillins (benzylpenicillin). [Moderate] Study
- **Leflunomide** is predicted to increase the exposure to pioglitazone. [Moderate] Study
- **Leflunomide** is predicted to decrease the exposure to pirfenidone. [Moderate] Theoretical
- **Leflunomide** is predicted to increase the exposure to quinolones (ciprofloxacin). [Moderate] Theoretical
- Rifamycins (rifampicin) might affect the exposure to leflunomide. [Moderate] Theoretical
- **Leflunomide** is predicted to increase the exposure to selexipag. Adjust **selexipag** dose, p. 209. [Moderate] Study

Leflunomide (continued)
▸ **Leflunomide** is predicted to decrease the exposure to SNRIs (duloxetine). Moderate Theoretical
▸ **Leflunomide** is predicted to increase the exposure to statins (atorvastatin, fluvastatin, pravastatin, simvastatin). Moderate Study
▸ **Leflunomide** is predicted to increase the exposure to statins (rosuvastatin). Adjust **rosuvastatin** dose, p. 235. Moderate Study
▸ **Leflunomide** is predicted to increase the exposure to sulfasalazine. Moderate Study → Also see **TABLE 14** p. 1575
▸ **Leflunomide** is predicted to increase the exposure to sulfonylureas (glibenclamide). Moderate Study
▸ **Leflunomide** is predicted to increase the exposure to talazoparib. Avoid or monitor. Moderate Theoretical → Also see **TABLE 14** p. 1575
▸ **Leflunomide** is predicted to increase the exposure to taxanes (docetaxel). Moderate Study → Also see **TABLE 14** p. 1575 → Also see **TABLE 11** p. 1574
▸ **Leflunomide** is predicted to increase the concentration of taxanes (paclitaxel). Severe Anecdotal → Also see **TABLE 14** p. 1575 → Also see **TABLE 11** p. 1574
▸ **Leflunomide** is predicted to increase the exposure to tenofovir alafenamide. Moderate Theoretical
▸ **Leflunomide** is predicted to increase the exposure to tenofovir disoproxil. Moderate Theoretical
▸ **Leflunomide** is predicted to decrease the exposure to theophylline. Adjust dose. Moderate Study
▸ **Leflunomide** moderately decreases the exposure to tizanidine. Mild Study
▸ **Leflunomide** is predicted to increase the exposure to topotecan. Moderate Study → Also see **TABLE 14** p. 1575
▸ **Leflunomide** is predicted to increase the exposure to tucatinib. Moderate Theoretical
▸ **Leflunomide** is predicted to increase the exposure to vadadustat. Moderate Study
▸ **Leflunomide** is predicted to increase the exposure to venetoclax. Avoid or monitor for toxicity. Severe Theoretical

Lenalidomide → see **TABLE 1** p. 1571 (hepatotoxicity), **TABLE 14** p. 1575 (myelosuppression), **TABLE 11** p. 1574 (peripheral neuropathy)
▸ **Combined hormonal contraceptives** are predicted to increase the risk of venous thromboembolism when given with **lenalidomide**. Avoid. Severe Theoretical
▸ **Hormone replacement therapy** is predicted to increase the risk of venous thromboembolism when given with **lenalidomide**. Moderate Theoretical

Leniolisib
▸ **Anti-androgens (apalutamide, enzalutamide)** are predicted to decrease the exposure to **leniolisib**. Avoid. Severe Theoretical
▸ **Antiarrhythmics (dronedarone)** are predicted to increase the exposure to **leniolisib**. Avoid. Moderate Study
▸ **Antiepileptics (carbamazepine, fosphenytoin, phenobarbital, phenytoin, primidone)** are predicted to decrease the exposure to **leniolisib**. Avoid. Severe Theoretical
▸ **Antifungals, azoles (fluconazole, isavuconazole, itraconazole, ketoconazole, posaconazole, voriconazole)** are predicted to increase the exposure to **leniolisib**. Avoid. Moderate Study
▸ **Leniolisib** is predicted to increase the exposure to antihistamines, non-sedating (fexofenadine). Avoid. Moderate Theoretical
▸ **Leniolisib** is predicted to increase the exposure to antipsychotics, second generation (clozapine). Avoid. Moderate Theoretical
▸ **Berotralstat** is predicted to increase the exposure to **leniolisib**. Avoid. Moderate Study
▸ **Calcium channel blockers (diltiazem, verapamil)** are predicted to increase the exposure to **leniolisib**. Avoid. Moderate Study
▸ **Cenobamate** is predicted to decrease the exposure to **leniolisib**. Avoid. Severe Theoretical
▸ **Ceritinib** is predicted to increase the exposure to **leniolisib**. Avoid. Moderate Study
▸ **Cobicistat** is predicted to increase the exposure to **leniolisib**. Avoid. Moderate Study
▸ **Crizotinib** is predicted to increase the exposure to **leniolisib**. Avoid. Moderate Study

▸ **Dabrafenib** is predicted to decrease the exposure to **leniolisib**. Avoid. Severe Theoretical
▸ **Encorafenib** is predicted to decrease the exposure to **leniolisib**. Avoid. Severe Theoretical
▸ **Endothelin receptor antagonists (bosentan)** are predicted to decrease the exposure to **leniolisib**. Avoid. Severe Theoretical
▸ **Leniolisib** is predicted to increase the exposure to endothelin receptor antagonists (bosentan). Avoid. Moderate Theoretical
▸ **Fedratinib** is predicted to increase the exposure to **leniolisib**. Avoid. Moderate Study
▸ **Grapefruit** juice is predicted to increase the exposure to **leniolisib**. Avoid. Moderate Theoretical
▸ **HIV-protease inhibitors** are predicted to increase the exposure to **leniolisib**. Avoid. Moderate Study
▸ **Idelalisib** is predicted to increase the exposure to **leniolisib**. Avoid. Moderate Study
▸ **Imatinib** is predicted to increase the exposure to **leniolisib**. Avoid. Moderate Study
▸ **Ivosidenib** is predicted to decrease the exposure to **leniolisib**. Avoid. Severe Theoretical
▸ **Letermovir** is predicted to increase the exposure to **leniolisib**. Avoid. Moderate Study
▸ **Lorlatinib** is predicted to decrease the exposure to **leniolisib**. Avoid. Severe Theoretical
▸ **Lumacaftor** is predicted to decrease the exposure to **leniolisib**. Avoid. Severe Theoretical
▸ **Macrolides (clarithromycin, erythromycin)** are predicted to increase the exposure to **leniolisib**. Avoid. Moderate Study
▸ **Leniolisib** is predicted to increase the exposure to meglitinides (repaglinide). Avoid. Moderate Theoretical
▸ **Leniolisib** is predicted to increase the exposure to melatonin. Avoid. Moderate Theoretical
▸ **Mitotane** is predicted to decrease the exposure to **leniolisib**. Avoid. Severe Theoretical
▸ **Modafinil** is predicted to decrease the exposure to **leniolisib**. Avoid. Severe Theoretical
▸ **Neurokinin-1 receptor antagonists (aprepitant, netupitant)** are predicted to increase the exposure to **leniolisib**. Avoid. Moderate Study
▸ **Nilotinib** is predicted to increase the exposure to **leniolisib**. Avoid. Moderate Study
▸ **NNRTIs (efavirenz, etravirine, nevirapine)** are predicted to decrease the exposure to **leniolisib**. Avoid. Severe Theoretical
▸ **Rifamycins (rifampicin)** are predicted to decrease the exposure to **leniolisib**. Avoid. Severe Theoretical
▸ **Leniolisib** is predicted to increase the exposure to SNRIs (duloxetine). Avoid. Moderate Theoretical
▸ **Sotorasib** is predicted to decrease the exposure to **leniolisib**. Avoid. Severe Theoretical
▸ **St John's wort** is predicted to decrease the exposure to **leniolisib**. Avoid. Severe Theoretical
▸ **Leniolisib** is predicted to increase the exposure to statins. Avoid. Moderate Theoretical
▸ **Leniolisib** is predicted to increase the exposure to sulfasalazine. Avoid. Moderate Theoretical
▸ **Leniolisib** is predicted to increase the exposure to sulfonylureas (glibenclamide). Avoid. Moderate Theoretical
▸ **Leniolisib** is predicted to increase the exposure to taxanes (docetaxel, paclitaxel). Avoid. Moderate Theoretical
▸ **Leniolisib** is predicted to increase the exposure to theophylline. Avoid. Moderate Theoretical
▸ **Leniolisib** is predicted to increase the exposure to tizanidine. Avoid. Moderate Theoretical
▸ **Leniolisib** is predicted to increase the exposure to topotecan. Avoid. Moderate Theoretical
▸ **Tucatinib** is predicted to increase the exposure to **leniolisib**. Avoid. Moderate Study

Lenograstim
▸ **Lenograstim** might increase the risk of pulmonary toxicity when given with bleomycin. Severe Theoretical

Lenvatinib → see **TABLE 8** p. 1573 (QT-interval prolongation), **TABLE 4** p. 1571 (antiplatelet effects)

Lercanidipine → see calcium channel blockers

Letermovir
- **Letermovir** is predicted to increase the exposure to abemaciclib. Moderate Study
- **Letermovir** is predicted to increase the exposure to acalabrutinib. Avoid or monitor. Severe Study
- **Letermovir** is predicted to increase the exposure to alpha blockers **(tamsulosin)**. Moderate Theoretical
- **Letermovir** is predicted to increase the concentration of antiarrhythmics **(amiodarone)**. Moderate Theoretical
- **Letermovir** is predicted to increase the exposure to antiarrhythmics **(propafenone)**. Monitor and adjust dose. Moderate Study
- Antiepileptics **(carbamazepine, phenobarbital, primidone)** are predicted to decrease the concentration of **letermovir**. Moderate Theoretical
- **Letermovir** is predicted to decrease the concentration of antiepileptics **(fosphenytoin, phenytoin)** and antiepileptics **(fosphenytoin, phenytoin)** are predicted to decrease the concentration of **letermovir**. Moderate Theoretical
- **Letermovir** is predicted to increase the exposure to antifungals, azoles **(isavuconazole)**. Moderate Theoretical
- **Letermovir** slightly decreases the exposure to antifungals, azoles **(voriconazole)**. Moderate Study
- **Letermovir** is predicted to increase the concentration of antihistamines, non-sedating **(fexofenadine)**. Moderate Theoretical
- **Letermovir** is predicted to increase the exposure to antihistamines, non-sedating **(mizolastine)**. Severe Theoretical
- **Letermovir** is predicted to increase the exposure to antihistamines, non-sedating **(rupatadine)**. Avoid. Moderate Study
- **Letermovir** is predicted to increase the exposure to antipsychotics, second generation **(cariprazine)**. Avoid. Severe Study
- **Letermovir** is predicted to increase the exposure to antipsychotics, second generation **(quetiapine)**. Avoid. Moderate Study
- **Letermovir** is predicted to increase the exposure to avapritinib. Avoid or adjust dose—consult product literature. Moderate Study
- **Letermovir** is predicted to increase the exposure to axitinib. Moderate Study
- **Letermovir** might increases the exposure to bedaquiline. Mild Theoretical
- **Letermovir** is predicted to increase the exposure to benzodiazepines **(alprazolam)**. Severe Study
- **Letermovir** is predicted to increase the exposure to benzodiazepines **(midazolam)**. Monitor adverse effects and adjust dose. Severe Study
- **Letermovir** is predicted to increase the exposure to bosutinib. Avoid or adjust dose. Severe Study
- **Letermovir** is predicted to increase the exposure to brigatinib. Moderate Study
- **Letermovir** is predicted to increase the exposure to buspirone. Use with caution and adjust dose. Moderate Study
- **Letermovir** is predicted to increase the exposure to cabozantinib. Moderate Study
- **Letermovir** is predicted to increase the exposure to calcium channel blockers **(amlodipine, felodipine, lacidipine, lercanidipine, nicardipine, nifedipine, nimodipine)**. Monitor and adjust dose. Moderate Study
- **Letermovir** is predicted to increase the exposure to capivasertib. Adjust dose. Moderate Study
- **Letermovir** is predicted to increase the exposure to ceritinib. Moderate Study
- **Letermovir** increases the exposure to ciclosporin and ciclosporin increases the exposure to **letermovir**. Monitor and adjust **letermovir** dose, p. 735. Severe Study
- **Letermovir** is predicted to increase the exposure to cobimetinib. Severe Study
- **Letermovir** is predicted to increase the exposure to colchicine. Adjust **colchicine** dose with moderate CYP3A4 inhibitors, p. 1279. Severe Study
- **Letermovir** is predicted to increase the exposure to corticosteroids **(methylprednisolone)**. Monitor and adjust dose. Moderate Study
- **Letermovir** is predicted to decrease the concentration of coumarins **(warfarin)**. Monitor and adjust dose. Moderate Theoretical
- **Letermovir** is predicted to increase the exposure to crizotinib. Moderate Study
- **Letermovir** is predicted to increase the exposure to dabrafenib. Moderate Study
- **Letermovir** is predicted to increase the exposure to daridorexant. Adjust **daridorexant** dose, p. 554. Severe Study
- **Letermovir** is predicted to increase the exposure to darifenacin. Moderate Study
- **Letermovir** is predicted to increase the exposure to dasatinib. Severe Study
- **Letermovir** is predicted to slightly increase the exposure to dienogest. Moderate Study
- **Letermovir** is predicted to increase the exposure to dipeptidylpeptidase-4 inhibitors **(saxagliptin)**. Mild Study
- **Letermovir** is predicted to increase the exposure to domperidone. Avoid. Severe Study
- **Letermovir** is predicted to increase the exposure to dopamine receptor agonists **(bromocriptine)**. Severe Theoretical
- **Letermovir** is predicted to increase the exposure to drospirenone. Severe Study
- **Letermovir** is predicted to moderately increase the exposure to dutasteride. Mild Study
- **Letermovir** is predicted to increase the exposure to elacestrant. Avoid moderate CYP3A4 inhibitors or adjust **elacestrant** dose, p. 1084. Severe Theoretical
- **Letermovir** is predicted to increase the exposure to elexacaftor. Adjust ivacaftor with tezacaftor and elexacaftor p. 337 dose with moderate CYP3A4 inhibitors. Severe Theoretical
- **Letermovir** is predicted to increase the exposure to eliglustat. Avoid or adjust dose—consult product literature. Severe Study
- Eltrombopag is predicted to increase the concentration of **letermovir**. Moderate Study
- **Letermovir** is predicted to moderately increase the exposure to encorafenib. Moderate Study
- **Letermovir** is predicted to increase the concentration of endothelin receptor antagonists **(bosentan)**. Moderate Theoretical
- **Letermovir** is predicted to increase the exposure to endothelin receptor antagonists **(macitentan)**. Manufacturer advises caution depending on other drugs taken—consult product literature. Moderate Theoretical
- **Letermovir** is predicted to increase the exposure to entrectinib. Avoid or adjust dose with moderate CYP3A4 inhibitors— consult product literature. Severe Theoretical
- **Letermovir** is predicted to increase the risk of ergotism when given with ergometrine. Severe Theoretical
- **Letermovir** is predicted to increase the exposure to erlotinib. Moderate Study
- **Letermovir** is predicted to increase the exposure to etrasimod. Avoid in poor CYP2C9 metabolisers. Severe Theoretical
- **Letermovir** is predicted to increase the concentration of everolimus. Avoid or adjust dose. Moderate Study
- **Letermovir** is predicted to increase the exposure to fedratinib. Monitor and adjust dose. Moderate Study
- **Letermovir** is predicted to increase the exposure to fesoterodine. Adjust **fesoterodine** dose with moderate CYP3A4 inhibitors in hepatic and renal impairment, p. 897. Mild Study
- Fibrates **(gemfibrozil)** are predicted to increase the concentration of **letermovir**. Moderate Study
- **Letermovir** is predicted to increase the exposure to gefitinib. Moderate Study
- **Letermovir** is predicted to increase the concentration of guanfacine. Adjust **guanfacine** dose, p. 407. Moderate Theoretical
- HIV-protease inhibitors **(atazanavir, lopinavir)** boosted with ritonavir are predicted to increase the concentration of **letermovir**. Moderate Study
- HIV-protease inhibitors **(ritonavir)** are predicted to decrease the concentration of **letermovir**. Moderate Theoretical
- **Letermovir** is predicted to increase the exposure to ibrutinib. Adjust dose with moderate CYP3A4 inhibitors—consult product literature. Severe Study
- **Letermovir** is predicted to increase the exposure to imatinib. Moderate Study

Letermovir (continued)

▸ **Letermovir** is predicted to increase the exposure to ivacaftor. Adjust dose with moderate CYP3A4 inhibitors, see ivacaftor p. 336, tezacaftor with ivacaftor p. 339, and ivacaftor with tezacaftor and elexacaftor p. 337. Moderate Study

▸ **Letermovir** is predicted to increase the exposure to ivosidenib. Monitor and adjust dose—consult product literature. Severe Study

▸ **Letermovir** is predicted to increase the exposure to lapatinib. Moderate Study

▸ **Letermovir** is predicted to increase the exposure to larotrectinib. Monitor and adjust dose. Moderate Theoretical

▸ **Leflunomide** is predicted to increase the concentration of **letermovir**. Moderate Study

▸ **Letermovir** is predicted to increase the exposure to leniolisib. Avoid. Moderate Study

▸ **Letermovir** is predicted to increase the exposure to lomitapide. Avoid. Moderate Theoretical

▸ **Macrolides (clarithromycin, erythromycin)** are predicted to increase the concentration of **letermovir**. Moderate Study

▸ **Letermovir** is predicted to increase the exposure to mavacamten. Adjust dose—consult product literature. Moderate Study

▸ **Letermovir** is predicted to increase the concentration of meglitinides **(repaglinide)**. Avoid. Moderate Theoretical

▸ **Letermovir** is predicted to increase the exposure to midostaurin. Moderate Theoretical

▸ **Letermovir** is predicted to increase the exposure to mineralocorticoid receptor antagonists **(eplerenone)**. Adjust **eplerenone** dose, p. 223. Severe Study

▸ **Letermovir** is predicted to increase the exposure to mineralocorticoid receptor antagonists **(finerenone)**. Severe Study

▸ **Letermovir** is predicted to increase the exposure to mobocertinib. Avoid or adjust dose and monitor ECG—consult product literature. Severe Study

▸ **Modafinil** is predicted to decrease the concentration of **letermovir**. Moderate Theoretical

▸ **Letermovir** is predicted to increase the exposure to naldemedine. Moderate Study

▸ **Letermovir** is predicted to increase the exposure to naloxegol. Adjust **naloxegol** dose and monitor adverse effects, p. 72. Moderate Study

▸ **Letermovir** is predicted to increase the exposure to neratinib. Avoid moderate CYP3A4 inhibitors or adjust dose and monitor for gastrointestinal adverse effects—consult product literature. Severe Study

▸ **Letermovir** is predicted to increase the exposure to nilotinib. Moderate Study

▸ **NNRTIs (efavirenz)** are predicted to decrease the concentration of **letermovir**. Moderate Theoretical

▸ **NNRTIs (etravirine)** are predicted to decrease the exposure to **letermovir**. Moderate Theoretical

▸ **Letermovir** is predicted to increase the exposure to olaparib. Avoid or adjust dose with moderate CYP3A4 inhibitors—consult product literature. Moderate Theoretical

▸ **Letermovir** is predicted to increase the exposure to opioids **(alfentanil, buprenorphine, fentanyl, oxycodone)**. Monitor and adjust dose. Moderate Study

▸ **Letermovir** is predicted to increase the exposure to opioids **(methadone, sufentanil)**. Moderate Theoretical

▸ **Letermovir** is predicted to increase the exposure to pazopanib. Moderate Study

▸ **Letermovir** is predicted to increase the exposure to pemigatinib. Severe Study

▸ **Letermovir** is predicted to increase the exposure to phosphodiesterase type-5 inhibitors **(avanafil)**. Adjust **avanafil** dose, p. 939. Moderate Theoretical

▸ **Letermovir** is predicted to increase the exposure to phosphodiesterase type-5 inhibitors **(sildenafil)**. Monitor or adjust **sildenafil** dose with moderate CYP3A4 inhibitors, p. 940. Moderate Study

▸ **Letermovir** is predicted to increase the exposure to phosphodiesterase type-5 inhibitors **(tadalafil)**. Severe Theoretical

▸ **Letermovir** is predicted to increase the exposure to phosphodiesterase type-5 inhibitors **(vardenafil)**. Adjust dose. Severe Theoretical

▸ **Letermovir** is predicted to increase the exposure to pimozide. Avoid. Severe Theoretical

▸ **Letermovir** is predicted to increase the exposure to ponatinib. Moderate Study

▸ **Letermovir** is predicted to increase the exposure to pralsetinib. Moderate Theoretical

▸ **Letermovir** is predicted to increase the exposure to ranolazine. Severe Study

▸ **Letermovir** is predicted to increase the exposure to regorafenib. Moderate Study

▸ **Letermovir** is predicted to increase the exposure to ribociclib. Moderate Study

▸ **Rifamycins (rifabutin)** are predicted to decrease the concentration of **letermovir**. Moderate Theoretical

▸ **Rifamycins (rifampicin)** are predicted to affect the concentration of **letermovir**. Severe Theoretical

▸ **Letermovir** is predicted to increase the exposure to rimegepant. Avoid another dose of rimegepant within 48 hours of concurrent use. Moderate Study

▸ **Letermovir** is predicted to increase the exposure to ruxolitinib. Moderate Study

▸ **Letermovir** is predicted to increase the exposure to selpercatinib. Moderate Study

▸ **Letermovir** is predicted to increase the exposure to selumetinib. Avoid or adjust dose—consult product literature. Severe Study

▸ **Letermovir** is predicted to increase the exposure to siponimod. Avoid depending on other drugs taken—consult product literature. Severe Study

▸ **Letermovir** increases the concentration of sirolimus. Monitor and adjust dose. Moderate Study

▸ **Letermovir** is predicted to increase the exposure to SSRIs **(dapoxetine)**. Adjust **dapoxetine** dose with moderate CYP3A4 inhibitors, p. 947. Moderate Theoretical

▸ **St John's wort** is predicted to decrease the concentration of **letermovir**. Moderate Theoretical

▸ **Letermovir** moderately increases the exposure to statins **(atorvastatin)**. Avoid or adjust **atorvastatin** dose, p. 234. Severe Study

▸ **Letermovir** is predicted to increase the exposure to statins **(fluvastatin)**. Monitor and adjust dose. Moderate Theoretical

▸ **Letermovir** is predicted to increase the exposure to statins **(pravastatin)**. Avoid or adjust dose. Moderate Theoretical

▸ **Letermovir** is predicted to increase the exposure to statins **(rosuvastatin, simvastatin)**. Avoid. Severe Study

▸ **Letermovir** is predicted to increase the concentration of sulfonylureas **(glibenclamide)**. Moderate Theoretical

▸ **Letermovir** is predicted to increase the exposure to sunitinib. Moderate Study

▸ **Letermovir** is predicted to increase the concentration of tacrolimus. Severe Study

▸ **Letermovir** is predicted to increase the exposure to taxanes **(cabazitaxel)**. Moderate Theoretical

▸ **Letermovir** is predicted to increase the exposure to taxanes **(docetaxel)**. Severe Study

▸ **Letermovir** is predicted to increase the exposure to taxanes **(paclitaxel)**. Moderate Anecdotal

▸ **Teriflunomide** is predicted to increase the concentration of **letermovir**. Moderate Study

▸ **Letermovir** is predicted to increase the exposure to tezacaftor. Adjust dose with moderate CYP3A4 inhibitors, see tezacaftor with ivacaftor p. 339 and ivacaftor with tezacaftor and elexacaftor p. 337. Severe Study

▸ **Letermovir** is predicted to decrease the concentration of thrombin inhibitors **(dabigatran)**. Avoid. Severe Theoretical

▸ **Letermovir** given with a potent CYP2C19 inhibitor is predicted to increase the exposure to tofacitinib. Adjust **tofacitinib** dose, p. 1265. Moderate Study

▸ **Letermovir** is predicted to increase the exposure to tolvaptan. Manufacturer advises caution or adjust **tolvaptan** dose with moderate CYP3A4 inhibitors, p. 767. Moderate Study

- **Letermovir** is predicted to increase the exposure to trazodone. Moderate Theoretical
- **Letermovir** is predicted to increase the exposure to ulipristal. Avoid if used for uterine fibroids. Moderate Study
- **Letermovir** is predicted to increase the exposure to vemurafenib. Severe Theoretical
- **Letermovir** is predicted to increase the exposure to venetoclax. Avoid or adjust dose—consult product literature. Severe Study
- **Letermovir** is predicted to increase the exposure to vinca alkaloids. Severe Theoretical
- **Letermovir** is predicted to increase the exposure to voclosporin. Adjust **voclosporin** dose, p. 973. Severe Study
- **Letermovir** is predicted to increase the exposure to zanubrutinib. Avoid or adjust dose with moderate CYP3A4 inhibitors—consult product literature. Severe Study
- **Letermovir** is predicted to increase the exposure to zopiclone. Adjust dose. Moderate Study

Levamisole
- Albendazole slightly decreases the exposure to **levamisole** and **levamisole** moderately decreases the exposure to albendazole. Moderate Study
- Alcohol potentially causes a disulfiram-like reaction when given with **levamisole**. Moderate Study
- **Levamisole** increases the exposure to ivermectin. Moderate Study

Levetiracetam → see antiepileptics
Levobunolol → see beta blockers, non-selective
Levobupivacaine → see anaesthetics, local
Levocetirizine → see antihistamines, non-sedating
Levodopa → see TABLE 7 p. 1572 (hypotension), TABLE 10 p. 1574 (CNS effects)
- Antiepileptics (fosphenytoin, phenytoin) decrease the effects of **levodopa**. Moderate Study → Also see TABLE 10 p. 1574
- Antipsychotics, second generation (amisulpride) are predicted to decrease the effects of **levodopa**. Avoid. Severe Theoretical → Also see TABLE 10 p. 1574
- Antipsychotics, second generation (aripiprazole, clozapine, lurasidone, paliperidone) are predicted to decrease the effects of **levodopa**. Severe Theoretical → Also see TABLE 7 p. 1572 → Also see TABLE 10 p. 1574
- Antipsychotics, second generation (asenapine) are predicted to decrease the effects of **levodopa**. Adjust dose. Severe Theoretical → Also see TABLE 7 p. 1572 → Also see TABLE 10 p. 1574
- Antipsychotics, second generation (olanzapine) decrease the effects of **levodopa**. Avoid or monitor worsening parkinsonian symptoms. Severe Anecdotal → Also see TABLE 7 p. 1572 → Also see TABLE 10 p. 1574
- Antipsychotics, second generation (quetiapine) decrease the effects of **levodopa**. Severe Anecdotal → Also see TABLE 7 p. 1572 → Also see TABLE 10 p. 1574
- Antipsychotics, second generation (risperidone) are predicted to decrease the effects of **levodopa**. Avoid or adjust dose. Severe Anecdotal → Also see TABLE 7 p. 1572 → Also see TABLE 10 p. 1574
- Baclofen is predicted to increase the risk of adverse effects when given with **levodopa**. Severe Anecdotal → Also see TABLE 7 p. 1572 → Also see TABLE 10 p. 1574
- Benperidol is predicted to decrease the effects of **levodopa**. Severe Study → Also see TABLE 7 p. 1572 → Also see TABLE 10 p. 1574
- Bupropion increases the risk of adverse effects when given with **levodopa**. Moderate Study
- Droperidol decreases the effects of **levodopa**. Severe Study → Also see TABLE 7 p. 1572 → Also see TABLE 10 p. 1574
- Drugs with antimuscarinic effects (see TABLE 9 p. 1573) might decrease the absorption of **levodopa**. Moderate Theoretical
- Entacapone increases the exposure to **levodopa**. Monitor adverse effects and adjust dose. Moderate Study
- Flupentixol decreases the effects of **levodopa**. Avoid or monitor worsening parkinsonian symptoms. Severe Theoretical → Also see TABLE 7 p. 1572 → Also see TABLE 10 p. 1574
- Haloperidol decreases the effects of **levodopa**. Severe Study → Also see TABLE 7 p. 1572 → Also see TABLE 10 p. 1574
- Oral iron decreases the absorption of oral **levodopa**. Moderate Study
- Isoniazid decreases the effects of **levodopa**. Moderate Study

- **Levodopa** is predicted to increase the risk of elevated blood pressure when given with linezolid. Avoid. Severe Theoretical
- Loxapine is predicted to decrease the effects of **levodopa**. Severe Theoretical → Also see TABLE 7 p. 1572 → Also see TABLE 10 p. 1574
- MAO-B inhibitors are predicted to increase the effects of **levodopa**. Adjust dose. Mild Study → Also see TABLE 7 p. 1572
- **Levodopa** increases the risk of a hypertensive crisis when given with MAOIs, irreversible. Avoid and for 14 days after stopping the MAOI. Severe Study → Also see TABLE 7 p. 1572
- Memantine is predicted to increase the effects of **levodopa**. Moderate Theoretical
- Metoclopramide decreases the effects of **levodopa**. Avoid. Moderate Study
- **Levodopa** increases the risk of adverse effects when given with moclobemide. Moderate Study
- Opicapone increases the exposure to **levodopa**. Adjust dose. Moderate Study
- Phenothiazines decrease the effects of **levodopa**. Avoid or monitor worsening parkinsonian symptoms. Severe Study → Also see TABLE 7 p. 1572 → Also see TABLE 10 p. 1574
- Pimozide decreases the effects of **levodopa**. Severe Theoretical → Also see TABLE 7 p. 1572 → Also see TABLE 10 p. 1574
- Sulpiride is predicted to decrease the effects of **levodopa**. Avoid. Severe Theoretical → Also see TABLE 7 p. 1572 → Also see TABLE 10 p. 1574
- Tetrabenazine is predicted to decrease the effects of **levodopa**. Use with caution or avoid. Moderate Theoretical → Also see TABLE 10 p. 1574
- Tolcapone increases the exposure to **levodopa**. Monitor and adjust dose. Moderate Study
- Tryptophan greatly decreases the concentration of **levodopa**. Moderate Study
- Zuclopenthixol is predicted to decrease the effects of **levodopa**. Avoid or monitor worsening parkinsonian symptoms. Severe Theoretical → Also see TABLE 7 p. 1572 → Also see TABLE 10 p. 1574

Levofloxacin → see quinolones
Levofolinic acid → see folates
Levomepromazine → see phenothiazines
Levonorgestrel
- Antiepileptics (carbamazepine, eslicarbazepine, fosphenytoin, oxcarbazepine, perampanel, phenobarbital, phenytoin, primidone, rufinamide, topiramate) are predicted to decrease the efficacy of some contraceptive methods containing **levonorgestrel**. For FSRH guidance, see Contraceptives, interactions p. 917. Severe Theoretical
- Antiepileptics (lamotrigine) might decrease the effects of **levonorgestrel**. For FSRH guidance, see Contraceptives, interactions p. 917. Moderate Theoretical
- Endothelin receptor antagonists (bosentan) are predicted to decrease the efficacy of some contraceptive methods containing **levonorgestrel**. For FSRH guidance, see Contraceptives, interactions p. 917. Severe Theoretical
- Glucagon-like peptide-1 receptor agonists (tirzepatide) might affect the absorption of oral **levonorgestrel**. Manufacturer advises precautions for those who are overweight or obese— see Conception and contraception p. 822. Moderate Study
- HIV-protease inhibitors (ritonavir) are predicted to decrease the efficacy of some contraceptive methods containing **levonorgestrel**. For FSRH guidance, see Contraceptives, interactions p. 917. Severe Theoretical
- Lumacaftor is predicted to decrease the efficacy of **levonorgestrel**. Use additional contraceptive precautions. Severe Theoretical
- Modafinil is predicted to decrease the efficacy of some contraceptive methods containing **levonorgestrel**. For FSRH guidance, see Contraceptives, interactions p. 917. Severe Theoretical
- Neurokinin-1 receptor antagonists (aprepitant, fosaprepitant) are predicted to decrease the efficacy of some contraceptive methods containing **levonorgestrel**. For FSRH guidance, see Contraceptives, interactions p. 917. Severe Theoretical
- NNRTIs (efavirenz, nevirapine) are predicted to decrease the efficacy of some contraceptive methods containing

Levonorgestrel (continued)
levonorgestrel. For FSRH guidance, see Contraceptives, interactions p. 917. Severe Theoretical

▶ NNRTIs (etravirine) might decrease the efficacy of some contraceptive methods containing **levonorgestrel**. Follow FSRH guidance for enzyme inducers, see Contraceptives, interactions p. 917. Severe Theoretical

▶ Rifamycins are predicted to decrease the efficacy of some contraceptive methods containing **levonorgestrel**. For FSRH guidance, see Contraceptives, interactions p. 917. Severe Theoretical

▶ St John's wort is predicted to decrease the efficacy of **levonorgestrel**. MHRA advises avoid. For FSRH guidance, see Contraceptives, interactions p. 917. Severe Theoretical

▶ Sugammadex is predicted to decrease the exposure to **levonorgestrel**. Use additional contraceptive precautions. Severe Theoretical

▶ **Levonorgestrel** might decrease the efficacy of ulipristal and ulipristal might decrease the efficacy of **levonorgestrel**. Avoid. Severe Theoretical

Levothyroxine → see thyroid hormones
Lidocaine → see antiarrhythmics
Linagliptin → see dipeptidylpeptidase-4 inhibitors
Linezolid → see TABLE 12 p. 1574 (serotonin syndrome)

FOOD AND LIFESTYLE Patients taking linezolid should avoid consuming large amounts of tyramine-rich foods (such as mature cheese, salami, pickled herring, *Bovril*®, *Oxo*®, *Marmite*® or any similar meat or yeast extract or fermented soya bean extract, and some beers, lagers or wines).

▶ Beta₂ agonists are predicted to increase the risk of elevated blood pressure when given with **linezolid**. Avoid. Severe Theoretical

▶ Bupropion is predicted to increase the risk of intraoperative hypertension when given with **linezolid**. Severe Anecdotal

▶ Buspirone is predicted to increase the risk of elevated blood pressure when given with **linezolid**. Avoid. Severe Theoretical

▶ Levodopa is predicted to increase the risk of elevated blood pressure when given with **linezolid**. Avoid. Severe Theoretical

▶ Macrolides (clarithromycin) increase the exposure to **linezolid**. Moderate Anecdotal

▶ MAO-B inhibitors (rasagiline, selegiline) are predicted to increase the risk of adverse effects when given with **linezolid**. Avoid and for 14 days after stopping the MAOI. Severe Theoretical → Also see TABLE 12 p. 1574

▶ MAO-B inhibitors (safinamide) are predicted to increase the risk of adverse effects when given with **linezolid**. Avoid and for 1 week after stopping **safinamide**. Severe Theoretical → Also see TABLE 12 p. 1574

▶ MAOIs, irreversible are predicted to increase the risk of adverse effects when given with **linezolid**. Avoid and for 14 days after stopping the MAOI. Severe Theoretical → Also see TABLE 12 p. 1574

▶ Methylphenidate might increase the risk of elevated blood pressure when given with **linezolid**. Avoid. Severe Theoretical

▶ Moclobemide is predicted to increase the risk of adverse effects when given with **linezolid**. Avoid and for 14 days after stopping **moclobemide**. Severe Theoretical → Also see TABLE 12 p. 1574

▶ Ozanimod might increase the risk of a hypertensive crisis when given with **linezolid**. Avoid. Severe Theoretical

▶ Reboxetine is predicted to increase the risk of a hypertensive crisis when given with **linezolid**. Avoid. Severe Theoretical

▶ Rifamycins (rifampicin) slightly decrease the exposure to **linezolid**. Moderate Study

▶ Sympathomimetics, inotropic are predicted to increase the risk of elevated blood pressure when given with **linezolid**. Avoid. Severe Theoretical

▶ Sympathomimetics, vasoconstrictor (adrenaline/epinephrine, ephedrine, isometheptene, noradrenaline/norepinephrine, phenylephrine) are predicted to increase the risk of elevated blood pressure when given with **linezolid**. Avoid. Severe Theoretical

▶ Sympathomimetics, vasoconstrictor (pseudoephedrine) increase the risk of elevated blood pressure when given with **linezolid**. Avoid. Severe Study

Linzagolix

▶ **Linzagolix** slightly increases the exposure to meglitinides (repaglinide). Avoid. Mild Study

▶ **Linzagolix** is predicted to increase the exposure to sorafenib. Avoid. Mild Theoretical

▶ **Linzagolix** is predicted to increase the exposure to taxanes (paclitaxel). Avoid. Mild Theoretical

Liothyronine → see thyroid hormones
Lipegfilgrastim

▶ **Lipegfilgrastim** might increase the risk of pulmonary toxicity when given with bleomycin. Severe Theoretical

Liraglutide → see glucagon-like peptide-1 receptor agonists
Lisdexamfetamine → see amfetamines
Lisinopril → see ACE inhibitors
Lithium → see TABLE 2 p. 1571 (nephrotoxicity), TABLE 12 p. 1574 (serotonin syndrome)

▶ ACE inhibitors are predicted to increase the concentration of **lithium**. Monitor and adjust dose. Severe Anecdotal → Also see TABLE 2 p. 1571

▶ Acetazolamide alters the concentration of **lithium**. Severe Anecdotal

▶ Aminophylline is predicted to decrease the concentration of **lithium**. Moderate Theoretical

▶ Angiotensin-II receptor antagonists potentially increase the concentration of **lithium**. Avoid or monitor. Severe Anecdotal

▶ Antiepileptics (carbamazepine, oxcarbazepine) are predicted to increase the risk of neurotoxicity when given with **lithium**. Severe Anecdotal

▶ Antipsychotics, second generation (quetiapine, risperidone) potentially increase the risk of neurotoxicity when given with **lithium**. Severe Anecdotal

▶ Calcitonins decrease the concentration of **lithium**. Adjust dose. Moderate Study

▶ Calcium channel blockers (diltiazem, verapamil) are predicted to increase the risk of neurotoxicity when given with **lithium**. Severe Anecdotal

▶ Loop diuretics increase the concentration of **lithium**. Monitor and adjust dose. Severe Study

▶ Methyldopa increases the risk of neurotoxicity when given with **lithium**. Severe Anecdotal

▶ Metronidazole is predicted to increase the concentration of **lithium**. Avoid or adjust dose. Severe Anecdotal

▶ Mexiletine potentially affects the exposure to **lithium**. Avoid. Unknown Theoretical

▶ Mineralocorticoid receptor antagonists (eplerenone) potentially increase the concentration of **lithium**. Avoid. Moderate Theoretical

▶ Mineralocorticoid receptor antagonists (spironolactone) potentially increase the concentration of **lithium**. Moderate Study

▶ NSAIDs increase the concentration of **lithium**. Monitor and adjust dose. Severe Study → Also see TABLE 2 p. 1571

▶ Phenothiazines potentially increase the risk of neurotoxicity when given with **lithium**. Severe Anecdotal

▶ Potassium-sparing diuretics (triamterene) potentially increase the clearance of **lithium**. Moderate Study

▶ Sodium bicarbonate decreases the concentration of **lithium**. Severe Anecdotal

▶ Sulpiride potentially increases the risk of neurotoxicity when given with **lithium**. Severe Anecdotal

▶ Tetracyclines are predicted to increase the risk of lithium toxicity when given with **lithium**. Avoid or adjust dose. Severe Anecdotal

▶ Theophylline is predicted to decrease the concentration of **lithium**. Monitor concentration and adjust dose. Moderate Anecdotal

▶ Thiazide diuretics increase the concentration of **lithium**. Avoid or adjust dose and monitor concentration. Severe Study

▶ Tricyclic antidepressants potentially increase the risk of neurotoxicity when given with **lithium**. Severe Anecdotal → Also see TABLE 12 p. 1574

▶ **Lithium** might decrease the antidiuretic and hypertensive effects of vasopressin. Moderate Theoretical

▶ Zuclopenthixol potentially increases the risk of neurotoxicity when given with **lithium**. Severe Anecdotal

Live vaccines

Bacillus Calmette-Guérin vaccine · cholera vaccine (live) · dengue vaccine · influenza vaccine (live) · measles, mumps and rubella vaccine · rotavirus vaccine · typhoid vaccine (live) · varicella-zoster vaccine · yellow fever vaccine

▸ Antibacterials might decrease the efficacy **cholera vaccine (live)**. Avoid concurrent use with, for 14 days before, and for 10 days after, giving cholera vaccine (live).

▸ **Typhoid vaccine (live)** is inactivated by concurrent administration of antibacterials or antimalarials: antibacterials should be avoided for 3 days before and after live typhoid vaccination; *mefloquine* should be avoided for at least 12 hours before or after live typhoid vaccination; for other antimalarials live typhoid vaccine vaccination should be completed at least 3 days before the first dose of the antimalarial (except proguanil hydrochloride with atovaquone, which can be given concurrently).

▸ **Live vaccines** are predicted to increase the risk of generalised infection (possibly life-threatening) when given with **abatacept**. UKHSA advises avoid (refer to Green Book). [Severe] Theoretical

▸ **Live vaccines** are predicted to increase the risk of generalised infection (possibly life-threatening) when given with **abrocitinib**. Avoid. [Severe] Theoretical

▸ **Live vaccines** are predicted to increase the risk of generalised infection (possibly life-threatening) when given with **alkylating agents**. UKHSA advises avoid (refer to Green Book). [Severe] Theoretical

▸ **Live vaccines** are predicted to increase the risk of generalised infection (possibly life-threatening) when given with **amsacrine**. UKHSA advises avoid (refer to Green Book). [Severe] Theoretical

▸ **Live vaccines** are predicted to increase the risk of generalised infection (possibly life-threatening) when given with **anakinra**. UKHSA advises avoid (refer to Green Book). [Severe] Theoretical

▸ **Live vaccines** are predicted to increase the risk of generalised infection (possibly life-threatening) when given with **anthracyclines**. UKHSA advises avoid (refer to Green Book). [Severe] Theoretical

▸ **Antimalarials (chloroquine)** might decrease the efficacy of **cholera vaccine (live)**. Avoid for at least 10 days before **chloroquine**. [Moderate] Study

▸ **Influenza vaccine (live)** might increase the risk of Reye's syndrome when given with **aspirin**. Avoid **aspirin** for 4 weeks after vaccination. [Severe] Theoretical

▸ **Varicella-zoster vaccine** might increase the risk of Reye's syndrome when given with **aspirin**. Avoid **aspirin** for 6 weeks after vaccination. [Severe] Theoretical

▸ **Live vaccines** are predicted to increase the risk of generalised infection (possibly life-threatening) when given with **azathioprine** (high-dose). UKHSA advises avoid (refer to Green Book). [Severe] Theoretical

▸ **Baloxavir marboxil** might decrease the efficacy of **influenza vaccine (live)**. [Moderate] Theoretical

▸ **Live vaccines** are predicted to increase the risk of generalised infection (possibly life-threatening) when given with **baricitinib**. Avoid. [Severe] Theoretical

▸ **Live vaccines** are predicted to increase the risk of generalised infection (possibly life-threatening) when given with **belatacept**. UKHSA advises avoid (refer to Green Book). [Severe] Theoretical

▸ **Live vaccines** are predicted to increase the risk of generalised infection (possibly life-threatening) when given with **bleomycin**. UKHSA advises avoid (refer to Green Book). [Severe] Theoretical

▸ **Live vaccines** are predicted to increase the risk of generalised infection (possibly life-threatening) when given with **capecitabine**. UKHSA advises avoid (refer to Green Book). [Severe] Theoretical

▸ **Live vaccines** are predicted to increase the risk of generalised infection (possibly life-threatening) when given with

▸ **ciclosporin**. UKHSA advises avoid (refer to Green Book). [Severe] Theoretical

▸ **Live vaccines** are predicted to increase the risk of generalised infection (possibly life-threatening) when given with **cladribine**. UKHSA advises avoid (refer to Green Book). [Severe] Theoretical

▸ **Live vaccines** are predicted to increase the risk of generalised infection (possibly life-threatening) when given with **clofarabine**. UKHSA advises avoid (refer to Green Book). [Severe] Theoretical

▸ **Live vaccines** are predicted to increase the risk of generalised infection (possibly life-threatening) when given with **corticosteroids** (high-dose). UKHSA advises avoid (refer to Green Book). [Severe] Theoretical

▸ **Live vaccines** are predicted to increase the risk of generalised infection (possibly life-threatening) when given with **cytarabine**. UKHSA advises avoid (refer to Green Book). [Severe] Theoretical

▸ **Live vaccines** are predicted to increase the risk of generalised infection (possibly life-threatening) when given with **dactinomycin**. UKHSA advises avoid (refer to Green Book). [Severe] Theoretical

▸ **Live vaccines** are predicted to increase the risk of generalised infection (possibly life-threatening) when given with **deucravacitinib**. Avoid. [Severe] Theoretical

▸ **Live vaccines** are predicted to increase the risk of generalised infection (possibly life-threatening) when given with **dimethyl fumarate**. UKHSA advises avoid (refer to Green Book). [Severe] Theoretical

▸ **Live vaccines** are predicted to increase the risk of generalised infection (possibly life-threatening) when given with **diroximel fumarate**. Use with caution or avoid. [Severe] Theoretical

▸ **Live vaccines** might increase the risk of generalised infection (possibly life-threatening) when given with **efgartigimod alfa**. Avoid. [Severe] Theoretical

▸ **Live vaccines** are predicted to increase the risk of generalised infection (possibly life-threatening) when given with **etanercept**. UKHSA advises avoid (refer to Green Book). [Severe] Theoretical

▸ **Live vaccines** are predicted to increase the risk of generalised infection (possibly life-threatening) when given with **etoposide**. UKHSA advises avoid (refer to Green Book). [Severe] Theoretical

▸ **Live vaccines** might increase the risk of generalised infection (possibly life-threatening) when given with **etrasimod**. Avoid and for at least 4 weeks before and 2 weeks after stopping **etrasimod**. [Severe] Theoretical

▸ **Live vaccines** are predicted to increase the risk of generalised infection (possibly life-threatening) when given with **everolimus**. UKHSA advises avoid (refer to Green Book). [Severe] Theoretical

▸ **Live vaccines** are predicted to increase the risk of generalised infection (possibly life-threatening) when given with **filgotinib**. Avoid. [Severe] Theoretical

▸ **Live vaccines** might increase the risk of generalised infection (possibly life-threatening) when given with **fingolimod**. UKHSA advises avoid (refer to Green Book). [Severe] Theoretical

▸ **Live vaccines** are predicted to increase the risk of generalised infection (possibly life-threatening) when given with **fludarabine**. UKHSA advises avoid (refer to Green Book). [Severe] Theoretical

▸ **Live vaccines** are predicted to increase the risk of generalised infection (possibly life-threatening) when given with **fluorouracil**. UKHSA advises avoid (refer to Green Book). [Severe] Theoretical

▸ **Live vaccines** are predicted to increase the risk of generalised infection (possibly life-threatening) when given with **gemcitabine**. UKHSA advises avoid (refer to Green Book). [Severe] Theoretical

▸ **Live vaccines** are predicted to increase the risk of generalised infection (possibly life-threatening) when given with **hydroxycarbamide**. UKHSA advises avoid (refer to Green Book). [Severe] Theoretical

Live vaccines (continued)

▶ **Immunoglobulins** are predicted to decrease the efficacy of live vaccines (**cholera vaccine (live), dengue vaccine, influenza vaccine (live), measles, mumps and rubella vaccine, rotavirus vaccine, typhoid vaccine (live), varicella-zoster vaccine**). Avoid and for 3 months after stopping **immunoglobulins**. Moderate Theoretical

▶ **Live vaccines** are predicted to increase the risk of generalised infection (possibly life-threatening) when given with irinotecan. UKHSA advises avoid (refer to Green Book). Severe Theoretical

▶ **Live vaccines** are predicted to increase the risk of generalised infection (possibly life-threatening) when given with iron chelators (**dexrazoxane**). Avoid. Severe Theoretical

▶ **Live vaccines** are predicted to increase the risk of generalised infection (possibly life-threatening) when given with leflunomide. UKHSA advises avoid (refer to Green Book). Severe Theoretical

▶ **Live vaccines** are predicted to increase the risk of generalised infection (possibly life-threatening) when given with mercaptopurine (high-dose). UKHSA advises avoid (refer to Green Book). Severe Theoretical

▶ **Live vaccines** are predicted to increase the risk of generalised infection (possibly life-threatening) when given with methotrexate (high-dose). UKHSA advises avoid (refer to Green Book). Severe Theoretical

▶ **Live vaccines** are predicted to increase the risk of generalised infection (possibly life-threatening) when given with mitomycin. UKHSA advises avoid (refer to Green Book). Severe Theoretical

▶ **Live vaccines** are predicted to increase the risk of generalised infection (possibly life-threatening) when given with monoclonal antibodies. UKHSA advises avoid (refer to Green Book). Severe Theoretical

▶ **Live vaccines** are predicted to increase the risk of generalised infection (possibly life-threatening) when given with mycophenolate. UKHSA advises avoid (refer to Green Book). Severe Theoretical

▶ Oseltamivir might decrease the efficacy of **influenza vaccine (live)**. Moderate Theoretical

▶ **Live vaccines** might increase the risk of generalised infection (possibly life-threatening) when given with ozanimod. Avoid and for 3 months after stopping **ozanimod**. Severe Theoretical

▶ **Live vaccines** are predicted to increase the risk of generalised infection (possibly life-threatening) when given with pemetrexed. UKHSA advises avoid (refer to Green Book). Severe Theoretical

▶ **Live vaccines** are predicted to increase the risk of generalised infection (possibly life-threatening) when given with platinum compounds. UKHSA advises avoid (refer to Green Book). Severe Theoretical

▶ **Live vaccines** might increase the risk of generalised infection (possibly life-threatening) when given with ponesimod. Avoid and for 1 week after stopping **ponesimod**. Severe Theoretical

▶ **Live vaccines** are predicted to increase the risk of generalised infection (possibly life-threatening) when given with procarbazine. UKHSA advises avoid (refer to Green Book). Severe Theoretical

▶ **Live vaccines** are predicted to increase the risk of generalised infection (possibly life-threatening) when given with raltitrexed. UKHSA advises avoid (refer to Green Book). Severe Theoretical

▶ **Live vaccines** are predicted to increase the risk of generalised infection (possibly life-threatening) when given with ritlecitinib. Avoid. Severe Theoretical

▶ **Live vaccines** might increase the risk of generalised infection (possibly life-threatening) when given with siponimod. Avoid and for 4 weeks after stopping **siponimod**. Severe Theoretical

▶ **Live vaccines** are predicted to increase the risk of generalised infection (possibly life-threatening) when given with sirolimus. UKHSA advises avoid (refer to Green Book). Severe Theoretical

▶ **Live vaccines** are predicted to increase the risk of generalised infection (possibly life-threatening) when given with streptozocin. UKHSA advises avoid (refer to Green Book). Severe Theoretical

▶ **Live vaccines** are predicted to increase the risk of generalised infection (possibly life-threatening) when given with tacrolimus. UKHSA advises avoid (refer to Green Book). Severe Theoretical

▶ **Live vaccines** are predicted to increase the risk of generalised infection (possibly life-threatening) when given with taxanes (**docetaxel, paclitaxel**). UKHSA advises avoid (refer to Green Book). Severe Theoretical

▶ **Live vaccines** are predicted to increase the risk of generalised infection (possibly life-threatening) when given with tegafur. UKHSA advises avoid (refer to Green Book). Severe Theoretical

▶ **Live vaccines** are predicted to increase the risk of generalised infection (possibly life-threatening) when given with temsirolimus. UKHSA advises avoid (refer to Green Book). Severe Theoretical

▶ **Live vaccines** are predicted to increase the risk of generalised infection (possibly life-threatening) when given with teriflunomide. UKHSA advises avoid (refer to Green Book). Severe Theoretical

▶ **Live vaccines** are predicted to increase the risk of generalised infection (possibly life-threatening) when given with tioguanine. UKHSA advises avoid (refer to Green Book). Severe Theoretical

▶ **Live vaccines** potentially increase the risk of generalised infection (possibly life-threatening) when given with tofacitinib. Avoid. Severe Theoretical

▶ **Live vaccines** are predicted to increase the risk of generalised infection (possibly life-threatening) when given with topotecan. UKHSA advises avoid (refer to Green Book). Severe Theoretical

▶ **Live vaccines** are predicted to increase the risk of generalised infection (possibly life-threatening) when given with trabectedin. UKHSA advises avoid (refer to Green Book). Severe Theoretical

▶ **Live vaccines** are predicted to increase the risk of generalised infection (possibly life-threatening) when given with upadacitinib. Avoid. Severe Theoretical

▶ Venetoclax potentially decreases the efficacy of **live vaccines**. Avoid. Severe Theoretical

▶ **Live vaccines** are predicted to increase the risk of generalised infection (possibly life-threatening) when given with vinca alkaloids. UKHSA advises avoid (refer to Green Book). Severe Theoretical

▶ **Live vaccines** are predicted to increase the risk of generalised infection (possibly life-threatening) when given with voclosporin. UKHSA advises avoid (refer to Green Book). Severe Theoretical

▶ Zanamivir might decrease the efficacy of **influenza vaccine (live)**. Moderate Theoretical

Lixisenatide → see glucagon-like peptide-1 receptor agonists

Lofepramine → see tricyclic antidepressants

Lofexidine → see TABLE 7 p. 1572 (hypotension), TABLE 10 p. 1574 (CNS effects)

Lomitapide → see TABLE 1 p. 1571 (hepatotoxicity)

FOOD AND LIFESTYLE Bitter (Seville) orange is predicted to increase the exposure to lomitapide; separate administration by 12 hours.

▶ Anti-androgens (**apalutamide, enzalutamide**) are predicted to decrease the exposure to **lomitapide**. Monitor and adjust dose. Moderate Theoretical

▶ Anti-androgens (**bicalutamide**) are predicted to increase the exposure to **lomitapide**. Separate administration by 12 hours. Moderate Theoretical

▶ Antiarrhythmics (**amiodarone**) are predicted to increase the exposure to **lomitapide**. Separate administration by 12 hours. Moderate Theoretical → Also see TABLE 1 p. 1571

▶ Antiarrhythmics (**dronedarone**) are predicted to increase the exposure to **lomitapide**. Avoid. Moderate Theoretical

▶ Antiepileptics (**carbamazepine, fosphenytoin, phenobarbital, phenytoin, primidone**) are predicted to decrease the exposure to **lomitapide**. Monitor and adjust dose. Moderate Theoretical

- Antifungals, azoles **(clotrimazole)** are predicted to increase the exposure to **lomitapide**. Separate administration by 12 hours. Moderate Theoretical
- Antifungals, azoles **(fluconazole, isavuconazole)** are predicted to increase the exposure to **lomitapide**. Avoid. Moderate Theoretical → Also see **TABLE 1** p. 1571
- Antifungals, azoles **(itraconazole, ketoconazole, posaconazole, voriconazole)** are predicted to markedly increase the exposure to **lomitapide**. Avoid. Severe Study → Also see **TABLE 1** p. 1571
- Benzodiazepines **(alprazolam)** are predicted to increase the exposure to **lomitapide**. Separate administration by 12 hours. Moderate Theoretical
- Berotralstat is predicted to increase the exposure to **lomitapide**. Avoid. Moderate Theoretical
- Calcium channel blockers **(amlodipine, lacidipine)** are predicted to increase the exposure to **lomitapide**. Separate administration by 12 hours. Moderate Theoretical
- Calcium channel blockers **(diltiazem, verapamil)** are predicted to increase the exposure to **lomitapide**. Avoid. Moderate Theoretical
- Cenobamate is predicted to decrease the exposure to **lomitapide**. Adjust dose. Moderate Theoretical
- Ceritinib is predicted to markedly increase the exposure to **lomitapide**. Avoid. Severe Study
- Ciclosporin is predicted to increase the exposure to **lomitapide**. Separate administration by 12 hours. Moderate Theoretical
- Cilostazol is predicted to increase the exposure to **lomitapide**. Separate administration by 12 hours. Moderate Theoretical
- Cobicistat is predicted to markedly increase the exposure to **lomitapide**. Avoid. Severe Study
- Oral combined hormonal contraceptives slightly increase the exposure to **lomitapide**. Separate administration by 12 hours. Moderate Theoretical
- **Lomitapide** increases the exposure to coumarins **(warfarin)**. Monitor INR and adjust dose. Severe Study
- Crizotinib is predicted to increase the exposure to **lomitapide**. Avoid. Moderate Theoretical
- **Lomitapide** might increase the exposure to digoxin. Adjust dose. Moderate Theoretical
- Dipeptidylpeptidase-4 inhibitors **(linagliptin)** are predicted to increase the exposure to **lomitapide**. Separate administration by 12 hours. Moderate Theoretical
- Encorafenib is predicted to decrease the exposure to **lomitapide**. Monitor and adjust dose. Moderate Theoretical
- Everolimus is predicted to increase the exposure to **lomitapide** and **lomitapide** might increase the exposure to everolimus. Adjust **everolimus** dose and separate administration by 12 hours, p. 1109. Moderate Theoretical
- Fedratinib is predicted to increase the exposure to **lomitapide**. Avoid. Moderate Theoretical
- Grapefruit juice is predicted to increase the exposure to **lomitapide**. Avoid. Mild Theoretical
- H₂ receptor antagonists **(cimetidine)** are predicted to increase the exposure to **lomitapide**. Separate administration by 12 hours. Mild Theoretical
- H₂ receptor antagonists **(ranitidine)** are predicted to increase the exposure to **lomitapide**. Separate administration by 12 hours. Moderate Theoretical
- HIV-protease inhibitors are predicted to markedly increase the exposure to **lomitapide**. Avoid. Severe Study → Also see **TABLE 1** p. 1571
- Idelalisib is predicted to markedly increase the exposure to **lomitapide**. Avoid. Severe Study
- Imatinib is predicted to increase the exposure to **lomitapide**. Avoid. Moderate Theoretical
- Isoniazid is predicted to increase the exposure to **lomitapide**. Separate administration by 12 hours. Unknown Theoretical → Also see **TABLE 1** p. 1571
- Ivacaftor is predicted to increase the exposure to **lomitapide**. Separate administration by 12 hours. Moderate Theoretical
- Ivosidenib is predicted to decrease the exposure to **lomitapide**. Monitor and adjust dose. Moderate Theoretical
- Lapatinib is predicted to increase the exposure to **lomitapide**. Separate administration by 12 hours. Mild Theoretical
- Letermovir is predicted to increase the exposure to **lomitapide**. Avoid. Moderate Theoretical

- Lumacaftor is predicted to decrease the exposure to **lomitapide**. Monitor and adjust dose. Moderate Theoretical
- Macrolides **(azithromycin)** are predicted to increase the exposure to **lomitapide**. Separate administration by 12 hours. Moderate Theoretical
- Macrolides **(clarithromycin)** are predicted to markedly increase the exposure to **lomitapide**. Avoid. Severe Study
- Macrolides **(erythromycin)** are predicted to increase the exposure to **lomitapide**. Avoid. Moderate Theoretical
- **Lomitapide** is predicted to increase the exposure to mavacamten. Monitor and adjust dose—consult product literature. Moderate Theoretical
- Mitotane is predicted to decrease the exposure to **lomitapide**. Monitor and adjust dose. Moderate Theoretical
- Neurokinin-1 receptor antagonists **(aprepitant, netupitant)** are predicted to increase the exposure to **lomitapide**. Avoid. Moderate Theoretical
- Neurokinin-1 receptor antagonists **(fosaprepitant)** are predicted to increase the exposure to **lomitapide**. Separate administration by 12 hours. Mild Theoretical
- Nilotinib is predicted to increase the exposure to **lomitapide**. Avoid. Moderate Theoretical
- Nirmatrelvir boosted with ritonavir is predicted to increase the concentration of **lomitapide**. Avoid. Severe Theoretical
- Pazopanib is predicted to increase the exposure to **lomitapide**. Separate administration by 12 hours. Mild Theoretical
- Peppermint oil is predicted to increase the exposure to **lomitapide**. Separate administration by 12 hours. Moderate Theoretical
- Propiverine is predicted to increase the exposure to **lomitapide**. Separate administration by 12 hours. Moderate Theoretical
- Ranolazine is predicted to increase the exposure to **lomitapide**. Separate administration by 12 hours. Mild Theoretical
- Rifamycins **(rifampicin)** are predicted to decrease the exposure to **lomitapide**. Monitor and adjust dose. Moderate Theoretical
- **Lomitapide** might increase the exposure to sirolimus. Adjust dose. Moderate Theoretical
- SSRIs **(fluoxetine)** are predicted to increase the exposure to **lomitapide**. Separate administration by 12 hours. Unknown Theoretical
- SSRIs **(fluvoxamine)** are predicted to increase the exposure to **lomitapide**. Separate administration by 12 hours. Mild Theoretical
- **Lomitapide** increases the exposure to statins **(atorvastatin)**. Adjust **lomitapide** dose or separate administration by 12 hours, p. 241. Mild Study → Also see **TABLE 1** p. 1571
- **Lomitapide** increases the exposure to statins **(simvastatin)**. Monitor and adjust **simvastatin** dose, p. 237. Moderate Study → Also see **TABLE 1** p. 1571
- Tacrolimus is predicted to increase the exposure to **lomitapide**. Separate administration by 12 hours. Moderate Theoretical
- **Lomitapide** might increase the exposure to talazoparib. Adjust dose. Moderate Theoretical
- **Lomitapide** might increase the exposure to taxanes **(paclitaxel)**. Adjust dose. Moderate Theoretical
- Ticagrelor is predicted to increase the exposure to **lomitapide**. Separate administration by 12 hours. Moderate Theoretical
- Tolvaptan is predicted to increase the exposure to **lomitapide**. Separate administration by 12 hours. Moderate Theoretical
- Tucatinib is predicted to markedly increase the exposure to **lomitapide**. Avoid. Severe Study

Lomustine → see alkylating agents

Loncastuximab tesirine → see monoclonal antibodies

Loop diuretics → see **TABLE 17** p. 1576 (hyponatraemia), **TABLE 7** p. 1572 (hypotension), **TABLE 18** p. 1576 (ototoxicity), **TABLE 16** p. 1575 (reduced serum potassium)

bumetanide · furosemide · torasemide

- Aliskiren slightly decreases the exposure to **furosemide**. Moderate Study → Also see **TABLE 7** p. 1572
- **Loop diuretics** increase the risk of nephrotoxicity when given with aminoglycosides. Avoid. Moderate Study → Also see **TABLE 18** p. 1576
- Antiepileptics **(fosphenytoin, phenytoin)** decrease the effects of **furosemide**. Moderate Study

Loop diuretics (continued)

▶ Intravenous **furosemide** potentially increases the risk of sweating, variable blood pressure, and tachycardia when given after chloral hydrate. Moderate Anecdotal

▶ **Loop diuretics** are predicted to increase the risk of adverse effects when given with immunoglobulins (cytomegalovirus immunoglobulin). Avoid. Moderate Theoretical

▶ **Loop diuretics** might increase the risk of adverse effects when given with immunoglobulins (hepatitis B immunoglobulin). Avoid. Moderate Theoretical

▶ **Loop diuretics** might increase the risk of adverse effects when given with immunoglobulins (normal immunoglobulin). Avoid. Moderate Theoretical

▶ Ivosidenib is predicted to increase the exposure to **furosemide**. Manufacturer advises caution or avoid—consult product literature. Moderate Theoretical

▶ Leflunomide is predicted to increase the exposure to **furosemide**. Moderate Study

▶ **Loop diuretics** increase the concentration of lithium. Monitor and adjust dose. Severe Study

▶ Nitisinone is predicted to increase the exposure to **furosemide**. Moderate Study

▶ Reboxetine is predicted to increase the risk of hypokalaemia when given with **loop diuretics**. Moderate Theoretical

▶ Selpercatinib is predicted to increase the exposure to torasemide. Avoid. Severe Study

▶ Teriflunomide is predicted to increase the exposure to **furosemide**. Moderate Study

▶ **Furosemide** might slightly decrease the clearance of treprostinil. Unknown Theoretical → Also see TABLE 7 p. 1572

▶ Vadadustat increases the exposure to **furosemide**. Monitor and adjust dose. Moderate Study

Loperamide

▶ Anti-androgens (apalutamide) are predicted to decrease the exposure to **loperamide**. Monitor and adjust dose. Moderate Study

▶ Antiarrhythmics (dronedarone) are predicted to increase the exposure to **loperamide**. Severe Theoretical

▶ Antipsychotics, second generation (clozapine) can cause constipation, as can **loperamide**; concurrent use might increase the risk of developing intestinal obstruction. Severe Anecdotal

▶ Ceritinib is predicted to increase the exposure to **loperamide**. Moderate Theoretical

▶ Danicopan is predicted to increase the exposure to **loperamide**. Moderate Study

▶ **Loperamide** greatly increases the absorption of oral desmopressin (and possibly sublingual). Moderate Study

▶ Eliglustat is predicted to increase the exposure to **loperamide**. Adjust dose. Moderate Study

▶ Glecaprevir is predicted to increase the exposure to **loperamide**. Severe Theoretical

▶ Ivosidenib is predicted to alter the exposure to **loperamide**. Moderate Theoretical

▶ Lapatinib is predicted to increase the exposure to **loperamide**. Moderate Theoretical

▶ Lorlatinib is predicted to decrease the exposure to **loperamide**. Moderate Study

▶ Mifepristone is predicted to increase the exposure to **loperamide**. Moderate Theoretical

▶ Mirabegron is predicted to increase the exposure to **loperamide**. Mild Theoretical

▶ Olaparib might increase the exposure to **loperamide**. Moderate Theoretical

▶ Opicapone is predicted to increase the exposure to **loperamide**. Avoid. Moderate Study

▶ Osimertinib is predicted to increase the exposure to **loperamide**. Moderate Study

▶ Pibrentasvir with glecaprevir is predicted to increase the exposure to **loperamide**. Moderate Study

▶ Pitolisant is predicted to decrease the exposure to **loperamide**. Mild Theoretical

▶ Selpercatinib is predicted to increase the exposure to **loperamide**. Moderate Study

▶ Tepotinib is predicted to increase the concentration of **loperamide**. Severe Study

▶ Velpatasvir is predicted to increase the exposure to **loperamide**. Severe Theoretical

▶ Vemurafenib might increase the exposure to **loperamide**. Use with caution and adjust dose. Moderate Theoretical

▶ Voxilaprevir with sofosbuvir and velpatasvir is predicted to increase the exposure to **loperamide**. Severe Theoretical

Lopinavir → see HIV-protease inhibitors

Loprazolam → see benzodiazepines

Loratadine → see antihistamines, non-sedating

Lorazepam → see benzodiazepines

Lorlatinib

▶ **Lorlatinib** is predicted to decrease the exposure to afatinib. Moderate Study

▶ **Lorlatinib** decreases the exposure to aliskiren. Moderate Study

▶ Anti-androgens (apalutamide, enzalutamide) are predicted to decrease the exposure to **lorlatinib**. Avoid. Severe Study

▶ **Lorlatinib** is predicted to decrease the exposure to anti-androgens (darolutamide). Avoid. Moderate Theoretical

▶ Antiepileptics (carbamazepine, fosphenytoin, phenobarbital, phenytoin, primidone) are predicted to decrease the exposure to **lorlatinib**. Avoid. Severe Study

▶ Antifungals, azoles (fluconazole) are predicted to increase the exposure to **lorlatinib**. Moderate Theoretical

▶ Antifungals, azoles (itraconazole, ketoconazole, posaconazole, voriconazole) are predicted to increase the exposure to **lorlatinib**. Avoid or adjust dose—consult product literature. Severe Study

▶ **Lorlatinib** is predicted to decrease the exposure to antifungals, azoles (isavuconazole). Avoid. Severe Theoretical

▶ **Lorlatinib** decreases the exposure to antihistamines, non-sedating (fexofenadine). Moderate Study

▶ **Lorlatinib** is predicted to decrease the exposure to antipsychotics, second generation (cariprazine). Avoid. Severe Theoretical

▶ **Lorlatinib** is predicted to decrease the exposure to antipsychotics, second generation (lurasidone). Monitor and adjust dose. Moderate Theoretical

▶ **Lorlatinib** is predicted to decrease the exposure to antipsychotics, second generation (quetiapine). Moderate Study

▶ **Lorlatinib** is predicted to decrease the exposure to avacopan. Severe Theoretical

▶ **Lorlatinib** is predicted to decrease the exposure to avapritinib. Avoid. Severe Study

▶ **Lorlatinib** is predicted to decrease the exposure to bedaquiline. Avoid. Severe Study

▶ **Lorlatinib** moderately decreases the exposure to benzodiazepines (midazolam). Avoid. Moderate Study

▶ **Lorlatinib** is predicted to decrease the concentration of berotralstat. Avoid. Severe Theoretical

▶ **Lorlatinib** is predicted to decrease the exposure to bosutinib. Avoid. Severe Study

▶ **Lorlatinib** is predicted to decrease the exposure to brigatinib. Avoid or adjust dose—consult product literature. Moderate Study

▶ **Lorlatinib** is predicted to decrease the exposure to cabozantinib. Moderate Study

▶ **Lorlatinib** is predicted to decrease the exposure to calcium channel blockers (amlodipine, felodipine, lacidipine, lercanidipine, nicardipine, nifedipine, nimodipine). Monitor and adjust dose. Moderate Theoretical

▶ **Lorlatinib** is predicted to decrease the exposure to calcium channel blockers (diltiazem, verapamil). Moderate Theoretical

▶ **Lorlatinib** is predicted to decrease the exposure to capivasertib. Avoid. Moderate Study

▶ Ceritinib is predicted to increase the exposure to **lorlatinib**. Avoid or adjust dose—consult product literature. Severe Study

▶ **Lorlatinib** is predicted to decrease the exposure to ciclosporin. Avoid. Moderate Theoretical

▶ Cobicistat is predicted to increase the exposure to **lorlatinib**. Avoid or adjust dose—consult product literature. Severe Study

▶ **Lorlatinib** is predicted to decrease the exposure to cobicistat. Avoid. Severe Theoretical

- ▶ **Lorlatinib** is predicted to decrease the exposure to cobimetinib. Avoid. [Severe] Theoretical
- ▶ **Lorlatinib** is predicted to decrease the exposure to colchicine. [Moderate] Theoretical
- ▶ **Lorlatinib** is predicted to decrease the exposure to combined hormonal contraceptives. Avoid. [Moderate] Theoretical
- ▶ **Lorlatinib** is predicted to decrease the exposure to coumarins. [Moderate] Theoretical
- ▶ **Lorlatinib** is predicted to decrease the exposure to crizotinib. Avoid. [Severe] Study
- ▶ **Lorlatinib** is predicted to decrease the exposure to daridorexant. [Severe] Study
- ▶ **Lorlatinib** is predicted to decrease the exposure to dasatinib. [Severe] Study
- ▶ **Lorlatinib** is predicted to decrease the exposure to digoxin. [Moderate] Study
- ▶ **Lorlatinib** is predicted to decrease the exposure to elacestrant. Avoid or adjust dose depending on duration—consult product literature. [Severe] Theoretical
- ▶ **Lorlatinib** is predicted to moderately decrease the exposure to elbasvir. Avoid. [Severe] Study
- ▶ **Lorlatinib** is predicted to decrease the concentration of elvitegravir. Avoid. [Severe] Theoretical
- ▶ **Encorafenib** is predicted to decrease the exposure to **lorlatinib**. Avoid. [Severe] Study
- ▶ **Lorlatinib** is predicted to decrease the exposure to encorafenib. [Moderate] Study
- ▶ **Lorlatinib** is predicted to decrease the exposure to entrectinib. Avoid. [Moderate] Theoretical
- ▶ **Lorlatinib** is predicted to decrease the exposure to erdafitinib. Adjust dose. [Moderate] Theoretical
- ▶ **Lorlatinib** is predicted to decrease the exposure to erlotinib. [Severe] Study
- ▶ **Lorlatinib** is predicted to decrease the concentration of everolimus. Avoid or adjust dose. [Severe] Study
- ▶ **Lorlatinib** is predicted to decrease the exposure to factor XA inhibitors (apixaban). Use with caution or avoid. [Severe] Study
- ▶ **Lorlatinib** is predicted to decrease the exposure to factor XA inhibitors (edoxaban). [Moderate] Study
- ▶ **Lorlatinib** is predicted to decrease the exposure to factor XA inhibitors (rivaroxaban). Avoid unless patient can be monitored for signs of thrombosis. [Severe] Study
- ▶ **Lorlatinib** is predicted to decrease the exposure to fedratinib. Avoid. [Moderate] Study
- ▶ **Lorlatinib** is predicted to decrease the exposure to fruquintinib. Avoid. [Moderate] Study
- ▶ **Lorlatinib** is predicted to decrease the exposure to gefitinib. Avoid. [Severe] Study
- ▶ **Lorlatinib** is predicted to decrease the exposure to glasdegib. Avoid or adjust dose—consult product literature. [Moderate] Theoretical
- ▶ **Lorlatinib** is predicted to decrease the exposure to glecaprevir. Avoid. [Severe] Study
- ▶ **Grapefruit** juice is predicted to increase the concentration of **lorlatinib**. Avoid. [Moderate] Theoretical
- ▶ **Lorlatinib** is predicted to markedly decrease the exposure to grazoprevir. Avoid. [Severe] Study
- ▶ **Lorlatinib** is predicted to decrease the concentration of guanfacine. Adjust dose. [Moderate] Theoretical
- ▶ **HIV-protease inhibitors** are predicted to increase the exposure to **lorlatinib**. Avoid or adjust dose—consult product literature. [Severe] Study
- ▶ **Idelalisib** is predicted to increase the exposure to **lorlatinib**. Avoid or adjust dose—consult product literature. [Severe] Study
- ▶ **Lorlatinib** is predicted to decrease the exposure to idelalisib. Avoid. [Moderate] Theoretical
- ▶ **Lorlatinib** is predicted to decrease the exposure to imatinib. [Moderate] Study
- ▶ **Ivosidenib** is predicted to decrease the exposure to **lorlatinib**. Avoid. [Severe] Study
- ▶ **Lorlatinib** is predicted to decrease the exposure to ixazomib. [Moderate] Theoretical
- ▶ **Lorlatinib** is predicted to decrease the exposure to lapatinib. Avoid. [Severe] Study

- ▶ **Lorlatinib** is predicted to decrease the exposure to larotrectinib. Avoid. [Moderate] Study
- ▶ **Lorlatinib** is predicted to decrease the exposure to ledipasvir. Avoid. [Severe] Study
- ▶ **Lorlatinib** is predicted to decrease the exposure to leniolisib. Avoid. [Severe] Theoretical
- ▶ **Lorlatinib** is predicted to decrease the exposure to loperamide. [Moderate] Study
- ▶ **Lumacaftor** is predicted to decrease the exposure to **lorlatinib**. Avoid. [Severe] Study
- ▶ **Macrolides (clarithromycin)** are predicted to increase the exposure to **lorlatinib**. Avoid or adjust dose—consult product literature. [Severe] Study
- ▶ **Lorlatinib** is predicted to decrease the exposure to mavacamten. Monitor and adjust dose—consult product literature. [Severe] Theoretical
- ▶ **Lorlatinib** is predicted to decrease the exposure to mifepristone. Adjust **mifepristone** dose, p. 954. [Severe] Study
- ▶ **Lorlatinib** is predicted to decrease the exposure to mineralocorticoid receptor antagonists (finerenone). Avoid. [Severe] Study
- ▶ **Mitotane** is predicted to decrease the exposure to **lorlatinib**. Avoid. [Severe] Study
- ▶ **Lorlatinib** is predicted to decrease the exposure to mobocertinib. Avoid. [Severe] Study
- ▶ **Lorlatinib** is predicted to decrease the exposure to naloxegol. [Moderate] Theoretical
- ▶ **Lorlatinib** is predicted to decrease the exposure to neratinib. Avoid. [Severe] Theoretical
- ▶ **Lorlatinib** is predicted to decrease the exposure to neurokinin-1 receptor antagonists (netupitant). [Moderate] Theoretical
- ▶ **Lorlatinib** is predicted to decrease the exposure to nilotinib. Avoid. [Severe] Theoretical
- ▶ **Lorlatinib** is predicted to decrease the exposure to nintedanib. [Moderate] Study
- ▶ **Lorlatinib** is predicted to decrease the exposure to NNRTIs (rilpivirine). Avoid. [Severe] Theoretical
- ▶ **Lorlatinib** is predicted to decrease the exposure to olaparib. Avoid. [Moderate] Theoretical
- ▶ **Lorlatinib** is predicted to decrease the exposure to opioids (alfentanil, fentanyl). Avoid. [Moderate] Theoretical
- ▶ **Lorlatinib** decreases the exposure to opioids (methadone). Monitor and adjust dose. [Severe] Study
- ▶ **Lorlatinib** is predicted to decrease the exposure to ospemifene. [Moderate] Study
- ▶ **Lorlatinib** is predicted to decrease the exposure to pazopanib. [Severe] Study
- ▶ **Lorlatinib** is predicted to decrease the exposure to pemigatinib. Avoid or monitor. [Severe] Study
- ▶ **Lorlatinib** is predicted to decrease the exposure to pibrentasvir. Avoid. [Severe] Study
- ▶ **Lorlatinib** is predicted to decrease the exposure to pimozide. Avoid. [Moderate] Theoretical
- ▶ **Lorlatinib** is predicted to decrease the exposure to ponatinib. [Severe] Study
- ▶ **Lorlatinib** is predicted to decrease the exposure to pralsetinib. [Moderate] Theoretical
- ▶ **Lorlatinib** is predicted to decrease the exposure to quizartinib. Avoid. [Severe] Study
- ▶ **Lorlatinib** is predicted to decrease the exposure to ranolazine. [Moderate] Theoretical
- ▶ **Rifamycins (rifampicin)** are predicted to decrease the exposure to **lorlatinib**. Avoid. [Severe] Study
- ▶ **Lorlatinib** is predicted to decrease the exposure to rimegepant. Avoid. [Moderate] Theoretical
- ▶ **Lorlatinib** is predicted to decrease the exposure to ripretinib. Avoid or adjust dose—consult product literature. [Moderate] Theoretical
- ▶ **Lorlatinib** is predicted to decrease the exposure to ruxolitinib. Monitor and adjust dose. [Moderate] Study
- ▶ **Lorlatinib** is predicted to decrease the exposure to selpercatinib. [Moderate] Study
- ▶ **Lorlatinib** is predicted to decrease the exposure to selumetinib. Avoid. [Severe] Study

Lorlatinib (continued)

▸ **Lorlatinib** is predicted to decrease the exposure to siponimod. Manufacturer advises caution depending on genotype—consult product literature. Moderate Theoretical

▸ **Lorlatinib** is predicted to decrease the exposure to sirolimus. Avoid. Moderate Theoretical

▸ **Lorlatinib** is predicted to decrease the exposure to sofosbuvir. Avoid. Severe Study

▸ **Lorlatinib** is predicted to decrease the exposure to sorafenib. Moderate Study

▸ St John's wort is predicted to decrease the exposure to lorlatinib. Avoid. Severe Theoretical

▸ **Lorlatinib** is predicted to decrease the exposure to statins (atorvastatin, simvastatin). Moderate Study

▸ **Lorlatinib** is predicted to decrease the exposure to sunitinib. Moderate Study

▸ **Lorlatinib** is predicted to decrease the exposure to tacrolimus. Avoid. Moderate Theoretical

▸ **Lorlatinib** is predicted to decrease the exposure to talazoparib. Moderate Study

▸ **Lorlatinib** is predicted to decrease the exposure to taxanes (docetaxel). Severe Theoretical

▸ **Lorlatinib** is predicted to decrease the exposure to taxanes (paclitaxel). Avoid. Severe Study

▸ **Lorlatinib** is predicted to decrease the concentration of temsirolimus. Avoid. Moderate Theoretical

▸ **Lorlatinib** is predicted to decrease the exposure to tenofovir alafenamide. Avoid. Moderate Theoretical

▸ **Lorlatinib** is predicted to decrease the exposure to thrombin inhibitors (dabigatran). Avoid. Severe Study

▸ **Lorlatinib** is predicted to decrease the exposure to ticagrelor. Moderate Theoretical

▸ **Lorlatinib** might decrease the exposure to tigecycline. Mild Theoretical

▸ **Lorlatinib** is predicted to decrease the exposure to tofacitinib. Severe Study

▸ Tucatinib is predicted to increase the exposure to lorlatinib. Avoid or adjust dose—consult product literature. Severe Study

▸ **Lorlatinib** is predicted to decrease the exposure to velpatasvir. Avoid. Moderate Theoretical

▸ **Lorlatinib** is predicted to decrease the exposure to venetoclax. Avoid. Severe Study

▸ **Lorlatinib** is predicted to decrease the concentration of voxilaprevir. Avoid. Severe Theoretical

▸ **Lorlatinib** is predicted to decrease the exposure to zanubrutinib. Avoid or adjust dose with moderate CYP3A4 inducers—consult product literature. Severe Theoretical

Lormetazepam → see benzodiazepines

Losartan → see angiotensin-II receptor antagonists

Low molecular-weight heparins → see TABLE 15 p. 1575 (increased serum potassium), TABLE 3 p. 1571 (anticoagulant effects)

bemiparin · dalteparin · enoxaparin · tinzaparin

▸ Andexanet alfa is predicted to affect the anticoagulant effect of **low molecular-weight heparins**. Avoid. Severe Theoretical

▸ Drugs that cause hepatotoxicity (see TABLE 1 p. 1571) might increase the risk of hepatotoxicity when given with **low molecular-weight heparins** (high-dose). Severe Theoretical

Loxapine → see TABLE 17 p. 1576 (hyponatraemia), TABLE 7 p. 1572 (hypotension), TABLE 9 p. 1573 (antimuscarinics), TABLE 10 p. 1574 (CNS effects)

▸ Antipsychotics, second generation (clozapine) can cause constipation, as can **loxapine**; concurrent use might increase the risk of developing intestinal obstruction. Severe Theoretical → Also see TABLE 17 p. 1576 → Also see TABLE 7 p. 1572 → Also see TABLE 9 p. 1573 → Also see TABLE 10 p. 1574

▸ Combined hormonal contraceptives is predicted to increase the exposure to **loxapine**. Avoid. Unknown Theoretical

▸ **Loxapine** is predicted to decrease the effects of dopamine receptor agonists. Moderate Theoretical → Also see TABLE 7 p. 1572 → Also see TABLE 9 p. 1573 → Also see TABLE 10 p. 1574

▸ **Loxapine** opposes the effects of the active metabolite of foslevodopa. Severe Theoretical → Also see TABLE 7 p. 1572 → Also see TABLE 10 p. 1574

▸ Givosiran is predicted to increase the exposure to **loxapine**. Avoid. Unknown Theoretical

▸ **Loxapine** is predicted to decrease the effects of levodopa. Severe Theoretical → Also see TABLE 7 p. 1572 → Also see TABLE 10 p. 1574

▸ Mexiletine is predicted to increase the exposure to **loxapine**. Avoid. Unknown Theoretical

▸ Osilodrostat is predicted to increase the exposure to **loxapine**. Avoid. Unknown Theoretical

▸ Quinolones (ciprofloxacin) are predicted to increase the exposure to **loxapine**. Avoid. Unknown Theoretical

▸ Rucaparib is predicted to increase the exposure to **loxapine**. Avoid. Unknown Theoretical

▸ SSRIs (fluvoxamine) are predicted to increase the exposure to **loxapine**. Avoid. Unknown Theoretical → Also see TABLE 17 p. 1576 → Also see TABLE 10 p. 1574

▸ Vemurafenib is predicted to increase the exposure to **loxapine**. Avoid. Unknown Theoretical

Lumacaftor

▸ **Lumacaftor** is predicted to decrease the exposure to 5-HT3-receptor antagonists (ondansetron). Moderate Study

▸ **Lumacaftor** is predicted to markedly decrease the exposure to abemaciclib. Avoid. Severe Study

▸ **Lumacaftor** is predicted to decrease the exposure to acalabrutinib. Avoid. Severe Study

▸ **Lumacaftor** is predicted to decrease the exposure to alpelisib. Avoid. Moderate Study

▸ **Lumacaftor** is predicted to decrease the exposure to anti-androgens (abiraterone). Avoid. Severe Study

▸ **Lumacaftor** is predicted to decrease the exposure to anti-androgens (darolutamide). Avoid. Moderate Study

▸ **Lumacaftor** is predicted to decrease the exposure to antiarrhythmics (disopyramide, dronedarone). Avoid. Severe Study

▸ **Lumacaftor** is predicted to decrease the efficacy of antiarrhythmics (propafenone). Moderate Study

▸ **Lumacaftor** is predicted to decrease the exposure to anticholinesterases, centrally acting (donepezil). Mild Study

▸ **Lumacaftor** is predicted to decrease the exposure to antiepileptics (carbamazepine, fosphenytoin, phenobarbital, phenytoin, primidone). Avoid. Severe Theoretical

▸ **Lumacaftor** is predicted to decrease the exposure to antiepileptics (perampanel). Monitor and adjust dose. Moderate Study

▸ **Lumacaftor** is predicted to decrease the exposure to antifungals, azoles (isavuconazole). Avoid. Severe Study

▸ **Lumacaftor** is predicted to decrease the exposure to antifungals, azoles (itraconazole, ketoconazole, posaconazole, voriconazole). Avoid or monitor efficacy. Moderate Theoretical

▸ **Lumacaftor** is predicted to decrease the exposure to antimalarials (artemether) with lumefantrine. Avoid. Severe Study

▸ **Lumacaftor** is predicted to moderately decrease the exposure to antipsychotics, second generation (aripiprazole). Adjust aripiprazole dose, p. 454. Moderate Study

▸ **Lumacaftor** is predicted to decrease the exposure to antipsychotics, second generation (cariprazine). Avoid. Severe Theoretical

▸ **Lumacaftor** is predicted to decrease the exposure to antipsychotics, second generation (lurasidone). Avoid. Moderate Study

▸ **Lumacaftor** is predicted to decrease the exposure to antipsychotics, second generation (paliperidone). Monitor and adjust dose. Severe Study

▸ **Lumacaftor** is predicted to decrease the exposure to antipsychotics, second generation (quetiapine). Moderate Study

▸ **Lumacaftor** is predicted to decrease the exposure to antipsychotics, second generation (risperidone). Adjust dose. Moderate Study

▸ **Lumacaftor** is predicted to decrease the exposure to avacopan. Avoid or monitor. Severe Study

▸ **Lumacaftor** is predicted to decrease the exposure to avapritinib. Avoid. Severe Study

▸ **Lumacaftor** is predicted to decrease the exposure to axitinib. Avoid or adjust dose. Moderate Study

▸ **Lumacaftor** decreases the exposure to bedaquiline. Avoid. Severe Study

- **Lumacaftor** is predicted to decrease the exposure to belumosudil. Adjust **belumosudil** dose, p. 979. Severe Study
- **Lumacaftor** is predicted to decrease the exposure to benzodiazepines **(alprazolam)**. Adjust dose. Moderate Theoretical
- **Lumacaftor** is predicted to decrease the exposure to benzodiazepines **(midazolam)**. Monitor and adjust dose. Severe Study
- **Lumacaftor** is predicted to decrease the exposure to bictegravir. Avoid. Moderate Study
- **Lumacaftor** slightly decreases the exposure to bortezomib. Avoid. Severe Study
- **Lumacaftor** is predicted to very markedly decrease the exposure to bosutinib. Avoid. Severe Study
- **Lumacaftor** is predicted to decrease the exposure to brigatinib. Avoid. Severe Study
- **Lumacaftor** is predicted to decrease the exposure to bupropion. Adjust dose. Moderate Theoretical
- **Lumacaftor** is predicted to decrease the exposure to buspirone. Use with caution and adjust dose. Severe Study
- **Lumacaftor** moderately decreases the exposure to cabozantinib. Avoid. Moderate Study
- **Lumacaftor** is predicted to decrease the exposure to calcium channel blockers **(amlodipine, felodipine, lacidipine, lercanidipine, nicardipine, nifedipine, nimodipine)**. Monitor and adjust dose. Moderate Study
- **Lumacaftor** is predicted to decrease the exposure to cannabidiol. Adjust dose. Moderate Study
- **Lumacaftor** is predicted to decrease the exposure to capivasertib. Avoid. Moderate Study
- **Lumacaftor** is predicted to decrease the exposure to ceritinib. Avoid. Severe Study
- **Lumacaftor** decreases the concentration of ciclosporin. Severe Study
- **Lumacaftor** is predicted to alter the effects of cilostazol. Moderate Theoretical
- **Lumacaftor** is predicted to decrease the exposure to cinacalcet. Monitor and adjust dose. Moderate Study
- **Lumacaftor** decreases the exposure to clomethiazole. Monitor and adjust dose. Moderate Study
- **Lumacaftor** is predicted to decrease the exposure to cobicistat. Avoid. Severe Study
- **Lumacaftor** is predicted to decrease the exposure to cobimetinib. Avoid. Severe Theoretical
- **Lumacaftor** is predicted to decrease the exposure to combined hormonal contraceptives. Use additional contraceptive precautions. Severe Theoretical
- **Lumacaftor** is predicted to decrease the exposure to corticosteroids **(budesonide, deflazacort, dexamethasone, fludrocortisone, hydrocortisone, methylprednisolone, prednisolone, triamcinolone)**. Monitor and adjust dose. Moderate Study
- **Lumacaftor** is predicted to decrease the exposure to corticosteroids **(fluticasone)**. Unknown Theoretical
- **Lumacaftor** is predicted to markedly decrease the exposure to crizotinib. Avoid. Severe Study
- **Lumacaftor** is predicted to decrease the exposure to dabrafenib. Avoid. Moderate Theoretical
- **Lumacaftor** is predicted to decrease the exposure to daridorexant. Severe Study
- **Lumacaftor** is predicted to decrease the exposure to darifenacin. Moderate Theoretical
- **Lumacaftor** is predicted to markedly decrease the exposure to dasatinib. Avoid. Severe Study
- **Lumacaftor** is predicted to slightly decrease the exposure to delamanid. Avoid. Moderate Study
- **Lumacaftor** might decrease the efficacy of desogestrel. Use additional contraceptive precautions. Severe Theoretical
- **Lumacaftor** is predicted to markedly decrease the exposure to dienogest. Severe Study
- **Lumacaftor** is predicted to decrease the exposure to dipeptidylpeptidase-4 inhibitors **(linagliptin)**. Moderate Study
- **Lumacaftor** is predicted to moderately decrease the exposure to dipeptidylpeptidase-4 inhibitors **(saxagliptin)**. Moderate Study
- **Lumacaftor** is predicted to decrease the exposure to dronabinol. Avoid or adjust dose. Mild Study

- **Lumacaftor** is predicted to decrease the efficacy of drospirenone. Use additional contraceptive precautions. Severe Theoretical
- **Lumacaftor** is predicted to decrease the exposure to elacestrant. Avoid or adjust dose depending on duration—consult product literature. Severe Study
- **Lumacaftor** is predicted to decrease the exposure to elbasvir. Avoid. Severe Study
- **Lumacaftor** is predicted to decreases the exposure to elexacaftor. Avoid. Severe Theoretical
- **Lumacaftor** is predicted to decrease the exposure to eliglustat. Avoid. Severe Study
- **Lumacaftor** is predicted to decrease the concentration of elvitegravir. Avoid. Severe Study
- **Lumacaftor** is predicted to decrease the exposure to encorafenib. Severe Theoretical
- **Lumacaftor** affects the exposure to endothelin receptor antagonists **(bosentan)**. Avoid. Severe Study
- **Lumacaftor** is predicted to decrease the exposure to endothelin receptor antagonists **(macitentan)**. Avoid. Severe Study
- **Lumacaftor** is predicted to decrease the exposure to the cytotoxic component of enfortumab vedotin. Moderate Theoretical
- **Lumacaftor** is predicted to decrease the exposure to entrectinib. Avoid. Severe Study
- **Lumacaftor** is predicted to decrease the exposure to erdafitinib. Avoid. Severe Study
- **Lumacaftor** is predicted to decrease the exposure to erlotinib. Avoid or adjust dose—consult product literature. Severe Study
- **Lumacaftor** is predicted to decrease the exposure to esketamine. Adjust dose. Mild Theoretical
- **Lumacaftor** is predicted to decrease the exposure to eszopiclone. Adjust dose. Moderate Theoretical
- **Lumacaftor** might decrease the efficacy of subdermal etonogestrel. Use additional contraceptive precautions. Severe Theoretical
- **Lumacaftor** is predicted to decrease the concentration of everolimus. Avoid or adjust dose. Severe Study
- **Lumacaftor** moderately decreases the exposure to exemestane. Moderate Study
- **Lumacaftor** is predicted to decrease the exposure to fedratinib. Avoid. Moderate Study
- **Lumacaftor** is predicted to decrease the exposure to fesoterodine. Avoid. Moderate Study
- **Lumacaftor** is predicted to decrease the exposure to fostamatinib. Avoid. Severe Study
- **Lumacaftor** is predicted to decrease the exposure to the active metabolite of fostemsavir. Avoid. Severe Study
- **Lumacaftor** is predicted to decrease the exposure to fruquintinib. Avoid. Moderate Study
- **Lumacaftor** is predicted to decrease the exposure to gefitinib. Avoid. Severe Study
- **Lumacaftor** is predicted to decrease the exposure to glasdegib. Avoid. Severe Study
- **Lumacaftor** potentially decreases the exposure to glecaprevir. Avoid. Severe Theoretical
- **Lumacaftor** is predicted to decrease the exposure to grazoprevir. Avoid. Severe Study
- **Lumacaftor** is predicted to decrease the concentration of guanfacine. Adjust **guanfacine** dose, p. 407. Moderate Study
- **Lumacaftor** decreases the concentration of haloperidol. Adjust dose. Moderate Study
- **Lumacaftor** is predicted to decrease the exposure to ibrutinib. Avoid or monitor. Severe Study
- **Lumacaftor** is predicted to decrease the exposure to idelalisib. Avoid. Severe Study
- **Lumacaftor** is predicted to decrease the exposure to imatinib. Avoid. Moderate Study
- **Lumacaftor** is predicted to decrease the exposure to irinotecan. Avoid. Severe Study
- **Lumacaftor** is predicted to decrease the exposure to ivabradine. Adjust dose. Moderate Theoretical
- **Lumacaftor** is predicted to decrease the exposure to ivacaftor. Avoid. Severe Study

Lumacaftor (continued)
- **Lumacaftor** is predicted to decrease the exposure to ixazomib. Avoid. Severe Study
- **Lumacaftor** is predicted to decrease the exposure to lapatinib. Avoid. Severe Study
- **Lumacaftor** is predicted to moderately decrease the exposure to larotrectinib. Avoid. Moderate Study
- **Lumacaftor** is predicted to decrease the exposure to leniolisib. Avoid. Severe Theoretical
- **Lumacaftor** is predicted to decrease the efficacy of levonorgestrel. Use additional contraceptive precautions. Severe Theoretical
- **Lumacaftor** is predicted to decrease the exposure to lomitapide. Monitor and adjust dose. Moderate Theoretical
- **Lumacaftor** is predicted to decrease the exposure to lorlatinib. Avoid. Severe Study
- **Lumacaftor** is predicted to decrease the exposure to macrolides (clarithromycin, erythromycin). Moderate Theoretical
- **Lumacaftor** is predicted to decrease the exposure to maraviroc. Adjust dose. Severe Study
- **Lumacaftor** is predicted to decrease the exposure to mavacamten. Monitor and adjust dose—consult product literature. Severe Theoretical
- **Lumacaftor** is predicted to decrease the exposure to meglitinides (repaglinide). Monitor blood glucose and adjust dose. Moderate Study
- **Lumacaftor** is predicted to decrease the exposure to midostaurin. Avoid. Severe Study
- **Lumacaftor** is predicted to decrease the exposure to mifepristone. Adjust **mifepristone** dose, p. 954. Severe Study
- **Lumacaftor** is predicted to decrease the exposure to mineralocorticoid receptor antagonists (eplerenone). Avoid. Moderate Theoretical
- **Lumacaftor** is predicted to decrease the exposure to mineralocorticoid receptor antagonists (finerenone). Avoid. Severe Study
- **Lumacaftor** is predicted to decrease the exposure to mirtazapine. Adjust dose. Moderate Study
- **Lumacaftor** is predicted to decrease the exposure to mobocertinib. Avoid. Severe Study
- **Lumacaftor** is predicted to decrease the exposure to monoclonal antibodies (polatuzumab vedotin). Moderate Theoretical
- **Lumacaftor** is predicted to decrease the exposure to the cytotoxic component of monoclonal antibodies (trastuzumab emtansine). Severe Theoretical
- **Lumacaftor** is predicted to decrease the exposure to montelukast. Mild Study
- **Lumacaftor** is predicted to markedly decrease the exposure to naldemedine. Avoid. Severe Study
- **Lumacaftor** is predicted to markedly decrease the exposure to naloxegol. Avoid. Moderate Study
- **Lumacaftor** is predicted to decrease the exposure to neratinib. Avoid. Severe Study
- **Lumacaftor** is predicted to markedly decrease the exposure to neurokinin-1 receptor antagonists (aprepitant). Avoid. Moderate Study
- **Lumacaftor** is predicted to decrease the exposure to neurokinin-1 receptor antagonists (fosaprepitant). Avoid. Moderate Theoretical
- **Lumacaftor** is predicted to decrease the exposure to neurokinin-1 receptor antagonists (netupitant). Avoid. Severe Study
- **Lumacaftor** is predicted to moderately decrease the exposure to nilotinib. Avoid. Severe Study
- **Lumacaftor** is predicted to decrease the exposure to nirmatrelvir boosted with ritonavir. Avoid. Severe Study
- **Lumacaftor** is predicted to decrease the exposure to nitisinone. Adjust dose. Moderate Theoretical
- **Lumacaftor** is predicted to decrease the exposure to NNRTIs (doravirine). Avoid. Severe Study
- **Lumacaftor** is predicted to decrease the exposure to NNRTIs (etravirine). Avoid. Severe Theoretical
- **Lumacaftor** markedly decreases the exposure to NNRTIs (rilpivirine). Avoid. Severe Study

- **Lumacaftor** might decrease the efficacy of norethisterone. Use additional contraceptive precautions. Severe Theoretical
- **Lumacaftor** is predicted to decrease the exposure to olaparib. Avoid. Moderate Theoretical
- **Lumacaftor** is predicted to decrease the exposure to opioids (alfentanil, fentanyl). Moderate Study
- **Lumacaftor** is predicted to decrease the exposure to opioids (buprenorphine). Monitor and adjust dose. Moderate Theoretical
- **Lumacaftor** decreases the exposure to opioids (methadone). Monitor and adjust dose. Severe Study
- **Lumacaftor** is predicted to decrease the exposure to opioids (oxycodone). Monitor and adjust dose. Moderate Study
- **Lumacaftor** is predicted to decrease the exposure to osilodrostat. Moderate Theoretical
- **Lumacaftor** is predicted to moderately decrease the exposure to osimertinib. Avoid. Moderate Study
- **Lumacaftor** is predicted to moderately decrease the exposure to ospemifene. Moderate Study
- **Lumacaftor** is predicted to decrease the exposure to palbociclib. Avoid. Severe Study
- **Lumacaftor** is predicted to decrease the exposure to panobinostat. Avoid. Moderate Theoretical
- **Lumacaftor** is predicted to decrease the exposure to pazopanib. Avoid. Severe Theoretical
- **Lumacaftor** is predicted to decrease the exposure to pemigatinib. Avoid. Severe Study
- **Lumacaftor** moderately decreases the exposure to phosphodiesterase type-4 inhibitors (apremilast). Avoid. Severe Study
- **Lumacaftor** is predicted to decrease the exposure to phosphodiesterase type-4 inhibitors (roflumilast). Avoid. Moderate Study
- **Lumacaftor** is predicted to decrease the exposure to phosphodiesterase type-5 inhibitors (avanafil, tadalafil). Avoid. Severe Study
- **Lumacaftor** is predicted to decrease the exposure to phosphodiesterase type-5 inhibitors (sildenafil, vardenafil). Moderate Theoretical
- **Lumacaftor** is predicted to moderately to markedly decrease the exposure to pibrentasvir. Avoid. Severe Study
- **Lumacaftor** is predicted to moderately decrease the exposure to pitolisant. Moderate Study
- **Lumacaftor** is predicted to decrease the exposure to ponatinib. Avoid. Moderate Theoretical
- **Lumacaftor** is predicted to decrease the exposure to pralsetinib. Avoid or adjust dose with potent CYP3A4 inducers—consult product literature. Moderate Study
- **Lumacaftor** is predicted to markedly decrease the exposure to praziquantel. Avoid. Moderate Study
- **Lumacaftor** is predicted to decrease the exposure to quizartinib. Avoid. Severe Study
- **Lumacaftor** is predicted to decrease the exposure to ranolazine. Avoid. Severe Study
- **Lumacaftor** is predicted to decrease the exposure to reboxetine. Moderate Anecdotal
- **Lumacaftor** is predicted to decrease the exposure to regorafenib. Avoid. Moderate Study
- **Lumacaftor** is predicted to markedly decrease the exposure to ribociclib. Avoid. Severe Study
- **Lumacaftor** is predicted to decrease the exposure to rifamycins (rifabutin). Adjust dose. Moderate Theoretical
- **Lumacaftor** is predicted to decrease the exposure to rimegepant. Avoid. Moderate Theoretical
- **Lumacaftor** is predicted to decrease the exposure to ripretinib. Avoid or adjust dose—consult product literature. Severe Study
- **Lumacaftor** is predicted to decrease the exposure to ruxolitinib. Monitor and adjust dose. Moderate Study
- **Lumacaftor** is predicted to decrease the exposure to selpercatinib. Avoid. Moderate Study
- **Lumacaftor** is predicted to decrease the exposure to selumetinib. Avoid. Severe Study
- **Lumacaftor** is predicted to decrease the exposure to siponimod. Manufacturer advises caution depending on genotype—consult product literature. Severe Study

- ▶ **Lumacaftor** is predicted to decrease the concentration of sirolimus. Avoid or monitor and adjust dose. [Severe] Study
- ▶ **Lumacaftor** is predicted to decrease the exposure to solifenacin. [Moderate] Theoretical
- ▶ **Lumacaftor** is predicted to decrease the exposure to sorafenib. [Moderate] Theoretical
- ▶ **Lumacaftor** is predicted to decrease the exposure to sotorasib. Avoid. [Severe] Study
- ▶ **Lumacaftor** is predicted to decrease the exposure to sunitinib. Avoid or adjust dose—consult product literature. [Moderate] Study
- ▶ **Lumacaftor** decreases the concentration of tacrolimus. Avoid or monitor and adjust dose. [Severe] Study
- ▶ **Lumacaftor** is predicted to decrease the exposure to taxanes (cabazitaxel). Avoid. [Moderate] Study
- ▶ **Lumacaftor** is predicted to decrease the exposure to taxanes (docetaxel). [Severe] Theoretical
- ▶ **Lumacaftor** is predicted to decrease the exposure to taxanes (paclitaxel). Avoid. [Severe] Study
- ▶ **Lumacaftor** is predicted to decrease the concentration of temsirolimus. Avoid. [Severe] Study
- ▶ **Lumacaftor** might decrease the exposure to tepotinib. Avoid. [Severe] Theoretical
- ▶ **Lumacaftor** is predicted to decrease the exposure to tetracyclines (eravacycline). Adjust **eravacycline** dose, p. 657. [Moderate] Study
- ▶ **Lumacaftor** is predicted to decrease the exposure to tezacaftor. Avoid. [Severe] Theoretical
- ▶ **Lumacaftor** is predicted to markedly decrease the exposure to ticagrelor. Avoid. [Severe] Study
- ▶ **Lumacaftor** is predicted to decrease the exposure to tivozanib. [Severe] Study
- ▶ **Lumacaftor** is predicted to decrease the exposure to tofacitinib. Avoid. [Severe] Study
- ▶ **Lumacaftor** is predicted to decrease the exposure to tolvaptan. Use with caution or avoid depending on indication. [Severe] Study
- ▶ **Lumacaftor** is predicted to decrease the exposure to toremifene. Adjust dose. [Moderate] Study
- ▶ **Lumacaftor** is predicted to decrease the exposure to trabectedin. Avoid. [Severe] Theoretical
- ▶ **Lumacaftor** is predicted to decrease the exposure to tucatinib. Avoid. [Severe] Study
- ▶ **Lumacaftor** is predicted to decrease the efficacy of ulipristal. Use additional contraceptive precautions. [Severe] Theoretical
- ▶ **Lumacaftor** is predicted to decrease the exposure to upadacitinib. [Moderate] Study
- ▶ **Lumacaftor** is predicted to decrease the exposure to vandetanib. Avoid. [Moderate] Study
- ▶ **Lumacaftor** is predicted to moderately decrease the exposure to velpatasvir. Avoid. [Severe] Study
- ▶ **Lumacaftor** is predicted to decrease the exposure to vemurafenib. Avoid. [Severe] Study
- ▶ **Lumacaftor** is predicted to decrease the exposure to venetoclax. Avoid. [Severe] Study
- ▶ **Lumacaftor** is predicted to decrease the exposure to vinca alkaloids (vinblastine, vincristine, vindesine). [Severe] Theoretical
- ▶ **Lumacaftor** is predicted to decrease the exposure to vinca alkaloids (vinorelbine). Use with caution or avoid. [Severe] Theoretical
- ▶ **Lumacaftor** is predicted to decrease the exposure to vismodegib. Avoid. [Moderate] Theoretical
- ▶ **Lumacaftor** is predicted to decrease the exposure to voclosporin. Avoid. [Severe] Study
- ▶ **Lumacaftor** is predicted to decrease the exposure to vortioxetine. Monitor and adjust dose. [Moderate] Study
- ▶ **Lumacaftor** is predicted to decrease the concentration of voxilaprevir. Avoid. [Severe] Study
- ▶ **Lumacaftor** is predicted to decrease the exposure to zanubrutinib. Avoid. [Severe] Study
- ▶ **Lumacaftor** is predicted to decrease the exposure to zopiclone. Adjust dose. [Moderate] Study

Lumefantrine → see antimalarials

Lurasidone → see antipsychotics, second generation

Lymecycline → see tetracyclines

Macitentan → see endothelin receptor antagonists

Macrogol 3350

> **SEPARATION OF ADMINISTRATION** Macrogol-containing preparations have been reported to decrease the efficacy of some drugs (such as antiepileptics) when given concurrently. Some manufacturers advise that other oral drugs should be avoided for 1 hour before, or 1 hour after, macrogol-containing preparations.

Macrolides → see TABLE 8 p. 1573 (QT-interval prolongation)

azithromycin · clarithromycin · erythromycin

> - ▶ Interactions do not generally apply to topical use of **azithromycin** unless specified.
> - ▶ Since systemic absorption can follow topical application of **erythromycin**, the possibility of interactions should be borne in mind.

- ▶ **Clarithromycin** is predicted to increase the exposure to abemaciclib. Avoid or adjust dose—consult product literature. [Severe] Study
- ▶ **Erythromycin** is predicted to increase the exposure to abemaciclib. [Moderate] Study
- ▶ **Clarithromycin** is predicted to increase the exposure to acalabrutinib. Avoid. [Severe] Study
- ▶ **Erythromycin** is predicted to increase the exposure to acalabrutinib. Avoid or monitor. [Severe] Study
- ▶ **Macrolides** are predicted to increase the exposure to afatinib. [Moderate] Study
- ▶ **Azithromycin** is predicted to increase the exposure to aliskiren. [Moderate] Theoretical
- ▶ Macrolides (clarithromycin, erythromycin) are predicted to increase the exposure to aliskiren. [Moderate] Study
- ▶ **Clarithromycin** is predicted to moderately increase the exposure to alpha blockers (alfuzosin, tamsulosin). Use with caution or avoid. [Moderate] Study
- ▶ **Clarithromycin** is predicted to increase the exposure to alpha blockers (doxazosin). [Moderate] Study
- ▶ **Erythromycin** is predicted to increase the exposure to alpha blockers (tamsulosin). [Moderate] Theoretical
- ▶ **Azithromycin** is predicted to increase the exposure to aminophylline. [Moderate] Theoretical
- ▶ **Clarithromycin** is predicted to increase the exposure to aminophylline. Adjust dose. [Moderate] Theoretical
- ▶ **Aminophylline** is predicted to decrease the exposure to erythromycin. Adjust dose. [Severe] Study
- ▶ Anti-androgens (enzalutamide) are predicted to affect the exposure to **clarithromycin**. Use with caution or avoid. [Moderate] Theoretical
- ▶ **Clarithromycin** is predicted to increase the exposure to anti-androgens (apalutamide). Monitor and adjust dose. [Mild] Study
- ▶ **Clarithromycin** is predicted to increase the exposure to anti-androgens (darolutamide). Monitor and adjust dose. [Moderate] Theoretical
- ▶ **Clarithromycin** is predicted to increase the exposure to antiarrhythmics (amiodarone). Avoid. [Moderate] Theoretical
- ▶ **Clarithromycin** very markedly increases the exposure to antiarrhythmics (dronedarone). Avoid. [Severe] Study
- ▶ **Erythromycin** is predicted to moderately increase the exposure to antiarrhythmics (dronedarone). Avoid. [Severe] Theoretical → Also see TABLE 8 p. 1573
- ▶ Macrolides (clarithromycin, erythromycin) are predicted to increase the exposure to antiarrhythmics (lidocaine). [Moderate] Theoretical
- ▶ **Clarithromycin** is predicted to increase the exposure to antiarrhythmics (propafenone). Monitor and adjust dose. [Severe] Study
- ▶ **Erythromycin** is predicted to increase the exposure to antiarrhythmics (propafenone). Monitor and adjust dose. [Moderate] Study
- ▶ **Clarithromycin** is predicted to increase the exposure to anticholinesterases, centrally acting (galantamine). Monitor and adjust dose. [Moderate] Study
- ▶ **Clarithromycin** slightly increases the concentration of antiepileptics (carbamazepine). Monitor concentration and adjust dose. [Severe] Study

Macrolides (continued)

▶ **Erythromycin** markedly increases the concentration of antiepileptics (carbamazepine). Monitor concentration and adjust dose. [Severe] Study

▶ **Clarithromycin** is predicted to very slightly increase the exposure to antiepileptics (perampanel). [Mild] Study

▶ **Clarithromycin** is predicted to increase the exposure to antifungals, azoles (isavuconazole). Avoid or monitor adverse effects. [Severe] Study

▶ **Erythromycin** is predicted to increase the exposure to antifungals, azoles (isavuconazole). [Moderate] Theoretical

▶ **Clarithromycin** is predicted to increase the exposure to antihistamines, non-sedating (fexofenadine). [Moderate] Theoretical

▶ **Clarithromycin** is predicted to increase the exposure to antihistamines, non-sedating (mizolastine). Avoid. [Severe] Study

▶ **Erythromycin** is predicted to increase the exposure to antihistamines, non-sedating (mizolastine). [Severe] Theoretical

▶ Macrolides **(clarithromycin, erythromycin)** are predicted to increase the exposure to antihistamines, non-sedating (rupatadine). Avoid. [Moderate] Study

▶ **Macrolides** might increase the risk of serious cardiovascular adverse effects when given with antimalarials (chloroquine). [Severe] Theoretical

▶ **Clarithromycin** is predicted to slightly increase the exposure to antipsychotics, second generation (aripiprazole). Adjust **aripiprazole** dose, p. 454. [Moderate] Study

▶ **Clarithromycin** is predicted to moderately increase the exposure to antipsychotics, second generation (cariprazine). Avoid. [Severe] Study

▶ **Erythromycin** is predicted to increase the exposure to antipsychotics, second generation (cariprazine). Avoid. [Severe] Study

▶ **Erythromycin** potentially increases the risk of toxicity when given with antipsychotics, second generation (clozapine). [Severe] Anecdotal

▶ **Erythromycin** is predicted to increase the exposure to antipsychotics, second generation (lurasidone). Adjust **lurasidone** dose. [Moderate] Study

▶ **Clarithromycin** is predicted to increase the exposure to antipsychotics, second generation (lurasidone, quetiapine). Avoid. [Severe] Study

▶ **Erythromycin** is predicted to increase the exposure to antipsychotics, second generation (quetiapine). Avoid. [Moderate] Study

▶ **Clarithromycin** is predicted to increase the exposure to antipsychotics, second generation (risperidone). Adjust dose. [Moderate] Study

▶ **Clarithromycin** is predicted to increase the exposure to atogepant. Adjust **atogepant** dose, p. 540. [Moderate] Study

▶ **Erythromycin** is predicted to increase the exposure to atogepant. Adjust **atogepant** dose, p. 540. [Moderate] Theoretical

▶ **Clarithromycin** is predicted to increase the exposure to avacopan. [Severe] Study

▶ **Clarithromycin** is predicted to increase the exposure to avapritinib. Avoid. [Moderate] Study

▶ **Erythromycin** is predicted to increase the exposure to avapritinib. Avoid or adjust dose—consult product literature. [Moderate] Study

▶ **Clarithromycin** is predicted to increase the exposure to axitinib. Avoid or adjust dose. [Moderate] Study

▶ **Erythromycin** is predicted to increase the exposure to axitinib. [Moderate] Study

▶ **Clarithromycin** might increases the exposure to bedaquiline. [Mild] Study

▶ **Erythromycin** might increases the exposure to bedaquiline. [Mild] Theoretical → Also see **TABLE 8** p. 1573

▶ **Clarithromycin** moderately increases the exposure to benzodiazepines (alprazolam). Avoid. [Moderate] Study

▶ **Erythromycin** is predicted to increase the exposure to benzodiazepines (alprazolam). [Severe] Study

▶ **Clarithromycin** is predicted to markedly to very markedly increase the exposure to benzodiazepines (midazolam). Avoid or adjust dose. [Severe] Study

▶ **Erythromycin** is predicted to increase the exposure to benzodiazepines (midazolam). Monitor adverse effects and adjust dose. [Severe] Study

▶ **Macrolides** are predicted to increase the exposure to beta blockers, non-selective (nadolol). [Moderate] Study

▶ **Clarithromycin** is predicted to increase the exposure to beta$_2$ agonists (salmeterol). Avoid. [Severe] Study

▶ **Macrolides** are predicted to increase the exposure to bictegravir. Use with caution or avoid. [Moderate] Theoretical

▶ **Clarithromycin** slightly increases the exposure to bortezomib. [Moderate] Study

▶ Macrolides **(clarithromycin, erythromycin)** are predicted to increase the exposure to bosutinib. Avoid or adjust dose. [Severe] Study → Also see **TABLE 8** p. 1573

▶ **Clarithromycin** is predicted to increase the exposure to brigatinib. Avoid or adjust dose—consult product literature. [Severe] Study

▶ **Erythromycin** is predicted to increase the exposure to brigatinib. [Moderate] Study

▶ **Clarithromycin** is predicted to increase the exposure to buspirone. Adjust **buspirone** dose, p. 396. [Severe] Study

▶ **Erythromycin** is predicted to increase the exposure to buspirone. Use with caution and adjust dose. [Moderate] Study

▶ Macrolides **(clarithromycin, erythromycin)** are predicted to increase the exposure to cabozantinib. [Moderate] Study → Also see **TABLE 8** p. 1573

▶ **Erythromycin** is predicted to increase the exposure to calcium channel blockers (amlodipine, felodipine, lacidipine, lercanidipine, nicardipine, nifedipine, nimodipine). Monitor and adjust dose. [Moderate] Study

▶ **Clarithromycin** is predicted to increase the exposure to calcium channel blockers (amlodipine, felodipine, lacidipine, nicardipine, nifedipine, nimodipine). Monitor and adjust dose. [Moderate] Study

▶ **Erythromycin** is predicted to increase the exposure to calcium channel blockers (diltiazem). [Severe] Theoretical

▶ **Clarithromycin** is predicted to increase the exposure to calcium channel blockers (diltiazem, verapamil). [Severe] Study

▶ **Clarithromycin** is predicted to markedly increase the exposure to calcium channel blockers (lercanidipine). Avoid. [Severe] Study

▶ **Erythromycin** is predicted to increase the exposure to calcium channel blockers (verapamil). [Severe] Study

▶ **Clarithromycin** is predicted to increase the exposure to cannabidiol. Avoid or adjust dose. [Mild] Study

▶ Macrolides **(clarithromycin, erythromycin)** are predicted to increase the exposure to capivasertib. Adjust dose. [Moderate] Study

▶ **Clarithromycin** is predicted to increase the exposure to ceritinib. Avoid or adjust dose—consult product literature. [Severe] Study

▶ **Erythromycin** is predicted to increase the exposure to ceritinib. [Moderate] Study → Also see **TABLE 8** p. 1573

▶ **Clarithromycin** increases the concentration of ciclosporin. [Severe] Study

▶ **Erythromycin** greatly increases the exposure to ciclosporin. Avoid or monitor. [Severe] Study

▶ **Clarithromycin** is predicted to moderately increase the exposure to cilostazol. Adjust **cilostazol** dose, p. 266. [Moderate] Study

▶ **Erythromycin** slightly increases the exposure to cilostazol. Adjust **cilostazol** dose, p. 266. [Moderate] Study

▶ **Clarithromycin** is predicted to moderately increase the exposure to cinacalcet. Adjust dose. [Moderate] Study

▶ **Cobicistat** is predicted to increase the concentration of erythromycin. [Moderate] Theoretical

▶ **Clarithromycin** is predicted to increase the exposure to cobimetinib. Avoid or monitor for toxicity. [Severe] Study

▶ **Erythromycin** is predicted to increase the exposure to cobimetinib. [Severe] Study

▶ **Azithromycin** is predicted to increase the exposure to colchicine. Avoid P-glycoprotein inhibitors or adjust **colchicine** dose, p. 1279. [Severe] Theoretical

▶ **Clarithromycin** is predicted to increase the exposure to colchicine. Avoid potent CYP3A4 inhibitors or adjust **colchicine** dose, p. 1279. [Severe] Study

- **Erythromycin** is predicted to increase the exposure to colchicine. Adjust **colchicine** dose with moderate CYP3A4 inhibitors, p. 1279. Severe Study
- **Clarithromycin** is predicted to increase the exposure to corticosteroids (beclometasone) (risk with beclometasone is likely to be lower than with other corticosteroids). Moderate Theoretical
- **Clarithromycin** is predicted to increase the exposure to corticosteroids (betamethasone, budesonide, ciclesonide, deflazacort, dexamethasone, fludrocortisone, fluticasone, hydrocortisone, methylprednisolone, mometasone, prednisolone, triamcinolone). Avoid or monitor adverse effects. Severe Study
- **Erythromycin** is predicted to increase the exposure to corticosteroids (methylprednisolone). Monitor and adjust dose. Moderate Study
- **Clarithromycin** is predicted to increase the exposure to corticosteroids (vamorolone). Adjust dose. Severe Study
- **Azithromycin** might increase the risk of bleeding events when given with coumarins. Severe Anecdotal
- Macrolides (clarithromycin, erythromycin) increase the anticoagulant effect of coumarins. Monitor INR and adjust dose. Severe Anecdotal
- Macrolides (clarithromycin, erythromycin) are predicted to increase the exposure to crizotinib. Avoid. Moderate Study → Also see **TABLE 8** p. 1573
- **Clarithromycin** is predicted to increase the exposure to dabrafenib. Use with caution or avoid. Moderate Study
- **Erythromycin** is predicted to increase the exposure to dabrafenib. Moderate Study
- **Clarithromycin** is predicted to increase the exposure to daridorexant. Avoid. Severe Study
- **Erythromycin** is predicted to increase the exposure to daridorexant. Adjust **daridorexant** dose, p. 554. Severe Study
- **Clarithromycin** is predicted to markedly to very markedly increase the exposure to darifenacin. Avoid. Severe Study
- **Erythromycin** slightly increases the exposure to darifenacin. Moderate Study
- **Clarithromycin** is predicted to increase the exposure to dasatinib. Avoid or adjust dose—consult product literature. Severe Study
- **Erythromycin** is predicted to increase the exposure to dasatinib. Severe Study → Also see **TABLE 8** p. 1573
- **Clarithromycin** very slightly increases the exposure to delamanid. Severe Study
- **Clarithromycin** is predicted to moderately increase the exposure to dienogest. Moderate Study
- **Erythromycin** is predicted to slightly increase the exposure to dienogest. Moderate Study
- **Macrolides** increase the concentration of digoxin. Severe Anecdotal
- **Clarithromycin** is predicted to increase the exposure to dipeptidylpeptidase-4 inhibitors (saxagliptin). Moderate Study
- **Erythromycin** is predicted to increase the exposure to dipeptidylpeptidase-4 inhibitors (saxagliptin). Mild Study
- Macrolides (clarithromycin, erythromycin) are predicted to increase the exposure to domperidone. Avoid. Severe Study
- **Clarithromycin** increases the exposure to dopamine receptor agonists (bromocriptine). Severe Study
- **Erythromycin** is predicted to increase the exposure to dopamine receptor agonists (bromocriptine). Severe Theoretical
- Macrolides (clarithromycin, erythromycin) are predicted to increase the concentration of dopamine receptor agonists (cabergoline). Avoid. Severe Study
- **Clarithromycin** is predicted to increase the exposure to dronabinol. Adjust dose. Mild Study
- Macrolides (clarithromycin, erythromycin) are predicted to increase the exposure to drospirenone. Severe Study
- **Clarithromycin** is predicted to increase the exposure to dutasteride. Monitor adverse effects and adjust dose. Moderate Theoretical
- **Erythromycin** is predicted to moderately increase the exposure to dutasteride. Mild Study

- **Clarithromycin** is predicted to increase the exposure to elacestrant. Avoid potent CYP3A4 inhibitors or adjust **elacestrant** dose, p. 1084. Severe Study
- **Erythromycin** is predicted to increase the exposure to elacestrant. Avoid moderate CYP3A4 inhibitors or adjust **elacestrant** dose, p. 1084. Severe Theoretical
- **Clarithromycin** is predicted to increase the exposure to elexacaftor. Adjust ivacaftor with tezacaftor and elexacaftor p. 337 dose with potent CYP3A4 inhibitors. Severe Study
- **Erythromycin** is predicted to increase the exposure to elexacaftor. Adjust ivacaftor with tezacaftor and elexacaftor p. 337 dose with moderate CYP3A4 inhibitors. Severe Theoretical
- Macrolides (clarithromycin, erythromycin) are predicted to increase the exposure to eliglustat. Avoid or adjust dose—consult product literature. Severe Study
- **Clarithromycin** is predicted to increase the exposure to encorafenib. Avoid or monitor. Severe Study
- **Erythromycin** is predicted to moderately increase the exposure to encorafenib. Moderate Study → Also see **TABLE 8** p. 1573
- **Clarithromycin** is predicted to increase the exposure to endothelin receptor antagonists (bosentan). Moderate Theoretical
- **Clarithromycin** is predicted to increase the exposure to endothelin receptor antagonists (macitentan). Moderate Study
- **Erythromycin** is predicted to increase the exposure to endothelin receptor antagonists (macitentan). Manufacturer advises caution depending on other drugs taken—consult product literature. Moderate Theoretical
- **Clarithromycin** is predicted to increase the exposure to the cytotoxic component of enfortumab vedotin. Severe Theoretical
- **Clarithromycin** is predicted to increase the exposure to entrectinib. Avoid or adjust dose with potent CYP3A4 inhibitors—consult product literature. Severe Study
- **Erythromycin** is predicted to increase the exposure to entrectinib. Avoid or adjust dose with moderate CYP3A4 inhibitors—consult product literature. Severe Theoretical → Also see **TABLE 8** p. 1573
- **Clarithromycin** is predicted to increase the exposure to erdafitinib. Adjust dose. Severe Study
- **Clarithromycin** is predicted to increase the risk of ergotism when given with ergometrine. Avoid. Severe Theoretical
- **Erythromycin** is predicted to increase the risk of ergotism when given with ergometrine. Severe Theoretical
- **Azithromycin** is predicted to increase the exposure to erlotinib. Moderate Theoretical
- **Clarithromycin** is predicted to increase the exposure to erlotinib. Use with caution and adjust dose. Severe Study
- **Erythromycin** is predicted to increase the exposure to erlotinib. Moderate Study
- **Clarithromycin** is predicted to increase the exposure to esketamine. Adjust dose. Moderate Study
- **Clarithromycin** is predicted to increase the exposure to eszopiclone. Adjust **eszopiclone** dose; avoid in the elderly, p. 554. Moderate Study
- **Clarithromycin** is predicted to increase the concentration of subdermal etonogestrel. Moderate Theoretical
- Macrolides (clarithromycin, erythromycin) are predicted to increase the exposure to etrasimod. Avoid in poor CYP2C9 metabolisers. Severe Theoretical
- **Clarithromycin** is predicted to increase the exposure to everolimus. Avoid. Severe Study
- **Erythromycin** is predicted to increase the concentration of everolimus. Avoid or adjust dose. Moderate Study
- **Clarithromycin** slightly increases the exposure to factor XA inhibitors (apixaban). Moderate Study
- Macrolides (azithromycin, erythromycin) are predicted to increase the exposure to factor XA inhibitors (apixaban). Moderate Theoretical
- **Erythromycin** slightly increases the exposure to factor XA inhibitors (edoxaban). Adjust **edoxaban** dose, p. 147. Severe Study
- Macrolides (azithromycin, clarithromycin) are predicted to increase the exposure to factor XA inhibitors (edoxaban). Severe Theoretical
- **Erythromycin** slightly increases the exposure to factor XA inhibitors (rivaroxaban). Mild Study

Macrolides (continued)

▸ **Clarithromycin** is predicted to increase the exposure to fedratinib. Adjust dose, but avoid depending on other drugs taken—consult product literature. Moderate Study

▸ **Erythromycin** is predicted to increase the exposure to fedratinib. Monitor and adjust dose. Moderate Study

▸ **Clarithromycin** is predicted to moderately increase the exposure to fesoterodine. Adjust **fesoterodine** dose with potent CYP3A4 inhibitors; avoid in hepatic and renal impairment, p. 897. Severe Study

▸ **Erythromycin** is predicted to increase the exposure to fesoterodine. Adjust **fesoterodine** dose with moderate CYP3A4 inhibitors in hepatic and renal impairment, p. 897. Mild Study

▸ **Macrolides** are predicted to increase the exposure to fidaxomicin. Avoid. Moderate Study

▸ **Clarithromycin** is predicted to increase the exposure to fostamatinib. Monitor adverse effects and adjust dose. Moderate Study

▸ **Clarithromycin** is predicted to increase the exposure to gefitinib. Severe Study

▸ **Erythromycin** is predicted to increase the exposure to gefitinib. Moderate Study

▸ **Clarithromycin** is predicted to increase the exposure to gilteritinib. Moderate Study

▸ **Macrolides (azithromycin, erythromycin)** are predicted to increase the exposure to gilteritinib. Moderate Theoretical

▸ **Clarithromycin** is predicted to increase the exposure to glasdegib. Use with caution or avoid. Severe Study

▸ **Clarithromycin** is predicted to moderately to markedly increase the exposure to grazoprevir. Avoid. Severe Study

▸ **Clarithromycin** is predicted to increase the exposure to guanfacine. Adjust **guanfacine** dose, p. 407. Moderate Study

▸ **Erythromycin** is predicted to increase the concentration of guanfacine. Adjust **guanfacine** dose, p. 407. Moderate Theoretical

▸ H₂ **receptor antagonists (cimetidine)** slightly increase the exposure to **erythromycin**. Moderate Study

▸ HIV-protease inhibitors (atazanavir) are predicted to increase the exposure to **clarithromycin**. Adjust dose in renal impairment. Severe Study

▸ HIV-protease inhibitors (darunavir, fosamprenavir, lopinavir) boosted with ritonavir are predicted to increase the exposure to **clarithromycin**. Adjust dose in renal impairment. Severe Study

▸ HIV-protease inhibitors (ritonavir) increase the exposure to **clarithromycin**. Adjust dose in renal impairment. Severe Study

▸ HIV-protease inhibitors are predicted to increase the exposure to **erythromycin**. Severe Theoretical

▸ **Macrolides** might increase the risk of serious cardiovascular adverse effects when given with hydroxychloroquine. Severe Theoretical → Also see TABLE 8 p. 1573

▸ **Clarithromycin** is predicted to increase the exposure to ibrutinib. Avoid or adjust dose with potent CYP3A4 inhibitors—consult product literature. Severe Study

▸ **Erythromycin** is predicted to increase the exposure to ibrutinib. Adjust dose with moderate CYP3A4 inhibitors—consult product literature. Severe Study

▸ **Macrolides** are predicted to increase the exposure to idelalisib. Moderate Theoretical

▸ **Clarithromycin** is predicted to increase the exposure to imatinib. Moderate Study

▸ **Erythromycin** is predicted to increase the exposure to imatinib. Moderate Theoretical

▸ **Clarithromycin** has been reported to cause hypoglycaemia when given with insulin. Severe Anecdotal

▸ **Clarithromycin** is predicted to increase the risk of toxicity when given with irinotecan. Avoid. Severe Study

▸ **Clarithromycin** is predicted to increase the exposure to ivabradine. Avoid. Severe Study

▸ **Erythromycin** is predicted to increase the exposure to ivabradine. Avoid. Severe Theoretical

▸ **Clarithromycin** is predicted to increase the exposure to ivacaftor. Adjust dose with potent CYP3A4 inhibitors, see ivacaftor p. 336, lumacaftor with ivacaftor p. 338, tezacaftor with ivacaftor p. 339, and ivacaftor with tezacaftor and elexacaftor p. 337. Severe Study

▸ **Erythromycin** is predicted to increase the exposure to ivacaftor. Adjust dose with moderate CYP3A4 inhibitors, see ivacaftor p. 336, tezacaftor with ivacaftor p. 339, and ivacaftor with tezacaftor and elexacaftor p. 337. Moderate Study

▸ **Macrolides (clarithromycin, erythromycin)** are predicted to increase the exposure to ivosidenib. Monitor and adjust dose—consult product literature. Severe Study → Also see TABLE 8 p. 1573

▸ **Clarithromycin** is predicted to increase the exposure to lapatinib. Avoid. Moderate Study

▸ **Erythromycin** is predicted to increase the exposure to lapatinib. Moderate Study → Also see TABLE 8 p. 1573

▸ **Clarithromycin** is predicted to moderately increase the exposure to larotrectinib. Avoid or adjust dose—consult product literature. Moderate Study

▸ **Erythromycin** is predicted to increase the exposure to larotrectinib. Monitor and adjust dose. Moderate Theoretical

▸ **Macrolides (clarithromycin, erythromycin)** are predicted to increase the exposure to leniolisib. Avoid. Moderate Study

▸ **Macrolides (clarithromycin, erythromycin)** are predicted to increase the concentration of letermovir. Moderate Study

▸ **Clarithromycin** increases the exposure to linezolid. Moderate Anecdotal

▸ **Azithromycin** is predicted to increase the exposure to lomitapide. Separate administration by 12 hours. Moderate Theoretical

▸ **Clarithromycin** is predicted to markedly increase the exposure to lomitapide. Avoid. Severe Study

▸ **Erythromycin** is predicted to increase the exposure to lomitapide. Avoid. Moderate Theoretical

▸ **Clarithromycin** is predicted to increase the exposure to lorlatinib. Avoid or adjust dose—consult product literature. Severe Study

▸ **Lumacaftor** is predicted to decrease the exposure to macrolides (clarithromycin, erythromycin). Moderate Theoretical

▸ **Clarithromycin** is predicted to markedly increase the exposure to maraviroc. Adjust dose. Severe Study

▸ **Clarithromycin** is predicted to increase the exposure to mavacamten. Avoid or monitor—consult product literature. Severe Study

▸ **Erythromycin** is predicted to increase the exposure to mavacamten. Adjust dose—consult product literature. Moderate Study

▸ **Clarithromycin** is predicted to increase the concentration of intramuscular medroxyprogesterone. Moderate Theoretical

▸ **Clarithromycin** might cause hypoglycaemia when given with meglitinides (repaglinide). Moderate Anecdotal

▸ **Clarithromycin** is predicted to increase the exposure to midostaurin. Avoid or monitor for toxicity. Severe Study

▸ **Erythromycin** is predicted to increase the exposure to midostaurin. Moderate Theoretical

▸ **Clarithromycin** is predicted to markedly increase the exposure to mineralocorticoid receptor antagonists (eplerenone). Avoid. Severe Study

▸ **Erythromycin** is predicted to increase the exposure to mineralocorticoid receptor antagonists (eplerenone). Adjust **eplerenone** dose, p. 223. Severe Study

▸ **Clarithromycin** is predicted to increase the exposure to mineralocorticoid receptor antagonists (finerenone). Avoid. Severe Study

▸ **Erythromycin** is predicted to increase the exposure to mineralocorticoid receptor antagonists (finerenone). Severe Study

▸ **Clarithromycin** is predicted to increase the exposure to mirabegron. Adjust **mirabegron** dose in hepatic and renal impairment, p. 901. Moderate Study

▸ **Clarithromycin** is predicted to increase the exposure to mirtazapine. Moderate Study

▸ **Clarithromycin** is predicted to increase the exposure to mobocertinib. Avoid. Severe Study

▸ **Erythromycin** is predicted to increase the exposure to mobocertinib. Avoid or adjust dose and monitor ECG—consult product literature. Severe Study → Also see TABLE 8 p. 1573

▸ **Clarithromycin** is predicted to increase the exposure to modafinil. Mild Theoretical

▸ Macrolides **(clarithromycin, erythromycin)** are predicted to increase the exposure to **momelotinib**. [Moderate] Study
▸ **Azithromycin** is predicted to increase the risk of neutropenia when given with monoclonal antibodies **(brentuximab vedotin)**. Monitor and adjust dose. [Severe] Theoretical
▸ **Clarithromycin** is predicted to increase the risk of neutropenia when given with monoclonal antibodies **(brentuximab vedotin)**. Monitor and adjust dose. [Severe] Study
▸ **Erythromycin** increases the risk of neutropenia when given with monoclonal antibodies **(brentuximab vedotin)**. Monitor and adjust dose. [Severe] Theoretical
▸ **Clarithromycin** is predicted to increase the exposure to monoclonal antibodies **(polatuzumab vedotin)**. [Moderate] Theoretical
▸ **Clarithromycin** is predicted to increase the exposure to the cytotoxic component of monoclonal antibodies **(trastuzumab emtansine)**. Avoid or monitor. [Severe] Theoretical
▸ **Clarithromycin** is predicted to increase the exposure to **naldemedine**. Avoid or monitor. [Moderate] Study
▸ Macrolides **(azithromycin, erythromycin)** are predicted to increase the exposure to naldemedine. [Moderate] Study
▸ **Clarithromycin** is predicted to markedly increase the exposure to **naloxegol**. Avoid. [Severe] Study
▸ **Erythromycin** is predicted to increase the exposure to naloxegol. Adjust **naloxegol** dose and monitor adverse effects, p. 72. [Moderate] Study
▸ **Azithromycin** is predicted to increase the exposure to **neratinib**. Avoid or adjust dose and monitor for gastrointestinal adverse effects—consult product literature. [Severe] Study
▸ **Clarithromycin** is predicted to increase the exposure to **neratinib**. Avoid or adjust dose with potent CYP3A4 inhibitors—consult product literature. [Severe] Study
▸ **Erythromycin** is predicted to increase the exposure to **neratinib**. Avoid moderate CYP3A4 inhibitors or adjust dose and monitor for gastrointestinal adverse effects—consult product literature. [Severe] Study
▸ **Clarithromycin** is predicted to markedly increase the exposure to neurokinin-1 receptor antagonists **(aprepitant)**. [Moderate] Study
▸ **Erythromycin** is predicted to increase the exposure to neurokinin-1 receptor antagonists **(aprepitant)**. [Moderate] Study
▸ **Clarithromycin** is predicted to increase the exposure to neurokinin-1 receptor antagonists **(fosaprepitant)**. [Moderate] Theoretical
▸ **Clarithromycin** is predicted to increase the exposure to neurokinin-1 receptor antagonists **(netupitant)**. [Moderate] Study
▸ **Clarithromycin** is predicted to increase the exposure to **nilotinib**. Avoid. [Severe] Study
▸ **Erythromycin** is predicted to increase the exposure to **nilotinib**. [Moderate] Study → Also see **TABLE 8** p. 1573
▸ **Macrolides** are predicted to increase the exposure to **nintedanib**. [Moderate] Study
▸ **Nirmatrelvir** boosted with ritonavir is predicted to increase the concentration of **clarithromycin**. Monitor; adjust dose in renal impairment. [Moderate] Theoretical
▸ **Nirmatrelvir** boosted with ritonavir is predicted to increase the concentration of **erythromycin**. [Moderate] Theoretical
▸ **Clarithromycin** is predicted to increase the exposure to **nitisinone**. Adjust dose. [Moderate] Theoretical
▸ NNRTIs **(efavirenz, nevirapine)** decrease the exposure to **clarithromycin**. [Moderate] Study
▸ NNRTIs **(etravirine)** decrease the exposure to **clarithromycin** and **clarithromycin** slightly increases the exposure to NNRTIs **(etravirine)**. [Severe] Study
▸ **Erythromycin** is predicted to increase the exposure to NNRTIs **(nevirapine)**. [Moderate] Theoretical
▸ **Clarithromycin** decreases the absorption of NRTIs **(zidovudine)**. Separate administration by 4 hours. [Moderate] Study
▸ **Clarithromycin** is predicted to increase the exposure to **olaparib**. Avoid or adjust dose with potent CYP3A4 inhibitors—consult product literature. [Moderate] Study
▸ **Erythromycin** is predicted to increase the exposure to olaparib. Avoid or adjust dose with moderate CYP3A4 inhibitors—consult product literature. [Moderate] Theoretical

▸ **Clarithromycin** is predicted to increase the exposure to opioids **(alfentanil, buprenorphine, fentanyl, oxycodone)**. Monitor and adjust dose. [Severe] Study
▸ **Erythromycin** is predicted to increase the exposure to opioids **(alfentanil, buprenorphine, fentanyl, oxycodone)**. Monitor and adjust dose. [Moderate] Study
▸ **Clarithromycin** is predicted to increase the concentration of opioids **(methadone)**. [Severe] Theoretical
▸ **Erythromycin** is predicted to increase the exposure to opioids **(methadone, sufentanil)**. [Moderate] Theoretical → Also see **TABLE 8** p. 1573
▸ **Clarithromycin** is predicted to increase the exposure to opioids **(sufentanil)**. [Moderate] Study
▸ **Clarithromycin** is predicted to increase the exposure to **osilodrostat**. [Moderate] Theoretical
▸ **Clarithromycin** is predicted to increase the exposure to **ospemifene**. Avoid in poor CYP2C9 metabolisers. [Moderate] Study
▸ **Clarithromycin** is predicted to increase the exposure to **oxybutynin**. [Mild] Study
▸ **Clarithromycin** is predicted to increase the exposure to **palbociclib**. Avoid or adjust dose—consult product literature. [Severe] Study
▸ **Clarithromycin** is predicted to increase the exposure to **panobinostat**. Adjust dose—consult product literature; in hepatic impairment avoid. [Moderate] Study
▸ Macrolides **(azithromycin, erythromycin)** are predicted to increase the exposure to **panobinostat**. Adjust dose. [Moderate] Theoretical → Also see **TABLE 8** p. 1573
▸ **Clarithromycin** is predicted to increase the exposure to **pazopanib**. Avoid or adjust dose—consult product literature. [Moderate] Study
▸ **Erythromycin** is predicted to increase the exposure to **pazopanib**. [Moderate] Study → Also see **TABLE 8** p. 1573
▸ **Clarithromycin** is predicted to increase the exposure to **pemigatinib**. Avoid or adjust dose—consult product literature. [Severe] Study
▸ **Erythromycin** is predicted to increase the exposure to **pemigatinib**. [Severe] Study
▸ **Azithromycin** might increase the risk of bleeding events when given with **phenindione**. [Severe] Theoretical
▸ **Erythromycin** is predicted to increase the exposure to phosphodiesterase type-5 inhibitors **(avanafil)**. Adjust **avanafil** dose, p. 939. [Moderate] Theoretical
▸ **Clarithromycin** is predicted to increase the exposure to phosphodiesterase type-5 inhibitors **(avanafil, vardenafil)**. Avoid. [Severe] Study
▸ **Clarithromycin** is predicted to increase the exposure to phosphodiesterase type-5 inhibitors **(sildenafil)**. Avoid potent CYP3A4 inhibitors or adjust **sildenafil** dose, p. 940. [Severe] Study
▸ **Erythromycin** is predicted to increase the exposure to phosphodiesterase type-5 inhibitors **(sildenafil)**. Monitor or adjust **sildenafil** dose with moderate CYP3A4 inhibitors, p. 940. [Moderate] Study
▸ **Clarithromycin** is predicted to increase the exposure to phosphodiesterase type-5 inhibitors **(tadalafil)**. Use with caution or avoid. [Severe] Study
▸ **Erythromycin** is predicted to increase the exposure to phosphodiesterase type-5 inhibitors **(tadalafil)**. [Severe] Theoretical
▸ **Erythromycin** is predicted to increase the exposure to phosphodiesterase type-5 inhibitors **(vardenafil)**. Adjust dose. [Severe] Theoretical → Also see **TABLE 8** p. 1573
▸ **Macrolides** are predicted to increase the exposure to **pibrentasvir**. [Moderate] Theoretical
▸ **Clarithromycin** is predicted to increase the exposure to **pimozide**. Avoid. [Severe] Study
▸ **Erythromycin** is predicted to increase the exposure to **pimozide**. Avoid. [Severe] Theoretical → Also see **TABLE 8** p. 1573
▸ **Clarithromycin** might cause hypoglycaemia when given with **pioglitazone**. [Moderate] Theoretical
▸ **Clarithromycin** is predicted to slightly increase the exposure to **ponatinib**. Monitor and adjust dose—consult product literature. [Moderate] Study
▸ **Erythromycin** is predicted to increase the exposure to **ponatinib**. [Moderate] Study

A1

Interactions | Appendix 1

Macrolides (continued)

▶ **Clarithromycin** is predicted to increase the exposure to **pralsetinib**. Avoid or adjust dose with potent CYP3A4 inhibitors—consult product literature. Moderate Study

▶ **Macrolides (azithromycin, erythromycin)** are predicted to increase the exposure to **pralsetinib**. Moderate Theoretical

▶ **Clarithromycin** is predicted to moderately increase the exposure to **praziquantel**. Mild Study

▶ **Clarithromycin** given with carbimazole is predicted to increase the exposure to **propiverine**. Adjust starting dose. Moderate Theoretical

▶ **Clarithromycin** is predicted to increase the exposure to **quizartinib**. Adjust dose—consult product literature. Severe Study

▶ **Clarithromycin** is predicted to increase the exposure to **ranolazine**. Avoid. Severe Study

▶ **Erythromycin** is predicted to increase the exposure to **ranolazine**. Severe Study → Also see **TABLE 8** p. 1573

▶ **Clarithromycin** is predicted to increase the exposure to **reboxetine**. Avoid. Moderate Study

▶ **Clarithromycin** is predicted to increase the exposure to **regorafenib**. Avoid. Moderate Study

▶ **Erythromycin** is predicted to increase the exposure to **regorafenib**. Moderate Study

▶ **Macrolides** are predicted to increase the exposure to **relugolix**. Avoid or take relugolix first and separate administration by at least 6 hours. Moderate Study

▶ **Clarithromycin** is predicted to increase the exposure to **retinoids (alitretinoin)**. Adjust **alitretinoin** dose, p. 1433. Moderate Theoretical

▶ **Clarithromycin** is predicted to increase the exposure to **ribociclib**. Avoid or adjust dose—consult product literature. Moderate Study

▶ **Erythromycin** is predicted to increase the exposure to **ribociclib**. Moderate Study → Also see **TABLE 8** p. 1573

▶ **Rifamycins (rifabutin)** have been reported to cause neutropenia when given with **azithromycin**. Severe Study

▶ **Rifamycins (rifabutin)** decrease the concentration of **clarithromycin** and **clarithromycin** increases the concentration of **rifamycins (rifabutin)**. Monitor and adjust dose. Severe Study

▶ **Rifamycins (rifampicin)** greatly decrease the concentration of **clarithromycin**. Severe Study

▶ **Erythromycin** is predicted to increase the concentration of **rifamycins (rifabutin)** and **rifamycins (rifabutin)** are predicted to decrease the concentration of **erythromycin**. Monitor and adjust dose. Severe Theoretical

▶ **Azithromycin** is predicted to increase the exposure to **rimegepant**. Avoid another dose of rimegepant within 48 hours of concurrent use. Moderate Theoretical

▶ **Clarithromycin** is predicted to increase the exposure to **rimegepant**. Avoid. Moderate Study

▶ **Erythromycin** is predicted to increase the exposure to **rimegepant**. Avoid another dose of rimegepant within 48 hours of concurrent use. Moderate Study

▶ **Macrolides (clarithromycin, erythromycin)** are predicted to increase the exposure to **ripretinib**. Moderate Theoretical

▶ **Clarithromycin** is predicted to increase the exposure to **ruxolitinib**. Adjust dose and monitor adverse effects. Moderate Study

▶ **Erythromycin** slightly increases the exposure to **ruxolitinib**. Mild Study

▶ **Clarithromycin** is predicted to increase the exposure to **selpercatinib**. Adjust dose—consult product literature. Moderate Study

▶ **Erythromycin** is predicted to increase the exposure to **selpercatinib**. Moderate Study → Also see **TABLE 8** p. 1573

▶ **Macrolides (clarithromycin, erythromycin)** are predicted to increase the exposure to **selumetinib**. Avoid or adjust dose—consult product literature. Severe Study

▶ **Clarithromycin** is predicted to increase the exposure to **siponimod**. Avoid depending on other drugs taken—consult product literature. Severe Theoretical

▶ **Erythromycin** is predicted to increase the exposure to **siponimod**. Avoid depending on other drugs taken—consult product literature. Severe Study

▶ **Clarithromycin** is predicted to increase the concentration of **sirolimus**. Avoid or monitor and adjust dose. Severe Study

▶ **Erythromycin** increases the concentration of **sirolimus**. Monitor and adjust dose. Moderate Study

▶ **Clarithromycin** is predicted to increase the exposure to **SNRIs (venlafaxine)**. Moderate Study

▶ **Clarithromycin** is predicted to increase the exposure to **solifenacin**. Adjust solifenacin p. 899 or tamsulosin with solifenacin p. 906 dose; avoid in hepatic and renal impairment. Severe Study

▶ **Clarithromycin** is predicted to moderately increase the exposure to **SSRIs (dapoxetine)**. Avoid potent CYP3A4 inhibitors or adjust **dapoxetine** dose, p. 947. Severe Study

▶ **Erythromycin** is predicted to increase the exposure to **SSRIs (dapoxetine)**. Adjust **dapoxetine** dose with moderate CYP3A4 inhibitors, p. 947. Moderate Theoretical

▶ **Clarithromycin** is predicted to increase the exposure to **statins (atorvastatin)**. Avoid or adjust dose and monitor rhabdomyolysis. Severe Study

▶ **Erythromycin** slightly increases the exposure to **statins (atorvastatin)**. Monitor and adjust dose. Severe Study

▶ **Clarithromycin** moderately increases the exposure to **statins (pravastatin)**. Severe Study

▶ **Erythromycin** slightly increases the exposure to **statins (pravastatin)**. Severe Study

▶ **Clarithromycin** is predicted to increase the exposure to **statins (simvastatin)**. Avoid. Severe Study

▶ **Erythromycin** markedly increases the exposure to **statins (simvastatin)**. Avoid. Severe Study

▶ **Clarithromycin** might increase the exposure to **sulfonylureas**. Moderate Theoretical

▶ **Clarithromycin** is predicted to increase the exposure to **sunitinib**. Avoid or adjust dose—consult product literature. Moderate Study

▶ **Erythromycin** is predicted to increase the exposure to **sunitinib**. Moderate Study → Also see **TABLE 8** p. 1573

▶ **Clarithromycin** is predicted to increase the concentration of **tacrolimus**. Monitor and adjust dose. Severe Study

▶ **Erythromycin** is predicted to increase the concentration of **tacrolimus**. Severe Study

▶ **Macrolides** are predicted to slightly increase the exposure to **talazoparib**. Avoid or adjust dose—consult product literature. Severe Study

▶ **Clarithromycin** is predicted to increase the exposure to **taxanes (cabazitaxel)**. Avoid or adjust dose—consult product literature. Severe Study

▶ **Erythromycin** is predicted to increase the exposure to **taxanes (cabazitaxel)**. Moderate Theoretical

▶ **Clarithromycin** is predicted to increase the exposure to **taxanes (docetaxel)**. Avoid or adjust dose. Severe Study

▶ **Erythromycin** is predicted to increase the exposure to **taxanes (docetaxel)**. Severe Study

▶ **Azithromycin** is predicted to increase the exposure to **taxanes (paclitaxel)**. Moderate Theoretical

▶ **Macrolides (clarithromycin, erythromycin)** are predicted to increase the exposure to **taxanes (paclitaxel)**. Moderate Anecdotal

▶ **Clarithromycin** is predicted to increase the concentration of **temsirolimus**. Avoid. Severe Theoretical

▶ **Erythromycin** is predicted to increase the concentration of **temsirolimus**. Use with caution or avoid. Moderate Theoretical

▶ **Clarithromycin** might increase the exposure to **tepotinib**. Avoid. Severe Theoretical

▶ **Clarithromycin** is predicted to increase the exposure to **tezacaftor**. Adjust dose with potent CYP3A4 inhibitors, see tezacaftor with ivacaftor p. 339 and ivacaftor with tezacaftor and elexacaftor p. 337. Severe Study

▶ **Erythromycin** is predicted to increase the exposure to **tezacaftor**. Adjust dose with moderate CYP3A4 inhibitors, see tezacaftor with ivacaftor p. 339 and ivacaftor with tezacaftor and elexacaftor p. 337. Severe Study

▶ **Erythromycin** decreases the clearance of **theophylline** and **theophylline** potentially decreases the clearance of **erythromycin**. Adjust dose. Severe Study

- Macrolides (**azithromycin, clarithromycin**) are predicted to increase the exposure to theophylline. Adjust dose. [Moderate] Anecdotal
- **Clarithromycin** increases the exposure to thrombin inhibitors (dabigatran). [Moderate] Study
- Macrolides (**azithromycin, erythromycin**) are predicted to increase the exposure to thrombin inhibitors (dabigatran). [Severe] Theoretical
- **Azithromycin** is predicted to increase the exposure to ticagrelor. Use with caution or avoid. [Severe] Study
- **Clarithromycin** is predicted to markedly increase the exposure to ticagrelor. Avoid. [Severe] Study
- **Macrolides** might increase the exposure to tigecycline. [Mild] Anecdotal
- **Clarithromycin** is predicted to increase the exposure to tofacitinib. Adjust **tofacitinib** dose, p. 1265. [Moderate] Study
- **Erythromycin** given with a potent CYP2C19 inhibitor is predicted to increase the exposure to tofacitinib. Adjust **tofacitinib** dose, p. 1265. [Moderate] Study
- **Clarithromycin** is predicted to increase the exposure to tolterodine. Avoid. [Severe] Study
- **Clarithromycin** is predicted to increase the exposure to tolvaptan. Manufacturer advises caution or adjust **tolvaptan** dose with potent CYP3A4 inhibitors, p. 767. [Severe] Study
- **Erythromycin** is predicted to increase the exposure to tolvaptan. Manufacturer advises caution or adjust **tolvaptan** dose with moderate CYP3A4 inhibitors, p. 767. [Moderate] Study
- **Macrolides** are predicted to increase the exposure to topotecan. [Severe] Study
- **Clarithromycin** is predicted to increase the exposure to toremifene. [Moderate] Theoretical
- **Clarithromycin** is predicted to increase the exposure to trabectedin. Avoid or adjust dose. [Severe] Theoretical
- **Macrolides** are predicted to increase the concentration of trametinib. [Moderate] Theoretical
- **Clarithromycin** is predicted to moderately increase the exposure to trazodone. Avoid or adjust dose. [Moderate] Study
- **Erythromycin** is predicted to increase the exposure to trazodone. [Moderate] Theoretical
- **Clarithromycin** increases the exposure to triptans (almotriptan). [Mild] Study
- **Clarithromycin** is predicted to markedly increase the exposure to triptans (eletriptan). Avoid. [Severe] Study
- **Erythromycin** moderately increases the exposure to triptans (eletriptan). Avoid. [Moderate] Study
- **Clarithromycin** is predicted to increase the exposure to ulipristal. Avoid if used for uterine fibroids. [Severe] Study
- **Erythromycin** moderately increases the exposure to ulipristal. Avoid if used for uterine fibroids. [Moderate] Study
- **Clarithromycin** is predicted to increase the exposure to upadacitinib. Manufacturer advises caution or avoid, or adjust **upadacitinib** dose depending on indication, p. 1267. [Severe] Study
- Macrolides (**clarithromycin, erythromycin**) are predicted to increase the exposure to vemurafenib. [Severe] Theoretical → Also see **TABLE 8** p. 1573
- Macrolides (**clarithromycin, erythromycin**) are predicted to increase the exposure to venetoclax. Avoid or adjust dose—consult product literature. [Severe] Study
- **Azithromycin** might increase the exposure to vinca alkaloids. [Severe] Theoretical
- Macrolides (**clarithromycin, erythromycin**) are predicted to increase the exposure to vinca alkaloids. [Severe] Theoretical
- **Clarithromycin** is predicted to increase the exposure to vitamin D substances (paricalcitol). [Moderate] Study
- **Clarithromycin** is predicted to increase the exposure to voclosporin. Avoid. [Severe] Study
- **Erythromycin** is predicted to increase the exposure to voclosporin. Adjust **voclosporin** dose, p. 973. [Severe] Study → Also see **TABLE 8** p. 1573
- **Clarithromycin** is predicted to increase the exposure to zanubrutinib. Avoid or adjust dose with potent CYP3A4 inhibitors—consult product literature. [Moderate] Study
- **Erythromycin** is predicted to increase the exposure to zanubrutinib. Avoid or adjust dose with moderate CYP3A4 inhibitors—consult product literature. [Severe] Study
- **Clarithromycin** is predicted to increase the exposure to zopiclone. Adjust dose. [Moderate] Theoretical
- **Erythromycin** is predicted to increase the exposure to zopiclone. Adjust dose. [Moderate] Study

Magnesium

> SEPARATION OF ADMINISTRATION **Magnesium-containing antacids** and other **oral magnesium preparations** should preferably not be taken at the same time as other drugs since they might impair absorption; some manufacturers suggest separating administration by several hours. **Magnesium-containing antacids** might damage enteric coatings designed to prevent dissolution in the stomach.

- Oral **magnesium** trisilicate decreases the absorption of oral antimalarials (chloroquine). Separate administration by at least 4 hours. [Moderate] Study
- Oral **magnesium** might decrease the concentration of the active metabolite of oral baloxavir marboxil. Avoid. [Severe] Theoretical
- Oral **magnesium** decreases the absorption of oral bisphosphonates (alendronate). Manufacturer advises take at least 30 minutes before magnesium. [Moderate] Study
- Oral **magnesium** decreases the absorption of oral bisphosphonates (clodronate). Avoid magnesium for 2 hours before or 1 hour after **clodronate**. [Moderate] Study
- Oral **magnesium** is predicted to decrease the absorption of oral bisphosphonates (ibandronate). Avoid for at least 6 hours before or 1 hour after **ibandronate**. [Moderate] Theoretical
- Oral **magnesium** decreases the absorption of oral bisphosphonates (risedronate). Separate administration by at least 2 hours. [Moderate] Study
- Intravenous **magnesium** potentially increases the risk of hypotension when given with calcium channel blockers (amlodipine, felodipine, lacidipine, lercanidipine, nicardipine, nifedipine, nimodipine, verapamil) in pregnant women. [Severe] Anecdotal
- Oral **magnesium** trisilicate is predicted to decrease the absorption of oral hydroxychloroquine. [Moderate] Theoretical
- Intravenous **magnesium** increases the effects of neuromuscular blocking drugs, non-depolarising. [Moderate] Study
- Oral **magnesium** trisilicate decreases the absorption of oral nitrofurantoin. [Moderate] Study
- **Magnesium** might decrease the exposure to roxadustat. Manufacturer advises take at least 1 hour after magnesium. [Moderate] Theoretical
- Intravenous **magnesium** is predicted to increase the effects of suxamethonium. [Moderate] Study
- Oral **magnesium** is predicted to decrease the exposure to oral vadadustat. Manufacturer advises take 1 hour before or 2 hours after magnesium. [Moderate] Theoretical

Mannitol → see **TABLE 17** p. 1576 (hyponatraemia)

MAO-B inhibitors → see **TABLE 5** p. 1572 (bradycardia), **TABLE 7** p. 1572 (hypotension), **TABLE 12** p. 1574 (serotonin syndrome)

rasagiline · safinamide · selegiline

> FOOD AND LIFESTYLE Hypertension is predicted to occur when high-dose **selegiline** is taken with tyramine-rich foods (such as mature cheese, salami, pickled herring, *Bovril*®, *Oxo*®, *Marmite*® or any similar meat or yeast extract or fermented soya bean extract, and some beers, lagers or wines).

- MAO-B inhibitors (**rasagiline, selegiline**) are predicted to increase the risk of severe hypertension when given with amfetamines. Avoid. [Severe] Theoretical → Also see **TABLE 12** p. 1574
- **Safinamide** is predicted to increase the risk of severe hypertension when given with amfetamines. [Severe] Theoretical → Also see **TABLE 12** p. 1574
- **Axitinib** is predicted to increase the exposure to rasagiline. [Moderate] Theoretical
- MAO-B inhibitors (**rasagiline, selegiline**) are predicted to increase the risk of severe hypertension when given with beta₂ agonists. Avoid. [Severe] Theoretical
- **Safinamide** is predicted to increase the risk of severe hypertension when given with beta₂ agonists. [Severe] Theoretical

MAO-B inhibitors (continued)

▶ **Bupropion** is predicted to increase the risk of severe hypertension when given with **MAO-B inhibitors**. Avoid. Moderate Theoretical

▶ **Combined hormonal contraceptives** slightly increases the exposure to **rasagiline**. Moderate Study

▶ **Combined hormonal contraceptives** increase the exposure to **selegiline**. Avoid. Severe Study

▶ **MAO-B inhibitors** are predicted to increase the dopaminergic effects of **foslevodopa**. Adjust dose. Mild Theoretical → Also see **TABLE 7** p. 1572

▶ **Givosiran** slightly increases the exposure to **rasagiline**. Moderate Study

▶ **Hormone replacement therapy** is predicted to increase the exposure to **selegiline**. Avoid. Moderate Study

▶ **MAO-B inhibitors** are predicted to increase the effects of **levodopa**. Adjust dose. Mild Study → Also see **TABLE 7** p. 1572

▶ MAO-B inhibitors (**rasagiline, selegiline**) are predicted to increase the risk of adverse effects when given with **linezolid**. Avoid and for 14 days after stopping the MAOI. Severe Theoretical → Also see **TABLE 12** p. 1574

▶ **Safinamide** is predicted to increase the risk of adverse effects when given with **linezolid**. Avoid and for 1 week after stopping **safinamide**. Severe Theoretical → Also see **TABLE 12** p. 1574

▶ MAO-B inhibitors (**rasagiline, selegiline**) are predicted to increase the risk of adverse effects when given with **MAOIs, irreversible**. Avoid and for 14 days after stopping the MAOI. Severe Theoretical → Also see **TABLE 7** p. 1572 → Also see **TABLE 12** p. 1574

▶ **Safinamide** is predicted to increase the risk of adverse effects when given with **MAOIs, irreversible**. Avoid and for 1 week after stopping **safinamide**. Severe Theoretical → Also see **TABLE 12** p. 1574

▶ **Rasagiline** is predicted to increase the risk of a hypertensive crisis when given with **methylphenidate**. Avoid. Severe Theoretical

▶ **Selegiline** might increase the risk of a hypertensive crisis when given with **methylphenidate**. Avoid. Severe Theoretical

▶ **Mexiletine** slightly increases the exposure to **rasagiline**. Moderate Study

▶ **Moclobemide** is predicted to increase the effects of MAO-B inhibitors (**rasagiline, selegiline**). Avoid. Severe Theoretical → Also see **TABLE 12** p. 1574

▶ **Moclobemide** is predicted to increase the risk of adverse effects when given with **safinamide**. Avoid and for 1 week after stopping **safinamide**. Severe Theoretical → Also see **TABLE 12** p. 1574

▶ **Rasagiline** is predicted to increase the risk of adverse effects when given with opioids (**pethidine**). Avoid and for 14 days after stopping **rasagiline**. Severe Theoretical → Also see **TABLE 12** p. 1574

▶ **Safinamide** is predicted to increase the risk of adverse effects when given with opioids (**pethidine**). Avoid and for 1 week after stopping **safinamide**. Severe Theoretical → Also see **TABLE 12** p. 1574

▶ **Selegiline** increases the risk of adverse effects when given with opioids (**pethidine**). Avoid. Severe Anecdotal → Also see **TABLE 12** p. 1574

▶ **Osilodrostat** slightly increases the exposure to **rasagiline**. Moderate Study

▶ **Ozanimod** might increase the risk of a hypertensive crisis when given with **MAO-B inhibitors** and **MAO-B inhibitors** might decrease the exposure to the active metabolites of **ozanimod**. Avoid. Severe Theoretical → Also see **TABLE 5** p. 1572

▶ **Quinolones (ciprofloxacin)** slightly increase the exposure to **rasagiline**. Moderate Study

▶ **Reboxetine** is predicted to increase the risk of a hypertensive crisis when given with MAO-B inhibitors (**rasagiline, selegiline**). Avoid. Severe Theoretical

▶ **Rucaparib** slightly increases the exposure to **rasagiline**. Moderate Study

▶ **Solriamfetol** is predicted to increase the risk of a hypertensive crisis when given with **MAO-B inhibitors**. Avoid and for 14 days after stopping **MAO-B inhibitors**. Severe Theoretical

▶ **Sympathomimetics, inotropic** are predicted to increase the risk of a hypertensive crisis when given with **MAO-B inhibitors**. Avoid. Severe Anecdotal

▶ **Sympathomimetics, vasoconstrictor** are predicted to increase the risk of a hypertensive crisis when given with **MAO-B inhibitors**. Avoid. Severe Anecdotal

▶ **Tetrabenazine** potentially increases the risk of CNS excitation and hypertension when given with **MAO-B inhibitors**. Severe Theoretical

▶ **Vemurafenib** slightly increases the exposure to **rasagiline**. Moderate Study

MAOIs, irreversible → see **TABLE 7** p. 1572 (hypotension), **TABLE 12** p. 1574 (serotonin syndrome)

isocarboxazid · phenelzine · tranylcypromine

FOOD AND LIFESTYLE Potentially life-threatening hypertensive crisis can develop in those taking MAOIs who eat tyramine-rich food (such as mature cheese, salami, pickled herring, *Bovril*®, *Oxo*®, *Marmite*® or any similar meat or yeast extract or fermented soya bean extract, and some beers, lagers or wines) or foods containing dopa (such as broad bean pods). Avoid tyramine-rich or dopa-rich food or drinks with, or for 2 to 3 weeks after stopping, the MAOI.

▶ **MAOIs, irreversible** are predicted to increase the effects of alpha blockers (**indoramin**). Avoid. Severe Theoretical → Also see **TABLE 7** p. 1572

▶ **Amfetamines** are predicted to increase the risk of a hypertensive crisis when given with **MAOIs, irreversible**. Avoid and for 14 days after stopping the MAOI. Severe Anecdotal → Also see **TABLE 12** p. 1574

▶ **Antiepileptics (carbamazepine)** are predicted to increase the risk of severe toxic reaction when given with **MAOIs, irreversible**. Avoid and for 14 days after stopping the MAOI. Severe Theoretical

▶ **Antiepileptics (phenobarbital, primidone)** are predicted to increase the effects of **MAOIs, irreversible**. Severe Theoretical

▶ **MAOIs, irreversible** are predicted to increase the risk of antimuscarinic adverse effects when given with **antihistamines, non-sedating**. Avoid. Severe Theoretical

▶ **MAOIs, irreversible** are predicted to increase the risk of antimuscarinic adverse effects when given with **antihistamines, sedating**. Avoid. Severe Theoretical

▶ **MAOIs, irreversible** are predicted to increase the risk of adverse effects when given with **atomoxetine**. Avoid and for 2 weeks after stopping the MAOI. Severe Theoretical

▶ **MAOIs, irreversible** are predicted to increase the risk of cardiovascular adverse effects when given with **beta$_2$ agonists**. Moderate Anecdotal

▶ **Bupropion** is predicted to increase the risk of severe hypertension when given with **MAOIs, irreversible**. Avoid and for 14 days after stopping the MAOI. Severe Theoretical

▶ **Buspirone** is predicted to increase the risk of elevated blood pressure when given with **MAOIs, irreversible**. Avoid. Severe Anecdotal

▶ **MAOIs, irreversible** are predicted to increase the effects of **doxapram**. Moderate Theoretical

▶ **Entacapone** is predicted to increase the risk of elevated blood pressure when given with **MAOIs, irreversible**. Avoid. Severe Theoretical

▶ **MAOIs, irreversible** might cause a hypertensive crisis when given with **foslevodopa**. Avoid and for 14 days after stopping the MAOI. Severe Theoretical → Also see **TABLE 7** p. 1572

▶ **Levodopa** increases the risk of a hypertensive crisis when given with **MAOIs, irreversible**. Avoid and for 14 days after stopping the MAOI. Severe Study → Also see **TABLE 7** p. 1572

▶ **MAOIs, irreversible** are predicted to increase the risk of adverse effects when given with **linezolid**. Avoid and for 14 days after stopping the MAOI. Severe Theoretical → Also see **TABLE 12** p. 1574

▶ MAO-B inhibitors (**rasagiline, selegiline**) are predicted to increase the risk of adverse effects when given with **MAOIs, irreversible**. Avoid and for 14 days after stopping the MAOI. Severe Theoretical → Also see **TABLE 7** p. 1572 → Also see **TABLE 12** p. 1574

▶ MAO-B inhibitors (**safinamide**) are predicted to increase the risk of adverse effects when given with **MAOIs, irreversible**. Avoid and for 1 week after stopping **safinamide**. Severe Theoretical → Also see **TABLE 12** p. 1574

▶ **MAOIs, irreversible** are predicted to alter the antihypertensive effects of methyldopa. Avoid. [Severe] Theoretical → Also see **TABLE 7** p. 1572

▶ Methylphenidate causes a hypertensive crisis when given with **MAOIs, irreversible**. Avoid and for 14 days after stopping the MAOI. [Severe] Theoretical

▶ Mianserin is predicted to increase the risk of toxicity when given with **MAOIs, irreversible**. Avoid and for 14 days after stopping the MAOI. [Severe] Theoretical

▶ Nefopam is predicted to increase the risk of serious elevations in blood pressure when given with **MAOIs, irreversible**. Avoid. [Severe] Theoretical

▶ Opicapone is predicted to increase the risk of elevated blood pressure when given with **MAOIs, irreversible**. Avoid. [Severe] Theoretical

▶ Opioids are predicted to increase the risk of CNS excitation or depression when given with **MAOIs, irreversible**. Avoid. [Severe] Study → Also see **TABLE 12** p. 1574

▶ Ozanimod might increase the risk of a hypertensive crisis when given with **MAOIs, irreversible**. Avoid. [Severe] Theoretical

▶ **MAOIs, irreversible** are predicted to increase the risk of neuroleptic malignant syndrome when given with phenothiazines. [Severe] Theoretical → Also see **TABLE 7** p. 1572

▶ Reboxetine is predicted to increase the risk of a hypertensive crisis when given with **MAOIs, irreversible**. Avoid. [Severe] Theoretical

▶ Solriamfetol is predicted to increase the risk of a hypertensive crisis when given with **MAOIs, irreversible**. Avoid and for 14 days after stopping the MAOI. [Severe] Theoretical

▶ Sympathomimetics, inotropic are predicted to increase the risk of a hypertensive crisis when given with **MAOIs, irreversible**. Avoid and for 14 days after stopping the MAOI. [Severe] Theoretical

▶ Sympathomimetics, vasoconstrictor are predicted to increase the risk of a hypertensive crisis when given with **MAOIs, irreversible**. Avoid and for 14 days after stopping the MAOI. [Severe] Study

▶ Tetrabenazine potentially increases the risk of CNS excitation and hypertension when given with **MAOIs, irreversible**. Avoid and for 14 days after stopping the MAOI. [Severe] Theoretical

▶ Tolcapone is predicted to increase the effects of **MAOIs, irreversible**. Avoid. [Severe] Theoretical

▶ Tricyclic antidepressants are predicted to increase the risk of severe toxic reaction when given with **MAOIs, irreversible**. Avoid and for 14 days after stopping the MAOI. [Severe] Theoretical → Also see **TABLE 7** p. 1572 → Also see **TABLE 12** p. 1574

▶ **MAOIs, irreversible** are predicted to increase the exposure to triptans (rizatriptan, sumatriptan). Avoid and for 14 days after stopping the MAOI. [Severe] Theoretical → Also see **TABLE 12** p. 1574

▶ **MAOIs, irreversible** are predicted to increase the exposure to triptans (zolmitriptan). [Severe] Theoretical → Also see **TABLE 12** p. 1574

▶ Tryptophan increases the risk of adverse effects when given with **MAOIs, irreversible**. [Severe] Anecdotal → Also see **TABLE 12** p. 1574

Maraviroc

▶ Anti-androgens (apalutamide, enzalutamide) are predicted to decrease the exposure to **maraviroc**. Adjust dose. [Severe] Study

▶ Antiepileptics (carbamazepine, fosphenytoin, phenobarbital, phenytoin, primidone) are predicted to decrease the exposure to **maraviroc**. Adjust dose. [Severe] Study

▶ Antifungals, azoles (itraconazole, ketoconazole, voriconazole) are predicted to markedly increase the exposure to **maraviroc**. Adjust dose. [Severe] Study

▶ Belzutifan is predicted to decrease the exposure to **maraviroc**. Avoid or adjust dose. [Severe] Theoretical

▶ Cenobamate is predicted to decrease the exposure to **maraviroc**. Adjust dose. [Moderate] Theoretical

▶ Cobicistat markedly increases the exposure to **maraviroc**. Refer to specialist literature. [Severe] Study

▶ Encorafenib is predicted to decrease the exposure to **maraviroc**. Adjust dose. [Severe] Study

▶ Endothelin receptor antagonists (bosentan) are predicted to decrease the exposure to **maraviroc**. Avoid. [Moderate] Theoretical

▶ HIV-protease inhibitors (atazanavir) moderately to markedly increase the exposure to **maraviroc**. Refer to specialist literature. [Severe] Study

▶ HIV-protease inhibitors (darunavir) boosted with ritonavir markedly increase the exposure to **maraviroc**. Refer to specialist literature. [Severe] Study

▶ HIV-protease inhibitors (lopinavir) boosted with ritonavir moderately increase the exposure to **maraviroc**. Refer to specialist literature. [Severe] Study

▶ HIV-protease inhibitors (ritonavir) markedly increase the exposure to **maraviroc**. Refer to specialist literature. [Severe] Study

▶ **Maraviroc** potentially decreases the exposure to HIV-protease inhibitors (fosamprenavir) and HIV-protease inhibitors (fosamprenavir) potentially decrease the exposure to **maraviroc**. Avoid. [Severe] Study

▶ Idelalisib markedly increases the exposure to **maraviroc**. Adjust dose. [Severe] Theoretical

▶ Ivosidenib is predicted to decrease the exposure to **maraviroc**. Adjust dose. [Severe] Study

▶ Lumacaftor is predicted to decrease the exposure to **maraviroc**. Adjust dose. [Severe] Study

▶ Macrolides (clarithromycin) are predicted to markedly increase the exposure to **maraviroc**. Adjust dose. [Severe] Study

▶ Mitotane is predicted to decrease the exposure to **maraviroc**. Adjust dose. [Severe] Study

▶ Neurokinin-1 receptor antagonists (aprepitant, netupitant) are predicted to increase the exposure to **maraviroc**. [Moderate] Study

▶ Nirmatrelvir boosted with ritonavir is predicted to increase the concentration of **maraviroc**. Refer to specialist literature. [Severe] Theoretical

▶ NNRTIs (efavirenz) decrease the exposure to **maraviroc**. Refer to specialist literature. [Severe] Theoretical

▶ NNRTIs (etravirine) slightly decrease the exposure to **maraviroc**. Refer to specialist literature. [Moderate] Study

▶ Rifamycins (rifampicin) are predicted to decrease the exposure to **maraviroc**. Adjust dose. [Severe] Study

▶ St John's wort is predicted to decrease the exposure to **maraviroc**. Avoid. [Severe] Theoretical

▶ Vemurafenib is predicted to increase the exposure to **maraviroc**. Use with caution or avoid. [Moderate] Theoretical

Maribavir

▶ Anti-androgens (apalutamide, enzalutamide) are predicted to decrease the exposure to **maribavir**. Avoid or adjust **maribavir** dose, p. 735. [Severe] Study

▶ Antiepileptics (carbamazepine, fosphenytoin, phenobarbital, phenytoin, primidone) are predicted to decrease the exposure to **maribavir**. Avoid or adjust **maribavir** dose, p. 735. [Severe] Study

▶ **Maribavir** is predicted to increase the exposure to ciclosporin. Monitor and adjust dose. [Severe] Theoretical

▶ Dabrafenib is predicted to decrease the exposure to **maribavir**. Avoid or adjust **maribavir** dose, p. 735. [Severe] Study

▶ **Maribavir** very slightly increases the exposure to digoxin. Monitor and adjust dose. [Moderate] Study

▶ Endothelin receptor antagonists (bosentan) are predicted to decrease the exposure to **maribavir**. Avoid or adjust **maribavir** dose, p. 735. [Severe] Study

▶ **Maribavir** increases the exposure to everolimus. Monitor and adjust dose. [Severe] Study

▶ **Maribavir** might decrease the efficacy of ganciclovir. Avoid. [Severe] Theoretical

▶ **Maribavir** is predicted to increase the exposure to gilteritinib. [Moderate] Theoretical

▶ **Maribavir** is predicted to increase the exposure to idelalisib. [Moderate] Theoretical

▶ Mitotane is predicted to decrease the exposure to **maribavir**. Avoid or adjust **maribavir** dose, p. 735. [Severe] Study

▶ NNRTIs (efavirenz, nevirapine) are predicted to decrease the exposure to **maribavir**. Avoid or adjust **maribavir** dose, p. 735. [Severe] Study

▶ NNRTIs (etravirine) are predicted to decrease the exposure to **maribavir**. Avoid or adjust **maribavir** dose, p. 735. [Severe] Theoretical

Maribavir (continued)

▸ Rifamycins **(rifabutin)** are predicted to decrease the exposure to **maribavir**. Avoid. [Severe] Theoretical

▸ Rifamycins **(rifampicin)** are predicted to decrease the exposure to **maribavir**. Avoid. [Severe] Study

▸ **Maribavir** is predicted to increase the exposure to **sirolimus**. Monitor and adjust dose. [Severe] Study

▸ St John's wort is predicted to decrease the exposure to **maribavir**. Avoid. [Severe] Study

▸ **Maribavir** is predicted to increase the exposure to statins **(rosuvastatin)**. [Moderate] Theoretical

▸ **Maribavir** is predicted to slightly increase the exposure to **tacrolimus**. Monitor and adjust dose. [Severe] Study

▸ **Maribavir** is predicted to increase the exposure to taxanes **(paclitaxel)**. Use with caution and adjust dose. [Unknown] Study

▸ **Maribavir** is predicted to decrease the exposure to **theophylline**. Avoid. [Mild] Theoretical

▸ **Maribavir** is predicted to increase the exposure to thrombin inhibitors **(dabigatran)**. [Moderate] Study

▸ **Maribavir** is predicted to decrease the exposure to **tizanidine**. Avoid. [Mild] Theoretical

▸ **Maribavir** might decrease the efficacy of **valganciclovir**. Avoid. [Severe] Theoretical

Mavacamten

▸ Anti-androgens **(apalutamide, enzalutamide)** are predicted to decrease the exposure to **mavacamten**. Monitor and adjust dose—consult product literature. [Severe] Theoretical

▸ Antiarrhythmics **(amiodarone)** are predicted to increase the exposure to **mavacamten**. Monitor and adjust dose—consult product literature. [Moderate] Theoretical

▸ Antiarrhythmics **(dronedarone)** are predicted to increase the exposure to **mavacamten**. Adjust dose—consult product literature. [Moderate] Study

▸ Antiepileptics **(carbamazepine, fosphenytoin, phenobarbital, phenytoin, primidone)** are predicted to decrease the exposure to **mavacamten**. Monitor and adjust dose—consult product literature. [Severe] Theoretical

▸ Antifungals, azoles **(fluconazole, isavuconazole)** are predicted to increase the exposure to **mavacamten**. Adjust dose—consult product literature. [Moderate] Study

▸ Antifungals, azoles **(itraconazole, ketoconazole, posaconazole, voriconazole)** are predicted to increase the exposure to **mavacamten**. Avoid or monitor—consult product literature. [Severe] Study

▸ Berotralstat is predicted to increase the exposure to **mavacamten**. Adjust dose—consult product literature. [Moderate] Study

▸ **Mavacamten** can cause negative inotropic effects, as can beta blockers, non-selective. [Severe] Theoretical

▸ **Mavacamten** can cause negative inotropic effects, as can beta blockers, selective. [Severe] Theoretical

▸ Calcium channel blockers **(diltiazem, verapamil)** are predicted to increase the exposure to **mavacamten**. Adjust dose—consult product literature. [Moderate] Study

▸ Cenobamate is predicted to decrease the exposure to **mavacamten**. Monitor and adjust dose—consult product literature. [Severe] Theoretical

▸ Ceritinib is predicted to increase the exposure to **mavacamten**. Avoid or monitor—consult product literature. [Severe] Study

▸ Cobicistat is predicted to increase the exposure to **mavacamten**. Avoid or monitor—consult product literature. [Severe] Study

▸ **Mavacamten** is predicted to affect the efficacy of some combined hormonal contraceptives. Use additional contraceptive precautions. [Severe] Theoretical

▸ Crizotinib is predicted to increase the exposure to **mavacamten**. Adjust dose—consult product literature. [Moderate] Study

▸ Dabrafenib is predicted to decrease the exposure to **mavacamten**. Monitor and adjust dose—consult product literature. [Severe] Theoretical

▸ Encorafenib is predicted to decrease the exposure to **mavacamten**. Monitor and adjust dose—consult product literature. [Severe] Theoretical

▸ Endothelin receptor antagonists **(bosentan)** are predicted to decrease the exposure to **mavacamten**. Monitor and adjust dose—consult product literature. [Severe] Theoretical

▸ Entrectinib is predicted to increase the exposure to **mavacamten**. Monitor and adjust dose—consult product literature. [Moderate] Theoretical

▸ Everolimus is predicted to increase the exposure to **mavacamten**. Monitor and adjust dose—consult product literature. [Moderate] Theoretical

▸ Fedratinib is predicted to increase the exposure to **mavacamten**. Adjust dose—consult product literature. [Moderate] Study

▸ Givosiran is predicted to increase the exposure to **mavacamten**. Monitor and adjust dose—consult product literature. [Moderate] Theoretical

▸ Grapefruit is predicted to increase the exposure to **mavacamten**. Monitor and adjust dose—consult product literature. [Moderate] Theoretical

▸ H_2 receptor antagonists **(cimetidine)** are predicted to increase the exposure to **mavacamten**. Monitor and adjust dose—consult product literature. [Moderate] Theoretical

▸ HIV-protease inhibitors are predicted to increase the exposure to **mavacamten**. Avoid or monitor—consult product literature. [Severe] Study

▸ Idelalisib is predicted to increase the exposure to **mavacamten**. Avoid or monitor—consult product literature. [Severe] Study

▸ Imatinib is predicted to increase the exposure to **mavacamten**. Adjust dose—consult product literature. [Moderate] Study

▸ Isoniazid is predicted to increase the exposure to **mavacamten**. Monitor and adjust dose—consult product literature. [Moderate] Theoretical

▸ Ivosidenib is predicted to decrease the exposure to **mavacamten**. Monitor and adjust dose—consult product literature. [Severe] Theoretical

▸ Lapatinib is predicted to increase the exposure to **mavacamten**. Monitor and adjust dose—consult product literature. [Moderate] Theoretical

▸ Larotrectinib is predicted to increase the exposure to **mavacamten**. Monitor and adjust dose—consult product literature. [Moderate] Theoretical

▸ Letermovir is predicted to increase the exposure to **mavacamten**. Adjust dose—consult product literature. [Moderate] Study

▸ Lomitapide is predicted to increase the exposure to **mavacamten**. Monitor and adjust dose—consult product literature. [Moderate] Theoretical

▸ Lorlatinib is predicted to decrease the exposure to **mavacamten**. Monitor and adjust dose—consult product literature. [Severe] Theoretical

▸ Lumacaftor is predicted to decrease the exposure to **mavacamten**. Monitor and adjust dose—consult product literature. [Severe] Theoretical

▸ Macrolides **(clarithromycin)** are predicted to increase the exposure to **mavacamten**. Avoid or monitor—consult product literature. [Severe] Study

▸ Macrolides **(erythromycin)** are predicted to increase the exposure to **mavacamten**. Adjust dose—consult product literature. [Moderate] Study

▸ Mitotane is predicted to decrease the exposure to **mavacamten**. Monitor and adjust dose—consult product literature. [Severe] Theoretical

▸ Moclobemide is predicted to increase the exposure to **mavacamten**. Adjust dose—consult product literature. [Severe] Theoretical

▸ Modafinil is predicted to increase the exposure to **mavacamten**. Monitor and adjust dose—consult product literature. [Moderate] Theoretical

▸ Neurokinin-1 receptor antagonists **(aprepitant, netupitant)** are predicted to increase the exposure to **mavacamten**. Adjust dose—consult product literature. [Moderate] Study

▸ Neurokinin-1 receptor antagonists **(fosaprepitant)** are predicted to increase the exposure to **mavacamten**. Monitor and adjust dose—consult product literature. [Moderate] Theoretical

▸ Nilotinib is predicted to increase the exposure to **mavacamten**. Adjust dose—consult product literature. [Moderate] Study

- NNRTIs **(efavirenz, etravirine, nevirapine)** are predicted to decrease the exposure to **mavacamten**. Monitor and adjust dose—consult product literature. [Severe] Theoretical
- **Osilodrostat** is predicted to increase the exposure to **mavacamten**. Monitor and adjust dose—consult product literature. [Moderate] Theoretical
- **Pazopanib** is predicted to increase the exposure to **mavacamten**. Monitor and adjust dose—consult product literature. [Moderate] Theoretical
- Proton pump inhibitors **(esomeprazole, omeprazole)** are predicted to increase the exposure to **mavacamten**. Adjust dose—consult product literature. [Severe] Theoretical
- Proton pump inhibitors **(pantoprazole)** might increase the exposure to **mavacamten**. Monitor and adjust dose—consult product literature. [Moderate] Theoretical
- **Ranolazine** is predicted to increase the exposure to **mavacamten**. Monitor and adjust dose—consult product literature. [Moderate] Theoretical
- Rifamycins **(rifampicin)** are predicted to decrease the exposure to **mavacamten**. Monitor and adjust dose—consult product literature. [Severe] Theoretical
- **Rucaparib** is predicted to increase the exposure to **mavacamten**. Monitor and adjust dose—consult product literature. [Moderate] Theoretical
- **Selpercatinib** is predicted to increase the exposure to **mavacamten**. Monitor and adjust dose—consult product literature. [Moderate] Theoretical
- **Sotorasib** is predicted to decrease the exposure to **mavacamten**. Monitor and adjust dose—consult product literature. [Severe] Theoretical
- SSRIs **(fluoxetine)** are predicted to increase the exposure to **mavacamten**. Adjust dose—consult product literature. [Severe] Theoretical
- SSRIs **(fluvoxamine)** are predicted to increase the exposure to **mavacamten**. Monitor and adjust dose—consult product literature. [Moderate] Theoretical
- **St John's wort** is predicted to decrease the exposure to **mavacamten**. Monitor and adjust dose—consult product literature. [Severe] Theoretical
- **Tucatinib** is predicted to increase the exposure to **mavacamten**. Avoid or monitor—consult product literature. [Severe] Study

Measles, mumps and rubella vaccine → see live vaccines

Mebendazole

- H₂ receptor antagonists **(cimetidine)** increase the concentration of **mebendazole**. [Moderate] Study

Medroxyprogesterone

- Antifungals, azoles **(itraconazole, ketoconazole, posaconazole, voriconazole)** are predicted to increase the concentration of intramuscular **medroxyprogesterone**. [Moderate] Theoretical
- **Ceritinib** is predicted to increase the concentration of intramuscular **medroxyprogesterone**. [Moderate] Theoretical
- **Cobicistat** is predicted to increase the concentration of intramuscular **medroxyprogesterone**. [Moderate] Theoretical
- **HIV-protease inhibitors** are predicted to increase the concentration of intramuscular **medroxyprogesterone**. [Moderate] Theoretical
- **Idelalisib** is predicted to increase the concentration of intramuscular **medroxyprogesterone**. [Moderate] Theoretical
- Macrolides **(clarithromycin)** are predicted to increase the concentration of intramuscular **medroxyprogesterone**. [Moderate] Theoretical
- **Sugammadex** is predicted to decrease the exposure to **medroxyprogesterone**. Use additional contraceptive precautions. [Severe] Theoretical
- **Tucatinib** is predicted to increase the concentration of intramuscular **medroxyprogesterone**. [Moderate] Theoretical

Mefenamic acid → see NSAIDs

Mefloquine → see antimalarials

Meglitinides → see **TABLE 13** p. 1575 (antidiabetic drugs)

  repaglinide

- Anti-androgens **(abiraterone)** are predicted to increase the exposure to **repaglinide**. [Moderate] Anecdotal
- Anti-androgens **(apalutamide, enzalutamide)** are predicted to decrease the exposure to **repaglinide**. Monitor blood glucose and adjust dose. [Moderate] Study
- Anti-androgens **(darolutamide)** are predicted to increase the concentration of **repaglinide**. [Moderate] Theoretical
- Antiepileptics **(carbamazepine, fosphenytoin, phenobarbital, phenytoin, primidone)** are predicted to decrease the exposure to **repaglinide**. Monitor blood glucose and adjust dose. [Moderate] Study
- **Belumosudil** is predicted to increase the exposure to **repaglinide**. Avoid or adjust dose. [Moderate] Study
- **Bulevirtide** is predicted to increase the exposure to **repaglinide**. Avoid or monitor. [Moderate] Theoretical
- **Ciclosporin** moderately increases the exposure to **repaglinide**. [Moderate] Study
- **Clopidogrel** increases the exposure to **repaglinide**. Avoid. [Severe] Study
- **Elexacaftor** is predicted to increase the exposure to **repaglinide**. [Moderate] Theoretical
- **Encorafenib** is predicted to decrease the exposure to **repaglinide**. Monitor blood glucose and adjust dose. [Moderate] Study
- **Fenfluramine** might decrease blood glucose concentrations when given with **meglitinides**. [Moderate] Theoretical
- Fibrates **(gemfibrozil)** increase the exposure to **repaglinide**. Avoid. [Severe] Study
- Iron chelators **(deferasirox)** moderately increase the exposure to **repaglinide**. Avoid. [Moderate] Study
- **Ivosidenib** is predicted to decrease the exposure to **repaglinide**. Monitor blood glucose and adjust dose. [Moderate] Study
- **Leflunomide** is predicted to increase the exposure to **repaglinide**. [Moderate] Study
- **Leniolisib** is predicted to increase the exposure to **repaglinide**. Avoid. [Moderate] Theoretical
- **Letermovir** is predicted to increase the concentration of **repaglinide**. Avoid. [Moderate] Theoretical
- **Linzagolix** slightly increases the exposure to **repaglinide**. Avoid. [Mild] Study
- **Lumacaftor** is predicted to decrease the exposure to **repaglinide**. Monitor blood glucose and adjust dose. [Moderate] Study
- Macrolides **(clarithromycin)** might cause hypoglycaemia when given with **repaglinide**. [Moderate] Anecdotal
- **Mifepristone** is predicted to increase the exposure to **repaglinide**. [Moderate] Theoretical
- **Mitotane** is predicted to decrease the exposure to **repaglinide**. Monitor blood glucose and adjust dose. [Moderate] Study
- **Opicapone** is predicted to increase the exposure to **repaglinide**. Avoid. [Moderate] Study
- **Pitolisant** is predicted to decrease the exposure to **repaglinide**. [Mild] Theoretical
- Rifamycins **(rifampicin)** are predicted to decrease the exposure to **repaglinide**. Monitor blood glucose and adjust dose. [Moderate] Study
- **Roxadustat** is predicted to increase the exposure to **repaglinide**. Monitor adverse effects and adjust dose. [Moderate] Study
- **Selpercatinib** increases the exposure to **repaglinide**. Avoid. [Moderate] Study
- **Somapacitan** might increase blood glucose concentrations, opposing the blood glucose-lowering effects of **meglitinides**. Adjust dose. [Moderate] Theoretical
- **Somatrogon** might increase blood glucose concentrations, opposing the blood glucose-lowering effects of **meglitinides**. Adjust dose. [Moderate] Theoretical
- Taxanes **(cabazitaxel)** are predicted to affect the exposure to **repaglinide**. Manufacturer advises take 12 hours before or 3 hours after **cabazitaxel**. [Moderate] Theoretical
- **Teriflunomide** is predicted to increase the exposure to **repaglinide**. [Moderate] Study
- **Trimethoprim** slightly increases the exposure to **repaglinide**. Avoid or monitor blood glucose. [Moderate] Study
- **Velpatasvir** is predicted to increase the exposure to **repaglinide**. [Moderate] Study
- **Venetoclax** is predicted to increase the exposure to **repaglinide**. [Moderate] Theoretical
- **Voclosporin** is predicted to increase the concentration of **repaglinide**. [Moderate] Theoretical

Meglitinides (continued)
- **Voxilaprevir** with sofosbuvir and velpatasvir is predicted to increase the exposure to **repaglinide**. Moderate Study

Melatonin → see TABLE 10 p. 1574 (CNS effects)
- Antiepileptics (phenytoin) are predicted to decrease the exposure to **melatonin**. Moderate Theoretical → Also see TABLE 10 p. 1574
- **Axitinib** is predicted to increase the exposure to **melatonin**. Moderate Theoretical
- **Combined hormonal contraceptives** is predicted to increase the exposure to **melatonin**. Moderate Theoretical
- **Givosiran** is predicted to increase the exposure to **melatonin**. Moderate Theoretical
- HIV-protease inhibitors (ritonavir) are predicted to decrease the exposure to **melatonin**. Moderate Theoretical
- **Leflunomide** is predicted to decrease the exposure to melatonin. Moderate Theoretical
- **Leniolisib** is predicted to increase the exposure to **melatonin**. Avoid. Moderate Theoretical
- **Mexiletine** is predicted to increase the exposure to **melatonin**. Moderate Theoretical
- **Osilodrostat** is predicted to increase the exposure to melatonin. Moderate Theoretical
- Quinolones (ciprofloxacin) are predicted to increase the exposure to **melatonin**. Moderate Theoretical
- Rifamycins (rifampicin) are predicted to decrease the exposure to **melatonin**. Moderate Theoretical
- **Rucaparib** is predicted to increase the exposure to **melatonin**. Moderate Theoretical
- SSRIs (fluvoxamine) very markedly increase the exposure to melatonin. Avoid. Severe Study → Also see TABLE 10 p. 1574
- **Teriflunomide** is predicted to decrease the exposure to melatonin. Moderate Theoretical
- **Vemurafenib** is predicted to increase the exposure to melatonin. Moderate Theoretical

Meloxicam → see NSAIDs
Melphalan → see alkylating agents
Memantine
- Dopamine receptor agonists (amantadine) increase the risk of CNS toxicity when given with **memantine**. Use with caution or avoid. Severe Theoretical
- **Memantine** is predicted to increase the effects of dopamine receptor agonists (apomorphine, bromocriptine, cabergoline, pramipexole, quinagolide, ropinirole, rotigotine). Moderate Theoretical
- **Memantine** is predicted to increase the risk of CNS adverse effects when given with ketamine. Avoid. Severe Theoretical
- **Memantine** is predicted to increase the effects of levodopa. Moderate Theoretical

Mepacrine
- **Mepacrine** is predicted to increase the concentration of antimalarials (primaquine). Avoid. Moderate Theoretical

Mepivacaine → see anaesthetics, local
Meptazinol → see opioids
Mercaptopurine → see TABLE 1 p. 1571 (hepatotoxicity), TABLE 14 p. 1575 (myelosuppression)
- **Allopurinol** potentially increases the risk of haematological toxicity when given with **mercaptopurine**. Adjust mercaptopurine dose, p. 1047. Severe Study
- **Mercaptopurine** decreases the anticoagulant effect of coumarins. Moderate Anecdotal
- **Febuxostat** is predicted to increase the exposure to mercaptopurine. Avoid. Severe Theoretical
- **Live vaccines** are predicted to increase the risk of generalised infection (possibly life-threatening) when given with mercaptopurine (high-dose). UKHSA advises avoid (refer to Green Book). Severe Theoretical
- **Trimethoprim** might increase the risk of haematological toxicity when given with **mercaptopurine** in renal transplant patients. Severe Theoretical

Meropenem → see carbapenems
Mesalazine → see TABLE 2 p. 1571 (nephrotoxicity)

ROUTE-SPECIFIC INFORMATION The manufacturers of some mesalazine gastro-resistant and modified-release medicines (*Asacol MR* tablets, *Ipocol*, *Salofalk* granules) suggest that preparations that lower stool pH (e.g. lactulose) might prevent the release of mesalazine.

Metaraminol → see sympathomimetics, vasoconstrictor
Metformin → see TABLE 13 p. 1575 (antidiabetic drugs)
- **Alcohol** (excessive consumption) potentially increases the risk of lactic acidosis when given with **metformin**. Avoid excessive alcohol consumption. Moderate Theoretical
- Antiepileptics (sultiame) might increase the risk of lactic acidosis when given with **metformin**. Severe Theoretical
- Antifungals, azoles (isavuconazole) are predicted to increase the exposure to **metformin**. Use with caution and adjust dose. Moderate Study
- Antimalarials (pyrimethamine) are predicted to increase the exposure to **metformin**. Use with caution and adjust dose. Moderate Study
- **Bictegravir** slightly increases the exposure to **metformin**. Moderate Study
- **Dolutegravir** is predicted to increase the exposure to **metformin**. Use with caution and adjust dose. Moderate Study
- **Fenfluramine** might decrease blood glucose concentrations when given with **metformin**. Moderate Theoretical
- **Givinostat** might increase the exposure to **metformin**. Moderate Theoretical
- **Guanfacine** is predicted to increase the concentration of **metformin**. Moderate Theoretical
- H_2 receptor antagonists (cimetidine) are predicted to increase the exposure to **metformin**. Use with caution and adjust dose. Moderate Study
- **Mexiletine** is predicted to affect the exposure to **metformin**. Unknown Theoretical
- **Pitolisant** is predicted to increase the exposure to **metformin**. Mild Theoretical
- **Ranolazine** is predicted to increase the exposure to **metformin**. Use with caution and adjust dose. Moderate Study
- **Ribociclib** is predicted to increase the exposure to **metformin**. Moderate Theoretical
- **Risdiplam** is predicted to increase the concentration of metformin. Monitor and adjust dose. Moderate Theoretical
- **Somapacitan** might increase blood glucose concentrations, opposing the blood glucose-lowering effects of **metformin**. Adjust dose. Moderate Theoretical
- **Somatrogon** might increase blood glucose concentrations, opposing the blood glucose-lowering effects of **metformin**. Adjust dose. Moderate Theoretical
- **Trimethoprim** is predicted to increase the exposure to metformin. Use with caution and adjust dose. Moderate Study
- **Vandetanib** is predicted to increase the exposure to **metformin**. Use with caution and adjust dose. Moderate Study

Methadone → see opioids
Methenamine
- **Acetazolamide** is predicted to decrease the efficacy of methenamine. Avoid. Moderate Theoretical
- **Potassium citrate** is predicted to decrease the efficacy of methenamine. Avoid. Moderate Theoretical
- **Sodium bicarbonate** is predicted to decrease the efficacy of methenamine. Avoid. Moderate Theoretical
- **Sodium citrate** is predicted to decrease the efficacy of methenamine. Avoid. Moderate Theoretical
- **Methenamine** might increase the risk of crystalluria when given with sulfonamides. Avoid. Severe Theoretical
- Thiazide diuretics (metolazone) are predicted to decrease the efficacy of **methenamine**. Moderate Theoretical

Methocarbamol → see TABLE 10 p. 1574 (CNS effects)
Methotrexate → see TABLE 1 p. 1571 (hepatotoxicity), TABLE 14 p. 1575 (myelosuppression), TABLE 2 p. 1571 (nephrotoxicity)
- **Acetazolamide** increases the urinary excretion of methotrexate. Moderate Study
- **Methotrexate** is predicted to decrease the clearance of aminophylline. Moderate Theoretical
- Anti-androgens (apalutamide) are predicted to decrease the exposure to **methotrexate**. Mild Study
- Anti-androgens (darolutamide) are predicted to increase the concentration of **methotrexate**. Moderate Theoretical
- Antiepileptics (levetiracetam) decrease the clearance of methotrexate. Severe Anecdotal

- **Antimalarials (pyrimethamine)** are predicted to increase the risk of adverse effects when given with **methotrexate**. Severe Theoretical
- **Asparaginase** affects the efficacy of **methotrexate**. Severe Anecdotal → Also see **TABLE 1** p. 1571 → Also see **TABLE 14** p. 1575
- **Aspirin** (high-dose) is predicted to increase the risk of toxicity when given with **methotrexate**. Severe Study → Also see **TABLE 2** p. 1571
- **Baricitinib** is predicted to enhance the risk of immunosuppression when given with **methotrexate**. Severe Study
- **Crisantaspase** affects the efficacy of **methotrexate**. Severe Anecdotal → Also see **TABLE 1** p. 1571 → Also see **TABLE 14** p. 1575
- **Eltrombopag** is predicted to increase the concentration of **methotrexate**. Moderate Theoretical
- **Methotrexate** potentially increases the risk of severe skin reaction when given with topical **fluorouracil**. Severe Anecdotal → Also see **TABLE 1** p. 1571 → Also see **TABLE 14** p. 1575
- **Ivosidenib** is predicted to increase the exposure to **methotrexate**. Use with caution or avoid. Moderate Theoretical
- **Leflunomide** is predicted to increase the exposure to **methotrexate**. Avoid. Severe Study → Also see **TABLE 14** p. 1575
- **Live vaccines** are predicted to increase the risk of generalised infection (possibly life-threatening) when given with **methotrexate** (high-dose). UKHSA advises avoid (refer to Green Book). Severe Theoretical
- **Nitisinone** is predicted to increase the exposure to **methotrexate**. Moderate Study
- **Nitrous oxide** potentially increases the risk of methotrexate toxicity when given with **methotrexate**. Avoid. Severe Study
- **NSAIDs** are predicted to increase the risk of toxicity when given with **methotrexate** (particularly high-dose). Severe Study → Also see **TABLE 2** p. 1571
- **Pegaspargase** affects the efficacy of **methotrexate**. Severe Anecdotal → Also see **TABLE 1** p. 1571 → Also see **TABLE 14** p. 1575
- **Penicillins** are predicted to increase the risk of toxicity when given with **methotrexate**. Severe Anecdotal
- **Potassium aminobenzoate** increases the concentration of **methotrexate**. Moderate Theoretical
- **Proton pump inhibitors** decrease the clearance of **methotrexate** (high-dose). Use with caution or avoid. Severe Study
- **Quinolones (ciprofloxacin)** potentially increase the risk of toxicity when given with **methotrexate**. Severe Anecdotal
- **Regorafenib** is predicted to increase the exposure to **methotrexate**. Moderate Theoretical → Also see **TABLE 14** p. 1575
- **Retinoids (acitretin)** are predicted to increase the concentration of **methotrexate**. Avoid. Moderate Anecdotal → Also see **TABLE 1** p. 1571
- **Methotrexate** is predicted to decrease the efficacy of **sapropterin**. Moderate Theoretical
- **Sulfonamides** are predicted to increase the exposure to **methotrexate**. Use with caution or avoid. Severe Theoretical
- **Tedizolid** is predicted to increase the exposure to **methotrexate**. Avoid. Moderate Theoretical
- **Methotrexate** is predicted to increase the risk of toxicity when given with **tegafur**. Severe Theoretical → Also see **TABLE 14** p. 1575
- **Teriflunomide** is predicted to increase the exposure to **methotrexate**. Moderate Study
- **Methotrexate** decreases the clearance of **theophylline**. Moderate Study
- **Trimethoprim** increases the risk of haematological side-effects (sometimes fatal) when given with **methotrexate**. Avoid. See methotrexate p. 1048 for further information. Severe Anecdotal → Also see **TABLE 2** p. 1571
- **Vadadustat** is predicted to increase the exposure to **methotrexate**. Monitor and adjust dose. Moderate Study

Methoxyflurane → see volatile halogenated anaesthetics

Methyldopa → see **TABLE 7** p. 1572 (hypotension)
- **Entacapone** is predicted to increase the exposure to **methyldopa**. Moderate Theoretical
- Oral **iron** decreases the effects of oral **methyldopa**. Moderate Study
- **Methyldopa** increases the risk of neurotoxicity when given with **lithium**. Severe Anecdotal
- **MAOIs, irreversible** are predicted to alter the antihypertensive effects of **methyldopa**. Avoid. Severe Theoretical → Also see **TABLE 7** p. 1572
- **Methyldopa** might enhance the antidiuretic and hypertensive effects of **vasopressin**. Moderate Theoretical

Methylphenidate
- **Alcohol** might increase the concentration of **methylphenidate**. Avoid. Moderate Study
- **Antiepileptics (carbamazepine)** might decrease the concentration of **methylphenidate**. Moderate Anecdotal
- **Antiepileptics (valproate)** might enhance the effects of **methylphenidate**. Severe Anecdotal
- **Methylphenidate** might increase the risk of dyskinesias when given with **antipsychotics, second generation (paliperidone)**. Severe Theoretical
- **Methylphenidate** increases the risk of dyskinesias when given with **antipsychotics, second generation (risperidone)**. Severe Anecdotal
- **Methylphenidate** is predicted to decrease the effects of **apraclonidine**. Avoid. Severe Theoretical
- **Methylphenidate** has been reported to cause psychotic symptoms when given with **disulfiram**. Severe Anecdotal
- **Methylphenidate** might increase the risk of elevated blood pressure when given with **linezolid**. Avoid. Severe Theoretical
- **MAO-B inhibitors (rasagiline)** are predicted to increase the risk of a hypertensive crisis when given with **methylphenidate**. Avoid. Severe Theoretical
- **MAO-B inhibitors (selegiline)** might increase the risk of a hypertensive crisis when given with **methylphenidate**. Avoid. Severe Theoretical
- **Methylphenidate** causes a hypertensive crisis when given with **MAOIs, irreversible**. Avoid and for 14 days after stopping the MAOI. Severe Theoretical
- **Methylphenidate** is predicted to cause a hypertensive crisis when given with **methylthioninium chloride**. Severe Theoretical
- **Methylphenidate** is predicted to cause a hypertensive crisis when given with **moclobemide**. Severe Theoretical
- **Nirmatrelvir** boosted with ritonavir is predicted to increase the concentration of **methylphenidate**. Severe Theoretical
- **Methylphenidate** is predicted to increase the risk of a hypertensive crisis when given with **ozanimod**. Severe Theoretical
- **Methylphenidate** might increase the concentration of **tricyclic antidepressants**. Use with caution and adjust dose. Moderate Study
- **Methylphenidate** might increase the risk of hypertension and arrhythmias when given with **volatile halogenated anaesthetics**. Avoid **methylphenidate** on day of surgery, p. 403. Severe Theoretical

Methylprednisolone → see corticosteroids

Methylthioninium chloride → see **TABLE 12** p. 1574 (serotonin syndrome)
- **Methylthioninium chloride** is predicted to increase the risk of severe hypertension when given with **bupropion**. Avoid. Severe Theoretical
- **Methylphenidate** is predicted to cause a hypertensive crisis when given with **methylthioninium chloride**. Severe Theoretical

Metoclopramide
- **Metoclopramide** potentially decreases the absorption of **antifungals, azoles (posaconazole)** oral suspension. Moderate Study
- **Metoclopramide** decreases the concentration of **antimalarials (atovaquone)**. Avoid. Moderate Study
- **Cilostazol** might increase the exposure to **metoclopramide**. Moderate Study
- **Metoclopramide** is predicted to decrease the effects of **dopamine receptor agonists (apomorphine, bromocriptine, cabergoline, pramipexole, quinagolide, ropinirole, rotigotine)**. Avoid. Moderate Study
- **Metoclopramide** might decrease the effects of **foslevodopa**. Moderate Theoretical
- **Metoclopramide** decreases the effects of **levodopa**. Avoid. Moderate Study

Metoclopramide (continued)

▶ **Metoclopramide** is predicted to increase the effects of neuromuscular blocking drugs, non-depolarising. Moderate Theoretical

▶ **Metoclopramide** increases the effects of suxamethonium. Moderate Study

Metolazone → see thiazide diuretics

Metoprolol → see beta blockers, selective

Metreleptin

▶ **Metreleptin** might alter the exposure to aminophylline. Severe Theoretical

▶ **Metreleptin** might alter the exposure to ciclosporin. Monitor concentration and adjust dose. Severe Theoretical

▶ **Metreleptin** might decrease the efficacy of combined hormonal contraceptives. Use additional contraceptive precautions. Severe Theoretical

▶ **Metreleptin** might alter the exposure to coumarins (warfarin). Monitor INR and adjust dose. Severe Theoretical

▶ **Metreleptin** is predicted to increase the risk of hypoglycaemia when given with insulin. Monitor blood glucose and adjust dose. Severe Theoretical

▶ **Metreleptin** is predicted to increase the risk of hypoglycaemia when given with sulfonylureas. Monitor blood glucose and adjust dose. Severe Theoretical

▶ **Metreleptin** might alter the exposure to theophylline. Monitor concentration and adjust dose. Severe Theoretical

Metronidazole → see TABLE 11 p. 1574 (peripheral neuropathy)

ROUTE-SPECIFIC INFORMATION Since systemic absorption can follow topical application, the possibility of interactions should be borne in mind.

▶ Alcohol potentially causes a disulfiram-like reaction when given with **metronidazole**. Avoid for at least 48 hours after stopping treatment. Moderate Study

▶ **Metronidazole** increases the risk of toxicity when given with alkylating agents (busulfan). Severe Study

▶ Antiepileptics (phenobarbital, primidone) are predicted to decrease the exposure to **metronidazole**. Moderate Study

▶ **Metronidazole** is predicted to increase the risk of capecitabine toxicity when given with capecitabine. Severe Theoretical

▶ **Metronidazole** increases the anticoagulant effect of coumarins. Monitor INR and adjust dose. Severe Study

▶ Disulfiram increases the risk of acute psychoses when given with **metronidazole**. Severe Study

▶ **Metronidazole** increases the risk of toxicity when given with fluorouracil. Severe Study

▶ **Metronidazole** is predicted to increase the concentration of lithium. Avoid or adjust dose. Severe Anecdotal

Metyrapone

▶ Antiepileptics (fosphenytoin, phenobarbital, phenytoin, primidone) are predicted to decrease the effects of metyrapone. Avoid. Moderate Study

▶ Antihistamines, sedating (cyproheptadine) decrease the effects of metyrapone. Avoid. Moderate Study

▶ Carbimazole decreases the effects of **metyrapone**. Avoid. Moderate Theoretical

▶ Combined hormonal contraceptives decrease the effects of metyrapone. Avoid. Moderate Theoretical

▶ Phenothiazines (chlorpromazine) decrease the effects of metyrapone. Avoid. Moderate Theoretical

▶ Propylthiouracil is predicted to decrease the effects of metyrapone. Avoid. Moderate Theoretical

▶ Tricyclic antidepressants (amitriptyline) decrease the effects of metyrapone. Avoid. Moderate Theoretical

Mexiletine

FOOD AND LIFESTYLE Dose adjustment might be necessary if smoking started or stopped during treatment.

▶ **Mexiletine** is predicted to increase the exposure to agomelatine. Moderate Study

▶ **Mexiletine** is predicted to increase the exposure to aminophylline. Adjust dose. Moderate Theoretical

▶ **Mexiletine** is predicted to increase the exposure to anaesthetics, local (ropivacaine). Moderate Theoretical

▶ **Mexiletine** is predicted to increase the exposure to anagrelide. Moderate Theoretical

▶ **Mexiletine** is predicted to increase the risk of torsade de pointes when given with antiarrhythmics. Avoid. Severe Theoretical

▶ Antiepileptics (phenytoin) are predicted to increase the clearance of **mexiletine**. Monitor and adjust dose. Moderate Study

▶ **Mexiletine** increases the concentration of antipsychotics, second generation (clozapine). Monitor adverse effects and adjust dose. Severe Study

▶ **Mexiletine** is predicted to increase the exposure to antipsychotics, second generation (olanzapine). Adjust dose. Moderate Anecdotal

▶ **Mexiletine** potentially increases the risk of cardiovascular adverse effects when given with beta blockers, non-selective. Avoid or monitor. Severe Theoretical

▶ **Mexiletine** potentially increases the risk of cardiovascular adverse effects when given with beta blockers, selective. Avoid or monitor. Severe Theoretical

▶ Bupropion is predicted to increase the exposure to **mexiletine**. Moderate Study

▶ **Mexiletine** increases the risk of cardiovascular adverse effects when given with calcium channel blockers (diltiazem). Avoid or monitor. Severe Theoretical

▶ **Mexiletine** potentially increases the risk of cardiovascular adverse effects when given with calcium channel blockers (verapamil). Avoid or monitor. Severe Theoretical

▶ Cinacalcet is predicted to increase the exposure to **mexiletine**. Moderate Study

▶ Cobicistat potentially increases the exposure to **mexiletine**. Severe Theoretical

▶ **Mexiletine** potentially affects the exposure to coumarins (warfarin). Avoid. Unknown Theoretical

▶ Dacomitinib is predicted to increase the exposure to mexiletine. Moderate Study

▶ **Mexiletine** is predicted to increase the exposure to dopamine receptor agonists (ropinirole). Adjust dose. Moderate Study

▶ **Mexiletine** are predicted to increases the exposure to erlotinib. Monitor adverse effects and adjust dose. Moderate Study

▶ **Mexiletine** is predicted to increase the exposure to fezolinetant. Avoid. Moderate Study

▶ HIV-protease inhibitors (ritonavir) are predicted to increase the clearance of **mexiletine**. Monitor and adjust dose. Moderate Study

▶ Leflunomide is predicted to increase the clearance of mexiletine. Monitor and adjust dose. Moderate Study

▶ **Mexiletine** potentially affects the exposure to lithium. Avoid. Unknown Theoretical

▶ **Mexiletine** is predicted to increase the exposure to loxapine. Avoid. Unknown Theoretical

▶ **Mexiletine** slightly increases the exposure to MAO-B inhibitors (rasagiline). Moderate Study

▶ **Mexiletine** is predicted to increase the exposure to melatonin. Moderate Theoretical

▶ **Mexiletine** is predicted to affect the exposure to metformin. Unknown Theoretical

▶ Opioids potentially decrease the absorption of oral **mexiletine**. Moderate Study

▶ **Mexiletine** is predicted to increase the exposure to phenothiazines (chlorpromazine). Moderate Theoretical

▶ **Mexiletine** is predicted to increase the exposure to phosphodiesterase type-4 inhibitors (roflumilast). Moderate Theoretical

▶ **Mexiletine** is predicted to increase the exposure to pirfenidone. Use with caution and adjust dose. Moderate Study

▶ Rifamycins (rifampicin) are predicted to increase the clearance of **mexiletine**. Monitor and adjust dose. Moderate Study

▶ **Mexiletine** is predicted to increase the exposure to riluzole. Moderate Theoretical

▶ **Mexiletine** is predicted to increase the exposure to SNRIs (duloxetine). Moderate Theoretical

▶ SSRIs (fluoxetine, fluvoxamine, paroxetine) are predicted to increase the exposure to **mexiletine**. Moderate Study

▶ Terbinafine is predicted to increase the exposure to **mexiletine**. Moderate Study

▸ **Teriflunomide** is predicted to increase the clearance of **mexiletine**. Monitor and adjust dose. Moderate Study
▸ **Mexiletine** is predicted to increase the exposure to **theophylline**. Monitor and adjust dose. Moderate Theoretical
▸ **Mexiletine** increases the exposure to **tizanidine**. Avoid. Moderate Study
▸ **Mexiletine** is predicted to increase the exposure to **triptans (zolmitriptan)**. Adjust **zolmitriptan** dose, p. 546. Moderate Theoretical

Mianserin → see TABLE 10 p. 1574 (CNS effects)
▸ **Antiepileptics (carbamazepine)** markedly decrease the exposure to **mianserin**. Adjust dose. Moderate Study
▸ **Antiepileptics (phenobarbital, primidone)** are predicted to decrease the exposure to **mianserin**. Moderate Study → Also see TABLE 10 p. 1574
▸ **Mianserin** is predicted to increase the risk of toxicity when given with **MAOIs, irreversible**. Avoid and for 14 days after stopping the MAOI. Severe Theoretical
▸ **Mianserin** is predicted to increase the risk of toxicity when given with **moclobemide**. Avoid and for 1 week after stopping **mianserin**. Severe Theoretical
▸ **Mianserin** is predicted to decrease the efficacy of **pitolisant**. Moderate Theoretical
▸ **Mianserin** decreases the effects of **sympathomimetics, vasoconstrictor (ephedrine)**. Severe Anecdotal

Micafungin → see TABLE 1 p. 1571 (hepatotoxicity)
▸ **Micafungin** slightly increases the exposure to **amphotericin B**. Avoid or monitor toxicity. Moderate Study

Miconazole → see antifungals, azoles

Midazolam → see benzodiazepines

Midodrine → see sympathomimetics, vasoconstrictor

Midostaurin
▸ **Anti-androgens (apalutamide, enzalutamide)** are predicted to decrease the exposure to **midostaurin**. Avoid. Severe Study
▸ **Antiarrhythmics (dronedarone)** are predicted to increase the exposure to **midostaurin**. Moderate Theoretical
▸ **Antiepileptics (carbamazepine, fosphenytoin, phenobarbital, phenytoin, primidone)** are predicted to decrease the exposure to **midostaurin**. Avoid. Severe Study
▸ **Antifungals, azoles (fluconazole, isavuconazole)** are predicted to increase the exposure to **midostaurin**. Moderate Theoretical
▸ **Antifungals, azoles (itraconazole, ketoconazole, posaconazole, voriconazole)** are predicted to increase the exposure to **midostaurin**. Avoid or monitor for toxicity. Severe Study
▸ **Berotralstat** is predicted to increase the exposure to **midostaurin**. Moderate Theoretical
▸ **Midostaurin** moderately decreases the exposure to the active metabolite of **bupropion**. Moderate Study
▸ **Calcium channel blockers (diltiazem, verapamil)** are predicted to increase the exposure to **midostaurin**. Moderate Theoretical
▸ **Ceritinib** is predicted to increase the exposure to **midostaurin**. Avoid or monitor for toxicity. Severe Study
▸ **Midostaurin** might increase the concentration of **ciclosporin**. Severe Anecdotal
▸ **Cobicistat** is predicted to increase the exposure to **midostaurin**. Avoid or monitor for toxicity. Severe Study
▸ **Crizotinib** is predicted to increase the exposure to **midostaurin**. Moderate Theoretical
▸ **Dabrafenib** is predicted to decrease the exposure to **midostaurin**. Severe Study
▸ **Elvitegravir** boosted with ritonavir is predicted to increase the exposure to **midostaurin**. Severe Theoretical
▸ **Encorafenib** is predicted to decrease the exposure to **midostaurin**. Avoid. Severe Study
▸ **Endothelin receptor antagonists (bosentan)** are predicted to decrease the exposure to **midostaurin** and **midostaurin** is predicted to increase the exposure to **endothelin receptor antagonists (bosentan)**. Severe Study
▸ **Fedratinib** is predicted to increase the exposure to **midostaurin**. Moderate Theoretical
▸ **Grapefruit** juice is predicted to increase the exposure to **midostaurin**. Moderate Theoretical
▸ **HIV-protease inhibitors** are predicted to increase the exposure to **midostaurin**. Avoid or monitor for toxicity. Severe Study

▸ **Idelalisib** is predicted to increase the exposure to **midostaurin**. Avoid or monitor for toxicity. Severe Study
▸ **Imatinib** is predicted to increase the exposure to **midostaurin**. Moderate Theoretical
▸ **Ivosidenib** is predicted to decrease the exposure to **midostaurin**. Avoid. Severe Study
▸ **Letermovir** is predicted to increase the exposure to **midostaurin**. Moderate Theoretical
▸ **Lumacaftor** is predicted to decrease the exposure to **midostaurin**. Avoid. Severe Study
▸ **Macrolides (clarithromycin)** are predicted to increase the exposure to **midostaurin**. Avoid or monitor for toxicity. Severe Study
▸ **Macrolides (erythromycin)** are predicted to increase the exposure to **midostaurin**. Moderate Theoretical
▸ **Mitotane** is predicted to decrease the exposure to **midostaurin**. Avoid. Severe Study
▸ **Neurokinin-1 receptor antagonists (aprepitant, netupitant)** are predicted to increase the exposure to **midostaurin**. Moderate Theoretical
▸ **Nilotinib** is predicted to increase the exposure to **midostaurin**. Moderate Theoretical
▸ **NNRTIs (efavirenz, etravirine, nevirapine)** are predicted to decrease the exposure to **midostaurin**. Severe Study
▸ **Rifamycins (rifampicin)** are predicted to decrease the exposure to **midostaurin**. Avoid. Severe Study
▸ **St John's wort** is predicted to decrease the exposure to **midostaurin**. Avoid. Severe Theoretical
▸ **Tucatinib** is predicted to increase the exposure to **midostaurin**. Avoid or monitor for toxicity. Severe Study

Mifamurtide → see TABLE 14 p. 1575 (myelosuppression)
▸ **Ciclosporin** is predicted to decrease the efficacy of **mifamurtide**. Avoid. Severe Theoretical
▸ **Corticosteroids** are predicted to decrease the efficacy of **mifamurtide**. Avoid. Severe Theoretical
▸ **NSAIDs** (high-dose) are predicted to decrease the efficacy of **mifamurtide**. Avoid. Severe Theoretical
▸ **Pimecrolimus** is predicted to decrease the efficacy of **mifamurtide**. Avoid. Severe Theoretical
▸ **Sirolimus** is predicted to decrease the efficacy of **mifamurtide**. Avoid. Severe Theoretical
▸ **Tacrolimus** is predicted to affect the efficacy of **mifamurtide**. Avoid. Severe Theoretical

Mifepristone
▸ **Anti-androgens (apalutamide, enzalutamide)** are predicted to decrease the exposure to **mifepristone**. Adjust **mifepristone** dose, p. 954. Severe Study
▸ **Antiepileptics (carbamazepine, fosphenytoin, phenobarbital, phenytoin, primidone)** are predicted to decrease the exposure to **mifepristone**. Adjust **mifepristone** dose, p. 954. Severe Study
▸ **Antifungals, azoles (posaconazole)** are predicted to increase the exposure to **mifepristone**. Moderate Theoretical
▸ **Mifepristone** is predicted to increase the exposure to **avatrombopag**. Moderate Theoretical
▸ **Mifepristone** is predicted to increase the exposure to **capivasertib**. Adjust dose. Moderate Theoretical
▸ **Cenobamate** is predicted to decrease the exposure to **mifepristone**. Adjust **mifepristone** dose, p. 954. Severe Study
▸ **Mifepristone** is predicted to decrease the efficacy of **corticosteroids**. Use with caution and adjust dose. Moderate Theoretical
▸ **Mifepristone** is predicted to increase the exposure to **coumarins (warfarin)**. Moderate Theoretical
▸ **Dabrafenib** is predicted to decrease the exposure to **mifepristone**. Adjust **mifepristone** dose, p. 954. Severe Study
▸ **Encorafenib** is predicted to decrease the exposure to **mifepristone**. Adjust **mifepristone** dose, p. 954. Severe Study
▸ **Endothelin receptor antagonists (bosentan)** are predicted to decrease the exposure to **mifepristone**. Adjust **mifepristone** dose, p. 954. Severe Study
▸ **Mifepristone** is predicted to increase the exposure to **everolimus**. Severe Theoretical
▸ **Grapefruit** juice is predicted to increase the exposure to **mifepristone**. Moderate Theoretical

Mifepristone (continued)

- **Ivosidenib** is predicted to decrease the exposure to mifepristone. Adjust **mifepristone** dose, p. 954. Severe Study
- **Mifepristone** is predicted to increase the exposure to loperamide. Moderate Theoretical
- **Lorlatinib** is predicted to decrease the exposure to mifepristone. Adjust **mifepristone** dose, p. 954. Severe Study
- **Lumacaftor** is predicted to decrease the exposure to mifepristone. Adjust **mifepristone** dose, p. 954. Severe Study
- **Mifepristone** is predicted to increase the exposure to meglitinides (repaglinide). Moderate Theoretical
- **Mitotane** is predicted to decrease the exposure to **mifepristone**. Adjust **mifepristone** dose, p. 954. Severe Study
- **Mifepristone** is predicted to increase the exposure to montelukast. Moderate Theoretical
- **NNRTIs** (efavirenz, etravirine, nevirapine) are predicted to decrease the exposure to **mifepristone**. Adjust **mifepristone** dose, p. 954. Severe Study
- **Mifepristone** is predicted to increase the exposure to opioids (alfentanil). Severe Theoretical
- **Mifepristone** is predicted to increase the exposure to pioglitazone. Moderate Theoretical
- **Rifamycins** (rifampicin) are predicted to decrease the exposure to **mifepristone**. Adjust **mifepristone** dose, p. 954. Severe Study
- **Mifepristone** is predicted to increase the exposure to siponimod. Moderate Theoretical
- **Mifepristone** is predicted to increase the exposure to sirolimus. Severe Theoretical
- **Sotorasib** is predicted to decrease the exposure to mifepristone. Adjust **mifepristone** dose, p. 954. Severe Study
- **St John's wort** is predicted to decrease the exposure to mifepristone. Adjust **mifepristone** dose, p. 954. Severe Study
- **Mifepristone** moderately increases the exposure to statins (fluvastatin). Moderate Study
- **Mifepristone** very markedly increases the exposure to statins (simvastatin). Severe Study
- **Mifepristone** is predicted to increase the exposure to sulfonylureas (glimepiride, tolbutamide). Moderate Theoretical
- **Mifepristone** is predicted to increase the exposure to temsirolimus. Severe Theoretical

Mineralocorticoid receptor antagonists → see TABLE 7 p. 1572 (hypotension), TABLE 15 p. 1575 (increased serum potassium)

eplerenone · finerenone · spironolactone

- Anti-androgens (apalutamide, enzalutamide) are predicted to decrease the exposure to **eplerenone**. Avoid. Moderate Theoretical
- Anti-androgens (apalutamide, enzalutamide) are predicted to decrease the exposure to **finerenone**. Avoid. Severe Study
- **Spironolactone** might oppose the effects of anti-androgens (abiraterone). Avoid. Severe Anecdotal
- Antiarrhythmics (amiodarone) are predicted to increase the exposure to **eplerenone**. Adjust **eplerenone** dose, p. 223. Severe Theoretical
- Antiarrhythmics (dronedarone) are predicted to increase the exposure to **eplerenone**. Adjust **eplerenone** dose, p. 223. Severe Study
- Antiarrhythmics (dronedarone) are predicted to increase the exposure to **finerenone**. Severe Study
- Antiepileptics (carbamazepine, fosphenytoin, phenobarbital, phenytoin, primidone) are predicted to decrease the exposure to **eplerenone**. Avoid. Moderate Theoretical
- Antiepileptics (carbamazepine, fosphenytoin, phenobarbital, phenytoin, primidone) are predicted to decrease the exposure to **finerenone**. Avoid. Severe Study
- Antifungals, azoles (fluconazole, isavuconazole) are predicted to increase the exposure to **eplerenone**. Adjust **eplerenone** dose, p. 223. Severe Study
- Antifungals, azoles (fluconazole, isavuconazole) are predicted to increase the exposure to **finerenone**. Severe Study
- Antifungals, azoles (itraconazole, ketoconazole, posaconazole, voriconazole) are predicted to markedly increase the exposure to **eplerenone**. Avoid. Severe Study
- Antifungals, azoles (itraconazole, ketoconazole, posaconazole, voriconazole) are predicted to increase the exposure to **finerenone**. Avoid. Severe Study

- **Berotralstat** is predicted to increase the exposure to eplerenone. Adjust **eplerenone** dose, p. 223. Severe Study
- **Berotralstat** is predicted to increase the exposure to finerenone. Severe Study
- Calcium channel blockers (diltiazem, verapamil) are predicted to increase the exposure to **eplerenone**. Adjust **eplerenone** dose, p. 223. Severe Study → Also see TABLE 7 p. 1572
- Calcium channel blockers (diltiazem, verapamil) are predicted to increase the exposure to **finerenone**. Severe Study → Also see TABLE 7 p. 1572
- **Cenobamate** is predicted to decrease the exposure to eplerenone. Adjust dose. Moderate Theoretical
- **Cenobamate** is predicted to decrease the exposure to finerenone. Avoid. Severe Study
- **Ceritinib** is predicted to markedly increase the exposure to eplerenone. Avoid. Severe Study
- **Ceritinib** is predicted to increase the exposure to **finerenone**. Avoid. Severe Study
- **Cobicistat** is predicted to markedly increase the exposure to eplerenone. Avoid. Severe Study
- **Cobicistat** is predicted to increase the exposure to **finerenone**. Avoid. Severe Study
- **Crizotinib** is predicted to increase the exposure to **eplerenone**. Adjust **eplerenone** dose, p. 223. Severe Study
- **Crizotinib** is predicted to increase the exposure to **finerenone**. Severe Study
- **Dabrafenib** is predicted to decrease the exposure to finerenone. Avoid. Severe Study
- **Eplerenone** very slightly increases the exposure to digoxin. Mild Study
- **Spironolactone** increases the concentration of digoxin. Monitor and adjust dose. Moderate Study
- **Encorafenib** is predicted to decrease the exposure to eplerenone. Avoid. Moderate Theoretical
- **Encorafenib** is predicted to decrease the exposure to finerenone. Avoid. Severe Study
- Endothelin receptor antagonists (bosentan) are predicted to decrease the exposure to **finerenone**. Avoid. Severe Study
- **Fedratinib** is predicted to increase the exposure to **eplerenone**. Adjust **eplerenone** dose, p. 223. Severe Study
- **Fedratinib** is predicted to increase the exposure to **finerenone**. Severe Study
- **Grapefruit** and grapefruit juice is predicted to increase the exposure to **finerenone**. Avoid. Moderate Theoretical
- **HIV-protease inhibitors** are predicted to markedly increase the exposure to **eplerenone**. Avoid. Severe Study
- **HIV-protease inhibitors** are predicted to increase the exposure to **finerenone**. Avoid. Severe Study
- **Idelalisib** is predicted to markedly increase the exposure to eplerenone. Avoid. Severe Study
- **Idelalisib** is predicted to increase the exposure to **finerenone**. Avoid. Severe Study
- **Imatinib** is predicted to increase the exposure to **eplerenone**. Adjust **eplerenone** dose, p. 223. Severe Study
- **Imatinib** is predicted to increase the exposure to **finerenone**. Severe Study
- **Ivosidenib** is predicted to decrease the exposure to **eplerenone**. Avoid. Moderate Theoretical
- **Ivosidenib** is predicted to decrease the exposure to **finerenone**. Avoid. Severe Study
- **Letermovir** is predicted to increase the exposure to **eplerenone**. Adjust **eplerenone** dose, p. 223. Severe Study
- **Letermovir** is predicted to increase the exposure to **finerenone**. Severe Study
- **Eplerenone** potentially increases the concentration of lithium. Avoid. Moderate Theoretical
- **Spironolactone** potentially increases the concentration of lithium. Moderate Study
- **Lorlatinib** is predicted to decrease the exposure to **finerenone**. Avoid. Severe Study
- **Lumacaftor** is predicted to decrease the exposure to eplerenone. Avoid. Moderate Theoretical
- **Lumacaftor** is predicted to decrease the exposure to finerenone. Avoid. Severe Study

- Macrolides (clarithromycin) are predicted to markedly increase the exposure to **eplerenone**. Avoid. Severe Study
- Macrolides (clarithromycin) are predicted to increase the exposure to **finerenone**. Avoid. Severe Study
- Macrolides (erythromycin) are predicted to increase the exposure to **eplerenone**. Adjust **eplerenone** dose, p. 223. Severe Study
- Macrolides (erythromycin) are predicted to increase the exposure to **finerenone**. Severe Study
- **Mitotane** is predicted to decrease the exposure to **eplerenone**. Avoid. Moderate Theoretical
- **Mitotane** is predicted to decrease the exposure to **finerenone**. Avoid. Severe Study
- **Spironolactone** is predicted to decrease the effects of mitotane. Avoid. Severe Anecdotal
- Neurokinin-1 receptor antagonists (aprepitant, netupitant) are predicted to increase the exposure to **eplerenone**. Adjust **eplerenone** dose, p. 223. Severe Study
- Neurokinin-1 receptor antagonists (aprepitant, netupitant) are predicted to increase the exposure to **finerenone**. Severe Study
- **Nilotinib** is predicted to increase the exposure to **eplerenone**. Adjust **eplerenone** dose, p. 223. Severe Study
- **Nilotinib** is predicted to increase the exposure to **finerenone**. Severe Study
- **Nirmatrelvir** boosted with ritonavir is predicted to increase the concentration of mineralocorticoid receptor antagonists (eplerenone, finerenone). Avoid. Severe Theoretical
- NNRTIs (efavirenz, etravirine, nevirapine) are predicted to decrease the exposure to **finerenone**. Avoid. Severe Study
- Rifamycins (rifampicin) are predicted to decrease the exposure to **eplerenone**. Avoid. Moderate Theoretical
- Rifamycins (rifampicin) are predicted to decrease the exposure to **finerenone**. Avoid. Severe Study
- **Sotorasib** is predicted to decrease the exposure to **finerenone**. Avoid. Severe Study
- St John's wort is predicted to slightly decrease the exposure to **eplerenone**. Avoid. Moderate Study
- St John's wort is predicted to decrease the exposure to **finerenone**. Avoid. Severe Study
- **Tucatinib** is predicted to markedly increase the exposure to **eplerenone**. Avoid. Severe Study
- **Tucatinib** is predicted to increase the exposure to **finerenone**. Avoid. Severe Study

Minocycline → see tetracyclines
Minoxidil → see TABLE 7 p. 1572 (hypotension)

> **ROUTE-SPECIFIC INFORMATION** Since systemic absorption can follow topical application, the possibility of interactions should be borne in mind.

Mirabegron

- **Mirabegron** is predicted to increase the exposure to aliskiren. Mild Theoretical
- Antifungals, azoles (itraconazole, ketoconazole, posaconazole, voriconazole) are predicted to increase the exposure to mirabegron. Adjust **mirabegron** dose in hepatic and renal impairment, p. 901. Moderate Study
- **Mirabegron** is predicted to increase the exposure to antihistamines, non-sedating (fexofenadine). Mild Theoretical
- **Mirabegron** is predicted to increase the exposure to beta blockers, selective (metoprolol). Moderate Study
- **Ceritinib** is predicted to increase the exposure to mirabegron. Adjust **mirabegron** dose in hepatic and renal impairment, p. 901. Moderate Study
- **Cobicistat** is predicted to increase the exposure to mirabegron. Adjust **mirabegron** dose in hepatic and renal impairment, p. 901. Moderate Study
- **Mirabegron** is predicted to increase the exposure to colchicine. Mild Theoretical
- **Mirabegron** slightly increases the exposure to digoxin. Monitor concentration and adjust dose. Severe Study
- **Mirabegron** is predicted to increase the exposure to eliglustat. Avoid or adjust dose—consult product literature. Severe Study
- **Mirabegron** is predicted to increase the exposure to everolimus. Mild Theoretical
- **Mirabegron** is predicted to increase the exposure to factor XA inhibitors (edoxaban). Mild Theoretical

- HIV-protease inhibitors are predicted to increase the exposure to **mirabegron**. Adjust **mirabegron** dose in hepatic and renal impairment, p. 901. Moderate Study
- **Idelalisib** is predicted to increase the exposure to **mirabegron**. Adjust **mirabegron** dose in hepatic and renal impairment, p. 901. Moderate Study
- **Mirabegron** is predicted to increase the exposure to loperamide. Mild Theoretical
- Macrolides (clarithromycin) are predicted to increase the exposure to **mirabegron**. Adjust **mirabegron** dose in hepatic and renal impairment, p. 901. Moderate Study
- **Mirabegron** is predicted to increase the exposure to sirolimus. Mild Theoretical
- **Mirabegron** is predicted to increase the exposure to taxanes (paclitaxel). Mild Theoretical
- **Mirabegron** is predicted to increase the exposure to thrombin inhibitors (dabigatran). Severe Theoretical
- **Tucatinib** is predicted to increase the exposure to **mirabegron**. Adjust **mirabegron** dose in hepatic and renal impairment, p. 901. Moderate Study

Mirikizumab → see monoclonal antibodies
Mirtazapine → see TABLE 17 p. 1576 (hyponatraemia), TABLE 12 p. 1574 (serotonin syndrome), TABLE 10 p. 1574 (CNS effects)

- Anti-androgens (apalutamide, enzalutamide) are predicted to decrease the exposure to **mirtazapine**. Adjust dose. Moderate Study
- Antiepileptics (carbamazepine, fosphenytoin, phenobarbital, phenytoin, primidone) are predicted to decrease the exposure to **mirtazapine**. Adjust dose. Moderate Study → Also see TABLE 17 p. 1576 → Also see TABLE 10 p. 1574
- Antifungals, azoles (itraconazole, ketoconazole, posaconazole, voriconazole) are predicted to increase the exposure to **mirtazapine**. Moderate Study
- **Ceritinib** is predicted to increase the exposure to **mirtazapine**. Moderate Study
- **Cobicistat** is predicted to increase the exposure to **mirtazapine**. Moderate Study
- **Encorafenib** is predicted to decrease the exposure to **mirtazapine**. Adjust dose. Moderate Study
- H$_2$ receptor antagonists (cimetidine) slightly increase the exposure to **mirtazapine**. Use with caution and adjust dose. Moderate Theoretical
- HIV-protease inhibitors are predicted to increase the exposure to **mirtazapine**. Moderate Study
- **Idelalisib** is predicted to increase the exposure to **mirtazapine**. Moderate Study
- **Ivosidenib** is predicted to decrease the exposure to **mirtazapine**. Adjust dose. Moderate Study
- **Lumacaftor** is predicted to decrease the exposure to **mirtazapine**. Adjust dose. Moderate Study
- Macrolides (clarithromycin) are predicted to increase the exposure to **mirtazapine**. Moderate Study
- **Mitotane** is predicted to decrease the exposure to **mirtazapine**. Adjust dose. Moderate Study
- **Mirtazapine** is predicted to decrease the efficacy of pitolisant. Moderate Theoretical
- Rifamycins (rifampicin) are predicted to decrease the exposure to **mirtazapine**. Adjust dose. Moderate Study
- **Tucatinib** is predicted to increase the exposure to **mirtazapine**. Moderate Study

Misoprostol

- **Misoprostol** can cause uterine contractions, as can oxytocin; concurrent use might increase the risk of developing this effect. Avoid and for 4 hours after stopping **misoprostol**. Severe Theoretical

Mitomycin → see TABLE 14 p. 1575 (myelosuppression)

- Live vaccines are predicted to increase the risk of generalised infection (possibly life-threatening) when given with **mitomycin**. UKHSA advises avoid (refer to Green Book). Severe Theoretical

Mitotane → see TABLE 14 p. 1575 (myelosuppression)

- **Mitotane** is predicted to decrease the exposure to 5-HT3-receptor antagonists (ondansetron). Moderate Study
- **Mitotane** is predicted to markedly decrease the exposure to abemaciclib. Avoid. Severe Study

Mitotane (continued)

▶ **Mitotane** is predicted to decrease the exposure to acalabrutinib. Avoid. [Severe] Study

▶ **Mitotane** is predicted to decrease the exposure to alpelisib. Avoid. [Moderate] Study

▶ **Mitotane** is predicted to decrease the exposure to anti-androgens (abiraterone). Avoid. [Severe] Study

▶ **Mitotane** is predicted to decrease the exposure to anti-androgens (darolutamide). Avoid. [Moderate] Study

▶ **Mitotane** is predicted to decrease the exposure to antiarrhythmics (disopyramide, dronedarone). Avoid. [Severe] Study

▶ **Mitotane** is predicted to decrease the efficacy of antiarrhythmics (propafenone). [Moderate] Study

▶ **Mitotane** is predicted to decrease the exposure to anticholinesterases, centrally acting (donepezil). [Mild] Study

▶ **Mitotane** is predicted to decrease the exposure to antiepileptics (perampanel). Monitor and adjust dose. [Moderate] Study

▶ **Mitotane** is predicted to decrease the exposure to antifungals, azoles (isavuconazole). Avoid. [Severe] Study

▶ **Mitotane** is predicted to decrease the exposure to antimalarials (artemether) with lumefantrine. Avoid. [Severe] Study

▶ **Mitotane** is predicted to moderately decrease the exposure to antipsychotics, second generation (aripiprazole). Adjust **aripiprazole** dose, p. 454. [Moderate] Study

▶ **Mitotane** is predicted to decrease the exposure to antipsychotics, second generation (cariprazine). Avoid. [Severe] Theoretical

▶ **Mitotane** is predicted to decrease the exposure to antipsychotics, second generation (lurasidone). Avoid. [Moderate] Study

▶ **Mitotane** is predicted to decrease the exposure to antipsychotics, second generation (paliperidone). Monitor and adjust dose. [Severe] Study

▶ **Mitotane** is predicted to decrease the exposure to antipsychotics, second generation (quetiapine). [Moderate] Study

▶ **Mitotane** is predicted to decrease the exposure to antipsychotics, second generation (risperidone). Adjust dose. [Moderate] Study

▶ **Mitotane** is predicted to decrease the exposure to avacopan. Avoid or monitor. [Severe] Study

▶ **Mitotane** is predicted to decrease the exposure to avapritinib. Avoid. [Severe] Study

▶ **Mitotane** is predicted to decrease the exposure to axitinib. Avoid or adjust dose. [Moderate] Study → Also see **TABLE 14** p. 1575

▶ **Mitotane** decreases the exposure to bedaquiline. Avoid. [Severe] Study

▶ **Mitotane** is predicted to decrease the exposure to belumosudil. Adjust **belumosudil** dose, p. 979. [Severe] Study

▶ **Mitotane** is predicted to decrease the exposure to benzodiazepines (alprazolam). Adjust dose. [Moderate] Theoretical

▶ **Mitotane** is predicted to decrease the exposure to benzodiazepines (midazolam). Monitor and adjust dose. [Severe] Study

▶ **Mitotane** is predicted to decrease the exposure to bictegravir. Avoid. [Moderate] Study

▶ **Mitotane** slightly decreases the exposure to bortezomib. Avoid. [Severe] Study → Also see **TABLE 14** p. 1575

▶ **Mitotane** is predicted to very markedly decrease the exposure to bosutinib. Avoid. [Severe] Study → Also see **TABLE 14** p. 1575

▶ **Mitotane** is predicted to decrease the exposure to brigatinib. Avoid. [Severe] Study

▶ **Mitotane** is predicted to decrease the exposure to buspirone. Use with caution and adjust dose. [Severe] Study

▶ **Mitotane** moderately decreases the exposure to cabozantinib. Avoid. [Moderate] Study → Also see **TABLE 14** p. 1575

▶ **Mitotane** is predicted to decrease the exposure to calcium channel blockers (amlodipine, felodipine, lacidipine, lercanidipine, nicardipine, nifedipine, nimodipine). Monitor and adjust dose. [Moderate] Study

▶ **Mitotane** is predicted to decrease the exposure to calcium channel blockers (diltiazem). [Severe] Study

▶ **Mitotane** is predicted to decrease the exposure to cannabidiol. Adjust dose. [Moderate] Study

▶ **Mitotane** is predicted to decrease the exposure to capivasertib. Avoid. [Moderate] Study

▶ **Mitotane** is predicted to decrease the exposure to ceritinib. Avoid. [Severe] Study → Also see **TABLE 14** p. 1575

▶ **Mitotane** decreases the concentration of ciclosporin. [Severe] Study

▶ **Mitotane** is predicted to alter the effects of cilostazol. [Moderate] Theoretical

▶ **Mitotane** is predicted to decrease the exposure to cinacalcet. Monitor and adjust dose. [Moderate] Study

▶ **Mitotane** decreases the exposure to clomethiazole. Monitor and adjust dose. [Moderate] Study

▶ **Mitotane** is predicted to decrease the exposure to cobicistat. Avoid. [Severe] Study

▶ **Mitotane** is predicted to decrease the exposure to cobimetinib. Avoid. [Severe] Theoretical

▶ **Mitotane** might decrease the efficacy of combined hormonal contraceptives. Use alternative methods with, and until concentrations are undetectable after stopping, **mitotane**. [Severe] Theoretical

▶ **Mitotane** is predicted to decrease the exposure to corticosteroids (budesonide, deflazacort, dexamethasone, fludrocortisone, hydrocortisone, methylprednisolone, prednisolone, triamcinolone). Monitor and adjust dose. [Moderate] Study

▶ **Mitotane** is predicted to decrease the exposure to corticosteroids (fluticasone). [Unknown] Theoretical

▶ **Mitotane** is predicted to markedly decrease the exposure to crizotinib. Avoid. [Severe] Study

▶ **Mitotane** is predicted to decrease the exposure to dabrafenib. Avoid. [Moderate] Theoretical

▶ **Mitotane** is predicted to decrease the exposure to daridorexant. [Severe] Study

▶ **Mitotane** is predicted to decrease the exposure to darifenacin. [Moderate] Theoretical

▶ **Mitotane** is predicted to markedly decrease the exposure to dasatinib. Avoid. [Severe] Study → Also see **TABLE 14** p. 1575

▶ **Mitotane** is predicted to slightly decrease the exposure to delamanid. Avoid. [Moderate] Study

▶ **Mitotane** is predicted to markedly decrease the exposure to dienogest. [Severe] Study

▶ **Mitotane** is predicted to decrease the exposure to dipeptidylpeptidase-4 inhibitors (linagliptin). [Moderate] Study

▶ **Mitotane** is predicted to moderately decrease the exposure to dipeptidylpeptidase-4 inhibitors (saxagliptin). [Moderate] Study

▶ **Mitotane** is predicted to decrease the exposure to dolutegravir. [Severe] Study

▶ **Mitotane** is predicted to decrease the exposure to dronabinol. Avoid or adjust dose. [Mild] Study

▶ **Mitotane** is predicted to decrease the exposure to elacestrant. Avoid or adjust dose depending on duration—consult product literature. [Severe] Study

▶ **Mitotane** is predicted to decrease the exposure to elbasvir. Avoid. [Severe] Study

▶ **Mitotane** is predicted to decreases the exposure to elexacaftor. Avoid. [Severe] Theoretical

▶ **Mitotane** is predicted to decrease the exposure to eliglustat. Avoid. [Severe] Study

▶ **Mitotane** is predicted to decrease the concentration of elvitegravir. Avoid. [Severe] Study

▶ **Mitotane** is predicted to decrease the exposure to encorafenib. [Severe] Theoretical

▶ **Mitotane** affects the exposure to endothelin receptor antagonists (bosentan). Avoid. [Severe] Study

▶ **Mitotane** is predicted to decrease the exposure to endothelin receptor antagonists (macitentan). Avoid. [Severe] Study

▶ **Mitotane** is predicted to decrease the exposure to the cytotoxic component of enfortumab vedotin. [Moderate] Theoretical

▶ **Mitotane** is predicted to decrease the exposure to entrectinib. Avoid. [Severe] Study

▶ **Mitotane** is predicted to decrease the exposure to erdafitinib. Avoid. [Severe] Study

▶ **Mitotane** is predicted to decrease the exposure to erlotinib. Avoid or adjust dose—consult product literature. [Severe] Study

- **Mitotane** is predicted to decrease the exposure to esketamine. Adjust dose. [Mild] Theoretical
- **Mitotane** is predicted to decrease the exposure to eszopiclone. Adjust dose. [Moderate] Theoretical
- **Mitotane** is predicted to decrease the concentration of everolimus. Avoid or adjust dose. [Severe] Study
- **Mitotane** moderately decreases the exposure to exemestane. [Moderate] Study
- **Mitotane** is predicted to decrease the exposure to factor XA inhibitors (apixaban). [Moderate] Study
- **Mitotane** is predicted to decrease the exposure to factor XA inhibitors (rivaroxaban). Avoid unless patient can be monitored for signs of thrombosis. [Severe] Study
- **Mitotane** is predicted to decrease the exposure to fedratinib. Avoid. [Moderate] Study
- **Mitotane** is predicted to decrease the exposure to fenfluramine. [Moderate] Theoretical
- **Mitotane** is predicted to decrease the exposure to fesoterodine. Avoid. [Moderate] Study
- **Mitotane** is predicted to decrease the exposure to fostamatinib. Avoid. [Severe] Study
- **Mitotane** is predicted to decrease the exposure to the active metabolite of fostemsavir. Avoid. [Severe] Study
- **Mitotane** is predicted to decrease the exposure to fruquintinib. Avoid. [Moderate] Study
- **Mitotane** is predicted to decrease the exposure to gefitinib. Avoid. [Severe] Study
- **Mitotane** is predicted to decrease the exposure to glasdegib. Avoid. [Severe] Study
- **Mitotane** is predicted to greatly decrease the concentration of glecaprevir. Avoid. [Severe] Study
- **Mitotane** is predicted to decrease the exposure to grazoprevir. Avoid. [Severe] Study
- **Mitotane** is predicted to decrease the concentration of guanfacine. Adjust **guanfacine** dose, p. 407. [Moderate] Study
- **Mitotane** decreases the concentration of haloperidol. Adjust dose. [Moderate] Study
- **Mitotane** is predicted to decrease the exposure to ibrutinib. Avoid or monitor. [Severe] Study → Also see TABLE 14 p. 1575
- **Mitotane** is predicted to decrease the exposure to idelalisib. Avoid. [Severe] Study
- **Mitotane** is predicted to decrease the exposure to imatinib. Avoid. [Moderate] Study → Also see TABLE 14 p. 1575
- **Mitotane** is predicted to decrease the exposure to irinotecan. Avoid. [Severe] Study → Also see TABLE 14 p. 1575
- **Mitotane** is predicted to decrease the exposure to ivabradine. Adjust dose. [Moderate] Theoretical
- **Mitotane** is predicted to decrease the exposure to ivacaftor. Avoid. [Severe] Study
- **Mitotane** is predicted to decrease the exposure to ivosidenib. Avoid. [Severe] Theoretical
- **Mitotane** is predicted to decrease the exposure to ixazomib. Avoid. [Severe] Study
- **Mitotane** is predicted to decrease the exposure to lapatinib. Avoid. [Severe] Study
- **Mitotane** is predicted to moderately decrease the exposure to larotrectinib. Avoid. [Moderate] Study
- **Mitotane** is predicted to decrease the exposure to leniolisib. Avoid. [Severe] Theoretical
- **Mitotane** is predicted to decrease the exposure to lomitapide. Monitor and adjust dose. [Moderate] Theoretical
- **Mitotane** is predicted to decrease the exposure to lorlatinib. Avoid. [Severe] Study
- **Mitotane** is predicted to decrease the exposure to maraviroc. Adjust dose. [Severe] Study
- **Mitotane** is predicted to decrease the exposure to maribavir. Avoid or adjust **maribavir** dose, p. 735. [Severe] Study
- **Mitotane** is predicted to decrease the exposure to mavacamten. Monitor and adjust dose—consult product literature. [Severe] Theoretical
- **Mitotane** is predicted to decrease the exposure to meglitinides (repaglinide). Monitor blood glucose and adjust dose. [Moderate] Study
- **Mitotane** is predicted to decrease the exposure to midostaurin. Avoid. [Severe] Study

- **Mitotane** is predicted to decrease the exposure to mifepristone. Adjust **mifepristone** dose, p. 954. [Severe] Study
- Mineralocorticoid receptor antagonists (spironolactone) are predicted to decrease the effects of **mitotane**. Avoid. [Severe] Anecdotal
- **Mitotane** is predicted to decrease the exposure to mineralocorticoid receptor antagonists (eplerenone). Avoid. [Moderate] Theoretical
- **Mitotane** is predicted to decrease the exposure to mineralocorticoid receptor antagonists (finerenone). Avoid. [Severe] Study
- **Mitotane** is predicted to decrease the exposure to mirtazapine. Adjust dose. [Moderate] Study
- **Mitotane** is predicted to decrease the exposure to mobocertinib. Avoid. [Severe] Study
- **Mitotane** is predicted to decrease the exposure to monoclonal antibodies (polatuzumab vedotin). [Moderate] Theoretical
- **Mitotane** is predicted to decrease the exposure to the cytotoxic component of monoclonal antibodies (trastuzumab emtansine). [Severe] Theoretical → Also see TABLE 14 p. 1575
- **Mitotane** is predicted to decrease the exposure to montelukast. [Mild] Study
- **Mitotane** is predicted to markedly decrease the exposure to naldemedine. Avoid. [Severe] Study
- **Mitotane** is predicted to markedly decrease the exposure to naloxegol. Avoid. [Moderate] Study
- **Mitotane** is predicted to decrease the exposure to neratinib. Avoid. [Severe] Study
- **Mitotane** is predicted to markedly decrease the exposure to neurokinin-1 receptor antagonists (aprepitant). Avoid. [Moderate] Study
- **Mitotane** is predicted to decrease the exposure to neurokinin-1 receptor antagonists (fosaprepitant). Avoid. [Moderate] Theoretical
- **Mitotane** is predicted to decrease the exposure to neurokinin-1 receptor antagonists (netupitant). Avoid. [Severe] Study
- **Mitotane** is predicted to moderately decrease the exposure to nilotinib. Avoid. [Severe] Study → Also see TABLE 14 p. 1575
- **Mitotane** is predicted to decrease the exposure to nirmatrelvir boosted with ritonavir. Avoid. [Severe] Study
- **Mitotane** is predicted to decrease the exposure to nitisinone. Adjust dose. [Moderate] Theoretical
- **Mitotane** is predicted to decrease the exposure to NNRTIs (doravirine). Avoid. [Severe] Study
- **Mitotane** is predicted to decrease the exposure to NNRTIs (etravirine). Avoid. [Severe] Theoretical
- **Mitotane** is predicted to decrease the exposure to NNRTIs (nevirapine). [Severe] Theoretical
- **Mitotane** markedly decreases the exposure to NNRTIs (rilpivirine). Avoid. [Severe] Study
- **Mitotane** is predicted to decrease the exposure to olaparib. Avoid. [Moderate] Theoretical → Also see TABLE 14 p. 1575
- **Mitotane** is predicted to decrease the exposure to opioids (alfentanil, fentanyl). [Moderate] Study
- **Mitotane** is predicted to decrease the exposure to opioids (buprenorphine). Monitor and adjust dose. [Moderate] Theoretical
- **Mitotane** decreases the exposure to opioids (methadone). Monitor and adjust dose. [Severe] Study
- **Mitotane** is predicted to decrease the exposure to opioids (oxycodone). Monitor and adjust dose. [Moderate] Study
- **Mitotane** is predicted to decrease the exposure to osilodrostat. [Moderate] Theoretical
- **Mitotane** is predicted to moderately decrease the exposure to osimertinib. Avoid. [Moderate] Study
- **Mitotane** is predicted to moderately decrease the exposure to ospemifene. [Moderate] Study
- **Mitotane** is predicted to decrease the exposure to palbociclib. Avoid. [Severe] Study → Also see TABLE 14 p. 1575
- **Mitotane** is predicted to decrease the exposure to panobinostat. Avoid. [Moderate] Theoretical → Also see TABLE 14 p. 1575
- **Mitotane** is predicted to decrease the exposure to pazopanib. Avoid. [Severe] Theoretical
- **Mitotane** is predicted to decrease the exposure to pemigatinib. Avoid. [Severe] Study

Mitotane (continued)
▶ **Mitotane** moderately decreases the exposure to phosphodiesterase type-4 inhibitors **(apremilast)**. Avoid. [Severe] Study
▶ **Mitotane** is predicted to decrease the exposure to phosphodiesterase type-4 inhibitors **(roflumilast)**. Avoid. [Moderate] Study
▶ **Mitotane** is predicted to decrease the exposure to phosphodiesterase type-5 inhibitors **(avanafil, tadalafil)**. Avoid. [Severe] Study
▶ **Mitotane** is predicted to decrease the exposure to phosphodiesterase type-5 inhibitors **(sildenafil, vardenafil)**. [Moderate] Theoretical
▶ **Mitotane** is predicted to moderately to markedly decrease the exposure to **pibrentasvir**. Avoid. [Severe] Study
▶ **Mitotane** is predicted to moderately decrease the exposure to **pitolisant**. [Moderate] Study
▶ **Mitotane** is predicted to decrease the exposure to **ponatinib**. Avoid. [Moderate] Theoretical
▶ **Mitotane** is predicted to decrease the exposure to **pralsetinib**. Avoid or adjust dose with potent CYP3A4 inducers—consult product literature. [Moderate] Study
▶ **Mitotane** is predicted to markedly decrease the exposure to **praziquantel**. Avoid. [Moderate] Study
▶ **Mitotane** is predicted to decrease the exposure to **quizartinib**. Avoid. [Severe] Study
▶ **Mitotane** is predicted to decrease the exposure to **ranolazine**. Avoid. [Severe] Study
▶ **Mitotane** is predicted to decrease the exposure to **reboxetine**. [Moderate] Anecdotal
▶ **Mitotane** is predicted to decrease the exposure to **regorafenib**. Avoid. [Moderate] Study → Also see **TABLE 14** p. 1575
▶ **Mitotane** is predicted to markedly decrease the exposure to **ribociclib**. Avoid. [Severe] Study → Also see **TABLE 14** p. 1575
▶ **Mitotane** is predicted to decrease the exposure to **rimegepant**. Avoid. [Moderate] Theoretical
▶ **Mitotane** is predicted to decrease the exposure to **ripretinib**. Avoid or adjust dose—consult product literature. [Severe] Study
▶ **Mitotane** is predicted to decrease the exposure to **ruxolitinib**. Monitor and adjust dose. [Moderate] Study → Also see **TABLE 14** p. 1575
▶ **Mitotane** is predicted to decrease the exposure to **selpercatinib**. Avoid. [Moderate] Study
▶ **Mitotane** is predicted to decrease the exposure to **selumetinib**. Avoid. [Severe] Study
▶ **Mitotane** is predicted to decrease the exposure to **siponimod**. Manufacturer advises caution depending on genotype— consult product literature. [Severe] Study
▶ **Mitotane** is predicted to decrease the concentration of **sirolimus**. Avoid or monitor and adjust dose. [Severe] Study
▶ **Mitotane** is predicted to decrease the exposure to **solifenacin**. [Moderate] Theoretical
▶ **Mitotane** is predicted to decrease the exposure to **sorafenib**. [Moderate] Theoretical → Also see **TABLE 14** p. 1575
▶ **Mitotane** is predicted to decrease the exposure to **sotorasib**. Avoid. [Severe] Study
▶ **Mitotane** is predicted to decrease the exposure to statins **(atorvastatin, simvastatin)**. [Moderate] Study
▶ **Mitotane** is predicted to decrease the exposure to **sunitinib**. Avoid or adjust dose—consult product literature. [Moderate] Study → Also see **TABLE 14** p. 1575
▶ **Mitotane** decreases the concentration of **tacrolimus**. Avoid or monitor and adjust dose. [Severe] Study
▶ **Mitotane** is predicted to decrease the exposure to taxanes **(cabazitaxel)**. Avoid. [Moderate] Study → Also see **TABLE 14** p. 1575
▶ **Mitotane** is predicted to decrease the exposure to taxanes **(docetaxel)**. [Severe] Theoretical → Also see **TABLE 14** p. 1575
▶ **Mitotane** is predicted to decrease the exposure to taxanes **(paclitaxel)**. Avoid. [Severe] Study → Also see **TABLE 14** p. 1575
▶ **Mitotane** is predicted to decrease the concentration of **temsirolimus**. Avoid. [Severe] Study → Also see **TABLE 14** p. 1575
▶ **Mitotane** might decrease the exposure to **tepotinib**. Avoid. [Severe] Theoretical
▶ **Mitotane** is predicted to decrease the exposure to tetracyclines **(eravacycline)**. Adjust **eravacycline** dose, p. 657. [Moderate] Study

▶ **Mitotane** is predicted to decrease the exposure to **tezacaftor**. Avoid. [Severe] Theoretical
▶ **Mitotane** is predicted to markedly decrease the exposure to **ticagrelor**. Avoid. [Severe] Study
▶ **Mitotane** is predicted to decrease the exposure to **tivozanib**. [Severe] Study
▶ **Mitotane** is predicted to decrease the exposure to **tofacitinib**. Avoid. [Severe] Study
▶ **Mitotane** is predicted to decrease the exposure to **tolvaptan**. Use with caution or avoid depending on indication. [Severe] Study
▶ **Mitotane** is predicted to decrease the exposure to **toremifene**. Adjust dose. [Moderate] Study
▶ **Mitotane** is predicted to decrease the exposure to **trabectedin**. Avoid. [Severe] Theoretical → Also see **TABLE 14** p. 1575
▶ **Mitotane** is predicted to decrease the exposure to **tucatinib**. Avoid. [Severe] Study
▶ **Mitotane** is predicted to decrease the efficacy of **uliprital**. Avoid and for 4 weeks after stopping **mitotane**. [Severe] Theoretical
▶ **Mitotane** is predicted to decrease the exposure to **upadacitinib**. [Moderate] Study
▶ **Mitotane** is predicted to decrease the exposure to **vandetanib**. Avoid. [Moderate] Study
▶ **Mitotane** is predicted to moderately decrease the exposure to **velpatasvir**. Avoid. [Severe] Study
▶ **Mitotane** is predicted to decrease the exposure to **vemurafenib**. Avoid. [Severe] Study
▶ **Mitotane** is predicted to decrease the exposure to **venetoclax**. Avoid. [Severe] Study
▶ **Mitotane** is predicted to decrease the exposure to vinca alkaloids **(vinblastine, vincristine, vindesine)**. [Severe] Theoretical → Also see **TABLE 14** p. 1575
▶ **Mitotane** is predicted to decrease the exposure to vinca alkaloids **(vinorelbine)**. Use with caution or avoid. [Severe] Theoretical → Also see **TABLE 14** p. 1575
▶ **Mitotane** is predicted to decrease the exposure to **vismodegib**. Avoid. [Moderate] Theoretical
▶ **Mitotane** is predicted to decrease the exposure to **voclosporin**. Avoid. [Severe] Study
▶ **Mitotane** is predicted to decrease the exposure to **vortioxetine**. Monitor and adjust dose. [Moderate] Study
▶ **Mitotane** is predicted to decrease the concentration of **voxilaprevir**. Avoid. [Severe] Study
▶ **Mitotane** is predicted to decrease the exposure to **zanubrutinib**. Avoid. [Severe] Study
▶ **Mitotane** is predicted to decrease the exposure to **zopiclone**. Adjust dose. [Moderate] Study

Mitoxantrone → see anthracyclines
Mivacurium → see neuromuscular blocking drugs, non-depolarising
Mizolastine → see antihistamines, non-sedating
Mobocertinib → see **TABLE 8** p. 1573 (QT-interval prolongation)
▶ Anti-androgens **(apalutamide, enzalutamide)** are predicted to decrease the exposure to **mobocertinib**. Avoid. [Severe] Study → Also see **TABLE 8** p. 1573
▶ Antiarrhythmics **(dronedarone)** are predicted to increase the exposure to **mobocertinib**. Avoid or adjust dose and monitor ECG—consult product literature. [Severe] Study → Also see **TABLE 8** p. 1573
▶ Antiepileptics **(carbamazepine, fosphenytoin, phenobarbital, phenytoin, primidone)** are predicted to decrease the exposure to **mobocertinib**. Avoid. [Severe] Study
▶ Antifungals, azoles **(fluconazole, isavuconazole)** are predicted to increase the exposure to **mobocertinib**. Avoid or adjust dose and monitor ECG—consult product literature. [Severe] Study → Also see **TABLE 8** p. 1573
▶ Antifungals, azoles **(itraconazole, ketoconazole, posaconazole, voriconazole)** are predicted to increase the exposure to **mobocertinib**. Avoid. [Severe] Study → Also see **TABLE 8** p. 1573
▶ **Berotralstat** is predicted to increase the exposure to **mobocertinib**. Avoid or adjust dose and monitor ECG—consult product literature. [Severe] Study
▶ Calcium channel blockers **(diltiazem, verapamil)** are predicted to increase the exposure to **mobocertinib**. Avoid or adjust dose and monitor ECG—consult product literature. [Severe] Study

- **Cenobamate** is predicted to decrease the exposure to mobocertinib. Avoid. Severe Study
- **Ceritinib** is predicted to increase the exposure to **mobocertinib**. Avoid. Severe Study → Also see **TABLE 8** p. 1573
- **Cobicistat** is predicted to increase the exposure to mobocertinib. Avoid. Severe Study
- **Mobocertinib** is predicted to decrease the exposure to combined hormonal contraceptives. Use alternative methods during treatment with, and for at least 28 days after stopping, mobocertinib. Moderate Theoretical
- **Crizotinib** is predicted to increase the exposure to mobocertinib. Avoid or adjust dose and monitor ECG—consult product literature. Severe Study → Also see **TABLE 8** p. 1573
- **Dabrafenib** is predicted to decrease the exposure to mobocertinib. Avoid. Severe Study
- **Encorafenib** is predicted to decrease the exposure to mobocertinib. Avoid. Severe Study → Also see **TABLE 8** p. 1573
- **Endothelin receptor antagonists (bosentan)** are predicted to decrease the exposure to **mobocertinib**. Avoid. Severe Study
- **Mobocertinib** is predicted to decrease the exposure to everolimus. Severe Theoretical
- **Fedratinib** is predicted to increase the exposure to mobocertinib. Avoid or adjust dose and monitor ECG—consult product literature. Severe Study
- **Grapefruit** and grapefruit juice are predicted to increase the exposure to **mobocertinib**. Avoid. Severe Theoretical
- **HIV-protease inhibitors** are predicted to increase the exposure to mobocertinib. Avoid. Severe Study
- **Idelalisib** is predicted to increase the exposure to mobocertinib. Avoid. Severe Study
- **Imatinib** is predicted to increase the exposure to **mobocertinib**. Avoid or adjust dose and monitor ECG—consult product literature. Severe Study
- **Ivosidenib** is predicted to decrease the exposure to mobocertinib. Avoid. Severe Study → Also see **TABLE 8** p. 1573
- **Letermovir** is predicted to increase the exposure to mobocertinib. Avoid or adjust dose and monitor ECG—consult product literature. Severe Study
- **Lorlatinib** is predicted to decrease the exposure to mobocertinib. Avoid. Severe Study
- **Lumacaftor** is predicted to decrease the exposure to mobocertinib. Avoid. Severe Study
- **Macrolides (clarithromycin)** are predicted to increase the exposure to **mobocertinib**. Avoid. Severe Study
- **Macrolides (erythromycin)** are predicted to increase the exposure to **mobocertinib**. Avoid or adjust dose and monitor ECG—consult product literature. Severe Study → Also see **TABLE 8** p. 1573
- **Mitotane** is predicted to decrease the exposure to mobocertinib. Avoid. Severe Study
- **Modafinil** is predicted to decrease the exposure to mobocertinib. Avoid. Severe Theoretical
- **Neurokinin-1 receptor antagonists (aprepitant, netupitant)** are predicted to increase the exposure to **mobocertinib**. Avoid or adjust dose and monitor ECG—consult product literature. Severe Study
- **Nilotinib** is predicted to increase the exposure to **mobocertinib**. Avoid or adjust dose and monitor ECG—consult product literature. Severe Study → Also see **TABLE 8** p. 1573
- **NNRTIs (efavirenz, etravirine, nevirapine)** are predicted to decrease the exposure to **mobocertinib**. Avoid. Severe Study → Also see **TABLE 8** p. 1573
- **Mobocertinib** is predicted to decrease the exposure to opioids (alfentanil). Moderate Theoretical
- **Rifamycins (rifabutin)** are predicted to decrease the exposure to mobocertinib. Avoid. Severe Theoretical
- **Rifamycins (rifampicin)** are predicted to decrease the exposure to mobocertinib. Avoid. Severe Study
- **Mobocertinib** is predicted to decrease the exposure to sirolimus. Severe Theoretical
- **Sotorasib** is predicted to decrease the exposure to mobocertinib. Avoid. Severe Study
- **St John's wort** is predicted to decrease the exposure to mobocertinib. Avoid. Severe Study

- **Mobocertinib** is predicted to decrease the exposure to temsirolimus. Severe Theoretical
- **Tucatinib** is predicted to increase the exposure to mobocertinib. Avoid. Severe Study

Moclobemide → see **TABLE 12** p. 1574 (serotonin syndrome)

FOOD AND LIFESTYLE Moclobemide is claimed to cause less potentiation of the pressor effect of tyramine than the traditional (irreversible) MAOIs, but patients should avoid consuming large amounts of tyramine-rich foods (such as mature cheese, salami, pickled herring, *Bovril*®, *Oxo*®, *Marmite*® or any similar meat or yeast extract or fermented soya bean extract, and some beers, lagers or wines).

- **Amfetamines** are predicted to increase the risk of a hypertensive crisis when given with **moclobemide**. Avoid. Severe Theoretical → Also see **TABLE 12** p. 1574
- **Anti-androgens (apalutamide)** are predicted to decrease the exposure to **moclobemide**. Avoid or monitor. Mild Study
- **Moclobemide** is predicted to increase the exposure to belzutifan. Monitor and adjust dose. Severe Theoretical
- **Moclobemide** potentially increases the exposure to benzodiazepines (clobazam). Adjust dose. Moderate Theoretical
- **Bupropion** is predicted to increase the risk of severe hypertension when given with **moclobemide**. Avoid. Severe Theoretical
- **Moclobemide** is predicted to increase the exposure to cannabidiol. Moderate Theoretical
- **Moclobemide** is predicted to increase the exposure to cilostazol. Moderate Theoretical
- **Moclobemide** is predicted to decrease the efficacy of clopidogrel. Avoid. Moderate Study
- **Moclobemide** is predicted to increase the exposure to eliglustat. Avoid or adjust dose—consult product literature. Severe Theoretical
- **Moclobemide** might increase the adverse effects of foslevodopa. Moderate Theoretical
- **H₂ receptor antagonists (cimetidine)** increase the exposure to moclobemide. Adjust **moclobemide** dose, p. 420. Mild Study
- **Levodopa** increases the risk of adverse effects when given with moclobemide. Moderate Study
- **Moclobemide** is predicted to increase the risk of adverse effects when given with linezolid. Avoid and for 14 days after stopping **moclobemide**. Severe Theoretical → Also see **TABLE 12** p. 1574
- **Moclobemide** is predicted to increase the effects of MAO-B inhibitors (rasagiline, selegiline). Avoid. Severe Theoretical → Also see **TABLE 12** p. 1574
- **Moclobemide** is predicted to increase the risk of adverse effects when given with MAO-B inhibitors (safinamide). Avoid and for 1 week after stopping safinamide. Severe Theoretical → Also see **TABLE 12** p. 1574
- **Moclobemide** is predicted to increase the exposure to mavacamten. Adjust dose—consult product literature. Severe Theoretical
- **Methylphenidate** is predicted to cause a hypertensive crisis when given with **moclobemide**. Severe Theoretical
- **Mianserin** is predicted to increase the risk of toxicity when given with **moclobemide**. Avoid and for 1 week after stopping mianserin. Severe Theoretical
- **Opicapone** is predicted to increase the risk of elevated blood pressure when given with **moclobemide**. Avoid. Severe Theoretical
- **Moclobemide** might cause serotonin syndrome, as can opioids (tramadol); concurrent use might increase the risk of developing this effect. Avoid. Severe Anecdotal → Also see **TABLE 12** p. 1574
- **Ozanimod** might increase the risk of a hypertensive crisis when given with **moclobemide**. Avoid. Severe Theoretical
- **Moclobemide** increases the risk of adverse effects when given with phenothiazines (levomepromazine). Moderate Study
- **Reboxetine** is predicted to increase the risk of a hypertensive crisis when given with **moclobemide**. Avoid. Severe Theoretical
- **Moclobemide** is predicted to increase the exposure to selumetinib. Avoid or adjust dose—consult product literature. Severe Theoretical

Moclobemide (continued)

▶ **Moclobemide** is predicted to increase the exposure to SSRIs (escitalopram). Use with caution and adjust dose. Severe Study → Also see **TABLE 12** p. 1574

▶ **Moclobemide** might cause serotonin syndrome, as can St John's wort; concurrent use might increase the risk of developing this effect. Avoid. Severe Theoretical → Also see **TABLE 12** p. 1574

▶ Sympathomimetics, vasoconstrictor (ephedrine, isometheptene, phenylephrine, pseudoephedrine) are predicted to increase the risk of a hypertensive crisis when given with **moclobemide**. Avoid. Severe Study

▶ Tetrabenazine potentially increases the risk of CNS excitation and hypertension when given with **moclobemide**. Severe Theoretical

▶ Tricyclic antidepressants are predicted to increase the risk of severe toxic reaction when given with **moclobemide**. Avoid. Severe Theoretical → Also see **TABLE 12** p. 1574

▶ **Moclobemide** slightly increases the exposure to triptans (almotriptan). Avoid. Severe Study → Also see **TABLE 12** p. 1574

▶ **Moclobemide** increases the concentration of triptans (eletriptan, frovatriptan, naratriptan). Avoid. Severe Study → Also see **TABLE 12** p. 1574

▶ **Moclobemide** moderately increases the exposure to triptans (rizatriptan, sumatriptan). Avoid. Severe Study → Also see **TABLE 12** p. 1574

▶ **Moclobemide** slightly increases the exposure to triptans (zolmitriptan). Avoid or adjust **zolmitriptan** dose, p. 546. Severe Study → Also see **TABLE 12** p. 1574

Modafinil

▶ **Modafinil** is predicted to decrease the efficacy of anti-androgens (cyproterone) with ethinylestradiol (co-cyprindiol). Use alternative methods during treatment with, and for 28 days after, the enzyme inducing drug is stopped. Severe Study

▶ Antiepileptics (carbamazepine, phenobarbital, primidone) are predicted to decrease the exposure to **modafinil**. Mild Theoretical

▶ Antiepileptics (fosphenytoin, phenytoin) are predicted to decrease the exposure to **modafinil** and **modafinil** is predicted to increase the concentration of antiepileptics (fosphenytoin, phenytoin). Monitor concentration and adjust dose. Moderate Theoretical

▶ Antifungals, azoles (itraconazole, ketoconazole, posaconazole, voriconazole) are predicted to increase the exposure to **modafinil**. Mild Theoretical

▶ **Modafinil** is predicted to decrease the exposure to avacopan. Severe Theoretical

▶ **Modafinil** is predicted to decrease the exposure to avapritinib. Avoid. Severe Theoretical

▶ **Modafinil** is predicted to decrease the exposure to bosutinib. Avoid. Severe Theoretical

▶ **Modafinil** is predicted to decrease the exposure to brigatinib. Avoid or adjust dose—consult product literature. Moderate Theoretical

▶ **Modafinil** is predicted to decrease the exposure to capivasertib. Avoid. Moderate Theoretical

▶ Ceritinib is predicted to increase the exposure to **modafinil**. Mild Theoretical

▶ Cobicistat is predicted to increase the exposure to **modafinil**. Mild Theoretical

▶ **Modafinil** is predicted to decrease the efficacy of combined hormonal contraceptives. For FSRH guidance, see Contraceptives, interactions p. 917. Severe Study

▶ **Modafinil** is predicted to decrease the efficacy of desogestrel. For FSRH guidance, see Contraceptives, interactions p. 917. Severe Theoretical

▶ **Modafinil** is predicted to decrease the efficacy of drospirenone. For FSRH guidance, see Contraceptives, interactions p. 917. Severe Theoretical

▶ **Modafinil** is predicted to decrease the exposure to elbasvir. Avoid. Unknown Theoretical

▶ **Modafinil** slightly decreases the exposure to encorafenib. Moderate Study

▶ **Modafinil** is predicted to decrease the exposure to erdafitinib. Adjust dose. Moderate Theoretical

▶ **Modafinil** is predicted to decrease the efficacy of estradiol. Moderate Theoretical

▶ **Modafinil** is predicted to decrease the efficacy of etonogestrel. For FSRH guidance, see Contraceptives, interactions p. 917. Severe Theoretical

▶ **Modafinil** is predicted to decrease the exposure to glasdegib. Avoid or adjust dose—consult product literature. Moderate Theoretical

▶ **Modafinil** is predicted to decrease the exposure to grazoprevir. Avoid. Severe Theoretical

▶ HIV-protease inhibitors are predicted to increase the exposure to **modafinil**. Mild Theoretical

▶ **Modafinil** is predicted to decrease the effects of hormone replacement therapy. Moderate Anecdotal

▶ Idelalisib is predicted to increase the exposure to **modafinil**. Mild Theoretical

▶ **Modafinil** is predicted to decrease the exposure to leniolisib. Avoid. Severe Theoretical

▶ **Modafinil** is predicted to decrease the concentration of letermovir. Moderate Theoretical

▶ **Modafinil** is predicted to decrease the efficacy of some contraceptive methods containing levonorgestrel. For FSRH guidance, see Contraceptives, interactions p. 917. Severe Theoretical

▶ Macrolides (clarithromycin) are predicted to increase the exposure to **modafinil**. Mild Theoretical

▶ **Modafinil** is predicted to increase the exposure to mavacamten. Monitor and adjust dose—consult product literature. Moderate Theoretical

▶ **Modafinil** is predicted to decrease the exposure to mobocertinib. Avoid. Severe Theoretical

▶ **Modafinil** is predicted to decrease the exposure to NNRTIs (doravirine). Avoid or adjust doravirine p. 741 or lamivudine with tenofovir disoproxil and doravirine p. 751 dose. Severe Theoretical

▶ **Modafinil** is predicted to decrease the efficacy of some contraceptive methods containing norethisterone. For FSRH guidance, see Contraceptives, interactions p. 917. Severe Anecdotal

▶ **Modafinil** is predicted to decrease the exposure to osimertinib. Use with caution or avoid. Severe Theoretical

▶ Rifamycins (rifampicin) are predicted to decrease the exposure to **modafinil**. Moderate Theoretical

▶ **Modafinil** is predicted to decrease the exposure to sofosbuvir. Avoid. Severe Theoretical

▶ Tucatinib is predicted to increase the exposure to **modafinil**. Mild Theoretical

▶ **Modafinil** decreases the efficacy of ulipristal. Avoid and for 4 weeks after stopping the enzyme inducing drug. For FSRH guidance, see Contraceptives, interactions p. 917. Severe Anecdotal

▶ **Modafinil** is predicted to decrease the exposure to velpatasvir. Avoid. Severe Theoretical

▶ **Modafinil** is predicted to decrease the concentration of voxilaprevir. Avoid. Severe Theoretical

▶ **Modafinil** is predicted to decrease the exposure to zanubrutinib. Avoid. Moderate Theoretical

Mogamulizumab → see monoclonal antibodies

Momelotinib

▶ Anti-androgens (darolutamide) are predicted to increase the exposure to **momelotinib**. Moderate Study

▶ Ciclosporin is predicted to increase the exposure to **momelotinib**. Moderate Study

▶ **Momelotinib** might decrease the efficacy of combined hormonal contraceptives. Additional non-hormonal contraception should be used for 7 days following administration. Severe Theoretical

▶ Eltrombopag is predicted to increase the exposure to **momelotinib**. Moderate Study

▶ Fibrates (gemfibrozil) are predicted to increase the exposure to **momelotinib**. Moderate Study

▶ HIV-protease inhibitors (atazanavir, lopinavir) are predicted to increase the exposure to **momelotinib**. Moderate Study

▶ Leflunomide is predicted to increase the exposure to **momelotinib**. Moderate Study

▶ Macrolides (clarithromycin, erythromycin) are predicted to increase the exposure to **momelotinib**. Moderate Study

▶ Rifamycins (rifampicin) are predicted to increase the exposure to **momelotinib**. Moderate Study

▶ **Momelotinib** increases the exposure to statins (rosuvastatin). Moderate Study

▶ Teriflunomide is predicted to increase the exposure to **momelotinib**. Moderate Study

▶ Velpatasvir is predicted to increase the exposure to **momelotinib**. Moderate Study

▶ Voxilaprevir is predicted to increase the exposure to **momelotinib**. Moderate Study

Mometasone → see corticosteroids

Monoclonal antibodies → see TABLE 14 p. 1575 (myelosuppression), TABLE 11 p. 1574 (peripheral neuropathy), TABLE 8 p. 1573 (QT-interval prolongation)

adalimumab · alemtuzumab · atezolizumab · avelumab · basiliximab · belimumab · bevacizumab · bimekizumab · blinatumomab · brentuximab vedotin · brodalumab · canakinumab · cemiplimab · certolizumab pegol · cetuximab · daratumumab · dinutuximab · dostarlimab · dupilumab · eculizumab · elotuzumab · elranatamab · golimumab · guselkumab · infliximab · inotuzumab ozogamicin · ipilimumab · ixekizumab · lebrikizumab · loncastuximab tesirine · mirikizumab · mogamulizumab · mosunetuzumab · natalizumab · nivolumab · obinutuzumab · ocrelizumab · ofatumumab · panitumumab · pembrolizumab · pertuzumab · polatuzumab vedotin · ramucirumab · risankizumab · rituximab · rozanolixizumab · sarilumab · satralizumab · secukinumab · siltuximab · spesolimab · tafasitamab · teclistamab · tezepelumab · tildrakizumab · tocilizumab · tralokinumab · trastuzumab · trastuzumab deruxtecan · trastuzumab emtansine · ublituximab · ustekinumab · vedolizumab

▶ **Certolizumab pegol** is predicted to increase the risk of generalised infection (possibly life-threatening) when given with abatacept. Avoid. Severe Theoretical

▶ Abatacept is predicted to increase the risk of generalised infection (possibly life-threatening) when given with monoclonal antibodies (adalimumab, golimumab, infliximab). Avoid. Severe Theoretical

▶ **Rozanolixizumab** might decrease the concentration of abatacept. Avoid and for 2 weeks after stopping rozanolixizumab. Moderate Theoretical

▶ **Rozanolixizumab** might decrease the concentration of aflibercept. Avoid and for 2 weeks after stopping rozanolixizumab. Moderate Theoretical

▶ **Blinatumomab** is predicted to transiently increase the exposure to aminophylline. Monitor and adjust dose. Moderate Theoretical

▶ **Sarilumab** potentially affects the exposure to aminophylline. Monitor and adjust dose. Moderate Theoretical

▶ **Tocilizumab** is predicted to decrease the exposure to aminophylline. Monitor and adjust dose. Moderate Theoretical

▶ **Certolizumab pegol** is predicted to increase the risk of generalised infection (possibly life-threatening) when given with anakinra. Avoid. Severe Theoretical

▶ Anakinra is predicted to increase the risk of generalised infection (possibly life-threatening) when given with golimumab. Avoid. Severe Theoretical

▶ Anthracyclines are predicted to increase the risk of cardiotoxicity when given with monoclonal antibodies (trastuzumab, trastuzumab emtansine). Avoid. Severe Theoretical → Also see TABLE 14 p. 1575

▶ Anthracyclines are predicted to increase the risk of cardiotoxicity when given with trastuzumab deruxtecan. Severe Theoretical → Also see TABLE 14 p. 1575

▶ Anti-androgens (apalutamide, enzalutamide) are predicted to decrease the exposure to polatuzumab vedotin. Moderate Theoretical

▶ Anti-androgens (apalutamide, enzalutamide) are predicted to decrease the exposure to the cytotoxic component of trastuzumab emtansine. Severe Theoretical

▶ Antiarrhythmics (amiodarone) are predicted to increase the risk of neutropenia when given with brentuximab vedotin. Monitor and adjust dose. Severe Theoretical → Also see TABLE 11 p. 1574

▶ Antiarrhythmics (dronedarone) increase the risk of neutropenia when given with brentuximab vedotin. Monitor and adjust dose. Severe Theoretical

▶ Antiepileptics (carbamazepine) are predicted to decrease the effects of brentuximab vedotin. Severe Theoretical

▶ Antiepileptics (carbamazepine, fosphenytoin, phenobarbital, phenytoin, primidone) are predicted to decrease the exposure to polatuzumab vedotin. Moderate Theoretical

▶ Antiepileptics (carbamazepine, fosphenytoin, phenobarbital, phenytoin, primidone) are predicted to decrease the exposure to the cytotoxic component of trastuzumab emtansine. Severe Theoretical

▶ **Tocilizumab** is predicted to decrease the exposure to antiepileptics (fosphenytoin, phenytoin). Monitor and adjust dose. Moderate Theoretical

▶ **Elranatamab** might affect the exposure to antiepileptics (phenytoin). Monitor and adjust dose. Moderate Theoretical

▶ Antifungals, azoles (itraconazole, ketoconazole, posaconazole, voriconazole) are predicted to increase the risk of neutropenia when given with brentuximab vedotin. Monitor and adjust dose. Severe Study

▶ Antifungals, azoles (itraconazole, ketoconazole, posaconazole, voriconazole) are predicted to increase the exposure to polatuzumab vedotin. Moderate Theoretical

▶ Antifungals, azoles (itraconazole, ketoconazole, posaconazole, voriconazole) are predicted to increase the exposure to the cytotoxic component of trastuzumab emtansine. Avoid or monitor. Severe Theoretical

▶ **Mosunetuzumab** is predicted to transiently increase the exposure to antifungals, azoles (voriconazole). Monitor and adjust dose. Moderate Theoretical

▶ **Rozanolixizumab** might decrease the concentration of belatacept. Avoid and for 2 weeks after stopping rozanolixizumab. Moderate Theoretical

▶ **Tocilizumab** is predicted to decrease the exposure to benzodiazepines (alprazolam, diazepam, midazolam). Monitor and adjust dose. Moderate Theoretical

▶ **Brentuximab vedotin** increases the risk of pulmonary toxicity when given with bleomycin. Avoid. Severe Study → Also see TABLE 14 p. 1575

▶ Calcium channel blockers (verapamil) increase the risk of neutropenia when given with brentuximab vedotin. Monitor and adjust dose. Severe Theoretical

▶ **Tocilizumab** is predicted to decrease the exposure to calcium channel blockers. Monitor and adjust dose. Moderate Theoretical

▶ Ceritinib is predicted to increase the risk of neutropenia when given with brentuximab vedotin. Monitor and adjust dose. Severe Study → Also see TABLE 14 p. 1575

▶ Ceritinib is predicted to increase the exposure to polatuzumab vedotin. Moderate Theoretical

▶ Ceritinib is predicted to increase the exposure to the cytotoxic component of trastuzumab emtansine. Avoid or monitor. Severe Theoretical → Also see TABLE 14 p. 1575

▶ Ciclosporin increases the risk of neutropenia when given with brentuximab vedotin. Monitor and adjust dose. Severe Theoretical

▶ **Elranatamab** might affect the exposure to ciclosporin. Monitor and adjust dose. Moderate Theoretical

▶ Monoclonal antibodies (blinatumomab, mosunetuzumab) are predicted to transiently increase the exposure to ciclosporin. Monitor and adjust dose. Moderate Theoretical

▶ **Sarilumab** potentially affects the exposure to ciclosporin. Monitor and adjust dose. Moderate Theoretical

▶ **Teclistamab** might affect the exposure to ciclosporin. Moderate Theoretical

▶ **Tocilizumab** is predicted to decrease the exposure to ciclosporin. Monitor and adjust dose. Moderate Theoretical

▶ Cobicistat is predicted to increase the risk of neutropenia when given with brentuximab vedotin. Monitor and adjust dose. Severe Study

▶ Cobicistat is predicted to increase the exposure to polatuzumab vedotin. Moderate Theoretical

▶ Cobicistat is predicted to increase the exposure to the cytotoxic component of trastuzumab emtansine. Avoid or monitor. Severe Theoretical

Monoclonal antibodies (continued)

‣ **Sarilumab** potentially decreases the exposure to combined hormonal contraceptives. [Severe] Theoretical

‣ **Corticosteroids** are predicted to increase the risk of immunosuppression when given with **dinutuximab**. Avoid except in life-threatening situations. [Severe] Theoretical

‣ **Corticosteroids** might affect the efficacy of monoclonal antibodies (**atezolizumab, pembrolizumab**). Use with caution or avoid. [Severe] Theoretical

‣ **Tocilizumab** is predicted to decrease the exposure to corticosteroids (**dexamethasone, methylprednisolone**). Monitor and adjust dose. [Moderate] Theoretical

‣ **Corticosteroids** might affect the efficacy of monoclonal antibodies (**ipilimumab, nivolumab**). Use with caution or avoid. [Severe] Theoretical

‣ **Corticosteroids** might increase the risk of generalised infection (possibly life-threatening) when given with **natalizumab**. Manufacturer advises short courses of corticosteroids can be taken. [Severe] Theoretical

‣ **Bimekizumab** might affect the exposure to coumarins (warfarin). [Moderate] Theoretical

‣ **Elranatamab** might affect the exposure to coumarins (warfarin). Monitor and adjust dose. [Moderate] Theoretical

‣ **Sarilumab** potentially affects the exposure to coumarins (warfarin). Monitor and adjust dose. [Severe] Theoretical

‣ **Tocilizumab** is predicted to decrease the exposure to coumarins (warfarin). Monitor and adjust dose. [Moderate] Theoretical

‣ Monoclonal antibodies (**blinatumomab, mosunetuzumab**) are predicted to transiently increase the exposure to coumarins (warfarin). Monitor and adjust dose. [Moderate] Theoretical

‣ **Crovalimab** increases the risk of hypersensitivity reactions when given with **eculizumab**. [Severe] Study

‣ Drugs with anticoagulant effects (see **TABLE 3** p. 1571) might increase the risk of gastrointestinal bleeding when given with **ipilimumab**. [Severe] Theoretical

‣ Drugs with anticoagulant effects (see **TABLE 3** p. 1571) cause bleeding, as can monoclonal antibodies (**bevacizumab, trastuzumab emtansine**); concurrent use might increase the risk of developing this effect. [Severe] Theoretical

‣ Drugs with antiplatelet effects (see **TABLE 4** p. 1571) cause bleeding, as can monoclonal antibodies (**bevacizumab, trastuzumab emtansine**); concurrent use might increase the risk of developing this effect. [Severe] Theoretical

‣ **Encorafenib** is predicted to decrease the exposure to **polatuzumab vedotin**. [Moderate] Theoretical

‣ **Encorafenib** is predicted to decrease the exposure to the cytotoxic component of **trastuzumab emtansine**. [Severe] Theoretical

‣ **Rozanolixizumab** might decrease the concentration of etanercept. Avoid and for 2 weeks after stopping rozanolixizumab. [Moderate] Theoretical

‣ **Sarilumab** might cause severe infection and neutropenia when given with etanercept. [Severe] Theoretical

‣ **Filgotinib** is predicted to increase the risk of immunosuppression when given with monoclonal antibodies (**adalimumab, certolizumab pegol, golimumab, infliximab, rituximab, sarilumab, secukinumab, tocilizumab**). Avoid. [Severe] Theoretical

‣ **Alemtuzumab** is predicted to increase the risk of generalised infection (possibly life-threatening) when given with fingolimod. Avoid. [Severe] Theoretical

‣ **Glecaprevir** is predicted to increase the risk of neutropenia when given with **brentuximab vedotin**. Monitor and adjust dose. [Severe] Theoretical

‣ **Rozanolixizumab** might decrease the concentration of glucagon-like peptide-1 receptor agonists (**dulaglutide**). Avoid and for 2 weeks after stopping rozanolixizumab. [Moderate] Theoretical

‣ **HIV-protease inhibitors** are predicted to increase the risk of neutropenia when given with **brentuximab vedotin**. Monitor and adjust dose. [Severe] Study

‣ **HIV-protease inhibitors** are predicted to increase the exposure to **polatuzumab vedotin**. [Moderate] Theoretical

‣ **HIV-protease inhibitors** are predicted to increase the exposure to the cytotoxic component of **trastuzumab emtansine**. Avoid or monitor. [Severe] Theoretical

‣ **Idelalisib** is predicted to increase the risk of neutropenia when given with **brentuximab vedotin**. Monitor and adjust dose. [Severe] Study

‣ **Idelalisib** is predicted to increase the exposure to **polatuzumab vedotin**. [Moderate] Theoretical

‣ **Idelalisib** is predicted to increase the exposure to the cytotoxic component of **trastuzumab emtansine**. Avoid or monitor. [Severe] Theoretical

‣ Immunoglobulins (normal immunoglobulin) are predicted to alter the effects of **dinutuximab**. Avoid. [Severe] Theoretical

‣ **Rozanolixizumab** might decrease the concentration of immunoglobulins. Avoid and for 2 weeks after stopping rozanolixizumab. [Moderate] Theoretical

‣ **Ivosidenib** is predicted to decrease the exposure to **polatuzumab vedotin**. [Moderate] Theoretical

‣ **Ivosidenib** is predicted to decrease the exposure to the cytotoxic component of **trastuzumab emtansine**. [Severe] Theoretical

‣ **Lapatinib** increases the risk of neutropenia when given with **brentuximab vedotin**. Monitor and adjust dose. [Severe] Theoretical

‣ **Live vaccines** are predicted to increase the risk of generalised infection (possibly life-threatening) when given with **monoclonal antibodies**. UKHSA advises avoid (refer to Green Book). [Severe] Theoretical

‣ **Lumacaftor** is predicted to decrease the exposure to **polatuzumab vedotin**. [Moderate] Theoretical

‣ **Lumacaftor** is predicted to decrease the exposure to the cytotoxic component of **trastuzumab emtansine**. [Severe] Theoretical

‣ Macrolides (**azithromycin**) are predicted to increase the risk of neutropenia when given with **brentuximab vedotin**. Monitor and adjust dose. [Severe] Theoretical

‣ Macrolides (**clarithromycin**) are predicted to increase the risk of neutropenia when given with **brentuximab vedotin**. Monitor and adjust dose. [Severe] Study

‣ Macrolides (**clarithromycin**) are predicted to increase the exposure to **polatuzumab vedotin**. [Moderate] Theoretical

‣ Macrolides (**clarithromycin**) are predicted to increase the exposure to the cytotoxic component of **trastuzumab emtansine**. Avoid or monitor. [Severe] Theoretical

‣ Macrolides (**erythromycin**) increase the risk of neutropenia when given with **brentuximab vedotin**. Monitor and adjust dose. [Severe] Theoretical

‣ **Mitotane** is predicted to decrease the exposure to **polatuzumab vedotin**. [Moderate] Theoretical

‣ **Mitotane** is predicted to decrease the exposure to the cytotoxic component of **trastuzumab emtansine**. [Severe] Theoretical → Also see **TABLE 14** p. 1575

‣ Monoclonal antibodies (**sarilumab**) might cause severe infection and neutropenia when given with monoclonal antibodies (**adalimumab, certolizumab pegol, infliximab**). [Severe] Theoretical

‣ Monoclonal antibodies (**sarilumab**) might cause the risk of severe infection and neutropenia when given with monoclonal antibodies (**golimumab**). [Severe] Theoretical

‣ **Alemtuzumab** is predicted to increase the risk of generalised infection (possibly life-threatening) when given with ozanimod. Avoid. [Severe] Theoretical

‣ **Pibrentasvir** is predicted to increase the risk of neutropenia when given with **brentuximab vedotin**. Monitor and adjust dose. [Severe] Theoretical

‣ **Alemtuzumab** is predicted to increase the risk of generalised infection (possibly life-threatening) when given with ponesimod. [Severe] Theoretical

‣ **Ranolazine** increases the risk of neutropenia when given with **brentuximab vedotin**. Monitor and adjust dose. [Severe] Theoretical

‣ Rifamycins (**rifampicin**) decrease the effects of **brentuximab vedotin**. [Severe] Study

‣ Rifamycins (**rifampicin**) are predicted to decrease the exposure to **polatuzumab vedotin**. [Moderate] Theoretical

- ▸ Rifamycins (rifampicin) are predicted to decrease the exposure to the cytotoxic component of **trastuzumab emtansine**. Severe Theoretical
- ▸ **Rozanolixizumab** might decrease the concentration of romiplostim. Avoid and for 2 weeks after stopping rozanolixizumab. Moderate Theoretical
- ▸ **Alemtuzumab** is predicted to increase the risk of generalised infection (possibly life-threatening) when given with siponimod. Avoid. Severe Theoretical
- ▸ **Elranatamab** might affect the exposure to sirolimus. Monitor and adjust dose. Moderate Theoretical
- ▸ **Sarilumab** potentially affects the exposure to sirolimus. Monitor and adjust dose. Moderate Theoretical
- ▸ **Sarilumab** is predicted to decrease the exposure to statins (atorvastatin, simvastatin). Moderate Study
- ▸ **Tocilizumab** is predicted to decrease the exposure to statins (atorvastatin, simvastatin). Monitor and adjust dose. Moderate Study
- ▸ **Sarilumab** potentially affects the exposure to tacrolimus. Monitor and adjust dose. Moderate Theoretical
- ▸ **Blinatumomab** is predicted to transiently increase the exposure to theophylline. Monitor and adjust dose. Moderate Theoretical
- ▸ **Sarilumab** potentially affects the exposure to theophylline. Monitor and adjust dose. Moderate Theoretical
- ▸ **Tocilizumab** is predicted to decrease the exposure to theophylline. Monitor and adjust dose. Moderate Theoretical
- ▸ **Tucatinib** is predicted to increase the risk of neutropenia when given with **brentuximab vedotin**. Monitor and adjust dose. Severe Study
- ▸ **Tucatinib** is predicted to increase the exposure to **polatuzumab vedotin**. Moderate Theoretical
- ▸ **Tucatinib** is predicted to increase the exposure to the cytotoxic component of **trastuzumab emtansine**. Avoid or monitor. Severe Theoretical
- ▸ **Velpatasvir** is predicted to increase the risk of neutropenia when given with **brentuximab vedotin**. Monitor and adjust dose. Severe Theoretical
- ▸ **Vemurafenib** increases the risk of neutropenia when given with **brentuximab vedotin**. Monitor and adjust dose. Severe Theoretical
- ▸ **Ipilimumab** might increase the risk of hepatotoxicity when given with vemurafenib. Avoid. Severe Study
- ▸ **Voxilaprevir** is predicted to increase the risk of neutropenia when given with **brentuximab vedotin**. Monitor and adjust dose. Severe Theoretical

Montelukast

- ▸ Anti-androgens (apalutamide, enzalutamide) are predicted to decrease the exposure to **montelukast**. Mild Study
- ▸ Antiepileptics (carbamazepine, fosphenytoin, phenobarbital, phenytoin, primidone) are predicted to decrease the exposure to **montelukast**. Mild Study
- ▸ Clopidogrel is predicted to moderately increase the exposure to **montelukast**. Moderate Study
- ▸ Encorafenib is predicted to decrease the exposure to **montelukast**. Mild Study
- ▸ Fibrates (gemfibrozil) are predicted to moderately increase the exposure to **montelukast**. Moderate Study
- ▸ Iron chelators (deferasirox) are predicted to increase the exposure to **montelukast**. Moderate Theoretical
- ▸ Ivosidenib is predicted to decrease the exposure to **montelukast**. Mild Study
- ▸ Leflunomide is predicted to increase the exposure to **montelukast**. Moderate Theoretical
- ▸ Lumacaftor is predicted to decrease the exposure to **montelukast**. Mild Study
- ▸ Mifepristone is predicted to increase the exposure to **montelukast**. Moderate Theoretical
- ▸ Mitotane is predicted to decrease the exposure to **montelukast**. Mild Study
- ▸ Opicapone is predicted to increase the exposure to **montelukast**. Avoid. Moderate Study
- ▸ Rifamycins (rifampicin) are predicted to decrease the exposure to **montelukast**. Mild Study

- ▸ Selpercatinib is predicted to increase the exposure to **montelukast**. Avoid. Moderate Study
- ▸ Teriflunomide is predicted to increase the exposure to **montelukast**. Moderate Theoretical

Morphine → see opioids

Mosunetuzumab → see monoclonal antibodies

Moxifloxacin → see quinolones

Moxonidine → see **TABLE 7** p. 1572 (hypotension), **TABLE 10** p. 1574 (CNS effects)

- ▸ Tricyclic antidepressants are predicted to decrease the effects of moxonidine. Avoid. Moderate Theoretical → Also see **TABLE 7** p. 1572 → Also see **TABLE 10** p. 1574

Mycophenolate

- ▸ **Mycophenolate** is predicted to increase the risk of haematological toxicity when given with aciclovir. Moderate Theoretical
- ▸ Oral antacids decrease the exposure to oral **mycophenolate**. Moderate Study
- ▸ Antifungals, azoles (isavuconazole) increase the exposure to **mycophenolate**. Moderate Study
- ▸ **Mycophenolate** is predicted to increase the risk of haematological toxicity when given with ganciclovir. Moderate Theoretical
- ▸ Live vaccines are predicted to increase the risk of generalised infection (possibly life-threatening) when given with **mycophenolate**. UKHSA advises avoid (refer to Green Book). Severe Theoretical
- ▸ Rifamycins (rifampicin) decrease the concentration of **mycophenolate**. Monitor and adjust dose. Severe Study
- ▸ **Mycophenolate** is predicted to increase the risk of haematological toxicity when given with valaciclovir. Moderate Theoretical
- ▸ **Mycophenolate** is predicted to increase the risk of haematological toxicity when given with valganciclovir. Moderate Theoretical

Nabilone → see **TABLE 10** p. 1574 (CNS effects)

- ▸ **Nabilone** is predicted to increase the risk of cardiovascular adverse effects when given with amfetamines. Severe Theoretical

Nabumetone → see NSAIDs

Nadolol → see beta blockers, non-selective

Naldemedine

- ▸ Anti-androgens (apalutamide, enzalutamide) are predicted to markedly decrease the exposure to **naldemedine**. Avoid. Severe Study
- ▸ Antiarrhythmics (amiodarone, dronedarone) are predicted to increase the exposure to **naldemedine**. Moderate Study
- ▸ Antiepileptics (carbamazepine, fosphenytoin, phenobarbital, phenytoin, primidone) are predicted to markedly decrease the exposure to **naldemedine**. Avoid. Severe Study
- ▸ Antifungals, azoles (fluconazole, isavuconazole) are predicted to increase the exposure to **naldemedine**. Moderate Study
- ▸ Antifungals, azoles (itraconazole, ketoconazole, posaconazole, voriconazole) are predicted to increase the exposure to **naldemedine**. Avoid or monitor. Moderate Study
- ▸ Berotralstat is predicted to increase the exposure to **naldemedine**. Moderate Study
- ▸ Calcium channel blockers (diltiazem, verapamil) are predicted to increase the exposure to **naldemedine**. Moderate Study
- ▸ Ceritinib is predicted to increase the exposure to **naldemedine**. Avoid or monitor. Moderate Study
- ▸ Ciclosporin is predicted to increase the exposure to **naldemedine**. Moderate Study
- ▸ Cobicistat is predicted to increase the exposure to **naldemedine**. Avoid or monitor. Moderate Study
- ▸ Crizotinib is predicted to increase the exposure to **naldemedine**. Moderate Study
- ▸ Encorafenib is predicted to markedly decrease the exposure to **naldemedine**. Avoid. Severe Study
- ▸ Fedratinib is predicted to increase the exposure to **naldemedine**. Moderate Study
- ▸ Grapefruit juice is predicted to increase the exposure to **naldemedine**. Avoid or monitor. Moderate Theoretical
- ▸ HIV-protease inhibitors are predicted to increase the exposure to **naldemedine**. Avoid or monitor. Moderate Study

Naldemedine (continued)
- **Idelalisib** is predicted to increase the exposure to **naldemedine**. Avoid or monitor. Moderate Study
- **Imatinib** is predicted to increase the exposure to **naldemedine**. Moderate Study
- **Ivosidenib** is predicted to markedly decrease the exposure to **naldemedine**. Avoid. Severe Study
- **Letermovir** is predicted to increase the exposure to **naldemedine**. Moderate Study
- **Lumacaftor** is predicted to markedly decrease the exposure to **naldemedine**. Avoid. Severe Study
- **Macrolides (azithromycin, erythromycin)** are predicted to increase the exposure to **naldemedine**. Moderate Study
- **Macrolides (clarithromycin)** are predicted to increase the exposure to **naldemedine**. Avoid or monitor. Moderate Study
- **Mitotane** is predicted to markedly decrease the exposure to **naldemedine**. Avoid. Severe Study
- **Neurokinin-1 receptor antagonists (aprepitant, netupitant)** are predicted to increase the exposure to **naldemedine**. Moderate Study
- **Nilotinib** is predicted to increase the exposure to **naldemedine**. Moderate Study
- **Ranolazine** is predicted to increase the exposure to **naldemedine**. Moderate Study
- **Rifamycins (rifampicin)** are predicted to markedly decrease the exposure to **naldemedine**. Avoid. Severe Study
- **St John's wort** is predicted to decrease the exposure to **naldemedine**. Avoid. Severe Study
- **Tucatinib** is predicted to increase the exposure to **naldemedine**. Avoid or monitor. Moderate Study
- **Vemurafenib** is predicted to increase the exposure to **naldemedine**. Moderate Study

Nalmefene
- **Nalmefene** is predicted to decrease the efficacy of **opioids**. Avoid except in an emergency situation—consult product literature. Severe Theoretical

Naloxegol
- **Anti-androgens (apalutamide, enzalutamide)** are predicted to markedly decrease the exposure to **naloxegol**. Avoid. Moderate Study
- **Antiarrhythmics (dronedarone)** are predicted to increase the exposure to **naloxegol**. Adjust **naloxegol** dose and monitor adverse effects, p. 72. Moderate Study
- **Antiepileptics (carbamazepine, fosphenytoin, phenobarbital, phenytoin, primidone)** are predicted to markedly decrease the exposure to **naloxegol**. Avoid. Moderate Study
- **Antifungals, azoles (fluconazole, isavuconazole)** are predicted to increase the exposure to **naloxegol**. Adjust **naloxegol** dose and monitor adverse effects, p. 72. Moderate Study
- **Antifungals, azoles (itraconazole, ketoconazole, posaconazole, voriconazole)** are predicted to markedly increase the exposure to **naloxegol**. Avoid. Severe Study
- **Berotralstat** is predicted to increase the exposure to **naloxegol**. Adjust **naloxegol** dose and monitor adverse effects, p. 72. Moderate Study
- **Calcium channel blockers (diltiazem, verapamil)** are predicted to increase the exposure to **naloxegol**. Adjust **naloxegol** dose and monitor adverse effects, p. 72. Moderate Study
- **Cenobamate** is predicted to decrease the exposure to **naloxegol**. Adjust dose. Moderate Theoretical
- **Ceritinib** is predicted to markedly increase the exposure to **naloxegol**. Avoid. Severe Study
- **Cobicistat** is predicted to markedly increase the exposure to **naloxegol**. Avoid. Severe Study
- **Crizotinib** is predicted to increase the exposure to **naloxegol**. Adjust **naloxegol** dose and monitor adverse effects, p. 72. Moderate Study
- **Dabrafenib** is predicted to decrease the exposure to **naloxegol**. Moderate Theoretical
- **Encorafenib** is predicted to markedly decrease the exposure to **naloxegol**. Avoid. Moderate Study
- **Endothelin receptor antagonists (bosentan)** are predicted to decrease the exposure to **naloxegol**. Moderate Theoretical

- **Fedratinib** is predicted to increase the exposure to **naloxegol**. Adjust **naloxegol** dose and monitor adverse effects, p. 72. Moderate Study
- **Grapefruit** juice is predicted to increase the exposure to **naloxegol**. Avoid. Moderate Theoretical
- **HIV-protease inhibitors** are predicted to markedly increase the exposure to **naloxegol**. Avoid. Severe Study
- **Idelalisib** is predicted to markedly increase the exposure to **naloxegol**. Avoid. Severe Study
- **Imatinib** is predicted to increase the exposure to **naloxegol**. Adjust **naloxegol** dose and monitor adverse effects, p. 72. Moderate Study
- **Ivosidenib** is predicted to markedly decrease the exposure to **naloxegol**. Avoid. Moderate Study
- **Letermovir** is predicted to increase the exposure to **naloxegol**. Adjust **naloxegol** dose and monitor adverse effects, p. 72. Moderate Study
- **Lorlatinib** is predicted to decrease the exposure to **naloxegol**. Moderate Theoretical
- **Lumacaftor** is predicted to markedly decrease the exposure to **naloxegol**. Avoid. Moderate Study
- **Macrolides (clarithromycin)** are predicted to markedly increase the exposure to **naloxegol**. Avoid. Severe Study
- **Macrolides (erythromycin)** are predicted to increase the exposure to **naloxegol**. Adjust **naloxegol** dose and monitor adverse effects, p. 72. Moderate Study
- **Mitotane** is predicted to markedly decrease the exposure to **naloxegol**. Avoid. Moderate Study
- **Neurokinin-1 receptor antagonists (aprepitant, netupitant)** are predicted to increase the exposure to **naloxegol**. Adjust **naloxegol** dose and monitor adverse effects, p. 72. Moderate Study
- **Nilotinib** is predicted to increase the exposure to **naloxegol**. Adjust **naloxegol** dose and monitor adverse effects, p. 72. Moderate Study
- **Nirmatrelvir** boosted with ritonavir is predicted to increase the concentration of **naloxegol**. Avoid. Severe Theoretical
- **NNRTIs (efavirenz, etravirine, nevirapine)** are predicted to decrease the exposure to **naloxegol**. Moderate Theoretical
- **Rifamycins (rifampicin)** are predicted to markedly decrease the exposure to **naloxegol**. Avoid. Moderate Study
- **Sotorasib** is predicted to decrease the exposure to **naloxegol**. Moderate Theoretical
- **St John's wort** is predicted to decrease the exposure to **naloxegol**. Avoid. Moderate Theoretical
- **Tucatinib** is predicted to markedly increase the exposure to **naloxegol**. Avoid. Severe Study

Naltrexone
- **Naltrexone** is predicted to decrease the efficacy of **opioids**. Avoid except in an emergency situation—consult product literature. Severe Theoretical

Naproxen → see NSAIDs
Naratriptan → see triptans
Natalizumab → see monoclonal antibodies
Nebivolol → see beta blockers, selective
Nefopam
- **Nefopam** is predicted to increase the risk of serious elevations in blood pressure when given with **MAOIs, irreversible**. Avoid. Severe Theoretical

Nelarabine → see TABLE 1 p. 1571 (hepatotoxicity), TABLE 14 p. 1575 (myelosuppression)
Neomycin → see TABLE 2 p. 1571 (nephrotoxicity), TABLE 18 p. 1576 (ototoxicity), TABLE 19 p. 1576 (neuromuscular blocking effects)

ROUTE-SPECIFIC INFORMATION Since systemic absorption can follow topical application of **neomycin**, the possibility of interactions should be borne in mind.

- **Neomycin** decreases the absorption of **digoxin**. Moderate Study
- **Neomycin** moderately decreases the exposure to **sorafenib**. Moderate Study

Neostigmine → see TABLE 5 p. 1572 (bradycardia)
- **Aminoglycosides** are predicted to decrease the effects of **neostigmine**. Moderate Theoretical

Nepafenac → see NSAIDs

Neratinib → see **TABLE 1** p. 1571 (hepatotoxicity)

> **FOOD AND LIFESTYLE** Avoid pomegranate, and pomegranate juice, as it might increase the concentration of neratinib.

▸ Oral **antacids** are predicted to decrease the exposure to oral **neratinib**. Separate administration by at least 3 hours. Mild Theoretical

▸ **Anti-androgens (apalutamide, enzalutamide)** are predicted to decrease the exposure to **neratinib**. Avoid. Severe Study

▸ **Antiarrhythmics (amiodarone)** are predicted to increase the exposure to **neratinib**. Avoid or adjust dose and monitor for gastrointestinal adverse effects—consult product literature. Severe Study → Also see **TABLE 1** p. 1571

▸ **Antiarrhythmics (dronedarone)** are predicted to increase the exposure to **neratinib**. Avoid moderate CYP3A4 inhibitors or adjust dose and monitor for gastrointestinal adverse effects—consult product literature. Severe Study

▸ **Antiepileptics (carbamazepine, fosphenytoin, phenobarbital, phenytoin, primidone)** are predicted to decrease the exposure to **neratinib**. Avoid. Severe Study

▸ **Antifungals, azoles (fluconazole, isavuconazole)** are predicted to increase the exposure to **neratinib**. Avoid moderate CYP3A4 inhibitors or adjust dose and monitor for gastrointestinal adverse effects—consult product literature. Severe Study → Also see **TABLE 1** p. 1571

▸ **Antifungals, azoles (itraconazole, ketoconazole, posaconazole, voriconazole)** are predicted to increase the exposure to **neratinib**. Avoid or adjust dose with potent CYP3A4 inhibitors—consult product literature. Severe Study → Also see **TABLE 1** p. 1571

▸ **Berotralstat** is predicted to increase the exposure to **neratinib**. Avoid moderate CYP3A4 inhibitors or adjust dose and monitor for gastrointestinal adverse effects—consult product literature. Severe Study

▸ **Calcium channel blockers (diltiazem, verapamil)** are predicted to increase the exposure to **neratinib**. Avoid moderate CYP3A4 inhibitors or adjust dose and monitor for gastrointestinal adverse effects—consult product literature. Severe Study

▸ Oral **calcium salts (calcium carbonate)** -containing antacids are predicted to decrease the exposure to oral **neratinib**. Separate administration by at least 3 hours. Mild Theoretical

▸ **Cenobamate** is predicted to decrease the exposure to **neratinib**. Avoid. Severe Theoretical

▸ **Ceritinib** is predicted to increase the exposure to **neratinib**. Avoid or adjust dose with potent CYP3A4 inhibitors—consult product literature. Severe Study

▸ **Ciclosporin** is predicted to increase the exposure to **neratinib**. Avoid or adjust dose and monitor for gastrointestinal adverse effects—consult product literature. Severe Study

▸ **Cobicistat** is predicted to increase the exposure to **neratinib**. Avoid or adjust dose with potent CYP3A4 inhibitors—consult product literature. Severe Study

▸ **Neratinib** might affect the efficacy of **combined hormonal contraceptives**. Use additional contraceptive precautions. Severe Theoretical

▸ **Crizotinib** is predicted to increase the exposure to **neratinib**. Avoid moderate CYP3A4 inhibitors or adjust dose and monitor for gastrointestinal adverse effects—consult product literature. Severe Study

▸ **Dabrafenib** is predicted to decrease the exposure to **neratinib**. Avoid. Severe Theoretical

▸ **Neratinib** slightly increases the exposure to **digoxin**. Moderate Study

▸ **Encorafenib** is predicted to decrease the exposure to **neratinib**. Avoid. Severe Study

▸ **Endothelin receptor antagonists (bosentan)** are predicted to decrease the exposure to **neratinib**. Avoid. Severe Theoretical

▸ **Neratinib** is predicted to increase the exposure to **erlotinib**. Moderate Theoretical

▸ **Neratinib** is predicted to increase the exposure to **everolimus**. Moderate Study

▸ **Neratinib** is predicted to increase the exposure to **factor XA inhibitors (apixaban)**. Moderate Theoretical

▸ **Fedratinib** is predicted to increase the exposure to **neratinib**. Avoid moderate CYP3A4 inhibitors or adjust dose and monitor for gastrointestinal adverse effects—consult product literature. Severe Study

▸ **Neratinib** is predicted to increase the exposure to **gilteritinib**. Moderate Theoretical

▸ **Glecaprevir** is predicted to increase the exposure to **neratinib**. Avoid or adjust dose and monitor for gastrointestinal adverse effects—consult product literature. Severe Study

▸ **Grapefruit** juice is predicted to increase the exposure to **neratinib**. Avoid. Severe Theoretical

▸ **H₂ receptor antagonists** are predicted to decrease the exposure to **neratinib**. Manufacturer advises take 2 hours before or 10 hours after **H₂ receptor antagonists**. Severe Study

▸ **HIV-protease inhibitors** are predicted to increase the exposure to **neratinib**. Avoid or adjust dose with potent CYP3A4 inhibitors—consult product literature. Severe Study → Also see **TABLE 1** p. 1571

▸ **Idelalisib** is predicted to increase the exposure to **neratinib**. Avoid or adjust dose with potent CYP3A4 inhibitors—consult product literature. Severe Study

▸ **Imatinib** is predicted to increase the exposure to **neratinib**. Avoid moderate CYP3A4 inhibitors or adjust dose and monitor for gastrointestinal adverse effects—consult product literature. Severe Study

▸ **Ivosidenib** is predicted to decrease the exposure to **neratinib**. Avoid. Severe Study

▸ **Letermovir** is predicted to increase the exposure to **neratinib**. Avoid moderate CYP3A4 inhibitors or adjust dose and monitor for gastrointestinal adverse effects—consult product literature. Severe Study

▸ **Lorlatinib** is predicted to decrease the exposure to **neratinib**. Avoid. Severe Theoretical

▸ **Lumacaftor** is predicted to decrease the exposure to **neratinib**. Avoid. Severe Study

▸ **Macrolides (azithromycin)** are predicted to increase the exposure to **neratinib**. Avoid or adjust dose and monitor for gastrointestinal adverse effects—consult product literature. Severe Study

▸ **Macrolides (clarithromycin)** are predicted to increase the exposure to **neratinib**. Avoid or adjust dose with potent CYP3A4 inhibitors—consult product literature. Severe Study

▸ **Macrolides (erythromycin)** are predicted to increase the exposure to **neratinib**. Avoid moderate CYP3A4 inhibitors or adjust dose and monitor for gastrointestinal adverse effects—consult product literature. Severe Study

▸ **Mitotane** is predicted to decrease the exposure to **neratinib**. Avoid. Severe Study

▸ **Neurokinin-1 receptor antagonists (aprepitant, netupitant)** are predicted to increase the exposure to **neratinib**. Avoid moderate CYP3A4 inhibitors or adjust dose and monitor for gastrointestinal adverse effects—consult product literature. Severe Study

▸ **Nilotinib** is predicted to increase the exposure to **neratinib**. Avoid moderate CYP3A4 inhibitors or adjust dose and monitor for gastrointestinal adverse effects—consult product literature. Severe Study

▸ **Nirmatrelvir** boosted with ritonavir is predicted to increase the concentration of **neratinib**. Avoid. Severe Theoretical

▸ **NNRTIs (efavirenz, etravirine, nevirapine)** are predicted to decrease the exposure to **neratinib**. Avoid. Severe Theoretical → Also see **TABLE 1** p. 1571

▸ **Pibrentasvir** is predicted to increase the exposure to **neratinib**. Avoid or adjust dose and monitor for gastrointestinal adverse effects—consult product literature. Severe Study

▸ **Proton pump inhibitors** are predicted to decrease the exposure to **neratinib**. Avoid. Severe Study

▸ **Ranolazine** is predicted to increase the exposure to **neratinib**. Avoid or adjust dose and monitor for gastrointestinal adverse effects—consult product literature. Severe Study

▸ **Rifamycins (rifampicin)** are predicted to decrease the exposure to **neratinib**. Avoid. Severe Study

▸ **Neratinib** is predicted to increase the exposure to the active component of **sacituzumab govitecan**. Severe Theoretical

▸ **Neratinib** is predicted to increase the exposure to **sirolimus**. Moderate Study

Neratinib (continued)

▸ Oral sodium bicarbonate -containing antacids are predicted to decrease the exposure to oral **neratinib**. Separate administration by at least 3 hours. Mild Theoretical

▸ Sotorasib is predicted to decrease the exposure to **neratinib**. Avoid. Severe Theoretical → Also see **TABLE 1** p. 1571

▸ St John's wort is predicted to decrease the exposure to **neratinib**. Avoid. Severe Theoretical

▸ **Neratinib** is predicted to increase the exposure to taxanes (paclitaxel). Moderate Study

▸ **Neratinib** might increase the exposure to tigecycline. Mild Anecdotal → Also see **TABLE 1** p. 1571

▸ Tucatinib is predicted to increase the exposure to **neratinib**. Avoid or adjust dose with potent CYP3A4 inhibitors—consult product literature. Severe Study

▸ Velpatasvir is predicted to increase the exposure to **neratinib**. Avoid or adjust dose and monitor for gastrointestinal adverse effects—consult product literature. Severe Study

▸ Vemurafenib is predicted to increase the exposure to **neratinib**. Avoid or adjust dose and monitor for gastrointestinal adverse effects—consult product literature. Severe Study

▸ **Neratinib** is predicted to increase the exposure to venetoclax. Avoid or monitor for toxicity. Severe Theoretical

▸ **Neratinib** might increase the exposure to vinca alkaloids. Severe Theoretical

▸ Voxilaprevir is predicted to increase the exposure to **neratinib**. Avoid or adjust dose and monitor for gastrointestinal adverse effects—consult product literature. Severe Study

Netilmicin → see aminoglycosides

Netupitant → see neurokinin-1 receptor antagonists

Neurokinin-1 receptor antagonists

aprepitant · fosaprepitant · netupitant

▸ Neurokinin-1 receptor antagonists (**aprepitant, netupitant**) are predicted to increase the exposure to abemaciclib. Moderate Study

▸ Neurokinin-1 receptor antagonists (**aprepitant, netupitant**) are predicted to increase the exposure to acalabrutinib. Avoid or monitor. Severe Study

▸ **Netupitant** very slightly increases the exposure to alkylating agents (cyclophosphamide). Moderate Study

▸ **Netupitant** is predicted to increase the exposure to alkylating agents (ifosfamide). Moderate Study

▸ Neurokinin-1 receptor antagonists (**aprepitant, fosaprepitant**) are predicted to increase the exposure to alkylating agents (ifosfamide). Severe Theoretical

▸ Neurokinin-1 receptor antagonists (**aprepitant, netupitant**) are predicted to increase the exposure to alpha blockers (tamsulosin). Moderate Theoretical

▸ Anti-androgens (apalutamide, enzalutamide) are predicted to markedly decrease the exposure to **aprepitant**. Avoid. Moderate Study

▸ Anti-androgens (apalutamide, enzalutamide) are predicted to decrease the exposure to **fosaprepitant**. Avoid. Moderate Theoretical

▸ Anti-androgens (apalutamide, enzalutamide) are predicted to decrease the exposure to **netupitant**. Avoid. Severe Study

▸ Neurokinin-1 receptor antagonists (**aprepitant, fosaprepitant**) are predicted to decrease the efficacy of anti-androgens (cyproterone) with ethinylestradiol (co-cyprindiol). Use alternative methods during treatment with, and for 28 days after, the enzyme inducing drug is stopped. Severe Study

▸ **Aprepitant** increases the exposure to antiarrhythmics (dronedarone). Severe Theoretical

▸ Neurokinin-1 receptor antagonists (**aprepitant, netupitant**) are predicted to increase the exposure to antiarrhythmics (propafenone). Monitor and adjust dose. Moderate Study

▸ Antiepileptics (carbamazepine, fosphenytoin, phenobarbital, phenytoin, primidone) are predicted to markedly decrease the exposure to **aprepitant**. Avoid. Moderate Study

▸ Antiepileptics (carbamazepine, fosphenytoin, phenobarbital, phenytoin, primidone) are predicted to decrease the exposure to **fosaprepitant**. Avoid. Moderate Theoretical

▸ Antiepileptics (carbamazepine, fosphenytoin, phenobarbital, phenytoin, primidone) are predicted to decrease the exposure to **netupitant**. Avoid. Severe Study

▸ Antifungals, azoles (fluconazole) are predicted to increase the exposure to **aprepitant**. Moderate Theoretical

▸ Antifungals, azoles (itraconazole, ketoconazole, posaconazole, voriconazole) are predicted to markedly increase the exposure to **aprepitant**. Moderate Study

▸ Antifungals, azoles (itraconazole, ketoconazole, posaconazole, voriconazole) are predicted to increase the exposure to **fosaprepitant**. Moderate Theoretical

▸ Antifungals, azoles (itraconazole, ketoconazole, posaconazole, voriconazole) are predicted to increase the exposure to **netupitant**. Moderate Study

▸ **Aprepitant** is predicted to increase the exposure to antifungals, azoles (isavuconazole). Moderate Theoretical

▸ **Netupitant** is predicted to decrease the exposure to antifungals, azoles (isavuconazole). Moderate Theoretical

▸ Neurokinin-1 receptor antagonists (**aprepitant, netupitant**) are predicted to increase the exposure to antihistamines, non-sedating (mizolastine). Severe Theoretical

▸ Neurokinin-1 receptor antagonists (**aprepitant, netupitant**) are predicted to increase the exposure to antihistamines, non-sedating (rupatadine). Avoid. Moderate Study

▸ Neurokinin-1 receptor antagonists (**aprepitant, netupitant**) are predicted to increase the exposure to antipsychotics, second generation (cariprazine). Avoid. Severe Study

▸ Neurokinin-1 receptor antagonists (**aprepitant, netupitant**) are predicted to increase the exposure to antipsychotics, second generation (lurasidone). Adjust **lurasidone** dose. Moderate Study

▸ Neurokinin-1 receptor antagonists (**aprepitant, netupitant**) are predicted to increase the exposure to antipsychotics, second generation (quetiapine). Avoid. Moderate Study

▸ Neurokinin-1 receptor antagonists (**aprepitant, netupitant**) are predicted to increase the exposure to avapritinib. Avoid or adjust dose—consult product literature. Moderate Study

▸ Neurokinin-1 receptor antagonists (**aprepitant, netupitant**) are predicted to increase the exposure to axitinib. Moderate Study

▸ Neurokinin-1 receptor antagonists (**aprepitant, netupitant**) might increase the exposure to bedaquiline. Mild Theoretical

▸ **Fosaprepitant** is predicted to increase the exposure to benzodiazepines (alprazolam). Moderate Study

▸ Neurokinin-1 receptor antagonists (**aprepitant, netupitant**) are predicted to increase the exposure to benzodiazepines (alprazolam). Severe Study

▸ **Fosaprepitant** slightly increases the exposure to benzodiazepines (midazolam). Moderate Study

▸ Neurokinin-1 receptor antagonists (**aprepitant, netupitant**) are predicted to increase the exposure to benzodiazepines (midazolam). Monitor adverse effects and adjust dose. Severe Study

▸ Neurokinin-1 receptor antagonists (**aprepitant, netupitant**) are predicted to increase the exposure to beta₂ agonists (salmeterol). Moderate Study

▸ **Fosaprepitant** is predicted to increase the exposure to bosutinib. Severe Theoretical

▸ Neurokinin-1 receptor antagonists (**aprepitant, netupitant**) are predicted to increase the exposure to bosutinib. Avoid or adjust dose. Severe Study

▸ Neurokinin-1 receptor antagonists (**aprepitant, netupitant**) are predicted to increase the exposure to brigatinib. Moderate Study

▸ Neurokinin-1 receptor antagonists (**aprepitant, netupitant**) are predicted to increase the exposure to buspirone. Use with caution and adjust dose. Moderate Study

▸ Neurokinin-1 receptor antagonists (**aprepitant, netupitant**) are predicted to increase the exposure to cabozantinib. Moderate Study

▸ Calcium channel blockers (diltiazem, verapamil) are predicted to increase the exposure to **aprepitant** and **aprepitant** is predicted to increase the exposure to calcium channel blockers (diltiazem, verapamil). Moderate Study

▸ Neurokinin-1 receptor antagonists (**aprepitant, netupitant**) are predicted to increase the exposure to calcium channel blockers (amlodipine, felodipine, lacidipine, lercanidipine, nicardipine, nifedipine, nimodipine). Monitor and adjust dose. Moderate Study

- Neurokinin-1 receptor antagonists **(aprepitant, netupitant)** are predicted to increase the exposure to capivasertib. Adjust dose. Moderate Study
- Cenobamate is predicted to decrease the exposure to **netupitant**. Moderate Theoretical
- Ceritinib is predicted to markedly increase the exposure to **aprepitant**. Moderate Study
- Fosaprepitant is predicted to increase the exposure to ceritinib. Severe Theoretical
- Ceritinib is predicted to increase the exposure to **fosaprepitant**. Moderate Theoretical
- Ceritinib is predicted to increase the exposure to **netupitant**. Moderate Study
- Neurokinin-1 receptor antagonists **(aprepitant, netupitant)** are predicted to increase the exposure to ceritinib. Moderate Study
- Neurokinin-1 receptor antagonists **(aprepitant, netupitant)** are predicted to increase the concentration of ciclosporin. Severe Study
- Cobicistat is predicted to markedly increase the exposure to **aprepitant**. Moderate Study
- Cobicistat is predicted to increase the exposure to **fosaprepitant**. Moderate Theoretical
- Cobicistat is predicted to increase the exposure to **netupitant**. Moderate Study
- Neurokinin-1 receptor antagonists **(aprepitant, netupitant)** are predicted to increase the exposure to cobimetinib. Severe Study
- Neurokinin-1 receptor antagonists **(aprepitant, netupitant)** are predicted to increase the exposure to colchicine. Adjust **colchicine** dose with moderate CYP3A4 inhibitors, p. 1279. Severe Study
- Neurokinin-1 receptor antagonists **(aprepitant, fosaprepitant)** are predicted to decrease the efficacy of combined hormonal contraceptives. For FSRH guidance, see Contraceptives, interactions p. 917. Severe Study
- Neurokinin-1 receptor antagonists **(aprepitant, netupitant)** are predicted to increase the exposure to oral corticosteroids (budesonide). Moderate Study
- Aprepitant moderately increases the exposure to corticosteroids (dexamethasone). Monitor and adjust dose. Moderate Study
- Netupitant moderately increases the exposure to corticosteroids **(dexamethasone)**. Adjust dose. Moderate Study
- Neurokinin-1 receptor antagonists **(aprepitant, netupitant)** are predicted to increase the exposure to corticosteroids (fluticasone). Moderate Study
- Neurokinin-1 receptor antagonists **(aprepitant, netupitant)** are predicted to increase the exposure to corticosteroids (methylprednisolone). Monitor and adjust dose. Moderate Study
- Aprepitant decreases the anticoagulant effect of coumarins. Moderate Study
- Fosaprepitant is predicted to decrease the anticoagulant effect of coumarins. Moderate Theoretical
- Netupitant is predicted to increase the exposure to crizotinib. Moderate Study
- Dabrafenib is predicted to decrease the exposure to **netupitant**. Moderate Theoretical
- Neurokinin-1 receptor antagonists **(aprepitant, netupitant)** are predicted to increase the exposure to dabrafenib. Moderate Study
- Neurokinin-1 receptor antagonists **(aprepitant, netupitant)** are predicted to increase the exposure to daridorexant. Adjust **daridorexant** dose, p. 554. Severe Study
- Neurokinin-1 receptor antagonists **(aprepitant, netupitant)** are predicted to increase the exposure to darifenacin. Moderate Study
- Neurokinin-1 receptor antagonists **(aprepitant, netupitant)** are predicted to increase the exposure to dasatinib. Severe Study
- Neurokinin-1 receptor antagonists **(aprepitant, fosaprepitant)** are predicted to decrease the efficacy of desogestrel. For FSRH guidance, see Contraceptives, interactions p. 917. Severe Theoretical
- Neurokinin-1 receptor antagonists **(aprepitant, netupitant)** are predicted to slightly increase the exposure to dienogest. Moderate Study

- Neurokinin-1 receptor antagonists **(aprepitant, netupitant)** are predicted to increase the exposure to dipeptidylpeptidase-4 inhibitors **(saxagliptin)**. Mild Study
- Neurokinin-1 receptor antagonists **(aprepitant, netupitant)** are predicted to increase the exposure to **domperidone**. Avoid. Severe Study
- Neurokinin-1 receptor antagonists **(aprepitant, netupitant)** are predicted to increase the exposure to dopamine receptor agonists **(bromocriptine)**. Severe Theoretical
- Neurokinin-1 receptor antagonists **(aprepitant, netupitant)** are predicted to increase the concentration of dopamine receptor agonists **(cabergoline)**. Moderate Anecdotal
- Netupitant is predicted to increase the exposure to drospirenone. Severe Study
- Neurokinin-1 receptor antagonists **(aprepitant, fosaprepitant)** are predicted to decrease the efficacy of drospirenone. For FSRH guidance, see Contraceptives, interactions p. 917. Severe Theoretical
- Neurokinin-1 receptor antagonists **(aprepitant, netupitant)** are predicted to moderately increase the exposure to dutasteride. Mild Study
- Neurokinin-1 receptor antagonists **(aprepitant, netupitant)** are predicted to increase the exposure to elacestrant. Avoid moderate CYP3A4 inhibitors or adjust **elacestrant** dose, p. 1084. Severe Theoretical
- Neurokinin-1 receptor antagonists **(aprepitant, netupitant)** are predicted to increase the exposure to elexacaftor. Adjust ivacaftor with tezacaftor and elexacaftor p. 337 dose with moderate CYP3A4 inhibitors. Severe Theoretical
- Neurokinin-1 receptor antagonists **(aprepitant, netupitant)** are predicted to increase the exposure to eliglustat. Avoid or adjust dose—consult product literature. Severe Study
- Encorafenib is predicted to markedly decrease the exposure to **aprepitant**. Avoid. Moderate Study
- Encorafenib is predicted to decrease the exposure to **fosaprepitant**. Avoid. Moderate Theoretical
- Encorafenib is predicted to decrease the exposure to **netupitant**. Avoid. Severe Study
- Neurokinin-1 receptor antagonists **(aprepitant, netupitant)** are predicted to moderately increase the exposure to encorafenib. Moderate Study
- Endothelin receptor antagonists **(bosentan)** are predicted to decrease the exposure to **aprepitant**. Moderate Study
- Endothelin receptor antagonists **(bosentan)** are predicted to decrease the exposure to neurokinin-1 receptor antagonists **(fosaprepitant, netupitant)**. Moderate Theoretical
- Neurokinin-1 receptor antagonists **(aprepitant, netupitant)** are predicted to increase the exposure to endothelin receptor antagonists **(macitentan)**. Manufacturer advises caution depending on other drugs taken—consult product literature. Moderate Theoretical
- Neurokinin-1 receptor antagonists **(aprepitant, netupitant)** are predicted to increase the exposure to entrectinib. Avoid or adjust dose with moderate CYP3A4 inhibitors—consult product literature. Severe Theoretical
- Neurokinin-1 receptor antagonists **(aprepitant, netupitant)** are predicted to increase the risk of ergotism when given with ergometrine. Severe Theoretical
- Neurokinin-1 receptor antagonists **(aprepitant, netupitant)** are predicted to increase the exposure to erlotinib. Moderate Study
- Neurokinin-1 receptor antagonists **(aprepitant, fosaprepitant)** are predicted to decrease the efficacy of estradiol. Moderate Theoretical
- Neurokinin-1 receptor antagonists **(aprepitant, fosaprepitant)** are predicted to decrease the efficacy of etonogestrel. For FSRH guidance, see Contraceptives, interactions p. 917. Severe Theoretical
- Netupitant slightly increases the exposure to etoposide. Moderate Study
- Neurokinin-1 receptor antagonists **(aprepitant, netupitant)** are predicted to increase the exposure to etrasimod. Avoid in poor CYP2C9 metabolisers. Severe Theoretical
- Neurokinin-1 receptor antagonists **(aprepitant, netupitant)** are predicted to increase the concentration of everolimus. Avoid or adjust dose. Moderate Study

Neurokinin-1 receptor antagonists (continued)

▸ Neurokinin-1 receptor antagonists **(aprepitant, netupitant)** are predicted to increase the exposure to fedratinib. Monitor and adjust dose. Moderate Study

▸ Neurokinin-1 receptor antagonists **(aprepitant, netupitant)** are predicted to increase the exposure to fesoterodine. Adjust **fesoterodine** dose with moderate CYP3A4 inhibitors in hepatic and renal impairment, p. 897. Mild Study

▸ Neurokinin-1 receptor antagonists **(aprepitant, netupitant)** are predicted to increase the exposure to gefitinib. Moderate Study

▸ **Fosaprepitant** is predicted to increase the concentration of guanfacine. Moderate Theoretical

▸ Neurokinin-1 receptor antagonists **(aprepitant, netupitant)** are predicted to increase the concentration of guanfacine. Adjust **guanfacine** dose, p. 407. Moderate Theoretical

▸ HIV-protease inhibitors are predicted to markedly increase the exposure to **aprepitant**. Moderate Study

▸ HIV-protease inhibitors are predicted to increase the exposure to **fosaprepitant**. Moderate Theoretical

▸ HIV-protease inhibitors are predicted to increase the exposure to **netupitant**. Moderate Study

▸ Neurokinin-1 receptor antagonists **(aprepitant, fosaprepitant)** are predicted to decrease the effects of hormone replacement therapy. Moderate Anecdotal

▸ **Fosaprepitant** is predicted to slightly increase the exposure to ibrutinib. Moderate Theoretical

▸ Neurokinin-1 receptor antagonists **(aprepitant, netupitant)** are predicted to increase the exposure to ibrutinib. Adjust dose with moderate CYP3A4 inhibitors—consult product literature. Severe Study

▸ Idelalisib is predicted to markedly increase the exposure to **aprepitant**. Moderate Study

▸ Idelalisib is predicted to increase the exposure to **fosaprepitant**. Moderate Theoretical

▸ Idelalisib is predicted to increase the exposure to **netupitant**. Moderate Study

▸ Neurokinin-1 receptor antagonists **(aprepitant, netupitant)** are predicted to increase the exposure to imatinib. Moderate Theoretical

▸ **Netupitant** is predicted to increase the exposure to irinotecan. Moderate Study

▸ Neurokinin-1 receptor antagonists **(aprepitant, fosaprepitant)** are predicted to increase the exposure to intravenous irinotecan. Severe Theoretical

▸ Neurokinin-1 receptor antagonists **(aprepitant, netupitant)** are predicted to increase the exposure to ivabradine. Adjust **ivabradine** dose, p. 245. Severe Theoretical

▸ Neurokinin-1 receptor antagonists **(aprepitant, netupitant)** are predicted to increase the exposure to ivacaftor. Adjust dose with moderate CYP3A4 inhibitors, see ivacaftor p. 336, tezacaftor with ivacaftor p. 339, and ivacaftor with tezacaftor and elexacaftor p. 337. Moderate Study

▸ Ivosidenib is predicted to markedly decrease the exposure to **aprepitant**. Avoid. Moderate Study

▸ Ivosidenib is predicted to decrease the exposure to **fosaprepitant**. Avoid. Moderate Theoretical

▸ Ivosidenib is predicted to decrease the exposure to **netupitant**. Avoid. Severe Study

▸ Neurokinin-1 receptor antagonists **(aprepitant, netupitant)** are predicted to increase the exposure to ivosidenib. Monitor and adjust dose—consult product literature. Severe Study

▸ Neurokinin-1 receptor antagonists **(aprepitant, netupitant)** are predicted to increase the exposure to lapatinib. Moderate Study

▸ Neurokinin-1 receptor antagonists **(aprepitant, netupitant)** are predicted to increase the exposure to larotrectinib. Monitor and adjust dose. Moderate Theoretical

▸ Neurokinin-1 receptor antagonists **(aprepitant, netupitant)** are predicted to increase the exposure to leniolisib. Avoid. Moderate Study

▸ Neurokinin-1 receptor antagonists **(aprepitant, fosaprepitant)** are predicted to decrease the efficacy of some contraceptive methods containing levonorgestrel. For FSRH guidance, see Contraceptives, interactions p. 917. Severe Theoretical

▸ **Fosaprepitant** is predicted to increase the exposure to lomitapide. Separate administration by 12 hours. Mild Theoretical

▸ Neurokinin-1 receptor antagonists **(aprepitant, netupitant)** are predicted to increase the exposure to lomitapide. Avoid. Moderate Theoretical

▸ Lorlatinib is predicted to decrease the exposure to **netupitant**. Moderate Theoretical

▸ Lumacaftor is predicted to markedly decrease the exposure to **aprepitant**. Avoid. Moderate Study

▸ Lumacaftor is predicted to decrease the exposure to **fosaprepitant**. Avoid. Moderate Theoretical

▸ Lumacaftor is predicted to decrease the exposure to **netupitant**. Avoid. Severe Study

▸ Macrolides **(clarithromycin)** are predicted to markedly increase the exposure to **aprepitant**. Moderate Study

▸ Macrolides **(clarithromycin)** are predicted to increase the exposure to **fosaprepitant**. Moderate Theoretical

▸ Macrolides **(clarithromycin)** are predicted to increase the exposure to **netupitant**. Moderate Study

▸ Macrolides **(erythromycin)** are predicted to increase the exposure to **aprepitant**. Moderate Study

▸ Neurokinin-1 receptor antagonists **(aprepitant, netupitant)** are predicted to increase the exposure to maraviroc. Moderate Study

▸ **Fosaprepitant** is predicted to increase the exposure to mavacamten. Monitor and adjust dose—consult product literature. Moderate Theoretical

▸ Neurokinin-1 receptor antagonists **(aprepitant, netupitant)** are predicted to increase the exposure to mavacamten. Adjust dose—consult product literature. Moderate Study

▸ Neurokinin-1 receptor antagonists **(aprepitant, netupitant)** are predicted to increase the exposure to midostaurin. Moderate Theoretical

▸ Neurokinin-1 receptor antagonists **(aprepitant, netupitant)** are predicted to increase the exposure to mineralocorticoid receptor antagonists **(eplerenone)**. Adjust **eplerenone** dose, p. 223. Severe Study

▸ Neurokinin-1 receptor antagonists **(aprepitant, netupitant)** are predicted to increase the exposure to mineralocorticoid receptor antagonists **(finerenone)**. Severe Study

▸ Mitotane is predicted to markedly decrease the exposure to **aprepitant**. Avoid. Moderate Study

▸ Mitotane is predicted to decrease the exposure to **fosaprepitant**. Avoid. Moderate Theoretical

▸ Mitotane is predicted to decrease the exposure to **netupitant**. Avoid. Severe Study

▸ Neurokinin-1 receptor antagonists **(aprepitant, netupitant)** are predicted to increase the exposure to mobocertinib. Avoid or adjust dose and monitor ECG—consult product literature. Severe Study

▸ Neurokinin-1 receptor antagonists **(aprepitant, netupitant)** are predicted to increase the exposure to naldemedine. Moderate Study

▸ Neurokinin-1 receptor antagonists **(aprepitant, netupitant)** are predicted to increase the exposure to naloxegol. Adjust **naloxegol** dose and monitor adverse effects, p. 72. Moderate Study

▸ Neurokinin-1 receptor antagonists **(aprepitant, netupitant)** are predicted to increase the exposure to neratinib. Avoid moderate CYP3A4 inhibitors or adjust dose and monitor for gastrointestinal adverse effects—consult product literature. Severe Study

▸ Neurokinin-1 receptor antagonists **(aprepitant, netupitant)** are predicted to increase the exposure to nilotinib. Moderate Study

▸ NNRTIs **(efavirenz, etravirine, nevirapine)** are predicted to decrease the exposure to **aprepitant**. Moderate Study

▸ NNRTIs **(etravirine)** are predicted to decrease the exposure to **netupitant**. Moderate Theoretical

▸ NNRTIs **(efavirenz, nevirapine)** are predicted to decrease the exposure to neurokinin-1 receptor antagonists **(fosaprepitant, netupitant)**. Moderate Theoretical

▸ Neurokinin-1 receptor antagonists **(aprepitant, fosaprepitant)** are predicted to decrease the efficacy of some contraceptive

methods containing norethisterone. For FSRH guidance, see Contraceptives, interactions p. 917. Severe Anecdotal
▶ Neurokinin-1 receptor antagonists (aprepitant, netupitant) are predicted to increase the exposure to olaparib. Avoid or adjust dose with moderate CYP3A4 inhibitors—consult product literature. Moderate Theoretical
▶ Neurokinin-1 receptor antagonists (aprepitant, netupitant) are predicted to increase the exposure to opioids (alfentanil, buprenorphine, fentanyl, oxycodone). Monitor and adjust dose. Moderate Study
▶ Neurokinin-1 receptor antagonists (aprepitant, netupitant) are predicted to increase the exposure to opioids (methadone, sufentanil). Moderate Theoretical
▶ Neurokinin-1 receptor antagonists (aprepitant, netupitant) are predicted to increase the exposure to pazopanib. Moderate Study
▶ Neurokinin-1 receptor antagonists (aprepitant, netupitant) are predicted to increase the exposure to pemigatinib. Severe Study
▶ Neurokinin-1 receptor antagonists (aprepitant, netupitant) are predicted to increase the exposure to phosphodiesterase type-5 inhibitors (avanafil). Adjust avanafil dose, p. 939. Moderate Theoretical
▶ Neurokinin-1 receptor antagonists (aprepitant, netupitant) are predicted to increase the exposure to phosphodiesterase type-5 inhibitors (sildenafil). Monitor or adjust sildenafil dose with moderate CYP3A4 inhibitors, p. 940. Moderate Study
▶ Neurokinin-1 receptor antagonists (aprepitant, netupitant) are predicted to increase the exposure to phosphodiesterase type-5 inhibitors (tadalafil). Severe Theoretical
▶ Neurokinin-1 receptor antagonists (aprepitant, netupitant) are predicted to increase the exposure to phosphodiesterase type-5 inhibitors (vardenafil). Adjust dose. Severe Theoretical
▶ **Neurokinin-1 receptor antagonists** are predicted to increase the exposure to pimozide. Avoid. Severe Theoretical
▶ Neurokinin-1 receptor antagonists (aprepitant, netupitant) are predicted to increase the exposure to ponatinib. Moderate Study
▶ Neurokinin-1 receptor antagonists (aprepitant, netupitant) are predicted to increase the exposure to pralsetinib. Moderate Theoretical
▶ Neurokinin-1 receptor antagonists (aprepitant, netupitant) are predicted to increase the exposure to ranolazine. Severe Study
▶ Neurokinin-1 receptor antagonists (aprepitant, netupitant) are predicted to increase the exposure to regorafenib. Moderate Study
▶ Neurokinin-1 receptor antagonists (aprepitant, netupitant) are predicted to increase the exposure to ribociclib. Moderate Study
▶ Rifamycins (rifampicin) are predicted to markedly decrease the exposure to aprepitant. Avoid. Moderate Study
▶ Rifamycins (rifampicin) are predicted to decrease the exposure to fosaprepitant. Avoid. Moderate Theoretical
▶ Rifamycins (rifampicin) are predicted to decrease the exposure to netupitant. Avoid. Severe Study
▶ Neurokinin-1 receptor antagonists (aprepitant, netupitant) are predicted to increase the exposure to rimegepant. Avoid another dose of rimegepant within 48 hours of concurrent use. Moderate Study
▶ Neurokinin-1 receptor antagonists (aprepitant, netupitant) are predicted to increase the exposure to ruxolitinib. Moderate Study
▶ Neurokinin-1 receptor antagonists (aprepitant, netupitant) are predicted to increase the exposure to selpercatinib. Moderate Study
▶ Neurokinin-1 receptor antagonists (aprepitant, netupitant) are predicted to increase the exposure to selumetinib. Avoid or adjust dose—consult product literature. Severe Study
▶ Neurokinin-1 receptor antagonists (aprepitant, netupitant) are predicted to increase the exposure to siponimod. Avoid depending on other drugs taken—consult product literature. Severe Study
▶ Neurokinin-1 receptor antagonists (aprepitant, netupitant) increase the concentration of sirolimus. Monitor and adjust dose. Moderate Study
▶ Sotorasib is predicted to decrease the exposure to netupitant. Moderate Theoretical

▶ Neurokinin-1 receptor antagonists (aprepitant, netupitant) are predicted to increase the exposure to SSRIs (dapoxetine). Adjust dapoxetine dose with moderate CYP3A4 inhibitors, p. 947. Moderate Theoretical
▶ St John's wort is predicted to decrease the exposure to netupitant. Moderate Theoretical
▶ St John's wort is predicted to decrease the exposure to neurokinin-1 receptor antagonists (aprepitant, fosaprepitant). Avoid. Moderate Theoretical
▶ Neurokinin-1 receptor antagonists (aprepitant, netupitant) are predicted to increase the exposure to statins (atorvastatin, simvastatin). Monitor and adjust dose. Severe Theoretical
▶ Neurokinin-1 receptor antagonists (aprepitant, netupitant) are predicted to increase the exposure to sunitinib. Moderate Study
▶ Neurokinin-1 receptor antagonists (aprepitant, netupitant) are predicted to increase the concentration of tacrolimus. Severe Study
▶ Neurokinin-1 receptor antagonists (aprepitant, netupitant) are predicted to increase the exposure to taxanes (cabazitaxel). Moderate Theoretical
▶ Neurokinin-1 receptor antagonists (aprepitant, netupitant) are predicted to increase the exposure to taxanes (docetaxel). Severe Study
▶ Neurokinin-1 receptor antagonists (aprepitant, netupitant) are predicted to increase the exposure to taxanes (paclitaxel). Moderate Anecdotal
▶ Neurokinin-1 receptor antagonists (aprepitant, netupitant) are predicted to increase the concentration of temsirolimus. Use with caution or avoid. Moderate Theoretical
▶ Neurokinin-1 receptor antagonists (aprepitant, netupitant) are predicted to increase the exposure to tezacaftor. Adjust dose with moderate CYP3A4 inhibitors, see tezacaftor with ivacaftor p. 339 and ivacaftor with tezacaftor and elexacaftor p. 337. Severe Study
▶ Neurokinin-1 receptor antagonists (aprepitant, netupitant) given with a potent CYP2C19 inhibitor are predicted to increase the exposure to tofacitinib. Adjust tofacitinib dose, p. 1265. Moderate Study
▶ Neurokinin-1 receptor antagonists (aprepitant, netupitant) are predicted to increase the exposure to tolvaptan. Manufacturer advises caution or adjust tolvaptan dose with moderate CYP3A4 inhibitors, p. 767. Moderate Study
▶ Neurokinin-1 receptor antagonists (aprepitant, netupitant) are predicted to increase the exposure to trazodone. Moderate Theoretical
▶ Neurokinin-1 receptor antagonists (aprepitant, netupitant) are predicted to increase the exposure to triptans (eletriptan). Moderate Study
▶ Tucatinib is predicted to markedly increase the exposure to aprepitant. Moderate Study
▶ Tucatinib is predicted to increase the exposure to fosaprepitant. Moderate Theoretical
▶ Tucatinib is predicted to increase the exposure to netupitant. Moderate Study
▶ **Netupitant** is predicted to increase the exposure to ulipristal. Avoid if used for uterine fibroids. Moderate Study
▶ Neurokinin-1 receptor antagonists (aprepitant, fosaprepitant) decrease the efficacy of ulipristal. Avoid and for 4 weeks after stopping the enzyme inducing drug. For FSRH guidance, see Contraceptives, interactions p. 917. Severe Anecdotal
▶ Neurokinin-1 receptor antagonists (aprepitant, netupitant) are predicted to increase the exposure to vemurafenib. Severe Theoretical
▶ Neurokinin-1 receptor antagonists (aprepitant, netupitant) are predicted to increase the exposure to venetoclax. Avoid or adjust dose—consult product literature. Severe Study
▶ **Neurokinin-1 receptor antagonists** are predicted to increase the exposure to vinca alkaloids. Severe Theoretical
▶ Neurokinin-1 receptor antagonists (aprepitant, netupitant) are predicted to increase the exposure to voclosporin. Adjust voclosporin dose, p. 973. Severe Study
▶ Neurokinin-1 receptor antagonists (aprepitant, netupitant) are predicted to increase the exposure to zanubrutinib. Avoid or adjust dose with moderate CYP3A4 inhibitors—consult product literature. Severe Study

Neurokinin-1 receptor antagonists (continued)
▶ Neurokinin-1 receptor antagonists **(aprepitant, netupitant)** are predicted to increase the exposure to zopiclone. Adjust dose. Moderate Study

Neuromuscular blocking drugs, non-depolarising → see TABLE 19 p. 1576 (neuromuscular blocking effects)

atracurium · cisatracurium · mivacurium · pancuronium · rocuronium · vecuronium

▶ Anticholinesterases, centrally acting are predicted to decrease the effects of **neuromuscular blocking drugs, non-depolarising.** Moderate Theoretical
▶ Antiepileptics (carbamazepine) are predicted to decrease the effects of (but acute use increases the effects of) neuromuscular blocking drugs, non-depolarising **(atracurium, cisatracurium, pancuronium, rocuronium, vecuronium).** Monitor and adjust dose. Moderate Study
▶ Antiepileptics (fosphenytoin, phenytoin) decrease the effects of (but acute use increases the effects of) neuromuscular blocking drugs, non-depolarising **(atracurium, cisatracurium, pancuronium, rocuronium, vecuronium).** Moderate Study
▶ Clindamycin increases the effects of **neuromuscular blocking drugs, non-depolarising.** Severe Anecdotal
▶ Corticosteroids are predicted to decrease the effects of neuromuscular blocking drugs, non-depolarising. Severe Anecdotal
▶ **Pancuronium** is predicted to increase the risk of cardiovascular adverse effects when given with digoxin. Severe Anecdotal
▶ Irinotecan is predicted to decrease the effects of neuromuscular blocking drugs, non-depolarising. Moderate Theoretical
▶ Intravenous magnesium increases the effects of **neuromuscular blocking drugs, non-depolarising.** Moderate Study
▶ Metoclopramide is predicted to increase the effects of neuromuscular blocking drugs, non-depolarising. Moderate Theoretical
▶ Penicillins (piperacillin) increase the effects of **neuromuscular blocking drugs, non-depolarising.** Moderate Study
▶ SSRIs potentially increase the risk of prolonged neuromuscular blockade when given with **mivacurium.** Unknown Theoretical

Nevirapine → see NNRTIs
Nicardipine → see calcium channel blockers
Nicorandil → see TABLE 7 p. 1572 (hypotension)
▶ Aspirin is predicted to increase the risk of gastrointestinal perforation when given with **nicorandil.** Severe Theoretical
▶ Corticosteroids increase the risk of gastrointestinal perforation when given with **nicorandil.** Severe Anecdotal
▶ **Nicorandil** is predicted to increase the risk of gastrointestinal perforation when given with NSAIDs. Severe Theoretical
▶ **Nicorandil** is predicted to increase the risk of hypotension when given with phosphodiesterase type-5 inhibitors. Avoid. Severe Theoretical → Also see TABLE 7 p. 1572

Nicotinic acid → see TABLE 1 p. 1571 (hepatotoxicity), TABLE 3 p. 1571 (anticoagulant effects)
▶ **Nicotinic acid** might increase the risk of rhabdomyolysis when given with statins. Use with caution or avoid. Severe Theoretical → Also see TABLE 1 p. 1571

Nifedipine → see calcium channel blockers
Nilotinib → see TABLE 14 p. 1575 (myelosuppression), TABLE 8 p. 1573 (QT-interval prolongation)
▶ **Nilotinib** is predicted to increase the exposure to abemaciclib. Moderate Study
▶ **Nilotinib** is predicted to increase the exposure to acalabrutinib. Avoid or monitor. Severe Study
▶ **Nilotinib** is predicted to increase the exposure to alpha blockers (tamsulosin). Moderate Theoretical
▶ Oral antacids might affect the absorption of oral **nilotinib.** Separate administration by at least 2 hours. Moderate Theoretical
▶ Anti-androgens (apalutamide, enzalutamide) are predicted to moderately decrease the exposure to **nilotinib.** Avoid. Severe Study → Also see TABLE 8 p. 1573
▶ **Nilotinib** is predicted to increase the exposure to antiarrhythmics (propafenone). Monitor and adjust dose. Moderate Study

▶ Antiepileptics (carbamazepine, fosphenytoin, phenobarbital, phenytoin, primidone) are predicted to moderately decrease the exposure to **nilotinib.** Avoid. Severe Study
▶ Antifungals, azoles (fluconazole, isavuconazole) are predicted to increase the exposure to **nilotinib.** Moderate Study → Also see TABLE 8 p. 1573
▶ Antifungals, azoles (itraconazole, ketoconazole, posaconazole, voriconazole) are predicted to increase the exposure to **nilotinib.** Avoid. Severe Study → Also see TABLE 8 p. 1573
▶ **Nilotinib** is predicted to increase the exposure to antihistamines, non-sedating (mizolastine). Severe Theoretical
▶ **Nilotinib** is predicted to increase the exposure to antihistamines, non-sedating (rupatadine). Avoid. Moderate Study
▶ **Nilotinib** is predicted to increase the exposure to antipsychotics, second generation (cariprazine). Avoid. Severe Study
▶ **Nilotinib** is predicted to increase the exposure to antipsychotics, second generation (lurasidone). Adjust **lurasidone** dose. Moderate Study
▶ **Nilotinib** is predicted to increase the exposure to antipsychotics, second generation (quetiapine). Avoid. Moderate Study
▶ **Nilotinib** is predicted to increase the exposure to avapritinib. Avoid or adjust dose—consult product literature. Moderate Study
▶ **Nilotinib** is predicted to increase the exposure to axitinib. Moderate Study → Also see TABLE 14 p. 1575
▶ **Nilotinib** might increases the exposure to bedaquiline. Mild Theoretical → Also see TABLE 8 p. 1573
▶ **Nilotinib** is predicted to increase the exposure to benzodiazepines (alprazolam). Severe Study
▶ **Nilotinib** is predicted to increase the exposure to benzodiazepines (midazolam). Monitor adverse effects and adjust dose. Severe Study
▶ **Nilotinib** is predicted to increase the exposure to bosutinib. Avoid or adjust dose. Severe Study → Also see TABLE 14 p. 1575 → Also see TABLE 8 p. 1573
▶ **Nilotinib** is predicted to increase the exposure to brigatinib. Moderate Study
▶ **Nilotinib** is predicted to increase the exposure to buspirone. Use with caution and adjust dose. Moderate Study
▶ **Nilotinib** is predicted to increase the exposure to cabozantinib. Moderate Study → Also see TABLE 14 p. 1575 → Also see TABLE 8 p. 1573
▶ Calcium channel blockers (diltiazem, verapamil) are predicted to increase the exposure to **nilotinib.** Moderate Theoretical
▶ **Nilotinib** is predicted to increase the exposure to calcium channel blockers (amlodipine, felodipine, lacidipine, lercanidipine, nicardipine, nifedipine, nimodipine). Monitor and adjust dose. Moderate Study
▶ Oral calcium salts (calcium carbonate) -containing antacids might affect the exposure to oral **nilotinib.** Separate administration by at least 2 hours. Moderate Study
▶ **Nilotinib** is predicted to increase the exposure to capivasertib. Adjust dose. Moderate Study
▶ Cenobamate is predicted to decrease the exposure to **nilotinib.** Avoid. Severe Theoretical
▶ Ceritinib is predicted to increase the exposure to **nilotinib.** Avoid. Severe Study → Also see TABLE 14 p. 1575 → Also see TABLE 8 p. 1573
▶ **Nilotinib** is predicted to increase the exposure to ceritinib. Moderate Study → Also see TABLE 14 p. 1575 → Also see TABLE 8 p. 1573
▶ **Nilotinib** is predicted to increase the concentration of ciclosporin. Severe Study
▶ Cobicistat is predicted to increase the exposure to **nilotinib.** Avoid. Severe Study
▶ **Nilotinib** is predicted to increase the exposure to cobimetinib. Severe Study
▶ **Nilotinib** is predicted to increase the exposure to colchicine. Adjust **colchicine** dose with moderate CYP3A4 inhibitors, p. 1279. Severe Study
▶ **Nilotinib** is predicted to increase the exposure to corticosteroids (methylprednisolone). Monitor and adjust dose. Moderate Study
▶ **Nilotinib** is predicted to increase the risk of bleeding events when given with coumarins. Severe Theoretical

- **Dabrafenib** is predicted to decrease the exposure to **nilotinib**. Avoid. Severe Theoretical
- **Nilotinib** is predicted to increase the exposure to dabrafenib. Moderate Study
- **Nilotinib** is predicted to increase the exposure to daridorexant. Adjust **daridorexant** dose, p. 554. Severe Study
- **Nilotinib** is predicted to increase the exposure to darifenacin. Moderate Study
- **Nilotinib** is predicted to increase the exposure to dasatinib. Severe Study → Also see **TABLE 14** p. 1575 → Also see **TABLE 8** p. 1573
- **Nilotinib** is predicted to slightly increase the exposure to dienogest. Moderate Study
- **Nilotinib** is predicted to increase the exposure to dipeptidylpeptidase-4 inhibitors (saxagliptin). Mild Study
- **Nilotinib** is predicted to increase the exposure to domperidone. Avoid. Severe Study
- **Nilotinib** is predicted to increase the exposure to dopamine receptor agonists (bromocriptine). Severe Theoretical
- **Nilotinib** is predicted to increase the concentration of dopamine receptor agonists (cabergoline). Moderate Anecdotal
- **Nilotinib** is predicted to increase the exposure to drospirenone. Severe Study
- **Nilotinib** is predicted to moderately increase the exposure to dutasteride. Mild Study
- **Nilotinib** is predicted to increase the exposure to elacestrant. Avoid moderate CYP3A4 inhibitors or adjust **elacestrant** dose, p. 1084. Severe Theoretical
- **Nilotinib** is predicted to increase the exposure to elexacaftor. Adjust ivacaftor with tezacaftor and elexacaftor p. 337 dose with moderate CYP3A4 inhibitors. Severe Theoretical
- **Nilotinib** is predicted to increase the exposure to eliglustat. Avoid or adjust dose—consult product literature. Severe Study
- **Encorafenib** is predicted to moderately decrease the exposure to **nilotinib**. Avoid. Severe Study → Also see **TABLE 8** p. 1573
- **Nilotinib** is predicted to moderately increase the exposure to encorafenib. Moderate Study → Also see **TABLE 8** p. 1573
- Endothelin receptor antagonists (bosentan) are predicted to decrease the exposure to **nilotinib**. Avoid. Severe Theoretical
- **Nilotinib** is predicted to increase the exposure to endothelin receptor antagonists (macitentan). Manufacturer advises caution depending on other drugs taken—consult product literature. Moderate Theoretical
- **Nilotinib** is predicted to increase the exposure to entrectinib. Avoid or adjust dose with moderate CYP3A4 inhibitors—consult product literature. Severe Theoretical → Also see **TABLE 8** p. 1573
- **Nilotinib** is predicted to increase the risk of ergotism when given with ergometrine. Severe Theoretical
- **Nilotinib** is predicted to increase the exposure to erlotinib. Moderate Study
- **Nilotinib** is predicted to increase the exposure to etrasimod. Avoid in poor CYP2C9 metabolisers. Severe Theoretical
- **Nilotinib** is predicted to increase the concentration of everolimus. Avoid or adjust dose. Moderate Study
- **Nilotinib** is predicted to increase the exposure to fedratinib. Monitor and adjust dose. Moderate Study
- **Nilotinib** is predicted to increase the exposure to fesoterodine. Adjust **fesoterodine** dose with moderate CYP3A4 inhibitors in hepatic and renal impairment, p. 897. Mild Study
- **Nilotinib** is predicted to increase the exposure to gefitinib. Moderate Study
- **Grapefruit** juice is predicted to increase the exposure to **nilotinib**. Avoid. Severe Theoretical
- **Nilotinib** is predicted to increase the concentration of guanfacine. Adjust **guanfacine** dose, p. 407. Moderate Theoretical
- H$_2$ receptor antagonists might affect the absorption of **nilotinib**. **H$_2$ receptor antagonists** should be taken 10 hours before or 2 hours after **nilotinib**. Mild Theoretical
- HIV-protease inhibitors are predicted to increase the exposure to **nilotinib**. Avoid. Severe Study
- **Nilotinib** is predicted to increase the exposure to ibrutinib. Adjust dose with moderate CYP3A4 inhibitors—consult product literature. Severe Study → Also see **TABLE 14** p. 1575
- **Idelalisib** is predicted to increase the exposure to **nilotinib**. Avoid. Severe Study

- **Nilotinib** is predicted to increase the exposure to imatinib. Moderate Study → Also see **TABLE 14** p. 1575
- **Nilotinib** is predicted to increase the exposure to ivabradine. Adjust **ivabradine** dose, p. 245. Severe Theoretical
- **Nilotinib** is predicted to increase the exposure to ivacaftor. Adjust dose with moderate CYP3A4 inhibitors, see ivacaftor p. 336, tezacaftor with ivacaftor p. 339, and ivacaftor with tezacaftor and elexacaftor p. 337. Moderate Study
- **Nilotinib** is predicted to increase the exposure to ivosidenib. Monitor and adjust dose—consult product literature. Severe Study → Also see **TABLE 8** p. 1573
- **Ivosidenib** is predicted to moderately decrease the exposure to **nilotinib**. Avoid. Severe Study → Also see **TABLE 8** p. 1573
- **Nilotinib** is predicted to increase the exposure to lapatinib. Moderate Study → Also see **TABLE 8** p. 1573
- **Nilotinib** is predicted to increase the exposure to larotrectinib. Monitor and adjust dose. Moderate Theoretical
- **Nilotinib** is predicted to increase the exposure to leniolisib. Avoid. Moderate Study
- **Letermovir** is predicted to increase the exposure to **nilotinib**. Moderate Study
- **Nilotinib** is predicted to increase the exposure to lomitapide. Avoid. Moderate Theoretical
- **Lorlatinib** is predicted to decrease the exposure to **nilotinib**. Avoid. Severe Theoretical
- **Lumacaftor** is predicted to moderately decrease the exposure to **nilotinib**. Avoid. Severe Study
- Macrolides (clarithromycin) are predicted to increase the exposure to **nilotinib**. Avoid. Severe Study
- Macrolides (erythromycin) are predicted to increase the exposure to **nilotinib**. Moderate Study → Also see **TABLE 8** p. 1573
- **Nilotinib** is predicted to increase the exposure to mavacamten. Adjust dose—consult product literature. Moderate Study
- **Nilotinib** is predicted to increase the exposure to midostaurin. Moderate Theoretical
- **Nilotinib** is predicted to increase the exposure to mineralocorticoid receptor antagonists (eplerenone). Adjust **eplerenone** dose, p. 223. Severe Study
- **Nilotinib** is predicted to increase the exposure to mineralocorticoid receptor antagonists (finerenone). Severe Study
- **Mitotane** is predicted to moderately decrease the exposure to **nilotinib**. Avoid. Severe Study → Also see **TABLE 14** p. 1575
- **Nilotinib** is predicted to increase the exposure to mobocertinib. Avoid or adjust dose and monitor ECG—consult product literature. Severe Study → Also see **TABLE 8** p. 1573
- **Nilotinib** is predicted to increase the exposure to naldemedine. Moderate Study
- **Nilotinib** is predicted to increase the exposure to naloxegol. Adjust **naloxegol** dose and monitor adverse effects, p. 72. Moderate Study
- **Nilotinib** is predicted to increase the exposure to neratinib. Avoid moderate CYP3A4 inhibitors or adjust dose and monitor for gastrointestinal adverse effects—consult product literature. Severe Study
- Neurokinin-1 receptor antagonists (aprepitant, netupitant) are predicted to increase the exposure to **nilotinib**. Moderate Study
- **Nirmatrelvir** boosted with ritonavir is predicted to increase the concentration of **nilotinib**. Avoid. Severe Theoretical
- NNRTIs (efavirenz, etravirine, nevirapine) are predicted to decrease the exposure to **nilotinib**. Avoid. Severe Theoretical → Also see **TABLE 8** p. 1573
- **Nilotinib** is predicted to increase the exposure to olaparib. Avoid or adjust dose with moderate CYP3A4 inhibitors—consult product literature. Moderate Theoretical → Also see **TABLE 14** p. 1575
- **Nilotinib** is predicted to increase the exposure to opioids (alfentanil, buprenorphine, fentanyl, oxycodone). Monitor and adjust dose. Moderate Study
- **Nilotinib** is predicted to increase the exposure to opioids (methadone, sufentanil). Moderate Theoretical → Also see **TABLE 8** p. 1573
- **Nilotinib** is predicted to increase the exposure to pazopanib. Moderate Study → Also see **TABLE 8** p. 1573
- **Nilotinib** is predicted to increase the exposure to pemigatinib. Severe Study

Nilotinib (continued)
▸ **Nilotinib** is predicted to increase the risk of bleeding events when given with phenindione. [Severe] Theoretical
▸ **Nilotinib** is predicted to increase the exposure to phosphodiesterase type-5 inhibitors (avanafil). Adjust **avanafil** dose, p. 939. [Moderate] Theoretical
▸ **Nilotinib** is predicted to increase the exposure to phosphodiesterase type-5 inhibitors (sildenafil). Monitor or adjust **sildenafil** dose with moderate CYP3A4 inhibitors, p. 940. [Moderate] Study
▸ **Nilotinib** is predicted to increase the exposure to phosphodiesterase type-5 inhibitors (tadalafil). [Severe] Theoretical
▸ **Nilotinib** is predicted to increase the exposure to phosphodiesterase type-5 inhibitors (vardenafil). Adjust dose. [Severe] Theoretical → Also see **TABLE 8** p. 1573
▸ **Nilotinib** is predicted to increase the exposure to pimozide. Avoid. [Severe] Theoretical → Also see **TABLE 8** p. 1573
▸ Pitolisant is predicted to decrease the exposure to **nilotinib**. Avoid. [Severe] Theoretical
▸ **Nilotinib** is predicted to increase the exposure to ponatinib. [Moderate] Study
▸ **Nilotinib** is predicted to increase the exposure to pralsetinib. [Moderate] Theoretical
▸ **Nilotinib** is predicted to increase the exposure to ranolazine. [Severe] Study → Also see **TABLE 8** p. 1573
▸ **Nilotinib** is predicted to increase the exposure to regorafenib. [Moderate] Study → Also see **TABLE 14** p. 1575
▸ **Nilotinib** is predicted to increase the exposure to ribociclib. [Moderate] Study → Also see **TABLE 14** p. 1575 → Also see **TABLE 8** p. 1573
▸ Rifamycins (rifampicin) are predicted to moderately decrease the exposure to **nilotinib**. Avoid. [Severe] Study
▸ **Nilotinib** is predicted to increase the exposure to rimegepant. Avoid another dose of rimegepant within 48 hours of concurrent use. [Moderate] Study
▸ **Nilotinib** is predicted to increase the exposure to ruxolitinib. [Moderate] Study → Also see **TABLE 14** p. 1575
▸ **Nilotinib** is predicted to increase the exposure to selpercatinib. [Moderate] Study → Also see **TABLE 8** p. 1573
▸ **Nilotinib** is predicted to increase the exposure to selumetinib. Avoid or adjust dose—consult product literature. [Severe] Study
▸ **Nilotinib** is predicted to increase the exposure to siponimod. Avoid depending on other drugs taken—consult product literature. [Severe] Study
▸ **Nilotinib** increases the concentration of sirolimus. Monitor and adjust dose. [Moderate] Study
▸ Oral sodium bicarbonate -containing antacids might affect the exposure to oral **nilotinib**. Separate administration by at least 2 hours. [Moderate] Study
▸ Sodium zirconium cyclosilicate is predicted to decrease the exposure to **nilotinib**. Separate administration by at least 2 hours. [Moderate] Theoretical
▸ Sotorasib is predicted to decrease the exposure to **nilotinib**. Avoid. [Severe] Theoretical
▸ **Nilotinib** is predicted to increase the exposure to SSRIs (dapoxetine). Adjust **dapoxetine** dose with moderate CYP3A4 inhibitors, p. 947. [Moderate] Theoretical
▸ St John's wort is predicted to decrease the exposure to **nilotinib**. Avoid. [Severe] Theoretical
▸ **Nilotinib** is predicted to increase the exposure to statins (atorvastatin). Monitor and adjust dose. [Moderate] Theoretical
▸ **Nilotinib** is predicted to increase the exposure to statins (simvastatin). Monitor and adjust dose. [Severe] Theoretical
▸ **Nilotinib** is predicted to increase the exposure to sunitinib. [Moderate] Study → Also see **TABLE 14** p. 1575 → Also see **TABLE 8** p. 1573
▸ **Nilotinib** is predicted to increase the concentration of tacrolimus. [Severe] Study
▸ **Nilotinib** is predicted to increase the exposure to taxanes (cabazitaxel). [Moderate] Theoretical → Also see **TABLE 14** p. 1575
▸ **Nilotinib** is predicted to increase the exposure to taxanes (docetaxel). [Severe] Study → Also see **TABLE 14** p. 1575
▸ **Nilotinib** is predicted to increase the exposure to taxanes (paclitaxel). [Moderate] Anecdotal → Also see **TABLE 14** p. 1575

▸ **Nilotinib** is predicted to increase the concentration of temsirolimus. Use with caution or avoid. [Moderate] Theoretical → Also see **TABLE 14** p. 1575
▸ **Nilotinib** is predicted to increase the exposure to tezacaftor. Adjust dose with moderate CYP3A4 inhibitors, see tezacaftor with ivacaftor p. 339 and ivacaftor with tezacaftor and elexacaftor p. 337. [Severe] Study
▸ **Nilotinib** given with a potent CYP2C19 inhibitor is predicted to increase the exposure to tofacitinib. Adjust **tofacitinib** dose, p. 1265. [Moderate] Study
▸ **Nilotinib** is predicted to increase the exposure to tolvaptan. Manufacturer advises caution or adjust **tolvaptan** dose with moderate CYP3A4 inhibitors, p. 767. [Moderate] Study
▸ **Nilotinib** is predicted to increase the exposure to trazodone. [Moderate] Theoretical
▸ Tucatinib is predicted to increase the exposure to **nilotinib**. Avoid. [Severe] Study
▸ **Nilotinib** is predicted to increase the exposure to ulipristal. Avoid if used for uterine fibroids. [Moderate] Study
▸ **Nilotinib** is predicted to increase the exposure to vemurafenib. [Severe] Theoretical → Also see **TABLE 8** p. 1573
▸ **Nilotinib** is predicted to increase the exposure to venetoclax. Avoid or adjust dose—consult product literature. [Severe] Study
▸ **Nilotinib** is predicted to increase the exposure to vinca alkaloids. [Severe] Theoretical → Also see **TABLE 14** p. 1575
▸ **Nilotinib** is predicted to increase the exposure to voclosporin. Adjust **voclosporin** dose, p. 973. [Severe] Study → Also see **TABLE 8** p. 1573
▸ **Nilotinib** is predicted to increase the exposure to zanubrutinib. Avoid or adjust dose with moderate CYP3A4 inhibitors—consult product literature. [Severe] Study
▸ **Nilotinib** is predicted to increase the exposure to zopiclone. Adjust dose. [Moderate] Study

Nimodipine → see calcium channel blockers

Nintedanib → see **TABLE 4** p. 1571 (antiplatelet effects)
▸ Antiarrhythmics (amiodarone, dronedarone) are predicted to increase the exposure to **nintedanib**. [Moderate] Study
▸ Antiepileptics (carbamazepine) are predicted to decrease the exposure to **nintedanib**. [Moderate] Study
▸ Antiepileptics (phenobarbital, phenytoin) are predicted to decrease the exposure to **nintedanib**. [Severe] Theoretical
▸ Antifungals, azoles (itraconazole, ketoconazole) are predicted to increase the exposure to **nintedanib**. [Moderate] Study
▸ Antifungals, azoles (voriconazole) are predicted to increase the exposure to **nintedanib**. [Moderate] Theoretical
▸ Calcium channel blockers (verapamil) are predicted to increase the exposure to **nintedanib**. [Moderate] Study
▸ Ciclosporin is predicted to increase the exposure to **nintedanib**. [Moderate] Study
▸ Cobicistat is predicted to increase the exposure to **nintedanib**. [Moderate] Study
▸ Glecaprevir is predicted to increase the exposure to **nintedanib**. [Moderate] Study
▸ HIV-protease inhibitors (atazanavir, darunavir, fosamprenavir) boosted with ritonavir are predicted to increase the exposure to **nintedanib**. [Moderate] Theoretical
▸ HIV-protease inhibitors (lopinavir, ritonavir) are predicted to increase the exposure to **nintedanib**. [Moderate] Study
▸ Lapatinib is predicted to increase the exposure to **nintedanib**. [Moderate] Study
▸ Lorlatinib is predicted to decrease the exposure to **nintedanib**. [Moderate] Study
▸ Macrolides are predicted to increase the exposure to **nintedanib**. [Moderate] Study
▸ Pibrentasvir is predicted to increase the exposure to **nintedanib**. [Moderate] Study
▸ Ranolazine is predicted to increase the exposure to **nintedanib**. [Moderate] Study
▸ Rifamycins (rifampicin) are predicted to decrease the exposure to **nintedanib**. [Moderate] Study
▸ St John's wort is predicted to decrease the exposure to **nintedanib**. [Moderate] Study
▸ Velpatasvir is predicted to increase the exposure to **nintedanib**. [Moderate] Study

► **Vemurafenib** is predicted to increase the exposure to nintedanib. Moderate Study
► **Voxilaprevir** is predicted to increase the exposure to nintedanib. Moderate Study

Niraparib → see TABLE 14 p. 1575 (myelosuppression)

Nirmatrelvir
► **Nirmatrelvir** boosted with ritonavir is predicted to increase the concentration of abemaciclib. Avoid or adjust dose—consult product literature. Severe Theoretical
► **Nirmatrelvir** boosted with ritonavir is predicted to increase the concentration of afatinib. Moderate Theoretical
► **Nirmatrelvir** boosted with ritonavir is predicted to increase the concentration of aliskiren. Avoid. Severe Theoretical
► **Nirmatrelvir** boosted with ritonavir is predicted to increase the concentration of alpha blockers (alfuzosin, tamsulosin). Avoid. Severe Theoretical
► **Nirmatrelvir** boosted with ritonavir is predicted to increase the concentration of amfetamines. Severe Theoretical
► **Nirmatrelvir** boosted with ritonavir is predicted to decrease the concentration of aminophylline. Adjust dose. Moderate Theoretical
► Anti-androgens (apalutamide, enzalutamide) are predicted to decrease the exposure to **nirmatrelvir** boosted with ritonavir. Avoid. Severe Study
► **Nirmatrelvir** boosted with ritonavir is predicted to increase the concentration of antiarrhythmics (amiodarone, dronedarone, flecainide, propafenone). Avoid. Severe Theoretical
► **Nirmatrelvir** boosted with ritonavir is predicted to increase the concentration of antiarrhythmics (disopyramide, lidocaine). Severe Theoretical
► Antiepileptics (carbamazepine, fosphenytoin, phenobarbital, phenytoin, primidone) are predicted to decrease the exposure to **nirmatrelvir** boosted with ritonavir. Avoid. Severe Study
► **Nirmatrelvir** boosted with ritonavir is predicted to decrease the concentration of antiepileptics (lamotrigine, valproate). Severe Theoretical
► **Nirmatrelvir** boosted with ritonavir is predicted to increase the concentration of antifungals, azoles (isavuconazole). Severe Theoretical
► **Nirmatrelvir** boosted with ritonavir increases the exposure to antifungals, azoles (itraconazole). Severe Study
► **Nirmatrelvir** boosted with ritonavir is predicted to increase the concentration of antifungals, azoles (ketoconazole). Adjust dose. Moderate Theoretical
► **Nirmatrelvir** boosted with ritonavir is predicted to decrease the concentration of antifungals, azoles (voriconazole). Avoid. Severe Theoretical
► **Nirmatrelvir** boosted with ritonavir is predicted to decrease the concentration of antimalarials (atovaquone). Moderate Theoretical
► **Nirmatrelvir** boosted with ritonavir is predicted to increase the concentration of antipsychotics, second generation (aripiprazole). Adjust dose. Moderate Theoretical
► **Nirmatrelvir** boosted with ritonavir is predicted to increase the concentration of antipsychotics, second generation (cariprazine). Avoid. Moderate Theoretical
► **Nirmatrelvir** boosted with ritonavir is predicted to increase the concentration of antipsychotics, second generation (clozapine). Avoid or adjust dose. Severe Theoretical
► **Nirmatrelvir** boosted with ritonavir is predicted to increase the concentration of antipsychotics, second generation (lurasidone, quetiapine). Avoid. Severe Theoretical
► **Nirmatrelvir** boosted with ritonavir is predicted to increase the concentration of antipsychotics, second generation (risperidone). Severe Theoretical
► **Nirmatrelvir** boosted with ritonavir is predicted to increase the concentration of bedaquiline. Avoid or monitor. Moderate Theoretical
► **Nirmatrelvir** boosted with ritonavir is predicted to increase the concentration of benzodiazepines (alprazolam). Moderate Theoretical
► **Nirmatrelvir** boosted with ritonavir is predicted to increase the concentration of benzodiazepines (clonazepam, diazepam, flurazepam). Monitor and adjust dose. Severe Theoretical

► **Nirmatrelvir** boosted with ritonavir very markedly increases the exposure to benzodiazepines (midazolam). Avoid or adjust dose. Severe Study
► **Nirmatrelvir** boosted with ritonavir is predicted to increase the concentration of beta₂ agonists (salmeterol). Avoid. Severe Theoretical
► **Nirmatrelvir** boosted with ritonavir is predicted to decrease the concentration of bupropion. Moderate Theoretical
► **Nirmatrelvir** boosted with ritonavir is predicted to increase the concentration of buspirone. Monitor and adjust dose. Moderate Theoretical
► **Nirmatrelvir** boosted with ritonavir is predicted to increase the concentration of calcium channel blockers. Severe Theoretical
► **Nirmatrelvir** boosted with ritonavir is predicted to increase the concentration of ceritinib. Avoid or adjust dose—consult product literature. Severe Theoretical
► **Nirmatrelvir** boosted with ritonavir is predicted to increase the concentration of ciclosporin. Avoid. Severe Theoretical
► **Nirmatrelvir** boosted with ritonavir is predicted to increase the concentration of cilostazol. Adjust dose. Moderate Theoretical
► **Nirmatrelvir** boosted with ritonavir is predicted to decrease the concentration of clopidogrel. Severe Theoretical
► **Nirmatrelvir** boosted with ritonavir is predicted to increase the concentration of colchicine. Avoid. Severe Theoretical
► **Nirmatrelvir** boosted with ritonavir is predicted to decrease the concentration of combined hormonal contraceptives (containing ethinylestradiol). Use additional contraceptive precautions. Moderate Theoretical
► **Nirmatrelvir** boosted with ritonavir is predicted to increase the concentration of corticosteroids (beclometasone) (risk with beclometasone is likely to be lower than with other corticosteroids). Moderate Theoretical
► **Nirmatrelvir** boosted with ritonavir is predicted to increase the concentration of corticosteroids (betamethasone, budesonide, ciclesonide, deflazacort, dexamethasone, fluticasone, hydrocortisone, methylprednisolone, mometasone, prednisolone, triamcinolone). Avoid or monitor adverse effects and consider beclomethasone as an alternative. Severe Theoretical
► **Nirmatrelvir** boosted with ritonavir is predicted to increase the concentration of corticosteroids (fludrocortisone, vamorolone). Avoid or monitor adverse effects. Severe Theoretical
► **Nirmatrelvir** boosted with ritonavir is predicted to affect the concentration of coumarins (warfarin). Moderate Theoretical
► **Nirmatrelvir** boosted with ritonavir is predicted to increase the concentration of darifenacin. Adjust dose. Severe Theoretical
► **Nirmatrelvir** boosted with ritonavir is predicted to increase the concentration of dasatinib. Avoid. Severe Theoretical
► **Nirmatrelvir** boosted with ritonavir is predicted to increase the concentration of delamanid. Severe Theoretical
► **Nirmatrelvir** boosted with ritonavir is predicted to increase the concentration of digoxin. Severe Theoretical
► **Nirmatrelvir** boosted with ritonavir is predicted to increase the concentration of dipeptidylpeptidase-4 inhibitors (saxagliptin). Adjust dose. Moderate Theoretical
► **Nirmatrelvir** boosted with ritonavir is predicted to increase the concentration of elexacaftor with tezacaftor and ivacaftor. Adjust dose. Severe Theoretical
► **Nirmatrelvir** boosted with ritonavir is predicted to increase the concentration of encorafenib. Avoid or monitor. Severe Theoretical
► Encorafenib is predicted to decrease the exposure to **nirmatrelvir** boosted with ritonavir. Avoid. Severe Study
► **Nirmatrelvir** boosted with ritonavir is predicted to increase the concentration of endothelin receptor antagonists (bosentan). Severe Theoretical
► **Nirmatrelvir** boosted with ritonavir is predicted to increase the concentration of ergometrine. Avoid. Severe Theoretical
► **Nirmatrelvir** boosted with ritonavir is predicted to increase the concentration of everolimus. Avoid. Severe Theoretical
► **Nirmatrelvir** boosted with ritonavir is predicted to increase the concentration of factor XA inhibitors (apixaban, rivaroxaban). Avoid. Severe Theoretical

Nirmatrelvir (continued)

▶ **Nirmatrelvir** boosted with ritonavir is predicted to increase the concentration of fostamatinib. Monitor adverse effects and adjust dose. Moderate Theoretical

▶ **Nirmatrelvir** boosted with ritonavir is predicted to increase the concentration of fusidate. Avoid. Moderate Theoretical

▶ **Nirmatrelvir** boosted with ritonavir is predicted to increase the concentration of glecaprevir. Avoid. Severe Theoretical

▶ **Nirmatrelvir** boosted with ritonavir is predicted to increase the concentration of grazoprevir. Severe Theoretical

▶ **Nirmatrelvir** boosted with ritonavir is predicted to increase the concentration of haloperidol. Severe Theoretical

▶ **Nirmatrelvir** boosted with ritonavir is predicted to increase the concentration of HIV-protease inhibitors (atazanavir, darunavir, fosamprenavir, lopinavir). Moderate Theoretical

▶ **Nirmatrelvir** boosted with ritonavir is predicted to increase the concentration of ibrutinib. Avoid or adjust dose—consult product literature. Severe Theoretical

▶ **Nirmatrelvir** boosted with ritonavir is predicted to increase the concentration of ivabradine. Avoid. Severe Theoretical

▶ **Nirmatrelvir** boosted with ritonavir is predicted to increase the concentration of ivacaftor. Adjust dose. Severe Theoretical

▶ **Nirmatrelvir** boosted with ritonavir is predicted to increase the concentration of ivosidenib. Monitor and adjust dose—consult product literature. Severe Theoretical

▶ Ivosidenib is predicted to decrease the exposure to **nirmatrelvir** boosted with ritonavir. Avoid. Severe Study

▶ **Nirmatrelvir** boosted with ritonavir is predicted to increase the concentration of lomitapide. Avoid. Severe Theoretical

▶ Lumacaftor is predicted to decrease the exposure to nirmatrelvir boosted with ritonavir. Avoid. Severe Study

▶ **Nirmatrelvir** boosted with ritonavir is predicted to increase the concentration of macrolides (clarithromycin). Monitor; adjust dose in renal impairment. Moderate Theoretical

▶ **Nirmatrelvir** boosted with ritonavir is predicted to increase the concentration of macrolides (erythromycin). Moderate Theoretical

▶ **Nirmatrelvir** boosted with ritonavir is predicted to increase the concentration of maraviroc. Refer to specialist literature. Severe Theoretical

▶ **Nirmatrelvir** boosted with ritonavir is predicted to increase the concentration of methylphenidate. Severe Theoretical

▶ **Nirmatrelvir** boosted with ritonavir is predicted to increase the concentration of mineralocorticoid receptor antagonists (eplerenone, finerenone). Avoid. Severe Theoretical

▶ Mitotane is predicted to decrease the exposure to **nirmatrelvir** boosted with ritonavir. Avoid. Severe Study

▶ **Nirmatrelvir** boosted with ritonavir is predicted to increase the concentration of naloxegol. Avoid. Severe Theoretical

▶ **Nirmatrelvir** boosted with ritonavir is predicted to increase the concentration of neratinib. Avoid. Severe Theoretical

▶ **Nirmatrelvir** boosted with ritonavir is predicted to increase the concentration of nilotinib. Avoid. Severe Theoretical

▶ **Nirmatrelvir** boosted with ritonavir is predicted to increase the concentration of NNRTIs (efavirenz, nevirapine). Moderate Theoretical

▶ **Nirmatrelvir** boosted with ritonavir is predicted to increase the concentration of opioids (buprenorphine). Monitor and adjust dose. Moderate Theoretical

▶ **Nirmatrelvir** boosted with ritonavir is predicted to increase the concentration of opioids (fentanyl, oxycodone, pethidine). Severe Theoretical

▶ **Nirmatrelvir** boosted with ritonavir is predicted to decrease the concentration of opioids (methadone). Adjust dose. Moderate Theoretical

▶ **Nirmatrelvir** boosted with ritonavir is predicted to decrease the concentration of opioids (morphine). Moderate Theoretical

▶ **Nirmatrelvir** boosted with ritonavir is predicted to increase the concentration of phosphodiesterase type-5 inhibitors (avanafil, vardenafil). Avoid. Severe Theoretical

▶ **Nirmatrelvir** boosted with ritonavir is predicted to increase the concentration of phosphodiesterase type-5 inhibitors (sildenafil, tadalafil). Avoid or adjust dose—consult product literature. Severe Theoretical

▶ **Nirmatrelvir** boosted with ritonavir is predicted to increase the concentration of pibrentasvir. Avoid. Severe Theoretical

▶ **Nirmatrelvir** boosted with ritonavir is predicted to increase the concentration of pimozide. Avoid. Severe Theoretical

▶ **Nirmatrelvir** boosted with ritonavir is predicted to increase the concentration of ranolazine. Avoid. Severe Theoretical

▶ Rifamycins (rifampicin) are predicted to decrease the exposure to **nirmatrelvir** boosted with ritonavir. Avoid. Severe Study

▶ **Nirmatrelvir** boosted with ritonavir is predicted to increase the concentration of rifamycins (rifabutin). Adjust dose. Severe Theoretical

▶ **Nirmatrelvir** boosted with ritonavir is predicted to increase the concentration of rimegepant. Avoid. Severe Theoretical

▶ **Nirmatrelvir** boosted with ritonavir is predicted to increase the concentration of riociguat. Adjust dose. Moderate Theoretical

▶ **Nirmatrelvir** boosted with ritonavir is predicted to increase the concentration of sirolimus. Avoid. Severe Theoretical

▶ St John's wort is predicted to decrease the exposure to nirmatrelvir boosted with ritonavir. Avoid. Severe Theoretical

▶ **Nirmatrelvir** boosted with ritonavir is predicted to increase the concentration of statins (atorvastatin, rosuvastatin). Adjust dose. Severe Theoretical

▶ **Nirmatrelvir** boosted with ritonavir is predicted to increase the concentration of statins (simvastatin). Avoid. Severe Theoretical

▶ **Nirmatrelvir** boosted with ritonavir is predicted to increase the concentration of tacrolimus. Avoid. Severe Theoretical

▶ **Nirmatrelvir** boosted with ritonavir is predicted to increase the concentration of tezacaftor with ivacaftor. Adjust dose. Severe Theoretical

▶ **Nirmatrelvir** boosted with ritonavir is predicted to decrease the concentration of theophylline. Adjust dose. Moderate Theoretical

▶ **Nirmatrelvir** boosted with ritonavir moderately increases the exposure to thrombin inhibitors (dabigatran). Avoid. Severe Study

▶ **Nirmatrelvir** boosted with ritonavir might decrease the efficacy of thyroid hormones (levothyroxine). Moderate Theoretical

▶ **Nirmatrelvir** boosted with ritonavir is predicted to increase the concentration of ticagrelor. Avoid. Severe Theoretical

▶ **Nirmatrelvir** boosted with ritonavir is predicted to increase the concentration of tofacitinib. Adjust dose. Severe Theoretical

▶ **Nirmatrelvir** boosted with ritonavir is predicted to increase the concentration of tolvaptan. Avoid. Severe Theoretical

▶ **Nirmatrelvir** boosted with ritonavir is predicted to increase the concentration of trazodone. Moderate Theoretical

▶ **Nirmatrelvir** boosted with ritonavir is predicted to increase the concentration of tricyclic antidepressants. Moderate Theoretical

▶ **Nirmatrelvir** boosted with ritonavir is predicted to increase the concentration of triptans (eletriptan). Avoid. Severe Theoretical

▶ **Nirmatrelvir** boosted with ritonavir is predicted to increase the concentration of upadacitinib. Adjust dose. Severe Theoretical

▶ **Nirmatrelvir** boosted with ritonavir is predicted to increase the concentration of venetoclax. Avoid or adjust dose—consult product literature. Severe Theoretical

▶ **Nirmatrelvir** boosted with ritonavir is predicted to increase the concentration of vinca alkaloids (vinblastine, vincristine). Severe Theoretical

▶ **Nirmatrelvir** boosted with ritonavir is predicted to increase the concentration of voclosporin. Avoid. Severe Theoretical

▶ **Nirmatrelvir** boosted with ritonavir is predicted to increase the concentration of zolpidem. Severe Theoretical

Nitisinone

▶ **Nitisinone** is predicted to increase the exposure to adefovir. Moderate Study

▶ Anti-androgens (apalutamide, enzalutamide) are predicted to decrease the exposure to **nitisinone**. Adjust dose. Moderate Theoretical

▶ Antiepileptics (carbamazepine, fosphenytoin, phenobarbital, phenytoin, primidone) are predicted to decrease the exposure to nitisinone. Adjust dose. Moderate Theoretical

▶ Antifungals, azoles (itraconazole, ketoconazole, posaconazole, voriconazole) are predicted to increase the exposure to nitisinone. Adjust dose. Moderate Theoretical

▶ **Nitisinone** is predicted to increase the exposure to baricitinib. Moderate Study

▶ **Nitisinone** is predicted to increase the exposure to cephalosporins (cefaclor). Moderate Study

▶ **Ceritinib** is predicted to increase the exposure to **nitisinone**. Adjust dose. Moderate Theoretical

▶ **Cobicistat** is predicted to increase the exposure to **nitisinone**. Adjust dose. Moderate Theoretical

▶ **Nitisinone** is predicted to increase the exposure to coumarins (warfarin). Moderate Study

▶ **Encorafenib** is predicted to decrease the exposure to **nitisinone**. Adjust dose. Moderate Theoretical

▶ **Nitisinone** is predicted to increase the exposure to ganciclovir. Moderate Study

▶ **Nitisinone** is predicted to increase the exposure to H_2 receptor antagonists (famotidine). Moderate Study

▶ **HIV-protease inhibitors** are predicted to increase the exposure to **nitisinone**. Adjust dose. Moderate Theoretical

▶ **Idelalisib** is predicted to increase the exposure to **nitisinone**. Adjust dose. Moderate Theoretical

▶ **Ivosidenib** is predicted to decrease the exposure to **nitisinone**. Adjust dose. Moderate Theoretical

▶ **Nitisinone** is predicted to increase the exposure to loop diuretics (furosemide). Moderate Study

▶ **Lumacaftor** is predicted to decrease the exposure to **nitisinone**. Adjust dose. Moderate Theoretical

▶ **Macrolides (clarithromycin)** are predicted to increase the exposure to **nitisinone**. Adjust dose. Moderate Theoretical

▶ **Nitisinone** is predicted to increase the exposure to methotrexate. Moderate Study

▶ **Mitotane** is predicted to decrease the exposure to **nitisinone**. Adjust dose. Moderate Theoretical

▶ **Nitisinone** is predicted to increase the exposure to NSAIDs (celecoxib). Moderate Study

▶ **Nitisinone** is predicted to increase the exposure to oseltamivir. Moderate Study

▶ **Nitisinone** is predicted to increase the exposure to penicillins (benzylpenicillin). Moderate Study

▶ **Nitisinone** is predicted to increase the exposure to quinolones (ciprofloxacin). Moderate Study

▶ **Rifamycins (rifampicin)** are predicted to decrease the exposure to **nitisinone**. Adjust dose. Moderate Theoretical

▶ **Nitisinone** is predicted to increase the exposure to sulfonylureas (glimepiride, tolbutamide). Moderate Study

▶ **Nitisinone** is predicted to increase the exposure to tenofovir alafenamide. Moderate Study

▶ **Nitisinone** is predicted to increase the exposure to tenofovir disoproxil. Moderate Study

▶ **Tucatinib** is predicted to increase the exposure to **nitisinone**. Adjust dose. Moderate Theoretical

Nitrates → see TABLE 7 p. 1572 (hypotension)

glyceryl trinitrate · isosorbide dinitrate · isosorbide mononitrate

PHARMACOLOGY Drugs with antimuscarinic effects can cause dry mouth, which can reduce the effectiveness of sublingual glyceryl trinitrate tablets.

▶ **Acetylcysteine** might increase the vasodilatory effects of **glyceryl trinitrate**. Moderate Theoretical

▶ **Nitrates** potentially increase the risk of hypotension when given with phosphodiesterase type-5 inhibitors. Avoid. Severe Study → Also see TABLE 7 p. 1572

Nitrazepam → see benzodiazepines

Nitrofurantoin → see TABLE 11 p. 1574 (peripheral neuropathy)

▶ **Acetazolamide** might decrease the efficacy of **nitrofurantoin**. Unknown Theoretical

▶ Oral magnesium trisilicate decreases the absorption of oral **nitrofurantoin**. Moderate Study

▶ **Potassium citrate** might decrease the efficacy of **nitrofurantoin**. Unknown Theoretical

▶ **Sodium bicarbonate** might decrease the efficacy of **nitrofurantoin**. Unknown Theoretical

▶ **Sodium citrate** might decrease the efficacy of **nitrofurantoin**. Unknown Theoretical

Nitroprusside → see TABLE 7 p. 1572 (hypotension)

Nitrous oxide → see TABLE 7 p. 1572 (hypotension), TABLE 10 p. 1574 (CNS effects)

▶ **Nitrous oxide** potentially increases the risk of methotrexate toxicity when given with methotrexate. Avoid. Severe Study

Nivolumab → see monoclonal antibodies

Nizatidine → see H_2 receptor antagonists

NNRTIs → see TABLE 1 p. 1571 (hepatotoxicity), TABLE 8 p. 1573 (QT-interval prolongation)

doravirine · efavirenz · etravirine · nevirapine · rilpivirine

▶ **Efavirenz** is predicted to decrease the exposure to abrocitinib. Avoid. Moderate Theoretical

▶ **NNRTIs (efavirenz, nevirapine)** are predicted to decrease the exposure to acalabrutinib. Severe Study

▶ Oral antacids are predicted to decrease the exposure to oral **rilpivirine**. Manufacturer advises take 4 hours before or 2 hours after antacids. Severe Theoretical

▶ **Anti-androgens (apalutamide, enzalutamide)** are predicted to decrease the exposure to **doravirine**. Avoid. Severe Study

▶ **Anti-androgens (apalutamide, enzalutamide)** are predicted to decrease the exposure to **etravirine**. Avoid. Severe Theoretical

▶ **Anti-androgens (apalutamide, enzalutamide)** are predicted to decrease the exposure to **nevirapine**. Severe Study

▶ **Anti-androgens (apalutamide, enzalutamide)** markedly decrease the exposure to **rilpivirine**. Avoid. Severe Study

▶ **NNRTIs (efavirenz, nevirapine)** are predicted to decrease the efficacy of anti-androgens (cyproterone) with ethinylestradiol (co-cyprindiol). Use alternative methods during treatment with, and for 28 days after, the enzyme inducing drug is stopped. Severe Study

▶ **NNRTIs (efavirenz, etravirine, nevirapine)** are predicted to decrease the exposure to anti-androgens (darolutamide). Avoid. Moderate Theoretical

▶ **NNRTIs (efavirenz, etravirine, nevirapine)** are predicted to decrease the exposure to antiarrhythmics (dronedarone). Severe Theoretical → Also see TABLE 8 p. 1573

▶ Antiepileptics (carbamazepine) slightly decrease the exposure to **efavirenz** and **efavirenz** slightly decreases the exposure to antiepileptics (carbamazepine). Severe Study

▶ Antiepileptics (carbamazepine, fosphenytoin, phenobarbital, phenytoin, primidone) are predicted to decrease the exposure to **doravirine**. Avoid. Severe Study

▶ Antiepileptics (carbamazepine, fosphenytoin, phenobarbital, phenytoin, primidone) are predicted to decrease the exposure to **etravirine**. Avoid. Severe Theoretical

▶ Antiepileptics (carbamazepine, fosphenytoin, phenobarbital, phenytoin, primidone) markedly decrease the exposure to **rilpivirine**. Avoid. Severe Study

▶ Antiepileptics (fosphenytoin, phenytoin) slightly decrease the exposure to **efavirenz** and **efavirenz** affects the concentration of antiepileptics (fosphenytoin, phenytoin). Severe Theoretical

▶ Antiepileptics (oxcarbazepine) are predicted to decrease the exposure to **doravirine**. Avoid. Severe Theoretical

▶ Antiepileptics (oxcarbazepine) are predicted to decrease the concentration of **rilpivirine**. Avoid. Severe Theoretical

▶ Antiepileptics (phenobarbital) are predicted to decrease the exposure to **efavirenz** and **efavirenz** affects the concentration of antiepileptics (phenobarbital). Severe Theoretical

▶ **Nevirapine** is predicted to decrease the concentration of antiepileptics (carbamazepine, fosphenytoin, phenobarbital, phenytoin, primidone) and antiepileptics (carbamazepine, fosphenytoin, phenobarbital, phenytoin, primidone) are predicted to decrease the concentration of **nevirapine**. Severe Study

▶ **Efavirenz** is predicted to affect the efficacy of antiepileptics (primidone) and antiepileptics (primidone) are predicted to slightly decrease the exposure to **efavirenz**. Severe Theoretical

▶ Antifungals, azoles (fluconazole) slightly to moderately increase the exposure to **nevirapine**. Moderate Study → Also see TABLE 1 p. 1571

▶ **NNRTIs (efavirenz, etravirine, nevirapine)** are predicted to decrease the exposure to antifungals, azoles (isavuconazole). Avoid. Severe Theoretical

▶ **Efavirenz** slightly decreases the exposure to antifungals, azoles (itraconazole). Avoid and for 14 days after stopping **efavirenz**. Moderate Study

▶ **Nevirapine** moderately decreases the exposure to antifungals, azoles (itraconazole). Avoid and for 14 days after stopping **nevirapine**. Moderate Study → Also see TABLE 1 p. 1571

▶ **Efavirenz** moderately decreases the exposure to antifungals, azoles (ketoconazole). Severe Study

NNRTIs (continued)

- **Nevirapine** moderately decreases the exposure to antifungals, azoles **(ketoconazole)**. Avoid. Severe Study
- **Efavirenz** slightly decreases the exposure to antifungals, azoles **(posaconazole)**. Avoid. Moderate Study
- **Efavirenz** moderately decreases the exposure to antifungals, azoles **(voriconazole)** and antifungals, azoles **(voriconazole)** slightly increase the exposure to **efavirenz**. Adjust dose. Severe Study → Also see **TABLE 8** p. 1573
- **Nevirapine** is predicted to decrease the exposure to antifungals, azoles **(voriconazole)** and antifungals, azoles **(voriconazole)** increase the exposure to **nevirapine**. Monitor and adjust dose. Severe Theoretical → Also see **TABLE 1** p. 1571
- **Efavirenz** decreases the concentration of antimalarials **(artemether)**. Severe Study → Also see **TABLE 8** p. 1573
- **Etravirine** decreases the exposure to antimalarials **(artemether)**. Moderate Study
- **Efavirenz** moderately decreases the exposure to antimalarials **(atovaquone)**. Avoid. Moderate Study
- **Efavirenz** affects the exposure to antimalarials **(proguanil)**. Avoid. Moderate Study
- NNRTIs **(efavirenz, etravirine, nevirapine)** are predicted to decrease the exposure to antipsychotics, second generation **(cariprazine)**. Avoid. Severe Theoretical
- NNRTIs **(efavirenz, etravirine, nevirapine)** are predicted to decrease the exposure to antipsychotics, second generation **(lurasidone)**. Monitor and adjust dose. Moderate Theoretical
- NNRTIs **(efavirenz, etravirine, nevirapine)** are predicted to decrease the exposure to antipsychotics, second generation **(quetiapine)**. Moderate Study
- NNRTIs **(efavirenz, etravirine, nevirapine)** are predicted to decrease the exposure to avacopan. Severe Theoretical
- NNRTIs **(efavirenz, etravirine, nevirapine)** are predicted to decrease the exposure to avapritinib. Avoid. Severe Study
- NNRTIs **(efavirenz, nevirapine)** are predicted to decrease the exposure to axitinib. Moderate Study
- NNRTIs **(efavirenz, etravirine, nevirapine)** are predicted to decrease the exposure to bedaquiline. Avoid. Severe Study → Also see **TABLE 8** p. 1573
- NNRTIs **(efavirenz, nevirapine)** are predicted to decrease the concentration of benzodiazepines **(alprazolam)**. Moderate Theoretical
- **Etravirine** has been reported to increase the concentration of benzodiazepines **(clobazam)**. Moderate Anecdotal
- **Nevirapine** is predicted to decrease the concentration of benzodiazepines **(clonazepam)** and benzodiazepines **(clonazepam)** are predicted to decrease the concentration of **nevirapine**. Moderate Theoretical
- **Etravirine** is predicted to increase the exposure to benzodiazepines **(diazepam)**. Avoid. Severe Theoretical
- **Efavirenz** is predicted to alter the effects of benzodiazepines **(midazolam)**. Avoid. Moderate Theoretical
- **Nevirapine** decreases the concentration of benzodiazepines **(midazolam)**. Monitor and adjust dose. Moderate Study
- NNRTIs **(efavirenz, etravirine, nevirapine)** are predicted to decrease the exposure to bosutinib. Avoid. Severe Study → Also see **TABLE 8** p. 1573
- NNRTIs **(efavirenz, etravirine, nevirapine)** are predicted to decrease the exposure to brigatinib. Avoid or adjust dose—consult product literature. Moderate Study
- **Efavirenz** is predicted to decrease the exposure to bupropion. Moderate Study
- NNRTIs **(efavirenz, etravirine, nevirapine)** are predicted to decrease the exposure to cabozantinib. Moderate Study → Also see **TABLE 8** p. 1573
- NNRTIs **(efavirenz, etravirine, nevirapine)** are predicted to decrease the exposure to calcium channel blockers **(amlodipine, felodipine, lacidipine, lercanidipine, nicardipine, nifedipine, nimodipine)**. Monitor and adjust dose. Moderate Theoretical
- NNRTIs **(efavirenz, etravirine, nevirapine)** are predicted to decrease the exposure to calcium channel blockers **(diltiazem, verapamil)**. Moderate Theoretical
- Oral calcium salts **(calcium carbonate)** -containing antacids are predicted to decrease the exposure to oral **rilpivirine**.

Manufacturer advises take 4 hours before or 2 hours after antacids. Severe Theoretical

- NNRTIs **(efavirenz, etravirine, nevirapine)** are predicted to decrease the exposure to capivasertib. Avoid. Moderate Study
- **Efavirenz** is predicted to decrease the concentration of caspofungin. Adjust dose. Moderate Study
- **Nevirapine** is predicted to decrease the concentration of caspofungin. Adjust dose. Moderate Theoretical → Also see **TABLE 1** p. 1571
- Cenobamate is predicted to decrease the exposure to rilpivirine. Avoid. Severe Theoretical
- **Etravirine** is predicted to decrease the exposure to ceritinib. Severe Theoretical
- NNRTIs **(efavirenz, nevirapine)** are predicted to decrease the exposure to ceritinib. Severe Study → Also see **TABLE 8** p. 1573
- **Efavirenz** decreases the concentration of ciclosporin. Monitor concentration and adjust dose. Moderate Study
- **Etravirine** is predicted to decrease the exposure to ciclosporin. Moderate Theoretical
- **Nevirapine** is predicted to decrease the concentration of ciclosporin. Moderate Study
- NNRTIs **(efavirenz, etravirine, nevirapine)** are predicted to decrease the exposure to cobicistat. Avoid. Severe Theoretical
- NNRTIs **(efavirenz, etravirine, nevirapine)** are predicted to decrease the exposure to cobimetinib. Avoid. Severe Theoretical
- **Etravirine** might decrease the efficacy of combined hormonal contraceptives. Follow FSRH guidance for enzyme inducers, see Contraceptives, interactions p. 917. Severe Theoretical
- NNRTIs **(efavirenz, nevirapine)** are predicted to decrease the efficacy of combined hormonal contraceptives. For FSRH guidance, see Contraceptives, interactions p. 917. Severe Study
- Corticosteroids **(dexamethasone)** are predicted to decrease the concentration of **rilpivirine**. Avoid multiple-dose dexamethasone. Severe Theoretical
- **Efavirenz** is predicted to affect the concentration of coumarins. Adjust dose. Moderate Theoretical
- **Etravirine** increases the anticoagulant effect of coumarins. Moderate Theoretical
- **Nevirapine** potentially alters the anticoagulant effect of coumarins. Severe Anecdotal
- NNRTIs **(efavirenz, etravirine, nevirapine)** are predicted to decrease the exposure to crizotinib. Avoid. Severe Study → Also see **TABLE 8** p. 1573
- Dabrafenib is predicted to decrease the exposure to **doravirine**. Avoid or adjust doravirine p. 741 or lamivudine with tenofovir disoproxil and doravirine p. 751 dose. Severe Theoretical
- NNRTIs **(efavirenz, nevirapine)** are predicted to decrease the exposure to dabrafenib. Moderate Study
- Dabrafenib is predicted to decrease the exposure to **rilpivirine**. Avoid. Severe Theoretical
- NNRTIs **(efavirenz, etravirine, nevirapine)** are predicted to decrease the exposure to daridorexant. Severe Study
- NNRTIs **(efavirenz, etravirine, nevirapine)** are predicted to decrease the exposure to dasatinib. Severe Study → Also see **TABLE 8** p. 1573
- **Etravirine** might decrease the efficacy of desogestrel. Follow FSRH guidance for enzyme inducers, see Contraceptives, interactions p. 917. Severe Theoretical
- NNRTIs **(efavirenz, nevirapine)** are predicted to decrease the efficacy of desogestrel. For FSRH guidance, see Contraceptives, interactions p. 917. Severe Theoretical
- **Efavirenz** moderately decreases the exposure to dolutegravir. Adjust **dolutegravir** dose, p. 739. Severe Study
- **Etravirine** moderately decreases the exposure to dolutegravir. Adjust **dolutegravir** dose unless given with atazanavir, darunavir, or lopinavir (all boosted with ritonavir), p. 739. Severe Study
- **Nevirapine** is predicted to decrease the exposure to dolutegravir. Adjust **dolutegravir** dose, p. 739. Severe Study
- **Etravirine** might decreases the efficacy of drospirenone. Follow FSRH guidance for enzyme inducers, see Contraceptives, interactions p. 917. Severe Theoretical
- NNRTIs **(efavirenz, nevirapine)** are predicted to decrease the efficacy of drospirenone. For FSRH guidance, see Contraceptives, interactions p. 917. Severe Theoretical

‣ **NNRTIs (efavirenz, etravirine, nevirapine)** are predicted to decrease the exposure to elacestrant. Avoid or adjust dose depending on duration—consult product literature. Severe Theoretical

‣ **NNRTIs (efavirenz, etravirine, nevirapine)** are predicted to moderately decrease the exposure to elbasvir. Avoid. Severe Study

‣ **NNRTIs (efavirenz, etravirine, nevirapine)** are predicted to decrease the exposure to eliglustat. Moderate Theoretical

‣ **NNRTIs (efavirenz, etravirine, nevirapine)** are predicted to decrease the concentration of elvitegravir. Avoid. Severe Theoretical

‣ Encorafenib is predicted to decrease the exposure to **doravirine**. Avoid. Severe Study

‣ Encorafenib is predicted to decrease the exposure to **etravirine**. Avoid. Severe Theoretical

‣ **NNRTIs (efavirenz, etravirine, nevirapine)** are predicted to decrease the exposure to encorafenib. Moderate Study → Also see **TABLE 8** p. 1573

‣ Encorafenib markedly decreases the exposure to **rilpivirine**. Avoid. Severe Study

‣ Endothelin receptor antagonists (bosentan) are predicted to decrease the exposure to **doravirine**. Avoid or adjust doravirine p. 741 or lamivudine with tenofovir disoproxil and doravirine p. 751 dose. Severe Theoretical

‣ Endothelin receptor antagonists (bosentan) are predicted to decrease the exposure to **nevirapine**. Severe Theoretical

‣ Endothelin receptor antagonists (bosentan) are predicted to decrease the exposure to **rilpivirine**. Avoid. Severe Theoretical

‣ **NNRTIs (efavirenz, etravirine, nevirapine)** are predicted to decrease the exposure to entrectinib. Avoid. Moderate Theoretical → Also see **TABLE 8** p. 1573

‣ **NNRTIs (efavirenz, etravirine, nevirapine)** are predicted to decrease the exposure to erdafitinib. Adjust dose. Moderate Theoretical

‣ **NNRTIs (efavirenz, etravirine, nevirapine)** are predicted to decrease the exposure to erlotinib. Severe Study

‣ **NNRTIs (efavirenz, nevirapine)** are predicted to decrease the efficacy of estradiol. Moderate Theoretical

‣ **Etravirine** might decrease the efficacy of etonogestrel. Follow FSRH guidance for enzyme inducers, see Contraceptives, interactions p. 917. Severe Theoretical

‣ **NNRTIs (efavirenz, nevirapine)** are predicted to decrease the efficacy of etonogestrel. For FSRH guidance, see Contraceptives, interactions p. 917. Severe Theoretical

‣ **NNRTIs (efavirenz, etravirine, nevirapine)** are predicted to decrease the concentration of everolimus. Avoid or adjust dose. Severe Study

‣ **Nevirapine** is predicted to decrease the exposure to factor XA inhibitors (rivaroxaban). Severe Anecdotal

‣ **NNRTIs (efavirenz, etravirine, nevirapine)** are predicted to decrease the exposure to fedratinib. Avoid. Moderate Study

‣ **NNRTIs (efavirenz, etravirine, nevirapine)** are predicted to decrease the exposure to fruquintinib. Avoid. Moderate Study

‣ **NNRTIs (efavirenz, etravirine, nevirapine)** are predicted to decrease the exposure to gefitinib. Avoid. Severe Study

‣ **NNRTIs (efavirenz, etravirine, nevirapine)** are predicted to decrease the exposure to glasdegib. Avoid or adjust dose—consult product literature. Moderate Theoretical → Also see **TABLE 8** p. 1573

‣ **NNRTIs (efavirenz, etravirine, nevirapine)** are predicted to decrease the exposure to glecaprevir. Avoid. Severe Study

‣ **NNRTIs (efavirenz, etravirine, nevirapine)** are predicted to markedly decrease the exposure to grazoprevir. Avoid. Severe Study

‣ **NNRTIs (efavirenz, etravirine, nevirapine)** are predicted to decrease the concentration of guanfacine. Adjust dose. Moderate Theoretical

‣ H$_2$ receptor antagonists are predicted to decrease the exposure to **rilpivirine**. H$_2$ receptor antagonists should be taken 12 hours before or 4 hours after **rilpivirine**. Severe Study

‣ **Efavirenz** decreases the exposure to HIV-protease inhibitors. Refer to specialist literature. Severe Study

‣ **Etravirine** increases the exposure to HIV-protease inhibitors (fosamprenavir) boosted with ritonavir. Refer to specialist literature. Moderate Study

‣ **Nevirapine** decreases the exposure to HIV-protease inhibitors. Refer to specialist literature. Moderate Study → Also see **TABLE 1** p. 1571

‣ **NNRTIs (efavirenz, nevirapine)** are predicted to decrease the effects of hormone replacement therapy. Moderate Anecdotal

‣ **NNRTIs (efavirenz, etravirine, nevirapine)** are predicted to decrease the exposure to ibrutinib. Avoid or monitor. Severe Study

‣ **NNRTIs (efavirenz, etravirine, nevirapine)** are predicted to decrease the exposure to idelalisib. Avoid. Moderate Theoretical

‣ **NNRTIs (efavirenz, etravirine, nevirapine)** are predicted to decrease the exposure to imatinib. Moderate Study

‣ **NNRTIs (efavirenz, nevirapine)** are predicted to decrease the exposure to ivacaftor. Moderate Study

‣ Ivosidenib is predicted to decrease the exposure to **doravirine**. Avoid. Severe Study

‣ Ivosidenib is predicted to decrease the exposure to **etravirine**. Avoid. Severe Theoretical

‣ Ivosidenib markedly decreases the exposure to **rilpivirine**. Avoid. Severe Study

‣ **NNRTIs (efavirenz, etravirine, nevirapine)** are predicted to decrease the exposure to ixazomib. Moderate Theoretical

‣ **NNRTIs (efavirenz, etravirine, nevirapine)** are predicted to decrease the exposure to lapatinib. Avoid. Severe Study → Also see **TABLE 8** p. 1573

‣ **NNRTIs (efavirenz, etravirine, nevirapine)** are predicted to decrease the exposure to larotrectinib. Avoid. Moderate Study

‣ **NNRTIs (efavirenz, etravirine, nevirapine)** are predicted to decrease the exposure to leniolisib. Avoid. Severe Theoretical

‣ **Efavirenz** is predicted to decrease the concentration of letermovir. Moderate Theoretical

‣ **Etravirine** is predicted to decrease the exposure to letermovir. Moderate Theoretical

‣ **Etravirine** might decrease the efficacy of some contraceptive methods containing levonorgestrel. Follow FSRH guidance for enzyme inducers, see Contraceptives, interactions p. 917. Severe Theoretical

‣ **NNRTIs (efavirenz, nevirapine)** are predicted to decrease the efficacy of some contraceptive methods containing levonorgestrel. For FSRH guidance, see Contraceptives, interactions p. 917. Severe Theoretical

‣ Lorlatinib is predicted to decrease the exposure to **rilpivirine**. Avoid. Severe Theoretical

‣ Lumacaftor is predicted to decrease the exposure to **doravirine**. Avoid. Severe Study

‣ Lumacaftor is predicted to decrease the exposure to **etravirine**. Avoid. Severe Theoretical

‣ Lumacaftor markedly decreases the exposure to **rilpivirine**. Avoid. Severe Study

‣ Macrolides (erythromycin) are predicted to increase the exposure to **nevirapine**. Moderate Theoretical

‣ **Etravirine** decreases the exposure to macrolides (clarithromycin) and macrolides (clarithromycin) slightly increase the exposure to **etravirine**. Severe Study

‣ **NNRTIs (efavirenz, nevirapine)** decrease the exposure to macrolides (clarithromycin). Moderate Study

‣ **Efavirenz** decreases the exposure to maraviroc. Refer to specialist literature. Severe Theoretical

‣ **Etravirine** slightly decreases the exposure to maraviroc. Refer to specialist literature. Moderate Study

‣ **Etravirine** is predicted to decrease the exposure to maribavir. Avoid or adjust **maribavir** dose, p. 735. Severe Theoretical

‣ **NNRTIs (efavirenz, nevirapine)** are predicted to decrease the exposure to maribavir. Avoid or adjust **maribavir** dose, p. 735. Severe Study

‣ **NNRTIs (efavirenz, etravirine, nevirapine)** are predicted to decrease the exposure to mavacamten. Monitor and adjust dose—consult product literature. Severe Theoretical

‣ **NNRTIs (efavirenz, etravirine, nevirapine)** are predicted to decrease the exposure to midostaurin. Severe Study

NNRTIs (continued)

▸ NNRTIs **(efavirenz, etravirine, nevirapine)** are predicted to decrease the exposure to **mifepristone**. Adjust **mifepristone** dose, p. 954. [Severe] Study

▸ NNRTIs **(efavirenz, etravirine, nevirapine)** are predicted to decrease the exposure to **mineralocorticoid receptor antagonists (finerenone)**. Avoid. [Severe] Study

▸ **Mitotane** is predicted to decrease the exposure to **doravirine**. Avoid. [Severe] Study

▸ **Mitotane** is predicted to decrease the exposure to **etravirine**. Avoid. [Severe] Theoretical

▸ **Mitotane** is predicted to decrease the exposure to **nevirapine**. [Severe] Theoretical

▸ **Mitotane** markedly decreases the exposure to **rilpivirine**. Avoid. [Severe] Study

▸ NNRTIs **(efavirenz, etravirine, nevirapine)** are predicted to decrease the exposure to **mobocertinib**. Avoid. [Severe] Study → Also see **TABLE 8** p. 1573

▸ **Modafinil** is predicted to decrease the exposure to **doravirine**. Avoid or adjust doravirine p. 741 or lamivudine with tenofovir disoproxil and doravirine p. 751 dose. [Severe] Theoretical

▸ NNRTIs **(efavirenz, etravirine, nevirapine)** are predicted to decrease the exposure to **naloxegol**. [Moderate] Theoretical

▸ NNRTIs **(efavirenz, etravirine, nevirapine)** are predicted to decrease the exposure to **neratinib**. Avoid. [Severe] Theoretical → Also see **TABLE 1** p. 1571

▸ NNRTIs **(efavirenz, etravirine, nevirapine)** are predicted to decrease the exposure to **neurokinin-1 receptor antagonists (aprepitant)**. [Moderate] Study

▸ NNRTIs **(efavirenz, nevirapine)** are predicted to decrease the exposure to **neurokinin-1 receptor antagonists (fosaprepitant, netupitant)**. [Moderate] Theoretical

▸ **Etravirine** is predicted to decrease the exposure to **neurokinin-1 receptor antagonists (netupitant)**. [Moderate] Theoretical

▸ NNRTIs **(efavirenz, etravirine, nevirapine)** are predicted to decrease the exposure to **nilotinib**. Avoid. [Severe] Theoretical → Also see **TABLE 8** p. 1573

▸ **Nirmatrelvir** boosted with ritonavir is predicted to increase the concentration of NNRTIs **(efavirenz, nevirapine)**. [Moderate] Theoretical

▸ NNRTIs **(efavirenz, nevirapine)** are predicted to decrease the exposure to NNRTIs **(doravirine)**. Avoid or adjust doravirine p. 741 or lamivudine with tenofovir disoproxil and doravirine p. 751 dose. [Severe] Theoretical

▸ NNRTIs **(etravirine)** are predicted to decrease the exposure to NNRTIs **(doravirine)**. Avoid. [Severe] Theoretical

▸ NNRTIs **(nevirapine)** decrease the concentration of NNRTIs **(efavirenz)**. Avoid. [Severe] Study

▸ NNRTIs **(efavirenz, etravirine, nevirapine)** are predicted to decrease the exposure to NNRTIs **(rilpivirine)**. Avoid. [Severe] Theoretical

▸ **Etravirine** might decrease the efficacy of some contraceptive methods containing **norethisterone**. Follow FSRH guidance for enzyme inducers, see Contraceptives, interactions p. 917. [Severe] Theoretical

▸ NNRTIs **(efavirenz, nevirapine)** are predicted to decrease the efficacy of some contraceptive methods containing **norethisterone**. For FSRH guidance, see Contraceptives, interactions p. 917. [Severe] Anecdotal

▸ **Nevirapine** is predicted to slightly decrease the exposure to NRTIs **(zidovudine)**. Refer to specialist literature. [Severe] Theoretical → Also see **TABLE 1** p. 1571

▸ NNRTIs **(efavirenz, etravirine, nevirapine)** are predicted to decrease the exposure to **olaparib**. Avoid. [Moderate] Theoretical

▸ **Efavirenz** moderately decreases the exposure to **opioids (buprenorphine)**. Adjust dose. [Moderate] Study

▸ NNRTIs **(efavirenz, etravirine, nevirapine)** decrease the exposure to **opioids (methadone)**. Monitor and adjust dose. [Severe] Study → Also see **TABLE 8** p. 1573

▸ **Etravirine** is predicted to decrease the exposure to **osimertinib**. Use with caution or avoid. [Severe] Theoretical

▸ NNRTIs **(efavirenz, nevirapine)** are predicted to decrease the exposure to **osimertinib**. Use with caution or avoid. [Severe] Study → Also see **TABLE 8** p. 1573

▸ NNRTIs **(efavirenz, etravirine, nevirapine)** are predicted to decrease the exposure to **ospemifene**. [Moderate] Study

▸ NNRTIs **(efavirenz, etravirine, nevirapine)** are predicted to decrease the exposure to **pazopanib**. [Severe] Study → Also see **TABLE 8** p. 1573

▸ **Efavirenz** is predicted to decrease the exposure to **pemigatinib** and **pemigatinib** might decrease the exposure to **efavirenz**. Avoid or monitor. [Severe] Study

▸ NNRTIs **(etravirine, nevirapine)** are predicted to decrease the exposure to **pemigatinib**. Avoid or monitor. [Severe] Study

▸ **Etravirine** moderately decreases the exposure to **phosphodiesterase type-5 inhibitors**. Adjust dose. [Moderate] Study

▸ NNRTIs **(efavirenz, nevirapine)** are predicted to decrease the exposure to **phosphodiesterase type-5 inhibitors**. [Moderate] Theoretical → Also see **TABLE 8** p. 1573

▸ NNRTIs **(efavirenz, etravirine, nevirapine)** are predicted to decrease the exposure to **pibrentasvir**. Avoid. [Severe] Study

▸ **Pitolisant** is predicted to decrease the exposure to **efavirenz**. [Mild] Theoretical

▸ NNRTIs **(efavirenz, etravirine, nevirapine)** are predicted to decrease the exposure to **ponatinib**. [Severe] Study

▸ NNRTIs **(efavirenz, nevirapine)** are predicted to decrease the exposure to **pralsetinib**. [Moderate] Theoretical

▸ **Proton pump inhibitors** are predicted to decrease the exposure to oral **rilpivirine**. Avoid. [Severe] Study

▸ NNRTIs **(efavirenz, etravirine, nevirapine)** are predicted to decrease the exposure to **quizartinib**. Avoid. [Severe] Study → Also see **TABLE 8** p. 1573

▸ NNRTIs **(efavirenz, etravirine, nevirapine)** are predicted to decrease the exposure to **regorafenib**. [Severe] Study

▸ **Efavirenz** is predicted to decrease the exposure to **relugolix**. Avoid or adjust dose depending on indication—consult product literature. [Moderate] Study

▸ NNRTIs **(efavirenz, etravirine, nevirapine)** are predicted to decrease the exposure to **ribociclib**. [Moderate] Study → Also see **TABLE 8** p. 1573

▸ **Rifamycins (rifabutin)** moderately decrease the exposure to **doravirine**. Adjust doravirine p. 741 or lamivudine with tenofovir disoproxil and doravirine p. 751 dose. [Moderate] Study

▸ **Rifamycins (rifabutin)** decrease the exposure to **etravirine**. [Moderate] Study

▸ **Rifamycins (rifabutin)** modestly decrease the exposure to **rilpivirine**. Avoid or adjust dose—consult product literature. [Severe] Study

▸ **Rifamycins (rifampicin)** are predicted to decrease the exposure to **doravirine**. Avoid. [Severe] Study

▸ **Rifamycins (rifampicin)** slightly decrease the exposure to **efavirenz**. Adjust dose. [Severe] Study

▸ **Rifamycins (rifampicin)** are predicted to decrease the exposure to **etravirine**. Avoid. [Severe] Theoretical

▸ **Rifamycins (rifampicin)** decrease the concentration of **nevirapine**. Avoid. [Severe] Study

▸ **Rifamycins (rifampicin)** markedly decrease the exposure to **rilpivirine**. Avoid. [Severe] Study

▸ **Efavirenz** slightly decreases the exposure to rifamycins **(rifabutin)**. Adjust dose. [Severe] Study

▸ NNRTIs **(efavirenz, etravirine, nevirapine)** are predicted to decrease the exposure to **rimegepant**. Avoid. [Moderate] Theoretical

▸ NNRTIs **(efavirenz, etravirine, nevirapine)** are predicted to decrease the exposure to **ripretinib**. Avoid or adjust dose—consult product literature. [Moderate] Theoretical

▸ NNRTIs **(efavirenz, etravirine, nevirapine)** are predicted to decrease the exposure to **ruxolitinib**. Monitor and adjust dose. [Moderate] Study

▸ NNRTIs **(efavirenz, etravirine, nevirapine)** are predicted to decrease the exposure to **selpercatinib**. [Moderate] Study → Also see **TABLE 8** p. 1573

▸ NNRTIs **(efavirenz, etravirine, nevirapine)** are predicted to decrease the exposure to **selumetinib**. Avoid. [Severe] Study

▸ NNRTIs **(efavirenz, etravirine, nevirapine)** are predicted to decrease the exposure to **siponimod**. Manufacturer advises caution depending on genotype—consult product literature. [Moderate] Theoretical

▶ **Doravirine** is predicted to decrease the exposure to sirolimus. Monitor **sirolimus** concentration and adjust dose, p. 968. Moderate Theoretical

▶ **Etravirine** is predicted to decrease the exposure to sirolimus. Monitor and adjust dose. Moderate Study

▶ NNRTIs **(efavirenz, nevirapine)** are predicted to decrease the concentration of sirolimus. Monitor and adjust dose. Moderate Theoretical

▶ Oral sodium bicarbonate -containing antacids are predicted to decrease the exposure to oral **rilpivirine**. Manufacturer advises take 4 hours before or 2 hours after antacids. Severe Theoretical

▶ **Efavirenz** is predicted to decrease the exposure to sodium glucose co-transporter 2 inhibitors (canagliflozin). Adjust **canagliflozin** dose, p. 824. Moderate Study

▶ **Sodium zirconium cyclosilicate** is predicted to decrease the exposure to rilpivirine. Separate administration by at least 2 hours. Moderate Theoretical

▶ NNRTIs **(efavirenz, etravirine, nevirapine)** are predicted to decrease the exposure to sorafenib. Moderate Study → Also see **TABLE 8** p. 1573

▶ **Sotorasib** is predicted to decrease the exposure to rilpivirine. Avoid. Severe Theoretical

▶ **St John's wort** is predicted to decrease the exposure to NNRTIs (doravirine, rilpivirine). Avoid. Severe Theoretical

▶ **St John's wort** is predicted to decrease the concentration of NNRTIs (efavirenz, nevirapine). Avoid. Severe Theoretical

▶ NNRTIs **(efavirenz, etravirine, nevirapine)** are predicted to decrease the exposure to statins (atorvastatin, simvastatin). Moderate Study → Also see **TABLE 1** p. 1571

▶ **Etravirine** is predicted to increase the exposure to statins (fluvastatin). Adjust dose. Severe Theoretical

▶ NNRTIs **(efavirenz, etravirine, nevirapine)** are predicted to decrease the exposure to sunitinib. Moderate Study → Also see **TABLE 8** p. 1573

▶ **Doravirine** is predicted to decrease the exposure to tacrolimus. Monitor **tacrolimus** concentration and adjust dose, p. 969. Moderate Theoretical

▶ **Etravirine** is predicted to decrease the exposure to tacrolimus. Monitor and adjust dose. Moderate Theoretical

▶ NNRTIs **(efavirenz, nevirapine)** are predicted to decrease the concentration of tacrolimus. Monitor and adjust dose. Moderate Theoretical

▶ NNRTIs **(efavirenz, etravirine, nevirapine)** are predicted to decrease the exposure to taxanes (cabazitaxel). Moderate Theoretical

▶ NNRTIs **(efavirenz, etravirine, nevirapine)** are predicted to decrease the exposure to taxanes (docetaxel). Severe Theoretical

▶ NNRTIs **(efavirenz, etravirine, nevirapine)** are predicted to decrease the exposure to taxanes (paclitaxel). Avoid. Severe Study

▶ **Telotristat ethyl** is predicted to decrease the exposure to **doravirine**. Avoid or adjust doravirine p. 741 or lamivudine with tenofovir disoproxil and doravirine p. 751 dose. Severe Theoretical

▶ NNRTIs **(efavirenz, etravirine, nevirapine)** are predicted to decrease the concentration of temsirolimus. Avoid. Moderate Theoretical

▶ NNRTIs **(efavirenz, etravirine, nevirapine)** are predicted to decrease the exposure to ticagrelor. Moderate Theoretical

▶ NNRTIs **(efavirenz, etravirine, nevirapine)** are predicted to decrease the exposure to tofacitinib. Severe Study

▶ **Etravirine** might decrease the efficacy of ulipristal. Avoid and for 4 weeks after stopping the enzyme inducing drug. For FSRH guidance, see Contraceptives, interactions p. 917. Severe Theoretical

▶ NNRTIs **(efavirenz, nevirapine)** decrease the efficacy of ulipristal. Avoid and for 4 weeks after stopping the enzyme inducing drug. For FSRH guidance, see Contraceptives, interactions p. 917. Severe Anecdotal

▶ NNRTIs **(efavirenz, etravirine, nevirapine)** are predicted to decrease the exposure to vandetanib. Moderate Study → Also see **TABLE 8** p. 1573

▶ NNRTIs **(efavirenz, etravirine, nevirapine)** are predicted to decrease the exposure to velpatasvir. Avoid. Moderate Theoretical

▶ NNRTIs **(efavirenz, etravirine, nevirapine)** are predicted to decrease the exposure to vemurafenib. Severe Study → Also see **TABLE 8** p. 1573

▶ NNRTIs **(efavirenz, etravirine, nevirapine)** are predicted to decrease the exposure to venetoclax. Avoid. Severe Study

▶ NNRTIs **(efavirenz, etravirine, nevirapine)** are predicted to decrease the exposure to voclosporin. Avoid. Severe Theoretical → Also see **TABLE 8** p. 1573

▶ NNRTIs **(efavirenz, etravirine, nevirapine)** are predicted to decrease the concentration of voxilaprevir. Avoid. Severe Theoretical

▶ NNRTIs **(efavirenz, etravirine, nevirapine)** are predicted to decrease the exposure to zanubrutinib. Avoid or adjust dose with moderate CYP3A4 inducers—consult product literature. Severe Theoretical

Noradrenaline/norepinephrine → see sympathomimetics, vasoconstrictor

Norethisterone

▶ Antiepileptics (carbamazepine, eslicarbazepine, fosphenytoin, oxcarbazepine, perampanel, phenobarbital, phenytoin, primidone, rufinamide, topiramate) are predicted to decrease the efficacy of some contraceptive methods containing **norethisterone**. For FSRH guidance, see Contraceptives, interactions p. 917. Severe Anecdotal

▶ Antiepileptics (lamotrigine) might decrease the effects of **norethisterone**. For FSRH guidance, see Contraceptives, interactions p. 917. Moderate Theoretical

▶ Endothelin receptor antagonists (bosentan) are predicted to decrease the efficacy of some contraceptive methods containing **norethisterone**. For FSRH guidance, see Contraceptives, interactions p. 917. Severe Anecdotal

▶ Glucagon-like peptide-1 receptor agonists (tirzepatide) might affect the absorption of oral **norethisterone**. Manufacturer advises precautions for those who are overweight or obese— see Conception and contraception p. 822. Moderate Study

▶ HIV-protease inhibitors (ritonavir) are predicted to decrease the efficacy of some contraceptive methods containing **norethisterone**. For FSRH guidance, see Contraceptives, interactions p. 917. Severe Anecdotal

▶ Lumacaftor might decrease the efficacy of **norethisterone**. Use additional contraceptive precautions. Severe Theoretical

▶ Modafinil is predicted to decrease the efficacy of some contraceptive methods containing **norethisterone**. For FSRH guidance, see Contraceptives, interactions p. 917. Severe Anecdotal

▶ Neurokinin-1 receptor antagonists (aprepitant, fosaprepitant) are predicted to decrease the efficacy of some contraceptive methods containing **norethisterone**. For FSRH guidance, see Contraceptives, interactions p. 917. Severe Anecdotal

▶ NNRTIs (efavirenz, nevirapine) are predicted to decrease the efficacy of some contraceptive methods containing **norethisterone**. For FSRH guidance, see Contraceptives, interactions p. 917. Severe Anecdotal

▶ NNRTIs (etravirine) might decrease the efficacy of some contraceptive methods containing **norethisterone**. Follow FSRH guidance for enzyme inducers, see Contraceptives, interactions p. 917. Severe Theoretical

▶ Rifamycins are predicted to decrease the efficacy of some contraceptive methods containing **norethisterone**. For FSRH guidance, see Contraceptives, interactions p. 917. Severe Anecdotal

▶ St John's wort is predicted to decrease the efficacy of **norethisterone**. MHRA advises avoid. For FSRH guidance, see Contraceptives, interactions p. 917. Severe Anecdotal

▶ Sugammadex is predicted to decrease the exposure to **norethisterone**. Use additional contraceptive precautions. Severe Theoretical

▶ **Norethisterone** might decrease the efficacy of ulipristal and ulipristal might decrease the efficacy of **norethisterone**. Avoid or use additional contraceptive precautions. Severe Theoretical

Normal immunoglobulin → see immunoglobulins

Nortriptyline → see tricyclic antidepressants

NRTIs → see **TABLE 1** p. 1571 (hepatotoxicity), **TABLE 11** p. 1574 (peripheral neuropathy)

abacavir · emtricitabine · lamivudine · zidovudine

- Antiepileptics **(carbamazepine, fosphenytoin, phenobarbital, phenytoin, primidone)** are predicted to decrease the exposure to **abacavir**. Moderate Theoretical
- Antiepileptics **(valproate)** slightly increase the exposure to **zidovudine**. Moderate Study → Also see TABLE 1 p. 1571
- Antifungals, azoles **(fluconazole)** slightly increase the exposure to **zidovudine**. Moderate Study → Also see TABLE 1 p. 1571
- Antimalarials **(pyrimethamine)** are predicted to increase the risk of adverse effects when given with **zidovudine**. Severe Theoretical
- **Zidovudine** increases the risk of haematological toxicity when given with **aspirin** (high-dose). Severe Study
- **Zidovudine** increases the risk of haematological toxicity when given with **flucytosine**. Monitor and adjust dose. Severe Theoretical
- **Leflunomide** is predicted to increase the exposure to **zidovudine**. Moderate Theoretical
- Macrolides **(clarithromycin)** decrease the absorption of **zidovudine**. Separate administration by 4 hours. Moderate Study
- NNRTIs **(nevirapine)** are predicted to slightly decrease the exposure to **zidovudine**. Refer to specialist literature. Severe Theoretical → Also see TABLE 1 p. 1571
- NRTIs **(zidovudine)** increase the risk of toxicity when given with NRTIs **(lamivudine)**. Severe Anecdotal
- **Zidovudine** increases the risk of haematological toxicity when given with **NSAIDs**. Severe Study
- Ribavirin increases the risk of anaemia and/or leucopenia when given with **zidovudine**. Avoid. Severe Study
- **Abacavir** might increase the exposure to riociguat. Adjust dose and monitor blood pressure. Moderate Study
- **Teriflunomide** is predicted to increase the exposure to **zidovudine**. Moderate Theoretical
- **Trimethoprim** slightly increases the exposure to **lamivudine**. Moderate Study
- **Vadadustat** is predicted to increase the exposure to **zidovudine**. Monitor and adjust dose. Moderate Study

NSAIDs → see TABLE 17 p. 1576 (hyponatraemia), TABLE 2 p. 1571 (nephrotoxicity), TABLE 15 p. 1575 (increased serum potassium), TABLE 4 p. 1571 (antiplatelet effects)

aceclofenac · benzydamine · bromfenac · celecoxib · dexketoprofen · diclofenac · etodolac · etoricoxib · felbinac · flurbiprofen · ibuprofen · indometacin · ketoprofen · ketorolac · mefenamic acid · meloxicam · nabumetone · naproxen · nepafenac · parecoxib · phenazone · piroxicam · sulindac · tenoxicam · tiaprofenic acid · tolfenamic acid

ROUTE-SPECIFIC INFORMATION Since systemic absorption can follow topical application of **NSAIDs**, the possibility of interactions should be borne in mind.

- **Celecoxib** is predicted to increase the exposure to antiarrhythmics **(flecainide, propafenone)**. Monitor and adjust dose. Moderate Theoretical
- Antifungals, azoles **(fluconazole)** moderately increase the exposure to **celecoxib**. Adjust **celecoxib** dose, p. 1295. Moderate Study
- Antifungals, azoles **(fluconazole)** increase the exposure to **parecoxib**. Monitor and adjust dose. Moderate Study
- Antifungals, azoles **(voriconazole)** slightly increase the exposure to **diclofenac**. Monitor and adjust dose. Moderate Study
- Antifungals, azoles **(voriconazole)** moderately increase the exposure to **ibuprofen**. Adjust dose. Moderate Study
- **NSAIDs** are predicted to increase the risk of gastrointestinal irritation when given with bisphosphonates **(alendronate, ibandronate)**. Moderate Study
- **NSAIDs** are predicted to increase the risk of renal impairment when given with bisphosphonates **(clodronate)**. Moderate Study
- **Ceritinib** is predicted to increase the exposure to NSAIDs **(celecoxib, diclofenac)**. Adjust dose. Moderate Theoretical
- **Ciclosporin** increases the concentration of **diclofenac**. Severe Study → Also see TABLE 2 p. 1571 → Also see TABLE 15 p. 1575
- **Sulindac** might increases the exposure to cladribine. Avoid or adjust dose. Moderate Theoretical
- **Etoricoxib** increases the exposure to combined hormonal contraceptives. Moderate Study

- **NSAIDs** increase the risk of gastrointestinal bleeding when given with corticosteroids. Severe Study
- **NSAIDs** increase the risk of renal impairment when given with daptomycin. Moderate Theoretical
- **Indometacin** increases the concentration of digoxin. Severe Study
- **Erlotinib** is predicted to increase the risk of gastrointestinal perforation when given with **NSAIDs**. Severe Theoretical
- **Etoricoxib** increases the exposure to hormone replacement therapy. Moderate Study
- **NSAIDs** are predicted to increase the risk of gastrointestinal bleeding when given with iron chelators **(deferasirox)**. Severe Theoretical → Also see TABLE 2 p. 1571
- **Diclofenac** is predicted to increase the exposure to iron chelators **(deferiprone)**. Moderate Theoretical
- **Leflunomide** is predicted to increase the exposure to NSAIDs **(indometacin, ketoprofen)**. Moderate Theoretical
- **NSAIDs** increase the concentration of lithium. Monitor and adjust dose. Severe Study → Also see TABLE 2 p. 1571
- **NSAIDs** are predicted to increase the risk of toxicity when given with methotrexate (particularly high-dose). Severe Study → Also see TABLE 2 p. 1571
- **NSAIDs** (high-dose) are predicted to decrease the efficacy of mifamurtide. Avoid. Severe Theoretical
- **Nicorandil** is predicted to increase the risk of gastrointestinal perforation when given with **NSAIDs**. Severe Theoretical
- **Nitisinone** is predicted to increase the exposure to celecoxib. Moderate Study
- NRTIs **(zidovudine)** increase the risk of haematological toxicity when given with **NSAIDs**. Severe Study
- **NSAIDs** are predicted to increase the exposure to pemetrexed. Use with caution or avoid. Severe Theoretical → Also see TABLE 2 p. 1571
- **NSAIDs** potentially increase the risk of seizures when given with quinolones. Severe Theoretical
- **Mefenamic acid** is predicted to increase the exposure to regorafenib. Avoid. Moderate Theoretical → Also see TABLE 4 p. 1571
- Rifamycins **(rifampicin)** moderately decrease the exposure to NSAIDs **(celecoxib, diclofenac, etoricoxib)**. Moderate Study → Also see TABLE 2 p. 1571
- **Teriflunomide** is predicted to increase the exposure to NSAIDs **(indometacin, ketoprofen)**. Moderate Theoretical
- **NSAIDs** increase the risk of acute renal failure when given with thiazide diuretics. Severe Theoretical → Also see TABLE 17 p. 1576
- **Indometacin** might prolong the antidiuretic effect of vasopressin. Moderate Study

Obeticholic acid
- **Obeticholic acid** decreases the anticoagulant effect of coumarins **(warfarin)**. Severe Study
- **Obeticholic acid** is predicted to increase the exposure to theophylline. Severe Theoretical
- **Obeticholic acid** is predicted to increase the exposure to tizanidine. Severe Theoretical

Obinutuzumab → see monoclonal antibodies
Ocrelizumab → see monoclonal antibodies
Octreotide
- **Octreotide** decreases the absorption of oral ciclosporin. Adjust ciclosporin dose, p. 966. Severe Anecdotal
- **Octreotide** (short-acting) decreases the exposure to telotristat ethyl. Telotristat ethyl should be taken at least 30 minutes before **octreotide**. Moderate Study

Ofatumumab → see monoclonal antibodies
Ofloxacin → see quinolones
Olanzapine → see antipsychotics, second generation
Olaparib → see TABLE 14 p. 1575 (myelosuppression)

FOOD AND LIFESTYLE Bitter (Seville) orange is predicted to increase the exposure to olaparib.

- **Olaparib** might increase the exposure to aliskiren. Moderate Theoretical
- Anti-androgens **(apalutamide, enzalutamide)** are predicted to decrease the exposure to **olaparib**. Avoid. Moderate Theoretical
- Antiarrhythmics **(dronedarone)** are predicted to increase the exposure to **olaparib**. Avoid or adjust dose with moderate CYP3A4 inhibitors—consult product literature. Moderate Theoretical

- Antiepileptics **(carbamazepine, fosphenytoin, phenobarbital, phenytoin, primidone)** are predicted to decrease the exposure to **olaparib**. Avoid. [Moderate] Theoretical
- Antifungals, azoles **(fluconazole, isavuconazole)** are predicted to increase the exposure to **olaparib**. Avoid or adjust dose with moderate CYP3A4 inhibitors—consult product literature. [Moderate] Theoretical
- Antifungals, azoles **(itraconazole, ketoconazole, posaconazole, voriconazole)** are predicted to increase the exposure to **olaparib**. Avoid or adjust dose with potent CYP3A4 inhibitors—consult product literature. [Moderate] Study
- **Olaparib** might increase the exposure to antihistamines, non-sedating **(fexofenadine)**. [Moderate] Theoretical
- **Olaparib** might alter the exposure to antipsychotics, second generation **(quetiapine)**. [Moderate] Theoretical
- **Berotralstat** is predicted to increase the exposure to **olaparib**. Avoid or adjust dose with moderate CYP3A4 inhibitors—consult product literature. [Moderate] Theoretical
- Calcium channel blockers **(diltiazem, verapamil)** are predicted to increase the exposure to **olaparib**. Avoid or adjust dose with moderate CYP3A4 inhibitors—consult product literature. [Moderate] Theoretical
- **Cenobamate** is predicted to decrease the exposure to **olaparib**. Avoid. [Moderate] Theoretical
- **Ceritinib** is predicted to increase the exposure to **olaparib**. Avoid or adjust dose with potent CYP3A4 inhibitors—consult product literature. [Moderate] Study → Also see **TABLE 14** p. 1575
- **Olaparib** might alter the exposure to ciclosporin. [Moderate] Theoretical
- **Cobicistat** is predicted to increase the exposure to **olaparib**. Avoid or adjust dose with potent CYP3A4 inhibitors—consult product literature. [Moderate] Study
- **Olaparib** might increase the exposure to colchicine. [Moderate] Theoretical
- **Olaparib** potentially affects the efficacy of combined hormonal contraceptives. Use additional contraceptive precautions. [Moderate] Theoretical
- **Crizotinib** is predicted to increase the exposure to **olaparib**. Avoid or adjust dose with moderate CYP3A4 inhibitors—consult product literature. [Moderate] Theoretical
- **Dabrafenib** is predicted to decrease the exposure to **olaparib**. Avoid. [Moderate] Theoretical
- **Olaparib** might increase the exposure to digoxin. [Moderate] Theoretical
- **Encorafenib** is predicted to decrease the exposure to **olaparib**. Avoid. [Moderate] Theoretical
- Endothelin receptor antagonists **(bosentan)** are predicted to decrease the exposure to **olaparib**. Avoid. [Moderate] Theoretical
- **Olaparib** might alter the exposure to ergometrine. [Moderate] Theoretical
- **Olaparib** might increase the exposure to everolimus. [Moderate] Theoretical
- **Olaparib** might increase the exposure to factor XA inhibitors **(edoxaban)**. [Moderate] Theoretical
- **Fedratinib** is predicted to increase the exposure to **olaparib**. Avoid or adjust dose with moderate CYP3A4 inhibitors—consult product literature. [Moderate] Theoretical
- **Grapefruit** juice is predicted to increase the exposure to **olaparib**. Avoid. [Moderate] Theoretical
- **HIV-protease inhibitors** are predicted to increase the exposure to **olaparib**. Avoid or adjust dose with potent CYP3A4 inhibitors—consult product literature. [Moderate] Study
- **Idelalisib** is predicted to increase the exposure to **olaparib**. Avoid or adjust dose with potent CYP3A4 inhibitors—consult product literature. [Moderate] Study
- **Imatinib** is predicted to increase the exposure to **olaparib**. Avoid or adjust dose with moderate CYP3A4 inhibitors—consult product literature. [Moderate] Theoretical → Also see **TABLE 14** p. 1575
- **Ivosidenib** is predicted to decrease the exposure to **olaparib**. Avoid. [Moderate] Theoretical
- **Letermovir** is predicted to increase the exposure to **olaparib**. Avoid or adjust dose with moderate CYP3A4 inhibitors—consult product literature. [Moderate] Theoretical

- **Olaparib** might increase the exposure to loperamide. [Moderate] Theoretical
- **Lorlatinib** is predicted to decrease the exposure to **olaparib**. Avoid. [Moderate] Theoretical
- **Lumacaftor** is predicted to decrease the exposure to **olaparib**. Avoid. [Moderate] Theoretical
- Macrolides **(clarithromycin)** are predicted to increase the exposure to **olaparib**. Avoid or adjust dose with potent CYP3A4 inhibitors—consult product literature. [Moderate] Study
- Macrolides **(erythromycin)** are predicted to increase the exposure to **olaparib**. Avoid or adjust dose with moderate CYP3A4 inhibitors—consult product literature. [Moderate] Theoretical
- **Mitotane** is predicted to decrease the exposure to **olaparib**. Avoid. [Moderate] Theoretical → Also see **TABLE 14** p. 1575
- Neurokinin-1 receptor antagonists **(aprepitant, netupitant)** are predicted to increase the exposure to **olaparib**. Avoid or adjust dose with moderate CYP3A4 inhibitors—consult product literature. [Moderate] Theoretical
- **Nilotinib** is predicted to increase the exposure to **olaparib**. Avoid or adjust dose with moderate CYP3A4 inhibitors—consult product literature. [Moderate] Theoretical → Also see **TABLE 14** p. 1575
- NNRTIs **(efavirenz, etravirine, nevirapine)** are predicted to decrease the exposure to **olaparib**. Avoid. [Moderate] Theoretical
- **Olaparib** might alter the exposure to opioids **(alfentanil)**. [Moderate] Theoretical
- **Olaparib** might alter the exposure to pimozide. [Moderate] Theoretical
- **Olaparib** might increase the exposure to pralsetinib. [Moderate] Theoretical
- **Olaparib** might increase the exposure to ranolazine. [Moderate] Theoretical
- Rifamycins **(rifampicin)** are predicted to decrease the exposure to **olaparib**. Avoid. [Moderate] Theoretical
- **Olaparib** might increase the exposure to rimegepant. [Moderate] Theoretical
- **Olaparib** might increase the exposure to sirolimus. [Moderate] Theoretical
- **Sotorasib** is predicted to decrease the exposure to **olaparib**. Avoid. [Moderate] Theoretical
- **St John's wort** is predicted to decrease the exposure to **olaparib**. Avoid. [Moderate] Theoretical
- **Olaparib** is predicted to increase the exposure to statins. [Moderate] Theoretical
- **Olaparib** might alter the exposure to tacrolimus. [Moderate] Theoretical
- **Olaparib** might increase the exposure to talazoparib. [Moderate] Theoretical → Also see **TABLE 14** p. 1575
- **Olaparib** might increase the exposure to taxanes **(paclitaxel)**. [Moderate] Theoretical → Also see **TABLE 14** p. 1575
- **Olaparib** might alter the exposure to temsirolimus. [Moderate] Theoretical → Also see **TABLE 14** p. 1575
- **Olaparib** might increase the exposure to thrombin inhibitors **(dabigatran)**. [Moderate] Theoretical
- **Tucatinib** is predicted to increase the exposure to **olaparib**. Avoid or adjust dose with potent CYP3A4 inhibitors—consult product literature. [Moderate] Study

Olmesartan → see angiotensin-II receptor antagonists

Olodaterol → see beta₂ agonists

Omega-3-acid ethyl esters → see **TABLE 4** p. 1571 (antiplatelet effects)
- **Omega-3-acid ethyl esters** might enhance the blood pressure-lowering effects of beta blockers, non-selective. [Moderate] Study
- **Omega-3-acid ethyl esters** might enhance the blood pressure-lowering effects of beta blockers, selective. [Moderate] Study

Omeprazole → see proton pump inhibitors

Ondansetron → see 5-HT3-receptor antagonists

Opicapone
- **Opicapone** might increase the exposure to the active metabolite of foslevodopa. Adjust dose. [Moderate] Theoretical
- **Opicapone** is predicted to increase the risk of cardiovascular adverse effects when given with isoprenaline. [Moderate] Theoretical

Opicapone (continued)

▶ **Opicapone** increases the exposure to levodopa. Adjust dose. Moderate Study
▶ **Opicapone** is predicted to increase the exposure to loperamide. Avoid. Moderate Study
▶ **Opicapone** is predicted to increase the risk of elevated blood pressure when given with MAOIs, irreversible. Avoid. Severe Theoretical
▶ **Opicapone** is predicted to increase the exposure to meglitinides (repaglinide). Avoid. Moderate Study
▶ **Opicapone** is predicted to increase the risk of elevated blood pressure when given with moclobemide. Avoid. Severe Theoretical
▶ **Opicapone** is predicted to increase the exposure to montelukast. Avoid. Moderate Study
▶ **Opicapone** is predicted to increase the exposure to pioglitazone. Avoid. Moderate Study
▶ **Opicapone** is predicted to increase the risk of cardiovascular adverse effects when given with sympathomimetics, inotropic. Severe Theoretical
▶ **Opicapone** is predicted to increase the risk of cardiovascular adverse effects when given with sympathomimetics, vasoconstrictor (adrenaline/epinephrine, noradrenaline/norepinephrine). Severe Theoretical

Opioids → see **TABLE 5** p. 1572 (bradycardia), **TABLE 17** p. 1576 (hyponatraemia), **TABLE 12** p. 1574 (serotonin syndrome), **TABLE 8** p. 1573 (QT-interval prolongation), **TABLE 10** p. 1574 (CNS effects)

alfentanil · buprenorphine · codeine · diamorphine · dihydrocodeine · diphenoxylate · dipipanone · fentanyl · hydromorphone · meptazinol · methadone · morphine · oxycodone · pentazocine · pethidine · remifentanil · sufentanil · tapentadol · tramadol

▶ **Alcohol** causes rapid release of opioids (hydromorphone, morphine) from extended-release preparations. Avoid. Severe Study → Also see **TABLE 10** p. 1574
▶ Anti-androgens (apalutamide, enzalutamide) are predicted to decrease the exposure to **buprenorphine**. Monitor and adjust dose. Moderate Theoretical
▶ Anti-androgens (apalutamide, enzalutamide) decrease the exposure to **methadone**. Monitor and adjust dose. Severe Study → Also see **TABLE 8** p. 1573
▶ Anti-androgens (apalutamide, enzalutamide) are predicted to decrease the exposure to **oxycodone**. Monitor and adjust dose. Moderate Study
▶ Anti-androgens (enzalutamide) are predicted to affect the exposure to **tramadol**. Use with caution or avoid. Moderate Theoretical
▶ Anti-androgens (apalutamide, enzalutamide) are predicted to decrease the exposure to opioids (alfentanil, fentanyl). Moderate Study
▶ Antiarrhythmics (amiodarone) are predicted to increase the concentration of **fentanyl**. Monitor and adjust dose. Moderate Theoretical → Also see **TABLE 5** p. 1572
▶ Antiarrhythmics (dronedarone) are predicted to increase the exposure to opioids (alfentanil, buprenorphine, fentanyl, oxycodone). Monitor and adjust dose. Moderate Study → Also see **TABLE 5** p. 1572
▶ Antiarrhythmics (dronedarone) are predicted to increase the exposure to opioids (methadone, sufentanil). Moderate Theoretical → Also see **TABLE 5** p. 1572 → Also see **TABLE 8** p. 1573
▶ Antiepileptics (carbamazepine) decrease the concentration of **tramadol**. Adjust dose. Severe Study → Also see **TABLE 17** p. 1576
▶ Antiepileptics (carbamazepine, fosphenytoin, phenobarbital, phenytoin, primidone) are predicted to decrease the exposure to **buprenorphine**. Monitor and adjust dose. Moderate Theoretical → Also see **TABLE 10** p. 1574
▶ Antiepileptics (carbamazepine, fosphenytoin, phenobarbital, phenytoin, primidone) decrease the exposure to **methadone**. Monitor and adjust dose. Severe Study → Also see **TABLE 10** p. 1574
▶ Antiepileptics (carbamazepine, fosphenytoin, phenobarbital, phenytoin, primidone) are predicted to decrease the exposure to **oxycodone**. Monitor and adjust dose. Moderate Study → Also see **TABLE 10** p. 1574

▶ Antiepileptics (carbamazepine, fosphenytoin, phenobarbital, phenytoin, primidone) are predicted to decrease the exposure to opioids (alfentanil, fentanyl). Moderate Study → Also see **TABLE 10** p. 1574
▶ Antifungals, azoles (itraconazole, ketoconazole, posaconazole, voriconazole) are predicted to increase the exposure to **sufentanil**. Moderate Study
▶ Antifungals, azoles (itraconazole, ketoconazole, voriconazole) are predicted to increase the exposure to **methadone**. Adjust dose. Severe Theoretical → Also see **TABLE 8** p. 1573
▶ Antifungals, azoles (miconazole) are predicted to increase the exposure to **alfentanil**. Use with caution and adjust dose. Moderate Theoretical
▶ Antifungals, azoles (fluconazole, isavuconazole) are predicted to increase the exposure to opioids (alfentanil, buprenorphine, fentanyl, oxycodone). Monitor and adjust dose. Moderate Study
▶ Antifungals, azoles (itraconazole, ketoconazole, posaconazole, voriconazole) are predicted to increase the exposure to opioids (alfentanil, buprenorphine, fentanyl, oxycodone). Monitor and adjust dose. Severe Study
▶ Antifungals, azoles (fluconazole, isavuconazole) are predicted to increase the exposure to opioids (methadone, sufentanil). Moderate Theoretical → Also see **TABLE 8** p. 1573
▶ Antipsychotics, second generation (clozapine) can cause constipation, as can **opioids**; concurrent use might increase the risk of developing intestinal obstruction. Severe Anecdotal → Also see **TABLE 17** p. 1576 → Also see **TABLE 10** p. 1574
▶ **Asciminib** is predicted to increase the exposure to **alfentanil**. Severe Theoretical
▶ **Berotralstat** is predicted to increase the exposure to opioids (alfentanil, buprenorphine, fentanyl, oxycodone). Monitor and adjust dose. Moderate Study
▶ **Berotralstat** is predicted to increase the exposure to opioids (methadone, sufentanil). Moderate Theoretical
▶ **Brigatinib** potentially decreases the concentration of opioids (alfentanil, fentanyl). Avoid. Moderate Theoretical → Also see **TABLE 5** p. 1572
▶ **Bulevirtide** is predicted to increase the exposure to **alfentanil**. Moderate Theoretical
▶ **Bupropion** is predicted to decrease the efficacy of **codeine**. Moderate Theoretical
▶ **Bupropion** is predicted to decrease the efficacy of **tramadol**. Severe Study
▶ Calcium channel blockers (nicardipine) are predicted to increase the exposure to **fentanyl**. Monitor and adjust dose. Moderate Theoretical
▶ Calcium channel blockers (diltiazem, verapamil) are predicted to increase the exposure to opioids (alfentanil, buprenorphine, fentanyl, oxycodone). Monitor and adjust dose. Moderate Study → Also see **TABLE 5** p. 1572
▶ Calcium channel blockers (diltiazem, verapamil) are predicted to increase the exposure to opioids (methadone, sufentanil). Moderate Theoretical → Also see **TABLE 5** p. 1572
▶ **Cenobamate** is predicted to decrease the exposure to **alfentanil**. Adjust dose. Moderate Theoretical → Also see **TABLE 10** p. 1574
▶ **Cenobamate** decreases the exposure to **methadone**. Monitor and adjust dose. Severe Study → Also see **TABLE 10** p. 1574
▶ **Ceritinib** is predicted to increase the exposure to opioids (alfentanil, buprenorphine, fentanyl, oxycodone). Monitor and adjust dose. Severe Study → Also see **TABLE 5** p. 1572
▶ **Ceritinib** is predicted to increase the exposure to **sufentanil**. Moderate Study → Also see **TABLE 5** p. 1572
▶ **Cinacalcet** is predicted to decrease the efficacy of **codeine**. Moderate Theoretical
▶ **Cinacalcet** is predicted to decrease the efficacy of **tramadol**. Severe Study
▶ **Cobicistat** is predicted to increase the exposure to opioids (alfentanil, buprenorphine, fentanyl, oxycodone). Monitor and adjust dose. Severe Study
▶ **Cobicistat** is predicted to increase the exposure to **sufentanil**. Moderate Study
▶ **Tramadol** might increase the anticoagulant effect of coumarins (acenocoumarol). Severe Study

A1

- **Tramadol** has been reported to increase the anticoagulant effect of coumarins **(warfarin)**. Severe Anecdotal
- **Crizotinib** is predicted to increase the exposure to opioids **(alfentanil, buprenorphine, fentanyl, oxycodone)**. Monitor and adjust dose. Moderate Study → Also see **TABLE 5** p. 1572
- **Crizotinib** is predicted to increase the exposure to opioids **(methadone, sufentanil)**. Moderate Theoretical → Also see **TABLE 5** p. 1572 → Also see **TABLE 8** p. 1573
- **Dabrafenib** decreases the exposure to **methadone**. Monitor and adjust dose. Severe Study
- **Dacomitinib** is predicted to decrease the efficacy of **codeine**. Moderate Theoretical
- **Dacomitinib** is predicted to decrease the efficacy of **tramadol**. Severe Study
- **Tapentadol** is predicted to increase the risk of serotonin syndrome when given with drugs that cause serotonin syndrome (see **TABLE 12** p. 1574). Severe Theoretical
- **Encorafenib** is predicted to decrease the exposure to **buprenorphine**. Monitor and adjust dose. Moderate Theoretical
- **Encorafenib** decreases the exposure to **methadone**. Monitor and adjust dose. Severe Study → Also see **TABLE 8** p. 1573
- **Encorafenib** is predicted to decrease the exposure to opioids **(alfentanil, fentanyl)**. Moderate Study
- **Encorafenib** is predicted to decrease the exposure to **oxycodone**. Monitor and adjust dose. Moderate Study
- Endothelin receptor antagonists **(bosentan)** decrease the exposure to **methadone**. Monitor and adjust dose. Severe Study
- **Fedratinib** is predicted to increase the exposure to opioids **(alfentanil, buprenorphine, fentanyl, oxycodone)**. Monitor and adjust dose. Moderate Study
- **Fedratinib** is predicted to increase the exposure to opioids **(methadone, sufentanil)**. Moderate Theoretical
- **Fostamatinib** is predicted to increase the exposure to **alfentanil**. Monitor and adjust dose. Moderate Theoretical
- **Givinostat** might increase the exposure to **alfentanil**. Moderate Study
- H_2 receptor antagonists **(cimetidine)** increase the concentration of **alfentanil**. Use with caution and adjust dose. Severe Study
- H_2 receptor antagonists **(cimetidine)** might increase the exposure to **fentanyl**. Monitor and adjust dose. Moderate Study
- **HIV-protease inhibitors** boosted with ritonavir are predicted to decrease the exposure to **methadone**. Moderate Study
- HIV-protease inhibitors **(ritonavir)** are predicted to decrease the concentration of **morphine**. Moderate Theoretical
- HIV-protease inhibitors **(ritonavir)** increase the risk of CNS toxicity when given with **pethidine**. Avoid. Severe Study
- **HIV-protease inhibitors** are predicted to increase the exposure to opioids **(alfentanil, buprenorphine, fentanyl, oxycodone)**. Monitor and adjust dose. Severe Study
- **HIV-protease inhibitors** are predicted to increase the exposure to **sufentanil**. Moderate Study
- **Idelalisib** is predicted to increase the exposure to **methadone**. Severe Theoretical
- **Idelalisib** is predicted to increase the exposure to opioids **(alfentanil, buprenorphine, fentanyl, oxycodone)**. Monitor and adjust dose. Severe Study
- **Idelalisib** is predicted to increase the exposure to **sufentanil**. Moderate Study
- **Imatinib** is predicted to increase the exposure to opioids **(alfentanil, buprenorphine, fentanyl, oxycodone)**. Monitor and adjust dose. Moderate Study
- **Imatinib** is predicted to increase the exposure to opioids **(methadone, sufentanil)**. Moderate Theoretical
- Interferons **(ropeginterferon alfa)** are predicted to increase the exposure to **methadone**. Moderate Theoretical
- **Ivosidenib** is predicted to decrease the exposure to **buprenorphine**. Monitor and adjust dose. Moderate Theoretical
- **Ivosidenib** decreases the exposure to **methadone**. Monitor and adjust dose. Severe Study → Also see **TABLE 8** p. 1573
- **Ivosidenib** is predicted to decrease the exposure to opioids **(alfentanil, fentanyl)**. Moderate Study
- **Ivosidenib** is predicted to decrease the exposure to **oxycodone**. Monitor and adjust dose. Moderate Study

- **Larotrectinib** is predicted to increase the exposure to opioids **(alfentanil, fentanyl)**. Use with caution and adjust dose. Mild Theoretical
- **Letermovir** is predicted to increase the exposure to opioids **(alfentanil, buprenorphine, fentanyl, oxycodone)**. Monitor and adjust dose. Moderate Study
- **Letermovir** is predicted to increase the exposure to opioids **(methadone, sufentanil)**. Moderate Theoretical
- **Lorlatinib** decreases the exposure to **methadone**. Monitor and adjust dose. Severe Study
- **Lorlatinib** is predicted to decrease the exposure to opioids **(alfentanil, fentanyl)**. Avoid. Moderate Theoretical
- **Lumacaftor** is predicted to decrease the exposure to **buprenorphine**. Monitor and adjust dose. Moderate Theoretical
- **Lumacaftor** decreases the exposure to **methadone**. Monitor and adjust dose. Severe Study
- **Lumacaftor** is predicted to decrease the exposure to opioids **(alfentanil, fentanyl)**. Moderate Study
- **Lumacaftor** is predicted to decrease the exposure to **oxycodone**. Monitor and adjust dose. Moderate Study
- Macrolides **(clarithromycin)** are predicted to increase the concentration of **methadone**. Severe Theoretical
- Macrolides **(clarithromycin)** are predicted to increase the exposure to **sufentanil**. Moderate Study
- Macrolides **(clarithromycin)** are predicted to increase the exposure to opioids **(alfentanil, buprenorphine, fentanyl, oxycodone)**. Monitor and adjust dose. Severe Study
- Macrolides **(erythromycin)** are predicted to increase the exposure to opioids **(alfentanil, buprenorphine, fentanyl, oxycodone)**. Monitor and adjust dose. Moderate Study
- Macrolides **(erythromycin)** are predicted to increase the exposure to opioids **(methadone, sufentanil)**. Moderate Theoretical → Also see **TABLE 8** p. 1573
- MAO-B inhibitors **(rasagiline)** are predicted to increase the risk of adverse effects when given with **pethidine**. Avoid and for 14 days after stopping **rasagiline**. Severe Theoretical → Also see **TABLE 12** p. 1574
- MAO-B inhibitors **(safinamide)** are predicted to increase the risk of adverse effects when given with **pethidine**. Avoid and for 1 week after stopping **safinamide**. Severe Theoretical → Also see **TABLE 12** p. 1574
- MAO-B inhibitors **(selegiline)** increase the risk of adverse effects when given with **pethidine**. Avoid. Severe Anecdotal → Also see **TABLE 12** p. 1574
- **Opioids** are predicted to increase the risk of CNS excitation or depression when given with **MAOIs, irreversible**. Avoid. Severe Study → Also see **TABLE 12** p. 1574
- **Opioids** potentially decrease the absorption of oral **mexiletine**. Moderate Study
- **Mifepristone** is predicted to increase the exposure to **alfentanil**. Severe Theoretical
- **Mitotane** is predicted to decrease the exposure to **buprenorphine**. Monitor and adjust dose. Moderate Theoretical
- **Mitotane** decreases the exposure to **methadone**. Monitor and adjust dose. Severe Study
- **Mitotane** is predicted to decrease the exposure to opioids **(alfentanil, fentanyl)**. Moderate Study
- **Mitotane** is predicted to decrease the exposure to **oxycodone**. Monitor and adjust dose. Moderate Study
- **Mobocertinib** is predicted to decrease the exposure to **alfentanil**. Moderate Theoretical
- **Moclobemide** might cause serotonin syndrome, as can **tramadol**; concurrent use might increase the risk of developing this effect. Avoid. Severe Anecdotal → Also see **TABLE 12** p. 1574
- **Nalmefene** is predicted to decrease the efficacy of **opioids**. Avoid except in an emergency situation—consult product literature. Severe Theoretical
- **Naltrexone** is predicted to decrease the efficacy of **opioids**. Avoid except in an emergency situation—consult product literature. Severe Theoretical
- Neurokinin-1 receptor antagonists **(aprepitant, netupitant)** are predicted to increase the exposure to opioids **(alfentanil, buprenorphine, fentanyl, oxycodone)**. Monitor and adjust dose. Moderate Study

Opioids (continued)

▸ Neurokinin-1 receptor antagonists **(aprepitant, netupitant)** are predicted to increase the exposure to opioids **(methadone, sufentanil)**. Moderate Theoretical

▸ **Nilotinib** is predicted to increase the exposure to opioids **(alfentanil, buprenorphine, fentanyl, oxycodone)**. Monitor and adjust dose. Moderate Study

▸ **Nilotinib** is predicted to increase the exposure to opioids **(methadone, sufentanil)**. Moderate Theoretical → Also see TABLE 8 p. 1573

▸ **Nirmatrelvir** boosted with ritonavir is predicted to increase the concentration of **buprenorphine**. Monitor and adjust dose. Moderate Theoretical

▸ **Nirmatrelvir** boosted with ritonavir is predicted to decrease the concentration of **methadone**. Adjust dose. Moderate Theoretical

▸ **Nirmatrelvir** boosted with ritonavir is predicted to decrease the concentration of **morphine**. Moderate Theoretical

▸ **Nirmatrelvir** boosted with ritonavir is predicted to increase the concentration of opioids **(fentanyl, oxycodone, pethidine)**. Severe Theoretical

▸ NNRTIs **(efavirenz)** moderately decrease the exposure to **buprenorphine**. Adjust dose. Moderate Study

▸ NNRTIs **(efavirenz, etravirine, nevirapine)** decrease the exposure to **methadone**. Monitor and adjust dose. Severe Study → Also see TABLE 8 p. 1573

▸ **Olaparib** might alter the exposure to **alfentanil**. Moderate Theoretical

▸ Opioids **(buprenorphine)** are predicted to increase the risk of opiate withdrawal when given with opioids **(alfentanil)**. Severe Theoretical → Also see TABLE 10 p. 1574

▸ Opioids **(meptazinol)** are predicted to increase the risk of opiate withdrawal when given with opioids **(alfentanil, codeine, diamorphine, dihydrocodeine, dipipanone, fentanyl, hydromorphone)**. Severe Theoretical → Also see TABLE 10 p. 1574

▸ Opioids **(pentazocine)** are predicted to increase the risk of opiate withdrawal when given with opioids **(alfentanil, codeine, diamorphine, dihydrocodeine, dipipanone, fentanyl, hydromorphone, methadone, morphine, oxycodone)**. Severe Theoretical → Also see TABLE 12 p. 1574 → Also see TABLE 10 p. 1574

▸ Opioids **(buprenorphine)** are predicted to increase the risk of opiate withdrawal when given with opioids **(codeine, diamorphine, dihydrocodeine, dipipanone, fentanyl, hydromorphone, methadone, morphine, oxycodone, pethidine, remifentanil, sufentanil, tapentadol, tramadol)**. Severe Theoretical → Also see TABLE 10 p. 1574

▸ Opioids **(meptazinol)** are predicted to increase the risk of opiate withdrawal when given with opioids **(methadone, morphine, oxycodone, pethidine, remifentanil, sufentanil, tapentadol, tramadol)**. Severe Theoretical → Also see TABLE 10 p. 1574

▸ Opioids **(pentazocine)** are predicted to increase the risk of opiate withdrawal when given with opioids **(pethidine, remifentanil, tapentadol, tramadol)**. Severe Theoretical → Also see TABLE 12 p. 1574 → Also see TABLE 10 p. 1574

▸ Opioids **(pentazocine)** are predicted to increase the risk of opiate withdrawal when given with opioids **(sufentanil)**. Severe Anecdotal → Also see TABLE 10 p. 1574

▸ **Opioids** might increase the risk of adverse effects when given with **ozanimod**. Severe Theoretical → Also see TABLE 5 p. 1572

▸ **Palbociclib** is predicted to increase the exposure to opioids **(alfentanil, fentanyl)**. Adjust dose. Moderate Theoretical

▸ **Pemigatinib** might decrease the exposure to **methadone**. Moderate Theoretical

▸ **Tramadol** might increase the anticoagulant effect of **phenindione**. Severe Anecdotal

▸ **Pitolisant** is predicted to decrease the exposure to **morphine**. Mild Theoretical

▸ **Ribociclib** is predicted to increase the exposure to opioids **(alfentanil, fentanyl)**. Use with caution and adjust dose. Moderate Theoretical

▸ Rifamycins **(rifampicin)** are predicted to decrease the exposure to **buprenorphine**. Monitor and adjust dose. Moderate Theoretical

▸ Rifamycins **(rifampicin)** decrease the exposure to **methadone**. Monitor and adjust dose. Severe Study

▸ Rifamycins **(rifampicin)** are predicted to decrease the exposure to **oxycodone**. Monitor and adjust dose. Moderate Study

▸ Rifamycins **(rifampicin)** are predicted to decrease the exposure to opioids **(alfentanil, fentanyl)**. Moderate Study

▸ Rifamycins **(rifampicin)** decrease the exposure to opioids **(codeine, morphine)**. Moderate Study

▸ **Ritlecitinib** is predicted to increase the exposure to **alfentanil**. Moderate Theoretical

▸ **Rucaparib** is predicted to increase the exposure to opioids **(alfentanil, fentanyl)**. Monitor and adjust dose. Moderate Study

▸ **Selpercatinib** is predicted to increase the exposure to opioids **(alfentanil, buprenorphine)**. Avoid. Moderate Study

▸ **Sotorasib** is predicted to decrease the exposure to **alfentanil**. Avoid or adjust dose. Moderate Theoretical

▸ **Sotorasib** decreases the exposure to **methadone**. Monitor and adjust dose. Severe Study

▸ SSRIs **(fluoxetine, paroxetine)** are predicted to decrease the efficacy of **codeine**. Moderate Theoretical → Also see TABLE 10 p. 1574

▸ SSRIs **(fluoxetine, paroxetine)** are predicted to decrease the efficacy of **tramadol**. Severe Study → Also see TABLE 17 p. 1576 → Also see TABLE 12 p. 1574 → Also see TABLE 10 p. 1574

▸ **St John's wort** decreases the exposure to **methadone**. Monitor and adjust dose. Severe Study → Also see TABLE 12 p. 1574

▸ **St John's wort** moderately decreases the exposure to **oxycodone**. Adjust dose. Moderate Study

▸ **Terbinafine** is predicted to decrease the efficacy of **codeine**. Moderate Theoretical

▸ **Terbinafine** is predicted to decrease the efficacy of **tramadol**. Severe Study

▸ **Tucatinib** is predicted to increase the exposure to opioids **(alfentanil, buprenorphine, fentanyl, oxycodone)**. Monitor and adjust dose. Severe Study

▸ **Tucatinib** is predicted to increase the exposure to **sufentanil**. Moderate Study

Opium → see interactions of codeine and morphine under opioids

Oritavancin

▸ **Oritavancin** might increase the exposure to coumarins **(warfarin)**. Moderate Theoretical

▸ **Oritavancin** might cause a falsely elevated aPTT when given with heparin. Avoid and for 120 hours after stopping **oritavancin**. Severe Theoretical

Orlistat

> **SEPARATION OF ADMINISTRATION** Orlistat might affect the absorption of concurrently administered oral drugs—consider separating administration. Particular care should be taken with antiepileptics, antiretrovirals, oral contraceptives, and drugs that have a narrow therapeutic index.

Orphenadrine → see TABLE 9 p. 1573 (antimuscarinics), TABLE 10 p. 1574 (CNS effects)

▸ Antipsychotics, second generation **(clozapine)** can cause constipation, as can **orphenadrine**; concurrent use might increase the risk of developing intestinal obstruction. Severe Theoretical → Also see TABLE 9 p. 1573 → Also see TABLE 10 p. 1574

Oseltamivir

▸ **Ivosidenib** is predicted to increase the exposure to the active metabolite of **oseltamivir**. Use with caution or avoid. Moderate Theoretical

▸ **Leflunomide** is predicted to increase the exposure to **oseltamivir**. Moderate Study

▸ **Oseltamivir** might decrease the efficacy of live vaccines **(influenza vaccine (live))**. Moderate Theoretical

▸ **Nitisinone** is predicted to increase the exposure to **oseltamivir**. Moderate Study

▸ **Teriflunomide** is predicted to increase the exposure to **oseltamivir**. Moderate Study

▸ **Vadadustat** is predicted to increase the exposure to the active metabolite of **oseltamivir**. Monitor and adjust dose. Moderate Study

Osilodrostat → see TABLE 8 p. 1573 (QT-interval prolongation)

▸ **Osilodrostat** is predicted to increase the exposure to agomelatine. Moderate Study

▸ **Osilodrostat** is predicted to increase the exposure to aminophylline. Adjust dose. Moderate Theoretical

- **Osilodrostat** is predicted to increase the exposure to anaesthetics, local **(ropivacaine)**. Moderate Theoretical
- **Osilodrostat** is predicted to increase the exposure to anagrelide. Moderate Theoretical → Also see **TABLE 8** p. 1573
- Anti-androgens **(apalutamide, enzalutamide)** are predicted to decrease the exposure to **osilodrostat**. Moderate Theoretical → Also see **TABLE 8** p. 1573
- Antiepileptics **(carbamazepine, fosphenytoin, phenobarbital, phenytoin, primidone)** are predicted to decrease the exposure to **osilodrostat**. Moderate Theoretical
- Antifungals, azoles **(itraconazole, ketoconazole, posaconazole, voriconazole)** are predicted to increase the exposure to **osilodrostat**. Moderate Theoretical → Also see **TABLE 8** p. 1573
- **Osilodrostat** increases the concentration of antipsychotics, second generation **(clozapine)**. Monitor adverse effects and adjust dose. Severe Study
- **Osilodrostat** is predicted to increase the exposure to antipsychotics, second generation **(olanzapine)**. Adjust dose. Moderate Anecdotal
- Ceritinib is predicted to increase the exposure to **osilodrostat**. Moderate Theoretical → Also see **TABLE 8** p. 1573
- Cobicistat is predicted to increase the exposure to **osilodrostat**. Moderate Theoretical
- **Osilodrostat** is predicted to increase the exposure to dopamine receptor agonists **(ropinirole)**. Adjust dose. Moderate Study
- Encorafenib is predicted to decrease the exposure to osilodrostat. Moderate Theoretical → Also see **TABLE 8** p. 1573
- **Osilodrostat** are predicted to increases the exposure to erlotinib. Monitor adverse effects and adjust dose. Moderate Study
- **Osilodrostat** is predicted to increase the exposure to fezolinetant. Avoid. Moderate Study
- HIV-protease inhibitors are predicted to increase the exposure to **osilodrostat**. Moderate Theoretical
- Idelalisib is predicted to increase the exposure to **osilodrostat**. Moderate Theoretical
- Ivosidenib is predicted to decrease the exposure to osilodrostat. Moderate Theoretical → Also see **TABLE 8** p. 1573
- **Osilodrostat** is predicted to increase the exposure to loxapine. Avoid. Unknown Theoretical
- Lumacaftor is predicted to decrease the exposure to osilodrostat. Moderate Theoretical
- Macrolides **(clarithromycin)** are predicted to increase the exposure to **osilodrostat**. Moderate Theoretical
- **Osilodrostat** slightly increases the exposure to MAO-B inhibitors **(rasagiline)**. Moderate Study
- **Osilodrostat** is predicted to increase the exposure to mavacamten. Monitor and adjust dose—consult product literature. Moderate Theoretical
- **Osilodrostat** is predicted to increase the exposure to melatonin. Moderate Theoretical
- Mitotane is predicted to decrease the exposure to **osilodrostat**. Moderate Theoretical
- **Osilodrostat** is predicted to increase the exposure to phenothiazines **(chlorpromazine)**. Moderate Theoretical → Also see **TABLE 8** p. 1573
- **Osilodrostat** is predicted to increase the exposure to phosphodiesterase type-4 inhibitors **(roflumilast)**. Moderate Theoretical
- **Osilodrostat** is predicted to increase the exposure to pirfenidone. Use with caution and adjust dose. Moderate Study
- Rifamycins **(rifampicin)** are predicted to decrease the exposure to **osilodrostat**. Moderate Theoretical
- **Osilodrostat** is predicted to increase the exposure to riluzole. Moderate Theoretical
- **Osilodrostat** is predicted to increase the exposure to SNRIs **(duloxetine)**. Moderate Theoretical
- **Osilodrostat** is predicted to increase the exposure to theophylline. Monitor and adjust dose. Moderate Theoretical
- **Osilodrostat** increases the exposure to tizanidine. Avoid. Moderate Study
- **Osilodrostat** is predicted to increase the exposure to triptans **(zolmitriptan)**. Adjust **zolmitriptan** dose, p. 546. Moderate Theoretical

- Tucatinib is predicted to increase the exposure to **osilodrostat**. Moderate Theoretical

Osimertinib → see **TABLE 8** p. 1573 (QT-interval prolongation)
- **Osimertinib** is predicted to increase the exposure to aliskiren. Moderate Study
- Anti-androgens **(apalutamide, enzalutamide)** are predicted to moderately decrease the exposure to **osimertinib**. Avoid. Moderate Study → Also see **TABLE 8** p. 1573
- Antiepileptics **(carbamazepine, fosphenytoin, phenobarbital, phenytoin, primidone)** are predicted to moderately decrease the exposure to **osimertinib**. Avoid. Moderate Study
- **Osimertinib** is predicted to increase the exposure to antihistamines, non-sedating **(fexofenadine)**. Moderate Study
- **Osimertinib** is predicted to increase the exposure to colchicine. Moderate Study
- Dabrafenib is predicted to decrease the exposure to osimertinib. Use with caution or avoid. Severe Study
- **Osimertinib** is predicted to increase the exposure to digoxin. Moderate Study
- Encorafenib is predicted to moderately decrease the exposure to **osimertinib**. Avoid. Moderate Study → Also see **TABLE 8** p. 1573
- Endothelin receptor antagonists **(bosentan)** are predicted to decrease the exposure to **osimertinib**. Use with caution or avoid. Severe Study
- **Osimertinib** is predicted to increase the exposure to everolimus. Moderate Study
- **Osimertinib** is predicted to increase the exposure to factor XA inhibitors **(edoxaban)**. Moderate Study
- Ivosidenib is predicted to moderately decrease the exposure to osimertinib. Avoid. Moderate Study → Also see **TABLE 8** p. 1573
- **Osimertinib** is predicted to increase the exposure to loperamide. Moderate Study
- Lumacaftor is predicted to moderately decrease the exposure to **osimertinib**. Avoid. Moderate Study
- Mitotane is predicted to moderately decrease the exposure to osimertinib. Avoid. Moderate Study
- Modafinil is predicted to decrease the exposure to **osimertinib**. Use with caution or avoid. Severe Theoretical
- NNRTIs **(efavirenz, nevirapine)** are predicted to decrease the exposure to **osimertinib**. Use with caution or avoid. Severe Study → Also see **TABLE 8** p. 1573
- NNRTIs **(etravirine)** are predicted to decrease the exposure to **osimertinib**. Use with caution or avoid. Severe Theoretical
- **Osimertinib** is predicted to increase the exposure to pralsetinib. Moderate Study
- **Osimertinib** is predicted to increase the exposure to ranolazine. Moderate Study → Also see **TABLE 8** p. 1573
- Rifamycins **(rifampicin)** are predicted to moderately decrease the exposure to **osimertinib**. Avoid. Moderate Study
- **Osimertinib** is predicted to increase the exposure to rimegepant. Moderate Study
- **Osimertinib** is predicted to increase the exposure to the active component of sacituzumab govitecan. Severe Theoretical
- **Osimertinib** is predicted to increase the exposure to sirolimus. Moderate Study
- St John's wort is predicted to decrease the exposure to osimertinib. Avoid. Severe Study
- **Osimertinib** causes a small increase in the exposure to statins **(rosuvastatin)**. Severe Study
- **Osimertinib** is predicted to increase the exposure to talazoparib. Moderate Study
- **Osimertinib** is predicted to increase the exposure to taxanes **(paclitaxel)**. Moderate Study
- **Osimertinib** is predicted to increase the exposure to thrombin inhibitors **(dabigatran)**. Moderate Study

Ospemifene
- Anti-androgens **(apalutamide, enzalutamide)** are predicted to moderately decrease the exposure to **ospemifene**. Moderate Study
- Antiepileptics **(carbamazepine, fosphenytoin, phenobarbital, phenytoin, primidone)** are predicted to moderately decrease the exposure to **ospemifene**. Moderate Study
- Antifungals, azoles **(fluconazole)** increase the exposure to **ospemifene**. Use with caution or avoid. Moderate Study

Ospemifene (continued)

▶ Antifungals, azoles **(itraconazole, ketoconazole, posaconazole, voriconazole)** are predicted to increase the exposure to **ospemifene**. Avoid in poor CYP2C9 metabolisers. [Moderate] Study

▶ **Cenobamate** is predicted to decrease the exposure to **ospemifene**. [Moderate] Study

▶ **Ceritinib** is predicted to increase the exposure to **ospemifene**. Avoid in poor CYP2C9 metabolisers. [Moderate] Study

▶ **Cobicistat** is predicted to increase the exposure to **ospemifene**. Avoid in poor CYP2C9 metabolisers. [Moderate] Study

▶ **Combined hormonal contraceptives** potentially oppose the effects of **ospemifene**. Avoid. [Severe] Theoretical

▶ **Dabrafenib** is predicted to decrease the exposure to **ospemifene**. [Moderate] Study

▶ **Encorafenib** is predicted to moderately decrease the exposure to **ospemifene**. [Moderate] Study

▶ Endothelin receptor antagonists **(bosentan)** are predicted to decrease the exposure to **ospemifene**. [Moderate] Study

▶ **HIV-protease inhibitors** are predicted to increase the exposure to **ospemifene**. Avoid in poor CYP2C9 metabolisers. [Moderate] Study

▶ **Hormone replacement therapy** potentially opposes the effects of **ospemifene**. Avoid. [Severe] Theoretical

▶ **Idelalisib** is predicted to increase the exposure to **ospemifene**. Avoid in poor CYP2C9 metabolisers. [Moderate] Study

▶ **Ivosidenib** is predicted to moderately decrease the exposure to **ospemifene**. [Moderate] Study

▶ **Lorlatinib** is predicted to decrease the exposure to **ospemifene**. [Moderate] Study

▶ **Lumacaftor** is predicted to moderately decrease the exposure to **ospemifene**. [Moderate] Study

▶ Macrolides **(clarithromycin)** are predicted to increase the exposure to **ospemifene**. Avoid in poor CYP2C9 metabolisers. [Moderate] Study

▶ **Mitotane** is predicted to moderately decrease the exposure to **ospemifene**. [Moderate] Study

▶ NNRTIs **(efavirenz, etravirine, nevirapine)** are predicted to decrease the exposure to **ospemifene**. [Moderate] Study

▶ Rifamycins **(rifampicin)** are predicted to moderately decrease the exposure to **ospemifene**. [Moderate] Study

▶ **Sotorasib** is predicted to decrease the exposure to **ospemifene**. [Moderate] Study

▶ **St John's wort** is predicted to decrease the exposure to **ospemifene**. [Moderate] Study

▶ **Tucatinib** is predicted to increase the exposure to **ospemifene**. Avoid in poor CYP2C9 metabolisers. [Moderate] Study

Oxaliplatin → see platinum compounds

Oxandrolone → see TABLE 1 p. 1571 (hepatotoxicity)

Oxazepam → see benzodiazepines

Oxcarbazepine → see antiepileptics

Oxybuprocaine → see anaesthetics, local

Oxybutynin → see TABLE 9 p. 1573 (antimuscarinics)

▶ **Oxybutynin** potentially increases the risk of overheating and dehydration when given with antiepileptics **(zonisamide)**. Avoid in children. [Severe] Theoretical

▶ Antifungals, azoles **(itraconazole, ketoconazole, posaconazole, voriconazole)** are predicted to increase the exposure to **oxybutynin**. [Mild] Study

▶ Antipsychotics, second generation **(clozapine)** can cause constipation, as can **oxybutynin**; concurrent use might increase the risk of developing intestinal obstruction. [Severe] Theoretical → Also see TABLE 9 p. 1573

▶ **Ceritinib** is predicted to increase the exposure to **oxybutynin**. [Mild] Study

▶ **Cobicistat** is predicted to increase the exposure to **oxybutynin**. [Mild] Study

▶ **HIV-protease inhibitors** are predicted to increase the exposure to **oxybutynin**. [Mild] Study

▶ **Idelalisib** is predicted to increase the exposure to **oxybutynin**. [Mild] Study

▶ Macrolides **(clarithromycin)** are predicted to increase the exposure to **oxybutynin**. [Mild] Study

▶ **Tucatinib** is predicted to increase the exposure to **oxybutynin**. [Mild] Study

Oxycodone → see opioids

Oxymetholone → see TABLE 1 p. 1571 (hepatotoxicity)

▶ **Oxymetholone** increases the anticoagulant effect of **coumarins**. [Severe] Anecdotal

▶ **Oxymetholone** increases the anticoagulant effect of **phenindione**. [Severe] Anecdotal

Oxytetracycline → see tetracyclines

Oxytocin → see TABLE 17 p. 1576 (hyponatraemia)

▶ **Misoprostol** can cause uterine contractions, as can **oxytocin**; concurrent use might increase the risk of developing this effect. Avoid and for 4 hours after stopping **misoprostol**. [Severe] Theoretical

Ozanimod → see TABLE 5 p. 1572 (bradycardia), TABLE 8 p. 1573 (QT-interval prolongation)

FOOD AND LIFESTYLE Tyramine-rich foods might increase the risk of hypertensive crisis when given ozanimod.

▶ **Clopidogrel** is predicted to increase the exposure to the active metabolites of **ozanimod**. [Moderate] Study

▶ Fibrates **(gemfibrozil)** are predicted to increase the exposure to the active metabolites of **ozanimod**. [Moderate] Study

▶ **Ozanimod** might increase the risk of a hypertensive crisis when given with **linezolid**. Avoid. [Severe] Theoretical

▶ **Live vaccines** might increase the risk of generalised infection (possibly life-threatening) when given with **ozanimod**. Avoid and for 3 months after stopping **ozanimod**. [Severe] Theoretical

▶ **Ozanimod** might increase the risk of a hypertensive crisis when given with **MAO-B inhibitors** and **MAO-B inhibitors** might decrease the exposure to the active metabolites of **ozanimod**. Avoid. [Severe] Theoretical → Also see TABLE 5 p. 1572

▶ **Ozanimod** might increase the risk of a hypertensive crisis when given with **MAOIs, irreversible**. Avoid. [Severe] Theoretical

▶ **Methylphenidate** is predicted to increase the risk of a hypertensive crisis when given with **ozanimod**. [Severe] Theoretical

▶ **Ozanimod** might increase the risk of a hypertensive crisis when given with **moclobemide**. Avoid. [Severe] Theoretical

▶ Monoclonal antibodies **(alemtuzumab)** are predicted to increase the risk of generalised infection (possibly life-threatening) when given with **ozanimod**. Avoid. [Severe] Theoretical

▶ **Opioids** might increase the risk of adverse effects when given with **ozanimod**. [Severe] Theoretical → Also see TABLE 5 p. 1572

▶ Rifamycins **(rifampicin)** moderately decrease the exposure to the active metabolites of **ozanimod**. Avoid. [Moderate] Study

▶ SNRIs **(duloxetine)** might increase the risk of adverse effects when given with **ozanimod**. [Severe] Theoretical

▶ **SSRIs** might increase the risk of adverse effects when given with **ozanimod**. [Severe] Theoretical

▶ **Sympathomimetics, vasoconstrictor** might increase the risk of a hypertensive crisis when given with **ozanimod**. [Severe] Theoretical

▶ **Tricyclic antidepressants** might increase the risk of adverse effects when given with **ozanimod**. [Severe] Theoretical

Paclitaxel → see taxanes

Palbociclib → see TABLE 14 p. 1575 (myelosuppression)

▶ Anti-androgens **(apalutamide, enzalutamide)** are predicted to decrease the exposure to **palbociclib**. Avoid. [Severe] Study

▶ Antiepileptics **(carbamazepine, fosphenytoin, phenobarbital, phenytoin, primidone)** are predicted to decrease the exposure to **palbociclib**. Avoid. [Severe] Study

▶ Antifungals, azoles **(itraconazole, ketoconazole, posaconazole, voriconazole)** are predicted to increase the exposure to **palbociclib**. Avoid or adjust dose—consult product literature. [Severe] Study

▶ **Palbociclib** increases the exposure to benzodiazepines **(midazolam)**. [Moderate] Study

▶ **Ceritinib** is predicted to increase the exposure to **palbociclib**. Avoid or adjust dose—consult product literature. [Severe] Study → Also see TABLE 14 p. 1575

▶ **Palbociclib** is predicted to increase the exposure to **ciclosporin**. Adjust dose. [Moderate] Theoretical

▶ **Cobicistat** is predicted to increase the exposure to **palbociclib**. Avoid or adjust dose—consult product literature. [Severe] Study

▶ **Encorafenib** is predicted to decrease the exposure to **palbociclib**. Avoid. [Severe] Study

- **Palbociclib** is predicted to increase the exposure to everolimus. Adjust dose. Moderate Theoretical
- **Grapefruit** juice is predicted to increase the exposure to **palbociclib**. Avoid. Severe Theoretical
- **HIV-protease inhibitors** are predicted to increase the exposure to **palbociclib**. Avoid or adjust dose—consult product literature. Severe Study
- **Idelalisib** is predicted to increase the exposure to **palbociclib**. Avoid or adjust dose—consult product literature. Severe Study
- **Ivosidenib** is predicted to decrease the exposure to **palbociclib**. Avoid. Severe Study
- **Lumacaftor** is predicted to decrease the exposure to **palbociclib**. Avoid. Severe Study
- **Macrolides (clarithromycin)** are predicted to increase the exposure to **palbociclib**. Avoid or adjust dose—consult product literature. Severe Study
- **Mitotane** is predicted to decrease the exposure to **palbociclib**. Avoid. Severe Study → Also see **TABLE 14** p. 1575
- **Palbociclib** is predicted to increase the exposure to opioids (alfentanil, fentanyl). Adjust dose. Moderate Theoretical
- **Palbociclib** is predicted to increase the exposure to pimozide. Adjust dose. Moderate Theoretical
- **Rifamycins (rifampicin)** are predicted to decrease the exposure to **palbociclib**. Avoid. Severe Study
- **Palbociclib** is predicted to increase the exposure to sirolimus. Adjust dose. Moderate Theoretical
- **St John's wort** is predicted to decrease the exposure to **palbociclib**. Avoid. Severe Theoretical
- **Palbociclib** is predicted to increase the exposure to tacrolimus. Adjust dose. Moderate Theoretical
- **Tucatinib** is predicted to increase the exposure to **palbociclib**. Avoid or adjust dose—consult product literature. Severe Study

Paliperidone → see antipsychotics, second generation

Palonosetron → see 5-HT3-receptor antagonists

Pamidronate → see bisphosphonates

Pancreatin
- **Pancreatin** is predicted to decrease the effects of acarbose. Avoid. Moderate Theoretical

Pancuronium → see neuromuscular blocking drugs, non-depolarising

Panitumumab → see monoclonal antibodies

Panobinostat → see **TABLE 14** p. 1575 (myelosuppression), **TABLE 8** p. 1573 (QT-interval prolongation)

FOOD AND LIFESTYLE Avoid pomegranate, pomegranate juice, and star fruit as they are predicted to increase panobinostat exposure.

- Anti-androgens (apalutamide, enzalutamide) are predicted to decrease the exposure to **panobinostat**. Avoid. Moderate Theoretical → Also see **TABLE 8** p. 1573
- Antiarrhythmics (amiodarone, dronedarone) are predicted to increase the exposure to **panobinostat**. Adjust dose. Moderate Theoretical → Also see **TABLE 8** p. 1573
- Antiepileptics (carbamazepine, fosphenytoin, phenobarbital, phenytoin, primidone) are predicted to decrease the exposure to **panobinostat**. Avoid. Moderate Theoretical
- Antifungals, azoles (itraconazole, ketoconazole, posaconazole, voriconazole) are predicted to increase the exposure to **panobinostat**. Adjust dose—consult product literature; in hepatic impairment avoid. Moderate Study → Also see **TABLE 8** p. 1573
- **Panobinostat** is predicted to increase the exposure to atomoxetine. Monitor and adjust dose. Severe Theoretical
- **Panobinostat** is predicted to increase the exposure to beta blockers, selective (metoprolol). Monitor and adjust dose. Moderate Theoretical
- **Panobinostat** is predicted to increase the exposure to beta blockers, selective (nebivolol). Monitor and adjust dose. Mild Theoretical
- Calcium channel blockers (verapamil) are predicted to increase the exposure to **panobinostat**. Adjust dose. Moderate Theoretical
- **Ceritinib** is predicted to increase the exposure to **panobinostat**. Adjust dose—consult product literature; in hepatic impairment avoid. Moderate Study → Also see **TABLE 14** p. 1575 → Also see **TABLE 8** p. 1573
- **Ciclosporin** is predicted to increase the exposure to **panobinostat**. Adjust dose. Moderate Theoretical

- **Cobicistat** is predicted to increase the exposure to panobinostat. Adjust dose—consult product literature; in hepatic impairment avoid. Moderate Study
- **Encorafenib** is predicted to decrease the exposure to panobinostat. Avoid. Moderate Theoretical → Also see **TABLE 8** p. 1573
- **Grapefruit** and grapefruit juice is predicted to increase the exposure to panobinostat. Avoid. Moderate Theoretical
- **HIV-protease inhibitors** are predicted to increase the exposure to panobinostat. Adjust dose—consult product literature; in hepatic impairment avoid. Moderate Study
- **Idelalisib** is predicted to increase the exposure to panobinostat. Adjust dose—consult product literature; in hepatic impairment avoid. Moderate Study
- **Ivosidenib** is predicted to decrease the exposure to panobinostat. Avoid. Moderate Theoretical → Also see **TABLE 8** p. 1573
- **Lapatinib** is predicted to increase the exposure to panobinostat. Adjust dose. Moderate Theoretical → Also see **TABLE 8** p. 1573
- **Lumacaftor** is predicted to decrease the exposure to panobinostat. Avoid. Moderate Theoretical
- Macrolides (azithromycin, erythromycin) are predicted to increase the exposure to panobinostat. Adjust dose. Moderate Theoretical → Also see **TABLE 8** p. 1573
- Macrolides (clarithromycin) are predicted to increase the exposure to panobinostat. Adjust dose—consult product literature; in hepatic impairment avoid. Moderate Study
- **Mitotane** is predicted to decrease the exposure to panobinostat. Avoid. Moderate Theoretical → Also see **TABLE 14** p. 1575
- **Panobinostat** is predicted to increase the exposure to pimozide. Avoid. Severe Theoretical → Also see **TABLE 8** p. 1573
- **Ranolazine** is predicted to increase the exposure to panobinostat. Adjust dose. Moderate Theoretical → Also see **TABLE 8** p. 1573
- Rifamycins (rifampicin) are predicted to decrease the exposure to panobinostat. Avoid. Moderate Theoretical
- **St John's wort** is predicted to decrease the exposure to panobinostat. Avoid. Moderate Theoretical
- **Tucatinib** is predicted to increase the exposure to panobinostat. Adjust dose—consult product literature; in hepatic impairment avoid. Moderate Study
- **Vemurafenib** is predicted to increase the exposure to panobinostat. Adjust dose. Moderate Theoretical → Also see **TABLE 8** p. 1573

Pantoprazole → see proton pump inhibitors

Paracetamol → see **TABLE 1** p. 1571 (hepatotoxicity)
- **Alcohol** (in those who drink heavily) causes severe liver damage when given with **paracetamol**. Severe Study
- **Paracetamol** is predicted to decrease the clearance of alkylating agents (busulfan). Moderate Theoretical
- Antiepileptics (carbamazepine, fosphenytoin, phenobarbital, phenytoin, primidone) decrease the exposure to **paracetamol**. Moderate Study
- **Paracetamol** increases the anticoagulant effect of coumarins. Moderate Study
- **Imatinib** increases the risk of hepatotoxicity when given with paracetamol. Severe Anecdotal
- **Paracetamol** has been reported to cause high anion gap metabolic acidosis when given with penicillins (flucloxacillin). Severe Anecdotal
- **Paracetamol** is predicted to increase the anticoagulant effect of phenindione. Severe Theoretical
- **Pitolisant** is predicted to decrease the exposure to paracetamol. Mild Theoretical
- Rifamycins (rifampicin) decrease the exposure to **paracetamol**. Moderate Study

Paraldehyde → see antiepileptics

Parathyroid hormone
- **Bisphosphonates** are predicted to decrease the effects of parathyroid hormone. Avoid. Moderate Study

Parecoxib → see NSAIDs

Paricalcitol → see vitamin D substances

Paroxetine → see SSRIs

Interactions | Appendix 1

Pasireotide → see TABLE 5 p. 1572 (bradycardia), TABLE 8 p. 1573 (QT-interval prolongation)
▶ **Pasireotide** is predicted to decrease the absorption of oral ciclosporin. Adjust dose. [Severe] Theoretical

Patiromer

SEPARATION OF ADMINISTRATION Manufacturer advises take 3 hours before, or after, other drugs.

Pazopanib → see TABLE 8 p. 1573 (QT-interval prolongation), TABLE 4 p. 1571 (antiplatelet effects)
▶ Oral antacids are predicted to decrease the absorption of oral **pazopanib**. Manufacturer advises take 1 hour before or 2 hours after antacids. [Moderate] Theoretical
▶ Anti-androgens (apalutamide, enzalutamide) are predicted to decrease the exposure to **pazopanib**. Avoid. [Severe] Theoretical → Also see TABLE 8 p. 1573
▶ Antiarrhythmics (dronedarone) are predicted to increase the exposure to **pazopanib**. [Moderate] Study → Also see TABLE 8 p. 1573
▶ Antiepileptics (carbamazepine, fosphenytoin, phenobarbital, phenytoin, primidone) are predicted to decrease the exposure to **pazopanib**. Avoid. [Severe] Theoretical
▶ Antifungals, azoles (fluconazole, isavuconazole) are predicted to increase the exposure to **pazopanib**. [Moderate] Study → Also see TABLE 8 p. 1573
▶ Antifungals, azoles (itraconazole, ketoconazole, posaconazole, voriconazole) are predicted to increase the exposure to **pazopanib**. Avoid or adjust dose—consult product literature. [Moderate] Study → Also see TABLE 8 p. 1573
▶ Berotralstat is predicted to increase the exposure to **pazopanib**. [Moderate] Study
▶ Calcium channel blockers (diltiazem, verapamil) are predicted to increase the exposure to **pazopanib**. [Moderate] Study
▶ Oral calcium salts (calcium carbonate) -containing antacids might decrease the absorption of oral **pazopanib**. Manufacturer advises take 1 hour before or 2 hours after antacids. [Moderate] Theoretical
▶ Cenobamate is predicted to decrease the exposure to **pazopanib**. [Severe] Study
▶ Ceritinib is predicted to increase the exposure to **pazopanib**. Avoid or adjust dose—consult product literature. [Moderate] Study → Also see TABLE 8 p. 1573
▶ Cobicistat is predicted to increase the exposure to **pazopanib**. Avoid or adjust dose—consult product literature. [Moderate] Study
▶ Crizotinib is predicted to increase the exposure to **pazopanib**. [Moderate] Study → Also see TABLE 8 p. 1573
▶ Dabrafenib is predicted to decrease the exposure to **pazopanib**. [Severe] Study
▶ Encorafenib is predicted to decrease the exposure to **pazopanib**. Avoid. [Severe] Theoretical → Also see TABLE 8 p. 1573
▶ Endothelin receptor antagonists (bosentan) are predicted to decrease the exposure to **pazopanib**. [Severe] Study
▶ Fedratinib is predicted to increase the exposure to **pazopanib**. [Moderate] Study
▶ Grapefruit juice is predicted to increase the exposure to **pazopanib**. Avoid. [Severe] Theoretical
▶ H₂ receptor antagonists are predicted to decrease the exposure to **pazopanib**. Manufacturer advises take 2 hours before or 10 hours after H₂ receptor antagonists. [Moderate] Theoretical
▶ HIV-protease inhibitors are predicted to increase the exposure to **pazopanib**. Avoid or adjust dose—consult product literature. [Moderate] Study
▶ Idelalisib is predicted to increase the exposure to **pazopanib**. Avoid or adjust dose—consult product literature. [Moderate] Study
▶ Imatinib is predicted to increase the exposure to **pazopanib**. [Moderate] Study → Also see TABLE 4 p. 1571
▶ Ivosidenib is predicted to decrease the exposure to **pazopanib**. Avoid. [Severe] Theoretical → Also see TABLE 8 p. 1573
▶ Lapatinib increases the exposure to **pazopanib**. Avoid. [Severe] Study → Also see TABLE 8 p. 1573
▶ Letermovir is predicted to increase the exposure to **pazopanib**. [Moderate] Study
▶ **Pazopanib** is predicted to increase the exposure to lomitapide. Separate administration by 12 hours. [Mild] Theoretical

▶ Lorlatinib is predicted to decrease the exposure to **pazopanib**. [Severe] Study
▶ Lumacaftor is predicted to decrease the exposure to **pazopanib**. Avoid. [Severe] Theoretical
▶ Macrolides (clarithromycin) are predicted to increase the exposure to **pazopanib**. Avoid or adjust dose—consult product literature. [Moderate] Study
▶ Macrolides (erythromycin) are predicted to increase the exposure to **pazopanib**. [Moderate] Study → Also see TABLE 8 p. 1573
▶ **Pazopanib** is predicted to increase the exposure to mavacamten. Monitor and adjust dose—consult product literature. [Moderate] Theoretical
▶ Mitotane is predicted to decrease the exposure to **pazopanib**. Avoid. [Severe] Theoretical
▶ Neurokinin-1 receptor antagonists (aprepitant, netupitant) are predicted to increase the exposure to **pazopanib**. [Moderate] Study
▶ Nilotinib is predicted to increase the exposure to **pazopanib**. [Moderate] Study → Also see TABLE 8 p. 1573
▶ NNRTIs (efavirenz, etravirine, nevirapine) are predicted to decrease the exposure to **pazopanib**. [Severe] Study → Also see TABLE 8 p. 1573
▶ **Pazopanib** is predicted to increase the risk of bleeding events when given with phenindione. [Severe] Theoretical
▶ Proton pump inhibitors are predicted to decrease the exposure to **pazopanib**. Avoid or administer concurrently without food. [Moderate] Study
▶ Rifamycins (rifampicin) are predicted to decrease the exposure to **pazopanib**. Avoid. [Severe] Theoretical
▶ Oral sodium bicarbonate -containing antacids might decrease the absorption of oral **pazopanib**. Manufacturer advises take 1 hour before or 2 hours after antacids. [Moderate] Theoretical
▶ Sotorasib is predicted to decrease the exposure to **pazopanib**. [Severe] Study
▶ St John's wort is predicted to decrease the exposure to **pazopanib**. [Severe] Study
▶ **Pazopanib** might affect the exposure to statins (atorvastatin, pravastatin, rosuvastatin). [Moderate] Theoretical
▶ **Pazopanib** might cause increased ALT concentrations when given with statins (simvastatin). [Moderate] Study
▶ Tucatinib is predicted to increase the exposure to **pazopanib**. Avoid or adjust dose—consult product literature. [Moderate] Study

Pegaspargase → see TABLE 1 p. 1571 (hepatotoxicity), TABLE 14 p. 1575 (myelosuppression), TABLE 3 p. 1571 (anticoagulant effects)
▶ **Pegaspargase** is predicted to increase the risk of hepatotoxicity when given with imatinib. [Severe] Theoretical → Also see TABLE 14 p. 1575
▶ **Pegaspargase** affects the efficacy of methotrexate. [Severe] Anecdotal → Also see TABLE 1 p. 1571 → Also see TABLE 14 p. 1575
▶ **Pegaspargase** potentially increases the risk of neurotoxicity when given with vinca alkaloids (vincristine). Vincristine should be taken 3 to 24 hours before **pegaspargase**. [Severe] Anecdotal → Also see TABLE 14 p. 1575

Pegfilgrastim
▶ **Pegfilgrastim** might increase the risk of pulmonary toxicity when given with bleomycin. [Severe] Theoretical

Peginterferon alfa → see interferons

Pembrolizumab → see monoclonal antibodies

Pemetrexed → see TABLE 1 p. 1571 (hepatotoxicity), TABLE 14 p. 1575 (myelosuppression), TABLE 2 p. 1571 (nephrotoxicity)
▶ Antimalarials (pyrimethamine) are predicted to increase the risk of adverse effects when given with **pemetrexed**. [Severe] Theoretical
▶ Aspirin (high-dose) potentially increases the exposure to **pemetrexed**. Use with caution or avoid. [Severe] Theoretical → Also see TABLE 2 p. 1571
▶ Live vaccines are predicted to increase the risk of generalised infection (possibly life-threatening) when given with **pemetrexed**. UKHSA advises avoid (refer to Green Book). [Severe] Theoretical
▶ NSAIDs are predicted to increase the exposure to **pemetrexed**. Use with caution or avoid. [Severe] Theoretical → Also see TABLE 2 p. 1571

Pemigatinib
- **Pemigatinib** might increase the exposure to the active metabolite of alkylating agents **(cyclophosphamide)**. Moderate Theoretical
- **Pemigatinib** might decrease the exposure to alkylating agents **(ifosfamide)**. Moderate Theoretical
- Anti-androgens **(apalutamide, enzalutamide)** are predicted to decrease the exposure to **pemigatinib**. Avoid. Severe Study
- Antiarrhythmics **(dronedarone)** are predicted to increase the exposure to **pemigatinib**. Severe Study
- Antiepileptics **(carbamazepine, fosphenytoin, phenobarbital, phenytoin, primidone)** are predicted to decrease the exposure to **pemigatinib**. Avoid. Severe Study
- Antifungals, azoles **(fluconazole, isavuconazole)** are predicted to increase the exposure to **pemigatinib**. Severe Study
- Antifungals, azoles **(itraconazole, ketoconazole, posaconazole, voriconazole)** are predicted to increase the exposure to **pemigatinib**. Avoid or adjust dose—consult product literature. Severe Study
- Berotralstat is predicted to increase the exposure to **pemigatinib**. Severe Study
- Calcium channel blockers **(diltiazem, verapamil)** are predicted to increase the exposure to **pemigatinib**. Severe Study
- Ceritinib is predicted to increase the exposure to **pemigatinib**. Avoid or adjust dose—consult product literature. Severe Study
- Cobicistat is predicted to increase the exposure to **pemigatinib**. Avoid or adjust dose—consult product literature. Severe Study
- Crizotinib is predicted to increase the exposure to **pemigatinib**. Severe Study
- Dabrafenib is predicted to decrease the exposure to **pemigatinib**. Avoid or monitor. Severe Study
- **Pemigatinib** might increase the exposure to digoxin. Separate administration by at least 6 hours. Moderate Theoretical
- Encorafenib is predicted to decrease the exposure to **pemigatinib**. Avoid. Severe Study
- Endothelin receptor antagonists **(bosentan)** are predicted to decrease the exposure to **pemigatinib**. Avoid or monitor. Severe Study
- **Pemigatinib** might increase the exposure to everolimus. Separate administration by at least 6 hours. Moderate Theoretical
- Fedratinib is predicted to increase the exposure to **pemigatinib**. Severe Study
- Grapefruit and grapefruit juice is predicted to increase the exposure to **pemigatinib**. Avoid. Severe Study
- HIV-protease inhibitors are predicted to increase the exposure to **pemigatinib**. Avoid or adjust dose—consult product literature. Severe Study
- Idelalisib is predicted to increase the exposure to **pemigatinib**. Avoid or adjust dose—consult product literature. Severe Study
- Imatinib is predicted to increase the exposure to **pemigatinib**. Severe Study
- Ivosidenib is predicted to decrease the exposure to **pemigatinib**. Avoid. Severe Study
- Letermovir is predicted to increase the exposure to **pemigatinib**. Severe Study
- Lorlatinib is predicted to decrease the exposure to **pemigatinib**. Avoid or monitor. Severe Study
- Lumacaftor is predicted to decrease the exposure to **pemigatinib**. Avoid. Severe Study
- Macrolides **(clarithromycin)** are predicted to increase the exposure to **pemigatinib**. Avoid or adjust dose—consult product literature. Severe Study
- Macrolides **(erythromycin)** are predicted to increase the exposure to **pemigatinib**. Severe Study
- Mitotane is predicted to decrease the exposure to **pemigatinib**. Avoid. Severe Study
- Neurokinin-1 receptor antagonists **(aprepitant, netupitant)** are predicted to increase the exposure to **pemigatinib**. Severe Study
- Nilotinib is predicted to increase the exposure to **pemigatinib**. Severe Study
- NNRTIs **(efavirenz)** are predicted to decrease the exposure to **pemigatinib** and **pemigatinib** might decrease the exposure to NNRTIs **(efavirenz)**. Avoid or monitor. Severe Study

- NNRTIs **(etravirine, nevirapine)** are predicted to decrease the exposure to **pemigatinib**. Avoid or monitor. Severe Study
- **Pemigatinib** might decrease the exposure to opioids **(methadone)**. Moderate Theoretical
- **Pemigatinib** is predicted to increase the risk of hyperphosphataemia when given with phosphate. Moderate Theoretical
- Proton pump inhibitors have been reported to decrease the exposure to **pemigatinib**. Avoid. Severe Anecdotal
- Rifamycins **(rifampicin)** are predicted to decrease the exposure to **pemigatinib**. Avoid. Severe Study
- **Pemigatinib** might increase the exposure to sirolimus. Separate administration by at least 6 hours. Moderate Theoretical
- Sotorasib is predicted to decrease the exposure to **pemigatinib**. Avoid or monitor. Severe Study
- St John's wort is predicted to decrease the exposure to **pemigatinib**. Avoid. Severe Study
- **Pemigatinib** might increase the exposure to talazoparib. Separate administration by at least 6 hours. Moderate Theoretical
- **Pemigatinib** might increase the exposure to taxanes **(paclitaxel)**. Separate administration by at least 6 hours. Moderate Theoretical
- Tucatinib is predicted to increase the exposure to **pemigatinib**. Avoid or adjust dose—consult product literature. Severe Study

Penicillamine
- Oral antacids decrease the absorption of oral **penicillamine**. Separate administration by 2 hours. Mild Study
- Antimalarials **(chloroquine)** are predicted to increase the risk of haematological toxicity when given with **penicillamine**. Avoid. Severe Theoretical
- **Penicillamine** potentially decreases the concentration of digoxin. Separate administration by 2 hours. Severe Anecdotal
- Hydroxychloroquine is predicted to increase the risk of haematological toxicity when given with **penicillamine**. Avoid. Severe Theoretical
- Oral iron is predicted to decrease the absorption of oral **penicillamine**. Separate administration by at least 2 hours. Mild Study
- Zinc is predicted to decrease the absorption of **penicillamine**. Mild Theoretical

Penicillins

> amoxicillin · ampicillin · benzathine benzylpenicillin · benzylpenicillin · flucloxacillin · phenoxymethylpenicillin · piperacillin · pivmecillinam · temocillin

- Allopurinol increases the risk of skin rash when given with penicillins **(amoxicillin, ampicillin)**. Moderate Study
- Antiepileptics **(valproate)** increase the risk of adverse effects when given with **pivmecillinam**. Avoid. Severe Anecdotal
- **Flucloxacillin** (particularly high-dose) might greatly decrease the concentration of antifungals, azoles **(isavuconazole)**. Moderate Anecdotal
- **Flucloxacillin** (particularly high-dose) might greatly decrease the concentration of antifungals, azoles **(posaconazole)**. Moderate Study
- **Flucloxacillin** (particularly high-dose) might greatly decrease the concentration of antifungals, azoles **(voriconazole)**. Avoid or monitor. Moderate Study
- **Penicillins** potentially alter the anticoagulant effect of coumarins. Monitor INR and adjust dose. Severe Anecdotal
- **Flucloxacillin** (high-dose) might decrease the exposure to everolimus. Moderate Study
- Ivosidenib is predicted to increase the exposure to benzylpenicillin. Use with caution or avoid. Moderate Theoretical
- Leflunomide is predicted to increase the exposure to benzylpenicillin. Moderate Study
- **Penicillins** are predicted to increase the risk of toxicity when given with methotrexate. Severe Anecdotal
- **Piperacillin** increases the effects of neuromuscular blocking drugs, non-depolarising. Moderate Study
- Nitisinone is predicted to increase the exposure to benzylpenicillin. Moderate Study

Penicillins (continued)
- **Paracetamol** has been reported to cause high anion gap metabolic acidosis when given with **flucloxacillin**. Severe Anecdotal
- **Penicillins** are predicted to increase the risk of bleeding events when given with **phenindione**. Severe Theoretical
- **Piperacillin** increases the effects of **suxamethonium**. Moderate Study
- **Flucloxacillin** (high-dose) might decrease the exposure to **tacrolimus**. Moderate Study
- **Teriflunomide** is predicted to increase the exposure to **benzylpenicillin**. Moderate Study
- **Benzylpenicillin** is predicted to increase the exposure to **vadadustat** and **vadadustat** is predicted to increase the exposure to **benzylpenicillin**. Moderate Study

Pentamidine → see TABLE 2 p. 1571 (nephrotoxicity), TABLE 8 p. 1573 (QT-interval prolongation), TABLE 15 p. 1575 (increased serum potassium)
- **Foscarnet** increases the risk of hypocalcaemia when given with **pentamidine**. Severe Anecdotal → Also see TABLE 2 p. 1571
- **Pentamidine** might enhance the antidiuretic and hypertensive effects of **vasopressin**. Moderate Theoretical

Pentazocine → see opioids

Pentosan → see TABLE 3 p. 1571 (anticoagulant effects)

Pentostatin → see TABLE 14 p. 1575 (myelosuppression)
- **Alkylating agents (cyclophosphamide)** (high-dose) increase the risk of toxicity when given with **pentostatin**. Avoid. Severe Anecdotal → Also see TABLE 14 p. 1575
- **Fludarabine** increases the risk of pulmonary toxicity when given with **pentostatin**. Avoid. Severe Study → Also see TABLE 14 p. 1575

Pentoxifylline
- **Pentoxifylline** is predicted to increase the concentration of **aminophylline**. Use with caution or avoid. Severe Theoretical
- **Quinolones (ciprofloxacin)** very slightly increase the exposure to **pentoxifylline**. Moderate Study
- **SSRIs (fluvoxamine)** are predicted to increase the exposure to **pentoxifylline**. Moderate Theoretical
- **Pentoxifylline** increases the concentration of **theophylline**. Monitor and adjust dose. Severe Study

Peppermint
- **Peppermint** oil is predicted to increase the exposure to **lomitapide**. Separate administration by 12 hours. Moderate Theoretical

Perampanel → see antiepileptics

Pericyazine → see phenothiazines

Perindopril → see ACE inhibitors

Pertuzumab → see monoclonal antibodies

Pethidine → see opioids

Phenazone → see NSAIDs

Phenelzine → see MAOIs, irreversible

Phenindione → see TABLE 3 p. 1571 (anticoagulant effects)

FOOD AND LIFESTYLE The effects of phenindione can be reduced or abolished by vitamin K, including that found in health foods, food supplements, enteral feeds, or large amounts of some green vegetables or green tea. Major changes in diet (especially involving salads and vegetables) and in alcohol consumption can affect anticoagulant control.

- **Antiarrhythmics (dronedarone)** might increase the anticoagulant effect of **phenindione**. Moderate Anecdotal
- **Antiarrhythmics (propafenone)** are predicted to increase the anticoagulant effect of **phenindione**. Monitor and adjust dose. Moderate Theoretical
- **Antifungals, azoles (miconazole)** greatly increase the anticoagulant effect of **phenindione**. Severe Theoretical
- **Cephalosporins (cefazolin, ceftriaxone)** potentially increase the risk of bleeding events when given with **phenindione**. Severe Anecdotal
- **Ceritinib** is predicted to increase the exposure to **phenindione**. Severe Theoretical
- **Corticosteroids** are predicted to increase the effects of **phenindione**. Moderate Anecdotal
- **Crizotinib** is predicted to increase the risk of bleeding events when given with **phenindione**. Severe Theoretical

- **Dabrafenib** is predicted to decrease the exposure to **phenindione**. Moderate Study
- **Disulfiram** is predicted to increase the anticoagulant effect of **phenindione**. Severe Theoretical
- **Enteral feeds** (vitamin-K containing) potentially decrease the effects of **phenindione**. Severe Theoretical
- **Erlotinib** is predicted to increase the risk of bleeding events when given with **phenindione**. Severe Theoretical
- **Fibrates** are predicted to increase the anticoagulant effect of **phenindione**. Monitor INR and adjust dose. Severe Study
- **Fostamatinib** might cause bleeding when given with **phenindione**. Moderate Theoretical
- **Gefitinib** is predicted to increase the risk of bleeding events when given with **phenindione**. Severe Theoretical
- **H_2 receptor antagonists (cimetidine)** increase the exposure to **phenindione**. Severe Anecdotal
- **Imatinib** is predicted to increase the risk of bleeding events when given with **phenindione**. Severe Theoretical
- **Lapatinib** is predicted to increase the risk of bleeding events when given with **phenindione**. Severe Theoretical
- **Macrolides (azithromycin)** might increase the risk of bleeding events when given with **phenindione**. Severe Theoretical
- **Nilotinib** is predicted to increase the risk of bleeding events when given with **phenindione**. Severe Theoretical
- **Opioids (tramadol)** might increase the anticoagulant effect of **phenindione**. Severe Anecdotal
- **Oxymetholone** increases the anticoagulant effect of **phenindione**. Severe Anecdotal
- **Paracetamol** is predicted to increase the anticoagulant effect of **phenindione**. Severe Theoretical
- **Pazopanib** is predicted to increase the risk of bleeding events when given with **phenindione**. Severe Theoretical
- **Penicillins** are predicted to increase the risk of bleeding events when given with **phenindione**. Severe Theoretical
- **Selumetinib** might increase the risk of bleeding when given with **phenindione**. Severe Theoretical
- **Statins (rosuvastatin)** are predicted to increase the anticoagulant effect of **phenindione**. Monitor INR and adjust dose. Severe Theoretical
- **Tetracyclines** are predicted to increase the anticoagulant effect of **phenindione**. Severe Theoretical
- **Tigecycline** is predicted to increase the anticoagulant effect of **phenindione**. Severe Theoretical
- **Tofacitinib** is predicted to increase the risk of bleeding when given with **phenindione**. Severe Theoretical
- **Vemurafenib** is predicted to increase the exposure to **phenindione**. Moderate Study

Phenobarbital → see antiepileptics

Phenothiazines → see TABLE 17 p. 1576 (hyponatraemia), TABLE 7 p. 1572 (hypotension), TABLE 8 p. 1573 (QT-interval prolongation), TABLE 9 p. 1573 (antimuscarinics), TABLE 10 p. 1574 (CNS effects)

chlorpromazine · levomepromazine · pericyazine · prochlorperazine · promazine · trifluoperazine

FOOD AND LIFESTYLE **Chlorpromazine** dose adjustment might be necessary if smoking started or stopped during treatment.

- **Phenothiazines** are predicted to decrease the effects of **amfetamines** and **amfetamines** are predicted to decrease the effects of **phenothiazines**. Moderate Study
- Oral **antacids** decrease the absorption of oral **phenothiazines**. Moderate Anecdotal
- **Chlorpromazine** decreases the concentration of **antiepileptics (phenobarbital, primidone)** and **antiepileptics (phenobarbital, primidone)** decrease the concentration of **chlorpromazine**. Moderate Study → Also see TABLE 10 p. 1574
- **Antipsychotics, second generation (clozapine)** can cause constipation, as can **phenothiazines**; concurrent use might increase the risk of developing intestinal obstruction. Severe Theoretical → Also see TABLE 17 p. 1576 → Also see TABLE 7 p. 1572 → Also see TABLE 9 p. 1573 → Also see TABLE 10 p. 1574
- **Combined hormonal contraceptives** is predicted to increase the exposure to **chlorpromazine**. Moderate Theoretical

▸ **Chlorpromazine** is predicted to increase the risk of hyponatraemia when given with desmopressin. Severe Theoretical → Also see **TABLE 17** p. 1576

▸ **Phenothiazines** are predicted to decrease the effects of dopamine receptor agonists. Avoid. Moderate Theoretical → Also see **TABLE 7** p. 1572 → Also see **TABLE 8** p. 1573 → Also see **TABLE 9** p. 1573 → Also see **TABLE 10** p. 1574

▸ **Phenothiazines** oppose the effects of the active metabolite of foslevodopa. Severe Theoretical → Also see **TABLE 7** p. 1572 → Also see **TABLE 10** p. 1574

▸ Givosiran is predicted to increase the exposure to **chlorpromazine**. Moderate Theoretical

▸ **Phenothiazines** decrease the effects of levodopa. Avoid or monitor worsening parkinsonian symptoms. Severe Study → Also see **TABLE 7** p. 1572 → Also see **TABLE 10** p. 1574

▸ **Phenothiazines** potentially increase the risk of neurotoxicity when given with lithium. Severe Anecdotal

▸ MAOIs, irreversible are predicted to increase the risk of neuroleptic malignant syndrome when given with **phenothiazines**. Severe Theoretical → Also see **TABLE 7** p. 1572

▸ **Chlorpromazine** decreases the effects of metyrapone. Avoid. Moderate Theoretical

▸ Mexiletine is predicted to increase the exposure to **chlorpromazine**. Moderate Theoretical

▸ Moclobemide increases the risk of adverse effects when given with **levomepromazine**. Moderate Study

▸ Osilodrostat is predicted to increase the exposure to **chlorpromazine**. Moderate Theoretical → Also see **TABLE 8** p. 1573

▸ Quinolones (ciprofloxacin) are predicted to increase the exposure to **chlorpromazine**. Moderate Theoretical

▸ Rucaparib is predicted to increase the exposure to **chlorpromazine**. Moderate Theoretical

▸ SSRIs (fluvoxamine) are predicted to increase the exposure to **chlorpromazine**. Moderate Theoretical → Also see **TABLE 17** p. 1576 → Also see **TABLE 10** p. 1574

▸ Vemurafenib is predicted to increase the exposure to **chlorpromazine**. Moderate Theoretical → Also see **TABLE 8** p. 1573

Phenoxymethylpenicillin → see penicillins

Phenylephrine → see sympathomimetics, vasoconstrictor

Phenytoin → see antiepileptics

Phosphate

▸ Pemigatinib is predicted to increase the risk of hyperphosphataemia when given with **phosphate**. Moderate Theoretical

Phosphodiesterase type-4 inhibitors

apremilast · roflumilast

▸ Aminophylline is predicted to slightly increase the exposure to **roflumilast**. Avoid. Moderate Theoretical

▸ Anti-androgens (apalutamide, enzalutamide) moderately decrease the exposure to **apremilast**. Avoid. Severe Study

▸ Anti-androgens (apalutamide, enzalutamide) are predicted to decrease the exposure to **roflumilast**. Avoid. Moderate Study

▸ Antiepileptics (carbamazepine, fosphenytoin, phenobarbital, phenytoin, primidone) moderately decrease the exposure to **apremilast**. Avoid. Severe Study

▸ Antiepileptics (carbamazepine, fosphenytoin, phenobarbital, phenytoin, primidone) are predicted to decrease the exposure to **roflumilast**. Avoid. Moderate Study

▸ Combined hormonal contraceptives is predicted to increase the exposure to **roflumilast**. Moderate Theoretical

▸ Encorafenib moderately decreases the exposure to **apremilast**. Avoid. Severe Study

▸ Encorafenib is predicted to decrease the exposure to **roflumilast**. Avoid. Moderate Study

▸ Givosiran is predicted to increase the exposure to **roflumilast**. Moderate Theoretical

▸ H_2 receptor antagonists (cimetidine) slightly increase the exposure to **roflumilast**. Moderate Study

▸ Ivosidenib moderately decreases the exposure to **apremilast**. Avoid. Severe Study

▸ Ivosidenib is predicted to decrease the exposure to **roflumilast**. Avoid. Moderate Study

▸ Lumacaftor moderately decreases the exposure to **apremilast**. Avoid. Severe Study

▸ Lumacaftor is predicted to decrease the exposure to **roflumilast**. Avoid. Moderate Study

▸ Mexiletine is predicted to increase the exposure to **roflumilast**. Moderate Theoretical

▸ Mitotane moderately decreases the exposure to **apremilast**. Avoid. Severe Study

▸ Mitotane is predicted to decrease the exposure to **roflumilast**. Avoid. Moderate Study

▸ Osilodrostat is predicted to increase the exposure to **roflumilast**. Moderate Theoretical

▸ Quinolones (ciprofloxacin) are predicted to increase the exposure to **roflumilast**. Moderate Theoretical

▸ Rifamycins (rifampicin) moderately decrease the exposure to **apremilast**. Avoid. Severe Study

▸ Rifamycins (rifampicin) are predicted to decrease the exposure to **roflumilast**. Avoid. Moderate Study

▸ Rucaparib is predicted to increase the exposure to **roflumilast**. Moderate Theoretical

▸ SSRIs (fluvoxamine) are predicted to increase the exposure to **roflumilast**. Moderate Study

▸ St John's wort is predicted to decrease the exposure to **apremilast**. Avoid. Severe Theoretical

▸ Theophylline is predicted to slightly increase the exposure to **roflumilast**. Avoid. Moderate Theoretical

▸ Vemurafenib is predicted to increase the exposure to **roflumilast**. Moderate Theoretical

Phosphodiesterase type-5 inhibitors → see **TABLE 7** p. 1572 (hypotension), **TABLE 8** p. 1573 (QT-interval prolongation)

avanafil · sildenafil · tadalafil · vardenafil

▸ Alpha blockers cause significant hypotensive effects when given with **phosphodiesterase type-5 inhibitors**. Patient should be stabilised on first drug then second drug should be added at the lowest recommended dose. Severe Study → Also see **TABLE 7** p. 1572

▸ Anti-androgens (apalutamide, enzalutamide) are predicted to decrease the exposure to phosphodiesterase type-5 inhibitors (avanafil, tadalafil). Avoid. Severe Study

▸ Anti-androgens (apalutamide, enzalutamide) are predicted to decrease the exposure to phosphodiesterase type-5 inhibitors (sildenafil, vardenafil). Moderate Theoretical → Also see **TABLE 8** p. 1573

▸ Antiarrhythmics (dronedarone) are predicted to increase the exposure to avanafil. Adjust **avanafil** dose, p. 939. Moderate Theoretical

▸ Antiarrhythmics (dronedarone) are predicted to increase the exposure to **sildenafil**. Monitor or adjust **sildenafil** dose with moderate CYP3A4 inhibitors, p. 940. Moderate Study

▸ Antiarrhythmics (dronedarone) are predicted to increase the exposure to **tadalafil**. Severe Theoretical

▸ Antiarrhythmics (dronedarone) are predicted to increase the exposure to **vardenafil**. Adjust dose. Severe Theoretical → Also see **TABLE 8** p. 1573

▸ Antiepileptics (carbamazepine, fosphenytoin, phenobarbital, phenytoin, primidone) are predicted to decrease the exposure to phosphodiesterase type-5 inhibitors (avanafil, tadalafil). Avoid. Severe Study

▸ Antiepileptics (carbamazepine, fosphenytoin, phenobarbital, phenytoin, primidone) are predicted to decrease the exposure to phosphodiesterase type-5 inhibitors (sildenafil, vardenafil). Moderate Theoretical

▸ Antifungals, azoles (fluconazole, isavuconazole) are predicted to increase the exposure to **avanafil**. Adjust **avanafil** dose, p. 939. Moderate Theoretical

▸ Antifungals, azoles (fluconazole, isavuconazole) are predicted to increase the exposure to **sildenafil**. Monitor or adjust **sildenafil** dose with moderate CYP3A4 inhibitors, p. 940. Moderate Study

▸ Antifungals, azoles (fluconazole, isavuconazole) are predicted to increase the exposure to **tadalafil**. Severe Theoretical

▸ Antifungals, azoles (fluconazole, isavuconazole) are predicted to increase the exposure to **vardenafil**. Adjust dose. Severe Theoretical → Also see **TABLE 8** p. 1573

▸ Antifungals, azoles (itraconazole, ketoconazole, posaconazole, voriconazole) are predicted to increase the exposure to **sildenafil**. Avoid potent CYP3A4 inhibitors or adjust **sildenafil** dose, p. 940. Severe Study

Phosphodiesterase type-5 inhibitors (continued)

▶ Antifungals, azoles **(itraconazole, ketoconazole, posaconazole, voriconazole)** are predicted to increase the exposure to **tadalafil**. Use with caution or avoid. [Severe] Study

▶ Antifungals, azoles **(miconazole)** are predicted to increase the exposure to **sildenafil**. Use with caution and adjust dose. [Severe] Theoretical

▶ Antifungals, azoles **(itraconazole, ketoconazole, posaconazole, voriconazole)** are predicted to increase the exposure to phosphodiesterase type-5 inhibitors **(avanafil, vardenafil)**. Avoid. [Severe] Study → Also see **TABLE 8** p. 1573

▶ **Berotralstat** is predicted to increase the exposure to **avanafil**. Adjust **avanafil** dose, p. 939. [Moderate] Theoretical

▶ **Berotralstat** is predicted to increase the exposure to **sildenafil**. Monitor or adjust **sildenafil** dose with moderate CYP3A4 inhibitors, p. 940. [Moderate] Study

▶ **Berotralstat** is predicted to increase the exposure to **tadalafil**. [Severe] Theoretical

▶ **Berotralstat** is predicted to increase the exposure to **vardenafil**. Adjust dose. [Severe] Theoretical

▶ Calcium channel blockers **(diltiazem, verapamil)** are predicted to increase the exposure to **avanafil**. Adjust **avanafil** dose, p. 939. [Moderate] Theoretical → Also see **TABLE 7** p. 1572

▶ Calcium channel blockers **(diltiazem, verapamil)** are predicted to increase the exposure to **sildenafil**. Monitor or adjust **sildenafil** dose with moderate CYP3A4 inhibitors, p. 940. [Moderate] Study → Also see **TABLE 7** p. 1572

▶ Calcium channel blockers **(diltiazem, verapamil)** are predicted to increase the exposure to **tadalafil**. [Severe] Theoretical → Also see **TABLE 7** p. 1572

▶ Calcium channel blockers **(diltiazem, verapamil)** are predicted to increase the exposure to **vardenafil**. Adjust dose. [Severe] Theoretical → Also see **TABLE 7** p. 1572

▶ **Cenobamate** is predicted to decrease the exposure to phosphodiesterase type-5 inhibitors **(avanafil, sildenafil, vardenafil)**. Adjust dose. [Moderate] Theoretical

▶ **Ceritinib** is predicted to increase the exposure to phosphodiesterase type-5 inhibitors **(avanafil, vardenafil)**. Avoid. [Severe] Study → Also see **TABLE 8** p. 1573

▶ **Ceritinib** is predicted to increase the exposure to **sildenafil**. Avoid potent CYP3A4 inhibitors or adjust **sildenafil** dose, p. 940. [Severe] Study

▶ **Ceritinib** is predicted to increase the exposure to **tadalafil**. Use with caution or avoid. [Severe] Study

▶ **Cobicistat** is predicted to increase the exposure to phosphodiesterase type-5 inhibitors **(avanafil, vardenafil)**. Avoid. [Severe] Study

▶ **Cobicistat** is predicted to increase the exposure to **sildenafil**. Avoid potent CYP3A4 inhibitors or adjust **sildenafil** dose, p. 940. [Severe] Study

▶ **Cobicistat** is predicted to increase the exposure to **tadalafil**. Use with caution or avoid. [Severe] Study

▶ **Crizotinib** is predicted to increase the exposure to **avanafil**. Adjust **avanafil** dose, p. 939. [Moderate] Theoretical

▶ **Crizotinib** is predicted to increase the exposure to **sildenafil**. Monitor or adjust **sildenafil** dose with moderate CYP3A4 inhibitors, p. 940. [Moderate] Study

▶ **Crizotinib** is predicted to increase the exposure to **tadalafil**. [Severe] Theoretical

▶ **Crizotinib** is predicted to increase the exposure to **vardenafil**. Adjust dose. [Severe] Theoretical → Also see **TABLE 8** p. 1573

▶ **Encorafenib** is predicted to decrease the exposure to phosphodiesterase type-5 inhibitors **(avanafil, tadalafil)**. Avoid. [Severe] Study

▶ **Encorafenib** is predicted to decrease the exposure to phosphodiesterase type-5 inhibitors **(sildenafil, vardenafil)**. [Moderate] Theoretical → Also see **TABLE 8** p. 1573

▶ Endothelin receptor antagonists **(bosentan)** decrease the exposure to **phosphodiesterase type-5 inhibitors**. [Moderate] Study

▶ **Fedratinib** is predicted to increase the exposure to **avanafil**. Adjust **avanafil** dose, p. 939. [Moderate] Theoretical

▶ **Fedratinib** is predicted to increase the exposure to **sildenafil**. Monitor or adjust **sildenafil** dose with moderate CYP3A4 inhibitors, p. 940. [Moderate] Study

▶ **Fedratinib** is predicted to increase the exposure to **tadalafil**. [Severe] Theoretical

▶ **Fedratinib** is predicted to increase the exposure to **vardenafil**. Adjust dose. [Severe] Theoretical

▶ **Givinostat** might increase the exposure to **sildenafil**. [Moderate] Study

▶ **Grapefruit** juice is predicted to increase the exposure to **phosphodiesterase type-5 inhibitors**. Use with caution or avoid. [Moderate] Study

▶ **HIV-protease inhibitors** are predicted to increase the exposure to phosphodiesterase type-5 inhibitors **(avanafil, vardenafil)**. Avoid. [Severe] Study

▶ **HIV-protease inhibitors** are predicted to increase the exposure to **sildenafil**. Avoid potent CYP3A4 inhibitors or adjust **sildenafil** dose, p. 940. [Severe] Study

▶ **HIV-protease inhibitors** are predicted to increase the exposure to **tadalafil**. Use with caution or avoid. [Severe] Study

▶ **Idelalisib** is predicted to increase the exposure to phosphodiesterase type-5 inhibitors **(avanafil, vardenafil)**. Avoid. [Severe] Study

▶ **Idelalisib** is predicted to increase the exposure to **sildenafil**. Avoid potent CYP3A4 inhibitors or adjust **sildenafil** dose, p. 940. [Severe] Study

▶ **Idelalisib** is predicted to increase the exposure to **tadalafil**. Use with caution or avoid. [Severe] Study

▶ **Imatinib** is predicted to increase the exposure to **avanafil**. Adjust **avanafil** dose, p. 939. [Moderate] Theoretical

▶ **Imatinib** is predicted to increase the exposure to **sildenafil**. Monitor or adjust **sildenafil** dose with moderate CYP3A4 inhibitors, p. 940. [Moderate] Study

▶ **Imatinib** is predicted to increase the exposure to **tadalafil**. [Severe] Theoretical

▶ **Imatinib** is predicted to increase the exposure to **vardenafil**. Adjust dose. [Severe] Theoretical

▶ **Ivosidenib** is predicted to decrease the exposure to phosphodiesterase type-5 inhibitors **(avanafil, tadalafil)**. Avoid. [Severe] Study

▶ **Ivosidenib** is predicted to decrease the exposure to phosphodiesterase type-5 inhibitors **(sildenafil, vardenafil)**. [Moderate] Theoretical → Also see **TABLE 8** p. 1573

▶ **Letermovir** is predicted to increase the exposure to **avanafil**. Adjust **avanafil** dose, p. 939. [Moderate] Theoretical

▶ **Letermovir** is predicted to increase the exposure to **sildenafil**. Monitor or adjust **sildenafil** dose with moderate CYP3A4 inhibitors, p. 940. [Moderate] Study

▶ **Letermovir** is predicted to increase the exposure to **tadalafil**. [Severe] Theoretical

▶ **Letermovir** is predicted to increase the exposure to **vardenafil**. Adjust dose. [Severe] Theoretical

▶ **Lumacaftor** is predicted to decrease the exposure to phosphodiesterase type-5 inhibitors **(avanafil, tadalafil)**. Avoid. [Severe] Study

▶ **Lumacaftor** is predicted to decrease the exposure to phosphodiesterase type-5 inhibitors **(sildenafil, vardenafil)**. [Moderate] Theoretical

▶ Macrolides **(clarithromycin)** are predicted to increase the exposure to **sildenafil**. Avoid potent CYP3A4 inhibitors or adjust **sildenafil** dose, p. 940. [Severe] Study

▶ Macrolides **(clarithromycin)** are predicted to increase the exposure to **tadalafil**. Use with caution or avoid. [Severe] Study

▶ Macrolides **(erythromycin)** are predicted to increase the exposure to **avanafil**. Adjust **avanafil** dose, p. 939. [Moderate] Theoretical

▶ Macrolides **(erythromycin)** are predicted to increase the exposure to **sildenafil**. Monitor or adjust **sildenafil** dose with moderate CYP3A4 inhibitors, p. 940. [Moderate] Study

▶ Macrolides **(erythromycin)** are predicted to increase the exposure to **tadalafil**. [Severe] Theoretical

▶ Macrolides **(erythromycin)** are predicted to increase the exposure to **vardenafil**. Adjust dose. [Severe] Theoretical → Also see **TABLE 8** p. 1573

▶ Macrolides **(clarithromycin)** are predicted to increase the exposure to phosphodiesterase type-5 inhibitors **(avanafil, vardenafil)**. Avoid. [Severe] Study

- **Mitotane** is predicted to decrease the exposure to phosphodiesterase type-5 inhibitors (**avanafil, tadalafil**). Avoid. [Severe] Study
- **Mitotane** is predicted to decrease the exposure to phosphodiesterase type-5 inhibitors (**sildenafil, vardenafil**). [Moderate] Theoretical
- Neurokinin-1 receptor antagonists (**aprepitant, netupitant**) are predicted to increase the exposure to **avanafil**. Adjust **avanafil** dose, p. 939. [Moderate] Theoretical
- Neurokinin-1 receptor antagonists (**aprepitant, netupitant**) are predicted to increase the exposure to **sildenafil**. Monitor or adjust **sildenafil** dose with moderate CYP3A4 inhibitors, p. 940. [Moderate] Study
- Neurokinin-1 receptor antagonists (**aprepitant, netupitant**) are predicted to increase the exposure to **tadalafil**. [Severe] Theoretical
- Neurokinin-1 receptor antagonists (**aprepitant, netupitant**) are predicted to increase the exposure to **vardenafil**. Adjust dose. [Severe] Theoretical
- **Nicorandil** is predicted to increase the risk of hypotension when given with **phosphodiesterase type-5 inhibitors**. Avoid. [Severe] Theoretical → Also see **TABLE 7** p. 1572
- **Nilotinib** is predicted to increase the exposure to **avanafil**. Adjust **avanafil** dose, p. 939. [Moderate] Theoretical
- **Nilotinib** is predicted to increase the exposure to **sildenafil**. Monitor or adjust **sildenafil** dose with moderate CYP3A4 inhibitors, p. 940. [Moderate] Study
- **Nilotinib** is predicted to increase the exposure to **tadalafil**. [Severe] Theoretical
- **Nilotinib** is predicted to increase the exposure to **vardenafil**. Adjust dose. [Severe] Theoretical → Also see **TABLE 8** p. 1573
- **Nirmatrelvir** boosted with ritonavir is predicted to increase the concentration of phosphodiesterase type-5 inhibitors (**avanafil, vardenafil**). Avoid. [Severe] Theoretical
- **Nirmatrelvir** boosted with ritonavir is predicted to increase the concentration of phosphodiesterase type-5 inhibitors (**sildenafil, tadalafil**). Avoid or adjust dose—consult product literature. [Severe] Theoretical
- **Nitrates** potentially increase the risk of hypotension when given with **phosphodiesterase type-5 inhibitors**. Avoid. [Severe] Study → Also see **TABLE 7** p. 1572
- NNRTIs (**efavirenz, nevirapine**) are predicted to decrease the exposure to **phosphodiesterase type-5 inhibitors**. [Moderate] Theoretical → Also see **TABLE 8** p. 1573
- NNRTIs (**etravirine**) moderately decrease the exposure to **phosphodiesterase type-5 inhibitors**. Adjust dose. [Moderate] Study
- Quinolones (**ciprofloxacin**) moderately increase the exposure to **sildenafil**. [Moderate] Theoretical
- **Ribociclib** is predicted to increase the exposure to **sildenafil**. Avoid. [Moderate] Theoretical
- Rifamycins (**rifampicin**) are predicted to decrease the exposure to phosphodiesterase type-5 inhibitors (**avanafil, tadalafil**). Avoid. [Severe] Study
- Rifamycins (**rifampicin**) are predicted to decrease the exposure to phosphodiesterase type-5 inhibitors (**sildenafil, vardenafil**). [Moderate] Theoretical
- **Phosphodiesterase type-5 inhibitors** are predicted to increase the risk of hypotension when given with sapropterin. [Moderate] Theoretical → Also see **TABLE 7** p. 1572
- St John's wort is predicted to decrease the exposure to **phosphodiesterase type-5 inhibitors**. [Moderate] Theoretical
- **Tucatinib** is predicted to increase the exposure to phosphodiesterase type-5 inhibitors (**avanafil, vardenafil**). Avoid. [Severe] Study
- **Tucatinib** is predicted to increase the exposure to **sildenafil**. Avoid potent CYP3A4 inhibitors or adjust **sildenafil** dose, p. 940. [Severe] Study
- **Tucatinib** is predicted to increase the exposure to **tadalafil**. Use with caution or avoid. [Severe] Study

Pibrentasvir

- **Pibrentasvir** is predicted to increase the exposure to afatinib. [Moderate] Study
- **Pibrentasvir** with glecaprevir is predicted to increase the exposure to aliskiren. [Moderate] Study

- Anti-androgens (**apalutamide, enzalutamide**) are predicted to moderately to markedly decrease the exposure to **pibrentasvir**. Avoid. [Severe] Study
- Antiarrhythmics (**amiodarone**) are predicted to increase the exposure to **pibrentasvir**. [Moderate] Theoretical
- Antiarrhythmics (**dronedarone**) potentially increase the exposure to **pibrentasvir**. [Moderate] Theoretical
- Antiepileptics (**carbamazepine, fosphenytoin, phenobarbital, phenytoin, primidone**) are predicted to moderately to markedly decrease the exposure to **pibrentasvir**. Avoid. [Severe] Study
- Antiepileptics (**eslicarbazepine, oxcarbazepine**) potentially decrease the exposure to **pibrentasvir**. Avoid. [Severe] Theoretical
- Antifungals, azoles (**itraconazole, ketoconazole**) are predicted to increase the exposure to **pibrentasvir**. [Moderate] Theoretical
- **Pibrentasvir** with glecaprevir is predicted to increase the exposure to antihistamines, non-sedating (**fexofenadine**). [Moderate] Study
- **Pibrentasvir** is predicted to increase the exposure to bictegravir. Use with caution or avoid. [Moderate] Theoretical
- Calcium channel blockers (**verapamil**) are predicted to increase the exposure to **pibrentasvir**. [Moderate] Theoretical
- **Cenobamate** is predicted to decrease the exposure to **pibrentasvir**. Avoid. [Severe] Study
- **Pibrentasvir** with glecaprevir is predicted to increase the exposure to colchicine. [Moderate] Study
- **Combined hormonal contraceptives** (containing ethinylestradiol) are predicted to increase the risk of increased ALT concentrations when given with **pibrentasvir**. Avoid. [Severe] Study
- **Crizotinib** potentially decreases the exposure to **pibrentasvir**. Avoid. [Severe] Theoretical
- **Dabrafenib** is predicted to decrease the exposure to **pibrentasvir**. Avoid. [Severe] Study
- **Pibrentasvir** with glecaprevir increases the exposure to digoxin. [Moderate] Study
- **Encorafenib** is predicted to moderately to markedly decrease the exposure to **pibrentasvir**. Avoid. [Severe] Study
- Endothelin receptor antagonists (**bosentan**) are predicted to decrease the exposure to **pibrentasvir**. Avoid. [Severe] Study
- **Pibrentasvir** with glecaprevir is predicted to increase the exposure to everolimus. [Moderate] Study
- **Pibrentasvir** with glecaprevir is predicted to increase the exposure to factor XA inhibitors (**edoxaban**). [Moderate] Study
- **Pibrentasvir** is predicted to increase the exposure to fidaxomicin. Avoid. [Moderate] Study
- HIV-protease inhibitors (**atazanavir, lopinavir**) boosted with ritonavir increase the exposure to **pibrentasvir**. Avoid. [Severe] Study
- HIV-protease inhibitors (**ritonavir**) potentially increase the exposure to **pibrentasvir**. [Severe] Theoretical
- **Ivosidenib** is predicted to moderately to markedly decrease the exposure to **pibrentasvir**. Avoid. [Severe] Study
- **Lapatinib** is predicted to increase the exposure to **pibrentasvir**. [Moderate] Theoretical
- **Pibrentasvir** with glecaprevir is predicted to increase the exposure to loperamide. [Moderate] Study
- **Lorlatinib** is predicted to decrease the exposure to **pibrentasvir**. Avoid. [Severe] Study
- **Lumacaftor** is predicted to moderately to markedly decrease the exposure to **pibrentasvir**. Avoid. [Severe] Study
- **Macrolides** are predicted to increase the exposure to **pibrentasvir**. [Moderate] Theoretical
- **Mitotane** is predicted to moderately to markedly decrease the exposure to **pibrentasvir**. Avoid. [Severe] Study
- **Pibrentasvir** is predicted to increase the risk of neutropenia when given with monoclonal antibodies (**brentuximab vedotin**). Monitor and adjust dose. [Severe] Theoretical
- **Pibrentasvir** is predicted to increase the exposure to neratinib. Avoid or adjust dose and monitor for gastrointestinal adverse effects—consult product literature. [Severe] Study
- **Pibrentasvir** is predicted to increase the exposure to nintedanib. [Moderate] Study
- **Nirmatrelvir** boosted with ritonavir is predicted to increase the concentration of **pibrentasvir**. Avoid. [Severe] Theoretical

Pibrentasvir (continued)

▸ NNRTIs (efavirenz, etravirine, nevirapine) are predicted to decrease the exposure to **pibrentasvir**. Avoid. [Severe] Study

▸ **Pibrentasvir** is predicted to increase the exposure to pralsetinib. [Moderate] Theoretical

▸ Ranolazine is predicted to increase the exposure to **pibrentasvir**. [Moderate] Theoretical

▸ **Pibrentasvir** is predicted to increase the exposure to relugolix. Avoid or take relugolix first and separate administration by at least 6 hours. [Moderate] Study

▸ Rifamycins (rifampicin) are predicted to moderately to markedly decrease the exposure to **pibrentasvir**. Avoid. [Severe] Study

▸ **Pibrentasvir** is predicted to increase the exposure to rimegepant. Avoid another dose of rimegepant within 48 hours of concurrent use. [Moderate] Theoretical

▸ **Pibrentasvir** with glecaprevir is predicted to increase the exposure to sirolimus. [Moderate] Study

▸ Sotorasib is predicted to decrease the exposure to **pibrentasvir**. Avoid. [Severe] Study

▸ St John's wort is predicted to decrease the exposure to **pibrentasvir**. Avoid. [Severe] Study

▸ **Pibrentasvir** with glecaprevir markedly increases the exposure to statins (atorvastatin). Avoid. [Severe] Study

▸ **Pibrentasvir** with glecaprevir is predicted to increase the exposure to statins (fluvastatin). [Moderate] Theoretical

▸ **Pibrentasvir** with glecaprevir moderately increases the exposure to statins (pravastatin). Use with caution and adjust pravastatin dose. [Moderate] Study

▸ **Pibrentasvir** with glecaprevir moderately increases the exposure to statins (rosuvastatin). Use with caution and adjust rosuvastatin dose, p. 235. [Moderate] Study

▸ **Pibrentasvir** with glecaprevir moderately increases the exposure to statins (simvastatin). Avoid. [Moderate] Study

▸ **Pibrentasvir** with glecaprevir slightly increases the exposure to tacrolimus. Monitor and adjust dose. [Mild] Study

▸ **Pibrentasvir** is predicted to slightly increase the exposure to talazoparib. Avoid or adjust dose—consult product literature. [Severe] Study

▸ **Pibrentasvir** with glecaprevir is predicted to increase the exposure to taxanes (paclitaxel). [Moderate] Study

▸ **Pibrentasvir** with glecaprevir increases the exposure to thrombin inhibitors (dabigatran). Avoid. [Moderate] Study

▸ **Pibrentasvir** is predicted to increase the exposure to topotecan. [Severe] Study

▸ **Pibrentasvir** is predicted to increase the concentration of trametinib. [Moderate] Theoretical

▸ Vemurafenib is predicted to increase the exposure to **pibrentasvir**. [Moderate] Theoretical

Pilocarpine

> **ROUTE-SPECIFIC INFORMATION** Since systemic absorption can follow topical application, the possibility of interactions should be borne in mind.

Pimecrolimus

▸ Alcohol increases the risk of facial flushing and skin irritation when given with topical **pimecrolimus**. [Moderate] Study

▸ **Pimecrolimus** is predicted to decrease the efficacy of mifamurtide. Avoid. [Severe] Theoretical

Pimozide → see TABLE 17 p. 1576 (hyponatraemia), TABLE 7 p. 1572 (hypotension), TABLE 8 p. 1573 (QT-interval prolongation), TABLE 9 p. 1573 (antimuscarinics), TABLE 10 p. 1574 (CNS effects)

▸ Antiarrhythmics (dronedarone) are predicted to increase the exposure to **pimozide**. Avoid. [Severe] Theoretical → Also see TABLE 8 p. 1573

▸ Antifungals, azoles (fluconazole, isavuconazole) are predicted to increase the exposure to **pimozide**. Avoid. [Severe] Theoretical → Also see TABLE 8 p. 1573

▸ Antifungals, azoles (itraconazole, ketoconazole, posaconazole, voriconazole) are predicted to increase the exposure to **pimozide**. Avoid. [Severe] Study → Also see TABLE 8 p. 1573

▸ Antifungals, azoles (miconazole) are predicted to increase the exposure to **pimozide**. Avoid. [Moderate] Theoretical

▸ Antipsychotics, second generation (clozapine) can cause constipation, as can **pimozide**; concurrent use might increase the risk of developing intestinal obstruction. [Severe]

Theoretical → Also see TABLE 17 p. 1576 → Also see TABLE 7 p. 1572 → Also see TABLE 9 p. 1573 → Also see TABLE 10 p. 1574

▸ Berotralstat is predicted to increase the exposure to **pimozide**. Avoid. [Severe] Theoretical

▸ Calcium channel blockers (diltiazem, verapamil) are predicted to increase the exposure to **pimozide**. Avoid. [Severe] Theoretical → Also see TABLE 7 p. 1572

▸ Ceritinib is predicted to increase the exposure to **pimozide**. Avoid. [Severe] Study → Also see TABLE 8 p. 1573

▸ Cobicistat is predicted to increase the exposure to **pimozide**. Avoid. [Severe] Study

▸ Crizotinib is predicted to increase the exposure to **pimozide**. Avoid. [Severe] Theoretical → Also see TABLE 8 p. 1573

▸ **Pimozide** is predicted to decrease the effects of dopamine receptor agonists. Avoid. [Moderate] Theoretical → Also see TABLE 7 p. 1572 → Also see TABLE 8 p. 1573 → Also see TABLE 9 p. 1573 → Also see TABLE 10 p. 1574

▸ Fedratinib is predicted to increase the exposure to **pimozide**. Avoid. [Severe] Theoretical

▸ **Pimozide** opposes the effects of the active metabolite of foslevodopa. [Severe] Theoretical → Also see TABLE 7 p. 1572 → Also see TABLE 10 p. 1574

▸ Grapefruit juice increases the exposure to **pimozide**. Avoid. [Severe] Theoretical

▸ HIV-protease inhibitors are predicted to increase the exposure to **pimozide**. Avoid. [Severe] Study

▸ Idelalisib is predicted to increase the exposure to **pimozide**. Avoid. [Severe] Study

▸ Imatinib is predicted to increase the exposure to **pimozide**. Avoid. [Severe] Theoretical

▸ Ivosidenib might decrease the exposure to **pimozide**. Avoid or monitor efficacy. [Moderate] Theoretical → Also see TABLE 8 p. 1573

▸ Larotrectinib is predicted to increase the exposure to **pimozide**. Use with caution and adjust dose. [Mild] Theoretical

▸ Letermovir is predicted to increase the exposure to **pimozide**. Avoid. [Severe] Theoretical

▸ **Pimozide** decreases the effects of levodopa. [Severe] Theoretical → Also see TABLE 7 p. 1572 → Also see TABLE 10 p. 1574

▸ Lorlatinib is predicted to decrease the exposure to **pimozide**. Avoid. [Moderate] Theoretical

▸ Macrolides (clarithromycin) are predicted to increase the exposure to **pimozide**. Avoid. [Severe] Study

▸ Macrolides (erythromycin) are predicted to increase the exposure to **pimozide**. Avoid. [Severe] Theoretical → Also see TABLE 8 p. 1573

▸ Neurokinin-1 receptor antagonists are predicted to increase the exposure to **pimozide**. Avoid. [Severe] Theoretical

▸ Nilotinib is predicted to increase the exposure to **pimozide**. Avoid. [Severe] Theoretical → Also see TABLE 8 p. 1573

▸ Nirmatrelvir boosted with ritonavir is predicted to increase the concentration of **pimozide**. Avoid. [Severe] Theoretical

▸ Olaparib might alter the exposure to **pimozide**. [Moderate] Theoretical

▸ Palbociclib is predicted to increase the exposure to **pimozide**. Adjust dose. [Moderate] Theoretical

▸ Panobinostat is predicted to increase the exposure to **pimozide**. Avoid. [Severe] Theoretical → Also see TABLE 8 p. 1573

▸ Pitolisant is predicted to decrease the exposure to **pimozide**. Avoid. [Severe] Theoretical

▸ Ribociclib (high-dose) is predicted to increase the exposure to **pimozide**. Avoid. [Moderate] Theoretical → Also see TABLE 8 p. 1573

▸ Ritlecitinib is predicted to increase the exposure to **pimozide**. [Moderate] Theoretical

▸ Rucaparib is predicted to increase the exposure to **pimozide**. Monitor and adjust dose. [Moderate] Study

▸ Tucatinib is predicted to increase the exposure to **pimozide**. Avoid. [Severe] Study

Pindolol → see beta blockers, non-selective

Pioglitazone → see TABLE 13 p. 1575 (antidiabetic drugs)

▸ Anti-androgens (abiraterone) slightly increase the exposure to **pioglitazone**. [Moderate] Study

▸ **Pioglitazone** potentially decreases the exposure to antifungals, azoles (isavuconazole). Use with caution or avoid. [Moderate] Theoretical

▸ **Clopidogrel** increases the exposure to **pioglitazone**. Monitor blood glucose and adjust dose. ⟨Severe⟩ Study
▸ **Fenfluramine** might decrease blood glucose concentrations when given with **pioglitazone**. ⟨Moderate⟩ Theoretical
▸ **Fibrates (gemfibrozil)** increase the exposure to **pioglitazone**. Monitor blood glucose and adjust dose. ⟨Severe⟩ Study
▸ **Iron chelators (deferasirox)** are predicted to increase the exposure to **pioglitazone**. ⟨Moderate⟩ Study
▸ **Ivosidenib** might decrease the exposure to **pioglitazone**. Avoid or monitor efficacy. ⟨Unknown⟩ Study
▸ **Leflunomide** is predicted to increase the exposure to **pioglitazone**. ⟨Moderate⟩ Study
▸ **Macrolides (clarithromycin)** might cause hypoglycaemia when given with **pioglitazone**. ⟨Moderate⟩ Theoretical
▸ **Mifepristone** is predicted to increase the exposure to **pioglitazone**. ⟨Moderate⟩ Theoretical
▸ **Opicapone** is predicted to increase the exposure to **pioglitazone**. Avoid. ⟨Moderate⟩ Study
▸ **Rifamycins (rifampicin)** moderately decrease the exposure to **pioglitazone**. Monitor and adjust dose. ⟨Moderate⟩ Study
▸ **Somapacitan** might increase blood glucose concentrations, opposing the blood glucose-lowering effects of **pioglitazone**. Adjust dose. ⟨Moderate⟩ Theoretical
▸ **Somatrogon** might increase blood glucose concentrations, opposing the blood glucose-lowering effects of **pioglitazone**. Adjust dose. ⟨Moderate⟩ Theoretical
▸ **St John's wort** slightly decreases the exposure to **pioglitazone**. ⟨Mild⟩ Study
▸ **Teriflunomide** is predicted to increase the exposure to **pioglitazone**. ⟨Moderate⟩ Study

Piperacillin → see penicillins

Pirfenidone

> **FOOD AND LIFESTYLE** Smoking increases pirfenidone clearance; patients should be encouraged to stop smoking before and during treatment with pirfenidone.

▸ **Antiepileptics (fosphenytoin, phenytoin)** are predicted to decrease the exposure to **pirfenidone**. ⟨Moderate⟩ Theoretical
▸ **Axitinib** is predicted to increase the exposure to **pirfenidone**. ⟨Moderate⟩ Theoretical
▸ **Combined hormonal contraceptives** is predicted to increase the exposure to **pirfenidone**. Use with caution and adjust dose. ⟨Moderate⟩ Study
▸ **Givosiran** is predicted to increase the exposure to **pirfenidone**. Use with caution and adjust dose. ⟨Moderate⟩ Study
▸ **HIV-protease inhibitors (ritonavir)** are predicted to decrease the exposure to **pirfenidone**. ⟨Moderate⟩ Theoretical
▸ **Leflunomide** is predicted to decrease the exposure to **pirfenidone**. ⟨Moderate⟩ Theoretical
▸ **Mexiletine** is predicted to increase the exposure to **pirfenidone**. Use with caution and adjust dose. ⟨Moderate⟩ Study
▸ **Osilodrostat** is predicted to increase the exposure to **pirfenidone**. Use with caution and adjust dose. ⟨Moderate⟩ Study
▸ **Quinolones (ciprofloxacin)** are predicted to increase the exposure to **pirfenidone**. Use with caution and adjust dose. ⟨Moderate⟩ Study
▸ **Rifamycins (rifampicin)** are predicted to decrease the exposure to **pirfenidone**. Avoid. ⟨Moderate⟩ Theoretical
▸ **Ritlecitinib** is predicted to increase the exposure to **pirfenidone**. Adjust dose. ⟨Moderate⟩ Theoretical
▸ **Rucaparib** is predicted to increase the exposure to **pirfenidone**. Use with caution and adjust dose. ⟨Moderate⟩ Study
▸ **SSRIs (fluvoxamine)** are predicted to moderately increase the exposure to **pirfenidone**. Avoid. ⟨Moderate⟩ Study
▸ **Teriflunomide** is predicted to decrease the exposure to **pirfenidone**. ⟨Moderate⟩ Theoretical
▸ **Vemurafenib** is predicted to increase the exposure to **pirfenidone**. Use with caution and adjust dose. ⟨Moderate⟩ Study

Piroxicam → see NSAIDs

Pitolisant

▸ **Pitolisant** is predicted to decrease the exposure to **aliskiren**. ⟨Mild⟩ Theoretical
▸ **Anti-androgens (apalutamide, enzalutamide)** are predicted to moderately decrease the exposure to **pitolisant**. ⟨Moderate⟩ Study

▸ **Antiepileptics (carbamazepine, fosphenytoin, phenobarbital, phenytoin, primidone)** are predicted to moderately decrease the exposure to **pitolisant**. ⟨Moderate⟩ Study
▸ **Pitolisant** is predicted to decrease the exposure to antihistamines, non-sedating **(fexofenadine)**. ⟨Mild⟩ Theoretical
▸ **Antihistamines, sedating** are predicted to decrease the efficacy of **pitolisant**. ⟨Moderate⟩ Theoretical
▸ **Pitolisant** is predicted to decrease the exposure to **bosutinib**. Avoid. ⟨Severe⟩ Theoretical
▸ **Bupropion** is predicted to moderately increase the exposure to **pitolisant**. Use with caution and adjust dose. ⟨Moderate⟩ Study
▸ **Pitolisant** is predicted to decrease the exposure to **ciclosporin**. Avoid. ⟨Severe⟩ Theoretical
▸ **Cinacalcet** is predicted to moderately increase the exposure to **pitolisant**. Use with caution and adjust dose. ⟨Moderate⟩ Study
▸ **Pitolisant** is predicted to decrease the exposure to **colchicine**. ⟨Mild⟩ Theoretical
▸ **Pitolisant** is predicted to decrease the efficacy of **combined hormonal contraceptives**. Avoid. ⟨Severe⟩ Theoretical
▸ **Pitolisant** is predicted to decrease the exposure to coumarins **(warfarin)**. ⟨Mild⟩ Theoretical
▸ **Pitolisant** is predicted to decrease the exposure to **crizotinib**. Avoid. ⟨Severe⟩ Theoretical
▸ **Dacomitinib** is predicted to moderately increase the exposure to **pitolisant**. Use with caution and adjust dose. ⟨Moderate⟩ Study
▸ **Pitolisant** is predicted to decrease the exposure to **dasatinib**. Avoid. ⟨Severe⟩ Theoretical
▸ **Pitolisant** is predicted to decrease the exposure to **digoxin**. ⟨Mild⟩ Theoretical
▸ **Encorafenib** is predicted to moderately decrease the exposure to **pitolisant**. ⟨Moderate⟩ Study
▸ **Pitolisant** is predicted to decrease the exposure to **everolimus**. Avoid. ⟨Severe⟩ Theoretical
▸ **Pitolisant** is predicted to decrease the exposure to factor XA inhibitors **(edoxaban)**. ⟨Mild⟩ Theoretical
▸ **Pitolisant** is predicted to decrease the exposure to **irinotecan**. ⟨Mild⟩ Theoretical
▸ **Ivosidenib** is predicted to moderately decrease the exposure to **pitolisant**. ⟨Moderate⟩ Study
▸ **Pitolisant** is predicted to decrease the exposure to **lapatinib**. Avoid. ⟨Severe⟩ Theoretical
▸ **Pitolisant** is predicted to decrease the exposure to **loperamide**. ⟨Mild⟩ Theoretical
▸ **Lumacaftor** is predicted to moderately decrease the exposure to **pitolisant**. ⟨Moderate⟩ Study
▸ **Pitolisant** is predicted to decrease the exposure to meglitinides **(repaglinide)**. ⟨Mild⟩ Theoretical
▸ **Pitolisant** is predicted to increase the exposure to **metformin**. ⟨Mild⟩ Theoretical
▸ **Mianserin** is predicted to decrease the efficacy of **pitolisant**. ⟨Moderate⟩ Theoretical
▸ **Mirtazapine** is predicted to decrease the efficacy of **pitolisant**. ⟨Moderate⟩ Theoretical
▸ **Mitotane** is predicted to moderately decrease the exposure to **pitolisant**. ⟨Moderate⟩ Study
▸ **Pitolisant** is predicted to decrease the exposure to **nilotinib**. Avoid. ⟨Severe⟩ Theoretical
▸ **Pitolisant** is predicted to decrease the exposure to NNRTIs **(efavirenz)**. ⟨Mild⟩ Theoretical
▸ **Pitolisant** is predicted to decrease the exposure to opioids **(morphine)**. ⟨Mild⟩ Theoretical
▸ **Pitolisant** is predicted to decrease the exposure to paracetamol. ⟨Mild⟩ Theoretical
▸ **Pitolisant** is predicted to decrease the exposure to **pimozide**. Avoid. ⟨Severe⟩ Theoretical
▸ **Rifamycins (rifampicin)** are predicted to moderately decrease the exposure to **pitolisant**. ⟨Moderate⟩ Study
▸ **Pitolisant** is predicted to decrease the exposure to **sirolimus**. Avoid. ⟨Severe⟩ Theoretical
▸ **SNRIs (duloxetine)** are predicted to increase the exposure to **pitolisant**. Use with caution and adjust dose. ⟨Moderate⟩ Study
▸ **SNRIs (venlafaxine)** are predicted to increase the exposure to **pitolisant**. Use with caution and adjust dose. ⟨Mild⟩ Theoretical

Pitolisant (continued)
- SSRIs **(fluoxetine, paroxetine)** are predicted to moderately increase the exposure to **pitolisant**. Use with caution and adjust dose. [Moderate] Study
- **St John's wort** is predicted to decrease the exposure to **pitolisant**. Monitor and adjust dose. [Moderate] Theoretical
- **Pitolisant** is predicted to decrease the exposure to **tacrolimus**. Avoid. [Severe] Theoretical
- **Pitolisant** is predicted to decrease the exposure to **taxanes (docetaxel)**. Avoid. [Severe] Theoretical
- **Pitolisant** is predicted to decrease the exposure to **taxanes (paclitaxel)**. [Mild] Theoretical
- **Pitolisant** is predicted to decrease the exposure to **temsirolimus**. Avoid. [Severe] Theoretical
- **Terbinafine** is predicted to moderately increase the exposure to **pitolisant**. Use with caution and adjust dose. [Moderate] Study
- **Pitolisant** is predicted to decrease the exposure to **thrombin inhibitors (dabigatran)**. [Mild] Theoretical
- **Tricyclic antidepressants** are predicted to decrease the efficacy of **pitolisant**. [Mild] Theoretical

Pivmecillinam → see penicillins

Pixantrone → see anthracyclines

Pizotifen → see antihistamines, sedating

Platinum compounds → see TABLE 17 p. 1576 (hyponatraemia), TABLE 14 p. 1575 (myelosuppression), TABLE 2 p. 1571 (nephrotoxicity), TABLE 18 p. 1576 (ototoxicity), TABLE 11 p. 1574 (peripheral neuropathy)

carboplatin · cisplatin · oxaliplatin

- **Cisplatin** increases the risk of pulmonary toxicity when given with **bleomycin**. [Severe] Study → Also see TABLE 14 p. 1575
- **Live vaccines** are predicted to increase the risk of generalised infection (possibly life-threatening) when given with **platinum compounds**. UKHSA advises avoid (refer to Green Book). [Severe] Theoretical

Polatuzumab vedotin → see monoclonal antibodies

Polymyxin b → see TABLE 19 p. 1576 (neuromuscular blocking effects)

ROUTE-SPECIFIC INFORMATION Since systemic absorption can follow topical application of **polymyxin B**, the possibility of interactions should be borne in mind.

Polystyrene sulfonate

SEPARATION OF ADMINISTRATION Manufacturers advise take other drugs at least 3 hours before or after calcium- or sodium-polystyrene sulfonate; a 6-hour separation should be considered in gastroparesis.

- Oral **antacids** increase the risk of metabolic alkalosis when given with oral **polystyrene sulfonate**. [Severe] Anecdotal

Pomalidomide → see TABLE 1 p. 1571 (hepatotoxicity), TABLE 14 p. 1575 (myelosuppression), TABLE 11 p. 1574 (peripheral neuropathy)

- **Combined hormonal contraceptives** are predicted to increase the risk of venous thromboembolism when given with **pomalidomide**. Avoid. [Severe] Theoretical
- **Hormone replacement therapy** is predicted to increase the risk of venous thromboembolism when given with **pomalidomide**. [Severe] Theoretical
- **Quinolones (ciprofloxacin)** are predicted to increase the exposure to **pomalidomide**. Adjust dose—consult product literature. [Moderate] Theoretical
- SSRIs **(fluvoxamine)** moderately increase the exposure to **pomalidomide**. Adjust dose—consult product literature. [Moderate] Study

Ponatinib → see TABLE 4 p. 1571 (antiplatelet effects)

- **Anti-androgens (apalutamide, enzalutamide)** are predicted to decrease the exposure to **ponatinib**. Avoid. [Moderate] Theoretical
- **Antiarrhythmics (dronedarone)** are predicted to increase the exposure to **ponatinib**. [Moderate] Study
- **Antiepileptics (carbamazepine, fosphenytoin, phenobarbital, phenytoin, primidone)** are predicted to decrease the exposure to **ponatinib**. Avoid. [Moderate] Theoretical
- **Antifungals, azoles (fluconazole, isavuconazole)** are predicted to increase the exposure to **ponatinib**. [Moderate] Study

- **Antifungals, azoles (itraconazole, ketoconazole, posaconazole, voriconazole)** are predicted to slightly increase the exposure to **ponatinib**. Monitor and adjust dose—consult product literature. [Moderate] Study
- **Berotralstat** is predicted to increase the exposure to **ponatinib**. [Moderate] Study
- **Calcium channel blockers (diltiazem, verapamil)** are predicted to increase the exposure to **ponatinib**. [Moderate] Study
- **Cenobamate** is predicted to decrease the exposure to **ponatinib**. [Severe] Study
- **Ceritinib** is predicted to slightly increase the exposure to **ponatinib**. Monitor and adjust dose—consult product literature. [Moderate] Study
- **Cobicistat** is predicted to slightly increase the exposure to **ponatinib**. Monitor and adjust dose—consult product literature. [Moderate] Study
- **Ponatinib** might affect the effects of **combined hormonal contraceptives**. Avoid or use additional contraceptive precautions. [Severe] Theoretical
- **Crizotinib** is predicted to increase the exposure to **ponatinib**. [Moderate] Study
- **Dabrafenib** is predicted to decrease the exposure to **ponatinib**. [Severe] Study
- **Encorafenib** is predicted to decrease the exposure to **ponatinib**. Avoid. [Moderate] Theoretical
- **Endothelin receptor antagonists (bosentan)** are predicted to decrease the exposure to **ponatinib**. [Severe] Study
- **Fedratinib** is predicted to increase the exposure to **ponatinib**. [Moderate] Study
- **Grapefruit** juice is predicted to increase the exposure to **ponatinib**. [Moderate] Theoretical
- **HIV-protease inhibitors** are predicted to slightly increase the exposure to **ponatinib**. Monitor and adjust dose—consult product literature. [Moderate] Study
- **Idelalisib** is predicted to slightly increase the exposure to **ponatinib**. Monitor and adjust dose—consult product literature. [Moderate] Study
- **Imatinib** is predicted to increase the exposure to **ponatinib**. [Moderate] Study → Also see TABLE 4 p. 1571
- **Ivosidenib** is predicted to decrease the exposure to **ponatinib**. Avoid. [Moderate] Theoretical
- **Letermovir** is predicted to increase the exposure to **ponatinib**. [Moderate] Study
- **Lorlatinib** is predicted to decrease the exposure to **ponatinib**. [Severe] Study
- **Lumacaftor** is predicted to decrease the exposure to **ponatinib**. Avoid. [Moderate] Theoretical
- **Macrolides (clarithromycin)** are predicted to slightly increase the exposure to **ponatinib**. Monitor and adjust dose—consult product literature. [Moderate] Study
- **Macrolides (erythromycin)** are predicted to increase the exposure to **ponatinib**. [Moderate] Study
- **Mitotane** is predicted to decrease the exposure to **ponatinib**. Avoid. [Moderate] Theoretical
- **Neurokinin-1 receptor antagonists (aprepitant, netupitant)** are predicted to increase the exposure to **ponatinib**. [Moderate] Study
- **Nilotinib** is predicted to increase the exposure to **ponatinib**. [Moderate] Study
- **NNRTIs (efavirenz, etravirine, nevirapine)** are predicted to decrease the exposure to **ponatinib**. [Severe] Study
- **Rifamycins (rifampicin)** are predicted to decrease the exposure to **ponatinib**. Avoid. [Moderate] Theoretical
- **Sotorasib** is predicted to decrease the exposure to **ponatinib**. [Severe] Study
- **St John's wort** is predicted to decrease the exposure to **ponatinib**. Avoid. [Severe] Theoretical
- **Tucatinib** is predicted to slightly increase the exposure to **ponatinib**. Monitor and adjust dose—consult product literature. [Moderate] Study

Ponesimod → see TABLE 5 p. 1572 (bradycardia), TABLE 8 p. 1573 (QT-interval prolongation)

- **Live vaccines** might increase the risk of generalised infection (possibly life-threatening) when given with **ponesimod**. Avoid and for 1 week after stopping **ponesimod**. [Severe] Theoretical

▶ Monoclonal antibodies **(alemtuzumab)** are predicted to increase the risk of generalised infection (possibly life-threatening) when given with **ponesimod**. Severe Theoretical

Posaconazole → see antifungals, azoles

Potassium aminobenzoate → see TABLE 15 p. 1575 (increased serum potassium)

▶ **Potassium aminobenzoate** increases the concentration of methotrexate. Moderate Theoretical

▶ **Potassium aminobenzoate** is predicted to affect the efficacy of sulfonamides. Avoid. Severe Theoretical

Potassium canrenoate → see TABLE 15 p. 1575 (increased serum potassium)

Potassium chloride → see TABLE 15 p. 1575 (increased serum potassium)

Potassium citrate

▶ **Potassium citrate** is predicted to decrease the efficacy of methenamine. Avoid. Moderate Theoretical

▶ **Potassium citrate** might decrease the efficacy of nitrofurantoin. Unknown Theoretical

▶ **Potassium citrate** increases the risk of adverse effects when given with sucralfate. Avoid. Moderate Theoretical

Potassium-sparing diuretics → see TABLE 17 p. 1576 (hyponatraemia), TABLE 15 p. 1575 (increased serum potassium)

amiloride · triamterene

▶ **Triamterene** potentially increases the clearance of lithium. Moderate Study

Pralsetinib

FOOD AND LIFESTYLE Bitter (Seville) orange is predicted to increase the exposure to pralsetinib. Avoid.

▶ Anti-androgens **(apalutamide, enzalutamide)** are predicted to decrease the exposure to **pralsetinib**. Avoid or adjust dose with potent CYP3A4 inducers—consult product literature. Moderate Study

▶ Antiarrhythmics **(amiodarone, dronedarone)** are predicted to increase the exposure to **pralsetinib**. Moderate Theoretical

▶ Antiepileptics **(carbamazepine, fosphenytoin, phenobarbital, phenytoin, primidone)** are predicted to decrease the exposure to **pralsetinib**. Avoid or adjust dose with potent CYP3A4 inducers—consult product literature. Moderate Study

▶ Antifungals, azoles **(fluconazole, isavuconazole)** are predicted to increase the exposure to **pralsetinib**. Moderate Theoretical

▶ Antifungals, azoles **(itraconazole, ketoconazole, posaconazole, voriconazole)** are predicted to increase the exposure to **pralsetinib**. Avoid or adjust dose with potent CYP3A4 inhibitors—consult product literature. Moderate Study

▶ Berotralstat is predicted to increase the exposure to **pralsetinib**. Moderate Theoretical

▶ Calcium channel blockers **(diltiazem, verapamil)** are predicted to increase the exposure to **pralsetinib**. Moderate Theoretical

▶ Cenobamate is predicted to decrease the exposure to **pralsetinib**. Moderate Theoretical

▶ Ceritinib is predicted to increase the exposure to **pralsetinib**. Avoid or adjust dose with potent CYP3A4 inhibitors—consult product literature. Moderate Study

▶ **Pralsetinib** might affect the exposure to ciclosporin and ciclosporin is predicted to increase the exposure to **pralsetinib**. Avoid. Moderate Theoretical

▶ Cobicistat is predicted to increase the exposure to **pralsetinib**. Avoid or adjust dose with potent CYP3A4 inhibitors—consult product literature. Moderate Study

▶ **Pralsetinib** might decrease the efficacy of combined hormonal contraceptives. Avoid or use additional contraceptive precautions. Severe Theoretical

▶ **Pralsetinib** might affect the exposure to coumarins **(warfarin)**. Avoid. Moderate Theoretical

▶ Crizotinib is predicted to increase the exposure to **pralsetinib**. Moderate Theoretical

▶ Dabrafenib is predicted to decrease the exposure to **pralsetinib**. Moderate Theoretical

▶ Danicopan is predicted to increase the exposure to **pralsetinib**. Moderate Study

▶ Eliglustat is predicted to increase the exposure to **pralsetinib**. Adjust dose. Moderate Study

▶ Encorafenib is predicted to decrease the exposure to **pralsetinib**. Avoid or adjust dose with potent CYP3A4 inducers—consult product literature. Moderate Study

▶ Endothelin receptor antagonists **(bosentan)** are predicted to decrease the exposure to **pralsetinib**. Moderate Theoretical

▶ Fedratinib is predicted to increase the exposure to **pralsetinib**. Moderate Theoretical

▶ Glecaprevir is predicted to increase the exposure to **pralsetinib**. Moderate Theoretical

▶ Grapefruit juice is predicted to increase the exposure to **pralsetinib**. Avoid. Moderate Study

▶ HIV-protease inhibitors are predicted to increase the exposure to **pralsetinib**. Avoid or adjust dose with potent CYP3A4 inhibitors—consult product literature. Moderate Study

▶ Idelalisib is predicted to increase the exposure to **pralsetinib**. Avoid or adjust dose with potent CYP3A4 inhibitors—consult product literature. Moderate Study

▶ Imatinib is predicted to increase the exposure to **pralsetinib**. Moderate Theoretical

▶ Ivosidenib is predicted to decrease the exposure to **pralsetinib**. Avoid or adjust dose with potent CYP3A4 inducers—consult product literature. Moderate Study

▶ Lapatinib is predicted to increase the exposure to **pralsetinib**. Moderate Theoretical

▶ Letermovir is predicted to increase the exposure to **pralsetinib**. Moderate Theoretical

▶ Lorlatinib is predicted to decrease the exposure to **pralsetinib**. Moderate Theoretical

▶ Lumacaftor is predicted to decrease the exposure to **pralsetinib**. Avoid or adjust dose with potent CYP3A4 inducers—consult product literature. Moderate Study

▶ Macrolides **(azithromycin, erythromycin)** are predicted to increase the exposure to **pralsetinib**. Moderate Theoretical

▶ Macrolides **(clarithromycin)** are predicted to increase the exposure to **pralsetinib**. Avoid or adjust dose with potent CYP3A4 inhibitors—consult product literature. Moderate Study

▶ Mitotane is predicted to decrease the exposure to **pralsetinib**. Avoid or adjust dose with potent CYP3A4 inducers—consult product literature. Moderate Study

▶ Neurokinin-1 receptor antagonists **(aprepitant, netupitant)** are predicted to increase the exposure to **pralsetinib**. Moderate Theoretical

▶ Nilotinib is predicted to increase the exposure to **pralsetinib**. Moderate Theoretical

▶ NNRTIs **(efavirenz, nevirapine)** are predicted to decrease the exposure to **pralsetinib**. Moderate Theoretical

▶ Olaparib might increase the exposure to **pralsetinib**. Moderate Theoretical

▶ Osimertinib is predicted to increase the exposure to **pralsetinib**. Moderate Study

▶ Pibrentasvir is predicted to increase the exposure to **pralsetinib**. Moderate Theoretical

▶ Ranolazine is predicted to increase the exposure to **pralsetinib**. Moderate Theoretical

▶ Rifamycins **(rifabutin)** are predicted to decrease the exposure to **pralsetinib**. Avoid or adjust dose—consult product literature. Moderate Study

▶ Rifamycins **(rifampicin)** are predicted to decrease the exposure to **pralsetinib**. Avoid or adjust dose with potent CYP3A4 inducers—consult product literature. Moderate Study

▶ Sotorasib is predicted to decrease the exposure to **pralsetinib**. Moderate Theoretical

▶ St John's wort is predicted to decrease the exposure to **pralsetinib**. Avoid or adjust dose—consult product literature. Moderate Study

▶ **Pralsetinib** might affect the exposure to taxanes **(paclitaxel)**. Avoid. Moderate Theoretical

▶ Tucatinib is predicted to increase the exposure to **pralsetinib**. Avoid or adjust dose with potent CYP3A4 inhibitors—consult product literature. Moderate Study

▶ Velpatasvir is predicted to increase the exposure to **pralsetinib**. Moderate Theoretical

▶ Vemurafenib is predicted to increase the exposure to **pralsetinib**. Moderate Theoretical

Pralsetinib (continued)
▶ **Voxilaprevir** is predicted to increase the exposure to pralsetinib. Moderate Theoretical

Pramipexole → see dopamine receptor agonists

Prasugrel → see TABLE 4 p. 1571 (antiplatelet effects)
▶ **Selumetinib** might increase the risk of bleeding when given with **prasugrel**. Severe Theoretical

Pravastatin → see statins

Praziquantel
▶ Anti-androgens **(apalutamide, enzalutamide)** are predicted to markedly decrease the exposure to **praziquantel**. Avoid. Moderate Study
▶ Antiepileptics **(carbamazepine, fosphenytoin, phenobarbital, phenytoin, primidone)** are predicted to markedly decrease the exposure to **praziquantel**. Avoid. Moderate Study
▶ Antifungals, azoles **(itraconazole, ketoconazole, posaconazole, voriconazole)** are predicted to moderately increase the exposure to **praziquantel**. Mild Study
▶ Antimalarials **(chloroquine)** moderately decrease the exposure to **praziquantel**. Use with caution and adjust dose. Moderate Study
▶ **Ceritinib** is predicted to moderately increase the exposure to **praziquantel**. Mild Study
▶ **Cobicistat** is predicted to moderately increase the exposure to **praziquantel**. Mild Study
▶ Corticosteroids **(dexamethasone)** decrease the exposure to **praziquantel**. Moderate Study
▶ **Encorafenib** is predicted to markedly decrease the exposure to **praziquantel**. Avoid. Moderate Study
▶ **Grapefruit** juice is predicted to increase the exposure to **praziquantel**. Moderate Study
▶ H₂ receptor antagonists **(cimetidine)** moderately increase the exposure to **praziquantel**. Moderate Study
▶ **HIV-protease inhibitors** are predicted to moderately increase the exposure to **praziquantel**. Mild Study
▶ **Idelalisib** is predicted to moderately increase the exposure to **praziquantel**. Mild Study
▶ **Ivosidenib** is predicted to markedly decrease the exposure to **praziquantel**. Avoid. Moderate Study
▶ **Lumacaftor** is predicted to markedly decrease the exposure to **praziquantel**. Avoid. Moderate Study
▶ Macrolides **(clarithromycin)** are predicted to moderately increase the exposure to **praziquantel**. Mild Study
▶ **Mitotane** is predicted to markedly decrease the exposure to **praziquantel**. Avoid. Moderate Study
▶ Rifamycins **(rifampicin)** are predicted to markedly decrease the exposure to **praziquantel**. Avoid. Moderate Study
▶ **Tucatinib** is predicted to moderately increase the exposure to **praziquantel**. Mild Study

Prazosin → see alpha blockers

Prednisolone → see corticosteroids

Pregabalin → see antiepileptics

Pridinol → see TABLE 9 p. 1573 (antimuscarinics)
▶ Antipsychotics, second generation **(clozapine)** can cause constipation, as can **pridinol**; concurrent use might increase the risk of developing intestinal obstruction. Severe Theoretical → Also see TABLE 9 p. 1573

Prilocaine → see anaesthetics, local

Primaquine → see antimalarials

Primidone → see antiepileptics

Procarbazine → see TABLE 14 p. 1575 (myelosuppression)

FOOD AND LIFESTYLE Procarbazine is a mild monoamine-oxidase inhibitor and might rarely interact with tyramine-rich foods (such as mature cheese, salami, pickled herring, *Bovril*®, *Oxo*®, *Marmite*® or any similar meat or yeast extract or fermented soya bean extract, and some beers, lagers or wines).

▶ **Alcohol** potentially causes a disulfiram-like reaction when given with **procarbazine**. Moderate Anecdotal
▶ Antiepileptics **(carbamazepine, phenobarbital, phenytoin, primidone)** are predicted to increase the risk of hypersensitivity reactions when given with **procarbazine**. Severe Anecdotal

▶ Antiepileptics **(fosphenytoin)** are predicted to increase the risk of hypersensitivity when given with **procarbazine**. Severe Anecdotal
▶ **Live vaccines** are predicted to increase the risk of generalised infection (possibly life-threatening) when given with **procarbazine**. UKHSA advises avoid (refer to Green Book). Severe Theoretical

Prochlorperazine → see phenothiazines

Procyclidine → see TABLE 9 p. 1573 (antimuscarinics), TABLE 10 p. 1574 (CNS effects)
▶ Antipsychotics, second generation **(clozapine)** can cause constipation, as can **procyclidine**; concurrent use might increase the risk of developing intestinal obstruction. Severe Theoretical → Also see TABLE 9 p. 1573 → Also see TABLE 10 p. 1574
▶ SSRIs **(paroxetine)** slightly increase the exposure to **procyclidine**. Monitor and adjust dose. Moderate Study → Also see TABLE 10 p. 1574

Proguanil → see antimalarials

Promazine → see phenothiazines

Promethazine → see antihistamines, sedating

Propafenone → see antiarrhythmics

Propantheline → see TABLE 9 p. 1573 (antimuscarinics)
▶ Antipsychotics, second generation **(clozapine)** can cause constipation, as can **propantheline**; concurrent use might increase the risk of developing intestinal obstruction. Severe Theoretical → Also see TABLE 9 p. 1573

Propiverine → see TABLE 9 p. 1573 (antimuscarinics)
▶ Antifungals, azoles **(itraconazole, ketoconazole, posaconazole, voriconazole)** given with carbimazole are predicted to increase the exposure to **propiverine**. Adjust starting dose. Moderate Theoretical
▶ Antipsychotics, second generation **(clozapine)** can cause constipation, as can **propiverine**; concurrent use might increase the risk of developing intestinal obstruction. Severe Theoretical → Also see TABLE 9 p. 1573
▶ **Carbimazole** given with a potent CYP3A4 inhibitor is predicted to increase the exposure to **propiverine**. Adjust starting dose. Moderate Theoretical
▶ **Ceritinib** given with carbimazole is predicted to increase the exposure to **propiverine**. Adjust starting dose. Moderate Theoretical
▶ **Cobicistat** given with carbimazole is predicted to increase the exposure to **propiverine**. Adjust starting dose. Moderate Theoretical
▶ **HIV-protease inhibitors** given with carbimazole are predicted to increase the exposure to **propiverine**. Adjust starting dose. Moderate Theoretical
▶ **Idelalisib** given with carbimazole is predicted to increase the exposure to **propiverine**. Adjust starting dose. Moderate Theoretical
▶ **Propiverine** is predicted to increase the exposure to **lomitapide**. Separate administration by 12 hours. Moderate Theoretical
▶ Macrolides **(clarithromycin)** given with carbimazole are predicted to increase the exposure to **propiverine**. Adjust starting dose. Moderate Theoretical
▶ **Tucatinib** given with carbimazole is predicted to increase the exposure to **propiverine**. Adjust starting dose. Moderate Theoretical

Propofol → see TABLE 5 p. 1572 (bradycardia), TABLE 7 p. 1572 (hypotension), TABLE 10 p. 1574 (CNS effects)
▶ Antiepileptics **(valproate)** potentially increase the concentration of **propofol**. Adjust dose. Severe Theoretical
▶ **Propofol** is predicted to increase the exposure to the active component of **sacituzumab govitecan**. Severe Theoretical

Propranolol → see beta blockers, non-selective

Propylthiouracil
▶ **Propylthiouracil** is predicted to decrease the effects of **metyrapone**. Avoid. Moderate Theoretical

Proton pump inhibitors

esomeprazole · lansoprazole · omeprazole · pantoprazole · rabeprazole

▶ **Pantoprazole** is predicted to increase the exposure to **alpelisib**. Moderate Theoretical

- Anti-androgens **(apalutamide)** markedly decrease the exposure to **omeprazole**. Avoid or monitor. [Moderate] Study
- Anti-androgens **(apalutamide)** are predicted to decrease the exposure to proton pump inhibitors **(lansoprazole, rabeprazole)**. Avoid or monitor. [Mild] Study
- Antifungals, azoles **(voriconazole)** increase the exposure to proton pump inhibitors **(esomeprazole, omeprazole)**. Adjust dose. [Moderate] Study
- **Proton pump inhibitors** decrease the absorption of antifungals, azoles **(itraconazole)**. Administer itraconazole capsules with an acidic beverage. [Moderate] Study
- **Proton pump inhibitors** decrease the absorption of antifungals, azoles **(ketoconazole)**. Administer ketoconazole with an acidic beverage. [Moderate] Study
- **Proton pump inhibitors** decrease the absorption of antifungals, azoles **(posaconazole)** oral suspension. Avoid. [Moderate] Study
- **Proton pump inhibitors** are predicted to decrease the exposure to belumosudil. Adjust **belumosudil** dose, p. 979. [Severe] Study
- Proton pump inhibitors **(esomeprazole, omeprazole)** are predicted to increase the exposure to belzutifan. Monitor and adjust dose. [Severe] Theoretical
- Proton pump inhibitors **(esomeprazole, omeprazole)** potentially increase the exposure to benzodiazepines **(clobazam)**. Adjust dose. [Moderate] Theoretical
- **Proton pump inhibitors** are predicted to decrease the absorption of bosutinib. [Moderate] Study
- **Esomeprazole** is predicted to increase the exposure to cannabidiol. [Moderate] Theoretical
- Cenobamate moderately increases the exposure to **omeprazole**. Adjust dose. [Moderate] Study
- **Proton pump inhibitors** are predicted to decrease the absorption of ceritinib. [Moderate] Theoretical
- **Esomeprazole** is predicted to increase the exposure to cilostazol. [Moderate] Theoretical
- **Omeprazole** is predicted to increase the exposure to cilostazol. Adjust **cilostazol** dose, p. 266. [Moderate] Study
- Proton pump inhibitors **(esomeprazole, omeprazole)** are predicted to decrease the efficacy of clopidogrel. Avoid. [Moderate] Study
- **Proton pump inhibitors** are predicted to decrease the exposure to dacomitinib. Avoid. [Moderate] Study
- **Proton pump inhibitors** are predicted to decrease the exposure to dasatinib. Avoid. [Severe] Study
- **Proton pump inhibitors** are predicted to decrease the absorption of dipyridamole (immediate release tablets). [Moderate] Theoretical
- **Proton pump inhibitors** are predicted to decrease the exposure to erlotinib. Avoid. [Moderate] Study
- Fedratinib moderately increases the exposure to **omeprazole**. Monitor and adjust dose. [Moderate] Study
- **Proton pump inhibitors** are predicted to decrease the exposure to gefitinib. [Severe] Theoretical
- **Proton pump inhibitors** decrease the exposure to HIV-protease inhibitors **(atazanavir)**. Avoid or adjust dose. [Severe] Study
- Ivosidenib might decrease the exposure to **omeprazole**. Avoid or monitor efficacy. [Unknown] Theoretical
- **Proton pump inhibitors** are predicted to decrease the exposure to ledipasvir. Adjust dose, see ledipasvir with sofosbuvir p. 724. [Moderate] Theoretical
- **Pantoprazole** might increase the exposure to mavacamten. Monitor and adjust dose—consult product literature. [Moderate] Theoretical
- Proton pump inhibitors **(esomeprazole, omeprazole)** are predicted to increase the exposure to mavacamten. Adjust dose—consult product literature. [Severe] Theoretical
- **Proton pump inhibitors** decrease the clearance of methotrexate (high-dose). Use with caution or avoid. [Severe] Study
- **Proton pump inhibitors** are predicted to decrease the exposure to neratinib. Avoid. [Severe] Study
- **Proton pump inhibitors** are predicted to decrease the exposure to oral NNRTIs **(rilpivirine)**. Avoid. [Severe] Study
- **Proton pump inhibitors** are predicted to decrease the exposure to pazopanib. Avoid or administer concurrently without food. [Moderate] Study

- **Proton pump inhibitors** have been reported to decrease the exposure to pemigatinib. Avoid. [Severe] Anecdotal
- **Proton pump inhibitors** are predicted to decrease the exposure to selpercatinib. Manufacturer advises take with food. [Moderate] Study
- Proton pump inhibitors **(esomeprazole, omeprazole)** are predicted to increase the exposure to selumetinib. Avoid or adjust dose—consult product literature. [Severe] Theoretical
- **Proton pump inhibitors** potentially decrease the exposure to sofosbuvir. Adjust dose, see ledipasvir with sofosbuvir p. 724, sofosbuvir with velpatasvir p. 725, and sofosbuvir with velpatasvir and voxilaprevir p. 726. [Moderate] Study
- **Proton pump inhibitors** are predicted to decrease the exposure to sotorasib. Manufacturer advises give **sotorasib** with an acidic beverage or use an antacid. [Moderate] Study
- **Esomeprazole** increases the exposure to SSRIs **(citalopram)**. Monitor and adjust dose. [Severe] Theoretical
- **Omeprazole** moderately increases the exposure to SSRIs **(citalopram)**. Monitor and adjust dose. [Severe] Study
- Proton pump inhibitors **(esomeprazole, omeprazole)** are predicted to increase the exposure to SSRIs **(escitalopram)**. Use with caution and adjust dose. [Severe] Study
- **Esomeprazole** might increase the concentration of SSRIs **(sertraline)**. [Moderate] Study
- **Proton pump inhibitors** might decrease the efficacy of ulipristal for emergency hormonal contraception. For FSRH guidance, see Contraceptives, interactions p. 917. [Unknown] Theoretical
- **Proton pump inhibitors** are predicted to decrease the concentration of velpatasvir. Adjust dose, see sofosbuvir with velpatasvir p. 725. [Moderate] Study
- **Proton pump inhibitors** are predicted to decrease the exposure to voxilaprevir. Adjust dose, see sofosbuvir with velpatasvir and voxilaprevir p. 726. [Moderate] Study

Proxymetacaine → see anaesthetics, local
Pseudoephedrine → see sympathomimetics, vasoconstrictor
Pyrazinamide → see TABLE 1 p. 1571 (hepatotoxicity)
- Allopurinol is predicted to increase the risk of hyperuricaemia when given with **pyrazinamide**. [Moderate] Theoretical
Pyridostigmine → see TABLE 5 p. 1572 (bradycardia)
- Aminoglycosides are predicted to decrease the effects of pyridostigmine. [Moderate] Theoretical
Pyrimethamine → see antimalarials
Quetiapine → see antipsychotics, second generation
Quinagolide → see dopamine receptor agonists
Quinapril → see ACE inhibitors
Quinine → see antimalarials
Quinolones → see TABLE 8 p. 1573 (QT-interval prolongation)

ciprofloxacin · delafloxacin · levofloxacin · moxifloxacin · ofloxacin

- Avoid concurrent administration of dairy products and mineral-fortified drinks with *oral* **ciprofloxacin** due to reduced exposure.
- Since systemic absorption can follow topical application of **ciprofloxacin, levofloxacin**, or **ofloxacin**, the possibility of interactions should be borne in mind.
- Interactions do not generally apply to topical use of **moxifloxacin** unless specified.

- **Ciprofloxacin** is predicted to increase the exposure to agomelatine. [Moderate] Study
- **Ciprofloxacin** is predicted to increase the exposure to aminophylline. Adjust dose. [Moderate] Theoretical
- **Ciprofloxacin** is predicted to increase the exposure to anaesthetics, local **(ropivacaine)**. [Moderate] Theoretical
- **Ciprofloxacin** is predicted to increase the exposure to anagrelide. [Moderate] Theoretical
- Oral antacids decrease the absorption of oral **quinolones**. Manufacturer advises take 2 hours before or 4 hours after antacids. [Moderate] Study
- **Ciprofloxacin** slightly increases the exposure to antiarrhythmics **(lidocaine)**. [Mild] Study
- **Ciprofloxacin** affects the concentration of antiepileptics **(fosphenytoin, phenytoin)**. Monitor concentration and adjust dose. [Severe] Study

Quinolones (continued)

‣ **Ciprofloxacin** increases the concentration of antipsychotics, second generation (clozapine). Monitor adverse effects and adjust dose. Severe Study

‣ **Ciprofloxacin** is predicted to increase the exposure to antipsychotics, second generation (olanzapine). Adjust dose. Moderate Anecdotal

‣ **Ciprofloxacin** might increase the exposure to bedaquiline. Mild Theoretical

‣ Oral calcium salts decrease the absorption of oral **ciprofloxacin**. Separate administration by 2 hours. Moderate Study

‣ **Ciprofloxacin** is predicted to increase the exposure to capivasertib. Adjust dose. Moderate Theoretical

‣ **Quinolones** increase the anticoagulant effect of coumarins. Severe Anecdotal

‣ **Ciprofloxacin** is predicted to increase the exposure to daridorexant. Adjust **daridorexant** dose, p. 554. Moderate Theoretical

‣ **Ciprofloxacin** is predicted to increase the exposure to dopamine receptor agonists (ropinirole). Adjust dose. Moderate Study

‣ **Ciprofloxacin** is predicted to increase the exposure to elacestrant. Avoid or adjust **elacestrant** dose, p. 1084. Severe Theoretical

‣ **Ciprofloxacin** is predicted to increase the exposure to eliglustat. Avoid or adjust dose—consult product literature. Severe Theoretical

‣ Enteral feeds decrease the exposure to **ciprofloxacin**. Moderate Study

‣ **Ciprofloxacin** are predicted to increases the exposure to erlotinib. Monitor adverse effects and adjust dose. Moderate Study

‣ **Ciprofloxacin** is predicted to increase the exposure to fezolinetant. Avoid. Moderate Study

‣ **Ciprofloxacin** is predicted to increase the concentration of guanfacine. Adjust **guanfacine** dose, p. 407. Moderate Theoretical

‣ **Ciprofloxacin** is predicted to increase the exposure to ibrutinib. Adjust dose—consult product literature. Severe Theoretical

‣ Oral iron decreases the exposure to oral **quinolones**. Separate administration by at least 2 hours. Moderate Study

‣ Lanthanum moderately decreases the exposure to **quinolones**. **Quinolones** should be taken 2 hours before or 4 hours after lanthanum. Moderate Study

‣ Leflunomide is predicted to increase the exposure to ciprofloxacin. Moderate Theoretical

‣ **Ciprofloxacin** is predicted to increase the exposure to loxapine. Avoid. Unknown Theoretical

‣ **Ciprofloxacin** slightly increases the exposure to MAO-B inhibitors (rasagiline). Moderate Study

‣ **Ciprofloxacin** is predicted to increase the exposure to melatonin. Moderate Theoretical

‣ **Ciprofloxacin** potentially increases the risk of toxicity when given with methotrexate. Severe Anecdotal

‣ Nitisinone is predicted to increase the exposure to ciprofloxacin. Moderate Study

‣ NSAIDs potentially increase the risk of seizures when given with **quinolones**. Severe Theoretical

‣ **Ciprofloxacin** very slightly increases the exposure to pentoxifylline. Moderate Study

‣ **Ciprofloxacin** is predicted to increase the exposure to phenothiazines (chlorpromazine). Moderate Theoretical

‣ **Ciprofloxacin** is predicted to increase the exposure to phosphodiesterase type-4 inhibitors (roflumilast). Moderate Theoretical

‣ **Ciprofloxacin** moderately increases the exposure to phosphodiesterase type-5 inhibitors (sildenafil). Moderate Theoretical

‣ **Ciprofloxacin** is predicted to increase the exposure to pirfenidone. Use with caution and adjust dose. Moderate Study

‣ **Ciprofloxacin** is predicted to increase the exposure to pomalidomide. Adjust dose—consult product literature. Moderate Theoretical

‣ **Ciprofloxacin** is predicted to increase the exposure to riluzole. Moderate Theoretical

‣ **Ciprofloxacin** is predicted to increase the exposure to ruxolitinib. Moderate Theoretical

‣ **Ciprofloxacin** is predicted to increase the exposure to SNRIs (duloxetine). Avoid. Moderate Theoretical

‣ Strontium is predicted to decrease the absorption of **quinolones**. Avoid. Moderate Theoretical

‣ Sucralfate decreases the exposure to **quinolones**. Separate administration by 2 hours. Moderate Study

‣ Teriflunomide is predicted to increase the exposure to ciprofloxacin. Moderate Theoretical

‣ **Ciprofloxacin** is predicted to increase the exposure to theophylline. Monitor and adjust dose. Moderate Theoretical

‣ **Ciprofloxacin** increases the exposure to tizanidine. Avoid. Moderate Study

‣ **Ciprofloxacin** is predicted to increase the exposure to tolvaptan. Use with caution and adjust **tolvaptan** dose, p. 767. Moderate Theoretical

‣ **Ciprofloxacin** is predicted to increase the exposure to triptans (zolmitriptan). Adjust **zolmitriptan** dose, p. 546. Moderate Theoretical

‣ Vadadustat is predicted to increase the exposure to ciprofloxacin. Monitor and adjust dose. Moderate Study

‣ **Ciprofloxacin** is predicted to increase the exposure to venetoclax. Avoid or adjust dose—consult product literature. Severe Theoretical

‣ **Ciprofloxacin** is predicted to increase the exposure to zanubrutinib. Avoid or adjust dose—consult product literature. Severe Theoretical

‣ Zinc is predicted to decrease the exposure to **quinolones**. Separate administration by 2 hours. Moderate Study

Quizartinib → see **TABLE 8** p. 1573 (QT-interval prolongation)

‣ Anti-androgens (apalutamide, enzalutamide) are predicted to decrease the exposure to **quizartinib**. Avoid. Severe Study → Also see **TABLE 8** p. 1573

‣ Antiepileptics (carbamazepine, fosphenytoin, phenobarbital, phenytoin, primidone) are predicted to decrease the exposure to **quizartinib**. Avoid. Severe Study

‣ Antifungals, azoles (itraconazole, ketoconazole, posaconazole, voriconazole) are predicted to increase the exposure to **quizartinib**. Adjust dose—consult product literature. Severe Study → Also see **TABLE 8** p. 1573

‣ Cenobamate is predicted to decrease the exposure to **quizartinib**. Avoid. Severe Study

‣ Ceritinib is predicted to increase the exposure to **quizartinib**. Adjust dose—consult product literature. Severe Study → Also see **TABLE 8** p. 1573

‣ Cobicistat is predicted to increase the exposure to **quizartinib**. Adjust dose—consult product literature. Severe Study

‣ Dabrafenib is predicted to decrease the exposure to **quizartinib**. Avoid. Severe Study

‣ Encorafenib is predicted to decrease the exposure to **quizartinib**. Avoid. Severe Study → Also see **TABLE 8** p. 1573

‣ Endothelin receptor antagonists (bosentan) are predicted to decrease the exposure to **quizartinib**. Avoid. Severe Study

‣ HIV-protease inhibitors are predicted to increase the exposure to **quizartinib**. Adjust dose—consult product literature. Severe Study

‣ Idelalisib is predicted to increase the exposure to **quizartinib**. Adjust dose—consult product literature. Severe Study

‣ Ivosidenib is predicted to decrease the exposure to **quizartinib**. Avoid. Severe Study → Also see **TABLE 8** p. 1573

‣ Lorlatinib is predicted to decrease the exposure to **quizartinib**. Avoid. Severe Study

‣ Lumacaftor is predicted to decrease the exposure to **quizartinib**. Avoid. Severe Study

‣ Macrolides (clarithromycin) are predicted to increase the exposure to **quizartinib**. Adjust dose—consult product literature. Severe Study

‣ Mitotane is predicted to decrease the exposure to **quizartinib**. Avoid. Severe Study

‣ NNRTIs (efavirenz, etravirine, nevirapine) are predicted to decrease the exposure to **quizartinib**. Avoid. Severe Study → Also see **TABLE 8** p. 1573

‣ Rifamycins (rifampicin) are predicted to decrease the exposure to **quizartinib**. Avoid. Severe Study

▶ **Sotorasib** is predicted to decrease the exposure to **quizartinib**. Avoid. [Severe] Study

▶ **St John's wort** is predicted to decrease the exposure to **quizartinib**. Avoid. [Severe] Study

▶ **Tucatinib** is predicted to increase the exposure to **quizartinib**. Adjust dose—consult product literature. [Severe] Study

Rabeprazole → see proton pump inhibitors

Rabies immunoglobulin → see immunoglobulins

Rabies vaccine

▶ **Antimalarials (chloroquine)** decrease the efficacy of **rabies vaccine** (intradermal). Avoid. [Moderate] Study

▶ **Hydroxychloroquine** is predicted to decrease efficacy **rabies vaccine**. [Moderate] Theoretical

Raloxifene

▶ **Combined hormonal contraceptives** potentially oppose the effects of **raloxifene**. Avoid. [Severe] Theoretical

▶ **Hormone replacement therapy** potentially opposes the effects of **raloxifene**. Avoid. [Severe] Theoretical

Raltegravir

▶ Oral **antacids** decrease the exposure to oral **raltegravir**. Avoid. [Moderate] Study

▶ **Antiepileptics (carbamazepine)** are predicted to affect the exposure to **raltegravir**. [Moderate] Theoretical

▶ **Antiepileptics (fosphenytoin, phenobarbital, phenytoin, primidone)** are predicted to affect the exposure to **raltegravir**. Use with caution or avoid. [Moderate] Theoretical

▶ **Belumosudil** is predicted to affect the exposure to **raltegravir**. [Moderate] Theoretical

▶ Oral **calcium salts (calcium carbonate)** -containing antacids greatly decrease the exposure to oral **raltegravir** (high-dose). Avoid. [Severe] Study

▶ **Encorafenib** is predicted to increase the exposure to **raltegravir**. [Moderate] Theoretical

▶ **HIV-protease inhibitors (atazanavir)** increase the exposure to **raltegravir** (high-dose). Avoid. [Moderate] Study

▶ **HIV-protease inhibitors (darunavir)** increase the risk of rash when given with **raltegravir**. [Moderate] Study

▶ **HIV-protease inhibitors (fosamprenavir)** boosted with ritonavir decrease the exposure to **raltegravir** and **raltegravir** decreases the exposure to **HIV-protease inhibitors (fosamprenavir)** boosted with ritonavir. Avoid. [Severe] Study

▶ Oral **iron** is predicted to decrease the exposure to oral **raltegravir**. Separate administration by at least 2 hours. [Moderate] Theoretical

▶ **Ivosidenib** might decrease the exposure to **raltegravir**. Avoid or monitor efficacy. [Unknown] Theoretical

▶ **Rifamycins (rifampicin)** slightly decrease the exposure to **raltegravir**. Avoid or adjust dose—consult product literature. [Moderate] Study

▶ **Sodium zirconium cyclosilicate** is predicted to decrease the exposure to **raltegravir**. Separate administration by at least 2 hours. [Moderate] Theoretical

Raltitrexed → see TABLE 14 p. 1575 (myelosuppression)

▶ **Folates** are predicted to alter the effects of **raltitrexed**. Avoid. [Moderate] Study

▶ **Live vaccines** are predicted to increase the risk of generalised infection (possibly life-threatening) when given with **raltitrexed**. UKHSA advises avoid (refer to Green Book). [Severe] Theoretical

Ramipril → see ACE inhibitors

Ramucirumab → see monoclonal antibodies

Ranibizumab

▶ **Drugs with anticoagulant effects** (see TABLE 3 p. 1571) cause bleeding, as can **ranibizumab**; concurrent use might increase the risk of developing this effect. [Severe] Theoretical

▶ **Drugs with antiplatelet effects** (see TABLE 4 p. 1571) cause bleeding, as can **ranibizumab**; concurrent use might increase the risk of developing this effect. [Severe] Theoretical

Ranitidine → see H$_2$ receptor antagonists

Ranolazine → see TABLE 8 p. 1573 (QT-interval prolongation)

▶ **Ranolazine** is predicted to increase the exposure to **afatinib**. [Moderate] Study

▶ **Ranolazine** is predicted to increase the exposure to **aliskiren**. [Moderate] Theoretical

▶ **Anti-androgens (apalutamide, enzalutamide)** are predicted to decrease the exposure to **ranolazine**. Avoid. [Severe] Study → Also see TABLE 8 p. 1573

▶ **Antiarrhythmics (dronedarone)** are predicted to increase the exposure to **ranolazine**. [Severe] Study → Also see TABLE 8 p. 1573

▶ **Antiepileptics (carbamazepine, fosphenytoin, phenobarbital, phenytoin, primidone)** are predicted to decrease the exposure to **ranolazine**. Avoid. [Severe] Study

▶ **Antifungals, azoles (fluconazole, isavuconazole)** are predicted to increase the exposure to **ranolazine**. [Severe] Study → Also see TABLE 8 p. 1573

▶ **Antifungals, azoles (itraconazole, ketoconazole, posaconazole, voriconazole)** are predicted to increase the exposure to **ranolazine**. Avoid. [Severe] Study → Also see TABLE 8 p. 1573

▶ **Ranolazine** is predicted to increase the exposure to **antihistamines, non-sedating (fexofenadine)**. [Moderate] Theoretical

▶ **Berotralstat** is predicted to increase the exposure to **ranolazine**. [Severe] Study

▶ **Ranolazine** is predicted to increase the exposure to **beta blockers, non-selective (nadolol)**. [Moderate] Study

▶ **Ranolazine** is predicted to increase the exposure to **bictegravir**. Use with caution or avoid. [Moderate] Theoretical

▶ **Calcium channel blockers (diltiazem, verapamil)** are predicted to increase the exposure to **ranolazine**. [Severe] Study

▶ **Ceritinib** is predicted to increase the exposure to **ranolazine**. Avoid. [Severe] Study → Also see TABLE 8 p. 1573

▶ **Ciclosporin** is predicted to increase the concentration of **ranolazine** and **ranolazine** is predicted to increase the concentration of **ciclosporin**. [Moderate] Theoretical

▶ **Cobicistat** is predicted to increase the exposure to **ranolazine**. Avoid. [Severe] Study

▶ **Ranolazine** is predicted to increase the exposure to **colchicine**. Avoid P-glycoprotein inhibitors or adjust **colchicine** dose, p. 1279. [Severe] Theoretical

▶ **Crizotinib** is predicted to increase the exposure to **ranolazine**. [Severe] Study → Also see TABLE 8 p. 1573

▶ **Danicopan** is predicted to increase the exposure to **ranolazine**. [Moderate] Study

▶ **Ranolazine** increases the concentration of **digoxin**. [Moderate] Study

▶ **Ranolazine** is predicted to increase the exposure to **dopamine receptor agonists (pramipexole)**. Adjust dose. [Moderate] Study

▶ **Eliglustat** is predicted to increase the exposure to **ranolazine**. Adjust dose. [Moderate] Study

▶ **Encorafenib** is predicted to decrease the exposure to **ranolazine**. Avoid. [Severe] Study → Also see TABLE 8 p. 1573

▶ **Ranolazine** is predicted to increase the exposure to **erlotinib**. [Moderate] Theoretical

▶ **Ranolazine** is predicted to increase the exposure to **factor XA inhibitors (apixaban)**. [Moderate] Theoretical

▶ **Ranolazine** is predicted to slightly increase the exposure to **factor XA inhibitors (edoxaban)**. [Severe] Theoretical

▶ **Fedratinib** is predicted to increase the exposure to **ranolazine**. [Severe] Study

▶ **Ranolazine** is predicted to increase the exposure to **fidaxomicin**. Avoid. [Moderate] Study

▶ **Ranolazine** is predicted to increase the exposure to **gilteritinib**. [Moderate] Theoretical

▶ **Glecaprevir** is predicted to increase the exposure to **ranolazine**. Adjust dose. [Severe] Theoretical

▶ **Grapefruit** juice is predicted to increase the concentration of **ranolazine**. Avoid. [Severe] Theoretical

▶ **HIV-protease inhibitors** are predicted to increase the exposure to **ranolazine**. Avoid. [Severe] Study

▶ **Idelalisib** is predicted to increase the exposure to **ranolazine**. Avoid. [Severe] Study

▶ **Imatinib** is predicted to increase the exposure to **ranolazine**. [Severe] Study

▶ **Ivosidenib** is predicted to decrease the exposure to **ranolazine**. Avoid. [Severe] Study → Also see TABLE 8 p. 1573

▶ **Lapatinib** is predicted to increase the exposure to **ranolazine**. [Moderate] Theoretical → Also see TABLE 8 p. 1573

▶ **Letermovir** is predicted to increase the exposure to **ranolazine**. [Severe] Study

Ranolazine (continued)
▸ **Ranolazine** is predicted to increase the exposure to lomitapide. Separate administration by 12 hours. Mild Theoretical
▸ Lorlatinib is predicted to decrease the exposure to **ranolazine**. Moderate Theoretical
▸ Lumacaftor is predicted to decrease the exposure to **ranolazine**. Avoid. Severe Study
▸ Macrolides (clarithromycin) are predicted to increase the exposure to **ranolazine**. Avoid. Severe Study
▸ Macrolides (erythromycin) are predicted to increase the exposure to **ranolazine**. Severe Study → Also see **TABLE 8** p. 1573
▸ **Ranolazine** is predicted to increase the exposure to mavacamten. Monitor and adjust dose—consult product literature. Moderate Theoretical
▸ **Ranolazine** is predicted to increase the exposure to metformin. Use with caution and adjust dose. Moderate Study
▸ Mitotane is predicted to decrease the exposure to **ranolazine**. Avoid. Severe Study
▸ **Ranolazine** increases the risk of neutropenia when given with monoclonal antibodies (brentuximab vedotin). Monitor and adjust dose. Severe Theoretical
▸ **Ranolazine** is predicted to increase the exposure to naldemedine. Moderate Study
▸ **Ranolazine** is predicted to increase the exposure to neratinib. Avoid or adjust dose and monitor for gastrointestinal adverse effects—consult product literature. Severe Study
▸ Neurokinin-1 receptor antagonists (aprepitant, netupitant) are predicted to increase the exposure to **ranolazine**. Severe Study
▸ Nilotinib is predicted to increase the exposure to **ranolazine**. Severe Study → Also see **TABLE 8** p. 1573
▸ **Ranolazine** is predicted to increase the exposure to nintedanib. Moderate Study
▸ Nirmatrelvir boosted with ritonavir is predicted to increase the concentration of **ranolazine**. Avoid. Severe Theoretical
▸ Olaparib might increase the exposure to **ranolazine**. Moderate Theoretical
▸ Osimertinib is predicted to increase the exposure to **ranolazine**. Moderate Study → Also see **TABLE 8** p. 1573
▸ **Ranolazine** is predicted to increase the exposure to panobinostat. Adjust dose. Moderate Theoretical → Also see **TABLE 8** p. 1573
▸ **Ranolazine** is predicted to increase the exposure to pibrentasvir. Moderate Theoretical
▸ **Ranolazine** is predicted to increase the exposure to pralsetinib. Moderate Theoretical
▸ **Ranolazine** is predicted to increase the exposure to relugolix. Avoid or take relugolix first and separate administration by at least 6 hours. Moderate Study
▸ Rifamycins (rifampicin) are predicted to decrease the exposure to **ranolazine**. Avoid. Severe Study
▸ **Ranolazine** is predicted to increase the exposure to rimegepant. Avoid another dose of rimegepant within 48 hours of concurrent use. Moderate Theoretical
▸ St John's wort is predicted to decrease the exposure to **ranolazine**. Avoid. Severe Study
▸ **Ranolazine** is predicted to increase the exposure to statins (atorvastatin). Moderate Theoretical
▸ **Ranolazine** slightly increases the exposure to statins (simvastatin). Adjust **simvastatin** dose, p. 237. Moderate Study
▸ **Ranolazine** increases the concentration of tacrolimus. Adjust dose. Severe Anecdotal
▸ **Ranolazine** is predicted to slightly increase the exposure to talazoparib. Avoid or adjust dose—consult product literature. Severe Study
▸ **Ranolazine** is predicted to increase the exposure to taxanes (paclitaxel). Severe Theoretical
▸ **Ranolazine** is predicted to increase the exposure to thrombin inhibitors (dabigatran). Severe Theoretical
▸ **Ranolazine** is predicted to increase the exposure to ticagrelor. Use with caution or avoid. Severe Study
▸ **Ranolazine** might increase the exposure to tigecycline. Mild Anecdotal
▸ **Ranolazine** is predicted to increase the exposure to topotecan. Severe Study

▸ **Ranolazine** is predicted to increase the concentration of trametinib. Moderate Theoretical
▸ Tucatinib is predicted to increase the exposure to **ranolazine**. Avoid. Severe Study
▸ Vemurafenib might increase the exposure to **ranolazine**. Use with caution or avoid. Moderate Theoretical → Also see **TABLE 8** p. 1573
▸ **Ranolazine** is predicted to increase the exposure to venetoclax. Avoid or monitor for toxicity. Severe Theoretical
▸ **Ranolazine** might increase the exposure to vinca alkaloids. Severe Theoretical
▸ Voxilaprevir with sofosbuvir and velpatasvir is predicted to increase the exposure to **ranolazine**. Adjust dose. Severe Theoretical

Rasagiline → see MAO-B inhibitors

Ravulizumab
▸ Crovalimab increases the risk of hypersensitivity reactions when given with **ravulizumab**. Severe Study

Reboxetine
▸ Anti-androgens (apalutamide, enzalutamide) are predicted to decrease the exposure to **reboxetine**. Moderate Anecdotal
▸ Antiepileptics (carbamazepine, fosphenytoin, phenobarbital, phenytoin, primidone) are predicted to decrease the exposure to **reboxetine**. Moderate Anecdotal
▸ Antifungals, azoles (itraconazole, ketoconazole, posaconazole, voriconazole) are predicted to increase the exposure to **reboxetine**. Avoid. Moderate Study
▸ Antifungals, azoles (miconazole) are predicted to increase the concentration of **reboxetine**. Use with caution and adjust dose. Moderate Theoretical
▸ Ceritinib is predicted to increase the exposure to **reboxetine**. Avoid. Moderate Study
▸ Cobicistat is predicted to increase the exposure to **reboxetine**. Avoid. Moderate Study
▸ Encorafenib is predicted to decrease the exposure to **reboxetine**. Moderate Anecdotal
▸ HIV-protease inhibitors are predicted to increase the exposure to **reboxetine**. Avoid. Moderate Study
▸ Idelalisib is predicted to increase the exposure to **reboxetine**. Avoid. Moderate Study
▸ Ivosidenib is predicted to decrease the exposure to **reboxetine**. Moderate Anecdotal
▸ **Reboxetine** is predicted to increase the risk of a hypertensive crisis when given with linezolid. Avoid. Severe Theoretical
▸ **Reboxetine** is predicted to increase the risk of hypokalaemia when given with loop diuretics. Moderate Theoretical
▸ Lumacaftor is predicted to decrease the exposure to **reboxetine**. Moderate Anecdotal
▸ Macrolides (clarithromycin) are predicted to increase the exposure to **reboxetine**. Avoid. Moderate Study
▸ **Reboxetine** is predicted to increase the risk of a hypertensive crisis when given with MAO-B inhibitors (rasagiline, selegiline). Avoid. Severe Theoretical
▸ **Reboxetine** is predicted to increase the risk of a hypertensive crisis when given with MAOIs, irreversible. Avoid. Severe Theoretical
▸ Mitotane is predicted to decrease the exposure to **reboxetine**. Moderate Anecdotal
▸ **Reboxetine** is predicted to increase the risk of a hypertensive crisis when given with moclobemide. Avoid. Severe Theoretical
▸ Rifamycins (rifampicin) are predicted to decrease the exposure to **reboxetine**. Moderate Anecdotal
▸ **Reboxetine** is predicted to increase the risk of hypokalaemia when given with thiazide diuretics. Moderate Anecdotal
▸ Tucatinib is predicted to increase the exposure to **reboxetine**. Avoid. Moderate Study

Regorafenib → see **TABLE 14** p. 1575 (myelosuppression), **TABLE 4** p. 1571 (antiplatelet effects)
▸ Anti-androgens (apalutamide, enzalutamide) are predicted to decrease the exposure to **regorafenib**. Avoid. Moderate Study
▸ Antiarrhythmics (dronedarone) are predicted to increase the exposure to **regorafenib**. Moderate Study
▸ Antiepileptics (carbamazepine, fosphenytoin, phenobarbital, phenytoin, primidone) are predicted to decrease the exposure to **regorafenib**. Avoid. Moderate Study

▶ Antifungals, azoles **(fluconazole, isavuconazole)** are predicted to increase the exposure to **regorafenib**. Moderate Study

▶ Antifungals, azoles **(itraconazole, ketoconazole, posaconazole, voriconazole)** are predicted to increase the exposure to **regorafenib**. Avoid. Moderate Study

▶ **Berotralstat** is predicted to increase the exposure to **regorafenib**. Moderate Study

▶ Calcium channel blockers **(diltiazem, verapamil)** are predicted to increase the exposure to **regorafenib**. Moderate Study

▶ **Ceritinib** is predicted to increase the exposure to **regorafenib**. Avoid. Moderate Study → Also see **TABLE** 14 p. 1575

▶ **Cobicistat** is predicted to increase the exposure to **regorafenib**. Avoid. Moderate Study

▶ **Crizotinib** is predicted to increase the exposure to **regorafenib**. Moderate Study

▶ **Dabrafenib** is predicted to decrease the exposure to **regorafenib**. Severe Study

▶ **Encorafenib** is predicted to decrease the exposure to **regorafenib**. Avoid. Moderate Study

▶ Endothelin receptor antagonists **(bosentan)** are predicted to decrease the exposure to **regorafenib**. Severe Study

▶ **Fedratinib** is predicted to increase the exposure to **regorafenib**. Moderate Study

▶ **Grapefruit** juice is predicted to increase the exposure to **regorafenib**. Avoid. Moderate Theoretical

▶ **HIV-protease inhibitors** are predicted to increase the exposure to **regorafenib**. Avoid. Moderate Study

▶ **Idelalisib** is predicted to increase the exposure to **regorafenib**. Avoid. Moderate Study

▶ **Imatinib** is predicted to increase the exposure to **regorafenib**. Moderate Study → Also see **TABLE 14** p. 1575 → Also see **TABLE 4** p. 1571

▶ **Ivosidenib** is predicted to decrease the exposure to **regorafenib**. Avoid. Moderate Study

▶ **Letermovir** is predicted to increase the exposure to **regorafenib**. Moderate Study

▶ **Lumacaftor** is predicted to decrease the exposure to **regorafenib**. Avoid. Moderate Study

▶ Macrolides **(clarithromycin)** are predicted to increase the exposure to **regorafenib**. Avoid. Moderate Study

▶ Macrolides **(erythromycin)** are predicted to increase the exposure to **regorafenib**. Moderate Study

▶ **Regorafenib** is predicted to increase the exposure to methotrexate. Moderate Theoretical → Also see **TABLE 14** p. 1575

▶ **Mitotane** is predicted to decrease the exposure to **regorafenib**. Avoid. Moderate Study → Also see **TABLE 14** p. 1575

▶ Neurokinin-1 receptor antagonists **(aprepitant, netupitant)** are predicted to increase the exposure to **regorafenib**. Moderate Study

▶ **Nilotinib** is predicted to increase the exposure to **regorafenib**. Moderate Study → Also see **TABLE 14** p. 1575

▶ NNRTIs **(efavirenz, etravirine, nevirapine)** are predicted to decrease the exposure to **regorafenib**. Severe Study

▶ NSAIDs **(mefenamic acid)** are predicted to increase the exposure to **regorafenib**. Avoid. Moderate Theoretical → Also see **TABLE 4** p. 1571

▶ Rifamycins **(rifampicin)** are predicted to decrease the exposure to **regorafenib**. Avoid. Moderate Study

▶ **Regorafenib** is predicted to increase the exposure to the active component of sacituzumab govitecan. Severe Theoretical

▶ **St John's wort** is predicted to decrease the exposure to **regorafenib**. Avoid. Severe Study

▶ **Regorafenib** is predicted to increase the exposure to statins **(atorvastatin, fluvastatin)**. Moderate Study

▶ **Regorafenib** moderately increases the exposure to statins **(rosuvastatin)**. Avoid or adjust **rosuvastatin** dose, p. 235. Moderate Study

▶ **Regorafenib** is predicted to increase the exposure to sulfasalazine. Moderate Study → Also see **TABLE 14** p. 1575

▶ **Regorafenib** is predicted to increase the exposure to topotecan. Moderate Study → Also see **TABLE 14** p. 1575

▶ **Tucatinib** is predicted to increase the exposure to **regorafenib**. Avoid. Moderate Study

Relugolix

▶ Aminoglycosides **(gentamicin)** are predicted to increase the exposure to **relugolix**. Avoid or take relugolix first and separate administration by at least 6 hours. Moderate Theoretical

▶ Anti-androgens **(apalutamide)** are predicted to decrease the exposure to **relugolix**. Avoid or adjust dose depending on indication—consult product literature. Moderate Study

▶ Antiarrhythmics **(amiodarone, dronedarone)** are predicted to increase the exposure to **relugolix**. Avoid or take relugolix first and separate administration by at least 6 hours. Moderate Study

▶ Antiarrhythmics **(propafenone)** are predicted to increase the exposure to **relugolix**. Avoid or take relugolix first and separate administration by at least 6 hours. Moderate Theoretical

▶ Antiepileptics **(carbamazepine, phenobarbital, phenytoin)** are predicted to decrease the exposure to **relugolix**. Avoid or adjust dose depending on indication—consult product literature. Moderate Study

▶ Antiepileptics **(oxcarbazepine, topiramate)** are predicted to decrease the exposure to **relugolix**. Avoid. Moderate Theoretical

▶ Antifungals, azoles **(itraconazole, ketoconazole)** are predicted to increase the exposure to **relugolix**. Avoid or take relugolix first and separate administration by at least 6 hours. Moderate Study

▶ Beta blockers, non-selective **(carvedilol)** are predicted to increase the exposure to **relugolix**. Avoid or take relugolix first and separate administration by at least 6 hours. Moderate Theoretical

▶ Calcium channel blockers **(verapamil)** are predicted to increase the exposure to **relugolix**. Avoid or take relugolix first and separate administration by at least 6 hours. Moderate Study

▶ **Ciclosporin** is predicted to increase the exposure to **relugolix**. Avoid or take relugolix first and separate administration by at least 6 hours. Moderate Study

▶ **Cobicistat** is predicted to increase the exposure to **relugolix**. Avoid or take relugolix first and separate administration by at least 6 hours. Moderate Study

▶ **Glecaprevir** is predicted to increase the exposure to **relugolix**. Avoid or take relugolix first and separate administration by at least 6 hours. Moderate Study

▶ **HIV-protease inhibitors (lopinavir, ritonavir)** are predicted to increase the exposure to **relugolix**. Avoid or take relugolix first and separate administration by at least 6 hours. Moderate Study

▶ **Lapatinib** is predicted to increase the exposure to **relugolix**. Avoid or take relugolix first and separate administration by at least 6 hours. Moderate Study

▶ **Macrolides** are predicted to increase the exposure to **relugolix**. Avoid or take relugolix first and separate administration by at least 6 hours. Moderate Study

▶ NNRTIs **(efavirenz)** are predicted to decrease the exposure to **relugolix**. Avoid or adjust dose depending on indication—consult product literature. Moderate Study

▶ **Pibrentasvir** is predicted to increase the exposure to **relugolix**. Avoid or take relugolix first and separate administration by at least 6 hours. Moderate Study

▶ **Ranolazine** is predicted to increase the exposure to **relugolix**. Avoid or take relugolix first and separate administration by at least 6 hours. Moderate Study

▶ **Rifamycins** are predicted to decrease the exposure to **relugolix**. Avoid or adjust dose depending on indication—consult product literature. Moderate Study

▶ **St John's wort** is predicted to decrease the exposure to **relugolix**. Avoid or adjust dose depending on indication—consult product literature. Moderate Study

▶ Tetracyclines **(tetracycline)** are predicted to increase the exposure to **relugolix**. Avoid or take relugolix first and separate administration by at least 6 hours. Moderate Theoretical

▶ **Velpatasvir** is predicted to increase the exposure to **relugolix**. Avoid or take relugolix first and separate administration by at least 6 hours. Moderate Study

▶ **Vemurafenib** is predicted to increase the exposure to **relugolix**. Avoid or take relugolix first and separate administration by at least 6 hours. Moderate Study

Relugolix (continued)

▶ **Voxilaprevir** is predicted to increase the exposure to **relugolix**. Avoid or take relugolix first and separate administration by at least 6 hours. Moderate Study

Remdesivir

▶ **Antimalarials (chloroquine)** might decrease the effects of **remdesivir**. Avoid. Moderate Theoretical

▶ **Hydroxychloroquine** might decrease the effects of **remdesivir**. Avoid. Moderate Theoretical

Remifentanil → see opioids

Remimazolam → see benzodiazepines

Repaglinide → see meglitinides

Retigabine → see antiepileptics

Retinoids → see TABLE 1 p. 1571 (hepatotoxicity), TABLE 14 p. 1575 (myelosuppression)

acitretin · adapalene · alitretinoin · bexarotene · isotretinoin · tretinoin

▶ Avoid concomitant use of keratolytics in patients taking **acitretin** or **isotretinoin**.

▶ Since systemic absorption can follow topical application of **isotretinoin** or **tretinoin**, the possibility of interactions should be borne in mind.

▶ **Alcohol** potentially increases the concentration of **acitretin**. Avoid and for 2 months after stopping **acitretin**. Moderate Study

▶ **Antiarrhythmics (amiodarone)** are predicted to increase the exposure to **alitretinoin**. Adjust **alitretinoin** dose, p. 1433. Moderate Theoretical

▶ **Antifungals, azoles (fluconazole, itraconazole, ketoconazole, miconazole, posaconazole, voriconazole)** are predicted to increase the exposure to **alitretinoin**. Adjust **alitretinoin** dose, p. 1433. Moderate Theoretical

▶ **Antifungals, azoles (fluconazole, ketoconazole, voriconazole)** are predicted to increase the risk of tretinoin toxicity when given with **tretinoin**. Moderate Study

▶ **Antifungals, azoles (posaconazole)** are predicted to increase the risk of tretinoin toxicity when given with **tretinoin**. Monitor and adjust dose. Severe Theoretical

▶ **Ceritinib** is predicted to increase the exposure to **alitretinoin**. Adjust **alitretinoin** dose, p. 1433. Moderate Theoretical

▶ **Clopidogrel** is predicted to increase the exposure to **alitretinoin**. Adjust **alitretinoin** dose, p. 1433. Moderate Theoretical

▶ **Cobicistat** is predicted to increase the exposure to **alitretinoin**. Adjust **alitretinoin** dose, p. 1433. Moderate Theoretical

▶ **Fibrates (gemfibrozil)** are predicted to increase the exposure to **alitretinoin**. Adjust **alitretinoin** dose, p. 1433. Moderate Theoretical

▶ **Fibrates (gemfibrozil)** increase the concentration of **bexarotene**. Avoid. Severe Study

▶ **HIV-protease inhibitors** are predicted to increase the exposure to **alitretinoin**. Adjust **alitretinoin** dose, p. 1433. Moderate Theoretical

▶ **Idelalisib** is predicted to increase the exposure to **alitretinoin**. Adjust **alitretinoin** dose, p. 1433. Moderate Theoretical

▶ **Macrolides (clarithromycin)** are predicted to increase the exposure to **alitretinoin**. Adjust **alitretinoin** dose, p. 1433. Moderate Theoretical

▶ **Acitretin** is predicted to increase the concentration of **methotrexate**. Avoid. Moderate Anecdotal → Also see TABLE 1 p. 1571

▶ **Retinoids (acitretin, alitretinoin, isotretinoin, tretinoin)** increase the risk of benign intracranial hypertension when given with **tetracyclines**. Avoid. Severe Anecdotal → Also see TABLE 1 p. 1571

▶ **Retinoids (acitretin, alitretinoin, isotretinoin, tretinoin)** increase the risk of benign intracranial hypertension when given with **tigecycline**. Avoid. Severe Anecdotal → Also see TABLE 1 p. 1571

▶ **Tucatinib** is predicted to increase the exposure to **alitretinoin**. Adjust **alitretinoin** dose, p. 1433. Moderate Theoretical

▶ **Bexarotene** is predicted to increase the risk of toxicity when given with **vitamin A**. Adjust dose. Moderate Theoretical → Also see TABLE 1 p. 1571

▶ **Retinoids (acitretin, alitretinoin, isotretinoin)** are predicted to increase the risk of vitamin A toxicity when given with **vitamin A**. Avoid. Severe Theoretical → Also see TABLE 1 p. 1571

▶ **Tretinoin** is predicted to increase the risk of vitamin A toxicity when given with **vitamin A**. Avoid. Severe Study

Ribavirin

▶ **Ribavirin** increases the risk of anaemia and/or leucopenia when given with NRTIs **(zidovudine)**. Avoid. Severe Study

Ribociclib → see TABLE 14 p. 1575 (myelosuppression), TABLE 8 p. 1573 (QT-interval prolongation)

FOOD AND LIFESTYLE Avoid concomitant use of pomegranate or pomegranate juice as it is predicted to increase ribociclib exposure.

▶ **Ribociclib** (high-dose) is predicted to increase the exposure to alpha blockers **(alfuzosin)**. Avoid. Moderate Theoretical

▶ **Anti-androgens (apalutamide, enzalutamide)** are predicted to markedly decrease the exposure to **ribociclib**. Avoid. Severe Study → Also see TABLE 8 p. 1573

▶ **Antiarrhythmics (dronedarone)** are predicted to increase the exposure to **ribociclib**. Moderate Study → Also see TABLE 8 p. 1573

▶ **Ribociclib** (high-dose) is predicted to increase the exposure to antiarrhythmics **(amiodarone)**. Avoid. Moderate Theoretical → Also see TABLE 8 p. 1573

▶ **Antiepileptics (carbamazepine, fosphenytoin, phenobarbital, phenytoin, primidone)** are predicted to markedly decrease the exposure to **ribociclib**. Avoid. Severe Study

▶ **Antifungals, azoles (fluconazole, isavuconazole)** are predicted to increase the exposure to **ribociclib**. Moderate Study → Also see TABLE 8 p. 1573

▶ **Antifungals, azoles (itraconazole, ketoconazole, posaconazole, voriconazole)** are predicted to increase the exposure to **ribociclib**. Avoid or adjust dose—consult product literature. Moderate Study → Also see TABLE 8 p. 1573

▶ **Ribociclib** (high-dose) is predicted to increase the exposure to antipsychotics, second generation **(quetiapine)**. Avoid. Moderate Theoretical

▶ **Ribociclib** moderately increases the exposure to benzodiazepines **(midazolam)**. Avoid. Moderate Study

▶ **Berotralstat** is predicted to increase the exposure to **ribociclib**. Moderate Study

▶ **Calcium channel blockers (diltiazem, verapamil)** are predicted to increase the exposure to **ribociclib**. Moderate Study

▶ **Ribociclib** is predicted to increase the exposure to capivasertib. Adjust dose. Moderate Theoretical

▶ **Ceritinib** is predicted to increase the exposure to **ribociclib**. Avoid or adjust dose—consult product literature. Moderate Study → Also see TABLE 14 p. 1575 → Also see TABLE 8 p. 1573

▶ **Ribociclib** is predicted to increase the exposure to ciclosporin. Use with caution and adjust dose. Moderate Theoretical

▶ **Cobicistat** is predicted to increase the exposure to **ribociclib**. Avoid or adjust dose—consult product literature. Moderate Study

▶ **Crizotinib** is predicted to increase the exposure to **ribociclib**. Moderate Study → Also see TABLE 8 p. 1573

▶ **Ribociclib** is predicted to increase the exposure to digoxin. Moderate Theoretical

▶ **Encorafenib** is predicted to markedly decrease the exposure to **ribociclib**. Avoid. Severe Study → Also see TABLE 8 p. 1573

▶ **Endothelin receptor antagonists (bosentan)** are predicted to decrease the exposure to **ribociclib**. Moderate Study

▶ **Ribociclib** is predicted to increase the exposure to everolimus. Use with caution and adjust dose. Moderate Theoretical

▶ **Fedratinib** is predicted to increase the exposure to **ribociclib**. Moderate Study

▶ **Grapefruit** juice is predicted to increase the exposure to **ribociclib**. Avoid. Moderate Theoretical

▶ **HIV-protease inhibitors** are predicted to increase the exposure to **ribociclib**. Avoid or adjust dose—consult product literature. Moderate Study

▶ **Idelalisib** is predicted to increase the exposure to **ribociclib**. Avoid or adjust dose—consult product literature. Moderate Study

▶ **Imatinib** is predicted to increase the exposure to **ribociclib**. Moderate Study → Also see TABLE 14 p. 1575

▶ **Ivosidenib** is predicted to markedly decrease the exposure to **ribociclib**. Avoid. Severe Study → Also see TABLE 8 p. 1573

▶ **Letermovir** is predicted to increase the exposure to **ribociclib**. Moderate Study

▶ **Lumacaftor** is predicted to markedly decrease the exposure to **ribociclib**. Avoid. Severe Study

▸ Macrolides **(clarithromycin)** are predicted to increase the exposure to **ribociclib**. Avoid or adjust dose—consult product literature. ⟨Moderate⟩ Study

▸ Macrolides **(erythromycin)** are predicted to increase the exposure to **ribociclib**. ⟨Moderate⟩ Study → Also see **TABLE 8** p. 1573

▸ **Ribociclib** is predicted to increase the exposure to metformin. ⟨Moderate⟩ Theoretical

▸ Mitotane is predicted to markedly decrease the exposure to **ribociclib**. Avoid. ⟨Severe⟩ Study → Also see **TABLE 14** p. 1575

▸ Neurokinin-1 receptor antagonists **(aprepitant, netupitant)** are predicted to increase the exposure to **ribociclib**. ⟨Moderate⟩ Study

▸ Nilotinib is predicted to increase the exposure to **ribociclib**. ⟨Moderate⟩ Study → Also see **TABLE 14** p. 1575 → Also see **TABLE 8** p. 1573

▸ NNRTIs **(efavirenz, etravirine, nevirapine)** are predicted to decrease the exposure to **ribociclib**. ⟨Moderate⟩ Study → Also see **TABLE 8** p. 1573

▸ **Ribociclib** is predicted to increase the exposure to opioids **(alfentanil, fentanyl)**. Use with caution and adjust dose. ⟨Moderate⟩ Theoretical

▸ **Ribociclib** is predicted to increase the exposure to phosphodiesterase type-5 inhibitors **(sildenafil)**. Avoid. ⟨Moderate⟩ Theoretical

▸ **Ribociclib** (high-dose) is predicted to increase the exposure to pimozide. Avoid. ⟨Moderate⟩ Theoretical → Also see **TABLE 8** p. 1573

▸ Rifamycins **(rifampicin)** are predicted to markedly decrease the exposure to **ribociclib**. Avoid. ⟨Severe⟩ Study

▸ **Ribociclib** is predicted to increase the exposure to sirolimus. Use with caution and adjust dose. ⟨Moderate⟩ Theoretical

▸ St John's wort is predicted to decrease the exposure to **ribociclib**. Avoid. ⟨Severe⟩ Study

▸ **Ribociclib** is predicted to increase the exposure to statins **(pravastatin, rosuvastatin)**. ⟨Moderate⟩ Theoretical

▸ **Ribociclib** (high-dose) is predicted to increase the exposure to statins **(simvastatin)**. Avoid. ⟨Moderate⟩ Theoretical

▸ **Ribociclib** is predicted to increase the exposure to tacrolimus. Use with caution and adjust dose. ⟨Moderate⟩ Theoretical

▸ Tucatinib is predicted to increase the exposure to **ribociclib**. Avoid or adjust dose—consult product literature. ⟨Moderate⟩ Study

Rifabutin → see rifamycins
Rifampicin → see rifamycins
Rifamycins → see **TABLE 2** p. 1571 (nephrotoxicity)

rifabutin · rifampicin

GENERAL INFORMATION Although some manufacturers class rifabutin as a potent inducer of CYP3A4, clinical data suggests it is potentially a weak inducer, and therefore the BNF does not extrapolate the interactions of potent CYP3A4 inducers to rifabutin. For those who wish to err on the side of caution, see the interactions of rifampicin but bear in mind other mechanisms might be involved.

▸ **Rifampicin** is predicted to decrease the exposure to 5-HT3-receptor antagonists **(ondansetron)**. ⟨Moderate⟩ Study

▸ **Rifampicin** is predicted to markedly decrease the exposure to abemaciclib. Avoid. ⟨Severe⟩ Study

▸ **Rifampicin** is predicted to decrease the exposure to abrocitinib. Avoid. ⟨Moderate⟩ Study

▸ **Rifampicin** is predicted to decrease the exposure to acalabrutinib. Avoid. ⟨Severe⟩ Study

▸ **Rifampicin** is predicted to decrease the exposure to afatinib. ⟨Moderate⟩ Study

▸ **Rifampicin** is predicted to decrease the exposure to agomelatine. ⟨Moderate⟩ Theoretical

▸ **Rifampicin** decreases the exposure to aliskiren. ⟨Moderate⟩ Study

▸ **Rifampicin** is predicted to decrease the exposure to alpelisib. Avoid. ⟨Moderate⟩ Study

▸ **Rifampicin** decreases the exposure to aminophylline. Adjust dose. ⟨Moderate⟩ Study

▸ **Rifampicin** is predicted to decrease the exposure to anaesthetics, local **(ropivacaine)**. ⟨Moderate⟩ Theoretical

▸ Oral **antacids** decrease the absorption of oral **rifampicin**. Manufacturer advises take 1 hour before antacids. ⟨Moderate⟩ Study

▸ **Rifampicin** is predicted to decrease the exposure to antiandrogens **(abiraterone)**. Avoid. ⟨Severe⟩ Study

▸ **Rifamycins** are predicted to decrease the efficacy of antiandrogens **(cyproterone)** with ethinylestradiol (co-cyprindiol). Use alternative methods during treatment with, and for 28 days after, the enzyme inducing drug is stopped. ⟨Severe⟩ Study

▸ **Rifampicin** is predicted to decrease the exposure to antiandrogens **(darolutamide)**. Avoid. ⟨Moderate⟩ Study

▸ **Rifampicin** is predicted to decrease the exposure to antiarrhythmics **(disopyramide, dronedarone)**. Avoid. ⟨Severe⟩ Study

▸ **Rifampicin** is predicted to decrease the efficacy of antiarrhythmics **(propafenone)**. ⟨Moderate⟩ Study

▸ **Rifampicin** is predicted to decrease the exposure to anticholinesterases, centrally acting **(donepezil)**. ⟨Mild⟩ Study

▸ Antiepileptics **(phenobarbital, primidone)** are predicted to decrease the exposure to **rifampicin** and **rifampicin** is predicted to decrease the exposure to antiepileptics **(phenobarbital, primidone)**. Use with caution and adjust dose. ⟨Moderate⟩ Study

▸ **Rifampicin** slightly decreases the exposure to antiepileptics **(brivaracetam)**. Adjust dose. ⟨Moderate⟩ Study

▸ **Rifampicin** decreases the concentration of antiepileptics **(fosphenytoin, phenytoin)**. Use with caution and adjust dose. ⟨Moderate⟩ Study

▸ **Rifampicin** markedly increases the clearance of antiepileptics **(lamotrigine)**. Adjust **lamotrigine** dose, p. 366. ⟨Moderate⟩ Study

▸ **Rifampicin** is predicted to decrease the exposure to antiepileptics **(perampanel)**. Monitor and adjust dose. ⟨Moderate⟩ Study

▸ **Rifampicin** is predicted to decrease the concentration of antiepileptics **(zonisamide)**. Monitor and adjust dose. ⟨Moderate⟩ Theoretical

▸ Antifungals, azoles **(fluconazole)** increase the risk of uveitis when given with **rifabutin**. Adjust dose. ⟨Severe⟩ Study

▸ Antifungals, azoles **(itraconazole, posaconazole)** increase the concentration of **rifabutin** and **rifabutin** decreases the concentration of antifungals, azoles **(itraconazole, posaconazole)**. Avoid. ⟨Severe⟩ Study

▸ Antifungals, azoles **(ketoconazole)** are predicted to increase the concentration of **rifabutin** and **rifabutin** is predicted to decrease the concentration of antifungals, azoles **(ketoconazole)**. Avoid. ⟨Severe⟩ Theoretical

▸ Antifungals, azoles **(miconazole)** are predicted to increase the concentration of **rifabutin**. Use with caution and adjust dose. ⟨Moderate⟩ Theoretical

▸ **Rifampicin** slightly decreases the exposure to antifungals, azoles **(fluconazole)**. Adjust dose. ⟨Moderate⟩ Study

▸ **Rifabutin** is predicted to decrease the exposure to antifungals, azoles **(isavuconazole)**. Avoid. ⟨Severe⟩ Theoretical

▸ **Rifampicin** is predicted to decrease the exposure to antifungals, azoles **(isavuconazole)**. Avoid. ⟨Severe⟩ Study

▸ **Rifampicin** markedly decreases the exposure to antifungals, azoles **(itraconazole)**. Avoid and for 14 days after stopping **rifampicin**. ⟨Moderate⟩ Study

▸ **Rifampicin** markedly decreases the exposure to antifungals, azoles **(ketoconazole)** and antifungals, azoles **(ketoconazole)** potentially decrease the exposure to **rifampicin**. Avoid. ⟨Moderate⟩ Study

▸ **Rifampicin** is predicted to decrease the exposure to antifungals, azoles **(posaconazole)**. Avoid. ⟨Moderate⟩ Anecdotal

▸ **Rifabutin** decreases the concentration of antifungals, azoles **(voriconazole)** and antifungals, azoles **(voriconazole)** increase the concentration of **rifabutin**. Avoid or adjust **voriconazole** dose, p. 695. ⟨Severe⟩ Study

▸ **Rifampicin** very markedly decreases the exposure to antifungals, azoles **(voriconazole)**. Avoid. ⟨Moderate⟩ Study

▸ **Rifampicin** is predicted to decrease the exposure to antihistamines, non-sedating **(bilastine)**. ⟨Moderate⟩ Theoretical

▸ **Rifampicin** increases the clearance of antihistamines, nonsedating **(fexofenadine)**. ⟨Moderate⟩ Study

▸ **Rifampicin** is predicted to decrease the exposure to antimalarials **(artemether)** with lumefantrine. Avoid. ⟨Severe⟩ Study

Rifamycins (continued)

▶ **Rifabutin** slightly decreases the exposure to antimalarials (atovaquone). Avoid. [Moderate] Study
▶ **Rifampicin** moderately decreases the exposure to antimalarials (atovaquone) and antimalarials (atovaquone) slightly increase the exposure to **rifampicin**. Avoid. [Moderate] Study
▶ **Rifampicin** moderately decreases the exposure to antimalarials (mefloquine). [Severe] Study
▶ **Rifampicin** decreases the exposure to antimalarials (quinine). [Severe] Study
▶ **Rifampicin** is predicted to moderately decrease the exposure to antipsychotics, second generation (aripiprazole). Adjust **aripiprazole** dose, p. 454. [Moderate] Study
▶ **Rifampicin** is predicted to decrease the exposure to antipsychotics, second generation (cariprazine). Avoid. [Severe] Theoretical
▶ **Rifampicin** decreases the exposure to antipsychotics, second generation (clozapine). [Severe] Anecdotal
▶ **Rifampicin** is predicted to decrease the exposure to antipsychotics, second generation (lurasidone). Avoid. [Moderate] Study
▶ **Rifampicin** is predicted to decrease the exposure to antipsychotics, second generation (olanzapine). Monitor and adjust dose. [Moderate] Study
▶ **Rifampicin** is predicted to decrease the exposure to antipsychotics, second generation (paliperidone). Monitor and adjust dose. [Severe] Study
▶ **Rifampicin** is predicted to decrease the exposure to antipsychotics, second generation (quetiapine). [Moderate] Study
▶ **Rifampicin** is predicted to decrease the exposure to antipsychotics, second generation (risperidone). Adjust dose. [Moderate] Study
▶ **Rifampicin** decreases the exposure to ataluren. [Moderate] Study
▶ **Rifampicin** (single-dose) increases the exposure to atogepant. Adjust **atogepant** dose, p. 540. [Moderate] Study
▶ **Rifampicin** is predicted to decrease the exposure to avacopan. Avoid or monitor. [Severe] Study
▶ **Rifampicin** is predicted to decrease the exposure to avapritinib. Avoid. [Severe] Study
▶ **Rifampicin** is predicted to decrease the exposure to avatrombopag. Adjust **avatrombopag** dose with moderate CYP2C9 inducers in chronic immune thrombocytopenia, p. 1169. [Moderate] Study
▶ **Rifampicin** is predicted to decrease the exposure to axitinib. Avoid or adjust dose. [Moderate] Study
▶ **Rifampicin** is predicted to decrease the exposure to bazedoxifene. [Moderate] Theoretical
▶ **Rifampicin** decreases the exposure to bedaquiline. Avoid. [Severe] Study
▶ **Rifampicin** is predicted to decrease the exposure to belumosudil. Adjust **belumosudil** dose, p. 979. [Severe] Study
▶ **Rifampicin** is predicted to decrease the exposure to benzodiazepines (alprazolam). Adjust dose. [Moderate] Theoretical
▶ **Rifampicin** is predicted to decrease the exposure to benzodiazepines (chlordiazepoxide). [Moderate] Theoretical
▶ **Rifampicin** moderately decreases the exposure to benzodiazepines (diazepam). Avoid. [Moderate] Study
▶ **Rifampicin** increases the clearance of benzodiazepines (lorazepam, nitrazepam). [Moderate] Study
▶ **Rifampicin** is predicted to decrease the exposure to benzodiazepines (midazolam). Monitor and adjust dose. [Severe] Study
▶ **Rifampicin** is predicted to decrease the concentration of berotralstat. Avoid. [Severe] Theoretical
▶ **Rifampicin** moderately decreases the exposure to beta blockers, non-selective (carvedilol). [Moderate] Study
▶ **Rifampicin** decreases the exposure to beta blockers, non-selective (propranolol). Monitor and adjust dose. [Moderate] Study
▶ **Rifampicin** slightly decreases the exposure to beta blockers, selective (bisoprolol, metoprolol). [Mild] Study
▶ **Rifampicin** moderately decreases the exposure to beta blockers, selective (celiprolol). [Moderate] Study
▶ **Rifabutin** slightly decreases the exposure to bictegravir. Avoid. [Mild] Study

▶ **Rifampicin** is predicted to decrease the exposure to bictegravir. Avoid. [Moderate] Study
▶ **Rifampicin** slightly decreases the exposure to bortezomib. Avoid. [Severe] Study
▶ **Rifampicin** is predicted to very markedly decrease the exposure to bosutinib. Avoid. [Severe] Study
▶ **Rifampicin** is predicted to decrease the exposure to brigatinib. Avoid. [Severe] Study
▶ **Rifampicin** is predicted to decrease the exposure to bupropion. [Moderate] Study
▶ **Rifampicin** is predicted to decrease the exposure to buspirone. Use with caution and adjust dose. [Severe] Study
▶ **Rifabutin** has been reported to cause a small decrease in the exposure to cabotegravir. Avoid intramuscular **cabotegravir**, p. 737. [Moderate] Study
▶ **Rifampicin** modestly decreases the exposure to cabotegravir. Avoid. [Severe] Study
▶ **Rifampicin** moderately decreases the exposure to cabozantinib. Avoid. [Moderate] Study
▶ **Rifampicin** is predicted to moderately increase the clearance of caffeine citrate. Monitor and adjust dose. [Moderate] Study
▶ **Rifampicin** is predicted to decrease the exposure to calcium channel blockers (amlodipine, felodipine, lacidipine, lercanidipine, nicardipine, nimodipine). Monitor and adjust dose. [Moderate] Study
▶ **Rifampicin** greatly decreases the exposure to calcium channel blockers (diltiazem, verapamil). [Severe] Study
▶ **Rifampicin** greatly decreases the exposure to calcium channel blockers (nifedipine). Avoid. [Severe] Study
▶ **Rifampicin** is predicted to decrease the exposure to cannabidiol. Adjust dose. [Moderate] Study
▶ **Rifabutin** is predicted to decrease the exposure to capivasertib. Avoid. [Moderate] Theoretical
▶ **Rifampicin** is predicted to decrease the exposure to capivasertib. Avoid. [Moderate] Study
▶ **Rifampicin** decreases the concentration of caspofungin. Adjust **caspofungin** dose, p. 687. [Moderate] Study
▶ **Rifampicin** is predicted to decrease the exposure to ceritinib. Avoid. [Severe] Study
▶ **Rifampicin** decreases the concentration of chloramphenicol. [Moderate] Study
▶ **Rifampicin** decreases the concentration of ciclosporin. [Severe] Study → Also see TABLE 2 p. 1571
▶ **Rifampicin** is predicted to alter the effects of cilostazol. [Moderate] Theoretical
▶ **Rifampicin** is predicted to decrease the exposure to cinacalcet. Monitor and adjust dose. [Moderate] Study
▶ **Rifampicin** decreases the exposure to clomethiazole. Monitor and adjust dose. [Moderate] Study
▶ **Rifampicin** moderately increases the exposure to the active metabolite of clopidogrel. Avoid. [Moderate] Study
▶ **Rifabutin** decreases the concentration of cobicistat and cobicistat increases the exposure to **rifabutin**. Avoid or adjust dose. [Severe] Study
▶ **Rifampicin** is predicted to decrease the exposure to cobicistat. Avoid. [Severe] Study
▶ **Rifampicin** is predicted to decrease the exposure to cobimetinib. Avoid. [Severe] Theoretical
▶ **Rifampicin** is predicted to decrease the exposure to colchicine. [Moderate] Theoretical
▶ **Rifamycins** are predicted to decrease the efficacy of combined hormonal contraceptives. For FSRH guidance, see Contraceptives, interactions p. 917. [Severe] Study
▶ **Rifampicin** is predicted to decrease the exposure to corticosteroids (budesonide, deflazacort, dexamethasone, fludrocortisone, hydrocortisone, methylprednisolone, prednisolone, triamcinolone). Monitor and adjust dose. [Moderate] Study
▶ **Rifampicin** is predicted to decrease the exposure to corticosteroids (fluticasone). [Unknown] Theoretical
▶ **Rifabutin** might decrease the anticoagulant effect of coumarins. [Moderate] Theoretical
▶ **Rifampicin** decreases the anticoagulant effect of coumarins. [Severe] Study

- **Rifampicin** is predicted to markedly decrease the exposure to crizotinib. Avoid. [Severe] Study
- **Rifampicin** is predicted to decrease the exposure to dabrafenib. Avoid. [Moderate] Theoretical
- **Rifamycins** decrease the exposure to dapsone. [Moderate] Study
- **Rifampicin** is predicted to decrease the exposure to daridorexant. [Severe] Study
- **Rifampicin** is predicted to decrease the exposure to darifenacin. [Moderate] Theoretical
- **Rifampicin** is predicted to markedly decrease the exposure to dasatinib. Avoid. [Severe] Study
- **Rifampicin** is predicted to slightly decrease the exposure to delamanid. Avoid. [Moderate] Study
- **Rifamycins** are predicted to decrease the efficacy of desogestrel. For FSRH guidance, see Contraceptives, interactions p. 917. [Severe] Theoretical
- **Rifampicin** is predicted to markedly decrease the exposure to dienogest. [Severe] Study
- **Rifampicin** decreases the concentration of digoxin. [Moderate] Study
- **Rifampicin** is predicted to decrease the exposure to dipeptidylpeptidase-4 inhibitors **(linagliptin)**. [Moderate] Study
- **Rifampicin** is predicted to moderately decrease the exposure to dipeptidylpeptidase-4 inhibitors **(saxagliptin)**. [Moderate] Study
- **Rifampicin** moderately decreases the exposure to dolutegravir. Adjust **dolutegravir** dose, p. 739. [Severe] Study
- **Rifampicin** is predicted to decrease the exposure to dronabinol. Avoid or adjust dose. [Mild] Study
- **Rifamycins** are predicted to decrease the efficacy of drospirenone. For FSRH guidance, see Contraceptives, interactions p. 917. [Severe] Theoretical
- **Rifampicin** is predicted to decrease the exposure to elacestrant. Avoid or adjust dose depending on duration—consult product literature. [Severe] Study
- **Rifampicin** is predicted to decrease the exposure to elbasvir. Avoid. [Severe] Study
- **Rifabutin** is predicted to decrease the exposure to elexacaftor. Avoid. [Severe] Theoretical
- **Rifampicin** is predicted to decreases the exposure to elexacaftor. Avoid. [Severe] Theoretical
- **Rifampicin** is predicted to decrease the exposure to eliglustat. Avoid. [Severe] Study
- **Rifampicin** is predicted to decrease the exposure to eltrombopag and **eltrombopag** is predicted to increase the concentration of **rifampicin**. [Moderate] Theoretical
- **Rifampicin** is predicted to decrease the concentration of elvitegravir. Avoid. [Severe] Study
- **Rifampicin** is predicted to decrease the exposure to encorafenib. [Severe] Theoretical
- **Rifampicin** transiently increases the exposure to endothelin receptor antagonists **(ambrisentan)**. [Moderate] Study
- **Rifampicin** affects the exposure to endothelin receptor antagonists **(bosentan)**. Avoid. [Severe] Study
- **Rifampicin** is predicted to decrease the exposure to endothelin receptor antagonists **(macitentan)**. Avoid. [Severe] Study
- **Rifampicin** is predicted to decrease the exposure to the cytotoxic component of **enfortumab vedotin**. [Moderate] Theoretical
- **Rifampicin** is predicted to decrease the exposure to entrectinib. Avoid. [Severe] Study
- **Rifabutin** is predicted to decrease the exposure to erdafitinib. Adjust dose. [Moderate] Theoretical
- **Rifampicin** is predicted to decrease the exposure to erdafitinib. Avoid. [Severe] Study
- **Rifampicin** is predicted to decrease the exposure to erlotinib. Avoid or adjust dose—consult product literature. [Severe] Study
- **Rifampicin** is predicted to decrease the exposure to esketamine. Adjust dose. [Mild] Theoretical
- **Rifamycins** are predicted to decrease the efficacy of estradiol. [Moderate] Theoretical
- **Rifampicin** is predicted to decrease the exposure to eszopiclone. Adjust dose. [Moderate] Theoretical
- **Rifamycins** are predicted to decrease the efficacy of etonogestrel. For FSRH guidance, see Contraceptives, interactions p. 917. [Severe] Theoretical

- **Rifampicin** slightly decreases the exposure to etrasimod. Avoid. [Severe] Study
- **Rifampicin** is predicted to decrease the concentration of everolimus. Avoid or adjust dose. [Severe] Study
- **Rifampicin** moderately decreases the exposure to exemestane. [Moderate] Study
- **Rifampicin** is predicted to decrease the exposure to factor XA inhibitors **(apixaban)**. Use with caution or avoid. [Severe] Study
- **Rifampicin** is predicted to decrease the exposure to factor XA inhibitors **(edoxaban)**. [Moderate] Study
- **Rifampicin** is predicted to decrease the exposure to factor XA inhibitors **(rivaroxaban)**. Avoid unless patient can be monitored for signs of thrombosis. [Severe] Study
- **Rifampicin** is predicted to decrease the exposure to fedratinib. Avoid. [Moderate] Study
- **Rifampicin** is predicted to decrease the concentration of fenfluramine. [Moderate] Theoretical
- **Rifampicin** is predicted to decrease the exposure to fesoterodine. Avoid. [Moderate] Study
- **Rifampicin** is predicted to decrease the exposure to fostamatinib. Avoid. [Severe] Study
- **Rifampicin** is predicted to decrease the exposure to the active metabolite of fostemsavir. Avoid. [Severe] Study
- **Rifampicin** is predicted to decrease the exposure to fruquintinib. Avoid. [Moderate] Study
- **Rifampicin** is predicted to decrease the exposure to gefitinib. Avoid. [Severe] Study
- **Rifampicin** moderately decreases the exposure to gilteritinib. Avoid. [Severe] Study
- **Rifampicin** is predicted to decrease the exposure to glasdegib. Avoid. [Severe] Study
- **Rifampicin** markedly affects the exposure to glecaprevir. Avoid. [Severe] Study
- **Rifampicin** is predicted to decrease the exposure to grazoprevir. Avoid. [Severe] Study
- **Rifampicin** is predicted to decrease the concentration of guanfacine. Adjust **guanfacine** dose, p. 407. [Moderate] Study
- **Rifampicin** decreases the concentration of haloperidol. Adjust dose. [Moderate] Study
- HIV-protease inhibitors **(atazanavir, darunavir, fosamprenavir, lopinavir)** boosted with ritonavir increase the exposure to **rifabutin**. Monitor and adjust dose. [Severe] Study
- HIV-protease inhibitors **(ritonavir)** markedly increase the exposure to **rifabutin**. Avoid or adjust dose. [Severe] Study
- **Rifampicin** is predicted to moderately to markedly decrease the exposure to HIV-protease inhibitors **(atazanavir, darunavir, fosamprenavir, lopinavir)**. Avoid. [Severe] Study
- **Rifampicin** slightly decreases the exposure to HIV-protease inhibitors **(ritonavir)**. [Severe] Study
- **Rifamycins** are predicted to decrease the effects of **hormone replacement therapy**. [Moderate] Anecdotal
- **Rifampicin** is predicted to decrease the exposure to ibrutinib. Avoid or monitor. [Severe] Study
- **Rifampicin** is predicted to decrease the exposure to idelalisib. Avoid. [Severe] Study
- **Rifampicin** is predicted to decrease the exposure to imatinib. Avoid. [Moderate] Study
- **Rifampicin** is predicted to decrease the exposure to iptacopan. Avoid or monitor. [Moderate] Theoretical
- **Rifampicin** is predicted to decrease the exposure to irinotecan. Avoid. [Severe] Study
- **Rifampicin** is predicted to decrease the exposure to iron chelators **(deferasirox)**. Monitor serum ferritin and adjust dose. [Moderate] Study → Also see **TABLE 2** p. 1571
- **Rifampicin** is predicted to decrease the exposure to ivabradine. Adjust dose. [Moderate] Theoretical
- **Rifampicin** is predicted to decrease the exposure to ivacaftor. Avoid. [Severe] Study
- **Rifampicin** is predicted to decrease the exposure to ivosidenib. Avoid. [Severe] Theoretical
- **Rifampicin** is predicted to decrease the exposure to ixazomib. Avoid. [Severe] Study
- **Rifampicin** is predicted to decrease the exposure to lapatinib. Avoid. [Severe] Study

Rifamycins (continued)

- **Rifampicin** is predicted to moderately decrease the exposure to larotrectinib. Avoid. Moderate Study
- **Rifabutin** is predicted to decrease the exposure to ledipasvir. Avoid. Severe Theoretical
- **Rifampicin** is predicted to decrease the exposure to ledipasvir. Avoid. Severe Study
- **Rifampicin** might affect the exposure to leflunomide. Moderate Theoretical
- **Rifampicin** is predicted to decrease the exposure to leniolisib. Avoid. Severe Theoretical
- **Rifabutin** is predicted to decrease the concentration of letermovir. Moderate Theoretical
- **Rifampicin** is predicted to affect the concentration of letermovir. Severe Theoretical
- **Rifamycins** are predicted to decrease the efficacy of some contraceptive methods containing levonorgestrel. For FSRH guidance, see Contraceptives, interactions p. 917. Severe Theoretical
- **Rifampicin** slightly decreases the exposure to linezolid. Moderate Study
- **Rifampicin** is predicted to decrease the exposure to lomitapide. Monitor and adjust dose. Moderate Theoretical
- **Rifampicin** is predicted to decrease the exposure to lorlatinib. Avoid. Severe Study
- Lumacaftor is predicted to decrease the exposure to **rifabutin**. Adjust dose. Moderate Theoretical
- Macrolides (erythromycin) are predicted to increase the concentration of **rifabutin** and **rifabutin** is predicted to decrease the concentration of macrolides (erythromycin). Monitor and adjust dose. Severe Theoretical
- **Rifabutin** has been reported to cause neutropenia when given with macrolides (azithromycin). Severe Study
- **Rifabutin** decreases the concentration of macrolides (clarithromycin) and macrolides (clarithromycin) increase the concentration of **rifabutin**. Monitor and adjust dose. Severe Study
- **Rifampicin** greatly decreases the concentration of macrolides (clarithromycin). Severe Study
- **Rifampicin** is predicted to decrease the exposure to maraviroc. Adjust dose. Severe Study
- **Rifabutin** is predicted to decrease the exposure to maribavir. Avoid. Severe Theoretical
- **Rifampicin** is predicted to decrease the exposure to maribavir. Avoid. Severe Study
- **Rifampicin** is predicted to decrease the exposure to mavacamten. Monitor and adjust dose—consult product literature. Severe Theoretical
- **Rifampicin** is predicted to decrease the exposure to meglitinides (repaglinide). Monitor blood glucose and adjust dose. Moderate Study
- **Rifampicin** is predicted to decrease the exposure to melatonin. Moderate Theoretical
- **Rifampicin** is predicted to increase the clearance of mexiletine. Monitor and adjust dose. Moderate Study
- **Rifampicin** is predicted to decrease the exposure to midostaurin. Avoid. Severe Study
- **Rifampicin** is predicted to decrease the exposure to mifepristone. Adjust **mifepristone** dose, p. 954. Severe Study
- **Rifampicin** is predicted to decrease the exposure to mineralocorticoid receptor antagonists (eplerenone). Avoid. Moderate Theoretical
- **Rifampicin** is predicted to decrease the exposure to mineralocorticoid receptor antagonists (finerenone). Avoid. Severe Study
- **Rifampicin** is predicted to decrease the exposure to mirtazapine. Adjust dose. Moderate Study
- **Rifabutin** is predicted to decrease the exposure to mobocertinib. Avoid. Severe Theoretical
- **Rifampicin** is predicted to decrease the exposure to mobocertinib. Avoid. Severe Study
- **Rifampicin** is predicted to decrease the exposure to modafinil. Moderate Theoretical
- **Rifampicin** is predicted to increase the exposure to momelotinib. Moderate Study

- **Rifampicin** decreases the effects of monoclonal antibodies (brentuximab vedotin). Severe Study
- **Rifampicin** is predicted to decrease the exposure to monoclonal antibodies (polatuzumab vedotin). Moderate Theoretical
- **Rifampicin** is predicted to decrease the exposure to the cytotoxic component of monoclonal antibodies (trastuzumab emtansine). Severe Theoretical
- **Rifampicin** is predicted to decrease the exposure to montelukast. Mild Study
- **Rifampicin** decreases the concentration of mycophenolate. Monitor and adjust dose. Severe Study
- **Rifampicin** is predicted to markedly decrease the exposure to naldemedine. Avoid. Severe Study
- **Rifampicin** is predicted to markedly decrease the exposure to naloxegol. Avoid. Moderate Study
- **Rifampicin** is predicted to decrease the exposure to neratinib. Avoid. Severe Study
- **Rifampicin** is predicted to markedly decrease the exposure to neurokinin-1 receptor antagonists (aprepitant). Avoid. Moderate Study
- **Rifampicin** is predicted to decrease the exposure to neurokinin-1 receptor antagonists (fosaprepitant). Avoid. Moderate Theoretical
- **Rifampicin** is predicted to decrease the exposure to neurokinin-1 receptor antagonists (netupitant). Avoid. Severe Study
- **Rifampicin** is predicted to moderately decrease the exposure to nilotinib. Avoid. Severe Study
- **Rifampicin** is predicted to decrease the exposure to nintedanib. Moderate Study
- Nirmatrelvir boosted with ritonavir is predicted to increase the concentration of **rifabutin**. Adjust dose. Severe Theoretical
- **Rifampicin** is predicted to decrease the exposure to nirmatrelvir boosted with ritonavir. Avoid. Severe Study
- **Rifampicin** is predicted to decrease the exposure to nitisinone. Adjust dose. Moderate Theoretical
- NNRTIs (efavirenz) slightly decrease the exposure to **rifabutin**. Adjust dose. Severe Study
- **Rifabutin** moderately decreases the exposure to NNRTIs (doravirine). Adjust doravirine p. 741 or lamivudine with tenofovir disoproxil and doravirine p. 751 dose. Moderate Study
- **Rifampicin** is predicted to decrease the exposure to NNRTIs (doravirine). Avoid. Severe Study
- **Rifampicin** slightly decreases the exposure to NNRTIs (efavirenz). Adjust dose. Severe Study
- **Rifabutin** decreases the exposure to NNRTIs (etravirine). Moderate Study
- **Rifampicin** is predicted to decrease the exposure to NNRTIs (etravirine). Avoid. Severe Theoretical
- **Rifampicin** decreases the concentration of NNRTIs (nevirapine). Avoid. Severe Study
- **Rifabutin** modestly decreases the exposure to NNRTIs (rilpivirine). Avoid or adjust dose—consult product literature. Severe Study
- **Rifampicin** markedly decreases the exposure to NNRTIs (rilpivirine). Avoid. Severe Study
- **Rifamycins** are predicted to decrease the efficacy of some contraceptive methods containing norethisterone. For FSRH guidance, see Contraceptives, interactions p. 917. Severe Anecdotal
- **Rifampicin** moderately decreases the exposure to NSAIDs (celecoxib, diclofenac, etoricoxib). Moderate Study → Also see **TABLE 2** p. 1571
- **Rifampicin** is predicted to decrease the exposure to olaparib. Avoid. Moderate Theoretical
- **Rifampicin** is predicted to decrease the exposure to opioids (alfentanil, fentanyl). Moderate Study
- **Rifampicin** is predicted to decrease the exposure to opioids (buprenorphine). Monitor and adjust dose. Moderate Theoretical
- **Rifampicin** decreases the exposure to opioids (codeine, morphine). Moderate Study
- **Rifampicin** decreases the exposure to opioids (methadone). Monitor and adjust dose. Severe Study
- **Rifampicin** is predicted to decrease the exposure to opioids (oxycodone). Monitor and adjust dose. Moderate Study
- **Rifampicin** is predicted to decrease the exposure to osilodrostat. Moderate Theoretical

- **Rifampicin** is predicted to moderately decrease the exposure to osimertinib. Avoid. Moderate Study
- **Rifampicin** is predicted to moderately decrease the exposure to ospemifene. Moderate Study
- **Rifampicin** moderately decreases the exposure to the active metabolites of ozanimod. Avoid. Moderate Study
- **Rifampicin** is predicted to decrease the exposure to palbociclib. Avoid. Severe Study
- **Rifampicin** is predicted to decrease the exposure to panobinostat. Avoid. Moderate Theoretical
- **Rifampicin** decreases the exposure to paracetamol. Moderate Study
- **Rifampicin** is predicted to decrease the exposure to pazopanib. Avoid. Severe Theoretical
- **Rifampicin** is predicted to decrease the exposure to pemigatinib. Avoid. Severe Study
- **Rifampicin** moderately decreases the exposure to phosphodiesterase type-4 inhibitors (apremilast). Avoid. Severe Study
- **Rifampicin** is predicted to decrease the exposure to phosphodiesterase type-4 inhibitors (roflumilast). Avoid. Moderate Study
- **Rifampicin** is predicted to decrease the exposure to phosphodiesterase type-5 inhibitors (avanafil, tadalafil). Avoid. Severe Study
- **Rifampicin** is predicted to decrease the exposure to phosphodiesterase type-5 inhibitors (sildenafil, vardenafil). Moderate Theoretical
- **Rifampicin** is predicted to moderately to markedly decrease the exposure to pibrentasvir. Avoid. Severe Study
- **Rifampicin** moderately decreases the exposure to pioglitazone. Monitor and adjust dose. Moderate Study
- **Rifampicin** is predicted to decrease the exposure to pirfenidone. Avoid. Moderate Theoretical
- **Rifampicin** is predicted to moderately decrease the exposure to pitolisant. Moderate Study
- **Rifampicin** is predicted to decrease the exposure to ponatinib. Avoid. Moderate Theoretical
- **Rifabutin** is predicted to decrease the exposure to pralsetinib. Avoid or adjust dose—consult product literature. Moderate Study
- **Rifampicin** is predicted to decrease the exposure to pralsetinib. Avoid or adjust dose with potent CYP3A4 inducers—consult product literature. Moderate Study
- **Rifampicin** is predicted to markedly decrease the exposure to praziquantel. Avoid. Moderate Study
- **Rifampicin** is predicted to decrease the exposure to quizartinib. Avoid. Severe Study
- **Rifampicin** slightly decreases the exposure to raltegravir. Avoid or adjust dose—consult product literature. Moderate Study
- **Rifampicin** is predicted to decrease the exposure to ranolazine. Avoid. Severe Study
- **Rifampicin** is predicted to decrease the exposure to reboxetine. Moderate Anecdotal
- **Rifampicin** is predicted to decrease the exposure to regorafenib. Avoid. Moderate Study
- **Rifamycins** are predicted to decrease the exposure to relugolix. Avoid or adjust dose depending on indication—consult product literature. Moderate Study
- **Rifampicin** is predicted to markedly decrease the exposure to ribociclib. Avoid. Severe Study
- **Rifampicin** is predicted to decrease the exposure to rimegepant. Avoid. Moderate Theoretical
- **Rifampicin** is predicted to decrease the exposure to ripretinib. Avoid or adjust dose—consult product literature. Severe Study
- **Rifampicin** might decrease the exposure to roxadustat. Monitor haemoglobin and adjust **roxadustat** dose, p. 1149. Moderate Study
- **Rifampicin** is predicted to decrease the exposure to ruxolitinib. Monitor and adjust dose. Moderate Study
- **Rifampicin** is predicted to decrease the exposure to the active component of sacituzumab govitecan. Severe Theoretical
- **Rifampicin** moderately decreases the exposure to the active metabolite of selexipag. Adjust dose. Moderate Study

- **Rifampicin** is predicted to decrease the exposure to selpercatinib. Avoid. Moderate Study
- **Rifampicin** is predicted to decrease the exposure to selumetinib. Avoid. Severe Study
- **Rifampicin** is predicted to decrease the exposure to siponimod. Manufacturer advises caution depending on genotype—consult product literature. Severe Study
- **Rifampicin** is predicted to decrease the concentration of sirolimus. Avoid or monitor and adjust dose. Severe Study
- **Rifampicin** is predicted to decrease the exposure to SNRIs (duloxetine). Moderate Theoretical
- **Rifampicin** moderately decreases the exposure to sodium glucose co-transporter 2 inhibitors (canagliflozin). Adjust **canagliflozin** dose, p. 824. Moderate Study
- **Rifampicin** might decrease the exposure to sodium glucose co-transporter 2 inhibitors (empagliflozin). Avoid or monitor diabetic control. Moderate Theoretical
- **Rifampicin** is predicted to decrease the exposure to sofosbuvir. Avoid. Severe Study
- **Rifampicin** is predicted to decrease the exposure to solifenacin. Moderate Theoretical
- **Rifampicin** is predicted to decrease the exposure to sorafenib. Moderate Theoretical
- **Rifampicin** is predicted to decrease the exposure to sotorasib. Avoid. Severe Study
- **Rifampicin** markedly decreases the exposure to statins (atorvastatin). Manufacturer advises take both drugs at the same time. Moderate Study
- **Rifampicin** moderately decreases the exposure to statins (fluvastatin). Monitor and adjust dose. Moderate Study
- **Rifampicin** very markedly decreases the exposure to statins (simvastatin). Moderate Study
- **Rifampicin** is predicted to decrease the exposure to sulfonylureas. Moderate Study
- **Rifampicin** is predicted to decrease the exposure to sunitinib. Avoid or adjust dose—consult product literature. Moderate Study
- **Rifampicin** decreases the concentration of tacrolimus. Avoid or monitor and adjust dose. Severe Study → Also see **TABLE 2** p. 1571
- **Rifampicin** markedly decreases the exposure to tamoxifen. Unknown Study
- **Rifabutin** is predicted to decrease the exposure to taxanes (cabazitaxel). Avoid. Moderate Theoretical
- **Rifampicin** is predicted to decrease the exposure to taxanes (cabazitaxel). Avoid. Moderate Study
- **Rifampicin** is predicted to decrease the exposure to taxanes (docetaxel). Severe Theoretical
- **Rifampicin** is predicted to decrease the exposure to taxanes (paclitaxel). Avoid. Severe Study
- **Rifampicin** is predicted to decrease the concentration of temsirolimus. Avoid. Severe Study
- **Rifamycins** are predicted to decrease the exposure to tenofovir alafenamide. Avoid. Moderate Theoretical
- **Rifampicin** might decrease the exposure to tepotinib. Avoid. Severe Theoretical
- **Rifampicin** decreases the exposure to terbinafine. Adjust dose. Moderate Study
- **Rifampicin** might affect the exposure to teriflunomide. Moderate Theoretical
- **Rifampicin** modestly decreases the exposure to tetracyclines (doxycycline). Adjust dose. Moderate Study
- **Rifampicin** is predicted to decrease the exposure to tetracyclines (eravacycline). Adjust **eravacycline** dose, p. 657. Moderate Study
- **Rifamycins** are predicted to decrease the exposure to tezacaftor. Avoid. Severe Theoretical
- **Rifampicin** is predicted to decrease the exposure to theophylline. Adjust dose. Moderate Study
- **Rifampicin** is predicted to decrease the exposure to thrombin inhibitors (dabigatran). Avoid. Severe Study
- **Rifampicin** is predicted to markedly decrease the exposure to ticagrelor. Avoid. Severe Study
- **Rifampicin** might decrease the exposure to tigecycline. Mild Theoretical

Rifamycins (continued)

▸ **Rifampicin** is predicted to decrease the exposure to tivozanib. [Severe] Study

▸ **Rifampicin** moderately decreases the exposure to tizanidine. [Mild] Study

▸ **Rifampicin** is predicted to decrease the exposure to tofacitinib. Avoid. [Severe] Study

▸ **Rifampicin** is predicted to decrease the exposure to tolvaptan. Use with caution or avoid depending on indication. [Severe] Study

▸ **Rifampicin** is predicted to decrease the exposure to toremifene. Adjust dose. [Moderate] Study

▸ **Rifampicin** is predicted to decrease the exposure to trabectedin. Avoid. [Severe] Theoretical

▸ **Rifampicin** slightly decreases the exposure to treprostinil. Adjust dose. [Mild] Study

▸ **Rifampicin** decreases the exposure to trimethoprim. [Moderate] Study → Also see **TABLE 2** p. 1571

▸ **Rifampicin** is predicted to decrease the exposure to tucatinib. Avoid. [Severe] Study

▸ **Rifamycins** decrease the efficacy of ulipristal. Avoid and for 4 weeks after stopping the enzyme inducing drug. For FSRH guidance, see Contraceptives, interactions p. 917. [Severe] Anecdotal

▸ **Rifampicin** is predicted to decrease the exposure to upadacitinib. [Moderate] Study

▸ **Rifampicin** is predicted to decrease the exposure to vandetanib. Avoid. [Moderate] Study

▸ **Rifampicin** is predicted to moderately decrease the exposure to velpatasvir. Avoid. [Severe] Study

▸ **Rifampicin** is predicted to decrease the exposure to vemurafenib. Avoid. [Severe] Study

▸ **Rifampicin** is predicted to decrease the exposure to venetoclax. Avoid. [Severe] Study

▸ **Rifampicin** is predicted to decrease the exposure to vinca alkaloids (vinblastine, vincristine, vindesine). [Severe] Theoretical

▸ **Rifampicin** is predicted to decrease the exposure to vinca alkaloids (vinorelbine). Use with caution or avoid. [Severe] Theoretical

▸ **Rifampicin** is predicted to decrease the exposure to vismodegib. Avoid. [Moderate] Theoretical

▸ **Rifampicin** is predicted to decrease the exposure to voclosporin. Avoid. [Severe] Study → Also see **TABLE 2** p. 1571

▸ **Rifampicin** potentially increases the risk of nephrotoxicity when given with volatile halogenated anaesthetics (methoxyflurane). Avoid. [Severe] Theoretical

▸ **Rifampicin** is predicted to decrease the exposure to vortioxetine. Monitor and adjust dose. [Moderate] Study

▸ **Rifabutin** is predicted to decrease the concentration of voxilaprevir. Avoid. [Severe] Theoretical

▸ **Rifampicin** is predicted to decrease the concentration of voxilaprevir. Avoid. [Severe] Study

▸ **Rifampicin** is predicted to decrease the exposure to zanubrutinib. Avoid. [Severe] Study

▸ **Rifampicin** moderately decreases the exposure to zolpidem. [Moderate] Study

▸ **Rifampicin** is predicted to decrease the exposure to zopiclone. Adjust dose. [Moderate] Study

Rifaximin

▸ **Ciclosporin** very markedly increases the exposure to **rifaximin**. [Severe] Study

▸ **Rifaximin** has been reported to decrease the anticoagulant effect of coumarins (warfarin). Monitor INR and adjust dose. [Severe] Anecdotal

Rilpivirine → see NNRTIs

Riluzole

FOOD AND LIFESTYLE Charcoal-grilled foods are predicted to decrease the exposure to riluzole.

▸ **Combined hormonal contraceptives** is predicted to increase the exposure to **riluzole**. [Moderate] Theoretical

▸ **Givosiran** is predicted to increase the exposure to **riluzole**. [Moderate] Theoretical

▸ **Mexiletine** is predicted to increase the exposure to **riluzole**. [Moderate] Theoretical

▸ **Osilodrostat** is predicted to increase the exposure to **riluzole**. [Moderate] Theoretical

▸ **Quinolones (ciprofloxacin)** are predicted to increase the exposure to **riluzole**. [Moderate] Theoretical

▸ **Rucaparib** is predicted to increase the exposure to **riluzole**. [Moderate] Theoretical

▸ **SSRIs (fluvoxamine)** are predicted to increase the exposure to **riluzole**. [Moderate] Theoretical

▸ **Vemurafenib** is predicted to increase the exposure to **riluzole**. [Moderate] Theoretical

Rimegepant

▸ **Anti-androgens (apalutamide, enzalutamide)** are predicted to decrease the exposure to **rimegepant**. Avoid. [Moderate] Theoretical

▸ **Antiarrhythmics (amiodarone)** are predicted to increase the exposure to **rimegepant**. Avoid another dose of rimegepant within 48 hours of concurrent use. [Moderate] Theoretical

▸ **Antiarrhythmics (dronedarone)** are predicted to increase the exposure to **rimegepant**. Avoid another dose of rimegepant within 48 hours of concurrent use. [Moderate] Study

▸ **Antiepileptics (carbamazepine, fosphenytoin, phenobarbital, phenytoin, primidone)** are predicted to decrease the exposure to **rimegepant**. Avoid. [Moderate] Theoretical

▸ **Antifungals, azoles (fluconazole, isavuconazole)** are predicted to increase the exposure to **rimegepant**. Avoid another dose of rimegepant within 48 hours of concurrent use. [Moderate] Study

▸ **Antifungals, azoles (itraconazole, ketoconazole, posaconazole, voriconazole)** are predicted to increase the exposure to **rimegepant**. Avoid. [Moderate] Study

▸ **Berotralstat** is predicted to increase the exposure to **rimegepant**. Avoid another dose of rimegepant within 48 hours of concurrent use. [Moderate] Study

▸ **Calcium channel blockers (diltiazem, verapamil)** are predicted to increase the exposure to **rimegepant**. Avoid another dose of rimegepant within 48 hours of concurrent use. [Moderate] Study

▸ **Cenobamate** is predicted to decrease the exposure to **rimegepant**. Avoid. [Moderate] Theoretical

▸ **Ceritinib** is predicted to increase the exposure to **rimegepant**. Avoid. [Moderate] Study

▸ **Ciclosporin** slightly increases the exposure to **rimegepant**. Avoid another dose of rimegepant within 48 hours of concurrent use. [Moderate] Study

▸ **Cobicistat** is predicted to increase the exposure to **rimegepant**. Avoid. [Moderate] Study

▸ **Crizotinib** is predicted to increase the exposure to **rimegepant**. Avoid another dose of rimegepant within 48 hours of concurrent use. [Moderate] Study

▸ **Dabrafenib** is predicted to decrease the exposure to **rimegepant**. Avoid. [Moderate] Theoretical

▸ **Danicopan** is predicted to increase the exposure to **rimegepant**. [Moderate] Study

▸ **Eliglustat** is predicted to increase the exposure to **rimegepant**. Adjust dose. [Moderate] Study

▸ **Encorafenib** is predicted to decrease the exposure to **rimegepant**. Avoid. [Moderate] Theoretical

▸ **Endothelin receptor antagonists (bosentan)** are predicted to decrease the exposure to **rimegepant**. Avoid. [Moderate] Theoretical

▸ **Fedratinib** is predicted to increase the exposure to **rimegepant**. Avoid another dose of rimegepant within 48 hours of concurrent use. [Moderate] Study

▸ **Glecaprevir** is predicted to increase the exposure to **rimegepant**. Avoid another dose of rimegepant within 48 hours of concurrent use. [Moderate] Theoretical

▸ **HIV-protease inhibitors** are predicted to increase the exposure to **rimegepant**. Avoid. [Moderate] Study

▸ **Idelalisib** is predicted to increase the exposure to **rimegepant**. Avoid. [Moderate] Study

▸ **Imatinib** is predicted to increase the exposure to **rimegepant**. Avoid another dose of rimegepant within 48 hours of concurrent use. [Moderate] Study

▸ **Ivosidenib** is predicted to decrease the exposure to **rimegepant**. Avoid. [Moderate] Theoretical

▶ **Lapatinib** is predicted to increase the exposure to **rimegepant**. Avoid another dose of rimegepant within 48 hours of concurrent use. Moderate Theoretical

▶ **Letermovir** is predicted to increase the exposure to **rimegepant**. Avoid another dose of rimegepant within 48 hours of concurrent use. Moderate Study

▶ **Lorlatinib** is predicted to decrease the exposure to **rimegepant**. Avoid. Moderate Theoretical

▶ **Lumacaftor** is predicted to decrease the exposure to **rimegepant**. Avoid. Moderate Theoretical

▶ **Macrolides (azithromycin)** are predicted to increase the exposure to **rimegepant**. Avoid another dose of rimegepant within 48 hours of concurrent use. Moderate Theoretical

▶ **Macrolides (clarithromycin)** are predicted to increase the exposure to **rimegepant**. Avoid. Moderate Study

▶ **Macrolides (erythromycin)** are predicted to increase the exposure to **rimegepant**. Avoid another dose of rimegepant within 48 hours of concurrent use. Moderate Study

▶ **Mitotane** is predicted to decrease the exposure to **rimegepant**. Avoid. Moderate Theoretical

▶ **Neurokinin-1 receptor antagonists (aprepitant, netupitant)** are predicted to increase the exposure to **rimegepant**. Avoid another dose of rimegepant within 48 hours of concurrent use. Moderate Study

▶ **Nilotinib** is predicted to increase the exposure to **rimegepant**. Avoid another dose of rimegepant within 48 hours of concurrent use. Moderate Study

▶ **Nirmatrelvir** boosted with ritonavir is predicted to increase the concentration of **rimegepant**. Avoid. Severe Theoretical

▶ **NNRTIs (efavirenz, etravirine, nevirapine)** are predicted to decrease the exposure to **rimegepant**. Avoid. Moderate Theoretical

▶ **Olaparib** might increase the exposure to **rimegepant**. Moderate Theoretical

▶ **Osimertinib** is predicted to increase the exposure to **rimegepant**. Moderate Study

▶ **Pibrentasvir** is predicted to increase the exposure to **rimegepant**. Avoid another dose of rimegepant within 48 hours of concurrent use. Moderate Theoretical

▶ **Ranolazine** is predicted to increase the exposure to **rimegepant**. Avoid another dose of rimegepant within 48 hours of concurrent use. Moderate Theoretical

▶ **Rifamycins (rifampicin)** are predicted to decrease the exposure to **rimegepant**. Avoid. Moderate Theoretical

▶ **Sotorasib** is predicted to decrease the exposure to **rimegepant**. Avoid. Moderate Theoretical

▶ **St John's wort** is predicted to decrease the exposure to **rimegepant**. Avoid. Moderate Theoretical

▶ **Tucatinib** is predicted to increase the exposure to **rimegepant**. Avoid. Moderate Study

▶ **Velpatasvir** is predicted to increase the exposure to **rimegepant**. Avoid another dose of rimegepant within 48 hours of concurrent use. Moderate Theoretical

▶ **Vemurafenib** is predicted to increase the exposure to **rimegepant**. Avoid another dose of rimegepant within 48 hours of concurrent use. Moderate Theoretical

▶ **Voxilaprevir** with sofosbuvir and velpatasvir is predicted to increase the exposure to **rimegepant**. Avoid another dose of rimegepant within 48 hours of concurrent use. Moderate Theoretical

Riociguat → see TABLE 7 p. 1572 (hypotension)

> **FOOD AND LIFESTYLE** Dose adjustment might be necessary if smoking is started or stopped during treatment.

▶ Oral **antacids** decrease the exposure to oral **riociguat**. Manufacturer advises take 1 hour before or 2 hours after antacids. Mild Study

▶ **Antifungals, azoles (itraconazole, posaconazole)** are predicted to increase the exposure to **riociguat**. Adjust **riociguat** dose and monitor blood pressure, p. 212. Moderate Theoretical

▶ **Antifungals, azoles (ketoconazole)** moderately increase the exposure to **riociguat**. Adjust **riociguat** dose and monitor blood pressure, p. 212. Moderate Study

▶ **Ciclosporin** is predicted to increase the exposure to **riociguat**. Moderate Theoretical

▶ **HIV-protease inhibitors (ritonavir)** are predicted to increase the exposure to **riociguat**. Adjust dose and monitor blood pressure. Moderate Theoretical

▶ **Nirmatrelvir** boosted with ritonavir is predicted to increase the concentration of **riociguat**. Adjust dose. Moderate Theoretical

▶ **NRTIs (abacavir)** might increase the exposure to **riociguat**. Adjust dose and monitor blood pressure. Moderate Study

Ripretinib

▶ **Anti-androgens (apalutamide, enzalutamide)** are predicted to decrease the exposure to **ripretinib**. Avoid or adjust dose—consult product literature. Severe Study

▶ **Antiepileptics (carbamazepine, fosphenytoin, phenobarbital, phenytoin, primidone)** are predicted to decrease the exposure to **ripretinib**. Avoid or adjust dose—consult product literature. Severe Study

▶ **Antifungals, azoles (itraconazole, ketoconazole, posaconazole, voriconazole)** are predicted to increase the exposure to **ripretinib**. Moderate Theoretical

▶ **Cenobamate** is predicted to decrease the exposure to **ripretinib**. Avoid or adjust dose—consult product literature. Moderate Theoretical

▶ **Ceritinib** is predicted to increase the exposure to **ripretinib**. Moderate Theoretical

▶ **Cobicistat** is predicted to increase the exposure to **ripretinib**. Moderate Theoretical

▶ **Dabrafenib** is predicted to decrease the exposure to **ripretinib**. Avoid or adjust dose—consult product literature. Moderate Theoretical

▶ **Encorafenib** is predicted to decrease the exposure to **ripretinib**. Avoid or adjust dose—consult product literature. Severe Study

▶ **Endothelin receptor antagonists (bosentan)** are predicted to decrease the exposure to **ripretinib**. Avoid or adjust dose—consult product literature. Moderate Theoretical

▶ **Grapefruit** juice is predicted to increase the exposure to **ripretinib**. Avoid. Mild Theoretical

▶ **HIV-protease inhibitors** are predicted to increase the exposure to **ripretinib**. Moderate Theoretical

▶ **Idelalisib** is predicted to increase the exposure to **ripretinib**. Moderate Theoretical

▶ **Ivosidenib** is predicted to decrease the exposure to **ripretinib**. Avoid or adjust dose—consult product literature. Severe Study

▶ **Lorlatinib** is predicted to decrease the exposure to **ripretinib**. Avoid or adjust dose—consult product literature. Moderate Theoretical

▶ **Lumacaftor** is predicted to decrease the exposure to **ripretinib**. Avoid or adjust dose—consult product literature. Severe Study

▶ **Macrolides (clarithromycin, erythromycin)** are predicted to increase the exposure to **ripretinib**. Moderate Theoretical

▶ **Mitotane** is predicted to decrease the exposure to **ripretinib**. Avoid or adjust dose—consult product literature. Severe Study

▶ **NNRTIs (efavirenz, etravirine, nevirapine)** are predicted to decrease the exposure to **ripretinib**. Avoid or adjust dose—consult product literature. Moderate Theoretical

▶ **Rifamycins (rifampicin)** are predicted to decrease the exposure to **ripretinib**. Avoid or adjust dose—consult product literature. Severe Study

▶ **Sotorasib** is predicted to decrease the exposure to **ripretinib**. Avoid or adjust dose—consult product literature. Moderate Theoretical

▶ **St John's wort** is predicted to decrease the exposure to **ripretinib**. Avoid or adjust dose—consult product literature. Moderate Theoretical

▶ **Tucatinib** is predicted to increase the exposure to **ripretinib**. Moderate Theoretical

Risankizumab → see monoclonal antibodies

Risdiplam

▶ **Risdiplam** is predicted to increase the concentration of **metformin**. Monitor and adjust dose. Moderate Theoretical

Risedronate → see bisphosphonates

Risperidone → see antipsychotics, second generation

Ritlecitinib

▶ **Ritlecitinib** moderately increases the exposure to **benzodiazepines (midazolam)**. Moderate Study

▶ **Ritlecitinib** is predicted to increase the exposure to **ciclosporin** and **ciclosporin** is predicted to increase the risk of generalised

Ritlecitinib (continued)
infection (possibly life-threatening) when given with **ritlecitinib**. Avoid. [Severe] Theoretical
▶ **Ritlecitinib** is predicted to increase the exposure to colchicine. Adjust dose. [Moderate] Theoretical
▶ **Ritlecitinib** is predicted to increase the exposure to everolimus. Adjust dose. [Moderate] Theoretical
▶ Live vaccines are predicted to increase the risk of generalised infection (possibly life-threatening) when given with **ritlecitinib**. Avoid. [Severe] Theoretical
▶ **Ritlecitinib** is predicted to increase the exposure to opioids (alfentanil). [Moderate] Theoretical
▶ **Ritlecitinib** is predicted to increase the exposure to pimozide. [Moderate] Theoretical
▶ **Ritlecitinib** is predicted to increase the exposure to pirfenidone. Adjust dose. [Moderate] Theoretical
▶ **Ritlecitinib** is predicted to increase the exposure to sirolimus. Adjust dose. [Moderate] Theoretical
▶ **Ritlecitinib** is predicted to increase the exposure to tacrolimus. Adjust dose. [Moderate] Theoretical
▶ **Ritlecitinib** is predicted to increase the exposure to temsirolimus. [Moderate] Theoretical
▶ **Ritlecitinib** is predicted to increase the exposure to theophylline. Adjust dose. [Moderate] Theoretical
▶ **Ritlecitinib** is predicted to increase the exposure to tizanidine. [Moderate] Theoretical

Ritonavir → see HIV-protease inhibitors
Rituximab → see monoclonal antibodies
Rivaroxaban → see factor XA inhibitors
Rivastigmine → see anticholinesterases, centrally acting
Rizatriptan → see triptans
Rocuronium → see neuromuscular blocking drugs, non-depolarising
Roflumilast → see phosphodiesterase type-4 inhibitors
Romiplostim
▶ Monoclonal antibodies (rozanolixizumab) might decrease the concentration of **romiplostim**. Avoid and for 2 weeks after stopping **rozanolixizumab**. [Moderate] Theoretical
Ropeginterferon alfa → see interferons
Ropinirole → see dopamine receptor agonists
Ropivacaine → see anaesthetics, local
Rosuvastatin → see statins
Rotavirus vaccine → see live vaccines
Rotigotine → see dopamine receptor agonists
Roxadustat
▶ Aluminium hydroxide might decrease the exposure to **roxadustat**. Manufacturer advises take at least 1 hour after aluminium-containing products. [Moderate] Theoretical
▶ Antacids might decrease the exposure to **roxadustat**. Manufacturer advises take at least 1 hour after antacids. [Moderate] Theoretical
▶ **Roxadustat** is predicted to increase the exposure to antihistamines, non-sedating (fexofenadine). Monitor adverse effects and adjust dose. [Moderate] Study
▶ Oral calcium salts minimally decrease the exposure to oral **roxadustat**. **Roxadustat** should be taken at least 1 hour after calcium. [Moderate] Study
▶ **Roxadustat** is predicted to increase the exposure to endothelin receptor antagonists (bosentan). Monitor adverse effects and adjust dose. [Moderate] Study
▶ Fibrates (gemfibrozil) moderately increase the exposure to **roxadustat**. Monitor haemoglobin and adjust dose. [Moderate] Study
▶ Iron might decrease the exposure to **roxadustat**. **Roxadustat** should be taken at least 1 hour after iron. [Moderate] Theoretical
▶ Magnesium might decrease the exposure to **roxadustat**. Manufacturer advises take at least 1 hour after magnesium. [Moderate] Theoretical
▶ **Roxadustat** is predicted to increase the exposure to meglitinides (repaglinide). Monitor adverse effects and adjust dose. [Moderate] Study
▶ Rifamycins (rifampicin) might decrease the exposure to **roxadustat**. Monitor haemoglobin and adjust **roxadustat** dose, p. 1149. [Moderate] Study

▶ Sevelamer modestly decreases the exposure to **roxadustat**. **Roxadustat** should be taken at least 1 hour after sevelamer. [Moderate] Study
▶ **Roxadustat** is predicted to increase the exposure to statins (atorvastatin, pravastatin, rosuvastatin, simvastatin). Monitor adverse effects and adjust dose. [Moderate] Study
▶ **Roxadustat** might increase the exposure to statins (fluvastatin). Monitor adverse effects and adjust dose. [Moderate] Theoretical
▶ **Roxadustat** might increase the exposure to sulfasalazine. Monitor adverse effects and adjust dose. [Moderate] Theoretical
▶ **Roxadustat** is predicted to increase the exposure to sulfonylureas (glibenclamide). Monitor adverse effects and adjust dose. [Moderate] Study
▶ **Roxadustat** is predicted to increase the exposure to taxanes (docetaxel, paclitaxel). Monitor adverse effects and adjust dose. [Moderate] Study
▶ **Roxadustat** might increase the exposure to topotecan. Monitor adverse effects and adjust dose. [Moderate] Theoretical
Rozanolixizumab → see monoclonal antibodies
Rucaparib → see TABLE 14 p. 1575 (myelosuppression)
▶ **Rucaparib** is predicted to increase the exposure to agomelatine. [Moderate] Study
▶ **Rucaparib** is predicted to increase the exposure to aminophylline. Adjust dose. [Moderate] Theoretical
▶ **Rucaparib** is predicted to increase the exposure to anaesthetics, local (ropivacaine). [Moderate] Theoretical
▶ **Rucaparib** is predicted to increase the exposure to anagrelide. [Moderate] Theoretical
▶ **Rucaparib** is predicted to increase the exposure to antiepileptics (phenytoin). Monitor and adjust dose. [Moderate] Study
▶ **Rucaparib** increases the concentration of antipsychotics, second generation (clozapine). Monitor adverse effects and adjust dose. [Severe] Study
▶ **Rucaparib** is predicted to increase the exposure to antipsychotics, second generation (olanzapine). Adjust dose. [Moderate] Anecdotal
▶ **Rucaparib** slightly increases the exposure to benzodiazepines (midazolam). Monitor and adjust dose. [Severe] Study
▶ **Rucaparib** is predicted to increase the exposure to ciclosporin. Monitor and adjust dose. [Moderate] Study
▶ **Rucaparib** slightly increases the exposure to coumarins (warfarin). Monitor and adjust dose. [Severe] Study
▶ **Rucaparib** is predicted to increase the exposure to dopamine receptor agonists (ropinirole). Adjust dose. [Moderate] Study
▶ **Rucaparib** are predicted to increases the exposure to erlotinib. Monitor adverse effects and adjust dose. [Moderate] Study
▶ **Rucaparib** is predicted to increase the exposure to fezolinetant. Avoid. [Moderate] Study
▶ **Rucaparib** is predicted to increase the exposure to gilteritinib. [Moderate] Theoretical
▶ **Rucaparib** is predicted to increase the exposure to idelalisib. [Moderate] Theoretical
▶ **Rucaparib** is predicted to increase the exposure to loxapine. Avoid. [Unknown] Theoretical
▶ **Rucaparib** slightly increases the exposure to MAO-B inhibitors (rasagiline). [Moderate] Study
▶ **Rucaparib** is predicted to increase the exposure to mavacamten. Monitor and adjust dose—consult product literature. [Moderate] Theoretical
▶ **Rucaparib** is predicted to increase the exposure to melatonin. [Moderate] Theoretical
▶ **Rucaparib** is predicted to increase the exposure to opioids (alfentanil, fentanyl). Monitor and adjust dose. [Moderate] Study
▶ **Rucaparib** is predicted to increase the exposure to phenothiazines (chlorpromazine). [Moderate] Theoretical
▶ **Rucaparib** is predicted to increase the exposure to phosphodiesterase type-4 inhibitors (roflumilast). [Moderate] Theoretical
▶ **Rucaparib** is predicted to increase the exposure to pimozide. Monitor and adjust dose. [Moderate] Study
▶ **Rucaparib** is predicted to increase the exposure to pirfenidone. Use with caution and adjust dose. [Moderate] Study
▶ **Rucaparib** is predicted to increase the exposure to riluzole. [Moderate] Theoretical

- **Rucaparib** is predicted to increase the exposure to sirolimus. Monitor and adjust dose. Moderate Study
- **Rucaparib** is predicted to increase the exposure to SNRIs (duloxetine). Monitor and adjust dose. Moderate Study
- **Rucaparib** is predicted to increase the exposure to tacrolimus. Monitor and adjust dose. Moderate Study
- **Rucaparib** is predicted to increase the exposure to theophylline. Monitor and adjust dose. Moderate Theoretical
- **Rucaparib** increases the exposure to tizanidine. Avoid. Moderate Study
- **Rucaparib** is predicted to increase the exposure to triptans (zolmitriptan). Adjust **zolmitriptan** dose, p. 546. Moderate Theoretical
- **Rucaparib** might increase the exposure to vinca alkaloids. Severe Theoretical → Also see **TABLE 14** p. 1575

Rufinamide → see antiepileptics

Rupatadine → see antihistamines, non-sedating

Ruxolitinib → see **TABLE 14** p. 1575 (myelosuppression)
- Anti-androgens (apalutamide, enzalutamide) are predicted to decrease the exposure to **ruxolitinib**. Monitor and adjust dose. Moderate Study
- Antiarrhythmics (dronedarone) are predicted to increase the exposure to **ruxolitinib**. Moderate Study
- Antiepileptics (carbamazepine, fosphenytoin, phenobarbital, phenytoin, primidone) are predicted to decrease the exposure to **ruxolitinib**. Monitor and adjust dose. Moderate Study
- Antifungals, azoles (fluconazole) are predicted to increase the exposure to **ruxolitinib**. Avoid or adjust dose. Moderate Theoretical
- Antifungals, azoles (isavuconazole) are predicted to increase the exposure to **ruxolitinib**. Moderate Study
- Antifungals, azoles (itraconazole, ketoconazole, posaconazole, voriconazole) are predicted to increase the exposure to **ruxolitinib**. Adjust dose and monitor adverse effects. Moderate Study
- Calcium channel blockers (diltiazem, verapamil) are predicted to increase the exposure to **ruxolitinib**. Moderate Study
- Cenobamate is predicted to decrease the exposure to **ruxolitinib**. Monitor and adjust dose. Moderate Study
- Ceritinib is predicted to increase the exposure to **ruxolitinib**. Adjust dose and monitor adverse effects. Moderate Study → Also see **TABLE 14** p. 1575
- Cobicistat is predicted to increase the exposure to **ruxolitinib**. Adjust dose and monitor adverse effects. Moderate Study
- Crizotinib is predicted to increase the exposure to **ruxolitinib**. Moderate Study
- Dabrafenib is predicted to decrease the exposure to **ruxolitinib**. Monitor and adjust dose. Moderate Study
- Drugs with anticoagulant effects (see **TABLE 3** p. 1571) cause bleeding, as can **ruxolitinib**; concurrent use might increase the risk of developing this effect. Severe Theoretical
- Drugs with antiplatelet effects (see **TABLE 4** p. 1571) cause bleeding, as can **ruxolitinib**; concurrent use might increase the risk of developing this effect. Severe Theoretical
- Encorafenib is predicted to decrease the exposure to **ruxolitinib**. Monitor and adjust dose. Moderate Study
- Endothelin receptor antagonists (bosentan) are predicted to decrease the exposure to **ruxolitinib**. Monitor and adjust dose. Moderate Study
- Grapefruit juice is predicted to increase the exposure to **ruxolitinib**. Severe Theoretical
- HIV-protease inhibitors are predicted to increase the exposure to **ruxolitinib**. Adjust dose and monitor adverse effects. Moderate Study
- Idelalisib is predicted to increase the exposure to **ruxolitinib**. Adjust dose and monitor adverse effects. Moderate Study
- Imatinib is predicted to increase the exposure to **ruxolitinib**. Moderate Study → Also see **TABLE 14** p. 1575
- Ivosidenib is predicted to decrease the exposure to **ruxolitinib**. Monitor and adjust dose. Moderate Study
- Letermovir is predicted to increase the exposure to **ruxolitinib**. Moderate Study
- Lorlatinib is predicted to decrease the exposure to **ruxolitinib**. Monitor and adjust dose. Moderate Study

- Lumacaftor is predicted to decrease the exposure to **ruxolitinib**. Monitor and adjust dose. Moderate Study
- Macrolides (clarithromycin) are predicted to increase the exposure to **ruxolitinib**. Adjust dose and monitor adverse effects. Moderate Study
- Macrolides (erythromycin) slightly increase the exposure to **ruxolitinib**. Mild Study
- Mitotane is predicted to decrease the exposure to **ruxolitinib**. Monitor and adjust dose. Moderate Study → Also see **TABLE 14** p. 1575
- Neurokinin-1 receptor antagonists (aprepitant, netupitant) are predicted to increase the exposure to **ruxolitinib**. Moderate Study
- Nilotinib is predicted to increase the exposure to **ruxolitinib**. Moderate Study → Also see **TABLE 14** p. 1575
- NNRTIs (efavirenz, etravirine, nevirapine) are predicted to decrease the exposure to **ruxolitinib**. Monitor and adjust dose. Moderate Study
- Quinolones (ciprofloxacin) are predicted to increase the exposure to **ruxolitinib**. Moderate Theoretical
- Rifamycins (rifampicin) are predicted to decrease the exposure to **ruxolitinib**. Monitor and adjust dose. Moderate Study
- Sotorasib is predicted to decrease the exposure to **ruxolitinib**. Monitor and adjust dose. Moderate Study
- St John's wort is predicted to decrease the exposure to **ruxolitinib**. Monitor and adjust dose. Moderate Study
- Tucatinib is predicted to increase the exposure to **ruxolitinib**. Adjust dose and monitor adverse effects. Moderate Study

Sacituzumab govitecan
- Afatinib is predicted to increase the exposure to the active component of **sacituzumab govitecan**. Severe Theoretical
- Antiepileptics (carbamazepine, fosphenytoin, phenytoin) are predicted to decrease the exposure to the active component of **sacituzumab govitecan**. Severe Theoretical
- Antifungals, azoles (ketoconazole) are predicted to increase the exposure to the active component of **sacituzumab govitecan**. Severe Theoretical
- Dacomitinib is predicted to increase the exposure to the active component of **sacituzumab govitecan**. Severe Theoretical
- Erlotinib is predicted to increase the exposure to the active component of **sacituzumab govitecan**. Severe Theoretical
- Gefitinib is predicted to increase the exposure to the active component of **sacituzumab govitecan**. Severe Theoretical
- HIV-protease inhibitors are predicted to decrease the exposure to the active component of **sacituzumab govitecan**. Severe Theoretical
- Lapatinib is predicted to increase the exposure to the active component of **sacituzumab govitecan**. Severe Theoretical
- Neratinib is predicted to increase the exposure to the active component of **sacituzumab govitecan**. Severe Theoretical
- Osimertinib is predicted to increase the exposure to the active component of **sacituzumab govitecan**. Severe Theoretical
- Propofol is predicted to increase the exposure to the active component of **sacituzumab govitecan**. Severe Theoretical
- Regorafenib is predicted to increase the exposure to the active component of **sacituzumab govitecan**. Severe Theoretical
- Rifamycins (rifampicin) are predicted to decrease the exposure to the active component of **sacituzumab govitecan**. Severe Theoretical
- Sorafenib is predicted to increase the exposure to the active component of **sacituzumab govitecan**. Severe Theoretical
- Vandetanib is predicted to increase the exposure to the active component of **sacituzumab govitecan**. Severe Theoretical

Sacubitril → see **TABLE 7** p. 1572 (hypotension)
- **Sacubitril** with valsartan increases the exposure to statins (atorvastatin). Moderate Study

Safinamide → see MAO-B inhibitors

Salbutamol → see beta$_2$ agonists

Salmeterol → see beta$_2$ agonists

Sapropterin → see **TABLE 7** p. 1572 (hypotension)
- Methotrexate is predicted to decrease the efficacy of **sapropterin**. Moderate Theoretical
- Phosphodiesterase type-5 inhibitors are predicted to increase the risk of hypotension when given with **sapropterin**. Moderate Theoretical → Also see **TABLE 7** p. 1572

Sapropterin (continued)
▶ **Trimethoprim** is predicted to decrease the efficacy of sapropterin. Moderate Theoretical
Sarilumab → see monoclonal antibodies
Satralizumab → see monoclonal antibodies
Saxagliptin → see dipeptidylpeptidase-4 inhibitors
Secukinumab → see monoclonal antibodies
Selegiline → see MAO-B inhibitors
Selenium

ROUTE-SPECIFIC INFORMATION Interactions do not generally apply to topical use unless specified.

▶ Oral **selenium** might decrease the concentration of the active metabolite of oral baloxavir marboxil. Avoid. Severe Theoretical
▶ Oral **selenium** is predicted to decrease the absorption of eltrombopag. **Eltrombopag** should be taken 2 hours before or 4 hours after **selenium**. Severe Theoretical
Selexipag
▶ Antiepileptics (carbamazepine, fosphenytoin, phenytoin) are predicted to decrease the exposure to the active metabolite of selexipag. Adjust dose. Moderate Study
▶ Antiepileptics (valproate) are predicted to increase the exposure to **selexipag**. Unknown Theoretical
▶ Antifungals, azoles (fluconazole) are predicted to increase the exposure to **selexipag**. Unknown Theoretical
▶ Clopidogrel is predicted to increase the exposure to **selexipag**. Adjust **selexipag** dose, p. 209. Moderate Study
▶ Fibrates (gemfibrozil) increase the exposure to **selexipag**. Avoid. Severe Study
▶ Iron chelators (deferasirox) are predicted to increase the exposure to **selexipag**. Adjust **selexipag** dose, p. 209. Moderate Study
▶ Leflunomide is predicted to increase the exposure to **selexipag**. Adjust **selexipag** dose, p. 209. Moderate Study
▶ Rifamycins (rifampicin) moderately decrease the exposure to the active metabolite of **selexipag**. Adjust dose. Moderate Study
▶ Selpercatinib is predicted to increase the exposure to selexipag. Avoid. Moderate Study
▶ Teriflunomide is predicted to increase the exposure to selexipag. Adjust **selexipag** dose, p. 209. Moderate Study
Selpercatinib → see TABLE 8 p. 1573 (QT-interval prolongation)
▶ Antacids are predicted to decrease the exposure to selpercatinib. Moderate Theoretical
▶ Anti-androgens (apalutamide, enzalutamide) are predicted to decrease the exposure to selpercatinib. Avoid. Moderate Study → Also see TABLE 8 p. 1573
▶ Antiarrhythmics (dronedarone) are predicted to increase the exposure to selpercatinib. Moderate Study → Also see TABLE 8 p. 1573
▶ Antiepileptics (carbamazepine, fosphenytoin, phenobarbital, phenytoin, primidone) are predicted to decrease the exposure to selpercatinib. Avoid. Moderate Study
▶ Antifungals, azoles (fluconazole, isavuconazole) are predicted to increase the exposure to selpercatinib. Moderate Study → Also see TABLE 8 p. 1573
▶ Antifungals, azoles (itraconazole, ketoconazole, posaconazole, voriconazole) are predicted to increase the exposure to selpercatinib. Adjust dose—consult product literature. Moderate Study → Also see TABLE 8 p. 1573
▶ Berotralstat is predicted to increase the exposure to selpercatinib. Moderate Study
▶ Calcium channel blockers (diltiazem, verapamil) are predicted to increase the exposure to selpercatinib. Moderate Study
▶ Ceritinib is predicted to increase the exposure to selpercatinib. Adjust dose—consult product literature. Moderate Study → Also see TABLE 8 p. 1573
▶ Cobicistat is predicted to increase the exposure to selpercatinib. Adjust dose—consult product literature. Moderate Study
▶ Crizotinib is predicted to increase the exposure to selpercatinib. Moderate Study → Also see TABLE 8 p. 1573
▶ Dabrafenib is predicted to decrease the exposure to selpercatinib. Moderate Study
▶ Selpercatinib is predicted to increase the exposure to digoxin. Moderate Study

▶ **Selpercatinib** is predicted to increase the exposure to dipeptidylpeptidase-4 inhibitors (saxagliptin). Moderate Study
▶ Encorafenib is predicted to decrease the exposure to selpercatinib. Avoid. Moderate Study → Also see TABLE 8 p. 1573
▶ Endothelin receptor antagonists (bosentan) are predicted to decrease the exposure to selpercatinib. Moderate Study
▶ **Selpercatinib** is predicted to increase the exposure to everolimus. Avoid. Moderate Study
▶ Fedratinib is predicted to increase the exposure to selpercatinib. Moderate Study
▶ H_2 receptor antagonists are predicted to decrease the exposure to selpercatinib. Manufacturer advises take 2 hours before or 10 hours after H_2 receptor antagonists. Moderate Study
▶ HIV-protease inhibitors are predicted to increase the exposure to selpercatinib. Adjust dose—consult product literature. Moderate Study
▶ Idelalisib is predicted to increase the exposure to selpercatinib. Adjust dose—consult product literature. Moderate Study
▶ Imatinib is predicted to increase the exposure to selpercatinib. Moderate Study
▶ Ivosidenib is predicted to decrease the exposure to selpercatinib. Avoid. Moderate Study → Also see TABLE 8 p. 1573
▶ Letermovir is predicted to increase the exposure to selpercatinib. Moderate Study
▶ **Selpercatinib** is predicted to increase the exposure to loop diuretics (torasemide). Avoid. Severe Study
▶ **Selpercatinib** is predicted to increase the exposure to loperamide. Moderate Study
▶ Lorlatinib is predicted to decrease the exposure to selpercatinib. Moderate Study
▶ Lumacaftor is predicted to decrease the exposure to selpercatinib. Avoid. Moderate Study
▶ Macrolides (clarithromycin) are predicted to increase the exposure to selpercatinib. Adjust dose—consult product literature. Moderate Study
▶ Macrolides (erythromycin) are predicted to increase the exposure to selpercatinib. Moderate Study → Also see TABLE 8 p. 1573
▶ **Selpercatinib** is predicted to increase the exposure to mavacamten. Monitor and adjust dose—consult product literature. Moderate Theoretical
▶ **Selpercatinib** increases the exposure to meglitinides (repaglinide). Avoid. Moderate Study
▶ Mitotane is predicted to decrease the exposure to selpercatinib. Avoid. Moderate Study
▶ **Selpercatinib** is predicted to increase the exposure to montelukast. Avoid. Moderate Study
▶ Neurokinin-1 receptor antagonists (aprepitant, netupitant) are predicted to increase the exposure to selpercatinib. Moderate Study
▶ Nilotinib is predicted to increase the exposure to selpercatinib. Moderate Study → Also see TABLE 8 p. 1573
▶ NNRTIs (efavirenz, etravirine, nevirapine) are predicted to decrease the exposure to selpercatinib. Moderate Study → Also see TABLE 8 p. 1573
▶ **Selpercatinib** is predicted to increase the exposure to opioids (alfentanil, buprenorphine). Avoid. Moderate Study
▶ Proton pump inhibitors are predicted to decrease the exposure to selpercatinib. Manufacturer advises take with food. Moderate Study
▶ Rifamycins (rifampicin) are predicted to decrease the exposure to selpercatinib. Avoid. Moderate Study
▶ **Selpercatinib** is predicted to increase the exposure to selexipag. Avoid. Moderate Study
▶ **Selpercatinib** is predicted to increase the exposure to sirolimus. Avoid. Moderate Study
▶ **Selpercatinib** is predicted to increase the exposure to sorafenib. Avoid. Severe Study → Also see TABLE 8 p. 1573
▶ Sotorasib is predicted to decrease the exposure to selpercatinib. Moderate Study
▶ St John's wort is predicted to decrease the exposure to selpercatinib. Avoid. Moderate Study
▶ **Selpercatinib** is predicted to increase the exposure to talazoparib. Moderate Study

- **Selpercatinib** is predicted to increase the exposure to temsirolimus. Avoid. [Moderate] Study
- **Selpercatinib** slightly increases the exposure to thrombin inhibitors (dabigatran). [Moderate] Study
- **Tucatinib** is predicted to increase the exposure to **selpercatinib**. Adjust dose—consult product literature. [Moderate] Study

Selumetinib

- Anti-androgens (apalutamide, enzalutamide) are predicted to decrease the exposure to **selumetinib**. Avoid. [Severe] Study
- Antiarrhythmics (dronedarone) are predicted to increase the exposure to **selumetinib**. Avoid or adjust dose—consult product literature. [Severe] Study
- Antiepileptics (carbamazepine, fosphenytoin, phenobarbital, phenytoin, primidone) are predicted to decrease the exposure to **selumetinib**. Avoid. [Severe] Study
- Antifungals, azoles (fluconazole, isavuconazole, itraconazole, ketoconazole, posaconazole, voriconazole) are predicted to increase the exposure to **selumetinib**. Avoid or adjust dose—consult product literature. [Severe] Study
- **Selumetinib** might increase the risk of bleeding when given with aspirin. [Severe] Theoretical
- Berotralstat is predicted to increase the exposure to **selumetinib**. Avoid or adjust dose—consult product literature. [Severe] Study
- Calcium channel blockers (diltiazem, verapamil) are predicted to increase the exposure to **selumetinib**. Avoid or adjust dose—consult product literature. [Severe] Study
- **Selumetinib** might increase the risk of bleeding when given with cangrelor. [Severe] Theoretical
- Cenobamate is predicted to decrease the exposure to **selumetinib**. Avoid. [Severe] Study
- Ceritinib is predicted to increase the exposure to **selumetinib**. Avoid or adjust dose—consult product literature. [Severe] Study
- **Selumetinib** might increase the risk of bleeding when given with cilostazol. [Severe] Theoretical
- **Selumetinib** might increase the risk of bleeding when given with clopidogrel. [Severe] Theoretical
- Cobicistat is predicted to increase the exposure to **selumetinib**. Avoid or adjust dose—consult product literature. [Severe] Study
- **Selumetinib** might increase the risk of bleeding when given with coumarins. [Severe] Theoretical
- Crizotinib is predicted to increase the exposure to **selumetinib**. Avoid or adjust dose—consult product literature. [Severe] Study
- Dabrafenib is predicted to decrease the exposure to **selumetinib**. Avoid. [Severe] Study
- **Selumetinib** might increase the risk of bleeding when given with dipyridamole. [Moderate] Theoretical
- Encorafenib is predicted to decrease the exposure to **selumetinib**. Avoid. [Severe] Study
- Endothelin receptor antagonists (bosentan) are predicted to decrease the exposure to **selumetinib**. Avoid. [Severe] Study
- Fedratinib is predicted to increase the exposure to **selumetinib**. Avoid or adjust dose—consult product literature. [Severe] Study
- Grapefruit juice is predicted to increase the exposure to **selumetinib**. Avoid. [Moderate] Theoretical
- HIV-protease inhibitors are predicted to increase the exposure to **selumetinib**. Avoid or adjust dose—consult product literature. [Severe] Study
- Idelalisib is predicted to increase the exposure to **selumetinib**. Avoid or adjust dose—consult product literature. [Severe] Study
- Imatinib is predicted to increase the exposure to **selumetinib**. Avoid or adjust dose—consult product literature. [Severe] Study
- Ivosidenib is predicted to decrease the exposure to **selumetinib**. Avoid. [Severe] Study
- Letermovir is predicted to increase the exposure to **selumetinib**. Avoid or adjust dose—consult product literature. [Severe] Study
- Lorlatinib is predicted to decrease the exposure to **selumetinib**. Avoid. [Severe] Study
- Lumacaftor is predicted to decrease the exposure to **selumetinib**. Avoid. [Severe] Study
- Macrolides (clarithromycin, erythromycin) are predicted to increase the exposure to **selumetinib**. Avoid or adjust dose—consult product literature. [Severe] Study

- Mitotane is predicted to decrease the exposure to **selumetinib**. Avoid. [Severe] Study
- Moclobemide is predicted to increase the exposure to **selumetinib**. Avoid or adjust dose—consult product literature. [Severe] Theoretical
- Neurokinin-1 receptor antagonists (aprepitant, netupitant) are predicted to increase the exposure to **selumetinib**. Avoid or adjust dose—consult product literature. [Severe] Study
- Nilotinib is predicted to increase the exposure to **selumetinib**. Avoid or adjust dose—consult product literature. [Severe] Study
- NNRTIs (efavirenz, etravirine, nevirapine) are predicted to decrease the exposure to **selumetinib**. Avoid. [Severe] Study
- **Selumetinib** might increase the risk of bleeding when given with phenindione. [Severe] Theoretical
- **Selumetinib** might increase the risk of bleeding when given with prasugrel. [Severe] Theoretical
- Proton pump inhibitors (esomeprazole, omeprazole) are predicted to increase the exposure to **selumetinib**. Avoid or adjust dose—consult product literature. [Severe] Theoretical
- Rifamycins (rifampicin) are predicted to decrease the exposure to **selumetinib**. Avoid. [Severe] Study
- Sotorasib is predicted to decrease the exposure to **selumetinib**. Avoid. [Severe] Study
- SSRIs (fluoxetine) are predicted to increase the exposure to **selumetinib**. Avoid or adjust dose—consult product literature. [Severe] Theoretical
- SSRIs (fluvoxamine) are predicted to increase the exposure to **selumetinib**. Avoid or monitor—consult product literature. [Severe] Theoretical
- St John's wort is predicted to decrease the exposure to **selumetinib**. Avoid. [Severe] Study
- **Selumetinib** might increase the risk of bleeding when given with ticagrelor. [Severe] Theoretical
- Tucatinib is predicted to increase the exposure to **selumetinib**. Avoid or adjust dose—consult product literature. [Severe] Study
- Vitamin E substances might increase the risk of bleeding when given with **selumetinib**. Avoid. [Severe] Theoretical

Semaglutide → see glucagon-like peptide-1 receptor agonists

Sertraline → see SSRIs

Sevelamer

> **SEPARATION OF ADMINISTRATION** Drugs for which a reduction in bioavailability could be clinically important should be administered at least 1 hour before, or 3 hours after, sevelamer; alternatively consider monitoring blood concentrations.

- **Sevelamer** modestly decreases the exposure to roxadustat. Roxadustat should be taken at least 1 hour after **sevelamer**. [Moderate] Study
- Oral **sevelamer** decreases the exposure to oral vadadustat. Manufacturer advises take 1 hour before or 2 hours after **sevelamer**. [Moderate] Study

Sevoflurane → see volatile halogenated anaesthetics

Sildenafil → see phosphodiesterase type-5 inhibitors

Siltuximab → see monoclonal antibodies

Silver sulfadiazine

> **PHARMACOLOGY** Silver might inactivate enzymatic debriding agents—concurrent use might not be appropriate.

Simvastatin → see statins

Siponimod → see TABLE 5 p. 1572 (bradycardia), TABLE 8 p. 1573 (QT-interval prolongation)

- Anti-androgens (apalutamide, enzalutamide) are predicted to decrease the exposure to **siponimod**. Manufacturer advises caution depending on genotype—consult product literature. [Severe] Study
- Antiarrhythmics (amiodarone, dronedarone) are predicted to increase the exposure to **siponimod**. Avoid depending on other drugs taken—consult product literature. [Severe] Study → Also see TABLE 5 p. 1572
- Antiepileptics (carbamazepine, fosphenytoin, phenobarbital, phenytoin, primidone) are predicted to decrease the exposure to **siponimod**. Manufacturer advises caution depending on genotype—consult product literature. [Severe] Study
- Antifungals, azoles (fluconazole, isavuconazole, miconazole) are predicted to increase the exposure to **siponimod**. Avoid

Interactions | Appendix 1

Siponimod (continued)

depending on other drugs taken—consult product literature. [Severe] Study

▶ Antifungals, azoles (itraconazole, ketoconazole, posaconazole, voriconazole) are predicted to increase the exposure to **siponimod**. Avoid depending on other drugs taken—consult product literature. [Severe] Theoretical

▶ Berotralstat is predicted to increase the exposure to **siponimod**. Avoid depending on other drugs taken—consult product literature. [Severe] Study

▶ Calcium channel blockers (diltiazem, verapamil) are predicted to increase the exposure to **siponimod**. Avoid depending on other drugs taken—consult product literature. [Severe] Study → Also see **TABLE 5** p. 1572

▶ Cenobamate is predicted to decrease the exposure to **siponimod**. Manufacturer advises caution depending on genotype—consult product literature. [Moderate] Theoretical

▶ Ceritinib is predicted to increase the exposure to **siponimod**. Avoid depending on other drugs taken—consult product literature. [Severe] Theoretical → Also see **TABLE 5** p. 1572

▶ Cobicistat is predicted to increase the exposure to **siponimod**. Avoid depending on other drugs taken—consult product literature. [Severe] Theoretical

▶ Crizotinib is predicted to increase the exposure to **siponimod**. Avoid depending on other drugs taken—consult product literature. [Severe] Study → Also see **TABLE 5** p. 1572

▶ Dabrafenib is predicted to decrease the exposure to **siponimod**. Manufacturer advises caution depending on genotype—consult product literature. [Moderate] Theoretical

▶ Encorafenib is predicted to decrease the exposure to **siponimod**. Manufacturer advises caution depending on genotype—consult product literature. [Severe] Study

▶ Endothelin receptor antagonists (bosentan) are predicted to decrease the exposure to **siponimod**. Manufacturer advises caution depending on genotype—consult product literature. [Moderate] Theoretical

▶ Fedratinib is predicted to increase the exposure to **siponimod**. Avoid depending on other drugs taken—consult product literature. [Severe] Study

▶ HIV-protease inhibitors are predicted to increase the exposure to **siponimod**. Avoid depending on other drugs taken—consult product literature. [Severe] Theoretical

▶ Idelalisib is predicted to increase the exposure to **siponimod**. Avoid depending on other drugs taken—consult product literature. [Severe] Theoretical

▶ Imatinib is predicted to increase the exposure to **siponimod**. Avoid depending on other drugs taken—consult product literature. [Severe] Study

▶ Ivosidenib is predicted to decrease the exposure to **siponimod**. Manufacturer advises caution depending on genotype—consult product literature. [Severe] Study

▶ Letermovir is predicted to increase the exposure to **siponimod**. Avoid depending on other drugs taken—consult product literature. [Severe] Study

▶ Live vaccines might increase the risk of generalised infection (possibly life-threatening) when given with **siponimod**. Avoid and for 4 weeks after stopping **siponimod**. [Severe] Theoretical

▶ Lorlatinib is predicted to decrease the exposure to **siponimod**. Manufacturer advises caution depending on genotype—consult product literature. [Moderate] Theoretical

▶ Lumacaftor is predicted to decrease the exposure to **siponimod**. Manufacturer advises caution depending on genotype—consult product literature. [Severe] Study

▶ Macrolides (clarithromycin) are predicted to increase the exposure to **siponimod**. Avoid depending on other drugs taken—consult product literature. [Severe] Theoretical

▶ Macrolides (erythromycin) are predicted to increase the exposure to **siponimod**. Avoid depending on other drugs taken—consult product literature. [Severe] Study

▶ Mifepristone is predicted to increase the exposure to **siponimod**. [Moderate] Theoretical

▶ Mitotane is predicted to decrease the exposure to **siponimod**. Manufacturer advises caution depending on genotype—consult product literature. [Severe] Study

▶ Monoclonal antibodies (alemtuzumab) are predicted to increase the risk of generalised infection (possibly life-threatening) when given with **siponimod**. Avoid. [Severe] Theoretical

▶ Neurokinin-1 receptor antagonists (aprepitant, netupitant) are predicted to increase the exposure to **siponimod**. Avoid depending on other drugs taken—consult product literature. [Severe] Study

▶ Nilotinib is predicted to increase the exposure to **siponimod**. Avoid depending on other drugs taken—consult product literature. [Severe] Study

▶ NNRTIs (efavirenz, etravirine, nevirapine) are predicted to decrease the exposure to **siponimod**. Manufacturer advises caution depending on genotype—consult product literature. [Moderate] Theoretical

▶ Rifamycins (rifampicin) are predicted to decrease the exposure to **siponimod**. Manufacturer advises caution depending on genotype—consult product literature. [Severe] Study

▶ Sotorasib is predicted to decrease the exposure to **siponimod**. Manufacturer advises caution depending on genotype—consult product literature. [Moderate] Theoretical

▶ St John's wort is predicted to decrease the exposure to **siponimod**. Manufacturer advises caution depending on genotype—consult product literature. [Moderate] Theoretical

▶ Tucatinib is predicted to increase the exposure to **siponimod**. Avoid depending on other drugs taken—consult product literature. [Severe] Theoretical

Sirolimus

▶ Abrocitinib might increase the exposure to **sirolimus**. [Moderate] Theoretical

▶ Anti-androgens (apalutamide, enzalutamide) are predicted to decrease the concentration of **sirolimus**. Avoid or monitor and adjust dose. [Severe] Study

▶ Antiarrhythmics (amiodarone) are predicted to increase the concentration of **sirolimus**. [Severe] Anecdotal

▶ Antiarrhythmics (dronedarone) increase the concentration of **sirolimus**. Monitor and adjust dose. [Moderate] Study

▶ Antiepileptics (carbamazepine, fosphenytoin, phenobarbital, phenytoin, primidone) are predicted to decrease the concentration of **sirolimus**. Avoid or monitor and adjust dose. [Severe] Study

▶ Antifungals, azoles (fluconazole, isavuconazole) increase the concentration of **sirolimus**. Monitor and adjust dose. [Moderate] Study

▶ Antifungals, azoles (itraconazole, ketoconazole, posaconazole, voriconazole) are predicted to increase the concentration of **sirolimus**. Avoid or monitor and adjust dose. [Severe] Study

▶ Antifungals, azoles (miconazole) are predicted to increase the concentration of **sirolimus**. Monitor and adjust dose. [Moderate] Study

▶ Asciminib is predicted to increase the exposure to **sirolimus**. [Severe] Theoretical

▶ Belumosudil might increase the exposure to **sirolimus**. Avoid or adjust dose. [Moderate] Theoretical

▶ Belzutifan is predicted to decrease the exposure to **sirolimus**. Avoid or adjust dose. [Severe] Theoretical

▶ Berotralstat increases the concentration of **sirolimus**. Monitor and adjust dose. [Moderate] Study

▶ Brigatinib potentially decreases the concentration of **sirolimus**. Avoid. [Moderate] Theoretical

▶ Bulevirtide is predicted to increase the exposure to **sirolimus**. [Moderate] Theoretical

▶ Calcium channel blockers (diltiazem, verapamil) increase the concentration of **sirolimus**. Monitor and adjust dose. [Moderate] Study

▶ Cannabidiol is predicted to increase the exposure to **sirolimus**. Monitor and adjust dose. [Moderate] Study

▶ Cenobamate is predicted to decrease the exposure to **sirolimus**. Adjust dose. [Moderate] Theoretical

▶ Ceritinib is predicted to increase the concentration of **sirolimus**. Avoid or monitor and adjust dose. [Severe] Study

▶ **Sirolimus** is predicted to affect the efficacy of chenodeoxycholic acid. Monitor and adjust dose. [Moderate] Theoretical

▶ Ciclosporin moderately increases the exposure to **sirolimus**. Separate administration by 4 hours. [Severe] Study

▶ **Cobicistat** is predicted to increase the concentration of **sirolimus**. Avoid or monitor and adjust dose. Severe Study

▶ **Crizotinib** increases the concentration of **sirolimus**. Monitor and adjust dose. Moderate Study

▶ **Danicopan** is predicted to increase the exposure to **sirolimus**. Moderate Study

▶ **Daridorexant** is predicted to increase the exposure to **sirolimus**. Moderate Study

▶ **Eliglustat** is predicted to increase the exposure to **sirolimus**. Adjust dose. Moderate Study

▶ **Encorafenib** is predicted to decrease the concentration of **sirolimus**. Avoid or monitor and adjust dose. Severe Study

▶ **Endothelin receptor antagonists (bosentan)** are predicted to decrease the concentration of **sirolimus** and **sirolimus** potentially increases the concentration of endothelin receptor antagonists (bosentan). Avoid. Severe Theoretical

▶ **Erdafitinib** is predicted to increase the exposure to **sirolimus**. Separate administration by at least 6 hours. Moderate Theoretical

▶ **Fedratinib** increases the concentration of **sirolimus**. Monitor and adjust dose. Moderate Study

▶ **Fostamatinib** is predicted to increase the exposure to **sirolimus**. Monitor and adjust dose. Moderate Theoretical

▶ **Givinostat** might increase the exposure to **sirolimus**. Moderate Study

▶ **Glecaprevir** is predicted to increase the exposure to **sirolimus**. Severe Theoretical

▶ **Grapefruit** juice increases the concentration of **sirolimus**. Avoid. Moderate Study

▶ **HIV-protease inhibitors** are predicted to increase the concentration of **sirolimus**. Avoid or monitor and adjust dose. Severe Study

▶ **Ibrutinib** might increase the exposure to **sirolimus**. Separate administration by at least 6 hours. Moderate Theoretical

▶ **Idelalisib** is predicted to increase the concentration of **sirolimus**. Avoid or monitor and adjust dose. Severe Study

▶ **Imatinib** increases the concentration of **sirolimus**. Monitor and adjust dose. Moderate Study

▶ **Ivacaftor** is predicted to increase the exposure to **sirolimus**. Moderate Study

▶ **Ivosidenib** is predicted to decrease the concentration of **sirolimus**. Avoid or monitor and adjust dose. Severe Study

▶ **Lapatinib** is predicted to increase the exposure to **sirolimus**. Moderate Theoretical

▶ **Larotrectinib** is predicted to increase the exposure to **sirolimus**. Use with caution and adjust dose. Mild Theoretical

▶ **Letermovir** increases the concentration of **sirolimus**. Monitor and adjust dose. Moderate Study

▶ **Live vaccines** are predicted to increase the risk of generalised infection (possibly life-threatening) when given with **sirolimus**. UKHSA advises avoid (refer to Green Book). Severe Theoretical

▶ **Lomitapide** might increase the exposure to **sirolimus**. Adjust dose. Moderate Theoretical

▶ **Lorlatinib** is predicted to decrease the exposure to **sirolimus**. Avoid. Moderate Theoretical

▶ **Lumacaftor** is predicted to decrease the concentration of **sirolimus**. Avoid or monitor and adjust dose. Severe Study

▶ **Macrolides (clarithromycin)** are predicted to increase the concentration of **sirolimus**. Avoid or monitor and adjust dose. Severe Study

▶ **Macrolides (erythromycin)** increase the concentration of **sirolimus**. Monitor and adjust dose. Moderate Study

▶ **Maribavir** is predicted to increase the exposure to **sirolimus**. Monitor and adjust dose. Severe Study

▶ **Sirolimus** is predicted to decrease the efficacy of mifamurtide. Avoid. Severe Theoretical

▶ **Mifepristone** is predicted to increase the exposure to **sirolimus**. Severe Theoretical

▶ **Mirabegron** is predicted to increase the exposure to **sirolimus**. Mild Theoretical

▶ **Mitotane** is predicted to decrease the concentration of **sirolimus**. Avoid or monitor and adjust dose. Severe Study

▶ **Mobocertinib** is predicted to decrease the exposure to **sirolimus**. Severe Theoretical

▶ **Monoclonal antibodies (elranatamab)** might affect the exposure to **sirolimus**. Monitor and adjust dose. Moderate Theoretical

▶ **Monoclonal antibodies (sarilumab)** potentially affect the exposure to **sirolimus**. Monitor and adjust dose. Moderate Theoretical

▶ **Neratinib** is predicted to increase the exposure to **sirolimus**. Moderate Study

▶ **Neurokinin-1 receptor antagonists (aprepitant, netupitant)** increase the concentration of **sirolimus**. Monitor and adjust dose. Moderate Study

▶ **Nilotinib** increases the concentration of **sirolimus**. Monitor and adjust dose. Moderate Study

▶ **Nirmatrelvir** boosted with ritonavir is predicted to increase the concentration of **sirolimus**. Avoid. Severe Theoretical

▶ **NNRTIs (doravirine)** are predicted to decrease the exposure to **sirolimus**. Monitor **sirolimus** concentration and adjust dose, p. 968. Moderate Theoretical

▶ **NNRTIs (efavirenz, nevirapine)** are predicted to decrease the concentration of **sirolimus**. Monitor and adjust dose. Moderate Theoretical

▶ **NNRTIs (etravirine)** are predicted to decrease the exposure to **sirolimus**. Monitor and adjust dose. Moderate Study

▶ **Olaparib** might increase the exposure to **sirolimus**. Moderate Theoretical

▶ **Osimertinib** is predicted to increase the exposure to **sirolimus**. Moderate Study

▶ **Palbociclib** is predicted to increase the exposure to **sirolimus**. Adjust dose. Moderate Theoretical

▶ **Pemigatinib** might increase the exposure to **sirolimus**. Separate administration by at least 6 hours. Moderate Theoretical

▶ **Pibrentasvir** with glecaprevir is predicted to increase the exposure to **sirolimus**. Moderate Study

▶ **Pitolisant** is predicted to decrease the exposure to **sirolimus**. Avoid. Severe Theoretical

▶ **Ribociclib** is predicted to increase the exposure to **sirolimus**. Use with caution and adjust dose. Moderate Theoretical

▶ **Rifamycins (rifampicin)** are predicted to decrease the concentration of **sirolimus**. Avoid or monitor and adjust dose. Severe Study

▶ **Ritlecitinib** is predicted to increase the exposure to **sirolimus**. Adjust dose. Moderate Theoretical

▶ **Rucaparib** is predicted to increase the exposure to **sirolimus**. Monitor and adjust dose. Moderate Study

▶ **Selpercatinib** is predicted to increase the exposure to **sirolimus**. Avoid. Moderate Study

▶ **Sotorasib** is predicted to decrease the exposure to **sirolimus**. Avoid or adjust dose. Severe Theoretical

▶ **St John's wort** is predicted to decrease the concentration of **sirolimus**. Monitor and adjust dose. Severe Theoretical

▶ **Sirolimus** is predicted to decrease the concentration of tacrolimus and tacrolimus increases the exposure to **sirolimus**. Severe Study

▶ **Tarlatamab** might affect the exposure to **sirolimus**. Monitor and adjust dose. Moderate Theoretical

▶ **Tepotinib** is predicted to increase the concentration of **sirolimus**. Severe Study

▶ **Tucatinib** is predicted to increase the concentration of **sirolimus**. Avoid or monitor and adjust dose. Severe Study

▶ **Velpatasvir** is predicted to increase the exposure to **sirolimus**. Severe Theoretical

▶ **Vemurafenib** is predicted to increase the exposure to **sirolimus**. Use with caution and adjust dose. Severe Theoretical

▶ **Venetoclax** is predicted to increase the exposure to **sirolimus**. Avoid or adjust dose. Severe Study

▶ **Voclosporin** is predicted to increase the exposure to **sirolimus**. Moderate Study

▶ **Voxilaprevir** with sofosbuvir and velpatasvir is predicted to increase the exposure to **sirolimus**. Severe Theoretical

Sitagliptin → see dipeptidylpeptidase-4 inhibitors

SNRIs → see TABLE 17 p. 1576 (hyponatraemia), TABLE 12 p. 1574 (serotonin syndrome), TABLE 4 p. 1571 (antiplatelet effects), TABLE 10 p. 1574 (CNS effects)

duloxetine · venlafaxine

- Antiepileptics **(phenytoin)** are predicted to decrease the exposure to **duloxetine**. [Moderate] Theoretical → Also see TABLE 10 p. 1574
- Antifungals, azoles **(itraconazole, ketoconazole, posaconazole, voriconazole)** are predicted to increase the exposure to **venlafaxine**. [Moderate] Study
- **Axitinib** is predicted to increase the exposure to **duloxetine**. [Moderate] Theoretical → Also see TABLE 4 p. 1571
- **Duloxetine** is predicted to increase the exposure to beta blockers, selective **(metoprolol)**. [Moderate] Study
- **Ceritinib** is predicted to increase the exposure to **venlafaxine**. [Moderate] Study
- **Cobicistat** is predicted to increase the exposure to **venlafaxine**. [Moderate] Study
- **Duloxetine** is predicted to increase the exposure to eliglustat. Avoid or adjust dose—consult product literature. [Severe] Study
- **Givosiran** is predicted to increase the exposure to **duloxetine**. Use with caution and adjust dose. [Moderate] Study
- H_2 receptor antagonists **(cimetidine)** slightly increase the exposure to **venlafaxine**. [Mild] Study
- **Venlafaxine** slightly increases the exposure to haloperidol. [Severe] Study → Also see TABLE 17 p. 1576 → Also see TABLE 10 p. 1574
- HIV-protease inhibitors **(ritonavir)** are predicted to decrease the exposure to **duloxetine**. [Moderate] Theoretical
- HIV-protease inhibitors are predicted to increase the exposure to **venlafaxine**. [Moderate] Study
- **Idelalisib** is predicted to increase the exposure to **venlafaxine**. [Moderate] Study
- **Leflunomide** is predicted to decrease the exposure to **duloxetine**. [Moderate] Theoretical
- **Leniolisib** is predicted to increase the exposure to **duloxetine**. Avoid. [Moderate] Theoretical
- Macrolides **(clarithromycin)** are predicted to increase the exposure to **venlafaxine**. [Moderate] Study
- **Mexiletine** is predicted to increase the exposure to **duloxetine**. [Moderate] Theoretical
- **Osilodrostat** is predicted to increase the exposure to **duloxetine**. [Moderate] Theoretical
- **Duloxetine** might increase the risk of adverse effects when given with ozanimod. [Severe] Theoretical
- **Duloxetine** is predicted to increase the exposure to pitolisant. Use with caution and adjust dose. [Moderate] Study
- **Venlafaxine** is predicted to increase the exposure to pitolisant. Use with caution and adjust dose. [Mild] Theoretical
- Quinolones **(ciprofloxacin)** are predicted to increase the exposure to **duloxetine**. Avoid. [Moderate] Theoretical
- Rifamycins **(rifampicin)** are predicted to decrease the exposure to **duloxetine**. [Moderate] Theoretical
- **Rucaparib** is predicted to increase the exposure to **duloxetine**. Monitor and adjust dose. [Moderate] Study
- SSRIs **(fluvoxamine)** markedly increase the exposure to **duloxetine**. Avoid. [Severe] Study → Also see TABLE 17 p. 1576 → Also see TABLE 12 p. 1574 → Also see TABLE 4 p. 1571 → Also see TABLE 10 p. 1574
- **Tacrolimus** potentially increases the risk of serotonin syndrome when given with **venlafaxine**. [Severe] Anecdotal
- **Teriflunomide** is predicted to decrease the exposure to **duloxetine**. [Moderate] Theoretical
- **Tucatinib** is predicted to increase the exposure to **venlafaxine**. [Moderate] Study
- **Vaborbactam** is predicted to increase the concentration of **venlafaxine**. [Unknown] Theoretical
- **Vemurafenib** is predicted to increase the exposure to **duloxetine**. Use with caution or avoid. [Moderate] Theoretical

Sodium bicarbonate

> **ROUTE-SPECIFIC INFORMATION** Interactions do not generally apply to topical use of **sodium bicarbonate** unless specified.

- Oral **sodium bicarbonate** decreases the absorption of oral antifungals, azoles **(ketoconazole)**. [Moderate] Study
- Oral **sodium bicarbonate** -containing antacids are predicted to decrease the absorption of oral bosutinib. Manufacturer advises take at least 12 hours before antacids. [Moderate] Theoretical
- Oral **sodium bicarbonate** -containing antacids are predicted to decrease the exposure to oral dasatinib. Separate administration by at least 2 hours. [Moderate] Study
- Oral **sodium bicarbonate** -containing antacids are predicted to decrease the absorption of oral erlotinib. Manufacturer advises take 2 hours before or 4 hours after antacids. [Moderate] Theoretical
- Oral **sodium bicarbonate** -containing antacids are predicted to decrease the exposure to oral gefitinib. [Moderate] Theoretical
- Oral **sodium bicarbonate** -containing antacids are predicted to decrease the absorption of oral lapatinib. Avoid. [Moderate] Theoretical
- **Sodium bicarbonate** decreases the concentration of lithium. [Severe] Anecdotal
- **Sodium bicarbonate** is predicted to decrease the efficacy of methenamine. Avoid. [Moderate] Theoretical
- Oral **sodium bicarbonate** -containing antacids are predicted to decrease the exposure to oral neratinib. Separate administration by at least 3 hours. [Mild] Theoretical
- Oral **sodium bicarbonate** -containing antacids might affect the exposure to oral nilotinib. Separate administration by at least 2 hours. [Moderate] Study
- **Sodium bicarbonate** might decrease the efficacy of nitrofurantoin. [Unknown] Theoretical
- Oral **sodium bicarbonate** -containing antacids are predicted to decrease the exposure to oral NNRTIs **(rilpivirine)**. Manufacturer advises take 4 hours before or 2 hours after antacids. [Severe] Theoretical
- Oral **sodium bicarbonate** -containing antacids might decrease the absorption of oral pazopanib. Manufacturer advises take 1 hour before or 2 hours after antacids. [Moderate] Theoretical
- Oral **sodium bicarbonate** is predicted to decrease the exposure to oral sotorasib. Manufacturer advises take 4 hours before or 10 hours after antacids. [Moderate] Theoretical

Sodium citrate

- **Sodium citrate** is predicted to decrease the efficacy of methenamine. Avoid. [Moderate] Theoretical
- **Sodium citrate** might decrease the efficacy of nitrofurantoin. [Unknown] Theoretical
- **Sodium citrate** is predicted to increase the risk of adverse effects when given with sucralfate. Avoid. [Moderate] Theoretical

Sodium glucose co-transporter 2 inhibitors → see TABLE 13 p. 1575 (antidiabetic drugs), TABLE 7 p. 1572 (hypotension)

canagliflozin · dapagliflozin · empagliflozin · ertugliflozin

- Antiepileptics **(carbamazepine, phenobarbital, phenytoin, primidone)** are predicted to decrease the exposure to canagliflozin. Adjust **canagliflozin** dose, p. 824. [Moderate] Study
- Antiepileptics **(fosphenytoin)** are predicted to decrease the exposure to **empagliflozin**. Avoid or monitor diabetic control. [Moderate] Theoretical
- Antiepileptics **(phenytoin)** might decrease the exposure to **empagliflozin**. Avoid or monitor diabetic control. [Moderate] Theoretical
- **Fenfluramine** might decrease blood glucose concentrations when given with **sodium glucose co-transporter 2 inhibitors**. [Moderate] Theoretical
- HIV-protease inhibitors **(ritonavir)** are predicted to decrease the exposure to **canagliflozin**. Adjust **canagliflozin** dose, p. 824. [Moderate] Study
- NNRTIs **(efavirenz)** are predicted to decrease the exposure to **canagliflozin**. Adjust **canagliflozin** dose, p. 824. [Moderate] Study
- Rifamycins **(rifampicin)** moderately decrease the exposure to **canagliflozin**. Adjust **canagliflozin** dose, p. 824. [Moderate] Study
- Rifamycins **(rifampicin)** might decrease the exposure to **empagliflozin**. Avoid or monitor diabetic control. [Moderate] Theoretical
- **Somapacitan** might increase blood glucose concentrations, opposing the blood glucose-lowering effects of **sodium glucose co-transporter 2 inhibitors**. Adjust dose. [Moderate] Theoretical
- **Somatrogon** might increase blood glucose concentrations, opposing the blood glucose-lowering effects of **sodium glucose co-transporter 2 inhibitors**. Adjust dose. [Moderate] Theoretical
- **St John's wort** is predicted to decrease the exposure to **canagliflozin**. Adjust **canagliflozin** dose, p. 824. [Moderate] Study

▶ **Empagliflozin** has been reported to increase the risk of muscle effects when given after statins (atorvastatin). [Moderate] Anecdotal

Sodium oxybate → see TABLE 7 p. 1572 (hypotension), TABLE 10 p. 1574 (CNS effects)

▶ Antiepileptics (valproate) increase the exposure to **sodium oxybate**. Adjust **sodium oxybate** dose, p. 558. [Moderate] Study

Sodium phenylbutyrate

▶ Antiepileptics (valproate) potentially decrease the effects of **sodium phenylbutyrate**. [Moderate] Anecdotal

▶ **Corticosteroids** potentially decrease the effects of **sodium phenylbutyrate**. [Moderate] Theoretical

▶ **Haloperidol** potentially decreases the effects of **sodium phenylbutyrate**. [Moderate] Anecdotal

Sodium picosulfate

▶ Oral **sodium picosulfate** might decrease the concentration of the active metabolite of oral baloxavir marboxil. [Severe] Theoretical

Sodium zirconium cyclosilicate

▶ **Sodium zirconium cyclosilicate** is predicted to decrease the exposure to antifungals, azoles. Separate administration by at least 2 hours. [Moderate] Theoretical

▶ **Sodium zirconium cyclosilicate** is predicted to decrease the exposure to dasatinib. Separate administration by at least 2 hours. [Moderate] Theoretical

▶ **Sodium zirconium cyclosilicate** is predicted to decrease the exposure to erlotinib. Separate administration by at least 2 hours. [Moderate] Theoretical

▶ **Sodium zirconium cyclosilicate** is predicted to decrease the exposure to HIV-protease inhibitors. Separate administration by at least 2 hours. [Moderate] Theoretical

▶ **Sodium zirconium cyclosilicate** is predicted to decrease the exposure to ledipasvir. Separate administration by at least 2 hours. [Moderate] Theoretical

▶ **Sodium zirconium cyclosilicate** is predicted to decrease the exposure to nilotinib. Separate administration by at least 2 hours. [Moderate] Theoretical

▶ **Sodium zirconium cyclosilicate** is predicted to decrease the exposure to NNRTIs (rilpivirine). Separate administration by at least 2 hours. [Moderate] Theoretical

▶ **Sodium zirconium cyclosilicate** is predicted to decrease the exposure to raltegravir. Separate administration by at least 2 hours. [Moderate] Theoretical

Sofosbuvir

▶ **Sofosbuvir** is predicted to increase the risk of severe bradycardia or heart block when given with antiarrhythmics (amiodarone). Refer to specialist literature. [Severe] Anecdotal

▶ Antiepileptics (carbamazepine) are predicted to decrease the exposure to **sofosbuvir**. Avoid. [Severe] Study

▶ Antiepileptics (fosphenytoin, oxcarbazepine, phenobarbital, phenytoin, primidone) are predicted to decrease the exposure to **sofosbuvir**. Avoid. [Severe] Theoretical

▶ H$_2$ receptor antagonists potentially decrease the exposure to **sofosbuvir**. Adjust dose, see ledipasvir with sofosbuvir p. 724, sofosbuvir with velpatasvir p. 725, and sofosbuvir with velpatasvir and voxilaprevir p. 726. [Moderate] Study

▶ Lorlatinib is predicted to decrease the exposure to **sofosbuvir**. Avoid. [Severe] Study

▶ Modafinil is predicted to decrease the exposure to **sofosbuvir**. Avoid. [Severe] Theoretical

▶ Proton pump inhibitors potentially decrease the exposure to **sofosbuvir**. Adjust dose, see ledipasvir with sofosbuvir p. 724, sofosbuvir with velpatasvir p. 725, and sofosbuvir with velpatasvir and voxilaprevir p. 726. [Moderate] Study

▶ Rifamycins (rifampicin) are predicted to decrease the exposure to **sofosbuvir**. Avoid. [Severe] Study

▶ St John's wort is predicted to decrease the exposure to **sofosbuvir**. Avoid. [Severe] Study

Solifenacin → see TABLE 9 p. 1573 (antimuscarinics)

▶ Anti-androgens (apalutamide, enzalutamide) are predicted to decrease the exposure to **solifenacin**. [Moderate] Theoretical

▶ Antiepileptics (carbamazepine, fosphenytoin, phenobarbital, phenytoin, primidone) are predicted to decrease the exposure to **solifenacin**. [Moderate] Theoretical

▶ Antifungals, azoles (itraconazole, ketoconazole, posaconazole, voriconazole) are predicted to increase the exposure to **solifenacin**. Adjust solifenacin p. 899 or tamsulosin with solifenacin p. 906 dose; avoid in hepatic and renal impairment. [Severe] Study

▶ Antipsychotics, second generation (clozapine) can cause constipation, as can **solifenacin**; concurrent use might increase the risk of developing intestinal obstruction. [Severe] Theoretical → Also see TABLE 9 p. 1573

▶ Ceritinib is predicted to increase the exposure to **solifenacin**. Adjust solifenacin p. 899 or tamsulosin with solifenacin p. 906 dose; avoid in hepatic and renal impairment. [Severe] Study

▶ Cobicistat is predicted to increase the exposure to **solifenacin**. Adjust solifenacin p. 899 or tamsulosin with solifenacin p. 906 dose; avoid in hepatic and renal impairment. [Severe] Study

▶ Encorafenib is predicted to decrease the exposure to **solifenacin**. [Moderate] Theoretical

▶ HIV-protease inhibitors are predicted to increase the exposure to **solifenacin**. Adjust solifenacin p. 899 or tamsulosin with solifenacin p. 906 dose; avoid in hepatic and renal impairment. [Severe] Study

▶ Idelalisib is predicted to increase the exposure to **solifenacin**. Adjust solifenacin p. 899 or tamsulosin with solifenacin p. 906 dose; avoid in hepatic and renal impairment. [Severe] Study

▶ Ivosidenib is predicted to decrease the exposure to **solifenacin**. [Moderate] Theoretical

▶ Lumacaftor is predicted to decrease the exposure to **solifenacin**. [Moderate] Theoretical

▶ Macrolides (clarithromycin) are predicted to increase the exposure to **solifenacin**. Adjust solifenacin p. 899 or tamsulosin with solifenacin p. 906 dose; avoid in hepatic and renal impairment. [Severe] Study

▶ Mitotane is predicted to decrease the exposure to **solifenacin**. [Moderate] Theoretical

▶ Rifamycins (rifampicin) are predicted to decrease the exposure to **solifenacin**. [Moderate] Theoretical

▶ Tucatinib is predicted to increase the exposure to **solifenacin**. Adjust solifenacin p. 899 or tamsulosin with solifenacin p. 906 dose; avoid in hepatic and renal impairment. [Severe] Study

Solriamfetol

▶ **Solriamfetol** is predicted to increase the risk of a hypertensive crisis when given with MAO-B inhibitors. Avoid and for 14 days after stopping MAO-B inhibitors. [Severe] Theoretical

▶ **Solriamfetol** is predicted to increase the risk of a hypertensive crisis when given with MAOIs, irreversible. Avoid and for 14 days after stopping the MAOI. [Severe] Theoretical

Somapacitan

▶ **Somapacitan** might increase blood glucose concentrations, opposing the blood glucose-lowering effects of acarbose. Adjust dose. [Moderate] Theoretical

▶ **Somapacitan** might decrease the exposure to antiepileptics (carbamazepine). [Moderate] Theoretical

▶ **Somapacitan** might decrease the exposure to ciclosporin. [Severe] Theoretical

▶ Corticosteroids might decrease the efficacy of **somapacitan**. Monitor and adjust dose. [Moderate] Theoretical

▶ **Somapacitan** might increase blood glucose concentrations, opposing the blood glucose-lowering effects of dipeptidylpeptidase-4 inhibitors. Adjust dose. [Moderate] Theoretical

▶ **Somapacitan** might increase blood glucose concentrations, opposing the blood glucose-lowering effects of glucagon-like peptide-1 receptor agonists. Adjust dose. [Moderate] Theoretical

▶ **Somapacitan** might increase blood glucose concentrations, opposing the blood glucose-lowering effects of insulin. Adjust dose. [Moderate] Theoretical

▶ **Somapacitan** might increase blood glucose concentrations, opposing the blood glucose-lowering effects of meglitinides. Adjust dose. [Moderate] Theoretical

▶ **Somapacitan** might increase blood glucose concentrations, opposing the blood glucose-lowering effects of metformin. Adjust dose. [Moderate] Theoretical

▶ **Somapacitan** might increase blood glucose concentrations, opposing the blood glucose-lowering effects of pioglitazone. Adjust dose. [Moderate] Theoretical

Somapacitan (continued)
▸ **Somapacitan** might increase blood glucose concentrations, opposing the blood glucose-lowering effects of sodium glucose co-transporter 2 inhibitors. Adjust dose. Moderate Theoretical
▸ **Somapacitan** might increase blood glucose concentrations, opposing the blood glucose-lowering effects of sulfonylureas. Adjust dose. Moderate Theoretical
▸ **Somapacitan** might decrease the concentration of testosterone. Moderate Theoretical
▸ **Somapacitan** might affect the efficacy of thyroid hormones. Monitor and adjust dose. Moderate Theoretical

Somatrogon
▸ **Somatrogon** might increase blood glucose concentrations, opposing the blood glucose-lowering effects of acarbose. Adjust dose. Moderate Theoretical
▸ **Somatrogon** might decreases the exposure to antiepileptics (carbamazepine). Moderate Theoretical
▸ **Somatrogon** might decrease the exposure to ciclosporin. Severe Theoretical
▸ Corticosteroids might decrease the efficacy of **somatrogon**. Monitor and adjust dose. Moderate Theoretical
▸ **Somatrogon** might increase blood glucose concentrations, opposing the blood glucose-lowering effects of dipeptidylpeptidase-4 inhibitors. Adjust dose. Moderate Theoretical
▸ **Somatrogon** might increase blood glucose concentrations, opposing the blood glucose-lowering effects of glucagon-like peptide-1 receptor agonists. Adjust dose. Moderate Theoretical
▸ **Somatrogon** might increase blood glucose concentrations, opposing the blood glucose-lowering effects of insulin. Adjust dose. Moderate Theoretical
▸ **Somatrogon** might increase blood glucose concentrations, opposing the blood glucose-lowering effects of meglitinides. Adjust dose. Moderate Theoretical
▸ **Somatrogon** might increase blood glucose concentrations, opposing the blood glucose-lowering effects of metformin. Adjust dose. Moderate Theoretical
▸ **Somatrogon** might increase blood glucose concentrations, opposing the blood glucose-lowering effects of pioglitazone. Adjust dose. Moderate Theoretical
▸ **Somatrogon** might increase blood glucose concentrations, opposing the blood glucose-lowering effects of sodium glucose co-transporter 2 inhibitors. Adjust dose. Moderate Theoretical
▸ **Somatrogon** might increase blood glucose concentrations, opposing the blood glucose-lowering effects of sulfonylureas. Adjust dose. Moderate Theoretical
▸ **Somatrogon** might decrease the concentration of testosterone. Moderate Theoretical
▸ **Somatrogon** might affect the efficacy of thyroid hormones. Adjust dose. Moderate Theoretical

Somatropin
▸ Corticosteroids are predicted to decrease the effects of somatropin. Moderate Theoretical

Sorafenib → see TABLE 14 p. 1575 (myelosuppression), TABLE 8 p. 1573 (QT-interval prolongation), TABLE 4 p. 1571 (antiplatelet effects)
▸ Anti-androgens (apalutamide, enzalutamide) are predicted to decrease the exposure to **sorafenib**. Moderate Theoretical → Also see TABLE 8 p. 1573
▸ Antiepileptics (carbamazepine, eslicarbazepine, fosphenytoin, phenobarbital, phenytoin, primidone) are predicted to decrease the exposure to **sorafenib**. Moderate Theoretical
▸ Antiepileptics (oxcarbazepine) are predicted to decrease the exposure to **sorafenib**. Moderate Study
▸ Cenobamate is predicted to decrease the exposure to **sorafenib**. Moderate Study
▸ Dabrafenib is predicted to decrease the exposure to **sorafenib**. Moderate Study
▸ Encorafenib is predicted to decrease the exposure to **sorafenib**. Moderate Theoretical → Also see TABLE 8 p. 1573
▸ Endothelin receptor antagonists (bosentan) are predicted to decrease the exposure to **sorafenib**. Moderate Study
▸ Ivosidenib is predicted to decrease the exposure to **sorafenib**. Moderate Theoretical → Also see TABLE 8 p. 1573

▸ Linzagolix is predicted to increase the exposure to **sorafenib**. Avoid. Mild Theoretical
▸ Lorlatinib is predicted to decrease the exposure to **sorafenib**. Moderate Study
▸ Lumacaftor is predicted to decrease the exposure to **sorafenib**. Moderate Theoretical
▸ Mitotane is predicted to decrease the exposure to **sorafenib**. Moderate Theoretical → Also see TABLE 14 p. 1575
▸ Neomycin moderately decreases the exposure to **sorafenib**. Moderate Study
▸ NNRTIs (efavirenz, etravirine, nevirapine) are predicted to decrease the exposure to **sorafenib**. Moderate Study → Also see TABLE 8 p. 1573
▸ Rifamycins (rifampicin) are predicted to decrease the exposure to **sorafenib**. Moderate Theoretical
▸ **Sorafenib** is predicted to increase the exposure to the active component of sacituzumab govitecan. Severe Theoretical
▸ Selpercatinib is predicted to increase the exposure to **sorafenib**. Avoid. Severe Study → Also see TABLE 8 p. 1573
▸ Sotorasib is predicted to decrease the exposure to **sorafenib**. Moderate Study
▸ St John's wort is predicted to decrease the exposure to **sorafenib**. Moderate Study

Sotalol → see beta blockers, non-selective

Sotorasib → see TABLE 1 p. 1571 (hepatotoxicity)
▸ Oral antacids are predicted to decrease the exposure to oral **sotorasib**. Manufacturer advises take 4 hours before or 10 hours after antacids. Moderate Theoretical
▸ Anti-androgens (apalutamide, enzalutamide) are predicted to decrease the exposure to **sotorasib**. Avoid. Severe Study
▸ **Sotorasib** is predicted to decrease the exposure to anti-androgens (darolutamide). Avoid. Moderate Theoretical
▸ Antiepileptics (carbamazepine, fosphenytoin, phenobarbital, phenytoin, primidone) are predicted to decrease the exposure to **sotorasib**. Avoid. Severe Study
▸ **Sotorasib** is predicted to decrease the exposure to antifungals, azoles (isavuconazole). Avoid. Severe Theoretical
▸ **Sotorasib** is predicted to decrease the exposure to antipsychotics, second generation (cariprazine). Avoid. Severe Theoretical
▸ **Sotorasib** is predicted to decrease the exposure to antipsychotics, second generation (lurasidone). Monitor and adjust dose. Moderate Theoretical
▸ **Sotorasib** is predicted to decrease the exposure to antipsychotics, second generation (quetiapine). Moderate Study
▸ **Sotorasib** is predicted to decrease the exposure to avacopan. Severe Theoretical
▸ **Sotorasib** is predicted to decrease the exposure to avapritinib. Avoid. Severe Study
▸ **Sotorasib** is predicted to decrease the exposure to bedaquiline. Avoid. Severe Study
▸ **Sotorasib** moderately decreases the exposure to benzodiazepines (midazolam). Moderate Study
▸ **Sotorasib** is predicted to decrease the exposure to bosutinib. Avoid. Severe Study
▸ **Sotorasib** is predicted to decrease the exposure to brigatinib. Avoid or adjust dose—consult product literature. Moderate Study
▸ **Sotorasib** is predicted to decrease the exposure to cabozantinib. Moderate Study
▸ **Sotorasib** is predicted to decrease the exposure to calcium channel blockers (amlodipine, felodipine, lacidipine, lercanidipine, nicardipine, nifedipine, nimodipine). Monitor and adjust dose. Moderate Theoretical
▸ **Sotorasib** is predicted to decrease the exposure to calcium channel blockers (diltiazem, verapamil). Moderate Theoretical
▸ Oral calcium salts (calcium carbonate) are predicted to decrease the exposure to oral **sotorasib**. Manufacturer advises take 4 hours before or 10 hours after antacids. Moderate Theoretical
▸ **Sotorasib** is predicted to decrease the exposure to capivasertib. Avoid. Moderate Study
▸ **Sotorasib** is predicted to decrease the exposure to cobicistat. Avoid. Severe Theoretical
▸ **Sotorasib** is predicted to decrease the exposure to cobimetinib. Avoid. Severe Theoretical

- **Sotorasib** is predicted to decrease the exposure to crizotinib. Avoid. Severe Study
- **Sotorasib** is predicted to decrease the exposure to daridorexant. Severe Study
- **Sotorasib** is predicted to decrease the exposure to dasatinib. Severe Study
- **Sotorasib** very slightly increases the exposure to digoxin. Avoid or adjust dose. Moderate Study
- **Sotorasib** is predicted to decrease the exposure to elacestrant. Avoid or adjust dose depending on duration—consult product literature. Severe Theoretical
- **Sotorasib** is predicted to moderately decrease the exposure to elbasvir. Avoid. Severe Study
- **Sotorasib** is predicted to decrease the concentration of elvitegravir. Avoid. Severe Theoretical
- Encorafenib is predicted to decrease the exposure to **sotorasib**. Avoid. Severe Study
- **Sotorasib** is predicted to decrease the exposure to encorafenib. Moderate Study
- **Sotorasib** is predicted to decrease the exposure to entrectinib. Avoid. Moderate Theoretical
- **Sotorasib** is predicted to decrease the exposure to erdafitinib. Adjust dose. Moderate Theoretical
- **Sotorasib** is predicted to decrease the exposure to erlotinib. Severe Study
- **Sotorasib** is predicted to decrease the concentration of everolimus. Avoid or adjust dose. Severe Study
- **Sotorasib** is predicted to decrease the exposure to fedratinib. Avoid. Moderate Study
- **Sotorasib** is predicted to decrease the exposure to fruquintinib. Avoid. Moderate Study
- **Sotorasib** is predicted to decrease the exposure to gefitinib. Avoid. Severe Study
- **Sotorasib** is predicted to decrease the exposure to glasdegib. Avoid or adjust dose—consult product literature. Moderate Theoretical
- **Sotorasib** is predicted to decrease the exposure to glecaprevir. Avoid. Severe Study
- **Sotorasib** is predicted to markedly decrease the exposure to grazoprevir. Avoid. Severe Study
- **Sotorasib** is predicted to decrease the concentration of guanfacine. Adjust dose. Moderate Theoretical
- H$_2$ receptor antagonists are predicted to decrease the exposure to **sotorasib**. Manufacturer advises give **sotorasib** with an acidic beverage or use an antacid. Moderate Study
- **Sotorasib** is predicted to decrease the exposure to idelalisib. Avoid. Moderate Theoretical
- **Sotorasib** is predicted to decrease the exposure to imatinib. Moderate Study
- Ivosidenib is predicted to decrease the exposure to **sotorasib**. Avoid. Severe Study
- **Sotorasib** is predicted to decrease the exposure to ixazomib. Moderate Theoretical
- **Sotorasib** is predicted to decrease the exposure to lapatinib. Avoid. Severe Study
- **Sotorasib** is predicted to decrease the exposure to larotrectinib. Avoid. Moderate Study
- **Sotorasib** is predicted to decrease the exposure to leniolisib. Avoid. Severe Theoretical
- Lumacaftor is predicted to decrease the exposure to **sotorasib**. Avoid. Severe Study
- **Sotorasib** is predicted to decrease the exposure to mavacamten. Monitor and adjust dose—consult product literature. Severe Theoretical
- **Sotorasib** is predicted to decrease the exposure to mifepristone. Adjust **mifepristone** dose, p. 954. Severe Study
- **Sotorasib** is predicted to decrease the exposure to mineralocorticoid receptor antagonists (finerenone). Avoid. Severe Study
- Mitotane is predicted to decrease the exposure to **sotorasib**. Avoid. Severe Study
- **Sotorasib** is predicted to decrease the exposure to mobocertinib. Avoid. Severe Study
- **Sotorasib** is predicted to decrease the exposure to naloxegol. Moderate Theoretical
- **Sotorasib** is predicted to decrease the exposure to neratinib. Avoid. Severe Theoretical → Also see **TABLE 1** p. 1571
- **Sotorasib** is predicted to decrease the exposure to neurokinin-1 receptor antagonists (netupitant). Moderate Theoretical
- **Sotorasib** is predicted to decrease the exposure to nilotinib. Avoid. Severe Theoretical
- **Sotorasib** is predicted to decrease the exposure to NNRTIs (rilpivirine). Avoid. Severe Theoretical
- **Sotorasib** is predicted to decrease the exposure to olaparib. Avoid. Moderate Theoretical
- **Sotorasib** is predicted to decrease the exposure to opioids (alfentanil). Avoid or adjust dose. Moderate Theoretical
- **Sotorasib** decreases the exposure to opioids (methadone). Monitor and adjust dose. Severe Study
- **Sotorasib** is predicted to decrease the exposure to ospemifene. Moderate Study
- **Sotorasib** is predicted to decrease the exposure to pazopanib. Severe Study
- **Sotorasib** is predicted to decrease the exposure to pemigatinib. Avoid or monitor. Severe Study
- **Sotorasib** is predicted to decrease the exposure to pibrentasvir. Avoid. Severe Study
- **Sotorasib** is predicted to decrease the exposure to ponatinib. Severe Study
- **Sotorasib** is predicted to decrease the exposure to pralsetinib. Moderate Theoretical
- Proton pump inhibitors are predicted to decrease the exposure to **sotorasib**. Manufacturer advises give **sotorasib** with an acidic beverage or use an antacid. Moderate Study
- **Sotorasib** is predicted to decrease the exposure to quizartinib. Avoid. Severe Study
- Rifamycins (rifampicin) are predicted to decrease the exposure to **sotorasib**. Avoid. Severe Study
- **Sotorasib** is predicted to decrease the exposure to rimegepant. Avoid. Moderate Theoretical
- **Sotorasib** is predicted to decrease the exposure to ripretinib. Avoid or adjust dose—consult product literature. Moderate Theoretical
- **Sotorasib** is predicted to decrease the exposure to ruxolitinib. Monitor and adjust dose. Moderate Study
- **Sotorasib** is predicted to decrease the exposure to selpercatinib. Moderate Study
- **Sotorasib** is predicted to decrease the exposure to selumetinib. Avoid. Severe Study
- **Sotorasib** is predicted to decrease the exposure to siponimod. Manufacturer advises caution depending on genotype—consult product literature. Moderate Theoretical
- **Sotorasib** is predicted to decrease the exposure to sirolimus. Avoid or adjust dose. Severe Theoretical
- Oral sodium bicarbonate is predicted to decrease the exposure to oral **sotorasib**. Manufacturer advises take 4 hours before or 10 hours after antacids. Moderate Theoretical
- **Sotorasib** is predicted to decrease the exposure to sorafenib. Moderate Study
- **Sotorasib** is predicted to decrease the exposure to statins (atorvastatin, simvastatin). Moderate Study → Also see **TABLE 1** p. 1571
- **Sotorasib** is predicted to increase the exposure to statins (fluvastatin, rosuvastatin). Monitor and adjust dose. Moderate Study → Also see **TABLE 1** p. 1571
- **Sotorasib** is predicted to increase the exposure to sulfasalazine. Monitor and adjust dose. Moderate Study
- **Sotorasib** is predicted to decrease the exposure to sunitinib. Moderate Study
- **Sotorasib** is predicted to decrease the exposure to tacrolimus. Monitor and adjust dose. Severe Theoretical
- **Sotorasib** is predicted to decrease the exposure to taxanes (docetaxel). Severe Theoretical
- **Sotorasib** is predicted to decrease the exposure to taxanes (paclitaxel). Avoid. Severe Study
- **Sotorasib** is predicted to decrease the concentration of temsirolimus. Avoid. Moderate Theoretical
- **Sotorasib** is predicted to decrease the exposure to ticagrelor. Moderate Theoretical

Sotorasib (continued)

▶ **Sotorasib** is predicted to decrease the exposure to tofacitinib. Severe Study

▶ **Sotorasib** is predicted to decrease the exposure to velpatasvir. Avoid. Moderate Theoretical

▶ **Sotorasib** is predicted to decrease the exposure to venetoclax. Avoid. Severe Study

▶ **Sotorasib** is predicted to decrease the concentration of voxilaprevir. Avoid. Severe Theoretical

▶ **Sotorasib** is predicted to decrease the exposure to zanubrutinib. Avoid or adjust dose with moderate CYP3A4 inducers—consult product literature. Severe Theoretical

Spesolimab → see monoclonal antibodies

Spironolactone → see mineralocorticoid receptor antagonists

SSRIs → see TABLE 17 p. 1576 (hyponatraemia), TABLE 12 p. 1574 (serotonin syndrome), TABLE 8 p. 1573 (QT-interval prolongation), TABLE 4 p. 1571 (antiplatelet effects), TABLE 10 p. 1574 (CNS effects)

citalopram · dapoxetine · escitalopram · fluoxetine · fluvoxamine · paroxetine · sertraline

▶ SSRIs **(fluoxetine, fluvoxamine)** are predicted to increase the exposure to abrocitinib. Adjust **abrocitinib** dose, p. 1430. Severe Study

▶ **Fluvoxamine** very markedly increases the exposure to agomelatine. Avoid. Severe Study → Also see TABLE 10 p. 1574

▶ SSRIs **(fluoxetine, paroxetine)** are predicted to increase the exposure to amfetamines. Severe Theoretical → Also see TABLE 12 p. 1574

▶ **Fluvoxamine** moderately to markedly increases the exposure to aminophylline. Avoid. Severe Study

▶ **Fluvoxamine** decreases the clearance of anaesthetics, local (ropivacaine). Avoid prolonged use. Moderate Study

▶ **Fluvoxamine** is predicted to increase the exposure to anagrelide. Moderate Theoretical → Also see TABLE 4 p. 1571

▶ Anti-androgens **(apalutamide)** are predicted to decrease the exposure to **citalopram**. Avoid or monitor. Mild Study → Also see TABLE 8 p. 1573

▶ Antiarrhythmics **(dronedarone)** are predicted to increase the exposure to **dapoxetine**. Adjust **dapoxetine** dose with moderate CYP3A4 inhibitors, p. 947. Moderate Theoretical

▶ Antiarrhythmics **(dronedarone)** are predicted to increase the exposure to SSRIs **(citalopram, escitalopram, fluoxetine, fluvoxamine, paroxetine, sertraline)**. Severe Theoretical → Also see TABLE 8 p. 1573

▶ **Fluvoxamine** is predicted to increase the exposure to antiarrhythmics **(propafenone)**. Monitor and adjust dose. Moderate Study

▶ SSRIs **(fluoxetine, paroxetine)** are predicted to increase the exposure to anticholinesterases, centrally acting (galantamine). Monitor and adjust dose. Moderate Study

▶ Antiepileptics **(fosphenytoin, phenytoin)** decrease the concentration of **paroxetine**. Moderate Study → Also see TABLE 10 p. 1574

▶ **Sertraline** potentially increases the risk of toxicity when given with antiepileptics **(fosphenytoin, phenytoin)**. Monitor concentration and adjust dose. Severe Anecdotal → Also see TABLE 10 p. 1574

▶ SSRIs **(fluoxetine, fluvoxamine)** are predicted to increase the concentration of antiepileptics **(fosphenytoin, phenytoin)**. Monitor and adjust dose. Severe Anecdotal → Also see TABLE 10 p. 1574

▶ Antifungals, azoles **(fluconazole, isavuconazole)** are predicted to increase the exposure to **dapoxetine**. Adjust **dapoxetine** dose with moderate CYP3A4 inhibitors, p. 947. Moderate Theoretical

▶ Antifungals, azoles **(fluconazole, voriconazole)** are predicted to increase the exposure to **escitalopram**. Use with caution and adjust dose. Severe Study → Also see TABLE 8 p. 1573

▶ Antifungals, azoles **(itraconazole, ketoconazole, posaconazole, voriconazole)** are predicted to moderately increase the exposure to **dapoxetine**. Avoid potent CYP3A4 inhibitors or adjust **dapoxetine** dose, p. 947. Severe Study

▶ Antifungals, azoles **(voriconazole)** are predicted to increase the exposure to **citalopram**. Severe Theoretical → Also see TABLE 8 p. 1573

▶ Antihistamines, sedating **(cyproheptadine)** potentially decrease the effects of **SSRIs**. Moderate Anecdotal → Also see TABLE 10 p. 1574

▶ SSRIs **(fluoxetine, paroxetine)** are predicted to moderately increase the exposure to antipsychotics, second generation **(aripiprazole)**. Adjust **aripiprazole** dose, p. 454. Moderate Study → Also see TABLE 17 p. 1576 → Also see TABLE 10 p. 1574

▶ **Fluvoxamine** increases the exposure to antipsychotics, second generation **(asenapine)**. Moderate Study → Also see TABLE 17 p. 1576 → Also see TABLE 10 p. 1574

▶ **Paroxetine** moderately increases the exposure to antipsychotics, second generation **(asenapine)**. Moderate Study → Also see TABLE 17 p. 1576 → Also see TABLE 10 p. 1574

▶ **Fluvoxamine** increases the concentration of antipsychotics, second generation **(clozapine)**. Monitor adverse effects and adjust dose. Severe Study → Also see TABLE 17 p. 1576 → Also see TABLE 10 p. 1574

▶ SSRIs **(fluoxetine, paroxetine)** are predicted to increase the exposure to antipsychotics, second generation **(clozapine)**. Use with caution and adjust dose. Severe Study → Also see TABLE 17 p. 1576 → Also see TABLE 10 p. 1574

▶ **Fluvoxamine** moderately increases the exposure to antipsychotics, second generation **(olanzapine)**. Adjust dose. Severe Anecdotal → Also see TABLE 17 p. 1576 → Also see TABLE 10 p. 1574

▶ SSRIs **(fluoxetine, paroxetine)** are predicted to increase the exposure to antipsychotics, second generation **(risperidone)**. Adjust dose. Moderate Study → Also see TABLE 17 p. 1576 → Also see TABLE 10 p. 1574

▶ SSRIs **(fluoxetine, paroxetine)** are predicted to markedly increase the exposure to **atomoxetine**. Adjust dose. Severe Study

▶ SSRIs **(fluoxetine, fluvoxamine)** are predicted to increase the exposure to belzutifan. Monitor and adjust dose. Severe Theoretical

▶ **Fluvoxamine** moderately increases the exposure to benzodiazepines **(alprazolam)**. Adjust dose. Moderate Study → Also see TABLE 10 p. 1574

▶ SSRIs **(fluoxetine, fluvoxamine)** potentially increase the exposure to benzodiazepines **(clobazam)**. Adjust dose. Moderate Theoretical → Also see TABLE 10 p. 1574

▶ **Fluvoxamine** moderately increases the exposure to benzodiazepines **(diazepam)**. Moderate Study → Also see TABLE 10 p. 1574

▶ **Berotralstat** is predicted to increase the exposure to **dapoxetine**. Adjust **dapoxetine** dose with moderate CYP3A4 inhibitors, p. 947. Moderate Theoretical

▶ **Fluvoxamine** moderately increases the concentration of beta blockers, non-selective **(propranolol)**. Moderate Study

▶ SSRIs **(fluoxetine, paroxetine)** are predicted to increase the exposure to beta blockers, selective **(metoprolol, nebivolol)**. Moderate Study

▶ **Bupropion** is predicted to increase the exposure to **dapoxetine**. Moderate Theoretical

▶ **Fluvoxamine** markedly decreases the clearance of **caffeine citrate**. Monitor and adjust dose. Severe Study

▶ Calcium channel blockers **(diltiazem, verapamil)** are predicted to increase the exposure to **dapoxetine**. Adjust **dapoxetine** dose with moderate CYP3A4 inhibitors, p. 947. Moderate Theoretical

▶ SSRIs **(fluoxetine, fluvoxamine)** are predicted to increase the exposure to cannabidiol. Moderate Theoretical → Also see TABLE 10 p. 1574

▶ **Fluvoxamine** is predicted to increase the exposure to capivasertib. Adjust dose. Moderate Theoretical

▶ **Cenobamate** is predicted to increase the exposure to **escitalopram**. Use with caution and adjust dose. Severe Study → Also see TABLE 10 p. 1574

▶ **Ceritinib** is predicted to moderately increase the exposure to **dapoxetine**. Avoid potent CYP3A4 inhibitors or adjust **dapoxetine** dose, p. 947. Severe Study

▶ SSRIs **(fluoxetine, fluvoxamine)** are predicted to increase the exposure to cilostazol. Adjust **cilostazol** dose, p. 266. Moderate Theoretical → Also see TABLE 4 p. 1571

▶ **Cinacalcet** is predicted to increase the exposure to **dapoxetine**. Moderate Theoretical

- **Fluvoxamine** is predicted to increase the exposure to cinacalcet. Adjust dose. [Moderate] Theoretical
- SSRIs **(fluoxetine, fluvoxamine)** are predicted to decrease the efficacy of clopidogrel. Avoid. [Severe] Theoretical → Also see **TABLE 4** p. 1571
- Cobicistat is predicted to moderately increase the exposure to **dapoxetine**. Avoid potent CYP3A4 inhibitors or adjust **dapoxetine** dose, p. 947. [Severe] Study
- Cobicistat is predicted to increase the exposure to SSRIs **(citalopram, escitalopram, fluoxetine, fluvoxamine, paroxetine, sertraline)**. Monitor and adjust dose. [Moderate] Theoretical
- Crizotinib is predicted to increase the exposure to **dapoxetine**. Adjust **dapoxetine** dose with moderate CYP3A4 inhibitors, p. 947. [Moderate] Theoretical
- Dacomitinib is predicted to increase the exposure to **dapoxetine**. [Moderate] Theoretical
- SSRIs **(fluoxetine, paroxetine)** are predicted to slightly increase the exposure to darifenacin. [Mild] Study
- **Fluvoxamine** is predicted to increase the exposure to dopamine receptor agonists **(ropinirole)**. Adjust dose. [Moderate] Study → Also see **TABLE 10** p. 1574
- **Fluvoxamine** is predicted to increase the exposure to elacestrant. Avoid or adjust **elacestrant** dose, p. 1084. [Severe] Theoretical
- SSRIs **(fluoxetine, paroxetine)** are predicted to increase the exposure to eliglustat. Avoid or adjust dose—consult product literature. [Severe] Study
- **Fluvoxamine** is predicted to increase the exposure to eltrombopag. [Moderate] Theoretical
- **Fluvoxamine** is predicted to increase the exposure to erlotinib. Monitor adverse effects and adjust dose. [Moderate] Theoretical
- Fedratinib is predicted to increase the exposure to **dapoxetine**. Adjust **dapoxetine** dose with moderate CYP3A4 inhibitors, p. 947. [Moderate] Theoretical
- Fedratinib is predicted to increase the exposure to escitalopram. Use with caution and adjust dose. [Severe] Study
- **Fluoxetine** is predicted to increase the exposure to fedratinib. Avoid depending on other drugs taken—consult product literature. [Moderate] Theoretical
- **Fluvoxamine** is predicted to increase the exposure to fedratinib. Avoid. [Moderate] Theoretical
- **Fluvoxamine** moderately increases the exposure to fenfluramine. [Moderate] Study → Also see **TABLE 12** p. 1574
- SSRIs **(fluoxetine, paroxetine)** are predicted to increase the exposure to fenfluramine. [Moderate] Study → Also see **TABLE 12** p. 1574
- SSRIs **(fluoxetine, paroxetine)** are predicted to increase the exposure to fesoterodine. Use with caution and adjust dose. [Mild] Theoretical
- **Fluvoxamine** is predicted to increase the exposure to fezolinetant. Avoid. [Moderate] Study
- SSRIs **(fluoxetine, paroxetine)** are predicted to increase the exposure to gefitinib. [Moderate] Theoretical
- Gilteritinib is predicted to decrease the efficacy of SSRIs **(escitalopram, fluoxetine, sertraline)**. Avoid. [Moderate] Theoretical
- Grapefruit juice moderately increases the exposure to **sertraline**. Avoid. [Moderate] Study
- H₂ receptor antagonists **(cimetidine)** slightly increase the exposure to SSRIs **(citalopram, escitalopram)**. Adjust dose. [Moderate] Study
- H₂ receptor antagonists **(cimetidine)** slightly increase the exposure to SSRIs **(paroxetine, sertraline)**. [Moderate] Study
- **Fluoxetine** increases the concentration of haloperidol. Adjust dose. [Moderate] Anecdotal → Also see **TABLE 17** p. 1576 → Also see **TABLE 10** p. 1574
- **Fluvoxamine** increases the concentration of haloperidol. Adjust dose. [Moderate] Study → Also see **TABLE 17** p. 1576 → Also see **TABLE 10** p. 1574
- HIV-protease inhibitors are predicted to moderately increase the exposure to **dapoxetine**. Avoid potent CYP3A4 inhibitors or adjust **dapoxetine** dose, p. 947. [Severe] Study
- Idelalisib is predicted to moderately increase the exposure to **dapoxetine**. Avoid potent CYP3A4 inhibitors or adjust **dapoxetine** dose, p. 947. [Severe] Study

- Imatinib is predicted to increase the exposure to **dapoxetine**. Adjust **dapoxetine** dose with moderate CYP3A4 inhibitors, p. 947. [Moderate] Theoretical → Also see **TABLE 4** p. 1571
- Letermovir is predicted to increase the exposure to **dapoxetine**. Adjust **dapoxetine** dose with moderate CYP3A4 inhibitors, p. 947. [Moderate] Theoretical
- **Fluoxetine** is predicted to increase the exposure to lomitapide. Separate administration by 12 hours. [Unknown] Theoretical
- **Fluvoxamine** is predicted to increase the exposure to lomitapide. Separate administration by 12 hours. [Mild] Theoretical
- **Fluvoxamine** is predicted to increase the exposure to loxapine. Avoid. [Unknown] Theoretical → Also see **TABLE 17** p. 1576 → Also see **TABLE 10** p. 1574
- Macrolides **(clarithromycin)** are predicted to moderately increase the exposure to **dapoxetine**. Avoid potent CYP3A4 inhibitors or adjust **dapoxetine** dose, p. 947. [Severe] Study
- Macrolides **(erythromycin)** are predicted to increase the exposure to **dapoxetine**. Adjust **dapoxetine** dose with moderate CYP3A4 inhibitors, p. 947. [Moderate] Theoretical
- **Fluoxetine** is predicted to increase the exposure to mavacamten. Adjust dose—consult product literature. [Severe] Theoretical
- **Fluvoxamine** is predicted to increase the exposure to mavacamten. Monitor and adjust dose—consult product literature. [Moderate] Theoretical
- **Fluvoxamine** very markedly increases the exposure to melatonin. Avoid. [Severe] Study → Also see **TABLE 10** p. 1574
- SSRIs **(fluoxetine, fluvoxamine, paroxetine)** are predicted to increase the exposure to mexiletine. [Moderate] Study
- Moclobemide is predicted to increase the exposure to escitalopram. Use with caution and adjust dose. [Severe] Study → Also see **TABLE 12** p. 1574
- Neurokinin-1 receptor antagonists **(aprepitant, netupitant)** are predicted to increase the exposure to **dapoxetine**. Adjust **dapoxetine** dose with moderate CYP3A4 inhibitors, p. 947. [Moderate] Theoretical
- **SSRIs** potentially increase the risk of prolonged neuromuscular blockade when given with neuromuscular blocking drugs, non-depolarising **(mivacurium)**. [Unknown] Theoretical
- Nilotinib is predicted to increase the exposure to **dapoxetine**. Adjust **dapoxetine** dose with moderate CYP3A4 inhibitors, p. 947. [Moderate] Theoretical
- SSRIs **(fluoxetine, paroxetine)** are predicted to decrease the efficacy of opioids **(codeine)**. [Moderate] Theoretical → Also see **TABLE 10** p. 1574
- SSRIs **(fluoxetine, paroxetine)** are predicted to decrease the efficacy of opioids **(tramadol)**. [Severe] Study → Also see **TABLE 17** p. 1576 → Also see **TABLE 12** p. 1574 → Also see **TABLE 10** p. 1574
- **SSRIs** might increase the risk of adverse effects when given with ozanimod. [Severe] Theoretical
- **Fluvoxamine** is predicted to increase the exposure to pentoxifylline. [Moderate] Theoretical
- **Fluvoxamine** is predicted to increase the exposure to phenothiazines **(chlorpromazine)**. [Moderate] Theoretical → Also see **TABLE 17** p. 1576 → Also see **TABLE 10** p. 1574
- **Fluvoxamine** is predicted to increase the exposure to phosphodiesterase type-4 inhibitors **(roflumilast)**. [Moderate] Study
- **Fluvoxamine** is predicted to moderately increase the exposure to pirfenidone. Avoid. [Moderate] Study
- SSRIs **(fluoxetine, paroxetine)** are predicted to moderately increase the exposure to pitolisant. Use with caution and adjust dose. [Moderate] Study
- **Fluvoxamine** moderately increases the exposure to pomalidomide. Adjust dose—consult product literature. [Moderate] Study
- **Paroxetine** slightly increases the exposure to procyclidine. Monitor and adjust dose. [Moderate] Study → Also see **TABLE 10** p. 1574
- Proton pump inhibitors **(esomeprazole)** increase the exposure to citalopram. Monitor and adjust dose. [Severe] Theoretical
- Proton pump inhibitors **(esomeprazole)** might increase the concentration of **sertraline**. [Moderate] Study

SSRIs (continued)

► Proton pump inhibitors (esomeprazole, omeprazole) are predicted to increase the exposure to **escitalopram**. Use with caution and adjust dose. Severe Study

► Proton pump inhibitors (omeprazole) moderately increase the exposure to **citalopram**. Monitor and adjust dose. Severe Study

► **Fluvoxamine** is predicted to increase the exposure to riluzole. Moderate Theoretical

► **Fluoxetine** is predicted to increase the exposure to selumetinib. Avoid or adjust dose—consult product literature. Severe Theoretical

► **Fluvoxamine** is predicted to increase the exposure to selumetinib. Avoid or monitor—consult product literature. Severe Theoretical

► **Fluvoxamine** markedly increases the exposure to SNRIs (duloxetine). Avoid. Severe Study → Also see TABLE 17 p. 1576 → Also see TABLE 12 p. 1574 → Also see TABLE 4 p. 1571 → Also see TABLE 10 p. 1574

► SSRIs (fluvoxamine) are predicted to increase the exposure to SSRIs (citalopram). Monitor and adjust dose. Severe Anecdotal → Also see TABLE 17 p. 1576 → Also see TABLE 12 p. 1574 → Also see TABLE 4 p. 1571 → Also see TABLE 10 p. 1574

► SSRIs (fluoxetine, paroxetine) are predicted to increase the exposure to SSRIs (dapoxetine). Moderate Theoretical → Also see TABLE 12 p. 1574 → Also see TABLE 4 p. 1571 → Also see TABLE 10 p. 1574

► SSRIs (fluoxetine, fluvoxamine) are predicted to increase the exposure to SSRIs (escitalopram). Use with caution and adjust dose. Severe Study → Also see TABLE 17 p. 1576 → Also see TABLE 12 p. 1574 → Also see TABLE 4 p. 1571 → Also see TABLE 10 p. 1574

► **SSRIs** potentially increase the risk of prolonged neuromuscular blockade when given with suxamethonium. Unknown Theoretical

► **Fluvoxamine** very slightly increases the exposure to talazoparib. Moderate Study

► SSRIs (fluoxetine, paroxetine) are predicted to decrease the efficacy of **tamoxifen**. Avoid. Severe Study

► Terbinafine is predicted to increase the exposure to **fluoxetine**. Adjust dose. Moderate Theoretical

► Terbinafine moderately increases the exposure to **paroxetine**. Moderate Study

► Terbinafine is predicted to increase the exposure to SSRIs (citalopram, dapoxetine, escitalopram, fluvoxamine, sertraline). Moderate Theoretical

► SSRIs (fluoxetine, paroxetine) are predicted to increase the exposure to the active metabolite of **tetrabenazine**. Moderate Study → Also see TABLE 10 p. 1574

► **Fluvoxamine** moderately to markedly increases the exposure to theophylline. Avoid. Severe Study

► **Fluvoxamine** very markedly increases the exposure to tizanidine. Avoid. Severe Study → Also see TABLE 10 p. 1574

► SSRIs (fluoxetine, fluvoxamine) given with a moderate CYP3A4 inhibitor are predicted to increase the exposure to **tofacitinib**. Adjust **tofacitinib** dose, p. 1265. Moderate Study

► SSRIs (fluoxetine, paroxetine) are predicted to increase the exposure to tricyclic antidepressants. Monitor for toxicity and adjust dose. Severe Study → Also see TABLE 17 p. 1576 → Also see TABLE 12 p. 1574 → Also see TABLE 10 p. 1574

► **Fluvoxamine** increases the exposure to tricyclic antidepressants (amitriptyline, imipramine). Adjust dose. Severe Study → Also see TABLE 17 p. 1576 → Also see TABLE 12 p. 1574 → Also see TABLE 10 p. 1574

► **Fluvoxamine** markedly increases the exposure to tricyclic antidepressants (clomipramine). Adjust dose. Severe Study → Also see TABLE 17 p. 1576 → Also see TABLE 12 p. 1574 → Also see TABLE 10 p. 1574

► **Fluvoxamine** increases the concentration of triptans (frovatriptan). Severe Study → Also see TABLE 12 p. 1574

► **Fluvoxamine** is predicted to increase the exposure to triptans (zolmitriptan). Adjust **zolmitriptan** dose, p. 546. Severe Theoretical → Also see TABLE 12 p. 1574

► Tucatinib is predicted to moderately increase the exposure to **dapoxetine**. Avoid potent CYP3A4 inhibitors or adjust **dapoxetine** dose, p. 947. Severe Study

► **SSRIs** might enhance the antidiuretic and hypertensive effects of vasopressin. Moderate Theoretical

► SSRIs (fluoxetine, paroxetine) are predicted to increase the exposure to vortioxetine. Monitor and adjust dose. Moderate Study → Also see TABLE 12 p. 1574 → Also see TABLE 4 p. 1571

St John's wort → see TABLE 12 p. 1574 (serotonin syndrome)

► **St John's wort** is predicted to decrease the exposure to abemaciclib. Avoid. Severe Study

► **St John's wort** is predicted to decrease the exposure to acalabrutinib. Avoid. Severe Study

► **St John's wort** is predicted to decrease the exposure to afatinib. Moderate Study

► **St John's wort** decreases the exposure to aliskiren. Moderate Study

► **St John's wort** is predicted to decrease the concentration of aminophylline. Severe Theoretical

► **St John's wort** is predicted to decrease the efficacy of anti-androgens (cyproterone) with ethinylestradiol (co-cyprindiol). Use alternative methods during treatment with, and for 28 days after, the enzyme inducing drug is stopped. Severe Study

► **St John's wort** is predicted to decrease the exposure to anti-androgens (darolutamide). Avoid. Moderate Theoretical

► **St John's wort** is predicted to decrease the exposure to antiarrhythmics (dronedarone). Avoid. Severe Theoretical

► **St John's wort** is predicted to decrease the exposure to antiepileptics (brivaracetam). Moderate Theoretical

► **St John's wort** is predicted to decrease the concentration of antiepileptics (carbamazepine). Monitor and adjust dose. Moderate Theoretical

► **St John's wort** is predicted to decrease the concentration of antiepileptics (fosphenytoin, phenobarbital, phenytoin, primidone). Avoid. Severe Theoretical

► **St John's wort** is predicted to decrease the exposure to antiepileptics (perampanel). Monitor and adjust dose. Moderate Theoretical

► **St John's wort** is predicted to decrease the exposure to antiepileptics (tiagabine). Avoid. Mild Theoretical

► **St John's wort** is predicted to decrease the exposure to antifungals, azoles (isavuconazole). Avoid. Severe Theoretical

► **St John's wort** moderately decreases the exposure to antifungals, azoles (voriconazole). Avoid. Moderate Study

► **St John's wort** is predicted to decrease the exposure to antipsychotics, second generation (cariprazine). Avoid. Severe Theoretical

► **St John's wort** is predicted to decrease the exposure to antipsychotics, second generation (lurasidone). Monitor and adjust dose. Moderate Theoretical

► **St John's wort** is predicted to decrease the exposure to antipsychotics, second generation (paliperidone). Severe Theoretical

► **St John's wort** is predicted to decrease the exposure to antipsychotics, second generation (quetiapine). Moderate Study

► **St John's wort** is predicted to decrease the exposure to avacopan. Severe Theoretical

► **St John's wort** is predicted to decrease the exposure to avapritinib. Avoid. Severe Study

► **St John's wort** is predicted to decrease the exposure to axitinib. Avoid or adjust dose. Moderate Study

► **St John's wort** is predicted to decrease the exposure to bedaquiline. Avoid. Severe Study

► **St John's wort** moderately decreases the exposure to benzodiazepines (alprazolam). Moderate Study

► **St John's wort** moderately decreases the exposure to benzodiazepines (midazolam). Monitor and adjust dose. Moderate Study

► **St John's wort** is predicted to decrease the concentration of berotralstat. Avoid. Severe Theoretical

► **St John's wort** is predicted to decrease the exposure to bictegravir. Avoid. Moderate Theoretical

► **St John's wort** is predicted to decrease the exposure to bosutinib. Avoid. Severe Study

► **St John's wort** is predicted to decrease the exposure to brigatinib. Avoid or adjust dose—consult product literature. Moderate Study

- **St John's wort** is predicted to decrease the exposure to cabozantinib. Moderate Study
- **St John's wort** is predicted to decrease the exposure to calcium channel blockers (amlodipine, felodipine, lacidipine, lercanidipine, nicardipine, nifedipine, nimodipine). Monitor and adjust dose. Moderate Theoretical
- **St John's wort** is predicted to decrease the exposure to calcium channel blockers (diltiazem, verapamil). Moderate Theoretical
- **St John's wort** is predicted to decrease the exposure to cannabidiol. Adjust dose. Mild Study
- **St John's wort** is predicted to decrease the exposure to capivasertib. Avoid. Moderate Study
- **St John's wort** is predicted to decrease the exposure to ceritinib. Avoid. Severe Theoretical
- **St John's wort** decreases the concentration of ciclosporin. Avoid. Moderate Study
- **St John's wort** is predicted to alter the effects of cilostazol. Moderate Theoretical
- **St John's wort** is predicted to decrease the exposure to cobicistat. Avoid. Severe Theoretical
- **St John's wort** is predicted to decrease the exposure to cobimetinib. Avoid. Severe Theoretical
- **St John's wort** is predicted to decrease the exposure to colchicine. Moderate Theoretical
- **St John's wort** decreases the efficacy of combined hormonal contraceptives. MHRA advises avoid. For FSRH guidance, see Contraceptives, interactions p. 917. Severe Anecdotal
- **St John's wort** decreases the anticoagulant effect of coumarins. Avoid. Severe Anecdotal
- **St John's wort** is predicted to decrease the exposure to crizotinib. Avoid. Severe Study
- **St John's wort** is predicted to decrease the exposure to dabrafenib. Avoid. Moderate Study
- **St John's wort** is predicted to decrease the exposure to daridorexant. Severe Study
- **St John's wort** is predicted to decrease the exposure to darifenacin. Moderate Theoretical
- **St John's wort** is predicted to decrease the exposure to dasatinib. Severe Study
- **St John's wort** is predicted to decrease the efficacy of desogestrel. MHRA advises avoid. For FSRH guidance, see Contraceptives, interactions p. 917. Severe Theoretical
- **St John's wort** decreases the concentration of digoxin. Avoid. Severe Anecdotal
- **St John's wort** is predicted to decrease the exposure to dolutegravir. Adjust **dolutegravir** dose, p. 739. Severe Study
- **St John's wort** is predicted to decrease the exposure to dronabinol. Avoid or adjust dose. Mild Study
- **St John's wort** is predicted to decrease the efficacy of drospirenone. For FSRH guidance, see Contraceptives, interactions p. 917. Severe Theoretical
- **St John's wort** is predicted to decrease the exposure to elacestrant. Avoid or adjust dose depending on duration—consult product literature. Severe Theoretical
- **St John's wort** is predicted to moderately decrease the exposure to elbasvir. Avoid. Severe Study
- **St John's wort** is predicted to decrease the exposure to elexacaftor. Avoid. Severe Theoretical
- **St John's wort** is predicted to increase the exposure to eliglustat. Avoid. Severe Study
- **St John's wort** is predicted to decrease the concentration of elvitegravir. Avoid. Severe Theoretical
- **St John's wort** is predicted to decrease the exposure to encorafenib. Severe Theoretical
- **St John's wort** is predicted to decrease the exposure to endothelin receptor antagonists (bosentan). Avoid. Moderate Theoretical
- **St John's wort** is predicted to decrease the exposure to endothelin receptor antagonists (macitentan). Avoid. Severe Theoretical
- **St John's wort** is predicted to decrease the exposure to the cytotoxic component of enfortumab vedotin. Moderate Theoretical
- **St John's wort** is predicted to decrease the exposure to entrectinib. Avoid. Moderate Theoretical

- **St John's wort** is predicted to decrease the exposure to erdafitinib. Avoid. Moderate Study
- **St John's wort** is predicted to decrease the exposure to erlotinib. Severe Study
- **St John's wort** is predicted to decrease the efficacy of estradiol. Moderate Theoretical
- **St John's wort** is predicted to decrease the exposure to eszopiclone. Adjust dose. Moderate Theoretical
- **St John's wort** is predicted to decrease the efficacy of etonogestrel. MHRA advises avoid. For FSRH guidance, see Contraceptives, interactions p. 917. Severe Theoretical
- **St John's wort** is predicted to decrease the concentration of everolimus. Avoid or adjust dose. Severe Study
- **St John's wort** is predicted to decrease the exposure to exemestane. Moderate Theoretical
- **St John's wort** is predicted to decrease the exposure to factor XA inhibitors (apixaban). Use with caution or avoid. Severe Study
- **St John's wort** is predicted to decrease the exposure to factor XA inhibitors (edoxaban). Moderate Study
- **St John's wort** is predicted to decrease the exposure to factor XA inhibitors (rivaroxaban). Avoid unless patient can be monitored for signs of thrombosis. Severe Study
- **St John's wort** is predicted to decrease the exposure to fedratinib. Avoid. Moderate Study
- **St John's wort** is predicted to decrease the exposure to fesoterodine. Avoid. Severe Theoretical
- **St John's wort** is predicted to decrease the exposure to fingolimod. Avoid. Moderate Theoretical
- **St John's wort** is predicted to decrease the exposure to the active metabolite of fostemsavir. Avoid. Severe Study
- **St John's wort** is predicted to decrease the exposure to fruquintinib. Avoid. Moderate Study
- **St John's wort** is predicted to decrease the exposure to gefitinib. Avoid. Severe Study
- **St John's wort** is predicted to decrease the exposure to gilteritinib. Avoid. Severe Study
- **St John's wort** is predicted to decrease the exposure to glasdegib. Avoid or adjust dose—consult product literature. Moderate Theoretical
- **St John's wort** is predicted to decrease the exposure to glecaprevir. Avoid. Severe Study
- **St John's wort** is predicted to markedly decrease the exposure to grazoprevir. Avoid. Severe Study
- **St John's wort** is predicted to decrease the concentration of guanfacine. Adjust dose. Moderate Theoretical
- **St John's wort** is predicted to decrease the exposure to HIV-protease inhibitors. Avoid. Severe Study
- **St John's wort** is predicted to decrease the efficacy of hormone replacement therapy. Moderate Theoretical
- **St John's wort** is predicted to decrease the exposure to ibrutinib. Avoid. Severe Theoretical
- **St John's wort** is predicted to decrease the exposure to idelalisib. Avoid. Moderate Theoretical
- **St John's wort** is predicted to decrease the exposure to imatinib. Moderate Study
- **St John's wort** slightly decreases the exposure to irinotecan. Avoid. Severe Study
- **St John's wort** decreases the exposure to ivabradine. Avoid. Moderate Study
- **St John's wort** is predicted to decrease the exposure to ivacaftor. Avoid. Severe Study
- **St John's wort** is predicted to decreases the exposure to ivosidenib. Avoid. Moderate Theoretical
- **St John's wort** is predicted to decrease the exposure to ixazomib. Avoid. Severe Theoretical
- **St John's wort** is predicted to decrease the exposure to lapatinib. Avoid. Severe Study
- **St John's wort** is predicted to decrease the exposure to larotrectinib. Avoid. Moderate Study
- **St John's wort** is predicted to decrease the exposure to ledipasvir. Avoid. Severe Study
- **St John's wort** is predicted to decrease the exposure to leniolisib. Avoid. Severe Theoretical
- **St John's wort** is predicted to decrease the concentration of letermovir. Moderate Theoretical

St John's wort (continued)
▶ St John's wort is predicted to decrease the efficacy of levonorgestrel. MHRA advises avoid. For FSRH guidance, see Contraceptives, interactions p. 917. Severe Theoretical
▶ St John's wort is predicted to decrease the exposure to lorlatinib. Avoid. Severe Theoretical
▶ St John's wort is predicted to decrease the exposure to maraviroc. Avoid. Severe Theoretical
▶ St John's wort is predicted to decrease the exposure to maribavir. Avoid. Severe Study
▶ St John's wort is predicted to decrease the exposure to mavacamten. Monitor and adjust dose—consult product literature. Severe Theoretical
▶ St John's wort is predicted to decrease the exposure to midostaurin. Avoid. Severe Theoretical
▶ St John's wort is predicted to decrease the exposure to mifepristone. Adjust **mifepristone** dose, p. 954. Severe Study
▶ St John's wort is predicted to slightly decrease the exposure to mineralocorticoid receptor antagonists **(eplerenone)**. Avoid. Moderate Study
▶ St John's wort is predicted to decrease the exposure to mineralocorticoid receptor antagonists **(finerenone)**. Avoid. Severe Study
▶ St John's wort is predicted to decrease the exposure to mobocertinib. Avoid. Severe Study
▶ **Moclobemide** might cause serotonin syndrome, as can St John's wort; concurrent use might increase the risk of developing this effect. Avoid. Severe Theoretical → Also see **TABLE 12** p. 1574
▶ St John's wort is predicted to decrease the exposure to naldemedine. Avoid. Severe Study
▶ St John's wort is predicted to decrease the exposure to naloxegol. Avoid. Moderate Theoretical
▶ St John's wort is predicted to decrease the exposure to neratinib. Avoid. Severe Theoretical
▶ St John's wort is predicted to decrease the exposure to neurokinin-1 receptor antagonists **(aprepitant, fosaprepitant)**. Avoid. Moderate Theoretical
▶ St John's wort is predicted to decrease the exposure to neurokinin-1 receptor antagonists **(netupitant)**. Moderate Theoretical
▶ St John's wort is predicted to decrease the exposure to nilotinib. Avoid. Severe Theoretical
▶ St John's wort is predicted to decrease the exposure to nintedanib. Moderate Study
▶ St John's wort is predicted to decrease the exposure to nirmatrelvir boosted with ritonavir. Avoid. Severe Theoretical
▶ St John's wort is predicted to decrease the exposure to NNRTIs **(doravirine, rilpivirine)**. Avoid. Severe Theoretical
▶ St John's wort is predicted to decrease the concentration of NNRTIs **(efavirenz, nevirapine)**. Avoid. Severe Theoretical
▶ St John's wort is predicted to decrease the efficacy of norethisterone. MHRA advises avoid. For FSRH guidance, see Contraceptives, interactions p. 917. Severe Anecdotal
▶ St John's wort is predicted to decrease the exposure to olaparib. Avoid. Moderate Theoretical
▶ St John's wort decreases the exposure to opioids **(methadone)**. Monitor and adjust dose. Severe Study → Also see **TABLE 12** p. 1574
▶ St John's wort moderately decreases the exposure to opioids **(oxycodone)**. Adjust dose. Moderate Study
▶ St John's wort is predicted to decrease the exposure to osimertinib. Avoid. Severe Study
▶ St John's wort is predicted to decrease the exposure to ospemifene. Moderate Study
▶ St John's wort is predicted to decrease the exposure to palbociclib. Avoid. Severe Theoretical
▶ St John's wort is predicted to decrease the exposure to panobinostat. Avoid. Moderate Theoretical
▶ St John's wort is predicted to decrease the exposure to pazopanib. Severe Study
▶ St John's wort is predicted to decrease the exposure to pemigatinib. Avoid. Severe Study
▶ St John's wort is predicted to decrease the exposure to phosphodiesterase type-4 inhibitors **(apremilast)**. Avoid. Severe Theoretical

▶ St John's wort is predicted to decrease the exposure to phosphodiesterase type-5 inhibitors. Moderate Theoretical
▶ St John's wort is predicted to decrease the exposure to pibrentasvir. Avoid. Severe Study
▶ St John's wort slightly decreases the exposure to pioglitazone. Mild Study
▶ St John's wort is predicted to decrease the exposure to pitolisant. Monitor and adjust dose. Moderate Theoretical
▶ St John's wort is predicted to decrease the exposure to ponatinib. Avoid. Severe Theoretical
▶ St John's wort is predicted to decrease the exposure to pralsetinib. Avoid or adjust dose—consult product literature. Moderate Study
▶ St John's wort is predicted to decrease the exposure to quizartinib. Avoid. Severe Study
▶ St John's wort is predicted to decrease the exposure to ranolazine. Avoid. Severe Study
▶ St John's wort is predicted to decrease the exposure to regorafenib. Avoid. Severe Study
▶ St John's wort is predicted to decrease the exposure to relugolix. Avoid or adjust dose depending on indication—consult product literature. Moderate Study
▶ St John's wort is predicted to decrease the exposure to ribociclib. Avoid. Severe Study
▶ St John's wort is predicted to decrease the exposure to rimegepant. Avoid. Moderate Theoretical
▶ St John's wort is predicted to decrease the exposure to ripretinib. Avoid or adjust dose—consult product literature. Moderate Theoretical
▶ St John's wort is predicted to decrease the exposure to ruxolitinib. Monitor and adjust dose. Moderate Study
▶ St John's wort is predicted to decrease the exposure to selpercatinib. Avoid. Moderate Study
▶ St John's wort is predicted to decrease the exposure to selumetinib. Avoid. Severe Study
▶ St John's wort is predicted to decrease the exposure to siponimod. Manufacturer advises caution depending on genotype—consult product literature. Moderate Theoretical
▶ St John's wort is predicted to decrease the concentration of sirolimus. Monitor and adjust dose. Severe Theoretical
▶ St John's wort is predicted to decrease the exposure to sodium glucose co-transporter 2 inhibitors **(canagliflozin)**. Adjust **canagliflozin** dose, p. 824. Moderate Study
▶ St John's wort is predicted to decrease the exposure to sofosbuvir. Avoid. Severe Study
▶ St John's wort is predicted to decrease the exposure to sorafenib. Moderate Study
▶ St John's wort is predicted to decrease the exposure to statins **(atorvastatin, simvastatin)**. Moderate Study
▶ St John's wort is predicted to decrease the exposure to sunitinib. Moderate Study
▶ St John's wort decreases the concentration of tacrolimus. Avoid. Severe Study
▶ St John's wort is predicted to decrease the exposure to taxanes **(cabazitaxel)**. Avoid. Severe Theoretical
▶ St John's wort is predicted to decrease the exposure to taxanes **(docetaxel)**. Severe Theoretical
▶ St John's wort is predicted to decrease the exposure to taxanes **(paclitaxel)**. Avoid. Severe Study
▶ St John's wort is predicted to decrease the concentration of temsirolimus. Avoid. Moderate Theoretical
▶ St John's wort is predicted to decrease the exposure to tenofovir alafenamide. Avoid. Moderate Theoretical
▶ **Tepotinib** might decrease the exposure to St John's wort. Avoid. Severe Theoretical
▶ St John's wort is predicted to decrease the exposure to tetracyclines **(eravacycline)**. Adjust **eravacycline** dose, p. 657. Moderate Theoretical
▶ St John's wort is predicted to decrease the exposure to tezacaftor. Avoid. Severe Theoretical
▶ St John's wort potentially decreases the exposure to theophylline. Severe Anecdotal
▶ St John's wort is predicted to decrease the exposure to thrombin inhibitors **(dabigatran)**. Avoid. Severe Study

- ▸ **St John's wort** is predicted to decrease the exposure to ticagrelor. Moderate Theoretical
- ▸ **St John's wort** might decrease the exposure to tigecycline. Mild Theoretical
- ▸ **St John's wort** is predicted to decrease the exposure to tivozanib. Avoid. Severe Study
- ▸ **St John's wort** is predicted to decrease the exposure to tofacitinib. Severe Study
- ▸ **St John's wort** is predicted to decrease the exposure to tolvaptan. Avoid. Moderate Theoretical
- ▸ **St John's wort** is predicted to decrease the exposure to topotecan. Severe Theoretical
- ▸ **St John's wort** is predicted to decrease the exposure to treprostinil. Adjust dose. Mild Theoretical
- ▸ **St John's wort** is predicted to decrease the exposure to tucatinib. Avoid. Severe Theoretical
- ▸ **St John's wort** is predicted to decrease the efficacy of ulipristal. For FSRH guidance, see Contraceptives, interactions p. 917. Severe Anecdotal
- ▸ **St John's wort** is predicted to decrease the exposure to vandetanib. Avoid. Severe Study
- ▸ **St John's wort** is predicted to decrease the exposure to velpatasvir. Avoid. Moderate Theoretical
- ▸ **St John's wort** is predicted to decrease the exposure to vemurafenib. Avoid. Severe Study
- ▸ **St John's wort** is predicted to decrease the exposure to venetoclax. Avoid. Severe Study
- ▸ **St John's wort** is predicted to decrease the exposure to vinca alkaloids. Severe Theoretical
- ▸ **St John's wort** is predicted to decrease the exposure to vismodegib. Avoid. Moderate Theoretical
- ▸ **St John's wort** is predicted to decrease the exposure to voclosporin. Avoid. Severe Theoretical
- ▸ **St John's wort** has been reported to cause severe hypotension when given with volatile halogenated anaesthetics. Severe Theoretical
- ▸ **St John's wort** is predicted to decrease the concentration of voxilaprevir. Avoid. Severe Theoretical
- ▸ **St John's wort** is predicted to decrease the exposure to zanubrutinib. Avoid or adjust dose with moderate CYP3A4 inducers—consult product literature. Severe Theoretical

Statins → see TABLE 1 p. 1571 (hepatotoxicity)

atorvastatin · fluvastatin · pravastatin · rosuvastatin · simvastatin

- ▸ **Acipimox** is predicted to increase the risk of rhabdomyolysis when given with **statins**. Severe Theoretical
- ▸ **Atorvastatin** slightly to moderately increases the exposure to aliskiren. Moderate Study
- ▸ Oral antacids decrease the absorption of oral **rosuvastatin**. Separate administration by 2 hours. Moderate Study
- ▸ Anti-androgens (apalutamide) are predicted to decrease the exposure to **atorvastatin**. Moderate Study
- ▸ Anti-androgens (apalutamide) are predicted to decrease the exposure to **fluvastatin**. Monitor and adjust dose. Mild Theoretical
- ▸ Anti-androgens (apalutamide) are predicted to decrease the exposure to **pravastatin**. Mild Study
- ▸ Anti-androgens (apalutamide) slightly decrease the exposure to **rosuvastatin**. Mild Study
- ▸ Anti-androgens (apalutamide) are predicted to decrease the exposure to **simvastatin**. Avoid or monitor. Moderate Study
- ▸ Anti-androgens (darolutamide) markedly increase the exposure to **rosuvastatin**. Avoid or adjust **rosuvastatin** dose, p. 235. Severe Study
- ▸ Anti-androgens (darolutamide) are predicted to increase the exposure to statins (**atorvastatin, fluvastatin**). Avoid. Severe Theoretical
- ▸ Anti-androgens (enzalutamide) are predicted to decrease the exposure to statins (**atorvastatin, simvastatin**). Moderate Study
- ▸ Anti-androgens (darolutamide) are predicted to increase the concentration of statins (**pravastatin, simvastatin**). Moderate Theoretical
- ▸ Antiarrhythmics (amiodarone) are predicted to increase the exposure to **atorvastatin**. Monitor and adjust dose. Moderate Theoretical → Also see TABLE 1 p. 1571

- ▸ Antiarrhythmics (amiodarone) are predicted to increase the exposure to **fluvastatin**. Moderate Study → Also see TABLE 1 p. 1571
- ▸ Antiarrhythmics (amiodarone) increase the exposure to **simvastatin**. Adjust **simvastatin** dose, p. 237. Severe Study → Also see TABLE 1 p. 1571
- ▸ Antiarrhythmics (dronedarone) slightly increase the exposure to **atorvastatin**. Monitor and adjust dose. Severe Study
- ▸ Antiarrhythmics (dronedarone) slightly increase the exposure to **rosuvastatin**. Adjust dose. Severe Study
- ▸ Antiarrhythmics (dronedarone) moderately increase the exposure to **simvastatin**. Monitor and adjust dose. Severe Study
- ▸ Antiepileptics (carbamazepine) are predicted to decrease the exposure to **atorvastatin**. Monitor and adjust dose. Moderate Study
- ▸ Antiepileptics (carbamazepine, eslicarbazepine) moderately decrease the exposure to **simvastatin**. Monitor and adjust dose. Moderate Study
- ▸ Antiepileptics (eslicarbazepine) are predicted to decrease the exposure to **atorvastatin**. Monitor and adjust dose. Moderate Theoretical
- ▸ Antiepileptics (eslicarbazepine) decrease the exposure to **rosuvastatin**. Moderate Study
- ▸ Antiepileptics (phenytoin) moderately decrease the exposure to **atorvastatin**. Moderate Study
- ▸ Antiepileptics (phenytoin) are predicted to decrease the exposure to **simvastatin**. Moderate Study
- ▸ Antiepileptics (fosphenytoin, phenobarbital, primidone) are predicted to decrease the exposure to statins (**atorvastatin, simvastatin**). Moderate Study
- ▸ Antiepileptics (oxcarbazepine) are predicted to decrease the exposure to statins (**atorvastatin, simvastatin**). Moderate Theoretical
- ▸ Antifungals, azoles (fluconazole, miconazole) are predicted to increase the exposure to **fluvastatin**. Moderate Study → Also see TABLE 1 p. 1571
- ▸ Antifungals, azoles (isavuconazole) slightly increase the exposure to **atorvastatin**. Moderate Study
- ▸ Antifungals, azoles (isavuconazole) are predicted to increase the exposure to **simvastatin**. Monitor and adjust dose. Severe Theoretical
- ▸ Antifungals, azoles (itraconazole, ketoconazole, posaconazole, voriconazole) are predicted to increase the exposure to **atorvastatin**. Avoid or adjust dose and monitor rhabdomyolysis. Severe Study → Also see TABLE 1 p. 1571
- ▸ Antifungals, azoles (itraconazole, ketoconazole, posaconazole, voriconazole) are predicted to increase the exposure to **simvastatin**. Avoid. Severe Study → Also see TABLE 1 p. 1571
- ▸ Antifungals, azoles (miconazole) (including the oral gel) might increase the exposure to **atorvastatin**. Moderate Theoretical
- ▸ Antifungals, azoles (miconazole) (including the oral gel) are predicted to increase the exposure to **simvastatin**. Avoid. Severe Anecdotal
- ▸ Antifungals, azoles (fluconazole) are predicted to increase the exposure to statins (**atorvastatin, simvastatin**). Monitor and adjust dose. Severe Anecdotal → Also see TABLE 1 p. 1571
- ▸ Antifungals, azoles (isavuconazole) are predicted to increase the exposure to statins (**fluvastatin, rosuvastatin**). Moderate Theoretical
- ▸ **Belumosudil** is predicted to increase the exposure to **fluvastatin**. Avoid or adjust dose. Moderate Theoretical
- ▸ **Belumosudil** is predicted to increase the exposure to statins (**atorvastatin, pravastatin, rosuvastatin, simvastatin**). Avoid or adjust dose. Moderate Study
- ▸ **Bempedoic acid** increases the exposure to **pravastatin**. Moderate Study
- ▸ **Bempedoic acid** increases the exposure to **simvastatin**. Adjust **simvastatin** dose, p. 237. Moderate Study
- ▸ **Bulevirtide** is predicted to increase the exposure to **statins**. Avoid or monitor. Moderate Theoretical
- ▸ Calcium channel blockers (amlodipine) cause a small increase in the exposure to **simvastatin**. Adjust **simvastatin** dose, p. 237. Moderate Study
- ▸ Calcium channel blockers (diltiazem) slightly increase the exposure to **atorvastatin**. Monitor and adjust dose. Severe Study

Statins (continued)

▶ Calcium channel blockers (diltiazem, verapamil) moderately increase the exposure to **simvastatin**. Monitor and adjust dose. [Severe] Study

▶ Calcium channel blockers (verapamil) are predicted to slightly to moderately increase the exposure to **atorvastatin**. Monitor and adjust dose. [Severe] Theoretical

▶ Cenobamate is predicted to decrease the exposure to statins (atorvastatin, simvastatin). [Moderate] Study

▶ Cephalosporins (ceftobiprole) are predicted to increase the concentration of **statins**. [Moderate] Theoretical

▶ Ceritinib is predicted to increase the exposure to **atorvastatin**. Avoid or adjust dose and monitor rhabdomyolysis. [Severe] Study

▶ Ceritinib is predicted to increase the exposure to **simvastatin**. Avoid. [Severe] Study

▶ Ciclosporin markedly to very markedly increases the exposure to **atorvastatin**. Avoid or adjust **atorvastatin** dose, p. 234. [Severe] Study

▶ Ciclosporin moderately increases the exposure to **fluvastatin**. [Severe] Study

▶ Ciclosporin markedly to very markedly increases the exposure to **pravastatin**. Adjust dose. [Severe] Study

▶ Ciclosporin markedly increases the exposure to **rosuvastatin**. Avoid. [Severe] Study

▶ Ciclosporin markedly to very markedly increases the exposure to **simvastatin**. Avoid. [Severe] Study

▶ Cilostazol is predicted to increase the exposure to **atorvastatin**. [Moderate] Theoretical

▶ Cilostazol slightly increases the exposure to **simvastatin**. [Moderate] Study

▶ Clopidogrel increases the exposure to **rosuvastatin**. Adjust **rosuvastatin** dose, p. 235. [Moderate] Study

▶ Cobicistat is predicted to increase the exposure to **atorvastatin**. Avoid or adjust dose and monitor rhabdomyolysis. [Severe] Study

▶ Cobicistat is predicted to increase the exposure to **simvastatin**. Avoid. [Severe] Study

▶ Colchicine has been reported to cause rhabdomyolysis when given with **statins**. [Severe] Anecdotal

▶ Statins (fluvastatin, rosuvastatin) increase the anticoagulant effect of coumarins. Monitor INR and adjust dose. [Severe] Study

▶ Crizotinib is predicted to increase the exposure to **atorvastatin**. Monitor and adjust dose. [Moderate] Theoretical

▶ Crizotinib is predicted to increase the exposure to **pravastatin**. [Moderate] Theoretical

▶ Crizotinib is predicted to increase the exposure to **simvastatin**. Monitor and adjust dose. [Severe] Theoretical

▶ Dabrafenib is predicted to decrease the exposure to statins (atorvastatin, simvastatin). [Moderate] Study

▶ Danicopan is predicted to increase the exposure to statins (atorvastatin, fluvastatin, rosuvastatin). [Moderate] Study

▶ Statins are predicted to increase the risk of rhabdomyolysis when given with daptomycin. [Severe] Theoretical

▶ Dasatinib is predicted to increase the exposure to **simvastatin**. [Moderate] Theoretical

▶ Elafibranor might increase the risk of muscle effects when given with **statins**. [Severe] Theoretical

▶ Elbasvir with grazoprevir slightly increases the exposure to **atorvastatin**. Adjust **atorvastatin** dose, p. 234. [Moderate] Study

▶ Elbasvir with grazoprevir is predicted to increase the exposure to **fluvastatin**. Adjust **fluvastatin** dose, p. 234. [Moderate] Theoretical

▶ Elbasvir with grazoprevir moderately increases the exposure to **rosuvastatin**. Adjust **rosuvastatin** dose, p. 235. [Moderate] Study

▶ Elbasvir with grazoprevir is predicted to increase the exposure to **simvastatin**. Adjust **simvastatin** dose, p. 237. [Moderate] Theoretical

▶ Elexacaftor is predicted to increase the exposure to statins (atorvastatin, pravastatin, rosuvastatin, simvastatin). [Moderate] Theoretical

▶ Eliglustat is predicted to increase the exposure to **pravastatin**. Adjust dose. [Moderate] Study

▶ Eltrombopag is predicted to increase the exposure to **statins**. Monitor and adjust dose. [Moderate] Study

▶ Encorafenib is predicted to increase the exposure to **atorvastatin**. [Mild] Theoretical

▶ Encorafenib is predicted to affect the exposure to **simvastatin**. [Mild] Theoretical

▶ Encorafenib is predicted to increase the exposure to statins (fluvastatin, pravastatin). [Mild] Study

▶ Endothelin receptor antagonists (bosentan) are predicted to decrease the exposure to statins (atorvastatin, simvastatin). [Moderate] Study

▶ Febuxostat increases the exposure to **rosuvastatin**. Adjust **rosuvastatin** dose, p. 235. [Moderate] Study

▶ Fibrates (bezafibrate, ciprofibrate) increase the risk of rhabdomyolysis when given with **pravastatin**. Avoid. [Severe] Study

▶ Fibrates (bezafibrate, ciprofibrate) increase the risk of rhabdomyolysis when given with **rosuvastatin**. Adjust **rosuvastatin** dose, p. 235. [Severe] Study

▶ Fibrates (bezafibrate, ciprofibrate) increase the risk of rhabdomyolysis when given with **simvastatin**. Adjust **simvastatin** dose, p. 237. [Severe] Study

▶ Fibrates (ciprofibrate) increase the risk of rhabdomyolysis when given with **atorvastatin**. Avoid or adjust dose. [Severe] Study

▶ Fibrates (ciprofibrate) increase the risk of rhabdomyolysis when given with **fluvastatin**. [Severe] Study

▶ Fibrates (fenofibrate) increase the risk of rhabdomyolysis when given with **atorvastatin**. Monitor and adjust **fenofibrate** dose, p. 231. [Severe] Anecdotal

▶ Fibrates (fenofibrate) are predicted to increase the risk of rhabdomyolysis when given with **fluvastatin**. Use with caution and adjust **fenofibrate** dose, p. 231. [Severe] Theoretical

▶ Fibrates (fenofibrate) are predicted to increase the risk of rhabdomyolysis when given with **pravastatin**. Avoid. [Severe] Theoretical

▶ Fibrates (fenofibrate) increase the risk of rhabdomyolysis when given with **rosuvastatin**. Adjust **fenofibrate** and **rosuvastatin** doses, p. 231, p. 235. [Severe] Anecdotal

▶ Fibrates (fenofibrate) increase the risk of rhabdomyolysis when given with **simvastatin**. Adjust **fenofibrate** dose, p. 231. [Severe] Anecdotal

▶ Fibrates (gemfibrozil) cause a small increase in the exposure to **atorvastatin**. Avoid. [Severe] Study

▶ Fibrates (gemfibrozil) increase the risk of rhabdomyolysis when given with **fluvastatin**. [Severe] Anecdotal

▶ Fibrates (gemfibrozil) modestly increase the exposure to **pravastatin**. Avoid or monitor. [Severe] Study

▶ Fibrates (gemfibrozil) cause a small increase in the exposure to **rosuvastatin**. Avoid or adjust **rosuvastatin** dose, p. 235. [Severe] Study

▶ Fibrates (gemfibrozil) modestly increase the exposure to **simvastatin**. Avoid. [Severe] Anecdotal

▶ Fibrates (bezafibrate) increase the risk of rhabdomyolysis when given with statins (atorvastatin, fluvastatin). [Severe] Study

▶ Fostamatinib moderately increases the exposure to **rosuvastatin**. Avoid or adjust **rosuvastatin** dose, p. 235. [Moderate] Study

▶ Fostamatinib slightly increases the exposure to **simvastatin**. Monitor adverse effects and adjust dose. [Moderate] Study

▶ Fostamatinib is predicted to increase the exposure to statins (atorvastatin, fluvastatin). Monitor and adjust dose. [Moderate] Theoretical

▶ Fostemsavir increases the exposure to **rosuvastatin**. Adjust starting dose and monitor. [Severe] Study

▶ Fostemsavir is predicted to increase the exposure to statins (atorvastatin, fluvastatin, simvastatin). Adjust starting dose and monitor. [Severe] Theoretical

▶ Fusidate has been reported to cause rhabdomyolysis when given with **statins**. Avoid. [Severe] Anecdotal

▶ Givinostat might increase the exposure to **simvastatin**. [Moderate] Study

▶ Glecaprevir with pibrentasvir markedly increases the exposure to **atorvastatin**. Avoid. [Severe] Study

▶ Glecaprevir with pibrentasvir is predicted to increase the exposure to **fluvastatin**. [Moderate] Theoretical

- **Glecaprevir** with pibrentasvir moderately increases the exposure to **pravastatin**. Use with caution and adjust **pravastatin** dose, p. 235. Moderate Study
- **Glecaprevir** with pibrentasvir moderately increases the exposure to **rosuvastatin**. Use with caution and adjust **rosuvastatin** dose, p. 235. Moderate Study
- **Glecaprevir** with pibrentasvir moderately increases the exposure to **simvastatin**. Avoid. Moderate Study
- **Grapefruit** juice increases the exposure to **atorvastatin**. Mild Study
- **Grapefruit** juice increases the exposure to **simvastatin**. Avoid. Severe Study
- **Grazoprevir** moderately increases the exposure to **atorvastatin**. Adjust **atorvastatin** dose, p. 234. Moderate Study
- **Grazoprevir** with elbasvir is predicted to increase the exposure to **fluvastatin**. Adjust **fluvastatin** dose, p. 234. Moderate Theoretical
- **Grazoprevir** with elbasvir moderately increases the exposure to **rosuvastatin**. Adjust **rosuvastatin** dose, p. 235. Moderate Study
- **Grazoprevir** with elbasvir is predicted to increase the exposure to **simvastatin**. Adjust **simvastatin** dose, p. 237. Moderate Theoretical
- **HIV-protease inhibitors** are predicted to increase the exposure to **atorvastatin**. Avoid or adjust dose and monitor rhabdomyolysis. Severe Study → Also see **TABLE 1** p. 1571
- **HIV-protease inhibitors** might affect the exposure to **pravastatin**. Moderate Study → Also see **TABLE 1** p. 1571
- **HIV-protease inhibitors (atazanavir, lopinavir)** boosted with ritonavir moderately increase the exposure to **rosuvastatin**. Avoid or adjust **rosuvastatin** dose, p. 235. Severe Study
- **HIV-protease inhibitors (darunavir, ritonavir)** are predicted to increase the exposure to **rosuvastatin**. Avoid or adjust dose. Severe Study → Also see **TABLE 1** p. 1571
- **HIV-protease inhibitors (fosamprenavir)** are predicted to increase the exposure to **rosuvastatin**. Use with caution and adjust dose. Severe Study
- **HIV-protease inhibitors** are predicted to increase the exposure to **simvastatin**. Avoid. Severe Study → Also see **TABLE 1** p. 1571
- **Idelalisib** is predicted to increase the exposure to **atorvastatin**. Avoid or adjust dose and monitor rhabdomyolysis. Severe Study
- **Idelalisib** is predicted to increase the exposure to **simvastatin**. Avoid. Severe Study
- **Imatinib** is predicted to increase the exposure to **atorvastatin**. Monitor and adjust dose. Severe Theoretical
- **Imatinib** moderately increases the exposure to **simvastatin**. Monitor and adjust dose. Severe Study
- **Ivosidenib** might affect the exposure to **simvastatin**. Avoid or monitor. Moderate Theoretical
- **Ivosidenib** is predicted to increase the exposure to statins (**atorvastatin, pravastatin, rosuvastatin**). Use with caution or avoid. Unknown Theoretical
- **Ledipasvir** with sofosbuvir is predicted to increase the exposure to **atorvastatin**. Monitor and adjust dose. Moderate Anecdotal
- **Ledipasvir** with sofosbuvir is predicted to increase the exposure to **rosuvastatin**. Avoid. Severe Theoretical
- **Ledipasvir** with sofosbuvir is predicted to increase the exposure to statins (**fluvastatin, pravastatin, simvastatin**). Monitor and adjust dose. Moderate Theoretical
- **Leflunomide** is predicted to increase the exposure to **rosuvastatin**. Adjust **rosuvastatin** dose, p. 235. Moderate Study
- **Leflunomide** is predicted to increase the exposure to statins (**atorvastatin, fluvastatin, pravastatin, simvastatin**). Moderate Study
- **Leniolisib** is predicted to increase the exposure to **statins**. Avoid. Moderate Theoretical
- **Letermovir** moderately increases the exposure to **atorvastatin**. Avoid or adjust **atorvastatin** dose, p. 234. Severe Study
- **Letermovir** is predicted to increase the exposure to **fluvastatin**. Monitor and adjust dose. Moderate Theoretical
- **Letermovir** is predicted to increase the exposure to **pravastatin**. Avoid or adjust dose. Moderate Theoretical
- **Letermovir** is predicted to increase the exposure to statins (**rosuvastatin, simvastatin**). Avoid. Severe Study

- **Lomitapide** increases the exposure to **atorvastatin**. Adjust **lomitapide** dose or separate administration by 12 hours, p. 241. Mild Study → Also see **TABLE 1** p. 1571
- **Lomitapide** increases the exposure to **simvastatin**. Monitor and adjust **simvastatin** dose, p. 237. Moderate Study → Also see **TABLE 1** p. 1571
- **Lorlatinib** is predicted to decrease the exposure to statins (**atorvastatin, simvastatin**). Moderate Study
- **Macrolides (clarithromycin)** are predicted to increase the exposure to **atorvastatin**. Avoid or adjust dose and monitor rhabdomyolysis. Severe Study
- **Macrolides (clarithromycin)** moderately increase the exposure to **pravastatin**. Severe Study
- **Macrolides (clarithromycin)** are predicted to increase the exposure to **simvastatin**. Avoid. Severe Study
- **Macrolides (erythromycin)** slightly increase the exposure to **atorvastatin**. Monitor and adjust dose. Severe Study
- **Macrolides (erythromycin)** slightly increase the exposure to **pravastatin**. Severe Study
- **Macrolides (erythromycin)** markedly increase the exposure to **simvastatin**. Avoid. Severe Study
- **Maribavir** is predicted to increase the exposure to **rosuvastatin**. Moderate Theoretical
- **Mifepristone** moderately increases the exposure to **fluvastatin**. Moderate Study
- **Mifepristone** very markedly increases the exposure to **simvastatin**. Severe Study
- **Mitotane** is predicted to decrease the exposure to statins (**atorvastatin, simvastatin**). Moderate Study
- **Momelotinib** increases the exposure to **rosuvastatin**. Moderate Study
- **Monoclonal antibodies (sarilumab)** are predicted to decrease the exposure to statins (**atorvastatin, simvastatin**). Moderate Study
- **Monoclonal antibodies (tocilizumab)** are predicted to decrease the exposure to statins (**atorvastatin, simvastatin**). Monitor and adjust dose. Moderate Study
- **Neurokinin-1 receptor antagonists (aprepitant, netupitant)** are predicted to increase the exposure to statins (**atorvastatin, simvastatin**). Monitor and adjust dose. Severe Theoretical
- **Nicotinic acid** might increase the risk of rhabdomyolysis when given with **statins**. Use with caution or avoid. Severe Theoretical → Also see **TABLE 1** p. 1571
- **Nilotinib** is predicted to increase the exposure to **atorvastatin**. Monitor and adjust dose. Moderate Theoretical
- **Nilotinib** is predicted to increase the exposure to **simvastatin**. Monitor and adjust dose. Severe Theoretical
- **Nirmatrelvir** boosted with ritonavir is predicted to increase the concentration of **simvastatin**. Avoid. Severe Theoretical
- **Nirmatrelvir** boosted with ritonavir is predicted to increase the concentration of statins (**atorvastatin, rosuvastatin**). Adjust dose. Severe Theoretical
- **NNRTIs (etravirine)** are predicted to increase the exposure to **fluvastatin**. Adjust dose. Severe Theoretical
- **NNRTIs (efavirenz, etravirine, nevirapine)** are predicted to decrease the exposure to statins (**atorvastatin, simvastatin**). Moderate Study → Also see **TABLE 1** p. 1571
- **Olaparib** is predicted to increase the exposure to **statins**. Moderate Theoretical
- **Osimertinib** causes a small increase in the exposure to **rosuvastatin**. Severe Study
- **Pazopanib** might cause increased ALT concentrations when given with **simvastatin**. Moderate Study
- **Pazopanib** might affect the exposure to statins (**atorvastatin, pravastatin, rosuvastatin**). Moderate Theoretical
- **Rosuvastatin** is predicted to increase the anticoagulant effect of **phenindione**. Monitor INR and adjust dose. Severe Theoretical
- **Pibrentasvir** with glecaprevir markedly increases the exposure to **atorvastatin**. Avoid. Severe Study
- **Pibrentasvir** with glecaprevir is predicted to increase the exposure to **fluvastatin**. Moderate Theoretical
- **Pibrentasvir** with glecaprevir moderately increases the exposure to **pravastatin**. Use with caution and adjust **pravastatin** dose, p. 235. Moderate Study

Statins (continued)

- **Pibrentasvir** with glecaprevir moderately increases the exposure to **rosuvastatin**. Use with caution and adjust **rosuvastatin** dose, p. 235. Moderate Study
- **Pibrentasvir** with glecaprevir moderately increases the exposure to **simvastatin**. Avoid. Moderate Study
- **Ranolazine** is predicted to increase the exposure to **atorvastatin**. Moderate Theoretical
- **Ranolazine** slightly increases the exposure to **simvastatin**. Adjust **simvastatin** dose, p. 237. Moderate Study
- **Regorafenib** moderately increases the exposure to **rosuvastatin**. Avoid or adjust **rosuvastatin** dose, p. 235. Moderate Study
- **Regorafenib** is predicted to increase the exposure to statins (**atorvastatin, fluvastatin**). Moderate Study
- **Ribociclib** (high-dose) is predicted to increase the exposure to **simvastatin**. Avoid. Moderate Theoretical
- **Ribociclib** is predicted to increase the exposure to statins (**pravastatin, rosuvastatin**). Moderate Theoretical
- **Rifamycins (rifampicin)** markedly decrease the exposure to **atorvastatin**. Manufacturer advises take both drugs at the same time. Moderate Study
- **Rifamycins (rifampicin)** moderately decrease the exposure to **fluvastatin**. Monitor and adjust dose. Moderate Study
- **Rifamycins (rifampicin)** very markedly decrease the exposure to **simvastatin**. Moderate Study
- **Roxadustat** might increase the exposure to **fluvastatin**. Monitor adverse effects and adjust dose. Moderate Theoretical
- **Roxadustat** is predicted to increase the exposure to statins (**atorvastatin, pravastatin, rosuvastatin, simvastatin**). Monitor adverse effects and adjust dose. Moderate Study
- **Sacubitril** with valsartan increases the exposure to **atorvastatin**. Moderate Study
- **Sodium glucose co-transporter 2 inhibitors (empagliflozin)** have been reported to increase the risk of muscle effects when given after **atorvastatin**. Moderate Anecdotal
- **Sotorasib** is predicted to decrease the exposure to statins (**atorvastatin, simvastatin**). Moderate Study → Also see TABLE 1 p. 1571
- **Sotorasib** is predicted to increase the exposure to statins (**fluvastatin, rosuvastatin**). Monitor and adjust dose. Moderate Study → Also see TABLE 1 p. 1571
- **St John's wort** is predicted to decrease the exposure to statins (**atorvastatin, simvastatin**). Moderate Study
- **Fluvastatin** slightly increases the exposure to sulfonylureas (glibenclamide). Mild Study
- **Tafamidis** slightly increases the exposure to **rosuvastatin**. Severe Study
- **Atorvastatin** very slightly increases the exposure to talazoparib. Moderate Study
- Taxanes (cabazitaxel) are predicted to affect the exposure to statins (**atorvastatin, pravastatin, rosuvastatin, simvastatin**). Manufacturer advises take 12 hours before or 3 hours after cabazitaxel. Moderate Theoretical
- **Tedizolid** is predicted to increase the exposure to statins (**atorvastatin, fluvastatin, rosuvastatin**). Avoid. Moderate Study
- **Tepotinib** might increase the exposure to statins (**atorvastatin, fluvastatin, rosuvastatin**). Moderate Theoretical
- **Teriflunomide** moderately increases the exposure to **rosuvastatin**. Adjust **rosuvastatin** dose, p. 235. Moderate Study
- **Teriflunomide** is predicted to increase the exposure to statins (**atorvastatin, fluvastatin, pravastatin, simvastatin**). Moderate Study
- **Ticagrelor** slightly to moderately increases the exposure to **simvastatin**. Adjust **simvastatin** dose, p. 237. Moderate Study
- **Tucatinib** is predicted to increase the exposure to **atorvastatin**. Avoid or adjust dose and monitor rhabdomyolysis. Severe Study
- **Tucatinib** is predicted to increase the exposure to **simvastatin**. Avoid. Severe Study
- **Vadadustat** increases the exposure to **simvastatin**. Monitor and adjust dose. Moderate Study
- **Vadadustat** is predicted to increase the exposure to statins (**atorvastatin, fluvastatin, rosuvastatin**). Monitor and adjust dose. Moderate Study

- **Velpatasvir** with sofosbuvir slightly increases the exposure to **atorvastatin**. Severe Study
- **Velpatasvir** moderately increases the exposure to **rosuvastatin**. Avoid or adjust **rosuvastatin** dose, p. 235. Severe Study
- **Velpatasvir** with sofosbuvir is predicted to increase the exposure to statins (**fluvastatin, simvastatin**). Monitor adverse effects and adjust dose. Severe Theoretical
- **Venetoclax** is predicted to increase the exposure to **atorvastatin**. Moderate Study
- **Venetoclax** is predicted to increase the exposure to statins (**fluvastatin, pravastatin, rosuvastatin, simvastatin**). Moderate Theoretical
- **Voclosporin** is predicted to increase the concentration of statins (**atorvastatin, pravastatin, rosuvastatin, simvastatin**). Moderate Theoretical
- **Voxilaprevir** with sofosbuvir and velpatasvir is predicted to increase the exposure to **atorvastatin**. Adjust **atorvastatin** dose, p. 234. Moderate Theoretical
- **Voxilaprevir** with sofosbuvir and velpatasvir moderately increases the exposure to **pravastatin**. Monitor and adjust **pravastatin** dose, p. 235. Moderate Study
- **Voxilaprevir** with sofosbuvir and velpatasvir markedly increases the exposure to **rosuvastatin**. Avoid. Severe Study
- **Voxilaprevir** with sofosbuvir and velpatasvir is predicted to increase the exposure to statins (**fluvastatin, simvastatin**). Avoid. Moderate Theoretical

Stiripentol → see antiepileptics

Streptokinase → see TABLE 3 p. 1571 (anticoagulant effects)

Streptomycin → see aminoglycosides

Streptozocin → see TABLE 1 p. 1571 (hepatotoxicity), TABLE 14 p. 1575 (myelosuppression), TABLE 2 p. 1571 (nephrotoxicity)

- **Live vaccines** are predicted to increase the risk of generalised infection (possibly life-threatening) when given with **streptozocin**. UKHSA advises avoid (refer to Green Book). Severe Theoretical

Strontium

- Oral antacids decrease the absorption of oral **strontium**. Separate administration by 2 hours. Moderate Study
- Oral calcium salts decrease the absorption of oral **strontium**. Separate administration by 2 hours. Moderate Study
- **Strontium** is predicted to decrease the absorption of quinolones. Avoid. Moderate Theoretical
- **Strontium** is predicted to decrease the absorption of tetracyclines. Avoid. Moderate Theoretical

Sucralfate

- **Sucralfate** is predicted to decrease the exposure to bictegravir. Avoid. Moderate Theoretical
- **Sucralfate** potentially decreases the effects of coumarins (warfarin). Separate administration by 2 hours. Moderate Anecdotal
- **Sucralfate** decreases the absorption of digoxin. Separate administration by 2 hours. Severe Anecdotal
- **Sucralfate** decreases the absorption of dolutegravir. Moderate Study
- **Sucralfate** increases the risk of blocked enteral or nasogastric tubes when given with enteral feeds. Separate administration by 1 hour. Moderate Study
- Potassium citrate increases the risk of adverse effects when given with **sucralfate**. Avoid. Moderate Theoretical
- **Sucralfate** decreases the exposure to quinolones. Separate administration by 2 hours. Moderate Study
- Sodium citrate is predicted to increase the risk of adverse effects when given with **sucralfate**. Avoid. Moderate Theoretical
- **Sucralfate** decreases the absorption of sulpiride. Separate administration by 2 hours. Moderate Study
- Oral **sucralfate** might decrease the absorption of oral tetracyclines. Moderate Theoretical
- **Sucralfate** potentially decreases the absorption of theophylline. Separate administration by at least 2 hours. Moderate Study
- **Sucralfate** decreases the absorption of thyroid hormones (levothyroxine). Separate administration by at least 4 hours. Moderate Study
- **Sucralfate** is predicted to decrease the absorption of tricyclic antidepressants. Moderate Study

Sucroferric oxyhydroxide → see interactions of iron
Sufentanil → see opioids
Sugammadex
▶ **Sugammadex** is predicted to decrease the exposure to combined hormonal contraceptives. Refer to patient information leaflet for missed pill advice. Severe Theoretical
▶ **Sugammadex** is predicted to decrease the exposure to desogestrel. Refer to patient information leaflet for missed pill advice. Severe Theoretical
▶ **Sugammadex** is predicted to decrease the exposure to drospirenone. Use additional contraceptive precautions. Severe Theoretical
▶ **Sugammadex** is predicted to decrease the efficacy of etonogestrel. Use additional contraceptive precautions. Severe Theoretical
▶ **Sugammadex** is predicted to decrease the exposure to levonorgestrel. Use additional contraceptive precautions. Severe Theoretical
▶ **Sugammadex** is predicted to decrease the exposure to medroxyprogesterone. Use additional contraceptive precautions. Severe Theoretical
▶ **Sugammadex** is predicted to decrease the exposure to norethisterone. Use additional contraceptive precautions. Severe Theoretical
Sulfadiazine → see sulfonamides
Sulfamethoxazole → see sulfonamides
Sulfasalazine → see TABLE 14 p. 1575 (myelosuppression), TABLE 2 p. 1571 (nephrotoxicity)
▶ Anti-androgens (apalutamide) are predicted to decrease the exposure to **sulfasalazine**. Mild Study
▶ Anti-androgens (darolutamide) are predicted to increase the exposure to **sulfasalazine**. Avoid. Severe Theoretical
▶ Antifungals, azoles (isavuconazole) are predicted to increase the exposure to **sulfasalazine**. Moderate Theoretical
▶ Belumosudil is predicted to increase the exposure to **sulfasalazine**. Avoid or adjust dose. Moderate Theoretical
▶ **Sulfasalazine** is predicted to affect the efficacy of bulevirtide. Avoid. Severe Theoretical
▶ Danicopan is predicted to increase the exposure to **sulfasalazine**. Moderate Study
▶ **Sulfasalazine** decreases the concentration of digoxin. Moderate Study
▶ Encorafenib is predicted to increase the exposure to **sulfasalazine**. Mild Study
▶ **Sulfasalazine** is predicted to decrease the absorption of folates. Moderate Study
▶ Fostamatinib is predicted to increase the exposure to **sulfasalazine**. Monitor and adjust dose. Moderate Theoretical
▶ Leflunomide is predicted to increase the exposure to **sulfasalazine**. Moderate Study → Also see TABLE 14 p. 1575
▶ Leniolisib is predicted to increase the exposure to **sulfasalazine**. Avoid. Moderate Theoretical
▶ Regorafenib is predicted to increase the exposure to **sulfasalazine**. Moderate Study → Also see TABLE 14 p. 1575
▶ Roxadustat might increase the exposure to **sulfasalazine**. Monitor adverse effects and adjust dose. Moderate Theoretical
▶ Sotorasib is predicted to increase the exposure to **sulfasalazine**. Monitor and adjust dose. Moderate Study
▶ Tedizolid is predicted to increase the exposure to **sulfasalazine**. Avoid. Moderate Study
▶ Tepotinib might increase the exposure to **sulfasalazine**. Moderate Theoretical
▶ Teriflunomide is predicted to increase the exposure to **sulfasalazine**. Moderate Study
▶ Vadadustat is predicted to increase the exposure to **sulfasalazine**. Monitor and adjust dose. Moderate Study
▶ Velpatasvir is predicted to increase the exposure to **sulfasalazine**. Moderate Theoretical
▶ Venetoclax is predicted to increase the exposure to **sulfasalazine**. Moderate Theoretical
▶ Voclosporin is predicted to increase the concentration of **sulfasalazine**. Moderate Theoretical → Also see TABLE 2 p. 1571
▶ Voxilaprevir is predicted to increase the concentration of **sulfasalazine**. Avoid. Severe Theoretical

Sulfonamides

sulfadiazine · sulfamethoxazole

▶ **Sulfadiazine** is predicted to increase the concentration of antiepileptics (fosphenytoin). Monitor and adjust dose. Moderate Study
▶ **Sulfadiazine** increases the concentration of antiepileptics (phenytoin). Monitor and adjust dose. Moderate Study
▶ Antimalarials (pyrimethamine) increase the risk of adverse effects when given with **sulfonamides**. Severe Study
▶ **Sulfonamides** might increase the risk of neutropenia when given with antipsychotics, second generation (clozapine). Avoid. Severe Theoretical
▶ Chloroprocaine is predicted to decrease the effects of **sulfonamides**. Avoid. Severe Theoretical
▶ **Sulfadiazine** is predicted to increase the anticoagulant effect of coumarins. Severe Theoretical
▶ **Sulfamethoxazole** increases the anticoagulant effect of coumarins. Severe Study
▶ Methenamine might increase the risk of crystalluria when given with **sulfonamides**. Avoid. Severe Theoretical
▶ **Sulfonamides** are predicted to increase the exposure to methotrexate. Use with caution or avoid. Severe Theoretical
▶ Potassium aminobenzoate is predicted to affect the efficacy of **sulfonamides**. Avoid. Severe Theoretical
▶ **Sulfonamides** are predicted to increase the exposure to sulfonylureas. Moderate Study
▶ **Sulfonamides** are predicted to increase the effects of thiopental. Moderate Theoretical

Sulfonylureas → see TABLE 13 p. 1575 (antidiabetic drugs)

glibenclamide · gliclazide · glimepiride · glipizide · tolbutamide

▶ Anti-androgens (apalutamide) are predicted to decrease the exposure to **glibenclamide**. Monitor and adjust dose. Mild Theoretical
▶ Anti-androgens (darolutamide) are predicted to increase the concentration of **glibenclamide**. Moderate Theoretical
▶ Antiarrhythmics (amiodarone) are predicted to increase the exposure to **sulfonylureas**. Use with caution and adjust dose. Moderate Study
▶ Antifungals, azoles (fluconazole, miconazole) are predicted to increase the exposure to **sulfonylureas**. Use with caution and adjust dose. Moderate Study
▶ Antifungals, azoles (voriconazole) are predicted to increase the concentration of **sulfonylureas**. Use with caution and adjust dose. Moderate Study
▶ Belumosudil is predicted to increase the exposure to **glibenclamide**. Avoid or adjust dose. Moderate Study
▶ Bulevirtide is predicted to increase the exposure to **glibenclamide**. Avoid or monitor. Moderate Theoretical
▶ Cephalosporins (ceftobiprole) are predicted to increase the concentration of **glibenclamide**. Moderate Theoretical
▶ Ceritinib is predicted to increase the exposure to **glimepiride**. Adjust dose. Moderate Theoretical
▶ Chloramphenicol is predicted to increase the exposure to **sulfonylureas**. Severe Study
▶ Ciclosporin is predicted to increase the exposure to **glibenclamide** and **glibenclamide** might increase the exposure to ciclosporin. Monitor and adjust **ciclosporin** dose, p. 966. Moderate Study
▶ Elexacaftor is predicted to increase the exposure to **glibenclamide**. Moderate Theoretical
▶ Encorafenib is predicted to increase the exposure to **glibenclamide**. Mild Study
▶ Endothelin receptor antagonists (bosentan) increase the risk of hepatotoxicity when given with **glibenclamide**. Avoid. Severe Study
▶ Fenfluramine might decrease blood glucose concentrations when given with **sulfonylureas**. Moderate Theoretical
▶ Fibrates are predicted to increase the risk of hypoglycaemia when given with **sulfonylureas**. Moderate Theoretical
▶ HIV-protease inhibitors (atazanavir, lopinavir) boosted with ritonavir are predicted to increase the exposure to **glibenclamide**. Moderate Theoretical
▶ Leflunomide is predicted to increase the exposure to **glibenclamide**. Moderate Study

Sulfonylureas (continued)

▸ **Leniolisib** is predicted to increase the exposure to glibenclamide. Avoid. Moderate Theoretical

▸ **Letermovir** is predicted to increase the concentration of glibenclamide. Moderate Theoretical

▸ **Macrolides (clarithromycin)** might increase the exposure to sulfonylureas. Moderate Theoretical

▸ **Metreleptin** is predicted to increase the risk of hypoglycaemia when given with sulfonylureas. Monitor blood glucose and adjust dose. Severe Theoretical

▸ **Mifepristone** is predicted to increase the exposure to sulfonylureas (glimepiride, tolbutamide). Moderate Theoretical

▸ **Nitisinone** is predicted to increase the exposure to sulfonylureas (glimepiride, tolbutamide). Moderate Study

▸ **Rifamycins (rifampicin)** are predicted to decrease the exposure to sulfonylureas. Moderate Study

▸ **Roxadustat** is predicted to increase the exposure to glibenclamide. Monitor adverse effects and adjust dose. Moderate Study

▸ **Somapacitan** might increase blood glucose concentrations, opposing the blood glucose-lowering effects of sulfonylureas. Adjust dose. Moderate Theoretical

▸ **Somatrogon** might increase blood glucose concentrations, opposing the blood glucose-lowering effects of sulfonylureas. Adjust dose. Moderate Theoretical

▸ **Statins (fluvastatin)** slightly increase the exposure to glibenclamide. Mild Study

▸ **Sulfonamides** are predicted to increase the exposure to sulfonylureas. Moderate Study

▸ **Taxanes (cabazitaxel)** are predicted to affect the exposure to glibenclamide. Manufacturer advises take 12 hours before or 3 hours after cabazitaxel. Moderate Theoretical

▸ **Teriflunomide** is predicted to increase the exposure to glibenclamide. Moderate Study

▸ **Velpatasvir** is predicted to increase the exposure to glibenclamide. Moderate Study

▸ **Venetoclax** is predicted to increase the exposure to glibenclamide. Moderate Theoretical

▸ **Voclosporin** is predicted to increase the concentration of glibenclamide. Moderate Theoretical

▸ **Voxilaprevir** with sofosbuvir and velpatasvir is predicted to increase the exposure to glibenclamide. Moderate Study

Sulindac → see NSAIDs

Sulpiride → see TABLE 17 p. 1576 (hyponatraemia), TABLE 7 p. 1572 (hypotension), TABLE 10 p. 1574 (CNS effects)

▸ Oral **antacids** decrease the absorption of oral sulpiride. Separate administration by 2 hours. Moderate Study

▸ **Sulpiride** is predicted to decrease the effects of dopamine receptor agonists. Avoid. Moderate Theoretical → Also see TABLE 7 p. 1572 → Also see TABLE 10 p. 1574

▸ **Sulpiride** opposes the effects of the active metabolite of foslevodopa. Severe Theoretical → Also see TABLE 7 p. 1572 → Also see TABLE 10 p. 1574

▸ **Sulpiride** is predicted to decrease the effects of levodopa. Avoid. Severe Theoretical → Also see TABLE 7 p. 1572 → Also see TABLE 10 p. 1574

▸ **Sulpiride** potentially increases the risk of neurotoxicity when given with lithium. Severe Anecdotal

▸ **Sucralfate** decreases the absorption of sulpiride. Separate administration by 2 hours. Moderate Study

Sultiame → see antiepileptics

Sumatriptan → see triptans

Sunitinib → see TABLE 14 p. 1575 (myelosuppression), TABLE 8 p. 1573 (QT-interval prolongation), TABLE 4 p. 1571 (antiplatelet effects)

▸ **Anti-androgens (apalutamide, enzalutamide)** are predicted to decrease the exposure to sunitinib. Avoid or adjust dose—consult product literature. Moderate Study → Also see TABLE 8 p. 1573

▸ **Antiarrhythmics (dronedarone)** are predicted to increase the exposure to sunitinib. Moderate Study → Also see TABLE 8 p. 1573

▸ **Antiepileptics (carbamazepine, fosphenytoin, phenobarbital, phenytoin, primidone)** are predicted to decrease the exposure to sunitinib. Avoid or adjust dose—consult product literature. Moderate Study

▸ **Antifungals, azoles (fluconazole, isavuconazole)** are predicted to increase the exposure to sunitinib. Moderate Study → Also see TABLE 8 p. 1573

▸ **Antifungals, azoles (itraconazole, ketoconazole, posaconazole, voriconazole)** are predicted to increase the exposure to sunitinib. Avoid or adjust dose—consult product literature. Moderate Study → Also see TABLE 8 p. 1573

▸ **Berotralstat** is predicted to increase the exposure to sunitinib. Moderate Study

▸ **Calcium channel blockers (diltiazem, verapamil)** are predicted to increase the exposure to sunitinib. Moderate Study

▸ **Cenobamate** is predicted to decrease the exposure to sunitinib. Moderate Study

▸ **Ceritinib** is predicted to increase the exposure to sunitinib. Avoid or adjust dose—consult product literature. Moderate Study → Also see TABLE 14 p. 1575 → Also see TABLE 8 p. 1573

▸ **Cobicistat** is predicted to increase the exposure to sunitinib. Avoid or adjust dose—consult product literature. Moderate Study

▸ **Crizotinib** is predicted to increase the exposure to sunitinib. Moderate Study → Also see TABLE 8 p. 1573

▸ **Dabrafenib** is predicted to decrease the exposure to sunitinib. Moderate Study

▸ **Elbasvir** is predicted to increase the concentration of sunitinib. Use with caution and adjust dose. Moderate Theoretical

▸ **Encorafenib** is predicted to decrease the exposure to sunitinib. Avoid or adjust dose—consult product literature. Moderate Study → Also see TABLE 8 p. 1573

▸ **Endothelin receptor antagonists (bosentan)** are predicted to decrease the exposure to sunitinib. Moderate Study

▸ **Fedratinib** is predicted to increase the exposure to sunitinib. Moderate Study

▸ **Grapefruit** juice is predicted to increase the exposure to sunitinib. Avoid. Moderate Theoretical

▸ **Grazoprevir** is predicted to increase the concentration of sunitinib. Use with caution and adjust dose. Moderate Theoretical

▸ **HIV-protease inhibitors** are predicted to increase the exposure to sunitinib. Avoid or adjust dose—consult product literature. Moderate Study

▸ **Idelalisib** is predicted to increase the exposure to sunitinib. Avoid or adjust dose—consult product literature. Moderate Study

▸ **Imatinib** is predicted to increase the exposure to sunitinib. Moderate Study → Also see TABLE 14 p. 1575 → Also see TABLE 4 p. 1571

▸ **Ivosidenib** is predicted to decrease the exposure to sunitinib. Avoid or adjust dose—consult product literature. Moderate Study → Also see TABLE 8 p. 1573

▸ **Letermovir** is predicted to increase the exposure to sunitinib. Moderate Study

▸ **Lorlatinib** is predicted to decrease the exposure to sunitinib. Moderate Study

▸ **Lumacaftor** is predicted to decrease the exposure to sunitinib. Avoid or adjust dose—consult product literature. Moderate Study

▸ **Macrolides (clarithromycin)** are predicted to increase the exposure to sunitinib. Avoid or adjust dose—consult product literature. Moderate Study

▸ **Macrolides (erythromycin)** are predicted to increase the exposure to sunitinib. Moderate Study → Also see TABLE 8 p. 1573

▸ **Mitotane** is predicted to decrease the exposure to sunitinib. Avoid or adjust dose—consult product literature. Moderate Study → Also see TABLE 14 p. 1575

▸ **Neurokinin-1 receptor antagonists (aprepitant, netupitant)** are predicted to increase the exposure to sunitinib. Moderate Study

▸ **Nilotinib** is predicted to increase the exposure to sunitinib. Moderate Study → Also see TABLE 14 p. 1575 → Also see TABLE 8 p. 1573

▸ **NNRTIs (efavirenz, etravirine, nevirapine)** are predicted to decrease the exposure to sunitinib. Moderate Study → Also see TABLE 8 p. 1573

▸ **Rifamycins (rifampicin)** are predicted to decrease the exposure to sunitinib. Avoid or adjust dose—consult product literature. Moderate Study

▸ **Sotorasib** is predicted to decrease the exposure to **sunitinib**. Moderate Study
▸ **St John's wort** is predicted to decrease the exposure to **sunitinib**. Moderate Study
▸ **Sunitinib** has been reported to cause hypothyroidism when given with thyroid hormones **(levothyroxine)**. Moderate Anecdotal
▸ **Tucatinib** is predicted to increase the exposure to **sunitinib**. Avoid or adjust dose—consult product literature. Moderate Study

Suxamethonium → see TABLE 5 p. 1572 (bradycardia), TABLE 15 p. 1575 (increased serum potassium), TABLE 19 p. 1576 (neuromuscular blocking effects)

▸ **Alkylating agents (cyclophosphamide)** increase the risk of prolonged neuromuscular blockade when given with **suxamethonium**. Moderate Study
▸ **Antiarrhythmics (lidocaine)** are predicted to increase the effects of **suxamethonium**. Moderate Study
▸ **Anticholinesterases, centrally acting** increase the effects of **suxamethonium**. Moderate Theoretical → Also see TABLE 5 p. 1572
▸ **Antiepileptics (carbamazepine)** increase the risk of prolonged neuromuscular blockade when given with **suxamethonium**. Moderate Study
▸ **Antiepileptics (fosphenytoin, phenytoin)** increase the effects of **suxamethonium**. Moderate Study
▸ **Suxamethonium** might increase the concentration of beta blockers, selective **(landiolol)** and beta blockers, selective **(landiolol)** might prolong the effects of **suxamethonium**. Moderate Study → Also see TABLE 5 p. 1572
▸ **Clindamycin** increases the effects of **suxamethonium**. Severe Anecdotal
▸ **Corticosteroids** are predicted to decrease the effects of **suxamethonium**. Severe Anecdotal
▸ **Suxamethonium** is predicted to increase the risk of cardiovascular adverse effects when given with digoxin. Severe Anecdotal → Also see TABLE 5 p. 1572
▸ **Irinotecan** is predicted to increase the risk of prolonged neuromuscular blockade when given with **suxamethonium**. Moderate Theoretical
▸ Intravenous **magnesium** is predicted to increase the effects of **suxamethonium**. Moderate Study
▸ **Metoclopramide** increases the effects of **suxamethonium**. Moderate Study
▸ **Penicillins (piperacillin)** increase the effects of **suxamethonium**. Moderate Study
▸ **SSRIs** potentially increase the risk of prolonged neuromuscular blockade when given with **suxamethonium**. Unknown Theoretical

Sympathomimetics, inotropic

dobutamine · dopamine

▸ **Sympathomimetics, inotropic** are predicted to decrease the effects of apraclonidine. Avoid. Severe Theoretical
▸ **Beta blockers, non-selective** increase the risk of hypertension and bradycardia when given with **dobutamine**. Severe Theoretical
▸ **Beta blockers, selective** increase the risk of hypertension and bradycardia when given with **dobutamine**. Moderate Theoretical
▸ **Entacapone** is predicted to increase the risk of cardiovascular adverse effects when given with **sympathomimetics, inotropic**. Moderate Theoretical
▸ **Ergometrine** potentially increases the risk of peripheral vasoconstriction when given with **dopamine**. Avoid. Severe Anecdotal
▸ **Sympathomimetics, inotropic** are predicted to increase the risk of elevated blood pressure when given with linezolid. Avoid. Severe Theoretical
▸ **Sympathomimetics, inotropic** are predicted to increase the risk of a hypertensive crisis when given with **MAO-B inhibitors**. Avoid. Severe Anecdotal
▸ **Sympathomimetics, inotropic** are predicted to increase the risk of a hypertensive crisis when given with **MAOIs, irreversible**. Avoid and for 14 days after stopping the MAOI. Severe Theoretical
▸ **Opicapone** is predicted to increase the risk of cardiovascular adverse effects when given with **sympathomimetics, inotropic**. Severe Theoretical

▸ **Tolcapone** is predicted to increase the risk of cardiovascular adverse effects when given with **sympathomimetics, inotropic**. Moderate Theoretical

Sympathomimetics, vasoconstrictor

adrenaline/epinephrine · ephedrine · isometheptene · metaraminol · midodrine · noradrenaline/norepinephrine · phenylephrine · pseudoephedrine · xylometazoline

ROUTE-SPECIFIC INFORMATION Since systemic absorption can follow topical application of **phenylephrine** or **xylometazoline**, the possibility of interactions should be borne in mind.

▸ **Ephedrine** increases the risk of adverse effects when given with aminophylline. Avoid in children. Moderate Study
▸ **Sympathomimetics, vasoconstrictor** are predicted to decrease the effects of apraclonidine. Avoid. Severe Theoretical
▸ **Atropine** increases the risk of severe hypertension when given with **phenylephrine**. Severe Study
▸ **Beta blockers, non-selective** are predicted to increase the risk of hypertension and bradycardia when given with sympathomimetics, vasoconstrictor **(adrenaline/epinephrine, noradrenaline/norepinephrine)**. Severe Study
▸ **Beta blockers, selective** are predicted to increase the risk of hypertension and bradycardia when given with sympathomimetics, vasoconstrictor **(adrenaline/epinephrine, noradrenaline/norepinephrine)**. Severe Study
▸ **Isometheptene** potentially increases the risk of adverse effects when given with dopamine receptor agonists **(bromocriptine)**. Avoid. Severe Anecdotal
▸ **Entacapone** is predicted to increase the risk of cardiovascular adverse effects when given with sympathomimetics, vasoconstrictor **(adrenaline/epinephrine, noradrenaline/norepinephrine)**. Moderate Study
▸ **Ergometrine** is predicted to increase the risk of peripheral vasoconstriction when given with **noradrenaline/norepinephrine**. Severe Anecdotal
▸ Sympathomimetics, vasoconstrictor **(adrenaline/epinephrine, noradrenaline/norepinephrine)** might increase the cardiovascular adverse effects of the active metabolite of foslevodopa. Moderate Theoretical
▸ **Pseudoephedrine** increases the risk of elevated blood pressure when given with linezolid. Avoid. Severe Study
▸ Sympathomimetics, vasoconstrictor **(adrenaline/epinephrine, ephedrine, isometheptene, noradrenaline/norepinephrine, phenylephrine)** are predicted to increase the risk of elevated blood pressure when given with linezolid. Avoid. Severe Theoretical
▸ **Sympathomimetics, vasoconstrictor** are predicted to increase the risk of a hypertensive crisis when given with **MAO-B inhibitors**. Avoid. Severe Anecdotal
▸ **Sympathomimetics, vasoconstrictor** are predicted to increase the risk of a hypertensive crisis when given with **MAOIs, irreversible**. Avoid and for 14 days after stopping the MAOI. Severe Study
▸ **Mianserin** decreases the effects of **ephedrine**. Severe Anecdotal
▸ Sympathomimetics, vasoconstrictor **(ephedrine, isometheptene, phenylephrine, pseudoephedrine)** are predicted to increase the risk of a hypertensive crisis when given with moclobemide. Avoid. Severe Study
▸ **Opicapone** is predicted to increase the risk of cardiovascular adverse effects when given with sympathomimetics, vasoconstrictor **(adrenaline/epinephrine, noradrenaline/norepinephrine)**. Severe Theoretical
▸ **Sympathomimetics, vasoconstrictor** might increase the risk of a hypertensive crisis when given with ozanimod. Severe Theoretical
▸ **Ephedrine** increases the risk of adverse effects when given with theophylline. Avoid in children. Moderate Study
▸ **Tolcapone** is predicted to increase the effects of sympathomimetics, vasoconstrictor **(adrenaline/epinephrine, noradrenaline/norepinephrine)**. Moderate Theoretical
▸ **Tricyclic antidepressants** are predicted to decrease the effects of **ephedrine**. Avoid. Severe Study
▸ **Tricyclic antidepressants** increase the effects of sympathomimetics, vasoconstrictor **(adrenaline/epinephrine,

Sympathomimetics, vasoconstrictor (continued)
noradrenaline/norepinephrine, phenylephrine). Avoid. Severe Study
▸ **Adrenaline/epinephrine** might increase the hypertensive effect of **vasopressin.** Moderate Theoretical
▸ **Noradrenaline/norepinephrine** might affect the hypertensive effect of **vasopressin.** Moderate Theoretical
▸ Volatile halogenated anaesthetics (sevoflurane) can cause hypertension, as can **ephedrine**. Avoid **ephedrine** for several days before surgery. Severe Theoretical
▸ Volatile halogenated anaesthetics (sevoflurane) can cause hypertension, as can **pseudoephedrine**. Avoid **pseudoephedrine** for several days before surgery. Severe Theoretical
▸ Volatile halogenated anaesthetics (sevoflurane) can cause hypertension, as can **xylometazoline**. Avoid **xylometazoline** for several days before surgery. Severe Theoretical

Tacalcitol → see vitamin D substances
Tacrolimus → see TABLE 2 p. 1571 (nephrotoxicity), TABLE 15 p. 1575 (increased serum potassium)

> ▸ Pomelo and pomegranate juices might greatly increase the concentration of tacrolimus.
> ▸ Since systemic absorption can follow topical application, the possibility of interactions should be borne in mind.

▸ **Tacrolimus** is predicted to increase the exposure to afatinib. Moderate Theoretical
▸ **Alcohol** increases the risk of facial flushing and skin irritation when given with topical **tacrolimus.** Moderate Study
▸ Anti-androgens (apalutamide, enzalutamide) decrease the concentration of **tacrolimus**. Avoid or monitor and adjust dose. Severe Study
▸ Antiarrhythmics (amiodarone) are predicted to increase the concentration of **tacrolimus**. Severe Anecdotal
▸ Antiarrhythmics (dronedarone) are predicted to increase the concentration of **tacrolimus**. Severe Study
▸ Antiepileptics (carbamazepine, fosphenytoin, phenobarbital, phenytoin, primidone) decrease the concentration of **tacrolimus**. Avoid or monitor and adjust dose. Severe Study
▸ Antifungals, azoles (fluconazole, isavuconazole) are predicted to increase the concentration of **tacrolimus**. Severe Study
▸ Antifungals, azoles (itraconazole, ketoconazole, posaconazole, voriconazole) are predicted to increase the concentration of **tacrolimus**. Monitor and adjust dose. Severe Study
▸ Antifungals, azoles (miconazole) are predicted to increase the concentration of **tacrolimus**. Monitor and adjust dose. Severe Theoretical
▸ **Baricitinib** is predicted to enhance the risk of immunosuppression when given with **tacrolimus.** Severe Theoretical
▸ **Berotralstat** is predicted to increase the concentration of **tacrolimus.** Severe Study
▸ **Brigatinib** potentially decreases the concentration of **tacrolimus**. Avoid. Moderate Theoretical
▸ **Bulevirtide** is predicted to increase the exposure to **tacrolimus.** Moderate Theoretical
▸ Calcium channel blockers (diltiazem, verapamil) are predicted to increase the concentration of **tacrolimus.** Severe Study
▸ Calcium channel blockers (nicardipine) potentially increase the concentration of **tacrolimus**. Monitor concentration and adjust dose. Severe Anecdotal
▸ **Cannabidiol** is predicted to increase the concentration of **tacrolimus**. Monitor and adjust dose. Moderate Theoretical
▸ **Ceritinib** is predicted to increase the concentration of **tacrolimus**. Monitor and adjust dose. Severe Study
▸ **Chloramphenicol** increases the concentration of **tacrolimus.** Severe Study
▸ **Ciclosporin** increases the concentration of **tacrolimus**. Avoid. Severe Study → Also see TABLE 2 p. 1571 → Also see TABLE 15 p. 1575
▸ **Cobicistat** is predicted to increase the concentration of **tacrolimus**. Monitor and adjust dose. Severe Study
▸ **Crizotinib** is predicted to increase the concentration of **tacrolimus.** Severe Study
▸ **Dabrafenib** is predicted to decrease the exposure to **tacrolimus**. Monitor and adjust dose. Moderate Theoretical

▸ **Danicopan** is predicted to increase the exposure to **tacrolimus.** Moderate Theoretical
▸ **Encorafenib** decreases the concentration of **tacrolimus**. Avoid or monitor and adjust dose. Severe Study
▸ Endothelin receptor antagonists (bosentan) are predicted to decrease the concentration of **tacrolimus** and **tacrolimus** potentially increases the concentration of endothelin receptor antagonists (bosentan). Avoid. Severe Theoretical
▸ **Fedratinib** is predicted to increase the concentration of **tacrolimus.** Severe Study
▸ **Filgotinib** is predicted to increase the risk of immunosuppression when given with **tacrolimus**. Avoid. Severe Theoretical
▸ **Givinostat** might increase the exposure to **tacrolimus.** Moderate Study
▸ **Glecaprevir** with pibrentasvir slightly increases the exposure to **tacrolimus**. Monitor and adjust dose. Mild Study
▸ **Grapefruit** juice greatly increases the concentration of **tacrolimus**. Avoid. Severe Study
▸ **Grazoprevir** increases the exposure to **tacrolimus.** Moderate Study
▸ **HIV-protease inhibitors** are predicted to increase the concentration of **tacrolimus**. Monitor and adjust dose. Severe Study
▸ **Idelalisib** is predicted to increase the concentration of **tacrolimus**. Monitor and adjust dose. Severe Study
▸ **Imatinib** is predicted to increase the concentration of **tacrolimus.** Severe Study
▸ Iron chelators (dexrazoxane) might increase the risk of immunosuppression when given with **tacrolimus**. Severe Theoretical
▸ **Ivacaftor** is predicted to increase the exposure to **tacrolimus.** Moderate Theoretical
▸ **Ivosidenib** decreases the concentration of **tacrolimus**. Avoid or monitor and adjust dose. Severe Study
▸ **Larotrectinib** is predicted to increase the exposure to **tacrolimus**. Use with caution and adjust dose. Mild Theoretical
▸ **Letermovir** is predicted to increase the concentration of **tacrolimus.** Severe Study
▸ **Live vaccines** are predicted to increase the risk of generalised infection (possibly life-threatening) when given with **tacrolimus**. UKHSA advises avoid (refer to Green Book). Severe Theoretical
▸ **Tacrolimus** is predicted to increase the exposure to lomitapide. Separate administration by 12 hours. Moderate Theoretical
▸ **Lorlatinib** is predicted to decrease the exposure to **tacrolimus**. Avoid. Moderate Theoretical
▸ **Lumacaftor** decreases the concentration of **tacrolimus**. Avoid or monitor and adjust dose. Severe Study
▸ Macrolides (clarithromycin) are predicted to increase the concentration of **tacrolimus**. Monitor and adjust dose. Severe Study
▸ Macrolides (erythromycin) are predicted to increase the concentration of **tacrolimus.** Severe Study
▸ **Maribavir** is predicted to slightly increase the exposure to **tacrolimus**. Monitor and adjust dose. Severe Study
▸ **Tacrolimus** is predicted to affect the efficacy of mifamurtide. Avoid. Severe Theoretical
▸ **Mitotane** decreases the concentration of **tacrolimus**. Avoid or monitor and adjust dose. Severe Study
▸ Monoclonal antibodies (sarilumab) potentially affect the exposure to **tacrolimus**. Monitor and adjust dose. Moderate Theoretical
▸ Neurokinin-1 receptor antagonists (aprepitant, netupitant) are predicted to increase the concentration of **tacrolimus**. Severe Study
▸ **Nilotinib** is predicted to increase the concentration of **tacrolimus.** Severe Study
▸ **Nirmatrelvir** boosted with ritonavir is predicted to increase the concentration of **tacrolimus**. Avoid. Severe Theoretical
▸ NNRTIs (doravirine) are predicted to decrease the exposure to **tacrolimus**. Monitor **tacrolimus** concentration and adjust dose, p. 969. Moderate Theoretical

▸ NNRTIs **(efavirenz, nevirapine)** are predicted to decrease the concentration of **tacrolimus**. Monitor and adjust dose. Moderate Theoretical

▸ NNRTIs **(etravirine)** are predicted to decrease the exposure to **tacrolimus**. Monitor and adjust dose. Moderate Theoretical

▸ Olaparib might alter the exposure to **tacrolimus**. Moderate Theoretical

▸ Palbociclib is predicted to increase the exposure to **tacrolimus**. Adjust dose. Moderate Theoretical

▸ Penicillins **(flucloxacillin)** (high-dose) might decrease the exposure to **tacrolimus**. Moderate Study

▸ Pibrentasvir with glecaprevir slightly increases the exposure to **tacrolimus**. Monitor and adjust dose. Mild Study

▸ Pitolisant is predicted to decrease the exposure to **tacrolimus**. Avoid. Severe Theoretical

▸ Ranolazine increases the concentration of **tacrolimus**. Adjust dose. Severe Anecdotal

▸ Ribociclib is predicted to increase the exposure to **tacrolimus**. Use with caution and adjust dose. Moderate Theoretical

▸ Rifamycins **(rifampicin)** decrease the concentration of **tacrolimus**. Avoid or monitor and adjust dose. Severe Study → Also see **TABLE 2** p. 1571

▸ Ritlecitinib is predicted to increase the exposure to **tacrolimus**. Adjust dose. Moderate Theoretical

▸ Rucaparib is predicted to increase the exposure to **tacrolimus**. Monitor and adjust dose. Moderate Study

▸ Sirolimus is predicted to decrease the concentration of **tacrolimus** and **tacrolimus** increases the exposure to sirolimus. Severe Study

▸ **Tacrolimus** potentially increases the risk of serotonin syndrome when given with SNRIs **(venlafaxine)**. Severe Anecdotal

▸ Sotorasib is predicted to decrease the exposure to **tacrolimus**. Monitor and adjust dose. Severe Theoretical

▸ St John's wort decreases the concentration of **tacrolimus**. Avoid. Severe Study

▸ Tarlatamab might affect the exposure to **tacrolimus**. Monitor and adjust dose. Moderate Theoretical

▸ **Tacrolimus** is predicted to increase the exposure to thrombin inhibitors **(dabigatran)**. Avoid. Severe Theoretical

▸ Tigecycline has been reported to increase the concentration of **tacrolimus**. Severe Anecdotal

▸ **Tacrolimus** increases the exposure to tofacitinib. Avoid. Severe Study

▸ Tucatinib is predicted to increase the concentration of **tacrolimus**. Monitor and adjust dose. Severe Study

Tadalafil → see phosphodiesterase type-5 inhibitors

Tafamidis

▸ **Tafamidis** slightly increases the exposure to statins **(rosuvastatin)**. Severe Study

Tafasitamab → see monoclonal antibodies

Talazoparib → see **TABLE 14** p. 1575 (myelosuppression)

▸ Anti-androgens **(apalutamide)** are predicted to decrease the exposure to **talazoparib**. Monitor and adjust dose. Moderate Study

▸ Anti-androgens **(enzalutamide)** moderately increase the exposure to **talazoparib**. Adjust starting dose. Moderate Study

▸ Antiarrhythmics **(amiodarone, dronedarone)** are predicted to slightly increase the exposure to **talazoparib**. Avoid or adjust dose—consult product literature. Severe Study

▸ Antiarrhythmics **(propafenone)** are predicted to increase the exposure to **talazoparib**. Avoid or adjust dose—consult product literature. Moderate Theoretical

▸ Antifungals, azoles **(itraconazole, ketoconazole)** are predicted to slightly increase the exposure to **talazoparib**. Avoid or adjust dose—consult product literature. Severe Study

▸ Belumosudil might increase the exposure to **talazoparib**. Avoid or adjust dose. Moderate Theoretical

▸ Berotralstat is predicted to increase the concentration of **talazoparib**. Monitor and adjust dose. Moderate Study

▸ Beta blockers, non-selective **(carvedilol)** cause a small increase in the bioavailability of **talazoparib**. Avoid or adjust dose—consult product literature. Moderate Study

▸ Calcium channel blockers **(diltiazem, felodipine)** very slightly increase the exposure to **talazoparib**. Moderate Study

▸ Calcium channel blockers **(verapamil)** are predicted to slightly increase the exposure to **talazoparib**. Avoid or adjust dose—consult product literature. Severe Study

▸ Cannabidiol is predicted to increase the exposure to **talazoparib**. Monitor and adjust dose. Moderate Study

▸ Ciclosporin is predicted to slightly increase the exposure to **talazoparib**. Avoid or adjust dose—consult product literature. Severe Study

▸ Cobicistat is predicted to slightly increase the exposure to **talazoparib**. Avoid or adjust dose—consult product literature. Severe Study

▸ Danicopan is predicted to increase the exposure to **talazoparib**. Moderate Study

▸ Daridorexant is predicted to increase the exposure to **talazoparib**. Moderate Study

▸ Eliglustat is predicted to increase the exposure to **talazoparib**. Adjust dose. Moderate Study

▸ Eltrombopag is predicted to increase the exposure to **talazoparib**. Avoid or monitor. Moderate Theoretical

▸ Erdafitinib is predicted to increase the exposure to **talazoparib**. Separate administration by at least 6 hours. Moderate Theoretical

▸ Glecaprevir is predicted to slightly increase the exposure to **talazoparib**. Avoid or adjust dose—consult product literature. Severe Study

▸ HIV-protease inhibitors **(darunavir)** are predicted to increase the exposure to **talazoparib**. Avoid or adjust dose—consult product literature. Moderate Theoretical

▸ HIV-protease inhibitors **(lopinavir, ritonavir)** are predicted to slightly increase the exposure to **talazoparib**. Avoid or adjust dose—consult product literature. Severe Study

▸ Ibrutinib might increase the exposure to **talazoparib**. Separate administration by at least 6 hours. Moderate Theoretical → Also see **TABLE 14** p. 1575

▸ Ivacaftor is predicted to increase the exposure to **talazoparib**. Moderate Study

▸ Ivosidenib is predicted to alter the exposure to **talazoparib**. Moderate Theoretical

▸ Lapatinib is predicted to slightly increase the exposure to **talazoparib**. Avoid or adjust dose—consult product literature. Severe Study

▸ Leflunomide is predicted to increase the exposure to **talazoparib**. Avoid or monitor. Moderate Theoretical → Also see **TABLE 14** p. 1575

▸ Lomitapide might increase the exposure to **talazoparib**. Adjust dose. Moderate Theoretical

▸ Lorlatinib is predicted to decrease the exposure to **talazoparib**. Moderate Study

▸ Macrolides are predicted to slightly increase the exposure to **talazoparib**. Avoid or adjust dose—consult product literature. Severe Study

▸ Olaparib might increase the exposure to **talazoparib**. Moderate Theoretical → Also see **TABLE 14** p. 1575

▸ Osimertinib is predicted to increase the exposure to **talazoparib**. Moderate Study

▸ Pemigatinib might increase the exposure to **talazoparib**. Separate administration by at least 6 hours. Moderate Theoretical

▸ Pibrentasvir is predicted to slightly increase the exposure to **talazoparib**. Avoid or adjust dose—consult product literature. Severe Study

▸ Ranolazine is predicted to slightly increase the exposure to **talazoparib**. Avoid or adjust dose—consult product literature. Severe Study

▸ Selpercatinib is predicted to increase the exposure to **talazoparib**. Moderate Study

▸ SSRIs **(fluvoxamine)** very slightly increase the exposure to **talazoparib**. Moderate Study

▸ Statins **(atorvastatin)** very slightly increase the exposure to **talazoparib**. Moderate Study

▸ Tepotinib is predicted to increase the concentration of **talazoparib**. Severe Study

▸ Teriflunomide is predicted to increase the exposure to **talazoparib**. Avoid or monitor. Moderate Theoretical

Talazoparib (continued)

▸ **Tucatinib** is predicted to increase the exposure to **talazoparib**. Use with caution and adjust dose. Moderate Theoretical

▸ **Velpatasvir** is predicted to slightly increase the exposure to **talazoparib**. Avoid or adjust dose—consult product literature. Severe Study

▸ **Vemurafenib** is predicted to slightly increase the exposure to **talazoparib**. Avoid or adjust dose—consult product literature. Severe Study

▸ **Voclosporin** is predicted to increase the exposure to **talazoparib**. Moderate Study

▸ **Voxilaprevir** is predicted to slightly increase the exposure to **talazoparib**. Avoid or adjust dose—consult product literature. Severe Study

Tamoxifen

▸ **Tamoxifen** (high-dose) might increase the concentration of antiepileptics (fosphenytoin) and antiepileptics (fosphenytoin) might decrease the concentration of **tamoxifen** (high-dose). Severe Theoretical

▸ **Tamoxifen** (high-dose) might increase the concentration of antiepileptics (phenytoin) and antiepileptics (phenytoin) might decrease the concentration of **tamoxifen** (high-dose). Severe Anecdotal

▸ **Tamoxifen** increases the risk of retinopathy when given with antimalarials (chloroquine). RCOphth guidance advises monitor. Severe Study

▸ **Bupropion** is predicted to decrease the efficacy of **tamoxifen**. Avoid. Severe Study

▸ **Cinacalcet** is predicted to decrease the efficacy of **tamoxifen**. Avoid. Severe Study

▸ **Tamoxifen** increases the anticoagulant effect of coumarins. Severe Study

▸ **Dacomitinib** is predicted to decrease the efficacy of **tamoxifen**. Avoid. Severe Study

▸ **Tamoxifen** increases the risk of retinopathy when given with hydroxychloroquine. RCOphth guidance advises monitor. Severe Study

▸ Rifamycins (rifampicin) markedly decrease the exposure to **tamoxifen**. Unknown Study

▸ SSRIs (fluoxetine, paroxetine) are predicted to decrease the efficacy of **tamoxifen**. Avoid. Severe Study

▸ **Terbinafine** is predicted to decrease the efficacy of **tamoxifen**. Avoid. Severe Study

Tamsulosin → see alpha blockers

Tapentadol → see opioids

Tarlatamab

▸ **Tarlatamab** might affect the exposure to sirolimus. Monitor and adjust dose. Moderate Theoretical

▸ **Tarlatamab** might affect the exposure to tacrolimus. Monitor and adjust dose. Moderate Theoretical

Taxanes → see TABLE 14 p. 1575 (myelosuppression), TABLE 11 p. 1574 (peripheral neuropathy)

cabazitaxel · docetaxel · paclitaxel

▸ **Cabazitaxel** is predicted to affect the exposure to angiotensin-II receptor antagonists (valsartan). Manufacturer advises take 12 hours before or 3 hours after **cabazitaxel**. Moderate Theoretical

▸ Anti-androgens (apalutamide, enzalutamide) are predicted to decrease the exposure to **cabazitaxel**. Avoid. Moderate Study

▸ Anti-androgens (apalutamide, enzalutamide) are predicted to decrease the exposure to **docetaxel**. Severe Theoretical

▸ Anti-androgens (apalutamide, enzalutamide) are predicted to decrease the exposure to **paclitaxel**. Avoid. Severe Study

▸ Anti-androgens (darolutamide) are predicted to increase the exposure to **paclitaxel**. Severe Theoretical

▸ Antiarrhythmics (amiodarone) are predicted to increase the exposure to **paclitaxel**. Severe Theoretical → Also see TABLE 11 p. 1574

▸ Antiarrhythmics (dronedarone) are predicted to increase the exposure to **cabazitaxel**. Moderate Theoretical

▸ Antiarrhythmics (dronedarone) are predicted to increase the exposure to **docetaxel**. Severe Study

▸ Antiarrhythmics (dronedarone) are predicted to increase the exposure to **paclitaxel**. Moderate Anecdotal

▸ Antiepileptics (carbamazepine, fosphenytoin, phenobarbital, phenytoin, primidone) are predicted to decrease the exposure to **cabazitaxel**. Avoid. Moderate Study → Also see TABLE 11 p. 1574

▸ Antiepileptics (carbamazepine, fosphenytoin, phenobarbital, phenytoin, primidone) are predicted to decrease the exposure to **docetaxel**. Severe Theoretical → Also see TABLE 11 p. 1574

▸ Antiepileptics (carbamazepine, fosphenytoin, phenobarbital, phenytoin, primidone) are predicted to decrease the exposure to **paclitaxel**. Avoid. Severe Study → Also see TABLE 11 p. 1574

▸ Antifungals, azoles (fluconazole, isavuconazole) are predicted to increase the exposure to **cabazitaxel**. Moderate Theoretical

▸ Antifungals, azoles (fluconazole, isavuconazole) are predicted to increase the exposure to **docetaxel**. Severe Study

▸ Antifungals, azoles (fluconazole, isavuconazole, itraconazole, ketoconazole, posaconazole, voriconazole) are predicted to increase the exposure to **paclitaxel**. Moderate Anecdotal

▸ Antifungals, azoles (itraconazole, ketoconazole, posaconazole, voriconazole) are predicted to increase the exposure to **cabazitaxel**. Avoid or adjust dose—consult product literature. Severe Study

▸ Antifungals, azoles (itraconazole, ketoconazole, posaconazole, voriconazole) are predicted to increase the exposure to **docetaxel**. Avoid or adjust dose. Severe Study

▸ Antifungals, azoles (miconazole) are predicted to increase the concentration of **docetaxel**. Use with caution and adjust dose. Moderate Theoretical

▸ **Cabazitaxel** is predicted to affect the exposure to antihistamines, non-sedating (fexofenadine). Manufacturer advises take 12 hours before or 3 hours after **cabazitaxel**. Moderate Theoretical

▸ **Belumosudil** is predicted to increase the exposure to taxanes (docetaxel, paclitaxel). Avoid or adjust dose. Moderate Study

▸ **Berotralstat** is predicted to increase the exposure to **cabazitaxel**. Moderate Theoretical

▸ **Berotralstat** is predicted to increase the exposure to **docetaxel**. Severe Study

▸ **Berotralstat** is predicted to increase the exposure to **paclitaxel**. Moderate Anecdotal

▸ **Bulevirtide** is predicted to increase the exposure to taxanes (docetaxel, paclitaxel). Avoid or monitor. Moderate Theoretical

▸ Calcium channel blockers (diltiazem, verapamil) are predicted to increase the exposure to **cabazitaxel**. Moderate Theoretical

▸ Calcium channel blockers (diltiazem, verapamil) are predicted to increase the exposure to **docetaxel**. Severe Study

▸ Calcium channel blockers (diltiazem, verapamil) are predicted to increase the exposure to **paclitaxel**. Moderate Anecdotal

▸ **Cannabidiol** is predicted to increase the exposure to **paclitaxel**. Monitor and adjust dose. Moderate Study

▸ **Cenobamate** is predicted to decrease the exposure to **docetaxel**. Severe Theoretical

▸ **Cenobamate** is predicted to decrease the exposure to **paclitaxel**. Avoid. Severe Study

▸ **Ceritinib** is predicted to increase the exposure to **cabazitaxel**. Avoid or adjust dose—consult product literature. Severe Study → Also see TABLE 14 p. 1575

▸ **Ceritinib** is predicted to increase the exposure to **docetaxel**. Avoid or adjust dose. Severe Study → Also see TABLE 14 p. 1575

▸ **Ceritinib** is predicted to increase the exposure to **paclitaxel**. Moderate Anecdotal → Also see TABLE 14 p. 1575

▸ **Ciclosporin** increases the concentration of **docetaxel** (oral). Unknown Study

▸ **Ciclosporin** increases the concentration of **paclitaxel**. Severe Study

▸ **Clopidogrel** is predicted to increase the concentration of **paclitaxel**. Severe Anecdotal

▸ **Cobicistat** is predicted to increase the exposure to **cabazitaxel**. Avoid or adjust dose—consult product literature. Severe Study

▸ **Cobicistat** is predicted to increase the exposure to **docetaxel**. Avoid or adjust dose. Severe Study

▸ **Cobicistat** is predicted to increase the exposure to **paclitaxel**. Moderate Anecdotal

▸ **Crizotinib** is predicted to increase the exposure to **cabazitaxel**. Moderate Theoretical

▸ **Crizotinib** is predicted to increase the exposure to **docetaxel**. Severe Study

- **Crizotinib** is predicted to increase the exposure to **paclitaxel**. Moderate Anecdotal
- **Dabrafenib** is predicted to decrease the exposure to **cabazitaxel**. Moderate Theoretical
- **Dabrafenib** is predicted to decrease the exposure to **docetaxel**. Severe Theoretical
- **Dabrafenib** is predicted to decrease the exposure to **paclitaxel**. Avoid. Severe Study
- **Danicopan** is predicted to increase the exposure to **paclitaxel**. Moderate Study
- **Daridorexant** is predicted to increase the exposure to **paclitaxel**. Moderate Study
- **Elexacaftor** is predicted to increase the exposure to taxanes (docetaxel, paclitaxel). Moderate Theoretical
- **Eliglustat** is predicted to increase the exposure to **paclitaxel**. Adjust dose. Moderate Study
- **Eltrombopag** is predicted to increase the exposure to taxanes (docetaxel, paclitaxel). Moderate Theoretical
- **Encorafenib** is predicted to decrease the exposure to **cabazitaxel**. Avoid. Moderate Study
- **Encorafenib** is predicted to decrease the exposure to **docetaxel**. Severe Theoretical
- **Encorafenib** is predicted to decrease the exposure to **paclitaxel**. Avoid. Severe Study
- **Endothelin receptor antagonists (bosentan)** are predicted to decrease the exposure to **cabazitaxel**. Moderate Theoretical
- **Endothelin receptor antagonists (bosentan)** are predicted to decrease the exposure to **docetaxel**. Severe Theoretical
- **Endothelin receptor antagonists (bosentan)** are predicted to decrease the exposure to **paclitaxel**. Avoid. Severe Study
- **Erdafitinib** is predicted to increase the exposure to **paclitaxel**. Separate administration by at least 6 hours. Moderate Theoretical
- **Fedratinib** is predicted to increase the exposure to **cabazitaxel**. Moderate Theoretical
- **Fedratinib** is predicted to increase the exposure to **docetaxel**. Severe Study
- **Fedratinib** is predicted to increase the exposure to **paclitaxel**. Moderate Anecdotal
- **Fibrates (gemfibrozil)** are predicted to increase the exposure to **docetaxel**. Moderate Theoretical
- **Fibrates (gemfibrozil)** are predicted to increase the concentration of **paclitaxel**. Severe Anecdotal
- **Glecaprevir** is predicted to increase the exposure to **paclitaxel**. Severe Theoretical
- **HIV-protease inhibitors** are predicted to increase the exposure to **cabazitaxel**. Avoid or adjust dose—consult product literature. Severe Study
- **HIV-protease inhibitors** are predicted to increase the exposure to **docetaxel**. Avoid or adjust dose. Severe Study
- **HIV-protease inhibitors** are predicted to increase the exposure to **paclitaxel**. Moderate Anecdotal
- **Ibrutinib** might increase the exposure to **paclitaxel**. Separate administration by at least 6 hours. Moderate Theoretical → Also see **TABLE 14** p. 1575
- **Idelalisib** is predicted to increase the exposure to **cabazitaxel**. Avoid or adjust dose—consult product literature. Severe Study
- **Idelalisib** is predicted to increase the exposure to **docetaxel**. Avoid or adjust dose. Severe Study
- **Idelalisib** is predicted to increase the exposure to **paclitaxel**. Moderate Anecdotal
- **Imatinib** is predicted to increase the exposure to **cabazitaxel**. Moderate Theoretical → Also see **TABLE 14** p. 1575
- **Imatinib** is predicted to increase the exposure to **docetaxel**. Severe Study → Also see **TABLE 14** p. 1575
- **Imatinib** is predicted to increase the exposure to **paclitaxel**. Moderate Anecdotal → Also see **TABLE 14** p. 1575
- **Iron chelators (deferasirox)** are predicted to increase the concentration of **paclitaxel**. Severe Anecdotal
- **Ivacaftor** is predicted to increase the exposure to **paclitaxel**. Moderate Study
- **Ivosidenib** is predicted to decrease the exposure to **cabazitaxel**. Avoid. Moderate Study
- **Ivosidenib** is predicted to decrease the exposure to **docetaxel**. Severe Theoretical

- **Ivosidenib** is predicted to decrease the exposure to **paclitaxel**. Avoid. Severe Study
- **Lapatinib** slightly increases the exposure to **paclitaxel**. Severe Study
- **Leflunomide** is predicted to increase the exposure to **docetaxel**. Moderate Study → Also see **TABLE 14** p. 1575 → Also see **TABLE 11** p. 1574
- **Leflunomide** is predicted to increase the concentration of **paclitaxel**. Severe Anecdotal → Also see **TABLE 14** p. 1575 → Also see **TABLE 11** p. 1574
- **Leniolisib** is predicted to increase the exposure to taxanes (docetaxel, paclitaxel). Avoid. Moderate Theoretical
- **Letermovir** is predicted to increase the exposure to **cabazitaxel**. Moderate Theoretical
- **Letermovir** is predicted to increase the exposure to **docetaxel**. Severe Study
- **Letermovir** is predicted to increase the exposure to **paclitaxel**. Moderate Anecdotal
- **Linzagolix** is predicted to increase the exposure to **paclitaxel**. Avoid. Mild Theoretical
- **Live vaccines** are predicted to increase the risk of generalised infection (possibly life-threatening) when given with taxanes (docetaxel, paclitaxel). UKHSA advises avoid (refer to Green Book). Severe Theoretical
- **Lomitapide** might increase the exposure to **paclitaxel**. Adjust dose. Moderate Theoretical
- **Lorlatinib** is predicted to decrease the exposure to **docetaxel**. Severe Theoretical
- **Lorlatinib** is predicted to decrease the exposure to **paclitaxel**. Avoid. Severe Study
- **Lumacaftor** is predicted to decrease the exposure to **cabazitaxel**. Avoid. Moderate Study
- **Lumacaftor** is predicted to decrease the exposure to **docetaxel**. Severe Theoretical
- **Lumacaftor** is predicted to decrease the exposure to **paclitaxel**. Avoid. Severe Study
- **Macrolides (azithromycin)** are predicted to increase the exposure to **paclitaxel**. Moderate Theoretical
- **Macrolides (clarithromycin)** are predicted to increase the exposure to **cabazitaxel**. Avoid or adjust dose—consult product literature. Severe Study
- **Macrolides (clarithromycin)** are predicted to increase the exposure to **docetaxel**. Avoid or adjust dose. Severe Study
- **Macrolides (clarithromycin, erythromycin)** are predicted to increase the exposure to **paclitaxel**. Moderate Anecdotal
- **Macrolides (erythromycin)** are predicted to increase the exposure to **cabazitaxel**. Moderate Theoretical
- **Macrolides (erythromycin)** are predicted to increase the exposure to **docetaxel**. Severe Study
- **Maribavir** is predicted to increase the exposure to **paclitaxel**. Use with caution and adjust dose. Unknown Study
- **Cabazitaxel** is predicted to affect the exposure to meglitinides (repaglinide). Manufacturer advises take 12 hours before or 3 hours after **cabazitaxel**. Moderate Theoretical
- **Mirabegron** is predicted to increase the exposure to **paclitaxel**. Mild Theoretical
- **Mitotane** is predicted to decrease the exposure to **cabazitaxel**. Avoid. Moderate Study → Also see **TABLE 14** p. 1575
- **Mitotane** is predicted to decrease the exposure to **docetaxel**. Severe Theoretical → Also see **TABLE 14** p. 1575
- **Mitotane** is predicted to decrease the exposure to **paclitaxel**. Avoid. Severe Study → Also see **TABLE 14** p. 1575
- **Neratinib** is predicted to increase the exposure to **paclitaxel**. Moderate Study
- **Neurokinin-1 receptor antagonists (aprepitant, netupitant)** are predicted to increase the exposure to **cabazitaxel**. Moderate Theoretical
- **Neurokinin-1 receptor antagonists (aprepitant, netupitant)** are predicted to increase the exposure to **docetaxel**. Severe Study
- **Neurokinin-1 receptor antagonists (aprepitant, netupitant)** are predicted to increase the exposure to **paclitaxel**. Moderate Anecdotal
- **Nilotinib** is predicted to increase the exposure to **cabazitaxel**. Moderate Theoretical → Also see **TABLE 14** p. 1575

Taxanes (continued)

▶ **Nilotinib** is predicted to increase the exposure to **docetaxel**. Severe Study → Also see **TABLE 14** p. 1575

▶ **Nilotinib** is predicted to increase the exposure to **paclitaxel**. Moderate Anecdotal → Also see **TABLE 14** p. 1575

▶ **NNRTIs (efavirenz, etravirine, nevirapine)** are predicted to decrease the exposure to **cabazitaxel**. Moderate Theoretical

▶ **NNRTIs (efavirenz, etravirine, nevirapine)** are predicted to decrease the exposure to **docetaxel**. Severe Theoretical

▶ **NNRTIs (efavirenz, etravirine, nevirapine)** are predicted to decrease the exposure to **paclitaxel**. Avoid. Severe Study

▶ **Olaparib** might increase the exposure to **paclitaxel**. Moderate Theoretical → Also see **TABLE 14** p. 1575

▶ **Osimertinib** is predicted to increase the exposure to **paclitaxel**. Moderate Study

▶ **Pemigatinib** might increase the exposure to **paclitaxel**. Separate administration by at least 6 hours. Moderate Theoretical

▶ **Pibrentasvir** with glecaprevir is predicted to increase the exposure to **paclitaxel**. Moderate Study

▶ **Pitolisant** is predicted to decrease the exposure to **docetaxel**. Avoid. Severe Theoretical

▶ **Pitolisant** is predicted to decrease the exposure to **paclitaxel**. Mild Theoretical

▶ **Pralsetinib** might affect the exposure to **paclitaxel**. Avoid. Moderate Theoretical

▶ **Ranolazine** is predicted to increase the exposure to **paclitaxel**. Severe Theoretical

▶ **Rifamycins (rifabutin)** are predicted to decrease the exposure to **cabazitaxel**. Avoid. Moderate Theoretical

▶ **Rifamycins (rifampicin)** are predicted to decrease the exposure to **cabazitaxel**. Avoid. Moderate Study

▶ **Rifamycins (rifampicin)** are predicted to decrease the exposure to **docetaxel**. Severe Theoretical

▶ **Rifamycins (rifampicin)** are predicted to decrease the exposure to **paclitaxel**. Avoid. Severe Study

▶ **Roxadustat** is predicted to increase the exposure to taxanes **(docetaxel, paclitaxel)**. Monitor adverse effects and adjust dose. Moderate Study

▶ **Sotorasib** is predicted to decrease the exposure to **docetaxel**. Severe Theoretical

▶ **Sotorasib** is predicted to decrease the exposure to **paclitaxel**. Avoid. Severe Study

▶ **St John's wort** is predicted to decrease the exposure to **cabazitaxel**. Avoid. Severe Theoretical

▶ **St John's wort** is predicted to decrease the exposure to **docetaxel**. Severe Theoretical

▶ **St John's wort** is predicted to decrease the exposure to **paclitaxel**. Avoid. Severe Study

▶ **Cabazitaxel** is predicted to affect the exposure to statins **(atorvastatin, pravastatin, rosuvastatin, simvastatin)**. Manufacturer advises take 12 hours before or 3 hours after **cabazitaxel**. Moderate Theoretical

▶ **Cabazitaxel** is predicted to affect the exposure to sulfonylureas **(glibenclamide)**. Manufacturer advises take 12 hours before or 3 hours after **cabazitaxel**. Moderate Theoretical

▶ **Tepotinib** is predicted to increase the concentration of **paclitaxel**. Severe Study

▶ **Teriflunomide** is predicted to increase the exposure to **docetaxel**. Moderate Study → Also see **TABLE 11** p. 1574

▶ **Teriflunomide** is predicted to increase the concentration of **paclitaxel**. Severe Anecdotal → Also see **TABLE 11** p. 1574

▶ **Tucatinib** is predicted to increase the exposure to **cabazitaxel**. Avoid or adjust dose—consult product literature. Severe Study

▶ **Tucatinib** is predicted to increase the exposure to **docetaxel**. Avoid or adjust dose. Severe Study

▶ **Tucatinib** is predicted to increase the exposure to **paclitaxel**. Moderate Anecdotal

▶ **Velpatasvir** is predicted to increase the exposure to **docetaxel**. Moderate Study

▶ **Velpatasvir** is predicted to increase the exposure to **paclitaxel**. Severe Theoretical

▶ **Vemurafenib** is predicted to increase the exposure to **paclitaxel**. Use with caution and adjust dose. Severe Theoretical

▶ **Voclosporin** is predicted to increase the exposure to **paclitaxel**. Moderate Study

▶ **Voxilaprevir** with sofosbuvir and velpatasvir is predicted to increase the exposure to taxanes **(docetaxel, paclitaxel)**. Moderate Study

Tebentafusp

▶ **Tebentafusp** is predicted to transiently increase the exposure to ciclosporin. Monitor and adjust dose. Moderate Theoretical

▶ **Tebentafusp** is predicted to transiently increase the exposure to coumarins **(warfarin)**. Monitor and adjust dose. Moderate Theoretical

Teclistamab → see monoclonal antibodies

Tedizolid

▶ **Tedizolid** is predicted to increase the exposure to imatinib. Avoid. Moderate Theoretical

▶ **Tedizolid** is predicted to increase the exposure to lapatinib. Avoid. Moderate Theoretical

▶ **Tedizolid** is predicted to increase the exposure to methotrexate. Avoid. Moderate Theoretical

▶ **Tedizolid** is predicted to increase the exposure to statins **(atorvastatin, fluvastatin, rosuvastatin)**. Avoid. Moderate Study

▶ **Tedizolid** is predicted to increase the exposure to sulfasalazine. Avoid. Moderate Study

▶ **Tedizolid** is predicted to increase the exposure to topotecan. Avoid. Moderate Study

Tegafur → see **TABLE 14** p. 1575 (myelosuppression)

▶ **Tegafur** potentially increases the concentration of antiepileptics **(fosphenytoin, phenytoin)**. Monitor concentration and adjust dose. Severe Anecdotal

▶ **Tegafur** increases the anticoagulant effect of coumarins. Moderate Theoretical

▶ Folates are predicted to increase the risk of toxicity when given with **tegafur**. Severe Theoretical

▶ H_2 receptor antagonists **(cimetidine)** are predicted to increase the risk of toxicity when given with **tegafur**. Severe Theoretical

▶ Live vaccines are predicted to increase the risk of generalised infection (possibly life-threatening) when given with **tegafur**. UKHSA advises avoid (refer to Green Book). Severe Theoretical

▶ Methotrexate is predicted to increase the risk of toxicity when given with **tegafur**. Severe Theoretical → Also see **TABLE 14** p. 1575

Teicoplanin

GENERAL INFORMATION If other nephrotoxic or neurotoxic drugs are given, monitor renal and auditory function on prolonged administration.

Telmisartan → see angiotensin-II receptor antagonists

Telotristat ethyl

▶ **Telotristat ethyl** decreases the exposure to benzodiazepines **(midazolam)**. Moderate Study

▶ **Telotristat ethyl** is predicted to decrease the exposure to capivasertib. Avoid. Moderate Theoretical

▶ **Telotristat ethyl** is predicted to decrease the exposure to erdafitinib. Adjust dose. Moderate Theoretical

▶ **Telotristat ethyl** is predicted to decrease the exposure to NNRTIs **(doravirine)**. Avoid or adjust doravirine p. 741 or lamivudine with tenofovir disoproxil and doravirine p. 751 dose. Severe Theoretical

▶ Octreotide (short-acting) decreases the exposure to **telotristat ethyl**. **Telotristat ethyl** should be taken at least 30 minutes before **octreotide**. Moderate Study

Temazepam → see benzodiazepines

Temocillin → see penicillins

Temozolomide → see alkylating agents

Temsirolimus → see **TABLE 14** p. 1575 (myelosuppression)

▶ ACE inhibitors are predicted to increase the risk of angioedema when given with **temsirolimus**. Moderate Theoretical

▶ Anti-androgens **(apalutamide, enzalutamide)** are predicted to decrease the concentration of **temsirolimus**. Avoid. Severe Study

▶ Antiarrhythmics **(dronedarone)** are predicted to increase the concentration of **temsirolimus**. Use with caution or avoid. Moderate Theoretical

▶ Antiepileptics **(carbamazepine, fosphenytoin, phenobarbital, phenytoin, primidone)** are predicted to decrease the concentration of **temsirolimus**. Avoid. Severe Study

▸ Antifungals, azoles (fluconazole, isavuconazole) are predicted to increase the concentration of **temsirolimus**. Use with caution or avoid. Moderate Theoretical

▸ Antifungals, azoles (itraconazole, ketoconazole, posaconazole, voriconazole) are predicted to increase the concentration of **temsirolimus**. Avoid. Severe Theoretical

▸ Asciminib is predicted to increase the exposure to **temsirolimus**. Severe Theoretical

▸ Belzutifan is predicted to decrease the exposure to **temsirolimus**. Avoid or adjust dose. Severe Theoretical

▸ Berotralstat is predicted to increase the exposure to **temsirolimus**. Use with caution or avoid. Moderate Study

▸ Bulevirtide is predicted to increase the exposure to **temsirolimus**. Moderate Theoretical

▸ Calcium channel blockers (diltiazem, verapamil) are predicted to increase the concentration of and the risk of angioedema when given with **temsirolimus**. Use with caution or avoid. Moderate Theoretical

▸ **Temsirolimus** is predicted to increase the risk of angioedema when given with calcium channel blockers (amlodipine, felodipine, lacidipine, lercanidipine, nicardipine, nifedipine, nimodipine). Moderate Theoretical

▸ Cenobamate is predicted to decrease the concentration of **temsirolimus**. Avoid. Moderate Theoretical

▸ Ceritinib is predicted to increase the concentration of **temsirolimus**. Avoid. Severe Theoretical → Also see **TABLE 14** p. 1575

▸ Cobicistat is predicted to increase the concentration of **temsirolimus**. Avoid. Severe Theoretical

▸ Crizotinib is predicted to increase the concentration of **temsirolimus**. Use with caution or avoid. Moderate Theoretical

▸ Dabrafenib is predicted to decrease the concentration of **temsirolimus**. Avoid. Moderate Theoretical

▸ Encorafenib is predicted to decrease the concentration of **temsirolimus**. Avoid. Severe Study

▸ Endothelin receptor antagonists (bosentan) are predicted to decrease the concentration of **temsirolimus**. Avoid. Moderate Theoretical

▸ Fedratinib is predicted to increase the exposure to **temsirolimus** (oral). Monitor and adjust dose. Moderate Theoretical

▸ Fostamatinib is predicted to increase the exposure to **temsirolimus**. Monitor and adjust dose. Moderate Theoretical

▸ Givinostat might increase the exposure to **temsirolimus**. Moderate Study

▸ Grapefruit juice is predicted to increase the concentration of **temsirolimus**. Use with caution or avoid. Moderate Theoretical

▸ HIV-protease inhibitors are predicted to increase the concentration of **temsirolimus**. Avoid. Severe Theoretical

▸ Idelalisib is predicted to increase the concentration of **temsirolimus**. Avoid. Severe Theoretical

▸ Imatinib is predicted to increase the concentration of **temsirolimus**. Use with caution or avoid. Moderate Theoretical → Also see **TABLE 14** p. 1575

▸ Ivosidenib is predicted to decrease the concentration of **temsirolimus**. Avoid. Severe Study

▸ Larotrectinib is predicted to increase the exposure to **temsirolimus**. Use with caution and adjust dose. Mild Theoretical

▸ Live vaccines are predicted to increase the risk of generalised infection (possibly life-threatening) when given with **temsirolimus**. UKHSA advises avoid (refer to Green Book). Severe Theoretical

▸ Lorlatinib is predicted to decrease the concentration of **temsirolimus**. Avoid. Moderate Theoretical

▸ Lumacaftor is predicted to decrease the concentration of **temsirolimus**. Avoid. Severe Study

▸ Macrolides (clarithromycin) are predicted to increase the concentration of **temsirolimus**. Avoid. Severe Theoretical

▸ Macrolides (erythromycin) are predicted to increase the concentration of **temsirolimus**. Use with caution or avoid. Moderate Theoretical

▸ Mifepristone is predicted to increase the exposure to **temsirolimus**. Severe Theoretical

▸ Mitotane is predicted to decrease the concentration of **temsirolimus**. Avoid. Severe Study → Also see **TABLE 14** p. 1575

▸ Mobocertinib is predicted to decrease the exposure to **temsirolimus**. Severe Theoretical

▸ Neurokinin-1 receptor antagonists (aprepitant, netupitant) are predicted to increase the concentration of **temsirolimus**. Use with caution or avoid. Moderate Theoretical

▸ Nilotinib is predicted to increase the concentration of **temsirolimus**. Use with caution or avoid. Moderate Theoretical → Also see **TABLE 14** p. 1575

▸ NNRTIs (efavirenz, etravirine, nevirapine) are predicted to decrease the concentration of **temsirolimus**. Avoid. Moderate Theoretical

▸ Olaparib might alter the exposure to **temsirolimus**. Moderate Theoretical → Also see **TABLE 14** p. 1575

▸ Pitolisant is predicted to decrease the exposure to **temsirolimus**. Avoid. Severe Theoretical

▸ Rifamycins (rifampicin) are predicted to decrease the concentration of **temsirolimus**. Avoid. Severe Study

▸ Ritlecitinib is predicted to increase the exposure to **temsirolimus**. Moderate Theoretical

▸ Selpercatinib is predicted to increase the exposure to **temsirolimus**. Avoid. Moderate Study

▸ Sotorasib is predicted to decrease the concentration of **temsirolimus**. Avoid. Moderate Theoretical

▸ St John's wort is predicted to decrease the concentration of **temsirolimus**. Avoid. Moderate Theoretical

▸ Tucatinib is predicted to increase the concentration of **temsirolimus**. Avoid. Severe Theoretical

Tenecteplase → see **TABLE 3** p. 1571 (anticoagulant effects)

Tenofovir alafenamide

▸ Anti-androgens (darolutamide) are predicted to increase the exposure to **tenofovir alafenamide**. Moderate Theoretical

▸ Antiepileptics (carbamazepine, fosphenytoin, oxcarbazepine, phenobarbital, phenytoin, primidone) are predicted to decrease the exposure to **tenofovir alafenamide**. Avoid. Moderate Theoretical

▸ Ciclosporin is predicted to increase the exposure to **tenofovir alafenamide**. Moderate Theoretical

▸ Eltrombopag is predicted to increase the exposure to **tenofovir alafenamide**. Moderate Theoretical

▸ Febuxostat is predicted to increase the exposure to **tenofovir alafenamide**. Moderate Theoretical

▸ Fostamatinib is predicted to increase the exposure to **tenofovir alafenamide**. Moderate Theoretical

▸ Fostemsavir is predicted to increase the exposure to **tenofovir alafenamide**. Adjust dose—consult product literature. Moderate Theoretical

▸ HIV-protease inhibitors (atazanavir, darunavir, lopinavir) increase the exposure to **tenofovir alafenamide**. Avoid or adjust dose. Moderate Study

▸ Leflunomide is predicted to increase the exposure to **tenofovir alafenamide**. Moderate Theoretical

▸ Lorlatinib is predicted to decrease the exposure to **tenofovir alafenamide**. Avoid. Moderate Theoretical

▸ Nitisinone is predicted to increase the exposure to **tenofovir alafenamide**. Moderate Study

▸ Rifamycins are predicted to decrease the exposure to **tenofovir alafenamide**. Avoid. Moderate Theoretical

▸ St John's wort is predicted to decrease the exposure to **tenofovir alafenamide**. Avoid. Moderate Theoretical

▸ Teriflunomide is predicted to increase the exposure to **tenofovir alafenamide**. Moderate Theoretical

▸ Vadadustat is predicted to increase the exposure to **tenofovir alafenamide**. Monitor and adjust dose. Moderate Study

▸ Velpatasvir is predicted to increase the exposure to **tenofovir alafenamide**. Moderate Theoretical

▸ Voxilaprevir is predicted to increase the exposure to **tenofovir alafenamide**. Moderate Theoretical

Tenofovir disoproxil → see **TABLE 2** p. 1571 (nephrotoxicity)

▸ Anti-androgens (darolutamide) are predicted to increase the exposure to **tenofovir disoproxil**. Moderate Theoretical

▸ Ciclosporin is predicted to increase the exposure to **tenofovir disoproxil**. Moderate Theoretical → Also see **TABLE 2** p. 1571

▸ Eltrombopag is predicted to increase the exposure to **tenofovir disoproxil**. Moderate Theoretical

Tenofovir disoproxil (continued)
- **Febuxostat** is predicted to increase the exposure to **tenofovir disoproxil**. [Moderate] Theoretical
- **Fostamatinib** is predicted to increase the exposure to **tenofovir disoproxil**. [Moderate] Theoretical
- **HIV-protease inhibitors (atazanavir, darunavir, lopinavir)** are predicted to increase the risk of renal impairment when given with **tenofovir disoproxil**. [Severe] Anecdotal
- **Ledipasvir** with sofosbuvir slightly increases the exposure to **tenofovir disoproxil**. [Moderate] Study
- **Leflunomide** is predicted to increase the exposure to **tenofovir disoproxil**. [Moderate] Theoretical
- **Nitisinone** is predicted to increase the exposure to **tenofovir disoproxil**. [Moderate] Study
- **Teriflunomide** is predicted to increase the exposure to **tenofovir disoproxil**. [Moderate] Theoretical
- **Vadadustat** is predicted to increase the exposure to **tenofovir disoproxil**. Monitor and adjust dose. [Moderate] Study
- **Velpatasvir** is predicted to increase the exposure to **tenofovir disoproxil**. [Moderate] Theoretical
- **Voxilaprevir** is predicted to increase the exposure to **tenofovir disoproxil**. [Moderate] Theoretical

Tenoxicam → see NSAIDs

Tepotinib
- **Tepotinib** is predicted to increase the concentration of aliskiren. [Severe] Study
- Anti-androgens **(apalutamide, enzalutamide)** might decrease the exposure to **tepotinib**. Avoid. [Severe] Theoretical
- Antiepileptics **(carbamazepine, fosphenytoin, phenobarbital, phenytoin, primidone)** might decrease the exposure to **tepotinib**. Avoid. [Severe] Theoretical
- Antifungals, azoles **(itraconazole, ketoconazole)** might increase the exposure to **tepotinib**. Avoid. [Severe] Theoretical
- **Tepotinib** is predicted to increase the concentration of antihistamines, non-sedating **(fexofenadine)**. [Severe] Study
- **Tepotinib** is predicted to increase the concentration of colchicine. [Severe] Study
- **Tepotinib** is predicted to increase the concentration of digoxin. [Severe] Study
- **Encorafenib** might decrease the exposure to **tepotinib**. Avoid. [Severe] Theoretical
- **Tepotinib** is predicted to increase the concentration of everolimus. [Severe] Study
- **Tepotinib** is predicted to increase the concentration of factor XA inhibitors **(edoxaban)**. [Severe] Study
- HIV-protease inhibitors **(lopinavir)** boosted with ritonavir might increase the exposure to **tepotinib**. Avoid. [Severe] Theoretical
- HIV-protease inhibitors **(ritonavir)** might increase the exposure to **tepotinib**. Avoid. [Severe] Theoretical
- **Ivosidenib** might decrease the exposure to **tepotinib**. Avoid. [Severe] Theoretical
- **Tepotinib** is predicted to increase the concentration of loperamide. [Severe] Study
- **Lumacaftor** might decrease the exposure to **tepotinib**. Avoid. [Severe] Theoretical
- **Macrolides (clarithromycin)** might increase the exposure to **tepotinib**. Avoid. [Severe] Theoretical
- **Mitotane** might decrease the exposure to **tepotinib**. Avoid. [Severe] Theoretical
- Rifamycins **(rifampicin)** might decrease the exposure to **tepotinib**. Avoid. [Severe] Theoretical
- **Tepotinib** is predicted to increase the concentration of sirolimus. [Severe] Study
- **Tepotinib** might decrease the exposure to St John's wort. Avoid. [Severe] Theoretical
- **Tepotinib** might increase the exposure to statins **(atorvastatin, fluvastatin, rosuvastatin)**. [Moderate] Theoretical
- **Tepotinib** might increase the exposure to sulfasalazine. [Moderate] Theoretical
- **Tepotinib** is predicted to increase the concentration of talazoparib. [Severe] Study
- **Tepotinib** is predicted to increase the concentration of taxanes **(paclitaxel)**. [Severe] Study
- **Tepotinib** slightly increases the exposure to thrombin inhibitors **(dabigatran)**. [Severe] Study

- **Tepotinib** might increase the exposure to topotecan. [Moderate] Theoretical

Terazosin → see alpha blockers

Terbinafine

> **ROUTE-SPECIFIC INFORMATION** Since systemic absorption can follow topical application, the possibility of interactions should be borne in mind.

- **Terbinafine** is predicted to increase the exposure to anticholinesterases, centrally acting **(galantamine)**. Monitor and adjust dose. [Moderate] Study
- **Terbinafine** is predicted to moderately increase the exposure to antipsychotics, second generation **(aripiprazole)**. Adjust **aripiprazole** dose, p. 454. [Moderate] Study
- **Terbinafine** is predicted to increase the exposure to antipsychotics, second generation **(clozapine)**. Use with caution and adjust dose. [Severe] Study
- **Terbinafine** is predicted to increase the exposure to antipsychotics, second generation **(risperidone)**. Adjust dose. [Moderate] Study
- **Terbinafine** is predicted to markedly increase the exposure to atomoxetine. Adjust dose. [Severe] Study
- **Terbinafine** is predicted to increase the exposure to beta blockers, selective **(metoprolol, nebivolol)**. [Moderate] Study
- **Terbinafine** is predicted to slightly increase the exposure to darifenacin. [Mild] Study
- **Terbinafine** is predicted to increase the exposure to eliglustat. Avoid or adjust dose—consult product literature. [Severe] Study
- **Terbinafine** is predicted to increase the exposure to fenfluramine. [Moderate] Study
- **Terbinafine** is predicted to increase the exposure to fesoterodine. Use with caution and adjust dose. [Mild] Theoretical
- **Terbinafine** is predicted to increase the exposure to gefitinib. [Moderate] Theoretical
- **Terbinafine** is predicted to increase the exposure to mexiletine. [Moderate] Study
- **Terbinafine** is predicted to decrease the efficacy of opioids **(codeine)**. [Moderate] Theoretical
- **Terbinafine** is predicted to decrease the efficacy of opioids **(tramadol)**. [Severe] Study
- **Terbinafine** is predicted to moderately increase the exposure to pitolisant. Use with caution and adjust dose. [Moderate] Study
- Rifamycins **(rifampicin)** decrease the exposure to **terbinafine**. Adjust dose. [Moderate] Study
- **Terbinafine** is predicted to increase the exposure to SSRIs **(citalopram, dapoxetine, escitalopram, fluvoxamine, sertraline)**. [Moderate] Theoretical
- **Terbinafine** is predicted to increase the exposure to SSRIs **(fluoxetine)**. Adjust dose. [Moderate] Theoretical
- **Terbinafine** moderately increases the exposure to SSRIs **(paroxetine)**. [Moderate] Study
- **Terbinafine** is predicted to decrease the efficacy of tamoxifen. Avoid. [Severe] Study
- **Terbinafine** is predicted to increase the exposure to the active metabolite of tetrabenazine. [Moderate] Study
- **Terbinafine** is predicted to increase the exposure to tricyclic antidepressants. Monitor for toxicity and adjust dose. [Severe] Study
- **Terbinafine** is predicted to increase the exposure to vortioxetine. Monitor and adjust dose. [Moderate] Study

Terbutaline → see beta₂ agonists

Teriflunomide → see TABLE 11 p. 1574 (peripheral neuropathy)
- **Teriflunomide** is predicted to increase the exposure to adefovir. [Moderate] Study
- **Teriflunomide** is predicted to decrease the exposure to agomelatine. [Moderate] Theoretical
- **Teriflunomide** is predicted to increase the exposure to alpelisib. [Moderate] Theoretical
- **Teriflunomide** decreases the exposure to aminophylline. Adjust dose. [Moderate] Study
- **Teriflunomide** is predicted to decrease the exposure to anaesthetics, local **(ropivacaine)**. [Moderate] Theoretical
- **Teriflunomide** is predicted to increase the exposure to anthracyclines **(daunorubicin, doxorubicin, mitoxantrone)**. [Moderate] Theoretical

▸ **Teriflunomide** is predicted to increase the exposure to antihistamines, non-sedating (fexofenadine). [Moderate] Study
▸ **Teriflunomide** is predicted to decrease the exposure to antipsychotics, second generation (clozapine). [Moderate] Theoretical
▸ **Teriflunomide** is predicted to decrease the exposure to antipsychotics, second generation (olanzapine). Monitor and adjust dose. [Moderate] Study
▸ **Teriflunomide** is predicted to increase the exposure to atogepant. Adjust **atogepant** dose, p. 540. [Moderate] Theoretical
▸ **Teriflunomide** is predicted to increase the exposure to baricitinib. [Moderate] Study
▸ **Teriflunomide** is predicted to moderately increase the clearance of caffeine citrate. Monitor and adjust dose. [Moderate] Study
▸ **Teriflunomide** is predicted to increase the exposure to cephalosporins (cefaclor). [Moderate] Study
▸ **Teriflunomide** is predicted to increase the exposure to cladribine. Avoid or adjust dose. [Moderate] Theoretical
▸ **Teriflunomide** affects the anticoagulant effect of coumarins. [Severe] Study
▸ **Teriflunomide** is predicted to increase the exposure to endothelin receptor antagonists (bosentan). [Moderate] Study
▸ **Teriflunomide** are predicted to increases the exposure to etrasimod. Avoid in poor CYP2C9 metabolisers. [Severe] Theoretical
▸ **Teriflunomide** is predicted to increase the exposure to ganciclovir. [Moderate] Study
▸ **Teriflunomide** is predicted to increase the exposure to H_2 receptor antagonists (famotidine). [Moderate] Study
▸ **Teriflunomide** is predicted to increase the concentration of letermovir. [Moderate] Study
▸ Live vaccines are predicted to increase the risk of generalised infection (possibly life-threatening) when given with **teriflunomide**. UKHSA advises avoid (refer to Green Book). [Severe] Theoretical
▸ **Teriflunomide** is predicted to increase the exposure to loop diuretics (furosemide). [Moderate] Study
▸ **Teriflunomide** is predicted to increase the exposure to meglitinides (repaglinide). [Moderate] Study
▸ **Teriflunomide** is predicted to decrease the exposure to melatonin. [Moderate] Theoretical
▸ **Teriflunomide** is predicted to increase the exposure to methotrexate. [Moderate] Study
▸ **Teriflunomide** is predicted to increase the clearance of mexiletine. Monitor and adjust dose. [Moderate] Study
▸ **Teriflunomide** is predicted to increase the exposure to momelotinib. [Moderate] Study
▸ **Teriflunomide** is predicted to increase the exposure to montelukast. [Moderate] Theoretical
▸ **Teriflunomide** is predicted to increase the exposure to NRTIs (zidovudine). [Moderate] Theoretical
▸ **Teriflunomide** is predicted to increase the exposure to NSAIDs (indometacin, ketoprofen). [Moderate] Theoretical
▸ **Teriflunomide** is predicted to increase the exposure to oseltamivir. [Moderate] Study
▸ **Teriflunomide** is predicted to increase the exposure to penicillins (benzylpenicillin). [Moderate] Study
▸ **Teriflunomide** is predicted to increase the exposure to pioglitazone. [Moderate] Study
▸ **Teriflunomide** is predicted to decrease the exposure to pirfenidone. [Moderate] Theoretical
▸ **Teriflunomide** is predicted to increase the exposure to quinolones (ciprofloxacin). [Moderate] Theoretical
▸ Rifamycins (rifampicin) might affect the exposure to **teriflunomide**. [Moderate] Theoretical
▸ **Teriflunomide** is predicted to increase the exposure to selexipag. Adjust **selexipag** dose, p. 209. [Moderate] Study
▸ **Teriflunomide** is predicted to decrease the exposure to SNRIs (duloxetine). [Moderate] Theoretical
▸ **Teriflunomide** is predicted to increase the exposure to statins (atorvastatin, fluvastatin, pravastatin, simvastatin). [Moderate] Study
▸ **Teriflunomide** moderately increases the exposure to statins (rosuvastatin). Adjust **rosuvastatin** dose, p. 235. [Moderate] Study

▸ **Teriflunomide** is predicted to increase the exposure to sulfasalazine. [Moderate] Study
▸ **Teriflunomide** is predicted to increase the exposure to sulfonylureas (glibenclamide). [Moderate] Study
▸ **Teriflunomide** is predicted to increase the exposure to talazoparib. Avoid or monitor. [Moderate] Theoretical
▸ **Teriflunomide** is predicted to increase the exposure to taxanes (docetaxel). [Moderate] Study → Also see **TABLE 11** p. 1574
▸ **Teriflunomide** is predicted to increase the concentration of taxanes (paclitaxel). [Severe] Anecdotal → Also see **TABLE 11** p. 1574
▸ **Teriflunomide** is predicted to increase the exposure to tenofovir alafenamide. [Moderate] Theoretical
▸ **Teriflunomide** is predicted to increase the exposure to tenofovir disoproxil. [Moderate] Theoretical
▸ **Teriflunomide** is predicted to decrease the exposure to theophylline. Adjust dose. [Moderate] Study
▸ **Teriflunomide** moderately decreases the exposure to tizanidine. [Mild] Study
▸ **Teriflunomide** is predicted to increase the exposure to topotecan. [Moderate] Study
▸ **Teriflunomide** is predicted to increase the exposure to tucatinib. [Moderate] Theoretical
▸ **Teriflunomide** is predicted to increase the exposure to vadadustat. [Moderate] Study
▸ **Teriflunomide** is predicted to increase the exposure to venetoclax. Avoid or monitor for toxicity. [Severe] Theoretical

Testosterone → see **TABLE 1** p. 1571 (hepatotoxicity)
▸ Somapacitan might decrease the concentration of **testosterone**. [Moderate] Theoretical
▸ Somatrogon might decrease the concentration of **testosterone**. [Moderate] Theoretical

Tetanus immunoglobulin → see immunoglobulins

Tetrabenazine → see **TABLE 8** p. 1573 (QT-interval prolongation), **TABLE 10** p. 1574 (CNS effects)
▸ Bupropion is predicted to increase the exposure to the active metabolite of **tetrabenazine**. [Moderate] Study
▸ Cinacalcet is predicted to increase the exposure to the active metabolite of **tetrabenazine**. [Moderate] Study
▸ Dacomitinib is predicted to increase the exposure to the active metabolite of **tetrabenazine**. [Moderate] Study
▸ **Tetrabenazine** is predicted to decrease the effects of levodopa. Use with caution or avoid. [Moderate] Theoretical → Also see **TABLE 10** p. 1574
▸ **Tetrabenazine** potentially increases the risk of CNS excitation and hypertension when given with MAO-B inhibitors. [Severe] Theoretical
▸ **Tetrabenazine** potentially increases the risk of CNS excitation and hypertension when given with MAOIs, irreversible. Avoid and for 14 days after stopping the MAOI. [Severe] Theoretical
▸ **Tetrabenazine** potentially increases the risk of CNS excitation and hypertension when given with moclobemide. [Severe] Theoretical
▸ SSRIs (fluoxetine, paroxetine) are predicted to increase the exposure to the active metabolite of **tetrabenazine**. [Moderate] Study → Also see **TABLE 10** p. 1574
▸ Terbinafine is predicted to increase the exposure to the active metabolite of **tetrabenazine**. [Moderate] Study

Tetracaine → see anaesthetics, local

Tetracycline → see tetracyclines

Tetracyclines → see **TABLE 1** p. 1571 (hepatotoxicity)

demeclocycline · doxycycline · eravacycline · lymecycline · minocycline · oxytetracycline · tetracycline

▸ Dairy products decrease the absorption of **demeclocycline** and **oxytetracycline**.
▸ Interactions do not generally apply to topical use of **oxytetracycline** unless specified.
▸ Dairy products decrease the exposure to **tetracycline**— manufacturer advises take 1 hour before or 2 hours after dairy products.
▸ Oral ACE inhibitors (quinapril) (magnesium carbonate-containing forms) might decrease the absorption of oral **tetracyclines**. Avoid. [Moderate] Study

Tetracyclines (continued)
- Oral antacids greatly decrease the absorption of oral **tetracyclines**. Separate administration by 2 to 3 hours. Moderate Study
- Anti-androgens (apalutamide, enzalutamide) are predicted to decrease the exposure to **eravacycline**. Adjust **eravacycline** dose, p. 657. Moderate Study
- Anti-androgens (enzalutamide) are predicted to affect the exposure to **doxycycline**. Use with caution or avoid. Moderate Theoretical
- Antiepileptics (carbamazepine, fosphenytoin, phenobarbital, phenytoin, primidone) are predicted to decrease the exposure to **eravacycline**. Adjust **eravacycline** dose, p. 657. Moderate Study
- Antiepileptics (carbamazepine, phenobarbital, phenytoin, primidone) decrease the concentration of **doxycycline**. Adjust dose. Moderate Study
- Antiepileptics (fosphenytoin) are predicted to decrease the concentration of **doxycycline**. Adjust dose. Moderate Theoretical
- **Tetracycline** decreases the concentration of antimalarials (atovaquone). Moderate Study
- Oral bismuth greatly decreases the absorption of oral **tetracyclines**. Separate administration by at least 2 to 3 hours. Moderate Study
- Oral calcium salts are predicted to decrease the absorption of oral **tetracyclines**. Separate administration by 2 to 3 hours. Moderate Theoretical
- **Doxycycline** is predicted to increase the concentration of ciclosporin. Severe Theoretical
- Combined hormonal contraceptives might exacerbate skin pigmentation when given with **minocycline**. Moderate Anecdotal
- **Tetracyclines** increase the anticoagulant effect of coumarins. Severe Anecdotal
- Encorafenib is predicted to decrease the exposure to **eravacycline**. Adjust **eravacycline** dose, p. 657. Moderate Study
- Oral iron decreases the absorption of oral **tetracyclines**. **Tetracyclines** should be taken 2 to 3 hours after iron. Moderate Study
- Ivosidenib is predicted to decrease the exposure to **eravacycline**. Adjust **eravacycline** dose, p. 657. Moderate Study
- Oral kaolin is predicted to decrease the absorption of oral **tetracyclines**. Moderate Theoretical
- Oral lanthanum might decrease the absorption of oral **tetracyclines**. Separate administration by 2 hours. Moderate Theoretical
- **Tetracyclines** are predicted to increase the risk of lithium toxicity when given with lithium. Avoid or adjust dose. Severe Anecdotal
- Lumacaftor is predicted to decrease the exposure to **eravacycline**. Adjust **eravacycline** dose, p. 657. Moderate Study
- Mitotane is predicted to decrease the exposure to **eravacycline**. Adjust **eravacycline** dose, p. 657. Moderate Study
- **Tetracyclines** are predicted to increase the anticoagulant effect of phenindione. Severe Theoretical
- **Tetracycline** is predicted to increase the exposure to relugolix. Avoid or take relugolix first and separate administration by at least 6 hours. Moderate Theoretical
- Retinoids (acitretin, alitretinoin, isotretinoin, tretinoin) increase the risk of benign intracranial hypertension when given with **tetracyclines**. Avoid. Severe Anecdotal → Also see **TABLE 1** p. 1571
- Rifamycins (rifampicin) modestly decrease the exposure to **doxycycline**. Adjust dose. Moderate Study
- Rifamycins (rifampicin) are predicted to decrease the exposure to **eravacycline**. Adjust **eravacycline** dose, p. 657. Moderate Study
- St John's wort is predicted to decrease the exposure to **eravacycline**. Adjust **eravacycline** dose, p. 657. Moderate Theoretical
- Strontium is predicted to decrease the absorption of **tetracyclines**. Avoid. Moderate Theoretical
- Oral sucralfate might decrease the absorption of oral **tetracyclines**. Moderate Theoretical
- **Demeclocycline** might decrease the antidiuretic and hypertensive effects of vasopressin. Moderate Theoretical
- Volatile halogenated anaesthetics (methoxyflurane) might increase the risk of nephrotoxicity when given with **tetracycline**. Severe Anecdotal

- Oral zinc is predicted to decrease the absorption of **tetracyclines**. Separate administration by 2 to 3 hours. Moderate Theoretical

Tezacaftor

FOOD AND LIFESTYLE Bitter (Seville) oranges might increase the exposure to tezacaftor.

- Anti-androgens (apalutamide, enzalutamide) are predicted to decrease the exposure to **tezacaftor**. Avoid. Severe Theoretical
- Antiarrhythmics (dronedarone) are predicted to increase the exposure to **tezacaftor**. Adjust dose with moderate CYP3A4 inhibitors, see tezacaftor with ivacaftor p. 339 and ivacaftor with tezacaftor and elexacaftor p. 337. Severe Study
- Antiepileptics (carbamazepine, fosphenytoin, phenobarbital, phenytoin, primidone) are predicted to decrease the exposure to **tezacaftor**. Avoid. Severe Theoretical
- Antifungals, azoles (fluconazole, isavuconazole) are predicted to increase the exposure to **tezacaftor**. Adjust dose with moderate CYP3A4 inhibitors, see tezacaftor with ivacaftor p. 339 and ivacaftor with tezacaftor and elexacaftor p. 337. Severe Study
- Antifungals, azoles (itraconazole, ketoconazole, posaconazole, voriconazole) are predicted to increase the exposure to **tezacaftor**. Adjust dose with potent CYP3A4 inhibitors, see tezacaftor with ivacaftor p. 339 and ivacaftor with tezacaftor and elexacaftor p. 337. Severe Study
- Berotralstat is predicted to increase the exposure to **tezacaftor**. Adjust dose with moderate CYP3A4 inhibitors, see tezacaftor with ivacaftor p. 339 and ivacaftor with tezacaftor and elexacaftor p. 337. Severe Study
- Calcium channel blockers (diltiazem, verapamil) are predicted to increase the exposure to **tezacaftor**. Adjust dose with moderate CYP3A4 inhibitors, see tezacaftor with ivacaftor p. 339 and ivacaftor with tezacaftor and elexacaftor p. 337. Severe Study
- Ceritinib is predicted to increase the exposure to **tezacaftor**. Adjust dose with potent CYP3A4 inhibitors, see tezacaftor with ivacaftor p. 339 and ivacaftor with tezacaftor and elexacaftor p. 337. Severe Study
- Cobicistat is predicted to increase the exposure to **tezacaftor**. Adjust dose with potent CYP3A4 inhibitors, see tezacaftor with ivacaftor p. 339 and ivacaftor with tezacaftor and elexacaftor p. 337. Severe Study
- Crizotinib is predicted to increase the exposure to **tezacaftor**. Adjust dose with moderate CYP3A4 inhibitors, see tezacaftor with ivacaftor p. 339 and ivacaftor with tezacaftor and elexacaftor p. 337. Severe Study
- Encorafenib is predicted to decrease the exposure to **tezacaftor**. Avoid. Severe Theoretical
- Fedratinib is predicted to increase the exposure to **tezacaftor**. Adjust dose with moderate CYP3A4 inhibitors, see tezacaftor with ivacaftor p. 339 and ivacaftor with tezacaftor and elexacaftor p. 337. Severe Study
- Grapefruit juice is predicted to increase the exposure to **tezacaftor**. Avoid. Severe Study
- HIV-protease inhibitors are predicted to increase the exposure to **tezacaftor**. Adjust dose with potent CYP3A4 inhibitors, see tezacaftor with ivacaftor p. 339 and ivacaftor with tezacaftor and elexacaftor p. 337. Severe Study
- Idelalisib is predicted to increase the exposure to **tezacaftor**. Adjust dose with potent CYP3A4 inhibitors, see tezacaftor with ivacaftor p. 339 and ivacaftor with tezacaftor and elexacaftor p. 337. Severe Study
- Imatinib is predicted to increase the exposure to **tezacaftor**. Adjust dose with moderate CYP3A4 inhibitors, see tezacaftor with ivacaftor p. 339 and ivacaftor with tezacaftor and elexacaftor p. 337. Severe Study
- Ivosidenib is predicted to decrease the exposure to **tezacaftor**. Avoid. Severe Theoretical
- Letermovir is predicted to increase the exposure to **tezacaftor**. Adjust dose with moderate CYP3A4 inhibitors, see tezacaftor with ivacaftor p. 339 and ivacaftor with tezacaftor and elexacaftor p. 337. Severe Study
- Lumacaftor is predicted to decrease the exposure to **tezacaftor**. Avoid. Severe Theoretical

▸ Macrolides (clarithromycin) are predicted to increase the exposure to **tezacaftor**. Adjust dose with potent CYP3A4 inhibitors, see tezacaftor with ivacaftor p. 339 and ivacaftor with tezacaftor and elexacaftor p. 337. Severe Study

▸ Macrolides (erythromycin) are predicted to increase the exposure to **tezacaftor**. Adjust dose with moderate CYP3A4 inhibitors, see tezacaftor with ivacaftor p. 339 and ivacaftor with tezacaftor and elexacaftor p. 337. Severe Study

▸ Mitotane is predicted to decrease the exposure to **tezacaftor**. Avoid. Severe Theoretical

▸ Neurokinin-1 receptor antagonists (aprepitant, netupitant) are predicted to increase the exposure to **tezacaftor**. Adjust dose with moderate CYP3A4 inhibitors, see tezacaftor with ivacaftor p. 339 and ivacaftor with tezacaftor and elexacaftor p. 337. Severe Study

▸ Nilotinib is predicted to increase the exposure to **tezacaftor**. Adjust dose with moderate CYP3A4 inhibitors, see tezacaftor with ivacaftor p. 339 and ivacaftor with tezacaftor and elexacaftor p. 337. Severe Study

▸ Nirmatrelvir boosted with ritonavir is predicted to increase the concentration of **tezacaftor** with ivacaftor. Adjust dose. Severe Theoretical

▸ Rifamycins are predicted to decrease the exposure to **tezacaftor**. Avoid. Severe Theoretical

▸ St John's wort is predicted to decrease the exposure to **tezacaftor**. Avoid. Severe Theoretical

▸ Tucatinib is predicted to increase the exposure to **tezacaftor**. Adjust dose with potent CYP3A4 inhibitors, see tezacaftor with ivacaftor p. 339 and ivacaftor with tezacaftor and elexacaftor p. 337. Severe Study

Tezepelumab → see monoclonal antibodies

Thalidomide → see **TABLE 5** p. 1572 (bradycardia), **TABLE 1** p. 1571 (hepatotoxicity), **TABLE 14** p. 1575 (myelosuppression), **TABLE 11** p. 1574 (peripheral neuropathy), **TABLE 10** p. 1574 (CNS effects)

▸ Combined hormonal contraceptives are predicted to increase the risk of venous thromboembolism when given with **thalidomide**. Avoid. Severe Study

▸ Hormone replacement therapy is predicted to increase the risk of venous thromboembolism when given with **thalidomide**. Severe Theoretical

Theophylline → see **TABLE 16** p. 1575 (reduced serum potassium)

FOOD AND LIFESTYLE Smoking can increase theophylline clearance and increased doses of theophylline are therefore required; dose adjustments are likely to be necessary if smoking started or stopped during treatment.

▸ Aciclovir is predicted to increase the exposure to **theophylline**. Monitor and adjust dose. Severe Theoretical

▸ **Theophylline** decreases the efficacy of antiarrhythmics (adenosine). Separate administration by 24 hours. Mild Study

▸ Antiepileptics (carbamazepine) potentially increase the clearance of **theophylline** and **theophylline** decreases the exposure to antiepileptics (carbamazepine). Adjust dose. Moderate Anecdotal

▸ Antiepileptics (fosphenytoin, phenytoin) are predicted to decrease the exposure to **theophylline**. Adjust dose. Moderate Study

▸ Antiepileptics (phenobarbital, primidone) are predicted to increase the clearance of **theophylline**. Adjust dose. Moderate Theoretical

▸ Antiepileptics (stiripentol) are predicted to increase the exposure to **theophylline**. Avoid. Moderate Theoretical

▸ Axitinib is predicted to increase the exposure to **theophylline**. Moderate Theoretical

▸ Beta blockers, non-selective are predicted to increase the risk of bronchospasm when given with **theophylline**. Avoid. Severe Theoretical

▸ Beta blockers, selective are predicted to increase the risk of bronchospasm when given with **theophylline**. Avoid. Severe Theoretical

▸ Caffeine citrate decreases the clearance of **theophylline**. Moderate Study

▸ Combined hormonal contraceptives is predicted to increase the exposure to **theophylline**. Monitor and adjust dose. Moderate Theoretical

▸ **Theophylline** increases the risk of agitation when given with doxapram. Moderate Study

▸ Enteral feeds decrease the exposure to **theophylline**. Moderate Study

▸ Esketamine is predicted to increase the risk of seizures when given with **theophylline**. Avoid. Severe Theoretical

▸ Givosiran is predicted to increase the exposure to **theophylline**. Monitor and adjust dose. Moderate Theoretical

▸ H₂ receptor antagonists (cimetidine) increase the concentration of **theophylline**. Adjust dose. Severe Study

▸ HIV-protease inhibitors (ritonavir) are predicted to decrease the exposure to **theophylline**. Adjust dose. Moderate Study

▸ Interferons slightly increase the exposure to **theophylline**. Adjust dose. Moderate Study

▸ Iron chelators (deferasirox) increase the exposure to **theophylline**. Avoid. Moderate Study

▸ Isoniazid is predicted to affect the clearance of **theophylline**. Severe Anecdotal

▸ Leflunomide is predicted to decrease the exposure to **theophylline**. Adjust dose. Moderate Study

▸ Leniolisib is predicted to increase the exposure to **theophylline**. Avoid. Moderate Theoretical

▸ **Theophylline** is predicted to decrease the concentration of lithium. Monitor concentration and adjust dose. Moderate Anecdotal

▸ Macrolides (azithromycin, clarithromycin) are predicted to increase the exposure to **theophylline**. Adjust dose. Moderate Anecdotal

▸ Macrolides (erythromycin) decrease the clearance of **theophylline** and **theophylline** potentially decreases the clearance of macrolides (erythromycin). Adjust dose. Severe Study

▸ Maribavir is predicted to decrease the exposure to **theophylline**. Avoid. Mild Theoretical

▸ Methotrexate decreases the clearance of **theophylline**. Moderate Study

▸ Metreleptin might alter the exposure to **theophylline**. Monitor concentration and adjust dose. Severe Theoretical

▸ Mexiletine is predicted to increase the exposure to **theophylline**. Monitor and adjust dose. Moderate Theoretical

▸ Monoclonal antibodies (blinatumomab) are predicted to transiently increase the exposure to **theophylline**. Monitor and adjust dose. Moderate Theoretical

▸ Monoclonal antibodies (sarilumab) potentially affect the exposure to **theophylline**. Monitor and adjust dose. Moderate Theoretical

▸ Monoclonal antibodies (tocilizumab) are predicted to decrease the exposure to **theophylline**. Monitor and adjust dose. Moderate Theoretical

▸ Nirmatrelvir boosted with ritonavir is predicted to decrease the concentration of **theophylline**. Adjust dose. Moderate Theoretical

▸ Obeticholic acid is predicted to increase the exposure to **theophylline**. Severe Theoretical

▸ Osilodrostat is predicted to increase the exposure to **theophylline**. Monitor and adjust dose. Moderate Theoretical

▸ Pentoxifylline increases the concentration of **theophylline**. Monitor and adjust dose. Severe Study

▸ **Theophylline** is predicted to slightly increase the exposure to phosphodiesterase type-4 inhibitors (roflumilast). Avoid. Moderate Theoretical

▸ Quinolones (ciprofloxacin) are predicted to increase the exposure to **theophylline**. Monitor and adjust dose. Moderate Theoretical

▸ Rifamycins (rifampicin) are predicted to decrease the exposure to **theophylline**. Adjust dose. Moderate Study

▸ Ritlecitinib is predicted to increase the exposure to **theophylline**. Adjust dose. Moderate Theoretical

▸ Rucaparib is predicted to increase the exposure to **theophylline**. Monitor and adjust dose. Moderate Theoretical

▸ SSRIs (fluvoxamine) moderately to markedly increase the exposure to **theophylline**. Avoid. Severe Study

▸ St John's wort potentially decreases the exposure to **theophylline**. Severe Anecdotal

Theophylline (continued)

▸ Sucralfate potentially decreases the absorption of **theophylline**. Separate administration by at least 2 hours. Moderate Study

▸ Sympathomimetics, vasoconstrictor (ephedrine) increase the risk of adverse effects when given with **theophylline**. Avoid in children. Moderate Study

▸ Teriflunomide is predicted to decrease the exposure to **theophylline**. Adjust dose. Moderate Study

▸ Valaciclovir is predicted to increase the exposure to **theophylline**. Severe Theoretical

▸ Vemurafenib is predicted to increase the exposure to **theophylline**. Monitor and adjust dose. Moderate Theoretical

Thiazide diuretics → see TABLE 17 p. 1576 (hyponatraemia), TABLE 7 p. 1572 (hypotension), TABLE 16 p. 1575 (reduced serum potassium)

bendroflumethiazide · chlorothiazide · chlortalidone · hydrochlorothiazide · hydroflumethiazide · indapamide · metolazone · xipamide

▸ **Thiazide diuretics** are predicted to increase the risk of hypersensitivity reactions when given with allopurinol. Severe Theoretical

▸ Aspirin (high-dose) increases the risk of acute renal failure when given with **thiazide diuretics**. Severe Theoretical

▸ **Thiazide diuretics** increase the risk of hypercalcaemia when given with calcium salts. Severe Anecdotal

▸ **Thiazide diuretics** increase the concentration of lithium. Avoid or adjust dose and monitor concentration. Severe Study

▸ Metolazone is predicted to decrease the efficacy of methenamine. Moderate Theoretical

▸ NSAIDs increase the risk of acute renal failure when given with **thiazide diuretics**. Severe Theoretical → Also see TABLE 17 p. 1576

▸ Reboxetine is predicted to increase the risk of hypokalaemia when given with **thiazide diuretics**. Moderate Anecdotal

▸ **Thiazide diuretics** are predicted to increase the risk of hypercalcaemia when given with toremifene. Severe Theoretical

▸ **Thiazide diuretics** increase the risk of hypercalcaemia when given with vitamin D substances. Moderate Theoretical

Thiopental → see TABLE 7 p. 1572 (hypotension), TABLE 10 p. 1574 (CNS effects)

▸ Sulfonamides are predicted to increase the effects of **thiopental**. Moderate Theoretical

▸ Tricyclic antidepressants increase the risk of cardiac arrhythmias and hypotension when given with **thiopental**. Moderate Study → Also see TABLE 7 p. 1572 → Also see TABLE 10 p. 1574

Thiotepa → see alkylating agents

Thrombin inhibitors → see TABLE 3 p. 1571 (anticoagulant effects)

argatroban · bivalirudin · dabigatran

▸ Abrocitinib slightly increases the exposure to **dabigatran**. Moderate Study

▸ Anti-androgens (apalutamide) are predicted to decrease the exposure to **dabigatran**. Mild Study

▸ Antiarrhythmics (amiodarone) increase the exposure to **dabigatran**. Monitor and adjust dose. Severe Study

▸ Antiarrhythmics (dronedarone) moderately increase the exposure to **dabigatran**. Avoid. Severe Study

▸ Antiepileptics (carbamazepine) are predicted to decrease the exposure to **dabigatran**. Avoid. Severe Study

▸ Antiepileptics (fosphenytoin, phenytoin) are predicted to decrease the exposure to **dabigatran**. Avoid. Severe Theoretical

▸ Antifungals, azoles (fluconazole, posaconazole) are predicted to increase the exposure to **dabigatran**. Severe Study

▸ Antifungals, azoles (isavuconazole) are predicted to increase the exposure to **dabigatran**. Monitor and adjust dose. Moderate Study

▸ Antifungals, azoles (itraconazole, ketoconazole) are predicted to increase the exposure to **dabigatran**. Avoid. Severe Study

▸ Asciminib is predicted to increase the exposure to **dabigatran**. Severe Theoretical

▸ Belumosudil increases the exposure to **dabigatran**. Avoid or adjust dose. Moderate Study

▸ Calcium channel blockers (verapamil) increase the exposure to **dabigatran**. Monitor and adjust dose. Severe Study

▸ Ceritinib is predicted to increase the exposure to **dabigatran**. Moderate Theoretical

▸ Ciclosporin is predicted to increase the exposure to **dabigatran**. Avoid. Severe Study

▸ Cobicistat moderately increases the exposure to **dabigatran**. Avoid. Severe Study

▸ Danicopan is predicted to increase the exposure to **dabigatran**. Moderate Study

▸ Elbasvir is predicted to increase the concentration of **dabigatran**. Moderate Theoretical

▸ Eliglustat is predicted to increase the exposure to **dabigatran**. Adjust dose. Moderate Study

▸ Erdafitinib is predicted to increase the exposure to **dabigatran**. Separate administration by at least 6 hours. Moderate Theoretical

▸ Glecaprevir with pibrentasvir increases the exposure to **dabigatran**. Avoid. Moderate Study

▸ HIV-protease inhibitors (atazanavir, darunavir, lopinavir) boosted with ritonavir are predicted to increase the exposure to **dabigatran**. Avoid. Severe Anecdotal

▸ HIV-protease inhibitors (fosamprenavir) boosted with ritonavir are predicted to increase the exposure to **dabigatran**. Avoid. Severe Theoretical

▸ HIV-protease inhibitors (ritonavir) are predicted to increase the exposure to **dabigatran**. Avoid. Severe Study

▸ Ivosidenib is predicted to alter the exposure to **dabigatran**. Avoid. Moderate Theoretical

▸ Lapatinib is predicted to increase the exposure to **dabigatran**. Severe Theoretical

▸ Ledipasvir is predicted to increase the exposure to **dabigatran**. Moderate Theoretical

▸ Letermovir is predicted to decrease the concentration of **dabigatran**. Avoid. Severe Theoretical

▸ Lorlatinib is predicted to decrease the exposure to **dabigatran**. Avoid. Severe Study

▸ Macrolides (azithromycin, erythromycin) are predicted to increase the exposure to **dabigatran**. Severe Theoretical

▸ Macrolides (clarithromycin) increase the exposure to **dabigatran**. Moderate Study

▸ Maribavir is predicted to increase the exposure to **dabigatran**. Moderate Study

▸ Mirabegron is predicted to increase the exposure to **dabigatran**. Severe Theoretical

▸ Nirmatrelvir boosted with ritonavir moderately increases the exposure to **dabigatran**. Avoid. Severe Study

▸ Olaparib might increase the exposure to **dabigatran**. Moderate Theoretical

▸ Osimertinib is predicted to increase the exposure to **dabigatran**. Moderate Study

▸ Pibrentasvir with glecaprevir increases the exposure to **dabigatran**. Avoid. Moderate Study

▸ Pitolisant is predicted to decrease the exposure to **dabigatran**. Mild Theoretical

▸ Ranolazine is predicted to increase the exposure to **dabigatran**. Severe Theoretical

▸ Rifamycins (rifampicin) are predicted to decrease the exposure to **dabigatran**. Avoid. Severe Study

▸ Selpercatinib slightly increases the exposure to **dabigatran**. Moderate Study

▸ St John's wort is predicted to decrease the exposure to **dabigatran**. Avoid. Severe Study

▸ Tacrolimus is predicted to increase the exposure to **dabigatran**. Avoid. Severe Theoretical

▸ Tepotinib slightly increases the exposure to **dabigatran**. Severe Study

▸ Ticagrelor increases the exposure to **dabigatran**. Monitor and adjust dose. Severe Study

▸ Velpatasvir increases the exposure to **dabigatran**. Avoid. Severe Study

▸ Vemurafenib is predicted to increase the exposure to **dabigatran**. Monitor and adjust dose. Severe Theoretical

▸ Venetoclax is predicted to increase the exposure to **dabigatran**. Avoid or adjust dose. Severe Study

▸ Voclosporin is predicted to increase the exposure to **dabigatran**. Mild Theoretical

▸ Voxilaprevir with sofosbuvir and velpatasvir increases the concentration of **dabigatran**. Avoid. [Severe] Study

Thyroid hormones

levothyroxine · liothyronine

FOOD AND LIFESTYLE Food, including dietary fibre, milk, soya products, and coffee, might decrease the absorption of levothyroxine.

▸ Oral **antacids** are predicted to decrease the absorption of oral **levothyroxine**. Separate administration by at least 4 hours. [Moderate] Anecdotal

▸ Anti-androgens **(apalutamide)** potentially decrease the exposure to **levothyroxine**. [Mild] Theoretical

▸ Anti-androgens **(enzalutamide)** are predicted to affect the exposure to **levothyroxine**. Use with caution or avoid. [Moderate] Theoretical

▸ Antiarrhythmics **(amiodarone)** are predicted to increase the risk of thyroid dysfunction when given with **thyroid hormones**. Avoid. [Moderate] Study

▸ Antiepileptics **(carbamazepine)** are predicted to increase the risk of hypothyroidism when given with **thyroid hormones**. Monitor and adjust dose. [Moderate] Study

▸ Antiepileptics **(fosphenytoin, phenytoin)** are predicted to increase the risk of hypothyroidism when given with **thyroid hormones**. [Moderate] Study

▸ Antiepileptics **(phenobarbital, primidone)** are predicted to decrease the effects of **thyroid hormones**. [Moderate] Theoretical

▸ Bulevirtide is predicted to increase the exposure to **thyroid hormones**. Avoid or monitor. [Moderate] Theoretical

▸ Oral **calcium salts** are predicted to decrease the absorption of oral **levothyroxine**. Separate administration by at least 4 hours. [Moderate] Anecdotal

▸ **Thyroid hormones** are predicted to affect the concentration of **digoxin**. Monitor and adjust dose. [Moderate] Theoretical

▸ Glucagon-like peptide-1 receptor agonists **(semaglutide)** slightly increase the exposure to **levothyroxine**. [Moderate] Study

▸ HIV-protease inhibitors **(ritonavir)** decrease the concentration of **levothyroxine**. MHRA advises monitor TSH for at least one month after starting or stopping ritonavir. [Moderate] Anecdotal

▸ Oral **hormone replacement therapy** is predicted to decrease the effects of **thyroid hormones**. [Moderate] Theoretical

▸ Imatinib causes hypothyroidism when given with **levothyroxine** in thyroidectomy patients. [Moderate] Study

▸ Oral **iron** decreases the absorption of oral **levothyroxine**. Separate administration by at least 4 hours. [Moderate] Study

▸ Lanthanum decreases the absorption of **thyroid hormones**. Separate administration by 2 hours. [Moderate] Study

▸ Nirmatrelvir boosted with ritonavir might decrease the efficacy of **levothyroxine**. [Moderate] Theoretical

▸ Somapacitan might affect the efficacy of **thyroid hormones**. Monitor and adjust dose. [Moderate] Theoretical

▸ Somatrogon might affect the efficacy of **thyroid hormones**. Adjust dose. [Moderate] Theoretical

▸ Sucralfate decreases the absorption of **levothyroxine**. Separate administration by at least 4 hours. [Moderate] Study

▸ Sunitinib has been reported to cause hypothyroidism when given with **levothyroxine**. [Moderate] Anecdotal

Tiagabine → see antiepileptics

Tiaprofenic acid → see NSAIDs

Ticagrelor → see **TABLE 5** p. 1572 (bradycardia), **TABLE 4** p. 1571 (antiplatelet effects)

▸ Anti-androgens **(apalutamide, enzalutamide)** are predicted to markedly decrease the exposure to **ticagrelor**. Avoid. [Severe] Study

▸ Antiarrhythmics **(amiodarone)** are predicted to increase the exposure to **ticagrelor**. Use with caution or avoid. [Severe] Study → Also see **TABLE 5** p. 1572

▸ Antiepileptics **(carbamazepine, fosphenytoin, phenobarbital, phenytoin, primidone)** are predicted to markedly decrease the exposure to **ticagrelor**. Avoid. [Severe] Study

▸ Antifungals, azoles **(itraconazole, ketoconazole, posaconazole, voriconazole)** are predicted to markedly increase the exposure to **ticagrelor**. Avoid. [Severe] Study

▸ Cenobamate is predicted to decrease the exposure to **ticagrelor**. [Moderate] Theoretical

▸ Ceritinib is predicted to markedly increase the exposure to **ticagrelor**. Avoid. [Severe] Study → Also see **TABLE 5** p. 1572

▸ Ciclosporin is predicted to increase the exposure to **ticagrelor**. Use with caution or avoid. [Severe] Study

▸ Cobicistat is predicted to markedly increase the exposure to **ticagrelor**. Avoid. [Severe] Study

▸ Dabrafenib is predicted to decrease the exposure to **ticagrelor**. [Moderate] Theoretical

▸ **Ticagrelor** increases the concentration of **digoxin**. [Moderate] Study → Also see **TABLE 5** p. 1572

▸ Encorafenib is predicted to markedly decrease the exposure to **ticagrelor**. Avoid. [Severe] Study

▸ Endothelin receptor antagonists **(bosentan)** are predicted to decrease the exposure to **ticagrelor**. [Moderate] Theoretical

▸ Grapefruit juice moderately increases the exposure to **ticagrelor**. [Moderate] Study

▸ HIV-protease inhibitors are predicted to markedly increase the exposure to **ticagrelor**. Avoid. [Severe] Study

▸ Idelalisib is predicted to markedly increase the exposure to **ticagrelor**. Avoid. [Severe] Study

▸ Ivosidenib is predicted to markedly decrease the exposure to **ticagrelor**. Avoid. [Severe] Study

▸ **Ticagrelor** is predicted to increase the exposure to **lomitapide**. Separate administration by 12 hours. [Moderate] Theoretical

▸ Lorlatinib is predicted to decrease the exposure to **ticagrelor**. [Moderate] Theoretical

▸ Lumacaftor is predicted to markedly decrease the exposure to **ticagrelor**. Avoid. [Severe] Study

▸ Macrolides **(azithromycin)** are predicted to increase the exposure to **ticagrelor**. Use with caution or avoid. [Severe] Study

▸ Macrolides **(clarithromycin)** are predicted to markedly increase the exposure to **ticagrelor**. Avoid. [Severe] Study

▸ Mitotane is predicted to markedly decrease the exposure to **ticagrelor**. Avoid. [Severe] Study

▸ Nirmatrelvir boosted with ritonavir is predicted to increase the concentration of **ticagrelor**. Avoid. [Severe] Theoretical

▸ NNRTIs **(efavirenz, etravirine, nevirapine)** are predicted to decrease the exposure to **ticagrelor**. [Moderate] Theoretical

▸ Ranolazine is predicted to increase the exposure to **ticagrelor**. Use with caution or avoid. [Severe] Study

▸ Rifamycins **(rifampicin)** are predicted to markedly decrease the exposure to **ticagrelor**. Avoid. [Severe] Study

▸ Selumetinib might increase the risk of bleeding when given with **ticagrelor**. [Severe] Theoretical

▸ Sotorasib is predicted to decrease the exposure to **ticagrelor**. [Moderate] Theoretical

▸ St John's wort is predicted to decrease the exposure to **ticagrelor**. [Moderate] Theoretical

▸ **Ticagrelor** slightly to moderately increases the exposure to statins **(simvastatin)**. Adjust **simvastatin** dose, p. 237. [Moderate] Study

▸ **Ticagrelor** increases the exposure to thrombin inhibitors **(dabigatran)**. Monitor and adjust dose. [Severe] Study

▸ Tucatinib is predicted to markedly increase the exposure to **ticagrelor**. Avoid. [Severe] Study

▸ Vemurafenib is predicted to increase the exposure to **ticagrelor**. Use with caution or avoid. [Severe] Study

Tigecycline → see **TABLE 1** p. 1571 (hepatotoxicity)

▸ Antiarrhythmics **(amiodarone, dronedarone)** might increase the exposure to **tigecycline**. [Mild] Anecdotal → Also see **TABLE 1** p. 1571

▸ Antiepileptics **(carbamazepine)** might decrease the exposure to **tigecycline**. [Mild] Theoretical

▸ Antifungals, azoles **(itraconazole, ketoconazole)** might increase the exposure to **tigecycline**. [Mild] Anecdotal → Also see **TABLE 1** p. 1571

▸ Calcium channel blockers **(verapamil)** might increase the exposure to **tigecycline**. [Mild] Anecdotal

▸ Ciclosporin might increase the exposure to **tigecycline** and **tigecycline** has been reported to increase the concentration of **ciclosporin**. [Severe] Anecdotal

▸ **Tigecycline** is predicted to alter the anticoagulant effect of **coumarins**. [Moderate] Anecdotal

▸ HIV-protease inhibitors **(lopinavir, ritonavir)** might increase the exposure to **tigecycline**. [Mild] Anecdotal → Also see **TABLE 1** p. 1571

Tigecycline (continued)

▶ **Ivacaftor** might increase the exposure to **tigecycline**. Mild Anecdotal

▶ **Lapatinib** might increase the exposure to **tigecycline**. Mild Anecdotal

▶ **Lorlatinib** might decrease the exposure to **tigecycline**. Mild Theoretical

▶ **Macrolides** might increase the exposure to **tigecycline**. Mild Anecdotal

▶ **Neratinib** might increase the exposure to **tigecycline**. Mild Anecdotal → Also see TABLE 1 p. 1571

▶ **Tigecycline** is predicted to increase the anticoagulant effect of **phenindione**. Severe Theoretical

▶ **Ranolazine** might increase the exposure to **tigecycline**. Mild Anecdotal

▶ **Retinoids (acitretin, alitretinoin, isotretinoin, tretinoin)** increase the risk of benign intracranial hypertension when given with **tigecycline**. Avoid. Severe Anecdotal → Also see TABLE 1 p. 1571

▶ **Rifamycins (rifampicin)** might decrease the exposure to **tigecycline**. Mild Theoretical

▶ **St John's wort** might decrease the exposure to **tigecycline**. Mild Theoretical

▶ **Tigecycline** has been reported to increase the concentration of **tacrolimus**. Severe Anecdotal

▶ **Vandetanib** might increase the exposure to **tigecycline**. Mild Anecdotal

▶ **Vemurafenib** might increase the exposure to **tigecycline**. Mild Anecdotal

Tildrakizumab → see monoclonal antibodies

Timolol → see beta blockers, non-selective

Tinzaparin → see low molecular-weight heparins

Tioguanine → see TABLE 1 p. 1571 (hepatotoxicity), TABLE 14 p. 1575 (myelosuppression)

▶ **Live vaccines** are predicted to increase the risk of generalised infection (possibly life-threatening) when given with **tioguanine**. UKHSA advises avoid (refer to Green Book). Severe Theoretical

Tiotropium → see TABLE 9 p. 1573 (antimuscarinics)

▶ **Antipsychotics, second generation (clozapine)** can cause constipation, as can **tiotropium**; concurrent use might increase the risk of developing intestinal obstruction. Severe Theoretical → Also see TABLE 9 p. 1573

Tirofiban → see TABLE 3 p. 1571 (anticoagulant effects)

Tirzepatide → see glucagon-like peptide-1 receptor agonists

Tivozanib

▶ **Anti-androgens (apalutamide, enzalutamide)** are predicted to decrease the exposure to **tivozanib**. Severe Study

▶ **Antiepileptics (carbamazepine, fosphenytoin, phenobarbital, phenytoin, primidone)** are predicted to decrease the exposure to **tivozanib**. Severe Study

▶ **Encorafenib** is predicted to decrease the exposure to **tivozanib**. Severe Study

▶ **Ivosidenib** is predicted to decrease the exposure to **tivozanib**. Severe Study

▶ **Lumacaftor** is predicted to decrease the exposure to **tivozanib**. Severe Study

▶ **Mitotane** is predicted to decrease the exposure to **tivozanib**. Severe Study

▶ **Rifamycins (rifampicin)** are predicted to decrease the exposure to **tivozanib**. Severe Study

▶ **St John's wort** is predicted to decrease the exposure to **tivozanib**. Avoid. Severe Study

Tizanidine → see TABLE 5 p. 1572 (bradycardia), TABLE 7 p. 1572 (hypotension), TABLE 10 p. 1574 (CNS effects)

▶ **Antiepileptics (fosphenytoin, phenytoin)** moderately decrease the exposure to **tizanidine**. Mild Study → Also see TABLE 10 p. 1574

▶ **Axitinib** is predicted to increase the exposure to **tizanidine**. Moderate Theoretical

▶ **Combined hormonal contraceptives** increases the exposure to **tizanidine**. Avoid. Moderate Study

▶ **Givosiran** increases the exposure to **tizanidine**. Avoid. Moderate Study

▶ **HIV-protease inhibitors (ritonavir)** moderately decrease the exposure to **tizanidine**. Mild Study

▶ **Iron chelators (deferasirox)** are predicted to increase the exposure to **tizanidine**. Avoid. Moderate Theoretical

▶ **Leflunomide** moderately decreases the exposure to **tizanidine**. Mild Study

▶ **Leniolisib** is predicted to increase the exposure to **tizanidine**. Avoid. Moderate Theoretical

▶ **Maribavir** is predicted to decrease the exposure to **tizanidine**. Avoid. Mild Theoretical

▶ **Mexiletine** increases the exposure to **tizanidine**. Avoid. Moderate Study

▶ **Obeticholic acid** is predicted to increase the exposure to **tizanidine**. Severe Theoretical

▶ **Osilodrostat** increases the exposure to **tizanidine**. Avoid. Moderate Study

▶ **Quinolones (ciprofloxacin)** increase the exposure to **tizanidine**. Avoid. Moderate Study

▶ **Rifamycins (rifampicin)** moderately decrease the exposure to **tizanidine**. Mild Study

▶ **Ritlecitinib** is predicted to increase the exposure to **tizanidine**. Moderate Theoretical

▶ **Rucaparib** increases the exposure to **tizanidine**. Avoid. Moderate Study

▶ **SSRIs (fluvoxamine)** very markedly increase the exposure to **tizanidine**. Avoid. Severe Study → Also see TABLE 10 p. 1574

▶ **Teriflunomide** moderately decreases the exposure to **tizanidine**. Mild Study

▶ **Vemurafenib** increases the exposure to **tizanidine**. Avoid. Moderate Study

Tobramycin → see aminoglycosides

Tocilizumab → see monoclonal antibodies

Tofacitinib

▶ **Anti-androgens (apalutamide, enzalutamide)** are predicted to decrease the exposure to **tofacitinib**. Avoid. Severe Study

▶ **Antiarrhythmics (dronedarone)** given with a potent CYP2C19 inhibitor are predicted to increase the exposure to **tofacitinib**. Adjust **tofacitinib** dose, p. 1265. Moderate Study

▶ **Antiepileptics (carbamazepine, fosphenytoin, phenobarbital, phenytoin, primidone)** are predicted to decrease the exposure to **tofacitinib**. Avoid. Severe Study

▶ **Antifungals, azoles (fluconazole)** increase the exposure to **tofacitinib**. Adjust **tofacitinib** dose, p. 1265. Moderate Study

▶ **Antifungals, azoles (isavuconazole)** given with a potent CYP2C19 inhibitor are predicted to increase the exposure to **tofacitinib**. Adjust **tofacitinib** dose, p. 1265. Moderate Study

▶ **Antifungals, azoles (itraconazole, ketoconazole, posaconazole, voriconazole)** are predicted to increase the exposure to **tofacitinib**. Adjust **tofacitinib** dose, p. 1265. Moderate Study

▶ **Calcium channel blockers (diltiazem, verapamil)** given with a potent CYP2C19 inhibitor are predicted to increase the exposure to **tofacitinib**. Adjust **tofacitinib** dose, p. 1265. Moderate Study

▶ **Cenobamate** is predicted to decrease the exposure to **tofacitinib**. Severe Study

▶ **Ceritinib** is predicted to increase the exposure to **tofacitinib**. Adjust **tofacitinib** dose, p. 1265. Moderate Study

▶ **Ciclosporin** increases the exposure to **tofacitinib**. Avoid. Severe Study

▶ **Cobicistat** is predicted to increase the exposure to **tofacitinib**. Adjust **tofacitinib** dose, p. 1265. Moderate Study

▶ **Tofacitinib** is predicted to increase the risk of bleeding when given with **coumarins**. Severe Theoretical

▶ **Crizotinib** given with a potent CYP2C19 inhibitor is predicted to increase the exposure to **tofacitinib**. Adjust **tofacitinib** dose, p. 1265. Moderate Study

▶ **Dabrafenib** is predicted to decrease the exposure to **tofacitinib**. Severe Study

▶ **Encorafenib** is predicted to decrease the exposure to **tofacitinib**. Avoid. Severe Study

▶ **Endothelin receptor antagonists (bosentan)** are predicted to decrease the exposure to **tofacitinib**. Severe Study

▶ **Filgotinib** is predicted to increase the risk of immunosuppression when given with **tofacitinib**. Avoid. Severe Theoretical

▶ **HIV-protease inhibitors** are predicted to increase the exposure to **tofacitinib**. Adjust **tofacitinib** dose, p. 1265. Moderate Study

▶ **Idelalisib** is predicted to increase the exposure to **tofacitinib**. Adjust **tofacitinib** dose, p. 1265. [Moderate] Study

▶ **Imatinib** given with a potent CYP2C19 inhibitor is predicted to increase the exposure to **tofacitinib**. Adjust **tofacitinib** dose, p. 1265. [Moderate] Study

▶ **Ivosidenib** is predicted to decrease the exposure to **tofacitinib**. Avoid. [Severe] Study

▶ **Letermovir** given with a potent CYP2C19 inhibitor is predicted to increase the exposure to **tofacitinib**. Adjust **tofacitinib** dose, p. 1265. [Moderate] Study

▶ **Live vaccines** potentially increase the risk of generalised infection (possibly life-threatening) when given with **tofacitinib**. Avoid. [Severe] Theoretical

▶ **Lorlatinib** is predicted to decrease the exposure to **tofacitinib**. [Severe] Study

▶ **Lumacaftor** is predicted to decrease the exposure to **tofacitinib**. Avoid. [Severe] Study

▶ **Macrolides (clarithromycin)** are predicted to increase the exposure to **tofacitinib**. Adjust **tofacitinib** dose, p. 1265. [Moderate] Study

▶ **Macrolides (erythromycin)** given with a potent CYP2C19 inhibitor are predicted to increase the exposure to **tofacitinib**. Adjust **tofacitinib** dose, p. 1265. [Moderate] Study

▶ **Mitotane** is predicted to decrease the exposure to **tofacitinib**. Avoid. [Severe] Study

▶ **Neurokinin-1 receptor antagonists (aprepitant, netupitant)** given with a potent CYP2C19 inhibitor are predicted to increase the exposure to **tofacitinib**. Adjust **tofacitinib** dose, p. 1265. [Moderate] Study

▶ **Nilotinib** given with a potent CYP2C19 inhibitor is predicted to increase the exposure to **tofacitinib**. Adjust **tofacitinib** dose, p. 1265. [Moderate] Study

▶ **Nirmatrelvir** boosted with ritonavir is predicted to increase the concentration of **tofacitinib**. Adjust dose. [Severe] Theoretical

▶ **NNRTIs (efavirenz, etravirine, nevirapine)** are predicted to decrease the exposure to **tofacitinib**. [Severe] Study

▶ **Tofacitinib** is predicted to increase the risk of bleeding when given with **phenindione**. [Severe] Theoretical

▶ **Rifamycins (rifampicin)** are predicted to decrease the exposure to **tofacitinib**. Avoid. [Severe] Study

▶ **Sotorasib** is predicted to decrease the exposure to **tofacitinib**. [Severe] Study

▶ **SSRIs (fluoxetine, fluvoxamine)** given with a moderate CYP3A4 inhibitor are predicted to increase the exposure to **tofacitinib**. Adjust **tofacitinib** dose, p. 1265. [Moderate] Study

▶ **St John's wort** is predicted to decrease the exposure to **tofacitinib**. [Severe] Study

▶ **Tacrolimus** increases the exposure to **tofacitinib**. Avoid. [Severe] Study

▶ **Tucatinib** is predicted to increase the exposure to **tofacitinib**. Adjust **tofacitinib** dose, p. 1265. [Moderate] Study

Tolbutamide → see sulfonylureas

Tolcapone

▶ **Tolcapone** might increase the exposure to the active metabolite of **foslevodopa**. Adjust dose. [Moderate] Theoretical

▶ **Tolcapone** is predicted to increase the risk of cardiovascular adverse effects when given with **isoprenaline**. [Moderate] Theoretical

▶ **Tolcapone** increases the exposure to **levodopa**. Monitor and adjust dose. [Moderate] Study

▶ **Tolcapone** is predicted to increase the effects of **MAOIs, irreversible**. Avoid. [Severe] Theoretical

▶ **Tolcapone** is predicted to increase the risk of cardiovascular adverse effects when given with **sympathomimetics, inotropic**. [Moderate] Theoretical

▶ **Tolcapone** is predicted to increase the effects of **sympathomimetics, vasoconstrictor (adrenaline/epinephrine, noradrenaline/norepinephrine)**. [Moderate] Theoretical

Tolfenamic acid → see NSAIDs

Tolterodine → see TABLE 8 p. 1573 (QT-interval prolongation), TABLE 9 p. 1573 (antimuscarinics)

▶ **Antifungals, azoles (itraconazole, ketoconazole, posaconazole, voriconazole)** are predicted to increase the exposure to **tolterodine**. Avoid. [Severe] Study → Also see TABLE 8 p. 1573

▶ **Antipsychotics, second generation (clozapine)** can cause constipation, as can **tolterodine**; concurrent use might increase the risk of developing intestinal obstruction. [Severe] Theoretical → Also see TABLE 9 p. 1573

▶ **Ceritinib** is predicted to increase the exposure to **tolterodine**. Avoid. [Severe] Study → Also see TABLE 8 p. 1573

▶ **Cobicistat** is predicted to increase the exposure to **tolterodine**. Avoid. [Severe] Study

▶ **Dacomitinib** is predicted to markedly increase the exposure to **tolterodine**. Avoid. [Severe] Study

▶ **Eliglustat** is predicted to increase the exposure to **tolterodine**. Adjust dose. [Moderate] Theoretical

▶ **HIV-protease inhibitors** are predicted to increase the exposure to **tolterodine**. Avoid. [Severe] Study

▶ **Idelalisib** is predicted to increase the exposure to **tolterodine**. Avoid. [Severe] Study

▶ **Macrolides (clarithromycin)** are predicted to increase the exposure to **tolterodine**. Avoid. [Severe] Study

▶ **Tucatinib** is predicted to increase the exposure to **tolterodine**. Avoid. [Severe] Study

Tolvaptan → see TABLE 15 p. 1575 (increased serum potassium)

GENERAL INFORMATION Avoid concurrent use of drugs that increase serum-sodium concentrations.

▶ **Anti-androgens (apalutamide, enzalutamide)** are predicted to decrease the exposure to **tolvaptan**. Use with caution or avoid depending on indication. [Severe] Study

▶ **Antiarrhythmics (dronedarone)** are predicted to increase the exposure to **tolvaptan**. Manufacturer advises caution or adjust **tolvaptan** dose with moderate CYP3A4 inhibitors, p. 767. [Moderate] Study

▶ **Antiepileptics (carbamazepine, fosphenytoin, phenobarbital, phenytoin, primidone)** are predicted to decrease the exposure to **tolvaptan**. Use with caution or avoid depending on indication. [Severe] Study

▶ **Antifungals, azoles (fluconazole, isavuconazole)** are predicted to increase the exposure to **tolvaptan**. Manufacturer advises caution or adjust **tolvaptan** dose with moderate CYP3A4 inhibitors, p. 767. [Moderate] Study

▶ **Antifungals, azoles (itraconazole, ketoconazole, posaconazole, voriconazole)** are predicted to increase the exposure to **tolvaptan**. Manufacturer advises caution or adjust **tolvaptan** dose with potent CYP3A4 inhibitors, p. 767. [Severe] Study

▶ **Berotralstat** is predicted to increase the exposure to **tolvaptan**. Manufacturer advises caution or adjust **tolvaptan** dose with moderate CYP3A4 inhibitors, p. 767. [Moderate] Study

▶ **Calcium channel blockers (diltiazem, verapamil)** are predicted to increase the exposure to **tolvaptan**. Manufacturer advises caution or adjust **tolvaptan** dose with moderate CYP3A4 inhibitors, p. 767. [Moderate] Study

▶ **Cenobamate** is predicted to decrease the exposure to **tolvaptan**. Adjust dose. [Moderate] Theoretical

▶ **Ceritinib** is predicted to increase the exposure to **tolvaptan**. Manufacturer advises caution or adjust **tolvaptan** dose with potent CYP3A4 inhibitors, p. 767. [Severe] Study

▶ **Cobicistat** is predicted to increase the exposure to **tolvaptan**. Manufacturer advises caution or adjust **tolvaptan** dose with potent CYP3A4 inhibitors, p. 767. [Severe] Study

▶ **Crizotinib** is predicted to increase the exposure to **tolvaptan**. Manufacturer advises caution or adjust **tolvaptan** dose with moderate CYP3A4 inhibitors, p. 767. [Moderate] Study

▶ **Tolvaptan** slightly increases the exposure to **digoxin**. [Moderate] Study

▶ **Encorafenib** is predicted to decrease the exposure to **tolvaptan**. Use with caution or avoid depending on indication. [Severe] Study

▶ **Fedratinib** is predicted to increase the exposure to **tolvaptan**. Manufacturer advises caution or adjust **tolvaptan** dose with moderate CYP3A4 inhibitors, p. 767. [Moderate] Study

▶ **Grapefruit** juice increases the exposure to **tolvaptan**. Avoid. [Moderate] Study

▶ **HIV-protease inhibitors** are predicted to increase the exposure to **tolvaptan**. Manufacturer advises caution or adjust **tolvaptan** dose with potent CYP3A4 inhibitors, p. 767. [Severe] Study

Tolvaptan (continued)

▸ **Idelalisib** is predicted to increase the exposure to **tolvaptan**. Manufacturer advises caution or adjust **tolvaptan** dose with potent CYP3A4 inhibitors, p. 767. [Severe] Study

▸ **Imatinib** is predicted to increase the exposure to **tolvaptan**. Manufacturer advises caution or adjust **tolvaptan** dose with moderate CYP3A4 inhibitors, p. 767. [Moderate] Study

▸ **Ivosidenib** is predicted to decrease the exposure to **tolvaptan**. Use with caution or avoid depending on indication. [Severe] Study

▸ **Letermovir** is predicted to increase the exposure to **tolvaptan**. Manufacturer advises caution or adjust **tolvaptan** dose with moderate CYP3A4 inhibitors, p. 767. [Moderate] Study

▸ **Tolvaptan** is predicted to increase the exposure to **lomitapide**. Separate administration by 12 hours. [Moderate] Theoretical

▸ **Lumacaftor** is predicted to decrease the exposure to **tolvaptan**. Use with caution or avoid depending on indication. [Severe] Study

▸ **Macrolides (clarithromycin)** are predicted to increase the exposure to **tolvaptan**. Manufacturer advises caution or adjust **tolvaptan** dose with potent CYP3A4 inhibitors, p. 767. [Severe] Study

▸ **Macrolides (erythromycin)** are predicted to increase the exposure to **tolvaptan**. Manufacturer advises caution or adjust **tolvaptan** dose with moderate CYP3A4 inhibitors, p. 767. [Moderate] Study

▸ **Mitotane** is predicted to decrease the exposure to **tolvaptan**. Use with caution or avoid depending on indication. [Severe] Study

▸ **Neurokinin-1 receptor antagonists (aprepitant, netupitant)** are predicted to increase the exposure to **tolvaptan**. Manufacturer advises caution or adjust **tolvaptan** dose with moderate CYP3A4 inhibitors, p. 767. [Moderate] Study

▸ **Nilotinib** is predicted to increase the exposure to **tolvaptan**. Manufacturer advises caution or adjust **tolvaptan** dose with moderate CYP3A4 inhibitors, p. 767. [Moderate] Study

▸ **Nirmatrelvir** boosted with ritonavir is predicted to increase the concentration of **tolvaptan**. Avoid. [Severe] Theoretical

▸ **Quinolones (ciprofloxacin)** are predicted to increase the exposure to **tolvaptan**. Use with caution and adjust **tolvaptan** dose, p. 767. [Moderate] Theoretical

▸ **Rifamycins (rifampicin)** are predicted to decrease the exposure to **tolvaptan**. Use with caution or avoid depending on indication. [Severe] Study

▸ **St John's wort** is predicted to decrease the exposure to **tolvaptan**. Avoid. [Moderate] Theoretical

▸ **Tucatinib** is predicted to increase the exposure to **tolvaptan**. Manufacturer advises caution or adjust **tolvaptan** dose with potent CYP3A4 inhibitors, p. 767. [Severe] Study

Topiramate → see antiepileptics

Topotecan → see TABLE 14 p. 1575 (myelosuppression)

▸ Anti-androgens **(apalutamide)** are predicted to decrease the exposure to **topotecan**. Monitor and adjust dose. [Moderate] Theoretical

▸ Anti-androgens **(darolutamide)** are predicted to increase the exposure to **topotecan**. Avoid. [Severe] Theoretical

▸ Antiarrhythmics **(amiodarone, dronedarone)** are predicted to increase the exposure to **topotecan**. [Severe] Study

▸ Antiepileptics **(fosphenytoin, phenytoin)** increase the clearance of **topotecan**. [Moderate] Study

▸ Antifungals, azoles **(isavuconazole)** are predicted to increase the exposure to **topotecan**. [Moderate] Theoretical

▸ Antifungals, azoles **(itraconazole, ketoconazole)** are predicted to increase the exposure to **topotecan**. [Severe] Study

▸ **Belumosudil** is predicted to increase the exposure to **topotecan**. Avoid or adjust dose. [Moderate] Theoretical

▸ Calcium channel blockers **(verapamil)** are predicted to increase the exposure to **topotecan**. [Severe] Study

▸ **Ceritinib** is predicted to increase the exposure to **topotecan**. [Moderate] Theoretical → Also see TABLE 14 p. 1575

▸ **Ciclosporin** is predicted to increase the exposure to **topotecan**. [Severe] Study

▸ **Cobicistat** is predicted to increase the exposure to **topotecan**. [Severe] Study

▸ **Danicopan** is predicted to increase the exposure to **topotecan**. [Moderate] Study

▸ **Eltrombopag** is predicted to increase the exposure to **topotecan**. [Moderate] Theoretical

▸ **Encorafenib** is predicted to increase the effects of **topotecan**. [Mild] Study

▸ **Febuxostat** is predicted to increase the exposure to **topotecan**. [Moderate] Theoretical

▸ **Fostamatinib** is predicted to increase the exposure to **topotecan**. Monitor and adjust dose. [Moderate] Theoretical

▸ **Glecaprevir** is predicted to increase the exposure to **topotecan**. [Severe] Study

▸ **HIV-protease inhibitors (lopinavir, ritonavir)** are predicted to increase the exposure to **topotecan**. [Severe] Study

▸ **Lapatinib** is predicted to increase the exposure to **topotecan**. [Severe] Study

▸ **Leflunomide** is predicted to increase the exposure to **topotecan**. [Moderate] Study → Also see TABLE 14 p. 1575

▸ **Leniolisib** is predicted to increase the exposure to **topotecan**. Avoid. [Moderate] Theoretical

▸ **Live vaccines** are predicted to increase the risk of generalised infection (possibly life-threatening) when given with **topotecan**. UKHSA advises avoid (refer to Green Book). [Severe] Theoretical

▸ **Macrolides** are predicted to increase the exposure to **topotecan**. [Severe] Study

▸ **Pibrentasvir** is predicted to increase the exposure to **topotecan**. [Severe] Study

▸ **Ranolazine** is predicted to increase the exposure to **topotecan**. [Severe] Study

▸ **Regorafenib** is predicted to increase the exposure to **topotecan**. [Moderate] Study → Also see TABLE 14 p. 1575

▸ **Roxadustat** might increase the exposure to **topotecan**. Monitor adverse effects and adjust dose. [Moderate] Theoretical

▸ **St John's wort** is predicted to decrease the exposure to **topotecan**. [Severe] Theoretical

▸ **Tedizolid** is predicted to increase the exposure to **topotecan**. Avoid. [Moderate] Study

▸ **Tepotinib** might increase the exposure to **topotecan**. [Moderate] Theoretical

▸ **Teriflunomide** is predicted to increase the exposure to **topotecan**. [Moderate] Study

▸ **Vadadustat** is predicted to increase the exposure to **topotecan**. Monitor and adjust dose. [Moderate] Study

▸ **Velpatasvir** is predicted to increase the exposure to **topotecan**. [Severe] Study

▸ **Vemurafenib** is predicted to increase the exposure to **topotecan**. [Severe] Study

▸ **Venetoclax** is predicted to increase the exposure to **topotecan**. [Moderate] Theoretical

▸ **Voxilaprevir** is predicted to increase the exposure to **topotecan**. [Severe] Study

Torasemide → see loop diuretics

Toremifene → see TABLE 8 p. 1573 (QT-interval prolongation)

▸ Anti-androgens **(apalutamide, enzalutamide)** are predicted to decrease the exposure to **toremifene**. Adjust dose. [Moderate] Study → Also see TABLE 8 p. 1573

▸ Antiepileptics **(carbamazepine, fosphenytoin, phenobarbital, phenytoin, primidone)** are predicted to decrease the exposure to **toremifene**. Adjust dose. [Moderate] Study

▸ Antifungals, azoles **(itraconazole, ketoconazole, posaconazole, voriconazole)** are predicted to increase the exposure to **toremifene**. [Moderate] Theoretical → Also see TABLE 8 p. 1573

▸ **Ceritinib** is predicted to increase the exposure to **toremifene**. [Moderate] Theoretical → Also see TABLE 8 p. 1573

▸ **Cobicistat** is predicted to increase the exposure to **toremifene**. [Moderate] Theoretical

▸ **Toremifene** is predicted to increase the anticoagulant effect of **coumarins**. [Severe] Theoretical

▸ **Encorafenib** is predicted to decrease the exposure to **toremifene**. Adjust dose. [Moderate] Study → Also see TABLE 8 p. 1573

▸ **HIV-protease inhibitors** are predicted to increase the exposure to **toremifene**. [Moderate] Theoretical

- ▸ **Idelalisib** is predicted to increase the exposure to **toremifene**. Moderate Theoretical
- ▸ **Ivosidenib** is predicted to decrease the exposure to **toremifene**. Adjust dose. Moderate Study → Also see **TABLE 8** p. 1573
- ▸ **Lumacaftor** is predicted to decrease the exposure to **toremifene**. Adjust dose. Moderate Study
- ▸ **Macrolides (clarithromycin)** are predicted to increase the exposure to **toremifene**. Moderate Theoretical
- ▸ **Mitotane** is predicted to decrease the exposure to **toremifene**. Adjust dose. Moderate Study
- ▸ **Rifamycins (rifampicin)** are predicted to decrease the exposure to **toremifene**. Adjust dose. Moderate Study
- ▸ **Thiazide diuretics** are predicted to increase the risk of hypercalcaemia when given with **toremifene**. Severe Theoretical
- ▸ **Tucatinib** is predicted to increase the exposure to **toremifene**. Moderate Theoretical

Trabectedin → see **TABLE 1** p. 1571 (hepatotoxicity), **TABLE 14** p. 1575 (myelosuppression)

- ▸ **Anti-androgens (apalutamide, enzalutamide)** are predicted to decrease the exposure to **trabectedin**. Avoid. Severe Theoretical
- ▸ **Antiepileptics (carbamazepine, fosphenytoin, phenobarbital, phenytoin, primidone)** are predicted to decrease the exposure to **trabectedin**. Avoid. Severe Theoretical
- ▸ **Antifungals, azoles (itraconazole, ketoconazole, posaconazole, voriconazole)** are predicted to increase the exposure to **trabectedin**. Avoid or adjust dose. Severe Theoretical → Also see **TABLE 1** p. 1571
- ▸ **Ceritinib** is predicted to increase the exposure to **trabectedin**. Avoid or adjust dose. Severe Theoretical → Also see **TABLE 14** p. 1575
- ▸ **Cobicistat** is predicted to increase the exposure to **trabectedin**. Avoid or adjust dose. Severe Theoretical
- ▸ **Encorafenib** is predicted to decrease the exposure to **trabectedin**. Avoid. Severe Theoretical
- ▸ **HIV-protease inhibitors** are predicted to increase the exposure to **trabectedin**. Avoid or adjust dose. Severe Theoretical → Also see **TABLE 1** p. 1571
- ▸ **Idelalisib** is predicted to increase the exposure to **trabectedin**. Avoid or adjust dose. Severe Theoretical
- ▸ **Ivosidenib** is predicted to decrease the exposure to **trabectedin**. Avoid. Severe Theoretical
- ▸ **Live vaccines** are predicted to increase the risk of generalised infection (possibly life-threatening) when given with **trabectedin**. UKHSA advises avoid (refer to Green Book). Severe Theoretical
- ▸ **Lumacaftor** is predicted to decrease the exposure to **trabectedin**. Avoid. Severe Theoretical
- ▸ **Macrolides (clarithromycin)** are predicted to increase the exposure to **trabectedin**. Avoid or adjust dose. Severe Theoretical
- ▸ **Mitotane** is predicted to decrease the exposure to **trabectedin**. Avoid. Severe Theoretical → Also see **TABLE 14** p. 1575
- ▸ **Rifamycins (rifampicin)** are predicted to decrease the exposure to **trabectedin**. Avoid. Severe Theoretical
- ▸ **Tucatinib** is predicted to increase the exposure to **trabectedin**. Avoid or adjust dose. Severe Theoretical

Tralokinumab → see monoclonal antibodies
Tramadol → see opioids
Trametinib

- ▸ **Antiarrhythmics (amiodarone, dronedarone)** are predicted to increase the concentration of **trametinib**. Moderate Theoretical
- ▸ **Antifungals, azoles (itraconazole, ketoconazole)** are predicted to increase the concentration of **trametinib**. Moderate Theoretical
- ▸ **Calcium channel blockers (verapamil)** are predicted to increase the concentration of **trametinib**. Moderate Theoretical
- ▸ **Ciclosporin** is predicted to increase the concentration of **trametinib**. Moderate Theoretical
- ▸ **Cobicistat** is predicted to increase the concentration of **trametinib**. Moderate Theoretical
- ▸ **Drugs with anticoagulant effects** (see **TABLE 3** p. 1571) cause bleeding, as can **trametinib**; concurrent use might increase the risk of developing this effect. Severe Theoretical
- ▸ **Drugs with antiplatelet effects** (see **TABLE 4** p. 1571) cause bleeding, as can **trametinib**; concurrent use might increase the risk of developing this effect. Severe Theoretical

- ▸ **Glecaprevir** is predicted to increase the concentration of **trametinib**. Moderate Theoretical
- ▸ **HIV-protease inhibitors (lopinavir, ritonavir)** are predicted to increase the concentration of **trametinib**. Moderate Theoretical
- ▸ **Lapatinib** is predicted to increase the concentration of **trametinib**. Moderate Theoretical
- ▸ **Macrolides** are predicted to increase the concentration of **trametinib**. Moderate Theoretical
- ▸ **Pibrentasvir** is predicted to increase the concentration of **trametinib**. Moderate Theoretical
- ▸ **Ranolazine** is predicted to increase the concentration of **trametinib**. Moderate Theoretical
- ▸ **Velpatasvir** is predicted to increase the concentration of **trametinib**. Moderate Theoretical
- ▸ **Vemurafenib** is predicted to increase the concentration of **trametinib**. Moderate Theoretical
- ▸ **Voxilaprevir** is predicted to increase the concentration of **trametinib**. Moderate Theoretical

Trandolapril → see ACE inhibitors
Tranylcypromine → see MAOIs, irreversible
Trastuzumab → see monoclonal antibodies
Trastuzumab deruxtecan → see monoclonal antibodies
Trastuzumab emtansine → see monoclonal antibodies
Trazodone → see **TABLE 17** p. 1576 (hyponatraemia), **TABLE 12** p. 1574 (serotonin syndrome), **TABLE 10** p. 1574 (CNS effects)

- ▸ **Antiarrhythmics (dronedarone)** are predicted to increase the exposure to **trazodone**. Moderate Theoretical
- ▸ **Antiepileptics (carbamazepine)** decrease the concentration of **trazodone**. Adjust dose. Moderate Anecdotal → Also see **TABLE 17** p. 1576
- ▸ **Antifungals, azoles (fluconazole, isavuconazole)** are predicted to increase the exposure to **trazodone**. Moderate Theoretical
- ▸ **Antifungals, azoles (itraconazole, ketoconazole, posaconazole, voriconazole)** are predicted to moderately increase the exposure to **trazodone**. Avoid or adjust dose. Moderate Study
- ▸ **Berotralstat** is predicted to increase the exposure to **trazodone**. Moderate Theoretical
- ▸ **Calcium channel blockers (diltiazem, verapamil)** are predicted to increase the exposure to **trazodone**. Moderate Theoretical
- ▸ **Ceritinib** is predicted to moderately increase the exposure to **trazodone**. Avoid or adjust dose. Moderate Study
- ▸ **Cobicistat** is predicted to moderately increase the exposure to **trazodone**. Avoid or adjust dose. Moderate Study
- ▸ **Crizotinib** is predicted to increase the exposure to **trazodone**. Moderate Theoretical
- ▸ **Fedratinib** is predicted to increase the exposure to **trazodone**. Moderate Theoretical
- ▸ **HIV-protease inhibitors** are predicted to moderately increase the exposure to **trazodone**. Avoid or adjust dose. Moderate Study
- ▸ **Idelalisib** is predicted to moderately increase the exposure to **trazodone**. Avoid or adjust dose. Moderate Study
- ▸ **Imatinib** is predicted to increase the exposure to **trazodone**. Moderate Theoretical
- ▸ **Letermovir** is predicted to increase the exposure to **trazodone**. Moderate Theoretical
- ▸ **Macrolides (clarithromycin)** are predicted to moderately increase the exposure to **trazodone**. Avoid or adjust dose. Moderate Study
- ▸ **Macrolides (erythromycin)** are predicted to increase the exposure to **trazodone**. Moderate Theoretical
- ▸ **Neurokinin-1 receptor antagonists (aprepitant, netupitant)** are predicted to increase the exposure to **trazodone**. Moderate Theoretical
- ▸ **Nilotinib** is predicted to increase the exposure to **trazodone**. Moderate Theoretical
- ▸ **Nirmatrelvir** boosted with ritonavir is predicted to increase the concentration of **trazodone**. Moderate Theoretical
- ▸ **Tucatinib** is predicted to moderately increase the exposure to **trazodone**. Avoid or adjust dose. Moderate Study

Tree pollen extract

> **GENERAL INFORMATION** Desensitising vaccines should be avoided in patients taking beta-blockers (adrenaline might be ineffective in case of a hypersensitivity reaction) or ACE inhibitors (risk of severe anaphylactoid reactions).

Treosulfan → see alkylating agents

Treprostinil → see TABLE 7 p. 1572 (hypotension), TABLE 4 p. 1571 (antiplatelet effects)

▸ **Antiepileptics (carbamazepine, phenobarbital, phenytoin)** are predicted to decrease the exposure to **treprostinil**. Adjust dose. Mild Theoretical

▸ **Clopidogrel** is predicted to increase the exposure to **treprostinil**. Adjust dose. Moderate Theoretical → Also see TABLE 4 p. 1571

▸ **Fibrates (gemfibrozil)** increase the exposure to **treprostinil**. Adjust dose. Moderate Study

▸ **Iron chelators (deferasirox)** are predicted to increase the exposure to **treprostinil**. Adjust dose. Moderate Theoretical

▸ **Loop diuretics (furosemide)** might slightly decrease the clearance of **treprostinil**. Unknown Theoretical → Also see TABLE 7 p. 1572

▸ **Rifamycins (rifampicin)** slightly decrease the exposure to **treprostinil**. Adjust dose. Mild Study

▸ **St John's wort** is predicted to decrease the exposure to **treprostinil**. Adjust dose. Mild Theoretical

▸ **Trimethoprim** is predicted to increase the exposure to **treprostinil**. Adjust dose. Moderate Theoretical

Tretinoin → see retinoids

Triamcinolone → see corticosteroids

Triamterene → see potassium-sparing diuretics

Tricyclic antidepressants → see TABLE 17 p. 1576 (hyponatraemia), TABLE 7 p. 1572 (hypotension), TABLE 12 p. 1574 (serotonin syndrome), TABLE 8 p. 1573 (QT-interval prolongation), TABLE 9 p. 1573 (antimuscarinics), TABLE 10 p. 1574 (CNS effects)

amitriptyline · clomipramine · dosulepin · doxepin · imipramine · lofepramine · nortriptyline · trimipramine

ROUTE-SPECIFIC INFORMATION Since systemic absorption can follow topical application, the possibility of interactions of topical **doxepin** should be borne in mind.

▸ **Antiarrhythmics (dronedarone)** are predicted to increase the exposure to **tricyclic antidepressants**. Avoid. Severe Theoretical → Also see TABLE 8 p. 1573

▸ **Antiarrhythmics (propafenone)** are predicted to increase the concentration of **tricyclic antidepressants**. Moderate Theoretical → Also see TABLE 9 p. 1573

▸ **Antiepileptics (carbamazepine)** decrease the exposure to **tricyclic antidepressants**. Adjust dose. Moderate Study → Also see TABLE 17 p. 1576

▸ **Antiepileptics (phenobarbital, primidone)** are predicted to decrease the exposure to **tricyclic antidepressants**. Moderate Study → Also see TABLE 10 p. 1574

▸ **Antiepileptics (valproate)** increase the concentration of **nortriptyline**. Severe Study → Also see TABLE 17 p. 1576

▸ **Tricyclic antidepressants (clomipramine, imipramine)** potentially increase the risk of overheating and dehydration when given with **antiepileptics (zonisamide)**. Avoid in children. Severe Theoretical

▸ **Antipsychotics, second generation (clozapine)** can cause constipation, as can **tricyclic antidepressants** ; concurrent use might increase the risk of developing intestinal obstruction. Severe Theoretical → Also see TABLE 17 p. 1576 → Also see TABLE 7 p. 1572 → Also see TABLE 9 p. 1573 → Also see TABLE 10 p. 1574

▸ **Berotralstat** is predicted to increase the exposure to **tricyclic antidepressants**. Monitor and adjust dose. Moderate Theoretical

▸ **Bupropion** is predicted to increase the exposure to **tricyclic antidepressants**. Monitor for toxicity and adjust dose. Severe Study

▸ **Cinacalcet** is predicted to increase the exposure to **tricyclic antidepressants**. Monitor for toxicity and adjust dose. Severe Study

▸ **Tricyclic antidepressants** decrease the antihypertensive effects of **clonidine**. Monitor and adjust dose. Moderate Anecdotal → Also see TABLE 7 p. 1572 → Also see TABLE 10 p. 1574

▸ **Cobicistat** is predicted to slightly increase the exposure to **tricyclic antidepressants**. Mild Study

▸ **Dacomitinib** is predicted to increase the exposure to **tricyclic antidepressants**. Monitor for toxicity and adjust dose. Severe Study

▸ **Darifenacin** (high-dose) is predicted to increase the exposure to **tricyclic antidepressants**. Moderate Study → Also see TABLE 9 p. 1573

▸ **Eliglustat** is predicted to increase the exposure to **nortriptyline**. Adjust dose. Moderate Theoretical

▸ **H₂ receptor antagonists (cimetidine)** increase the exposure to **tricyclic antidepressants**. Moderate Study

▸ **HIV-protease inhibitors (ritonavir)** are predicted to increase the exposure to **tricyclic antidepressants**. Moderate Theoretical

▸ **Tricyclic antidepressants** potentially increase the risk of neurotoxicity when given with **lithium**. Severe Anecdotal → Also see TABLE 12 p. 1574

▸ **Tricyclic antidepressants** are predicted to increase the risk of severe toxic reaction when given with **MAOIs, irreversible**. Avoid and for 14 days after stopping the MAOI. Severe Theoretical → Also see TABLE 7 p. 1572 → Also see TABLE 12 p. 1574

▸ **Methylphenidate** might increase the concentration of **tricyclic antidepressants**. Use with caution and adjust dose. Moderate Study

▸ **Amitriptyline** decreases the effects of **metyrapone**. Avoid. Moderate Theoretical

▸ **Tricyclic antidepressants** are predicted to increase the risk of severe toxic reaction when given with **moclobemide**. Avoid. Severe Theoretical → Also see TABLE 12 p. 1574

▸ **Tricyclic antidepressants** are predicted to decrease the effects of **moxonidine**. Avoid. Moderate Theoretical → Also see TABLE 7 p. 1572 → Also see TABLE 10 p. 1574

▸ **Nirmatrelvir** boosted with ritonavir is predicted to increase the concentration of **tricyclic antidepressants**. Moderate Theoretical

▸ **Tricyclic antidepressants** might increase the risk of adverse effects when given with **ozanimod**. Severe Theoretical

▸ **Tricyclic antidepressants** are predicted to decrease the efficacy of **pitolisant**. Mild Theoretical

▸ **SSRIs (fluoxetine, paroxetine)** are predicted to increase the exposure to **tricyclic antidepressants**. Monitor for toxicity and adjust dose. Severe Study → Also see TABLE 17 p. 1576 → Also see TABLE 12 p. 1574 → Also see TABLE 10 p. 1574

▸ **SSRIs (fluvoxamine)** markedly increase the exposure to **clomipramine**. Adjust dose. Severe Study → Also see TABLE 17 p. 1576 → Also see TABLE 12 p. 1574 → Also see TABLE 10 p. 1574

▸ **SSRIs (fluvoxamine)** increase the exposure to tricyclic antidepressants **(amitriptyline, imipramine)**. Adjust dose. Severe Study → Also see TABLE 17 p. 1576 → Also see TABLE 12 p. 1574 → Also see TABLE 10 p. 1574

▸ **Sucralfate** is predicted to decrease the absorption of **tricyclic antidepressants**. Moderate Study

▸ **Tricyclic antidepressants** increase the effects of sympathomimetics, vasoconstrictor **(adrenaline/epinephrine, noradrenaline/norepinephrine, phenylephrine)**. Avoid. Severe Study

▸ **Tricyclic antidepressants** are predicted to decrease the effects of sympathomimetics, vasoconstrictor **(ephedrine)**. Avoid. Severe Study

▸ **Terbinafine** is predicted to increase the exposure to **tricyclic antidepressants**. Monitor for toxicity and adjust dose. Severe Study

▸ **Tricyclic antidepressants** increase the risk of cardiac arrhythmias and hypotension when given with **thiopental**. Moderate Study → Also see TABLE 7 p. 1572 → Also see TABLE 10 p. 1574

▸ **Tricyclic antidepressants** might enhance the antidiuretic and hypertensive effects of **vasopressin**. Moderate Theoretical

Trientine

▸ Oral **trientine** potentially decreases the absorption of oral **iron**. Moderate Theoretical

▸ **Trientine** potentially decreases the absorption of **zinc**. Moderate Theoretical

Trifluoperazine → see phenothiazines

Trihexyphenidyl → see TABLE 9 p. 1573 (antimuscarinics), TABLE 10 p. 1574 (CNS effects)

▸ **Antipsychotics, second generation (clozapine)** can cause constipation, as can **trihexyphenidyl**; concurrent use might increase the risk of developing intestinal obstruction. Severe Theoretical → Also see TABLE 9 p. 1573 → Also see TABLE 10 p. 1574

Interactions | Appendix 1   A1

Trimethoprim → see **TABLE 2** p. 1571 (nephrotoxicity), **TABLE 15** p. 1575 (increased serum potassium)
▶ **Trimethoprim** increases the concentration of antiepileptics (fosphenytoin, phenytoin). [Moderate] Study
▶ Antimalarials (pyrimethamine) increase the risk of adverse effects when given with **trimethoprim**. [Severe] Study
▶ **Trimethoprim** might increase the risk of neutropenia when given with antipsychotics, second generation (clozapine). Avoid. [Severe] Theoretical
▶ **Trimethoprim** might increase the risk of haematological toxicity when given with azathioprine in renal transplant patients. [Severe] Anecdotal
▶ **Trimethoprim** is predicted to increase the anticoagulant effect of coumarins. [Severe] Study
▶ Dapsone increases the exposure to **trimethoprim** and **trimethoprim** increases the exposure to dapsone. [Severe] Study
▶ **Trimethoprim** increases the concentration of digoxin. [Moderate] Study
▶ **Trimethoprim** is predicted to increase the exposure to dopamine receptor agonists (pramipexole). Adjust dose. [Moderate] Study
▶ **Trimethoprim** slightly increases the exposure to meglitinides (repaglinide). Avoid or monitor blood glucose. [Moderate] Study
▶ **Trimethoprim** might increase the risk of haematological toxicity when given with mercaptopurine in renal transplant patients. [Severe] Theoretical
▶ **Trimethoprim** is predicted to increase the exposure to metformin. Use with caution and adjust dose. [Moderate] Study
▶ **Trimethoprim** increases the risk of haematological side-effects (sometimes fatal) when given with methotrexate. Avoid. See methotrexate p. 1048 for further information. [Severe] Anecdotal → Also see **TABLE 2** p. 1571
▶ **Trimethoprim** slightly increases the exposure to NRTIs (lamivudine). [Moderate] Study
▶ Rifamycins (rifampicin) decrease the exposure to **trimethoprim**. [Moderate] Study → Also see **TABLE 2** p. 1571
▶ **Trimethoprim** is predicted to decrease the efficacy of sapropterin. [Moderate] Theoretical
▶ **Trimethoprim** is predicted to increase the exposure to treprostinil. Adjust dose. [Moderate] Theoretical

Trimipramine → see tricyclic antidepressants
Triptans → see **TABLE 12** p. 1574 (serotonin syndrome)

almotriptan · eletriptan · frovatriptan · naratriptan · rizatriptan · sumatriptan · zolmitriptan

▶ Anti-androgens (enzalutamide) are predicted to decrease the exposure to **eletriptan**. [Severe] Study
▶ Antifungals, azoles (itraconazole, ketoconazole, posaconazole, voriconazole) increase the exposure to **almotriptan**. [Mild] Study
▶ Antifungals, azoles (itraconazole, ketoconazole, posaconazole, voriconazole) are predicted to markedly increase the exposure to **eletriptan**. Avoid. [Severe] Study
▶ Beta blockers, non-selective (propranolol) slightly to moderately increase the exposure to **rizatriptan**. Adjust **rizatriptan** dose and separate administration by at least 2 hours, p. 545. [Moderate] Study
▶ Cenobamate is predicted to decrease the exposure to **eletriptan**. Adjust dose. [Moderate] Theoretical
▶ Ceritinib increases the exposure to **almotriptan**. [Mild] Study
▶ Ceritinib is predicted to markedly increase the exposure to **eletriptan**. Avoid. [Severe] Study
▶ Cobicistat increases the exposure to **almotriptan**. [Mild] Study
▶ Cobicistat is predicted to markedly increase the exposure to **eletriptan**. Avoid. [Severe] Study
▶ Combined hormonal contraceptives is predicted to increase the exposure to **zolmitriptan**. Adjust **zolmitriptan** dose, p. 546. [Moderate] Theoretical
▶ Givinostat might increase the exposure to **eletriptan**. [Moderate] Study
▶ Givosiran is predicted to increase the exposure to **zolmitriptan**. Adjust **zolmitriptan** dose, p. 546. [Moderate] Theoretical
▶ H_2 receptor antagonists (cimetidine) slightly increase the exposure to **zolmitriptan**. Adjust **zolmitriptan** dose, p. 546. [Mild] Study
▶ HIV-protease inhibitors increase the exposure to **almotriptan**. [Mild] Study

▶ HIV-protease inhibitors are predicted to markedly increase the exposure to **eletriptan**. Avoid. [Severe] Study
▶ Idelalisib increases the exposure to **almotriptan**. [Mild] Study
▶ Idelalisib is predicted to markedly increase the exposure to **eletriptan**. Avoid. [Severe] Study
▶ Ivosidenib might decrease the exposure to **eletriptan**. Avoid or monitor. [Moderate] Theoretical
▶ Macrolides (clarithromycin) increase the exposure to **almotriptan**. [Mild] Study
▶ Macrolides (clarithromycin) are predicted to markedly increase the exposure to **eletriptan**. Avoid. [Severe] Study
▶ Macrolides (erythromycin) moderately increase the exposure to **eletriptan**. Avoid. [Moderate] Study
▶ MAOIs, irreversible are predicted to increase the exposure to triptans (rizatriptan, sumatriptan). Avoid and for 14 days after stopping the MAOI. [Severe] Theoretical → Also see **TABLE 12** p. 1574
▶ MAOIs, irreversible are predicted to increase the exposure to **zolmitriptan**. [Severe] Theoretical → Also see **TABLE 12** p. 1574
▶ Mexiletine is predicted to increase the exposure to **zolmitriptan**. Adjust **zolmitriptan** dose, p. 546. [Moderate] Theoretical
▶ Moclobemide slightly increases the exposure to **almotriptan**. Avoid. [Severe] Study → Also see **TABLE 12** p. 1574
▶ Moclobemide increases the concentration of triptans (eletriptan, frovatriptan, naratriptan). Avoid. [Severe] Study → Also see **TABLE 12** p. 1574
▶ Moclobemide moderately increases the exposure to triptans (rizatriptan, sumatriptan). Avoid. [Severe] Study → Also see **TABLE 12** p. 1574
▶ Moclobemide slightly increases the exposure to **zolmitriptan**. Avoid or adjust **zolmitriptan** dose, p. 546. [Severe] Study → Also see **TABLE 12** p. 1574
▶ Neurokinin-1 receptor antagonists (aprepitant, netupitant) are predicted to increase the exposure to **eletriptan**. [Moderate] Study
▶ Nirmatrelvir boosted with ritonavir is predicted to increase the concentration of **eletriptan**. Avoid. [Severe] Theoretical
▶ Osilodrostat is predicted to increase the exposure to **zolmitriptan**. Adjust **zolmitriptan** dose, p. 546. [Moderate] Theoretical
▶ Quinolones (ciprofloxacin) are predicted to increase the exposure to **zolmitriptan**. Adjust **zolmitriptan** dose, p. 546. [Moderate] Theoretical
▶ Rucaparib is predicted to increase the exposure to **zolmitriptan**. Adjust **zolmitriptan** dose, p. 546. [Moderate] Theoretical
▶ SSRIs (fluvoxamine) increase the concentration of **frovatriptan**. [Severe] Study → Also see **TABLE 12** p. 1574
▶ SSRIs (fluvoxamine) are predicted to increase the exposure to **zolmitriptan**. Adjust **zolmitriptan** dose, p. 546. [Severe] Theoretical → Also see **TABLE 12** p. 1574
▶ Tucatinib increases the exposure to **almotriptan**. [Mild] Study
▶ Tucatinib is predicted to markedly increase the exposure to **eletriptan**. Avoid. [Severe] Study
▶ Vemurafenib is predicted to increase the exposure to **zolmitriptan**. Adjust **zolmitriptan** dose, p. 546. [Moderate] Theoretical

Tropicamide → see **TABLE 9** p. 1573 (antimuscarinics)
▶ Antipsychotics, second generation (clozapine) can cause constipation, as can **tropicamide**; concurrent use might increase the risk of developing intestinal obstruction. [Severe] Theoretical → Also see **TABLE 9** p. 1573

Trospium → see **TABLE 9** p. 1573 (antimuscarinics)
▶ Antipsychotics, second generation (clozapine) can cause constipation, as can **trospium**; concurrent use might increase the risk of developing intestinal obstruction. [Severe] Theoretical → Also see **TABLE 9** p. 1573

Tryptophan → see **TABLE 12** p. 1574 (serotonin syndrome)
▶ **Tryptophan** greatly decreases the concentration of levodopa. [Moderate] Study
▶ **Tryptophan** increases the risk of adverse effects when given with MAOIs, irreversible. [Severe] Anecdotal → Also see **TABLE 12** p. 1574

Tucatinib

▶ **Tucatinib** is predicted to increase the exposure to abemaciclib. Avoid or adjust dose—consult product literature. Severe Study

▶ **Tucatinib** is predicted to increase the exposure to acalabrutinib. Avoid. Severe Study

▶ **Tucatinib** is predicted to moderately increase the exposure to alpha blockers (alfuzosin, tamsulosin). Use with caution or avoid. Moderate Study

▶ **Tucatinib** is predicted to increase the exposure to alpha blockers (doxazosin). Moderate Study

▶ Anti-androgens (apalutamide, enzalutamide) are predicted to decrease the exposure to **tucatinib**. Avoid. Severe Study

▶ **Tucatinib** is predicted to increase the exposure to anti-androgens (apalutamide). Monitor and adjust dose. Mild Study

▶ **Tucatinib** very markedly increases the exposure to antiarrhythmics (dronedarone). Avoid. Severe Study

▶ **Tucatinib** is predicted to increase the exposure to antiarrhythmics (propafenone). Monitor and adjust dose. Severe Study

▶ **Tucatinib** is predicted to increase the exposure to anticholinesterases, centrally acting (galantamine). Monitor and adjust dose. Moderate Study

▶ Antiepileptics (carbamazepine, fosphenytoin, phenobarbital, phenytoin, primidone) are predicted to decrease the exposure to **tucatinib**. Avoid. Severe Study

▶ **Tucatinib** is predicted to very slightly increase the exposure to antiepileptics (perampanel). Mild Study

▶ **Tucatinib** is predicted to increase the exposure to antifungals, azoles (isavuconazole). Avoid or monitor adverse effects. Severe Study

▶ **Tucatinib** is predicted to increase the exposure to antihistamines, non-sedating (mizolastine). Avoid. Severe Study

▶ **Tucatinib** is predicted to increase the exposure to antihistamines, non-sedating (rupatadine). Avoid. Moderate Study

▶ **Tucatinib** is predicted to slightly increase the exposure to antipsychotics, second generation (aripiprazole). Adjust **aripiprazole** dose, p. 454. Moderate Study

▶ **Tucatinib** is predicted to moderately increase the exposure to antipsychotics, second generation (cariprazine). Avoid. Severe Study

▶ **Tucatinib** is predicted to increase the exposure to antipsychotics, second generation (lurasidone, quetiapine). Avoid. Severe Study

▶ **Tucatinib** is predicted to increase the exposure to antipsychotics, second generation (risperidone). Adjust dose. Moderate Study

▶ **Tucatinib** is predicted to increase the exposure to atogepant. Adjust **atogepant** dose, p. 540. Moderate Study

▶ **Tucatinib** is predicted to increase the exposure to avacopan. Severe Study

▶ **Tucatinib** is predicted to increase the exposure to avapritinib. Avoid. Moderate Study

▶ **Tucatinib** is predicted to increase the exposure to axitinib. Avoid or adjust dose. Moderate Study

▶ **Tucatinib** might increases the exposure to bedaquiline. Mild Study

▶ **Tucatinib** moderately increases the exposure to benzodiazepines (alprazolam). Avoid. Moderate Study

▶ **Tucatinib** is predicted to markedly to very markedly increase the exposure to benzodiazepines (midazolam). Avoid or adjust dose. Severe Study

▶ **Tucatinib** is predicted to increase the exposure to beta₂ agonists (salmeterol). Avoid. Severe Study

▶ **Tucatinib** slightly increases the exposure to bortezomib. Moderate Study

▶ **Tucatinib** is predicted to increase the exposure to bosutinib. Avoid or adjust dose. Severe Study

▶ **Tucatinib** is predicted to increase the exposure to brigatinib. Avoid or adjust dose—consult product literature. Severe Study

▶ **Tucatinib** is predicted to increase the exposure to buspirone. Adjust **buspirone** dose, p. 396. Severe Study

▶ **Tucatinib** is predicted to increase the exposure to cabozantinib. Moderate Study

▶ **Tucatinib** is predicted to increase the exposure to calcium channel blockers (amlodipine, felodipine, lacidipine, nicardipine, nifedipine, nimodipine). Monitor and adjust dose. Moderate Study

▶ **Tucatinib** is predicted to increase the exposure to calcium channel blockers (diltiazem, verapamil). Severe Study

▶ **Tucatinib** is predicted to markedly increase the exposure to calcium channel blockers (lercanidipine). Avoid. Severe Study

▶ **Tucatinib** is predicted to increase the exposure to cannabidiol. Avoid or adjust dose. Mild Study

▶ **Tucatinib** is predicted to increase the exposure to capivasertib. Adjust dose. Moderate Study

▶ **Tucatinib** is predicted to increase the exposure to ceritinib. Avoid or adjust dose—consult product literature. Severe Study

▶ **Tucatinib** increases the concentration of ciclosporin. Severe Study

▶ **Tucatinib** is predicted to moderately increase the exposure to cilostazol. Adjust **cilostazol** dose, p. 266. Moderate Study

▶ **Tucatinib** is predicted to moderately increase the exposure to cinacalcet. Adjust dose. Moderate Study

▶ Clopidogrel is predicted to increase the exposure to **tucatinib**. Avoid or adjust dose—consult product literature. Severe Study

▶ **Tucatinib** is predicted to increase the exposure to cobimetinib. Avoid or monitor for toxicity. Severe Study

▶ **Tucatinib** is predicted to increase the exposure to colchicine. Avoid potent CYP3A4 inhibitors or adjust **colchicine** dose, p. 1279. Severe Study

▶ **Tucatinib** is predicted to increase the exposure to corticosteroids (beclometasone) (risk with beclometasone is likely to be lower than with other corticosteroids). Moderate Theoretical

▶ **Tucatinib** is predicted to increase the exposure to corticosteroids (betamethasone, budesonide, ciclesonide, deflazacort, dexamethasone, fludrocortisone, fluticasone, hydrocortisone, methylprednisolone, mometasone, prednisolone, triamcinolone). Avoid or monitor adverse effects. Severe Study

▶ **Tucatinib** is predicted to increase the exposure to corticosteroids (vamorolone). Adjust dose. Severe Study

▶ **Tucatinib** is predicted to increase the exposure to crizotinib. Avoid. Moderate Study

▶ **Tucatinib** is predicted to increase the exposure to dabrafenib. Use with caution or avoid. Moderate Study

▶ **Tucatinib** is predicted to increase the exposure to daridorexant. Avoid. Severe Study

▶ **Tucatinib** is predicted to markedly to very markedly increase the exposure to darifenacin. Avoid. Severe Study

▶ **Tucatinib** is predicted to increase the exposure to dasatinib. Avoid or adjust dose—consult product literature. Severe Study

▶ **Tucatinib** very slightly increases the exposure to delamanid. Severe Study

▶ **Tucatinib** is predicted to moderately increase the exposure to dienogest. Moderate Study

▶ **Tucatinib** slightly increases the exposure to digoxin. Use with caution and adjust dose. Moderate Study

▶ **Tucatinib** is predicted to increase the exposure to dipeptidylpeptidase-4 inhibitors (saxagliptin). Moderate Study

▶ **Tucatinib** is predicted to increase the exposure to domperidone. Avoid. Severe Study

▶ **Tucatinib** increases the exposure to dopamine receptor agonists (bromocriptine). Severe Study

▶ **Tucatinib** is predicted to increase the exposure to dronabinol. Adjust dose. Mild Study

▶ **Tucatinib** is predicted to increase the exposure to dutasteride. Monitor adverse effects and adjust dose. Moderate Theoretical

▶ **Tucatinib** is predicted to increase the exposure to elacestrant. Avoid potent CYP3A4 inhibitors or adjust **elacestrant** dose, p. 1084. Severe Study

▶ **Tucatinib** is predicted to increase the exposure to elexacaftor. Adjust ivacaftor with tezacaftor and elexacaftor p. 337 dose with potent CYP3A4 inhibitors. Severe Study

▶ **Tucatinib** is predicted to increase the exposure to eliglustat. Avoid or adjust dose—consult product literature. Severe Study

▶ Encorafenib is predicted to decrease the exposure to **tucatinib**. Avoid. Severe Study

▶ **Tucatinib** is predicted to increase the exposure to encorafenib. Avoid or monitor. Severe Study

▸ **Tucatinib** is predicted to increase the exposure to endothelin receptor antagonists **(macitentan)**. Moderate Study
▸ **Tucatinib** is predicted to increase the exposure to the cytotoxic component of enfortumab vedotin. Severe Theoretical
▸ **Tucatinib** is predicted to increase the exposure to entrectinib. Avoid or adjust dose with potent CYP3A4 inhibitors—consult product literature. Severe Study
▸ **Tucatinib** is predicted to increase the exposure to erdafitinib. Adjust dose. Severe Study
▸ **Tucatinib** is predicted to increase the risk of ergotism when given with ergometrine. Avoid. Severe Theoretical
▸ **Tucatinib** is predicted to increase the exposure to erlotinib. Use with caution and adjust dose. Severe Study
▸ **Tucatinib** is predicted to increase the exposure to esketamine. Adjust dose. Moderate Study
▸ **Tucatinib** is predicted to increase the exposure to eszopiclone. Adjust **eszopiclone** dose; avoid in the elderly, p. 554. Moderate Study
▸ **Tucatinib** is predicted to increase the concentration of subdermal etonogestrel. Moderate Theoretical
▸ **Tucatinib** is predicted to increase the exposure to etrasimod. Avoid in poor CYP2C9 metabolisers. Severe Theoretical
▸ **Tucatinib** is predicted to increase the exposure to everolimus. Avoid. Severe Study
▸ **Tucatinib** is predicted to increase the exposure to fedratinib. Adjust dose, but avoid depending on other drugs taken—consult product literature. Moderate Study
▸ **Tucatinib** is predicted to moderately increase the exposure to fesoterodine. Adjust **fesoterodine** dose with potent CYP3A4 inhibitors; avoid in hepatic and renal impairment, p. 897. Severe Study
▸ Fibrates **(gemfibrozil)** are predicted to increase the exposure to **tucatinib**. Avoid or adjust dose—consult product literature. Severe Study
▸ **Tucatinib** is predicted to increase the exposure to fostamatinib. Monitor adverse effects and adjust dose. Moderate Study
▸ **Tucatinib** is predicted to increase the exposure to gefitinib. Severe Study
▸ **Tucatinib** is predicted to increase the exposure to gilteritinib. Moderate Study
▸ **Tucatinib** is predicted to increase the exposure to glasdegib. Use with caution or avoid. Severe Study
▸ **Tucatinib** is predicted to moderately to markedly increase the exposure to grazoprevir. Avoid. Severe Study
▸ **Tucatinib** is predicted to increase the exposure to guanfacine. Adjust **guanfacine** dose, p. 407. Moderate Study
▸ **Tucatinib** is predicted to increase the exposure to ibrutinib. Avoid or adjust dose with potent CYP3A4 inhibitors—consult product literature. Severe Study
▸ **Tucatinib** is predicted to increase the exposure to idelalisib. Moderate Theoretical
▸ **Tucatinib** is predicted to increase the exposure to imatinib. Moderate Study
▸ **Tucatinib** is predicted to increase the risk of toxicity when given with irinotecan. Avoid. Severe Study
▸ Iron chelators **(deferasirox)** are predicted to increase the exposure to **tucatinib**. Moderate Theoretical
▸ **Tucatinib** is predicted to increase the exposure to ivabradine. Avoid. Severe Study
▸ **Tucatinib** is predicted to increase the exposure to ivacaftor. Adjust dose with potent CYP3A4 inhibitors, see ivacaftor p. 336, lumacaftor with ivacaftor p. 338, tezacaftor with ivacaftor p. 339, and ivacaftor with tezacaftor and elexacaftor p. 337. Severe Study
▸ Ivosidenib is predicted to decrease the exposure to **tucatinib**. Avoid. Severe Study
▸ **Tucatinib** is predicted to increase the exposure to lapatinib. Avoid. Moderate Study
▸ **Tucatinib** is predicted to moderately increase the exposure to larotrectinib. Avoid or adjust dose—consult product literature. Moderate Study
▸ Leflunomide is predicted to increase the exposure to **tucatinib**. Moderate Theoretical
▸ **Tucatinib** is predicted to increase the exposure to leniolisib. Avoid. Moderate Study

▸ **Tucatinib** is predicted to markedly increase the exposure to lomitapide. Avoid. Severe Study
▸ **Tucatinib** is predicted to increase the exposure to lorlatinib. Avoid or adjust dose—consult product literature. Severe Study
▸ Lumacaftor is predicted to decrease the exposure to **tucatinib**. Avoid. Severe Study
▸ **Tucatinib** is predicted to increase the exposure to mavacamten. Avoid or monitor—consult product literature. Severe Study
▸ **Tucatinib** is predicted to increase the concentration of intramuscular medroxyprogesterone. Moderate Theoretical
▸ **Tucatinib** is predicted to increase the exposure to midostaurin. Avoid or monitor for toxicity. Severe Study
▸ **Tucatinib** is predicted to markedly increase the exposure to mineralocorticoid receptor antagonists **(eplerenone)**. Avoid. Severe Study
▸ **Tucatinib** is predicted to increase the exposure to mineralocorticoid receptor antagonists **(finerenone)**. Avoid. Severe Study
▸ **Tucatinib** is predicted to increase the exposure to mirabegron. Adjust **mirabegron** dose in hepatic and renal impairment, p. 901. Moderate Study
▸ **Tucatinib** is predicted to increase the exposure to mirtazapine. Moderate Study
▸ Mitotane is predicted to decrease the exposure to **tucatinib**. Avoid. Severe Study
▸ **Tucatinib** is predicted to increase the exposure to mobocertinib. Avoid. Severe Study
▸ **Tucatinib** is predicted to increase the exposure to modafinil. Mild Theoretical
▸ **Tucatinib** is predicted to increase the risk of neutropenia when given with monoclonal antibodies **(brentuximab vedotin)**. Monitor and adjust dose. Severe Study
▸ **Tucatinib** is predicted to increase the exposure to monoclonal antibodies **(polatuzumab vedotin)**. Moderate Theoretical
▸ **Tucatinib** is predicted to increase the exposure to the cytotoxic component of monoclonal antibodies **(trastuzumab emtansine)**. Avoid or monitor. Severe Theoretical
▸ **Tucatinib** is predicted to increase the exposure to naldemedine. Avoid or monitor. Moderate Study
▸ **Tucatinib** is predicted to markedly increase the exposure to naloxegol. Avoid. Severe Study
▸ **Tucatinib** is predicted to increase the exposure to neratinib. Avoid or adjust dose with potent CYP3A4 inhibitors—consult product literature. Severe Study
▸ **Tucatinib** is predicted to markedly increase the exposure to neurokinin-1 receptor antagonists **(aprepitant)**. Moderate Study
▸ **Tucatinib** is predicted to increase the exposure to neurokinin-1 receptor antagonists **(fosaprepitant)**. Moderate Theoretical
▸ **Tucatinib** is predicted to increase the exposure to neurokinin-1 receptor antagonists **(netupitant)**. Moderate Study
▸ **Tucatinib** is predicted to increase the exposure to nilotinib. Avoid. Severe Study
▸ **Tucatinib** is predicted to increase the exposure to nitisinone. Adjust dose. Moderate Theoretical
▸ **Tucatinib** is predicted to increase the exposure to olaparib. Avoid or adjust dose with potent CYP3A4 inhibitors—consult product literature. Moderate Study
▸ **Tucatinib** is predicted to increase the exposure to opioids **(alfentanil, buprenorphine, fentanyl, oxycodone)**. Monitor and adjust dose. Severe Study
▸ **Tucatinib** is predicted to increase the exposure to opioids **(sufentanil)**. Moderate Study
▸ **Tucatinib** is predicted to increase the exposure to osilodrostat. Moderate Theoretical
▸ **Tucatinib** is predicted to increase the exposure to ospemifene. Avoid in poor CYP2C9 metabolisers. Moderate Study
▸ **Tucatinib** is predicted to increase the exposure to oxybutynin. Mild Study
▸ **Tucatinib** is predicted to increase the exposure to palbociclib. Avoid or adjust dose—consult product literature. Severe Study
▸ **Tucatinib** is predicted to increase the exposure to panobinostat. Adjust dose—consult product literature; in hepatic impairment avoid. Moderate Study

Tucatinib (continued)

▶ **Tucatinib** is predicted to increase the exposure to pazopanib. Avoid or adjust dose—consult product literature. Moderate Study

▶ **Tucatinib** is predicted to increase the exposure to pemigatinib. Avoid or adjust dose—consult product literature. Severe Study

▶ **Tucatinib** is predicted to increase the exposure to phosphodiesterase type-5 inhibitors (avanafil, vardenafil). Avoid. Severe Study

▶ **Tucatinib** is predicted to increase the exposure to phosphodiesterase type-5 inhibitors (sildenafil). Avoid potent CYP3A4 inhibitors or adjust **sildenafil** dose, p. 940. Severe Study

▶ **Tucatinib** is predicted to increase the exposure to phosphodiesterase type-5 inhibitors (tadalafil). Use with caution or avoid. Severe Study

▶ **Tucatinib** is predicted to increase the exposure to pimozide. Avoid. Severe Study

▶ **Tucatinib** is predicted to slightly increase the exposure to ponatinib. Monitor and adjust dose—consult product literature. Moderate Study

▶ **Tucatinib** is predicted to increase the exposure to pralsetinib. Avoid or adjust dose with potent CYP3A4 inhibitors—consult product literature. Moderate Study

▶ **Tucatinib** is predicted to moderately increase the exposure to praziquantel. Mild Study

▶ **Tucatinib** given with carbimazole is predicted to increase the exposure to propiverine. Adjust starting dose. Moderate Theoretical

▶ **Tucatinib** is predicted to increase the exposure to quizartinib. Adjust dose—consult product literature. Severe Study

▶ **Tucatinib** is predicted to increase the exposure to ranolazine. Avoid. Severe Study

▶ **Tucatinib** is predicted to increase the exposure to reboxetine. Avoid. Moderate Study

▶ **Tucatinib** is predicted to increase the exposure to regorafenib. Avoid. Moderate Study

▶ **Tucatinib** is predicted to increase the exposure to retinoids (alitretinoin). Adjust **alitretinoin** dose, p. 1433. Moderate Theoretical

▶ **Tucatinib** is predicted to increase the exposure to ribociclib. Avoid or adjust dose—consult product literature. Moderate Study

▶ Rifamycins (rifampicin) are predicted to decrease the exposure to **tucatinib**. Avoid. Severe Study

▶ **Tucatinib** is predicted to increase the exposure to rimegepant. Avoid. Moderate Study

▶ **Tucatinib** is predicted to increase the exposure to ripretinib. Moderate Theoretical

▶ **Tucatinib** is predicted to increase the exposure to ruxolitinib. Adjust dose and monitor adverse effects. Moderate Study

▶ **Tucatinib** is predicted to increase the exposure to selpercatinib. Adjust dose—consult product literature. Moderate Study

▶ **Tucatinib** is predicted to increase the exposure to selumetinib. Avoid or adjust dose—consult product literature. Severe Study

▶ **Tucatinib** is predicted to increase the exposure to siponimod. Avoid depending on other drugs taken—consult product literature. Severe Theoretical

▶ **Tucatinib** is predicted to increase the concentration of sirolimus. Avoid or monitor and adjust dose. Severe Study

▶ **Tucatinib** is predicted to increase the exposure to SNRIs (venlafaxine). Moderate Study

▶ **Tucatinib** is predicted to increase the exposure to solifenacin. Adjust solifenacin p. 899 or tamsulosin with solifenacin p. 906 dose; avoid in hepatic and renal impairment. Severe Study

▶ **Tucatinib** is predicted to moderately increase the exposure to SSRIs (dapoxetine). Avoid potent CYP3A4 inhibitors or adjust **dapoxetine** dose, p. 947. Severe Study

▶ St John's wort is predicted to decrease the exposure to **tucatinib**. Avoid. Severe Theoretical

▶ **Tucatinib** is predicted to increase the exposure to statins (atorvastatin). Avoid or adjust dose and monitor rhabdomyolysis. Severe Study

▶ **Tucatinib** is predicted to increase the exposure to statins (simvastatin). Avoid. Severe Study

▶ **Tucatinib** is predicted to increase the exposure to sunitinib. Avoid or adjust dose—consult product literature. Moderate Study

▶ **Tucatinib** is predicted to increase the concentration of tacrolimus. Monitor and adjust dose. Severe Study

▶ **Tucatinib** is predicted to increase the exposure to talazoparib. Use with caution and adjust dose. Moderate Theoretical

▶ **Tucatinib** is predicted to increase the exposure to taxanes (cabazitaxel). Avoid or adjust dose—consult product literature. Severe Study

▶ **Tucatinib** is predicted to increase the exposure to taxanes (docetaxel). Avoid or adjust dose. Severe Study

▶ **Tucatinib** is predicted to increase the exposure to taxanes (paclitaxel). Moderate Anecdotal

▶ **Tucatinib** is predicted to increase the concentration of temsirolimus. Avoid. Severe Theoretical

▶ Teriflunomide is predicted to increase the exposure to **tucatinib**. Moderate Theoretical

▶ **Tucatinib** is predicted to increase the exposure to tezacaftor. Adjust dose with potent CYP3A4 inhibitors, see tezacaftor with ivacaftor p. 339 and ivacaftor with tezacaftor and elexacaftor p. 337. Severe Study

▶ **Tucatinib** is predicted to markedly increase the exposure to ticagrelor. Avoid. Severe Study

▶ **Tucatinib** is predicted to increase the exposure to tofacitinib. Adjust **tofacitinib** dose, p. 1265. Moderate Study

▶ **Tucatinib** is predicted to increase the exposure to tolterodine. Avoid. Severe Study

▶ **Tucatinib** is predicted to increase the exposure to tolvaptan. Manufacturer advises caution or adjust **tolvaptan** dose with potent CYP3A4 inhibitors, p. 767. Severe Study

▶ **Tucatinib** is predicted to increase the exposure to toremifene. Moderate Theoretical

▶ **Tucatinib** is predicted to increase the exposure to trabectedin. Avoid or adjust dose. Severe Theoretical

▶ **Tucatinib** is predicted to moderately increase the exposure to trazodone. Avoid or adjust dose. Moderate Study

▶ **Tucatinib** increases the exposure to triptans (almotriptan). Mild Study

▶ **Tucatinib** is predicted to markedly increase the exposure to triptans (eletriptan). Avoid. Severe Study

▶ **Tucatinib** is predicted to increase the exposure to upadacitinib. Manufacturer advises caution or avoid, or adjust **upadacitinib** dose depending on indication, p. 1267. Severe Study

▶ **Tucatinib** is predicted to increase the exposure to vemurafenib. Severe Theoretical

▶ **Tucatinib** is predicted to increase the exposure to venetoclax. Avoid or adjust dose—consult product literature. Severe Study

▶ **Tucatinib** is predicted to increase the exposure to vinca alkaloids. Severe Theoretical

▶ **Tucatinib** is predicted to increase the exposure to vitamin D substances (paricalcitol). Moderate Study

▶ **Tucatinib** is predicted to increase the exposure to voclosporin. Avoid. Severe Study

▶ **Tucatinib** is predicted to increase the exposure to zanubrutinib. Avoid or adjust dose with potent CYP3A4 inhibitors—consult product literature. Moderate Study

▶ **Tucatinib** is predicted to increase the exposure to zopiclone. Adjust dose. Moderate Theoretical

Typhoid vaccine (live) → see live vaccines

Ublituximab → see monoclonal antibodies

Ulipristal

▶ Antacids might decrease the efficacy of **ulipristal** for emergency hormonal contraception. For FSRH guidance, see Contraceptives, interactions p. 917. Unknown Theoretical

▶ Anti-androgens (apalutamide) are predicted to decrease the efficacy of **ulipristal**. Avoid and for 4 weeks after stopping **apalutamide**. Severe Theoretical

▶ Anti-androgens (enzalutamide) are predicted to decrease the efficacy of **ulipristal**. Avoid and for 4 weeks after stopping **enzalutamide**. Severe Theoretical

▶ Antiarrhythmics (dronedarone) are predicted to increase the exposure to **ulipristal**. Avoid if used for uterine fibroids. Moderate Study

▶ Antiepileptics (carbamazepine, eslicarbazepine, fosphenytoin, oxcarbazepine, perampanel, phenobarbital, phenytoin, primidone, rufinamide, topiramate) decrease the efficacy of **ulipristal**. Avoid and for 4 weeks after stopping the enzyme inducing drug. For FSRH guidance, see Contraceptives, interactions p. 917. Severe Anecdotal

▶ Antifungals, azoles (fluconazole, isavuconazole, posaconazole) are predicted to increase the exposure to **ulipristal**. Avoid if used for uterine fibroids. Moderate Study

▶ Antifungals, azoles (itraconazole, ketoconazole, voriconazole) are predicted to increase the exposure to **ulipristal**. Avoid if used for uterine fibroids. Severe Study

▶ Calcium channel blockers (diltiazem, verapamil) are predicted to increase the exposure to **ulipristal**. Avoid if used for uterine fibroids. Moderate Study

▶ Calcium salts (calcium carbonate) -containing antacids might decrease the efficacy of **ulipristal** for emergency hormonal contraception. For FSRH guidance, see Contraceptives, interactions p. 917. Unknown Theoretical

▶ Cobicistat is predicted to increase the exposure to **ulipristal**. Avoid if used for uterine fibroids. Severe Study

▶ Combined hormonal contraceptives might decrease the efficacy of **ulipristal** and **ulipristal** might decrease the efficacy of combined hormonal contraceptives. Avoid or use additional contraceptive precautions. Severe Theoretical

▶ Crizotinib is predicted to increase the exposure to **ulipristal**. Avoid if used for uterine fibroids. Moderate Study

▶ Dabrafenib is predicted to decrease the efficacy of **ulipristal**. Avoid and for 4 weeks after stopping **dabrafenib**. Severe Theoretical

▶ Desogestrel might decrease the efficacy of **ulipristal** and **ulipristal** might decrease the efficacy of desogestrel. Avoid or use additional contraceptive precautions. Severe Theoretical

▶ Drospirenone might decreases the efficacy of **ulipristal** and **ulipristal** might decreases the efficacy of drospirenone. Avoid. Severe Theoretical

▶ Endothelin receptor antagonists (bosentan) decrease the efficacy of **ulipristal**. Avoid and for 4 weeks after stopping the enzyme inducing drug. For FSRH guidance, see Contraceptives, interactions p. 917. Severe Anecdotal

▶ Etonogestrel might decrease the efficacy of **ulipristal** and **ulipristal** might decrease the efficacy of etonogestrel. Avoid. Severe Theoretical

▶ Grapefruit juice is predicted to increase the exposure to **ulipristal**. Avoid if used for uterine fibroids. Moderate Theoretical

▶ H₂ receptor antagonists might decrease the efficacy of **ulipristal** for emergency hormonal contraception. For FSRH guidance, see Contraceptives, interactions p. 917. Unknown Theoretical

▶ HIV-protease inhibitors (atazanavir, darunavir, fosamprenavir, lopinavir) boosted with ritonavir are predicted to increase the exposure to **ulipristal**. Avoid if used for uterine fibroids. Severe Study

▶ HIV-protease inhibitors (ritonavir) decrease the efficacy of **ulipristal**. Avoid and for 4 weeks after stopping the enzyme inducing drug. For FSRH guidance, see Contraceptives, interactions p. 917. Severe Anecdotal

▶ Idelalisib is predicted to increase the exposure to **ulipristal**. Avoid if used for uterine fibroids. Severe Study

▶ Imatinib is predicted to increase the exposure to **ulipristal**. Avoid if used for uterine fibroids. Moderate Study

▶ Letermovir is predicted to increase the exposure to **ulipristal**. Avoid if used for uterine fibroids. Moderate Study

▶ Levonorgestrel might decrease the efficacy of **ulipristal** and **ulipristal** might decrease the efficacy of levonorgestrel. Avoid. Severe Theoretical

▶ Lumacaftor is predicted to decrease the efficacy of **ulipristal**. Use additional contraceptive precautions. Severe Theoretical

▶ Macrolides (clarithromycin) are predicted to increase the exposure to **ulipristal**. Avoid if used for uterine fibroids. Severe Study

▶ Macrolides (erythromycin) moderately increase the exposure to **ulipristal**. Avoid if used for uterine fibroids. Moderate Study

▶ Mitotane is predicted to decrease the efficacy of **ulipristal**. Avoid and for 4 weeks after stopping **mitotane**. Severe Theoretical

▶ Modafinil decreases the efficacy of **ulipristal**. Avoid and for 4 weeks after stopping the enzyme inducing drug. For FSRH guidance, see Contraceptives, interactions p. 917. Severe Anecdotal

▶ Neurokinin-1 receptor antagonists (aprepitant, fosaprepitant) decrease the efficacy of **ulipristal**. Avoid and for 4 weeks after stopping the enzyme inducing drug. For FSRH guidance, see Contraceptives, interactions p. 917. Severe Anecdotal

▶ Neurokinin-1 receptor antagonists (netupitant) are predicted to increase the exposure to **ulipristal**. Avoid if used for uterine fibroids. Moderate Study

▶ Nilotinib is predicted to increase the exposure to **ulipristal**. Avoid if used for uterine fibroids. Moderate Study

▶ NNRTIs (efavirenz, nevirapine) decrease the efficacy of **ulipristal**. Avoid and for 4 weeks after stopping the enzyme inducing drug. For FSRH guidance, see Contraceptives, interactions p. 917. Severe Anecdotal

▶ NNRTIs (etravirine) might decrease the efficacy of **ulipristal**. Avoid and for 4 weeks after stopping the enzyme inducing drug. For FSRH guidance, see Contraceptives, interactions p. 917. Severe Theoretical

▶ Norethisterone might decrease the efficacy of **ulipristal** and **ulipristal** might decrease the efficacy of norethisterone. Avoid or use additional contraceptive precautions. Severe Theoretical

▶ Proton pump inhibitors might decrease the efficacy of **ulipristal** for emergency hormonal contraception. For FSRH guidance, see Contraceptives, interactions p. 917. Unknown Theoretical

▶ Rifamycins decrease the efficacy of **ulipristal**. Avoid and for 4 weeks after stopping the enzyme inducing drug. For FSRH guidance, see Contraceptives, interactions p. 917. Severe Anecdotal

▶ St John's wort is predicted to decrease the efficacy of **ulipristal**. For FSRH guidance, see Contraceptives, interactions p. 917. Severe Anecdotal

Umeclidinium → see TABLE 9 p. 1573 (antimuscarinics)

▶ Antipsychotics, second generation (clozapine) can cause constipation, as can **umeclidinium**; concurrent use might increase the risk of developing intestinal obstruction. Severe Theoretical → Also see TABLE 9 p. 1573

Upadacitinib

▶ Anti-androgens (apalutamide, enzalutamide) are predicted to decrease the exposure to **upadacitinib**. Moderate Study

▶ Antiepileptics (carbamazepine, fosphenytoin, phenobarbital, phenytoin, primidone) are predicted to decrease the exposure to **upadacitinib**. Moderate Study

▶ Antifungals, azoles (itraconazole, ketoconazole, posaconazole, voriconazole) are predicted to increase the exposure to **upadacitinib**. Manufacturer advises caution or avoid, or adjust **upadacitinib** dose depending on indication, p. 1267. Severe Study

▶ Ceritinib is predicted to increase the exposure to **upadacitinib**. Manufacturer advises caution or avoid, or adjust **upadacitinib** dose depending on indication, p. 1267. Severe Study

▶ Cobicistat is predicted to increase the exposure to **upadacitinib**. Manufacturer advises caution or avoid, or adjust **upadacitinib** dose depending on indication, p. 1267. Severe Study

▶ Encorafenib is predicted to decrease the exposure to **upadacitinib**. Moderate Study

▶ Filgotinib is predicted to increase the risk of immunosuppression when given with **upadacitinib**. Avoid. Severe Theoretical

▶ Grapefruit is predicted to increase the exposure to **upadacitinib**. Avoid. Moderate Theoretical

▶ HIV-protease inhibitors are predicted to increase the exposure to **upadacitinib**. Manufacturer advises caution or avoid, or adjust **upadacitinib** dose depending on indication, p. 1267. Severe Study

▶ Idelalisib is predicted to increase the exposure to **upadacitinib**. Manufacturer advises caution or avoid, or adjust **upadacitinib** dose depending on indication, p. 1267. Severe Study

▶ Ivosidenib is predicted to decrease the exposure to **upadacitinib**. Moderate Study

▶ Live vaccines are predicted to increase the risk of generalised infection (possibly life-threatening) when given with **upadacitinib**. Avoid. Severe Theoretical

Upadacitinib (continued)
- ▶ Lumacaftor is predicted to decrease the exposure to **upadacitinib**. Moderate Study
- ▶ Macrolides (clarithromycin) are predicted to increase the exposure to **upadacitinib**. Manufacturer advises caution or avoid, or adjust **upadacitinib** dose depending on indication, p. 1267. Severe Study
- ▶ Mitotane is predicted to decrease the exposure to **upadacitinib**. Moderate Study
- ▶ Nirmatrelvir boosted with ritonavir is predicted to increase the concentration of **upadacitinib**. Adjust dose. Severe Theoretical
- ▶ Rifamycins (rifampicin) are predicted to decrease the exposure to **upadacitinib**. Moderate Study
- ▶ Tucatinib is predicted to increase the exposure to **upadacitinib**. Manufacturer advises caution or avoid, or adjust **upadacitinib** dose depending on indication, p. 1267. Severe Study

Urokinase → see TABLE 3 p. 1571 (anticoagulant effects)

Ursodeoxycholic acid
- ▶ Oral antacids are predicted to decrease the absorption of oral **ursodeoxycholic acid**. Separate administration by 2 hours. Moderate Theoretical
- ▶ **Ursodeoxycholic acid** affects the concentration of ciclosporin. Use with caution and adjust dose. Severe Anecdotal
- ▶ Fibrates are predicted to decrease the efficacy of **ursodeoxycholic acid**. Avoid. Severe Theoretical

Ustekinumab → see monoclonal antibodies

Vaborbactam
- ▶ **Vaborbactam** is predicted to increase the concentration of beta blockers, selective (metoprolol). Unknown Theoretical
- ▶ **Vaborbactam** is predicted to increase the concentration of SNRIs (venlafaxine). Unknown Theoretical

Vadadustat
- ▶ Oral aluminium hydroxide is predicted to decrease the exposure to oral **vadadustat**. Manufacturer advises take 1 hour before or 2 hours after aluminium-containing products. Moderate Theoretical
- ▶ **Vadadustat** is predicted to increase the exposure to angiotensin-II receptor antagonists (olmesartan). Monitor and adjust dose. Moderate Study
- ▶ **Vadadustat** is predicted to increase the exposure to baricitinib. Monitor and adjust dose. Moderate Study
- ▶ Oral calcium salts (calcium acetate) decrease the exposure to oral **vadadustat**. Manufacturer advises take 1 hour before or 2 hours after calcium acetate. Moderate Study
- ▶ Oral calcium salts (calcium carbonate) are predicted to decrease the exposure to oral **vadadustat**. Manufacturer advises take 1 hour before or 2 hours after calcium carbonate. Moderate Theoretical
- ▶ **Vadadustat** is predicted to increase the exposure to cephalosporins (cefaclor). Monitor and adjust dose. Moderate Study
- ▶ **Vadadustat** is predicted to increase the exposure to dipeptidylpeptidase-4 inhibitors (sitagliptin). Monitor and adjust dose. Moderate Study
- ▶ **Vadadustat** is predicted to increase the exposure to ganciclovir. Monitor and adjust dose. Moderate Study
- ▶ **Vadadustat** is predicted to increase the exposure to H_2 receptor antagonists (famotidine). Monitor and adjust dose. Moderate Study
- ▶ Oral iron decreases the exposure to oral **vadadustat**. Manufacturer advises take 1 hour before **vadadustat**. Moderate Study
- ▶ Oral lanthanum is predicted to decrease the exposure to oral **vadadustat**. Manufacturer advises take 1 hour before or 2 hours after lanthanum. Moderate Theoretical
- ▶ Leflunomide is predicted to increase the exposure to **vadadustat**. Moderate Study
- ▶ **Vadadustat** increases the exposure to loop diuretics (furosemide). Monitor and adjust dose. Moderate Study
- ▶ Oral magnesium is predicted to decrease the exposure to oral **vadadustat**. Manufacturer advises take 1 hour before or 2 hours after magnesium. Moderate Theoretical
- ▶ **Vadadustat** is predicted to increase the exposure to methotrexate. Monitor and adjust dose. Moderate Study

- ▶ **Vadadustat** is predicted to increase the exposure to NRTIs (zidovudine). Monitor and adjust dose. Moderate Study
- ▶ **Vadadustat** is predicted to increase the exposure to the active metabolite of oseltamivir. Monitor and adjust dose. Moderate Study
- ▶ Penicillins (benzylpenicillin) are predicted to increase the exposure to **vadadustat** and **vadadustat** is predicted to increase the exposure to penicillins (benzylpenicillin). Moderate Study
- ▶ **Vadadustat** is predicted to increase the exposure to quinolones (ciprofloxacin). Monitor and adjust dose. Moderate Study
- ▶ Oral sevelamer decreases the exposure to oral **vadadustat**. Manufacturer advises take 1 hour before or 2 hours after sevelamer. Moderate Study
- ▶ **Vadadustat** is predicted to increase the exposure to statins (atorvastatin, fluvastatin, rosuvastatin). Monitor and adjust dose. Moderate Study
- ▶ **Vadadustat** increases the exposure to statins (simvastatin). Monitor and adjust dose. Moderate Study
- ▶ **Vadadustat** is predicted to increase the exposure to sulfasalazine. Monitor and adjust dose. Moderate Study
- ▶ **Vadadustat** is predicted to increase the exposure to tenofovir alafenamide. Monitor and adjust dose. Moderate Study
- ▶ **Vadadustat** is predicted to increase the exposure to tenofovir disoproxil. Monitor and adjust dose. Moderate Study
- ▶ Teriflunomide is predicted to increase the exposure to **vadadustat**. Moderate Study
- ▶ **Vadadustat** is predicted to increase the exposure to topotecan. Monitor and adjust dose. Moderate Study

Valaciclovir → see TABLE 2 p. 1571 (nephrotoxicity)
- ▶ **Valaciclovir** is predicted to increase the exposure to aminophylline. Severe Anecdotal
- ▶ Mycophenolate is predicted to increase the risk of haematological toxicity when given with **valaciclovir**. Moderate Theoretical
- ▶ **Valaciclovir** is predicted to increase the exposure to theophylline. Severe Theoretical

Valganciclovir → see TABLE 14 p. 1575 (myelosuppression), TABLE 2 p. 1571 (nephrotoxicity)
- ▶ **Valganciclovir** is predicted to increase the risk of seizures when given with carbapenems (imipenem). Avoid. Severe Anecdotal
- ▶ Maribavir might decrease the efficacy of **valganciclovir**. Avoid. Severe Theoretical
- ▶ Mycophenolate is predicted to increase the risk of haematological toxicity when given with **valganciclovir**. Moderate Theoretical

Valproate → see antiepileptics

Valsartan → see angiotensin-II receptor antagonists

Vamorolone → see corticosteroids

Vancomycin → see TABLE 2 p. 1571 (nephrotoxicity), TABLE 18 p. 1576 (ototoxicity)

Vandetanib → see TABLE 8 p. 1573 (QT-interval prolongation)
- ▶ Anti-androgens (apalutamide, enzalutamide) are predicted to decrease the exposure to **vandetanib**. Avoid. Moderate Study → Also see TABLE 8 p. 1573
- ▶ Antiepileptics (carbamazepine, fosphenytoin, phenobarbital, phenytoin, primidone) are predicted to decrease the exposure to **vandetanib**. Avoid. Moderate Study
- ▶ Dabrafenib is predicted to decrease the exposure to **vandetanib**. Moderate Study
- ▶ **Vandetanib** very slightly increases the exposure to digoxin. Moderate Study
- ▶ **Vandetanib** is predicted to increase the exposure to dopamine receptor agonists (pramipexole). Adjust dose. Moderate Study
- ▶ Encorafenib is predicted to decrease the exposure to **vandetanib**. Avoid. Moderate Study → Also see TABLE 8 p. 1573
- ▶ Endothelin receptor antagonists (bosentan) are predicted to decrease the exposure to **vandetanib**. Moderate Study
- ▶ **Vandetanib** is predicted to increase the exposure to erlotinib. Moderate Theoretical
- ▶ **Vandetanib** is predicted to increase the exposure to factor XA inhibitors (apixaban). Moderate Theoretical
- ▶ **Vandetanib** is predicted to increase the exposure to gilteritinib. Moderate Theoretical

▸ **Vandetanib** is predicted to increase the exposure to idelalisib. Moderate Theoretical

▸ Ivosidenib is predicted to decrease the exposure to **vandetanib**. Avoid. Moderate Study → Also see TABLE 8 p. 1573

▸ Lumacaftor is predicted to decrease the exposure to **vandetanib**. Avoid. Moderate Study

▸ **Vandetanib** is predicted to increase the exposure to metformin. Use with caution and adjust dose. Moderate Study

▸ Mitotane is predicted to decrease the exposure to **vandetanib**. Avoid. Moderate Study

▸ NNRTIs (efavirenz, etravirine, nevirapine) are predicted to decrease the exposure to **vandetanib**. Moderate Study → Also see TABLE 8 p. 1573

▸ Rifamycins (rifampicin) are predicted to decrease the exposure to **vandetanib**. Avoid. Moderate Study

▸ **Vandetanib** is predicted to increase the exposure to the active component of sacituzumab govitecan. Severe Theoretical

▸ St John's wort is predicted to decrease the exposure to **vandetanib**. Avoid. Severe Study

▸ **Vandetanib** might increase the exposure to tigecycline. Mild Anecdotal

▸ **Vandetanib** might increase the exposure to vinca alkaloids. Severe Theoretical

Vardenafil → see phosphodiesterase type-5 inhibitors

Varicella-zoster immunoglobulin → see immunoglobulins

Varicella-zoster vaccine → see live vaccines

Vasopressin

▸ ACE inhibitors (enalapril) might enhance the antidiuretic and hypertensive effects of **vasopressin**. Moderate Theoretical

▸ Alcohol might decrease the antidiuretic effect of **vasopressin**. Moderate Theoretical

▸ Alkylating agents (cyclophosphamide, ifosfamide) might enhance the antidiuretic and hypertensive effects of **vasopressin**. Moderate Theoretical

▸ Antiepileptics (carbamazepine) might enhance the antidiuretic effect of **vasopressin**. Moderate Theoretical

▸ Antipsychotics, second generation (clozapine) might decrease the antidiuretic and hypertensive effects of **vasopressin**. Moderate Theoretical

▸ Corticosteroids (fludrocortisone) might enhance the antidiuretic effect of **vasopressin**. Moderate Theoretical

▸ Foscarnet might decrease the antidiuretic and hypertensive effects of **vasopressin**. Moderate Theoretical

▸ Haloperidol might enhance the antidiuretic and hypertensive effects of **vasopressin**. Moderate Theoretical

▸ Heparin might decrease the antidiuretic effect of **vasopressin**. Moderate Theoretical

▸ Lithium might decrease the antidiuretic and hypertensive effects of **vasopressin**. Moderate Theoretical

▸ Methyldopa might enhance the antidiuretic and hypertensive effects of **vasopressin**. Moderate Theoretical

▸ NSAIDs (indometacin) might prolong the antidiuretic effect of **vasopressin**. Moderate Study

▸ Pentamidine might enhance the antidiuretic and hypertensive effects of **vasopressin**. Moderate Theoretical

▸ SSRIs might enhance the antidiuretic and hypertensive effects of **vasopressin**. Moderate Theoretical

▸ Sympathomimetics, vasoconstrictor (adrenaline/epinephrine) might increase the hypertensive effect of **vasopressin**. Moderate Theoretical

▸ Sympathomimetics, vasoconstrictor (noradrenaline/norepinephrine) might affect the hypertensive effect of **vasopressin**. Moderate Theoretical

▸ Tetracyclines (demeclocycline) might decrease the antidiuretic and hypertensive effects of **vasopressin**. Moderate Theoretical

▸ Tricyclic antidepressants might enhance the antidiuretic and hypertensive effects of **vasopressin**. Moderate Theoretical

▸ Vinca alkaloids (vincristine) might enhance the antidiuretic and hypertensive effects of **vasopressin**. Moderate Theoretical

Vecuronium → see neuromuscular blocking drugs, non-depolarising

Vedolizumab → see monoclonal antibodies

Velpatasvir

▸ **Velpatasvir** is predicted to increase the exposure to afatinib. Moderate Study

▸ **Velpatasvir** is predicted to increase the exposure to aliskiren. Severe Theoretical

▸ **Velpatasvir** is predicted to increase the exposure to alpelisib. Moderate Theoretical

▸ Oral antacids are predicted to decrease the concentration of oral **velpatasvir**. Separate administration by 4 hours. Moderate Theoretical

▸ Anti-androgens (apalutamide, enzalutamide) are predicted to moderately decrease the exposure to **velpatasvir**. Avoid. Severe Study

▸ Antiarrhythmics (amiodarone) are predicted to increase the concentration of **velpatasvir**. Avoid or monitor. Moderate Theoretical

▸ Antiepileptics (carbamazepine, fosphenytoin, phenobarbital, phenytoin, primidone) are predicted to moderately decrease the exposure to **velpatasvir**. Avoid. Severe Study

▸ Antiepileptics (oxcarbazepine) are predicted to decrease the exposure to **velpatasvir**. Avoid. Severe Theoretical

▸ **Velpatasvir** is predicted to increase the exposure to antihistamines, non-sedating (fexofenadine). Severe Theoretical

▸ **Velpatasvir** is predicted to increase the exposure to bictegravir. Use with caution or avoid. Moderate Theoretical

▸ Oral calcium salts (calcium carbonate) -containing antacids are predicted to decrease the concentration of oral **velpatasvir**. Separate administration by 4 hours. Moderate Theoretical

▸ Cenobamate is predicted to decrease the exposure to **velpatasvir**. Avoid. Moderate Theoretical

▸ **Velpatasvir** is predicted to increase the exposure to cladribine. Avoid or adjust dose. Moderate Theoretical

▸ **Velpatasvir** is predicted to increase the exposure to colchicine. Severe Theoretical

▸ Dabrafenib is predicted to decrease the exposure to **velpatasvir**. Avoid. Moderate Theoretical

▸ **Velpatasvir** is predicted to increase the exposure to digoxin. Severe Study

▸ Encorafenib is predicted to moderately decrease the exposure to **velpatasvir**. Avoid. Severe Study

▸ Endothelin receptor antagonists (bosentan) are predicted to decrease the exposure to **velpatasvir**. Avoid. Moderate Theoretical

▸ **Velpatasvir** is predicted to increase the exposure to everolimus. Severe Theoretical

▸ **Velpatasvir** is predicted to increase the exposure to factor XA inhibitors (edoxaban). Severe Theoretical

▸ **Velpatasvir** is predicted to increase the exposure to fidaxomicin. Avoid. Moderate Study

▸ H₂ receptor antagonists are predicted to decrease the concentration of **velpatasvir**. Adjust dose, see sofosbuvir with velpatasvir p. 725. Moderate Study

▸ Ivosidenib is predicted to moderately decrease the exposure to **velpatasvir**. Avoid. Severe Study

▸ **Velpatasvir** is predicted to increase the exposure to loperamide. Severe Theoretical

▸ Lorlatinib is predicted to decrease the exposure to **velpatasvir**. Avoid. Moderate Theoretical

▸ Lumacaftor is predicted to moderately decrease the exposure to **velpatasvir**. Avoid. Severe Study

▸ **Velpatasvir** is predicted to increase the exposure to meglitinides (repaglinide). Moderate Study

▸ Mitotane is predicted to moderately decrease the exposure to **velpatasvir**. Avoid. Severe Study

▸ Modafinil is predicted to decrease the exposure to **velpatasvir**. Avoid. Severe Theoretical

▸ **Velpatasvir** is predicted to increase the exposure to momelotinib. Moderate Study

▸ **Velpatasvir** is predicted to increase the risk of neutropenia when given with monoclonal antibodies (brentuximab vedotin). Monitor and adjust dose. Severe Theoretical

▸ **Velpatasvir** is predicted to increase the exposure to neratinib. Avoid or adjust dose and monitor for gastrointestinal adverse effects—consult product literature. Severe Study

▸ **Velpatasvir** is predicted to increase the exposure to nintedanib. Moderate Study

Velpatasvir (continued)

▸ NNRTIs (efavirenz, etravirine, nevirapine) are predicted to decrease the exposure to **velpatasvir**. Avoid. Moderate Theoretical

▸ **Velpatasvir** is predicted to increase the exposure to pralsetinib. Moderate Theoretical

▸ Proton pump inhibitors are predicted to decrease the concentration of **velpatasvir**. Adjust dose, see sofosbuvir with velpatasvir p. 725. Moderate Study

▸ **Velpatasvir** is predicted to increase the exposure to relugolix. Avoid or take relugolix first and separate administration by at least 6 hours. Moderate Study

▸ Rifamycins (rifampicin) are predicted to moderately decrease the exposure to **velpatasvir**. Avoid. Severe Study

▸ **Velpatasvir** is predicted to increase the exposure to rimegepant. Avoid another dose of rimegepant within 48 hours of concurrent use. Moderate Theoretical

▸ **Velpatasvir** is predicted to increase the exposure to sirolimus. Severe Theoretical

▸ Sotorasib is predicted to decrease the exposure to **velpatasvir**. Avoid. Moderate Theoretical

▸ St John's wort is predicted to decrease the exposure to **velpatasvir**. Avoid. Moderate Theoretical

▸ **Velpatasvir** with sofosbuvir slightly increases the exposure to statins (atorvastatin). Severe Study

▸ **Velpatasvir** with sofosbuvir is predicted to increase the exposure to statins (fluvastatin, simvastatin). Monitor adverse effects and adjust dose. Severe Theoretical

▸ **Velpatasvir** moderately increases the exposure to statins (rosuvastatin). Avoid or adjust **rosuvastatin** dose, p. 235. Severe Study

▸ **Velpatasvir** is predicted to increase the exposure to sulfasalazine. Moderate Theoretical

▸ **Velpatasvir** is predicted to increase the exposure to sulfonylureas (glibenclamide). Moderate Study

▸ **Velpatasvir** is predicted to slightly increase the exposure to talazoparib. Avoid or adjust dose—consult product literature. Severe Study

▸ **Velpatasvir** is predicted to increase the exposure to taxanes (docetaxel). Moderate Study

▸ **Velpatasvir** is predicted to increase the exposure to taxanes (paclitaxel). Severe Theoretical

▸ **Velpatasvir** is predicted to increase the exposure to tenofovir alafenamide. Moderate Theoretical

▸ **Velpatasvir** is predicted to increase the exposure to tenofovir disoproxil. Moderate Theoretical

▸ **Velpatasvir** increases the exposure to thrombin inhibitors (dabigatran). Avoid. Severe Study

▸ **Velpatasvir** is predicted to increase the exposure to topotecan. Severe Study

▸ **Velpatasvir** is predicted to increase the concentration of trametinib. Moderate Theoretical

Vemurafenib → see TABLE 8 p. 1573 (QT-interval prolongation)

▸ **Vemurafenib** is predicted to increase the exposure to afatinib. Moderate Study

▸ **Vemurafenib** is predicted to increase the exposure to agomelatine. Moderate Study

▸ **Vemurafenib** is predicted to increase the exposure to aliskiren. Use with caution and adjust dose. Moderate Theoretical

▸ **Vemurafenib** is predicted to increase the exposure to aminophylline. Adjust dose. Moderate Theoretical

▸ **Vemurafenib** is predicted to increase the exposure to anaesthetics, local (ropivacaine). Moderate Theoretical

▸ **Vemurafenib** is predicted to increase the exposure to anagrelide. Moderate Theoretical → Also see TABLE 8 p. 1573

▸ Anti-androgens (apalutamide, enzalutamide) are predicted to decrease the exposure to **vemurafenib**. Avoid. Severe Study → Also see TABLE 8 p. 1573

▸ Antiarrhythmics (dronedarone) are predicted to increase the exposure to **vemurafenib**. Severe Theoretical → Also see TABLE 8 p. 1573

▸ Antiepileptics (carbamazepine, fosphenytoin, phenobarbital, phenytoin, primidone) are predicted to decrease the exposure to **vemurafenib**. Avoid. Severe Study

▸ Antifungals, azoles (fluconazole, isavuconazole, itraconazole, ketoconazole, posaconazole, voriconazole) are predicted to increase the exposure to **vemurafenib**. Severe Theoretical → Also see TABLE 8 p. 1573

▸ **Vemurafenib** is predicted to increase the exposure to antihistamines, non-sedating (fexofenadine). Use with caution and adjust dose. Severe Theoretical

▸ **Vemurafenib** increases the concentration of antipsychotics, second generation (clozapine). Monitor adverse effects and adjust dose. Severe Study

▸ **Vemurafenib** is predicted to increase the exposure to antipsychotics, second generation (olanzapine). Adjust dose. Moderate Anecdotal

▸ **Vemurafenib** slightly to moderately decreases the exposure to benzodiazepines (midazolam). Moderate Study

▸ Berotralstat is predicted to increase the exposure to **vemurafenib**. Severe Theoretical

▸ **Vemurafenib** is predicted to increase the exposure to beta blockers, non-selective (nadolol). Moderate Study

▸ **Vemurafenib** is predicted to increase the exposure to bictegravir. Use with caution or avoid. Moderate Theoretical

▸ **Vemurafenib** is predicted to decrease the concentration of bupropion. Moderate Theoretical

▸ Calcium channel blockers (diltiazem, verapamil) are predicted to increase the exposure to **vemurafenib**. Severe Theoretical

▸ Ceritinib is predicted to increase the exposure to **vemurafenib**. Severe Theoretical → Also see TABLE 8 p. 1573

▸ Ciclosporin might affect the exposure to **vemurafenib**. Severe Theoretical

▸ Cobicistat is predicted to increase the exposure to **vemurafenib**. Severe Theoretical

▸ **Vemurafenib** is predicted to increase the exposure to colchicine. Avoid P-glycoprotein inhibitors or adjust **colchicine** dose, p. 1279. Severe Theoretical

▸ **Vemurafenib** might decrease the efficacy of combined hormonal contraceptives. Use additional contraceptive precautions. Severe Theoretical

▸ **Vemurafenib** is predicted to increase the exposure to coumarins. Moderate Study

▸ Crizotinib is predicted to increase the exposure to **vemurafenib**. Severe Theoretical → Also see TABLE 8 p. 1573

▸ Dabrafenib is predicted to decrease the exposure to **vemurafenib**. Severe Study

▸ **Vemurafenib** slightly increases the exposure to digoxin. Use with caution and adjust dose. Severe Study

▸ **Vemurafenib** is predicted to increase the exposure to dipeptidylpeptidase-4 inhibitors (sitagliptin). Use with caution or avoid. Moderate Theoretical

▸ **Vemurafenib** is predicted to increase the exposure to dopamine receptor agonists (ropinirole). Adjust dose. Moderate Study

▸ Encorafenib is predicted to decrease the exposure to **vemurafenib**. Avoid. Severe Study → Also see TABLE 8 p. 1573

▸ Endothelin receptor antagonists (bosentan) are predicted to decrease the exposure to **vemurafenib**. Severe Study

▸ **Vemurafenib** is predicted to increase the exposure to endothelin receptor antagonists (ambrisentan). Use with caution or avoid. Moderate Theoretical

▸ **Vemurafenib** are predicted to increases the exposure to erlotinib. Monitor adverse effects and adjust dose. Moderate Study

▸ **Vemurafenib** is predicted to increase the exposure to everolimus. Use with caution and adjust dose. Severe Theoretical

▸ **Vemurafenib** is predicted to increase the exposure to factor XA inhibitors (apixaban). Moderate Theoretical

▸ **Vemurafenib** is predicted to slightly increase the exposure to factor XA inhibitors (edoxaban). Severe Theoretical

▸ Fedratinib is predicted to increase the exposure to **vemurafenib**. Severe Theoretical

▸ **Vemurafenib** is predicted to increase the exposure to fezolinetant. Avoid. Moderate Study

▸ **Vemurafenib** is predicted to increase the exposure to fidaxomicin. Avoid. Moderate Study

▸ Gefitinib might affect the exposure to **vemurafenib**. Moderate Theoretical

‣ **Vemurafenib** is predicted to increase the exposure to gilteritinib. Moderate Theoretical
‣ **HIV-protease inhibitors** are predicted to increase the exposure to **vemurafenib**. Severe Theoretical
‣ **Idelalisib** is predicted to increase the exposure to **vemurafenib**. Severe Theoretical
‣ **Imatinib** is predicted to increase the exposure to **vemurafenib**. Severe Theoretical
‣ **Ivosidenib** is predicted to decrease the exposure to **vemurafenib**. Avoid. Severe Study → Also see **TABLE 8** p. 1573
‣ **Letermovir** is predicted to increase the exposure to **vemurafenib**. Severe Theoretical
‣ **Vemurafenib** might increase the exposure to loperamide. Use with caution and adjust dose. Moderate Theoretical
‣ **Vemurafenib** is predicted to increase the exposure to loxapine. Avoid. Unknown Theoretical
‣ **Lumacaftor** is predicted to decrease the exposure to **vemurafenib**. Avoid. Severe Study
‣ **Macrolides (clarithromycin, erythromycin)** are predicted to increase the exposure to **vemurafenib**. Severe Theoretical → Also see **TABLE 8** p. 1573
‣ **Vemurafenib** slightly increases the exposure to MAO-B inhibitors (rasagiline). Moderate Study
‣ **Vemurafenib** is predicted to increase the exposure to maraviroc. Use with caution or avoid. Moderate Theoretical
‣ **Vemurafenib** is predicted to increase the exposure to melatonin. Moderate Theoretical
‣ **Mitotane** is predicted to decrease the exposure to **vemurafenib**. Avoid. Severe Study
‣ **Monoclonal antibodies (ipilimumab)** might increase the risk of hepatotoxicity when given with **vemurafenib**. Avoid. Severe Study
‣ **Vemurafenib** increases the risk of neutropenia when given with monoclonal antibodies (brentuximab vedotin). Monitor and adjust dose. Severe Theoretical
‣ **Vemurafenib** is predicted to increase the exposure to naldemedine. Moderate Study
‣ **Vemurafenib** is predicted to increase the exposure to neratinib. Avoid or adjust dose and monitor for gastrointestinal adverse effects—consult product literature. Severe Study
‣ **Neurokinin-1 receptor antagonists (aprepitant, netupitant)** are predicted to increase the exposure to **vemurafenib**. Severe Theoretical
‣ **Nilotinib** is predicted to increase the exposure to **vemurafenib**. Severe Theoretical → Also see **TABLE 8** p. 1573
‣ **Vemurafenib** is predicted to increase the exposure to nintedanib. Moderate Study
‣ **NNRTIs (efavirenz, etravirine, nevirapine)** are predicted to decrease the exposure to **vemurafenib**. Severe Study → Also see **TABLE 8** p. 1573
‣ **Vemurafenib** is predicted to increase the exposure to panobinostat. Adjust dose. Moderate Theoretical → Also see **TABLE 8** p. 1573
‣ **Vemurafenib** is predicted to increase the exposure to phenindione. Moderate Study
‣ **Vemurafenib** is predicted to increase the exposure to phenothiazines (chlorpromazine). Moderate Theoretical → Also see **TABLE 8** p. 1573
‣ **Vemurafenib** is predicted to increase the exposure to phosphodiesterase type-4 inhibitors (roflumilast). Moderate Theoretical
‣ **Vemurafenib** is predicted to increase the exposure to pibrentasvir. Moderate Theoretical
‣ **Vemurafenib** is predicted to increase the exposure to pirfenidone. Use with caution and adjust dose. Moderate Study
‣ **Vemurafenib** is predicted to increase the exposure to pralsetinib. Moderate Theoretical
‣ **Vemurafenib** might increase the exposure to ranolazine. Use with caution or avoid. Moderate Theoretical → Also see **TABLE 8** p. 1573
‣ **Vemurafenib** is predicted to increase the exposure to relugolix. Avoid or take relugolix first and separate administration by at least 6 hours. Moderate Study
‣ **Rifamycins (rifampicin)** are predicted to decrease the exposure to **vemurafenib**. Avoid. Severe Study

‣ **Vemurafenib** is predicted to increase the exposure to riluzole. Moderate Theoretical
‣ **Vemurafenib** is predicted to increase the exposure to rimegepant. Avoid another dose of rimegepant within 48 hours of concurrent use. Moderate Theoretical
‣ **Vemurafenib** is predicted to increase the exposure to sirolimus. Use with caution and adjust dose. Severe Theoretical
‣ **Vemurafenib** is predicted to increase the exposure to SNRIs (duloxetine). Use with caution or avoid. Moderate Theoretical
‣ **St John's wort** is predicted to decrease the exposure to **vemurafenib**. Avoid. Severe Study
‣ **Vemurafenib** is predicted to slightly increase the exposure to talazoparib. Avoid or adjust dose—consult product literature. Severe Study
‣ **Vemurafenib** is predicted to increase the exposure to taxanes (paclitaxel). Use with caution and adjust dose. Severe Theoretical
‣ **Vemurafenib** is predicted to increase the exposure to theophylline. Monitor and adjust dose. Moderate Theoretical
‣ **Vemurafenib** is predicted to increase the exposure to thrombin inhibitors (dabigatran). Monitor and adjust dose. Severe Theoretical
‣ **Vemurafenib** is predicted to increase the exposure to ticagrelor. Use with caution or avoid. Severe Study
‣ **Vemurafenib** might increase the exposure to tigecycline. Mild Anecdotal
‣ **Vemurafenib** increases the exposure to tizanidine. Avoid. Moderate Study
‣ **Vemurafenib** is predicted to increase the exposure to topotecan. Severe Study
‣ **Vemurafenib** is predicted to increase the concentration of trametinib. Moderate Theoretical
‣ **Vemurafenib** is predicted to increase the exposure to triptans (zolmitriptan). Adjust **zolmitriptan** dose, p. 546. Moderate Theoretical
‣ **Tucatinib** is predicted to increase the exposure to **vemurafenib**. Severe Theoretical
‣ **Vemurafenib** is predicted to increase the exposure to venetoclax. Avoid or monitor for toxicity. Severe Theoretical
‣ **Vemurafenib** might increase the exposure to vinca alkaloids. Severe Theoretical

Venetoclax

FOOD AND LIFESTYLE Avoid bitter (Seville) orange and star fruit as they might increase the exposure to venetoclax.

‣ **Anti-androgens (apalutamide, enzalutamide)** are predicted to decrease the exposure to **venetoclax**. Avoid. Severe Study
‣ **Antiarrhythmics (amiodarone)** are predicted to increase the exposure to **venetoclax**. Avoid or monitor for toxicity. Severe Theoretical
‣ **Antiarrhythmics (dronedarone)** are predicted to increase the exposure to **venetoclax**. Avoid or adjust dose—consult product literature. Severe Study
‣ **Antiepileptics (carbamazepine, fosphenytoin, phenobarbital, phenytoin, primidone)** are predicted to decrease the exposure to **venetoclax**. Avoid. Severe Study
‣ **Antifungals, azoles (fluconazole, isavuconazole, itraconazole, ketoconazole, posaconazole, voriconazole)** are predicted to increase the exposure to **venetoclax**. Avoid or adjust dose—consult product literature. Severe Study
‣ **Venetoclax** is predicted to increase the exposure to antihistamines, non-sedating (fexofenadine). Moderate Theoretical
‣ **Berotralstat** is predicted to increase the exposure to **venetoclax**. Avoid or adjust dose—consult product literature. Severe Study
‣ **Calcium channel blockers (diltiazem, verapamil)** are predicted to increase the exposure to **venetoclax**. Avoid or adjust dose—consult product literature. Severe Study
‣ **Cenobamate** is predicted to decrease the exposure to **venetoclax**. Avoid. Severe Study
‣ **Ceritinib** is predicted to increase the exposure to **venetoclax**. Avoid or adjust dose—consult product literature. Severe Study
‣ **Ciclosporin** is predicted to increase the exposure to **venetoclax**. Avoid or monitor for toxicity. Severe Theoretical
‣ **Cobicistat** is predicted to increase the exposure to **venetoclax**. Avoid or adjust dose—consult product literature. Severe Study

Venetoclax (continued)

▸ **Venetoclax** is predicted to increase the exposure to colchicine. Avoid or adjust dose. [Severe] Study

▸ **Venetoclax** slightly increases the exposure to coumarins (warfarin). [Moderate] Study

▸ Crizotinib is predicted to increase the exposure to **venetoclax**. Avoid or adjust dose—consult product literature. [Severe] Study

▸ Dabrafenib is predicted to decrease the exposure to **venetoclax**. Avoid. [Severe] Study

▸ **Venetoclax** increases the exposure to digoxin. Avoid or adjust dose. [Severe] Study

▸ Eltrombopag is predicted to increase the exposure to **venetoclax**. Avoid or monitor for toxicity. [Severe] Theoretical

▸ Encorafenib is predicted to decrease the exposure to **venetoclax**. Avoid. [Severe] Study

▸ Endothelin receptor antagonists (bosentan) are predicted to decrease the exposure to **venetoclax**. Avoid. [Severe] Study

▸ **Venetoclax** is predicted to increase the exposure to endothelin receptor antagonists (bosentan). [Moderate] Theoretical

▸ **Venetoclax** is predicted to increase the exposure to everolimus. Avoid or adjust dose. [Severe] Study

▸ **Venetoclax** is predicted to increase the exposure to factor XA inhibitors (edoxaban, rivaroxaban). Avoid or adjust dose. [Severe] Study

▸ Fedratinib is predicted to increase the exposure to **venetoclax**. Avoid or adjust dose—consult product literature. [Severe] Study

▸ Grapefruit juice is predicted to increase the exposure to **venetoclax**. Avoid. [Severe] Theoretical

▸ HIV-protease inhibitors are predicted to increase the exposure to **venetoclax**. Avoid or adjust dose—consult product literature. [Severe] Study

▸ Idelalisib is predicted to increase the exposure to **venetoclax**. Avoid or adjust dose—consult product literature. [Severe] Study

▸ Imatinib is predicted to increase the exposure to **venetoclax**. Avoid or adjust dose—consult product literature. [Severe] Study

▸ Ivacaftor is predicted to increase the exposure to **venetoclax**. Avoid or monitor for toxicity. [Severe] Theoretical

▸ Ivosidenib is predicted to decrease the exposure to **venetoclax**. Avoid. [Severe] Study

▸ Lapatinib is predicted to increase the exposure to **venetoclax**. Avoid or monitor for toxicity. [Severe] Theoretical

▸ Leflunomide is predicted to increase the exposure to **venetoclax**. Avoid or monitor for toxicity. [Severe] Theoretical

▸ Letermovir is predicted to increase the exposure to **venetoclax**. Avoid or adjust dose—consult product literature. [Severe] Study

▸ **Venetoclax** potentially decreases the efficacy of live vaccines. Avoid. [Severe] Theoretical

▸ Lorlatinib is predicted to decrease the exposure to **venetoclax**. Avoid. [Severe] Study

▸ Lumacaftor is predicted to decrease the exposure to **venetoclax**. Avoid. [Severe] Study

▸ Macrolides (clarithromycin, erythromycin) are predicted to increase the exposure to **venetoclax**. Avoid or adjust dose—consult product literature. [Severe] Study

▸ **Venetoclax** is predicted to increase the exposure to meglitinides (repaglinide). [Moderate] Theoretical

▸ Mitotane is predicted to decrease the exposure to **venetoclax**. Avoid. [Severe] Study

▸ Neratinib is predicted to increase the exposure to **venetoclax**. Avoid or monitor for toxicity. [Severe] Theoretical

▸ Neurokinin-1 receptor antagonists (aprepitant, netupitant) are predicted to increase the exposure to **venetoclax**. Avoid or adjust dose—consult product literature. [Severe] Study

▸ Nilotinib is predicted to increase the exposure to **venetoclax**. Avoid or adjust dose—consult product literature. [Severe] Study

▸ Nirmatrelvir boosted with ritonavir is predicted to increase the concentration of **venetoclax**. Avoid or adjust dose—consult product literature. [Severe] Theoretical

▸ NNRTIs (efavirenz, etravirine, nevirapine) are predicted to decrease the exposure to **venetoclax**. Avoid. [Severe] Study

▸ Quinolones (ciprofloxacin) are predicted to increase the exposure to **venetoclax**. Avoid or adjust dose—consult product literature. [Severe] Theoretical

▸ Ranolazine is predicted to increase the exposure to **venetoclax**. Avoid or monitor for toxicity. [Severe] Theoretical

▸ Rifamycins (rifampicin) are predicted to decrease the exposure to **venetoclax**. Avoid. [Severe] Study

▸ **Venetoclax** is predicted to increase the exposure to sirolimus. Avoid or adjust dose. [Severe] Study

▸ Sotorasib is predicted to decrease the exposure to **venetoclax**. Avoid. [Severe] Study

▸ St John's wort is predicted to decrease the exposure to **venetoclax**. Avoid. [Severe] Study

▸ **Venetoclax** is predicted to increase the exposure to statins (atorvastatin). [Moderate] Study

▸ **Venetoclax** is predicted to increase the exposure to statins (fluvastatin, pravastatin, rosuvastatin, simvastatin). [Moderate] Theoretical

▸ **Venetoclax** is predicted to increase the exposure to sulfasalazine. [Moderate] Theoretical

▸ **Venetoclax** is predicted to increase the exposure to sulfonylureas (glibenclamide). [Moderate] Theoretical

▸ Teriflunomide is predicted to increase the exposure to **venetoclax**. Avoid or monitor for toxicity. [Severe] Theoretical

▸ **Venetoclax** is predicted to increase the exposure to thrombin inhibitors (dabigatran). Avoid or adjust dose. [Severe] Study

▸ **Venetoclax** is predicted to increase the exposure to topotecan. [Moderate] Theoretical

▸ Tucatinib is predicted to increase the exposure to **venetoclax**. Avoid or adjust dose—consult product literature. [Severe] Study

▸ Vemurafenib is predicted to increase the exposure to **venetoclax**. Avoid or monitor for toxicity. [Severe] Theoretical

Venlafaxine → see SNRIs

Verapamil → see calcium channel blockers

Vericiguat → see TABLE 7 p. 1572 (hypotension)

Vernakalant → see antiarrhythmics

Verteporfin

GENERAL INFORMATION Caution on concurrent use with other photosensitising drugs.

Vigabatrin → see antiepileptics

Vilanterol → see beta₂ agonists

Vildagliptin → see dipeptidylpeptidase-4 inhibitors

Vinblastine → see vinca alkaloids

Vinca alkaloids → see TABLE 17 p. 1576 (hyponatraemia), TABLE 14 p. 1575 (myelosuppression), TABLE 18 p. 1576 (ototoxicity), TABLE 11 p. 1574 (peripheral neuropathy)

vinblastine · vincristine · vindesine · vinorelbine

▸ Anti-androgens (apalutamide, enzalutamide) are predicted to decrease the exposure to **vinorelbine**. Use with caution or avoid. [Severe] Theoretical

▸ Anti-androgens (apalutamide, enzalutamide) are predicted to decrease the exposure to vinca alkaloids (vinblastine, vincristine, vindesine). [Severe] Theoretical

▸ Antiarrhythmics (amiodarone) might increase the exposure to **vinca alkaloids**. [Severe] Theoretical → Also see TABLE 11 p. 1574

▸ Antiarrhythmics (dronedarone) are predicted to increase the exposure to **vinca alkaloids**. [Severe] Theoretical

▸ Antiepileptics (carbamazepine, fosphenytoin, phenobarbital, phenytoin, primidone) are predicted to decrease the exposure to **vinorelbine**. Use with caution or avoid. [Severe] Theoretical → Also see TABLE 17 p. 1576 → Also see TABLE 11 p. 1574

▸ Antiepileptics (carbamazepine, fosphenytoin, phenobarbital, phenytoin, primidone) are predicted to decrease the exposure to vinca alkaloids (vinblastine, vincristine, vindesine). [Severe] Theoretical → Also see TABLE 17 p. 1576 → Also see TABLE 11 p. 1574

▸ Antifungals, azoles (fluconazole, isavuconazole, itraconazole, ketoconazole, posaconazole, voriconazole) are predicted to increase the exposure to **vinca alkaloids**. [Severe] Theoretical

▸ Antifungals, azoles (miconazole) are predicted to increase the concentration of **vinca alkaloids**. Use with caution and adjust dose. [Moderate] Theoretical

▸ Asparaginase potentially increases the risk of neurotoxicity when given with **vincristine**. **Vincristine** should be taken 3 to 24 hours before **asparaginase**. [Severe] Anecdotal → Also see TABLE 14 p. 1575

▸ Berotralstat is predicted to increase the exposure to **vinca alkaloids**. [Severe] Theoretical

▸ Calcium channel blockers (diltiazem, verapamil) are predicted to increase the exposure to **vinca alkaloids**. [Severe] Theoretical

▸ **Ceritinib** is predicted to increase the exposure to **vinca alkaloids**. [Severe] Theoretical → Also see **TABLE 14** p. 1575

▸ **Ciclosporin** might increase the exposure to **vinca alkaloids**. [Severe] Theoretical

▸ **Cobicistat** is predicted to increase the exposure to **vinca alkaloids**. [Severe] Theoretical

▸ **Crisantaspase** potentially increases the risk of neurotoxicity when given with **vincristine**. **Vincristine** should be taken 3 to 24 hours before **crisantaspase**. [Severe] Anecdotal → Also see **TABLE 14** p. 1575

▸ **Crizotinib** is predicted to increase the exposure to **vinca alkaloids**. [Severe] Theoretical

▸ **Encorafenib** is predicted to decrease the exposure to vinca alkaloids (**vinblastine, vincristine, vindesine**). [Severe] Theoretical

▸ **Encorafenib** is predicted to decrease the exposure to **vinorelbine**. Use with caution or avoid. [Severe] Theoretical

▸ **Fedratinib** is predicted to increase the exposure to **vinca alkaloids**. [Severe] Theoretical

▸ **HIV-protease inhibitors** are predicted to increase the exposure to **vinca alkaloids**. [Severe] Theoretical

▸ **Idelalisib** is predicted to increase the exposure to **vinca alkaloids**. [Severe] Theoretical

▸ **Imatinib** is predicted to increase the exposure to **vinca alkaloids**. [Severe] Theoretical → Also see **TABLE 14** p. 1575

▸ **Ivacaftor** might increase the exposure to **vinca alkaloids**. [Severe] Theoretical

▸ **Ivosidenib** is predicted to decrease the exposure to vinca alkaloids (**vinblastine, vincristine, vindesine**). [Severe] Theoretical

▸ **Ivosidenib** is predicted to decrease the exposure to **vinorelbine**. Use with caution or avoid. [Severe] Theoretical

▸ **Lapatinib** might increase the exposure to **vinca alkaloids**. [Severe] Theoretical

▸ **Letermovir** is predicted to increase the exposure to **vinca alkaloids**. [Severe] Theoretical

▸ **Live vaccines** are predicted to increase the risk of generalised infection (possibly life-threatening) when given with **vinca alkaloids**. UKHSA advises avoid (refer to Green Book). [Severe] Theoretical

▸ **Lumacaftor** is predicted to decrease the exposure to vinca alkaloids (**vinblastine, vincristine, vindesine**). [Severe] Theoretical

▸ **Lumacaftor** is predicted to decrease the exposure to **vinorelbine**. Use with caution or avoid. [Severe] Theoretical

▸ **Macrolides (azithromycin)** might increase the exposure to **vinca alkaloids**. [Severe] Theoretical

▸ **Macrolides (clarithromycin, erythromycin)** are predicted to increase the exposure to **vinca alkaloids**. [Severe] Theoretical

▸ **Mitotane** is predicted to decrease the exposure to vinca alkaloids (**vinblastine, vincristine, vindesine**). [Severe] Theoretical → Also see **TABLE 14** p. 1575

▸ **Mitotane** is predicted to decrease the exposure to **vinorelbine**. Use with caution or avoid. [Severe] Theoretical → Also see **TABLE 14** p. 1575

▸ **Neratinib** might increase the exposure to **vinca alkaloids**. [Severe] Theoretical

▸ **Neurokinin-1 receptor antagonists** are predicted to increase the exposure to **vinca alkaloids**. [Severe] Theoretical

▸ **Nilotinib** is predicted to increase the exposure to **vinca alkaloids**. [Severe] Theoretical → Also see **TABLE 14** p. 1575

▸ **Nirmatrelvir** boosted with ritonavir is predicted to increase the concentration of vinca alkaloids (**vinblastine, vincristine**). [Severe] Theoretical

▸ **Pegaspargase** potentially increases the risk of neurotoxicity when given with **vincristine**. **Vincristine** should be taken 3 to 24 hours before **pegaspargase**. [Severe] Anecdotal → Also see **TABLE 14** p. 1575

▸ **Ranolazine** might increase the exposure to **vinca alkaloids**. [Severe] Theoretical

▸ **Rifamycins (rifampicin)** are predicted to decrease the exposure to **vinorelbine**. Use with caution or avoid. [Severe] Theoretical

▸ **Rifamycins (rifampicin)** are predicted to decrease the exposure to vinca alkaloids (**vinblastine, vincristine, vindesine**). [Severe] Theoretical

▸ **Rucaparib** might increase the exposure to **vinca alkaloids**. [Severe] Theoretical → Also see **TABLE 14** p. 1575

▸ **St John's wort** is predicted to decrease the exposure to **vinca alkaloids**. [Severe] Theoretical

▸ **Tucatinib** is predicted to increase the exposure to **vinca alkaloids**. [Severe] Theoretical

▸ **Vandetanib** might increase the exposure to **vinca alkaloids**. [Severe] Theoretical

▸ **Vincristine** might enhance the antidiuretic and hypertensive effects of **vasopressin**. [Moderate] Theoretical

▸ **Vemurafenib** might increase the exposure to **vinca alkaloids**. [Severe] Theoretical

Vincristine → see vinca alkaloids

Vindesine → see vinca alkaloids

Vinorelbine → see vinca alkaloids

Vismodegib

▸ **Anti-androgens (apalutamide, enzalutamide)** are predicted to decrease the exposure to **vismodegib**. Avoid. [Moderate] Theoretical

▸ **Antiepileptics (carbamazepine, fosphenytoin, phenobarbital, phenytoin, primidone)** are predicted to decrease the exposure to **vismodegib**. Avoid. [Moderate] Theoretical

▸ **Encorafenib** is predicted to decrease the exposure to **vismodegib**. Avoid. [Moderate] Theoretical

▸ **Ivosidenib** is predicted to decrease the exposure to **vismodegib**. Avoid. [Moderate] Theoretical

▸ **Lumacaftor** is predicted to decrease the exposure to **vismodegib**. Avoid. [Moderate] Theoretical

▸ **Mitotane** is predicted to decrease the exposure to **vismodegib**. Avoid. [Moderate] Theoretical

▸ **Rifamycins (rifampicin)** are predicted to decrease the exposure to **vismodegib**. Avoid. [Moderate] Theoretical

▸ **St John's wort** is predicted to decrease the exposure to **vismodegib**. Avoid. [Moderate] Theoretical

Vitamin A → see **TABLE 1** p. 1571 (hepatotoxicity)

▸ **Retinoids (acitretin, alitretinoin, isotretinoin)** are predicted to increase the risk of vitamin A toxicity when given with **vitamin A**. Avoid. [Severe] Theoretical → Also see **TABLE 1** p. 1571

▸ **Retinoids (bexarotene)** are predicted to increase the risk of toxicity when given with **vitamin A**. Adjust dose. [Moderate] Theoretical → Also see **TABLE 1** p. 1571

▸ **Retinoids (tretinoin)** are predicted to increase the risk of vitamin A toxicity when given with **vitamin A**. Avoid. [Severe] Study

Vitamin D substances

alfacalcidol · calcifediol · calcipotriol · calcitriol · colecalciferol · ergocalciferol · paricalcitol · tacalcitol

ROUTE-SPECIFIC INFORMATION Since systemic absorption can follow topical application, the possibility of interactions with topical **calcitriol** should be borne in mind.

▸ **Antiepileptics (carbamazepine)** are predicted to decrease the effects of **vitamin D substances**. [Moderate] Study

▸ **Antiepileptics (fosphenytoin, phenytoin)** decrease the effects of **vitamin D substances**. [Moderate] Study

▸ **Antiepileptics (phenobarbital, primidone)** are predicted to decrease the effects of **vitamin D substances**. [Moderate] Theoretical

▸ **Antifungals, azoles (clotrimazole, ketoconazole)** are predicted to decrease the exposure to **colecalciferol**. [Moderate] Theoretical

▸ **Antifungals, azoles (itraconazole, ketoconazole, posaconazole, voriconazole)** are predicted to increase the exposure to **paricalcitol**. [Moderate] Study

▸ **Ceritinib** is predicted to increase the exposure to **paricalcitol**. [Moderate] Study

▸ **Cobicistat** is predicted to increase the exposure to **paricalcitol**. [Moderate] Study

▸ **Vitamin D substances** are predicted to increase the risk of toxicity when given with **digoxin**. [Severe] Theoretical

▸ **HIV-protease inhibitors** are predicted to increase the exposure to **paricalcitol**. [Moderate] Study

▸ **Idelalisib** is predicted to increase the exposure to **paricalcitol**. [Moderate] Study

▸ **Macrolides (clarithromycin)** are predicted to increase the exposure to **paricalcitol**. [Moderate] Study

▸ **Thiazide diuretics** increase the risk of hypercalcaemia when given with **vitamin D substances**. [Moderate] Theoretical

Vitamin D substances (continued)

▶ **Tucatinib** is predicted to increase the exposure to **paricalcitol**. Moderate Study

Vitamin E substances

▶ **Vitamin E substances** affect the exposure to ciclosporin. Moderate Study

▶ **Vitamin E substances** might increase the risk of bleeding when given with selumetinib. Avoid. Severe Theoretical

Voclosporin → see TABLE 2 p. 1571 (nephrotoxicity), TABLE 15 p. 1575 (increased serum potassium), TABLE 8 p. 1573 (QT-interval prolongation)

▶ Anti-androgens (apalutamide, enzalutamide) are predicted to decrease the exposure to **voclosporin**. Avoid. Severe Study → Also see TABLE 8 p. 1573

▶ Antiarrhythmics (dronedarone) are predicted to increase the exposure to **voclosporin**. Adjust **voclosporin** dose, p. 973. Severe Study → Also see TABLE 8 p. 1573

▶ Antiepileptics (carbamazepine, fosphenytoin, phenobarbital, phenytoin, primidone) are predicted to decrease the exposure to **voclosporin**. Avoid. Severe Study

▶ Antifungals, azoles (fluconazole, isavuconazole) are predicted to increase the exposure to **voclosporin**. Adjust **voclosporin** dose, p. 973. Severe Study → Also see TABLE 8 p. 1573

▶ Antifungals, azoles (itraconazole, ketoconazole, posaconazole, voriconazole) are predicted to increase the exposure to **voclosporin**. Avoid. Severe Study → Also see TABLE 8 p. 1573

▶ **Voclosporin** is predicted to increase the exposure to antihistamines, non-sedating (fexofenadine). Mild Theoretical

▶ **Berotralstat** is predicted to increase the exposure to **voclosporin**. Adjust **voclosporin** dose, p. 973. Severe Study

▶ Calcium channel blockers (diltiazem, verapamil) are predicted to increase the exposure to **voclosporin**. Adjust **voclosporin** dose, p. 973. Severe Study

▶ **Cenobamate** is predicted to decrease the exposure to **voclosporin**. Adjust dose. Moderate Theoretical

▶ **Ceritinib** is predicted to increase the exposure to **voclosporin**. Avoid. Severe Study → Also see TABLE 8 p. 1573

▶ **Cobicistat** is predicted to increase the exposure to **voclosporin**. Avoid. Severe Study

▶ **Crizotinib** is predicted to increase the exposure to **voclosporin**. Adjust **voclosporin** dose, p. 973. Severe Study → Also see TABLE 8 p. 1573

▶ **Dabrafenib** is predicted to decrease the exposure to **voclosporin**. Avoid. Severe Theoretical

▶ **Voclosporin** slightly increases the exposure to digoxin. Moderate Study

▶ **Encorafenib** is predicted to decrease the exposure to **voclosporin**. Avoid. Severe Study → Also see TABLE 8 p. 1573

▶ Endothelin receptor antagonists (bosentan) are predicted to decrease the exposure to **voclosporin** and **voclosporin** is predicted to increase the concentration of endothelin receptor antagonists (bosentan). Avoid. Severe Theoretical

▶ **Voclosporin** is predicted to increase the exposure to everolimus. Moderate Study

▶ **Fedratinib** is predicted to increase the exposure to **voclosporin**. Adjust **voclosporin** dose, p. 973. Severe Study

▶ **Voclosporin** is predicted to increase the exposure to gilteritinib. Moderate Theoretical

▶ **Grapefruit** and grapefruit juice are predicted to increase the exposure to **voclosporin**. Avoid. Moderate Theoretical

▶ **HIV-protease inhibitors** are predicted to increase the exposure to **voclosporin**. Avoid. Severe Study

▶ **Idelalisib** is predicted to increase the exposure to **voclosporin**. Avoid. Severe Study

▶ **Imatinib** is predicted to increase the exposure to **voclosporin**. Adjust **voclosporin** dose, p. 973. Severe Study

▶ **Ivosidenib** is predicted to decrease the exposure to **voclosporin**. Avoid. Severe Study → Also see TABLE 8 p. 1573

▶ **Letermovir** is predicted to increase the exposure to **voclosporin**. Adjust **voclosporin** dose, p. 973. Severe Study

▶ **Live vaccines** are predicted to increase the risk of generalised infection (possibly life-threatening) when given with **voclosporin**. UKHSA advises avoid (refer to Green Book). Severe Theoretical

▶ **Lumacaftor** is predicted to decrease the exposure to **voclosporin**. Avoid. Severe Study

▶ Macrolides (clarithromycin) are predicted to increase the exposure to **voclosporin**. Avoid. Severe Study

▶ Macrolides (erythromycin) are predicted to increase the exposure to **voclosporin**. Adjust **voclosporin** dose, p. 973. Severe Study → Also see TABLE 8 p. 1573

▶ **Voclosporin** is predicted to increase the concentration of meglitinides (repaglinide). Moderate Theoretical

▶ **Mitotane** is predicted to decrease the exposure to **voclosporin**. Avoid. Severe Study

▶ Neurokinin-1 receptor antagonists (aprepitant, netupitant) are predicted to increase the exposure to **voclosporin**. Adjust **voclosporin** dose, p. 973. Severe Study

▶ **Nilotinib** is predicted to increase the exposure to **voclosporin**. Adjust **voclosporin** dose, p. 973. Severe Study → Also see TABLE 8 p. 1573

▶ **Nirmatrelvir** boosted with ritonavir is predicted to increase the concentration of **voclosporin**. Avoid. Severe Theoretical

▶ NNRTIs (efavirenz, etravirine, nevirapine) are predicted to decrease the exposure to **voclosporin**. Avoid. Severe Theoretical → Also see TABLE 8 p. 1573

▶ Rifamycins (rifampicin) are predicted to decrease the exposure to **voclosporin**. Avoid. Severe Study → Also see TABLE 2 p. 1571

▶ **Voclosporin** is predicted to increase the exposure to sirolimus. Moderate Study

▶ **St John's wort** is predicted to decrease the exposure to **voclosporin**. Avoid. Severe Theoretical

▶ **Voclosporin** is predicted to increase the concentration of statins (atorvastatin, pravastatin, rosuvastatin, simvastatin). Moderate Theoretical

▶ **Voclosporin** is predicted to increase the concentration of sulfasalazine. Moderate Theoretical → Also see TABLE 2 p. 1571

▶ **Voclosporin** is predicted to increase the concentration of sulfonylureas (glibenclamide). Moderate Theoretical

▶ **Voclosporin** is predicted to increase the exposure to talazoparib. Moderate Study

▶ **Voclosporin** is predicted to increase the exposure to taxanes (paclitaxel). Moderate Study

▶ **Voclosporin** is predicted to increase the exposure to thrombin inhibitors (dabigatran). Mild Theoretical

▶ **Tucatinib** is predicted to increase the exposure to **voclosporin**. Avoid. Severe Study

Volanesorsen

▶ Drugs with anticoagulant effects (see TABLE 3 p. 1571) cause bleeding, as can **volanesorsen**; concurrent use might increase the risk of developing this effect. Avoid depending on platelet count—consult product literature. Severe Theoretical

▶ Drugs with antiplatelet effects (see TABLE 4 p. 1571) cause bleeding, as can **volanesorsen**; concurrent use might increase the risk of developing this effect. Avoid depending on platelet count—consult product literature. Severe Theoretical

Volatile halogenated anaesthetics → see TABLE 7 p. 1572 (hypotension), TABLE 8 p. 1573 (QT-interval prolongation), TABLE 10 p. 1574 (CNS effects)

desflurane · isoflurane · methoxyflurane · sevoflurane

▶ **Sevoflurane** can cause hypertension, as can amfetamines. Avoid **amfetamines** for several days before surgery. Severe Theoretical

▶ Antiepileptics (phenobarbital, primidone) potentially increase the risk of nephrotoxicity when given with **methoxyflurane**. Avoid. Severe Theoretical → Also see TABLE 10 p. 1574

▶ **Isoniazid** potentially increases the risk of nephrotoxicity when given with **methoxyflurane**. Avoid. Severe Theoretical

▶ **Isoniazid** might increase the risk of sevoflurane toxicity when given with **sevoflurane**. Avoid isoniazid from 1 week before, until 15 days after, surgery. Moderate Theoretical

▶ **Methylphenidate** might increase the risk of hypertension and arrhythmias when given with **volatile halogenated anaesthetics**. Avoid **methylphenidate** on day of surgery. Severe Theoretical

▶ Rifamycins (rifampicin) potentially increase the risk of nephrotoxicity when given with **methoxyflurane**. Avoid. Severe Theoretical

- **St John's wort** has been reported to cause severe hypotension when given with **volatile halogenated anaesthetics**. [Severe] Theoretical
- **Sevoflurane** can cause hypertension, as can sympathomimetics, vasoconstrictor **(ephedrine)**. Avoid **ephedrine** for several days before surgery. [Severe] Theoretical
- **Sevoflurane** can cause hypertension, as can sympathomimetics, vasoconstrictor **(pseudoephedrine)**. Avoid **pseudoephedrine** for several days before surgery. [Severe] Theoretical
- **Sevoflurane** can cause hypertension, as can sympathomimetics, vasoconstrictor **(xylometazoline)**. Avoid **xylometazoline** for several days before surgery. [Severe] Theoretical
- **Methoxyflurane** might increase the risk of nephrotoxicity when given with tetracyclines **(tetracycline)**. [Severe] Anecdotal

Voriconazole → see antifungals, azoles

Vortioxetine → see TABLE 12 p. 1574 (serotonin syndrome), TABLE 4 p. 1571 (antiplatelet effects)
- Anti-androgens **(apalutamide, enzalutamide)** are predicted to decrease the exposure to **vortioxetine**. Monitor and adjust dose. [Moderate] Study
- Antiepileptics **(carbamazepine, fosphenytoin, phenobarbital, phenytoin, primidone)** are predicted to decrease the exposure to **vortioxetine**. Monitor and adjust dose. [Moderate] Study
- **Bupropion** is predicted to increase the exposure to **vortioxetine**. Monitor and adjust dose. [Moderate] Study
- **Cinacalcet** is predicted to increase the exposure to **vortioxetine**. Monitor and adjust dose. [Moderate] Study
- **Dacomitinib** is predicted to increase the exposure to **vortioxetine**. Monitor and adjust dose. [Moderate] Study
- **Encorafenib** is predicted to decrease the exposure to **vortioxetine**. Monitor and adjust dose. [Moderate] Study
- Interferons **(ropeginterferon alfa)** are predicted to increase the exposure to **vortioxetine**. [Moderate] Theoretical
- **Ivosidenib** is predicted to decrease the exposure to **vortioxetine**. Monitor and adjust dose. [Moderate] Study
- **Lumacaftor** is predicted to decrease the exposure to **vortioxetine**. Monitor and adjust dose. [Moderate] Study
- **Mitotane** is predicted to decrease the exposure to **vortioxetine**. Monitor and adjust dose. [Moderate] Study
- Rifamycins **(rifampicin)** are predicted to decrease the exposure to **vortioxetine**. Monitor and adjust dose. [Moderate] Study
- SSRIs **(fluoxetine, paroxetine)** are predicted to increase the exposure to **vortioxetine**. Monitor and adjust dose. [Moderate] Study → Also see TABLE 12 p. 1574 → Also see TABLE 4 p. 1571
- **Terbinafine** is predicted to increase the exposure to **vortioxetine**. Monitor and adjust dose. [Moderate] Study

Voxilaprevir
- **Voxilaprevir** is predicted to increase the exposure to afatinib. [Moderate] Study
- **Voxilaprevir** with sofosbuvir and velpatasvir is predicted to increase the exposure to aliskiren. [Severe] Theoretical
- **Voxilaprevir** is predicted to increase the exposure to alpelisib. [Moderate] Theoretical
- Anti-androgens **(apalutamide, enzalutamide)** are predicted to decrease the concentration of **voxilaprevir**. Avoid. [Severe] Study
- Antiepileptics **(carbamazepine, fosphenytoin, phenobarbital, phenytoin, primidone)** are predicted to decrease the concentration of **voxilaprevir**. Avoid. [Severe] Study
- Antiepileptics **(oxcarbazepine)** are predicted to decrease the concentration of **voxilaprevir**. Avoid. [Severe] Theoretical
- **Voxilaprevir** with sofosbuvir and velpatasvir is predicted to increase the exposure to antihistamines, non-sedating **(fexofenadine)**. [Moderate] Study
- **Voxilaprevir** is predicted to increase the exposure to bictegravir. Use with caution or avoid. [Moderate] Theoretical
- **Bulevirtide** is predicted to increase the exposure to **voxilaprevir**. Avoid or monitor. [Moderate] Theoretical
- **Cenobamate** is predicted to decrease the concentration of **voxilaprevir**. Avoid. [Severe] Theoretical
- **Ciclosporin** increases the concentration of **voxilaprevir**. Avoid. [Severe] Study
- **Voxilaprevir** is predicted to increase the exposure to cladribine. Avoid or adjust dose. [Moderate] Theoretical
- **Voxilaprevir** with sofosbuvir and velpatasvir is predicted to increase the exposure to colchicine. Avoid P-glycoprotein inhibitors or adjust **colchicine** dose, p. 1279. [Severe] Theoretical
- **Combined hormonal contraceptives** (containing ethinylestradiol) are predicted to increase the risk of increased ALT concentrations when given with **voxilaprevir** with sofosbuvir and velpatasvir. Avoid. [Severe] Study
- **Dabrafenib** is predicted to decrease the concentration of **voxilaprevir**. Avoid. [Severe] Theoretical
- **Voxilaprevir** with sofosbuvir and velpatasvir is predicted to increase the exposure to digoxin. Monitor and adjust dose. [Severe] Theoretical
- **Encorafenib** is predicted to decrease the concentration of **voxilaprevir**. Avoid. [Severe] Study
- Endothelin receptor antagonists **(bosentan)** are predicted to decrease the concentration of **voxilaprevir**. Avoid. [Severe] Theoretical
- **Voxilaprevir** with sofosbuvir and velpatasvir is predicted to increase the exposure to everolimus. [Severe] Theoretical
- **Voxilaprevir** with sofosbuvir and velpatasvir is predicted to increase the concentration of factor XA inhibitors **(edoxaban)**. Avoid. [Severe] Theoretical
- **Voxilaprevir** is predicted to increase the exposure to fidaxomicin. Avoid. [Moderate] Study
- HIV-protease inhibitors **(atazanavir)** boosted with ritonavir increase the concentration of **voxilaprevir**. Avoid. [Severe] Study
- HIV-protease inhibitors **(lopinavir)** boosted with ritonavir are predicted to increase the concentration of **voxilaprevir**. Avoid. [Severe] Theoretical
- **Ivosidenib** is predicted to decrease the concentration of **voxilaprevir**. Avoid. [Severe] Study
- **Voxilaprevir** with sofosbuvir and velpatasvir is predicted to increase the exposure to loperamide. [Severe] Theoretical
- **Lorlatinib** is predicted to decrease the concentration of **voxilaprevir**. Avoid. [Severe] Theoretical
- **Lumacaftor** is predicted to decrease the concentration of **voxilaprevir**. Avoid. [Severe] Study
- **Voxilaprevir** with sofosbuvir and velpatasvir is predicted to increase the exposure to meglitinides **(repaglinide)**. [Moderate] Study
- **Mitotane** is predicted to decrease the concentration of **voxilaprevir**. Avoid. [Severe] Study
- **Modafinil** is predicted to decrease the concentration of **voxilaprevir**. Avoid. [Severe] Theoretical
- **Voxilaprevir** is predicted to increase the exposure to momelotinib. [Moderate] Study
- **Voxilaprevir** is predicted to increase the risk of neutropenia when given with monoclonal antibodies **(brentuximab vedotin)**. Monitor and adjust dose. [Severe] Theoretical
- **Voxilaprevir** is predicted to increase the exposure to neratinib. Avoid or adjust dose and monitor for gastrointestinal adverse effects—consult product literature. [Severe] Study
- **Voxilaprevir** is predicted to increase the exposure to nintedanib. [Moderate] Study
- NNRTIs **(efavirenz, etravirine, nevirapine)** are predicted to decrease the concentration of **voxilaprevir**. Avoid. [Severe] Theoretical
- **Voxilaprevir** is predicted to increase the exposure to pralsetinib. [Moderate] Theoretical
- **Proton pump inhibitors** are predicted to decrease the exposure to **voxilaprevir**. Adjust dose, see sofosbuvir with velpatasvir and voxilaprevir p. 726. [Moderate] Study
- **Voxilaprevir** with sofosbuvir and velpatasvir is predicted to increase the exposure to ranolazine. Adjust dose. [Severe] Theoretical
- **Voxilaprevir** is predicted to increase the exposure to relugolix. Avoid or take relugolix first and separate administration by at least 6 hours. [Moderate] Study
- Rifamycins **(rifabutin)** are predicted to decrease the concentration of **voxilaprevir**. Avoid. [Severe] Theoretical
- Rifamycins **(rifampicin)** are predicted to decrease the concentration of **voxilaprevir**. Avoid. [Severe] Study
- **Voxilaprevir** with sofosbuvir and velpatasvir is predicted to increase the exposure to rimegepant. Avoid another dose of

Voxilaprevir (continued)
rimegepant within 48 hours of concurrent use. Moderate Theoretical
‣ **Voxilaprevir** with sofosbuvir and velpatasvir is predicted to increase the exposure to sirolimus. Severe Theoretical
‣ Sotorasib is predicted to decrease the concentration of **voxilaprevir**. Avoid. Severe Theoretical
‣ St John's wort is predicted to decrease the concentration of **voxilaprevir**. Avoid. Severe Theoretical
‣ **Voxilaprevir** with sofosbuvir and velpatasvir is predicted to increase the exposure to statins (atorvastatin). Adjust **atorvastatin** dose, p. 234. Moderate Theoretical
‣ **Voxilaprevir** with sofosbuvir and velpatasvir is predicted to increase the exposure to statins (fluvastatin, simvastatin). Avoid. Moderate Theoretical
‣ **Voxilaprevir** with sofosbuvir and velpatasvir moderately increases the exposure to statins (pravastatin). Monitor and adjust **pravastatin** dose. Moderate Study
‣ **Voxilaprevir** with sofosbuvir and velpatasvir markedly increases the exposure to statins (rosuvastatin). Avoid. Severe Study
‣ **Voxilaprevir** is predicted to increase the concentration of sulfasalazine. Avoid. Severe Theoretical
‣ **Voxilaprevir** with sofosbuvir and velpatasvir is predicted to increase the exposure to sulfonylureas (glibenclamide). Moderate Study
‣ **Voxilaprevir** is predicted to slightly increase the exposure to talazoparib. Avoid or adjust dose—consult product literature. Severe Study
‣ **Voxilaprevir** with sofosbuvir and velpatasvir is predicted to increase the exposure to taxanes (docetaxel, paclitaxel). Moderate Study
‣ **Voxilaprevir** is predicted to increase the exposure to tenofovir alafenamide. Moderate Theoretical
‣ **Voxilaprevir** is predicted to increase the exposure to tenofovir disoproxil. Moderate Theoretical
‣ **Voxilaprevir** with sofosbuvir and velpatasvir increases the concentration of thrombin inhibitors (dabigatran). Avoid. Severe Study
‣ **Voxilaprevir** is predicted to increase the exposure to topotecan. Severe Study
‣ **Voxilaprevir** is predicted to increase the concentration of trametinib. Moderate Theoretical

Warfarin → see coumarins

Wasp venom extract

GENERAL INFORMATION Desensitising vaccines should be avoided in patients taking beta-blockers (adrenaline might be ineffective in case of a hypersensitivity reaction) or ACE inhibitors (risk of severe anaphylactoid reactions).

Xipamide → see thiazide diuretics
Xylometazoline → see sympathomimetics, vasoconstrictor
Yellow fever vaccine → see live vaccines

Zanamivir
‣ **Zanamivir** might decrease the efficacy of live vaccines (influenza vaccine (live)). Moderate Theoretical

Zanubrutinib → see TABLE 4 p. 1571 (antiplatelet effects)

FOOD AND LIFESTYLE Bitter (Seville) orange is predicted to increase the exposure to zanubrutinib.

‣ Anti-androgens (apalutamide, enzalutamide) are predicted to decrease the exposure to **zanubrutinib**. Avoid. Severe Study
‣ Antiarrhythmics (dronedarone) are predicted to increase the exposure to **zanubrutinib**. Avoid or adjust dose with moderate CYP3A4 inhibitors—consult product literature. Severe Study
‣ Antiepileptics (carbamazepine, fosphenytoin, phenobarbital, phenytoin, primidone) are predicted to decrease the exposure to **zanubrutinib**. Avoid. Severe Study
‣ Antifungals, azoles (fluconazole, isavuconazole) are predicted to increase the exposure to **zanubrutinib**. Avoid or adjust dose with moderate CYP3A4 inhibitors—consult product literature. Severe Study
‣ Antifungals, azoles (itraconazole, ketoconazole, posaconazole, voriconazole) are predicted to increase the exposure to **zanubrutinib**. Avoid or adjust dose with potent CYP3A4 inhibitors—consult product literature. Moderate Study

‣ Berotralstat is predicted to increase the exposure to **zanubrutinib**. Avoid or adjust dose with moderate CYP3A4 inhibitors—consult product literature. Severe Study
‣ Calcium channel blockers (diltiazem, verapamil) are predicted to increase the exposure to **zanubrutinib**. Avoid or adjust dose with moderate CYP3A4 inhibitors—consult product literature. Severe Study
‣ Cenobamate is predicted to decrease the exposure to **zanubrutinib**. Avoid or adjust dose with moderate CYP3A4 inducers—consult product literature. Severe Theoretical
‣ Ceritinib is predicted to increase the exposure to **zanubrutinib**. Avoid or adjust dose with potent CYP3A4 inhibitors—consult product literature. Moderate Study
‣ Cobicistat is predicted to increase the exposure to **zanubrutinib**. Avoid or adjust dose with potent CYP3A4 inhibitors—consult product literature. Moderate Study
‣ Crizotinib is predicted to increase the exposure to **zanubrutinib**. Avoid or adjust dose with moderate CYP3A4 inhibitors—consult product literature. Severe Study
‣ Dabrafenib is predicted to decrease the exposure to **zanubrutinib**. Avoid or adjust dose with moderate CYP3A4 inducers—consult product literature. Severe Theoretical
‣ Encorafenib is predicted to decrease the exposure to **zanubrutinib**. Avoid. Severe Study
‣ Endothelin receptor antagonists (bosentan) are predicted to decrease the exposure to **zanubrutinib**. Avoid or adjust dose with moderate CYP3A4 inducers—consult product literature. Severe Theoretical
‣ Fedratinib is predicted to increase the exposure to **zanubrutinib**. Avoid or adjust dose with moderate CYP3A4 inhibitors—consult product literature. Severe Study
‣ Grapefruit juice is predicted to increase the exposure to **zanubrutinib**. Moderate Theoretical
‣ HIV-protease inhibitors are predicted to increase the exposure to **zanubrutinib**. Avoid or adjust dose with potent CYP3A4 inhibitors—consult product literature. Moderate Study
‣ Idelalisib is predicted to increase the exposure to **zanubrutinib**. Avoid or adjust dose with potent CYP3A4 inhibitors—consult product literature. Moderate Study
‣ Imatinib is predicted to increase the exposure to **zanubrutinib**. Avoid or adjust dose with moderate CYP3A4 inhibitors—consult product literature. Severe Study → Also see TABLE 4 p. 1571
‣ Ivosidenib is predicted to decrease the exposure to **zanubrutinib**. Avoid. Severe Study
‣ Letermovir is predicted to increase the exposure to **zanubrutinib**. Avoid or adjust dose with moderate CYP3A4 inhibitors—consult product literature. Severe Study
‣ Lorlatinib is predicted to decrease the exposure to **zanubrutinib**. Avoid or adjust dose with moderate CYP3A4 inducers—consult product literature. Severe Theoretical
‣ Lumacaftor is predicted to decrease the exposure to **zanubrutinib**. Avoid. Severe Study
‣ Macrolides (clarithromycin) are predicted to increase the exposure to **zanubrutinib**. Avoid or adjust dose with potent CYP3A4 inhibitors—consult product literature. Moderate Study
‣ Macrolides (erythromycin) are predicted to increase the exposure to **zanubrutinib**. Avoid or adjust dose with moderate CYP3A4 inhibitors—consult product literature. Severe Study
‣ Mitotane is predicted to decrease the exposure to **zanubrutinib**. Avoid. Severe Study
‣ Modafinil is predicted to decrease the exposure to **zanubrutinib**. Avoid. Moderate Theoretical
‣ Neurokinin-1 receptor antagonists (aprepitant, netupitant) are predicted to increase the exposure to **zanubrutinib**. Avoid or adjust dose with moderate CYP3A4 inhibitors—consult product literature. Severe Study
‣ Nilotinib is predicted to increase the exposure to **zanubrutinib**. Avoid or adjust dose with moderate CYP3A4 inhibitors—consult product literature. Severe Study
‣ NNRTIs (efavirenz, etravirine, nevirapine) are predicted to decrease the exposure to **zanubrutinib**. Avoid or adjust dose with moderate CYP3A4 inducers—consult product literature. Severe Theoretical

- Quinolones **(ciprofloxacin)** are predicted to increase the exposure to **zanubrutinib**. Avoid or adjust dose—consult product literature. Severe Theoretical
- Rifamycins **(rifampicin)** are predicted to decrease the exposure to **zanubrutinib**. Avoid. Severe Study
- Sotorasib is predicted to decrease the exposure to **zanubrutinib**. Avoid or adjust dose with moderate CYP3A4 inducers—consult product literature. Severe Theoretical
- St John's wort is predicted to decrease the exposure to **zanubrutinib**. Avoid or adjust dose with moderate CYP3A4 inducers—consult product literature. Severe Theoretical
- Tucatinib is predicted to increase the exposure to **zanubrutinib**. Avoid or adjust dose with potent CYP3A4 inhibitors—consult product literature. Moderate Study

Zidovudine → see NRTIs

Zinc

> ROUTE-SPECIFIC INFORMATION Interactions do not generally apply to topical use unless specified.

- Oral **zinc** might decrease the concentration of the active metabolite of oral baloxavir marboxil. Avoid. Severe Theoretical
- Oral **zinc** decreases the absorption of oral bisphosphonates (alendronate). **Alendronate** should be taken at least 30 minutes before **zinc**. Moderate Study
- Oral **zinc** decreases the absorption of oral bisphosphonates (clodronate). Avoid **zinc** for 2 hours before or 1 hour after **clodronate**. Moderate Study
- Oral **zinc** is predicted to decrease the absorption of oral bisphosphonates (ibandronate). Avoid **zinc** for at least 6 hours before or 1 hour after **ibandronate**. Moderate Theoretical
- Oral **zinc** decreases the absorption of oral bisphosphonates (risedronate). Separate administration by at least 2 hours. Moderate Study
- Oral calcium salts decrease the absorption of oral **zinc**. Moderate Study
- Oral **zinc** is predicted to decrease the absorption of eltrombopag. **Eltrombopag** should be taken 2 hours before or 4 hours after **zinc**. Severe Theoretical
- Oral **zinc** is predicted to decrease the efficacy of oral iron and oral iron is predicted to decrease the efficacy of oral **zinc**. Moderate Study
- Oral **zinc** is predicted to decrease the absorption of oral iron chelators (deferiprone). Moderate Theoretical
- **Zinc** is predicted to decrease the absorption of penicillamine. Mild Theoretical
- **Zinc** is predicted to decrease the exposure to quinolones. Separate administration by 2 hours. Moderate Study
- Oral **zinc** is predicted to decrease the absorption of tetracyclines. Separate administration by 2 to 3 hours. Moderate Theoretical
- Trientine potentially decreases the absorption of **zinc**. Moderate Theoretical

Zoledronate → see bisphosphonates

Zolmitriptan → see triptans

Zolpidem → see TABLE 10 p. 1574 (CNS effects)

- Anti-androgens (enzalutamide) are predicted to affect the exposure to **zolpidem**. Use with caution or avoid. Moderate Theoretical
- Antiepileptics (carbamazepine) moderately decrease the exposure to **zolpidem**. Moderate Study
- Idelalisib is predicted to increase the exposure to **zolpidem**. Monitor and adjust dose. Moderate Theoretical
- Nirmatrelvir boosted with ritonavir is predicted to increase the concentration of **zolpidem**. Severe Theoretical
- Rifamycins **(rifampicin)** moderately decrease the exposure to **zolpidem**. Moderate Study

Zonisamide → see antiepileptics

Zopiclone → see TABLE 10 p. 1574 (CNS effects)

- Anti-androgens (apalutamide, enzalutamide) are predicted to decrease the exposure to **zopiclone**. Adjust dose. Moderate Study

- Antiarrhythmics **(dronedarone)** are predicted to increase the exposure to **zopiclone**. Adjust dose. Moderate Study
- Antiepileptics (carbamazepine, fosphenytoin, phenobarbital, phenytoin, primidone) are predicted to decrease the exposure to **zopiclone**. Adjust dose. Moderate Study → Also see TABLE 10 p. 1574
- Antifungals, azoles (fluconazole, isavuconazole) are predicted to increase the exposure to **zopiclone**. Adjust dose. Moderate Study
- Antifungals, azoles (itraconazole, ketoconazole, posaconazole, voriconazole) are predicted to increase the exposure to **zopiclone**. Adjust dose. Moderate Theoretical
- Berotralstat is predicted to increase the exposure to **zopiclone**. Adjust dose. Moderate Study
- Calcium channel blockers (diltiazem, verapamil) are predicted to increase the exposure to **zopiclone**. Adjust dose. Moderate Study
- Ceritinib is predicted to increase the exposure to **zopiclone**. Adjust dose. Moderate Theoretical
- Cobicistat is predicted to increase the exposure to **zopiclone**. Adjust dose. Moderate Theoretical
- Crizotinib is predicted to increase the exposure to **zopiclone**. Adjust dose. Moderate Study
- Encorafenib is predicted to decrease the exposure to **zopiclone**. Adjust dose. Moderate Study
- Fedratinib is predicted to increase the exposure to **zopiclone**. Adjust dose. Moderate Study
- HIV-protease inhibitors are predicted to increase the exposure to **zopiclone**. Adjust dose. Moderate Theoretical
- Idelalisib is predicted to increase the exposure to **zopiclone**. Adjust dose. Moderate Theoretical
- Imatinib is predicted to increase the exposure to **zopiclone**. Adjust dose. Moderate Study
- Ivosidenib is predicted to decrease the exposure to **zopiclone**. Adjust dose. Moderate Study
- Letermovir is predicted to increase the exposure to **zopiclone**. Adjust dose. Moderate Study
- Lumacaftor is predicted to decrease the exposure to **zopiclone**. Adjust dose. Moderate Study
- Macrolides (clarithromycin) are predicted to increase the exposure to **zopiclone**. Adjust dose. Moderate Theoretical
- Macrolides (erythromycin) are predicted to increase the exposure to **zopiclone**. Adjust dose. Moderate Study
- Mitotane is predicted to decrease the exposure to **zopiclone**. Adjust dose. Moderate Study
- Neurokinin-1 receptor antagonists (aprepitant, netupitant) are predicted to increase the exposure to **zopiclone**. Adjust dose. Moderate Study
- Nilotinib is predicted to increase the exposure to **zopiclone**. Adjust dose. Moderate Study
- Rifamycins **(rifampicin)** are predicted to decrease the exposure to **zopiclone**. Adjust dose. Moderate Study
- Tucatinib is predicted to increase the exposure to **zopiclone**. Adjust dose. Moderate Theoretical

Zuclopenthixol → see TABLE 17 p. 1576 (hyponatraemia), TABLE 7 p. 1572 (hypotension), TABLE 9 p. 1573 (antimuscarinics), TABLE 10 p. 1574 (CNS effects)

- Antipsychotics, second generation (clozapine) can cause constipation, as can **zuclopenthixol**; concurrent use might increase the risk of developing intestinal obstruction. Severe Theoretical → Also see TABLE 17 p. 1576 → Also see TABLE 7 p. 1572 → Also see TABLE 9 p. 1573 → Also see TABLE 10 p. 1574
- **Zuclopenthixol** is predicted to decrease the effects of dopamine receptor agonists. Avoid. Moderate Theoretical → Also see TABLE 7 p. 1572 → Also see TABLE 9 p. 1573 → Also see TABLE 10 p. 1574
- **Zuclopenthixol** opposes the effects of the active metabolite of foslevodopa. Severe Theoretical → Also see TABLE 7 p. 1572 → Also see TABLE 10 p. 1574
- **Zuclopenthixol** is predicted to decrease the effects of levodopa. Avoid or monitor worsening parkinsonian symptoms. Severe Theoretical → Also see TABLE 7 p. 1572 → Also see TABLE 10 p. 1574
- **Zuclopenthixol** potentially increases the risk of neurotoxicity when given with lithium. Severe Anecdotal

Appendix 2
Borderline substances

CONTENTS

In certain conditions some foods (and toilet preparations) have characteristics of drugs and the Advisory Committee on Borderline Substances (ACBS) advises as to the circumstances in which such substances may be regarded as drugs. Prescriptions issued in accordance with the Committee's advice and endorsed 'ACBS' will normally not be investigated.

Information

General Practitioners are reminded that the ACBS recommends products on the basis that they may be regarded as drugs for the management of specified conditions. Doctors should satisfy themselves that the products can safely be prescribed, that patients are adequately monitored and that, where necessary, expert hospital supervision is available.

Foods which may be prescribed on FP10, GP10 (Scotland), or WP10 (Wales)

All the food products listed in this appendix have ACBS approval. The clinical condition for which the product has been approved is included with each entry.
Note Foods included in this appendix may contain cariogenic sugars and patients should be advised to take appropriate oral hygiene measures.

Enteral feeds and oral nutritional supplements

For most enteral feeds and oral nutritional supplements, the main source of **carbohydrate** is either maltodextrin or glucose syrup; other carbohydrate sources are listed in the relevant entry. Products containing residual lactose (less than 1 g lactose/100 mL formula) are described as 'clinically lactose-free' or 'lactose-free' by some manufacturers. The presence of lactose (including residual lactose) is indicated in the relevant entry. The primary sources of **protein** or **amino acids** are included with each product entry. The **fat** or **oil** content is derived from a variety of sources such as vegetables, soya bean, corn, palm nuts, and seeds; where the fat content is derived from animal or fish sources, this information is included in the relevant product entry. The presence of medium chain triglycerides (MCT) is also noted where the quantity exceeds 30% of the fat content. Enteral feeds and oral nutritional supplements can contain varying amounts of **vitamins**, **minerals**, and **trace elements**—the manufacturer's product literature should be consulted for more detailed information. Products containing vitamin K may affect the INR in patients receiving warfarin.
The suitability of food products for patients requiring a vegan, kosher, halal, or other compliant diet should be confirmed with individual manufacturers.

Note Feeds containing more than 6 g/100 mL protein or
2 g/100 mL fibre should be avoided in children unless
recommended by an appropriate specialist or dietician.

Nutritional values

Representative values for enteral feeds and oral nutritional
supplements are included where nutritional values vary
between flavour or pack size, and are usually based on
neutral or vanilla flavour.

For details of all presentations of a product range, consult
product literature.

Other conditions for which ACBS products can be prescribed

Clinical conditions for which the ACBS has approved toilet
preparations.

Dermatitis, Eczema and Pruritus
See Emollient and barrier preparations p. 1387

**Disfiguring skin lesions (birthmarks, mutilating
lesions, scars, vitiligo)**
See Camouflages p. 1455

Disinfectants (antiseptics)
See Skin cleansers, antiseptics and desloughing agents
p. 1450

Photodermatoses (skin protection in)
See Sunscreen p. 1455

Standard ACBS indications: Disease-related malnutrition,
intractable malabsorption, pre-operative preparation of
malnourished patients, dysphagia, proven inflammatory
bowel disease, following total gastrectomy, short-bowel
syndrome, bowel fistula

Table 1 Enteral nutrition
Tube feeds: Additional protein fortifiers

1 kcal/mL higher protein

Product	Formulation	Energy	Protein	Carbohydrate	Fat	Fibre	Special Characteristics	ACBS Indications	Presentation & Flavour
Nutrison® Protein Shot (Nutricia Ltd)	Liquid (tube feed) per 100 mL	480 kJ (113 kcal)	27.5 g whey protein hydrolysate	0.6 g	0.1 g	Nil	Contains beef derivatives, residual lactose	Disease related malnutrition for tube fed patients with increased protein requirements.	Nutrison Protein Shot liquid: 240 ml = £9.36
Not suitable for use in child under 3 years									
ProSource® TF (Nutrinovo Ltd)	Liquid (tube feed) per 100 mL	373 kJ (98 kcal)	24.4 g collagen protein, protein equivalent (amino acids)	2.2 g (sugars Nil)	Less than 1 g	Less than 1 g	Contains bovine derivatives. Gluten-free, lactose-free	Hypoproteinaemia.	ProSource TF liquid 45ml sachets: 100 sachet = £159.12
Not recommended for child under 3 years									
ProSource® TF ENFit (Nutrinovo Ltd)	Liquid (tube feed) per 100 mL	530 kJ (127 kcal)	33.3 g collagen protein, protein equivalent (amino acids)	0.55 g (sugars 0.55 g)	0.2 g	0.33 g	Contains bovine derivatives. Gluten-free, lactose-free	Hypoproteinaemia.	ProSource TF ENFit liquid 60ml sachets: 50 sachet = £133.34
Not recommended for child under 3 years									

2 kcal/mL higher protein

Product	Formulation	Energy	Protein	Carbohydrate	Fat	Fibre	Special Characteristics	ACBS Indications	Presentation & Flavour
ProSource® TF plant (Nutrinovo Ltd)	Liquid (tube feed) per 100 mL	837 kJ (200 kcal)	33 g pea protein hydrolysate	12 g (sugars less than 1 g)	1.1 g	1.5 g	Gluten-free, lactose-free	Hypoproteinaemia.	ProSource TF plant liquid 45ml sachets: 50 sachet = £119.63
Not recommended for child under 3 years									

Tube feeds: Critically ill

1.5 kcal/mL peptide based, higher protein

Product	Formulation	Energy	Protein	Carbohydrate	Fat	Fibre	Special Characteristics	ACBS Indications	Presentation & Flavour
Peptamen® AF (Nestle Health Science)	Liquid (tube feed) per 100 mL	638 kJ (152 kcal)	9.4 g whey protein	14 g (sugars 1.4 g)	6.5 g (MCT 52 %)	Nil	Contains fish oil, residual lactose, soya. Gluten-free	Borderline substances standard ACBS indications p. 1879 except dysphagia.	Peptamen AF liquid: 500 ml = £11.12
Suitable for over 3 years									

Tube feeds: Impaired gastro-intestinal function or malabsorption

1 to less than 1.5 kcal/mL peptide based

Product	Formulation	Energy	Protein	Carbohydrate	Fat	Fibre	Special Characteristics	ACBS Indications	Presentation & Flavour
Nutrison® Peptisorb (Nutricia Ltd)	Liquid (tube feed) per 100 mL	425 kJ (100 kcal)	4 g whey protein hydrolysate	17.6 g (sugars 1.7 g)	1.7 g (MCT 47 %)	Nil	Contains residual lactose, soya. Gluten-free	Borderline substances standard ACBS indications p. 1879; also growth failure.	Nutrison Peptisorb liquid: 500 ml = £12.17
Not suitable for use in child under 1 year; not recommended for child 1–6 years									
Peptamen® HN (Nestle Health Science)	Liquid (sip or tube feed) per 100 mL	559 kJ (133 kcal)	6.6 g whey protein hydrolysate	16 g (sugars 1.4 g)	4.9 g (MCT 69%)	Nil	Contains meat derivatives, residual lactose, soya. Gluten-free	Impaired gastrointestinal function, short bowel syndrome, intractable malabsorption, proven inflammatory bowel disease and bowel fistula or with higher nutritional requirements.	Peptamen HN liquid: 500 ml = £10.17; 1000 ml = £19.09
Not suitable for use in child under 3 years									
Peptamen® tube feed (Nestle Health Science)	Liquid (sip or tube feed) per 100 mL	421 kJ (100 kcal)	4 g whey protein	13 g (sugars 0.48 g)	3.7 g (MCT 70 %)	Nil	Contains residual lactose, soya. Gluten-free	Short bowel syndrome, intractable malabsorption, proven inflammatory bowel disease, bowel fistulae.	Peptamen tube feed liquid unflavoured: 500 ml = £9.46; 1000 ml = £17.75
Not suitable for use in child under 3 years; not recommended for child under 5 years									
Perative® (Abbott Laboratories Ltd)	Liquid (sip or tube feed) per 100 mL	552 kJ (131 kcal)	6.7 g caseinates, whey protein hydrolysate	17.7 g (sugars 0.45 g)	3.7 g (MCT 37%)	Nil	Contains residual lactose, soya. Gluten-free	Borderline substances standard ACBS indications p. 1879 except dysphagia.	Perative liquid: 500 ml = £11.97; 1000 ml = £22.11
Not suitable for use in child under 1 year; not recommended for use in children									
Survimed® OPD HN (Fresenius Kabi Ltd)	Liquid (tube feed) per 100 mL	560 kJ (133 kcal)	6.7 g whey protein hydrolysate	18.3 g (sugars 1.33 g)	3.7 g (MCT 52%)	Less than or equal to 0.1 g	Contains fish oil, residual lactose. Gluten-free	Borderline substances standard ACBS indications p. 1879; also haemodialysis and continuous ambulatory peritoneal dialysis.	Survimed OPD HN liquid: 500 ml = £10.15
Not suitable for use in child under 3 years; use with caution in child under 6 years									
Survimed® OPD tube feed (Fresenius Kabi Ltd)	Liquid (tube feed) per 100 mL	420 kJ (100 kcal)	4.5 g whey protein hydrolysate	14.3 g (sugars 1.1 g)	2.8 g (MCT 51%)	Less than or equal to 0.1 g	Contains fish oil, residual lactose. Gluten-free	Borderline substances standard ACBS indications p. 1879	Survimed OPD tube feed liquid: 500 ml = £10.47; 1000 ml = £19.81
Not suitable for use in child under 3 years; use with caution in child under 6 years									

1.5 kcal/mL or more peptide based

Product	Formulation	Energy	Protein	Carbohydrate	Fat	Fibre	Special Characteristics	ACBS Indications	Presentation & Flavour
Nutrison® Peptisorb Plus HEHP (Nutricia Ltd)	Liquid (tube feed) per 100 ml	631 kJ (150 kcal)	7.5 g whey protein hydrolysate	18.7 g (sugars 1.4 g)	5 g (MCT 60%)	Less than 0.5 g	Contains residual lactose, soya. Gluten-free	Borderline substances standard ACBS indications p. 1879 except dysphagia.	Nutrison Peptisorb Plus HEHP liquid: 500 ml = £12.13; 1000 ml = £22.83
Not suitable for use in child under 1 year; not recommended for child 1–6 years									
Vital® 1.5kcal tube feed (Abbott Laboratories Ltd)	Liquid (tube feed) per 100 mL	631 kJ (150 kcal)	6.75 g caseinates, whey protein hydrolysate	18.4 g (sugars 3.5 g)	5.5 g (MCT 64%)	Nil	Contains residual lactose. Gluten-free	Borderline substances standard ACBS indications p. 1879 except dysphagia.	Vital 1.5kcal tube feed liquid vanilla: 1000 ml = £24.27
Not recommended for use in children									

Tube feeds: Non-milk based feeds

1 kcal/mL soya based

Product	Formulation	Energy	Protein	Carbohydrate	Fat	Fibre	Special Characteristics	ACBS Indications	Presentation & Flavour
Nutrison® PlantBased Soya (Nutricia Ltd)	Liquid (tube feed) per 100 mL	420 kJ (100 kcal)	4 g soya protein	12.3 g (sugars 0.97 g)	3.9 g	Nil	Contains residual lactose, soya. Gluten-free	Borderline substances standard ACBS indications p. 1879; also cow's milk protein and lactose intolerance.	Nutrison PlantBased Soya liquid: 1000 ml = £16.71

Not suitable for use in child under 3 years; use with caution in child over 3 years

1 kcal/mL soya based with fibre

Product	Formulation	Energy	Protein	Carbohydrate	Fat	Fibre	Special Characteristics	ACBS Indications	Presentation & Flavour
Fresubin® Soya Fibre (Fresenius Kabi Ltd)	Liquid (tube feed) per 100 mL	420 kJ (100 kcal)	3.8 g soya protein	12.1 g (sugars 4.1 g)	3.6 g	2 g	Contains fish oil, soya. Gluten-free, lactose-free	Borderline substances standard ACBS indications p. 1879 except dysphagia. Also cow's milk protein intolerance, lactose intolerance.	Fresubin Soya Fibre liquid: 500 ml = £7.15
Nutrison® PlantBased Soya Multi Fibre (Nutricia Ltd)	Liquid (tube feed) per 100 mL	430 kJ (103 kcal)	4 g soya protein	12.3 g (sugars 0.7 g)	3.9 g	1.5 g	Contains residual lactose, soya. Gluten-free	Borderline substances standard ACBS indications p. 1879; also cows' milk protein and lactose intolerance.	Nutrison PlantBased Soya Multi Fibre liquid: 1500 ml = £27.80

Not suitable for use in child under 3 years; use with caution in child under 6 years

Tube feeds: Renal failure

1.8 kcal/mL

Product	Formulation	Energy	Protein	Carbohydrate	Fat	Fibre	Special Characteristics	ACBS Indications	Presentation & Flavour
Nepro® HP tube feed (Abbott Laboratories Ltd)	Liquid (tube feed) per 100 mL	752 kJ (180 kcal)	8.1 g caseinates, milk protein isolate	14.7 g (sugars 3.2 g)	9.77 g	1.26 g	Contains residual lactose, soya. Gluten-free Minerals/100 mL: Na 3.04 mmol K 2.71 mmol Ca 2.64 mmol P 2.32 mmol	Patients with chronic renal failure who are on haemodialysis or complete ambulatory peritoneal dialysis (CAPD), or patients with cirrhosis or other conditions requiring a high energy, low fluid, low electrolyte diet.	Nepro HP tube feed liquid vanilla: 500 ml = £11.58

Not recommended for use in children

Tube feeds: Standard feeds

Less than 1 kcal/mL with fibre, higher protein

Product	Formulation	Energy	Protein	Carbohydrate	Fat	Fibre	Special Characteristics	ACBS Indications	Presentation & Flavour
Nutrison® 800 Complete Multi Fibre (Nutricia Ltd)	Liquid (tube feed) per 100 mL	345 kJ (83 kcal)	5.5 g caseinate, pea, soya, whey proteins	8.8 g (sugars 0.6 g)	2.5 g	1.5 g	Contains fish oil, residual lactose, soya. Gluten-free	Borderline substances standard ACBS indications p. 1879 except bowel fistula.	Nutrison 800 Complete Multi Fibre liquid: 1000 ml = £16.44

Not suitable for use in child under 6 years; not recommended for child under 12 years

1 to less than 1.5 kcal/mL

Product	Formulation	Energy	Protein	Carbohydrate	Fat	Fibre	Special Characteristics	ACBS Indications	Presentation & Flavour
Fresubin® Original tube feed (Fresenius Kabi Ltd)	Liquid (tube feed) per 100 mL	420 kJ (100 kcal)	3.8 g milk, soya proteins	13.8 g (sugars 0.85 g)	3.4 g	Nil	Contains fish oil, residual lactose, soya. Gluten-free	Borderline substances standard ACBS indications p. 1879; also Refsum's Disease.	Fresubin Original tube feed liquid: 500 ml = £7.04; 1000 ml = £11.92; 1500 ml = £18.46
Not suitable for use in child under 3 years; use with caution in child under 6 years									
Nutrison® (Nutricia Ltd)	Liquid (tube feed) per 100 mL	420 kJ (100 kcal)	4 g cow's milk, pea, soya, whey proteins	12.4 g (sugars 0.81 g)	3.9 g	Nil	Contains fish oil, residual lactose, soya. Gluten-free	Borderline substances standard ACBS indications p. 1879.	Nutrison liquid: 500 ml = £7.72; 1000 ml = £13.57; 1500 ml = £20.38
Not suitable for use in child under 3 years; use with caution in child over 3 years									
Osmolite® (Abbott Laboratories Ltd)	Liquid (tube feed) per 100 mL	424 kJ (101 kcal)	4 g caseinates, soya protein isolate	13.6 g (sugars 0.6 g)	3.4 g	Nil	Contains residual lactose, soya. Gluten-free	Borderline substances standard ACBS indications p. 1879.	Osmolite liquid: 500 ml = £7.77; 1000 ml = £13.66
Not suitable for use in child under 1 year; not recommended for use in children									

1 to less than 1.5 kcal/mL higher protein

Product	Formulation	Energy	Protein	Carbohydrate	Fat	Fibre	Special Characteristics	ACBS Indications	Presentation & Flavour
Nutrison® Protein Plus (Nutricia Ltd)	Liquid (tube feed) per 100 mL	525 kJ (125 kcal)	6.3 g caseinates, pea, soya, whey proteins	14.2 g (sugars 0.9 g)	4.9 g	Less than 0.1 g	Contains fish oil, residual lactose, soya. Gluten-free	Disease related malnutrition.	Nutrison Protein Plus liquid: 500 ml = £8.33; 1000 ml = £16.13
Not suitable for use in child under 1 year; not recommended for child 1–6 years									
Osmolite® Plus (Abbott Laboratories Ltd)	Liquid (tube feed) per 100 mL	508 kJ (121 kcal)	5.6 g caseinates	15.8 g (sugars 0.42 g)	3.9 g	Nil	Contains residual lactose, soya. Gluten-free	Borderline substances standard ACBS indications p. 1879.	Osmolite Plus liquid: 500 ml = £8.45; 1000 ml = £15.38
Not suitable for use in child under 1 year; not recommended for use in children									

1 to less than 1.5 kcal/mL with fibre

Product	Formulation	Energy	Protein	Carbohydrate	Fat	Fibre	Special Characteristics	ACBS Indications	Presentation & Flavour
Compleat® (Nestle Health Science)	Liquid (tube feed) per 100 mL	461 kJ (110 kcal)	4.4 g chicken, milk proteins	14 g (sugars 1.4 g)	3.7 g	1.4 g	Contains fish oil, meat derivatives, residual lactose. Gluten-free	Borderline substances standard ACBS indications p. 1879; also feeding intolerance, and developmental disabilities.	Compleat tube feed liquid: 1000 ml = £14.38
Suitable from 3 years									
Fresubin® 1500 Complete (Fresenius Kabi Ltd)	Liquid (tube feed) per 100 mL	420 kJ (100 kcal)	3.8 g milk, soya proteins	13 g (sugars 0.9 g)	3.4 g	1.5 g	Contains fish oil, residual lactose, soya. Gluten-free	Borderline substances standard ACBS indications p. 1879 except bowel fistula and pre-operative preparation of malnourished patients.	Fresubin 1500 Complete liquid: 1.5 litre = £20.64
Not suitable for use in child under 3 years; use with caution in child under 6 years									

1 to less than 1.5 kcal/mL with fibre (product list continued)

Product	Formulation	Energy	Protein	Carbohydrate	Fat	Fibre	Special Characteristics	ACBS Indications	Presentation & Flavour
Fresubin® Original Fibre (Fresenius Kabi Ltd)	Liquid (tube feed) per 100 mL	420 kJ (100 kcal)	3.8 g milk, soya proteins	13.0 g (sugars 0.9 g)	3.4 g	1.5 g	Contains fish oil, residual lactose, soya. Gluten-free	Borderline substances standard ACBS indications p. 1879 except bowel fistula and pre-operative preparation of malnourished patients.	Fresubin Original Fibre liquid: 500 ml = £7.16; 1000 ml = £13.78
Not suitable for use in child under 3 years; use with caution in child under 6 years									
Jevity® (Abbott Laboratories Ltd)	Liquid (tube feed) per 100 mL	449 kJ (107 kcal)	4 g caseinates	14.1 g (sugars 0.25 g)	3.47 g	1.76 g	Contains residual lactose, soya. Gluten-free	Borderline substances standard ACBS indications p. 1879 except bowel fistula.	Jevity liquid: 500 ml = £8.40; 1000 ml = £15.86; 1500 ml = £23.76
Not suitable for use in child under 1 year; not recommended for use in children									
Nutrison® Multi Fibre (Nutricia Ltd)	Liquid (tube feed) per 100 mL	433 kJ (103 kcal)	4 g caseinate, pea, soya, whey proteins	12.3 g (sugars 0.88 g)	3.9 g	1.5 g	Contains fish oil, residual lactose, soya. Gluten-free	Borderline substances standard ACBS indications p. 1879.	Nutrison Multi Fibre liquid: 500 ml = £8.35; 1000 ml = £15.71; 1500 ml = £23.55;
Not suitable for use in child under 3 years; use with caution in child over 3 years									

1 to less than 1.5 kcal/mL with fibre, higher protein

Product	Formulation	Energy	Protein	Carbohydrate	Fat	Fibre	Special Characteristics	ACBS Indications	Presentation & Flavour
Fresubin® 1000 Complete (Fresenius Kabi Ltd)	Liquid (tube feed) per 100 mL	418 kJ (100 kcal)	5.5 g milk protein	12.5 g (sugars 1.1 g)	2.7 g	2 g	Contains fish oil, residual lactose, soya lecithin. Gluten-free	Borderline substances standard ACBS indications p. 1879	Fresubin 1000 Complete liquid: 1 litre = £14.88
Not suitable for use in child under 3 years; use with caution in child under 6 years									
Fresubin® 1200 Complete (Fresenius Kabi Ltd)	Liquid (tube feed) per 100 mL	504 kJ (120 kcal)	6 g milk protein	14 g (sugars 1.17 g)	4.1 g	2 g	Contains fish oil, residual lactose, soya lecithin. Gluten-free	Borderline substances standard ACBS indications p. 1879 except dysphagia.	Fresubin 1200 Complete liquid: 1 litre = £17.45
Not suitable for use in child under 3 years; use with caution in child under 6 years									
Fresubin® 1800 Complete (Fresenius Kabi Ltd)	Liquid (tube feed) per 100 mL	504 kJ (120 kcal)	6 g milk protein	14 g (sugars 1.17 g)	4.1 g	2 g	Contains fish oil, residual lactose, soya lecithin. Gluten-free	Borderline substances standard ACBS indications p. 1879 except dysphagia.	Fresubin 1800 Complete liquid: 1.5 litre = £18.55
Not suitable for use in child under 3 years; use with caution in child under 6 years									
Jevity® Plus (Abbott Laboratories Ltd)	Liquid (tube feed) per 100 mL	514 kJ (122 kcal)	5.6 g caseinates, soya protein isolate	15.1 g (sugars 0.75 g)	3.9 g	2.2 g	Contains residual lactose, soya. Gluten-free	Borderline substances standard ACBS indications p. 1879.	Jevity Plus liquid: 500 ml = £10.07; 1000 ml = £18.37; 1500 ml = £27.50
Not recommended for use in children									
Jevity® Plus HP (Abbott Laboratories Ltd)	Liquid (tube feed) per 100 mL	551 kJ (131 kcal)	8.1 g caseinates, milk, soya protein isolates	14.2 g (sugars 0.7 g)	4.3 g	1.5 g	Contains residual lactose, soya. Gluten-free	Borderline substances standard ACBS indications p. 1879; also CAPD, haemodialysis.	Jevity Plus HP gluten free liquid: 500 ml = £9.87
Not suitable for use in child under 2 years; not recommended for use in children									

Product	Formulation	Energy	Protein	Carbohydrate	Fat	Fibre	Special Characteristics	ACBS Indications	Presentation & Flavour
Jevity® Promote (Abbott Laboratories Ltd)	Liquid (tube feed) per 100 mL	434 kJ (103 kcal)	5.6 g caseinates, soya protein isolate	12 g (sugars 0.52 g)	3.3 g	1.7 g	Contains residual lactose, soya. Gluten-free	Borderline substances standard ACBS indications p. 1879.	Jevity Promote liquid: 1 litre = £17.57
Not suitable for use in child under 2 years; not recommended for use in children									
Nutrison® 1000 Complete Multi Fibre (Nutricia Ltd)	Liquid (tube feed) per 100 mL	440 kJ (104 kcal)	5.5 g caseinate, pea, soya, whey proteins	11.3 g (sugars 0.8 g)	3.7 g	2 g	Contains fish oil, residual lactose, soya. Gluten-free	Disease related malnutrition in patients with low energy and/or low fluid requirements.	Nutrison 1000 Complete Multi Fibre liquid: 1000 ml = £17.45
Not suitable for use in child under 1 year; not recommended for child under 12 years									
Nutrison® 1200 Complete Multi Fibre (Nutricia Ltd)	Liquid (tube feed) per 100 mL	525 kJ (124 kcal)	5.5 g caseinates, pea, soya, whey proteins	15 g (sugars 1 g)	4.3 g	2 g	Contains fish oil, residual lactose, soya. Gluten-free	Borderline substances standard ACBS indications p. 1879 except bowel fistula.	Nutrison 1200 Complete Multi Fibre liquid: 1000 ml = £18.45; 1500 ml = £27.72
Not suitable for use in child under 1 year; not recommended for child under 12 years									
Nutrison® Protein Plus Multifibre (Nutricia Ltd)	Liquid (tube feed) per 100 mL	535 kJ (128 kcal)	6.3 g caseinates, pea, soya, whey proteins	14.1 g (sugars 1 g)	4.9 g	1.5 g	Contains fish oil, residual lactose, soya. Gluten-free	Disease related malnutrition.	Nutrison Protein Plus Multifibre liquid: 500 ml = £9.25; 1000 ml = £17.98
Not suitable for use in child under 1 year; not recommended in child 1–6 years									

1.5 to less than 2 kcal/mL

Product	Formulation	Energy	Protein	Carbohydrate	Fat	Fibre	Special Characteristics	ACBS Indications	Presentation & Flavour
Fresubin® Energy tube feed (Fresenius Kabi Ltd)	Liquid (tube feed) per 100 mL	630 kJ (150 kcal)	5.6 g milk protein, whey protein	18.8 g (sugars 1.15 g)	5.8 g	Nil	Contains fish oil, residual lactose, soya. Gluten-free	Borderline substances standard ACBS indications p. 1879.	Fresubin Energy tube feed liquid unflavoured: 500 ml = £7.57; 1000 ml = £14.46; 1500 ml = £22.25
Not suitable for use in child under 3 years; use with caution in child under 6 years									
Nutrison® Energy (Nutricia Ltd)	Liquid (tube feed) per 100 mL	630 kJ (150 kcal)	6 g caseinate, pea, soya, whey proteins	18.5 g (sugars 1.2 g)	5.8 g	Nil	Contains fish oil, residual lactose, soya. Gluten-free	Borderline substances standard ACBS indications p. 1879.	Nutrison Energy liquid: 500 ml = £9.01; 1000 ml = £16.93; 1500 ml = £25.36
Not suitable for use in child under 3 years; use with caution in child over 3 years									
Osmolite® 1.5kcal (Abbott Laboratories Ltd)	Liquid (tube feed) per 100 mL	634 kJ (151 kcal)	6.3 g caseinates, soya protein isolate	20.4 g (sugars 1.2 g)	4.9 g	Nil	Contains residual lactose, soya. Gluten-free	Borderline substances standard ACBS indications p. 1879; also continuous ambulatory peritoneal dialysis (CAPD), and haemodialysis.	Osmolite 1.5kcal tube feed liquid: 500 ml = £9.04; 1000 ml = £17.08; 1500 ml = £25.57
Not suitable for use in child under 1 year; not recommended for use in children									

1.5 to less than 2 kcal/mL higher protein

Product	Formulation	Energy	Protein	Carbohydrate	Fat	Fibre	Special Characteristics	ACBS Indications	Presentation & Flavour
Fresubin® HP Energy (Fresenius Kabi Ltd)	Liquid (tube feed) per 100 mL	630 kJ (150 kcal)	7.5 g milk protein	17 g (sugars 1 g)	5.8 g (MCT 57 %)	Nil	Contains fish oil, residual lactose, soya. Gluten-free	Borderline substances standard ACBS indications p. 1879; also CAPD and haemodialysis.	Fresubin HP Energy liquid: 500 ml = £7.96; 1000 ml = £14.98
Not suitable for use in child under 1 year; use with caution in child under 6 years									
Jevity® Advance (Abbott Laboratories Ltd)	Liquid (tube feed) per 100 mL	631 kJ (150 kcal)	8 g milk protein, soya protein isolate	18 g (sugars 1.31 g)	4.85 g	0.75 g	Contains soya. Gluten-free	Malnourished or nutritionally-at-risk older adults.	Jevity Advance liquid: 500 ml = £8.60
Not recommended for use in children									
Nutrison® Protein Plus Energy (Nutricia Ltd)	Liquid (tube feed) per 100 mL	630 kJ (150 kcal)	7.5 g caseinates, pea, soya, whey proteins	16.9 g (sugars 3.3 g)	5.8 g	Less than 0.1 g	Contains fish oil, residual lactose, soya. Gluten-free	Borderline substances standard ACBS indications p. 1879.	Nutrison Protein Plus Energy liquid: 500 ml = £9.01; 1000 ml = £16.94
Not suitable for use in child under 1 year; not recommended for child 1-6 years									

1.5 to less than 2 kcal/mL with fibre

Product	Formulation	Energy	Protein	Carbohydrate	Fat	Fibre	Special Characteristics	ACBS Indications	Presentation & Flavour
Fresubin® 2250 Complete (Fresenius Kabi Ltd)	Liquid (tube feed) per 100 mL	630 kJ (150 kcal)	5.6 g milk, soya proteins	18 g (sugars 1.2 g)	5.8 g	1.5 g	Contains fish oil, residual lactose, soya. Gluten-free	Borderline substances standard ACBS indications p. 1879	Fresubin 2250 Complete liquid: 1.5 litre = £22.48
Not suitable for use in child under 3 years; not recommended for child under 6 years									
Fresubin® Energy Fibre tube feed (Fresenius Kabi Ltd)	Liquid (tube feed) per 100 mL	630 kJ (150 kcal)	5.6 g milk, soya proteins	18.8 g (sugars 1.2 g)	5.8 g	1.5 g	Contains fish oil, residual lactose, soya. Gluten-free	Borderline substances standard ACBS indications p. 1879.	Fresubin Energy Fibre tube feed liquid unflavoured: 500 ml = £8.11; 1000 ml = £15.59
Not suitable for use in child under 3 years; use with caution in child under 6 years									
Jevity® 1.5kcal (Abbott Laboratories Ltd)	Liquid (tube feed) per 100 mL	649 kJ (154 kcal)	6.38 g caseinates, soya protein isolate	20.1 g (sugars 1.3 g)	4.9 g	2.2 g	Contains residual lactose, soya. Gluten-free	Borderline substances standard ACBS indications p. 1879.	Jevity 1.5kcal liquid: 500 ml = £10.05; 1000 ml = £18.97; 1500 ml = £29.30
Not recommended for use in children									
Nutrison® Energy Multi Fibre (Nutricia Ltd)	Liquid (tube feed) per 100 mL	643 kJ (153 kcal)	6 g caseinates, pea, soya, whey proteins	18.4 g (sugars 2.6 g)	5.8 g	1.5 g	Contains fish oil, residual lactose, soya. Gluten-free	Borderline substances standard ACBS indications p. 1879.	Nutrison Energy Multi Fibre liquid: 500 ml = £9.99; 1000 ml = £18.80; 1500 ml = £29.02
Not suitable for use in child under 3 years; use with caution in child over 3 years									
Nutrison® Energy Multi Fibre Vanilla (Nutricia Ltd)	Liquid (tube feed) per 100 mL	645 kJ (154 kcal)	6 g milk protein	18.4 g (sugars 6.8 g)	5.8 g	2.2 g	Contains residual lactose, soya. Gluten-free	Borderline substances standard ACBS indications p. 1879.	Nutrison Energy Multi Fibre Vanilla liquid: 200 ml = £3.36
Not suitable for use in child under 3 years; not recommended for child under 6 years									

1.5 to less than 2 kcal/mL with fibre, higher protein

Product	Formulation	Energy	Protein	Carbohydrate	Fat	Fibre	Special Characteristics	ACBS Indications	Presentation & Flavour
Compleat® 1.5 HP (Nestle Health Science)	Liquid (tube feed) per 100 mL	626 kJ (150 kcal)	7.5 g chicken, milk protein	12.7 g (sugars 1.4 g)	7.3 g	1.5 g	Contains fish oil, meat derivatives, residual lactose, soya oil. Gluten-free	Borderline substances standard ACBS indications p. 1879; also feeding intolerance, and developmental disabilities.	Compleat 1.5 HP tube feed liquid: 500 ml = £9.53
Fresubin® HP Energy Fibre (Fresenius Kabi Ltd)	Liquid (tube feed) per 100 mL	630 kJ (150 kcal)	7.5 g milk protein	16.2 g (sugars 1.11 g)	5.8 g (MCT 57%)	1.5 g	Contains fish oil, residual lactose, soya. Gluten-free	Borderline substances standard ACBS indications p. 1879 except dysphagia. Also CAPD and haemodialysis.	Fresubin HP Energy Fibre liquid: 500 ml = £8.67; 1000 ml = £16.52

Not suitable for use in child under 3 years; use with caution in child under 6 years

2 kcal/mL or more higher protein

Product	Formulation	Energy	Protein	Carbohydrate	Fat	Fibre	Special Characteristics	ACBS Indications	Presentation & Flavour
Fresubin® 2kcal HP (Fresenius Kabi Ltd)	Liquid (tube feed) per 100 mL	838 kJ (200 kcal)	10 g milk protein	18 g (sugars 2.7 g)	10 g	Nil	Contains fish oil, residual lactose, soya lecithin. Gluten-free	Disease-related malnutrition requiring a high energy and protein supply within a low volume, including patients with chronic diseases e.g. cancer, cardiac failure, COPD, renal and liver disease.	Fresubin 2kcal HP tube liquid feed: 500 ml = £10.11

Not suitable for use in child under 3 years; use with caution in child under 6 years

2 kcal/mL or more with fibre

Product	Formulation	Energy	Protein	Carbohydrate	Fat	Fibre	Special Characteristics	ACBS Indications	Presentation & Flavour
TwoCal® (Abbott Laboratories Ltd)	Liquid (tube feed) per 100 mL	837 kJ (200 kcal)	8.4 g casein, milk protein isolate	21 g hydrolysed corn starch (sugars 4.7 g)	8.9 g	1 g	Contains residual lactose, soya. Gluten-free	Adults with or at risk of disease-related malnutrition, catabolic or fluid-restricted patients, and other patients requiring a 2 kcal/mL feed.	TwoCal liquid: 1 litre = £24.83

Not recommended for use in children

Product	Formulation	Energy	Protein	Carbohydrate	Fat	Fibre	Special Characteristics	ACBS Indications	Presentation & Flavour
TwoCal® Bolus (Abbott Laboratories Ltd)	Liquid (tube feed) per 100 mL	837 kJ (200 kcal)	8.4 g casein, milk protein isolate	21 g hydrolysed corn starch (sugars 4.65 g)	8.9 g	1 g	Contains residual lactose, soya. Gluten-free	Adults with or at risk of disease-related malnutrition, catabolic or fluid-restricted patients, and other patients requiring a 2 kcal/mL feed.	TwoCal Bolus liquid: 200 ml = £4.45

Not recommended for use in children

2 kcal/mL or more with fibre, higher protein

Product	Formulation	Energy	Protein	Carbohydrate	Fat	Fibre	Special Characteristics	ACBS Indications	Presentation & Flavour
Fresubin® 2kcal HP Fibre (Fresenius Kabi Ltd)	Liquid (tube feed) per 100 mL	840 kJ (200 kcal)	10 g milk protein	16.7 g (sugars 2.53 g)	10 g	1.5 g	Contains fish oil, residual lactose, soya lecithin. Gluten-free	Disease-related malnutrition requiring a high energy and protein supply within a low volume, including patients with chronic diseases e.g. cancer, cardiac failure, COPD, renal and liver disease.	Fresubin 2kcal HP Fibre tube feed liquid: 500 ml = £11.99

Not suitable for use in child under 3 years; use with caution in child under 6 years

2 kcal/mL or more with fibre, higher protein (product list continued)

Product	Formulation	Energy	Protein	Carbohydrate	Fat	Fibre	Special Characteristics	ACBS Indications	Presentation & Flavour
Nutrison® PlantBased 2kcal HP Multi Fibre (Nutricia Ltd)	Liquid (tube feed) per 100 mL	839 kJ (200 kcal)	10 g pea protein isolate, soya protein	18.5 g sugars (1.3 g)	9.3 g	1.5 g	Contains residual lactose, soya. Gluten-free	Borderline substances standard ACBS indications p. 1879	Nutrison PlantBased 2kcal HP Multi Fibre liquid: 500 ml = £13.19

Not suitable for use in child under 3 years; use with caution in child 3-17 years

Table 2 Oral nutrition

Oral nutritional supplements: Cancer (ready to serve)

1.5 kcal/mL milkshake

Product	Formulation	Energy	Protein	Carbohydrate	Fat	Fibre	Special Characteristics	ACBS Indications	Presentation & Flavour
Supportan® (Fresenius Kabi Ltd)	Liquid (sip feed) per 100 mL	630 kJ (150 kcal)	10 g milk protein	11.6 g sucrose (sugars 7.5 g)	6.7 g	1.5 g	Contains fish oil, residual lactose, soya lecithin. Gluten-free Minerals/100 mL: Na 2.1 mmol K 3.3 mmol Ca 5.1 mmol P 3.9 mmol	Patients with pancreatic cancer or patients with lung cancer undergoing chemotherapy.	Supportan drink tropical fruits: 800 ml = £16.18

Not suitable for use in child under 3 years; use with caution in child under 6 years

Oral nutritional supplements: Dysphagia (ready to serve)

1.3 kcal/g dessert style (fruit based)

Product	Formulation	Energy	Protein	Carbohydrate	Fat	Fibre	Special Characteristics	ACBS Indications	Presentation & Flavour
Nutilis® Fruit Dessert Level 4 (Nutricia Ltd)	Semi-solid per 100 g	575 kJ (137 kcal)	6.9 g whey protein isolate	17 g (sugars 11.5 g)	4 g	2.6 g	Contains residual lactose, soya. Gluten-free	Borderline substances standard ACBS indications p. 1879 except bowel fistula; also CAPD, haemodialysis.	Nutilis Fruit Dessert Level 4: apple 450 gram = £10.08; strawberry 450 gram = £10.08

Not suitable for use in child under 3 years; not recommended for child under 6 years

1.5 kcal/mL milkshake higher protein, pre-thickened

Product	Formulation	Energy	Protein	Carbohydrate	Fat	Fibre	Special Characteristics	ACBS Indications	Presentation & Flavour
Fresubin® Thickened (Fresenius Kabi Ltd)	Liquid (sip feed) per 100 mL	630 kJ (150 kcal)	10 g milk protein	12 g sucrose (sugars 7.3 g)	6.7 g	0.83 g	Contains soya lecithin, residual lactose. Gluten-free	Dysphagia or disease-related malnutrition.	Fresubin Thickened Level 2: wild strawberry 800 ml = £10.87; vanilla 800 ml = £10.87; Fresubin Thickened Level 3: wild strawberry 800 ml = £10.87; vanilla 800 ml = £10.87

Not suitable for use in child under 3 years; use with caution in child under 6 years

2.4 kcal/g dessert style (milk based)

Product	Formulation	Energy	Protein	Carbohydrate	Fat	Fibre	Special Characteristics	ACBS Indications	Presentation & Flavour
Nutilis® Complete Creme Level 3 (Nutricia Ltd)	Semi-solid per 100 g	1030 kJ (245 kcal)	9.6 g milk protein	29.1 g (sugars 11.8 g)	9.4 g	3.2 g	Contains residual lactose, soya. Gluten-free	Borderline substances standard ACBS indications p. 1879.	Nutilis Complete Creme Level 3 custard: strawberry 500 gram = £11.48; vanilla 500 gram = £11.48; chocolate 500 gram = £11.48

Not suitable for use in child under 3 years; not recommended for child under 6 years

2.4 kcal/mL milkshake lower volume

Product	Formulation	Energy	Protein	Carbohydrate	Fat	Fibre	Special Characteristics	ACBS Indications	Presentation & Flavour
Nutilis® Complete Drink Level 3 (Nutricia Ltd)	Liquid (sip feed) per 100 mL	1025 kJ (245 kcal)	9.6 g caseinates, milk proteins	29.1 g (sugars 5.4 g)	9.3 g	3.2 g	Contains residual lactose, soya. Gluten-free	Borderline substances standard ACBS indications p. 1879	Nutilis Complete Drink Level 3 liquid: strawberry 500 ml = £11.48; *mango & passionfruit* 500 ml = £11.48; lemon tea 500 ml = £11.48; chocolate 500 ml = £11.48; vanilla 500 ml = £11.48

Not suitable for use in child under 3 years; not recommended for child under 6 years

Oral nutritional supplements: Impaired gastro-intestinal function or malabsorption (powder)

4.4 kcal/g amino acid based with MCT

Product	Formulation	Energy	Protein	Carbohydrate	Fat	Fibre	Special Characteristics	ACBS Indications	Presentation & Flavour
Emsogen® (Nutricia Ltd)	Standard dilution (20 % w/v) of powder per 100 mL	368 kJ (88 kcal)	2.5 g protein equivalent (essential and nonessential amino acids)	12.0 g (sugars 1.6 g)	3.3 g (MCT 83 %)	Nil		Short-bowel syndrome, intractable malabsorption, proven inflammatory bowel disease, bowel fistula.	Emsogen powder unflavoured: 100 gram = £11.09

Powder provides: protein 12.5 g, carbohydrate 60.0 g, fat 16.4 g, energy 1839 kJ (438 kcal)/100 g
Not suitable for use in child under 1 year; not recommended for use in child under 5 years

4.4 kcal/g juice style

Product	Formulation	Energy	Protein	Carbohydrate	Fat	Fibre	Special Characteristics	ACBS Indications	Presentation & Flavour
Elemental 028® Extra powder (Nutricia Ltd)	Standard dilution (20% w/v) of powder per 100 mL	374 kJ (89 kcal)	2.5 g protein equivalent (essential and nonessential amino acids)	12 g (sugars 1.1 g)	3.5 g (MCT 35%)	Nil	Gluten-free, lactose-free	Short bowel syndrome, intractable malabsorption, proven inflammatory bowel disease, bowel fistulae.	Elemental 028 Extra powder: orange 100 gram = £10.77; plain 100 gram = £10.77; banana 100 gram = £10.77

Powder provides: protein 12.5 g, carbohydrate 59 g, fat 17.5 g, energy 1871 kJ (443 kcal)/100 g
Not suitable for use in child under 1 year; not recommended for child 1-5 years

5 kcal/g milkshake

Product	Formulation	Energy	Protein	Carbohydrate	Fat	Fibre	Special Characteristics	ACBS Indications	Presentation & Flavour
Modulen IBD® (Nestle Health Science)	Standard dilution (20 % w/v) of powder (sip feed) per 100 mL	414 kJ (100 kcal)	3.6 g casein	11 g (sugars 4.2 g)	4.6 g	Nil	Contains residual lactose, soya. Gluten-free Minerals/100 mL: Na 1.5 mmol K 3 mmol Ca 2.2 mmol P 1.9 mmol	Sole source of nutrition during active phase of Crohn's disease, and nutritional support during remission phase for malnourished patients.	Modulen IBD powder: 350 gram = £17.82

Powder provides: protein 18 g, carbohydrate 54 g, fat 23 g, energy 2070 kJ (500 kcal)/100 g
Not suitable for use in child under 6 years

Oral nutritional supplements: Impaired gastro-intestinal function or malabsorption (ready to serve)

0.9 kcal/mL juice style

Product	Formulation	Energy	Protein	Carbohydrate	Fat	Fibre	Special Characteristics	ACBS Indications	Presentation & Flavour
Elemental 028® Extra liquid (Nutricia Ltd)	Liquid (sip feed) per 100 mL	360 kJ (86 kcal)	2.5 g protein equivalent (essential and nonessential amino acids)	11 g (sugars 4.7 g)	3.5 g (MCT 35%)	Nil	Gluten-free, lactose-free	Short bowel syndrome, intractable malabsorption, proven inflammatory bowel disease, bowel fistulae.	Elemental 028 Extra liquid: orange & pineapple 250 ml = £5.52; summer fruits 250 ml = £5.52; grapefruit 250 ml = £5.52

Not suitable for use in child under 1 year; not recommended for child 1-5 years

1 kcal/mL milkshake

Product	Formulation	Energy	Protein	Carbohydrate	Fat	Fibre	Special Characteristics	ACBS Indications	Presentation & Flavour
Peptamen® (Nestle Health Science)	Liquid (sip feed) per 100 mL	421 kJ (100 kcal)	4 g whey protein	12.7 g (sugars 3.3 g)	3.7 g (MCT 68 %)	Nil	Contains residual lactose, soya	Short bowel syndrome, intractable malabsorption, proven inflammatory bowel disease, bowel fistulae.	Peptamen liquid vanilla: 800 ml = £16.84

Not suitable for use in child under 3 years; not recommended for child under 5 years

Product	Formulation	Energy	Protein	Carbohydrate	Fat	Fibre	Special Characteristics	ACBS Indications	Presentation & Flavour
Survimed® OPD (Fresenius Kabi Ltd)	Liquid (sip feed) per 100 mL	420 kJ (100 kcal)	4.65 g whey protein hydrolysate	14.1 g (sugars 5 g)	2.8 g (MCT 48%)	Less than 0.1 g	Contains residual lactose. Gluten-free	Borderline substances standard ACBS indications p. 1879	Survimed OPD liquid: 800 ml = £15.27

Not suitable for use in child under 3 years; use with caution in child under 6 years

1.5 kcal/mL milkshake higher protein, higher energy

Product	Formulation	Energy	Protein	Carbohydrate	Fat	Fibre	Special Characteristics	ACBS Indications	Presentation & Flavour
Peptisip Energy HP (Nutricia Ltd)	Liquid (sip feed) per 100 mL	634 kJ (150 kcal)	7.5 g whey protein hydrolysate	18.8 g (sugars 4.1 g)	5 g (MCT 60 %)	0.28 g	Contains residual lactose, soya lecithin	Disease-related malnutrition in patients with malabsorption and/or maldigestion.	Peptisip Energy HP liquid: 200 ml = £3.93

Not suitable for use in child under 3 years; use with caution in child 3-6 years

Product	Formulation	Energy	Protein	Carbohydrate	Fat	Fibre	Special Characteristics	ACBS Indications	Presentation & Flavour
Survimed® OPD 1.5kcal (Fresenius Kabi Ltd)	Liquid (sip feed) per 100 mL	630 kJ (150 kcal)	7.5 g whey protein hydrolysate	20.6 g (sugars 7.4 g)	4.2 g (MCT 50%)	Less than 0.1 g	Contains residual lactose. Gluten-free	Borderline substances standard ACBS indications p. 1879 except dysphagia.	Survimed OPD 1.5kcal drink: vanilla 200 ml = £3.82; cappuccino 200 ml = £3.82

Not suitable for use in child under 3 years; use with caution in child under 6 years

| Vital® 1.5kcal (Abbott Laboratories Ltd) | Liquid (sip feed) per 100 mL | 631 kJ (150 kcal) | 6.8 g caseinates, whey protein hydrolysate | 18.4 g (sugars 3.5 g) | 5.5 g (MCT 64%) | Nil | Contains residual lactose. Gluten-free | Borderline substances standard ACBS indications p. 1879 except dysphagia. | Vital 1.5kcal liquid: vanilla 200 ml = £4.71; mixed berry 200 ml = £4.71; cafe latte 200 ml = £4.71 |

Not recommended for use in children

Oral nutritional supplements: Renal failure (powder)

3.7 kcal/g energy and protein fortifier

Product	Formulation	Energy	Protein	Carbohydrate	Fat	Fibre	Special Characteristics	ACBS Indications	Presentation & Flavour
Renapro® (Stanningley Pharma Ltd)	Powder per 100 g	1611 kJ (385 kcal)	90 g whey protein	3.4 g	1 g	Nil	Gluten-free Minerals/100 g: Na 300 mg K 310 mg Ca 340 mg P 140 mg	Dialysis and hypoproteinaemia.	Renapro powder 20g sachets: 30 sachet = £69.60

Powder 20 g reconstituted with 60-100 mL cold water provides: protein 18 g, carbohydrate 0.7 g, fat less than 0.2 g, energy 322 kJ (77 kcal)
Not suitable for use in child under 1 year

4.8 kcal/g milk replacer

Product	Formulation	Energy	Protein	Carbohydrate	Fat	Fibre	Special Characteristics	ACBS Indications	Presentation & Flavour
Renamil® (Stanningley Pharma Ltd)	Powder per 100 g	2012 kJ (479 kcal)	5 g milk protein, whey protein isolate	71.2 g (sugars 6.8 g)	19.3 g	Nil	Contains lactose, soya. Gluten-free Minerals/100 mL: Na 3 mmol K 0.1 mmol Ca 3.7 mmol P 0.8 mmol	Chronic renal failure.	Renamil powder 100g sachets: 10 sachet = £31.75

Not suitable for use in child under 1 year

Oral nutritional supplements: Renal failure (ready to serve)

1.8 kcal/mL milkshake

Product	Formulation	Energy	Protein	Carbohydrate	Fat	Fibre	Special Characteristics	ACBS Indications	Presentation & Flavour
Nepro® HP (Abbott Laboratories Ltd)	Liquid (sip or tube feed) per 100 mL	752 kJ (180 kcal)	8.1 g caseinates, milk protein isolate	14.7 g (sugars 3.2 g)	9.8 g	1.3 g	Contains meat derivatives, residual lactose, soya. Gluten-free Minerals/100 mL: Na 3 mmol K 2.7 mmol Ca 2.6 mmol P 2.3 mmol	Patients with chronic renal failure who are on haemodialysis or complete ambulatory peritoneal dialysis (CAPD), or patients with cirrhosis or other conditions requiring a high energy, low fluid, low electrolyte diet.	Nepro HP liquid: strawberry 220 ml = £5.04; vanilla 220 ml = £5.04

Not recommended for use in children

2 kcal/mL milkshake lower volume

Product	Formulation	Energy	Protein	Carbohydrate	Fat	Fibre	Special Characteristics	ACBS Indications	Presentation & Flavour
Renastep® (Vitaflo International Ltd)	Liquid (sip or tube feed) per 100 mL	836 kJ (200 kcal)	4 g milk protein	21 g (sugars 3.4 g)	11.1 g	Nil	Contains fish oil Minerals/100 mL: Na 3.6 mmol K 0.9 mmol Ca 1.2 mmol P 1.1 mmol	Renal failure.	Renastep liquid: 125 ml = £6.49

Not suitable for use in child under 3 years

Product	Formulation	Energy	Protein	Carbohydrate	Fat	Fibre	Special Characteristics	ACBS Indications	Presentation & Flavour
Renilon® 7.5 (Nutricia Ltd)	Liquid (sip feed) per 100 mL	835 kJ (199 kcal)	7.3 g milk protein	20 g (sugars 4.8 g)	10 g	Nil	Contains residual lactose, soya Minerals/100 mL: Na 2.7 mmol K 0.9 mmol Ca less than 0.27 mmol P less than 0.29 mmol	Borderline substances standard ACBS indications p. 1879 except dysphagia.	Renilon 7.5 liquid: caramel 500 ml = £13.44; apricot 500 ml = £13.44

Not suitable for use in child under 3 years; not recommended for child under 6 years

Oral nutritional supplements: Standard feeds (powder)

1 - 2.2 kcal/mL soup

Product	Formulation	Energy	Protein	Carbohydrate	Fat	Fibre	Special Characteristics	ACBS Indications	Presentation & Flavour
Aymes® ActaSolve Savoury (Aymes International Ltd)	Powder per 100 g	1844 kJ (438 kcal)	15.9 g milk protein	60.3 g (sugars 11.9-22.6 g)	14.7 g	0.5 g	Contains celery (vegetable flavour only), lactose, meat derivatives (chicken flavour only). Gluten-free	Borderline substances standard ACBS indications p. 1879 except dysphagia.	Aymes ActaSolve Savoury Starter Pack powder: 3 sachet = £2.78; Aymes ActaSolve Savoury powder 57g sachets: potato & leek 7 sachet = £6.49; chicken 7 sachet = £6.49; vegetable 7 sachet = £6.49

Powder 57 g reconstituted with 200 mL water provides: protein 9.1 g, carbohydrate 34.4 g, fat 8.4 g, energy 1051 kJ (250 kcal)
Not suitable for use in child under 3 years; use with caution in child under 6 years

1.4 - 1.6 kcal/mL milkshake

Product	Formulation	Energy	Protein	Carbohydrate	Fat	Fibre	Special Characteristics	ACBS Indications	Presentation & Flavour
Aymes® Shake (Aymes International Ltd)	Powder per 100 g	1871 kJ (445 kcal)	21 g milk protein	57 g (sugars 31.5 g)	14.8 g	0.2 g	Contains lactose, soya. Gluten-free	Borderline substances standard ACBS indications p. 1879	Aymes Shake powder: banana 1600 gram = £15.96; chocolate 1600 gram = £15.96; neutral 1600 gram = £15.96; strawberry 1600 gram = £15.96; vanilla 1600 gram = £15.96; Aymes Shake Starter Pack powder: 6 sachet = £4.57; Aymes Shake powder 57g sachets: strawberry 7 sachet = £3.99; ginger 7 sachet = £3.99; vanilla 7 sachet = £3.99; banana 7 sachet = £3.99; chocolate 7 sachet = £3.99; neutral 7 sachet = £3.99

Powder 57 g reconstituted with 200 mL whole milk provides: protein 19 g, carbohydrate 42 g, fat 15.8 g, energy 1618 kJ (383 kcal)
Not suitable for use in child under 3 years; use with caution in child under 6 years

Product	Dilution/form	Energy	Protein	Carbohydrate	Fat	Fibre	Special characteristics	Presentation	Price
Complan® Shake (Nutricia Ltd)	Standard dilution (24% w/v) of powder per 100 mL	673 kJ (160 kcal)	6.5 g cow's milk	18.9 g (sugars 11.6 g)	6.6 g	Less than 0.04 g	Contains lactose. Gluten-free	Borderline substances standard ACBS indications p. 1879.	Complan Shake Starter Pack sachets: 5 sachet = £3.70; Complan Shake oral powder 57g sachets: chocolate 4 sachet = £2.12; vanilla 4 sachet = £2.12; banana 4 sachet = £2.12; milk 4 sachet = £2.12; strawberry 4 sachet = £2.12

Powder provides: protein 15.4 g, carbohydrate 62.5 g, fat 14.8 g, energy 1870kJ (445 kcal)/100 g
Not suitable for use in child under 3 years; not recommended for child 3-6 years

Product	Dilution/form	Energy	Protein	Carbohydrate	Fat	Fibre	Special characteristics	Presentation	Price
EnergieShake® Powder (Anaiah Healthcare PVT Ltd)	Powder per 100 g	1849 kJ (439 kcal)	16.5 g milk protein	62.1 g (sugars 26.8 g)	13.9 g	Less than 1 g	Contains lactose, soya	Borderline substances standard ACBS indications p. 1879.	EnergieShake Powder Starter Pack oral powder sachets: 285 gram = £2.88; EnergieShake Powder oral powder 57g sachets: neutral 4 sachet = £1.76; 7 sachet = £3.08; banana 4 sachet = £1.76; 7 sachet = £3.08; strawberry 4 sachet = £1.76; 7 sachet = £3.08; chocolate 4 sachet = £1.76; 7 sachet = £3.08; vanilla 4 sachet = £1.76; 7 sachet = £3.08

Powder 57 g reconstituted with 200 mL water provides: protein 9.4 g, carbohydrate 35.4 g, fat 7.9 g, energy 1054 kJ (250 kcal)
Not recommended for use in child under 6 years

Product	Dilution/form	Energy	Protein	Carbohydrate	Fat	Fibre	Special characteristics	Presentation	Price
Ensure® Shake (Abbott Laboratories Ltd)	Powder per 100 g	1852 kJ (443 kcal)	17.8 g milk, whey proteins	59 g (sugars 33.7 g)	15.1 g	Nil	Contains lactose, soya. Gluten-free	Borderline substances standard ACBS indications p. 1879.	Ensure Shake oral powder 57g sachets: chocolate 7 sachet = £4.56; strawberry 7 sachet = £4.56; banana 7 sachet = £4.56; vanilla 7 sachet = £4.56

Powder 57 g reconstituted with 200 mL whole milk provides: protein 17 g, carbohydrate 43.2 g, fat 16.6 g, energy 1626 kJ (389 kcal)
Not suitable for use in child under 1 year; not recommended for use in children

Product	Dilution/form	Energy	Protein	Carbohydrate	Fat	Fibre	Special characteristics	Presentation	Price
Foodlink® Complete (Nualtra Ltd)	Powder per 100 g	1869 kJ (444 kcal)	21 g milk protein	56 g (sugars 43 g)	15 g	Nil	Contains lactose, soya. Gluten-free	Borderline substances standard ACBS indications p. 1879	Foodlink Complete powder: banana 1596 gram = £16.24; chocolate 1596 gram = £16.24; natural 1596 gram = £16.24; strawberry 1596 gram = £16.24; vanilla 1596 gram = £16.24; Foodlink Complete Starter Pack powder: 5 sachet = £4.60; Foodlink Complete powder 57g sachets: chocolate 7 sachet = £4.06; vanilla 7 sachet = £4.06; natural 7 sachet = £4.06; strawberry 7 sachet = £4.06; banana 7 sachet = £4.06

Powder 57 g reconstituted with 200 ml whole milk provides: protein 19 g, carbohydrate 41 g, fat 16 g, energy 1611 kJ (383 kcal)
Not suitable for use in child under 3 years; not recommended in child 3-6 years

1.4 - 1.6 kcal/mL milkshake (product list continued)

Product	Formulation	Energy	Protein	Carbohydrate	Fat	Fibre	Special Characteristics	ACBS Indications	Presentation & Flavour
Fresubin® Powder Extra (Fresenius Kabi Ltd)	Powder per 100 g	1764 kJ (420 kcal)	17.5 g milk, whey proteins	63 g (sugars 18.6 g)	10.9 g	Nil	Contains lactose. Gluten-free	Borderline substances standard ACBS indications p. 1879.	Fresubin Powder Extra oral powder 62g sachets: chocolate 7 sachet = £5.11; strawberry 7 sachet = £5.11; neutral 7 sachet = £5.11; vanilla 7 sachet = £5.11

Powder 62 g reconstituted with 200 ml whole milk provides: protein 17.7 g, carbohydrate 48.5 g, fat 14.8 g, energy 1658 kJ (397 kcal)
Not suitable for use in child under 3 years; use with caution in child under 6 years

1.5 kcal/mL smoothie

Product	Formulation	Energy	Protein	Carbohydrate	Fat	Fibre	Special Characteristics	ACBS Indications	Presentation & Flavour
Aymes® ActaSolve Smoothie (Aymes International Ltd)	Powder per 100 g	1892 kJ (450 kcal)	16.2 g soya protein isolate	62.8 g (sugars 24.8 g)	14.6 g	0.7 g	Contains soya. Gluten-free	Borderline substances standard ACBS indications p. 1879 except dysphagia.	Aymes ActaSolve Smoothie Starter Pack powder: 4 sachet = £5.93; Aymes ActaSolve Smoothie powder 66g sachets: strawberry & cranberry 7 sachet = £7.56; pineapple 7 sachet = £7.56; peach 7 sachet = £7.56; mango 7 sachet = £7.56

Powder 66 g reconstituted with 150ml water provides: protein 10.7 g, carbohydrate 41.5 g, fat 9.7 g, energy 1249 kJ (297 kcal)
Not suitable for use in child under 3 years; use with caution in child under 6 years

Product	Formulation	Energy	Protein	Carbohydrate	Fat	Fibre	Special Characteristics	ACBS Indications	Presentation & Flavour
Foodlink® Smoothie (Nualtra Ltd)	Powder per 100 g	1810 kJ (435 kcal)	15 g soya protein isolate	69 g (sugars 24 g)	11 g	Nil	Contains soya. Gluten-free, lactose-free	Disease-related malnutrition.	Foodlink Smoothie Starter Pack sachets: 4 sachet = £4.60; Foodlink Smoothie powder 66g sachets: orange & mango 7 sachet = £7.77; tropical 7 sachet = £7.77; red berry 7 sachet = £7.77; peach 7 sachet = £7.77

Powder 66 g reconstituted with 150 mL water provides: protein 10 g, carbohydrate 45 g, fat 7 g, energy 1195 kJ (287 kcal)
Not suitable for use in child under 3 years; use with caution in child under 6 years

1.6 kcal/mL milkshake with fibre

Product	Formulation	Energy	Protein	Carbohydrate	Fat	Fibre	Special Characteristics	ACBS Indications	Presentation & Flavour
Aymes® Shake Fibre (Aymes International Ltd)	Powder per 100 g	1793 kJ (427 kcal)	21 g milk protein	48.1 g (sugars 34.2 g)	14.8 g	8.8 g	Contains lactose, soya. Gluten-free	Borderline substances standard ACBS indications p. 1879 except dysphagia.	Aymes Shake Fibre Starter Pack powder: 5 sachet = £4.35; Aymes Shake Fibre powder 57g sachets: neutral 7 sachet = £6.10; banana 7 sachet = £6.10; chocolate 7 sachet = £6.10; strawberry 7 sachet = £6.10; vanilla 7 sachet = £6.10

Powder 57 g reconstituted with 200 mL whole milk provides: protein 19 g, carbohydrate 36.9 g, fat 15.8 g, energy 1573 kJ (375 kcal)
Not suitable for use in child under 3 years; use with caution in child under 6 years

	Formulation	Energy	Protein	Carbohydrate	Fat	Fibre	Special Characteristics	ACBS Indications	Presentation & Flavour
Foodlink® Complete with Fibre (Nualtra Ltd)	Powder per 100 g	1779 kJ (423 kcal)	19 g milk, soya proteins	52 g (sugars 40 g)	14 g	7.2 g	Contains lactose, soya. Gluten-free	Borderline substances standard ACBS indications p. 1879	Foodlink Complete powder with fibre 63g sachets: vanilla 7 sachet = £6.86; strawberry 7 sachet = £6.86; chocolate 7 sachet = £6.86; natural 7 sachet = £6.86; banana 7 sachet = £6.86; Foodlink Complete powder with fibre Starter Pack: 5 sachet = £5.10

Powder 63 g reconstituted with 200 ml whole milk provides: protein 19 g, carbohydrate 42 g, fat 16 g, energy 1667 kJ (397 kcal)
Not suitable for use in child under 3 years; not recommended for child 3-6 years

2 kcal/mL milkshake higher volume, higher energy

Product	Formulation	Energy	Protein	Carbohydrate	Fat	Fibre	Special Characteristics	ACBS Indications	Presentation & Flavour
Aymes® ActaSolve High Energy (Aymes International Ltd)	Powder per 100 g	2105 kJ (503 kcal)	4.8 g milk protein	63.8 g (sugar 22.5 g)	25.3 g	0.40 g	Contains lactose, soya. Gluten-free	Borderline substances standard ACBS indications p. 1879 except dysphagia.	Aymes ActaSolve High Energy Starter Pack powder: 4 sachet = £8.96; Aymes ActaSolve High Energy powder 85g sachets: vanilla 6 sachet = £9.62; banana 6 sachet = £9.62; chocolate 6 sachet = £9.62; strawberry 6 sachet = £9.62

Powder 85 g reconstituted with 240 ml whole milk provides: protein 12.3 g, carbohydrate 65.6 g, fat 30.4 g, energy 2451 kJ (586 kcal)
Not suitable for use in child under 3 years; use with caution in child under 6 years

| Calshake® powder (Fresenius Kabi Ltd) | Standard dilution (28% w/v) of powder per 100 mL | 795 kJ (190 kcal) | 3.8 g milk protein | 22.2 g dextrose and maltodextrin (sugars 7-14.1 g) | 9.5 g | Less than 0.15 g | Contains lactose. Gluten-free. | Disease related malnutrition, malabsorption states or other conditions requiring fortification with a fat/carbohydrate supplement. | Calshake powder 87g sachets: neutral 7 sachet = £21.83; vanilla 7 sachet = £21.83; strawberry 7 sachet = £21.83; banana 7 sachet = £21.83; Calshake powder 90g sachets chocolate: 7 sachet = £21.83 |

Powder provides: protein 4.3 g, carbohydrate 67.3 g, fat 24.1 g, energy 2100 kJ (500 kcal)/100 g
Not suitable for use in child under 3 years; neutral flavour not suitable for use in child under 1 year; use with caution in child under 6 years

| Enshake® (Abbott Laboratories Ltd) | Standard dilution (31.1% w/v) of powder per 100 mL | 815 kJ (194 kcal) | 5.2 g caseinate, milk, soya protein isolates | 25.5 g 24.7 g corn syrup (sugars 7.4 g) | 8 g | Nil | Contains residual lactose, soya. Gluten-free | Disease-related malnutrition, malabsorption states or other conditions requiring fortification with a fat/carbohydrate supplement. | Enshake oral powder 96.5g sachets: chocolate 6 sachet = £22.02; strawberry 6 sachet = £22.02; banana 6 sachet = £22.02; vanilla 6 sachet = £22.02 |

Powder provides: protein 8.4 g, carbohydrate 69.5 g, fat 15.6 g, energy 1902 kJ (452 kcal)/100 g
Not suitable for use in child under 1 year; not recommended for use in children

| Foodlink® Extra (Nualtra Ltd) | Powder per 100 g | 2186 kJ (523 kcal) | 4.9 g milk protein | 60 g (sugars 15 g) | 30 g | Nil | Contains lactose. Gluten-free | Disease-related malnutrition. | Foodlink Extra Starter Pack sachets: 4 sachet = £6.60; Foodlink Extra powder 85g sachets: strawberry 7 sachet = £11.20; banana 7 sachet = £11.20; vanilla 7 sachet = £11.20; chocolate 7 sachet = £11.20 |

Powder 85 g reconstituted with 240 mL whole milk provides: protein 13 g, carbohydrate 62 g, fat 35 g, energy 2513 kJ (601 kcal)
Not suitable for use in child under 3 years; use with caution in child under 6 years

2 kcal/mL milkshake higher volume, higher energy (product list continued)

Product	Formulation	Energy	Protein	Carbohydrate	Fat	Fibre	Special Characteristics	ACBS Indications	Presentation & Flavour
Scandishake® Mix (Nutricia Ltd)	Powder per 100 g	2120 kJ (507 kcal)	4.8 g caseinates	67 g (sugars 20.5 g)	24.5 g	Nil	Contains lactose, soya.	Disease-related malnutrition, malabsorption states or other conditions requiring fortification with a fat / carbohydrate supplement.	Scandishake Mix oral powder 85g sachets: banana 6 sachet = £21.42; vanilla 6 sachet = £21.42; chocolate 6 sachet = £21.42; caramel 6 sachet = £21.42; strawberry 6 sachet = £21.42; unflavoured 6 sachet = £21.42

Powder 85 g reconstituted with 240 mL whole milk provides: protein 12.1 g, carbohydrate 68.2 g, fat 29.6 g, energy 2460 kJ (587 kcal)
Not suitable for use in child under 3 years

2.3 - 2.4 kcal/mL milkshake lower volume

Product	Formulation	Energy	Protein	Carbohydrate	Fat	Fibre	Special Characteristics	ACBS Indications	Presentation & Flavour
Aymes® Shake Compact (Aymes International Ltd)	Powder per 100 g	1862 kJ (442 kcal)	15.5 g milk protein	61.7 g (sugars 35 g)	14.8 g	0.2 g	Contains lactose, soya. Gluten-free	Borderline substances standard ACBS indications p. 1879 except dysphagia.	Aymes Shake Compact Starter Pack powder: 6 sachet = £4.57; Aymes Shake Compact powder 57g sachets: strawberry 7 sachet = £3.99; chocolate 7 sachet = £3.99; vanilla 7 sachet = £3.99; neutral 7 sachet = £3.99; banana 7 sachet = £3.99; ginger 7 sachet = £3.99

Powder 57 g reconstituted with 100 ml milk provides: protein 12.2 g, carbohydrate 39.7 g, fat 12.4 g, energy 1343 kJ (320 kcal)
Not suitable for child under 1 year, not recommended for child under 6 years

Product	Formulation	Energy	Protein	Carbohydrate	Fat	Fibre	Special Characteristics	ACBS Indications	Presentation & Flavour
Foodlink® Complete Compact (Nualtra Ltd)	Powder per 100 g	1869 kJ (444 kcal)	21 g milk protein	56 g (sugars 43 g)	15 g	Nil	Contains lactose, soya. Gluten-free	Disease-related malnutrition.	Foodlink Complete Compact Starter Pack sachets: 5 sachet = £4.60; Foodlink Complete Compact powder 57g sachets: strawberry 7 sachet = £4.06; vanilla 7 sachet = £4.06; banana 7 sachet = £4.06; natural 7 sachet = £4.06; chocolate 7 sachet = £4.06

Powder 57 g reconstituted with 100 ml whole milk provides: protein 15 g, carbohydrate 37 g, fat 12 g, energy 1338 kJ (318 kcal)
Not suitable for use in children under 3 years; not recommended for child 3-6 years

2.4 kcal/mL milkshake lower volume, higher protein

Product	Formulation	Energy	Protein	Carbohydrate	Fat	Fibre	Special Characteristics	ACBS Indications	Presentation & Flavour
Aymes® ActaSolve Protein Compact (Aymes International Ltd)	Powder per 100 g	1843 kJ (437 kcal)	29.7 g milk, soya proteins	53.2 g (sugars 22.1 g)	11.6 g	0.40 g	Contains soya. Gluten-free	Borderline substances standard ACBS indications p. 1879 except dysphagia.	Aymes ActaSolve Protein Compact Starter Pack powder: 5 sachet = £5.82; Aymes ActaSolve Protein Compact powder 57g sachets: chocolate 7 sachet = £8.16; banana 7 sachet = £8.16; neutral 7 sachet = £8.16; vanilla 7 sachet = £8.16; strawberry 7 sachet = £8.16

Powder 57 g reconstituted with 100 mL whole milk provides: protein 20.4 g, carbohydrate 35.1 g, fat 10.3 g, energy 1326 kJ (315 kcal)
Not suitable for use in child under 3 years; use with caution in child under 6 years

2.6 kcal/g dessert style (milk based)

Product	Formulation	Energy	Protein	Carbohydrate	Fat	Fibre	Special Characteristics	ACBS Indications	Presentation & Flavour
Aymes® ActaSolve Delight (Aymes International Ltd)	Powder per 100 g	1857 kJ (441 kcal)	15.2 g milk protein	62 g (sugars 38.6 g)	14.5 g	0.9 g	Contains lactose, soya	Borderline substances standard ACBS indications p. 1879 except dysphagia.	Aymes ActaSolve Delight Starter Pack powder: 3 sachet = £4.15; Aymes ActaSolve Delight powder 57g sachets: mixed berries 7 sachet = £8.02; butterscotch 7 sachet = £8.02; lemon 7 sachet = £8.02

Powder 57 g reconstituted with 75 ml milk provides: protein 11.2 g, carbohydrate 38.7 g, fat 11.3 g, energy 1270 kJ (302 kcal)
Not suitable for use in child under 1 year, not recommended for child under 6 years

Oral nutritional supplements: Standard feeds (ready to serve)

1 - 1.3 kcal/mL milkshake lower energy

Product	Formulation	Energy	Protein	Carbohydrate	Fat	Fibre	Special Characteristics	ACBS Indications	Presentation & Flavour
EnergieShake® Advance 1.3kcal (Anaiah Healthcare PVT Ltd)	Liquid (sip feed) per 100 mL	544 kJ (130 kcal)	7 g milk protein	13 g (sugars 0.85 g)	5 g	2 g	Contains fish oil, soya. Gluten-free	Dietary management of patients with or at risk of disease-related malnutrition, or nutritionally at-risk older adults. Suitable for frail elderly (over 65 years of age, with a BMI under 23 kg/m^2), where clinical assessment and screening shows the individual to be at risk of under-nutrition.	EnergieShake Advance 1.3kcal oral liquid: chocolate 200 ml = £1.25; vanilla 200 ml = £1.25

Not recommended for use in children

Product	Formulation	Energy	Protein	Carbohydrate	Fat	Fibre	Special Characteristics	ACBS Indications	Presentation & Flavour
Ensure® (Abbott Laboratories Ltd)	Liquid (sip or tube feed) per 100 mL	423 kJ (100 kcal)	4 g caseinates, soya protein isolate	13.6 g (sugars 3.8 g)	3.4 g	Nil	Contains residual lactose, soya. Gluten-free.	Disease-related malnutrition, intractable malabsorption, total gastrectomy, proven inflammatory bowel disease, and pre-operative preparation of patients who are undernourished.	Ensure liquid: chocolate 250 ml = £3.42; vanilla 250 ml = £3.42

Not suitable for use in child under 1 year; not recommended for use in children

Product	Formulation	Energy	Protein	Carbohydrate	Fat	Fibre	Special Characteristics	ACBS Indications	Presentation & Flavour
Fresubin® Original (Fresenius Kabi Ltd)	Liquid (sip feed) per 100 mL	420 kJ (100 kcal)	3.8 g milk, soya proteins	13.8 g (sugars 3.5 g)	3.4 g	Nil	Contains residual lactose, soya. Gluten-free	Borderline substances standard ACBS indications p. 1879; also Refsum's Disease.	Fresubin Original drink: vanilla 200 ml = £3.31; chocolate 200 ml = £3.31; peach 200 ml = £3.31

Not suitable for use in child under 3 years; use with caution in child under 6 years

1.4 - 2 kcal/g dessert style (milk based)

Product	Formulation	Energy	Protein	Carbohydrate	Fat	Fibre	Special Characteristics	ACBS Indications	Presentation & Flavour
Aymes® ActaCal Creme (Aymes International Ltd)	Semi-solid per 100 g	632 kJ (150 kcal)	7.5 g caseinates, milk protein	19 g (sugars 8.1 g)	4.9 g	Nil	Contains residual lactose. Gluten-free.	Borderline substances standard ACBS indications p. 1879 except dysphagia.	Aymes ActaCal Creme Starter Pack dessert: 250 gram = £3.02; Aymes ActaCal Creme dessert: vanilla 500 gram = £6.16; chocolate 500 gram = £6.16

Not suitable for use in child under 3 years; not recommended for child under 6 years

1.4 - 2 kcal/g dessert style (milk based) (product list continued)

Product	Formulation	Energy	Protein	Carbohydrate	Fat	Fibre	Special Characteristics	ACBS Indications	Presentation & Flavour
EnergieShake® dessert (Anaiah Healthcare PVT Ltd)	Semi-solid per 100 g	632 kJ (150 kcal)	7.5 g caseinates, milk protein isolate	19 g (sugars 8.1 g)	4.9 g	Nil	Contains residual lactose. Gluten-free	Borderline substances standard ACBS indications p. 1879 except dysphagia.	EnergieShake dessert: caramel 375 gram = £3.30; chocolate 375 gram = £3.30
Not suitable for use in child under 3 years									
Forticreme® Complete (Nutricia Ltd)	Semi-solid per 100 g	675 kJ (160 kcal)	9.5 g milk proteins	19.2 g (sugars 10.6 g)	5 g	Less than 0.5 g	Contains residual lactose. Gluten-free	Borderline substances standard ACBS indications p. 1879; also continuous ambulatory peritoneal dialysis (CAPD), haemodialysis.	Forticreme Complete dessert: forest fruits 500 gram = £10.40; banana 500 gram = £10.40; vanilla 500 gram = £10.40; chocolate 500 gram = £10.40
Not suitable for use in child under 3 years; not recommended for child under 6 years									
Fresubin® 2kcal Creme (Fresenius Kabi Ltd)	Semi-solid per 100 g	840 kJ (200 kcal)	10 g milk protein	22.5 g sucrose (sugars 13.4 g)	7.8 g	Nil	Contains residual lactose, soya	Borderline substances standard ACBS indications p. 1879, continuous ambulatory peritoneal dialysis (CAPD) and haemodialysis.	Fresubin 2kcal Creme dessert: chocolate 500 gram = £8.40; vanilla 500 gram = £8.40; wild strawberry 500 gram = £8.40; praline 500 gram = £8.40; cappuccino 500 gram = £8.40
Not suitable for use in child under 3 years; not recommended for child under 6 years									
Fresubin® YOcrème (Fresenius Kabi Ltd)	Semi-solid per 100 g	630 kJ (150 kcal)	7.5 g milk, whey proteins	19.3 g sucrose (sugars 17.4 g)	4.7 g	0.4 g	Contains lactose, soya lecithin. Gluten-free	Patients with or at risk of malnutrition in particular with increased energy or protein needs or dysphagia.	Fresubin YOcreme dessert: raspberry 500 gram = £11.11; lemon 500 gram = £11.11; biscuit 500 gram = £11.11; apricot-peach 500 gram = £11.11
Not suitable for use in child under 3 years; use with caution in child under 6 years									
Nutricrem® (Nualtra Ltd)	Semi-solid per 100 g	756 kJ (180 kcal)	10 g caseinates, milk protein, soya protein	18.8 g (sugars 9.7 g)	7.2 g	Nil	Contains residual lactose, soya. Gluten-free	Borderline substances standard ACBS indications p. 1879.	Nutricrem Starter Pack dessert: 500 gram = £9.16; Nutricrem dessert: chocolate orange 500 gram = £9.48; vanilla 500 gram = £9.48; mint chocolate 500 gram = £9.48; strawberry 500 gram = £9.48
Not suitable for use in child under 3 years; not recommended for child under 6 years									

1.5 kcal/mL juice style

Product	Formulation	Energy	Protein	Carbohydrate	Fat	Fibre	Special Characteristics	ACBS Indications	Presentation & Flavour
Altrajuce® (Nualtra Ltd)	Liquid (sip feed) per 100 mL	636 kJ (150 kcal)	3.9 g milk protein	33.5 g (sugars 13.5 g)	Nil	Nil	Contains residual lactose. Gluten-free	Borderline substances standard ACBS indications p. 1879 except dysphagia.	Altrajuce Starter Pack liquid: 800 ml = £9.20; Altrajuce liquid: blackcurrant 200 ml = £1.89; orange 200 ml = £1.89; strawberry 200 ml = £1.89; apple 200 ml = £1.89
Not suitable for use in child under 3 years; not recommended for child under 6 years									

| Aymes® Actagain Juce (Aymes International Ltd) | Liquid (sip feed) per 100 mL | 638 kJ (150 kcal) | 5 g milk protein | 32.5 g (sugars 13.5 g) | Nil | Nil | Gluten-free | Borderline substances standard ACBS indications p. 1879 except dysphagia. | Aymes Actagain Juce Starter Pack liquid: 1000 ml = £9.50; Aymes Actagain Juce liquid berry medley: 200 ml = £1.80; Aymes Actagain Juce liquid exotic fruit: 200 ml = £1.80; Aymes Actagain Juce liquid juicy peach: 200 ml = £1.80; Aymes Actagain Juce liquid juicy apple: 200 ml = £1.80; Aymes Actagain Juce liquid zesty orange: 200 ml = £1.80 |

Not suitable for use in child under 6 years; use with caution in child under 11 years

| Ensure® Plus Juce (Abbott Laboratories Ltd) | Liquid (sip or tube feed) per 100 mL | 638 kJ (150 kcal) | 4.8 g whey protein isolate | 32.7 g (sugars 9.4 g) | Nil | Nil | Contains residual lactose. Gluten-free | Borderline substances standard ACBS indications p. 1879 | Ensure Plus Juce Starter Pack liquid: 1320 ml = £14.82; Ensure Plus Juce liquid: strawberry 220 ml = £2.75; orange 220 ml = £2.75; fruit punch 220 ml = £2.75; peach 220 ml = £2.75; lemon & lime 220 ml = £2.75; apple 220 ml = £2.75 |

Not suitable for use in child under 1 year; use with caution in child under 5 years

| Fortijuce® (Nutricia Ltd) | Liquid (sip feed) per 100 mL | 635 kJ (150 kcal) | 3.9 g milk protein | 33.5 g (sugars 13.1 g) | Nil | Nil | Contains residual lactose. Gluten-free | Borderline substances standard ACBS indications p. 1879; except dysphagia. | Fortijuce Starter Pack liquid: 800 ml = £7.20; Fortijuce liquid: tropical 200 ml = £1.80; lemon 200 ml = £1.80; orange 200 ml = £1.80; apple 200 ml = £1.80; strawberry 200 ml = £1.80 |

Not suitable for use in child under 1 year; not recommended for child 1–5 years

| Fresubin® Jucy (Fresenius Kabi Ltd) | Liquid (sip feed) per 100 mL | 630 kJ (150 kcal) | 4 g whey protein | 33.5 g (sugars 8 g) | Nil | Nil | Contains residual lactose. Gluten-free | Borderline substances standard ACBS indications p. 1879; also CAPD and haemodialysis. | Fresubin Jucy drink: starter pack 1200 ml = £12.45; pineapple 800 ml = £7.57; apple 800 ml = £7.57; orange 800 ml = £7.57; cherry 800 ml = £7.57; blackcurrant 800 ml = £7.57 |

Not suitable for use in child under 3 years; use with caution in child under 6 years

1.5 kcal/mL milkshake

Product	Formulation	Energy	Protein	Carbohydrate	Fat	Fibre	Special Characteristics	ACBS Indications	Presentation & Flavour
Altraplen® Energy (Nualtra Ltd)	Liquid (sip feed) per 100 mL	640 kJ (150 kcal)	6 g milk protein	18.5 g (sugars 6.5 g)	5.8 g	Nil	Gluten-free	Disease related malnutrition.	Altraplen Energy Starter Pack liquid: 800 ml = £4.88; Altraplen Energy liquid: banana 200 ml = £0.99; chocolate 200 ml = £0.99; vanilla 200 ml = £0.99; strawberry 200 ml = £0.99

Not suitable for use in child under 3 years; not recommended for child 3-6 years

1.5 kcal/mL milkshake (product list continued)

Product	Formulation	Energy	Protein	Carbohydrate	Fat	Fibre	Special Characteristics	ACBS Indications	Presentation & Flavour
Aymes® Actagain 1.5 Complete (Aymes International Ltd)	Liquid (sip feed) per 100 mL	630 kJ (150 kcal)	7 g milk protein	17 g (sugars 6.8 g)	6 g	Nil	Contains residual lactose. Gluten-free	Borderline substances standard ACBS indications p. 1879.	Aymes Actagain 1.5 Complete Starter Pack liquid: 800 ml = £5.94; Aymes Actagain 1.5 Complete liquid: smooth vanilla 200 ml = £1.11; strawberry burst 200 ml = £1.11; banana milkshake 200 ml = £1.11; double chocolate 200 ml = £1.11
Not suitable for use in child under 3 years; not suitable as a sole source of nutrition in child under 11 years									
Aymes® Actagain 1.5 Plant Powered (Aymes International Ltd)	Liquid (sip feed) per 100 mL	631 kJ (150 kcal)	6.7 g faba protein isolate	17 g (sugars 4.3 g)	6 g	0.1 g	Gluten-free, lactose-free	Borderline substances standard ACBS indications p. 1879 except dysphagia.	Aymes Actagain 1.5 Plant Powered Starter Pack liquid: 600 ml = £4.62; Aymes Actagain 1.5 Plant Powered liquid: cafe latte 200 ml = £1.54; salted caramel 200 ml = £1.54; madagascan vanilla 200 ml = £1.54
Not suitable for use in child under 3 years; use with caution in child over 3 years									
EnergieShake® Complete 1.5kcal (Anaiah Healthcare PVT Ltd)	Liquid (sip feed) per 100 mL	630 kJ (150 kcal)	6 g milk proteins	18 g (sugars 6.5 g)	6 g	Nil	Contains lactose, soya. Gluten-free	Borderline substances standard ACBS indications p. 1879, CAPD and haemodialysis.	EnergieShake Complete 1.5kcal liquid: chocolate 200 ml = £0.89; vanilla 200 ml = £0.89; strawberry 200 ml = £0.89; banana 200 ml = £0.89
Not suitable for use in child under 3 years; not recommended for child under 11 years									
Ensure® Plus milkshake style (Abbott Laboratories Ltd)	Liquid (sip or tube feed) per 100 mL	632 kJ (150 kcal)	6.3 g caseinates, milk protein isolate, soya protein isolate	20.2 g (sugars 6.5 g)	4.9 g	Nil	Contains residual lactose, soya. Gluten-free	Borderline substances standard ACBS indications p. 1879; also continuous ambulatory peritoneal dialysis (CAPD), haemodialysis.	Ensure Plus Commence liquid assorted: 2000 ml = £15.48; Ensure Plus milkshake style liquid: coffee 200 ml = £1.52; strawberry 200 ml = £1.52; chocolate 200 ml = £1.52; banana 200 ml = £1.52; fruits of the forest 200 ml = £1.52; vanilla 200 ml = £1.52; neutral 200 ml = £1.52; peach 200 ml = £1.52
Not suitable for use in child under 1 year; not recommended for use in children									
Fortisip® Bottle (Nutricia Ltd)	Liquid (sip feed) per 100 mL	625 kJ (150 kcal)	5.9 g milk proteins	18.4 g (sugars 6.7 g)	5.8 g	Nil	Contains residual lactose, soya.	Borderline substances standard ACBS indications p. 1879	Fortisip Bottle: chocolate 200 ml = £1.45; vanilla 200 ml = £1.45; strawberry 200 ml = £1.45; banana 200 ml = £1.45; neutral 200 ml = £1.45; 200 ml = £1.45
Not suitable for use in child under 3 years									
Fortisip® PlantBased 1.5kcal (Nutricia Ltd)	Liquid (sip feed) per 100 mL	630 kJ (150 kcal)	6.0 g pea protein isolate, soy protein isolate	18.6 g (sugars 9.4 g)	5.8 g	0.05 g	Contains soya. Lactose-free	Borderline substances standard ACBS indications p. 1879 except dysphagia.	Fortisip PlantBased 1.5kcal liquid: mango passionfruit 200 ml = £1.60; mocha 200 ml = £1.60
Not suitable for use in child under 3 years; use with caution in child over 3 years									

Product	Formulation	Energy	Protein	Carbohydrate	Fat	Fibre	Special Characteristics	ACBS Indications	Presentation & Flavour
Fresubin® Energy (Fresenius Kabi Ltd)	Liquid (sip feed) per 100 mL	630 kJ (150 kcal)	5.6 g milk protein	18.8 g (sugars 3.9-6.3 g)	5.8 g	Nil	Contains residual lactose, soya lecithin. Gluten-free	Borderline substances standard ACBS indications p. 1879.	Fresubin Energy liquid: tropical fruits 200 ml = £1.53; lemon 200 ml = £1.53; blackcurrant 200 ml = £1.53; cappuccino 200 ml = £1.53; chocolate 200 ml = £1.53; strawberry 200 ml = £1.53; vanilla 200 ml = £1.53; banana 200 ml = £1.53

Not suitable for use in child under 3 years; use with caution in child under 6 years

Product	Formulation	Energy	Protein	Carbohydrate	Fat	Fibre	Special Characteristics	ACBS Indications	Presentation & Flavour
Fresubin® Plant-Based drink (Fresenius Kabi Ltd)	Liquid (sip feed) per 100 mL	630 kJ (150 kcal)	7.5 g soya protein	16.1 g sugars (6.3 g)	5.7 g	2.3 g	Contains soya. Gluten-free, lactose-free	Borderline substances standard ACBS indications p. 1879	Fresubin Plant-Based drink: 200 ml = £1.60

Not suitable for use in child under 3 years; use with caution in child under 6 years

Product	Formulation	Energy	Protein	Carbohydrate	Fat	Fibre	Special Characteristics	ACBS Indications	Presentation & Flavour
Resource® Energy (Nestle Health Science)	Liquid (sip feed) per 100 mL	637 kJ (151 kcal)	5.6 g milk protein	21 g (sugars 5.7 g)	5 g	Less than 0.5 g	Contains residual lactose, soya. Gluten-free	Borderline substances standard ACBS indications p. 1879 except bowel fistula.	Resource Energy liquid: strawberry & raspberry 800 ml = £10.63; vanilla 800 ml = £10.63; chocolate 800 ml = £10.63

Not suitable for use in child under 3 years

1.5 kcal/mL yoghurt style drink

Product	Formulation	Energy	Protein	Carbohydrate	Fat	Fibre	Special Characteristics	ACBS Indications	Presentation & Flavour
Fresubin® YoDrink (Fresenius Kabi Ltd)	Liquid (sip feed) per 100 mL	630 kJ (150 kcal)	7.5 g milk, whey proteins	19.5 g sucrose (sugars 15.4 g)	4.7 g	0.1 g	Contains lactose, soya. Gluten-free	Dietary management of patients with or at risk of malnutrition who are not able to meet their nutritional requirements from ordinary foods alone. Includes elderly patients, patients with chronic wasting disease (cancer, HIV/AIDS), peri-operative patients, further patients with evidence based indication for oral nutritional supplementation (eg pre- and post-organ transplantation, inflammatory bowel disease).	Fresubin YoDrink: apricot-peach 200 ml = £1.92; lemon 200 ml = £1.92; raspberry 200 ml = £1.92

Not suitable for use in child under 3 years; not recommended for child under 6 years

1.5 - 1.6 kcal/mL milkshake higher protein

Product	Formulation	Energy	Protein	Carbohydrate	Fat	Fibre	Special Characteristics	ACBS Indications	Presentation & Flavour
Altraplen® Protein (Nualtra Ltd)	Liquid (sip feed) per 100 mL	632 kJ (150 kcal)	10 g milk, soya proteins	15 g (sugars 4.6 g)	5.6 g	Nil	Contains residual lactose, soya. Gluten-free	Borderline substances standard ACBS indications p. 1879.	Altraplen Protein Starter Pack liquid: 400 ml = £4.60; Altraplen Protein liquid: vanilla 800 ml = £9.52; strawberry 800 ml = £9.52

Not suitable for use in child under 3 years; not recommended for child under 6 years

1.5 - 1.6 kcal/mL milkshake higher protein (product list continued)

Product	Formulation	Energy	Protein	Carbohydrate	Fat	Fibre	Special Characteristics	ACBS Indications	Presentation & Flavour
Ensure® Plus Advance (Abbott Laboratories Ltd)	Liquid (sip or tube feed) per 100 mL	631 kJ (150 kcal)	9.1 g caseinates, milk protein isolate, soya protein isolate, whey protein.	16.8 g sucrose (sugars 6.8 g)	4.8 g	0.75 g	Contains soya. Gluten-free	Frail elderly people (this is defined as older than 65 years with BMI less than or equal to 23 kg/m^2 where clinical assessment and nutritional screening show the individual to be at risk of undernutrition).	Ensure Plus Advance liquid: strawberry 220 ml = £2.38; coffee 220 ml = £2.38; banana 220 ml = £2.38; chocolate 220 ml = £2.38; vanilla 220 ml = £2.38

Not recommended for use in children

Product	Formulation	Energy	Protein	Carbohydrate	Fat	Fibre	Special Characteristics	ACBS Indications	Presentation & Flavour
Fortisip® Extra (Nutricia Ltd)	Liquid (sip feed) per 100 mL	670 kJ (159 kcal)	9.8 g milk proteins	18.1 g (sugars 9 g)	5.3 g	Nil	Contains lactose, soya. Gluten-free	Borderline substances standard ACBS indications p. 1879	Fortisip Extra liquid: vanilla 200 ml = £1.65; strawberry 200 ml = £1.65

Not suitable for use in child under 3 years

Product	Formulation	Energy	Protein	Carbohydrate	Fat	Fibre	Special Characteristics	ACBS Indications	Presentation & Flavour
Fresubin® Protein Energy (Fresenius Kabi Ltd)	Liquid (sip feed) per 100 mL	630 kJ (150 kcal)	10 g milk protein	12.4 g maltodextrin and sucrose (sugars 6.5-7.4 g)	6.7 g	Nil	Contains residual lactose, soya lecithin. Gluten-free	Borderline substances standard ACBS indications p. 1879; also CAPD, haemodialysis.	Fresubin Protein Energy drink: wild strawberry 200 ml = £2.45; cappuccino 200 ml = £2.45; chocolate 200 ml = £2.45; vanilla 200 ml = £2.45; tropical fruits 200 ml = £2.45

Not suitable for use in child under 3 years; use with caution in child under 6 years

1.5 - 1.6 kcal/mL milkshake with fibre

Product	Formulation	Energy	Protein	Carbohydrate	Fat	Fibre	Special Characteristics	ACBS Indications	Presentation & Flavour
Ensure® Plus Fibre (Abbott Laboratories Ltd)	Liquid (sip feed) per 100 mL	652 kJ (155 kcal)	6.25 g caseinates, milk protein isolate, soya protein isolate	20.2 g sucrose (sugars 4.9 g)	4.92 g	2.5 g	Contains residual lactose, soya. Gluten-free	Borderline substances standard ACBS indications p. 1879; also CAPD, haemodialysis.	Ensure Plus Fibre liquid: vanilla 200 ml = £3.05; banana 200 ml = £3.05; strawberry 200 ml = £3.05; chocolate 200 ml = £3.05; raspberry 200 ml = £3.05

Not suitable for child under 1 year; not recommended for use in children.

Product	Formulation	Energy	Protein	Carbohydrate	Fat	Fibre	Special Characteristics	ACBS Indications	Presentation & Flavour
Fresubin® Energy Fibre (Fresenius Kabi Ltd)	Liquid (sip feed) per 100 mL	630 kJ (150 kcal)	5.6 g milk protein	17.8 g (sugars 5-6.4 g)	5.8 g	2 g	Contains residual lactose, soya lecithin. Gluten-free	Borderline substances standard ACBS indications p. 1879.	Fresubin Energy Fibre liquid: strawberry 200 ml = £2.76; chocolate 200 ml = £2.76; caramel 200 ml = £2.76; vanilla 200 ml = £2.76; cherry 200 ml = £2.76; banana 200 ml = £2.76

Not suitable for use in child under 3 years; use with caution in child under 6 years

1.6 kcal/g dessert style (fruit based)

Product	Formulation	Energy	Protein	Carbohydrate	Fat	Fibre	Special Characteristics	ACBS Indications	Presentation & Flavour
Fresubin® Dessert Fruit Puree (Fresenius Kabi Ltd)	Semi-solid per 100 g	670 kJ (160 kcal)	7 g whey protein	18.7 g sucrose (sugars 16.2 g)	5.6 g	3.5 g	Contains residual lactose, soya lecithin. Gluten-free	Borderline substances standard ACBS indications p. 1879 except intractable malabsorption.	Fresubin Dessert Fruit Puree: 500 gram = £11.23

Not suitable for use in child under 3 years; use with caution in child under 6 years

2 kcal/mL milkshake higher protein, higher energy with fibre

Product	Formulation	Energy	Protein	Carbohydrate	Fat	Fibre	Special Characteristics	ACBS Indications	Presentation & Flavour
Aymes® Actagain 2.0 Fibre (Aymes International Ltd)	Liquid (sip feed) per 100 mL	855 kJ (204 kcal)	10 g milk protein	21.5 g (sugars 7.5 g)	8.1 g	2.5 g	Contains residual lactose, soya. Gluten-free	Borderline substances standard ACBS indications p. 1879 except dysphagia.	Aymes Actagain 2.0 Fibre Starter Pack liquid: 600 ml = £6.20; Aymes Actagain 2.0 Fibre liquid: cafe latte 200 ml = £2.10; strawberry burst 200 ml = £2.10; smooth vanilla 200 ml = £2.10
Not suitable for use in child under 6 years; use with caution in child under 11 years									
Fresubin® 2kcal Fibre (Fresenius Kabi Ltd)	Liquid (sip feed) per 100 mL	840 kJ (200 kcal)	10 g milk protein	21.8 g (sugars 3.3-5.9 g)	7.8 g	1.5 g	Contains residual lactose, soya lecithin. Gluten-free	Borderline substances standard ACBS indications p. 1879; also CAPD, haemodialysis.	Fresubin 2kcal Fibre drink: vanilla 200 ml = £2.50; chocolate 200 ml = £2.50; lemon 200 ml = £2.50; apricot-peach 200 ml = £2.50; neutral 200 ml = £2.50; cappuccino 200 ml = £2.50
Not suitable for use in child under 3 years; use with caution in child under 6 years									
Resource® 2.0 Fibre (Nestle Health Science)	Liquid (sip or tube feed) per 100 mL	835 kJ (200 kcal)	9 g milk protein	20 g (sugars 6 g)	8.7 g	2.5 g	Contains residual lactose. Gluten-free	Borderline substances standard ACBS indications p. 1879.	Resource Fibre 2.0 liquid: vanilla 200 ml = £2.61; strawberry 200 ml = £2.61
Not suitable for use in child under 6 years; use with caution in child under 10 years									

2 - 2.4 kcal/mL milkshake higher protein, higher energy

Product	Formulation	Energy	Protein	Carbohydrate	Fat	Fibre	Special Characteristics	ACBS Indications	Presentation & Flavour
Aymes® Actagain 2.0 (Aymes International Ltd)	Liquid (sip feed) per 100 mL	857 kJ (200 kcal)	10 g milk protein	23 g (sugars 7.5 g)	8 g	Nil	Contains residual lactose. Gluten-free	Borderline substances standard ACBS indications p. 1879 except dysphagia.	Aymes Actagain 2.0 Starter Pack liquid: 1200 ml = £12.60; Aymes Actagain 2.0 liquid: golden apricot 200 ml = £2.10; cafe latte 200 ml = £2.10; berry medley 200 ml = £2.10; smooth vanilla 200 ml = £2.10; neutral 200 ml = £2.10; dulce de leche 200 ml = £2.10
Not suitable for use in child under 6 years; use with caution in child under 11 years									
Aymes® Actagain 2.4 (Aymes International Ltd)	Liquid (sip feed) per 100 mL	1008 kJ (240 kcal)	9.6 g milk protein	29 g (sugars 8 g)	9.6 g	Nil	Contains residual lactose. Gluten-free	Borderline substances standard ACBS indications p. 1879 except dysphagia.	Aymes Actagain 2.4 Starter Pack liquid: 600 ml = £5.18; Aymes Actagain 2.4 liquid: banana milkshake 200 ml = £1.72; strawberry burst 200 ml = £1.72; smooth vanilla 200 ml = £1.72
Not suitable for use in child under 6 years; use with caution in child under 11 years									
EnergieShake® 2.0kcal (Anaiah Healthcare PVT Ltd)	Liquid (sip feed) per 100 mL	840 kJ (200 kcal)	9.6 g milk protein	21.7 g (sugars 10.1 g)	8.2 g	Nil	Contains residual lactose. Gluten-free	Borderline substances standard ACBS indications p. 1879; also CAPD and haemodialysis.	EnergieShake 2.0kcal liquid: strawberry 200 ml = £1.52; banana 200 ml = £1.52; vanilla 200 ml = £1.52
Not suitable for use in child under 6 years; not recommended for child 6-11 years									

2 - 2.4 kcal/mL milkshake higher protein, higher energy (product list continued)

Product	Formulation	Energy	Protein	Carbohydrate	Fat	Fibre	Special Characteristics	ACBS Indications	Presentation & Flavour
Ensure® TwoCal (Abbott Laboratories Ltd)	Liquid (sip or tube feed) per 100 mL	837 kJ (200 kcal)	8.4 g caseinates, milk protein	21 g (sugars 5 g)	8.9 g	1 g	Contains soya. Gluten-free	Borderline substances standard ACBS indications p. 1879; also haemodialysis and CAPD.	Ensure TwoCal liquid: neutral 200 ml = £2.99; banana 200 ml = £2.99; vanilla 200 ml = £2.99; strawberry 200 ml = £2.99
Not suitable for use in child under 1 year; not recommended for use in children									
Fortisip® 2kcal (Nutricia Ltd)	Liquid (sip feed) per 100 mL	839 kJ (201 kcal)	10.1 g milk proteins	20.6 g (sugars 15.4 g)	8.6 g	Nil	Contains residual lactose, soya.	Borderline substances standard ACBS indications p. 1879 except dysphagia; also CAPD and haemodialysis.	Fortisip 2kcal liquid: vanilla 200 ml = £2.50; strawberry 200 ml = £2.50; forest fruit 200 ml = £2.50; chocolate-caramel 200 ml = £2.50; mocha 200 ml = £2.50
Not suitable for use in child under 3 years; use with caution in child 3-6 years									
Fresubin® 2kcal (Fresenius Kabi Ltd)	Liquid (sip feed) per 100 mL	840 kJ (200 kcal)	10 g milk protein	22.5 g (sugars 3.2-5.8 g)	7.8 g	Nil	Contains residual lactose, soya. Gluten-free	Borderline substances standard ACBS indications p. 1879; also CAPD, haemodialysis.	Fresubin 2kcal drink: toffee 200 ml = £2.40; cappuccino 200 ml = £2.40; vanilla 200 ml = £2.40; apricot-peach 200 ml = £2.40; neutral 200 ml = £2.40; fruits of the forest 200 ml = £2.40
Not suitable for use in child under 3 years; use with caution in child under 6 years									

2 - 2.4 kcal/mL milkshake lower volume

Product	Formulation	Energy	Protein	Carbohydrate	Fat	Fibre	Special Characteristics	ACBS Indications	Presentation & Flavour
Altraplen® Compact (Nualtra Ltd)	Liquid (sip feed) per 100 mL	1008 kJ (240 kcal)	9.6 g milk, soya proteins	28.8 g (sugars 11.6 g)	9.6 g	Nil	Contains residual lactose, soya. Gluten-free	Borderline substances standard ACBS indications p. 1879.	Altraplen Compact Starter Pack liquid: 500 ml = £8.24; Altraplen Compact liquid: hazel chocolate 500 ml = £6.44; vanilla 500 ml = £6.44; strawberry 500 ml = £6.44; banana 500 ml = £6.44
Not suitable for use in child under 3 years; not recommended for child under 6 years									
Ensure® Compact (Abbott Laboratories Ltd)	Liquid (sip feed) per 100 mL	1008 kJ (240 kcal)	10.2 g caseinates, milk protein isolate	28.8 g corn syrup (sugars 6.2 g)	9.35 g	Nil	Contains lactose, soya. Gluten-free	Disease-related malnutrition.	Ensure Compact Starter Pack liquid: 500 ml = £6.43; Ensure Compact liquid: strawberry 500 ml = £7.13; cafe latte 500 ml = £7.13; banana 500 ml = £7.13; vanilla 500 ml = £7.13
Not recommended for use in children									
Fortisip® Compact (Nutricia Ltd)	Liquid (sip feed) per 100 mL	1010 kJ (240 kcal)	9.6 g milk proteins	29.6 g (sugars 15.5 g)	9.3 g	Nil	Contains residual lactose, soya	Borderline substances standard ACBS indications p. 1879 except dysphagia.	Fortisip Compact Starter Pack liquid: 750 ml = £9.90; Fortisip Compact liquid: neutral 500 ml = £6.60; mocha 500 ml = £6.60; strawberry 500 ml = £6.60; banana 500 ml = £6.60; vanilla 500 ml = £6.60; chocolate 500 ml = £6.60
Not suitable for use in child under 3 years; use with caution in child 3-6 years									

| Fresubin® 2kcal Mini (Fresenius Kabi Ltd) | Liquid (sip feed) per 100 mL | 840 kJ (200 kcal) | 10 g milk protein | 22.5 g (sugars 5.3-5.8 g) | 7.8 g | Nil | Contains residual lactose, soya lecithin. Gluten-free | Borderline substances standard ACBS indications p. 1879; also CAPD, haemodialysis. | Fresubin 2kcal Mini drink: vanilla 500 ml = £5.80; fruits of the forest 500 ml = £5.80; apricot-peach 500 ml = £5.80 |

Not suitable for use in child under 3 years; use with caution in child under 6 years

2 - 2.4 kcal/mL milkshake lower volume with fibre

Product	Formulation	Energy	Protein	Carbohydrate	Fat	Fibre	Special Characteristics	ACBS Indications	Presentation & Flavour
Fortisip® Compact Fibre (Nutricia Ltd)	Liquid (sip feed) per 100 mL	1007 kJ (240 kcal)	9.5 g cow's milk	25.4 g (sugars 13.4 g)	10.4 g	3.6 g	Contains residual lactose, soya	Borderline substances standard ACBS indications p. 1879 except dysphagia.	Fortisip Compact Fibre liquid: mocha 500 ml = £11.48; strawberry 500 ml = £11.48; vanilla 500 ml = £11.48

Not suitable for use in child under 3 years; use with caution in child 3-6 years

| Fresubin® 2kcal Fibre Mini (Fresenius Kabi Ltd) | Liquid (sip feed) per 100 mL | 840 kJ (200 kcal) | 10 g milk protein | 21.8 g (sugars 5.9 g) | 7.8 g | 1.5 g | Contains residual lactose, soya lecithin. Gluten-free | Borderline substances standard ACBS indications p. 1879; also CAPD, haemodialysis. | Fresubin 2kcal Fibre Mini drink: vanilla 500 ml = £6.24; chocolate 500 ml = £6.24 |

Not suitable for use in child under 3 years; use with caution in child under 6 years

2.4 kcal/mL milkshake higher volume

Product	Formulation	Energy	Protein	Carbohydrate	Fat	Fibre	Special Characteristics	ACBS Indications	Presentation & Flavour
Altraplen® Compact Daily (Nualtra Ltd)	Liquid (sip feed) per 100 mL	1008 kJ (240 kcal)	9.6 g milk protein, soya protein	28.8 g (sugars 11.3 g)	9.6 g	Nil	Contains residual lactose, soya. Gluten-free	Disease related malnutrition.	Altraplen Compact Daily Starter Pack liquid: 1000 ml = £7.16; Altraplen Compact Daily liquid: strawberry 250 ml = £1.60; vanilla 250 ml = £1.60; banana 250 ml = £1.60

Not suitable for use in child under 3 years; use with caution in child under 6 years

| Aymes® Actagain 2.4 Daily (Aymes International Ltd) | Liquid (sip feed) per 100 mL | 1008 kJ (240 kcal) | 9.6 g milk protein | 29 g (sugars 8 g) | 9.6 g | Nil | Contains residual lactose. Gluten-free | Borderline substances standard ACBS indications p. 1879 except dysphagia. | Aymes Actagain 2.4 Daily Starter Pack liquid: 750 ml = £4.80; Aymes Actagain 2.4 Daily liquid: smooth vanilla 250 ml = £1.60; banana milkshake 250 ml = £1.60; strawberry burst 250 ml = £1.60 |

Not suitable for use in child under 6 years; use with caution in child under 11 years

2.4 kcal/mL milkshake lower volume, higher protein

Product	Formulation	Energy	Protein	Carbohydrate	Fat	Fibre	Special Characteristics	ACBS Indications	Presentation & Flavour
Fortisip® Compact Protein (Nutricia Ltd)	Liquid (sip feed) per 100 mL	1029 kJ (245 kcal)	14.6 g milk proteins	25.1 g (sugars 13.7 g)	9.6 g	Nil	Contains residual lactose, soya. Gluten-free	Borderline substances standard ACBS indications p. 1879 except dysphagia.	Fortisip Compact Protein Starter Pack liquid: 1000 ml = £20.80; Fortisip Compact Protein liquid: vanilla 500 ml = £10.40; banana 500 ml = £10.40; cool red fruits 500 ml = £10.40; mocha 500 ml = £10.40; hot tropical ginger 500 ml = £10.40; berries 500 ml = £10.40; neutral 500 ml = £10.40; peach & mango 500 ml = £10.40; strawberry 500 ml = £10.40
Not suitable for use in child under 6 years; use with caution in child 6-10 years									
Fresubin® 3.2kcal (Fresenius Kabi Ltd)	Liquid (sip feed) per 100 mL	1344 kJ (320 kcal)	16 g collagen, milk proteins	28 g (sugars 11 g)	16 g	0.4 g	Contains residual lactose, soya lecithin. Gluten-free	Borderline substances standard ACBS indications p. 1879.	Fresubin 3.2kcal drink: mango 500 ml = £10.24; vanilla-caramel 500 ml = £10.24; hazelnut 500 ml = £10.24; cappuccino 500 ml = £10.24
Not suitable for use in child under 3 years; use with caution in child under 6 years									
Fresubin® Pro Compact (Fresenius Kabi Ltd)	Liquid (sip feed) per 100 mL	1008 kJ (240 kcal)	14.4 g milk protein	24 g (sugars 4.5 g)	9.4 g	Nil	Contains residual lactose, soya lecithin. Gluten-free	Borderline substances standard ACBS indications p. 1879 except dysphagia.	Fresubin Pro Compact drink: vanilla 125 ml = £1.69; cappuccino 125 ml = £1.69; apricot-peach 125 ml = £1.69
Not suitable for use in child under 7 years; use with caution in child under 10 years									

Table 3 Energy, protein, and fibre fortifiers

Energy (carbohydrate) fortifiers

Product	Formulation	Energy	Protein	Carbohydrate	Fat	Fibre	Special Characteristics	ACBS Indications	Presentation & Flavour
Duocal® Super Soluble (Nutricia Ltd)	Powder per 100 g	2061 kJ (492 kcal)	Nil	72.7 g (sugars 6.5 g)	22.3 g (MCT 38 %)	Nil		Disease related malnutrition, malabsorption states or other conditions requiring fortification with a fat/carbohydrate supplement.	Duocal Super Soluble powder: 400 gram = £27.28
Maxijul® Super Soluble (Nutricia Ltd)	Powder per 100 g	1615 kJ (380 kcal)	Nil	95 g (sugars 8.6 g)	Nil	Nil	Gluten-free, lactose-free	Disease-related malnutrition, malabsorption states or other conditions requiring fortification with a high or readily available carbohydrate supplement.	Maxijul Super Soluble: powder 132g sachets 4 sachet = £9.68; powder 200 gram = £3.90; 25000 gram = £234.85
Polycal® liquid (Nutricia Ltd)	Liquid (sip feed) per 100 mL	1050 kJ (247 kcal)	Nil	61.9 g (sugars 12.2 g)	Nil	Nil		Disease related malnutrition, malabsorption states or other conditions requiring fortification with a high or readily available carbohydrate supplement.	Polycal liquid neutral: 200 ml = £2.66
Not suitable for use in child under 3 years									

Product	Formulation	Energy	Protein	Carbohydrate	Fat	Fibre	Special Characteristics	ACBS Indications	Presentation & Flavour
Polycal® powder (Nutricia Ltd)	Powder per 100 g	1630 kJ (384 kcal)	Nil	96 g (sugars 6 g)	Nil	Nil		Disease-related malnutrition, malabsorption states or other conditions requiring fortification with a high or readily available carbohydrate supplement.	Polycal powder: 400 gram = £6.73

Not suitable for infants; use with caution in child 1-6 years

Product	Formulation	Energy	Protein	Carbohydrate	Fat	Fibre	Special Characteristics	ACBS Indications	Presentation & Flavour
Vitajoule® (Vitaflo International Ltd)	Powder per 100 g	1615 kJ (380 kcal)	Nil	95 g (sugars 9 g)	Nil	Nil		Disease related malnutrition, malabsorption states, other conditions requiring fortification with carbohydrate and as a carbohydrate source in modular feeds.	Vitajoule powder: 500 gram = £6.87

Suitable from birth

Energy (fat) fortifiers

Product	Formulation	Energy	Protein	Carbohydrate	Fat	Fibre	Special Characteristics	ACBS Indications	Presentation & Flavour
Calogen® (Nutricia Ltd)	Liquid (sip or tube feed) per 100 mL	1850 kJ (450 kcal)	Nil	0.1 g (sugars Nil)	50 g	Nil		Disease-related malnutrition, malabsorption states, or other conditions requiring fortification with a high fat supplement, with or without fluid and electrolyte restrictions.	Calogen emulsion: strawberry 200 ml = £6.84; neutral 200 ml = £6.84; 500 ml = £16.84

Use with caution in child under 6 years; strawberry flavour not suitable for child under 3 years

Product	Formulation	Energy	Protein	Carbohydrate	Fat	Fibre	Special Characteristics	ACBS Indications	Presentation & Flavour
Fresubin® 5kcal shot (Fresenius Kabi Ltd)	Liquid (sip feed) per 100 mL	2100 kJ (500 kcal)	Nil	4 g sucrose (sugars 4 g)	53.8 g	0.4 g	Gluten-free, lactose-free	Disease related malnutrition malabsorption states or other conditions requiring fortification with a high fat supplement with or without fluid or electrolyte restrictions.	Fresubin 5kcal shot drink: neutral 480 ml = £14.20; lemon 480 ml = £14.20

Not suitable for use in child under 3 years

Energy and protein fortifiers

Product	Formulation	Energy	Protein	Carbohydrate	Fat	Fibre	Special Characteristics	ACBS Indications	Presentation & Flavour
Altrashot® (Nualtra Ltd)	Liquid (sip feed) per 100 mL	1451 kJ (350 kcal)	5 g milk protein isolate	17 g (sugars 6.1 g)	29.1 g	Nil	Contains residual lactose. Gluten-free	Disease-related malnutrition.	Altrashot 120ml bottles: neutral 4 bottle = £11.30; strawberry 4 bottle = £12.00; vanilla 4 bottle = £12.00; Altrashot Starter Pack liquid: 2 bottle = £5.98

Not suitable for use in child under 3 years; not recommended for child under 6 years

Product	Formulation	Energy	Protein	Carbohydrate	Fat	Fibre	Special Characteristics	ACBS Indications	Presentation & Flavour
Calogen® Extra (Nutricia Ltd)	Liquid (sip or tube feed) per 100 mL	1650 kJ (400 kcal)	5 g caseinates, whey protein hydrolysate	4.5 g (sugars 3.5 g)	40.3 g	Nil	Contains residual lactose. Gluten-free	Disease related malnutrition, malabsorption states or other conditions requiring fortification with a high fat supplement with or without fluid restriction.	Calogen Extra Shots emulsion: strawberry 240 ml = £7.20; neutral 240 ml = £7.20; Calogen Extra emulsion: neutral 200 ml = £6.03; strawberry 200 ml = £6.03

Not suitable for use in child under 3 years; use with caution in child 3-6 years

Energy and protein fortifiers (product list continued)

Product	Formulation	Energy	Protein	Carbohydrate	Fat	Fibre	Special Characteristics	ACBS Indications	Presentation & Flavour
MCTprocal® (Vitaflo International Ltd)	Powder per 100 g	2907 kJ (703 kcal)	12.2 g caseinates	20.6 g (sugars 3.1 g)	63.5 g (MCT 96%)	Nil	Contains lactose	Disorders of long chain fatty acid oxidation, fat malabsorption and other disorders requiring a low LCT, high MCT supplement.	MCTprocal oral powder 16g sachets: 30 sachet = £37.45
Suitable from 3 years									
Pro-Cal® powder (Vitaflo International Ltd)	Powder per 100 g	2744 kJ (662 kcal)	13.5 g milk protein	26 g (sugars 20 g)	56 g	Nil	Contains residual lactose. Gluten-free	Disease-related malnutrition, malabsorption states or other conditions requiring fortification with a fat / carbohydrate supplement (with protein).	Pro-Cal powder: 510 gram = £23.11; 1500 gram = £47.12; 12500 gram = £335.14; Pro-Cal powder: starter pack 8 sachet = £7.86; 15g sachets 30 sachet = £29.71
Powder 15 g reconstituted with 100 ml water provides: protein 2 g, carbohydrate 3.9 g, fat 8.4 g, energy 412 kJ (100 kcal) Suitable from 3 years									
Pro-Cal® Shot (Vitaflo International Ltd)	Liquid (sip feed) per 100 mL	1385 kJ (334 kcal)	6.7 g caseinates, milk protein	13.4 g lactose (sugars 13.3 g)	28.2 g	Nil	Contains lactose, soya. Gluten-free	Disease-related malnutrition, malabsorption states or other conditions requiring fortification with a fat/carbohydrate supplement (with protein).	Pro-Cal: shot starter pack 360 ml = £10.94; shot neutral 720 ml = £21.91; shot strawberry 720 ml = £21.91; shot banana 720 ml = £21.91
Suitable from 3 years									

Energy and higher protein fortifiers

Product	Formulation	Energy	Protein	Carbohydrate	Fat	Fibre	Special Characteristics	ACBS Indications	Presentation & Flavour
Altrapro (Nualtra Ltd)	Liquid (sip feed) per 100 mL	574 kJ (135 kcal)	33.3 g milk protein	0.09 g (sugars 0.03 g)	0.04 g	Nil	Gluten-free, lactose-free	Disease-related malnutrition in patients with higher protein needs.	Altrapro liquid: lemon & lime 60 ml = £1.75; berry 60 ml = £1.75
Not suitable for use in child under 3 years; use with caution in child under 6 years									
Aymes® Actagain Protein Shot (Aymes International Ltd)	Liquid (sip or tube feed) per 100 mL	644 kJ (154 kcal)	37 g collagen protein	2 g fructose (sugars 2 g)	Nil	Nil	Contains bovine derivatives. Gluten-free, lactose-free	Hypoproteinaemia.	Aymes Actagain Protein: Shot mixed berry 60 ml = £1.75; Shot tropical fruit 60 ml = £1.75
Not suitable for use in child under 3 years; use with caution in child under 7 years									
ProSource® 20 (Nutrinovo Ltd)	Liquid (sip and tube feed) per 100 mL	628 kJ (150 kcal)	33.3 g collagen protein, whey protein isolate	3.33 g (sugars Nil)	Nil	Nil	Contains beef derivatives, residual lactose. Gluten-free	Hypoproteinaemia.	ProSource 20 liquid: 60 ml = £2.32
Not recommended for child under 3 years									
ProSource® liquid (Nutrinovo Ltd)	Liquid (sip or tube feed) per 100 mL	1400 kJ (333 kcal)	33.3 g collagen protein, whey protein isolate	50 g (sugars 26.7 g)	Less than 1 g	Less than 1 g	Contains residual lactose, porcine derivatives. Gluten-free	Biochemically proven hypoproteinaemia.	ProSource liquid 30ml sachets: neutral 100 sachet = £148.10; citrus berry 100 sachet = £148.10; orange creme 100 sachet = £148.10
Not recommended for child under 3 years									

Product	Formulation	Energy	Protein	Carbohydrate	Fat	Fibre	Special Characteristics	ACBS Indications	Presentation & Flavour
ProSource® Plus (Nutrinovo Ltd)	Liquid (sip and tube feed) **per 100 mL**	1400 kJ (333 kcal)	50 g collagen protein, whey protein isolate	36.7 g sucrose (sugars 33.3 g)	Less than 1 g	Less than 1 g	Contains porcine derivatives, residual lactose. Gluten-free	Hypoproteinaemia.	ProSource Plus liquid 30ml sachets: orange creme 50 sachet = £99.27; 100 sachet = £198.54; citrus berry 50 sachet = £99.27; 100 sachet = £198.54; neutral 50 sachet = £99.27; 100 sachet = £198.54; ProSource Plus liquid citrus berry: 887 ml = £58.70; ProSource Plus liquid orange creme: 887 ml = £58.70; ProSource Plus liquid neutral: 887 ml = £58.70
Not recommended for child under 3 years									
Protifar® (Nutricia Ltd)	Powder **per 100 g**	1560 kJ (368 kcal)	87.2 g cow's milk	1.5 g	1.6 g	Nil	Contains lactose, soya. Gluten-free	Hypoproteinaemia.	Protifar powder: 225 gram = £13.70
Powder 2.5 g provides: protein 2.2 g, carbohydrate 0.04 g, fat 0.04 g, energy 39 kJ (9 kcal) Not suitable for use in child under 3 years									
Renapro® Shot (Stanningley Pharma Ltd)	Liquid (sip or tube feed) **per 100 mL**	711 kJ (167 kcal)	33 g collagen protein	4.9 g fructose (sugars 4.9 g)	Less than 0.5 g	Nil	Contains beef derivatives. Gluten-free, lactose-free	Hypoproteinaemia.	Renapro Shot 60ml bottles: wild berry 30 bottle = £69.60; apple 30 bottle = £69.60; pineapple & coconut 30 bottle = £69.60; cola 30 bottle = £69.60; peach 30 bottle = £69.60
Not suitable for use in child under 3 years									

Higher protein fortifiers

Product	Formulation	Energy	Protein	Carbohydrate	Fat	Fibre	Special Characteristics	ACBS Indications	Presentation & Flavour
ProSource® jelly (Nutrinovo Ltd)	Semi-solid **per 100 mL**	315 kJ (75 kcal)	16.9 g collagen protein, whey protein isolate	Less than 1 g	Nil	Less than 1 g	Contains porcine derivatives, residual lactose. Gluten-free	Hypoproteinaemia.	ProSource jelly: blackcurrant 118 ml = £2.74; lime 118 ml = £2.74; fruit punch 118 ml = £2.74; orange 118 ml = £2.74
Not recommended for child under 3 years									

Fibre fortifiers

Product	Formulation	Energy	Protein	Carbohydrate	Fat	Fibre	Special Characteristics	ACBS Indications	Presentation & Flavour
HyFiber® (Nutrinovo Ltd)	Liquid (sip or tube feed) **per 100 mL**	484 kJ (119 kcal)	Nil	10.4 g (sugars 10.4 g)	Nil	39 g	Gluten-free, lactose-free	Bowel transit disorders.	HyFiber: liquid 30ml sachets 100 sachet = £112.94; liquid 887 ml = £33.05
Not recommended for child under 3 years									
Optifibre® (Nestle Health Science)	Powder **per 100 g**	816 kJ (202 kcal)	Less than 1.5 g	6 g partially hydrolysed guar gum (sugars 6 g)	Nil	86 g	Contains residual lactose. Gluten-free	Borderline substances standard ACBS indications p. 1879 except dysphagia.	Optifibre: powder 5g sachets 16 sachet = £5.78; powder 250 gram = £14.27
Not suitable for use in child under 5 years									

Flavour additives
Flavour additive powders

FlavourPac ®
▶ For use with Vitaflo's inborn error range of protein substitutes. Not suitable for use in child under 3 years.
POWDER

FlavourPac oral powder 4g sachets blackcurrant (Vitaflo International Ltd)
30 sachet (ACBS) · NHS indicative price = £21.72

FlavourPac oral powder 4g sachets orange (Vitaflo International Ltd)
30 sachet (ACBS) · NHS indicative price = £21.72

FlavourPac oral powder 4g sachets raspberry (Vitaflo International Ltd)
30 sachet (ACBS) · NHS indicative price = £21.72

FlavourPac oral powder 4g sachets tropical (Vitaflo International Ltd)
30 sachet (ACBS) · NHS indicative price = £21.72

Nutricia Flavour Modjul ®
▶ For use with a range of unflavoured amino acid and peptide based foods for special medical purposes. Not suitable for use in child under 6 months.
POWDER

Nutricia Flavour Modjul powder blackcurrant (Nutricia Ltd)
100 gram (ACBS) · NHS indicative price = £18.35

Nutricia Flavour Modjul powder orange (Nutricia Ltd)
100 gram (ACBS) · NHS indicative price = £18.35

Nutricia Flavour Modjul powder pineapple (Nutricia Ltd)
100 gram (ACBS) · NHS indicative price = £18.35

Foods for special diets
Gluten-free foods

ACBS indications: coeliac disease and dermatitis herpetiformis.

Bread

Genius ® Loaves
GLUTEN-FREE

Genius gluten free brown sandwich bread sliced (Genius Foods Ltd)
535 gram (ACBS) · NHS indicative price = £4.97

Genius gluten free seeded brown farmhouse loaf sliced (Genius Foods Ltd)
535 gram (ACBS) · NHS indicative price = £4.92

Genius gluten free white sandwich bread sliced (Genius Foods Ltd)
535 gram (ACBS) · NHS indicative price = £4.98

Glutafin ® Loaves
GLUTEN-FREE

Glutafin gluten free fibre loaf sliced (Dr Schar UK Ltd)
300 gram (ACBS) · NHS indicative price = £3.34

Glutafin gluten free high fibre loaf sliced (Dr Schar UK Ltd)
350 gram (ACBS) · NHS indicative price = £3.89

Glutafin gluten free white loaf sliced (Dr Schar UK Ltd)
300 gram (ACBS) · NHS indicative price = £3.34

Glutafin ® Select Loaves
GLUTEN-FREE

Glutafin gluten free Select fibre loaf sliced (Dr Schar UK Ltd)
400 gram (ACBS) · NHS indicative price = £3.97

Glutafin gluten free Select fresh brown loaf sliced (Dr Schar UK Ltd)
400 gram (ACBS) · NHS indicative price = £4.04

Glutafin gluten free Select fresh white loaf sliced (Dr Schar UK Ltd)
400 gram (ACBS) · NHS indicative price = £4.04

Glutafin gluten free Select seeded loaf sliced (Dr Schar UK Ltd)
400 gram (ACBS) · NHS indicative price = £4.30

Glutafin gluten free Select white loaf sliced (Dr Schar UK Ltd)
400 gram (ACBS) · NHS indicative price = £3.97

Juvela ® Loaf
GLUTEN-FREE

Juvela gluten free fibre loaf sliced (Juvela Ltd)
400 gram (ACBS) · NHS indicative price = £4.10

Juvela gluten free fibre loaf unsliced (Juvela Ltd)
400 gram (ACBS) · NHS indicative price = £4.10

Juvela gluten free fresh fibre loaf sliced (Juvela Ltd)
400 gram (ACBS) · NHS indicative price = £4.10

Juvela gluten free fresh white loaf sliced (Juvela Ltd)
400 gram (ACBS) · NHS indicative price = £4.10

Juvela gluten free loaf sliced (Juvela Ltd)
400 gram (ACBS) · NHS indicative price = £4.10

Juvela gluten free loaf unsliced (Juvela Ltd)
400 gram (ACBS) · NHS indicative price = £4.10

Juvela gluten free part baked fibre loaf (Juvela Ltd)
400 gram (ACBS) · NHS indicative price = £4.50

Juvela gluten free part baked loaf (Juvela Ltd)
400 gram (ACBS) · NHS indicative price = £4.50

Warburtons ® Loaf
GLUTEN-FREE

Warburtons gluten free brown bread sliced (Warburtons Ltd)
400 gram (ACBS) · NHS indicative price = £3.34

Warburtons gluten free white bread sliced (Warburtons Ltd)
400 gram (ACBS) · NHS indicative price = £3.34

Flour type mixes

Finax ® Flour mixes
GLUTEN-FREE

Finax gluten free coarse flour mix (Drossa (London) Ltd)
900 gram (ACBS) · NHS indicative price = £9.97

Finax gluten free fibre bread mix (Drossa (London) Ltd)
1000 gram (ACBS) · NHS indicative price = £11.45

Finax gluten free flour mix (Drossa (London) Ltd)
900 gram (ACBS) · NHS indicative price = £9.97

Glutafin ® Flour mixes
GLUTEN-FREE

Glutafin gluten free bread mix (Dr Schar UK Ltd)
500 gram (ACBS) · NHS indicative price = £7.71

Glutafin gluten free fibre bread mix (Dr Schar UK Ltd)
500 gram (ACBS) · NHS indicative price = £7.71

Glutafin gluten free multipurpose white mix (Dr Schar UK Ltd)
500 gram (ACBS) · NHS indicative price = £7.71

Glutafin gluten free wheat free fibre mix (Dr Schar UK Ltd)
500 gram (ACBS) · NHS indicative price = £7.71

Glutafin ® Select Flour mix
GLUTEN-FREE

Glutafin gluten free Select bread mix (Dr Schar UK Ltd)
500 gram (ACBS) · NHS indicative price = £7.71

Glutafin gluten free Select fibre bread mix (Dr Schar UK Ltd)
500 gram (ACBS) · NHS indicative price = £7.71

Glutafin gluten free Select multipurpose fibre mix (Dr Schar UK Ltd)
500 gram (ACBS) · NHS indicative price = £7.71

Glutafin gluten free Select multipurpose white mix (Dr Schar UK Ltd)
500 gram (ACBS) · NHS indicative price = £7.71

Juvela ® Flour mixes
GLUTEN-FREE

Juvela gluten free fibre mix (Juvela Ltd)
500 gram (ACBS) · NHS indicative price = £8.25

Juvela gluten free harvest mix (Juvela Ltd)
500 gram (ACBS) · NHS indicative price = £8.25

Juvela gluten free mix (Juvela Ltd)
500 gram (ACBS) · NHS indicative price = £8.25

Rolls and baguettes

Glutafin ® Rolls and baguettes
GLUTEN-FREE

Glutafin gluten free 4 white rolls (Dr Schar UK Ltd)
200 gram (ACBS) · NHS indicative price = £4.26

Glutafin gluten free baguettes (Dr Schar UK Ltd)
350 gram (ACBS) · NHS indicative price = £4.06

Glutafin gluten free part baked 2 long white rolls (Dr Schar UK Ltd)
150 gram (ACBS) · NHS indicative price = £3.25

Glutafin gluten free part baked 4 fibre rolls (Dr Schar UK Ltd)
200 gram (ACBS) · NHS indicative price = £4.26

Glutafin gluten free part baked 4 white rolls (Dr Schar UK Ltd)
200 gram (ACBS) · NHS indicative price = £4.26

Juvela ® Rolls
GLUTEN-FREE

Juvela gluten free bread rolls (Juvela Ltd)
425 gram (ACBS) · NHS indicative price = £5.60

Juvela gluten free fibre bread rolls (Juvela Ltd)
425 gram (ACBS) · NHS indicative price = £5.60

Juvela gluten free fresh fibre rolls (Juvela Ltd)
425 gram (ACBS) · NHS indicative price = £5.25

Juvela gluten free fresh white rolls (Juvela Ltd)
425 gram (ACBS) · NHS indicative price = £5.25

Juvela gluten free part baked fibre bread rolls (Juvela Ltd)
375 gram (ACBS) · NHS indicative price = £5.60

Juvela gluten free part baked white bread rolls (Juvela Ltd)
375 gram (ACBS) · NHS indicative price = £5.60

Proceli ® Baguettes
GLUTEN-FREE

Proceli gluten free part baked baguettes (Ambe Ltd)
250 gram (ACBS) · NHS indicative price = £2.75

Warburtons ® Rolls
GLUTEN-FREE

Warburtons gluten free brown rolls (Warburtons Ltd)
232 gram (ACBS) · NHS indicative price = £2.80

Warburtons gluten free white rolls (Warburtons Ltd)
232 gram (ACBS) · NHS indicative price = £2.80

Low-protein foods

ACBS indications: inherited metabolic disorders, renal or liver failure, requiring a low-protein diet.

Bread, rolls, and baguettes

Juvela ® Bread and rolls
LOW-PROTEIN

Juvela low protein bread rolls (Juvela Ltd)
350 gram (ACBS) · NHS indicative price = £5.50

Juvela low protein loaf sliced (Juvela Ltd)
400 gram (ACBS) · NHS indicative price = £4.50

Mevalia ® Bread and rolls
LOW-PROTEIN

Mevalia low protein ciabattine (Vitaflo International Ltd)
260 gram (ACBS) · NHS indicative price = £4.59

Mevalia low protein pan carre (Vitaflo International Ltd)
300 gram (ACBS) · NHS indicative price = £3.36

Mevalia low protein pane casereccio (Vitaflo International Ltd)
220 gram (ACBS) · NHS indicative price = £2.97

Promin ® Bread and rolls
LOW-PROTEIN

Promin low protein breadcrumbs (Firstplay Dietary Foods Ltd)
300 gram (ACBS) · NHS indicative price = £8.00

Promin low protein croutons 40g sachets (Firstplay Dietary Foods Ltd)
4 sachet (ACBS) · NHS indicative price = £7.75

Promin low protein farmhouse loaf (Firstplay Dietary Foods Ltd)
400 gram (ACBS) · NHS indicative price = £4.65

Promin low protein fresh baked bread buns (Firstplay Dietary Foods Ltd)
450 gram (ACBS) · NHS indicative price = £6.70

Promin low protein fresh baked bread sliced (Firstplay Dietary Foods Ltd)
800 gram (ACBS) · NHS indicative price = £8.65

Promin low protein fresh baked brown bread sliced (Firstplay Dietary Foods Ltd)
400 gram (ACBS) · NHS indicative price = £4.10

Breakfast cereals

Loprofin ® Cereals
LOW-PROTEIN

Loprofin low protein breakfast flakes chocolate (Nutricia Ltd)
375 gram (ACBS) · NHS indicative price = £11.37

Loprofin low protein breakfast flakes strawberry (Nutricia Ltd)
375 gram (ACBS) · NHS indicative price = £11.37

Loprofin low protein breakfast loops (Nutricia Ltd)
375 gram (ACBS) · NHS indicative price = £11.78

Promin ® Cereals
LOW-PROTEIN

Promin low protein cereal chocolate (Firstplay Dietary Foods Ltd)
340 gram (ACBS) · NHS indicative price = £8.40

Promin low protein hot breakfast powder 56g sachets original (Firstplay Dietary Foods Ltd)
6 sachet (ACBS) · NHS indicative price = £10.55

Promin low protein hot breakfast powder 57g sachets apple & cinnamon (Firstplay Dietary Foods Ltd)
6 sachet (ACBS) · NHS indicative price = £10.55

Promin low protein hot breakfast powder 57g sachets banana (Firstplay Dietary Foods Ltd)
6 sachet (ACBS) · NHS indicative price = £10.55

Promin low protein hot breakfast powder 57g sachets chocolate (Firstplay Dietary Foods Ltd)
6 sachet (ACBS) · NHS indicative price = £10.55

Cake, confectionery, and sweet biscuits

metaX Sweet biscuits
LOW-PROTEIN

metaX low protein lemon wafers (metaX Institut fuer Diaetetik GmbH)
100 gram (ACBS) · NHS indicative price = £5.52

Mevalia ® Cake, confectionery, and sweet biscuits
LOW-PROTEIN

Mevalia low protein chocotino bars (Vitaflo International Ltd)
100 gram (ACBS) · NHS indicative price = £6.67

Mevalia low protein cookies (Vitaflo International Ltd)
200 gram (ACBS) · NHS indicative price = £9.12

Mevalia low protein frollini biscuits (Vitaflo International Ltd)
200 gram (ACBS) · NHS indicative price = £10.03

Mevalia low protein fruit bar (Vitaflo International Ltd)
125 gram (ACBS) · NHS indicative price = £6.39

Promin ® Cake, confectionery, and sweet biscuits
LOW-PROTEIN

Promin low protein 40g breakfast bars apple & cinnamon (Firstplay Dietary Foods Ltd)
6 pack (ACBS) · NHS indicative price = £12.65

Promin low protein 40g breakfast bars banana (Firstplay Dietary Foods Ltd)
6 pack (ACBS) · NHS indicative price = £12.65

Promin low protein 40g breakfast bars chocolate & cranberry (Firstplay Dietary Foods Ltd)
6 pack (ACBS) · NHS indicative price = £12.65

Promin low protein 40g breakfast bars cranberry (Firstplay Dietary Foods Ltd)
6 pack (ACBS) · NHS indicative price = £12.65

Promin low protein fresh baked fruit loaf (Firstplay Dietary Foods Ltd)
800 gram (ACBS) · NHS indicative price = £7.65

Taranis ® Cake, confectionery, and sweet biscuits
LOW-PROTEIN

Taranis low protein apricot cake (Lactalis Nutrition Sante)
240 gram (ACBS) · NHS indicative price = £6.80

Taranis low protein biscuits with caramel shards (Lactalis Nutrition Sante)
120 gram (ACBS) · NHS indicative price = £5.80

Taranis low protein chocolate chip biscuits (Lactalis Nutrition Sante)
120 gram (ACBS) · NHS indicative price = £5.95

Taranis low protein chocolate chip cookies (Lactalis Nutrition Sante)
160 gram (ACBS) · NHS indicative price = £11.67

Taranis low protein lemon cake (Lactalis Nutrition Sante)
240 gram (ACBS) · NHS indicative price = £6.80

Taranis low protein raspberry shortbread biscuits (Lactalis Nutrition Sante)
120 gram (ACBS) · NHS indicative price = £5.95

Taranis low protein shortbread biscuits (Lactalis Nutrition Sante)
120 gram (ACBS) · NHS indicative price = £5.30

VitaBite ® Confectionery
LOW-PROTEIN

VitaBite bar (Vitaflo International Ltd)
175 gram (ACBS) · NHS indicative price = £13.54

Cake and flour type mixes

Fate ® Cake and flour type mixes
LOW-PROTEIN

Fate low protein all purpose mix (Fate Special Foods)
500 gram (ACBS) · NHS indicative price = £8.69

Fate low protein chocolate cake mix (Fate Special Foods)
500 gram (ACBS) · NHS indicative price = £8.69

Fate low protein plain cake mix (Fate Special Foods)
500 gram (ACBS) · NHS indicative price = £8.69

Juvela ® Low Protein flour mixes
LOW-PROTEIN

Juvela low protein mix (Juvela Ltd)
500 gram (ACBS) · NHS indicative price = £9.25

Loprofin ® Cake and flour type mixes
LOW-PROTEIN

Loprofin low protein chocolate flavour cake mix (Nutricia Ltd)
500 gram (ACBS) · NHS indicative price = £12.71

Loprofin low protein mix (Nutricia Ltd)
500 gram (ACBS) · NHS indicative price = £11.84

Mevalia ® Cake and flour type mixes
LOW-PROTEIN

Mevalia low protein bread mix (Vitaflo International Ltd)
500 gram (ACBS) · NHS indicative price = £8.14

Promin ® Cake and flour type mixes
LOW-PROTEIN

Promin low protein all purpose baking mix (Firstplay Dietary Foods Ltd)
1000 gram (ACBS) · NHS indicative price = £14.95

Promin low protein chocolate cake mix (Firstplay Dietary Foods Ltd)
500 gram (ACBS) · NHS indicative price = £7.15

Promin low protein classic cake mix (Firstplay Dietary Foods Ltd)
500 gram (ACBS) · NHS indicative price = £7.15

Promin low protein potato cake mix (Firstplay Dietary Foods Ltd)
300 gram (ACBS) · NHS indicative price = £7.15

Promin low protein sweet pancake mix (Firstplay Dietary Foods Ltd)
300 gram (ACBS) · NHS indicative price = £4.65

Taranis ® Cake and flour type mixes
LOW-PROTEIN

Taranis low protein natural cake mix (Lactalis Nutrition Sante)
300 gram (ACBS) · NHS indicative price = £4.95

Taranis low protein pancakes and waffles mix (Lactalis Nutrition Sante)
300 gram (ACBS) · NHS indicative price = £4.95

Desserts

Promin ® Desserts
LOW-PROTEIN

Promin low protein dessert 36.5g sachets caramel (Firstplay Dietary Foods Ltd)
6 sachet (ACBS) · NHS indicative price = £8.25

Promin low protein dessert 36.5g sachets chocolate & banana (Firstplay Dietary Foods Ltd)
6 sachet (ACBS) · NHS indicative price = £8.25

Promin low protein dessert 36.5g sachets custard (Firstplay Dietary Foods Ltd)
6 sachet (ACBS) · NHS indicative price = £8.25

Promin low protein dessert 36.5g sachets strawberry & vanilla (Firstplay Dietary Foods Ltd)
6 sachet (ACBS) · NHS indicative price = £8.25

Promin low protein imitation rice pudding 69g sachets apple (Firstplay Dietary Foods Ltd)
4 sachet (ACBS) · NHS indicative price = £8.40

Promin low protein imitation rice pudding 69g sachets banana (Firstplay Dietary Foods Ltd)
4 sachet (ACBS) · NHS indicative price = £8.40

Promin low protein imitation rice pudding 69g sachets original (Firstplay Dietary Foods Ltd)
4 sachet (ACBS) · NHS indicative price = £8.40

Promin low protein imitation rice pudding 69g sachets strawberry (Firstplay Dietary Foods Ltd)
4 sachet (ACBS) · NHS indicative price = £8.40

Taranis ® Pause Desserts
LOW-PROTEIN

Taranis Pause low protein dessert caramel (Lactalis Nutrition Sante)
500 gram (ACBS) · NHS indicative price = £12.30

Taranis Pause low protein dessert strawberry (Lactalis Nutrition Sante)
500 gram (ACBS) · NHS indicative price = £12.30

YoguMaxx ® Dessert
LOW-PROTEIN

YoguMaxx low protein instant powder (Firstplay Dietary Foods Ltd)
400 gram (ACBS) · NHS indicative price = £20.45

Egg replacers

Loprofin ® Egg replacers
LOW-PROTEIN

Loprofin low protein egg replacer (Nutricia Ltd)
500 gram (ACBS) · NHS indicative price = £22.10

Loprofin low protein egg white replacer (Nutricia Ltd)
100 gram (ACBS) · NHS indicative price = £14.19

Promin ® Egg replacer
LOW-PROTEIN

Promin low protein scrambled egg & omelette mix (Firstplay Dietary Foods Ltd)
500 gram (ACBS) · NHS indicative price = £10.85

Meat and fish replacers

Promin ® Meat replacers
LOW-PROTEIN

Promin low protein burger mix 62g sachets lamb & mint (Firstplay Dietary Foods Ltd)
4 sachet (ACBS) · NHS indicative price = £17.00

Promin low protein burger mix 62g sachets original (Firstplay Dietary Foods Ltd)
4 sachet (ACBS) · NHS indicative price = £17.00

Promin low protein chicken burger mix 62g sachets (Firstplay Dietary Foods Ltd)
4 sachet (ACBS) · NHS indicative price = £15.25

Promin low protein sausage mix 30g sachets apple & sage (Firstplay Dietary Foods Ltd)
4 sachet (ACBS) · NHS indicative price = £9.55

Promin low protein sausage mix 30g sachets original (Firstplay Dietary Foods Ltd)
4 sachet (ACBS) · NHS indicative price = £9.55

Promin low protein sausage mix 30g sachets tomato & basil (Firstplay Dietary Foods Ltd)
4 sachet (ACBS) · NHS indicative price = £9.55

Taranis ® Fish substitute
LOW-PROTEIN

Taranis low protein fish substitute (Lactalis Nutrition Sante)
248 gram (ACBS) · NHS indicative price = £14.35

Milk replacers

Loprofin ® Drinks
LOW-PROTEIN

Loprofin drink LQ (Nutricia Ltd)
200 ml (ACBS) · NHS indicative price = £1.04

Loprofin SNO-PRO drink (Nutricia Ltd)
200 ml (ACBS) · NHS indicative price = £1.76

ProZero ® Drink
LOW-PROTEIN

ProZero liquid chocolate (Vitaflo International Ltd)
250 ml (ACBS) · NHS indicative price = £2.25

ProZero liquid unflavoured (Vitaflo International Ltd)
250 ml (ACBS) · NHS indicative price = £2.25 | 1000 ml (ACBS)
· NHS indicative price = £9.06

Taranis ® Milk substitutes
LOW-PROTEIN

Taranis Dalia low protein milk (Lactalis Nutrition Sante)
200 ml (ACBS) · NHS indicative price = £1.34

Taranis low protein Dalia milk substitute powder (Lactalis Nutrition
Sante)
400 gram (ACBS) · NHS indicative price = £9.50

Pasta and pizza bases

Loprofin ® Pasta
LOW-PROTEIN

Loprofin low protein pasta animal shapes (Nutricia Ltd)
500 gram (ACBS) · NHS indicative price = £12.10

Loprofin low protein pasta fusilli (Nutricia Ltd)
500 gram (ACBS) · NHS indicative price = £12.53

Loprofin low protein pasta lasagne (Nutricia Ltd)
250 gram (ACBS) · NHS indicative price = £6.10

Loprofin low protein pasta macaroni (Nutricia Ltd)
250 gram (ACBS) · NHS indicative price = £6.03

Loprofin low protein pasta penne (Nutricia Ltd)
500 gram (ACBS) · NHS indicative price = £12.53

Loprofin low protein pasta spaghetti (Nutricia Ltd)
500 gram (ACBS) · NHS indicative price = £12.53

Loprofin low protein pasta tagliatelle (Nutricia Ltd)
250 gram (ACBS) · NHS indicative price = £6.03

Mevalia ® Pasta and pizza bases
LOW-PROTEIN

Mevalia low protein fusilli (Vitaflo International Ltd)
500 gram (ACBS) · NHS indicative price = £8.54

Mevalia low protein pasta ditali (Vitaflo International Ltd)
500 gram (ACBS) · NHS indicative price = £8.54

Mevalia low protein penne (Vitaflo International Ltd)
500 gram (ACBS) · NHS indicative price = £8.54

Mevalia low protein pizza base (Vitaflo International Ltd)
300 gram (ACBS) · NHS indicative price = £8.06

Mevalia low protein spaghetti (Vitaflo International Ltd)
500 gram (ACBS) · NHS indicative price = £8.55

Promin ® Pasta
LOW-PROTEIN

Promin low protein lasagne sheets (Firstplay Dietary Foods Ltd)
200 gram (ACBS) · NHS indicative price = £3.55

Promin low protein pastameal (Firstplay Dietary Foods Ltd)
500 gram (ACBS) · NHS indicative price = £8.25

Promin low protein pasta alphabets (Firstplay Dietary Foods Ltd)
500 gram (ACBS) · NHS indicative price = £8.25

Promin low protein pasta flat noodles (Firstplay Dietary Foods Ltd)
500 gram (ACBS) · NHS indicative price = £8.05

Promin low protein pasta macaroni (Firstplay Dietary Foods Ltd)
500 gram (ACBS) · NHS indicative price = £8.25

Promin low protein pasta shells (Firstplay Dietary Foods Ltd)
500 gram (ACBS) · NHS indicative price = £8.25

Promin low protein pasta short cut spaghetti (Firstplay Dietary
Foods Ltd)
500 gram (ACBS) · NHS indicative price = £8.25

Promin low protein pasta spirals (Firstplay Dietary Foods Ltd)
500 gram (ACBS) · NHS indicative price = £8.25

Promin low protein tricolour pasta alphabets (Firstplay Dietary
Foods Ltd)
500 gram (ACBS) · NHS indicative price = £8.25

Promin low protein tricolour pasta shells (Firstplay Dietary Foods
Ltd)
500 gram (ACBS) · NHS indicative price = £8.25

Promin low protein tricolour pasta spirals (Firstplay Dietary Foods
Ltd)
500 gram (ACBS) · NHS indicative price = £8.25

Ready meals

Promin ® Ready meals
LOW-PROTEIN

Promin low protein Mac Pot cheese (Firstplay Dietary Foods Ltd)
244 gram (ACBS) · NHS indicative price = £24.50

Promin low protein Mac Pot tomato (Firstplay Dietary Foods Ltd)
244 gram (ACBS) · NHS indicative price = £24.50

Promin low protein pasta in sauce 66g sachets cheese & broccoli
(Firstplay Dietary Foods Ltd)
4 sachet (ACBS) · NHS indicative price = £9.95

**Promin low protein pasta in sauce 72g sachets tomato, pepper &
herb** (Firstplay Dietary Foods Ltd)
4 sachet (ACBS) · NHS indicative price = £11.10

**Promin low protein pasta spirals in Moroccan type sauce 72g
sachets** (Firstplay Dietary Foods Ltd)
4 sachet (ACBS) · NHS indicative price = £11.10

Promin low protein potato pot with croutons cabbage & bacon
(Firstplay Dietary Foods Ltd)
200 gram (ACBS) · NHS indicative price = £21.70

Promin low protein potato pot with croutons onion (Firstplay
Dietary Foods Ltd)
200 gram (ACBS) · NHS indicative price = £21.70

Promin low protein potato pot with croutons sausage (Firstplay
Dietary Foods Ltd)
200 gram (ACBS) · NHS indicative price = £21.70

Promin low protein X-Pot all day scramble (Firstplay Dietary Foods
Ltd)
240 gram (ACBS) · NHS indicative price = £27.10

Promin low protein X-Pot beef & tomato (Firstplay Dietary Foods Ltd)
240 gram (ACBS) · NHS indicative price = £27.10

Promin low protein X-Pot chip shop curry (Firstplay Dietary Foods
Ltd)
240 gram (ACBS) · NHS indicative price = £27.10

Promin low protein X-Pot rogan style curry (Firstplay Dietary Foods
Ltd)
240 gram (ACBS) · NHS indicative price = £27.10

Rice and cous cous replacers

Loprofin ® Rice replacer
LOW-PROTEIN

Loprofin low protein rice replacer (Nutricia Ltd)
500 gram (ACBS) · NHS indicative price = £12.19

Mevalia ® Rice replacer
LOW-PROTEIN

Mevalia low protein rice replacer (Vitaflo International Ltd)
400 gram (ACBS) · NHS indicative price = £7.04

Promin ® Rice and cous cous replacers
LOW-PROTEIN

Promin low protein cous cous (Firstplay Dietary Foods Ltd)
500 gram (ACBS) · NHS indicative price = £8.25

Promin low protein imitation rice (Firstplay Dietary Foods Ltd)
500 gram (ACBS) · NHS indicative price = £8.25

Taranis ® Rice replacer
LOW-PROTEIN

Taranis low protein risotto substitute (Lactalis Nutrition Sante)
1200 gram (ACBS) · NHS indicative price = £31.85

Sauces

Promin ® Sauce mix
LOW-PROTEIN

Promin low protein cheese sauce mix (Firstplay Dietary Foods Ltd)
225 gram (ACBS) · NHS indicative price = £6.70

Savoury biscuits and snacks

Loprofin ® Savoury biscuits and snacks
LOW-PROTEIN

Loprofin low protein crackers (Nutricia Ltd)
150 gram (ACBS) · NHS indicative price = £5.13

Loprofin low protein herb crackers (Nutricia Ltd)
150 gram (ACBS) · NHS indicative price = £5.13

Promin ® Savoury biscuits and snacks
LOW-PROTEIN

Promin low protein Snax (Firstplay Dietary Foods Ltd)
12 sachet (ACBS) · NHS indicative price = £14.20

Promin low protein Snax cheese & onion 25g sachets (Firstplay Dietary Foods Ltd)
3 sachet · No NHS indicative price available | 12 sachet (ACBS) · NHS indicative price = £14.20

Promin low protein Snax jalapeno 25g sachets (Firstplay Dietary Foods Ltd)
3 sachet · No NHS indicative price available | 12 sachet (ACBS) · NHS indicative price = £14.20

Promin low protein Snax ready salted 25g sachets (Firstplay Dietary Foods Ltd)
3 sachet · No NHS indicative price available | 12 sachet (ACBS) · NHS indicative price = £14.20

Promin low protein Snax salt & vinegar 25g sachets (Firstplay Dietary Foods Ltd)
3 sachet · No NHS indicative price available | 12 sachet (ACBS) · NHS indicative price = £14.20

Vitaflo Choices ® Snacks
LOW-PROTEIN

Vitaflo Choices mini crackers (Vitaflo International Ltd)
40 gram (ACBS) · NHS indicative price = £1.32

Soups

Promin ® Soups
LOW-PROTEIN

Promin low protein soup with croutons oral powder 28g sachets creamy chicken (Firstplay Dietary Foods Ltd)
4 sachet (ACBS) · NHS indicative price = £6.70

Promin low protein soup with croutons oral powder 23g sachets creamy tomato (Firstplay Dietary Foods Ltd)
4 sachet (ACBS) · NHS indicative price = £6.70

Promin low protein soup with croutons oral powder 28g sachets minestrone (Firstplay Dietary Foods Ltd)
4 sachet (ACBS) · NHS indicative price = £6.70

Promin low protein soup with croutons oral powder 23g sachets pea and mint (Firstplay Dietary Foods Ltd)
4 sachet (ACBS) · NHS indicative price = £6.70

Spreads

Taranis ® Spreads
LOW-PROTEIN

Taranis low protein hazelnut spread (Lactalis Nutrition Sante)
230 gram (ACBS) · NHS indicative price = £10.00

Ketogenic diet

Medium chain triglycerides (MCT) liquid

K.Quik ®
▶ Ketogenic diet or conditions requiring a source of MCT. Suitable from 3 years.
LIQUID (SIP FEED), medium chain triglycerides (MCT) 20 g, energy 777 kJ (189 kcal)/100 mL.

K.Quik liquid (Vitaflo International Ltd)
225 ml (ACBS) · NHS indicative price = £5.02

K.Vita ®
▶ For the dietary management of drug resistant epilepsy. Suitable from 3 years.
LIQUID (SIP OR TUBE FEED), medium chain triglycerides (MCT) 33.5 g, energy 1265 kJ (308 kcal)/100 mL.

K.Vita liquid (Vitaflo International Ltd)
120 ml (ACBS) · NHS indicative price = £18.52

Kanso ® MCT Oil 100%
▶ Intractable epilepsy, pyruvate dehydrogenase deficiency, glucose transporter type 1 deficiency syndrome and other conditions where a ketogenic diet is indicated.
LIQUID, medium chain triglycerides (MCT) 91 g, energy 3367 kJ (819 kcal)/100 mL.

Kanso MCT Oil 100% liquid (Dr Schar UK Ltd)
500 ml (ACBS) · NHS indicative price = £16.63

Liquigen ®
▶ Steatorrhoea associated with cystic fibrosis of the pancreas, intestinal lymphangiectasia, surgery of the intestine, chronic liver disease, liver cirrhosis, other proven malabsorption syndromes, a ketogenic diet in the management of epilepsy and in type 1 hyperlipoproteinaemia.
LIQUID (SIP OR TUBE FEED), medium chain triglycerides (MCT) 49.1 g, energy 1865 kJ (454 kcal)/100 mL.

Liquigen emulsion (Nutricia Ltd)
250 ml (ACBS) · NHS indicative price = £13.97

MCT Oil
▶ Steatorrhoea associated with cystic fibrosis of the pancreas, intestinal lymphangiectasia, surgery of the intestine, chronic liver disease, liver cirrhosis, other proven malabsorption syndromes, in a ketogenic diet in the management of epilepsy and in type 1 hyperlipoproteinaemia.
LIQUID, medium chain triglycerides (MCT) 95 g, energy 3515 kJ (855 kcal)/100 mL.

MCT oil (Nutricia Ltd)
500 ml (ACBS) · NHS indicative price = £22.15

Powder

KetoCal ® 4:1
▶ For use as part of the ketogenic diet in the management of epilepsy resistant to drug therapy. Only to be prescribed on the advice of a secondary care physician with experience of the ketogenic diet. Suitable from 1 year.
POWDER, protein 14.4 g, carbohydrate 2.9 g, fat 69.2 g, fibre 5.4 g, energy 2897 kJ (703 kcal)/100 g.

KetoCal 4:1 powder unflavoured (Nutricia Ltd)
300 gram (ACBS) · NHS indicative price = £45.99

KetoCal 4:1 powder vanilla (Nutricia Ltd)
300 gram (ACBS) · NHS indicative price = £45.99

Ready to serve

K.Flo ® 4:1
▶ Epilepsy, neurometabolic disorders (e.g. glut 1 deficiency syndrome) and other conditions requiring a ketogenic diet. Suitable from 3 years.
LIQUID (SIP OR TUBE FEED), protein 3.4 g, carbohydrate 0.35 g, fat 14.7 g, fibre 1.4 g, energy 619 kJ (150 kcal)/100 mL.

K.Flo liquid (Vitaflo International Ltd)
250 ml (ACBS) · NHS indicative price = £7.64

K.Yo ® 3:1
▶ Epilepsy in a ketogenic diet, glut 1 deficiency syndrome or other conditions requiring a ketogenic diet. Suitable from 3 years.
SEMI-SOLID, protein 8 g, carbohydrate 1.5 g, fat 30 g, fibre Nil, energy 1272 kJ (308 kcal)/100 g.

K.Yo semi-solid food 100g pots chocolate (Vitaflo International Ltd)
4 pot (ACBS) · NHS indicative price = £37.16 | 36 pot (ACBS) · NHS indicative price = £250.88

K.Yo semi-solid food 100g pots vanilla (Vitaflo International Ltd)
4 pot (ACBS) · NHS indicative price = £37.16 | 36 pot (ACBS) · NHS indicative price = £250.88

KetoCal ® 2.5:1 LQ
▶ Drug resistant epilepsy or other conditions for which the ketogenic diet is indicated. Only to be prescribed on the advice of a specialist with experience of the ketogenic diet. Not suitable for use in child under 8 years.
LIQUID (SIP OR TUBE FEED), protein 4.5 g, carbohydrate 1.1 g, fat 14.3 g, fibre 1.1 g, energy 637 kJ (153 kcal)/100 mL.

KetoCal 2.5:1LQ liquid (Nutricia Ltd)
200 ml (ACBS) · NHS indicative price = £6.53

KetoCal ® 4:1 LQ
▶ Drug resistant epilepsy or other conditions for which a ketogenic diet is indicated. Suitable from 1 year.
LIQUID (SIP OR TUBE FEED), protein 3.09 g, carbohydrate 0.61 g, fat 14.8 g, fibre 1.12 g, energy 620 kJ (150 kcal)/100 mL.

KetoCal 4:1LQ liquid unflavoured (Nutricia Ltd)
200 ml (ACBS) · NHS indicative price = £6.18

KetoCal 4:1LQ liquid vanilla (Nutricia Ltd)
200 ml (ACBS) · NHS indicative price = £6.18

KetoVie ® 4:1
▶ Intractable epilepsy and other conditions where a ketogenic diet is indicated. Not suitable for use in child under 3 years.
LIQUID (SIP OR TUBE FEED), protein 3.4 g, carbohydrate 0.2 g, fat 14 g, fibre 1.8 g, energy 602 kJ (144 kcal)/100 mL.

KetoVie 4:1 liquid chocolate (Cambrooke UK Ltd)
250 ml (ACBS) · NHS indicative price = £7.52

KetoVie 4:1 liquid vanilla (Cambrooke UK Ltd)
250 ml (ACBS) · NHS indicative price = £7.52

KetoVie ® Peptide 4:1
▶ Intractable epilepsy and other conditions where a ketogenic diet is indicated. Not suitable for use in child under 3 years.
LIQUID (SIP OR TUBE FEED), protein 3.2 g, carbohydrate 0.33 g, fat 15 g, fibre 1.1 g, energy 632 kJ (151 kcal)/100 mL.

KetoVie Peptide 4:1 liquid (Cambrooke UK Ltd)
250 ml (ACBS) · NHS indicative price = £7.28

Specialist food replacers

Kanso ® 4.8:1 DeliMCT CacaoBar
▶ Intractable epilepsy when following a ketogenic diet, pyruvate dehydrogenase deficiency, glucose transporter type 1 deficiency syndrome or other conditions requiring a ketogenic diet. Suitable from 3 years.
SOLID, protein 7.1 g, carbohydrate 15.4 g, fat 55.4 g (MCT 38 %), fibre 18.9 g, energy 2394 kJ (582 kcal)/100 g.

Kanso DeliMCT CacaoBar (Dr Schar UK Ltd)
100 gram (ACBS) · NHS indicative price = £6.08

KetoClassic ® 3:1 Bar
▶ Intractable epilepsy, pyruvate dehydrogenase deficiency, glucose transporter type 1 deficiency and other conditions where a ketogenic diet is indicated. Suitable from 3 years.
SOLID, protein 10.8 g, carbohydrate 3.3 g, fat 43.6 g, fibre 28.7 g, energy 2082 kJ (498 kcal)/100 g.

KetoClassic 3:1 Bar (KetoCare Foods Ltd)
420 gram (ACBS) · NHS indicative price = £30.38

KetoClassic ® 3:1 Bisk
▶ Intractable epilepsy, pyruvate dehydrogenase deficiency, glucose transporter type 1 deficiency and other conditions where a ketogenic diet is indicated. Suitable from 3 years.
SOLID, protein 10.7 g, carbohydrate 4.6 g, fat 47.1 g, fibre 23.3 g, energy 2206 kJ (534 kcal)/100 g.

KetoClassic 3:1 Bisk (KetoCare Foods Ltd)
420 gram (ACBS) · NHS indicative price = £28.65

KetoClassic ® 3:1 Breakfast Muesli
▶ Intractable epilepsy, pyruvate dehydrogenase deficiency, glucose transporter type 1 deficiency and other conditions where a ketogenic diet is indicated. Suitable from 3 years.
SOLID, protein 11 g, carbohydrate 7.5 g, fat 57.1 g, fibre 17.5 g, energy 2569 kJ (623 kcal)/100 g.

KetoClassic 3:1 Breakfast muesli (KetoCare Foods Ltd)
600 gram (ACBS) · NHS indicative price = £48.57

KetoClassic ® 3:1 Breakfast Porridge
▶ Intractable epilepsy, pyruvate dehydrogenase deficiency, glucose transporter type 1 deficiency and other conditions where a ketogenic diet is indicated. Suitable from 3 years.
SOLID, protein 11.7 g, carbohydrate 7.8 g, fat 59.1 g, fibre 16.7 g, energy 2649 kJ (643 kcal)/100 g.

KetoClassic 3:1 Breakfast porridge (KetoCare Foods Ltd)
600 gram (ACBS) · NHS indicative price = £48.57

KetoClassic ® 3:1 Meal
▶ Intractable epilepsy, pyruvate dehydrogenase deficiency, glucose transporter type 1 deficiency and other conditions where a ketogenic diet is indicated. Suitable from 3 years.
SEMI-SOLID, protein 5.1-5.2 g, carbohydrate 2-3.7 g, fat 21.7-26.7 g, fibre 0.4-2.1 g, energy 936-1182 kJ (224-287 kcal)/100 g.

KetoClassic 3:1 Meal bolognese 130g pouches (KetoCare Foods Ltd)
14 pouch (ACBS) · NHS indicative price = £105.64

KetoClassic 3:1 Meal chicken 135g pouches (KetoCare Foods Ltd)
14 pouch (ACBS) · NHS indicative price = £106.91

KetoClassic ® 3:1 Savoury Bread
▶ Intractable epilepsy, pyruvate dehydrogenase deficiency, glucose transporter type 1 deficiency and other conditions where a ketogenic diet is indicated. Suitable from 3 years.
SOLID, protein 9 g, carbohydrate 7.3 g, fat 48.7 g, fibre 13.7 g, energy 2190 kJ (531 kcal)/100 g.

KetoClassic 3:1 Savoury meal (KetoCare Foods Ltd)
840 gram (ACBS) · NHS indicative price = £60.30

KetoVie ® 4:1 Kwik Mix
▶ Intractable epilepsy and other conditions where a ketogenic diet is indicated. Suitable from 3 years.
POWDER, protein 5.1 g, carbohydrate 5.8 g, fat 44 g, fibre 36 g, energy 2122 kJ (507 kcal)/100 g.

KetoVie Kwik Mix baking mix (Cambrooke UK Ltd)
680 gram (ACBS) · NHS indicative price = £42.48

Nutritional products for inherited metabolic disorders

Glutaric aciduria type 1

5 g protein equivalent

GA amino5 ®
▶ Nutritional supplement for the dietary management of glutaric aciduria type 1 (GA1).
POWDER, protein equivalent 83 g, carbohydrate Nil, fat Nil, energy 1411 kJ (332 kcal)/100 g

GA amino5 oral powder 6g sachets (Vitaflo International Ltd)
30 sachet (ACBS) · NHS indicative price = £159.25

Glycogen storage disease

Slow-release carbohydrate supplements

Glycosade ®
▶ Nutritional supplement for the dietary management of hepatic glycogen storage disease. Unflavoured suitable from 2 years; lemon flavour suitable from 3 years.
POWDER, protein Nil, carbohydrate 88 g, fat Nil, energy 1496 kJ (352 kcal)/100 g

Glycosade oral powder 60g sachets lemon (Vitaflo International Ltd)
30 sachet (ACBS) · NHS indicative price = £176.17

Glycosade oral powder 60g sachets unflavoured (Vitaflo International Ltd)
30 sachet (ACBS) · NHS indicative price = £176.17

Homocystinuria

10 g protein equivalent

HCU cooler ® 10

▶ Nutritional supplement for the dietary management of homocystinuria. Suitable from 3 years. Includes added vitamins A, B, C, D, E and K.
LIQUID, protein equivalent 11.5 g, carbohydrate 5.1 g, fat 0.9 g, energy 316 kJ (75 kcal)/100 mL.

HCU red cooler10 liquid (Vitaflo International Ltd)
87 ml (ACBS) · NHS indicative price = £10.81

HCU Lophlex ® LQ 10

▶ Nutritional supplement for the dietary management of proven homocystinuria. Suitable from 4 years. Includes added vitamins A, B, C, D, E and K.
LIQUID, protein 16 g, carbohydrate 7 g, fat 0.35 g, energy 407 kJ (96 kcal)/100 mL.

HCU Lophlex LQ 10 liquid (Nutricia Ltd)
62.5 ml (ACBS) · NHS indicative price = £11.72

15 g protein equivalent

HCU cooler ® 15

▶ Nutritional supplement for the dietary management of homocystinuria. Suitable from 3 years. Includes added vitamins A, B, C, D, E and K.
LIQUID, protein equivalent 11.5 g, carbohydrate 5.1 g, fat 0.9 g, energy 316 kJ (75 kcal)/100 ml.

HCU orange cooler15 liquid (Vitaflo International Ltd)
130 ml (ACBS) · NHS indicative price = £17.68

HCU red cooler15 liquid (Vitaflo International Ltd)
130 ml (ACBS) · NHS indicative price = £17.68

HCU express ® 15

▶ Nutritional supplement for the dietary management of homocystinuria. Suitable from 8 years. Includes added vitamins A, B, C, D, E and K.
POWDER, protein equivalent 60 g, carbohydrate 13.7 g, fat 0.2 g, energy 1260 kJ (297 kcal)/100 g.

HCU express15 oral powder 25g sachets (Vitaflo International Ltd)
30 sachet (ACBS) · NHS indicative price = £520.85

20 g protein equivalent

HCU cooler ® 20

▶ Nutritional supplement for the dietary management of homocystinuria. Suitable from 3 years. Includes added vitamins A, B, C, D, E and K.
LIQUID, protein equivalent 11.5 g, carbohydrate 5.1 g, fat 0.9 g, energy 316 kJ (75 kcal)/100 mL.

HCU red cooler20 liquid (Vitaflo International Ltd)
174 ml (ACBS) · NHS indicative price = £22.61

HCU express ® 20

▶ Nutritional supplement for the dietary management of homocystinuria. Suitable from 8 years. Includes added vitamins A, B, C, D, E and K.
POWDER, protein equivalent 60 g, carbohydrate 13.7 g, fat 0.2 g, energy 1260 kJ (297 kcal)/100 g.

HCU express20 oral powder 34g sachets (Vitaflo International Ltd)
30 sachet (ACBS) · NHS indicative price = £672.92

HCU Lophlex ®

▶ Nutritional supplement for the dietary management of homocystinuria. Suitable from 3 years. Includes added vitamins A, B, C, D, E and K.
POWDER, protein 68.9 g, carbohydrate 13.4 g, fat 1.4 g, energy 1430 kJ (338 kcal)/100 g.

HCU Lophlex powder 29g sachets (Nutricia Ltd)
30 sachet (ACBS) · NHS indicative price = £651.00

HCU Lophlex ® LQ 20

▶ Nutritional supplement for the dietary management of proven homocystinuria. Suitable from 4 years. Includes added vitamins A, B, C, D, E and K.
LIQUID, protein 16 g, carbohydrate 7 g, fat 0.35 g, energy 407 kJ (96 kcal)/100 mL.

HCU Lophlex LQ 20 liquid (Nutricia Ltd)
125 ml (ACBS) · NHS indicative price = £24.18

HCU-LV ®

▶ Nutritional supplement for the dietary management of hypermethioninaemia or vitamin B6 non-responsive homocystinuria. Suitable from 8 years. Includes added vitamins A, B, C, D, E and K.
POWDER, protein 72 g, carbohydrate 5 g, fat 0.7 g, energy 1335 kJ (314 kcal)/100 g.

HCU-LV oral powder 27.8g sachets tropical (Nutricia Ltd)
30 sachet (ACBS) · NHS indicative price = £743.70

Powder protein source

HCU Maxamum ®

▶ Nutritional supplement for the dietary management of hypermethioninaemia, homocystinuria. Suitable from 8 years. Includes added vitamins A, B, C, D, E and K.
POWDER, protein 39 g, carbohydrate 34 g, fat less than 0.5 g, energy 1260 kJ (297 kcal)/100 g.

HCU Maxamum powder (Nutricia Ltd)
500 gram (ACBS) · NHS indicative price = £237.60

Homocystinuria or hypermethioninaemia

Powder protein source

XMET Homidon ®

▶ Nutritional supplement for the dietary management of homocystinuria or hypermethioninaemia.
POWDER, protein 77 g, carbohydrate 4.5 g, fat Nil, energy 1386 kJ (326 kcal)/100 g.

XMET Homidon powder (Nutricia Ltd)
500 gram (ACBS) · NHS indicative price = £280.81

Maple syrup urine disease

5 g protein equivalent

MSUD amino5 ®

▶ Nutritional supplement for the dietary management of maple syrup urine disease (MSUD).
POWDER, protein equivalent 83 g, carbohydrate Nil, fat Nil, energy 1411 kJ (332 kcal)/100 g

MSUD amino5 oral powder 6g sachets (Vitaflo International Ltd)
30 sachet (ACBS) · NHS indicative price = £159.25

10 g protein equivalent

MSUD cooler ® 10

▶ Nutritional supplement for the dietary management of maple syrup urine disease. Suitable from 3 years. Includes added vitamins A, B, C, D, E and K.
LIQUID, protein equivalent 11.5 g, carbohydrate 5.1 g, fat 0.9 g, energy 316 kJ (75 kcal)/100 mL.

MSUD red cooler10 liquid (Vitaflo International Ltd)
87 ml (ACBS) · NHS indicative price = £10.81

MSUD Lophlex ® LQ 10

▶ Nutritional supplement for the dietary management of maple syrup urine disease. Includes added vitamins A, B, C, D, E and K.
LIQUID, protein 16 g, carbohydrate 7 g, fat 0.35 g, energy 407 kJ (96 kcal)/100 mL.

MSUD Lophlex LQ 10 liquid (Nutricia Ltd)
62.5 ml (ACBS) · NHS indicative price = £11.72

15 g protein equivalent

MSUD cooler ® 15

▶ Nutritional supplement for the dietary management of maple syrup urine disease. Suitable from 3 years. Includes added vitamins A, B, C, D, E and K.
LIQUID, protein equivalent 11.5 g, carbohydrate 5.1 g, fat 0.9 g, energy 316 kJ (75 kcal)/100 mL.

MSUD orange cooler15 liquid (Vitaflo International Ltd)
130 ml (ACBS) · NHS indicative price = £17.68

MSUD red cooler15 liquid (Vitaflo International Ltd)
130 ml (ACBS) · NHS indicative price = £17.68

MSUD express ® 15
▸ Nutritional supplement for the dietary management of maple syrup urine disease. Suitable from 8 years. Includes added vitamins A, B, C, D, E, K.
POWDER, protein equivalent 60 g, carbohydrate 13.7 g, fat 0.2 g, energy 1260 kJ (297 kcal)/100 g.

MSUD express15 oral powder 25g sachets (Vitaflo International Ltd)
30 sachet (ACBS) · NHS indicative price = £520.85

20 g protein equivalent

MSUD cooler ® 20
▸ Nutritional supplement for the dietary management of maple syrup urine disease. Suitable from 3 years. Includes added vitamins A, B, C, D, E and K.
LIQUID, protein equivalent 11.5 g, carbohydrate 5.1 g, fat 0.9 g, energy 316 kJ (75 kcal)/100 mL.

MSUD red cooler20 liquid (Vitaflo International Ltd)
174 ml (ACBS) · NHS indicative price = £22.61

MSUD express ® 20
▸ Nutritional supplement for the dietary management of maple syrup urine disease. Suitable from 8 years. Includes added vitamins A, B, C, D, E and K.
POWDER, protein equivalent 60 g, carbohydrate 13.7 g, fat 0.2 g, energy 1260 kJ (297 kcal)/100 g.

MSUD express20 oral powder 34g sachets (Vitaflo International Ltd)
30 sachet (ACBS) · NHS indicative price = £672.92

MSUD Lophlex ®
▸ Nutritional supplement for the dietary management of maple syrup urine disease. Suitable from 3 years. Includes added vitamins A, B, C, D, E and K.
POWDER, protein 71.4 g, carbohydrate 15 g, fat 1.5 g, energy 1530 kJ (355 kcal)/100 g.

MSUD Lophlex powder 28g sachets (Nutricia Ltd)
30 sachet (ACBS) · NHS indicative price = £651.00

MSUD Lophlex ® LQ 20
▸ Nutritional supplement for the dietary management of maple syrup urine disease. Includes added vitamins A, B, C, D, E and K.
LIQUID, protein 16 g, carbohydrate 7 g, fat 0.35 g, energy 407 kJ (96 kcal)/100 mL.

MSUD Lophlex LQ 20 liquid (Nutricia Ltd)
125 ml (ACBS) · NHS indicative price = £24.18

Powder protein source

MSUD Aid III ®
▸ Nutritional supplement for the dietary management of maple syrup urine disease (MSUD) and related conditions when it is necessary to limit the intake of branched chain amino acids.
POWDER, protein 77 g, carbohydrate 4.5 g, fat Nil, energy 1386 kJ (326 kcal)/100 g.

MSUD Aid 111 powder (Nutricia Ltd)
500 gram (ACBS) · NHS indicative price = £280.81

MSUD Maxamum ®
▸ Nutritional supplement for the dietary management of maple syrup urine disease. Suitable from 8 years. Includes added vitamins A, B, C, D, E and K.
POWDER, protein equivalent (essential and non-essential amino acids) 39 g, carbohydrate 34 g, fat less than 0.5 g, energy 1260 kJ (297 kcal)/100 g.

MSUD Maxamum powder orange (Nutricia Ltd)
500 gram (ACBS) · NHS indicative price = £237.60

MSUD Maxamum powder unflavoured (Nutricia Ltd)
500 gram (ACBS) · NHS indicative price = £237.60

Methylmalonic or propionic acidaemia
5 g protein equivalent

MMA/PA amino5 ®
▸ Nutritional supplement for the dietary management of the organic acidaemias, methylmalonic acidaemia (MMA) and the propionic acidaemia (PA).
POWDER, protein equivalent 83 g, carbohydrate Nil, fat Nil, energy 1411 kJ (332 kcal)/100 g

MMA / PA amino5 oral powder 6g sachets (Vitaflo International Ltd)
30 sachet (ACBS) · NHS indicative price = £159.25

Powder protein source

MMA/PA Maxamum ®
▸ Nutritional supplement for the dietary management of methylmalonic acidaemia or propionic acidaemia. Suitable from 8 years. Includes added vitamins A, B, C, D, E and K.
POWDER, protein 39 g, carbohydrate 34 g, fat less than 0.5 g, energy 1260 kJ (297 kcal)/100 g.

MMA / PA Maxamum powder (Nutricia Ltd)
500 gram (ACBS) · NHS indicative price = £237.60

XMTVI Asadon ®
▸ Nutritional supplement for the dietary management of methylmalonic acidaemia or propionic acidaemia.
POWDER, protein 77 g, carbohydrate 4.5 g, fat Nil, energy 1386 kJ (326 kcal)/100 g.

XMTVI Asadon powder (Nutricia Ltd)
200 gram (ACBS) · NHS indicative price = £112.33

Non-specific inherited metabolic disorders
Energy (carbohydrate) fortifiers

S.O.S. ®
▸ Nutritional supplement for the dietary management of inherited metabolic disorders.
POWDER, protein Nil, carbohydrate 95 g, fat Nil, energy 1615 kJ (380 kcal)/100 g.

S.O.S10 oral powder 21g sachets (Vitaflo International Ltd)
30 sachet (ACBS) · NHS indicative price = £11.51

S.O.S15 oral powder 31g sachets (Vitaflo International Ltd)
30 sachet (ACBS) · NHS indicative price = £17.00

S.O.S20 oral powder 42g sachets (Vitaflo International Ltd)
30 sachet (ACBS) · NHS indicative price = £23.05

S.O.S25 oral powder 52g sachets (Vitaflo International Ltd)
30 sachet (ACBS) · NHS indicative price = £28.50

Energy (carbohydrate and fat) fortifiers

Basecal200 ®
▸ Nutritional supplement for the dietary management of inborn errors of protein metabolism requiring a low protein diet. Suitable from 3 years. Includes added vitamins A, B, C, D, E and K.
POWDER, protein equivalent Nil, carbohydrate 69.8 g, fat 20.7 g, energy 1952 kJ (465 kcal)/100 g.

Basecal200 oral powder 43g sachets (Vitaflo International Ltd)
30 sachet (ACBS) · NHS indicative price = £107.47

Essential fatty acid supplements

KeyOmega ®
▸ Nutritional supplement for the dietary management of inborn errors of metabolism. Includes added vitamin C.
POWDER, protein 4.4 g, carbohydrate 70 g, fat 19 g, energy 1999 kJ (476 kcal)/100 g.

KeyOmega oral powder 4g sachets (Vitaflo International Ltd)
30 sachet (ACBS) · NHS indicative price = £63.01

Single L-amino acid supplements

Cystine500 ®
▸ Nutritional supplement for the dietary management of inborn errors of amino acid metabolism. Suitable from 3 years.

POWDER, protein equivalent 11.6 g, carbohydrate 82.5 g, fat Nil, energy 1600 kJ (376 kcal)/100 g.

Cystine500 oral powder sachets (Vitaflo International Ltd)
30 sachet (ACBS) · NHS indicative price = £85.15

Isoleucine50 ®
▸ Nutritional supplement for the dietary management of inborn errors of amino acid metabolism.
POWDER, protein equivalent 1 g, carbohydrate 95 g, fat Nil, energy 1632 kJ (384 kcal)/100 g.

Isoleucine50 oral powder 4g sachets (Vitaflo International Ltd)
30 sachet (ACBS) · NHS indicative price = £85.15

L-Tyrosine
▸ Nutritional supplement for the dietary management of maternal phenylketonuria in patients with low plasma tyrosine levels.
POWDER, protein 90.1 g, carbohydrate Nil, fat Nil, energy 1532 kJ (360 kcal)/100 g.

L-Tyrosine powder (Nutricia Ltd)
100 gram (ACBS) · NHS indicative price = £33.06

Leucine100 ®
▸ Nutritional supplement for the dietary management of inborn errors of amino acid metabolism.
POWDER, protein equivalent 2.2 g, carbohydrate 92.5 g, fat Nil, energy 1610 kJ (379 kcal)/100 g.

Leucine100 oral powder sachets (Vitaflo International Ltd)
30 sachet (ACBS) · NHS indicative price = £85.15

Phenylalanine50 ®
▸ Nutritional supplement for the dietary management of inborn errors of amino acid metabolism.
POWDER, protein equivalent 1.1 g, carbohydrate 95 g, fat Nil, energy 1634 kJ (384 kcal)/100 g.

Phenylalanine50 oral powder sachets (Vitaflo International Ltd)
30 sachet (ACBS) · NHS indicative price = £82.68

Tyrosine1000 ®
▸ Nutritional supplement for the dietary management of inborn errors of amino acid metabolism. Not suitable for use in child under 3 years.
POWDER, protein equivalent 22.5 g, carbohydrate 72.5 g, fat Nil, energy 1615 kJ (380 kcal)/100 g.

Tyrosine1000 oral powder 4g sachets (Vitaflo International Ltd)
30 sachet (ACBS) · NHS indicative price = £7.59

Valine50 ®
▸ Nutritional supplement for the dietary management of inborn errors of amino acid metabolism.
POWDER, protein equivalent 1 g, carbohydrate 95 g, fat Nil, energy 1632 kJ (384 kcal)/100 g.

Valine50 oral powder 4g sachets (Vitaflo International Ltd)
30 sachet (ACBS) · NHS indicative price = £85.15

Phenylketonuria

10 g GMP protein equivalent

Glytactin ® **Build 10**
▸ Nutritional supplement for the dietary management of phenylketonuria. Suitable from 3 years. Includes added vitamins A, B, C, D, E and K.
POWDER, protein equivalent 67 g, carbohydrate 2.4 g, fat 4.2 g, energy 1400 kJ (335 kcal)/100 g.

Glytactin Build 10 oral powder 16g sachets (Cambrooke UK Ltd)
30 sachet (ACBS) · NHS indicative price = £229.17

PKU GMPro ®
▸ Nutritional supplement for the dietary management of phenylketonuria. Suitable from 3 years; use with caution in child 3–6 years. Includes added vitamins A, B, C, D, E and K.
POWDER, protein 30 g, carbohydrate 37.5 g, fat 11.7 g, energy 1616 kJ (384 kcal)/100 g.

PKU GMPro oral powder 33.3g sachets (Nutricia Ltd)
16 sachet (ACBS) · NHS indicative price = £122.72

PKU GMPro ® **LQ**
▸ Nutritional supplement for the dietary management of phenylketonuria. Suitable from 3 years; use with caution in child 3–6 years. Includes added vitamins A, B C, D, E and K.
LIQUID, protein equivalent 4 g, carbohydrate 3.4 g, fat 1.6 g, energy 188 kJ (45 kcal)/100 mL

PKU GMPro LQ liquid (Nutricia Ltd)
250 ml (ACBS) · NHS indicative price = £7.68

PKU GMPro ® **Mix-In**
▸ Nutritional supplement for the dietary management of phenylketonuria. Not suitable for use in child under 3 years.
POWDER, protein 80 g, carbohydrate 3.4 g, fat nil, energy 1418 kJ (334 kcal)/100 g.

PKU GMPro Mix-In oral powder 12.5g sachets (Nutricia Ltd)
30 sachet (ACBS) · NHS indicative price = £188.40

10 g protein equivalent

Mevalia ® **PKU Motion 10**
▸ Nutritional supplement for the dietary management of phenylketonuria. Suitable from 3 years. Includes added vitamins A, B, C, D, E and K.
LIQUID, protein equivalent 14 g, carbohydrate 5 g, fat Nil, energy 328 kJ (77 kcal)/100 mL.

Mevalia PKU Motion 10 liquid red fruits (Vitaflo International Ltd)
70 ml (ACBS) · NHS indicative price = £5.48

Mevalia PKU Motion 10 liquid tropical (Vitaflo International Ltd)
70 ml (ACBS) · NHS indicative price = £5.48

Phlexy-10 ® **drink mix**
▸ Nutritional supplement for the dietary management of phenylketonuria. Suitable from 1 year.
POWDER, protein 41.7 g, carbohydrate 44 g, fat Nil, energy 1456 kJ (343 kcal)/100 g.

Phlexy-10 drink mix 20g sachets apple & blackcurrant (Nutricia Ltd)
30 sachet (ACBS) · NHS indicative price = £187.20

Phlexy-10 drink mix 20g sachets citrus burst (Nutricia Ltd)
30 sachet (ACBS) · NHS indicative price = £187.20

Phlexy-10 drink mix 20g sachets tropical surprise (Nutricia Ltd)
30 sachet (ACBS) · NHS indicative price = £187.20

PKU cooler ® **10**
▸ Nutritional supplement for the dietary management of phenylketonuria. Suitable from 3 years. Includes added vitamins A, B, C, D, E and K.
LIQUID, protein equivalent 11.5 g, carbohydrate 5.1 g, fat 0.9 g, energy 316 kJ (75 kcal)/100 mL.

PKU orange cooler10 liquid (Vitaflo International Ltd)
87 ml (ACBS) · NHS indicative price = £7.19

PKU purple cooler10 liquid (Vitaflo International Ltd)
87 ml (ACBS) · NHS indicative price = £7.19

PKU red cooler10 liquid (Vitaflo International Ltd)
87 ml (ACBS) · NHS indicative price = £7.19

PKU white cooler10 liquid (Vitaflo International Ltd)
87 ml (ACBS) · NHS indicative price = £7.19

PKU yellow cooler10 liquid (Vitaflo International Ltd)
87 ml (ACBS) · NHS indicative price = £7.19

PKU Lophlex ® **LQ 10**
▸ Nutritional supplement for the dietary management of proven phenylketonuria. Suitable from 4 years. Includes added vitamins A, B, C, D, E and K.
LIQUID, protein 16 g, carbohydrate 7 g, fat Nil, energy 391 kJ (92 kcal)/100 mL.

PKU Lophlex LQ 10 liquid berry (Nutricia Ltd)
62.5 ml (ACBS) · NHS indicative price = £7.36

PKU Lophlex LQ 10 liquid juicy berries (Nutricia Ltd)
62.5 ml (ACBS) · NHS indicative price = £7.36

PKU Lophlex LQ 10 liquid juicy citrus (Nutricia Ltd)
62.5 ml (ACBS) · NHS indicative price = £7.36

PKU Lophlex LQ 10 liquid juicy orange (Nutricia Ltd)
62.5 ml (ACBS) · NHS indicative price = £7.36

PKU Lophlex LQ 10 liquid juicy tropical (Nutricia Ltd)
62.5 ml (ACBS) · NHS indicative price = £7.36

XPhe ® jump 10
▸ Nutritional supplement for the dietary management of phenylketonuria (PKU) or hyperphenylalaninemia (HPA). Suitable from 3 years. Includes added vitamins A, B, C, D, E and K.
LIQUID, protein equivalent 16 g, carbohydrate 9 g, fat less than 0.1 g, energy 376 kJ (89 kcal)/100 mL.

XPhe jump 10 liquid cola (metaX Institut fuer Diaetetik GmbH)
63 ml (ACBS) · NHS indicative price = £4.79

XPhe jump 10 liquid neutral (metaX Institut fuer Diaetetik GmbH)
63 ml (ACBS) · NHS indicative price = £4.79

XPhe jump 10 liquid orange (metaX Institut fuer Diaetetik GmbH)
63 ml (ACBS) · NHS indicative price = £4.79

XPhe jump 10 liquid tropical (metaX Institut fuer Diaetetik GmbH)
63 ml (ACBS) · NHS indicative price = £4.79

XPhe jump 10 liquid vanilla (metaX Institut fuer Diaetetik GmbH)
63 ml (ACBS) · NHS indicative price = £4.79

XPhe jump 10 liquid wild berries (metaX Institut fuer Diaetetik GmbH)
63 ml (ACBS) · NHS indicative price = £4.79

15 g GMP protein equivalent

Glytactin ® Complete 15
▸ Nutritional supplement for the dietary management of phenylketonuria. Suitable from 3 years. Includes added vitamins A, B, C, D, E and K.
SOLID, protein equivalent 19 g, carbohydrate 43 g, fat 15 g, energy 1705 kJ (407 kcal)/100 g.

Glytactin Complete 15 81g bars fruit frenzy (Cambrooke UK Ltd)
7 bar (ACBS) · NHS indicative price = £80.13

Glytactin Complete 15 81g bars peanut butter (Cambrooke UK Ltd)
7 bar (ACBS) · NHS indicative price = £80.13

Glytactin ® RTD 15
▸ Nutritional supplement for the dietary management of phenylketonuria. Suitable for over 3 years. Includes added vitamins A, B, C, D, E and K.
LIQUID, protein equivalent 6 g, carbohydrate 9.2 g, fat 2 g, energy 335 kJ (80 kcal)/100 mL.

Glytactin RTD 15 liquid chocolate (Cambrooke UK Ltd)
250 ml (ACBS) · NHS indicative price = £11.45

Glytactin RTD 15 liquid original (Cambrooke UK Ltd)
250 ml (ACBS) · NHS indicative price = £11.45

Glytactin ® RTD Lite 15
▸ Nutritional supplement for the dietary management of phenylketonuria. Suitable for over 3 years. Includes added vitamins A, B, C, D, E and K.
LIQUID, protein 6 g, carbohydrate 3 g, fat 1.4 g, energy 201 kJ (48 kcal)/100 mL.

Glytactin RTD Lite 15 liquid coffee mocha (Cambrooke UK Ltd)
250 ml (ACBS) · NHS indicative price = £11.54

Glytactin RTD Lite 15 liquid vanilla (Cambrooke UK Ltd)
250 ml (ACBS) · NHS indicative price = £11.54

PKU sphere ® 15
▸ Nutritional supplement for the dietary management of phenylketonuria. Suitable from 4 years. Includes added vitamins A, B, C, D, E and K.
POWDER, protein 56 g, carbohydrate 18 g, fat 4.7 g, energy 1432 kJ (338 kcal)/100 g.

PKU sphere15 oral powder 27g sachets chocolate (Vitaflo International Ltd)
30 sachet (ACBS) · NHS indicative price = £351.44

PKU sphere15 oral powder 27g sachets red berry (Vitaflo International Ltd)
30 sachet (ACBS) · NHS indicative price = £351.44

PKU sphere15 oral powder 27g sachets vanilla (Vitaflo International Ltd)
30 sachet (ACBS) · NHS indicative price = £351.44

15 g protein equivalent

PKU Air ® 15
▸ Nutritional supplement for the dietary management of phenylketonuria. Suitable from 3 years. Includes added vitamins A, B, C, D, E and K.
LIQUID, protein equivalent 11.5 g, carbohydrate 1.5 g, fat 0.6 g, energy 243 kJ (57 kcal)/100 mL.

PKU Air15 gold liquid (Vitaflo International Ltd)
130 ml (ACBS) · NHS indicative price = £10.34

PKU Air15 green liquid (Vitaflo International Ltd)
130 ml (ACBS) · NHS indicative price = £10.34

PKU Air15 red liquid (Vitaflo International Ltd)
130 ml (ACBS) · NHS indicative price = £10.34

PKU Air15 white liquid (Vitaflo International Ltd)
130 ml (ACBS) · NHS indicative price = £10.34

PKU Air15 yellow liquid (Vitaflo International Ltd)
130 ml (ACBS) · NHS indicative price = £10.34

PKU cooler ® 15
▸ Nutritional supplement for the dietary management of phenylketonuria. Suitable from 3 years. Includes added vitamins A, B, C, D, E and K.
LIQUID, protein equivalent 11.5 g, carbohydrate 5.1 g, fat 0.9 g, energy 316 kJ (75 kcal)/100 mL.

PKU orange cooler15 liquid (Vitaflo International Ltd)
130 ml (ACBS) · NHS indicative price = £10.71

PKU purple cooler15 liquid (Vitaflo International Ltd)
130 ml (ACBS) · NHS indicative price = £10.71

PKU red cooler15 liquid (Vitaflo International Ltd)
130 ml (ACBS) · NHS indicative price = £10.71

PKU white cooler15 liquid (Vitaflo International Ltd)
130 ml (ACBS) · NHS indicative price = £10.71

PKU yellow cooler15 liquid (Vitaflo International Ltd)
130 ml (ACBS) · NHS indicative price = £10.71

PKU Easy ® Shake and Go
▸ Nutritional supplement for the dietary management of phenylketonuria. Suitable from 3 years. Includes added vitamins A, B, C, D, E and K.
POWDER, protein 45 g, carbohydrate 42 g, fat 0.4 g, energy 1559 kJ (367 kcal)/100 g.

PKU Easy Shake & Go oral powder 34g sachets (Galen Ltd)
30 sachet (ACBS) · NHS indicative price = £213.90

PKU express ® plus15
▸ Nutritional supplement for the dietary management of phenylketonuria. Suitable from 3 years. Includes added vitamins A, B, C, D, E and K.
POWDER, protein equivalent 60 g, carbohydrate 14 g, fat 2.2 g, energy 1339 kJ (316 kcal)/100 g.

PKU express plus15 powder 25g sachets lemon (Vitaflo International Ltd)
30 sachet (ACBS) · NHS indicative price = £309.74

PKU express plus15 powder 25g sachets orange (Vitaflo International Ltd)
30 sachet (ACBS) · NHS indicative price = £309.74

PKU express plus15 powder 25g sachets tropical (Vitaflo International Ltd)
30 sachet (ACBS) · NHS indicative price = £309.74

PKU express plus15 powder 25g sachets unflavoured (Vitaflo International Ltd)
30 sachet (ACBS) · NHS indicative price = £309.74

20 g GMP protein equivalent

PKU GMPro ® Ultra
▸ Nutritional supplement for the dietary management of phenylketonuria. Suitable from 3 years; use with caution in child 3–6 years. Includes added vitamins A, B, C, D, E and K.
POWDER, protein 60 g, carbohydrate 14.7 g, fat 2.2 g, energy 1356 kJ (320 kcal)/100 g.

PKU GMPro Ultra oral powder 33.4g sachets lemonade (Nutricia Ltd)
30 sachet (ACBS) · NHS indicative price = £377.10

PKU GMPro Ultra oral powder 33.4g sachets vanilla (Nutricia Ltd)
30 sachet (ACBS) · NHS indicative price = £377.10

PKU sphere ® 20
▸ Nutritional supplement for the dietary management of phenylketonuria. Suitable from 4 years. Includes added vitamins A, B, C, D, E and K.
POWDER, protein 56 g, carbohydrate 18 g, fat 4.7 g, energy 1432 kJ (338 kcal)/100 g.

PKU sphere20 oral powder 35g sachets banana (Vitaflo International Ltd)
30 sachet (ACBS) · NHS indicative price = £490.98

PKU sphere20 oral powder 35g sachets chocolate (Vitaflo International Ltd)
30 sachet (ACBS) · NHS indicative price = £490.98

PKU sphere20 oral powder 35g sachets lemon (Vitaflo International Ltd)
30 sachet (ACBS) · NHS indicative price = £490.98

PKU sphere20 oral powder 35g sachets red berry (Vitaflo International Ltd)
30 sachet (ACBS) · NHS indicative price = £490.98

PKU sphere20 oral powder 35g sachets vanilla (Vitaflo International Ltd)
30 sachet (ACBS) · NHS indicative price = £490.98

PKU sphere ® 20 liquid
▸ Nutritional supplement for the dietary management of phenylketonuria. Suitable from 3 years. Includes added vitamins A, B, C, D, E and K.
LIQUID, protein 8.3 g, carbohydrate 2.8 g, fat 0.5 g, energy 207 kJ (50 kcal)/100 mL.

PKU sphere20 liquid chocolate (Vitaflo International Ltd)
237 ml (ACBS) · NHS indicative price = £15.66

PKU sphere20 liquid vanilla (Vitaflo International Ltd)
237 ml (ACBS) · NHS indicative price = £15.66

20 g protein equivalent

Easiphen ®
▸ Nutritional supplement for the dietary management of phenylketonuria. Suitable from 8 years. Includes added vitamins A, B, C, D, E and K.
LIQUID, protein equivalent 6.7 g, carbohydrate 5.1 g, fat 2 g, energy 275 kJ (65 kcal)/100 mL

Easiphen liquid (Nutricia Ltd)
250 ml (ACBS) · NHS indicative price = £14.09

Glytactin ® Build 20/20
▸ Nutritional supplement for the dietary management of phenylketonuria. Suitable from 3 years. Includes added vitamins A, B, C, D, E and K.
POWDER, protein equivalent 67 g, carbohydrate 2.4 g, fat 4.2 g, energy 1400 kJ (335 kcal)/100 g.

Glytactin Build 20/20 oral powder 32g sachets chocolate (Cambrooke UK Ltd)
30 sachet (ACBS) · NHS indicative price = £451.00

Glytactin Build 20/20 oral powder 30g sachets neutral (Cambrooke UK Ltd)
30 sachet (ACBS) · NHS indicative price = £457.92

Glytactin Build 20/20 oral powder 31g sachets raspberry lemonade (Cambrooke UK Ltd)
30 sachet (ACBS) · NHS indicative price = £451.00

Glytactin Build 20/20 oral powder 31.2g sachets smooth (Cambrooke UK Ltd)
30 sachet (ACBS) · NHS indicative price = £451.00

Glytactin Build 20/20 oral powder 33g sachets vanilla (Cambrooke UK Ltd)
30 sachet (ACBS) · NHS indicative price = £451.00

Mevalia ® PKU Motion 20
▸ Nutritional supplement for the dietary management of phenylketonuria. Suitable from 3 years. Includes added vitamins A, B, C, D, E and K.
LIQUID, protein equivalent 14 g, carbohydrate 5 g, fat Nil, energy 328 kJ (77 kcal)/100 mL.

Mevalia PKU Motion 20 liquid red fruits (Vitaflo International Ltd)
140 ml (ACBS) · NHS indicative price = £10.96

Mevalia PKU Motion 20 liquid tropical (Vitaflo International Ltd)
140 ml (ACBS) · NHS indicative price = £10.96

PKU Air ® 20
▸ Nutritional supplement for the dietary management of phenylketonuria. Suitable from 3 years. Includes added vitamins A, B, C, D, E and K.
LIQUID, protein equivalent 11.5 g, carbohydrate 1.5 g, fat 0.6 g, energy 243 kJ (57 kcal)/100 mL.

PKU Air20 gold liquid (Vitaflo International Ltd)
174 ml (ACBS) · NHS indicative price = £13.87

PKU Air20 green liquid (Vitaflo International Ltd)
174 ml (ACBS) · NHS indicative price = £13.87

PKU Air20 red liquid (Vitaflo International Ltd)
174 ml (ACBS) · NHS indicative price = £13.87

PKU Air20 white liquid (Vitaflo International Ltd)
174 ml (ACBS) · NHS indicative price = £13.87

PKU Air20 yellow liquid (Vitaflo International Ltd)
174 ml (ACBS) · NHS indicative price = £13.87

PKU cooler ® 20
▸ Nutritional supplement for the dietary management of phenylketonuria. Suitable from 3 years. Includes added vitamins A, B, C, D, E and K.
LIQUID, protein equivalent 11.5 g, carbohydrate 5.1 g, fat 0.9 g, energy 316 kJ (75 kcal)/100 mL.

PKU orange cooler20 liquid (Vitaflo International Ltd)
174 ml (ACBS) · NHS indicative price = £14.40

PKU purple cooler20 liquid (Vitaflo International Ltd)
174 ml (ACBS) · NHS indicative price = £14.40

PKU red cooler20 liquid (Vitaflo International Ltd)
174 ml (ACBS) · NHS indicative price = £14.40

PKU white cooler20 liquid (Vitaflo International Ltd)
174 ml (ACBS) · NHS indicative price = £14.40

PKU yellow cooler20 liquid (Vitaflo International Ltd)
174 ml (ACBS) · NHS indicative price = £14.40

PKU express ® plus20
▸ Nutritional supplement for the dietary management of phenylketonuria. Suitable from 3 years. Includes added vitamins A, B, C, D, E and K.
POWDER, protein equivalent 60 g, carbohydrate 14 g, fat 2.2 g, energy 1339 kJ (316 kcal)/100 g.

PKU express plus20 powder 34g sachets lemon (Vitaflo International Ltd)
30 sachet (ACBS) · NHS indicative price = £412.99

PKU express plus20 powder 34g sachets orange (Vitaflo International Ltd)
30 sachet (ACBS) · NHS indicative price = £412.99

PKU express plus20 powder 34g sachets tropical (Vitaflo International Ltd)
30 sachet (ACBS) · NHS indicative price = £412.99

PKU express plus20 powder 34g sachets unflavoured (Vitaflo International Ltd)
30 sachet (ACBS) · NHS indicative price = £412.99

PKU Lophlex ®
▸ Nutritional supplement for the dietary management of proven phenylketonuria. Not suitable for use in child under 3 years. Includes added vitamins A, B, C, D, E and K.
POWDER, protein 71.4 g, carbohydrate 13.6 g, fat 1.5 g, energy 1487 kJ (350 kcal)/100 g.

PKU Lophlex powder 28g sachets berries (Nutricia Ltd)
30 sachet (ACBS) · NHS indicative price = £412.50

PKU Lophlex powder 28g sachets neutral (Nutricia Ltd)
30 sachet (ACBS) · NHS indicative price = £412.50

PKU Lophlex powder 28g sachets orange (Nutricia Ltd)
30 sachet (ACBS) · NHS indicative price = £412.50

PKU Lophlex ® LQ 20
▸ Nutritional supplement for the dietary management of proven phenylketonuria. Suitable from 4 years. Includes added vitamins A, B, C, D, E and K.

LIQUID, protein 16 g, carbohydrate 7 g, fat Nil, energy 391 kJ (92 kcal)/100 mL.

PKU Lophlex LQ 20 liquid berry (Nutricia Ltd)
125 ml (ACBS) · NHS indicative price = £14.71

PKU Lophlex LQ 20 liquid juicy berries (Nutricia Ltd)
125 ml (ACBS) · NHS indicative price = £14.71

PKU Lophlex LQ 20 liquid juicy citrus (Nutricia Ltd)
125 ml (ACBS) · NHS indicative price = £14.71

PKU Lophlex LQ 20 liquid juicy orange (Nutricia Ltd)
125 ml (ACBS) · NHS indicative price = £14.71

PKU Lophlex LQ 20 liquid juicy tropical (Nutricia Ltd)
125 ml (ACBS) · NHS indicative price = £14.71

PKU Lophlex LQ 20 liquid orange (Nutricia Ltd)
125 ml (ACBS) · NHS indicative price = £14.71

PKU Lophlex ® Select 20
▸ Nutritional supplement for the dietary management of phenylketonuria. Suitable from 4 years. Includes added vitamins A, B, C, D, E and K.
LIQUID, protein 16 g, carbohydrate 4.1 g, fat 0.3 g, energy 342 kJ (81.7 kcal)/100 mL.

PKU Lophlex Select 20 liquid (Nutricia Ltd)
125 ml (ACBS) · NHS indicative price = £13.03

PKU Lophlex ® Sensation 20
▸ Nutritional supplement for the dietary management of phenylketonuria. Suitable from 4 years. Includes added vitamins A, B, C, D, E and K.
SEMI-SOLID, protein 18.3 g, carbohydrate 18.5 g, fat 0.34 g, energy 648 kJ (152 kcal)/100 g.

PKU Lophlex Sensation 20 berries (Nutricia Ltd)
327 gram (ACBS) · NHS indicative price = £47.02

PKU Maxamum ® sachets
▸ Nutritional supplement for the dietary management of phenylketonuria. Suitable from 8 years. Includes added vitamins A, B, C, D, E and K.
POWDER, protein 39 g, carbohydrate 34 g, fat less than 0.5 g, energy 1260 kJ (297 kcal)/100 g.

PKU Maxamum oral powder 50g sachets orange (Nutricia Ltd)
30 sachet (ACBS) · NHS indicative price = £393.60

PKU Maxamum oral powder 50g sachets unflavoured (Nutricia Ltd)
30 sachet (ACBS) · NHS indicative price = £393.60

PKU Synergy ®
▸ Nutritional supplement for the dietary management of phenylketonuria and hyperphenylalaninaemia. Suitable from 10 years. Includes added vitamins A, B, C, D, E and K.
POWDER, protein equivalent 60.6 g, carbohydrate 10.7 g, fat 1 g, energy 1238 kJ (296 kcal)/100 g.

PKU Synergy oral powder 33g sachets (Nutricia Ltd)
30 sachet (ACBS) · NHS indicative price = £453.00

XPhe ® jump 20
▸ Nutritional supplement for the dietary management of phenylketonuria (PKU) or hyperphenylalaninemia (HPA). Suitable from 3 years. Includes added vitamins A, B, C, D, E and K.
LIQUID, protein equivalent 16 g, carbohydrate 9 g, fat less than 0.1 g, energy 376 kJ (89 kcal)/100 mL.

XPhe jump 20 liquid cola (metaX Institut fuer Diaetetik GmbH)
125 ml (ACBS) · NHS indicative price = £9.55

XPhe jump 20 liquid neutral (metaX Institut fuer Diaetetik GmbH)
125 ml (ACBS) · NHS indicative price = £9.55

XPhe jump 20 liquid orange (metaX Institut fuer Diaetetik GmbH)
125 ml (ACBS) · NHS indicative price = £9.55

XPhe jump 20 liquid tropical (metaX Institut fuer Diaetetik GmbH)
125 ml (ACBS) · NHS indicative price = £9.55

XPhe jump 20 liquid vanilla (metaX Institut fuer Diaetetik GmbH)
125 ml (ACBS) · NHS indicative price = £9.55

XPhe jump 20 liquid wild berries (metaX Institut fuer Diaetetik GmbH)
125 ml (ACBS) · NHS indicative price = £9.55

Powder protein source

PK Aid 4 ®
▸ Nutritional supplement for the dietary management of phenylketonuria.
POWDER, protein 79 g, carbohydrate 4.5 g, fat Nil, energy 1420 kJ (334 kcal)/100 g.

PK Aid 4 powder (Nutricia Ltd)
500 gram (ACBS) · NHS indicative price = £209.11

PKU Maxamum ®
▸ Nutritional supplement for the dietary management of phenylketonuria. Suitable from 8 years. Includes added vitamins A, B, C, D, E and K.
POWDER, protein 39 g, carbohydrate 34 g, fat less than 0.5 g, energy 1260 kJ (297 kcal)/100 g.

PKU Maxamum powder orange (Nutricia Ltd)
500 gram (ACBS) · NHS indicative price = £131.39

PKU Maxamum powder unflavoured (Nutricia Ltd)
500 gram (ACBS) · NHS indicative price = £131.39

Tablet protein source

Phlexy-10 ® tablets
▸ Nutritional supplement for the dietary management of phenylketonuria. Suitable from 8 years.
SOLID, protein 56.4 g, carbohydrate 4.4 g, fat 2.6 g, energy 1310 kJ (307 kcal)/100 g.

Phlexy-10 tablets (Nutricia Ltd)
75 tablet (ACBS) · NHS indicative price = £40.74

PKU Easy ® microtabs
▸ Nutritional supplement for the dietary management of phenylketonuria. Suitable from 8 years.
SOLID, protein equivalent (essential and non-essential amino acids) 70.8 g, carbohydrate 13 g, fat 3.6 g, energy 1678 kJ (396 kcal)/100 g.

PKU Easy microtabs (Galen Ltd)
440 gram (ACBS) · NHS indicative price = £227.83

XPhe ® minis
▸ Nutritional supplement for the dietary management of phenylketonuria and hyperphenylalaninemia. Suitable from 7 years. Includes added vitamins A, B, C, D, E and K.
SOLID, protein 62 g, carbohydrate nil, fat 2 g, energy 1175 kJ (278 kcal)/100 g.

XPhe minis tablets (metaX Institut fuer Diaetetik GmbH)
720 tablet (ACBS) · NHS indicative price = £165.00

Pyridoxine-dependent epilepsy
5 g protein equivalent

PDE reach ® 5
▸ Nutritional supplement for the dietary management of pyridoxine-dependent epilepsy. Suitable from 1 year. Includes added vitamins A, B, C, D, E and K.
POWDER, protein equivalent 28 g, carbohydrate 58 g, fat 0.4 g, energy 1477 kJ (348 kcal)/100 g.

PDE reach5 oral powder 18g sachets (Vitaflo International Ltd)
30 sachet (ACBS) · NHS indicative price = £170.42

Sucrase-isomaltase deficiency
Carbohydrate supplements

Glucose powder
▸ For use as an energy supplement in sucrose-isomaltase deficiency.
POWDER, contains dextrose monohydrate.

Glucose powder for oral use BP 1980 (Thornton & Ross Ltd)
500 gram (ACBS) · NHS indicative price = £2.41 · Drug Tariff (Part VIIIA Category C) price = £2.41

Tyrosinaemia

10 g protein equivalent

TYR cooler ® 10
▸ Nutritional supplement for the dietary management of tyrosinaemia. Suitable from 3 years. Includes added vitamins A, B, C, D, E and K.
LIQUID, protein equivalent 11.5 g, carbohydrate 5.1 g, fat 0.9 g, energy 316 kJ (75 kcal)/100 mL.

TYR red cooler10 liquid (Vitaflo International Ltd)
87 ml (ACBS) · NHS indicative price = £10.81

TYR Lophlex ® LQ 10
▸ Nutritional supplement for the dietary management of proven tyrosinaemia. Includes added vitamins A, B, C, D, E and K.
LIQUID, protein 16 g, carbohydrate 7 g, fat 0.35 g, energy 407 kJ (96 kcal)/100 mL.

TYR Lophlex LQ 10 liquid (Nutricia Ltd)
62.5 ml (ACBS) · NHS indicative price = £11.72

15 g protein equivalent

TYR cooler ® 15
▸ Nutritional supplement for the dietary management of tyrosinaemia. Suitable from 3 years. Includes added vitamins A, B, C, D, E and K.
LIQUID, protein equivalent 11.5 g, carbohydrate 5.1 g, fat 0.9 g, energy 316 kJ (75 kcal)/100 mL.

TYR orange cooler15 liquid (Vitaflo International Ltd)
130 ml (ACBS) · NHS indicative price = £17.68

TYR red cooler15 liquid (Vitaflo International Ltd)
130 ml (ACBS) · NHS indicative price = £17.68

TYR Easy ® Shake and Go
▸ Nutritional supplement for the dietary management of tyrosinaemia. Suitable from 3 years. Includes added vitamins A, B, C, D, E and K.
POWDER, protein equivalent 45 g, carbohydrate 38 g, fat less than 0.5 g, energy 1542 kJ (363 kcal)/100 g.

TYR Easy Shake & Go oral powder 34g sachets (Galen Ltd)
30 sachet (ACBS) · NHS indicative price = £362.00

TYR express ® 15
▸ Nutritional supplement for the dietary management of tyrosinaemia. Suitable from 8 years. Includes added vitamins A, B, C, D, E and K.
POWDER, protein equivalent 60 g, carbohydrate 13.7 g, fat 0.2 g, energy 1260 kJ (297 kcal)/100 g.

TYR express15 oral powder 25g sachets (Vitaflo International Ltd)
30 sachet (ACBS) · NHS indicative price = £520.85

20 g GMP protein equivalent

TYR sphere ® 20
▸ Nutritional supplement for the dietary management of tyrosinaemia. Suitable from 3 years. Includes added vitamins A, B, C, D, E and K.
POWDER, protein 56 g, carbohydrate 17 g, fat 4.7 g, energy 1415 kJ (335 kcal)/100 g.

TYR sphere20 oral powder 35g sachets red berry (Vitaflo International Ltd)
30 sachet (ACBS) · NHS indicative price = £718.66

TYR sphere20 oral powder 35g sachets vanilla (Vitaflo International Ltd)
30 sachet (ACBS) · NHS indicative price = £718.66

20 g protein equivalent

TYR cooler ® 20
▸ Nutritional supplement in the dietary management of tyrosinaemia. Suitable from 3 years. Includes added vitamins A, B, C, D, E and K.
LIQUID, protein equivalent 11.5 g, carbohydrate 5.1 g, fat 0.9 g, energy 316 kJ (75 kcal)/100 mL.

TYR red cooler20 liquid (Vitaflo International Ltd)
174 ml (ACBS) · NHS indicative price = £22.61

TYR express ® 20
▸ Nutritional supplement for the dietary management of tyrosinaemia. Suitable from 8 years. Includes added vitamins A, B, C, D, E and K.
POWDER, protein equivalent 60 g, carbohydrate 13.7 g, fat 0.2 g, energy 1260 kJ (297 kcal)/100 g.

TYR express20 oral powder 34g sachets (Vitaflo International Ltd)
30 sachet (ACBS) · NHS indicative price = £672.92

TYR Lophlex ®
▸ Nutritional supplement for the dietary management of tyrosinaemia. Suitable from 3 years. Includes added vitamins A, B, C, D, E and K.
POWDER, protein 71.4 g, carbohydrate 13.7 g, fat 1.5 g, energy 1488 kJ (350 kcal)/100 g.

TYR Lophlex powder 28g sachets (Nutricia Ltd)
30 sachet (ACBS) · NHS indicative price = £651.00

TYR Lophlex ® LQ 20
▸ Nutritional supplement for the dietary management of proven tyrosinaemia. Includes added vitamins A, B, C, D, E and K.
LIQUID, protein 16 g, carbohydrate 7 g, fat 0.35 g, energy 407 kJ (96 kcal)/100 mL.

TYR Lophlex LQ 20 liquid (Nutricia Ltd)
125 ml (ACBS) · NHS indicative price = £24.18

Powder protein source

XPHEN TYR Tyrosidon ®
▸ Nutritional supplement for the dietary management of tyrosinaemia where plasma methionine levels are normal.
POWDER, protein 77 g, carbohydrate 4.5 g, fat Nil, energy 1386 kJ (326 kcal)/100 g.

XPHEN TYR Tyrosidon Free AA Mix powder (Nutricia Ltd)
500 gram (ACBS) · NHS indicative price = £280.81

Tablet protein source

TYR Easy ®
▸ Nutritional supplement for the dietary management of tyrosinaemia. Suitable from 8 years.
SOLID, protein equivalent 73.0 g, carbohydrate 8.7 g, fat 3.2 g, energy 1703 kJ (402 kcal)/100 g.

TYR Easy tablets (Galen Ltd)
462 tablet (ACBS) · NHS indicative price = £372.65

Urea cycle disorders

5 g protein equivalent

EAA ® Supplement
▸ Nutritional supplement for the dietary management of disorders of protein metabolism including urea cycle disorders. Suitable from 3 years. Includes added vitamins A, B, C, D, E and K.
POWDER, protein equivalent 40 g, carbohydrate 26 g, fat 0.1 g, energy 1126 kJ (265 kcal)/100 g.

EAA Supplement oral powder 12.5g sachets (Vitaflo International Ltd)
30 sachet (ACBS) · NHS indicative price = £192.81

UCD amino5 ®
▸ Nutritional supplement for the dietary management of urea cycle disorders (UCD).
POWDER, protein equivalent 75.4 g, carbohydrate Nil, fat Nil, energy 1282 kJ (302 kcal)/100 g.

UCD amino5 oral powder 6.6g sachets (Vitaflo International Ltd)
30 sachet (ACBS) · NHS indicative price = £159.25

Powder protein source

Dialamine ®
▸ Nutritional supplement for oral feeding where essential amino acid supplements are required, for example chronic renal failure, hypoproteinaemia, wound fistula leakage with excessive protein loss, conditions requiring a controlled nitrogen intake and haemodialysis. Suitable from 6 months. Includes added vitamin C.

POWDER, protein 25 g, carbohydrate 65 g, fat Nil, energy 1530 kJ (360 kcal)/100 g.

Dialamine powder (Nutricia Ltd)
400 gram (ACBS) · NHS indicative price = £110.85

Thickeners and pre-thickened drinks
Thickeners: gum based powder

Instant Carobel ®
▸ For thickening of liquids or foods in the treatment of vomiting.
POWDER, contains maltodextrin, carob bean gum, calcium carbonate, iron sulfate, zinc sulfate. Contains residual lactose.

Instant Carobel powder (Nutricia Ltd)
135 gram (ACBS) · NHS indicative price = £3.98

Nutilis ® **Clear**
▸ For thickening of liquids or foods in dysphagia. Not suitable for use in child under 3 years.
POWDER, contains guar gum, maltodextrin, xanthan gum. Gluten-free, lactose-free.

Nutilis Clear powder (Nutricia Ltd)
175 gram (ACBS) · NHS indicative price = £10.54

Nutilis Clear powder 1.25g sachets (Nutricia Ltd)
50 sachet (ACBS) · NHS indicative price = £14.50

Osmosip ® **Clear and Thick Instant Thickener**
▸ For thickening of liquids or foods in dysphagia. Not suitable for use in child under 3 years.
POWDER, contains maltodextrin (corn, potato), potassium chloride, xanthan gum. Gluten-free.

Osmosip Clear & Thick Instant Thickener powder (Spectral Pharmaceuticals Ltd)
133 gram (ACBS) · NHS indicative price = £3.95

Resource ® **ThickenUp** ® **Clear**
▸ For thickening of liquids or foods in dysphagia. Not suitable for use in child under 3 years.
POWDER, contains maltodextrin (corn, potato), potassium chloride, residual lactose (tin only), xanthan gum. Gluten-free.

Resource ThickenUp Clear powder (Nestle Health Science)
215 gram (ACBS) · NHS indicative price = £15.27

Resource ThickenUp Clear powder 1.2g sachets (Nestle Health Science)
24 sachet (ACBS) · NHS indicative price = £5.28

Swalloweze ® **Clear Instant Food & Fluid Thickener**
▸ For thickening of liquids or foods in dysphagia. Not suitable for use in child under 3 years.
POWDER, contains erythritol (E968), maltodextrin, xanthan gum (E415). Gluten-free, lactose-free.

Swalloweze Clear Instant Food & Fluid Thickener powder (Nualtra Ltd)
165 gram (ACBS) · NHS indicative price = £5.50

Swalloweze Clear Instant Food & Fluid Thickener powder 1.6g sachets (Nualtra Ltd)
48 sachet (ACBS) · NHS indicative price = £9.60

Thick and Easy ® **Clear**
▸ For thickening of liquids or foods in dysphagia, and for the dietary management of conditions such as stroke, Parkinson's disease, muscular dystrophy, motor neurone disease, multiple sclerosis, malignancies of the oral cavity and throat, neurological disorders caused by injury or disease. Not suitable for use in child under 3 years.
POWDER, contains maltodextrin,xanthan gum, carrageenan, erythritol. Gluten-free, lactose-free.

Thick & Easy Clear powder (Fresenius Kabi Ltd)
126 gram (ACBS) · NHS indicative price = £6.69

Thick & Easy Clear powder 1.4g sachets (Fresenius Kabi Ltd)
100 sachet (ACBS) · NHS indicative price = £25.21

Thickeners: starch based powder

Thick and Easy ® **Original**
▸ For thickening of liquids or foods in dysphagia. Not suitable for use in child under 3 years.
POWDER, contains maltodextrin, modified maize starch (E1442). Gluten-free, lactose-free.

Thick & Easy Original powder (Fresenius Kabi Ltd)
225 gram (ACBS) · NHS indicative price = £6.27 | 4540 gram (ACBS) · NHS indicative price = £131.73

Thixo-D ® **Original**
▸ For thickening of liquids or foods in dysphagia. Not recommended for child under 1 year.
POWDER, contains modified maize starch. Gluten-free, lactose-free.

Thixo-D Original powder (Ecogreen Technologies Ltd)
375 gram (ACBS) · NHS indicative price = £9.05

Vitamin and mineral supplements
Cystic fibrosis

DEKAs ® **Essential capsules**
▸ Vitamin supplement in cystic fibrosis on the specific recommendation of a cystic fibrosis specialist. Suitable from 4 years.
CAPSULES, containing vitamins A, D, E and K.

DEKAs Essential capsules (Alveolus Biomedical B.V.)
60 capsule (ACBS) · NHS indicative price = £40.70

DEKAs ® **Plus chewable tablets**
▸ Vitamin and mineral supplement in cystic fibrosis on the specific recommendation of a cystic fibrosis specialist. Suitable from 4 years.
CHEWABLE TABLETS, containing vitamins A, B, C, D, E and K, minerals, and trace elements.

DEKAs Plus chewable tablets (Alveolus Biomedical B.V.)
60 tablet (ACBS) · NHS indicative price = £47.45

DEKAs ® **Plus softgels capsules**
▸ Vitamin and mineral supplement in cystic fibrosis on the specific recommendation of a cystic fibrosis specialist. Suitable from 10 years.
CAPSULES, containing vitamins A, B, C, D, E and K, minerals, and trace elements.

DEKAs Plus softgels capsules (Alveolus Biomedical B.V.)
60 capsule (ACBS) · NHS indicative price = £47.45

Paravit ®**-CF capsules**
▸ Vitamin supplement in cystic fibrosis on the specific recommendation of a cystic fibrosis specialist. Suitable from 3 years.
CAPSULES, containing vitamins A, D, E and K.

Paravit-CF capsules (Nordic Pharma Ltd)
60 capsule (ACBS) · NHS indicative price = £42.93

Paravit ®**-CF liquid**
▸ Vitamin supplement in cystic fibrosis on the specific recommendation of a cystic fibrosis specialist.
LIQUID, containing vitamins A, D, E and K.

Paravit-CF liquid (Nordic Pharma Ltd)
7 ml (ACBS) · NHS indicative price = £34.01

Paravit ®**-Mod capsules**
▸ Vitamin supplement in cystic fibrosis on the specific recommendation of a cystic fibrosis specialist. Suitable from 3 years.
CAPSULES, containing vitamins A, D, E and K.

Paravit-Mod capsules (Nordic Pharma Ltd)
60 capsule (ACBS) · NHS indicative price = £41.80

Paravit ®**-Mod liquid**
▸ Vitamin supplement in cystic fibrosis on the specific recommendation of a cystic fibrosis specialist.
LIQUID, containing vitamins A, D, E and K.

Paravit-Mod liquid (Nordic Pharma Ltd)
7 ml (ACBS) · NHS indicative price = £33.12

Renal failure

Renavit ®

▸ Dietary management of water-soluble vitamin deficiency in renal failure patients on dialysis. Not suitable for use in children.
TABLETS, containing vitamins B and C.

Renavit tablets (Stanningley Pharma Ltd)
100 tablet (ACBS) · NHS indicative price = £16.78

Restrictive therapeutic diet

Phlexy-Vits ® powder

▸ Vitamin and mineral supplement in phenylketonuria and similar amino acid abnormalities. Suitable from 11 years.
POWDER, containing vitamins A, B, C, D, E and K, minerals, and trace elements.
Powder also provides protein 0.3 g, carbohydrate 0.5 g, fat Nil, energy 63 kJ (15 kcal)/100 g. Powder 7 g sachet provides protein 0.02 g, carbohydrate 0.04 g, fat Nil, energy 4 kJ (1 kcal)

Phlexy-Vits powder 7g sachets (Nutricia Ltd)
30 sachet (ACBS) · NHS indicative price = £103.50

Phlexy-Vits ® tablets

▸ Vitamin and mineral supplement in phenylketonuria and similar amino acid abnormalities. Suitable from 11 years.
TABLETS, containing vitamins A, B, C, D, E and K, minerals, and trace elements.

Phlexy-Vits tablets (Nutricia Ltd)
180 tablet (ACBS) · NHS indicative price = £119.35

Appendix 3
Cautionary and advisory labels for dispensed medicines

Guidance for cautionary and advisory labels

Medicinal forms within BNF publications include code numbers of the cautionary labels that pharmacists are recommended to add when dispensing. It is also expected that pharmacists will counsel patients and carers when necessary.

Counselling needs to be related to the age, experience, background, and understanding of the individual patient or carer. The pharmacist should ensure understanding of how to take or use the medicine and how to follow the correct dosage schedule. Any effects of the medicine on co-ordination, performance of skilled tasks (e.g. driving or work), any foods or medicines to be avoided, and what to do if a dose is missed should also be explained. Other matters, such as the possibility of staining of the clothes or skin, or discolouration of urine or stools by a medicine should also be mentioned.

For some medicines there is a special need for counselling, such as an unusual method or time of administration or a potential interaction with a common food or domestic remedy, and this should be mentioned where necessary.

Original packs

Most preparations are dispensed in unbroken original packs that include further advice for the patient in the form of patient information leaflets. Label 10 may be of value where appropriate. More general leaflets advising on the administration of preparations such as eye drops, eye ointments, inhalers, and suppositories are also available.

Scope of labels

In general no label recommendations have been made for injections on the assumption that they will be administered by a healthcare professional or a well-instructed patient. The labelling is not exhaustive and pharmacists are recommended to use their professional discretion in labelling new preparations and those for which no labels are shown.

Individual labelling advice is not given on the administration of the large variety of antacids. In the absence of instructions from the prescriber, and if on enquiry the patient has had no verbal instructions, the directions given under 'Dose' should be used on the label.

It is recognised that there may be occasions when pharmacists will use their knowledge and professional discretion and decide to omit one or more of the recommended labels for a particular patient. In this case counselling is of the utmost importance. There may also be an occasion when a prescriber does not wish additional cautionary labels to be used, in which case the prescription should be endorsed 'NCL' (no cautionary labels). The exact wording that is required instead should then be specified on the prescription.

Pharmacists label medicines with various wordings in addition to those directions specified on the prescription. Such labels include 'Shake the bottle', 'For external use only', and 'Store in a cool place', as well as 'Discard.... days after opening' and 'Do not use after....', which apply particularly to antibiotic mixtures, diluted liquid and topical preparations, and to eye-drops. Although not listed in the BNF these labels should continue to be used when appropriate; indeed, 'For external use only' is a legal requirement on external liquid preparations, while 'Keep out of the reach of children' is a legal requirement on all dispensed medicines. Care should be taken not to obscure other relevant information with adhesive labelling.

It is the usual practice for patients to take standard tablets with water or other liquid and for this reason no separate label has been recommended.

The label wordings recommended by the BNF apply to medicines dispensed against a prescription. Patients should be aware that a dispensed medicine should never be taken by, or shared with, anyone other than for whom the prescriber intended it. Therefore, the BNF does not include warnings against the use of a dispensed medicine by persons other than for whom it was specifically prescribed.

The label or labels for each preparation are recommended after careful consideration of the information available. However, it is recognised that in some cases this information may be either incomplete or open to a different interpretation. The BNF will therefore be grateful to receive any constructive comments on the labelling suggested for any preparation.

Recommended label wordings

For BNF 61 (March 2011), a revised set of cautionary and advisory labels were introduced. All of the existing labels were user-tested, and the revised wording selected reflects terminology that is better understood by patients.

Wordings which can be given as separate warnings are labels 1–19, 29–30, and 32. Wordings which can be incorporated in an appropriate position in the directions for dosage or administration are labels 21–28. A label has been omitted for number 20; labels 31 and 33 no longer apply to any medicines in the BNF and have therefore been deleted.

If separate labels are used it is recommended that the wordings be used without modification.

Welsh labels

Comprehensive Welsh translations are available for each cautionary and advisory label.

Labels

1 **Warning: This medicine may make you sleepy**

   Rhybudd: Gall y feddyginiaeth hon eich gwneud yn gysglyd
   To be used on *preparations for children* containing antihistamines, or other preparations given to children where the warnings of label 2 on driving or alcohol would not be appropriate.

2 **Warning: This medicine may make you sleepy. If this happens, do not drive or use tools or machines. Do not drink alcohol**

   Rhybudd: Gall y feddyginiaeth hon eich gwneud yn gysglyd. Peidiwch â gyrru, defnyddio offer llaw neu beiriannau os yw hyn yn digwydd. Peidiwch ag yfed alcohol
   To be used on *preparations for adults that can cause drowsiness*, thereby affecting coordination and the ability to drive and operate hazardous machinery; label 1 is more appropriate for children. *It is an offence to drive while under the influence of drink or drugs.*

   Some of these preparations only cause drowsiness in the first few days of treatment and some only cause drowsiness in higher doses.

   In such cases the patient should be told that the advice applies until the effects have worn off. However many of these preparations can produce a slowing of reaction time and a loss of mental concentration that can have the same effects as drowsiness.

   Avoidance of alcoholic drink is recommended because the effects of CNS depressants are enhanced by alcohol. Strict prohibition however could lead to some patients not taking the medicine. Pharmacists should therefore explain the risk and encourage compliance, particularly in patients who may think they already tolerate the effects of alcohol (see also label 3). Queries from patients with epilepsy regarding fitness to drive should be referred back to the patient's doctor.

Side-effects unrelated to drowsiness that may affect a patient's ability to drive or operate machinery safely include *blurred vision, dizziness, or nausea.* In general, no label has been recommended to cover these cases, but the patient should be suitably counselled.

3   **Warning: This medicine may make you sleepy. If this happens, do not drive or use tools or machines**

Rhybudd: Gall y feddyginiaeth hon eich gwneud yn gysglyd. Peidiwch â gyrru, defnyddio offer llaw neu beiriannau os yw hyn yn digwydd

To be used on *preparations containing monoamine-oxidase inhibitors*; the warning to avoid alcohol and dealcoholised (low alcohol) drink is covered by the patient information leaflet.

Also to be used as for label 2 but where alcohol is not an issue.

4   **Warning: Do not drink alcohol**

Rhybudd: Peidiwch ag yfed alcohol

To be used on *preparations where a reaction such as flushing may occur if alcohol is taken* (e.g. metronidazole). Alcohol may also enhance the hypoglycaemia produced by some oral antidiabetic drugs but routine application of a warning label is not considered necessary.

Patients should be advised not to drink alcohol for as long as they are receiving/using a course of medication, and in some cases for a period of time after the course is finished.

5   **Do not take indigestion remedies 2 hours before or after you take this medicine**

Peidiwch â chymryd meddyginiaethau camdreuliad 2 awr cyn neu ar ôl y feddyginiaeth hon

To be used with label 25 on *preparations coated to resist gastric acid* (e.g. enteric-coated tablets). This is to avoid the possibility of premature dissolution of the coating in the presence of an alkaline pH.

Label 5 also applies to drugs such as gabapentin *where the absorption is significantly affected by antacids.* Pharmacists will be aware (from a knowledge of physiology) that the usual time during which indigestion remedies should be avoided is at least 2 hours before and after the majority of medicines have been taken; when a manufacturer advises a different time period, this can be followed, and should be explained to the patient.

6   **Do not take indigestion remedies, or medicines containing iron or zinc, 2 hours before or after you take this medicine**

Peidiwch â chymryd meddyginiaethau camdreuliad neu feddyginiaethau sy'n cynnwys haearn neu sinc, 2 awr cyn neu ar ôl y feddyginiaeth hon

To be used on *preparations containing ofloxacin and some other quinolones, doxycycline, lymecycline, minocycline, and penicillamine.* These drugs chelate calcium, iron, and zinc and are less well absorbed when taken with calcium-containing antacids or preparations containing iron or zinc. Pharmacists will be aware (from a knowledge of physiology) that these incompatible preparations should be taken at least 2 hours apart for the majority of medicines; when a manufacturer advises a different time period, this can be followed, and should be explained to the patient.

7   **Do not take milk, indigestion remedies, or medicines containing iron or zinc, 2 hours before or after you take this medicine**

Peidiwch â chymryd llaeth, meddyginiaethau camdreuliad, neu feddyginiaeth sy'n cynnwys haearn neu sinc, 2 awr cyn neu ar ôl cymryd y feddyginiaeth hon

To be used on *preparations containing ciprofloxacin, norfloxacin, or tetracyclines that chelate calcium, iron, magnesium, and zinc,* and are thus less available for absorption. Pharmacists will be aware (from a knowledge of physiology) that these incompatible preparations should be taken at least 2 hours apart for the majority of medicines;

when a manufacturer advises a different time period, this can be followed, and should be explained to the patient. Doxycycline, lymecycline, and minocycline are less liable to form chelates and therefore only require label 6 (see above).

8   **Warning: Do not stop taking this medicine unless your doctor tells you to stop**

Rhybudd: Peidiwch â stopio cymryd y feddyginiaeth hon, oni bai fod eich meddyg yn dweud wrthych am stopio

To be used on *preparations that contain a drug which is required to be taken over long periods without the patient necessarily perceiving any benefit* (e.g. antituberculous drugs).

Also to be used on *preparations that contain a drug whose withdrawal is likely to be a particular hazard* (e.g. clonidine for hypertension). Label 10 (see below) is more appropriate for corticosteroids.

9   **Space the doses evenly throughout the day. Keep taking this medicine until the course is finished, unless you are told to stop**

Gadewch yr un faint o amser rhwng pob dôs yn ystod y dydd. Parhewch i gymryd y feddyginiaeth nes bod y cyfan wedi'i orffen, oni bai eich bod yn cael cyngor i stopio

To be used on *preparations where a course of treatment should be completed* to reduce the incidence of relapse or failure of treatment.

The preparations are antimicrobial drugs given by mouth. Very occasionally, some may have severe side-effects (e.g. diarrhoea in patients receiving clindamycin) and in such cases the patient may need to be advised of reasons for stopping treatment quickly and returning to the doctor.

The pharmacist should omit the first sentence of the label for antimicrobial drugs that are given once daily, and the patient should be suitably counselled.

10   **Warning: Read the additional information given with this medicine**

Rhybudd: Darllenwch y wybodaeth ychwanegol gyda'r feddyginiaeth hon

To be used particularly on *preparations containing anticoagulants, lithium, and oral corticosteroids.* The appropriate treatment card should be given to the patient and any necessary explanations given.

This label may also be used on other preparations to remind the patient of the instructions that have been given.

11   **Protect your skin from sunlight—even on a bright but cloudy day. Do not use sunbeds**

Diogelwch eich croen rhag golau'r haul, hyd yn oed ar ddiwrnod braf ond cymylog. Peidiwch â defnyddio gwely haul

To be used on *preparations that may cause phototoxic or photoallergic reactions* if the patient is exposed to ultraviolet radiation. Exposure to high intensity ultraviolet radiation from sunray lamps and sunbeds is particularly likely to cause reactions.

12   **Do not take anything containing aspirin while taking this medicine**

Peidiwch â chymryd unrhyw beth sy'n cynnwys aspirin gyda'r feddyginiaeth hon

To be used on *preparations containing sulfinpyrazone* whose activity is reduced by aspirin.

Label 12 should not be used for anticoagulants since label 10 is more appropriate.

13   **Dissolve or mix with water before taking**

Gadewch i doddi mewn dŵr cyn ei gymryd

To be used on *preparations that are intended to be dissolved in water* (e.g. soluble tablets) or *mixed with water* (e.g. powders, granules) before use. In a few cases other liquids such as fruit juice or milk may be used.

14   **This medicine may colour your urine. This is harmless**

Gall y feddyginiaeth hon liwio eich dŵr. Nid yw hyn yn arwydd o ddrwg

To be used on *preparations that may cause the patient's urine to turn an unusual colour.* These include triamterene (blue under some lights), levodopa (dark reddish), and rifampicin (red).

15   **Caution: flammable. Keep your body away from fire or flames after you have put on the medicine**

Rhybudd: Fflamadwy. Ar ôl rhoi'r feddyginiaeth ymlaen, cadwch yn glir o dân neu fflamau

To be used on *preparations containing sufficient flammable solvent to render them flammable if exposed to a naked flame.*

16   **Dissolve the tablet under your tongue–do not swallow. Store the tablets in this bottle with the cap tightly closed. Get a new supply 8 weeks after opening**

Rhowch y dabled i ddoddi dan eich tafod - peidiwch â'i lyncu. Cadwch y tabledi yn y botel yma gyda'r caead wedi'i gau yn dynn. Gofynnwch am dabledi newydd 8 wythnos ar ôl ei hagor

To be used on *glyceryl trinitrate tablets* to remind the patient not to transfer the tablets to plastic or less suitable containers.

17   **Do not take more than... in 24 hours**

Peidiwch â chymryd mwy na... mewn 24 awr

To be used on *preparations for the treatment of acute migraine* except those containing ergotamine, for which label 18 is used. The dose form should be specified, e.g. tablets or capsules.

    It may also be used on preparations for which no dose has been specified by the prescriber.

18   **Do not take more than... in 24 hours. Also, do not take more than... in any one week**

Peidiwch â chymryd mwy na... mewn 24 awr. Hefyd, peidiwch â chymryd mwy na... mewn wythnos

To be used on preparations containing ergotamine. The dose form should be specified, e.g. tablets or suppositories.

19   **Warning: This medicine makes you sleepy. If you still feel sleepy the next day, do not drive or use tools or machines. Do not drink alcohol**

Rhybudd: Bydd y feddyginiaeth hon yn eich gwneud yn gysglyd. Os ydych yn dal i deimlo'n gysglyd drannoeth, peidiwch â gyrru, defnyddio offer llaw neu beiriannau. Peidiwch ag yfed alcohol

To be used on *preparations containing hypnotics (or some other drugs with sedative effects) prescribed to be taken at night.* On the rare occasions when hypnotics are prescribed for daytime administration (e.g. nitrazepam in epilepsy), this label would clearly not be appropriate. Also to be used as an *alternative to the label 2 wording* (the choice being at the discretion of the pharmacist) *for anxiolytics prescribed to be taken at night.*

    It is hoped that this wording will convey adequately the problem of residual morning sedation after taking 'sleeping tablets'.

21   **Take with or just after food, or a meal**

Cymerwch gyda neu ar ôl bwyd

To be used on *preparations that are liable to cause gastric irritation, or those that are better absorbed with food.*

    Patients should be advised that a *small amount of food is sufficient.*

22   **Take 30 to 60 minutes before food**

Cymerwch 30 i 60 munud cyn bwyd

To be used on some preparations *whose absorption is thereby improved.*

    Most oral antibacterials require label 23 instead (see below).

23   **Take this medicine when your stomach is empty. This means an hour before food or 2 hours after food**

Cymerwch y feddyginiaeth hon ar stumog wag. Mae hyn yn golygu awr cyn, neu 2 awr ar ôl bwyd

To be used on *oral antibacterials whose absorption may be reduced by the presence of food and acid in the stomach.*

24   **Suck or chew this medicine**

Bydd angen cnoi neu sugno'r feddyginiaeth hon

To be used on *preparations that should be sucked or chewed.*

    The pharmacist should use discretion as to which of these words is appropriate.

25   **Swallow this medicine whole. Do not chew or crush**

Llyncwch yn gyfan. Peidiwch â chnoi neu falu'n fân

To be used on *preparations that are enteric-coated or designed for modified-release.*

    Also to be used on *preparations that taste very unpleasant or may damage the mouth* if not swallowed whole.

    Patients should be advised (where relevant) that some modified-release preparations can be broken in half, but that the halved tablet should still be swallowed whole, and not chewed or crushed.

26   **Dissolve this medicine under your tongue**

Gadewch i'r feddyginiaeth hon ddoddi o dan y tafod

To be used on *preparations designed for sublingual use.* Patients should be advised to hold under the tongue and avoid swallowing until dissolved. The buccal mucosa between the gum and cheek is occasionally specified by the prescriber.

27   **Take with a full glass of water**

Cymerwch gyda llond gwydr o ddŵr

To be used on *preparations that should be well diluted* (e.g. chloral hydrate), *where a high fluid intake is required* (e.g. sulfonamides), or *where water is required to aid the action* (e.g. methylcellulose). The patient should be advised that 'a full glass' means at least 150 mL. In most cases fruit juice, tea, or coffee may be used.

28   **Spread thinly on the affected skin only**

Taenwch yn denau ar y croen sydd wedi'i effeithio yn unig

To be used on *external preparations* that should be applied sparingly (e.g. corticosteroids, dithranol).

29   **Do not take more than 2 at any one time. Do not take more than 8 in 24 hours**

Peidiwch â chymryd mwy na 2 ar unrhyw un adeg. Peidiwch â chymryd mwy nag 8 mewn 24 awr

To be used on containers of dispensed *solid dose preparations containing paracetamol for adults when the instruction on the label indicates that the dose can be taken on an 'as required' basis.* The dose form should be specified, e.g. tablets or capsules.

    This label has been introduced because of the serious consequences of overdosage with paracetamol.

30   **Contains paracetamol. Do not take anything else containing paracetamol while taking this medicine. Talk to a doctor at once if you take too much of this medicine, even if you feel well**

Yn cynnwys paracetamol. Peidiwch â chymryd unrhyw beth arall sy'n cynnwys paracetamol tra'n cymryd y feddyginiaeth hon. Siaradwch gyda'ch meddyg ar unwaith os ydych yn cymryd gormod, hyd yn oed os ydych yn teimlo'n iawn

To be used on all containers of dispensed *preparations containing paracetamol.*

32   **Contains aspirin. Do not take anything else containing aspirin while taking this medicine**

Yn cynnwys aspirin. Peidiwch â chymryd unrhyw beth arall sy'n cynnwys aspirin tra'n cymryd y feddyginiaeth hon

To be used on containers of dispensed *preparations containing aspirin when the name on the label does not include the word 'aspirin'.*

Appendix 4
Wound management products and elasticated garments

CONTENTS

The correct dressing for wound management depends not only on the type of wound but also on the stage of the healing process. The principal stages of healing are: cleansing, removal of debris; granulation, vascularisation; epithelialisation. The ideal dressing for moist wound healing needs to ensure that the wound remains: moist with exudate, but not macerated; free of clinical infection and excessive slough; free of toxic chemicals, particles or fibres; at the optimum temperature for healing; undisturbed by the need for frequent changes; at the optimum pH value. As wound healing passes through its different stages, different types of dressings may be required to satisfy better one or other of these requirements. Under normal circumstances, a moist environment is a necessary part of the wound healing process; exudate provides a moist environment and promotes healing, but excessive exudate can cause maceration of the wound and surrounding healthy tissue. The volume and viscosity of exudate changes as the wound heals. There are certain circumstances where moist wound healing is not appropriate (e.g. gangrenous toes associated with vascular disease).

Advanced wound dressings are designed to control the environment for wound healing, for example to donate fluid (hydrogels), maintain hydration (hydrocolloids), or to absorb wound exudate (alginates, foams).

Practices such as the use of irritant cleansers and desloughing agents may be harmful and are largely obsolete; removal of debris and dressing remnants should need minimal irrigation with lukewarm sterile sodium chloride 0.9% solution or water.

Hydrogel, hydrocolloid, and medical grade honey dressings can be used to deslough wounds by promoting autolytic

debridement; there is insufficient evidence to support any particular method of debridement for difficult-to-heal surgical wounds. Sterile larvae (maggots) are also available for biosurgical removal of wound debris.

There have been few clinical trials able to establish a clear advantage for any particular product. The choice between different dressings depends not only on the type and stage of the wound, but also on patient preference or tolerance, site of the wound, and cost. For further information, see Buyers' Guide: Advanced wound dressings (October 2008); NHS Purchasing and Supply Agency, Centre for Evidence-based Purchasing.

Prices quoted in Appendix 4 are basic NHS net prices; for further information see *Prices in the BNF* under How to use the BNF.

The table below gives suggestions for choices of primary dressing depending on the type of wound (a secondary dressing may be needed in some cases).

Basic wound contact dressings

Absorbent dressings

Perforated film absorbent dressings are suitable only for wounds with mild to moderate amounts of exudate; they are not appropriate for leg ulcers or for other lesions that produce large quantities of viscous exudate. Dressings with an absorbent cellulose or polymer wadding layer are suitable for use on moderately to heavily exuding wounds.

Wound contact material for different types of wounds

Wound PINK (epithelialising)

Low Exudate	Moderate Exudate
Low adherence p. 1930 Vapour-permeable films and membranes p. 1931 Soft polymer p. 1933 Hydrocolloid p. 1934	Soft polymer p. 1933 Foam, low absorbent p. 1935 Alginate p. 1936

Wound RED (granulating)
Symptoms or signs of infection, see Wounds with signs of infection

Low Exudate	Moderate Exudate	Heavy Exudate
Low adherence p. 1930 Soft polymer p. 1933 Hydrocolloid p. 1934 Foam, low absorbent p. 1935	Hydrocolloid-fibrous p. 1934 Foam p. 1935 Alginate p. 1936	Foam with extra absorbency p. 1935 Hydrocolloid-fibrous p. 1934 Alginate p. 1936

Wound YELLOW (Sloughy) (granulating)
Symptoms or signs of infection, see Wounds with signs of infection

Low Exudate	Moderate Exudate	Heavy Exudate
Hydrogel p. 1931 Hydrocolloid p. 1934	Hydrocolloid-fibrous p. 1934 Alginate p. 1936	Hydrocolloid-fibrous p. 1934 Alginate p. 1936 Capillary-acting p. 1937

Wound BLACK (Necrotic/ Eschar)
Consider mechanical debridement alongside autolytic debridement

Low Exudate	Moderate Exudate	Heavy Exudate
Hydrogel p. 1931 Hydrocolloid p. 1934	Hydrocolloid p. 1934 Hydrocolloid-fibrous p. 1934 Foam p. 1935	Seek advice from wound care specialist

Wounds with signs of infection
Consider systemic antibacterials if appropriate; also consider odour-absorbent dressings.
For malodourous wounds with slough or necrotic tissue, consider mechanical or autolytic debridement

Low Exudate	Moderate Exudate	Heavy Exudate
Low adherence with honey p. 1937 Low adherence with iodine p. 1938 Low adherence with silver p. 1939	Foam with silver p. 1940 Alginate with silver p. 1939 Honey-topical p. 1938 Cadexomer-iodine p. 1938	Foam extra absorbent, with silver p. 1940 Alginate with honey p. 1937 Alginate with silver p. 1939

Note In each section of this table the dressings are listed in order of increasing absorbency.
Some wound contact (primary) dressings require a secondary dressing

Absorbent cellulose dressings
CelluDress
Absorbent cellulose dressing with fluid repellent backing
CelluDress dressing (Medicareplus International Ltd) 10cm × 10cm= £0.19, 10cm × 15cm= £0.20, 10cm × 20cm= £0.22, 15cm × 20cm= £0.30, 20cm × 25cm= £0.40, 20cm × 30cm= £0.85

Eclypse
Absorbent cellulose dressing with fluid repellent backing
Eclypse (Advancis Medical) Boot dressing 55cm × 47cm= £11.04, 60cm × 70cm=£15.65, 71cm × 80cm=£22.77, dressing 10cm × 10cm=£0.82, 10cm × 20cm=£1.02, 15cm × 15cm=£1.10, 20cm × 20cm=£1.58, 20cm × 30cm=£2.43, 60cm × 40cm=£9.26

Exu-Dry
Absorbent cellulose dressing with fluid repellent backing
Exu-Dry dressing (Smith & Nephew Healthcare Ltd) 10cm × 15cm= £1.24, 15cm × 23cm= £2.53, 23cm × 38cm= £5.87

Mesorb
Cellulose wadding pad with gauze wound contact layer and non-woven repellent backing
Mesorb dressing (Molnlycke Health Care Ltd) 10cm × 10cm= £0.67, 10cm × 15cm= £0.88, 10cm × 20cm= £1.08, 15cm × 20cm= £1.54, 20cm × 25cm= £2.43, 20cm × 30cm= £2.76

Zetuvit E
Absorbent cellulose dressing with fluid repellent backing; sterile or non-sterile
Zetuvit E (Paul Hartmann Ltd) non-sterile dressing 10cm × 10cm= £0.07, 10cm × 20cm=£0.10, 20cm × 20cm= £0.16, 20cm × 40cm= £0.30, sterile dressing 10cm × 10cm= £0.24, 10cm × 20cm= £0.27, 20cm × 20cm= £0.43, 20cm × 40cm= £1.22

Absorbent perforated dressings
Adpore
Low-adherence primary dressing consisting of viscose and rayon absorbent pad with adhesive border
Adpore dressing (Medicareplus International Ltd) 10cm × 10cm= £0.10, 10cm × 15cm= £0.16, 10cm × 20cm= £0.30, 10cm × 25cm= £0.34, 10cm × 30cm= £0.42, 10cm × 35cm= £0.50, 7cm × 8cm= £0.08

Cosmopor E
Low-adherence primary dressing consisting of viscose and rayon absorbent pad with adhesive border
Cosmopor E dressing (Paul Hartmann Ltd) 10cm × 20cm= £0.50, 10cm × 25cm= £0.62, 10cm × 35cm= £0.86, 5cm × 7.2cm= £0.09, 8cm × 10cm= £0.19, 8cm × 15cm= £0.31

Cutiplast Steril
Low-adherence primary dressing consisting of viscose and rayon absorbent pad with adhesive border
Cutiplast Steril dressing (Smith & Nephew Healthcare Ltd) 10cm × 20cm= £0.34, 10cm × 25cm= £0.35, 10cm × 30cm= £0.47, 5cm × 7.2cm= £0.06, 8cm × 10cm= £0.12, 8cm × 15cm= £0.27

Leukomed
Low-adherence primary dressing consisting of viscose and rayon absorbent pad with adhesive border
Leukomed dressing (Essity UK Ltd) 10cm × 20cm= £0.47, 10cm × 25cm= £0.53, 10cm × 30cm= £0.69, 10cm × 35cm= £0.79, 5cm × 7.2cm= £0.09, 8cm × 10cm= £0.20, 8cm × 15cm= £0.36

Medipore + Pad

Low-adherence primary dressing consisting of viscose and rayon absorbent pad with adhesive border

Medipore + Pads dressing (3M Health Care Ltd) 10cm × 10cm= £0.16, 10cm × 15cm= £0.26, 10cm × 20cm= £0.40, 10cm × 25cm= £0.49, 10cm × 35cm= £0.68, 5cm × 7.2cm= £0.08

Medisafe

Low-adherence primary dressing consisting of viscose and rayon absorbent pad with adhesive border

Medisafe dressing (Neomedic Ltd) 6cm × 8cm= £0.08, 8cm × 10cm= £0.13, 8cm × 12cm= £0.23, 9cm × 15cm= £0.29, 9cm × 20cm= £0.34, 9cm × 25cm= £0.36

Mepore

Low-adherence primary dressing consisting of viscose and rayon absorbent pad with adhesive border

Mepore dressing (Molnlycke Health Care Ltd) 10cm × 11cm= £0.23, 11cm × 15cm= £0.39, 7cm × 8cm= £0.12, 9cm × 20cm= £0.48, 9cm × 25cm= £0.65, 9cm × 30cm= £0.75, 9cm × 35cm= £0.82

PremierPore

Low-adherence primary dressing consisting of viscose and rayon absorbent pad with adhesive border

PremierPore dressing (Mediq Healthcare UK Ltd) 10cm × 10cm= £0.12, 10cm × 15cm= £0.18, 10cm × 20cm= £0.32, 10cm × 25cm= £0.36, 10cm × 30cm= £0.45, 10cm × 35cm= £0.52, 5cm × 7cm= £0.05

Primapore

Low-adherence primary dressing consisting of viscose and rayon absorbent pad with adhesive border

Primapore dressing (Smith & Nephew Healthcare Ltd) 10cm × 20cm= £0.48, 10cm × 25cm= £0.55, 10cm × 30cm= £0.69, 10cm × 35cm= £1.06, 6cm × 8.3cm= £0.20, 8cm × 10cm= £0.21, 8cm × 15cm= £0.36

Softpore

Low-adherence primary dressing consisting of viscose and rayon absorbent pad with adhesive border

Softpore dressing (Richardson Healthcare Ltd) 10cm × 10cm= £0.14, 10cm × 15cm= £0.21, 10cm × 20cm= £0.38, 10cm × 25cm= £0.43, 10cm × 30cm= £0.53, 10cm × 35cm= £0.62, 6cm × 7cm= £0.06

Absorbent perforated plastic film faced dressings

Absopad

Low-adherence primary dressing consisting of 3 layers— perforated polyester film wound contact layer, absorbent cotton pad, and hydrophobic backing

Absopad dressing (Medicareplus International Ltd) 10cm × 10cm= £0.13, 20cm × 10cm= £0.28, 5cm × 5cm= £0.07

Askina Pad

Low-adherence primary dressing consisting of 3 layers— perforated polyester film wound contact layer, absorbent cotton pad, and hydrophobic backing

Askina Pad dressing (B.Braun Medical Ltd) 10cm × 10cm= £0.23

Melolin

Low-adherence primary dressing consisting of 3 layers— perforated polyester film wound contact layer, absorbent cotton pad, and hydrophobic backing

Melolin dressing (Smith & Nephew Healthcare Ltd) 10cm × 10cm= £0.30, 20cm × 10cm= £0.59, 5cm × 5cm= £0.19

Skintact

Low-adherence primary dressing consisting of 3 layers— perforated polyester film wound contact layer, absorbent cotton pad, and hydrophobic backing

Skintact dressing (Robinson Healthcare) 10cm × 10cm= £0.17, 20cm × 10cm= £0.34, 5cm × 5cm= £0.10

Solvaline N

Low-adherence primary dressing consisting of 3 layers— perforated polyester film wound contact layer, absorbent cotton pad, and hydrophobic backing

Solvaline N dressing (Lohmann & Rauscher) 10cm × 10cm= £0.20, 20cm × 10cm= £0.39, 5cm × 5cm= £0.11

Super absorbent cellulose and polymer primary dressings

Curea P1

Super absorbent cellulose and polymer primary dressing

Curea P1 dressing (Regen Medical Ltd) 10cm × 10cm square= £1.56, 10cm × 20cm rectangular= £2.08, 10cm × 30cm rectangular= £3.32, 12cm × 12cm square= £2.67, 15cm × 15cm square= £3.38, 20cm × 20cm square= £4.03, 20cm × 30cm rectangular= £4.68, 7.5cm × 7.5cm square= £1.50

Curea P2

Super absorbent cellulose and polymer primary dressing (non-adherent)

Curea P2 dressing (Regen Medical Ltd) 10cm × 20cm rectangular= £3.12, 11cm × 11cm square= £2.12, 15cm × 15cm square= £4.94, 20cm × 20cm square= £5.59, 20cm × 30cm rectangular= £7.28

DryMax Super

Super absorbent cellulose and polymer primary dressing

DryMax Super dressing (C D Medical Ltd) 10cm × 11cm rectangular= £0.91, 11cm × 20cm rectangular= £1.09, 20cm × 20cm square= £1.93, 20cm × 30cm rectangular= £2.44, 37cm × 56cm rectangular= £5.02

Zetuvit Plus

Super absorbent cellulose primary dressing

Zetuvit Plus Superabsorber dressing (Paul Hartmann Ltd) 10cm × 10cm= £0.90, 10cm × 20cm= £1.24, 15cm × 20cm= £1.43, 20cm × 25cm= £1.95, 20cm × 40cm= £3.02

Super absorbent hydroconductive dressings

Drawtex

Super absorbent hydroconductive dressing with absorbent, cross-action structures of viscose, polyester and cotton

Drawtex dressing (Martindale Pharmaceuticals Ltd) 10cm × 1.3m= £16.00, 10cm × 10cm= £2.24, 10cm × 1m= £16.00, 15cm × 20cm= £6.00, 20cm × 1m= £25.00, 20cm × 20cm= £6.98, 5cm × 5cm= £0.95, 7.5cm × 1m= £15.50, 7.5cm × 7.5cm= £1.77

Low adherence dressings

Low adherence dressings are used as interface layers under secondary absorbent dressings. Placed directly on the wound bed, non-absorbent, low adherence dressings are suitable for clean, granulating, lightly exuding wounds without necrosis, and protect the wound bed from direct contact with secondary dressings. Care must be taken to avoid granulation tissue growing into the weave of these dressings. Tulle dressings are manufactured from cotton or viscose fibres which are impregnated with white or yellow soft paraffin to prevent the fibres from sticking, but this is only partly successful and it may be necessary to change the dressings frequently. The paraffin reduces absorbency of the dressing. Dressings with a reduced content (light loading) of soft paraffin are less liable to interfere with absorption; dressings with 'normal loading' (such as *Jelonet* ®) have been used for skin graft transfer. Knitted viscose primary dressing is an alternative to tulle dressings for exuding wounds; it can be used as the initial layer of multi-layer compression bandaging in the treatment of venous leg ulcers.

Knitted polyester primary dressings

Atrauman

Non-adherent knitted polyester primary dressing impregnated with neutral triglycerides

Atrauman dressing (Paul Hartmann Ltd) 10cm × 20cm= £0.97, 20cm × 30cm= £2.65, 5cm × 5cm= £0.41, 7.5cm × 10cm= £0.42

Knitted viscose primary dressings

N-A Ultra

Warp knitted fabric manufactured from a bright viscose monofilament

N-A Ultra dressing (Systagenix Wound Management Ltd) 19cm × 9.5cm= £0.66, 9.5cm × 9.5cm= £0.35

Profore

Warp knitted fabric manufactured from a bright viscose monofilament

Profore (Smith & Nephew Healthcare Ltd) wound contact layer 14cm × 20cm= £0.35

Paraffin gauze dressings
Cuticell
(Tulle Gras). Fabric of leno weave, weft and warp threads of cotton and/or viscose yarn, impregnated with white or yellow soft paraffin; for light or normal loading
Cuticell (Essity UK Ltd) Classic dressing 10cm × 10cm= £0.32

Jelonet
(Tulle Gras). Fabric of leno weave, weft and warp threads of cotton and/or viscose yarn, impregnated with white or yellow soft paraffin; for light or normal loading
Jelonet (Smith & Nephew Healthcare Ltd) dressing 10cm × 10cm= £0.45

Neotulle
(Tulle Gras). Fabric of leno weave, weft and warp threads of cotton and/or viscose yarn, impregnated with white or yellow soft paraffin; for light or normal loading
Neotulle (Neomedic Ltd) dressing 10cm × 10cm= £0.29

Advanced wound dressings

Advanced wound dressings can be used for both acute and chronic wounds. These dressings are classified according to their primary component; some dressings are comprised of several components.

Hydrogel dressings
Hydrogel dressings are most commonly supplied as an amorphous, cohesive topical application that can take up the shape of a wound. A secondary, non-absorbent dressing is needed. These dressings are generally used to donate liquid to dry sloughy wounds and facilitate autolytic debridement of necrotic tissue; some also have the ability to absorb very small amounts of exudate. Hydrogel products that do not contain propylene glycol should be used if the wound is to be treated with larval therapy. Hydrogel sheets have a fixed structure and limited fluid-handling capacity; hydrogel sheet dressings are best avoided in the presence of infection, and are unsuitable for heavily exuding wounds.

Hydrogel applications (amorphous)
ActivHeal Hydrogel
Hydrogel containing guar gum and propylene glycol
ActivHeal Hydrogel (Advanced Medical Solutions Ltd) dressing= £1.46

Cutimed
Hydrogel
Cutimed (Essity UK Ltd) Gel dressing= £3.32

Flexigran
Hydrogel containing modified starch and glycerol
Flexigran (A1 Pharmaceuticals) Gel dressing= £1.90

GranuGEL
Hydrogel containing carboxymethylcellulose, pectin and propylene glycol
GranuGEL (ConvaTec Ltd) Hydrocolloid Gel dressing= £2.56

Intrasite Gel
Hydrogel containing modified carmellose polymer and propylene glycol
IntraSite Gel (Smith & Nephew Healthcare Ltd) dressing= £3.94

Nu-Gel
Hydrogel containing alginate and propylene glycol
Nu-Gel (Systagenix Wound Management Ltd) dressing= £2.25

Purilon Gel
Hydrogel containing carboxymethylcellulose and calcium alginate
Purilon Gel (Coloplast Ltd) dressing= £2.49

Hydrogel sheet dressings
Aquaflo
Hydrogel dressing
Aquaflo sheet (Covidien (UK) Commercial Ltd) 12cm discs= £5.37, 7.5cm discs= £2.60

Coolie
Hydrogel dressing (without adhesive border)
Coolie sheet (Zeroderma Ltd) 7cm discs= £1.96

Gel FX
Hydrogel dressing (without adhesive border)
Gel FX sheet (Synergy Health (UK) Ltd) 10cm × 10cm square= £1.60, 15cm × 15cm square= £3.20

Geliperm
Hydrogel sheets
Geliperm sheet (Geistlich Sons Ltd) 10cm × 10cm square= £2.53

Intrasite Conformable
Soft non-woven dressing impregnated with *Intrasite* ® gel
IntraSite Conformable dressing (Smith & Nephew Healthcare Ltd) 10cm × 10cm square= £1.98, 10cm × 20cm rectangular= £2.68, 10cm × 40cm rectangular= £4.78

Novogel
Glycerol-based hydrogel sheets (standard or thin)
Novogel sheet (Ford Medical Associates Ltd) 10cm × 10cm square= £3.18, 15cm × 20cm rectangular= £6.07, 20cm × 40cm rectangular= £11.56, 30cm × 30cm (0.15cm thickness) square= £12.71, (0.30cm thickness) square= £13.47, 5cm × 7.5cm rectangular= £1.99, 7.5cm diameter circular= £5.84

SanoSkin NET
Hydrogel sheet (without adhesive border)
SanoSkin NET sheet (Ideal Medical Solutions Ltd) 8.5cm × 12cm rectangular= £2.28

Vacunet
Non-adherent, hydrogel coated polyester net dressing
Vacunet dressing (Protex Healthcare Ltd) 10cm × 10cm square= £1.93, 10cm × 15cm rectangular= £2.86

Vapour-permeable films and membranes
Vapour-permeable films and membranes allow the passage of water vapour and oxygen but are impermeable to water and micro-organisms, and are suitable for lightly exuding wounds. They are highly conformable, provide protection, and a moist healing environment; transparent film dressings permit constant observation of the wound. Water vapour loss can occur at a slower rate than exudate is generated, so that fluid accumulates under the dressing, which can lead to tissue maceration and to wrinkling at the adhesive contact site (with risk of bacterial entry). Newer versions of these dressings have increased moisture vapour permeability. Despite these advances, vapour-permeable films and membranes are unsuitable for infected, large heavily exuding wounds, and chronic leg ulcers. Vapour-permeable films and membranes are suitable for partial-thickness wounds with minimal exudate, or wounds with eschar. Most commonly, they are used as a secondary dressing over alginates or hydrogels; film dressings can also be used to protect the fragile skin of patients at risk of developing minor skin damage caused by friction or pressure.

Vapour-permeable adhesive film dressings (semi-permeable adhesive dressings)
Dressfilm
Extensible, waterproof, water vapour-permeable polyurethane film coated with synthetic adhesive mass; transparent. Supplied in single-use pieces
Dressfilm dressing (St Georges Medical Ltd) 15cm × 20cm= £1.90

Hydrofilm
Extensible, waterproof, water vapour-permeable polyurethane film coated with synthetic adhesive mass; transparent. Supplied in single-use pieces
Hydrofilm dressing (Paul Hartmann Ltd) 10cm × 12.5cm= £0.46, 10cm × 15cm= £0.58, 10cm × 25cm= £0.90, 12cm × 25cm= £0.95, 15cm × 20cm= £1.07, 20cm × 30cm= £1.77, 6cm × 7cm= £0.25

Hypafix Transparent
Extensible, waterproof, water vapour-permeable polyurethane film coated with synthetic adhesive mass; transparent. Supplied in single-use pieces
Hypafix Transparent dressing (Essity UK Ltd) 10cm × 2m= £9.43

A4

Wound management | Appendix 4

Leukomed T

Extensible, waterproof, water vapour-permeable polyurethane film coated with synthetic adhesive mass; transparent. Supplied in single-use pieces

Leukomed T dressing (Essity UK Ltd) 10cm × 12.5cm= £1.13, 11cm × 14cm= £1.36, 15cm × 20cm= £2.61, 15cm × 25cm= £2.79, 7.2cm × 5cm= £0.41, 8cm × 10cm= £0.77

Mepitel Film

Extensible, waterproof, water vapour-permeable polyurethane film coated with synthetic adhesive mass; transparent. Supplied in single-use pieces

Mepitel Film dressing (Molnlycke Health Care Ltd) 10.5cm × 12cm= £1.42, 10.5cm × 25cm= £2.75, 15.5cm × 20cm= £3.50, 6cm × 7cm= £0.50

Mepore Film

Extensible, waterproof, water vapour-permeable polyurethane film coated with synthetic adhesive mass; transparent. Supplied in single-use pieces

Mepore Film dressing (Molnlycke Health Care Ltd) 10cm × 12cm= £1.30, 10cm × 25cm= £2.53, 15cm × 20cm= £3.21, 6cm × 7cm= £0.48

OpSite Flexifix

Extensible, waterproof, water vapour-permeable polyurethane film coated with synthetic adhesive mass; transparent. Supplied in single-use pieces

OpSite Flexifix dressing (Smith & Nephew Healthcare Ltd) 10cm × 1m= £7.25, 5cm × 1m= £4.30

OpSite Flexigrid

Extensible, waterproof, water vapour-permeable polyurethane film coated with synthetic adhesive mass; transparent. Supplied in single-use pieces

OpSite Flexigrid dressing (Smith & Nephew Healthcare Ltd) 12cm × 12cm= £1.24, 15cm × 20cm= £3.13, 6cm × 7cm= £0.44

ProtectFilm

Extensible, waterproof, water vapour-permeable polyurethane film coated with synthetic adhesive mass; transparent. Supplied in single-use pieces

ProtectFilm dressing (Wallace, Cameron & Company Ltd) 10cm × 12cm= £0.20, 15cm × 20cm= £0.40, 6cm × 7cm= £0.11

Tegaderm Film

Extensible, waterproof, water vapour-permeable polyurethane film coated with synthetic adhesive mass; transparent. Supplied in single-use pieces

Tegaderm Film dressing (3M Health Care Ltd) 12cm × 12cm= £1.17, 15cm × 20cm= £2.55, 6cm × 7cm= £0.41

Vellafilm

Extensible, waterproof, water vapour-permeable polyurethane film coated with synthetic adhesive mass; transparent. Supplied in single-use pieces

Vellafilm dressing (Advancis Medical) 12cm × 12cm= £1.28, 12cm × 35cm= £3.19, 15cm × 20cm= £2.44

Vapour-permeable adhesive film dressings with absorbent pad

Adpore Ultra

Film dressing with absorbent pad

Adpore Ultra dressing (Medicareplus International Ltd) 10cm × 10cm= £0.14, 10cm × 15cm= £0.22, 10cm × 20cm= £0.33, 10cm × 25cm= £0.35, 10cm × 30cm= £0.52, 7cm × 8cm= £0.12

Alldress

Film dressing with absorbent pad

Alldress dressing (Molnlycke Health Care Ltd) 10cm × 10cm= £1.04, 15cm × 15cm= £2.27, 15cm × 20cm= £2.80

Clearpore

Film dressing with absorbent pad

Clearpore dressing (Richardson Healthcare Ltd) 10cm × 10cm= £0.21, 10cm × 15cm= £0.26, 10cm × 20cm= £0.39, 10cm × 25cm= £0.43, 10cm × 30cm= £0.70, 6cm × 10cm= £0.16, 6cm × 7cm= £0.13

Cosmopor Transparent

Film dressing with absorbent pad

Cosmopor Transparent dressing (Paul Hartmann Ltd) 10cm × 20cm= £0.51, 10cm × 25cm= £0.67, 10cm × 30cm= £0.76, 7.2cm × 5cm= £0.20, 9cm × 10cm= £0.30, 9cm × 15cm= £0.33

Leukomed T Plus

Film dressing with absorbent pad

Leukomed T plus dressing (Essity UK Ltd) 10cm × 20cm= £1.48, 10cm × 25cm= £1.66, 10cm × 30cm= £2.79, 10cm × 35cm= £3.38, 7.2cm × 5cm= £0.30, 8cm × 10cm= £0.59, 8cm × 15cm= £0.89

Mepore Film & Pad

Film dressing with absorbent pad

Mepore Film & Pad dressing (Molnlycke Health Care Ltd) 4cm × 5cm= £0.26, 5cm × 7cm= £0.26, 9cm × 10cm= £0.67, 9cm × 15cm= £0.99, 9cm × 20cm= £1.47, 9cm × 25cm= £1.62, 9cm × 30cm= £2.18, 9cm × 35cm= £2.71

Mepore Ultra

Film dressing with absorbent pad

Mepore Ultra dressing (Molnlycke Health Care Ltd) 10cm × 11cm= £0.87, 11cm × 15cm= £1.27, 7cm × 8cm= £0.44, 9cm × 20cm= £1.63, 9cm × 25cm= £1.80, 9cm × 30cm= £2.98

OpSite Plus

Film dressing with absorbent pad

OpSite Plus dressing (Smith & Nephew Healthcare Ltd) 10cm × 12cm= £1.32, 10cm × 20cm= £2.22, 10cm × 35cm= £3.67, 6.5cm × 5cm= £0.36, 8.5cm × 9.5cm= £0.97

OpSite Post-Op

Film dressing with absorbent pad

OpSite Post-Op dressing (Smith & Nephew Healthcare Ltd) 10cm × 12cm= £1.29, 10cm × 20cm= £2.17, 10cm × 25cm= £2.74, 10cm × 30cm= £3.24, 10cm × 35cm= £3.61, 8.5cm × 15.5cm= £1.32, 8.5cm × 9.5cm= £0.95

Pharmapore-PU

Film dressing with absorbent pad

Pharmapore-PU dressing (Wallace, Cameron & Company Ltd) 10cm × 25cm= £0.38, 10cm × 30cm= £0.58, 8.5cm × 15.5cm= £0.20

PremierPore VP

Film dressing with absorbent pad

PremierPore VP dressing (Mediq Healthcare UK Ltd) 10cm × 10cm= £0.16, 10cm × 15cm= £0.24, 10cm × 20cm= £0.36, 10cm × 25cm= £0.38, 10cm × 30cm= £0.57, 10cm × 35cm= £0.70, 5cm × 7cm= £0.13

Tegaderm + Pad

Film dressing with absorbent pad

Tegaderm + Pad dressing (3M Health Care Ltd) 5cm × 7cm= £0.28, 9cm × 10cm= £0.70, 9cm × 15cm= £1.02, 9cm × 20cm= £1.50, 9cm × 25cm= £1.69, 9cm × 35cm= £2.80

Tegaderm Absorbent Clear

Film dressing with clear acrylic polymer oval-shaped pad or rectangular-shaped pad

Tegaderm Absorbent Clear Acrylic dressing (3M Health Care Ltd) 11.1cm × 12.7cm oval= £4.42, 14.2cm × 15.8cm oval= £6.22, 14.9cm × 15.2cm rectangular= £9.32, 20cm × 20.3cm rectangular= £14.96, 7.6cm × 9.5cm oval= £3.41

Vapour-permeable transparent adhesive film dressings

IV3000

For intravenous and subcutaneous catheter sites

IV3000 dressing (Smith & Nephew Healthcare Ltd) 10cm × 12cm= £1.54, 11cm × 14cm= £1.78, 5cm × 6cm= £0.46, 6cm × 7cm= £0.61, 7cm × 9cm= £0.80, 9cm × 12cm= £1.59

Mepore IV

For intravenous and subcutaneous catheter sites

Mepore IV dressing (Molnlycke Health Care Ltd) 10cm × 11cm= £1.14, 5cm × 5.5cm= £0.33, 8cm × 9cm= £0.42

Pharmapore-PU IV

For intravenous and subcutaneous catheter sites

Pharmapore-PU-I.V dressing (Wallace, Cameron & Company Ltd) 6cm × 7cm= £0.08, 7cm × 8.5cm= £0.07, 7cm × 9cm= £0.17

Tegaderm IV Advanced

For intravenous and subcutaneous catheter sites

Tegaderm IV Advanced dressing with securing tapes (3M Health Care Ltd) 10cm × 15.5cm= £1.76, 7cm × 8.5cm= £0.63

Vapour-permeable transparent film dressings with adhesive foam border
EasI-V
For intravenous and subcutaneous catheter sites
EasI-V (ConvaTec Ltd) dressing 7cm × 7.5cm= £0.38

Soft polymer dressings

Dressings with soft polymer, often a soft silicone polymer, in a non-adherent or gently adherent layer are suitable for use on lightly to moderately exuding wounds. For moderately to heavily exuding wounds, an absorbent secondary dressing can be added, or a soft polymer dressing with an absorbent pad can be used. Wound contact dressings coated with soft silicone have gentle adhesive properties and can be used on fragile skin areas or where it is beneficial to reduce the frequency of primary dressing changes. Soft polymer dressings should not be used on heavily bleeding wounds; blood clots can cause the dressing to adhere to the wound surface. For silicone keloid dressings see under Specialised dressings.

Cellulose dressings
Sorbion Sachet EXTRA
Absorbent polymers in cellulose matrix, hypoallergenic polypropylene envelope
Cutimed Sorbion Sachet Extra dressing (Essity UK Ltd) 10cm × 10cm= £2.47, 20cm × 10cm= £4.10, 20cm × 20cm= £7.70, 30cm × 20cm= £10.98, 5cm × 5cm= £1.59, 7.5cm × 7.5cm= £1.96

Sorbion Sachet Multi Star
Absorbent polymers in cellulose matrix, hypoallergenic polypropylene envelope
Cutimed Sorbion Sachet Multi Star dressing (Essity UK Ltd) 14cm × 14cm= £5.38, 8cm × 8cm= £3.29

Sorbion Sachet S Drainage
Absorbent polymers in cellulose matrix, hypoallergenic polypropylene envelope ('v' shaped dressing)
Cutimed Sorbion Sachet S drainage dressing (Essity UK Ltd) 10cm × 10cm= £2.90

Suprasorb X
Biosynthetic cellulose fibre dressing
Suprasorb X dressing (Lohmann & Rauscher) 14cm × 20cm rectangular= £9.31, 2cm × 21cm rope= £7.23, 5cm × 5cm square= £2.26, 9cm × 9cm square= £4.70

Soft polymer dressings with absorbent pad
Advazorb Border
Soft silicone wound contact dressing with polyurethane foam film backing and adhesive border
Advazorb Border dressing (Advancis Medical) 10cm × 10cm= £2.36, 10cm × 20cm= £3.27, 10cm × 30cm= £4.79, 12.5cm × 12.5cm= £2.91, 15cm × 15cm= £3.55, 20cm × 20cm= £6.15, 7.5cm × 7.5cm= £1.34

Advazorb Border Lite
Soft silicone wound contact dressing with polyurethane foam film backing and adhesive border
Advazorb Border Lite dressing (Advancis Medical) 10cm × 10cm= £2.13, 10cm × 20cm= £2.94, 10cm × 30cm= £4.31, 12.5cm × 12.5cm= £2.62, 15cm × 15cm= £3.19, 20cm × 20cm= £5.53, 7.5cm × 7.5cm= £1.21

Advazorb Silfix
Soft silicone wound contact dressing with polyurethane foam film backing
Advazorb Silfix dressing (Advancis Medical) 10cm × 10cm= £2.08, 10cm × 20cm= £3.58, 12.5cm × 12.5cm= £2.92, 15cm × 15cm= £3.78, 20cm × 20cm= £5.61, 7.5cm × 7.5cm= £1.12

Allevyn Gentle
Soft silicone wound contact dressing, with polyurethane foam film backing
Allevyn Gentle dressing (Smith & Nephew Healthcare Ltd) 20cm × 50cm= £22.54

Allevyn Gentle Border
Silicone gel wound contact dressing, with polyurethane foam film backing

Allevyn Gentle Border (Smith & Nephew Healthcare Ltd) Heel dressing 23cm × 23.2cm= £10.59, dressing 10cm × 10cm= £2.41, 10cm × 20cm= £3.87, 10cm × 25cm= £4.90, 10cm × 30cm= £5.91, 12.5cm × 12.5cm= £2.94, 15cm × 15cm= £4.40, 17.5cm × 17.5cm= £5.81, 7.5cm × 7.5cm= £1.64

Allevyn Gentle Border Lite
Silicone gel wound contact dressing, with polyurethane foam film backing
Allevyn Gentle Border Lite dressing (Smith & Nephew Healthcare Ltd) 10cm × 10cm= £2.37, 10cm × 20cm= £3.87, 15cm × 15cm= £4.18, 5.5cm × 12cm= £2.03, 5cm × 5cm= £0.99, 7.5cm × 7.5cm= £1.52, 8cm × 15cm= £3.77, 15.2cm × 13.1cm oval= £3.98, 8.6cm × 7.7cm oval= £1.70

Allevyn Life
Soft silicone wound contact dressing, with central mesh screen, polyurethane foam film backing and adhesive border
Allevyn Life dressing (Smith & Nephew Healthcare Ltd) 10.3cm × 10.3cm= £1.86, 12.9cm × 12.9cm= £2.72, 15.4cm × 15.4cm= £3.33, 21cm × 21cm= £6.56

Cutimed Siltec
Soft silicone wound contact dressing, with polyurethane foam film backing
Cutimed Siltec (Essity UK Ltd) Sacrum dressing 17.5cm × 17.5cm= £4.90, 23cm × 23cm= £6.69, dressing 10cm × 10cm= £2.44, 10cm × 20cm= £4.03, 15cm × 15cm= £4.55, 20cm × 20cm= £6.91, 5cm × 6cm= £1.31

Cutimed Siltec B
Soft silicone wound contact dressing, with polyurethane foam film backing, with adhesive border, for lightly to moderately exuding wounds
Cutimed Siltec B dressing (Essity UK Ltd) 12.5cm × 12.5cm= £2.48, 15cm × 15cm= £3.30, 17.5cm × 17.5cm= £5.34, 22.5cm × 22.5cm= £6.52, 7.5cm × 7.5cm= £1.46

Cutimed Siltec L
Soft silicone wound contact dressing, with polyurethane foam film backing, for lightly to moderately exuding wounds
Cutimed Siltec L dressing (Essity UK Ltd) 10cm × 10cm= £1.69, 15cm × 15cm= £3.72, 5cm × 6cm= £1.15

Cutimed Sorbion Sana
Non-adherent polyethylene wound contact dressing with absorbent core
Cutimed Sorbion Sana Gentle dressing (Essity UK Ltd) 12cm × 12cm= £2.74, 12cm × 22cm= £4.94, 22cm × 22cm= £8.78, 32cm × 22cm= £12.08, 8.5cm × 8.5cm= £2.19

Eclypse Adherent
Soft silicone wound contact layer with absorbent pad and film backing
Eclypse Adherent dressing (Advancis Medical) 10cm × 10cm= £3.40, 10cm × 20cm= £4.27, 15cm × 15cm= £5.67, 20cm × 30cm= £11.35, 17cm × 19cm sacral= £4.37, 22cm × 23cm sacral= £7.24

Kliniderm Foam Silicone
Absorbent soft silicone dressing with polyurethane foam film backing
kliniderm Foam Silicone (Mediq Healthcare UK Ltd) Heel dressing 10cm × 17.5cm= £3.14, dressing 10cm × 10cm= £1.74, 10cm × 20cm= £2.60, 15cm × 15cm= £3.13, 20cm × 20cm= £4.59, 5cm × 5cm= £0.78

Kliniderm Foam Silicone Border
Absorbent soft silicone dressing with polyurethane foam film backing and adhesive border
kliniderm Foam Silicone (Mediq Healthcare UK Ltd) Border dressing 10cm × 10cm= £1.27, 10cm × 20cm= £3.26, 10cm × 30cm= £4.79, 12.5cm × 12.5cm= £1.85, 15cm × 15cm= £2.79, 15cm × 20cm= £4.81, 7.5cm × 7.5cm= £0.97, Heel Border dressing 20cm × 20.8cm= £5.69, Sacrum Border dressing 15cm × 15cm= £3.12, 18cm × 18cm= £3.75, 22.5cm × 22.5cm= £5.58

Kliniderm Foam Silicone Lite
Thin absorbent soft silicone dressing with polyurethane foam film backing
kliniderm Foam Silicone Lite dressing (Mediq Healthcare UK Ltd) 10cm × 10cm= £1.58, 15cm × 15cm= £3.72, 20cm × 50cm= £19.42, 6cm × 8.5cm= £1.28

Kliniderm Foam Silicone Lite Border
Thin absorbent soft silicone dressing with polyurethane foam film backing and adhesive border
Kliniderm Foam Silicone Lite Border dressing (Mediq Healthcare UK Ltd) 10cm × 10cm= £1.06, 15cm × 15cm= £3.52, 4cm × 5cm= £0.60, 5cm × 12.5cm= £1.51, 7.5cm × 7.5cm= £0.99

Mepilex
Absorbent soft silicone dressing with polyurethane foam film backing
Mepilex (Molnlycke Health Care Ltd) Heel dressing 13cm × 20cm= £5.70, 15cm × 22cm= £6.67, dressing 11cm × 20cm= £4.60, 20cm × 21cm= £7.63, 20cm × 50cm= £31.13, 5cm × 5cm= £1.31

Mepilex Border
Absorbent soft silicone dressing with polyurethane foam film backing and adhesive border
Mepilex Border (Molnlycke Health Care Ltd) Heel dressing 22cm × 23cm= £8.00, Sacrum dressing 15cm × 15cm= £3.53, 16cm × 20cm= £4.92, 22cm × 25cm= £8.02

Mepilex Lite
Thin absorbent soft silicone dressing with polyurethane foam film backing
Mepilex Lite dressing (Molnlycke Health Care Ltd) 10cm × 10cm= £2.33, 15cm × 15cm= £4.53, 20cm × 50cm= £28.61, 6cm × 8.5cm= £1.95

Mepilex Transfer
Soft silicone exudate transfer dressing
Mepilex Transfer dressing (Molnlycke Health Care Ltd) 10cm × 12cm= £3.80, 15cm × 20cm= £11.50, 20cm × 50cm= £29.39, 7.5cm × 8.5cm= £2.41

Mepilex XT
Absorbent soft silicone dressing with polyurethane foam film backing
Mepilex XT dressing (Molnlycke Health Care Ltd) 10cm × 11cm= £2.81, 11cm × 20cm= £4.64, 15cm × 16cm= £5.09, 20cm × 21cm= £7.69

UrgotulDuo
Non-adherent soft polymer wound contact dressing with absorbent pad
UrgotulDuo dressing (Urgo Ltd) 10cm × 12cm= £4.16, 15cm × 20cm= £9.66, 5cm × 10cm= £2.69

Vliwasorb Adhesive
Absorbent polymer dressing with non-adherent wound contact layer and adhesive border
Vliwasorb Adhesive dressing (Lohmann & Rauscher) 12cm × 12cm square= £3.64, 15cm × 15cm square= £4.92, 15cm × 25cm rectangular= £7.11

Soft polymer dressings without absorbent pad
Adaptic Touch
Non-adherent soft silicone wound contact dressing
Adaptic Touch dressing (Systagenix Wound Management Ltd) 12.7cm × 15cm= £4.91, 20cm × 32cm= £13.20, 5cm × 7.6cm= £1.19, 7.6cm × 11cm= £2.38

Askina SilNet
Soft silicone-coated wound contact dressing
Askina SilNet dressing (B.Braun Medical Ltd) 10cm × 18cm= £5.47

Kliniderm Silicone
Soft silicone, thin, transparent wound contact dressing
Kliniderm Silicone wound contact layer dressing (Mediq Healthcare UK Ltd) 10cm × 18cm= £4.33, 12cm × 15cm= £4.33, 20cm × 30cm= £12.52, 24cm × 27.5cm= £13.03, 5cm × 7.5cm= £1.11, 7.5cm × 10cm= £2.00

Mepitel
Soft silicone, semi-transparent wound contact dressing
Mepitel dressing (Molnlycke Health Care Ltd) 12cm × 15cm= £5.91, 20cm × 32cm= £16.69, 5cm × 7cm= £1.48, 8cm × 10cm= £2.96

Mepitel One
Soft silicone, thin, transparent wound contact dressing
Mepitel One dressing (Molnlycke Health Care Ltd) 13cm × 15cm= £5.22, 24cm × 27.5cm= £14.92, 27.5cm × 50cm= £40.36, 6cm × 7cm= £1.28, 9cm × 10cm= £2.52

Silflex
Soft silicone-coated polyester wound contact dressing
Silflex dressing (Advancis Medical) 12cm × 15cm= £5.32, 20cm × 30cm= £13.70, 35cm × 60cm= £45.97, 5cm × 7cm= £1.29, 8cm × 10cm= £2.65

Silon-TSR
Soft silicone polymer wound contact dressing
Silon-TSR dressing (Bio Med Sciences) 13cm × 13cm= £3.52, 13cm × 25cm= £5.47, 28cm × 30cm= £7.37

Tegaderm Contact
Non-adherent soft polymer wound contact dressing
Tegaderm Contact dressing (3M Health Care Ltd) 20cm × 25cm= £11.06, 7.5cm × 10cm= £2.32

Urgotul
Non-adherent soft polymer wound contact dressing
Urgotul dressing (Urgo Ltd) 10cm × 10cm= £3.18, 10cm × 40cm= £10.68, 15cm × 15cm= £6.75, 15cm × 20cm= £8.99, 20cm × 30cm= £14.45, 5cm × 5cm= £1.59

Hydrocolloid dressings
Hydrocolloid dressings are usually presented as a hydrocolloid layer on a vapour-permeable film or foam pad. Semi-permeable to water vapour and oxygen, these dressings form a gel in the presence of exudate to facilitate rehydration in lightly to moderately exuding wounds and promote autolytic debridement of dry, sloughy, or necrotic wounds; they are also suitable for promoting granulation. Hydrocolloid-fibrous dressings made from modified carmellose fibres resemble alginate dressings; hydrocolloid-fibrous dressings are more absorptive and suitable for moderately to heavily exuding wounds.

Hydrocolloid dressings with adhesive border
Biatain Super
Semi-permeable hydrocolloid dressing; with adhesive border
Biatain Super dressing (adhesive) (Coloplast Ltd) 10cm × 10cm square= £2.39, 12.5cm × 12.5cm square= £3.95, 12cm × 20cm rectangular= £3.96, 15cm × 15cm square= £4.76, 20cm × 20cm square= £7.43

Granuflex Bordered
Hydrocolloid wound contact layer bonded to plastic foam layer, with outer semi-permeable polyurethane film
Granuflex Bordered dressing (ConvaTec Ltd) 10cm × 10cm square= £3.66, 10cm × 13cm triangular= £4.32, 15cm × 15cm square= £6.99, 6cm × 6cm square= £1.93

Hydrocoll Border
Hydrocolloid dressing with adhesive border and absorbent wound contact pad
Hydrocoll Border (bevelled edge) dressing (Paul Hartmann Ltd) 10cm × 10cm square= £2.67, 12cm × 18cm sacral= £4.00, 15cm × 15cm square= £5.02, 5cm × 5cm square= £1.12, 7.5cm × 7.5cm square= £1.83, 8cm × 12cm concave= £2.35

Tegaderm Hydrocolloid
Hydrocolloid dressing with adhesive border; normal or thin
Tegaderm Hydrocolloid (3M Health Care Ltd) Thin dressing 10cm × 12cm oval= £1.62, 13cm × 15cm oval= £3.03, dressing 10cm × 12cm oval= £2.44, 13cm × 15cm oval= £4.55, 17.1cm × 16.1cm sacral= £5.09

Hydrocolloid dressings without adhesive border
Biatain Super
Semi-permeable, hydrocolloid film dressing without adhesive border
Biatain Super dressing (non-adhesive) (Coloplast Ltd) 10cm × 10cm square= £2.39, 12.5cm × 12.5cm square= £3.95, 12cm × 20cm rectangular= £3.96, 15cm × 15cm square= £4.76, 20cm × 20cm square= £7.43

Comfeel Plus
Hydrocolloid dressings containing carmellose sodium and calcium alginate
Comfeel Plus dressing (Coloplast Ltd) 10cm × 10cm square= £2.73, 15cm × 15cm square= £5.85, 17cm × 17cm sacral= £6.18, 20cm × 20cm square= £8.42, 4cm × 6cm rectangular= £1.07

Comfeel Plus Contour
Hydrocolloid dressings containing carmellose sodium and calcium alginate
Comfeel Plus Contour dressing (Coloplast Ltd) 6cm × 8cm= £2.47, 9cm × 11cm= £4.29

Comfeel Plus Transparent
Hydrocolloid dressings containing carmellose sodium and calcium alginate
Comfeel Plus Transparent dressing (Coloplast Ltd) 10cm × 10cm square= £1.42, 15cm × 15cm square= £3.72, 15cm × 20cm rectangular= £3.77, 20cm × 20cm square= £3.80, 5cm × 15cm rectangular= £1.77, 5cm × 25cm rectangular= £2.87, 5cm × 7cm rectangular= £0.75, 9cm × 14cm rectangular= £2.71, 9cm × 25cm rectangular= £3.85

DuoDERM Extra Thin
Semi-permeable hydrocolloid dressing
DuoDERM Extra Thin dressing (ConvaTec Ltd) 10cm × 10cm square= £1.45, 15cm × 15cm square= £3.13, 5cm × 10cm rectangular= £0.85, 7.5cm × 7.5cm square= £0.88, 9cm × 15cm rectangular= £1.94, 9cm × 25cm rectangular= £3.10, 9cm × 35cm rectangular= £4.33

DuoDERM Signal
Semi-permeable hydrocolloid dressing with 'Time to change' indicator
DuoDERM Signal dressing (ConvaTec Ltd) 10cm × 10cm square= £2.33, 14cm × 14cm square= £4.08, 20cm × 20cm square= £8.11

Flexigran
Semi-permeable hydrocolloid dressing without adhesive border; normal or thin
Flexigran (A1 Pharmaceuticals) Thin dressing 10cm × 10cm square= £1.08, dressing 10cm × 10cm square= £2.19

Granuflex
Hydrocolloid wound contact layer bonded to plastic foam layer, with outer semi-permeable polyurethane film
Granuflex (modified) dressing (ConvaTec Ltd) 10cm × 10cm square= £3.07, 15cm × 15cm square= £5.83, 20cm × 20cm square= £8.77

Hydrocoll Basic
Hydrocolloid dressing with absorbent wound contact pad
Hydrocoll Basic dressing (Paul Hartmann Ltd) 10cm × 10cm square= £2.72

Hydrocoll Thin Film
Thin hydrocolloid dressing with absorbent wound contact pad
Hydrocoll Thin Film dressing (Paul Hartmann Ltd) 10cm × 10cm square= £1.28, 15cm × 15cm square= £2.88, 7.5cm × 7.5cm square= £0.77

Nu-Derm
Semi-permeable hydrocolloid dressing; normal and thin
Nu-Derm dressing (Systagenix Wound Management Ltd) 10cm × 10cm square= £1.57, 15cm × 15cm square= £3.21, 15cm × 18cm sacral= £4.56, 20cm × 20cm square= £6.41, 5cm × 5cm square= £0.86, 8cm × 12cm heel/elbow= £3.21, thin 10cm × 10cm square= £1.07

Tegaderm Hydrocolloid
Hydrocolloid dressing without adhesive border; normal and thin
Tegaderm Hydrocolloid (3M Health Care Ltd) Thin dressing 10cm × 10cm square= £1.63, dressing 10cm × 10cm square= £2.49

Hydrocolloid-fibrous dressings
Aquacel
Soft non-woven pad containing hydrocolloid fibres
Aquacel Ribbon dressing (ConvaTec Ltd) 1cm × 45cm= £2.05, 2cm × 45cm= £2.69

Aquacel Foam
Soft non-woven pad containing hydrocolloid fibres with foam layer; with or without adhesive border
Aquacel Foam dressing (ConvaTec Ltd) (adhesive) 10cm × 10cm= £2.35, 10cm × 20cm= £2.91, 10cm × 30cm= £5.44, 12.5cm × 12.5cm= £2.91, 15cm × 15cm= £4.17, 17.5cm × 17.5cm= £5.83, 19.8cm × 14cm heel= £5.96, 20cm × 16.9cm sacral= £5.35, 21cm × 21cm= £8.53, 24cm × 21.5cm sacral= £5.98, 25cm × 30cm=

£11.04, 8cm × 13cm= £2.50, 8cm × 8cm= £1.52, (non-adhesive) 10cm × 10cm= £2.78, 10cm × 20cm= £3.85, 15cm × 15cm= £4.67, 15cm × 20cm= £6.51, 20cm × 20cm= £7.62, 5cm × 5cm= £1.47

UrgoClean Pad
Pad, hydrocolloid fibres coated with soft-adherent lipo-colloidal wound contact layer
UrgoClean Pad dressing (Urgo Ltd) 10cm × 10cm square= £2.31, 15cm × 15cm square= £4.18, 20cm × 15cm rectangular= £4.34, 6cm × 6cm square= £1.04

UrgoClean Rope
Rope, non-woven rope containing hydrocolloid fibres
UrgoClean Rope dressing (Urgo Ltd) 2.5cm × 40cm= £2.59, 5cm × 40cm= £3.43

Polyurethane matrix dressings
Cutinova Hydro
Polyurethane matrix with absorbent particles and waterproof polyurethane film
Cutinova Hydro dressing (Smith & Nephew Healthcare Ltd) 10cm × 10cm square= £2.79, 15cm × 20cm rectangular= £5.91, 5cm × 6cm rectangular= £1.39

Foam dressings
Dressings containing hydrophilic polyurethane foam (adhesive or non-adhesive), with or without plastic film-backing, are suitable for all types of exuding wounds, but not for dry wounds; some foam dressings have a moisture-sensitive film backing with variable permeability dependant on the level of exudate. Foam dressings vary in their ability to absorb exudate; some are suitable only for lightly to moderately exuding wounds, others have greater fluid-handling capacity and are suitable for heavily exuding wounds. Saturated foam dressings can cause maceration of healthy skin if left in contact with the wound. Foam dressings can be used in combination with other primary wound contact dressings. If used under compression bandaging or compression garments, the fluid-handling capacity of the foam dressing may be reduced. Foam dressings can also be used to provide a protective cushion for fragile skin. A foam dressing containing ibuprofen is available and may be useful for treating painful exuding wounds.

Polyurethane foam dressings
Cutimed Cavity
Cutimed Cavity dressing (Essity UK Ltd) 10cm × 10cm= £3.43, 15cm × 15cm= £5.15, 5cm × 6cm= £2.06

Polyurethane foam film dressings with adhesive border
ActivHeal Foam Adhesive
ActivHeal Foam Adhesive dressing (Advanced Medical Solutions Ltd) 10cm × 10cm square= £1.69, 12.5cm × 12.5cm square= £1.74, 15cm × 15cm square= £2.23, 20cm × 20cm square= £4.67, 7.5cm × 7.5cm square= £1.22

Allevyn Adhesive
Allevyn Adhesive dressing (Smith & Nephew Healthcare Ltd) 10cm × 10cm square= £2.40, 12.5cm × 12.5cm square= £2.94, 12.5cm × 22.5cm rectangular= £4.57, 17.5cm × 17.5cm square= £5.79, 17cm × 17cm anatomically shaped sacral= £4.35, 22.5cm × 22.5cm square= £8.43, 22cm × 22cm anatomically shaped sacral= £6.27, 7.5cm × 7.5cm square= £1.64

Biatain Adhesive
Biatain Adhesive dressing (Coloplast Ltd) 10cm × 10cm square= £1.92, 12.5cm × 12.5cm square= £2.80, 15cm × 15cm square= £4.17, 17cm diameter contour= £5.44, 17cm × 17cm sacral= £2.55, 18cm × 18cm square= £5.66, 18cm × 28cm rectangular= £8.38, 19cm × 20cm heel= £5.66, 23cm × 23cm sacral= £4.84, 7.5cm × 7.5cm square= £1.16

Biatain Silicone
Biatain Silicone dressing (Coloplast Ltd) 10cm × 10cm= £2.35, 10cm × 20cm= £2.97, 10cm × 30cm= £5.72, 12.5cm × 12.5cm= £2.88, 15cm × 15cm= £4.28, 17.5cm × 17.5cm= £5.68, 7.5cm × 7.5cm= £1.60

PolyMem

PolyMem dressing (Mediq Healthcare UK Ltd) (adhesive) 5cm × 5cm square= £0.57, 8.9cm × 11.4cm rectangular= £2.39, 16.5cm × 20.9cm oval= £7.42, 18.4cm × 20cm sacral= £4.99, 5cm × 7.6cm oval= £1.27, 8.8cm × 12.7cm oval= £2.26

PolyMem Max

PolyMem Max dressing (Mediq Healthcare UK Ltd) 13.3cm × 13.3cm square= £3.21

PolyMem Silicone Border

PolyMem Silicone Border dressing (Mediq Healthcare UK Ltd) 16.5cm × 20.9cm oval= £9.70, 5cm × 7.6cm oval= £1.84, 8.8cm × 12.7cm oval= £3.55

Tegaderm Foam Adhesive

Tegaderm Foam dressing (adhesive) (3M Health Care Ltd) 10cm × 11cm oval= £2.48, 13.9cm × 13.9cm circular (heel)= £4.54, 14.3cm × 14.3cm square= £3.81, 14.3cm × 15.6cm oval= £4.57, 19cm × 22.2cm oval= £7.49, 6.9cm × 6.9cm soft cloth border= £1.84, 6.9cm × 7.6cm oval= £1.57

Polyurethane foam film dressings without adhesive border

ActivHeal Non-Adhesive Foam

ActivHeal Non-Adhesive Foam polyurethane dressing (Advanced Medical Solutions Ltd) 10cm × 10cm square= £1.17, 10cm × 20cm rectangular= £2.43, 20cm × 20cm square= £4.07, 5cm × 5cm square= £0.77

Advazorb

Advazorb (Advancis Medical) Heel dressing 17cm × 21cm= £5.26, dressing 10cm × 10cm square= £1.22, 10cm × 20cm rectangular= £3.77, 12.5cm × 12.5cm square= £1.79, 15cm × 15cm square= £2.36, 20cm × 20cm square= £4.23, 5cm × 5cm square= £0.72, 7.5cm × 7.5cm square= £0.88

Allevyn Non-Adhesive

Allevyn dressing (non-adhesive) (Smith & Nephew Healthcare Ltd) 10.5cm × 13.5cm heel (cup shaped)= £5.61, 10cm × 10cm square= £2.74, 10cm × 20cm rectangular= £4.40, 20cm × 20cm square= £7.36, 5cm × 5cm square= £1.38

Askina Foam

Askina Foam (B.Braun Medical Ltd) dressing 10cm × 10cm square= £2.41, Heel dressing 12cm × 20cm= £5.14

Biatain Non-Adhesive

Biatain Non-Adhesive dressing (Coloplast Ltd) 10cm × 10cm square= £2.61, 10cm × 20cm rectangular= £4.31, 15cm × 15cm square= £4.81, 20cm × 20cm square= £7.14, 5cm × 7cm rectangular= £1.44

Biatain-Ibu Non-Adhesive

Biatain-Ibu Non-Adhesive dressing (Coloplast Ltd) 10cm × 12cm rectangular= £3.63, 10cm × 22.5cm rectangular= £5.72, 15cm × 15cm square= £5.72, 20cm × 20cm square= £9.72, 5cm × 7cm rectangular= £1.89

Biatain-Ibu Soft-Hold

Biatain-Ibu Soft-Hold dressing (Coloplast Ltd) 10cm × 12cm rectangular= £3.63, 10cm × 22.5cm rectangular= £5.72, 15cm × 15cm square= £5.72

Kerraheel

Kerraheel (Crawford Healthcare Ltd) dressing 12cm × 20cm heel= £4.78

PermaFoam

PermaFoam (Paul Hartmann Ltd) Classic dressing (non-adhesive) 8cm × 8cm square (fenestrated) = £1.39

PolyMem

PolyMem dressing (Mediq Healthcare UK Ltd) 7cm × 7cm tube= £1.89, 9cm × 9cm tube= £2.40, finger/toe size 1= £2.75, 2= £2.75, 3= £2.75, 4= £3.29, 5= £3.57

PolyMem Max

PolyMem Max dressing (Mediq Healthcare UK Ltd) 11cm × 11cm square= £3.26, 20cm × 20cm square= £12.87

PolyMem Non-Adhesive

PolyMem dressing (non-adhesive) (Mediq Healthcare UK Ltd) 10cm × 10cm square= £2.72, 10cm × 61cm roll= £14.43, 13cm × 13cm square= £4.54, 17cm × 19cm rectangular= £6.70, 20cm × 60cm roll= £34.04, 8cm × 8cm square= £1.75

PolyMem WIC

PolyMem WIC dressing (Mediq Healthcare UK Ltd) 8cm × 8cm= £4.07

Tegaderm Foam

Tegaderm Foam dressing (3M Health Care Ltd) 10cm × 10cm square= £2.35, 10cm × 20cm rectangular= £3.99, 10cm × 60cm rectangular= £12.77, 20cm × 20cm square= £6.37, 8.8cm × 8.8cm square (fenestrated)= £2.40

Transorbent

Transorbent dressing (B.Braun Medical Ltd) (adhesive) 10cm × 10cm square= £2.13, 15cm × 15cm square= £3.91, 20cm × 20cm square= £6.25, 5cm × 7cm rectangular= £1.13

UrgoTul Absorb

UrgoTul Absorb dressing (Urgo Ltd) 10cm × 10cm= £2.52, 15cm × 20cm= £4.44, 6cm × 6cm= £1.28, 12cm × 19cm heel= £5.07

Alginate dressings

Non-woven or fibrous, non-occlusive, alginate dressings, made from calcium alginate, or calcium sodium alginate, derived from brown seaweed, form a soft gel in contact with wound exudate. Alginate dressings are highly absorbent and suitable for use on exuding wounds, and for the promotion of autolytic debridement of debris in very moist wounds. Alginate dressings also act as a haemostatic, but caution is needed because blood clots can cause the dressing to adhere to the wound surface. Alginate dressings should not be used if bleeding is heavy and extreme caution is needed if used for tumours with friable tissue. Alginate sheets are suitable for use as a wound contact dressing for moderately to heavily exuding wounds and can be layered into deep wounds; alginate rope can be used in sinus and cavity wounds to improve absorption of exudate and prevent maceration. If the dressing does not have an adhesive border or integral adhesive plastic film backing, a secondary dressing will be required.

ActivHeal Alginate

Calcium sodium alginate dressing

ActivHeal Alginate (Advanced Medical Solutions Ltd) Rope dressing 2.5cm × 30cm= £2.21, dressing 10cm × 10cm= £1.19, 10cm × 20cm= £2.94, 5cm × 5cm= £0.61

ActivHeal Aquafiber

Non-woven, calcium sodium alginate dressing

ActivHeal Aquafiber (Advanced Medical Solutions Ltd) Rope dressing 2cm × 42cm= £1.88, dressing 10cm × 10cm= £1.54, 15cm × 15cm= £2.89, 5cm × 5cm= £0.64

Algisite M

Calcium alginate fibre, non-woven dressing

Algisite M (Smith & Nephew Healthcare Ltd) Rope dressing 2cm × 30cm= £3.81, dressing 10cm × 10cm= £2.10, 15cm × 20cm= £5.64, 5cm × 5cm= £1.02

Biatain Alginate

Alginate and carboxymethylcellulose dressing, highly absorbent, gelling dressing

Biatain Alginate dressing (Coloplast Ltd) 10cm × 10cm= £2.53, 15cm × 15cm= £4.81, 44cm= £2.99, 5cm × 5cm= £1.07

Cutimed Alginate

Calcium sodium alginate dressing

Cutimed Alginate dressing (Essity UK Ltd) 10cm × 10cm= £1.72, 10cm × 20cm= £3.23, 5cm × 5cm= £0.82

Kaltostat

Calcium alginate fibre, non-woven

Kaltostat dressing (ConvaTec Ltd) 10cm × 20cm= £4.48, 15cm × 25cm= £7.70, 2g= £4.20, 5cm × 5cm= £1.05, 7.5cm × 12cm= £2.28

Melgisorb

Calcium sodium alginate fibre, highly absorbent, gelling dressing, non-woven

Melgisorb Cavity dressing (Molnlycke Health Care Ltd) 2.2cm × 32cm= £3.55

Sorbsan Flat

Calcium alginate fibre, highly absorbent, flat non-woven pads

Sorbsan Flat dressing (Aspen Medical Europe Ltd) 10cm × 10cm= £1.72, 10cm × 20cm= £3.22, 5cm × 5cm= £0.82

Sorbsan Ribbon
Alginate dressing bonded to a secondary absorbent viscose pad
Sorbsan Ribbon dressing (Aspen Medical Europe Ltd) 40cm= £2.06

Sorbsan Surgical Packing
Alginate dressing bonded to a secondary absorbent viscose pad
Sorbsan Packing dressing (Aspen Medical Europe Ltd) 2g= £3.50

Suprasorb A
Calcium alginate dressing
Suprasorb A (Lohmann & Rauscher) alginate dressing 10cm × 10cm= £1.35, 5cm × 5cm= £0.69, cavity dressing 2g= £2.51

Tegaderm Alginate
Calcium alginate dressing
Tegaderm Alginate dressing (3M Health Care Ltd) 10cm × 10cm= £1.82, 2cm × 30.4cm= £2.96, 5cm × 5cm= £0.86

Urgosorb
Alginate and carboxymethylcellulose dressing without adhesive border
Urgosorb (Urgo Ltd) Pad dressing 10cm × 10cm= £2.32, 10cm × 20cm= £4.25, 5cm × 5cm= £0.97, Rope dressing 30cm= £3.04

Capillary-acting dressings
Vacutex
Low-adherent dressing consisting of two external polyester wound contact layers with central wicking polyester/cotton mix absorbent layer
Vacutex dressing (Richardson Healthcare Ltd) 10cm × 10cm= £1.70, 10cm × 15cm= £2.29, 10cm × 20cm= £2.75, 5cm × 5cm= £0.96

Odour absorbent dressings
Dressings containing activated charcoal are used to absorb odour from wounds. The underlying cause of wound odour should be identified. Wound odour is most effectively reduced by debridement of slough, reduction in bacterial levels, and frequent dressing changes. Fungating wounds and chronic infected wounds produce high volumes of exudate which can reduce the effectiveness of odour absorbent dressings. Many odour absorbent dressings are intended for use in combination with other dressings; odour absorbent dressings with a suitable wound contact layer can be used as a primary dressing.

Askina Carbosorb
Activated charcoal and non-woven viscose rayon dressing
Askina Carbosorb dressing (B.Braun Medical Ltd) 10cm × 10cm= £1.62, 10cm × 20cm= £2.31

CarboFLEX
Dressing in 5 layers: wound-facing absorbent layer containing alginate and hydrocolloid; water-resistant second layer; third layer containing activated charcoal; non-woven absorbent fourth layer; water-resistant backing layer
CarboFlex dressing (ConvaTec Ltd) 10cm × 10cm= £3.56, 15cm × 20cm= £8.10, 8cm × 15cm oval= £4.28

Carbopad VC
Activated charcoal non-absorbent dressing
Carbopad VC dressing (Synergy Health (UK) Ltd) 10cm × 10cm= £1.62, 10cm × 20cm= £2.19

CliniSorb Odour Control Dressings
Activated charcoal cloth enclosed in viscose rayon with outer polyamide coating
CliniSorb dressing (CliniMed Ltd) 10cm × 10cm= £2.07, 10cm × 20cm= £2.76, 15cm × 25cm= £4.44

Antimicrobial dressings
Spreading infection at the wound site requires treatment with systemic antibacterials. For local wound infection, a topical antimicrobial dressing can be used to reduce the level of bacteria at the wound surface but will not eliminate a spreading infection. Some dressings are designed to release the antimicrobial into the wound, others act upon the bacteria after absorption from the wound. The amount of exudate present and the level of infection should be taken into account when selecting an antimicrobial dressing. Medical grade honey has antimicrobial and anti-inflammatory properties. Dressings impregnated with iodine can be used to treat clinically infected wounds. Dressings containing silver should be used only when clinical signs or symptoms of infection are present. Dressings containing other antimicrobials such as polihexanide (polyhexamethylene biguanide) or dialkylcarbamoyl chloride are available for use on infected wounds. Although hypersensitivity is unlikely with chlorhexidine impregnated tulle dressing, the antibacterial efficacy of these dressings has not been established.

Honey dressings
Medical grade honey has antimicrobial and anti-inflammatory properties and can be used for acute or chronic wounds. Medical grade honey has osmotic properties, producing an environment that promotes autolytic debridement; it can help control wound malodour. Honey dressings should not be used on patients with extreme sensitivity to honey, bee stings or bee products. Patients with diabetes should be monitored for changes in blood-glucose concentrations during treatment with topical honey or honey-impregnated dressings.
For *Actilite*®, *Activon Tulle*® and *Revamil*®, where no size is stated by the prescriber the 5 cm size is to be supplied. *Medihoney*® *Antimicrobial Wound Gel* is not recommended for use in deep wounds or body cavities where removal of waxes may be difficult.

Honey sheet dressings
Actilite
Knitted viscose impregnated with medical grade manuka honey and manuka oil
Actilite gauze dressing (Advancis Medical) 10cm × 10cm= £1.28, 10cm × 20cm= £2.48, 20cm × 30cm= £6.99, 30cm × 30cm= £11.57, 30cm × 60cm= £19.99, 5cm × 5cm= £0.74

Activon Tulle
Knitted viscose impregnated with medical grade manuka honey
Activon Tulle gauze dressing (Advancis Medical) 10cm × 10cm= £3.87, 5cm × 5cm= £2.35

Algivon
Absorbent, non-adherent calcium alginate dressing impregnated with medical grade manuka honey
Algivon dressing (Advancis Medical) 10cm × 10cm= £4.44, 5cm × 5cm= £2.59

Algivon Plus
Reinforced calcium alginate dressing impregnated with medical grade manuka honey
Algivon Plus (Advancis Medical) Ribbon dressing 2.5cm × 20cm= £4.38, dressing 10cm × 10cm= £4.38, 5cm × 5cm= £2.56

L-Mesitran Border
Hydrogel, semi-permeable dressing impregnated with medical grade honey, with adhesive border
L-Mesitran Border sheet (Mediq Healthcare UK Ltd) 10cm × 10cm square= £2.78

L-Mesitran Hydro
Hydrogel, semi-permeable dressing impregnated with medical grade honey, without adhesive border
L-Mesitran Hydro sheet (Mediq Healthcare UK Ltd) 10cm × 10cm square= £2.66

L-Mesitran Net
Hydrogel, non-adherent wound contact layer, without adhesive border
L-Mesitran Net sheet (Mediq Healthcare UK Ltd) 10cm × 10cm square= £2.57

Medihoney Antibacterial Honey Apinate
Non-adherent calcium alginate dressing, impregnated with medical grade honey

Medihoney Antibacterial Honey Apinate (Integra NeuroSciences Ltd) dressing 10cm × 10cm square= £3.57, 5cm × 5cm square= £2.10, rope dressing 1.9cm × 30cm= £4.41

Medihoney Antibacterial Honey Tulle
Woven fabric impregnated with medical grade manuka honey
Medihoney Tulle dressing (Integra NeuroSciences Ltd) 10cm x10cm= £3.13, 5cm × 5cm= £1.78

Medihoney Gel Sheet
Sodium alginate dressing impregnated with medical grade honey
Medihoney Gel Sheet dressing (Integra NeuroSciences Ltd) 10cm × 10cm= £4.41, 5cm × 5cm= £1.84

Medihoney HCS
Hydrogel colloidal dressing impregnated with medical grade manuka honey 63%, with adhesive border
Medihoney HCS dressing with adhesive border (Integra NeuroSciences Ltd) 11cm × 11cm square= £3.21, 15cm × 15cm square= £6.08

Medihoney HCS
Hydrogel colloidal dressing impregnated with medical grade manuka honey 63%, without adhesive border
Medihoney HCS dressing (Integra NeuroSciences Ltd) 11cm × 11cm square= £4.69, 20cm × 20cm square= £18.95, 20cm × 30cm rectangular= £29.48, 6cm × 6cm square= £2.35

Medihoney HCS Surgical
Hydrogel colloidal dressing impregnated with medical grade manuka honey, with adhesive border
Medihoney HCS Surgical dressing with adhesive border (Integra NeuroSciences Ltd) 7.5cm × 20cm = £3.20

Melladerm Plus Tulle
Knitted viscose impregnated with medical grade honey (Bulgarian, mountain flower) 45% in a basis containing polyethylene glycol
Melladerm Plus Tulle dressing (SanoMed Manufacturing BV) 10cm × 10cm= £2.10

Revamil
Polyacetate dressing impregnated with medical grade honey
Revamil dressing (Oswell Penda Pharmaceutical Ltd) 10cm × 10cm= £3.02, 10cm × 20cm= £5.52, 5cm × 5cm= £1.79, 8cm × 8cm= £3.04

Honey-based topical applications
Activon Honey
Medical grade manuka honey
Activon (Advancis Medical) Medical Grade Manuka Honey dressing= £2.89

L-Mesitran Ointment
Medical grade honey 48%
L-Mesitran (Mediq Healthcare UK Ltd) ointment dressing= £9.96

L-Mesitran SOFT
Medical grade honey 40%
L-Mesitran SOFT (Mediq Healthcare UK Ltd) ointment dressing= £3.64

MANUKApli Honey
Medical grade manuka honey
MANUKApli (Dot Medical Ltd) dressing= £5.90

Medihoney Antibacterial Medical Honey
Medical grade manuka honey
Medihoney Antibacterial Medical Honey (Integra NeuroSciences Ltd) dressing= £4.16

Medihoney Antibacterial Wound Gel
Medical grade manuka honey 80% in natural waxes and oils
Medihoney Antibacterial Wound Gel (Integra NeuroSciences Ltd) dressing= £4.22

Melladerm Plus Honey
Medical grade; Bulgarian (mountain flower) 45% in basis containing polyethylene glycol
Melladerm Plus (SanoMed Manufacturing BV) dressing= £8.50

Melloxy
Medical grade honey 40% in a basis containing propylene glycol

Melloxy (SanoMed Manufacturing BV) dressing= £8.76

Revamil Balm
Medical grade honey-based ointment
Revamil Balm (Oswell Penda Pharmaceutical Ltd) dressing= £7.88

Revamil Wound Gel
Medical grade honey
Revamil Wound Gel (Oswell Penda Pharmaceutical Ltd) dressing= £3.63

Iodine dressings
Cadexomer–iodine, like povidone–iodine, releases free iodine when exposed to wound exudate. The free iodine acts as an antiseptic on the wound surface, the cadexomer absorbs wound exudate and encourages de-sloughing. Two-component hydrogel dressings containing glucose oxidase and iodide ions generate a low level of free iodine in the presence of moisture and oxygen. Povidone–iodine fabric dressing is a knitted viscose dressing with povidone–iodine incorporated in a hydrophilic polyethylene glycol basis; this facilitates diffusion of the iodine into the wound and permits removal of the dressing by irrigation. The iodine has a wide spectrum of antimicrobial activity but it is rapidly deactivated by wound exudate. Systemic absorption of iodine may occur, particularly from large wounds or with prolonged use.
Iodoflex® and *Iodosorb*® are used for the treatment of chronic exuding wounds; max. single application 50 g, max. weekly application 150 g; max. duration up to 3 months in any single course of treatment. They are contra-indicated in patients receiving lithium, in thyroid disorders, in pregnancy and breast feeding, and in children; they should be used with caution in patients with severe renal impairment or history of thyroid disorder.
Iodozyme® is an antimicrobial dressing used for lightly to moderately exuding wounds. It is contra-indicated in thyroid disorders and in patients receiving lithium; it should be used with caution in children and in women who are pregnant or breast-feeding.
Oxyzyme® is used for non-infected, dry to moderately exuding wounds. It is contra-indicated in thyroid disorders and in patients receiving lithium; it should be used with caution in children and in women who are pregnant or breast-feeding.
Povidone-iodine Fabric Dressing is used as a wound contact layer for abrasions and superficial burns. It is contra-indicated in patients with severe renal impairment and in women who are pregnant or breast-feeding; it should be used with caution in patients with thyroid disease and in children under 6 months.

Iodoflex Paste
Iodine 0.9% as cadexomer–iodine in a paste basis with gauze backing
Iodoflex paste (Smith & Nephew Healthcare Ltd) dressing= £9.07

Iodosorb Ointment
Iodine 0.9% as cadexomer–iodine in an ointment basis
Iodosorb ointment (Smith & Nephew Healthcare Ltd) dressing= £5.01

Iodosorb Powder
Iodine 0.9% as cadexomer–iodine microbeads, 3-g sachet
Iodosorb powder (Smith & Nephew Healthcare Ltd) dressing sachets= £2.15

Povidone-iodine fabric dressings
Inadine
(Drug Tariff specification 43). Knitted viscose primary dressing impregnated with povidone–iodine ointment 10%
Inadine dressing (Systagenix Wound Management Ltd) 5cm × 5cm= £0.35, 9.5cm × 9.5cm= £0.51

Povitulle
(Drug Tariff specification 43). Non-adherent sterile gauze dressing impregnated with povidone–iodine 10%
Povitulle dressing (C D Medical Ltd) 5cm × 5cm= £0.29, 9.5cm × 9.5cm= £0.43

Other antimicrobial dressings

Cutimed Siltec Sorbact

Polyurethane foam dressing with acetate fabric coated with dialkylcarbamoyl chloride, with adhesive border

Cutimed Siltec Sorbact B dressing (Essity UK Ltd) 12.5cm × 12.5cm= £7.08, 15cm × 15cm= £8.78, 17.5cm × 17.5cm= £12.28, 22.5cm × 22.5cm= £18.68, 7.5cm × 7.5cm= £2.76, 17.5cm × 17.5cm sacral= £8.88, 23cm × 23cm sacral= £13.34

Cutimed Sorbact

Low adherence acetate tissue impregnated with dialkylcarbamoyl chloride; dressing pad, swabs, or ribbon gauze, cotton

Cutimed Sorbact (Essity UK Ltd) Contact swab 4cm × 6cm= £1.81, 7cm × 9cm= £3.02, Pad dressing 10cm × 10cm= £6.04, 10cm × 20cm= £9.43, 7cm × 9cm= £3.87, Ribbon dressing 2cm × 50cm= £4.43, 5cm × 200cm= £8.74

Cutimed Sorbact Gel

Hydrogel dressing impregnated with dialkylcarbamoyl chloride

Cutimed Sorbact Hydro dressing (Essity UK Ltd) 7.5cm × 15cm rectangular= £4.92, 7.5cm × 7.5cm square= £2.92

Cutimed Sorbact Hydroactive

Non-adhesive gel dressing with hydropolymer matrix and acetate fabric coated with dialkylcarbamoyl chloride

Cutimed Sorbact Hydroactive dressing (Essity UK Ltd) 14cm × 14cm= £5.90, 14cm × 24cm= £9.45, 19cm × 19cm= £11.11, 24cm × 24cm= £16.83, 7cm × 8.5cm= £4.04

Cutimed Sorbact Hydroactive B

Gel dressing with hydropolymer matrix and acetate fabric coated with dialkylcarbamoyl chloride, with adhesive border

Cutimed Sorbact Hydroactive B dressing (Essity UK Ltd) 10cm × 10cm= £7.79, 10cm × 20cm= £12.48, 15cm × 15cm= £14.66, 5cm × 6.5cm= £4.37

Cutimed Sorbion Sorbact

Wound contact layer coated with dialkylcarbamoyl chloride, with superabsorbent core and water repellent backing

Cutimed Sorbion Sorbact dressing (Essity UK Ltd) 10cm × 10cm square= £6.21, 10cm × 20cm rectangular= £9.70, 20cm × 20cm square= £16.78, 20cm × 30cm rectangular= £25.18

Flaminal Forte gel

Alginate with glucose oxidase and lactoperoxidase

Flaminal Forte gel (Flen Health UK Ltd) dressing= £8.58

Flaminal Hydro gel

Alginate with glucose oxidase and lactoperoxidase

Flaminal Hydro gel (Flen Health UK Ltd) dressing= £8.58

Kendall AMD

Foam dressing with polihexanide, without adhesive border

Kendall AMD Antimicrobial foam dressing (Mediq Healthcare UK Ltd) 10cm × 10cm square= £4.85, 10cm × 20cm rectangular= £9.19, 15cm × 15cm square= £9.19, 20cm × 20cm square= £13.46, 5cm × 5cm square= £2.57, 8.8cm × 7.5cm rectangular (fenestrated)= £4.36

Octenilin Wound Gel

Wound gel, hydroxyethylcellulose and propylene glycol, with octenidine hydrochloride

Octenilin Wound Gel (Schulke & Mayr UK Ltd) dressing= £5.15

Prontosan Wound Gel

Hydrogel containing betaine surfactant and polihexanide

Prontosan Wound Gel (B.Braun Medical Ltd) gel dressing= £7.01

Suprasorb X + PHMB

Biosynthetic cellulose fibre dressing with polihexanide

Suprasorb X + PHMB dressing (Lohmann & Rauscher) 14cm × 20cm rectangular= £12.80, 2cm × 21cm rope= £7.97, 5cm × 5cm square= £2.83, 9cm × 9cm square= £5.63

Chlorhexidine gauze dressings

Bactigras

Fabric of leno weave, weft and warp threads of cotton and/or viscose yarn, impregnated with ointment containing chlorhexidine acetate

Bactigras gauze dressing (Smith & Nephew Healthcare Ltd) 10cm × 10cm, 5cm × 5cm

Irrigation fluids

Octenilin Wound irrigation solution

Aqueous solution containing glycerol, ethylhexylglycerin and octenidine hydrochloride

Octenilin irrigation solution (Schulke & Mayr UK Ltd) 350ml bottles= £4.95

Prontosan Wound Irrigation Solution

Aqueous solution containing betaine surfactant and polihexanide

Prontosan irrigation solution (B.Braun Medical Ltd) 350ml bottles= £5.25, 40ml unit dose= £15.58

Silver dressings

Antimicrobial dressings containing silver should be used only when infection is suspected as a result of clinical signs or symptoms (see also Antimicrobial dressings p. 1937). Silver ions exert an antimicrobial effect in the presence of wound exudate; the volume of wound exudate as well as the presence of infection should be considered when selecting a silver-containing dressing. Silver-impregnated dressings should not be used routinely for the management of uncomplicated ulcers. It is recommended that these dressings should not be used on acute wounds as there is some evidence to suggest they delay wound healing. Dressings impregnated with silver sulfadiazine have broad antimicrobial activity; if silver sulfadiazine is applied to large areas, or used for prolonged periods, there is a risk of blood disorders and skin discoloration. The use of silver sulfadiazine-impregnated dressings is contra-indicated in neonates, in pregnancy, and in patients with significant renal or hepatic impairment, sensitivity to sulfonamides, or G6PD deficiency. Large amounts of silver sulfadiazine applied topically may interact with other drugs—see Appendix 1 (sulfonamides).

Alginate dressings with silver

ActivHeal Aquafiber Ag

Calcium alginate and carboxymethylcellulose dressing, with silver

ActivHeal Aquafiber Ag dressing (Advanced Medical Solutions Ltd) 10cm × 10cm square= £4.13, 15cm × 15cm square= £7.78, 2.7cm × 32cm rope= £4.20, 5cm × 5cm square= £1.73

Algicell Ag

Calcium alginate dressing, with silver

Algicell Ag (Gentell UK Ltd) dressing 10.1cm × 20.3cm= £7.08, 10.8cm × 10.8cm= £3.56, 20.3cm × 30.5cm= £19.00, 5cm × 5cm= £1.23, rope dressing 1.9cm × 30.5cm= £4.50

Algisite Ag

Calcium alginate dressing, with silver

Algisite Ag dressing (Smith & Nephew Healthcare Ltd) 10cm × 10cm= £4.54, 10cm × 20cm= £8.35, 2g= £6.27, 5cm × 5cm= £1.82

Askina Calgitrol Thin

Calcium alginate and silver alginate matrix, for use with absorptive secondary dressings

Askina Calgitrol Thin dressing (B.Braun Medical Ltd) 5cm × 5cm square= £2.16

Biatain Alginate Ag

Alginate and carboxymethylcellulose dressing, with ionic silver

Biatain Alginate Ag dressing (Coloplast Ltd) 10cm × 10cm= £4.36, 15cm × 15cm= £7.13, 3cm × 44cm= £4.71, 5cm × 5cm= £1.78

Melgisorb Ag

Alginate and carboxymethylcellulose dressing, with ionic silver

Melgisorb Ag (Molnlycke Health Care Ltd) Cavity dressing 3cm × 44cm= £4.95, dressing 10cm × 10cm= £3.97, 15cm × 15cm= £8.40, 5cm × 5cm= £1.98

Silvercel

Alginate and carboxymethylcellulose dressing impregnated with silver

Silvercel dressing (Systagenix Wound Management Ltd) 10cm × 20cm rectangular= £8.26, 11cm × 11cm square= £4.45, 2.5cm × 30.5cm rectangular= £4.79, 5cm × 5cm square= £1.80

Silvercel Non-Adherent

Alginate and carboxymethylcellulose dressing with film wound contact layer, impregnated with silver

Silvercel Non-Adherent (Systagenix Wound Management Ltd) cavity dressing 2.5cm × 30.5cm= £4.21, dressing 10cm × 20cm rectangular= £7.74, 11cm × 11cm square= £4.15, 5cm × 5cm square= £1.73

Sorbsan Silver Flat

Calcium alginate dressing, with ionic silver

Sorbsan Silver Flat dressing (Aspen Medical Europe Ltd) 10cm × 10cm= £4.00, 10cm × 20cm= £7.31, 5cm × 5cm= £1.58

Sorbsan Silver Ribbon

With silver

Sorbsan Silver Ribbon dressing (Aspen Medical Europe Ltd) 1g= £4.18

Sorbsan Silver Surgical Packing

With silver

Sorbsan Silver Packing dressing (Aspen Medical Europe Ltd) 2g= £5.80

Suprasorb A + Ag

Calcium alginate dressing, with silver

Suprasorb A + Ag (Lohmann & Rauscher) dressing 10cm × 10cm= £4.52, 10cm × 20cm= £8.35, 5cm × 5cm= £1.80, rope dressing 2g= £6.69

Urgosorb Silver

Alginate and carboxymethylcellulose dressing, impregnated with silver

Urgosorb Silver (Urgo Ltd) Rope dressing 2.5cm × 30cm= £4.03, dressing 10cm × 10cm= £4.01, 10cm × 20cm= £7.55, 5cm × 5cm= £1.68

Foam dressings with silver
Acticoat Moisture Control

Three-layer polyurethane dressing consisting of a silver-coated layer, a foam layer, and a waterproof layer

Acticoat Moisture Control dressing (Smith & Nephew Healthcare Ltd) 10cm × 10cm square= £18.44, 10cm × 20cm rectangular= £35.92, 5cm × 5cm square= £7.88

Allevyn Ag

Silver sulfadiazine-impregnated polyurethane foam film dressing, with or without adhesive border

Allevyn Ag (Smith & Nephew Healthcare Ltd) Adhesive dressing 10cm × 10cm square= £6.04, 12.5cm × 12.5cm square= £7.94, 17.5cm × 17.5cm square= £15.27, 17cm × 17cm sacral= £11.92, 22cm × 22cm sacral= £15.98, 7.5cm × 7.5cm square= £3.84, Heel Non-Adhesive dressing 10.5cm × 13.5cm= £11.82, Non-Adhesive dressing 10cm × 10cm square= £6.75, 15cm × 15cm square= £12.79, 20cm × 20cm square= £18.73, 5cm × 5cm square= £3.58

Biatain Ag

Silver-impregnated polyurethane foam film dressing, with or without adhesive border

Biatain Ag dressing (Coloplast Ltd) 10cm × 10cm square= £8.87, 10cm × 20cm rectangular= £16.30, 15cm × 15cm square= £17.80, 20cm × 20cm square= £25.11, 5cm × 7cm rectangular= £3.64

Biatain Silicone Ag

Silver-impregnated polyurethane foam film dressing, with silicone adhesive border

Biatain Silicone Ag dressing (Coloplast Ltd) 10cm × 10cm= £5.71, 10cm × 20cm= £9.66, 10cm × 30cm= £14.50, 12.5cm × 12.5cm= £7.47, 15cm × 15cm= £12.31, 17.5cm × 17.5cm= £13.62, 7.5cm × 7.5cm= £3.63, 15cm × 19cm sacral= £11.21, 18cm × 18cm heel= £15.05, 25cm × 25cm sacral= £24.04

PolyMem Silver

Silver-impregnated polyurethane foam film dressing, with or without adhesive border

PolyMem Silver (Mediq Healthcare UK Ltd) WIC dressing 8cm × 8cm= £7.77, dressing 10.8cm × 10.8cm square= £9.76, 12.7cm × 8.8cm oval= £6.17, 17cm × 19cm rectangular= £19.56, 5cm × 7.6cm oval= £2.51

Low adherence dressings with silver
Acticoat

Three-layer antimicrobial barrier dressing consisting of a polyester core between low adherent silver-coated high density polyethylene mesh (for 3-day wear)

Acticoat dressing (Smith & Nephew Healthcare Ltd) 10cm × 10cm square= £9.41, 10cm × 20cm rectangular= £14.71, 20cm × 40cm rectangular= £50.33, 5cm × 5cm square= £3.85

Acticoat 7

Five-layer antimicrobial barrier dressing consisting of a polyester core between low adherent silver-coated high density polyethylene mesh (for 7-day wear)

Acticoat 7 dressing (Smith & Nephew Healthcare Ltd) 10cm × 12.5cm rectangular= £19.94, 15cm × 15cm square= £35.85, 5cm × 5cm square= £6.69

Acticoat Flex 3

Conformable antimicrobial barrier dressing consisting of a polyester core between low adherent silver-coated high density polyethylene mesh (for 3-day wear)

Acticoat Flex 3 dressing (Smith & Nephew Healthcare Ltd) 10cm × 10cm square= £9.61, 10cm × 20cm rectangular= £15.02, 20cm × 40cm rectangular= £51.41, 5cm × 5cm square= £3.94

Acticoat Flex 7

Conformable antimicrobial barrier dressing consisting of a polyester core between low adherent silver-coated high density polyethylene mesh (for 7-day wear)

Acticoat Flex 7 dressing (Smith & Nephew Healthcare Ltd) 10cm × 12.5cm rectangular= £20.37, 15cm × 15cm square= £36.63, 2.5cm × 60cm= £10.31, 5cm × 5cm square= £6.84

Atrauman Ag

Non-adherent polyamide fabric impregnated with silver and neutral triglycerides

Atrauman Ag dressing (Paul Hartmann Ltd) 10cm × 10cm= £1.39, 10cm × 20cm= £2.72, 5cm × 5cm= £0.57

Silverlon Flex

Silver-plated nylon wound contact dressing (for 7-day wear)

Silverlon Flex dressing (Griffiths and Nielsen Ltd) 10cm × 10cm square= £6.60, 10cm × 20cm rectangular= £10.35, 20cm × 20cm square= £18.78, 5cm × 5cm square= £3.36

Odour absorbent dressings with silver
Actisorb Silver 220

Knitted fabric of activated charcoal, with one-way stretch, with silver residues, within spun-bonded nylon sleeve

Actisorb Silver 220 dressing (Systagenix Wound Management Ltd) 10.5cm × 10.5cm= £2.78, 10.5cm × 19cm= £5.05, 6.5cm × 9.5cm= £1.77

Soft polymer dressings with silver
Allevyn Ag Gentle

Soft polymer wound contact dressing, with silver sulfadiazine impregnated polyurethane foam layer, with or without adhesive border

Allevyn Ag Gentle (Smith & Nephew Healthcare Ltd) Border dressing 10cm × 10cm= £6.99, 12.5cm × 12.5cm= £8.98, 17.5cm × 17.5cm= £17.12, 7.5cm × 7.5cm= £4.65, dressing 10cm × 10cm= £6.75, 10cm × 20cm= £11.15, 15cm × 15cm= £12.55, 20cm × 20cm= £18.58, 5cm × 5cm= £3.62

Mepilex Ag

Soft silicone wound contact dressing with polyurethane foam film backing, with silver, with or without adhesive border

Mepilex Ag (Molnlycke Health Care Ltd) dressing 10cm × 10cm= £6.51, 10cm × 20cm= £10.99, 15cm × 15cm= £12.38, 20cm × 20cm= £18.34, 20cm × 50cm= £68.82, Border Ag dressing 10cm × 12.5cm= £6.71, 10cm × 20cm= £9.77, 10cm × 25cm= £12.23, 10cm × 30cm= £14.66, 15cm × 17.5cm= £12.32, 17cm × 20cm= £15.96, 7cm × 7.5cm= £3.71, Border Sacrum Ag dressing 18cm × 18cm= £12.57, 20cm × 20cm= £15.28, 23cm × 23cm= £20.07, Heel Ag dressing 13cm × 20cm= £13.92, 15cm × 22cm= £15.59

Urgotul Silver

Non-adherent soft polymer wound contact dressing, with silver

Wound management | Appendix 4

Urgotul Silver dressing (Urgo Ltd) 10cm × 12cm= £3.39, 15cm × 20cm= £9.59

Specialised dressings

Protease-modulating matrix dressings

Cadesorb Ointment
Cadesorb (Smith & Nephew Healthcare Ltd) ointment= £10.13

Catrix
Catrix dressing (Cranage Healthcare Ltd) sachets= £3.80

Kliniderm
Four-layer cellulose and polymer primary dressing
kliniderm superabsorbent dressing (Mediq Healthcare UK Ltd) 10cm × 10cm square= £0.51, 10cm × 15cm rectangular= £0.71, 10cm × 20cm rectangular= £0.88, 20cm × 20cm square= £1.02, 20cm × 30cm rectangular= £1.54, 20cm × 40cm rectangular= £2.05

Promogran
Collagen and oxidised regenerated cellulose matrix, applied directly to wound and covered with suitable dressing
Promogran dressing (Systagenix Wound Management Ltd) 123 square cm= £16.81, 28 square cm= £5.58

Promogran Prisma Matrix
Collagen, silver and oxidised regenerated cellulose matrix, applied directly to wound and covered with suitable dressing
Promogran Prisma dressing (Systagenix Wound Management Ltd) 123 square cm= £19.34, 28 square cm= £6.79

UrgoStart
Soft adherent polymer matrix containing nano-oligosaccharide factor (NOSF), with polyurethane foam film backing
UrgoStart dressing (Urgo Ltd) 10cm × 10cm= £6.70, 15cm × 20cm= £12.05, 6cm × 6cm= £4.84, 12cm × 19cm heel= £9.23

UrgoStart Contact
Non-adherent soft polymer wound contact dressing containing nano-oligosaccharide factor (NOSF)
UrgoStart Contact dressing (Urgo Ltd) 10cm × 10cm= £4.45, 15cm × 20cm= £10.62, 5cm × 7cm= £3.15

Silicone keloid dressings
Silicone gel and gel sheets are used to reduce or prevent hypertrophic and keloid scarring. They should not be used on open wounds. Application times should be increased gradually. Silicone sheets can be washed and reused.

Silicone gels
Bapscarcare
Silicone gel
Bapscarcare (Espere Healthcare Ltd) gel= £18.18

Ciltech
Silicone gel
Ciltech (Su-Med International (UK) Ltd) gel= £50.00

Dermatix
Silicone gel
Dermatix (Meda Pharmaceuticals Ltd) gel = £60.53

Kelo-cote UV
Silicone gel with SPF 30 UV protection
Kelo-cote UV (Alliance Pharmaceuticals Ltd) gel= £18.32

Kelo-cote gel
Silicone gel
Kelo-cote (Alliance Pharmaceuticals Ltd) gel= £52.26

Kelo-cote spray
Silicone spray
Kelo-cote (Alliance Pharmaceuticals Ltd) spray= £52.26

ScarSil
Silicone gel
ScarSil (Medigarments Ltd) gel= £16.92

Silgel STC-SE
Silicone gel
Silgel STC-SE (Nagor Ltd) gel= £19.00

Silicone sheets
Advasil Conform
Self-adhesive silicone gel sheet with polyurethane film backing
Advasil Conform sheet (Advancis Medical) 10cm × 10cm square= £6.04, 15cm × 10cm rectangular= £10.66

Bapscarcare T
Self-adhesive silicone gel sheet
Bapscarcare T sheet (Espere Healthcare Ltd) 10cm × 15cm rectangular= £9.62, 5cm × 30cm rectangular= £9.62, 5cm × 7cm rectangular= £3.37

Cica-Care
Soft, self-adhesive, semi-occlusive silicone gel sheet with backing
Cica-Care sheet (Smith & Nephew Healthcare Ltd) 15cm × 12cm rectangular= £31.34, 6cm × 12cm rectangular= £16.08

Ciltech
Silicone gel sheet
Ciltech sheet (Su-Med International (UK) Ltd) 10cm × 10cm square= £7.50, 10cm × 20cm rectangular= £12.50, 15cm × 15cm square= £14.00

Dermatix
Self-adhesive silicone gel sheet (clear- or fabric-backed)
Dermatix (Meda Pharmaceuticals Ltd) Clear sheet 13cm × 13cm square= £15.79, 13cm × 25cm rectangular= £28.53, 20cm × 30cm rectangular= £51.97, 4cm × 13cm rectangular= £6.88, Fabric sheet 13cm × 13cm square= £15.79, 13cm × 25cm rectangular= £28.53, 20cm × 30cm rectangular= £51.97, 4cm × 13cm rectangular= £6.88

Mepiform
Self-adhesive silicone gel sheet with polyurethane film backing
Mepiform sheet (Molnlycke Health Care Ltd) 4cm × 31cm rectangular= £12.01, 5cm × 7cm rectangular= £3.80, 9cm × 18cm rectangular= £14.87

Scar FX
Self-adhesive, transparent, silicone gel sheet
Scar Fx sheet (Medigarments Ltd) 10cm × 20cm rectangular= £18.60, 22.5cm × 14.5cm shaped= £13.95, 25.5cm × 30.5cm rectangular= £69.75, 3.75cm × 22.5cm rectangular= £13.95, 7.5cm diameter shaped= £9.88

Silgel
Silicone gel sheet
Silgel sheet (Nagor Ltd) 10cm × 10cm square= £13.50, 10cm × 30cm rectangular= £31.50, 10cm × 5cm rectangular= £7.50, 15cm × 10cm rectangular= £19.50, 20cm × 20cm square= £40.00, 25cm × 15cm shaped= £21.12, 30cm × 5cm rectangular= £19.50, 40cm × 40cm square= £144.00, 46cm × 8.5cm shaped= £39.46, 5.5cm diameter shaped= £4.00

Adjunct dressings and appliances

Surgical absorbents
Surgical absorbents applied directly to the wound have many disadvantages—dehydration of and adherence to the wound, shedding of fibres, and the leakage of exudate ('strike through') with an associated risk of infection. Gauze and cotton absorbent dressings can be used as secondary layers in the management of heavily exuding wounds (but see also Capillary-action dressings). Absorbent cotton gauze fabric can be used for swabbing and cleaning skin. Ribbon gauze can be used post-operatively to pack wound cavities, but adherence to the wound bed will cause bleeding and tissue damage on removal of the dressing—an advanced wound dressing (e.g. hydrocolloid-fibrous, foam, or alginate) layered into the cavity is often more suitable.

Cotton
Absorbent Cotton, BP
Carded cotton fibres of not less than 10 mm average staple length, available in rolls and balls
Absorbent cotton BP 1988 (Robert Bailey & Son Plc)

Absorbent Cotton, Hospital Quality
As for absorbent cotton but lower quality materials, shorter staple length etc.
Absorbent cotton hospital quality (Robert Bailey & Son Plc)

Gauze and cotton tissue
Gamgee Tissue (blue)
Consists of absorbent cotton enclosed in absorbent cotton gauze type 12 or absorbent cotton and viscose gauze type 2
Gamgee tissue blue label (Robinson Healthcare)

Gamgee Tissue (pink)
Consists of absorbent cotton enclosed in absorbent cotton gauze type 12 or absorbent cotton and viscose gauze type 2
Gamgee tissue pink label DT (Robinson Healthcare)

Gauze and tissue
Absorbent Cotton Gauze, BP 1988
Cotton fabric of plain weave, in rolls and as swabs (see below), usually Type 13 light, sterile
Absorbent cotton BP 1988 (Robert Bailey & Son Plc)
Alvita absorbent cotton BP 1988 (Alliance Healthcare (Distribution) Ltd)
Clini absorbent cotton BP 1988 (Clinisupplies Ltd)

Absorbent Cotton and Viscose Ribbon Gauze, BP 1988
Woven fabric in ribbon form with fast selvedge edges, warp threads of cotton, weft threads of viscose or combined cotton and viscose yarn, sterile
Vernaid Fast Edge ribbon gauze sterile (Vernacare International Ltd) 1.25cm, 2.5cm

Lint
Absorbent Lint, BPC
Cotton cloth of plain weave with nap raised on one side from warp yarns
Absorbent lint (Robinson Healthcare)
Alvita absorbent lint BPC (Alliance Healthcare (Distribution) Ltd)
Clini absorbent lint BPC (Clinisupplies Ltd)

Pads
Drisorb
Absorbent dressing pads, sterile
Drisorb dressing pad (Synergy Health (UK) Ltd) 10cm × 20cm= £0.17

PremierPad
Absorbent dressing pads, sterile
PremierPad dressing pad (Mediq Healthcare UK Ltd) 10cm × 20cm= £0.18, 20cm × 20cm= £0.25

Xupad
Absorbent dressing pads, sterile
Xupad dressing pad (Richardson Healthcare Ltd) 10cm × 12cm= £0.17, 10cm × 20cm= £0.19, 20cm × 20cm= £0.32, 20cm × 40cm= £0.48

Wound drainage pouches
Wound drainage pouches can be used in the management of wounds and fistulas with significant levels of exudate.

Eakin Access window
For use with *Eakin*® pouches
Eakin access window (Pelican Healthcare Ltd) large= £41.47, small= £41.04

Eakin Wound pouch, bung closure
Wound pouch, bung closure
Eakin wound drainage bag with bung closure (Pelican Healthcare Ltd) large= £112.56, medium= £82.94, small= £59.24, small plus= £69.87, and access window for horizontal wounds, extra large= £112.56, vertical wounds, extra large= £110.63, for horizontal wounds, extra large= £100.72, for vertical incision wounds, extra large= £100.72, for vertical wounds, extra large= £100.72, large= £73.08

Eakin Wound pouch, fold and tuck closure
Wound pouch, fold and tuck closure
Eakin wound drainage bag with fold and tuck closure (Pelican Healthcare Ltd) large= £100.72, medium= £77.02, small= £53.32, extra large= £88.87

Option Wound Manager
Wound drainage bag

Option wound manager bag (Oakmed Ltd) large= £172.87, medium= £145.04, oblong= £125.98, small= £141.89, square= £151.34, extra small= £127.57

Option Wound Manager with access port
Wound drainage bag, with access port
Option wound manager bag with access port (Oakmed Ltd) large= £184.79, medium= £151.34, oblong= £137.75, small= £148.19, square= £157.65, extra small= £139.49

Option Wound Manager, cut to fit
Wound drainage bag, cut to fit
Option wound manager bag (Oakmed Ltd) large= £90.88, medium= £86.77, small= £78.32

Welland Fistula bag
Wound drainage bag, cut to fit
Welland Fistula wound drainage bag (Welland Medical Ltd) = £90.17

Physical debridement pads
DebriSoft® is a pad that is used for the debridement of superficial wounds containing loose slough and debris, and for the removal of hyperkeratosis from the skin. *DebriSoft*® must be fully moistened with a wound cleansing solution before use and is not appropriate for use as a wound dressing.

DebriSoft Pad
Polyester fibres with bound edges and knitted outer surface coated with polyacrylate
Debrisoft pad (Lohmann & Rauscher) 10cm × 10cm= £7.10

Complex adjunct therapies

Topical negative pressure therapy
Topical negative pressure therapy accessories
Renasys
Soft port and connector
Renasys (Smith & Nephew Healthcare Ltd) Soft Port= £12.33, connector for use with soft port= £3.57

V.A.C.
Drape, gel for canister, Sensa T.R.A.C. Pad
SensaT.R.A.C.(KCI Medical Ltd) pad= £11.45
T.R.A.C.(KCI Medical Ltd) connector= £3.36
V.A.C.(KCI Medical Ltd) drape= £10.02, gel strips= £4.10

WoundASSIST gel strip
WoundASSIST (Huntleigh Healthcare Ltd) TNP gel strip= £3.37

Vacuum assisted closure products
Exsu-Fast kit 1
Dressing kit
Exsu-Fast (Synergy Health (UK) Ltd) dressing kit 1= £28.04

Exsu-Fast kit 2
Dressing kit
Exsu-Fast (Synergy Health (UK) Ltd) dressing kit 2= £35.83

Exsu-Fast kit 3
Dressing kit
Exsu-Fast (Synergy Health (UK) Ltd) dressing kit 3= £35.83

Exsu-Fast kit 4
Dressing kit
Exsu-Fast (Synergy Health (UK) Ltd) dressing kit 4= £28.04

V.A.C GranuFoam
Polyurethane foam dressing (with adhesive drapes and pad connector); with or without silver
V.A.C. GranuFoam (KCI Medical Ltd) Bridge dressing kit= £34.94, Silver with SensaT.R.A.C dressing kit medium= £40.80, small= £35.17, dressing kit large= £34.56, medium= £29.79, small= £25.03

V.A.C Simplace
Spiral-cut polyurethane foam dressings, vapour-permeable adhesive film dressings (with adhesive drapes and pad connector)
V.A.C. Simplace EX dressing kit (KCI Medical Ltd) medium= £31.98, small= £29.01

V.A.C WhiteFoam
Polyvinyl alcohol foam dressing or dressing kit

V.A.C. WhiteFoam dressing (KCI Medical Ltd) large= £18.58, small= £11.61, kit large= £35.98, small= £27.80

WoundASSIST
Wound pack and channel drain
WoundASSIST TNP dressing pack (Huntleigh Healthcare Ltd) medium/large= £23.85, small/medium= £20.81, channel drain medium/large= £23.85, small/medium= £20.81, extra large= £34.05

Wound drainage collection devices
ActiV.A.C.
Canister with gel
ActiV.A.C (KCI Medical Ltd) canister with gel= £30.99

S-Canister
Canister kit
S-Canister (Smith & Nephew Healthcare Ltd) kit= £19.00

V.A.C Freedom
Canister with gel
V.A.C. Freedom (KCI Medical Ltd) Canister with gel= £31.46

Venturi
Canister kit with solidifier
Venturi (Talley Group Ltd) Compact canister kit= £12.81, canister kit= £12.81

WoundASSIST
Canister
WoundASSIST (Huntleigh Healthcare Ltd) TNP canister= £20.30

Wound care accessories

Dressing packs
The role of dressing packs is very limited. They are used to provide a clean or sterile working surface; some packs shown below include cotton wool balls, which are not recommended for use on wounds.

Multiple Pack Dressing No. 1
Contains absorbent cotton, absorbent cotton gauze type 13 light (sterile), open-wove bandages (banded)
Vernaid (Synergy Health (UK) Ltd) multiple pack dressing

Non-drug tariff specification sterile dressing packs
Dressit
Vitrex gloves, large apron, disposable bag, paper towel, softswabs, adsorbent pad, sterile field
Dressit sterile dressing pack (Richardson Healthcare Ltd) medium/large gloves= £0.70, small/medium gloves= £0.70

Nurse It
Contains latex-free, powder-free nitrile gloves, sterile laminated paper sheet, large apron, non-woven swabs, paper towel, disposable bag, compartmented tray, disposable forceps, paper measuring tape
Nurse It sterile dressing pack (Medicareplus International Ltd) medium/large gloves= £0.73, small/medium gloves= £0.73

Polyfield Nitrile Patient Pack
Contains powder-free nitrile gloves, laminate sheet, non-woven swabs, towel, polythene disposable bag, apron
Polyfield Nitrile Patient Pack (Mediq Healthcare UK Ltd) large gloves= £0.52, medium gloves= £0.52, small gloves= £0.52

Sterile dressing packs
Vernaid
(Drug Tariff specification 10). Contains gauze and cotton tissue pad, gauze swabs, absorbent cotton wool balls, absorbent paper towel, water repellent inner wrapper
Vernaid (Synergy Health (UK) Ltd) sterile dressing pack

Sterile dressing packs with non-woven pads
Vernaid
(Drug Tariff specification 35). Contains non-woven fabric covered dressing pad, non-woven fabric swabs, absorbent cotton wool balls, absorbent paper towel, water repellent inner wrapper
Vernaid (Synergy Health (UK) Ltd) sterile dressing pack with non-woven pads

Woven and fabric swabs
Gauze Swab, PB 1988
Consists of absorbent cotton gauze type 13 light or absorbent cotton and viscose gauze type 1 folded into squares or rectangles of 8-ply with no cut edges exposed, sterile or non-sterile
Alvita gauze swab 8ply (Alliance Healthcare (Distribution) Ltd) non-sterile 10cm × 10cm, sterile 7.5cm × 7.5cm
CS gauze swab 8ply (Clinisupplies Ltd) non-sterile 10cm × 10cm
Clini gauze swab 8ply (Clinisupplies Ltd) non-sterile 10cm × 10cm, sterile 7.5cm × 7.5cm
Gauze swab 8ply (Robert Bailey & Son Plc) non-sterile 10cm × 10cm
MeCoBo gauze swab 8ply (MeCoBo Ltd) non-sterile 10cm × 10cm, sterile 7.5cm × 7.5cm
Sovereign gauze swab 8ply (Waymade Healthcare Plc) sterile 7.5cm × 7.5cm
Steraid gauze swab 8ply (Robert Bailey & Son Plc) sterile 7.5cm × 7.5cm
Vernaid gauze swab 8ply (Synergy Health (UK) Ltd) non-sterile 10cm × 10cm, sterile 7.5cm × 7.5cm

Non-woven Fabric Swab
(Drug Tariff specification 28). Consists of non-woven fabric folded 4-ply; alternative to gauze swabs, type 13 light, sterile or non-sterile
CS non-woven fabric swab 4ply (Clinisupplies Ltd) non-sterile 10cm × 10cm
Clini non-woven fabric swab 4ply (Clinisupplies Ltd) non-sterile 10cm × 10cm, sterile 7.5cm × 7.5cm
CliniMed non-woven fabric swab 4ply (CliniMed Ltd) non-sterile 10cm × 10cm
MeCoBo non-woven fabric swab 4ply (MeCoBo Ltd) non-sterile 10cm × 10cm
Sofsorb non-woven fabric swab 4ply (Vernacare International Ltd) non-sterile 10cm × 10cm, sterile 7.5cm × 7.5cm
Softswab non-woven fabric swab 4ply (Richardson Healthcare Ltd) non-sterile 10cm × 10cm, sterile 7.5cm × 7.5cm
Topper 8 non-woven fabric swab 4ply (Systagenix Wound Management Ltd) non-sterile 10cm × 10cm

Filmated non-woven fabric swabs
Regal
(Drug Tariff specification 29). Film of viscose fibres enclosed within non-woven viscose fabric folded 8-ply, non-sterile
Regal filmated swab 8ply (Systagenix Wound Management Ltd) 10cm × 10cm

Surgical adhesive tapes
Adhesive tapes are useful for retaining dressings on joints or awkward body parts. These tapes, particularly those containing rubber, can cause irritant and allergic reactions in susceptible patients; synthetic adhesives have been developed to overcome this problem, but they, too, may sometimes be associated with reactions. Synthetic adhesive, or silicon adhesive, tapes can be used for patients with skin reactions to plasters and strapping containing rubber, or undergoing prolonged treatment.
Adhesive tapes that are occlusive may cause skin maceration. Care is needed not to apply these tapes under tension, to avoid creating a tourniquet effect. If applied over joints they need to be orientated so that the area of maximum extensibility of the fabric is in the direction of movement of the limb.

Occlusive adhesive tapes
Blenderm
(Impermeable Plastic Synthetic Adhesive Tape, BP 1988). Extensible water-impermeable plastic film spread with a polymeric adhesive mass
Blenderm (3M Health Care Ltd) tape 5cm= £3.58

Leukoplast Sleek
(Impermeable Plastic Adhesive Tape, BP 1988). Extensible water-impermeable plastic film spread with an adhesive mass
Leukoplast Sleek tape (Essity UK Ltd) 2.5cm, 5cm, 7.5cm

Permeable adhesive tapes

3M Micropore Silicone Tape
Soft silicone, water-resistant, knitted fabric, polyurethane film adhesive tape
3M Micropore Silicone tape (3M Health Care Ltd) 2.5cm= £3.71, 5cm= £6.71

Clinipore
(Permeable Non-Woven Synthetic Adhesive Tape, BP 1988). Backing of paper-based or non-woven textile material spread with a polymeric adhesive mass
Clinipore tape (Clinisupplies Ltd) 1.25cm= £0.37, 2.5cm= £0.76, 5cm= £1.04

Hypafix
(Permeable, Apertured Non-Woven Synthetic Adhesive Tape, BP 1988). Non-woven fabric with a polyacrylate adhesive
Hypafix tape (Essity UK Ltd) 10cm= £5.02, 15cm= £7.43, 2.5cm= £1.81, 20cm= £9.85, 30cm= £14.24, 5cm= £2.87

Insil
Soft silicone, water-resistant, knitted fabric, polyurethane film adhesive tape
Insil tape (Insight Medical Products Ltd) 2cm= £5.86, 4cm= £5.86

Leukofix
(Permeable Non-Woven Synthetic Adhesive Tape, BP 1988). Backing of paper-based or non-woven textile material spread with a polymeric adhesive mass
Leukofix tape (Essity UK Ltd) 1.25cm= £0.60, 2.5cm= £0.97, 5cm= £1.70

Leukopor
(Permeable Non-Woven Synthetic Adhesive Tape, BP 1988). Backing of paper-based or non-woven textile material spread with a polymeric adhesive mass
Leukopor tape (Essity UK Ltd) 1.25cm= £0.53, 2.5cm= £0.82, 5cm= £1.45

Mediplast
(Permeable Non-Woven Synthetic Adhesive Tape, BP 1988). Backing of paper-based or non-woven textile material spread with a polymeric adhesive mass
Mediplast tape (Neomedic Ltd) 1.25cm= £0.30, 2.5cm= £0.50

Mediplast
Fabric, plain weave, warp and weft of cotton and/or viscose, spread with an adhesive containing zinc oxide
Mediplast Zinc Oxide plaster (Neomedic Ltd) 1.25cm= £0.82, 2.5cm= £1.19, 5cm= £1.99, 7.5cm= £2.99

Mefix
(Permeable, Apertured Non-Woven Synthetic Adhesive Tape, BP 1988). Non-woven fabric with a polyacrylate adhesive
Mefix tape (Molnlycke Health Care Ltd) 10cm= £3.14, 15cm= £4.27, 2.5cm= £1.11, 20cm= £5.48, 30cm= £7.86, 5cm= £1.96

Mepitac
Soft silicone, water-resistant, knitted fabric, polyurethane film adhesive tape
Mepitac tape (Molnlycke Health Care Ltd) 2cm= £7.53, 4cm= £7.53

Micropore
(Permeable Non-Woven Synthetic Adhesive Tape, BP 1988). Backing of paper-based or non-woven textile material spread with a polymeric adhesive mass
Micropore tape (3M Health Care Ltd) 1.25cm= £0.66, 2.5cm= £0.97, 5cm= £1.72

Omnifix
(Permeable, Apertured Non-Woven Synthetic Adhesive Tape, BP 1988). Non-woven fabric with a polyacrylate adhesive
Omnifix tape (Paul Hartmann Ltd) 10cm= £4.49, 15cm= £6.62, 5cm= £2.66

OpSite Flexifix Gentle
Soft silicone, water-resistant, knitted fabric, polyurethane film adhesive tape
OpSite Flexifix Gentle tape (Smith & Nephew Healthcare Ltd) 2.5cm= £11.46, 5cm= £21.48

Primafix
(Permeable, Apertured Non-Woven Synthetic Adhesive Tape, BP 1988). Non-woven fabric with a polyacrylate adhesive
Primafix tape (Smith & Nephew Healthcare Ltd) 10cm= £2.56, 15cm= £3.79, 20cm= £4.66, 5cm= £1.75

Scanpor
(Permeable Non-Woven Synthetic Adhesive Tape, BP 1988). Backing of paper-based or non-woven textile material spread with a polymeric adhesive mass
Scanpor tape (Bio-Diagnostics Ltd) 1.25cm= £0.58, 2.5cm= £0.96, 5cm= £1.83, 7.5cm= £2.68

Siltape
Soft silicone, water-resistant, knitted fabric, polyurethane film adhesive tape
Siltape (Advancis Medical) 2cm= £6.51, 4cm= £6.51

Tensoplast
(Elastic Adhesive Tape, BP 1988). Woven fabric, elastic in warp (crepe-twisted cotton threads), weft of cotton and/or viscose threads, spread with adhesive mass containing zinc oxide
Tensoplast (Essity UK Ltd) elastic adhesive tape 2.5cm

Transpore
(Permeable Non-Woven Synthetic Adhesive Tape, BP 1988). Backing of paper-based or non-woven textile material spread with a polymeric adhesive mass
Transpore (3M Health Care Ltd) tape 5cm= £1.57

Zinc Oxide Adhesive Tape, BP 1988
Fabric, plain weave, warp and weft of cotton and/or viscose, spread with an adhesive containing zinc oxide
Fast Aid zinc oxide adhesive tape (Robinson Healthcare) 1.25cm, 2.5cm, 5cm, 7.5cm

Skin closure dressings
Skin closure strips are used as an alternative to sutures for minor cuts and lacerations. Skin tissue adhesive can be used for closure of minor skin wounds and for additional suture support.

Skin closure strips, sterile

Leukostrip
Drug Tariff specifies that these are specifically for personal administration by the prescriber
Leukostrip (Smith & Nephew Healthcare Ltd) skin closure strips 6.4mm × 76mm= £6.94

Omnistrip
Drug Tariff specifies that these are specifically for personal administration by the prescriber
Omnistrip (Paul Hartmann Ltd) skin closure strips sterile 6mm × 76mm= £26.77

Steri-strip
Drug Tariff specifies that these are specifically for personal administration by the prescriber
Steri-strip (3M Health Care Ltd) skin closure strips 6mm × 75mm= £9.31

Bandages

Non-extensible bandages
Skin closure strips are used as an alternative to sutures for minor cuts and lacerations. Skin tissue adhesive can be used for closure of minor skin wounds and for additional suture support.

Open-wove Bandage, Type 1 BP 1988
Cotton cloth, plain weave, warp of cotton, weft of cotton, viscose, or combination, one continuous length
Clini open wove bandage Type 1 BP 1988 (Clinisupplies Ltd) 10cm × 5m, 2.5cm × 5m, 5cm × 5m, 7.5cm × 5m
Vernaid white open wove bandage (Synergy Health (UK) Ltd) 10cm × 5m, 2.5cm × 5m, 5cm × 5m, 7.5cm × 5m
White open wove bandage (Robert Bailey & Son Plc) 10cm × 5m, 2.5cm × 5m, 5cm × 5m, 7.5cm × 5m

Triangular Calico Bandage, BP 1980
Unbleached calico right-angled triangle
Clini triangular calico bandage BP 1980 (Clinisupplies Ltd) 90cm × 127cm
Triangular calico bandage (Essity UK Ltd) 90cm × 127cm

Light-weight conforming bandages

Lightweight conforming bandages are used for dressing retention, with the aim of keeping the dressing close to the wound without inhibiting movement or restricting blood flow. The elasticity of conforming-stretch bandages (also termed contour bandages) is greater than that of cotton conforming bandages.

Easifix
Fabric, plain weave, warp of polyamide filament, weft of cotton or viscose, fast edges, one continuous length, 4 m stretched (all)
Easifix bandage (Essity UK Ltd) 10cm × 4m= £0.55, 15cm × 4m= £0.94, 5cm × 4m= £0.38, 7.5cm × 4m= £0.46

Easifix K
Fabric, knitted warp of polyamide filament, weft of cotton or viscose, fast edges, one continuous length. 4 m stretched
Easifix K bandage (Essity UK Ltd) 10cm × 4m= £0.20, 15cm × 4m= £0.35, 2.5cm × 4m= £0.10, 5cm × 4m= £0.12, 7.5cm × 4m= £0.18

Hospiform
Fabric, plain weave, warp of polyamide, weft of viscose
Hospiform bandage (Paul Hartmann Ltd) 10cm × 4m= £0.21, 12cm × 4m= £0.26, 6cm × 4m= £0.15, 8cm × 4m= £0.19

K-Band
Fabric, knitted warp of polyamide filament, weft of cotton or viscose, fast edges, one continuous length. 4 m stretched
K-Band bandage (Urgo Ltd) 10cm × 4m= £0.31, 15cm × 4m= £0.54, 5cm × 4m= £0.22, 7cm × 4m= £0.28

Knit Fix
Fabric, knitted warp of polyamide filament, weft of cotton or viscose, fast edges, one continuous length. 4 m stretched
Knit Fix bandage (Robert Bailey & Son Plc) 10cm × 4m= £0.17, 15cm × 4m= £0.33, 5cm × 4m= £0.12, 7cm × 4m= £0.17

Knit-Band
Fabric, knitted warp of polyamide filament, weft of cotton or viscose, fast edges, one continuous length. 4 m stretched
Knit-Band bandage (Clinisupplies Ltd) 10cm × 4m= £0.18, 15cm × 4m= £0.32, 5cm × 4m= £0.11, 7cm × 4m= £0.16

Kontour
Fabric, plain weave, warp of polyamide filament, weft of cotton or viscose, fast edges, one continuous length, 4 m stretched (all)
Kontour bandage (Easigrip Ltd) 10cm × 4m= £0.40, 15cm × 4m= £0.66, 5cm × 4m= £0.28, 7.5cm × 4m= £0.35

Mollelast
Fabric, plain weave, warp of polyamide filament, weft of cotton or viscose, fast edges, one continuous length, 4 m stretched (all)
Mollelast bandage (Lohmann & Rauscher) 4cm × 4m= £0.33

Peha-haft
Polyamide and cellulose contour bandage, cohesive, latex-free
Peha-haft bandage (Paul Hartmann Ltd) 10cm × 4m= £0.84, 12cm × 4m= £1.00, 2.5cm × 4m= £0.81, 4cm × 4m= £0.52, 6cm × 4m= £0.62, 8cm × 4m= £0.74

Stayform
Fabric, plain weave, warp of polyamide filament, weft of cotton or viscose, fast edges, one continuous length, 4 m stretched (all)
Stayform bandage (Robinson Healthcare) 10cm × 4m= £0.40, 15cm × 4m= £0.69, 5cm × 4m= £0.29, 7.5cm × 4m= £0.36

Tubular bandages and garments

Tubular bandages are available in different forms, according to the function required of them. Some are used under orthopaedic casts and some are suitable for protecting areas to which creams or ointments (other than those containing potent corticosteroids) have been applied. The conformability of the elasticated versions makes them particularly suitable for retaining dressings on difficult parts of the body or for soft tissue injury, but their use as the only means of applying pressure to an oedematous limb or to a varicose ulcer is not appropriate, since the pressure they exert is inadequate. Compression hosiery reduces the recurrence of venous leg ulcers and should be considered for use after wound healing. Silk clothing is available as an alternative to elasticated viscose stockinette garments, for use in the management of severe eczema and allergic skin conditions.

Elasticated Surgical Tubular Stockinette, Foam padded is used for relief of pressure and elimination of friction in relevant area; porosity of foam lining allows normal water loss from skin surface.

For *Elasticated Tubular Bandage, BP 1993*, where no size stated by the prescriber, the 50 cm length should be supplied and width endorsed.

Non-elasticated Cotton Stockinette, Bleached, BP 1988 1m lengths is used as basis (with wadding) for Plaster of Paris bandages etc.; 6 m length, compression bandage.

For *Non-elasticated Ribbed Cotton and Viscose Surgical Tubular Stockinette, BP 1988*, the Drug Tariff specifies various combinations of sizes to provide sufficient material for part or full body coverage. It is used as protective dressings with tar-based and other steroid ointments.

Elasticated bandages and garments

Acti-Fast
(Drug Tariff specification 46). Lightweight plain-knitted elasticated tubular bandage
Acti-Fast 2-way stretch stockinette (L&R Medical UK Ltd) 10.75cm= £6.09, 17.5cm= £1.96, 20cm= £3.31, 3.5cm= £0.60, 5cm= £0.62, 7.5cm= £0.82

CliniFast
(Drug Tariff specification 46). Lightweight plain-knitted elasticated tubular bandage; various colours and sizes
CliniFast stockinette (Clinisupplies Ltd) 10.75cm= £6.27, 17.5cm= £1.90, 3.5cm= £0.58, 5cm= £0.60, 7.5cm= £0.80, clava 5-14 years= £7.10, 6 months-5 years= £6.16, cycle shorts large adult= £17.23, medium adult= £15.11, small adult= £13.25, gloves large adult= £5.29, large child/small adult= £5.29, gloves medium adult= £5.29, medium child= £5.29, gloves small child= £5.29, leggings (Blue, Pink, White) 11-14 years= £12.50, 2-5 years= £10.00, 5-8 years= £11.25, 8-11 years= £12.50, large adult= £17.45, medium adult= £15.30, small adult= £13.42, mittens 2-8 years= £3.13, 8-14 years= £3.13, up to 24 months= £3.13, socks 8-14 years= £3.15, up to 8 years= £3.13, tights (Blue, Pink, White) 6-24 months= £7.50, vest long sleeve (Blue, Pink, White) 11-14 years= £12.50, 2-5 years= £10.00, 5-8 years= £11.25, 6-24 months= £7.50, 8-11 years= £12.50, large adult= £17.45, medium adult= £15.30, small adult= £13.42, vest short sleeve large adult= £17.23, medium adult= £15.11, small adult= £13.25

Comfifast
(Drug Tariff specification 46). Lightweight plain-knitted elasticated tubular bandage; various colours and sizes
Comfifast stockinette (Vernacare International Ltd) 10.75cm= £6.04, 17.5cm= £1.83, 3.5cm= £0.56, 5cm= £0.58, 7.5cm= £0.77

Comfifast Easywrap
(Drug Tariff specification 46). Lightweight plain-knitted elasticated tubular bandage; various colours and sizes
Comfifast Easywrap stockinette (Vernacare International Ltd) clava 5-14 years= £6.75, 6 months-5 years= £5.85, leggings 11-14 years= £11.88, 2-5 years= £9.50, 5-8 years= £10.69, 8-11 years= £11.88, large adult= £16.58, medium adult= £14.54, small adult= £12.75, mittens 2-8 years= £2.97, 8-14 years= £2.97, up to 24 months= £2.97, socks 8-14 years= £2.97, up to 8 years= £2.97, tights 6-24 months= £7.13, vest long sleeve 11-14 years= £11.88, 2-5 years= £9.50, 5-8 years= £10.69, 6-24 months= £7.13, 8-11years= £11.88, large adult= £16.58, medium adult= £14.54, small adult= £12.75

Comfifast MultiStretch

(Drug Tariff specification 46). Lightweight plain-knitted elasticated tubular bandage; various colours and sizes

Comfifast MultiStretch 2-way stretch stockinette (Vernacare International Ltd) 10.75cm= £6.45, 17.5cm= £2.49, 3.5cm= £0.61, 5cm= £0.63, 7.5cm= £0.83

Easifast

(Drug Tariff specification 46). Lightweight plain-knitted elasticated tubular bandage; various colours and sizes

Easifast stockinette (Easigrip Ltd) 10.75cm= £7.23, 17.5cm= £1.91, 3.5cm= £0.65, 5cm= £0.69, 7.5cm= £0.94

Elasticated Tubular Bandage, BP 1993

(Drug Tariff specification 25). Fabric as for Elasticated Tubular Bandage with polyurethane foam lining; lengths 50 cm and 1 m

CLINIgrip bandage (Clinisupplies Ltd) 10cm size F= £0.78, 12cm size G= £0.81, 17.5cm size J= £0.98, 4.5cm size A= £0.65, 6.25cm size B= £0.65, 6.75cm size C= £0.69, 7.5cm size D= £0.70, 8.75cm size E= £0.78

Comfigrip bandage (Vernacare International Ltd) 10cm size F= £0.74, 12cm size G= £0.77, 6.25cm size B= £0.61, 6.75cm size C= £0.65, 7.5cm size D= £0.66, 8.75cm size E= £0.74

Surgrip bandage (Sigma Pharmaceuticals Plc) 10cm size F= £0.71, 12cm size G= £0.74, 6.25cm size B= £0.58, 6.75cm size C= £0.62, 7.5cm size D= £0.63, 8.75cm size E= £0.71

Tubigrip bandage (Molnlycke Health Care Ltd) 10cm size F= £2.20, 12cm size G= £2.54, 6.25cm size B= £1.92, 6.75cm size C= £2.03, 7.5cm size D= £2.03, 8.75cm size E= £2.20

easiGRIP bandage (Easigrip Ltd) 10cm size F= £0.75, 12cm size G= £0.78, 6.25cm size B= £0.62, 6.75cm size C= £0.66, 7.5cm size D= £0.68, 8.75cm size E= £0.75

Skinnies

(Drug Tariff specification 46). Lightweight plain-knitted elasticated tubular bandage; various colours and sizes

Skinnies Viscose stockinette (Dermacea Ltd) body suit (Blue, Ecru, Pink) 3-6 months= £18.24, 6-12 months= £20.54, up to 3 months= £18.24, clava (Blue, Ecru, Pink) 5-14 years= £8.72, 6 months-5 years= £7.60, gloves large (Beige, Blue, Ecru, Grey, Pink) adult= £6.02, child= £6.02, gloves medium (Beige, Blue, Ecru, Grey, Pink) adult= £6.02, child= £6.02, gloves small (Beige, Blue, Ecru, Grey, Pink) adult= £5.97, child= £5.97, knee length shorts (White) 11-14 years= £19.27, 2-5 years= £15.37, 5-8 years= £17.38, 6-24 months= £11.71, 8-11 years= £19.27, large adult= £28.23, medium adult= £26.05, small adult= £23.87, knee socks extra large (Black, Natural, White) adult 11+= £15.72, knee socks large (Black, Natural, White) adult 8-11= £15.72, child 2-4= £15.72, knee socks medium (Black, Natural, White) adult 6-8= £15.72, child 1-2= £15.72, knee socks small (Black, Natural, White) adult 4-6= £15.72, child 0-1= £15.72, leggings (Beige, Black, Blue, Ecru, Grey, Pink) 11-14 years= £19.39, 2-5 years= £15.49, 5-8 years= £17.50, 6-24 months= £11.81, 8-11 years= £19.39, large adult= £28.34, medium adult= £26.17, small adult= £23.98, mittens (Blue, Ecru, Pink) 2-8 years= £4.36, 8-14 years= £4.36, up to 24 months= £4.36, socks (Blue, Ecru, Pink) 6 months-8 years= £4.82, 8-14 years= £4.82, vest long sleeve (Beige, Black, Blue, Ecru, Grey, Pink) 11-14 years= £19.39, 2-5 years= £15.49, 5-8 years= £17.50, 6-24 months= £11.81, 8-11 years= £19.39, large adult= £28.34, medium adult= £26.17, small adult= £23.98, vest short sleeve (White) 11-14 years= £19.27, 2-5 years= £15.37, 5-8 years= £17.33, 6-24 months= £11.71, 8-11 years= £19.27, large adult= £28.23, medium adult= £26.05, small adult= £23.87, vest sleeveless (White) 11-14 years= £19.27, 2-5 years= £15.37, 5-8 years= £17.38, 6-24 months= £11.71, 8-11 years= £19.27, large adult= £28.23, medium adult= £26.05, small adult= £23.87

Tubifast 2-way stretch

(Drug Tariff specification 46). Lightweight plain-knitted elasticated tubular bandage; various colours and sizes

Tubifast 2-way stretch stockinette (Molnlycke Health Care Ltd) 10.75cm= £6.09, 20cm= £3.40, 3.5cm= £0.65, 5cm= £0.67, 7.5cm= £0.82, gloves extra small child= £6.15, medium/large adult= £6.15, small child= £6.15, small/medium adult, medium/large child= £6.15, leggings 11-14 years= £20.46, 2-5 years= £16.37, 5-8 years= £18.41, 8-11 years= £20.46, socks (one size)= £5.18,

tights 6-24 months= £11.83, vest long sleeve 11-14 years= £20.46, 2-5 years= £16.37, 5-8 years= £18.41, 6-24 months= £12.27, 8-11 years= £20.46

Non-elasticated bandages and garments

Cotton Stockinette, Bleached, BP 1988

Knitted fabric, cotton yarn, tubular length, 1m

Cotton stockinette bleached heavyweight (E Sallis Ltd) 10cm, 2.5cm, 5cm, 7.5cm

Silk clothing

DermaSilk

Knitted silk fabric, hypoallergenic, sericin-free

DermaSilk (Espere Healthcare Ltd) body suit 0-3 months= £41.20, 12-18 months= £43.66, 18-24 months= £44.75, 24-36 months= £44.84, 3-4 years= £46.02, 3-6 months= £41.29, 6-9 months= £42.47, 9-12 months= £43.57, boxer shorts male adult extra large/XX large= £44.99, medium/large= £44.99, extra small/small= £44.99, briefs 3-6 years boy= £23.45, girl= £23.45, briefs 7-10 years boy= £23.45, girl= £23.45, briefs female adult extra large-XX large= £33.47, medium-large= £33.47, extra small-small= £33.47, comfort socks adult 11 - 13= £19.77, 5 - 6 1/2= £19.77, 7 - 8 1/2= £19.77, 9 - 10 1/2= £19.77, eye mask= £10.87, facial mask adult= £22.60, child= £17.72, infant= £17.72, teen= £22.60, fingerless gloves 3-4 years= £15.77, 5-9 years= £15.77, XX large adult= £22.13, extra large adult= £22.13, large adult= £22.13, medium adult= £22.13, small adult= £22.13, gloves extra large adult= £22.34, gloves large adult= £22.39, gloves medium adult= £22.39, child= £15.95, gloves small adult= £22.39, child= £15.95, infant hat 0-3 months= £18.32, 12-24 months= £18.32, 3-12 months= £18.32, knee length undersocks longer length= £26.18, standard length= £26.18, leggings 0-3 months= £29.42, leggings 12-18 months= £31.84, leggings 18-24 months= £32.97, leggings 24-36 months= £33.02, leggings 3-4 years= £34.20, leggings 3-6 months= £29.48, leggings 6-9 months= £30.66, leggings 9-12 months= £31.78, leggings adult female XX large= £84.62, extra large= £84.62, large= £84.62, medium= £84.62, small= £84.62, leggings adult male XX large= £84.62, extra large= £84.62, large= £84.62, medium= £84.62, small= £84.62, mini shorts extra large-XX large adult female= £35.61, extra small-small adult female= £35.61, mini shorts medium-large adult female= £35.61, pyjamas 10-12 years= £88.55, 3-4 years= £76.74, 5-6 years= £81.46, 7-8 years= £85.01, roll neck shirt 10-12 years= £58.81, 3-4 years= £50.88, 5-6 years= £54.28, 7-8 years= £56.54, round neck shirt adult female XX large= £83.64, extra large= £83.64, large= £83.64, medium= £83.64, small= £83.64, round neck shirt adult male XX large= £83.64, extra large= £83.64, large= £83.64, medium= £83.64, small= £83.64, soft cup bra extra large-XX large= £41.01, medium-large= £41.01, extra small-small= £41.01, thigh length undersocks longer length= £37.28, standard length= £37.28, tubular sleeves= £29.48, sleeves= £44.92, sleeves= £36.38, undersocks adult 11-13= £19.91, 5 1/2 - 6 1/2= £19.91, 7 - 8 1/2= £19.91, 9 - 10 1/2= £19.91, undersocks child 2-5= £19.91, 3-8= £19.91, 9-1= £19.91, unisex roll neck shirt adult XX large= £83.64, extra large= £83.64, large= £83.64, medium= £83.64, small= £83.64

DreamSkin

Knitted silk fabric, hypoallergenic, sericin-free, with methyacrylate copolymer and zinc-based antibacterial

DreamSkin (DreamSkin Health Ltd) baby leggings with foldaway feet 0-3 months= £25.92, 12-18 months= £28.89, 18-24 months= £29.43, 24-36 months= £29.96, 3-4 years= £31.04, 3-6 months= £26.44, 6-9 months= £27.82, 9-12 months= £28.36, body suit 0-3 months= £36.52, 12-18 months= £39.61, 18-24 months= £40.15, 24-36 months= £40.68, 3-4 years= £41.76, 3-6 months= £37.04, 6-9 months= £38.54, 9-12 months= £39.10, boxer shorts 11-12 years= £22.02, boxer shorts 3-4 years= £22.02, boxer shorts 5-6 years= £22.02, boxer shorts 7-8 years= £22.02, boxer shorts 9-10 years= £22.02, boxer shorts male adult XX large= £34.63, extra large= £34.63, large= £34.63, medium= £34.63, small= £34.63, briefs 11-12 years= £22.02, briefs 3-4 years= £22.02, briefs 5-6 years= £22.02, briefs 7-8 years= £22.02, briefs 9-10 years= £22.02, briefs female adult XX large= £32.53, extra large= £32.53, large= £32.53, medium= £32.53, small= £32.53, eye mask= £10.46, footless leggings 11-12 years= £34.15, footless leggings 3-4 years= £31.04, footless leggings 5-6 years= £32.57, footless leggings 7-8 years= £33.10, footless leggings 9-10 years= £33.62, footless leggings adult female XX large= £78.55, extra large= £78.55, large= £78.55, medium= £78.55, small= £78.55, footless leggings adult male XX large= £78.55, extra large= £78.55, large= £78.55, medium= £78.55, small= £78.55, gloves extra large adult= £20.62, gloves large adult= £20.62, gloves medium adult= £20.62, child= £14.69, gloves small adult= £20.62, child= £14.69, head mask child= £16.08, infant= £16.08, teenager= £20.98, head/facial mask adult= £20.98, heel-less undersocks= £24.30, liner socks adult female 4 - 5 1/2= £18.48, 6 - 8 1/2= £18.48, liner socks adult male 6 - 8 1/2= £18.48, 9 - 11= £18.48, liner socks child 12 1/2 - 3 1/2= £18.48, 3 - 5 1/2= £18.48, 4 - 5 1/2= £18.48, 6 - 8 1/2= £18.48, 9 - 12= £18.48, polo neck shirt 11-12 years= £54.59, polo neck shirt 3-4 years= £47.23, polo neck shirt 5-6 years= £50.39, polo neck shirt 7-8 years= £52.49, polo neck shirt 9-10 years= £53.54, polo neck shirt adult female XX large= £77.64, extra large= £77.64, large= £77.64, medium= £77.64, small= £77.64, polo neck shirt adult male XX large= £77.64, extra large= £77.64, large= £77.64, medium= £77.64, small= £77.64, pyjamas 11-12 years= £80.35, 3-4 years= £69.63, 5-6 years= £73.92, 7-8 years= £77.13, 9-10 years= £78.77, round neck shirt 11-12 years= £53.55, round neck shirt 3-4 years= £47.24, round neck shirt 5-6 years= £49.34, round neck shirt 7-8 years= £51.45, round neck shirt 9-10 years= £52.50, round neck shirt adult female XX large= £77.64, extra large= £77.64, large= £77.64, medium= £77.64, small= £77.64, round neck shirt adult male XX large= £77.64, extra large= £77.64, large= £77.64, medium= £77.64, small= £77.64, tubular sleeves-50cm = £33.77, tubular sleeves-33cm= £27.15

Support bandages

Light support bandages, which include the various forms of crepe bandage, are used in the prevention of oedema; they are also used to provide support for mild sprains and joints but their effectiveness has not been proven for this purpose. Since they have limited extensibility, they are able to provide light support without exerting undue pressure. For a warning against injudicious compression see Compression bandages.

Cotton Crepe Bandage, BP 1988
Fabric, plain weave, warp of crepe-twisted cotton threads, weft of cotton and/or viscose threads; stretch bandage. 4.5 m stretched (both)
Elastocrepe bandage (Essity UK Ltd) 10cm × 4.5m, 7.5cm × 4.5m
Flexocrepe bandage (Robinson Healthcare) 10cm × 4.5m, 7.5cm × 4.5m
Sterocrepe bandage (Steroplast Healthcare Ltd) 10cm × 4.5m, 7.5cm × 4.5m

Crepe Bandage, BP 1988
Fabric, plain weave, warp of wool threads and crepe-twisted cotton threads, weft of cotton threads; stretch bandage; 4.5 m stretched
Alvita crepe bandage (Alliance Healthcare (Distribution) Ltd) 10cm × 4.5m, 15cm × 4.5m, 5cm × 4.5m, 7.5cm × 4.5m
Clinicrepe bandage (Clinisupplies Ltd) 10cm × 4.5m, 15cm × 4.5m, 5cm × 4.5m, 7.5cm × 4.5m
Crepe bandage (Robert Bailey & Son Plc) 10cm × 4.5m, 15cm × 4.5m, 5cm × 4.5m, 7.5cm × 4.5m
Propax crepe bandage (Essity UK Ltd) 10cm × 4.5m, 15cm × 4.5m, 5cm × 4.5m, 7.5cm × 4.5m

Elset
Knitted fabric, viscose and elastomer yarn. Type 2 (light support bandage)
Elset (Molnlycke Health Care Ltd) S bandage 15cm × 12m= £6.06, bandage 10cm × 6m= £2.82, 10cm × 8m= £3.61, 15cm × 6m= £3.02

Hospilite
Fabric, cotton, polyamide, and elastane; light support bandage (Type 2), 4.5 m stretched (all)
Hospilite bandage (Paul Hartmann Ltd) 10cm × 4.5m= £0.68, 15cm × 4.5m= £1.00, 5cm × 4.5m= £0.40, 7.5cm × 4.5m= £0.56

K-Lite
Knitted fabric, viscose and elastomer yarn. Type 2 (light support bandage)

K-Lite (Urgo Ltd) Long bandage 10cm × 5.25m= £1.25, bandage 10cm × 4.5m= £1.09, 15cm × 4.5m= £1.58, 5cm × 4.5m= £0.60, 7cm × 4.5m= £0.83

K-Plus
Knitted fabric, viscose and elastomer yarn. Type 3a (light support bandage)
K-Plus (Urgo Ltd) Long bandage 10cm × 10.25m= £2.86, bandage 10cm × 8.7m= £2.47

Knit-Firm
Knitted fabric, viscose and elastomer yarn. Type 2 (light support bandage)
Knit-Firm bandage (Millpledge Healthcare) 10cm × 4.5m= £0.66, 15cm × 4.5m= £0.96, 5cm × 4.5m= £0.36, 7cm × 4.5m= £0.51

L3
Knitted fabric, viscose and elastomer yarn. Type 2 (light support bandage)
L3 (Smith & Nephew Healthcare Ltd) bandage 10cm × 8.6m= £2.41

Neosport
Fabric, cotton, polyamide, and elastane; light support bandage (Type 2), 4.5 m stretched (all)
Neosport bandage (Neomedic Ltd) 10cm × 4.5m= £0.91, 15cm × 4.5m= £1.12, 5cm × 4.5m= £0.54, 7.5cm × 4.5m= £0.73

Profore #2
Fabric, cotton, polyamide, and elastane; light support bandage (Type 2), 4.5 m stretched (all)
Profore #2 (Smith & Nephew Healthcare Ltd) latex free bandage 10cm × 4.5m= £1.57

Profore #3
Knitted fabric, viscose and elastomer yarn. Type 2 (light support bandage)
Profore #3 (Smith & Nephew Healthcare Ltd) latex free bandage 10cm × 8.7m= £4.68

Soffcrepe
Fabric, cotton, polyamide, and elastane; light support bandage (Type 2), 4.5 m stretched (all)
Soffcrepe bandage (Essity UK Ltd) 10cm × 4.5m= £1.36, 15cm × 4.5m= £1.98, 5cm × 4.5m= £0.76, 7.5cm × 4.5m= £1.08

Adhesive bandages

Elastic adhesive bandages are used to provide compression in the treatment of varicose veins and for the support of injured joints; they should no longer be used for the support of fractured ribs and clavicles. They have also been used with zinc paste bandage in the treatment of venous ulcers, but they can cause skin reactions in susceptible patients and may not produce sufficient pressures for healing (significantly lower than those provided by other compression bandages).

Elastic Adhesive Bandage, BP 1993
Woven fabric, elastic in warp (crepe-twisted cotton threads), weft of cotton and/or viscose threads spread with adhesive mass containing zinc oxide. 4.5 m stretched
Tensoplast bandage (Essity UK Ltd) 10cm × 4.5m, 5cm × 4.5m, 7.5cm × 4.5m

Cohesive bandages

Cohesive bandages adhere to themselves, but not to the skin, and are useful for providing support for sports use where ordinary stretch bandages might become displaced and adhesive bandages are inappropriate. Care is needed in their application, however, since the loss of ability for movement between turns of the bandage to equalise local areas of high tension carries the potential for creating a tourniquet effect. Cohesive bandages can be used to support sprained joints and as an outer layer for multi-layer compression bandaging; they should not be used if arterial disease is suspected.

Cohesive extensible bandages
Profore #4
Bandage
Profore #4 (Smith & Nephew Healthcare Ltd) latex free bandage 10cm × 2.5m= £3.87

Ultra Fast
Bandage
Ultra Fast (Robinson Healthcare) cohesive bandage 10cm × 6.3m= £2.62

Compression bandages

High compression products are used to provide the high compression needed for the management of gross varices, post-thrombotic venous insufficiency, venous leg ulcers, and gross oedema in average-sized limbs. Their use calls for an expert knowledge of the elastic properties of the products and experience in the technique of providing careful graduated compression. Incorrect application can lead to uneven and inadequate pressures or to hazardous levels of pressure. In particular, injudicious use of compression in limbs with arterial disease has been reported to cause severe skin and tissue necrosis (in some instances calling for amputation). Doppler testing is required before treatment with compression. Oral pentoxifylline p. 267 can be used as adjunct therapy if a chronic venous leg ulcer does not respond to compression bandaging [unlicensed indication].

High compression bandages
High Compression Bandages
Cotton, viscose, nylon, and *Lycra*® extensible bandage, 3 m (unstretched)
K-ThreeC (Urgo Ltd) bandage 10cm × 3m= £3.08

PEC High Compression Bandages
Polyamide, elastane, and cotton compression (high) extensible bandage, 3.5 m unstretched
Setopress (Molnlycke Health Care Ltd) bandage 10cm × 3.5m= £3.84

Short stretch compression bandages
Actico
Bandage
Actico bandage (L&R Medical UK Ltd) 10cm × 6m= £3.67, 12cm × 6m= £4.68, 4cm × 6m= £2.63, 6cm × 6m= £3.08, 8cm × 6m= £3.54

Comprilan
Bandage
Comprilan bandage (Essity UK Ltd) 10cm × 5m= £3.71, 12cm × 5m= £4.51, 6cm × 5m= £2.93, 8cm × 5m= £3.44

Rosidal K
Bandage
Rosidal K bandage (Lohmann & Rauscher) 10cm × 10m= £6.63, 10cm × 5m= £3.81, 12cm × 5m= £4.62, 6cm × 5m= £2.92, 8cm × 5m= £3.49

Sub-compression wadding bandages
Cellona Undercast Padding
Padding
Cellona Undercast padding bandage (Lohmann & Rauscher) 10cm × 2.7m= £0.52, 15cm × 2.7m= £0.67, 5cm × 2.7m= £0.34, 7.5cm × 2.7m= £0.42

Flexi-Ban
Padding
Flexi-Ban (L&R Medical UK Ltd) bandage 10cm × 3.5m= £0.55

K-Soft
Padding
K-Soft (Urgo Ltd) Long bandage 10cm × 4.5m= £0.62, bandage 10cm × 3.5m= £0.49

Ortho-Band Plus
Padding
Ortho-Band Plus (Millpledge Healthcare) bandage 10cm × 3.5m= £0.37

Profore #1
Padding
Profore #1 (Smith & Nephew Healthcare Ltd) latex free bandage 10cm × 3.5m= £0.83

Ultra Soft
Padding
Ultra Soft (Robinson Healthcare) wadding bandage 10cm × 3.5m= £0.39

Velband
Padding
Velband (Essity UK Ltd) absorbent padding bandage 10cm × 4.5m= £0.80

Multi-layer compression bandaging

Multi-layer compression bandaging systems are an alternative to High Compression Bandages for the treatment of venous leg ulcers. Compression is achieved by the combined effects of two or three extensible bandages applied over a layer of orthopaedic wadding and a wound contact dressing.

Four layer bandaging systems
K-Four
Multi-layer compression bandaging kit, four layer system
K-Four (Urgo Ltd) Reduced Compression multi-layer compression bandage kit 18cm+ ankle circumference = £4.87, multi-layer compression bandage kit 18cm-25cm ankle circumference= £7.44, 25cm-30cm ankle circumference= £7.44, greater than 30cm ankle circumference= £10.25, less than 18cm ankle circumference= £7.78

Profore
Multi-layer compression bandaging kit, four layer system
Profore (Smith & Nephew Healthcare Ltd) Lite latex free multi-layer compression bandage kit= £6.53, latex free multi-layer compression bandage kit 18cm-25cm ankle circumference = £11.11

Ultra Four
Multi-layer compression bandaging kit, four layer system
Ultra Four (Robinson Healthcare) Reduced Compression multi-layer compression bandage kit= £4.19, multi-layer compression bandage kit 18cm-25cm ankle circumference= £5.73, up to 18cm ankle circumference= £6.48

Two layer bandaging systems
Andoflex
Multi-layer compression bandaging kit, two layer system (latex-free, foam bandage and cohesive compression bandage)
AndoFlex TLC (Creed Medical Ltd) -XL latex free multi-layer compression bandage kit= £8.76, Calamine Lite latex free multi-layer compression bandage kit 10cm= £9.78, 7.62cm= £8.64, Calamine latex free multi-layer compression bandage kit 10cm= £9.78, 7.62cm= £8.64, Lite latex free multi-layer compression bandage kit= £7.47, Zinc Lite latex free multi-layer compression bandage kit 10cm= £6.52, 7.5cm= £5.39, latex free multi-layer compression bandage kit= £7.47

Coban 2
Multi-layer compression bandaging kit, two layer system (latex-free, foam bandage and cohesive compression bandage)
Coban 2 (3M Health Care Ltd) Lite multi-layer compression bandage kit= £8.61, multi-layer compression bandage kit 10cm × 3.5m= £8.61, 10cm × 4.5m= £12.30, 5cm × 2.7m= £5.25

UrgoKTwo
Multi-layer compression bandaging kit, two layer system
UrgoKTwo (Urgo Ltd) Reduced latex free multi-layer compression bandage kit (10cm) 18cm-25cm ankle circumference= £9.26, 25cm-32cm ankle circumference= £10.12, Reduced multi-layer compression bandage kit 18cm-25cm ankle circumference= £8.72, 25cm-32cm ankle circumference= £9.53, latex free multi-layer compression bandage kit (10cm) 18cm-25cm ankle circumference= £9.26, 25cm-32cm ankle circumference= £10.12, multi-layer compression bandage kit (10cm) 18cm-25cm ankle circumference= £8.72, 25cm-32cm ankle circumference= £9.53, multi-layer compression bandage kit (12cm) 18cm-25cm ankle circumference= £10.99, 25cm-32cm ankle circumference= £12.02, multi-layer compression bandage kit (8cm) 18cm-25cm ankle circumference= £8.23, 25cm-32cm ankle circumference= £8.95, with UrgoStart multi-layer compression bandage kit 18cm-25cm ankle circumference= £10.87, 25cm-32cm ankle circumference= £11.59

Medicated bandages

Zinc Paste Bandage has been used with compression bandaging for the treatment of venous leg ulcers. However, paste bandages are associated with hypersensitivity reactions and should be used with caution. Zinc paste bandages are also used with coal tar or ichthammol in chronic lichenified skin conditions such as chronic eczema (ichthammol often being preferred since its action is considered to be milder). They are also used with calamine in milder eczematous skin conditions.

Zipzoc® can be used under appropriate compression bandages or hosiery in chronic venous insufficiency.

Zinc Paste Bandage, BP 1993

Cotton fabric, plain weave, impregnated with suitable paste containing zinc oxide; requires additional bandaging
Excipients: may include cetostearyl alcohol, hydroxybenzoates

Viscopaste (Evolan Pharma AB) PB7 bandage 7.5cm × 6m= £3.99

Zinc Paste and Ichthammol Bandage, BP 1993

Cotton fabric, plain weave, impregnated with suitable paste containing zinc oxide and ichthammol; requires additional bandaging
Excipients: may include cetostearyl alcohol

Ichthopaste (Evolan Pharma AB) bandage 7.5cm × 6m= £4.03

Zipzoc

Sterile rayon stocking impregnated with ointment containing zinc oxide 20%

Zipzoc (Evolan Pharma AB) stockings= £55.29

Compression hosiery and garments

Compression (elastic) hosiery is used to treat conditions associated with chronic venous insufficiency, to prevent recurrence of thrombosis, or to reduce the risk of further venous ulceration after treatment with compression bandaging. Doppler testing to confirm arterial sufficiency is required before recommending the use of compression hosiery.

Before elastic hosiery can be dispensed, the quantity (single or pair), article (including accessories), and compression class must be specified by the prescriber. There are different compression values for graduated compression hosiery and lymphoedema garments (see below). All dispensed elastic hosiery articles must state on the packaging that they conform with Drug Tariff technical specification No. 40, for further details see Drug Tariff.

Graduated Compression hosiery, Class 1 Light Support is used for superficial or early varices, varicosis during pregnancy.
Graduated Compression hosiery, Class 2 Medium Support is used for varices of medium severity, ulcer treatment and prophylaxis, mild oedema, varicosis during pregnancy.
Graduated Compression hosiery, Class 3 Strong Support is used for gross varices, post thrombotic venous insufficiency, gross oedema, ulcer treatment and prophylaxis.

Compression values for hosiery and lymphoedema garments

Class 1: compression hosiery (British standard) 14–17 mmHg, lymphoedema garments (European classification) 18–21 mmHg.
Class 2: compression hosiery (British standard) 18–24 mmHg, lymphoedema garments (European classification) 23–32 mmHg.
Class 3: compression hosiery (British standard) 25–35 mmHg, lymphoedema garments (European classification) 34–46 mmHg.
Class 4: compression hosiery (British standard)—not available, lymphoedema garments (European classification) 49–70 mmHg.
Class 4 super: compression hosiery (British standard)—not available, lymphoedema garments (European classification) 60–90 mmHg.

Graduated compression hosiery

Class 1 Light Support
Hosiery, compression at ankle 14–17 mmHg, thigh length or below knee with knitted in heel

Class 2 Light Support
Hosiery, compression at ankle 14–17 mmHg, thigh length or below knee with knitted in heel

Compression hosiery – anklets
Class 2 Medium Support
Anklets, compression 18–24 mmHg, circular knit (standard and made-to-measure)

Class 3 Strong Support
Anklets, compression 18–24 mmHg, circular knit (standard and made-to-measure)

Compression hosiery – kneecaps
Class 2 Medium Support
Kneecaps, compression 18–24 mmHg, circular knit (standard and made-to-measure)

Class 3 Strong Support
Kneecaps, compression 18–24 mmHg, circular knit (standard and made-to-measure)

Hosiery accessories
Suspender
Suspender, for thigh stockings

Lymphoedema garments

Lymphoedema compression garments are used to maintain limb shape and prevent additional fluid retention. Either flat-bed or circular knitting methods are used in the manufacture of elasticated compression garments. Seamless, circular-knitted garments (in standard sizes) can be used to prevent swelling if the lymphoedema is well controlled and if the limb is in good shape and without skin folds. Flat-knitted garments (usually made-to-measure) with a seam, provide greater rigidity and stiffness to maintain reduction of lymphoedema following treatment with compression bandages.

A standard range of light, medium, or high compression garments are available, as well as low compression (12–16 mmHg) armsleeves, made-to-measure garments up to compression 90 mmHg, and accessories—see Drug Tariff for details. Note, there are different compression values for lymphoedema garments and graduated compression hosiery, see Compression hosiery and garments above.

Dental Practitioners' Formulary

List of Dental Preparations

The following list has been approved by the appropriate Secretaries of State, and the preparations therein may be prescribed by dental practitioners on form FP10D (GP14 in Scotland, WP10D in Wales).

Licensed **sugar-free** versions, where available, are preferred. Licensed **alcohol-free** mouthwashes, where available, are preferred.

Aciclovir Cream, BP
Aciclovir Oral Suspension, BP, 200 mg/5 mL
Aciclovir Tablets, BP, 200 mg
Aciclovir Tablets, BP, 800 mg
Amoxicillin Capsules, BP
Amoxicillin Oral Powder, DPF
Amoxicillin Oral Suspension, BP
Artificial Saliva Gel, DPF
Artificial Saliva Oral Spray, DPF
Artificial Saliva Pastilles, DPF
Artificial Saliva Protective Spray, DPF
Artificial Saliva Substitutes as listed below (to be prescribed only for indications approved by ACBS (patients suffering from dry mouth as a result of having or, having undergone, radiotherapy or sicca syndrome):
   BioXtra® Gel Mouthspray
   Glandosane®
   Saliveze®
Artificial Saliva Substitute Spray, DPF
Aspirin Tablets, Dispersible, BP
Azithromycin Capsules, 250 mg, DPF
Azithromycin Oral Suspension, 200 mg/5 mL, DPF
Azithromycin Tablets, 250 mg, DPF
Azithromycin Tablets, 500 mg, DPF
Beclometasone Pressurised Inhalation, BP, 50 micrograms/metered inhalation, CFC-free, as:
   Clenil Modulite®
Benzydamine Mouthwash, BP 0.15%
Benzydamine Oromucosal Spray, BP 0.15%
Betamethasone Soluble Tablets, 500 micrograms, DPF
Carbamazepine Tablets, BP
Cefalexin Capsules, BP
Cefalexin Oral Suspension, BP
Cefalexin Tablets, BP
Cefradine Capsules, BP
Cetirizine Oral Solution, BP, 5 mg/5 mL
Cetirizine Tablets, BP, 10 mg
Chlorhexidine Gluconate Gel, BP
Chlorhexidine Mouthwash, BP
Chlorhexidine Oral Spray, DPF
Chlorphenamine Oral Solution, BP
Chlorphenamine Tablets, BP
Choline Salicylate Dental Gel, BP
Clarithromycin Oral Suspension, 125 mg/5 mL, DPF
Clarithromycin Oral Suspension, 250 mg/5 mL, DPF
Clarithromycin Tablets, BP
Clindamycin Capsules, BP
Co-amoxiclav Tablets, BP, 250/125 (amoxicillin 250 mg as trihydrate, clavulanic acid 125 mg as potassium salt)
Co-amoxiclav Oral Suspension, BP, 125/31 (amoxicillin 125 mg as trihydrate, clavulanic acid 31.25 mg as potassium salt)/5 mL
Co-amoxiclav Oral Suspension, BP, 250/62 (amoxicillin 250 mg as trihydrate, clavulanic acid 62.5 mg as potassium salt)/5 mL
Diazepam Oral Solution, BP, 2 mg/5 mL
Diazepam Tablets, BP
Diclofenac Sodium Tablets, Gastro-resistant, BP
Dihydrocodeine Tablets, BP, 30 mg
Doxycycline Tablets, Dispersible, BP
Doxycycline Capsules, BP, 100 mg
Doxycycline Tablets, 20 mg, DPF
Ephedrine Nasal Drops, BP
Erythromycin Ethyl Succinate Oral Suspension, BP
Erythromycin Ethyl Succinate Tablets, BP
Erythromycin Stearate Tablets, BP
Erythromycin Tablets, Gastro-resistant, BP
Fluconazole Capsules, 50 mg, DPF
Fluconazole Oral Suspension, 50 mg/5 mL, DPF
Hydrocortisone Cream, BP, 1%
Hydrocortisone Oromucosal Tablets, BP
Hydrogen Peroxide Mouthwash, BP, 6%
Ibuprofen Oral Suspension, BP, sugar-free
Ibuprofen Tablets, BP
Lansoprazole Capsules, Gastro-resistant, BP
Lidocaine Ointment, BP, 5%
Lidocaine Spray 10%, DPF
Loratadine Syrup, 5 mg/5 mL, DPF
Loratadine Tablets, BP, 10 mg
Menthol and Eucalyptus Inhalation, BP 1980
Metronidazole Oral Suspension, BP
Metronidazole Tablets, BP
Miconazole Cream, BP
Miconazole Oromucosal Gel, BP
Miconazole and Hydrocortisone Cream, BP
Miconazole and Hydrocortisone Ointment, BP
Nystatin Oral Suspension, BP
Omeprazole Capsules, Gastro-resistant, BP
Oxytetracycline Tablets, BP
Paracetamol Oral Suspension, BP
Paracetamol Tablets, BP
Paracetamol Tablets, Soluble, BP
Phenoxymethylpenicillin Oral Solution, BP
Phenoxymethylpenicillin Tablets, BP
Promethazine Hydrochloride Tablets, BP
Promethazine Oral Solution, BP
Saliva Stimulating Tablets, DPF
Sodium Chloride Mouthwash, Compound, BP
Sodium Fluoride Mouthwash, BP
Sodium Fluoride Oral Drops, BP
Sodium Fluoride Tablets, BP
Sodium Fluoride Toothpaste 0.619%, DPF
Sodium Fluoride Toothpaste 1.1%, DPF
Sodium Fusidate Ointment, BP
Temazepam Oral Solution, BP
Temazepam Tablets, BP
Tetracycline Tablets, BP

Preparations in this list which are not included in the BP or BPC are described under Details of DPF preparations. For details of preparations that can be prescribed, see individual entries under the relevant drug monographs throughout the BNF publications.

Details of DPF preparations

Preparations on the List of Dental Preparations which are specified as DPF are described as follows in the DPF. Although brand names have sometimes been included for identification purposes preparations on the list should be prescribed by non-proprietary name.

Amoxicillin Oral Powder
amoxicillin (as trihydrate) 3 g sachet

Artificial Saliva Gel
(proprietary products: *BioXtra Dry Mouth Oral Gel*; *Oralieve Moisturising Mouth Gel*) consists of lactoperoxidase, lactoferrin, glucose oxidase, xylitol, and other ingredients, in a gel basis

Artificial Saliva Oral Spray
(proprietary products: *Xerotin*) consists of water, sorbitol, carmellose (carboxymethylcellulose), potassium chloride, sodium chloride, potassium phosphate, magnesium chloride, calcium chloride and other ingredients, pH neutral

Artificial Saliva Pastilles
(proprietary product: *Salivix*), consists of acacia, malic acid, and other ingredients

Artificial Saliva Protective Spray
(proprietary product: *Aequasyal*) consists of oxidised glycerol triesters, silicon dioxide, flavouring agents, aspartame

Artificial Saliva Substitute Spray
(proprietary product: *AS Saliva Orthana Spray*) consists of mucin, methylparaben, benzalkonium chloride, EDTA, xylitol, peppermint oil, spearmint oil, mineral salts

Azithromycin Capsules
azithromycin 250 mg

Azithromycin Oral Suspension 200 mg/5 mL
azithromycin 200 mg/5 mL when reconstituted with water

Azithromycin Tablets
azithromycin 250 mg and 500 mg

Betamethasone Soluble Tablets 500 micrograms
betamethasone (as sodium phosphate) 500 micrograms

Chlorhexidine Oral Spray
(proprietary product: *Corsodyl Oral Spray*), chlorhexidine gluconate 0.2%

Clarithromycin Oral Suspension 125 mg/5 mL
clarithromycin 125 mg/5 mL when reconstituted with water

Clarithromycin Oral Suspension 250 mg/5 mL
clarithromycin 250 mg/5 mL when reconstituted with water

Doxycycline Tablets 20 mg
(proprietary product: *Periostat*), doxycycline (as hyclate) 20 mg

Fluconazole Capsules 50 mg
fluconazole 50 mg

Fluconazole Oral Suspension 50 mg/5 mL
(proprietary product: *Diflucan*), fluconazole 50 mg/5 mL when reconstituted with water

Lidocaine Spray 10%
(proprietary product: *Xylocaine Spray*), lidocaine 10% supplying 10 mg lidocaine/spray

Loratadine Syrup 5 mg/5 mL
loratadine 5 mg/5 mL

Saliva Stimulating Tablets
(proprietary product: *SST*), citric acid, malic acid and other ingredients in a sorbitol base

Sodium Fluoride Toothpaste 0.619%
(proprietary product: *Duraphat '2800 ppm' Toothpaste*), sodium fluoride 0.619%

Sodium Fluoride Toothpaste 1.1%
(proprietary product: *Duraphat '5000 ppm' Toothpaste*), sodium fluoride 1.1%

Approved list for prescribing by Community Practitioner Nurse Prescribers (NPF)

Nurse Prescribers' Formulary for Community Practitioners

The Nurse Prescribers' Formulary for Community Practitioners is for use by District Nurses and Specialist Community Public Health Nurses (including Health Visitors) who have received nurse prescriber training. It provides a list of preparations approved by the Secretary of State that can be prescribed for patients receiving NHS treatment on form FP10P (form HS21(N) in Northern Ireland, form GP10(N) in Scotland, forms WP10CN and WP10PN in Wales). Community practitioner nurse prescribers should only prescribe items appearing in the nurse prescribers' list set out below (for the indications specified). Most medicinal preparations should be prescribed generically, except where this would not be clinically appropriate or where there is no approved generic name—see individual entries for further information.

The Nurse Prescribers' Advisory Group p. vii oversees the preparation of the NPF and advises UK health ministers on the list of preparations that may be prescribed by community practitioner nurse prescribers. Feedback from nurse prescribers is welcome and will be taken into account when reviewing this list; comments and constructive criticism should be sent to editor@bnf.org.

How to use the NPF

The list of medicinal preparations includes:
- Links to BNF monographs to allow full prescribing information for each preparation to be accessed;
- Details of the indications for which each medicinal preparation can be prescribed;
- Signposting to doses for community practitioner nurse prescribers where these differ from those in the BNF for the specified indications;
- Additional information that should be considered before prescribing certain preparations.

The NPF should be used in conjunction with BNF monographs to ensure that all relevant prescribing information is considered when prescribing decisions are made; links to the relevant BNF monographs allow quick access to this prescribing information. Most of the doses that can be prescribed by nurse prescribers for the specified indications are in line with those in BNF monographs, so the BNF doses for those indications can be used. If doses that can be prescribed by nurse prescribers differ from those in the BNF, specific indications and doses have been added to BNF monographs. These can be found towards the bottom of indication and dose sections of the relevant monographs with the statement "dose approved for use by community practitioner nurse prescribers" following the indication; individual preparation entries signpost to these doses.

General guidance for community practitioner nurse prescribers (Nurse Prescribers' Formulary—General guidance) includes information on prescribing for nurse prescribers and can be found in online versions of the BNF and the BNF app. Treatment summaries for nurse prescribers (e.g. Nurse Prescribers' Formulary—Analgesics) can also be found in online versions of the BNF and the BNF app; these provide an overview of the drug management or prophylaxis of conditions that are commonly managed by nurse prescribers and/or information on the use of appliances, such as stoma appliances. In order to select safe and effective medicines for individual patients, information in the treatment summaries must be used in conjunction with other prescribing details about the drugs and knowledge of the patient's medical and drug history.

Medicinal Preparations

Preparations on this list which are not included in the BP or BPC are described under Details of NPF preparations.
- **Almond oil ear drops p. 1365, BP**
  - *Removal of ear wax*
- **Arachis oil enema p. 66, NPF**
  - *To soften impacted faeces*
- **Aspirin tablets, dispersible, 300 mg p. 142, BP** (max. 96 tablets; max. pack size 32 tablets)
  - *Mild to moderate pain| Pyrexia* (for both indications, see doses for community practitioner nurse prescribers)
- **Bisacodyl suppositories p. 67, BP** (includes 5-mg and 10-mg strengths)
  - *Constipation* (see dose for community practitioner nurse prescribers)
- **Bisacodyl tablets p. 67, BP**
  - *Constipation* (see dose for community practitioner nurse prescribers)
- **Catheter maintenance solutions, sodium chloride p. 911, NPF**
  - *For removal of clots and other debris, to be instilled as required*
- **Catheter maintenance solutions, 'Solution G' p. 911, NPF**
  - *For prevention of catheter encrustation and crystallisation; in very severe cases use 'Solution R'*
- **Catheter maintenance solutions p. 911, 'Solution R', NPF**
  - *For prevention of catheter encrustation and dissolution of crystallisation if 'Solution G' unsuccessful*
- **Chlorhexidine gluconate alcoholic solutions** containing at least 0.05%, see chlorhexidine p. 1452 and chlorhexidine gluconate with isopropyl alcohol p. 1453
  - *Skin disinfection*
- **Chlorhexidine gluconate aqueous solutions p. 1452** containing at least 0.05%
  - *Skin disinfection*
- **Choline salicylate dental gel p. 1382, BP**
  - *Mild oral and perioral lesions*
- **Clotrimazole cream 1% p. 1399, BP**
  - *Fungal skin infections*
- **Co-danthramer capsules, NPF** [discontinued]
- **Co-danthramer capsules, strong, NPF** [discontinued]
- **Co-danthramer oral suspension p. 67, NPF**
  - *In consultation with doctor, constipation in palliative care*
- **Co-danthramer oral suspension, strong p. 67, NPF**
  - *In consultation with doctor, constipation in palliative care*
- **Co-danthrusate capsules, BP** [discontinued]
- **Co-danthrusate oral suspension p. 68, NPF**
  - *In consultation with doctor, constipation in palliative care*
- **Crotamiton cream p. 1437, BP**
  - *Pruritus (including pruritus after scabies)*

Nurse Prescribers' Formulary (NPF)

- **Crotamiton lotion, BP** [discontinued]
- **Dimeticone barrier creams** containing at least 10%, see barrier creams and ointments p. 1388
  - *For use as a barrier preparation*
- **Dimeticone lotion p. 1403, NPF**
  - *Head lice*
- **Docusate sodium capsules p. 66, BP**
  - *Chronic constipation*
- **Docusate sodium enema p. 66, NPF**
  - *Chronic constipation*
- **Docusate sodium oral solution p. 66, BP**
  - *Chronic constipation*
- **Docusate sodium oral solution, paediatric p. 66, BP**
  - *Chronic constipation*
- **Econazole nitrate cream 1% p. 1400, BP**
  - *Fungal skin infections*

Emollient creams and ointments, paraffin-containing p. 1392 as listed below:
- *Dry skin conditions| Eczema| Psoriasis| Ichthyosis| Pruritus*
- **Cetraben® emollient cream**
- **Dermamist®**
- **Diprobase® cream**
- **Diprobase® ointment**
- **Doublebase®**
- **Doublebase® Dayleve gel**
- **E45® cream**
- **Emulsifying ointment, BP**
- **Hydromol® cream**
- **Hydrous ointment, BP**
- **Lipobase®**
- **Liquid and white soft paraffin ointment, NPF**
- **Neutrogena® Norwegian Formula Dermatological cream** [discontinued]
- **Oilatum® cream**
- **Oilatum® Junior cream**
- **Paraffin, white soft, BP**
- **Paraffin, yellow soft, BP**
- **Ultrabase®**
- **Unguentum M®**

Emollients, urea-containing p. 1394 as listed below:
- **Aquadrate® 10% w/w cream**
  - *Dry, scaling, and itching skin*
- **Balneum® Plus cream**
  - *Dry, scaling, and itching skin*
- **E45® Itch Relief cream**
  - *Dry, scaling, and itching skin*
- **Eucerin® Intensive 10% w/w urea treatment cream**
  - *Dry skin conditions including eczema, ichthyosis, xeroderma, and hyperkeratosis*
- **Eucerin® Intensive 10% w/w urea treatment lotion**
  - *Dry skin conditions including eczema, ichthyosis, xeroderma, and hyperkeratosis*
- **Hydromol® Intensive**
  - *Dry, scaling, and itching skin*
- **Nutraplus® cream**
  - *Dry, scaling, and itching skin*

Emollient bath and shower products, paraffin-containing p. 1389 as listed below:
- **Aqueous cream, BP**
  - *Dry skin conditions*
- **Cetraben® emollient bath additive**
  - *Dry skin conditions, including eczema*
- **Dermalo® bath emollient**
  - *Dermatitis| Dry skin conditions, including ichthyosis| Pruritus of the elderly*
- **Doublebase® emollient bath additive**
  - *Dry skin conditions, including dermatitis and ichthyosis| Pruritus of the elderly*
- **Doublebase® emollient shower gel**
  - *Dry, chapped, or itchy skin conditions*
- **Doublebase® emollient wash gel**
  - *Dry, chapped, or itchy skin conditions*

- **Hydromol® bath and shower emollient**
  - *Dry skin conditions| Eczema| Ichthyosis| Pruritus of the elderly*
- **Oilatum® emollient**
  - *Dry skin conditions including dermatitis and ichthyosis| Pruritus of the elderly*
- **Oilatum® gel** [discontinued]
- **Oilatum® Junior bath additive**
  - *Dry skin conditions including dermatitis and ichthyosis| Pruritus of the elderly*
- **Zerolatum® emollient medicinal bath oil**
  - *Dry skin conditions| Dermatitis| Ichthyosis*

Emollient bath and shower products, soya-bean oil-containing p. 1391 as listed below:
- **Balneum®** (except pack sizes that are not to be prescribed under the NHS (see Part XVIIIA of the Drug Tariff, Part XI of the Northern Ireland Drug Tariff))
  - *Dry skin conditions including those associated with dermatitis and eczema*
- **Balneum Plus® bath oil** (except pack sizes that are not to be prescribed under the NHS (see Part XVIIIA of the Drug Tariff, Part XI of the Northern Ireland Drug Tariff))
  - *Dry skin conditions including those associated with dermatitis and eczema where pruritus also experienced*
- **Folic acid tablets 400 micrograms p. 1161, BP**
  - *Prevention of neural tube defects (in those at a low risk of conceiving a child with a neural tube defect)*
- **Glycerol suppositories p. 68, BP**
  - *Constipation*
- **Ibuprofen oral suspension p. 1302, BP** (except for indications and doses that are prescription-only)
  - *Pain and inflammation in rheumatic disease and other musculoskeletal disorders| Mild to moderate pain including dysmenorrhoea| Migraine| Dental pain| Headache| Fever| Symptoms of colds and influenza| Neuralgia| Mild to moderate pain| Pain and inflammation of soft-tissue injuries| Pyrexia with discomfort| Post-immunisation pyrexia in infants (for all indications, see doses for community practitioner nurse prescribers)*
- **Ibuprofen tablets p. 1302, BP** (except for indications and doses that are prescription-only)
  - *Pain and inflammation in rheumatic disease and other musculoskeletal disorders| Mild to moderate pain including dysmenorrhoea| Migraine| Dental pain| Headache| Fever| Symptoms of colds and influenza| Neuralgia| Mild to moderate pain| Pain and inflammation of soft-tissue injuries| Pyrexia with discomfort (for all indications, see doses for community practitioner nurse prescribers)*
- **Ispaghula husk granules p. 60, BP**
  - *Constipation* (see dose for community practitioner nurse prescribers)
- **Ispaghula husk granules, effervescent p. 60, BP**
  - *Constipation* (see dose for community practitioner nurse prescribers)
- **Ispaghula husk oral powder, BP** [discontinued]
- **Lactulose solution p. 61, BP**
  - *Constipation* (see dose for community practitioner nurse prescribers)
- **Lidocaine hydrochloride ointment p. 1547, BP**
  - *Sore nipples from breast-feeding*
- **Lidocaine and chlorhexidine gel, BP**, see chlorhexidine with lidocaine p. 911
  - *Surface anaesthesia* (see dose for community practitioner nurse prescribers)
- **Macrogol oral liquid, compound, NPF**, see macrogol 3350 with potassium chloride, sodium bicarbonate and sodium chloride p. 62
  - *Chronic constipation*
- **Macrogol oral powder, compound, NPF**, see macrogol 3350 with potassium chloride, sodium bicarbonate and sodium chloride p. 62

▶ *Chronic constipation| Faecal impaction (important: initial assessment by doctor; usual max. duration of treatment 3 days)*
● **Macrogol oral powder, compound, half-strength, NPF**, see macrogol 3350 with potassium chloride, sodium bicarbonate and sodium chloride p. 62
▶ *Chronic constipation| Faecal impaction (important: initial assessment by doctor; usual max. duration of treatment 3 days)*
● **Magnesium hydroxide mixture p. 64, BP**
▶ *Constipation*
● **Magnesium sulfate paste, BP**
▶ *Adjunct in management of boils, apply under dressing; stir before use*
● **Malathion aqueous lotions p. 1404** containing at least 0.5%
▶ *Head lice| Scabies*
● **Mebendazole oral suspension p. 701, NPF**
▶ *Threadworm infections* (see dose for community practitioner nurse prescribers)
● **Mebendazole tablets p. 701, NPF**
▶ *Threadworm infections* (see dose for community practitioner nurse prescribers)
● **Methylcellulose tablets, BP**[discontinued]
▶ *Constipation*
● **Miconazole cream 2% p. 1400, BP**
▶ *Fungal skin infections*
● **Miconazole oromucosal gel p. 1384, BP**
▶ *Prevention and treatment of oral candidiasis* (see dose for community practitioner nurse prescribers)
● **Mouthwash solution-tablets, NPF**
● **Nicotine inhalation cartridge for oromucosal use p. 567, NPF**
▶ *Nicotine replacement therapy*
● **Nicotine lozenge p. 567, NPF**
▶ *Nicotine replacement therapy*
● **Nicotine medicated chewing gum p. 567, NPF**
▶ *Nicotine replacement therapy in individuals who smoke fewer than 20 cigarettes each day| Nicotine replacement therapy in individuals who smoke more than 20 cigarettes each day or who require more than 15 pieces of 2-mg strength gum each day*
● **Nicotine nasal spray p. 567, NPF**
▶ *Nicotine replacement therapy*
● **Nicotine oral spray p. 567, NPF**
▶ *Nicotine replacement therapy*
● **Nicotine sublingual tablets p. 567, NPF**
▶ *Nicotine replacement therapy in individuals who smoke fewer than 20 cigarettes each day| Nicotine replacement therapy in individuals who smoke more than 20 cigarettes each day*
● **Nicotine transdermal patches p. 567, NPF**
▶ *Nicotine replacement therapy*
● **Nystatin oral suspension p. 1385, BP**
▶ *Oral and perioral fungal infections* (see dose for community practitioner nurse prescribers)
● **Olive oil ear drops p. 1365, BP**
▶ *Removal of earwax* (see dose for community practitioner nurse prescribers)
● **Paracetamol oral suspension p. 507, BP** (includes 120 mg/5 mL and 250 mg/5 mL strengths—both of which are available as sugar-free formulations)
▶ *Mild to moderate pain (in adults)| Pyrexia (in adults)| Pain (in children)| Pyrexia with discomfort (in children)| Post-immunisation pyrexia in infants (refer to doctor if pyrexia persists)*
● **Paracetamol tablets p. 507, BP** (max. 96 tablets; max. pack size 32 tablets)
▶ *Mild to moderate pain (in adults)| Pyrexia (in adults)| Pain (in children)| Pyrexia with discomfort (in children)*
● **Paracetamol tablets, soluble p. 507, BP** (max. 96 tablets; max. pack size 32 tablets)

▶ *Mild to moderate pain (in adults)| Pyrexia (in adults)| Pain (in children)| Pyrexia with discomfort (in children)*
● **Permethrin cream p. 1404, NPF**
▶ *Scabies*
● **Phosphates enema, BP**, see sodium acid phosphate with sodium phosphate p. 64
▶ *Constipation, using Phosphates enema BP Formula B| Constipation, using Phosphates enema (Cleen Ready-to-Use)* (for both indications, see doses for community practitioner nurse prescribers)
● **Povidone-iodine solution p. 1451, BP**
▶ *Skin disinfection*
● **Senna oral solution p. 69, NPF**
▶ *Constipation* (see dose for community practitioner nurse prescribers)
● **Senna tablets p. 69, BP**
▶ *Constipation* (see dose for community practitioner nurse prescribers)
● **Senna with ispaghula husk granules p. 69, NPF**
▶ *Constipation*
● **Sodium chloride solution, sterile, BP**, see Irrigation solutions p. 1454
▶ *Skin cleansing*
● **Sodium citrate compound enema p. 909, NPF**
▶ *Constipation* (see dose for community practitioner nurse prescribers)
● **Sodium picosulfate capsules, NPF** [discontinued]
● **Sodium picosulfate elixir p. 70, NPF**
▶ *Constipation* (see dose for community practitioner nurse prescribers)
● **Spermicidal contraceptive: Gygel ® contraceptive jelly**, see nonoxinol p. 938
▶ *Spermicidal contraceptive in conjunction with barrier methods of contraception such as diaphragms or caps*
● **Sterculia granules p. 61, NPF**
▶ *Constipation*
● **Sterculia with frangula granules p. 61, NPF**
▶ *Constipation*
● **Titanium ointment, BP**, see barrier creams and ointments p. 1388
▶ *For use as a barrier preparation*
● **Water for injections, BP**; available as 2-mL ampoules, 5-mL ampoules, 10-mL ampoules, 10-mL vials, 20-mL ampoules, and 100-mL vials
● **Zinc and castor oil ointment, BP**, see barrier creams and ointments p. 1388
▶ *For use as a barrier preparation*
● **Zinc oxide and dimeticone spray, NPF**, see barrier creams and ointments p. 1388
▶ *For use as a barrier preparation*
● **Zinc oxide impregnated medicated bandage, NPF**, see Medicated bandages p. 1949
● **Zinc oxide impregnated medicated stocking, NPF**, see Medicated bandages p. 1949
● **Zinc paste bandage, BP 1993**, see Medicated bandages p. 1949
● **Zinc paste and ichthammol bandage, BP 1993**, see Medicated bandages p. 1949

Appliances and Reagents (including Wound Management Products)

Community Practitioner Nurse Prescribers in England, Wales and Northern Ireland can prescribe any appliance or reagent in the relevant Drug Tariff. In the Scottish Drug Tariff, Appliances and Reagents which may **not** be prescribed by Nurses are annotated **Nx**.

Appliances (including Contraceptive Devices) as listed in Part IXA of the Drug Tariff (Part III of the Northern Ireland Drug Tariff, Part 3 (Appliances) and Part 2 (Dressings) of the Scottish Drug Tariff). (Where it is not appropriate for nurse prescribers in family planning clinics to prescribe contraceptive devices using form FP10(P) (forms WP10CN and WP10PN in Wales), they may prescribe using the same system as doctors in the clinic.)

Incontinence Appliances as listed in Part IXB of the Drug Tariff (Part III of the Northern Ireland Drug Tariff, Part 5 of the Scottish Drug Tariff.)

Stoma Appliances and Associated Products as listed in Part IXC of the Drug Tariff (Part III of the Northern Ireland Drug Tariff, Part 6 of the Scottish Drug Tariff).

Chemical Reagents as listed in Part IXR of the Drug Tariff (Part II of the Northern Ireland Drug Tariff, Part 9 of the Scottish Drug Tariff).

The Drug Tariffs can be accessed online at:

National Health Service Drug Tariff for England and Wales: www.nhsbsa.nhs.uk/pharmacies-gp-practices-and-appliance-contractors/drug-tariff

Health and Personal Social Services for Northern Ireland Drug Tariff: www.hscbusiness.hscni.net/services/2034.htm

Scottish Drug Tariff: publichealthscotland.scot/resources-and-tools/medical-practice-and-pharmaceuticals/scottish-drug-tariff/

Details of NPF preparations

Preparations on the Nurse Prescribers' Formulary which are not included in the BP or BPC are described as follows in the Nurse Prescribers' Formulary. Although brand names have sometimes been included for identification purposes, it is recommended that non-proprietary names should be used for prescribing medicinal preparations in the NPF except where a non-proprietary name is not available.

- **Arachis oil enema**
- arachis oil 100%
- **Catheter maintenance solution, sodium chloride**
- (proprietary products: *OptiFlo S; Uro-Tainer Sodium Chloride; Uriflex-S*), sodium chloride 0.9%
- **Catheter maintenance solution, 'Solution G'**
- (proprietary products: *OptiFlo G; Uro-Tainer Suby G; Uriflex G*), citric acid 3.23%, magnesium oxide 0.38%, sodium bicarbonate 0.7%, disodium edetate 0.01%
- **Catheter maintenance solution, 'Solution R'**
- (proprietary products: *OptiFlo R; Uro-Tainer Solutio R; Uriflex R*), citric acid 6%, gluconolactone 0.6%, magnesium carbonate 2.8%, disodium edetate 0.01%
- **Chlorhexidine gluconate alcoholic solutions**
- (proprietary products: *ChloraPrep; Hydrex Solution; Hydrex spray*), chlorhexidine gluconate in alcoholic solution
- **Chlorhexidine gluconate aqueous solutions**
- (proprietary product: *Unisept*), chlorhexidine gluconate in aqueous solution
- **Co-danthramer capsules** PoM
- co-danthramer 25/200 (dantron 25 mg, poloxamer '188' 200 mg)
- **Co-danthramer capsules, strong** PoM
- co-danthramer 37.5/500 (dantron 37.5 mg, poloxamer '188' 500 mg)
- **Co-danthramer oral suspension** PoM
- co-danthramer 25/200 in 5 mL (dantron 25 mg, poloxamer '188' 200 mg/5 mL)
- **Co-danthramer oral suspension, strong** PoM
- co-danthramer 75/1000 in 5 mL (dantron 75 mg, poloxamer '188' 1 g/5 mL)
- **Co-danthrusate oral suspension** PoM
- (proprietary product: *Normax*), co-danthrusate 50/60 (dantron 50 mg, docusate sodium 60 mg/5 mL)
- **Dimeticone barrier creams**
- (proprietary products *Conotrane Cream*, dimeticone '350' 22%; *Siopel Barrier Cream*, dimeticone '1000' 10%), dimeticone 10–22%
- **Dimeticone lotion**
- (proprietary product: *Hedrin*), dimeticone 4%
- **Docusate enema**
- (proprietary product: *Norgalax Micro-enema*), docusate sodium 120 mg in 10 g

- **Liquid and white soft paraffin ointment**
- liquid paraffin 50%, white soft paraffin 50%
- **Macrogol oral liquid, compound**
- (proprietary product: *Movicol Liquid*), macrogol '3350' (polyethylene glycol '3350') 13.125 g, sodium bicarbonate 178.5 mg, sodium chloride 350.7 mg, potassium chloride 46.6 mg/25 mL
- **Macrogol oral powder, compound**
- (proprietary products: *Laxido Orange, Molaxole, Movicol*), macrogol '3350' (polyethylene glycol '3350') 13.125 g, sodium bicarbonate 178.5 mg, sodium chloride 350.7 mg, potassium chloride 46.6 mg/sachet; (amount of potassium chloride varies according to flavour of *Movicol*® as follows: plain-flavour (sugar-free) = 50.2 mg/sachet; lime and lemon flavour = 46.6 mg/sachet; chocolate flavour = 31.7 mg/sachet. 1 sachet when reconstituted with 125 mL water provides K$^+$ 5.4 mmol/litre)
- **Macrogol oral powder, compound, half-strength**
- (proprietary product: *Movicol-Half*), macrogol '3350' (polyethylene glycol '3350') 6.563 g, sodium bicarbonate 89.3 g, sodium chloride 175.4 mg, potassium chloride 23.3 mg/sachet
- **Malathion aqueous lotions**
- (proprietary products: *Derbac-M Liquid*), malathion 0.5% in an aqueous basis
- **Mebendazole oral suspension** PoM
- (proprietary product: *Vermox*), mebendazole 100 mg/5 mL
- **Mebendazole tablets** PoM
- (proprietary products: *Ovex, Vermox*), mebendazole 100 mg (can be supplied for oral use in the treatment of enterobiasis in adults and children over 2 years provided its container or package is labelled to show a max. single dose of 100 mg and it is supplied in a container or package containing not more than 800 mg)
- **Mouthwash solution-tablets**
- consist of tablets which may contain antimicrobial, colouring and flavouring agents in a suitable soluble effervescent basis to make a mouthwash
- **Nicotine inhalation cartridge for oromucosal use**
- (proprietary products: *NicAssist Inhalator, Nicorette Inhalator*), nicotine 15 mg (for use with inhalation mouthpiece; to be prescribed as either a starter pack (6 cartridges with inhalator device and holder) or refill pack (42 cartridges with inhalator device)
- **Nicotine lozenge**
- nicotine (as bitartrate) 1 mg or 2 mg (proprietary product: *Nicorette Mint Lozenge, Nicotinell Mint Lozenge*), or nicotine (as resinate) 1.5 mg, 2 mg, or 4 mg (proprietary product: *NiQuitin Lozenges, NiQuitin Minis, NiQuitin Pre-quit*)
- **Nicotine medicated chewing gum**
- (proprietary products: *NicAssist Gum, Nicorette Gum, Nicotinell Gum, NiQuitin Gum*), nicotine 2 mg or 4 mg
- **Nicotine nasal spray**
- (proprietary product: *NicAssist Nasal Spray, Nicorette Nasal Spray*), nicotine 500 micrograms/metered spray
- **Nicotine oral spray**
- (proprietary product: *Nicorette Quickmist*), nicotine 1 mg/metered spray
- **Nicotine sublingual tablets**
- (proprietary product: *NicAssist Microtab, Nicorette Microtab*), nicotine (as a cyclodextrin complex) 2 mg (to be prescribed as either a starter pack (2 × 15-tablet discs with dispenser) or refill pack (7 × 15-tablet discs))
- **Nicotine transdermal patches**
- releasing in each 16 hours, nicotine approx. 5 mg, 10 mg, or 15 mg (proprietary products: *Boots NicAssist Patch, Nicorette Patch*), or releasing in each 16 hours approx. 10 mg, 15 mg, or 25 mg (proprietary products: *NicAssist Translucent Patch, Nicorette Invisi Patch*), or releasing in each 24 hours nicotine approx. 7 mg, 14 mg, or 21 mg (proprietary products: *Nicopatch, Nicotinell TTS, NiQuitin,*

NiQuitin Clear) (prescriber should specify the brand to be dispensed)

- **Permethrin cream**
  - ▸ (proprietary product: *Lyclear Dermal Cream*), permethrin 5%
- **Senna oral solution**
  - ▸ (proprietary product: *Senokot Syrup*), sennosides 7.5 mg/5 mL
- **Senna and ispaghula granules**
  - ▸ (proprietary product: *Manevac Granules*), senna fruit 12.4%, ispaghula 54.2%
- **Sodium citrate compound enema**
  - ▸ (proprietary products: *Micolette Micro-enema; Micralax Micro-enema; Relaxit Micro-enema*), sodium citrate 450 mg with glycerol, sorbitol and an anionic surfactant
- **Sodium picosulfate capsules**
  - ▸ (proprietary products: *Dulcolax Perles*), sodium picosulfate 2.5 mg
- **Sodium picosulfate elixir**
  - ▸ (proprietary product: *Dulcolax Liquid*), sodium picosulfate 5 mg/5 mL
- **Sterculia granules**
  - ▸ (proprietary product: *Normacol Granules*), sterculia 62%
- **Sterculia and frangula granules**
  - ▸ (proprietary product: *Normacol Plus Granules*), sterculia 62%, frangula (standardised) 8%
- **Zinc oxide and dimeticone spray**
  - ▸ (proprietary product: *Sprilon*), dimeticone 1.04%, zinc oxide 12.5% in a pressurised aerosol unit
- **Zinc oxide impregnated medicated bandage**
  - ▸ (proprietary product: *Steripaste*), sterile cotton bandage impregnated with paste containing zinc oxide 15%
- **Zinc oxide impregnated medicated stocking**
  - ▸ (proprietary product: *Zipzoc*), sterile rayon stocking impregnated with ointment containing zinc oxide 20%

Non-medical prescribing

Overview

A range of non-medical healthcare professionals can prescribe medicines for patients as either Independent or Supplementary Prescribers.

Independent prescribers are practitioners responsible and accountable for the assessment of patients with previously undiagnosed or diagnosed conditions and for decisions about the clinical management required, including prescribing. They are recommended to prescribe generically, except where this would not be clinically appropriate or where there is no approved non-proprietary name.

Supplementary prescribing is a partnership between an independent prescriber (a doctor or a dentist) and a supplementary prescriber to implement an agreed Clinical Management Plan for an individual patient with that patient's agreement.

Independent and Supplementary Prescribers are identified by an annotation next to their name in the relevant professional register.

Information and guidance on non-medical prescribing is available on the Department of Health website at www.dh.gov.uk/health/2012/04/prescribing-change.

For information on the mixing of medicines by Independent and Supplementary Prescribers, see *Mixing of medicines prior to administration in clinical practice: medical and non-medical prescribing*, National Prescribing Centre, May 2010 (available at www.gov.uk/government/publications/mixing-of-medicines-prior-to-administration-in-clinical-practice-medical-and-non-medical-prescribing).

For information on the supply and administration of medicines to groups of patients using Patient Group Directions see Guidance on prescribing p. 1.

In order to protect patient safety, the initial prescribing and supply of medicines prescribed should normally remain separate functions performed by separate healthcare professionals.

Nurses

Nurse Independent Prescribers (formerly known as Extended Formulary Nurse Prescribers) are able to prescribe any medicine for any medical condition. Unlicensed medicines are excluded from the Nurse Prescribing Formulary in Scotland.

Nurse Independent Prescribers are able to prescribe, administer, and give directions for the administration of Schedule 2, 3, 4, and 5 Controlled Drugs. This extends to diamorphine hydrochloride p. 518, dipipanone, or cocaine for treating organic disease or injury, but not for treating addiction.

Nurse Independent Prescribers must work within their own level of professional competence and expertise.

The Approved list for prescribing by Community Practitioner Nurse Prescribers (NPF) p. 1953 for Community Practitioners provides information on prescribing.

Pharmacists

Pharmacist Independent Prescribers can prescribe any medicine for any medical condition. This includes unlicensed medicines, subject to accepted clinical good practice.

They are also able to prescribe, administer, and give directions for the administration of Schedule 2, 3, 4, and 5 Controlled Drugs. This extends to diamorphine hydrochloride p. 518, dipipanone, or cocaine for treating organic disease or injury, but not for treating addiction.

Pharmacist Independent Prescribers must work within their own level of professional competence and expertise.

Physiotherapists

Physiotherapist Independent Prescribers can prescribe any medicine for any medical condition. This includes "off-label" medicines subject to accepted clinical good practice. They are also allowed to prescribe the following Controlled Drugs: oral or injectable morphine p. 525, transdermal fentanyl p. 520 and oral diazepam p. 398, dihydrocodeine tartrate p. 518, lorazepam p. 393, oxycodone hydrochloride p. 528 or temazepam p. 552.

Physiotherapist Independent Prescribers must work within their own level of professional competence and expertise.

Therapeutic radiographers

Therapeutic Radiographer Independent Prescribers can prescribe any medicine for any medical condition. This includes "off-label" medicines subject to accepted clinical good practice. Prescribing of Controlled Drugs is subject to legislative changes. Therapeutic Radiographer Independent Prescribers must work within their own level of professional competence and expertise.

Optometrists

Optometrist Independent Prescribers can prescribe any licensed medicine for ocular conditions affecting the eye and the tissues surrounding the eye, except Controlled Drugs or medicines for parenteral administration. Optometrist Independent Prescribers must work within their own level of professional competence and expertise.

Podiatrists

Podiatrist Independent Prescribers can prescribe any medicine for any medical condition. This includes "off-label" medicines subject to accepted clinical good practice. They are also allowed to prescribe the following Controlled Drugs for oral administration: diazepam p. 398, dihydrocodeine tartrate p. 518, lorazepam p. 393 and temazepam p. 552.

Podiatrist Independent Prescribers must work within their own level of professional competence and expertise.

Paramedics

Paramedic Independent Prescribers can prescribe any medicine for any medical condition. This includes "off-label" medicines subject to accepted clinical good practice. Prescribing of Controlled Drugs is subject to legislative changes. Paramedic Independent Prescribers must work within their own level of professional competence and expertise.

Further Information

For further details about the different types of prescribers, see *Medicines, Ethics and Practice*, London, Pharmaceutical Press (always consult latest edition).

Index of manufacturers

The following is an alphabetical list of manufacturers and other companies referenced in the BNF, with their medicines information or general contact details. For information on 'special-order' manufacturers and specialist importing companies see Special-order manufacturers p. 1967.

3M Health Care Ltd, Tel: 01509 611611

AAH Pharmaceuticals Ltd, Tel: 03445 612 266

A. Menarini Farmaceutica Internazionale SRL, Tel: 0800 0858678, menarini@medinformation.co.uk

A1 Pharmaceuticals, Tel: 01708 528900, enquiries@a1plc.co.uk

Abbott Healthcare Products Ltd, Tel: 0800 1701177, ukabbottnutrition@abbott.com

AbbVie Ltd, Tel: 01628 561092, ukmedinfo@abbvie.com

Accord Healthcare Ltd, Tel: 01271 385257, medinfo@accord-healthcare.com

Advanced Medical Solutions Ltd, Tel: 01606 863500

Advancis Medical, Tel: 01623 751500

Advanz Pharma, Tel: 08700 703033, medicalinformation@advanzpharma.com

AFT Pharma UK Ltd, Tel: 0203 6707602, customer.service@aftpharm.com

AgaMatrix Europe Ltd, Tel: 0800 0931812, info@agamatrix.co.uk

Agepha Pharma s.r.o., Tel: +42 1692054363, office@agepha.com

Aguettant Ltd, Tel: 01275 463691, info@aguettant.co.uk

AJ Vaccines, Tel: +45 7229 7000, ajvaccines@ajvaccines.com

Alan Pharmaceuticals, Tel: 020 72842887, info@alanpharmaceuticals.com

Alcon Eye Care Ltd, Tel: 0345 2669363, gb.medicaldepartment@alcon.com

Alexion Pharma UK Ltd, Tel: 0800 028 4394, medinfo.EMEA@alexion.com

Alimera Sciences Ltd, Tel: 0800 0191253, medicalinformation@alimerasciences.com

Alissa Healthcare Research Ltd, Tel: 01489 564069, enquiries@alissahealthcare.com

ALK-Abello Ltd, Tel: 0118 9037940, info@uk.alk-abello.com

Allergan Ltd, Tel: 01628 494026, UK_MedInfo@Allergan.com

Allergy Therapeutics (UK) Ltd, Tel: 01903 844702, infoservices@allergytherapeutics.com

Alliance Pharmaceuticals Ltd, Tel: 01249 466966, medinfo@alliancepharma.co.uk

Almirall Ltd, Tel: 0800 0087399, Almirall@EU.ProPharmaGroup.com

Almus Pharmaceuticals Ltd, Tel: 0800 9177983, med.info@almus.co.uk

Alnylam UK Ltd, Tel: 0800 1412569, medinfo@alnylam.com

Altacor Ltd, Tel: 01182 210150, info@altacor-pharma.com

Alturix Ltd, Tel: 0845 5191609, medinfo@alturix.com

Alveolus Biomedical B.V., Tel: 07879 427173, info@alveolus.nl

Ambe Ltd, Tel: 01732 760900, info@ambemedical.com

Amgen Ltd, Tel: 01223 436441, gbinfoline@amgen.com

Amicus Therapeutics UK Ltd, Tel: 0808 2346864, PhV.Migalastat_SO@Quintiles.com

AMO UK Ltd, Tel: 01344 864042, crc@its.jnj.com

Amring Pharmaceuticals Ltd, Tel: +33 1 58 28 16 80, infomed.france@amringpharma.com

Amryt Pharma, Tel: 01604 549952, medinfo@amrytpharma.com

AOP Orphan Pharmaceuticals AG, Tel: 0121 2624119, office.uk@aoporphan.com

Aristo Pharma Ltd, Tel: 01353 887100, contactus@aristo-pharma.co.uk

Arjun Products Ltd, Tel: 0800 0157806, info@arjunproducts.co.uk

Ascot Laboratories Ltd, Tel: 01923 711971, specials@ascotpharma.com

Aspar Pharmaceuticals Ltd, Tel: 020 82059846, info@aspar.co.uk

Aspen Pharma Trading Ltd, Tel: 0800 0087392, aspenmedinfo@professionalinformation.co.uk

Aspire Pharma Ltd, Tel: 01730 231148, medinfo@aspirepharma.co.uk

Astellas Pharma Ltd, Tel: 0800 7835018, medinfo.gb@astellas.com

AstraZeneca UK Ltd, Tel: 0800 7830033, medical.informationuk@astrazeneca.com

Atnahs Pharma UK Ltd, Tel: 01279 406759, atnahspv@diamondpharmaservices.com

Axunio Pharma GmbH, Tel: + 49 40 38 02 32 14, medinfo@axunio.eu

AYMES International Ltd, Tel: 0845 6805496, info@aymes.com

B. Braun Medical Ltd, Tel: 0800 298 0299, medinfo.bbmuk@bbraun.com

B. Braun Melsungen AG, Tel: +49 5661 710, info@bbraun.com

Bard Ltd, Tel: 01293 527888, customer.services@crbard.com

Bausch & Lomb UK Ltd, Tel: 0800 041 8721, UKMedInformation@bausch.com

Baxter Healthcare Ltd, Tel: 01635 206345, medinfo_uki@baxter.com

Bayer Plc, Tel: 0118 206 3116, medical.information@bayer.co.uk

BBI Healthcare Ltd, Tel: 01656 868930, info@bbihealthcare.com

Becton, Dickinson UK Ltd, Tel: 0800 0437 546, SafetyInformation@bd.com

Beiersdorf UK Ltd, Tel: 0121 329 8800

Bell, Sons & Co (Druggists) Ltd, Tel: 0151 4221200, Med-info@bells-healthcare.com

Besins Healthcare (UK) Ltd, Tel: 01748 828 789, besins@eu.propharmagroup.com

BHR Pharmaceuticals Ltd, Tel: 02476 377210

BIAL Pharma UK Ltd, Tel: 01753 916010, medinfo.uk@bial.com

Bio Med Sciences, Tel: +1 610 5303193, info@silon.com

Bio Products Laboratory Ltd, Tel: 020 89572255, medinfo@bpl.co.uk

BioCare Ltd, Tel: 01214 338702, clinicalnutrition@biocare.co.uk

Bio-Diagnostics Ltd, Tel: 01684 592262, enquiries@bio-diagnostics.co.uk

Biogen Idec Ltd, Tel: 0800 0087401, MedInfoUKI@biogen.com

Biolitec Pharma Ltd, Tel: +49 3641 5195330, medinfo@biolitecpharma.com

BioMarin Europe Ltd, Tel: 0845 0177013, medinfoeu@bmrn.com

Bioprojet UK Ltd, Tel: 01722 742900, medicalinformation@bioprojet.uk

Bio-Tech Pharmacal Inc, Tel: +1 800 3451199, customerservice@bio-tech-pharm.com

Biotest (UK) Ltd, Tel: 0845 241 3090, medinfo.uk@grifols.com

Blackrock Pharmaceuticals Ltd, Tel: 0115 9890841, safety.uk@lambda-cro.com

Blueprint Medicines (UK) Ltd, Tel: +31 85 064 4001, medinfoeurope@blueprintmedicines.com

BOC Ltd, Tel: 0800 136603, healthcare.home-uk@boc.com

Boehringer Ingelheim Ltd, Tel: 01344 742579, medinfo@bra.boehringer-ingelheim.com

Bowmed Ibisqus Ltd, Tel: 01483 212151, medinfo@bowmed.com

Brancaster Pharma Ltd, Tel: 01737 243407, safety@brancasterpharma.com

Bray Group Ltd, Tel: 01367 240736, info@bray-healthcare.com

Bristol Laboratories Ltd, Tel: 01442 200922, info@bristol-labs.co.uk

Bristol-Myers Squibb Pharmaceuticals Ltd, Tel: 0800 7311736, medical.information@bms.com

Britannia Pharmaceuticals Ltd, Tel: 0808 196 8585, medinfo@britannia-pharm.com

Brown & Burk UK Ltd, Tel: 0203 384 7188, bbukqa@bbukltd.com

BSN Medical Ltd, Tel: 01482 670100, orders.uk@bsnmedical.com

C D Medical Ltd, Tel: 01942 813933

Cambridge Healthcare Supplies Ltd, Tel: 0330 1359434, medinfo@cambridge-healthcare.co.uk

Cambridge Sensors Ltd, Tel: 0800 0883920, info@microdotcs.com

Cambrooke Therapeutics, Tel: 0161 9627377, Tel: 07950 716133, ukinfo@cambrooke.com

Camurus AB, medicalinfo@camurus.com

CD Pharma Srl, Tel: +39 02 43980539, info@cdpharmagroup.one

Celltrion Healthcare UK Ltd, Tel: 01753 983500, UKMedical@celltrionhc.com

Chemidex Pharma Ltd, Tel: 01784 477167, info@chemidex.co.uk

Chiesi Ltd, Tel: 01748 827 271, medinfo.uk@chiesi.com

Chugai Pharma UK Ltd, Tel: 020 89875600, medinfo@chugai-pharm.co.uk

Special-order manufacturers

Unlicensed medicines are available from 'special-order' manufacturers and specialist-importing companies; the MHRA maintains a register of these companies at www.gov.uk/government/publications/human-and-veterinary-medicines-register-of-licensed-manufacturing-sites.

Licensed **hospital manufacturing units** also manufacture 'special-order' products as unlicensed medicines, the principal NHS units are listed below. A database (*Pro-File*; www.pro-file.nhs.uk) provides information on medicines manufactured in the NHS; access is restricted to NHS pharmacy staff.

The Association of Pharmaceutical Specials Manufacturers may also be able to provide further information about commercial companies (www.apsm-uk.com).

The MHRA recommends that an unlicensed medicine should only be used when a patient has special requirements that cannot be met by use of a licensed medicine.

As well as being available direct from the hospital manufacturer(s) concerned, many NHS-manufactured Specials may be bought from the Oxford Pharmacy Store, owned and operated by Oxford Health NHS Foundation Trust.

England

London

Barts Health NHS Trust

T. Patel, Head of Pharmacy, Shared Services
Pharmacy Technical Services Unit
First Floor, Pathology and Pharmacy Building
80 Newark Street
London
E1 2ES
(020) 3246 0397 (order/enquiry)
tejal.patel5@nhs.net

Guy's and St. Thomas' NHS Foundation Trust

Mr P. Forsey, Associate Chief Pharmacist
Guy's and St. Thomas' NHS Foundation Trust
Guy's Hospital
Pharmacy Department
Great Maze Pond
London
SE1 9RT
(020) 7188 4992 (order)
(020) 7188 5003 (enquiry)
Fax: (020) 7188 5013
paul.forsey@gstt.nhs.uk

London North West Healthcare NHS Trust

Mr K. Wong,
London North West Healthcare NHS Trust
Pharmacy Technical Services Department
Northwick Park Hospital
Watford Road
Harrow
Middlesex
HA1 3UJ
(020) 8869 2295 (order/enquiry)
Fax: (020) 8869 2370
LNWH-tr.nphmanufacturing@nhs.net (enquiry)
kwong@nhs.net

Royal Free London NHS Foundation Trust

Mr M. Baker, Head of Pharmacy Manufacturing Unit
Royal Free Specials Pharmaceuticals
Royal Free London NHS Foundation Trust
Pond Street
Hampstead
London
NW3 2QG
(020) 7830 2424 (order/enquiry)
rf.specials@nhs.net (order/enquiry)
marc.baker@nhs.net

St George's Healthcare NHS Trust

Mr V. Kumar, Chief Pharmacist
St George's University Hospitals
NHS Foundation Trust
Ground Floor, Lanesborough Wing
Blackshaw Road
London
SW17 0QT
(020) 8725 1378
vinodh.kumar@stgeorges.nhs.uk

University College Hospital NHS Foundation Trust

Mr T. Murphy, Production Manager
University College Hospital
235 Euston Road
London
NW1 2BU
(020) 7380 9723 (order)
(020) 7380 9472 (enquiry)
Fax: (020) 7380 9726
tony.murphy@uclh.nhs.uk

Midlands and Eastern

Barking, Havering and Redbridge University Trust

Mr N. Fisher, Senior Principal Pharmacist
Queen's Hospital
Pharmacy Department
Romford
Essex
RM7 0AG
(01708) 435 463 (order)
(01708) 435 042 (enquiry)
neil.fisher@bhrhospitals.nhs.uk

Burton Hospitals NHS Foundation Trust

Mr D. Raynor, Head of Pharmacy Manufacturing Unit
Queens Hospital
Burton Hospitals NHS Foundation Trust
Pharmacy Manufacturing Unit
Belvedere Road
Burton-on-Trent
DE13 0RB
(01283) 511 511 ext: 5275 (order/enquiry)
Fax: (01283) 593 036
david.raynor@burtonft.nhs.uk

East Suffolk and North Essex NHS Foundation Trust (Colchester site)

Mr S. Pullen, Head of Pharmacy Production
Colchester Hospital
Pharmacy Manufacturing Unit
Turner Road
Colchester
Essex
CO4 5JL
(01206) 742 007 (order)
(01206) 744 208 (enquiry)
Pharmacy.Stores@esneft.nhs.uk (order)
PSU.Enquiries@esneft.nhs.uk (enquiry)

East Suffolk and North Essex NHS Foundation Trust (Ipswich site)

Mr B. Tabrizi, Deputy Head of Production
Ipswich Hospital
Pharmacy Manufacturing Unit
Heath Road
Ipswich
Suffolk
IP4 5PD
(01473) 703 440 (order)
(01473) 703 603 (enquiry)
pharmacy.manufacture@esneft.nhs.uk (order/enquiry)
behnam.tabrizi@esneft.nhs.uk

Nottingham University Hospitals NHS Trust

Mr J. Graham, Senior Pharmacist, Production
Queens Medical Centre Campus
Pharmacy Production
Derby Road
Nottingham
NG7 2UH
(0115) 924 9924 ext: 87516 (order/enquiry)
jeff.graham@nuh.nhs.uk

North East

The Newcastle upon Tyne Hospitals NHS Foundation Trust

Mr Y. Hunter-Blair, Production Manager
Royal Victoria Infirmary
Newcastle Specials
Pharmacy Production Unit
Queen Victoria Road
Newcastle-upon-Tyne
NE1 4LP
(0191) 282 0395 (order)
(0191) 282 0389 (enquiry)
Fax: (0191) 282 0469
yan.hunter-blair@nuth.nhs.uk

North West

Preston Pharmaceuticals

J. Parrington, Head of Production
Preston Pharmaceuticals
Pharmacy Manufacturing Unit
Royal Preston Hospital
Sharoe Green Lane
Fulwood
Preston
PR2 9HT
(01772) 523 617 (order/enquiry)
prestonpharmaceuticals@lthtr.nhs.uk (order/enquiry)
janet.parrington@lthtr.nhs.uk

Stockport Pharmaceuticals

Mr A. Singleton, Head of Production
Stepping Hill Hospital
Stockport NHS Foundation Trust
Stockport Pharmaceuticals
Poplar Grove
Stockport
SK2 7JE
(0161) 419 5666 (order/enquiry)
Fax: (0161) 419 5426
sppu.orders@stockport.nhs.uk
andrew.singleton@stockport.nhs.uk

South

Portsmouth Hospitals University NHS Trust

Mr R. Lucas, Quality Assurance Manager
Portsmouth Hospitals University NHS Trust
Pharmacy Manufacturing Unit
Unit D2, Railway Triangle
Walton Road
Farlington
Portsmouth
PO6 1TF
(02392) 389 078 (order/enquiry)
PMU.office@porthosp.nhs.uk (order)
robert.lucas@porthosp.nhs.uk

South West

Torbay Pharmaceuticals

Mr L. Rudd, Commercial Strategy Director
Torbay and South Devon NHS Foundation Trust
Torbay Pharmaceuticals
Wilkins Drive
Paignton
TQ4 7FG
(01803) 664 707 (order/enquiry)
Fax: (01803) 231 121
torbaypharmaceuticals@nhs.net
leon.rudd@nhs.net

Yorkshire

Calderdale and Huddersfield NHS Foundation Trust

Dr B. Grewal, Managing Director
Calderdale and Huddersfield NHS Foundation
Trust
Huddersfield Pharmacy Specials
Gate 2 - Acre Mills, School Street West
Huddersfield
HD3 3ET
(01484) 355 388 (order/enquiry)
hps.orders@cht.nhs.uk

Northern Ireland

Victoria Pharmaceuticals

Mr S. Cameron, Production Manager -
Pharmacy
Victoria Pharmaceuticals
Royal Hospitals
Plenum Building
Grosvenor Road
Belfast
BT12 6BA
(028) 9615 1000 (order/enquiry)
samuel.cameron@belfasttrust.hscni.net

Scotland

NHS Scotland Pharmaceutical 'Specials' Service

Mr S. Bath, Production Manager
Ninewells Hospital
James Arrott Drive
Dundee
DD2 1UB
(01382) 496702 (order/enquiry)
(01382) 496730 (technical enquiry)
Fax: (01382) 496703 (order)
tay.pssoffice@nhs.scot (order/enquiry)
simond.bath@nhs.scot (technical enquiry)

Wales

Cardiff and Vale University Health Board

Ms A. Jones, Principal Pharmacist - Head of
Technical Services
Cardiff and Vale University Health Board
20 Fieldway
Cardiff
CF14 4HY
(029) 2184 8120 (order/enquiry)
Fax: (029) 2184 8130
contact@smpu.co.uk

Index

Recommended wording of cautionary and advisory labels

For details including Welsh Language translation see p. 1925

1　Warning: This medicine may make you sleepy

2　Warning: This medicine may make you sleepy. If this happens, do not drive or use tools or machines. Do not drink alcohol

3　Warning: This medicine may make you sleepy. If this happens, do not drive or use tools or machines

4　Warning: Do not drink alcohol

5　Do not take indigestion remedies 2 hours before or after you take this medicine

6　Do not take indigestion remedies, or medicines containing iron or zinc, 2 hours before or after you take this medicine

7　Do not take milk, indigestion remedies, or medicines containing iron or zinc, 2 hours before or after you take this medicine

8　Warning: Do not stop taking this medicine unless your doctor tells you to stop

9　Space the doses evenly throughout the day. Keep taking this medicine until the course is finished, unless you are told to stop

10　Warning: Read the additional information given with this medicine

11　Protect your skin from sunlight—even on a bright but cloudy day. Do not use sunbeds

12　Do not take anything containing aspirin while taking this medicine

13　Dissolve or mix with water before taking

14　This medicine may colour your urine. This is harmless

15　Caution: flammable. Keep your body away from fire or flames after you have put on the medicine

16　Dissolve the tablet under your tongue—do not swallow. Store the tablets in this bottle with the cap tightly closed. Get a new supply 8 weeks after opening

17　Do not take more than... in 24 hours

18　Do not take more than... in 24 hours. Also, do not take more than... in any one week

19　Warning: This medicine makes you sleepy. If you still feel sleepy the next day, do not drive or use tools or machines. Do not drink alcohol

21　Take with or just after food, or a meal

22　Take 30 to 60 minutes before food

23　Take this medicine when your stomach is empty. This means an hour before food or 2 hours after food

24　Suck or chew this medicine

25　Swallow this medicine whole. Do not chew or crush

26　Dissolve this medicine under your tongue

27　Take with a full glass of water

28　Spread thinly on the affected skin only

29　Do not take more than 2 at any one time. Do not take more than 8 in 24 hours

30　Contains paracetamol. Do not take anything else containing paracetamol while taking this medicine. Talk to a doctor at once if you take too much of this medicine, even if you feel well

32　Contains aspirin. Do not take anything else containing aspirin while taking this medicine

Approximate Conversions and Units

Conversion of pounds to kilograms

lb	kg
1	0.45
2	0.91
3	1.36
4	1.81
5	2.27
6	2.72
7	3.18
8	3.63
9	4.08
10	4.54
11	4.99
12	5.44
13	5.90
14	6.35

Conversion of stones to kilograms

stones	kg
1	6.35
2	12.70
3	19.05
4	25.40
5	31.75
6	38.10
7	44.45
8	50.80
9	57.15
10	63.50
11	69.85
12	76.20
13	82.55
14	88.90
15	95.25

Conversion from millilitres to fluid ounces

mL	fl oz
50	1.8
100	3.5
150	5.3
200	7.0
500	17.6
1000	35.2

Length

1 metre (m) = 1000 millimetres (mm)
1 centimetre (cm) = 10 mm
1 inch (in) = 25.4 mm
1 foot (ft) = 12 inches
12 inches = 304.8 mm

Mass

1 kilogram (kg) = 1000 grams (g)
1 gram (g) = 1000 milligrams (mg)
1 milligram (mg) = 1000 micrograms
1 microgram = 1000 nanograms
1 nanogram = 1000 picograms

Volume

1 litre = 1000 millilitres (mL)
1 millilitre (1 mL) = 1000 microlitres
1 pint ≈ 568 mL

Other units

1 kilocalorie (kcal) = 4186.8 joules (J)
1000 kilocalories (kcal) = 4.1868 megajoules (MJ)
1 megajoule (MJ) = 238.8 kilocalories (kcal)
1 millimetre of mercury (mmHg) = 133.3 pascals (Pa)
1 kilopascal (kPa) = 7.5 mmHg (pressure)

Plasma-drug concentrations

Plasma-drug concentrations in BNF publications are expressed in mass units per litre (e.g. mg/litre). The approximate equivalent in terms of amount of substance units (e.g. micromol/litre) is given in brackets.

Prescribing for children: weight, height, and sex

The table below shows the **mean values** for weight, height, and sex by age; these values have been derived from the UK-WHO growth charts 2009 and UK 1990 standard centile charts, by extrapolating the 50th centile, and may be used to calculate doses in the absence of measurements. However, an individual's weight and height might vary considerably from the values in the table and it is important to ensure that the value chosen is appropriate. In most cases the actual measurement should be obtained as soon as possible and the dose re-calculated.

Age	Weight (kg)	Height (cm)
Full-term neonate	3.5	51
1 month	4.3	55
2 months	5.4	58
3 months	6.1	61
4 months	6.7	63
6 months	7.6	67
1 year	9	75
3 years	14	96
5 years	18	109
7 years	23	122
10 years	32	138
12 years	39	149
14 year old boy	49	163
14 year old girl	50	159
Adult male	68	176
Adult female	58	164

Abbreviations and Symbols

Internationally recognised units and symbols are used in the BNF publications where possible.

ACBS	Advisory Committee on Borderline Substances, *see* Borderline Substances
ACE	Angiotensin-converting enzyme
ADHD	Attention deficit hyperactivity disorder
AIDS	Acquired immunodeficiency syndrome
approx.	approximately
AV	atrioventricular
AWMSG	All Wales Medicines Strategy Group
BAN	British Approved Name
BMI	body mass index
BP	British Pharmacopoeia 2013, unless otherwise stated
BPC	British Pharmaceutical Codex 1973 and Supplement 1976, unless otherwise stated
BRCA	breast cancer gene
CAPD	Continuous ambulatory peritoneal dialysis
CD1	preparation in Schedule 1 of the Misuse of Drugs Regulations 2001 (and subsequent amendments). For regulations *see* Controlled drugs and drug dependence p. 7.
CD2	preparation in Schedule 2 of the Misuse of Drugs Regulations 2001 (and subsequent amendments). For regulations *see* Controlled drugs and drug dependence p. 7.
CD3	preparation in Schedule 3 of the Misuse of Drugs Regulations 2001 (and subsequent amendments). For regulations *see* Controlled drugs and drug dependence p. 7.
CD4–1	preparation in Schedule 4 (Part I) of the Misuse of Drugs Regulations 2001 (and subsequent amendments). For regulations *see* Controlled drugs and drug dependence p. 7.
CD4–2	preparation in Schedule 4 (Part II) of the Misuse of Drugs Regulations 2001 (and subsequent amendments). For regulations *see* Controlled drugs and drug dependence p. 7.
CD5	preparation in Schedule 5 of the Misuse of Drugs Regulations 2001 (and subsequent amendments). For regulations *see* Controlled drugs and drug dependence p. 7.
CHM	Commission on Human Medicines
CHMP	Committee for Medicinal Products for Human Use
CNS	central nervous system
CSM	Committee on Safety of Medicines (now subsumed under Commission on Human Medicines)
d. c.	direct current
DMARD	Disease-modifying antirheumatic drug
DPF	Dental Practitioners' Formulary
DT	Drug Tariff price
e/c	enteric-coated (termed gastro-resistant in BP)
ECG	electrocardiogram
EEG	electro-encephalogram
eGFR	estimated glomerular filtration rate, *see* Prescribing in renal impairment p. 21
EMA	European Medicines Agency
FSRH	Faculty of Sexual and Reproductive Healthcare
G6PD	glucose 6-phosphate dehydrogenase
GSL	general sales list
HDL-cholesterol	high-density lipoprotein cholesterol
HIV	Human immunodeficiency virus
HRT	Hormone replacement therapy
i/m	intramuscular
i/v	intravenous
INR	international normalised ratio
JCVI	Joint Committee on Vaccination and Immunisation
LDL-cholesterol	low-density lipoprotein cholesterol
MAOI	Monoamine-oxidase inhibitor
max.	maximum
MHRA	Medicines and Healthcare products Regulatory Agency
NCL	no cautionary labels (prescription endorsement made by prescriber when recommended cautionary labels are not required)
NHS	National Health Service
NICE	National Institute for Health and Care Excellence
NPF	Nurse Prescribers' Formulary
NSAID	Non-steroidal anti-inflammatory drug
NSTEMI	non-ST-segment elevation myocardial infarction
P	pharmacy only medicine
PARP	poly (ADP-ribose) polymerase
PGD	patient group direction
PHE	Public Health England (formerly Health Protection Agency (HPA))
PoM	prescription-only medicine, *see* Fig. 1 *How to use BNF publications*
®	registered trade mark
rINN	Recommended International Non-proprietary Name
RSV	respiratory syncytial virus
SF	sugar-free
SIGN	Scottish Intercollegiate Guidelines Network
SLS	Selected List Scheme
SMC	Scottish Medicines Consortium
SPC	Summary of Product Characteristics
spp.	species
SSRI	Selective serotonin reuptake inhibitor
STEMI	ST-segment elevation myocardial infarction
UK	United Kingdom
UKHSA	United Kingdom Health Security Agency (formerly Public Health England (PHE))
Units	for SI units *see* Prescription writing p. 4
WHO	World Health Organization
▼	limited experience of the use of this product and the MHRA requests that all suspected adverse reactions should be reported, *see* Adverse reactions to drugs p. 11
🔁	drug-class monograph, *see* How to use BNF Publications, p. x
F1234	drug monograph has a corresponding drug-class monograph; the page number of the class monograph is indicated within the tab, *see* How to use BNF Publications, p. x
EvGr	precedes evidence graded content, *see* How BNF Publications are constructed p. viii
Ⓐ to Ⓔ	symbols will be displayed - grades reflect the strengths of recommendations in evidence graded content, *see* How BNF Publications are constructed p. viii
Ⓜ	indicates manufacturer information, see How BNF Publications are constructed p. viii
🚫	no price available

Latin abbreviations

Directions should be in English without abbreviation. However, Latin abbreviations have been used when prescribing.

The following is a list of appropriate abbreviations. It should be noted that the English version is not always an exact translation.

a. c.	=	ante cibum (before food)
b. d.	=	bis die (twice daily)
o. d.	=	omni die (every day)
o. m.	=	omni mane (every morning)
o. n.	=	omni nocte (every night)
p. c.	=	post cibum (after food)
p. r. n.	=	pro re nata (when required)
q. d. s.	=	quater die sumendum (to be taken four times daily)
q. q. h.	=	quarta quaque hora (every four hours)
stat	=	immediately
t. d. s.	=	ter die sumendum (to be taken three times daily)
t.i.d.	=	ter in die (three times daily)

E numbers

The following is a list of common E numbers and the inactive ingredients to which they correspond.

E102	Tartrazine
E104	Quinoline Yellow
E110	Sunset Yellow FCF
E123	Amaranth
E124	Ponceau 4R
E127	Erythrosine BS
E132	Indigo Carmine
E142	Green S
E171	Titanium Dioxide
E172	Iron oxides, iron hydroxides
E200	Sorbic Acid
E211	Sodium Benzoate
E223	Sodium Metabisulfite
E320	Butylated Hydroxyanisole
E321	Butylated Hydroxytoluene
E322	Lecithins
E420	Sorbitol
E421	Mannitol
E422	Glycerol
E901	Beeswax (white and yellow)
E1520	Propylene Glycol

Medical emergencies in the community

15-Jan-2025

Overview

Drug treatment outlined below is intended for use by **appropriately qualified healthcare professionals**. Only drugs that are used for immediate relief are shown; advice on supporting care is not given. Where the patient's condition requires investigation and further treatment, the patient should be transferred to hospital promptly.

Acute coronary syndromes

▶ **ANGINA: UNSTABLE**

Aspirin dispersible tablets p. 142 (75 mg, 300 mg)

BY MOUTH (DISPERSED IN WATER OR CHEWED)

▸ Adult: 300 mg

▶ **PLUS**

▶ **EITHER Glyceryl trinitrate aerosol spray p. 252**
(400 micrograms/metered dose)

SUBLINGUALLY

▸ Adult: 1–2 sprays, dose may be repeated at 5 minute intervals if symptoms have not resolved, up to a maximum of 3 sprays in total

▶ OR **Glyceryl trinitrate tablets** (500 micrograms, 600 micrograms)

SUBLINGUALLY

▸ Adult: 1 tablet, dose may be repeated at 5 minute intervals if symptoms have not resolved, up to a maximum of 3 tablets in total

NOTE Seek urgent medical attention if symptoms have not resolved 5 minutes after the second dose of glyceryl trinitrate, or earlier if the pain is intensifying or the person is unwell.

▶ **MYOCARDIAL INFARCTION: NON-ST-SEGMENT ELEVATION**

Treat as for Angina: unstable

▶ **MYOCARDIAL INFARCTION: ST-SEGMENT ELEVATION**

Aspirin dispersible tablets (75 mg, 300 mg)

BY MOUTH (DISPERSED IN WATER OR CHEWED)

▸ Adult: 300 mg

Glyceryl trinitrate aerosol spray (400 micrograms/metered dose)

SUBLINGUALLY

▸ Adult: 1–2 sprays, dose may be repeated at 5 minute intervals if symptoms have not resolved, up to a maximum of 3 sprays in total

▶ OR **Glyceryl trinitrate tablets** (500 micrograms, 600 micrograms)

SUBLINGUALLY

▸ Adult: 1 tablet, dose may be repeated at 5 minute intervals if symptoms have not resolved, up to a maximum of 3 tablets in total

NOTE Seek urgent medical attention if symptoms have not resolved 5 minutes after the second dose of glyceryl trinitrate, or earlier if the pain is intensifying or the person is unwell.

Metoclopramide hydrochloride injection p. 494 (5 mg/mL)

BY INTRAVENOUS INJECTION

▸ Adult 18-19 years (body-weight up to 60 kg): 5 mg
▸ Adult 18-19 years (body-weight 60 kg and over): 10 mg
▸ Adult over 19 years: 10 mg

Diamorphine hydrochloride injection p. 518 (5 mg powder for reconstitution)

BY SLOW INTRAVENOUS INJECTION (1–2 MG/MINUTE)

▸ Adult: 5 mg followed by a further 2.5–5 mg if necessary
▸ Elderly or frail patients: reduce dose by half

▶ OR **Morphine sulfate injection p. 525** (10 mg/mL)

BY SLOW INTRAVENOUS INJECTION (1–2 MG/MINUTE)

▸ Adult: 5–10 mg followed by a further 5–10 mg if necessary
▸ Elderly or frail patients: reduce dose by half

Oxygen, if appropriate

Airways disease, obstructive

▶ **ASTHMA: ACUTE**

[EvGr] Emergency asthma consultations should be regarded as being for severe acute asthma until shown otherwise. Patients with features of severe or life-threatening acute asthma, and patients who fail to respond adequately at any time should be referred to hospital immediately. Acute asthma in children aged under 2 years should be managed in hospital. Ⓐ

High-flow **oxygen** should be given if available (via tight-fitting face mask in children) to achieve and maintain an SpO_2 level of 94-98%.

Salbutamol aerosol inhaler p. 287 (100 micrograms/dose inhaler)

BY INHALATION OF AEROSOL VIA A SPACER
(AND A CLOSE-FITTING FACE MASK IF CHILD UNDER 3 YEARS)

▸ Child 1-17 years: 100 micrograms every 0.5–1 minute for up to 10 doses; each dose is to be inhaled separately; repeat every 10–20 minutes or when required
▸ Adult: 100 micrograms every 0.5–1 minute for up to 10 doses; each dose is to be inhaled separately; repeat every 10–20 minutes or when required

▶ OR **Salbutamol dry powder inhaler** (100 micrograms/dose inhaler, 200 micrograms/dose inhaler)

BY INHALATION OF DRY POWDER

▸ Child 6-17 years: 100 micrograms every 0.5–1 minute for up to 10 doses, *or alternatively* 200 micrograms every 0.5–1 minute for up to 5 doses; each dose is to be inhaled separately; repeat every 10–20 minutes or when required
▸ Adult: 100 micrograms every 0.5–1 minute for up to 10 doses, *or alternatively* 200 micrograms every 0.5–1 minute for up to 5 doses; each dose is to be inhaled separately; repeat every 10–20 minutes or when required

▶ OR **Salbutamol nebuliser solution** (1 mg/mL, 2 mg/mL)

BY INHALATION OF NEBULISED SOLUTION (VIA OXYGEN-DRIVEN NEBULISER IF AVAILABLE)

▸ Child 1-4 years: 2.5 mg; repeat every 20–30 minutes or when required
▸ Child 5-17 years: 2.5–5 mg; repeat every 20–30 minutes or when required
▸ Adult: 2.5–5 mg; repeat every 15–30 minutes or when required

▶ OR **Terbutaline sulfate nebuliser solution p. 290** (2.5 mg/mL)

BY INHALATION OF NEBULISED SOLUTION (VIA OXYGEN-DRIVEN NEBULISER IF AVAILABLE)

▸ Child 4 years and below: 5 mg every 20–30 minutes or as necessary

- Child 5-11 years: 5–10 mg every 20–30 minutes or as necessary
- Child 12-17 years: 10 mg every 20–30 minutes or as necessary
- Adult: 10 mg every 20–30 minutes or as necessary

▶ PLUS **(in all cases)**
▶ EITHER **Prednisolone tablets p. 791 (*or* prednisolone soluble tablets)** (5 mg)
BY MOUTH
- Child 11 years and below: 1–2 mg/kg (max. 40 mg) once daily for up to 3 days or longer if necessary; if child has been taking an oral corticosteroid for more than a few days, give prednisolone 2 mg/kg (max. 60 mg) once daily
- Child 12-17 years: 40–50 mg once daily for at least 5 days
- Adult: 40–50 mg once daily for at least 5 days

▶ OR **Hydrocortisone p. 787 (preferably as sodium succinate)**
BY INTRAVENOUS INJECTION
- Child 17 years and below: 4 mg/kg (max. 100 mg) every 6 hours until conversion to oral prednisolone is possible; alternative dose if weight unavailable:
  - Child 1 year and below: 25 mg
  - Child 2-4 years: 50 mg
  - Child 5-17 years: 100 mg
- Adult: 100 mg every 6 hours until conversion to oral prednisolone is possible

Monitor response 15 to 30 minutes after nebulisation; if any signs of acute asthma persist, arrange hospital admission. While awaiting ambulance, repeat **nebulised beta₂ agonist** (as above) and give with

Ipratropium bromide nebuliser solution p. 281
(250 micrograms/mL)
BY INHALATION OF NEBULISED SOLUTION (VIA OXYGEN-DRIVEN NEBULISER IF AVAILABLE)
- Child 11 years and below: 250 micrograms, repeated every 20–30 minutes for the first 2 hours, then every 4–6 hours as necessary
- Child 12-17 years: 500 micrograms every 4–6 hours as necessary
- Adult: 500 micrograms every 4–6 hours as necessary

▶ **CROUP**
Dexamethasone oral solution p. 786 (2 mg/5 mL)
BY MOUTH
- Child 1 month-2 years: 150 micrograms/kg as a single dose

Anaphylaxis

▶ **ANAPHYLAXIS**
Adrenaline/epinephrine injection p. 256 (1 mg/mL (1 in 1000))
BY INTRAMUSCULAR INJECTION
- Child up to 6 months: 100–150 micrograms (0.1–0.15 mL), repeated after 5 minutes if necessary
- Child 6 months-5 years: 150 micrograms (0.15 mL), repeated after 5 minutes if necessary
- Child 6-11 years: 300 micrograms (0.3 mL), repeated after 5 minutes if necessary
- Child 12-17 years: 500 micrograms (0.5 mL), repeated after 5 minutes if necessary; 300 micrograms (0.3 mL) should be given if child is small or prepubertal
- Adult: 500 micrograms (0.5 mL), repeated after 5 minutes if necessary

If life-threatening features persist, further doses of intramuscular adrenaline/epinephrine can be given every 5 minutes until specialist critical care available.

High-flow **oxygen** should be given as soon as available. For guidance on other treatment that may be used for the management of anaphylaxis, *see* Antihistamines, allergen immunotherapy and allergic emergencies p. 316.

Bacterial infection

▶ **SUSPECTED MENINGOCOCCAL DISEASE, AND SUSPECTED BACTERIAL MENINGITIS (WHERE THERE IS LIKELY TO BE A CLINICALLY SIGNIFICANT DELAY IN TRANSFER TO HOSPITAL)**
NOTE Administer a single dose before urgent transfer to hospital, unless this will delay transfer.

Benzylpenicillin sodium injection p. 633 (600 mg, 1.2 g)
BY INTRAVENOUS INJECTION (OR BY INTRAMUSCULAR INJECTION IF VENOUS ACCESS NOT AVAILABLE)
- Child 1 month-11 months: 300 mg
- Child 1-9 years: 600 mg
- Child 10-17 years: 1.2 g
- Adult: 1.2 g

▶ OR **Ceftriaxone injection p. 609** (250 mg, 1 g, 2 g)
BY DEEP INTRAMUSCULAR INJECTION
- Child 1 month: 250 mg
- Child 2-11 months: 500 mg
- Child 1-4 years: 1g
- Child 5-8 years: 1.5g
- Child 9-11 years: 2 g
BY INTRAVENOUS INJECTION OR BY DEEP INTRAMUSCULAR INJECTION
- Child 12-17 years: 2 g
- Adult: 2 g

Do not administer antibacterial treatment outside of hospital if history of severe allergy to a beta-lactam antibacterial.
See also Central nervous system infections, antibacterial therapy p. 580.

▶ **SUSPECTED MENINGOCOCCAL DISEASE**
Benzylpenicillin sodium injection (600 mg, 1.2 g)
BY INTRAVENOUS INJECTION (OR BY INTRAMUSCULAR INJECTION IF VENOUS ACCESS NOT AVAILABLE)
- Neonate: 300 mg
NOTE Administer a single dose before urgent transfer to hospital, unless this will delay transfer.

Hypoglycaemia

▶ **DIABETIC HYPOGLYCAEMIA**
Fast-acting carbohydrate (glucose p. 1182 is preferred)
CHILD UP TO 5 YEARS
By mouth
- 5 g (20 mL *Lift*® (previously *Glucojuice*®) oral glucose liquid *or* 1.5 glucose tablets *or* half a tube of glucose 40% oral gel *or* 1 teaspoonful of sugar dissolved in an appropriate volume of water), repeated after 15 minutes if necessary
Or by buccal administration [in conscious but uncooperative children]
- 5 g (half a tube of glucose 40% oral gel), repeated after 15 minutes if necessary
CHILD 5-11 YEARS
By mouth
- 10 g (40 mL *Lift*® (previously *Glucojuice*®) oral glucose liquid *or* 3 glucose tablets *or* 1 tube of glucose 40% oral gel *or* 2 teaspoonfuls of sugar dissolved in an appropriate volume of water), repeated after 15 minutes if necessary
Or by buccal administration [in conscious but uncooperative children]
- 10 g (1 tube of glucose 40% oral gel), repeated after 15 minutes if necessary
CHILD 12-17 YEARS
By mouth
- 15 g (60 mL *Lift*® (previously *Glucojuice*®) oral glucose liquid *or* 4 glucose tablets *or* 1.5 tubes of glucose 40% oral gel *or* 3 teaspoonfuls of sugar dissolved in an appropriate volume of water), repeated after 15 minutes if necessary
Or by buccal administration [in conscious but uncooperative children]
- 15 g (1.5 tubes of glucose 40% oral gel), repeated after 15 minutes if necessary

ADULT

By mouth

▸ 15–20 g (60–80 mL *Lift* ® (previously *Glucojuice* ®) oral glucose liquid *or* 4–5 glucose tablets *or* 1.5–2 tubes of glucose 40% oral gel *or* 150–200 mL pure fruit juice *or* 3–4 heaped teaspoonfuls of sugar dissolved in an appropriate volume of water), repeated after 15 minutes if necessary

Or by buccal administration [in conscious but uncooperative patients]

▸ 15–20 g (1.5–2 tubes of glucose 40% oral gel), repeated after 15 minutes if necessary

NOTE Examples of glucose preparations which can be used to give oral doses are based on the use of oral liquid containing glucose 250 mg/mL and tablets containing glucose 4 g per tablet. Buccal dosing is based on tubes of 40% oral gel containing glucose 10 g per tube.

▸ OR **if hypoglycaemia unresponsive *or* if oral route cannot be used**

Glucagon injection p. 845 (*GlucaGen* ® 1 mg/mL)

BY INTRAMUSCULAR INJECTION

▸ Child 8 years and below or body-weight up to 25 kg: 500 micrograms (0.5 mL)

▸ Child 9-17 years or body-weight 25 kg and over: 1 mg (1 mL)

▸ Adult: 1 mg (1 mL)

▸ OR **if hypoglycaemia prolonged *or* unresponsive to glucagon after 10 minutes**

Glucose 10% intravenous infusion

BY INTRAVENOUS INJECTION INTO LARGE VEIN

▸ Child: 5 mL/kg (glucose 500 mg/kg)

▸ Adult: 150–200 mL infused over 15 minutes

▸ OR **Glucose 20% intravenous infusion**

BY INTRAVENOUS INJECTION INTO LARGE VEIN

▸ Adult: 75–100 mL infused over 15 minutes

Seizures

▸ **CONVULSIVE (INCLUDING FEBRILE) SEIZURES LASTING 5 MINUTES OR LONGER, OR RECURRENT SEIZURES WITHOUT RECOVERY IN BETWEEN**

▸ EITHER **Diazepam rectal solution p. 398** (2 mg/mL, 4 mg/mL)

BY RECTUM

▸ Neonate: 1.25–2.5 mg, repeated once after 5–10 minutes if necessary

▸ Child 1 month-1 year: 5 mg, repeated once after 5–10 minutes if necessary

▸ Child 2-11 years: 5–10 mg, repeated once after 5–10 minutes if necessary

▸ Child 12-17 years: 10–20 mg, repeated once after 5–10 minutes if necessary

▸ Adult: 10–20 mg, repeated once after 5–10 minutes if necessary

▸ Elderly: 10 mg, repeated once after 5–10 minutes if necessary

▸ OR **Midazolam oromucosal solution p. 394**

BY BUCCAL ADMINISTRATION

▸ Neonate: 300 micrograms/kg, repeated once after 5–10 minutes if necessary [unlicensed]

▸ Child 1-2 months: 300 micrograms/kg (max. 2.5 mg), repeated once after 5–10 minutes if necessary [unlicensed]

▸ Child 3 months-11 months: 2.5 mg, repeated once after 5–10 minutes if necessary

▸ Child 1-4 years: 5 mg, repeated once after 5–10 minutes if necessary

▸ Child 5-9 years: 7.5 mg, repeated once after 5–10 minutes if necessary

▸ Child 10-17 years: 10 mg, repeated once after 5–10 minutes if necessary

▸ Adult: 10 mg, repeated once after 5–10 minutes if necessary [unlicensed]